Harrison's

PRINCIPLES OF INTERNAL MEDICINE

EDITORS OF PREVIOUS EDITIONS

T. R. Harrison, Editor-in-Chief, Editions 1, 2, 3, 4, 5

W. R. Resnik, Editor, Editions 1, 2, 3, 4, 5

M. M. Wintrobe, Editor, Editions 1, 2, 3, 4, 5
Editor-in-Chief, Editions 6, 7

G. W. Thorn, Editor, Editions 1, 2, 3, 4, 5, 6, 7
Editor-in-Chief, Edition 8

R. D. Adams, Editor, Editions 2, 3, 4, 5, 6, 7, 8, 9, 10

P. B. Beeson, Editor, Editions 1, 2

I. L. Bennett, Jr., Editor, Editions 3, 4, 5, 6

E. Braunwald, Editor, Editions 6, 7, 8, 9, 10

K. J. Isselbacher, Editor, Editions 6, 7, 8, 10
Editor-in-Chief, Edition 9

R. G. Petersdorf, Editor, Editions 6, 7, 8, 9
Editor-in-Chief, Edition 10

J. D. Wilson, Editor, Editions 9, 10

J. B. Martin, Editor, Edition 10

Harrison's

PRINCIPLES OF INTERNAL MEDICINE

Eleventh Edition

Editors

EUGENE BRAUNWALD, A.B., M.D., M.A. (Hon.), M.D. (Hon.) Hersey Professor of the Theory and Practice of Physic and Herrman Ludwig Blumgart Professor of Medicine, Harvard Medical School; Chairman, Department of Medicine, Brigham and Women's and Beth Israel Hospitals, Boston

KURT J. ISSELBACHER, A.B., M.D. Mallinckrodt Professor of Medicine, Harvard Medical School; Physician and Chief, Gastrointestinal Unit, Massachusetts General Hospital, Boston

ROBERT G. PETERSDORF, A.B., M.D., M.A. (Hon.), D.Sc. (Hon.), M.D. (Hon.), L.H.D. (Hon.) Professor of Medicine, Dean and Vice Chancellor, Health Sciences, University of California School of Medicine, San Diego, La Jolla

JEAN D. WILSON, M.D. Professor of Internal Medicine, The University of Texas Southwestern Medical School, Dallas

JOSEPH B. MARTIN, M.D., Ph.D., F.R.C.P.(C), M.A. (Hon.) Julieanne Dorn Professor of Neurology, Harvard Medical School; Chief, Neurology Service, Massachusetts General Hospital, Boston

ANTHONY S. FAUCI, M.D. Chief, Laboratory of Immunoregulation and Director, National Institute of Allergy and Infectious Diseases, National Institutes of Health, Bethesda

McGRAW-HILL BOOK COMPANY *New York St. Louis San Francisco Auckland Bogotá Hamburg Johannesburg London Madrid Mexico Milan Montreal New Delhi Panama Paris São Paulo Singapore Sydney Tokyo Toronto*

NOTICE

Medicine is an ever-changing science. As new research and clinical experience broaden our knowledge, changes in treatment and drug therapy are required. The editors and the publisher of this work have made every effort to ensure that the drug dosage schedules herein are accurate and in accord with the standards accepted at the time of publication. Readers are advised, however, to check the product information sheet included in the package of each drug they plan to administer to be certain that changes have not been made in the recommended dose or in the contraindications for administration. This recommendation is of particular importance in regard to new or infrequently used drugs.

Harrison's

Principles of Internal Medicine

3 4 5 6 7 8 9 0 DOW DOW 8 9

Foreign Editions

FRENCH (Eleventh Edition)—Flammarion, © 1988 (est.)
GERMAN (Tenth Edition)—Schwabe and Company, Ltd., © 1986
GREEK (Tenth Edition)—Parissianos, © 1986
ITALIAN (Eleventh Edition)—McGraw-Hill Libri Italia S.r.l. © 1987 (est.)
JAPANESE (Tenth Edition)—Hirokawa, © 1985
PORTUGUESE (Eleventh Edition)—Editora Guanabara Koogan, S.A., © 1987 (est.)
SPANISH (Tenth Edition)—Libros McGraw-Hill de Mexico, S.A., © 1986

This book was set in Times Roman by Monotype Composition Company.
The editors were J. Dereck Jeffers, Eileen J. Scott, and Mariapaz Ramos-Englis
The indexer was Philip James; the production supervisor was Ave McCracken; the cover was designed by Edward R. Schultheis
R. R. Donnelley & Sons Company was printer and binder.

Library of Congress Cataloging-in-Publication Data

Principles of internal medicine.
Harrison's principles of internal medicine.

Also issued in 2 v.
Includes bibliographies and index.
1. Internal medicine. I. Harrison, Tinsley Randolph, Date. II. Braunwald, Eugene, Date.
III. Title. [DNLM: 1. Internal Medicine. WB 115 P957]
RC46.P895 1987 616 86-14383
ISBN 0-07-007261-2 (1-vol. ed.)
ISBN 0-07-079454-5 (2-vol. ed. : set)

A salute to George W. Thorn by the editors of Harrison's

George W. Thorn, one of the founding editors of *Harrison's* and Editor-in-Chief of the eighth edition, has enjoyed a long association with this book. He has had an enormous impact on the book and thereby on the education of countless thousands of physicians and medical students. His incisiveness, inventiveness, and originality, coupled with his broad knowledge of clinical medicine and medical science and his unswerving dedication to the application of techniques of contemporary science to the advance of clinical medicine, have played a vital role in the basic organization of this textbook. Thorn has always championed the view that students, residents, and practicing physicians require more of a textbook of medicine than discussions of clinical disorders, but that their understanding of and ability to deal with patients is enhanced by a detailed appreciation of how the sciences fundamental to medicine affect the clinical process.

George Thorn began his remarkable career in endocrinologic research as a medical student at the University of Buffalo School of Medicine. Following a stint in general practice, which subsequently served him well as an educator, clinical investigator, and consultant, he obtained research training and held faculty positions at several institutions. He became Harvard's eighth Hersey Professor of Medicine and the Brigham's third Physician-in-Chief at the age of 36. During the three decades in which he filled these positions with distinction he created a model academic medical unit. During the 1950s and 1960s, the halcyon years of post-World War II academic medicine, the education of the physician-scientist, the highest standard of clinical care, and the conduct of exciting clinical research on his service were inextricably intertwined and mutually reinforcing. Thorn's personal investigative interests focused on the adrenal cortex and the kidney. He developed techniques for the diagnosis of adrenal disease which are still in wide use today. He characterized salt-losing nephritis and catalyzed the development of renal dialysis and the work that led to the development of renal transplantation.

George Thorn has played many leadership roles in medicine and medical science. As a member of the governing board of the Massachusetts Institute of Technology (MIT) he was instrumental in the development of the Harvard-MIT program in Health Science and Technology. Under his leadership the Howard Hughes Medical Institute has become a major force in the conduct of the fundamental and clinical research which is certain to improve the care of patients in the twenty-first century.

George Thorn has influenced most profoundly a number of institutions—Harvard, the Brigham, MIT, and the Hughes Institute. To these, and to *Harrison's,* he has brought a unique blend of ebullience, imagination, curiosity, personal leadership, good humor, optimism, warmth, and compassion, which has inspired generations of Harvard medical students, Brigham residents and research fellows, and colleagues. Therefore, the present editors are pleased to express their admiration and affection for this medical giant and beloved friend by dedicating this edition of *Harrison's* to George W. Thorn.

ABBREVIATED CONTENTS

CONTENTS

Section 4: Mycobacterial diseases

Section 5: Spirochetal diseases

Section 6: Viral diseases

Section 7: Infections caused by higher bacteria and fungi

Section 8: Rickettsia, *mycoplasma*, and *chlamydia*

Section 9: Protozoal and helminthic infections

Section 10: Disorders caused by environmental agents

PART FOUR DISORDERS OF THE CARDIOVASCULAR SYSTEM

Section 1: Disorders of the heart

LIST OF CONTRIBUTORS

RAYMOND D. ADAMS, B.A., M.A., M.D., M.A. (Hon.), D.Sc. (Hon.), M.D. (Hon.)
Bullard Professor of Neuropathology, Emeritus, Harvard Medical School; Consultant Neurologist and formerly Chief of Neurology Service, Massachusetts General Hospital; Emeritus Director, Eunice K. Shriver Research Center, Boston; Médicin Adjoint, L'Hôpital Cantonale de Lausanne, Lausanne

JOHN W. ADAMSON, M.D.
Professor of Medicine and Head, Division of Hematology, Department of Medicine, University of Washington School of Medicine, Seattle

ELLIOT ALPERT, M.D.
Professor of Medicine and Chief, Division of Gastroenterology, Baylor College of Medicine, Houston

JOSEPH S. ALPERT, M.D.
Professor of Medicine, University of Massachusetts Medical School; Director, Division of Cardiovascular Medicine, University of Massachusetts Medical Center, Worcester

ROBERT J. ANDERSON, M.D.
Associate Professor of Medicine, University of Colorado Health Sciences Center, Denver

JACK P. ANTEL, M.D.
Associate Professor of Neurology, University of Chicago Pritzker School of Medicine, Chicago

BARRY G. W. ARNASON, M.D.
Professor and Chairman, Department of Neurology, University of Chicago Pritzker School of Medicine, Chicago

PAUL M. ARNOW, M.D.
Associate Professor of Medicine, Section of Infectious Disease, University of Chicago Hospital and Clinics, Chicago

ARTHUR K. ASBURY, M.D.
Ruth Wagner Van Meter and J. Ray Van Meter Professor of Neurology, University of Pennsylvania School of Medicine and Hospital of the University of Pennsylvania, Philadelphia

K. FRANK AUSTEN, M.D.
Theodore B. Bayles Professor of Medicine, Harvard Medical School; Physician-in-Chief, Robert B. Brigham Division and Chairman, Department of Rheumatology and Immunology, Brigham and Women's Hospital, Boston

ROBERT AUSTRIAN, M.D., D.Sc. (Hon.)
John Herr Musser Professor and Chairman, Department of Research Medicine, University of Pennsylvania School of Medicine, Philadelphia

BERNARD M. BABIOR, M.D., Ph.D.
Head, Division of Biochemistry, Department of Basic and Clinical Research, Scripps Clinic and Research Foundation, La Jolla

JEFFREY P. BAKER, M.D., F.R.C.P. (C)
Assistant Professor of Medicine, University of Toronto; Consultant Staff Gastroenterologist, Toronto Western Hospital, Toronto

M. FLINT BEAL, M.D.
Assistant Professor, Harvard Medical School; Assistant Neurologist, Massachusetts General Hospital, Boston

HARRY N. BEATY, M.D.
Professor of Medicine and Dean, Northwestern University Medical School, Chicago

ARTHUR L. BEAUDET, M.D.
Investigator, Howard Hughes Medical Institute; Professor of Pediatrics and Cell Biology, Baylor College of Medicine, Houston

JOHN E. BENNETT, M.D.
Head, Clinical Mycology Section, National Institute of Allergy and Infectious Diseases, National Institutes of Health, Bethesda

JEFFREY D. BERNHARD, M.D.
Assistant Professor of Medicine, Director, Division of Dermatology, and Director of Phototherapy Center, Department of Medicine, University of Massachusetts Medical Center, Worcester

EDWIN L. BIERMAN, M.D.
Professor of Medicine and Chief, Division of Metabolism, Endocrinology, and Nutrition, University of Washington School of Medicine, Seattle

ALAN B. BISNO, M.D.
Professor of Medicine and Chief, Division of Infectious Diseases, University of Tennessee Center for the Health Sciences, Memphis

HENRY R. BOURNE, M.D.
Chairman, Department of Pharmacology, School of Medicine, University of California, San Francisco

WALTER G. BRADLEY, D.M., F.R.C.P.
Chairman and Professor of Neurology, University of Vermont College of Medicine; Chairman, Department of Neurology, University Health Center, Burlington

DAVID L. BRAFF, M.D.
Associate Professor, Department of Psychiatry, School of Medicine, University of California at San Diego; Director, Psychiatric Inpatient Services, U.C.S.D. Medical Center, San Diego

EUGENE BRAUNWALD, A.B., M.D., M.A. (Hon.), M.D. (Hon.)
Hersey Professor of the Theory and Practice of Physic and Herrman Ludwig Blumgart Professor of Medicine, Harvard Medical School; Chairman, Department of Medicine, Brigham and Women's and Beth Israel Hospitals, Boston

BARRY M. BRENNER, B.S., M.D., M.A. (Hon.)
Samuel A. Levine Professor of Medicine, Harvard Medical School; Senior Physician and Director, Renal Division, Brigham and Women's Hospital, Boston

KAREN THATCHER BRITTON, M.D., Ph.D.
Assistant Professor of Psychiatry, School of Medicine, University of California at San Diego, La Jolla

SAMUEL BRODER, M.D.
Associate Director, Clinical Oncology Program, Division of Cancer Treatment and Deputy Clinical Director, National Cancer Institute, National Institutes of Health, Bethesda

MICHAEL S. BROWN, M.D.
Paul J. Thomas Professor, Department of Molecular Genetics, The University of Texas Health Science Center, Dallas

H. FRANKLIN BUNN, M.D.
Professor of Medicine, Harvard Medical School; Senior Physician and Director, Hematology Research, Brigham and Women's Hospital; Investigator, Howard Hughes Medical Institute, Boston

JOHN R. BURTON, M.D.
Associate Professor of Medicine, Johns Hopkins University School of Medicine; Deputy Director of Department of Medicine, Director of Division of Geriatric Medicine, Francis Scott Key Medical Center, Baltimore

ALFRED E. BUXTON, M.D.
Assistant Professor of Medicine, University of Pennsylvania School of Medicine; Director, Cardiac Electrophysiology Laboratory, Hospital of the University of Pennsylvania, Philadelphia

CHARLES B. CARPENTER, M.D.
Professor of Medicine, Harvard Medical School; Senior Physician, Brigham and Women's Hospital, Boston

CHARLES C. J. CARPENTER, M.D.
Professor of Medicine, Brown University; Physician-in-Chief, The Miriam Hospital, Providence

BRUCE R. CARR, M.D.
Associate Professor, Department of Obstetrics and Gynecology and Cecil and Ida Green Center for Reproductive Biology Sciences, The University of Texas Health Science Center, Dallas

EDWIN CASSEM, M.D.
Associate Professor of Psychiatry, Harvard Medical School; Chief, Psychiatric Consultation–Liason Service, Massachusetts General Hospital, Boston

RICHARD CHAMPLIN, M.D.
Associate Professor of Medicine and Director, Leukemia/Bone Marrow Transplant Service, School of Medicine, University of California at Los Angeles

KEITH H. CHIAPPA, M.D.
Assistant Professor of Neurology, Harvard Medical School; Director, EEG and Evoked Potentials Unit of the Clinical Neurophysiology Laboratory and Department of Neurology, Massachusetts General Hospital, Boston

WALLACE A. CLYDE, JR., M.D.
Professor of Pediatrics and Microbiology, University of North Carolina School of Medicine, Chapel Hill

FREDRIC L. COE, M.D.
Professor of Medicine and Physiology and Chief, Nephrology Program, University of Chicago Pritzker School of Medicine, Chicago

ALAN S. COHEN, M.D.
Chief of Medicine and Director, Thorndike Memorial Laboratory, Boston City Hospital; Conrad Wesselhoeft Professor of Medicine, Boston University School of Medicine, Boston

HARVEY R. COLTEN, M.D.
Professor and Chairman, Department of Pediatrics, Washington University School of Medicine, St. Louis

WILSON S. COLUCCI, M.D.
Assistant Professor of Medicine, Harvard Medical School; Associate Physician, Brigham and Women's Hospital, Boston

PATRICIA C. COME, M.D.
Assistant Professor of Medicine, Harvard Medical School; Director, Noninvasive Cardiovascular Diagnostic Laboratory, Beth Israel Hospital, Boston

MAX D. COOPER, M.D.
Professor of Pediatrics and Microbiology, Cellular Immunobiology Unit, The University of Alabama in Birmingham, Birmingham

RICHARD A. COOPER, M.D.
Dean and Professor of Medicine, Medical College of Wisconsin, Milwaukee

LAWRENCE COREY, M.D.
Professor of Laboratory Medicine and Microbiology and Adjunct Professor of Medicine and Pediatrics, University of Washington School of Medicine, Seattle

RONALD G. CRYSTAL, M.D.
Chief, Pulmonary Branch, National Heart, Lung and Blood Institute, National Institutes of Health, Bethesda

JOHN J. CUSH, M.D.
Fellow in Rheumatology, Department of Internal Medicine, The University of Texas Health Science Center, Dallas

DAVID C. DALE, M.D.
Professor of Medicine and Dean, University of Washington School of Medicine, Seattle

JAMES E. DALEN, M.D.
Professor and Chairman, Department of Medicine, University of Massachusetts Medical School; Physician-in-Chief, University of Massachusetts Hospital, Worcester

THOMAS M. DANIEL, M.D.
Professor of Medicine, Case Western Reserve University School of Medicine; Physician, University Hospitals of Cleveland, Cleveland

GILBERT H. DANIELS, M.D.
Associate Professor of Medicine, Thyroid Unit, Massachusetts General Hospital, Boston

ROBERT B. DAROFF, M.D.
Gilbert W. Humphrey Professor and Chairman, Case Western Reserve University School of Medicine, Director, Department of Neurology, University Hospitals of Cleveland; Neurology Service, Cleveland Veterans Administration Medical Center, Cleveland

JOHN R. DAVID, M.D.
Professor of Medicine, Harvard Medical School; Chief, Division of Tropical Medicine, Robert B. Brigham Division of Brigham and Women's Hospital; John LaPorte Given Professor and Chairman, Department of Tropical Public Health, Harvard School of Public Health, Boston

G. ROBERT DELONG, M.D.
Assistant Professor of Neurology, Harvard Medical School; Associate Neurologist and Associate Pediatrician, Massachusetts General Hospital, Boston

VINCENT T. DEVITA, JR., M.D.
Director, National Cancer Institute, National Institutes of Health, Bethesda

MARC A. DICHTER, M.D., Ph.D.
Professor of Neurology, University of Pennsylvania School of Medicine, Philadelphia

JULES L. DIENSTAG, M.D.
Associate Professor of Medicine, Harvard Medical School; Assistant Physician, Massachusetts General Hospital, Boston

ROBERT G. DLUHY, M.D.
Associate Professor of Medicine, Harvard Medical School; Associate Program Director of the Clinical Research Center, Brigham and Women's Hospital, Boston

RAPHAEL DOLIN, M.D.
Professor of Medicine and Head, Infectious Diseases Unit, University of Rochester School of Medicine and Dentistry, Rochester

ANDREW G. ENGEL, M.D.
Professor of Neurology, Mayo Medical School; Department of Neurology, Mayo Clinic, Rochester

KENNETH H. FALCHUK, M.D.
Associate Professor of Medicine, Harvard Medical School; Brigham and Women's Hospital, Boston

ANTHONY S. FAUCI, M.D.
Chief, Laboratory of Immunoregulation and Director, National Institute of Allergy and Infectious Diseases, National Institutes of Health, Bethesda

MURRAY J. FAVUS, M.D.
Associate Professor of Medicine, University of Chicago Pritzker School of Medicine, Chicago

RALPH D. FEIGIN, M.D.
Professor and Chairman, Department of Pediatrics, Baylor College of Medicine; Physician-in-Chief, Texas Children's Hospital, Houston

BERNARD N. FIELDS, M.D.
Adele Lehman Professor and Chairman, Department of Microbiology and Molecular Genetics, Harvard Medical School; Professor of Medicine, Division of Infectious Diseases, Brigham and Women's Hospital, Boston

ALFRED P. FISHMAN, M.D.
William Maul Measey Professor of Medicine, University of Pennsylvania; Director, Cardiovascular-Pulmonary Division, Hospital of the University of Pennsylvania, Philadelphia

THOMAS B. FITZPATRICK, M.D., Ph.D.
Edward Wigglesworth Professor of Dermatology and Chairman, Department of Dermatology, Harvard Medical School; Chief, Dermatology Service, Massachusetts General Hospital, Boston

DANIEL W. FOSTER, M.D.
Professor of Internal Medicine, The University of Texas Health Science Center, Dallas

MICHAEL M. FRANK, M.D.
Chief, Laboratory of Clinical Investigation and Clinical Director, National Institute of Allergy and Infectious Diseases, National Institutes of Health, Bethesda

STANLEY D. FREEDMAN, M.D.
Head, Division of Infectious Diseases, Scripps Clinic and Research Foundation; Associate Clinical Professor of Medicine, University of California at San Diego, La Jolla

LAURENCE S. FRIEDMAN, M.D.
Assistant Professor of Medicine, Jefferson Medical College and Thomas Jefferson University Hospital, Philadelphia

PAUL A. FRIEDMAN, M.D.
Associate Professor of Medicine and Pharmacology, Harvard Medical School; Associate Physician, Beth Israel Hospital, Boston

WILLIAM F. FRIEDMAN, M.D.
J. H. Nicholson Professor of Pediatrics (Cardiology) and Executive Chairman, Department of Pediatrics, University of California at Los Angeles School of Medicine and Medical Center, Los Angeles

LAWRENCE A. FROHMAN, M.D.
Professor of Medicine, Director of Division of Endocrinology and Metabolism, University of Cincinnati College of Medicine, Cincinnati

JOHN I. GALLIN, M.D.
Scientific Director, National Institute of Allergy and Infectious Diseases, National Institutes of Health, Bethesda

ROBERT C. GALLO, M.D.
Chief, Laboratory of Tumor Cell Biology, Division of Cancer Treatment, National Cancer Institute, National Institutes of Health, Bethesda

PIERCE GARDNER, M.D.
Professor of Medicine and Pediatrics, University of Chicago Pritzker School of Medicine; Director, Infectious Diseases Training Program, University of Chicago Medical Center, Chicago

MARC B. GARNICK M.D.
Associate Professor of Medicine, Dana-Farber Cancer Institute, Harvard Medical School; Associate Physician, Brigham and Women's Hospital, Boston

JAMES L. GERMAN III, M.D.
Professor (Genetics), Department of Pediatrics, Cornell University Medical College; Senior Investigator and Director, Laboratory of Human Genetics, The New York Blood Center, New York

ELOISE R. GIBLETT, M.D.
Research Professor of Medicine, University of Washington School of Medicine; Executive Director, Puget Sound Blood Center, Seattle

BRUCE C. GILLILAND, M.D.
Professor of Medicine and Laboratory Medicine, University of Washington School of Medicine; Chief of Medicine, Pacific Medical Center, Seattle

J. CHRISTIAN GILLIN, M.D.
Professor of Psychiatry, University of California at San Diego, La Jolla

SID GILMAN, M.D.
Professor and Chairman, Department of Neurology, The University of Michigan Medical Center, Ann Arbor

RICHARD J. GLASSOCK, M.D.
Professor of Medicine, School of Medicine, University of California at Los Angeles; Chairman, Department of Medicine, Harbor-UCLA Medical Center, Torrance

ROBERT M. GLICKMAN, M.D.
Samuel Bard Professor of Medicine, Columbia University College of Physicians and Surgeons; Director, Medical Service, Presbyterian Hospital, New York

DAVID W. GOLDE, M.D.
Professor of Medicine and Chief, Division of Hematology/Oncology, School of Medicine, University of California at Los Angeles, Los Angeles

STEPHEN E. GOLDFINGER, M.D.
Associate Professor of Medicine and Associate Dean of Continuing Education, Harvard Medical School; Physician, Gastrointestinal Unit, Massachusetts General Hospital, Boston

PAUL GOLDHABER, D.D.S.
Dean and Professor of Periodontology, Harvard School of Dental Medicine, Boston

LEE GOLDMAN, M.D.
Associate Professor of Medicine, Harvard Medical School; Assistant Physician-in-Chief, Brigham and Women's Hospital, Boston

JOSEPH L. GOLDSTEIN, M.D.
Paul J. Thomas Professor and Chairman, Department of Molecular Genetics, The University of Texas Health Science Center, Dallas

RAJ K. GOYAL, M.D.
Rabb Professor of Medicine, Harvard Medical School; Chief, Division of Gastroenterology, Beth Israel Hospital, Boston

JOHN W. GRAEF, M.D.
Assistant Clinical Professor, Harvard Medical School; Director, The Lead/Toxicology Clinic, The Children's Hospital, Boston

IGOR GRANT, M.D.
Professor of Psychiatry, School of Medicine, University of California at San Diego, La Jolla

HARRY B. GREENBERG, M.D.
Associate Professor of Medicine, Department of Medicine, Stanford University Medical School; Palo Alto Veterans Administration Medical Center, Palo Alto

NORTON J. GREENBERGER, M.D.
Peter T. Bohan Professor and Chairman, Department of Medicine, University of Kansas School of Medicine, Kansas City

JAMES E. GRIFFIN III, M.D.
Associate Professor of Internal Medicine, The University of Texas Health Science Center, Dallas

ROBERT C. GRIGGS, M.D.
Professor of Neurology and Medicine, University of Rochester School of Medicine and Dentistry, University of Rochester Medical Center, Rochester

JOHN H. GROWDON, M.D.
Associate Professor of Neurology, Harvard Medical School; Associate Neurologist, Massachusetts General Hospital, Boston

RICHARD L. GUERRANT, M.D.
Professor of Medicine and Head, Division of Geographic Medicine, University of Virginia School of Medicine, Charlottesville

BEVRA HANNAHS HAHN, M.D.
Professor of Medicine and Chief of Rheumatology, University of California, Los Angeles

ROBERT I. HANDIN, M.D.
Associate Professor of Medicine, Harvard Medical School; Director, Hematology Division, Brigham and Women's Hospital, Boston

H. HUNTER HANDSFIELD, M.D.
Director, Sexually Transmitted Disease Control Program, Seattle-King County Department of Public Health; Associate Professor of Medicine, University of Washington School of Medicine, Seattle

JAMES P. HARNISCH, M.D.
Clinical Associate Professor of Medicine, University of Washington School of Medicine; Chief of Dermatology, Pacific Medical Center, Seattle

DONALD H. HARTER, M.D.
Benjamin and Virginia T. Boshes Professor of Neurology and Chairman, Department of Neurology, Northwestern University Medical School; Chairman, Department of Neurology, Northwestern Memorial Hospital, Chicago

BARTON F. HAYNES, M.D.
Associate Professor of Medicine and Assistant Professor of Microbiology and Immunology, Duke University School of Medicine, Durham

HARLEY A. HAYNES, M.D.
Associate Professor of Dermatology, Harvard Medical School; Director, Dermatology Division, Department of Medicine, Brigham and Women's Hospital; Chief, Dermatology, West Roxbury Veterans Administration Hospital, Boston

WILLIAM R. HAZZARD, M.D.
Professor and Chair, Department of Medicine, Bowman-Gray School of Medicine, Wake Forest University; Chief of Medicine, North Carolina Baptist Hospital, Winston-Salem

STEVEN C. HEBERT, M.D.
Assistant Professor of Medicine, Harvard Medical School; Associate Physician, Brigham and Women's Hospital, Boston

FRED J. HENDLER, M.D., Ph.D.
Assistant Professor of Internal Medicine, Division of Hematology/Oncology, The University of Texas Health Science Center, Dallas

JANE ELLEN HENNEY, M.D.
Associate Vice Chancellor and Associate Professor of Medicine, Division of Clinical Oncology, Department of Medicine, University of Kansas Medical Center, Kansas City

RAYMOND L. HINTZ, M.D.
Professor of Pediatrics and Head, Division of Pediatric Endocrinology, Stanford University School of Medicine, Stanford

MARTIN S. HIRSCH, M.D.
Associate Professor, Harvard Medical School; Associate Physician, Infectious Disease Unit, Massachusetts General Hospital, Boston

JAN V. HIRSCHMANN, M.D.
Assistant Chief, Medical Service, Seattle Veterans Administration Medical Center; Associate Professor of Medicine, University of Washington School of Medicine, Seattle

FRED HOCHBERG, M.D.
Associate Professor of Neurology, Harvard Medical School; Associate Neurologist, Massachusetts General Hospital, Boston

PAUL D. HOEPRICH, M.D.
Professor of Medicine and Chief, Section of Medical Mycology, Department of Internal Medicine, Division of Infectious and Immunologic Diseases, School of Medicine, University of California, Davis

JOHN H. HOLBROOK, M.D.
Associate Professor of Medicine, Division of General Internal Medicine, Department of Medicine, University of Utah Medical Center, Salt Lake City

MICHAEL F. HOLICK, M.D., Ph.D.
Professor of Physiology and Nutrition and Director of Vitamin D and Bone Metabolism Laboratory, U.S. Department of Agriculture/Human Nutrition Research Center, Tufts University, Boston

NORMAN K. HOLLENBERG, M.D.
Professor of Radiology, Harvard Medical School; Physician, Brigham and Women's Hospital, Boston

KING K. HOLMES, M.D., Ph.D.
Professor and Vice Chairman, Department of Medicine, University of Washington School of Medicine; Chief of Medicine, Harborview Medical Center, Seattle

THOMAS M. HOSTETTER, M.D.
Associate Professor of Medicine, University of Minnesota School of Medicine; Director, Division of Renal Diseases, University Hospital, Minneapolis

LEIGHTON Y. HUEY, M.D.
Associate Professor of Psychiatry, University of California at San Diego; Chief of Psychiatry Service, San Diego Veterans Administration Medical Center, San Diego

GARY W. HUNNINGHAKE, M.D.
Professor of Internal Medicine and Director, Pulmonary Division, University of Iowa College of Medicine, Iowa City

SIDNEY H. INGBAR, M.D., D.Sc.
William Bosworth Castle Professor of Medicine, Harvard Medical School; Director, Thorndike Laboratory, Beth Israel Hospital, Boston

ROLAND H. INGRAM, JR., M.D.
Parker B. Francis Professor of Medicine, Harvard Medical School; Director, Respiratory Division, Brigham and Women's Hospital, Boston

KURT J. ISSELBACHER, A.B., M.D.
Mallinckrodt Professor of Medicine, Harvard Medical School; Physician and Chief, Gastrointestinal Unit, Massachusetts General Hospital, Boston

KHURSHEED N. JEEJEEBHOY, M.B.B.S., Ph.D., F.R.C.P. (Lond.), F.R.C.P. (Edin.), F.R.C.P. (C).
Professor of Medicine, University of Toronto; Director, Division of Gastroenterology, Toronto General Hospital, Toronto

MARK E. JOSEPHSON, M.D.
Professor of Medicine, University of Pennsylvania School of Medicine; Chief, Cardiovascular Section, Hospital of the University of Pennsylvania, Philadelphia

LEWIS L. JUDD, M.D.
Professor and Chairman, Department of Psychiatry, School of Medicine, University of California at San Diego, La Jolla

DENNIS L. KASPER, M.D.
Professor of Medicine, Harvard Medical School; Chief, Division of Infectious Diseases, Beth Israel Hospital; Associate Director, Channing Laboratory, Brigham and Women's Hospital, Boston

SATISH KATHPALIA, M.D.
Assistant Professor of Medicine, University of Chicago Pritzker School of Medicine; Attending Physician, Michael Reese Hospital and Medical Center, Chicago

DONALD KAYE, M.D., F.A.C.P.
Professor and Chairman, Department of Medicine, Medical College of Pennsylvania; Chief of Medicine, Hospital of the Medical College of Pennsylvania, Philadelphia

WILLIAM N. KELLEY, M.D.
John G. Searle Professor and Chairman, Department of Internal Medicine, University of Michigan Medical School, Ann Arbor

PHILIP KIRBY, M.D.
Instructor in Medicine, Division of Dermatology, University of Washington School of Medicine, Seattle

J. PHILLIP KISTLER, M.D.
Associate Professor of Neurology, Harvard Medical School; Associate Neurologist, Massachusetts General Hospital, Boston

RAYMOND S. KOFF, M.D.
Professor of Medicine, Boston University School of Medicine; Chief of Hepatology Section, Boston University Medical Center; Chief of Medicine, Framingham Union Hospital, Framingham

WILLIAM J. KOVACS, M.D.
Assistant Professor of Medicine, Division of Endocrinology, Vanderbilt University School of Medicine, Nashville

STEPHEN M. KRANE, M.D.
Professor of Medicine, Harvard Medical School; Physician and Chief, Arthritis Unit, Massachusetts General Hospital, Boston

J. THOMAS LAMONT, M.D.
Professor of Medicine, Boston University Medical Center; Chief, Gastrointestinal Section, University Hospital, Boston

LEWIS LANDSBERG, M.D.
Professor of Medicine, Harvard Medical School; Director, Division of Endocrinology and Metabolism, Beth Israel Hospital, Boston

H. CLIFFORD LANE, M.D.
Senior Investigator, Laboratory of Immunoregulation and Deputy Clinical Director, National Institute of Allergy and Infectious Diseases, National Institutes of Health, Bethesda

THOMAS J. LAWLEY, M.D.
Senior Investigator, Dermatology Branch, National Cancer Institute, National Institutes of Health, Bethesda

ALEXANDER R. LAWTON, M.D.
Professor of Pediatrics and Microbiology, Division of Pediatric Immunology, Vanderbilt University School of Medicine, Nashville

J. MICHAEL LAZARUS, M.D.
Associate Professor of Medicine, Harvard Medical School; Physician, Brigham and Women's Hospital, Boston

NORMAN G. LEVINSKY, M.D.
Wade Professor and Chairman, Division of Medicine, Boston University School of Medicine; Physician-in-Chief and Director, Evans Memorial Department of Clinical Research, University Hospital, Boston

PETER E. LIPSKY, M.D.
Professor of Internal Medicine and Microbiology and Chief, Division of Immunologic and Rheumatologic Diseases, Department of Internal Medicine; Director, Harold C. Simmons Arthritis Research Center, The University of Texas Health Science Center, Dallas

RICHARD M. LOCKSLEY, M.D.
Assistant Professor of Medicine, University of San Francisco; Chief of Infectious Diseases, University of San Francisco Medical Center, Moffitt-Long Hospital, San Francisco

DAN L. LONGO, M.D.
Associate Director, Biological Response Modifiers Program, Division of Biology and Diagnosis, National Cancer Institute-Frederick Cancer Research Facility, Frederick

FREDERICK H. LOVEJOY, Jr., M.D.
Associate Professor, Harvard Medical School; Associate Physician-in-Chief, The Children's Hospital; Director, Massachusetts Poison Control System, Boston

SHEILA A. LUKEHART, Ph.D.
Research Assistant Professor, Division of Infectious Diseases, University of Washington School of Medicine, Seattle

WALTER C. MacDONALD, M.D.
Chairman, GI Tumor Group, Cancer Control Agency of British Columbia, Vancouver

RAYMOND MACIEWICZ, M.D.
Assistant Professor of Neurology, Harvard Medical School; Assistant Neurologist, Massachusetts General Hospital, Boston

HENRY J. MANKIN, M.D.
Edith M. Ashley Professor of Orthopedic Surgery, Harvard Medical School; Chief, Orthopedic Services, Massachusetts General Hospital, Boston

FRANCIS E. MARCHLINSKI, M.D.
Assistant Professor of Medicine, University of Pennsylvania School of Medicine; Director, Arrhythmia Evaluation Center, Hospital of the University of Pennsylvania, Philadelphia

JOSEPH B. MARTIN, M.D., Ph.D., F.R.C.P. (C), M.A. (Hon.)
Julieanne Dorn Professor of Neurology, Harvard Medical School; Chief, Neurology Service, Massachusetts General Hospital, Boston

HENRY MASUR, M.D.
Deputy Chief, Critical Care Medicine, Clinical Center, National Institutes of Health, Bethesda

ROGER J. MAY, M.D.
Instructor in Medicine, Harvard Medical School; Assistant in Medicine, Beth Israel Hospital, Boston

E.R. McFADDEN, Jr., M.D.
Argyl J. Beams Professor of Medicine and Director, Asthma and Allergic Disease Center, Case Western Reserve University, Cleveland

JAMES E. McGUIGAN, M.D.
Chairman, Department of Medicine, University of Florida College of Medicine, Gainesville

RIMA McLEOD, M.D.
Associate Professor of Medicine, University of Chicago Pritzker School of Medicine; Attending Physician, Michael Reese Hospital and Medical Center, Chicago

MARK S. McPHEE, M.D.
Clinical Associate Professor of Medicine and Director, Gastrointestinal Endoscopy Unit, University of Kansas, Kansas City

NANCY K. MELLO, Ph.D.
Professor of Psychology, Department of Psychiatry, Harvard Medical School; Co-Director, Alcohol and Drug Abuse Research Center, McLean Hospital, Belmont

JERRY R. MENDELL, M.D.
Professor of Neurology, Ohio State University College of Medicine, Columbus

JOHN MENDELSOHN, M.D.
Chairman, Department of Medicine and Head, Division of Medical Oncology, Memorial Sloan-Kettering Cancer Center; Professor of Medicine, Cornell University Medical College, New York

JACK H. MENDELSON, M.D.
Professor of Psychiatry, Harvard Medical School; Co-Director, Alcohol and Drug Abuse Research Center, McLean Hospital, Belmont

URS A. MEYER, M.D.
Professor of Pharmacology and Chairman, Department of Pharmacology, Biocenter of the University of Basel, Basel, Switzerland

MARTIN C. MIHM, Jr., M.D.
Professor of Pathology, Harvard Medical School; Chief, Dermatopathology Unit, Massachusetts General Hospital, Boston

EDGAR L. MILFORD, M.D.
Assistant Professor of Medicine, Harvard Medical School; Associate Physician, Brigham and Women's Hospital, Boston

MYRON MILLER, M.D.
Professor of Medicine, State University of New York Upstate Medical Center; Chief of Gerontology, Veterans Administration Medical Center, Syracuse

RICHARD A. MILLER, M.D.
Assistant Professor of Medicine, University of Washington School of Medicine; Division of Infectious Diseases, Pacific Medical Center, Seattle

JOHN D. MINNA, M.D.
Chief, NCI-Navy Medical Oncology Branch, National Cancer Institute, National Institutes of Health; Professor of Medicine, Uniformed Services University for the Health Sciences, Naval Hospital, Bethesda

JAY P. MOHR, M.D.
Sciarra Professor of Clinical Neurology, College of Physicians and Surgeons of Columbia University Neurological Institute, New York

KENNETH M. MOSER, M.D.
Professor of Medicine, School of Medicine, University of California at San Diego; Director, Pulmonary and Critical Care Division, U.C.S.D. Medical Center, San Diego

ARNOLD M. MOSES, M.D.
Professor of Medicine and Director, Clinical Research Center, State University of New York Upstate Medical Center; Chief, Endocrinology Section, Veterans Administration Medical Center, Syracuse

DAVID B. MOSHER, M.D.
Clinical Instructor in Dermatology, Harvard Medical School; Assistant in Dermatology, Massachusetts General Hospital, Boston

HARALAMPOS M. MOUTSOPOULOS, M.D., F.A.C.P.
Professor and Head of Medicine, Medical School, University of Ioannina, Ioannina, Greece

FREDERICK M. MURPHY, M.D.
Fellow in Neonatology, Baylor School of Medicine, Houston

JOHN F. MURRAY, M.D., D.Sc. (Hon.)
Professor of Medicine, University of California at San Francisco; Chief, Chest Service, San Francisco General Hospital, San Francisco

ROBERT J. MYERBURG, M.D.
Professor of Medicine and Physiology and Director, Division of Cardiology, University of Miami Medical Center, Miami

THEODORE E. NASH, M.D.
Senior Scientist, Laboratory of Parasitic Diseases, National Institute of Allergy and Infectious Diseases, National Institutes of Health, Bethesda

PAUL NEIMAN, M.D.
Professor of Medicine, University of Washington School of Medicine; Member and Associate Director for Basic Sciences, Fred Hutchinson Cancer Research Center, Seattle

HAROLD C. NEU, M.D.
Professor of Medicine and Pharmacology and Chief, Division of Infectious Diseases, College of Physicians and Surgeons, Columbia University, New York

JOHN A. OATES, M.D.
Professor and Chairman, Department of Medicine, Vanderbilt University School of Medicine; Physician-in-Chief, Vanderbilt University Hospital, Nashville

JERROLD M. OLEFSKY, M.D.
Professor of Medicine and Head, Division of Endocrinology and Metabolism, School of Medicine, University of California at San Diego, La Jolla

ROBERT A. O'ROURKE, M.D.
Charles Conrad and Anna Sahm Brown Professor of Medicine, University of Texas; Director, Division of Cardiovascular Diseases, The University of Texas Health Science Center, San Antonio

THOMAS D. PALELLA, M.D.
Assistant Professor of Internal Medicine, Division of Rheumatology, University of Michigan Medical School, Ann Arbor

DARWIN L. PALMER, M.D.
Professor of Medicine and Chief, Division of Infectious Disease, University of New Mexico School of Medicine; Chief, Infectious Disease Section, Veterans Administration Medical Center, Albuquerque

JOHN A. PARRISH, M.D.
Professor of Dermatology, Harvard Medical School; Director, Wellman Research Laboratory, Massachusetts General Hospital, Boston

A. WILLIAM PASCULLE, D.Sc.
Associate Professor of Pathology, University of Pittsburgh School of Medicine; Associate Director of Microbiology, Presbyterian-University Hospital, Pittsburgh

RICHARD C. PASTERNAK, M.D.
Assistant Professor of Medicine, Harvard Medical School; Assistant Physician and Director, Coronary Care Unit, Beth Israel Hospital, Boston

MADHUKAR A. PATHAK, M.S., Ph.D.
Senior Associate in Dermatology, Harvard Medical School; Dermatology Service, Massachusetts General Hospital, Boston

RICHARD D. PEARSON, M.D.
Associate Professor of Medicine and Pathology, Division of Geographic Medicine, University of Virginia School of Medicine, Charlottesville

LAWRENCE L. PELLETIER, Jr., M.D.
Professor of Medicine, University of Kansas School of Medicine; Chief, Medical Service, Wichita Veterans Administration Medical Center, Wichita

PETER L. PERINE, M.D., M.P.H.
Professor and Director, Division of Tropical Public Health and Professor of Medicine, Uniformed Services University of the Health Sciences School of Medicine, Bethesda

ROBERT G. PETERSDORF, M.D., M.A. (Hon.), D.Sc. (Hon.), M.D. (Hon.), L.H.D. (Hon.)
Dean and Professor of Medicine and Vice Chancellor, Health Sciences, School of Medicine, University of California at San Diego, La Jolla

KIRK L. PETERSON, M.D.
Professor of Medicine, University of California at San Diego; Director, Cardiology Service, U.C.S.D. Medical Center, San Diego

JAMES J. PLORDE, M.D.
Professor, Departments of Medicine and Laboratory Medicine and Chief, Clinical Microbiology Laboratory, Veterans Administration Medical Center, Seattle

FRANCIS ALLAN PLUMMER, M.D., F.R.C.P. (C)
Assistant Professor, Departments of Medicine and Medical Microbiology and Division of Community Medicine, University of Manitoba, Winnipeg

DANIEL K. PODOLSKY, M.D.
Associate Professor of Medicine, Harvard Medical School; Assistant Physician, Gastrointestinal Unit, Massachusetts General Hospital, Boston

JOHN T. POTTS, Jr., M.D.
Jackson Professor of Clinical Medicine, Harvard Medical School; Chief of the General Medical Service, Massachusetts General Hospital, Boston

LAWRIE W. POWELL, M.D.
Professor of Medicine, University of Queensland; Physician, Royal Brisbane Hospital, Brisbane, Australia

DARWIN J. PROCKOP, M.D., Ph.D.
Professor and Chairman, Department of Biochemistry, Jefferson Medical College of Thomas Jefferson University; Director, Department of Biochemistry, Jefferson Institute of Molecular Medicine, Philadelphia

AMY PRUITT, M.D.
Assistant Professor of Neurology, Harvard Medical School; Associate Neurologist, Massachusetts General Hospital, Boston

PAUL G. RAMSEY, M.D.
Associate Professor of Medicine, Department of Medicine, University of Washington School of Medicine, Seattle

JOEL M. RAPPEPORT, M.D.
Associate Professor of Medicine, Harvard Medical School; Physician, Brigham and Women's Hospital, Boston

C. GEORGE RAY, M.D.
Professor of Pathology and Pediatrics and Chief, Clinical Virology-Serology and Pediatrics Infectious Diseases Sections, University of Arizona College of Medicine, Tucson

PETER REICH, M.D.
Professor of Psychiatry, Harvard Medical School; Chief of Psychiatry, Brigham and Women's Hospital, Boston

RICHARD C. REICHMAN, M.D.
Associate Professor of Medicine, Infectious Diseases Unit, University of Rochester School of Medicine and Dentistry, Rochester

JACK S. REMINGTON, M.D.
Chairman, Department of Immunology and Infectious Diseases, Research Institute, Palo Alto Medical Foundation; Professor of Medicine, Division of Infectious Diseases, Stanford University School of Medicine, Palo Alto

EDWARD P. RICHARDSON, Jr., M.D.
Bullard Professor of Neuropathology, Harvard Medical School; Neurologist, Massachusetts General Hospital, Boston

HAL B. RICHERSON, M.D.
Professor of Internal Medicine and Director, Allergy-Immunology Division, University of Iowa College of Medicine, Iowa City

JAMES M. RICHTER, M.D.
Assistant Professor of Medicine, Harvard Medical School, Assistant Physician, Gastrointestinal Unit, Massachusetts General Hospital, Boston

CRAIG RISCH, M.D.
Associate Professor of Psychiatry, School of Medicine, University of California at San Diego, La Jolla

L. JACKSON ROBERTS II, M.D.
Associate Professor of Medicine, Pharmacology, and Clinical Pharmacology, Vanderbilt University School of Medicine, Nashville

R. PAUL ROBERTSON, M.D.
Professor of Medicine, Director of Clinical Research Center, and Director, Diabetes Center, University of Minnesota, Minneapolis

ALLAN R. RONALD, M.D.
H.F. Sellers Professor and Chairman, Department of Medicine, University of Manitoba; Physician-in-Chief, Department of Medicine, Health Sciences Centre, Winnipeg

RICHARD K. ROOT, M.D.
Professor and Chairman, Department of Medicine, University of California, San Francisco

ALLAN H. ROPPER, M.D.
Associate Professor of Neurology, Harvard Medical School; Director of Neurological/Neurosurgical Intensive Care Unit and Assistant Neurologist, Massachusetts General Hospital, Boston

LEON E. ROSENBERG, M.D.
Dean and C.N.H. Long Professor of Human Genetics, Medicine, and Pediatrics, Yale University School of Medicine, New Haven

MICHAEL ROSENBLATT, M.D.
Vice President for Biological Research, Merck, Sharp and Dohme Research Laboratories, West Point

JOHN ROSS, Jr., M.D.
Professor of Medicine and Head, Division of Cardiology, School of Medicine, University of California at San Diego; Attending Physician, U.C.S.D. Medical Center, San Diego

ARTHUR H. RUBENSTEIN, M.D.
Professor and Chairman, Department of Medicine, University of Chicago Pritzker School of Medicine, Chicago

CYRUS E. RUBIN, M.D.
Professor of Medicine and Adjunct Professor of Pathology, Division of Gastroenterology, University of Washington School of Medicine, Seattle

DANIEL RUDMAN, M.D.
Chief, Geriatric Medicine Division and Chief of Staff, Veterans Administration Medical Center; Professor of Medicine, University Health Science Center, Chicago Medical School, Chicago

ARTHUR I. SAGALOWSKY, M.D.
Associate Professor of Urology and Surgical Director of Renal Transplantation, The University of Texas Health Science Center, Dallas

JAY P. SANFORD, M.D.
Professor of Medicine and Dean, F. Edward Hebert School of Medicine; President, Uniformed Services University of the Health Sciences, Bethesda

DENNIS R. SCHABERG, M.D.
Associate Professor of Medicine, University of Michigan, Ann Arbor

ANDREW I. SCHAFER, M.D.
Assistant Professor of Medicine, Harvard Medical School; Associate Physician, Brigham and Women's Hospital, Boston

I. HERBERT SCHEINBERG, M.D.
Professor of Medicine and Head, Division of Genetic Medicine, Albert Einstein College of Medicine; Attending Physician, Hospital of the Albert Einstein College of Medicine, New York

ALAN L. SCHILLER, M.D.
Associate Professor of Pathology, Harvard Medical School; Associate Pathologist and Chief, Autopsy Pathology and Bone Laboratory, Massachusetts General Hospital, Boston

RUDI SCHMID, M.D.
Professor of Medicine and Dean, School of Medicine, University of California, San Francisco

R. NEIL SCHIMKE, M.D.
Professor of Pediatrics and Internal Medicine and Director, Division of Metabolism, Endocrinology, and Genetics, The University of Kansas College of Health Sciences, Kansas City

ROBERT T. SCHOOLEY, M.D.
Assistant Professor of Medicine, Harvard Medical School; Massachusetts General Hospital, Boston

ROBERT W. SCHRIER, M.D.
Professor and Chairman, Department of Medicine, University of Colorado School of Medicine, Denver

MARC A. SCHUCKIT, M.D.
Professor of Psychiatry, School of Medicine, University of California at San Diego; Director, Alcohol Research Center, San Diego Veterans Administration Medical Center, San Diego

WILLIAM J. SCHWARTZ, M.D.
Assistant Professor of Neurology, Harvard Medical School; Assistant Neurologist, Massachusetts General Hospital, Boston

DAVID S. SEGAL, Ph.D.
Professor of Psychiatry, School of Medicine, University of California at San Diego, La Jolla

JULIAN L. SEIFTER, M.D.
Assistant Professor of Medicine, Harvard Medical School; Associate Physician, Brigham and Women's Hospital, Boston

ANDREW P. SELWYN, M.D.
Associate Professor of Medicine, Harvard Medical School; Director, Cardiac Catheterization Laboratory, Brigham and Women's Hospital, Boston

BHAGWAN T. SHAHANI, M.B., B.S.
Associate Professor of Neurology, Harvard Medical School; Associate Neurologist, Massachusetts General Hospital, Boston

GORDON C. SHARP, M.D.
Professor of Medicine and Pathology and Director, Division of Rheumatology, University of Missouri-Columbia School of Medicine, Columbia

ELIZABETH M. SHORT, M.D.
Director, Division of Biomedical Research and Faculty Development, American Association of Medical Colleges, Washington, DC

WILLIAM SILEN, M.D.
Johnson and Johnson Professor of Surgery, Harvard Medical School; Surgeon-in-Chief, Department of Surgery, Beth Israel Hospital, Boston

FRED E. SILVERSTEIN, M.D.
Associate Professor of Medicine, Division of Gastroenterology, University of Washington School of Medicine, Seattle

JAMES B. SNOW, JR., M.D.
Professor and Chairman, Department of Otorhinolaryngology and Human Communication, University of Pennsylvania School of Medicine, Philadelphia

BURTON E. SOBEL, M.D.
Lewin Professor of Medicine, Washington University School of Medicine; Director, Cardiovascular Division, Barnes Hospital, St. Louis

ARTHUR J. SOBER, M.D.
Associate Professor of Dermatology, Harvard Medical School; Associate Dermatologist, Massachusetts General Hospital, Boston

FRANK E. SPEIZER, M.D.
Professor of Medicine, Harvard Medical School; Director, Occupational and Environmental Health Center, Brigham and Women's Hospital, Boston

JOHN W. STAKES, M.D.
Instructor in Neurology, Harvard Medical School; Assistant Neurologist, Massachusetts General Hospital, Boston

WALTER E. STAMM, M.D.
Professor of Medicine, University of Washington School of Medicine; Head, Division of Infectious Disease, Harborview Medical Center, Seattle

ALLEN C. STEERE, M.D.
Associate Professor of Medicine, Yale University School of Medicine, New Haven

KARI STEFANSSON, M.D.
Assistant Professor of Neurology and Pathology (Neuropathology), University of Chicago Pritzker School of Medicine, Chicago

GENE H. STOLLERMAN, M.D.
Professor of Medicine, Boston University School of Medicine; Attending Physician, University Hospital, Boston

D. E. STRANDNESS, JR., M.D.
Professor of Surgery, University of Washington School of Medicine; University Hospital, Seattle

DAVID H. P. STREETEN, M.B., D. Phil, F.R.C.P.
Professor of Medicine and Head, Section of Endocrinology, State University of New York Upstate Medical Center, Syracuse

E. DONNALL THOMAS, M.D.
Professor, Department of Medicine, University of Washington School of Medicine; Associate Director for Clinical Programs, Fred Hutchinson Cancer Research Center, Seattle

GENNARO M. TISI, M.D.
Professor of Medicine, Pulmonary and Critical Care Division, School of Medicine, University of California at San Diego; U.C.S.D. Medical Center, San Diego

PHILLIP P. TOSKES, M.D.
Professor of Medicine and Director, Division of Gastroenterology, Hepatology, and Nutrition, University of Florida College of Medicine; Veterans Administration Medical Center, Gainesville

MARVIN TURCK, M.D.
Professor of Medicine and Associate Dean, University of Washington School of Medicine; Medical Director, Harborview Medical Center, Seattle

KENNETH L. TYLER, M.D.
Assistant Professor of Neurology, Harvard Medical School; Clinical Assistant in Neurology, Massachusetts General Hospital, Boston

JOHN E. ULTMANN, M.D.
Professor of Medicine, Department of Medicine; Director, University of Chicago, Cancer Research Center; Dean for Research and Development, Division of the Biological Sciences, University of Chicago Pritzker School of Medicine, Chicago

MAURICE VICTOR, M.D.
Professor of Neurology, Case Western Reserve University School of Medicine; Director, Neurology Service, Cleveland Metropolitan General Hospital, Cleveland

JAMES F. WALLACE, M.D.
Professor of Medicine, University of Washington School of Medicine; Associate Physician-in-Chief, University Hospital, Seattle

PATRICK C. WALSH, M.D.
David Hall McConnell Professor and Director, Department of Urology, The Johns Hopkins University School of Medicine; Urologist-in-Chief, James Buchanan Brady Urological Institute, The Johns Hopkins Hospital, Baltimore

PETER D. WALZER, M.D.
Associate Professor of Medicine, University of Cincinnati College of Medicine; Chief, Infectious Diseases Section, Cincinnati Veterans Administration Medical Center, Cincinnati

JACK R. WANDS, M.D.
Associate Professor of Medicine, Harvard Medical School; Associate Physician, Gastrointestinal Unit, Massachusetts General Hospital, Boston

LOUIS WEINSTEIN, M.D., Ph.D., Sc.D. (Hon.)
Lecturer in Medicine, Harvard Medical School; Senior Consultant in Medicine, Brigham and Women's Hospital, Boston

JOHN B. WEST, M.D., Ph.D., D.Sc., F.R.C.P., F.R.A.C.P.
Professor of Medicine and Physiology, School of Medicine, University of California at San Diego; Physician, U.C.S.D. Medical Center, San Diego

NICHOLAS J. WHITE, M.D., M.R.C.P
Tropical Medicine Unit, Nuffield Department of Clinical Medicine, Oxford University, England; Faculty of Tropical Medicine, Mahidol University, Bangkok, Thailand

RICHARD J. WHITLEY, M.D.
Professor of Pediatrics and Microbiology, School of Medicine, University of Alabama in Birmingham, Birmingham

GRANT R. WILKINSON, M.D.
Professor of Pharmacology, Vanderbilt University School of Medicine, Nashville

GORDON H. WILLIAMS, M.D.
Professor of Medicine, Harvard Medical School; Chief, Endocrinology-Hypertension Division, Brigham and Women's Hospital, Boston

JEAN D. WILSON, M.D.
Professor of Internal Medicine, The University of Texas Health Science Center, Dallas

SHELDON M. WOLFF, M.D.
Endicott Professor and Chairman, Department of Medicine, Tufts University School of Medicine; Physician-in-Chief, New England Medical Center, Boston

ALASTAIR J. J. WOOD, M.D., M.B., Ch.B., M.R.C.P.
Associate Professor of Medicine and Associate Professor of Pharmacology, Vanderbilt University School of Medicine; Attending Physician, Vanderbilt University Hospital, Nashville

THEODORE E. WOODWARD, B.S., M.D., D.Sc. (Hon.)
Professor of Medicine Emeritus, University of Maryland School of Medicine; Distinguished Physician, Veterans Administration Hospital, Baltimore

SHIRLEY H. WRAY, M.D., Ph.D., F.R.C.P.
Associate Professor of Neurology, Harvard Medical School; Director, Unit for Neurovisual Disorders, Department of Neurology, Massachusetts General Hospital, Boston

JOSHUA WYNNE, M.D.
Professor of Internal Medicine and Chief, Division of Cardiology, Wayne State University School of Medicine; Chief, Section of Cardiology, Harper-Grace Hospitals, Detroit

JAMES B. YOUNG, M.D.
Professor of Medicine, Harvard Medical School; Associate Physician, Beth Israel Hospital, Boston

ROBERT R. YOUNG, M.D.
Professor of Neurology, Harvard Medical School; Neurologist and Director, Clinical Neurophysiology Laboratory, Massachusetts General Hospital, Boston

PREFACE

In this, the eleventh edition of *Harrison's Principles of Internal Medicine,* the editors have attempted to incorporate the latest advances in the biology, pathophysiology, diagnosis, and treatment of disease. The objective has been to provide appropriate bridges between the basic sciences and clinical medicine and to emphasize those advances in biomedical research which are of clinical importance, while retaining those facts which, while not new, remain clinically useful.

In adherence to the principles of those who founded the book, Part One, "Cardinal Manifestations of Disease," remains a mainstay of this edition. Its 54 chapters form a comprehensive introduction to clinical medicine with an emphasis on the pathophysiology of disease and the mechanisms of symptoms. The chapters in Part Two, "Biologic Considerations in the Approach to Clinical Medicine," focus on disorders which usually affect multiple organ systems, including genetic diseases, immune disturbances, disorders of nutrition, neoplasia, and geriatric medicine. In this section the interface between the "new biology" and clinical medicine receives major emphasis. These multisystem disorders are then followed, in Part Three, by a predominantly etiologically oriented section on infections, while the diseases of the major organ systems are discussed in the remaining ten parts of the book.

The eleventh edition also pays close attention to updated and current references. Although space constraints require that references be kept to a modest number, the editors have made particular efforts to include papers that were published in 1984, 1985, and even 1986. Although this has required omission of some important older papers, these almost always appear in the bibliographies of the newer ones. The reverse is, of course, not the case and hence our effort to keep the references up-to-date.

Cognizant of the current requirements for continuing education for licensure and relicensure, as well as the emphasis on certification and recertification, a revision of the *PreTest Self-Assessment and Review* appears in conjunction with this edition. *PreTest Self-Assessment and Review* consists of several hundred questions based upon the textbook, along with answers and explanations for the answers.

The rapid developments in clinical medicine and in the basic sciences on which it rests have mandated more extensive changes in the preparation of this edition of *Harrison's* than of any other edition.

Although we cannot highlight in this short preface all of the new and extensively updated parts of the eleventh edition, we would like to call the reader's attention to several of these:

- A new chapter attempts to demonstrate how rigorous quantitative methods may be applied in clinical reasoning and decision making.
- The genetics section has been reorganized and expanded to emphasize the relevance of molecular genetics to medicine in general and of oncogenes to the understanding of neoplasia.
- The endocrinology and metabolism section contains new comprehensive chapters on neuroendocrine and anterior pituitary disease, on disorders of growth, and on hereditable disorders of connective tissue. The chapter on diabetes mellitus has been extensively revised to take into account advances in the nosology and etiology of the disease. The section on disorders of bone and mineral metabolism has been extensively revised and contains a new chapter on hypercalcemic and hypocalcemic disorders.
- The autonomic nervous system is recognized to play a key role in many disease states, and drugs which affect this system are of increasing importance in many areas of clinical medicine. The normal and abnormal physiology and the pharmacology of this system are discussed in an expanded chapter.
- In the area of infectious diseases, more than a third of the chapters are new. Among these, the following are of particular importance: The chapter on *infections in the compromised host* has been completely revised and includes the most current understanding of the mechanisms of host defenses and their relationship to protection from infectious disease. The significance of *skin rashes* in infections is covered both in the text and in the expanded color atlas. There is an extensive update on *antibiotics,* including agents that are still under investigation, but are likely to become available in the near future; there is a new chapter on *antiviral chemotherapy.* In view of the growing importance of *sexually transmitted diseases,* there is considerable expansion of these chapters. The section on *virology* has been entirely revamped, with particular emphasis on the molecular biology of viral diseases. The chapters on cytomegalovirus infection and Epstein-Barr virus infection include the most current understanding of the relationship of these infections to modulation of the immune system. The chapter on *Pneumocystis carinii pneumonia* has been revised, particularly with regard to the newly appreciated importance of this infection in patients with AIDS. New chapters on *schistosomiasis* and such new parasitic pathogens as *cryptosporidiosis* have been added. An extensive and up-to-date description of Lyme arthritis is provided.
- The major advances in cardiology that are emphasized in new or radically revised chapters include noninvasive methods of cardiac examination, electrophysiologic approaches to the diagnosis and treatment of cardiac arrhythmias, percutaneous transluminal angioplasty, and thrombolytic treatment of acute myocardial infarction.
- There has been considerable progress in understanding the pathogenesis and management of cystic fibrosis, hypersensitivity pneumonitis, and interstitial lung disease. The section on respiratory disease includes new chapters on these important disorders.
- Major revisions have been made in the gastrointestinal section with special emphasis on gastrointestinal endoscopy. New color plates of the appropriate endoscopic findings of various gastrointestinal disorders are included.
- The entire section on liver diseases has undergone major revision with a totally new chapter on viral as well as on drug-induced hepatitis, including the approach to the diagnosis of non-A, non-B hepatitis and the delta agent. Similarly, the important area of cirrhosis has also been revised. There is a new chapter on liver transplantation.
- The sections on disorders of the immune system and disorders of immune-mediated injury have been rewritten almost completely. These chapters now represent the most updated understanding of the relationship between aberrancies of immune function and immune-mediated diseases. Of particular note is the chapter on the acquired immunodeficiency syndrome which provides an in-depth understanding of all aspects of this syndrome. Also of note in this section is the much expanded chapter on the vasculitic syndromes. This chapter provides a coherent organization of these complex diseases and a better understanding of pathogenesis as well as the most modern approaches toward therapy.
- In the section on hematology there are new chapters on the anemias due to bone marrow failure and bone marrow transplantation. The chapters on platelets and blood coagulation are completely new with a new author for this important section. The chapter on enlargement of lymph nodes and spleen has been expanded to include a detailed description of the multiple mechanisms of lymph node and spleen enlargement, while the chapter on disorders of the phagocytic cells includes the most updated understanding of the metabolism of functional capabilities of phagocytic cells.
- The rapid advances in oncology are reflected in new chapters on the basic principles of neoplasia, carcinoma of the ovary and testis, the endocrine manifestations of neoplasia, and neurologic manifestations of neoplastic disorders. The chapter on the human T-lymphotropic virus is a comprehensive and authoritative treatise on the role of these important retroviruses in human diseases, an observation which has only recently been made and which has important potential implications in understanding the role of viruses

in neoplastic as well as nonneoplastic diseases. The new chapter on the leukemias includes the modern classification of these important disorders.

- The neurology section, long a key component of *Harrison's*, has undergone substantial change. There are new chapters on acute and chronic pain, on dizziness and vertigo, ataxia and disorders of equilibrium and gait, the peripheral neuropathies, cerebrovascular diseases, and brain trauma. A radically revised chapter on the degenerative diseases of the nervous system with particular focus on Alzheimer's disease and Parkinson's disease brings the latest information about the neurochemistry, neuropathology, and management of these important disorders.
- The entire section on psychiatry has been rewritten and represents a major addition to this edition.

One of the strengths of *Harrison's* has been the close-knit relationships among the editors. Dr. Joseph Martin, the Julieanne Dorn Professor of Neurology at Harvard Medical School and Chief of the Neurological Services of the Massachusetts General Hospital, worked together with his distinguished predecessor, Dr. Raymond D. Adams on the tenth edition. With the latter's retirement from the textbook, Dr. Martin assumed sole editorial responsibility for the sections on neurology, myology, and psychiatry in the eleventh edition. He has been an important addition to the editorial group.

The editors warmly welcome Dr. Anthony S. Fauci, Director of the National Institute of Allergy and Infectious Diseases and Chief of its Laboratory of Immunoregulation, to *Harrison's*. Dr. Fauci is one of the leading clinical immunologists in the world. He has made a profound contribution to this edition with his expertise in this critically important area of biology and his ability to describe its impact on many areas of internal medicine.

We also wish to express our appreciation to our many associates and colleagues who, as experts in their fields, have helped us with constructive and valuable criticisms of the chapters in the eleventh edition. We wish to thank the following for many helpful suggestions: Drs. Stuart Aaronson, Raymond D. Adams, John W. Adamson, John F. Alksne, Ronald J. Anderson, Elliott M. Antman, Gust H. Bardy, Robert C. Bast, John E. Bennett, David Bilheimer, Harry G. Bluestein, Neil Breslau, Oscar L. Bronsther, Michael S. Brown, Robert H. Brown, George P. Canellos, Antonino Catanzaro, Bayard D. Catherwood, Bruce A. Chabner, Robert M. Chanock, Harold A. Chapman, Thomas N. Chase, William W. Chin, Mario Chojkier, Charles G. Cochrane, David I. Cohen, Steven E. Come, Rex William Cowdry, Clyde S. Crumpacker, Gilbert H. Daniels, Charles E. Davis, David M. Dawson, Leonard J. Deftos, Thomas L. Delbanco, Robert O. Dillman, Robert G. Dluhy, William P. Docken, Jeffrey M. Drazen, David M. Eddy, Leonard Ellman, Arthur S. Elstein, Darrell D. Fanestil, Alvan R. Feinstein, Mark Feldman, Joshua Fierer, Brian G. Firth, Daniel W. Foster, Fred H. Frankel, Lawrence S. Friedman, Paul A. Friedman, Peter Friedman, Theodore Friedmann, Gary R. Fujimoto, Harris H. Funkenstein, Ary L. Goldberger, Joseph L. Goldstein, John L. Gollan, Harvey H. Gralnick, Mark R. Green, James E. Griffin, Robert C. Griggs, Richard H. Haas, Ivan R. Harwood, Fred Hendler, Martin S. Hirsch, Stephen B. Howell, Gary W. Hunninghake, Jon I. Isenberg, Stephen P. James, Kenneth Lee Jones, Lewis L. Judd, Albert Z. Kapikian, Dennis L. Kasper, Barrett Katz, Robert Katzman, Robert S. Kauffman, Martin J. Kelly, Anthony L. Komaroff, Conrad V. Kufta, Randi Y. Leavitt, Mark Leshin, Ronald Levy, Matthew H. Liang, Markku Linnoila, John D. Loeser, Kenneth Luskey, Paula Macrae, John A. Mannick, Lawrence F. Marshall, Henry Masur, J. Allen McCutchan, Henry F. McFarland, Dale E. McFarlin, George R. Merriam, Edgar L. Milford, Brian R. Murphy, James R. Nelson, Anne Nicholson-Weller, Michael R. Oxman, Charles Y. C. Pak, Alan G. Palestine, Sebastian Palmeri, Alfred F. Parisi, Joseph E. Parillo, Stephen G. Pauker, Alan S. Pearlman, James E. Pennington, Candace B. Pert, Marion Peters, Kirk L. Peterson, Willy F. Piessens, Richard Platt, Robert M. Post, William Z. Potter, Joe W. Ramsdell, Samuel I. Rapaport, Peter Reich, Michael Ronthal, Richard K. Root, Allan H. Ropper, Saul W. Rosen, David S. Rosenthal, John F. Rothrock, Daniel Rotrosen, John W. Rowe, John D. Rutherford, John E. Salvaggio, Martin A. Samuels, Stephen Scharfstein, Joseph D. Schmidt, Brian Schmitt, Edward L. Schneider, Lowell E. Schnipper, Peter H. Schur, John D. Schwankhaus, William J. Schwartz, Dennis J. Selkoe, Larry J. Shapiro, Clifford W. Shults, Cecelia M. Smith, Stephen A. Spector, Frank E. Speizer, Stephen E. Straus, Michael R. Swenson, Raymond Taetle, Ira B. Tager, Michael D. Tharp, David E. Trentham, Jerry S. Trier, H. Richard Tyler, Athol J. Ware, Steven E. Weinberger, Michael E. Weinblatt, Michael H. Weisman, Peter F. Weller, Alison Wichman, Robert F. Wilkens, Shirley H. Wray, Neal S. Young, Randall K. Young, Robert C. Young, Robert R. Young, and Elizabeth J. Ziegler.

This book could not have been edited without the dedicated help of our coworkers in the editorial offices of the individual editors. We are especially indebted to Patricia A. Clougherty, Patricia E. DeLosh, Lourdes C. Felix, Hilda Gardner, Brenda Hennis, Mary Jackson, Ann C. London, Lucy Renzi, Darlene Reynolds, Janice Stearns, and Michéle M. Stewart.

Finally, we need to say a word of thanks to our colleagues at McGraw-Hill, Dereck Jeffers, Executive Editor, and Eileen Scott, Development Editor. They formed a most effective team who gave the editors constant encouragement, and were of enormous help in the countless efforts involved in bringing this complex effort to fruition.

THE EDITORS

Harrison's
PRINCIPLES OF INTERNAL MEDICINE

COLOR ATLASES

Atlas 1 Atlas of common lesions encountered during the physical examination of the skin

The skin and mucous membrane may frequently contain a variety of lesions that are rarely a major complaint (see Fig. 47-1). They are, therefore, incidental findings in the general physical examination. The recognition of "bumps and blemishes" is a necessary first step for physicians inasmuch as they will be required to distinguish the trivial from the serious and important skin changes. For example, such a serious lesion as a malignant melanoma may be incidentally discovered during a routine physical examination (see Figs. A1-30 to A1-32 and the discussion in Chap. 302).

The common disorders of the skin that every physician should be able to recognize are presented in this series of color photographs (Figs. A1-1 to A1-23).

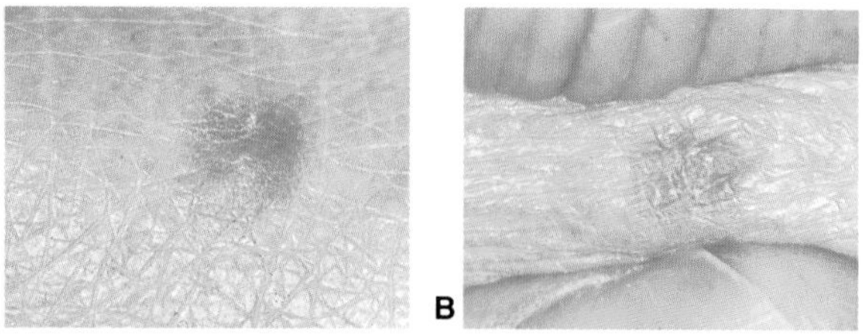

A B

A1-1 **Dermatofibroma** is especially common in middle life and in women. The lesions, when pigmented, are occasionally confused with malignant melanoma. They appear as isolated, slightly elevated, hard, button-like nodules (*A*). In fair-skinned persons, the lesions are not usually skin color, but are pink or dark red, yellowish brown, or gray-black. They are usually less than 1 cm in diameter. A diagnostic sign is that a dermatofibroma dimples or becomes depressed (*B*) when it is laterally compressed; melanocytic nevus and melanoma, however, with which dermatofibroma may be easily confused, become elevated with lateral compression.

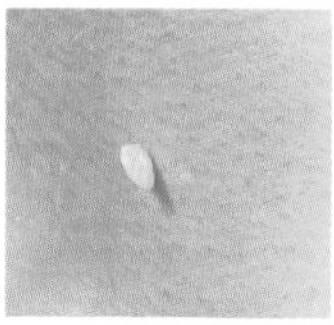

A1-2 **Acrochordon** (skin tag) is very common after middle life and appears on the neck, especially in women, in the axillae, and on the upper part of the trunk. The lesions are small (1 to 5 mm), soft, pedunculated papules, usually of normal skin color.

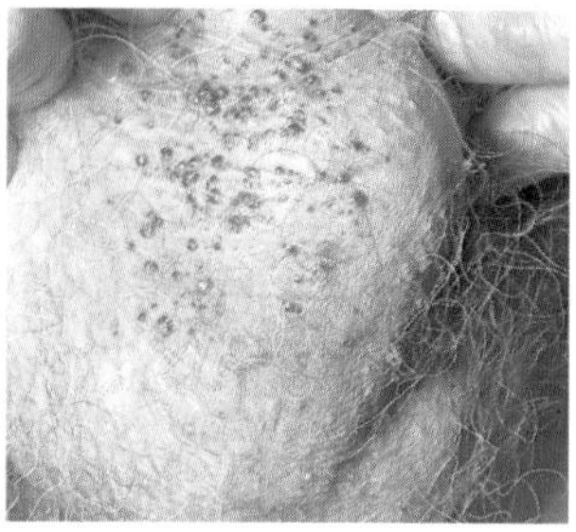

A1-3 **Angiokeratomas** are bizarre vascular dilatations that occur under the tongue and on the scrotum and consist of myriads of 2- to 3-mm purplish red papules. They are of no known significance. When they occur on the trunk and extremities, a biopsy is indicated to rule out glycolipid lipidosis or Fabry's disease.

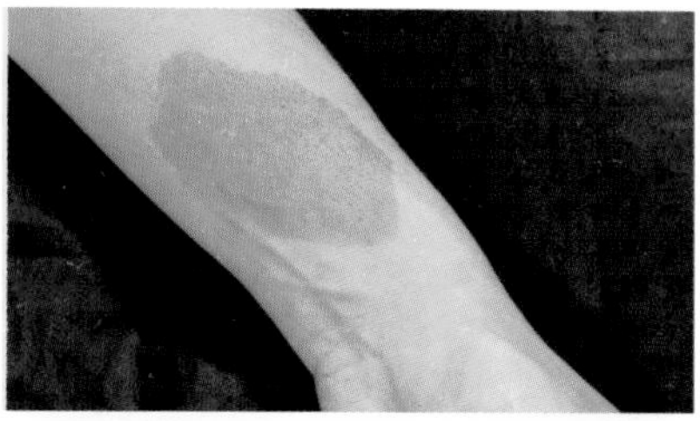

A1-4 **Café au lait macules** are found in about 10 percent of the normal population and, in fair-skinned persons, are light yellowish brown macules, which may also be markers of neurofibromatosis and polyostotic fibrous dysplasia (Albright's syndrome). The presence of six or more café au lait macules with a diameter of 1.5 cm or greater is diagnostic of neurofibromatosis.

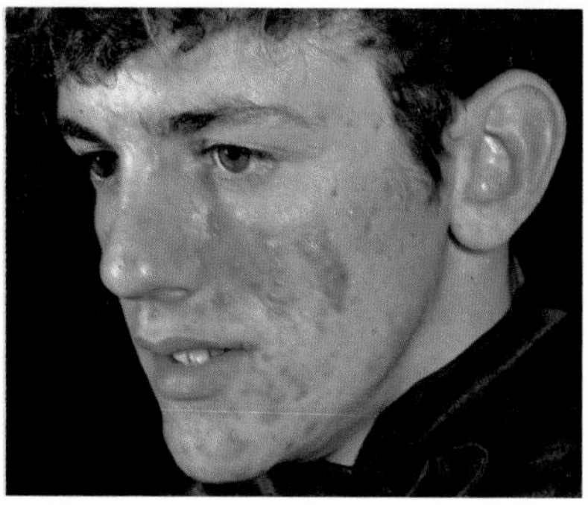

A1-5 **Acne** is a condition in which the most characteristic lesion is the comedo, or "blackhead," that later becomes a conical erythematous papule or pustule. A third type of lesion is the "blind boil," which is a dermal cyst without an orifice. This lesion is often associated with atrophic or hypertrophic scarring. Cystic acne may appear with only a very few comedones; also, comedo-like acne may occur with few cysts or erythematous papules.

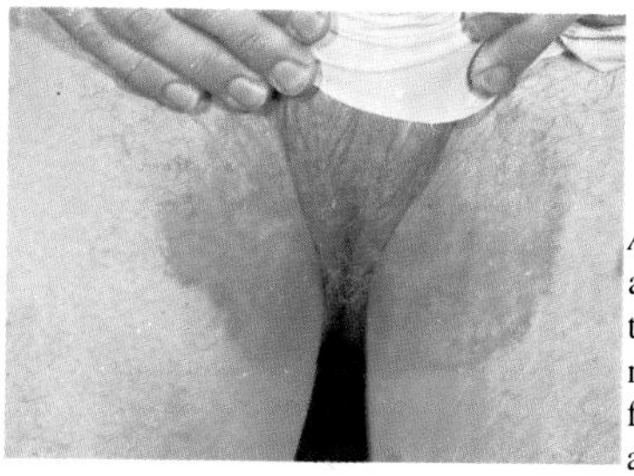

A1-6 **Dermatophytosis** is identified by the striking polycyclic, annular shape of the scaling, especially on the feet and hands, where there is often a scalloped pattern. A positive diagnosis of dermatophytosis is quickly established by direct examination of scales from the advancing border; the mycelia are revealed when the scales are immersed in 10% potassium hydroxide or Swartz stain.

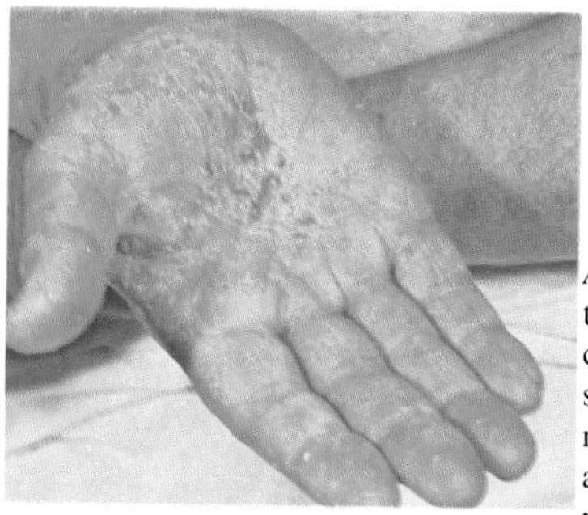

A1-7 **Eczematous dermatitis** is a very common cutaneous reaction that is localized to the hands of housewives, to the legs in patients with chronic venous insufficiency, and behind the ears in patients with seborrheic dermatitis. In subacute eczematous dermatitis, there are mild erythema, dry scales, and often small red papules, many of which are excoriated. In chronic eczematous dermatitis, lichenification is the most prominent feature.

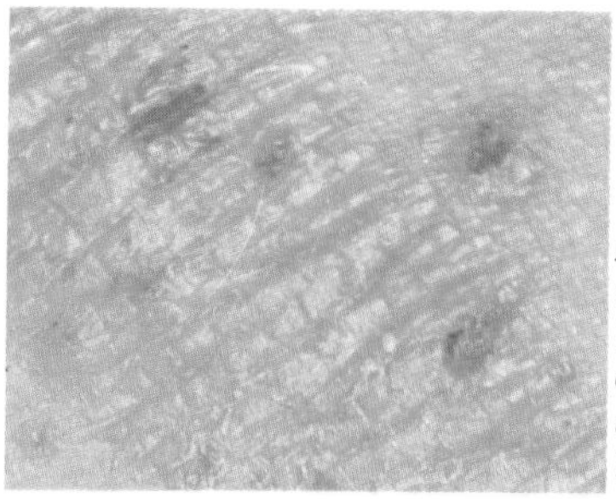

A1-8 **Localized lichenification** results from repeated rubbing of the skin and consists of isolated, circumscribed plaques. These single lesions vary in size from 2 to 10 cm and occur most often on the extensor aspect of the forearm and in the scrotal, nuchal, inguinal, and anogenital areas. The perianal and vulvar areas may become diffusely lichenified. Lichenification is thought to be more frequent in persons with an atopic background.

A1-9 **Melasma (chloasma)** is the so-called "mask" of pregnancy, but it also occurs in men and in women taking progestational agents. The pigmentation is uniform and is limited to the exposed areas of the face. There is no scaling or epidermal change. In fair-skinned persons, the pigment may be any shade from light tan to a very dark brown. It is most often seen on the cheek and upper lip, as here, and on the forehead.

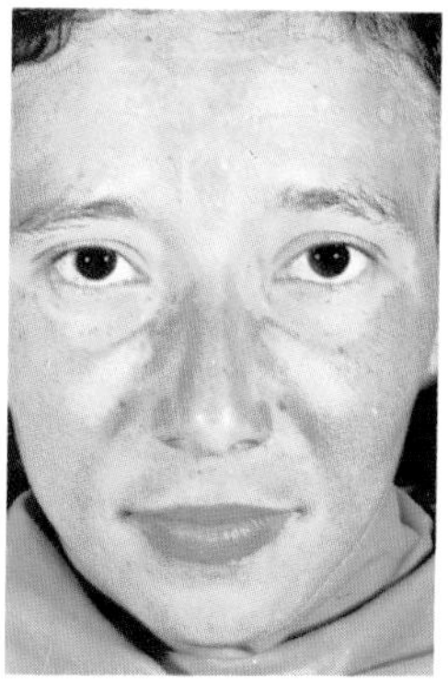

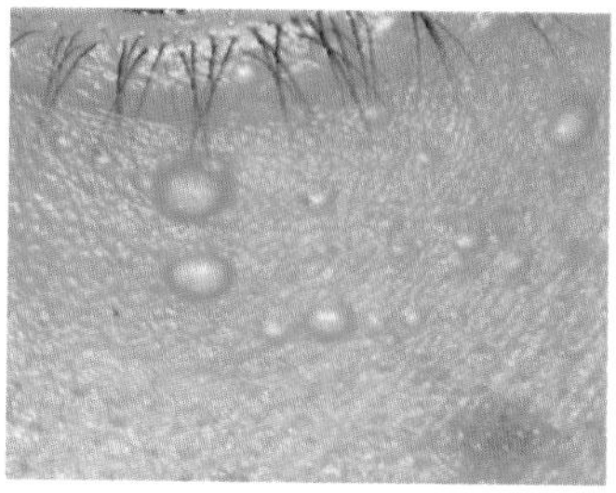

A1-10 **Milia** are a collection of lesions, occurring most commonly on the face, and consist of tiny (1 to 2 mm), white, hard, rounded, superficial papules. There is no orifice, and the keratinous contents are easily expressed by lateral compression after the making of a tiny incision in the dome of the lesion.

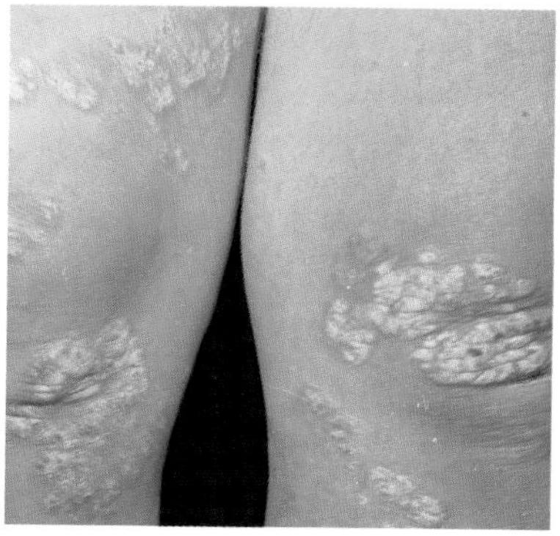

A1-11 **Psoriasis,** affecting more than 2 percent of the population, consists of isolated scaling papules or plaques and is quite commonly observed in the routine physical examination. The lesions occur most frequently on the scalp, elbows, and knees. The color and type of scales are the identifying features of the lesions. The scales are either dense and lamellated with peripherally detached edges or loose and branny. The plaques are pink to deep red, and the borders are distinct.

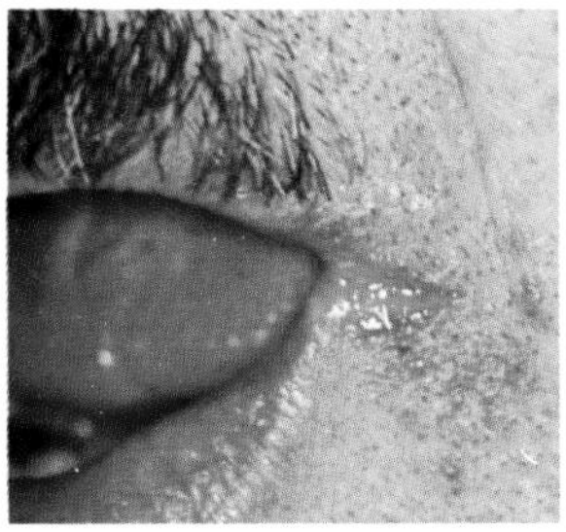

A1-12 **Perlèche** consists of painful small fissures at the angles of the mouth, often covered with yellow crusts. Perlèche most often occurs with poorly fitting dentures and in moniliasis and secondary syphilis.

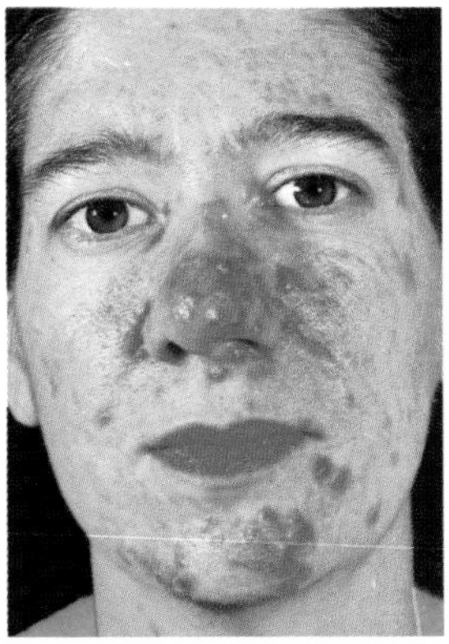

A1-13 **Rosacea,** usually limited to the face, consists of tiny, erythematous papules and pustules 1 to 5 mm in size. The pustules, often tiny and sometimes hardly visible, sit on the dome of the papules. The diffuse redness of the face is due to vasodilatation, as well as to myriad telangiectases. In men, rhinophyma, a disfiguring enlargement of the nose, may occur.

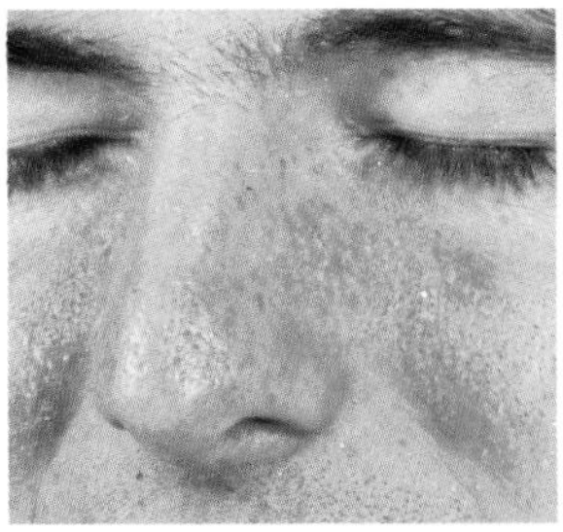

A1-14 **Seborrheic dermatitis,** a common disorder found in all age groups, occurs most frequently on the scalp, eyebrows, and nasolabial folds and behind the ears. Scaling is the prominent feature and is loose and branny; it may be yellow and oily or dry and white. The lesion may become exudative and crusted or eczematous.

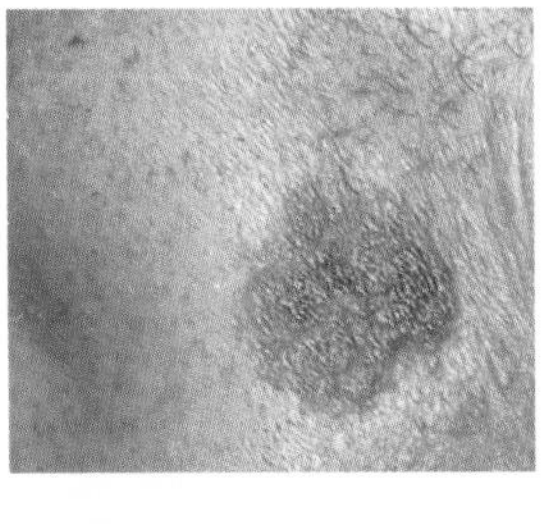

A1-15 **Seborrheic keratosis** appears in middle life and may occur on exposed or unexposed areas but is especially common on the trunk. The lesions are irregularly round or oval flat-topped papules or plaques that seem "stuck" on the skin. The margins are distinct, and the surface is often warty or consists of multiple tiny projections (vegetation). In fair-skinned persons, the lesions are light brown at first but, enlarging, become more heavily pigmented and may be confused with malignant melanoma.

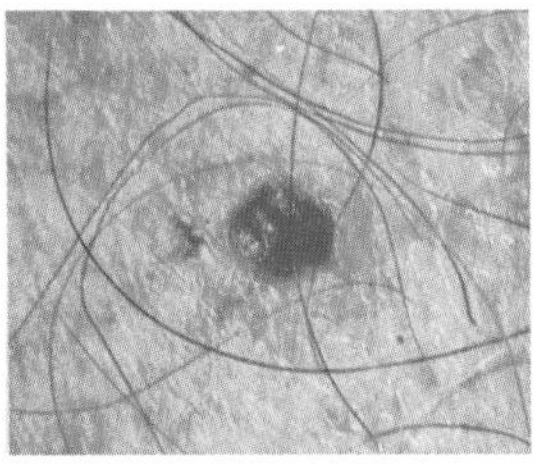

A1-16 **Senile angioma ("cherry red spot")** appears in the third decade. On the lip, the lesion is usually singular and consists of a bluish red round nodule. On the trunk, the lesions are small (2 to 3 mm), bright red, globular papules.

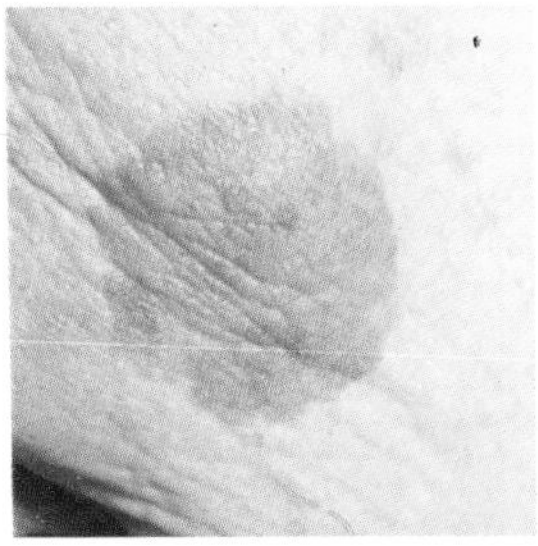

A1-17 **Senile lentigo** occurs as a single macule or as a group of isolated, sharply circumscribed macules on the exposed areas, especially on the dorsal surfaces of the hands and arms and on the forehead and cheeks. The macules are usually light yellowish brown, but may be dark brown; the color is somewhat variegated, rather than uniform as it is in a café au lait macule. Rarely, dark brown *papules* develop in these lesions, and then the condition is called *lentigo maligna,* which may slowly develop, over a period of years, into a melanoma (lentigo maligna melanoma).

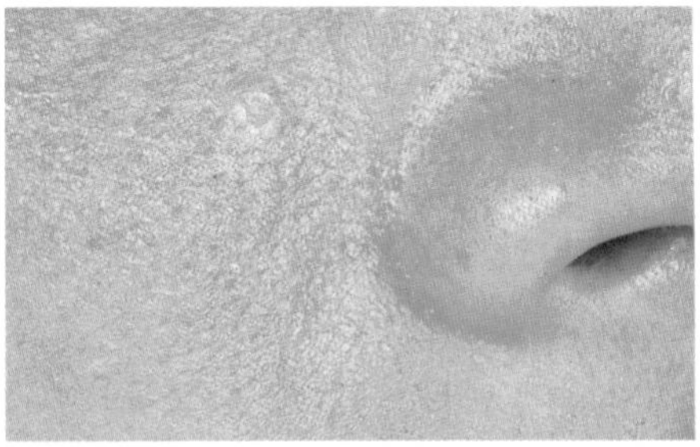

A1-18 **Senile sebaceous adenoma** occurs on the face in patients over 40 and is often diagnosed as basal-cell carcinoma. The lesions are soft, small, flat-topped papules, varying in size from 1 to 8 mm, and are characterized by a minute central depression from which sebaceous material can be exuded by lateral compression.

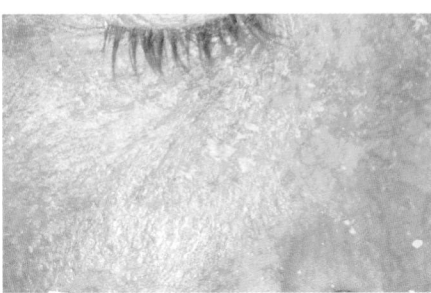

A1-19 **Solar keratosis** (1) occurs usually in persons with light skin prone to sunburn or with darker skin after chronic excessive exposure; (2) is strictly limited to exposed skin, especially on the face and dorsal surfaces of the hands; (3) is more easily felt than seen (gritty and sandpaperish); (4) in fair-skinned persons, consists of skin-colored or light brown macules or slightly raised papules with superficial adherent scales not easily removed; and (5) is associated with marked wrinkling, telangiectasia, and often diffuse, tiny, pale yellow papules indicating solar degeneration of connective tissue ("turkey skin").

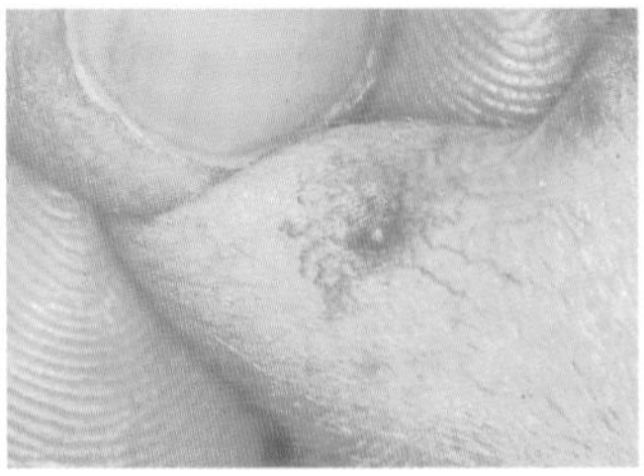

A1-20 **Spider nevus** consists of a central, punctate, bright red macule or papule (the body) from which fine red lines radiate like spider legs. There is often a red flare between the radiating vessels. On diascopy, the central body pulsates.

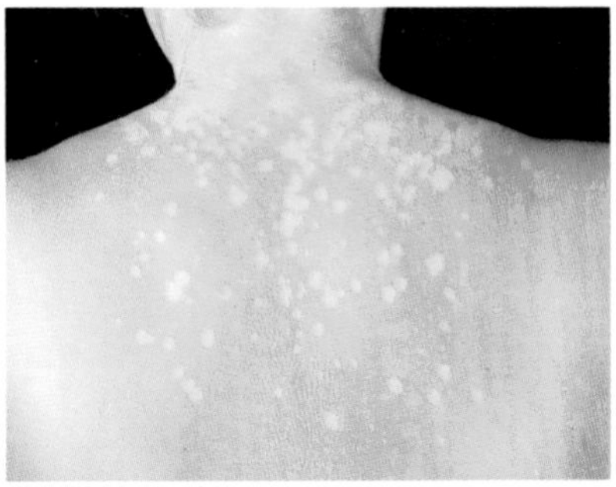

A1-21 **Tinea versicolor** is a relatively common disorder occurring primarily on the trunk and appearing in two forms: as scattered, 3- to 5-mm, very slightly scaling brown macules or as whitish macules that may be confused with vitiligo. The fungal spores and hyphae can be easily demonstrated on direct examination of the scales using Swartz stain.

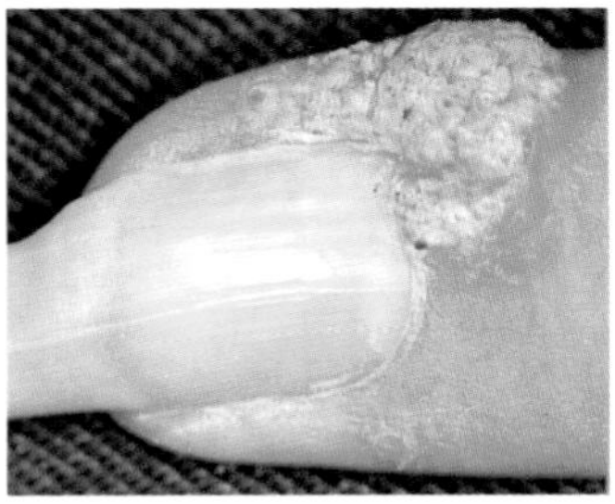

A1-22 **Verruca vulgaris** may occur at any age, but it is most common in children. The lesions, which vary in size from 0.5 to 2.0 cm, are round or oval, firm, skin colored papules with multiple tiny keratotic, rounded or filiform projections covering the surface (vegetation). They occur most frequently on the hands and soles.

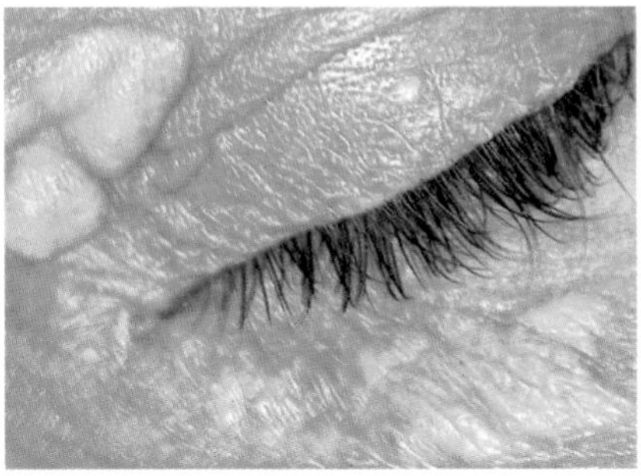

A1-23 **Xanthelasma** consists of one or more bright yellow, sharply marginated plaques with no epidermal change, usually occurring on the eyelids. All patients with xanthelasma should be investigated for evidence of plasma lipid abnormalities.

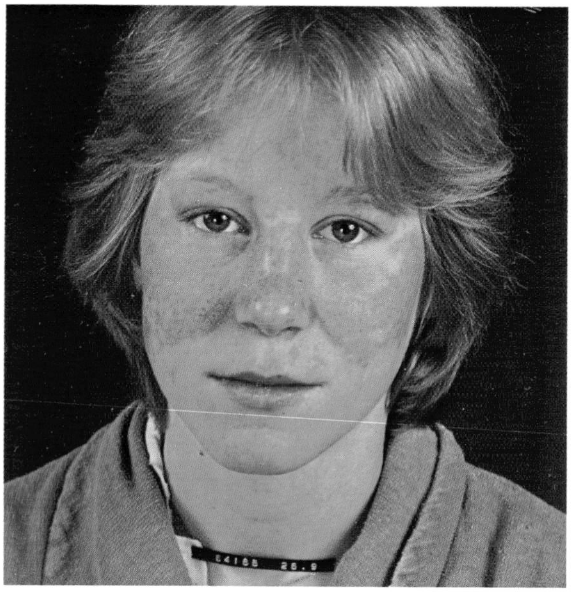

A1-24 **Systemic lupus erythematosus.** Erythematous, confluent, butterfly-like eruption with fine scaling.

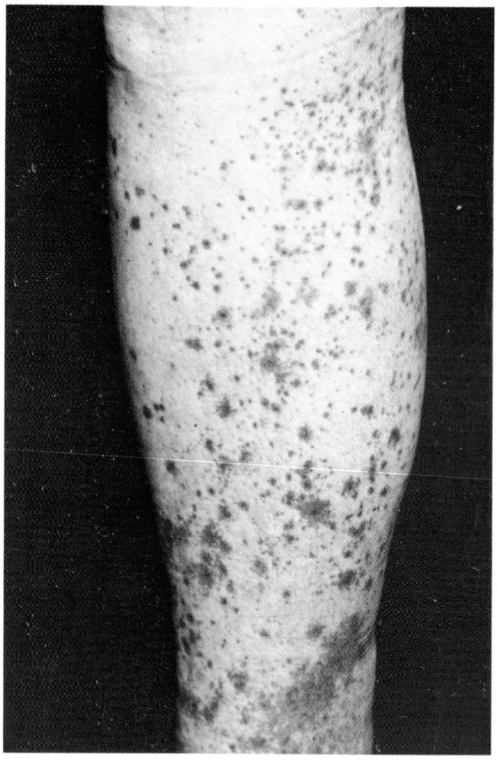

A1-25 **Necrotizing vasculitis syndrome.** Scattered discrete, purpuric eruption on the legs. The purpura is "palpable."

A

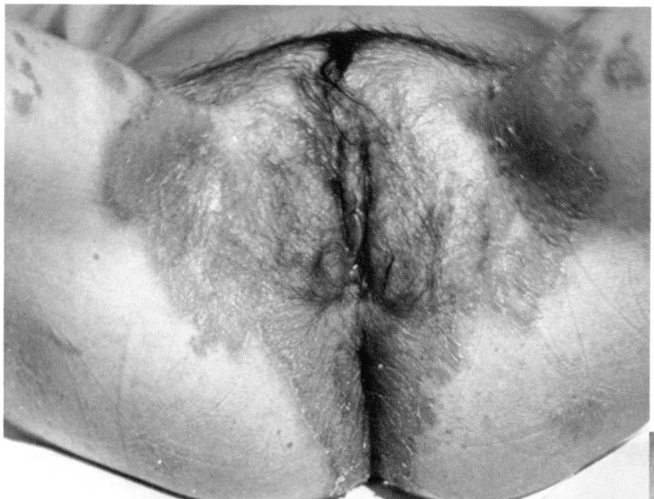

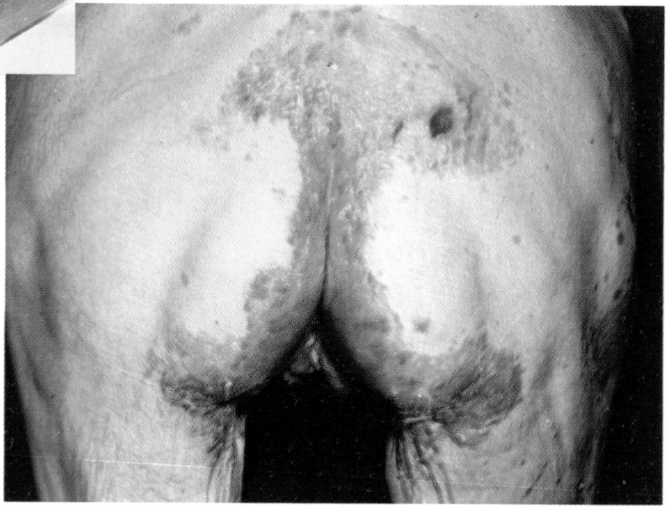

B

A1-26 **Glucagonoma** (*A*) and **acquired zinc deficiency** (*B*). Circinate and gyrate areas of blistering, erosion, and maceration. The eruption is often mistaken for psoriasis or mucocutaneous moniliasis.

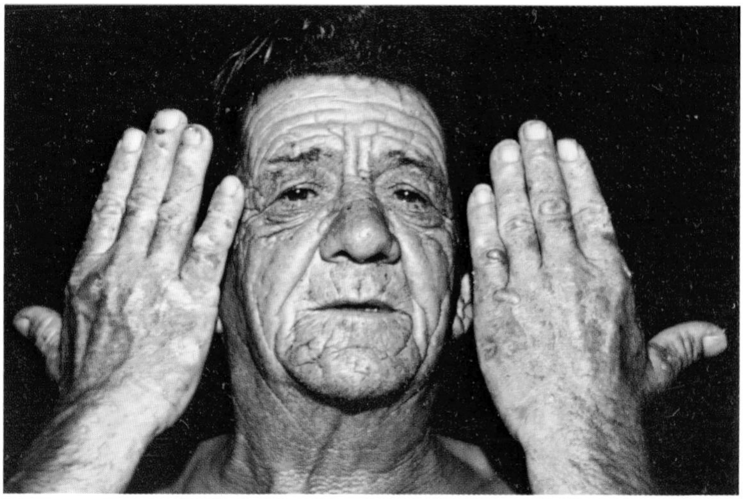

A1-27 **Porphyria cutanea tarda.** Violaceous suffusion in the periorbital skin is evident. There are erosions and pink atrophic scars at sites of previous bullae on the dorsa of the hands.

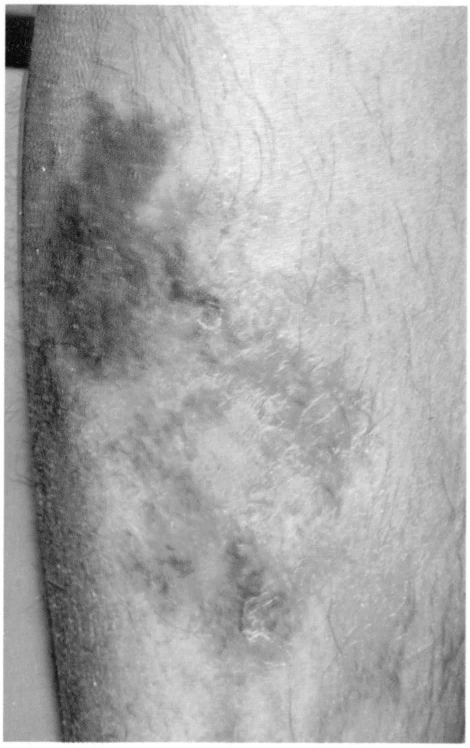

A1-28 **Necrobiosis lipoidica.** The lesion often begins as a small, dusky red, elevated nodule with a sharp border. It slowly enlarges, becomes flattened and eventually depressed as the dermis becomes atrophic. The color becomes brownish yellow except for the border, which may remain reddened. Delicate vessels can be seen through the atrophic epidermis.

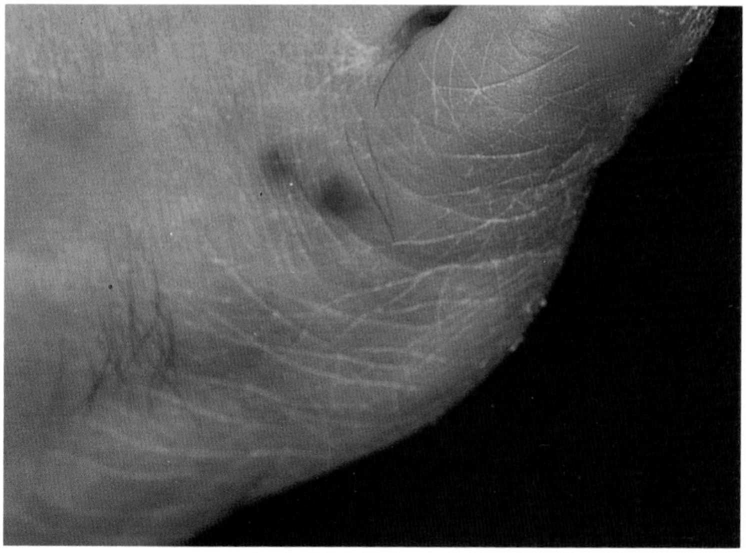

A1-29 Two purplish red nodules of **Kaposi's sarcoma** in a patient with AIDS.

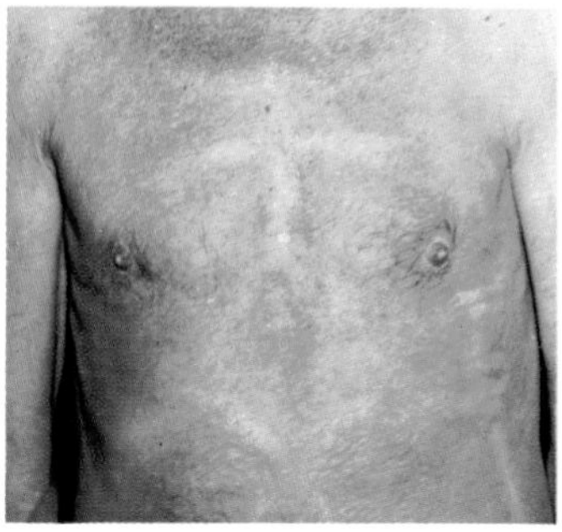

A1-30 **Carcinoid** showing the effect of stroking. In contrast to the flushing that occurs in other disorders, the flush in carcinoid is typically a panorama of colors, ranging from bizarre pinkish orange to bright red to violaceous to blanching white. The flush (which lasts only a few minutes) spreads from the face to the neck, shoulders, chest, and arms.

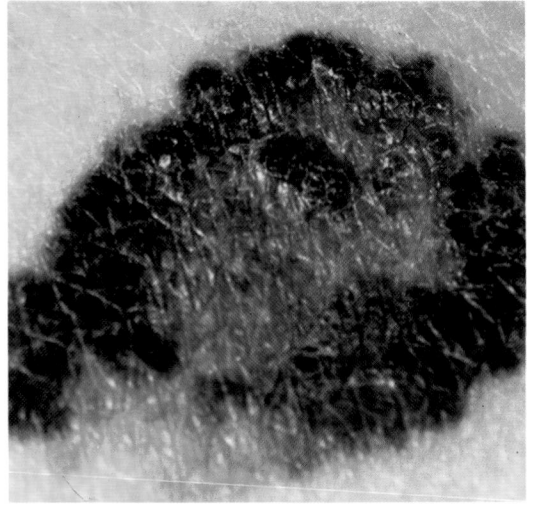

A

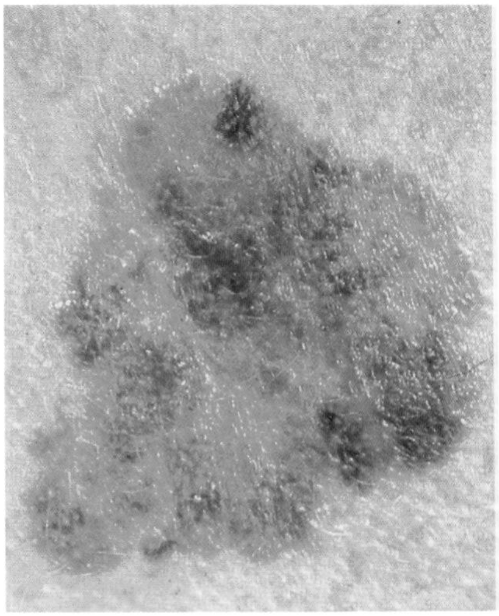

B

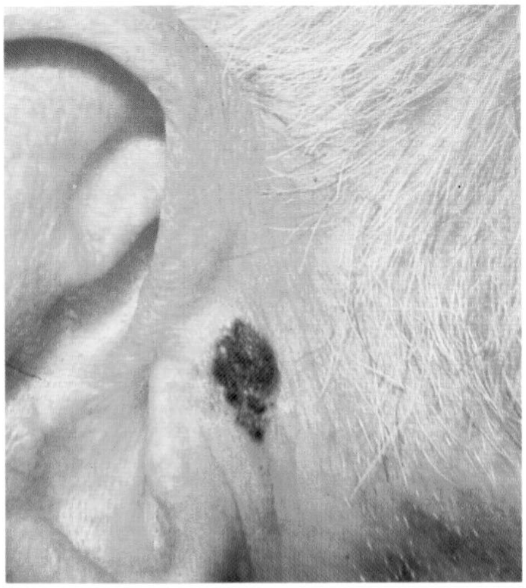

C

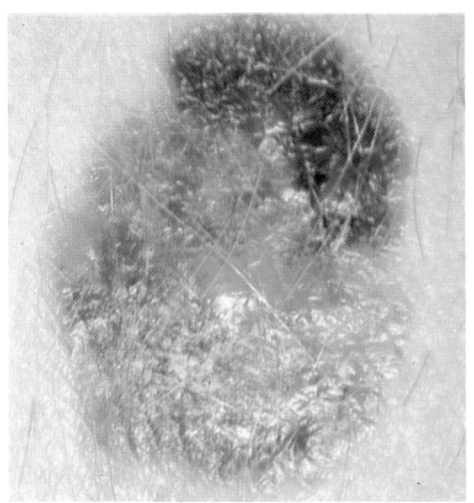

D

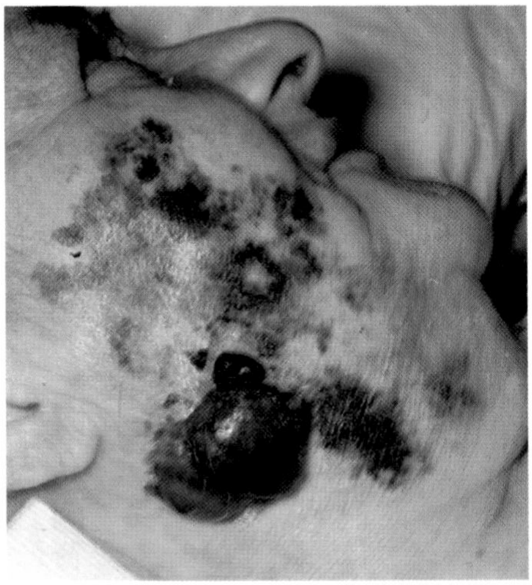

E

A1-31 **Malignant melanoma.** On close inspection melanomas shown are characterized by irregular surface (*A*), irregular border and notching (*B*), and nodularity (*C*). Also shown are a reniform melanoma (*D*), an extensive lentigo maligna on face of patient (*E*) and a regressive melanoma characterized by grayish color infiltrated with pink areas (*F*). (From Hospital Practice, January 1982, with permission.)

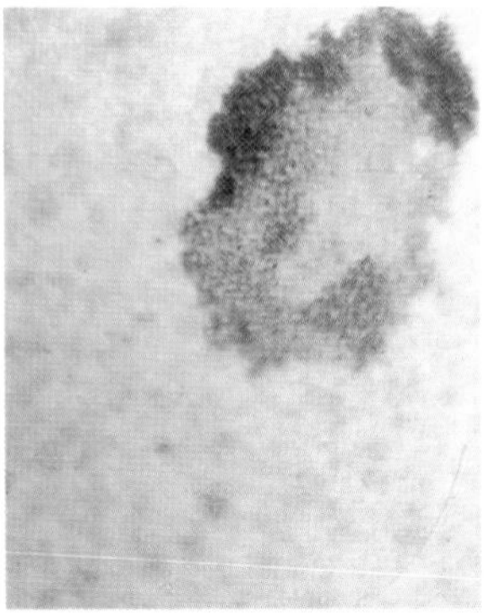

F

A

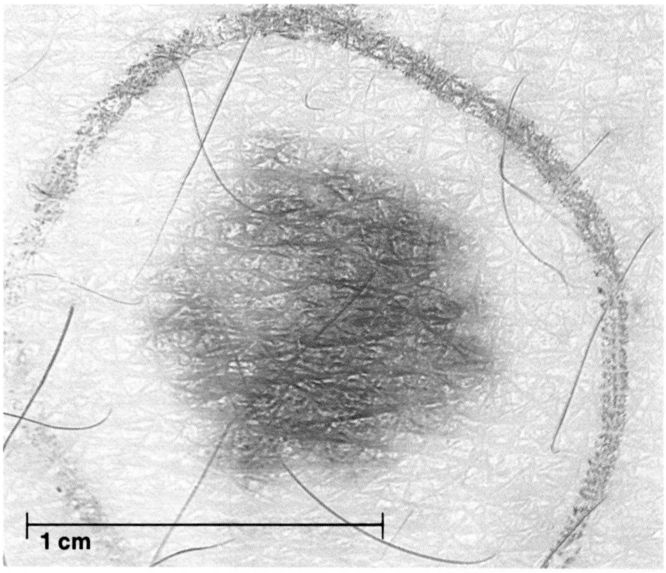

B

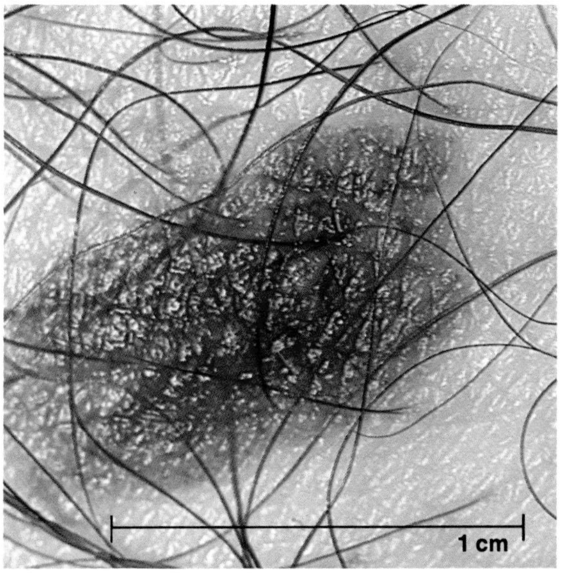

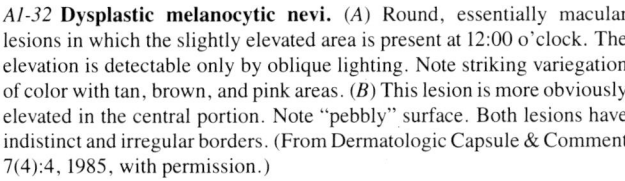

A1-32 **Dysplastic melanocytic nevi.** (*A*) Round, essentially macular lesions in which the slightly elevated area is present at 12:00 o'clock. The elevation is detectable only by oblique lighting. Note striking variegation of color with tan, brown, and pink areas. (*B*) This lesion is more obviously elevated in the central portion. Note "pebbly" surface. Both lesions have indistinct and irregular borders. (From Dermatologic Capsule & Comment 7(4):4, 1985, with permission.)

A1-33 **Malignant melanoma – dysplastic nevus syndrome.** This 28-year-old woman gave a history of a rapidly growing (3 to 6 months), asymptomatic lesion on her right scapular area. Her mother had melanoma and both mother and siblings had many dark "moles." Diagnosis: (1) Superficial spreading melanoma, level IV, 4.75 mm. (2) Regional nodes – of 32 removed, 1 was positive. (3) Dysplastic nevus syndrome with family history of melanoma. Note primary lesion and many dark "moles" on back (*A*) and dysplastic nevi on untanned areas under the bathing suit straps (*B*). (From Dermatologic Capsule & Comment 6(4):3, 1984, with permission.)

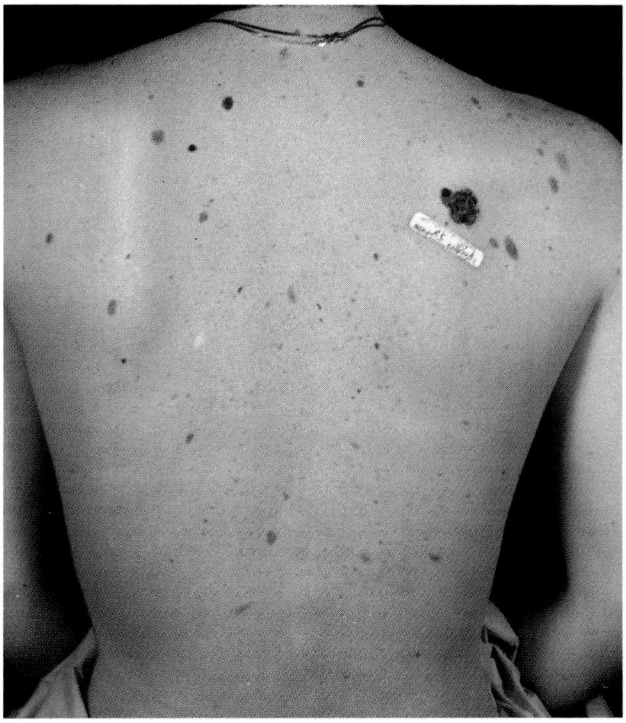

A

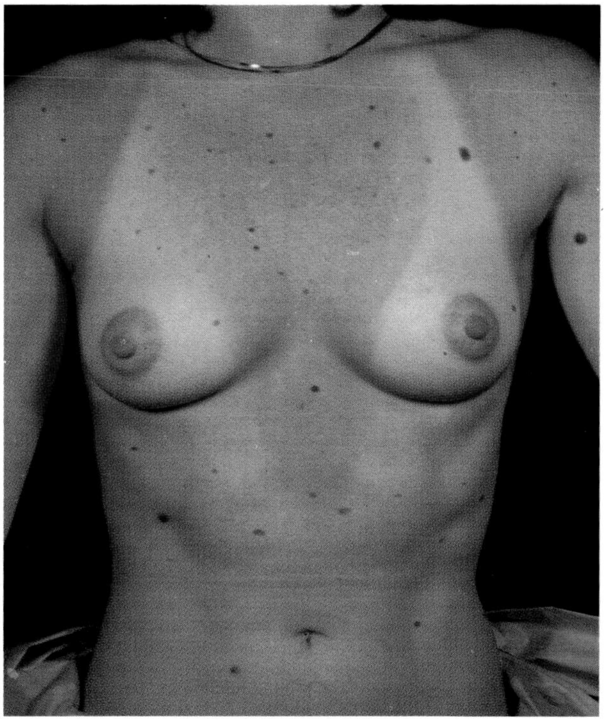

B

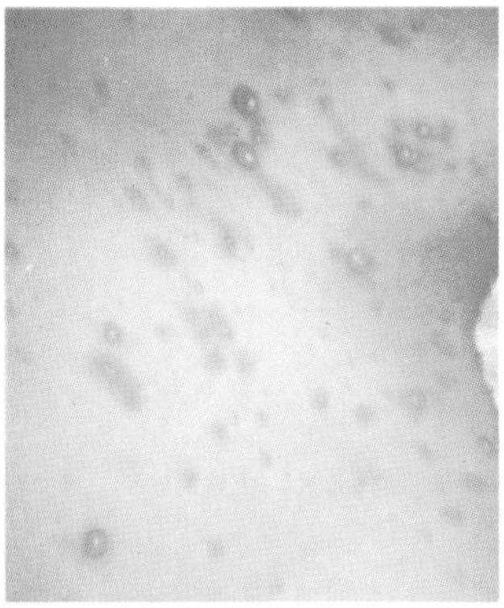

A2-1 **Varicella** (chickenpox).[3]

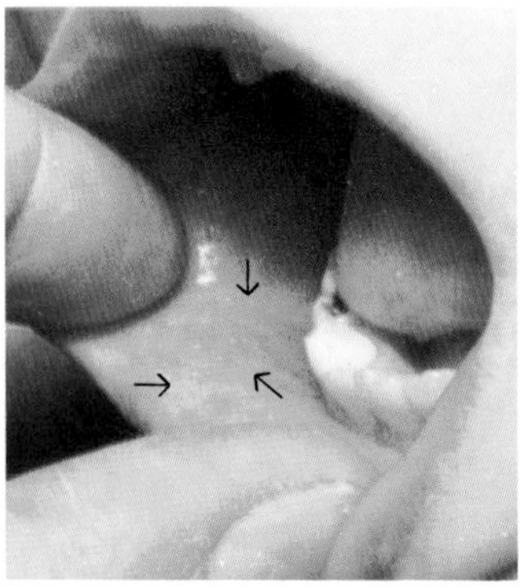

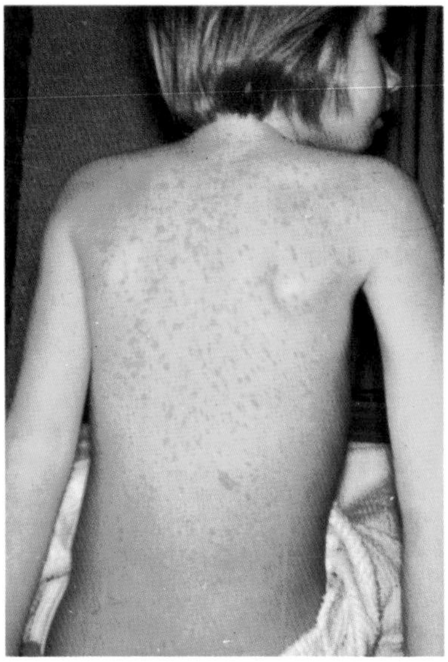

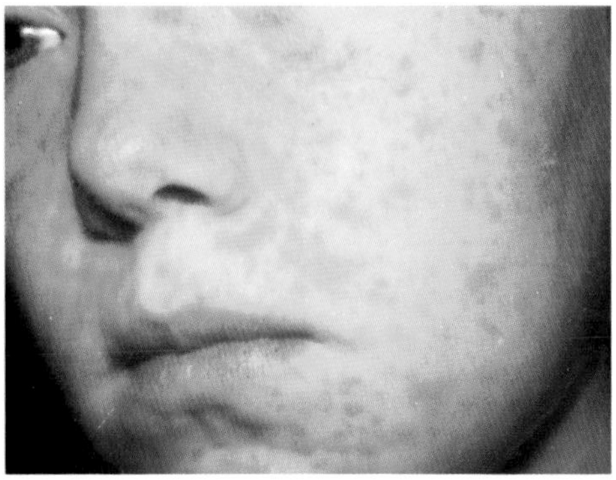

A2-2 **Measles** (rubeola).[3]

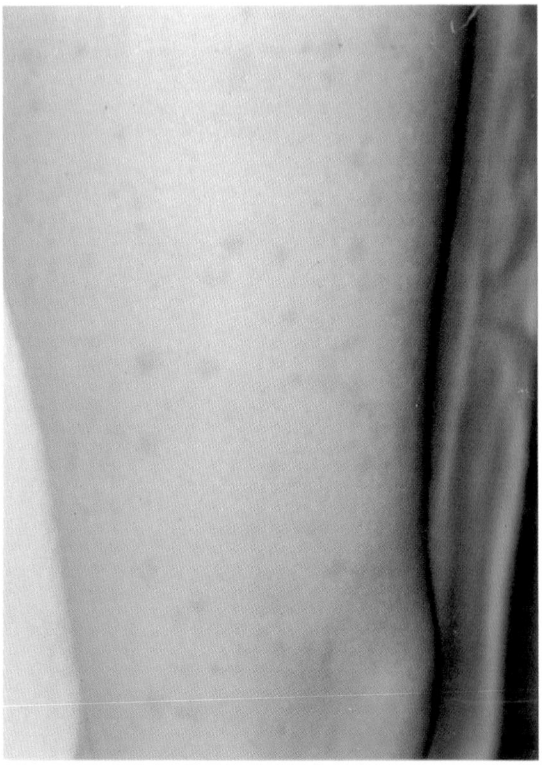

A2-3 **Rocky Mountain spotted fever** – early rash.[2]

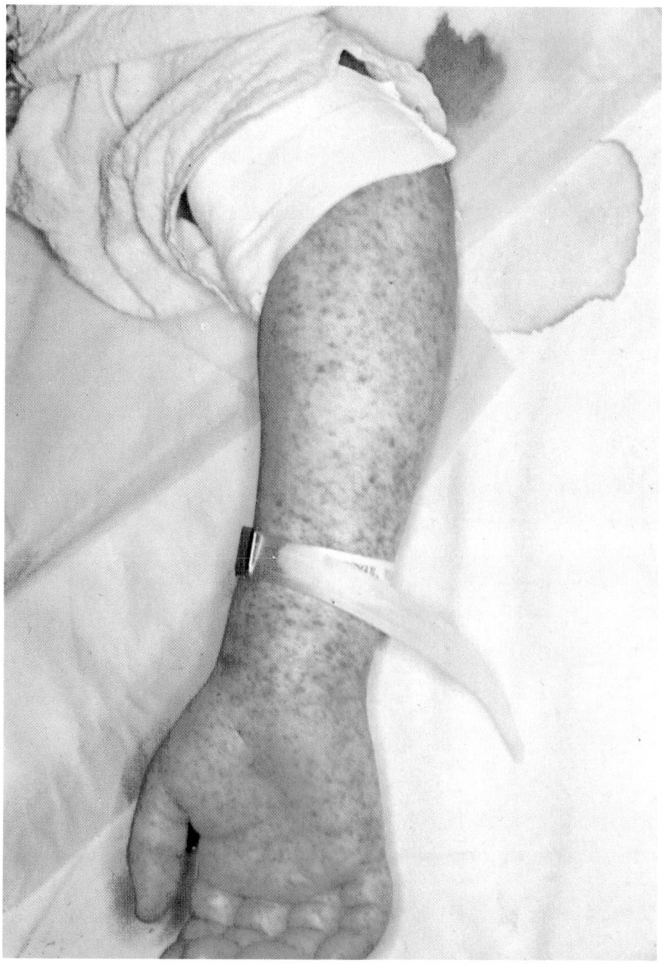

A2-4 **Rocky Mountain spotted fever** – late rash.[2]

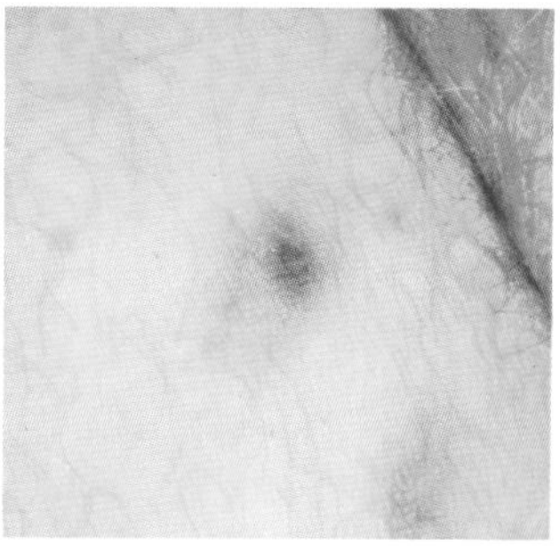

A2-7 **Pseudomonas septicemia**.[3]

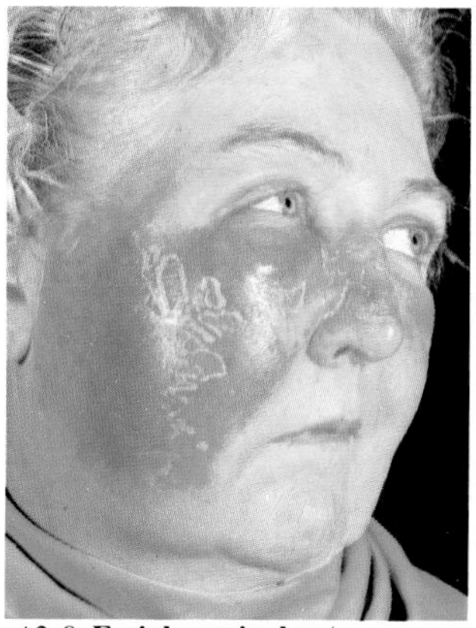

A2-8 **Facial erysipelas**.[3]

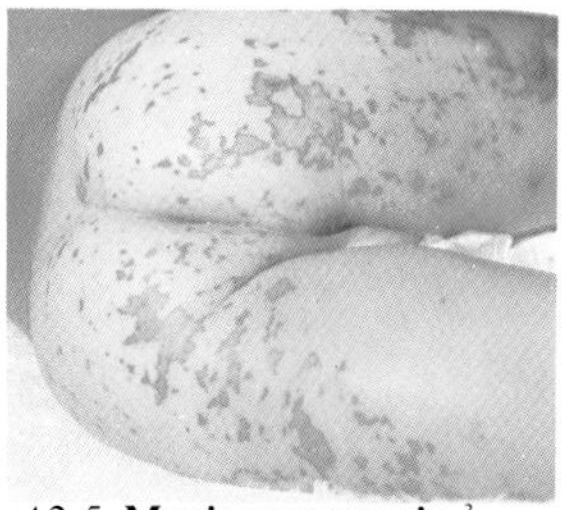

A2-5 **Meningococcemia**.[3]

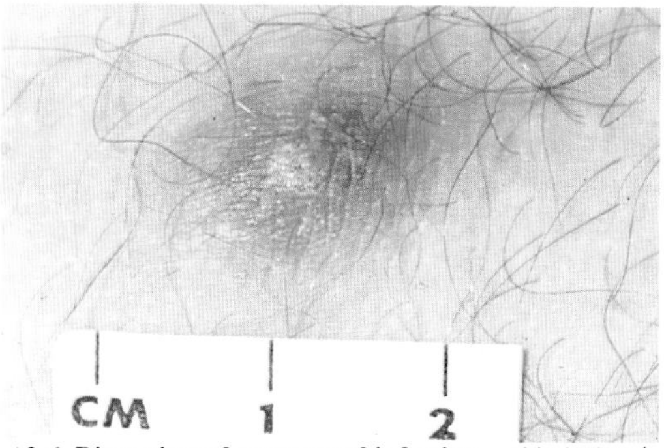

A2-6 **Disseminated gonococcal infection** – skin lesion.[4]

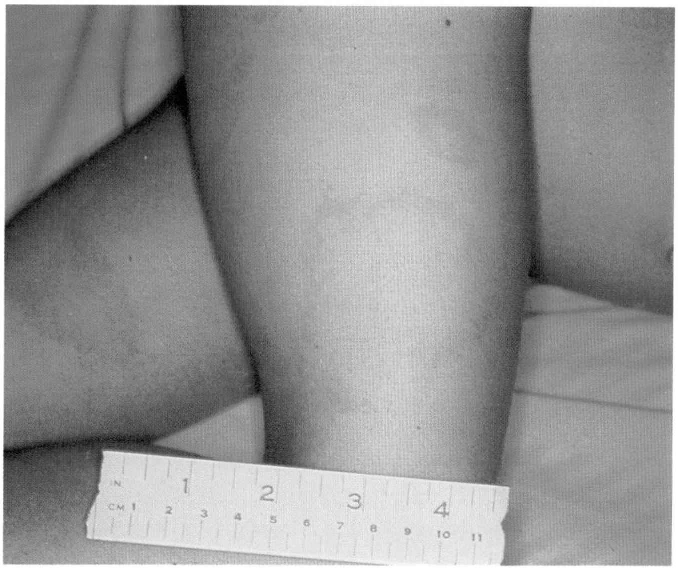

A2-9 **Lyme disease: erythema chronicum migrans** – secondary lesion.[5]

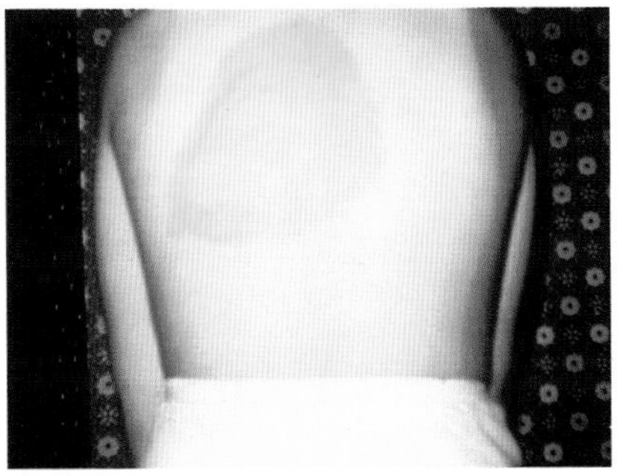

A2-10 **Lyme disease: erythema chronicum migrans** – primary lesion.[5]

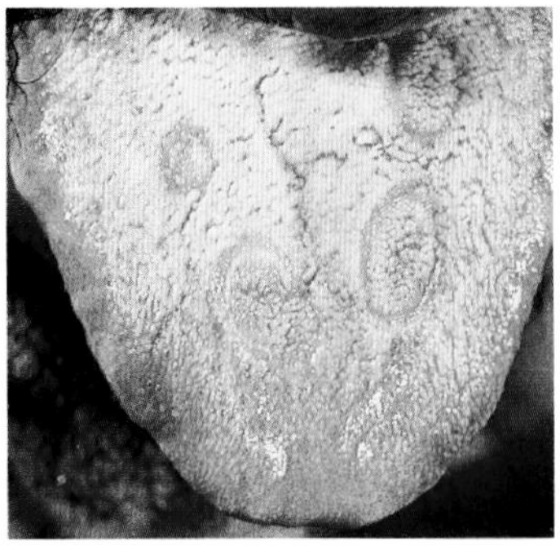

A2-11 Mucous patches involving the tongue in **secondary syphilis**.[4]

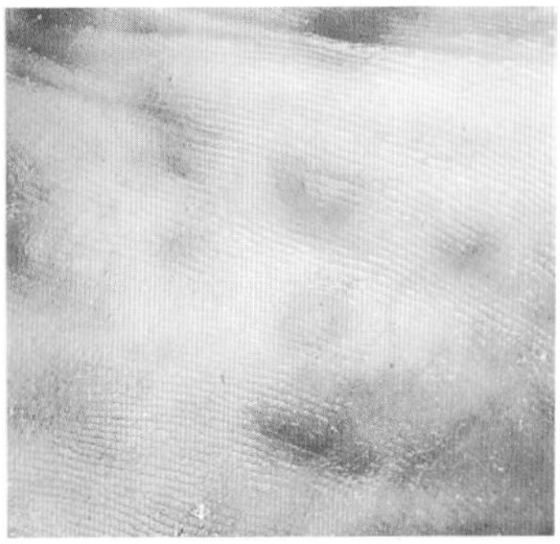

A2-12 **Papulosquamous lesions of secondary syphilis** on the sole of the foot.[4]

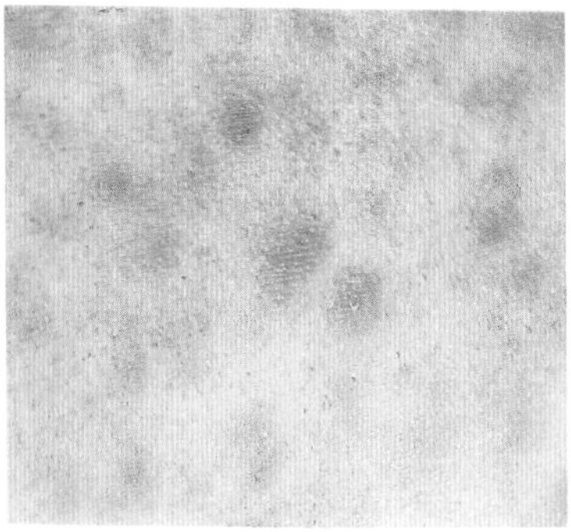

A2-13 **Macular syphilids** in early secondary syphilis.[4]

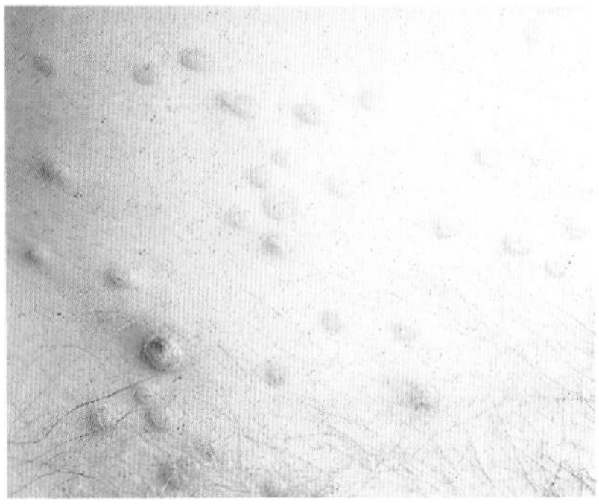

A2-14 **Molluscum contagiosum** of the lower abdomen in a patient with coexisting genital molluscum lesions. Note central umbilication and pale-salmon color.[4]

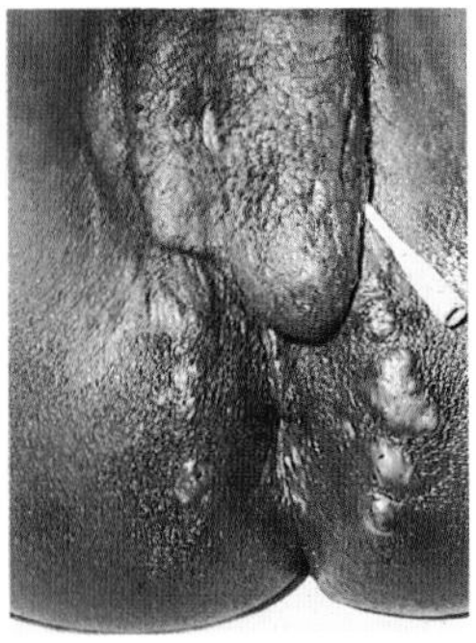

A2-15 **Esthiomene** due to lymphogranuloma venereum.[4]

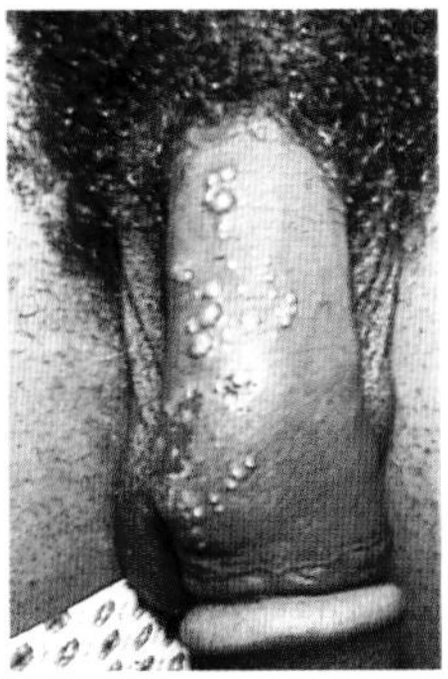

A2-16 **Severe primary HSV* infection** with extensive vesicles, ulcerations, and penile edema.[4]

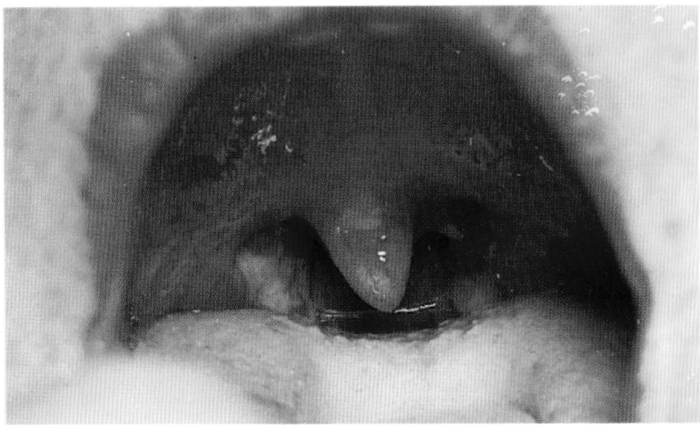

A2-17 **Primary HSV* pharyngitis** showing ulcerative lesions on the uvula and palate together with exudative tonsillitis. HSV-2 was recovered from pharyngeal and genital lesions.[4]

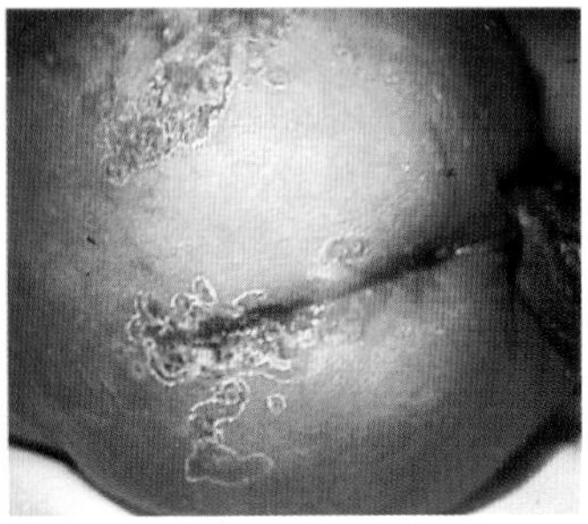

A2-18 **Neonatal HSV* infection.** Ulcers and crusting lesions on the buttocks.[4]

*Herpes Simplex Virus

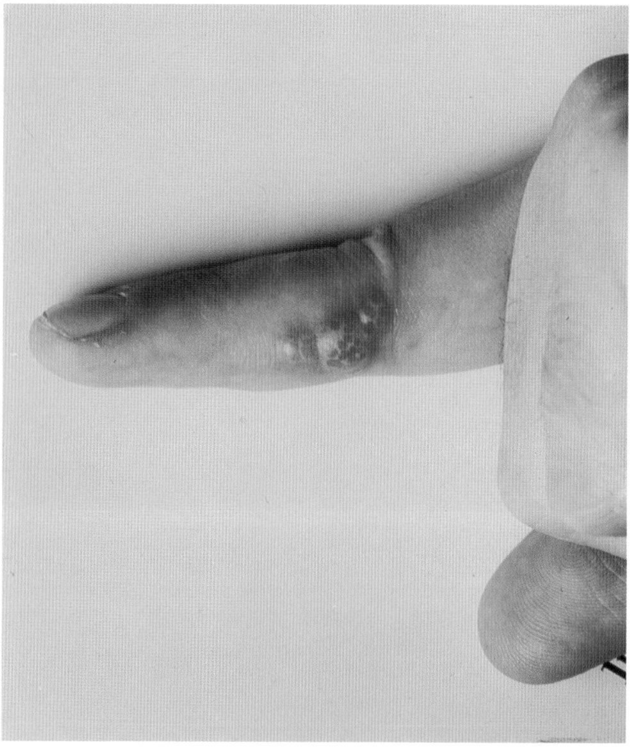

A2-19 **Herpetic whitlow.**[1]

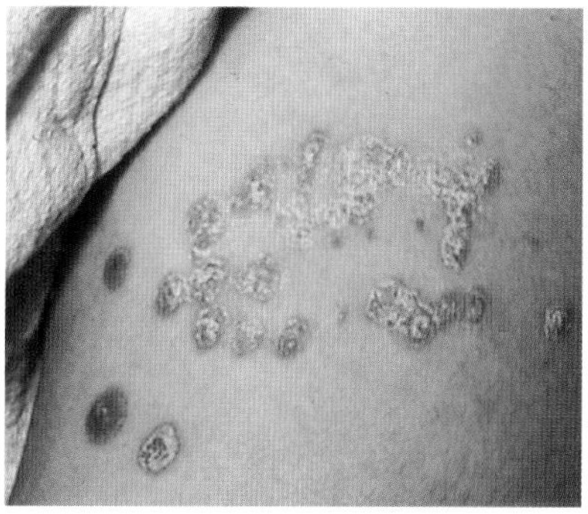

A2-20 **Keratodermia blenorrhagica** in Reiter's syndrome.[4]

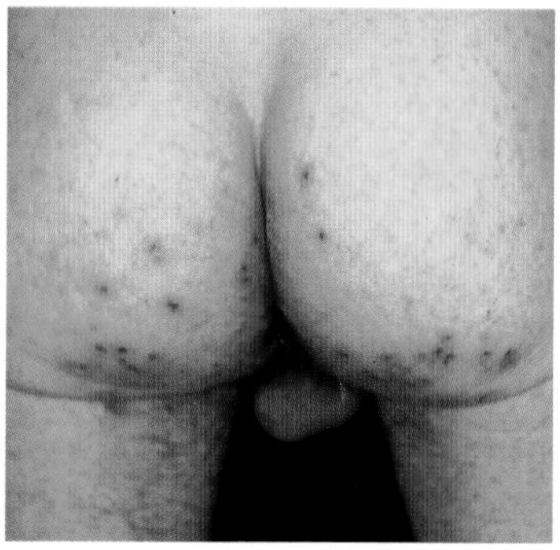

A2-21 Grouped excoriations due to **scabies** on the lower buttocks, simulating dermatitis herpetiformis.[4]

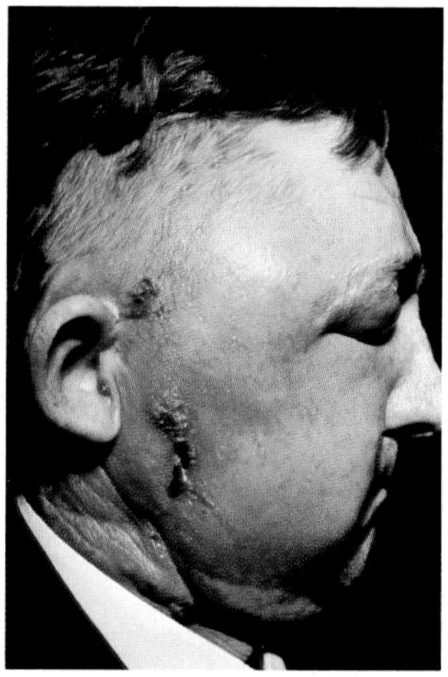

A2-22 **Cervicofacial actinomycosis.**[3]

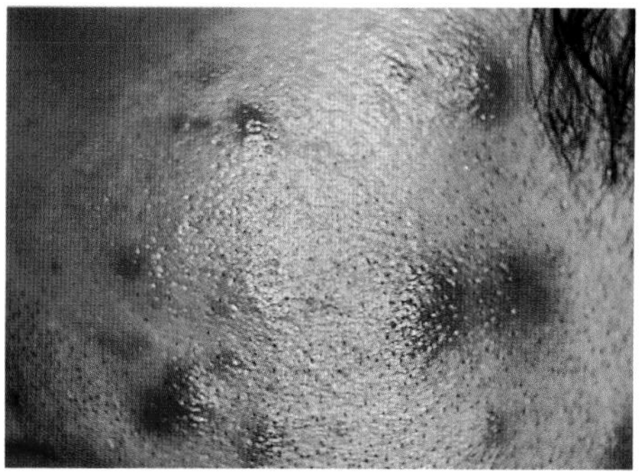

A2-23 Lesions of **Kaposi's sarcoma** on the cheek of a homosexually active man.[4]

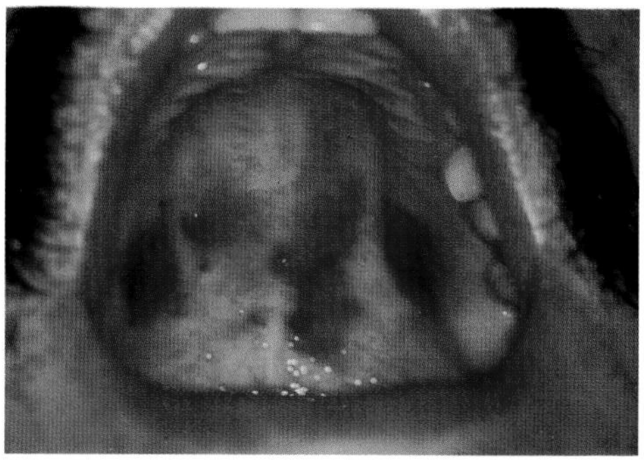

A2-24 **Kaposi's sarcoma** involving the palate of a homosexually active man.[4]

Sources

1 Courtesy of Lawrence Corey, M.D.
2 Courtesy of Theodore E. Woodward, M.D.
3 Fitzpatrick TB et al: *Dermatology in General Medicine*, 2nd ed. New York, McGraw-Hill, 1984
4 Holmes KK et al: *Sexually Transmitted Diseases*. New York, McGraw-Hill, 1984
5 Steere AC et al: Ann Intern Med 86:685, 1977 (reprinted with permission)

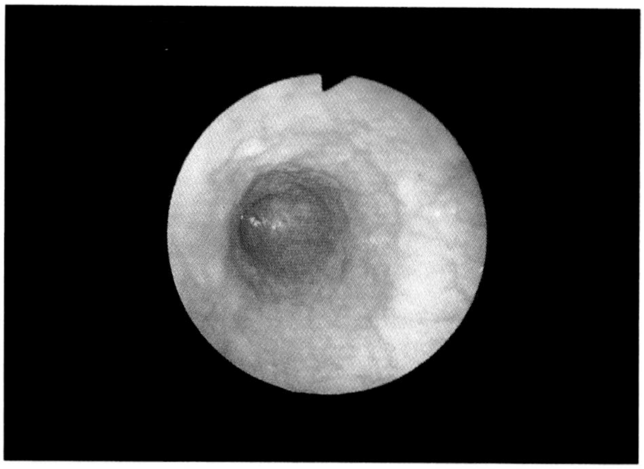

A3-1 **Normal esophagus;** normal fine vasculature can be seen.

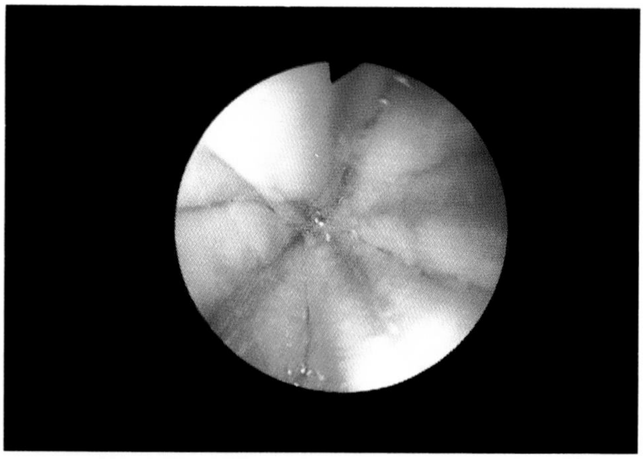

A3-2 **Peptic regurgitant esophagitis;** linear red streaks with a central white streak are noted extending up the esophagus.

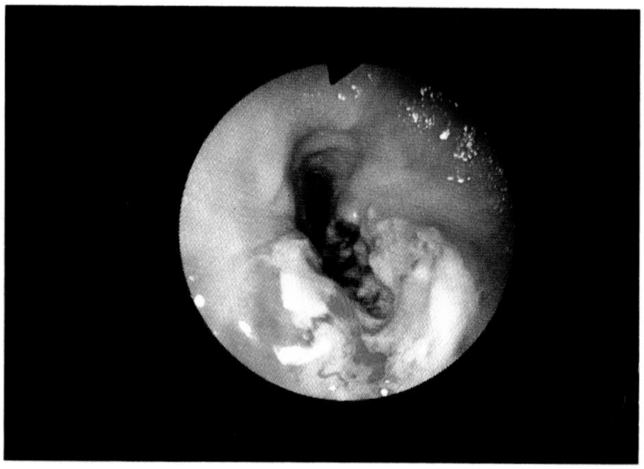

A3-3 **Ulcerated squamous cell carcinoma,** with a depressed center, involving one wall of the esophagus.

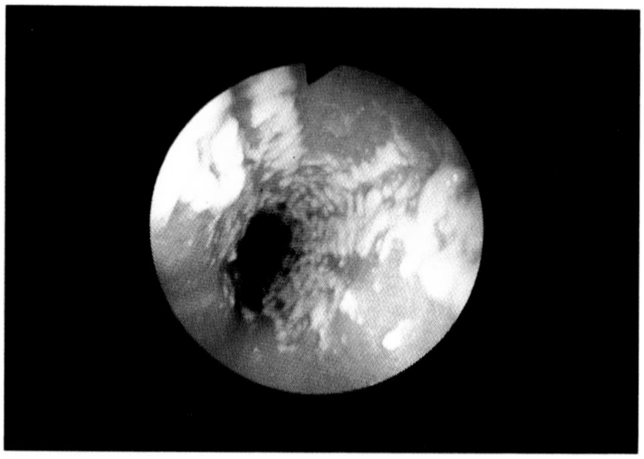

A3-4 **Moniliasis of the esophagus.** A white exudate is seen with underlying erythematous mucosa.

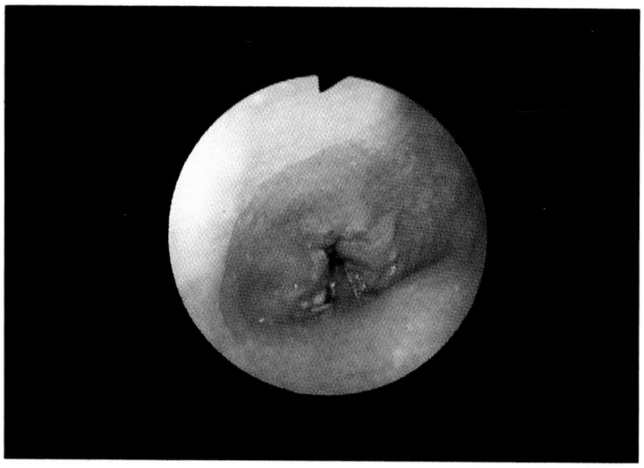

A3-5 **Barrett's metaplasia of the esophagus with an adenocarcinoma.** The squamo-columnar junction is noted in the proximal esophagus. A mucosal irregularity in the center of the photograph was an adenocarcinoma.

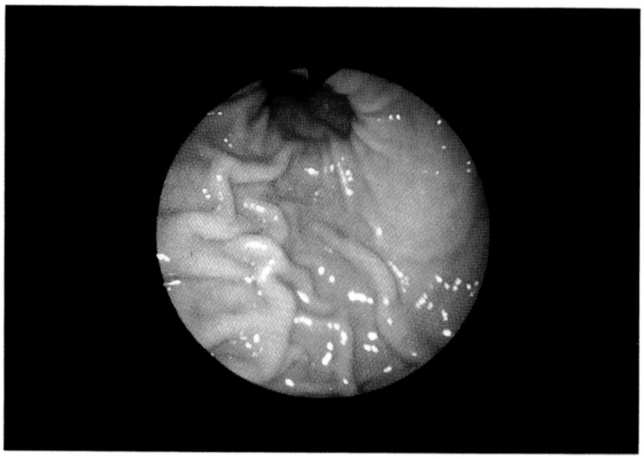

A3-6 **Normal body of the stomach with rugal folds.**

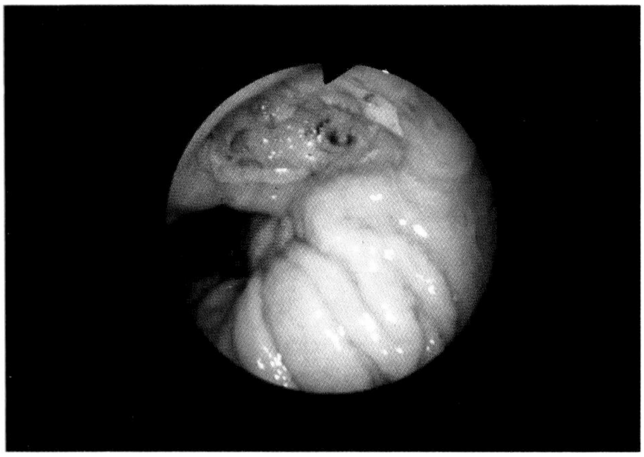

A3-7 **Large, benign, lesser curve, gastric ulcer.** The folds end at the ulcer margin.

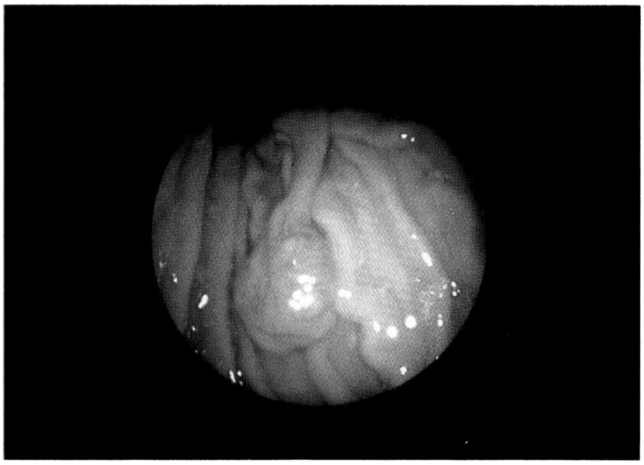

A3-8 **Gastric polyp.** The histologic type must be determined by excision and pathologic examination.

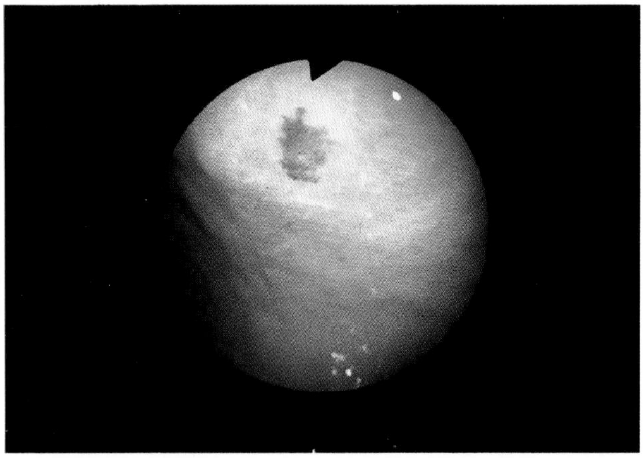

A3-9 **Arteriovenous malformation of the gastric mucosa.**

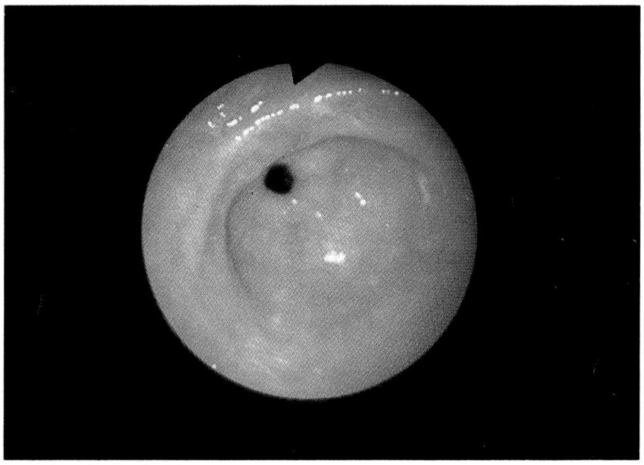

A3-10 **Normal pylorus.** Note the absence of gastric rugal folds in the antrum proximal to the pylorus.

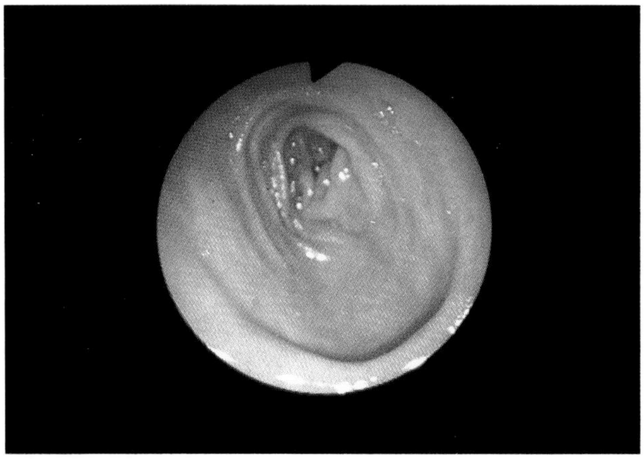

A3-11 **Normal duodenal bulb.**

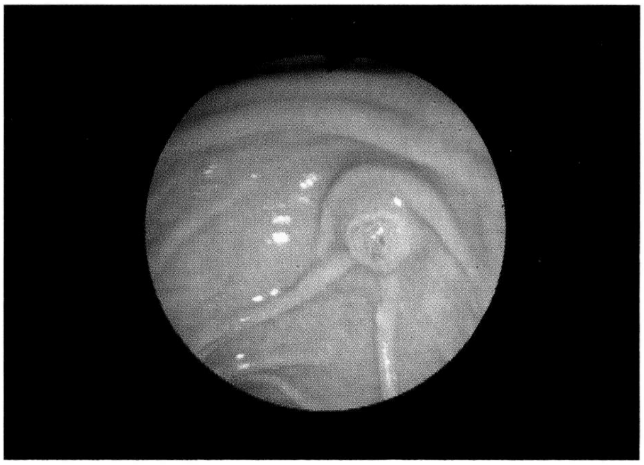

A3-12 **Normal papilla of Vater.** The fold pattern surrounding the papilla is normal; bile is seen adjacent to the papilla.

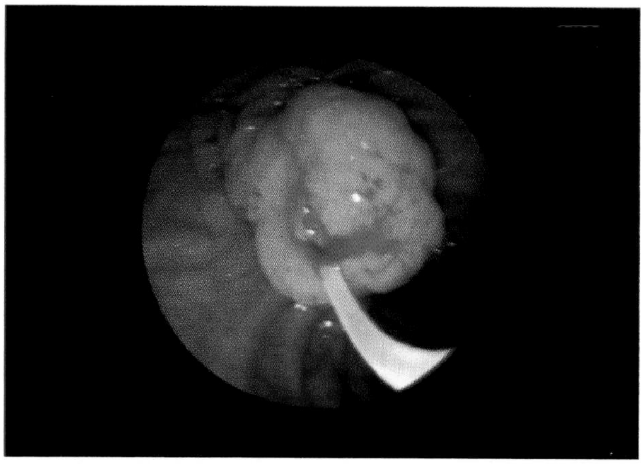

A3-13 **Periampullary carcinoma.** The mass at the papilla of Vater has been catheterized during ERCP.

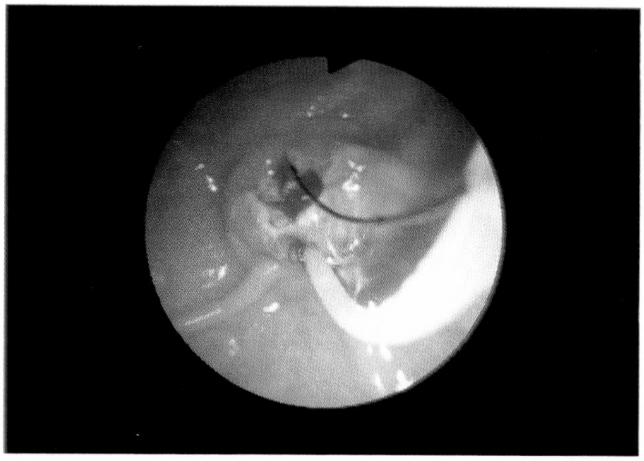

A3-14 **Endoscopic papillotomy.** A papillotome has been passed into the papilla, the wire bowed, and an incision made, with electrosurgical current, in the superior aspect of the papilla.

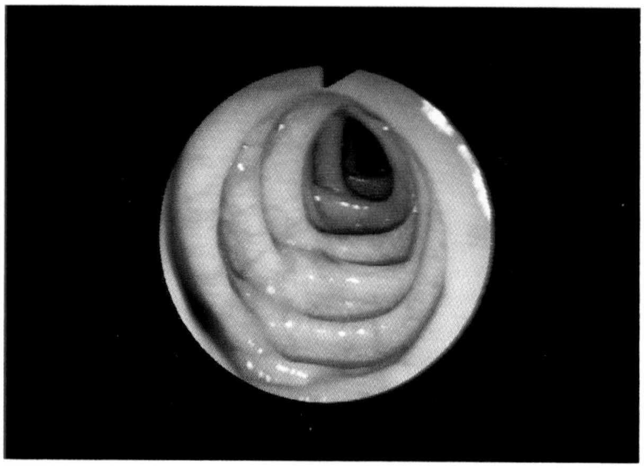

A3-15 **Normal colon;** typical haustral folds and a normal vascular pattern can be seen.

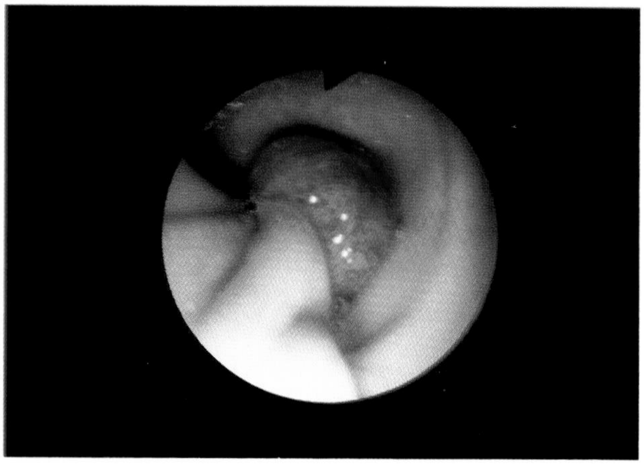

A3-16 **Colonic adenomatous polyp.** The polyp is erythematous; a stalk is seen covered with normal mucosa.

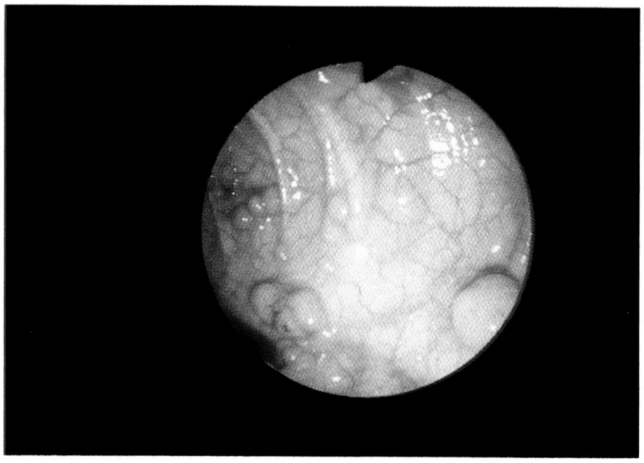

A3-17 **Multiple, small, colonic adenomatous polyps** in a case of familial polyposis coli. This colon must be removed to prevent the development of cancer.

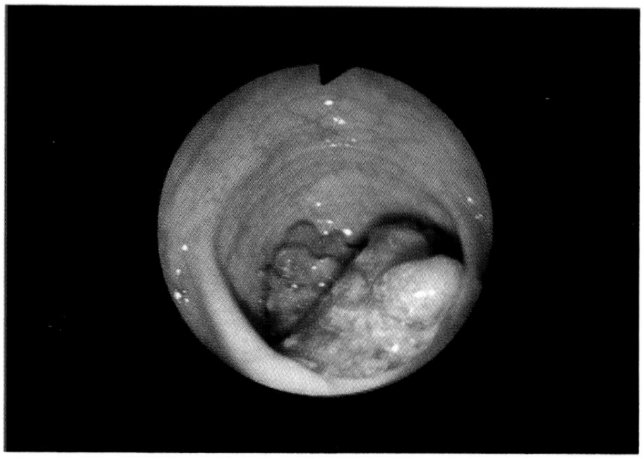

A3-18 **Colon adenocarcinoma.** The cancer is multilobed and growing into the lumen.

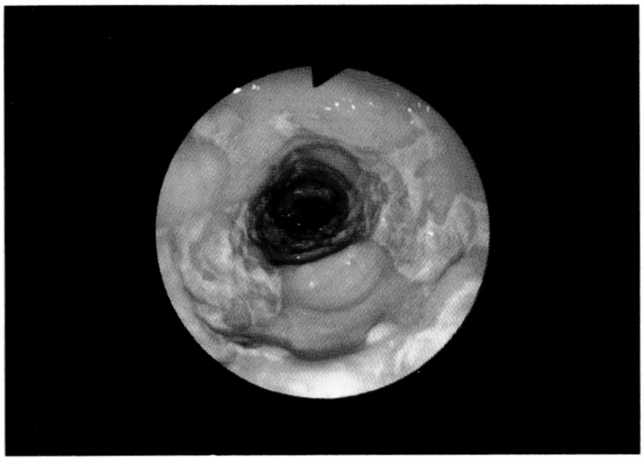

A3-19 **Crohn's colitis** with linear, serpiginous, white-based ulcers surrounded by colonic mucosa which is relatively normal.

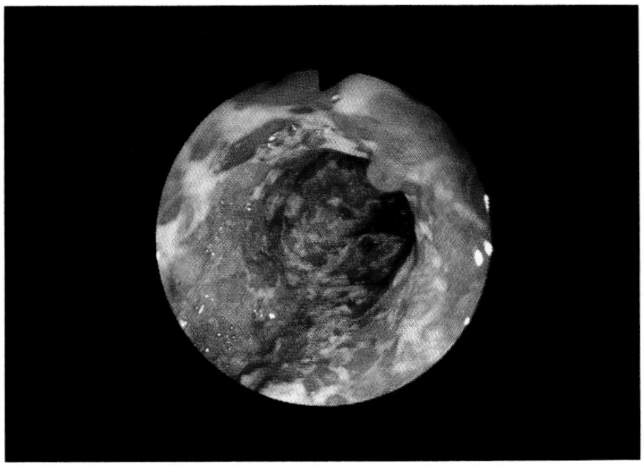

A3-20 **Severe ulcerative colitis** with diffuse ulceration, bleeding, and exudation.

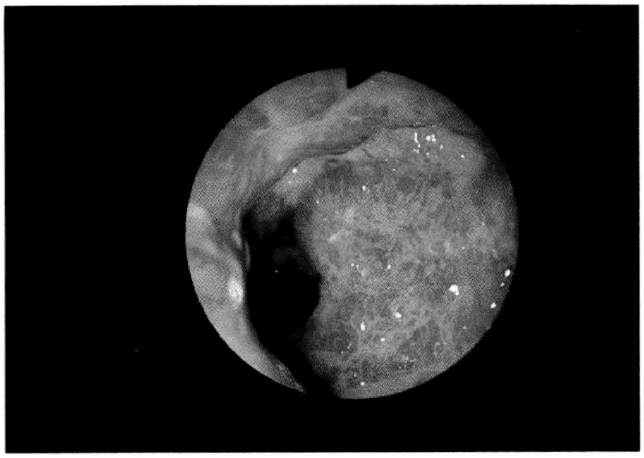

A3-21 **Kaposi's sarcoma involving the colon** in a patient with AIDS. The erythematous lesions involve most of the colonic mucosa in the photograph.

Source: Courtesy of FE Silverstein and GN Tytgat: *Atlas of Gastrointestinal Endoscopy.* Gower Medical Publishing, New York, 1987.

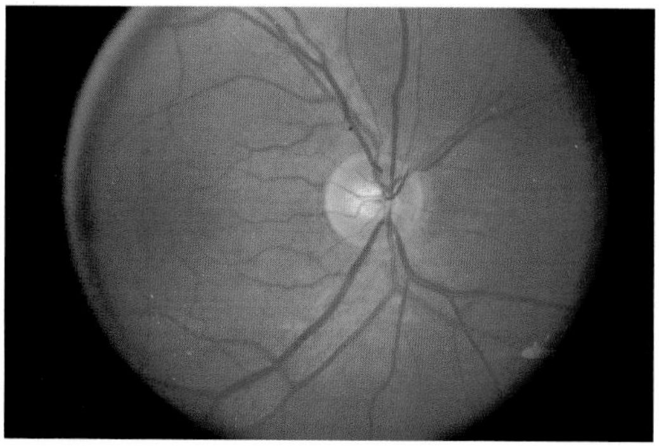

A4-1 **Normal optic nerve and retina.**

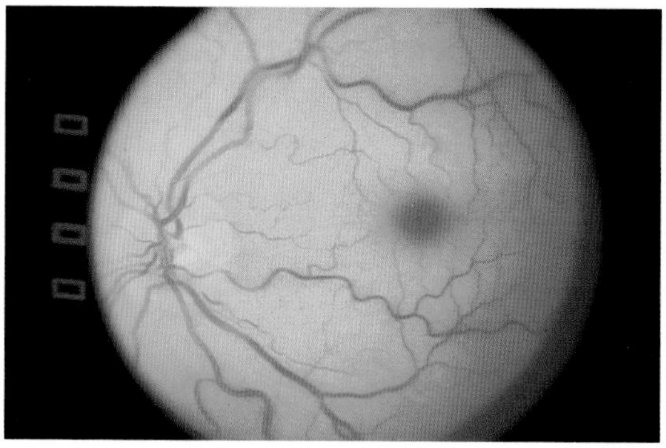

A4-2 **Central retinal artery occlusion.**

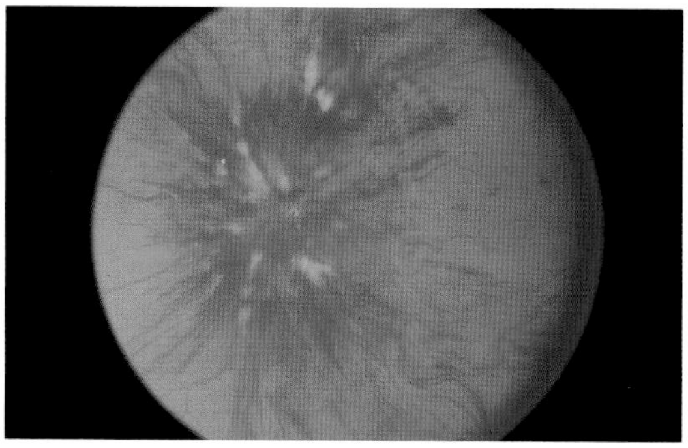

A4-3 **Central retinal vein occlusion.**

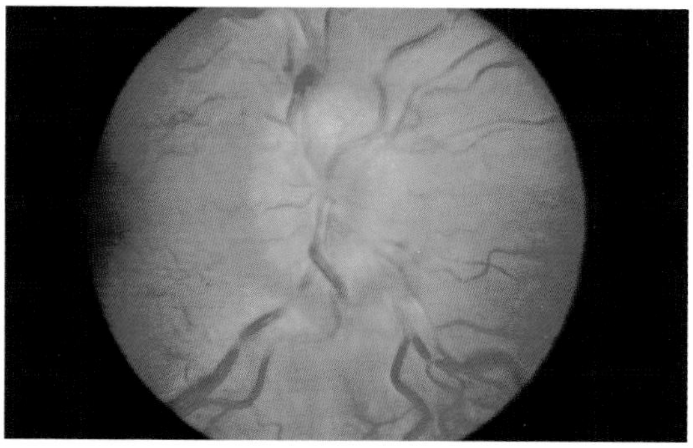

A4-4 **Early papilledema.**

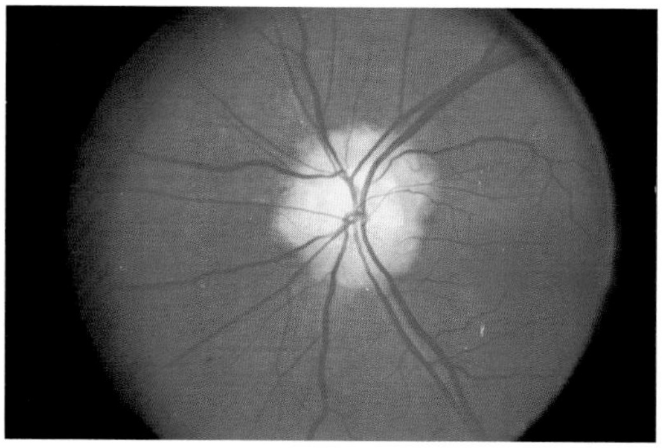

A4-5 **Drusen of the optic nerve head.**

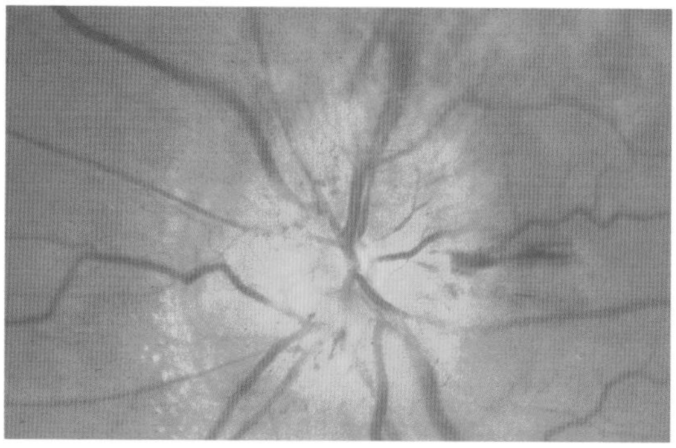

A4-6 **Anterior ischemic optic neuropathy.**

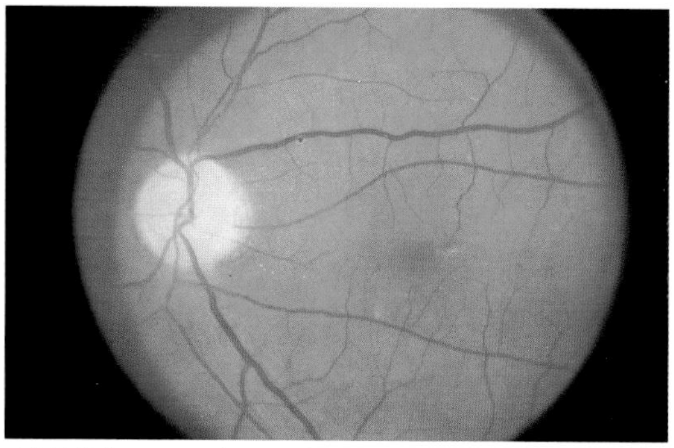

A4-7 **Primary optic atrophy.**

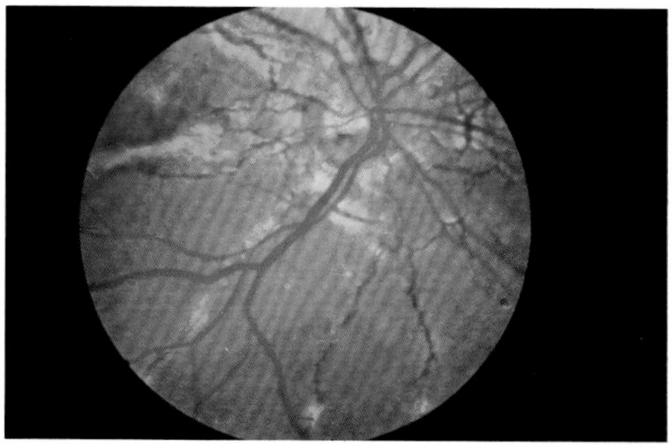

A4-8 **Angioid streaks.**

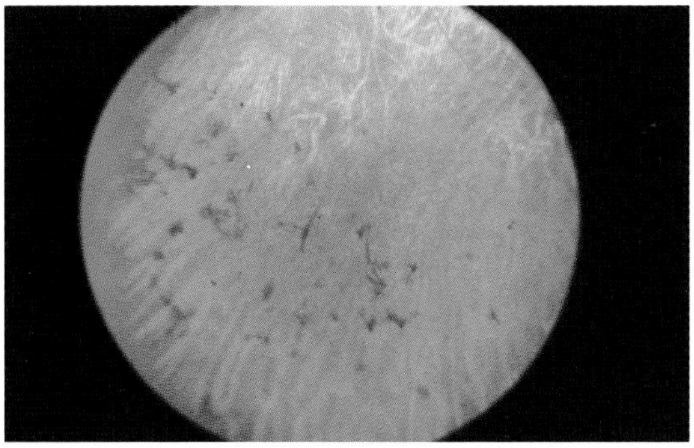

A4-9 **Retinitis pigmentosa.**

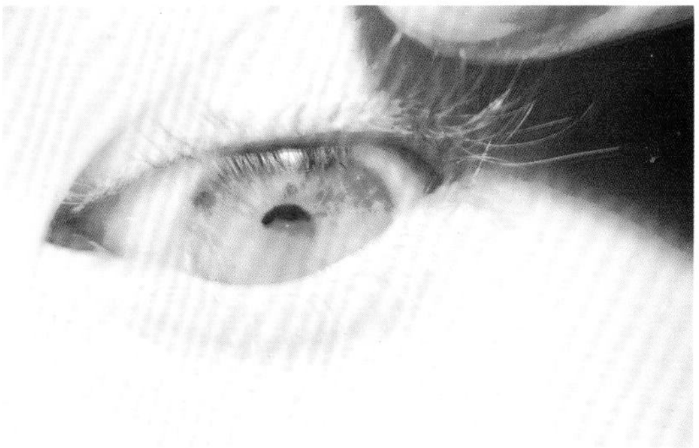

A4-10 **Band keratopathy.**

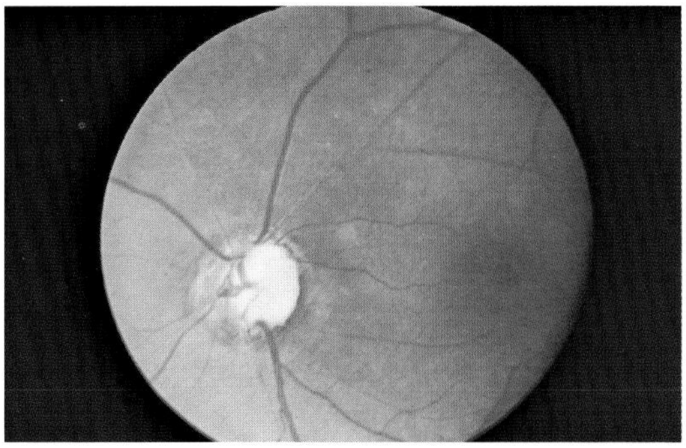

A4-11 **Glaucomatous optic disk with secondary atrophy.**

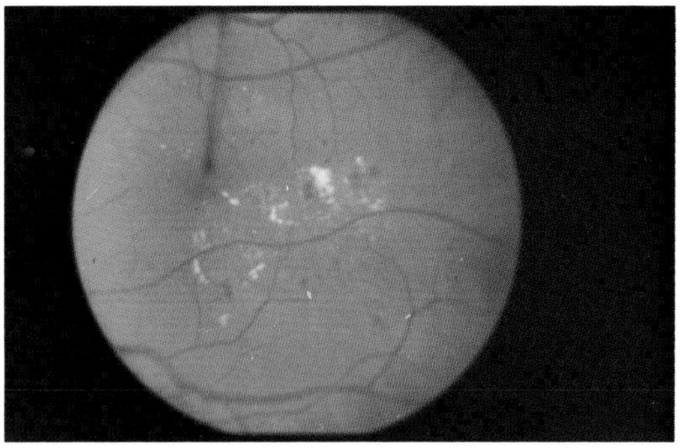

A4-12 **Diabetic retinopathy with microaneurysms.**

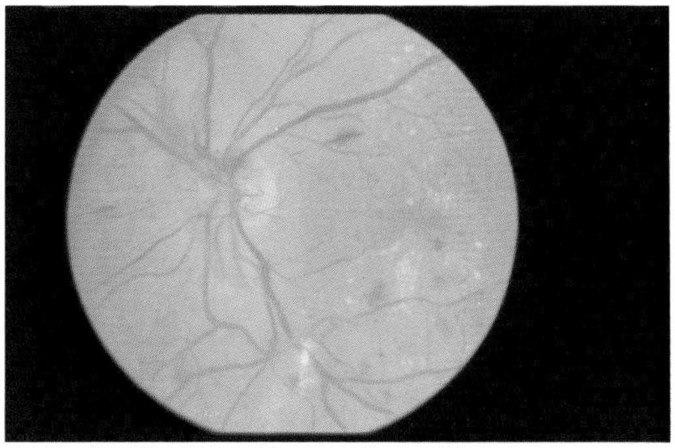

A4-13 **Proliferative diabetic retinopathy.**

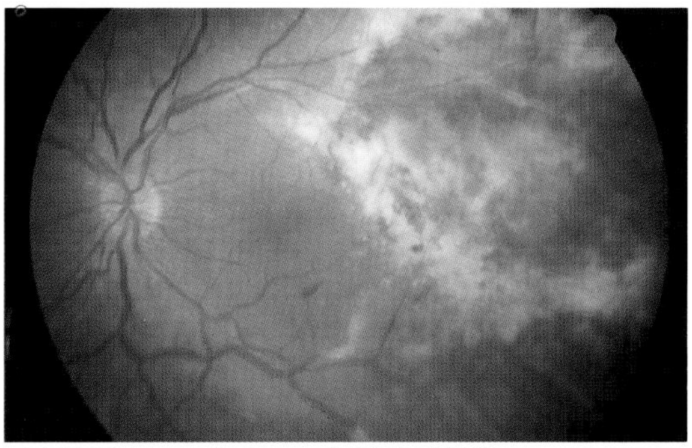

A4-14 **Cytomegalovirus retinitis in AIDS.**
(Courtesy of Donald J. D'Amico, M.D.)

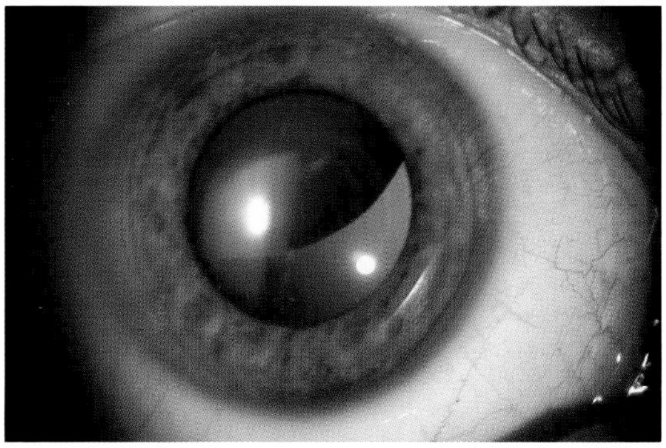

A4-15 **Dislocated lens in Marfan's disease.**
(Courtesy of S. Fourman, M.D.)

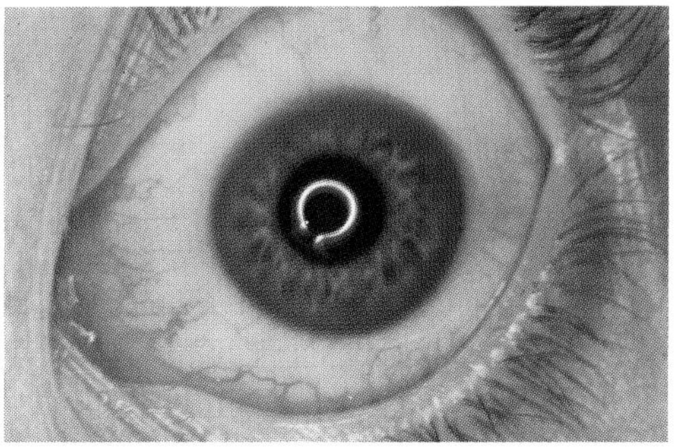

A4-16 **Kayser-Fleischer ring in Wilson's disease.**
(Note: The ring is the golden brown pigment at the periphery of the cornea and is characteristically broader superiorly and inferiorly than it is medially and laterally.)

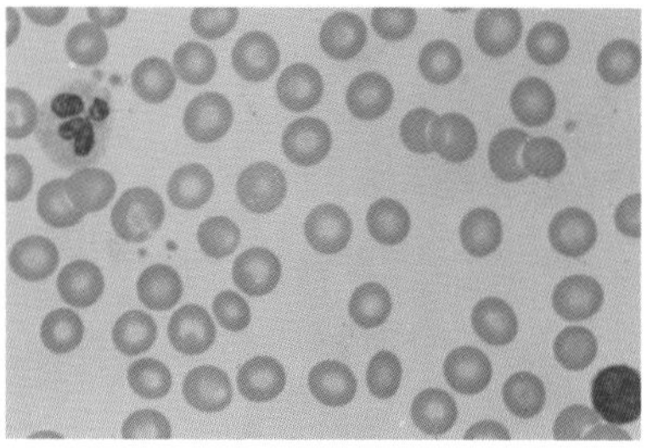

A5-1 **Normal blood smear.** Normal red blood cells are round, possess an area of central pallor, appear slightly smaller than the nucleus of a mature lymphocyte, and vary little in size (anisocytosis) or in shape (poikilocytosis).

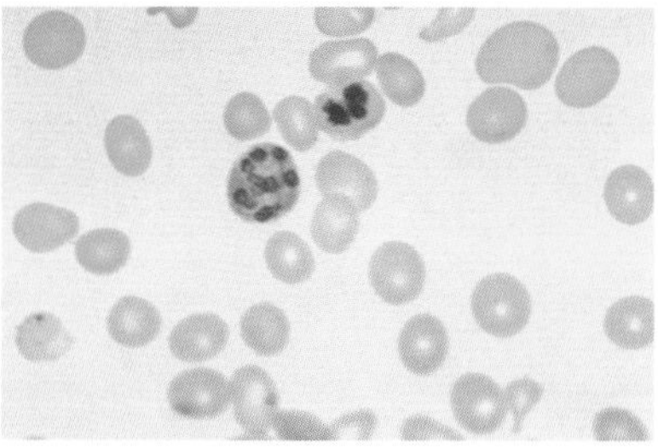

A5-2 **Megaloblastic anemia.** Oval macrocytes, well filled with hemoglobin, are admixed with lesser numbers of small teardrop-shaped red blood cells. Note also hypersegmented granulocyte.

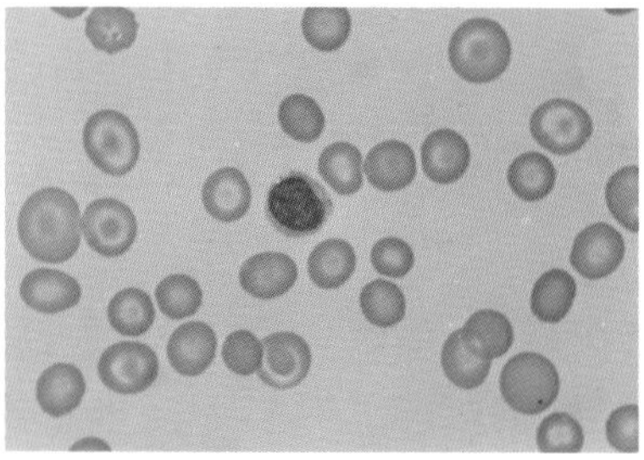

A5-3 **Liver disease.** Round macrocytes of rather uniform size are seen. Many of the macrocytes are also target cells.

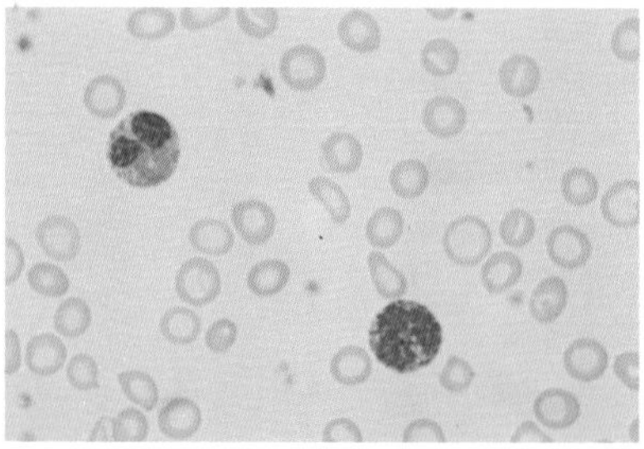

A5-4 **Iron-deficiency anemia.** In severe iron deficiency, the red blood cells are smaller than normal (microcytosis), and their central area of pallor is expanded (hypochromia) so that the cells appear to have only a thin rim of hemoglobin.

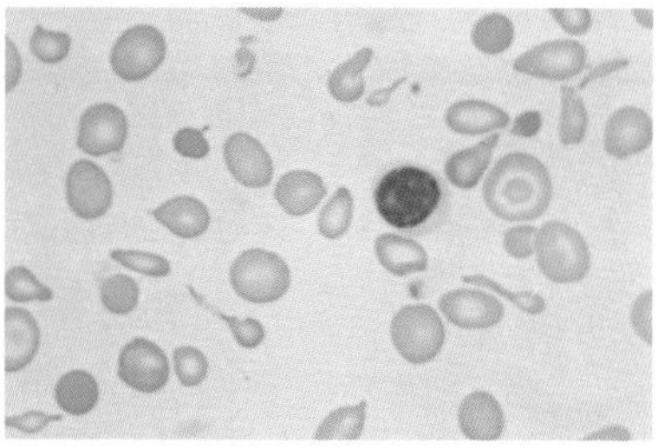

A5-5 **β thalassemia intermedia.** Microcytic and hypochromic red blood cells are seen that resemble the red blood cells of severe iron deficiency anemia shown in Fig. A5-4. Many elliptical and teardrop-shaped red blood cells are noted.

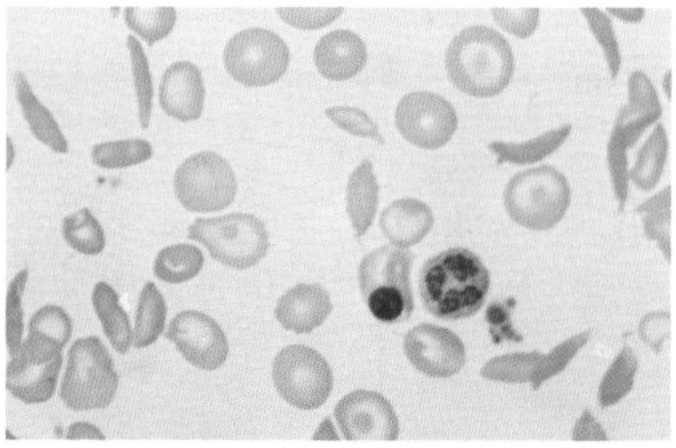

A5-6 **Sickle cell anemia.** The elongated and crescent-shaped red blood cells seen on this smear represent circulating irreversible sickled cells. Target cells and a nucleated red blood cell are also seen.

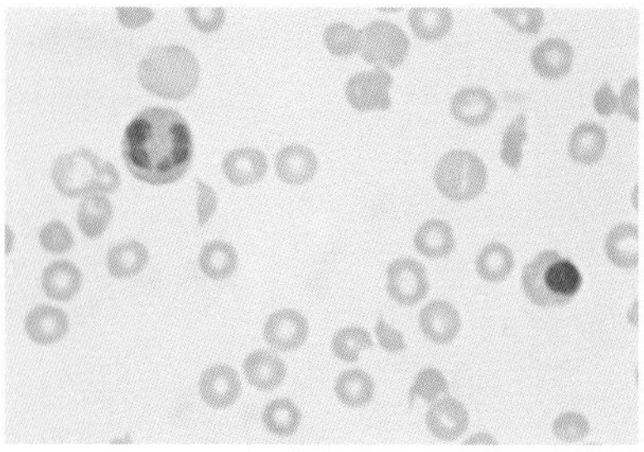

A5-7 **Traumatic hemolysis.** The helmet-shaped red blood cell and the small triangular-shaped red blood cells seen on this smear represent morphologic evidence of mechanical damage to red blood cells within the circulatory tree.

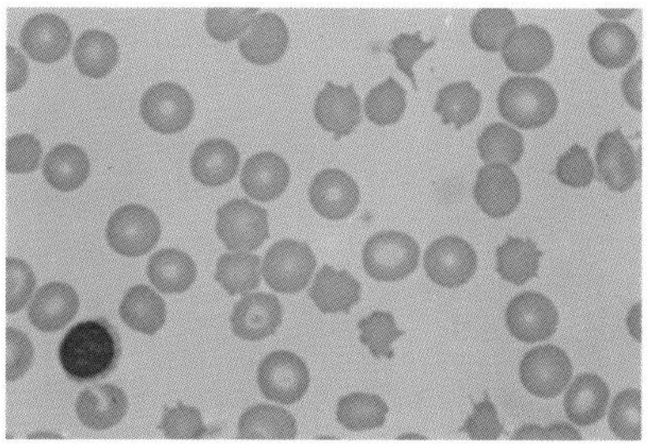

A5-8 **Spur cell anemia.** Spur cells are recognized as distorted red blood cells containing several irregularly distributed thornlike projections. Cells with this morphologic abnormality are also called acanthocytes.

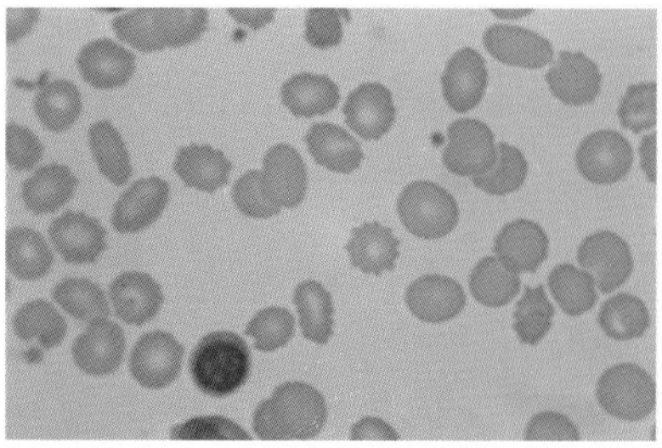

A5-9 **Uremia.** The red blood cells in uremia may acquire numerous, regularly spaced, small spiny projections. Such cells, called burr cells or echinocytes, are readily distinguishable from the irregularly spiculated acanthocytes shown in Fig. A5-8.

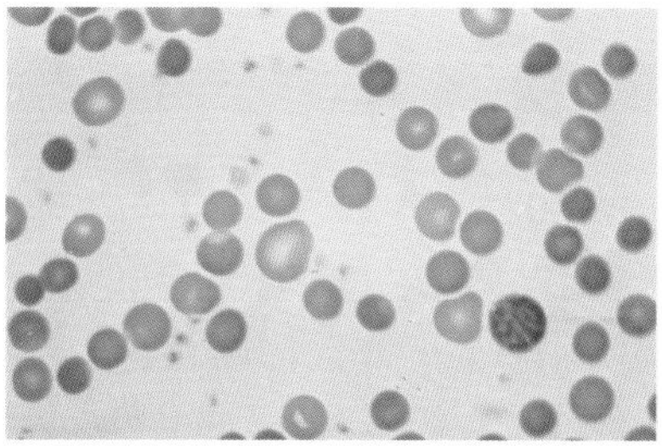

A5-10 **Hereditary spherocytosis.** Small, densely staining red blood cells are seen that have lost their central area of pallor (microspherocytes). Microspherocytes may also be found in other hemolytic disorders (Fig. A5-11).

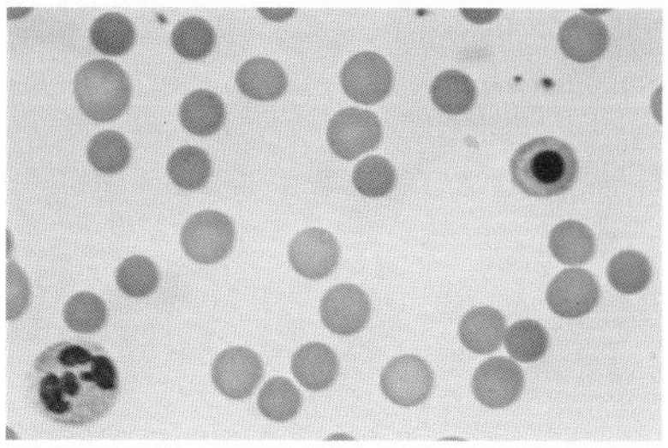

A5-11 **Immunohemolytic anemia.** Microspherocytes are seen on this blood smear along with several macrocytes with a slight purple tinge (polychromasia). The latter represent new red blood cells released early from the bone marrow. The microspherocytes seen in immunohemolytic anemia may be indistinguishable from the microspherocytes seen in hereditary spherocytosis (Fig. A5-10).

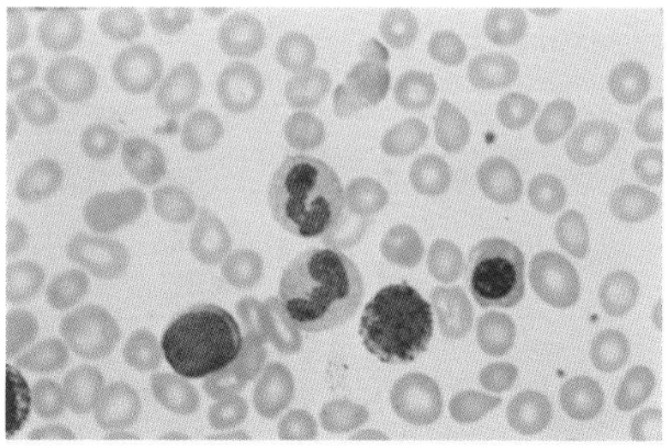

A5-12 **Myeloid metaplasia.** Teardrop-shaped red blood cells, a nucleated red blood cell, and immature myeloid cells are seen on this blood smear.

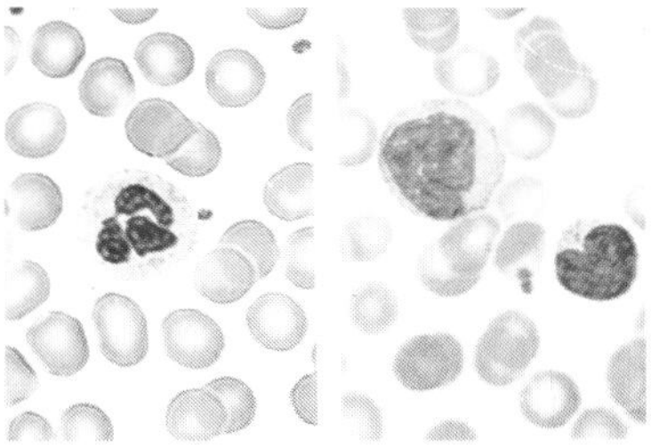

A **B**

A5-13 *A*. **Normal granulocyte.** The normal granulocyte has a segmented nucleus with heavy, clumped chromatin; fine neutrophilic granules are dispersed throughout its cytoplasm. *B*. **Normal monocyte and lymphocyte.** The normal monocyte is a large cell with an indented or folded nucleus containing loose, strandlike chromatin; the cytoplasm is a blue-gray color and usually contains fine azurophilic granules. The normal lymphocyte is a smaller cell. Its nucleus is usually round but may be indented, as in the cell shown in this plate. The nuclear chromatin has a smudgy appearance; the cytoplasm is a blue color.

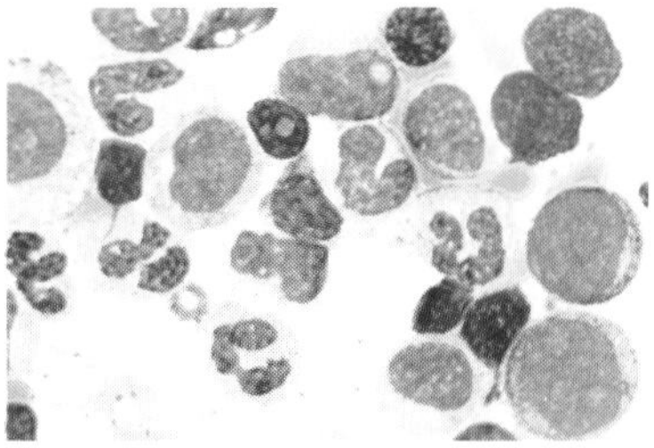

A5-15 **Normal granulocyte precursors in marrow.** The earliest granulocytic precursor (myeloblast) possesses a round nucleus with fine, punctate chromatin and one or more nucleoli; the cytoplasm is blue. As nuclear differentiation proceeds, the nucleoli disappear, the chromatin coarsens, and the nucleus becomes increasingly indented and finally segmented. As cytoplasmic differentiation proceeds, azurophilic granules appear and the cytoplasm changes color from blue to the yellow-pink-gray hue of the mature granulocyte, and as this occurs the azurophilic granules become obscured by fine neutrophilic granules.

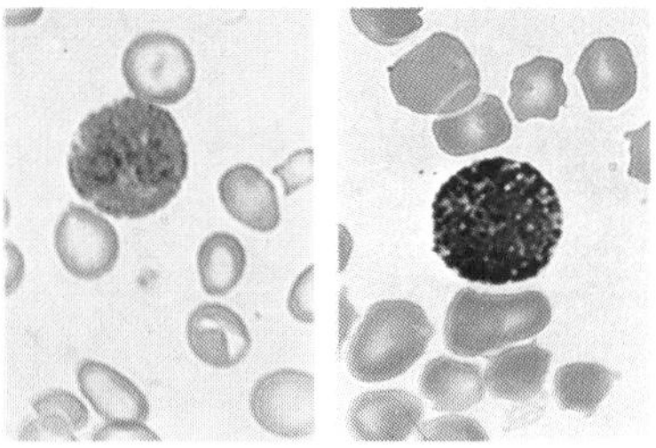

A **B**

A5-14 *A*. **Normal eosinophil.** The eosinophil contains large, bright-orange granules; the nucleus is bilobed. *B*. **Basophil.** The basophil contains large purple-black granules which fill the cell and obscure the nucleus.

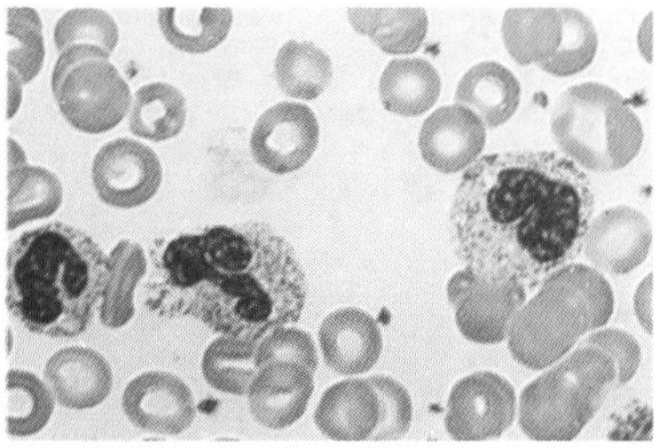

A5-16 **Neutrophils with toxic granulation.** In infection and other toxic states, azurophilic granules may become visible in mature granulocytes as coarse, dark-staining cytoplasmic granules.

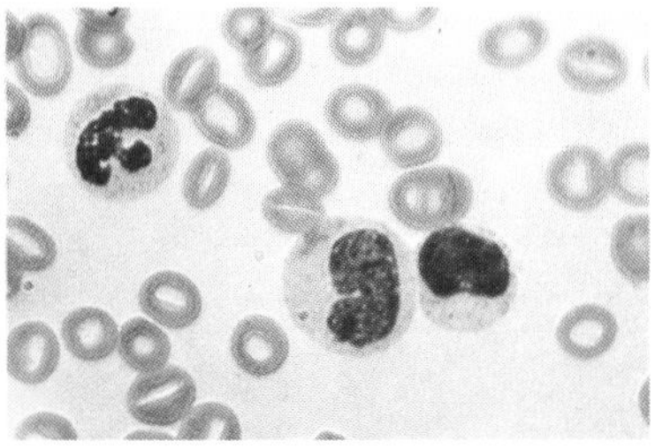

A5-17 **Band with Döhle body** (center). Döhle bodies are discrete, blue-staining, nongranular areas found in the periphery of the cytoplasm of the neutrophil in infections and other toxic states. They represent aggregates of rough endoplasmic reticulum.

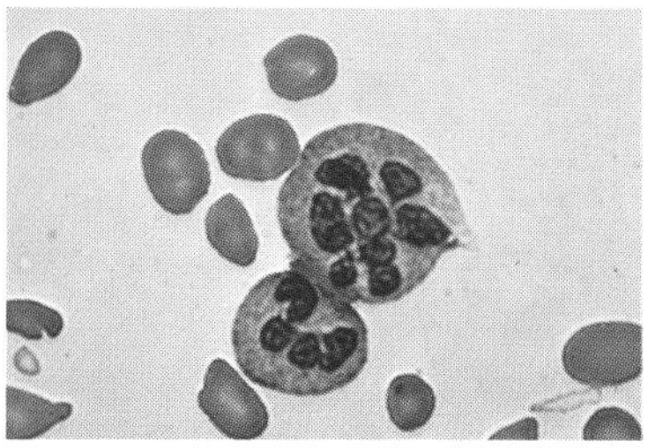

A5-18 **Hypersegmentation.** Frequent five-lobed granulocytes on a blood smear or granulocytes with more than five lobes are evidence of hypersegmentation, an important clue to the diagnosis of megaloblastic anemia.

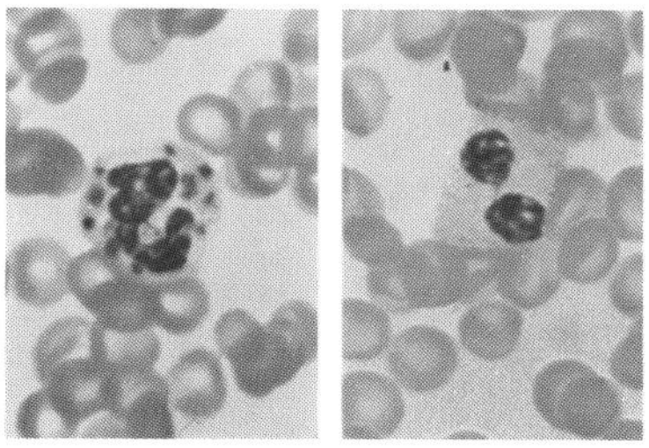

A B

A5-19 A. **Chédiak-Higashi anomaly.** In this ultimately fatal disorder, the granulocytes contain huge cytoplasmic granules, formed from aggregation and fusion of azurophilic and specific granules. Large, abnormal granules are found in other granule-containing cells throughout the body. *B*. **Pelger-Hüet anomaly.** In this benign disorder, the majority of granulocytes are bilobed. The nucleus frequently has a spectacle-like or "pince-nez" configuration.

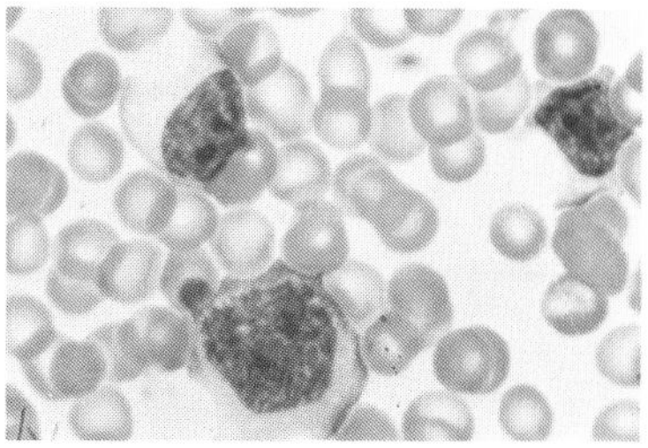

A5-20 **Reactive lymphocytes** (infectious mononucleosis). Reactive lymphocytes are usually large, cytoplasmic lymphocytes. The nucleus may be eccentrically placed and may have irregular borders and indentations (not seen on this plate). The cytoplasm contains areas that stain a darker blue due to their increased content of RNA. The cytoplasm may be indented where it abuts against a red blood cell.

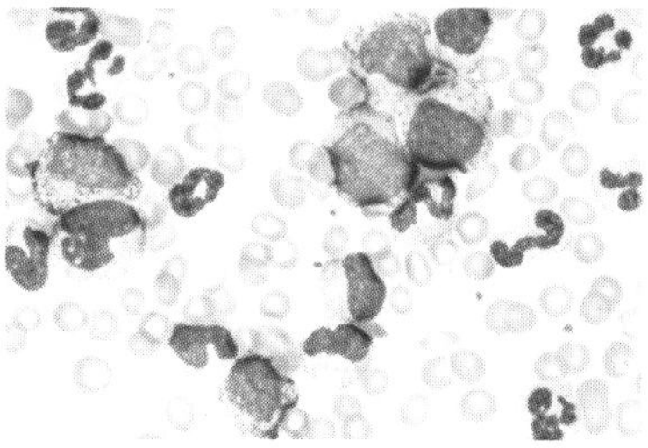

A5-21 **Chronic granulocytic leukemia.** The peripheral blood WBC count is high due to increased numbers of granulocytes and their precursors. The majority of the WBCs are segmented granulocytes or band forms, but as seen on this plate, myelocytes and promyeloblasts (not seen on this plate) may also be found on review of the blood smear.

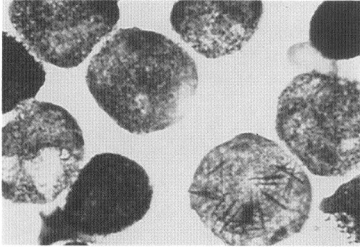

A5-22 **Leukemic cell in acute promyelocytic leukemia.** Note multiple Auer rods.

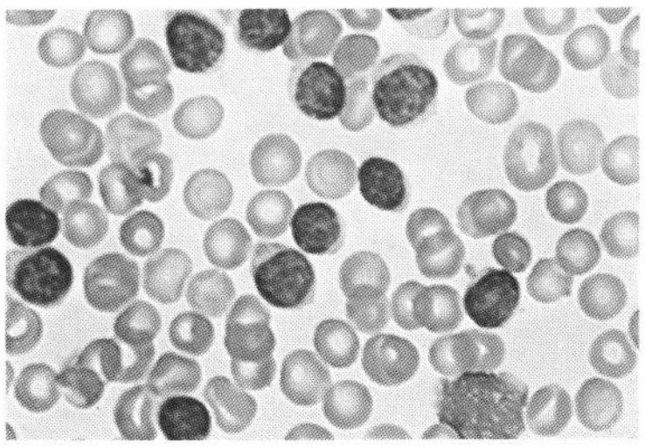

A5-23 **Chronic lymphocytic leukemia.** The peripheral blood WBC count is high due to increased numbers of small, well-differentiated lymphocytes. However, the leukemic lymphocytes are fragile, and substantial numbers of broken, smudged cells are usually also present on the blood smear.

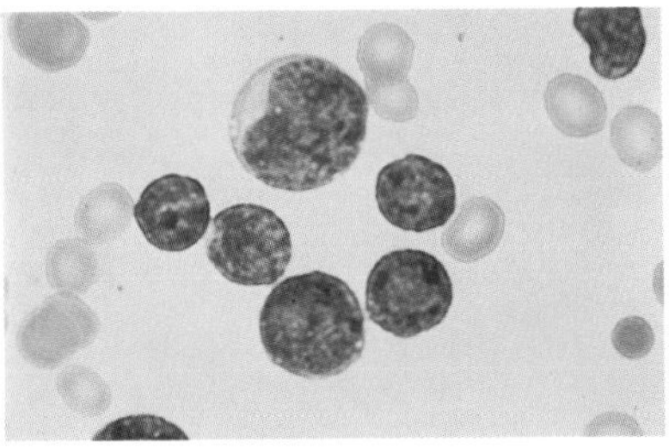

A5-24 **Leukemic cells in acute lymphoblastic leukemia** characterized by round or convoluted nuclei, high nuclear/cytoplasmic ratio and absence of cytoplasmic granules.

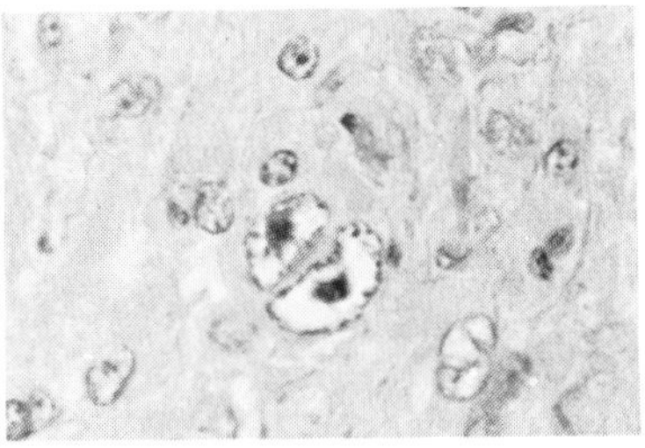

A5-25 **Hodgkin's disease:** Reed-Sternberg cell in marrow (center). The Reed-Sternberg cell is recognized by its bilobed, mirror-image nucleus, which contains in each lobe a giant, inclusion body–like nucleolus. The cytoplasmic borders of the cell cannot be identified on this plate.

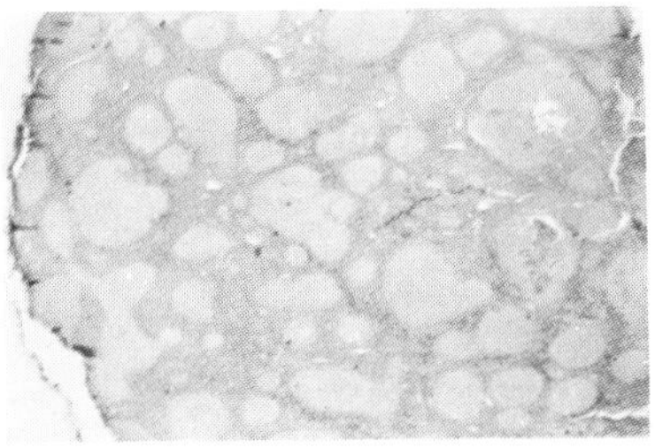

A5-26 **Non-Hodgkin's nodular lymphoma** (lymph node). This low-power view illustrates that a proliferative process has caused the normal architecture of the lymph node to be replaced by multiple nodules of varying size that extend throughout the entire lymph node.

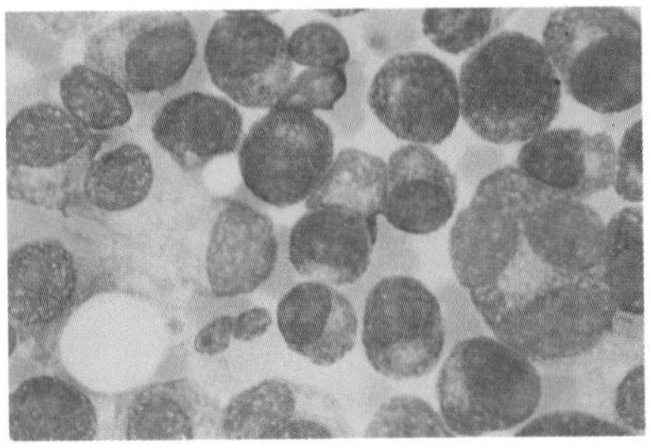

A5-27 **Multiple myeloma** (marrow). The cells bear the characteristic morphologic features of plasma cells, round or oval cells with an eccentric nucleus composed of coarsely clumped chromatin, a densely basophilic cytoplasm, and a perinuclear clear zone (hof) containing the Golgi apparatus. Binucleate and multinucleate malignant plasma cells can also be seen.

Harrison's

PRINCIPLES OF INTERNAL MEDICINE

Eleventh Edition

VOLUME 1

PART ONE
THROUGH
PART FOUR

INTRODUCTION TO CLINICAL MEDICINE

1 THE PRACTICE OF MEDICINE

THE EDITORS

WHAT IS EXPECTED OF THE PHYSICIAN The practice of medicine combines both science and art. The role of science in medicine is clear. Technology based on science is the foundation for the solution to many clinical problems; the dazzling advances in biochemical methodology and in biophysical imaging techniques that allow access to the remotest recesses of the body are the products of science. So too are the therapeutic maneuvers which increasingly are a major part of medical practice. Yet skill in the most sophisticated application of laboratory technology or the use of the latest therapeutic modality alone does not make a good physician. The ability to extract from a mass of contradictory physical signs and from the crowded computer printouts of laboratory data those items that are of crucial significance, to know in a difficult case whether to "treat" or to "watch," to determine when a clinical clue is worth pursuing or when to dismiss it as a "red herring," and to estimate in any given patient whether a proposed treatment entails a greater risk than the disease are all involved in the decisions which the clinician, skilled in the practice of medicine, must make many times each day. This combination of medical knowledge, intuition, and judgment is termed the *art of medicine*. It is as necessary to the practice of medicine as a sound scientific base.

However much the knowledge base of medicine has expanded and will continue to expand, the fundamental commitment of the physician to the care of the patient remains unaltered. The editors of the first edition of *Harrison's Principles of Internal Medicine* put it so eloquently that their words bear repeating:

Tact, sympathy and understanding are expected of the physician, for the patient is no mere collection of symptoms, signs, disordered functions, damaged organs, and disturbed emotions. He is human, fearful, and hopeful, seeking relief, help and reassurance. To the physician, as to the anthropologist, nothing human is strange or repulsive. The misanthrope may become a smart diagnostician of organic disease, but he can scarcely hope to succeed as a physician. The true physician has a Shakespearean breadth of interest in the wise and the foolish, the proud and the humble, the stoic hero and the whining rogue. He cares for people.

THE PATIENT-PHYSICIAN RELATIONSHIP It may be trite to emphasize that physicians need to approach patients not as "cases" or "diseases" but as individuals whose problems all too often transcend the complaints which bring them to the doctor. Most patients are anxious and frightened. Often they go to great ends to convince themselves that illness does not exist, or unconsciously they set up elaborate defenses to divert attention from the real problem that they perceive to be serious or life-threatening. Some patients use illness to gain attention or to serve as a crutch to extricate themselves from an emotionally stressful situation; some even feign physical illness. Whatever the patient's attitude, the physician needs to consider the terrain in which an illness occurs—in terms not only of the patients themselves but also of their families and social backgrounds. All too often medical workups and records fail to include essential information about the patient's origins, schooling, job, home and family, hopes and fears. Without this knowledge it is difficult for the physician to gain rapport with the patient or to develop insight into the patient's illness. Such a relationship must be based on thorough knowledge of the patient and on mutual trust and the ability to communicate with one another.

The direct, one-to-one patient-physician relationship which traditionally has characterized the practice of medicine is changing, primarily because of the changing setting in which medicine is being practiced. Often the management of the individual patient requires the active participation of a variety of trained professional personnel as well as several physicians. In most instances, health care is a team effort. The patient can benefit greatly from such collaboration, but it is the duty of the primary physician to guide the patient through an illness. To carry out this increasingly difficult task, this physician must have some familiarity with the techniques, skills, and objectives of specialist physicians as well as colleagues in the fields allied to medicine. In giving the patient an opportunity to receive all the benefits of the important advances of science, the primary physician must, in the last analysis, retain responsibility for the major decisions concerning diagnosis and treatment.

Increasingly, patients are being cared for by groups of physicians, clinics, hospitals, and health-maintenance organizations (HMOs) rather than by individual independent practitioners. There are many potential advantages in the use of such organized medical groups, but there are also potential drawbacks, the chief of which is a loss of identity of the physician who is primarily and continuously responsible for the patient. It is essential, even in the group setting, that each patient have a physician who has an overview of the patient's problems and who maintains familiarity with the patient's reaction to his or her illness, to the drugs given, and to the challenges of daily living. Moreover, because a number of physicians may, at any one time, contribute to the care of a particular patient, accurate and detailed medical records are essential to good patient care.

In the United States in particular, but to a progressively greater extent throughout the world, the modern hospital poses a particularly intimidating environment for most patients. Lying in a bed surrounded by air jets, buttons, and lights; invaded by tubes and wires; beset by the numerous members of the health care team—nurses, nurses' aides, physicians' assistants, social workers, technologists, physical therapists, medical students, house officers, attending and consulting physicians, and many others; transported to special laboratories and x-ray chambers replete with machines with blinking lights and strange sounds, it is little wonder that patients lose their sense of reality. In fact, the patient's physician is often the only tenuous link between the patient and the real world. A strong personal relationship with the physician is essential in order to sustain the patient in such a stressful situation.

Many influences in contemporary society have the potential of leading to the impersonalization of medical care. Some of these have been mentioned already and include (1) vigorous efforts to reduce the escalating costs of health care; (2) the increasing reliance on technologic advances and computerization for many aspects of diagnosis and treatment; (3) the increased geographic mobility of both patients and physicians; (4) the growing number of "closed-system" arrangements, such as health maintenance organizations, in which the patient has little if any choice in selecting a physician; (5) the need for more than a single physician to be involved in the care of most patients who are seriously ill; and (6) an increasing reliance by patients on legal means to express their disappointments with the health care system (i.e., by malpractice litigation). Given these changes in the medical care system, maintaining the humanistic aspects of medical care and the humanistic qualities of the physician is a particular challenge. It is now more important than ever that the physician consider each patient to be a unique individual deserving of humane treatment, regardless of personal or financial circumstances.

The American Board of Internal Medicine has defined humanistic qualities as encompassing integrity, respect, and compassion. Availability, the expression of sincere concern, the willingness to take the time to explain all aspects of the patient's illness, and an attitude of being nonjudgmental with patients who have lifestyles, attitudes, and values which are different from the physician's own and which he or she may in some instances even find repugnant are just a few of the characteristics of the humane physician. Every physician will, at times, be challenged by patients who evoke strongly negative (and occasionally strongly positive) emotional responses. Physicians should be alert to their own reactions to such patients and situations and consciously monitor and control their behavior so that the patients' best interests remain the principal motivation for their actions at all times.

The famous statement of Dr. Francis Peabody is even more relevant today than when delivered more than a half century ago:

The significance of the intimate personal relationship between physician and patient cannot be too strongly emphasized, for in an extraordinarily large number of cases both the diagnosis and treatment are directly dependent on it. One of the essential qualities of the clinician is interest in humanity, for the secret of the care of the patient is in caring for the patient.

CLINICAL SKILLS **History taking** The written history of an illness should embody all the facts of medical significance in the life of the patient. If the history is recorded in chronologic order, recent events should be given the most attention. Likewise, if a problem-oriented approach is used, the problems that are clinically dominant should be listed first. Ideally, the narration of symptoms or problems should be in the patient's own words. However, few patients have sufficient powers of observation or recall to give a history without some guidance from the physician, who must be careful not to suggest the answers to the questions being posed. Often a symptom which has concerned a patient has little significance, while a seemingly minor complaint may be of considerable importance. Therefore, the physician must be constantly alert to the possibility that any event related by the patient, however trivial or apparently remote, may be the key to the solution of the medical problem.

An informative history is more than an orderly listing of symptoms. Something is always gained by listening to patients and noting the way in which they talk about their symptoms. Inflections of voice, facial expression, and attitude may betray important clues to the meaning of the symptoms to the patient. In listening to the history, the physician discovers not only something about the disease but also something about the patient.

With experience, the pitfalls of history taking become apparent. What patients relate for the most part consists of subjective phenomena colored by past experience. Patients obviously differ widely in their responses to the same stimuli and in their coping mechanisms. Their attitudes are variably influenced by fear of disability and death and by concern over the consequences of their illness to their families. Sometimes the accuracy of the history is affected by language or sociologic barriers, by failing intellectual powers which interfere with recall, or by disorders of consciousness that make them unaware of their illness. It is not surprising, then, that even the most careful physician may at times despair of collecting factual data and be forced to proceed with evidence that represents little more than an approximation of the truth. It is in obtaining the history that the physician's skill, knowledge, and experience are most clearly in evidence.

The family history serves several functions. First, in rare single-gene defects a positive family history of a similarly affected individual or a history of consanguinity may have important diagnostic implications. Second, in diseases of multifactorial etiology that have a familial aggregation, it may be possible to identify patients at risk for disease and to intervene prior to development of overt manifestations. For example, recent weight gain is a more ominous development in a woman who has a family history of diabetes than in one who does not. In certain situations the family history has major implications for preventive medicine. When a diagnosis of a hereditary condition known to predispose to cancer is made, it is the physician's obligation to follow up this possibility carefully in the patient, to survey the family, and to educate them about the need for long-term follow-up.

However accurate and complete, the medical history does much more than provide facts of critical importance. The very act of taking the history provides the physician with the opportunity to establish or enhance the unique bond that is the basis for the critically important patient-physician relationship. An effort should be made to place the patient at ease, regardless of the circumstances of the encounter. The patient should, at some point, have the opportunity to tell his or her own story of the illness without frequent interruption and, when appropriate, should receive expression of interest, encouragement, and empathy from the physician. It is often enlightening to develop an appreciation of the patient's own perception of the illness and the patient's expectations of the physician and the medical care system. The patient's financial status, at least as it relates to the ability to pay for the costs of care, should also be discussed. The confidentiality of the patient-physician relationship should be emphasized, and the patient should be given the opportunity to identify those aspects of the history which he or she wishes not to be disclosed to anyone else.

Physical examination Physical signs are the objective and verifiable marks of disease and represent solid, indisputable facts. Their significance is enhanced when they confirm a functional or structural change already suggested by the patient's history. At times, the physical signs may be the only evidence of disease, especially when the history has been inconsistent, confused, or lacking altogether.

The physical examination should be performed methodically and thoroughly, with due regard for the patient's comfort and modesty. Although attention has often been directed by the history to the diseased organ or part of the body, the examination must extend from head to toe in an objective search for abnormalities. Unless the examination procedure is systematic, important parts of it may be omitted, an error which is common even among the most skilled clinicians. The results of the examination, like the details of the history, should be recorded at the time they are elicited, not hours later when they are subject to the distortions of memory. Many inaccuracies stem from the careless practice of writing or dictating notes long after the examination has been concluded. Skill in physical diagnosis is acquired with experience, but it is not merely technique that determines success in eliciting signs. The detection of a few scattered petechiae, a faint diastolic murmur, or a small mass in the abdomen is not a question of keener eyes and ears or more sensitive fingers but of a mind prepared to be alert to these findings. Skill in physical diagnosis reflects a way of thinking more than a way of doing. Physical findings are subject to change. Just because the examination is normal on one occasion does not guarantee that this will be the case on subsequent examinations. It is important, therefore, to repeat pertinent parts of the physical examination as long as the clinical situation warrants.

Laboratory tests The marked increase in the number and availability of laboratory tests has inevitably resulted in increasing reliance being placed on knowledge gained from these studies in the solution of clinical problems. It is essential, however, to bear in mind the limitations of such procedures, which by virtue of their impersonal quality and complexity often gain an aura of authority regardless of the fallibility of the tests themselves, of the individuals doing or interpreting them, or of their instruments. More importantly, the accumulation of laboratory data cannot relieve the physician from the responsibility of careful observation and study of the patient. Physicians also must weigh carefully the hazards and the expense involved in the laboratory procedures they order. Moreover, laboratory tests are rarely ordered and reported singly. Rather, they are produced as "batteries." Some laboratories now perform batteries of 24 and even 40 tests. The various combinations of laboratory tests are often useful. For example, they may provide the clue to such nonspecific symptoms as generalized weakness and increased fatigability by revealing abnormalities of hepatic function together with elevated levels of serum IgG which, in turn, would suggest the diagnosis of chronic liver disease. Sometimes a single abnormality, such as an elevated serum calcium, points to a specific disease, such as hyperparathyroidism.

The thoughtful use of screening tests should not be confused with indiscriminate laboratory testing. The use of screening tests is based on the fact that a group of laboratory determinations can be carried out conveniently on a single specimen of blood at relatively low cost. Biochemical measurements, together with simple laboratory examinations such as blood count, urinalysis, and sedimentation rate, often provide the major clue to the presence of a pathologic process. At the same time the physican must learn to evaluate occasional abnormalities among the screening tests that may not necessarily connote significant disease. There is nothing more wasteful and unproductive than an in-depth workup following a report of an isolated laboratory abnormality in a patient who is otherwise well. Among the more than 40 tests that are performed on many patients, one is often slightly abnormal. If there is no clinical suspicion of an underlying illness, the test is ordinarily repeated to ensure that the abnormality does not represent a laboratory error. If the abnormality is confirmed it is important to distinguish a minor one (less than two standard deviations) from a major one (more than two standard deviations). Even in the case of the latter, the decision of whether to proceed with further workup is a test of the physician's clinical judgment.

Newer imaging techniques The last decade and a half have seen the arrival of ultrasonography, a variety of isotopic scans that employ new isotopes to visualize organs heretofore inaccessible, computerized tomography with its varying permutations, and magnetic resonance imaging. Aside from opening up new diagnostic vistas, this new, highly sophisticated technology benefits patients because it has frequently supplanted invasive techniques which require surgical biopsy or the insertion of tubes, wires, or catheters into the body—procedures which are often painful and sometimes risky. While the enthusiasm for noninvasive technology is understandably justified, all too often the results have not been validated properly before they are disseminated as clinical dogma. Moreover, the expense entailed in performing these imaging tests is often substantial and is not always considered when ordering them. There is no question that a tool like computerized tomography has led to a reassessment of the problem of adrenal tumors, just as routine measurement of calcium caused a redefinition of hyperparathyroidism. The principles being espoused here are simply to use these examinations judiciously, preferably in lieu of, not in addition to, the invasive maneuvers they are meant to replace.

THE DIAGNOSIS OF DISEASE Accurate diagnosis requires, first of all, the collection of accurate data. But much more is required in making a diagnosis. Each item of data must be interpreted in the light of what is known about the structure and function of the involved organ(s). Knowledge of anatomy, physiology, and biochemistry must be combined into a plausible pathophysiologic mechanism.

Clinical diagnosis requires both aspects of logic—analysis and synthesis—and the more difficult the clinical problem, the more important is a logical approach to it. Such an approach requires that the physician list carefully each problem suggested by the patient's symptoms and physical and laboratory findings and seek answers to each. Most physicians attempt consciously or unconsciously to fit a given problem into one of a series of syndromes. *The syndrome is a group of symptoms and signs of disordered function, related to one another by means of some anatomic, physiologic, or biochemical peculiarity.* It embodies a hypothesis concerning the deranged function of an organ, organ system, or tissue. Congestive heart failure, Cushing's syndrome, and dementia are examples. In congestive heart failure dyspnea, orthopnea, cyanosis, dependent edema, engorged neck veins, pleural effusion, rales, and hepatomegaly are known to be connected by a single pathophysiologic mechanism—insufficiency of the cardiac pump mechanism. In Cushing's syndrome the moon facies, hypertension, diabetes, and osteoporosis are the recognized effects of excess glucocorticoids acting on many target organs. In dementia, deterioration of memory, incoherent thinking, impaired language functions, visual-spatial disorientation, and faulty judgment are related to destruction of the association areas of the cerebrum.

A syndrome usually does not identify the precise cause of an illness, but it greatly narrows the number of possibilities and often suggests certain special clinical and laboratory studies. The derangements of each organ system in humans are reducible to a relatively small number of syndromes. The diagnosis is simplified greatly if a clinical problem conforms neatly to a well-defined syndrome, because only a few diseases need to be considered in the differential diagnosis. In contrast, the search for the cause of an illness that does not conform to a syndrome is more difficult because a much greater number of diseases have to be sought. Even here an orderly approach which proceeds from symptom to sign to laboratory findings will result in the diagnosis most of the time.

CARING FOR THE PATIENT The care of the patient begins with the development of a personal relationship between the patient and the physician. In the absence of a sense of trust and confidence on the part of the patient, the effectiveness of most therapeutic measures is diminished. In many instances, when there is confidence in the physician, reassurance is the best treatment and is all that is needed. Likewise, in those cases which do not lend themselves to easy solutions or for which no effective treatment is available, a feeling on the part of the patient that the physician is doing all that is possible is one of the most important therapeutic measures that can be provided. An important aspect of clinical decision making and patient care involves the "quality of life," a subjective assessment of what each patient values most. Such an assessment requires detailed, sometimes intimate knowledge of the patient, which can usually be obtained only through deliberate, unhurried, and often repeated conversation. In situations where complete freedom from signs and symptoms of disease is impossible, maximization of the quality of life becomes the major goal of therapy.

Drug therapy With each succeeding year, more drugs are released, every one with the hope and the promise that it is an improvement over its predecessor. Although the pharmaceutical industry must be given most of the credit for advances in drug therapy, it is also true that many new drugs have only a marginal advantage over the agents they are aimed to replace. The barrage of new information with which practitioners are deluged does little to provide a clear picture of clinical pharmacology; on the contrary, to most physicians new drugs are confusing. With some exceptions, however, the approach to a new drug should be one of caution. Unless the new agent is established beyond doubt to be a real advance, it is wiser to use well-tested and well-established agents which are not only efficacious but whose safety has been well-established.

Iatrogenic disorders An iatrogenic disorder occurs when the deleterious effects of a procedure or drug produce pathology independent of the condition for which the drug is given. No matter what the clinical situation, it is the responsibility of the physician to use new and powerful therapeutic measures wisely, with due regard to their action, potential dangers, and cost. Every medical procedure, whether diagnostic or therapeutic, has the potential for harm, but it would be impossible to afford the patient all the benefits of modern scientific medicine if reasonable steps in diagnosis and therapy were withheld because of possible risks. "Reasonable" implies that the physician has weighed the pros and cons of a procedure and has concluded on rational grounds that it is advisable or essential for the relief of discomfort or the cure or amelioration of disease. For example, the use of glucocorticoids to arrest progressive disseminated lupus erythematosus may produce Cushing's syndrome. In this instance, the benefits usually exceed the untoward side effects. However, much harm can result when the deleterious effects of a procedure or a drug exceed any possible advantages that might have been anticipated. Examples include the dangerous or fatal drug reactions that occasionally follow the use of antibiotics given for trivial respiratory infections, the gastric hemorrhage or perforation caused by glucocorticoid administration for mild arthritis, or the occurrence of fatal hepatitis that may follow needless transfusions of blood or plasma.

But the harm that a physician can do to a patient is not limited to the imprudent use of medication. Equally important are ill-considered or unjustified remarks. Many a patient has developed a cardiac neurosis because the physician ventured a grave prognosis on the basis of a misinterpreted electrocardiogram. Not only the treatment itself but the physician's words and behavior are capable of causing injury.

The physician must never become so absorbed in the disease as to forget the patient who is its victim. As the science of medicine advances, it is all too easy to become so fascinated by the manifestations of disease that the ailing person's fears and concerns about job and family, the cost of medical care, and the specter of economic insecurity are disregarded. Treatment of a patient consists of more than the dispassionate confrontation of a disease. It embodies also the exercise of warmth, compassion, and understanding.

Informed consent In an era of rapidly advancing technology, patients will require diagnostic and therapeutic procedures that are painful and that pose some risk. These include all surgical procedures, e.g., biopsies of tissues, radiographic maneuvers involving the insertion of catheters, endoscopy, and many others. In most American hospitals and clinics, patients undergoing such procedures are required to sign a form consenting to them. More important, however, is the notion that the patient must understand clearly the risk entailed in these procedures; this is the definition of *informed consent*. It is incumbent upon the physician to explain to the patient, in a clearly understandable fashion, the procedures which he or she faces. By doing this conscientiously much of the dread of the unknown that is inherent in hospitalization will be mitigated.

Accountability Throughout the world physicians, once licensed to practice medicine, have not had to account for their actions except to their peers. In the United States, however, during the past decade and a half, there have been increasing demands for physicians to account for the way in which they practice medicine by meeting certain standards prescribed by federal and state governments. Hospitalized patients whose health care is reimbursed by the government (Medicare and Medicaid) and other third parties have been subjected to utilization review. This means that the physician must defend the cause for and duration of a patient's hospitalization if it falls outside certain "average" standards. In some instances a second opinion is necessary before a patient can be admitted to the hospital for elective surgery. The purpose of these regulations is to contain spiraling health care costs. It is likely that this type of review will be extended to all phases of medical practice and will inevitably alter the practice of medicine.

Physicians also may be expected to give account of their continuing competence by mandatory continuing education, patient record audit, recertification by examination, or relicensure. While these measures probably enhance the physician's factual knowledge, there is no evidence that they have a similar effect on the quality of practice.

Cost-effectiveness in medical care As the cost of medical care continues to rise, it has become necessary to establish stringent priorities in the expenditure of health care dollars. In some instances, preventive measures offer the greatest return per dollar; outstanding examples include vaccination, immunization, reduction in accidents and occupational hazards, and improved environmental control. The cost of "newborn screening" for metabolic diseases is being evaluated. For example, the detection of phenylketonuria by screening of large populations may result in a net saving of many thousands of dollars.

As resources become more and more constrained, it will be necessary to weigh the justifiability of performing prohibitively costly operations that provide only a limited life expectancy against the pressing need for more primary care for those persons who do not have adequate access to medical services. At the level of the individual patient it is important to minimize costly hospital admissions as far as possible, if total health care is to be provided at an expense which most can afford. This, of course, implies and depends upon a close cooperative effort between patients, their physicians, their employers, third-party carriers, and government, along with constant surveillance of those types of procedures which can be conducted safely and effectively on an ambulatory basis. Equally important in reducing total health care expenditures is the need for individual physicians to monitor carefully both the cost and effectiveness of the drugs they prescribe. In the last analysis the medical profession should provide leadership and guidance to the public in matters of cost control, and the medical profession must take this responsibility seriously without being or seeming to be self-serving. It is important, however, that these significant socioeconomic aspects of health care delivery not be permitted to interfere with the concern of physicians for the welfare of their patients. The patient must be able to rely on the individual physician as his or her principal advocate in matters of health care.

Research and teaching The title "doctor" is derived from the Latin *docere,* "to teach," and the physician should share information and medical knowledge with others and be willing to teach what he or she has learned to colleagues as well as to students of medicine and related professions. The practice of medicine is dependent on the sum total of medical knowledge, which in turn is based on an unending chain of scientific discovery, clinical observation, analysis, and interpretation. Advances in medicine depend on the acquisition of new information, i.e., on research, which must often involve patients; improved medical care requires the transmission of this information. As part of broader societal responsibilities, the physician should encourage patients to participate in ethical and properly approved clinical investigations if they do not impose undue hazard, discomfort, or inconvenience.

Incurability and death No problem is more distressing than that presented by the patient with an incurable disease, particularly when premature death is inevitable. What should the patient and family be told, what measures should be taken to maintain life, and how is death to be defined?

Although some would argue otherwise, there is no ironclad rule that the patient must be told "everything," even if the patient is an adult and the head of a family. How much the patient is told should depend upon the patient's ability and capacity to deal with the possibility of imminent death; often this capacity grows with time and, whenever possible, gradual rather than abrupt disclosure is the best strategy. This decision may also take into consideration the patient's religious beliefs, financial and business affairs, and to some extent the wishes of the family. The patient must be given an opportunity to talk with the physician and ask questions. Patients may find it easier to share their feelings about death with their physician, who is likely to be more objective and less emotional than family members.

One thing is certain; it is not for you to don the black cap and, assuming the judicial function, take hope away from any patient . . . hope that comes to us all.

William Osler

Even when the patient directly inquires, "Doctor, am I dying?" the physician must attempt to determine whether this is a request for information, a demand for reassurance, or even an expression of hostility. Most would agree that only open communication between the patient and the physician can resolve these questions and guide the physician in what to say and how to say it.

The physician should provide or arrange for emotional, physical, and spiritual support, and must be compassionate, unhurried, and open. Pain should be adequately controlled, human dignity maintained, and isolation from family avoided. The last two in particular tend to be overlooked in hospitals, where the intrusion of life-sustaining apparatus can so easily detract from attention to the whole person and concentrate instead on the life-threatening disease. The physician must also prepare to deal with guilt feelings on the part of the family when a member becomes gravely or hopelessly ill. It is important for the doctor to reassure the family that everything possible has been done.

The President's Committee for the Study of Ethical Problems in Medicine defined death as (1) irreversible cessation of circulatory and respiratory function, or (2) irreversible cessation of all functions of the entire brain, including the brain stem. Clinical and electroencephalographic criteria are at hand which permit the reliable diagnosis of cerebral death. According to the criteria adopted by the staff of the Massachusetts General Hospital and the Harvard Committee on Brain Death, death occurs when all signs of receptivity and responsivity are absent, including all brainstem reflexes (pupillary reactions, ocular movement, blinking, swallowing, breathing), and the electroencephalogram is isoelectric. Occasionally, intoxications and metabolic disorders may simulate this state; hence the diagnosis requires expert evaluation. Under the aforementioned circumstances, to continue with heroic, highly costly supportive measures merely for the purpose of preserving cardiac function is against the best interests of patient, family, and society. In such instances, the dilemma of continuing care could be avoided if the medical profession, in accord with social sanction, can be brought to redefine life and death by these criteria.

A practice which has proved acceptable in many settings is as follows:

1 The diagnosis of brain death, based on the above criteria, should be corroborated by another physician and confirmed by clinical examination and EEG, repeated one or more times.

2 The family should be informed of the irreversibility of brain function but should not be requested to ratify the decision of whether the medical treatment should be discontinued. An exception to this limited decision-making power of the family might apply where the patient has directed the family that he or she wishes them to make the decision.

3 The physician, after consultation with a professional colleague, may withdraw supportive measures, assuming that nothing more can be offered. This interpretation is in general agreement with that of most religions.

4 The possibility that such patients may become sources of organs for grafting should not enter into the aforementioned decisions, although prior to the cessation of heart action the family may be asked whether this would be their wish, or the family may suggest that organs be used for this purpose.

"Do not resuscitate" orders and cessation of therapy When carried out in a timely and expert manner, cardiopulmonary resuscitation is often useful in the prevention of sudden, unexpected death. However, unless there are reasons to the contrary it should not ordinarily be carried out when it merely prolongs life in a patient with terminal, incurable disease. The decision not to resuscitate a patient and decisions about the intensity of therapy and, indeed, whether or not treatment is to be delivered at all to patients who are incurably and terminally ill must be reviewed frequently and must take into consideration any unexpected changes in the patient's condition. These decisions must take into account both the underlying medical condition and the wishes of the patient or if these cannot or have not been ascertained directly, those of a close relative or other surrogate who can be relied upon to transmit the patient's feelings and to be guided by the patient's best interests. Legal rulings, reflecting societal views, increasingly support the view that medical interventions of any kind which only sustain biologic functions in the hopelessly ill are futile and unnecessary gestures.

The issues involving death and dying are among the most difficult in medicine. In approaching them rationally and consistently, the physician must combine the art of medicine with the science.

2 QUANTITATIVE ASPECTS OF CLINICAL REASONING

LEE GOLDMAN

The process of clinical reasoning is poorly understood but is based upon factors such as experience and learning, inductive and deductive reasoning, interpretation of evidence that itself varies in reproducibility and validity, and intuition that often is difficult to define. In an effort to improve clinical reasoning, a number of attempts have been made to analyze quantitatively the many factors involved, including defining the cognitive approaches that clinicians apply to difficult problems, devising computerized decision support systems that are designed to emulate certain features of decision making, and applying decision theory to understand how judgments should be reached. While each of these approaches has advanced the understanding of the diagnostic process, all have practical and/or theoretical problems that limit their direct applicability to the care of the individual patient.

Nevertheless, these preliminary attempts to apply the rigor and logic inherent in the quantitative method have provided significant insights into the process by which clinical reasoning is accomplished, have identified ways in which the process may be improved, and have made it possible to minimize certain features of the workup that are not cost-effective. Thus, while clinical reasoning cannot be reduced to probabilities or numbers, attempts at quantitative analysis of the process may improve the ways in which the problems of individual patients are approached and solved.

In a simplified model, quantitative clinical reasoning includes five phases. It begins with an investigation of the chief complaint through key questions that are included in the history of the present illness (Table 2-1). These questions are supplemented by the past medical history and by a physical examination that emphasizes detailed investigation of potential key organ systems. In the second phase, the physician may select an array of diagnostic tests, each with its own accuracy and usefulness for investigating the possibilities raised in the differential diagnosis. Since each test costs something, and some entail discomfort and risk as well, the physician must ask whether the history and physical examination are sufficiently diagnostic before ordering tests. Third, the clinical data must be integrated with test results to estimate the likelihood of conditions in the differential diagnosis. Fourth, the comparative risks and benefits of

TABLE 2-1 Phases of clinical reasoning and decision making

1 Investigation of the complaint by means of clinical examination (history and physical examination)
2 Ordering of diagnostic tests, each with its own intrinsic accuracy and usefulness
3 Integration of clinical findings with test results to assess diagnostic probabilities
4 Weighing of comparative risks and benefits of alternative courses of action
5 Determination of patient's preferences and development of a therapeutic plan

further diagnostic and therapeutic options must be weighed to reach a recommendation for the patient. Finally, this recommendation is presented to the patient, and after appropriate discussion of the options, a therapeutic plan is initiated. Each of the five steps in this simplified model of the clinical reasoning process can be analyzed individually.

HISTORY AND PHYSICAL EXAMINATION It originally had been assumed that physicians begin investigating a patient's chief complaint by obtaining a comprehensive history, which includes many if not most of the questions included in a full review of systems, and by performing an all-inclusive physical examination. However, experienced clinicians begin to form hypotheses based on the chief complaint and on the responses to initial questioning, and they ask further questions in a sequence that allows them to evaluate the initial hypotheses and, if necessary, shorten or amend the list of possibilities. Only a limited number of diagnostic hypotheses can be entertained at any one time, and information is used to build a case for or against the most likely. In such a way, high-priority questions are selected from the almost limitless number that might be asked, and these specific questions are incorporated into the history of the present illness. Often, a key response, such as a history of melena, will be selected, a list of potential explanations for it will be formulated, and this list will then be trimmed, based on the response to more probing questions, so that a principal diagnosis can be selected and then tested. This process, termed *iterative hypothesis testing*, is an efficient approach to diagnosis and is preferable to attempts to gather every conceivable piece of information prior to formulating a differential diagnosis.

Advocacy of iterative hypothesis testing does not argue against the need for a systematic, thorough, and complete history of the present illness, past medical history, review of systems, family history, social history, and physical examination. For example, if a patient presents with abdominal pain, the physician may gather information regarding its location and quality as well as the factors that precipitate and/or relieve it. The physician then asks questions relating to the diagnoses that may be suspected based on the response to the initial questions. If the pain is suggestive of pancreatitis, the clinician might ask about alcohol intake, the use of thiazide diuretics or glucocorticosteroids, symptoms suggestive of concomitant gallbladder disease, a family history of pancreatitis, and questions aimed at uncovering the possibility of a posterior penetrating ulcer. Alternatively, if the discomfort seems more typical of reflux esophagitis, a different sequence of questions would be triggered. The use of iterative hypothesis testing encourages the physician to elicit detailed information in high-yield areas, without forgoing a systematic and thorough approach to the patient. Findings on the history and physical examination should influence each other. The history focuses the physical examination on certain organs, and findings on physical examination should encourage more detailed review of certain systems.

As physicians proceed through this reasoning process with both the history and physical examination, a variety of issues may influence the accuracy of the decision-making process. First is the potential for some historical information to be poorly reproducible, either because the patient's responses vary or because different physicians ask questions differently or vary in the way they interpret the answers. For example, in one study, two physicians' estimates of functional cardiac class agreed only about half of the time. When a subjective scale was replaced by a more specific series of precisely worded questions, both reproducibility and validity improved significantly, although some patients still gave frankly conflicting responses to the same question when asked by different interviewers on the same day. The careful use of clear, and when possible, precise questions can increase the reproducibility and validity of the medical history, but still cannot eliminate all variability.

When assessing the reproducibility of findings on the physical examination, two observers frequently agree that an uncommon abnormality such as an enlarged spleen is not present but agree less often when one of them thinks that it is present in a patient in whom it would not usually be expected. This principle can best be demonstrated by understanding that some agreement always occurs by chance, and the likelihood of chance agreement is higher if the finding is either very common or very uncommon. For example, if two physicians each consider 90 percent of patients to be abnormal in some manner, such as having a systolic heart murmur, they will agree 81 percent of the time by chance alone. In some studies of the reproducibility of common signs and symptoms, such as whether or not a liver was enlarged, actual agreement rates have not been substantially better than chance. Disagreement rates may be reduced by emphasizing physical examination skills during medical training, by looking for other correlative physical findings, and by learning how physical findings correlate with the results of diagnostic tests. Therefore, when a clinician notes an unexpected and somewhat subjective abnormality for which there may be a high rate of interobserver disagreement, such as an unexpectedly enlarged spleen, other abnormalities that may often be associated with it, such as hepatomegaly or lymphadenopathy, should be sought to increase the likelihood that the spleen would be expected to be abnormal. In some situations, ordering a diagnostic test, such as a liver and spleen scan, to assess the finding more objectively should be considered if the test is sufficiently reliable.

These comments about the factors that limit the reproducibility and validity of the medical history and physical examination do not denigrate their critical importance in clinical reasoning. Rather, they emphasize that care and diligence in the application of these skills are necessary.

When physicians use the history and the physical examination to arrive at a diagnosis, they are rarely certain of it. Therefore, it would be better to assess the likelihood of the diagnosis in terms of probabilities. All too frequently, this probability is not expressed as an actual percentage but rather in such terms as "nearly always," "commonly," "sometimes," or "rarely." Since different physicians may assign different probabilities to the same terms, these imprecise words frequently lead to major misunderstandings among physicians or between the physician and the patient. Physicians should be as rigorous and quantitative as possible in their assessments, and when feasible, a quantitative expression of probability should be used. For example, rather than saying that it is unlikely that a radiographic pattern is indicative of a carcinoma of the colon, it would be preferable, if possible, to provide a more precise indication of the probability of carcinoma with this radiographic pattern. A 10 to 15 percent probability of carcinoma may be interpreted as "unlikely," but from a clinical perspective usually warrants further evaluation because of the serious consequences of missing a potentially resectable tumor.

Although such quantitative estimates would be desirable, they usually are not available in practice. Even experienced physicians often are unable to estimate accurately the likelihood of particular conditions. There is a tendency to overestimate the likelihood of relatively uncommon conditions, and physicians are especially poor at quantifying probabilities that are very high or very low. For example, a physician may not know whether the probability of bacterial meningitis or of another disease that could be diagnosed by a lumbar puncture in a patient with a severe headache is 1 in 20 or 1 in 200. In both situations, the probability is low, but the decision as to whether a lumbar puncture should be performed may depend on this estimate.

Since the establishment of valid diagnostic probabilities is a cornerstone to clinical reasoning, accumulated clinical experience, often in the form of computerized data banks, has been used to generate statistical approaches for improving diagnostic predictions. In such research, it is common to identify factors that have a univariate correlation with the diagnosis in question. Then, these univariate correlates may be included in a multivariate analysis to determine which of them are significant independent predictors of the diagnosis.

Some analyses may identify the important predictive factors and then assign them "weights," which can be transformed to calculate a probability. Alternatively, the analysis may result in a limited number of categories of patients, each with a discrete probability of the diagnosis.

These quantitative approaches to the estimation of various diagnostic probabilities, which are often termed "prediction rules," are especially helpful if they are in a format that is readily usable by the clinician and if they have been validated prospectively on a sufficient number and spectrum of patients. For example, by carefully defining the key historical questions and findings on physical examination that might predict the causes of common acute complaints observed in ambulatory patients, algorithms have been devised to guide nonphysicians on the ordering of diagnostic tests and the need for an examination by a physician; nonphysicians aided by these algorithms, and working under the general supervision of a physician, can provide care that is less costly and as effective as that provided by unaided physicians.

For such prediction rules to be useful to the clinician, they must be derived from relevant patient populations and use tests that are reproducible and readily available, so that the results can be extrapolated to local medical practice. Since only a minority of published prediction rules have adhered to rigid criteria as to the number and spectrum of patients examined and their prospective validation, most are not yet suitable for routine clinical application. Furthermore, many prediction rules cannot evaluate the probability of each of the diagnoses or outcomes that the clinician must consider.

As was emphasized in Chap. 1, the history and physical examination have other important purposes. They allow the physician to evaluate the emotional status of the patient and to understand how the present problems fit into the context of the patient's social and family life, and they encourage the development in the patient of confidence in the physician, which is so necessary for reaching an agreement on the coming plan of action.

DIAGNOSTIC TESTS: INDICATIONS, ACCURACY, AND USEFULNESS A diagnostic test should be ordered for specified clinical indications, be sufficiently accurate to be efficacious for such indications, and be the least expensive and/or risky of the available efficacious tests. No diagnostic test is totally accurate, and physicians often have difficulty interpreting test results. It is therefore critical to understand several commonly used terms in test analysis and epidemiology, including prevalence, sensitivity, specificity, positive predictive value, and negative predictive value (Table 2-2).

Although reports of the accuracies of diagnostic tests are commonly expressed in terms of positive and negative predictive values, these calculated values are dependent on the prevalence of the disease in the population being studied (Table 2-3). A test with a particular sensitivity and specificity has different positive and negative predictive values when used in groups that have different prevalences of disease. For example, a mildly abnormal alkaline phosphatase level in a young adult with a known lymphoma suggests hepatic involvement by the tumor, i.e., it is likely to be a *true positive*, while the same alkaline phosphatase level as part of a routine screening battery of blood tests in an asymptomatic person of the same age is unlikely to be due to tumor, i.e., in this setting it is more likely to be a *false positive*.

Although the sensitivity and specificity of a test do not depend on the prevalence (or percentage of patients being tested who have the disease), they do depend on the spectrum of patients in whom the test is being evaluated. For example, a technetium pyrophosphate scintiscan for diagnosing myocardial infarction (Chap. 179) will appear to have a nearly perfect sensitivity and specificity if the diseased population has a history typical of myocardial infarction, electrocardiographic changes of transmural infarction, and clear-cut elevations of the MB isoenzyme of creatine kinase (CK) and the nondiseased population is composed of normal medical students. If, however, without changing the prevalence of disease in the population being tested, the spectrum of the diseased and nondiseased patients is altered by including patients with other characteristics, i.e., if the population of patients with myocardial infarction were composed principally of those with non-Q-wave infarctions and small or borderline elevations of CK-MB, while the population without acute infarction included patients with old infarcts and unstable angina pectoris, the sensitivity and specificity might change dramatically. In the latter situation, the sensitivity and specificity of the technetium pyrophosphate scintiscan are not only lower than in the first example, because the spectrum of diseased and nondiseased patients has been changed, but, more importantly, they are so low that the test has little clinical value. This example also demonstrates the methodologic problems encountered when applying data from one study to a different type of patient or when pooling data from studies of different subsets of patients.

In some situations, uncertainty about the sensitivity and specificity of the test in the type of patient being assessed may limit its clinical value. Since the physician rarely knows (or can know) the population on which every test which is ordered has been standardized, the results provide information that is far less decisive than usually thought. Furthermore, it may be quite difficult to distinguish random laboratory errors from test results that might be falsely positive or negative because of coexistence of a process that can affect the test, such as the finding of an elevated level of CK in a patient who has undergone strenuous exercise and is being evaluated for chest pain.

Because no single value or cutoff point of an individual test can be expected to have both a perfect sensitivity and a perfect specificity, it is often necessary to determine which value or cutoff point is the most appropriate to guide decision making. A graph (Fig. 2-1) of the test's *receiver operating characteristic curve*, which displays the inevitable trade-off between emphasizing a high sensitivity, such as defining an exercise electrocardiogram as abnormal if it shows ≥0.5 mm of ST-segment depression, versus emphasizing a high specificity, such as defining an exercise electrocardiogram as abnormal only if it shows ≥2.0 mm of ST-segment depression, can help the clinician understand the implications of various definitions of a "positive" test result. Such a graph demonstrates that different definitions of

TABLE 2-2 Definitions of commonly used terms in epidemiology and decision making

Test result	Disease state: Present	Disease state: Absent
Positive	a (true positive)	b (false positive)
Negative	c (false negative)	d (true negative)

Prevalence (prior probability)	=	(a+c)/(a+b+c+d)	=	all patients with the disease/all patients tested
Sensitivity	=	a/(a+c)	=	true-positive test results/all patients with the disease
Specificity	=	d/(b+d)	=	true-negative test results/all patients without the disease
False-negative rate	=	c/(a+c)	=	false-negative test results/all patients with the disease
False-positive rate	=	b/(b+d)	=	false-positive test results/all patients without the disease
Positive predictive value	=	a/(a+b)	=	true-positive test results/all positive test results
Negative predictive value	=	d/(c+d)	=	true-negative test results/all patients with negative results
Overall accuracy	=	(a+d)/(a+b+c+d)	=	true-positive + true-negative test results/all tests

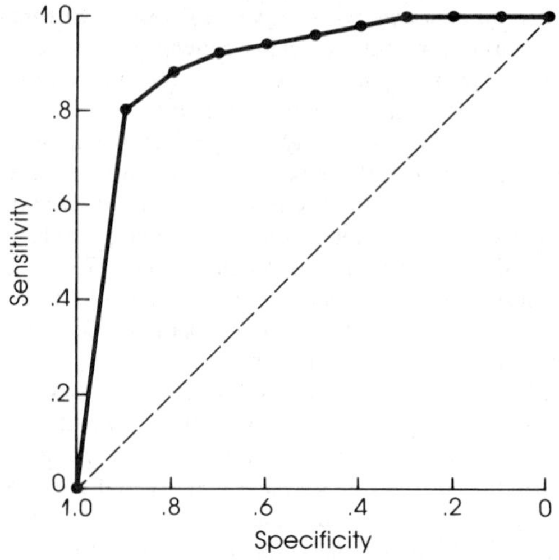

FIGURE 2-1 *The inherent trade-off between sensitivity and specificity. For any diagnostic test, an increase in sensitivity will be associated with a decline in specificity. The closer this curve comes to the upper-left-hand corner, the more useful the test; the closer to the broken line, the less useful it is. When deciding on the cutoff between normal versus abnormal, one must determine what sensitivity and specificity are most useful clinically.*

normal versus abnormal may be appropriate depending on whether one wishes to rule in the disease with a test result that has a high specificity or to exclude the disease with a test result that has a high sensitivity. Different tests may have different sensitivities and specificities, and better tests may have both a higher sensitivity and a higher specificity than poorer tests.

One example of a sensitive test is an M-mode echocardiogram to exclude severe aortic stenosis in adults: the sensitivity of the test for aortic stenosis is close to 100 percent, and a normal aortic valve echogram virtually excludes the diagnosis of severe aortic stenosis in the adult. Unfortunately, this sensitive test is not very specific, and many patients who have abnormal aortic valves on echocardiogram do not have severe aortic stenosis and require further testing (e.g., with Doppler echocardiography and perhaps cardiac catheterization) to establish the diagnosis (Chap. 187). A common example of a reasonably specific test would be an electrocardiogram to diagnose acute myocardial infarction. While the precise specificity depends on the spectrum of patients being tested, the presence of new ST-segment elevations exceeding 1.0 mm in two or more adjacent leads in patients who present to an emergency room with prolonged acute chest pain consistent with myocardial ischemia is sufficiently specific, i.e., sufficiently unlikely to be a false positive, that admission to an intensive care unit is virtually always recommended. However, this test is not sensitive, and if admission to the unit were restricted to patients with this electrocardiographic finding, almost half of patients with myocardial infarctions presenting to hospital emergency rooms would be missed.

To optimize the clinical value of a diagnostic test, it is helpful to obtain local experience with it; oftentimes, its value will differ from that reported in the literature. Reports of the efficacy of a test should emphasize its accuracy when compared to an independent standard, and the test must be evaluated in a spectrum of patients with varying severities of the disease in question and in patients who have conditions that are part of the same differential diagnosis. The reproducibility of the test should be known, and the "normal limits" of the test should be clear and appropriate. In some instances, the test or procedure required to establish the validity of a diagnostic test is so risky that only a skewed sample of patients are included in a study, as, for example, in the analysis of the usefulness of the abdominal CT scan in patients with suspected pancreatic carcinoma. If patients with "negative" CT scan results never come to laparotomy or postmortem examination, neither the sensitivity nor specificity of the CT scan for pancreatic carcinoma can be assessed. In such situations, an estimated value of the diagnostic test may be inaccurate because it has not been validated.

INTEGRATION OF CLINICAL DATA AND TEST RESULTS Although, as we have seen, neither clinical data nor test results may be entirely accurate, the integration of the two can lead to better diagnostic predictions than either alone. By knowing the probability that the patient has a particular condition before a test is performed (the prior, or pretest, probability), and by knowing the sensitivity and the specificity of the test, the posttest probability can be calculated. A common mathematical technique for integrating clinical data and a test result is the odds-likelihood form of Bayesian analysis (Table 2-4). A pretest probability can be expressed as odds (as in a horse race for example) and multiplied by the likelihood ratio (which is the sensitivity of the test divided by 1 minus the specificity of the test) to yield the posttest odds, which may be transformed back into a posttest probability. This approach can be employed in any situation in which the physician can use clinical findings to estimate a pretest

TABLE 2-3 How the positive and negative predictive values of the same test vary depending on the prior probability of disease

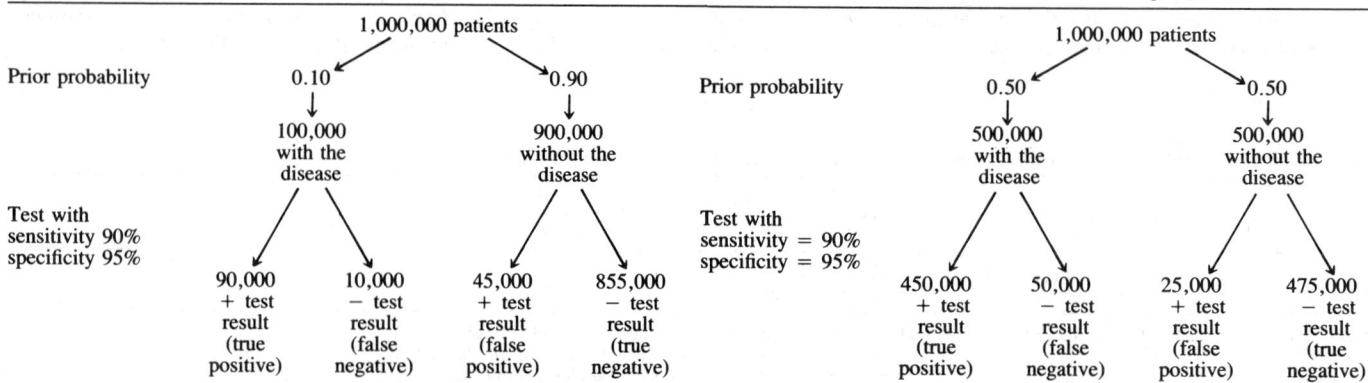

INTERPRETATION OF THE TEST RESULT WHEN 10% OF THE PATIENTS BEING TESTED HAVE THE DISEASE (PRIOR PROBABILITY = 10%)

1,000,000 patients

Prior probability: 0.10 → 100,000 with the disease; 0.90 → 900,000 without the disease

Test with sensitivity 90% specificity 95%

90,000 + test result (true positive)	10,000 − test result (false negative)	45,000 + test result (false positive)	855,000 − test result (true negative)

The probability of disease in a patient with a positive test result (positive predictive value) = 90,000/135,000 = 67%

The probability of no disease in a patient with a negative test result (negative predictive value) = 855,000/865,000 = 99%

INTERPRETATION OF THE TEST RESULT WHEN 50% OF THE PATIENTS BEING TESTED HAVE THE DISEASE (PRIOR PROBABILITY = 50%)

1,000,000 patients

Prior probability: 0.50 → 500,000 with the disease; 0.50 → 500,000 without the disease

Test with sensitivity = 90% specificity = 95%

450,000 + test result (true positive)	50,000 − test result (false negative)	25,000 + test result (false positive)	475,000 − test result (true negative)

The probability of disease in a patient with a positive test result (positive predictive value) = 450,000/475,000 = 95%

The probability of no disease in a patient with a negative test result (negative predictive value) = 475,000/525,000 = 90%

TABLE 2-4 Example of the use of Bayesian analysis to integrate the pretest probability with the test result to calculate a posttest probability

Example 1: Prior probability of disease = 25%; a test with a sensitivity (true-positive rate) of 90% and a specificity of 80% (which implies a false-positive rate of 20%) gives a positive result

Clinical data

↓

Prior probability → prior odds

25% 1:3

$\frac{0.90}{0.20} \leftarrow \frac{\text{sensitivity*}}{(1-\text{specificity})\dagger} \leftarrow$ positive test

Posttest odds

$(1{:}3) \times \frac{0.90}{0.20} = 4.5{:}3$

Posttest probability

$\frac{4.5}{7.5} = 60\%$

Example 2: Same pretest probability and test, but now the test gives a negative result. Here the true-negative rate would be 80% and the false negative rate (which is 1 − sensitivity) would be 10%.

Clinical data

↓

Prior probability → prior odds

25% 1:3

$\frac{0.10}{0.80} \leftarrow \frac{(1-\text{sensitivity})\ddagger}{\text{specificity}\S} \leftarrow$ negative test

Posttest odds

$(1{:}3) \times \frac{0.10}{0.80} = 0.125{:}3 = 1{:}24$

Posttest probability

$\frac{1}{25} = 4\%$

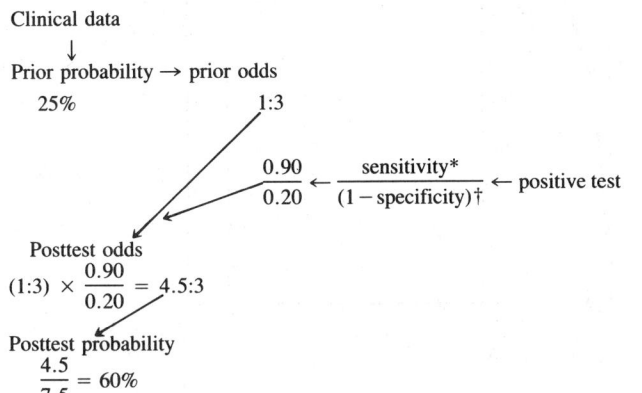

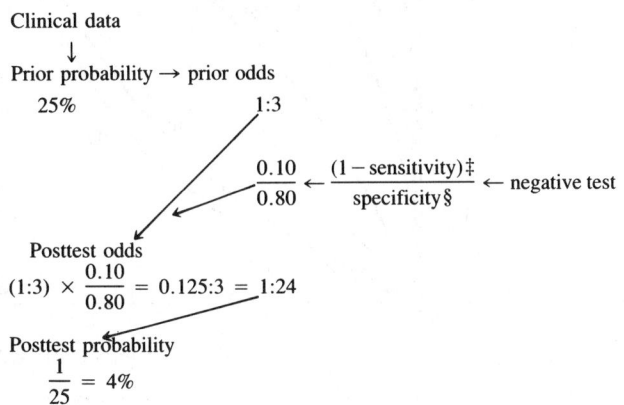

* *Sensitivity = probability of a positive test result in a patient with the disease*
† *(1 − Specificity) = probability of a positive test result in a patient without the disease*
‡ *(1 − Sensitivity) = probability of a negative test result in a patient with the disease*
§ *Specificity = probability of a negative test result in a patient without the disease*

diagnostic probability and integrate this with the result as well as the sensitivity and specificity of the diagnostic test. Many clinical situations may be so complex that it is not practical to estimate the prior probabilities of all likely diagnoses or to know the sensitivities and specificities of each of the tests that might be performed individually or in sequence. Nevertheless, attempts in this direction will stimulate critical thinking, expose uncertainties, and generate ideas for original investigations or a review of past experiences to facilitate the application of Bayesian analysis to the integration of clinical data and laboratory tests.

The results of Bayesian analyses often can be expressed in graphic form, such as the value of exercise electrocardiograms for predicting the presence of coronary artery disease (Fig. 2-2; also see Chap. 189). This series of curves also demonstrates how to consider a test whose result may be in the "gray zone" rather than clearly positive or clearly negative.

One of the key assumptions inherent in most such analyses is that the correlation between the pretest probability and the test result is no greater than expected by chance. If the diagnostic test simply duplicates information that has already been obtained by the clinical examination, it will not have any additional benefit for predicting whether or not the disease is present. For example, in trying to determine whether or not a patient with carcinoma of the colon has hepatic metastases, the finding of jaundice on physical examination should be a strong predictor. The degree of hyperbilirubinemia can also be measured, but the bilirubin level in a patient with clinical jaundice does not add substantial *independent* information to that obtained by a careful physical examination. When integrating a diagnostic test with clinical information, such a test is helpful only when it adds incremental information to what can be inferred based on the history and physical examination and on prior less costly or less risky diagnostic tests. If a diagnostic test (such as a retrograde cholangiogram in the patient with hyperbilirubinemia) provides information that cannot be inferred directly, it is less likely that its results are associated with pretest probabilities to an extent greater than would be expected by chance.

A diagnostic test has an impact on the evaluation of a specific patient only if it changes the diagnostic probability to the extent that the new probability dictates a change in the diagnostic strategy or therapeutic plans or if the test serves as part of a sequence of tests that moves the probability across such a threshold. An example is a patient suspected of having a pulmonary embolism, with an estimated probability of 50 percent based on clinical data alone. A "low probability" pulmonary ventilation-perfusion scan may reduce the probability of pulmonary embolism, but if the goal is to exclude pulmonary embolism with the highest possible degree of certainty, a pulmonary angiogram would be required (Chap. 211).

Because diagnostic tests oftentimes do not provide important new information even when their results are accurate, several questions should be considered in deciding when to order diagnostic tests. First, how likely is the disease in question? Second, what would be the clinical consequences if the diagnosis were missed or if the patient were mistakenly treated for a disease that is not present? Third, what is the likelihood that the diagnostic test will change the probability sufficiently to have an effect on either diagnosis or therapy? The physician should consider the probabilities, the risks, the likelihood and costs of obtaining new information, and the adverse consequences of delay, because observation and follow-up are always among the available diagnostic options.

COMPARING RISKS AND BENEFITS: DECISION ANALYSIS Inherent in the concept that probabilities can guide decision making is the assumption that one can arrive at a reasonable threshold by knowing the relative risks (or costs) and benefits of various options and deciding at what probability this ratio changes to favor an alternative strategy. Decision analysis is an organized process for evaluating such situations and identifies the key issues and problems.

One problem with applying decision-analysis techniques to difficult clinical problems is that the decision analysis is no better than the data on which it is based. In some instances, an attempted decision analysis of a complex clinical problem may yield no more information than that the critical data required for the analysis are missing and that more research in the field needs to be performed. In addition, when clinicians are uncertain about diagnostic or therapeutic strategies, formal analyses may indicate that the differences in outcome among various strategies are very small. In such cases, the formal analysis may have such inherent error that it is not dependable. Even when decision analysis is potentially helpful, it may not be feasible to complete the detailed estimations and calculations within the time constraints of bedside decision making. Nevertheless, the value of the analytic approach to decision making is that it integrates available data, mandates rigorous thinking, and exposes areas of uncertainty or ignorance.

Decision analysis depicts graphically two types of issues in the decision making process: first, the decisions (or choices) available to the physician and second, the probabilities of all of the events that may result from each decision. To illustrate how this process works, a decision analysis of whether to biopsy the brain, treat, or wait in suspected herpes encephalitis (Chap. 136) may be considered. Figure 2-3 depicts the decision tree for this problem. The square box or

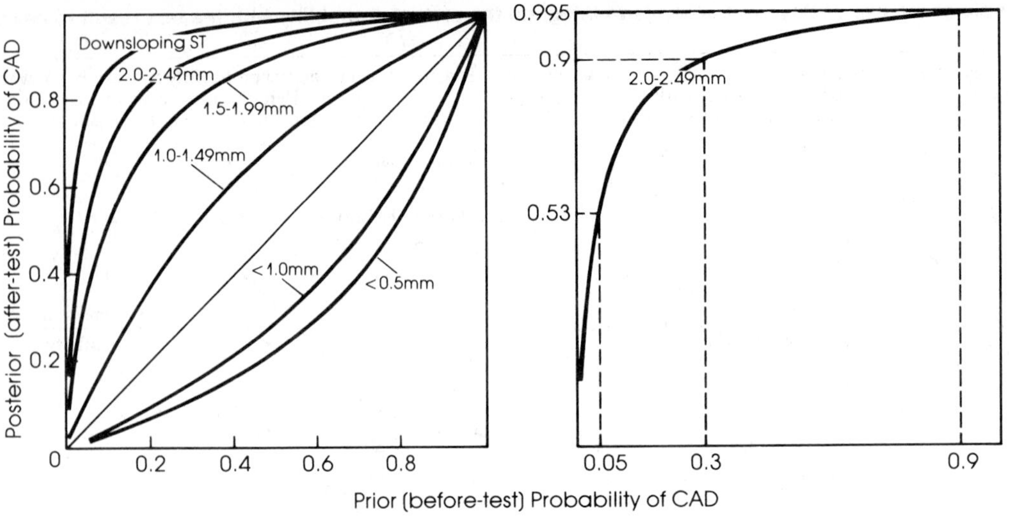

FIGURE 2-2 *How the exercise tolerance test affects the probability of coronary artery disease. The prior, or before-test, probability of coronary artery disease (CAD) will be modified by the result of the exercise electrocardiogram to yield a posterior, or after-test, probability of CAD. Note that the finding of <1 mm of ST depression will reduce the probability of CAD, whereas ≥1 mm of ST depression will increase the probability. For example, if a patient with a before-test probability of CAD of 90 percent, which is about the probability in a middle-aged man with very typical anginal symptoms, had 2 to 2.49 mm of ST depression of exercise testing, the after-test probability of CAD would be 99.5 percent. In contrast the same exercise test result in a patient with 30 percent before-test probability of CAD, which is about what one would expect in a patient with atypical anginal symptoms, would yield an after-test probability of about 90 percent. In an asymptomatic patient, with a before-test probability of about 5 percent, the same exercise test result would yield an after-test probability of 53 percent. Thus, the same test yields different after-test probabilities in patients with different before-test probabilities. (Adapted, with permission of the New England Journal of Medicine, from RD Rifkin, WB Hood: Bayesian analysis of electrocardiographic exercise stress testing. N Engl J Med 297:684, 1977.)*

''node'' labeled A indicates a decision that the physician must make. The circular nodes, labeled B through I, indicate where different outcomes, each of which has an estimatable probability, could occur. In this analysis, the initial choices were to treat with vidarabine (a relatively toxic drug), not to treat with vidarabine, or to perform a brain biopsy and use its results to guide the treatment decision. The use of vidarabine may or may not result in complications of therapy, and a biopsy itself may or may not be associated with a complication.

Each of the possible outcomes for a patient is typically assigned a ''utility,'' which is the relative preference for the outcome, where 1.0 is a perfect outcome and 0 is the worst possible outcome. Each terminal branch of the decision tree is assigned the utility corresponding to its outcome, and the ''expected value'' of each terminal branch is calculated by multiplying its probability by its utility. To calculate the ''expected value'' of each of the three possible courses of action (see Fig. 2-3, node A), the expected values of each of the terminal branches that originate from it would be summed. The preferred course of action is the one which, when all possible outcomes are considered, yields the highest expected value, which is the sum of the product of the probability multiplied by the utility for each of its possible outcomes.

In performing any decision analysis, the relevant probabilities

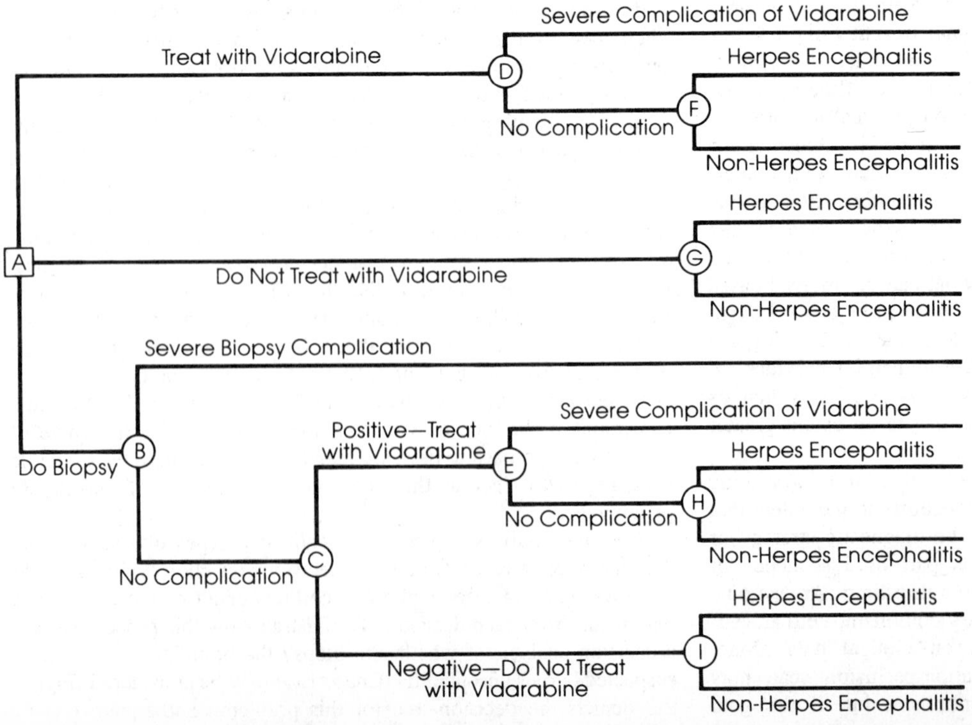

FIGURE 2-3 *Decision tree for diagnosis and treatment of suspected herpes simplex encephalitis. The square node represents the decision point, and the round nodes denote chance events. See text for details. (Reprinted with permission from M Barza, SG Pauker, The decision to biopsy, treat, or wait in suspected herpes encephalitis, Ann Intern Med 92:644, 1980.)*

must be known or estimated, a process that sometimes requires guesswork. Next, utilities could be assigned to each of these outcomes. A major practical limitation of decision analysis is the subjective judgment often required to estimate utilities. It is also difficult to adjust future years of life for their quality in any numerical fashion, for example, in considering how drug toxicity or the disability resulting from disease or treatment lowers the quality of future years of life.

The results and usefulness of a decision analysis depend on the probabilities and utilities that are used in the calculation, and it is imperative for decision analyses to include a *sensitivity analysis*, in which various estimates for each probability are included in the analysis to determine if the conclusions would be changed. For example, in the analysis in Fig. 2-3, some range of probabilities must be assumed for vidarabine toxicity, for serious complications of brain biopsy, and for the likelihood of false-positive or false-negative biopsy results. The authors of this particular analysis concluded that waiting, i.e., neither treating nor performing a biopsy, was the preferable course of action when the likelihood of herpes encephalitis is less than 3 percent. At probabilities between 3 and 42 percent, the analysis favored brain biopsy, but at probabilities above 42 percent, it favored immediate treatment with vidarabine. However, it is uncommon for any patient to have substantially greater than a 42 percent probability of herpes encephalitis, and hence it would be unusual for empiric vidarabine treatment ever to be preferred over brain biopsy. The authors demonstrated that these conclusions did not change when they varied the assumptions about the probabilities of several relevant events. If the conclusions of an analysis were altered by relatively minor changes in the assumptions on which it was based, the analysis would not be sufficiently reliable to become the basis for decision making.

Decision analysis sometimes demonstrates a clear and dramatic advantage with one particular option. In other circumstances, there may be little difference between two options; either option may be reasonable, or secondary issues that cannot be taken into account in the formal analysis, such as the patient's feelings about taking risks or the recent local experience with particular interventions, should be the final determinants in the decision. Physicians who perform a decision analysis therefore must determine the probabilities of each of the possible events by reviewing the pertinent patient experience at their own institution or practice, or by reviewing the pertinent literature. Even when the outcome of the analysis seems clear, the physician or the patient may believe that the situation in question is an exception to the rule. Furthermore, even the best analyses, like all clinical intuition, are based on assumptions that may be open to debate.

In the preceding example, the management of an individual patient with possible herpes encephalitis, decision analysis indicated the preferred strategy in terms of outcome but did not consider the costs at which such benefits might be achieved. In determining health policy, a formal cost-effectiveness analysis can be performed to determine how many dollars must be spent to achieve a unit of benefit, often defined as a life saved, a year of life saved, or a quality-adjusted year of life saved, in which the years are adjusted to take into account the quality of life during that time. For example, 1 year of in-center hemodialysis can be estimated to cost about $35,000 in 1986 dollars; this figure includes only the direct medical costs and not indirect costs related to issues such as time lost or travel, or any benefits in terms of a patient's ability to work. In some situations, the ability of the patient to maintain gainful employment may offset some or all of the direct medical expenses.

Although many analyses are now expressed in terms of cost-effectiveness, where dollars spent are compared to lives or years of life gained, some studies have utilized cost-benefit analyses in which a dollar value is placed on the life that is saved. For example, an analysis of the rubella vaccination, which attempted to place a dollar value on the vaccine's ability to prevent the congenital rubella syndrome and the resulting expenses, concluded that the optimal national policy would be to vaccinate all females at age 12.

ETHICS AND PATIENT INPUT In both quantitative and nonquantitative clinical reasoning, the physician must consider ethical issues as well as the patient's values and preferences. While a detailed discussion of these issues is beyond the scope of this chapter, it is important to emphasize that patients' preferences for alternate therapies may not agree with the preferences that the physicians propose on the basis of their own clinical judgment or the results of a decision-analysis approach. For example, many patients with carcinoma of the larynx may prefer radiation therapy, with a lower cure rate but a higher likelihood of maintaining speech, to extirpative surgery. It is imperative that physicians assess those characteristics of life that the patient prizes most (the elusive "quality of life") prior to basing controversial decisions solely on quantitative approaches, the physicians' own subjective impressions of the likely medical benefits, their own personal preferences, or their assumptions about the patient's preferences. Therefore, the final plan should reflect an agreement between a well-informed patient and a sympathetic physician who has detailed knowledge of the relevant medical issues and of the impact of the various possible outcomes on the specific patient.

REFERENCES

ELSTEIN AS et al: *Medical Problem Solving. An Analysis of Clinical Reasoning.* Cambridge, Harvard University, 1978

GOLDMAN L et al: Comparative reproducibility and validity of systems for assessing cardiovascular functional class: Advantages of a new specific activity scale. Circulation 64:1227, 1981

GREENFIELD S et al: Efficiency and cost of primary care by nurses and physician assistants. N Engl J Med 298:305, 1978

MCNEIL BJ et al: Speech and survival: Trade offs between quality and quantity of life in laryngeal cancer. N Engl J Med 305:982, 1981

RANSOHOFF DF, FEINSTEIN AR: Problems of spectrum and bias in evaluating the efficacy of diagnostic tests. N Engl J Med 299:926, 1978

ROBERTS SD et al: Cost-effective care of end-stage renal disease: A billion dollar question. Ann Intern Med 92:243, 1980

SCHOENBAUM SC et al: Benefit-cost analysis of rubella vaccination policy. N Engl J Med 294:303, 1976

WEINSTEIN MC, FINEBERG HV: *Clinical Decision Analysis.* Philadelphia, Saunders, 1980

PART ONE CARDINAL MANIFESTATIONS OF DISEASE

section 1 Pain

3 PAIN: PATHOPHYSIOLOGY AND MANAGEMENT

RAYMOND MACIEWICZ / JOSEPH B. MARTIN

Pain is the most common symptom of disease. Although the nature, location, and etiology of pain differ in each case, approximately half of all patients who visit a physician have a primary complaint of pain. For most patients, correct treatment of a self-evident, limited disease process (such as a broken bone) alleviates the pain. In many, however, the symptom of pain itself must be carefully assessed and evaluated to interpret its significance and to establish an approach for its treatment. In some patients uncontrolled pain continues as a major problem. The cost of medical treatment of patients with chronic pain is in excess of $50 billion annually, and low back pain alone accounts for the loss of 100 million work days each year. Chronic pain is therefore not only a difficult medical management problem but also an issue of major social concern.

The evaluation of the patient with pain is frequently complex, partially because pain is a perception rather than a sensation. A person's physical state, past experience, and anticipation all influence the way a given sensory input is interpreted. For example, soldiers and athletes may deny pain despite an acute injury, while certain patients with chronic pain may continue to suffer despite the lack of an obvious nociceptive stimulus. Our knowledge of pain and most of our treatments for it focus on decreasing the nociceptive sensory input; however, a patient's interpretation of a sensation, the affective reaction, and the behavioral response are equally important factors that deserve the physician's careful attention.

ORGANIZATION OF PAIN PATHWAYS Nociceptive afferents Sensory stimuli of potentially tissue-damaging intensity activate free nerve endings in skin, underlying tissue, and viscera. Nociceptive signals are conveyed to the spinal cord by unmyelinated and small myelinated sensory axons. In humans, stimulation of individual small sensory axons can evoke the report of pain in the area of skin supplied by that fiber, clearly demonstrating that under certain conditions even single axons can transmit activity that is interpreted as "pain" by the brain.

Many unmyelinated nociceptive afferents exhibit "polymodal" responses. Such fibers can be activated by intense mechanical stimulation, potentially tissue-damaging thermal stimulation, and chemical stimulation by substances injected into skin. Any intense stimulus applied to normal skin can produce a "triple response" that consists of a red flush at the site of stimulation, a surrounding red flare due to arterial dilatation, and local edema caused by increased vascular permeability. Many substances likely play an important role in this response. Some of these agents are released by damaged tissue (potassium, histamine, serotonin, prostaglandins), while others enter from the circulation (bradykinin) or come from local nerve endings themselves (substance P). Certain of these substances also activate free nerve endings, and their long-lasting effects may partially explain the hypersensitivity of the skin that often follows a noxious stimulus.

Dorsal horn Sensory fibers extend distally and proximally from cells located in the segmental dorsal root ganglia. Nociceptive afferents enter the spinal cord through the dorsal root to terminate on dorsal horn neurons (Fig. 3-1*A*). Many of the fine afferents ending in these regions contain neuropeptides, including substance P, cholecystokinin, and somatostatin. There is increasing evidence that these peptides play an important role in normal sensory transmission. Chemical destruction of substance P fibers in animals produces analgesia in certain tests for pain and there is also a marked decrease in substance P terminal staining in the dorsal horn in patients with congenital neuropathies that are associated with decreased sensitivity to pain.

The spinal dorsal horn can be divided into a series of layers based on cell morphology and arrangement. Neurons that process nociceptive information are found in several of these layers. The output neurons that project to brainstem and thalamus are found principally in layers I and V, zones where many small-caliber afferents terminate. The axons of these dorsal horn neurons form a crossed pathway that ascends in the ventrolateral quadrant of the spinal cord, the spinothalamic tract.

Spinothalamic system The axons of nociceptive dorsal horn neurons that form the spinothalamic tracts terminate in several brainstem and thalamic nuclei. The spinothalamic tract can be divided conceptually into two systems based on these connections: a direct spinothalamic system that carries sensory discriminative information about pain to thalamic levels, and a phylogenetically older spinoreticulothalamic system that terminates more diffusely in brainstem reticular nuclei.

The direct spinothalamic system that ends in the thalamus may be important for the conscious perception of nociceptive sensations. This system terminates in an orderly fashion within the *nucleus ventralis posterolateralis* (VPL). The terminal field of the spinothalamic tract in VPL overlaps the dorsal column–medial lemniscal input that relays light touch and joint sensation. The organized pattern of terminations and the convergence of light touch and pain information within VPL may be important for perception of the sensory discriminative aspects of pain, including the location, nature, and intensity of a noxious input. Consistent with this view, cells in VPL project principally to primary somatosensory cortex.

The more diffuse spinoreticulothalamic system may mediate aspects of the autonomic and affective reactions to pain. Ascending spinoreticular fibers terminate at several levels of the brainstem reticular formation, forming part of a polysynaptic system that terminates in the medial thalamic nuclei (*nucleus centralis lateralis* and *nucleus parafascicularis*). Cells throughout the spinoreticulothalamic system have large, bilateral sensory receptive fields that can include the entire body surface. These cells often respond best to noxious sensory input. Such cells are unlikely to be important for sensory discrimination or localization; they probably are important for arousal or orientation to a painful stimulus.

Under normal conditions, there appears to be a balance between the precise, specific information channeled through VPL and the more generalized alerting effects mediated through the medial thalamus. Clinical disorders that partially destroy the lateral thalamus including VPL can result in a syndrome of continuous, burning pain involving the contralateral side of the body (the thalamic syndrome of Déjerine and Roussy); the pain frequently has an exaggerated emotional or autonomic component. This condition may be due to an unrestricted flow of sensory information through the medial thalamus which is interpreted as pain by the brain. The fact that in some patients surgical lesions of the medial thalamus may relieve this type of continuous central pain is consistent with this idea.

Descending analgesic pathways In addition to the major ascending pain pathways outlined above, the brain contains powerful descending circuits that suppress nociceptive inputs (Fig. 3-1*B*). In animals, electrical stimulation of the midbrain periaqueductal gray region can produce generalized analgesia without other obvious sensory or motor responses. A similar system may exist in humans, as stimulation of the nearby periventricular gray is reported to relieve clinical pain. This effect appears to be at least partly mediated at the spinal level, since it can be blocked in animals by cutting pathways that carry descending projections from the brainstem to the dorsal horn. However, few periaqueductal gray cells project directly to the spinal cord. Instead, the descending pathway important for analgesia appears to first synapse in the midline raphe nuclei of the medulla (principally *nucleus raphe magnus*). Raphe neurons in turn project to the spinal cord where they inhibit the nociceptive response of dorsal horn neurons. This descending system can potentially gate the flow of nociceptive information from the level of the first synapse in the dorsal horn.

The periaqueductal gray region, the medullary raphe, and the dorsal horn all contain a high density of endogenous opiate peptides and opiate receptors. Systemic narcotic analgesics may in part work by activating the descending analgesia system at these sites. High densities of opiate receptors are also found in the medial thalamus and limbic forebrain; these structures may play an additional, important role in the analgesic response to, and the addictive potential of, systemically administered narcotics.

Biogenic amines represent another class of neurotransmitters found in the descending pathways that modulate nociception. Serotonin is contained in many of the raphe neurons that end in the dorsal horn, and some serotonergic axon terminals end directly on spinothalamic tract neurons. A major descending inhibitory pathway containing norepinephrine also arises in the *nucleus locus coeruleus* of the pons; this system appears to inhibit the nociceptive responses of dorsal horn neurons by an alpha-adrenergic mechanism. Drugs that potentiate the central effects of biogenic amines, such as the tricyclic antidepressants, may therefore be effective analgesic adjuvants that work by enhancing the effects of these descending pathways.

EVALUATION OF THE PATIENT WITH PAIN **Somatic pain** Pain usually occurs when a potentially tissue-damaging stimulus excites peripheral nociceptive afferents. When a noxious stimulus activates receptors in skin, muscle, or joint, the somatic pain that results is usually well-localized and easily described by the patient (see Table 3-1). In contrast, pain of visceral origin is often poorly localized and may be referred to an area of skin supplied by the same sensory roots that innervate the diseased visceral organ. For example, myocardial pain activates visceral afferents terminating in the upper four thoracic segments of the spinal cord. This nociceptive information converges on the same neurons that receive cutaneous input from the T1 to T4 dermatomes, and the reported pain is frequently referred to this region of otherwise normal skin or underlying tissue. Visceral pain originating in the gallbladder or kidney will similarly refer pain to the corresponding dermatome.

Both cutaneous and visceral pain are common experiences and do not always signal a disease process. The somatic pain resulting from a new injury or illness is therefore generally familiar to the patient and described in the context of prior similar pains. Somatic pain due to activation of normal nociceptive mechanisms is usually effectively relieved by a brief course of an appropriate analgesic.

Neuropathic pain Pain can also result from injury to, or chronic changes in, peripheral or central somatosensory pathways. This may be due to the induced abnormal pattern of afferent neuronal activity that reaches the dorsal horn and more central structures. Damage to sensory pathways may also decrease the inhibitory controls that are normally activated by a peripheral input. Neuropathic pain that follows damage to sensory pathways can develop and persist without a demonstrable primary nociceptive stimulus. In contrast to most somatic pain, neuropathic pain is frequently poorly localized. The patient often uses unusual terms to describe the pain, emphasizing the distinction between perception of normal somatic pains and neuropathic sensations (Table 3-1).

The sensory symptoms in neuropathic pain can be either focal or

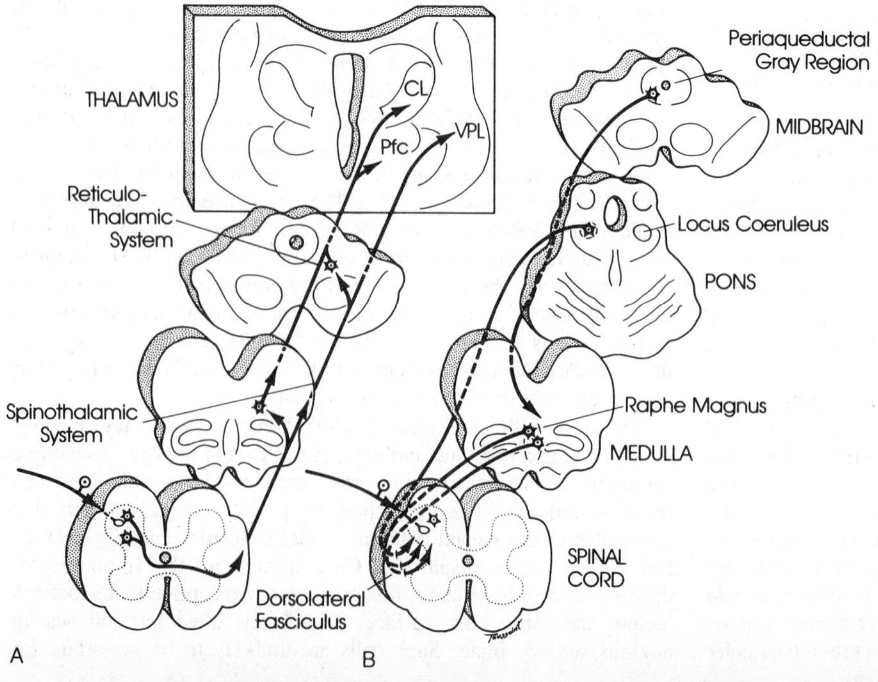

FIGURE 3-1 *A. Ascending nociceptive pathways. The direct spinothalamic tract terminates in the* nucleus ventroposterolateralis *(VPL). The indirect, spinoreticulothalamic pathway relays through the brainstem reticular formation and ends in nuclei of the medial and intralaminar thalamus [*nuclei parafascicularis *(Pfc) and* centralis lateralis *(CL)]. B. Descending analgesia pathways. Periaqueductal gray neurons project to* nucleus raphe magnus. *A descending projection from* raphe magnus *inhibits the nociceptive responses of dorsal horn neurons. A separate inhibitory pathway from the* nucleus locus coeruleus *also directly ends in dorsal horn.*

more generalized. Trauma or irritation to a peripheral nerve may result in a *neuralgia,* which is defined as pain in the distribution of a single nerve; the pain is often (but not always) accompanied by signs of nerve dysfunction, such as sensory loss or weakness of muscles innervated by the nerve. Frequently the pain consists of a background spontaneous burning or aching sensation (*dysesthesia*) that can be associated with paroxysmal jabs of sharp pain within the affected region. Despite an elevated sensory detection threshold, patients will often have an exaggerated response to a nociceptive stimulus (*hyperalgesia*) or to touch (*hyperesthesia*) or perceive a non-nociceptive stimulus as painful (*allodynia*). These terms for altered hypersensitivity to sensory stimuli are commonly grouped under the term *hyperpathia.*

In some forms of neuralgia (such as trigeminal neuralgia) paroxysmal, lancinating pain predominates without other signs of nerve dysfunction. In contrast, *causalgia* following nerve injury is characterized by a continuous, severe burning pain, allodynia, and evident sympathetic dysfunction. Pain can also be a feature of more generalized neuropathies associated with the degeneration of small caliber axons. In such cases there can be multiple locations for the pain as well as a variety of types of pain. In diffuse sensory or sensorimotor neuropathies, the pain is usually symmetric and distal, affecting the feet and, with progression, the hands. As with more focal neuralgias, the pain often consists of a spontaneous aching or burning sensation with superimposed paroxysmal jabs of pain. Allodynia and hyperalgesia are common features during acute, painful phases of the disease.

Pain may also be a debilitating symptom following damage to central somatosensory pathways. Lesions of the ascending somatosensory pathways at the level of the cord, brainstem, thalamus, or cortex can result in a syndrome of continuous spontaneous pain that is referred to the periphery, often with superimposed sensory abnormalities as discussed above.

TABLE 3-1 Characteristics of somatic and neuropathic pain

SOMATIC PAIN	
1	Nociceptive stimulus usually evident.
2	Pain is usually well localized; visceral pain may be referred.
3	Pain is similar to other somatic pains in the patient's experience.
4	Pain is relieved by anti-inflammatory or narcotic analgesics.
NEUROPATHIC PAIN	
1	No obvious nociceptive stimulus.
2	Pain is often poorly localized.
3	Pain is unusual, dissimilar from somatic pain.
4	Pain is only partially relieved by narcotic analgesics.

Psychological aspects of pain In certain pain patients, particularly those with chronic pain, there is often little correlation between the severity of active disease and the amount of pain behavior. Social and psychological factors may be important dimensions that exacerbate and perpetuate pain complaints in such patients. An appraisal by a psychiatrist or a psychologist should therefore be part of the complete evaluation of most patients with persistent pain complaints. Psychological tests, including the Minnesota Multiphasic Personality Profile, can form an important part of this evaluation.

Several categories of psychological diagnoses can be associated with chronic pain syndromes. The two most common presentations are patients with depression and patients with somatoform disorders.

DEPRESSION Depressive symptoms are common in patients with chronic pain, and depressive illness is found in approximately 30 percent. Many pain patients deny depression and do not show a depressed affect. In such patients vegetative signs of insomnia, diminished libido, and lack of energy may be present.

The relationship between pain and depression is complex. The pain threshold is lowered in clinically depressed patients, and pain is a common complaint among patients with primary depression. Patients with pain associated with chronic somatic disease also frequently develop depressive symptoms. However, the incidence of depression defined by strict clinical criteria is not clearly different in chronic pain patients when compared to medically ill patients without pain.

In an effort to delineate more clearly the relationship between pain and depression, a subgroup of chronic pain patients with a "pain-prone" disorder has been described. Such patients tend to have a hypochondriacal preoccupation with their pain. The pain is often continuous in nature and obscure in origin. Associated with the pain complaint, the patient may have depressive symptoms of insomnia, fatigue, and despair. Pain-prone individuals have developmental histories characterized by stress and unmet dependency needs. There may be a family history of depression, alcoholism, or physical abuse. Before the onset of their pain, however, such individuals have an idealized view of themselves and their family relations, denying conflicts. They may also have compulsive work records and hold several jobs. Chronic pain in this group of individuals may be associated in part with unresolved personal or interpersonal conflicts.

Consistent with the association of pain and depression, antidepressant drugs can stabilize the sleep pattern and improve the dysphoric symptoms of patients with chronic pain. There is often a reduction in the intensity of reported pain that may be associated with a decrease in the requirement for analgesics. Antidepressants may therefore have an important role in the management of chronic pain, although it is still uncertain whether these drugs act primarily to potentiate analgesics or to relieve subclinical depression.

SOMATOFORM DISORDERS Patients with somatoform disorders have symptoms that suggest an organic disease but have no evidence of a physical disorder that might explain these symptoms. The heading "somatoform disorders" includes patients with somatization disorder, conversion disorder, hypochondriasis, or psychogenic pain disorder. Although symptoms of chronic pain are often part of the presentation of a somatoform disorder, patients with this diagnosis are not clinically depressed and do not usually respond to antidepressants. However, such patients seek out doctors and undergo repetitive tests to evaluate vague complaints. A variety of analgesics, anxiolytics, and muscle relaxants are usually prescribed with little or no benefit. Surgical procedures are often performed for pain relief without success.

Patients with somatoform disorders need frequent reassurance that their pain is benign; the management of these conditions is therefore primarily supportive. These patients should have careful follow-up from a small number of care givers to minimize unnecessary tests and reduce the amount of medication prescribed. In this group of patients diagnosing new pains that signal true organic pathology can be a clinical challenge.

MANAGEMENT OF PATIENTS WITH PAIN Acute somatic pain is usually effectively treated with nonnarcotic analgesic agents which decrease pain without causing an alteration in the level of consciousness (Table 3-2). Aspirin, 300 to 600 mg, or acetaminophen, 600 mg, orally every 4 h is often effective. Other nonsteroidal anti-inflammatory agents, including phenacetin, naproxen, sulindac, or ibuprofen, may be used; however, there is little evidence that these agents are clearly better than the less expensive analgesics aspirin and acetaminophen. All nonsteroidal anti-inflammatory drugs have side effects of gastrointestinal irritation and may cause allergic reactions. The side effects of aspirin, particularly dyspepsia, gastrointestinal bleeding, and inhibition of platelet aggregation, are not observed with acetaminophen; however, acetaminophen does not have anti-inflammatory properties. Aspirin and acetaminophen in combination are not more effective than either one alone, but either in combination with codeine is more effective than codeine alone.

Narcotic analgesics are usually required for relief of severe pain. In general, patients should be treated with only one narcotic agent at a time, and therapy should be begun with an intermediate strength narcotic such as codeine, 30 mg every 4 to 6 h. In oral doses, codeine is relatively safe, potent, and well tolerated. However, if codeine,

TABLE 3-2 Drugs used to relieve pain

NONNARCOTIC ANALGESICS: EQUIVALENT DOSES AND INTERVALS

Generic Name	Dose, mg	Interval
Aspirin	750–1250	q 3 h
Phenacetin	750–1000	q 3 h
Acetaminophen	600–800	q 3 h
Phenylbutazone	200–400	q 4 h
Indomethacin	50–75	q 4 h
Ibuprofen	200–400	q 4 h
Naproxen	250–500	q 4 h
Nefopam	60–120	q 4 h

NARCOTIC ANALGESICS COMPARED TO 10 MG MORPHINE SULFATE (MS)

Generic Name	IM Dose, mg	PO dose, mg	Differences from MS
Oxymorphine	1	6	None
Hydromorphine	1.5	7.5	Shorter acting
Levorphanol	2	4	Good PO-IM potency
Heroin	4		Short-acting
Methadone	10	20	Good PO-IM potency
Morphine	10	60	
Oxycodone	15	30	Short-acting
Meperidine	75	300	None
Pentazocine	60	180	Agonist-antagonist
Codeine	130	200	More toxic

ANTICONVULSANTS

Generic Name	PO Dose, mg	Interval
Phenytoin	100	q 6–8 h
Carbamazepine	200	q 6 h
Clonazepam	1	q 6 h

ANTIDEPRESSANTS

Generic name	PO Dose, mg	Range, mg/day
Doxepin	200	75–400
Amitriptyline	150	75–300
Imipramine	200	75–400
Nortriptyline	100	40–150
Desipramine	150	75–300
Amoxapine	200	75–300
Trazodone	150	50–600

60 mg orally every 4 h, fails to provide relief, then it should be discontinued in favor of a higher potency narcotic, such as morphine or meperidine in the appropriate dosage and frequency. Increasing doses of codeine well above the recommended range will increase the frequency of side effects without clearly adding to its analgesic effectiveness.

Patients with pain due to evident organic disease are frequently treated with parenteral narcotic analgesics such as morphine or meperidine on an "every 6 h when necessary" basis. Effective analgesia from such drugs usually lasts only 2 to 3 h, allowing the patient to reexperience pain before the next dose. Analgesics given on a when necessary basis are also rarely administered as frequently as ordered, resulting in periods of inadequate analgesia; this produces a situation that reinforces "pain behavior," potentially delaying recovery. Inadequate analgesia in postoperative patients reduces the tidal volume due to splinting and delays patient mobilization. When indicated, narcotic analgesics should be given frequently enough and in high enough doses to alleviate pain. Pain medication should be offered the patient on a routine rather than a when necessary basis, with the understanding that the patient can refuse the drug if the level of analgesia is sufficient. Changes in analgesic doses and the need to taper narcotics as the acute phase of pain passes should be understood by the patient.

Chronic diseases usually cause recurrent bouts of acute pain rather than continuous discomfort. The management of acute painful exacerbations should be the same as the treatment of any new, acute pain. Analgesics should be available to the patient when pain is present, with the understanding between patient and physician that the drugs will be discontinued as the acute episode subsides.

Patients with terminal diseases such as metastatic cancer often suffer from continuous or recurrent acute pain. In such patients, tolerance to medications becomes an important factor. Increasing doses of narcotic analgesics may be necessary in such patients to maintain satisfactory analgesia, although the underlying disease process remains essentially unchanged. As the narcotic dose is increased, the frequency of side effects including sedation, dysphoric reactions, and constipation may also increase. In selected patients with terminal disease, morphine injections through spinal epidural or intrathecal catheters can provide substantial analgesia with potentially few side effects. For most patients, however, a change in drug, dose, or the addition of an adjuvant analgesic can often improve pain relief while minimizing adverse reactions.

Management of neuropathic pain Neuropathic pain is often a chronic disabling condition that can involve pathophysiologic changes at many levels of the nervous system. The medical management of neuropathic pain is disappointing, however, and patients rarely achieve substantial, lasting improvement with any single therapy. For patients with neuropathic pain, conventional analgesics are only rarely effective. The search for improved forms of treatment in such patients has resulted in a number of approaches.

ANTICONVULSANTS In patients with neuropathic pain with little or no evidence of sympathetic dysfunction, anticonvulsants and antidepressant drugs are frequently prescribed, although there is only limited evidence that such medications are effective.

Phenytoin, carbamazepine, or clonazepam may be helpful in certain patients with painful neuropathies or neuralgias. Anticonvulsants are particularly effective in treating the sharp, lancinating pains associated with focal neuralgias such as trigeminal neuralgia. They are less effective for the more constant dull, burning sensations that are a major component of conditions such as postherpetic neuralgia or diabetic neuropathy.

ANTISYMPATHETIC AGENTS In some patients, traumatic neuralgias can present with spontaneous burning pain and evidence of sympathetic dysfunction in the affected limb. This condition is termed *causalgia* and may be a distinct form of sympathetic dystrophy. Associated with the sensory changes in causalgia are disturbances in the sympathetic innervation of the affected limb. Sympathectomy by either surgery or local anesthetic block frequently relieves the pain in causalgia, and in the opinion of a number of authors pain relief by sympathetic block is an essential part of the diagnosis.

When pain relief follows a sympathetic block, treatment with intravenous regional or systemic antisympathetic drugs such as guanethidine may provide sustained relief in some patients.

TRICYCLIC ANTIDEPRESSANTS Antidepressant drugs are frequently used to treat pain following peripheral nerve injury. Tricyclic iminodibenzyl derivatives are the most commonly used drugs. Their pharmacologic effects include facilitation of monoamine transmission by inhibition of transmitter reuptake at the synapse and changes in pre- and postsynaptic adrenergic receptor sensitivity. The important site of action of tricyclic antidepressants for pain relief is not clear. However, they may act to potentiate the brainstem inhibition of nociceptive transmission at the level of the dorsal horn. Tricyclic antidepressants also have major effects on ascending monoaminergic systems that project into the forebrain. It seems probable that these ascending systems are also important in pain perception, although how antidepressant drugs influence sensory pathways at the level of the thalamus and cortex remains speculative.

TRANSCUTANEOUS ELECTRICAL NERVE STIMULATION (TENS) Electrical stimulation with a TENS unit applied to the painful region or over the proximal nerve may provide substantial pain relief in patients with painful nerve injuries. However, the duration of the effect is usually limited to the period of stimulation. After a period of days to months, in many patients the analgesic response to TENS habituates, and electrical stimulation may actually worsen the patient's pain.

Management of chronic pain Unrelieved pain that has continued to be a major, disabling condition for a minimum of 6 months is usually referred to as "chronic" pain. Patients with chronic pain often present special problems in evaluation and management.

When patients with long-standing chronic pain are seen for a new evaluation, they often have unrealistic expectations of the physician. Frequently they state that none of their prior physicians was competent and that this is their last hope for relief from their suffering. A detailed medical history will often reveal poor compliance with previous treatment recommendations made by other physicians.

To avoid another treatment failure, the chronic pain patient should be evaluated by a multidisciplinary group of specialists skilled in managing chronic pain complaints. The specialists composing this group may vary, depending on the nature of the pain complaint and the resources available at an institution. At a minimum, however, a patient should receive a medical, psychological, neurologic, and physical therapy evaluation. A group approach avoids potential confrontation between patient and physician that may stall progress; it also enhances the credibility of the treatment group, increasing the likelihood of patient compliance. The goal of this evaluation is to establish a treatment plan with specific objectives. Each objective should be accomplished according to a timetable mutually agreed on by the patient and the treatment team.

In general, three main goals should be emphasized. First, drug treatment should be simplified and minimized. In many chronic pain patients, common analgesics and muscle relaxants are only minimally effective. The patient therefore tends to increase the dosage in the hope of enhancing pain relief. With the patient's understanding, the number of medications should be reduced by eliminating redundant or ineffective drugs. The dosages of the remaining medications should then be decreased systematically to a point where the patient is taking only drugs that have a definite beneficial effect with minimal side effects.

The second goal of therapy is to assist the patient in developing a better understanding of the pain and the factors that exacerbate it. The psychological significance of the pain and its relationship to developmental or interpersonal factors may be worth exploring with individual patients. Antidepressant medications also have a role in the management of affective symptoms in certain chronic pain patients.

The third goal of therapy should be to increase mobilization and functional ability. Under the direction of a specialist in rehabilitation medicine, a program of physical treatments for pain relief (TENS, massage, etc.) should be coupled with an exercise program to increase pain-free movement. Realistic timetables should be set for a return to self-care and independent function.

Social and interpersonal factors may perseverate pain; certain chronic pain patients are therefore refractory to treatment on an out-patient basis. Admission to an in-patient multidisciplinary pain treatment facility can provide an opportunity for an intensive program of evaluation and treatment of such patients. Standards for such in-patient units have been established by the Committee on Standards of Pain Treatment Facilities of the American Pain Society. Studies of the effectiveness of pain treatment units demonstrate a decreased report of pain, decreased drug use, and increased functional ability in the majority of patients completing this type of program. However, the ultimate success of such programs depends on maintained functional improvement in patients over long periods following discharge. Careful follow-up and reevaluation of successfully managed chronic pain patients, as with all medical patients, becomes a priority.

REFERENCES

Aronoff GM: Psychological aspects of nonmalignant chronic pain, in *Evaluation and Treatment of Chronic Pain,* GM Aronoff (ed). Baltimore, Urban and Schwarzenberg, 1985

Asbury A, Fields HL: Pain due to peripheral nerve damage: An hypothesis. Neurology 34:1587–1590, 1984

Basbaum AI, Fields HL: Endogenous pain control systems: Brainstem spinal pathways and endorphin circuitry. Ann Rev Neurosci 7:309–338, 1984

Blumer D, Heilbronn: Chronic pain as a variant of depressive disease. J Nerv Ment Dis 170:381–406, 1982

Fields HL: Pain II: New approaches to management. Ann Neurol 9:101, 1981

Hackett TP: The pain patient: Evaluation and treatment, in *Massachusetts General Hospital Handbook of General Hospital Psychiatry,* TP Hackett (ed). pp 41–63, 1978

Hannington-Kiff JG: Antisympathetic drugs in limbs. In *Textbook of Pain,* PD Wall, R Melzack (ed). Edinburgh, Churchill Livingstone, 1983

Maciewicz R, Fields HL: Pain pathways, in *Diseases of the Nervous System,* A Asbury, G McKann (ed). London, Saunders, 1986

Sweet WH, Poletti CE: Causalgia, in *Evaluation and Treatment of Chronic Pain,* GM Aronoff (ed). Baltimore, Urban and Schwarzenberg, 1985

Tasker RR: Deafferentation, in *Textbook of Pain,* P Wall (ed). Edinburgh, Churchill Livingstone, 1984, pp 119–132

Taub A, Collins WF: Observations on the treatment of denervation dysesthesia with psychotropic drugs: Postherpetic neuralgia, anesthesia dolorosa, peripheral neuropathy, in *Advances in Neurology,* JJ Bonica (ed). New York, Raven, 1974, pp 309–315

White JC, Sweet WH: *Pain and the Neurosurgeon—A Forty Year's Experience.* Springfield, Illinois, Charles C Thomas, 1969

Yaksh TL, Hammond DL: Peripheral and central substrates involved in the rostrad transmission of nociceptive information. Pain 13:1–85, 1982

4 CHEST DISCOMFORT AND PALPITATION

EUGENE BRAUNWALD

CHEST DISCOMFORT

Chest discomfort is one of the most frequent complaints for which patients seek medical attention; the potential benefit (or harm) resulting from the proper (or improper) assessment and management of the patient with this complaint is enormous. An incorrect diagnosis of a potentially hazardous condition such as angina pectoris is likely to have harmful psychologic and economic consequences and may lead to unnecessary complex procedures, such as cardiac catheterization and coronary arteriography, while failure to recognize a serious disorder, such as ischemic heart disease or mediastinal tumor, may result in the dangerous delay of much-needed treatment. There is little relation between the severity of chest discomfort and the gravity of its cause. Therefore, a frequent problem in patients who complain of chest discomfort or pain is distinguishing trivial disorders from coronary artery disease and other serious disorders.

The radiation of pain arising in the thoracic viscera can usually be explained in terms of the known facts concerning nerve supply (Chap. 3). One occasionally sees a patient with extension of discomfort to a location which cannot be logically explained. In most instances, such a person will be found to have more than one disorder capable of causing chest discomfort. The presence of one condition may affect the radiation of the pain produced by the other disorder. For example, when the discomfort of transient myocardial ischemia, i.e., angina pectoris, extends to the back or abdomen, the patient may be found to have also a significant degree of spinal arthritis or an upper abdominal disorder, such as hiatus hernia, disease of the gallbladder, pancreatitis, or peptic ulcer. Pain impulses which enter one cord segment may spill over and excite nearby cord segments. In this manner, the pain of myocardial ischemia may be referred to the epigastrium in a patient with chronic cholecystitis.

It should not be assumed that the presence of an objective abnormality, such as a hiatus hernia or an electrocardiographic abnormality, necessarily means that an *atypical* chest pain arises in the stomach or the heart. Such an assumption is justified only if a careful clinical examination, if necessary supported by appropriate laboratory tests, indicates that the behavior of the discomfort is compatible with the site of origin suggested by the objective finding.

THE LEFT-ARM MYTH There is a long tradition, widely accepted by physicians and nonphysicians alike, that discomfort in the left arm, especially when appearing in conjunction with chest discomfort, has a unique and ominous significance as being almost certain evidence of the presence of ischemic heart disease. This is a myth that has neither theoretic nor clinical foundation. Impulses from somatic structures, such as the skin, and visceral structures, such as the esophagus and heart, converge on a common pool of neurons in the posterior horn of the spinal cord. Their origin may be confused by the cerebral cortex. Also, stimulation of one of the thoracic nerves that also innervates the heart by, for example, protrusion of an intervertebral disk, may be misinterpreted as pain originating from the heart.

From a theoretic standpoint, *any* disorder involving the deep afferent fibers of the left upper thoracic region should be capable of causing discomfort in the chest, the left arm, or both areas. Hence almost any condition capable of causing chest discomfort may induce radiation to the left arm. Such localization is common not only in patients with coronary disease but also in those with numerous other types of chest pain. Although discomfort due to myocardial ischemia most frequently is substernal, radiates down the ulnar aspect of the left arm (Chap. 189), and is pressing and constricting in nature, the location, radiation, and quality of the discomfort are of less diagnostic significance than its behavior in terms of the conditions which induce it and relieve it.

Most persons also believe that cardiac pain is situated in the region of the left breast, and therefore left inframammary pain is one of the common symptoms that brings the patient to seek medical advice. It differs radically from the discomfort due to myocardial ischemia, i.e., angina pectoris. The left inframammary discomfort is either a momentary, sharp and lancinating pain, or a long-lasting, dull ache, occasionally accentuated by sharp stabs. Relief of non-anginal discomfort is often sudden, or occurs slowly and after prolonged rest, and may not be temporally related to nitroglycerin administration. In contrast to angina pectoris, such precordial pain usually has *no* relationship to exertion, may be accompanied by tenderness over the precordium and is frequently observed in patients who are tense, easily fatigued, unusually anxious, or psychoneurotic. Angina pectoris, on the other hand, is usually described as a *discomfort* rather than frank *pain* in the chest and is characteristically substernal rather than precordial. It is further characterized on page 19.

DISCOMFORT DUE TO MYOCARDIAL ISCHEMIA Physiologic considerations of the coronary circulation Discomfort due to myocardial ischemia occurs when the oxygen supply to the heart is deficient in relation to the oxygen need. The oxygen consumption of this organ is closely related to the physiologic effort made during contraction. It is dependent primarily on three factors: (1) the tension developed by the myocardium, (2) the contractile (inotropic) state of the myocardium, and (3) the heart rate. When these three factors remain relatively constant, an elevation of stroke volume produces an efficient type of response because it leads to an increase in the external work of the heart (i.e., in the product of cardiac output and arterial pressure) with little accompanying augmentation of myocardial oxygen requirements. Thus, a rise in flow load (unless it raises intraventricular wall tension markedly by increasing preload substantially) causes less increment in myocardial oxygen consumption than does a comparable increase in cardiac work brought about by elevation either of pressure or of heart rate. The net effects of the changes in these hemodynamic variables depend not on oxygen need alone, but rather on the balance between the demand for and the supply of oxygen. The heart is always active, and the coronary venous blood is normally much more desaturated than that draining other areas of the body. Thus the removal of more oxygen from each unit of blood, which is one of the adjustments commonly utilized by exercising skeletal muscle, is already employed in the heart in the basal state. Therefore, the heart must rely primarily on an increase in the coronary blood flow for obtaining additional oxygen.

The blood flow through the coronary arteries is directly proportional to the pressure gradient between the aorta and the ventricular myocardium during systole and the ventricular cavity during diastole, but is also proportional to the fourth power of the radius of the coronary arteries. Thus a relatively slight alteration in coronary diameter below a critical level of coronary luminal diameter can produce a large change in coronary flow, provided that other factors remain constant. Coronary blood flow occurs primarily during diastole, when it is unopposed by systolic myocardial compression of the coronary vessels. Coronary flow is regulated primarily by myocardial oxygen needs, probably through the release of vasodilator metabolites, such as adenosine, and through variations in myocardial P_{O_2}. Control of the lumen of the coronary arterial bed through autonomic nerves and by hydraulic factors constitute additional important mechanisms of regulation of coronary blood flow.

When the epicardial coronary arteries are narrowed critically (>70 percent stenosis of the luminal diameter), the intramyocardial coronary arterioles dilate in an effort to maintain total coronary blood flow at a level that will avert myocardial ischemia at rest. Further dilatation which normally occurs during exercise is therefore not possible. Thus, any condition in which increased heart rate, arterial pressure, or myocardial contractility occurs in the presence of coronary obstruction tends to precipitate anginal attacks by increasing myocardial oxygen needs in the face of a fixed supply. Bradycardia, when not severe, usually has the opposite effects, and this apparently explains the rarity of angina in patients with complete heart block, even when this disorder is associated with coronary disease.

Causes of myocardial ischemia By far the most frequent underlying cause is organic narrowing of the coronary arteries secondary to coronary atherosclerosis. A *dynamic* component of increased coronary vascular resistance, secondary to spasm of the major epicardial vessels, often near an atherosclerotic placque, or to constriction of smaller coronary arterioles is present in many, perhaps the majority, of patients with chronic angina pectoris. Less frequently, narrowing of the coronary orifices due to syphilitic aortitis or to distortion by an aortic dissection may be responsible. There is no evidence that systemic arterial constriction or increased cardiac contractile activity (rise in heart rate or blood pressure, or increase in contractility due to liberation of catecholamines or adrenergic activity) due to emotion can precipitate angina unless there is also narrowing of the coronary vessels.

Aside from conditions which narrow the lumen of the coronary arteries, the only other frequent causes of myocardial ischemia are disorders, such as aortic stenosis and/or regurgitation (Chap. 187), which cause a marked disproportion between the perfusion pressure and the heart's oxygen requirements. Under such conditions the rise in left ventricular systolic pressure is not, as in hypertensive states, balanced by a corresponding elevation of aortic perfusion pressure.

An increase in heart rate is especially harmful in patients with coronary atherosclerosis and with aortic stenosis, because on the one hand it increases myocardial oxygen needs, and on the other it shortens diastole more than systole and thereby decreases the total available perfusion time per minute.

Patients with marked *right ventricular hypertension* may have exertional pain which is quite similar to that of the common type of angina. It is likely that this discomfort results from relative ischemia of the right ventricle brought about by the increased oxygen needs and by the elevated intramural resistance, with reduction of the normally large systolic pressure gradient which perfuses this chamber. Angina is common in patients with *syphilitic aortitis,* in whom the relative roles of aortic regurgitation and of coronary ostial narrowing are difficult to assess. The importance of tachycardia, decline in arterial pressure, thyrotoxicosis, or diminution in arterial oxygen content (such as occurs in anemia or arterial hypoxia) in the production of myocardial hypoxia will be apparent from the above discussion. However, these are precipitating and aggravating factors rather than the underlying cause of angina; as already noted, the latter is, in almost all instances, coronary arterial narrowing.

Effects of myocardial ischemia A common manifestation of ischemia is *anginal discomfort*, considered in some detail in Chap. 189. Usually it is described as a heavy pressure or squeezing, a sensation of strangling or constriction in the chest, a "burning" or "heavy feeling," or difficulty in breathing, and it occurs particularly on walking, especially after meals, on cold days, against a wind or uphill. Typically it develops gradually during exertion, after heavy meals, and with anger, excitement, frustration, and other emotional states; it is not precipitated by coughing or respiratory movements or other motion. When angina is induced by walking, it forces the patient to stop or to reduce speed; it is characteristically relieved by rest and nitroglycerin. The exact mechanism of the stimulus for anginal discomfort is still unknown, but it is probably related to an accumulation of metabolites within the heart muscle. Angina occurs most typically in the substernal region, anteriorly across the midthorax; it may radiate to or rarely occur alone in the interscapular region, in the arms, shoulders, teeth, and abdomen. It rarely radiates to below the umbilicus or to the back of the neck or the occiput. The more severe the attack, the greater the radiation from the substernal areas to the left arm, especially its ulnar aspect.

Myocardial infarction is usually associated with a discomfort similar in quality and distribution to that of angina but of longer duration (usually 30 min) and of sufficient intensity that it qualifies as true *pain*. In contrast to angina, the pain of myocardial infarction is not relieved by rest or by coronary dilator drugs and may require large doses of narcotics. It may be accompanied by diaphoresis, nausea, and hypotension (Chap. 190).

A second effect of myocardial ischemia consists of *electrocardiographic changes* (Chaps. 178, 189, and 190). Many patients with angina have normal tracings between attacks, and the record may even remain normal during the episode of pain. However, depression of the ST segments, caused by myocardial ischemia, typically occurs during exertion and is accompanied by anginal discomfort; moreover, electrocardiographic evidence of myocardial ischemia may occur at rest and with or without accompanying chest discomfort. The finding of flat or downsloping ST-segment depressions of 0.1 mV or greater during an attack of pain, with a return to normal after the pain subsides, strongly suggests that the pain is anginal in origin. The value and limitation of electrocardiographic changes occurring after exercise in the diagnosis of angina pectoris are discussed in Chap. 189.

A third effect of myocardial ischemia is impairment of *myocardial contraction*. The left ventricular end-diastolic and pulmonary vascular pressures may rise during anginal attacks, particularly if they are prolonged and are caused, presumably, by the decreased contractility and reduced distensibility of the ischemic areas. A fourth heart sound is also frequently heard during the anginal episode; paradoxic pulsations may be evident on palpation of the precordium and can be recorded by apex cardiography. Two-dimensional echocardiography or left ventricular angiography carried out during myocardial ischemia often reveals left ventricular dysfunction, i.e., hypokinesis or akinesis (Chap. 179) in the territory of the obstructed vessel(s).

Another characteristic effect of myocardial ischemia is liability to sudden death (Chap. 30). This may never occur, despite thousands of anginal episodes. However, it may supervene early in the disease and even in the first attack. The usual mechanism is probably ischemia-induced ventricular fibrillation, but occasionally sudden death may be due to ventricular standstill in patients with impaired atrioventricular conduction.

PAIN DUE TO IRRITATION OF SEROUS MEMBRANES OR JOINTS **Pericarditis** The visceral surface of the pericardium ordinarily is insensitive to pain, as is the parietal surface, except in its lower portion, which has a relatively small number of pain fibers carried in the phrenic nerves. The pain associated with pericarditis is believed to be due to inflammation of the adjacent parietal pleura. These observations explain why noninfectious pericarditis (e.g., that associated with uremia and with myocardial infarction) and cardiac tamponade with relatively mild inflammation are usually painless or accompanied by only mild pain, whereas infectious pericarditis, being nearly always more intense and spreading to the neighboring pleura, is usually associated with pain having some pleuritic features, i.e., it is aggravated by breathing, coughing, etc. Since the central part of the diaphragm receives its sensory supply from the phrenic nerve (which arises from the third to fifth cervical segments of the spinal cord), pain arising from the lower parietal pericardium and central tendon of the diaphragm is felt characteristically at the tip of the shoulder, the adjoining trapezius ridge, and the neck. Involvement of the more lateral part of the diaphragmatic pleura, supplied by branches from the sixth to ninth intercostal nerves, causes pain not only in the anterior part of the chest but also in the upper part of the abdomen or corresponding region of the back, sometimes simulating the pain of acute cholecystitis or pancreatitis.

Pericarditis causes two distinct types of pain (Chap. 194). The commonest is pleuritic pain, related to respiratory movements and aggravated by cough and/or deep inspiration. It is sometimes brought on by swallowing, because the esophagus lies just beyond the posterior portion of the heart and is often altered by a change of bodily position, becoming sharper and more left-sided in the supine position and reduced when the patient sits upright, leaning forward. It is frequently referred to the neck and lasts longer than the pain of angina pectoris. This type of pain is due to the pleuritic component of infectious pleuropericarditis.

The second form of pericardial pain is the steady, crushing substernal pain which mimics that of acute myocardial infarction. The mechanism of this steady substernal pain is not certain, but it may arise from marked inflammation of the relatively sensitive inner parietal surface of the pericardium, or from irritated afferent cardiac nerve fibers lying in the periadventitial layers of the superficial coronary arteries. Occasionally both types of pain may be present simultaneously.

The painful syndromes which may follow trauma to or operations on the heart (i.e., the postcardiotomy syndrome) or myocardial infarction are discussed in later chapters (Chaps. 190 and 194). Such pain often but not always arises in the pericardium.

Pleural pain is very common; it generally results from stretching of inflamed parietal pleura and may be identical in character with that of pericarditis. It occurs in fibrinous pleurisy, as well as when pneumonic processes reach the periphery of the lung. Pneumothorax and tumors involving the pleural space may also irritate the parietal pleura and cause pleural pain; the latter is sharp, knifelike, superficial in quality, and its aggravation by each breath and by coughing distinguishes it from the deep, dull, relatively steady pain of myocardial ischemia.

The pain resulting from *pulmonary embolism* may resemble that of acute myocardial infarction, and in massive embolism it is located substernally. In patients with smaller emboli the pain is located more laterally, is pleuritic in nature, and may be associated with hemoptysis (Chap. 211). Massive pulmonary emboli and other causes of acute pulmonary hypertension may cause severe, persistent substernal pain, presumably due to distention of the pulmonary artery. The pain of *mediastinal emphysema* (Chap. 214) may be intense and sharp and may radiate from the substernal region to the shoulders; often a distinct crepitus is heard. The pain associated with *mediastinitis* and *mediastinal tumors* usually resembles that of pleuritis but is more likely to be maximal in the substernal region, and the associated feeling of constriction or oppression may cause confusion with myocardial infarction. The pain due to *acute dissection of the aorta* or to an expanding aortic aneurysm results from stimulation of the adventitia; it is usually extremely severe, is localized to the center of the chest, lasts for hours, and requires unusually large amounts of analgesics for relief. It often radiates into the back but is not aggravated by changes in position or respiration (Chap. 197).

The *costochondral and chondrosternal articulations* are the commonest sites of anterior chest pain. Objective signs in the form of swelling (Tietze's syndrome), redness, and heat are rare, but sharply localized tenderness is common. The pain may be darting and lasting for only a few seconds, or a dull ache enduring for hours or days. An associated feeling of tightness due to muscle spasm (see below) is frequent. When the discomfort persists for a few days only, a story of minor trauma or of some unaccustomed physical effort can often be obtained. *Pressure on the chondrosternal and costochondral junctions is an essential part of the examination of every patient with chest pain* and will reproduce the pain arising from these tissues. A large percentage of patients with costochondral pain, especially those who also have minor and innocent T-wave alterations, are erroneously labeled as having coronary disease, sometimes with dire consequences. Pain in the xiphoid (xiphodynia) can also be reproduced by pressure on the xiphisternum.

Pain secondary to *subacromial bursitis* and *arthritis of the shoulder and spine* may be precipitated by exercise of the local area but not by general exertion. It may be brought about by passive movement of the involved area as well as by coughing. Other forms of chest pain include the "precordial catch," which may be associated with poor posture and characteristically lasts only a few seconds. Myofascitis of the pectoral muscle or biceps tendonitis may be confused with angina pectoris but may be reproduced by squeezing the pectoral muscles or the head of the biceps.

PAIN DUE TO TISSUE DISRUPTION Rupture or tear of a structure may give rise to pain that sets in abruptly and reaches its peak of intensity almost instantly. Such a story should arouse the suspicion of aortic dissection, pneumothorax, mediastinal emphysema, a cervical disk syndrome, or rupture of the esophagus. However, the patient may be too ill to recall the precise circumstances, or the pain may be atypical and increase gradually in severity. Likewise, other and more benign conditions, such as a slipped costal cartilage or an intercostal muscle cramp, may also produce pain with an abrupt onset.

CLINICAL ASPECTS OF THE COMMONER CAUSES OF CHEST PAIN The more serious causes of chest pain such as myocardial ischemia, aortic dissection, pericarditis, and disorders of the pleura, esophagus, stomach, duodenum, and pancreas are considered in the appropriate chapters dealing with these problems.

Pain arising in the chest wall or upper extremity This may develop as a result of muscle or ligament strains brought on by unaccustomed exercise and felt in the costochondral or chondrosternal junctions or in the chest wall muscles. Other causes are *osteoarthritis* of the dorsal or thoracic spine and *ruptured cervical disks.* Pain in the left upper extremity and precordium may be due to compression of portions of the brachial plexus by a cervical rib or by spasm and shortening of the scalenus anticus muscle secondary to high fixation of the ribs and sternum. Finally, pains in the upper extremity (shoulder-hand syndrome) and in the pectoral muscles may, through unknown mechanisms, occur in patients following myocardial infarction.

Pain arising in the chest wall or shoulder girdles or arms is usually recognized by the presence of localized tenderness of the affected area and the clear relation between pain and motion. Deep breathing, turning or twisting of the chest, and movements of the shoulder girdle and arm may elicit and duplicate the pain of which the patient complains. The pain may be very brief, lasting only a few seconds, or full and aching and enduring for hours. The duration is, therefore, likely to be either longer or shorter than untreated angina pectoris, which usually lasts for only a few minutes.

These skeletal pains often have a sharp or sticking quality. In addition, there is frequently a feeling of tightness, which is probably due to associated spasm of intercostal or pectoral muscles. This may produce the "morning stiffness" seen in so many skeletal disorders. The discomfort is unaffected by nitroglycerin but often is abolished by infiltration of the painful areas with procaine. When chest wall pain is of recent origin and follows trauma, strain, or some unusual activity involving the pectoral muscles, it presents no problem in diagnosis. However, since both disorders are common, long-standing skeletal pain is frequent in persons who also have angina pectoris. This coexistence of the two different types of chest pain in the same patient is frequently confusing because in the patient's mind the anginal needle may be hidden in the skeletal haystack. Thus every middle-aged or elderly patient who has long-standing anterior chest wall pain merits careful study for the presence of ischemic heart disease.

The confusion created by the presence of innocent skeletal pain impairs the reliability of the history and is probably the commonest cause of errors—both positive and negative—in the diagnosis of angina pectoris. It may be necessary also to learn by direct observation whether exercise alone or postprandial exertion is capable of producing the pain. Repeated tests may be required, comparing the relative effects of preceding placebos and nitroglycerin on the amount of exertion required to induce the pain. When the history is inconclusive, the exercise electrocardiogram, or in patients with equivocal or nondiagnostic tests, the exercise stress test with thallium scintigraphy (Chap. 179), may furnish useful information concerning the existence of myocardial ischemia. In rare instances coronary arteriography may be required.

Esophageal pain This usually presents as deep thoracic pain; it results from chemical (acid) irritation of the esophageal mucosa secondary to acid reflux or from spasm of the esophageal muscle and characteristically follows deglutition. The sudden relief of pain by one or two swallows of food or water suggests esophageal pain. Accompanying dysphagia, regurgitation of undigested food, and weight loss direct attention to the esophagus (see Chaps. 32 and 234). The Bernstein acid perfusion test, in which an attempt is made to reproduce the pain by infusing 0.1 *M* HCl into the esophagus, is helpful in establishing acid gastric reflux into the esophagus as the cause of pain. Esophageal manometry and measurement of lower esophageal sphincter pressure, sometimes with ergonovine stimulation, are useful in identifying esophageal spasm as the origin of the pain.

Emotional disorders These are also common causes of chest pain. Usually, the discomfort is experienced as a sense of "tightness," sometimes called "aching," and occasionally it may be sufficiently severe as to be designated a pain of considerable magnitude. Since the discomfort has almost always the additional quality of tightness or constriction, and is often localized at least in part beneath the sternum, it is not surprising that this type of discomfort is frequently confused with that of myocardial ischemia. Ordinarily, it lasts for a half hour or more and may persist for a day or less with slow fluctuation of intensity. The association with fatigue or emotional strain is usually clear, although this may not be recognized by the patient until called to his or her attention. The pain probably develops through unconscious and prolonged increase of muscle tone, perhaps enhanced by accompanying hyperventilation (by causing a contraction of the chest wall muscles similar to the painful tetany of the extremities). When the hyperventilation and/or the associated adrenergic effect due to anxiety also causes innocent changes in the T waves and ST segments, the confusion with coronary disease is strengthened. However, the long duration of the pain, the lack of any relation to exertion but association rather with fatigue or tension, and the usually periodic occurrence on successive days without any limitation of capacity for exercise usually make the differentiation from ischemic pain quite clear.

Other causes of chest pain The several *abdominal disorders* which may at times mimic anginal pain may usually be suspected from the history, which, as in esophageal pain, ordinarily indicates some relationship to swallowing, eating, belching, etc. Pain resulting from gastric or duodenal ulcer (Chap. 235) is epigastric or substernal, commences about 1 to $1\frac{1}{2}$ h after meals, and is usually promptly relieved by antacids or milk. The gastrointestinal roentgenogram is of crucial significance, and roentgenographic examination is also often helpful in differentiating biliary, gastrointestinal, aortic, pulmonary, and skeletal disease pain from angina pectoris. The demonstration of the presence of a coexistent abdominal disorder such as a hiatus hernia does not constitute proof that the chest pain of which the patient complains is due to this. Such disorders are frequently asymptomatic and are not at all uncommon in patients who also have angina pectoris.

Substernal discomfort also frequently occurs in the presence of *tracheobronchitis;* it is described as a burning sensation accentuated by coughing. A variety of *disorders involving the breast,* including inflammatory breast disease, benign and malignant tumors, as well as mastodynia, are common causes of thoracic pain. The localization in the breast and superficial swelling and tenderness of this organ are of diagnostic importance. A number of other causes of thoracic pain or discomfort including spinal arthritis, herpes zoster, anterior scalene and hyperabduction syndromes, compression of the cervical roots, malignant disease of the ribs, while less common, can usually be readily recognized after appropriate observation.

APPROACH TO THE PATIENT WITH CHEST DISCOMFORT Most persons with this complaint will fall into one of two general groups. The first consists of persons with prolonged and often severe pain without obvious initiating factors. Such persons will frequently be seriously ill. The problem is that of differentiating such serious conditions as myocardial infarction, aortic dissection, and pulmonary embolism from each other and from less grave causes. In some such instances, a careful history and physical examination will provide significant clues, which can then be followed up by appropriate laboratory tests [electrocardiogram, serum enzymes, various forms of diagnostic imaging] which will commonly provide the correct answer.

The second group of patients comprises those who have brief episodes of pain and are otherwise in apparently excellent health. Here, the resting electrocardiogram will rarely supply decisive information, but records taken during or immediately after exercise or pain will often reveal characteristic changes (Chap. 189). Radionuclide scintigraphy at rest and during exercise (Chap. 179) is often helpful as well. However, in many instances it is the study of the subjective phenomenon, i.e., of the pain itself, that will lead to the diagnosis. Of the several methods of investigation which are available for such patients, three are of cardinal importance.

A detailed and *meticulous history* of the behavior of the pain is the most important method. The location, radiation, quality, intensity, and duration of the episodes are important. Even more so is the story of the aggravating and alleviating factors. A history of sharp aggravation by breathing, coughing, or other respiratory movements will usually point toward the pleura and pericardium or mediastinum as the site, although chest wall pain is likewise affected by respiratory motions. Similarly, a pain which regularly appears on rapid walking and vanishes within a few minutes upon standing still suggests the diagnosis of angina pectoris, although a similar story will occasionally be obtained from patients with skeletal disorders.

When the history is inconclusive, the *study of the patient at the time of the spontaneous episode* will often supply crucial information. For example, the electrocardiogram, which may be normal both at rest and even during or after exercise in the absence of pain, will occasionally demonstrate striking changes when recorded during an anginal episode. Similarly, radiographic study of the esophagus or of the stomach may show no evidence of cardiospasm or of hiatal hernia except when the observation is made during the pain.

The third method of study represents the *attempt to produce and alleviate the pain at will.* This procedure is necessary only when doubt exists following the history or when needed for psychotherapeutic purposes. Thus the demonstration that a localized pain, which can be reproduced by pressure on the chest, is completely relieved by local infiltration with procaine will often be of conclusive importance in convincing the patient that the heart is not the site. When the pain is precipitated by intravenous injections of ergonovine and this is accompanied by electrocardiographic ST-segment elevations and coronary spasm on arteriography, the diagnosis of Prinzmetal's angina can be made.

When, as is often the case, the history is atypical, the correct diagnosis of angina pectoris may be aided by noting the response to nitroglycerin. Relief of pain after its sublingual administration does not necessarily prove that there is a cause-and-effect relationship. It is necessary to be certain that the pain vanishes more rapidly (usually within 5 min) and more completely when the drug is used than when it is not employed. A false-negative impression concerning the effect of nitroglycerin may be the result of the use of a deteriorated preparation which has been exposed to light. In doubtful instances, repeated exercise tests, with and without preceding administration of nitroglycerin, may be necessary. The demonstration that the time required for a given exercise to produce pain is consistently and considerably longer when it is undertaken within a few minutes after a sublingual nitroglycerin pill than after a placebo may, in some instances, represent powerful clinical evidence for the recognition of angina pectoris. A completely negative response to such repeated tests constitutes powerful evidence against angina. Angina is rarely relieved within a few seconds of lying down, nor is angina suddenly precipitated by stooping forward.

In patients in whom the question of whether there is coronary disease cannot be resolved despite the aforementioned clinical and laboratory tests, including exercise electrocardiography (Chap. 178) and nuclear scintigraphy (Chap. 179), cardiac catheterization and coronary arteriography may be required. A useful stress test that can be carried out at the time of catheterization is to elevate the heart rate in stepwise fashion by electrical pacing; the development of ST-segment depressions on the electrocardiogram and the reproduction of the pain support the diagnosis of myocardial ischemia. Coronary arteriography will show critical (more than 70 percent) reduction of the luminal diameter in at least one major vessel in patients with obstructive coronary artery disease (Chaps. 180 and 189).

PALPITATION

Palpitation is a common, disagreeable symptom which may be defined as an awareness of the beating of the heart, an awareness most commonly brought about by a change in the heart's rhythm or rate or by an augmentation of its contractility. Palpitation is not pathognomonic of any particular group of disorders; indeed, often it signifies not a primary physical disorder but rather a psychological disturbance. Even when it occurs as a more or less prominent complaint, the diagnosis of the underlying disease is made largely on the basis of other associated symptoms and data. Nevertheless, palpitation is frequently of considerable importance in the minds of patients, who fear that it may indicate heart disease. Concern is all the more pronounced in patients who have been told that they *may* have heart disease; to them palpitation may seem to be an omen of impending disaster. Since the resulting anxiety may be associated with increased activity of the autonomic nervous system, with consequent increases of the cardiac rate and rhythm and the vigor of contraction, the patient's awareness of these changes may then lead to a vicious cycle, which may ultimately be responsible for incapacitation.

Palpitation may be described by the patient in various terms, such as "pounding," "fluttering," "flopping," and "skipping," and in most cases it will be obvious that the complaint is of a sensation of disturbed heartbeat. The sensitivity to alterations in cardiac activity among different individuals varies widely. Some patients seem to be unaware of the most serious and chaotic dysrhythmias; others are seriously troubled by an occasional extrasystole. Patients with anxiety states often exhibit a lowered threshold at which disorders of rate and rhythm result in palpitation. The awareness of the heartbeat also tends to be more common at night and during introspective moments, but is less marked during activity. Patients with organic heart disease and chronic disorders of cardiac rate, rhythm, or stroke volume tend to accommodate to these abnormalities and are often less sensitive than normal persons to such events. Persistent tachycardia and/or atrial fibrillation may not be accompanied by continuous palpitation, in contrast to a sudden, brief alteration in cardiac rate or rhythm which often causes considerable subjective discomfort. Palpitation is particularly prominent when the precipitating cause for increased heart rate or contractility or arrhythmia is recent, transient, and episodic. Conversely, in emotionally well-adjusted individuals palpitation becomes progressively less disconcerting as the cause (e.g., anemia, frequent extrasystoles, complete atrioventricular block) persists.

PATHOGENESIS OF PALPITATION Under ordinary circumstances the rhythmic heartbeat is imperceptible to the healthy individual of placid or even average temperament. Palpitation may be experienced by normal persons who have engaged in strenuous physical effort or have been aroused emotionally or sexually. This type of palpitation is physiologic and represents the normal awareness of an overactive heart—i.e., a heart that is beating at a rapid rate and with an increased contractility. Palpitation due to overactivity of the heart may also occur in certain pathologic states, e.g., fever, acute or severe anemia, or thyrotoxicosis.

When palpitation is heavy and regular, it is usually caused by an augmented stroke volume, and it should raise the question of aortic regurgitation or of a variety of hyperkinetic circulatory states (anemia, arteriovenous fistula, thyrotoxicosis, and the so-called idiopathic hyperkinetic heart syndrome). It may also occur immediately after the onset of cardiac slowing, as with the sudden development of complete atrioventricular block, or upon the conversion from atrial fibrillation to sinus rhythm. Unusual movements of the heart within the thorax are also frequently the mechanism of palpitation. Thus, the ectopic beat and/or the compensatory pause may be appreciated, since both are associated with alterations in cardiac motion.

IMPORTANT CAUSES OF PALPITATION See also Chap. 184.

Extrasystoles In most cases the diagnosis will be suggested by the patient's story. The premature contraction and postpremature beat are often described as a "flopping," or the patient may say that it feels as if "the heart were turning over." The pause following the premature contraction may be felt as an actual cessation of the heartbeat. The first ventricular contraction succeeding the pause may be felt as an unusually vigorous beat and will be described as "pounding" or "thudding."

When extrasystoles are numerous, clinical differentiation from atrial fibrillation can be made by any procedure that will bring about a definite increase in the ventricular rate; at increasingly rapid heart rates, the extrasystoles usually diminish in frequency and then disappear, whereas the ventricular irregularity of atrial fibrillation increases.

Ectopic tachycardias These conditions, which are considered in detail in Chap. 184, are common and medically important causes of palpitation. Ventricular tachycardia, one of the most serious arrhythmias, rarely is manifested as palpitation; this may be related to the abnormal sequence, and hence impaired coordination and vigor, of ventricular contraction. If the patient is seen between attacks, the diagnosis of ectopic tachycardia and its type will have to depend on the history, but the precise diagnosis can be made only when an electrocardiogram and observations on the effect of carotid sinus pressure are made during the episode. The mode of onset and offset gives the most important lead in distinguishing sinus from one of the various forms of ectopic tachycardias; sinus tachycardia commences and ceases over the course of minutes or seconds, but not instantaneously as is characteristic of ectopic rhythms. Continuous ambulatory (Holter) electrocardiography and asking the patient to record the time of onset and cessation of the palpitations in a diary are extremely helpful in determining the cause of this symptom.

Other causes These include thyrotoxicosis (Chap. 324), hypoglycemia (Chap. 329), pheochromocytoma (Chap. 326), fever (Chap. 9), and drugs. The relationship between the development of palpitation and the use of tobacco, coffee, tea, alcohol, epinephrine, ephedrine, aminophylline, atropine, or thyroid extract is usually obvious.

Palpitation as a manifestation of the anxiety state Persons who are healthy physically and well adjusted emotionally may have palpitation under certain circumstances. During or immediately after vigorous physical exertion or during sudden emotional tension, palpitation is common and is usually associated with sinus tachycardia. In poorly conditioned persons without organic heart disease, the sinus tachycardia of exercise may be excessive and associated with palpitation.

In some persons, palpitation may be one of the outstanding manifestations of an episode of acute anxiety. In others the palpitation may, with other symptoms, represent prolonged anxiety neurosis or a lifelong disorder characterized by volatile autonomic function. Whether these illnesses are simply an expression of a chronic, deep-seated anxiety state superimposed on a normal autonomic nervous system or whether they depend on instability of the autonomic nervous system is not clear. At any rate, the clinical significance of the differentiation between the transitory and the enduring forms is that the former is often dissipated by firm reassurance from the physician, whereas the latter is usually resistant even to the most thorough and expert psychiatric care. In the latter case, the patient must be treated with most carefully planned psychological support and tranquilizing medications. This chronic form of palpitation is known by various names such as *Da Costa's syndrome, soldier's heart, effort syndrome, irritable heart, neurocirculatory asthenia,* and *functional cardiovascular disease*. Aside from palpitation, the chief symptoms are those of an anxiety state.

Physical examination usually reveals the typical findings of the hyperkinetic syndrome. These include a left parasternal lift, a precordial or apical systolic murmur, a wide pulse pressure, rapidly rising pulse, and excessive perspiration. The electrocardiogram may display minor depressions of the ST junction and inversion of T waves and so occasionally lead to a mistaken diagnosis of coronary disease; this is particularly likely to occur when these findings are associated with complaints by the patients of an aching feeling of substernal tightness, commonly present in emotional stress. The presence of any kind of organic disease is one of the commonest causes of the underlying anxiety which frequently precipitates this functional syndrome. Thus, even when a patient presents undoubted objective evidence of organic cardiac disease, the possibility that a superimposed anxiety state may be responsible for the symptoms described above should be considered. Palpitation associated with organic cardiac disease is nearly always accompanied by arrhythmia or tachycardia, whereas the symptom may exist with regular rhythm and with a heart rate of 80 beats per minute or less in patients with the anxiety state. An anxiety state, in contrast to heart disease, causes a sighing type of dyspnea. Also pain localized to the apex, either brief and lancinating in character or lasting for hours or days and

TABLE 4-1 Items to be covered in history

Does the palpitation occur:	If so, suspect:
As isolated "jumps" or "skips"?	Extrasystoles
In attacks, known to be of abrupt beginning, with a heart rate of 120 beats per minute or over, with regular or irregular rhythm?	Paroxysmal rapid heart action
Independent of exercise or excitement adequate to account for the symptom?	Atrial fibrillation, atrial flutter, thyrotoxicosis, anemia, febrile states, hypoglycemia, anxiety state
In attacks developing rapidly though not absolutely abruptly, unrelated to exertion or excitement?	Hemorrhage, hypoglycemia, tumor of the adrenal medulla
In conjunction with the taking of drugs?	Tobacco, coffee, tea, alcohol, epinephrine, ephedrine, aminophylline, atropine, thyroid extract, monoamine oxidase inhibitors
On standing?	Postural hypotension
In middle-aged women, in conjunction with flushes and sweats?	Menopausal syndrome
When the rate is known to be normal and the rhythm regular?	Anxiety state

accompanied by hyperesthesia, is due usually to an anxiety state, not to structural cardiac disease. Giddiness due to this syndrome can usually be reproduced by hyperventilation or by change from the recumbent to the erect posture.

The *treatment* of the anxiety state with palpitation is difficult and depends on removal of the cause. In many instances a thorough examination of the heart and a statement that it is normal will suffice. Instructions to take more rather than less physical exercise will reinforce these statements. When the anxiety state is a manifestation of chronic anxiety neurosis or related emotional disorder, the symptoms are more likely to persist.

Table 4-1 summarizes the main points of information to be ascertained in the history in elucidating the significance of palpitation. The recording of an ambulatory electrocardiogram and the precise temporal correlation of the cardiac rate and rhythm with the presence of palpitation are extremely useful in the identification or exclusion of an arrhythmia if the symptom does not occur when the patient is under direct observation. The effectiveness of antiarrhythmia treatment can also be assessed objectively in this manner, without the necessity of relying only on the patient's subjective symptoms. Beta-adrenergic blockade with propranolol, beginning with 40 mg per day in divided doses, and ranging as high as 400 mg per day, can be extremely effective in patients with palpitation and sinus rhythm or sinus tachycardia.

One point merits special emphasis. *As a rule palpitation produces anxiety and fear out of all proportion to its seriousness.* When the cause has been accurately determined and its significance explained to patients, their concern is often ameliorated and may disappear entirely.

REFERENCES

ARESKOG NH, TIBBLING L (eds): Differential diagnostic aspects of chest pain. Acta Med Scand (suppl):644, 1980

BRAUNWALD E: Control of myocardial oxygen consumption: Physiologic and clinical considerations. Am J Cardiol 27:416, 1971

CHRISTIE LG et al: Systematic approach to evaluation of angina-like chest pain: Pathophysiology and clinical testing with emphasis on objective documentation of myocardial ischemia. Am Heart J 102:897, 1981

COHN PF, BRAUNWALD E: Chronic ischemic heart disease, in *Heart Disease,* 2d ed, E Braunwald (ed). Philadelphia, Saunders, 1984, chap 39, p 1334

CONSTANT J: The clinical diagnosis of nonanginal chest pain: The differentiation of angina from nonanginal chest pain by history. Clin Cardiol 6:11, 1983

DEMEESTER et al: Esophageal function in patients with angina-type chest pain and normal coronary angiograms. Ann Surg 196:488, 1982

DRESSLER W: *Clinical Aids in Cardiac Diagnosis.* New York, Grune & Stratton, 1970

GOLDSCHLAGER N: Use of the treadmill test in the diagnosis of coronary artery disease in patients with chest pain. Ann Intern Med 97:383, 1982

HURST JW et al: The history: Past events and symptoms related to cardiovascular disease, in *The Heart,* 6th ed, JW Hurst (ed). New York, McGraw-Hill, 1986, p 113

LEVENE DL: *Chest Pain.* Philadelphia, Lea & Febiger, 1977, p 203

PATTERSON DR: Diffuse esophageal spasm in patients with undiagnosed chest pain. J Clin Gastroenterol 4:415, 1982

5 ABDOMINAL PAIN

WILLIAM SILEN

The correct interpretation of acute abdominal pain is one of the most challenging demands made of any physician. Since proper therapy often requires urgent action, the luxury of the leisurely approach suitable for the study of other conditions is frequently denied. Few other clinical situations demand greater experience and judgment, because the most catastrophic of events may be forecast by the subtlest of symptoms and signs. Nowhere in medicine is a meticulously executed, detailed history and physical examination of greater importance. The etiologic classification in Table 5-1, although not complete, forms a useful frame of reference for the evaluation of patients with abdominal pain.

TABLE 5-1 Some important causes of abdominal pain

- *I* Pain originating in the abdomen
  - *A* Parietal peritoneal inflammation
    - *1* Bacterial contamination, e.g., perforated appendix, pelvic inflammatory disease
    - *2* Chemical irritation, e.g., perforated ulcer, pancreatitis, mittelschmerz
  - *B* Mechanical obstruction of hollow viscera
    - *1* Obstruction of the small or large intestine
    - *2* Obstruction of the biliary tree
    - *3* Obstruction of the ureter
  - *C* Vascular disturbances
    - *1* Embolism or thrombosis
    - *2* Vascular rupture
    - *3* Pressure or torsional occlusion
    - *4* Sickle cell anemia
  - *D* Abdominal wall
    - *1* Distortion or traction of mesentery
    - *2* Trauma or infection of muscles
  - *E* Distention of visceral surfaces, e.g., hepatic or renal capsules
- *II* Pain referred from extraabdominal sources
  - *A* Thorax, e.g., pneumonia, referred pain from coronary occlusion
  - *B* Spine, e.g., radiculitis from arthritis
  - *C* Genitalia, e.g., torsion of the testicle
- *III* Metabolic causes
  - *A* Exogenous
    - *1* Black widow spider bite
    - *2* Lead poisoning and others
  - *B* Endogenous
    - *1* Uremia
    - *2* Diabetic ketoacidosis
    - *3* Porphyria
    - *4* Allergic factors (C′1 esterase inhibitor deficiency)
- *IV* Neurogenic causes
  - *A* Organic
    - *1* Tabes dorsalis
    - *2* Herpes zoster
    - *3* Causalgia and others
  - *B* Functional

The diagnosis of ''acute or surgical abdomen'' so often heard in emergency wards is not an acceptable one because of its often misleading and erroneous connotation. The most obvious of ''acute abdomens'' may not require operative intervention, and the mildest of abdominal pains may herald the onset of an urgently correctable lesion. Any patient with abdominal pain of recent onset requires early and thorough evaluation with specific attempts at accurate diagnosis.

SOME MECHANISMS OF PAIN ORIGINATING IN THE ABDOMEN

Inflammation of the parietal peritoneum The pain of parietal peritoneal inflammation is steady and aching in character and is located directly over the inflamed area, its exact reference being possible because it is transmitted by overlapping somatic nerves supplying the parietal peritoneum. The intensity of the pain is dependent upon the type and amount of foreign substance to which the peritoneal surfaces are exposed in a given period of time. For example, the sudden release into the peritoneal cavity of a small quantity of *sterile* acid gastric juice causes much more pain than the same amount of grossly contaminated neutral fecal material. Enzymatically active pancreatic juice incites more pain and inflammation than does the same amount of sterile bile containing no potent enzymes. Blood and urine are often so bland as to go undetected if exposure of the peritoneum has not been sudden and massive. In the case of bacterial contamination, such as in pelvic inflammatory disease, the pain is frequently of low intensity early in the illness until bacterial multiplication has caused the elaboration of irritating substances.

So important is the rate at which the irritating material is applied to the peritoneum that cases of perforated peptic ulcer may be associated with entirely different clinical pictures dependent only upon the rapidity with which the gastric juice enters the peritoneal cavity.

The pain of peritoneal inflammation is invariably accentuated by pressure or changes in tension of the peritoneum, whether produced by palpation or by movement, as in coughing or sneezing. Consequently, the patient with peritonitis lies quietly in bed, preferring to avoid motion, in contrast to the patient with colic, who may writhe incessantly.

Another of the characteristic features of peritoneal irritation is tonic reflex spasm of the abdominal musculature, localized to the involved body segment. The intensity of the tonic muscle spasm accompanying peritoneal inflammation is dependent upon the location of the inflammatory process, the rate at which it develops, and the integrity of the nervous system. Spasm over a perforated retrocecal appendix or perforated ulcer into the lesser peritoneal sac may be minimal or absent because of the protective effect of overlying viscera. As in pain of peritoneal inflammation, a slowly developing process often greatly attenuates the degree of muscle spasm. Catastrophic abdominal emergencies such as a perforated ulcer have been repeatedly associated with minimal or occasionally no detectable pain or muscle spasm in obtunded, seriously ill, debilitated elderly patients or in psychotic patients.

Obstruction of hollow viscera The pain of obstruction of hollow abdominal viscera is classically described as intermittent, or colicky. Yet the lack of a truly cramping character should not be misleading, because distention of a hollow viscus may produce steady pain with only very occasional exacerbations. Although not nearly as well localized as the pain of parietal peritoneal inflammation, some useful generalities can be made concerning its distribution.

The colicky pain of obstruction of small intestine is usually periumbilical or supraumbilical and is poorly localized. As the intestine becomes progressively dilated with loss of muscular tone, the colicky nature of the pain may become less apparent. With superimposed strangulating obstruction, pain may spread in the lower lumbar region if there is traction on the root of the mesentery. The colicky pain of colonic obstruction is of lesser intensity than that of the small intestine and is often located in the infraumbilical area. Lumbar radiation of pain is common in colonic obstruction.

Sudden distention of the biliary tree produces a steady rather than colicky type of pain; hence the term *biliary colic* is misleading. Acute distention of the gallbladder usually causes pain in the right upper quadrant with radiation to the right posterior region of the thorax or to the tip of the right scapula, and distention of the common bile duct is often associated with pain in the epigastrium radiating to the upper part of the lumbar region. Considerable variation is common, however, so that differentiation between these may be impossible. The typical subscapular pain or lumbar radiation is frequently absent. Gradual dilatation of the biliary tree as in carcinoma of the head of the pancreas may cause no pain or only a mild aching sensation in the epigastrium or right upper quadrant. The pain of distention of the pancreatic ducts is similar to that described for distention of the common bile duct but in addition is very frequently accentuated by recumbency and relieved by the upright position.

Obstruction of the urinary bladder results in dull suprapubic pain, usually low in intensity. Restlessness without specific complaint of pain may be the only sign of a distended bladder in an obtunded patient. In contrast, acute obstruction of the intravesicular portion of the ureter is characterized by severe suprapubic and flank pain which radiates to the penis, scrotum, or inner aspect of the upper region of the thigh. Obstruction of the ureteropelvic junction is felt as pain in the costovertebral angle, whereas obstruction of the remainder of the ureter is associated with flank pain, which often extends into the corresponding side of the abdomen.

Vascular disturbances A frequent misconception, despite abundant experience to the contrary, is that pain associated with intraabdominal vascular disturbances is sudden and catastrophic in nature. The pain of embolism or thrombosis of the superior mesenteric artery or that of impending rupture of an abdominal aortic aneurysm certainly may be severe and diffuse. Yet just as frequently, the patient with occlusion of the superior mesenteric artery has only mild continuous diffuse pain for 2 or 3 days before vascular collapse or findings of peritoneal inflammation appear. The early, seemingly insignificant discomfort is caused by hyperperistalsis rather than peritoneal inflammation. Indeed, absence of tenderness and rigidity in the presence of continuous, diffuse pain in a patient likely to have vascular disease is quite characteristic of occlusion of the superior mesenteric artery. Abdominal pain with radiation to the sacral region, flank, or genitalia should always signal the possible presence of a rupturing abdominal aortic aneurysm. This pain may persist over a period of several days before rupture and collapse occur.

Abdominal wall Pain arising from the abdominal wall is usually constant and aching. Movement and pressure accentuate the discomfort and muscle spasm. In the case of hematoma of the rectus sheath, now most frequently encountered in association with anticoagulant therapy, a mass may be present in the lower quadrants of the abdomen. Simultaneous involvement of muscles in other parts of the body usually serves to differentiate myositis of the abdominal wall from an intraabdominal process which might cause pain in the same region.

REFERRED PAIN IN ABDOMINAL DISEASES Pain referred to the abdomen from the thorax, spine, or genitalia may prove a vexing problem in differential diagnosis, because diseases of the upper part of the abdominal cavity such as acute cholecystitis, perforated ulcer, or subphrenic abscesses are frequently associated with intrathoracic complications. A most important, yet often forgotten, dictum is that the possibility of intrathoracic disease must be considered in every patient with abdominal pain, especially if the pain is in the upper part of the abdomen. Systematic questioning and examination directed toward detecting the presence or absence of myocardial or pulmonary infarction, pneumonia, pericarditis, or esophageal disease (the intrathoracic diseases which most often masquerade as abdominal emergencies) will often provide sufficient clues to establish the proper diagnosis. Diaphragmatic pleuritis resulting from pneumonia or pulmonary infarction may cause pain in the right upper quadrant and pain in the supraclavicular area, the latter radiation to be sharply distinguished from the referred subscapular pain caused by acute distention of the extrahepatic biliary tree. The ultimate decision as to the origin of abdominal pain may require deliberate and planned observation over a period of several hours, during which time repeated questioning and examination will provide the proper explanation.

Referred pain of thoracic origin is often accompanied by splinting of the involved hemithorax with respiratory lag and decrease in excursion more marked than that seen in the presence of intraabdominal disease. In addition, apparent abdominal muscle spasm caused by referred pain will diminish during the inspiratory phase of respiration, whereas it is persistent throughout both respiratory phases if it is of abdominal origin. Palpation over the area of referred pain in the abdomen also does not usually accentuate the pain and in many instances actually seems to relieve it. The frequent coexistence of thoracic and abdominal disease may be misleading and confusing, so that differentiation might be difficult or impossible. For example, the patient with known biliary tract disease often has epigastric pain during myocardial infarction, or biliary colic may be referred to the precordium or left shoulder in a patient who has suffered previously from angina pectoris. For the explanation of the radiation of pain to a previously diseased area, see Chap. 3.

Referred pain from the spine, which usually involves compression or irritation of nerve roots, is characteristically intensified by certain motions such as cough, sneeze, or strain and is associated with hyperesthesia over the involved dermatomes. Pain referred to the abdomen from the testicles or seminal vesicles is generally accentuated by the slightest pressure on either of these organs. The abdominal discomfort is of dull aching character and is poorly localized.

METABOLIC ABDOMINAL CRISES Pain of metabolic origin may simulate almost any other type of intraabdominal disease. Here several mechanisms may be at work. In certain instances, such as hyperlipemia, the metabolic disease itself may be accompanied by an intraabdominal process such as pancreatitis, which can lead to unnecessary laparotomy unless recognized. C'l esterase deficiency associated with angioneurotic edema is also often associated with episodes of severe abdominal pain. Whenever the cause of abdominal pain is obscure, a metabolic origin must always be considered. Abdominal pain is also the hallmark of familial Mediterranean fever (Chap. 271).

The problem of differential diagnosis is often not readily resolved. The pain of porphyria and of lead colic usually is difficult to distinguish from that of intestinal obstruction, because severe hyperperistalsis is a prominent feature of both. The pain of uremia or diabetes is nonspecific, and the pain and tenderness frequently shift in location and intensity. Diabetic acidosis may be precipitated by acute appendicitis or intestinal obstruction, so that if prompt resolution of the abdominal pain does not result from correction of the metabolic abnormalities, an underlying organic problem should be suspected. Black widow spider bites produce intense pain and rigidity of the abdominal muscles and of the back, an area infrequently involved in disease of intraabdominal origin.

NEUROGENIC CAUSES Causalgic pain may occur in diseases which injure nerves of sensory type. It has a burning character and is usually limited to the distribution of a given peripheral nerve. Normal stimuli such as touch or change in temperature may be transformed into this type of pain, which is also frequently present in a patient at rest. A helpful finding is the demonstration that cutaneous pain spots are now irregularly spaced, and this may be the only indication of an old nerve lesion underlying causalgic pain. Even though the pain may be precipitated by gentle palpation, rigidity of the abdominal muscles is absent, and the respirations are not disturbed. Distention of the abdomen is uncommon, and the pain has no relationship to the intake of food.

Pain arising from spinal nerves or roots comes and goes suddenly and is of a lancinating type (see Chap. 7). It may be caused by herpes zoster, impingement by arthritis, tumors, herniated nucleus pulposus, diabetes, or syphilis. Again, it is not associated with food intake, abdominal distention, or changes in respiration. Severe muscle spasm, as in the gastric crises of tabes dorsalis, is common but is either relieved or is not accentuated by abdominal palpation. The pain is made worse by movement of the spine and is usually confined to a few dermatome segments. Hyperesthesia is very common.

Psychogenic pain conforms to none of the aforementioned patterns of disease. Here the mechanism is hard to define. The most common problem is the hysterical adolescent or young woman who develops abdominal pain; she frequently loses an appendix and other organs because of it. Ovulation or some other natural event that causes brief mild abdominal discomfort may sometimes be experienced as an abdominal catastrophe.

Psychogenic pain varies enormously in type and location but usually has no relation to meals. It is often at its onset markedly accentuated during the night. Nausea and vomiting are rarely observed, although occasionally the patient reports these symptoms. Spasm is seldom induced in the abdominal musculature and if present does not persist, especially if the attention of the patient can be distracted. Persistent localized tenderness is rare, and if found, the muscle spasm in the area is inconsistent and often absent. Restriction of the depth of respiration is the most common respiratory abnormality, but this is in the nature of a smothering or choking sensation and is part of an anxiety state (see Chap. 11). It occurs in the absence of thoracic splinting or change in the respiratory rate.

APPROACH TO THE PATIENT WITH ABDOMINAL PAIN There are few abdominal conditions which require such urgent operative intervention that an orderly approach need be abandoned, no matter how ill the patient. Only those patients with exsanguinating hemorrhage must be rushed to the operating room immediately, but in such instances only a few minutes are required to assess the critical nature of the problem. Under these circumstances, all obstacles must be swept aside, adequate access for intravenous fluid replacement obtained, and the operation begun. Many patients of this type have died in the radiology department or the emergency room while awaiting such unnecessary examinations as electrocardiograms or films of the abdomen. *There are no contraindications to operation when massive hemorrhage is present.* Although exceedingly important, this situation fortunately is relatively rare.

Nothing will supplant an orderly, painstakingly *detailed history,* which is far more valuable than any laboratory or roentgenologic examination. This kind of history is laborious and time-consuming, making it not especially popular even though a reasonably accurate diagnosis can be made on the basis of the history alone in the majority of cases. In cases of *acute* abdominal pain, a diagnosis is readily established in most instances, whereas success is not so frequently achieved in patients with *chronic* pain. Since the irritable bowel syndrome is one of the most common causes of abdominal pain, the possibility of this diagnosis must always be kept in mind (see Chap. 239). The *chronological sequence of events* in the patient's history is often more important than emphasis on the location of pain. If the examiner is sufficiently open-minded and unhurried, asks the proper questions, and listens, the patient will often provide the diagnosis. Careful attention should be paid to the extraabdominal regions which may be responsible for abdominal pain. An accurate menstrual history in a female patient is essential. Narcotics or analgesics should be withheld until a definitive diagnosis or a definitive plan has been formulated, because these agents often make it more difficult to secure and to interpret the history and physical findings.

In the examination, simple critical inspection of the patient, e.g., of facies, position in bed, and respiratory activity, may provide valuable clues. The amount of information to be gleaned is directly proportional to the *gentleness* and thoroughness of the examiner. Once a patient with peritoneal inflammation has been examined in a brusque manner, accurate assessment by the next examiner becomes almost impossible. For example, eliciting rebound tenderness by sudden release of a deeply palpating hand in a patient with suspected peritonitis is cruel and unnecessary. The same information can be obtained by gentle percussion of the abdomen (rebound tenderness on a miniature scale), a maneuver which can be far more precise and localizing. Asking the patient to cough will elicit true rebound tenderness without the need for placing a hand on the abdomen. Furthermore, the brusque demonstration of rebound tenderness will startle and induce protective spasm in a nervous or worried patient in whom true rebound tenderness is not present. A palpable gallbladder will be missed if palpation is so brusque that voluntary muscle spasm becomes superimposed upon involuntary muscular rigidity.

As in history taking, there is no substitute for sufficient time spent in the examination. It is important to remember that abdominal signs may be minimal but nevertheless, if accompanied by consistent symptoms, may be exceptionally meaningful when carefully assessed. Signs may be virtually or actually totally absent in cases of pelvic peritonitis, so that careful *pelvic and rectal examinations are mandatory in every patient with abdominal pain.* The presence of tenderness on pelvic or rectal examination in the absence of other abdominal signs must not lead the examiner to exclude such important operative indications as perforated appendicitis, diverticulitis, twisted ovarian cyst, and many others.

Much attention has been paid to the presence or absence of peristaltic sounds, their quality, and their frequency. Auscultation of the abdomen is probably one of the least rewarding aspects of the physical examination of a patient with abdominal pain. Severe catastrophes, such as strangulating small-intestinal obstruction or perforated appendicitis, may occur in the presence of normal peristalsis. Conversely, when the proximal part of the intestine above an obstruction becomes markedly distended and edematous, peristaltic sounds may lose the characteristics of borborygmi and become weak or absent even when peritonitis is not present. It is usually the severe chemical peritonitis of sudden onset which is associated with the truly silent abdomen. Assessment of the patient's state of hydration is important. The hematocrit and urinalysis permit an accurate estimate of the severity of dehydration, so that adequate replacement can be carried out.

Laboratory examinations may be of enormous value in the assessment of the patient with abdominal pain, yet with but a few exceptions they rarely establish a diagnosis. Leukocytosis should never be the single deciding factor as to whether or not operation is indicated. A white blood cell count greater than 20,000 per cubic millimeter may be observed with perforation of a viscus, but pancreatitis, acute cholecystitis, pelvic inflammatory disease, and intestinal infarction may be associated with marked leukocytosis. A normal white blood cell count is by no means rare in cases of perforation of abdominal viscera. The diagnosis of anemia may be more helpful than the white blood cell count, especially when combined with the history.

The urinalysis is also of great value in indicating to some degree the state of hydration or to rule out severe renal disease, diabetes, or urinary infection. Determination of the blood urea nitrogen, blood sugar, and serum bilirubin levels may also be helpful. The serum amylase determination is overrated, since in carefully controlled series of patients with proven pancreatitis where the determination has been done within the first 72 h, amylase was less than 200 Somogyi units in one-third of the cases, between 200 and 500 in another one-third of the cases, and greater than 500 in one-third. Since many diseases other than pancreatitis, e.g., perforated ulcer, strangulating intestinal obstruction, and acute cholecystitis, may be associated with very marked increase in the serum amylase, great care must be exercised in denying an operation to a patient solely on the basis of an elevated serum amylase level. The determination of the serum lipase may have a somewhat greater accuracy than the serum amylase.

Peritoneal lavage is a safe and effective diagnostic maneuver in patients with acute abdominal pain. It is of special value in patients with blunt trauma to the abdomen in whom evaluation of the abdomen may be difficult because of other multiple injuries to the spine, pelvis, or ribs and in whom blood in the peritoneal cavity produces only a very mild peritoneal reaction. The gallbladder is the only organ which may continue to seep fluid following accidental perforation, so that the region of this organ must be assiduously avoided. Determination of the pH of the aspirated fluid to ascertain the site of a perforation is misleading, because even highly acid gastric juice is rapidly buffered by peritoneal exudate.

Plain and upright or lateral decubitus roentgenograms of the abdomen may be of the greatest value. They are usually unnecessary in patients with acute appendicitis or strangulated external hernias. However, in cases of intestinal obstruction, perforated ulcer, and a variety of other conditions, films may be diagnostic. During a search for free air, the patient should be kept in the decubitus or upright position for at least 10 min before the appropriate film is taken lest a small pneumoperitoneum be missed. In rare instances, barium or water-soluble medium examination of the upper part of the gastrointestinal tract may demonstrate partial intestinal obstruction which may elude diagnosis by other means. If there is any question of obstruction of the colon, oral administration of barium sulfate should be avoided. On the other hand, barium enema is of inestimable value in cases of colonic obstruction and should be used with greater frequency where the possibility of perforation does not exist. Ultrasound recently has proved to be useful in detecting an enlarged gallbladder or pancreas, the presence of gallstones, or a localized collection of fluid or pus. Radioisotopic scans (HIDA) may help differentiate acute cholecystitis from acute pancreatitis.

Sometimes, even under the best of circumstances with all available auxiliary aids and with the greatest of clinical skill, a definitive diagnosis cannot be established at the time of the initial examination. Nevertheless, despite lack of a clear anatomic diagnosis it may be abundantly clear to an experienced and thoughtful physician and surgeon that on clinical grounds alone operation is indicated. Should that decision be questionable, watchful waiting with repeated questioning and examination will often elucidate the true nature of the illness and indicate the proper course of action.

REFERENCES

De Dombal FT: Acute abdominal pain. Scand J Gastroenterol (Suppl) 14:29, 1979

Lee PWR: The plain x-ray in the acute abdomen: A surgeon's evaluation. Br J Surg 63:763, 1976

Leek BF: Abdominal and pelvic visceral receptors. Br Med Bull 33:163, 1977

Silen W: *Cope's Early Diagnosis of the Acute Abdomen*, 16th ed. London, Oxford Press, 1983

Staniland JR et al: Clinical presentation of acute abdomen: Study of 600 patients. Br Med J 2:393, 1972

Valman HB: Acute abdominal pain. Br Med J 282:1858, 1981

6 HEADACHE

RAYMOND D. ADAMS / JOSEPH B. MARTIN

The term *headache* should encompass all aches and pains located in the head, but in common language its application is restricted to unpleasant sensations in the region of the cranial vault. Facial, pharyngeal, laryngeal, and cervical pain are described in Chaps. 7 and 352. (See also Table 6-1.)

Headache represents one of the most frequent human discomforts. Its significance is often abstruse, for it may signal serious disease or represent only tension or fatigue. Fortunately, in most instances it reflects the latter, and only exceptionally does it warn of an intracranial abnormality. But it is this dual significance, the benign and the potentially malignant, that should keep the physician on the alert. Systematic approach to the headache problem necessitates a broad knowledge of medical and surgical diseases of which it is a symptom and a clinical methodology which leaves none of the common and treatable causes unexplored.

GENERAL CONSIDERATIONS The quality, location, duration, and time course of the headache and conditions which produce, exacerbate, or relieve it should be carefully reviewed. Unfortunately, except in special circumstances such as temporal arteritis, physical examination of the head itself is seldom useful.

The patient is rarely helpful in describing the *quality* of cephalic pain. In fact persistent questioning on that point occasions surprise, for the patient usually assumes that the word *headache* conveys adequate information about the nature of the discomfort. Most headaches are dull, deeply located, and of aching character. Occasionally superficial burning or stinging pain localized to the skin is reported. The patient may make allusion to tightness, pressure, or a bursting feeling, terms which may give clues to muscular tension or psychologic state.

Queries about the *intensity* of the pain are seldom of value since they reflect more the patient's attitude toward the condition than the true severity. The stoical person tends to minimize discomfort, whereas the neurotic or depressed patient dramatizes it. Degree of incapacity is a better index. A severe migraine attack seldom allows performance of the day's work. The pain which awakens the patient from sleep at night, or prevents sleep, is also more likely to have a demonstrable organic basis. As a rule, the most intense cranial pains are those that accompany subarachnoid hemorrhage and meningitis, which have grave implications, or migraine and paroxysmal nocturnal *cluster* headaches, which are benign.

Data regarding *location* of the headache are often informative. If the source is in extracranial structures, as is usually the case, the correspondence with the site of the pain is fairly precise. Inflammation of an extracranial artery causes pain localized to the site of the vessel. Lesions of paranasal sinuses, teeth, eyes, and upper cervical vertebrae induce a less sharply localized pain, but one that is still referred in a regional distribution that is fairly constant. Intracranial lesions in the posterior fossa cause pain in the occipital-nuchal region, homolateral if the lesion is one-sided. Supratentorial lesions induce frontotemporal pains, again homolateral to the lesion if it is on one side. But localization can also be very uninformative or misleading. Ear pain, for example, although it may mean disease in the ear, more often is referred from other regions such as the neck, and eye pain may be referred to the occiput or cervical spine.

Duration and *time-intensity curve* of headaches both during the attack itself and in their life profile are most useful. The headache of bacterial meningitis or subarachnoid hemorrhage occurs usually in single attacks over a period of days. Single, brief, momentary (1 to 2 s) pains in the cranium (icepick-like headaches) are common but uninterpretable and rarely indicate serious underlying disease. Migraine of the classic type has its onset in the early morning hours or daytime, reaches its peak of severity in a half hour or so, lasts, unless treated, for several hours up to 1 to 2 days, is often accompanied by nausea or vomiting, and is terminated by sleep. A frequency of more than a single attack every few weeks is exceptional. A migraine patient having several attacks per week usually proves to have a combination of migraine and tension headaches. In contrast to this is the nightly occurrence (2 to 3 h after onset of sleep) over a period of several weeks to months of the rapidly peaking, nonthrobbing orbital or supraorbital pain of cluster headache, which tends to dissipate within an hour. The headache of intracranial tumor characteristically can occur at any time of day or night, can interrupt sleep, varies in intensity, and lasts a few minutes to hours. The natural history is one of increasing frequency and intensity over a period of months. Tension headache, once commenced, may persist continuously for weeks or months, often waxing and waning from hour to hour or day to day.

Headache that bears a more or less constant relationship to certain biologic events and also to physical environmental changes may prove to be informative. Premenstrual headaches, most typically of migrainous or tension type, may occur as part of the premenstrual syndrome; they usually vanish after the first day of vaginal bleeding. The headaches of cervical arthritis are most typically intense after a period of inactivity, and the first movements in the morning are both difficult and painful. Hypertensive headaches, like those of cerebral tumor, tend to occur on waking in the morning, but, as with all vascular headaches, excitement and tension may provoke them. Headache from infection of nasal sinuses may appear, with clocklike regularity, upon awakening and in midmorning, and is characteristically worsened by stooping and jarring of the head. Eyestrain headaches naturally follow prolonged use of the eyes, as in reading, peering for a long time against glaring headlights in traffic, or watching a movie. Atmospheric cold may evoke pain in the so-called fibrositic or nodular headache or when the underlying condition is arthritic or neuralgic. Anger, excitement, or irritation may initiate common migraine in certain disposed persons; this is more typical of common migraine than of the classic type. Change of position, stooping, straining, cough, and sexual intercourse are each known to produce a special type of headache, described below. Exertional headaches, another well-known type, are usually benign (only 1 in 10 will have an intracranial lesion) and disappear within weeks to months.

PAIN-SENSITIVE STRUCTURES OF THE HEAD Understanding of headache has been greatly augmented by observations made during surgery of pain-sensitive structures. The following are sensitive to mechanical stimulation: (1) skin, subcutaneous tissue, muscles, arteries, and periosteum of skull; (2) tissues of the eye, ear, and nasal and sinus cavities; (3) intracranial venous sinuses and their tributary veins; (4) parts of the dura at the base of the brain and the arteries within the dura mater and pia-arachnoid; and (5) the trigeminal, glossopharyngeal, vagus, and first three cervical nerves. Interestingly, pain is practically the only sensation produced by stimulation of these structures. The bony skull, much of the pia-arachnoid and dura, and the parenchyma of the brain lack sensitivity.

Sensory stimuli from the head are conveyed to the central nervous system via the trigeminal nerves for structures above the tentorium in the anterior and middle fossae of the skull, and the first three cervical nerves for those in the posterior fossa and infradural structures. The ninth and tenth cranial nerves supply part of the posterior fossa and refer the pain to the ear and throat. The pain of intracranial disease is commonly referred to a part of the cranium lying within the areas supplied by these nerves. There may be associated local tenderness of the scalp at the site of reference. Dental or jaw pain may also have cranial reference. The pain of disease in other parts of the body is not referred to the head, although it may initiate headache by other means.

Headache can occur as a result of (1) distention, traction, or dilatation of intracranial or extracranial arteries, (2) traction or displacement of large intracranial veins or of their dural envelope, (3) compression, traction, or inflammation of cranial and spinal nerves, (4) voluntary or involuntary spasm, inflammation, and trauma to cranial and cervical muscles, and (5) meningeal irritation and raised intracranial pressure. More specifically, intracranial mass lesions cause headache only if they deform, displace, or exert traction on vessels, dural structures, or cranial nerves at the base of the brain, and this may happen long before intracranial pressure rises. Raised intracranial pressure causes headache in a bioccipital or bifrontal distribution which is rapidly relieved by lumbar puncture and lowering of the cerebrospinal fluid (CSF) pressure.

Dilatation of the extracranial, temporal, and intracranial *arteries* with stretching of surrounding sensitive structures is believed to be the mechanism of most of the pain of migraine. Extracranial, temporal, and occipital arteries, when involved in giant cell arteritis (cranial or "temporal" arteritis), a disease which usually afflicts individuals over 50 years of age, give rise to headache of dull aching and throbbing type, at first localized and then more diffuse. Characteristically it is severe and persistent over a period of weeks or months. The offending artery, strangely, is not always tender to pressure, yet section of it, as in biopsy, may relieve the pain (Chap. 269). Evolving atherosclerotic thrombosis of internal carotid, anterior, and middle cerebral arteries is sometimes accompanied by pain in the forehead or temple; with vertebral artery thrombosis the pain is postauricular, and basilar artery thrombosis causes referred pain in the occiput and sometimes the forehead.

In *infection or blockage of paranasal sinuses,* pain is usually felt over the antrum or in the forehead; with the *ethmoid* and *sphenoid sinuses,* the pain localizes around the eyes on one or both sides or in the vertex. Usually it is associated with tenderness of the skin in the same distribution. The pain may have two remarkable properties: (1) When throbbing, it may be abolished by compressing the carotid artery on the same side. (2) It tends to recur and subside at the same hours, i.e., on awakening, with gradual disappearance when the person is upright, and coming again in the late morning hours. The time relations are believed to yield information concerning the mechanism; morning pain is ascribed to the sinuses filling at night, and its relief on arising to emptying after the erect posture has been assumed. Stooping, blowing the nose, and jarring the head intensify the pain; and inhalant sympathomimetic drugs such as phenylephrine, which reduce swelling and congestion, tend to relieve the pain. Sinus pain may persist after all purulent secretions have disappeared, probably because of persistent blockage of the draining orifices eliciting a vacuum or suction effect on the sinus wall (*vacuum sinus headaches*). The condition is relieved when aeration is restored. During air flights both earache and sinus headache tend to occur on descent, when the relative pressure in the blocked viscus falls.

Headache of ocular origin is usually located in the orbit, forehead, or temple, and has a steady, aching quality which may follow prolonged use of the eyes in close work. Ocular muscle imbalance, hyperopia, astigmatism, and impaired convergence and accommodation may give rise to sustained contraction of extraocular as well as frontal, temporal, and even occipital muscles. Raised intraocular pressure in acute glaucoma or iridocyclitis causes steady, aching pain felt in the eye. When intense, it may radiate throughout the distribution of the ophthalmic division of the trigeminal nerve. The pain of diabetic third nerve palsy, intracranial aneurysm, pituitary tumor,

TABLE 6-1 Common types of headache

Type	Site	Age and sex	Clinical characteristics	Diurnal pattern	Life profile
Common migraine	Frontotemporal Uni- or bilateral	Children, young to middle-aged adults, both sexes, female > male	Throbbing and/or dull ache; worse behind one eye or ear, nausea or vomiting Becomes generalized	Upon awakening or later in day Duration: hours to 1–2 days	Irregular interval, weeks to months Tends to disappear in middle age and during pregnancy
Classic migraine	Same as above	Same as above	Same as above; visual prodrome common.	Same as above	Same as above
Cluster, histamine headache, or migrainous neuralgia	Orbital Temporal Unilateral	Adolescent and adult males (80–90%)	Intense, nonthrobbing pain	Usually nocturnal; occurs one or more hours after falling asleep Rarely diurnal	Nightly for several weeks to months (cluster) Recurrence: years later
Tension headaches	Generalized	Children, adolescents, and adults, both sexes	Pressure (nonthrobbing); tightness Aching	Continuous, variable intensity, for weeks and months	One or more periods of months to years
Meningeal irritation (meningitis, subarachnoid hemorrhage)	Generalized	Any age, both sexes	Intense, steady deep pain, may be worse in neck	Duration: days to a week or more	Single episode
Brain tumor	(See text)	Any age, both sexes	Variable in intensity May awaken patient Steady pain	Lasts minutes to hours; increasing severity	Once in a lifetime: weeks to months
Temporal arteritis	Unilateral, temporal, or occipital	Over 50 years, either sex	Persistent burning, aching	Continuous or intermittent	Persists for weeks to a few months

SOURCE: *After J Patten, Neurological Differential Diagnosis, London, Harold Starke, Springer-Verlag, 1977.*

cavernous sinus thrombosis, and Raeder's paratrigeminal syndrome is often referred to the eye.

The *headaches accompanying disease of ligaments, muscles, and apophyseal joints* in the upper part of the spine, which are referred to occipital and upper cervical regions, are difficult to separate from the more common muscular contraction (tension) headaches. Such referred pains are especially frequent in middle and late adult life in patients with rheumatoid arthritis and cervical spondylosis and tend also to occur after whiplash injuries to the neck. If the pain is articular or synovial in origin, the first movements after being still for some hours are both stiff and painful. In fact, evocation of pain by active and passive motion of the spine should indicate traumatic or other disease of movable parts. The pain of *myofibrositis,* evidenced by tender nodules near the cranial insertion of cervical and other muscles, is more obscure. There are no pathologic data as to the nature of these vaguely palpable lesions, and it is uncertain whether the pain actually arises in them. They may represent only the deep tenderness felt in the region of referred pain or the involuntary secondary protective spasm of muscles. Characteristically, the pain is steady (nonthrobbing) and spreads from one to both sides of the head. Exposure to cold or draft may precipitate it. Though severe at times, it seldom prevents sleep. Massage of muscles and heat have unpredictable effects but relieve the pain in some cases.

The *headache of meningeal irritation* (infection or hemorrhage) is acute in onset, severe, generalized, deep-seated, constant, especially intense at the base of the skull, and associated with stiffness of neck on bending forward. Dilatation and congestion of inflamed meningeal vessels are likely the main cause of the pain.

Lumbar puncture headache is characterized by a steady occipital-nuchal or bifrontal pain that comes on a few minutes after arising from a recumbent position and is relieved within a few minutes by lying down. Its cause is persistent leakage of CSF into the lumbar tissues through the needle site. The CSF pressure is low. The headache is usually increased by compression of the jugular veins and is unaffected by digital obliteration of one carotid artery. It is probable that in the upright position a low intraspinal and negative intracranial pressure exerts traction on dural attachments and dural sinuses by caudal displacement of the brain. Understandably, then, headache following cisternal puncture is rare. As soon as the leakage of CSF stops and CSF pressure is gradually restored (usually from a few days up to a week or so), the headache disappears. "Spontaneous" low-pressure headache may also follow a sneeze or strain, presumably because of rupture of the spinal arachnoid along a nerve root.

The mechanism of the *throbbing or steady headache which accompanies febrile illnesses,* located in frontal or occipital regions or generalized, is probably vascular. It is much like histamine headache in being relieved on one side by carotid artery compression and on both sides by jugular vein compression or the subarachnoid injection of saline solution. It is increased by shaking the head. It seems probable that the meningeal vessels pulsate unduly and stretch pain-sensitive structures around the base of the brain. In certain cases, however, the pain may be lessened by compression of temporal arteries, and in these cases a component of the headache seems to be derived from the walls of extracranial arteries, as in migraine.

The so-called *tension headaches* of patients with anxiety states and depression are allegedly due to chronic spasm of cranial and cervical muscles. Combinations of the tension and vascular headaches give rise to the "mixed headaches" so common in many patients.

PRINCIPAL CLINICAL VARIETIES OF HEADACHE Usually there is no difficulty in diagnosing the headache of glaucoma, purulent sinusitis, bacterial meningitis, and brain tumor, and a fuller account of these special headaches will be found where these diseases are described in other sections of the book. It is when headache is

Provoking factors	Associated features	Treatment
Bright light, noise, tension, alcohol Dark room and sleep relieve Scalp sensitive Pressure helps	Nausea in some cases	Ergot preparation at onset Phenergan in established phase Inderal and Bellergal Methysergide for prevention
Same as above	Blindness and scintillating lights Unilateral numbness Disturbed speech Vertigo Confusion	Same as above
Alcohol in some	Lacrimation, congested eye	Ergot preparation at bedtime Amitriptyline and lithium carbonate for prevention
Fatigue and nervous strain	Depression, nervousness, anxiety, insomnia	Antianxiety and antidepressant drugs
None	Neck stiff on forward bending Kernig and Brudzinski signs	For meningitis or bleeding (see text)
None Sometimes position	Papilledema Vomiting Slow mentation	Corticosteroids Mannitol Glycerol Treatment of tumor
Scalp sensitive Tender arteries	Intermittent or permanent loss of sight Rheumatic myalgia Fever	Corticosteroid therapy

chronic, recurrent, and unattended by other important signs of disease that the physician faces one of the most difficult medical problems.

The types of headache subsequently described should then be considered.

Migraine The term *migraine* refers to periodic, hemicranial, throbbing headaches often accompanied by nausea and vomiting which usually begin in childhood, adolescence, or early adult life and recur in diminishing number and intensity during advancing years. Migraine is frequent, with a prevalence of 20 to 30 percent in the population. Women are affected three times as often as men. There is a tendency for the headaches to occur during the period of premenstrual tension and fluid retention and to decrease during pregnancy. The immediate family history is positive for migraine in over 60 percent of cases. Migraine or vascular headaches present in one of four clinical patterns: (1) classic migraine, (2) common migraine, (3) complicated migraine, and (4) cluster headache.

Classic migraine begins with a prodrome of prominent neurologic symptoms such as visual scintillations, dazzling zigzag lines (fortification spectra), photophobia and spreading scotomas, or dizziness and tinnitus. Classic migraine may be heralded hours before the attack by premonitory symptoms, most commonly a feeling of elation, excessive energy, thirst, a craving for sweet foods, or drowsiness. At other times, there may be a slowing of mentation or a feeling of impending doom or of depression, or there may be no warning whatsoever. The disturbance of vision that commences the attack may be followed by homonymous hemianopic field defects; sometimes they are bilateral, and even total blindness may rarely occur.

In *common migraine* there is an unheralded onset of headache, often with nausea and sometimes vomiting, following the same temporal pattern but without the antecedent neurologic symptoms.

Both of these headache syndromes respond to ergot preparations, if administered early in the attack. A genetic basis is suggested by history of headaches in near relatives in over 50 percent of cases.

Complicated migraine refers to headaches accompanied by neurologic symptoms that may either precede or accompany the headache. Numbness and tingling of the lips, face, hand, and leg on one side may occur, sometimes in combination with an aphasic disorder. The arm and leg may become weak or paralyzed on one side, mimicking a stroke. The numbness or weakness spreads from one part of the body to another slowly over a period of minutes. Full recovery usually occurs. However, permanent deficits consisting of hemianopia (lesion in distribution of the posterior cerebral artery), hemiplegia or hemianesthesia (lesion in territory of middle cerebral artery), or ophthalmoplegia (usually third nerve lesion) may occur.

Several other neurologic syndromes have been delineated in association with complicated migraine. Bickerstaff first called attention to *basilar migraine,* in which the visual disorder and paresthesias are bilateral and are accompanied by confusion, stupor, rarely coma, aggressive outbursts, vertigo, diplopia, and dysarthria. While the full syndrome is infrequent, partial basilar syndromes are found in some 30 percent of children with migraine. Alternating hemiplegias in children have also been attributed to basilar migraine but could as well be due to alternating involvement of the middle cerebral arteries.

It is also recognized that neurologic syndromes may occur due to migraine which are not followed by headache. In children, abdominal pain and vomiting, sometimes cyclical, may occur without headache as the sole expression of migraine; the same is true of some cases of paroxysmal vertigo in children. Such *migraine equivalents* may be manifest as pain localized in the thorax, pelvis, or extremities; bouts of fever; paroxysmal vertigo; transient disturbances in mood (psychic equivalents). The first neurologic syndrome due to migraine may occur in late adult life in a person not previously known to have migraine. Fisher refers to these as *transient migrainous accompaniments* to distinguish them from transient cerebral ischemic attacks (TIAs).

Cluster headache, also called paroxysmal nocturnal cephalalgia, migrainous neuralgia, histamine headache, and Horton's syndrome, has a fourfold higher incidence in men than in women. It is characterized by constant, unilateral orbital pain, with onset usually within 2 or 3 h after falling asleep. It tends to occur during the phase of rapid eye movement (REM) sleep. The pain is intense and steady (nonthrobbing) with lacrimation, blocked nostril, then rhinorrhea, and sometimes miosis, ptosis, flush, and edema of cheek, all lasting approximately an hour or two. It tends to recur nightly for several weeks or a few months (hence the term *cluster*), followed by complete freedom for years. The pain of a given attack may leave as rapidly as it began. Clusters may recur over the years, being possibly more likely in times of stress, prolonged strain, overwork, and with upsetting emotional experiences. Episodes of cluster headache lasting 2 to 3 weeks may recur several times over a lifetime. Often the pain involves the same orbit in each cluster. Occasionally alcohol, nitroglycerin, or tyramine-containing foods precipitate an attack. Rarely, the condition may occur in daytime and may not cluster but continue for years. The picture is so characteristic that its presentation is diagnostic, though to those unfamiliar with it the possibility of a carotid aneurysm, hemangioma, brain tumor, or sinusitis may be suggested.

The relationship of the cluster headache to migraine remains conjectural. A portion of the cases have a background of migraine, which led to the earlier postulation of migrainous neuralgia, but the majority do not.

MECHANISM AND PATHOPHYSIOLOGY A satisfactory theory of the pathophysiology of migraine has eluded clinical investigators. Certain facts appear indisputable; the symptoms of migraine are associated with changes in cerebral blood flow, presumably secondary to changes in vessel caliber; the prodromal phase with neurologic symptoms is accompanied by arteriolar constriction and decreased cerebral blood flow beginning most often in the posterior part of the brain; the decrease in cerebral blood flow in migraine proceeds at a rate of about 2 mm/min, resembling the spreading depression originally described by Leão, which is characterized by a transient self-propagating perturbation of brain electrical activity followed by hypoperfusion. Less certain is the assumption that the headache that follows is due to vascular dilatation, since direct measurements of cerebral blood flow during the headache phase fail to show significant increases. In the studies reported by Lauritzen and coworkers regional cerebral blood flow, measured by xenon 133, showed oligemic regions of cortex during migraine attacks with diminished reactivity to carbon dioxide, suggesting an abnormality of vessel responses. Between attacks of migraine, patients had normal regulation of brain circulation.

The factors that elicit these changes in cerebral blood flow are unknown. Two general hypotheses about the cause of migraine have emerged. The first is that it is due to a central nervous system neurovascular disorder that triggers alterations in vasomotor regulation. The premonitory symptoms of changes in mood, appetite, and thirst have led some to consider a central hypothalamic disorder to be the cause. The second considers migraine to be a systemic metabolic disregulation with attacks elicited secondary to intravascular events associated with changes in serotonin metabolism. Changes in platelet serotonin levels, shown to fall during the attack, accompanied by increased urinary excretion of serotonin and of 5-hydroxyindoleacetic acid support the contention that migraine is a systemic disorder. Further support for a role of serotonin comes from observations that reserpine, which triggers serotonin release, causes migraine in some patients and that antiserotonin drugs, like methysergide, show some success in its treatment. However, there is difficulty in understanding how changes in intravascular serotonin, which has little direct effect on vessel contraction, can induce the changes of migraine. Lance considers the mechanism of migraine to involve changes in biogenic amine or neuropeptide neurotransmitters in the central nervous system, associated with or followed by platelet release reactions. Recent work has focused on the neurotransmitters found in nerve fibers that innervate cerebral blood vessels. Moskowitz has demonstrated that cerebral vessels are innervated by nerves that contain substance P, a peptide important for pain transmission (see Chap. 3) and also thought to be capable of eliciting local tissue reactions resembling inflammation. Other neuropeptides found in cerebral blood vessels and known to affect vascular tone include vasoactive intestinal polypeptide, neurotensin, and neuropeptide Y.

There is persistent debate concerning factors that trigger the migraine attacks. Dietary factors are likely important in some patients. Monro and coworkers identified sensitivity to milk and wheat products in patients with severe refractory migraine. Many patients learn to avoid alcohol (particularly red wine), chocolate, coffee, tea, or other agents with pharmacologically active ingredients. How these substances elicit the attacks is unknown. Some patients describe exposure to sunlight, exercise, tension, or the use of oral contraceptives as increasing the frequency and severity of migraine.

DIFFERENTIAL DIAGNOSIS Classic migraine usually causes no difficulty in diagnosis. Difficulties arise from two sources: (1) ignorance of the fact that a progressively unfolding neurologic syndrome may be migrainous in origin, and (2) lack of appreciation that the neurologic disorder may occur without headache.

The neurologic symptoms of the migraine syndrome may resemble focal epilepsy, the clinical picture of a vascular malformation such as an angioma or aneurysm, or some other vascular disease such as a thrombotic or embolic stroke. The pace of the neurologic symptoms of migraine, rather than their character, reliably distinguishes them from epilepsy. The clinical profile of the aura of epilepsy is measured in seconds, for it depends on spreading neural excitation, in contrast to the slow progression of migraine, which is based on spreading depression of nervous tissue. Nevertheless, there are instances where episodes of coma with electroencephalogram (EEG) abnormality may be either migraine or epilepsy. Furthermore, a seizure is often followed by a generalized headache.

Ophthalmoplegic migraine always suggests a carotid aneurysm, and carotid arteriography may be necessary to exclude it. Despite many claims that vascular malformations may cause hemicranial pain occurring invariably on the same side of the head (unlike migraine), larger series of cases have shown this only rarely to be the case. Focal epilepsy, protracted headache, stiff neck and bloody CSF, a persistent neurologic deficit, and cranial bruit are indicative of a vascular type of headache associated with angioma or aneurysm. Only in the earlier stages, when periodic throbbing headache is the sole symptom, are these conditions confused with true migraine.

Tension headache The tension headache is usually bilateral, often with diffuse extension over the top of the cranium. Occipital-nuchal or bifrontal localization is common. Although the sensation may be described as pain, close questioning may uncover other sensations, viz., fullness, tightness, or pressure (as if the head is surrounded by a band or in a vise), on which waves of aching pain are superimposed. The onset of a given attack is more gradual than in migraine and not infrequently a throbbing "vascular" type of headache is described. Tension headache may occur acutely under conditions of emotional duress or intense worry and lasts for hours or a day or two. More often it persists unremittingly for weeks or months. In fact, this is the only type of headache that exhibits the peculiarity of being absolutely continuous day and night for long periods of time. Although sleep may be possible, whenever the patient awakens, the headache is present; a common feature is the finding that analgesic remedies have relatively little effect in alleviating the pain. In contrast to migraine, in which pain is periodic and lifelong, with tendency to lessen in late adult years, tension headache occurs more often in middle age and may persist for many years.

It is unlikely that the origin of the pain is sustained muscle activity, since electromyographic (EMG) investigations show no changes in forehead or neck muscles. On the other hand, elicitation of headache after administration of amyl nitrite, a vasodilator, in about 50 percent of patients suggests a vascular contribution to the pain. Histamine can also cause headaches in these patients.

It is a common experience for both tension headache and common migraine to coexist in the same patient. The management of such patients may require therapy of both types of headache.

Psychologic studies of groups of patients with tension headaches have revealed prominent symptoms of depression, anxiety, and in some hypochrondriasis. Kudrow records that 65 percent of depressed patients have this type of headache and that over 60 percent of his patients with tension headaches were depressed.

Headache of angioma and aneurysm The temporal profile of any given attack shows the onset to be sudden or very acute, with the pain reaching a peak within minutes. Neurologic disturbances such as defects in vision, unilateral numbness, weakness, or aphasia may precede or occur after the onset of headache and outlast it. Should hemorrhage occur, the headache is often extremely severe and localizes in the occiput and neck, lasting many days in association with stiff neck. A cranial or cervical bruit and the presence of blood in the CSF establish the diagnosis. The claim that vascular malformations may give rise to migraine is probably untenable. Statistical data show migraine to be no more frequent in this group of patients than in the general population. Vascular lesions may exist for long periods of time without headache, or headache may develop many years after other manifestations such as epilepsy and hemiplegia (see Chap. 343).

Traumatic headaches Severe, chronic, continuous, or intermittent headaches often associated with giddiness, vertigo, or tinnitus appear as the cardinal symptoms of the posttraumatic syndrome. The cause of the headache is unknown, but it is a clear-cut disorder unrelated in most instances to medicolegal issues of compensation. *Posttraumatic dysautonomic cephalalgia* is a term given by Vijayan and Dreyfus to severe, episodic, throbbing, unilateral headaches accompanied by ipsilateral mydriasis and excessive facial sweating. The condition follows injury to the neck in the region of the carotid sheath. It was postulated that the sympathetic nervous supply of the cranium had been disinhibited, and there was clinical and pharmacologic evidence of sympathetic dysfunction (see Chap. 344).

Headache and dizziness of fluctuating severity, followed by drowsiness, stupor, coma, and hemiparesis, are the usual manifestations of *chronic subdural hematoma.* The head injury may have been minor and forgotten by patient and family. The headaches are deep-seated, steady, unilateral or generalized, and respond to the usual analgesic drugs. The typical attack profile of the headache and other symptoms is one of increasing frequency and severity over several weeks or months. Diagnosis is established by computerized tomography (CT) scan and arteriography (see Chap. 344).

Headaches of brain tumor Headache is the outstanding symptom of cerebral tumor. Unfortunately, the quality of the pain has no specific feature. It tends to be deep-seated, nonthrobbing (or throbbing), and aching or bursting. Attacks last a few minutes to an hour or more and occur once or many times during the day. Activity and, frequently, change in the position of the head may provoke pain, while rest in bed diminishes its frequency. Nocturnal awakening because of pain, although typical, is by no means diagnostic. Unexpected forceful (projectile) vomiting may punctuate the illness in its later stages. As the tumor grows, the pain becomes more frequent and severe; it sometimes is nearly continuous terminally. If unilateral, the headache is homolateral to the tumor in 9 out of 10 patients. Supratentorial tumors are felt anterior to the interauricular circumference of the skull; posterior fossa tumors behind this line. Bifrontal and bioccipital headache, coming on after unilateral headache, signifies the development of increased intracranial pressure.

Headaches related to medical disorders Experienced physicians are aware of many conditions in which headache figures as a dominant symptom. These include fevers of any cause, carbon monoxide exposure, chronic lung disease with hypercapnia (headaches often nocturnal), hypothyroidism, Cushing's syndrome, withdrawal of corticosteroid medication, chronic nitrite or ergot exposure, occasionally Addison's disease, aldosterone-producing adrenal tumors, use of contraceptive medications, acute rises in blood pressure, e.g., from pheochromocytoma, and acute anemia with hemoglobin below 10 g. Hypertension per se is an uncommon cause of headache.

Unusual types of headache Sharp, jabbing pains in the head (icepick-like pains) last a second or two, and have no clinical significance. They are reported in up to 3 percent of the normal population and in 46 percent of migrainous patients. The pain is usually felt in the temporal or orbital region.

Cough and exertional headache or headache brought on by stooping follows the initiating action by a few seconds and lasts a minute or two. Usually no explanation is apparent, but exceptionally it occurs in patients with arteriovenous malformations, Paget's disease of the skull, Arnold-Chiari malformation, or an intracranial tumor. In a series of 103 patients followed for 3 years or longer by Rooke only 10 developed neurologic signs. The mechanism of this headache may be venous distention, for jugular compression has induced it in some of our patients. Lance has described a generalized headache that begins suddenly during coitus usually at the time of orgasm. It may last minutes or hours. Most of his 21 patients were males.

Erythrocyanotic headache is a rare form of generalized throbbing headache which occurs in conjunction with flushing of the face and hands and numbness of the fingers (erythromelalgia). The condition has been reported in association with (a) mastocytosis (infiltration of tissues with mast cells, which elaborate histamine, heparin, and serotonin); (b) carcinoid tumors; (c) some tumors of pancreatic islets; (d) pheochromocytoma.

HEADACHE AND FACIAL PAIN The facial neuralgias are discussed in Chap. 352 (see Table 6-2).

APPROACH TO THE PATIENT WITH HEADACHE Obviously very different possibilities are raised by a patient who presents for the first time with severe headache and a patient who has had recurrent headache over a period of years. The chances of uncovering the cause in the first instance are much greater than in the second and in the former the underlying conditions (meningitis, subarachnoid hemorrhage, epidural or subdural hematoma, glaucoma, and purulent sinusitis) often are more serious. In general, severe, persistent headache with stiff neck and fever means meningitis, and the same combination without fever, subarachnoid hemorrhage. A lumbar puncture is mandatory. Acute persistent headache over a period of hours or days may occur in systemic infections such as influenza (febrile) or as a manifestation of an acute tension state. If there is a diagnosable febrile disease and no stiffness of the neck, lumbar puncture may be deferred. The first attack of migraine may also present in this way, but of course there is no fever.

In searching for the cause of recurrent headache one should investigate the status of cardiovascular and renal systems by blood pressure and urine examination, eyes by fundoscopy, intraocular pressure, and refraction, the sinuses by transillumination and x-rays, the cranial arteries by palpation (and biopsy?), the cervical spine by the effect of passive movement of the head and x-rays, the nervous system by neurologic examination, and psychic function by mental status.

Hypertension is frequent in the general population and is not often a cause of recurrent headaches. Severe hypertension with diastolic blood pressures of over 110 mmHg may be associated with headache. If headache is severe and frequent, the possibilities of underlying anxiety or tension state or a common migraine syndrome should be considered.

The adolescent with daily frontal headaches represents a special type of problem. Often the relationship of the headaches to eyestrain is unclear, and refraction of the eyes and new eyeglasses do not relieve the condition. Anxiety or tension is probably a factor in such cases, but it is difficult to be certain of a causal relationship. Some of the most persistent and inexplicable headaches, which have led to a survey by a battery of diagnostic procedures for tumor, have proved in the end to be associated with endogenous depression.

Equally puzzling is the somber, tense adult whose primary complaint is headache, or the migrainous person who in late life or at menopause begins to have daily headaches. Here it becomes important to assess mental status along the lines suggested in Chaps. 11 and 23, looking for evidences of anxiety, depression, and hypochondriasis. The quality and persistence of the headache are suggestive of the possibility of psychiatric illness. Sometimes a direct question as to the patient's idea of what is the matter may elicit suspicion and fear of brain tumor. Antidepressant drugs given as an empirical test may relieve the headache, thus clarifying the diagnosis.

The most worrisome type of patient is the one who has headache of increasing frequency and severity over a period of months or a year or so. Since an intracranial mass lesion (tumor, abscess, subdural hematoma) is a leading possibility, a complete neurologic survey, including careful inspection of optic discs, CT scan, and electroencephalogram, should be performed.

Every person over 50 to 55 years with severe headache of some few days' or weeks' duration should be considered as possibly having cranial arteritis (see Chap. 269). The overall incidence in patients over 50 years is 1 in 750; that of polymyalgia rheumatica in the same age group is 1 in 200. Women are more often affected than men (4:1), and there is an associated polymyalgia in 25 percent of cases. Conversely, in 50 percent of polymyalgia rheumatica patients there is a cranial arteritis. Increased sedimentation rate, fever, and anemia may occur. The findings of a thickened, tender temporal artery and claudication of jaw muscles from involvement of facial arteries are important. The disease may cause blindness and/or ophthalmoplegia but rarely involves intracranial arteries. Arterial biopsy and response to corticosteroids establish the diagnosis.

TREATMENT The most important steps in the treatment of headache are those measures which uncover and remove the underlying disease or functional disturbance.

For the *common everyday headache* due to fatigue, acute stress, or excessive use of alcohol and tobacco, the physician advises

TABLE 6-2 Types of facial pain

Types	Site	Clinical characteristics	Aggravating-relieving factors	Diseases	Treatment
Trigeminal neuralgia (tic douloureux)	Second to third division of trigeminal nerve, unilateral	Men : women = 1:3 Over 50 years Paroxysms (10–30 s) of stabbing, burning pain Trigger points, intermittent ache No sensory or motor paralysis	Touching face, chewing, smiling, talking, blowing nose	Idiopathic If in young adults unilateral or bilateral, multiple sclerosis Vascular anomaly Tumor of fifth cranial nerve	Carbamazepine (Tegretol) Phenytoin Radiofrequency lesion of ganglion
Atypical facial neuralgia	Unilateral or bilateral	Predominantly female 30–50 years Continuous intolerable pain Mainly maxillary areas	None	Depressive and anxiety states Hysteria Idiopathic	Antidepressant and antianxiety medication
Supraorbital ciliary, infraorbital, sphenopalatine neuralgias	Unilateral in eye, cheek, ear, neck	Persistent, aching pain	Occasional nasal obstruction	Idiopathic Paranasal sinus disease	Decongestant nasal medication ?Nerve section and injection
Postzoster neuralgia	Unilateral Any one of trigeminal divisions	History of zoster Aching, burning pain; jabs of pain Paresthesia, slight sensory loss Dermal scars	Contact, movement	Herpes zoster	Carbamazepine and phenytoin and antidepressants
Costen's syndrome	Unilateral, near temporomandibular joints	Elderly females Severe aching pain, intensified by chewing Tenderness over joints Malocclusion	Chewing, pressure over temporomandibular joint	Loss of teeth, rheumatoid arthritis	Bite correction and surgery
Tolosa-Hunt syndrome	Unilateral, mainly orbital	Intense sharp, aching pain; associated ophthalmoplegias of varying degree Pupil inequality, sensory loss	None	?Arteritis and granulomatous lesions	Corticosteroids
Raeder's paratrigeminal syndrome	Unilateral, frontotemporal and maxilla	Intense sharp, aching pain Pupil inequality, sensory loss	None	Tumors, granulomatous lesions, injuries	Depends on type of lesion

SOURCE: *After J Patten, Neurological Differential Diagnosis, London, Harold Starke, Springer-Verlag, 1977.*

avoidance of the offending activity or agent, and symptomatic therapy in the form of aspirin, 0.6 g, or acetaminophen, 0.6 g, given every 6 to 8 h. Chronic headaches falling into the common migraine or tension category are much more difficult to manage. Analgesics may alleviate the pain, but rarely abolish it. Patients commonly self-administer four to eight tablets daily for years despite acknowledging minimal benefit. Such headaches often respond to amitriptyline given in gradually increased doses to 100 to 150 mg preferably administered as a single bedtime dose. *Premenstrual headache,* if troublesome, can usually be helped by the use of a diuretic compound for the week preceding the menstrual period and a mixture of mild analgesic and sedative medications (aspirin or acetaminophen, 0.6 g, and barbiturate). If the headaches are severe and incapacitating, they should be treated as common migraine.

Migraine may require no treatment at all, other than an explanation of its nature to the patient and a reassurance that it will do no harm. Some patients know, or allege to know, that certain factors induce attacks, and these should be avoided. In some patients alcoholic drinks, particularly red wine, are invariably followed by a migraine. Others claim reduction of attacks of headache by an elimination diet, correction of refractive error, or by psychotherapy. Biofeedback can reduce the number of migraine attacks in some patients, and practiced relaxation is beneficial in others.

Drugs used for treatment of migraine can be separated into agents used for the acute attack and those administered for prophylaxis. Patients who experience more than two or three severe attacks each month should be considered for preventive treatment. Treatment of the neurologic aura of migraine is rarely required or possible because of its brevity. If the deficits are lasting, inhalation of an ampul of amyl nitrite can be tried as a preventive measure; it should be used at the first premonition of the attack. The time to initiate treatment of the oncoming headache is during the neurologic disorder. If many of the headaches are mild, the patient may already have learned that 0.6 g aspirin or acetaminophen will control the pain. A combination of analgesic and soporific medicine such as Fiorinal or Bellergal may be helpful. If severe disabling attacks are expected, they too may respond to simple analgesic medication and rest in a quiet, darkened room. Some patients find relief with ergot preparations given orally, 1 to 3 mg held under the tongue until dissolved, or ergotamine tartrate, 0.25 mg by intravenous injection. These treatments if given early will abort a classic migraine attack in 80 to 90 percent of patients. Sometimes the combination of caffeine, 100 mg with 1 mg ergotamine, is preferred. It may be taken in the form of a tablet (two at the onset of headache and a third in half an hour) or as a rectal suppository (2 mg ergotamine and 100 mg caffeine) if vomiting prevents oral administration.

Because of the danger of prolonged vascular spasm in patients who have vascular disease or are pregnant, ergot preparations must be used cautiously, if at all. Even in healthy individuals more than 10 to 15 mg ergotamine per week is risky, for it may in itself produce headache. Hakkareinen et al. report that tolfenamic acid, an anti-inflammatory agent that blocks prostaglandin receptors in oral doses of 200 mg, was found to be as effective as ergotamine tartrate. For the frequent atypical migraine headaches, some of which respond poorly to ergot, one should prescribe a preparation containing 150 mg aspirin, 160 mg phenacetin, and dextroamphetamine sulfate,

5 mg, with phenobarbital, 30 mg. This can be repeated once or twice in a severe attack. Once the headache has become intense (after 30 min), ergot is of little help, and one must resort to codeine sulfate, 30 mg, or meperidine, 50 mg, as the only means of terminating the pain. If sleep customarily terminates headache, 50 mg of promethazine orally is helpful; it also relieves vomiting.

In individuals with frequent migrainous attacks (more than one to three a month), efforts at prevention are worthwhile. Some success has been obtained with preparations of ergot, 0.5 mg, atropine, 0.3 mg, and phenobarbital, 15 mg, two or three times a day for a few weeks. Propranolol, 40 mg three times a day, has been effective in reducing the frequency and intensity of attacks in approximately two-thirds of cases. For the most severe forms of the disorder, methysergide in a dose of 6 to 8 mg per day given for several weeks or months has proved to be most promising in reducing the frequency of or abolishing attacks. The main adverse effect has been retroperitoneal and pulmonary fibrosis; this complication has been reported in several dozen cases when the patient has been treated continuously for more than 6 months. Discontinuing treatment for 1 month out of every 6 has greatly reduced the incidence of this complication. Recently, claims have been made for pizotifen (a histamine- and serotonin-blocking agent), for amitriptyline, apart from its antidepressant action, for phenelzine, a monoamine oxidase inhibitor, and for calcium channel blockers. Severe attacks of migraine lasting for several days or even weeks have been treated successfully with chlorpromazine in large doses of 50 to 100 mg daily. Prednisone in divided doses of 20 mg three or four times a day is also effective in some severe cases.

All experienced physicians appreciate the importance of helping patients rearrange their schedules so as to control the tensions and hard-driving ways of living so often a feature of many migrainous patients. There is no one way of accomplishing this, but in general, long and costly psychotherapy has not been helpful, or at least one can say there are no substantial data as to its value.

Cluster headaches have proved to be most resistant to treatment. One capsule of Cafergot or 1.0 mg of ergotamine tartrate at bedtime is most widely recommended. However, if the headaches are frequent, severe, and diurnal as well as nocturnal, the intake of ergot may reach dangerous levels. Success has also been claimed for amitriptyline, 25 to 100 mg three times a day, and methysergide, 6 to 8 mg per day, as means of interrupting a cluster. Lance recommends prednisone, 40 mg daily for 5 days then reduced to an amount necessary to control headaches. Lithium carbonate in an initial dose of 250 mg three times a day is said to give relief in 80 to 90 percent of cases. Histamine desensitization, originally proposed by Horton, has been little used in recent years because of inconsistent results. In rare cases of persistent cluster headaches lasting for 10 to 20 years spectacular success has been obtained by indomethacin.

Hypertensive headaches respond to agents which lower blood pressure and relieve muscle tension. Chlorothiazide, 250 to 500 mg twice a day, and methyldopa, 250 to 500 mg per day, when combined with a small amount of phenobarbital, 15 mg three times a day, or propranolol, 40 mg three times a day, have given satisfactory results. Meprobamate, 200 mg three times a day, or chlordiazepoxide hydrochloride, 5 mg three times a day, may be administered in place of phenobarbital.

The *muscle tension headaches* respond best to massage, relaxation, and a combination of drugs which relieve depression (e.g., amitriptyline or imipramine) and anxiety (e.g., meprobamate and chlordiazepoxide hydrochloride). Pain-relieving medicine of non-habit-forming type (e.g., aspirin and propoxyphene hydrochloride) should be added when throbbing headache is present. Stronger analgesic medication (codeine or meperidine hydrochloride) should be avoided. Psychotherapy may be helpful in this group of patients.

The headache of the *posttraumatic syndrome* requires supportive psychotherapy in the form of reassurance and frequent explanation of its benign and transient nature, a program of increasing physical activity, and drugs which allay anxiety and depression. However, the tricyclic antidepressants are generally less effective than in the mixed tension and throbbing headaches of anxious depressions. Tender scars from scalp laceration may be novocainized repeatedly (subcutaneous injection of 5 mL of 1% procaine) with some degree of success. Settlement of litigation as soon as possible works to the patient's advantage.

Heat, massage, salicylates, and indomethacin or phenylbutazone usually effect some improvement in those arthritic diseases of the cervical spine which are associated with cervicocranial pain (see Chaps. 263 and 274). A soft collar and traction may be beneficial.

Corticosteroid therapy is indicated in *cranial arteritis* to prevent disastrous blindness by occlusion of the ophthalmic arteries, which occurs in 50 percent of untreated patients. Prednisone should be given in full doses (40 to 60 mg per day) for at least a month and continued until all symptoms and laboratory abnormalities have disappeared. The headaches of cranial tumor often respond promptly to large doses of corticosteroids.

In conclusion, it is well to mention the importance of general hygienic measures. Young physicians in particular are apt to seek a specific therapy for each headache syndrome and give little thought to the general health of the patient. We have observed that most of the recurrent and chronic headaches are likely to be more severe and disabling whenever the patient becomes nervous, sick, and tired. A well-rounded diet, adequate rest, a reasonable amount of physical exercise, and a balanced view of the sources of daily anxieties and how to cope with them should be the goal of all therapeutic programs.

REFERENCES

APPENZELLER O: *Pathogenesis and Treatment of Headache*. New York, Spectrum, 1976

BICKERSTAFF ER: Basilar artery migraine. Lancet 1:15, 1961

BOGDUK N, LANCE JW: Pain and pain syndrome including headache, in *Current Neurology*, SF Appel (ed). New York, Wiley, 1981, vol 3, chap 14

CAVINESS VS, O'BRIEN P: Headache. N Engl J Med 302:446, 1980

COUCH JR, HASSANEIM RS: Platelet aggregability in migraine. Neurology 27:843, 1977

CRITCHLEY M et al (eds): *Advances in Neurology*, vol. 33: *Headache: Physiopathological and Clinical Aspects*. New York, Raven Press, 1982

DIAMOND S: Prolonged benign exertional headache. Headache 22:96, 1982

EHYAI A, FENICHEL GM: Natural history of acute confusional migraine. Arch Neurol 35:368, 1978

FISHER CM: Transient migrainous accompaniments of late onset. Stroke 10:96, 1979

GELMERS HJ: Nimodipine, a new calcium antagonist, in the prophylactic treatment of migraine. *Headache* 23(3):106, 1983

HAKKAREINEN H et al: Tolfenamic acid is as effective as ergotamine during migraine attacks. Lancet 2:326, 1979

HOCKADAY JM: Basilar migraine in children. Dev Med Child Neurol 21:455, 1979

KAYAN A, HOOD JD: Neuro-otological manifestations of migraine. Brain 107:1123, 1984

LAKE A, RAINEY J, PAPSDORF JD: Biofeedback and rational-emotive therapy in the management of migraine headache. Appl Behav Anal 12:127, 1979

LANCE JW: Headache. Ann Neurol 10:1, 1981

———: Headaches related to sexual activity. J Neurol Neurosurg Psychiat 39:1226, 1976

MOSKOWITZ M: Neurobiology of vascular head pain. Ann Neurol 16:157, 1984

OLESON J et al: Focal hyperemia followed by spreading oligemia in classic migraine. Ann Neurol 9:344, 1981

PEROUTKA J: The pharmacology of calcium channel antagonists: Novel class of anti-migraine agents? Headache 23:278, 1983

RASKIN NH, SCHWARTZ RK: Icepick-like pain. Neurology 29:550, 1979

VIJAYAN N, DREYFUS PM: Posttraumatic dysautonomic cephalalgia: Clinical observations and treatment. Arch Neurol 32:649, 1976

VINKEN PJ, BRUYN GW (eds): *Handbook of Clinical Neurology*, vol 5: *Headache and Cranial Neuralgias*. Amsterdam, North-Holland, 1968.

7 PAIN IN THE BACK AND NECK

HENRY J. MANKIN / RAYMOND D. ADAMS

ANATOMY AND PHYSIOLOGY OF THE LOWER PART OF THE BACK

The bony spine is a complex structure, anatomically divisible into two parts. The anterior part consists of a series of cylindrical vertebral bodies connected to one another by the intervertebral disks and held together by the anterior and posterior longitudinal ligaments. The posterior part consists of more delicate elements that extend from the vertebral body as pedicles and broaden posteriorly to form laminae, which together with ligamentous structures form the vertebral canal. The posterior elements are joined to adjacent vertebrae by two small facetal synovial joints which allow a range of motion (Fig. 7-1). Stout transverse and spinous bony processes project laterally and posteriorly and serve as the attachments of muscles which move, support, and protect the vertebral column. The stability of the spine depends on two types of support: that provided by the bony articulations (principally by the diskal joints and the synovial articulations of the posterior elements) and a second type provided by the ligamentous (passive) and muscular (active) supporting structures. The ligamentous structures are quite strong, but because neither they nor the vertebral body–disk complexes have sufficient integral strength to resist the enormous forces acting on the column during even simple movements, voluntary and reflex contractions of the sacrospinalis, abdominal, gluteal, psoas, and hamstring muscles afford most of the stability.

The vertebral and paravertebral structures derive their innervation from the recurrent branches of the spinal nerves. Pain endings and fibers have been demonstrated in the ligaments, muscles, periosteum of bone, outer layers of annulus fibrosus, and synovium of the articular facets. The sensory fibers from these structures and the sacroiliac and lumbosacral joints join to form the sinovertebral nerves which pass via the recurrent branches of the spinal nerves of the first sacral and the fifth to first lumbar vertebrae into the gray matter of the corresponding segments of the spinal cord. Efferent fibers emerge from these segments and extend to the muscles through the same nerves.

The parts of the back that possess the greatest freedom of movement, and hence are most frequently subject to injury, are the lumbar and cervical regions. In addition to the voluntary motions required for bending, twisting, and other movements, many actions of the spine are reflex in nature and are the basis of posture.

FIGURE 7-1 *Left: Superior view of a stripped lumbar vertebra. Right: Lateral view of two articulated lumbar vertebrae. B = body; SC = spinal canal; IVF = intervertebral foramen; IF = inferior articular facet; SF = superior articular facet; P = pedicle; TP = transverse process; SP = spinous process; L = lamina. (Adapted from DB Levine, in Arthritis and Allied Conditions: A Textbook of Rheumatology, 10th ed, DJ McCarty (ed), Philadelphia, Lea & Febiger, 1985.)*

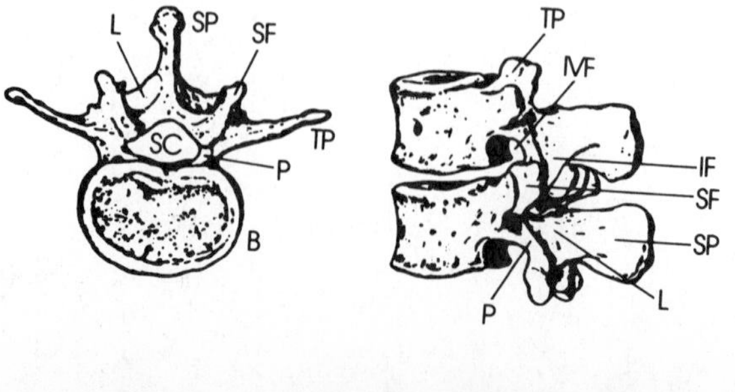

GENERAL CLINICAL CONSIDERATIONS

TYPES OF LOW BACK PAIN Four types of pain may be differentiated: local, referred, radicular, and that arising from secondary (protective) muscular spasm.

Local pain is caused by any pathologic process which impinges upon or irritates sensory endings. Involvement of structures which contain no sensory endings is painless. The central, medullary portion of the vertebral body may be destroyed by tumor, for example, without evocation of pain, whereas cortical fractures, or tears and distortions of the periosteum, synovial membranes, muscles, annulus fibrosus, and ligaments are often exquisitely painful. Although painful states are often accompanied by swelling of the affected tissues, this may not be apparent if a deep structure of the back is the site of disease. Local pain is often described as steady but may be intermittent, varying considerably with position or activity. The pain may be sharp or dull and although often diffuse is always felt in or near the affected part of the spine. Reflex splinting of the spine segments by paravertebral muscles is frequently noted, and certain movements or postures that alter the position of the injured tissues aggravate the pain. Firm pressure or percussion upon superficial structures in the region involved usually evokes tenderness, which is of aid in identifying the site of the abnormality.

Referred pain is of two types: that projected from the spine into regions lying within the area of the lumbar and upper sacral dermatomes and that projected from the pelvic and abdominal viscera to the spine. Pain due to diseases of the upper part of the lumbar spine is usually referred to the anterior aspects of the thighs and legs; that from the lower lumbar and sacral segments is referred to the gluteal regions, posterior thighs, calves, and sometimes feet. Pain of this type, although of deep, aching quality and rather diffuse, tends at times to be superficially projected. In general the referred pain parallels in intensity the local pain in the back. In other words, maneuvers which alter local pain have a similar effect on referred pain, though not with such precision and immediacy as in radicular, or "root," pain. Referred pain may be confused with pain from visceral disease, but the latter is usually described as "deep" and tends to radiate from the abdomen through to the back. Also, visceral pain is usually unaffected by movement of the spine, does not improve with recumbency, and may be modified by the activity of the involved viscus.

Radicular, or "root," *pain* has some of the characteristics of referred pain but differs in its greater intensity, distal radiation, circumscription to the territory of a root, and the factors which excite it. The mechanism is distortion, stretching, irritation, or compression of a spinal root, most often central to the intervertebral foramen. Although the pain itself is often dull or aching, various maneuvers which increase the irritation of the root may greatly intensify the pain, eliciting a lancinating quality. Nearly always the radiation of pain is from a central position near the spine to some part of the lower extremity. Cough, sneeze, and strain are characteristically evocative maneuvers; but since they may also jar or move the spine, they may aggravate local pain as well. Any motion which stretches the nerve, e.g., forward bending with the knees extended or "straight-leg raising," in disease of the lower part of the lumbar spine excites radicular pain; jugular vein compression, which raises intraspinal pressure and may cause a shift in the position of or pressure on the root, may have a similar effect. The fourth and fifth lumbar and first sacral roots, which form the sciatic nerve, cause pain which extends mainly down the posterior aspects of thigh, the postero- and antero-lateral aspects of the leg, and into the foot, in the distribution of this nerve—so called sciatica. Tingling, paresthesias, and numbness or sensory impairment of the skin, soreness of the skin, and tenderness along the nerve usually accompany radicular pain. Reflex loss, weakness, atrophy, fascicular twitching, and occasionally stasis edema may occur if motor fibers of the anterior root are involved.

Pain resulting from muscular spasm is usually mentioned in relation to local pain. Muscle spasm may be associated with many disorders of the spine and can produce significant distortions of the normal posture. Chronic tension in muscles may give rise to a dull and sometimes cramping ache. One can in this instance feel the tautness of the sacrospinalis and gluteal muscles and demonstrate by palpation that the pain is localized to these structures.

Other pains often of undetermined origin are sometimes described by patients with chronic disease of the lower part of the back. In the legs, drawing, pulling, cramping sensations (without involuntary muscle spasm), tearing, throbbing, or jabbing pains, or feelings of burning or coldness are difficult to interpret and, like paresthesias and numbness, should always suggest the possibility of nerve or root disease.

In addition to assessing the character and location of the pain, one should determine the factors which aggravate and relieve it, its constancy, and its relationship to recumbency and such stereotypical movements and maneuvers as forward bending, cough, sneeze, and strain. Frequently the most important lead comes from the knowledge of the mode of onset and circumstances which initiated the pain. Inasmuch as many painful afflictions of the back are the result of injury incurred during work or in an accident, the possibility of exaggeration or prolongation of pain for purposes of compensation or other personal reasons, or because of hysteria or malingering, must always be kept in mind.

EXAMINATION OF THE LOWER PART OF THE BACK

Inspection of the normal spine shows a dorsal kyphosis and lumbar lordosis in the sagittal plane, which in some individuals may be exaggerated (swayback). In spinal disorders, one should observe the spine closely for excessive curvature, flattening of the normal lumbar arch, presence of a gibbus (a short, sharp, kyphotic angulation usually indicative of a fracture or congenital abnormality), pelvic tilt or obliquity, or asymmetry of the paravertebral or gluteal musculature. In severe sciatica, one may observe abnormalities of posture of the affected leg, presumably to reduce tension on the irritated part.

The spine, hips, and legs should be observed during certain motions. No advantage accrues from trying to find out how much the patient can be hurt. Instead, it is much more important to determine when and under what conditions the pain commences. One looks for limitation of the natural motions of the patient while he or she is disrobing, standing, and reclining. When standing, the motion of forward bending normally produces flattening and reversal of the lumbar lordotic curve and exaggeration of the dorsal curve. With lesions of the lumbosacral region which involve the posterior ligaments, articular facets, or sacrospinalis muscle and with ruptured lumbar disks, protective reflexes prevent stretching of these structures. As a consequence, the sacrospinalis muscles remain taut and limit motion in the lumbar part of the spine. Forward bending then occurs at the hips and at the lumbar-thoracic junction. With disease of the lumbosacral joints and spinal roots, the patient bends in such a way as to avoid tensing the hamstring muscles and putting undue leverage upon the pelvis. In unilateral "sciatica," with its increased curvature toward the side of the lesion, lumbar and lumbosacral motions are splinted, and bending is mainly at the hips; at a certain point the knee on the affected side is flexed to relieve hamstring spasm and tilting of the pelvis occurs to slacken the lumbosacral roots and sciatic nerve.

In unilateral ligamentous or muscular strain, bending to the opposite side aggravates the pain by stretching the damaged tissues. Moreover, in lateral disk lesions, bending of the spine toward the side of the lesion is restricted. In diseases of the lower part of the spine, flexion while sitting with the hips and knees flexed can normally be performed easily, even to the point of bringing the knees in contact with the chest. The reason is that knee flexion relaxes the tightened hamstring muscles and also relieves stretch of the sciatic nerve.

With lumbosacral lesions and sciatica, passive lumbar flexion in the supine position causes little pain and is not limited as long as the hamstrings are relaxed and there is no stretching of the sciatic nerve. With lumbosacral and lumbar spine disease (e.g., arthritis), passive flexion of the hips is free, whereas flexion of the lumbar spine may be impeded and painful. Passive straight-leg raising (possible in most normal individuals up to 80 to 90° except in those who have unusually tight hamstrings), like forward bending in the standing posture with the legs straight, places the sciatic nerve and its roots under tension, thereby producing pain. It may also cause an anterior rotation of the pelvis around a transverse axis, increasing stress on the lumbosacral joint, and thus causing pain if this segment is arthritic or otherwise impaired. Consequently, in diseases of the lumbosacral joints and lumbosacral roots, this movement is limited on the affected side and to a lesser extent on the opposite side. Lasègue's sign (pain and limitation of movement during flexion of the hip when the knee is extended) is a useful test of this condition. Straight-leg raising of the opposite leg may also cause contralateral pain but of lesser degree and is believed by some to be a sign of a more extensive lesion, such as an extruded disk fragment, rather than a simple prolapse or protrusion. It is important to remember, however, that the evoked pain is always referred to the diseased side, no matter which leg is flexed.

Hyperextension is best performed with the patient standing or lying prone. If the condition causing back pain is acute, it may be difficult to extend the spine in the standing position. A patient with lumbosacral strain or disk disease can usually extend or hyperextend the spine without aggravation of pain. If the lesion is in the upper lumbar segments or if an active inflammatory process or fracture of the vertebral body or posterior elements is present, hyperextension may be markedly limited.

Palpation and percussion of the spine are the last steps in the examination. It is preferable to palpate first those regions which are the least likely to evoke pain. At all times the examiner should know what structures are being palpated (see Fig. 7-2). Localized tenderness

FIGURE 7-2 *(1) Costovertebral angle. (2) Spinous process and interspinous ligament. (3) Region of the articular fifth lumbar to the first sacral facet. (4) Dorsum of sacrum. (5) Region of iliac crest. (6) Iliolumbar angle. (7) Spinous processes of fifth lumbar to first sacral vertebrae (tenderness = faulty posture or occasionally spina bifida occulta). (8) Region between posterior superior and posterior inferior spines. Sacroiliac ligaments (tenderness = sacroiliac sprain, often tender with fifth lumbar to first sacral disk). (9) Sacrococcygeal junction (tenderness = sacrococcygeal injury, i.e., sprain or fracture). (10) Region of sacrosciatic notch (tenderness = fourth to fifth lumbar disk rupture and sacroiliac sprain). (11) Sciatic nerve trunk (tenderness = ruptured lumbar disk or sciatic nerve lesion).*

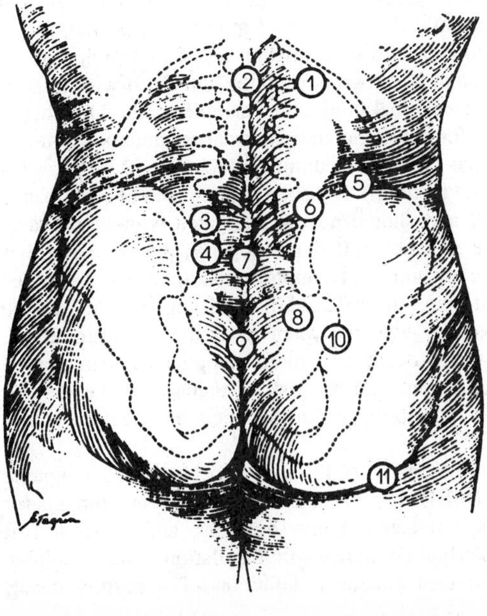

is seldom pronounced in disease of the spine because the involved structures are so deep that they rarely give rise to surface tenderness. Mild superficial and poorly localized tenderness signifies only a disease process within the affected segment of the body, i.e., dermatome.

Tenderness over the costovertebral angle often indicates renal disease, adrenal disease, or an injury to the transverse processes of the first or second lumbar vertebra. Hypersensitivity on palpation of the transverse processes of the other lumbar vertebrae as well as the overlying sacrospinalis muscles may signify fracture of the transverse process or a strain of muscle attachments. Tenderness of a spinous process or aggravation of pain by the jarring of gentle percussion may be nonspecific but frequently indicates the presence of a disk lesion at the site deep to it, inflammation (as in disk space infection), or fracture. Tenderness in the region of the articular facets between the fifth lumbar and first sacral vertebrae is consistent with disease of a lumbosacral disk [Fig. 7-2 (3)]. It is also frequent in rheumatoid arthritis.

In palpation of the spinous processes, it is important to note any deviation in the lateral plane (this may be indicative of fracture or arthritis) or in the anteroposterior plane. A "step-off" forward displacement of the spinous process may be an important clue to a spondylolisthesis, one segment below the displaced level.

Abdominal, rectal, and pelvic examination and assessment of the status of the peripheral vascular system are important parts of the examination of the patient with complaints in the lower back and should not be omitted. They may provide evidence for vascular, visceral, neoplastic, or inflammatory disorders which may extend to the spine or cause pain to be referred to this region.

Finally, a careful neurologic examination should be performed, with special attention given to motor, reflex, and sensory changes (see "Protrusion of Lumbar Intervertebral Disks," below), particularly in the lower extremities.

SPECIAL LABORATORY PROCEDURES Useful laboratory tests, depending on the nature of the problem and the circumstances, include a complete blood count, erythrocyte sedimentation rate (especially helpful in screening for infection or myeloma), measurement of serum calcium, phosphorus, alkaline phosphatase, acid phosphatase (the last mentioned is of importance if one suspects metastatic carcinoma from the prostate), protein electrophoresis, immunoglobulin electrophoresis, and tests for rheumatoid. Roentgenograms of the lumbar part of the spine should be taken in every case of low back pain and sciatica in the anteroposterior, lateral, and oblique planes. Special spot views or stereoscopic or laminographic films may provide further information in certain cases. Bone scans are of aid in revealing some fractures and neoplastic and inflammatory lesions.

Examination of the spinal canal with a contrast medium is often of great value, especially if a spinal cord tumor is suspected or if a patient is thought to have a disk herniation and fails to improve on a conservative regimen. Myelography can be combined with tests of dynamics of the cerebrospinal fluid, and a sample of the fluid should always be removed for cytologic and chemical examination prior to the instillation of the contrast medium (Pantopaque, Myodil, or a water-soluble contrast medium). Injection and removal of Pantopaque require special skill and should not be attempted without previous experience with the procedure. If done properly, the procedure has a very low incidence of significant complications. Injection of contrast medium directly into the intervertebral disk (diskograms) has waxed and waned in popularity over the years and remains controversial. The technique of this procedure is more complicated than that of myelographic examination, and the risk of damage to the disk or nerve roots and the possibility of introduction of infection is not inconsiderable.

Computerized tomography (CT) and more recently, magnetic resonance imaging (MRI) have become very valuable instruments for the study of the spinal canal, bony segments, and adjacent soft tissues. CT, particularly if combined with instillation of water-soluble contrast media, provides excellent definition of a narrow canal, destructive lesions of the vertebral bodies and posterior elements, presence of a paravertebral soft tissue mass, and by appropriate computerized reconstruction techniques can also identify disk herniations, sometimes with greater accuracy than the myelogram. Even without radiopaque material in the canal, the reconstructed CT scans have a high resolution and provide a noninvasive method of study of disk disease with a relatively low level of radiation.

Confirmation of proximal motor and sensory nerve and root disease can be obtained by nerve conduction studies, H and F responses, and electromyography (see Chap. 354).

PRINCIPAL CONDITIONS WHICH GIVE RISE TO DISABLING PAIN IN THE LOWER PART OF THE BACK

CONGENITAL ANOMALIES OF THE LUMBAR SPINE One of the most common disorders is a failure of fusion of the laminae of the neural arch (spina bifida) of one or several of the lumbar vertebrae or of the sacrum. Hypertrichosis or hyperpigmentation in the sacral area may betray the condition, but in most patients the spine defect remains entirely occult until disclosed by x-ray. The anomaly has greater potentiality for pain if accompanied by malformation of vertebral joints. Usually the pain is induced by injury. Other congenital anomalies that affect the lower lumbar vertebrae such as asymmetrical facetal joints, abnormalities of the transverse processes, sacralization of the fifth lumbar vertebra (in which L5 is firmly fixed to the sacrum), or lumbarization of the first sacral vertebra (in which the first sacral resembles a sixth lumbar) are rarely the cause of specific symptomatology.

Spondylolysis consists of a bony defect probably caused by trauma to a congenitally abnormal segment in the pars interarticularis (a segment near the junction of the pedicle with the lamina) of the lower lumbar area. The defect is best visualized on oblique projections. In some individuals the defect is bilateral. Under the circumstance of single or multiple injuries, the vertebral body, pedicle, and superior articular facet move anteriorly, leaving the posterior elements behind. This latter abnormality, known as *spondylolisthesis,* usually results in symptoms. The patient complains of pain in the low back radiating into the thighs, and there is limitation of motion. Often tenderness is elicited near the segment which has "slipped" forward (most often L5 on S1 or occasionally L4 on L5), and one can feel a "step" on deep palpation of the posterior elements. The pelvis is sometimes rotated and hip flexion limited by hamstring spasm; a variety of neurologic deficits indicative of radiculopathy complete the clinical syndrome. In exceptionally severe degrees of spondylolisthesis the trunk may be shortened and the abdomen protuberant, both the result of the extreme forward displacement of L5 on S1.

TRAUMATIC AFFLICTIONS OF THE LOWER PART OF THE BACK Trauma constitutes the most frequent cause of low back pain. In severe acute injuries, the examining physician must be careful to avoid further damage. In tests of mobility, all movements must be kept to a minimum until a diagnosis has been made and adequate measures have been instituted for the proper care of the patient. A patient complaining of back pain and inability to move the legs may have a fractured spine. The neck should not be flexed, nor should the patient be allowed to sit up. (See Chap. 353 for further discussion of spinal cord injury.)

Sprains, strains, and derangements The terms lumbosacral *sprain* and *strain* are often used loosely by physicians, and do not clearly relate to a known anatomic lesion. The authors prefer the term *low back derangement* or *strain* for minor, self-limited injuries usually associated with lifting a heavy object, a fall, or a sudden deceleration as may occur in an automobile accident. Occasionally, these syndromes are more chronic in nature, suggesting that diskal or arthritic factors may play a role. The patients with low back derangement are often acutely discomfited and may assume unusual postures related to spasm of the sacrospinalis muscles. The pain is usually confined to the lower back and is almost invariably relieved by rest within a few days. More extensive or longer lasting problems, formerly classified as sacroiliac strain or sprain are now known to be due to disk disease in most instances (see below).

Vertebral fractures Most fractures of the lumbar vertebral body are the result of flexion injuries and consist of anterior wedging or compression. With more severe trauma the patient may sustain a fracture dislocation, ''bursting'' fracture, or asymmetrical fracture involving not only the body but the posterior elements. The initiating trauma which causes fractures of the vertebrae is usually a fall from a height (in which case the calcanei may also be fractured) or may result from an automobile accident or other violence. When fractures occur with minimal trauma (or spontaneously), the bone is presumed to have been previously weakened by some pathologic process. Most of the time, particularly in older individuals, the cause of such an event is idiopathic osteoporosis, but there are many other underlying systemic disorders such as osteomalacia, hyperparathyroidism, hyperthyroidism, multiple myeloma, metastatic carcinoma, and a large number of local conditions that may play a role in weakening the vertebral body. Spasm of the lower lumbar muscles, limitation of motion of the lumbar section of the spine, and the roentgenographic appearance of the damaged lumbar segment (with or without neurologic abnormalities) are the basis of clinical diagnosis. The pain is usually immediate, though occasionally it may be delayed in onset for a few days. The patient may develop a mild paralytic ileus or urinary retention during the acute period.

Fractures of the transverse processes are almost always associated with tearing of the paravertebral muscles, principally the psoas. They may cause significant retroperitoneal hemorrhage resulting in a marked depression in hematocrit and, in extensive fractures, hypovolemic shock. Such injuries may be diagnosed by the finding of deep tenderness at the site of the injury, local muscle spasm on one side, and limitation of all movements which stretch the lumbar muscles. Radiologic evidence including bone scans, body CT, or MRI scanning provides the final confirmation. Fractures of multiple transverse processes, although seemingly trivial, should be the object of considerable concern, and the patient should be carefully watched for internal hemorrhage.

Protrusion of lumbar intervertebral disks This condition is the major cause of severe and chronic or recurrent low back and leg pain. It is most likely to occur between the fifth lumbar and first sacral vertebrae, and, with lessening frequency, between the fourth and fifth lumbar, the third and fourth lumbar, the second and third lumbar, and rarely, between the first and second lumbar vertebrae. Rare in the thoracic portion of the spine, it is next most frequent between the sixth and seventh and fifth and sixth cervical vertebrae. The cause is usually a flexion injury, but in many cases no trauma is recalled. Degeneration of the posterior longitudinal ligaments and the annulus fibrosus, which occurs in most adults of middle and advanced years, may have taken place silently or have been manifested by mild, recurrent lumbar ache. A sneeze, lurch, or other trivial movement may then cause the nucleus pulposus to prolapse, pushing the frayed and weakened annulus posteriorly. In more severe cases of disk disease, the nucleus may protrude through the annulus or become extruded to lie as a free fragment in the vertebral canal.

The fully developed syndrome of ruptured lumbar intervertebral disk consists of backache, abnormal posture, and limitation of motion of the spine (particularly flexion). Nerve root involvement is indicated by radicular pain, sensory disturbances (paresthesias, hyper- and hyposensitivity in dermatome pattern), coarse twitching and fasciculation, muscle spasms, and impairment of a tendon reflex. Motor abnormalities (weakness and muscle atrophy) may also occur but are usually less prominent than the pain and sensory disorder. Since herniation of the intervertebral lumbar disks most often occurs between the fourth and fifth lumbar vertebrae and the fifth lumbar and first sacral vertebrae with irritation and compression of the fifth lumbar and first sacral roots, respectively, it is important to recognize the clinical characteristics of lesions of these two roots. *Lesions of the fifth lumbar root* produce pain in the region of the hip, groin, posterolateral thigh, lateral calf to the external malleolus, dorsal surface of the foot, and the first or second and third toes. Paresthesias may be in the entire territory or only in the distal parts of these territories. The tenderness is in the lateral gluteal region and near the head of the fibula. Weakness, if present, involves the extensor of the great toe and less often of the foot. The knee and ankle reflexes are seldom altered, although occasionally the ankle jerk is moderately depressed. Walking on the heels may be more difficult, because of weakness of dorsiflexion of the foot, and more uncomfortable than walking on the toes. In *lesions of the first sacral root* the pain is felt in the midgluteal region, posterior part of the thigh, posterior region of the calf to the heel, and the plantar surface of the foot and fourth and fifth toes. Tenderness is most pronounced over the midgluteal region (sacroiliac joint), posterior thigh area, and calf. Rarely it may be referred to the rectum, testicles, or labia. Paresthesias and sensory loss are mainly in the lower leg and outer toes, and weakness, if present, involves the flexor muscles of the foot and toes, abductors of the toes, and hamstring muscles. The ankle reflex is diminished or absent in the majority of cases. Walking on the toes is more difficult, because of weakness of plantar flexors, and more uncomfortable than walking on the heel. With lesions of either root there may be limitation of straight-leg raising during the acute, painful stages.

Degeneration of the intervertebral disk without frank extrusion of a fragment of disk tissue may give rise to low back pain, or the disk may herniate into the adjacent vertebral body, giving rise to a Schmorl's node, usually visualized by x-ray. Such cases often show no signs of nerve root involvement though the back pain may be referred to the thigh and leg.

The rarer *lesions of the fourth and third lumbar roots* give rise to pain in the anterior part of the thigh and knee, with corresponding sensory loss. The knee jerk is diminished or abolished. An inverted Lasègue sign (pain with hypertension of the limb in relation to the trunk, best elicited with the patient in the prone position) is positive when the third lumbar root is affected.

The lumbar disk syndromes are usually unilateral. Only with massive derangements of the disk or the extrusion of a large, free fragment into the canal do bilateral symptoms and signs occur, and these may sometimes be associated with paralysis of the sphincters. The pain may be mild or severe. All or part of the above syndrome may be present. There may be back pain with little or no leg pain, and occasionally the patient experiences leg pain with little or no discomfort in the back. The rupture of multiple lumbar or lumbar and cervical disks is not infrequent, suggesting a diffuse disorder of the connective tissue of the disks, including both the annulus fibrosus and the nucleus pulposus.

When all components of the syndrome are present, the diagnosis is easy; when only one part is present (particularly backache), it may be difficult, especially if there has not been a clearly remembered initiating traumatic event. Since similar symptoms may occur without demonstrable disk rupture, other diagnostic procedures are required. Plain roentgenograms usually show no abnormality or at most a narrowing of the intervertebral space, sometimes more on the side of the rupture. Traction spurs, which are indicative of disk degeneration, may be present; in extreme cases, there may be a ''vacuum'' disk sign, in which a gas-density shadow is present in the intervertebral space, usually on lateral roentgenogram. Frequently, however, one must resort to Pantopaque or soluble contrast media myelography, which in most cases will reveal an indentation of the lumbar subarachnoid space or deformity of the root sleeve. Occasionally, with large lesions there is a complete interruption of the flow of contrast material. In some patients, CT with or without contrast material may show the disk herniation clearly even when it is small or laterally placed. A small ruptured disk may not show any abnormality in the CT scan or myelogram, especially at the fifth lumbar to first sacral level where there is a large space between the spinal canal and dura. Some clinics use diskograms (opaque material is injected directly into the disk) to reveal any evidence of extrusion, but the procedure is risky, and the results are difficult to interpret. The electromyogram is helpful in showing denervation of paravertebral and leg muscles (see Chap. 354). The protein level of the cerebrospinal fluid may be elevated in some instances.

Tumor of the spinal canal, epidural or intradural, may produce a syndrome similar to that of ruptured disk (see Chap. 353).

OTHER CAUSES OF LOW BACK PAIN AND SCIATICA A large experience with lumbar back pain, gluteal neuralgia, and sciatica in a medical referral center has impressed the authors with the sizable number of patients whose symptoms cannot be ascribed to a ruptured disk. Often the patients have had an operation for diskogenic disease with or without attempted fusion of the lumbar vertebrae, but the pain has not remitted. The indications for the original surgery may have been questionable; only a disk bulge (''hard disk'') without definite neurologic signs. To explain these chronic pain states a number of new pathologic entities, some of uncertain status, have been introduced. Entrapment of one or more nerve roots may be the consequence not only of a disk but also of spondylotic spurs with variable stenosis of the lateral recess and intervertebral canal, hypertrophy of apophyseal facets, or ''spinal arachnoiditis.''

Spondylotic spurs and stenosis of the lateral recess and intervertebral foramen have been distinguished clinically from ruptured disk. The pain involves one or both legs on standing and walking and is relieved by squatting or lying down. In the 35 cases reported by Mikhael et al. motor, reflex, and sensory changes were present. Radiologically, there was stenosis at one vertebral level. Most often the superior facet at L5 had narrowed the lateral recess at the upper border of the pedicle, compressing the L5 root and sometimes S1, as well. By polytomography the lateral recess was seen to be reduced to less than 3 mm. A more proper designation for this condition is *unilateral spondylosis,* and in some instances *spondylolysis*. In this condition, the adjacent articular capsule may suffer injury and add direct and referred pain to a radicular syndrome (see below and Chap. 353 for further discussion of the lumbar stenosis or claudication syndrome).

The *unilateral facet syndrome* is closely related. Reynolds et al. have reported 22 cases in which a lumbar monoradiculopathy had simulated that of a ruptured disk: 16 had an L5 radiculopathy, 3 an S1 radiculopathy, and 3 an L4 radiculopathy. Coexisting back pain was present in 15 of the cases. No disk rupture was found by myelography. At operation the spinal root was compressed against the floor or roof of the intervertebral canal by an enlarged superior or inferior facet. Foraminotomy and facetectomy relieved the symptoms in 12 of the 15 operated cases. Denervation of the lumbar facets by radiofrequency electrodes (percutaneous rhizolysis) of nerves supplying the zygoapophyseal joints has been utilized by Collier, who obtained relief of the patients' symptoms in 35 of 122 cases. But there is doubt as to whether the favorable results were due to the rhizolysis or to some other factor.

In some cases myelography has revealed a loculated, cystlike expansion of the perineurial sheath. It may extend beyond the intervertebral canal. Multiple cervical or lumbar spinal nerves may be involved. There are numerous surgical reports of relief of radicular pain and other symptoms by opening the cysts. The authors find it difficult to evaluate the results.

Lumbar adhesive arachnoiditis with radiculopathy is receiving increasing attention. This is an ambiguous entity in which patients after multiple lumbar operations and myelograms are left with backache and leg pain in combination with motor, sensory, and reflex changes. The arachnoidal membrane is thickened and opaque, adherent to dura, and tightly bound to pia and roots. The contrast medium during myelography does not fill the root sheaths and tends to be irregularly loculated. According to a British survey lumbar arachnoiditis was found in only 80 of 7600 myelograms, but judging from the American literature it is much more frequent. In our case material, disk rupture, multiple Pantopaque myelograms, operative procedures, infection, and subarachnoid hemorrhage, in various combinations, are factors which favor its development. Treatment is unsatisfactory; lysis of adhesions and intrathecal steroid therapy have been of no value.

In patients with persistent chronic low back pain and sciatica after failed disk surgery, or due to spondylitic spurs, spondylolysis, facetal joint degeneration, or arachnoiditis, some surgeons have attributed the disability in part, at least, to ''instability'' of the lumbar segments and the perpetuation of the pain to excessive or abnormal movements of the lumbar vertebral segments. For such patients spinal fusion is occasionally advocated and can in certain circumstances provide a measure of relief. A posterior arthrodesis of the fourth and fifth lumbar segments to the sacrum may reduce motion at these parts and decrease pressure on the nerve roots associated with abnormal movements. More often than not, however, the patient continues to have pain (although often reduced in degree), and the procedure should not be regarded as a panacea. The authors rarely advocate such an operative intervention, unless clear anatomic evidence exists for a mechanical problem which could be alleviated by stabilization of the spine.

ARTHRITIS Arthritis of the spine is a major cause of backache, cervical pain, and occipital headache.

Osteoarthritis (see also Chap. 274) This more frequent type of osteoarthritic spinal disease occurs usually in later life and may involve any part of the spine. It is most prevalent in the cervical and lumbar regions, however, and the exact location determines the localization of the symptoms. Patients often complain of pain centered in the spine which is increased by motion and is almost invariably associated with complaints of stiffness and limitation of motion. There is a notable absence of systemic symptoms such as fatigue, malaise, and fever, and the pain usually can be relieved by rest. The severity of the symptoms often bears little relation to the radiologic findings; pain may be present when there are minimal findings on an x-ray, and, conversely, marked osteophytic overgrowth with spur formation, ridging, and bridging of vertebrae can be seen in asymptomatic patients in middle and later life. Osteoarthropathic changes in the cervical spine and to a lesser extent in the lumbar spine may by their location compress roots or even the cauda equina or spinal cord, giving rise to the spondylitic form of myelopathy (see Chaps. 353 and 354).

Multiple spondylitic caudal radiculopathy (SCR) is another variant of hypertrophic arthritis. A congenital smallness of the lumbar canal, especially at the L4 to L5 level, renders the individual susceptible to either a rupture of an intervertebral disk or arthrosis. The latter condition further narrows the anteroposterior diameter of the canal and leads to compression of lumbosacral roots and even to a block of the spinal canal. The roots are actually caught between the posterior surface of the vertebral body and the ligamentum flavum posterolaterally. Lumbosacral pains are followed by weakening of the lower legs, impairment of ankle and knee reflexes, and numbness and paresthesia in the feet and legs. Extension of the lumbar spine during walking and standing produces or aggravates the neurologic symptoms, and flexion relieves them. The clinical picture and its intermittency correspond to the so-called intermittent claudication of the spinal cord. The diagnosis may be suspected on the basis of history and radiographic findings but may be confirmed by myelography, CT, or MRI scan, which will demonstrate the narrowed lumbar canal. Decompression of the spinal canal relieves the symptoms in a considerable proportion of the cases but should be approached with caution since it may lead to instability, necessitating an arthrodesis. SCR is the lumbar equivalent of spondylitic cervical myelopathy (SCM), described below. SCR is a cauda equina syndrome, and its differential diagnosis is discussed in Chap. 353.

Rheumatoid arthritis and ankylosing spondylitis (see also Chaps. 263 and 267) Arthritic disease of the spine takes two distinct forms, ankylosing spondylitis (the more common) and rheumatoid arthritis.

Patients with *ankylosing spondylitis* (also called Marie-Strümpell arthritis) are usually young men who complain of mild to moderate pain which early in the course of the disease is centered in the back and on occasion radiates to the back of the thighs. The symptoms may be vague at first (tired back, "catches" up and down the back, sore back) and the diagnosis may be overlooked for a considerable period. Although the pain is often intermittent, the finding of limitation of movement is constant and progressive and over a period of time tends to dominate the picture. Early in the course, this finding is described as "morning stiffness" or increasing stiffness after periods of inactivity, and may be present long before radiologic changes are manifest. Limitation of chest expansion, tenderness over the sternum, and decreased motion and flexion contractures of the hips may also be present early in the course. The radiologic hallmarks of the disease are destruction and subsequent obliteration of the sacroiliac joints, development of syndesmophytes on the margins of the vertebral bodies, followed by bridging by bone to produce the characteristic "bamboo spine." The entire spine becomes immobilized, often in a flexed position, and usually the pain then subsides. Patterns of restricted movement, indistinguishable from those of ankylosing spondylitis, may accompany Reiter's syndrome, psoriatic arthritis, and chronic inflammatory bowel diseases. Patients with these disorders rarely show the joint manifestations of peripheral rheumatoid arthritis, and seldom do they display involvement of the hips or knees. The rheumatoid factor is usually absent, but the sedimentation rate is often rapid, and many of the patients are found to have an HLA-B27 antigen.

Occasionally ankylosing spondylitis is complicated by progressively destructive vertebral lesions. This complication should be suspected whenever the pain returns, after a period of quiescence, or becomes localized. The etiology of these lesions is not known, but they may represent an exaggerated healing response to fracture or excessive production of fibrous inflammatory tissues. Rarely they may result in collapse of a segment of the spine and compression of the spinal cord. Another complication of severe ankylosing spondylitis is bilateral ankylosis of the ribs to the spine, which, coupled with a decrease in the height of axial thoracic structures, causes marked impairment of respiratory function.

Spinal rheumatoid arthritis tends to be localized to the cervical apophyseal joints and atlantoaxial articulation; the pain, stiffness, and limitation of motion are then in the neck and back of the head. Unlike ankylosing spondylitis, rheumatoid arthritis is rarely confined to the spine, and it does not lead to significant degrees of intervertebral bridging. Because of major affection of other joints, the diagnosis is relatively easy to make, but significant involvement of the neck may be overlooked. In the advanced stages of the disease, one or several of the vertebrae may be displaced anteriorly, or a synovitis of the atlantoaxial joint may damage the transverse ligament of the atlas, resulting in forward displacement of the atlas on the axis, i.e., atlantoaxial subluxation. In either instance serious and even life-threatening compression of the spinal cord may occur gradually or suddenly (see Chaps. 263 and 353). Lateral roentgenograms in flexion and extension, performed cautiously, are necessary to visualize dislocation or subluxation.

OTHER DESTRUCTIVE DISEASES Neoplastic, infectious, and metabolic diseases Metastatic carcinoma (breast, lung, prostate, thyroid, kidney, gastrointestinal tract), multiple myeloma, and non-Hodgkin's and Hodgkin's lymphomas are the malignant tumors which most frequently involve the spine. Since the primary site may be overlooked or asymptomatic, the presenting complaint in such patients may be pain in the back. The pain tends to be constant and dull, and is often unrelieved by rest. Indeed, it may be worse at night. Radiographic changes may be absent early in the disease, but when they appear, usually are manifest as destructive lesions in one or several vertebral bodies with little or limited involvement of the disk space, even in the face of a compression fracture. A ^{99m}Tc diphosphonate bone scan is helpful in demonstrating "hot spots," indicating areas of increased blood flow and reactive bone formation associated with destructive, inflammatory, or arthritic lesions. It should be noted, however, that myeloma and sometimes metastatic thyroid carcinoma may fail to show increased activity on a bone scan.

Infection of the vertebral column is usually the result of pyogenic organisms (staphylococci or coliform bacilli) or tubercule bacilli and is often diffcult to distinguish on the basis of clinical findings. Patients complain of pain in the back of subacute or chronic nature that is exacerbated by motion but not materially relieved by rest. There is limitation of motion, tenderness over the spine of the involved segments, and pain with jarring of the spine, such as occurs with walking on the heels. Usually, these patients are afebrile and often do not have a leukocytosis although the erythrocyte sedimentation rate is almost invariably elevated. Radiographs may demonstrate narrowing of a disk space with erosion and destruction of the two adjacent vertebrae. A paravertebral soft tissue mass may be present, indicating an abscess, which may in the case of tuberculosis drain spontaneously, at sites quite remote from the vertebral column. In addition to a bone scan, a gallium scan is sometimes helpful in identifying a soft tissue inflammatory or infectious lesion even when overt bone destruction is not visible in x-rays.

Special mention should be made of the spinal *epidural abscess* (usually staphylococcal), which necessitates urgent surgical treatment. The symptoms are a localized pain, occurring spontaneously, aggravated by percussion and palpation. The patient is febrile and usually has severe radicular complaints, often bilateral, progressing rapidly to a flaccid paraplegia (see Chaps. 340 and 353).

In so-called metabolic bone diseases (osteoporosis or osteomalacia) a considerable degree of loss of bone substance may occur without any symptoms whatsoever. Many patients with such conditions do, however, complain of aching in the lumbar or thoracic area. This is most likly to occur following an injury, sometimes of trivial degree, which leads to collapse or wedging of a vertebra. Certain movements greatly enhance the pain, and certain positions relieve it. One or more spinal roots may be involved. Paget's disease of the spine is nearly always painless but may lead to compression of the spinal cord or roots because of encroachment on the canal or foramina by the pagetoid bone. The recognition of these bone disorders is discussed in some detail elsewhere (Chaps. 337 and 338).

In general, patients thought to have neoplastic, infectious, or metabolic disease of the spine should be thoroughly evaluated by means of radiographs, bone scans, CT scans, and appropriate laboratory studies (see above).

REFERRED PAIN FROM VISCERAL DISEASE The pain of disease of the pelvic, abdominal, or thoracic viscera is often felt in the region of the spine; i.e., it is referred to the posterior parts of the spinal segment which innervates the diseased organ. Occasionally back pain may be the first and only sign. The general rule is that pelvic diseases are referred to the sacral region, lower abdominal diseases to the lumbar region (centering around the second to fourth lumbar vertebrae), and upper abdominal diseases to the lower thoracic spine (eighth thoracic to the first and second lumbar vertebrae). Characteristically there are no local signs or stiffness of the back, and motion is of full range without augmentation of the pain. However, some positions, e.g., flexion of the lumbar area of the spine in the lateral recumbent position, may be more comfortable than others.

Low thoracic and upper lumbar pain in abdominal disease Peptic ulceration or tumor of the wall of the stomach and of the duodenum most typically induces pain in the epigastrium (see Chaps. 235 and 255); but if the posterior wall is involved, and particularly if there is retroperitoneal extension, the pain may be felt in the region of the spine. The pain may be central in location or more intense on one side, or it may be felt in both locations. If very intense, it may seem to encircle the body. It tends to retain the characteristics of pain from the affected organ; e.g., if due to peptic ulceration, it appears about 2 h after a meal and is relieved by food and antacids.

Diseases of the pancreas (peptic ulceration with extension to the pancreas, cholecystitis with pancreatitis, cyst, or tumor) are apt to cause pain in the back, being more to the right of the spine if the head of the pancreas is involved and to the left if the body and tail are implicated.

Diseases of retroperitoneal structures, e.g., lymphomas, sarcomas, and carcinomas, may evoke pain in this part of the spine with some tendency toward radiation to the lower part of the abdomen, groin, and anterior thighs. A secondary tumor of the iliopsoas region on one side often produces a unilateral lumbar ache with radiation toward the groin and labia or testicle; there may also be signs of involvement of the upper lumbar spinal roots. An aneurysm of the abdominal aorta may induce pain which is localized to this region of the spine but may be felt higher or lower, depending on the location of the lesion.

The sudden appearance of obscure lumbar pain in a patient receiving anticoagulants should arouse the suspicion of retroperitoneal bleeding.

Lumbar pain with lower abdominal diseases Inflammatory diseases of segments of the colon (colitis, diverticulitis) or tumor of the colon cause pain which may be felt in the lower part of the abdomen between the umbilicus and pubis, in the midlumbar region, or in both places. If very intense, the pain may have a beltlike distribution around the body. A lesion in the transverse colon or first part of the descending colon may be central or left-sided, and its level of reference to the back is to the second to third lumbar vertebrae. If the sigmoid colon is implicated, the pain is lower, in the upper sacral region and anteriorly in the midline suprapubic region or left lower quadrant of the abdomen.

Sacral pain in pelvic (urologic and gynecologic) diseases The pelvis is seldom the site of a disease which causes obscure low back pain although gynecologic disorders may manifest themselves in this manner. Of painful pelvic lesions less than a third are due to inflammatory disease; other more hypothetical entities, such as relaxation of uterine supporting structures, retroversion of uterus, pelvic varicosities, and adnexal edema, have been largely discredited. Recently, diagnostic laparoscopy has been recommended as a valuable supplement to rectal and pelvic examinations, sigmoidoscopy, and intravenous pyelography. The importance of psychiatric illness in the majority of undiagnosed cases has been stressed.

Menstrual pain itself may be felt in the sacral region. It is rather poorly localized, tends to radiate down the legs, and is of a crampy nature. The most important source of chronic back pain from the pelvic organs, however, is the uterosacral ligaments. Endometriosis or carcinoma of the uterus (body or cervix) may invade these structures, while malposition of the uterus may pull on them. The pain is localized centrally in the sacrum below the lumbosacral joint but may be more on one side. In endometriosis the pain begins during the premenstrual phase and often continues until it merges with menstrual pain. Malposition of the uterus (retroversion, descensus, and prolapse) is thought by some to lead to sacral pain, especially after the patient has been standing for several hours. One may observe the effect of postural influences here as when a fibroma of the uterus pulls on the uterosacral ligaments. Carcinomatous pain due to involvement of nerve plexuses is continuous and becomes progressively more severe; it tends to be more intense at night. The primary lesion may be inconspicuous, being overlooked upon pelvic examination. Papanicolaou smears, pyelogram, and CT scan are the most useful diagnostic procedures. X-ray therapy of these tumors may produce sacral pain consequent to necrosis of tissue and injury to nerve roots. Low back pain with radiation into one or both thighs is a common phenomenon during the last weeks of pregnancy.

Chronic prostatitis, evidenced by prostatic discharge, burning and frequency of urination, and slight reduction in sexual potency, may be attended by a nagging sacral ache; it may be mainly on one side, with radiation into one leg if the seminal vesicle is involved on that side. Carcinoma of the prostate with metastases to the lower part of the spine is another more common cause of sacral or lumbar pain. It may be present without urinary frequency or burning. Spinal nerves may be infiltrated by tumor cells, or the spinal cord itself may be compressed if the epidural space is invaded. The diagnosis is established by rectal examination, roentgenograms and bone scans of the spine, and measurement of acid phosphatase (particularly the prostatic phosphatase fraction). Lesions of the bladder and testes are usually not accompanied by back pain. When the kidney is the site of disease, the pain is ipsilateral, being felt in the flank or lumbar region.

Visceral derangements of whatever type may intensify the pain of arthritis, and the presence of arthritis may alter the distribution of visceral pain. With disease of the spine in the lumbosacral region, for example, distention of the ampulla of the sigmoid by feces or a bout of colitis may aggravate the arthritic pain. In patients with arthritis of the cervical or thoracic spine the pain of myocardial ischemia may radiate to the back.

OBSCURE TYPES OF LOW BACK PAIN AND THE QUESTION OF PSYCHIATRIC DISEASE The practitioner is frequently consulted by persons who complain of low back pain of obscure origin. Usually the disorder is benign in nature and results from some minor derangement, muscular strain, or diskal prolapse. This is particularly true for those lesions which are of acute onset, aggravated by motion, and relieved by rest. Considerably more difficult are patients with chronic pain, especially those who have had prior back surgery or chronic visceral disease, or those who have severe and progressive pain in which neoplasia or infection is considered.

Even when exhaustive studies have been performed, there remains a group of patients in whom no anatomic or pathologic lesion can be found. These patients generally fall into two categories: those with postural back pain and those with psychiatric illness.

Postural back pain Many slender asthenic individuals and some obese middle-aged individuals have discomfort in the back. Their backs ache much of the time, and the pain interferes with effective work. The physical examination is negative except for slack musculature and poor posture. The pain is diffuse in the mid or low region of the back and characteristically is relieved by bed rest and induced by the maintenance of a particular posture over a period of time. Pain in the neck and between the shoulder blades is a common complaint among thin, tense, active women and seems to be related to taut trapezius muscles.

Psychiatric illness Low back pain may be encountered in compensation hysteria and malingering, in anxiety or neurocirculatory asthenia (formerly called neurasthenia), in depression and hypochondriasis, and in many nervous persons whose symptoms and complaints do not fall within any category of psychiatric illness. It is probably correct to assume that pain in the back in such patients usually signifies diseases of the spine and adjacent structures, and one should always search for a specific cause. However, even when organic factors are found, the pain may be exaggerated, prolonged, or woven into a pattern of invalidism or disability because of coexistent psychological factors. This is especially true when there is the possibility of secondary gain (notably compensation).

PAIN IN THE NECK AND SHOULDER

It is useful to distinguish three major categories of painful disease—of the spine, brachial plexus (thoracic outlet), and shoulder. Although pain in these three regions of the body may overlap, the patient usually can indicate the site of origin. Pain arising from the cervical spine is felt in the neck and back of the head (though it may often be projected to the shoulder and arm), is evoked or enhanced by certain movements or positions of the neck, and is accompanied by tenderness and limitation of motions of the neck. Similarly, pain resulting from abnormalities of the thoracic outlet is experienced in and around the shoulder in the supraclavicular region, or between the shoulders; is induced by the performance of certain tasks and by certain positions; and is associated with tenderness of structures above the clavicle. There may be a palpable abnormality above the clavicle (aneurysms of the subclavian artery, tumor, cervical rib). The combination of circulatory symptoms and signs referable to the lower part of the brachial plexus, manifested in the hand by obliteration of pulse when the patient holds a full breath with the head tilted back or turned (Adson's test), unilateral Raynaud's phenomenon, trophic changes in the fingers, and sensory loss over the ulnar side of the hand with or without interosseous atrophy complete the clinical picture. Roentgenograms showing a cervical rib, deformed thoracic outlet, or superior sulcus tumor of the lung (Pancoast's syndrome) corroborate disease in this location. Electromyography and conduction studies along the plexus from points stimulated above and below the clavicle, and studies of arterial and venous circulation (venograms, noninvasive Doppler techniques) are especially helpful in evaluating this problem.

Pain localized to the shoulder region, often worse at night, associated with tenderness and aggravated by abduction, internal rotation, and extension points toward a lesion of the tendinous structures about the shoulder. Most often these are in the form of a tendonitis or bursitis (sometimes calcific) usually affecting the supraspinatus tendon and the adjacent subdeltoid bursa; occasionally the lesion is more extensive and consists of a rupture of the rotator cuff, in which case the patient may have weakness on abduction and forward flexion. In some such patients there is an adhesive capsulitis, leading to profound limitation of motion, designated as a "frozen shoulder." Shoulder pain may radiate into the arm or hand, but the sensory, motor, and reflex changes which indicate disease of nerve roots, plexus, or peripheral nerves are absent.

Osteoarthritis of the cervical part of the spine may cause pains which radiate into the back of the head, shoulders, and arms on one or both sides of the thorax. Coincident involvement of nerve roots is manifested by paresthesias, sensory loss, weakness, or deep tendon reflex change. Should bony ridges form in the spinal canal (spondylosis) the spinal cord may be compressed (see Chap. 353). A myelogram or CT scan may reveal the degree of encroachment on the spinal canal (narrowing of the canal to less than 11 mm in the anteroposterior diameter) at the level at which the spinal cord is affected. The authors have experienced difficulty in distinguishing spondylosis with or without disk rupture and spinal cord compression from primary neurologic diseases (syringomyelia, amyotrophic lateral sclerosis, or tumor) with an unrelated osteoarthritis of the cervical portion of the spine, particularly at the fifth to sixth and sixth to seventh cervical vertebrae, where the disk spaces are often narrowed in the adult. A combination of anxiety with osteoarthritis of the cervical part of the spine or a painful injury to ligaments and muscles after an accident in which the neck is forcibly extended and flexed (e.g., "whiplash" injury to spine) may be a difficult diagnostic problem, particularly if in the course of the injury a cerebral concussion has occurred. If the pain is persistent and limited to the neck, the problem will sometimes prove to have been due to disruption of a disk, but it is often complicated by psychological factors.

RUPTURED CERVICAL DISKS One of the commonest causes of neck, shoulder, and arm pain is disk herniation in the lower cervical region. As with rupture of the lumbar disks, the complete syndrome includes the disorder of spinal function and evidence of neural involvement. It may develop after trauma either major or minor (sudden hyperextension of the neck, diving, forceful manipulations, etc.). Virtually every patient exhibits an abnormality in range of motion of the neck (limitation and pain). Hyperextension is the movement that most consistently aggravates the pain, although one occasionally sees patients whose principal limitation is in flexion. Rotation and lateral movements are often moderately restricted by pain. With laterally situated disk lesions between the fifth and sixth cervical vertebrae, the symptoms and signs are referred to the sixth cervical roots. The full syndrome is characterized by pain felt at the trapezius ridge, tip of the shoulder, anterior upper part of the arm, radial forearm, and often in the thumb; paresthesias and sensory impairment or hypersensitivity in the same regions; tenderness in the area above the spine of the scapula and in the supraclavicular and biceps regions; weakness in flexion of the forearm; diminished to absent biceps and supinator reflexes (triceps retained or exaggerated). When the protruded disk lies between the sixth and seventh cervical vertebrae, the seventh cervical root is involved. Under these circumstances, in the patient with the complete syndrome, the pain is in the region of the shoulder blade, pectoral region and medial axilla, posterolateral upper arm, elbow and dorsal forearm, index and middle fingers, or all the fingers; tenderness is most pronounced over the medial aspect of the shoulder blade opposite the third to fourth thoracic spinous processes, in the supraclavicular area and triceps region; paresthesias and sensory loss are most pronounced in the second and third fingers or tips of all the fingers; weakness is seen in extension of the forearm, in the extension of the wrist, and in the hand grip; the triceps reflex is diminished to absent, and the biceps and supinator reflexes are preserved. Either of these syndromes may be incomplete in that only one of several of the typical findings (e.g., pain) is present. Usually the patient states that cough, sneeze, and downward pressure on the head in the hyperextension position exacerbate pain and traction (even manual) tends to relieve it.

Unlike lumbar disks, the cervical ones, if large and centrally situated, may result in compression of the spinal cord (central disk, all the cord; paracentral disk, part of the cord). The central disk is often nearly painless, and the cord syndrome may simulate a degenerative disease (amyotrophic lateral sclerosis, combined system disease). A common error is to fail to think of a ruptured disk in the cervical region in patients with obscure symptoms in the legs. The diagnosis of ruptured cervical disk should be confirmed by the same laboratory procedures that were mentioned under "Spondylosis," above.

OTHER CONDITIONS Metastases to the cervical spine are fortunately less common than to other parts of the vertebral column. They are frequently painful and the cause of disordered root function. Compression fractures or extension of the tumor posteriorly may lead to rapid development of quadriplegia.

Shoulder injuries (rotator cuff), subacromial or subdeltoid bursitis, the frozen shoulder (periarthritis or capsulitis), tendonitis, and arthritis may develop in patients who are otherwise well, but these conditions are also frequent in hemiplegics or in individuals suffering from coronary heart disease. The pain is often severe and extends toward the neck and down the arm into the hand. The dorsum of the latter may tingle without other signs of nerve involvement. Vasomotor and arthropathic changes also may occur in the hand (shoulder-hand syndrome, reflex dystrophy), and after a time, osteoporosis and atrophy of cutaneous and subcutaneous structures occur (Sudeck's atrophy or Sudeck-Leriche syndrome). These conditions fall more within the province of orthopedics than of medicine and are not discussed here in detail. The physician, however, must know that they can often be prevented by proper exercises (Chap. 198).

The *carpal tunnel syndrome,* with paresthesias and numbness in palmar distribution of the median nerve and aching pain which extends up into the forearm, may be mistaken for disease of the shoulder or neck. Similarly, other less common forms of nerve entrapment may involve the ulnar, radial, or median nerves and lead to a mistaken diagnosis of brachial plexus lesion or cervical syndrome. Electromyography and conduction studies are especially helpful in such conditions (Chap. 354).

MANAGEMENT OF BACK AND NECK PAIN

Without doubt the preventive aspects of back pain are important. There would be far fewer back problems if adults kept their trunk muscles in optimal condition by regular exercise such as swimming, bicycle riding, walking briskly, running, or calisthenic programs. A regular exercise program to strengthen abdominal and paraspinal muscles is frequently very beneficial for patients with chronic low back discomfort. Morning is the ideal time since the back of the older adult tends to stiffen during the night because of inactivity. This happens regardless of whether a bed board or a stiff mattress is used. Sleeping with back hyperextended and sitting for long times in an overstuffed chair or a badly designed auto seat commonly cause difficulties for the patient with low back problems. It is estimated that pressures between disks are increased 200 percent by changing from a recumbent to a standing position and by 400 percent by sitting slumped in an easy chair. Correct sitting posture lessens this. Long trips in a car or plane without change in position put maximal strain on disk and ligamentous structures in the spine. Lifting from a position of flexed trunk, as in removing a suitcase from the trunk of a car, is dangerous (always lift with the object close to the body). Sudden strenuous activity without conditioning and warm-up also is likely to cause trouble to disks and their ligamentous envelopes (the commonest sources of back pain); certain families seem disposed.

Muscular and ligamentous strains and minor disk prolapses are usually self-limited, responding to simple measures in a relatively short period of time. The basic principle of therapy is rest in a recumbent position for several days to weeks. When weight bearing is resumed, a light lumbosacral support is usually helpful in continuing the immobilization until the patient is restored to full health. Physical measures such as heat, cold, diathermy, or massage are of limited value; of considerably greater importance are active exercises to both reduce the spasm and improve muscle tone. Analgesic medication should be given liberally during the first few days: codeine, 30 mg, and aspirin, 0.6 g, or pentazocine, 50 mg, propoxyphene, 65 mg, or meperidine, 50 mg. Muscle relaxants are often a valuable adjunct, particularly in that such drugs as diazepam, 8 to 40 mg in divided doses may make bed rest more tolerable. If an inflammatory component is suspected, indomethacin, 75 mg per day (in divided doses), or ibuprofen, 600 mg 3 or 4 times daily, may be helpful.

In the treatment of an acute or chronic rupture of a lumbar or cervical disk, complete bed rest is essential, at least initially, and strong analgesic medication may be required. Traction is of little value in lumbar disk disease, and it is best to permit the patient to find the most comfortable position. Cervical traction with a halter may be of considerable benefit to patients with cervical disk syndrome. It can be administered with the patient in recumbency, or after sufficient improvement to allow ambulation, can be performed intermittently in the erect position using special equipment. During the recumbent phase of treatment of lumbar disk disease, exercises to reduce spasm, muscle relaxants, and anti-inflammatory agents as described above may be of considerable value. After 2 to 3 weeks in bed, the patient can be allowed to slowly resume activities, usually with the protection of a brace or light spinal support. Exercise programs designed to increase the strength of the abdominal and paraspinal muscles are helpful at this point. The patient may suffer some minor recurrence of the pain but be able to carry on his or her usual activities, and eventually most individuals will recover. If the pain and neurologic findings do not disappear on prolonged, conservative management, or if the patient suffers frequently recurring acute episodes, surgical management may be indicated. This should always be preceded by a myelogram and a computerized reconstructed body scan to localize the lesion (and rule out the presence of intra- or extradural tumors). The surgical procedure most often indicated is a hemilaminectomy with excision of the disk involved. Arthrodesis of the involved segments is indicated only in cases in which there is extraordinary instability usually related to an anatomic abnormality (such as spondylolysis) or in the cervical region when an extensive laminectomy has rendered the spine unstable. The results of conservative management of so-called sciatica cases in the controlled study of Coxhead et al. was approximately 80 percent improved at the end of 4 weeks, regardless of whether traction, exercises, manipulation, or corset, or some combination thereof, was used.

Over the past two decades, orthopedists and neurosurgeons have performed several trials of intradiskal administration of the enzyme chymopapain in the treatment of disk disease. The theoretical advantages of such a technique are clear; if the lesion can be sharply localized by myelography and diskography and the disk space injected with this potent proteoglycanolytic agent, the patient should get relief of localized back and radicular pain within a short period of time and be spared the risk, disability, and prolonged convalescence of an operative procedure. It has become apparent during these trials, however, that the use of this agent is not always effective; and, more importantly, its use is not without some rather spectacular complications which are not entirely predictable and may seriously threaten the patient's well-being. A small but significant number of patients develop an anaphylactoid response to the agent and many experience severe spasms of the low back and legs immediately after the procedure. Of greater concern is a very small number of patients who have developed an irreversible transverse myelitis or other major neurologic problems following the procedure. Although the authors have not encountered these complications, we currently do not advocate the procedure except in individuals in whom the pain fails to respond to conservative management and for whom open surgery is contraindicated.

Spondylosis of the cervical spine, if painful, is helped by bed rest and traction; if signs of spinal cord involvement are present, a collar to limit movement may lead to improvement. Decompressive laminectomy or anterior fusion is reserved for severe instances of the disease with advancing neurologic symptoms. The shoulder-hand syndrome may benefit from stellate ganglion blocks or ganglionectomy, but the basic treatment is physiotherapy, with or without prednisone, and surgical procedures are used only as measures of last resort.

The management of patients with thoracic outlet syndrome is complex and requires first a careful study to be certain that the cause of the lesion is really a mechanical encroachment of the brachial plexus in the interspace between the clavicle and first rib. Exercises to reduce the tension in this region are mainly designed to strengthen the clavicular musculature and improve posture, thus opening the outlet. Many patients benefit from change of work circumstances, and for women with pendulous breasts, a better designed brassiere is sometimes helpful. Nonsteroidal anti-inflammatory agents are sometimes beneficial, as are muscle relaxants such as diazepam. In the event that the patient's difficulties are intractable or the root compression causes neurologic deficits, exploration of the anterior scalene triangle with resection of the first rib is advocated with usually excellent results.

REFERENCES

Armstrong JR: *Lumbar Disc Lesions,* 3d ed. Baltimore, Williams & Wilkins, 1965

Bogduk N: The innervation of the lumbar spine. Spine 8:286, 1983

Brady LP et al: An evaluation of the electromyogram in the diagnosis of lumbar disk lesion. J Bone Joint Surg 51A:539, 1969

Chevetz NI et al: Recognition of lumbar disk herniation with NMR. Am J Radiol 141: 1153, 1983

Collier B: Treatment for lumbar sciatic pain in posterior articular lumbar joint syndrome. Anesthesia 34:202, 1979

Coxhead CE et al: Multicenter trial of physiotherapy in the management of sciatic symptoms. Lancet 1:1065, 1981

Edeiken J, Pitt MJ: The radiologic diagnoses of disk disease. Orthop Clin North Am 2:405, 1971

Friedenberg AB, Miller WT: Degenerative disk disease of the cervical spine. J Bone Joint Surg 45A:1171, 1963

Grabias SL, Mankin HJ: Pain in lower back. Bull Rheum Dis 30:1040, 1980

Mikhael MH et al: Neurologic evaluation of lateral recess syndrome. Radiology 140:97, 1981

Murphy RW: Nerve roots and spinal nerves in degenerative disk disease. Clin Orthop 129:46, 1977

Naylor A: The changes in the human intervertebral disk in degeneration and nuclear prolapse. Orthop Clin North Am 2:343, 1971

Raskin SP: Computerized tomographic findings in lumbar disk disease. Orthopedics 5:419, 1981

Reynolds AV et al: Lumbar monoradiculopathy due to unilateral facet hypertrophy. Neurosurgery 10:480, 1982

Rothman RC, Simeone F: *Lumbar Disc Disease.* Philadelphia, Saunders, 1975, pp 443–458

Williams AL et al: Computed tomography in the diagnosis of herniated nucleus pulposus. Radiology 135:95, 1980

Wilson ES, Brill RF: Spinal stenosis: The narrow lumbar canal syndrome. Clin Orthop 122:244, 1977

section 2 Alterations in body temperature

8 DISTURBANCES OF HEAT REGULATION

ROBERT G. PETERSDORF / RICHARD K. ROOT

CONTROL OF BODY TEMPERATURE In health, the body temperature of humans is maintained within a narrow range despite extremes in environmental conditions and physical activity. This is also true for most birds and mammals, and such animals are termed *homeothermic,* or warm-blooded. An almost invariable accompaniment of systemic illness is a disturbance in temperature regulation, usually an abnormal elevation, or *fever.* In fact, fever is such a sensitive and reliable indicator of the presence of disease that thermometry is probably the commonest clinical procedure in use. Even in the absence of a frank febrile response, interference with heat regulation by disease is evident. This may take the form of flushing, pallor, sweating, shivering, and abnormal sensations of cold or warmth, or it may consist of erratic fluctuations of body temperature within normal limits when a patient is at bed rest.

Heat production The major source of basal heat production is through thyroid thermogenesis and the action of adenosine triphosphatase (ATPase) on the sodium pump of all membranes. The muscles are most important in promoting increased heat production through increased shivering. Heat production by muscle is of particular importance because the quantity can be varied according to the need. In most circumstances this variation consists of small increases and decreases in the number of nerve impulses to the muscles, causing inapparent tensing or relaxing. When, however, there is a strong stimulus for heat production, muscle activity may increase to the point of shivering, or even to a generalized rigor. During digestion of food, gastrointestinal production of heat is significant.

Heat loss Heat is lost from the body in several ways. Small amounts are used in warming food or drink and in the evaporation of moisture from the respiratory tract. Most heat is lost from the surface of the body by *convection,* i.e., the transfer of heat to a fluid medium. Heat loss by convection depends on the existence of a temperature gradient between the body surface and the ambient air. A second mechanism for heat loss is *radiation,* which may be defined as an exchange of electromagnetic energy between the body and the radiant environment. *Evaporation* is the third major mechanism for dissipating heat and is particularly important when the ambient temperature exceeds that of the body, or when core temperatures are increased by vigorous exercise.

The principal method of regulating heat loss is by varying the volume of blood flowing to the surface of the body. A rich circulation in the skin and subcutaneous tissues carries heat to the surface, where it can escape. In addition, sweating increases heat loss by providing water to be vaporized. The sweat, or eccrine, glands are under the control of the sympathetic nerves which, in this instance, mediate cholinergic stimuli. Heat loss by sweating may be tremendous, and as much as 1 liter per hour of sweat may be evaporated. The amount of heat loss through sweating is also dependent upon the humidity in the air. The greater the humidity, the less the ability to lose heat through sweat.

When there is need for conservation of heat, adrenergic autonomic stimuli cause a sharp reduction in the blood flow to the surface. This causes vasoconstriction and transforms the skin and subcutaneous tissue into layers of insulation.

Heat transfer within the body This depends upon *conduction,* i.e., the transfer of heat between adjacent organs, and upon *circulatory convection,* which is governed by bulk movement of body fluids and which is responsible for the transfer of heat between the cells and the bloodstream. It is useful, although oversimplified, to visualize the body as a central core at uniform temperatures surrounded by an insulating shell. The role of the shell as a mediator for heat conservation and heat loss is determined in part by its blood supply and by vasoconstriction or vasodilatation. Although insulation is relatively uniform throughout the body, some parts, such as the digits, are particularly susceptible to cold because of the increased surface-to-volume ratio. Moreover, blood that reaches the digits has already been cooled on the way. Insulation may be enhanced by the addition of clothing.

Neural control of temperature The control of body temperature, integrating the various physical and chemical processes for heat production or heat loss, is a function of cerebral centers located in the hypothalamus. A high-decerebrate animal has a normal temperature if the hypothalamus is left intact. On the other hand, an animal whose brainstem has been sectioned loses ability to control body temperature, which consequently tends to vary with the environment, a condition referred to as *poikilothermia.* Animal experiments suggest that the preoptic anterior hypothalamus and some centers in the spinal cord have neurons which respond directly to local temperature and act as a sensor for internal temperature. This function is distinct from the integrative function which responds to temperature-sensitive structures all over the body.

FACTORS AFFECTING NEURAL CONTROL OF TEMPERATURE The temperature-regulating system is a negative feedback control system, and possesses three elements essential to such a system: (1) receptors which sense the existing central temperatures; (2) effector mechanisms, consisting of the vasomotor, sudomotor, and metabolic effectors; and (3) integrative structures which determine whether the existing temperature is too high or too low and which activate the appropriate motor response. It is a negative feedback system because a rise in central temperature initiates mechanisms for losing heat while a fall in central temperature activates mechanisms for heat production and heat conservation. The activation of these effector responses is governed by a central integrative mechanism which may be compared with a thermostat and which responds to a variety of stimuli, such as the sensory impulses engendered in flushing or sweating, behavioral impulses, exercise, endocrine influences, and probably the temperature of the blood circulating through the hypothalamic centers. In a sense all these stimuli reset the thermostat, thereby activating compensatory heat loss or heat conservation mechanisms.

A classic example of the endocrine influence on temperature is the effect of menstruation. The mean body temperature of women is higher during the second half of the menstrual cycle than it is between the onset of menstruation and the time of ovulation. The sensations of intense heat followed by diaphoresis that characterize the vasomotor instability experienced by some women at the menopause are undoubtedly the result of endocrine imbalance. The activation of the adrenal medulla in response to cold is another example of the relationship between the endocrine system and the thermoregulatory apparatus.

Normal body temperature It is not practical to designate an exact upper level of normal body temperature because there are small differences among normal persons. There are rare individuals whose temperatures are always elevated slightly above accepted "normal" levels, and there is considerable variation in temperature in a given individual. In general, however, it is safe to regard an oral temperature above 99°F (37.2°C) in a person at bed rest as probable indication of disease. The temperature may be as low as 96.5°F (35.8°C) in healthy persons. Rectal temperature is usually 0.5 to 1.0°F higher than oral temperature. In very hot weather the body temperature may be elevated by 0.5 or even 1.0°F.

There is a distinct diurnal variation in body temperature in healthy human beings. Oral readings of 97°F (36.1°C) are relatively common on arising in the morning. Body temperature rises steadily through the day, reaches a peak of 99°F (37.2°C) or greater between 6 P.M. and 10 P.M., and then drops slowly to reach a minimum at 2 A.M. to 4 A.M. Although it has been postulated that this diurnal variation is dependent upon increasing activity during the day and rest at night, the pattern is not reversed in individuals who work at night and sleep during the day for long periods of time. The febrile patterns of most human diseases also tend to follow this normal diurnal pattern. Fevers tend to be higher, to "spike," in the evening, and many patients with febrile disease have relatively normal temperatures in the early morning hours.

Body temperature is more labile in young children, and transient elevations after relatively slight exertion in warm weather are frequently observed in them.

Severe or prolonged exercise can produce considerable elevation in body temperature. For example, marathon runners often have temperatures between 103.2 and 105.8°F (39 and 41°C). Although this marked increase in temperature with exercise tends to be balanced by compensatory cutaneous vasodilatation, resulting in loss of heat, and hyperventilation, these compensatory mechanisms may fail, leading to hyperpyrexia and, if uncontrolled, to heat stroke. Many of the adverse effects of long-distance running can be prevented by holding races only if the ambient temperature is below 82°F (27.8°C), preferably in the early morning or early evening, and by ensuring ample fluid intake both before and during a race.

Disordered thermoregulation In exercise, there is a temporary imbalance between heat production and heat loss with prompt reestablishment of normal temperatures at rest due to continuing activation of heat loss mechanisms. In fact, in prolonged exercise, cutaneous vasodilatation in response to an increase in central body temperature stops in order to preserve central temperature. Less adaptation occurs in fever because once a stable body temperature is reached, heat production equals heat loss, but both are greater than in the basal state. Cutaneous blood flow plays a greater role in controlling heat production and heat loss in fever than does sweating. At the beginning of fever, the body temperature as sensed by the thermoreceptors is low and the individual responds physiologically as if he or she were cold. *Heat production* is increased by shivering, and *heat loss* is decreased by vasoconstriction. These events explain the sensation of cold or chills that characterizes the beginning of fever. Conversely, when the cause of fever is removed, the temperature returns to normal, and the individual responds as if warm. Cutaneous vasodilatation, sweating, and inhibition of shivering are the compensatory responses.

Deviations of 5°F (approximately 3.5°C) from the normal body temperature do not interfere appreciably with most bodily functions. Convulsions are common at temperatures higher than 106°F (41.1°C) in children, and irreversible brain damage, presumably due to protein denaturation (impairment of normal enzymic functions), is common when temperatures of 108°F (42.2°C) are reached. Fortunately, when hyperthermia reaches dangerous levels, the mechanisms for heat loss are suddenly activated; consequently, oral temperatures above 106°F (41.1°C) are relatively rare in humans. Conversely, when temperatures are lowered to 91°F (32.8°C), loss of consciousness occurs; at 86°F (30°C) poikilothermia sets in, and between 83 and 84°F (28.5°C) slow atrial fibrillation supervenes. Ventricular fibrillation occurs at extremely hypothermic temperatures.

The systemic symptoms accompanying deviations in temperature are poorly understood. For example at temperatures of 102°F (39°C) many patients have malaise, drowsiness, weakness, and generalized aches and pains. Many others, however, feel entirely well. Why some individuals are able to tolerate fever so well while others become markedly ill remains an enigma. Perhaps the inciting stimulus rather than fever per se is the major determinant of systemic complaints. The macrophage product, endogenous pyrogen/interleukin-1 (IL-1), may also play a role in the systemic symptoms accompanying fever.

DISEASES OF THE NERVOUS SYSTEM Disease of the regulatory centers in the hypothalamus may affect body temperature. Cases have been observed in which there was destruction of the centers controlling heat-conserving mechanisms, with resulting hypothermia. More commonly, cerebral lesions are manifested by hyperthermia; this may occur with tumors, degenerative diseases, vascular accidents, particularly cerebral hemorrhage, or infections involving the hypothalamus, such as encephalitis. All these may result in loss of neurons and gliosis. Central fever is accompanied by lack of a diurnal variation, absence of sweating, resistance to antipyretic drugs, excessive response to external cooling, and loss of consciousness.

There are several diseases, of which heat stroke is the cardinal example, in which the central mechanisms for cooling suddenly fail and the patient ceases to sweat, despite the fact that his or her temperature is rising. Some of the highest temperatures ever observed in human beings [112 to 113°F (44.4°C)] have been in cases of heat stroke. A temperature higher than 114°F (45.6°C) is probably not compatible with life.

INCREASED HEAT PRODUCTION Patients with thyrotoxicosis show exaggerated heat production, and their temperature is often 1 to 2°F above the normal range.

IMPAIRMENT OF HEAT LOSS Patients with *congestive heart failure* often have an elevation of body temperature between 0.5 and 1.5°F. Perhaps this elevation is caused by impairment of heat dissipation as a result of diminished cardiac output, decline in cutaneous blood flow (with increasing insulation of the central temperature core), the insulating effect of edema, and the increased heat production incident to the muscular activity of dyspnea. On the other hand, patients with congestive heart failure are likely to have other causes of fever, such as venous thrombosis, pulmonary embolism and infarction, myocardial infarction, pneumonia, and urinary tract infection. However, since slight fever is so regularly present even in the absence of such complications, the circulatory disturbance may be responsible.

Patients with skin disorders such as *ichthyosis* and *congenital absence of sweat glands* may have fever in a warm environment because of inability to lose heat from the surface of the body. Individuals with congenitally absent sweat glands lack the ability of active cutaneous vasodilatation and hence are unable to dissipate heat by at least two mechanisms. Drugs which impair sweating, such as atropine, scopolamine, phenothiazines, monoamine oxidase inhibitors, glutethimide, lysergic acid diethylamide (LSD), amphetamines, and inhalation anesthetics, may result in elevated temperatures.

Patients with severe burns tend to be hyperthermic, probably because occlusive dressings interfere with heat loss despite large areas of denuded skin; they are also hypermetabolic, and heat production is increased.

PATHOGENESIS OF FEVER Fever may be produced by many stimuli, including bacteria and their endotoxins; viruses; yeasts; spirochetes; immune reactions; hormonal substances, exemplified by progesterone; drugs; and synthetic polynucleotides like poly I:poly C. These substances, which have been termed collectively *exogenous pyrogens,* are both diverse and complex. It has been postulated that they act through an intermediary substance termed *endogenous pyrogen* (EP). Most of the knowledge concerning EP has come from work in experimental animals.

EP is now known to be identical to interleukin-1 (IL-1), a product of monocytes and macrophages which initiates many of the reactions termed collectively the "acute phase response." EP/IL-1 is a polypeptide of about 15,000 molecular weight that is synthesized in response to exogenous pyrogens. In addition to temperature-regulating centers in the anterior hypothalamus, other targets for EP/IL-1 include B and T lymphocytes, myeloid cells in the bone marrow, mature neutrophils, fibroblasts, striated muscle, hepatocytes, and cerebral neurons responsible for slow-wave sleep signals. The action of EP/IL-1 at each of these sites is quite different and with some targets involves an intermediate role for specific prostaglandin metabolites.

When EP/IL-1 engages thermosensitive neurons in the preoptic region of the hypothalamus, an abrupt increase in muscular heat production (rigors) occurs, accompanied by decreased heat loss (cutaneous vasoconstriction, and "goose flesh," i.e., "chills"). The core body temperature increases until a higher stable point is reached in the balance between heat production and heat loss. The temperature of the blood bathing the hypothalamus is equivalent to the new "set point."

Within the hypothalamus EP/IL-1 appears to act by inducing the synthesis of prostaglandins of the E series using arachidonate released from target cell membranes. In particular, prostaglandin E_1 (PGE_1) activates heat generating and conserving mechanisms by inducing synthesis of cyclic adenyl monophosphate (cyclic AMP). The precise chemical events remain to be elucidated; however, the antipyretic actions of aspirin and nonsteroidal anti-inflammatory drugs can be ascribed to their inhibition of cyclooxygenase and resultant blockade of PGE_1 and PGE_2 synthesis. Glucocorticoids are antipyretic through more complex mechanisms including inhibition of EP/IL-1 production peripherally and arachidonate release centrally. Fever contrasts with hyperthermia of other causes in which there is no resetting of the central thermostat by EP/IL-1; core temperatures are increased because heat loss mechanisms fail to balance heat production.

EP/IL-1 plays a key role in initiating the immune response by activating helper/inducer T cells to synthesize the polypeptide interleukin-2 (IL-2), which causes clonal expansion of responding T cells. Furthermore, T-cell mitogenesis in response to IL-2 is enhanced at febrile temperatures reaching an optimum at 103.1°F (39.5°C). By this means, fever induction appears to exert a positive feedback in the specific immune response. B-cell proliferation and specific antibody production are also enhanced by IL-1.

EP/IL-1 mobilizes myeloid cells from marrow storage pools, has chemotactic activity for neutrophils and monocytes and induces lysosomal discharge in neutrophils. It also stimulates neutrophil microbicidal oxidative metabolism. Hence, key nonspecific inflammatory mechanisms which can eradicate microorganisms are promoted by the action of EP/IL-1.

Other less well defined actions of EP/IL-1 appear to contribute to antimicrobial and protective mechanisms during infection. These include induction of hypoferremia and a fall in plasma zinc concentrations. Iron is an essential growth factor for many microorganisms. Hepatic synthesis of acute phase proteins is augmented. These include complement factors and C-reactive protein, which may participate directly in antimicrobial events as well as haptoglobin, ceruloplasmin, certain protease inhibitors, fibrinogen, and serum amyloid A protein. The precise role of many of these proteins in host defense requires elucidation, but some, at least, have the capacity to regulate inflammatory mechanisms triggered during infection.

EP/IL-1 mobilizes amino acids from muscle through a proteolytic mechanism mediated by cyclooxygenase and PGE_1. Mobilization can be inhibited by cyclooxygenase inhibitors and presumably functions to supply amino acids as nutrients for other cells. PGE_1 production and muscle degradation are enhanced at febrile body temperatures, indicative of a positive feedback in this event as there is for stimulation of immune responses. Muscle wasting in febrile states can be profound and lead to weight loss of up to a kilogram per day. Myalgias experienced during fever are relieved by aspirin and other antipyretics and may reflect inhibition of muscle catabolism by lysosomal proteases.

EP/IL-1 activates fibroblasts to synthesize collagen. This presumably contributes to tissue reparative responses during infection. Production of IL-1 at local sites may contribute to site-specific inflammatory processes such as joint injury in rheumatoid arthritis, periodontal disease, and even sunburn (ultraviolet-induced keratinocyte production of IL-1).

Finally, EP/IL-1 contained and released by astrocytes in the brain may not only cause fever during cerebral hemorrhage but activates slow-wave sleep–inducing neurons. The drowsiness and prolonged sleep characteristic of febrile illnesses may have their basis in the action of EP/IL-1 and serve as additional protective mechanisms.

Both fever and specific events mediated by the fever-producing molecule EP/IL-1 have a broad and highly integrated role in the characteristic responses to infection and/or acute inflammation. Some of these responses may be viewed as protective, whereas others contribute to deleterious symptoms and signs. Given this complexity it is not surprising that conflict surrounds the need to treat fever with antipyretics or by other means. While symptomatology might be relieved, the cost could be interference with normally protective mechanisms including the specific immune response and the mobilization of nutrients necessary to promote a successful recovery.

DISORDERS ASSOCIATED WITH HIGH TEMPERATURES Heat syndromes Four clinical syndromes are associated with high environmental temperature: *heat cramps, heat exhaustion, exertional heat injury,* and *heat stroke.* Although each of these entities may be separated from the other on clinical grounds, there is considerable overlap between them, and they may be considered as a series of syndromes along a single spectrum. The incidence of heat syndromes is unknown, but during an ordinary summer about 200 cases of heat stroke are reported. During the heat wave of June 1984, there was a 35 percent increase in mortality in New York City almost exclusively due to a rise in deaths in elderly persons living at home. Heat syndromes occur primarily at elevated temperatures (>90°F) and at high relative humidities (>60%); and elderly individuals, those with mental illness or alcoholism or who receive antipsychotic drugs, diuretics, and anticholinergics, or those who reside in poorly ventilated places without air conditioning are most susceptible. Heat syndromes are especially prevalent during the first days of a heat wave before effective acclimatization can occur. Prophylaxis by augmenting fluid intake prior to exposure and by ensuring that susceptible individuals, particularly the elderly or the very young, wear light clothing, take frequent cool baths, remain in a cool environment, and avoid strenuous physical activity can help prevent the full-blown syndrome, especially heat stroke.

ACCLIMATIZATION The basic mechanism by which humans accommodate to excessive temperatures is unknown. Acclimatization does not increase the threshold for sweating. However, sweating is the most effective natural means of combating heat stress and can occur with little or no change in the core temperature of the body. As long as sweating continues, humans can withstand remarkably high temperatures, provided water and sodium chloride, the most important physiologic constituents of sweat, are replaced. The concentration of sodium chloride varies between that of interstitial fluid and very low concentrations and the ability to secrete sweat with low sodium chloride content, as well as to increase the quantity of sweat, is a major mechanism for the conservation of salt in hot weather. Dilatation of the peripheral blood vessels in an attempt to dissipate heat is another major way for the body to acclimatize to hot temperatures. Other alterations include a decrease in total circulating blood volume, a decrease in renal blood flow, an increase of antidiuretic hormone (ADH) as well as aldosterone, a decrease in urine sodium, and an increase in respiratory and pulse rates. Ordinarily, acclimatization takes from 4 to 7 days. The hyperaldosteronism may result in potassium loss, which may be aggravated by replacement of sodium without concomitant repletion of potassium. Initially there is an increase in cardiac output but as heat stress persists, venous return diminishes and heart failure may occur. If environmental temperatures in excess of the body's temperature persist, heat is retained and hyperpyrexia develops.

HEAT CRAMPS Heat cramps, called "miner's cramps" and "stoker's cramps," are the most benign heat syndrome. Cramps are characterized by painful spasms of the voluntary muscles and usually follow strenuous exercise. In general, only individuals in good physical condition develop this syndrome. External temperatures need not exceed the body temperature, and direct exposure to the sun is not necessary. The body temperature is usually not elevated. Muscle cramps usually occur after excessive sweating and may even be precipitated by strenuous exercise in cold environments in untrained persons heavily clothed. Muscles of the extremities bear the brunt of physical activity and hence show the highest incidence of cramps. Physical examination of the patient is normal between the paroxysms. Examination of the blood reveals a concentration of the formed elements and a decreased sodium chloride concentration. Excretion of these ions in the urine is characteristically low. Treatment consists of sodium chloride; cessation of cramps with replacement of sodium chloride and water is striking and supports the hypothesis that the cause of heat cramps is depletion of these essential electrolytes. Occasionally cramps involve the abdominal musculature, mimicking an intraabdominal emergency. Such patients have had mistaken exploratory surgery performed, often with disastrous results. Replacement of saline prior to surgery would have obviated such operations.

HEAT EXHAUSTION Heat prostration, or heat collapse, is probably the most common heat syndrome. It represents a failure of the cardiovascular responses to high external temperatures and is particularly common in elderly individuals who are receiving diuretics. Weakness, vertigo, headache, anorexia, nausea, vomiting, the urge to defecate, and faintness may precede collapse. Heat collapse occurs in both physically active and sedentary individuals. The onset is usually sudden and the duration of collapse brief. During the acute stage, the patient looks ashen-gray. The skin is cold and clammy. The pupils are dilated. The blood pressure may be low and the pulse pressure elevated. Since prostration develops before exposure to heat is prolonged, body temperature is subnormal or normal. The duration of exposure and the extent to which sweat is lost determine the degree of hemoconcentration. Treatment consists of removal of the patient to a cool area and placing him or her in the recumbent position. Spontaneous recovery then usually takes place. Intravenous administration of saline solution or whole blood is necessary only rarely. Although the pathogenetic mechanism of heat prostration is not primarily a depletion of water and salt, it is likely that maintenance of these electrolytes will prevent heat prostration in individuals exposed to high temperatures.

EXERTIONAL HEAT INJURY This syndrome occurs in individuals who are exerting themselves in hot ambient temperatures (about 80°F) when the relative humidity is high. It is particularly common in runners who enter races with insufficient acclimatization, inadequate conditioning, or improper hydration (before and during the race). Obesity, age, and previous heat stroke are contributing predisposing factors. In contrast to classic heat stroke, individuals with exertional heat injury usually sweat freely, and their temperatures are lower (102 to 104°F as opposed to 106°F and higher in heat stroke). Symptoms consist of headache, piloerection (gooseflesh) on the chest and upper arms, chills, overbreathing, nausea, vomiting, muscle cramps, ataxia, unsteady gait, and incoherent speech. In some individuals, loss of consciousness occurs. Physical examination shows tachycardia, hypotension, and evidence of low peripheral resistance. Laboratory data show hemoconcentration, hypernatremia, abnormal liver and muscle enzymes, hypocalcemia, hypophosphatemia, and, in some instances, hypoglycemia. An occasional patient has thrombocytopenia, hemolysis, disseminated intravascular coagulation, rhabdomyolysis, myoglobinuria, and acute tubular necrosis. Injury to the vascular endothelium may be widespread and contribute to these manifestations as well as organ failure. These severe complications can be avoided by prompt treatment, which consists of placing the victim under wet cold sheets to lower core temperature to 100.4°F (38°C) as quickly as possible, massaging the extremities to improve blood flow from the core to the periphery, and infusing fluids consisting primarily of hypotonic glucose-saline. Patients should be hospitalized for 36 h of observation.

Exertional heat injury can be prevented by (1) running races early in the morning (before 8 A.M.) when the temperature and humidity are likely to be low, (2) educating runners to enter a race well hydrated by drinking 300 mL of water 10 min before a race and 250 mL every 3 to 4 km (salt and glucose solutions should be avoided), (3) placing aid stations at 5-km intervals, (4) instructing runners not to increase their pace after most of the race has been run, and (5) avoiding alcohol before a race.

HEAT STROKE Heat hyperpyrexia, heat stroke, or sunstroke is most common in elderly individuals with preexisting chronic disease. Among these are arteriosclerosis and congestive heart failure, particularly when patients receive diurectics. Other predisposing factors include diabetes mellitus, alcoholism, the use of anticholinergic drugs, and skin disorders in which it may be difficult to lose heat such as ectodermal dysplasia, congenital absence of the sweat glands, or severe scleroderma. Heat stroke is also common in military recruits undergoing basic training, and in an occasional long-distance runner. The mechanism for heat stroke is not known. Although most patients with heat stroke cease sweating, in some sweating is preserved. The vasoconstriction that accompanies heat stroke prevents dissipation of heat from the core, but whether this vasoconstriction is cause or effect is not clear. Direct exposure to the sun is not a necessary prerequisite.

There may be few premonitory symptoms of heat stroke, and loss of consciousness may be the first sign. Other patients may complain of headache, vertigo, faintness, abdominal distress, confusion, or hyperpnea. Delirium may develop in more severe cases.

Pyrexia and prostration are the significant findings on physical examination. A rectal temperature greater than 106°F (41.1°C) is common and internal body temperatures as high as 112 to 113°F (44.4°C) have been recorded. The skin is hot and dry, and, in most cases, sweating is absent. The pulse rate is increased, and respirations are rapid and weak. The blood pressure is usually low. The muscles are flaccid, and tendon reflexes may be diminished. Lethargy, stupor, or coma, depending on the severity, is present. Shock is common in fatal cases.

Examination of the blood and urine may show few abnormalities. Hemoconcentration is common. Leukocytosis is characteristic as are proteinuria, cylindruria, and an elevation in BUN. There is usually a respiratory alkalosis which is followed by a metabolic acidosis. Lactacidemia is common. Serum potassium is normal or low and there are usually hypocalcemia and hypophosphatemia. The electrocardiogram may show, in addition to tachycardia and sinus arrhythmia, flattening and subsequent inversion of the T wave and depression of the ST segment. Diffuse myocardial necrosis with ECG evidence of myocardial infarction has been reported. Other major laboratory abnormalities include thrombocytopenia; prolonged bleeding, clotting, and prothrombin times; afibrinogenemia and fibrinolysis; and disseminated intravascular coagulation. All these may be responsible for diffuse bleeding. Liver damage is common; it appears 24 to 36 h after admission and is characterized by clinically apparent jaundice and, often, by abnormalities in hepatocellular enzymes. Renal failure is a common complication of heat stroke.

Patients with heat stroke may die within a few hours after being discovered, or may die of complications such as acute renal failure. However, a number of patients will die several weeks after the acute episode, usually of myocardial infarction, heart failure, renal failure, bronchopneumonia, or complicating bacteremia. In them autopsy may show extensive parenchymal damage to various organs, either from hyperpyrexia per se or from petechial hemorrhages in the brain, heart, kidneys, or liver.

Heat stroke requires heroic emergency measures. Time is most important. The patient should be placed in a cool place with adequate circulation of fresh air and with most of the clothing removed. Because the pathogenesis of heat stroke involves failure of the heat-regulating mechanism with cessation of sweating, external means of heat dissipation must be employed. The most effective measure is to immerse the patient in an ice-water bath, and there is no effective substitute for this seemingly drastic treatment. An ice-water bath does not induce shock or stimulate significant cutaneous vasoconstriction. The bath should be given with a minimum of delay. The patient should be watched constantly by a nurse or physician and the rectal temperature monitored. The bath may be discontinued when the rectal temperature falls below 101°F (38.3°C), but treatment should be resumed if there is a febrile rebound. Compared with immersion in ice water, other forms of therapy are less effective, but covering the patient with cold wet towels under a fan may be satisfactory if a bath is not available. After the bath the patient should be placed in a cool, well-ventilated room. Massage of the skin should be employed along with cooling because it stimulates return of the cool peripheral blood to the overheated brain and viscera and aids acceleration of heat loss. The patient should be well hydrated with hypotonic crystalloid solutions. Phenothiazine may be helpful in reducing shivering. Stimulants such as epinephrine and narcotics are contraindicated. A Swan-Ganz catheter should be inserted, and urinary output needs to be monitored. Prompt ice-bath cooling, massage of the limbs, and vigorous hydration, along with establishment of a proper airway, avoidance of aspiration, treating coma and convulsions, and watching for arrhythmia, will lead to survival of most patients, particularly if they are young and were previously well. Unfortunately, the poor, ill, and elderly who are often not discovered until heat hyperpyrexia has been present for some hours have a much less favorable outcome. Both dehydration and heart failure must be avoided. Fresh blood should be given in case of bleeding, and clear-cut evidence of disseminated intravascular coagulation calls for heparin (7500 units per hour). Persistent oliguria is an indication for early dialysis.

Malignant hyperthermia ETIOLOGY Malignant hyperthermia (MH) consists of a group of inherited disorders that are characterized by a rapid increase in temperature to 102.2 to 107.6°F (39 to 42°C) in response to inhalational anesthetics such as halothane, methoxyflurane, cyclopropane, and ethyl ether or muscle relaxants, notably succinylcholine. In one form of the disease where the mechanism of inheritance is autosomal dominant, the individuals are normal between attacks although about 50 percent have an elevation in creatine phosphokinase (CPK), and in 90 percent, muscle from susceptible individuals contracts on exposure to concentrations of caffeine, halothane, or hexamethonium that cause only minimal changes in normal muscle. A second recessive form occurs in young boys and, less commonly, girls, with a number of congenital abnormalities including short stature, undescended testes, lumbar lordosis, thoracic kyphosis, pectus carinatum, webbed neck, winged scapulae, small chin, low-set ears, and an antimongoloid obliquity of the palpebral fissures. This form is called the *King syndrome*. MH has also been described in several other myopathies including myotonia congenita, central core disease, and Duchenne's muscular dystrophy. The incidence of the autosomal dominant form is 1:50,000 to 1:100,000.

PATHOGENESIS The triggering anesthetic releases calcium from the membrane of the muscle cell's sarcoplasmic reticulum, which is defective in storing this ion. The result is a sudden increase in myoplasmic calcium. The calcium activates myosin ATPase, which converts adenosine triphosphate (ATP) to adenosine diphosphate, phosphate, and heat. There are also inhibition of tropanin, uncoupling of oxidative phosphorylation, activation of phosphorylase kinase, and increased glycolysis. Muscular contraction occurs and it, as well as the chemical events, leads to production of heat.

MANIFESTATIONS Existence of malignant hyperthermia can be suspected if less relaxation is noted during induction of anesthesia and muscle fasciculations become evident when succinylcholine is given. In some patients trismus during intubation is the first sign of a muscle disorder. Although the elevation in temperature is the result of muscular contraction, it may rise very rapidly, and if the temperature is not monitored, the first signs may be a hot skin and tachycardia or a cardiac arrhythmia. In addition to the high fever, there is muscle rigidity, hypotension, and mottled cyanosis.

Early laboratory abnormalities include respiratory and metabolic acidosis, hyperkalemia and hypermagnesemia, and elevation in blood lactate and pyruvate. Late complications include massive skeletal muscle swelling, pulmonary edema, disseminated intravascular coagulation, and acute renal failure.

TREATMENT Malignant hyperthermia is a medical emergency. Surgery must be interrupted and the patient cooled with ice. One hundred percent oxygen should be given, along with sodium bicarbonate, to combat the severe metabolic acidosis. A diuresis should be induced with fluids and diuretics to reduce myoglobinemia and hyperkalemia. Specific treatment consists of dantrolene sodium, 1 mg/kg, by rapid intravenous infusion. The drug should be continued until symptoms have begun to subside or up to a maximum single dose of 10 mg/kg. The regimen can be repeated if symptoms recur. Procainamide to combat arrhythmias, in dosage of 0.5 to 1 (mg/kg)/min with ECG monitoring, should be administered as well.

PREVENTION Because of the tendency of this syndrome to run in families, its detection is essential. This can be achieved by monitoring the temperature of all patients under anesthesia; the best way to avert it altogether is to take a thorough family history. Examining patients preoperatively is often not helpful because between attacks persons susceptible to malignant hyperthermia may be entirely normal. Some have increased muscle bulk, some have localized areas of muscle weakness, some have spontaneous muscle cramps, and a few have generalized muscle weakness. In some of these patients, the CPK is elevated, but in many this test is entirely normal. Prophylactic dantrolene orally has not been successful in preventing MH. In susceptible patients, surgery should be performed under spinal, epidural, or regional anesthesia. If this is not possible, a combination of Pentothal and diazepam is probably safest. Phosphorylase A and adenylate cyclase are elevated in muscles of MH patients and along with their increased contractility provide useful biochemical markers of MH.

Neuroleptic malignant syndrome (NMS) This syndrome is characterized by muscular rigidity, hyperthermia, altered consciousness, and autonomic dysfunction. Rigidity and akinesia develop concomitantly with fever as high as 106°F (41°C). Consciousness fluctuates from alertness to coma. Autonomic dysfunction is manifested by tachycardia, labile blood pressure, profuse sweating, dyspnea, and incontinence. Laboratory abnormalities consist of leukocytosis (15,000 to 30,000) and elevation in CPK. The syndrome occurs after use of potent neuroleptics in therapeutic doses. Most cases have been reported after haloperidol, thiothixene, or piperazine phenothiazine. Young adult males predominate. The NMS lasts 5 to 10 days after administration of oral neuroleptics is discontinued, and longer after depot injection. The overall mortality is 20 percent and fatalities have occurred as late as 30 days after onset and have been due to renal failure or arrhythmias. Although the etiology of NMS is unknown, its similarity to malignant hyperthermia is striking, and the fact that MH has occurred in the wake of neuroleptic drugs strengthens the hypothesis that NMS may be a variant of MH. No specific treatment for NMS has been described, although dantrolene sodium may be worth trying if supportive measures, cooling, and drug withdrawal do not result in improvement.

DISORDERS ASSOCIATED WITH LOW TEMPERATURES **Cold acclimatization** The state of increased resistance to cold injury is the result of exposure to a cold but tolerable environment. Adaptive responses consist of circulatory adjustments protecting the temperatures of exposed portions of the body, metabolic adaptation providing greater heat production to compensate for increased heat loss, and behavioral and neural adaptations minimizing either the actual cold stress or the discomfort resulting from physiologically tolerable hypothermia. In contrast with heat acclimatization, it is not possible to delineate adaptive physiologic changes to cold. Nevertheless, primitive people live at zero temperatures wearing little or no clothing; pain perception is less in persons, such as fishermen, who work periodically with their hands in ice water; and military personnel shiver less during cold exposure after training in the Arctic. Adaptation may take place either by shivering, with production of excess heat, or, as is the case with Australian aborigines, by a drop of internal temperature with only minimal shivering.

Hypothermia Although far less common than is elevation in temperature, hypothermia is of considerable importance because it can represent a medical emergency which lends itself to treatment.

ACCIDENTAL HYPOTHERMIA This is a well-known complication of exposure and has been reported frequently during the winter months. It usually occurs in elderly or inebriated individuals after prolonged exposure, not necessarily to excessively low external temperatures. It is true, however, that both of these groups detect low temperatures less well than normal. The diagnosis of hypothermia may prove elusive because *clinical thermometers do not record temperatures below 95°F (35°C). Whenever a patient presents with a temperature below this level, the true temperature should be determined with an incubator thermometer or a thermocouple.* Accidental hypothermia has been found in association with myxedema, pituitary insufficiency, Addison's disease, hypoglycemia, cerebrovascular disease, Wernicke's encephalopathy, myocardial infarction, cirrhosis, pancreatitis, and ingestion of drugs or alcohol. For example, it is not uncommon to find a derelict in a railroad yard or under a bridge following an alcoholic debauch with a temperature between 85 and 90°F (28.5 and 32.3°C) or lower. These patients usually appear cold and pale and, when their temperatures are very low, give the appearance of having rigor mortis, so stiff is their musculature. Patients with temperatures less than 80°F (26.7°C) are usually unconscious. The pupils are usually miotic, respirations tend to be shallow and slow, there is bradycardia, and most patients are hypotensive. Generalized edema is often present. When the temperature falls below 77°F (25°C), coma, areflexia, and lack of pupillary response are present. Laboratory data tend to show hemoconcentration, mild azotemia, and metabolic acidosis. The acidosis is due to lactacidemia which is, in part, a result of hypoxemia in peripheral tissues. At cold temperatures, the hemoglobin dissociation curve is shifted to the left, and there is decreased unloading of oxygen in the peripheral tissues. Some patients have hypoglycemia while others have hyperglycemia. Thyroid function tests may give results typical of myxedema. Some patients have elevations in serum amylase, and a few show pancreatitis at autopsy. The electrocardiogram is distorted by muscular tremors and may show bradycardia or slow atrial fibrillation and a characteristic J wave (occurring at the junction of the QRS complex and ST segment). Other arrythmias are common; ventricular fibrillation is usually a terminal event. The mortality rate is five times higher in people over 75.

Hypothermia is a medical emergency, and therapy should be instituted at once. The following steps are indicated:

1 An airway must be established and maintained, and the patient should be well oxygenated. Warmed oxygen may be helpful.
2 Blood gases should be monitored; they should be corrected for temperature.
3 Blood volume should be expanded with glucose and saline, low-molecular-weight dextran, or albumin. Maintenance of blood volume is necessary to prevent the infarctions which have been a hallmark in fatal cases and to avert "rewarming shock."
4 Because of the tendency to arrythmias, serum potassium should be monitored carefully; a transvenous pacemaker may be indicated.
5 Sodium bicarbonate should be given if pH is less than 7.25.
6 Although external rewarming with blankets or placing the patient in a warm room is appropriate in patients with mild hypothermia, patients who are moderately hypothermic require reestablishment of core temperature. This can be done effectively by placing the patient in a warm bath or a Hubbard tank at 104 to 108°F (40 to 42°C). This maneuver must be carried out cautiously; physiologic monitoring may be difficult, and if an arrhythmia occurs, resuscitation is hampered. Nevertheless, external warming tends to dilate the constricted peripheral blood vessels and to divert blood from the visceral organs. In severely hypothermic patients, this may result in rewarming shock and does not lead to sufficient restoration of the core temperature to warm the myocardium sufficiently to make it responsive to antiarrhythmic agents. In this situation hemodialysis, during which the blood is warmed externally, or peritoneal dialysis, during which the dialysate is warmed to 98.6°F (37°C), are the methods of choice. It is particularly important to rewarm the myocardium because in cases of ventricular fibrillation defibrillation will not be successful until myocardial temperature is raised to near normal levels.
7 There is a tendency for these patients to develop pneumonia, which should be treated promptly with antibiotics.
8 Finally, resuscitative efforts should be vigorous and prolonged despite the poor prognosis which is related primarily to the advanced age and associated debilitating disease of these patients. In younger individuals, some remarkable rescues have been recorded; one young woman was resuscitated even after her temperature had dropped to 69°F (20.6°C). *Authorities agree that hypothermia victims without vital signs (prolonged asystole) should not be pronounced dead until they have been rewarmed to 96.8°F (36°C) and remain unresponsive to CPR at that temperature.*

HYPOTHERMIA SECONDARY TO ACUTE ILLNESS There is a group of patients who develop moderate hypothermia in association with acute diseases including congestive heart failure, uremia, diabetes mellitus, drug overdose, acute respiratory failure, and hypoglycemia. These patients are generally elderly and upon admission to the hospital are found to have temperatures of 92 to 93.9°F (33.3 to 34.4°C). They also have a severe metabolic acidosis, due to increased production of lactic acid, and cardiac arrhythmias. Most of these patients are comatose. This entity differs from accidental hypothermia only in the absence of exposure; these cases have all occurred at normal ambient temperatures. The mechanism appears to be an acute failure of thermoregulation; shivering did not occur in any of these patients. Usually these patients have been rewarmed within a few hours by means of an alcohol-circulating blanket. Upon return to normal temperature, cardiac arrythmias, which were present in most of these patients, responded to treatment, and the sensorium returned to normal. With the exception that core rewarming is established by external means, other facets of therapy should follow the steps outlined above. In addition, treatment of the underlying disease such as diabetes with insulin, uremia with dialysis, or congestive heart failure with appropriate cardiac drugs and diuretics is essential. The prognosis is good provided the syndrome is recognized early and treatment is instituted at once.

IMMERSION HYPOTHERMIA Responses to cold-water immersion may be classified as (1) stimulatory, with deep body temperature normal to 95°F (35°C); (2) depressant, with deep body temperature 95 to 86°F (35 to 30°C); and (3) critical, with deep body temperature 86 to 77°F (30 to 25°C).

The long-distance swimmer is able to maintain a normal body temperature for periods of 15 to 25 h or more in water that may plunge skin temperature to 59°F (15°C) or lower, which is some 28°F below deep body temperature, lending support to the concept of a body core insulated by a body shell. The vasoconstriction operative in cold water greatly reduces heat loss. However, there is great individual variability in heat loss in cold water. The relatively obese swimmer may maintain a normal rectal temperature for 2 h without shivering in 61°F (16°C) water. A lean person under the same conditions, despite violent shivering, may experience a fall in rectal temperature of several degrees and become incapacitated from the rigor. In hypersensitive persons, immersion in cold water may be followed by vascular spasm, vomiting, and syncope.

Other compensatory responses include bradycardia, a slight rise in blood pressure, and an early rise in rectal temperature followed by a fall. At 86°F (30°C), atrial fibrillation is common.

Rewarming in warm water has been recommended as the treatment of immersion hypothermia. In severe cases, hemodialysis or peritoneal dialysis should be instituted.

Local cold injuries MECHANISMS OF FREEZING INJURY These can be divided into phenomena which affect cells and extracellular fluids (direct effects) and those which disrupt the function of organized tissues and the integrity of the circulation (indirect effects).

When tissue freezes, ice crystals form and, concomitantly, solutes in the residual liquid become concentrated. The physical dislocation during slow freezing is extreme. Ice crystals many times the size of individual cells form but only in the extracellular spaces. Large ice crystals can develop between cells in soft tissue without producing irreversible injury as long as the percentage of water frozen does not exceed a critical amount. A major source of damage to living cells during freezing and thawing appears to be the strong salt solutions which develop during formation and dissolution of ice; changes in the proportions of lipids and phospholipids in the cell membrane are also of great importance.

The fulminating vascular reaction and stasis which supervene are associated with production of histamine-like substances which increase the permeability of the capillary bed. Within blood vessels, cellular elements aggregate. Irreversible occlusion of small blood vessels by cell masses has been demonstrated in thawed tissue following freezing injury. The damaged frozen tissue simulates tissue damage produced by burns.

MANIFESTATIONS The mildest form of cold injury is called *frostnip* and tends to occur in organs farthest removed from the core of the body such as the earlobes, nose, cheeks, fingers and toes, and hands and feet. It can be prevented by warm clothing and treated with simple rewarming. More consequential local cold injuries may be divided into freezing (frostbite) and nonfreezing (immersion-foot) injuries. The two types may be observed in the same extremity or in different extremities in the same individual.The diagnosis of freezing versus nonfreezing injury generally can be made on the basis of history and clinical manifestations.

Immersion foot is an entity observed in shipwreck survivors or in soldiers (trench foot) whose feet have been wet but not freezing cold for prolonged periods. There is primarily injury to nerve and muscle tissue, but no gross or irreparable pathologic changes occur in blood vessels and skin. The clinical picture reflects primary hypoxic trauma giving rise to three clearly recognizable conditions: (1) *ischemia*, denoted by a pale, pulseless extremity; (2) *hyperemia*, characterized by a bounding pulsatile circulation in red, swollen, painful feet; and (3) the *posthyperemic* or recovery period. The initial cold-induced vasoconstriction, increased blood viscosity, and impaired oxygen transport in the ischemic state are aggravated by such factors as malnutrition, general hypothermia, dehydration, and trauma from relatively fixed, pendant extremities. The problem of rewarming is critical in these patients during the stage of ischemia, when overheating of tissue may lead to gangrene. In the state of hyperemia, the red, swollen feet require judicious cooling. Severe cases may show muscular weakness, atrophy, ulceration, and gangrene of superficial areas. Sensitivity to cold and pain on weight bearing, which may cause discomfort for many years, are sequelae even of milder injuries.

Frostbite stands in contrast with immersion foot because the blood vessels may be severely and irreparably injured, the circulation of blood ceases, and the vascular bed of the frozen tissue is occluded by agglutinated cell aggregates and thrombi. The cutaneous injury consists in part of separation of the epidermal-dermal interface. Early, the intravascular clumping is reversible. However, with the passage of time, clumped red blood cells within vessels in injured tissue lose their morphologic identity and take on the appearance of a homogenous, hyalinaceous plug. It has been shown in some, but not all, experimental studies that much of the intravascular aggregation following freezing injury can be reversed and microcirculatory perfusion improved if low-molecular-weight dextran is given intravenously shortly after injury, but the data in humans are less convincing. Frostbitten tissues unfortunately are often neglected and with thawing become macerated; if this is the situation, the method of rewarming is not important. The method of rewarming has been a matter of controversy. It seems most rational to warm the core of the body before treating the local area of frostbite. Following restoration of the core temperature to normal, warming of a frostbitten limb should begin in water at 50 to 59°F (10 to 15°C), which is then increased 9°F (5°C) every 5 min to a maximum of 104°F (40°C).

Once the frostbitten limb has been rewarmed, treatment should be conservative and consists of bed rest, elevation of the injured part, tetanus toxoid administration, and use of antibiotics if infection is present; early drainage of blebs and bullae; daily washes with chlorhexidine or an iodophor; and early institution of physiotherapy. Alcohol and cigarettes are strongly contraindicated. Surgical amputation and reconstruction is usually not necessary. Regional sympathectomy performed 24 to 48 h after thawing has not been of value in acute frostbite although it has prevented some late complications, and recurrent episodes of cold injury in individuals who have been reexposed. The effect of regional sympathectomy is probably due to ablation of persistent vasospasm and to restoration of cold perception. Intraarterial reserpine has effects similar to sympathectomy.

Some patients with frostbite have residua consisting of excessive sweating, pain, cold feet, numbness, abnormal color, and pain in the joints. The symptoms are generally worse in the winter and following exposure to cold. These patients also often show abnormal nails, discoloration and pigmentation, hyperhydrosis, and, by x-ray, osteoporosis and cystic defects near the joints. These abnormalities tend to be milder in patients who have had sympathetic blockade. Most cold injuries are preventable by graded exposure to cold, as well as appropriate clothing in freezing temperatures.

REFERENCES

Temperature regulation

ATKINS E: Fever: The old and the new. J Infect Dis 149:339, 1984

BARACOS V et al: Stimulation of muscle protein degradation and prostaglandin E_2 release by leukocytic pyrogen (interleukin-1): A mechanism for increased degradation of muscle during fever. N Engl J Med 308:553, 1983

BULLEN JJ: The significance of iron in infection. Rev Infect Dis 3:1127, 1981

DINARELLO CA: Interleukin-1 and the pathogenesis of the acute phase response. N Engl J Med 311:1413, 1984

———: Interleukin 1. Rev Infect Dis 6:41, 1984

KREUGER JM et al: Sleep promoting effects of endogenous pyrogen (interleukin-1). Am J Physiol (in press)

Heat injury

BRITT BA: Etiology and pathophysiology of malignant hyperthermia. Fed Proc 38:44, 1979

CLOWES GHA JR, O'DONNEL TF JR: Current concepts: Heat stroke. N Engl J Med 291:564, 1974

COSTRINI AM et al: Cardiovascular and metabolic manifestations of heat stroke and severe heat exhaustion. Am J Med 66:296, 1979

DOWNEY GP et al: Neuroleptic malignant syndrome. Patient with unique clinical and physiologic features. Am J Med 77:338, 1984

GRONERT GA: Malignant hyperthermia. Anesthesiology 53:395, 1980

HANSON PG, ZIMMERMAN SW: Exertional heat stroke in novice runners. JAMA 242:159, 1979

MCPHERSON EW, TAYLOR CA JR: The King syndrome: Malignant hyperthermia, myopathy and multiple anomalies. Am J Med Genet 8:159, 1981

SHIBOLET S et al: Heat stroke: A review. Aviat Space Environ Med 47:280, 1976

SPRUNG CL et al: The metabolic and respiratory alterations of heat stroke. Arch Intern Med 140:665, 1980

WILLNER JH et al: Increased myophosphorylase A in malignant hyperthermia. N Engl J Med 303:138, 1980

——— et al: High skeletal muscle adenylate cyclase in malignant hyperthermia. J Clin Invest 68:1119, 1981

WYNDHAM CH: Heat stroke and hyperthermia in marathon runners. Ann NY Acad Sci 301:128, 1977

Cold injury

BOUWMAN DL et al: Early sympathetic blockade for frostbite—Is it of value? J Trauma 20:744, 1980
GAGE AM: Frostbite. Trauma and Emergency Med 7:25, 1981
MACLEAN D et al: Metabolic aspects of spontaneous recovery in accidental hypothermia and hypothermic myxedema. Q J Med (n.s.) 43:371, 1974
SOUTHWICK FS, DALGLISH PH JR: Recovery after prolonged asystolic cardiac arrest in profound hypothermia. JAMA 243:1250, 1980
VAUGHN PB: Local cold injury—Menace to military operations: A review. Military Med 143:305, 1980
WHITTLE JL, BATES JH: Thermoregulatory failure secondary to acute illness: Complications and treatment. Arch Intern Med 139:418, 1979
WICKSTROM P et al: Accidental hypothermia. Am J Surg 131:622, 1976

9 CHILLS AND FEVER

ROBERT G. PETERSDORF / RICHARD K. ROOT

Omitting disorders which may involve cerebral thermoregulatory centers directly, such as brain tumors, intracranial hemorrhage or thrombosis, or heat stroke, the following disease states may be accompanied by fever:

1 All *infections,* whether caused by bacteria, rickettsias, chlamydia, viruses, or parasites, can cause fever.
2 *Mechanical trauma,* e.g., a crushing injury, frequently gives rise to fever lasting 1 or 2 days. Not infrequently, however, complicating infection sets in.
3 Many *neoplastic diseases* are associated with fever. In most patients, fever in patients with cancer is related to obstruction or infection produced by the tumor. In some solid tumors, however, fever may be due to the tumor per se, particularly following metastasis to the liver. Tumors which are associated with fever include hypernephroma, carcinoma of the pancreas, lung, or bone, and hepatoma. In tumors of the reticuloendothelial system, including Hodgkin's disease, non-Hodgkin's lymphoma, acute leukemias, and malignant histiocytosis, fever may be one of the prominent early manifestations. The production of endogenous pyrogen/interleukin-1 (EP/IL-1) by these tumors is responsible for fever production.
4 *Hematopoietic disorders,* e.g., acute hemolytic episodes, may be characterized by pyrexia.
5 *Vascular accidents* of any magnitude, e.g., myocardial, pulmonary, and cerebral infarctions, nearly always cause fever.
6 *Diseases due to immune mechanisms* are often febrile. These include the connective tissue diseases, drug fevers, and fever due to other immunologic abnormalities.
7 Certain *acute metabolic disorders,* such as gout, porphyria, hypertriglyceridemia, Fabry's disease, and Addisonian or thyroid crises, sometimes are associated with fever. The pathogenesis varies from activation of the inflammatory response (EP/IL-1 production) to alterations in thermogenesis and heat regulation (hyperthyroidism).

ACCOMPANIMENTS OF FEVER **Systemic symptoms** The perception of fever by patients varies enormously. Some persons can tell with considerable accuracy whether their body temperatures are elevated; others with chronic febrile illnesses (e.g., patients with tuberculosis) may be wholly unaware of body temperature as high as 103°F (39.4°C). Often, patients may pay no attention to fever because of other unpleasant symptoms such as headache and pleuritic pain. Pain in the back, generalized myalgias, and arthralgia without arthritis are commonly associated with fever. Whether these symptoms reflect the presence of an infectious agent or are merely a manifestation of IL-1 activity is not clear (see Chap. 8).

Chills Abrupt onset of fever with a *chill* or *rigor* is characteristic of some diseases and, in the absence of antipyretic drugs, rare in others. Although repeated rigors are typical of pyogenic infection with bacteremia, a similar pattern of fever may occur in noninfectious diseases such as lymphoma. It is important to differentiate a true chill, which is accompanied by teeth chattering and bed shaking, from the chilly sensation which occurs in almost all fevers, particularly those in viral infections. In some instances, however, a true rigor occurs in viremia. Chills may be evoked or perpetuated by the intermittent administration of aspirin or other antipyretics. These agents may cause a sharp depression in temperature, which is followed by compensatory involuntary muscular contractions, i.e., a chill. This unpleasant side effect of antipyretic drugs can be averted by administering these agents no less frequently than every 3 h, around the clock, rather than by prescribing them only for elevations in temperature above a certain level.

Herpes labialis So-called fever blisters result from activation of latent herpes simplex virus infection by elevations in temperature. For reasons which are obscure, fever blisters are common in pneumococcal infections, streptococcosis, malaria, meningococcemia, and rickettsioses but are rare in mycoplasma pneumonia, tuberculosis, brucellosis, smallpox, and typhoid.

Delirium This may result from elevation of body temperature and is particularly common in patients with alcoholism, cerebrovascular disease, or senility.

Convulsions Some febrile children, especially those with a family history of epilepsy, develop seizures with fever. Febrile convulsions do not, in general, reflect serious cerebral disease.

CLINICAL IMPORTANCE OF FEVER The temperature is a simple, objective, and accurate indicator of a physiologic state and is much less subject to external and psychogenic stimuli than the other vital signs, such as pulse, respiratory rate, and blood pressure. For these reasons, determination of the body temperature assists in estimating the severity of an illness, its course and duration, and the effect of therapy, or even in deciding whether a person has an organic illness.

Benefit of fever There are a few infections of humans in which pyrexia appears definitely to be beneficial to the host, such as neurosyphilis, some forms of chronic arthritis, and widespread cancer. Certain other diseases, such as uveitis and rheumatoid arthritis, sometimes improve after fever therapy. Specific immune responses are accelerated at febrile body temperatures, as are catabolic processes involving mobilization of amino acids from muscle. These events are mediated by EP/IL-1 and may involve synthesis of prostaglandins of the E series. In humans, the benefits of fever on other host defense mechanisms other than the multiple actions of EP/IL-1 (see Chap. 8) are not as apparent as in cold-blooded animals. In these species higher ambient temperatures augment the acute inflammatory response. Minor increases in phagocytosis and chemotaxis by human polymorphonuclear leukocytes have been observed at febrile incubation temperatures. Aged and debilitated patients with infection may have little or no fever, and this is generally interpreted as a bad prognostic sign.

Detrimental aspects of fever Fever accelerates many metabolic processes and is accompanied by EP/IL-1–mediated muscle wasting and weight loss. The work and the rate of the heart are increased. Sweating aggravates loss of salt and water. There may be discomfort due to headache, photophobia, general malaise, or an unpleasant sensation of warmth. Fever may precipitate seizures in epileptic patients. The rigors and profuse sweats of hectic fevers are particularly unpleasant for the patient. In elderly individuals with overt or potential cardiac or cerebral vascular disease, fever may be particularly deleterious.

MANAGEMENT OF FEVER Since fever ordinarily does little harm, imposes no great discomfort, and may have benefits to host defense mechanisms, antipyretic drugs are rarely essential to patient welfare and may obfuscate the effect of a specific therapeutic agent or of the natural course of the disease. There are situations, however, in which lowering of the body temperature is of vital importance; e.g., heat stroke, postoperative hyperthermia, delirium due to hyperpyrexia, epileptic seizures, or shock associated with fever and heart failure. Under these circumstances lowering the temperature is indicated. Cooling blankets which can be set at hypothermic temperatures are a highly effective means for external cooling. Alternatively, sponging the body surface with cool saline solution or the application of cool compresses to the skin and forehead may be employed. There is no advantage in sponging with alcohol, which, because of its pungent odor, makes some patients ill. When high internal temperature is combined with cutaneous vasoconstriction, as in heat stroke or postoperative hyperthermia, the cooling measures should be combined with massage of the skin in order to bring blood to the surface, where it may be cooled. Immediate immersion in a tub of ice water should be considered a lifesaving emergency procedure in patients with heat stroke if the internal body temperature is in excess of 108°F (42.2°C). If cooling blankets are available, they are preferable to immersion in ice in most instances.

Antipyretic drugs, such as aspirin (0.3 to 0.6 g) or acetaminophen (0.5 g), are often employed in lowering temperature, particularly if patients are uncomfortable or if fever poses a high risk to them, as is the case in patients with heart failure, febrile seizures (usually children), head injury, mental disorders, or pregnancy. Antipyretics are sometimes associated with unpleasant diaphoresis, an alarming fall in blood pressure, and the subsequent return of fever occasionally accompanied by a chill. These can be mitigated by enforcing a liberal fluid intake and by administering the drugs regularly and frequently at 2- to 3-h intervals. Although glucocorticosteroids are also potent antipyretics, they must be used with caution because of their tendency to precipitate abrupt falls in temperature accompanied by hypotension. The capacity of these drugs to mask other manifestations of infection also constitutes a relative contraindication to their use. In contrast to other antipyretics, glucocorticoids inhibit EP/IL-1 production and may thereby diminish beneficial actions induced by this molecule (see Chap. 8).

The discomfort of a rigor can be alleviated in many patients by the intravenous injection of calcium salts. This procedure will stop the shivering and chilliness but has no influence on the ultimate height of the fever. Severe disruptive rigors sometimes need to be abolished with morphine sulfate (10 to 15 mg subcutaneously) or with parenteral chlorpromazine.

DIAGNOSTIC CONSIDERATIONS IN FEVER In many illnesses fever is the most prominent and often the only manifestation of disease. It is not an indication of any particular type of disease; rather it should be considered a reaction to injury comparable with an elevated leukocyte count or a rapid erythrocyte sedimentation rate.

Definitions of fever Fever is classically described as intermittent, remittent, sustained, or relapsing. In *intermittent fever* the temperature falls to normal each day. When the variation between the peak and the nadir is very large, the fever is called *hectic* or *septic*. Intermittent fevers are characteristic in pyogenic infections, particularly abscesses, lymphomas, and miliary tuberculosis. In *remittent fever* the temperature falls each day but does not return to normal. Most fevers are remittent, and this type of febrile response is not characteristic of any disease. A *sustained fever* is characterized by persistent elevation without significant diurnal variation. It is exemplified by the fever of untreated typhoid or typhus. With *relapsing fever* short febrile periods occur between one or several days of normal temperature. Examples of relapsing fever are the following:

Malaria (see Chap. 154) had vanished from the United States almost completely, but for several years Vietnam war veterans constituted an important and sizable reservoir of this infection, as do other persons recently arrived from foreign countries. It is most unusual, however, for malaria to recur after a symptom-free interval of 1 year or more. Febrile bouts recur at 2- or 3-day intervals, or more irregularly in falciparum infections, depending on the maturation cycle of the parasite. The diagnosis depends on demonstration of the parasites in the blood.

Relapsing fever (see Chap. 126) occurs in the southwest part of the United States, as far east as Texas, the Pacific Northwest, and in many other parts of the world. The recurrences are related to the cyclic development of parasites. Diagnosis is by demonstration of the spirochetal organisms in stained films of the blood.

Rat-bite fever (see Chap. 125) is brought about by two agents—*Spirillum minus* and *Streptobacillus moniliformis,* both transmitted by the bite of a rat. Both may cause an illness characterized by periodic exacerbations of fever. The clue to the diagnosis depends on obtaining a history of rat bite 1 to 10 weeks prior to the onset of symptoms. The cause can be established by appropriate laboratory procedures.

Localized *pyogenic infections* in rare instances give rise to periodic bouts of fever separated by afebrile and relatively symptom-free intervals. The so-called Charcot's intermittent biliary fever, i.e., cholangitis with biliary obstruction due to stones, is an example. *Urinary tract infection,* with episodes of ureteral obstruction due to small stones or inspissated pus, can also cause recurrent fever.

A few patients with Hodgkin's disease at some time have so-called Pel-Ebstein fever—bouts of fever lasting 3 to 10 days, separated by afebrile and asymptomatic periods of 3 to 10 days. These cycles may be repeated regularly over a period of several months. In rare instances this periodicity of the fever has been sufficiently striking to suggest the correct diagnosis before lymphadenopathy or splenomegaly became evident. However, relapsing fevers indistinguishable from Pel-Ebstein fever usually have causes other than Hodgkin's disease.

Epidemiology of fever The diagnosis of febrile illnesses must take into consideration the context of the epidemiologic setting. For example, an acute febrile illness in southeast Asia or Africa is probably due to one of the arboviruses (see Chap. 143) or malaria (see Chap. 154); in a college student in the United States it may result from infectious mononucleosis or some other viral infection; and in an octogenarian following prostatectomy it is probably an indication of urinary tract infection, wound infection, pulmonary infarction, or aspiration pneumonia. In children, infections are more likely to be responsible for prolonged fevers than in adults. Likewise, travelers returning from short trips to foreign countries are much more likely to have febrile illnesses indigenous to their home than to the foreign country they have visited. Patients whose host defenses are altered by malignancy, cytotoxic or steroid therapy, or congenital or acquired immune deficiency are much more likely to have unusual infections as a cause for fever than are normal hosts.

Rare versus common diseases Most of the time fever is a manifestation of a common disease, and fever associated with a pulmonary infiltrate is much more likely to be due to pneumococcal than to *Pneumocystis* pneumonia. Failure to appreciate this cardinal principle has led to many prolonged and futile diagnostic workups.

Febrile illnesses of short duration Acute febrile illnesses of less than 2 weeks' duration are common in medical practice. In many instances they run their course, progressing to complete recovery, and a precise diagnosis is not made. In most instances, however, it is safe to assume that the illness is of infectious origin. Although short febrile illnesses may be noninfectious (e.g., allergic fevers due to drugs, thromboembolic disease, hemolytic crises, or gout), these are decidedly in the minority.

Most undiagnosed acute febrile infectious diseases are probably viral and remain undiagnosed because diagnostic methods are unavailable, cumbersome, or not cost-effective. It is not practical to carry out tests needed to identify all the known viruses, and, furthermore, there must be a considerable number of still unidentified viruses pathogenic for humans. In bacterial infections, on the other hand, laboratory diagnosis is simpler, and these infections are often rapidly controlled with chemotherapy.

The following characteristics, though not restricted solely to acute infections, are highly suggestive that infection is present:

1 Abrupt onset
2 High fever, i.e., 102 to 105°F (38.9 to 40.6°C), with or without chills
3 Respiratory symptoms—sore throat, coryza, cough
4 Severe malaise, with muscle or joint pain, photophobia, pain on movement of the eyes, headache
5 Nausea, vomiting, or diarrhea
6 Acute enlargement of lymph nodes or spleen
7 Meningeal signs, with or without spinal fluid pleocytosis
8 Leukocyte count above 12,000 or below 5000 per cubic millimeter
9 Dysuria, frequency, and flank pain

None of the symptoms or signs listed is encountered only in infection. Many of these features could be seen in acute leukemia or in disseminated lupus erythematosus. Nevertheless, in a given instance of acute febrile illness with some of or all the manifestations listed, the probabilities strongly favor infection, and the patient may be given reasonable reassurance that he or she will probably recover in a week or two, regardless of a precise diagnosis.

It is desirable, of course, to establish an accurate diagnosis, and whatever steps are practicable in the circumstances to establish the cause should be taken. Cultures of the throat, blood, urine, or feces should be obtained before institution of antibacterial chemotherapy. Skin and/or serologic tests should be carried out when indicated.

There is a tendency to rely immediately and excessively on the laboratory in ascertaining the cause of fever. In many instances, a thorough history and a complete and, if necessary, repeated physical examination, along with a complete blood count (CBC), urinalysis, and sedimentation rate will provide the answer. Often a little patience, in the form of watchful waiting, before plunging into an expensive and extensive laboratory workup, will lead to the diagnosis.

Prolonged febrile illnesses Some of the knottiest problems in medicine are found in cases of prolonged fever in which the diagnosis remains obscure for weeks or even months. Eventually, however, the true nature of the illness usually reveals itself, since a disease which causes injury sufficient to evoke temperature elevations to 101°F (38.3°C) or higher for several weeks does not often subside without leaving some clue as to its nature. The elucidation of problems of this sort calls for skillful application of all diagnostic methods—careful history, thorough physical examination, and the carefully considered use of laboratory examinations and imaging techniques.

FEVER OF UNKNOWN ORIGIN In some patients fever becomes the dominant sign or symptom in a patient's illness, and when its cause escapes detection, it is defined as fever of unknown origin (FUO). It is appropriate to use this term only in patients who have elevations in temperature [>101°F (38.3°C)] for a prolonged period (at least 2, and preferably 3, weeks) and in whom the diagnosis cannot be made during at least 1 week of intensive study. These rigid criteria eliminate from this diagnostic category patients with common bacterial or viral infections, those in whom the diagnosis is obvious, and those whose fever is due to a sequential occurrence of etiologically unrelated diseases. An example is a patient who is febrile following a myocardial infarction, who then develops thrombophlebitis that is associated with fever, and in whom this is followed by multiple pulmonary emboli, also a febrile disease. Much of the confusion in the literature concerning causes of FUO is due to failure to define the criteria employed in classifying patients who have had fever of unknown origin.

DISEASES CAUSING PROLONGED FEVERS Table 9-1 lists some of the diseases responsible for prolonged fever. Some of these disorders must initially be considered to be FUO; in others the diagnosis comes to mind readily.

Infections Infections occupy a less prominent position among causes of prolonged fever now than formerly because of the common practice of administering antibiotics to any patient in whom fever persists for more than a few days. Consequently, many infections are eradicated by more or less "blind" therapy without accurate determination of their nature or location. In the 1950s, patients with infections comprised about 40 percent of patients with FUO, but in a comparable series collected in the 1970s this figure had fallen to 32 percent, while neoplasms had risen from 20 to 33 percent. Many of these infections are relatively resistant to rapid eradication by host defenses (e.g., localized pyogenic infections or intracellular infections), which allows them to pursue a chronic or subacute course.

ABSCESSES (see Chap. 87) Abscesses are the most common form of infection presenting as FUO and are important because they can be cured with early diagnosis and treatment, while failure to make the diagnosis may eventuate fatally. These abscesses usually arise in the abdomen or pelvis including the subphrenic space, the liver or spleen, or a ruptured diverticulum or appendix. Ultrasonography, liver-spleen scan, or CT scan should provide the diagnosis in most instances. Laparotomy is usually necessary to confirm the diagnosis and to achieve cure.

MYCOBACTERIAL INFECTIONS Although less common than formerly, mycobacterial infections, such as tuberculosis (see Chap. 119) and, less commonly, atypical mycobacterial infections (see Chap. 121), cause FUO. These infections are more common among blacks, native Americans, southeast Asians, and individuals from outside the United States. In patients with the acquired immunodeficiency syndrome, disseminated infection due to *Mycobacterium-avium-intracellulare* (MAI) is a common preterminal event. Most of these infections are extrapulmonary and involve the bones, lymph nodes, genital or urinary organs, peritoneum, or liver. Extrapulmonary or miliary tuberculosis may not be detectable by x-ray until late in the course. Many of these patients are debilitated and have overwhelming disease. Despite this, the diagnosis, which is usually made by biopsy of lymph nodes or involved tissue, is essential because patients with *Mycobacterium tuberculosis* infection respond well to treatment, particularly with bactericidal drugs such as isoniazid and rifampin. In contrast, infection with MAI is often resistant to treatment.

RENAL INFECTIONS Ordinary pyelonephritis is rarely accompanied by prolonged fever; if pyrexia occurs in these patients, intrarenal or extrarenal obstruction should be considered. Ureteral obstruction by either a mass of leukocytes or renal epithelium, as in papillary necrosis, may be accompanied by prolonged fever. Prostatic abscess should be considered in males. These patients may not have dysuria or rectal pain. Occasionally, focal pyelonephritis may cause prolonged fever.

OTHER BACTERIAL INFECTIONS These include sinusitis, vertebral osteomyelitis (usually occurring in association with chronic bacteriuria, and most easily diagnosed by bone scan), infected intravenous or intraarterial catheters, and retroperitoneal infection such as aneurysms that have become filled with organizing clot and debris that have become secondarily infected. Enteric pathogens (including *Escherichia coli, Bacteroides,* and *Salmonella*) have been isolated frequently from patients with such infections. Surgery is mandatory for both diagnosis and therapy. In addition, some patients with dissecting aneurysms have fever without superimposed infections.

BACTERIAL ENDOCARDITIS Perhaps because of a high index of suspicion, the ubiquitous use of blood cultures, and the indiscriminate use of antibiotics, which must cure some patients, bacterial endocarditis has become a rare cause of FUO. Similarly, bacteremia due to *Neisseria, Salmonella,* and *Brucella* rarely causes FUO, but must be considered in the proper epidemiologic setting.

IATROGENIC INFECTIONS These include catheter infections, infected arteriovenous fistulas, and sometimes ordinary wound infections in obscure locations. Usually, their cure requires removal of a foreign body in addition to antimicrobial therapy. Infection of intravascular grafts constitutes a particularly difficult management problem which may give rise to prolonged bacteremia.

VIRAL, RICKETTSIAL, AND CHLAMYDIAL INFECTIONS These are rarely the cause of prolonged fevers, but occasionally patients with Epstein-

TABLE 9-1 Common disease entities in the United States causing prolonged fever

- *I* Infections
  - *A* Granulomatous infections
    - *1* Tuberculosis
    - *2* Deep-seated fungus infections
    - *3* Atypical mycobacterial infections
  - *B* Pyogenic infections
    - *1* Upper abdominal infections
      - *a* Cholecystitis (stone), empyema of gallbladder
      - *b* Cholangitis
      - *c* Liver abscess
      - *d* Lesser sac abscess
      - *e* Subphrenic abscess
      - *f* Splenic abscess
    - *2* Lower abdominal infections
      - *a* Diverticulitis (± abscess)
      - *b* Appendicitis
    - *3* Pelvic inflammatory disease
    - *4* Urinary tract infections
      - *a* Pyelonephritis (rare)
      - *b* Intrarenal abscess
      - *c* Perinephric abscess
      - *d* Ureteral obstruction
      - *e* Prostatic abscess
    - *5* Sinusitis
    - *6* Osteomyelitis
  - *C* Intravascular infections
    - *1* Bacterial endocarditis (acute and subacute)
    - *2* Intravascular catheter infections
  - *D* Bacteremias without overt primary focus
    - *1* Meningococcemia
    - *2* Gonococcemia
    - *3* Vibriosis
    - *4* Listeriosis
    - *5* Brucellosis
    - *6* Coliform bacteremia in patients with cirrhosis
  - *E* Viral, rickettsial, and chlamydial infections
    - *1* Infectious mononucleosis
    - *2* Cytomegalovirus
    - *3* Hepatitis
    - *4* Group B coxsackievirus diseases
    - *5* Q fever (including endocarditis)
    - *6* Psittacosis
  - *F* Parasitic diseases
    - *1* Amebiasis
    - *2* Malaria
    - *3* Trichinosis
  - *G* Spirochetal infections
    - *1* Leptospirosis
    - *2* Relapsing fever
- *II* Neoplasms
  - *A* Solid (localized)
    - *1* Kidney
    - *2* Lung
    - *3* Pancreas
    - *4* Liver
    - *5* Large bowel
    - *6* Atrial myxoma
  - *B* Metastatic
    - *1* From gastrointestinal tract
    - *2* From lung, kidneys, bone, cervix, ovary
    - *3* Melanoma
    - *4* Sarcoma
  - *C* Tumors of the reticuloendothelial system
    - *1* Hodgkin's disease
    - *2* Non-Hodgkin's lymphoma
    - *3* Malignant histiocytosis
    - *4* Immunoblastic lymphadenopathy
    - *5* Lymphomatoid granulomatosis
    - *6* Mucocutaneous lymph node syndrome (children)
- *III* Connective tissue disease
  - *A* Rheumatic fever
  - *B* Systemic lupus erythematosus
  - *C* Rheumatoid arthritis (particularly Still's disease)
  - *D* Giant cell arteritis (polymyalgia rheumatica)
  - *E* Hypersensitivity vasculitis
  - *F* Periarteritis nodosa
  - *G* Wegener's granulomatosis
  - *H* Panaortitis
- *IV* Granulomatus diseases
  - *A* Crohn's disease (regional enteritis)
  - *B* Granulomatous hepatitis
  - *C* Sarcoidosis
  - *D* Erythema nodosum
- *V* Miscellaneous
  - *A* Drug fever
  - *B* Pulmonary emboli
  - *C* Thyroiditis
  - *D* Hemolytic states
  - *E* Cryptic trauma with bleeding into enclosed spaces (hematomas)
  - *F* Dissecting aneurysm (with or without infection)
  - *G* Whipple's disease
- *VI* Metabolic and inherited diseases
  - *A* Familial Mediterranean fever
  - *B* Hypertriglyceridemia and hypercholesterolemia
  - *C* Fabry's disease
- *VII* Psychogenic fevers
  - *A* Habitual hyperthermia
  - *B* Factitious fever
- *VIII* Periodic fevers (e.g., cyclic neutropenia)
- *IX* Thermoregulatory disorders
- *X* Undiagnosed
  - *A* Resolved
    - *1* Without treatment
    - *2* With antibiotics
    - *3* With anti-inflammatory drugs
  - *B* Recurrent
    - *1* Suppressed with steroids

Barr or cytomegalovirus infections may have febrile illnesses, which are often characterized by spontaneous remissions and exacerbations. Cytomegalovirus (with or without *Pneumocystis*) is becoming a progressively more common cause of prolonged fever in immunocompromised hosts. In them, it should not pose a diagnostic problem, but an infectious mononucleosis–like syndrome or postperfusion fever in otherwise healthy patients may be difficult diagnostic dilemmas. Since these patients are generally not very ill and improve spontaneously, they should not be subjected to prolonged, expensive FUO workups. *Psittacosis* may look much like typhoid fever, and *Q-fever endocarditis* has been a particularly puzzling and lethal illness that must be treated both with antibiotics and valve replacement.

PARASITIC DISEASES Amebiasis can present as an FUO, either in the form of diffuse hepatitis or liver abscess. The diagnosis of malaria demands a history of recent exposure.

Neoplasms HODGKIN'S DISEASE Fever may be the principal symptom and only objective finding early in the course of Hodgkin's disease, especially because patients with this disease who present with FUO may have only intraabdominal or retroperitoneal disease or involvement of the bone marrow. The diagnosis is usually made by biopsy or staging laparotomy. It is important to arrive at the diagnosis early because, with proper chemotherapy, prolonged remissions and even cure may be achieved.

LYMPHOMA-LIKE SYNDROMES Several disease entities have been described which are clinically and histologically similar to non-Hodgkin's lymphoma but which may have a better prognosis or respond differently to steroids and antitumor agents. Among these entities, all of which may present as FUOs, are immunoblastic lymphadenopathy, lymphadenoid granulomatosis, acute megakaryocytic myelosis, and, in children, the mucocutaneous lymph node syndrome (Kawasaki's disease). These diseases are discussed more fully in Chap. 55.

NON-HODGKIN'S LYMPHOMA These illnesses usually present with fever, nonspecific symptoms, and lymphadenopathy which the patient recognizes. Hepatosplenomegaly and bone pain and tenderness are common. The laboratory findings usually consist of anemia, leukocytosis, and atypical lymphocytosis. The diagnosis is usually made by lymph node biopsy, but biopsies can be mistaken for reactive hyperplasia or atypical lymphocytic infiltrates, at least initially. Improvements in chemotherapy have led to prolonged remissions.

MALIGNANT HISTIOCYTOSIS This is a rare infiltrative disease secondary to malignant proliferation of cutaneous Langerhans cells. A poor prognosis presenting with fever, wasting, generalized lymphadenopathy, and hepatosplenomegaly is characteristic. The bone marrow, lung, and skin may also be involved by this rapidly progressing illness. There tends to be anemia, leukopenia, and thrombocytopenia, or a combination of the three. Biopsied tissue is often difficult to diagnose definitively but a rapidly progressive febrile illness, and the presence of large, malignant, primitive reticuloendothelial cells with histiocytic predominance and erythrophagocytosis should yield the answer.

LEUKEMIAS It is not uncommon for acute leukemia to be mistaken for acute infection at the onset. The acute leukemias are nearly always accompanied by fever, sometimes as high as 105°F (40.6°C). The diagnosis is characteristically delayed by the absence of blast cells in the blood or bone marrow. However, the patients are usually anemic and leukopenic and often have been labeled as having preleukemia. Chronic lymphatic or granulocytic leukemia may be characterized by fever, but such fever is usually due to concomitant infection. Because of the typical changes in circulating leukocytes, fever does not often cause a diagnostic problem. Before it is assumed that fever in a patient with leukemia is due to the blood dyscrasia, infection must be ruled out by appropriate tests and cultures, and attempts to treat the "most likely" pathogen must be made.

SOLID TUMORS An invariable feature of solid tumors causing FUO is the presence of metastatic cancer in the abdomen. These patients are usually older; the diagnosis is characteristically made by laparotomy which is directed to the proper location on the basis of history, physical examination, and noninvasive studies. The sites of the primary vary widely and include the kidney, liver, pancreas, stomach, pleura, lung, and bowel. Not surprisingly, survival is short.

ATRIAL MYXOMA Patients with changing heart murmurs, peripheral embolic phenomena, and joint pains are usually suspected of having bacterial endocarditis, rheumatic fever, or occasionally some other connective tissue disease. In the face of persistence of these symptoms and signs without a positive diagnosis, two-dimensional echocardiography and, if the echocardiogram is positive, angiography should be performed with the possibility that an atrial myxoma may be responsible.

Connective tissue disease RHEUMATIC FEVER Perhaps because of the common use of immunologic diagnostic tests, connective tissue diseases now form a smaller part of FUO series. The incidence of rheumatic fever in North America and Europe has decreased dramatically. Systemic lupus erythematosus often presents with fever, but is usually diagnosed promptly.

RHEUMATOID ARTHRITIS In its classic form, this disease is not difficult to recognize, but in certain patients who initially have FUO, arthritis is absent early in the course of the illness; these patients have primarily fever, hepatosplenomegaly, lymphadenopathy, evanescent rashes, anemia, and leukocytosis. Joint changes do not appear until late in the disease. This disease usually occurs in young adults and may be considered the adult counterpart of juvenile rheumatoid disease. The diagnosis is made usually only after prolonged observation, in part because serologic tests for rheumatoid disease are characteristically negative. The prognosis is generally good, and patients respond well to aspirin, nonsteroidal anti-inflammatory drugs, or steroids. Arthritis and a characteristic skin rash (erythema chronicum migrans) caused by infection with *Borrelia burgdorferi* (Lyme disease) may cause confusion in the diagnosis (see Chap. 278).

GIANT CELL ARTERITIS (POLYMYALGIA RHEUMATICA) This is a disease of elderly persons, who complain of fever, headache, and pain in the muscles and joints. Overt arthritis is unusual. At times, fever is the only symptom, and there are no abnormal physical findings. The sedimentation rate tends to be very rapid, and there may be anemia, leukocytosis, or eosinophilia. Occasionally, the temporal or occipital arteries are inflamed and tender, but usually they are normal. In either instance, the diagnosis can be made by temporal artery biopsy. There may be accompanying visual defects or blindness because of involvement of the retinal artery. This disease responds extremely well to low doses of steroids, which may be used as a therapeutic trial.

OTHER CONNECTIVE TISSUE DISEASES These include classical periarteritis nodosa, with or without hepatitis B infection, a disease that involves small and medium-sized arteries as well as the aorta and its main branches (see Chap. 269).

Granulomatous diseases SARCOIDOSIS Ordinarily, fever is not characteristic of sarcoidosis, but it is prominent in a minority of cases, especially those characterized by arthralgia, hilar lymphadenopathy, and cutaneous lesions resembling erythema nodosum, or in those with extensive hepatic lesions. The diagnosis is suggested by lymphoid enlargement, ocular lesions, and hyperglobulinemia and is clinched by biopsy of skin, lymph nodes, muscle, and liver. Serum angiotensin–converting enzyme activity is increased (see Chap. 270). The diagnosis may be obfuscated by the presence of erythema nodosum or other vascular rashes long before granulomas are found.

REGIONAL ENTERITIS Inflammatory lesions of the large and small intestine rarely present as FUO, but an occasional patient who has only fever, abdominal pain, recurrent bouts of diarrhea, or subtle changes in bowel habits which may indicate low-grade obstruction will be found to have regional enteritis. Likewise, Whipple's disease may make itself known by fever, without arthritis or malabsorption.

GRANULOMATOUS HEPATITIS This disease of unknown etiology is a relatively common cause of FUO. It is probably a manifestation of hypersensitivity, although the responsible antigens are rarely identified. Liver biopsy typically shows noncaseating granulomas. Specific diseases which can cause this reaction must be excluded and include tuberculosis, Hodgkin's disease, histoplasmosis, sarcoidosis, drug reactions, primary biliary cirrhosis, and schistosomiasis, to name only some. The fever generally subsides spontaneously over a period of weeks or months. Sometimes defervescence can be achieved with anti-inflammatory drugs or steroids, but because the diagnosis of tuberculosis cannot be ruled out completely, patients to whom steroid therapy is given should also be given antituberculous medication.

Miscellaneous causes of fever DRUG FEVER This is an important cause of cryptic fever; a careful history of drug intake should be taken in every patient with unexplained fever. Fever due to allergy to one of the antibiotics may become superimposed on the fever of the infection for which the drug was given, resulting in a very confused picture. Often, fever is due to common drugs, including sulfonamides, bromides, arsenicals, iodides, thiouracils, barbiturates, and laxatives, especially those containing phenolphthalein. Any questions of drug fever can be resolved rapidly by discontinuing all medications. The diagnosis can be further substantiated by giving a test dose of the drug after fever has subsided, but this may result in a very unpleasant or even dangerous reaction.

MULTIPLE PULMONARY EMBOLI Multiple pulmonary emboli are decreasing as a cause of FUO; in fact, in one series, they were overdiagnosed. Nevertheless, symptomless thrombosis of deep calf or pelvic veins may cause prolonged febrile illness either because of the thrombophlebitis or as a result of repeated small pulmonary emboli. These emboli may not be manifested by pleuritic pain or hemoptysis, but cough, dyspnea, and vague thoracic discomfort are likely to be present. Lung scans and venography should reveal the diagnosis. Sometimes these patients present with a nephrotic syndrome due to renal vein thrombosis. Pelvic thrombophlebitis with or without pulmonary emboli is an important cause of FUO in postpartum patients.

HEMOLYTIC EPISODES Most hemolytic diseases are characterized by bouts of fever, and acute hemolytic crises may give rise to shaking chills and marked elevations of temperature. The difficulty sometimes encountered in differentiating sickle cell disease from acute rheumatic fever is well known. The presence of these hemolytic disorders is suggested by the more rapid development of anemia than occurs in other febrile illnesses and by the usual accompaniment of reticulocytosis and jaundice. Fever is not characteristic of severe anemia due to external blood loss or of the anemia of uremia.

CRYPTIC HEMATOMAS Accumulation of old blood in closed spaces, for instance, at sites of remote trauma, particularly in the perisplenic area, in the pericardium, or in the retroperitoneal area, particularly in patients receiving anticoagulants, has resulted in prolonged fever. The diagnosis is important because evacuation of the clot is often curative. Fever often accompanies intraluminal dissection of the aorta.

NONSPECIFIC PERICARDITIS Occasionally, this entity escapes diagnosis and presents as an FUO.

FAMILIAL MEDITERRANEAN FEVER (see Chap. 271) Either the disease is decreasing in incidence, or it is being recognized more readily.

THERMOREGULATORY DISORDERS Rare patients have fever due to an abnormality in their temperature-regulating mechanism. They may be febrile without any other cause or may have exaggerated responses in temperature during the course of other fever-producing diseases. The diagnosis is made by exclusion. Some patients have responded to chlorpromazine.

Psychogenic fever HABITUAL HYPERTHERMIA Not infrequently, a patient, while not appearing acutely ill, has been subject to elevation of body temperature above the "normal" range level, i.e., temperatures in the range of 99.0 to 100.5°F (37.2 to 38°C). Prolonged low-grade fever may be a manifestation of serious illness, or it may be a matter of no real consequence. Possibly there are some persons whose "normal" temperatures are in this range. However, there is no certain way of identifying such individuals. The possibilities to be considered in such cases vary considerably according to the age groups concerned. A special problem termed *habitual hyperthermia* is encountered in young females. The patient may have temperatures ranging from 99.0 to 100.5°F (37.2 to 38.0°C) regularly or intermittently for years and also usually has a variety of complaints characteristic of psychoneurosis, such as fatigability, insomnia, bowel distress, vague aches, and headache. Prolonged careful study and observation fail to reveal evidence of organic disease. Unfortunately, many of these people go from physician to physician and are subjected to a variety of unpleasant, expensive, and even harmful tests, treatments, and operations. The diagnosis of this syndrome can be made with reasonable certainty after a suitable period of observation and study, and if the patient can be convinced of its validity, a real service will have been rendered.

In a patient past middle age, even low-grade fever should always be regarded as a probable indication of organic disease. The possibilities to be considered in this age group are the same as those discussed earlier under "Prolonged Febrile Illness."

FACTITIOUS FEVER Occasionally, patients will produce purposeful false elevations in temperature. Many of these patients are young women, who are often allied health professionals. Some are schoolchildren wishing to avoid school. They fall into two groups—one infects itself with bacteria or other contaminated materials and the second finds a way to cause the thermometer to register higher than the true temperature. If malingering is suspected, all that is necessary to prove it is to repeat the temperature determination immediately after a high reading has been obtained, with someone remaining at the bedside while the thermometer is in place. Other clues to false elevations in the temperature are a dissociation between pulse and temperature, and excessively high fevers [greater than 106°F (41.1°C) in adults] and the absence of chills, sweats, or tachycardia. These patients fall into the psychiatric diagnostic category of "borderline syndrome," a state between neurosis and psychosis, in which the prognosis is guarded. Others, mostly young girls, falsify their temperatures as a means of asking for psychiatric help and do well with psychotherapy.

Patients with FUO who remain undiagnosed These patients divide themselves into several groups. Some have a self-limited, prolonged viral infection that resembles infectious mononucleosis, cytomegalovirus, hepatitis virus, or adenovirus infection, but in which these agents are never isolated. They recover spontaneously. Others appear to have responded to antibiotics and can be presumed to have had a cryptic bacterial infection. A third group has a steroid-responsive fever which resembles, but is not diagnostic of, immunologically mediated diseases. Some of these patients eventually no longer require steroids for suppression of fever, but some do not stay free of pyrexia or other inflammatory symptoms without steroids. An occasional elderly patient looks like an example of a superannuated juvenile rheumatoid arthritis (Still's disease).

DIAGNOSTIC PROCEDURES IN FEVER OF UNKNOWN ORIGIN

With so large a number of possibilities, it is obvious that no single plan can be outlined for the systematic study of every problem in unexplained fever. In any given patient, the history, physical examination, and, most importantly, epidemiologic setting must determine the diagnostic approach. If the features suggest infectious disease, the main dependence will be upon microbiologic methods, whereas when a person in the "cancer age group" has an obscure febrile disorder, the best chance of early diagnosis may lie in x-ray studies, scans, and biopsy.

History Careful attention to the patient's past history and the chronologic development of symptoms may provide important leads. Places of recent residence, contact with domestic or wild animals and birds, preceding acute infectious diseases such as diarrheal illness or boils, and contact with persons with tuberculosis may provide clues to infection. Localizing symptoms may provide a lead to the affected organ system. It is important to query the patient repeatedly. All too often facts of historical importance do not come to light until several interviews have been held.

Physical examination Careful search should be made for skin lesions and for petechial hemorrhages in the ocular fundi, conjunctivas, nail beds, and skin. The lymph nodes should be carefully palpated, with special attention given to the supraclavicular, axillary, and epitrochlear areas. The finding of a heart murmur may be important, particularly if it occurs in diastole. Detection of an abdominal mass may be the first lead to the diagnosis of neoplastic disease. Palpable enlargement of the spleen suggests infection, leukemia, or lymphoma and points away from a diagnosis of solid tumors. Enlargement of the liver and spleen suggests lymphoma, leukemia, chronic infection, or cirrhosis. A large liver without a palpable spleen points to liver abscess or metastatic cancer. The rectum and the female pelvic organs may reveal masses or abscesses; the testicles may reveal tumor or tuberculosis.

Laboratory tests Patients with FUO are subjected to a large number of laboratory tests, often repeatedly and to excess. The following may be useful guidelines in the use of these tests.

HEMATOLOGY These tests are often abnormal, showing anemia, leukopenia, thrombocytopenia or thrombocytosis, and elevation in the sedimentation rate. They are rarely specific. Blood smears for morphology show many abnormalities but, by virtue of the type of patient who presents with FUO, are rarely diagnostic.

CHEMISTRY Unless specific organ dysfunction is defined, these tests are rarely useful. Even serum enzymes indicating hepatic infiltrative disease such as the alkaline phosphatase or 5′-nucleotidase may be normal in the presence of liver disease.

IMMUNOLOGIC TESTS These are most helpful in the diagnosis of fevers caused by connective tissue disorders or, occasionally, because of secondary immune complex disease or infectious endocarditis.

MICROBIOLOGY In the initial evaluation of prolonged fever, blood cultures are indicated. However, in no instance should more than six blood cultures (which are expensive) be performed on any one patient. Smears and cultures of pus are useful but in sick patients should not delay institution of therapy. Anaerobic cultures should be performed in all abscesses. Mycobacterial cultures continue to be the mainstay in the diagnosis of acid-fast disease. Cultures and special stains or biopsies of suspected tissues are often required to diagnose disseminated fungal infections.

SEROLOGY Serologic testing is useful in Epstein-Barr virus and occasionally cytomegalovirus infections and in amebiasis. Routine febrile agglutinins are rarely helpful, but may reveal brucellosis.

SKIN TESTS These are rarely helpful, due to anergy or nonspecificity for acute infection. Many patients with far-advanced neoplasia are anergic. Not all patients with disseminated tuberculosis have positive tuberculin tests. Patients with disseminated histoplasmosis are usually skin test–negative.

Imaging techniques ROENTGENOGRAMS Chest x-rays and, when urinary tract involvement is suspected, intravenous urograms are the most valuable films in the diagnosis of FUO. Review of earlier films, including those performed at other institutions, often turns up important clues when viewed by a fresh observer. Conversely, there is nothing to be gained by repeating earlier films that are technically satisfactory, provided such films were obtained within a reasonable period of time. Sinus and bone films are also often useful. In contrast, gastrointestinal x-rays; oral, intravenous, transhepatic, or retrograde endoscopic cholangiograms; aortograms; and lymphangiograms are helpful only if there are clues that clearly indicate the likelihood of an abnormality in the organ or organ system to be imaged.

ULTRASONOGRAPHY This technique has come into vogue to detect abdominal, renal, retroperitoneal, or pelvic mass lesions. While both false-positive and false-negative results are common, the techniques are still evolving and with further improvement will provide relatively inexpensive, noninvasive screening for masses. It is probably the method of choice for imaging the gallbladder and biliary tree.

RADIONUCLIDE SCANS Of all nuclide scans, the technetium sulfocolloid liver-spleen scan remains the most useful. Gallium scanning, on the other hand, is subject to many false-positive and false-negative tests and has been overrated. Indium 111 leukocyte scanning may be more reliable in the diagnosis of intraabdominal abscesses. Lung scans may reveal pulmonary emboli, and simultaneous liver and lung scans are useful in delineating subphrenic abscess. Bone scans may detect osseous metastases or osteomyelitis more readily than x-rays. Renal scans are helpful in the diagnosis of hypernephroma.

COMPUTERIZED TOMOGRAPHY (CT) SCANS CT scans are very useful in the detection of subphrenic, abdominal, and pelvic abscesses and are the most effective method for imaging the retroperitoneum, which is often the site of the cause of FUO in the form of retroperitoneal lymph nodes, tumors, abscesses, or hematomas. CT scanning is excellent for detecting space-occupying lesions in the liver, although some feel that ultrasound is more effective for visualizing the gallbladder and biliary tree.

Biopsies Often the best means of definitive diagnosis is a biopsy.

Bone marrow biopsy may be helpful not only in clarifying the histologic nature of the marrow but also for occasional demonstration of other disease processes such as metastatic carcinoma or granulomas and for culture. Bone marrow is one location where blind sampling is productive.

Needle biopsy of the liver, while often abnormal, has a low diagnostic yield. It may be particularly helpful in granulomatous diseases. It rarely yields the diagnosis if there are no abnormalities in liver function tests.

Biopsies of other tissues that appear abnormal on physical examination or by noninvasive imaging tests are more likely to be helpful in the diagnosis than of tissues that are biopsied blindly. These include biopsies of the lung, muscle, skin, gastrointestinal mucosa, bone, and arteries. Occasionally, "blind biopsies" of muscle or temporal artery will yield abnormalities, but even here tenderness of the affected part makes finding an abnormality much more likely.

Lymph node biopsy is helpful in the diagnosis of many diseases, including the lymphomas, metastatic cancer, tuberculosis, and mycotic infections. Inguinal nodes are notoriously unsatisfactory for biopsy and are too frequently chosen because of their easy accessibility. Axillary, cervical, and supraclavicular nodes are much more likely to yield helpful information, and the node excised need not necessarily be large.

Exploratory laparotomy Exploratory laparotomy has been advocated as the most definitive diagnostic maneuver in FUO but is valuable only when other investigations, including history, physical examination, noninvasive imaging techniques, and laboratory data point to the abdomen as a possible source of disease. Laparotomies are most helpful in patients with solid tumors or intraabdominal abscesses. The clues to intraabdominal disease are often subtle, but they are present nonetheless. Blind exploration of the abdomen simply because the diagnosis is obscure is poor practice.

Therapeutic trials It is common practice to give a trial of antibiotics to patients with unidentified febrile disorders. Occasionally, this kind of marksmanship is effective, but in general, blind therapy does more harm than good. Undesirable features include drug toxicity, superinfection due to resistant pathogenic bacteria, and interference with accurate diagnosis by cultural methods. Furthermore, a coincidental fall in temperature not due to therapy is likely to be interpreted as response to treatment, with the conclusion that an infectious disease is present. If therapeutic trials are instituted, they should be as specific as possible. Examples are *isoniazid* and *ethambutol* or *rifampin* for tuberculosis; *aspirin* for rheumatic fever; *metronidazole* for hepatic amebiasis; *penicillin* and *gentamicin* for enterococcal endocarditis; and *chloramphenicol* for *Salmonella* bacteremia. Relatively few trials with antibiotics will be successful; those with aspirin, nonsteroidal anti-inflammatory agents, and steroids are more likely to be effective, but these drugs should be used with caution and only in patients in whom the likelihood of connective tissue disease is high and in whom granulomas, infection, and cancer have been ruled out as definitively as possible.

Prognosis in FUO The intelligent application of appropriate diagnostic maneuvers should provide the answer in approximately 90 percent of patients with prolonged obscure febrile illness. The mortality rate in patients with FUO is high among elderly patients, particularly since cancer is the most likely cause of the fever in this age group. Fortunately, most of the remaining patients respond to medical or surgical treatment or recover spontaneously. Of those who do come to autopsy (about 10 percent), fewer than half have had potentially curable disease.

A brief philosophy about patients with FUO Many patients are placed in the FUO category because attending physicians overlook, disregard, or reject an obvious clue. This statement implies no malice; it simply means that physicians, being human instruments, are far from perfect. No algorithms or computers are likely to reverse this trend; moreover, even the new technology is not sufficiently sophisticated to sort out the causes of fever in these patients who often present in very atypical fashion.

In order to mitigate these human errors, clinicians have to work harder. This requires repeated histories and physical examinations, frequent chart reviews to look for the "clue" that is there but has not been appreciated, extensive discussion of the problem with colleagues, and last but not least, time spent in quiet contemplation of the clinical enigma. It does not mean yet another barrage of tests, some of which might be painful and all of which are likely to be expensive, or dousing the patient with more drugs, or, in the absence of corroborating data and as a last resort, subjecting the patient to exploratory surgery. Physicians who care for patients with FUO need to observe them, to talk to them, and to think about them. There are no substitutes for these simple clinical principles.

REFERENCES

ADUAN RP et al: Factitious fever and self-induced infection. Ann Intern Med 90:230, 1979

BUJAK JS et al: Juvenile rheumatoid arthritis present in the adult as fever of unknown origin. Medicine 52:431, 1973

DINARELLO CA, WOLFF SM: *Fever. Current Concepts.* Kalamazoo, The Upjohn Company, 1980, pp 3–38
FAUCI AS et al: The spectrum of vasculitis: Clinical pathologic, immunologic and therapeutic considerations. Ann Intern Med 89:660, 1978
GHOSE MK et al: Arteritis of the aged (giant cell arteritis) and fever of unexplained origin. Am J Med 60:429, 1976
JACOBY GA, SWARTZ MN: Fever of undetermined origin. N Engl J Med 289:1407, 1973
KLATSKIN G: Hepatic granulomata: Problems in interpretation. Mt Sinai J Med 44:798, 1977
LARSON EB et al: Fever of undetermined origin: Diagnosis and follow-up of 105 cases, 1970–1980. Medicine 61:269, 1982
MALMVALL BE et al: The clinical pictures of giant cell arteritis: Temporal arteritis, polymyalgia rheumatica and fever of unknown origin. Postgrad Med 67:141, 1980
MCDOUGALL IR et al: Evaluation of ^{111}In leukocyte whole body scanning. Am J Roentgenol 133:849, 1979
MCNEIL BJ et al: A prospective study of computed tomography, ultrasound and gallium imaging in patients with fever. Radiology 139:647, 1981
MITCHELL DP et al: Fever of unknown origin: Assessment of the value of percutaneous liver biopsy. Arch Intern Med 137:1001, 1977
PETERSDORF RG, BEESON PB: Fever of unexplained origin: Report of 100 cases. Medicine 40:1, 1961
QUINN MJ et al: Computed tomography of the abdomen in evaluation of patients with fever of unknown origin. Radiology 136:407, 1980
SIMON HB, WOLFF SM: Granulomatous hepatitis and prolonged fever of unknown origin: A study of 13 patients. Medicine 52:1, 1973
WOLFF SM et al: Unusual etiologies of fever and their evaluation. Ann Rev Med 26:277, 1975

section 3 Alterations in nervous system function

10 APPROACH TO THE PATIENT WITH NERVOUS SYSTEM DISEASE

JOSEPH B. MARTIN

The symptoms and signs of disordered nervous system function, to be described in the following chapters, are among the most frequent and complex in clinical medicine. Because neurologic disorders may affect higher cortical function with disturbances in language, perception, and memory, as well as produce specific symptoms referable to subcortical structures, spinal cord, peripheral nerve, or muscle, the array of symptoms experienced by the patient is numerous and diverse. Such symptoms are common, not only because diseases that primarily affect various parts of the nervous system occur frequently, but also because many systemic diseases may at one time or another cause disorders of the nervous system. A careful assessment of the character and pattern of the symptoms, their temporal profile, and associated complaints, together with a focused neurologic examination, permit a conclusion to be reached among various alternatives.

These considerations are made more complicated by the difficulties that often arise in distinguishing so-called neurologic from psychiatric diseases. In general, the neurologist has defined disease of the nervous system as any condition that produces a visible anatomic or definable biochemical lesion. However, it is now recognized that many primary neurologic disorders, which present with severe clinical manifestations, fail to show any demonstrable neuropathologic or neurochemical abnormality, even when scrutinized by the most modern techniques of neurobiology. The conditions of dystonia musculorum deformans, spasmodic torticollis, tardive dyskinesia, and Gilles de la Tourette's syndrome, for example, are considered to be neurologic disorders, yet no defined structural abnormality has been reported. The possibility that such disorders are caused by abnormalities of neurotransmitter release or of receptor function is currently viewed as likely because of their partial response to various neuropharmacologic drugs. In other disorders traditionally treated by the psychiatrist, in particular the major psychoses of schizophrenia and of manic-depressive disease, accumulated evidence based on genetic analysis, responses to neuroactive agents, and documented neuroendocrine-biochemical abnormalities suggest that these, too, are primary disorders of nervous system function. This conclusion is supported further by observations that similar psychotic symptoms can be observed in patients with readily identifiable lesions of the nervous system (chronic temporal lobe seizures, brain tumor) or after the administration of certain drugs, such as lysergic acid or amphetamines.

Despite the importance of these areas of overlap between neurology and psychiatry, most neurologic conditions for which a patient seeks general medical care are due to readily demonstrated disease processes. It is the task of the clinician to develop a neurologic method of analysis that will result in accurate diagnosis of the site of the disorder and of its likely cause. Only then can effective approaches to management and treatment be developed.

In this volume, the sections on neurology and psychiatry are considered separately because many of the approaches to diagnosis and treatment remain distinct. In this and the chapters that follow are described the approach to neurologic and psychiatric disorders and a discussion of the manifestations of neurologic diseases as they present to the neurologist or general internist. The aim in these introductory chapters is lucid description of each of the major symptoms and signs of disordered nervous system function. Currently accepted explanations in terms of anatomy, physiology, pharmacology, and chemistry are offered. Sections on specific neurologic diseases are found in Chaps. 341 to 359 and those of psychiatric disorders in Chaps. 360 to 367.

THE NEUROLOGIC METHOD OF CLINICAL EVALUATION The strategy used in evaluating a patient with neurologic illness is to begin with the question, Where is the lesion? The first clues to answering this question appear in the history, and the examination is then "tailor-made" to clarify uncertainties or to make distinctions suggested by the history. Thus, optokinetic nystagmus might be an important part of the examination in a patient with a left hemiparesis and dressing apraxia, but irrelevant to the examination of a patient complaining of burning feet. In a patient who presents with the history of ascending paresthesia and weakness, the examination must be *directed* to deciding, among other things, if the location of the lesion is the spinal cord or a peripheral nerve. Notations regarding muscle stamina or endurance might be crucial to the examination of a patient with myasthenia gravis, as opposed to the usual tests of peak muscle power. What one does with the neurologic examination depends on what the questions are; the questions are formulated by a properly taken history.

Deciding "where the lesion is" accomplishes the task of delimiting the number of possible etiologies to a manageable, finite size. In addition, this strategy safeguards against making really tragic errors. Symptoms of recurrent vertigo, diplopia, and nystagmus should not trigger "multiple sclerosis" as an answer (etiology), but "brainstem" or "pons" (location); then a diagnosis of brainstem arteriovenous malformation will not be missed because it is not considered. The combination of optic neuritis and spastic, ataxic paraparesis should not be memorized as "multiple sclerosis"; then central nervous system syphilis and vitamin B_{12} deficiency (both treatable) will not be overlooked.

Only after the clinician decides "where the lesion is," should the question "what the lesion is" be asked.

The neurologic history A bewildering array of clinical abnormalities require documentation and interpretation during the neurologic evaluation of a patient. The analysis becomes difficult because similar symptoms and signs may present in a patient with any of several disorders. A number of general principles relevant to obtaining a complete neurologic history are important for the physician, whether a generalist or a specialist. Careful attention to the description of the symptoms as experienced by the patient and substantiated by family members or friends permits, in many instances, an accurate localization and determination of the probable cause of the complaints even before an examination of the patient has been undertaken. Two principles should be followed. First, each complaint ought to be chased down as far as possible in an effort to delineate (before the examination) where the lesion might be or, more importantly, *to formulate a set of questions to be answered by the examination.* A patient complains of weakness of the right upper limb. What are the associated features? Is this weakness for brushing the hair or opening a twist-top can? Second, in neurology—where many of the diseases are due to *anatomically restricted* lesions—*negative* associations may be crucial. A patient with a right hemiparesis without a language deficit likely has a different lesion (and likely etiology) than a patient with a right hemiparesis and aphasia. Several of the important factors that aid greatly in defining the nature of the neurologic disorder include:

1 *Temporal course of the illness.* It is particularly important to ascertain the precise rate of appearance and progression of the symptoms experienced by the patient. A paroxysmal onset of a neurologic complaint, occurring within seconds or minutes, usually indicates a cerebrovascular lesion or a seizure. Attention to the temporal march of symptoms may help define a focal seizure, a transient cerebral ischemic attack (TIA), or the onset of a migraine. For example, the onset of sensory symptoms located in one extremity that spreads over a few seconds to adjacent portions of that extremity and then to the other limb or to the face suggests a seizure. A more gradual onset involving less discrete regions of the extremities points to the possibility of a TIA. A similar, but slower progression of sensory change occurring in a young person together with other symptoms of headache, nausea, or visual disturbance suggest migraine. In general, the march of a migraine is slower than that of seizure, and a TIA tends to be more generalized in location on the side of the body or extremities. The presence of positive sensory symptoms or motor movements suggests a seizure; in contrast, transient loss of a function (negative symptom) suggests a TIA. A stuttering onset where symptoms appear, stabilize, regress, and then progress over hours or days also suggests the presence of impending vascular ischemia. In some cases, a demyelinating process may produce new symptoms over the course of a few hours. Progressing symptoms associated with the systemic manifestation of fever, stiff neck, and altered level of consciousness or awareness suggest the possibility of an infectious process. The course of the illness over years in terms of remissions and exacerbations offers additional clues to the nature of the process. Recurrent neurologic symptoms involving any level of the neuraxis with partial or complete recovery suggest the possibility of multiple sclerosis. Slowly progressive disorders without remissions tend to be characteristic of the neurodegenerative processes that affect the nervous system.

2 *Subjective descriptions of the complaint.* It is wise for the physician to recall that patient vocabularies are limited and that symptoms are interpreted within the experience of the patient. Descriptions are highly introspective and subject to the patient's degree of intelligence and general familiarity with medical terminology. The same words often mean very different things to individual patients. For example, dizziness may be a description applied by the patient to impending syncope, to a sense of giddiness, or to true vertigo. Numbness may mean a complete loss of feeling, a positive sensation of tingling, or paralysis. Blurring of vision may be used to describe unilateral visual loss, as in amaurosis fugax, or diplopia. It is important to determine the level of understanding that the patient exhibits with respect to the complaint in order to assess accurately the precise significance of the symptom.

3 *Corroboration of the history by other close associates.* It is often useful to obtain additional information from family, friends, or observers to corroborate or expand the patient's description. Memory loss, personality change, drug abuse, excess alcohol intake, and other factors may severely impair the ability of patients to describe accurately their subjective experiences or prevent them from being completely open and forthright about the factors that have contributed to the illness. Complaints of loss of consciousness which may be due to syncope or seizures necessitate seeking details from patients and family to ascertain the exact circumstances. It is often important to recognize the major manifestations of depression and anxiety which may mask or color the presentation given by the patient. Failure to note these underlying factors which interfere with the patient's performance may result in the incorrect interpretation that a variety of complaints are actually due to structural disease of the brain.

4 *Family history.* Many neurologic disorders, particularly those presenting in childhood or early adulthood, are familial or inherited conditions. It is important to ascertain the familial frequency of occurrence of systemic diseases such as hypertension, heart disease, or stroke, which may affect the nervous system. It is essential to inquire about the possibility of consanguinity of the parents or of the existence of similar symptoms in other members of the family. These may provide clues to a propensity toward a hereditary neurologic condition. It is critical to distinguish between a *negative* family history and an *incomplete* family history. It is insufficient to simply ask, Is there any similar illness in any member of your family? A negative response to such an inquiry may mean that there is, in fact, no such illness in the patient's family, but it may also mean that the patient is unfamiliar with relatives or their medical histories. It is wise to elicit specific positive or negative data about relatives as follows: Are your parents living? If so, are they well? If not, what illness did they have and how did they die? It should always be remembered that maternity is a fact, but paternity is only an assumption.

It is also important to elicit family history data regarding all illnesses rather than just neurologic and psychiatric disorders. Many familial neurologic illnesses are associated with signs and symptoms in other systems (e.g., the phakomatoses, hepatocerebral disorders, neuroophthalmic syndromes, etc.).

5 *Medical illnesses.* Many neurologic illnesses occur in the context of systemic disorders. A history of allergy and asthma may suggest the onset of polyarteritis, with mononeuritis multiplex. Previous or current medical illnesses such as diabetes mellitus, hypertension, and abnormalities of blood lipids may be relevant to evolving symptoms that affect the nervous system. Similarly, the presence of systemic diseases that have an increased association with peripheral neuropathy should be explored. Most patients with coma in a hospital setting can be shown to have a metabolic, toxic, or infectious process.

6 *The patient's perception of the disease.* It is frequently helpful to ask patients what they perceive to be wrong. Do they have a particular fear about a disease like Alzheimer's disease, a brain tumor, or multiple sclerosis? Increasingly, patients who complain of failing memory are concerned about early symptoms of Alzheimer's disease. Patients with headaches may fear that a tumor or an impending stroke is a possibility. Patients with sensory

symptoms frequently are concerned about the possibility of multiple sclerosis. Or the patient may seek attention because a relative or friend has been diagnosed with a serious neurologic illness. More often, however, patients are concerned only about the discomfort and disability caused by a chronic headache or low back pain which persists despite repeated attempts at diagnosis and treatment.

7 *Drug use and abuse and toxin exposure*. It is essential to inquire about the history of drug use, both prescribed and illicit. Complaints of yellow vision may occur with digitalis administration. Excessive vitamin administration may lead to peripheral neuropathy, as has been recently demonstrated in the case of pyridoxine. Aminoglycoside antibiotics may exacerbate symptoms of weakness in patients with disorders of neuromuscular transmission, such as myasthenia gravis. Dizziness may be secondary to ototoxicity caused by the aminoglycosides. In eliciting a history of drug use it is often necessary to be quite specific and to use lay terminology. Most patients are, for example, unaware that over-the-counter sleeping pills, cold preparations, and diet pills are actually drugs. Alcohol, the most prevalent neurotoxin, is often not recognized as such by patients. History of environmental or industrial exposure to neurotoxins may provide the essential clue; consultation with the patient's family or employer may be required.

8 *History of malignancy*. Because malignant tumors may present with nervous system metastases or occasionally with any of several paraneoplastic syndromes, it is important to determine whether any history of malignancy exists and whether chemotherapy or radiotherapy was given. Patients with prior malignancy can present with unexpected and unusual neurologic complications.

9 *Formulating an impression of the patient*. Use the opportunity while taking the history to form an impression of the patient. Is there evidence of anxiety, depression, hypochondriasis? Are there any clues to defects of language, memory, inappropriate behavior, or secondary gain? The neurologic assessment begins as soon as the patient walks into the room and the first introduction is made.

The neurologic examination After obtaining a complete medical and neurologic history, the physician should have reliable clues to the portions of the nervous system to be examined. By the elicitation of specific signs it is then determined whether the nervous system is affected, and, if so, to what degree and which part. The anatomic localization of the lesion assumes special significance in neurology, as certain diseases are known to affect certain regions of the nervous system and not to involve others. Recognition of a constellation of symptoms and signs (a syndrome) points to the possible existence of certain diseases and to the exclusion of others. *Anatomic diagnosis in neurology is ordinarily the most important first step in the diagnostic workup*.

A systematic neurologic examination should encompass a survey of all functions from the cerebrum to peripheral nerve and muscle, i.e., from the mental status examination to the simplest reflexes. Such a detailed examination requires the performance of a series of physical tests aimed at eliciting the functional capacities of each part of the nervous system. The examiner must acquire skills that come only from the repeated use of the same techniques and instruments on a large number of normal and abnormal individuals. Errors and serious omissions are avoided if the examination procedure is orderly and systemic, beginning with mental (cerebral) functions and continuing with cranial nerves, then with motor, reflex, and sensory functions of the arms, trunk, and legs, and finishing with an analysis of posture and gait.

The mental status is already appreciated while the history is being taken. But rather profound disorders of recent memory or of spatial organization may be missed unless specifically tested for. Faults of memory, incoherence of thought, dominating ideas, peculiarities of mood and outlook, aphasic errors, problems of articulation, and loss of insight and judgment should be sought. If abnormalities are noted, a more formal analysis of these functions is undertaken along the lines suggested in Chaps. 11, 22, 23, and 24. The function of each cranial nerve is then examined in order, beginning with olfaction (see Chaps. 13, 14, 19, and 352). Examination of the motor system should include estimates of power of each of the major muscle groups, evidence of atrophy or fasciculation, and assessment of the tone of the musculature during passive manipulations, looking for signs of spasticity, rigidity, or hypotonia (as outlined in Chap. 15). Speed and coordination of the limbs are assessed. Next, prevailing postures and the stance and gait are evaluated (Chap. 16). The tendon reflexes are examined for evidence of increased or decreased (or absent) response or of asymmetry between right and left sides or between arms and legs. The superficial cutaneous reflexes, abdominal and plantar, are then evaluated. Touch, pain, vibration, and joint-position sense are tested as the final part of the examination (see Chap. 18).

This detailed neurologic examination is undertaken only if there are symptoms of disturbed nervous system functioning. If none are present, it suffices to do an abbreviated examination which includes evaluation only of pupils, ocular movements, optic fundi, facial movements, speech, strength of arm and leg muscles, tendon and plantar reflexes, pain and vibratory sensation in hands and feet, and gait. All of this can be completed in 3 to 5 min. The findings, even in the short examination, should be recorded in the patient's record for future reference.

Two additional points about the examination are worth noting. First, in recording observations it is important for the physician to describe what is found, rather than to apply a poorly defined medical term (i.e., "patient groans to sternal rub" rather than "obtunded"). Second, if the patient's complaint is brought out by some activity, reproduce the activity in the office. If the complaint is of dizziness when raising the right arm and turning the head to the left, have the patient do it. If pain occurs after walking two blocks, have the patient demonstrate it and repeat the examination.

Experience teaches that the neurologic examination may be normal even in patients with a serious neurologic disease, such as one which causes seizures or syncope. Or the patient may arrive in a coma with no available history, and the examination proceeds along the lines described in Chap. 21. An inadequate history may to some extent be replaced by a succession of examinations from which the course of the illness may be plotted.

The formulation of the problem and establishment of an etiologic diagnosis The clinical data obtained from the history and the examination are assembled into one of the known syndromes and are interpreted and translated in terms of neuroanatomy and neurophysiology. From the syndrome the physician should be able to determine the anatomic localization(s) that best explains the clinical findings. The anatomic localization, mode of onset and course of illness, other medical data, and laboratory findings are then integrated. Finally, the etiologic diagnosis is reached, and therapy appropriate for the disorder is proposed.

The proper selection of laboratory tests which will assist in arriving at an anatomic, but more particularly at an etiologic, diagnosis poses another set of problems for the clinician. In Chaps. 341 and 354 are described the principal tests and when they should be used. Radiologic imaging techniques, utilizing computerized tomography (CT) scanning, and magnetic resonance imaging (MRI) have had a major impact on the neurologic assessment. It cannot be overemphasized, however, that the anatomic method of physical diagnosis should proceed together with imaging studies for localization of the site of the disorder. There are commonly great discrepancies between the findings on examination and on brain imaging which are resolved only after continued careful assessment of the patient, together with further radiologic study. Assiduous attention to the clinical method in neurology remains as important today as it ever was.

In some neurologic and in most psychiatric diseases, there are no available specific laboratory tests, so one must rely primarily on the history and physical examination. The physician must reject the tendency to label as hysterical or malingering those symptoms that are not readily interpretable.

The application of the neurologic method described above offers an assured and rational approach to the majority of neurologic diseases and conditions. Some problems seen daily in a general hospital defy solution. Sometimes, one reaches an anatomic diagnosis without being able to determine etiologic diagnosis, and one must wait patiently for further developments. Because of the irreversibility of lesions that destroy neurons, a major objective of the neurologic method is diagnosis and treatment at the earliest stage of disease or, even better, the prevention of it. For the clinical investigator the diagnosis of untreatable disease is equally important, for the identification of a disease entity is the first step in its scientific study.

REFERENCES

ADAMS RD, VICTOR M: *Principles of Neurology*, 3d ed. New York, McGraw-Hill, 1985
DEJONG RN: *The Neurologic Examination*. New York, Harper and Row, 1979
SWANSON PD: *Symptoms and Signs in Neurology*. Philadelphia, Lippincott, 1984

11 APPROACH TO THE PATIENT WITH MENTAL AND EMOTIONAL COMPLAINTS

EDWIN H. CASSEM

Physicians see many patients with subjective complaints that are difficult to ascribe to a given clinical disorder; fatigue, tension, nervousness, listlessness, anxiety, depression, giddiness. One patient may complain that he is constantly "on edge," another that her thoughts are being broadcast through the local television station, a third that she has lost all interest in living since the birth of her last child. With other complaints the symptom itself is somatic—dizziness, shortness of breath, unsteadiness, or pain (headache, backache, cramps), but the intensity of the complaint is out of proportion to the physical findings, if any. In such patients, it is the anxiety, tears, look of despair, or a shirt soaked in the axillary area despite a cool room that catch the physician's eye. Or perhaps use of a handkerchief to open the office door, virtual absence of eye contact, a condescending manner with secretaries, or repeated demands for analgesic prescriptions may be the clue to a clinical disorder. Strictly, these behaviors are not "complaints" and when asked about them, the patient may indignantly deny them or have a ready excuse ("The secretary made me stand there for 5 minutes"; "My infant son flushed my Demerol tablets down the toilet"). Nevertheless, such behaviors are important for the examining physician to recognize since they are often relevant to the diagnosis.

Whenever somatic complaints are vague, unexplained by the physical examination or unaccompanied by signs of emotional upset, the physician can inquire about stress. "Sometimes the wear and tear of our daily lives can produce symptoms very much like yours. Have you been under much pressure lately?" is a question which may lead to a lucid account of a recent death in the family, financial loss, or job stress that began or worsened shortly before the patient's symptoms. Often the discussion of such life stresses and emotionally generated symptoms can make the patient feel better. Such interactions are taken for granted in this chapter, since careful observation and listening are basic components of the medical examination.

When are mental and emotional disturbances "abnormal"? No person escapes stress of some sort in daily life. Anxiety or despondency may be a normal response to a threat or disappointment. Few people go through life without some idiosyncracy of manner. Psychiatry, like the rest of medicine, does not focus on the normal. Disease is the formal object of the physician's diagnostic quest. In all clinical encounters with patients complaining of or demonstrating abnormalities of thought, feeling, or behavior, the physician's primary question is not about "mental health" (impossible to define) but whether these symptoms and signs are manifestations of a psychiatric *disorder*.

When symptoms are vague and unexplained by the physical examination, and when the patient denies any psychological cause ("I'm not depressed; I'd be fine if I could only get rid of these headaches"), discovery of a diagnosis that explains them may be difficult. Many of these complaints are caused by common and treatable psychiatric disorders like the anxiety and affective disorders which affect 8.3 and 6 percent of American adults, respectively (Robins et al, 1984). The physician, with the mistaken notion that psychiatric diagnoses are only subjective, lack defining criteria, or are diagnoses of exclusion, may fail to include these common disorders in the differential diagnosis of patient complaints. Another common difficulty arises when the patient has an obvious disorder, such as Parkinson's disease, appropriate treatment is prescribed which leads to significant improvement in the core symptoms of rigidity and bradykinesia, yet the patient continues to complain of exhaustion, insomnia and inability to concentrate. In this case, the patient suffers from both Parkinson's disease and major depression and requires treatment for both conditions. On the other hand, this same patient could have presented to the physician with the primary complaint of exhaustion and "inability to get going." This could be misconstrued as an emotional complaint, and the diagnosis of Parkinson's disease overlooked.

This chapter formulates an approach to the diagnosis of mental, emotional, and behavioral complaints and abnormalities. The classification of such symptoms, as defined in the Diagnostic and Statistical Manual of Mental Disorders (DSM III), is organized to ascertain whether the patient's complaints and findings meet diagnostic criteria for psychiatric disorders.

THE HISTORY OF THE COMPLAINT Chapter 10 discussed the approach to the patient with nervous system disease. Examination of the patient with psychiatric symptoms or signs must be equally careful and systematic. Historical information provides the foundation for the diagnostic formulation. Five factors must be included.

Onset Was the onset of problems sudden or gradual? Did the feelings of depression follow a loss, childbirth, initiation of medication, beginning of a systemic illness (stroke, infectious mononucleosis, or malignancy), stopping a medication or illicit drug (benzodiazepine or cocaine)?

Longitudinal course Is this the first such event? Onset of clinical hypomania in a 70-year-old man, for example, with no prior history of depression or mania, strongly suggests the presence of an organic disorder. Is the symptom recurrent with remissions of normal function or has it been sustained? Recurrent paranoid episodes with remissions or fully normal function make depressive illness more likely than schizophrenia. Did the patient ever consult anyone about the symptoms? Were any treatments attempted and with what success?

Family history Do these symptoms or any other psychiatric disorder appear in the patient's family? Inquiries about depression, mania, panic attacks, phobia, alcoholism, psychosis, and epilepsy should always be solicited directly. Major depression is a familial disorder. Drugs which were successfully used to treat a first-degree relative may be specifically helpful to the patient being examined, should diagnosis prove to be similar.

Premorbid functioning Quality of function will help distinguish some disorders. The chronic schizophrenic, for example, usually has a history of poor interpersonal relations and premorbid difficulty more often than the manic-depressive patient, who may report having been successful in academic, extracurricular, athletic, and interpersonal activities before entering a sustained interval of psychiatric disorder. The patient with antisocial personality disorder always has a history of a rather dramatic constellation of disruptive behaviors (e.g., truancy, theft, vandalism, lying) before the age of 15. As with other medical conditions, these elements of past and family history may not be given willingly by the patient and must be sought from family and other professionals who have treated the patient in the past. Patients with psychiatric disorders may be unable (because of psychosis, memory impairment, or sheer lack of insight) or unwilling (because of embarrassment, wish to deceive, or fear of not being taken seriously) to provide past history.

Hypochondriasis, conversion disorders, substance abuse disorders, somatization disorder and factitious disorders are conditions in which the patient's past medical record is often the most important historical clue to the diagnosis.

Current symptoms and signs When seen by the physician, patients demonstrate what their conditions look like in cross-sectional view. Examination may reveal a person with a major depressive episode; yet a past history of a hypomanic episode or a family history of bipolar illness may suggest that lithium will be the drug of choice. Drugs and other substances can produce severe and distressing symptoms; drug and substance use is an essential component of every history.

TABLE 11-1 General inspection of the patient

Appearance
Dress (jewelry, colors)
Skin (tattoos, hirsutism)
Posture
Grooming
Body build
Thin (anorexic)
Obese
Eye contact
Speech
Quantity
Quality (loud, articulate, fluent)
Content (logic, ability to name)
Motor activity
Quantity (over- or underactive)
Quality (tic-ridden, clumsy, choreoid)
Consciousness
Alert
Not alert: clouded, stuporous
Mood
General cognition
Cooperativeness

THE PSYCHIATRIC EXAMINATION Since mental and emotional symptoms may be the first and even the only symptoms of a medical illness, the physician must be cautious in "jumping to conclusions." A systematic psychiatric examination is the best guarantee that a correct diagnosis will be made. The assessment of patients with psychiatric disorders is described in detail in Chaps. 360 to 367.

The general inspection of the patient should include the factors listed in Table 11-1. Although not an exhaustive list, it demonstrates that the psychiatric examination cannot be limited to inferences based on "hunches" or "intuition," but must be systematic and thorough, going beyond examination of verbal productions of the patient.

Psychiatric disorders involve five spheres; cognition, emotion, behavior, perception, and memory. Just as the internist examines organ systems sequentially—heart, lungs, liver, kidneys, etc., the psychiatrist examines thought, feeling, and behavior.

Cognition Cognition includes orientation, level of awareness, thought, attention, language, judgment, and insight into illness. Whenever defects are found in this realm which are not due to some other medical illness, the diagnosis is usually among the neurologic disorders, including the dementias or the psychoses (see Chaps. 23 and 364). Memory evaluation is of particular importance. A patient may state "I am losing my mind," focusing specifically on an inability to remember names and details. Examination of memory may indicate that concentration and attention are primarily disordered, such that the patient performs accurately only when stimulated or even provoked. The misnomer "*pseudodementia* of depression" is often given to such a condition. Although it can be difficult at times to sort out the cognitive defects in depressed patients, major depression alone does not directly impair memory. Difficulty concentrating, along with the other diagnostic criteria for major depression, point to a diagnosis of depression. With treatment of the depression and restoration of the ability to concentrate (as well as the capacity to take interest in the topic), the "memory" defect disappears. If, on the other hand, a patient with such a complaint reveals a history of insidious, increasing difficulty with simple monetary transactions, following directions, and interpersonal relations, and examination shows some trouble naming, memory impairment, mild apraxia, and difficulty with abstraction, dementia is then highly likely. Depression and dementia can, of course, coexist. In such a case, when the depression is treated, the patient's mental functioning is noticeably improved—but any improvement in memory will be due to improvement in concentration, attentiveness, and motivation, not to improvement in recent recall, which is permanently impaired in dementia.

Emotion Feelings can be reduced to four basic states, each with its variation of intensity: depression (sadness, grief), elation (joy, mania), anxiety (fear, panic), and anger (irritation, rage). Some persons quite accurately perceive their feelings, others seem completely out of touch with them. Facial expression, raised voice, grimacing, gritted teeth, a clenched fist, darting eyes, sweating, tears, and many other clues indicate not only the presence of emotion but often the general category to which it belongs. When patients put their feet on the physician's desk or repeatedly drop ashes on the carpet, they are most likely hostile—even though their response to inquiry about feelings of anger may include fervent protestations that they were unaware these behaviors might adversely affect the physician. A patient can weep profusely when mentioning the death of a spouse or parent yet deny depression. "That's all in the past" shows only the discrepancy between the subjective evaluation and the objective behavior displayed. Psychiatric disorders with disturbed emotions are commonly the affective and the anxiety disorders (Chaps. 360 and 361).

Behavior Behavioral disturbances may be either motor or interpersonal in form. Automatisms, stereotypy, and compulsions are gross examples which usually appear in the history or examination. Examination of interpersonal behavior should include the patient's family, work, and play histories, as well as past interactions with physicians. Disorders of thought and emotion regularly interfere with these dimensions of a person's life, at least temporarily. With psychosis or severe depression patients commonly lose ability to function effectively in any of these areas. When the physician can find no disorder of thought or emotion, it is the behavioral history which may provide the clue. The patient may present such a problem as a chief complaint, like premature ejaculation. This is classified as a sexual dysfunction and can occur without any other psychiatric disorder. At other times the patient either cannot or will not specify the behavioral problem. The personality disorders may have their only manifestations in the behavioral realm. For example, after an illness the dependent personality may continue to complain of symptoms because the illness brought so much caring attention. The patient is not depressed and may appear anxious but fits no psychiatric diagnosis of anxiety disorder. Examination may show that symptoms worsen only when the spouse returns home. The patient with hypochondriasis may have a thick medical chart which documents visits to a dozen prior physicians for a variety of symptoms, but always with the fear that there is an underlying malignancy. The examinations reveal no structural pathology, so the patient seeks another opinion, genuinely convinced that cancer is present.

Perception Disorders of perception include hallucinatory or illusory abnormalities, which can involve any of the primary sensory modalities, alone or in combination. Hearing accusatory voices when no one is present is common in psychotic depression, while hearing one's thoughts broadcast to all the other shoppers in the supermarket is more characteristic of schizophrenia. Visual hallucinations should alert the physician to the likelihood of an organic illness: temporal lobe epilepsy, alcohol withdrawal, or digitalis intoxication are examples of conditions associated with these phenomena.

Memory Memory is the process by which information is stored by the brain for later recall. For clinical purposes it is divided into present and past memory. There is an important interaction with attention and concentration which must be considered when memory is tested. Present memory is tested by asking the patient to recall a list of items or a story. Inability to do so is commonly associated with dementia, chronic alcohol abuse, and drug abuse. Disorders of past memory are sometimes also referred to as *amnesia*. Past memory is impaired in progressive dementia, but when a patient with a normal memory complains of an amnesic episode, the cause may be either organic, as with transient global amnesia, or functional, as with a hysterical fugue episode. Such a patient typically may have disappeared, assumed a new identity, and been unable to recall the past. Psychogenic amnesia occurs when a patient has no apparent ability to recall a traumatic event, such as a sexual molestation by a parent in childhood. A patient may also lie about inability to recall a past event, which is called *malingering*. Memory can also be distorted by a number of abnormal processes. Sometimes false details may be added to a true event, as a "fish story" grows with time. Commonly seen in patients with organic brain disease is *confabulation,* in which the patient attempts to fill in memory defects by telling a plausible but false story in answer to specific questions. *Déjà vu* distorts a present new situation so that it seems to the subject to be the exact repetition of an event that occurred in the past.

FORMULATION OF THE PROBLEM Proceeding in a manner similar to that for any nonpsychiatric symptom, the physician considers the past, present, and family history, the past medical history, the current medications, and the current examination with relevant laboratory tests, and makes a differential diagnosis. The differential diagnosis for psychiatric symptoms has two basic steps: exclusion of organic disease and psychiatric differential diagnosis. Every physician is encouraged to approach psychiatric presentations in this manner.

Exclusion of organic disease Even when the symptoms suggest a psychiatric origin, the physician begins the differential diagnostic process by giving thought to those medical illnesses that might give rise to the constellation of symptoms and signs elicited during the patient examination. The more vague and diffuse the symptoms, the harder it is to be confident that an underlying systemic illness is not the culprit. One need only consider how dramatically disordered thought, feeling, and behavior can be in cases of severe hypoglycemia, hypertensive encephalopathy, Wernicke's encephalopathy, acute hypoxia, subarachnoid hemorrhage, meningitis, or a drug overdose. Many a hypoglycemic diabetic has been initially mistaken for a drunk because of clouded consciousness, slurred speech, and abusive behavior. The fear of the physician is that carelessness or trusting too much in clinical "intuition" might cause a premature dismissal of the symptoms without that sort of careful, systematic diagnostic thinking that insists on further history, vital signs, and laboratory tests to confirm or reject critical hypotheses. This entire textbook is devoted to equipping the physician with more comprehensive knowledge of diseases. The reminder here, however, is that systemic medical illnesses have *psychiatric* symptomatology in many cases. Syphilis has been called "the great imitator" because its manifestations are protean. When a patient with neurosyphilis presents with a manic psychosis, only the physician who includes this diagnosis in a systematic differential diagnosis will never miss it.

Psychiatric-like symptoms can be categorized as depressive, anxious, psychotic, confusional, and euphoric/irritable. The same set of symptoms can be caused by two or more diseases. Just because the patient fully meets the diagnostic criteria for major depression is no guarantee that the cause is not a prescribed drug or a disease like myxedema.

Symptoms of depression Complaints of fatigue, weakness, insomnia, and poor concentration can be caused by many exogenous substances and endogenous diseases. Alcohol, antihypertensive medications—reserpine, alphamethyldopa, and beta-adrenergic blocking agents—and corticosteroids, are frequently implicated in causing depression. Cimetidine, more often a cause of confusion, can produce a strikingly "pure" clinical picture of depression. Use of cocaine, barbiturates, and amphetamines are often associated with a depressive syndrome. Hypothyroidism, hyperparathyroidism, Cushing's and Addison's diseases, and subcortical dementias like Huntington's and Parkinson's diseases are often *heralded* by depression. Anemia, hypo- and hyperglycemia, hyponatremia, hypercalcemia, hypokalemia, encephalitis, and an occult malignancy regularly produce symptoms of weakness and fatigue that can mistakenly be ascribed to depression. An apathetic state, mistakenly labeled by family or nursing staff as depression, can be due to frontal lobe disease or a right hemisphere stroke.

Symptoms of anxiety Few symptoms are more challenging to the diagnostician than anxiety. The feeling state itself, in its "pure" mental denotation, is often defined by somatic symptoms: "butterflies" or a knot in the stomach, sweating, tremulousness, palpitations, flushing, breathlessness, numbness, muscular tension, pallor, dry mouth, urinary frequency. The normal diet contains caffeine and monosodium glutamate, each capable of inducing acute and, in the case of caffeine, chronic anxiety. Withdrawal from alcohol, barbiturates, meprobamate, and benzodiazepines can produce dramatic anxiety, occasionally progressing to a life-threatening medical emergency. Diseases that cause the physical symptoms of anxiety commonly frighten the patient, who may be unaware of the underlying disease. Any event or disorder causing episodic tachycardia or adrenergic arousal, such as hyperthyroidism, paroxysmal atrial tachycardia, mitral valve prolapse, pheochromocytoma, insulinoma, myocardial infarction, or hypoglycemia can produce symptoms of anxiety. Ingestion of excess thyroid medication, sympathomimetic amines, and bronchodilators like theophylline can produce tachycardia and, with it, anxiety. Pulmonary diseases causing breathlessness regularly make the patient anxious: asthma, obstructive pulmonary disease, pneumothorax, pulmonary embolism. Pulmonary edema and congestive heart failure do the same. These conditions are not often mistaken for an emotional disorder unless they are subtle—as occult, intermittent showers of pulmonary emboli may be.

Fear is the commonest emotion produced by a complex partial seizure. Carcinoid tumor, the commonest endocrine neoplasm of the digestive tract, is of special interest because its clinical episodes of flushing and tachycardia may be triggered by intense emotion. In such a case a patient may relate that anger caused the feeling of being "on fire." Patients who receive neuroleptic medications occasionally develop *akathisia,* a side effect characterized by extreme restlessness, inability to remain seated (which gives the condition its name), and a state hard to distinguish from anxious agitation. Failure to recognize this side effect may cause the physician to increase the dose of the neuroleptic, which only worsens the akathisia. Paradoxically, even though depression and anxiety are classified as two separate categories of psychiatric disorder, anxiety is one of the most common and most severe features of major depression. Unless the physician includes depression in the differential diagnosis of the symptoms of anxiety the diagnosis will be missed.

Psychosis with a clear sensorium Psychosis generally refers to a state in which cognition is disorderd by delusions, hallucinations, or both. Schizophrenia, perhaps because it is such a dramatically disabling disorder, retains a premier position as the "hallmark" of psychotic disorders, but it is far from being their commonest cause. The more bizarre delusions are patently absurd, such as those of being controlled, of thought broadcasting, or of thought insertion. These are commonly, but by no means always, associated with schizophrenia. Manic psychosis often presents with similar bizarre delusions. Somatic delusions (that one's body is rotting or giving off a foul odor), grandiose delusions (that one has discovered the secret to world peace), paranoid delusions, and hallucinations of any kind (auditory, visual, olfactory, tactile) require a systematic differential diagnosis. All of these symptoms are commonly found in confusional states, but even when the patient is alert and fully oriented, they may be due to medical illness or exogenous agents. Amphetamine and cocaine abuse tend to produce paranoid states. L-Dopa, administered to patients with Parkinson's disease, may produce paranoid, manic, or confusional states. Lysergic acid (LSD), mescaline, phencyclidine (PCP), and other psychotomimetic agents may produce isolated hallucinations or delusions or both; PCP is particularly associated with severe confusional states marked by agitation and violence. Characteristic organic delusions are described with neurologic disorders, such as denial of blindness after bilateral occipital lobe lesions (Anton's syndrome) or the denial of hemiparesis after a parietal lobe injury. This latter lesion may be associated with the delusion that the involved side of the body has multiple limbs. Another neurologic "delusion," *reduplicative paramnesia,* is a state in which the patient is convinced that he or she is simultaneously in two different places. Such patients may be mentally clear in all other aspects. Ideas of reference, e.g., a sudden intense belief that the television news commentator is referring to oneself, may be the result of a complex partial seizure. Psychosis indistinguishable from functional psychosis can also occur with complex partial seizures.

Delusions with paranoid and depressive content are most commonly associated with depressive disorder. Other delusions, such as those occurring in elderly persons who believe they are infested by parasites and in younger persons who believe that their noses (males) or breasts (females) are too large, are classified as monosymptomatic hypochondriacal psychosis. The younger persons are exceedingly difficult to help, but the older patients with delusions of parasitosis often respond to the dopamine antagonist pimozide. Diffuse brain disease of structural (such as Alzheimer's disease) or toxic/metabolic etiology may be associated with psychotic manifestations, and it may be the psychotic manifestation that first leads to a consultation with the physician.

Hallucinations are often associated with organic conditions. Visual hallucinations ought to be considered as due to an organic etiology until proven otherwise. Alcoholic hallucinosis, as distinguished from delirium tremens, is unique in usually being *auditory,* with a paranoid theme (accusatory voices). The sensorium is clear, there is often no tremor, and it occurs during drinking, not withdrawal (see Chap. 365). It usually occurs after many years of drinking. Withdrawal from addicting substances, especially alcohol, can produce formed visual hallucinations. Formed visual hallucinations have also been reported with digoxin and pentazocine, viral encephalitis, Creutzfeldt-Jakob disease, and sensory deprivation. Macropsia, micropsia (the illusion of objects expanding or shrinking in size), formed visual hallucinations, olfactory hallucinations, déjà vu or jamais vu, and amnesic episodes are symptoms common to focal epilepsy of the temporal lobe or subcortical limbic structures.

Confusion and delirium Confusional states are defined as global dysfunctional states characterized by abnormal orientation, attention, arousal, thought, and memory (see Chap. 23). The findings may be subtle, as when a patient labeled as depressed by the family turns out on examination to have Alzheimer's disease, or dramatic, like delirium tremens. When the state is acute in onset, a toxic state is more likely to prove to be the cause. Whenever mental functions are globally impaired, medications must be considered as potential causes, due either to toxic side effects or abrupt withdrawal. Abrupt cessation of alcohol, barbiturates, meprobamate, benzodiazepines, other sedative hypnotics, and opiates regularly produce an adrenergic, hyperarousal state with symptoms of tremor, tachycardia, mydriasis, sweating, insomnia, and agitation progressing to delirium. Withdrawal of barbiturate anticonvulsants in children can cause similar acute symptoms. In the adult, abrupt withdrawal of tricyclic antidepressants can produce acute symptoms of insomnia, nightmares, gastrointestinal symptoms, and movement disorder with bradykinesia and rigidity. These symptoms are thought to be caused by "cholinergic overdrive," which results when these highly anticholinergic substances are stopped. For the same reason, sudden withdrawal of the anticholinergic neuroleptic thioridazine may cause the same symptoms. Rebound mania may occur after abrupt withdrawal of an antidepressant in manic-depressive patients. In its most severe form it can be difficult to distinguish from delirium. Rebound mania has also been observed following sudden cessation of phenelzine, a monoamine oxidase inhibitor devoid of anticholinergic activity.

More often, confusion is caused directly by a medication prescribed for the patient. Common culprits include anticholinergic drugs (atropine, scopolamine, tricyclic antidepressants) anti-parkinsonian drugs, barbiturates, long-acting benzodiazepines, and bromides. Lithium, essential for treatment of mania or depression, in excessive doses can cause confusion. Almost every drug has been reported on occasion to cause confusion; narcotics, antiarrhythmic agents, antibiotics, digoxin and other digitalis preparations, cimetidine, beta-adrenergic blocking agents, alphamethyldopa, metrizamide, prostaglandin synthetase inhibitors, theophylline, L-dopa, bromocriptine, and clonidine have all been frequent offenders. Antineoplastic agents such as procarbazine, methotrexate, cytosine arabinoside, and occasionally vincristine and vinblastine may cause confusion or delirium. Cyclosporine, so important in protecting transplanted organs from rejection, has also produced confusion in rare cases.

Drugs of abuse, including PCP and other hallucinogens, cocaine, and amphetamines, and combinations of many drugs with alcohol must be considered when a delirious patient is brought to the emergency ward.

Delirious and confusional states are common manifestations of neurologic disorders (see Chap. 23). Trauma, cerebral hypoxia, brain tumor, complex partial status epilepticus, viral encephalitis or meningitis, and Creutzfeldt-Jakob disease may cause an acute confusional state. Acute confusional states occur commonly in demented patients hospitalized for medical illnesses.

Systemic disorders may cause similar adverse results on general mentation; hypercarbia, hypoxemia, renal failure, liver failure, and electrolyte imbalances may present first with alterations in cognition (see Chap. 349). Deficiencies of thiamine, B_{12}, folate, and niacin can produce confusional states. Endocrine disorders, hyper- and hypothyroidism, hyper- and hypoparathyroidism, Cushing's and Addison's diseases, panhypopituitarism, the disorders of glucose metabolism, systemic lupus erythematosus, and hypertensive encephalopathy can cause confusion.

Surgical procedures quite remote from the CNS can produce a setting for unexpected encephalopathy. Most common is the delirium that begins on the third or fourth day after cardiac surgery, which may last several days. No specific cause may be identified. Morbidly obese patients treated with jejunoileostomy have been reported to experience confusional states after ingesting a high carbohydrate diet, thought to be associated with elevated concentration of D-lactate in blood.

Euphoria/irritability Patients who appear "hyper"—expansive, elated, hypertalkative, egotistical, distractable, and boundlessly energetic with a decreased need for sleep—may be manifesting a lifelong personality style or be either manic or hypomanic; or they may be medically ill. If ill, the cause is either drug ingestion or brain disease. The drugs most commonly associated with manic-like symptoms are corticosteroids and ACTH, stimulants like cocaine, amphetamines, sympathomimetics, and excessive thyroid replacement substances, antidepressants and anti-parkinsonian agents.

Rarely brain tumor, ACTH-producing tumors, viral encephalitis, temporal lobe seizures, neurosyphilis, multiple sclerosis, Huntington's disease, uremia, hyperthyroidism, B_{12} deficiency, carcinoid syndrome, and dialysis dementia syndrome can cause mania. Whenever manic symptoms appear in a patient over 50 years of age who has no prior history of either mania or depression, the abnormal state is almost always "secondary" to one of the conditions listed above and not a "primary" psychiatric disorder.

Psychiatric differential diagnosis The general physician, cannot be expected to become an expert in psychiatric disorders. Some disorders, however, are so common that general physicians not only see them frequently but see more of their total number than do psychiatrists. This is most often the case, for example, with major depression. Estimates suggest that up to 60 percent of depressed patients are seen by general physicians and internists and 20 percent by psychiatrists or other mental health professionals, while 20 percent consult no professional for help with their disorder. The general physician who includes depression in the differential diagnosis is in an excellent position to recognize this disorder when it appears and to treat it appropriately.

What does this mean in practical terms? Two psychiatric disorders, major depression and panic disorder serve as examples (Chaps. 360 and 361). For purposes of brevity, we can say that to make the diagnosis of depression the physician needs to find that the patient has at least four of eight symptoms, and for the diagnosis of panic disorder four of twelve (different) symptoms. Since these are common disorders in the general population, these two symptom constellations should be known and readily available for the process of differential diagnosis. Were this the case, differential diagnosis could proceed as follows: When a patient complained of severe anxiety, restlessness, and inability to concentrate, the history, physical, and laboratory exams could be conducted to exclude any likely medical illness. At any time during this process, the physician, noting that the patient already had two (psychomotor agitation and poor concentration) of the eight symptoms of a major depressive episode, would inquire about the other six (sleep or appetite disturbance, blunted interests, decreased energy, guilt, and recurrent thoughts of death or suicide). Should the patient have four or more of these symptoms, qualifying for the diagnosis, major depression might from the outset seem the most likely diagnosis. Even so, a careful approach would mandate the quick but systematic review of illnesses capable of causing a similar symptom constellation. If confident that the patient had no such occult medical illness, the physician could treat the patient's depression.

What if this process has been carefully completed, and there remains neither medical nor psychiatric diagnosis? The term *neurotic*, or *psychoneurotic*, while descriptive of certain conflicts that patients may have, is no longer a psychiatric diagnosis. Certain other terms, like *neurasthenia*, *psychasthenia*, *neurocirculatory asthenia*, and *soldier's heart* have also been eliminated from lists of psychiatric diagnoses because more precise diagnostic categories have replaced them. Because medicine's basic activities are diagnosis and treatment, attempts to specify thought, feeling, or behavior as abnormal are valuable as long as there is an effort to make a diagnosis. Then the physician can prescribe treatment and alleviate the distress that caused the patient to seek medical help.

REFERENCES

AMERICAN PSYCHIATRIC ASSOCIATION: Diagnostic and Statistic Manual of Mental Disorders (DSM III), 3d ed, Washington, 1980

CUMMINGS JL: Organic delusions: Phenomenology, anatomical correlations, and review. Br J Psychiatr 146:184, 1985

GREDEN JF: Laboratory tests in psychiatry, in HI Kaplan, BJ Sadock (eds), *Comprehensive Textbook of Psychiatry IV*. Baltimore, Williams & Wilkins, 1985, vol II, pp 2028–2033

KAPLAN HI, SADOCK BJ: Typical signs and symptoms of psychiatric illness, HI Kaplan, BJ Sadock (eds), *Comprehensive Textbook of Psychiatry IV*. Baltimore, Williams & Wilkins, 1985, vol I, pp 499–501

LUDWIG AM: *Principles of Clinical Psychiatry*. New York, Free Press, 1980

ROBINS LN et al: Lifetime prevalence of specific psychiatric disorders in three sites. Arch Gen Psychiatry 41:949, 1984

12 FAINTNESS, SYNCOPE, AND SEIZURES

RAYMOND D. ADAMS / JOSEPH B. MARTIN

Episodic faintness, light-headedness or giddiness, and reduced alertness are frequently difficult to distinguish, tending to shade into one another. The difference between faintness and frank syncope is often only quantitative. Types of episodic weakness, such as myasthenia gravis, cataplexy, and familial periodic paralysis, which cause striking reduction of muscular strength but no impairment of consciousness, should be set apart (see Chaps. 358 and 359). Seizures, an important cause of altered consciousness, usually differ from syncope, but in some instances their distinction may be difficult. The features that distinguish seizures from syncope are discussed at the end of this chapter and in Chap. 342.

SYNCOPE AND FAINTNESS

Syncope comprises a generalized weakness of muscles, with loss of postural tone, inability to stand upright, and a loss of consciousness. The term *faintness,* in contrast, refers to lack of strength, with sensation of impending loss of consciousness. At the beginning of a syncopal attack the patient is nearly always in the upright position, either sitting or standing [the Stokes-Adams attack (see Chap. 183) is exceptional in this respect]. Usually the patient is warned of the impending faint by a sense of "feeling bad." A sense of giddiness and movement or swaying of the floor or surrounding objects ensues. The senses become confused; the patient yawns or gapes, there are spots before the eyes, vision may dim, and the ears may ring. Nausea and sometimes vomiting accompany these symptoms. There is a striking pallor or ashen gray color of the face, and very often the face and body are bathed in cold perspiration. The deliberate onset may often allow the patient time for protection against injury; a hurtful fall is exceptional. If the patient can lie down promptly, the attack may be averted without complete loss of consciousness.

The depth and duration of unconsciousness vary. Sometimes the patient is not completely oblivious of the surroundings, or there may be profound coma with complete lack of awareness and of capacity to respond. The patient may remain in this state for seconds to minutes or even as long as half an hour. Usually the patient lies motionless with skeletal muscles relaxed, but a few clonic jerks of the limbs and face may occur shortly after the beginning of the unconsciousness. Sphincter control is usually maintained. The pulse is feeble or cannot be felt; the blood pressure may be low and breathing may be almost imperceptible. Once the patient is in a horizontal position, perhaps from having fallen, gravitation no longer hinders the flow of blood to the brain. The strength of the pulse then improves, color begins to return to the face, breathing becomes quicker and deeper, and consciousness is regained. There is from this moment onward a correct perception of the environment. The patient is, nevertheless, keenly aware of physical weakness, and rising too soon may precipitate another faint. Headache and drowsiness, which, with mental confusion, are the usual sequelae of a convulsion, do not follow a syncopal attack.

ETIOLOGY The list of causes in Table 12-1 is based on established or assumed physiologic mechanisms. The commoner types of faint are reducible to a few simple mechanisms. Syncope results from a sudden impairment of brain metabolism usually brought about by hypotension with reduction of cerebral blood flow.

Nature has provided humans with several mechanisms by which circulation adjusts to the upright posture. Approximately three-fourths of the systemic blood volume is contained in the venous bed, and any interference with venous return may lead to a reduction in cardiac output. Cerebral blood flow may still be maintained, as long as systemic arterial vasoconstriction occurs; but when this adjustment fails, serious hypotension with resultant cerebral underperfusion to less than half of normal results in syncope. Normally, the pooling of blood in the lower parts of the body is prevented by (1) pressor reflexes which induce constriction of peripheral arterioles and venules, (2) reflex acceleration of the heart by means of aortic and carotid reflexes, and (3) improvement of venous return to the heart by activity of the muscles of the limbs. Placing a normal person on a tilt table to relax the muscles and tilting upright slightly diminishes cardiac output, and allows the blood to accumulate in the legs to a slight degree. This may then be followed by a slight transitory fall in systolic arterial pressure and, in patients with defective vasomotor reflexes, may be a means of producing faints.

TYPES OF SYNCOPE Vasovagal (vasodepressor) syncope This syncope is the common faint that may be experienced by normal persons; it is frequently recurrent and tends to take place during emotional stress (especially in a warm, crowded room), after an injurious, shocking accident, and during pain. Mild blood loss, poor physical condition, prolonged bed rest, anemia, fever, organic heart disease, and fasting are other factors which increase the possibility of fainting in susceptible individuals. A short premonitory phase is characterized by nausea, perspiration, yawning, epigastric distress, hyperpnea, tachypnea, weakness, confusion, tachycardia, and pupillary dilatation. Physiologically, there is first a marked fall in arterial pressure and systemic vascular resistance which is most notable in the skeletal muscular beds. Cardiac output may be within normal limits but fails to exhibit the expected increase which normally occurs with hypotension. Output declines when vagal activity leads to marked bradycardia, replacing tachycardia, resulting in further lowering of arterial pressure and reduction of cerebral perfusion. Assumption of the supine posture with elevation of the legs and removal of the offending stimulus will rapidly restore consciousness.

Postural hypotension with syncope This type of syncope affects persons who have a chronic defect in, or variable instability of, vasomotor reflexes. The fall in blood pressure on assumption of upright posture is due to a loss of vasoconstriction reflexes in resistance and capacitance vessels of the lower extremities. Though the character of the syncopal attack differs little from that of the vasovagal or vasodepressor type, the effect of posture is its cardinal feature; sudden arising from a recumbent position or standing still are the circumstances under which it is most likely to happen.

Postural syncope tends to occur under the following conditions:

1 In otherwise normal persons who for some unknown reason have defective postural reflexes (this may be familial). In such individuals fainting may occur when tilted on a table. Under such circumstances it has been found that at first the blood pressure diminishes slightly and then stabilizes at a lower level. Shortly thereafter, the compensatory reflexes suddenly fail and the arterial pressure falls precipitously.

2 In *primary autonomic insufficiency* and in the *dysautonomias*. At least three syndromes have been delineated.

a Acute or subacute dysautonomia. In this disease an otherwise healthy adult or child is afflicted over a period of a few days or weeks with a partial or complete paralysis of the parasympathetic and sympathetic nervous systems. Pupillary reflexes are lost, as are lacrimation, salivation, and sweating, and there is impotence, paresis of bladder and bowel musculature, and orthostatic hypotension. The CSF protein is increased. Sensory and motor nerve fibers are demonstrably intact, but nonmedullated autonomic ones have degenerated. Recovery occurs within a few months, possibly hastened by prednisone therapy. The disease is believed to represent a variant of acute idiopathic polyneuritis, akin to Landry-Guillain-Barré syndrome.

b Chronic postganglionic autonomic insufficiency. This is a disease of middle-aged and elderly individuals who gradually develop chronic orthostatic hypotension, sometimes in conjunction with impotence and sphincter disturbances. Upon standing for 5 to 10 min, the blood pressure decreases at least 35 mmHg and the pulse pressure narrows, both without increase in pulse rate, pallor, or nausea. Men are more often affected than women. The condition is relatively benign and seemingly irreversible.

c Chronic preganglionic autonomic insufficiency. In this condition orthostatic hypotension with variable anhidrosis, impotence, and sphincter disturbances is combined with any one of three or more disorders of the central nervous system. These include (1) tremor, extrapyramidal rigidity, and akinesia (Shy-Drager syndrome); (2) progressive cerebellar degeneration, some instances of which are familial; and (3) a more variable extrapyramidal and cerebellar disorder (striatonigral degeneration). These syndromes lead to disability and often death within a few years. (See Chap. 350.)

The differentiation of the chronic peripheral postganglionic and central preganglionic insufficiency is based on pathologic and pharmacologic evidence. In the postganglionic type, neurons of the sympathetic ganglia degenerate, whereas in the central type, the lateral horn cells of the thoracic spinal cord degenerate. In the postganglionic peripheral type, the resting levels of norepinephrine are subnormal because of failure to release norepinephrine from postganglionic endings, and there is hypersensitivity to injected norepinephrine. In the central type, resting levels of norepinephrine are normal. On standing, unlike the reaction in the normal individual, there is little if any rise in norepinephrine levels in either type. And in both types, the levels of plasma dopamine β-hydroxylase (the enzyme that converts dopamine to norepinephrine) are subnormal.

The distinction between the various types of orthostatic hypotension has therapeutic significance. In the peripheral postgan-

TABLE 12-1 Causes of recurrent weakness, faintness, and disturbances of consciousness

I Circulatory (reduced cerebral blood flow)
- *A* Inadequate vasoconstrictor mechanisms
  - *1* Vasovagal (vasodepressor)
  - *2* Postural hypotension
  - *3* Primary autonomic insufficiency
  - *4* Sympathectomy (pharmacologic due to antihypertensive medications such as alphamethyldopa and hydralazine, or surgical)
  - *5* Diseases of central and peripheral nervous systems, including autonomic nerves (Chap. 355)
  - *6* Carotid sinus syncope (see also "Bradyarrhythmias," below)
  - *7* Hyperbradykininemia
- *B* Hypovolemia
  - *1* Blood loss—gastrointestinal hemorrhage
  - *2* Addison's disease
- *C* Mechanical reduction of venous return
  - *1* Valsalva maneuver
  - *2* Cough
  - *3* Micturition
  - *4* Atrial myxoma, ball valve thrombus
- *D* Reduced cardiac output
  - *1* Obstruction to left ventricular outflow: aortic stenosis, hypertrophic subaortic stenosis
  - *2* Obstruction to pulmonary flow: pulmonic stenosis, primary pulmonary hypertension, pulmonary embolism
  - *3* Myocardial: massive myocardial infarction with pump failure
  - *4* Pericardial: cardiac tamponade
- *E* Arrhythmias (Chaps. 183 and 184)
  - *1* Bradyarrhythmias
    - *a* Atrioventricular (AV) block (second- and third-degree), with Stokes-Adams attacks
    - *b* Ventricular asystole
    - *c* Sinus bradycardia, sinoatrial block, sinus arrest, sick-sinus syndrome
    - *d* Carotid sinus syncope (see also inadequate vasoconstrictor mechanisms, above)
    - *e* Glossopharyngeal neuralgia (and other painful states)
  - *2* Tachyarrhythmias
    - *a* Episodic ventricular fibrillation with or without associated bradyarrhythmias
    - *b* Ventricular tachycardia
    - *c* Supraventricular tachycardia without AV block

II Other causes of weakness and episodic disturbances of consciousness
- *A* Altered state of blood to the brain
  - *1* Hypoxia
  - *2* Anemia
  - *3* Diminished carbon dioxide due to hyperventilation (faintness common, syncope seldom occurs)
  - *4* Hypoglycemia (episodic weakness common, faintness occasional, syncope rare)
- *B* Cerebral
  - *1* Cerebrovascular disturbances (cerebral ischemic attacks, see Chap. 343)
    - *a* Extracranial vascular insufficiency (vertebral-basilar, carotid)
    - *b* Diffuse spasm of cerebral arterioles (hypertensive encephalopathy)
  - *2* Emotional disturbances, anxiety attacks, and hysterical seizures (see Chap. 11)

glionic type, the most effective treatment is 9α-fluorohydrocortisone (oral dose 0.1 to 0.2 mg per day) and salt loading to increase blood volume, supplemented by mechanical devices to prevent pooling of blood in the legs and lower trunk (g suit). However, salt together with mineralocorticoids may induce serious supine hypertension, and the dose of the drug must be adjusted for this. For the central preganglionic type, there has been greater success with use of a sympathomimetic amine such as tyramine (which releases norepinephrine from intact postganglionic endings) supplemented by a monoamine oxidase inhibitor (to prevent destruction of the amine), and possibly propranolol. Levodopa has been effective in some cases. In the postganglionic type, judicious use of phenylephrine or ephedrine may be beneficial. Initial reports of the effectiveness of indomethacin in chronic orthostatic hypotension have not been substantiated.

3 After physical deconditioning, e.g., after prolonged illness with recumbency, especially in elderly individuals with reduced muscle tone.
4 After a sympathectomy that has abolished vasopressor reflexes.
5 In diabetic, alcoholic, and other neuropathies; syringomyelia; and diseases of the nervous system which cause muscular atrophy and paralysis of vasopressor reflexes. The most common form of neurogenic orthostatic hypotension is that which accompanies diseases of the peripheral nervous system. Diabetic polyneuropathy, beriberi, amyloid polyneuropathy, and the Adie syndrome are examples. Usually the orthostatic hypotension is associated with disturbances in sweating, impotence, and sphincter difficulties. Presumably the lesion involves postganglionic, nonmedullated fibers in peripheral nerves.
6 In patients receiving antihypertensive and vasodilator drugs as well as those who may be hypovolemic because of diuretics, excessive sweating, or adrenal insufficiency.

Micturition syncope, a condition usually seen in the elderly during or after urination, particularly after arising from the recumbent position, is probably a special type of postural syncope. It has been suggested that release of intravesicular pressure causes sudden vasodilatation, augmented by standing, and that vagally mediated bradycardia is a contributory factor.

Hyperbradykininemia Deficient kinin-inactivating enzymes with apparently normal sympathetic function may result in symptoms of faintness or syncope on assumption of upright posture. Hyperbradykininemia causes arteriolar and venular dilatation giving rise to postural hypotension and syncope with tachycardia. The pathophysiology of this condition remains uncertain. Treatment with beta-receptor antagonists has been beneficial.

Syncope of cardiac origin (cardiac syncope) Cardiac syncope results from a sudden reduction in cardiac output, caused most commonly by a cardiac arrhythmia. In normal individuals slow ventricular rates, but above 35 to 40 beats per minute, and fast ones not exceeding 180 beats per minute do not reduce cerebral blood flow, especially if the person is in the supine position, but changes in pulse rate outside these limits may impair cerebral circulation and function. The upright posture, cerebrovascular disease, anemia, and coronary, myocardial, or valvular disease all reduce the tolerance to alterations in rate.

Complete atrioventricular block is the commonest arrhythmia that leads to fainting, and syncopal episodes associated with this arrhythmia are known as the Stokes-Adams-Morgagni syndrome. The etiology of disturbances in atrioventricular conduction is considered elsewhere (Chap. 183), but in patients with these attacks the block may be persistent or intermittent; it is often preceded or followed by disturbed conduction in one or two of the three fascicles through which the ventricles are normally activated, by second-degree atrioventricular block (Mobitz type II), or bifascicular or trifascicular block. When the block is complete and the pacemaker below the block fails to function, syncope occurs. A brief bout of ventricular tachycardia or fibrillation may also be responsible for the syncopal episode (Chap. 184). Recurrent syncope due to ventricular fibrillation, characterized by a prolonged QT interval (sometimes associated with congenital deafness), has been reported; this condition may be familial or sporadic.

Stokes-Adams attacks occur usually without more than a momentary sense of weakness, the patient suddenly losing consciousness. After cardiac standstill of more than several seconds, the patient turns pale, falls unconscious, and, as in other types of fainting, may exhibit a few clonic jerks. With longer periods of asystole, the ashen gray pallor gives way to cyanosis, stertorous breathing, fixed pupils, incontinence, and bilateral Babinski signs. Prolonged confusion and neurologic signs due to cerebral ischemia may occur in some patients, and permanent impairment of mental function may result, although focal neurologic signs are rare. Cardiac faints of this type may recur several times a day. Occasionally the heart block is transitory, and the electrocardiogram taken later may not show any arrhythmia.

Less commonly, a decreased rate of discharge of the sinoatrial node leads to syncope. Recurrent attacks of tachyarrhythmias—including atrial flutter and paroxysmal atrial and ventricular tachycardia with normal AV conduction—may also suddenly reduce cardiac output to a degree sufficient to cause syncope.

In another form of cardiac syncope the heart block is reflexive and is due to irritation of the vagus nerves. Examples of this phenomenon have been observed in patients with esophageal diverticula, mediastinal tumors, gallbladder disease, carotid sinus disease, glossopharyngeal neuralgia, and pleural and pulmonary irritation. However, in these conditions reflex bradycardia is more commonly of the sinoatrial than the atrioventricular type.

Cardiac syncope may also result from *acute massive myocardial infarction,* particularly when associated with cardiogenic shock. *Aortic stenosis* often sets the stage for exertional syncope, most commonly by limiting cardiac output in the face of peripheral vasodilatation, but sometimes during exertion, with resultant myocardial and cerebral ischemia and occasionally arrhythmias. *Idiopathic hypertrophic subaortic stenosis* may also lead to exertional syncope, because of intensified obstruction and/or ventricular arrhythmias (Chap. 192). In *primary pulmonary hypertension* a relatively fixed cardiac output and bouts of acute right ventricular failure may be associated with syncope (Chap. 191). However, vagal reflexes may be involved in this condition as well as in the syncope that occurs with *pulmonary embolism.* Ball valve thrombus in the left atrium, left atrial myxoma, or thrombosis or malfunction of a prosthetic valve may produce sudden mechanical obstruction of the circulation and syncope. *Tetralogy of Fallot* is the congenital cardiac malformation most commonly responsible for syncope. In this condition systemic vasodilatation, perhaps associated with infundibular spasm, greatly increases the right-to-left shunt and produces arterial hypoxia, which leads to syncope (Chap. 185).

Carotid sinus syncope The carotid sinus is normally sensitive to stretch and gives rise to sensory impulses carried via the nerve of Hering, a branch of the glossopharyngeal nerve, to the medulla oblongata. Massage of one or both of the carotid sinuses, particularly in elderly persons, causes (1) a reflex cardiac slowing (sinus bradycardia, sinus arrest, or even atrioventricular block), the so-called vagal type of response and (2) a fall of arterial pressure without cardiac slowing, the so-called depressor type of response. Both types of carotid sinus response may coexist.

Syncope due to carotid sinus sensitivity may be initiated by turning of the head to one side, by a tight collar, or, as in a few reported cases, by shaving over the region of the sinus. But the absence of such stimuli is of no aid in diagnosis, since spontaneous attacks may occur. The attack nearly always begins when the patient is in an upright position, usually when standing. The period of unconsciousness seldom lasts longer than a few minutes. The sensorium is immediately clear when consciousness is regained. The majority of the reported cases have been in men. In a patient displaying faintness on compression of one carotid sinus, it is important to distinguish between the benign disorder (hypersensitivity of one carotid sinus) and a much more serious condition—atheromatous narrowing of the opposite carotid or of the basilar artery (see Chap. 343).

Other forms of vasovagal syncope have been described. Exceptionally intense pain of visceral origin may inhibit cardiac action through vagal stimulation, e.g., cardiac standstill during an attack of gallbladder colic, a lesion of the esophagus or mediastinum, bronchoscopy, pleural or peritoneal taps, intense vertigo from labyrinthine or vestibular disease, and needling of body cavities. Occasionally, a patient with a severe migraine attack will sustain a syncopal episode.

Vagal and glossopharyngeal neuralgia Occasionally this induces a reflex type of fainting. Again the sequence is always pain, then syncope; in this instance the pain is localized to the base of the tongue, pharynx or larynx, tonsillar area, and ear. It may be triggered by pressure at these sites. Section of the appropriate branches of the ninth or tenth cranial nerve relieves the condition. The cardiovascular effects are attributable to excitation of the dorsal motor nucleus of the vagus via collateral fibers from the nucleus of the tractus solitarius.

Tussive syncope (laryngeal vertigo) This is a rare condition that results from a paroxysm of coughing, usually in men with chronic bronchitis. After hard coughing the patient suddenly becomes weak and loses consciousness momentarily. The intrathoracic pressure becomes elevated and interferes with the venous return to the heart, as does the Valsalva maneuver (exhaling against a closed glottis).

Syncope associated with cerebrovascular disease This is usually caused by partial or complete occlusion of the large arteries in the neck. Physical activity may then critically reduce blood flow to the upper part of the brainstem, causing abrupt loss of consciousness (see Chap. 343).

PATHOPHYSIOLOGY OF SYNCOPE The loss of consciousness in each type of syncope is caused by reduction of oxygenation to those parts of the brain which subserve consciousness. During syncopal attacks, there are demonstrable reductions in cerebral blood flow, cerebral oxygen utilization, and cerebrovascular resistance. The electroencephalogram reveals high-voltage slow waves, two to five per second, coincident with the loss of consciousness. If the ischemia lasts only a few minutes, there are no lasting effects on the brain. If it persists for a longer time, it may result in necrosis of brain tissue in the border zones of perfusion between the vascular territories of the major cerebral and cerebellar arteries.

When faintness is related to reduced cerebral blood flow resulting directly from a disorder of cardiac function, there is likely to be a combination of pallor and cyanosis. When, on the other hand, the peripheral circulation is at fault, pallor is usually striking but is not accompanied by cyanosis or respiratory disturbances. When the primary disturbance lies in the cerebral circulation, the face is likely to be florid and the breathing slow and stertorous. During the attack a heart rate faster than 150 beats per minute indicates an ectopic cardiac rhythm, while a striking bradycardia (rate of less than 40 beats per minute) suggests complete heart block. In a patient with faintness or syncope attended by bradycardia, one has to distinguish that due to failure of neurogenic reflexes from that due to a cardiogenic (Stokes-Adams) attack. The electrocardiogram is decisive, but even without it, the Stokes-Adams attacks can be recognized clinically by their longer duration, by the greater constancy of the slow heart rate, by the presence of audible sounds synchronous with atrial contractions, by atrial contraction (A) waves in the jugular venous pulse, and by marked variation in intensity of the first sound, despite the regular rhythm (Chap. 183).

DIFFERENTIAL DIAGNOSIS OF CONDITIONS INVOLVING EPISODIC WEAKNESS AND FAINTNESS BUT NOT SYNCOPE *Anxiety attacks and the hyperventilation syndrome* are discussed in detail in Chaps. 11 and 360. The giddiness of anxiety is frequently interpreted as a feeling of faintness without actual loss of consciousness. Such symptoms are not accompanied by facial pallor and are not relieved by recumbency. The diagnosis is made on the basis of symptoms, and part of the attack can be reproduced by hyperventilation. Two of the mechanisms known to be involved in the attacks are reduction in carbon dioxide as the result of hyperventilation and the release of epinephrine. Hyperventilation results in hypocapnia, alkalosis, increased cerebrovascular resistance, and decreased cerebral blood flow.

Hypoglycemia, when severe, is usually traceable to a serious disease, such as a tumor of the islets of Langerhans or advanced adrenal, pituitary, or hepatic disease, or to excessive administration of insulin. The clinical picture is one of confusion or even a loss of consciousness. When mild, as is usually the case, hypoglycemia is often of the reactive type (Chap. 329), occurring 2 to 5 h after eating, and is not usually associated with a disturbance of consciousness. The diagnosis depends on the history and the documentation of reduced blood sugar during an attack.

Acute hemorrhage, usually within the gastrointestinal tract, is an occasional cause of syncope. In the absence of pain and hematemesis the cause of the weakness, faintness, or even unconsciousness may remain obscure until the passage of a black stool.

Cerebral ischemic attacks occur in some patients with arteriosclerotic narrowings or occlusion of the major arteries of the brain. The main symptoms vary from patient to patient and include dim vision, hemiparesis or sudden drop attacks, numbness of one side of the body, dizziness, and thick speech. In any one patient all attacks are of identical type and indicate a temporary deficit of function in a certain region of the brain due to inadequate circulation.

Hysterical fainting is rather frequent and usually occurs under dramatic circumstances. The attack is unattended by any outward display of anxiety. The evident lack of change in pulse and blood pressure or color of the skin and mucous membranes distinguishes it from the vasodepressor faint. The diagnosis is based on the bizarre nature of the attack in a person who exhibits the general personality and behavioral characteristics of the hysteric.

Type of onset When the attack begins over the period of a few seconds, carotid sinus syncope, postural hypotension, sudden atrioventricular block, ventricular standstill, or fibrillation is likely. When the symptoms develop gradually during a period of several minutes, hyperventilation or hypoglycemia should be considered. Onset of syncope during or immediately after exertion suggests aortic stenosis, idiopathic hypertrophic subaortic stenosis or excessive bradycardia, and, in elderly subjects, postural hypotension. Exertional syncope is seen occasionally in persons with aortic insufficiency and with severe occlusive disease of cerebral arteries. In patients with ventricular standstill or ventricular fibrillation, loss of consciousness occurs several seconds later, followed rapidly by cessation of electroencephalographic activity and then often by brief clonic muscle contractions.

Position at onset of attack Epilepsy and syncopal attacks due to hypoglycemia, hyperventilation, or heart block are likely to be independent of posture. Faintness associated with a decline in blood pressure (including carotid sinus attacks) and with ectopic tachycardia usually occurs only in the sitting or standing position, whereas faintness resulting from orthostatic hypotension is apt to set in shortly after change from the recumbent to the standing position.

Associated symptoms such as palpitation are likely to be present when the attack is due to anxiety or hyperventilation, to ectopic tachycardia, or to hypoglycemia. Numbness and tingling in the hands and face are frequent accompaniments of hyperventilation. Genuine convulsions during the attack may occasionally occur with heart block, ventricular standstill, or fibrillation. When *duration of attack* is very brief, i.e., a few seconds to a few minutes, carotid sinus syncope or one of the several forms of postural hypotension is most likely. A duration of more than a few minutes but less than an hour suggests hypoglycemia or hyperventilation.

SPECIAL METHODS OF EXAMINATION In many patients who complain of recurrent weakness or syncope but do not have a spontaneous attack while under observation, an attempt to reproduce attacks is of great assistance in diagnosis.

When hyperventilation is accompanied by faintness, the pattern of symptoms can be reproduced readily by having the subject breathe rapidly and deeply for 2 to 3 min. This test is often of therapeutic value also, because the underlying anxiety tends to be lessened when the patient learns that the symptoms can be produced and alleviated at will simply by controlling breathing.

Among other conditions in which the diagnosis is commonly clarified by reproducing the attacks are carotid sinus hypersensitivity (massage of one or the other carotid sinus), orthostatic hypotension and orthostatic tachycardia (observations of pulse rate, blood pressure, and symptoms in the recumbent and standing positions), and tussive syncope (by inducing the Valsalva maneuver). In all these instances the crucial point is not whether symptoms are produced (the procedures mentioned frequently induce symptoms in healthy persons) but whether the exact pattern of symptoms that occurs in the spontaneous attacks is reproduced in the artificial ones. Careful, continuous Holter monitoring of the electrocardiogram in the hospital or the recording of the electrocardiogram over 1 or 2 days using a portable lightweight tape recorder in an ambulatory patient may be extremely useful in identifying an arrhythmia responsible for the syncopal episode. Monitoring is most helpful if it shows that the syncopal episode is characterized by a bout of cardiac standstill, extreme bradycardia, or tachyarrhythmia.

In cases of recurrent syncope of unknown cause, the use of intracardiac electrophysiologic techniques with programmed stimulation can be helpful in determining cardiac abnormalities and in establishing effective treatment. During stimulation, up to two-thirds of such patients can be shown to have rapid ventricular tachycardia, His bundle conduction delays, atrial flutter, sick-sinus syndrome, or hypervagotonia.

The electroencephalogram may be helpful in differentiating syncope from seizures. In the interval between epileptic seizures it may show some degree of abnormality in 40 to 80 percent of cases. In the interval between syncopal attacks it should be normal.

TREATMENT In most instances fainting is relatively benign. In dealing with patients who have fainted, the physician should think first of those causes of fainting that constitute a therapeutic emergency. Among them are massive internal hemorrhage and myocardial infarction, which may be painless, and cardiac arrhythmias. In elderly persons a sudden faint, without obvious cause, should arouse the suspicion of complete heart block, even though all findings are negative when the patient is seen.

Patients seen during the preliminary stages of fainting or after they have lost consciousness should be placed in a position which permits maximal cerebral blood flow, i.e., with head lowered between the knees, if sitting, or in the supine position. All tight clothing and other constrictions should be loosened and the head turned so that the tongue does not fall back into the throat, blocking the airway. Peripheral irritation, such as sprinkling or dashing cold water on the face and neck or the application of cold moist towels, is helpful. If the temperature is subnormal, the body should be covered with a warm blanket. Since emesis is frequent, aspiration should be prevented. The head should be turned to the side and nothing should be given by mouth until the patient has regained consciousness. Patients should not be permitted to rise until the sense of physical weakness has passed, and they should be watched carefully for a few minutes after rising.

The *prevention* of fainting depends on the mechanisms involved. In the usual vasovagal faint of adolescents, which tends to occur in periods of emotional excitement, fatigue, hunger, etc., it is enough to advise the patient to avoid such circumstances. In postural hypotension, patients should be cautioned against arising suddenly from bed. Instead, they should first exercise their legs for a few seconds, then sit on the edge of the bed and make sure they are not light-headed or dizzy before starting to walk. Sleeping with the headposts of the bed elevated on wooden blocks 8 to 12 in high and wearing snug elastic abdominal binder and elastic stockings are often helpful. Drugs of the ephedrine group may be useful if they do not cause insomnia. If there are no contraindications, a high intake of sodium chloride, which expands the extracellular fluid volume, may be beneficial.

In the syndrome of chronic orthostatic hypotension, special corticosteroid preparations (fludrocortisone acetate tablets, 0.1 to 0.2 mg per day in divided doses) have given relief in some cases. Binding of the legs (g suit) and sleeping with head and shoulders elevated are helpful.

The treatment of carotid sinus syncope involves first of all instructing the patient in measures that minimize the hazards of a fall (see below). Loose collars should be worn, and the patient should learn to turn the whole body, rather than the head alone, when looking to one side. Atropine or the ephedrine group of drugs should be used, respectively, in patients with pronounced bradycardia or hypotension during attacks. If atropine is not successful, a demand pacemaker should be inserted into the right ventricle. Radiation or surgical denervation of the carotid sinus has apparently yielded favorable results in some patients, but it is rarely necessary. Once it has been concluded that the attacks are due to a narrowing of major cerebral arteries, some of the surgical measures discussed in Chap. 343 must be considered.

The treatment of the various cardiac arrhythmias which may induce syncope is discussed in Chap. 183. The treatment of hypoglycemia will be found in Chap. 329 and of the hyperventilation syndrome and hysterical fainting in Chap. 11.

The chief hazard of a faint in most elderly persons is not the underlying disease but fracture or other trauma due to the fall. Therefore, patients subject to recurrent syncope should cover the bathroom floor and bathtub with rubber mats and should have as much of their home carpeted as is feasible. Especially important is the floor space between the bed and the bathroom, because faints are common in elderly persons when walking from bed to toilet. Outdoor walking should be on soft ground rather than hard surfaces, and the patient should avoid standing still, which is more likely than walking to induce an attack.

SEIZURES

A seizure or convulsion is defined as an abrupt alteration in cortical electrical activity manifested clinically by a change in consciousness or by a motor, sensory, or behavioral symptom. Seizures, which may be due to a variety of causes, become important in the differential diagnosis of syncope when the episode occurs with minimal or no warning and results in only a brief loss of consciousness. *Epilepsy* (discussed in Chap. 342) is the term used to describe recurrent seizures present over months or years, often with a stereotyped clinical pattern.

CLINICAL CHARACTERISTICS OF SEIZURES A detailed account of the types of seizures, of their pathophysiology, and of their treatment is found in Chap. 342. The purpose here is to recount briefly the varieties of seizures that occur (Table 12-2), and to outline their clinical presentation, particularly with respect to their distinction from syncope. A single seizure may occur during the course of many medical illnesses; its importance derives from the fact that it signifies involvement of the central nervous system by the disease process.

Partial seizures (focal seizures) The appearance of focal motor or sensory manifestations provides clinical documentation of the localization of the cerebral lesion. Deviation of the eyes and head to one side (aversive seizure) usually points to an irritative focus in the opposite prefrontal region. A Jacksonian seizure begins as a clonic movement in one portion of the body, often the thumb, the corner of the mouth, or the great toe, and spreads to adjacent muscular groups over a few seconds or minutes. The seizure may progress to involve the entire side or become generalized with attendant loss of consciousness.

Jacksonian seizures almost always are accompanied by an abnormal interictal EEG.

Complex partial seizures (temporal lobe or psychomotor seizures) These differ from generalized motor seizures by (1) the frequent occurrence of an aura that arises from discharges in the autonomic, visceral, and olfactory portions of the temporal lobe and limbic system; and (2) loss of awareness or contact with the environment, often associated with behavioral or complex motor movements for which the patient is amnesic after the attack. Subjective experiences of the aura include hallucinations (olfactory, gustatory, visual, or auditory), illusions (spatial distortions, shrinkage, or angulation), aberrations in cognition (déjà vu, a sense of familiarity; jamais vu, a sense of unfamiliarity; or recurrent memory), and affective changes (anxiety, fear, and, very rarely, rage). The seizure may terminate with only the subjective component or may progress to the motor phase which is often evident by repetitive motor acts like smacking the lips, swallowing, undressing, and incoherent or dysphasic speech.

The abrupt onset of complex partial seizures often indicates a disorder of the temporal lobe and its connection to the limbic system. Complete investigation in search of the cause is indicated.

Tonic-clonic (grand mal) seizure The abrupt presentation, without warning, of a generalized motor seizure is one of the commonest indications of involvement of the cerebral cortex by a disease process. Grand mal seizures usually begin with opening of the eyes and mouth, flexion and abduction of the arms, and extension of the legs. The *tonic* phase of the seizure is often heralded by contraction of the respiratory muscles resulting in a vocalization. These motor signs are followed by closure of the jaw, often with laceration of the tongue, respiratory arrest with plethora and cyanosis, and urinary, or less commonly, fecal incontinence. The tonic phase of the seizure, which usually persists for only 15 to 30 s, is followed immediately by the *clonic* phase, characterized by violent rhythmic muscular contractions affecting the whole body including the muscles of respiration. Eye movements, facial grimacing, and persistence of respiratory apnea are evident. The clonic movements subside in amplitude and frequency and the seizure terminates, usually within 1 to 2 min. Normal respiration resumes and the patient falls asleep; arousal may occur in a few minutes but lethargy, fatigue, and postseizure (postictal) confusion are common and may persist for several hours. Postictal headache is also common.

The generalized seizure occurring in the course of a major medical illness signifies involvement of the central nervous system by the disorder and requires careful assessment and investigation. Such a seizure may accompany high fever, hyponatremia, metabolic acidosis, alcohol or drug withdrawal, and renal or liver failure, indicating the presence of a *metabolic encephalopathy,* without requiring the postulation of another separate neurologic illness. The determination that a metabolic encephalopathy may be responsible is dependent upon documentation of the systemic illness and careful attention to the exclusion of an additional infectious, vascular, or neoplastic lesion in the nervous system. Central nervous system evaluation should include a careful history, a detailed neurologic examination searching for focal neurologic deficit, and, in many cases, electroencephalography and computerized tomography (CT) scan. If infection is suspected, an examination of the cerebrospinal fluid is mandatory. Recurrent seizures (status epilepticus) indicate a serious compromise of cerebral cortical function and require vigorous treatment to prevent hypoxic damage to the brain and, following termination of the seizures, a thorough investigation of the cause.

An isolated generalized seizure occurring in an otherwise healthy, asymptomatic patient when observed by family or other bystanders is not difficult to distinguish from syncope. More difficult to assess is the circumstance of sudden loss of consciousness occurring without warning and unwitnessed by an observer or an akinetic "drop-seizure" (atypical petit mal). The latter may be indistinguishable from syncope. Postictal confusion or drowsiness, injury such as laceration of the tongue, urinary or fecal incontinence, or muscle soreness suggests that a convulsion has occurred. One common clinical presentation is the sudden occurrence of a brief clonic seizure during a minor surgical or dental procedure. The patient is usually in a seated position and the episode is considered to be due to cerebral ischemia associated with systemic hypotension and bradycardia accompanying vasovagal syncope. There are usually only two or three clonic movements, without a prior tonic phase, and recovery is rapid without postictal symptoms. Such patients should have a neurologic examination and an EEG and, if these are normal, be treated with reassurance and not given anticonvulsants. There is no evidence to indicate an underlying cerebral lesion in such patients.

Generalized seizures may be preceded by a specific warning or *aura,* and attention to these symptoms may be important in aiding in the localization of the seizure focus and can assist in distinguishing the episode from syncope. Tingling or numbness points to involvement of the parietal lobe, and visual or auditory sensations suggest occipitotemporal localization. More complex psychological and cognitive sensations may accompany temporal lobe seizures. Such symptoms may also accompany transient cerebral ischemic attacks (see Chap. 343), but in this case the symptoms usually persist for many minutes or hours.

Absence (petit mal) seizures Absence seizures, in contrast to grand mal, are noted for their brevity and for the degree of loss of awareness accompanied by minimal motor manifestations. They are abrupt in onset and are often evident only by a stare or cessation of ongoing behavior; they may be accompanied by fluttering of the eyelids or by a few facial twitches. Full recovery occurs in 5 to 10 s, and the episode may go unnoticed by the patient, the family, or the teacher. Loss of postural tone (atonic or akinetic seizure) with falling is uncommon but when present requires distinction from syncope. The EEG is diagnostic in such cases, consisting of three-per-second spike and wave discharges. This condition, which indicates a specific generalized disorder of cerebral electrical activity, is responsive to specific drug treatments (see Chap. 342).

DIFFERENTIAL DIAGNOSIS OF SEIZURES AND SYNCOPE Syncope must be distinguished from disturbances of cerebral function, caused by a seizure. A seizure may occur day or night, regardless of the position of the patient; syncope rarely appears when the patient is recumbent, the only common exception being the Stokes-Adams attack. The patient's color may not change in seizures, though there may be cyanosis; pallor is an early and invariable finding in all types of syncope, except chronic orthostatic hypotension and hysteria, and it precedes unconsciousness. Seizures are often heralded by an aura, which is caused by a focal seizure discharge and hence has brain localizing significance. It is usually followed by rapid return to normal or by loss of consciousness. The onset of syncope is usually more deliberate and without aura. Injury from falling is frequent in a seizure and rare in syncope, for the reason that only in seizures are protective reflexes abolished instantaneously. Tonic-convulsive movements with upturning eyes are a feature of seizures and usually do not occur with syncope, although, as stated above, brief tonic clonic seizure-like activity can accompany fainting episodes. The period of unconsciousness tends to be longer in seizures than in syncope. Urinary incontinence is frequent in seizures and rare in syncope. The return of consciousness is prompt in syncope, slow after a seizure. Mental confusion, headache, and drowsiness are common sequelae of seizures; physical weakness with a clear sensorium characterizes

TABLE 12-2 Classification of seizures

I Partial or focal seizures
- *A* Simple partial seizures (with motor, sensory, autonomic, or psychic signs)
- *B* Complex partial seizures (psychomotor or temporal lobe seizures)
- *C* Secondary generalized partial seizures

II Primary generalized seizures
- *A* Tonic clonic (grand mal)
- *B* Absence (petit mal)
- *C* Myoclonic
- *D* Atonic or akinetic

the postsyncopal state. Repeated spells of unconsciousness in a young person at a rate of several per day or month are more suggestive of epilepsy than of syncope. No one of these points will absolutely differentiate a seizure from syncope, but taken as a group and supplemented by electroencephalograms, they provide a means of distinguishing the two conditions.

REFERENCES

CRILL WE: Neuronal mechanisms of seizure initiation, in *Antiepileptic Drugs: Mechanisms of Action,* GH Glaser et al (eds). New York, Raven Press, 1980, p 169

DAY SC: et al: Evaluation and outcome of emergency room patients with transient loss of consciousness. Am J Med 73:15, 1982

DIMARCO JP et al: Intracardiac electrophysiologic techniques in recurrent syncope of unknown cause. Ann Intern Med 95:542, 1981

ECTOR H et al: Bradycardia, ventricular pauses, syncope, and sports. Lancet 1:591, 1984

EWING DJ et al: The natural history of diabetic autonomic neuropathy. Q J Med 49:95, 1980

HICKLER R: Fainting, in *Signs and Symptoms,* 6th ed, RS Blacklow (ed). Philadelphia, Lippincott, 1977, chap 33

JOHNSON RH, SPAULDING JMK: *Disorders of the Autonomic Nervous System.* Philadelphia, Davis, 1974

KAPOOR WN et al: A prospective evaluation and follow-up of patients with syncope. N Engl J Med 309:197, 1983

LEE JE et al: Episodic unconsciousness, in *Diagnostic Approaches to Presenting Syndromes,* JA Barondess (ed). Baltimore, Williams & Wilkins, 1971, pp 133–167

POLINSKY RJ et al: Pharmacologic distinction of different orthostatic hypotension syndromes. Neurology 31:1, 1981

RICHARDS AM et al: Syncope in aortic valvular stenosis. Lancet 1:1113, 1984

SILVERSTEIN MD et al: Patients with syncope admitted to medical intensive care units. JAMA 248:1185, 1982

STREETER DHP et al: Hyperbradykininism: A new orthostatic syndrome. Lancet 2:1048, 1972

SUTHERLAND JM, EADIE MJ: *The Epilepsies,* 3d ed. Edinburgh, Churchill Livingstone, 1980

WEISSLER AM, WARREN, JV: Syncope and shock, in *The Heart,* 4th ed, JW Hurst et al (eds). New York, McGraw-Hill, 1978, p 705

WRIGHT KE JR, MCINTOSH MD: Syncope: Review of pathophysiological mechanisms. Prog Cardiovasc Dis 13:580, 1971

YOUNG RR et al: Pure pandysautonomia with recovery. Description and discussion of diagnostic criteria. Brain 98:613, 1975

13 DISTURBANCES OF VISION AND OCULAR MOVEMENTS

SHIRLEY H. WRAY

The eye, if not the window of the soul, is the mirror reflecting the body's health. No clinician can afford not to examine an organ which gives so many clues to systemic disorders, and one that is the only part of the body where vascular and neural tissue can be viewed directly.

Rose

The eye is a sensory optical organ designed to focus light on a highly photosensitive neuronal membrane, the retina. Light entering the eye passes through the cornea, aqueous humor, lens, and vitreous humor before traversing the transparent layers of the retina to reach photoreceptors in the outer nuclear layer.

The amount of light entering the lens for imaging on the retina is controlled by the iris diaphragm. Its opening, the pupil, can be constricted or dilated by the action of the muscles of the iris. At the start of the visual process light is detected by photoreceptor cells called rods and cones. These neurons contain visual pigments that enable them to capture units of light, called photons. A physiologic interaction involving both excitation and inhibition takes place at progressively more complex synaptic levels among the multiple cell types in the retina. This permits characteristics of incident light striking the eye to be analyzed in terms of spatial, luminous, spectral, and temporal functions.

Rods and cones differ in their capabilities. Rods detect light at low intensity (scotopic condition), have poor image discrimination, and do not detect color. Cones function at high light intensity (photopic condition), have good image resolution, and mediate color vision. Cones are abundant at the center of the retina, in the macula. The macula contains the thin fovea and the tiny circular foveola. The fovea lies 3 mm temporal to the margin of the optic disc. It is the site of maximum acuity (normal 20/20). Visual acuity drops off rapidly in the paramacular areas, where cone concentration drops off abruptly. Rods outnumber cones in the human retina (100 million rods to 60 million cones). They are absent in the foveola and peak in concentration at 20° from the fovea, gradually diminishing peripherally.

The distribution of the retinal ganglion cells parallels that of the cones. In the foveola a single ganglion cell connects via a bipolar cell to an individual cone, a 1:1 ratio that maximizes visual discrimination. Once the initial processing of visual information is completed by the retina, the analysis is relayed as electrical impulses from the ganglion cells through their nerve fibers in the optic nerve, to the lateral geniculate nucleus. After synaptic relay, fibers project via the geniculocalcarine pathway to the visual cortex. Visual function is classified under the terms *form sense, color sense,* and *light sense.*

FORM SENSE Form sense in clinical practice is tested by the determination of visual acuity, a test of macular function. This should be part of any complete medical examination, regardless of symptomatology or lack thereof. The Snellen chart, commonly used for distance vision, is placed 20 feet (approximately 6 meters) away from the patient. The chart consists of letters of graduated sizes; the distance at which each size subtends an angle of 5′ is indicated along the side of the chart. A patient with a corrected refractive error should wear eyeglasses for the test. The vision of a normal eye is 20/20. If the patient is able to read down only to the 20/30 line, the vision is recorded as 20/30. If the patient is unable to read even the large E at the top, he or she may be moved closer so that the distance is changed. The visual acuity may then be recorded as 10/400, for instance, if the patient is able to read this letter at 10 feet from the chart. Pinhole vision should be tested if the patient is unable to read the 20/30 line. A patient whose visual loss is secondary to a refractive error should read close to 20/20 through the pinhole because of the narrow alignment of light rays transmitted through the hole. If the pinhole fails to improve the visual acuity score, the examiner should suspect another cause for the reduced vision, such as opacities in the ocular media or macular or optic nerve disease. Visual acuity corrected by glasses or contact lenses only to 20/200 or less in both eyes or visual fields less than 10° centrally constitutes legal blindness in the United States, and the patient should be registered by the Commission for the Blind in the patient's home state.

COLOR SENSE Many abnormalities of visual function are characterized by acquired defects in color vision. For example, red and green often cannot be distinguished, although the vision for white is normal, in some types of macular disease (due to toxic or degenerative causes), and in optic nerve disease (due to multiple sclerosis, toxins, drugs, or nutritional deficiencies, such as occurs in tobacco-alcohol amblyopia). The most commonly used quantitative tests for color sense are the polychromatic plates of Ishihara, which identify defects in red-green discrimination, and the Hardy-Rand-Ritler (HRR) figures, which are useful in detecting red-green and blue-yellow defects. Demonstration of adequate color vision is mandatory for certain jobs. Hereditary red-green and other types of inherited color blindness are reviewed in the *Manual of Ocular Diagnosis and Therapy* (see references).

LIGHT SENSE Light sense is assessed by visual field examination. Abnormalities indicate damage to a portion of the visual pathway from the retina to the visual cortex. A conventional method of testing visual fields is called kinetic perimetry (Goldmann hemispheric perimeter), which consists of moving a target to identify points of equal sensitivity in the two fields (Anderson). The patient signals when the target is seen, indicating when it disappears and when it reappears. In this way the visual fields can be charted accurately for defects from the periphery into central or foveal fixation. Monocular confrontation visual field testing with a cotton pledget or white-headed pin compares the periphery of the patient's visual field with that of the examiner. The visual field is considered normal if the patient sees the target 90° temporally, 50° nasally, 50° upward, and 65 ° downward.

Each of these indices of visual function may be affected singly or in combination. Failing eyesight may thus be due to an abnormality of the refractive media of the eye, or to a lesion of the retina, the optic nerve, or those parts of the brain with which they are connected.

DISORDERS OF VISION AND THE VISUAL PATHWAY

THE CORNEA The cornea, the main refracting surface of the eye, is vulnerable to environmental hazards including exposure (direct trauma, drying, radiant and ionizing energy), infectious agents (bacteria, viruses—notably herpes simplex and herpes zoster—fungi, and parasites), and inflammation, sometimes in association with systemic dermatologic disorders such as atopic dermatitis, cicatricial pemphigoid, and erythema multiforme (Stevens-Johnson syndrome). *Keratitis* is an inflammation or infection of the cornea. It is often associated with inflammation of the iris (iritis) or of the uveal tract—the iris, ciliary body, and choroid (uveitis). Keratitis combined with uveitis or iritis is seen commonly in Reiter's disease and occasionally in Behçet's disease. Keratitis and uveitis may also occur with herpes simplex infection, in sarcoidosis (Chap. 270), and in collagen vascular diseases (Chap. 269). Metabolic disorders can also cause opacification of the cornea since the cornea can store material present in excess in the body. In hypercalcemia secondary to sarcoid (Chap. 270), hyperparathyroidism (Chap. 336), and vitamin D intoxication (Chap. 337), calcium phosphates and carbonates precipitate beneath the corneal epithelium in a plane corresponding to the interpalpebral fissure, so-called band keratopathy: cystine crystals are deposited in cystinosis (Chap. 308), cholesterol esters in hypercholesterolemia (arcus senilis) (Chap. 315), chloroquine crystals in treatment of discoid lupus, polysaccharides in Hurler's disease (Chap. 319), and copper in hepatolenticular degeneration (Kayser-Fleischer ring) (Chap. 311). Keratoplasty (transplantation) for restoration of sight may be warranted when the cornea is sufficiently scarred and/or opaque.

THE PUPIL Normal pupil size is determined by the level of light entering the eye. Slight degrees of pupil asymmetry (anisocoria) with equal pupil reflexes to light and accommodation can be normal. Pathologic anisocoria occurs with lesions of the sympathetic (Horner's syndrome) or parasympathetic (internal ophthalmoplegia) innervation of the eye. Horner's syndrome is characterized by an ipsilateral normal-reacting miotic pupil, partial ptosis, and, occasionally, impaired facial sweating. An internal ophthalmoplegia (third nerve) causes a fixed or poorly responsive dilated pupil which constricts with 1% pilocarpine eyedrops. The use of different concentrations of topical pilocarpine allows the physician to distinguish between a third nerve palsy, a drug-induced (atropine) mydriasis, and the myotonic pupil of Adie. The test is detailed in the reference by Rose.

AQUEOUS HUMOR AND GLAUCOMA Glaucoma is a condition in which elevated intraocular pressure (IOP) transmitted through the aqueous humor damages the optic nerve. Aqueous humor, formed by secretion of the epithelium of the ciliary body, functions to support metabolism of the avascular lens and cornea. The level of IOP represents a balance between the rate of aqueous humor formation and the resistance to its outflow through the trabecular meshwork to the canal of Schlemm and the aqueous veins. Glaucoma is caused in most cases by an abnormality in outflow from the anterior chamber, not from an increased rate of aqueous humor formation.

Glaucoma is the second leading cause of blindness in the United States; approximately 1 of 50 individuals over age 35 have the condition. About 1 million persons in the United States are estimated to have glaucoma without being aware of it. Detection of glaucoma is, therefore, a major public health problem; measurement of eye pressure should be part of any routine eye examination. An IOP greater than 22 mmHG (Schiötz tonometry) is abnormal, but since considerable diurnal variation of IOP may occur in patients with glaucoma, including normal values, it is important to inspect the optic disc for evidence of glaucoma. The cup usually enlarges vertically before visual field loss occurs, and asymmetry of the optic disc cup may be an early sign. With progressive glaucomatous damage to the nerve, there is loss of nerve tissue and optic atrophy develops, with changes in both contour (cupping) and color (pallor) changes in the disc.

The major types of glaucoma are open-angle, angle-closure, congenital, and secondary.

Open-angle glaucoma Open-angle glaucoma arises as a complication of chronic obstruction of aqueous humor reabsorption in the trabecular meshwork. Open-angle glaucoma is usually asymptomatic and only rarely causes ocular pain or corneal edema. Visual loss occurs first in the peripheral fields and visual acuity remains normal until late in the course of the disorder.

Diagnosis depends on measurement of elevated IOP, and direct visualization (gonioscopy) of the structures at the angle. Management consists initially of careful follow-up with repeated measurements of IOP, visual field assessment, and careful funduscopic evaluation for disc cupping.

The treatment of open-angle glaucoma is primarily medical. Cholinergic drugs (pilocarpine or carbachol) and beta-adrenergic blockers (timolol) decrease IOP after topical application. Carbonic anhydrase inhibitors (acetazolamide or methazolamide) may be beneficial.

Surgery to prevent permanent visual loss is necessary in only a minority of patients. *Laser trabeculoplasty* or creation of a fistula from the anterior chamber to the subconjunctival space are the techniques used.

Angle-closure glaucoma Angle-closure glaucoma develops when aqueous outflow is impeded by a narrow anterior chamber. Tissue in the periphery of the iris covers the trabecular meshwork, preventing egress of aqueous humor. The obstruction may occur acutely, usually in one eye. The eye is red and painful and the pupil may be dilated and nonreactive to light. Vision is impaired. Chronic angle-closure glaucoma may present with visual loss, pupillary dilation, and pain. Gonioscopy is necessary to distinguish open-angle from angle-closure glaucoma in cases with chronic or subacute onset.

Angle-closure glaucoma can be precipitated by administration of drugs to dilate the pupil. Because a narrow angle predisposes to this complication, it is important, particularly in patients over age 50, to examine the anterior chamber of the eye before pharmacologic dilation.

The treatment of acute angle-closure glaucoma is a medical emergency. Intravenous mannitol, parenteral acetazolamide, and topical pilocarpine or timolol are used to counteract the acute increase in IOP. Surgical treatment may be required after acute medical management to create a communication between the anterior and posterior chambers.

Congenital glaucoma This is a rare cause of open-angle glaucoma arising from dysgenesis of structures in the angle of the eye. It may lead to visual loss, enlargement of the eye, and corneal damage. Early recognition is important, followed by medical and surgical management.

Secondary glaucoma Secondary glaucoma can occur as a complication of a systemic disease, or result from a local disorder of the eye. Systemic diseases and drugs that may be associated with glaucoma are (1) hematologic diseases: leukemia, sickle cell disease, Waldenström's macroglobulinemia; (2) collagen diseases: ankylosing spondylitis, rheumatoid arthritis, sarcoidosis; (3) diseases of the skin:

atopic diseases (corticosteroid use), nevus of Ota; (4) infectious diseases: congenital rubella, onchocerciasis; (5) metabolic diseases: amyloidosis, Marchesani's syndrome; (6) musculoskeletal disorders: Conradi's syndrome, osteogenesis imperfecta; (7) neoplastic disease: metastases to the trabecular meshwork; (8) phacomatoses: neurofibromatosis, Sturge-Weber syndrome; (9) pulmonary diseases: asthma and emphysema (corticosteroid use); (10) renal diseases: Lowe's syndrome (aminoaciduria), Wilms's tumor, renal transplantation (corticosteroid use); (11) toxic substances: amphetamines, corticosteroids, hexamethonium, reserpine; and (12) anticholinergic drugs. Local eye disorders causing glaucoma include ocular trauma and dislocation of the lens, as occurs in homocystinuria and Marfan's syndrome.

THE LENS AND CATARACT A cataract is an opacity of the lens; the opacity may be located in the center of the lens (nuclear), in the superficial cortical region, or in the posterior subcapsular area. Cataracts may be congenital or acquired. Lens fibers opacify in response to alterations of the physical and chemical milieu within the semipermeable lens capsule.

Congenital cataracts occur in rubella, herpes simplex, syphilis, and cytomegalic inclusion disease. Acquired cataracts can result from trauma, radiation, drugs, metabolic disorders or aging (senile cataracts). Two types of cataracts are described in diabetes mellitus: metabolic (or snowflake) and senile. Snowflake cataracts are common in insulin-dependent diabetics and begin in the subcapsular region. Senile cataracts occur at an earlier age in diabetics than in control subjects and mature more rapidly. Other metabolic disorders frequently complicated by cataracts include hypocalcemia (Chap. 366), galactosemia (Chap. 314), and hypoglycemia. Cataracts located in the posterior lens occur in more than one-third of patients with myotonic dystrophy. Systemic corticosteroid treatment promotes formation of posterior subcapsular cataracts. Cataracts may also be associated with the following: (1) chromosomal disorders: Alport's syndrome, cri-du-chat syndrome, Conradi's syndrome, Crouzon's syndrome, Turner's syndrome; (2) metabolic and nutritional diseases: aminoaciduria (Lowe's syndrome), Fabry's disease, hypervitaminosis D, hypoparathyroidism, hypothyroidism, mucopolysaccharidoses, Wilson's disease; (3) infectious diseases: acquired cysticercosis, leprosy, onchocerciasis, and toxoplasmosis; (4) toxic substances: corticosteroids, haloperidol, and miotics.

Visual symptoms of cataract include glare, image blur for near visual tasks, image duplication (monocular diplopia), altered color perception, and impaired visual acuity. Cataract extraction may lead to complete visual rehabilitation.

Dislocation or subluxation of the lens (ectopia lentis) can occur in homocystinuria (Chap. 306) and in Marfan's syndrome (Chap. 319) (Fig. A4-15). Dislocation may precipitate glaucoma in these conditions.

VITREOUS HUMOR The vitreous humor undergoes significant physical and biochemical changes with aging. The commonest vitreous opacities are benign "floaters" which appear to patients as gray or black spots or elongated, irregular objects that move with eye movement. Vitreous hemorrhage usually arises from retinal vessels; it may be diffusely dispersed in the vitreous cavity. Massive hemorrhages may reduce vision severely. Vitreous hemorrhage and membrane formation are seen in diabetic retinopathy, retinal vein occlusion, sickle cell retinopathy, congenital retinal vascular anomalies, trauma, disciform macular lesions, choroidal malignant melanoma, and subarachnoid hemorrhage. Asteroid hyalitis (Benson's disease) is characterized by tiny yellow vitreous opacities containing calcium soaps (palmitate and stearate). This condition, which represents dystrophy of the vitreous, can occur in diabetics, but is also a frequent finding in patients with no known ocular disease. Vitreous opacifications can also occur in primary amyloidosis. In reticulum cell sarcoma and retinoblastoma, tumor cells may be seen floating freely in the vitreous. Vitrectomy, the most significant advance in the treatment of vitreous disease, is used to clear vitreous opacities and relieve or prevent vitreoretinal traction. Vitreous biopsy may be useful in establishing the diagnosis in suspected amyloidosis or reticulum cell sarcoma.

THE RETINA Retinal vasculopathies that are potentially blinding are associated with many major medical conditions. The severity of the arterial changes in hypertensive retinopathy, for example, correlates closely with the level of systemic hypertension. Grade I shows moderate arteriolar attenuation and a silver-wire arteriolar reflex; grade II is characterized by arteriovenous crossing defects, hard exudates, and splinter hemorrhages; grade III includes retinal edema, hemorrhages, and cotton-wool spots, the latter due to focal ischemia in the nerve fiber layer; grade IV combines all the signs of grade III plus papilledema, often with a macular star of hard exudates.

Cotton-wool spots are the hallmark of malignant hypertension, but they are also found in anemia, leukemia, collagen vascular diseases, dysproteinemia, infective endocarditis, and diabetes mellitus. They are the most common ophthalmic lesion in acquired immunodeficiency syndrome (AIDS); other retinal manifestations in AIDS may include cytomegalovirus retinitis and retinal periphlebitis.

Diabetic retinopathy is classified into two groups: (1) background retinopathy characterized by microaneurysms, hemorrhages, cotton-wool spots, hard exudates, intraretinal microvascular shunt vessels, and venous bleeding; and (2) proliferative retinopathy characterized by neovascularization and macular edema, which commonly leads to a decrease in visual acuity to 20/200 or worse. Panretinal photocoagulation is beneficial in delaying blindness in such patients.

Permanent blindness can result if the retina is infarcted due to occlusion of the central retinal artery (CRA). Funduscopic examination shows boxcar segmentation of blood flow in the retinal veins, an opaque milky white retina and a central cherry red spot due to visualization of the vascular choroid (Fig. A4-2). CRA occlusion is an ophthalmic emergency and paracentesis of aqueous humor to reduce IOP is the best method to increase blood flow. Embolization of the CRA should be suspected in cases where atheroma is present in the ipsilateral internal carotid artery, aorta, or heart. Other causes of CRA occlusion include giant cell (temporal) arteritis, arteriosclerosis, collagen vascular disease, and hyperviscosity states. Monocular transient blurring of vision (amaurosis fugax) may herald CRA occlusion and/or an impending stroke. Patients with this symptom need urgent attention (see Chaps. 343 and 352).

Venous retinopathies can also threaten vision. Central retinal vein (Fig. A4-3) and branch vein occlusion (common in hypertension) and low-pressure venous stasis retinopathy due to impaired retinal perfusion may occur in carotid occlusive disease, pulseless disease, macroglobulinemia, and polycythemia.

The systemic coagulopathies (thrombocytopenia and disseminated intravascular coagulopathy) may cause retinal hemorrhages or clotting in the submacular choriocapillaries, sometimes associated with choroidal hemorrhage and detachment of the retina. Patients complain of blurred vision due to a focal loss of vision (scotoma). Retinal vascular anomalies are rare. They include retinal telangiectasia (Coat's disease), retinal angiomatosis (von Hippel's disease, Chap. 351) and arteriovenous cirsoid aneurysm (Wyburn-Mason syndrome).

Aside from the visible vascular lesions, other alterations of the retina may also impair vision. The most important of these are detachment or tears of the retina. Retinal degeneration can take several forms:

Retinal degeneration Degeneration of the outer receptor layer and subjacent pigment epithelium occurs as a hereditary trait in retinitis pigmentosa. This condition presents with loss of night vision followed by deficits in peripheral and eventually central vision. Multisystem disorders that include retinal degeneration are abetalipoproteinemia (Bassen-Kornzweig syndrome, Chap. 355), neuronal lipofuscinosis (Batten-Mayou disease, Chap. 350), Refsum's disease Chap. 355), and the Kearns-Sayre syndrome (Chap. 357).

Degeneration of Bruch's membrane Bruch's membrane supports the layer of pigment epithelium adjacent to the rods and cones.

Degeneration results in angioid streaks (breaks) which extend from the disc to the equator. Angioid streaks signify the frequent association of widespread degenerative changes involving elastic tissue elsewhere, such as occur in pseudoxanthoma elasticum, Paget's disease, lead poisoning, and familial hyperphosphatemia.

Degeneration of the outer retinal layers This may occur as a toxic side effect of phenothiazine drugs. These drugs conjugate with the melanin of the pigment layer and should be used in the lowest therapeutic dosages possible. Central visual fields should be tested at 3-month intervals with small red and white test objects in patients receiving chronic therapy with these agents.

Degeneration of the inner retinal layers This may occur as a toxic side effect of chloroquine and hydroxychloroquine.

THE CHOROID Diseases affecting the choroid are uncommon and are discussed in the *Manual of Ocular Diagnosis and Therapy*.

THE OPTIC DISC Elevation or swelling of the optic disc occurs in papilledema (Fig. A4-4), papillitis, optic disc drusen (Fig. A4-5), infiltration of the nerve head by malignant cells, and many other conditions.

True papilledema due to axonal swelling and axoplasmic stasis is caused by elevation of the intracranial cerebrospinal fluid (CSF) pressure which is transmitted to the subarachnoid space around the optic nerves. Visual acuity is minimally affected at first except for transient visual obscurations, constriction of the visual fields, and enlargement of the blind spots (Fig. 13-1*C*). Vascular changes, i.e., hyperemia, venous congestion, and hemorrhage, are secondary phenomena in papilledema. As a general rule, the presence of spontaneous venous pulsations on the disc indicates that the CSF pressure is not elevated. The term *pseudopapilledema* refers to congenitally elevated discs secondary to hyaloid tissue (drusen) or hyperopia.

Papillitis is the term used to describe disc swelling associated with optic neuritis and is accompanied by early visual loss. Papillitis can occur with inflammation, demyelination of the optic nerve (multiple sclerosis, neuromyelitis optica), degeneration (Leber's optic neuropathy), malignant cell infiltration, or vascular disorders of the nerve head. It is important to distinguish this condition from *retrobulbar optic neuritis,* which is characterized by demyelinative lesions of the nerve that intitially show no abnormality in the fundus or disc. Retrobulbar neuritis causes visual loss and an afferent pupillary constriction defect in the light reflex. A comparison of the direct response of the pupil to light in each eye with that elicited indirectly (consensual response) is important to localize the side of the afferent defect. The test to determine this is sometimes called the swinging flashlight test. A Marcus Gunn pupil is a pupil that shows a better constriction to an indirect response than to direct light.

Retrobulbar optic neuritis must be differentiated from hysterical visual loss (steropsis intact, no afferent pupil defect). A history of trauma, drug abuse, toxic exposure, or alcoholism is important to the diagnosis. In young adults, with idiopathic optic neuritis (papillitis or retrobulbar), the risk of developing multiple sclerosis is approximately 30 to 40 percent (Chap. 348). In elderly patients, on the other hand, a common cause of loss of visual acuity and field defects is infarction of the optic nerve (anterior ischemic optic neuropathy) (Fig. A4-6) due to giant cell (temporal) arteritis, nonarteritic arteriosclerosis, or emboli to the posterior ciliary circulation.

Optic disc pallor (Fig. A4-7) is the sequel to most optic nerve lesions, and three etiologic processes are recognized: (1) heredofamilial optic atrophy (Fig. A4-7); (2) primary optic atrophy consequent to death of retinal ganglion cells and axons, and (3) secondary optic atrophy following papillitis and chronic papilledema.

THE CENTRAL VISUAL PATHWAY Visual disturbances can be caused by defects in the retina, optic nerve, chiasm, and tracts, lateral geniculate nucleus, geniculocalcarine path, and striate cortex of the occipital lobes. Retinal lesions cause arcuate scotomas defined as islands of impaired vision within the visual field that point directly to or emanate from the blind spot (Fig. 13-1*A*). Arcuate (nerve fiber bundle) defects have a sharp border on the horizontal meridian and when extensive produce an altitudinal defect (Fig. 13-1*B*). Damage to the papillomacular bundle which subserves foveal visual fixation produces central (involving the fixation point) (Fig. 13-1*D*) or centrocecal (involving both the fixation point and the blind spot) scotomas (Fig. 13-1*E*). Small central scotomas in macular disease often cause distorted vision, particularly for straight lines (metamorphopsia), which aids in the distinction between a macular lesion and one in the optic nerve. A centrocecal scotoma (Fig. 13-1*E*) is a specific and common sign of optic nerve disease due to intrinsic (demyelinative, infiltrative, degenerative) and occasionally to extrinsic compressive lesions (aneurysms, tumor). Toxic states (methyl alcohol, quinine, and certain phenothiazine tranquilizing drugs) and nutritional disorders (tobacco-alcohol amblyopia) are characterized by relatively symmetric bilateral central or centrocecal scotomas. Progressive generalized constriction of peripheral isopters with relative sparing of central vision (Fig. 13-1*G*) may occur with circumferential compression by a tumor, e.g., a perioptic sheath meningioma.

FIGURE 13-1 *Types of monocular visual field loss in left eye. A. Superior arcuate scotoma (inferior nerve fiber bundle defect). B. Inferior altitudinal field defect respecting the horizontal meridian (superior nerve fiber bundle defect). C. Enlargement of the blind spot in the left eye. D. Central scotoma, normal blind spot. E. Centrocecal scotoma. F. Temporal hemianopsia respecting the vertical meridian but with involvement of central vision. G. Generalized constriction of the visual field to 2 isopters. H. Nonorganic "corkscrew" field defect to 1 isopter. (From Wray, 1985; by permission.)*

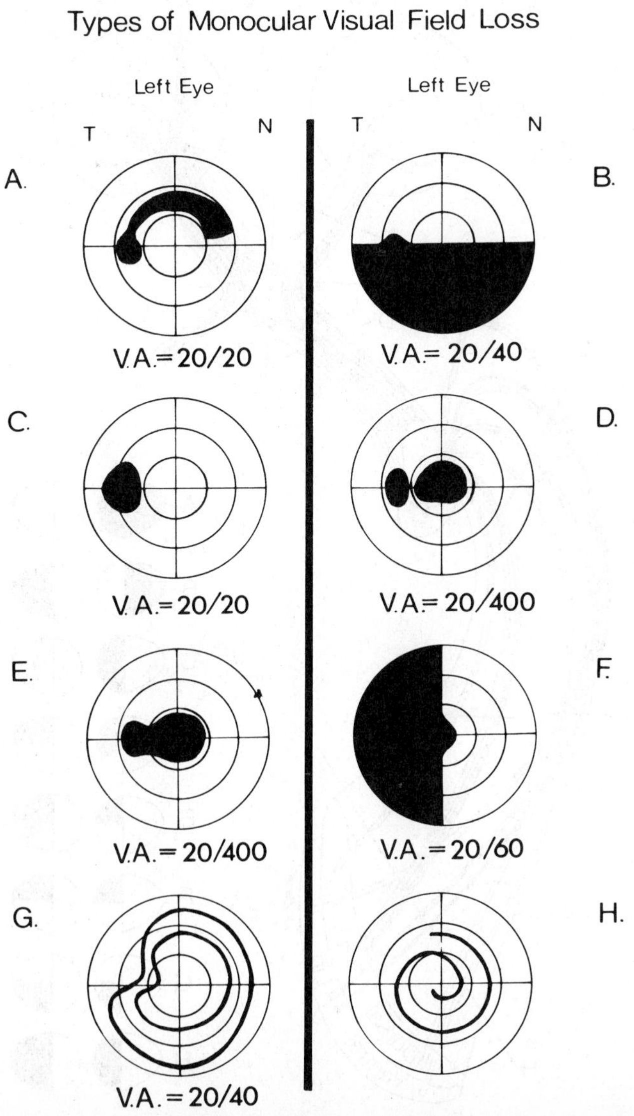

Nonorganic (hysteria, malingerer) corkscrew constriction (Fig. 13-1*H*) or tubular fields persist despite the distance tested. In organic defects, the outer circumference of the field loss will enlarge in a physiologic manner as the distance between the eye and the test object is increased. Hemianopsia means blindness in one-half of the visual field. The defect has a sharp border aligned to the vertical meridian (Figs. 13-1*F*, 13-2*B*, and 13-2*C*). Bitemporal hemianopsia (Fig. 13-2*B*) indicates a lesion of the decussating nasal retinal fibers of the optic chiasm and is due usually to compression of the chiasm (pituitary tumor, craniopharyngioma, meningioma of the diaphragm of the sella, suprasellar aneurysm of the circle of Willis). Homonymous hemianopsia (a loss of vision in corresponding halves of the visual fields) (Fig. 13-2*D* to *H*) signifies a lesion of the visual pathway behind the chiasm and, if complete, gives no more information than that. Incomplete homonymous hemianopsia has more localizing value: if the field defects in the two eyes are identical (congruous), the lesion is likely to be in the calcarine cortex; if incongruous, the visual fibers in the optic tract or lateral geniculate nucleus or in the parietal or temporal radiations are more likely to be implicated.

FIGURE 13-2 *Diagram showing the nerve fiber anatomy of the visual pathways from retina to occipital cortex. The effect on the fields of vision produced by lesions at various points along the optic pathway is shown on the right. A. complete blindness in left eye. B. Bitemporal hemianopsia. C. Nasal hemianopsia of left eye. D and E. Right incongruous homonymous hemianopsia. F and G. Right upper and lower homonymous quadrantanopia. H. complete right homonymous hemianopsia. Courtesy of DD Donaldson. (From Wray, 1985; by permission.)*

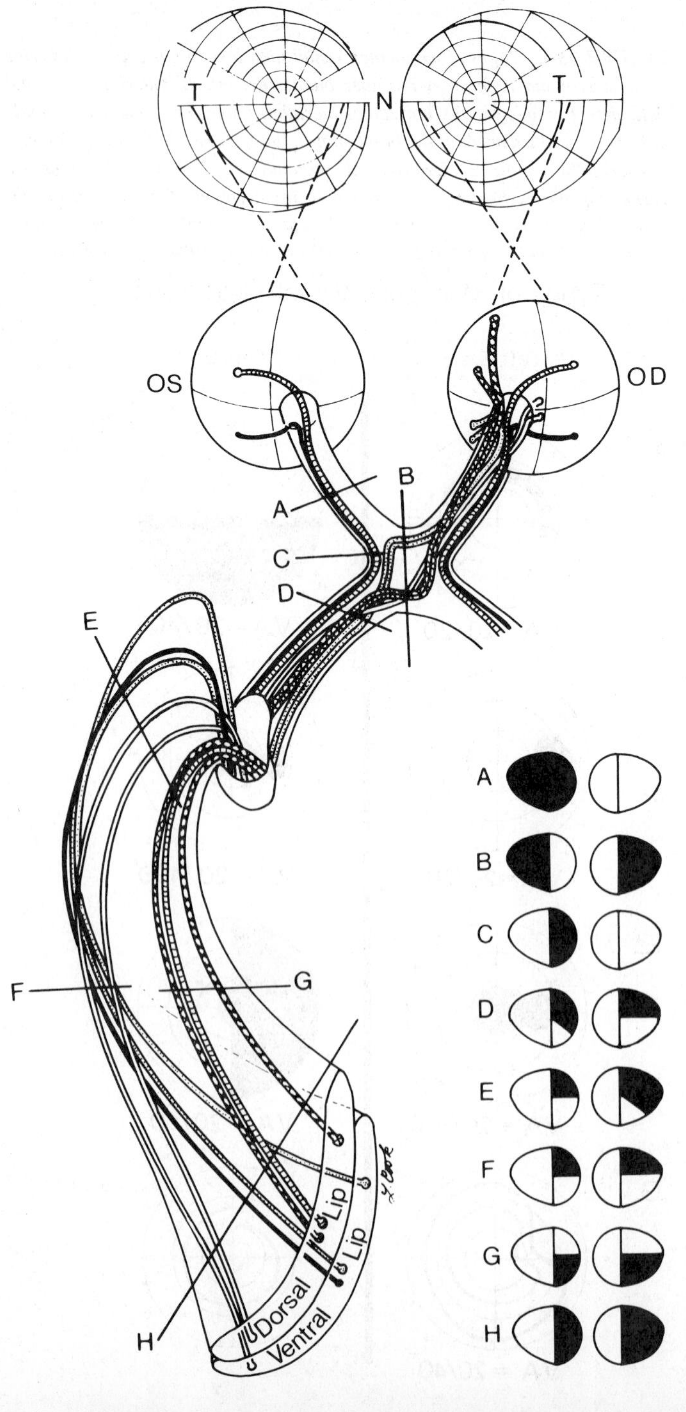

In optic tract lesions, incongruous homonymous hemianopsia is characteristic. Chronic tract lesions are accompanied by an afferent pupil defect and transverse band optic atrophy in the contralateral eye. In postgeniculate lesions (Fig. 13-2*B* to *H*) the pupil reflexes are normal. Fibers from the lower quadrants of the retina extend for a variable distance into the temporal lobe; hence, lesions of this lobe may be accompanied by an homonymous upper quadrantic field defect (Fig. 13-2*E* to *F*). Parietal lobe lesions may affect the lower quadrants more than the upper (Fig. 13-2*G*), or cause a complete hemianopic defect due to inattention. A complete homonymous hemianopsia with splitting of the macula fibers results if the entire calcarine cortex is destroyed on one side (Fig. 13-2*H*). Macular sparing is frequently due to imperfect fixation. Bilateral homonymous hemianopsia results from bilateral, usually ischemic lesions of the visual cortex supplied by the posterior cerebral arteries. Permanent cortical blindness may result, and such patients may show *Anton's syndrome:* bilateral blindness, denial of blindness, normal pupil reflexes, and bilateral occipitoparietal infarcts.

Other disturbances of central vision include various types of distortion in which the perceived objects appear too small (micropsia), too large (macropsia), or askew. When bilateral, such phenomena suggest disease of the temporal lobes, in which case the visual disturbances tend to occur in attacks and may be accompanied by complex visual hallucinations, or other manifestations of temporal lobe seizures (Chap. 342).

In addition to the visual field examination, electrophysiologic techniques are valuable in the analysis of lesions of the anterior visual pathways—especially the flash electroretinogram (ERG), the pattern electroretinogram (P-ERG), and the pattern stimulus visual evoked response (VER) (see Chap. 341). The ERG measures the chain of graded electrical responses from each layer of the retina and can detect retinal disease before funduscopic changes are evident, e.g., in retinitis pigmentosa. However, the ERG is normal in diseases of the retinal ganglion cells and afferent visual pathways. The P-ERG is used as a marker of ganglion cell activity. Such activity is impaired or absent in disorders of the optic nerve secondary to retrograde ganglion cell loss (Leber's optic atrophy, demyelination). The VER is a macular dominant response recorded at the occipital pole of the cerebral cortex (Chap. 341). In the absence of retinal disease it evaluates primarily the function of the anterior visual pathways and particularly the optic nerve. The VER has been useful in establishing the diagnosis of multiple sclerosis by providing objective evidence of an optic nerve lesion even when other clinical signs of visual impairment are lacking (Chap. 348).

DISORDERS OF EYE MOVEMENT

THE ANATOMY OF EYE MOVEMENTS: THIRD, FOURTH, AND SIXTH NERVES AND CENTRAL CONNECTIONS Cranial nerves III, IV, and VI innervate the eye muscles. The oculomotor (third nerve) nuclear complex lies on either side of the midline in the rostral midbrain. It supplies five extraocular muscles including the levator muscle of the eyelid and contains the parasympathetic neurons (Edinger-Westphal nucleus) mediating pupillary constriction and accommodation. Subnuclear groups of motor neurons for individual eye muscles are anatomically distinct within the complex. Those for the medial rectus, inferior oblique, and inferior rectus are ipsilateral to the eye they innervate. The subnucleus for the superior rectus is contralateral to its muscle. The levator palpebrae superioris is innervated by a central group of cells. The motor neurons of the fourth nerve (trochlear) are continuous with the larger oculomotor complex. The left trochlear nucleus innervates the right superior oblique muscle and vice versa. The motor neurons of the sixth nerve (abducens), which innervates the ipsilateral lateral rectus muscle, lie in the abducens nuclei in the caudal pons. All three oculomotor nerves, after leaving the brainstem, pass through the cavernous sinus and enter the orbit through the superior orbital fissure. Accurate binocular vision is achieved by the associated action of individual ocular muscles which yoke the two eyes together.

Conjugate eye movements are controlled by supranuclear gaze centers and their connections. Functionally, there are five distinct supranuclear systems for gaze: *saccadic, pursuit, vergence, position maintenance fixation,* and *vestibular*. Ipsilateral *saccadic* (rapid) eye movements originate in the contralateral frontal cortical eye field (area 8), except for fovea-initiated movements occurring in response to visual stimuli, which arise from the occipitoparietal region. These frontal and occipital control centers project bilaterally to supranuclear brainstem centers, whose function is also modulated by inputs from the cerebellum and the vestibular complex. The paramedian pontine reticular formation (PPRF) acts as the brainstem center for conjugate saccadic eye movements. Simultaneous innervation of one medial rectus and the opposite lateral rectus, during horizontal gaze, is mediated through the medial longitudinal fasciculus (MLF) which connects one abducens nucleus with the contralateral medial rectus subnucleus in the oculomotor complex. Bilateral cortical input to the PPRF is required to initiate vertical saccades. The PPRF relays signals up the brainstem to the supranuclear vertical gaze center—the rostral interstitial nucleus of the medial longitudinal fasciculus (RiMLF)—located in the mesencephalon.

The cortical center for smooth *pursuit* or tracking motions of the eyes is located in the occipitoparietal region. The control is ipsilateral; i.e., the right occipitoparietal region controls smooth pursuit to the right. The control for *vergence* movements is less well understood, but the vergence neurons are known to be located in the mesencephalic reticular formation surrounding the oculomotor complex. They project to the motor neurons of the medial rectus muscle.

A brainstem center called the neural integrator is responsible for *position maintenance of fixation* (gaze-holding). This center converts eye velocity signals into eye position signals. Neurons with this dynamic property lie in the pons caudal to the abducens nucleus.

Coordination of eye movements in response to changes in gravitation and acceleration is mediated by the *vestibular system* (vestibular-ocular reflex) (see Chaps. 14 and 21). Diplopia develops if binocular fusion is impaired since images then fall on disparate (noncorresponding) parts of the two retinas. In *congenital strabismus* or squint, a muscle imbalance that results in improper alignment of the two eyes (nonparalytic strabismus) may result in the brain suppressing one image. The resulting diminished visual acuity in the nonfixing eye is called *amblyopia ex anopsia.* In *paralytic strabismus,* diplopia is due to paralysis of an eye muscle, usually secondary to a lesion of one of the third, fourth, or sixth cranial nerves.

OCULAR MUSCLE AND GAZE PALSIES There are three types of paralysis of extraocular muscles: (1) paralysis of isolated ocular muscles, (2) paralysis of conjugate movements (gaze), and (3) mixed ocular and gaze paralysis.

Paralysis of isolated ocular muscles Characteristic clinical disturbances result from single lesions of the third, fourth, and sixth cranial nerves. A complete third nerve lesion causes ptosis (paresis of levator palpebrae) and inability to turn the eye upward, downward, or inward; a divergent strabismus due to unopposed action of the lateral rectus muscle; a dilated nonreactive pupil (iridoplegia); and paralysis of accommodation (cycloplegia). When only the muscles of the iris and ciliary body are paralyzed, the condition is termed *internal ophthalmoplegia.* Fourth nerve lesions (superior oblique palsy) result in extorsion of the eye and a weakness of downward gaze most marked when the eye is turned inward. Diplopia is corrected by head tilt to the opposite shoulder, which causes a compensatory intorsion of the unaffected eye.

A sixth nerve palsy results in paralysis of abduction and a convergent strabismus, owing to the unopposed action of the medial rectus muscle. With incomplete sixth nerve palsies, the patient may turn the head toward the side of the paretic muscle to overcome diplopia by compensating for the paretic lateral rectus muscle. The foregoing signs may occur with variable degrees of completeness, depending on the severity and site of the lesion or lesions.

Paralysis of conjugate gaze The term conjugate gaze refers to the simultaneous movement of the two eyes in the same direction. An acute lesion in one frontal lobe, as occurs in infarction, may cause a transient paralysis of voluntary contralateral horizontal gaze with preservation of the full range of ocular movement elicited by doll's-head maneuver of passive head turning, or by a caloric stimulus (Chap. 21). A unilateral caudal PPRF lesion, at the level of the abducens nucleus, causes a permanent horizontal gaze palsy to the ipsilateral side and absent oculocephalic reflex movements. Lesions of the RiMLF in the rostral midbrain and/or a lesion of the posterior commissure produce a supranuclear paralysis of conjugate upward gaze and light-near dissociation of the pupils (pupils are sluggish in response to light but constrict briskly to near vision or accommodation). Occasionally, paralysis of convergence is also present. This grouping of signs, called Parinaud's syndrome, is seen in pineal region tumors, and occasionally with infarction, multiple sclerosis, or hydrocephalus. Isolated paralysis of downward gaze is rare. When it occurs, it is usually due to occlusion of a midline penetrating artery and bilateral midbrain infarction. With certain extrapyramidal degenerative disorders, e.g., Huntington's chorea and progressive supranuclear palsy, ocular movements may be limited in all directions, especially upward (Chap. 350).

Mixed gaze and ocular muscle paralyses A combination of gaze paralysis and ocular muscle paralysis is usually a sign of mesencephalic or pontine disease. A lesion of the lower pons affecting the abducens nucleus may cause an ipsilateral horizontal saccadic palsy and sixth nerve palsy. Lesions of the MLF (internuclear ophthalmoplegia) interfere with horizontal gaze in a different way. Unilateral lesions caused by an infarct or demyelination of the MLF cause failure of full adduction of the eye. This may be observed as a complete paralysis with failure to adduct the eye past the midline, or as a mild subclinical paresis characterized by a decrease in the velocity of adducting saccades (adduction lag). In the eye contralateral to the MLF lesion, the main abnormality is abducting nystagmus: a gaze-evoked nystagmus on abduction with a slow centripetal drift toward the midline followed by rapid horizontal corrective saccades. *Skew deviation,* a vertical misalignment of the eyes, is common with unilateral internuclear ophthalmoplegia. The higher eye (hypertropia) is ipsilateral to the side of the lesion. Bilateral internuclear ophthalmoplegia caused by demyelination, tumor, infarct, or an arteriovenous malformation causes a more complete ocular motility syndrome characterized by bilateral adduction weakness, bilateral abduction nystagmus, and impaired vertical, vestibular, and pursuit eye movements. Impairment of ability to maintain vertical gaze is observed with an upbeat nystagmus on looking up and a downbeat (gaze-evoked) nystagmus on looking down. Convergence may be impaired in rostral midbrain MLF lesions.

NYSTAGMUS AND OTHER ENTITIES THAT MIMIC NYSTAGMUS Nystagmus is a repetitive, to-and-fro movement of the eyes. The term includes two types of movements: *pendular nystagmus,* smooth sinusoidal oscillations, and *jerk nystagmus,* alternation of slow drift and corrective quick phase. Normal subjects show nystagmus in response to vestibular and optokinetic stimuli. Identification of the cause of a patient's nystagmus requires historical information (especially drug use, alcohol) and a complete ocular motor evaluation.

Pathologic nystagmus is due to disorders of the mechanisms that maintain fixation. The vestibular, optokinetic, and pursuit systems each act to hold images steady on the retina, and a neural integrator enables the subject to hold eccentric positions of gaze. Disorders of these systems create nystagmus. The most important types of nystagmus are now discussed.

CONGENITAL NYSTAGMUS Long-standing horizontal pendular or jerk nystagmus is characteristic. Occasionally congenital nystagmus is accompanied by anomalies of the visual pathways and impaired vision. The mechanism and site of the abnormality are unknown.

LABYRINTHINE-VESTIBULAR NYSTAGMUS Disease of the vestibular apparatus causes constant velocity slow-phase drifts with corrective quick phases that create a "saw-tooth" jerk nystagmus (see also Chap. 14). Such unidirectional slow-phase drifts reflect an imbalance in the tonic neural activity of the vestibular nuclei. If, for example, disease occurs in one semicircular canal, there results a slow deviation of the eyes to the side of the lesion, followed by a quick corrective movement directed away from the side of the lesion. The abnormality is the slow drift to one side, but by convention the side of the nystagmus is designated by the direction of the quick corrective saccade (fast phase). Such an imbalance of vestibular tone usually causes *vertigo* and *oscillopsia* (illusory movement of the environment) (see Chap. 14). In peripheral vestibular disease, since more than one labyrinthine canal is nearly always affected, an imbalance results between inputs from individual semicircular canals, and the nystagmus is usually of mixed type. For example, in *benign positional nystagmus*, a mixed vertical-torsional nystagmus is common. In unilateral labyrinthine destruction, a mixed horizontal-torsional nystagmus occurs. Peripheral vestibular nystagmus is suppressed by fixation and exacerbated by changes in head position. With disturbances of central vestibular connections, there occurs a central imbalance between semicircular canal inputs, and disruption of ascending vestibular or cerebellar-vestibular connections. Central vestibular nystagmus may mimic nystagmus caused by disease of one semicircular canal, but purely bilateral vertical (upbeat, downbeat), torsional, or horizontal nystagmus is probably more common. This type of nystagmus is poorly suppressed by fixation, but exacerbated or induced by change in head position (Chap. 14). Three forms of labyrinthine-vestibular nystagmus are of clinical importance because of their anatomic localizing value—downbeat, upbeat, and horizontal (sidebeat) nystagmus.

Downbeat nystagmus is usually present in the primary position and is accentuated on lateral gaze. It occurs in posterior fossa anomalies such as the Arnold-Chiari malformation and basilar invagination, and in multiple sclerosis, cerebellar atrophy, hydrocephalus, metabolic disorders, familial periodic ataxia, or as a toxic side effect of anticonvulsant drugs. *Upbeat nystagmus* in the primary position occurs with lesions localized anatomically to the anterior vermis of the cerebellum. It occurs with diffuse brainstem disease (Wernicke's encephalopathy, meningitis, drug side effect). *Horizontal (sidebeat) primary position nystagmus* is usually due to peripheral vestibular disease and only rarely to a posterior fossa tumor, or Arnold-Chiari malformation.

GAZE-EVOKED NYSTAGMUS This type of nystagmus is elicited by the eye assuming an eccentric position in the orbit. It implies a weakness in holding the eyes in the desired position due to defect in the neural integrator in the brainstem. Asymmetric but conjugate horizontal gaze–evoked nystagmus occurs with unilateral cerebellar disease and cerebello–pontine angle tumors (acoustic neuroma). A common cause is drugs (sedatives, anticonvulsants). Horizontal gaze nystagmus in which the quick phases of the adducting eye are slower than the abducting eye (dissociated nystagmus) is characteristic of internuclear ophthalmoplegia.

CONVERGENCE-RETRACTION NYSTAGMUS This movement, stimulated by attempting to look up, is characterized by opposed adducting saccades that converge and retract the eyes. It is usually accompanied by other dorsal midbrain signs (Parinaud's syndrome).

PERIODIC ALTERNATING NYSTAGMUS In this condition, horizontal nystagmus occurs in the primary position but reverses direction periodically, usually every 1 to 2 min. Gaze-evoked and downbeat nystagmus may accompany it. It occurs in a congenital form, with craniocervical junction anomalies, in multiple sclerosis, and with anticonvulsant intoxication. Baclofen usually abolishes the nystagmus and oscillopsia in acquired cases.

SEESAW NYSTAGMUS The eyes show alternating movements. As one eye rises and intorts, the other falls and extorts. Seesaw nystagmus reflects an abnormality of the mesencephalic reticular nuclei including the interstitial nucleus of Cajal. It occurs with suprasellar tumors (craniopharyngioma), head trauma, and rarely with infarcts. Bitemporal hemianopsia frequently coexists.

OTHER ENTITIES THAT MIMIC NYSTAGMUS A variety of motility disorders can mimic nystagmus. These include square-wave jerks (small horizontal saccades away from fixation and back), ocular flutter (horizontal oscillations), opsoclonus (back-to-back saccadic oscillations), superior oblique myokymia (monocular torsional-vertical movements), ocular bobbing (rapid downward deviation of the eyes with slow drift up), and ping-pong gaze (periodic horizontal deviation of the eyes changing direction every few seconds. These conditions are discussed in detail by Leigh and Zee.

This chapter began with an analogy—the eye as a mirror reflecting the body's health. It closes with an analogy that is less passive: that disturbances of vision and ocular movement are in fact diagnostic distress flags whose recognition can significantly expand the physician's understanding. Those internists who truly are alert to the signals the eye can send will not only recognize them, they will read them.

REFERENCES

ANDERSON DR: *Testing the Field of Vision*. St. Louis, Mosby, 1982

BURDE RM et al: *Clinical Decisions in Neuro-ophthalmology*. St. Louis, Mosby, 1985

COGAN D: *Ophthalmic Manifestations of Systemic Vascular Disease*, vol 3. Philadelphia, Saunders, 1974

LEIGH RJ, ZEE DS: *The Neurology of Eye Movement*. Philadelphia, Davis, 1983

PAVAN-LANGSTON D (ed): *Manual of Ocular Diagnosis and Therapy*, 2d ed. Boston, Little, Brown, 1985

ROSE CF: *The Eye in General Medicine*. London, Chapman & Hall, 1983

WALL M, WRAY SH: The one-and-a-half syndrome—a unilateral disorder of the pontine tegmentum: A study of 20 cases and a review of the literature. Neurology 33:971, 1983

WRAY SH: Neuro-ophthalmologic diseases, in *The Clinical Neurosciences*, RN Rosenberg et al (eds). New York, Churchill Livingstone, 1983

WRAY SH: Neuro-ophthalmology: Visual fields, optic nerve, and pupil, in *Manual of Ocular Diagnosis and Therapy*, 2d ed, D Pavan-Langston (ed). Boston, Little, Brown, 1985

14 DIZZINESS AND VERTIGO

ROBERT B. DAROFF

Dizziness is a common and often vexing symptom. Patients use the term to encompass a variety of sensations including those which seem semantically appropriate (e.g., lightheadedness, fainting, spinning, giddiness, etc.) as well as those which are seemingly inappropriate, such as blurred vision, blindness, headache, tingling, "walking on cotton," etc. Moreover, some patients with gait disturbances will describe their problem as "dizziness." A careful history is necessary to determine exactly what a patient who states, "Doctor, I'm dizzy," is experiencing.

After eliminating misleading sensations such as blurred vision, "dizziness" usually means either *faintness* (analogous to the feelings that precede syncope) or *vertigo* (an illusory sense of environmental or bodily movement). In other instances, none of these terms accurately describes a patient's symptoms, and the explanation may only become apparent when the neurologic examination reveals spasticity, parkinsonism, or other ambulation disturbances as the cause of the complaint. Operationally, dizziness is classified into four categories: (1) faintness, (2) vertigo, (3) miscellaneous head sensation, and (4) gait disturbances.

FAINTNESS Fainting (syncope) is a loss of consciousness secondary to cerebral ischemia, more specifically ischemia to the brainstem (see Chap. 12). Prior to the actual faint, there are often prodromal symptoms (*faintness*) reflecting ischemia to a degree insufficient to impair consciousness. The sequence of symptoms is reasonably stereotyped and includes increasing lightheadedness, visual blurring proceeding to blindness, and heaviness in the lower limbs progressing to postural sway. The symptoms increase in severity until consciousness is lost or the ischemia is corrected, often by assumption of the recumbent position. True vertigo almost never occurs during the presyncopal state.

The causes of faintness are described in Chap. 12 and include the multiple etiologies of decreased cardiac output, postural (orthostatic) hypotension, and mimics such as vertebrobasilar insufficiency and seizures.

VERTIGO Vertigo is an illusion of self- or environmental movement, most commonly a feeling of spinning, usually due to a disturbance in the vestibular system. The end organs of this system, situated in the bony labyrinths of the inner ears, consist of the three semicircular canals and the otolithic apparatus (utricle and saccule) on each side. The canals transduce angular acceleration while the otoliths transduce linear acceleration and static gravitational forces, the latter providing a sense of head position in space. The neural output of the end organs is conveyed to the vestibular nuclei in the brainstem via the eighth cranial nerves. The principal projections from the vestibular nuclei are to the nuclei of cranial nerves III, IV, and VI, the spinal cord, cerebral cortex, and cerebellum. The vestibuloocular reflex serves to maintain visual stability during head movement and depends upon direct projections from the vestibular nuclei to the sixth cranial nerve (abducens) nuclei in the pons and, via the medial longitudinal fasciculus, to the third (oculomotor) and fourth (trochlear) cranial nerve nuclei in the midbrain. These connections account for the nystagmus (to-and-fro oscillation of the eyes) which is an almost invariable accompaniment of vestibular dysfunction. The vestibulospinal pathways assist in the maintenance of postural stability. Projections to the cerebral cortex, via the thalamus, provide conscious awareness of head position and movement. The vestibular nerves and nuclei project to areas of the cerebellum (primarily the flocculus and nodulus) which modulate the vestibuloocular reflex.

The vestibular system is one of three sensory systems subserving spatial orientation and posture; the other two are the visual system (retina to occipital cortex) and the somatosensory system that conveys peripheral information from skin, joint, and muscle receptors. The three stabilizing systems overlap sufficiently to compensate (partially or completely) for each other's deficiencies. Vertigo may represent either physiologic stimulation or pathologic dysfunction in any of the three systems.

Physiologic vertigo This occurs when (1) the brain is confronted with a mismatch among the three stabilizing systems or (2) the vestibular system is subjected to unfamiliar head movements to which it has never adapted, such as in seasickness. Intersensory mismatch explains carsickness, height vertigo, and the visual vertigo most commonly experienced during motion picture chase scenes; in the latter the visual sensation of environmental movement is unaccompanied by concomitant vestibular and somatosensory movement cues. *Space sickness*, a frequent transient effect of active head movement in the weightless zero-gravity environment, is another example of physiologic vertigo.

Pathologic vertigo This results from lesions of the visual, somatosensory, or vestibular systems. Visual vertigo is caused by new or incorrect spectacles or by the sudden onset of an extraocular muscle paresis with diplopia; in either instance, central nervous system compensation rapidly counteracts the vertigo. Somatosensory vertigo, rare in isolation, is usually due to a peripheral neuropathy which reduces the sensory input necessary for central compensation when there is dysfunction of the vestibular or visual systems.

The most common cause of pathologic vertigo is vestibular dysfunction. The vertigo is frequently accompanied by nausea, jerk nystagmus, postural unsteadiness, and gait ataxia.

LABYRINTHINE DYSFUNCTION This causes severe rotational or linear vertigo with the illusion of movement, whether of environment or self, directed away from the side of the lesion. The fast phases of nystagmus beat away from the lesion side, and the tendency to fall is toward the side of the lesion.

When the head is straight and immobile, the vestibular end organs generate a tonic resting firing frequency which is equal from the two sides. With any rotational acceleration, the anatomic positions of the semicircular canals on each side necessitate an increased firing rate from one and a commensurate decrease from the other. This change in neural activity is ultimately projected to the cerebral cortex where it is summed with inputs from the visual and somatosensory systems to produce the appropriate conscious sense of rotational movement. The end organs' response to deceleration continues for some time after cessation of prolonged rotation. The side with the initially increased firing rate decreases below the steady state level and the other side increases. A sense of rotation in the opposite direction is experienced; since there is no actual head movement, this illusory sensation is *vertigo*. Any disease state that changes the firing frequency of an end organ, producing unequal neural input to the brainstem and ultimately the cerebral cortex, causes vertigo. The symptom can be conceptualized as the cortex inappropriately interpreting the abnormal neural input from the brainstem as indicating actual head rotation. Transient deficits produce short-lived symptoms. With a fixed unilateral deficit, central compensatory mechanisms ultimately diminish the vertigo. Since compensation depends upon plasticity of connections between the vestibular nuclei and cerebellum, patients with brainstem or cerebellar disease have diminished adaptive capacity and symptoms may persist indefinitely. Compensation is always inadequate for severe fixed bilateral lesions despite normal cerebellar connections; these patients are symptomatic indefinitely.

Acute unilateral labyrinthine dysfunction is caused by infection, trauma, ischemia, and toxins (usually drugs or alcohol). Often, no specific etiology is uncovered and the nonspecific term *acute labyrinthitis* or, preferably, *acute peripheral vestibulopathy* is used to describe the event. It is impossible to determine whether a patient recovering from the first bout of vertigo will have recurrent episodes.

Schwannomas involving the eighth cranial nerve (*acoustic neuroma*) grow slowly and produce such a gradual reduction of labyrinthine output that central compensatory mechanisms usually prevent or minimize the vertigo; auditory symptoms of hearing loss and tinnitus are the most common manifestations. While lesions of the brainstem or cerebellum can cause acute vertigo, associated signs and symptoms permit distinction from a labyrinthine etiology (Table 14-1). Rarely, an acute lesion of the vestibulocerebellum may present with monosymptomatic vertigo indistinguishable from a labyrinthopathy.

Recurrent unilateral labyrinthine dysfunction, in association with signs and symptoms of cochlear disease (progressive hearing loss and tinnitus), is usually due to Ménière's disease. When auditory manifestations are absent, the term *vestibular neuronitis* denotes recurrent monosymptomatic vertigo. Transient ischemic attacks of the posterior cerebral circulation (vertebrobasilar insufficiency) almost never cause recurrent vertigo without concomitant motor, sensory, cranial nerve, or cerebellar signs.

Positional vertigo is precipitated by a recumbent head position, either to the right or to the left. Benign paroxysmal positional vertigo

TABLE 14-1 Differentiation of peripheral and central vertigo

Sign or symptom	Peripheral (labyrinth)	Central (brainstem or cerebellum)
Direction of associated nystagmus	Unidirectional; fast phase opposite lesion*	Bidirectional or unidirectional
Purely horizontal nystagmus without torsional component	Uncommon	Common
Vertical or purely torsional nystagmus	Never present	May be present
Visual fixation	Inhibits nystagmus and vertigo	No inhibition
Severity of vertigo	Marked	Often mild
Direction of spin	Toward fast phase	Variable
Direction of fall	Toward slow phase	Variable
Duration of symptoms	Finite (minutes, days, weeks) but recurrent	May be chronic
Tinnitus and/or deafness	Often present	Usually absent
Associated central abnormalities	None	Extremely common
Common causes	Infection (labyrinthitis), Ménière's, neuronitis, ischemia, trauma, toxin	Vascular or demyelinating disease, neoplasm, trauma

* *In Ménière's disease, the fast phase is variable in direction.*

(BPPV) is particularly common. Although the condition may be due to head trauma, usually no precipitating factors are identified. It generally abates spontaneously after weeks or months. The vertigo and accompanying nystagmus have a distinct pattern of latency, fatigability, and habituation that differs from the less common central positional vertigo (Table 14-2) due to lesions in and around the fourth ventricle.

Position*al* must be distinguished from position*ing* vertigo. The latter is provoked by head movement rather than head position and is an invariable feature of *all* vestibulopathies, central or peripheral. Since vertigo increases with quick head movements, patients tend to hold their heads still.

Vestibular epilepsy, vertigo secondary to temporal lobe epileptic activity, is rare, and almost always intermixed with other epileptic manifestations.

Psychogenic vertigo, usually a concomitant of agoraphobia (fear of large open spaces, crowds, or leaving the safety of home), should be suspected in patients so ''incapacitated'' by their symptoms that they adopt a prolonged housebound status. Despite their discomfort, most patients with organic vertigo attempt to function. Vertigo should be accompanied by nystagmus; a psychogenic etiology is almost certain when nystagmus is absent during a vertiginous episode.

EVALUATION OF PATIENTS WITH PATHOLOGIC VESTIBULAR VERTIGO The evaluation depends upon whether a central etiology is suspected (Table 14-1). If so, computerized tomography, with emphasis upon the posterior fossa, is mandatory. Such an examination is rarely helpful in cases of recurrent monosymptomatic vertigo with a normal neurologic examination. BPPV requires no investigation after the diagnosis is made (Table 14-2).

Vestibular function tests serve to (1) demonstrate an abnormality when the distinction between organic and psychogenic is uncertain, (2) establish the side of the abnormality, and (3) distinguish between peripheral and central etiologies. The standard test is electronystagmography (ENG) where warm and cold water (or air) is applied, in a prescribed fashion, to the tympanic membranes, and the slow phase velocities of the resultant nystagmus from the right and left ears are compared. A velocity decrease from one side indicates hypofunction (''canal paresis''). An inability to induce nystagmus with ice water denotes a ''dead labyrinth.'' Some institutions have the capability of quantitatively determining various aspects of the vestibuloocular reflex using computer-driven rotational chairs and precise oculographic recording of eye movements.

Treatment of acute vertigo consists of bed rest and vestibular suppressant drugs such as antihistaminics (meclizine, dimenhydrinate, promethazine), centrally acting anticholinergics (scopolamine) or a tranquilizer with GABA-ergic effects (diazepam). If the vertigo persists beyond a few days, most authorities advise ambulation in an attempt to induce central compensatory mechanisms, despite the short-term discomfiture to the patient. Chronic vertigo of labyrinthine origin may be treated with a systematized exercise program to facilitate compensation.

Prophylactic measures to prevent recurrent vertigo are variably effective. Antihistamines are commonly utilized. Ménière's disease may respond to a low-salt diet combined with a diuretic. The unusual examples of persisting (beyond 4 to 6 weeks) BPPV respond dramatically, usually within 7 to 10 days, to a specific exercise program.

There are a variety of surgical procedures for all forms of refractory chronic or recurrent vertigo, but these are only rarely necessary.

MISCELLANEOUS HEAD SENSATIONS This designation is used, primarily for purposes of initial classification, to describe dizziness which is neither faintness nor vertigo. However, cephalic ischemia or vestibular dysfunction may be of such low intensity that the usual symptomology is not clearly identified. For example, a small decrease in blood pressure or a slight vestibular imbalance may cause sensations different than distinct faintness or vertigo but which may be identified properly during provocative testing techniques. Other causes of dizziness in this category are hyperventilation syndrome, hypoglycemia, and the somatic symptoms of a clinical depression. All these patients should have normal neurologic examinations.

GAIT DISTURBANCES Some individuals with gait disorders complain of dizziness despite the absence of vertigo or other abnormal cephalic sensations. The causes include peripheral neuropathy, myelopathy, spasticity, parkinsonian rigidity, and cerebellar ataxia. In this context, the term dizziness is being used to describe disturbed mobility. There may be associated lightheadedness, particularly with impaired sensation from the feet or poor vision; this is known as *multiple sensory defect dizziness* and occurs in elderly individuals who complain of dizziness only during ambulation. Decreased position sense (secondary to neuropathy or myelopathy) and poor vision (from cataracts or retinal degeneration) create an overreliance on the aging vestibular apparatus. A less precise, but sometimes comforting, designation is *benign dysequilibrium of aging*.

EVALUATION OF THE DIZZY PATIENT The most important diagnostic tool is a careful history focused upon the meaning of ''dizziness'' to the patient. Is it faintness? Is there a sensation of spinning? If either of these is affirmed, and the neurologic examination is normal, appropriate investigations for the multiple etiologies of cephalic ischemia or vestibular dysfunction are undertaken.

When the source of the dizziness is uncertain, provocative tests may be helpful. These office procedures simulate either cephalic ischemia or vestibular dysfunction. The former becomes obvious if the dizziness is duplicated during orthostatic hypotension. Further

TABLE 14-2 Benign paroxysmal positional (BPPV) and central positional vertigo

Features	BPPV	Central
Latency*	3–40 s	None: immediate vertigo and nystagmus
Fatigability†	Yes	No
Habituation‡	Yes	No
Intensity of vertigo	Severe	Mild
Reproducibility§	Variable	Good

* *Time between attaining head position and onset of symptoms.*
† *Disappearance of symptoms with maintenance of offending position.*
‡ *Lessening of symptoms with repeated trials.*
§ *Likelihood of symptom production during any examination session.*

provocation involves the Valsalva maneuver, which decreases cerebral blood flow and should reproduce ischemic symptoms.

The simplest provocative test for vestibular dysfunction is rapid rotation and abrupt cessation of movement in a swivel chair. This always induces vertigo which the patient can compare to his or her symptomatic dizziness. The intense induced vertigo may be unlike the spontaneous symptoms but shortly thereafter, when the vertigo has all but subsided, a lightheadedness supervenes which may be identified as "my dizziness." When this occurs, the dizzy patient, originally classified as suffering from "miscellaneous head sensations," is now properly diagnosed as having mild vertigo secondary to a vestibulopathy.

Another technique for provoking vertigo is with caloric testing. A tympanic membrane is irrigated with cold water until vertigo is induced; the sensation is then compared to the patient's complaint. Since visual fixation inhibits the caloric response, provocative caloric testing (as distinct from the diagnostic quantitative calorics of ENG) is best performed with the eyes closed or using special spectacles which preclude visual fixation (Frenzel lenses). Patients with symptoms of positional vertigo should be appropriately tested (Table 14-2); as with provocative calorics, positional testing is more sensitive when visual fixation is eliminated.

A final provocative test, requiring the use of Frenzel lenses, is vigorous head shaking in the horizontal plane for about 10 s. If nystagmus develops after the shaking stops, even in the absence of vertigo, vestibular dysfunction is demonstrated. The maneuver can then be repeated in the vertical plane. If the provocative tests establish the dizziness as a vestibular symptom, the previously described evaluation of vestibular vertigo is undertaken.

Hyperventilation is the cause of dizziness in many anxious individuals; tingling of the hands and face may be absent. Two minutes of forced hyperventilation is indicated for patients with enigmatic dizziness and normal neurologic examinations. Similarly, depressive symptoms (which patients usually insist are "secondary" to the dizziness) must alert the examiner to a clinical depression as the *cause*, rather than the effect, of the dizziness.

Central nervous system disease can produce dizzy sensations of all types. Consequently, a neurologic examination is always required even if the history or provocative tests suggest a cardiac, peripheral vestibular, or psychogenic etiology. Any abnormality on the neurologic examination should prompt appropriate neurodiagnostic studies.

REFERENCES

BALOH RW: *Dizziness, Hearing Loss, and Tinnitus: The Essentials of Neurotology*. Philadelphia, Davis, 1984

BRANDT T, DAROFF RB: The multisensory physiological and pathological vertigo syndromes. Ann Neurol 7:195, 1980

HINCHCLIFFE FR: *Hearing and Balance in the Elderly*. New York, Churchill Livingston, 1983, section II, pp 227–488

LEIGH RJ, ZEE DS: *The Neurology of Eye Movements*. Philadelphia, Davis, 1984, Chaps 2 and 9

OOSTERVELD WJ: Vertigo—Current concepts in management. Drugs 30:275, 1985

15 PARALYSIS AND OTHER DISORDERS OF MOVEMENT

JOHN H. GROWDON / ROBERT R. YOUNG

Impairments of motor function may be subdivided into (1) paralysis due to disorders of bulbar or spinal motor neurons, (2) paralysis due to lesions of corticospinal, corticobulbar, or brainstem descending (subcorticospinal) neurons, (3) abnormalities of coordination (ataxia) due to lesions in the cerebellar system, including its inputs and outputs, (4) abnormalities of movement and posture due to disease of the extrapyramidal motor system, and (5) apraxic or nonparalytic disturbances of purposive movement due to involvement of the cerebrum. This chapter reviews those symptoms and signs which result from lesions of lower motor neurons, descending corticospinal and other tracts, and the extrapyramidal system. It also includes consideration of apraxic disorders. The cerebellar system is discussed in Chap. 16.

THE MOTOR SYSTEM

DEFINITIONS When applied to voluntary muscles, *paralysis* means loss of contraction due to interruption of one or more motor pathways from the cerebrum to the muscle fiber. In everyday medical parlance motor paralysis usually stands for either partial or complete loss of function; it is preferable to use *paresis* for slight and *paralysis* or *plegia* for severe loss of motor function. In addition to weakness, lack of facility of movement is an important functional deficit.

PARALYSIS DUE TO DISEASE OF THE LOWER MOTOR NEURONS Each motor nerve cell, through the extensive arborization of the terminal part of its fiber, comes into contact with hundreds of muscle fibers; altogether they constitute "the motor unit." All variations in force and type of movement are determined by differences in the number and size of motor units called into activity, the frequency of their actions, and the patterns of activity in different muscles. Feeble movements recruit few units, stronger ones many more units of increasing size. Motor units involved in tonic contractions (type I) have muscle fibers rich in oxidative enzymes and mitochondria, and those involved in powerful, phasic contractions (type II) are anaerobic. When a motor neuron becomes diseased, as in progressive muscular atrophy, its axon may manifest increased irritability, and all the muscle fibers that it controls may discharge sporadically, in isolation from other units. The result of the contraction of one or several such units is a visible twitch, or *fasciculation,* which can be recorded in the electromyogram (EMG). If the motor neuron or its axon is destroyed, all the muscle fibers to which it is attached undergo a profound denervation atrophy. Individual denervated muscle fibers begin to be hypersensitive and to contract spontaneously, though they can no longer do so in response to a nerve impulse. Isolated activity of individual muscle fibers is called *fibrillation;* it is so fine that it cannot be seen through the intact skin and can be recorded only as a short-duration spike potential in the EMG. Motor nerve fibers of each anterior root intermingle with those from adjacent roots and join to form plexuses. Although the innervation of muscles is roughly according to segments of the spinal cord, each large muscle is supplied by two or more roots. In contrast, a single peripheral nerve usually provides the complete motor innervation of a muscle or group of muscles. For this reason the distribution of paralysis due to disease of the anterior horn cells or anterior roots differs from that which follows a lesion of a peripheral nerve.

Lower motor neuron paralysis is the direct result of physiologic block or destruction of anterior horn cells or their axons in anterior roots and nerves. The signs and symptoms vary according to the location of the lesion. Probably the most important question for clinical purposes is whether sensory changes coexist. The combination of flaccid, areflexic paralysis and sensory loss usually indicates involvement of mixed motor and sensory nerves or affection of both anterior and posterior roots. If sensory changes are absent, the lesion must be situated in the gray matter of the spinal cord, in the anterior roots, in a purely motor branch of a peripheral nerve, or in motor axons alone. The distinction between nuclear (spinal) and anterior root (radicular) lesions may at times be impossible to make.

All motor activity, even of the most elementary reflex type, requires the cooperation of several muscles. Analysis of a relatively simple movement, such as clenching the fist, affords some idea of the complexity of the underlying neural arrangements. In this act the primary movement is a contraction of the flexor muscles of the fingers, the flexor digitorum sublimis and profundus, the flexor pollicis longus and brevis, and the adductor pollicis brevis. These muscles act as *agonists,* or *prime movers,* in this act. In order for flexion to be smooth and forceful, finger extensor muscles (antagonists) must relax at the same rate at which the flexors contract. The muscles which flex the fingers also tend to flex the wrist; and since that weakens the grip, muscles which extend the wrist must be brought into play to prevent its flexion. The action of the wrist extensors is *synergic,* and these muscles are called synergists in this particular act. The elbow and shoulder must be stabilized by appropriate flexor and extensor muscles, which serve as *fixators.* The coordination of agonists, antagonists, synergists, and fixators involves reciprocal innervation and is managed entirely by segmental spinal mechanisms with guidance from proprioceptive input. Only the agonist movement in a voluntary act is believed to be initiated at a cortical level.

In addition, there are many basic motor activities, such as the maintenance of certain postures and stepping movements where agonists and antagonists contract simultaneously (see Chap. 16). The alternating movements of spinal stepping represent an even more elaborate type of coordination. Also, in the support of the body in an upright posture, when the limb must be as rigid as a pillar, and in shivering, the agonists and antagonists must act together. In general, the more delicate the movement, the more precise the coordination between agonist and antagonist muscles.

If all or practically all peripheral motor nerves supplying a muscle are destroyed, voluntary, postural, and reflex movements are abolished. The muscle becomes soft and yields excessively to passive stretching, a condition known as *flaccidity.* Muscle tone—the slight resistance that normal relaxed muscle offers to passive movement—is reduced (*hypotonia* or *atonia*). The denervated muscles undergo extreme atrophy, usually being reduced to 20 to 30 percent of their original bulk within 4 months. The reflex reaction of the muscle to sudden stretch, as by tapping its tendon, is lost. If only a few motor units in the muscles are affected, partial paralysis will ensue. With partial denervation, EMG evidence of fibrillations may also be obtained.

Muscle tone and tendon reflexes are known to depend on muscle spindles and the afferent fibers to which they give origin. A tap on a tendon, by stimulating muscle spindles, activates afferent neurons which transmit impulses to alpha motor neurons. The result is the familiar brief muscle contraction or tendon reflex.

PARALYSIS DUE TO DISEASE OF CORTICOSPINAL, CORTICOBULBAR, AND SUBCORTICOSPINAL NEURONS The corticospinal tract at the level of the medulla contains approximately 1 million axons. Many fibers arise not only from the giant Betz cells of the motor cortex (area 4 of Brodmann) but also from the smaller Betz cells of area 4, cells of the adjacent precentral cortex (area 6), and those of the secondary motor cortex in the superior frontal convolution and postcentral cortex (areas 1, 2, 3, 5, 7). The corticospinal tract is the only direct connection from the cerebrum to the spinal cord. At the level of the internal capsule these corticospinal fibers are intermingled with many others destined to end in the striatum, globus pallidus, substantia nigra, red nucleus, and reticular substance and with others ascending from the thalamus. Fibers to the cranial nerve nuclei become separated at about the level of the midbrain, where they cross the midline to the contralateral cranial nerve nuclei. These fibers form the corticomesencephalic, corticopontine, and corticobulbar tracts, and since they have functions similar to those of the corticospinal tract, they may be included in the pyramidal system of motor neurons. The decussation of the corticospinal tract at the lower end of the medulla is variable. Most of the crossing fibers come to occupy a position in the posterolateral part of the lateral funiculus; a few cross to form an anterior fasciculus. A small number of fibers, 10 to 20 percent, do not cross but descend ipsilaterally as the uncrossed corticospinal tract. Exceptionally, all of them cross; rarely, none. The termination of the corticospinal tract is predominantly upon interneurons in the intermediate zone of spinal gray matter, and not more than 25 percent establish direct synaptic connection with anterior horn cells (Fig. 15-1).

The motor area of the cerebral cortex includes that part of the precentral convolution which contains Betz cells (area 4), but it also extends anteriorly into area 6 and the secondary motor area of the superior frontal convolution and posteriorly into the anterior parietal lobe, where it overlaps the sensory areas. Physiologically it is defined as the region of electrically excitable cortex from which isolated movements can be evoked by stimuli of minimal intensity. The muscle groups of the contralateral face, arm, trunk, and leg are represented in the motor cortex, those of the face being at the lower end of the precentral convolution and those of the leg in the paracentral lobule on the medial surface of the cerebral hemisphere. The parts of the body capable of the most delicate movements have, in general, the largest cortical representation. One of the functions of the motor cortex is to synthesize simple movements into an infinite variety of finely graded, highly differentiated patterns.

Corticospinal paralysis may be due to lesions in the cerebral cortex, subcortical white matter, internal capsule, brainstem, or spinal cord. Almost always much more is involved than the corticospinal,

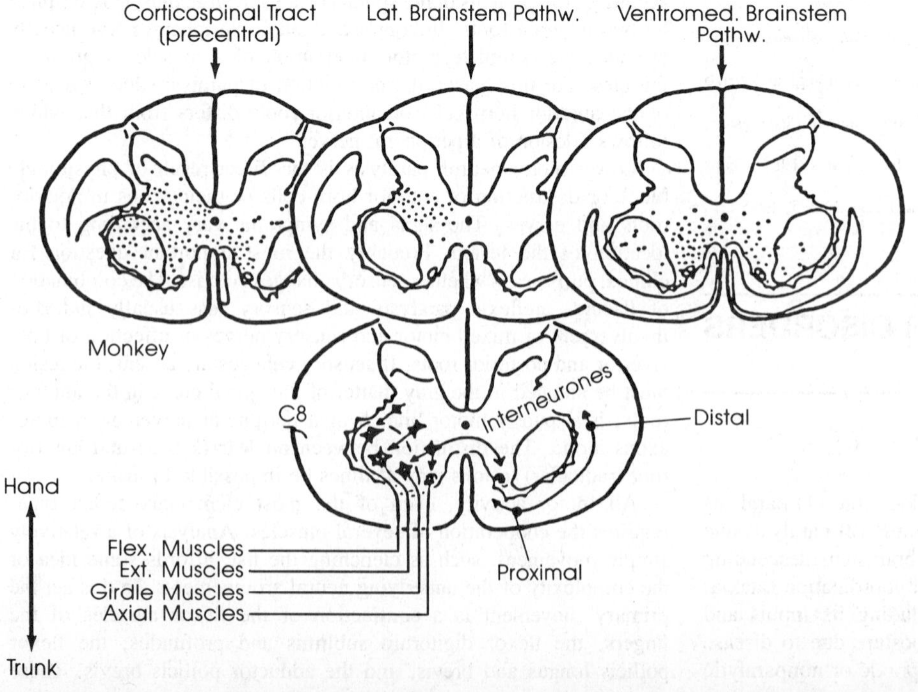

FIGURE 15-1 *The distribution of terminations of cortical and brainstem descending pathways (dots) in the spinal intermediate zone and motor neuronal cell groups in rhesus monkey. Note that lateral brainstem pathways (arising from the magnocellular red nucleus and the ventrolateral pontine tegmentum) end on interneurons concerned principally with hand muscles. Ventromedial brainstem pathways (from the superior colliculus, interstitial nucleus of Cajal, pontine, medullary and mesencephalic medial reticular formation, and vestibular nuclei) end on interneurons concerned with trunkal and limb girdle muscles. [From HGJM Kuypers, in JE Desmedt (ed). New Developments in Electromyography and Clinical Neurophysiology, Basel, Karger, 1973, vol. 3.]*

or pyramidal, tract. The effects of a pure lesion of the corticospinal system are considerably less than are typically seen with a hemiplegia due to a vascular lesion or other cause. Where only the pyramid of the medulla is destroyed on one side, there is a remarkable degree of recovery of motor function in the contralateral arm and leg, leaving only slight spasticity, an increase in phasic myotatic or tendon reflexes, and an inverted plantar reflex (Babinski's sign). This recovery may be due to preservation of a few fibers in the pyramid or to preservation of lateral brainstem pathways, but the more important idea revealed by such cases is that complete spastic hemiplegias in humans involve interruption not only of the corticospinal tract but of other descending fibers from the cerebral cortex (corticorubral, corticostriatal, corticopallidal, corticopontine, and corticoreticular) and from the brainstem (reticulospinal, vestibulospinal, and rubrospinal). The influence of these nonpyramidal fibers not only is reflected in the degree of paralysis but also in the status of the disconnected segmental motor neurons subserving reflex, postural, and locomotory functions. It is therefore unwise to refer to spastic hemiplegia as "the pyramidal syndrome." Hemiplegic dystonia (see below) involves some dysfunction of ventromedial brainstem pathways (Fig. 15-1).

With corticospinal lesions in humans the distribution of the paralysis varies with the locale of the lesion, but there are certain common features. Paralysis due to a lesion of these upper motor neurons always involves a group of muscles, never individual muscles. Concerning whatever volitional movement remains, the maximum effort is attained more slowly than in the normal limb, fewer motor units are recruited, and the frequency of their discharge is reduced. The paralysis never involves all the muscles on one side of the body, even with a complete hemiplegia. Movements that are invariably bilateral, such as those of the eyes, jaw, pharynx, larynx, neck, thorax, and abdomen, are little if at all affected. The hand and arm muscles suffer most severely, the leg muscles next, and of the cranial musculature only the muscles of the lower part of the face and tongue are involved to any significant degree. The cortical control of all movements is to some extent bilateral. Examples that prove this are hemiplegias that worsen when the contralateral motor system is interrupted by disease. Corticospinal motor paralysis is rarely complete for any long period of time; in this respect it differs from the total and absolute paralysis due to a complete destruction or interruption of anterior horn cells and their axons. The paralyzed arm may suddenly move during yawning and stretching, and various spinal reflexes can be elicited at all times.

Acute lesions of the corticospinal and subcorticospinal motor systems, at lower levels, such as the cervical cord, may not only cause a paralysis of voluntary movement but may also abolish temporarily the spinal reflexes subserved by segments below the lesion. This condition is known as *spinal shock*. After a few days to weeks the shock disappears if the patient is otherwise healthy and gives way to a phenomenon known as *spasticity*. The latter is a feature of all lesions of the motor system at cerebral, capsular, midbrain, and pontine levels. In cerebral and brainstem lesions it does not usually appear immediately, and in exceptional cases the paralyzed limbs remain flaccid but with lively reflexes. Spasticity is related to the excessive activity of the released or disinhibited spinal motor neurons. It is defined as a motor disorder characterized by a velocity-dependent increase in tonic stretch reflexes ("muscle tone") with exaggerated tendon jerks, resulting from hyperexcitability of the stretch reflex; it is one component of the "upper motor neuron" syndrome. The postures of the arm and leg inform us that certain spinal neurons are more active than others. With supraspinal lesions, the arm is maintained in a pronated, flexed position and the leg in an adducted, extended position. Any attempts to extend the arm or flex the leg passively will encounter, after a brief free interval, a resistance which increases and then may yield (clasp-knife phenomenon). When the limb is left in the new position, the resistance reappears (lengthening and shortening reactions). Actually the clasp-knife type of spasticity is infrequent. It is more usual for combined lesions of corticospinal and other suprasegmental tracts to produce a sustained resistance to movement. The nocifensive spinal flexion reflexes, of which Babinski's sign is a part, are also released and the cutaneomuscular abdominal and cremasteric reflexes abolished. With cerebral lesions exaggerated stretch and cutaneous reflexes can also be elicited in cranial as well as limb and trunk muscles, and when the corticospinal disorder is bilateral, there is pseudobulbar paralysis (dysarthria, dysphonia, and dysphagia with bifacial paralysis) accompanied commonly by "emotional lability." Prolonged flexor and extensor spasms occur with lesions of the spinal cord; they are due to a release of cutaneous reflexes. Retention of reflexes and spasticity in muscles weakened by a spinal lesion point to a lesion of the descending motor tracts and integrity of the segments below the level of the lesion.

Spasticity may be present when the limbs are not paralyzed but only paretic, and it is then associated with interesting abnormalities of voluntary movements. In general, all attempts by the patient to move the hemiparetic extremities appear to be hampered. Discrete movements of individual fingers and finely coordinated movements of the hand are lost. Proximal muscles are under better voluntary control. Synergies of movements eventually appear. For example, in the upper extremity a flexion synergy consisting of finger flexion, wrist flexion and pronation, elbow flexion, and shoulder elevation and abduction is produced in a slow, massive, stereotyped fashion upon attempted grasp of an object. Attempts to push with the hand result in a weaker pronation of the hand, extension or flexion of the fingers, extension of the wrist and elbow, adduction of the upper arm, and lowering of the shoulder. In the lower extremity the extensor synergy (thigh adduction, thigh and knee extension, and plantar flexion of the toes and foot) is more powerful than the flexor synergy of hip abduction, hip and knee flexion, and dorsiflexion and inversion of toes and foot. The latter part of this flexion synergy is called Strumpell's tibialis sign, which appears during attempts to elevate a paretic leg. A bias toward extensor synergy facilitates weight-bearing and walking, which are eventually achieved by nearly all hemiplegic patients. These synergies indicate that there is not only a diminution in voluntary anterior horn cell activation (the negative effect of a motor lesion), but excessive reflex and synergistic discharges in the same motor neuron pools (positive effects of the lesion). Strong-willed effort to move the paretic limb may also evoke symmetric associated (mirror) movements in the normal limb.

The neurotransmitters for excitation and inhibition of spinal motor neurons by the corticospinal, rubrospinal, vestibulospinal, and reticulospinal tracts, or by peripheral sensory afferents, have not been fully elucidated. At least five neurotransmitters—acetylcholine (ACh), noradrenaline, serotonin, glycine, and γ-aminobutyric acid (GABA) have been identified. Some, such as ACh, are excitatory; others, like glycine and GABA, are inhibitory. But their precise localizations have not been established. Even in spasticity, where the neurons responsible for excitation of the extensor muscles of the leg and flexors of the arm are overactive, it is not known whether there is a functional excess of excitatory neurotransmitters or a deficiency of inhibitory transmitter *or both*. Current evidence indicates that drugs that decrease spasticity act at the spinal cord level to alter neurotransmitter function. Baclofen interferes with release of excitatory neurotransmitters and diazepam facilitates GABA-mediated presynaptic inhibition.

Table 15-1 shows the main differences between corticospinal and lower motor neuron syndromes.

APRAXIC OR NONPARALYTIC DISORDERS OF MOTOR FUNCTION Aside from upper and lower motor neuron paralysis with cerebral lesions, there may be loss of learned movement that can simulate paresis of a limb. This is called *apraxia;* it can be defined as a disorder of learned movement that is not due to weakness, incoordination, sensory loss, or failure to comprehend commands. Actions acquired by learning or practice depend on the formation of movement patterns, particularly gestures and those actions which involve the use of tools and instruments. Once established, they are

TABLE 15-1 Differences between paralysis due to lesions of upper versus lower motor neurons

Upper motor neuron paralysis	Lower motor neuron paralysis
Muscle groups affected diffusely, never individual muscles	Individual muscles may be affected
Atrophy slight	Atrophy pronounced, 70 to 80 percent of total bulk
Spasticity with hyperactivity of the tendon reflexes	Flaccidity and hypotonia of affected muscles with loss of tendon reflexes
Extensor plantar reflex, Babinski's sign	Plantar reflex, if present, is of normal flexor type
Fascicular twitches not produced	Fasciculations may be present
	Electromyogram reveals reduced numbers of motor units and fibrillations

remembered and may be reproduced under the proper circumstances. Any purposive act of these types may be conceived as occurring in several stages. The idea of an act must be aroused in the mind of the subject by an appropriate stimulus situation, perhaps by a spoken command to do something. In right-handed and most left-handed persons the neural mechanisms for the comprehension and formulation of an idea of an act (motor schema or image) in response to a spoken command or a verbal stimulus and its reproduction are located posteriorly at the junction of the left parietal and temporal lobes; this region (Wernicke's area) is connected with the left premotor regions for the control of the right hand and thence through the corpus callosum with the motor areas of the right cerebral hemisphere for the control of the left side. Disconnection of Wernicke's area from motor areas of the right hemisphere (most commonly by lesions of the midcorpus callosum) results in *apraxia* of left limbs when tested by response to verbal commands.

A failure to execute certain acts in the correct context while retaining the ability to carry out the individual movements upon which such acts depend is the main feature of apraxia. The most adequate clinical test of motor deficits of this type is to observe a series of self-initiated actions such as using a comb, a razor, a toothbrush, or a common tool, or gesturing, e.g., waving goodbye, saluting, shaking the fist as though angry, or blowing a kiss. These actions can be normally elicited by a command or a request to imitate the examiner. Of course, failure to follow a spoken or written request may be due to an aphasia that prevents understanding of what is asked, or an agnosia may prevent recognition of the tool or object to be used. But when these difficulties are excluded, there remains a peculiar motor deficit in which the patient appears to understand but has lost the memory of how to perform a given act, especially if it is called for in an unnatural setting. The patient may have the idea of what to do but cannot translate the idea of the sequence of movements into a precise, well-executed act. This apraxic deficit may be evident both after a spoken command and in requests to imitate the gestures of the examiner. Sometimes these two conditions may be dissociated; the patient, while not aphasic, cannot execute a spoken command but can still imitate the act if it is called forth by gesture. Also, if merely given the tool, the patient may use it properly in an automatic fashion.

DIFFERENTIAL DIAGNOSIS OF PARALYSIS The diagnostic consideration of paralysis may be simplified by the following subdivisions, which relate to the location and distribution of weakness.

Monoplegia The examination of patients who complain of weakness of one extremity often discloses an unnoticed weakness in another limb, and the condition is actually hemiplegia or paraplegia. Or instead of weakness of all the muscles in a limb, only isolated groups are found to be affected. Ataxia, sensory disturbances, or pain in an extremity will often be interpreted by the patient as weakness, as will the mechanical limitation resulting from arthritis or the rigidity of parkinsonism.

In general, the presence or absence of atrophy of muscles in a monoplegic limb can be of diagnostic help.

PARALYSIS WITH LITTLE OR NO ATROPHY Long-continued disuse of a limb may lead to atrophy, but this is usually not so marked as in diseases that denervate muscles; the tendon reflexes are normal, and the response of the muscles to electric stimulation and on EMG are unaltered.

The most frequent cause of monoplegia without muscular wasting is a lesion of the cerebral cortex. Rarely does it occur in diseases which interrupt the corticospinal tract at the level of the internal capsule, brainstem, or spinal cord because fibers to arm and leg are very close together there. A cortical vascular lesion (thrombosis or embolus) is the commonest cause, but a discrete traumatic lesion, tumor, or abscess may have the same effect. Multiple sclerosis and spinal cord tumor, early in their course, may cause weakness of one extremity, usually the leg. Weakness due to damage to the corticospinal and subcorticospinal system is usually accompanied by spasticity, increased reflexes, and an extensor plantar reflex (Babinski's sign). However, acute diseases that destroy the motor tracts in the spinal cord may at first (for several days) reduce the tendon reflexes and cause hypotonia (*spinal shock*). This does not occur in partial or slowly evolving lesions and occurs only to minimal degree, if at all, in lesions of brainstem and cerebrum. In acute diseases affecting the lower motor neurons the tendon reflexes are always reduced or abolished, but atrophy may not appear for several weeks. Hence one must take into account the mode of onset and the duration of the disease in evaluating the tendon reflexes, muscle tone, and degree of atrophy before reaching an anatomic diagnosis.

PARALYSIS WITH MUSCULAR ATROPHY In addition to the paralysis, reduced or abolished tendon reflexes, and decreased tone, there may be visible fasciculations. The EMG shows reduced numbers of motor units (often of large size), fasciculations at rest, and fibrillations. The lesion may be in the spinal cord, spinal roots, or peripheral nerves. Its location can usually be decided by the distribution of the palsied muscles (whether the pattern is one of nerve, spinal root, or spinal cord involvement), by the associated neurologic symptoms and signs, and by special tests (cerebrospinal fluid examination, CT or magnetic resonance imaging (MRI) scans of the spine, and myelogram).

Brachial atrophic monoplegia (affecting the arm) is relatively rare, and when present, it should suggest in an infant brachial plexus trauma, in a child poliomyelitis, in an adult poliomyelitis, syringomyelia, amyotrophic lateral sclerosis, or other brachial plexus lesions. Crural monoplegia (affecting the leg) is more frequent and may be caused by any lesion of thoracic or lumbar cord, i.e., trauma, tumor, myelitis, multiple sclerosis, etc. Multiple sclerosis almost never causes atrophy, and ruptured intervertebral disk and the many varieties of neuritis rarely paralyze all or most of the muscles of a limb. Muscle dystrophy may begin in one limb, but by the time the patient is seen the typical more or less symmetric pattern of proximal limb and trunk involvement is evident. A unilateral retroperitoneal tumor may paralyze the leg by implicating the lumbosacral plexus.

Hemiplegia Loss of strength in the arm, leg, and sometimes face on one side of the body is the most frequent distribution of paralysis in humans. With rare exceptions (a few unusual cases of poliomyelitis or motor system disease) this pattern of paralysis is due to involvement of the descending motor tracts.

LOCATION OF LESION-PRODUCING HEMIPLEGIA The site or level of the lesion can usually be deduced from the associated neurologic findings. Diseases localized in the cerebral cortex, cerebral white matter (corona radiata), and internal capsule usually evoke weakness or paralysis of the face, arm, and leg on the opposite side. The occurrence of convulsive seizures or the presence of a defect in speech (aphasia), a cortical type of sensory loss (astereognosis, loss of two-point discrimination, etc.), anosognosia, or defects in the visual fields suggest a cortical or subcortical location. A pure, isolated hemiplegia affecting simultaneously the face, arm, and leg indicates a lesion in the posterior limb of the internal capsule, often a vascular lacune.

Damage to the corticospinal and corticobulbar tracts in the upper portion of the brainstem will cause paralysis of the face, arm, and leg on the opposite side. The lesion in such cases is localized by the presence of a paralysis of the muscles supplied by the oculomotor nerve on the same side as the lesion (Weber's syndrome) or other neurologic findings. With low pontine lesions an ipsilateral abducens or facial palsy is combined with a contralateral weakness or paralysis of the arm and leg (Millard-Gubler syndrome). Lesions of the lowermost part of the brainstem, i.e., in the medulla, affect the tongue and sometimes the pharynx and larynx on one side and arm and leg on the other side. These "crossed paralyses," so common in brainstem diseases, are described in Chap. 343. Ataxic hemiplegia with or without dysarthria also indicates a lesion in the contralateral basis pons.

Rarely, a homolateral hemiplegia (sparing cranial muscles) may be caused by a lesion in the lateral column of the cervical spinal cord. At this level, however, the pathologic process often induces bilateral signs, with resulting quadriparesis or quadriplegia. Homolateral paralysis, if combined with a loss of vibratory and position sense on the same side and a contralateral loss of pain and temperature (Brown-Séquard syndrome), signifies unilateral disease of the spinal cord (Chap. 353).

Muscle atrophy of minor degree often is associated with a hemiplegia but never reaches the proportions seen in diseases of the lower motor neurons. The former atrophy is largely due to disuse. When the motor cortex and adjacent parts of the parietal lobe are damaged in infancy or childhood, the normal development of the muscles and the skeletal system in the affected limbs is retarded. The palsied limbs and even the trunk on one side are small. This does not occur if the paralysis begins after the greater part of skeletal growth is attained (after puberty). In the hemiplegia due to spinal cord injury, muscles at the level of the lesion may undergo atrophy if there is associated damage to anterior horn cells or ventral roots.

CAUSES OF HEMIPLEGIA Vascular diseases of the cerebrum and brainstem exceed all others as causes of hemiplegia. Trauma (brain contusion, epidural and subdural hemorrhage) ranks second, and other diseases such as brain tumor, brain abscess and encephalitis, demyelinative diseases, and complications of meningitis, tuberculosis, and syphilis are less important.

Paraplegia Paralysis of both lower extremities may occur in diseases of the spinal cord and the spinal roots or of the peripheral nerves. Parasagittal tumors and hydrocephalus can, on occasion, cause leg weakness. If the onset is acute, it may be difficult to distinguish spinal from neural paralysis, for in any acute myelopathy spinal shock may result in abolition of reflexes and flaccidity. As a rule, in acute spinal cord diseases the paralysis affects all muscles below a given level; often, if the white matter is extensively damaged, sensory loss below a particular level (loss of pain and temperature sense—lateral spinothalamic tracts and loss of vibratory and position sense—posterior columns) is conjoined. Also, in bilateral disease of the spinal cord the bladder and bowel sphincters are paralyzed. Alterations of cerebrospinal fluid (dynamic block, increase in protein or cells) are frequent. In peripheral nerve diseases both sensory loss and motor loss tend to involve the distal muscles of the legs more than the proximal ones (an exception is acute idiopathic polyneuritis), and the sphincters are spared or only briefly deranged in function. Sensory loss, if present, is more likely to consist of distal impairment of touch, vibration, and position sense, with pain and temperature sense spared in many instances. The cerebrospinal fluid protein level may be normal or elevated. Studies of nerve conduction through spinal roots (F waves) are always abnormal.

Acute paraplegia (except that due to trauma or metastatic tumor) is relatively infrequent. Rarely it may be due to a medial pontine lesion affecting the leg fibers which are near to the midline (as in pontine infarction or central pontine myelinolysis). Spontaneous hematomyelia with bleeding from a vascular malformation (angioma, telangiectasis), thrombosis of a spinal artery with infarction (myelomalacia), and dissecting aortic aneurysm or atherosclerotic occlusion of nutrient spinal arteries arising from the aorta with resulting infarction (myelomalacia) are the commonest varieties of sudden paraplegia (or quadriplegia, if the cervical cord is involved). Postinfectious or postvaccinial myelitis, acute demyelinative myelitis (Devic's disease if the optic nerves are affected), necrotizing myelitis, and epidural abscess or hemorrhage with spinal cord compression tend to develop somewhat more slowly, over a period of hours or days, but they may have an acute onset. Poliomyelitis, in those countries where immunization is incomplete, presents as a purely motor disorder with meningitis, and must be distinguished from the other acute myelopathies.

In adult life subacute or chronic paraplegia can occur in multiple sclerosis, subacute combined degeneration, spinal cord tumor, ruptured cervical disk and cervical spondylosis, syphilitic meningomyelitis, chronic epidural infections (fungus and other granulomatous diseases), motor system disease, familial spastic paraplegia, and syringomyelia. (See Chap. 353 for discussion of these spinal cord diseases.) The several varieties of polyneuritis and polymyositis must be considered in their differential diagnosis, for they, too, may cause paraparesis. Friedreich's ataxia and familial paraplegia, progressive muscular dystrophy, and the chronic varieties of polyneuritis tend to appear during late childhood and adolescence and are slowly progressive.

Paraplegia (or paraparesis) may be due to a lesion of the leg areas of the motor cortex. Arterial (anterior cerebral arteries) or venous (superior sagittal sinus and tributary cerebral veins) distribution cerebral infarction are causes of acute paraplegia; parasagittal meningioma is a cause of asymmetric chronic paraplegia. Usually other signs such as confusion, stupor, or seizures indicate the cerebral localization, and differential diagnosis is not a problem.

Quadriplegia All that has been written about the common causes of paraplegia applies to quadriplegia except that the lesion is in the cervical rather than the thoracic or lumbar segments of the spinal cord. If it is situated in the low cervical segments and involves the anterior half of the spinal cord, as in occlusion of the anterior spinal artery, the arm paralysis may be flaccid and areflexic and the leg paralysis spastic (anterior spinal syndrome). There are only a few points of difference between the common paraplegic and quadriplegic syndromes. Repeated cerebral vascular accidents may lead to bilateral hemiplegia, usually accompanied by pseudobulbar palsy.

Isolated paralysis Paralysis of isolated muscle groups usually indicates a lesion of one or more peripheral nerves. The diagnosis of a lesion of an individual peripheral nerve is based on the presence of weakness or paralysis of the muscle or group of muscles and impairment or loss of sensation in the distribution of the nerve in question (Chap. 355). Complete transection or severe injury to a peripheral nerve is usually followed by atrophy of the muscles it innervates and by loss of their tendon reflexes. Trophic changes in the skin, nails, and subcutaneous tissue may also occur. It is of considerable importance to decide whether the lesion is only a temporary one (conduction block), or whether there has been a dissolution of axonal continuity, requiring nerve regeneration for recovery. EMG is of value here.

EXAMINATION SCHEME FOR MOTOR PARALYSIS AND APRAXIA The first step is to inspect the paralyzed limb, taking note of its posture and of the presence or absence of muscle atrophy, hypertrophy, and fascicular twitchings. Slight atrophy may be due to disuse from any cause, i.e., pain, fixation as the result of a cast, or any type of paralysis. Pronounced atrophy usually occurs only with denervation of several weeks' or months' standing. The patient is then called upon to move each muscle group, and the power and facility of movement are graded and recorded. The range of passive movement is then determined by moving all the joints. This provides information concerning alterations of muscle tone, i.e., hypotonia, spasticity, and rigidity. Dislocations, diseased joints, and ankyloses may also be revealed by these same maneuvers. The tendon reflexes are then tested. The usual routine is to try to elicit the jaw jerk (increased in pseudobulbar palsy) and the supinator, biceps, triceps, quadriceps, and Achilles tendon reflexes. Two cutaneous reflexes are then tested, the abdominal and plantar reflexes.

If there is no evidence of upper or lower motor neuron disease, but certain acts are nonetheless imperfectly performed, one should look for a disorder of postural sensibility, cerebellar incoordination, or rigidity with abnormality of posture and movement due to disease of the basal ganglia. In the absence of these disorders, the possibility of an apraxic disorder may be investigated by watching the patient's own movements and those called forth by specific command and gesture.

Hysterical paralysis may pose problems. Usually it is easily distinguished from chronic lower motor neuron disease by absence of areflexia and severe atrophy. Diagnostic difficulty arises only in certain acute cases of upper motor neuron disease that lack all the usual changes in reflexes and muscle tone. In hysterical paralysis one arm or one leg or all one side of the body may be affected. The hysterical gait is sometimes diagnostic (Chap. 16). Often there is loss of all forms of sensation (touch, pain, smell, vision, and hearing) on the paralyzed side, a group of sensory changes that is never seen in organic brain disease. The patient should be asked to move the affected limbs; the movement is seen to be slow and jerky, often with contraction of both agonist and antagonist muscles simultaneously or intermittently. Hoover's sign and Babinski's combined leg flexion test are helpful in distinguishing hysterical from organic hemiplegia. To elicit Hoover's sign, the patient, lying on the back, is asked to raise one leg from the bed against resistance; in a normal individual the back of the heel of the contralateral leg presses firmly down, and the same is true when the patient with organic hemiplegia attempts to lift the paralyzed leg. The hysteric will press down the supposedly paralyzed leg more strongly under these circumstances than when asked to do so directly. To carry out Babinski's combined leg flexion test, a patient with an organic hemiplegia is asked to sit up without using the arms; in doing this, the paralyzed or weak leg flexes at the hip and the heel is lifted from the bed, while the heel of the sound leg is pressed into the bed. This sign is absent in hysterical hemiplegia.

THE BASAL GANGLIA

The basal ganglia subserve motor functions that are distinct from those attributed to the pyramidal (corticospinal) tract. The term *extrapyramidal* underscores this distinction and calls attention to a set of neurologic illnesses caused by lesions that affect the basal ganglia. Familiar examples include Parkinson's disease, Huntington's disease, and Wilson's disease. This section reviews the basal ganglia and describes the clinical symptoms and signs that arise from their dysfunction.

ANATOMIC CONNECTIONS AND NEURONAL TRANSMITTERS IN THE BASAL GANGLIA The basal ganglia are paired subcortical masses of gray matter that form anatomically distinct nuclear groups. The major nuclei are the caudate and the putamen (which together are called the striatum), the internal and external segments of the globus pallidus, the subthalamic nucleus, and the substantia nigra (Fig. 15-2). The striatum receives afferent inputs from many sources, including the cerebral cortex, thalamic nuclei, brainstem raphe nuclei, and the substantia nigra. Cortical neurons that project to the striatum release the excitatory amino acid glutamate. Neurons that project to the striatum from the raphe nuclei synthesize and release serotonin (5-HT). Neurons in the pars compacta of the substantia nigra synthesize and release dopamine (DA), which acts as an inhibitory neurotransmitter on striatal neurons. Transmitters released by thalamic projections are unknown. The striatum contains two distinct classes of cells: local circuit neurons, whose axons do not project beyond the confines of the nucleus, and other neurons whose axons project to the globus pallidus and substantia nigra. Local circuit neurons synthesize and release acetylcholine (ACh), gamma aminobutyric acid (GABA), and neuropeptides, including somatostatin and vasoactive intestinal polypeptide. Striatal neurons that inhibit the pars reticulata of the substantia nigra release GABA, whereas those that excite the nigra release substance P (Fig. 15-3). Transmitters released in the striatal projections to the globus pallidus include GABA, the enkephalins, and substance P.

Axons that originate in the internal segment of the globus pallidus form the main efferent projection from the basal ganglia. There is a massive projection around and through the internal capsule (the ansa and fasciculus lenticularis that pass through the fields of Forel) to the ventral anterior and ventral lateral thalamus as well as to intralaminar thalamic nuclei, including the centromedian nucleus. Chemical transmitters released by this pathway are unknown. Other efferent projections from the basal ganglia include direct dopaminergic connections from the substantia nigra to regions of limbic and frontal cerebral cortex; the pars reticulata of the substantia nigra also sends a projection to thalamic nuclei and to the superior colliculus.

Recent anatomic studies have clarified the cortical distribution of ascending thalamic fibers. Ventral thalamic neurons project to premotor and motor cerebral cortices; medial thalamic nuclei project primarily to prefrontal cortex. The supplementary motor cortex receives a prominent input from the basal ganglia, including a dopaminergic projection from the substantia nigra, whereas the

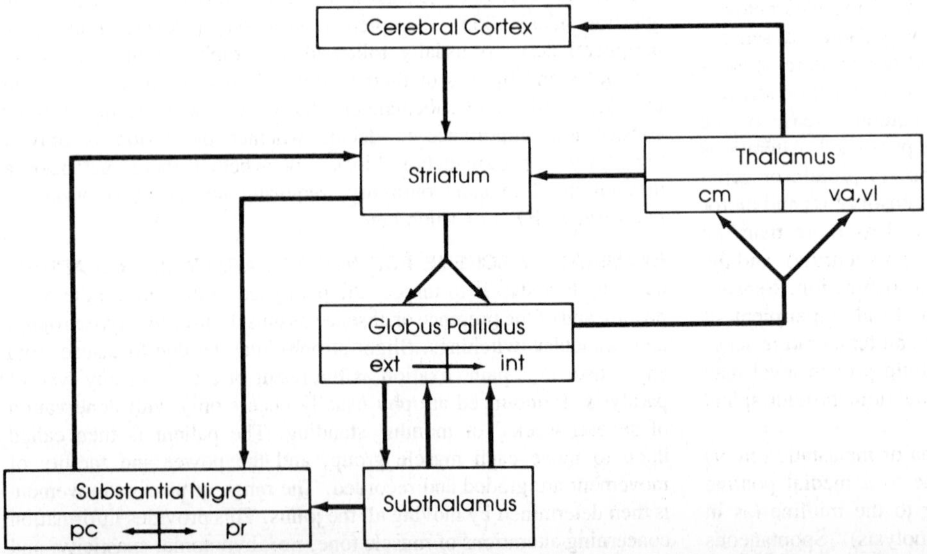

FIGURE 15-2 *Simplified schematic diagram of the major neuronal connections between the basal ganglia, thalamus, and cerebral cortex. The projection from the internal segment of the globus pallidus constitutes the principal efferent pathway from the basal ganglia. Abbreviations: ext = external, int = internal, pc = pars compacta, pr = pars reticulata, cm = centromedian, va = ventroanterior, vl = ventrolateral.*

primary motor and premotor cortex receives a major input from the cerebellum. Thus there are a series of parallel loops reciprocally linking specific basal ganglionic structures and cerebral cortical regions. Although the exact mechanism whereby these various inputs are translated into coordinated volitional acts remains uncertain, it is clear that most of the basal ganglionic and cerebellar influences on the motor system are funneled through this ventral plane of thalamic nuclei. The major cerebellar output, which exits from the cerebellum through the superior cerebellar peduncle, terminates with the pallidal-thalamic fibers in the ventroanterior and ventrolateral thalamic nuclei. This region of the thalamus forms an essential link in the ascending fiber systems from both the basal ganglia and the cerebellum to the motor cortex. Despite the apparently crucial nature of these structures, lesions placed stereotactically in the ventral thalamus can abolish essential-familial tremor or the rigidity and tremor in Parkinson's disease without producing functional deficits. Ascending thalamocortical fibers pass through the internal capsule and cerebral white matter, so lesions in these parts or in the cortex may simultaneously affect both corticospinal and extrapyramidal systems.

Axons from some cortical neurons form the internal capsule (the corticobulbar and corticospinal tracts); these and others also project to the striatum. This forms a complete loop—from cerebral cortex to striatum, to globus pallidus, to thalamus, to cerebral cortex. Axons that originate in the centromedian nucleus of the thalamus project back to the striatum, thus completing a subcortical loop from striatum to globus pallidus, to centromedian nucleus, to striatum. There is another subcortical loop between the striatum and the substantia nigra: Dopaminergic neurons in the pars compacta of substantia nigra project to the striatum, and separate striatal neurons that release GABA and substance P send projections to the pars reticulata of the substantia nigra. There are reciprocal connections between the pars reticulata and pars compacta of the substantia nigra; the pars reticulata sends projections to ventral thalamus, superior colliculus, and brainstem reticular formation structures as well. The subthalamic nucleus receives fibers from the neocortex and from the external segment of the globus pallidus; neurons within the subthalamic nucleus form reciprocal connections with the external segment of the globus pallidus and also send axons to the internal segment of the globus pallidus and pars reticulata of the substantia nigra. The neurochemicals involved in these pathways remain unknown, although GABA has been implicated.

PHYSIOLOGY OF THE BASAL GANGLIA Recordings from neurons in the globus pallidus and substantia nigra in awake, performing primates confirm the main motor function of the basal ganglia. Cells within these regions clearly participate in the initiation of movement, since they increase their firing rates before movement is observed clinically or detected by EMG. Discharges in the basal ganglia are related principally to contralateral rather than ipsilateral limb movements. Many neurons increase their firing rates during slow (ramp) movements, but some others discharge during more rapid (ballistic) movements. There is somatotopic localization of leg, arm, and face within the internal segment of the globus pallidus and pars reticulata of the substantia nigra. This observation provides a possible explanation for the occurrence of restricted dyskinesias: Focal dystonia and buccal-lingual-masticatory tardive dyskinesia may result from localized pallidal or nigral biochemical lesions that affect only regions with hand or face representation.

Although the basal ganglia are motor nuclei, it is not possible to identify a specific type of basal ganglia movement. Hypotheses about the function of the basal ganglia in human beings derive from correlations between clinical signs and sites of pathologic lesions in patients with extrapyramidal diseases. The basal ganglia are a constellation of nuclei centered around the globus pallidus, through which impulses are channeled to the thalamus and onward to the cerebral cortex (Fig. 15-2). Neurons in each satellite nucleus contribute excitatory and inhibitory impulses, and the sum of these influences on the main pathway from basal ganglia to thalamus and cerebral cortex, modified by the cerebellum, determine smooth motor function as expressed through the corticospinal and other descending cortical tracts. If one or more of the supporting nuclei is damaged, the sum of the impulses to the globus pallidus changes and disordered mobility can occur. Hemiballismus is the most dramatic of these; damage to the subthalamic nucleus apparently removes inhibitory influences on the substantia nigra and globus pallidus, which results in violent, involuntary, rotatory flinging movements of the contralateral arm and leg. Similarly, damage to the caudate nucleus often results in chorea, whereas the opposite phenomenon, akinesia, typically occurs when dopamine-producing cells in the substantia nigra degenerate, releasing the intact caudate nucleus from inhibition. Lesions restricted to the globus pallidus often cause flexion dystonia and impaired postural reflexes.

NEUROPHARMACOLOGY OF THE BASAL GANGLIA: GENERAL PRINCIPLES Transfer of information from one cell to another in the mammalian nervous system usually involves one or more chemicals released from the first neuron to a specific receptor site on a second neuron, thereby altering the biochemical and physical properties of the second neuron. These chemicals taken together are called neuroregulators. There are three distinct classes of neuroregulators: neurotransmitters, neuromodulators, and neurohormones. Neurotransmitters, such as the catecholamines, GABA, and ACh, are the best

FIGURE 15-3 *Schematic diagram of the excitatory and inhibitory effects of neuroregulators released by neurons in the basal ganglia pathways. The area (enclosed by dashed lines) in the striatum indicates neurons with efferent projection systems. The other striatal transmitters are present in intrinsic neurons. Plus sign (+) indicates an excitatory postsynaptic effect. Minus sign (−) indicates an inhibitory effect. Abbreviations: cm = centromedian nucleus, GABA = gamma aminobutyric acid, TRH = thyrotropin releasing hormone, va/vl = ventroanterior and ventrolateral.*

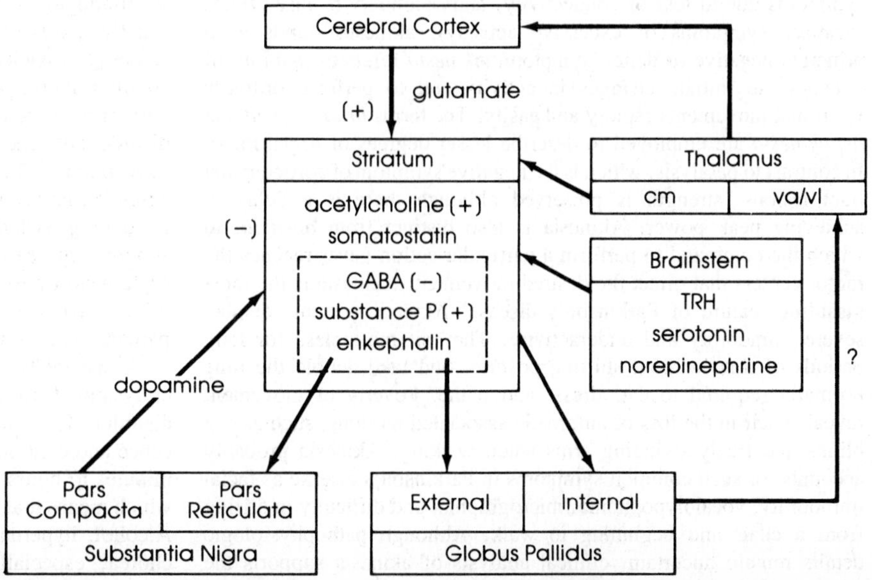

known and clinically most important class of neuroregulators. They cause short-latency, brief postsynaptic effects (e.g., depolarization) close to their point of release. Neuromodulators, such as the endorphins, somatostatin, and substance P, also exert effects close to the point of release but generally do not initiate neuronal depolarization. The neuromodulators apparently can enhance or diminish effects of the classic neurotransmitters. Many neurons that contain classic neurotransmitters also contain neuromodulator peptides. Substance P coexists within raphe neurons that synthesize 5-HT, for example, and vasoactive intestinal polypeptide coexists with ACh in many cortical cholinergic neurons. Neurohormones, such as vasopressin and angiotensin II, differ from other regulators because they are released into the bloodstream and are transported to remote receptors. Their effects are slow in onset and have a long duration of action. The distinction between the various classes of neuroregulators is not absolute. DA, for example, acts as a neurotransmitter in the caudate nucleus but is believed to act as a neurohormone in the hypothalamus.

Neuroregulators of the neurotransmitter class are the best-studied transmitters in the basal ganglia and the ones on which most drugs exert their effects. Neurotransmitters are synthesized in the presynaptic terminals of neurons and some, like the catecholamines and ACh, are stored in vesicles. Following the arrival of an electric impulse, neurotransmitters are released from the presynaptic terminal into the synaptic cleft, diffuse across the synaptic gap, and combine with specific receptor sites on the postsynaptic cell. This initiates a series of biochemical and biophysical changes; the sum of all postsynaptic excitatory and inhibitory influences determines the likelihood that a given neuron will discharge. The biogenic amines DA, norepinephrine (NE), and 5-HT are inactivated by uptake into the presynaptic terminals; ACh is inactivated by intrasynaptic hydrolysis. There are also receptor sites on the presynaptic terminal, called autoreceptors, and their stimulation generally causes a decrease in synthesis and release of the transmitter. The affinity of an autoreceptor for its neurotransmitter is often much greater than that of the postsynaptic receptor. Drugs that stimulate DA autoreceptors can be expected to decrease dopaminergic transmission and possibly be useful in the treatment of hyperkinetic movement disorders such as Huntington's disease and tardive dyskinesia. Receptors may be further subdivided based on response to pharmacologic agents. There are at least two separate populations of DA receptors, for example: Stimulation of D-1 sites activates adenylate cyclase, whereas D-2 receptor stimulation does not. The ergot alkaloid bromocriptine, used in the treatment of Parkinson's disease, stimulates D-2 but blocks D-1 receptors; most neuroleptics block D-2 receptors.

CLINICAL MANIFESTATIONS OF LESIONS OF THE BASAL GANGLIA

Akinesia When extrapyramidal diseases are analyzed along classic neurologic lines into primary functional deficits (negative symptoms due to loss of connectivity) and secondary release effects (positive symptoms of excessive activity), akinesia stands as a principal negative or deficit symptom. *Akinesia* refers to inability of a patient to initiate changes in activity and to perform ordinary volitional movements rapidly and easily. The terms *bradykinesia* and *hypokinesia* are employed to describe lesser degrees of impairment. In contrast to paralysis, which is the negative symptom of corticospinal tract lesions, strength is preserved although there is a delay in achieving peak power. Akinesia is also distinct from *apraxia,* in which the command to perform a particular action never reaches the motor centers that direct the desired movement. Akinesia is the most disabling feature of Parkinson's disease. Akinetic patients display severe immobility and underactivity. They sit motionless for long periods of time without shifting postures and take double the time normally required to eat, dress, and bathe. Poverty of movement reveals itself in the loss of automatic associated motions, such as eye blinks and freely swinging arms when walking. Akinesia probably accounts for such common symptoms in Parkinson's disease as facial immobility, vocal hypophonia, micrographia, and difficulty in arising from a chair and beginning to walk. Although pathophysiologic details remain uncertain, clinical analysis of akinesia supports the hypothesis that the basal ganglia are mainly responsible for initiation and automatic execution of learned motor plans. Neuropharmacologic evidence suggests that akinesia itself results from DA deficiency.

Rigidity *Muscle tone* is defined as the amount of resistance encountered when a relaxed limb is moved passively. In rigidity, the muscles are in continuous contraction and resistance to passive movement is constant. Rigidity secondary to extrapyramidal disorders may superficially resemble spasticity due to corticospinal tract lesions in that both produce increases in muscular tone. A few clinical guidelines provide help in distinguishing these conditions at the bedside. The distribution of increased tone often differs in rigidity and spasticity. Although rigidity is present in both flexor and extensor muscle groups, it tends to be more prominent in those that maintain a flexed posture. Rigidity is easy to detect in large muscle groups, but smaller muscles of the face, tongue, and larynx are also often affected. In contrast to rigidity, spasticity usually produces increased tone in the extensor muscles of the legs and the flexor musculature of the arms. The quality of hypertonus can also be used to distinguish the two conditions. Resistance to passive movements is constant in rigidity, accounting for terms such as "lead pipe" and "plastic" resistance. In spasticity, there may be a free interval followed classically by the clasp-knife phenomenon; muscles do not contract until they are stretched a bit, and later during stretch the augmentation in muscle tone quickly subsides. Deep tendon reflexes are normal in rigidity but increased in spastic states. Spasticity results from hyperactivity of the stretch reflex arc due to central changes but without increased sensitivity of the muscle spindle; spasticity can be abolished by sectioning posterior spinal roots. Rigidity has less relationship with hyperactivity of segmental reflex arcs and depends more upon heightened discharge of alpha motor neurons. A special type of rigidity is the cogwheel phenomenon, which is especially common in Parkinson's disease. When the hypertonic muscle is passively stretched, the resistance may be rhythmically jerky, as though the resistance of the limb were controlled by a ratchet.

Chorea Derived from the Greek word meaning "dance," chorea refers to widespread arrhythmic movements of a forcible, rapid, jerky, restless type. Choreic movements are noted for their irregularity and variability; they are generally continuous, may be simple or quite elaborate, and affect any part of the body. They may resemble voluntary movement in complexity, but they are never combined into a coordinated act unless the patient incorporates them into a deliberate movement in order to make them less noticeable. Normal volitional movements are possible because there is no paralysis, but they may be excessively quick, poorly sustained, and deformed by choreic movements. Chorea may be generalized or limited to one side of the body. Generalized chorea is the predominant involuntary movement in Huntington's disease and in rheumatic (Sydenham's) chorea, and usually involves the face, trunk, and limbs; it is often seen with levodopa toxicity in patients with Parkinson's disease. Another common choreiform disorder, tardive dyskinesia, occurs in association with chronic neuroleptic administration. Choreic movements in this disorder are generally restricted to the buccal, lingual, and mandibular musculature, although trunk and limbs may be involved in severe cases. Sedatives such as phenobarbital or a benzodiazepine are used in treating Sydenham's chorea; neuroleptics are commonly used to suppress chorea in Huntington's disease. Drugs that increase cholinergic neurotransmission, such as phosphatidylcholine and physostigmine, have been used to suppress chorea in about 30 percent of patients with tardive dyskinesia.

A special type of paroxysmal chorea, sometimes with athetosis or dystonic features, occurs sporadically, or as an autosomal dominant disorder. These disorders usually appear during childhood or adolescence and continue throughout life; patients have paroxysms that last minutes to hours. In one special subtype, the chorea is kinesogenic, which means that it may be initiated by a sudden voluntary movement. Alcohol, hypernatremia, and phenytoin may precipitate paroxysmal chorea, especially in patients who have Sydenham's chorea in childhood. In some cases, anticonvulsant drugs, including phenobarbital and clonazepam, and in other instances levodopa have prevented attacks.

Athetosis This term is from a Greek word meaning "unfixed" or "changeable." Athetosis is characterized by an inability to sustain the muscles of the fingers, toes, tongue or any other group of muscles in one position. The maintained posture is interrupted by continuous slow, purposeless movements. These are most pronounced in the digits and hands and consist of extension, pronation, flexion, and supination of the arm with alternating flexion and extension of the fingers. Athetotic movements are slower than those associated with chorea, but gradations are commonly seen and termed *choreoathetosis* when it is impossible to distinguish between the two. Generalized athetosis may be seen in children with static encephalopathy (cerebral palsy); it can also occur in Wilson's disease, in torsion dystonia, and following cerebral anoxia. Posthemiplegic athetosis is unilateral and occurs especially in children who have suffered a stroke. Patients whose athetosis is due to cerebral palsy or cerebral anoxia have variable degrees of additional motor deficit due to associated corticospinal tract disease. Discrete individual movements of the tongue, lips, and hands are often impossible, and attempts to perform such voluntary movements result in contraction of all the muscles in the limb and other parts of the body. Variable degrees of rigidity are generally associated with all forms of athetosis and may account for the slower quality of movement in this disorder in contrast to chorea. Treatment of athetosis is generally unsatisfactory, although some patients improve with the drugs used to suppress chorea and dystonia.

The dystonias Dystonia refers to abnormally increased muscular tone that causes fixed abnormal postures. Some patients with dystonia also have shifting postures resulting from irregular, forceful twisting movements that affect trunk and extremities and produce bizarre, grotesque movements and positions of the body. The mobile spasms of dystonia are similar to those of athetosis but are generally slower and involve axial (trunk) rather than appendicular (extremity) muscles. Dystonic movements increase during volitional motor activity, nervousness, and emotional stress; they diminish during relaxation and, like most extrapyramidal movement disorders, disappear completely during sleep. *Primary torsion dystonia,* formerly known as dystonia musculorum deformans, is frequently inherited as an autosomal recessive characteristic in Ashkenazic Jews and as an autosomal dominant trait in non-Jewish families. Spontaneous cases are also common. Manifestations of dystonia usually begin in the first two decades of life, but adult forms are recognized. Generalized torsion spasms can also occur in children with kernicterus and after cerebral hypoxia.

"Dystonia" is also used in another sense, to describe any fixed posture which may be the end result of a motor system disease. For example, dystonia secondary to a stroke (flexed arm and extended leg) is often called hemiplegic dystonia, and that associated with parkinsonism called flexion dystonia. In contrast to these permanent dystonic states, drugs such as the neuroleptics, and levodopa in patients with parkinsonism, can induce dystonic postures and spasms that subside once the offending medication is discontinued.

Secondary or *focal dystonias* are more common than torsion dystonia and include such disorders as spasmodic torticollis, writer's cramp, blepharospasm, spastic dystonia, and Meige's syndrome. In the focal dystonias as a group, symptoms tend to be highly localized, to remain stable, and not to spread to involve other body parts. Focal dystonias occur more frequently in adults and most often arise spontaneously without known genetic transmission or antecedent illness. Spasmodic torticollis is the most common focal dystonia. There are intermittent or continuous spasms of the sternocleidomastoid, trapezius, and other neck muscles, usually more prominent on one side than the other, that cause turning or tipping of the head. Torticollis is involuntary and cannot be inhibited, and thereby differs from habit spasm or tic. Torticollis is worse when the patient sits, stands, or walks; placing a finger to the chin or side of the jaw often alleviates the muscle imbalance. Women are affected twice as often as men; the average age of onset is 40.

Torsion dystonia is classified as an extrapyramidal disease even though no pathologic lesions have been observed in the basal ganglia or elsewhere in the brain. Development of rational therapy is further impaired by the lack of information regarding possible neurotransmitter abnormalities. Effective treatment of secondary dystonias is no more satisfactory than that of torsion dystonia. Symptomatic relief is sometimes achieved with sedatives such as the benzodiazepines and high doses of anticholinergic drugs; levodopa has been helpful in some instances. Biofeedback therapy has sometimes been beneficial but psychiatric treatment is ineffectual. When spasmodic torticollis is severe, surgical denervation of the affected muscles (C1 to C3 bilaterally and C4 on one side) has given favorable results in most patients. Blepharospasm has been successfully treated by injecting a dilute solution of botulinum toxin into periocular muscles. The toxin produces a mild neuromuscular blockade; its effect is transient and treatment must be repeated every 2 or 3 months.

Myoclonus This is a descriptive term for very brief, involuntary, random muscular contractions. Myoclonus can occur spontaneously at rest, in response to sensory stimuli, or with voluntary movements. Myoclonus may involve a single motor unit and simulate a fasciculation, or it may simultaneously involve groups of muscles that displace the limb or distort its voluntary movement. Myoclonus is a symptom that occurs in a wide variety of generalized metabolic and neurologic disorders collectively called the myoclonias. Posthypoxic intention myoclonus is a special myoclonic syndrome that occurs as a sequel to transient cerebral anoxia such as might occur, for example, during a brief cardiorespiratory arrest. Cognitive abilities are usually preserved; however, there are cerebellar signs, and voluntary movements are marred by action myoclonus involving the extremities, facial muscles, and even the voice. Action myoclonus deforms all movement and severely limits the patient's ability to eat, talk, write, or even walk. Myoclonus may also result from lipid storage disease, encephalitis, Creutzfeldt-Jakob disease, or metabolic encephalopathies due to respiratory failure, chronic renal failure, hepatic failure, or electrolyte imbalance. Posthypoxic intention myoclonus and idiopathic myoclonus may be treated with the 5-HT precursor 5-hydroxytryptophan (Fig. 15-4); alternate therapies include baclofen, clonazepam, and valproic acid.

Asterixis Quick arrhythmic movements that occur due to brief interruptions in background tonic muscular contractions are called asterixis; in a sense, asterixis may be considered as negative myoclonus. Asterixis may be observed in any voluntary muscle during contraction but is usually demonstrated clinically as a brief lapse of posture with prompt restoration during voluntary extension of the limb with dorsiflexion of the wrist or ankle. Asterixis is characterized by 50- to 200-ms silent periods in ongoing EMG activity in all muscle groups in one limb (Fig. 15-5). This results in the wrist or ankle moving down before muscular activity resumes and restores the limb to its original position. Asterixis is commonly observed bilaterally in metabolic encephalopathies, and its description in hepatic failure accounted for the original term "liver flap." Asterixis may be caused by drugs, including all anticonvulsants and the radiographic contrast agent metrizamide. Unilateral asterixis can occur after brain lesions in the distributions of the anterior or posterior cerebral arteries. The smallest brain lesion that can cause unilateral asterixis involves structures that are destroyed during stereotactic ventrolateral thalamotomy.

Hemiballismus Hemiballismus is a hyperkinetic movement disorder characterized by violent flinging motions in the arm contralateral to a lesion (usually vascular) in or near the subthalamic nucleus. The movements in ballism also have a rotary component at the shoulder and hip; there may be concomitant flexion and extension movements in the hand and foot as well. The involuntary motions persist throughout the day but generally attenuate during sleep. Strength and muscle tone may be slightly decreased in the affected extremities and

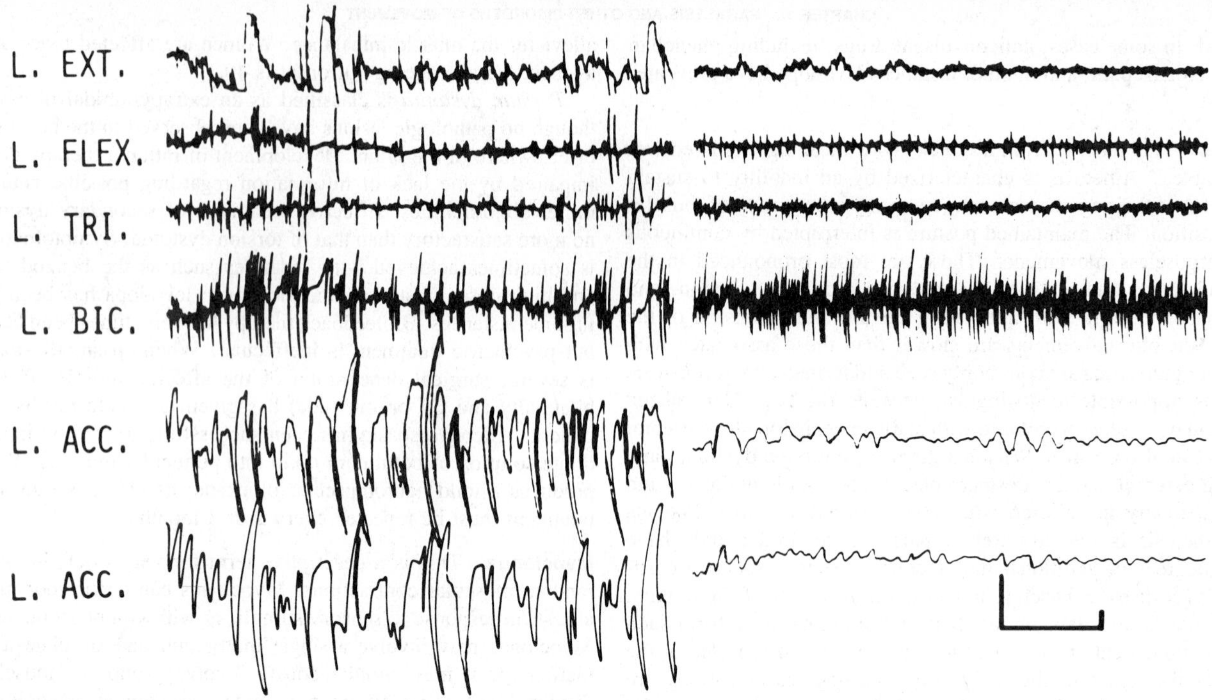

FIGURE 15-4 *Recordings from the left arm of a patient with posthypoxic intention myoclonus (A) before and (B) during treatment with 5-hydroxytryptophan. In both, the arm was held out horizontally from the shoulder. The upper four traces are EMGs from wrist extensors, wrist flexors, triceps, and biceps. The lower two traces are from accelerometers at right angles to one another on the hand. The horizontal calibration is 1 s. A. The continuous, large, jerky movements during voluntary activity are produced by arrhythmic bursts of EMG activity interspersed with irregular periods of EMG silence. The former positive and latter negative abnormalities occurred synchronously in antagonistic muscle groups. B. Only a little irregular tremor remains, and the EMG is much more continuous. (From JH Growdon et al, Neurology 26:1135, 1976.)*

FIGURE 15-5 *Asterixis recorded from the outstretched left arm of a patient with metrizamide-induced encephalopathy. The upper four EMG traces are identical to those in Fig. 15-4. The bottom trace is from an accelerometer on the dorsum of the hand. Calibration is 1 s. Note the continuous voluntary EMG interrupted at the arrow by a brief involuntary silent period in all four muscles. This silent period is followed by a lapse of posture and its jerky restitution, which is recorded by the accelerometer.*

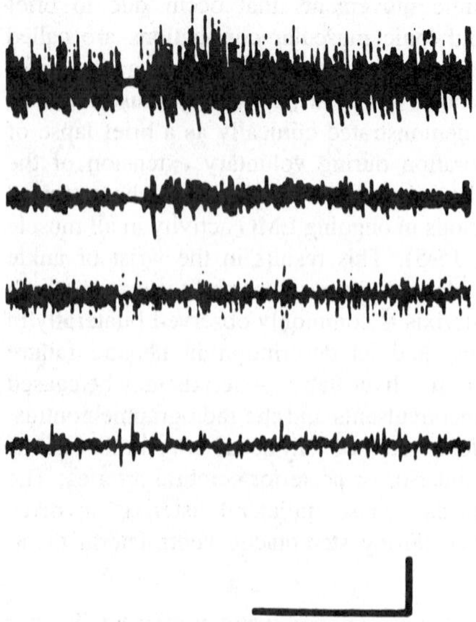

accurate movements are impaired, but patients with hemiballismus are not paralyzed. Both experimental and clinical observations indicate that the subthalamic nucleus probably exerts a controlling influence on the globus pallidus. Damage to the subthalamic nucleus destroys this restraining influence and results in hemiballismus. The exact biochemical consequences of these lesions remain unclear, but indirect evidence suggests that there is an increase in dopaminergic tone in the remaining basal ganglia structures. Medical treatment with neuroleptic drugs given to block DA receptors are generally effective in suppressing ballismus. Surgery is reserved for refractory cases; a stereotactic lesion placed in the ipsilateral globus pallidus, thalamic fasciculus, or ventrolateral thalamus can also abolish hemiballismus and restore normal function. Although recovery can be complete, many patients are left with variable amounts of hemichorea involving the hand and foot.

Tremor This common symptom consists of a rhythmic oscillation of a part of the body around a fixed point. Tremors usually involve the distal parts of limbs; the head, tongue, or jaw; and rarely the trunk. There are several different types of tremor, and each has its own clinical setting, pathophysiology, and therapeutic requirements. Often several different tremors exist in the same patient and must be treated individually. In a general hospital, most patients who appear tremulous actually have asterixis as a manifestation of one or another metabolic encephalopathy. Tremors may be subdivided clinically according to their distribution, amplitude, and relationship to volitional movement.

Tremor at rest is a coarse tremor with an average rate of four to five beats per second. It is most often localized in one or both hands and, occasionally, in the jaw or tongue. It is frequently a feature of Parkinson's disease. It characteristically occurs when there is postural (tonic) contraction of axial and limb girdle musculature when the limb is in an attitude of repose; willed movement temporarily suppresses it (Fig. 15-6). If the proximal muscles are completely relaxed, the tremor usually disappears, but the average patient rarely achieves this state. In some cases the tremor is constant; in others it varies from time to time and may extend from one group of muscles to another as the disease progresses. In some patients with Parkinson's disease there is no tremor; in others the tremor tends to be rather gentle and more or less limited to the distal muscles, whereas in a minority of parkinsonian patients and in patients with Wilson's disease (hepatolenticular degeneration) it often has a wider range and involves proximal muscles. In many cases there is a variable degree of rigidity of a plastic type in the tremulous limb or elsewhere. Although it is a source of great embarrassment and often is deemed responsible for all of a patient's motor difficulties, this type of tremor interferes with voluntary movements surprisingly little: It is not uncommon to see a patient who has been trembling violently raise a full glass of water to the lips and drain the contents without spilling a drop. The handwriting of these patients is often small and cramped (micrographia). The gait may be of festinating type. It is the combination of tremor at rest, slowness of movement, rigidity, flexed postures without true paralysis, and postural instability that constitutes Parkinson's syndrome. Often patients with Parkinson's disease also suffer from the tremor of stage fright (one of the enhanced physiologic tremors—see below) or from essential-familial tremor. Both may be exaggerated by increased levels of catecholamines in the blood stream and may be suppressed by drugs, such as propranolol, that block beta-adrenergic receptors.

The exact pathologic anatomy of *tremor at rest* is unknown. In Parkinson's disease, the visible lesions are predominantly in the substantia nigra. In Wilson's disease, in which tremor is mixed with cerebellar ataxia, the lesions are diffuse. Elderly persons may develop resting tremor without rigidity, slowness of movement, flexed postures, or masked facies. Unlike patients with parkinsonism, individuals with this syndrome do not progress to motor disability; their tremor does not respond to anti-parkinsonian drugs. In any given case it is not predictable whether a tremor is the initial sign of Parkinson's disease. Patients with titubation and a proximal tremor at rest (rubral tremor) as a symptom of cerebellar system dysfunction can be differentiated by the presence of ataxia and dysmetria from those with Parkinson's disease.

Action tremor refers to tremors present when the limbs are active, either when maintained in a certain position, as when outstretched, or throughout voluntary movement. Tremor amplitude may increase slightly as the action of the limbs becomes more precise, but it never approaches the degree of augmentation seen with cerebellar ataxia/dysmetria. Action tremors are easily made to disappear when the limbs are relaxed. Some of the action tremors are an exaggeration of normal *physiologic tremor;* such enhanced physiologic tremors are extremely common. They are experienced occasionally by all normal persons as well as by patients with essential-familial tremor or Parkinson's disease. They involve the outstretched hand as well as head, lips, and tongue. In general, they are due to a hyperadrenergic state and sometimes are iatrogenic (Table 15-2). Activation of $beta_2$ receptors in muscle alters the mechanical properties of muscle, eliciting action tremor. These alterations are reflected in discharges of muscle spindle afferents which modify the timing of activity around the stretch reflex arc and serve to augment the amplitude of preexisting physiologic tremor. Only patients without functional stretch reflex arcs are immune to these tremors. Peripherally active drugs that block $beta_2$ adrenergic receptors diminish enhanced physiologic tremors. This type of tremor is seen in numerous medical, neurologic, and psychiatric diseases and is therefore more difficult to interpret than tremor at rest.

There is another, somewhat slower action tremor which may occur as the only neurologic abnormality either sporadically or in several members of a family. It is known as *essential-familial tremor* (Fig. 15-7). It may begin in childhood but usually comes on later and persists throughout adult life. It becomes a source of embarrassment because it suggests to the onlooker that the patient is nervous. A curious fact about this tremor is that one or two drinks of an alcoholic beverage may abolish it but it will become worse after the effects of

TABLE 15-2 Conditions that enhance physiologic tremors

HYPERADRENERGIC STATES
Anxiety
Bronchodilators and other beta agonists
Excitement
Hypoglycemia
Hyperthyroidism
Pheochromocytoma
Peripheral metabolites of levodopa
Stage fright
POSSIBLE HYPERADRENERGIC STATES
Amphetamines
Antidepressants
Withdrawal from alcohol or opiates
Xanthines in tea and coffee
STATES OF UNCERTAIN ETIOLOGY
Corticosteroid therapy
Exercise
Fatigue
Lithium therapy

FIGURE 15-6 *Tremor at rest in a patient with Parkinson's disease. The upper two traces are surface EMG recordings from extensors and flexors of the left wrist; the lower trace is from an accelerometer attached to the left hand. The horizontal calibration denotes 1 s. Note the tremor at rest results from alternating contractions of antagonistic muscles at approximately 5 Hz. At the arrow, the patient is asked to dorsiflex the left wrist, and the tremor at rest disappears.*

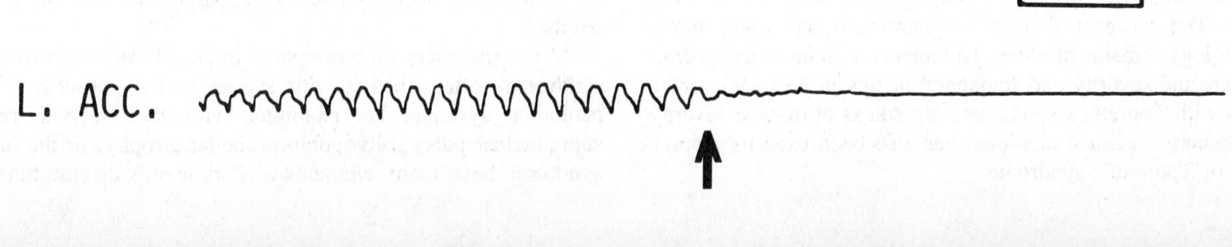

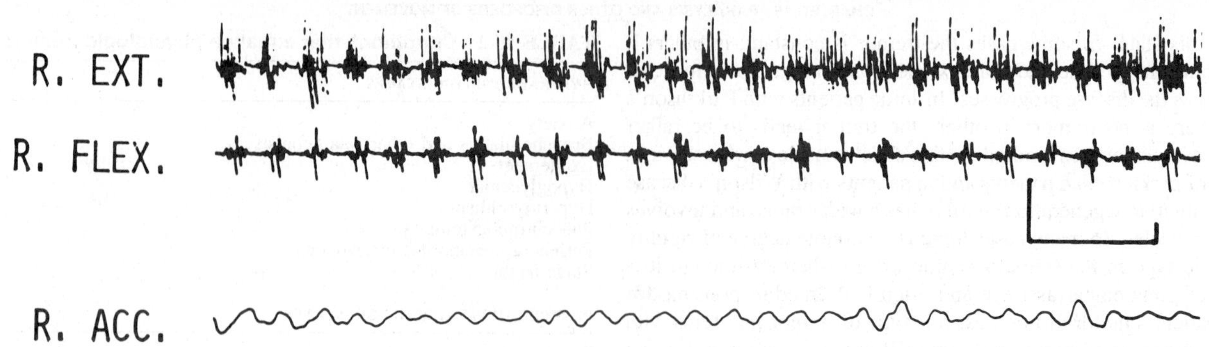

FIGURE 15-7 *Action tremor in a patient with essential-familial tremor. Recordings from the right upper extremity are with the hand actively dorsiflexed; otherwise, traces are similar to Fig. 15-4. The horizontal calibration denotes 500 ms. Note that during this action tremor, bursts of EMG activity at approximately 8 Hz occur synchronously in antagonistic muscles.*

the alcohol have worn off. Essential-familial tremors are suppressed by primidone or CNS-active beta-adrenergic blocking agents such as propranolol.

Intention tremor is an ambiguous term: The abnormal movements are certainly not intentional, and the abnormality is best described as an oscillatory ataxia generated proximally rather than as tremor. True tremors tend to affect distal musculature and the movements are more rhythmic and tend to be in one plane. Cerebellar ataxia, in which the direction of abnormal movement varies from second to second, requires for its full expression the performance of an exacting, precise, willed movement. The ataxia is absent when the limbs are inactive and during the first part of a voluntary movement, but as the action continues and greater precision is demanded (e.g., in touching a target such as the patient's nose or the examiner's finger), a jerky, somewhat rhythmic interruption of forward progression, with side-to-side oscillation, appears. It continues for a fraction of a second or so after the act is completed. Such dysmetria may seriously interfere with the patient's performance of skilled acts. Sometimes the head is involved (titubation). This movement disorder invariably indicates disease of the cerebellar system including its connections. When the disease is very severe, every movement, even the lifting of a limb, results in a wide-ranging oscillation of such violence as to throw the patient off balance. This state is occasionally seen in multiple sclerosis, Wilson's disease, and vascular, traumatic, and other lesions of the tegmentum of the midbrain and subthalamus but not of the cerebellum.

Habit spasms and tics Many individuals develop habitual movements that persist unchanged throughout life. Common examples include sniffing, clearing the throat, protruding the chin, and pulling on the collar. These are called habit spasms. These individuals admit that the movements are voluntary, but that they feel compelled to make them in order to relieve tension. Habit spasms can be inhibited for a time by a willful effort but reappear when attention is diverted. In certain cases, they become so ingrained that the person is unaware of them and unable to control them. Children between 5 and 10 years of age are especially likely to have habit spasms.

Tics are characterized by stereotyped, purposeless, and irregularly repetitive movements. Gilles de la Tourette syndrome is the most common and severe form of multiple tic disorder. This syndrome is a neuropsychiatric disorder with motor and behavior abnormalities; it usually begins in the first two decades of life and affects boys four times more frequently than girls. Motor symptoms include multiple brief muscular spasms, known as convulsive tics, in the face, neck, and shoulders. Vocal tics, including grunts and barking sounds, are also common. Behavioral abnormalities include coprolalia (swearing and repeating other vile utterances) and repeating the words of others (echolalia). The cause of Tourette's syndrome is unknown, and its pathophysiology remains obscure. Treatments with neuroleptic drugs will decrease the severity and frequency of tics in 75 to 90 percent of patients with Tourette's syndrome, regardless of disease severity. The noradrenergic agonist clonidine has also been used to suppress symptoms of Tourette's syndrome.

EXAMINATION AND DIFFERENTIAL DIAGNOSIS OF EXTRAPYRAMIDAL SYNDROMES In broad terms, all of the extrapyramidal disorders should be viewed in terms of primary deficit (negative symptoms) and of the new phenomena (abnormal postures and involuntary movements) that have appeared. The positive symptoms are ascribed to release from inhibition or disequilibrium of undamaged motor parts of the nervous system. The physician must cultivate the habit of accurately observing and describing abnormalities of movement and must not be content merely to give the condition a name or to force it into some superficial category. The fully developed extrapyramidal motor syndromes can be recognized without difficulty once the physician has become familiar with the typical pictures. A mental picture of Parkinson's disease, with its slowness of movement, poverty of facial expression, tremor at rest, and rigidity, should be fixed in mind. Similarly, the gross distortions of postural abnormalities in dystonia, whether widespread in trunk muscles or involving only neck muscles as in spasmodic torticollis, should be easily recognized. Athetosis, with its instability of postures, ceaseless movements of finger and hands, and intention spasm; chorea, with its rapid and complicated movements; myoclonus, with its abrupt movements that flit over the body, are other standard syndromes. There tends to be a mild defect in the voluntary use of the affected parts in all extrapyramidal syndromes.

Early or mild forms of these conditions, like all medical diseases, may offer special difficulties in diagnosis. Cases of Parkinson's disease, seen before the appearance of tremor, are often overlooked. Uncertainty of balance and short gait (*marche à petit pas*) in the elderly is often incorrectly attributed to loss of confidence and fear of falling. Patients may complain of being nervous and restless and describe a stiffness and aching in parts of the body. Because there is no weakness or change in reflexes, the disorder may then be considered rheumatic or even psychogenic. Parkinson's disease often begins in a hemiplegic distribution, and for this reason, the illness may be misdiagnosed as cerebral thrombosis or tumor. Facial immobility, a suggestion of a limp, mild rigidity, failure of an arm to swing naturally in walking, or loss of certain movements of cooperation will help in diagnosis at this time. Every case presenting with atypical extrapyramidal symptoms should be surveyed for Wilson's disease in order to avoid missing a treatable illness. Mild or early chorea is often mistaken for simple nervousness. Observing the patient at rest as well as in action is critical to the diagnosis. There are instances, nonetheless, in which it is impossible to distinguish simple fidgets from early chorea, especially in children, and there are no laboratory tests to aid in the diagnosis. The first postural manifestations of dystonia may suggest hysteria, and it is only later when the fixity of the postural abnormality becomes apparent that accurate diagnosis is reached.

Motor disorders seldom appear in pure form, and extrapyramidal syndromes often coexist with lesions in the corticospinal tract or cerebellar systems. For example, syndromes such as progressive supranuclear palsy, olivopontocerebellar atrophy, or the Shy-Drager syndrome have many elements of Parkinson's disease but also have paralysis of voluntary eye movements, ataxia, apraxia, postural hypotension, or spasticity with bilateral Babinski signs. Wilson's disease usually displays tremor at rest, rigidity, slowness of movement, and flexion dystonia of the trunk, but exceptionally there are athetosis, dystonia, and intention tremor. Emotional or cognitive abnormalities may be the presenting signs in Wilson's disease. Hallervorden-Spatz disease may take the form of universal rigidity and flexion dystonia, but choreoathetosis is sometimes observed. In some forms of Huntington's disease, particularly with juvenile onset, rigidity replaces choreoathetosis. Corticospinal and various extrapyramidal disorders may be associated in patients with cerebral diplegia. Some of the neurodegenerative diseases in which corticospinal tract and basal ganglia lesions coexist are described in Chap. 350.

Anatomic and neuropathologic studies of the basal ganglia, coupled with biochemical analyses of neurotransmitter content and behavioral responses to neuropharmacologic agents, provide the basis for understanding disorders involving the basal ganglia and for guiding their treatment. This is most clearly seen in Parkinson's disease and Huntington's disease. In Parkinson's disease, the DA content of the striatum is depleted owing to a loss of neurons in the substantia nigra and degeneration of their axonal projection to the striatum. As a result of decreased DA release, neurons within the striatum that synthesize ACh are released from inhibition. This results in the preponderance of cholinergic neurotransmission relative to dopaminergic transmission that accounts for most of the symptoms in Parkinson's disease. Recognition of this imbalance provides the basis for rational pharmacologic treatments. According to this formulation, drugs that increase dopaminergic neurotransmission, such as levodopa or bromocriptine, would be expected to rectify the imbalance between cholinergic and dopaminergic tone. These drugs, often prescribed in combination with anticholinergic drugs, are now standard therapy in Parkinson's disease. Excess levodopa or bromocriptine in patients with Parkinson's disease may induce a wide variety of abnormal movements that result from excessive stimulation of DA receptors in the striatum. The most frequent of these is craniofacial choreoathetosis, but more generalized choreoathetosis, facial and cervical spasms, dystonic postures, and myoclonic jerks may also occur. On the other hand, administration of drugs that block DA receptors (such as the neuroleptics) or deplete DA storage (such as reserpine or tetrabenazine) may produce a parkinsonian syndrome in an otherwise normal individual.

Huntington's disease is in many ways the clinical and pharmacologic opposite of Parkinson's disease. In Huntington's disease, characterized by personality change and dementia, gait abnormality, and chorea, there is a loss of neurons within the caudate and putamen, with resultant depletion of GABA and ACh but preserved DA content. The symptoms of chorea are believed to result from relative excess of DA compared with other transmitters in the striatum; drugs that block DA receptors, such as the neuroleptics, generally suppress chorea, whereas levodopa administration increases it. Similarly, physostigmine, given to increase cholinergic neurotransmission, may suppress chorea, whereas anticholinergic drugs enhance it.

These examples of clinical pharmacology further confirm the existence of delicate balances between excitatory and inhibitory impulses in the basal ganglia. In any one patient, the variable clinical manifestations seen during therapy are due to alterations in the neurochemical environment; the anatomic lesions remain unchanged. These examples illustrate the power of neuropharmacologic therapy in basal ganglia disease and provide the basis for optimism regarding the future ability of drugs to benefit patients with extrapyramidal movement disorders.

REFERENCES

DeLong MR, Georgopoulos AP: Motor functions of the basal ganglia, in *Handbook of Physiology*, Section I, *The Nervous System*, vol II: *Motor Control, Part 2*, VB Brooks (ed). Bethesda, American Physiological Society, 1981, pp 1017–1062

Delwaide PJ, Young RR (eds): *Restorative Neurology*, vol. 1: *Clinical Neurophysiology in Spasticity*. Amsterdam, Elsevier, 1985

Emson PC (ed): *Chemical Neuroanatomy*. New York, Raven Press, 1983

Feldman RG et al (eds): *Spasticity: Disordered Motor Control*. Chicago, Year Book Medical Publishers, 1980

Geschwind N: The apraxias: Neural mechanisms of disorders of learned movement. Am Sci 63:188, 1975

Growdon JH, Scheife RT: Medical treatment of extrapyramidal diseases, in *Update III: Harrison's Principles of Internal Medicine*, KJ Isselbacher et al (eds). New York, McGraw-Hill, 1982, pp 185–208

Kuypers HGJM: Anatomy of the descending pathways, in *Handbook of Physiology*, Section I, *The Nervous System*, vol II: *Motor Control, Part 1*, VB Brooks (ed). Bethesda, American Physiological Society, 1981, pp 597–666

Lawrence DG, Kuypers HGJM: The functional organization of the motor system in the monkey. Brain 91:1, 1968

Marsden CD: The mysterious motor function of the basal ganglia. Neurology 32:514, 1982

Martin JB: Huntington's disease: New approaches to an old problem. Neurology 34:1059, 1984

Young RR, Shahani BT: Asterixis: One type of negative myoclonus, in *Myoclonus*, S Fahn et al (eds). New York, Raven Press, 1985, pp 12–30

Young RR, Delwaide PJ: Drug therapy: Spasticity. N Engl J Med 304:28, 1981

16 ATAXIA AND DISORDERS OF EQUILIBRIUM AND GAIT

SID GILMAN

In the assessment of patients with neurologic disorders, it is important to inquire when taking the history about posture and gait and to examine these functions routinely as part of the neurologic examination. Abnormalities of posture and gait can result from disorders of several levels of the nervous system, and the type of abnormality observed clinically often indicates the site affected.

NEURAL STRUCTURES REQUIRED FOR STANDING AND WALKING The structures in the central nervous system that control standing and walking are the basal ganglia, a "locomotor region" in the mesencephalon, the cerebellum, and the spinal cord. The cerebral cortex doubtless is important in many aspects of standing and walking, but in experimental animals, complete removal of the cerebral cortex during the neonatal period, preserving the basal ganglia, thalamus, and lower structures, leaves stance and locomotion essentially normal. If the cerebral cortex, basal ganglia, and thalamus are removed, leaving the mesencephalon and lower brainstem intact, standing and walking are still possible. Electrical stimulation in a region of the mesencephalon termed the "locomotor region" evokes walking motions, and the speed and form of locomotion can be modified from a slow walk to a trot or gallop with changes in stimulation strength. This region receives projections from the basal ganglia, including the subthalamic and endopeduncular nuclei and the substantia nigra.

The spinal cord contains neural circuitry that coordinates the muscles for locomotion. After experimental transection of the spinal cord in the midthoracic region, the hindlimbs maintain the capacity to perform coordinated walking movements when placed on a moving treadmill. With increased treadmill speed, walking movements can switch to simultaneous movements of the hindlimbs, as in a gallop. After a high spinal transection, both the forelimbs and the hindlimbs can generate alternating movements and the sets of limbs remain coordinated. Thus, neural circuitry in the spinal cord can coordinate movements among all four limbs. The cerebellum controls many of the movements required for walking. Ablation of the cerebellum results in severe disorders of standing and walking.

In summary, walking is the result of integrated activity of the basal ganglia, mesencephalon, cerebellum, and spinal cord. Sensory inputs from movements of joints and muscle afferents provide important components for the control of walking. Without appropriate sensory feedback information, the pattern of walking is severely disrupted.

THE CEREBELLUM The cerebellum does not initiate movements, but it works closely with the motor cortex, basal ganglia, and many brainstem structures in executing a variety of movements. The cerebellum is needed to maintain proper posture and balance for walking and running; to perform fine voluntary movements such as those needed for writing, dressing, and eating; to carry out rapidly alternating and repetitive movements as in playing a musical instrument or working with a computer; and to coordinate smooth tracking movements of the eyes. The cerebellum is able to control certain properties of movements, including trajectory, velocity, and acceleration. Voluntary movements can be performed in the absence of cerebellar function, but the movements are clumsy and disorganized. The disturbances of movement from cerebellar dysfunction are termed *dyssynergia* (also *asynergia* or *ataxia*).

The cerebellum consists of a midline vermal region and two hemispheres which are attached to the medulla, pons, and midbrain by three peduncles on each side. A layer of gray matter, the cerebellar cortex, covers the cerebellar surface and encloses an internal core of white matter. Three pairs of deep cerebellar nuclei are buried within the cerebellum. From medial to lateral these consist of the fastigial, interposed (globose and emboliform), and dentate nuclei.

The cerebellum consists of three lobes. The *flocculonodular lobe*, which is the oldest part of the cerebellum phylogenetically (archicerebellum), consists of the paired flocculi and the nodulus. It receives input principally from the vestibular nuclei. The *anterior lobe*, the second oldest part (paleocerebellum), consists of vermal and paravermal structures in the anterior superior portion of the cerebellum. It receives input chiefly from the spinal cord. The *posterior lobe* is the largest and phylogenetically newest part of the cerebellum (neocerebellum) and is located between the other two lobes. The posterior lobe receives projections from the cerebral hemispheres via the pontine nuclei.

The cerebellar cortex contains three layers: an outermost *molecular layer*, a middle *Purkinje cell layer*, and an inner *granular layer*. The afferent fibers reaching the cerebellar cortex send collateral projections to the deep cerebellar nuclei and terminate either in the granule cell layer as *mossy fibers* or upon the dendrites of Purkinje cells as *climbing fibers*. Mossy fiber afferents are derived from the spinal cord, pontine nuclei, vestibular receptors and nuclei, trigeminal nuclei, reticular nuclei, and deep cerebellar nuclei. Climbing fiber afferents are derived exclusively from the inferior olive. Both mossy fiber and climbing fiber inputs are excitatory to the deep cerebellar nuclei and the cortex. Purkinje cells provide the only route for all information exiting from the cerebellar cortex and are inhibitory to the deep cerebellar and vestibular nuclei.

Projections to the cerebellum also originate in the locus coeruleus and the raphe nuclei of the brainstem. The afferents to the cerebellum from the locus coeruleus are noradrenergic; those from the raphe nuclei are serotonergic; and both sets of afferents are inhibitory. Several amino acids have been identified as putative neurotransmitters in the cerebellum. These include glutamate, which is used by granule cells; aspartate, which is used by climbing fibers; and γ-aminobutyric acid, which is used by Purkinje cells, Golgi cells, and basket cells.

The *inferior cerebellar peduncle* (*restiform body*) consists chiefly of afferent fibers. The peduncle contains a single efferent tract, the fastigiobulbar tract, which projects to the vestibular nuclei and completes a vestibular circuit through the cerebellum. Afferent fibers enter the inferior cerebellar peduncle from at least six sources (Fig. 16-1): (1) fibers from the vestibular nerve and nuclei; (2) olivocerebellar fibers from the inferior olivary nuclei; (3) the dorsal spinocerebellar tract; (4) some of the fibers from the dorsal spinocerebellar tract; (5) the cuneocerebellar tract from the accessory cuneate nuclei in the medulla; and (6) reticulocerebellar fibers. *The middle cerebellar peduncle* (*brachium pontis*) consists almost entirely of crossed afferent fibers from the pontine nuclei in the gray substance of the basal part of the pons (pontocerebellar or transverse pontine fibers) (Fig. 16-2). The major projections to the pontine nuclei originate within the cerebral cortex. The *superior cerebellar peduncle* (*brachium conjunctivum*) consists principally of efferent projections from the cerebellum. Rubral, thalamic, and reticular projections arise from the dentate and interposed nuclei. Some of the fastigiobulbar tract fibers also run with the superior penduncle for a short distance before they enter the inferior cerebellar peduncle. The superior cerebellar peduncle contains afferent projections from the ventral spinocerebellar tract, a portion of the rostral spinocerebellar tract, and trigeminocerebellar projections.

Except for direct projections of Purkinje cells onto vestibular nuclei, the efferent pathways of the cerebellum begin with the deep nuclei. The fastigial nucleus sends fibers to the reticular and vestibular nuclei of the brainstem. These nuclei project into the spinal cord and are concerned with posture and balance. The interposed nuclei of each side of the cerebellum project axons through the superior cerebellar peduncle to the red nucleus of the contralateral side. The red nucleus projects into the spinal cord via the rubrospinal tract (Fig. 16-2). This tract crosses the midline and descends into the spinal cord. The origin of this pathway in the interposed nuclei and the terminal portion in the spinal cord are on the same side of the body. Both the dentate and the interposed nuclei send fibers through the superior cerebellar peduncle to the contralateral ventrolateral nucleus of the thalamus. The ventrolateral nucleus relays fibers to

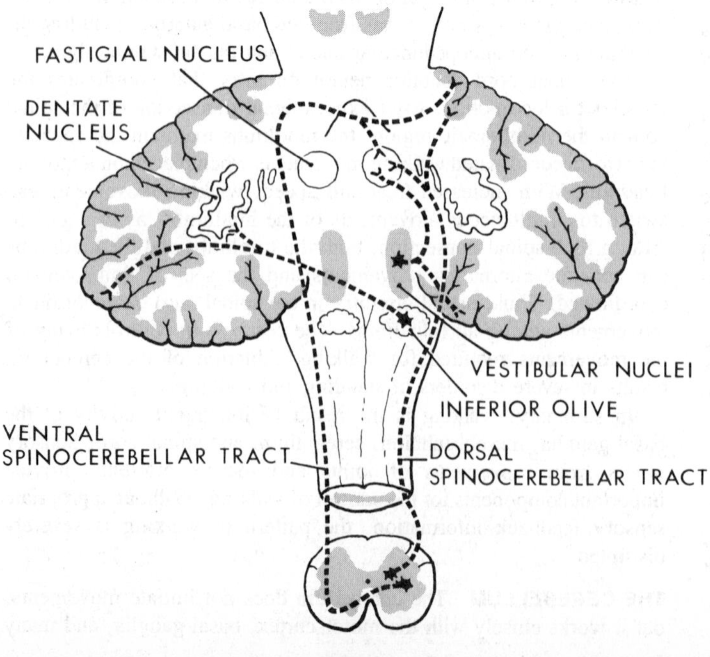

FIGURE 16-1 *The central nervous system connections of the dorsal and ventral spinocerebellar tracts, the fastigial nuclei, and the vestibular nuclei. (Adapted from S Gilman and SS Winans, in Manter & Gatz's Essentials of Clinical Neuroanatomy and Neurophysiology, 6th ed, Philadelphia, Davis Co, 1982.)*

the motor regions of the ipsilateral frontal lobe. The thalamic endings in the cerebral cortex make connection with corticospinal neurons whose efferent fibers pass through the pyramidal tract and cross to the contralateral side of the spinal cord. Thus, the origin of the cerebellothalamocortical pathway in the dentate and interposed nuclei and its termination in the spinal cord are on the same side of the body (Fig. 16-2).

For clinical purposes, a useful method of describing the cerebellum is based upon the existence of longitudinal sagittal zones. Each half of the cerebellum is subdivided into three longitudinal strips arranged from medial to lateral, including the cerebellar cortex, underlying white matter, and deep cerebellar nuclei: (1) a midline zone consisting of the vermal region with the fastigial nucleus; (2) an intermediate zone, the paravermal region, with the interposed nuclei; and (3) a lateral zone consisting of the cerebellar hemisphere with the dentate nucleus. Lesions of the midline zone cause disorders of stance and gait, truncal ataxia and titubation, and rotated or tilted postures of the head. Lesions of the lateral zone lead to disturbances in coordinated limb movement (ataxia), dysarthria, hypotonia, nystagmus, and kinetic tremor. Lesions of the intermediate zone cause symptoms characteristic of involvement of both the midline and lateral zones.

Ataxia is the result of dysmetria and decomposition of movement. *Dysmetria* is a disturbance of the trajectory or placement of a limb during active movement in which the limb falls short of its target (*hypometria*) or extends beyond its target (*hypermetria*). *Decomposition of movement* refers to errors in the sequence and speed of the component parts of a movement. The result is a lack of speed and skill in acts requiring the smoothly coordinated activity of several muscles. Movements previously fluid and accurate become halting and imprecise. *Ataxia* presents clinically as a disturbance in the rate and extent of an individual movement and commonly occurs from lesions of the cerebellum or of the sensory systems. Ataxia of gait consists of irregularities in the rate, length, and consistency of walking movements with veering to one side or the other.

PHYSIOLOGIC RESPONSES IMPORTANT IN STANDING AND WALKING Maintenance of the upright posture results from the actions of a number of postural reflex responses: (1) local static reactions acting on individual limbs; (2) segmental static reactions linking the extremities together; and (3) general static reactions resulting from the position of the head in space. *Local static reactions* include the stretch reflex and the positive supporting reaction. The simplest *stretch reflex* is illustrated by the muscle stretch response (deep tendon reflex), a brief muscle twitch evoked by rapid stretch of the muscle's tendon. Maintenance of muscle extension results in sustained contraction of that muscle through the stretch reflex. The *positive supporting reaction*, as elucidated in animal studies, results from a light cutaneous contact of the skin of the foot and also by proprioceptive stimulation owing to stretch of the interosseous muscles. The result of these stimuli is an extensor thrust by the limb.

The *segmental static reactions* include the crossed extension reflex and interlimb coordination. In the crossed extension reflex, application of noxious stimulation to an extremity results in flexion of that limb and simultaneous extension of the contralateral limb. With stronger stimulation, the crossed extension reflex triggered from a hindlimb can induce flexion in the contralateral forelimb and extension in the ipsilateral forelimb. Thus, the whole body moves along a diagonal path through the extended contralateral hindlimb and ipsilateral

FIGURE 16-2 *The central nervous system connections of the dentate nucleus and interposed (emboliform and globose) nuclei. (Adapted from S Gilman and SS Winans, in Manter & Gatz's Essentials of Clinical Neuroanatomy and Neurophysiology, 6th ed, Philadelphia, Davis Co, 1982.)*

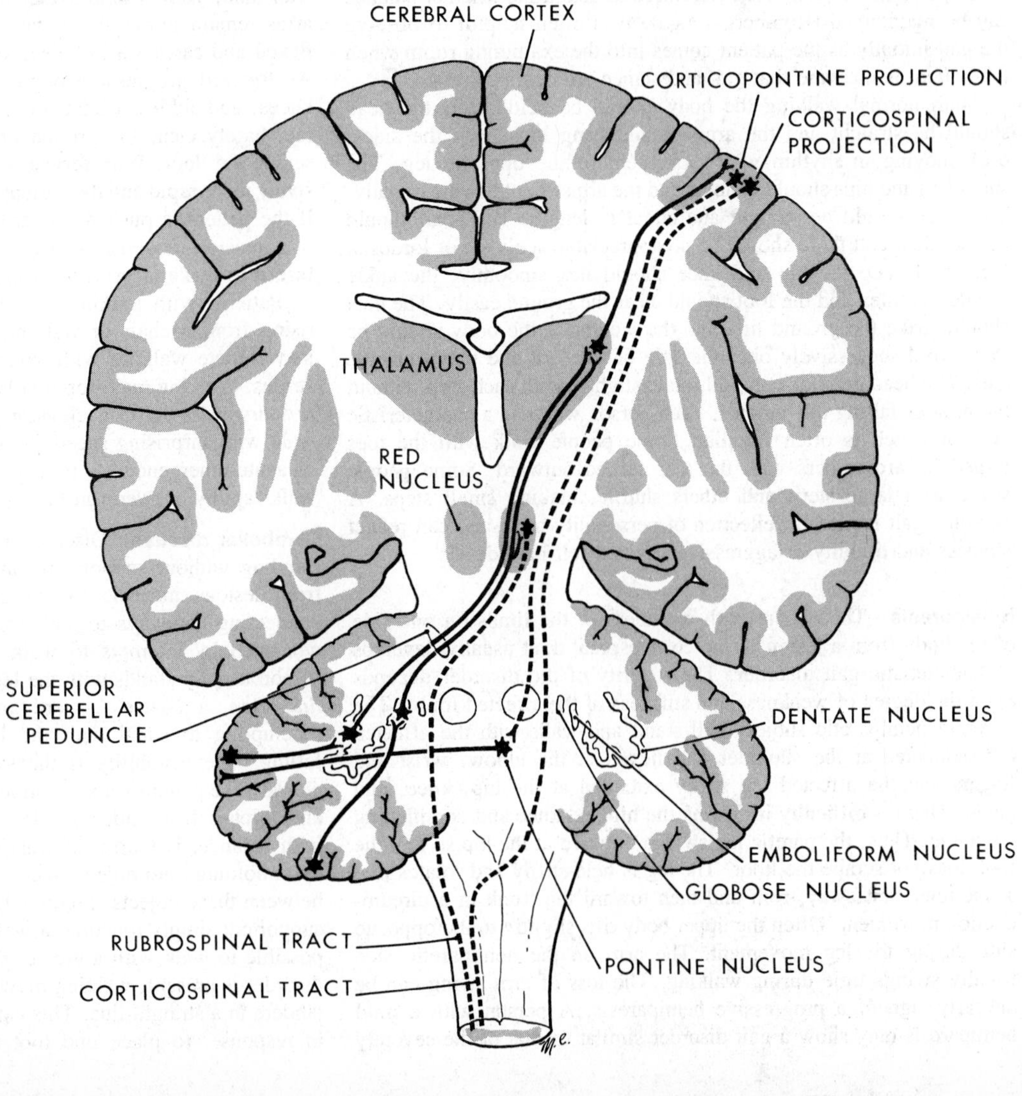

forelimb, thereby removing the stimulated limb from the source of noxious stimulation. This diagonal pattern of interlimb coordination also provides postural adjustments in various situations.

The *general static reactions* consist of two general types. The first, the *tonic neck* and *labyrinthine reflexes*, function together to adjust body posture when the head moves relative to the trunk in space. The second, the *righting reflex*, is triggered by labyrinthine, neck, and visual stimuli and helps the animal to regain an upright position after a fall. The *grasp reflex* is a component of the righting reflex. Other forms of general static reactions include the placing and hopping reactions as well as adjustment of body postures during limb movements.

CLINICAL APPROACH TO DISORDERS OF EQUILIBRIUM AND GAIT When evaluating a disorder of gait, the physician should inquire whether the disturbance occurs more in the dark than in the light; whether there is any accompanying vertigo, giddiness, or lightheadedness; and whether there is pain, numbness, tingling, or other type of paresthesias of the limbs. Inquiry should search for weakness, bowel and bladder dysfunction, and limb stiffness or rigidity. The physician should ask whether there is difficulty in the initiation or termination of walking.

Examination of stance and gait is performed best in a setting in which the physician can observe the patient walk from the front, back, and sides. The patient should rise quickly from a chair, walk normally at a slow pace, then more rapidly, and then turn around. Walking should be examined on the heels, on the toes, and in tandem, placing the heel of one foot directly in front of the toes of the opposite foot, attempting to progress in a straight line. The patient should stand erect with the feet together and the head straight, first with the eyes open and then with the eyes closed to determine whether balance can be maintained (Romberg's sign). It is often helpful to observe the gait initially as the patient comes into the examining room when the patient is unaware that gait and stance are being examined.

With normal walking the body should be held erect, the head should be straight and the arms should hang loosely at the sides, each moving in rhythm with movement of the opposite leg. The shoulders and hips should be level and the arms should swing equally. The steps should be straight and equal in length. The head should not be tilted and there should be no appreciable scoliosis or lordosis. With each step the hip and knee should flex smoothly, the ankle should dorsiflex and the foot should clear the ground easily. The heel should strike the ground first and the weight of the body should be transferred successively onto the sole of the foot and then onto the toes. The head and body should rotate slightly with each step without lurching or falling movements. Each person walks in a characteristic fashion which is often familial. Some people walk with the toes turned inward, others with the toes turned outward. Some people stride with large steps and others shuffle, making small steps. A person's gait is often a reflection of personality traits and can reflect shyness and timidity or aggressiveness and self-confidence.

Hemiparesis The patient with weakness of the limbs on one side of the body from a lesion of the corticospinal tract usually develops a characteristic gait disorder. The severity of the disorder depends upon the degree of weakness and stiffness of the affected limbs. The severely hemiparetic subject will stand and walk with the affected arm adducted at the shoulder and flexed at the elbow, wrist and fingers and the affected leg stiffly extended at the hip, knee, and ankle. There is difficulty in flexing the hip and knee and dorsiflexing the ankle. Thus, the paretic leg swings outward at the hip so that the foot does not scrape the floor. The leg is held stiffly and rotates in a semicircle, first away from and then toward the trunk in a circumduction movement. Often the upper body tilts slightly to the opposite side during the leg movement. The arm on the hemiparetic side usually swings little during walking. The loss of arm swing can be an early sign of a progressive hemiparesis. A person with a mild hemiparesis may show a gait disorder similar to that of the severely hemiparetic individual, but with a lesser degree of abnormality. In this case, a decrease in arm swing may be associated with subtle circumduction of the leg, without clear stiffness or weakness of the affected limbs.

Paraparesis Diseases of the spinal cord that affect leg function produce a characteristic gait resulting from a combination of spasticity and weakness of the lower extremities. Walking requires considerable effort and consists of slow, stiff movements at the hips and knees. The legs are usually maintained extended or slightly flexed at the hips and knees and adducted at the hips. In some people with paraparesis the legs may cross with each step, producing a scissoring motion. The steps usually are regular and short, and the patient may move the trunk from side to side, attempting to compensate for the stiff movements of the legs. The legs circumduct at the hips and the feet scrape along the floor so that the soles of the shoes become worn at the toes.

Parkinsonism Patient's with Parkinson's disease have a characteristic posture and gait. The severely affected individual stands in a posture of flexion, with the thoracic spine bent forward, the head bent downward, the arms moderately flexed at the elbows and the legs slightly flexed at the hips and knees. The patient sits or stands with striking immobility, showing a fixed facial expression with infrequent blinking and making few automatic movements of the limbs. The patient seldom crosses the legs or adjusts body posture when seated in a chair. Although the arms are held immobile, often a tremor involves the fingers and wrists at four to five cycles per second. In some people the tremor also occurs at the elbows and even at the shoulders. In advanced cases there may be drooling and a rhythmic tremor of the jaw. The patient usually gets up slowly to walk and, with walking, the trunk bends even farther forward, the arms remain immobile at the sides of the body or become further flexed and carried a bit ahead of the body. The arms fail to swing. As forward progression begins, the legs remain bent at the hips, knees, and ankles. Characteristically, the steps are short so that the feet barely clear the ground and the soles of the feet shuffle and scrape the floor. With forward locomotion the steps become successively more rapid and the patient may fall unless assisted (*festination*). If the patient is pushed forward or backward, compensatory flexion or extension movements of the trunk fail to occur and the patient is forced to make a series of propulsive or retropulsive steps.

Patients with Parkinson's disease often have great difficulty in rising from a chair or walking after standing still. The individual may initiate walking with several small steps before taking longer strides. Walking may stop involuntarily with attempts to pass through a doorway or into an elevator. Parkinsonian patients at times can walk with surprising speed and dexterity for brief intervals. In times of acute emergency, as in a fire, a person previously immobile can walk rapidly or even run briefly.

Cerebellar disease Disease of the cerebellum causes difficulty in standing without support and in walking. The disorder may result from lesions intrinsic to the cerebellum or from lesions in the connecting pathways to and from the cerebellum. The difficulty is worsened by attempts to walk with a narrow base. The affected person usually stands with the legs apart, and standing may provoke *titubation*, a coarse forward and backward tremor of the trunk. Attempting to stand with the feet together provokes swaying or falling. The instability is the same whether the eyes are open or closed. The patient walks cautiously, taking steps of varying lengths, and lurches from side to side. The patient complains of difficulty with balance, is fearful of walking without support, and may insist upon holding onto objects such as a bed or chair, moving cautiously between these objects. Frequently the individual does not need to be supported; simply touching a wall or an object in the room makes it possible to walk with a greater sense of security. When a mild gait disorder is present, walking may deteriorate with attempts to walk in tandem in a straight line. This causes the patient to lose balance and, in response, to place one foot to the side to avoid falling. With unilateral lesions of the cerebellum, balance is lost toward the side of the lesion.

When disease is restricted to the midline (vermal) portions of the cerebellum, as occurs in alcoholic cerebellar degeneration, disorders of stance and gait may develop without other signs of cerebellar dysfunction such as limb ataxia or nystagmus. In contrast, disease of the cerebellar hemispheres, either unilaterally or bilaterally, often causes marked limb ataxia and nystagmus in association with a gait disorder. With a lesion confined to one cerebellar hemisphere, ipsilateral disturbances of posture and movement commonly accompany the gait disorder. The patient usually stands with the shoulder on the side of the lesion lower than the other, and there may be an accompanying scoliosis. The limbs on the side of the cerebellar lesion show diminished resistance to passive manipulation (hypotonia). On walking the patient staggers and deviates toward the affected side. This can be demonstrated by asking the patient to walk around a chair. Rotation toward the affected side results in a fall into the chair, and rotation toward the normal side causes movement away from the chair in a spiral. The affected arm and leg show marked ataxia in tests of coordinated movement such as successively touching the patient's nose and then the examiner's finger or running the heel of the affected leg down the shin of the opposite leg.

Sensory ataxia A characteristic gait disorder results from loss of sensation in the lower extremities due to disease processes in the peripheral nerves, dorsal roots, dorsal columns of the spinal cord, or medial lemnisci. The most disabling component of the sensory disorder is the loss of joint position sense, but loss of input from muscle spindle receptors, vibration detectors, and cutaneous receptors also contributes to the disability. People with sensory ataxia are unaware of the position of the lower extremities and consequently have difficulty in both standing and walking. The patient usually stands with the legs spread widely apart. The patient remains stable if asked to stand with the feet together and the eyes open, but sways and often falls (positive Romberg's sign) when the eyes are closed. The test for Romberg's sign cannot be performed if the patient is unsteady when standing with the feet together and the eyes open, as may occur with cerebellar disease.

The patient with sensory ataxia walks with the legs spread widely apart, watching the ground carefully. The legs are lifted higher than necessary at the hips and are flung forward and outward in abrupt motions. The steps vary in length and the feet make characteristic slapping sounds as they contact the floor. The patient usually holds the body somewhat flexed at the hips, often using a cane for support. If vision is impaired or the patient attempts to walk in the dark, the gait disturbance worsens. The patient becomes unsteady and often falls when attempting to wash the face because of the temporary loss of visual compensation occurring with closure of the eyes.

Cerebral palsy This term encompasses a number of different motor abnormalities, most of them resulting from hypoxic-ischemic injury to the central nervous system in the perinatal period. The severity of the gait disturbance varies with the nature and extent of the lesion. Mild limited lesions can lead to increased deep tendon reflexes and extensor plantar responses with a slight degree of talipes equinovarus, without a clear gait disorder. More severe and extensive lesions commonly lead to bilateral hemiparesis. The patient stands and walks with a paraparetic posture and gait. The arms are adducted at the shoulders and flexed at the elbows and wrists.

Movement disorders commonly alter the gait in patients with cerebral palsy. Athetosis occurs frequently and consists of slow or moderately rapid serpentine movements of the arms and legs, with postures alternating between the extremes of flexion with supination and extension with pronation. On walking, patients with athetotic cerebral palsy show involuntary limb movements that are accompanied by rotary movements of the neck and frequent facial grimacing. The arms are usually flexed and the legs are extended, but asymmetric limb postures can occur with ambulation. For example, one arm may flex and supinate and the other may extend and pronate. Asymmetric limb postures commonly occur as the head rotates from side to side. Usually when the chin turns to one side, the arm on that side extends and the opposite arm flexes.

Chorea Patients with choreic movements often develop a characteristic gait disorder. Chorea occurs most frequently in children with Sydenham's chorea, in adults with Huntington's disease, and occasionally in adults with Parkinson's disease treated with excessive amounts of dopamine agonist medications. Choreic movements consist of intermittent rapid movements of the face, trunk, neck, and limbs. Flexion, extension, and rotary movements of the neck occur along with grimacing movements of the face, twisting movements of the trunk and limbs, and rapid piano-playing movements of the digits. Frequently, in early chorea, flexion and extension movements of the hips occur so that the patient constantly seems to be crossing and uncrossing the legs. The patient may scowl, frown, and smile involuntarily. Walking usually accentuates the choreic movements. Sudden forward or sideward thrusting movements of the pelvis and rapid twisting movements of the trunk and limbs result in a gait that resembles a series of dance steps. The steps are usually irregular in size, and the patient has difficulty walking in a straight line. The rate of progression varies from slow to rapid owing to variability in the rate and amplitude of each step.

Dystonia This is an involuntary postural and movement disorder affecting children (dystonia musculorum deformans or torsion dystonia) and adults (dystonia of adult onset). The condition may occur sporadically without known cause, as a genetic disorder, or as part of another process such as Wilson's disease. In dystonia musculorum deformans, which commonly begins in children, the first symptom often consists of an abnormal gait. Characteristically the patient will walk with one foot inverted at the ankle, placing weight on the lateral side of the foot; as the disease progresses, this problem worsens and other postural abnormalities develop. These include elevation of one shoulder, elevation of a hip, twisted postures of the trunk, and excessive flexion of the wrist and fingers of one upper limb. Intermittent spasms of the trunk and limbs may interfere with walking. Eventually torticollis, tortipelvis, lordosis, and scoliosis may supervene. In extreme cases, the patient becomes unable to walk. Adult onset dystonia often results in a similar progression of movement disorders.

Muscular dystrophy Marked weakness of the muscles of the trunk and proximal portions of the legs causes a characteristic stance and gait. In attempting to rise from a seated position, the affected person bends forward, flexing the trunk at the hips, places the hands on the knees, and pushes the trunk upward by working the hands up the thighs. Standing occurs with exaggerated lumbar lordosis and a protuberant abdomen owing to weakness of the abdominal and paravertebral muscles. The patient walks with the legs spread widely apart and develops a waddling motion of the pelvis because of weakness of the gluteal muscles. The shoulders often slope forward, and winging of the scapulae may be seen with walking.

Frontal lobe disease Bilateral frontal lobe disease causes a characteristic gait disorder which is usually associated with dementia and frontal lobe release signs including grasp, suck, and snout reflexes. The patient characteristically stands with the feet spread widely apart and takes a first step only after a long delay. This hesitancy is followed by very small shuffling steps and then by a few steps of moderate amplitude after which time the patient freezes, unable to continue walking. The cycle then is repeated. Affected individuals usually do not show muscular weakness, abnormalities of the deep tendon reflexes, sensory changes, or extensor plantar reflex responses. Usually the patient can perform the individual limb movements required for walking if asked to mimic walking movements while lying supine. The gait disorder with frontal lobe disease is a form of apraxia, i.e., a disturbance in the performance of a motor function in the absence of weakness of the muscles required for the function.

Normal-pressure hydrocephalus Normal-pressure hydrocephalus (NPH) is a disorder characterized by dementia, gait apraxia, and urinary incontinence. Computerized axial tomography reveals large cerebral ventricles, widening of the callosal angle, and lack of filling with cerebospinal fluid of the subarachnoid space over the cerebral hemispheres. Injection of radioactive isotope into the lumbar subarachnoid space demonstrates pathologic reflux of the isotope into the ventricular system and inadequate penetration into the cortical subarachnoid spaces.

The gait in NPH resembles that seen in apraxia from frontal lobe disease, consisting of a series of small, shuffling steps making it appear that the feet are glued to the floor. Initiation of walking is impaired, and slow and small angular displacements of the hip, knee, and ankle joints occur along with low clearance of the foot from the floor so that the patient appears to be sliding the feet along the floor. There is continuous contraction of the antigravity muscles of the legs but low muscle activity in the calf muscles. The gait disorder in NPH is thought to result from impaired function of the frontal lobes. In about half the patients with NPH the gait is improved by surgical shunting of cerebrospinal fluid from the cerebral ventricles into the venous system.

Aging Changes in gait and difficulties with balance occur with aging. Elderly men develop forward flexion of the upper portion of the trunk with flexion of the arms and knees, decreased arm swing, and shortening of step length. Elderly women develop a waddling gait with shortening of step length. Abnormalities of gait and balance predispose the elderly to falls. About half the falls in the aged result from environmental factors, including poor illumination, stairs, and uneven or slippery surfaces. Other causes of falls include drop attacks, orthostatic hypotension, turning movements of the head, and vertigo.

Lower motor neuron disorders Diseases of the lower motor neurons or peripheral nerves characteristically cause distal limb weakness. Foot drop is a common manifestation. In the case of lower motor neuron disease, the limb weakness occurs in association with fasciculations and muscle atrophy. The patient usually cannot dorsiflex the foot and compensates by raising the knees higher than usual, thereby walking with a "steppage gait." If proximal muscles are affected, the gait also can take on a waddling quality.

Hysterical gait disorders Hysterical disorders of gait commonly appear in association with hysterical paralysis of one or more limbs. Usually the gait is bizarre, easily recognized as hysterical and unlike any disorder of gait evoked by organic disease. In other instances, however, hysterical gait disorders may resemble organic gait disorders and can be difficult to identify. Hysterical gait disorders can occur in men or women and can appear in youth, young adulthood, and middle age.

In hysterical hemiplegia, the patient drags the affected leg along the ground behind the body and does not circumduct the leg or use it to support the body weight. At times the hemiplegic leg may be pushed ahead of the patient and used mainly for support. The arm on the affected side often remains limp, hanging uselessly beside the body and does not develop the flexed posture commonly seen in hemiplegia from organic causes. The patient with hysterical hemiplegia usually shows "give way" weakness. This is tested by asking the patient to make a maximum contraction of a set of muscles in an affected limb. Initially a strong contraction may occur, but as the examiner attempts to oppose the contracting muscles, the contraction suddenly gives way. Hysterical patients also commonly contract their muscles very slowly upon request, displaying great concentration and effort to evoke the contraction. Objective signs of neurologic disease are absent; the affected limbs show normal resistance to passive manipulation, the deep tendon reflexes are equal on the two sides of the body, and the plantar responses are downgoing.

In hysterical paraplegia, the patient usually walks with one or two crutches or lies in bed with the legs maintained either completely limp or stiffly extended. The term *astasia-abasia* refers to patients who cannot stand or walk but who can carry out natural movements of the limbs when lying in bed. Some patients with hysterical paraparesis walk with seeming difficulty but show normal power and coordination when lying in bed. On walking, the hysterical person clings to the bed or the furnishings of the room. If asked to walk without support the patient may lurch forward dramatically, veering from side to side at regular intervals. The patient can manage feats of extraordinary balance to avoid falling and may assume a variety of postures, walking with the legs in stiff extension, as if the legs are granite pillars, or walking with the legs in flexion and teetering from side to side. The hysterical patient may fall with walking, but only when a nearby physician or family member can catch the patient or when soft objects are available to cushion the fall. The gait disturbance is usually dramatic when an audience is present, and the patient can display remarkable agility in the rapid postural adjustments that occur.

REFERENCES

GILMAN S: Gait disorders, in *Merritt's Textbook of Neurology*, LP Rowland (ed). Philadelphia, Lea & Febiger, 1984, pp 44–48

——— et al: *Disorders of the Cerebellum*. Philadelphia, Davis, 1981

GRILLNER S: Neurobiological bases of rhythmic motor acts in vertebrates. Science 228: 143, 1985

ITO M: *The Cerebellum and Neural Control*. New York, Raven, 1984

KATZMAN R, TERRY R: *The Neurology of Aging*. Philadelphia, Davis, 1983

KNUTSSON E, LYING-TUNELL U: Gait apraxia in normal-pressure hydrocephalus: Patterns of movement and muscle activation. Neurology 35:155, 1985

17 MUSCLE PAINS, SPASMS, CRAMPS, AND EPISODIC WEAKNESS

ROBERT C. GRIGGS

Spontaneous or exercise-related discomfort from muscles or joints is usually benign and does not signal neuromuscular disease. Such symptoms may, however, provide clues to disabling disorders that too often evade diagnosis. The terms pain, spasm, and cramp are often used interchangeably by patients to describe symptoms referable to muscles. Other terms, including aching, heaviness, stiffness, and rheumatism, are also used, and usually connote less certainty about the source or localization of the discomfort. In clinical terminology, *spasm* refers to a brief, unsustained contraction of a single or multiple muscles. *Cramp* is a paroxysmal, spontaneous, prolonged, and painful contraction of one or more muscles.

SPASMS Abnormal movements of muscle may arise from abnormal electrical activity of the central nervous system mediated via the motor neuron, or occur within the muscle fiber itself. It may be difficult on clinical grounds alone to determine the precise site of origin of the abnormal motor activity. In general, movements originating in the central nervous system affect the entire side of the body, an entire limb, or a group of muscles. Central disorders may be rhythmic or intermittent; those arising in the periphery are usually random. The electroencephalogram may provide evidence for altered cortical activity in some conditions with a central nervous system etiology. The electromyogram (EMG) is less helpful because it reflects motor activity from any cause. EMG evidence of an underlying nerve disease may, however, be helpful in diagnosis (see Chap. 354) and certain abnormal muscle contractions have characteristic EMG features.

Intermittent, nonrhythmic movements of an entire limb, of the trunk, or of a portion of the face may result from cerebral seizure activity (Chap. 342) or from myoclonus (Chap. 15). Flexor and extensor spasms of an entire side or of the lower limbs result from a loss of motor inhibition within the central nervous system (Chap. 15). *Segmental myoclonus* results from focal disease within the brainstem or spinal cord that causes an abnormal discharge of groups of motor neurons. Localized vascular disease, tumor, or another lesion may be implicated.

Abnormal facial movements *Hemifacial spasm* results from paroxysmal facial nerve activity, sometimes triggered by pressure from a tortuous blood vessel adjacent to the facial nerve as it leaves the brainstem. Hemifacial spasm commonly occurs in muscles about the eye, but may also involve or spread to the entire side of the face. Symptoms are often intermittent and intensified when patients are using facial muscles in activities such as speaking. Hemifacial spasm is painless but embarrassing, especially to individuals dealing with the public. Since it is often intensified and more severe when the patient is in stressful situations, an erroneous diagnosis of tic (habit spasm) is often made. Cerebellopontine angle lesions can occasionally produce a similar disorder. Neuroradiologic investigation is indicated in patients with facial hemispasm. Anticonvulsant medications occasionally alleviate the spasms, but surgical exploration and shielding of the facial nerve from the adjacent vessel is curative.

Facial *tics* (habit spasms) are stereotyped movements of the face such as eyeblinking, headturning, or grimacing that are under voluntary control but may be suppressed only by effort and anxiety on the part of the subject (see Chap. 15). Some tics are so frequently encountered as to be considered mannerisms, analogous to excessive clearing of the throat. The repetitious elevation of the eyebrows by frontalis muscle contraction is an example. Certain hereditary movement disorders such as Gilles de la Tourette syndrome are characterized by multiple tics (Chap. 15).

Synkinesias of the face result from aberrant regeneration of the facial nerve following facial paralysis from Bell's palsy or other facial nerve lesions. Nearly 50 percent of patients who recover from Bell's palsy display such movements; an example is *jawwinking*, where voluntary movements of the lower face elicit contraction of the orbicularis oculi muscle with eye closure.

Trigeminal neuralgia (tic douloureux) is characterized by brief, paroxysmal, lancinating pain in one side of the face (see Chap. 352). Although the portion of the nerve involved is almost exclusively sensory, the severity of the pain causes involuntary contraction of facial muscles; hence the name tic. Abnormal movements do not occur in the absence of pain.

Facial myokymia refers to a nearly continuous, fine or coarse rippling and fascicular twitching of facial muscles. Although often benign it may result from lesions of the pons such as a neoplasm or multiple sclerosis. Similar movements occur in motor neuron diseases such as amyotrophic lateral sclerosis or occasionally as an isolated, hereditary condition.

Abnormal limb movements No movement should be visible in totally relaxed muscles. Diseases of motor neurons or their proximal axons are often associated with *fasciculations*, the spontaneous firing of an entire motor unit. Fasciculations are visible on inspection of muscle or perceived by the patient as a pulsation or quivering within muscle. Fasciculations occur at times in most normal individuals and unless weakness is present are seldom of any significance. Fasciculations are normal if observed in incompletely relaxed muscles. *Myokymia*, consisting of numerous, repetitive fasciculations, may also occur in limb muscles, giving a writhing appearance. Myokymia disappears with neuromuscular blockade, proving that the activity originates in anterior horn cells or in peripheral nerve. In patients with long-standing muscle denervation and reinnervation, motor unit size enlarges and fasciculations may be so large as to produce movement of the limbs, particularly of the fingers, a condition termed *minipolymyoclonus*. Similarly, the enlarged motor units of chronic denervation may be associated with a tremor of the fingers on extension.

Certain conditions are characterized by a compulsion to move the extremities. *Akathisia* or motor restlessness occurs in Parkinson's disease and other disorders of the basal ganglia including drug-induced movement disorders. The *restless legs syndrome* describes an uncomfortable sensation in muscles, usually in the legs and thighs, which occurs most commonly in middle-aged women. Patients feel they need to move their legs to relieve the abnormal sensation. The restless leg syndrome is frequent in uremia and may occur in other neuropathies, suggesting that the sensation is caused by an underlying neuropathy. It may also be familial and detailed study of such patients has failed to demonstrate any evidence of neuropathy. The restless sensation may be accompanied by myoclonic jerks of muscle often occurring during sleep. These myoclonic jerks are similar to the myoclonus observed in normal individuals entering REM sleep (see Chap. 20).

These forms of muscle spasm and myoclonus are somewhat similar to a group of unusual and unexplained *startle* syndromes or *hyperekplexias* characterized by sudden jerking of limbs or occasionally of trunk muscles. Sudden noise or touch may cause a patient to jump or to fling an extremity. Their cause is unknown.

SUSTAINED MUSCLE CONTRACTIONS Distinguishing central from peripheral causes of sustained muscle contraction is often difficult. Abnormal muscle contractions with increased muscle tone usually result from central nervous system disease. Thus, loss or disturbance of central nervous system inhibition may lead to abnormal muscle contraction characteristic of spasticity, rigidity, or "paratonic" rigidity. In most instances there is other evidence of central nervous system disorder (Chap. 15). Diseases of the basal ganglia, presumably resulting from altered neurotransmitter release, may lead to dystonia (Chaps. 15 and 16).

Abnormal muscle contractions may also arise from repetitive depolarization of the component portions of the motor unit: the motor neuron; the peripheral axon of the neuron; the neuromuscular junction; or muscle fibers. Electrically inactive contractions may arise from disorders of the muscle contractile system.

Motor neuron disorders *Cramp* is a term often used by patients to refer to a painful, involuntary contraction of a single muscle or a muscle group. Muscle cramps can arise from spontaneous firing of groups of anterior horn cells followed by contraction of many motor units. EMG recordings indicate that motor units fire at a rate of up to 300 per second, much higher than occurs with voluntary contraction. Cramps occur frequently in the legs in elderly patients and when severe are followed by residual tenderness and evidence of muscle fiber necrosis including elevation of serum creatine kinase. Cramps in the calf muscles are so common as to be considered normal, but more generalized cramps may be a sign of chronic disease of the motor neuron such as amyotrophic lateral sclerosis. They may be particularly troublesome during pregnancy, in patients with electrolyte disturbances (hyponatremia), and in patients on hemodialysis. When recurrent and localized to one muscle group they suggest nerve root disease. In many instances, however, it is impossible to determine the cause of cramps. Benign cramps, occurring commonly at night, may be relieved by quinine sulfate. Other causes of contractions arising from the motor neuron include *tetanus* (Chap. 99) and the *stiff-man syndrome*. In both disorders a loss of inhibitory neuronal input to anterior horn cells may result in repeated firing of motor neurons, producing severe, painful muscle contraction. A similar clinical picture may occur acutely with *strychnine poisoning*. Diazepam improves these spasms but may cause respiratory depression in doses sufficient to alleviate muscle contraction.

Peripheral nerve *Tetany* is characterized by contractions of predominantly distal muscles, particularly in the hand (carpal spasm) and feet (pedal spasm). Laryngospasm may also occur. Tetany results from increased excitability of peripheral nerves. The muscle contractions are initially painless, but if sustained may cause muscle damage with pain. Severe tetany may involve spine musculature to produce opisthotonus. Tetany is usually caused by hypocalcemia, but may occur with hypomagnesemia or severe respiratory alkalosis (see Chap. 336). Idiopathic normocalcemic tetany, *spasmophilia*, occurs in both hereditary and sporadic forms.

Muscle MYOTONIA Repetitive depolarization of muscle cells can cause muscle contraction resulting in muscle stiffness and impaired relaxation. Myotonia is usually painless, but may disable patients by interfering with fine hand movements or by slowing ambulation. Myotonic dystrophy is the commonest disorder associated with myotonia although other manifestations of the disease such as cataracts and muscle weakness are usually more symptomatic (see Chap. 357). Myotonia congenita and paramyotonia congenita are less common, but more troublesome in terms of severity of myotonia. Myotonia is often worsened by cold and characteristically is attenuated by "warm-ups," decreasing with repeated activity. *Paradoxical myotonia* worsens with repeated activity and is characteristic of paramyotonia congenita; these patients also suffer from episodic and cold-induced weakness (Chap. 377). Impaired muscle relaxation that is electrically inactive is characteristic of the delayed relaxation of myxedema. This delay produces the characteristic "hung-up" ankle reflexes but is essentially asymptomatic.

CONTRACTURE Muscle contracture is a painful shortening of a muscle unassociated with muscle membrane depolarization. It occurs in disorders where a metabolic defect such as myophosphorylase deficiency limits the production of high-energy phosphates. Contractures are precipitated by exercise and are usually intensely painful. This use of the term *contracture* is confusing since the same word is used to describe the unrelated limitation of joint movement by shortening of muscle tendons seen in rheumatologic disorders, cerebral palsy, or chronic myopathies. Muscle rigidity from metabolic contracture can occur in the malignant hyperthermia syndrome, usually associated with general anesthesia. In the hyperthermia of the neuroleptic malignant syndrome, muscle rigidity arises from central nervous system overactivity, and intense electrical activity is present in muscle.

MUSCLE PAIN, ACHING, AND TENDERNESS Painful muscles do not always imply muscle disease. Joint and bone disease frequently produce complaints of muscle pain and may further confuse the anatomic localization of symptoms by resulting in disuse atrophy and moderate muscle weakness. Pain from disease of overlying subcutaneous tissue or fascia and of tendons may also be referred to muscle. Additionally, disease of major peripheral nerves or of their small intramuscular branches may produce both muscle pain and weakness. Muscle pain may be a major symptom in inflammatory, metabolic, endocrine, and toxic myopathies (Chaps. 356 and 357).

Muscle trauma Vigorous activity, even in conditioned athletes may be associated with muscle and tendon tears which lead to temporary acute muscle pain, swelling, and tenderness. Rupture of muscle tendons such as the biceps or gastrocnemius muscle may produce visible muscle shortening.

The almost-pleasurable ache and fatigue of muscles after strenuous activity is separable only by degree from more severe, but still normal pain following severe, unaccustomed activity. Such symptoms are often associated with laboratory evidence of profound muscle damage including a rise in serum enzymes (creatine kinase) and widespread muscle necrosis on biopsy. Myoglobinemia and myoglobinuria may occur. Particularly likely to produce muscle pain and necrosis are certain types of exercise: brief periods of contracting a muscle while it is lengthening (eccentric contractions); and prolonged exercise such as marathon running. The point at which such symptoms become abnormal is not clear. Many patients have pain with moderate activity. Such exertional muscle pain is also characteristic of metabolic disorders of muscle including carnitine palmityl transferase deficiency and myoadenylate deaminase deficiency; deficiencies of enzymes of glycolysis are more commonly associated with contractures. The majority of patients with exertional and postexertional muscle pain do not have a definable abnormality.

Diffuse myalgias Muscle pain in the absence of muscle weakness can occur in acute infections caused by influenza and Coxsackie viruses. Fibrositis, fibromyalgia, and fibromyositis are synonyms for a disorder associated with pain and tenderness of muscle and adjacent connective tissue. Focal "trigger points" of tenderness can be identified and systemic symptoms such as fatigue, insomnia, and depression are frequently present (see Chap. 356). Although patients often identify painful swellings, histologic evaluation discloses no abnormality of muscle or connective tissue. Symptoms may respond partially to nonsteroidal anti-inflammatory agents, but the disorder tends to be chronic and unrelenting. Patients whose symptoms persist for months or years are often considered to have a psychiatric disorder, but its nature has not been defined.

Polymyalgia rheumatica occurs in patients over age 50 and is characterized by stiffness and pain in shoulder and hip musculature. Despite symptoms of pain localized to muscles, there is convincing evidence that the disease includes a proximal, inflammatory arthritis; joint effusions are often present in knees and other peripheral joints as well. Patients often develop profound disuse atrophy of muscles and complain of weakness, giving rise to a suspicion of polymyositis. However, creatine kinase levels are usually normal, and muscle biopsy shows atrophy without evidence of muscle necrosis or inflammation. The erythrocyte sedimentation rate is elevated in most patients, and giant cell arteritis may be present. Treatment with nonsteroidal anti-inflammatory agents is advocated except in patients with giant cell artertis, for whom prednisone (50 to 100 mg daily) is recommended. Patients with polymyalgia rheumatica who fail to respond to nonsteroidal anti-inflammatory agents may require low-dose prednisone (10 to 20 mg daily). Myalgias are also frequent in other rheumatologic disorders including rheumatoid arthritis, systemic lupus erythematosus, polyarteritis nodosa, scleroderma, and the mixed connective tissue syndrome. When muscle pain occurs as an early symptom, it may erroneously suggest a primary muscle disease, and the myalgia may be due to inflammatory muscle involvement that can occur in each of these conditions (see Chap. 356). Patients with polymyositis and dermatomyositis may have myalgias, although in the majority, muscle pain is lacking or minimal (Chap. 356).

EPISODIC WEAKNESS The term *weakness* is often used by a patient to describe a loss of stamina or decreased "energy." Even careful efforts at eliciting a history of true as opposed to subjective weakness may fail to distinguish the two conditions. The most helpful strategy is to ask the patient to identify whether a discrete loss of function has occurred and to elicit the circumstances in which symptoms are noted.

Weakness whether true or perceived may be due to disorders of the central or peripheral nervous system. Weakness from central nervous system disorders such as transient cerebral ischemia is usually associated with a change in level of consciousness or cognition, with increased muscle tone and muscle stretch reflexes, and often with alterations of sensation. Most neuromuscular causes of intermittent weakness are associated with normal mental function but with diminished muscle tone and muscle stretch reflexes. The major causes of intermittent weakness are listed in Table 17-1. Central causes are considered in Chap. 343.

EPISODIC ASTHENIA Patients who describe intermittent "weakness" as *fatigue* and loss of *stamina* suffer from asthenia, which can be separated from true weakness by the fact that patients do not lack the ability to do a task but rather the ability to perform it repetitively. Asthenia is a major problem in many patients with serious renal, hepatic, cardiac, or pulmonary disease. Examination of such patients usually confirms their ability to do all functional activities at least once, such as rising from a knee bend, climbing stairs, or rising from a chair. Fatigue is also characteristic of relatively selective damage to central nervous system descending motor tracts, in which signs of neurologic abnormality may be minimal.

Intermittent weakness due to peripheral neuromuscular disease may result from abrupt changes in peripheral nerve function; intermittent destruction of muscle; alterations of electrophysiologic properties of muscle from abnormalities of blood electrolytes; and intermittent failure of neuromuscular transmission.

FAILURE OF PERIPHERAL NERVE CONDUCTION A number of uncommon peripheral neuropathies are associated with recurrent weakness. *Hereditary liability to pressure palsies*, often termed *tomaculous* neuropathy because of the sausage-like appearance of myelin on nerve biopsy, is an autosomal dominant disorder characterized by abrupt paralysis following compression of a peripheral nerve. The paralysis is usually self-limited, lasting days to weeks. Other types of peripheral neuropathy may also predispose to the development of reversible, compressive neuropathies (see Chap. 355).

DISORDERED NEUROMUSCULAR JUNCTION TRANSMISSION *Myasthenia gravis*, particularly in its initial manifestations, is characterized by transient weakness. Cranial muscles are usually affected first, causing double vision, ptosis, dysphagia, and dysarthria. Rarely, limb weakness may herald the onset of myasthenia gravis and in the absence of cranial muscle dysfunction may escape diagnosis for months. Diurnal variation in strength is typical, and reflexes are preserved. Other, less-common defects of the neuromuscular junction such as the Eaton-Lambert syndrome may also present with intermittent weakness (see Chap. 358).

INTERMITTENT ALTERATIONS IN ELECTROLYTES Transient shifts in serum potassium are associated with profound alterations in muscle strength. Although the primary periodic paralyses (hypo- and hyperkalemic periodic paralysis) spring to mind in a patient with weakness and an abnormality in serum potassium, other causes of abnormal serum potassium more frequently result in episodic weakness (see Chap. 359). Familial periodic paralysis seldom presents after age 30; other causes are usually present in older patients. Hypokalemic periodic paralysis may occur in patients with hyperthyroidism. Episodic weakness due to hypokalemia may occur with renal or gastrointestinal potassium loss; major causes include renal tubular acidosis, diuretic-induced hypokalemia, hyperaldosteronism, Bartter's syndrome, and villous adenoma of the colon.

Hyperkalemic weakness occurs in chronic renal or adrenal insufficiency, with hyporeninemic hypoaldosteronism, and on an iatrogenic basis from injudicious administration of oral potassium preparations alone or in combination with potassium-sparing diuretics such as triamterene, amiloride, and spironolactone. The use of potassium salts as a substitute for table salt may cause hyperkalemia in patients with impaired potassium excretion.

Other electrolyte disturbances may occasionally produce intermittent weakness as the initial clinical manifestation of a severe metabolic abnormality. These include elevation or depression of serum sodium, calcium, or magnesium as well as hypophosphatemia.

METABOLIC MUSCLE DISEASE (see Chap. 347) A number of uncommon defects in glycogen and lipid utilization are associated with impaired energy production by muscle and cause intermittent weakness, usually accompanied by muscle pain. Carnitine palmityl transferase deficiency is one such condition. Other metabolic defects of muscle such as mitochondrial disorders and the purine nucleotide cycle defect, myoadenylate deaminase deficiency, may also cause episodic weakness. This latter disorder occurs in approximately 1 percent of the population but inexplicably causes symptoms in a small proportion of subjects deficient in the enzyme.

Recurrent attacks of a feeling of "weakness" often occur in patients with the *hyperventilation syndrome*; such patients are, however, of normal strength when tested. Similarly, *recurrent hypoglycemic episodes* are associated with subjective weakness though hypoglycemia is uncommon as the cause of this symptom. Central nervous system disorders infrequently cause generalized weakness without an associated alteration of consciousness. *Drop attacks* resulting from impaired blood supply to the motor pathways of the brainstem cause sudden paraparesis or quadriparesis, usually lasting only a few seconds. Patients with narcolepsy may have sudden loss of muscle strength and tone during episodes of *cataplexy*. A disorder of the reticular activating system is responsible for these episodes as well as for *sleep paralysis* that occurs as narcoleptic patients are falling asleep or awakening (see Chap. 20).

TABLE 17-1 Causes of episodic generalized weakness

Electrolyte disturbances
Hypokalemia: Primary hyperaldosteronism (Conn's syndrome); barium poisoning; primary renal tubular acidosis; renal tubular acidosis secondary to amphotericin B or toluene abuse; juxtaglomerular apparatus hyperplasia (Bartter's syndrome); villous adenoma of colon; alcoholism; diuretics; licorice; para-aminosalicylic acid; corticosteroids
Hyperkalemia: Addison's disease; chronic renal failure; hyporeninemic hypoaldosteronism; recurrent rhabdomyolysis
Hypercalcemia
Hypocalcemic tetany
Hyponatremia
Hypophosphatemia
Hypermagnesemia
Neuromuscular junction disorders
Myasthenia gravis
Eaton-Lambert syndrome
Central nervous system causes
Cataplexy and sleep paralysis associated with narcolepsy
Multiple sclerosis
Transient ischemic attacks
Disorders with only subjective weakness: hyperventilation, hypoglycemia

REFERENCES

AUGER RG et al: Hereditary form of sustained muscle activity of peripheral nerve origin causing generalized myokymia and muscle stiffness. Ann Neurol 15:13 1984

CLARK S et al: Clinical characteristics of fibrositis. II. A "blinded," controlled study using standard psychological tests. Arthritis Rheum 28:132, 1985

GRIGGS RC: The myotonic disorders and the periodic paralyses. Adv Neurol 17:143, 1977

LAYZER RB: Muscle pain, cramps and fatigue, in AG Engel, BQ Banker (eds), *Myology*. New York, McGraw-Hill, 1986

SAENZ-LOPE E et al: Hyperekplexia: A syndrome of pathological startle responses. Ann Neurol 15:36, 1985

18 NUMBNESS, TINGLING, AND OTHER ABNORMALITIES OF SENSATION

ARTHUR K. ASBURY

Normal somatic sensation is a continuous process occupying a considerable proportion of moment-to-moment nervous system activity. Little of the activity intrudes upon consciousness or exacts notice. In contrast, disordered sensation, particularly pains and paresthesias, may be highly intrusive, alarming, and tenacious and may dominate attention. Abnormalities of sensation tend to bring patients quickly to medical attention. The physician must have a framework of knowledge in order to assess abnormal sensations, estimate their likely site of origin, and recognize their implications. When abnormal sensations are perceived as painful, medical advice is even more quickly sought. For a consideration of pain, see Chap. 3.

POSITIVE AND NEGATIVE PHENOMENA It is useful to divide all abnormal sensory phenomena into two great categories, positive and negative. Positive phenomena include tingling, pins-and-needles, pricking, bandlike sensations, lightning-like shooting feelings (lancinations), aching, and knifelike, twisting, drawing, pulling, tightening, burning, searing, electrical, and raw sensations. These descriptors are frequently the actual words used by patients. Such sensations may or may not be experienced as painful. It is thought that the pathophysiologic basis of positive phenomena resides in the ectopic generation of volleys of impulses at some site of lowered neural threshold along the sensory pathways, either in peripheral or central sensory fibers. Such trains of ectopically generated afferent impulses arising from sites other than normal peripheral nerve receptors determine the quality of the abnormal sensation experienced, depending upon the number, rate, and distribution of impulses and the type and size of nerve fibers in which they arise.

Positive phenomena represent heightened activity in sensory pathways; therefore they are not in and of themselves necessarily associated with any demonstrable sensory deficit upon examination, an important point for the examiner to bear in mind.

Negative phenomena result from loss of sensory function and are characterized by numbness, or diminution or absence of feeling in a particular distribution. Negative phenomena, in contrast to positive phenomena, are accompanied by abnormal findings on sensory examination. In disorders affecting peripheral sensation, it is estimated that at least one-half of afferent fibers innervating a given site must be lost or functionless in order for sensory deficit to be demonstrated. This estimate probably varies according to how rapidly sensory fibers have lost function. If the rate of loss is slow and chronic, lack of cutaneous feeling may be difficult to demonstrate on examination, even though few sensory fibers are functioning. Rapidly evolving sensory abnormality usually evokes positive phenomena of some type and is more readily recognized by patients than insidious deafferentation. Subclinical degrees of sensory dysfunction not demonstrable on clinical sensory examination may be revealed by sensory nerve conduction studies or somatosensory cerebral evoked potentials (see Chaps. 341 and 354).

Terminology Two general types of medical terms are used to characterize abnormal sensation, those referring to symptoms of which patients complain (both positive and negative phenomena) and those describing abnormalities found on examination (only negative phenomena). *Paresthesia* and *dysesthesia* are terms used to denote positive phenomena. Paresthesia carries the implication that the abnormal sensation is perceived without an apparent stimulus; whereas dysesthesia is a more general term used to describe all types of positive sensations whether stimulus-generated or not. Abnormalities on examination are denoted by *hypesthesia* or *hypoesthesia* (reduction of cutaneous sensation to a specific type of testing such as pressure, light touch, and warm or cold stimuli), *anesthesia* (complete absence of skin sensation to the same stimuli plus pinprick), and *hypalgesia* (referring to loss of pain perception, i.e., nociception, such as the pricking quality elicited by a pin). *Hyperesthesia* connotes exaggerated perception of sensations in response to light touch or stroking of the skin. Similarly *allodynia* describes the situation in which an ordinarily nonpainful stimulus, once perceived, is experienced as painful, even excruciating. An example is elicitation of a painful sensation by application of a vibrating tuning fork. *Hyperalgesia* denotes an exaggerated response to a noxious stimulus, and *hyperpathia,* a broad term, encompasses the phenomena implied by hyperesthesia, allodynia, and hyperalgesia.

Disorders of deep sensation, arising from muscle spindles, tendons, and joints, deserve special comment. Normally these afferents subserve proprioception (position sense) and the moment-to-moment sense of the state of muscle contraction. If a significant number of these special nerve endings become denervated, the resulting manifestations include imbalance, particularly with eyes closed or in the dark, clumsiness of precision movements, and unsteadiness of gait, all of which is referred to as *sensory ataxia* (see Chap. 16). Other findings on examination are reduced or absent joint position and vibratory sensibility in the affected limbs. Romberg's sign is positive, which means that the patient sways or topples when asked to stand with feet close together and eyes closed.

In severe states of deafferentation involving deep sensation, the patient cannot walk or stand unaided, or even sit unsupported. Continuous, sometimes wormlike involuntary movements, called *pseudoathetosis,* of the hands and arms occur, particularly with eyes closed. Such patients are severely disabled.

Normal sensation Cutaneous afferent innervation is subserved by a rich variety of receptors, both naked endings (nociceptors and thermoreceptors) and encapsulated terminals (mechanoreceptors). Each has its own set of sensitivities to specific stimuli (see Table 18-1), size and distinctness of receptive fields, and adaptational qualities. Much of the knowledge about these receptors has come from the development of techniques to study single intact nerve fibers intraneurally in alert unanesthetized human subjects. It is possible not only to record from single nerve fibers, large or small, but also to stimulate single fibers in isolation. A single impulse, whether elicited by a natural stimulus or evoked ty electrical microstimulation, in a large myelinated afferent fiber may be both perceived and localized.

Afferent fibers in peripheral nerve trunks sort themselves into topographically coherent patterns as they approach the dorsal roots and enter the dorsal horn of the spinal cord. From there, the polysynaptic projections of the smaller fibers (unmyelinated and small myelinated), which in general subserve nociception and temperature sensibility, cross and ascend in the contralateral spinothalamic tract through spinal cord, through brainstem, to the ventral posterolateral nucleus (VPL) of the thalamus, and ultimately project to the postcentral gyrus of the parietal cortex (see Chap. 3). The larger fibers which subserve tactile and position sense and kinesthesia project rostrally in the ipsilateral posterior column of the spinal cord and finally make their first synapse in the gracile or cuneate nuclei of the lower medulla (see Fig. 18-1). The second-order neuron decussates and ascends in the medial lemniscus located medially in the medulla and in the tegmentum of the pons and midbrain, and synapses in VPL. The third-order neuron projects to parietal cortex; this system is referred to as *lemniscal.*

Although the fiber types and functions which make up the spinothalamic and lemniscal systems are relatively well known, it has been found that many other fibers, particularly those associated with touch, pressure, and position sense, ascend in a diffusely distributed pattern both ipsilaterally and contralaterally in the anterolateral quadrants of the spinal cord. These anatomic facts explain why an individual with a known complete lesion of the posterior columns of the spinal cord may have little sensory deficit on examination.

EXAMINATION OF SENSATION The initial step in examination of the somatosensory system is to do the tests of primary sensation,

TABLE 18-1 Human cutaneous sensory receptors*

Receptor type	Location	Activating stimulus	Afferent nerve fiber	Sensation evoked	Central pathway
Meissner's corpuscle	S	Light pressure, once or repetitive	LM	Tapping, fluttering	
Merkel's disk	S	Sustained pressure	LM	Sense of pressure	
Pacinian corpuscle	D	Light touch, once or repetitive	LM	Sense of vibration	Lemiscal
Ruffini's ending	D	Sustained, angulated pressure	LM	None, thought to be proprioceptive	
Naked ending	S	Noxious	SM	Sharp pain	
Naked ending	S	Noxious	UM	Dull pain, itch	Spinothalamic
Naked ending	S	Thermal; 34–50°C	UM	Warmth	
Naked ending	S	Thermal, range uncertain	SM	Coldness	

* *LM = large myelinated fiber; SM = small myelinated fiber; UM = unmyelinated fiber; D = deep; S = superficial.*
SOURCE: *After Lindblom and Ochoa, 1986.*

TABLE 18-2 Testing primary sensation

Sense	Test device	Endings activated	Fiber size mediating	Central pathway*
Pain	Pinprick	Cutaneous nociceptors	Small	SpTh, also D
Temperature, heat	Flask with warm water	Cutaneous thermoreceptors for hot	Small	SpTh
Temperature, cold	Flask with cold water	Cutaneous thermoreceptors for cold	Small	SpTh
Touch	Cotton wisp, fine brush	Cutaneous mechanoreceptors, also naked endings	Large and small	Lem, also D and SpTh
Vibration	Tuning fork, 128 Hz	Mechanoreceptors, especially pacinian corpuscles	Large	Lem, also D
Joint position	Passive movement of specific joints	Joint capsule and tendon endings, muscle spindles	Large	Lem, also D

* *D = diffuse ascending projections in ipsilateral and contralateral anteriolateral columns; SpTh = spinothalamic projection, contralateral; Lem = posterior column and lemniscal projection, ipsilateral.*

which by convention include the sense of pain, touch, vibration, joint position, and thermal sensation, both hot and cold. These tests have gradually become codified through tradition, but they do appear to assess, if crudely, the major afferent functions and pathways (see Table 18-2). Testing of both primary sensation and cortical sensory function can be carried out in the office or at the bedside with a minimum of special equipment.

Some general principles pertain to the sensory examination. First, it should be remembered that the examiner is depending upon subjective patient response; therefore, discriminating responses depend upon the level of alertness, motivation, and intelligence of the patient and also upon the skill with which the examiner has made the task clear. In a stupefied or obtunded patient, the examiner is reduced to observing the briskness of withdrawal and the complexity of defensive movements of the patient in response to a pinch or other noxious stimulus. In the alert but uncooperative patient, it is often possible to get some idea of proprioceptive function by observing the patient's best performance in casually observed movements requiring balance and precision, but cutaneous sensation may be unexaminable. Second, sensory examination should not be pressed if the patient is fatigued. An abbreviated survey will suffice until a more extensive examination can be carried out in the rested patient. Third, sensory examination in a patient who has no neurologic complaints should be quite abbreviated and may consist of pin, touch, and vibration testing in the hands and feet plus evaluation of station and gait including Romberg's maneuver, which also tests the integrity of motor and cerebellar systems. Fourth, patients should be tested with their eyes closed or covered during both primary sensation and cortical sensory function examination.

Primary sensation (see Table 18-2) The sense of pain is usually tested with a pin, asking the patient to focus on the pricking or unpleasant quality of the stimulus and not just the pressure or touch sensation elicited. Areas of hypalgesia should be mapped by proceeding from the most hypalgesic zones to less affected ones (see Figs. 18-2 and 18-3).

Temperature sensation, both to hot and to cold, is probably best tested by touching the skin for a couple of seconds with a water flask filled with water of the desired temperature, using a thermometer to verify the temperature. For most purposes, it is satisfactory if a patient can identify as warm the flask which is 35 or 36°C and as cool the one which is at 28 to 32°C. Between 28 and 32°C, most individuals can distinguish temperature differences in 1°C steps. Both cold and warm should be tested because different receptors respond to each.

Touch is usually tested with a wisp of cotton or a fine camel's hair brush. In general, it is better to avoid testing touch on hairy skin because of the profusion of sensory endings which surround each hair follicle. The patients, whose eyes are covered, should be asked to say "now" each time they feel the stimulus. They may also be asked to point to the site where the stimulus was felt, although this tests not only the sense of touch but also touch localization (see cortical sensory testing below).

Joint position testing is a measure of proprioception, one of the most important functions of the sensory system. Joint position is usually tested first in the great toe and in the fingers. Patients are asked to keep their eyes closed and to relax completely the part to be examined. In the case of the great toe, one starts with the toe in a neutral position and grasps it lightly between the thumb and the forefinger on either side of the toe (not top and bottom) and then the toe is moved a few degrees either in a dorsal or a plantar direction, and the patient is asked to say whether the movement was up or down. One must make sure that the patient understands that it is the direction of movement which is being tested and not the direction the toe is pointing when it stops. A patient with absence of position sense in the part being tested will have a 50 percent error rate because only two choices are available. Answers which are consistently greater

FIGURE 18-1 *Schematic diagram of lemniscal system which subserves proprioception and discriminative touch.*

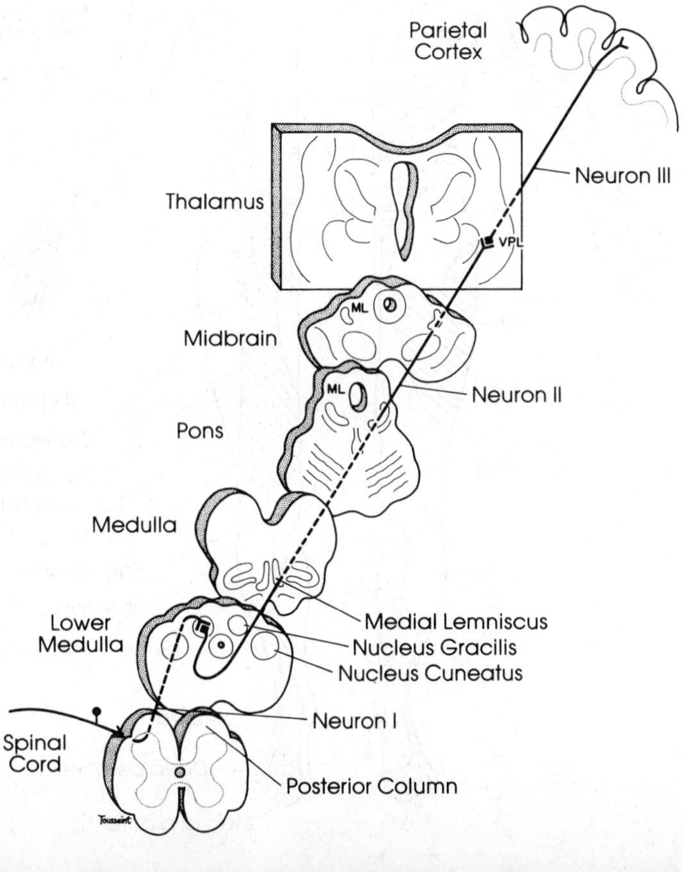

than 50 percent in error should be viewed with skepticism. If errors are made in recognizing the direction of passive movements of the toe, then passive movements of the ankle or even of the knee should be undertaken in the same way. Similarly, position sense at the proximal interphalangeal joint of the index finger may be tested, and if abnormal, other finger joints and the wrist and elbow joints should also be tested. A test of proximal joint position sense, primarily at the shoulder, can be carried out by asking the patient to bring the two index fingers together with the arms extended and the eyes closed. Normal individuals should be able to do this quite accurately with errors of a centimeter of less.

The sense of vibration is tested with a tuning fork, preferably a large one which vibrates at 128 Hz. The decay of vibration using this fork is slow enough to be of quantitative use because it requires between 15 and 20 s to decay below the threshold of perceptibility. Vibration is usually tested at bony prominences, specifically the malleoli at the ankles, the patella, the anterior iliac spine, the spinous processes of the vertebral bodies, the metacarpal-phalangeal joints (knuckles), the styloid process of the ulna, the elbow, and the acromion of the shoulder. Control sites at which to test vibration are the sternum and on the forehead. The examiner can compare the threshold at a given site for both patient and self. A crude approximation of degree of vibratory sense loss can be made by counting the seconds that the examiner can feel the sense of vibration longer than the patient. It must be clear to the patient that it is the sense of vibration and not just the pressure of the end of the tuning fork to which attention is directed.

Cortical sensation Cortical sensory testing includes two-point discrimination, touch localization, stereognosis, graphesthesia, and bilateral simultaneous stimulation, to name the most commonly used methods. Abnormalities of these sensory tests, in the presence of normal primary sensation and an alert cooperative patient, signifies a lesion of the parietal cortex or thalamocortical projections to the parietal lobe. If primary sensation is altered, it is not possible to test for these cortical discriminative functions.

Two-point discrimination is tested by special calipers whose points may be set from 2 mm to several centimeters apart and then applied simultaneously to the site to be tested. The pulp of the fingertips is a common site to test; a normal individual can distinguish about 3-mm separation of points there. One can distinguish more closely set points on the tongue and lips, but the threshold for discriminating two points may be centimeters at other sites on the body. Comparisons should always be made between analogous sites on the two sides of the body, since the deficit, with a specific parietal lesion, is likely to be hemilateral. This point holds true for all cortical sensory testing.

Touch localization is usually carried out by light pressure with the examiner's fingertip, asking the patient, whose eyes are closed, to identify the site of touch. It is usual to ask the patient to touch the same site with a fingertip. Bilateral simultaneous stimulation at

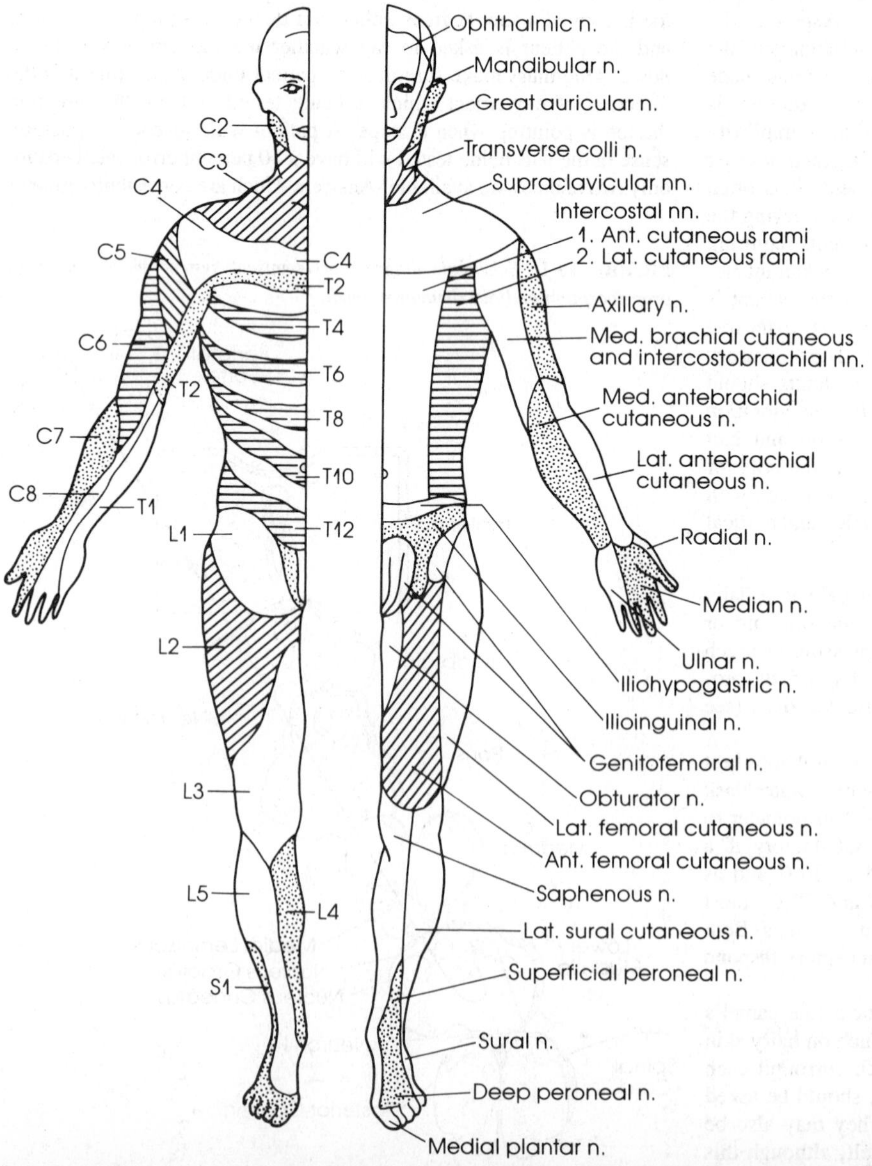

FIGURE 18-2 *Anterior view of dermatomes (left) and cutaneous areas supplied by individual peripheral nerves (right). (From MB Carpenter and J Sutin, in Human Neuroanatomy, 8th ed, Baltimore, Williams & Wilkins, 1983.)*

analogous sites (e.g., the dorsa of both hands) can be carried out to determine whether the perception of touch is extinguished consistently on one side or the other. The phenomenon is referred to as extinction on bilateral simultaneous stimulation.

Graphesthesia means the capacity to recognize letters or numbers drawn by the examiner's fingertip on various parts of the body while the patient maintains eyes closed. The usual comparison is the palm of one hand versus the palm of the other. Numbers should be drawn large enough to occupy most of the palm. Once again, the comparison of one side to the other is of prime importance. Failure to recognize numbers or letters is termed *agraphesthesia*.

Stereognosis refers to the ability to identify common objects by palpation, recognizing their shape, texture, and size. Common standard objects are the best test objects, such as a marble, a paper clip, a small rubber ball, or coins. Patients with normal stereognosis should be able to distinguish a dime from a penny and certainly a nickel from a quarter. Patients should only be allowed to feel the object with one hand at time. If they are unable to identify it in one hand, it should be placed in the other for comparison. Individuals unable to identify common objects and coins in one hand who can do so in the other are said to have *astereognosis* of the abnormal hand. Note that the major comparison is one side of the body with the other.

Localization of sensory abnormalities Peripheral neuropathies are generally graded, distal, and symmetric in their distribution of deficit. Although most peripheral neuropathies are pansensory and affect all modalities of sensation, selective sensory dysfunction according to nerve fiber size may occur. In small fiber neuropathies, the hallmark is burning, painful dysesthesias with reduced pinprick and thermal sensation but with sparing of proprioception, motor function, and even deep tendon jerks. Touch is variably involved, but when spared, the sensory pattern is referred to as sensory dissociation (see below). In contrast to small fiber neuropathies, large fiber neuropathies are characterized by position sense deficit, imbalance, absent tendon jerks, variable motor dysfunction, but preservation of most cutaneous sensation and few or no dysesthesias.

Paresthesias and dysesthesias may be of either peripheral nerve or spinal cord origin, and probably can arise in the brainstem, but in every instance are thought to represent abnormal showers of impulses generated from an ectopic focus or foci. By themselves, paresthesias may not be localizable, but when accompanied by other signs of neuropathy or of myelopathy, the correct site of origin may be deduced.

Dissociated sensory deficit patterns, in which pinprick and thermal sensation is lost but touch is spared, are usually a sign of spinothalamic tract involvement in the spinal cord, especially if the deficit is unilateral and has an upper level on the torso. Bilateral spinothalamic tract involvement occurs with lesions affecting the center of the spinal cord, such as happens with expansion of the central canal in hydromyelia or syringomyelia. Sensory dissociation may also occur

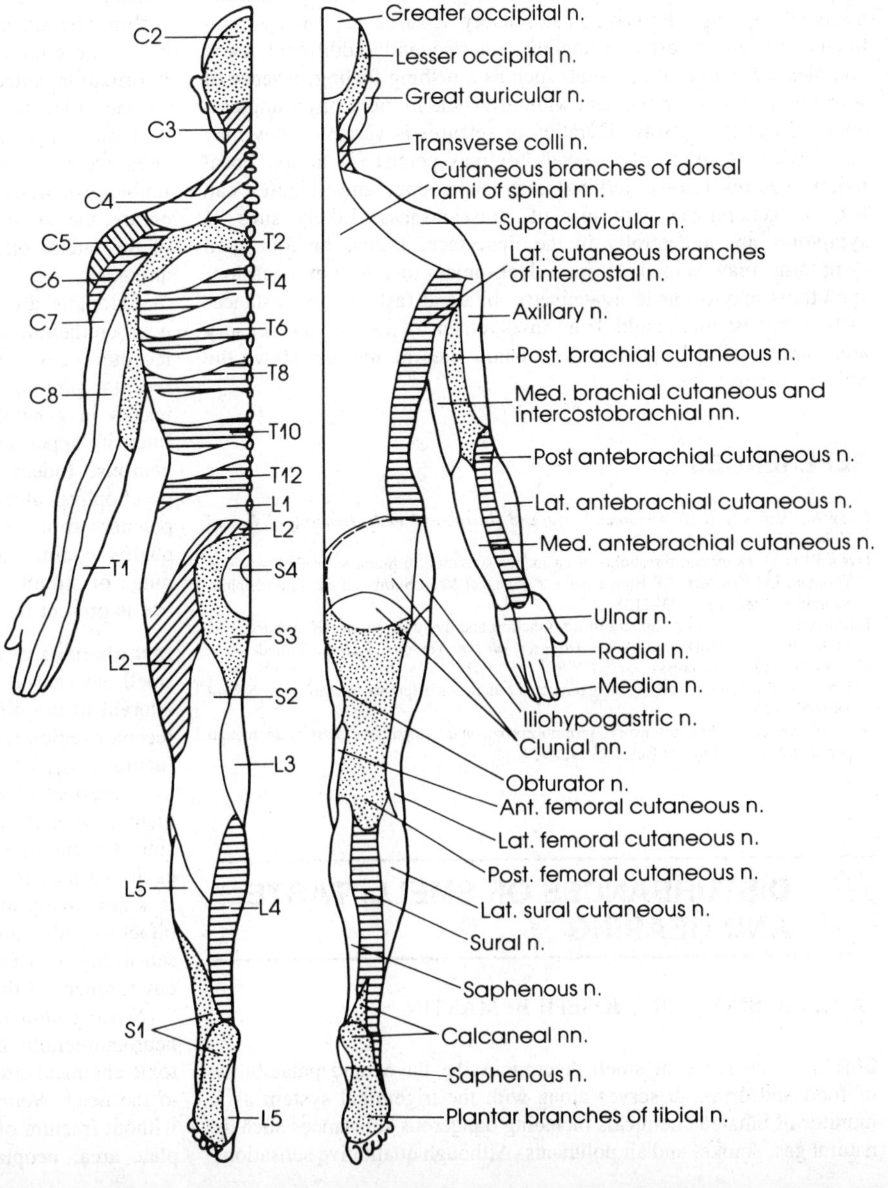

FIGURE 18-3 *Posterior view of dermatomes (left) and cutaneous areas supplied by individual peripheral nerves (right). (From MB Carpenter and J Sutin, in Human Neuroanatomy, 8th ed, Baltimore, Williams & Wilkins, 1983.)*

in peripheral neuropathies in which afferent cutaneous nerve fibers of small diameter are preferentially affected. Neuropathies in which sensory dissociation may occur include leprous neuritis, hereditary sensory neuropathy, and certain cases of amyloid and diabetic polyneuropathy (see Chap. 355).

Hemisensory disturbance with tingling numbness from head to foot is usually thalamic in origin. If abrupt in onset, the thalamic lesion is likely to be due to a small stroke (lacunar infarction). Occasionally, with lesions affecting the posterolateral thalamus (VPL) or adjacent white matter, a syndrome of thalamic pain, also called Déjerine-Roussy syndrome, may ensue. This is a persistent unrelenting hemipainful state often described in dramatic terms such as ''like the flesh is being torn from my limbs'' or ''as though that side is bathed in acid'' (see Chap. 3). Harlequin patterns of sensory disturbance, in which one side of the face and the opposite side of the body are affected, localize to the lateral medulla where a small lesion may damage both the ipsilateral descending trigeminal tract and ascending spinothalamic fibers (lateral lemniscus) subserving the opposite arm, leg, and hemitorso (see ''Lateral Medulla Syndrome,'' Chap. 343).

With lesions of the parietal lobe, either of the cortex or subjacent white matter, the most prominent symptoms are contralateral hemineglect, hemi-inattention, and a tendency not to use the opposite hand and arm. Tests of primary sensation are usually normal or minimally altered, but tests of cortical sensation are often severely abnormal (see Chap. 24). Dysesthesias or even a sense of numbness are unusual except in the special circumstance of focal sensory seizures. These are generally due to lesions in or near the postcentral gyrus. Symptoms of focal somatosensory seizures are usually combinations of numbness and tingling, but frequently additional, more complex sensations are present, such as a rushing feeling, a sense of warmth, a sense of movement without visible motion, or an unpleasantly dysesthetic quality. Duration of seizures is variable; they may be transient, lasting only seconds, or may persist for hours. Focal motor features (clonic jerking) may supervene, and seizures can become generalized with loss of consciousness. Likely sites of symptoms are unilaterally in the lips, face, digits, or foot, and symptoms may spread as in a Jacksonian march. On occasion, symptoms may occur in a symmetric bilateral fashion, for instance, in both hands; this results from involvement of the second sensory area (unilaterally) located in the rolandic area at and just above the Sylvian fissure.

REFERENCES

Culp W, Ochoa JL (eds): *Abnormal Nerves and Muscles as Impulse Generators*. Oxford University, New York, 1982

Dyck PJ et al: Detection thresholds of cutaneous sensation in humans, in PJ Dyck, PK Thomas, EH Lambert, RP Bunge (eds), *Peripheral Neuropathy*, 2d ed. Philadelphia, Saunders, 1984, pp 1103–1138

Lindblom U, Ochoa JL: Somatosensory function and dysfunction; in AK Asbury, GM McKhann, WI McDonald (eds), *Diseases of the Nervous System*, Philadelphia, Saunders, 1986, (in press)

Mackel R: Single unit analysis of regenerated cutaneous afferents in man. Ann Neurol 18:165, 1985

Vallbo AB et al: Somatosensory, proprioceptive, and sympathetic activity in human peripheral nerve. Physiol Rev 59:919, 1979

19 DISTURBANCES OF SMELL, TASTE, AND HEARING

JAMES B. SNOW, JR. / JOSEPH B. MARTIN

SMELL The sense of smell determines the flavor and palatability of food and drink. It serves along with the trigeminal system as a monitor of inhaled chemicals including dangerous substances such as natural gas, smoke, and air pollutants. Although qualitative sensations of smell are subserved by the olfactory neuroepithelium, many substances are capable of producing somatic sensations of coolness, warmth, and irritation through the trigeminal, facial, glossopharyngeal, and vagal afferents in the nose, oral cavity, tongue, pharynx, and larynx. The sense of smell should be considered as one of several chemosensory systems since most chemical substances initiate olfactory, trigeminal, and taste perceptions.

The *olfactory neuroepithelium* is located in the superior part of the nasal cavities. It contains an orderly arrangement of bipolar olfactory receptor cells, microvillar cells, sustentacular cells, and basal cells. The dendritic process of the bipolar cell has a bulb-shaped knob or vesicle that projects into the mucous layer and bears 10 to 20 cilia. The receptor sites for odorant molecules are located on the cilia. The microvillar cells are located adjacent to the receptor cells on the surface of the neuroepithelium. The sustentacular cells, unlike their counterparts in the respiratory epithelium, are not specialized to secrete mucus. Their function is unknown. The basal cells are progenitors of other cell types in the olfactory neuroepithelium including the bipolar receptor cells. There is a regular turnover of the bipolar receptor cells, which function as the primary sensory neurons. In addition with injury to the cell body or its axon, the receptor cell is replaced by a basal cell which reestablishes a central neural connection. *Hence, these primary sensory neurons are unique among sensory systems in that they are regularly replaced and regenerate after injury.*

The unmyelinated axons of the receptor cells form the fila of the olfactory nerve, pass through the cribriform plate, and terminate within spherical masses of neuropil, termed glomeruli, in the olfactory bulb. The glomeruli are a focus of a high degree of convergence of information, since many more fibers enter than leave them. The main second-order neurons are the mitral cells. The primary dendrite of each mitral cell extends into a single glomerulus. Axons of the mitral cells project along with the axons of adjacent tufted cells to the limbic system, including the anterior olfactory nucleus, the prepiriform cortex, the periamygdaloid cortex, the olfactory tubercle, the nucleus of the lateral olfactory tract, and the corticomedial nucleus of the amygdala.

Odorants are absorbed into the mucus overlying the olfactory neuroepithelium, diffuse to the cilia, and reversibly bind to membrane receptor sites. The process causes conformational changes in the receptor proteins which induce a chain of biochemical events that results in generation of action potentials in the primary neurons. Intensity appears to be coded by the amount of firing in the afferent neurons. Indeed, a clear relationship exists in humans between psychophysical measures of intensity and the magnitude of the evoked potential from the olfactory neuroepithelium. Little is known about quality coding. Individual receptor cells are responsive to a wide range of stimuli. It is thought that more than one type of receptor site is present on each cell.

Disturbances of the sense of smell Disturbances of the sense of smell are caused by conditions that interfere with the access of the odorant to the olfactory neuroepithelium (transport loss), injure the receptor region (sensory loss), or damage central olfactory pathways (neural loss).

Transport olfactory loss can result from swollen nasal mucous membrane in acute viral upper respiratory infections, bacterial rhinitis, sinusitis, and allergic rhinitis and with structural changes in the nasal cavity such as deviations of the nasal septum, polyps, and neoplasms. It is also likely that abnormalities of mucous secretion in which the olfactory cilia are immersed could result in a loss of olfactory sensitivity. Currently little is known about alterations in the mucous environment of the olfactory neuroepithelium.

Sensory olfactory losses are caused by destruction of the olfactory neuroepithelium by viral infections, neoplasms, the inhalation of toxic chemicals, drugs that affect cell turnover, and radiation therapy to the head. *Neural olfactory losses* occur in head trauma, with or without fracture of the base of the anterior cranial fossa or cribriform plate area, neoplasms of the anterior cranial fossa, neurosurgical procedures, administration of neurotoxic drugs, and in some congenital disorders such as Kallmann's syndrome.

From the psychophysical point of view, disturbances of the sense of smell may be categorized by either the patient's complaint or the objective sensory measurements as *total anosmia* (general anosmia)—inability to detect any qualitative olfactory sensations; *partial anosmia*—ability to detect some, but not all, qualitative olfactory sensations; *specific anosmia*—loss of ability to appreciate only one or a very limited number of odorants; *total hyposmia* (general hyposmia)—decreased sensitivity to all odorants; *partial hyposmia*—decreased sensitivity to some odorants; dysosmia (cacosmia or paraosmia)—distortion in the perception of an odor, that is, the perception of an unpleasant odor when a pleasant odorant is being presented or the perception of an odor when there is no odorant in the environment; *total hyperosmia* (general hyperosmia)—increased sensitivity to all odorants; *partial hyperosmia*—increased sensitivity to some odorants; and *agnosia*—inability to classify, contrast, or identify odor sensations verbally, even though the ability to distinguish between odorants or to recognize them may be normal.

CLINICAL EVALUATION The history of the onset and development of the disturbance of the sense of smell may be of paramount importance in making an etiologic diagnosis. Unilateral anosmia is rarely a complaint. Only by separate testing of smell in each nasal cavity can it be recognized. Bilateral anosmia, on the other hand, does bring patients to medical attention. The usual complaint is of a loss of taste, because taste to a large extent depends on the volatile substances in food, and the sensation of flavor is a combination of smell and taste. The physical examination should include a complete examination of the ears, upper respiratory tract, and head and neck. A neurologic examination emphasizing the cranial nerves is essential. Computerized tomography scans of the head with enhancement is required to rule out neoplasms of the anterior cranial fossa, unsuspected fractures of the anterior cranial fossa, paranasal sinusitis, and neoplasms of the nasal cavity and paranasal sinuses.

The sensory evaluation of olfactory function is necessary for corroboration of the patient's complaint, evaluation of the efficacy of treatment, and determination of the degree of permanent impairment. The first step in the sensory evaluation is to determine the degree to which qualitative sensations are present. For this assessment, a smell identification test is used that consists of a 40-item, forced choice, microencapsulated odor, scratch-and-sniff paradigm. For example, one of the items reads, "This odor smells most like (a) chocolate, (b) banana, (c) onion, or (d) fruit punch," and the patient is instructed to answer one of the alternatives. The test is highly reliable (short-term test-retest reliability $r = 0.95$) and is sensitive to age and sex differences (Fig. 19-1). It is an accurate quantitative determination of the relative degree of olfactory deficit. Persons with a total loss of smell function score in the range of 7 to 19 out of 40. The average score for total anosmics is slightly higher than that expected on the basis of chance because of the inclusion of some odorants which act by trigeminal stimulation.

The second step is to establish a detection threshold for the odorant phenylethyl alcohol, using a graduated stimulus. Although the detection threshold usually agrees with the results of the smell identification test, in some instances patients who fail the smell identification test perform well on the threshold test. However, the reverse is much less common. Since the threshold test can be influenced by trigeminal and nonolfactory nerve clues, the results of the smell identification test are relied upon more heavily in the sensory evaluation.

Techniques have been developed to biopsy the olfactory neuroepithelium but in view of the widespread degeneration of the olfactory neuroepithelium and intercalation of respiratory epithelium in the olfactory area of adults with no apparent olfactory dysfunction, biopsy material must be interpreted cautiously.

DIFFERENTIAL DIAGNOSIS At the present time there are no psychophysical methods to differentiate sensory from neural olfactory losses. Fortunately, the history of the disease provides important clues to the cause. The leading causes of olfactory disorders are head trauma and viral infections. Head trauma is a more frequent cause of anosmia in children and young adults, and viral infections are more important causes of anosmia in older adults.

Cranial trauma is followed by uni- or bilateral impairment of smell in 5 to 10 percent of cases. Frontal injuries and fractures disrupt the cribriform plate and olfactory axons which perforate it. Sometimes there is an associated cerebrospinal fluid (CSF) rhinorrhea resulting from a tearing of the dura overlying the paranasal sinuses. If the anosmia is unilateral, it is usually on the side of the CSF leak, and this fact aids in localization of the fistula. Anosmia may also follow blows to the occiput. Once traumatic anosmia develops, it is usually permanent; only about 10 percent of patients ever improve or recover. Perversion of the sense of smell may occur as a phase in the recovery process.

The occurrence of a permanent hyposmia or anosmia may follow viral infections and is called *postviral anosmia*. In this instance the sensory epithelium of the olfactory zone is destroyed by the virus and replaced by respiratory epithelial and goblet cells and scar tissue. The congenital anosmias, one type of which is associated with a

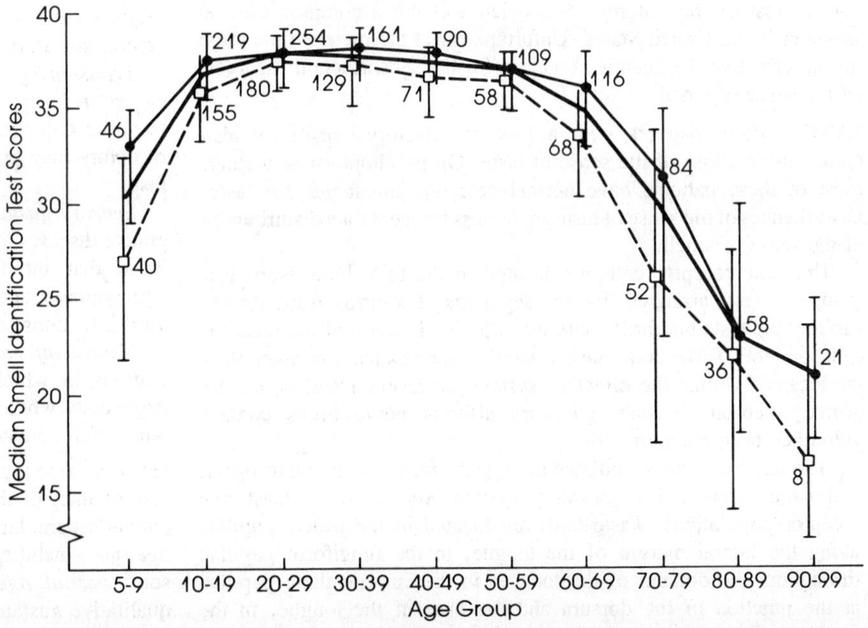

FIGURE 19-1 *Smell identification test. Scores for a group of male and female subjects 5 to 99 years in age are shown.* ●——●*: Females (n = 1158);* □-----□*: males (n = 797);* ——*: total group (n = 1955). (Reprinted with permission from RL Doty et al. Copyright 1984 by the AAAS.)*

hypothalamic defect (Kallmann's syndrome, or congenital anosmia with hypogonadotropic hypogonadism), are rare but important causes of anosmia or hyposmia. Anosmia can also occur in albinos. The receptor cells are present but hypoplastic, lack cilia, and do not project above the surrounding supporting cells.

Meningioma of the inferior frontal region is the most frequent neoplastic cause of anosmia; rarely anosmia can occur with glioma of the frontal lobe. Occasionally pituitary adenomas, craniopharyngiomas, suprasellar meningiomas, and aneurysms of the anterior part of the circle of Willis extend forward and damage olfactory structures. These tumors and hamartomas may also induce seizures with olfactory hallucinations, indicating involvement of the uncus.

Paraosmia and dysosmia, subjective distortions of olfactory perception, may occur with intranasal disease that partially impairs smell, or may represent a phase in the recovery from a neurogenic anosmia. Most paraosmic disturbances consist of disagreeable or foul odors, and they may be accompanied by distortions of taste. Dysosmia may also be a symptom in elderly patients with depression. Every article of food has an extremely unpleasant odor (cacosmia). Sensations of disagreeable taste are often noted (cacogeusia).

Olfactory hallucinations are descriptions of smelling an odor that no one else can smell. They occur in alcohol withdrawal, in which olfactory hallucinations are occasionally associated with other types of hallucinations, and in uncal seizures, which are brief and clearly related to a derangement of consciousness and other epileptic components. In other settings, olfactory hallucinations usually signify a psychiatric disease. A huge range of odors may be reported, most of them foul. Some patients perceive the smell as emanating from themselves (intrinsic); others perceive the source to be external (extrinsic). Most are associated with schizophrenia and depressive illnesses.

TREATMENT Therapy for patients with transport olfactory losses due to allergic rhinitis, bacterial rhinitis and sinusitis, polyps, neoplasms, and structural abnormalities of the nasal cavities can be undertaken rationally and with a high chance of improvement. Allergic management, antibiotic therapy, topical and systemic corticosteroid therapy, and operations for nasal polyps, deviation of the nasal septum, and chronic hyperplastic sinusitis are frequently effective in restoring the sense of smell.

There is no treatment with demonstrated efficacy for sensorineural olfactory losses. Fortunately spontaneous recovery often occurs. Zinc and vitamin therapy are advocated by some. Profound zinc deficiency can undoubtedly result in losses and distortion of the sense of smell, but it is not a clinical problem except in very limited geographic areas. Vitamin therapy has mainly been in the form of vitamin A. The epithelial degeneration associated with vitamin A deficiency can cause anosmia, but vitamin A deficiency is not a common clinical problem in the United States. Unfortunately at the present time there are no effective therapeutic strategies for the sensorineural disorders of the sense of smell.

TASTE Many patients with a loss of olfactory sensitivity also complain of a loss of the sense of taste. On psychophysical testing, most of these patients have normal detection thresholds for taste. Disturbances of the sense of taste are far less frequent than disturbances of the sense of smell.

The taste receptor cells are located in the taste buds, spherical groups of cells arranged like the segments of a citrus fruit. At the surface, the taste bud has a pore into which microvilli of the receptor cells project. Taste buds have a similar appearance wherever they are located. Unlike the olfactory system the receptor cell is not the primary neuron. Instead, gustatory afferent nerve fibers contact individual taste receptor cells.

The sense of taste is mediated through the facial, glossopharyngeal, and vagal nerves. The gustatory system consists of at least five receptor populations. Taste buds are located in the foliate papillae along the lateral margin of the tongue, in the fungiform papillae throughout the dorsum of the tongue, in the circumvallate papillae at the junction of the dorsum and the base of the tongue, in the palate, and in the epiglottis. The chorda tympani branch of the facial nerve subserves taste from the lateral margin of the tongue, while the greater superficial petrosal branch of the facial nerve carries the taste afferents from the dorsum of the tongue and the palate. The lingual branch of the glossopharyngeal nerve subserves taste from the circumvallate papillae, and the internal branch of the superior laryngeal nerve of the vagus nerve contains the taste afferents from the epiglottis.

The central connections of the nerves terminate in the brainstem in the nucleus of the tractus solitarius. The fibers of the chorda tympani and greater superficial petrosal nerves go to the cephalic portion of the nucleus. The glossopharyngeal gustatory fibers go to the middle, and the superior laryngeal nerve fibers to the caudal portion of the nucleus. The central pathway from the nucleus of the tractus solitarius projects to the ipsilateral parabrachial nuclei of the pons. Two divergent pathways project from the parabrachial nuclei. One ascends to the gustatory relay in the dorsal thalamus, synapses, and continues to the cortex of the insula. There is also evidence for a direct pathway from the parabrachial nuclei to the cortex. (Olfaction and taste appear to be unique among sensory systems in that at least some fibers bypass the thalamus.) The other pathway from the parabrachial nuclei goes to the ventral forebrain including the lateral hypothalamus, substantia innominata, central nucleus of the amygdala, and the stria terminalis.

Tastants gain access to the receptor cells through the taste pore. Four classes of taste are recognized: sweet, salt, sour, and bitter. Individual gustatory afferent fibers almost always respond to a number of different chemicals. Response patterns of gustatory afferent axons can be grouped into classes based on the stimulus chemical that produces the largest response. For example, for sucrose-best response neurons, the second-best stimulus is almost always sodium chloride. The fact that individual gustatory afferent fibers respond to a large number of different chemicals led to the *across-fiber-pattern* theory of gustatory coding, while the best-stimulus analysis led to the concept of *labeled* afferents. It appears that labeled fibers are important for establishing gross quality, but the across-fiber-pattern within a best-stimulus category, and perhaps among categories, is needed for discriminating chemicals within qualities. For example, sweetness may be carried by sucrose-best neurons, but the differentiation of sucrose and fructose may require a comparison of the relative activity among sucrose-best, salt-best, and quinine-best neurons. As with olfaction and other sensory systems, intensity appears to be encoded by the quantity of neural activity.

Disturbances of the sense of taste Disturbances of the sense of taste are caused by conditions that interfere with the access of the tastant to the receptor cells in the taste bud (transport loss), injure receptor cells (sensory loss), or damage gustatory afferent nerves and central gustatory pathways (neural loss).

Transport gustatory losses result from xerostomia due to many causes including Sjögren's syndrome, heavy metal intoxication, and bacterial colonization of the taste pore. The salivary milieu of the receptors may prove to be important to diverse causes of gustatory loss.

Sensory gustatory losses are caused by inflammatory and degenerative diseases in the oral cavity, a vast number of drugs, particularly those that interfere with cell turnover such as antithyroid and antineoplastic agents, radiation therapy to the oral cavity and pharynx, viral infections, endocrine disorders, neoplasms, and aging.

Neural olfactory losses occur with neoplasms, trauma, and operations in which the gustatory afferents are injured. Taste buds degenerate when their gustatory afferents are transected but remain when their somatosensory afferents are severed.

CLINICAL MANIFESTATIONS From the psychophysical point of view disturbances of the sense of taste may be categorized by either the patient's complaint or the objective sensory measurements as *total ageusia*—inability to detect the qualities of sweet, salty, bitter, or sour; *partial ageusia*—ability to detect some but not all of the qualitative gustatory sensations; *specific ageusia*—inability to detect the taste quality of certain substances; *total hypoguesia*—decreased sensitivity to all tastants; *partial hypogeusia*—decreased sensitivity to some tastants; *dysgeusia*—distortion in the perception of a tastant, that is, the perception of the wrong quality when a tastant is presented or the perception of a taste when there has been no tastant ingested. Confusions of sour and bitter are common and, at times, may be semantic misunderstandings. Frequently, however, they have physiologic or pathophysiologic bases.

It may be possible to differentiate between the loss of flavor recognition in patients with olfactory losses who complain of a loss of taste as well as smell by asking if they are able to taste sweetness in sodas, saltiness in potato chips, etc.

Patients who complain of loss of taste should be evaluated psychophysically for gustatory function in addition to being evaluated for olfactory function. The first step is to perform suprathreshold whole-mouth taste testing for quality, intensity, and pleasantness perception with sucrose, citric acid, quinine hydrochloride, and sodium chloride. In the quantification of the sense of taste, detection thresholds are obtained by applying graduated dilutions to the tongue quadrants or by whole-mouth sips. Finally suprathreshold magnitude estimation may be used to shed further light on the patient's complaint. Electric taste testing (electrogustometry) lacks sufficient specificity, validity, and reliability for routine clinical taste evaluations at the present time.

Biopsy of the foliate or fungiform papillae for histopathologic study of taste buds remains experimental but holds promise of shedding light on the categorization of taste disorders.

DIFFERENTIAL DIAGNOSIS As with olfaction, psychophysical methods for differentiating transport, sensory, and neural gustatory losses are not available. Once there is objective evidence of a disorder of taste, it is important to establish, as is done in other neurologic deficits, an anatomic diagnosis before proceeding to an etiologic diagnosis. The history of the disease often provides important clues to the cause. For example, absence of taste on the anterior two-thirds of the tongue associated with a facial paralysis indicates that the lesion is proximal to the point of junction of the chorda tympani branch with the facial nerve (near the inner ear).

TREATMENT Therapy for gustatory losses remains limited. Artifical saliva benefits some patients with a disturbed salivary milieu. Treatment for bacterial and fungal infections of the oral cavity are appropriate and may be helpful. Withdrawal of drugs affecting cell turnover are usually helpful if the patient's general condition permits. Zinc and vitamin therapy for gustatory losses are advocated by some, but lack demonstrated efficacy. No therapeutic strategies exist for the sensorineural disorders of taste.

HEARING Hearing occurs by air conduction and bone conduction. In air conduction, sound waves reach the ear by propagation in air, enter the external auditory canal, and set the tympanic membrane in motion, which in turn moves the malleus, incus, and stapes. Movement of the footplate of the stapes causes pressure changes in the fluid-filled inner ear eliciting a traveling wave in the basilar membrane of the cochlea. The traveling wave moves from the base to the apex of the cochlea. Hairs of the hair cells of the organ of Corti, which rests on the basilar membrane, are imbedded in the tectorial membrane and are deformed by the traveling wave. A point of maximal displacement of the basilar membrane determined by the frequency of the stimulating tone occurs with each traveling wave. High-frequency tones cause maximal displacement of the basilar membrane near the base of the cochlea. As the frequency of the stimulating tone decreases, the point of maximal displacement moves toward the apex of the cochlea. Hearing by bone conduction occurs when the sounding source, in contact with the head, results in vibration of the bones of the skull including the temporal bone, producing a traveling wave in the basilar membrane.

The deformation of the hairs of the hair cells produces several bioelectric phenomena. The cochlear microphonic, an alternating current response that faithfuly represents the frequency and intensity of the stimulating tone, occurs about 0.5 ms prior to the eighth nerve action potential. This latency is taken as evidence for release of an as yet unidentified neurotransmitter at the hair cell and cochlear nerve dendrite interface. Each of the cochlear nerve neurons can be activated at a frequency and intensity specific for that cell. This phenomenon of the characteristic or best frequency occurs at each point of the central auditory pathway: superior olivary complex, lateral lemniscus, inferior colliculus, medial geniculate body, and auditory cortex. At low frequencies, individual auditory nerve fibers can respond more or less synchronously with the stimulating tone. At higher frequencies, phase-locking occurs so that neurons take turns in responding to particular phases of the cycle of the sound wave. Intensity is encoded by the amount of neural activity in individual neurons, the number of neurons that are active, and the specific neurons that are activated.

Disturbances of the sense of hearing A loss of hearing can result from lesions in the external auditory canal, middle ear, inner ear, or central auditory pathways. Lesions in the external auditory canal or the middle ear cause conductive hearing losses while lesions in the inner ear or eighth nerve cause sensorineural hearing losses.

Conductive hearing losses result from obstruction of the external auditory canal by cerumen, debris and foreign bodies, swelling of the lining of the canal, and stenosis and neoplasms of the canal. Perforations of the tympanic membrane, as in chronic otitis media, disruption of the ossicular chain, as occurs with necrosis of the long process of the incus in trauma or infection, fixation of the ossicles as in otosclerosis, and fluid, scarring, or neoplasms in the middle ear also result in conductive hearing losses. *Sensory hearing losses* are due principally to damage to the hair cells of the organ of Corti caused by intense noise, viral infections, ototoxic drugs, fractures of the temporal bone, meningitis, cochlear otosclerosis, Ménière's disease, and aging. Neural hearing losses are due mainly to cerebellar angle tumors such as acoustic neurinomas, but may also result from any neoplastic, vascular, demyelinating, or degenerative disease affecting the central auditory pathways.

CLINICAL EVALUATION OF HEARING The physical examination should evaluate the external ear canal and tympanic membrane. Careful inspection of the nose, nasopharynx, and the upper respiratory tract is indicated. The other nerves should be carefully evaluated. Conductive and sensorineural hearing losses can be differentiated by comparing the threshold of hearing by air conduction with that elicited by bone conduction. Testing the hearing by air conduction is accomplished by presenting the stimulus in air. Hearing by air conduction is affected by the patency of the external auditory canal, the efficiency of the middle ear, and the integrity of the inner ear, eighth nerve, and the central auditory pathways. Testing the hearing by bone conduction is accomplished by placing an oscillator or the stem of a vibrating tuning fork in contact with the head. Hearing by bone conduction bypasses the external auditory canal and middle ear and tests the integrity of the inner ear, eighth nerve, and central auditory pathways. If air conduction thresholds are elevated and bone conduction thresholds are in the normal range, the lesion causing hearing loss is in the external auditory canal or middle ear. If both air conduction and bone conduction thresholds are elevated, the lesion is in the inner ear, eighth nerve, or central auditory pathways. Of course, conductive and sensorineural hearing losses can coexist, in which case both the air conduction and bone conduction thresholds are elevated, but in this case, air conduction thresholds are elevated more than bone conduction thresholds.

The Weber and Rinne tuning fork tests are used to differentiate conductive from sensorineural hearing losses. Weber's test is performed by placing the stem of a vibrating tuning fork on the head in the midline and asking the patient whether the tone is heard in both ears or better in one ear than in the other. With a unilateral conductive hearing loss, the tone is perceived in the affected ear. With a unilateral sensorineural hearing loss, the tone is perceived in the unaffected ear. Rinne's test compares the ability to hear by air conduction with the ability to hear by bone conduction. The tines of a vibrating tuning fork are held near the opening of the external auditory canal and then the stem is placed on the mastoid process. The patient is asked to indicate whether the tone is louder by air conduction or bone conduction. Normally a tone is heard louder by air conduction than by bone conduction. With a conductive hearing loss, the bone conduction stimulus is perceived as louder than the air conduction stimulus. With sensorineural hearing losses, both air and bone conduction perception are reduced, but the air conduction stimulus is perceived as louder, as it is in normal hearing. The combined information from the Weber and Rinne tests permits a tentative conclusion as to whether a conductive or sensorineural hearing loss is present.

Measurement of hearing Quantification of hearing loss is obtained with an audiometer, an electronic device that allows the presentation of specific frequencies at specific intensities to each ear by either air or bone conduction. The testing is done in a sound-attenuated chamber, and masking, usually with broad-spectrum noise, is presented to the nontest ear so that responses are based on perception from the ear under test. Frequencies from 250 to 8000 Hz are used in clinical testing. The responses are measured in decibels. A decibel (dB) is equal to 10 times the logarithm of the ratio of the acoustic power required to achieve threshold in the patient to the acoustic power required to achieve threshold in a normal hearing person. An audiogram is a plot of intensity in decibels versus frequency.

The audiometric pattern of hearing loss is often of diagnostic value. Conductive hearing losses usually have a fairly equal threshold elevation for each frequency. Conductive hearing losses with a large mass component, as is often seen in middle ear effusions, have a greater elevation of thresholds in the higher frequencies. Conductive hearing losses with a large stiffness component, as in fixation of the footplate of the stapes in early otosclerosis, have a greater elevation of thresholds in the lower frequencies. In general, sensorineural hearing losses tend to have a greater threshold elevation at each higher frequency. Interesting exceptions to this generalization are noise-induced hearing loss, in which the loss at 4000 Hz is greater than it is at higher frequencies, and in Ménière's disease, particularly in the early stages of the disease, where thresholds are elevated more in lower than in higher frequencies.

Speech audiometry provides essential additional information. The *spondee threshold*, defined as the intensity at which speech is recognized as a meaningful symbol, is obtained by presenting through an audiometer two-syllable words with an equal accent on each syllable. The intensity at which the patient can repeat 50 percent of the words correctly is the spondee threshold and usually approximates the average threshold at the speech frequencies (500, 1000, and 2000 Hz). Once the spondee threshold is determined, the discrimination ability is tested by presenting one-syllable words at 25 to 40 dB above the spondee threshold. An individual with normal hearing can repeat 90 to 100 percent of the words correctly. Likewise, individuals with a conductive hearing loss do well in discrimination testing. On the other hand, patients with a sensorineural hearing loss have a loss of discrimination attributable to the loss of peripheral analysis of sound in the inner ear or eighth nerve. With a lesion in the inner ear, the discrimination is moderately affected, usually in the 50 to 80 percent range, while with neural lesions the discrimination is severely affected, often in the 0 to 50 percent range.

The discrimination testing may then be done at higher intensities than 25 to 40 dB above the spondee threshold to determine the performance-intensity function. A deterioration in discrimination ability at higher intensities suggests a lesion in the eighth nerve or central auditory pathways.

Tympanometry measures the impedance of the middle ear to sound. A sounding source and microphone are introduced into the ear canal with an airtight seal. The amount of sound that is absorbed through the middle ear or reflected from the middle ear is measured at the microphone. In conductive hearing losses, more sound is reflected than in the normal middle ear. The pressure in the ear canal can be increased or decreased from atmospheric pressure. Normallly the middle ear is most compliant at atmospheric pressure. With a negative pressure in the middle ear as with eustachian tube obstruction, the point of maximal compliance occurs with negative pressure in the ear canal. With discontinuity of the ossicular chain, no point of maximal compliance can be obtained. Tympanometry is particularly useful in the identification and diagnosis of middle ear effusions in children.

During tympanometry, an intense tone (80 dB above the hearing threshold) elicits contraction of the stapedius muscle. The change in compliance of the middle ear with contraction of the stapedius muscle can be detected. The presence or absence of this *acoustic reflex* is important in the anatomic localization of facial nerve paralysis. The presence or absence of *acoustic reflex decay* helps differentiate sensory from neural hearing losses. In neural hearing loss, the reflex adapts or decays with time.

In order to evaluate a patient with a loss of hearing the minimum audiologic assessment should include the measurement of pure tone air and bone conduction thresholds, spondee threshold, discrimination score, performance-intensity function, tympanometry, acoustic reflexes, and acoustic reflex decay. This information provides a comprehensive screening evaluation of the whole auditory system and allows one to determine whether further differentiation of a sensory from a neural hearing loss is indicated.

In addition to these tests, testing for recruitment, the short increment sensitivity index, tone decay, Békésy audiometry, and brainstem auditory evoked responses (BAERs) help differentiate sensory from neural hearing losses. Of these, BAERs are the most powerful means of differentiating the site of sensorineural hearing loss (see Chap. 341). In response to sound, five distinct waves can be recorded with computer averaging from scalp surface electrodes. Poor or absent waveforms, abnormal latency of waves, and abnormal interwave latency are evidence of lesions in the eighth nerve and brainstem. In addition BAERs are valuable in situations in which patients cannot or will not give reliable voluntary thresholds. It also is used to monitor the integrity of the auditory nerve and brainstem intraoperatively and in determination of brain death.

CLINICAL ASSESSMENT OF A COMPLAINT OF HEARING LOSS In evaluating patients who complain of loss of hearing, associated symptoms of tinnitus, vertigo, earache, otorrhea, and aural fullness should be sought along with a careful reconstruction of the history of evolution of the hearing deficit. A sudden onset of unilateral hearing loss, with or without tinnitus, may represent a viral infection in the inner ear. Gradual progression in a hearing deficit is common with otosclerosis, schwannoma of the acoustic nerve, or Ménière's disease. In the latter case, intermittent tinnitus and dizziness are usual. Hearing loss can occur with demyelinative lesions in the brainstem. Hearing loss is a hallmark of several genetic diseases, some with onset at birth, others occurring in children or adults (see Konigsmark for review).

Tinnitus is defined as the perception of a sound when there is no sound in the environment. It may have a buzzing, roaring, or ringing quality and may be pulsatile (synchronous with the heartbeat). Tinnitus is usually associated with a conductive or sensorineural loss of hearing. The pathophysiology of tinnitus is not well understood. The cause of the tinnitus can usually be determined by finding the cause of the associated hearing loss. Tinnitus may be the first symptom of a serious condition such as an acoustic schwannoma. Pulsatile tinnitus requires evaluation of the vascular system of the head to exclude vascular tumors such as glomus jugulare tumors, aneurysms, and stenotic lesions.

DIFFERENTIAL DIAGNOSIS Most patients with conductive and unilateral or asymmetric sensorineural hearing losses should have CT scans of the temporal bone. Patients with sensorineural hearing losses should have the vestibular system evaluated with electronystagmography and caloric testing (see Chap. 14).

TREATMENT Most patients with conductive hearing losses can be treated with middle ear reconstruction using procedures such as tympanoplasty after chronic otitis media and trauma, and stapedectomy for otosclerosis. Tympanostomy tubes allow the prompt return of hearing to normal in children and adults with middle ear effusions. Hearing aids are effective and well-tolerated for patients with conductive hearing losses. Patients with mild, moderate, and severe sensorineural hearing losses are regularly rehabilitated with hearing aids of varying configuration and strength. The profoundly deaf may benefit from cochlear implants.

The treatment of tinnitus is particularly problematic. The frequency range and intensity of tinnitus can often be matched with the use of an audiometer. Relief of the tinnitus may be obtained by masking it with background music. Hearing aids also are helpful in tinnitus suppression, as are tinnitus maskers, devices that present a sound to the affected ear which is more pleasant to listen to than the tinnitus. The use of a tinnitus masker is often followed by several hours of inhibition of the tinnitus.

REFERENCES

DALLOS P: *The Auditory Periphery: Biophysics and Physiology*. New York, Academic Press, 1973

DOTY RL: A review of olfactory dysfunctions in man. Am J Otolaryngol 1:57, 1979

——— et al: Smell identification ability: Changes with age. Science 226:1441, 1984

JERGER JR: *Modern Developments in Audiology*, 2d ed. New York, Academic Press, 1973

KONIGSMARK BW: Hereditary diseases of the nervous system with hearing loss, in PJ Vinken, GW Bruyn (eds), *Handbook of Clinical Neurology*. Elsevier, Amsterdam, 1975, vol 22, chap 23, pp 499–526

NAKASHIMA T et al: Structure of human fetal and adult olfactory neuroepithelium. Arch Otolaryngol 110:641, 1984

NORGREN R: The gustatory system in mammals. Am J Otolaryngol 4:234, 1983

RINTELMAN WF: *Hearing Assessment*. Baltimore, Baltimore University, 1979

SNOW JB: Sudden deafness, in MM Paprella, DA Shumrick (eds), *Otolaryngology*, 2d ed. Philadelphia, Saunders, 1980, pp 1751–1767

——— et al: Central auditory imperception. Laryngoscope 87:1450, 1977

———: Clinical problems in chemosensory distrubances. Am J Otolaryngol 4:224 1983

20 THE SLEEP-WAKE CYCLE AND DISORDERS OF SLEEP

WILLIAM J. SCHWARTZ / JOHN W. STAKES / JOSEPH B. MARTIN

The outward appearance of sleep—its passivity, relative immobility, and decreased sensitivity to external stimuli—belies an underlying organized brain activity both complex and heterogeneous. The operating characteristics and input-output relationships of physiologic systems change dramatically from wakefulness to sleep, and many systems which function normally during the day can decompensate during the night. Sleep pathology may present merely as an unrefreshing night's sleep or may masquerade as misleading symptoms of headache, lethargy, or unsatisfactory daytime performance. All these complaints must be pursued and addressed by the physician, not overlooked or pharmacologically suppressed.

Sleep length and depth vary markedly between healthy individuals. The average total sleep period is 7.5 h and ranges from 4 to 10 h. Sleep duration and organization also vary within individuals as a function of age. Total sleep time is highest in infancy, decreases to adult levels after completion of body growth, and declines with old age. Therefore, "how much sleep is enough" must be judged empirically. Sleep should be both *efficient*, resulting in few nocturnal arousals and minimal diurnal sleepiness, and *effective*, permitting maximal daytime function.

SLEEP STAGES AND CYCLES *Polysomnography*, the use of continuous recordings of brain waves (electroencephalogram, EEG), muscle electrical activity (electromyogram, EMG), and eye movements (electrooculogram, EOG), together with measurements of the respiratory rate, blood pressure, and heart rate, has provided important information about normal patterns of sleep and given clues to the nature of sleep disorders. For such studies, EEG electrodes are attached to the scalp, EOG electrodes to the skin at the outer canthus of both eyes, and EMG electrodes to the skin overlying the chin (mentalis) muscle.

The characteristic EEG pattern during wakefulness, with the eyes closed, is a sinusoidal posterior alpha rhythm of 8 to 12 Hz combined with low-voltage fast (beta) activity of mixed frequency (13 to 22 Hz). The EMG shows high-amplitude tonic activity. There are two defined states of sleep, *non-rapid eye movement* (NREM) sleep, and *rapid eye movement* (REM) sleep. NREM sleep is divided into four stages. Stage I sleep is characterized by low-voltage, mixed-frequency EEG activity, accompanied by slow eye movements recorded on the EOG. The EMG shows continuous high-amplitude discharges, which are decreased in size from those of the waking stage. Stage II sleep is represented by a moderately low-voltage EEG, interspersed with brief, generalized high-voltage discharges (K complexes), vertex waves, and low- to moderate-amplitude discharges of 12 to 15 Hz (sleep spindles). Stage III sleep consists of high-amplitude background activity of theta (5 to 7 Hz) and delta (1 to 3 Hz) slow waves, as well as K complexes and sleep spindles. Such high-voltage, slow-wave activity is present for 20 to 50 percent of the record. Stage IV sleep consists of high-voltage (75 μV or greater) delta waves present for 50 percent or more of the record. Spindles are rare. Low-voltage muscle potentials persist during each NREM sleep stage. Eye movements are infrequent or absent in stages III and IV. Delta sleep is the deepest (highest threshold to arousal) of the NREM stages.

The transition to REM sleep consists of a change in the EEG to low-voltage, fast-frequency (6 to 22 Hz) activity which resembles that seen during waking or stage I sleep. Moderately high amplitude, 3- to 5-Hz triangular-shaped waveforms (sawtooth waves) are also commonly observed. The EOG shows clusters of fast conjugate eye movements (REM activity). EMG activity becomes either totally absent or markedly suppressed, an effect due to descending inhibition of motor neurons from the brainstem reticular formation. The deep tendon and H reflexes are also absent. Upon awakening from REM sleep, subjects commonly recall vivid, hallucinatory dreams, but such cognitive activity is not restricted to this stage.

REM sleep alternates with NREM sleep approximately every 90 to 100 min, the first REM period usually occurring about 90 to 100 min after the onset of sleep. The full sequence of transition through stages I, II, III, and IV of NREM typically occurs after first going to sleep (Fig. 20-1). The sequence is then reversed through stages IV, III, and II, and REM sleep appears. A normal night's sleep consists of four to five such alternating cycles, characterized as the night progresses by an increasing duration and percentage of REM-sleep episodes. Stages III and IV occur predominantly during the first one-third of the sleep period. Stage I sleep normally occupies approximately 5 to 10 percent of total sleep, stage II about 50 percent, stage III approximately 15 percent, stage IV about 10 percent, and REM sleep approximately 20 percent.

Although NREM and REM sleep are defined by electrical recordings, they are characterized as *states* by a constellation of physiologic events. Blood pressure and heart and respiratory rates decrease during progressive stages of NREM sleep and fluctuate abruptly during REM sleep. During REM sleep, penile erections occur, effective thermoregulation is absent, and ventilatory responses to CO_2 are depressed. A number of endocrine functions are temporally associated with sleep. There is a major surge of growth hormone secretion during the first 2 h of sleep that is commonly, but not exclusively, associated with stages III and IV sleep. Adrenocorticotropic hormone (ACTH)–cortisol secretion occurs as a series of individual surges during the latter half of night sleep. Prolactin secretion in both men and women also increases during the night, especially immediately after sleep onset. Increased sleep-associated luteinizing hormone secretion has been shown to occur during puberty in boys and girls.

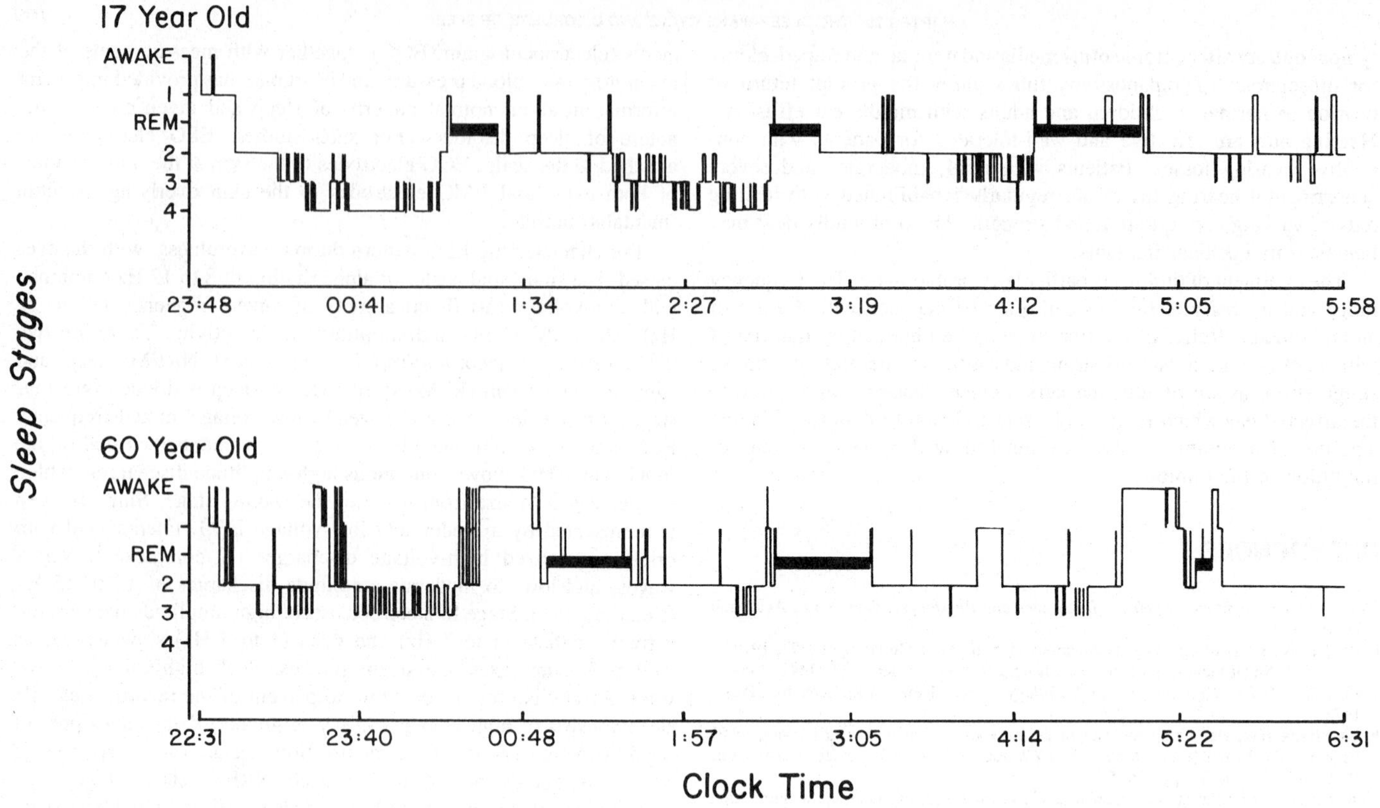

FIGURE 20-1 *Plots of the four stages of NREM sleep and REM sleep (solid bars) over the course of an entire night's sleep for a representative young (upper panel) and aged (lower panel) adult. In the elderly, there is diminished delta sleep and frequent spontaneous awakenings. Actual histograms are from the Sleep-Wake Disorders Unit, Massachusetts General Hospital.*

NEUROBIOLOGY OF SLEEP Although numerous theories have been proposed, the function(s) of sleep is unknown. Answering this question is likely to be as difficult and complex as investigating the ''function'' of wakefulness. The notion has emerged that NREM sleep serves some restorative, recuperative functions for the brain, although the nature, purpose, or necessity for such ''rest'' is unclear. REM sleep, with its intense neural activity generated independent of sensory input and uncoupled from motor output, is thought to play some as yet undefined rejuvenative role essential for the proper operation of higher neocortical activity during wakefulness.

A focus of contemporary sleep research has been to localize the brain mechanisms responsible for generating NREM-REM cycles. Especially implicated is the pontine tegmentum and the neurotransmitters norepinephrine, serotonin, and acetylcholine located in the locus coeruleus, dorsal raphe nucleus, and gigantocellular tegmental field. Over the course of development, a different neural mechanism matures to consolidate and restrict the expression of these sleep cycles to the nighttime portion of the 24-h day. An important component of this endogenous timekeeping mechanism (''circadian clock'') is the suprachiasmatic nucleus of the anterior hypothalamus. The coupling of these mechanisms is unknown but has stimulated the characterization of endogenous sleep-inducing substances. This research is in its infancy, but apparent sleep-promoting peptides have been isolated from the body fluids of both sleep-deprived and sleeping animals.

An obvious approach for assessing the function of sleep is to prevent its occurrence and search for resulting deficits. Healthy adults can tolerate 10 or more days of sleep deprivation without overt medical impairment. Performance on simple, subject-paced, short-duration tasks is unaffected. There is no evidence that selective REM deprivation leads to psychological instability or psychosis. With prolonged deprivation, subjects experience increasing fatigue, irritability, lapses of attention, and diminished motivation. Performance of tasks deteriorates, apparently due to transient and intrusive ''microsleep'' episodes. The frustration and difficulty of this research is epitomized by the facetious statement that the principal effect of sleep deprivation is to make people sleepy.

Recovery after prolonged sleep deprivation shows that the amount of sleep restored is not equal to the amount lost. During the first recovery sleep period the subject rapidly falls into stage IV of NREM sleep, often with ''supernormal'' slow waves in the EEG, and remains there at the expense of stage II sleep; REM sleep is decreased. By the second night, there is some REM sleep ''rebound'' which exceeds that of the predeprivation period.

SLEEP DISORDERS Disorders of sleep are common. Between 8 and 15 percent of the adult population in the United States have frequent and chronic complaints about the quality and the amount of their sleep. From 3 to 11 percent of adults use sedative-hypnotic drugs, and the percentage increases with age.

Sleep disorders can occur at any period of life. Some are peculiar to specific age groups, such as nocturnal enuresis, night terrors, and somnambulism in children and adolescents, and insomnia and hypersomnia in middle and old age. Others, such as the narcolepsy-cataplexy syndrome, may begin in childhood and persist throughout life.

The classification of sleep disorders is still evolving. Recently, a committee of the Association of Sleep Disorders Centers proposed a classification based principally on clinical symptomatology (see Table 20-1 and descriptions in references by Hauri and Weitzman).

Insomnias Insomnia, defined as want of sleep, is used popularly to indicate any impairment in duration, depth, or restorative properties of sleep. Insomnia may occur as a primary disorder; as a secondary manifestation of psychiatric illness, anxiety, drug use, or medical conditions; and in association with other disorders of sleep such as sleep apnea.

In order to understand the cause of insomnia, it is important to document the patient's sleep disturbance. A sleep log provided by the patient and observations by the bed partner of snoring, partial arousals, or kicking may suggest a more specific diagnosis. The history may determine whether sleep is disturbed by irregular sleep-wake schedules and wake-up times, afternoon naps, excessive nighttime noise or heat, self-medication by over-the-counter preparations, or consumption of alcohol, tobacco, or caffeine and its derivatives. The nature of the sleep complaint may also furnish etiologic clues. Inability to fall asleep or awakening 2 to 3 h after sleep onset may occur with the use of drugs or alcohol, painful or debilitating medical illness, periodic movements of sleep, or nonobstructive sleep apnea. Other patients go to sleep promptly and sleep well most of the night, only to awaken too early in the morning. Frequently in this category are individuals with depression or anxiety, or older persons who spontaneously go to bed and arise early in the day.

PSYCHOPHYSIOLOGIC INSOMNIA Situational insomnias are defined as lasting less than 3 weeks, usually with a suggested emotional cause. Symptoms include difficulty falling asleep, frequent arousals, or persistent early morning awakening, each contributing to feelings of chronic fatigue and irritability. Such symptoms may become persistent or worsened by worry about sleep loss. Anxiously lying awake at night and angrily trying to fall asleep, such patients often estimate 1 to 2 h sleep loss as 3 to 4 h. Such individuals may show no evidence of anxiety or depressive disorder.

Benzodiazepines are currently the hypnotic drugs of choice for the short-term management of insomnia. The effectiveness of long-term use (greater than 30 days) of any hypnotic has not been established. Flurazepam, 15 to 60 mg before going to bed, is the most frequently prescribed hypnotic in the United States. Older sedatives include chloral hydrate and barbiturates, but tolerance and withdrawal limits their use. L-Tryptophan, 1 to 5 g, has been advocated by some investigators, but its clinical effectiveness has not been conclusively demonstrated.

The widespread use of benzodiazepines as nighttime sedatives is now complicated by recognition of certain undesirable properties. First, they are mildly addictive and show cross-tolerance with each other and with alcohol. Second, rebound insomnia may occur with tolerance to or withdrawal from these agents (see below). Third, active metabolites of flurazepam and certain other benzodiazepines have biologic effects lasting 36 to 48 h (or longer in the elderly).

When psychophysiologic insomnia becomes chronic, pharmacologic therapy alone is rarely efficacious. A vicious cycle develops as the patient's conditioned arousal at bedtime and fear over sleep loss aggravate the insomnia. This can be one of the most difficult problems in office practice and requires combined psychosocial and behavioral approaches in addition to hypnotics.

INSOMNIA ASSOCIATED WITH THE AFFECTIVE PSYCHIATRIC DISORDERS The sleep abnormalities found in the affective disorders consist of chronic or recurrent inability to maintain sleep through the expected sleep period. Patients complain of persistent restlessness at night and of a tired, apathetic feeling during the day. More frequent arousal throughout the night, failure to "sleep deeply," and early morning awakening complete the clinical picture.

The affective disorders have been divided into major depressive and bipolar (manic-depressive) disorders (see Chap. 360). The sleep disorder in unipolar depression is characterized by repeated awakenings with a shortened REM latency (time from sleep onset to first episode of REM sleep) and decreased stages III and IV NREM sleep. Patients with bipolar depression also show these polysomnographic features, but they often have excessive daytime sleepiness (take naps) and have extended sleep periods at night. During periods of hypomania, partial or total sleeplessness may occur, lasting for several days.

Treatment is directed to the underlying psychiatric disorder and may include nighttime administration of tricyclic antidepressants or monoamine oxidase inhibitors. Several new nonpharmacologic treatments for depression are currently under study, including manipulation of the timing of sleep within the 24-h day. REM sleep deprivation or progressive phase advance of sleep onset have been reported to reverse the depressive phase of bipolar illness in some patients.

INSOMNIA ASSOCIATED WITH THE USE OF DRUGS AND ALCOHOL The widespread use and abuse of central nervous system depressants (hypnotic and sedative drugs, tranquilizers, or bedtime use of alcohol) is well documented and may produce an insomnia syndrome. As tolerance develops with continued use, the sleep-promoting properties of such drugs are lost, and the patient and the physician tend to increase the dosage. Specific sleep-disturbing symptoms caused by partial withdrawal can develop, even though administration of the drug is continued. The resulting early morning arousal is often misinterpreted, and dosage is increased further. In patients who regularly and chronically use hypnotic agents, sleep is interrupted by frequent awakenings lasting more than 5 min, especially during the second half of the night. Stages III and IV and REM sleep are decreased, and sleep-stage demarcations are less clear. These observations point to a considerable degree of sleep disorganization.

After rapid or acute withdrawal from hypnotic agents used chronically in high daily doses, the percentage of REM sleep greatly increases. Sleep-related periodic movements (nocturnal myoclonus) may also occur during the withdrawal period. In addition, daytime symptoms appear, including restlessness, nervousness, myalgias, and, in severe cases, drug withdrawal symptoms, including confusion, hallucinations, and grand mal convulsions. These complications are most common after barbiturate and glutethimide withdrawal, but may be seen with benzodiazepines as well. In patients who are chronic high-dose users of multiple hypnotic drugs, withdrawal should be gradual and supervised by a clinician. Many patients then show substantial improvement in both objective and subjective sleep patterns, although they may not return immediately to a fully normal sleep.

Heavy and sustained ingestion of alcohol severely disrupts sleep-stage organization. REM sleep periods are shortened and nightly awakenings occur. Acute withdrawal from alcohol in the chronic alcoholic leads to a lengthening of the latency to sleep onset, a decrease in NREM sleep, and an increase in REM sleep with shortened latency. If severe, acute toxic withdrawal syndrome (delirium tremens) may develop. In the abstaining alcoholic, abnormal sleep patterns may persist for many weeks, although normal sleep usually returns within 2 weeks.

INSOMNIA ASSOCIATED WITH SLEEP-RELATED MYOCLONUS In some patients with primary insomnia and in many with other forms of

TABLE 20-1 Classification of sleep disorders

I Insomnias: Disorders of initiating and maintaining sleep
- *A* Psychophysiologic—situational or persistent
- *B* Associated with psychiatric disorders, particularly affective disorders
- *C* Associated with drugs and alcohol
  - *1* Tolerance to or withdrawal from CNS depressants
  - *2* Sustained use of CNS stimulants
  - *3* Sustained use of or withdrawal from other drugs
  - *4* Chronic alcoholism
- *D* Associated with sleep-induced respiratory impairment
  - *1* Sleep apnea syndrome
  - *2* Alveolar hypoventilation syndrome
- *E* Associated with sleep-related (nocturnal) myoclonus and "restless legs"
- *F* Miscellaneous—other medical, toxic, or environmental conditions

II Hypersomnias: Disorders of excessive somnolence
- *A* Psychophysiologic—situational or persistent
- *B* Associated with psychiatric disorders, particularly affective disorders
- *C* Associated with drugs and alcohol
- *D* Associated with sleep-induced respiratory impairment (as in *D* above)
- *E* Narcolepsy-cataplexy
- *F* Miscellaneous—other medical, toxic, environmental, or idiopathic conditions

III Disorders of the sleep-wake schedule
- *A* Transient—jet lag, work shift
- *B* Persistent
  - *1* Delayed sleep phase syndrome
  - *2* Advanced sleep phase syndrome
  - *3* Non-24-h sleep-wake syndrome

IV Parasomnias: Dysfunctions associated with sleep, sleep stages, or partial arousal
- *A* Sleepwalking
- *B* Sleep terrors and dream anxiety attacks
- *C* Enuresis
- *D* Nocturnal seizures
- *E* Other sleep-related dysfunctions

insomnia, *periodic movements of sleep* (PMS) occur, usually during NREM sleep. The movements consist of stereotyped, repetitive dorsiflexion of the foot and big toe and sometimes flexion of the knee and hip. Movements recur every 20 to 30 s and last about 2 s each. They are to be distinguished from the common and benign "night starts" which occur at the onset of sleep. Sleep recordings indicate that PMS occur in a wide variety of sleep disorders in middle-aged persons, including narcolepsy-cataplexy, sleep apnea, and drug-dependency insomnia. The symptoms thus appear to be secondary to a chronic sleep-wake disturbance rather than representing a primary disorder. Although the neurophysiologic mechanisms responsible for PMS are unknown, modest therapeutic successes have been reported with clonazepam, 1 mg before bedtime.

In *restless legs syndrome,* the affected individual feels an irresistible urge to move the legs, generally when sitting or lying down, especially prior to sleep. There is a discomfort deep inside the calves which is alleviated by moving, exercising, or walking about. This interferes with sleep onset and may recur during the night. Usually by morning the restless legs symptoms have diminished, and the patient may be able to fall asleep. PMS is present in all cases of restless legs syndrome studied polygraphically.

MISCELLANEOUS CAUSES OF INSOMNIA Patients with sleep apnea or hypopnea, especially the nonobstructive type, may be frequently awakened and complain of unrefreshing sleep (see below). Poor sleep may occur in persons with a debilitating or painful illness which generates more pain and restlessness as muscles relax to leave painful areas unsplinted. Medical disorders such as paroxysmal nocturnal dyspnea, nocturnal asthma, and rheumatic or gastrointestinal illness may cause insomnia.

Hypersomnias These disorders are typified by inappropriate sleepiness leading to sleep during a time when the patient wishes to be awake. The patient complains of an irresistible urge to sleep during the day, decreased concentration, excessive yawning, and an increase in total sleep time over a 24-h period. The complaint of excessive sleep need should be distinguished from self-imposed sleep deprivation and from other symptoms of lethargy, fatigue, and apathy that commonly accompany anxiety or depression.

A classification of disorders of excessive daytime somnolence is given in Table 20-1. In clinical practice two major disorders, sleep-induced respiratory impairment and the narcolepsy-cataplexy syndrome, account for about 80 percent of patients with complaints of hypersomnia.

SLEEP-INDUCED RESPIRATORY IMPAIRMENT (THE SLEEP APNEA–HYPERSOMNIA SYNDROME) Excessive daytime somnolence is the usual complaint. In addition, disturbing nighttime symptoms include intermittent inspiratory snoring alternating with periods of apnea lasting from 10 to 120 s. Episodes begin with increasing snoring over 20 to 60 s, culminating in a loud gasp. Brief arousal followed by a variable period of apnea recurs cyclically. In serious cases, more than 500 apneas may occur per night. The patient often talks during sleep (somniloquy) and awakens in the morning unrefreshed, still sleepy, and often with a generalized headache. Polysomnography shows that the periods of apnea may result in oxygen desaturation (often below 50% saturation), occasional bradycardia alternating with tachycardia, and cardiac arrhythmias. Stages III and IV of NREM sleep are decreased.

The ratio of men to women with the sleep apnea–hypersomnia syndrome is 20:1, and the age range is the fourth to sixth decade. Approximately two-thirds of the patients are obese. A rapid weight gain may precipitate or increase the severity of the symptoms. Hypertension and signs of right heart failure may be associated.

In *obstructive apnea,* there is absent airflow despite respiratory effort. Direct endoscopic observations of the airway during the apneic episode show that the site of obstruction is in the oral pharynx at the level of the velopharyngeal sphincter. Obstruction is caused by apposition of the lateral pharyngeal walls and by posterior movement of the base of the tongue. Narrowing of the upper airway may be secondary to enlarged tonsils or adenoids, mandibular abnormalities, or pharyngeal soft tissue alterations in acromegaly and hypothyroid myxedema. Apnea may also result from cessation of respiratory movements (central or *nonobstructive apnea*). Neuromuscular disorders with respiratory muscle weakness have been associated with this condition. An initial nonobstructive apnea may be followed by obstruction (*mixed apnea*). Also, oxygen desaturation and arousals may be seen with a variety of other respiratory disturbances including hypopneas and partial obstructions. Each of these patterns may be present in an individual patient.

Treatment should begin with weight loss, but many individuals require tracheostomy to establish an adequate airway during sleep. Other treatments for milder forms have included tricyclic antidepressants (e.g., protriptyline HCl), oral progesterone, and continuous nasal positive airway pressure.

NARCOLEPSY-CATAPLEXY The narcolepsy-cataplexy syndrome is characterized by recurrent episodes of irresistible daytime sleepiness associated with abnormal manifestations of REM sleep. The "sleep attacks" appear as clinically normal sleep, are characteristically brief (about 15 min), and are often precipitated by boredom, but also occur inappropriately during coitus, athletics, or while driving an automobile. Patients usually awake refreshed, and there is a refractory period of from one to a few hours before the next attack occurs. Between attacks the patient is sleepy and inattentive; waking behaviors may become automatic and interrupted by "microsleeps." This can be quantitated using a multiple sleep latency test. Nocturnal sleep is usually also disturbed by frequent awakenings.

In about 80 percent of cases, there is also a history of *cataplexy,* characterized by sudden, brief episodes of loss of muscle tone without loss of consciousness. Cataplexy is commonly triggered by an emotional event such as laughter, anger, fear, or surprise. In its most severe form, the cataplectic attack results in total flaccid paralysis (with sparing of diaphragmatic and extraocular eye muscle movements), and collapse to the floor. Less severe symptoms may consist of sagging of the jaw or head, speechlessness, or a feeling of weakening of the knees. Full recovery occurs within a minute or two, or sleep may supervene. Two other symptoms complete the clinical tetrad of the narcolepsy-cataplexy syndrome. *Sleep paralysis* is a frightening sensation of inability to move the voluntary muscles, occurring at the transition of sleep onset or at awakening. *Vivid hallucinations* (usually visual) may occur either at sleep onset (hypnagogic) or on awakening (hypnopompic).

The disorder occurs with a prevalence of 40 per 100,000 population and has a genetic predisposition. It affects men and women equally, usually begins in adolescence with daytime sleepiness, and is a lifelong illness. The condition has severe psychosocial consequences. Symptoms often pass unrecognized, and poor school performance is ascribed to laziness; in adults, accidents, job disruptions, and depression may occur.

Narcolepsy is believed to represent a disorder of the REM sleep process. Polygraphic sleep recordings show that narcoleptics frequently begin their sleep with an REM period (sleep-onset REM). The sleep attacks that occur suddenly during the waking state are often sleep-onset REM attacks, and cataplexy, with loss of muscle tone, appears to be the quiescent state of the EMG during REM sleep. Hypnagogic hallucinations and sleep paralysis are the subjective equivalents of dreaming and muscle paralysis, respectively, which occur at the waking-sleeping interphase as manifestations of the activated REM state. Animal models of this disorder have been recently described in dogs and horses.

The treatment of narcolepsy is symptomatic. Two separate classes of drugs are effective in the management of narcolepsy and cataplexy, respectively. Narcoleptics may show improvement with strategically timed naps (during lunch hour or after meals), but most require administration of central adrenergic stimulant drugs. Methylphenidate, 10 mg two to three times daily, or amphetamine sulfate, 5 to 10 mg three to four times daily, are given to sustain the patient through the most difficult periods of the day. Late afternoon or evening administration should be avoided since it may interfere with night sleep. Cataplexy responds best to imipramine or desipramine, in doses ranging from 75 to 200 mg daily. These drugs suppress REM sleep by facilitation of adrenergic transmission and inhibition of cholinergic systems. Each class of drug should be titrated separately to achieve best results for the symptoms of narcolepsy and cataplexy, respectively.

OTHER CONDITIONS ASSOCIATED WITH EXCESSIVE DAYTIME SOMNOLENCE The *Kleine-Levin syndrome* (periodic hypersomnia) is a rare disorder that first presents between the ages of 12 and 20. It is more common in men but is also described in women. Recurrent periods of hypersomnolence lasting from a few days to several weeks alternate with asymptomatic intervals of months or years.

During a bout of hypersomnolence, the patients develop a voracious appetite and may exhibit disturbances in mood, show sexual hyperactivity and exhibitionism, and have hallucinations, disorientation, and memory deficits. The condition is usually self-limited, rarely occurring beyond the fourth or fifth decade. The etiology is unknown, and no specific neuropathology has been associated, although the disorder has been postulated to be a dysfunction of limbic and hypothalamic rhythms. Rarely, cerebrospinal fluid pleocytosis has been found, which suggests that an episode of encephalitis may underlie the disorder in some cases.

Excessive somnolence is a feature of many endocrine and metabolic disorders, including uremia, liver failure, hypothyroidism (severe, with myxedema), chronic pulmonary disease (with hypercapnia), and diabetes mellitus with incipient coma or with severe hypoglycemia. Sleep-onset REM can be rarely observed following sleep deprivation or withdrawal from REM-suppressant drugs. In addition, hypersomnolence may occur in central nervous system disorders, such as a tumor in the area of the third ventricle, obstructive hydrocephalus, and meningoencephalitis. Finally, there is a category of hypersomnolence (idiopathic central nervous system hypersomnolence) for which no etiology has been identified. Such patients respond to stimulant medications. In all of the above conditions, it is important to distinguish complaints of tiredness, fatigue, and apathy secondary to metabolic, endocrine, neurologic, and psychiatric disease from sleepiness per se.

Disorders of the sleep-wake schedule Sleep is one of many daily rhythms synchronized to the earth's 24-h geophysical cycle. Normal humans studied in controlled laboratory conditions in the absence of environmental time cues show that the endogenous length of the "free-running" circadian period for humans is approximately 25 h. Under such time-isolated conditions, the normal coupling of the rhythms of body temperature, plasma hormone levels, and sleep cycles is lost as the phase relationships between them become desynchronized.

Disorders of the circadian sleep-wake cycle are classified under two categories, transient and persistent. The transient dyssomnia of a rapid time-zone change ("jet lag") is very familiar, as is that found after an acute work-shift change. The sleep disturbance that results is due to both sleep deprivation and the circadian phase-shift change. The symptoms include an inability to sustain sleep with frequent arousals and sleepiness at inopportune clock times. Resynchronization takes several days to 2 weeks.

Persistent disorders of the sleep-wake cycle include (1) delayed sleep phase syndrome, (2) advanced sleep phase syndrome, and (3) non-24-h sleep-wake syndrome. The delayed sleep phase syndrome is a sleep disorder that can be differentiated from other forms of insomnia. Patients cannot fall asleep at the desired clock time required to meet work or study schedules; typically, they finally fall asleep at 2 to 6 A.M. However, when not required to maintain a strict schedule (e.g., weekends, holidays, and vacation periods), the patient will sleep normally if allowed to retire and awaken spontaneously. These individuals have normal sleep duration and architecture, but the *timing* of their sleep period within the 24-h day is abnormal. Such patients have been successfully treated by a progressive phase delay of their sleep times (chronotherapy). By delaying the time of going to sleep by 3 h each day (i.e., a 27-h sleep-wake cycle) the patient's sleep can be "reset" to occur at a socially acceptable clock time.

The advanced sleep phase syndrome describes individuals with normal sleep duration and architecture but with inappropriate early sleep onset and wake times. These "early to bed, early to rise" people rarely seek medical help. The process of aging leads to a characteristic change in the timing of sleep such that older individuals spontaneously awaken earlier in the morning and become sleepy and go to sleep earlier in the evening.

The non-24-h sleep-wake (hypernychthermal) syndrome is characterized by an inability to be entrained to society's 24-h day. These individuals develop a 25- to 27-h biologic day length in spite of all social cues. Blindness or a personality disorder may predispose to this condition.

Parasomnias A number of undesirable behavioral and physiologic events occur in association with sleep or specific sleep stages. Since their etiologies and interrelationships are uncertain, they are usually listed as individual clinical entities.

SLEEPWALKING (SOMNAMBULISM) In this condition, individuals suddenly sit up in bed, walk, or carry out automatic and semipurposeful complex motor activities. Patients remain unconscious and will resist being aroused. On occasion, dangerous acts, such as climbing out a window, can occur. The episode lasts less than 15 min and is finished by returning to bed or spontaneous arousal (without dream report). Sleepwalking occurs in stage III or IV of NREM sleep. There is no evidence of seizure activity either preceding or during the episode, although clinically it must be distinguished from a nocturnal seizure disorder originating in the temporal lobes.

This condition occurs normally in children and adolescents; 15 percent of all children have one or more episodes. A small percent of children (1 to 6 percent) have frequent attacks (at times, nightly). Psychopathology may be found if the episodes begin or persist into adulthood.

SLEEP TERRORS AND DREAM ANXIETY ATTACKS Sleep terrors (pavor nocturnus, incubus) commonly occur in children. The attacks occur within the first 1 to 2 h of the night, during stage III or IV of NREM sleep. With a frightened scream, the child sits up in bed, agitated and panicked. Autonomic changes appear, including sweating, tachycardia, hyperventilation, and pupillary dilation. It may be difficult to arouse the child fully, and the attack may persist for several minutes before sleep returns. There is no report of dream imagery after the attack and no memory for the event the following morning. Night terrors are almost always benign and time-limited so that reassurance is both adequate and sufficient.

Dream anxiety attacks (nightmares) occur later in the night during REM sleep. Screams are uncommon, and arousal is rapid. Vivid hallucinatory and emotionally charged dreams are usually recounted. Recurrent nightmares may reflect underlying psychological conflicts.

SLEEP-RELATED ENURESIS Bed-wetting occurs during stage III and IV of NREM sleep, usually during the first third of the night. Primary enuresis is the persistence of bed-wetting from infancy to childhood, whereas secondary enuresis occurs after a period of successful toilet training. Both need to be distinguished from symptomatic enuresis, which is caused by a known organic lesion affecting bladder regulation. All forms need to be separated from nocturnal seizures associated with incontinence.

NOCTURNAL SEIZURES Paroxysmal abnormalities of brain electrical activity of the type seen in seizure disorders sometimes occur in epileptic patients during or shortly after the onset of sleep. Up to 25 percent of subjects with grand mal attacks have them only at night during sleep. Seizures are often accompanied by tongue biting and incontinence and by muscle soreness the following day. Other seizures may mimic somnambulism, sleep terrors, and enuresis, or may present as fragmented, unrefreshing sleep periods.

OTHER SLEEP-RELATED DYSFUNCTIONS The list of such disturbances is growing and includes bruxism, head banging (jactatio capitis nocturnus), sleep-related painful erections, cluster headaches, gastroesophageal reflux, paroxysmal nocturnal hemoglobinuria, and sleep palsies due to compression of peripheral nerves.

REFERENCES

COLEMAN R et al: Sleep-wake disorders based on a polysomnographic diagnosis. JAMA 247:997, 1982

GUILLEMINAULT C (ed): *Sleeping and Waking Disorders: Indications and Techniques.* Menlo Park, Calf, Addison-Wesley, 1981

HAURI P: *The Sleep Disorders.* Kalamazoo, Mich, Upjohn, 1977

HOBSON JA, BRAZIER MAB (eds): *The Reticular Formation Revisited.* New York, Raven, 1980

KALES A et al: Insomnia and other sleep disorders. Med Clin North Am 66:971, 1982

MCGINTY DJ, SIEGEL JM: Sleep States, in *Handbook of Behavioral Neurobiology,* vol 6, *Motivation,* E Satinoff and P Teitelbaum (eds). New York, Plenum, 1983, p 105

MOORE-EDE MC et al: Circadian timekeeping in health and disease. N Engl J Med 309:469, 530, 1983

OREM J, BARNES CD (eds): *Physiology in Sleep.* New York, Academic, 1980

ROFFWARG H: Diagnostic classification of sleep and arousal disorders. Sleep 2:1, 1979

WEITZMAN ED: Sleep and its disorders. Ann Rev Neurosci 4:381, 1981

21 COMA AND OTHER DISORDERS OF CONSCIOUSNESS

ALLAN H. ROPPER / JOSEPH B. MARTIN

Coma is a common problem in general medicine; it is estimated that up to 3 percent of admissions to the emergency ward of large municipal hospitals are due to diseases that cause a disorder of consciousness. The importance of this class of neurologic disorders points to the necessity of acquiring a systematic approach to their diagnosis and management.

The increased availability of computerized tomography (CT) has resulted in an artificial orientation to the diagnosis of coma by focusing attention on lesions that are detectable by CT (e.g., hemorrhages, tumors, or hydrocephalus). This approach, although at times expedient, is often imprudent because most coma is metabolic or toxic in origin. The physician confronted with an unresponsive patient should formulate a differential diagnosis based on the history and the clinical signs before leaving the bedside. Certain signs observed during general and neurologic examination allow the physician to decide which of several generic diseases is responsible for coma, thus limiting the diagnostic possibilities. A rational approach to the precise diagnosis and subsequent management can then be planned and clinical changes anticipated. The clinical approach must be coupled to knowledge of the pathologic entities that cause coma. This chapter describes a practical approach to coma based on the anatomy and physiology of consciousness and a consideration of the general and neurologic examination and CT.

Coma is epitomized by unresponsiveness and as such is easily recognized. The interesting and sometimes subtle distinctions made between coma, stupor, and drowsiness are largely semantic because there is no anatomic or physiologic basis for distinguishing them except as relative degrees of unresponsiveness. A narrative description of the clinical state of the patient and of responses evoked by various stimuli, precisely as they are observed at the bedside, remains the optimal way to characterize coma and related disturbances of consciousness. Such a description is preferable to summary terms such as *stupor, semicoma,* or *obtundation,* which are often ambiguous and commonly differ between observers. *Stupor,* as currently used, implies a state in which the patient can be aroused by vigorous stimuli but verbal responses are slow or absent; *semicoma* suggests a state of unsustained stirring, moaning, or agitation in response to stimulation.

Although the definition of consciousness is a psychological and philosophical matter, the distinction between *level* of consciousness, or wakefulness, and *content* of consciousness, or awareness, has physiologic significance. Wakefulness or alertness is maintained by a diffuse system of upper brainstem and thalamic neurons, the reticular activating system (RAS), and its connections to the cerebral hemispheres as a whole. Therefore, depression of either hemispheral or RAS activity may cause reduced wakefulness. Awareness is dependent on integrated and organized material thoughts, subjective experience, emotions, and mental processes, each of which resides to some extent in anatomically defined regions of the brain. The inability to maintain a coherent sequence of thoughts and actions is called *confusion* and is a disorder of content of consciousness. Reduced wakefulness often precludes evaluation of content of consciousness, but content of consciousness can be severly impaired, as in confusion, without affecting arousal. Confusion is used to describe a state of inattention, and lack of clarity in thinking. In special cases it is accompanied by illusions (misperceptions of environmental sight, sound, or touch) or hallucinations (spontaneous endogenous perceptions). Psychiatrists often use the term *delirium* for any confusion, but delirium should be reserved as a description for an agitated, hypersympathotonic, frequently hallucinatory state most often due to specific causes such as alcohol or drug withdrawal. Usually, the confused patient is subdued, not inclined to speak, and less active physically than usual. Many processes that ultimately lead to coma begin with confusion, and diagnostic considerations should address the primary problem as an alteration in the level of consciousness. Confusion alone generally indicates a metabolic derangement, although focal cerebral lesions that cause deficits in language, orientation, or memory may make the patient appear to be confused.

ANATOMIC CORRELATES OF CONSCIOUSNESS A normal level of consciousness (wakefulness) depends upon activation of the cerebral hemispheres by groups of neurons located in the brainstem RAS. Both of the cerebral hemispheres, the RAS, and the connections between them must be preserved for normal consciousness. The principal causes of coma are, therefore, (1) bilateral hemispheral damage or suppression by drugs or toxins and (2) a brainstem lesion or metabolic derangement that damages or suppresses the RAS. There is some evidence that large, purely unilateral hemispheral lesions particularly on the left may cause drowsiness (though not coma), even in the absence of damage to the opposite hemisphere or RAS.

Reticular activating system The RAS is best defined as a physiologic system, not an anatomic one. It is contained within the reticular formation, which consists of loosely grouped neurons located bilaterally in the medial tegmental gray matter of the brainstem extending from the medulla to the posterior diencephalon. These neurons have been shown in neuroanatomic studies to span long rostrocaudal distances within the reticular formation. Animal experiments and human clinical-neuropathologic observations have established that the *neurons located in the region extending from the rostral pons to the caudal diencephalon are of primary importance for maintaining wakefulness.* Lesions here that produce coma also commonly affect adjacent brainstem structures concerned with control of pupillary constriction and mechanisms for eye movements (Fig. 21-1). Abnormalities in these systems on physical examination provide signposts of brainstem damage. Lesions confined to the cerebral hemispheres do not directly affect the brainstem RAS, though secondary derangement may result from midline compression due to shifts in a cerebral hemisphere.

Brainstem RAS neurons project rostrally to the cortex, primarily via "nonspecific" thalamic relay nuclei which exert a tonic influence on the activity of the cerebral cortex. Experimental work suggests that the brainstem RAS indirectly affects the level of consciousness by suppressing the activity of the nonspecific nuclei. Electrical stimulation of the pontine and midbrain RAS desynchronizes the electroencephalogram (EEG), a pattern associated with behavioral arousal. Stimulation of the thalamic relay nuclei opposes this activity, resulting in synchronization and slowing of the EEG. The basis of behavioral arousal by environmental stimuli (somesthetic, auditory, and visual) depends on the rich innervation of the RAS by each sensory system.

The relay between the RAS and thalamic and cortical areas is accomplished by neurotransmitters. Of these, the influence of acetylcholine and norepinephrine on arousal is the best established. Cholinergic fibers connect the midbrain to other areas of the upper brainstem, thalamus, and cortex. These pathways are thought to mediate the clinical and EEG arousal observed after administration of cholinergic drugs such as physostigmine. Noradrenergic neurons in the locus coeruleus and serotonergic cells of the raphe nucleus of the pons are known to project diffusely to the cortex. Serotonin and norepinephrine subserve important functions in the regulation of the sleep-wake cycle (see Chap. 20). Their roles in arousal and coma have not been clearly established, although the alerting effects of amphetamines are likely to be mediated by catecholamine release.

Cerebral hemispheres and consciousness The specialized functions of the cerebral cortex in language, control of movement, and perception are regionalized (see Chaps. 22 to 24). In contrast, wakefulness is related in a semiquantitative way to the total mass of functioning cortex (and RAS connections) and is not focally represented in any region of the hemispheres. Hemispheral lesions may cause coma in one of three ways: (1) most commonly, bilateral, generalized hemispheral lesions or metabolic derangements such as occur in encephalitis, generalized epilepsy, drug ingestion, ischemia, and hypoglycemia interfere with awareness in a graded fashion as more cortical territory is damaged or rendered functionally inactive; (2) rarely, enlarging masses or secondary brain swelling initially confined to one side of the brain may compress the contralateral hemisphere, effectively creating bilateral hemispheral lesions; and (3) large lesions in one or both hemispheres may compress the brainstem and diencephalon causing coma indirectly by damaging the RAS. *The degree of decrease in alertness is often related to the acuteness of onset of the cortical dysfunction.*

The concept of *transtentorial herniation* with progressive brainstem compression has dominated thinking about neurologic signs in coma caused by supratentorial mass lesions. Herniation refers to displacement of brain tissue away from a mass, past a less mobile structure such as dura, and into a space that it normally does not occupy. Herniation suggests a degree of irreversibility because the tissue is trapped in its new location. The common herniations seen at postmortem are transfalcial (under the falx in the anterior midline), transtentorial (into the tentorial opening), and cerebellar tonsillar (into the foramen magnum). Uncal transtentorial herniation, or impaction of the uncal gyrus into the cistern between the free edge of the tentorium and lateral edge of the midbrain, causes compression of the third nerve with pupillary dilation and subsequent coma due to midbrain compression. Central transtentorial herniation denotes downward movement of the diencephalon (thalamic region) through the tentorial opening in the midline and is said to be heralded by miotic pupils and drowsiness. In both cases an orderly progression of rostral to caudal compression of first the midbrain, then pons, and finally medulla leads to the sequential appearance of neurologic signs and progressively diminished alertness. However, many patients with supratentorial masses do not follow these stereotypic patterns; an orderly progression of signs from midbrain to medulla is rarely seen in catastrophic lesions where all brainstem functions are lost almost simultaneously. Furthermore, stupor typically occurs with only moderate lateral shifts at the level of the diencephalon (4 to 8 mm) before actual herniation is evident on a CT scan.

PATHOPHYSIOLOGY OF COMA The pathophysiologic basis of coma is either mechanical destruction of crucial areas of the brainstem or cerebral cortex (anatomic coma) or global disruption of brain metabolic processes (metabolic coma). Coma of metabolic origin may be produced by interruption of energy substrate delivery (hypoxia, ischemia, hypoglycemia) or by alteration of the neurophysiologic responses of neuronal membranes (drug or alcohol intoxication, epilepsy, or acute head injury).

The brain is markedly dependent on continuous blood flow and delivery of oxygen and glucose, which are consumed at rates of 3.5 mL per 100 g per minute and 5 mg per 100 g per minute, respectively. Brain stores of glucose provide energy for approximately 2 min after blood flow is interrupted, although consciousness is lost within 8 to 10 s. When hypoxia occurs simultaneously with ischemia, available glucose is exhausted more rapidly. Normal resting cerebral blood flow (CBF) is approximately 75 mL per 100 g per minute in gray matter and 30 mL per 100 g per minute in white matter (mean = 55 mL per 100 g per minute). This provides for adequate metabolic supplies with a modest safety factor to accommodate most physiologic changes. When mean CBF diminishes to 25 mL per 100 g per minute, the EEG becomes diffusely slowed (typical of metabolic encepha-

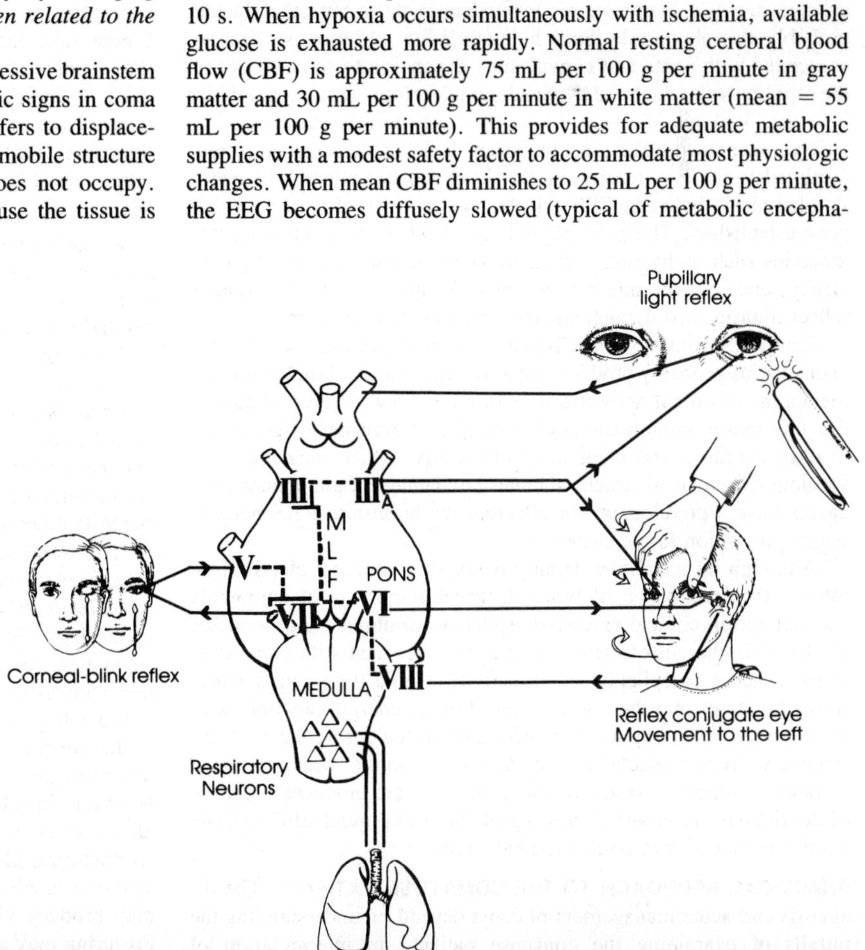

FIGURE 21-1 *Brainstem reflexes in the coma examination. Midbrain and third nerve function are tested by pupillary reaction to light, pontine function by spontaneous and reflex eye movements and corneal responses, and medullary function by respiratory and pharyngeal responses.*

Reflex conjugate, horizontal eye movements are dependent upon the medial longitudinal fasciculus (MLF) interconnecting the sixth and contralateral third nerve nuclei. Eye movements are elicited by head rotation (oculocephalic reflex) or caloric stimulation of the labyrinths (oculovestibular or vestibuloocular reflex). These reflex movements are suppressed in the awake patient by the cerebral hemispheres via their connections to the brainstem.

lopathies), and at 15 mL per 100 g per minute brain electrical activity ceases. If all other conditions such as temperature and arterial oxygenation remain normal, CBF less than 10 mL per 100 g per minute causes irrevocable brain damage.

Coma due to hyponatremia, hyperosmolarity, hypercapnia, and the encephalopathies of hepatic and renal failure are associated with a variety of metabolic derangements of neurons and astrocytes. The toxic effects of these conditions on the brain are frequently multifactorial, producing impaired energy supplies, changes in resting membrane potentials, neurotransmitter abnormalities, and in some instances morphologic changes. For example, hepatic coma may be related in part to a high brain ammonia concentration which interferes with cerebral energy metabolism and the Na^+,K^+-ATPase pump. The increased number and size of astrocytes seen in the brains of patients who die as a result of hepatic encephalopathy may contribute to neurologic symptoms. This change may be due to the need to detoxify ammonia. In addition, abnormalities of neurotransmitters have been found in experimental hepatic coma, including possible "false" neurotransmitters, which may act competitively at monoaminergic receptor sites.

The exact cause of the encephalopathy of renal failure is also poorly understood. Urea itself does not produce nervous system toxicity. A multifactorial cause is likely, including increased permeability of the blood-brain barrier to toxic substances such as organic acids and an increase in brain calcium or cerebrospinal fluid (CSF) phosphate content. Cellular membrane potentials change in uremia due to brain potassium shifts, but the magnitude of this effect is small and unlikely to account for neurologic symptoms. Parathyroid hormone excess may also play a part in uremic encephalopathy.

Abnormalities of osmolarity are involved in the coma and seizures caused by several medical disorders including diabetic ketoacidosis, the nonketotic hyperosmolar state, and hyponatremia. In hyperosmolarity, brain volume is reduced while hypoosmolarity leads to brain swelling. Brain water volume correlates best with level of consciousness in hyponatremic-hypoosmolar states but other factors probably also play a role. Sodium levels below 115 meq per liter are associated with coma and convulsions, depending to some extent on the rapidity with which the hyponatremia develops. Serum osmolarity is generally above 350 mosmol per liter in hyperosmolar coma.

Hypercapnia produces a diminished level of consciousness proportional to the P_{CO_2} tension in the blood and to acuteness of onset. A relationship between CSF acidosis and severity of symptoms has been established. The pathophysiology of other metabolic encephalopathies such as hypercalcemia, hypothyroidism, vitamin B_{12} deficiency, and hypothermia are incompletely understood but probably reflect multifaceted derangements of cerebral biochemistry.

Central nervous system (CNS) depressant drugs and some endogenous toxins probably produce coma by suppression of metabolic and membrane electrical activities in both the RAS and cerebral cortex. For this reason combinations of cortical and brainstem signs occur in drug overdose and other metabolic comas which may lead to a specious diagnosis of structural brainstem damage. Certain anesthetic agents have a predilection for affecting the brainstem RAS neurons out of proportion to the cortex.

Although all metabolic derangements alter neuronal electrophysiology, the disturbance of brain electrical activity most commonly encountered in clinical practice is epilepsy. Continuous, generalized electrical discharges of the cortex may be associated with coma even in the absence of epileptic motor activity. Coma following seizures (postictal state) may be due to exhaustion of energy metabolites or be secondary to locally toxic molecules produced during the seizures. Recovery from postictal unresponsiveness occurs when neuronal metabolic balance is restored. The postictal state produces a pattern of continuous, generalized slowing of the background EEG activity similar to that of metabolic encephalopathy.

PRACTICAL APPROACH TO THE COMATOSE PATIENT The diagnosis and acute management of coma depend on understanding the pitfalls of examining the comatose patient, an interpretation of brainstem reflexes, and on the wise use of selected diagnostic tests. Respiratory and cardiovascular problems should be attended to prior to neurologic diagnosis. The general medical evaluation, except for the vital signs and examination for nuchal rigidity, should be deferred until the neurologic evaluation has established the severity and nature of coma.

History In many cases the cause of coma is immediately evident (e.g., trauma, cardiac arrest, and known drug ingestion). However, in the remainder, historical information about the onset of coma is often sparse. The most useful historical points, when obtainable, are (1) the circumstances and temporal profile of the onset of neurologic symptoms, (2) the precise details of preceding neurologic symptoms (weakness, headaches, seizures, dizziness, diplopia, or vomiting), (3) the use of drugs or alcohol, (4) history of liver, kidney, lung, heart, or other medical disease. Telephone calls to family and observers on the scene are an important part of the initial evaluation of coma.

PHYSICAL EXAMINATION AND GENERAL OBSERVATIONS The temperature, pulse, respiratory rate and pattern, and blood pressure should be measured. Fever suggests systemic infection, bacterial meningitis, or a brain lesion that has disturbed the temperature-regulating centers. High body temperature, 42 to 44°C, associated with dry skin should arouse the suspicion of heat stroke. Hypothermia is observed with bodily exposure; alcoholic, barbiturate, or phenothiazine intoxication; hypoglycemia; peripheral circulatory failure; or myxedema. Hypothermia causes coma directly only when the temperature is below 31°C. Aberrant respiratory patterns commonly reflect brainstem disorders and are discussed below. A change of pulse rate combined with hyperventilation and hypertension may signal an increase in intracranial pressure. Marked hypertension occurs in patients with hypertensive encephalopathy, cerebral hemorrhage, and, at times, in those with other causes of increased intracranial pressure. Hypotension may occur in the coma of alcohol or barbiturate intoxication, internal hemorrhage, myocardial infarction, gram-negative bacillary septicemia, and Addisonian crisis. The funduscopic examination is useful in detecting subarachnoid hemorrhage (subhyaloid hemorrhages), hypertensive encephalopathy (exudates, hemorrhages, vessel-crossing changes), and increased intracranial pressure (papilledema). Generalized cutaneous petechiae suggest thrombotic thrombocytopenic purpura or a bleeding diathesis causing intracerebral hemorrhage.

General neurologic assessment An exact description of spontaneous and elicited movements in coma is of great value in establishing the level of neurologic dysfunction. The patient's state is observed first without examiner intervention. The nature of respirations, similarity to sleep, and spontaneous movements are observed. Patients who toss about, reach up toward the face, cross the midline with an arm, cross their legs, yawn, swallow, cough, or moan are closest to being awake. Adventitious movements or postures may be subtle and must be specifically sought. For example, the only sign of seizures may be small excursion twitching of a foot, finger, or facial muscle. An outturned leg at rest or lack of restless movements on one side suggests a hemiparesis.

The terms *decorticate* and *decerebrate rigidity* or "posturing" have been adapted from animal experiments to describe stereotyped tonic flexor and extensor arm movements, respectively, with extension of the legs. Spontaneous flexion of the elbows and wrists and arm supination (decortication) suggest severe bilateral damage in the hemispheres above the midbrain, while extension of the elbows and wrists with pronation (decerebration) suggests damage in the midbrain or diencephalon. Arm extension with weak leg flexion or flaccid legs has been associated with lesions in the low pons. Acute lesions, however, frequently cause limb extension regardless of location, and almost all extensor posturing becomes flexor in nature as time passes, so posturing alone cannot be depended upon to make an accurate anatomic localization. Metabolic coma, especially after acute hypoxia, may produce vigorous spontaneous extensor (decerebrate) rigidity. Posturing may alternate or coexist with purposeful limb movements, usually reflecting subtotal damage to the motor system. Multifocal myoclonus is almost always an indication of metabolic disorder, particularly azotemia, or drug ingestion. The later stages of Creutzfeldt-Jakob disease may also produce coma with myoclonus that is stimulus-sensitive. In an awake, confused patient, asterixis is a certain sign of metabolic encephalopathy.

Elicited movements and level of arousal A sequence of increasingly intense stimuli is used to determine the patient's best level of arousal and the optimal motor response of each limb. If the patient is not aroused by conversational voice, shouting should be tried. Shaking the patient is attempted next, then painful pressure on the limbs. Nasal tickle with a cotton wisp is a strong arousal stimulus. Deep pressure on the knuckles or bony prominences is the preferred and humane form of noxious stimulus. Pinching the skin over the face or chest may cause unsightly ecchymoses and is rarely necessary.

Responses to noxious stimuli should be appraised critically. Abduction avoidance of a limb is a purposeful, cortically derived movement and denotes an intact corticospinal system to that limb. If abduction is present in all limbs, it is a reliable sign of only minimal motor dysfunction. Stereotyped posturing following stimulation of a limb indicates severe dysfunction of the corticospinal system. Adduction and flexion of the stimulated limbs may occur as reflex movements and do not imply an intact corticospinal system. Brief oscillatory limb movements frequently occur at the end of elicited extensor posturing excursions and should not be mistaken for seizures.

Brainstem reflexes Brainstem signs are the key to the localization of the causative lesion in coma (Fig. 21-1). As a rule, coma associated with normal brainstem function indicates widespread and bilateral hemispheral disease. The brainstem contains several intrinsic reflexes that are convenient to examine. Normal pupillary symmetry, size, shape, and reaction to light indicate intact functioning of the midbrain and efferent parasympathetic fibers of the third cranial nerve responsible for pupillary constriction. The afferent component of the light reflex utilizes the optic nerve. Pupillary reaction should be examined with a bright diffuse light and, if absent, confirmed with a magnifying lens. Excessive room lighting mutes pupillary reactivity. Equal and reactive round pupils (2.5 to 5 mm in diameter) usually exclude midbrain damage as the cause of coma. An enlarged (greater than 5 mm) and unreactive or poorly reactive pupil can result either from an intrinsic midbrain lesion (on the same side) or, more commonly, be secondary to compression of the midbrain and/or third nerve as occurs in transtentorial herniation. Unilateral pupillary enlargement usually denotes an ipsilateral mass but rarely can occur contralaterally by compression of the cerebral peduncle of the midbrain against the opposite tentorial margin. Oval and slightly eccentric pupils (corectopia) often accompany early midbrain–third nerve compression. Bilaterally dilated and unreactive pupils indicate severe midbrain damage, usually from secondary compression by transtentorial herniation or metabolically by ingestion of drugs with anticholinergic activity. The unannounced use of mydriatic eye drops by a previous examiner or direct ocular trauma may cause misleading pupillary enlargement. Reactive and bilaterally small but not pinpoint pupils (1 to 2.5 mm) are most commonly seen in metabolic encephalopathy or after deep bilateral hemispheral lesions such as hydrocephalus or thalamic hemorrhage. This has been attributed to dysfunction of sympathetic nervous system efferents emerging from the posterior hypothalamus. Profound barbiturate-induced coma may produce similar-sized pupils. Very small but reactive pupils (less than 1 mm) denote narcotic overdose but may also occur with acute, extensive bilateral pontine damage. The response to naloxone and the presence of reflex eye movements (see below) distinguishes these. The unilaterally small pupil of a Horner's syndrome is rare in coma but may occur ipsilateral to a large cerebral hemorrhage.

Eye movements are the foundation of physical diagnosis in coma because their examination permits exploration of a large portion of the rostrocaudal extent of the brainstem. The eyes are first observed by elevating the lids and noting the resting position and spontaneous movements of the globes. Horizontal divergence of the eyes at rest is normally observed in drowsiness. As patients either awaken or slip deeper into coma, the ocular axes become parallel again. An adducted eye at rest indicates lateral rectus paresis (weakness) due to a sixth nerve lesion and may indicate damage to the pons. However, sixth nerve paresis, often bilateral, occurs with increased intracranial pressure and is not a localizing sign. An abducted eye at rest indicates medial rectus paresis due to third nerve paresis. With few exceptions, vertical separation of the ocular axes, or *skew deviation,* results from pontine or cerebellar lesions. In hydrocephalus with dilatation of the third ventricle, the eye globes frequently rest below the horizontal meridian.

When spontaneous eye movements are present in coma, they generally take the form of conjugate horizontal roving. This motion exonerates the midbrain and pons and has the same meaning as normal reflex eye movements (see below). Cyclic vertical downward movements are seen in specific circumstances. "Ocular bobbing" describes a brisk conjugate downward and slow upward movement of the globes in situations in which horizontal eye movement mechanisms have been disrupted and is diagnostic of bilateral pontine damage. "Ocular dipping" is a slow downward movement followed by a faster upward movement in patients with normal reflex horizontal gaze. Dipping occurs particularly in patients with diffuse anoxic damage to the cerebral cortex and may be preceded by sustained up or down gaze. The eyes may turn down and inward in thalamic and upper midbrain lesions. Conjugate ocular deviation at rest is discussed below.

Doll's-eye, or *oculocephalic,* movements are tested by moving the head from side to side or vertically, first slowly then briskly. Reflex eye movements are evoked in the opposite direction to head turning (Fig. 21-1). These responses are mediated by brainstem mechanisms originating in the labyrinths and vestibular nuclei and cervical proprioceptors. They are normally suppressed by visual fixation mediated by the cerebral hemispheres in awake patients. The neuronal pathways for reflex horizontal eye movements require integrity of the region surrounding the sixth nerve nucleus and are yoked to the contralateral third nerve via the medial longitudinal fasciculus (MLF) (Fig. 21-1). Two disparate pieces of information can be obtained from the reflex eye movements. *First,* in coma resulting from bihemispheral disease or early metabolic or drug depression, the eyes move easily or "loosely" from side to side in a direction opposite to the direction of head turning. The ease with which the globes move toward the opposite side is a reflection of disinhibition of brainstem reflexes by damaged cerebral hemispheres. In drowsy patients, the first two or three head rotations cause opposite conjugate eye movements following which the maneuver itself usually causes arousal and the reflex movements stop. *Second,* full conjugate oculocephalic movements require integrity of the brainstem pathways extending from the high cervical spinal cord and medulla, where vestibular and proprioceptive input from head turning originates, to the midbrain, where the third nerve originates, and the MLF running between these regions. Thus, the oculocephalic maneuver is a convenient way to demonstrate the functional integrity of a large segment of brainstem pathways and to exclude a lesion in the brainstem as the cause of coma. Faulty abduction of an eye suggests a sixth nerve lesion, due either to ipsilateral pontine damage or the distant effects of increased intracranial pressure. Lack of complete adduction indicates an ipsilateral midbrain (third nerve) lesion or, alternatively, damage to the pathways mediating reflex eye movements in the MLF (i.e., internuclear ophthalmoplegia). Third nerve damage is usually associated with an enlarged pupil and horizontal ocular divergence at rest, whereas MLF destruction shows neither. Adduction of the globes is by nature more difficult to obtain with head turning than abduction, and subtle symmetric abnormalities in the doll's-eye maneuver should be interpreted with caution.

Caloric stimulation of the vestibular apparatus (*oculovestibular* or *vestibuloocular response*) is a useful adjunct to the oculocephalic test and acts as a stronger stimulus to reflex eye movements. Irrigation of the external auditory canal with ice-cold water causes convection currents in the endolymph of the labyrinths of the inner ear. With the head placed at 30° elevation from the supine position, endolymph movement is induced primarily in the horizontal semicircular canals. An intact brainstem response is indicated by tonic deviation of both eyes (lasting 30 to 120 s) to the side of cold-water irrigation. Bilateral conjugate eye movements have the same significance as full oculocephalic responses. If the cerebral hemispheres are intact, a rapid corrective conjugate movement is generated away from the side of tonic deviation. The absence of this saccadic, nystagmus-like quick phase signifies damage to the opposite cerebral hemisphere.

Conjugate ocular deviation at rest or incomplete conjugate eye movements with head turning indicates damage in the pons on the side of the gaze paresis or frontal lobe damage on the opposite side. This phenomenon may be summarized by the phrase "the eyes look toward a hemispheral lesion and away from a brainstem lesion." It is usually possible to overcome the ocular deviation associated with frontal lobe damage by brisk head turning. Seizures may also cause aversive (opposite) eye deviation with rhythmic, jerky movements to the side of gaze. On rare occasions, the eyes may turn paradoxically away from the side of a deep hemispheral lesion ("wrong-way eyes").

A major pitfall in coma diagnosis may occur when reflex eye movements are suppressed by drugs. The eyes often move with the head as it is turned as if locked in place, thus spuriously suggesting anatomic brainstem damage. Overdoses of phenytoin, tricyclic antidepressants, and barbiturates are commonly implicated as well as, on occasion, alcohol, phenothiazines, diazepam, and neuromuscular blockers such as succinylcholine. The presence of normal pupillary size and light reaction will distinguish most drug-induced coma from brainstem damage (except for pontine infarction or hemorrhage in which the pupils remain small). Both absent oculocephalic responses and dilated, fixed pupils may occur with glutethimide intoxication. Small to midposition, nonreactive pupils may also occur with very high serum levels of barbiturates or secondary to hydrocephalus (see below).

Although the *corneal reflexes* are rarely useful alone, they may corroborate eye movement abnormalities because they also depend on the integrity of pontine pathways. By touching the cornea with a wisp of cotton, a response consisting of brief bilateral lid closure may be observed. The corneal response may be lost when the afferent fifth nerve, the efferent seventh nerve, or their reflex connections within the pons are damaged. The normal efferent response is bilateral, with closure of both eyelids. Nervous system depressant drugs diminish or eliminate the corneal responses soon after the reflex eye movements become paralyzed but before the pupils become unreactive to light.

Respiration Respiratory patterns have received much attention in coma diagnosis but are of inconsistent localizing value. Shallow, slow, but well-timed regular breathing suggests metabolic or drug depression. Rapid, deep (Kussmaul) breathing usually implies metabolic acidosis but may also occur with pontomesencephalic lesions. Cheyne-Stokes respiration in its classic cyclic form, ending with a brief apneic period, signifies mild bihemispheral damage or metabolic suppression and commonly accompanies light coma. Gasps, held in inspiration, reflect bilateral lower brainstem damage and are well known as the terminal respiratory pattern of severe brain damage. In brain-dead patients, shallow respiratory-like movements with irregular, nonrepetitive back arching may be stimulated by hypercapnia or hypoxia and are probably generated by the surviving cervical spinal cord and lower medulla. Other cyclic breathing variations are not usually diagnostic of specific local lesions.

COMA-LIKE SYNDROMES AND RELATED STATES The simple observation of inability to arouse a patient characterizes most comatose states. Several syndromes, however, appear to render patients unresponsive or insensate but are considered separately because of their unusual features. The *vegetative state* occurs in patients who were earlier comatose but whose eyes have subsequently opened giving the appearance of being awake. There may be yawning, grunting, picking with the hands, and random limb and head movements. These are associated with signs of extensive damage to both cerebral hemispheres, i.e., Babinski signs, decerebrate or decorticate posturing, absence of response to visual stimuli, and absent corrective nystagmus on vestibuloocular testing. Autonomic nervous system functions such as cardiovascular and thermoregulatory and neuroendocrine control are preserved and may be subject to periods of overactivity. The syndrome is best viewed as a severe dementia resulting from global damage to the cerebral cortex and differs somewhat from akinetic mutism (described below) because of a complete inability to respond to commands or communicate. *Akinetic mutism,* or coma vigil, refers to the appearance of a partially or fully awake patient who is immobile and silent. The state may result from hydrocephalus or may occur with masses in the region of the third ventricle or with lesions in the cingulate gyrus or other portions of both frontal lobes. *Abulia* is a mild form of akinetic mutism in which the patient is hypokinetic and slow to respond but generally gives correct answers. Lesions in the periaqueductal or low diencephalic regions may cause a similar state in which hypophonia is prominent. The *locked-in syndrome* (pseudocoma) describes patients who are awake but selectively deefferented, i.e., have no means of producing speech or limb, face, or pharyngeal movements. This results from infarction or hemorrhage of the ventral pons which transects all descending corticospinal and corticobulbar pathways but spares the RAS arousal system. Vertical eye movements and blinking are generally normal because these midbrain functions are outside the field of infarction in basilar artery thrombosis. Such movements can be used by the patient to signal to the examiner. A similar awake state simulating unresponsiveness may occur in severe cases of acute polyneuritis or myasthenia gravis as a result of total paralysis of limb and bulbar musculature. Unlike basilar artery stroke, vertical eye movements are not selectively spared in these nerve and muscle diseases.

Certain psychiatric states mimic coma because they produce apparent unresponsiveness. *Catatonia* is a generic term for peculiar motor activities associated with major psychosis. In the typical hypomobile form catatonic patients appear awake with eyes open but make no voluntary or responsive movements, though they blink spontaneously and may not appear distressed. There may be associated "waxy flexibility" in which limbs maintain their posture when lifted by the examiner. Upon recovery, such patients have full memory of events that occurred during their catatonic stupor. Patients with *pseudocoma conversion* states (trance) have signs which indicate voluntary attempts to appear comatose. They may resist eyelid elevation, blink to threat when the lids are held open, and move the eyes concomitantly with head rotation, all signs belying brain damage.

LABORATORY EXAMINATION IN COMA Four laboratory tests are used most frequently in the diagnosis of coma: chemical-toxicologic analysis of blood and urine, CT or MRI, EEG, and cerebral spinal fluid (CSF) examination.

Chemical blood determinations are routinely made to investigate metabolic, toxic, or drug-induced encephalopathies. The major metabolic aberrations encountered in clinical practice are those of electrolytes, calcium, blood urea nitrogen (BUN), glucose, and hepatic dysfunction. Toxicologic analysis is of great value in any case of coma where the diagnosis is not immediately clear. However, the presence of exogenous drugs or toxins, especially alcohol, does not ensure that other factors, particularly head trauma, may not also contribute to the clinical state.

The notion that a normal CT scan excludes anatomic lesions as the cause of coma is erroneous. Early hemisphere infarction, small brainstem lesions, encephalitis, mechanical shearing of axons as a result of closed head trauma, absent cerebral perfusion associated with brain death, sagittal sinus thrombosis, and subdural hematomas which are isodense to adjacent brain are some of the lesions which may be overlooked by CT. Nevertheless, in coma of unknown etiology, a CT scan should be obtained early in the evaluation. In those cases in which the etiology is clinically apparent, the CT provides verification and defines the extent of the lesion.

The EEG is rarely diagnostic in coma, with the occasional exceptions of coma due to ongoing clinically unrecognized seizures, herpes virus encephalitis, and Creutzfeldt-Jakob disease. Examination of the EEG does, however, provide important information about the general electrophysiologic state of the cortex, and asymmetries may point to unilateral lesions not visualized on the CT scan. The amount of background slowing of the EEG is useful for gauging and following the severity of any diffuse encephalopathy. The EEG pattern of "alpha coma" deserves separate mention. It is defined by widespread, invariant 8- to 12-Hz activity superficially resembling the normal alpha rhythm of waking, but which is unresponsive to environmental stimuli. Alpha coma results from either high pontine or diffuse cortical damage and is associated with a poor prognosis. Coma due to persistent epileptic discharges that are not clinically manifested may be revealed by EEG recordings. Normal alpha activity on the EEG may also alert the clinician to the "locked-in" syndrome. Evoked potential recordings (auditory and somatosensory) are currently under investigation as additional methods of coma diagnosis and monitoring.

Lumbar puncture is now used more judiciously than previously because the CT scan excludes intracerebral hemorrhages and most subarachnoid hemorrhages. The use of lumbar puncture in coma is limited to diagnosis of meningitis-encephalitis, occasional cases of subarachnoid hemorrhage, and cases with normal CT in which the origin of coma is obscure. If the CT is normal or unavailable and suspicion of meningeal infection or subarachnoid hemorrhage remains, then the CSF should be examined for white cells, microorganisms, and blood. Xanthochromia is documented by spinning the CSF in a large tube and comparing the supernatant to water. Yellow coloration indicates preexisting blood in the CSF and permits exclusion of a traumatic puncture. In addition, initial and final tubes should be inspected for a decrement in the number of erythrocytes, indicating traumatic puncture.

DIFFERENTIAL DIAGNOSIS OF COMA In most instances, coma is part of an obvious medical problem such as known drug ingestion, hypoxia, stroke, trauma, or liver or kidney failure. Attention is appropriately focused on the primary illness. A complete listing of all diseases which cause coma would serve little purpose since it would not aid diagnosis. Some general rules, however, are helpful. Illnesses which cause sudden or acute coma are due to drug ingestion or to one of the catastrophic brain lesions—hemorrhage, trauma, or hypoxia. Coma which appears subacutely is usually related to preceding medical or neurologic problems, including the secondary brain swelling which surrounds a preexisting lesion. Coma diagnosis, therefore, requires familiarity with the common intracerebral catastrophies. These are described in more detail in Chap. 343, but may be summarized as follows: (1) basal ganglia and thalamic hemorrhage (acute but not instantaneous onset, vomiting, headache, hemiplegia, and characteristic eye signs); (2) subarachnoid hemorrhage (instantaneous onset, severe headache, neck stiffness, vomiting, third or sixth nerve lesions, transient loss of consciousness, or sudden coma with vigorous extensor posturing); (3) pontine hemorrhage (sudden onset, pinpoint pupils, loss of reflex eye movements and corneal responses, ocular bobbing, posturing, hyperventilation, and sweating); (4) cerebellar hemorrhage (occipital headache, vomiting, gaze paresis, and inability to stand); (5) basilar artery thrombosis (neurologic prodrome or warning spells, diplopia, dysarthria, vomiting, eye movement and corneal response abnormalities, and asymmetric limb paresis). The commonest stroke, namely, infarction in the territory of the middle cerebral artery, does not cause coma acutely. The syndrome of acute hydrocephalus causing coma may accompany many intracranial catastrophes, including subarachnoid hemorrhage, or obstructive lesions of the cerebral aqueduct in the midbrain, due to cerebellar hemorrhage, tumors, or cysts. Acute symmetric enlargement of both lateral ventricles causes headache and vomiting. Further ventricular enlargement leads to drowsiness that may progress quickly to coma, with extensor posturing of the limbs, bilateral Babinski signs, often small (1 mm diameter) nonreactive pupils, and impaired vertical oculocephalic movements.

If the history and examination are not typical for any neurologic diagnosis, and metabolic or drug causes are excluded, then information obtained from CT may be used as outlined in Table 21-1. The neurologic examination remains preeminent because it allows localization of lesions to one or both hemispheres or to the brainstem (with the exceptions noted above). The CT scan is useful to focus the differential diagnosis, and because of its accuracy and general availability, the diagnoses which it facilitates are listed in the table. The majority of medical causes of coma are established without a CT or with the study being normal.

COMA AFTER HEAD TRAUMA Concussion is a common form of transient coma which probably results from torsion of the hemispheres about the midbrain-diencephalic junction with brief interruption of RAS function. Persistent coma after head trauma presents a more complex and serious problem. (Chap. 344).

EMERGENCY TREATMENT OF THE COMATOSE PATIENT The immediate goal in acute coma is prevention of further nervous system damage. Hypotension, hypoglycemia, hypoxia, hypercapnia, and hyperthermia should be rapidly and assiduously corrected. An oro-

TABLE 21-1 Approach to the differential diagnosis of coma

I Normal brainstem reflexes, no lateralizing signs
- *A* Anatomic lesions of hemisphere found
  - *1* Hydrocephalus
  - *2* Bilateral subdural hematomas
  - *3* Bilateral contusions, edema, or axonal shearing of hemispheres due to closed head trauma, subarachnoid hemorrhage
- *B* Bilateral hemispheral dysfunction without mass lesion (CT normal)
  - *1* Drug-toxin ingestion (toxicologic analysis)
  - *2* Endogenous metabolic encephalopathy (glucose, ammonia, calcium, osmolarity, P_{O_2}, P_{CO_2}, urea, sodium)
  - *3* Shock, hypertensive encephalopathy
  - *4* Meningitis (CSF analysis)
  - *5* Nonherpetic viral encephalitis (CSF analysis)
  - *6* Epilepsy (EEG)
  - *7* Reye's syndrome (ammonia, increased intracranial pressure)
  - *8* Fat embolism
  - *9* Subarachnoid hemorrhage with normal CT (CSF analysis)
  - *10* Acute disseminated encephalomyelitis (CSF analysis)
  - *11* Acute hemorrhagic leukoencephalitis
  - *12* Advanced Alzheimer's and Creutzfeldt-Jakob disease

II Normal brainstem reflexes (with or without unilateral compressive third nerve palsy), lateralizing motor signs (CT abnormal)
- *A* Unilateral mass lesion found
  - *1* Cerebral hemorrhage (basal ganglia, thalamus)
  - *2* Large infarction with surrounding brain edema
  - *3* Herpes virus encephalitis (temporal lobe lesion)
  - *4* Subdural or epidural hematoma
  - *5* Tumor with edema
  - *6* Brain abscess with edema
  - *7* Vasculitis with multiple infarctions
  - *8* Metabolic encephalopathy superimposed on preexisting focal lesions (i.e., stroke)
  - *9* Pituitary apoplexy
- *B* Asymmetric signs accompanied by diffuse hemispheral dysfunction
  - *1* Metabolic encephalopathies with asymmetric signs (blood chemical determinations)
  - *2* Isodense subdural hematoma (brain scan, angiogram)
  - *3* Thrombotic thrombocytopenic purpura (blood smear, platelet count)
  - *4* Epilepsy with focal seizures or postictal state (EEG)

III Multiple brainstem reflex abnormalities
- *A* Anatomic lesions in brainstem found
  - *1* Pontine, midbrain hemorrhage
  - *2* Cerebellar hemorrhage, tumor, abscess
  - *3* Cerebellar infarction with brainstem compression
  - *4* Mass in hemisphere causing advanced bilateral brainstem compression
  - *5* Brainstem tumor or demyelination
  - *6* Traumatic brainstem contusion-hemorrhage (clinical signs, auditory-evoked potentials)
- *B* Brainstem dysfunction without mass lesion
  - *1* Basilar artery thrombosis causing brainstem stroke (clinical signs, angiogram)
  - *2* Severe drug overdose (toxicologic analysis)
  - *3* Brainstem encephalitis
  - *4* Basilar artery migraine
  - *5* Brain death

pharyngeal airway is adequate to keep the pharynx open in drowsy patients who are breathing normally. Tracheal intubation is indicated if there is obvious apnea, hypoventilation, or emesis, or if the patient is liable to aspirate. Mechanical ventilation is required if the patient is apneic or hypoventilating or if there is an intracranial mass and hypocapnia is therapeutically necessary. An intravenous access is established and naloxone and dextrose administered if narcotic overdose or hypoglycemia are even remote possibilities. Thiamine is generally administered with glucose in order to prevent an exacerbation of Wernicke's encephalopathy. The veins of intravenous drug abusers may be difficult to cannulate; in such cases, naloxone can be injected sublingually through a small-gauge needle. In cases of suspected basilar thrombosis with brainstem ischemia, intravenous heparin is administered after obtaining a CT scan, keeping in mind that cerebellar and pontine hemorrhages bear some resemblance to the syndrome of basilar occlusion. Physostigmine, when used by experienced physicians with careful monitoring, may awaken patients with anticholinergic-type drug overdose, but many physicians believe that this is justified only if cardiac arrhythmias are a problem. Intravenous fluid administration should be carefully monitored in any serious acute nervous system illness because of the potential for exacerbating brain swelling. Neck injuries must not be overlooked, particularly prior to attempting the oculocephalic maneuver. Headache accompanied by fever and meningismus indicate need for examination of the CSF to diagnose meningitis, and *lumbar puncture should not be delayed while awaiting a CT scan.*

Enlargement of one pupil usually indicates secondary midbrain compression by a hemispheral mass and demands immediate reduction of intracranial pressure. Intravenous fluids are slowed to the minimum necessary to support blood pressure. Therapeutic hyperventilation is then used to achieve an arterial P_{CO_2} of 28 to 32 mmHg. This acts rapidly to reduce intracranial pressure, but the beneficial effect rarely lasts more than 2 h. Hyperosmolar therapy with mannitol may be used simultaneously with hyperventilation in critical cases, but its effects are not apparent for several minutes. It is generally best to administer mannitol before attempting to intubate a patient with suspected, impending herniation. A ventricular puncture may be necessary to decompress the intracranial compartment by removing CSF if medical measures fail. Virtually all patients who survive to arrive in an emergency room can be protected from further brain damage by these means until definitive therapy is possible. The use of high-dose barbiturates soon after cardiac arrest has not been shown in clinical studies to be beneficial, although they may still be useful in lowering intracranial pressure acutely under special circumstances.

BRAIN DEATH Brain death results from total cessation of cerebral blood flow and global infarction of the brain at a time when cardiovascular and respiratory functions remain preserved, the latter requiring artificial support. It is the only type of irrevocable loss of brain function recognized by law as death. Many sets of roughly equivalent criteria have been advanced for the diagnosis of brain death, and it is essential to adhere to those approved locally and recognized as standard practice. Ideal criteria are ones that are simple and conducted at the bedside and which allow no chance of diagnostic error. Widespread cortical destruction is usually shown by an isoelectric EEG and unresponsiveness to the environment, midbrain damage by absent pupillary light reaction, pontine damage by absent oculovestibular and corneal reflexes, and medullary dysfunction by apnea. Some period of observation, usually 6 to 24 h, is desirable during which this state is shown to be sustained. The pupils need not be fully dilated but should not be constricted. The absence of spinal reflexes is not required since the spinal cord remains functional in many cases. The possibility of profound drug-induced or hypothermic nervous system depression should always be excluded.

The demonstration of apnea generally requires that the P_{CO_2} be high enough to stimulate respiration. This can be safely accomplished in most patients by removing the respirator and using diffusion oxygenation sustained by a tracheal cannula connected to an oxygen supply. In brain-dead patients, CO_2 tension increases approximately 2 mmHg/min during apnea. At the end of an appropriate interval, arterial P_{CO_2} should be at least above 50 mmHg (higher limits have been suggested) for the test to be valid. Large posterior fossa lesions that compress the brainstem, nervous system–depressant drugs, and profound hypothermia can simulate brain death, but adherence to recognized protocols for diagnosis will prevent these errors. Radionuclide brain scanning or cerebral angiography may be used to demonstrate the absence of cerebral blood flow in brain death. These techniques have the virtue of rapidity but are often cumbersome and expensive and have not been extensively correlated with pathologic material.

There is no implicit pressure to make the diagnosis of brain death except when organ transplantation or difficult resource allocation (intensive care) issues are involved. Although it is eminently reasonable to disconnect the respirator from a brain-dead patient after proper explanations to the family, there is no obligation to do so and some physicians prefer to await the inevitable cardiovascular failure that follows brain death if full medical support is omitted, usually within a week.

PROGNOSIS OF COMA Interest in predicting the outcome of coma is oriented toward allocating medical resources and limiting the support of hopeless cases. To date, no collection of clinical signs except those of brain death assuredly predicts coma outcome. Children and young adults may have ominous, early clinical findings such as abnormal brainstem reflexes and yet recover. All schemes for prognosis should, therefore, be taken as only approximate indicators, and medical judgments must be conservatively tempered by other factors such as age, underlying disease, general medical condition, and the previously expressed wishes of the patient. In an attempt to collect prognostic information from large numbers of patients with head injury, a "coma scale" scoring system has been devised which empirically has predictive value in cases of brain trauma (see Chap. 344). Major points include a 95 percent death rate in patients whose pupillary reaction or reflex eye movements were absent 6 h after onset of coma, and a 91 percent death rate if the pupils were unreactive at 24 h (though 4 percent made a good recovery).

Prognostication of nontraumatic coma is more difficult because of the heterogeneity of contributing diseases. Unfavorable signs in the first hours after admission have been reported to be the absence of any two of pupillary reaction, corneal reflex, or the oculovestibular response. One day after the onset of coma, the above signs, in addition to absence of eye opening and muscle tone, predicted death or severe disability and the same signs at 3 days strengthened the prediction of a poor outcome. In many patients precise combinations of predictive signs do not occur and coma scales lose their value. The use of evoked potentials has recently been shown to aid prognostication in head-injured and postcardiac arrest patients. Bilateral absence of cortical somatosensory evoked potentials is associated with death or a vegetative state in most cases. It may be wisest to fully support all but those patients whose extreme signs convincingly suggest a poor outcome. Medical practitioners are becoming less reluctant to withdraw support from brain-dead patients as predictions become more reliable and resources more limited.

REFERENCES

FINKLESTEIN S, ROPPER A: The diagnosis of coma: Its pitfalls and limitations. Heart Lung 8:1059, 1979

FISHER CM: The neurological examination of the comatose patient. Acta Neurol Scand 45 (Suppl 6):1, 1969

IVAN L, BRUCE D: *Coma*. Springfield, Ill, Charles C Thomas, 1982

JENNET B et al: Prognosis of patients with severe head injury. Neurosurgery 4:283, 1979

LEVY D et al: Prognosis in non-traumatic coma. Ann Intern Med 94:229, 1981

PLUM F, POSNER J: *The Diagnosis of Stupor and Coma*, 3d ed. Philadelphia, Davis, 1980

ROPPER AH: Coma and acutely raised intracranial pressure, in *Diseases of the Nervous System*, A Asbury, G McKhann, I McDonald (eds). Philadelphia, Saunders, 1986

22 DISORDERS OF SPEECH AND LANGUAGE

JAY P. MOHR / RAYMOND D. ADAMS

Language and speech are fundamental both to social intercourse and to intellectual life. When disordered as a consequence of disease of the brain, the loss exceeds blindness, deafness, or paralysis in gravity.

The terms *speech* and *language* refer to complex and poorly understood activities of the cerebrum. The terms are not synonymous. *Speech* involves the execution of acquired skills of the vocal, manual, auditory, and visual systems in communication. These skills include pronunciation of words; variations in stress, intonation, and melody; the production of graphic marks in the accepted spatial orientation; the auditory discrimination of spoken speech and its classification as to speaker; the visual discrimination of handwritten or printed speech; the visual search patterns involved in scanning a text; and the use of other, less specifiable behaviors. Deficiencies in these skills impede communication apart from any separate impairment in language usage; when intact, these skills suffice only for elemental communication, such as that between two individuals who speak languages unfamiliar to each other.

Language has a wider connotation and refers to the selection and serial ordering of individual words according to rules that permit a person using the speech modalities to modify the behavior of another and to express that poorly understood cerebral activity termed *thinking*. A disturbance of language usage, usually accompanied by a disturbance in speech from cerebral dysfunction, is referred to as *aphasia*, or more properly as *dysphasia*.

CEREBRAL DOMINANCE AND ITS RELATIONSHIP TO SPEECH AND HANDEDNESS

The dominant side is inferred from which eye, hand, or foot is chosen preferentially for intricate, complex acts. Such preference is more complete in some persons than in others. The reason for preference of a hand, foot, or eye depends on hereditary and anatomic factors and is partly acquired. Over 90 percent of people are right-handed. Left-handedness may be hereditary or may result from disease of the left cerebral hemisphere in early life. Handedness and cerebral dominance may fail to develop in some individuals and in certain families.

Anatomic differences exist between the dominant and the minor cerebral hemispheres. The planum temporale, a part of Wernicke's language zone, is larger in the left hemisphere in right-handed individuals. Many children are shifted at an early age from left to right (shifted sinistrals) because it is a handicap to be left-handed in a right-handed world. A disturbance in language is produced in almost all right-handers by unilateral brain damage that affects the left hemisphere. Lesions in the left cerebral hemisphere also account for most language disturbances in left-handed individuals, implying that cerebral dominance can differ for different functions.

LANGUAGE DISORDERS IN MEDICAL PRACTICE

Language disorders may be divided into four categories:

1. *Aphasia* is defined as a state in which there is a loss more or less exclusively of the production and/or comprehension of speech and language from an acquired cerebral lesion. The more limited term, dysphasia, is commonly used.
2. *Dysarthria* is a defect in articulation. These defects are pure motor disorders of the muscles of articulation in the presence of intact mental functions and may be due to flaccid or spastic paralysis, rigidity, repetitive spasms (stuttering), or ataxia.
3. *Aphonia or dysphonia* is the loss of voice due to a disease of the larynx or its innervation.
4. *Disturbances of language* occur with diseases that produce delirium and dementia (see Chap. 23). Speech is seldom lost, and language is deranged as part of a general impairment of cerebral functions.

APHASIA OR DYSPHASIA As a general orientation, most lesions that lead to aphasia occur in the perisylvian regions (frontal, temporal, and parietal) of the dominant cerebral hemisphere, i.e., the left side in right-handed individuals. The anatomic site of the lesion can usually be characterized by computerized tomography (CT scan) or magnetic resonance imaging (MRI).

Diseases of the cerebral surface gray matter produce a more significant deficit than those confined to the white matter: tumors, located largely in the white matter, usually reach a large size before causing a speech or language deficit. Infarcts or traumatic lesions of one or more centimeters in diameter are usually associated with an evanescent deficit that fades to functional insignificance within weeks or months.

Deficits due to acute lesions are most easily demonstrated in the acute phase. Improvements over weeks to months occur in all but the largest vascular lesions, but those due to tumors show progression. The site is more significant than the size of the lesion: the former determines the qualitative features of the deficit, while size determines the severity of the syndrome. Furthermore, deficits in speech function predominate in smaller lesions, while major disturbances in language are superimposed on the speech disturbance in the larger lesions.

Anteriorly placed sylvian lesions mainly disturb the acts of speaking, ranging from mutism, through impaired articulation, to disordered transitions from syllable to syllable, to abnormalities in phrasing, intonation, and melody. Lesions more posterior produce malpositioning of the tongue, lips, and other structures in the oropharynx with errors from some anticipatory syllables occurring out of sequence. Lesions grouped around the posterior sylvian fissure including the superior temporal lobe and its auditory gyri are manifested by disordered understanding of spoken words, resulting in poor repetition of speech sounds.

The language deficits that are superimposed on the speech disturbances are less well correlated with anatomic pathology. Language disturbances can be separated by pathoanatomic considerations into two large groups. Large anterior lesions involving the bulk of the frontal operculum (that region which lies above the insula) and the insula itself result in agrammatism, featuring sharply contracted sentence structure, absence of most small words, and a preservation of words serving mainly a predicative, interjectional, or substantive function. The patient may only be able to say "hi," "no," "hello" or to use simple nouns, i.e., ball, top, key. Large posterior sylvian lesions show almost the opposite, with simple speech elements missing or replaced by substitutions in which the desired response is only approximated (*paraphasias*). These latter may consist of faulty pronunciations (*literal paraphasias*) or faulty word selections (*verbal paraphasias*). Verbal paraphasias may approximate the desired word with a similarity of sound or of spelling (*formal verbal paraphasias*), such as "stock" for "stop" or by similarity of meaning (*semantic verbal paraphasias*) such as "slow" for "stop." Disturbances in understanding language, both auditory and visual speech, occur in both types of major paraphasias.

Lesions well away from the sylvian region either cause no disturbance of human communicative skills or alter them only secondarily. An example of the latter is the lesion of the anterior frontal lobes, especially the medial and orbital parts, that impairs all motor activities and often results in lack of attention and responsiveness (abulia), verging on the akinetic mute state (see Chap. 21). The speech is laconic with long pauses between utterances, and there is an inability to sustain monologue and narrative. Extensive occipital lesions impair reading and reduce the utilization of all visual, lexical stimuli. Thalamic and deep cerebral lesions impair alertness and cause fluctuating states or inattention and disorientation, thereby inducing fragmentation of words (neologisms) and phrases, and protracted uncontrollable talking (logorrhea). Strong stimulation to increase momentarily the level of awareness and altertness will show that such patients have intact language mechanisms.

The nondominant hemisphere provides the substratum for several types of behavior: motor responses of mimicry, social anticipation (smiling, handshaking, modesty reactions), and self-care (washing and feeding); avoidance behavior to noxious stimuli; and the capability of cross matching visually when presented simple words with pictures. It follows that tests which elicit these behaviors are no guide to functions of the hemisphere dominant for language.

Lesions of the frontal (motor) regions are generally believed to produce syndromes independent from those of the posterior (sensory) regions; the dysphasias can be classified as motor (Broca's) or sensory (Wernicke's) and can be further specified as subcortical, cortical, or transcortical in location. Subcortical lesions are believed to cut off the main efferent or afferent projections of the cortical "center"; cortical lesions involve the centers themselves; transcortical lesions isolate the centers from one another, i.e., a kind of "conduction" aphasia, or from other regions of the brain related to speech. These basic concepts provide a useful framework for the classification of the aphasias but are inadequate as guides to the lesions site and size.

TYPES OF APHASIA Disturbances of speech and language can result from several abnormalities. Classifications have been based upon the predominant form, the presumed physiologic or psychological bases, and the anatomy of the underlying diseases. The classification utilized here has been formulated on the basis of the anatomic localization and the clinical presentation (see Table 22-1). The prognoses are helpful in management, particularly in the choice of corrective measures in therapy. Aphasias may also be classified according to the severity of impediment to speech production and flow. *Fluent aphasias* are characterized by runs of well-articulated speech, of basically normal rhythm and flow, although lacking in language meaning. The defect is usually a lesion in the dominant parietal or temporal lobe. *Nonfluent aphasias* are characterized by slow, incorrectly articulated words and sentences. The lesion usually lies in the dominant frontal lobe.

Complete (global) aphasia In complete, or global, aphasia the causative lesion destroys a large part of the speech and language areas of the major cerebral hemisphere, producing the maximal aphasic deficit and has the least chance of improvement of any aphasic syndrome. Infarction from occlusion of the left internal or the middle cerebral artery at its origin, or a large hemorrhage, major tumor, or trauma is most often responsible. In the rare instances of rapid improvement, the main cause is transitory ischemia from a fragmenting embolus, posttraumatic edema, or postconvulsive paralysis; rarely, hyperthermia, infection, or hyponatremia may transiently cause a temporary relapse of aphasia due to an old lesion.

Most patients with total aphasia say at most a few words; they do not read or write, and they understand only a few words and phrases of the speech of others. Related signs include right hemiplegia, hemianesthesia, and homonymous hemianopsia. The state of consciousness may vary from full alertness to semicoma. The alert patient

TABLE 22-1 Classification of aphasic disorders

	Anatomic location	Clinical manifestations	Etiology	Associated clinical symptoms
MAJOR SYNDROMES				
Global aphasia	Large lesion of dominant frontal, parietal, and superior temporal lobe	Minimal speech; nonfluent aphasia; comprehension poor for spoken and written language	Infarction in distribution of internal carotid or middle cerebral artery; trauma; tumor	Contralateral hemiplegia; hemisensory loss; hemianopsia
Broca's aphasia	Cortical and subcortical lesion of prefrontal and frontal regions	Nonfluent aphasia; agrammatic sentences; poor articulation; dysprosody; may be mute	Infarction in distribution of superior frontal branch middle cerebral artery; hemorrhage; tumor	Contralateral hemiparesis; minor or no sensory loss; no visual field disturbance; oral dyspraxia; cortical dysarthria; severe impairment in writing
Wernicke's aphasia (central or sensory aphasia)	Posterior perisylvian structures of the parietal and temporal lobe	Fluent speech; total incomprehension of spoken speech; inability to read or to repeat sounds or words; alexia, agraphia, paraphasia common	Infarction in distribution of lower division of middle cerebral artery; tumor; herpes simplex encephalitis	Parietal lobe sensory deficits; hemianopsia; no motor disturbance
MINOR CENTRAL APHASIA SYNDROMES				
Conduction aphasia	Upper bank of sylvian fissure; inferior parietal lobule	Paraphasia; difficulty in repetition of speech and in reading aloud; aware of deficit; adequate comprehension of written and spoken words	Embolic occlusion of posterior branches of middle cerebral artery	Contralateral hemihypesthesia or homonymous hemianopsia; abnormal optokinetic nystagmus
Mainly auditory (pure word deafness)	Lesion in superior temporal gyrus	Impaired auditory comprehension; inability to repeat a sentence or write a dictation	Infarction; tumor; abscess	Rare deafness
Mainly visual (dyslexia with dysgraphia)	Parietooccipital lesion	Visual language compromised more than auditory; cannot read or write	Infarction; tumor, lobar hemorrhage	Hemianopsia
OTHER SYNDROMES				
Pure word blindness	Left occipito-striate cortex, adjacent association cortex, and posterior corpus callosum (splenium)	Normal spoken language and writing, with inability to read	Infarction in distribution of posterior cerebral artery; tumor, lobar hemorrhage	Hemianopsia
Isolation of speech areas	Ischemic infarction in border (watershed) zones between anterior, middle and posterior cerebral artery distributions	Parrot-like speech; echolalia	Systemic hypotension or hypoxia; cardiac arrest	Decreased alertness and responsiveness; bilateral leg weakness
Amnesic-dysnomic aphasia	Deep temporal lobe lesions, parahippocampal, hippocampal gyrus	Inability to recall names of objects or parts of objects; difficulty with recent memory	Tumor; Alzheimer's disease; infarction in distribution posterior cerebral artery; herpes simplex encephalitis	Apraxia; dementia; no motor or sensory abnormalities; upper quadrantic visual field defect

may participate in common gestures of greeting, may show modesty and avoidance reactions, and is able to engage in self-help activities. The early appearance of clearly vocalized stereotyped words, such as "hi" and "yes," are often falsely encouraging signs; they may reflect the uninhibited function of the right hemisphere. With the passage of time some degree of understanding of spoken speech may be evident, and a few spoken words may emerge.

Broca's aphasia (major motor aphasia) This term is used to designate a complex syndrome, which features failure of motor aspects of speaking and writing, accompanied by agrammatism with a less obvious impairment in language comprehension. Although formerly thought to be due to a circumscribed lesion in the inferior frontal convolution (Broca's area), the syndrome is the result of a much larger lesion involving cortical and subcortical structures along the frontal and superior sylvian fissure and the insula. This region may not be well visualized by CT scan since the tissue defect may seem to merge with the sylvian fissure.

The syndrome is most often due to embolic occlusions of the upper division of the left middle cerebral artery; major putaminal hypertensive hemorrhage, huge frontal lobe tumor or abscess, metastatic lesions, subdural hematoma, and encephalitis are less common causes.

The lesions are smaller than those causing complete aphasia and usually involve the sensorimotor rolandic region, producing an accompanying persisting hemiparesis and hemisensory syndrome. Initially, a transient ipsilateral deviation of the eyes is observed, due to the frontal infarction.

In the acute phase, the entire language mechanism appears to be inactivated, and the helplessly mute, noncommunicative, and uncomprehending patient presents the syndrome of complete or global aphasia, indistinguishable by present methods from that resulting from infarction of the whole left middle cerebral artery territory. Within weeks to years, the disorder of comprehension abates somewhat but remains detected by formal testing. The improvement in comprehension exceeds that in speaking and writing, leaving a syndrome that conforms to the traditional motor aphasia.

For a time, despite a satisfactory comprehension of spoken words and the ability to read simple commands, an apraxia of the lingual and oropharyngeal apparatus retards efforts to make purposeful or commanding movements. Imitation of the examiner's actions may be better performed than execution of acts on command, and self-initiated actions are often, but not always, normal. Certain stereotyped and simple phrases or curses are uttered more easily, such as "hi," "good morning," "how are you," and the words of popular songs may be sung surprisingly well. The patient's efforts to speak and facial expressions suggest an awareness of his or her own ineptitudes and mistakes, and an accompanying exasperation and despair are common.

As improvement occurs, particularly in the milder forms of motor aphasia, the patient is able to speak aloud to some degree. Words are enunciated slowly and laboriously. Articulation and the melody of speech (prosody) are impaired. This dysfluency takes the form of improper accent on stress on certain syllables, incorrect phrasing of words in a series and pacing of the speed of word sequences, and even a stammering quality to the uttered phrases. Speech is sparse and consists mainly of nouns, transitive verbs, and important adjectives; many of the small words (articles, prepositions, conjunctions) are omitted, giving the speech an *agrammatic* and telegraphic character. The preservation of substantive words allows the patients to communicate despite the gross mechanical and language difficulties. Once fully established, these speech impediments persist and improve only slightly despite years of therapy.

Most patients with Broca's aphasia have a correspondingly severe impairment in writing. Should their right hand be paralyzed, they cannot print with their left one; if manual mobility is spared, they fail as completely in writing out their commands or replies to questions as in speaking them. Writing from dictation is severly impaired, though letters and words can still be copied. On careful testing, however, communication by writing is superior to that of speaking, suggesting a certain independence between these two acts as vehicles of language.

Minor motor aphasia More circumscribed focal lesions along the anterior and superior sylvian operculum and insula produce remarkably discrete effects on the mechanical elaboration of speech. The important point with minor motor aphasias is that they at first may resemble major motor aphasia except for the satisfactory understanding of spoken and written words. The prognosis for nearly full recovery is excellent. Indeed, *none of these focal lesions produces significant or lasting deficits in language usage*. However, in the acute phase the experienced listener can easily detect the error patterns in speech and, through them, discern the nature of the communicative difficulties of the sufferer, who is acutely aware of and discouraged by the deficit.

The effects of speech or focal lesions take several forms. *Broca's area infarction* involves the lower premotor cortex adjacent to the motor cortex for the oropharynx, larynx, and respiratory apparatus; the infarct interrupts skilled movements of these muscle groups, and the resultant dyspraxia in speech takes the form of impaired transitions between syllables and words and disruption of the melodic intonation of phrases (dysprosody). Involvement of this region alone is insufficient to produce the major syndrome referred to as Broca's aphasia. *Rolandic infarction* involves the sensorimotor cortex itself; either the syndrome of dysprosody occurs or speech has poor articulation and lowered volume and pitch, while a nasal quality to the voice reveals the paresis of the nasopharyngeal musculature. *Postcentral, anterior parietal infarction* is associated with errors in the positioning of the oral cavity for individual sounds, syllables, and whole words; the acoustic features of the utterance are often distorted by these malpositions of the oral cavity and strike the ear as literal paraphasias. Since they are easily produced in tests of repeating, reading aloud, and occur in conversation, the patient could be mislabeled as having "conduction" aphasia.

Lesions in the lateral parts of the dominant frontal lobe, sparing Broca's area may also cause an aphasic disorder. Usually speech output is reduced and nonfluent, and auditory comprehension is intact. Repetition of words spoken by the examiner is preserved. This condition has been called *transcortical motor aphasia*. It must be distinguished from a closely related condition in which spontaneous speech is lacking (mutism) and all motor activity is reduced (akinesia). What is lacking is the impulse to speak or to move. The causative lesions are more widespread—in the medial part of the frontal lobe, the supplementary motor area, and the cingulate gyrus.

Most such focal lesions are due to emboli to the sequential branches of the upper division of the middle cerebral artery. Deeper, larger lesions or larger emboli involving the stem of the upper division can cause several types of deficit in a single patient, making these individual distinctions less clear and blending with the major syndrome of Broca's aphasia. Facial, lingual, and sometimes brachial paresis and ideomotor dyspraxia of the face and left, nondominant limbs commonly accompany the speech disorder. Most of these syndromes recede within weeks or months.

Wernicke's aphasia (major central or sensory aphasia) This term encompasses a range of syndromes that arise from lesions of the posterior perisylvian structures or the posterior temporal, parietal, and occipital regions supplied by the lower division of the middle cerebral artery. There is disruption of the whole array of language behavior. When restricted to the temporal lobe, the main disturbance is most evident in language tasks involving words heard; and when more parietal and occipital, in words seen.

Spoken and written efforts in communication as well as in auditory and visual comprehension are affected, a combination that justifies the term *central aphasia*. The term *sensory aphasia* was formerly used to accentuate the contrast with motor (Broca's) aphasia. Instead of the difficult articulation, faulty transitions, dysmelodic speaking, and disproportionate condensation of grammatical forms that characterize Broca's aphasia, the speech of Wernicke's aphasia is fluent, hence the name *fluent aphasia*.

In severe cases, the patients utters a series of incomprehensible syllables, makes illegible marks on a page in attempts at writing, cannot be made to repeat aloud or copy correctly at sight, and treats the examiner's attempts at written and verbal communication as if they were in a wholly unfamiliar foreign language. In less severe cases, the patient can repeat aloud and copy but echoes the words heard with faulty pronunciation or copies the words in a slavish manner, imitating even the examiner's handwriting style, as though the test words were unfamiliar. The disturbance in language does not simply reflect a disturbance in hearing or in vision. In the mildest cases, the deficits are manifested in errors in word comprehension and usage. The patient may choose words that show approximation to the desired response, the words often belonging to the same functional class [i.e., *cow* for *pig*, but not *cow* for *yellow* (such errors are labeled *semantic verbal paraphasias*)]; or they may be similar in sound or shape (*formal verbal paraphasias*) such as "flee" for "tree"; there may be errors in word structure, with improper tenses, prefixes, suffixes (i.e., *beautifuling*); or other errors that resemble those of normal people unfamiliar with the language in question. Some such patients pass for normal in brief or casual conversation. In its milder form or later in the course of the illness, the speech resembles that of a person tired or distracted, and the abnormality is detected only on tests of complex language function.

CT scanning and MRI are the best methods to delineate the topography of the lesion. Arteriographic findings are an unreliable basis of correlation because the vascular occlusions, most often due to cerebral embolism, frequently fail to show the embolus because it has disintegrated or drifted distally into one or more smaller branches. Radionuclide brain scanning is useful only for the largest lesions.

Minor central aphasia syndromes In time, Wernicke's aphasia improves, and a number of lesser syndromes appear. These latter, however, may be present in comparatively pure form from the beginning, when only a small, restricted lesion involves some part of the territory of the lower division of the middle cerebral artery.

The posterior sylvian region, comprising posterosuperior temporal, opercular, supramarginal, and posterior insular gyri, appears to encompass a variety of language functions. Seemingly minor changes in size and locale of the lesion are associated with important variations in the elements of Wernicke's aphasia. Depending on the location of the lesion, language behavior dependent on auditory function (hearing spoken words, echoing sounds and speech, relating the spoken to the written word, and finally repeating and writing it) may be deranged partially or completely. The same is true of language behavior dependent upon visual function, when the left posterior parietal lobe is involved. These partial syndromes are termed conduction aphasia, pure word deafness, dyslexia with dysgraphia, and pure word blindness.

CONDUCTION APHASIA: SEPARATION OF WERNICKE'S AND BROCA'S LANGUAGE AREAS The principal abnormality resembles Wernicke's aphasia. There is the same degree of paraphasia in self-initiated speech, in repeating what is heard, and in reading aloud. However, little or no difficulty is encountered in comprehending words that are heard or seen. Because the motor regions are unaffected, no element of dysarthria or dysprosody occurs. The patient is alert and unaware of the deficit. The mistakes take the form of literal paraphasia; i.e., errors in oropharyngeal positioning produce detectably different sounds from those intended. The disorder in repeating from dictation becomes more apparent when the rate of presentation of auditory material is increased, the uttered words are polysyllabic, or when words are unfamiliar, e.g., sets of nonsense syllables. Since nouns are usually the longest words in sentences, one may gain an impression that they are specifically affected.

The lesion at autopsy is located in the cortex and subcortical white matter in the upper bank of the sylvian fissure, involving the supramarginal gyrus of the inferior parietal lobule. The posterior part of the superior temporal region is occasionally affected. The usual cause is an embolus in the ascending parietal or posterior temporal branch of the middle cerebral artery. Deeper, larger lesions that interrupt the arcuate fasciculus connecting the temporal and frontal lobes may produce the syndrome, but usually they involve other pathways as well, giving rise to a more extensive speech deficit (Wernicke's aphasia or amnesic aphasia). However, these latter types of aphasia, as they regress, may resolve into conduction aphasia. More anterior insular lesions usually include some degree of Broca's aphasia.

PURE WORD DEAFNESS Instead of a disturbance confined to auditory comprehension, this more inclusive syndrome is the auditory form of Wernicke's aphasia. The most obvious findings are an impaired auditory comprehension and inability to repeat what is said or to write to dictation. Spoken language is less impaired but rarely normal, and occasionally the patient is initially diagnosed as having Wernicke's aphasia. By audiometric testing no hearing defect is found, or minor abnormalities appear that reveal the underlying deficit in individual cases. Ordinary sounds can be distinguished. The patient is forced to depend heavily on visual cues in understanding the remarks of others and frequently uses these cues well enough to obviate much of the difficulty. Tests that prevent the use of visual cues readily uncover the deficit. Comprehension of visually presented material such as printed matter, although not normal, is better than auditory comprehension. There may be full preservation of reading skill, in which instance one is justified in using the traditional term *pure word deafness.*

In most autopsy studies a lesion is embolic, bilateral in the superior temporal gyrus, in position to damage the primary auditory cortex in the transverse gyrus of Heschl and to impair its relation to the associated areas of the superior, posterior part of the temporal lobe. The occasional unilateral lesions are localized in this part of the major (dominant) temporal lobe and encroach on those regions whose involvement precipitates the larger syndrome of Wernicke's aphasia.

DYSLEXIA WITH DYSGRAPHIA This language disturbance is often a late sequela of the larger syndrome of Wernicke's aphasia, most evident in reading and writing. The syndrome is the visual form of Wernicke's aphasia. Errors occur in response to lexical stimuli. Auditory comprehension, while not normal, is less impaired than visual comprehension. Since conversational testing is frequently the only type of clinical evaluation in such patients, satisfactory auditory comprehension, ability to repeat aloud, and mild paraphasic errors in spontaneous speech frequently lead to a misdiagnosis of mild Wernicke's aphasia. Detailed testing of reading aloud and reading for comprehension and tests of spontaneous writing and of writing in response to dictated and visually presented material reveal a greater disturbance in these tasks and expose the syndrome.

The parietal and occipital region is usually affected. Although a discrete embolism is unusual, a small clot may pass through the more proximal territory and lodge distally. Tumors, abscess, and lobar hemorrhages usually disrupt other structures as well, and this syndrome is often a less conspicuous part of a larger clinical picture. Systemic hypotension and hypoxia may leave dyslexia with dysgraphia as a residual impairment, but more often they produce a more severe defect, described below under "Isolation of speech areas."

PURE WORD BLINDNESS In the fully developed syndrome, the victims lose the ability to read and usually to name colors. The patient is unable to name or point to a letter or word on command. However, understanding spoken language, repetition of what is heard, writing to dictation, and conversation are all intact. Because the victim may be unaware the deficit exists, the examiner is often required to test for its presence, rather than simply assume the complaint will be volunteered. In the most severe alexics, the actual letter or name responses have little connection with the presented stimuli. The response may be corrected and the defect obscured if other visual cues are available, such as the bottle on which the words Coca-Cola appear. The naming of common colors presented singly and of objects is also impaired. In lesser degrees of the affection, reading is impaired mainly in the affected visual field, producing a dyslexia for the letters on the affected side of the longer words (so-called hemidyslexia). The condition is also sometimes termed *dyslexia without dysgraphia*.

Right homonymous hemianopsia, an amnesic defect (see Chap. 23), and a hemisensory defect on the right reflect the involvement of the left occipital lobe, the left fornix and its decussation, and the left thalamus, respectively, a combination that nearly always signifies thrombosis or embolism of the left posterior cerebral artery, placing the origin of this syndrome rather remote from the main language zone supplied by the middle cerebral artery territory.

Autopsy usually demonstrates a lesion that destroys the left visual striate cortex (area 17) and visual association areas (18 and 19), as well as the connections of the right visual cortex and association areas with the temporoparietal region. This latter "disconnection" usually is due to interruption of the fibers passing through the posterior part (splenium) of the corpus callosum, which connect the visual association areas of the two hemispheres. A lesion deep in the left parietooccipital region may also prevent visual information from both occipital lobes reaching the left angular gyrus. In this case the right homonymous hemianopsia may be absent. With purely left cerebral lesions, aside from infarction, there may be a primary or secondary tumor, or, rarely, multifocal leukoencephalopathy.

Isolation of speech areas Following prolonged hypoxia, widespread cerebral ischemia can affect the vascular anatomic border zones linking the major cerebral arteries and their distal branches on the cerebral surfaces and spread centripetally into their adjacent territories. The central fields of supply of these arteries may be spared. In the middle cerebral artery territory, this sparing leaves largely intact the sylvian region and its speech areas. With much of the rest of the brain out of action in patients who survive such episodes, the speech mechanism can be activated by spoken words. There is parrotlike repetition of words and sounds (echolalia) and similar findings which indicate that the auditory-vocal loop is functional. Scant evidence of comprehension or self-initiated conversation is present, reflecting the widespread injury outside the speech regions. The syndrome is common following cardiac arrest.

Amnesic-dysnomic aphasia This may be a relatively early or an isolated manifestation of disease of the nervous system. The patient loses only the ability to produce names on demand, including nouns, adjectives, and other descriptive parts of speech. There are typical pauses in speech, groping for words, and substitution of another word or phrase that conveys the meaning (circumlocution). When shown a series of common objects, the patient may tell of their use instead of giving their names. The difficulty applies not only to objects seen but to the names of things heard or felt. By contrast, other verbal tasks, including recall of the names of the letters and digits, reading, writing, spelling, etc., are almost invariably preserved. That the deficit is principally one of naming is shown by the patient's correct use of the object and, usually, by an ability to point to the correct object on hearing or seeing the name. There is a tendency among patients to attribute the failure to forgetfulness or to give some other excuse for the disability, suggesting that they are not completely aware of the nature of their difficulty.

The causative lesion is usually deep in the temporal lobe, presumably interrupting connections of sensory speech areas with the hippocampal-parahippocampal regions concerned with learning and memory. Masses such as a tumor or abscess are the most frequent; as they enlarge, an upper contralateral quadrantic visual field defect or Wernicke's aphasia is added. Dysnomia may be part of the syndromes produced by occlusion of the temporal branches of the posterior cerebral artery. Alzheimer's disease may begin with a dysnomic or amnesic type of aphasia; by the time the patient's difficulty is fully recognized, other disorders of speech and indifference, apathy, and abulia are conjoined. Dysnomia may also be present in confusional states caused by metabolic, infectious, intoxicative, or other acute medical illnesses, but then it has no certain localizing value.

The combination of dysnomia and major impairment of auditory comprehension with a remarkable retention of the ability to repeat what is heard is called *transcortical sensory aphasia*. The causative lesion spares the auditory cortex and Wernicke area and involves the inferior temporal cortices, particularly area 37.

DISORDERS OF ARTICULATION AND PHONATION In simple dysarthria there is no abnormality of the cortical centers. Dysarthric patients are able to understand what they hear, to read, and to write, even though they are unable to utter a single intelligible word.

The highly coordinated act of speaking involves the larynx, pharynx, palate, tongue, lips, and respiratory musculature, which are innervated by the hypoglossal, vagal, facial, and phrenic nerves. Their nuclei are controlled through the corticobulbar tracts by both motor cortices and by extrapyramidal influences from the cerebellum and basal ganglia. The current of air is produced by expiration and is finely regulated by the activity of the various muscles engaged in speech. *Phonation*, or the production of vocal sounds, is a function of the larynx. Changes in the size and shape of the glottis and in the length and tension of the vocal cords are controlled by the laryngeal muscles, which transmit their vibrations to the column of air passing over the vocal cords. Sounds thus formed are modified as they pass through the nasopharynx and mouth, which act as resonators. Articulation consists of contractions of the tongue, lips, pharynx, and palate, which interrupt or alter the vocal sounds. Vowels are of laryngeal origin, as are some consonants, but the latter are formed for the most part during articulation. For instance, the consonants *m*, *b*, and *p* are labial; *l* and *t* are lingual; and *nk* and *ng* are nasoguttural.

Disorders of phonation prompt examination of the vocal cords, tongue, palate, and pharynx. Defects in articulation can be subdivided into paretic dysarthria; spastic and rigid dysarthria; choreic, myoclonic, and ataxic dysarthria.

Paretic dysarthria This is due to a neural or bulbar (medullary) weakness or paralysis of the articulatory muscles (lower motor neuron paralysis). There is a special difficulty in the correct utterance of vibratives, such as *r*; the voice develops a nasal quality due to palatal weakness; as the paralysis becomes more complete, lingual and labial consonants are not pronounced. In the advanced stages, the shriveled tongue lies inert on the floor of the mouth, and the lips are relaxed and tremulous. Saliva collects in the mouth because of dysphagia and spills over the lips causing drooling. Bulbar palsy, peripheral neuropathies, and muscle diseases, including myasthenia gravis, are common causes.

Spastic and rigid dysarthria These are more frequent than the paralytic variety. Diseases that involve the corticobulbar tracts, usually from vascular disease or motor system disease, either simultaneously or in stages, cause pseudobulbar palsy. In the past, the patient may have had a minor stroke affecting the corticobulbar fibers on one side; but since the bulbar muscles are probably represented in both motor cortices, there is no impairment in speech or swallowing from a unilateral lesion. Should another stroke then occur, involving the other corticobulbar tract and possibly the corticospinal tract at the pontine, midbrain, or capsular level, the patient becomes anarthric or dysarthric and dysphagic. Often the muscles of facial expression on both sides are weakened as well. Unlike bulbar paralysis due to lower neuron involvement, this condition entails no atrophy or fasciculation of the paralyzed muscles; the jaw jerk and other facial reflexes are exaggerated; the palatal reflexes are retained; emotional control is poor (pathologic laughter and crying); and sometimes breathing is periodic (Cheyne-Stokes). When the frontal operculum alone is involved, the speech deficit may be a pure dysarthria but usually without the impairment in emotional control. In the beginning, the patient may be totally anarthric and aphonic, but when improvement occurs or when the patient has a milder version of the same condition, speech is notably slow, thick, and indistinct, much like that of partial bulbar paralysis.

An extrapyramidal disturbance of articulation occurs in Parkinson's syndrome. The patient speaks hastily and articulates poorly, slurring over many syllables and trailing the ends of sentences. The voice is low-pitched, monotonous, and lacking in inflection; voice volume diminishes. In advanced cases speech is almost unintelligible; only whispering is possible.

In many cases of capsular hemiplegia or partially recovered Broca's aphasia, residual dysarthria may be difficult to distinguish from a pure articulatory defect.

Choreic and myoclonic dysarthria In chorea and myoclonus, speech may also be characteristic. Unlike the defect of pseudobulbar palsy or parkinsonism, chorea and myoclonus abruptly interrupt the pronunciation of words by the abnormal movements. Grimacing and other characteristic motor signs suggest the diagnosis.

Ataxic dysarthria This is characteristic of acute and chronic cerebellar lesions and may be observed in multiple sclerosis, Friedreich's ataxia, cerebellar atrophy, and heat stroke. The principal speech abnormality is slowness; imprecise enunciation, monotony, and unnatural, irregular separation of the syllables of words (scanning) are additional features. Coordination of speech and respiration are poor. There may not be enough breath to utter certain words, and others may be ejaculated explosively. Myoclonic jerks involving the speech musculature may be superimposed on cerebellar ataxia in a number of diseases.

APHONIA AND DYSPHONIA Some speech disorders involve disturbances of voice. Paresis of the respiratory movements, as in poliomyelitis and acute infectious polyneuritis, or incoordination as part of extrapyramidal disease may affect the voice because insufficient air is provided for phonation and speech. Reduced volume of speech due to limited excursion of the breathing muscles is common; the patient is unable to speak above a whisper or to shout. Whispering speech is also a feature of stupor, but strong stimulation may make the voice audible.

Paresis of both vocal cords causes complete aphonia. There is no voice, and the patient can speak only in whispers. Since the vocal cords normally separate during inspiration, their failure to do so when paralyzed may result in an inspiratory stridor. If one vocal cord is paralyzed, the voice becomes hoarse, low-pitched, and rasping. Involvement of one of the tenth cranial nerves by tumor, for example, may also cause a nasal voice because the posterior nares do not close during phonation. Consonants such as *b, p, n,* and *k* are followed by escape of air into the nasal passages. The abnormality may be less pronounced in recumbency and may increase when the head is thrown forward. Hoarseness may also be due to structural changes in the vocal cords caused by cigarette smoking, chronic inflammation, polyps, etc.

Spastic dysphonia is a poorly understood neurologic disorder similar to dystonia. Many patients, middle-aged or elderly, otherwise healthy, gradually lose the ability to speak quietly and fluently. Any effort to speak results in contraction of the speech musculature so that the voice is strained and phonation is labored. The patients are not neurotic, and psychotherapy and speech therapy are ineffective. The condition differs from the stridor caused by spasm of the laryngeal muscles in tetany. It is nonprogressive but may be combined with restricted extrapyramidal disorders such as blepharospasm and spasmodic torticollis. Surgical section of the superior laryngeal nerve on one side has been found to at least partially diminish the rigidity.

CLINICAL APPROACH TO LANGUAGE DISORDERS Aphasia In investigating aphasia, it is first necessary to enquire into the patient's native language, handedness, and previous education. Some left-handed children are trained to use their right hand for writing; therefore, one must ask which hand is used for throwing a ball; threading a needle; or using a spoon, hammer, or saw. It is important to establish that the patient is alert and can participate reliably in testing, because assessment of language depends on these factors, as does determining whether the patient has other signs of cerebral disease such as hemiplegia, facial weakness, homonymous hemianopsia, or cortical sensory loss. When hemiplegia, hemianesthesia, and homonymous hemianopsia coexist, the aphasic disorder is usually complete or global. Such major neurologic signs are seldom associated with the less complete forms of language disorder, the posterior sylvian syndromes, or the dissociative syndromes, though one defect may exceed others. Dyspraxia of limbs and speech musculature, in response to spoken commands or to visual mimicry, is generally associated with Broca's aphasia and sometimes with Wernicke's aphasia. Bilateral or unilateral homonymous hemianopsia without motor weakness is often linked with pure word blindness (alexia or dyslexia) or to amnesic-dysnomic aphasia. Bilateral hemiplegias due to extensive frontal lesions are accompanied not infrequently by pure word muteness. The special types of aphasia—alexia, pure word deafness, etc.—are often associated with evidence of embolism to other parts of the brain or other organs.

Conversational testing permits quick assessment of the motor aspects of speech (praxis and prosody), apparent language formulation, and auditory comprehension. Disabilities in the purely motor aspects of speech suggest a motor aphasia, and this possibility can be pursued by tests of repeating from dictation and by tests of praxis of the oropharyngeal and respiratory apparatus. Disabilities in language formulation such as literal paraphasias with impaired comprehension are indicative of Wernicke's aphasia. Disorders confined to naming, generally without paraphasias, when other language functions (reading, writing, spelling, etc.) are adequate, are diagnostic of amnesic dysnomia.

When conversation shows virtually no disabilities, other tests may be revealing. Reading aloud single letters, words, and text may reveal pure word blindness, while tests of writing in this syndrome are normal. Literal and verbal paraphasic errors may appear in milder cases of Wernicke's aphasia as the patient reads aloud from text or from words in the examiner's handwriting. Similar errors occur more frequently when the patient is asked to explain the text, read aloud, or give explanations in writing. Adequacy of response channels is determined by presenting tasks that permit a response physically identical with the test stimulus, such as copying visual stimuli and repeating aloud from auditory stimuli. Inadequacy of receptive or response channels precludes further analysis of the deficit involving that channel in more complex types of tests, except in the unlikely instance that the more complex test is better performed. If reception and response channels are adequate in these initial tests, they may then be used in tests requiring all types of language function, such as writing from dictation, vocal naming of visual stimuli, matching physically dissimilar stimuli having a name in common (e.g., the word *cow* and a picture of a cow). By utilizing the same test material used in the earlier tests, direct comparison of performances in spoken naming, written naming, and matching can be compared from visual, auditory, and palpated stimuli. A performance profile can be constructed separately for each type of stimulus material tested (objects, pictures, words, letters, numbers, colors, etc.) The resultant profile can then be used to determine whether the main deficits fall across one or more input or response channels. These data provide a baseline against which later changes may be compared.

Articulatory-phonation disorders Disturbances of articulation point to involvement of a different set of neural structures, such as the motor cortices; the corticobulbar pathways; the seventh, ninth, and tenth nuclei; the brainstem; and extrapyramidal nuclei and tracts. It may be necessary to use other neurologic findings to decide which of these are implicated. It is particularly important to distinguish between the pseudobulbar or supranuclear palsies and the bulbar palsies. The information obtained by separating these two types of dysarthria is particularly helpful in differential diagnosis.

Dysphonia should lead to an investigation of laryngeal disease, either primary or secondary to an abnormality of innervation. Inspection of the vocal cords is necessary.

TREATMENT Except for almost pure motor defects, most patients show remarkably little concern over the sudden loss of speech. The very lesion that deprives them of speech also appears to cause a partial loss of insight into the disability. For example, in Wernicke's aphasia patients may become indignant when others cannot understand their jargon. Nonetheless, as improvement occurs, many patients become discouraged. Reassurance and a positive program of speech rehabilitation are the best ways of helping the patient at this stage.

Most aphasias are due to vascular disease of the brain, and some degree of spontaneous improvement usually occurs over days to months after the stroke. Sometimes recovery is complete within hours or days; at times not more than a few words are regained after a year or two of assiduous speech training. Nevertheless, many experts in the field believe that speech training is worthwhile.

As a rule, speech therapy is not advisable in the first few days of an aphasic illness, because one does not know how lasting it will be. Also, if a global aphasia is present, the speech therapist is helpless. Under such circumstances, it is preferable to wait until some of the language function has begun to return. Then the physician may begin to encourage and help the patient to use the function to a maximal degree. In milder aphasic disorders speech therapy can be begun as soon as the illness is stabilized. Although speech therapy has not been proved, in controlled studies, to be of benefit to recovery, its value in terms of support for the patient and the family needs to be emphasized. The methods of speech training are specialized, and it is advisable to consult an expert in this field.

There is no special treatment for the dysarthric disturbance of speech.

PROGNOSIS The outcome depends on the underlying disease and the magnitude of the lesion within the speech areas. Global aphasias lasting more than a week or two usually have a bad outcome. Seldom is there enough recovery of communicative speech to permit resumption of occupation or profession. Partial aphasias frequently improve, sometimes to a gratifying degree, if of vascular or encephalitic origin. Aphasias due to embolism, whether global or restricted, may disappear in hours to days or may persist.

REFERENCES

ALBERT ML et al: *Clinical Aspects of Dysphasia.* New York, Springer-Verlag, 1981

DAMASIO AR, GESCHWIND N: The neural basis of language. Ann Rev Neurosci 7:127, 1984

GESCHWIND N: Disconnection syndromes in animals and man. Brain 88:237, 585, 1965

KERTESZ A: *Localization in Neuropsychology.* New York, Academic, 1983

LECOURS AR et al: *Aphasiology.* London, Bailliere Tindall, 1983

MOHR JP: Broca's area and Broca's aphasia, in *Studies in Neurolinguistics,* H Whitaker (ed). New York, Academic, 1975, chap 6

———, SIDMAN M: Aphasia: Behavioral aspects, in *American Handbook of Psychiatry,* vol 4, M Reiser (ed). New York, Basic Books, 1975, pp 279–298

23 CONFUSION, DELIRIUM, AMNESIA, AND DEMENTIA

MAURICE VICTOR / RAYMOND D. ADAMS

All physicians must be able to assess with complete objectivity the patient's character, intellectual function, mood, memory, judgment, and other attributes of personality and behavior. Examination of these affective and cognitive functions permits the physician to reach certain conclusions regarding the patient's *mental status.* Without such data, errors will be made in evaluating the patient's history, in diagnosing the neurologic or psychiatric disease from which he or she suffers, and in conducting an appropriate therapeutic program.

DEFINITION OF TERMS

The definition of normal and abnormal states of mind is difficult because the terms used to describe these states have been given so many different meanings in both medical and nonmedical writings (see also Chap. 11). Compounding the difficulty is the fact that the pathophysiology of the confusional states, delirium, and dementia, is not fully understood, and the definitions depend on their clinical relationships, with the lack of precision which this entails. The following nomenclature, though tentative, has been found useful by the authors and will be employed throughout this textbook.

Confusion is a general term denoting an incapacity of the patient to think with customary speed and clarity. This abnormality may depend on any one of several factors or conditions. At certain stages in the evolution or devolution of stupor and coma, as indicated in Chap. 21, confusion is aligned with a disorder of conscious awareness and perception. In patients with dementia, confusion is related to a derangement of intellectual function, i.e., an inability to learn, remember, calculate, make appropriate deductions from given premises, or reason abstractly. In toxic psychosis, inattention, impairment of perception, and the intrusion of illusory and hallucinatory experiences are mainly responsible for the confusional state. Intense anxiety and other emotional experiences may temporarily interfere with coherence of thinking.

The term *delirium* is used here to denote a special type of confusional state, acute in onset and transient in nature. It is characterized by gross disorientation in the presence of heightened alertness, i.e., an increased readiness to respond to stimuli; a disorder of perception in which illusions and vivid hallucinations are prominent; and overactivity of psychomotor and autonomic nervous functions. Implicit in the definition are certain nonmedical connotations of the term—agitation, excitement, vivid dreams, and creations of the imagination. Most stuporous and many demented patients, in contrast to those with delirium, show a *reduced* state of arousal, alertness, and attentiveness; *decreased* psychomotor activity; and a *relatively slight* tendency to hallucinate. For these reasons, and also because of the particular clinical settings in which they occur, it seems worthwhile to set the delirious states apart from those of depressed consciousness on the one hand and of dementia and amnesia on the other. Such a concept is far from new. To a greater or lesser extent, the terms *symptomatic psychosis, toxic psychosis, infective-exhaustive psychosis,* and *drug, traumatic,* or *febrile delirium* all have reference to the syndrome of delirium. Each of these terms conveys the idea of an acute and transient (reversible) confusional state, occurring in a particular clinical setting and carrying a serious prognosis by virtue of adding its burden to an already serious medical illness.

It should be pointed out that not all psychiatrists agree with our distinction between delirium and other confusional states. Some, such as Lipowski and Engel and Romano, use the term *delirium* in reference to confusional states of all types. Our insistence on their separation is based on the differences in their clinical manifestations and in the clinical settings in which they occur.

The term *amnesia,* in the clinical sense, refers to the inability of the patient to remember past events, coupled with an inability to form new memories, i.e., to learn. The term presupposes an alert state of mind and ability to grasp the problem, to comprehend and use language normally, and to maintain adequate motivation. The failure is mainly one of retention, recall, and reproduction. It should be distinguished from the impairment or loss of memory that accompanies states of drowsiness and acute confusion, in which information seems never to have been adequately assimilated or registered in the first place.

The term *dementia* literally means a loss of mind and, more particularly, means a deterioration of all intellectual and cognitive functions (see above), without disturbance of consciousness, awareness, or perception. Implied in this designation is a gradual and in most instances irreversible enfeeblement of mental powers in a person who formerly possessed a normal mind. *Amentia,* by contrast, indicates a developmental failure to achieve normal intellectual capacity, i.e., mental retardation.

OBSERVABLE ASPECTS OF BEHAVIOR

The components of mentation and behavior that lend themselves to bedside examination are (1) the processes of sensation and perception; (2) the capacity for memorizing; (3) the ability to think and reason; (4) temperament, mood, and emotion; (5) initiative, impulse, and drive; and (6) insight. Of these, (1) is sensorial, (2) and (3) are cognitive, (4) is affective, and (5) is volitional or conative. Insight (6) includes all introspective observations made by patients concerning their own normal or disordered functioning. Each of these components has its objective side, expressed in behavioral responses that are produced by certain stimuli, and its subjective side, expressed in what the patient thinks and feels in relation to the stimuli.

DISTURBANCES OF PERCEPTION Perception, i.e., the processes utilized in acquiring through the senses a knowledge of the "world about" or of one's own body, involves a number of psychological mechanisms in addition to a simple awareness of the attributes of a stimulus. It includes the maintenance of attention, the selective focusing on a stimulus, the elimination of all extraneous stimuli, and the identification of the stimulus by recognizing its relationship to personal, remembered experience. The perception of a stimulus undergoes predictable types of derangement in disease affecting the cerebrum. Commonly, there is a reduction in the number of perceptions in a given unit of time and a failure to synthesize them properly and to relate them to the ongoing activities of the mind. There may be inattention or fluctuations of attention, distraction (pertinent and irrelevant stimuli have equal value), and inability to persist in an assigned task. Qualitative changes also appear, mainly in the form of sensory distortions, causing misinterpretation of sounds and objects and misidentification of persons (illusions). These changes form the basis for certain hallucinatory experiences in which the patient reports and reacts inappropriately to stimuli present in the environment. There is also an inability to perceive simultaneously all elements of a complex of stimuli, which has been referred to as a *failure of subjective reorganization*. These major disturbances in the perceptual sphere, sometimes called *clouding of the sensorium,* occur most often in deliria and other acute confusional states, but a quantitative deficiency may also become evident in amentia and in the advancing stages of dementia.

DISTURBANCES OF MEMORY Memory, the retention of learned experiences, is involved in all mental activities. It may be arbitrarily subdivided into several parts: (1) registration, which includes all that was mentioned under perception; (2) mnemonic integration and retention; (3) recall; and (4) reproduction. In severe disturbances of perception and attention there may be a complete failure of learning and consequently, of memory, because the material to be learned was never registered and assimilated. In Korsakoff's amnesic syndrome (see below), newly presented material appears to be temporarily registered but cannot be retained for more than a few minutes, and there is always an associated defect in the recall and reproduction of memories that had been formed some days, weeks, or even years before the onset of the illness (*retrograde amnesia*). Proof of the integrity of immediate memory, i.e., registration, is the ability to repeat phrases or numbers to be learned. Normal retention with failure of recall is at times a normal state ("tip of the tongue" syndrome, benign forgetfulness); when it is severe and extends to all events of past life, including personal identity, it is usually due to hysteria or malingering. Proof that the processes of registration and retention are intact under the latter circumstances comes from hypnosis and suggestion and from questioning under amobarbital or thiopental sodium narcosis, whereby the lost items are fully recalled and reproduced. Since some aspect of memory is involved.to some extent in all mental processes, it becomes the most testable component of mentation and behavior.

DISTURBANCES OF THINKING Thinking, which is central to practically all intellectual activity, remains the most elusive of all mental operations. If by thinking we mean the selective ordering of symbols for problem solving and the capacity to reason and form sound judgments (the usual definition), then the working units of this type of mental activity are mainly words and numbers. The substitution of words and numbers for the objects for which they stand (symbolization) is a fundamental part of the process. The formation of these symbols into ideas or concepts and the arrangement of new and remembered ideas into certain orders or relationships, according to the rules of logic, constitute other intricate parts of thought. One test of logical thinking is problem solving—the capacity to formulate a problem into several hypotheses, to analyze critically the evidence for and against each hypothesis, and to make a correct choice. In a general way one may examine thinking for speed and efficiency, ideational content, coherence and logical relationships of ideas, quantity and quality of associations with a given idea, and the propriety of the feeling and behavior engendered by an idea.

Information concerning the thought processes and associative functions is best obtained by analyzing the patient's spontaneous verbal productions and by engaging him or her in conversation. If the patient is taciturn or mute, one may have to depend on the responses to direct questions or upon written material, e.g., letters, etc. One notes the prevailing trends of the patient's thoughts; whether the ideas are to the point, reasonable, and coherent or vague, circumstantial, tangential, and irrelevant; and whether the thought processes are shallow and fragmented. Disorders of thinking are observed regularly in deliria and other confusional states and in dementia and schizophrenia. Incoherence of thinking characterizes confusional states of all types. The patient may be excessively critical, rationalizing, and hairsplitting; this type of thinking is often manifest in depressive psychosis. Derangement of thinking may also take the form of a flight of ideas; the patient moves nimbly from one thought to another, and associations are numerous and loosely linked. This is a common feature of hypomanic or manic states. The opposite condition, poverty of ideas, is characteristic both of depression, in which it is combined with gloomy thoughts, and of dementing diseases, in which it is part of a general reduction in intellectual activity. Thinking may be distorted in such a way that patients fail to check their ideas against reality. When a belief is maintained in spite of convincing contradictory evidence, the patient is said to have a *delusion.* Delusions are common in many psychiatric illnesses, particularly manic-depressive and schizophrenic states, but may also occur in dementing illnesses and in chronic infections of the central nervous system.

DISTURBANCES OF EMOTION, MOOD, AND AFFECT The emotional life of the patient is expressed in a variety of ways. In the first place, rather marked individual differences in basic temperament are observed in otherwise normal persons; some persons are throughout life cheerful, gregarious, optimistic, and free from worry, whereas others are just the opposite. Strong emotional states such as fear and anxiety are more easily induced in some individuals than others; they are normal reactions to life situations and may be accompanied by derangements of visceral function. If disproportionate to the stimulus and persistent, they are usually manifestations of an anxiety disorder or depression. Emotional responses that are excessively labile and poorly controlled or uninhibited are a common manifestion of many cerebral diseases, particularly those involving the corticopontine and corticobulbar pathways. Such responses then constitute a part of the syndrome of pseudobulbar palsy.

Temperament, mood, and other emotional experiences are evaluated by the appearance of the patient and by verbalized accounts of his or her feelings. For these purposes some psychiatrists divide emotionality into mood and feeling (affect). By *mood* is meant the prevailing emotional state of the individual without reference to impinging stimuli. It may be cheerful or melancholic. Language, e.g., the adjectives used, and facial expressions, attitudes, postures, and speed of movement most reliably betray the patient's mood. By contrast, *feelings* (or *affect*) are said to be emotional experiences evoked by particular stimuli.

DISTURBANCES IN IMPULSE (CONATION) Impulse, that basic biologic urge, driving force, or purpose by which every organism is directed to reach its objectives, is another important and observable, though somewhat neglected, dimension of behavior. Again, one notes wide normal variations in strength of impulse to action and thought, and these individual differences are present throughout life. Many types of cerebral diseases (particularly those which involve the medial-orbital parts of the frontal lobes) cause a reduction in impulse coupled with an indifference or lack of concern about the consequences of actions. In such cases all other measurable aspects of psychic function may be normal. Pathologic lack of impulse, or *abulia,* may reach an extreme degree—to the point of mutism and immobility, a state sometimes called *akinetic mutism. Psychomotor retardation* is a lesser degree of the same state and is a feature of both cerebral disease and depression.

LOSS OF INSIGHT Insight, the state of being fully aware of the nature and degree of one's deficits, becomes manifestly impaired or abolished in all types of cerebral disease that cause complex disorders of behavior. Rarely does the patient with such a disorder seek advice or help for the illness. Instead, the family usually brings the individual to the physician. Thus, diseases which produce high-order or complex mental abnormalities not only evoke observable changes in mentation and behavior but also alter or reduce the patient's capacity for self-observation.

APPROACH TO THE PATIENT

Confronted by a patient with one of these disorders, the physician must adopt an examination technique designed to expose fully the perceptual and intellectual defect. Abnormalities of posture, movement, sensation, and reflexes cannot be relied upon for the full demonstration of the neurologic deficit, for it must be remembered that the association and limbic areas of the brain may be severely damaged without demonstrable neurologic signs of these types.

The initial assessment of the patient should include (1) a reliable history of the illness; (2) findings on mental examination, i.e., so-called mental status; (3) findings on the rest of the neurologic examination; and (4) application of special laboratory procedures, including endocrine, biochemical, and toxic studies, CT scanning or MRI imaging, lumbar puncture, electroencephalogram, and sometimes angiography.

The history should always be supplemented by information obtained from a person other than the patient. Through lack of insight, patients are often unaware of their illness; indeed, they may be ignorant even of their chief complaint. Special inquiry should be made about the patient's general behavior, social adjustment, capacity for work, personal habits, and family history.

A systemic examination of the mental status should provide answers to the following questions:

1 Insight (patient's replies to questions about the chief symptoms): What is your difficulty? Are you ill? When did your illness begin?

2 Orientation:

- *a* Knowledge of personal identity and present situation: What is your name? What is your occupation? Where do you live? Are you married? What are you doing now?
- *b* Place: What is the name of the place where you are now? How did you get here? What floor is it on? Where is the secretary's or nurses' desk or the bathroom?
- *c* Time: What is the date today? What day of the week is it? What is the time of day? What meals have you had? When was the last holiday?

3 Memory:

- *a* Remote: Tell me the names of your children and their birth dates. When were you married? What was your mother's maiden name? What was the name of your first school teacher? What jobs have you held?
- *b* Recent past: Tell me about your recent illness (compare with previous statements). What did you have for breakfast today? What is my name or the nurse's name? When did you see me for the first time? What tests were done yesterday? What were the headlines in the newspaper today? Give patient a simple story, oral or written, and ask her or him to recall it after 3 to 5 min.
- *c* Immediate recall (short-term memory): Repeat these numbers after me (give a series of three, four, five, six, seven and then eight digits at the speed of one per second). Now when I give a series of numbers, repeat them in reverse order.
- *d* Visual span: Show patient a picture of several objects; ask him or her to name what has been seen and note any inaccuracies.

4 General information: Ask about the names of presidents, well-known historic dates, or the names of large rivers or cities. Ask the patient to give the names of 10 fruits, 10 flowers, or 10 vegetables as quickly as possible.

5 Capacity for sustained mental activity:

- *a* Calculation: Test ability to add, subtract, multiply, and divide. Serial subtraction of 7s or 3s from 100 is a good test of calculation as well as of concentration.
- *b* Abstract thinking: See if patient can detect similarities and differences between classes of objects or explain a proverb of a fable.

6 General behavior (attitudes, general bearing, attentiveness, manner of dress, etc.):

- *a* Content of thought: What ideas occupy the patient's thoughts? Does the patient believe that his or her thoughts and actions are being controlled or broadcasted to others? Are there hallucinations and/or delusions? Is there a press of speech or lack of speech?
- *b* Mood: Do patients appear cheerful or sad? How do they feel? Are they nervous, worried, or apprehensive? What feeling is revealed through speech, attitude, and facial expression?

7 Special tests of localized cerebral functions: Tests for grasping and sucking; tests for aphasia, praxis with both hands, cortical sensory function, and visual field defects; tests of ability in drawing clock face, map of United States or Europe, floor plan of patient's house, etc.

In order to enlist the full cooperation of patients, physicians must prepare them for questions of this type. Otherwise, the patient's first reaction will be one of embarrassment or anger because of the implication that his or her mind is not sound. Reassurance that these are not tests of intelligence or of sanity is helpful.

More formal methods of examining the mental capacity of adults, such as the Wechsler Adult Intelligence Scale (WAIS), are widely available. Discrepancies between vocabulary, picture-completion, and object-assembly tests as a group (which correlate well with premorbid intelligence and are relatively resistant to dementing brain disease) and arithmetic, block design, digit span, and digit symbol tests (which decline in dementia) provide an index of deterioration. The Wechsler Memory Scale is a reliable method for quantitating the degree of impairment of retentive memory. Characteristically, in patients with Korsakoff's amnesic syndrome there is a striking discrepancy between performance on the WAIS and that on the Wechsler Memory Scale.

COMMON SYNDROMES

DELIRIUM Clinical features These are most perfectly depicted in the alcoholic patient. The symptoms usually develop over a period of 2 or 3 days. The first indications of the approaching attack are difficulty in concentrating, restless irritability, tremulousness, insomnia, and poor appetite. One or several generalized convulsions are the initial major symptom in almost 30 percent of the cases. The patient's rest becomes troubled by unpleasant and terrifying dreams or by hallucinations. There may be momentary disorientation as revealed by an occasional inappropriate remark.

These initial symptoms rapidly give way to a clinical picture which, in severe cases, is one of the most colorful and dramatic in medicine. The state of consciousness becomes altered (sensorium is "clouded") in that the patient is inattentive and unable to perceive all elements of the situation. The patient may talk incessantly and incoherently and look distressed and perplexed; the facial expression is in keeping with vague notions of being annoyed or threatened. From the patient's manner and speech content it is evident that he or she misinterprets the meaning of ordinary objects and ambient sounds and has vivid visual, auditory, and tactile hallucinations, often of a most unpleasant type. At first the patient can be brought momentarily in touch with reality and may in fact answer questions correctly, but almost at once there is a relapse into the preoccupied, confused state; the patient gives wrong answers, is unable to think coherently, and is incapable of self-orientation. Before long the patient is unable to shake off the hallucinations even for a second and does not recognize family or physician. Coarse tremor and restless movements are usually present. Sleep is impossible or occurs only in brief naps. The countenance is flushed, the pupils are dilatated, and the conjunctivas are injected; the pulse is rapid, and the temperature may be raised. There is much sweating, and the urine is scanty and of high specific gravity. The signs of overactivity of the autonomic nervous system, more than any other signs, distinguish delirium from all other confusional states.

In most patients the symptoms abate after 3 to 5 days, although in a few they may persist for several weeks. The most certain indication of the end of the attack is the occurrence of sound sleep and of lucid intervals of increasing length. Recovery is usually complete. The most severe form ends fatally in a small percentage of patients.

Delirium is subject to all degrees of variability, not only from patient to patient but in the same patient from day to day and hour to hour. The entire syndrome may be observed in one patient and only one or two components in another. In its mildest form, as so often occurs in febrile diseases, it consists of an occasional wandering of the mind and incoherence of verbal expression, interrupted by periods of lucidity. This form, lacking motor and autonomic overactivity, is sometimes referred to as a *quiet delirium* (or *hypokinetic delirium*) and is difficult to distinguish from other confusional states. Agitation and excitement resembling delirium can also occur in hepatic encephalopathy, hyponatremia, and, transiently, in hypoglycemia.

Morbid anatomy and pathophysiology The brains of patients who have died in delirium tremens usually show no pathologic changes of significance. Those diseases that give rise to local lesions in the brain that may cause delirium include focal embolic encephalitis, viral encephalitis, and trauma. The topography of these lesions is of particular interest. They tend to be localized in the high midbrain and subthalamus and in the temporal lobes, where they involve the reticular activating and limbic systems.

Penfield's studies of the human cortex during surgical exploration indicate the importance of the temporal lobe in producing visual, auditory, and olfactory hallucinations. With subthalamic and midbrain lesions there may be visual hallucinations that are pleasant, animated, and accompanied by good insight (the peduncular hallucinosis of Lhermitte).

The electroencephalogram in delirium may show nonfocal theta activity (5 to 7 Hz) with return to normal as the delirium clears. In other patients only low-voltage, fast activity (11 to 20 Hz) is seen, and in milder degrees of delirium there is usually no abnormality at all.

An analysis of the several conditions conducive to delirium suggests at least three different physiologic mechanisms. First, the withdrawal of alcohol, barbiturates, or other sedative-hypnotic drugs, following a period of chronic intoxication, is the most common cause of delirium. These drugs have a strong depressant effect on certain areas of the central nervous system; presumably the release and overactivity of these parts, after withdrawal of the drug, are the basis of the delirium. Second, in the case of bacterial infections, toxic encephalopathies, or drug-induced delirium such as occurs with atropine or scopolamine, the delirious state probably results from the direct action of the toxin or chemical agent on these same parts of the brain. Third, destructive lesions, such as those of the temporal lobes in trauma or herpes simplex encephalitis, may cause delirium by disturbing the function of these particular areas.

ACUTE CONFUSIONAL STATES ASSOCIATED WITH REDUCED ALERTNESS AND DECREASED PSYCHOMOTOR ACTIVITY **Clinical features** In the most typical examples of these states, all mental functions are reduced to some degree but alertness, attentiveness, and the ability to grasp all elements of the immediate situation suffer most. In the mildest form the patient may pass for normal; only failure to recollect and reproduce happenings of the past few hours or days reveals the inadequacy of mental function. The more obviously confused patient spends much time in idleness, and what the patient does may be inappropriate. Only the more automatic acts and verbal responses are properly performed, but these may permit the examiner to obtain from the patient a number of relevant and accurate replies to questions about age, occupation, and residence. Reactions are slow and indecisive, and it is difficult for the patient to sustain a conversation. The patient may fall asleep during the interview and if left alone sleeps more hours each day than is natural. Responses tend to be rather abrupt, brief, and mechanical. Disturbances of perception are frequent, causing misinterpretation of voices, common objects, and the actions of other persons. Often one cannot discern whether the patient is hallucinating, i.e., hearing and seeing things that do not exist, or merely misinterpreting stimuli in the environment. Inadequate perception and forgetfulness result in a constant state of bewilderment. Failing to recognize the surroundings and having lost all sense of time, the patient repeats the same question and makes the same remarks over and over again. Irritability may or may not be present. Some patients are extremely suspicious, demanding, and aggressive; in fact, a paranoid trend may be the most pronounced and troublesome feature of the illness.

As the confusion deepens, conversation becomes more difficult, and at a certain stage the patient no longer notices or responds to much of what is occurring. Questions may be answered with a single word or a short phrase spoken in a soft, tremulous voice or whisper, or the patient may be mute. In its most advanced stages confusion gives way to stupor and finally to coma. As the patient improves, there may again be a stage of stupor and confusion, occurring in the reverse order. This informs us that at least one category of confusion is a manifestation of the disease processes which, in their severest form, cause coma.

In the most typical cases, this type of confusional state is readily distinguished from delirium; in others, with more than the usual degree of irritability and restlessness, one cannot fail to notice the resemblance of one to the other. Similarly, when a delirium is complicated by an illness that superimposes stupor (e.g., delirium tremens with pneumonia, meningitis, or hepatic encephalopathy), it may be difficult to distinguish the delirium from other confusional states.

When clouding of consciousness is minimal and the confusion is of insidious onset and several weeks' duration, it may mimic dementia. Lipowski has called this "reversible dementia," claiming that it is an intermediate state between delirium and dementia and still potentially reversible. We would classify it as a protracted confusional state.

Morbid anatomy and pathophysiology Confusional states are so diverse and are associated with such a wide variety of diseases that one would hardly expect a common anatomy or pathophysiologic basis. In general there is a more frequent occurrence with lesions of the right (nondominant) hemisphere, especially its posterior parts. Large ischemic and other acute lesions of the parietal lobe tend to render patients underactive, apathetic, and unaware of their neurologic disabilities; disorientation and inattentiveness are often associated (see Chap. 24). Only if the lesion is large enough to cause a hemiplegia, hemisensory disorder, or homonymous hemianopsia will the focal nature of the lesion be appreciated. Infarction of the thalamus, particularly of the dominant side, is commonly associated with a confusional state with recent memory impairment. This condition may persist for days or weeks, but usually clears.

More frequently, the basis of the confusional state is an acute metabolic disease, and the pathologic changes, if detectable, are bilateral and diffuse. Hypoxia, hyperglycemia, uremia, metabolic acidosis or alkalosis, hepatic stupor, hyponatremia, and certain drug intoxications are the commonly recognized causes which are readily corroborated by appropriate biochemical analyses of blood, urine, and cerebrospinal fluid. Clues to these biochemical derangements are often provided by alterations of respiration and the presence of asterixis, myoclonus, and tremor, with preserved pupillary reflexes. Correction of the biochemical derangements may result in rapid improvements in the patient's condition. Table 23-1 is a classification of the conditions that cause delirium and confusion.

DEMENTIA The term *dementia,* in current neurologic parlance, usually denotes a clinical syndrome composed of failing memory and loss of other intellectual functions due to chronic progressive degenerative disease of the brain. Such a definition is too narrow. The syndrome of dementia is characterized not only by intellectual deterioration but also by certain behavioral abnormalities and changes in personality. Moreover, it is illogical to set apart any one constellation of cerebral symptoms on the basis of their tempo of evolution and duration. Since there are several states of dementia of multiple causation and mechanism and because chronic degeneration of neurons is only one of the many causes, it is more correct to speak of the *dementias* or the *dementing diseases.*

Another concept that requires qualification is that of dementia as a global loss, in which all intellectual functions are affected more or less equally. When the latter are carefully analyzed they are found to include several separable though related functions, such as memory, verbal facility, and the ability to deal with mathematical symbols, to perceive visuospatial relationships, and to think abstractly and solve problems. Each of these functions (except thinking) has a definable anatomy in the cerebrum and can therefore be affected individually by a disease. For example, retentive memory involves neural mechanisms located bilaterally in the inferomedial parts of the temporal lobes, and the language mechanisms lie in the para-Sylvian region of the left (dominant) hemisphere. It comes as no surprise, therefore, that the dementing illnesses may affect certain intellectual functions predominantly or in various combinations and sequences.

Another point of importance is that most dementing diseases appear during the senium and many others during late adult life. In 17 series comprising 15,000 persons over the age of 60 years, the mean incidence of moderate to severe dementia was found to be 4.8 percent. In 1983, according to Terry and Katzman, there were in the United States about 1.3 million patients with severe dementia, and an additional 2.8 million with mild to moderate intellectual impairment. Since the elderly population in the western world is increasing both in percentage of the population and in absolute numbers, the magnitude of the medical problems they will present reaches an alarming dimension. Finally, it needs to be emphasized that the dementias of the elderly are to be regarded not as merely the inevitable consequences of growing old but as age-linked diseases, some 15 percent of which are treatable (Wells, 1981).

Clinical features These clinical features are observed most commonly and prototypically in patients with Alzheimer's disease. The earliest signs of dementia may be so subtle as to escape the notice of even the most discerning physician. Often an observant relative of the patient or an employer is the first to become aware of a certain lack of initiative, irritability, loss of interest, forgetfulness, and inability to perform up to the usual standard. Later there is distractibility and inattentiveness; inability to think with accustomed clarity; reduced general comprehension; perseveration in speech, action, and thought; and defective memory, especially for recent events. Frequently, a change in mood becomes apparent, taking the form more often of apathy than of depression or elation. Excessive lability of mood may be observed, i.e,. easy fluctuation from laughter to tears on slight provocation. Lapses in social graces and conduct occur and judgment becomes impaired, early in some cases and late in others. Paranoid ideas, delusions, and sometimes hallucinations may develop. As a rule, the patient has little or no realization of these changes in behavior and lacks insight into their meaning. However, early in the disease the patient may be aware of his or her declining capacities and become depressed on this account.

As the condition progresses, particularly in the degenerative diseases, there is loss of almost all intellectual faculties. Speech and language disturbances are almost invariable. The proper word or name cannot be found. Words are misspelled. Reading and auditory comprehension fail. Later, sphincteric incontinence, reduced responsivity, and finally mutism may be added to the clinical picture. Secondary physical deterioration eventually takes place. Food intake, which may be increased in the beginning of the illness, is in the end usually limited, with resulting emaciation. Locomotion fails; voluntary movements become poorly coordinated. Any febrile illness or metabolic upset induces a marked increase in confusion and even stupor or coma, indicating the precarious state of cerebral compensation. Finally, the patient remains in bed most of the time and dies of pneumonia or some other intercurrent infection. This whole process may evolve over a period of months or years, usually the latter.

Many of the alterations of behavior are the direct result (i.e., primary symptoms) of disease of the nervous system; others are

TABLE 23-1 Classification of delirium and acute confusional states

I Delirium
- *A* In a medical or surgical illness (no focal or lateralizing neurologic signs; cerebrospinal fluid usually clear)
  - *1* Postoperative (hypoxia) and postconcussive states
  - *2* Febrile illness: pneumonia, typhoid fever, malaria, septicemia from streptococcus, rheumatic fever
  - *3* Thyrotoxicosis and ACTH intoxication (rare)
- *B* In neurologic disease that causes focal or lateralizing signs or changes in the cerebrospinal fluid
  - *1* Vascular, neoplastic, or traumatic lesions, particularly those involving the temporal lobes and upper part of the brainstem
  - *2* Acute bacterial and tuberculous meningitis
  - *3* Subarachnoid hemorrhage
  - *4* Viral encephalitis or meningoencephalitis, particularly herpes simplex encephalitis
- *C* In the abstinence states, exogenous intoxications, and postconvulsive states (signs of other medical, surgical, and neurologic illnesses absent or coincidental)
  - *1* Withdrawal of alcohol (delirium tremens), barbiturates, and nonbarbiturate sedative drugs following chronic intoxication
  - *2* Drug intoxications: amphetamine, camphor, caffeine, ergot, scopolamine, atropine, etc.
  - *3* Postconvulsive delirium

II Acute confusional states associated with psychomotor underactivity
- *A* Associated with a medical or surgical disease (no focal lateralizing neurologic signs; cerebrospinal fluid clear)
  - *1* Metabolic disorders: hepatic stupor, uremia, hypoxia, hypercapnea, hypoglycemia, porphyria, electrolyte imbalance
  - *2* Febrile illnesses
  - *3* Congestive heart failure, with hypoxia
  - *4* Postoperative and posttraumatic states
- *B* Associated with drug intoxication (no focal or lateralizing signs; cerebrospinal fluid clear): opiates, barbiturates and other sedatives, trihexyphenidyl, etc.
- *C* Associated with diseases of the nervous system (the focal or lateralizing neurologic signs and cerebrospinal fluid changes are commoner in these conditions than in delirium)
  - *1* Cerebral vascular disease, tumor, abscess
  - *2* Subdural hematoma
  - *3* Meningitis
  - *4* Encephalitis
  - *5* Senile or other brain disease in combination with infective fevers, drug reactions, heart failure, or other medical or surgical disease ("beclouded dementia")

secondary, i.e., they are reactions to the catastrophe of losing one's mind. For example, the dement is said to seek solitude to hide the affliction and may thus appear asocial or apathetic. Again, excessive orderliness may be an attempt to compensate for failing memory; apprehension, gloom, or irritability may reflect general dissatisfaction with a necessarily restricted life. It would appear that even in a state of fairly advanced deterioration the patient is still capable of reacting to the illness and to the persons who provide care.

Degenerative diseases may terminate in virtually complete decortication. The patient lies with eyes open but is unaware of what is happening. He or she no longer speaks or responds to spoken commands. There is no interest in food or drink, though they are swallowed if placed in the mouth. The facial and limb muscles are stiff with increased tendon reflexes and occasionally Babinski's signs are present. Grasping and sucking are prominent. The sphincters are incontinent.

Morbid anatomy and pathophysiology Dementia is usually related to obvious structural disease of the cerebrum and the diencephalon. In some, such as the Alzheimer–senile dementia complex and Pick's disease, the main process appears to be a degeneration and loss of nerve cells in the association areas of the cerebral cortex, with secondary changes in the cerebral white matter. A degeneration of neurons confined to the thalamus may also cause dementia. In others, such as Huntington's chorea and certain of the spinocerebellar and cerebral-basal ganglionic degenerations, dementia is associated with a degeneration of neurons in the putamen and caudate nuclei. Arteriosclerotic vascular disease may result in multiple foci of infarction throughout the thalami, basal ganglia, brainstem, and cerebrum with dementia. Cerebral involvement may include the motor, sensory, or visual projection areas as well as the association areas. This condition, in the relatively rare instances in which mental deterioration dominates the clinical picture, is called *multi-infarct dementia.* Trauma may cause contusions of cerebral convolutions, particularly of the inferior and anterior parts of the frontal and temporal lobes, as well as necroses and hemorrhages in the midbrain, lesions which are responsible for protracted stupor, coma, or dementia. Most diseases that produce dementia are quite extensive, and the frontal and temporal lobes are affected more often than other parts of the cerebrum.

Mechanisms other than the destruction of brain tissue may be operative in some cases. Chronic increased intracranial pressure or chronic hydrocephalus (with large ventricles the pressure may not exceed 180 mmHg), regardless of cause, is often associated with a general impairment of mental function. Gait is usually also impaired. Compression of cerebral white matter is the main factor. The compression of one or both of the cerebral hemispheres by chronic subdural hematomas may cause a widespread disturbance of cortical function. A diffuse inflammatory process is at least in part the basis for dementia in syphilis and in certain virus infections such as herpes simplex encephalitis. Lastly, several of the toxic and metabolic diseases discussed in Chaps. 349 and 350 may interfere with nervous function over a period of time and create a clinical picture similar, if not identical, to that of dementia. One must suppose that the altered biochemical environment has affected neuronal function.

TABLE 23-2 Bedside classification of dementia

I Diseases in which dementia is usually the only evidence of neurologic or medical disease
- *A* Alzheimer's disease and senile dementia
- *B* Pick's disease

II Diseases in which dementia is associated with other neurologic signs but not with other obvious medical disease
- *A* Invariably associated with other neurologic signs
  - *1* Huntington's chorea (choreoathetosis)
  - *2* Leukodystrophies: Schilder's disease, adrenoleukodystrophy, metachromatic leukodystrophy, and related demyelinative diseases (spastic weakness, pseudobulbar palsy, blindness, deafness)
  - *3* Lipofuscinosis and other lipid storage diseases (myoclonic seizures, blindness, spasticity, cerebellar ataxia)
  - *4* Myoclonic epilepsy (diffuse myoclonus, generalized seizures, cerebellar ataxia)
  - *5* Creutzfeldt-Jakob disease (diffuse myoclonus and cerebellar ataxia)
  - *6* Cerebrocerebellar degeneration (cerebellar ataxia of olivopontocerebellar type and others)
  - *7* Cerebral-basal ganglionic degenerations (apraxia, rigidity) and supranuclear palsy (paralysis of vertical gaze, neck dystonia)
  - *8* Dementia with spastic paraplegia
  - *9* Basal ganglia calcification (idiopathic and hypoparathyroidism)
  - *10* Hallervorden-Spatz disease (pyramidal and extrapyramidal signs)
  - *11* Dementia with Parkinson's disease (tremor, rigidity, bradykinesia)
- *B* Often associated with other neurologic signs
  - *1* Cerebral arteriosclerosis and ischemic infarction
  - *2* Brain tumor, especially gliomas of frontal and temporal lobes and corpus callosum
  - *3* Brain trauma (cerebral contusions, midbrain hemorrhages, chronic subdural hematoma)
  - *4* Marchiafava-Bignami disease (apraxia and other frontal lobe signs)
  - *5* Normal-pressure hydrocephalus (nearly always with ataxia of gait and often with sphincteric incontinence)
  - *6* Chronic CNS infections: cryptococcosis, toxoplasmosis, dementia associated with acquired immunodeficiency syndrome (AIDS)

III Diseases in which dementia is usually associated with clinical and laboratory signs of other medical disease
- *A* Hypothyroidism
- *B* Cushing's disease
- *C* Nutritional deficiency states such as pellagra, the Wernicke-Korsakoff syndrome, and subacute combined degeneration of spinal cord and brain (vitamin B_{12} deficiency)
- *D* Neurosyphilis: general paresis and meningovascular syphilis
- *E* Hepatolenticular degeneration, familial and acquired
- *F* Chronic drug intoxication (barbiturates and other sedative drugs)

Classification of dementia Not all of the diseases listed in Table 23-2 are of equal importance as causes of dementia. Some are rare. In a series of 84 patients with established presenile dementia (at less than 65 years of age) admitted to a British neurologic center, 58 percent had brain atrophy, probably of the Alzheimer type, and 10 percent had multi-infarct dementia. Because this was a primary neurologic referral hospital, the incidence of tumors was high, nearly 10 percent. Normal-pressure hydrocephalus, alcoholic dementia, Creutzfeldt-Jakob disease, Huntington's chorea, posttraumatic sequelae, and alcoholism accounted for the remaining 30 percent. In an older population (over 65 years), brain atrophy was found in approximately 80 percent and multi-infarct dementia in 15 percent (Tomlinson). Probably the statistics amassed by Wells from a survey of patients with dementia entering a university hospital are the most representative. These are presented in Table 23-3.

The degenerative diseases that cause dementia are discussed further in Chap. 350. The special features of the dementias that accompany arteriosclerotic, syphilitic, traumatic, nutritional, and metabolic diseases are discussed in the appropriate chapters.

Differential diagnosis The first task in dealing with this class of patients is to make sure that the central probem is one of progressive general deterioration of intellect and personality change. It may be necessary to examine the patient several times before one is confident of the clinical findings. In this regard, use of standardized scales for assessment of dementia, such as the Blessed scale, may be useful.

An easy mistake is to assume that mental function is normal if patients complain only of nervousness, fatigue, insomnia, or vague somatic symptoms, and to label the illnesses as psychiatric disorders. *This will be avoided if one keeps in mind that such disorders rarely begin in middle or late adult life.* A practical rule is to assume that all mental illnesses beginning during this period are due either to structural disease of the brain or to a depressive psychosis.

A mild aphasia must not be mistaken for dementia. Aphasic patients appear uncertain of themselves, and their speech may be incoherent. Furthermore, they may be anxious and depressed over this ineptitude. Careful attention to the language performance of these patients will lead to the correct diagnosis in most instances, and further observation will disclose that their behavior, except that which is related to the language disorder, is within normal limits.

Depressed patients present another type of problem. They may remark that their mental function is poor or that they are forgetful and cannot concentrate. Scrutiny of these remarks will show, however, that they can actually remember details of their history and that no qualitative change in cognitive function has occurred. Their difficulty is either a lack of energy and interest or an anxiety that prevents the focusing of attention on anything except their own problems. Even during mental tests their performance may be impaired by their emotional state in much the same way as the performance of a worried student is impaired during examinations. When patients are calmed by reassurance and given more time in the performance of tests, mental function improves, indicating that intellectual deterioration has not occurred. Hypomanic patients may fail in tests of intellectual function because of restlessness and distractibility. It is helpful to remember that demented patients, except in the early phases of their illness, rarely have sufficient insight to complain of mental deterioration; those who admit to poor memory seldom realize the degree of their disability. The physician must never rely on the patient's statements concerning the efficiency of mental function and must always evaluate a poor performance on tests in the light of the emotional state and motivation at the time the test is given. Especially difficult is the mildly demented patient who is also depressed and whose CT scan shows some degree of ventricular enlargement—even to a degree that raises the question of normal-pressure hydrocephalus. Sometimes the contribution of depression can only be ascertained by an empirical trial of antidepressant drugs.

Certain metabolic or endocrine disorders, i.e., hypothyroidism, ACTH therapy, Cushing's disease, or Addison's disease, or the postpartum state may create difficulties in diagnosis because of the wide variety of clinical pictures by which they manifest themselves. Some such patients appear to be suffering from a dementia, others from an acute confusional psychosis; if mood change or delusions predominate, a manic-depressive psychosis or schizophrenia is suggested. In these conditions, some degree of confusion can usually be recognized, and on this basis one can exclude schizophrenia and manic-depressive psychosis. It is well to remember that acute onset of mental symptoms always suggests a confusional state of delirium; inasmuch as these conditions are generally reversible, they must be distinguished from the dementing diseases (see preceding sections).

Once it is decided that the patient suffers from a dementing disease, the next step is to determine, by careful physical examination, whether there are other signs or indications of neurologic or medical disease. This enables the physician to place the case in one of the three categories of the bedside classification (Table 23-2). CT scans, MRI, EEG, lumbar puncture, and toxic metabolic studies are obtained. The final step is to determine, from the total clinical picture, the particular disease within any one category. This may sometimes be difficult. If the dementia is of recent onset, complicated by the use of drugs, or associated with temporal lobe seizures or an endocrine disease, a period of observation may be required before the diagnosis can be settled. Finally, it is important to keep in mind that the correct diagnosis of treatable forms of mental disease (e.g., general paresis, subdural hematoma, brain tumor, chronic drug intoxication, normal-pressure hydrocephalus, pellagra and other deficiency states, and hypothyroidism) is of greater practical importance than the diagnosis of the untreatable ones.

SENILE DEMENTIA AND OTHER CEREBRAL DISEASES COMPLICATED BY MEDICAL OR SURGICAL ILLNESS (BECLOUDED DEMENTIA) Many elderly patients who enter the hospital with a medical or surgical illness are mentally confused. Presumably this deterioration is determined by preexisting brain disease, in most instances senile dementia of the Alzheimer type, which may or may not have been obvious to the family before the onset of the complicating illness. Other cerebral diseases (vascular, neoplastic, or demyelinative) may have the same effect.

All the clinical features that one observes in the acute confusional states may be present. The severity varies greatly. The confusion may be reflected only in the patient's inability to relate sequentially the history of the illness, or it may be so severe that the patient is virtually *non compos mentis*.

Although almost any complicating illness may bring out the confusion, it is particularly frequent with infectious diseases; with posttraumatic and postoperative states, notably after concussive brain injuries and the removal of cataracts (in which case the confusion is probably related to being temporarily deprived of vision); and with congestive heart failure, chronic respiratory disease, and severe anemia, especially pernicious anemia. Often it is difficult to determine which of several possible factors is responsible for the confusion, and there may be more than one. In a cardiac patient with a confusional psychosis, for example, there may be low-grade fever, a marginally reduced cerebral blood flow, intoxication with one or more drugs, marginal renal function, and water and electrolyte imbalance.

When these patients recover from their medical or surgical illness, they usually return to their premorbid state, though their shortcomings, now drawn to the attention of the family and physician, may be more obvious than before.

THE AMNESIC SYNDROME The *amnesic syndrome, the amnestic-confabulatory syndrome,* and *Korsakoff's psychosis* are terms used interchangeably to designate a unique but common disorder of cognitive function in which memory is deranged out of all proportion to other components of mentation and behavior. It possesses two salient features which may vary in severity but are always conjoined: (1) an impaired ability to recall events and other information that had been recorded before the onset of the illness (retrograde amnesia), and (2) an impaired ability to acquire new information, i.e., to learn or to form new memories (anterograde amnesia). Other cognitive functions (particularly the capacity for concentration, spatial organization, and visual and verbal abstraction), which depend little or not at all on memory, are also impaired but to a relatively minor degree. The patient tends to lack initiative and spontaneity and is usually complacent. Ability to repeat a series of numbers or a spoken sentence (immediate memory) is intact. Recent memories are affected more than remote ones, but the extent of this varies with the nature and severity of the disease. *Confabulation,* meaning the fabrication of ready answers or the recital of fictitious experiences, is variably present. The latter is observed mainly in the acute phase of the illness.

The definition of Korsakoff's psychosis is predicated also upon the intactness of certain aspects of behavior and mental function. The patient should be alert, attentive, responsive, and capable of understanding the written and spoken word, capable of making appropriate deductions from given premises, and capable of solving such problems as can be concluded within his or her forward memory span. These "negative" features are of particular importance because they help to distinguish Korsakoff's psychosis from a number of other disorders in which the basic defect is not in retentive memory but in some

TABLE 23-3 Frequency of dementing cerebral diseases (417 patients)

	Number	Percent
Dementia of unknown cause*	199	47.7
Alcoholic dementia (Korsakoff's syndrome)	42	10.0
Multi-infarct dementia	39	9.4
Normal-pressure hydrocephalus	25	6.0
Intracranial masses	20	4.8
Huntington's chorea	12	2.9
Drug toxicity	10	2.4
Posttraumatic dementia	7	1.7
Other identified cerebral diseases (subarachnoid hemorrhage, hypo- and hyperthyroidism, encephalitis, hypoxia, pernicious anemia, etc.)	28	6.7
Pseudodementias:		5.5
Schizophrenia	5	
Depression	16	
Mania	2	
Other:		2.6
No diagnosis	7	
No dementia	4	

* *The majority of patients in this group are assumed to have Alzheimer's disease.*
SOURCE: *Wells, 1977.*

other psychological mechanism, e.g., in attention and perception (as in the delirious, confused, or stuporous patient), in recall (as in the hysterical patient), or in volition (as in the abulic patient with frontal lobe disease).

Pathologic anatomy The anatomic structures of particular importance in memory function are the diencephalon (specifically the medial portions of the medial dorsal nuclei of the thalamus) and the inferomedial portions of the temporal lobes, particularly the hippocampal formations and underlying white matter. Bilaterally placed lesions in either of these regions derange memory and learning out of all proportion to other cognitive functions, and even a unilateral lesion in the dominant thalamus or hippocampus produces the same effect to a lesser degree. It would appear that the aforementioned anatomic structures are involved in all forms of learning and integration of newly formed memories, and that they form a tenuous but vital link between the high brainstem reticular formation (the integrity of which is necessary to maintain an alert state of mind, a prerequisite for any learning) and the cerebral cortex, which is the locus for special memories, i.e., memories for words, geometric figures, numbers, and so forth.

Classification of diseases characterized by an amnesic syndrome A classification of these diseases is given in Table 23-4. Some of these amnesic syndromes are unique. For example, in *transient global amnesia,* described originally by Fisher and Adams, an elderly person (usually over 50 years) will suddenly become bewildered, being uncertain as to his or her whereabouts, the time of day, and what he or she is doing. If told, the patient quickly forgets and asks the same questions repeatedly. In contrast to the patient having a temporal lobe seizure, the patient with transient global amnesia is in contact with the environment and can reply to complex questions, read, calculate, and perform routine tasks. There is also a loss of memory for events that had occurred hours or days before the attack began. During the episode of amnesia, there is no evidence of pallor, twitching, or altered consciousness. Within a few hours the patient makes a complete recovery but is left with a gap in memory that covers the period of the attack and a short period before its onset. During the attack, an EEG may disclose minor changes in the temporal regions. An ischemic attack due to occlusive disease of the temporal branches of the posterior cerebral arteries is one postulated cause. Most patients have only a single attack and no treatment is necessary. Second, third, or several attacks may occur, however, and nothing is known about how to prevent them.

Herpes simplex encephalitis is a common cause of an amnesic state, because of its tendency to localize in the medial parts of the temporal lobes (see Chap. 347). In some patients with carcinomatosis, a limbic encephalitis of unknown etiology has been found (see Chap. 304). Some gliomas infiltrate the temporal lobes, fornices, and thalamus over a period of weeks to months, resulting in a characteristic syndrome.

In many of these diseases other components of intellectual function are impaired and other neurologic disorders are conjoined. Lack of impulse—a psychomotor retardation—is the most frequent.

TABLE 23-4 Classification of diseases characterized by an amnesic syndrome

I Amnesic syndrome of sudden onset, usually with gradual but incomplete recovery
- *A* Bilateral or unilateral (dominant) hippocampal infarction due to atherosclerotic-thrombotic or embolic occlusion of the posterior cerebral arteries or their inferior temporal branches
- *B* Trauma to the diencephalic or inferomedial temporal regions
- *C* Spontaneous subarachnoid hemorrhage
- *D* Carbon monoxide poisoning and other hypoxic states (rare)

II Amnesia of sudden onset and brief duration with full recovery
- *A* Temporal lobe seizures
- *B* Postconcussive states
- *C* Transient global amnesia

III Amnesic syndrome of subacute onset with varying degrees of recovery, usually leaving permanent residue
- *A* Wernicke-Korsakoff disease
- *B* Herpes simplex encephalitis
- *C* Tuberculous and other forms of meningitis characterized by a granulomatous exudate at the base of the brain

IV Slowly progressive amnesic states
- *A* Tumors involving the walls of the third ventricle and temporal lobes
- *B* Alzheimers disease and other degenerative disorders (early stage only)

OTHER BEHAVIORAL DISORDERS ASSOCIATED WITH CEREBRAL DISEASE When one attempts to categorize all the patients with relatively acute or subacute disorders of mentation and behavior under the types of syndromes above, there are still a considerable number that remain difficult to classify. They present themselves as an almost infinite variety of syndromes in which the following abnormalities of function may occur: reduced or increased levels of speech, thought, and action; disorientation as to time and place; loss of initiative and lack of interest; loss of spontaneity and sense of humor; muteness and hypokinesia, resistiveness and negativism; hostility, lack of observance of social customs, and use of abusive and vulgar language; inexplicable fright, euphoria, or lack of proper concern; complaints of visual distortion or of excess sensitivity to sounds; distortions of smell and taste; inability to find the names of objects, to follow a conversation, and to think coherently; sexual indiscretion, lack of modesty, and other signs of disinhibition; seizures; and disturbances of sleep. Obviously these many symptoms do not all have the same basic significance, and the majority possess only relative localizing value. They may be associated with definite hemiparesis, hemihypesthesia, frank aphasia, or homonymous hemianopsia, but even without these lateralizing signs they point to the existence of cerebral disease.

Syndromes comprising these elements may be observed in subacute sclerosing panencephalitis, listeriosis with meningoencephalitis, Behçet's meningoencephalitis, adult toxoplasmosis, infectious mononucleosis, acute or subacute demyelinative diseases (acute or subacute recurrent multiple sclerosis), granulomatous and other forms of angiitis, gliomatosis cerebri, carcinomatosis with encephalopathy of multifocal type, multiple tumor metastases, acute and subacute bacterial endocarditis, and thrombotic thrombocytopenia. Fuller accounts of some of the cerebral symptoms enumerated above are found in chapters dealing with these diseases.

PATIENT MANAGEMENT

CARE OF THE DELIRIOUS AND CONFUSED PATIENT The primary therapeutic effort is directed to the control of the underlying medical disease. Other important objectives are to quiet the patient and protect him or her against injury. A private nurse, an attendant, or a member of the family should be with the patient at all times, if this can be arranged. Depending on the degree of the patient's activity, a locked room, screened windows, and a low bed should be arranged. It is preferable that the patient be allowed to walk about the room rather than be tied into bed, which may provoke him or her to struggle to the point of exhaustion and collapse. If less active, the patient can be kept in bed by leather wrist restraints, a restraining sheet, or a net thrown over the bed. The patient should be permitted to sit up or walk part of the day, unless this is contraindicated by the primary disease.

Any drug that can possibly be responsible for the acute confusional state or delirium should be discontinued (unless withdrawal effects are believed to underlie the illness). In these circumstances, chlordiazepoxide, chlorpromazine, and diazepam are the drugs favored by most physicians, but the older sedatives—paraldehyde and chloral hydrate—are equally safe and effective if given in full doses. Whichever drug is used should be given until natural sleep is restored. In the case of severe delirium, drugs must be used with caution. One should not attempt to suppress agitation completely; to accomplish this may require very large doses of drugs, and vital functions may then be dangerously impaired. The purpose of sedation is to blunt the agitation so that the patient does not become exhausted and nursing care is facilitated.

Confusional states related to antidepressant drugs, e.g., amitriptyline, are said to be reversed by a 2-mg dose of physostigmine.

A fluid intake and output chart should be kept, and any fluid and electrolyte deficit should be corrected. The pulse and blood pressure should be recorded at frequent intervals in anticipation of circulatory collapse. Transfusions of whole blood and vasopressor drugs may be lifesaving if shock develops.

Finally, the physician should be aware of many small therapeutic measures that may allay fear and suspicion and reduce the tendency toward hallucinations. The room should be kept dimly lighted at night, and if possible the patient should not be moved from one room to another. Every procedure should be explained in detail, even such simple ones as the taking of blood pressure or temperature. The presence of a member of the family may enable the patient to maintain contact with reality.

Most delirious patients tend to recover if they receive competent medical and nursing care. The family should be reassured on this point and must also understand that the abnormal behavior and irrational actions of the patient are not willful but rather are symptomatic of a brain disease. Once recovered, the patient will be at least partly amnesic for the period of confusion; the gap must be filled by information provided by physician and family.

MANAGEMENT OF THE PATIENT WITH DEMENTIA AND THE AMNESIC STATE These major mental derangements are clinical states of the most serious nature, and usually it is worthwhile to admit the patient to the hospital for a period of observation. The physician then has an opportunity to see the patient several times in a neutral and fairly constant hospital environment, and certain special procedures such as CT scan, MRI, lumbar puncture and EEG as well as analysis of blood for endocrine state, toxic or metabolic abnormalities, and drugs can be carried out.

Once it is established that the patient has an untreatable dementing or amnesic brain disease, a responsible member of the family should be apprised of the medical facts. The patient should be told that he or she has a neurologic condition for which rest and treatment has been prescribed; often little is accomplished by telling more. The family should be given the diagnosis and prognosis if these are sufficiently certain for this to be done. If the abnormalities are slight and circumstances are suitable, the patient should remain at home, continue customary activities, and receive appropriate medication. If the patient becomes demented while still at work, plans for occupational retirement should be carried out. In more advanced stages of disease, mental and physical enfeeblement become pronounced and institutional care should be advised. Seizures should be treated symptomatically. Nerve tonics, vitamins, and hormones are of no value in the treatment of dementia. They may, however, offer some support to the patient and family. Sometimes, stimulants in the form of dextroamphetamine, caffeine, and nicotinic acid cause transitory improvement in mental function. Undesirable restlessness, nocturnal wandering, belligerency, or anxiety may be reduced by appropriate sedative drugs. Drugs advocated for specific treatment of dementia are currently under investigation.

REFERENCES

ADAMS RD, VICTOR M: *Principles of Neurology*, 3d ed. New York, McGraw-Hill, 1985

BENSON FD, BLUMER D: *Psychiatric Aspects of Neurologic Disease*. New York, Grune & Stratton, 1975, chap 2

BLESSED, G et al: The association between quantitative measures of dementia and of senile change in the cerebral grey matter of elderly subjects. Brit J Psychiat 114:797, 1968

BUTTERS N, MILIOTIS, P: Amnesic disorders, in *Clinical Neuropsychology*, K Heilman and E Valenstein (eds). London, Oxford, 1985, pp 403–451

ENGEL GL, ROMANO J: Delirium, a syndrome of cerebral insufficiency. J Chronic Dis 9:260, 1959

FISHER CM, ADAMS RD: Episodic global amnesia. Acta Neurol Scand 40:Suppl 9, 1964

GRAFF-RADFORD, NR et al: Nonhaemorrhagic thalamic infarction: Clinical, neuropsychological and electrophysiological findings in four anatomical groups defined by computerized tomography. Brain 108:485, 1985

LIPOWSKI ZJ: *Delirium: Acute Brain Failure in Man*. Springfield, Ill., Charles C Thomas, 1980

LISHMAN WA: *Organic Psychiatry: The Psychological Consequences of Cerebral Disorders*. Oxford, Blackwell, 1978

TERRY RD, KATZMAN R: Senile dementia of the Alzheimer type. Ann Neurol 14:497, 1983

TOMLINSON BE: The pathology of dementia, in *Dementia*, CE Wells (ed). Philadelphia, Davis, 1977, chap 6

WELLS CE: *Dementia*, 2d ed. Philadelphia, Davis, 1977

WELLS CE: Treatable forms of dementia, in *Update II: Harrison's Principles of Internal Medicine*, KJ Isselbacher et al (eds). New York, McGraw-Hill, 1981

24 SYNDROMES DUE TO FOCAL CEREBRAL LESIONS

RAYMOND D. ADAMS / MAURICE VICTOR

In addition to the general syndromes described in Chap. 23, there are many others which relate to lesions of particular parts of the cerebrum. Recognition of these constitutes irrefutable evidence that all parts of the cerebrum are not functionally equivalent. Some of the symptoms and signs which make up these syndromes have the same diagnostic value as a hemiplegia, and, once identified, require the same type of clinical analysis as to cause and pathophysiologic mechanism.

These focal syndromes will be described in terms of the conventional anatomic divisions of the cerebrum, but it will be obvious that most diseases do not respect these boundaries. Hence the syndromes may overlap or occur in a number of combinations.

FRONTAL LOBES In Fig. 24-1, it is seen that the frontal lobes lie anterior to the central (rolandic) sulcus and superior to the Sylvian

FIGURE 24-1 *Diagram to show cortical areas, numbered according to the scheme of Brodmann. The speech areas are in black, the three main ones of which are 39, 41, and 45. The zone marked by vertical stripes in the superior frontal convolution is the secondary motor area which, like Broca's area 45, if stimulated causes vocal arrest. (After Handbuch der Inneren Medizin, Berlin, Springer-Verlag, 1939.)*

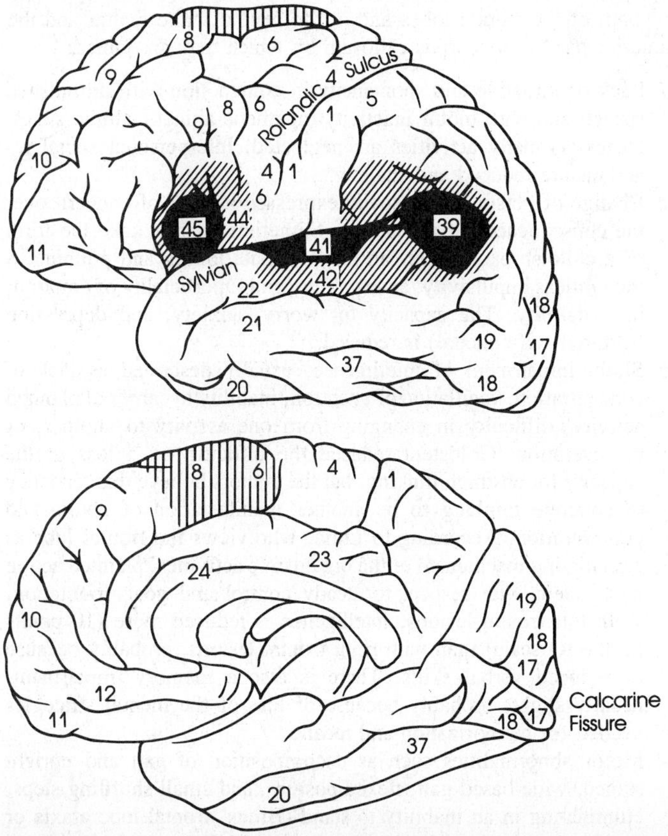

fissure. They consist of several functionally different parts, which are conventionally designated in the neurologic literature by numbers (according to the scheme devised by Brodmann) or by letters (according to the scheme of von Economo and Koskinas).

The posterior parts, areas 4 and 6 of Brodmann, are specifically related to motor function. There is also a secondary motor area in the posterior part of the superior frontal convolution. Voluntary movement in humans depends on the integrity of these areas, and lesions in them produce spastic paralysis of the contralateral face, arm, and leg. This is discussed in Chap. 15. A lesion limited more or less to the premotor area (area 6) is accompanied by a contralateral grasp reflex, and bilateral lesions are accompanied by a suck reflex. A lesion in area 8 of Brodmann interferes with the mechanism concerned with turning the head and eyes contralaterally. A lesion of the left supplementary motor area can result in mutism at its onset; in time the condition resolves to a state of transcortical motor aphasia with reduced language output with preserved repetition and naming. There may be hypokinesia of the arms, especially on the right. Lesions of the left premotor area in many instances result in a phonetic-articulatory defect (*cortical dysarthria*) and verbal perseveration. Agrammatism, with retention of "content words" but not of functional connecting words, is characteristic (see Chap. 22). A lesion in area 44 (Broca's area) of the dominant cerebral hemisphere, usually the left one, results in at least a temporary loss of verbal expression. Lesions of the anterior cingulate gyrus, in the acute stages, may cause a speechless, aphonic state; with recovery, speech returns through whispering and hoarseness rather than dysarthria and aphasia, according to Brown. Lesions in the medial limbic or piriform cortex (areas 23 and 24), where the mechanisms controlling respiration, circulation, and micturition are organized bilaterally, have relatively unclear clinical effects.

The remaining parts of the frontal lobes (areas 9 to 12 of Brodmann), sometimes called the *prefrontal areas,* have less specific and measurable functions. In contrast to the motor areas of the frontal lobes and other areas of the brain, stimulation of the prefrontal areas in humans has yielded a paucity of findings. Many patients with gunshot wounds of these areas have shown only mild and inconsistent abnormalities of behavior. Nevertheless, the following groups of symptoms have been observed in patients with large lesions of one or both of the frontal lobes and of the central white matter and the anterior part of the corpus callosum by which they are joined:

1 Lack of initiative and spontaneity in conjunction with diminished speech and with motor inactivity (apathetic-akinetic-abulic state). Necessary daily activities are neglected. Interpersonal social reactions are reduced and shallow.

2 Change of personality, usually expressed as lack of concern over the consequences of any action. Sometimes it may take the form of a childish excitement, an inappropriate joking and punning, a thoughtless impulsivity, an instability and superficiality of emotion, or irritability. The capacity for worry, anxiety, and depression (tortured self-concern) is reduced.

3 Slight impairment of intelligence, usually described as lack of concentration, vacillation of attention, inability to carry out planned activity, difficulty in changing from one activity to another, or perseveration. Goldstein reduced the difficulty to a loss of the capacity for abstract thinking, but the authors believe this tendency to concrete thinking to be another manifestation of abulia and perseveration. According to Luria, who views the frontal lobe as a regulating mechanism of the organism's activities, planned action is deficient with respect to steady control and goal orientation. With left frontal lesions, intelligence is reduced more (10 points on the IQ scale) than with right frontal lesions, probably because of reduced verbal skills. There is also a memory impairment, usually slight, probably because of loss of the mental strategies needed for memorization and recall.

4 Motor abnormalities such as decomposition of gait and upright stance, wide-based gait, flexed posture, and small shuffling steps, culminating in an inability to stand (Bruns' frontal lobe ataxia or gait apraxia) accompanied by abnormal postures, reflex grasping or sucking, and incontinence of sphincters.

Some differences have been noted between the dominant (left) and right frontal lobes. In psychological tests, left frontal lesions impair verbal fluency and cause a greater degree of perseveration, and right frontal lesions impair the learning of visual spatial patterns and cause impersistence (see Hecaen and Albert, and Luria for details). From these comments it should be evident that the frontal lobes have not a unitary function, but participate in a number of interconnected functional components, each subserving a different component of behavior

TEMPORAL LOBES The boundaries of the temporal lobes are illustrated in Fig. 24-1. The Sylvian fissure separates the superior surface of each temporal lobe from the frontal lobe and anterior part of the parietal lobe. There is no definite anatomic boundary between the temporal and occipital lobes or the posterior temporal and parietal lobes. The temporal lobe includes the superior, middle, and inferior temporal, fusiform, and hippocampal convolutions and the transverse convolutions of Heschl, which are the auditory receptive area, present on the superior surface within the Sylvian fissure. The hippocampal convolution was once believed to be related to olfactory function, but now it is known that lesions here do not cause anosmia. Only the medial and anterior parts of the temporal lobes (uncal regions) are related to smell. The lower fibers of the geniculocalcarine pathway (from the inferior retina) swing in a wide arc over the temporal horn of the ventricle into the white matter of the temporal lobe en route to the occipital lobes, and lesions which interrupt them characteristically produce a contralateral upper homonymous quadrantanopsia. Hearing, localized in the superior surfaces of the temporal lobes (Heschl's gyri), is bilaterally represented, which accounts for the fact that both temporal lobes need to be affected to cause deafness. Loss of equilibrium has not been observed with temporal lobe lesions. Disease in the superior convolution of the left temporal lobe and adjacent inferior parietal lobule in right-handed individuals results in a Wernicke's aphasia. This syndrome, discussed in Chap. 22, consists of paraphasic speech or jargon aphasia and inability to read, write, repeat, or understand the meaning of spoken words.

Between the auditory and olfactory projection areas there is a large expanse of temporal lobe which subserves three specific functional systems. In the inferolateral parts (areas 20, 21, and 37) are located some of the visual-associated projections. In the superior-lateral parts (areas 22, 41, and 42) are the primary and secondary areas for acoustic perception. In the mediobasal parts are the limbic structures (amygdaloid nuclei and hippocampi) where the neural organizations for emotional and memory processes lie. Bilateral lesions of the visual parts result in cortical blindness; visual and limbic disorders contribute to the Klüver-Bucy syndrome. Bilateral hippocampal/parahippocampal lesions produce a deficit in which the patient is unable to record events and information, i.e., has a loss of memory, in both its general and specific aspects (see Chap. 23). Lastly, the temporal lobes include a large part of the limbic system, which subserves the emotional and motivational aspects of behavior and vegetative functions ("visceral brain").

Apart from aphasia, psychological studies have shown a difference between the effects of dominant and nondominant temporal lobe lesions. With dominant lesions there is impairment in learning auditorially presented verbal material; with nondominant lesions there is a failure in learning visually presented nonverbal material. In addition, about 20 percent of patients with either a right or left lobectomy have shown an alteration of personality similar to that described after lesions in the prefrontal parts of the brain (see above).

The study of patients with uncinate epilepsy, with the characteristic dreamy state, olfactory or gustatory hallucinations, and masticatory movements, suggests that all these functions are organized through the temporal lobes. Stimulation of the posterior parts of the temporal lobes of fully conscious epileptic patients during surgical procedures has brought to light the interesting fact that complex memories and visual and auditory images, some with strong emotional content, can be aroused. Studies of the effects of stimulation of the amygdaloid nucleus, which is in the anterior and medial part of the temporal lobe, have shed additional light on this subject. Some symptoms like those of schizophrenia and mania may be evoked. Complex emotional experiences that had occurred previously may be revived. There are also remarkable autonomic effects: the blood pressure rises, pulse increases, respirations increase in frequency and depth, and the patient looks frightened. In temporal lobe epilepsy, there may be an intensification of the patient's emotional reactions, vague preoccupation with moral and religious issues, a tendency to write excessively, and sometimes aggressiveness. Ablation of the amygdaloid nuclei has eliminated uncontrollable rage reactions in psychotic patients. Hippocampal and adjacent convolutions have been excised bilaterally, with a disastrous loss of ability to learn or to establish new memories (Korsakoff psychosis).

Bilateral destruction of the temporal lobes in both humans and monkeys results in placidity, loss of visual recognition, tendency to examine objects by touch and mouthing, and hypersexuality. This is called the Klüver-Bucy syndrome.

The abnormalities consequent upon lesions of the temporal lobes may be summarized as follows:

1 Effects of unilateral disease of the dominant temporal lobe
- *a* Upper homonymous quadrantanopsia
- *b* Wernicke's aphasia
- *c* Impairment in tests of verbal material presented through the auditory sense
- *d* Dysnomia or amnesic aphasia
- *e* Amusia (inability to name scores and read and write music)

2 Effects of unilateral disease of nondominant temporal lobe
- *a* Upper homonymous quadrantanopsia
- *b* Inability to judge spatial relationships in rare cases
- *c* Impairment in tests of nonverbal visually presented material
- *d* Agnosia for nonlexical qualities of music

3 Effects of disease of either temporal lobe
- *a* Auditory illusions and hallucinations
- *b* Psychotic behavior (aggressivity)

4 Effects of bilateral disease
- *a* Korsakoff amnesic defect
- *b* Apathy and placidity } Klüver-Bucy syndrome
- *c* Increased sexual activity } Klüver-Bucy syndrome
- *d* Sham rage
- *e* Cortical deafness
- *f* Loss of other unilateral functions

PARIETAL LOBES The postcentral convolution is the terminus of somatic sensory pathways from the opposite half of the body. However, destructive lesions here do not abolish cutaneous sensation but cause mainly a defect in sensory discrimination with variable impairment of primary sensation. In other words, the perception of painful, tactile, thermal, and vibratory stimuli is affected little or not at all, whereas stereognosis, sense of position, distinction between single and double contacts (two-point threshold), and the localization of sensory stimuli are impaired or lost (atopognosia). There is also the phenomenon of extinction, i.e., if a stimulus (tactile, painful, visual) is delivered simultaneously to both sides of the body, only the stimulus on the normal side is perceived. This type of sensory disturbance, sometimes called *cortical sensory defect,* is discussed in Chap. 18. Extensive lesions deep in the white matter of the parietal lobes produce an impairment of all forms of sensation contralaterally, and if these lesions encroach upon the uppermost part of the temporal lobe, there may be a contralateral homonymous hemianopsia, often incongruous and greater in the inferior quadrants. Lesions of the angular gyrus of the dominant hemisphere result in an inability to read (alexia).

More recent investigations have centered on the function of the parietal lobes in the perception of one's position in space, the interrelationships of objects in space, and the relationship of the various parts of the body to one another. Since the time of Babinski it has been known that patients with large lesions of the minor parietal lobe are often unaware of their hemiplegias and hemianesthesias. Babinski called this condition *anosognosia.* Related psychological disorders are lack of recognition of the left arm and leg, neglect of the left side of the body (as in dressing) and of the external space on the left side, and constructional apraxia (an inability to construct simple figures). All of these disorders may occur with left-sided lesions as well but are observed only infrequently, in part because the aphasia that occurs with lesions of the left hemisphere makes it difficult to adequately test other parietal lobe functions.

Another frequent constellation of symptoms, usually referred to as *Gerstmann's syndrome,* occurs only with lesions of the dominant parietal lobe. This consists of inability to write (agraphia), calculate (acalculia), distinguish right from left, and identify fingers (finger agnosia). This syndrome is a true *agnosia,* since it represents a defect in the formulation and use of symbolic concepts, including the significance of numbers and letters and the names of parts of the body. An ideomotor apraxia may or may not be associated. *Apraxia* and *agnosia* are discussed in Chaps. 15 and 18.

The effects of disease of the parietal lobes may be organized into three major categories:

1 Effects of unilateral disease of the parietal lobe, right or left
- *a* Cortical sensory syndrome and sensory extinction (or total hemianesthesia with large acute lesions of white matter)
- *b* In children, mild contralateral hemiparesis and hemiatrophy
- *c* Visual inattention or, less often, homonymous hemianopsia, and sometimes anosognosia, neglect of the opposite one-half of the body and extrapersonal space (more frequent with right than with left parietal lesions)
- *d* Abolition of optokinetic nystagmus to one side

2 Effects of unilateral disease of the dominant parietal lobe (left hemisphere in right-handed patients), additional phenomena
- *a* Disorders of language (especially alexia)
- *b* Gerstmann's syndrome
- *c* Bimanual astereognosis (tactile agnosia)
- *d* Bilateral apraxia of the ideomotor type

3 Effects of lesions of the nondominant parietal lobe, additional phenomena
- *a* Disorders of location and orientation, and constructional apraxia
- *b* Unawareness of paralysis (anosognosia) and misidentification of left arm and leg
- *c* Dressing apraxia
- *d* Bland mood, indifference to illness or neurologic defects

In all these lesions, if sufficiently extensive, there may be a reduction in the capacity to think clearly, inattentiveness, and impaired memory.

OCCIPITAL LOBES The occipital lobes are the termini of the geniculocalcarine pathways and are essential for visual sensation and perception. Destructive lesions in one occipital lobe result in a contralateral homonymous hemianopsia, i.e., a loss of vision in part or all of the homonymous fields. Occasionally patients complain of changes in the form and contour of visually perceived objects (metamorphopsia), as well as illusory displacement of images from one side of the visual field to another (visual allesthesia), or of abnormal persistence of the visual image after the object has been removed (palinopsia). Visual illusions and elementary (unformed) hallucinations may also occur. Bilateral lesions cause "cortical" blindness, a state of blindness without change in optic fundi or pupillary reflexes.

Lesions in Brodmann's areas 18 and 19 of the dominant hemisphere (Fig. 24-1) cause a loss of recognition of objects presented visually, despite the ability to see, at least to some degree—a state termed *visual object agnosia.* In the classic form of this disorder, individuals with intact mental powers are unable to recognize objects visually, even though by tests of visual acuity and perimetry they appear to see sufficiently well to do so; they are able to recognize objects by tactile or other nonvisual senses. In these terms, *alexia,* or inability to read, represents a visual verbal agnosia or "word blindness." Patients can see letters and words but do not know their meaning, although they can still recognize them through tactile or auditory senses. Other types of agnosia, for recognition of faces (prosopagnosia), for a complex of objects the elements of which are perceived but not the whole (simultanagnosia), and for color, and Balint's syndrome (inability to look at and grasp an object, visual ataxia, and visual inattention) are observed with bilateral occipital lesions.

The details of these syndromes of the different lobes of the cerebrum can be found in the textbook of Adams and Victor and the monograph by Walsh.

CORPUS CALLOSUM AND THE DISCONNECTION SYNDROMES Considerable attention has been devoted to the study of each of the two cerebral hemispheres in isolation. This is possible only when the corpus callosum, which forms a bridge between the two hemispheres, is surgically sectioned (for epilepsy) or destroyed by infarction or tumors. From these studies emerges the well-known fact that the left hemisphere is dominant in all language functions and auditory perception and the right hemisphere is superior in spatial and visual perception. Partial lesions of the corpus callosum or of the long tracts in the cerebral white matter are found to be associated with a number of interesting syndromes (commissural and intrahemispheric) which will be described below.

When the corpus callosum is sectioned by a surgical procedure or destroyed by an anterior cerebral artery occlusion (anterior four-fifths), the language and perceptual areas of the left hemisphere are isolated from the sensory and motor areas of the right hemisphere. These patients, if blindfolded, are then unable to match an object held in one hand with an identical object in the other hand. Further, they cannot match an object seen in the right half of the visual field with one in the left half. If given verbal commands, they perform correctly with the right hand but not with the left. Without vision, objects placed in the right hand are named correctly, but not those in the left. In lesions confined to the posterior fifth of the corpus callosum (splenium), only the visual part of the disconnection syndrome occurs. Occlusion of the left posterior cerebral artery provides the best examples of this. Infarction of the left occipital lobe cause a right homonymous hemianopsia, as a consequence of which all visual information needed for activating the speech areas of the left hemisphere must come from the right occipital lobe, across the splenium of the corpus callosum. If there is a lesion in the corpus callosum (or in other portions of the crossing fibers), the patient cannot read or name colors because the visual information cannot reach the left angular gyrus. There is no difficulty in copying words, though the patient cannot read what he or she has written; matching colors without naming them is done without error. Apparently the visual information for activating the left motor area crosses the corpus callosum more anteriorly. A disconnection in the anterior third of the corpus callosum, where fiber systems between the right and left premotor areas must pass, results only in failure of the left hand to obey commands, the right one performing perfectly (left-sided apraxia). The left hand can still imitate the examiner's movements or carry out the patient's intention.

There are also intrahemispheric disconnections, of which the most important are the following:

1 *Conduction aphasia* (also called *central* aphasia). The patient has fluent but paraphasic speech and writing with nearly perfect comprehension of spoken or written language. Repetition of what is heard or read is, however, severely impaired. The lesion is presumably in the arcuate fasciculus, which connects Wernicke's area with Broca's area.
2 *Pure word deafness.* Although the patient is able to hear and identify nonverbal sounds, there is a loss of ability to comprehend spoken language. The patient's speech remains normal. The defect has been attributed to a subcortical lesion, undercutting Wernicke's area.

The reader is referred to Geschwind and to Dimond for further details on the disconnection syndromes.

DIAGNOSIS AND MANAGEMENT OF PATIENTS WITH FOCAL CEREBRAL LESIONS These involve the same principles described in Chap. 23. Special tests, mostly of the psychological type, are available for each of the focal cerebral syndromes (Walsh). The investigation and care of individual patients will, of course, also be governed by the underlying disease.

REFERENCES

Adams RD, Victor M: *Principles of Neurology,* 3d ed. New York, McGraw-Hill, 1985
Brodal A: *Neurological Anatomy in Relation to Clinical Medicine,* 3d ed. New York, Oxford University Press, 1981
Brown JW: Frontal lobe syndromes, in *Handbook of Clinical Neurology,* JAM Frederiks (ed). Amsterdam, Elsevier Science, 1985, vol 45, chap 3
Dimond SJ: The disconnection syndromes, in *Modern Trends in Neurology,* D. Williams (ed). London, Butterworth, 1975
Geschwind N: Disconnection syndromes in animals and man. Brain 88:237, 585, 1965
Hacaen H, Albert ML: Disorders of mental functioning related to the frontal lobes, in *Modern Trends in Neurology,* D Williams (ed). London, Butterworth, 1975
Luria AR: *The Working Brain: An Introduction to Neuropsychology.* New York, Basic Books (translation Penguin Books Ltd), 1973
Walsh KW: *Neuropsychology: A Clinical Approach.* London, Churchill Livingstone, 1978

section 4 Alterations in circulatory and respiratory function

25 COUGH AND HEMOPTYSIS

GENNARO M. TISI / EUGENE BRAUNWALD

COUGH

Cough, one of the most frequent cardiorespiratory symptoms, is an explosive expiration which provides a means of clearing the tracheobronchial tree of secretions and foreign bodies.

MECHANISM Coughing may be initiated either voluntarily or reflexly. As a defensive reflex it has both afferent and efferent pathways. The *afferent limb* includes cough receptors within the sensory distribution of the trigeminal, glossopharyngeal, superior laryngeal, and vagus nerves. The *efferent limb* includes the recurrent laryngeal nerve (which causes glottic closure) and the spinal nerves (which cause contraction of the thoracic and abdominal musculature). The *sequence of a cough* includes an appropriate stimulus which initiates a deep inspiration. This is followed by glottic closure, relaxation of the diaphragm, and muscle contraction against a closed glottis so as to produce maximally positive intrathoracic and intraairway pressures.

These positive intrathoracic pressures result in a narrowing of the trachea, produced by an infolding of its more compliant posterior membrane. Once the glottis opens, the combination of a large pressure differential between the airways and the atmosphere coupled with this tracheal narrowing produces flow rates through the trachea close to the speed of sound. The shearing forces which are developed aid in the elimination of mucus and foreign materials. A tracheostomy short-circuits glottic closure and therefore decreases the effectiveness of the cough mechanism.

ETIOLOGY Cough is produced by inflammatory, mechanical, chemical, and thermal stimulation of the cough receptors. *Inflammatory* stimuli are initiated by edema and hyperemia of the respiratory mucous membranes, and by irritation from exudative processes. Such stimuli may arise either in the airways (as in laryngitis, tracheitis, bronchitis, and bronchiolitis) or in the alveoli (as in pneumonitis and lung abscess). *Mechanical* stimuli are produced by inhalation of particulate matter, such as dust particles, and by compression of the air passages and pressure or tension upon these structures. Lesions associated with airway compression may be either extramural or intramural in type. The former include aortic aneurysms, granulomas, pulmonary neoplasms, and mediastinal tumors; intramural lesions include bronchogenic carcinoma, bronchial adenoma, foreign bodies, granulomatous endobronchial involvement, and contraction of airway smooth muscle (bronchial asthma). Pressure or tension upon the air passages is usually produced by lesions associated with a decrease in pulmonary compliance. Examples of specific causes include acute and chronic interstitial fibrosis (Chap. 209), pulmonary edema, and atelectasis. *Chemical* stimuli may result from inhalation of irritant gases, including cigarette smoke and chemical fumes. Finally, *thermal* stimuli may be produced by inhalation of either very hot or cold air.

Cough is commonly associated with episodic wheezing secondary to bronchoconstriction in symptomatic patients with bronchial asthma (Chap. 202). Recent reports have drawn attention to patients with chronic, persistent cough as the *sole* presenting manifestation of bronchial asthma, (''cough asthma''). Such patients are characterized by (1) absence of a history of episodic wheezing and (2) no evidence of expiratory airflow obstruction by spirometry, but (3) hyperreactive airways (characteristic of asthma) when challenged with a cholinergic agent, methacholine.

DIAGNOSTIC EVALUATION When one is considering the above list of causes, answers to the following general questions will significantly narrow the diagnostic possibilities: Is the cough acute or chronic? Is it productive of sputum or nonproductive?

Features of the history, physical examination, chest roentgenogram, screening pulmonary function studies (static lung volumes and dynamic flow rates), and sputum examination may indicate a specific cause. The *history* may indicate specific diagnoses. Acute episodes of cough may be associated with such viral infections as acute tracheobronchitis or pneumonitis or with bacterial bronchopneumonia. Cough associated with an acute febrile episode and associated with hoarseness is usually produced by viral laryngotracheobronchitis. Postnasal drip is also a common cause of chronic cough.

The character of the cough may suggest the anatomic site of involvement: the patient with a ''barking'' type of cough may have epiglottal involvement, (i.e., ''whooping cough'' due to *Haemophilus pertussis* infection in young children), while the cough associated with tracheal or major airway involvement is often loud and ''brassy.'' Cough associated with generalized wheezing may be produced by acute bronchospasm. The time of occurrence of a cough may indicate a specific cause: a cough which occurs selectively at night suggests congestive heart failure; one related to meals suggests a tracheoesophageal fistula, a hiatal hernia, or an esophageal diverticulum; a cough precipitated by a change in position suggests a lung abscess or a localized area of bronchiectasis. The description of sputum or secretions produced in conjunction with the cough may also be helpful: putrid sputum suggests a lung abscess; bloody sputum, bleeding (see ''Hemoptysis,'' below); frothy and pink-tinged sputum, pulmonary edema; mucoid and massive sputum, alveolar cell carcinoma; purulent and/or large amounts of sputum, lung abscess and bronchiectasis.

On *physical examination* the character of the auscultatory findings may suggest the site of disease: inspiratory stridor and wheezing may be present in laryngeal disease, inspiratory and expiratory rhonchi favor tracheal and major airway involvement, coarse subcrepitant inspiratory rales may indicate interstitial fibrosis and/or edema, fine crepitant rales may indicate a process such as pneumonitis or pulmonary edema, which fills the alveoli with fluid. The *chest roentgenogram* may reveal the cause of the cough; it may show an intrapulmonary mass lesion which may be either central or peripheral (Chap. 213), an alveolar filling process which may be pneumonic or nonpneumonic, an area of honeycombing and cyst formation which may indicate an area of localized bronchiectasis, or bilateral hilar adenopathy which may indicate sarcoidosis or a lymphoma.

Screening pulmonary function studies (Chap. 200) may also indicate specific diagnoses. Significant expiratory obstruction to airflow (as determined from a forced expiratory flow maneuver), coupled with a history of cough and significant sputum production, suggests that irrespective of other lesions the patient has significant bronchitis. Decreased lung volume (as determined from the static lung volumes) indicates that a restrictive type of lung disease is present—reduction of lung volumes produced by thoracic, pleural, alveolar, or interstitial disease. Finally, a careful *sputum examination* may be more enlightening than a patient's description of the character of the sputum. Examination shows whether the sputum is thin or viscid, purulent or not, foul-smelling or not, blood-tinged or not, scant or copious. In pneumococcal pneumonia the sputum has a ''rusty'' color, while in *Klebsiella* pneumonia it may look like ''currant jelly.'' Gram stain and culture of the deep-cough specimen may reveal a specific bacterial, fungal, or mycoplasmal causation, while sputum cytology may result in a positive diagnosis of a pulmonary neoplasm.

Two features of cough should be highlighted: (1) A cough is often so common in the cigarette smoker as to be ignored or minimized. *Any change in the nature or character of a chronic cigarette cough should initiate immediate diagnostic evaluation, with particular attention directed to detection of bronchogenic carcinoma.* (2) Female patients are inclined to swallow sputum and not to expectorate as male patients do. This tendency may lead to the incorrect conclusion that a cough in a female patient is irritative and nonproductive.

COMPLICATIONS Three complications may be produced by the coughing mechanism: paroxysms of coughing may precipitate syncope (cough syncope, Chap. 12), and strenuous coughing may produce rupture of an emphysematous bleb and rib fractures. A potential mechanism for cough syncope includes the development of markedly positive intrathoracic and alveolar pressures which decrease venous return, producing a decrease in cardiac output and resultant syncope. Although cough fractures of the ribs may occur in otherwise normal patients, their occurrence should at least raise the possibility of pathologic fractures, which are seen in multiple myeloma, osteoporosis, and osteolytic metastases.

THERAPY Definitive treatment of cough depends on determining its precise cause and then initiating specific therapy for the underlying cause. Symptomatic therapy should be considered when the cause of the cough is idiopathic and the cough performs no useful function or represents a potential hazard to the patient. An irritative, nonproductive cough may be suppressed by an antitussive agent, such as codeine or dextromethorphan, 15 mg qid. These drugs are particularly useful in interrupting prolonged, self-perpetuating paroxysms. However, a cough productive of significant quantities of sputum should not be suppressed, since retention of sputum in the tracheobronchial tree may interfere with the distribution of ventilation, alveolar aeration, and the ability of the lung to resist infection. When secretions are tenacious and thick, adequate hydration, expectorants, and humidification of the air with an ultrasonic nebulizer may be helpful.

Ipratropium (a new class of bronchodilator with antimuscarinic actions) may prove especially useful in patients with cough asthma.

HEMOPTYSIS

For purposes of definition hemoptysis includes both blood-streaked sputum and gross hemoptysis. It is apparent that any patient with gross hemoptysis should be given appropriate diagnostic tests so that a specific cause may be found. The patient with blood-streaked sputum should also be studied unless one can be certain that this type of hemoptysis is due to a benign condition. A major pitfall in dealing with hemoptysis is to ascribe recurrent episodes to a previously established diagnosis, such as chronic bronchiectasis or bronchitis. Such an approach may result in missing a serious but potentially treatable lesion. The safest approach to a recurrent episode of hemoptysis is to treat it as if it were the initial episode and proceed with a complete diagnostic evaluation.

ETIOLOGY AND INCIDENCE Prior to embarking upon an extensive diagnostic workup of hemoptysis, it is essential to determine that the blood is in fact coming from the respiratory tract, not from the nasopharynx or gastrointestinal tract. Distinguishing hemoptysis from hematemesis is difficult at times. In hemoptysis, the prodrome is usually a tingling in the throat or a desire to cough, the blood is coughed up, and it is usually bright-red and *frothy*; in hematemesis, the prodrome includes nausea and abdominal discomfort, the blood is vomited, and it is usually *magenta* in color. Once this point is established, the diagnostic tests for hemoptysis may proceed. Although there are numerous single case reports of diseases which have been associated with hemoptysis, Table 25-1 presents the more common disorders.

The incidence of the diagnoses listed in Table 25-1 depends upon the nature of the series reported and whether one includes both gross bleeding and blood streaking of the sputum. If both types of bleeding are included, then the major causes (approximately 60 to 70 percent) are chronic bronchitis and bronchiectasis. If the definition is restricted to gross bleeding (greater than several tablespoons) then the incidence depends upon the type of series reported. Surgical series favor the incidence of mass lesions and operable lesions (carcinoma, 20 percent; localized, segmental, or lobar bronchiectasis, 30 percent). Those from centers with a large tuberculosis population favor this condition (incidence varying between 2 and 40 percent). Combined medical-surgical series include a wider representation of those lesions which present with hemoptysis (carcinoma, 20 percent; bronchiectasis, 30 percent; bronchitis, 15 percent; other inflammatory lesions including tuberculosis, 10 to 20 percent; other lesions including the vascular, traumatic, and hemorrhagic etiologies listed in Table 25-1, 10 percent). Despite the most extensive of evaluations, 5 to 15 percent of cases entailing gross hemoptysis remain undiagnosed.

TABLE 25-1 Causes of hemoptysis

1 Inflammatory
- *a* Bronchitis
- *b* Bronchiectasis
- *c* Tuberculosis
- *d* Lung abscess
- *e* Pneumonia, particularly *Klebsiella*

2 Neoplastic
- *a* Lung cancer: squamous cell, adenocarcinoma, oat cell
- *b* Bronchial adenoma

3 Other
- *a* Pulmonary thromboembolism
- *b* Left ventricular failure
- *c* Mitral stenosis
- *d* Traumatic, including foreign body and lung contusion
- *e* Primary pulmonary hypertension; arteriovenous malformation; Eisenmenger's syndrome; pulmonary vasculitis including Wegener's granulomatosis and Goodpasture's syndrome; idiopathic pulmonary hemosiderosis; and amyloid
- *f* Hemorrhagic diathesis including anticoagulant therapy

Two points should be highlighted with reference to diseases associated with hemoptysis: (1) *hemoptysis is rare in metastatic carcinoma to the lung*; (2) *although hemoptysis may occur at some time during the course of a viral or pneumococcal pneumonia, it is usually scanty and its occurrence should always raise the question of a more serious underlying process.*

DIAGNOSIS The *history* may suggest specific diagnoses: recurrent, chronic hemoptysis in a young, otherwise asymptomatic female favors the diagnosis of a bronchial adenoma; recurrent hemoptysis with chronic, marked sputum production associated with ring shadows, tram lines (abnormal air bronchograms), and cyst formation on the roentgenogram suggests a diagnosis of bronchiectasis; putrid sputum production suggests a lung abscess; weight loss and anorexia in a male smoker over the age of 40 raise the possibility of a bronchogenic carcinoma; a recent history of blunt trauma to the chest suggests a lung contusion; and acute pleuritic chest pain raises the possibility of pulmonary embolism with infarction or some other pleurally based lesion (lung abscess, coccidioidomycosis cavity, and vasculitis). Several findings on the *physical examination* may also suggest a specific diagnosis: a pleural friction rub suggests those diagnoses just mentioned in connection with pleuritic pain; the findings of pulmonary hypertension raise the diagnostic possibilities of primary pulmonary hypertension, mitral stenosis, recurrent or chronic thromboembolism, and Eisenmenger's syndrome; a localized wheeze over a major lobar airway suggests an intramural lesion such as a bronchogenic carcinoma or a foreign body; systemic arteriovenous communications or the presence of a murmur over the lung fields suggest the diagnosis of Osler-Rendu-Weber disease with pulmonary arteriovenous malformation; evidence of significant expiratory obstruction to airflow coupled with sputum production suggests that whatever other lesion may be present, the patient has significant bronchitis. Finally, the *chest roentgenogram* is critical to diagnosis. The presence of ring shadows favors a diagnosis of bronchiectasis; an air-fluid level, the diagnosis of a lung abscess; and a mass lesion, the diagnosis of a central or peripheral pulmonary neoplasm. A mass lesion which may cause hemoptysis should be distinguished from an area of blood pneumonitis caused by aspiration of blood into contiguous areas.

One of the most demanding diagnostic problems is the identification of the site of bleeding in a patient with normal findings on physical examination and a normal roentgenogram of the chest. A patient with hemoptysis tends to keep the bleeding side dependent. Otherwise, gravitational drainage would cause aspiration into the noninvolved dependent lung. The patient may also be able to give a history of a burning or deep pain which may localize the side of bleeding; bronchoscopy may then be useful. This procedure generally is most helpful when the bleeding is scant, and of least help when the bleeding is massive, since blood may be aspirated into contiguous airways. Such aspiration may produce alveolar filling (i.e., a "blood pneumonitis") that may obscure the etiology of the hemoptysis on the initial chest roentgenogram. Blood pneumonitis usually clears within a week, and once clearing has occurred, a repeat chest roentgenogram may disclose the origin of the hemoptysis.

Following the history and physical examination, the diagnostic approach to a patient with hemoptysis includes whatever specialized studies and procedures are required to make a specific diagnosis. The first step is to obtain a roentgenogram. Usually bronchoscopy is the procedure employed next. Rigid bronchoscopy permits visualization of the more central airways. It is of particular value when the source of bleeding is in this portion of the airway system, the degree of hemoptysis is massive, and selective endobronchial intubation is being considered. Fiberoptic bronchoscopy (Chap. 201) includes within the range of visualization airways as small as several millimeters in diameter. This endoscopic technique may provide definitive visual, biopsy, or cytologic information. Since direct visualization of more peripheral portions of the airway system is now possible, the indications for bronchography in the evaluation of hemoptysis are being modified. The principal indications for bronchography in such patients are (1) to establish the presence of localized bronchiectasis (including a sequestered lobe) and (2) to rule out the presence of more generalized bronchiectasis in a patient with localized disease who is regarded as a surgical candidate because of either repetitive hemoptysis or recurrent infections. The majority of patients with bronchiectasis have a normal chest roentgenogram. If bronchoscopy in such patients is also negative, bronchography is the only means of establishing an anatomic diagnosis of bronchiectasis. If the chest roentgenogram is abnormal, revealing either ring shadows or tram lines, a diagnosis of bronchiectasis may be made without the need for bronchography.

THERAPY Since hemoptysis is such an alarming symptom, there is a tendency to overtreat the patient. Usually hemoptysis is scant and will stop spontaneously without specific therapy. If the hemoptysis is substantial, the mainstays of therapy include keeping the patient calm, instituting complete bed rest, excluding unnecessary diagnostic procedures until the hemoptysis has begun to subside, and suppressing cough if it is present and an aggravating feature of the hemoptysis. The emergency care of such a patient demands that intubation and suctioning equipment be at the bedside. In patients in danger of asphyxiation by flooding of the lung contralateral to the site of hemorrhage, intubation by a technique which isolates the hemorrhaging lung and prevents contralateral aspiration of blood should be carried out. This can be accomplished by strategic location of a balloon catheter whose introduction into the bronchus in question is facilitated by direct visualization through a fiberoptic bronchoscope.

The management of potentially lethal massive hemoptysis remains controversial. The choice between a medical approach and surgical intervention hinges on the words *potentially lethal*. Massive hemoptysis, usually defined as greater than 600 to 800 mL in 24 h, is an alarming clinical situation in which asphyxiation due to aspiration of blood represents the principal threat to life. The choice between surgical and medical management relates most often to the anatomic basis for the massive hemoptysis. In patients with cavitary tuberculosis, anaerobic lung abscess, and lung cancer, the risk of mortality is far greater than when the cause of the hemoptysis is bronchitis or bronchiectasis. Operation may occasionally be necessary in the former, but virtually never in the latter group. In either case the initial management should include the conservative measures suggested above. With such management, spontaneous cessation of bleeding usually occurs. Surgical intervention should be considered in that small group of patients with a definable lesion on chest roentgenogram (i.e., cavitary disease, lung abscess, lung cancer) who have evidence of uncontrollable respiratory or hemodynamic compromise. If a patient is a surgical candidate, bronchoscopy should be performed to identify the specific site of bleeding. Otherwise bronchoscopy should be deferred for several days because of the tendency of this procedure to aggravate cough and thereby perpetuate the hemoptysis. Bronchial arterial catheterization and embolization are new modalities of treatment currently under evaluation for the nonsurgical control of massive hemoptysis, especially in patients with nonresectable lung cancer. Laser (neodymium YAG—yttrium aluminum garnet) therapy should also be considered as a palliative modality for massive hemoptysis in such patients.

REFERENCES

Adelman M et al: Cryptogenic hemoptysis: Clinical features, bronchoscopic findings, and natural history in 67 patients. Ann Intern Med 102:829, 1985

Boushey HA et al: Medical staff conference: Evaluating and treating intractable cough. West J Med 143:223, 1985

Conlan AA: Massive hemoptysis: Diagnostic and therapeutic implications. Surg Ann 17:337, 1985

Corrao WMC et al: Chronic cough as the sole presenting manifestation of bronchial asthma. N Engl J Med 300:633, 1979

Gross NJ et al: Anticholinergic, antimuscarinic bronchodilators. Am Rev Resp Dis 129:856, 1984

Irwin RS et al: Persistent cough in the adult: The spectrum and frequency of causes and successful outcome of specific therapy. Am Rev Resp Dis 123:413, 1981

Leith DE: The development of cough. Am Rev Respir Dis 131:S39, 1985

Williams MH: Management of massive hemoptysis. Pulmonary Perspectives, a publication of the American College of Chest Physicians 1:3, 1984

26 DYSPNEA AND PULMONARY EDEMA

ROLAND H. INGRAM, JR. / EUGENE BRAUNWALD

DYSPNEA

The breathing pattern is controlled by a series of higher central and peripheral mechanisms which can increase ventilation in excess of metabolic demands in conditions such as anxiety and fear, and can increase ventilation appropriate to increased metabolic demands during physical activity. A normal resting person is unaware of the act of breathing, and while he or she may become conscious of breathing during mild to moderate exertion, no discomfort is experienced. However, during and following exhausting exertion an individual may become unpleasantly aware of breathing, yet feel reasonably assured that the sensation will be transitory and is appropriate to the level of exercise. Therefore, as a cardinal symptom of diseases affecting the cardiorespiratory system, dyspnea is defined as an *abnormally uncomfortable awareness of breathing*.

Although dyspnea is not painful in the usual sense of the word, it is, like pain, involved with both the perception of a sensation and the reaction to that perception. Patients experience a number of uncomfortable sensations related to breathing and use an even larger number of verbal expressions to describe these sensations, such as "cannot get enough air," "air does not go all the way down," "smothering feeling in the chest," "tightness in the chest," "fatigue in the chest," and a "choking sensation." It may be necessary, therefore, to review meticulously the patient's history in order to ascertain whether the more abstruse descriptions do, in fact, represent dyspnea. Once it is established that a patient does have dyspnea, it is of paramount importance to define the circumstances in which it occurs and to assess associated symptoms. There are situations in which breathing appears labored but in which dyspnea does not occur. For example, the hyperventilation in association with metabolic acidemia is rarely accompanied by dyspnea. On the other hand, patients with apparently normal breathing patterns may complain of shortness of breath.

QUANTITATION OF DYSPNEA The gradation of dyspnea may usefully be based upon the amount of physical exertion required to produce the sensation. In actual practice the major functional classifications of patients with heart or lung disease are based largely on dyspnea in relation to degree of exertion. However, in assessing the severity of dyspnea, it is important to obtain a clear understanding of the patient's general physical condition, work history, and recreational habits. For example, the development of dyspnea in a trained runner upon running 2 mi may signify a more serious disturbance than a similar degree of breathlessness in a sedentary person upon running a fraction of this distance. Some patients with lung or heart disease may have such reduced capabilities due to other disease (e.g., peripheral vascular insufficiency or severe osteoarthritis of the hips or knees) that exertional dyspnea is precluded despite serious impairment of pulmonary or cardiac function.

Some patterns of dyspnea are not directly related to physical exertion. Sudden and unexpected dyspneic episodes at rest can be associated with pulmonary emboli, spontaneous pneumothorax, or anxiety. Nocturnal episodes of severe paroxysmal dyspnea are characteristic of left ventricular failure. Dyspnea upon assuming the supine posture, *orthopnea* (see below), thought to be mainly characteristic of congestive heart failure, may also occur in some patients with asthma and chronic obstruction of the airways and is a regular finding in the rare occurrence of bilateral diaphragmatic paralysis. *Trepopnea* is used to describe the unusual circumstance in which dyspnea occurs only in the left or right lateral decubitus position, most often in patients with heart disease, while *platypnea* is dyspnea which occurs only in the upright position. Both of these patterns remain to be fully explained but may be related to positional alterations in ventilation-perfusion relations (Chap. 200).

MECHANISMS OF DYSPNEA Physicians usually relate the symptom of dyspnea to a process such as obstruction of the airways or congestive heart failure and generally proceed with further diagnostic and/or therapeutic attempts, having satisfied themselves that they understand the mechanism of the dyspnea. In fact, elucidation of the *actual* mechanism(s) of dyspnea has eluded clinical investigators.

Dyspnea occurs whenever the work of breathing is excessive. Increased force generation is required of the respiratory muscles to produce a given volume change if the chest wall or lungs are less compliant or if resistance to airflow is increased. Increased work of breathing also occurs when the ventilation is excessive for the level of activity. Although an individual is more apt to become dyspneic when the work of breathing is increased, the work theory does not account for the perceptual difference between a deep breath with a normal mechanical load and a normal-sized breath with an increased mechanical load. The work might be the same with both breaths, but the normal one with the increased load will be associated with discomfort. In fact, with respiratory loading, such as adding a resistance at the mouth, there is an increase in respiratory center output, as gauged by newer indexes, that is disproportionate to the increase in work of breathing. Hence, a more appealing theory is one that links inappropriate length to tension in the respiratory muscles. Campbell has proposed that a sense of discomfort arises when there is misalignment of the nerve spindles, which are sensing tension, in relation to muscle length. This misalignment would lead to the sensation that a person is getting an insufficient breath for the tension generated by the respiratory muscles. Such a theory is difficult to test and, if tested and proved in some circumstances, would still not explain why patients who are completely paralyzed, either by cord transections or neuromuscular blockade, experience dyspnea although aided by a mechanical ventilator. It is probable, in these circumstances, that signals from the lungs and/or airways travel via the vagus nerve to the central nervous system to account for the sensation.

In all likelihood several different mechanisms operate to different degrees in the various clinical situations in which dyspnea occurs. Perhaps, in some circumstances, dyspnea is evoked by stimulation of receptors in the upper respiratory tract; in others it may originate from receptors in the lungs, airways, respiratory muscles, or some combination of those structures. In any event, dyspnea is characterized by an excessive or abnormal activation of the respiratory centers in the brainstem. This activation comes about from stimuli transmitted from or through a variety of structures and pathways including (1) intrathoracic receptors via the vagi; (2) afferent somatic nerves, particularly from the respiratory muscles and chest wall, but also from other skeletal muscles and joints; (3) chemoreceptors in the brain, aortic and carotid bodies, and elsewhere in the circulation; (4) higher (cortical) centers; and perhaps (5) afferent fibers in the phrenic nerves. In general, there is a reasonably good correlation between the severity of dyspnea and the disturbances of pulmonary or cardiac function which are responsible.

DIFFERENTIAL DIAGNOSIS **Obstructive disease of airways** (see also Chaps. 202 and 208) Obstruction to airflow can be present anywhere from the extrathoracic airways out to the small airways in the periphery of the lung. Large extrathoracic airway obstruction can occur acutely, as with aspiration of food or a foreign body or with angioneurotic edema of the glottis. Circumstantial evidence or testimony from witnesses should cause the physician to suspect aspiration, and an allergic history together with a few scattered hives should raise the possibility of glottic edema. The acute form of upper airway obstruction is a medical emergency. More chronic forms can occur with tumors or with fibrotic stenosis following tracheostomy or prolonged endotracheal intubation. Whether acute or chronic, the cardinal symptom is dyspnea, and the characteristic signs are stridor and retraction of the supraclavicular fossae with inspiration.

Obstruction of intrathoracic airways can occur acutely and intermittently or can be present chronically with worsening during respiratory infections. Acute intermittent obstruction with wheezing is typical of *asthma*. Chronic cough with expectoration is typical of *chronic bronchitis* and *bronchiectasis*. Most often there is a prolongation of expiration and coarse rhonchi which are generalized in chronic bronchitis and may be localized in the case of bronchiectasis. Intercurrent infection results in worsening of the cough, increased expectoration of purulent sputum, and more severe dyspnea. During such episodes the patient may complain of nocturnal paroxysms of dyspnea with wheezing relieved by cough and expectoration of sputum.

Many years of exertional dyspnea progressing to dyspnea at rest characterize the patient with predominant *emphysema* (Chap. 208). Although a parenchymal disease by definition, emphysema is invariably accompanied by obstruction of airways.

Diffuse parenchymal lung diseases (see also Chap. 209) This category includes a large number of diseases ranging from acute pneumonia to chronic disorders such as sarcoidosis and the various forms of *pneumoconiosis*. History, physical findings, and radiographic abnormalities often provide clues to the diagnosis. The patients are often tachypneic with arterial P_{CO_2} and P_{O_2} values below normal. Exertion often further reduces the arterial P_{O_2}. Lung volumes are decreased and the lungs are stiffer, i.e., less compliant than normal.

Pulmonary vascular occlusive diseases (see also Chap. 211) Repeated episodes of dyspnea at rest often occur with recurrent pulmonary emboli. A source for emboli, such as phlebitis of a lower extremity or the pelvis, is quite helpful in leading the physician to suspect the diagnosis. Arterial blood gases are almost invariably abnormal, but lung volumes are frequently normal or only minimally abnormal.

Diseases of the chest wall or respiratory muscles (see also Chap. 215) The physical examination establishes the presence of a chest wall disease such as severe kyphoscoliosis, pectus excavatum, or spondylitis. Although all three of these deformities may be associated with dyspnea, only severe kyphoscoliosis regularly interferes with ventilation sufficiently to produce chronic cor pulmonale and respiratory failure. Even though vital capacity, lung volumes, and airflow rates are normal with pectus excavatum, there is some evidence that cardiac compression from the posteriorly displaced sternum interferes with diastolic filling of the ventricle during the increased demands of exercise. Hence a cardiogenic component to the dyspnea may be present in this condition.

Both weakness and paralysis of respiratory muscles can lead to respiratory failure and dyspnea (Chap. 215), but most often the signs and symptoms of the neurologic or muscular disorder are more prominently manifested in other systems.

Heart disease In patients with cardiac disease exertional dyspnea occurs most commonly as a consequence of an elevated pulmonary capillary pressure; aside from uncommon causes such as obstructive disease of the pulmonary veins (Chap. 185), pulmonary capillary hypertension is a consequence of left atrial hypertension, which in turn may be due to left ventricular dysfunction (Chaps. 181 and 182), reduced left ventricular compliance, and mitral stenosis. The elevation of hydrostatic pressure in the pulmonary vascular bed tends to upset the Starling equilibrium (see "Pulmonary Edema," below) with resulting transudation of liquid into the interstitial space, reducing the compliance of the lungs and stimulating J (juxtacapillary) receptors in the alveolar interstitial space. When prolonged, pulmonary venous hypertension results in thickening of pulmonary vessels and an increase in perivascular cells and fibrous tissue, causing a further reduction in compliance. The competition for space between vessels, airways, and increased liquid within the interstitial space compromises the lumina of small airways, increasing the airways' resistance. Diminution in compliance and an increase in airways' resistance increase the work of breathing which, to some degree, is minimized by a reduction in tidal volume which is compensated for by an increase in frequency of respiration. In severe heart disease, usually involving elevation of both pulmonary and systemic venous pressures, hydrothorax may develop, further interfering with pulmonary function and intensifying dyspnea. In patients with heart failure and a severely diminished cardiac output, dyspnea may also be related to fatigue of the respiratory muscles as a consequence of their reduced perfusion. The metabolic acidosis characteristic of severe heart failure may play a contributory role. Dyspnea may also be associated with severe systemic and cerebral anoxia, as occurs during exertion in patients with congenital heart disease and right-to-left shunts.

Cardiac dyspnea usually begins as breathlessness on strenuous exertion and, over the course of months or years, progresses until the patient is dyspneic at rest. Occasionally, a nonproductive cough developing in the recumbent position, particularly at night, may be the first complaint.

Orthopnea, i.e., dyspnea in the recumbent position and *paroxysmal nocturnal dyspnea*, i.e., attacks of shortness of breath which usually occur at night and awaken the patient from sleep, are characteristic of more advanced forms of heart failure associated with elevations of pulmonary venous and capillary pressures and are discussed in Chap. 182. Orthopnea is the result of the alteration of gravitational forces when the recumbent position is assumed. This augmentation of intrathoracic blood volume elevates pulmonary venous and capillary pressures which increases the pulmonary closing volume (Chap. 200) and reduces the vital capacity. An additional factor associated with recumbency is the elevation of the diaphragm, which results in a lower end-expiratory lung volume. This combination of lower end-expiratory lung volume and increase in closing volume results in a significant alteration of alveolar-capillary gas exchange.

PAROXYSMAL (NOCTURNAL) DYSPNEA Also known as *cardiac asthma*, this condition is characterized by attacks of severe shortness of breath which generally occur at night and usually awaken the patient from sleep. The attack is precipitated by stimuli which aggravate the previously existing pulmonary congestion; frequently the total blood volume is augmented at night because of the reabsorption of edema from dependent portions of the body during recumbency; the redistribution of blood volume which takes place results in an increase in intrathoracic blood volume and therefore produces pulmonary congestion. A sleeping patient can tolerate relatively severe pulmonary engorgement and may awaken only when actual pulmonary edema and bronchospasm have developed, with the feeling of suffocation and with wheezing respirations.

CHEYNE-STOKES RESPIRATION See Chap. 182.

DIAGNOSIS The diagnosis of cardiac dyspnea depends on the recognition of heart disease on the basis of the history and physical examination. There may be a history of antecedent myocardial infarction, third and fourth heart sounds may be audible, and/or there may be evidence of left ventricular enlargement, jugular neck vein distention, and/or peripheral edema. Often there are radiographic signs of heart failure, with evidence of interstitial edema, pulmonary vascular redistribution, and accumulation of liquid in the septal planes and pleural cavity. Cardiomegaly is often present, but the overall heart size may be normal, particularly in patients with dyspnea due to acute myocardial infarction or mitral stenosis; an enlarged left atrium is usually evident in the latter condition. The electrocardiogram (Chap. 178) is rarely specific for heart disease and cannot specifically indicate whether a patient's dyspnea is caused by heart disease; however, it is rarely normal in patients with cardiac dyspnea.

Differentiation between cardiac and pulmonary dyspnea In most patients with dyspnea there is obvious clinical evidence of disease of either heart or lungs. The dyspnea of chronic obstructive lung disease tends to develop more gradually than that of heart diseases; exceptions, of course, occur in patients with obstructive lung disease who develop an episode of infectious bronchitis, pneumonia, or pneumothorax, or an exacerbation of asthma. Like patients with cardiac dyspnea, patients with chronic obstructive lung disease may also waken at night with dyspnea, but this is usually associated with sputum production; the dyspnea is relieved after these patients rid themselves of secretions.

The difficulty in the distinction between cardiac and pulmonary dyspnea may be compounded by the coexistence of diseases involving both organ systems. Patients with a history of chronic bronchitis or asthma who develop left ventricular failure tend to develop recurrences of bronchoconstriction and wheezing in association with bouts of paroxysmal nocturnal dyspnea and pulmonary edema. This condition, i.e., cardiac asthma, usually occurs in patients with overt clinical evidence of heart disease. Acute cardiac asthma is further differentiated from acute attacks of bronchial asthma by the presence of diaphoresis, more bubbly airway sounds, and the more common occurrence of cyanosis.

It is desirable to carry out pulmonary function testing in patients in whom the etiology of dyspnea is not clear, for these tests should be helpful in determining whether dyspnea is produced by heart disease, lung disease, abnormalities of the chest wall, or anxiety. In addition to the usual means of assessing patients for heart disease (Chap. 176), determination of the ejection fraction at rest and during exercise by radionuclide ventriculography (Chap. 179) is helpful in the differential diagnosis of dyspnea; the left ventricular ejection fraction is depressed in left ventricular failure while the right ventricular ejection fraction may be low at rest or may decline during exercise in patients with severe lung disease; both ejection fractions are normal both at rest and during exercise in dyspnea due to anxiety or malingering. Careful observation during the performance of an exercise treadmill test will often help in the identification of the patient who is malingering or whose dyspnea is secondary to anxiety. Under these circumstances the patient usually complains of severe shortness of breath but appears to be breathing either effortlessly or totally irregularly.

Anxiety neurosis Dyspnea experienced by someone with an anxiety neurosis is a difficult symptom to evaluate. The signs and symptoms of acute and chronic hyperventilation do not serve to distinguish between anxiety neurosis and other processes, such as recurrent pulmonary emboli. Another potentially confusing situation is seen when chest pain and electrocardiographic changes accompany the hyperventilation syndrome. When present and attributable to this condition, often referred to as *neurocirculatory asthenia* (Chap. 4), the chest pain is often sharp, fleeting, and in various loci, and the electrocardiographic changes are most often seen during repolarization; yet occasional ventricular ectopic activity can be seen as well. A rather extensive series of pulmonary and cardiac function tests, carried out both at rest and during exercise, may be needed to be certain that anxiety is, in fact, the cause of the dyspnea. Certain clues are helpful in leading one to suspect a psychogenic origin. Frequent sighing respirations and a bizarre, irregular breathing pattern are helpful. Often the breathing pattern returns to normal during sleep.

PULMONARY EDEMA

CARDIOGENIC PULMONARY EDEMA An increase in pulmonary venous pressure, which results initially in the engorgement of the pulmonary vasculature, is common in most instances of dyspnea in association with congestive heart failure. The lungs become less compliant, the resistance of small airways increases, and there is an increase in lymphatic flow which apparently serves to maintain a constant pulmonary extravascular liquid volume. At this early stage there is usually mild tachypnea, and if arterial blood gases are measured, the arterial P_{O_2} and P_{CO_2} are both lowered with an increase in the alveolar-to-arterial oxygen difference. Tachypnea itself, which might result from stimulation of receptors in the pulmonary interstitium, apparently increases lymphatic flow by augmenting ventilatory pumping of lymphatic vessels. The changes described are seen well in advance of auscultatory findings or radiographic signs pointing to congestive heart failure. If sufficient both in magnitude and duration, the increase in intravascular pressure results in a net gain of liquid in the extravascular space despite further increases in lymphatic flow. It is at this point that symptoms worsen, tachypnea increases, gas exchange deteriorates further, and radiographic changes, such as Kerley B lines and loss of distinct vascular margins, are seen. Even at this intermediate stage, the capillary endothelial intercellular junctions have been shown to widen and allow passage of macromolecules into the interstices. Up to and including this stage, the edema is purely *interstitial*. Sufficient further elevations in intravascular pressure result in disruption of the tighter junctions between alveolar lining cells, and alveolar edema ensues with outpouring of liquid, which contains both red blood cells and macromolecules. At this point *alveolar edema* is present. Although originally considered an early and subtle radiographic sign of interstitial edema, recent evidence suggests that an antigravity redistribution of pulmonary blood flow occurs only after the onset of alveolar edema. With yet more severe disruption of the alveolar-capillary membrane, edematous liquid floods the alveoli and airways. At this point, full-blown clinical pulmonary edema with bilateral wet rales and rhonchi will occur, and the chest radiograph may show diffuse haziness of the lung fields with greater density in the more proximal hilar regions. Typically, the patient is anxious and perspires freely, and the sputum is frothy and blood-tinged. Gas exchange is more severely compromised with worsening hypoxia and possibly hypercapnia. Without effective treatment (Chap. 182) progressive acidemia, hypoxia, and respiratory arrest ensue.

The earlier sequence of fluid accumulation described above follows the Starling law of capillary–interstitial fluid exchange:

$$\text{Fluid accumulation} = K[(P_c - P_{IF}) - \sigma(\pi_{pl} - \pi_{IF})] - Q_{lymph}$$

where K = permeability coefficient
P_c = mean intracapillary pressure
π_{IF} = oncotic pressure of interstitial fluid
σ = reflection coefficient of macromolecules
P_{IF} = mean interstitial liquid pressure
π_{pl} = oncotic pressure of the plasma
Q_{lymph} = lymphatic flow

The pressures tending to move liquid out of the vessel are P_c and π_{IF}, which are normally more than offset by pressures tending to move liquid back into the vasculature, i.e., the algebraic sum of P_{IF} and π_{pl}. Implicit in the above equation is that lymphatic flow can increase in the case of imbalance of forces and result in no net accumulation of interstitial fluid. However, in later sequences, with opening of first the endothelial and then the alveolar intercellular junctions, the permeability and reflection coefficients change strikingly. Thus, the initial process of hemodynamic pulmonary edema is one of liquid filtration and clearance. With further increasing pressures, disruption of both the structure and the function of the alveolar-capillary membrane occurs.

NONCARDIOGENIC PULMONARY EDEMA There are several clinical conditions which are associated with pulmonary edema based upon an imbalance of Starling forces other than through primary elevations of pulmonary capillary pressure. Although diminished plasma oncotic pressure in hypoalbuminemic states (e.g., severe liver disease, nephrotic syndrome, protein-losing enteropathy) might be expected to lead to pulmonary edema, the balance of forces normally so strongly favors resorption that even under these conditions some elevation of capillary pressure is necessary before interstitial edema develops. Increased negativity of interstitial pressure has been implicated in the genesis of unilateral pulmonary edema following rapid evacuation of a large pneumothorax. In this situation the findings are apparent only by radiography. It has been recently proposed that large negative intrapleural pressures during acute severe asthma may be associated with the development of interstitial edema. If this proposal can be supported by sufficient clinical data, then asthma would represent an additional example of edema due to increased negativity of interstitial pressure. Lymphatic blockade secondary to fibrotic and inflammatory diseases or lymphangitic carcinomatosis may lead to interstitial edema. In such instances both clinical and radiographic manifestations are dominated by the underlying disease process.

There are other conditions characterized by increases in the interstitial liquid content of the lungs which begin neither with an imbalance between intravascular and interstitial forces nor with alterations in lymphatics, but rather appear to be associated primarily with disruption of the alveolar-capillary membranes. Experimentally the prototype for such conditions is the pulmonary edema following alloxan administration. Any number of spontaneously occurring or environmental toxic insults, including diffuse pulmonary infections, aspiration, shock (particularly due to gram-negative septicemia and hemorrhagic pancreatitis, and following cardiopulmonary bypass), are associated with diffuse pulmonary edema which clearly does not have a hemodynamic origin. These conditions, which may lead to the adult respiratory distress syndrome, are discussed in Chap. 216.

Other forms of pulmonary edema There are three forms of pulmonary edema which have not been clearly related to increased permeability, inadequate lymphatic flow, or an imbalance of Starling forces; hence their precise mechanism remains unexplained. *Narcotic overdose* is a well-recognized antecedent to pulmonary edema. Although illicit use of parenteral heroin has been the most frequent cause, parenteral and oral overdoses of legitimate preparations of morphine, methadone, and dextropropoxyphene have also been associated with pulmonary edema. Thus the earlier idea that injected impurities lead to the disorder is untenable. Available evidence suggests that there are alterations in the permeability of alveolar and capillary membranes rather than elevation of pulmonary capillary pressure.

Exposure to high altitude in association with severe physical exertion is a well-recognized setting for pulmonary edema in unacclimatized, yet otherwise healthy, persons. Recent data show that acclimatized high-altitude natives also develop this syndrome upon return to high altitude after a relatively brief sojourn at low altitudes. The syndrome is far more common in persons under the age of 25 years. The mechanism for high-altitude pulmonary edema remains obscure, and studies have been conflicting, some suggesting pulmonary venous constriction and others indicating pulmonary arteriolar constriction as the prime mechanisms. A role for hypoxia at altitude is suggested by the fact that patients respond to the administration of oxygen and/or return to lower altitudes. Hypoxia per se does not alter permeability of the alveolar-capillary membrane. Hence, increased cardiac output and pulmonary arterial pressures with exercise combined with hypoxic pulmonary arteriolar constriction, which is more prominent in young persons, may combine to make this an example of prearteriolar, high-pressure pulmonary edema.

Neurogenic pulmonary edema has been suspected in patients with central nervous system disorders and without apparent preexisting left ventricular dysfunction. Although most experimental equivalents have implicated sympathetic nervous system activity, the mechanism whereby sympathetic efferent activity leads to pulmonary edema is a matter of speculation. It is known that a massive adrenergic discharge leads to peripheral vasoconstriction with elevation of blood pressure and shifts of blood to the central circulation. In addition, it is probable that a decrease in left ventricular compliance also occurs, and both factors serve to increase left atrial pressures sufficiently to induce pulmonary edema on a hemodynamic basis. Recent experimental evidence suggests that stimulation of adrenergic receptors increases capillary permeability directly, but this effect is relatively minor as compared to the imbalance of Starling forces.

TREATMENT OF PULMONARY EDEMA See Chap. 182.

REFERENCES

AYRES SM: Mechanism and consequences of pulmonary edema: Cardiac lung, shock lung, and principles of ventilatory therapy in adult respiratory distress syndrome. Am Heart J 103:97, 1982

FISHMAN AP, RENKIN EM (eds): *Pulmonary Edema*. Washington, DC, American Physiological Society, 1979

INGRAM RH JR, BRAUNWALD E: Pulmonary edema: Cardiogenic and noncardiogenic, in *Heart Disease*, E. Braunwald (ed). Philadelphia, Saunders, 1984, p 560

KILLIAN KJ, CAMPBELL EJM: Dyspnea and exercise. Ann Rev Physiol 45:465, 1983

MALIK AB: Mechanisms of neurogenic pulmonary edema. Circ Res 57:1, 1985

MCFADDEN ER, INGRAM RH JR: Relationship between diseases of the heart and lungs, in *Heart Disease*, E Braunwald (ed). Philadelphia, Saunders, 1984, p 1782

RASANEN J et al: Continuous positive airway pressure by face mask in acute cardiogenic pulmonary edema. Am J Cardiol 55:296, 1985

ROUSSOS C, MACKLEM PT: Disorders of the respiratory muscle function, in *Update III: Harrison's Principles of Internal Medicine*, KJ Isselbacher et al (eds). New York, McGraw-Hill, 1982, p 83

SCHOENE RB et al: High altitude pulmonary edema and exercise at 4400 meters on Mount McKinley: Effect of expiratory positive airway pressure. Chest 87:330, 1985

SNIDERMAN A et al: Pulmonary blood flow: A potential factor in the pathogenesis of pulmonary edema. J Thorac Cardiovasc Surg 87:130, 1984

SPRUNG CL et al: The spectrum of pulmonary edema: Differentiation of cardiogenic, intermediate, and noncardiogenic forms of pulmonary edema. Am Rev Resp Dis 124:718, 1981

STAUB NC: The pathogenesis of pulmonary edema. Prog Cardiovasc Dis 23:53, 1980

ZEMA MJ et al: Dyspnea: The heart or the lungs? Differentiation at bedside by use of the simple valsalva maneuver. Chest 85:59, 1984

27 CYANOSIS, HYPOXIA, AND POLYCYTHEMIA

EUGENE BRAUNWALD

CYANOSIS

Cyanosis refers to a bluish color of the skin and mucous membranes resulting from an increased amount of reduced hemoglobin, or of hemoglobin derivatives, in the small blood vessels of those areas. It is usually most marked in the lips, nail beds, ears, and malar eminences. The "red cyanosis" of polycythemia vera (Chap. 289) must be distinguished from the true cyanosis discussed here. A cherry-colored flush, rather than cyanosis, is caused by carboxyhemoglobin (Chap. 171). The degree of cyanosis is modified by the quality of cutaneous pigment, the color of the blood plasma, and the thickness of the skin, as well as by the state of the cutaneous capillaries. The accurate clinical detection of the presence and degree of cyanosis is difficult, as proved by oximetric studies. In some instances central cyanosis can be reliably detected when the arterial saturation has fallen to 85 percent; in others it may not be detected until the saturation has reached 75 percent.

The increase in the quantity of reduced hemoglobin in the cutaneous vessels which produces cyanosis may be brought about either by an increase in the quantity of venous blood in the skin as the result of dilatation of the venules and venous ends of the capillaries, or by a decrease in the oxygen saturation in the capillary blood. In general, cyanosis becomes apparent when the mean capillary concentration of reduced hemoglobin exceeds 5 g/dL. It is the *absolute* rather than the *relative* amount of reduced hemoglobin which is important in producing cyanosis. Thus, in a patient with severe anemia the relative amount of reduced hemoglobin in the venous blood may be very large when considered in relation to the total amount of hemoglobin. However, since the latter is markedly lowered, the absolute amount of reduced hemoglobin may still be small, and therefore patients with severe anemia and even marked arterial desaturation do not display cyanosis. Conversely, the higher the total hemoglobin content, the greater the tendency toward cyanosis; thus, patients with marked polycythemia tend to be cyanotic at higher levels of arterial oxygen saturation than patients with normal hematocrit values. Likewise, local passive congestion, which causes an increase in the total amount of reduced hemoglobin in the vessels in a given area, may cause cyanosis. Cyanosis also is observed when nonfunctional hemoglobin is present in the blood; as little as 1.5 g/dL methemoglobin or 0.5 g sulfhemoglobin is sufficient to produce cyanosis.

Cyanosis may be subdivided into *central* and *peripheral* categories. In the *central* type, there is arterial blood unsaturation or an abnormal hemoglobin derivative, and the mucous membranes and skin are both affected. *Peripheral* cyanosis is due to a slowing of blood flow to an area and abnormally great extraction of oxygen from normally saturated arterial blood. It results from vasoconstriction and diminished peripheral blood flow, such as occurs in cold exposure, shock, congestive failure, and peripheral vascular disease. Often, in these conditions the mucous membranes of the oral cavity or those beneath the tongue may be spared. Clinical differentiation between central and peripheral cyanosis may not always be simple, and in conditions such as cardiogenic shock with pulmonary edema there may be a mixture of both types.

DIFFERENTIAL DIAGNOSIS (See Table 27-1) **Central cyanosis** Decreased arterial oxygen saturation results from a marked reduction in the oxygen tension in the arterial blood. This may be brought about by a decline in the tension of oxygen in the inspired air without sufficient compensatory alveolar hyperventilation to maintain alveolar oxygen tension. Cyanosis does not occur in a significant degree in an ascent to an altitude of 8000 ft but is marked in a further ascent to 16,000 ft. The reason for this becomes clear on studying the *S* shape of the oxygen dissociation curve (Fig. 283-4). At 8000 ft the tension of oxygen in the inspired air is about 120 mmHg, the alveolar tension is approximately 80 mmHg, and the hemoglobin is nearly completely saturated. However, at 16,000 ft the oxygen tensions in atmospheric air and alveolar air are about 85 and 50 mmHg, respectively, and the oxygen dissociation curve shows that the arterial blood is only about 75 percent saturated. This leaves 25 percent of the hemoglobin in the reduced form, an amount likely to be associated with cyanosis in the absence of anemia. Similarly, a mutant hemoglobin with a low affinity for oxygen (Hb Kansas) causes lowered arterial oxygen saturation and resultant central cyanosis (Chap. 288).

Seriously *impaired pulmonary function,* through alveolar hypoventilation or perfusion of unventilated or poorly ventilated areas of the lung, is a common cause of central cyanosis (Chap. 200). This may occur acutely, as in extensive pneumonia or pulmonary edema, or with chronic pulmonary diseases (e.g., emphysema). In the last situation polycythemia is generally present and clubbing of the fingers may occur. However, in many types of chronic pulmonary disease

TABLE 27-1 Causes of cyanosis

I Central cyanosis
- *A* Decreased arterial oxygen saturation
  - *1* Decreased atmospheric pressure—high altitude
  - *2* Impaired pulmonary function
    - *a* Alveolar hypoventilation
    - *b* Uneven relationships between pulmonary ventilation and perfusion
    - *c* Impaired oxygen diffusion
  - *3* Anatomic shunts
    - *a* Certain types of congenital heart disease
    - *b* Pulmonary arteriovenous fistulas
    - *c* Multiple small intrapulmonary shunts
  - *4* Hemoglobin with low affinity for oxygen
- *B* Hemoglobin abnormalities
  - *1* Methemoglobinemia—hereditary, acquired
  - *2* Sulfhemoglobinema—acquired
  - *3* Carboxyhemoglobinemia (not true cyanosis)

II Peripheral cyanosis
- *A* Reduced cardiac output
- *B* Cold exposure
- *C* Redistribution of blood flow from extremities
- *D* Arterial obstruction
- *E* Venous obstruction

with fibrosis and obliteration of the capillary vascular bed, cyanosis does not occur because there is relatively little perfusion of underventilated areas.

Another cause of decreased arterial oxygen saturation is *shunting of systemic venous blood into the arterial circuit.* Certain forms of congenital heart disease are associated with cyanosis (Chap. 185). Since blood normally flows from a high-pressure to a low-pressure region, in order for a cardiac defect to result in a right-to-left shunt, it must ordinarily be combined with an obstructive lesion distal to the defect or with elevated pulmonary vascular resistance. The commonest congenital cardiac lesion associated with cyanosis in the adult is the combination of ventricular septal defect and pulmonary outflow tract obstruction (tetralogy of Fallot). The more severe the obstruction, the greater the degree of right-to-left shunting and resultant cyanosis. The mechanisms for the elevated pulmonary vascular resistance which may produce cyanosis in the presence of intra- and extracardiac communications without pulmonic stenosis are discussed elsewhere (Chap. 185). In patients with patent ductus arteriosus, pulmonary hypertension, and right-to-left shunt, *differential cyanosis* results; i.e., cyanosis occurs in the lower extremities but not in the upper extremities.

Pulmonary arteriovenous fistulas may be congenital or acquired, solitary or multiple, microscopic or massive. The degree of cyanosis produced by these fistulas depends upon their size and number. They occur with some frequency in hereditary hemorrhagic telangiectasia (Chap. 280). Arterial oxygen unsaturation also occurs in some patients with cirrhosis, presumably as a consequence of pulmonary arteriovenous fistulas or portal vein–pulmonary vein anastomoses.

In patients with cardiac or pulmonary right-to-left shunts, the presence and severity of cyanosis depend on the size of the shunt relative to the systemic flow as well as on the oxyhemoglobin saturation of the venous blood. In patients with central cyanosis due to arterial oxygen unsaturation, the severity of cyanosis increases with exercise. With increased extraction of oxygen from the blood by the exercising muscles, the venous blood returning to the right side of the heart is more unsaturated than at rest, and shunting of this blood or its passage through lungs incapable of normal oxygenation intensifies the cyanosis. Also, since the systemic vascular resistance normally decreases with exercise, the right-to-left shunt is augmented by exercise in patients with congenital heart disease and communications between the two sides of the heart. Secondary polycythemia occurs frequently in patients with arterial unsaturation and contributes to the cyanosis.

Cyanosis can be caused by small amounts of circulating methemoglobin and by even smaller amounts of sulfhemoglobin (Chap. 288). Although they are uncommon causes of cyanosis, these abnormal hemoglobin pigments should be sought by spectroscopy when cyanosis is not readily explained by malfunction of the circulatory or respiratory systems. Generally, clubbing does not occur with them. The diagnosis of methemoglobinemia can be suspected, if, on mixing the patient's blood in a test tube and exposing it to air, it remains brown.

Peripheral cyanosis Probably the most common cause of peripheral cyanosis is generalized vasoconstriction resulting from exposure to cold air or water. This is a normal response. When cardiac output is low, as in severe congestive heart failure or shock, cutaneous vasoconstriction occurs as a compensatory mechanism, so that blood is diverted to more vital areas [central nervous system, heart (Chap. 182)], and intense cyanosis associated with cool extremities may result. Even though the arterial blood is normally saturated, the reduced volume flow through the skin and the reduced oxygen tension at the venous end of the capillary result in cyanosis.

Arterial obstruction to an extremity, as with an embolus, or arteriolar constriction, as in cold-induced vasospasm (Raynaud's phenomenon, Chap. 198), generally results in pallor and coldness, but there may be associated slight cyanosis. If there is venous obstruction, the extremity is usually congested and also cyanotic, and there is true stagnation of blood flow. Venous hypertension, which may be local (as in thrombophlebitis) or generalized (as in tricuspid valve disease or constrictive pericarditis), dilates the subpapillary venous plexuses and intensifies cyanosis.

APPROACH TO THE PATIENT WITH CYANOSIS Certain features are important in arriving at the proper cause of cyanosis:

1 The history, particularly the duration (cyanosis present since birth is usually due to congenital heart disease); possible exposure to drugs or chemicals which may produce abnormal types of hemoglobin.
2 Clinical differentiation of central as opposed to peripheral cyanosis. Objective evidence by physical or radiographic examination of disorders of the respiratory or cardiovascular systems. Massage or gentle warming of a cyanotic extremity will increase peripheral blood flow and abolish peripheral but not central cyanosis.
3 The presence or absence of clubbing of the fingers. Clubbing without cyanosis is frequent in patients with infective endocarditis and in association with ulcerative colitis, it may occasionally occur in healthy persons, and in some instances it may be occupational, e.g., in jackhammer operators. Slight cyanosis of the lips and cheeks, without clubbing of the fingers, is common in patients with well-compensated mitral stenosis and is probably due to minimal arterial hypoxia resulting from fibrotic changes in the lungs secondary to long-standing congestion combined with reduction of cardiac output (Chap. 187). The combination of cyanosis and clubbing is frequent in many patients with certain types of congenital cardiac disease and is seen occasionally in persons with pulmonary disease such as lung abscess or pulmonary arteriovenous shunts. On the other hand, peripheral cyanosis or acutely developing central cyanosis is not associated with clubbed fingers.
4 Determination of arterial blood oxygen tension or oxygen saturation, spectroscopic and other examinations of the blood for abnormal types of hemoglobin.

CLUBBING Clubbing is the selective bullous enlargement of the distal segment of a digit due to an increase in soft tissue. It may be hereditary or idiopathic, or acquired and associated with a variety of disorders, including cyanotic heart disease, infective endocarditis, and a variety of pulmonary conditions (among them, primary and metastatic lung cancer, bronchiectasis, lung abscess, and mesothelioma), as well as with some gastrointestinal diseases (including regional enteritis, chronic ulcerative colitis, and hepatic cirrhosis). Primary lung cancer, mesothelioma, neurogenic diaphragmatic tumors, and rarely cyanotic congenital heart disease may be associated with hypertrophic osteoarthropathy, the subperiosteal formation of new bone in the distal diaphyses of the long bones of the extremities. Although the mechanism of clubbing is unclear, it appears to be secondary to a (presumably humoral) substance, which causes dilation of the vessels of the fingertip.

HYPOXIA

The fundamental purpose of the cardiorespiratory system is to deliver oxygen (and substrates) to the cells and to remove carbon dioxide (and other metabolic products) from them. Proper maintenance of this function depends on intact cardiovascular and respiratory systems and a supply of inspired gas containing adequate oxygen. Changes in oxygen and in carbon dioxide tension as well as changes in the intraerythrocytic concentration of certain *organic phosphate compounds,* especially 2,3-diphosphoglyceric acid (2,3-DPG), cause shifts in the oxygen dissociation curve. These are discussed in detail in Chap. 283 and are illustrated in Fig. 283-4. When hypoxia results as a consequence of respiratory failure, arterial P_{CO_2} usually rises (Chaps. 208 and 216), and the oxygen dissociation curve tends to be displaced to the right. Under these conditions the percentage saturation of the hemoglobin in the arterial blood at a given level of alveolar oxygen tension declines. Thus arterial hypoxia and cyanosis are likely to be more marked in proportion to the degree of depression of alveolar oxygen tension when such depression results from pulmonary disease than when the depression occurs as the result of a decline in the partial pressure of oxygen in the inspired air, in which case arterial P_{CO_2} falls and the oxygen dissociation curve is displaced to the left.

DIFFERENTIAL DIAGNOSIS Anemic hypoxia Any decrease in hemoglobin concentration is attended by a corresponding decline in the oxygen-carrying capacity. The P_{O_2} in the arterial blood remains normal, but the absolute amount of oxygen transported per unit volume of blood is diminished. As the anemic blood passes through the capillaries, and the usual amount of oxygen is removed from it, the P_{O_2} in the venous blood declines to a greater degree than would normally be the case.

Circulatory hypoxia As in anemic hypoxia, arterial P_{O_2} is normal, but venous and tissue P_{O_2} are reduced as a consequence of reduced tissue perfusion in the face of normal tissue oxygen consumption. For this reason the term *stagnant hypoxia* may be used for this condition. Generalized circulatory hypoxia occurs in heart failure (Chap. 182), and in most forms of shock (Chap. 29).

Specific organ hypoxia Decreased circulation to a specific organ resulting in localized stagnant hypoxia may be due to organic arterial or venous obstruction or may occur as a consequence of vasoconstriction. The latter may occur in the upper extremities in Raynaud's phenomenon. Reduced circulation may occur in all limbs in patients with heart failure or hypovolemic shock in an attempt to maintain adequate perfusion to more vital organs. When organic arterial obliterative disease develops, ischemic hypoxia results, with accompanying pallor. Localized hypoxia may also result from venous obstruction which results in congestion. Edema, which increases the distance through which oxygen diffuses before it reaches the cells, can also cause localized hypoxia.

Increased oxygen requirements Even if oxygen diffusion into blood perfusing the pulmonary capillary bed is unhampered and the hemoglobin is qualitatively and quantitatively normal, the P_{O_2} in venous blood (hence, capillary and tissue P_{O_2}) may be reduced if the oxygen consumption of the tissues is elevated without a corresponding increase in volume flow per unit of time. Such a situation may be encountered when fever or thyrotoxicosis occurs in patients in whom the cardiac output cannot rise normally. Under such conditions the circulation may be considered deficient relative to the metabolic requirements.

Ordinarily, the clinical picture of patients with hypoxia due to an elevated basal metabolic rate is quite different from that in other types of hypoxia; the skin is warm and flushed, owing to increased cutaneous blood flow which dissipates the excessive heat produced, and cyanosis is absent in these patients.

Exercise is a classic example of increased tissue oxygen requirements. The increased demands are normally met by several mechanisms: (1) increasing the cardiac output and ventilation and thus oxygen delivery to the tissues; (2) preferentially directing the blood to the exercising muscles and away from resting muscles (by changing vascular resistances in various circulatory beds, directly and/or reflexly); (3) increasing oxygen extraction from the delivered blood and widening the arteriovenous oxygen differences; (4) reducing the pH of the tissues and capillary blood, thereby unloading more oxygen from hemoglobin. If the capacity of these mechanisms is exceeded, then hypoxia, especially of the exercising muscles, will result.

Carbon monoxide intoxication (Chap. 171) This condition is analogous to anemic hypoxia in that the hemoglobin which is combined with the carbon monoxide (carboxyhemoglobin) is unavailable for oxygen transport. In addition, the presence of carboxyhemoglobin shifts the dissociation curve of hemoglobin to the left, so that the oxygen can be unloaded only at lower tensions. By such formation of carboxyhemoglobin a given degree of reduction in oxygen-carrying power produces a far greater degree of tissue hypoxia than the equivalent reduction in hemoglobin due to simple anemia.

Improper oxygen utilization Cyanide (Chap. 171) and several other similarly acting poisons cause a paradoxic state in which the tissues are unable to utilize oxygen and as a consequence the venous blood tends to have a high oxygen tension. This condition has been termed *histotoxic hypoxia*. Cyanide produces cellular hypoxia by paralyzing the electron-transfer function of cytochrome oxidase so that it cannot pass electrons to oxygen, whereas diphtheria toxin is believed to inhibit the synthesis of one of the cytochromes and thus interfere with oxygen consumption and energy production by the cells involved.

EFFECTS OF HYPOXIA Changes in the central nervous system, particularly the higher centers, are especially important. Acute hypoxia produces impaired judgment, motor incoordination, and a clinical picture closely resembling that of acute alcoholism. When hypoxia is long-standing, the symptoms consist of fatigue, drowsiness, apathy, inattentiveness, delayed reaction time, and reduced work capacity. As hypoxia becomes more severe, the centers of the brainstem are affected, and death usually results from respiratory failure. With reduction of arterial oxygen tension, cerebrovascular resistance decreases and cerebral blood flow increases, which tends to reduce the cerebral hypoxia. On the other hand when the reduction of arterial P_{O_2} is accompanied by hyperventilation and diminution of P_{CO_2}, cerebrovascular resistance rises, blood flow falls, and hypoxia is enhanced. Compared with the brain, the phylogenetically older spinal cord and peripheral nerves are relatively insensitive to hypoxia. Hypoxia also causes pulmonary arterial constriction, which serves the useful function of shunting blood away from poorly ventilated areas toward better-ventilated portions of the lung. However, it has the disadvantage of causing increased pulmonary vascular resistance and an increased burden on the right ventricle.

A complex disturbance of cellular functions results from the metabolic effects of severe acute hypoxia. In liver and muscles the breakdown of the primary foodstuff, carbohydrate, normally proceeds anaerobically (i.e., without oxidation) to the stage of formation of pyruvic acid. The breakdown of pyruvate requires oxygen, and when this is deficient, increasing proportions of pyruvate are reduced to lactic acid, which cannot be broken down further (Chap. 328). Hence, there is an increase in the blood lactate, with decrease in bicarbonate and a corresponding acidosis. Under these circumstances the total energy obtained from foodstuff breakdown is greatly reduced, and the amount of energy available for continuing resynthesis of energy-rich phosphate compounds becomes inadequate, leading to a complex disturbance of cellular function.

Most of the useful respiratory response to hypoxia originates in special chemosensitive cells in the carotid and aortic bodies, although the respiratory center is also stimulated directly by oxygen lack. The resultant increase in ventilation, with loss of carbon dioxide, leads to respiratory alkalosis. On the other hand, the diffusion of additional quantities of lactic acid from the tissues into the blood tends to produce metabolic acidosis. In either case the total amount of bicarbonate, and hence the carbon dioxide–combining power, tends to be diminished.

Diminished oxygen tension in any tissue results in local vasodilatation, and the diffuse vasodilatation which occurs in generalized hypoxia causes an elevation of total cardiac output (Fig. 283-5). In patients with preexisting heart disease, particularly coronary artery disease, the combination of hypoxia and the requirements of the peripheral tissues for an increase of cardiac output may precipitate congestive heart failure. Prolonged or severe hypoxia may also impair hepatic and renal function.

One of the important mechanisms of compensation for prolonged hypoxia is an increase in the quantity of hemoglobin in the blood (Fig. 283-5). This is due not to direct stimulation of the bone marrow but to the effect of erythropoietin, which originates primarily in the kidneys. Assayable levels of erythropoietin are increased by hypoxia, and its production has been found to be regulated by the balance between tissue oxygen supply and demand.

TABLE 27-2 Differential diagnosis of erythrocytosis

ABSOLUTE (↑ RED CELL MASS)

I Autonomous erythroid proliferation (↓ EP*); polycythemia vera
II Secondary erythroid proliferation
- *A* Autonomous or inappropriate increase in EP
  - *1* Neoplasm
  - *2* Renal lesions
  - *3* Familial erythrocytosis (autosomal recessive inheritance)
- *B* Secondary increase in EP
  - *1* Hypoxia (↓ arterial P_{O_2})
    - *a* High altitude
    - *b* Alveolar hypoventilation
    - *c* Pulmonary disease
    - *d* Cardiac right-to-left shunt
  - *2* Abnormal hemoglobin function (normal arterial P_{O_2})
    - *a* High-affinity variants (autosomal dominant inheritance)
    - *b* Congenital methemoglobinemia
    - *c* Carboxyhemoglobin (smokers')
- *C* Hormonal stimulus to erythropoiesis
  - *1* Cushing's syndrome
  - *2* Androgen or corticosteroid administration

RELATIVE (REDUCED PLASMA VOLUME, NORMAL RED CELL MASS)

I Dehydration
II Stress erythrocytosis

* *Erythropoietin.*
SOURCE: *Adapted from HF Bunn et al, Human Hemoglobins, Philadelphia, Saunders, 1977.*

POLYCYTHEMIA (See also Chap. 289)

The term *polycythemia* signifies an increase above the normal in the number of red blood cells in the circulating blood. This increase is usually, though not always, accompanied by a corresponding increase in the quantity of hemoglobin and in the hematocrit. The increase may or may not be associated with an increase in the total quantity of red blood cells in the body. It is important to distinguish between *absolute* polycythemia (an increase in the total red cell mass) and *relative* polycythemia, which occurs when, through loss of blood plasma, the concentration of the red cells becomes greater than normal in the circulating blood. This may be the consequence of abnormally lowered fluid intake, of the loss of plasma into the interstitial fluid, or of the marked loss of body fluids, such as occurs in persistent vomiting, severe diarrhea, copious sweating, or acidosis.

Because the term polycythemia is used loosely to refer to all varieties of increase in the number of red corpuscles, the terms *erythrocytosis* and *erythremia* are preferred in referring to two forms of *absolute* polycythemia. Erythrocytosis denotes absolute polycythemia which occurs in response to some known stimulus (secondary polycythemia); erythremia (polycythemia vera) refers to the disease of unknown etiology (Chap. 289). An approach to the differential diagnosis of erythrocytosis should begin with a consideration of its mechanisms (Table 27-2). Erythrocytosis develops as a consequence of a variety of factors and represents a physiologic response to conditions of hypoxia.

FIGURE 27-1 *Relationship between mean arterial oxygen saturation (percent) and the mean hemoglobin content (grams per deciliter) in healthy male residents at various altitudes. (From Hurtado, by permission of Annals of Internal Medicine.)*

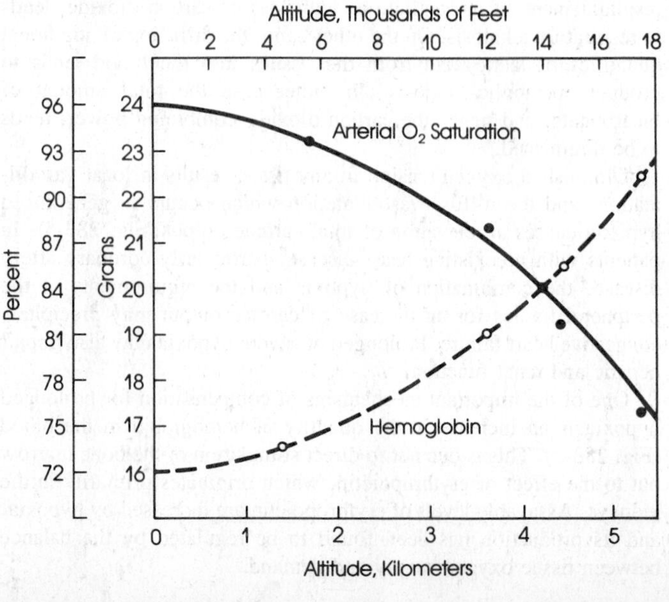

Sojourn at high altitudes leads to defective saturation of arterial blood with oxygen and stimulates the production of more red cells. The oxygen saturation, rather than oxygen tension, appears to be the more important determinant of the erythropoietic response to chronic hypoxia (Fig. 27-1). A disorder may set in insidiously after several years of continued residence at high altitudes, leading to the development of a condition known as *chronic mountain sickness* or *seroche* (Monge's disease), which appears to be caused by the development of alveolar hypoventilation superimposed on a lowered inspired O_2 concentration. Prominent manifestations are a florid color which turns to cyanosis on mild exertion, mental torpor, fatigue, and headache. Those affected are usually in the fourth to sixth decades. Return to sea level promptly relieves the symptoms. Living at high altitudes also evokes a number of compensatory reactions which act to increase oxygen delivery to the tissues. These include hyperventilation, which reduces the oxygen gradient between ambient and alveolar air, an augmentation of pulmonary capillary blood volume, an increase of diffusing capacity, and an increase in cardiac output.

Any pulmonary disease which produces chronic hypoxia may lead to erythrocytosis. The increased blood viscosity secondary to the polycythemia elevates pulmonary arterial pressure and, combined with the elevation of pulmonary vascular resistance resulting from hypoxia, further elevates right ventricular pressure, contributing to the development or intensification of cor pulmonale (Chap. 191). The *abnormal ventilatory conditions* present in very obese individuals may cause alveolar hypoventilation and result in arterial unsaturation, erythrocytosis, hypercapnia, and somnolence (the Pickwickian syndrome, Chap. 215). This syndrome is observed less commonly in nonobese persons (sleep-apnea syndrome), in whom decreased sensitivity of the respiratory center to CO_2 may play a role (Chap. 215).

The partial shunting of blood from the pulmonary circuit, such as occurs in *congenital heart disease,* causes the most striking erythrocytosis resulting from abnormalities in the heart or lungs (Chap. 185). Erythrocyte counts as high as 13 million per cubic millimeter, which are possible only when the red corpuscles are smaller than normal, have been observed in such patients, with volumes of packed red blood cells even as high as 86 mL/dL of blood. As the polycythemia develops, there is a progressive rise in blood viscosity, which begins to rise logarithmically when the volume of packed red blood cells exceeds 55 percent. The commonest defects producing such polycythemia in the adult are tetralogy of Fallot and Eisenmenger's complex. Other conditions include transposition of the great arteries, tricuspid atresia, and persistent truncus arteriosus. The polycythemia of cyanotic congenital heart disease may lead to spontaneous thrombosis at any site, including the central nervous system. The increase in hematocrit and the sharp increase in viscosity which occur when these patients become dehydrated are particularly hazardous. This condition may also be accompanied by a variety of blood coagulation defects, including reduced fibrinogen and prothrombin concentrations, as well as thrombocytopenia. Reduction in red blood cell volume (phlebotomy with reinfusion of the plasma) is sometimes performed in severely symptomatic patients with extremely high hematocrit levels, but it must be carried out slowly and with caution. It results in a reduction of the elevated blood viscosity which improves blood flow.

The excessive use of coal-tar derivatives and other forms of chronic poisoning, by producing abnormal hemoglobin pigments such as *methemoglobin* and *sulfhemoglobin* (Chap. 288), also may cause erythrocytosis. Patients with abnormal hemoglobins which displace the oxygen dissociation curve to the left and interfere with oxygen unloading in the tissues stimulate the production of erythropoietin and a secondary erythrocytosis unassociated with leukocytosis or thrombocytosis (Chap. 288).

Mild erythrocytosis is sometimes found in *Cushing's syndrome* and can be produced by the administration of large amounts of adrenocortical steroids. Androgens also exert an erythropoietic effect and when administered to normal individuals can produce erythrocytosis. Especially intriguing are the instances of erythrocytosis observed in association with various *tumors* which produce erythropoietin or an erythropoietin-like substance. These have been chiefly of two varieties, *infratentorial* and *renal*. The tumors in the posterior fossa have usually been vascular (hemangioblastomas). The renal tumors have included hypernephroma, adenoma, and sarcoma. Other tumors that have been associated with erythrocytosis include uterine myoma, hepatic carcinoma, and pheochromocytoma. Erythrocytosis also has been reported in association with solitary and polycystic disease of the kidneys, with hydronephrosis, and with renal artery stenosis. However, only a small proportion of the various renal disorders mentioned above have been associated with polycythemia. Plasma erythropoietin levels have been found to be elevated in a number of these patients. Erythropoietin-like activity has been demonstrated in tumor extracts and in renal cyst fluid, and erythrocytosis has disappeared after the associated tumor was removed.

The term *stress erythrocytosis* has been applied to the polycythemia seen occasionally in very active, hard-working, middle-aged white males who are typically hypertensive and overweight and in a state of anxiety, who appear florid but who have none of the other characteristic signs of polycythemia vera—no splenomegaly or leukocytosis with immature cells in the blood. In such persons the total red blood cell mass is normal, and the plasma volume is below normal. Thus, they have an elevated hematocrit and *relative* polycythemia. *Smokers' polycythemia* is a closely related condition, but the high carboxyhemoglobin concentration may cause a small absolute increase in red cell mass which is often asssociated with a reduced plasma volume.

The *clinical features* of polycythemia include, in addition to the symptoms of the underlying condition (in the secondary forms), a characteristic "ruddy" cyanosis, dizziness, headache, epistaxes, and an increased incidence of thrombotic complications.

The *differential diagnosis* of absolute polycythemia is discussed in Chap. 289. In polycythemia vera, erythropoietin levels are usually absent, leukocyte alkaline phosphatase and vitamin B_{12} levels and platelet and total white blood cells are usually elevated, and splenomegaly is common; the bone marrow shows hyperplasia of all elements. In secondary polycythemia with hypoxia, arterial P_{CO_2} is reduced, erythropoietin levels are elevated, while levels of leukocyte alkaline phosphatase, serum vitamin B_{12}, platelet, total white blood cell, and differential counts are all normal, and the liver and spleen are not enlarged; the bone marrow shows only erythroid hyperplasia. In the absence of features of either polycythemia vera or polycythemia secondary to hypoxia or to a tumor, a hemoglobin with a high affinity for oxygen should be sought for.

REFERENCES

DOLL DC, GREENBERG BR: Cerebral thrombosis in smokers' polycythemia. Ann Intern Med 102:786, 1985

ERSLEV AJ: Erythrocytosis (sec 17, Chaps 73–75), in *Hematology*, 3d ed, WJ Williams (ed). New York, McGraw-Hill, 1983, p 673.

HURTADO A: Some clinical aspects of life at high altitudes. Ann Intern Med 53:247, 1960

LANKEN PN, FISHMAN AP: Clubbing and hypertrophic osteoarthropathy, in *Pulmonary Diseases and Disorders*, AP Fishman (ed). New York, McGraw-Hill, 1980, p 84

LUPINETTI FM et al: Pathophysiology of chronic cyanosis in a canine model. Functional and metabolic response to global ischemia. J Thorac Cardiovasc Surg 90:291, 1985

ROSENTHAL A, TYLER DC: Effect of red cell volume reduction or pulmonary blood flow in polycythemia of cyanotic congenital heart disease. Am J Cardiol 33:410, 1974

SMITH JR, LANDAW SA: Smokers' polycythemia. N Engl J Med 298:6, 1978

28 EDEMA

EUGENE BRAUNWALD

Edema is defined as an increase in the extravascular (interstitial) component of the extracellular fluid volume, which may expand by several liters before the abnormality is recognized. Therefore, a weight gain of several kilograms usually precedes overt manifestations of edema, and a similar weight loss from diuresis can be induced in a slightly edematous patient before "dry weight" is achieved. *Ascites* (Chap. 39) and *hydrothorax* refer to accumulation of excess fluid in the peritoneal and pleural cavities, respectively, and are considered to be special forms of edema. *Anasarca* refers to gross, generalized edema. Depending on its etiology and mechanism, edema may be localized or have a generalized distribution; it is recognized in its generalized form by puffiness of the face, which is most readily apparent in the periorbital areas, and by the persistence of an indentation of the skin following pressure; this is known as "pitting" edema. In its more subtle form, it may be detected by the fact that the rim of the bell of the stethoscope leaves an indentation on the skin of the chest that lasts a few minutes. One of the early symptoms a patient may note is the ring on a finger fitting more snugly than in the past, or difficulty in putting on shoes, particularly in the evening.

PATHOGENESIS (See also Chap. 41) About one-third of the total body water is confined to the extracellular space. This compartment, in turn, is composed of the plasma volume and the interstitial space. Under ordinary circumstances the plasma volume represents about 25 percent of the extracellular space, and the remainder is interstitial fluid. The forces that regulate the disposition of fluid between these two components of the extracellular compartment are frequently referred to as the Starling forces (page 144). In general terms, the hydrostatic pressure within the vascular system and the colloid oncotic pressure in the interstitial fluid tend to promote movement of fluid from the vascular to the extravascular space. In contrast, the colloid oncotic pressure contributed by the plasma proteins and the hydrostatic pressure within the interstitial fluid, referred to as the *tissue tension,* promote a movement of fluid into the vascular compartment. As a consequence of these forces there is a movement of water and diffusible solutes from the vascular space at the arteriolar end of the capillaries. Fluid is returned from the interstitial space into the vascular system by way of the lymphatics, and unless these channels are obstructed, lymph flow tends to increase if there is net movement of fluid from the vascular compartment to the interstitium. These forces are usually balanced so that a steady state exists in the size of the intravascular and interstitial compartments, and yet a large exchange between them is permitted. However, should any one of these forces be altered significantly, a net movement of fluid from one component of the extracellular space to the other will occur.

An increase in capillary pressure may result from an increase in venous pressure due to local obstruction in venous drainage, to congestive heart failure, or rarely to the simple expansion of the vascular volume by the administration of large volumes of fluid at a rate in excess of the ability of the kidneys to excrete them. The colloid oncotic pressure of the plasma may be reduced, owing to any factor that may induce hypoalbuminemia, such as malnutrition, liver disease, loss of protein into the urine or into the gastrointestinal tract, or a severe catabolic state.

Edema may also result from damage to the capillary endothelium, which increases their permeability and permits the transfer to the interstitial compartment of fluid containing more protein than usual. Injury to the capillary walls can result from chemical, bacterial, thermal, or mechanical agents. Increased capillary permeability may also be a consequence of a hypersensitivity reaction and is characteristic of immune injury. Damage to the capillary endothelium is presumably responsible for inflammatory edema, which is nonpitting, usually localized, and accompanied by other signs of inflammation—redness, heat, and tenderness.

To formulate a hypothesis about the pathophysiology of an edematous state, it is important to discriminate between the *primary* events, such as venous or lymphatic obstruction, reduction of cardiac output, hypoalbuminemia, trapping of fluid in spaces such as the peritoneal cavity, or an increase in capillary permeability, and the predictable *secondary* consequences, which include the renal retention of salt and water. There are instances in which an abnormal positive balance of salt and water may, in fact, be the primary disturbance. In these circumstances the edema is a secondary manifestation of the generalized increase in extracellular fluid volume. These special instances are usually related to conditions characterized by an acute reduction in renal function, such as acute tubular necrosis or acute glomerulonephritis (Fig. 28-1).

These circumstances aside, a hypothesis can be advanced, which, although incomplete, leads to improved understanding of the events and enhances the perception of the pathophysiology. The basic premise is that the primary disorder concerns one or more alterations in the Starling forces so that there is a net movement of fluid from the vascular system into the interstitium or into a "third space" or from the arterial compartment of the vascular space into the chambers of the heart or into the venous circulation itself. The *effective arterial blood volume,* an as yet poorly defined parameter of the filling of the arterial tree, is reduced, and as a consequence a series of physiologic responses designed to restore it to normal are set into motion. A key element of these responses is the retention of an increment of salt and therefore of water, and in many instances this repairs the deficit of the effective arterial blood volume; often this occurs without the development of overt edema. If, however, the retention of salt and water is insufficient to restore and maintain the effective arterial blood volume, the stimuli are not dissipated, the retention of salt and water continues, and edema develops. This sequence of events is operative in dehydration and hemorrhage. Although, in these conditions there is a reduction of effective arterial blood volume and activation of the entire sequence shown on the right side of Fig. 28-1, including the diminished excretion of salt and water, edema does not occur because the net sodium and water balance is negative. In most conditions that lead to edema the mechanisms responsible for maintaining a normal effective osmolality in the body fluids operate efficiently so that sodium retention promotes thirst and secretion of the antidiuretic hormone, which, in turn, lead to the ingestion and retention of approximately 1 liter of water for each 140 mmol sodium retained. Similarly, measures that promote the loss of sodium into the urine, such as the administration of diuretics, are accompanied by the net loss of an equivalent volume of water from the body.

A reduction of cardiac output, whatever the cause, is associated with a reduction of the effective arterial blood volume as well as of renal blood flow and an elevation of the filtration fraction, i.e., the ratio of glomerular filtration rate to renal plasma flow. In severe heart failure the blood flow to the outer renal cortex, in particular, is reduced with less depression in the more central regions of the kidney, and there is a reduction in the glomerular filtration rate. This constriction of renal cortical vessels plays an important role in the retention of salt and water and in the formation of edema in heart failure. At different stages of heart failure, activation of the sympathetic nervous system or of the renin-angiotensin systems is responsible for renal vasoconstriction. Activation of the former can be counteracted by the administration of alpha-adrenergic blocking agents, a finding which indicates that the elevated renal vascular resistance in heart failure is mediated, at least in part, by sympathetic stimuli. The augmented renal blood flow and profound diuresis induced by treatment with angiotensin-converting enzyme inhibitors points to the

FIGURE 28-1 *Sequence of events leading to the formation and retention of salt and water and the development of edema. ANF, atrial natriuretic factor; -------, inhibits renal vasoconstriction.*

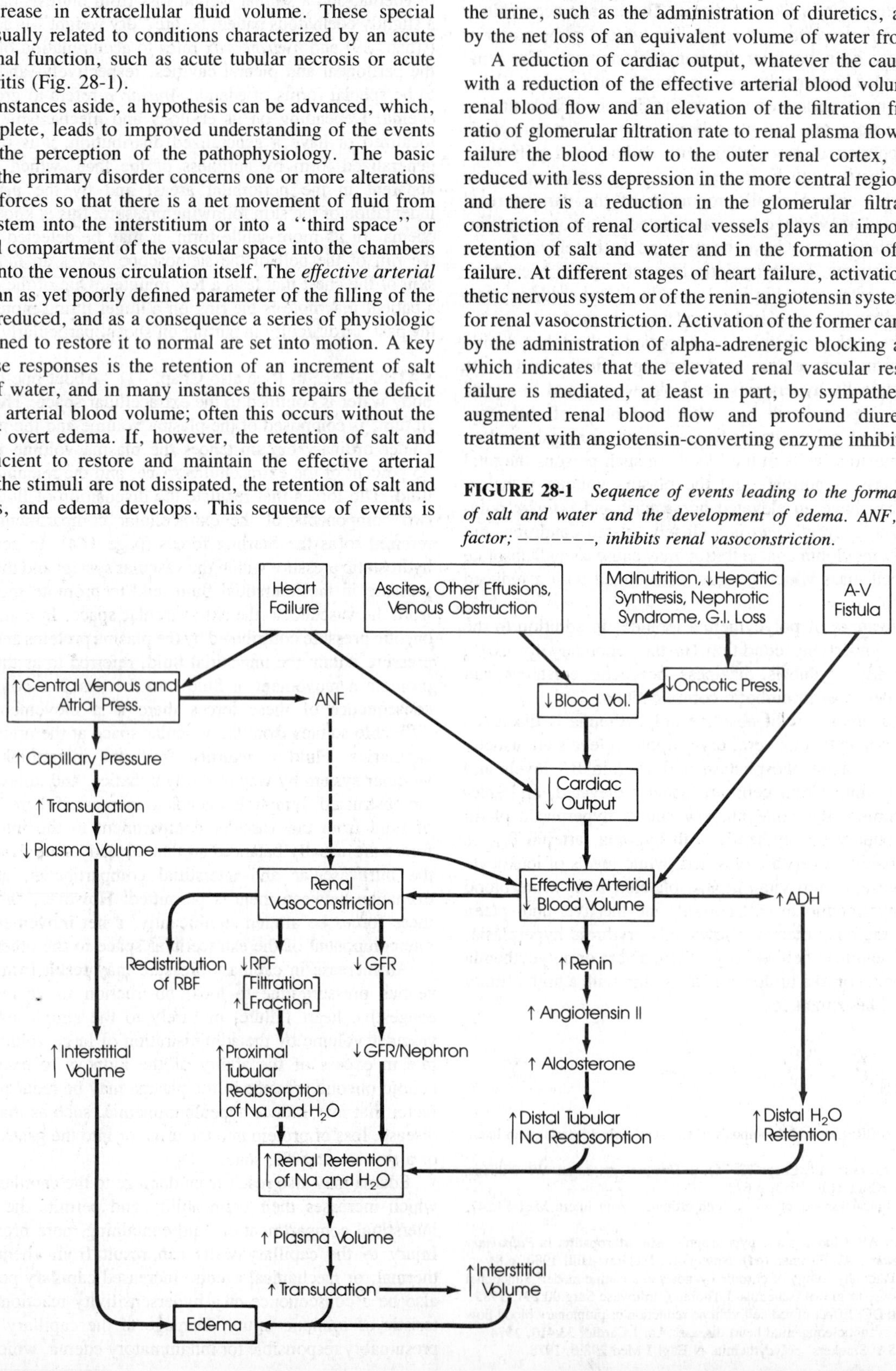

involvement of the renin-angiotensin system in the retention of salt and water in heart failure.

An increase in the tubular reabsorption of glomerular filtrate plays a principal role in the salt and water retention of heart failure. However, the precise sites(s) in the renal tubules, loops of Henle, and collecting ducts which are involved is not clear, nor have the responsible mechanism(s) been identified. Alterations in intrarenal hemodynamics appear to play a significant role. Heart failure, by augmenting renal arteriolar constriction, reduces the hydrostatic pressure and raises the colloid osmotic pressure in the peritubular capillaries, thus enhancing salt and water reabsorption in the proximal tubule. The aforementioned distribution of intrarenal blood flow characteristic of heart failure may be responsible for augmentation of sodium reabsorption in the ascending limb of the loop of Henle.

In addition, the diminished renal blood flow characteristic of states in which the effective arterial blood volume is reduced is translated by the renal juxtaglomerular cells into a signal for increased renin release (Chap. 325). The specific nature of the signal is complex. One factor involves a baroreceptor mechanism, in which reduced renal perfusion results in incomplete filling of the renal arterioles and diminished stretch of the juxtaglomerular cells, a signal that provides for the elaboration or release, or both, of renin. A second mechanism involves the macula densa; as a result of reduced glomerular filtration the sodium load reaching the distal renal tubules is reduced. This is sensed by the macula densa, which in an undefined manner signals the neighboring juxtaglomerular cells to secrete renin. A third mechanism involves the sympathetic nervous system and circulating catecholamines. Activation of the beta-adrenergic receptors in the juxtaglomerular cells stimulates renin release. These three mechanisms generally act in concert.

Renin, an enzyme with a molecular weight of about 40,000, acts on its substrate, angiotensinogen, an alpha$_2$ globulin synthesized by the liver to release angiotensin I, a decapeptide, which is broken down to angiotensin II, an octapeptide with vasoconstrictor properties. The intrarenal production of angiotensin II may also contribute to renal vasoconstriction and to the salt and water retention in heart failure. Angiotensin II also enters the circulation and stimulates the production of aldosterone by the zona glomerulosa of the adrenal cortex. In patients with heart failure, not only is aldosterone secretion elevated, but the biologic half-life of aldosterone is prolonged, which further increases the plasma level of the hormone. A depression of hepatic blood flow, particularly during exercise, secondary to a reduction in cardiac output, is responsible for the reduced hepatic catabolism of aldosterone.

Although increased quantities of aldosterone are secreted in heart failure and in other edematous states and although blockade of the action of aldosterone by spironolactone often induces a moderate diuresis in edematous states, augmented levels of aldosterone (or other mineralocorticoids) do not always promote accumulation of edema, as witnessed by the lack of striking fluid retention in most instances of primary aldosteronism (Chap. 325). Furthermore, although normal subjects retain some salt and water under the influence of a potent mineralocorticoid, such as deoxycorticosterone acetate or fludrocortisone, the accumulation is self-limiting, despite continued exposure to the steroid and to salt and water. The failure of normal subjects to accumulate large quantities of fluid is probably a consequence of an increase in glomerular filtration rate, other hemodynamic influences, and most importantly the increase in volume which promotes an increased excretion of salt that is independent of the filtered load of sodium, i.e., through the action of natriuretic substance(s). The role of aldosterone in the accumulation of fluid in edematous states may be more important because these patients are unable to repair the deficit in effective arterial blood volume.

Atrial distention and/or a sodium load cause release into the circulation of atrial natriuretic factor (ANF), a polypeptide whose active fraction contains 21 to 33 amino acids; a high-molecular-weight precursor of ANF is stored in secretory granules within atrial myocytes. Release of ANF causes (1) excretion of sodium and water by augmenting glomerular filtration rate and inhibiting release of renin and aldosterone; and (2) arteriolar and venous dilatation. Thus, ANF has the capacity to oppose sodium retention and arterial pressure elevation in states characterized by hypervolemia. There is also some evidence for the existence of a distinctly different natriuretic factor, a low-molecular-weight substance that is activated or released as a result of the expansion of the extracellular fluid and causes natriuresis by inhibiting renal sodium reabsorption through inhibiting ouabain-sensitive Na^+,K^+-ATPase. The role of this factor and of ANF in normal and pathophysiologic conditions requires clarification.

Obstruction of venous and lymphatic drainage of a limb In this condition the hydrostatic pressure in the capillary bed upstream to the obstruction increases so that more fluid than normal is transferred from the vascular to the interstitial space; since the alternate route (i.e., the lymphatic channels) is obstructed as well, this event causes an increased volume of interstitial fluid in the limb, i.e., a trapping of fluid in the extremity, at the expense of the blood volume in the remainder of the body, thereby reducing effective arterial blood volume and leading to the consequences shown in Fig. 28-1.

As fluid accumulates in the interstitium of the limb in which venous and lymphatic drainage are obstructed, tissue tension rises until it counterbalances the primary alterations in the Starling forces, at which time no further fluid accumulates in that limb. At this point the additional accumulation of fluid repairs the deficit in plasma volume, and the stimuli to retain more salt and water are dissipated. The net effect is an increase in the volume of interstitial fluid in a local area, and the secondary responses repair the plasma volume deficit incurred by the primary event. This same sequence occurs in ascites and hydrothorax in which fluid is trapped or accumulates in the interstitial space, depleting the intravascular volume and leading to secondary salt and fluid retention as already described.

Congestive heart failure (see also Chap. 182) In this disorder the defective systolic emptying of the chambers of the heart promotes an accumulation of blood in the heart and venous circulation at the expense of the arterial volume, and the aforementioned sequence of events (Fig. 28-1) is initiated. In many instances of mild heart failure, a small increment of volume may repair the volume deficit and establish a new steady state because, through the operation of Starling's law of the heart, up to a point, an increase in the volume of blood within the chambers of the heart promotes a more forceful contraction and may thereby increase the cardiac output (Fig. 181-4). However, if the cardiac disorder is more severe, retention of fluid cannot repair the deficit in effective arterial blood volume. The increment accumulates in the venous circulation, and the increase in hydrostatic pressure therein promotes the formation of edema. The formation of edema in the lungs (Chap. 26) impairs gas exchange and may induce hypoxia, which embarrasses cardiac function still further.

In addition to the sequence shown on the right-hand side of Fig. 28-1, incomplete ventricular emptying leads to an elevation of ventricular diastolic pressure. If the impairment of cardiac function involves the right ventricle, then incomplete ventricular emptying leads to an elevation of right ventricular diastolic volume and pressure; as a consequence pressures in the systemic veins and capillaries also rise, thereby augmenting transudation of fluid into the interstitial space and enhancing the likelihood of peripheral edema. The elevated systemic venous pressure is transmitted to the thoracic duct with consequent reduction of lymph drainage, further increasing edema formation. If the impairment of cardiac function involves the left ventricle, then pulmonary venous and capillary pressures rise [leading in some instances to pulmonary edema (Chap. 26)], as does pulmonary artery pressure; this in turn interferes with the systolic emptying of the right ventricle, leading to an elevation of right ventricular diastolic and central and systemic venous pressures, enhancing the likelihood of formation of systemic edema.

Nephrotic syndrome and other hypoalbuminic states (see also Chap. 223) The primary alteration in this disorder is a diminished colloid oncotic pressure due to massive losses of protein into the urine. This promotes a net movement of fluid into the interstitium, causes hypovolemia, and initiates the sequence of events described above. As long as the hypoalbuminemia is severe, the salt and water retained cannot be restrained within the vascular compartment, and hence the stimuli to retain salt and water are not abated. A similar sequence of events occurs in other conditions which lead to severe hypoalbuminemia, including severe nutritional deficiency states, protein-losing enteropathy, congenital hypoalbuminemia, and severe, chronic liver disease.

Cirrhosis (see also Chaps. 39 and 249) The total blood volume in cirrhosis of the liver is commonly increased when the disorder is accompanied by a system of dilated venous radicles and multiple small arteriovenous fistulas. Effective systemic perfusion, the effective arterial blood volume, and the intrathoracic blood volume appear to be diminished, probably as a consequence of the passage of blood through these fistulas, as well as from the portal venous hypertension and the obstruction of the lymphatic drainage of the liver. These alterations are frequently complicated by reduced serum albumin, which reduces the effective arterial blood volume even further, leading to activation of the renin-angiotensin-aldosterone system and other salt- and water-retaining mechanisms. Initially, the excess interstitial fluid is localized preferentially behind the congested portal venous system and obstructed hepatic lymphatics, i.e., in the peritoneal cavity. In late stages of the disease, particularly when there is hypoalbuminemia, peripheral edema may also be noted.

Idiopathic edema This syndrome, which occurs almost exclusively in women, often with psychosocial difficulties, is characterized by periodic episodes of edema, frequently accompanied by abdominal distention. Fairly large, diurnal alterations in weight occur, so that the patient may weigh several pounds more after having been in the upright posture for several hours. Such large diurnal weight changes suggest an increase in capillary permeability which appears to fluctuate in severity and is aggravated by hot weather. The fact that it occurs most commonly in women, appears to be most prominent during the premenstrual period, and may be improved by progesterone administration suggests that there may be a hormonal effect on the permeability of the vessels that permits the loss of plasma volume into the interstitial space in the upright position and that leads in turn to a contraction in plasma volume and the subsequent retention of salt and water.

The treatment of idiopathic cyclic edema includes a reduction in salt intake, education in the use of rest in the supine position for several hours each day, the wearing of elastic stockings which are put on before arising in the morning, and an attempt to understand any underlying emotional problems. The angiotensin-converting enzyme inhibitor captopril, progesterone, the dopamine receptor agonist bromocriptine, and the sympathomimetic amine dextroamphetamine have all been reported to be useful when administered to patients who do not respond to simpler measures. Diuretics are initially useful but may lose their effectiveness with continuous administration; accordingly, they should be employed sparingly, if at all.

DIFFERENTIAL DIAGNOSIS As a rule, localized edema can be readily differentiated from generalized edema. The great majority of patients with noninflammatory generalized edema of significant degree suffer from advanced cardiac, renal, hepatic, or nutritional disorders. Consequently, the differential diagnosis of generalized edema should be directed toward implicating or excluding these several conditions.

Localized edema Edema originating from inflammation or hypersensitivity is usually readily identified. Localized edema due to venous or lymphatic obstruction may be caused by thrombophlebitis, chronic lymphangitis, resection of regional lymph nodes, filariasis, etc. Lymphedema is particularly intractable because restriction of lymphatic flow results in increased protein concentration in the interstitial fluid, a circumstance which severely impedes removal of retained fluid.

Edema of heart failure Evidence of heart disease, as manifested by cardiac enlargement and gallop rhythm together with evidence of cardiac failure, such as dyspnea, basilar rales, venous distention, and hepatomegaly, usually provides an indication on clinical examination of the pathogenesis of edema resulting from heart failure. Noninvasive tests such as echocardiography and radionuclide angiography may be helpful in establishing the diagnosis of heart failure (see also Chaps. 179 and 182).

Edema of the nephrotic syndrome Massive proteinuria, (> 3.5 g per day), severe hypoalbuminemia, and in some instances hypercholesterolemia are present. This syndrome may occur during the course of a variety of kidney diseases, which include glomerulonephritis, diabetic glomerulosclerosis, and hypersensitivity reactions. A history of previous renal disease may or may not be elicited (see also Chap. 223).

Edema of acute glomerulonephritis The edema occurring during the acute phases of glomerulonephritis is characteristically associated with hematuria, proteinuria, and hypertension. Although some evidence supports the view that the fluid retention is due to increased capillary permeability, in most instances the edema in this disease results from primary retention of sodium and water by the kidneys owing to renal insufficiency. This state differs from congestive heart failure in that it is characterized by a normal or increased cardiac output, normal or diminished circulation time, a reduction in the hematocrit, and a normal arterial–mixed venous oxygen difference. Patients commonly have evidence of pulmonary congestion on chest roentgenograms before cardiac enlargement is significant and do not develop orthopnea (see also Chap. 223).

Edema of cirrhosis Ascites and evidence of hepatic disease (collateral venous channels, jaundice, and spider angiomas) characterize edema of hepatic origin. The ascites is frequently refractory to treatment because it collects as a result of a combination of obstruction of hepatic lymphatic drainage, portal hypertension, and hypoalbuminemia. Edema may also occur in other parts of the body in these patients as a result of hypoalbuminemia. Furthermore, the sizable accumulation of ascitic fluid may increase intraabdominal pressure and impede venous return from the lower extremities; hence, it tends to promote accumulation of edema in this region as well (see also Chap. 249).

Edema of nutritional origin An inadequate diet over a prolonged period may produce hypoproteinemia and edema, which may be intensified by beriberi heart disease, in which multiple peripheral arteriovenous fistulas result in reduced effective systemic perfusion and effective arterial blood volume, thereby enhancing edema formation (Chap. 193). More striking edema is commonly observed when these famished subjects are provided with an adequate diet. The ingestion of more food may increase the quantity of salt ingested, which is then retained along with water. In addition to hypoalbuminemia, hypokalemia and caloric deficits may be involved in the edema of starvation.

Other causes of edema These include hypothyroidism in which myxedema may be located typically in the pretibial region and which may also be associated with periorbital puffiness. Exogenous hyperadrenocortism, pregnancy, and administration of estrogens and vasodilators may also all cause edema.

Distribution The distribution of edema is an important guide to the cause. Thus, edema of one leg or of one or both arms is usually the result of venous and/or lymphatic obstruction. Edema resulting from hypoproteinemia characteristically is generalized, but it is especially evident in the very soft tissues of the eyelids and face and tends to be most pronounced in the morning because of the recumbent posture assumed during the night. Edema associated with heart failure, on the other hand, tends to be more extensive in the legs and to be accentuated in the evening, a feature also determined largely by posture. In the rare types of cardiac disease, such as tricuspid stenosis and constrictive pericarditis, in which orthopnea may be absent and the patient actually prefers the recumbent posture, the factor of gravity may be equalized and facial edema observed. Less common causes of facial edema include trichinosis, allergic reactions, and myxedema. Unilateral edema occasionally results from lesions in the central nervous system affecting the vasomotor fibers on one side of the body; paralysis also reduces lymphatic and venous drainage on the affected side.

Additional factors in diagnosis The color, thickness, and sensitivity of the skin are significant. Local tenderness and increase in temperature suggest inflammation. Local cyanosis may signify a venous obstruction. In individuals who have had repeated episodes of prolonged edema, the skin over the involved areas may be thickened, hard, and often red.

Measurement of the venous pressure is of importance in evaluating edema. Elevation in an isolated part of the body usually reflects localized venous obstruction. Generalized elevation of systemic venous pressure usually suggests the presence of congestive heart failure, although it may occur with the hypervolemia that accompanies acute renal insufficiency. Ordinarily, significant increase in venous pressure can be recognized by the level at which cervical veins collapse; in doubtful cases and for accurate recording, the central venous pressure should be measured. In patients with obstruction of the superior vena cava, edema is confined to the face, neck, and upper extremities, where the venous pressure is elevated compared with that in the lower extremities. Measurement of venous pressure in the upper extremities is also useful in patients with massive edema of the lower extremities and ascites; it is elevated when the edema is on a cardiac basis (e.g., constrictive pericarditis or tricuspid stenosis) but is normal when it is secondary to cirrhosis.

Determination of the concentration of serum proteins, and especially of serum albumin, identifies those patients in whom edema is due, at least in part, to diminished intravascular colloid oncotic pressure. The presence of proteinuria affords useful clues. The complete absence of protein in the urine is evidence against renal disease as a cause of edema. Slight to moderate proteinuria is the rule in patients with heart failure, whereas persistent massive proteinuria is usually due to the nephrotic syndrome.

APPROACH TO THE PATIENT WITH EDEMA A significant question to ask is whether the edema is localized or generalized. If it is localized, those phenomena that may be responsible should be concentrated upon. In this context, localized edema may include hydrothorax, ascites, or both, in the absence of congestive heart failure or hypoalbuminemia. Either of these collections may be a consequence of local venous or lymphatic obstruction, as in inflammatory disease or carcinoma.

If the edema is generalized, it should be determined, first, if there is hypoalbuminemia of significant degree, e.g., serum albumin concentration less than 2.5 g/dL. If there is, the history, physical examination, urinalysis, and other laboratory data will help evaluate the question of cirrhosis, severe malnutrition, protein-losing gastroenteropathy, or the nephrotic syndrome as the underlying disorder. If hypoalbuminemia is not present, it should be determined if there is evidence of congestive heart failure of a severity to promote generalized edema. Finally, it should be ascertained whether the patient has an adequate urine output, or if there is significant oliguria or even anuria. These abnormalities are discussed in Chaps. 40, 219, and 220. The major differential diagnosis in these instances is frequently the discrimination between primary renal retention of salt and water and congestive heart failure.

REFERENCES

BUCKALEW VM JR, GRUBER KA: Natriuretic hormone. Ann Rev Physiol 46:343, 1984

GOLDEN MHN: Protein deficiency, energy deficiency, and the oedema of malnutrition. Lancet 1:1261, 1982

HRICIK DE, KASSIRER JP: The nephrotic syndrome, in *Disease-A-Month,* NJ Cotsonas et al (eds). Chicago, Year Book Medical, 1982, p 5

NEEDLEMAN P et al: Atriopeptins as cardiac hormones. Hypertension 7:469, 1985

SEIFTER JL et al: Control of extracellular fluid volume and pathophysiology of edema formation, in BM Brenner, FC Rector (eds): *The Kidney,* 3d ed. Philadelphia, Saunders, 1986, p 343

SKORECKI KL, BRENNER BM: Body fluid homeostasis in congestive heart failure cirrhosis with ascites. Am J Med 72:325, 1982

STAUB NC, TAYLOR AE (eds): *Edema.* New York, Raven, 1984

STREETEN DHP: Idiopathic edema: Pathogenesis, clinical features, and treatment. Metabolism 27:353, 1978

SUZUKI H et al: Effect of the angiotensin converting enzyme inhibitor, captopril (SQ14,225), on orthostatic sodium and water retention in patients with idiopathic edema. Nephron 39:244, 1985

29 ALTERATIONS IN ARTERIAL PRESSURE AND THE SHOCK SYNDROME

EUGENE BRAUNWALD / GORDON H. WILLIAMS

CONTROL AND MEASUREMENT OF ARTERIAL PRESSURE

Arterial pressure must be maintained at levels sufficient to permit adequate perfusion of the capillary networks in the systemic vascular bed. The pressure in the central arterial bed is dependent on the product of two factors—the volume of blood ejected by the left ventricle per unit of time, i.e., the cardiac output, and the resistance to blood flow offered by the vessels in the peripheral vascular bed. The resistance of a blood vessel, in turn, varies inversely as the fourth power of its radius, and at any given level of cardiac output arterial pressure is therefore largely dependent upon the degree of constriction of the smooth muscle in the walls of the arterioles. Though resistance to flow also varies with the viscosity of the fluid and the length of the vessels, alterations in these factors are ordinarily of only secondary importance.

Cardiac output is controlled largely by factors which regulate ventricular end-diastolic volume (preload), the level of myocardial contractility, the impedance against which the left ventricle ejects (afterload), and heart rate (Chap. 181). The autonomic nervous system (Chap. 66) plays a major role in the maintenance of arterial pressure by its influences on all four determinants of cardiac output through activation of adrenergic receptors in the sinoatrial node, myocardium, smooth muscle in the walls of the arterioles, venules, and veins. The afferent limbs of the autonomic reflex arcs regulating arterial pressure acutely arise in stretch receptors in the carotid sinuses, the aortic arch, the chambers of the heart, and the lungs. Impulses are transmitted along afferent fibers in the glossopharyngeal and vagus nerves to extensive central autonomic connections in the medulla. Synapses connect not only the sympathetic and parasympathetic nuclei and efferent arcs, but also the cerebral cortex and hypothalamic nuclei which control hormonal secretion via the pituitary gland.

A rapid reduction of arterial pressure diminishes the stimulation of pressoreceptors, which in turn activates sympathetic outflow and inhibits parasympathetic activity. As a result, the vascular smooth muscle in arterioles and veins constricts, while heart rate and myocardial contractility are augmented. In addition, as arterial pressure falls, adrenal medullary secretion increases, along with the output of antidiuretic hormone (ADH), adrenocorticotropic hormone (ACTH), renin, and aldosterone; all these effects act to restore the arterial pressure to control levels. Opposite changes occur if arterial pressure is raised acutely. Thus, the operation of the pressoreceptor and a number of humoral systems normally serve to buffer the body from a variety of influences which would otherwise produce marked alterations in arterial pressure.

MEASUREMENT OF ARTERIAL PRESSURE Arterial pressure is determined clinically with a pneumatic cuff; ordinarily, this indirect method provides slight underestimation of the true arterial pressure. However, considerable error may be introduced if proper precautions are not taken in determining blood pressure by this method. The arterial pressure may be significantly underestimated if the air in the cuff is released too rapidly, especially in the presence of bradycardia or an irregular rhythm, or if inadequate inflation of the cuff does not result in complete vascular occlusion. This indirect method is most accurate when, in normal-sized adults with arm circumferences between 24 and 32 cm, a "standard adult" cuff is employed. However, when a cuff of this size is used on children or adults with unusually thin arms, blood pressure may be seriously underestimated, or conversely, it may be overestimated when employed on an arm or thigh greater than 33 cm in girth. Sphygmomanometers for adults are available in four sizes. The proper size should be employed in any given patient. Marked vasoconstriction resulting in severely attenuated limb blood flow and/or marked reductions in pulse pressure may also result in serious underestimation of arterial pressure by the auscultatory method. Under these circumstances direct intraarterial recordings may reveal a normal or even an elevated pressure, while the absence of Korotkoff sounds makes the pressure unobtainable by the indirect methods. Diastolic pressure usually corresponds closely to the disappearance (phase V) of the Korotkoff sounds, but in severe aortic regurgitation it corresponds with the muffling (phase IV) of the sounds.

THE "NORMAL" BLOOD PRESSURE The "normal" blood pressure is difficult to define. Traditional statistical approaches define normality on the basis of values included within two standard deviations of the mean of pressures obtained in a large population of presumably healthy individuals. However, a better definition of abnormality would be based on demonstrated deleterious effects of blood pressure levels exceeding certain limits. If such criteria are used, chronic *hypotension* would seem to occur very rarely. However, the incidence of hypertension based on casual blood pressure levels exceeding 140/90 (widely accepted as hazardous because it is associated with increased risk of cardiovascular mortality which can be reduced by therapy) is estimated to be approximately 20 percent in the adult population of the United States, the incidence in the black population exceeding that in the nonblacks by 50 to 100 percent. Even these statistics may understate the prevalence of hypertension if one accepts the validity of actuarial data indicating that longevity is shortened progressively in adults whose blood pressures exceed 100/60 (see Chap. 196).

TABLE 29-1 Etiologic factors in shock

- *I* Hypovolemia
  - *A* External fluid losses
    - *1* Hemorrhage
    - *2* Gastrointestinal
      - *a* Vomiting (pyloric stenosis, intestinal obstruction)
      - *b* Diarrhea
    - *3* Renal
      - *a* Diabetes mellitus
      - *b* Diabetes insipidus
      - *c* Excessive use of diuretics
    - *4* Cutaneous
      - *a* Burns
      - *b* Exudative lesions
      - *c* Perspiration and insensible water loss without replacement
  - *B* Internal sequestration
    - *1* Fractures
    - *2* Ascites (peritonitis, pancreatitis, cirrhosis)
    - *3* Intestinal obstruction
    - *4* Hemothorax
    - *5* Hemoperitoneum
- *II* Cardiogenic
  - *A* Myocardial infarction
  - *B* Arrhythmia (paroxysmal tachycardia or fibrillation, severe bradycardia)
  - *C* Severe congestive heart failure with low cardiac output
  - *D* Cardiac mechanical factors
    - *1* Acute mitral or aortic regurgitation
    - *2* Rupture of interventricular septum
- *III* Obstruction to blood flow
  - *A* Pulmonary embolus
  - *B* Tension pneumothorax
  - *C* Cardiac tamponade
  - *D* Dissecting aortic aneurysm
  - *E* Intracardiac (ball valve thrombus, atrial myxoma)
- *IV* Neuropathic
  - *A* Drug induced
    - *1* Anesthesia
    - *2* Ganglion-blocking or other antihypertensive drugs
    - *3* "Ingestion" (barbiturates, glutethimide, phenothiazines)
  - *B* Spinal cord injury
  - *C* Orthostatic hypotension (primary autonomic insufficiency, peripheral neuropathies)
- *V* Other
  - *A* Infection
    - *1* Gram-negative septicemia (endotoxin)
    - *2* Other septicemias
  - *B* Anaphylaxis
  - *C* Endocrine failure (Addison's disease, myxedema)
  - *D* Anoxia

ACUTE HYPOTENSION AND SHOCK

Hypotension and shock are not synonymous; although shock is usually associated with hypotension, a previously hypertensive patient may be in shock despite an arterial pressure within normal limits, and hypotension may occur in the absence of shock. *Shock* may be defined as a state in which there is widespread, serious reduction of tissue perfusion, which, if prolonged, leads to generalized impairment of cellular function.

CAUSES The most common clinical causes of shock are listed in Table 29-1. Since arterial pressure is dependent on the product of cardiac output and systemic vascular resistance, marked reductions in either of these variables without a compensatory elevation of the other results in systemic hypotension. Reduction of cardiac output may be due to (1) hypovolemia, with volume loss being external (e.g., hemorrhage or diarrhea) or endogenous (e.g., anaphylaxis); (2) myocardial failure (e.g., cardiogenic shock); (3) circulatory obstruction (e.g., pulmonary embolism); (4) redistribution of blood into the venous capacitance bed ("distributive shock," e.g., septic shock); and (5) reduction of peripheral vasomotor tone, caused, for example, by acute spinal cord injury, which results in reduced systemic vascular resistance and venous dilatation, the latter causing reduced venous return and cardiac output. In many patients, particularly in the late stages of shock, multiple factors are involved simultaneously regardless of the inciting event.

Hypovolemia has been studied much more extensively than any other cause of shock; the mechanism of development is usually readily evident and well understood, and therapy, i.e., restoration of blood volume, is both simple and effective if applied before irreversible tissue damage occurs. Whether the primary insult is the external loss of blood, plasma, or water and salt or the internal sequestration of these fluids in a hollow viscus or body cavity, the general effect is similar, i.e., reduced venous return and decreased cardiac output. This leads to a set of reflex responses designed to maintain the supply of oxygen to critical organs, such as the brain and heart. However, these responses may so limit perfusion of other organs, such as the gut, as to produce necrosis. For purposes of a general discussion of shock, hemorrhagic hypovolemia will be used as the model, but the consequences of general reduced tissue perfusion are similar in other forms of shock.

Stages of hypovolemic shock Depending upon the severity and rate of development of hypovolemia, the shock syndrome may develop abruptly or evolve gradually. If the precipitating factors progress unabated, the endogenous defense mechanisms, while initially competent to maintain adequate circulation, eventually are extended beyond their capacity for compensation. The development of the shock syndrome may be thought to evolve through several stages which merge with one another. The first is the period in which the blood volume deficit is relatively minor and in which the patient may be asymptomatic. In a previously healthy individual compensation for an acute blood loss of as much as 10 percent of the normal blood volume (as with venesection of 500 mL blood from a donor) is achieved acutely by constriction of the arteriolar bed and an augmentation of heart rate, effects mediated by reflex increases in the release of norepinephrine from sympathetic nerve endings and of both norepinephrine and epinephrine from the adrenal medulla. Other responses with more gradual effects include the increased secretion of antidiuretic hormone and the activation of the renin-angiotensin-aldosterone axis (Chap. 325). Arterial pressure is maintained and cardiac output is normal, or only slightly reduced, primarily as a consequence of selective reductions of blood flow to the skin and muscle beds. Heart rate may rise and arterial pressure decline modestly when the patient assumes the erect posture. Hemorrhage may be associated with thrombocytosis, increased platelet adhesiveness, and resultant stasis in blood flow in some capillary beds.

During the second stage, with a reduction in blood volume of 15 to 25 percent, cardiac output falls markedly, even in the recumbent position, and is redistributed with larger fractions going to the liver, heart, and brain and smaller fractions to the kidney, gut, and skin. Despite intense arteriolar constriction in most vascular beds, systolic arterial pressure declines by 10 to 20 mmHg in previously normotensive individuals, although it falls proportionately less than cardiac output. Generalized venoconstriction occurs, increasing the fraction of the total blood volume in the central circulation and tending to sustain venous return. Fluid moves from the interstitial to the intravascular compartment and the hematocrit falls. There is a massive reflex adrenergic discharge accompanied by tachycardia, tachypnea, intense cutaneous vasoconstriction, pallor, cold distal extremities, diaphoresis, piloerection, oliguria, apprehension, and restlessness. The latter mental signs relate to a reduction in cerebral circulation due to decreased perfusion pressure rather than to local vasoconstriction. Angina may occur in patients who have intrinsic coronary vascular disease. Reduced availability of oxygen to tissues activates anaerobic glycolysis, plasma lactate levels rise, and a metabolic acidosis develops. Tachypnea causes a compensatory respiratory alkalosis.

Once the patient has achieved this state of maximal mobilization of compensatory mechanisms, small additional losses of blood result in the third stage characterized by rapid deterioration of the circulation, with life-threatening reductions of cardiac output, blood pressure, and tissue perfusion. The duration of this shock state, the severity of tissue anoxia, and the age and underlying physical state of the patient are of primary importance in determining the ultimate outcome. If tissue perfusion is restored rapidly, recovery may be expected. However, if shock persists, severe vasoconstriction, a compensatory mechanism which aids in the maintenance of arterial pressure, may itself become a complicating factor, and by reducing tissue perfusion even further may initiate a vicious cycle leading to an irreversible state due to widespread cellular injury. Blood flow to the brain, heart, and kidneys is further reduced, and severe ischemia of these vital organs leads to irreversible tissue damage which may result in impaired function of the organ and, eventually, death. Impaired coronary perfusion depresses cardiac function, particularly in patients with some coronary vascular obstruction, and this may lead to further lowering of cardiac output, thus perpetuating a vicious cycle. Cardiac function may also be depressed by the release of a myocardial *depressant factor* from the hypoperfused pancreas. Reduced flow to the medullary vasomotor center late in the stage of shock depresses the activity of compensatory reflexes. Anoxia, hypercapnia, and lactic acidosis result from hypoperfusion of tissues and anaerobic metabolism. These metabolic derangements ultimately result in failure of the energy-requiring active transport systems of cell membranes. The cellular high-energy phosphate reserves are depleted. The integrity of the cells is compromised, and potassium ions, intracellular lysosomal enzymes, peptides, and other vasoactive compounds are released into the circulation. The integrity of capillary membranes is disrupted, and fluid, proteins, and cellular constituents of the blood seep into the extravascular space of tissues.

In profound shock from any cause, an additional important factor which may exacerbate the status of the microcirculation is platelet aggregation and widespread disseminated intravascular coagulation (DIC, Chap. 281) in the bowel, kidney, and other organs. The resultant ischemia produced in the bowel may further complicate the circulatory compensation as a result of breakdown of the mucosal barrier, leading to entry of bacteria and toxic bacterial products into the circulation. Similar changes in the capillary network of the lungs result in interstitial and alveolar edema (noncardiogenic pulmonary edema), impaired respiratory gas transfer, and ultimately development of the adult respiratory distress syndrome (ARDS, Chap. 216), a common lethal complication of shock. Acute tubular necrosis, caused by prolonged renal hypoperfusion, may result in prolonged postshock renal insufficiency (Chap. 219). Because many bacterial substances are potent vasodilators, vasoconstrictor mechanisms may be inhibited, with a further decrease in blood pressure despite intense sympathetic activity. The release of oxygen-derived free radicals may occur during treatment and may be responsible for severe postischemic tissue injury.

Just as tissue perfusion may fall to dangerous or even fatal levels because of actual fluid losses or sequestration with diminished venous return, acute cardiac failure (cardiogenic shock) or a massive pulmonary embolus may have similar effects. Furthermore, even in the presence of a normal blood volume and cardiac function, "vasomotor collapse" due to drug-induced or neuropathic failure of sympathetic vasomotor activity can result in shock because of reduction of peripheral resistance, the pooling of blood in the venous bed, and reduction of cardiac output.

Other forms of shock A complex form of shock may result from infection, especially gram-negative bacteremia with endotoxin release (Chap. 86). This form of shock is associated in its early stage with fever, arteriovenous shunting, low systemic vascular resistance and arterial pressure, and an elevated cardiac output, with warm, dry skin, and in its late stages with vascular pooling, diminished venous return, reduced cardiac output, and hypotension despite increased vascular resistance, and with activation of complement leading to further cell damage. In anaphylactic shock (Chap. 260), release of histamine, leukotrienes, prostaglandins, and other mediators causes arteriolar dilatation as well as increased capillary permeability with loss of intravascular volume, and an attendant reduction in venous return and cardiac output, leading to a marked reduction in arterial pressure, and reductions in central venous and pulmonary capillary wedge pressures and hemoconcentration.

TREATMENT This should be directed toward the rapid restoration of cardiac output and tissue perfusion. The patient should be treated in a properly equipped intensive care unit, where continuous monitoring of intraarterial, pulmonary artery wedge, and central venous pressures is possible. Frequent determinations of arterial blood gases, pH, and serum electrolytes are necessary. However, general supportive measures must be undertaken immediately, even before transfer to the unit. Whether shock results from decreased cardiac output due to a primary reduction in intravascular volume or from a reduction of "effective blood volume" with pooling of blood in the venous bed, the most effective means of restoring adequate circulation is by the rapid infusion of volume-expanding fluids (whole blood, plasma, plasma substitutes, or isotonic electrolyte solutions) to restore systolic arterial pressure to above 100 mmHg in a previously normotensive person, with central venous and pulmonary artery wedge pressures below approximately 15 and 20 mmHg, respectively.

However, when shock is secondary to, or is accompanied by, cardiac failure with increased pulmonary vascular and central venous pressures, the infusion of volume-expanding fluids may result in pulmonary edema. Here attention must be directed toward restoring cardiac function with cardiotonic drugs such as digitalis glycosides and isoproterenol (Chap. 182), and an attempt should be made to support arterial pressure at levels sufficient to maintain the coronary perfusion pressure (Chap. 190). Intraaortic balloon counterpulsation, together with augmentation of contractility with a sympathomimetic amine, and adjustment of preload to an optimal level of left ventricular filling pressure (approximately 20 mmHg) may be used to treat this state. Arrhythmias, which may also contribute to the low cardiac output, should be corrected (Chaps. 183 and 184).

The appearance of the external jugular veins may be helpful in differentiating between shock with high or low central venous pressure. However, catheters inserted into the superior vena cava and, if possible, into the pulmonary artery (a Swan-Ganz balloon-tipped catheter) are the best means for continuously monitoring ventricular filling pressure and of considerable value in guiding therapy. Serial measurements of central venous pressure, urine flow rate, heart rate, and the clinical and mental state of the patient often provide more important indexes of the efficacy of therapy than arterial pressure changes do. In patients with cardiogenic shock, the balloon-tipped catheter "floated" into the pulmonary artery at the bedside without the aid of fluoroscopy is essential in guiding treatment (Chap. 190). Shock secondary to cardiac tamponade may be recognized by the presence of a paradoxical pulse, jugular venous distention, and pericardial fluid detected by echocardiography (Chap. 194). Pericardiocentesis may be life-saving. Adequate ventilation with 100% O_2 must be assured. In patients with infection, appropriate antibiotics and, if necessary, surgical debridement are required.

There is considerable debate concerning the efficacy of vasoconstrictor drugs in shock. In patients with severe peripheral constriction these agents are often ineffective and may actually reduce the already impaired tissue perfusion. However, these drugs may be helpful in patients with inadequate vasoconstrictor responses who are not in heart failure. The use of alpha-adrenergic blocking agents or massive doses of adrenal glucocorticoids in shock secondary to gram-negative septicemia with endotoxin release is also a matter of considerable controversy. The release of the endogenous opiate β-endorphin in many forms of stress has led to trials with the specific opiate antagonist naloxone, with favorable responses having been reported in patients with septic shock.

Following immediate attention to improvement of perfusion in patients with shock, efforts should be directed to treating the underlying etiologic factors, such as gastrointestinal hemorrhage, diabetic acidosis, or septicemia (Table 29-1). Normal pH and serum electrolyte patterns should be restored. After hypovolemia has been corrected, consideration must also be given to the function of other organ systems, particularly the lungs and kidneys, with treatment of ARDS and acute tubular necrosis as outlined elsewhere (Chaps. 216 and 219, respectively). It should be remembered that death secondary to failure of the lungs, kidney, and/or liver occurs not infrequently in patients whose circulation has been restored after they have experienced prolonged shock.

CHRONIC HYPOTENSION

Although many patients have been treated for chronic "low blood pressure," most of them, with systolic pressures in the range of 90 to 110 mmHg, are normal and may actually have a greater life expectancy than those with "normal" pressures. Patients with true chronic hypotension may complain of lethargy, weakness, easy fatigability, and dizziness or faintness, especially if arterial pressure is lowered further when the erect position is assumed. These symptoms are presumably due to a decrease in perfusion of the brain, heart, skeletal muscle, and other organs.

Chronic hypotension occasionally results from severe reductions of the cardiac output. The major endocrine causes of chronic hypotension are associated with deficient gluco- and mineralocorticoid secretion and resultant reductions of the extracellular fluid volume. Hypotension is usually more pronounced in patients with primary adrenocortical insufficiency than in those with hypopituitarism because secretion of the salt-retaining adrenocortical hormone, aldosterone, is partially preserved in pituitary insufficiency (Chap. 325).

Malnutrition, cachexia, chronic bed rest, and a variety of neurologic disorders may result in chronic hypotension, especially in the standing position. Interference with the neural pathways anywhere between the vasomotor center and the efferent sympathetic nerve endings on the blood vessels or heart may prevent the vasoconstriction and increase in cardiac output which occur as a normal response to a reduction in arterial pressure. Multiple sclerosis, amyotrophic lateral sclerosis, subacute combined sclerosis, syringomyelia, tabes dorsalis, peripheral neuropathies, spinal cord section, diabetic neuropathy, extensive lumbodorsal sympathectomy, and the administration of drugs interfering with nerve transmission in the sympathetic nervous system are all associated with orthostatic hypotension.

IDIOPATHIC ORTHOSTATIC HYPOTENSION (PRIMARY AUTONOMIC INSUFFICIENCY) This is a rare condition occurring mostly in older men in which there is degeneration of central and/or peripheral autonomic nervous structures, which may result in such severe orthostatic hypotension that syncope or seizures occur when the patient arises from recumbency. This condition is progressive and characterized by ascending anhydrosis and loss of hair, decreased basal metabolic rate (BMR), reduced norepinephrine production, deficient secretion of lacrimal and salivary glands, ileus, bladder atony, and absence of tachycardia on standing despite marked reduction of blood pressure. Hypertension may occur in the supine position.

Those patients with orthostatic hypotension and central nervous system disease (*Shy-Drager syndrome*) have degeneration of the extrapyramidal tracts, the basal ganglia, and the dorsal nucleus of the vagus and have normal resting plasma norepinephrine levels, while those with only peripheral autonomic disease have depressed levels at rest. Both groups fail to increase their circulating concentrations of the neurotransmitter normally during standing and exercise. Thus, it appears that patients with orthostatic hypotension and central nervous system disease have an intact peripheral sympathetic nervous system, but are unable to activate it, while those without central disease have true insufficiency of the peripheral autonomic nervous system with depletion of norepinephrine in sympathetic nerve endings.

Specific therapy is not available for most of the neurologic causes of orthostatic hypotension, and treatment with sympathomimetic drugs has not proved effective over prolonged periods. However, the expansion of extracellular volume, which may be achieved with a high-salt diet (10 to 20 g per day), and/or the potent synthetic salt-retaining steroid, 9α-fluorohydrocortisone (0.1 to 0.5 mg per day) may be useful but often results in hypertension when the patient is supine. Tight, full-length elastic supportive hose to reduce orthostatic pooling of blood in the legs may also be helpful in sustaining arterial pressure, and in the most severe cases pressurized aviator suits may be necessary to permit ambulation. Occasionally, favorable results may be achieved with sympathomimetic amines such as dihydroergotamine, hydroxyamphetamine, or L-dopa in combination with a monoamine oxidase inhibitor, such as tranylcypromine, with indomethacin or propranolol.

HYPERTENSION (See also Chap. 196)

DIAGNOSIS Patients with elevations of arterial pressure are usually asymptomatic, and the blood pressure abnormality often arouses attention only incidentally during military, life insurance, or other periodic physical examinations. Because hypertension results in secondary organ damage and a reduced life span, it should be evaluated and, when appropriate, treated.

Often, however, the first question is whether patients with a moderately elevated routine blood pressure recording are truly hypertensive. It is well established that anxiety, discomfort, physical activity, or other stress can acutely and transiently raise arterial pressure. Arterial pressure should be measured with the patient sitting comfortably and having been at rest for at least 5 min. Most persons have a higher pressure when initially examined than after several measurements made in the course of a single visit; in order to establish the diagnosis of hypertension, it is necessary to document in the course of at least two separate examinations in each of which arterial pressure is measured at least twice, that arterial pressure remains elevated. This precaution need not be taken in patients with markedly elevated blood pressure and/or in those in whom significant target organ damage is already manifest. Patients with transient or ''labile'' hypertension may not require immediate treatment but should be reexamined periodically, since over the course of time they may develop sustained hypertension. A diastolic pressure that is consistently ≥90 mmHg is considered to be abnormal; in the presence of a normal diastolic pressure, a systolic pressure ≥160 mmHg represents isolated systolic hypertension.

MECHANISM Regardless of the primary cause, the hemodynamic abnormality in most patients with fixed hypertension is increased vascular resistance, especially at the level of the smaller muscular arteries and arterioles, though some patients may have an increased cardiac output, particularly in the early stages of the illness.

Peripheral resistance is determined by the intrinsic physical characteristics of the resistance vessels, i.e., the ratio of lumen to wall thickness, as well as the neurohumoral influences that act on vascular smooth muscle; the latter include the neurotransmitters norepinephrine, a vasoconstrictor, and in some vessels, acetylcholine, a vasodilator. Humoral and locally acting substances include angiotensin II and vasopressin (vasoconstrictors) and prostaglandins and kinins (vasodilators). Hypoxia and products of metabolism, such as H^+, lactic acid, and, perhaps most important, adenosine, also exert potent *local* vasodilating influences.

Systolic hypertension is most commonly seen in elderly patients with decreased compliance of the aortic wall and, like diastolic hypertension, is a risk factor for the development of atherosclerosis. When systolic hypertension is due to an elevated stroke volume, as in patients with severe bradycardia, thyrotoxicosis, severe anemia, aortic valvular regurgitation, arteriovenous shunts or fistulas, patent ductus arteriosus, or the hyperkinetic heart syndrome, it is usually accompanied by a reduced diastolic pressure and a normal mean pressure, and under these circumstances it does not appear to be a risk factor for atherosclerosis.

ETIOLOGY A specific cause for the elevated arterial pressure cannot be defined for most patients with hypertension. The percentage of patients with so-called idiopathic, essential, or primary hypertension is high, varying from 80 to 95 percent depending on both the patient population and how extensive the ''routine'' evaluation is. More specific etiologic relationships have been established for a smaller group of patients with systemic hypertension, i.e., secondary hypertension (Table 196-1). Primary renal vascular and renal parenchymal diseases associated with the development of serious hypertension (as distinguished from renal damage secondary to hypertension) are well recognized, as are a number of endocrine disorders, including Cushing's syndrome, primary hyperaldosteronism (Chap. 325), acromegaly (Chap. 321), and pheochromocytoma (Chap. 326).

EFFECTS OF HYPERTENSION Patients with untreated hypertension die prematurely, most commonly due to heart disease (Chaps. 182 and 196), with strokes (Chap. 343) and renal failure (Chap. 227) also frequently occurring.

APPROACH TO THE PATIENT WITH HYPERTENSION The physician's first task is to determine whether or not a patient with a given level of arterial pressure has hypertension. Then, determinations of the extent of pretreatment evaluation, whether or not to treat, how to treat, and how frequently to reevaluate are necessary. In general, it is preferable to measure arterial pressure on several occasions prior to starting therapy. Initial history, physical examination, and laboratory evaluation should be directed at uncovering correctable secondary forms of hypertension (Table 196-1).

An assessment of the following areas in the medical history is particularly important: family or personal history of hypertension; drugs or dietary factors which may aggravate the hypertension, e.g., high salt intake, oral contraceptives, and hormones; cardiovascular risk factors including diabetes mellitus, smoking, lipid abnormalities, or strokes; cardiac or renal disease; and symptoms suggestive of secondary forms of hypertension, e.g., muscle cramps and weakness associated with primary aldosteronism (Chap. 325) or episodic headaches, palpitations, and sweating associated with pheochromocytoma (Chap. 326).

The *physical examination* should include a standing blood pressure, height, weight, funduscopic examination, assessment of thyroid size, bruits in neck or abdomen, peripheral pulses including determination of synchrony between upper and lower extremities, examination of the heart for size, rate, murmurs, gallops, auscultation of the lungs, examination of the abdomen for masses, and particularly kidney size, and a neurologic examination to assess the presence of deficits associated with a stroke.

The basic *laboratory evaluation* should consist of hematocrit, urinalysis, blood urea nitrogen or creatinine, serum potassium, ECG, and chest x-ray. Often blood glucose, uric acid, and cholesterol determinations and a blood count are also useful, particularly since they may be part of a battery of automated blood tests that as a group are about the same price as the individual tests listed above. Other studies to identify secondary forms of hypertension may be indicated on the basis of the response to initial therapy or physical examination.

If the diastolic pressure is consistently higher than 90 mmHg, therapy is almost always indicated unless contraindications exist.

Therapy should be directed at reducing the arterial pressure to or near normal levels, since studies have documented that morbidity and mortality are reduced. Ideally, this will be accomplished with agents directed at correcting the underlying mechanism(s) responsible for the elevated blood pressure in the individual patient. When the underlying mechanism(s) is(are) unknown or no specific therapy is available, then a ''stepcare approach'' has been advocated to achieve this goal. The principle involves initiating therapy with a small dose of a single drug, either a thiazide diuretic or a beta-adrenergic blocker, if necessary increasing the dose of that drug, and then adding the other drug and, if necessary, other agents one at a time (Chap. 196). The therapeutic regimen should be revised as dictated by the arterial pressure measured at periodic intervals. The frequency of reevaluation should be as often as weekly while blood pressure is being lowered in patients with initial diastolic pressures greater than 115 mmHg, and approximately every 4 months in symptom-free patients on stable treatment programs.

The specific drugs are discussed elsewhere (Chap. 196). However, it is important to emphasize here that control of arterial pressure is a lifelong endeavor, the success of which is often dependent on the physician's ability to motivate the patient to adhere to the therapeutic program and to recognize the pharmacologic interactions and adverse reactions of antihypertensive agents.

REFERENCES

ABBOUD FM: Pathophysiology of hypotension and shock, in Hurst JW (ed): *The Heart*, 6th ed. New York, McGraw-Hill, 1986, p 370

ABBRUZZESE JL et al: Postural hypotension. Johns Hopkins Med J 148:127, 1981

BERNTON EW et al: Opioids and neuropeptides: Mechanisms in circulatory shock. Fed Proc 44:290, 1985

GENEST J (ed): *Hypertension: Physiopathology and Treatment*, 2d ed. New York, McGraw-Hill, 1983

GUYTON AC: Circulatory shock and physiology of its treatment, in *Textbook of Medical Physiology*, 7th ed. Philadelphia, Saunders, 1986, p 326

———: Arterial pressure regulation, in *Textbook of Medical Physiology*, 7th ed. Philadelphia, Saunders, 1986, p 244

HOLCROFT JW, BLAISDELL FW: Shock: Causes and management of circulatory collapse, in *Davis-Christopher Textbook of Surgery*, 13th ed, DC Sabiston Jr (ed). Philadelphia, Saunders, 1986, p 38

THE JOINT NATIONAL COMMITTEE ON DETECTION, EVALUATION AND TREATMENT OF HIGH BLOOD PRESSURE: The 1984 Report of the Joint National Committee on Detection, Evaluation, and Treatment of High Blood Pressure. Arch Intern Med 144:1045, 1984

KAPLAN NM: Systemic hypertension: Therapy, in *Heart Disease*, 2d ed, E Braunwald (ed). Philadelphia, Saunders, 1984, p 902

KIRKENDALL WM et al: AHA Committee Report: Recommendations for human blood pressure determination by sphygmomanometers. Circulation 62:1146A, 1980
LEDINGHAM IM et al: Prognosis in severe shock. Brit Heart J 284:443, 1982
MANNING DM et al: Miscuffing: Inappropriate blood pressure cuff application. Circulation 68:763, 1983
ROCK P et al: Efficacy and safety of naloxone in septic shock. Crit Care Med 13:28, 1985
SOBEL BE: Cardiac and noncardiac forms of acute circulation failure (shock), in *Heart Disease*, 2d ed, E Braunwald (ed). Philadelphia, Saunders, 1984, p 578
———, ROBERTS R: Hypotension and syncope, in *Heart Disease*, 2d ed, E Braunwald (ed). Philadelphia, Saunders, 1984, p 928
ZIEGLER MG et al: The sympathetic nervous system defect in primary orthostatic hypotension. N Engl J Med 296:293, 1977

30 SUDDEN CARDIOVASCULAR COLLAPSE AND DEATH

BURTON E. SOBEL / EUGENE BRAUNWALD

Sudden cardiac death claims approximately 400,000 lives annually in the United States alone, a frequency on the order of one death per minute. Definitions vary, but most include death occurring unexpectedly and instantaneously or within 1 h of the onset of symptoms in a subject with or without known preexisting heart disease. Usually only several minutes elapse between sudden cardiovascular collapse (without effective cardiac output) and irreversible ischemic changes in the central nervous system. Nevertheless, prolonged survival without functional impairment may result from prompt treatment of certain forms of cardiovascular collapse.

CAUSES

MECHANISMS Sudden cardiovascular collapse may be due to (1) arrhythmia (Chaps. 183 and 184)—(*a*) most commonly, ventricular fibrillation or tachycardia, sometimes occurring following a bradyarrhythmia, or (*b*) severe bradycardia or ventricular asystole, factors generally presaging failure of resuscitative efforts; (2) a marked, abrupt reduction in cardiac output, such as occurs with mechanical blockade of the circulation; massive pulmonary thromboembolism (Chap. 211) and cardiac tamponade are two examples of this form; (3) sudden ventricular (pump) failure, which may occur in the presence of acute myocardial infarction (''nonarrhythmic cardiac death'') with or without ventricular rupture (Chap. 190) or critical aortic stenosis (Chap. 187); (4) activation of vasodepressor reflexes, which may contribute to sudden reductions in arterial pressure and heart rate, and which are activated in diverse conditions, including pulmonary thromboembolism, the hypersensitive carotid sinus syndrome (Chap. 12), and primary pulmonary hypertension (Chap. 210). Among the primary electrophysiologic disturbances, the relative incidences of ventricular fibrillation, ventricular tachycardia, and severe bradyarrhythmia or asystole are approximately 75, 10, and 25 percent.

SUDDEN DEATH AND CORONARY ATHEROSCLEROSIS Sudden death is primarily a complication of severe, multivessel coronary atherosclerosis. Fresh coronary thrombi have been found in a variable percentage of patients, ranging from 25 to 75 percent, studied at postmortem. Plaque fissures causing obstruction have been found in some patients without thrombosis; thus, it appears likely that an acute obstructive event triggers sudden death in the majority of patients with coronary artery disease. In other patients, sudden death may result from functional electrophysiologic instability, detectable with provocative, invasive electrophysiologic testing and persisting for prolonged intervals or indefinitely after myocardial infarction. In victims of sudden death less than 45 years of age, platelet thrombi in the coronary microcirculation are often seen. Approximately 60 percent of patients who die of acute myocardial infarction succumb before they reach the hospital. In fact, in 25 percent of patients with coronary artery disease, death is the first indication of the presence of the disorder (Chap. 190). By extrapolation from experience in coronary care units, in which control of electrical activity of the heart has affected the mortality rate favorably, it would appear that the incidence of sudden death in the community might be reduced substantially by prophylactic therapy in populations at particularly high risk, if such therapy could be demonstrated to be effective, of low toxicity, and convenient to the patient. However, sudden death may be but one mode of expression of coronary artery disease, and effective prevention of sudden death will almost certainly require reduction in the incidence and severity of atherosclerosis. The risk of sudden death, when it is a manifestation of remote, prior infarction, is increased in patients with severe left ventricular dysfunction, complex ventricular ectopic activity, and particularly both.

FACTORS ASSOCIATED WITH INCREASED RISK OF SUDDEN DEATH IN NONHOSPITALIZED PERSONS When electrocardiograms are recorded for 24 h during the course of normal activities, supraventricular premature contractions are found to occur in most American men over 50 years of age, and ventricular premature contractions occur in almost two-thirds. Simple ventricular premature beats in patients with otherwise normal hearts are not associated with increased risk of sudden death, but conduction abnormalities and couplets or high-grade ventricular ectopic beats (repetitive forms, or R-on-T complexes) are associated with an increased risk, particularly among patients who suffered a myocardial infarction during the preceding year. Among patients with acute myocardial infarction, ventricular ectopic beats occurring late in the cardiac cycle are particularly prone to be associated with malignant ventricular arrhythmia. High-frequency, low-amplitude potentials occurring during the inscription of the terminal portion of the QRS complex and ST segment, detectable by frequency analysis of signal-averaged electrocardiogram (ECG) recordings, may also identify patients at increased risk.

Ventricular premature beats may trigger ventricular fibrillation, particularly in the presence of myocardial ischemia. On the other hand, they may be manifestations of common fundamental electrophysiologic disturbances which predispose to both ventricular premature beats and ventricular fibrillation, or they may be totally independent phenomena associated with electrophysiologic mechanisms different from those responsible for fibrillation. Their role may differ in different persons. Ambulatory electrocardiographic monitoring has revealed that a several hour period of increasingly frequent or complex ventricular arrhythmias often precedes ventricular fibrillation.

In general, ventricular arrhythmias are of greater significance and more ominous in the presence of acute ischemia and of severe left ventricular dysfunction secondary to ischemic heart disease or cardiomyopathy than in their absence.

Severe coronary artery disease, not necessarily accompanied by morphologic evidence of an acute infarction, hypertension, or diabetes mellitus, is present in more than 75 percent of persons dying suddenly, and perhaps more significantly, the incidence of sudden death in persons with at least one of the three abnormalities is substantially increased. More than 75 percent of men without known prior coronary artery disease who die suddenly exhibit at least two of the following four risk factors for the development of atherosclerosis: hypercholesterolemia, hypertension, hyperglycemia, and cigarette smoking. Obesity and electrocardiographic criteria of left ventricular hypertrophy are also associated with an increased incidence. The incidence of sudden death is higher in cigarette smokers than in nonsmokers, perhaps because of the elevation of circulating catecholamines and fatty acids and the production of increased circulating carboxyhemoglobin with consequently diminished oxygen-carrying capacity by the blood. The proclivity of cigarette smoking to cause sudden death is not cumulative and appears to be reversible when smoking is discontinued.

Cardiovascular collapse on exertion occurs only rarely in patients with ischemic heart disease undergoing exercise testing, and with appropriate personnel and facilities these episodes respond promptly to electrical defibrillation. Rarely, acute emotional stress may precipitate acute myocardial infarction and sudden death, a finding which is in keeping with recent clinical observations of an association of these events with type A personality and experimental observations of increased susceptibility to ventricular tachycardia and ventricular fibrillation after coronary occlusion in emotionally stressed animals or those with augmented sympathetic activity, and protection of experimental animals with selected central nervous system neurotransmitter precursors.

Two major clinical syndromes may be recognized in patients who die suddenly and unexpectedly; both are generally associated with ischemic heart disease. In the larger group, the arrhythmia occurs totally unexpectedly and without preceding symptoms or prodromata. This form is *not* associated with acute myocardial infarction although most patients afflicted exhibit criteria of remote myocardial infarction or other types of organic heart disease. After resuscitation, there is a propensity for early recurrence, probably reflecting the myocardial electrical instability responsible for the intitial episode, and a relatively high 2-year mortality rate (approximately 50 percent). Clearly, these patients can be salvaged only by a rapidly responsive system and aggressive evaluation and management with drugs, surgery, implantable defibrillators, or programmable pacing devices. Pharmacologic prophylaxis probably enhances survival. The second, smaller group consists of patients who, following resuscitation, exhibit evidence of acute myocardial infarction. These patients often exhibit prodromal symptoms—chest pain, dyspnea, and syncope—and show a much lower recurrence and 2-year mortality rate (15 percent). Survival in this subgroup is similar to that following resuscitation from ventricular fibrillation complicating acute myocardial infarction in the coronary care unit. The propensity for developing ventricular fibrillation at the time of acute infarction is of short duration, in contrast to the prolonged interval of high risk among patients in whom fibrillation occurs without acute infarction. However, the risk of sudden death remains particularly high among some survivors of infarction. Risk factors include extensive infarction; severe impairment of ventricular function; persistent, complex ventricular ectopic activity; QT prolongation after the acute episode; loss of the normal hypertensive response to exercise after convalescence; and persistently positive myocardial infarct scintigrams.

OTHER CAUSES OF SUDDEN DEATH Sudden cardiovascular collapse may result from a number of disorders other than coronary atherosclerosis (Table 30-1). Severe aortic stenosis (congenital or acquired) with sudden arrhythmias or pump failure, hypertrophic cardiomyopathy, and myocarditis or cardiomyopathy associated with arrhythmia may be responsible. Massive pulmonary embolism leads to circulatory collapse and death within minutes in approximately 10 percent of patients; some of the remainder succumb gradually with progressive right ventricular failure and hypoxia. Acute circulatory collapse may be presaged by smaller emboli occurring at variable intervals before the lethal attack. Accordingly, implementation of therapy during the premonitory sublethal phase, including anticoagulant administration, may be lifesaving (Chap. 211). Cardiovascular collapse and sudden death are rare but always potential complications of infective endocarditis (Chap. 188).

A number of less common causes of sudden death have been recognized increasingly in recent years. Sudden cardiac death has been associated with liquid-protein, modified-fast diet programs. Distinguishing features include QT prolongation as well as the less specific morphologic cardiac lesions typical of cachexia seen in autopsied cases. Primary degeneration of the atrioventricular conduction system, with or without deposition of calcium or cartilage, may lead to sudden death in the absence of severe coronary atherosclerosis. Trifascicular atrioventricular (AV) block is often seen in these conditions, which account for more than two-thirds of the cases of chronic AV block in adults (Chap. 183). However, the risk of sudden death is substantially greater with impaired conduction associated with ischemic heart disease than that due to primary conduction system disease itself. Electrocardiographic QT-interval prolongation, nerve deafness, and autosomal recessive inheritance (the Jervell and Lange-Nielsen syndrome) are associated with a high proportion of cases of ventricular fibrillation. The same electrocardiographic abnormality and electrophysiologic instability without nerve deafness (the Romano-Ward syndrome) appears to be inherited in an autosomal dominant mode. Electrocardiographic changes in these disorders may be manifest only after exercise. The overall risk of sudden death in afflicted subjects is approximately 1 percent per year. Congenital deafness, history of syncope, female gender, and documented torsades de pointes (see below) or ventricular fibrillation are independent risk factors for sudden cardiac death. Although left stellate ganglionectomy exerts transitory prophylactic benefit, long-term salutary effects have not been substantiated.

Other conditions with QT prolongation and increased temporal dispersion of repolarization, such as hypothermia and a number of drugs (including quinidine, disopyramide, procainamide, the phenothiazines and tricyclic antidepressants), hypokalemia, hypomagnesemia, and acute myocarditis, have been associated with sudden death, particularly when preceded by episodes of torsades de pointes, a form of rapid ventricular tachycardia with distinctive electrocardiographic and pathophysiologic features (Chap. 184). Sinoatrial arrest or block with depression of lower pacemakers or the sick sinus syndrome, usually accompanied by conduction system dysfunction as well, may also lead to asystole. Rarely, fibromas or inflammatory processes in the region of the sinus or AV nodes and conduction system elements (ganglionitis and neuritis) may precipitate sudden death in subjects without prior manifestations of heart disease. Sudden rupture of a papillary muscle, the ventricular septum, or free wall, usually occurring within the first few days following acute myocardial infarction, occasionally causes sudden death (Chap. 190). Sudden cardiovascular collapse is also a major, and frequently the terminal, event in patients with major cerebrovascular accidents, particularly subarachnoid hemorrhage, sudden alterations of intracranial pressure, or lesions affecting the brainstem. It may also occur with asphyxia. Digitalis toxicity may result in life-threatening arrhythmias, leading to sudden cardiovascular collapse and, if treatment is not immediate, to death (Chap. 182). Paradoxically, antiarrhythmic drugs may exacerbate arrhythmia or predispose to ventricular fibrillation in as many as 15 percent of patients.

TABLE 30-1 Conditions associated with cardiovascular collapse and sudden death in adults

Ischemic heart disease secondary to coronary atherosclerosis (including acute myocardial infarction)
Prinzmetal's variant angina; coronary artery spasm
Congenital coronary artery disease (including anomalous origins, coronary arteriovenous fistula)
Coronary embolism
Acquired, nonatherosclerotic coronary disease (including aneurysms occurring with Kawasaki's disease)
Myocardial bridges that demonstrably impair perfusion
Wolff-Parkinson-White syndrome
Hereditary or acquired QT-interval prolongation (with or without congenital deafness)
Sinoatrial node disease
Atrioventricular block (Stokes-Adams syndrome)
Secondary disease of the conduction system (e.g., amyloid, sarcoid, hemochromatosis, thrombotic thrombocytopenic purpura, myotonia dystrophica)
Drug toxicity or idiosyncrasy (e.g., digitalis, quinidine)
Electrolyte derangements (with myocardial magnesium and potassium deficiencies having been implicated)
Valvular heart disease, especially aortic stenosis
Infective endocarditis
Myocarditis
Cardiomyopathies, particularly idiopathic hypertrophic subaortic stenosis
Liquid-protein, modified-fast diet programs
Pericardial tamponade
Mitral valve prolapse (extremely uncommon cause of sudden death)
Cardiac tumor
Ruptured or dissecting aortic aneurysm
Pulmonary thromboembolism
Cerebrovascular accident, particularly hemorrhage

ELECTROPHYSIOLOGIC MECHANISMS Potentially lethal ventricular arrhythmias in patients with acute myocardial infarction may result from reentry, derangements of automaticity, or both. It would appear that reentry plays a dominant role in early arrhythmia, for example, within the first hour, and that derangements of automaticity are an important contributing factor later.

Several factors appear to set the stage for ventricular fibrillation and other rhythms dependent upon reentry early after the onset of ischemia (see also Chap. 184). Local accumulation of hydrogen ions, an increased ratio of extra- to intracellular potassium, and regional adrenergic stimulation tend to shift diastolic transmembrane potentials toward zero and elicit anomalous depolarizations possibly mediated by calcium currents or indicative of depressed, fast sodium-mediated depolarizations. This type of depolarization appears to contribute to slowed conduction required for the development of reentry early after the onset of ischemia.

Another mechanism implicated in reentry early after ischemia is focal reexcitation. Anoxia results in abbreviation of the duration of the action potential. Accordingly, during electrical systole, cells within an ischemic zone may be repolarized before cells in adjacent nonischemic tissue. The consequent disparity between prevailing transmembrane potentials may give rise to an uneven depolarization of adjacent cells and hence contribute to arrhythmia dependent upon reentry. Concomitant pharmacologic or metabolic factors may predispose toward reentry. For example, quinidine may depress conduction velocity disproportionately to its prolongation of refractoriness, thereby facilitating arrhythmias dependent upon reentry early after the onset of ischemia.

The so-called vulnerable period, corresponding to the ascending limb of the T wave, represents that portion of the cardiac cycle when temporal dispersion of ventricular refractoriness is maximum and, accordingly, when reentrant rhythms leading to sustained, repetitive activity can be initiated most readily. In patients with severe myocardial ischemia, the vulnerable period is prolonged and the intensity of stimulus required to evoke repetitive tachycardia or ventricular fibrillation is reduced. Temporal dispersion of refractoriness may be increased in nonischemic tissue in the presence of a slow heart rate. Accordingly, profound bradycardia due to decreased automaticity of the sinus node or AV block may also be particularly dangerous in patients with acute myocardial infarction since it may potentiate reentry.

Ventricular tachycardia occurring more than 8 to 12 h after the onset of ischemia appears to be dependent in part on derangements of automaticity or triggered activity of Purkinje fibers and possibly of myocardial cells as well. This rhythm resembles the slow ventricular tachycardia often occurring between a few hours and a day after coronary ligation in experimental animals. It does not generally degenerate into ventricular fibrillation or other malignant arrhythmia. Reduction of diastolic transmembrane potential in response to regional biochemical alterations induced by ischemia may contribute to the derangements of automaticity by facilitating repetitive depolarizations of Purkinje fibers triggered by a single depolarization. Since catecholamines facilitate propagation of such slow-current responses, enhanced regional adrenergic stimulation may be an important contributing factor. The apparent efficacy of beta-adrenergic blockade in suppressing some ventricular arrhythmias and the relative inefficacy of conventional antiarrhythmic agents such as lidocaine in patients with sympathetic hyperactivity may be reflections of the importance of regional adrenergic stimulation to enhanced automaticity.

Asystole and/or profound bradycardia are less common electrophysiologic mechanisms underlying sudden death caused by coronary atherosclerosis. They may be manifestations of complete right coronary artery occlusion and usually presage failure of resuscitative efforts. They often result from failure of impulse formation in the sinus node, AV block, and failure of subsidiary pacemakers to function effectively. Sudden death associated with these manifestations is usually a consequence of diffuse myocardial disease in most patients rather than the AV block per se.

TREATMENT AND PREVENTION

IDENTIFICATION OF HIGH-RISK SUBJECTS The difficulties entailed in ambulatory electrocardiographic monitoring or other procedures for mass screening to detect candidates at risk for sudden death are formidable, since the population at risk comprises more than one-third of all men 35 to 74 years of age, and since ventricular ectopic activity occurs so commonly and is so variable from day to day in the same subject. At greatest risk are the following: (1) patients who have previously experienced primary ventricular fibrillation without associated acute myocardial infarction; (2) patients with ischemic heart disease who exhibit bouts of rapid ventricular tachycardia; (3) patients seen within 6 months after recovery from acute myocardial infarction with frequent, early, or multifocal ventricular premature contractions at rest, during physical activity, or during psychological stress, particularly those who also have severe left ventricular dysfunction with ejection fraction <40 percent or overt heart failure; (4) patients with prolonged QT intervals and frequent premature contractions, particularly those who present with a history of syncope. Although identification of patients at high risk is particularly important, selection of an effective prophylactic regimen remains difficult, and none has clearly demonstrated effectiveness in reducing the risk. For survivors of sustained ventricular tachycardia or fibrillation, induction of the arrhythmia by ventricular stimulation techniques with catheter electrodes and selection of a pharmacologic regimen based on abolition of subsequent induction of the arrhythmia appear to be predictive of the efficacy of specific pharmacologic regimens for preventing or interrupting recurrent malignant arrhythmia, particularly ventricular tachycardia. In addition, it identifies patients refractory to conventional management and facilitates selection of candidates for aggressive measures such as administration of investigational drugs, implantation of automatic defibrillators, or cardiac surgery (Chap. 184).

PHARMACOLOGIC THERAPY Treatment with antiarrhythmic drugs in doses sufficient to maintain "therapeutic" drug levels has been claimed to be effective in reducing recurrent ventricular tachycardia and/or fibrillation in survivors of sudden death, if during acute drug testing advanced grades of ventricular premature contraction (early or repetitive forms) can be eliminated or reduced. For those survivors of sudden cardiac death who exhibit frequent and complex ventricular ectopic activity occurring between episodes of ventricular tachycardia and/or fibrillation (approximately 30 percent), prophylactic treatment should be employed on an individual basis, with pharmacologic efficacy defined by suppression of the intercedent arrhythmia. Conventional doses of long-acting procainamide (30 to 50 mg/kg per day by mouth in divided doses every 6 h), quinidine gluconate (15 mg/kg per day by mouth in divided doses every 6 h), or disopyramide (6 to 10 mg/kg per day by mouth in divided doses every 6 h) may be effective in suppressing these arrhythmias. Dosage of quinidine may be increased up to 3 g per day if found necessary, unless gastrointestinal disturbances or electrocardiographic evidence of toxicity occurs. Amiodarone (an investigational drug in the United States, 5 mg/kg intravenously over 5 to 15 min or 300 to 800 mg per day by mouth with or without a loading dose of 1200 to 2000 mg per day in divided doses for 1 to 4 weeks) has striking antifibrillatory actions but a very slow rate of onset with peak effects seen only after several days or weeks of administration. Toxicity may occur both acutely and with chronic administration (Chap. 184). Although amiodarone is an unequivocally effective antifibrillatory drug, its use should be reserved for conditions refractory to less toxic agents or alternative approaches.

For most survivors of sudden cardiac death, frequent or complex ventricular ectopic activity is manifest only rarely or not at all between episodes of ventricular tachycardia and/or fibrillation. For such patients, selection of an appropriate prophylactic regimen should be based upon favorable responses to specific regimens reflected by results of provocative, invasive electrophysiologic testing, as described in Chap. 184. Ambulatory electrocardiographic monitoring with or without exercise stress may be particularly helpful in documenting the efficacy of treatment, since the incomplete knowledge regarding the pathogenesis of sudden death makes rational prophylactic drug selection and dosage difficult and a stereotyped regimen for all patients impractical. However, because of the marked variability of spontaneous arrhythmias on Holter recordings, which should be characterized for each subject, profound reduction of ectopic activity (at least 80 percent over a 24-h period) must be documented before attributing pharmacologic efficacy to a specific regimen. Even when such efficacy is demonstrable, it does not necessarily imply comparable protection against ventricular fibrillation. Some patients require concomitant administration of multiple drugs. Since the fundamental electrophysiologic derangements underlying ventricular fibrillation and premature beats may not be the same, even documented suppression of premature beats, while desirable, provides no reassurance of prevention of sudden death.

Decreased incidence of sudden death in a random selection of patients surviving acute myocardial infarction has been documented in several prospective double-blind studies utilizing beta-adrenergic blocking agents, although the effect of treatment on arrhythmia was not quantified and the mechanism of apparent protection has not yet been identified. The incidence of sudden cardiac death was significantly decreased, in proportion to an overall decrease in mortality, during follow-up intervals of several years among survivors of myocardial infarction by treatment with beta blockers initiated several days after the infarct.

Delays by the patient, physician, and transportation system and in the emergency room after the occurrence of acute myocardial infarction are significant impediments to prevention of sudden death. The median elapsed time between onset of symptoms of acute infarction and hospitalization averages 3 to 5 h in most areas of the United States. Denial by the patient of the seriousness of the condition and indecision by both the patient and physician contribute most to total delay.

SURGICAL APPROACHES In carefully selected survivors of sudden cardiac death with recurrent malignant arrhythmia, described in Chap. 184, surgical approaches may be indicated. In some patients prophylaxis with an automatic implantable defibrillator may enhance survival, although the unpleasant nature of the discharges of the device and the possibility of physiologically inappropriate discharges are serious disadvantages.

COMMUNITY EFFORTS Experience gained in Seattle, Washington, has shown that in order to deal effectively on a communitywide basis with the problem of sudden cardiovascular collapse and death, it is necessary to develop a system that provides rapid and effective response for these emergencies. Important elements of the system include a citywide emergency call number through which the system can be activated, a well-trained group of paramedical personnel such as fire fighters to respond, a short average time of response (under 4 min), and a large number of lay people trained in techniques of resuscitation. Clearly, the success in immediate resuscitation and for long-term survival is directly related to how soon following collapse resuscitation efforts are initiated. The availability of special ambulances (mobile coronary care units) equipped and staffed to handle acute cardiac emergencies appears to reduce delay by increasing community and physician awareness of the urgency of prompt medical attention. Such a system can be effective in resuscitating more than 40 percent of patients who have undergone cardiovascular collapse. Involvement of well-trained citizens in a communitywide program of "bystander cardiopulmonary resuscitation" appears to increase the likelihood that resuscitation will lead to a favorable outcome, reflected by an increased fraction of successful hospital discharges among patients sustaining prehospital cardiac arrest (30 to 35 percent compared with 10 to 15 percent in the absence of such a program). Long-term survival may be increased also from a 50 percent 2-year rate to 70 percent or more. Advocates of bystander resuscitation are presently exploring the use of portable home defibrillators designed for safe use by lay persons with only a modicum of training required.

PATIENT EDUCATION Providing instructions to susceptible persons on how to seek medical care on an emergency basis upon the development of symptoms of myocardial infarction is of great importance in the prevention of sudden cardiac death. This strategy includes instructing the patient that prompt entry into an effective emergency care system is not only urgent but also what the physician expects of the patient, regardless of whether symptoms suggestive of myocardial infarction occur during the day or night (Chap. 190); this concept also means instructing the patient to bypass the physician and to contact the emergency care system directly. Unsupervised physical stress, such as jogging, should be discouraged in patients with known ischemic heart disease and prohibited in those at high risk of sudden death, as defined above.

APPROACH TO THE PATIENT WITH SUDDEN CARDIOVASCULAR COLLAPSE

Sudden death can often be averted even when cardiovascular collapse has occurred. When a patient under close medical observation develops sudden collapse from arrhythmia, the immediate goal must be restoration of effective cardiac rhythm. Circulatory collapse must be recognized and confirmed immediately. Its cardinal features are (1) loss of consciousness and seizures; (2) absent peripheral arterial pulses; and (3) absent heart sounds. Since external cardiac massage provides only limited cardiac output, presently no more than 30 percent of the lower limit of normal, definitive restoration of effective rhythm should be the immediate goal, and in the absence of evidence to the contrary, abrupt circulatory collapse should be assumed to be due to ventricular fibrillation. If the physician sees the patient within 1 min of the collapse, time should not be wasted by attempting to achieve oxygenation. An immediate blow to the precordium ("thump version") may be attempted, since this is occasionally effective and takes only seconds. Rarely, when circulatory collapse is due to ventricular tachycardia and the patient is still conscious when first seen, a vigorous cough may terminate the arrhythmia. In the absence of immediate restoration of the circulation, electrical defibrillation (Chap. 184) should be attempted immediately thereafter, without necessarily even pausing first to record an electrocardiogram on separate equipment, although use of portable defibrillators capable of electrocardiographic recording directly from the defibrillating electrodes may be helpful. Maximum electrical output of conventionally available equipment (320 W·s) is generally adequate, even for obese patients, and should be used. Efficacy is potentiated by application of the electrode paddles with firm pressure, and delivery of the electrical discharge promptly and before the energy requirements for defibrillation increase with the duration of ventricular fibrillation. Devices with automated impedance adjustment are promising because they can minimize the hazards of unnecessarily high energy discharges while avoiding ineffectively low discharges for patients with higher-than-anticipated impedance. If these immediate attempts are unsuccessful, external cardiac massage and complete cardiopulmonary resuscitation with prompt establishment and maintenance of a good airway should be implemented.

If collapse is due to unequivocal asystole, transthoracic or transvenous electrical pacing should be implemented immediately. Intracardiac epinephrine, 5 to 10 mL of 1:10,000 solution, may facilitate the heart's response to artificial pacing or be helpful when a slow ventricular focus is present but ineffective. If these initial definitive measures fail despite adequate technical performance, prompt restitution of a favorable metabolic milieu and monitoring are necessary. This is best accomplished by these three procedures:

1 External cardiac massage.
2 Correction of acid-base balance, often requiring intravenous sodium bicarbonate administration in an initial dose of 1 meq/kg. One-

half the dose should be repeated every 10 to 12 min as needed based on frequent determinations of arterial pH.

3 Assessment and correction of electrolyte imbalance. Definitive efforts to restore an effective cardiac rhythm should be attempted again as soon as possible, certainly within minutes. When effective cardiac rhythm is restored but rapidly degenerates again into ventricular tachycardia or fibrillation, lidocaine should be administered as a bolus, 1 mg/kg intravenously, then continued by intravenous infusion at a rate up to 1 to 5 (mg/kg)/h, and countershock repeated.

CARDIAC MASSAGE (Fig. 30-1) External cardiac massage was designed by Kouwenhoven and coworkers to establish perfusion of vital organs by sequential, manual compression of the chest. Adherence to several aspects of technique is essential. (1) If efforts to rouse the patient by shaking the shoulders and calling fail, the patient should be placed supine on a firm surface (a wooden board serves well). (2) An open airway should be established by a maneuver such as chin lift, performed by tilting the patient's head backward with firm pressure applied to the forehead while bringing the mandible anteriorly with the fingers of the other hand under the chin. (3) If a carotid pulse is not palpable during a 5-s observation interval, compression of the chest should be performed with the heel of one hand at the midsternal region with the inferior portion two fingerbreadths cephalad to the xiphoid process (to avoid lacerations of the liver) and the other hand applied with the fingers locked on top of the first. (4) Chest compression of 3 to 5 cm should be delivered at a frequency of one per second to permit adequate time for ventricular filling. (5) The resuscitator's waist must be higher than the patient's chest to permit application of the approximately 50-kg force required, and the elbows should be straight. (6) Depression and release of the chest wall should each occupy 50 percent of the cycle. Sudden compression may elicit a pressure wave palpable at the femoral or carotid artery but one able to eject little blood. (7) Massage should not be interrupted, even for a moment, because cardiac output increases cumulatively during the first 8 to 10 compressions, and even brief interruptions are detrimental. (8) Effective ventilation must be maintained throughout at a rate of approximately 12 breaths per minute and monitored by arterial blood gas analyses. If the latter are clearly abnormal, endotracheal intubation should be carried out expeditiously with no more than a 20-s pause in the external chest compression sequence.

FIGURE 30-1 *Cardiopulmonary resuscitation (CPR) and external chest compression. A diagrammatic representation of the steps required for resuscitation by a single rescuer. [Modified from Standards and guidelines for cardiopulmonary resuscitation (CPR) and emergency cardiac care (ECC). JAMA 244:453, 1980.]*

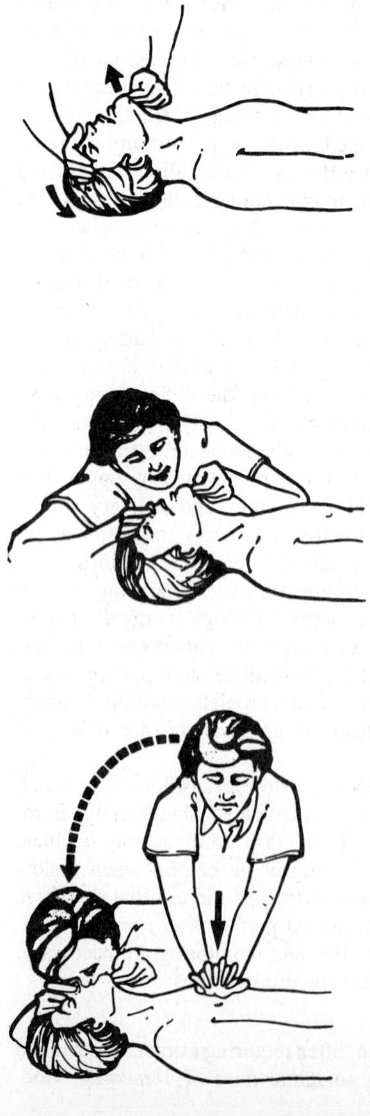

Each external cardiac compression unavoidably limits venous return, to some extent. Thus, the optimal anticipated cardiac index during external massage approximates only 40 percent of the lower limit of normal, well below that seen in most patients after spontaneous ventricular contractions have returned. Therefore, prompt restoration of effective cardiac rhythm is essential.

It is likely that some modifications of the classical technique of cardiopulmonary resuscitation (CPR) will become established in the near future aimed at (1) augmenting intrathoracic pressure during compression (positive airway pressure, simultaneous ventilation and compression, abdominal binding, initiating compression at end-inspiration), (2) reducing intrathoracic pressure during relaxation (negative airway pressure during this phase), and (3) reducing intrathoracic aortic and systemic arterial collapse during compression (augmentation of vascular volume and antishock inflatable trousers). One application of these concepts that has already been employed is "cough CPR," a technique with which a still-conscious patient can maintain cardiac output despite ventricular fibrillation, at least for brief intervals, by repetitive, rhythmic coughing which phasically augments intrathoracic pressure, simulating the changes induced by conventional chest compression. Because of effects of CPR on blood flow, needed drugs should be given intravenously via upper extremity or central (not femoral) lines and generally by bolus injection rather than by continuous infusion. Isotonic agents can be given after dilution in saline by injection into the endotracheal tube because absorption occurs through the bronchial circulation.

Rarely, organized electrocardiographic activity unaccompanied by effective cardiac contraction (electromechanical dissociation) may occur. Intracardiac epinephrine (5 to 10 mL of 1:10,000 solution) or calcium gluconate (1 g) may be helpful in restoring mechanical function. Alternatively, calcium chloride (10%) can be given intravenously in a dose of 5 to 7 mg/kg. Refractory or repetitively recurrent ventricular fibrillation may respond to lidocaine, 1 mg/kg followed by 0.5 mg/kg at 10- to 12-min intervals to a maximum of 225 mg; procainamide, 20 mg every 5 min to a maximum of 1000 mg followed by an infusion of 2 to 6 mg/min; or bretylium tosylate, 5 to 12 mg/kg given over several minutes followed by infusion of 1 to 2 mg/kg per minute. Cardiac massage should be terminated as soon as effective cardiac contractions serve to produce a detectable pulse and systemic arterial blood pressure.

The therapeutic approach outlined above is based on several considerations: (1) irreversible brain damage often occurs after a few (approximately 4) minutes of circulatory collapse; (2) the likelihood of restoring effective cardiac rhythm and successfully resuscitating the patient diminishes rapidly with time; (3) 80 to 90 percent survival can be anticipated in patients developing primary ventricular fibrillation, as when undergoing cardiac catheterization or exercise testing, in whom definitive treatment is prompt; (4) survival rates in the general hospital setting are much lower, approximately 20 percent, depending in part on the coexisting or underlying disease process; (5) survival rates in the community approach zero, unless special emergency care systems have been perfected, probably because of unavoidable delays in initiating definitive therapy and limitations of equipment and available personnel; and (6) external cardiac massage can provide only a limited cardiac output. When ventricular fibrillation occurs, the earliest application of electrical countershock is the one most likely to succeed. Thus, when circulatory collapse is a primary event, therapy must be directed toward prompt restoration of effective cardiac rhythm.

COMPLICATIONS External cardiac massage is not free from significant complications, including rib fracture, hemopericardium and tamponade, hemothorax, pneumothorax, liver laceration, fat embolus, and ruptured spleen with late, occult blood loss. However, these complications can be minimized by proper technique and, if appropriately considered, can be readily recognized and often managed effectively. The decision to terminate unsuccessful cardiopulmonary resuscitation is always difficult. In general, if effective cardiac rhythm has not been restored and if the patient's pupils are fixed and dilated despite 30 min or more of cardiac massage, a successful resuscitation cannot be expected.

REFERENCES

Beta-Blocker Heart Attack Trial Research Group: A randomized trial of propranolol in patients with acute myocardial infarction. I. Mortality results. JAMA 247:1707, 1982

Bigger JT Jr et al: The Multicenter Post-Infarction Research Group: The relationships among ventricular arrhythmias, left ventricular dysfunction, and mortality in the 2 years after myocardial infarction. Circulation 62:250, 1984

Chandra N et al: Simultaneous chest compression and ventilation at high airway pressure during cardiopulmonary resuscitation. Lancet 1:175, 1980

Cobb LA et al: Sudden cardiac death. A decade's experience with out-of-hospital resuscitation. Mod Concepts Cardiovasc Dis 49:31, 1980

Davies MJ, Thomas AC: Thrombosis and acute coronary-artery lesions in sudden cardiac ischemic death. N Engl J Med 310:1137, 1984

———, ———: Plaque fissuring: The cause of acute myocardial infarction, sudden ischaemic death, and crescendo angina. Br Heart J 53:363, 1985

Echt DA et al: Clinical experience, complications, and survival in 70 patients with the automatic implantable cardioverter/defibrillator. Circulation 71:289, 1985

Halperin HR et al: The determinants of vital organ flow during cardiac arrest in dogs. Circulation, vol. 73, March, 1986

James TN (ed): *15th Bethesda Conference Report: Sudden Cardiac Death.* J Am Coll Cardiol 5(Suppl):1B, 1985

Lever HM et al: Sudden death in hypertrophic cardiomyopathy. Clev Clin Quart 51:65, 1984

Lewis BH et al: Detailed analysis of 24 hour ambulatory electrocardiographic recordings during ventricular fibrillation of torsade de pointes. J Am Coll Cardiol 2:426, 1983

Lewis RP et al: Reduction of mortality from prehospital myocardial infarction by prudent patient activation of mobile coronary care system. Am Heart J 103:123, 1982

McIntyre KM, Lewis AJ (eds): *Textbook of Advanced Cardiac Life Support.* Dallas, American Heart Association, 1981

Miller JM et al: Subendocardial resection for ventricular tachycardia: Predictors of surgical success. Circulation 70:624, 1984

Roth R et al: Out-of-hospital cardiac arrest: Factors associated with survival. Ann Emerg Med 13:237, 1984

Smith WM, Gallagher JJ: "Les Torsades de Pointes": An unusual ventricular arrhythmia. Ann Intern Med 93:578, 1980

Tresch DD et al: Long-term survival after prehospital sudden cardiac death. Am Heart J 108:1, 1984

Vincent R et al: A community training scheme in cardiopulmonary resuscitation. Brit Med J 288:617, 1984

Weaver WD et al: Improved neurologic recovery and survival after early defibrillation. Circulation 69:943, 1984

section 5 Alterations in gastrointestinal function

31 ORAL MANIFESTATIONS OF DISEASE

PAUL GOLDHABER

DISTURBANCES OF THE TEETH AND DENTAL TISSUES

DENTAL CARIES, PULPAL AND PERIAPICAL INFECTION, AND SEQUELAE Dental caries, the principal cause of tooth loss up to the fourth decade of life, is characterized by a bacteria-induced progressive destruction of the mineral and organic components of the outer enamel and underlying dentin. Numerous long-term studies have clearly shown that the artificial fluoridation of drinking water supplies to a level of 1 part per million leads to a 50 to 75 percent reduction in the occurrence of dental caries in permanent teeth of children, presumably because of an alteration of the developing enamel crystals during tooth formation which makes them more resistant to acid dissolution.

If the carious lesion progresses unchecked, there is eventual infection of the dental pulp, giving rise to an *acute pulpitis.* During the early stages of pulpitis moderately severe pain may result from thermal changes, particularly with cold drinks. As more of the pulp becomes involved because of advanced caries, heat or reclining may stimulate the onset of even more severe and continuous pain. At this stage, damage to the pulp is irreversible, and treatment consists of either extraction or thorough removal of the remaining contents of the pulp chamber and root canals followed by sterilization and filling with an inert material (root canal therapy).

If the pulpitis is not treated, infection may spread beyond the apex of the tooth into the periodontal ligament, giving rise to pain on chewing or percussion. The most common manifestation of periapical disease is the *periapical granuloma,* a localized mass of chronic granulation tissue which slowly expands at the expense of the surrounding alveolar bone. The *chronic periapical granuloma* may present the above symptoms or may be asymptomatic. If allowed to persist untreated, the periapical granuloma may give rise to a *periapical cyst* or a *periapical abscess*—all three lesions appearing as radiolucent areas on roentgenograms. The acute periapical abscess may extend into the surrounding bone marrow, resulting in an *osteomyelitis.* More frequently, the abscess perforates the cortical plate and, following the path of least resistance, spreads through various tissue spaces, giving rise to cellulitis and bacteremia, or discharges into the oral cavity, into the maxillary sinus, or through the skin.

The symptoms produced by cellulitis depend on which tissue space is affected. For example, *Ludwig's angina* originates from an infected mandibular molar, involves the submaxillary space, and subsequently extends into the sublingual and submental spaces. Clinically, this is manifested by swelling of the floor of the mouth, elevation of the tongue, and difficulty in swallowing and breathing. With continued swelling, there may be edema of the glottis, necessitating an emergency tracheotomy. Spread of the infection to the parapharyngeal spaces may lead to cavernous sinus thrombosis.

EFFECT OF SYSTEMIC FACTORS ON TEETH Systemic factors, occurring in utero or in infancy during the stages of crown formation, may influence the development and structure of the teeth. *Enamel hypoplasia* of the primary and/or permanent teeth, manifested by alterations ranging from white spots to gross defects in the surface structure of the crowns, may be caused by disturbances of calcium and phosphate metabolism such as are found in vitamin D-refractory rickets, hypoparathyroidism, gastroenteritis, and celiac disease. Premature birth or high fevers may also give rise to enamel hypoplasia. Tetracycline, given during the last half of pregnancy, infancy, and childhood up to 8 years of age, causes both a permanent discoloration of the teeth and enamel hypoplasia. Daily ingestion of more than 1.5 mg fluoride can result in enamel discoloration (mottling). Prenatal factors appear to influence crown size. Larger teeth are associated with maternal diabetes, maternal hypothyroidism, and large birth size. Tooth size is reduced in *Down's syndrome*. Premature loss of the deciduous dentition is frequently the first symptom in *juvenile hypophosphatasia*. Systemic disease may give rise to pain that simulates pulpal disease. *Maxillary sinusitis* is frequently manifested by pain in the maxillary teeth, including sensitivity to thermal changes and percussion. *Cardiac disease* with *angina pectoris* may result in referred pain to the lower jaw.

PERIODONTAL DISEASE

After the third decade chronic destructive periodontal disease *(periodontitis)* is responsible for the loss of more teeth than dental caries. It begins as a marginal inflammation of the gingivae (gingivitis), which slowly spreads to involve the underlying alveolar bone and periodontal ligament. As the disease progresses, the alveolar bone is resorbed, resulting in loss of periodontal ligament fiber attachment from the tooth to the bone. The separation of the soft tissue from the tooth surface results in "pocket" formation, the inner aspect of which bleeds readily on probing or spontaneously during chewing. Frank pus sometimes exudes from under the gingival margin, accounting for the use of the now outmoded term *pyorrhea*. With continued loss of alveolar bone the involved teeth become mobile. As the periodontal pockets deepen, the pocket orifice may become occluded, leading to the formation of a *periodontal abscess*. The prognosis for teeth with advanced bone loss, extreme mobility, and recurrent abscess formation is usually poor or hopeless, and the usual treatment is extraction.

The most important local etiologic factors associated with this disease are thought to be *poor oral hygiene,* resulting in the accumulation of grossly visible adherent masses of bacteria *(bacterial plaque),* calculus (mineralized bacterial plaque), and food impaction. The margins of overextended fillings also play a role as local irritating factors. Occlusal trauma, particularly trauma due to grinding and clenching habits, may be involved. Therapy is aimed at elimination of these factors and the development of a local environment which can be maintained in health by good oral hygiene. It appears that specific groups of organisms found subgingivally correlate with the different types and severity of periodontal disease. In advanced periodontitis, the flora is dominated by motile rods and spirochetes.

Systemic factors are thought to modify the response of the host to the local factors, but their nature is more obscure. Reduced neutrophil functions, such as chemotaxis and phagocytosis, appear to predispose to *juvenile periodontitis,* a form of periodontitis characterized by early and severe alveolar bone loss and a familial pattern of occurrence. Of possible etiologic importance is the finding that a sonic extract of *Actinobacillus actinomycetemcomitans,* a microorganism consistently isolated from patients with juvenile periodontitis, contains a leukotoxin which specifically kills human polymorphonuclear leukocytes and monocytes. *Capnocytophaga,* another organism implicated in periodontal disease, has also been reported to be associated with morphologic and functional abnormalities of neutrophils. On the other hand, patients with IgA deficiency and agammaglobulinemia have less periodontal disease and dental caries than matched immunocompetent controls. Individuals with *Down's syndrome* seem to be particularly susceptible to periodontal disease and may demonstrate advanced alveolar bone loss around the permanent mandibular incisors and maxillary first molars. Severe chronic periodontal disease may be present in uncontrolled *diabetes mellitus*. In some instances, however, there are characteristic alterations in the gingiva in response to a number of specific systemic conditions. For example, during *pregnancy* the gingiva may become edematous and friable, with a raspberry-like appearance of the interdental papillae. Occasionally, a tumorlike mass may develop in an interdental area; this usually regresses following parturition. Oral contraceptives may lead to an increase in gingival inflammation. The use of the anticonvulsant drug *phenytoin* (Dilantin) frequently results in fibrous hyperplasia of the gingiva, which may actually cover the teeth, interfere with mastication, and cause a serious aesthetic problem. A similar clinical picture, although usually more generalized and extensive, occurs in *idiopathic familial fibromatosis*. The latter condition appears to be hereditary.

A relatively common gingival disease, found predominantly in young adults, is *acute necrotizing ulcerative gingivitis* (Vincent's infection, trench mouth). This disease is characterized by tender or painful gingivae, bleeding on pressure, and the pathognomonic sign of papillary or marginal gingival necrosis and ulceration. Clinical evidence suggests that the cause of this disease has a psychosomatic component. Vincent's infection differs from *acute herpetic gingivostomatitis,* with which it is most frequently confused, because fever or malaise rarely develops, and patients respond rapidly to penicillin or broad-spectrum antibiotics.

It should be noted that both infected periapical lesions and periodontal disease provide potential sources of infection which may spread to other sites. Transient bacteremias have been demonstrated after simple massage of inflamed gingivae or use of an oral irrigative device, as well as during tooth extraction. The frequent association of tooth extraction with the subsequent occurrence of subacute bacterial endocarditis has led to the prophylactic use of antibiotics in dental patients with a history of rheumatic fever or other evidence of valvular disease. Similar precautions should be taken with dental patients having heart valve or joint prostheses. Prophylactic extraction of healthy teeth in leukemic patients is not justified.

DISEASES OF THE ORAL MUCOSA AND TONGUE

HEMATOLOGIC DISTURBANCES Oral manifestations are common in both the acute and chronic forms of all types of leukemia, particularly *monocytic leukemia*. They consist of local gingival bleeding, enlargement, and necrosis. Petechiae and ulceration of the oral mucosa may also be evident. Extensive ulcerations of the gingivae, buccal mucosa, lips, soft palate, pharynx, and tonsils may also occur in *agranulocytosis*. In thrombocytopenic states multiple petechiae, ecchymoses, and bleeding gingivae may be observed. The mucous membranes of the oral cavity, including the papillae of the tongue, are atrophic in the *Plummer-Vinson syndrome* (see Chaps. 32 and 234). As a result, the tongue is red, smooth, and sore, and there is difficulty in swallowing. Of interest is the finding that the atrophic mucous membranes have a predisposition toward the development of oral carcinoma. The oral symptoms in *pernicious anemia* are similar (see Chap. 285). Ulceration, mucositis, xerostomia, and infection (bacterial or fungal) are relatively common oral complications among patients receiving chemotherapy and/or radiotherapy for malignancies not involving the head or neck.

VITAMIN DEFICIENCIES *The oral effects of deficiency of the B group of vitamins* involve the soft tissues primarily, giving rise to reddening and ulceration of the oral mucosa and tongue, swelling and burning of the tongue, and fissuring at the corners of the lips (*angular cheilosis*). Severe vitamin C deficiency (*scurvy*) is manifested by petechiae in the oral mucosa; swollen, ulcerated, bleeding gingivae; and loosening of teeth.

PIGMENTATIONS (See Table 31-1) The spread of irregular spots or blotches or brown pigment throughout the oral mucosa, primarily the buccal mucosa, may be the first sign of *Addison's disease*. The pigmentation associated with the *Peutz-Jeghers syndrome* is readily differentiated because of its characteristic distribution around the lips, eyes, and nostrils, as well as its intraoral distribution. Both *lead poisoning* and *bismuth poisoning* may be manifested by a dark line along the gingival margin, particularly in individuals who have poor oral hygiene. Bismuth poisoning may also demonstrate pigmented patches elsewhere in the oral mucosa.

INFECTIONS See Tables 31-2 and 31-3.

DERMATOLOGIC DISEASES See Tables 31-2 and 31-3 and Chaps. 47 to 52.

TONGUE ALTERATIONS See Table 31-4.

MALODOROUS BREATH A distinctly unpleasant odor of the breath (halitosis) may emanate from any patient with *infections of the upper part of the respiratory tract,* especially in bronchiectasis and lung abscess. Halitosis may occur with oral sepsis as in *stomatitis, gingivitis,* or extensive *caries*. Some persons who smoke excessively may have halitosis. Occasionally otherwise normal persons will have halitosis without obvious cause. The primary oral sources of bad breath are inflamed periodontal pockets and the coating on the dorsoposterior surface of the tongue. A *fishy odor* of the breath is found in patients with hepatic failure (fetor hepaticus), an *ammoniacal* or *urinary odor* is found in azotemia, and a *sweet, fruity odor* is typical of diabetic ketoacidosis.

DISEASES OF THE SALIVARY GLANDS

Conditions affecting the salivary glands include mumps parotitis (Chap. 141), Mikulicz's disease, Sjögren's syndrome (Chap. 266), and sarcoidosis. Inflammation of the salivary glands (*sialadenitis*) is usually associated with the presence of a salivary stone (*sialolithiasis*) in the duct of one of the major salivary glands. The classic history of pain and swelling of the gland at mealtimes is due to the partial blockage of salivary flow by the stone. Localization of the stone may be accomplished by palpation or by roentgenograms with or without the use of an intraductal injection of radiopaque material (*sialography*). Acute or recurrent parotitis, with or without a defined microorganism, may occur in children and is marked by sudden onset of swelling of the whole gland or side of the face, accompanied by suppuration from Stensen's duct.

Xerostomia, or dryness of the mouth, is due to salivary gland dysfunction and may be temporary or permanent. Among the factors which cause temporary dryness are emotional factors (such as fear), infection of the glands, and administration of drugs such as atropine, antihistamines, or tricyclic antidepressants and phenothiazines. Radiation of the area may produce a more permanent xerostomia because of atrophy of the glands. A similar dryness may occur in Sjögren's syndrome. The dry mouth may give rise to rampant caries, particularly if sugar-containing candies are sucked in an attempt to stimulate salivary flow. Other symptoms may include disturbances in taste, difficulty in speech or swallowing, and inflammation of the oral mucosa. Altered taste (dysgeusia) may also be due to central nervous system diseases or trauma. Extensive dental caries, especially around the gum margins of the teeth, may be seen in drug addicts and alcoholics, presumably due to xerostomia and lack of oral hygiene and dental care. Xerostomia-induced caries may be prevented or arrested by the daily topical application of a 1% sodium fluoride gel. The soft tissue complications may be relieved by the utilization of an artificial saliva or by oral administration of pilocarpine.

Benign or malignant tumors may arise in the major or minor salivary glands. The benign *mixed tumor* accounts for the vast majority of all salivary gland tumors and has a relatively high recurrence rate. Malignant tumors of the parotid gland may affect the facial nerve.

ORAL CANCER

Oral cancer constitutes more than 5 percent of all human cancers. *Squamous cell carcinoma* is the most common malignant oral tumor, accounting for approximately 90 to 95 percent of all oral malignant tumors. Most of these tumors occur on the lips, primarily the lower lip, rather than intraorally. About half the intraoral tumors involve the tongue, primarily the posterior two-thirds and the lateral borders. The major etiologic factor in lip cancer appears to be exposure to intense sunlight. Predisposing factors for intraoral carcinoma include tobacco (usually in the form of cigar or pipe smoking, or snuff placed in the mucobuccal fold), excessive consumption of alcohol, syphilitic glossitis, and the atrophic mucosa of the Plummer-Vinson syndrome. Although numerous instances of carcinoma of the tongue adjacent to a sharp tooth or dental appliance have been reported, animal studies with chronic irritation per se, as well as epidemiologic studies, cast doubt on this apparent relationship. The most common *precancerous lesion* in the oral cavity is *leukoplakia,* a whitish patch on the mucosa that histologically shows hyperkeratosis, acanthosis, and dyskeratosis.

TABLE 31-1 Pigmented lesions of the oral mucosa

Condition	Usual location	Clinical features	Course
Black, hairy tongue	Dorsum of tongue	Elongation of filiform papillae of tongue, which take on a brown to black coloration	Long-lasting but may disappear spontaneously
Heavy metal pigmentation (bismuth, mercury, lead)	Gingival margin	Thin blue-black pigmented line along gingival margin due to prior treatment for syphilis with bismuth or mercury or from accidental absorption of lead	Long-lasting
Drug ingestion (tranquilizers, oral contraceptives, antimalarials)	Any area in mouth	Brown, black, or gray areas of pigmentation	Disappears following cessation of drug
Amalgam tattoo	Gingiva and mucobuccal fold	Small blue-black pigmented areas associated with embedded amalgam particles in soft tissues; these will show up on radiographs as radiopaque particles	Remains indefinitely
Fordyce's disease	Buccal and labial mucosa	Aggregation of numerous, small yellowish spots just beneath mucosal surface; no subjective symptoms	Remains without apparent change indefinitely
Addison's disease	Any area in mouth but mostly on buccal mucosa	Blotches or spots of bluish-black to dark-brown pigmentation occurring early in the disease, accompanied by diffuse pigmentation of skin; other symptoms of adrenal insufficiency	Condition controlled by steroid therapy
Peutz-Jeghers syndrome	Any area in mouth	Dark brown spots on lips, buccal mucosa, and palate with characteristic distribution of pigment around lips, nose, eyes, and on hands; concomitant intestinal polyposis	Lesions remaining indefinitely
Malignant melanoma	Any area in mouth	May appear as a raised, painless, brown-black lesion or may be amelanotic; may be ulcerated and infected	Early metastasis leading to death

TABLE 31-2 Vesicular, bullous, or ulcerative lesions of the oral mucosa

Condition	Usual location	Clinical features	Course
VIRAL DISEASES			
Acute herpetic gingivostomatitis (herpes simplex, type 1)	Lip and oral mucosa	Labial vesicles which rupture and crust, and intraoral vesicles which quickly ulcerate; extremely painful to pressure; acute gingivitis, fever, malaise, foul odor, and cervical lymphadenopathy; occurs primarily in infants and children	Heals spontaneously in 10–14 days unless secondarily infected
Recurrent herpes labialis	Mucocutaneous junction of lip	Eruption of groups of vesicles which may coalesce, then rupture and crust; painful to pressure or spicy foods	Lasts about 1 week, but condition may be prolonged if secondary infection occurs
Primary herpes, type 2	Mouth, oral pharynx, and genitalia	Large, painful, discrete vesicles on zone of erythema; anterior cervical glands enlarged	Lasts several weeks; may recur
Herpangina (coxsackievirus A; also possibly coxsackievirus B and echovirus)	Oral mucosa, pharynx, tongue	Sudden onset of fever, sore throat, and oropharyngeal vesicles usually in children under 4 years, during summer months; diffuse pharyngeal injection and vesicles (1–2 mm), grayish white surrounded by red areola; vesicles enlarge and ulcerate	Incubation period 2–9 days; fever for 1–4 days; recovery uneventful
Hand, foot, and mouth disease (type A coxsackieviruses)	Oral mucosa, pharynx, palms, and soles	Fever, malaise, headache with oropharyngeal vesicles which become painful, shallow ulcers	Incubation period 2–18 days; lesions heal spontaneously in 2–4 weeks
Chickenpox	Gingiva and oral mucosa	Skin lesions may be accompanied by small vesicles on oral mucosa that rupture to form shallow ulcers; may coalesce to form large bullous lesions that ulcerate; mucosa may have generalized erythema	Lesions heal spontaneously within 2 weeks
Herpes zoster	Cheek, tongue, gingiva, or palate	Unilateral vesicular eruption and ulceration in linear pattern following sensory distribution of trigeminal nerve	Gradual healing without scarring
Infectious mononucleosis	Oral mucosa	Fatigue, sore throat, malaise, low-grade fever, and enlarged cervical lymph nodes; numerous small ulcers usually appear several days before lymphadenopathy; gingival bleeding and multiple petechiae at junction of hard and soft palates	Oral lesions disappear during convalescence
Warts	Any place on skin and oral mucosa, primarily lips and vestibule	Single or multiple papillary lesions, with thick, white, keratinized surfaces containing many pointed projections	Lesions grow rapidly and spread
BACTERIAL OR FUNGAL DISEASES			
Acute necrotizing ulcerative gingivitis (''trench mouth,'' Vincent's infection)	Gingiva	Painful, bleeding gingiva characterized by necrosis and ulceration of gingival papillae and margins plus lymphadenopathy and foul odor	Continued destruction of tissue followed by remission, but may recur
Prenatal (congenital) syphilis	Palate, jaws, tongue, and teeth	Gummatous involvement of palate, jaws, and facial bones; Hutchinson's incisors, mulberry molars, glossitis, mucous patches, and fissures of corners of mouth	Tooth deformities in permanent dentition irreversible
Primary syphilis (chancre)	Lesion appears where organism enters body; may occur on lips, tongue, or tonsillar area	Small papule developing rapidly into a large, painless ulcer with indurated border; unilateral lymphadenopathy; chancre and lymph nodes containing spirochetes; serologic tests positive by third to fourth weeks	Healing of chancre in 1–2 months, followed by secondary syphilis in 6–8 weeks
Secondary syphilis	Oral mucosa frequently involved with mucous patches, primarily on palate but also at commissures of mouth	Maculopapular lesions of oral mucosa, about 5–10 mm in diameter with central ulceration covered by grayish membrane; eruptions occurring on various mucosal surfaces and skin accompanied by fever, malaise, and sore throat	Lesions may persist from several weeks to a year
Tertiary syphilis	Palate and tongue	Gummatous infiltration of palate or tongue followed by ulceration and fibrosis; atrophy of tongue papillae may produce characteristic bald tongue and glossitis	Gumma may destroy palate, causing complete perforation
Gonorrhea	Lesions may occur in mouth at site of inoculation or secondarily by hematogenous spread from a primary focus elsewhere	Earliest symptoms are burning or itching sensation, dryness, or heat in mouth followed by acute pain on eating or speaking; tonsils and oropharynx most frequently involved; oral tissues may be diffusely inflamed or ulcerated; saliva develops increased viscosity and fetid odor; submaxillary lymphadenopathy with fever in severe cases	Lesions resolve with appropriate antibiotic therapy
Tuberculosis	Tongue, tonsillar area, soft palate	A solitary, irregular ulcer covered by a persistent exudate; ulcer has an undermined, indurated border	Lesion may persist
Cervicofacial actinomycosis	Swellings in region of face, neck, and floor of mouth	Infection may be associated with an extraction, jaw fracture, or eruption of molar tooth; in acute form resembles an acute pyogenic abscess, but contains yellow ''sulfur granules'' (gram-positive mycelia and their hyphae)	Acute form may last a few weeks; chronic form lasts months or years; prognosis excellent; actinomycetes respond to antibiotics (tetracyclines or penicillin) but not to antifungal drugs
Histoplasmosis	Any area in mouth, particularly tongue, gingiva, or palate	Numerous small nodules which may ulcerate; hoarseness and dysphagia may occur because of lesions in larynx, usually associated with fever and malaise	May be fatal

TABLE 31-2 Vesicular, bullous, or ulcerative lesions of the oral mucosa *(Continued)*

Condition	Usual location	Clinical features	Course
DERMATOLOGIC DISEASES			
Mucous membrane pemphigoid	Primarily mucous membranes of the oral cavity, but may also involve the eyes, urethra, vagina, and rectum	Painful, grayish white collapsed vesicles or bullae with peripheral erythematous zone; gingival lesions desquamate, leaving ulcerated area	Protracted course with remissions and exacerbations; involvement of different sites occurs slowly; corticosteroids may control severe cases
Erythema multiforme (Stevens-Johnson syndrome)	Primarily the oral mucosa and skin of hands and feet	Intraoral ruptured bullae surrounded by an inflammatory area; lips may show hemorrhagic crusts; the "iris," or "target" lesion, on the skin is pathognomonic; patient may have severe signs of toxicity	Onset very rapid; condition may last 1–2 weeks; may be fatal
Pemphigus vulgaris	Oral mucosa and skin	Ruptured bullae and ulcerated oral areas; mostly in older adults	With repeated recurrence of bullae, toxicity may lead to cachexia, infection, and death within 2 years
NEOPLASTIC DISEASES			
Squamous cell carcinoma	Any area in mouth, most commonly on lower lip, tongue, and floor of mouth	Ulcer with elevated, indurated border; failure to heal, pain not prominent; lesions tend to arise in areas of leukoplakia or in smooth or atrophic tongue	Invades and destroys underlying tissues or may metastasize to regional lymph nodes
Acute leukemia	Gingiva	Gingival swelling and superficial ulcerations followed by hyperplasia of gingiva with extensive necrosis and hemorrhage; deep ulcers may occur elsewhere on the mucosa complicated by secondary infection	Fatal
Lymphoma	Gingiva, palate, tongue, and tonsillar area	Elevated, ulcerated area which may proliferate rapidly, giving the appearance of a traumatic inflammatory lesion; swelling of regional lymph nodes	Fatal
Metastatic tumors	Deep in jaw bone, usually in premolar-molar area of mandible	May arise from carcinoma of distant organ, such as breast, lung, or kidney; advanced lesion may expand and destroy bone, loosen and spread teeth, involve inferior alveolar nerve, cause pain and numbness of lower lip	Fatal
OTHER CONDITIONS			
Recurrent aphthous stomatitis	Any place on oral mucosa	Single or clusters of painful ulcers with surrounding erythematous border, found anywhere on mucosa; lesions may be 1–15 mm in diameter	Lesions heal in 1–2 weeks but may recur monthly or several times a year. Topical corticosteroid ointments give symptomatic relief in mild cases. Systemic corticosteroids are used in severe cases. A tetracycline oral suspension may decrease ulcer severity.
Behçet's syndrome	Oral mucosa, eyes, and genitalia	Multiple aphthouslike ulcers in mouth; inflammatory ocular changes and ulcerative lesions on genitalia	Ulcers may persist for several weeks and heal without scarring
Traumatic ulcers	Any place on oral mucosa; dentures frequently responsible for ulcers in vestibule	Localized, discrete ulcerated lesion with red border; produced by accidental biting of mucosa, penetration by a foreign object, or chronic irritation by a denture	Lesion usually heals in 7–10 days when irritant is removed, unless secondarily infected

TABLE 31-3 White lesions of oral mucosa

Condition	Usual location	Clinical features	Course
Pachyderma oralis	Any area in mouth	Elevated white lesion due to hyperkeratosis and thickening of the oral epithelium secondary to chronic irritation	Removal of irritant leads to healing in 2–3 weeks
Leukoplakia	Any area in mouth	White patch or raised plaque with sharply defined borders; in more severe cases the lesion is indurated and rough, and may be fissured and eroded; pain not present in early lesions	Carcinoma frequently arises in the more severe type of lesion
Lichen planus	Any area in mouth but most often on buccal mucosa	Varied appearance of lesion due to arrangement of grayish-white papules which coalesce to make up the pattern; a reticular network is most common; oral lesions may precede skin lesions; lichenoid lesions may be drug-induced	May disappear spontaneously
Candidiasis (moniliasis, thrush)	Any area in mouth	Creamy white curdlike patches which reveal a raw, bleeding surface when scraped; found in sick infants, debilitated elderly patients, patients receiving high doses of corticosteroids or broad-spectrum antibiotics, or in patients with acquired immunodeficiency syndrome (AIDS)	Responds favorably to antifungal therapy after correction of predisposing causes
Chemical burns	Any area in mouth	White slough due to necrosis of epithelium and underlying connective tissue caused by contact with agents (e.g., aspirin) applied locally or the use of undiluted sodium perborate or hydrogen peroxide as a mouthwash; removal of slough leaves a raw, painful surface	Lesion heals in several weeks if not secondarily infected

Nodular leukoplakias have a much higher potential for malignant transformation than homogeneous leukoplakias. Recent evidence suggests that the asymptomatic, red velvety (erythroplastic) lesion of the floor of the mouth, ventrolateral aspect of the tongue, or soft palate–anterior pillar complex is more likely to be carcinoma in situ or invasive carcinoma than is the white lesion. *All chronic ulcerative lesions which fail to heal within 1 to 2 weeks should be considered potentially malignant* and must be biopsied in order to make the definitive diagnosis. It is noteworthy that in their early stages intraoral epidermoid carcinomas are rarely painful, in contrast to similar-appearing inflammatory lesions.

The prognosis for patients with carcinoma of the lip is usually good, since these malignant tumors are noted sooner and apparently metastasize later. Patients with carcinoma of the tongue have a poorer prognosis, particularly as the tumor occurs more posteriorly on the tongue. Intraoral carcinomas may spread by direct invasion to the underlying bone. Depending on the site of origin of the intraoral carcinoma, metastases usually spread to the submaxillary or cervical lymph nodes. Death may result from recurrent or uncontrollable disease above the clavicles; metastatic disease beyond the neck; treatment complications; or a second primary cancer, usually in the oral cavity or the upper parts of the gastrointestinal or respiratory tract. Metastatic tumors to the jaw may occur from carcinomas of the lung, breast, kidney, or gastrointestinal tract.

NEUROLOGIC DISTURBANCES

A number of neurologic disturbances have a direct effect on oral and paraoral structures. *Trigeminal neuralgia* (tic douloureux) is an example of a syndrome involving the trigeminal nerve. It is characterized by extremely severe, unilateral, lancinating pain of the face occurring spontaneously or set off by pressure on a "trigger zone" on the face (see Chap. 352). In some cases of idiopathic trigeminal neuralgia, dental and oral pathoses, primarily in the form of jawbone cavities at sites of previous extractions, may be major etiologic factors. Facial palsy is a unilateral disturbance of the motor branch of the facial nerve due to either trauma, surgical sectioning, or tumor involvement. When it is of acute onset and unknown cause, possibly a localized infection in the nerve, it is called *Bell's palsy*. It may be due to cranial herpes zoster in some instances. The condition is manifested by drooping of the corner of the mouth, inability to close the eye on the same side, and difficulty in speech and eating. In mild cases the symptoms may disappear spontaneously within a month. Alteration in taste sensation in the anterior two-thirds of the tongue due to disturbance of the sensory component of the facial nerve occurs in some cases and indicates a more central location of the lesion in the nerve (see Chap. 352). Taste acuity declines with age for salty and bitter, but not for sour and sweet. This change may be associated in part with the number of missing teeth and the size of any artificial prosthesis used, thereby influencing food preferences, palatability, intake, and nutritional status of the elderly.

The pain associated with the *glossopharyngeal neuralgia syndrome* is similar in type and intensity to that found in trigeminal neuralgia, being set off by a trigger zone in the pharynx and affecting the posterior region of the tongue, pharynx, soft palate, and ear. Disturbance of the hypoglossal nerve leads to dysfunction of the tongue musculature and atrophy. Bilateral nerve involvement prevents protrusion of the tongue; unilateral involvement leads to deviation of the protruded tongue toward the affected side.

TABLE 31-4 Alterations of the tongue

Type of change	Clinical features
SIZE OR MORPHOLOGY CHANGES	
Macroglossia	Enlarged tongue which may be part of a syndrome found in developmental conditions such as Down's syndrome; may be due to tumor (hemangioma or lymphangioma), metabolic disease (such as primary amyloidosis), or endocrine disturbance (such as acromegaly or cretinism)
Fissured ("scrotal") tongue	Dorsal surface and sides of tongue covered by painless shallow or deep fissures which may collect debris and become irritated
Median rhomboid glossitis	Congenital abnormality of tongue with ovoid, denuded area in the median posterior portion of the tongue
COLOR CHANGES	
"Geographic" tongue ("wandering rash")	Asymptomatic inflammatory condition of the tongue, with rapid loss and regrowth of filiform papillae, leading to appearance of denuded red patches "wandering" across the surface of the tongue
Hairy tongue	Elongation of filiform papillae of the medial dorsal surface area due to failure of keratin layer of the papillae to desquamate normally; brownish-black coloration may be due to staining by tobacco, food, or chromogenic organisms
"Strawberry" and "raspberry" tongue	Appearance of tongue during scarlet fever due to the hypertrophy of fungiform papillae plus changes in the filiform papillae
"Bald" tongue	Complete atrophy of papillae which may occur in pernicious anemia, severe iron-deficiency anemia, pellagra, or syphilis; may be accompanied by painful, burning sensations

DISTURBANCES OF THE TEMPOROMANDIBULAR JOINT

Pain in the area of the temporomandibular joint frequently causes the patient to seek therapy. It may be due to posterior displacement of the condyle in the fossa leading to displacement of the meniscus and chronic trauma. *Dislocation of the condyle anteriorly* beyond the articular eminence due to sudden stretching or tearing of the capsular ligament may result in a locking of the mandible in an open position. In *osteoarthritis* the clinical signs and symptoms may be minimal despite extensive changes in the condyle. Temporomandibular joint involvement occurs less frequently in *rheumatoid arthritis*. When affected, the joints are swollen and painful, leading to limitation of movement, particularly on arising in the morning. In children the disease may lead to malocclusion. *Ankylosis* of the joint may occur eventually, necessitating a condylectomy (see Chap. 263).

The myofascial pain syndrome, the most common disorder of the temporomandibular joint, is characterized by facial pain and mandibular dysfunction in the absence of clinical or radiologic evidence of organic disease. The pain is often localized in the ear or jaw and may extend to the neck and shoulder. The mandibular dysfunction is manifested by limitation of movement, particularly an inability to open the jaw to the fullest extent. It is thought that such patients have increased musculature tension and hyperexcitable reflexes related to emotional tension. The precipitating factor appears to be the stretching of an abnormal focus of pain which initiates a self-sustaining pain-spasm-pain cycle. Treatment of the pain-dysfunction syndrome involves emotional support, stress reduction, and the use of drugs to relieve the pain, lessen cortical excitability, and relax the muscles. Local heat therapy, elimination of gross occlusal discrepancies, and jaw-opening exercises are also used. Local anesthetics are used intramuscularly in the region of the trigger zone or as superficial sprays in an attempt to break the pain-spasm-pain cycle.

REFERENCES

BEITMAN RG: Oral manifestations of gastrointestinal disease. Dig Dis Sci 26:741, 1981

GOLDMAN HS, MARDER MZ: *Physician's Guide to Disease of the Oral Cavity*. Oradell, NJ, Medical Economics, 1982

LYNCH MA et al: *Burket's Oral Medicine, Diagnosis, and Treatment*, 8th ed. Philadelphia, Lippincott, 1984

ROSE LF, KAYE D: *Internal Medicine for Dentistry*. St. Louis, Mosby, 1983

SHAFER WG et al: *A Textbook of Oral Pathology*, 4th ed. Philadelphia, Saunders, 1983
SHKLAR G: *Oral Cancer: The Diagnosis, Therapy, Management, and Rehabilitation of the Oral Cancer Patient*. Philadelphia, Saunders, 1984
SONIS ST et al: *Principles and Practice of Oral Medicine*. Philadelphia, Saunders, 1984
WOOD NK, GOAZ PW: *Differential Diagnosis of Oral Lesions*. St. Louis, Mosby, 1980

32 DYSPHAGIA

RAJ K. GOYAL

Dysphagia is defined as a sensation of "sticking" or obstruction of the passage of food through the mouth, pharynx, or the esophagus.

Dysphagia should be distinguished from other symptoms related to swallowing. *Aphagia* signifies complete esophageal obstruction which is usually due to bolus impaction and represents a medical emergency. *Difficulty in initiating a swallow* occurs in disorders of the voluntary phase of swallowing. Once initiated, however, swallowing is completed normally. *Odynophagia* means painful swallowing. Frequently, odynophagia and dysphagia occur together. *Globus hystericus* is the sensation of a lump lodged in the throat. No difficulty, however, is encountered when actual swallowing is performed. *Phagophobia,* meaning fear of swallowing, and *refusal to swallow* may occur in hysteria, rabies, tetanus, and pharyngeal paralysis due to fear of aspiration. Painful inflammatory lesions that cause odynophagia may also cause refusal to swallow. Some patients may feel the food as it goes down the esophagus. This esophageal sensitivity is not associated with sticking of the food or obstruction, however. Similarly, the *feeling of fullness in the epigastrium* that occurs after a meal or after swallowing air should not be confused with dysphagia.

PHYSIOLOGY OF SWALLOWING The process of swallowing begins with a voluntary (oral) phase during which a bolus of food is pushed backward into the pharynx. The bolus activates oropharyngeal sensory receptors which initiate the involuntary (pharyngeal and esophageal) phase, or deglutition reflex. The deglutition reflex is a complex series of events which serves both to propel food through the pharynx and the esophagus and to prevent its entry into the airway. At the same time as the bolus is propelled backward by the tongue, the larynx moves forward and the upper esophageal sphincter opens. As the bolus moves into the pharynx, contraction of the superior pharyngeal constrictor against the contracted soft palate initiates a peristaltic contraction that proceeds rapidly downward to move the bolus through the pharynx and the esophagus. The lower esophageal sphincter opens as the food enters the esophagus and remains open until the peristaltic contraction has swept the bolus into the stomach. Peristaltic contraction in response to a swallow involves the entire swallowing passages and is called *primary peristalsis*. Local distention of the esophagus due to food activates intramural reflexes in the smooth muscle which result in *secondary peristalsis,* limited to the lower esophagus. *Tertiary contractions* are nonperistaltic as they occur simultaneously over a long segment of the esophagus. Tertiary contractions may occur in response to a swallow or esophageal distention, or they may occur spontaneously.

PATHOPHYSIOLOGY OF DYSPHAGIA The normal transport of an ingested bolus through the swallowing passage depends on (1) the size of the ingested bolus, (2) the luminal diameter of the swallowing passage, (3) the peristaltic contraction, and (4) deglutitive inhibition, which includes normal relaxation of upper and lower esophageal sphincters during swallowing and inhibition of persisting contractions in the esophageal body, for example, due to an immediately preceding swallow. Dysphagia caused by a large bolus or luminal narrowing is called *mechanical dysphagia,* while dysphagia due to incoordination or weakness of peristaltic contractions or to impaired deglutitive inhibition is called *motor dysphagia*.

Mechanical dysphagia Mechanical dysphagia could be caused by luminal factors, intrinsic narrowing or extrinsic compression of the lumen. In an adult, the esophageal lumen can distend to a diameter of well over 4 cm because of the elasticity of the esophageal wall. When the esophagus cannot dilate to more than 2.5 cm in diameter, dysphagia can occur, but it is always present when it cannot distend beyond 1.3 cm. Circumferential lesions produce dysphagia more consistently than eccentric lesions. Eccentric benign tumors and lesions causing extrinsic compression cause dysphagia infrequently. The causes of mechanical dysphagia are listed in Table 32-1. Common causes are carcinoma, peptic and other benign strictures, and lower esophageal ring.

Motor dysphagia Motor dysphagia may result from difficulty in initiating a swallow or abnormalities in peristalsis and deglutitive inhibition due to diseases of the esophageal skeletal or smooth muscle.

Diseases of the skeletal muscle involve the pharynx, upper esophageal sphincter, and the upper part of the esophagus. The striated muscle is innervated by a somatic component of the vagus with cell bodies of the lower motor neurons located in the nucleus ambiguus. These neurons are cholinergic and excitatory and are the sole determinant of the muscle activity. Peristalsis in the skeletal muscle segment is due to sequential central activation of neurons innervating muscles at different levels. Motor dysphagia of the pharynx results from neuromuscular disorders causing muscle paralysis, simultaneous nonperistaltic contraction, or loss of opening of

TABLE 32-1 Causes of mechanical dysphagia

I Luminal
- *A* Large bolus
- *B* Foreign body

II Intrinsic narrowing
- *A* Inflammatory condition causing edema and swelling
  - *1* Stomatitis
  - *2* Pharyngitis, epiglottitis
  - *3* Esophagitis (e.g., viral, monilial)
- *B* Webs
  - *1* Pharyngeal (Plummer-Vinson syndrome)
  - *2* Esophageal
- *C* Lower esophageal ring
  - *1* Mucosal ring (Schatzki ring)
- *D* Benign strictures
  - *1* Peptic
  - *2* Caustic and drug-induced
  - *3* Inflammatory (Crohn's disease, moniliasis, epidermolysis bullosa)
  - *4* Ischemic
  - *5* Postoperative, postirradiation
  - *6* Congenital
- *E* Malignant tumors
  - *1* Primary carcinoma
    - *a* Squamous cell carcinoma
    - *b* Adenocarcinoma
    - *c* Carcinosarcoma
    - *d* Pseudosarcoma
    - *e* Lymphoma
    - *f* Melanoma
  - *2* Metastatic carcinoma
- *F* Benign tumors
  - *1* Leiomyoma
  - *2* Lipoma
  - *3* Angioma
  - *4* Inflammatory fibroid polyp
  - *5* Epithelial papilloma

III Extrinsic compression
- *A* Cervical spondylitis
- *B* Vertebral osteophytes
- *C* Retropharyngeal abscess and masses
- *D* Enlarged thyroid gland
- *E* Zenker's diverticulum
- *F* Vascular compression
  - *1* Aberrant right subclavian artery
  - *2* Right-sided aorta
  - *3* Left atrial enlargement
  - *4* Aortic aneurysm
- *G* Posterior mediastinal masses
- *H* Pancreatic tumor, pancreatitis
- *I* Postvagotomy hematoma and fibrosis

NOTE: *Some lesions can occur anywhere along the swallowing passages while others occur in a specific location.*

the upper esophageal sphincter. Loss of opening of the upper sphincter is caused by paralysis of geniohyoid and other suprahyoid muscles or loss of deglutitive inhibition of the cricopharyngeus muscle. Because each side of the pharynx is innervated by ipsilateral nerves, a lesion of motor neurons occurring only on one side leads to unilateral pharyngeal paralysis. Although lesions of skeletal muscle also involve the upper part of the esophagus, the clinical manifestations of pharyngeal dysfunction usually overshadow the manifestations due to esophageal involvement.

Diseases of the smooth muscle segment involve the lower part of the esophagus and the lower esophageal sphincter. This smooth muscle is innervated by the parasympathetic component of the vagal preganglionic fibers and postganglionic noncholinergic neurons in the myenteric ganglia. These nerves exert a predominantly inhibitory influence on the lower esophageal sphincter and cause inhibition followed by contraction in the esophageal body. Peristalsis in this segment is due to neuromuscular mechanisms in the wall of the esophagus itself. Dysphagia results when the peristaltic contractions are weak or nonperistaltic or when the lower sphincter fails to open normally. Loss of contractile power occurs due to muscle weakness, as in scleroderma, or to loss of myenteric neurons, as in achalasia. The cause of simultaneous onset of contractions, typically seen in diffuse esophageal spasm, is not understood. Impairment of deglutitive inhibition of the lower esophageal sphincter is associated with a defect in inhibitory nerves to the sphincter and is the major cause of dysphagia in achalasia.

The causes of motor dysphagia are listed in Table 32-2. The important causes are achalasia, diffuse esophageal spasm and related motor disorders, pharyngeal paralysis, cricopharyngeal achalasia, and scleroderma of the esophagus.

TABLE 32-2 Causes of motor (neuromuscular) dysphagia

I Difficulty in initiating swallowing reflex
- *A* Oral lesions and paralysis of tongue
- *B* Oropharyngeal anesthesia
- *C* Lack of saliva
- *D* Lesions of sensory components of vagus and glossopharyngeal nerves
- *E* Lesions of swallowing center

II Disorders of pharyngeal and esophageal skeletal muscle
- *A* Muscle weakness
  - *1* Lower motor neuron lesion (bulbar paralysis)
    - *a* Cerebrovascular accident
    - *b* Motor neuron disease
    - *c* Poliomyelitis
    - *d* Polyneuritis
    - *e* Amyotrophic lateral sclerosis
    - *f* Familial dysautonomia
  - *2* Neuromuscular
    - *a* Myasthenia gravis
  - *3* Muscle disorders
    - *a* Polymyositis
    - *b* Dermatomyositis
    - *c* Myopathies (myotonic dystrophy, oculopharyngeal myopathy)
- *B* Simultaneous onset contractions or impaired deglutitive inhibition
  - *1* Pharynx and upper esophagus
    - *a* Rabies
    - *b* Stiff-man syndrome
    - *c* Extrapyramidal tract disease
    - *d* Upper motor neuron lesions (pseudobulbar paralysis)
  - *2* Upper esophageal sphincter (UES)
    - *a* Paralysis of suprahyoid muscles (causes same as paralysis of pharyngeal musculature)
    - *b* Cricopharyngeal achalasia

III Disorders of esophageal smooth muscle
- *A* Paralysis of esophageal body causing weak contractions
  - *1* Scleroderma and related collagen vascular diseases
  - *2* Myotonic dystrophy
  - *3* Metabolic neuromyopathy (amyloid, alcohol?, diabetes?)
  - *4* Achalasia (classical)
- *B* Simultaneous-onset contractions or impaired deglutitive inhibition
  - *1* Esophageal body
    - *a* Diffuse esophageal spasm
    - *b* Achalasia (vigorous)
    - *c* Variants of diffuse esophageal spasm
  - *2* Lower esophageal sphincter (LES)
    - *a* Achalasia
      - *(1)* Primary
      - *(2)* Secondary
        - *(a)* Chagas' disease
        - *(b)* Carcinoma
        - *(c)* Lymphoma
        - *(d)* Intestinal pseudoobstruction syndrome
        - *(e)* Toxins and drugs
        - *(f)* Irradiation
    - *b* Lower esophageal muscular (contractile) ring

APPROACH TO THE PATIENT WITH DYSPHAGIA **History** The history can provide a correct presumptive diagnosis in over 80 percent of patients. The type of food causing dysphagia provides useful information. Difficulty only with solids implies mechanical dysphagia with a lumen that is not severely narrowed. The impacted bolus may be forced through the narrowed area by drinking liquids. In advanced obstruction dysphagia occurs with liquids as well as solids. In contrast, motor dysphagia due to achalasia and diffuse esophageal spasm is equally affected by solids and liquids from the very onset. Patients with scleroderma have dysphagia to solids that is unrelated to posture and to liquids in the recumbent but not in the upright posture. When peptic stricture develops in these patients dysphagia becomes more persistent.

The duration and course of dysphagia are helpful in diagnosis. Transient dysphagia of short duration may be due to an inflammatory process. Progressive dysphagia of a few weeks' to a few months' duration is suggestive of carcinoma of the esophagus. Episodic dysphagia to solids of several years' duration indicates a benign disease and is characteristic of a lower esophageal ring.

The localization of dysphagia is helpful when it is described in the chest, where the site of dysphagia generally correlates with the site of esophageal obstruction. However, localization of dysphagia to the neck is of no diagnostic value because lesions of the pharynx, cervical esophagus, and even lower esophagus may cause dysphagia to be perceived in the neck.

Associated symptoms provide important diagnostic clues. Nasal regurgitation and tracheobronchial aspiration with swallowing are hallmarks of pharyngeal paralysis or a tracheoesophageal fistula. Tracheobronchial aspiration unrelated to swallowing may be secondary to achalasia, a Zenker's diverticulum, or gastroesophageal reflux. Severe weight loss out of proportion to the degree of dysphagia is highly suggestive of carcinoma. When hoarseness precedes dysphagia, the primary lesion is usually in the larynx. Hoarseness following dysphagia may suggest involvement of the recurrent laryngeal nerve by extension of esophageal carcinoma beyond the walls of the esophagus. Sometimes hoarseness may be due to laryngitis secondary to gastroesophageal reflux. Association of laryngeal symptoms and dysphagia also occurs in various neuromuscular disorders. Hiccups suggest a lesion in the distal portion of the esophagus. Unilateral wheezing with dysphagia indicates a mediastinal mass involving the esophagus and a large bronchus. Chest pain with dysphagia occurs in diffuse esophageal spasm and in related motor disorders. Chest pain resembling diffuse esophageal spasms also may occur in acute aphagia due to a large bolus. A prolonged history of heartburn and reflux preceding dysphagia indicates peptic stricture. Similarly, a history of prolonged nasogastric intubation, ingestion of caustic agents, previous radiation therapy, or associated mucocutaneous diseases may provide the cause of esophageal stricture. If odynophagia is present, monilial or herpes esophagitis should be suspected, particularly in debilitated patients with carcinoma or those receiving immunosuppressive therapy.

Physical examination Physical examination is important in motor dysphagia due to skeletal muscle, neurologic, and oropharyngeal diseases. Signs of bulbar or pseudobulbar palsy, including dysarthria, dysphonia, ptosis, tongue atrophy, and hyperactive jaw jerk, in addition to evidence of generalized neuromuscular disease, should be carefully searched for. The neck should be examined for thyromegaly or a spinal abnormality. A careful inspection of the mouth and pharynx should disclose lesions that may cause interference with passage of food from the mouth or esophagus because of pain or obstruction. Changes in the skin and extremities may suggest a diagnosis of scleroderma and other collagen vascular diseases, or mucocutaneous diseases such as pemphigoid or epidermolysis bullosa which may involve the esophagus. Metastatic diseases to lymph nodes and liver may be evident. Pulmonary complications of acute aspiration pneumonia or chronic aspiration may be present.

Diagnostic procedures Dysphagia is one of the major symptoms of esophageal disease, and a cause for this symptom can invariably be determined. Therefore, all patients with dysphagia must be thoroughly investigated until a specific cause is determined. This is particularly important because the treatment depends upon the underlying cause of dysphagia. Barium swallow with cineradiography, esophagogastroscopy with biopsy and exfoliative cytology, and esophageal motility study are the main diagnostic procedures (see Chap. 234).

REFERENCES

CASTELL DO, JOHNSON LF (eds): *Esophageal Function in Health and Disease*. New York, Elsevier Biomedical, 1983

ENTERLINE H, THOMPSON, J: *Pathology of the Esophagus*. New York, Springer-Verlag, 1984

GIDDA JS, GOYAL RK: Regional gradient of initial inhibition and refractoriness in esophageal smooth muscle. Gastroenterology 89:843, 1985

GOYAL RK, COBB BW: Motility of pharynx, esophagus and esophageal sphincter, in *Physiology of the Gastrointestinal Tract*, LR Johnson (ed). New York, Raven Press, 1981, pp 359–391

SCHULZE-DELNIEU K, CHRISTENSEN J: The esophagus, in *The Gastroenterology Annual*, F Kern, A Blum (eds). New York, Elsevier Science, 1984, pp 1–28

33 INDIGESTION

LAWRENCE S. FRIEDMAN / KURT J. ISSELBACHER

Indigestion, or *dyspepsia*, is a term frequently used by patients to describe a variety of symptoms generally appreciated as distress associated with the intake of food. The term is nonspecific and may not have the same meaning for the patient and physician. Thus, in approaching the patient with indigestion, it is important for the physician first to elicit a precise description of this complaint. To some patients indigestion refers to actual abdominal pain, pressure, or heartburn. Others may use the term to describe a sense of abdominal fullness or a vague feeling that digestion has not proceeded naturally. Still others may use it to describe belching, a feeling of excessive gas, or flatulence. These complaints are considered in this chapter. Discussed elsewhere are the closely related symptoms of dysphagia, anorexia, and nausea and vomiting (Chaps. 32 and 34).

After having ascertained the patient's definition of indigestion, it is important to determine (1) the location and duration of the discomfort, (2) the temporal relation of the symptoms to the ingestion of food, and (3) the possible relation of the symptoms to the ingestion of specific types of food (e.g., milk, fatty foods) or drugs.

Indigestion may occur in association with diseases of the gastrointestinal tract or pathologic states in other organ systems. As a result of a systematic clinical and laboratory investigation, a definable pathophysiologic process often can be shown to be responsible for the symptoms in a given case of indigestion. Frequently, however, a clear etiologic explanation for the patient's complaint of indigestion is not established. Such cases are often designated as "functional indigestion," with a strong implication that psychosomatic factors underlie the complaint. Although it is clear that psychological factors may lead to symptoms of indigestion, the designation of "functional indigestion" is rarely a satisfactory explanation, serving only to rephrase the patient's description of the symptoms. Moreover, on the basis of electrophysiologic studies of the intestine it appears likely that some cases of functional indigestion result from subtle disturbances of gastrointestinal motility. Indeed, some patients with functional indigestion also have other features of the irritable bowel syndrome, suggesting a diffuse motility disturbance of the gastrointestinal tract (see Chap. 239).

SYNDROMES COMMONLY DESCRIBED AS INDIGESTION

PAIN Pain patterns A careful elucidation of the pattern of pain may provide important diagnostic information. True visceral abdominal pain is mediated by visceral afferent nerves which accompany the abdominal sympathetic pathways (see Chap. 5). Visceral pain is generally described as dull and aching in nature, with a diffuse midline localization, or as fullness or pressure. The location of the discomfort corresponds generally to the segmental level of neural innervation of the affected organ. Abdominal visceral pain can be produced experimentally by artificially increasing pressure in a hollow viscus. Usually this pain is the result of distention or exaggerated muscular contraction of a viscus. Inflammation generally lowers the threshold for pain from such stimuli.

The visceral pain of indigestion should be distinguished from the sharp, localized pain patterns of many acute abdominal processes involving the peritoneum. In contrast to true visceral pain, this pain is mediated by cerebrospinal afferent nerves.

In view of the diffuse nature of true visceral abdominal pain, the main clue to the cause comes from the *location of the pain* and the corresponding segmental level of neural innervation; however, in any given segmental region there is no way of determining which of several viscera is the source of the pain (Table 33-1). The following rules, already described in Chap. 5, are useful: *Substernal pain* of gastrointestinal origin usually arises from disorders of the esophagus or cardia of the stomach. Because pain in this area frequently emanates from the heart, cardiac disease must be carefully considered and excluded. *Epigastric pain* is generally of gastric, duodenal, biliary, or pancreatic origin. (The epigastrium is also a frequent location for "functional" pain.) As pathologic processes in the biliary tract or pancreas become more intense, pain may lateralize and localize, e.g., biliary pain to the right upper quadrant and tip of the scapula and pancreatic pain to the left upper quadrant and back. *Periumbilical pain* is generally associated with disease involving the small intestine. *Pain below the umbilicus* is often of appendiceal, colonic, or pelvic origin.

Temporal relationships The unraveling of the *temporal relationships* of the patient's symptoms often provides additional diagnostic

TABLE 33-1 Distribution of visceral pain and examples of disorders frequently involving the specific organ

Organ	Location of pain	Examples of disorders
Esophagus	Substernum, epigastrium	Peptic esophagitis, stricture, esophageal spasm, carcinoma
Stomach	Epigastrium	Gastritis, gastric ulcer, carcinoma
Duodenum (first and second portions)	Epigastrium	Duodenal ulcer
Small intestine (excluding first and second portions of duodenum)	Periumbilical	Infectious gastroenteritis, regional enteritis, lymphoma, intestinal obstruction
Gallbladder	Epigastrium, right upper quadrant, right upper back	Cholelithiasis, cholecystitis
Pancreas	Epigastrium, left upper quadrant, left side of back	Pancreatitis, pancreatic carcinoma
Liver	Right upper quadrant	Hepatitis, cirrhosis, passive congestion
Colon	Below umbilicus	Infectious colitis, ulcerative colitis, carcinoma, partial obstruction

clues. It is important to ascertain whether the symptoms are *constant* (continually present over extended periods of time), as may occur, for example, with an infiltrating gastric carcinoma, or *intermittent,* as in acute gastritis or biliary colic. The symptoms may have a *diurnal* pattern as in the case of reflux esophagitis in which pain often occurs nocturnally and with recumbency. Pain that awakens the patient from a sound sleep occurs most often with duodenal ulcer. Occasionally symptoms are *seasonal,* as in peptic ulcer disease, in which some patients experience more discomfort in the spring and autumn than at other times.

Another helpful diagnostic feature is the relation of pain to the *ingestion of food. Early postprandial symptoms* may reflect esophageal disease, acute gastritis, or gastric carcinoma. *Late postprandial indigestion,* i.e., that occurring several hours after eating, may reflect failure of the stomach to empty adequately, as in gastric outlet obstruction or atony, or duodenal ulcer, in which case pain results from exposure of ulcerated mucosa to acid secreted by the stomach and unbuffered by food. Conversely, the relief of pain following ingestion of food or antacids is characteristic of duodenal ulcer and is presumably due to the neutralization of the acid. Late postprandial indigestion also may result from impaired digestive and absorptive processes, as in pancreatic insufficiency.

It is important to recognize that the pain patterns and relationships to the intake of food described above are generalizations, and many cases do not conform to classic "textbook" descriptions. For example, although pain limited to the right upper quadrant is often caused by gallbladder disease, about half of patients with this condition experience only epigastric pain. Similarly, there are some patients with peptic ulcer whose pain is not relieved by antacids, while there are other patients with functional indigestion and even gastric carcinoma whose pain improves with antacids.

HEARTBURN Heartburn, or pyrosis, is a sensation of warmth or burning located substernally or high in the epigastrium with radiation into the neck and occasionally to the arms. Occasional heartburn is common in normal persons, but frequent and severe heartburn is generally a manifestation of esophageal dysfunction. Heartburn may result from abnormal motor activity or distention of the esophagus, reflux of acid or bile into the esophagus, or direct esophageal mucosal irritation (esophagitis).

Heartburn is most often associated with gastroesophageal reflux (see Chap. 234). In this setting, heartburn occurs after a large meal, with stooping or bending, or when the patient is supine. It may be accompanied by the spontaneous appearance in the mouth of fluid which may be salty ("water brash"), sour (gastric contents), or bitter and green or yellow (bile). Heartburn may arise following the ingestion of certain foods (e.g., citrus fruit juices) or drugs (e.g., alcohol and aspirin). Characteristically heartburn is alleviated promptly, even if only temporarily, by antacids.

Heartburn may also occur in the absence of a demonstrable or motor pathologic condition. In this setting, it is frequently accompanied by aerophagia, which may represent an attempt by the patient to relieve discomfort, and is often attributed to psychological factors for lack of other explanation.

FOOD INTOLERANCE In some persons specific foods or types of foods appear to be related to indigestion. Careful documentation of this relationship is sometimes of great help in arriving at an etiologic diagnosis.

Some foods may be poorly tolerated because of their consistency. Patients with esophageal stricture or carcinoma may tolerate liquids well but may experience discomfort, especially substernal distress, after ingesting solids (see Chap. 234). Certain foods may be tolerated poorly because of impaired intestinal digestion or absorption. This condition may occur following the ingestion of fatty foods in patients with pancreatic or biliary tract disease. Citrus fruits, with their relatively low pH, often provoke symptoms in patients with peptic ulcer disease or peptic esophagitis.

Persons may have a congenital or acquired *lack or deficiency of a specific enzyme* required for intestinal absorption of a certain nutrient. One example is the deficiency of lactase, the intestinal mucosal enzyme which catalyzes the hydrolysis of lactose. In persons who are lactase-deficient, the ingestion of milk (which contains lactose) results in abdominal cramps, distention, diarrhea, and flatulence (Chap. 237). Also, certain substances may lead to profound systemic effects because of *biochemical defects* in the patient which render the substances particularly hazardous. An example of the latter is galactose intolerance in persons with galactosemia (see Chap. 314).

There are a number of other conditions in which specific foods are tolerated poorly. For example, some foods may initiate *allergic reactions,* which should be suspected when symptoms occur immediately after ingestion of the food, recur on challenge testing, and are associated with other features of an allergic reaction, such as lip swelling, urticaria, angioedema, asthma, or rarely anaphylactic shock. Other foods may exert *toxic effects* on the intestinal tracts of susceptible persons (e.g., gluten in patients with celiac sprue).

The mechanisms described above do not explain the majority of clinical situations in which indigestion is associated with the ingestion of specific foods. For example, a history of fatty food intolerance or an inability to eat spicy foods is commonly obtained from patients with indigestion. However, the mechanisms underlying the production of symptoms in these circumstances are still unclear.

AEROPHAGIA, GASEOUSNESS, FLATULENCE A number of common clinical syndromes which may be described by the patient as indigestion appear to be related to increased quantities of or sensitivity to gas in the intestinal tract.

Aerophagia Patients with a complaint of *chronic, repetitive eructation* (belching) can be observed to precede each belch with a swallow of air, most of which passes only partway down the esophagus and is then regurgitated. Thus, excessive eructation results from *aerophagia,* or air swallowing, not from excessive gas production in the stomach or the intestine. A degree of aerophagia occurs in normal persons, but some individuals gulp air excessively because of chronic anxiety, rapid eating, drinking carbonated beverages, gum chewing, postnasal drip, or poorly fitting dentures. Because eructation which follows aerophagia may provide a temporary sense of relief to the patient, a vicious cycle of aerophagia and eructation may ensue.

About 20 to 60 percent of intestinal gas represents swallowed air. Because N_2 (nitrogen) and O_2 (oxygen) are the only gases present in the atmosphere in appreciable concentrations and because they are not produced in the gastrointestinal tract, the detection of these gases on gas chromatographic analysis of intestinal gas indicates that swallowed air must be the source. Swallowed air that is not eructated passes on to the stomach and intestinal tract. Accumulation of swallowed air in the stomach may lead to postprandial fullness and pressure and the finding on an abdominal radiograph of a large amount of air in the gastric fundus. This symptom complex, referred to as the *magenblase* (i.e., gastric bubble) *syndrome,* may occur when a patient lies supine after a large meal so that the gastric air is "trapped" below the gastroesophageal junction by overlying fluid and cannot be eructated. Acute gastric distention by swallowed air can occasionally produce sharp pains which may mimic angina pectoris. Swallowed air which successfully passes the stomach may either produce diffuse abdominal distention or become trapped in the splenic flexure of the colon. The latter condition, known as the *splenic flexure syndrome,* is characterized by a sensation of left upper quadrant fullness and pressure with radiation to the left side of the chest. Relief of pain often follows defecation or the expulsion of flatus. The diagnosis is suggested by the finding of increased tympany in the extreme left lateral portion of the upper abdomen on physical examination or of large amounts of air in the splenic flexure of the colon on a plain abdominal radiograph.

Gaseousness, bloating, and flatulence Despite the widely held belief that feelings of *diffuse abdominal pain and bloating* are often caused by excessive quantities of intestinal gas, studies employing an intestinal gas wash-out technique suggest that patients complaining of excessive gas have normal volumes of intestinal gas. The primary abnormality causing functional bloating and pain in such persons appears to be a motility disturbance that causes the patient to perceive pain with an intestinal gas volume that is well tolerated by normal subjects. Alternatively, intestinal motility may be normal in such persons, but they may be excessively responsive to normal impulses arising from the intestinal tract.

A major source of intestinal gas is the fermentative action of intestinal bacteria on carbohydrates and proteins within the lumen. Normally such bacteria are limited to the colon, and the principal gases produced are CO_2 (carbon dioxide) and H_2 (hydrogen) (in addition to minute quantities of odoriferous gases which give flatus its characteristic odor). In the upper small bowel CO_2 is also produced when hydrochloric acid from the stomach or ingested fatty acids are neutralized by bicarbonate. (This may explain, in part, indigestion associated with fatty foods.) In addition, about one-third of the adult population produces appreciable quantities of CH_4 (methane) in the colon, a characteristic which appears to be a familial trait and unrelated to food ingestion. An increase in intraluminal gas production with resulting *abdominal distention, bloating,* and *flatulence* occurs following the ingestion of certain foods, such as legumes and some grains, which contain significant quantities of nonabsorbable carbohydrates that pass into the colon where they supply gas-forming substrate for the colonic bacteria. The best studied example of this is the case of beans, which contain the oligosaccharides stachyose and raffinose that cannot be split by the mucosal enzymes of the small intestine. As stated above, increased intraluminal gas production may also occur in patients with carbohydrate malabsorption states, such as lactose malabsorption due to intestinal lactase deficiency. Abnormal bacterial colonization of the small intestine (bacterial overgrowth syndrome) or infection with *Giardia lamblia* may also lead to an increase in intraluminal gas production, resulting in distention, pain, diarrhea, and flatulence.

INDIGESTION DUE TO DISEASE OUTSIDE THE INTESTINAL TRACT

A number of extraintestinal diseases may result in indigestion by mechanisms which are poorly understood, For example, indigestion may be the presenting complaint in congestive heart failure, pulmonary tuberculosis, neoplastic disease, and uremia. Also, a variety of drugs such as aspirin, nonsteroidal anti-inflammatory agents, and corticosteroids may cause symptoms of indigestion because of their ulcerogenic properties.

DIAGNOSTIC APPROACH TO THE PATIENT WITH INDIGESTION

Indigestion represents a challenging and difficult diagnostic problem because of the nonspecific nature of its manifestations. The cornerstone of the evaluation of indigestion is obtaining a clear and detailed description of the specific symptoms, particularly the patient's definition of the term *indigestion.* The nature of the distress, its frequency and time of occurrence, its relationship to meals, and the special circumstances which lead to its exacerbation or relief should be elicited. Associated intestinal symptoms such as nausea and vomiting, abnormal bowel habits, diarrhea, steatorrhea, and melena should be sought, and an assessment of nutritional status, appetite, and changes in weight should be made. A careful history should also include an assessment of the patient's general health, including the possible presence of extraintestinal disorders which may produce indigestion. A careful evaluation of psychological factors is crucial, because they often play an etiologic or contributory role to the patient's problems. Of particular importance are anxiety, depressive symptoms, and hysteria (see Chap. 11).

Physical examination rarely establishes the specific diagnosis, but it may be useful in detecting diseases in other organ systems which can affect intestinal function (e.g., congestive heart failure). Stools should be examined for appearance and occult blood.

Whether further diagnostic studies are indicated depends on the specific nature of the patient's complaints and the patient's age (concern about the possibility of gastrointestinal malignancy being greater in older patients). Abdominal pain may be evaluated with radiologic studies of the esophagus, stomach, small intestine, colon, pancreas, and biliary tract. Esophagogastroscopy, endoscopic cholangiopancreatography, sigmoidoscopy, or colonoscopy may also be helpful or necessary. On the other hand, in patients under age 30 with epigastric pain typical of acid-peptic disease, routine diagnostic studies are unlikely to disclose serious diseases (such as gastric carcinoma) and are often negative; thus, an empiric trial of antacids or possibly H_2-blocking drugs may be appropriate before proceeding with further diagnostic tests. In individuals complaining of excessive eructation, a simple demonstration that aerophagia reproduces the symptoms may suffice to confirm the diagnosis and break the patient of the habit. Patients complaining of excessive gas, bloating, distention, and flatulence must be questioned carefully about dietary preferences and the relation of symptoms to specific foods. In some cases elimination of certain foods (e.g., milk) from the diet followed by rechallenge may confirm the role of that food in producing the patient's symptoms. In other cases a more detailed evaluation, including stool examination for fat and muscle fibers and for parasites such as *Giardia lamblia,* breath tests to detect carbohydrate malabsorption, and intestinal motility studies, may be helpful.

Even after completion of careful diagnostic studies, many cases of indigestion will turn out to have no clear explanation. Some of these are psychogenic and may respond to appropriate psychiatric measures. Others represent subtle physiologic derangements which are undetectable by currently available diagnostic methods. In some such instances, an empiric trial of dopamine antagonists, such as metoclopramide, which augment gastrointestinal motility may be beneficial. Still other cases represent early stages of actual disease processes which may only be diagnosable by conventional methods at a later date. The ultimate evaluation of indigestion requires, therefore, the utmost in sensitivity, diligence, and concern on the part of the examining physician.

REFERENCES

BOND JH, LEVITT MD: Gaseousness and intestinal gas. Med Clin North Am 62:155, 1978

HEALTH AND PUBLIC POLICY COMMITTEE, American College of Physicians: Endoscopy in the evaluation of dyspepsia. Ann Intern Med 102:266, 1985

HORROCKS JC, DEDOMBAL FT: Clinical presentation of patients with "dyspepsia." Gut 19:19, 1978

LASSER RB et al: The role of intestinal gas in functional abdominal pain. N Engl J Med 293:524, 1975

LEVITT MD: Intestinal gas production—recent advances in flatology. N Engl J Med 302:1474, 1980

MEAD GM et al: Use of barium meal examination in dyspeptic patients under 50. Br Med J 1:1460, 1977

34 ANOREXIA, NAUSEA, AND VOMITING

KURT J. ISSELBACHER

ANOREXIA Anorexia, or loss of the desire to eat, is a prominent symptom in a wide variety of intestinal and extraintestinal disorders. It must be clearly differentiated from satiety and from specific food intolerance. Anorexia occurs in many disorders and as a result *by itself is of little specific diagnostic value.* The mechanisms whereby hunger and appetite are modified in various disease states are poorly understood. Normally food intake is regulated by two hypothalamic centers—a lateral "feeding center" and a ventromedial "satiety center.'' The latter inhibits the feeding center following a meal, leading to the sensation of satiety. There is some evidence to suggest that the brain-gut peptide cholecystokinin (CCK) has a satiety effect and is involved in the regulation of feeding behavior.

Anorexia is commonly seen in diseases of the gastrointestinal tract and liver. For example, it may precede the appearance of jaundice in hepatitis, or it may be a prominent symptom in gastric carcinoma. In the setting of intestinal disease, anorexia should be clearly differentiated from *sitophobia,* or fear of eating because of subsequent or associated discomfort. In such circumstances, appetite may persist, but the ingestion of food is curtailed nonetheless. Sitophobia may be seen, for example, in regional enteritis (especially with partial obstruction) or in patients with gastric ulcer following partial or total gastrectomy.

Anorexia may also be a prominent feature of severe extraintestinal diseases. For example, anorexia may be profound in severe congestive heart failure and is often associated with cardiac glycoside intoxication. It may be a major symptom in patients with uremia, pulmonary failure, and various endocrinopathies (e.g., hyperparathyroidism, Addison's disease, and panhypopituitarism). Anorexia also often accompanies psychogenic disturbances, such as anxiety or depression. For a discussion of anorexia nervosa, see Chap. 73.

NAUSEA AND VOMITING Nausea and vomiting may occur independently of each other, but generally they are so closely allied that they may conveniently be considered together. *Nausea* denotes the feeling of the imminent desire to vomit, usually referred to the throat or epigastrium. *Vomiting* refers to the forceful oral expulsion of gastric contents; *retching* denotes the labored rhythmic respiratory activity that frequently precedes emesis. Extremely forceful *projectile vomiting* is a special form of vomiting which has significance because it may connote the presence of increased intracranial pressure.

Nausea often precedes or accompanies vomiting. It is usually associated with diminished functional activity of the stomach and alterations of the motility of the duodenum and small intestine. Accompanying severe nausea there is often evidence of altered autonomic (especially parasympathetic) activity: pallor of the skin, increased perspiration, hypersalivation, and the occasional association of hypotension and bradycardia (vasovagal syndrome). Anorexia is also often present.

Following a period of nausea and a brief interval of retching, a sequence of involuntary visceral and somatic motor events occurs, resulting in emesis. The stomach plays a relatively passive role in the vomiting process, the major ejection force being provided by the abdominal musculature. With relaxation of the gastric fundus and gastroesophageal sphincter, a sharp increase in intraabdominal pressure is brought about by forceful contraction of the diaphragm and abdominal wall. This, together with concomitant annular contraction of the gastric pylorus, results in the expulsion of gastric contents into the esophagus. Increased intrathoracic pressure results in the further movement of esophageal contents into the mouth. Reversal of the normal direction of esophageal peristalsis may play a role in this process. Reflex elevation of the soft palate during the vomiting act prevents the entry of the material into the nasopharynx, whereas reflex closure of the glottis and inhibition of respiration help to prevent pulmonary aspiration.

Repeated emesis may have deleterious effects in a number of different ways. The process of vomiting, if forceful, may lead to pressure rupture of the esophagus (Boerhaave's syndrome) or linear mucosal tears in the region of the cardioesophageal junction, resulting in massive hematemesis (Mallory-Weiss syndrome). Prolonged vomiting may lead to dehydration and the loss of gastric secretions (especially hydrochloric acid), resulting in metabolic alkalosis with hypokalemia. Finally, in states of central nervous system depression (coma, etc.), gastric contents may be aspirated into the lungs, with a resulting aspiration pneumonitis.

Vomiting mechanism The act of vomiting is under the control of two functionally distinct medullary centers: the *vomiting center* and the *chemoreceptor trigger zone.* They lie close to each other near other brainstem centers regulating vasomotor and autonomic functions. The vomiting center controls and integrates the actual act of emesis. It receives afferent stimuli from the intestinal tract and other parts of the body, from higher cortical centers, especially the labyrinthine apparatus, and from the chemoreceptor trigger zone. The important efferent pathways in vomiting are the phrenic nerves (to the diaphragm), the spinal nerves (to the abdominal musculature), and visceral efferent nerves (to the stomach and esophagus).

The chemoreceptor trigger zone is also located in the medulla but by itself is incapable of mediating the act of vomiting. Activation of this zone results in efferent impulses to the medullary vomiting center, which in turn initiates the act of emesis. Dopamine receptors in the chemoreceptor trigger zone can be activated by many stimuli, including drugs such as apomorphine and levodopa, after decarboxylation to dopamine.

Phenothiazine derivatives such as prochlorperazine and metoclopramide inhibit cerebral dopamine receptors and can be effective against both nausea and vomiting. Metoclopramide is the prototype of selective dopamine antagonists called *substituted benzamides.* In contrast to the phenothiazines, which have anticholinergic effects, metoclopramide has powerful cholinergic effects. These effects, together with its dopamine antagonism, have made metoclopramide a useful agent equal or superior to drugs such as prochlorperazine in the treatment of nausea and vomiting. The usual oral dosage is 10 mg four times daily. Metoclopramide is also effective in hastening esophageal clearance, accelerating gastric emptying, and shortening small-bowel transit. It may be used intravenously in doses up to 1 to 3 mg/kg as prophylaxis prior to potent chemotherapy agents (e.g., cisplatin).

Clinical classification Nausea and vomiting are common manifestations of organic and functional disorders. The precise mechanisms triggering vomiting in the various clinical states are poorly understood, making classification of mechanisms difficult. The categories mentioned below serve to illustrate some of the many disorders which may be accompanied by nausea and vomiting.

Many *acute abdominal emergencies* which lead to the ''surgical abdomen'' are associated with nausea and vomiting. Notably, vomiting may be seen with inflammation of a viscus as in acute appendicitis or acute cholecystitis, obstruction of the intestine, or acute peritonitis (see Chap. 5).

In many of the disorders involving *chronic indigestion* (see Chap. 33) nausea and vomiting may be prominent. Emesis may be either spontaneous or self-induced and may lead to relief of symptoms, as, for example, in uncomplicated peptic ulcer. Nausea and vomiting may accompany the distention and pain seen in the aerophagic syndromes. Often in patients with chronic indigestion, nausea and vomiting may be provoked by specific foods (e.g., fatty foods), for reasons that are poorly understood.

Acute systemic infections with fever, especially in young children, are frequently accompanied by vomiting and often by severe diarrhea. The mechanism whereby infections remote from the gastrointestinal tract produce these manifestations is unclear. Viral, bacterial, and parasitic infections of the intestinal tract may be associated with severe nausea and vomiting, often with diarrhea. Severe nausea and vomiting may be prominent in viral hepatitis, even before the appearance of jaundice.

Central nervous system disorders which lead to increased intracranial pressure may be accompanied by vomiting, often projectile. Brain swelling due to inflammation, anoxemia, acute hydrocephalus, neoplasms, etc., may thus be complicated by vomiting. Disorders of the labyrinthine apparatus and its central connections which underlie vertigo may be accompanied by vomiting with nausea and retching. Acute labyrinthitis and Ménière's disease are examples of such disturbances. Migraine headaches, tabetic crises, and acute meningitis are additional examples of disorders of the nervous system which may lead to vomiting. In the reactive phase of hypotension with syncope, there may also be nausea and vomiting.

Severe nausea and vomiting may be present in *acute myocardial infarction,* especially of the posterior wall of the heart. Nausea and vomiting may also be seen in *congestive heart failure,* perhaps in relation to congestion of the liver. The possibility that these symptoms may be due to drugs (e.g., opiates or digitalis) should always be borne in mind in patients with cardiac disease.

Nausea and vomiting commonly accompany several *endocrinologic disorders,* including diabetic acidosis and adrenal insufficiency, especially adrenal crisis. The morning sickness of early pregnancy is another instance of nausea and vomiting possibly related to hormonal changes.

The *side effects of many drugs and chemicals* include nausea and vomiting. In some instances this is because of gastric irritation which stimulates the medullary vomiting center. The ingestion of a *toxin* (e.g., food poisoning) may also cause acute vomiting.

Psychogenic vomiting means vomiting which may occur as part of any emotional upset on a transitory basis or more persistently as part of a psychic disturbance. Close observation will usually disclose the condition to be one of regurgitation rather than of vomiting, and weight loss may not correspond at all to the patient's description of the frequency and severity of vomiting. As discussed in Chap. 73, anorexia nervosa is an emotional disturbance which may be associated not only with anorexia but also with vomiting. Often patients with emotional disorders and vomiting maintain a relatively normal state of nutrition because a relatively small amount of the ingested food is vomited.

Differential diagnosis Vomiting should be distinguished from *regurgitation,* which refers to the expulsion of food in the absence of nausea and without abdominal diaphragmatic muscular contraction which is part of vomiting. Regurgitation of esophageal contents may occur with esophageal stricture or diverticula. Regurgitation of gastric contents is generally seen with gastroesophageal sphincter incompetence, especially with hiatus hernia or in association with peptic ulcer, usually when pylorospasm supervenes.

The temporal relationships of vomiting to eating may be of help diagnostically. Vomiting which occurs predominantly in the morning is often seen early in pregnancy and uremia. Alcoholic gastritis is commonly accompanied by early-morning emesis, the so-called dry heaves. Vomiting which occurs shortly after eating may suggest pylorospasm or gastritis. On the other hand, vomiting which occurs 4 to 6 h or longer after eating and involves the elimination of large quantities of undigested food often indicates gastric retention (e.g., diabetic gastric atony or pyloric obstruction). However, with gastric retention vomiting may also occur early (e.g., 30 to 90 min) after a meal.

The character of the vomitus offers clues to the diagnosis. If the vomitus contains free hydrochloric acid, the obstruction may be due to an ulcer; absence of free hydrochloric acid is more compatible with gastric malignancy. A feculent or putrid odor reflects the results of bacterial action on the intestinal contents. Such vomiting may be seen with low-intestinal obstruction, peritonitis, or gastrocolic fistula. Bile is commonly present in gastric contents whenever vomiting is prolonged. It has no significance unless constantly present in large quantities, when it may signify an obstructive lesion below the ampulla of Vater. The presence of blood in the gastric contents usually denotes bleeding from the esophagus, stomach, or duodenum.

REFERENCES

FELDMAN M: Nausea and vomiting, in *Gastrointestinal Disease,* 3d ed, MH Sleisenger, JS Fordtran (eds). Philadelphia, Saunders, 1983, pp 160–177

HERZOG DB, COPELAND PM: Eating disorders. N Engl J Med 313:295, 1985

SMITH GP: Satiety effect of gastrointestinal hormones, in *Polypeptide Hormones,* RF Beers, EG Bassett (eds). New York, Raven Press, 1980, pp 413–420

WESER E: Anorexia and obesity in *Gastrointestinal Disease,* 3d ed, MH Sleisenger, JS Fordtran (eds). Philadelphia, Saunders, 1983, pp 135–144

35 GAIN AND LOSS IN WEIGHT

DANIEL W. FOSTER

GENERAL PRINCIPLES In normal persons weight is stable because caloric intake is matched to caloric expenditure by the coordinated activity of "feeding" and "satiety" centers presumably located in the hypothalamus. The signals that regulate the interactions of these centers are not known; regulation is probably multifactorial, and both short- and long-term controls are thought to be operative. Whatever the mechanisms the system is normally efficient over periods of months to years.

Gain or loss in tissue mass is determined by the net balance between caloric intake and caloric expenditure. Caloric intake is determined by availability and attractiveness of food and by emotional and physical factors. The bulk of energy expenditure is due to basal metabolism and physical activity. The former is defined as the total caloric requirement when the body is in the supine position, motionless except for quiet respiration, e.g., the energy required to maintain structural and functional integrity of the organism in the absence of physical activity. About half the total daily caloric intake is normally consumed by basal processes. Active persons spend about 40 percent of calories in physical activity; athletes may utilize 50 percent or more of ingested energy in exercise. Persons sedentary because of habit, illness, or obesity may expend far less in activity. In nonobese, nonsedentary subjects 10 percent of ingested calories is released as heat associated with the absorption of food, a process called dietary thermogenesis. This fraction, previously designated specific dynamic action, is usually considered a separate component of energy costs. Heat generated during and after exercise and that released for maintenance of body temperature (regulatory thermogenesis) are included in the energy costs of physical activity and basal metabolism, respectively.

Change in body weight as a consequence of voluntary alteration in diet or exercise is never worrisome; change in weight that is not deliberately sought, on the other hand, is a frequent reason for consultation with the physician and often indicates the presence of disease. Changes in weight may reflect alteration in either tissue mass or body fluid content. Rapid swings usually indicate the latter. Even when tissue mass is changing, fluid loss or gain plays a major role in the measured change in weight, particularly over the short run. This point is illustrated in Table 35-1, where the composition of weight loss was estimated during a 24-day period of semistarvation in 13 normal men (daily intake, 1010 kcal). During the first 3 days 70 percent of the decrease in weight was due to water loss, while in subsequent stages a diminution of protein and fat accounted for essentially all the weight loss. This varying contribution of fluid explains why a fixed formula cannot be used for predicting weight loss or gain. It is frequently stated that a net change of 7700 kcal will be accompanied by a 1-kg change in body mass (3500 kcal/lb). While this estimate is reasonable for long-term changes in caloric intake, the apparent caloric cost per kilogram of weight lost or gained varies with the accompanying fluid shifts. In the experiment summarized in Table 35-1, for example, a negative balance of only 2596

TABLE 35-1 Percentage composition of mean daily weight loss in 13 young men during caloric restriction for 24 days

Days	Mean weight loss, kg/day	Water, %	Fat, %	Protein, %	Calorie equivalents of weight loss, kcal/kg
1–3	0.80	70	25	5	2596
11–13	0.23	19	69	12	7043
22–24	0.17	0	85	15	8700

SOURCE: *After Brožek et al.*

kcal resulted in the loss of a kilogram of weight between days 1 and 3, while between days 22 and 24, loss of a kilogram required a deficit of 8700 kcal. In general if weight loss or gain has occurred over a period of weeks or months, it is safe to assume that change in tissue mass has occurred; weight loss or gain limited to a several-day period may be due to fluid shifts alone. Occasionally true loss of tissue mass is obscured by fluid retention as in the case of the cirrhotic patient who develops ascites or the patient with anorexia nervosa who has significant edema.

WEIGHT GAIN

While obesity is a major public health concern (see Chap. 317), its diagnosis is usually uncomplicated. Obese subjects often deny overeating, but the true situation can be assessed either by tabulating actual food intake and determining its caloric content from standard tables or by interviewing the patient's family and friends.

Regardless of history, excess caloric intake is the cause of obesity in the majority of cases. Pathologic causes are rare. In the adult, Cushing's syndrome can result in acquired obesity in a previously nonobese patient, but usually the diagnosis is suggested by the pattern of fat distribution and the clinical picture. Other endocrine diseases such as hypothyroidism, hypogonadism, and insulin-secreting tumors are frequently listed in the differential diagnosis of obesity but do not represent significant diagnostic problems. Congenital diseases that cause obesity such as the Prader-Willi, Laurence-Moon-Biedl, and Alström syndromes are readily recognizable and appear early in life. Rarely, a disease involving the hypothalamus, particularly craniopharyngioma, may cause acquired obesity. Extensive workup of the central nervous system in obesity is not indicated, however, in the absence of suspicious symptoms (headache, visual difficulties, vomiting, or endocrine changes).

WEIGHT LOSS

Weight loss in the absence of deliberate dieting is a more serious problem than weight gain because there is a high chance that organic disease is present. Mechanisms include decreased appetite, accelerated metabolism, and loss of calories in urine or stool, acting singly or in combination. No attempt will be made to list all diseases capable of causing weight loss, but in one prospective study 26 percent of patients had no identifiable physical or psychiatric illness to which the weight loss could be attributed. If uncontrolled and symptomatic, any serious illness can cause weight loss; the usual mechanism is anorexia due either to direct pathophysiologic consequences (e.g., congestion of the liver and gastrointestinal tract in right-sided heart failure) or malaise and depression. The following categories are singled out for special comment because the primary illness may be masked at the time of initial presentation.

DIABETES MELLITUS Initial weight loss with the onset of diabetes is largely fluid and is due to the osmotic diuresis induced by hyperglycemia. Subsequently, loss of tissue mass occurs in the insulin-dependent form of the disease as a result of caloric wastage (the consequence of glycosuria) and of the hormonal abnormalities that characterize the illness. Insulin deficiency and glucagon excess result in impaired synthesis of protein and fat and simultaneously cause accelerated proteolysis and lipolysis such that the net energy state is catabolic. Weight loss in diabetes is frequently associated with increased food intake.

ENDOCRINE DISEASE While weight loss is not inevitable (indeed, thyrotoxicosis may rarely be found in a patient who has gained weight), it is common in hyperthyroidism. Increased appetite and food intake are the rule, and patients often consume a high-carbohydrate diet. Caloric expenditure is enormous, primarily because of an increased metabolic rate, but increased motor activity also plays a role. The molecular mechanism whereby thyrotoxicosis causes weight loss is not settled, but thyroid hormone is thought to increase sodium-potassium adenosine triphosphatase (ATPase) activity in many tissues, suggesting that the diminished efficiency of ingested calories is due to futile cycle of adenosine triphosphate (ATP) synthesis and breakdown with energy lost as heat. In ''apathetic'' hyperthyroidism weight loss and weakness may predominate with little evidence of nervousness or other symptoms. Another cause of weight loss due to hypermetabolism is pheochromocytoma, the inducing agent being catecholamine release. Panhypopituitarism and adrenal insufficiency may also be associated with weight loss, largely as a consequence of diminished appetite secondary to cortisol deficiency.

GASTROINTESTINAL DISEASE Overt or occult steatorrhea due to sprue, chronic pancreatitis, or cystic fibrosis may produce wasting despite major increases in food intake. Chronic diarrhea due to inflammatory bowel disease (with or without fistulas) or parasites, esophageal disease with reflux or vomiting, and even ordinary peptic ulcer have to be considered in the differential diagnosis. The mechanism of weight loss in alimentary tract disease is generally either decreased food intake or malabsorption, though inflammation per se probably plays a role in the weight loss of ulcerative colitis and regional enteritis.

INFECTION Hidden infection must always be sought in patients with unexplained weight loss. Tuberculosis, fungal disease, amebic abscess, and subacute bacterial endocarditis should be high on the list of suspects. The mechanism probably involves both anorexia and inflammation-induced acceleration of cellular metabolic demands. Glucagon may play a role in the negative nitrogen balance and tissue wastage of inflammation, but the catabolic state probably also requires changes in other hormones.

MALIGNANCY Occult malignancy is probably the most common cause of weight loss in the absence of major signs and symptoms. In the search for malignancy particular emphasis must be placed on the gastrointestinal tract, pancreas, and liver. Lymphoma and leukemia should also be considered. While silent (except for weight loss) malignancy can occur in any organ, the gastrointestinal tract is the most common site. Mechanisms of weight loss in cancer vary, and more than one factor often plays a role. For example, although anorexia is almost invariably present in carcinoma of the pancreas, malabsorption appears to play the predominant role, with weight gain frequently occurring when pancreatic enzymes are provided. In other tumors, particularly lymphomas and leukemias, the mechanism appears to be increased metabolism with caloric wastage.

PSYCHIATRIC DISEASE The classic psychiatric illness associated with profound weight loss is anorexia nervosa (Chap. 73). Conversion disorders, schizophrenia, and depression may also cause weight loss due to decreased food intake. While organic disease causing both anorexia and depression has to be ruled out, ordinarily the psychiatric nature of the problem will be clear.

RENAL DISEASE One of the earliest manifestations of uremia is anorexia. As a consequence all patients with unexplained weight loss should be given screening renal function tests.

SUMMARY

Weight loss is more often a diagnostic problem than weight gain and more often a sign of serious organic illness. If the weight loss is associated with increased food intake, the diagnosis is likely diabetes, thyrotoxicosis, or malabsorption; less frequently, leukemias, lymphomas, or pheochromocytoma cause weight loss in the presence of increased food intake. If food intake is normal or decreased, malignancy, infection, renal disease, psychiatric syndromes, or endocrine deficiency is more common.

REFERENCES

BROŽEK J et al: Changes in body weight and body dimensions in men performing work on a low calorie carbohydrate diet. J Appl Physiol 10:412, 1957

FOSTER DW: Eating disorders: Obesity and anorexia nervosa, in *Williams Textbook of Endocrinology,* 7th ed, JD Wilson, DW Foster (eds). Philadelphia, Saunders, 1985, p 1081

GARFINKEL PE et al: Differential diagnosis of emotional disorders that cause weight loss. Can Med Assoc J 129:939, 1983

KHOURY P et al: Weight change since age 18 years in 30- to 55-year-old whites and blacks. Associations with lipid values, lipoprotein levels, and blood pressure. JAMA 250:3179, 1983

KONISHI F: Food energy equivalents of various activities. J Am Diet Assoc 46:186, 1965

MARTON KI et al: Involuntary weight loss: Diagnostic and prognostic significance. Ann Intern Med 95:568, 1981

PEREZ MM et al: Assessment of weight loss, food intake, fat metabolism, malabsorption, and treatment of pancreatic insufficiency in pancreatic cancer. Cancer 52:346, 1983

RUNCIE J, HILDITCH TE: Energy provision, tissue utilization and weight loss in prolonged starvation. Br Med J 2:352, 1974

YANG M-U, VAN ITALLIE TB: Composition of weight loss during short-term weight reduction. Metabolic responses of obese subjects to starvation and low calorie ketogenic and non-ketogenic diets. J Clin Invest 58:722, 1976

36 CONSTIPATION, DIARRHEA, AND DISTURBANCES OF ANORECTAL FUNCTION

STEPHEN E. GOLDFINGER

NORMAL COLONIC FUNCTION Each day approximately 9 liters of fluid enters the digestive tract; 2 liters represents ingested fluids and the remainder comes from salivary, gastric, biliary, pancreatic, and intestinal secretions that are needed to provide an appropriate milieu for food digestion. Most of this fluid is absorbed in the upper bowel. Approximately 1 liter containing undigested dietary residue and cellular debris passes across the ileocecal valve to the colon. Little of nutritional value remains following the extensive digestive processing and absorption that occurs in the small intestine. The colon's principal function is to convert this liquid ileal effluent to solid feces before it is advanced to the rectum and evacuated. Several important physiologic processes underlie normal colonic function; among these are *absorption* of fluid and electrolytes; *peristaltic contractions* that facilitate mixing, dessication, and passage of feces to the rectum; and, finally, *defecation*.

Absorption of fluid and electrolytes (see also Chap. 237) In western societies where dietary fiber content is relatively low, the average daily stool weight is less than 200 g, of which 60 to 80 percent is water. Thus, the colon normally absorbs approximately 80 to 90 percent of the fluid it receives, and this occurs well within its absorptive capacity of 6 liters water and 800 meq sodium per day. Fluid and electrolyte absorption occurs primarily in the ascending and transverse colon. Water absorption occurs passively, osmotically following the active transport of sodium and chloride ions. In addition, bicarbonate is secreted in exchange for chloride. The secreted bicarbonate is converted, in part, to carbon dioxide by reacting with acids produced by colonic bacteria.

The term *diarrhea* generally connotes *frequent* or *loose* stools. Based on physiologic events described above, diarrhea may be defined more quantitatively as a fecal output exceeding 200 g per day when dietary fiber content is low. Diarrhea can be further classified on the basis of underlying mechanisms (see Table 36-1). In *secretory diarrhea*, fecal fluid rich in sodium and potassium is lost as a consequence of impaired absorption and/or excessive secretion of electrolytes by the bowel. In *osmotic diarrhea*, absorption of water is decreased by the osmotic effect of nonabsorbable, intraluminal molecules. *Exudative diarrhea* is caused by an outpouring of necrotic mucosa, colloid, fluid, and electrolytes from an inflamed colon which, in addition, is less able to carry out its normal absorptive function. Increased amounts of arachidonic acid metabolites present in inflamed mucosa may also promote increased ion secretion. *Anatomic derangements* of the bowel and *motility disorders* cause diarrhea by reducing the surface area or the contact time necessary for adequate absorption to occur.

Colonic innervation and motility The colon and rectum are innervated by fibers that release norepinephrine, acetylcholine, and a variety of other neurotransmitters, which may include bioactive amines, peptides, and nucleotides. Signals transmitted by autonomic nervous system fibers originating centrally, local reflex arcs confined to the autonomous "enteric nervous system," and intrinsic contractile responses of smooth muscle all play a part in the coordination of colonic motility. Parasympathetic nerves, which stimulate peristaltic contraction as well as electrolyte secretion, dominate the neurogenic regulation of colonic motor activity; adrenergic tone inhibits cholinergic stimulation and also increases electrolyte absorption. The precise integration of all neural and nonneural mediators of colonic motility and ion transport remains poorly understood.

The basal motor activity of the colon corresponds to the function of its various segments. In the ascending colon, where most fluid absorption occurs, rhythmic, retrograde contractions occur to prolong fecal contact time. In the midcolon, segmental contractions continue the process of absorption while feces are gradually advanced to the left colon. The most distal portion of the colon, which is under the greatest neurogenic control, propels feces caudally in preparation for defecation. In addition, massive peristalsis occurs several times per day.

Since colonic motility plays an important role in both absorption and movement of contents to the rectum, alterations of bowel tone occurring as a result of disease, stress, or various drugs tend to have an important influence on bowel movements. In view of the number of pharmacologic agents that may influence smooth muscle contractility, it is essential to take a careful drug history when evaluating patients with constipation or diarrhea of recent onset.

Defecation The defecatory reflex is initiated by acute distention of the rectum. When it is allowed to progress by supraspinal centers, sigmoidal and rectal contractions heighten the pressure within the rectum and also obliterate the rectosigmoidal angle. Concomitant relaxation of the internal and external anal sphincters then permits the evacuation of feces. This can be augmented by an increase in intraabdominal pressure created by the Valsalva maneuver. Conversely, defecation may be consciously prevented by the voluntary contraction of the striated muscles of the pelvic diaphragm and

TABLE 36-1 Classification of diarrhea

Type	Mechanism	Stool characteristics	Examples
Secretory	↑ Secretion of electrolytes ↓ Absorption of electrolytes	Clear $Na^+ + K^+ \simeq 2 \times$ osmolality No polymorphs	Cholera Diarrheogenic islet cell tumors Bile salt enteropathy
Exudative	Impaired colonic absorption; outpouring of cells and colloid	Purulent Polymorphs present Gross or occult blood	Ulcerative colitis Shigellosis Amebiasis
Decreased absorption			
Osmotic	Nonabsorbable intraluminal molecules	Clear $Na^+ + K^+ \simeq 2 \times$ osmolality No polymorphs	Lactase deficiency Mg^{2+}-containing cathartics
Anatomic derangement	Decreased absorption surface	Variable	Subtotal colectomy Gastrocolic fistula
Motility disorder	Decreased contact time	Variable	Hyperthyroidism Irritable bowel syndrome

external anal sphincter. The functional value of voluntary control of defecation requires little elaboration, but the opportunity for individuals to resist the defecatory urge, when abused, may lead to chronic rectal distention, reduced afferent signals, lax tone, and chronic constipation.

DIARRHEA AND CONSTIPATION The bowel habits of apparently healthy persons vary widely. For this reason, the complaint of *diarrhea* and *constipation* should be evaluated in terms of the degree of change from an individual's customary pattern. Reasonably detailed information is important in either abnormality. When patients complain of diarrhea, it is important to obtain an estimate of the volume as well as frequency of fecal output and, whenever possible, to examine directly a stool sample for consistency, blood, oiliness, and malodor. For example, the repeated elimination of small quantities of solid material admixed with gas, so typical in the irritable bowel syndrome, has a far different connotation than the same number of movements of liquid, blood-tinged feces. It is also useful to learn if fecal incontinence is present. Involuntary loss of feces may be an embarrassing complaint for a patient to verbalize, but such information may point to a potentially correctable anal sphincter abnormality. The term *constipation* may be used by the patient to refer to a variety of changes including reduction in frequency of defecation, a constant sensation of rectal fullness with incomplete evacuation of feces, and sometimes painful defecation due to hard stools or perianal pathology. Excessively hard stools are usually due to increased absorption of fluid as a result of prolonged contact of the luminal contents with the colonic mucosa consequent to delayed transit. In an assessment of complaints of diarrhea or constipation, it is important to consider the patient's emotional state since in many instances the recent onset of psychological stress is the major reason for altered bowel habits. However, it can be hazardous to assume this to be the case, even when the relationship seems convincing. For this reason, the judicious use of laboratory, proctoscopic, and radiologic procedures is recommended to make certain that organic disease will not be overlooked.

Acute diarrhea Diarrhea of abrupt onset occurring in otherwise healthy persons is usually due to an infectious cause. A variety of accompanying symptoms are often observed, including fever, headache, anorexia, vomiting, malaise, and myalgia, but they cannot be used to distinguish with certainty among viral, bacterial, and protozoal causes. Because bacterial and protozoal pathogens are usually not recovered from the feces, so-called nonspecific diarrhea is often considered to be of viral etiology. However, the demonstration of enterotoxins produced by strains of *Escherichia coli*, which are not distinguishable from "normal flora" on routine culture, suggests that these bacteria may account for a number of cases that are usually ascribed to viral infection.

Acute diarrhea presumed to be of viral etiology typically persists for a period of 1 to 3 days; death is extremely rare except in previously debilitated individuals who become severely dehydrated. When human volunteers have been infected with the Norwalk virus, which is believed to account for approximately one-third of epidemics of acute viral diarrhea in American adults, transient malabsorption of fat and xylose has been described. Changes in the small intestine include abnormalities of intestinal cell morphology such as villous shortening, an increase in the number of crypt cells, and increased cellularity of the lamina propria. The colonic mucosa is unaffected in viral diarrhea; this is consistent with the absence of polymorphonuclear leukocytes when fresh stool is examined microscopically after preparation with Loeffler's methylene blue.

Bacterial diarrhea may be suspected if there is a history of a similar and simultaneous illness in individuals who have shared contaminated food with the patient. Diarrhea developing within 12 h of the meal is most likely due to ingestion of a preformed toxin (e.g., staphylococcal exotoxin). A lag period of up to 3 days after consumption of contaminated food can occur with salmonellosis. The pathogenesis of bacterial diarrhea is due to two principal mechanisms, *mucosal invasion* and *enterotoxin-induced hypersecretion*. Bacterial invasion of the colonic wall leads to mucosal hyperemia, edema, leukocytic infiltration, and frank ulceration. Lower abdominal cramps and tenderness are prominent, as are tenesmus and rectal urgency. In severe cases the stool is grossly bloody. At other times, microscopic examination of the stool will reveal erythrocytes along with pus cells. In *shigellosis*, diarrhea is mainly due to mucosal destruction by the invading microorganisms, but small intestinal hypersecretion may also occur in the early stage of enteritis caused by some enterotoxin-producing strains of *Shigella*. The prototype of hypersecretory bacterial diarrhea is *cholera*, in which the organism *Vibrio cholerae* adheres to, but does not invade, the surface epithelial cells and releases an enterotoxin which stimulates massive secretion of fluid and electrolytes by the small intestine. This may be produced experimentally in animals by placing the enterotoxin, free of the organism itself, into isolated intestinal loops. Hypersecretion reaches a peak at 4 to 6 h and is mediated by the stimulation of mucosal adenylate cyclase by the toxin. It should be emphasized that in cholera, mucosal morphology is essentially normal and intestinal absorptive capacity is preserved. This provides the basis for oral rehydration therapy with solutions containing simple sugars and sodium chloride, the former stimulating absorption of the latter. Because other species of bacteria, such as *E. coli, Clostridium,* and *Salmonella*, have been shown to produce enterotoxins, the finding of an exudate-free stool does not preclude bacterial infection as the cause of diarrhea.

Protozoal infections may also be responsible for acute diarrhea. *Entamoeba histolytica*, prevalent in some areas of the United States and in the homosexual male population, produces an inflammatory colitis which can closely mimic idiopathic ulcerative colitis. Giardiasis is a cause of prolonged, watery diarrhea that often afflicts travelers returning from endemic areas where the water supply has been contaminated. *Cryptosporidial* infection, initially described as occurring in immunocompromised patients, has also been linked to diarrheal illness in otherwise normal persons. Careful microscopic examination of fresh stools by experienced personnel is required for the diagnosis of protozoal infection. Duodenal samples in the form of aspirate and biopsy touch preparations may be necessary to make the diagnosis of giardiasis and cryptosporidiosis (see Chaps. 160, 161).

Travelers' diarrhea may result from any one or several of the pathogens described above. When no specific agent is identified, the etiology is usually assumed to be due to enterotoxin-producing coliform organisms or viruses; both Norwalk virus and rotavirus have been implicated. Not infrequently prolonged bowel irregularity will occur following the acute illness.

Ulcerative colitis and *Crohn's disease* may begin as acute diarrhea (Chap. 238). Bloody stools, abdominal cramping, tenderness, and fever are often observed. When Crohn's disease is limited to the small bowel (regional enteritis), the diarrhea tends to be milder, is often nonbloody, and is associated with right lower quadrant pain and tenderness. Diarrhea may be caused by a variety of *drugs*, including cholinergic agents, magnesium-containing antacids, antimetabolites used in cancer chemotherapy, and many antibiotics. A necrolytic toxin produced by *Clostridium difficile* is the cause of pseudomembranous colitis occurring during or after antibiotic use. Diarrhea due to *diverticulitis* is usually accompanied by fever, tenesmus, and rectal urgency, together with cramps and tenderness in the left lower quadrant (Chap. 239). When there is no evidence of acute inflammation, diarrhea in the presence of colonic diverticula is probably due to a spastic (irritable) colon, a disorder which may set the stage for the development of diverticula. In elderly and debilitated individuals with *fecal impaction*, the presenting symptom may be the frequent expulsion of small amounts of liquid stool overflowing from colonic distention behind the impaction. This is sometimes termed *paradoxical diarrhea*. Fecal incontinence due to anal sphincter impairment is a problem that may be encountered in certain neurologic disorders or following local surgical procedures (e.g., hemorrhoidectomy, episiotomy). Acute *psychological stress* can cause diarrhea at any age.

DIAGNOSTIC APPROACH The appropriate tempo and approach in the evaluation of acute diarrhea depend so heavily on the clinical setting in which it occurs that only very general guidelines can be offered. It is entirely reasonable to withhold studies in mild, self-limited cases such as are seen as part of an epidemic viral illness. When dealing with sporadic severe diarrhea or when a suggestive epidemiologic history is obtained, bacterial cultures and microscopic examination of the stool for parasites and inflammatory cells are appropriate. Proctoscopy is generally reserved for patients with bloody diarrhea, or those who do not show improvement within 10 days. Likewise, radiologic studies should usually be deferred until the initial course of the illness has been observed. In cases of massive fluid loss, measurement of serum electrolytes is useful to aid in determining replacement therapy.

TREATMENT General and nonspecific treatment of acute diarrhea includes rest, encouragement of fluid intake, and prescription of opiate-containing agents by mouth. Intravenous fluid and electrolyte replacement may be desirable and necessary in infants and the elderly. As a result of success achieved with cholera patients, the use of oral sugar-electrolyte solutions is being extended to the treatment of patients with acute diarrhea considered to be due to other enterotoxin-producing bacteria. Biofeedback therapy has proved helpful for some patients who suffer from fecal incontinence due to anal sphincter impairment.

Chronic diarrhea Diarrhea persisting for weeks or months, whether constant or intermittent, may be a functional symptom or a manifestation of serious illness. For this reason, it is incumbent upon the physician to search carefully for evidence of organic disease, such as fever, weight loss, malnutrition, or anemia. Abdominal tenderness and fever suggest the presence of inflammation. When there is involvement of the large bowel, the major diseases to be considered include ulcerative colitis, Crohn's disease of the colon, amebiasis, and diverticulitis. Crohn's disease of the small intestine may involve one or more of its segments. The ileum is most frequently affected. Other diarrheal conditions which may resemble Crohn's disease radiographically include tuberculous and fungal enteritis, lymphoma, amyloidosis, and argentaffin (carcinoid) tumors of the small bowel.

Prolonged diarrhea without evidence of inflammation may reflect impairments of absorption, secretion, or digestion. Selective derangements, such as those due to *bile salt enteropathy* and *lactase deficiency*, are usually not accompanied by weight loss or malnutrition. *Mucosal disorders,* best exemplified by sprue, are frequently associated with weight loss, malodorous stools, abdominal distention, and anemia, and, when more severe, with osteomalacia, bleeding due to hypoprothrombinemia, avitaminotic neuropathies, and tetany. *Pancreatic insufficiency* resulting from chronic pancreatitis, carcinoma, resection, or cystic fibrosis produces steatorrhea and weight loss of varying severity. A number of mechanisms may be responsible for *postgastrectomy diarrhea* (see Chap. 235). These include the dumping syndrome, postvagotomy motility derangements, inadequate stimulation of pancreatic digestive enzymes, and incomplete mixing of these enzymes with food. On rare occasions severe postgastrectomy diarrhea and malnutrition are due to the inadvertent creation by the surgeon of a gastroileostomy instead of a gastrojejunostomy. *Bacterial overgrowth* in the small intestine, as may occur with extensive diverticulosis and prolonged bowel stasis secondary to disorders of peristalsis (e.g., scleroderma, diabetic visceral neuropathy), can also lead to chronic diarrhea and weight loss. This has been attributed to bacterial deconjugation of bile salts and hydroxylation of long-chain fatty acids, to consumption of nutrients by the organisms, and to mucosal abnormalities believed to be caused by bacteria or their metabolites (see Chap. 237). At times, diarrhea may accompany stasis in the absence of bacterial overgrowth.

Endocrine disorders that may be accompanied by chronic diarrhea include thyrotoxicosis, diabetes mellitus, adrenal insufficiency, and hypoparathyroidism. The release of potent secretagogues from neoplastic tissue in the Zollinger-Ellison syndrome (gastrin), medullary carcinoma of the thyroid (calcitonin, prostaglandins), and pancreatic cholera syndrome (vasoactive intestinal peptide) makes diarrhea a prominent feature of these disorders. *Rectal villous adenomas* may secrete large quantities of fluid and electrolytes, which are promptly evacuated as a clear, odorless liquid. When marked fluid loss occurs, hypokalemia and dehydration may result.

Habitual *cathartic abuse* must be suspected when the cause of prolonged diarrhea remains perplexing. Even if this is denied by the patient, a stool sample should be alkalinized with sodium hydroxide; this will produce a lavender color if phenolphthalein-containing laxatives have been surreptitiously ingested. The observation of melanosis coli by sigmoidoscopy indicates chronic usage of anthraquinone laxatives.

Constipation Constipation is a common complaint often resulting from the inordinate expectation of "regularity" in bowel-conscious individuals. Stools are described as infrequent, incomplete, or unduly hard; unusual straining may be required to achieve defecation. A review of the patient's habits often reveals contributory and correctable causes, such as insufficient dietary roughage, lack of exercise, suppression of defecatory urges arising at inconvenient moments, inadequate allotment of time for full defecation, and prolonged travel. Appropriate adjustments of these patterns and reassurance are preferable to the prescription of laxatives and may be all that is required for improvement. When the patient also has symptoms such as fatigue, malaise, headaches, or anorexia, the possibility should be considered that such symptoms reflect an underlying depression of which constipation is but one component. Decreased colonic motility is responsible for the constipation associated with the use of parasympatholytic drugs, spinal cord injury, scleroderma, and Hirschsprung's disease.

Hemorrhoids, anal fissures, perineal abscesses, and rectal strictures often prevent easy and adequate stool evacuation. When constipation and tenesmus of recent onset are reported, the possibility of carcinoma of the rectum or sigmoid colon must be seriously considered. In such instances sigmoidoscopic and barium enema examinations should be obtained early and are virtually obligatory if fecal blood has been observed or if occult blood is detected on any of three successive stool specimens. Stools of abnormally thin caliber occur in patients with rectal or sigmoid colon carcinoma but are even more commonly due to a spastic colon. Other mechanical causes of constipation include volvulus of the sigmoid colon, diverticulitis, intussusception, and hernias. A variety of metabolic abnormalities, such as hypothyroidism, hypercalcemia, hypokalemia, porphyria, lead poisoning, and dehydration are often associated with constipation. Prolonged fecal retention, leading to impaction, may occur in certain neurologic disorders (e.g., spinal cord injury, multiple sclerosis, cerebral palsy, senility), and in these instances, when autonomous regulation of evacuation is unachievable, vigorous and sustained enema programs are often necessary.

IRRITABLE BOWEL The irritable bowel syndrome (also referred to as *spastic colon* and *mucous colitis*) is one of the most frequent gastrointestinal disorders (see Chap. 239). This condition is characterized by periodic or chronic bowel symptoms which include diarrhea, constipation, and abdominal pain. These symptoms are often secondary to mental distress, but the anxiety produced by the bowel disturbance is sometimes regarded by the patient as the fundamental cause of the emotional upset. During periods of discomfort, stools are apt to become thin, fragmented, or pelletlike, and accompanied by excessive mucus and gas. Efforts to ameliorate symptoms with mild cathartics or antispasmodic drugs may yield adverse and exaggerated responses. A variety of therapeutic approaches, including the avoidance of foods which tend to upset the patient, addition of bulk-forming agents, judicious use of antispasmodics and tranquilizers, and psychotherapy may provide some degree of relief. If the patient's life goals can be shifted away from the quixotic search for the perfect stool, much can be accomplished. At the same time, it must be remembered that such individuals are not exempt from developing bowel cancer, and any worrisome deviation from their general pattern of derangement must be seriously evaluated.

FLATULENCE A significant amount of flatus is passed each day by normal persons, and the complaint of flatulence often reflects a heightened and embarrassing awareness of this natural occurrence. Excessive quantities of flatus may be caused by aerophagia or the formation of increased amounts of gas by intestinal bacteria. The latter process can be associated with malabsorption syndromes but is more frequently a consequence of eating foods such as beans, broccoli, and cabbage which have a high content of nondigestible polysaccharides. The oligosaccharides stachyose and raffinose, isolated from beans, are particularly effective substrates for fermentation to carbon dioxide, hydrogen, and methane by colonic flora. Chromatographic analysis of a sample of flatus will show these gases to predominate, in contrast to the high nitrogen levels that occur when excessive flatus is caused by aerophagia. The treatment of flatulence is generally undertaken to reduce embarrassment and consists of measures to decrease aerophagia along with avoidance of foods that cause excessive gas.

REFERENCES

BLACKLOW NR, CUKOR GC: Viral gastroenteritis. N Engl J Med 304:397, 1981

CHRISTENSEN J: Motility of the colon, in *Physiology of the Gastrointestinal Tract*, LR Johnson et al (eds). New York, Raven Press, 1981, vol 1, chap 14

DROSSMAN DA et al: The irritable bowel syndrome. Gastroenterology 73:811, 1977

FIELD M et al (eds): *Secretory Diarrhea*, Clinical Physiology Series. Bethesda, Md, American Physiological Society, 1980

GERSHON MD, ERDE SM: The nervous system of the gut. Gastroenterology 80:1571, 1981

LIEBERMAN DA: Common anorectal disorders. Ann Intern Med 101:837, 1984

PLOTKIN GR et al: Gastroenteritis: Etiology, pathophysiology and clinical manifestations. Medicine 58:95, 1979

READ NW et al: Chronic diarrhea of unknown origin. Gastroenterology 78:2644, 1980

SCHULTZ SG: Ion transport by mammalian large intestine, in *Physiology of the Gastrointestinal Tract*, LR Johnson et al (eds). New York, Raven Press, 1981, vol 2, chap 38

SNOOKS SJ et al: Damage to the innervation of the pelvic floor musculature in chronic constipation. Gastroenterology 89:977, 1985

WOLFSON JS et al: Cryptosporidiosis in immunocompetent patients. N Engl J Med 312:1278, 1985

37 HEMATEMESIS, MELENA, AND HEMATOCHEZIA

KURT J. ISSELBACHER / JAMES M. RICHTER

Hematemesis is defined as the vomiting of blood, and *melena* as the passage of stools rendered black and tarry by the presence of altered blood. These symptoms of gastrointestinal hemorrhage should bring the patient to medical attention and, within certain limits, suggest the anatomic site of bleeding. Exsanguinating gastrointestinal hemorrhage will rarely occur without the appearance of altered or gross blood passed by mouth or rectum. The color of vomited blood will vary depending on the concentration of hydrochloric acid in the stomach and its admixture with the blood. Thus, if vomiting occurs shortly after the onset of bleeding, the vomitus appears red; if there is a delay in vomiting, the appearance will be dark red, brown, or black. Precipitated blood clots in the vomitus will produce a characteristic "coffee grounds" appearance. Hematemesis usually indicates bleeding proximal to the ligament of Treitz, since blood entering the gastrointestinal tract below the duodenum rarely enters the stomach.

While bleeding sufficient to produce hematemesis usually results in melena, less than half of patients with melena have hematemesis. *Melena* usually denotes bleeding from the esophagus, stomach, or duodenum, but lesions in the jejunum, ileum, and even ascending colon may cause melena provided the gastrointestinal transit time is sufficiently prolonged. Approximately 60 mL of blood is required to produce a single black stool; acute blood loss greater than this may produce melena for up to 3 days. After the stool color returns to normal, tests for occult blood may remain positive for up to a week or longer.

The black color of stools secondary to intestinal bleeding results from contact of the blood with hydrochloric acid to produce hematin. Characteristically, such stools are tarry ("sticky"). This tarry consistency is in contrast to black or dark stools occurring after the ingestion of iron, bismuth, or licorice. Similarly, red stools may result from the ingestion of beets or intravenous administration of sulfobromophthalein. Gastrointestinal bleeding, even if detected only by positive tests for occult blood, indicates potentially serious disease and must be further investigated.

Hematochezia, the passage of bright-red blood per rectum, generally signifies bleeding from a source distal to the ligament of Treitz. However, since blood must remain in the gut for approximately 8 h to produce melena, rapid hemorrhage into the esophagus, stomach, or duodenum may also result in hematochezia.

The clinical manifestations of gastrointestinal bleeding depend upon the extent and rate of hemorrhage, and the presence of coincidental diseases. Blood loss of less than 500 mL is rarely associated with systemic signs; exceptions include bleeding in the elderly or in the anemic patient in whom smaller amounts of blood loss may produce hemodynamic alterations. Rapid hemorrhage of greater volume results in decreased venous return to the heart, decreased cardiac output, and increased peripheral resistance due to reflex vasoconstriction. Orthostatic hypotension greater than 10 mmHg usually indicates a 20 percent or greater reduction in blood volume. Concomitant symptoms include syncope, lightheadedness, nausea, sweating, and thirst. When blood loss approaches 40 percent of blood volume, shock frequently ensues with pronounced tachycardia and hypotension. Pallor is prominent, and the skin is cool.

It is important to recognize that the hematocrit, when determined immediately after the onset of bleeding, may not accurately reflect blood loss, since equilibration with extravascular fluid and hemodilution require several hours. Common laboratory findings include mild leukocytosis and thrombocytosis which develop within 6 h after the onset of bleeding. The blood urea nitrogen may be mildly elevated, particularly in upper gastrointestinal bleeding, due to breakdown of blood proteins to urea by intestinal bacteria as well as from a mild reduction in the glomerular filtration rate.

ETIOLOGY OF UPPER GASTROINTESTINAL BLEEDING A careful history and physical examination of the oropharynx and nasal cavity should serve to exclude swallowed blood as a source of hematemesis or melena.

The four most common causes of upper gastrointestinal hemorrhage are (1) peptic ulceration, (2) erosive gastritis, (3) variceal bleeding, and (4) Mallory-Weiss syndrome. These entities account for up to 90 percent of all cases of upper gastrointestinal hemorrhage in which a definite lesion can be found.

Peptic ulcer Peptic ulcer is probably the most common cause of upper gastrointestinal bleeding; the majority of such ulcers are found in the duodenum. Approximately 20 to 30 percent of patients with documented ulcers will have significant bleeding sometime during the course of their disease. Because hemorrhage may be the initial manifestation of a peptic ulcer, this lesion should be seriously considered even when a history characteristic of ulcer disease is not obtained.

Gastritis Gastritis may be associated with recent alcohol ingestion or with the use of anti-inflammatory drugs, such as aspirin or indomethacin. Gastric erosions also frequently develop in patients with major trauma, surgery, and severe systemic disease, particularly burn victims and patients with increased intracranial pressure. Because there are no characteristic physical findings, the diagnosis of gastritis must be suspected when the appropriate clinical setting is encountered.

When a specific diagnosis is required, gastroscopy is usually needed to confirm the diagnosis since radiologic examination generally lacks the sensitivity required to detect gastritis.

Variceal bleeding Variceal bleeding is characteristically abrupt and massive; chronic gastrointestinal blood loss is unusual. Bleeding from esophageal or gastric varices is usually the result of portal hypertension, secondary to cirrhosis. Although alcoholic cirrhosis is the most prevalent cause of esophageal varices in the United States, any condition producing portal hypertension, even in the absence of hepatic disease (i.e., portal vein thrombosis or idiopathic portal hypertension), may result in variceal bleeding. Further, while the presence of varices usually connotes long-standing portal hypertension, acute hepatitis or severe fatty infiltration of the liver may occasionally produce varices which disappear once the hepatic abnormality resolves. It should be emphasized that although upper gastrointestinal bleeding in a patient with cirrhosis suggests a variceal source, approximately half those patients will be bleeding from other lesions (e.g., gastritis, ulcers). Consequently, it is essential to exclude nonvariceal causes of bleeding so that the appropriate treatment can be instituted.

MALLORY-WEISS SYNDROME With the advent of esophagogastroduodenoscopy, the Mallory-Weiss syndrome has been demonstrated with increasing frequency as a cause of acute upper gastrointestinal hemorrhage (see also Chap. 34). This syndrome refers to a mucosal laceration in the region of the esophagogastric junction which is often characterized historically by retching or nonbloody vomiting followed by hematemesis.

OTHER LESIONS Less common bleeding esophageal lesions include esophagitis and carcinoma; these generally cause chronic blood loss and rarely produce massive bleeding.

Gastric carcinoma may result in chronic gastrointestinal bleeding. Lymphoma, polyps, and other tumors of the stomach and small bowel are uncommon and, consequently, are infrequent causes of hemorrhage. Leiomyoma and leiomyosarcoma are likewise rare, but they can lead to massive hemorrhage. Bleeding from duodenal and jejunal diverticula is relatively unusual. Vascular insufficiency of the mesenteric vessels, including occlusive and nonocclusive disease, may lead to bloody diarrhea.

Arteriosclerotic aortic aneurysms may rupture into the small intestine; such an event is almost always fatal. Rupture may also occur following arterial reconstructive surgery with fistula formation between synthetic graft and bowel lumen. A small or herald bleed may precede a sudden massive hemorrhage from an aortoenteric fistula. Sudden bleeding may also occur after trauma resulting in hepatic laceration; this may result in blood loss into the bile ducts (i.e., hemobilia).

Primary blood dyscrasias, including leukemia, thrombocytopenic states, the hemophilias, and disseminated intravascular coagulation may result in significant gastrointestinal bleeding. Polycythemia vera may be associated with an increased incidence of peptic ulceration, and may also result in gastrointestinal bleeding due to mesenteric or portal vein thrombosis. Periarteritis nodosa, Henoch-Schönlein purpura, and other forms of vasculitis may lead to gastrointestinal blood loss. Gastrointestinal bleeding may be seen with amyloidosis, Osler-Weber-Rendu disease, other arteriovenous malformations, pseudoxanthoma elasticum, Turner's syndrome, intestinal hemangiomas, neurofibromatosis, Kaposi's sarcoma, and Peutz-Jeghers syndrome. Uremia may produce gastrointestinal blood loss; the most common presentation is chronic, occult bleeding from diffuse involvement of the mucosa of the stomach and small bowel.

ETIOLOGY OF LOWER GASTROINTESTINAL BLEEDING **Anal and rectal lesions** Small amounts of bright red-blood on the surface of the stool and toilet tissue are often caused by hemorrhoids; such bleeding is generally precipitated by the strained passage of a hard stool. Anal fissures and fistulas may present in a similar fashion. Proctitis is another source of rectal bleeding; it is frequently seen in young adults, especially in male homosexuals. In the latter situation, proctitis may be due to gonorrheal or mycoplasma infections or may be idiopathic. Rectal trauma is a cause of hematochezia, and the placement of foreign objects in the rectal vault may precipitate perforation as well as acute rectal hemorrhage. It must be emphasized that anal pathology does not preclude other sources of blood loss, and these must be sought and excluded.

Colonic lesions Carcinoma of the colon, as well as colonic polyps, may produce chronic blood loss. Angiodysplastic lesions, usually involving the ascending colon, are a major source of acute or chronic bleeding in elderly patients; such vascular lesions can be identified by angiography or colonoscopy. Frankly bloody diarrhea is common and may be the presenting symptom in patients with ulcerative colitis; it is less frequent in granulomatous colitis, but occult blood may be present in the stool. Bleeding may also accompany diarrhea due to infections such as shigellosis, amebiasis, campylobacterosis, and rarely, salmonellosis. In the elderly patient, ischemic colitis may be a cause of bloody diarrhea; this lesion may also be seen in younger women who use oral contraceptive agents.

Diverticula Colonic diverticula are most often located in the sigmoid colon; however, diverticular bleeding may originate anywhere in the colon. Bleeding from colonic diverticula is a cause of massive lower gastrointestinal hemorrhage. The usual presentation of a diverticular hemorrhage is that of painless passage of a maroon-colored stool. Meckel's diverticulum, a congenital anomaly of the distal ileum, is present in about 2 percent of the population and may cause bleeding. Although only about 15 percent of these diverticula contain gastric mucosa, half of the lesions which cause acute bleeding contain gastric mucosa. This anomaly is an important cause of acute hemorrhage in children and young adults.

APPROACH TO THE PATIENT WITH GASTROINTESTINAL BLEEDING The approach to the bleeding patient depends upon the site, extent, and rate of bleeding. Patients with hematemesis have usually bled greater amounts (often greater than 1000 mL) than those who have melena alone (usually 500 mL or less), and mortality with the former is about twice that of the latter. When first seen, the patient may be in shock. Prior to taking a history and performing a thorough physical examination, vital signs should be noted, blood sent for typing and cross-matching, and a large-bore intravenous line placed for infusion of saline or other plasma expanders. The physician initiating the evaluation of the bleeding patient must be aware that the primary consideration is the necessity of maintaining adequate intravascular volume and hemodynamic stability during the diagnostic workup.

History A history or symptoms suggestive of prior ulcer disease may provide a useful clue. Similarly, recent abuse of alcohol or ingestion of anti-inflammatory drugs should make erosive gastritis more suspect. If alcohol abuse has been long-standing, esophageal varices may be a more likely source of hemorrhage. Aspirin use may also cause gastroduodenitis, peptic ulceration, and bleeding. Prior history of gastrointestinal bleeding may be helpful, as may a family history of intestinal disease or hemorrhagic diathesis. Recent retching followed by hematemesis should suggest the possibility of the Mallory-Weiss syndrome. The acute onset of bloody diarrhea may indicate the presence of inflammatory bowel disease or an infectious colitis. It is also important to exclude associated systemic illnesses or recent trauma, since bleeding from erosive gastritis is frequently seen under such conditions.

Physical examination Following evaluation for orthostatic changes in pulse and blood pressure and institution of volume repletion, the patient should be examined for clues to the underlying illness. A nonintestinal bleeding source should be excluded by careful examination of the oral cavity and nasopharynx. Dermatologic examination may disclose the characteristic telangiectasia of Osler-Weber-Rendu disease (although these will not be visible if severe anemia is present), the perioral pigmentation of Peutz-Jeghers syndrome, the dermal fibromas of neurofibromatosis, the sebaceous cysts and bony tumors of Gardner's syndrome, the palpable purpura frequently seen with vasculitis, or the diffuse pigmentation seen in hemochromatosis. Stigmata of chronic liver disease such as spider angiomata, gynecomastia, testicular atrophy, jaundice, ascites, and hepatosplenomegaly should suggest portal hypertension resulting in bleeding from esophageal or gastric varices. Significant lymph node enlargement or abdominal masses may reflect underlying intraabdominal malignancy. Careful rectal examination is important to exclude local pathology as well as to observe the color of the stool.

Laboratory studies Initial studies should include the hematocrit, hemoglobin, careful assessment of red blood cell morphologic features (hypochromic, microcytic red blood cells suggest that blood loss is chronic), white blood cell count, differential, and platelet count. Prothrombin time, partial thromboplastin time, and other coagulation studies may be in order to exclude primary or secondary clotting defects. A radiograph of the abdomen is rarely helpful in establishing a diagnosis unless a perforated viscus is suspected. Though the initial studies are valuable and essential, repeated evaluation of the laboratory data is important as one follows the clinical course of the bleeding.

Diagnostic and therapeutic approach The diagnostic approach to the patient with gastrointestinal hemorrhage must be individualized. The initial management of gastrointestinal bleeding may be under the direction of the internist, but it is prudent to consult a surgeon in the event that surgery is required.

When there is a history of melena or hematemesis or the suspicion of bleeding from the upper part of the gastrointestinal tract, the patient should have a nasogastric tube passed to empty the stomach and to determine whether the bleeding is in the upper part of the gastrointestinal tract. If the initial nasogastric aspirate is clear, the tube should be left in place for several hours, since active duodenal bleeding may occur with an initially clear nasogastric aspirate. If the aspirate is negative for blood during a period of active bleeding, it is reasonable to conclude that active bleeding is not occurring in the gastroduodenal region, and the nasogastric tube can be removed. However, if there is no evidence of active bleeding at the time the nasogastric tube is placed, one cannot assume bleeding did not come from the stomach or duodenum and endoscopy may be required.

If red blood or "coffee grounds" material is aspirated from the nasogastric tube, saline irrigation of the stomach should be initiated. Irrigation serves two purposes: it provides the clinician with an assessment of the rapidity of the bleeding, and clears the stomach of old blood prior to possible endoscopy. Subsequent diagnostic maneuvers will depend on whether bleeding continues; this can be assessed by vital signs, transfusion requirements, and the number and consistency of stools. Most medical centers now have available experienced endoscopists as well as radiologists with facilities for selective arteriography so that it is possible to have emergency endoscopic or angiographic studies performed within hours of the patient's admission to the hospital. It must be emphasized that demonstration of a lesion in a patient with gastrointestinal bleeding should also be accompanied by evidence that this lesion is the site of bleeding (Fig. 37-1).

If the bleeding has stopped, and the patient is stable, one may proceed with either esophagogastroduodenoscopy or upper gastrointestinal barium studies. Although *endoscopy* provides a higher diagnostic yield, it has not been proved conclusively that survival is increased by early endoscopy. *Barium examination* may identify a potential source of hemorrhage, but there are important limitations to such x-rays. First, lesions such as erosive gastritis and Mallory-Weiss lacerations are not visualized by x-ray. Second, if the patient rebleeds following a barium exam, the retained contrast material will make endoscopy difficult and angiography impossible. Clearly the approach in this setting must be individualized. The decision to employ esophagogastroduodenoscopy or barium studies will depend on several variables, including the availability of an experienced endoscopist and the condition of the patient. Although studies have shown that emergency endoscopy and a vigorous diagnostic approach do not generally decrease patient morbidity or mortality, emergency endoscopy may be important in planning therapy in certain patients with cirrhosis or previous gastric surgery. By identifying other patients with visible vessels and thus a high risk for recurrent bleeding, possible complications can be anticipated. Newer techniques for coagulation of bleeding ulcers or sclerosis of varices via the endoscope may broaden the indications for and utility of early endoscopy in the future.

Persistent upper gastrointestinal hemorrhage must be viewed differently, and most clinicians would proceed immediately to esophagogastroduodenoscopy. Determination of the site and cause of bleeding is essential to plan for appropriate therapy, particularly if varices are suspected. Thus, anticipation of surgery, angiography, or the suspicion of bleeding varices are strong indications for esophagogastroduodenoscopy in the evaluation of the patient with persistent upper gastrointestinal bleeding. In contrast, esophagogastroduodenoscopy is more difficult in the evaluation of *massive* hemorrhage, since large amounts of blood obscure visualization of mucosal pathology, and angiography may be required in addition to endoscopy.

Should bleeding continue and endoscopy fail to reveal the bleeding source, the site of hemorrhage may be beyond the ligament of Treitz. In this situation angiography is frequently valuable in establishing a diagnosis. Angiographic demonstration of the bleeding site requires blood loss at a rate of at least 0.5 mL/min. Clinical correlates reflecting this degree of blood loss include postural hypotension and the necessity for blood transfusion to maintain stable vital signs. Emergency angiography may localize the site of bleeding; however, the cause of the bleeding may not be determined unless varices, vascular malformations, or aneurysms are present.

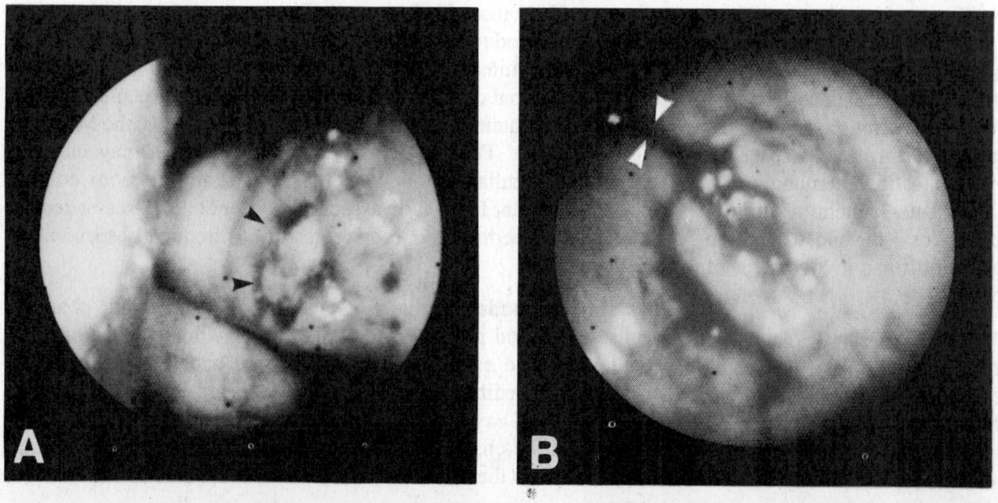

FIGURE 37-1 *Endoscopic photographs from a patient with hematemesis. A. A gastric ulcer along the lesser curvature of the stomach is identified (arrows). B. The same ulcer is bleeding actively from a spurting artery (arrows).*

Therapeutic angiography is a helpful approach to the control of persistent hemorrhage. Continuous intraarterial infusion of vasoconstrictor agents, such as vasopressin, is often successful in controlling hemorrhage due to gastric ulcer or Mallory-Weiss tear. Additionally, embolic material may be injected directly into the artery perfusing the bleeding site. However, intravenous infusions of vasopressin and endoscopic sclerosis for control of variceal bleeding are more valuable than angiographic techniques.

If bleeding esophageal varices are identified on upper endoscopy, peripheral infusions of vasopressin may control the bleeding. The response to such therapy depends upon the general condition of the patient as assessed by clinical and laboratory parameters. It has been shown that intraarterial vasopressin is no more effective than intravenous administration in the control of variceal bleeding. Varices may also be controlled by balloon tamponade with a Sengstaken-Blakemore tube. Unlike vasopressin, this technique is generally used as a preoperative stabilizing measure which should be followed by definitive therapy within 48 h whenever possible. Endoscopic sclerosis of varices has emerged as an effective therapy for bleeding esophageal varices and when available should be attempted prior to surgery.

In the evaluation of *lower gastrointestinal bleeding* the most important procedures are the digital examination, anoscopy, and sigmoidoscopy. The last of these may identify a bleeding site or document bleeding coming from above the range of the instrument. Colonoscopy is a valuable technique for the evaluation of patients with small to moderate lower gastrointestinal bleeds. Preparation of the colon with saline lavage solutions permits a colonoscopic evaluation of the bowel within hours. Most colonic abnormalities, including angiodysplasia, can be detected and treated with polypectomy or electrocoagulation. If brisk bleeding continues, arteriography may serve to localize the bleeding site and allow local infusion of vasoconstrictor agents to control bleeding. Because arteriography detects actively bleeding lesions only when blood loss exceeds 0.5 mL/min and gastrointestinal bleeding tends to be intermittent, arteriography is often nondiagnostic. Radiolabeled erythrocyte scanning is more sensitive than arteriography in detecting blood loss of 0.1 mL/min and may be used to investigate less severe bleeding. However, bleeding scans are less specific than arteriography, generally localizing the lesion and seldom making a discrete diagnosis. Bleeding scans are most helpful in detecting active, low-grade, or intermittent bleeding in order to better time arteriography and obtain the maximal diagnostic yield. Finally, a barium enema has a limited role in the evaluation of acute rectal bleeding. Although it may localize potential bleeding sources, it will not define the bleeding site. Furthermore, if brisk bleeding recurs, subsequent colonoscopy or angiography will be difficult to interpret due to retained contrast material. Therefore, it is advisable to withhold barium studies of both the upper and lower bowel for at least 48 h after the cessation of active bleeding.

REFERENCES

ATHANASOULIS CA: Angiography. Its contribution to the emergency management of gastrointestinal hemorrhage. Radiol Clin North Am 14:265, 1976

CELLO JP et al: Endoscopic sclerotherapy versus portocaval shunt in patients with severe cirrhosis and variceal hemorrhage. N Engl J Med 311:1589, 1984

CHOJKIER M et al: A controlled comparison of continuous intra-arterial and intravenous infusions of vasopressin in hemorrhage from esophageal varices. Gastroenterology 77:540, 1979

FLEISCHER D: Endoscopic therapy of upper gastrointestinal bleeding. Gastroenterology 90:217, 1986

LICHTENSTEIN JL: Accuracy and reliability of endoscopy and x-ray in upper gastrointestinal bleeding. Dig Dis Sc 26:70s, 1981

LUK GD et al: Gastric aspiration in localization of gastrointestinal hemorrhage. JAMA 241:576, 1979

PETERSON WL et al: Routine early endoscopy in upper gastrointestinal tract bleeding: A randomized, controlled trial. N Engl J Med 304:925, 1981

PRIEBE HJ et al: Antacid versus cimetidine in preventing acute gastrointestinal bleeding. A randomized trial in 75 critically ill patients. N Engl J Med 302:426, 1980

RICHTER JM et al: Angiodysplasia: Clinical presentation and colonoscopic diagnosis. Dig Dis Sci 29:481, 1984

STEER ML, SILEN W: Diagnostic procedures in gastrointestinal hemorrhage. N Engl J Med 309:646, 1983

38 JAUNDICE AND HEPATOMEGALY

KURT J. ISSELBACHER

JAUNDICE

Jaundice, or *icterus,* refers to the yellow pigmentation of the skin or scleras by bilirubin. This in turn is a result of elevated levels of bilirubin in the bloodstream. Jaundice may be brought to clinical attention by a darkening of the urine or a yellow discoloration of the skin or sclera; the latter often is the site where clinical icterus may first be detected. Scleral pigmentation is attributed to richness of this tissue in elastin, which has a special affinity for bilirubin. Jaundice must be distinguished from other causes of yellow pigmentation such as carotenemia (see Chaps. 51 and 76), which is due to carotenoid pigments in the bloodstream and is associated with a yellowish discoloration of the skin but not of the sclera.

Normal serum bilirubin concentrations range from 0.3 to 1.0 mg/dL (or 5.1 to 17 μmol per liter), and normally most of this is unconjugated (see Fig. 38-1). The precise level at which jaundice becomes clinically evident varies, but it can usually be recognized when the total serum bilirubin exceeds 2 to 2.5 mg/dL. With pronounced jaundice the skin may take on a greenish hue because of

FIGURE 38-1 *The sources and precursors of bilirubin and steps in its subsequent metabolism and excretion.*

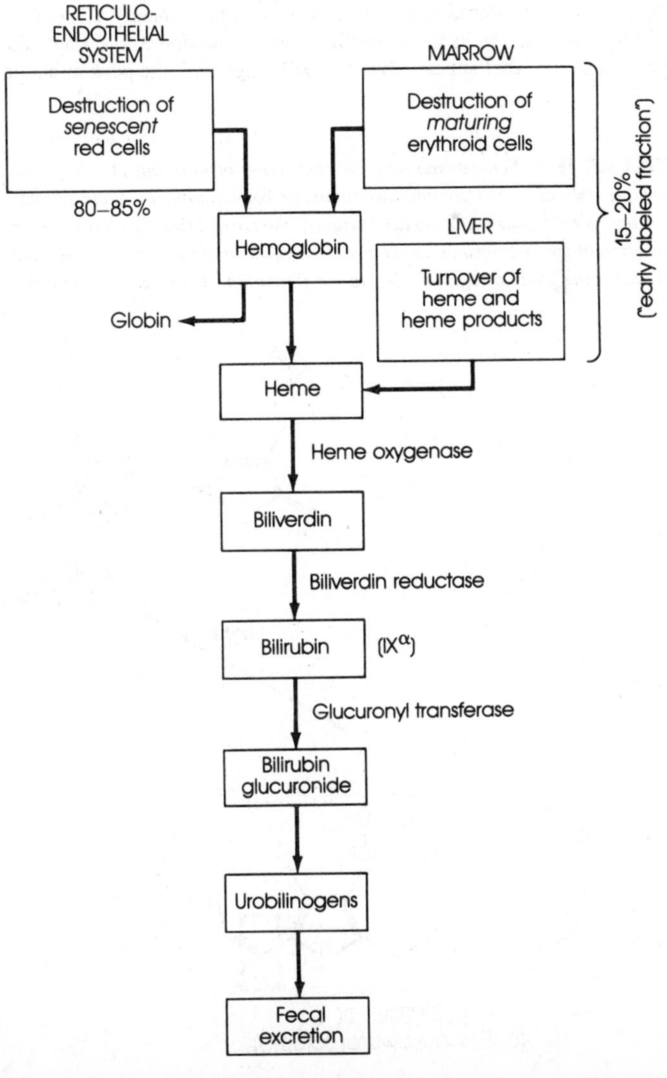

the conversion of bilirubin to biliverdin, an oxidation product of bilirubin. Oxidation occurs more readily with conjugated bilirubin, and hence a greenish hue is seen more frequently in conditions with pronounced conjugated hyperbilirubinemia. When bilirubin is exposed to visible blue light (430 to 470 nm), metastable isomers of bilirubin are produced. These photoisomers are polar (because they permit no intramolecular hydrogen bonding) and can be excreted by the liver into bile without having to be conjugated (see below and Fig. 38-2).

PRODUCTION AND METABOLISM OF BILIRUBIN **Normal sources of bilirubin** (Fig. 38-2) Most bilirubin is derived from the catabolism of hemoglobin present in senescent red blood cells. This normally accounts for about 80 to 85 percent of the daily bilirubin production. When a circulating red blood cell reaches the end of its normal life span of approximately 120 days, it is destroyed in the reticuloendothelial system. In the catabolism of hemoglobin, globin is first dissociated from heme, after which the heme moiety (ferroprotoporphyrin IX) is oxidatively cleaved and converted to biliverdin by a microsomal heme oxygenase. This enzyme system requires oxygen and a cofactor, reduced nicotinamide adenine dinucleotide phosphate (NADPH). Bilirubin (in the chemical form of bilirubin IXα) is then formed from biliverdin by biliverdin reductase.

About 15 to 20 percent of the bilirubin is derived from sources other than senescent erythrocytes. One source is the *destruction of maturing erythroid cells in the bone marrow,* or so-called ineffective erythropoiesis (see Chap. 287). The other is *nonerythroid components,* especially in the liver, and involves the turnover of heme and heme proteins (such as cytochrome, myoglobin, and heme-containing enzymes). These two sources of bilirubin are collectively referred to as the *early labeled fraction,* a term derived from experiments with labeled glycine and Δ-aminolevulinic acid (ALA). Thus when labeled glycine is administered to a normal subject, approximately 15 percent of the label appears in stool urobilinogens in the first 3 to 5 days; 85 percent of the label appears over a broad range with the peak at about 120 days and reflects bilirubin produced from the normal destruction of senescent red blood cells.

Transport of bilirubin Following liberation of unconjugated bilirubin into the plasma, virtually all the pigment is tightly *bound to albumin.* The maximum binding capacity is 2 mol bilirubin per mole of albumin in a reversible, noncovalent manner. Certain organic anions, such as sulfonamides and salicylates, compete with bilirubin for common binding sites on albumin and may displace bilirubin from albumin, permitting it to enter tissues such as the central nervous system. Most of the evidence for albumin binding has been obtained from studies using unconjugated bilirubin. Conjugated bilirubin is also bound to albumin, but in both a reversible and an irreversible manner. The reversible binding is similar to the noncovalent binding of unconjugated bilirubin, but the binding is much weaker. The second type involves a very tight, irreversible albumin-bilirubin complex that appears in the serum when hepatic excretion of bilirubin is impaired (i.e., with cholestasis). Due to the nature of the binding, the complex does *not* appear in urine. Also this bilirubin-albumin conjugate may remain detectable in the serum for several weeks after the relief of the obstruction or during recovery from hepatocellular jaundice.

Bilirubin is found in body fluids (cerebrospinal fluid, joint effusions, cysts, etc.) in proportion to the albumin content of the fluids and is absent from true secretions such as tears, saliva, and pancreatic juice. The appearance of jaundice is also influenced by blood flow and edema. Paralyzed extremities and edematous areas tend to remain uncolored, and "unilateral" jaundice in patients with hemiplegia and edema may be seen if jaundice develops.

Hepatic metabolism of bilirubin (Fig. 38-3) The liver occupies a central role in the metabolism of the bile pigments. Three distinct phases are recognized: (1) *hepatic uptake,* (2) *conjugation,* and (3) *excretion* into bile. Of these three steps, excretion appears to be the

FIGURE 38-2 *Scheme showing the conversion of bilirubin IXα to water-soluble derivatives by photoisomerization or conjugation. In A the normal, unconjugated pigment Z-Z isomer is shown; the dashed line shows the* upright *position of the hydrogen at the methene bridges linking the pyrrole molecules. B shows the effect of light leading to the formation of the water-soluble E-E isomer; the dashed-line box serves to emphasize the inversion of the hydrogens at the methene bridges between the pyrrole molecules. C shows the formation of water-soluble bilirubin diglucuronide formation; the dashed-line box encloses one of the two glucuronic acid moieties.*

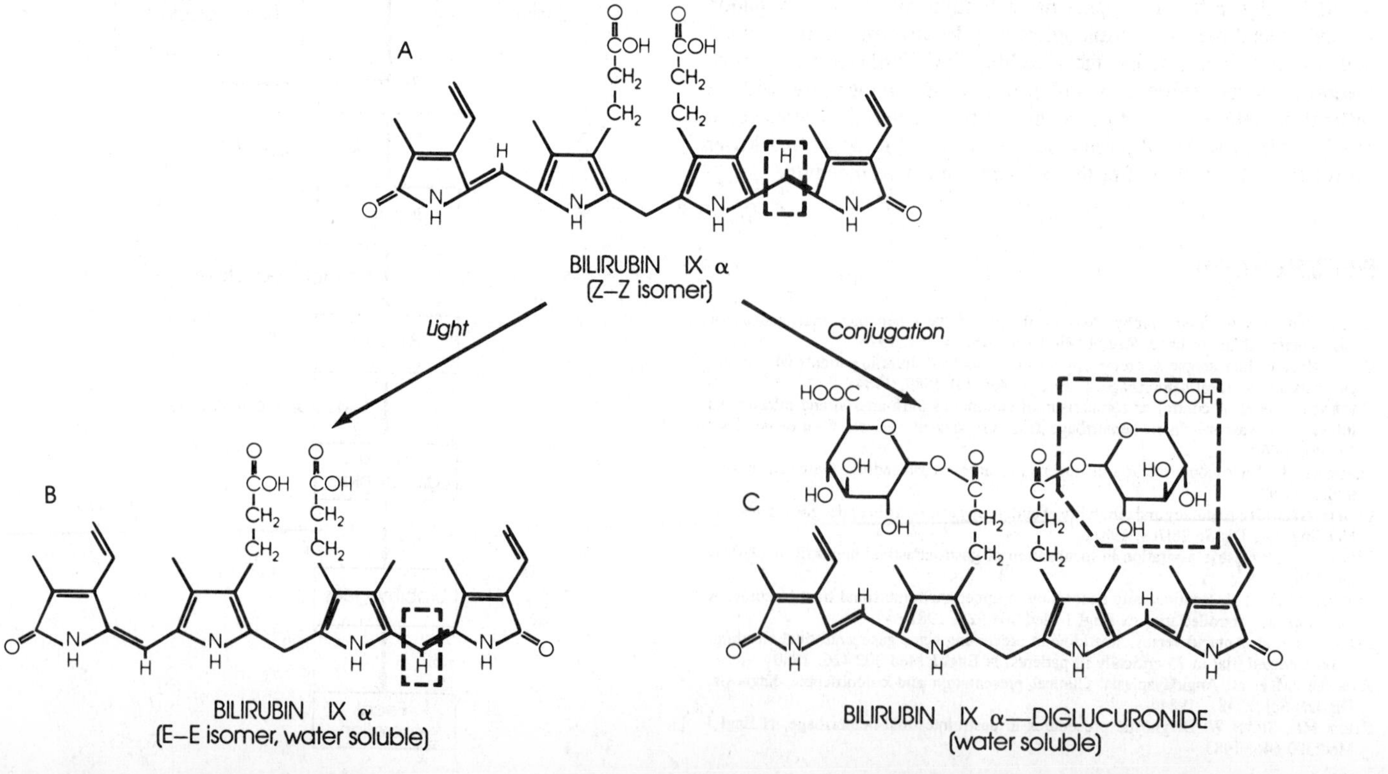

rate-limiting step and the one most susceptible to impairment when the liver cell is damaged.

UPTAKE Unconjugated bilirubin bound to albumin is presented to the liver cell, and upon entry the pigment and albumin become dissociated. The uptake phase and subsequent hepatocyte storage of bilirubin involves binding of bilirubin to certain cytoplasmic anionic binding proteins, especially ligandin. This binding may prevent efflux of bilirubin back into the plasma.

CONJUGATION Unconjugated bilirubin is water-insoluble and must be converted to a *water-soluble derivative* in order to be excreted by the liver cell into bile. This is accomplished by conjugation whereby bilirubin is predominantly converted to bilirubin glucuronide. The reaction occurs in the endoplasmic reticulum of the hepatocytes by action of bilirubin glucuronyl transferase. As shown in Fig. 38-3, this appears to be a two-step reaction, resulting first in the formation of the monoglucuronide followed by the production of the diglucuronide. Normally, bile contains 85 percent of bilirubin diconjugates and 15 percent monoconjugates. Unconjugated bilirubin usually is *not* excreted by the liver into the bile (except following photooxidation, see below).

EXCRETION OR SECRETION INTO BILE Normally, for bilirubin to be excreted into bile, *the pigment must be in the conjugated form.* Although the overall process is not well understood, the excretion of conjugated bilirubin into bile appears to be an energy-dependent and *rate-limiting* step in the hepatic metabolism of bilirubin. When this step is compromised, two consequences occur: (1) decreased excretion of bilirubin into the bile, and (2) "regurgitation," or reentry of conjugated bilirubin from the liver cells into the bloodstream.

As indicated above, bilirubin IXα can exist as four geometric isomers. The naturally occurring isomer is the Z-Z form (see Fig. 38-2), which permits intramolecular hydrogen bonding, making the molecule hydrophobic. The other isomers (Z-E, E-Z, and E-E, depending on the position of the hydrogens at the two bridge double bonds) can be formed upon exposure to blue light and are unstable. They are *water-soluble* because their geometric configuration prevents intramolecular hydrogen bonding. Thus, these isomers (photoisomers) can be *excreted* into bile *without having to be conjugated.* The natural Z-Z isomer is also rendered water-soluble by conjugation with glucuronic acid. Bilirubin glucuronide formation prevents intramolecular hydrogen bonding, makes the molecule polar, and permits excretion of the pigment into bile (Fig. 38-2).

Intestinal phase of bilirubin metabolism After its appearance in the intestinal lumen, bilirubin glucuronide may be excreted in the stool or metabolized to urobilinogen and related products. Because of its polarity, *conjugated bilirubin is not reabsorbed* by the intestinal mucosa, a mechanism which may serve to rid the body of this pigment. The formation of urobilinogen from conjugated bilirubin requires the action of bacteria and occurs in the lower part of the small intestine and colon.

In contrast to conjugated bilirubin, *urobilinogen is reabsorbed* from the small intestine into the portal blood and is thus subject to the enterohepatic circulation. Some urobilinogen is reexcreted by the liver into the bile; the rest is excreted in the urine in an amount usually not exceeding 4 mg daily. When the hepatic excretory mechanism is impaired (e.g., in hepatocellular disease) or the production of bilirubin is greatly increased (e.g., in hemolytic anemia), the urinary urobilinogen may increase significantly.

The normal output of fecal urobilinogen ranges from 50 to 280 mg per day. Under conditions of decreased excretion of conjugated bilirubin into the intestine (e.g., liver disease, bile duct obstruction) or suppression of intestinal flora by antibiotics, fecal output will be diminished. In hemolytic anemia, urinary and fecal urobilinogen excretion is greatly increased.

In a normal person with a blood volume of 5 liters and a hemoglobin concentration of 15 g/dL, the total circulating hemoglobin is 750 g. Because approximately 0.8 percent of the red blood cells are destroyed daily, 6.3 g hemoglobin is released for catabolism.

Renal excretion of bilirubin Normally the urine contains no bilirubin that can be detected by the methods usually employed, although traces may be detectable by sensitive spectrophotometric procedures. Unconjugated bilirubin, being tightly bound to albumin, is not filtered by the renal glomeruli, and because there is no tubular secretory process for bilirubin, *unconjugated bilirubin (as the IXα, Z-Z isomer) is not excreted in urine.* On the other hand, conjugated bilirubin is less tightly bound to albumin, and a small fraction (about 5 percent) is unbound. The unbound fraction is dialyzable and is filtered by the renal glomeruli. Thus, in contrast to the unconjugated pigment, a fraction of plasma *conjugated bilirubin appears in the urine.* Bile salts enhance the dialyzability of conjugated bilirubin, and in obstructive jaundice, the elevated level of plasma bile acids may account for an increased renal excretion of conjugated bilirubin. This may also explain why in biliary tract obstruction, serum conjugated bilirubin levels tend to plateau and not to exceed 30 to 40 mg/dL, while with severe hepatocellular injury bilirubin levels higher than this may occur.

CHEMICAL TESTS FOR BILE PIGMENTS The most widely employed chemical test for the bile pigments in serum is the van den Bergh reaction. In this reaction the bilirubin pigments are diazotized with sulfanilic acid, and the chromogenic products are measured colorimetrically. The van den Bergh reaction can be used to distinguish between unconjugated and conjugated bilirubin because of the different solubility properties of the pigments. When the reaction is carried out in an *aqueous* medium, the water-soluble conjugated bilirubin reacts to give the so-called direct van den Bergh reaction. When the reaction is carried out in *methanol,* the intramolecular hydrogen bonds

FIGURE 38-3 *Scheme of bilirubin uptake, conjugation, and excretion by the liver cell. Although the conversion of BMG to BDG appears to be catalyzed by glucuronyl transferase, some have also postulated its formation by a plasma membrane transglucuronidase. B = bilirubin; BMG = bilirubin monoglucuronide; BDG = bilirubin diglucuronide; UDP = uridine diphosphate.*

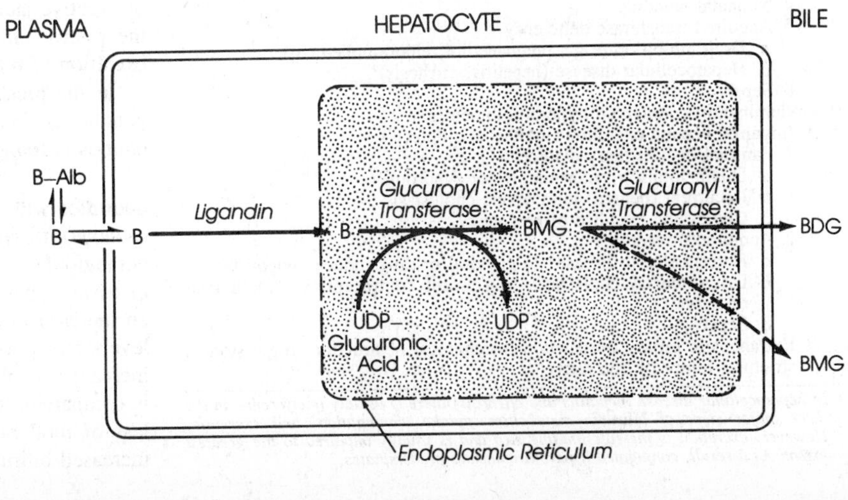

of unconjugated bilirubin are broken; thus both conjugated and unconjugated pigments react, giving a measure of the *total* bilirubin level. The total minus the direct-reacting bilirubin give the *indirect* value, which is a measure of the unconjugated bilirubin level.

In the direct van den Bergh reaction, the most accurate measurements are those carried out at 1 min. If the reaction is allowed to proceed longer, a small amount of the unconjugated pigment may begin to react in the aqueous medium. As a result, if the reaction is carried out at 30 min in a patient with unconjugated hyperbilirubinemia, falsely low values for the indirect-reacting bilirubin may be obtained. This serves to emphasize that the direct and indirect van den Bergh reactions represent *approximations* (not absolute measurements) of the conjugated and unconjugated pigments.

The most accurate method for measuring bilirubin in biologic fluids involves the formation of bilirubin methyl esters (by alkaline methanolysis) and measuring the products by high-performance liquid chromatography (HPLC). Studies with this procedure show that *normal serum contains mostly unconjugated bilirubin* with less than 4 percent of the total bilirubin being conjugated. This confirms the long-held suspicion that the small amount of "direct-reacting" bilirubin measured by the van den Bergh method (0.1 to 0.3 mg/dL) is not correct and is an overestimate of the amount of conjugated bilirubin actually present in normal serum. The HPLC method also shows that in patients with liver disease and conjugated hyperbilirubinemia, the serum contains significant amounts of *monoconjugates as well as diconjugates.* A summary of the key differences in the properties and reactions of the bilirubin pigments is presented in Table 38-1.

The qualitative measurement of bilirubin in the urine may be carried out with Ictotest tablets or the dipstick method. The foam test is also a simple and qualitatively valid procedure. When normal urine is vigorously shaken in a test tube, the foam is absolutely white. In urine containing bilirubin, the foam will be yellow. This difference may be subtle and may become evident only by comparing a normal urine specimen and one containing bilirubin side by side.

Except for concentrated urine, the most common cause of a deep-yellow-brown or dark urine is bilirubinuria. However, other mechanisms and diseases associated with a dark urine need to be considered. These include yellow urine due to drugs (e.g., sulfasalazine); red urine due to porphyria, hemoglobinuria, myoglobinuria, or drugs (e.g., pyridium); and dark-brown or black urine due to homogentisic acid (in ochronosis) or melanin (with melanoma).

TABLE 38-1 Comparison of the major differences between conjugated and unconjugated bilirubin

Properties and reactions	Unconjugated*	Conjugated
Water solubility	0	+
Affinity for lipids	+	0
Renal excretion	0	+
van den Bergh reaction	Indirect (total minus direct)	Direct
Binding to serum albumin (reversible)	+ + +	+
Formation of bilirubin-albumin complex (irreversible)	0	+†

* *These properties apply to the naturally occurring bilirubin IXα. Other geometric and photoisomers behave like conjugated bilirubin. See text for details.*
† *Detectable in plasma under conditions of cholestasis (see text).*

TABLE 38-2 Classification of jaundice based on underlying derangement of bilirubin metabolism

I Predominantly *unconjugated* hyperbilirubinemia
- *A* Overproduction
  - *1* Hemolysis (intra- and extravascular)
  - *2* Ineffective erythropoiesis
- *B* Decreased hepatic uptake
  - *1* Drugs (e.g., flavaspidic acid)
  - *2* Prolonged fasting (< 300 cal per day)
  - *3* Sepsis
- *C* Decreased bilirubin conjugation (decreased glucuronyl transferase activity)
  - *1* Gilbert's syndrome (*mild* decrease in transferase)
  - *2* Crigler-Najjar type II (*moderate* decrease in transferase)
  - *3* Crigler-Najjar type I (*absent* transferase)
  - *4* Neonatal jaundice
  - *5* Acquired transferase deficiency
    - *a* Drug inhibition (e.g., pregnanediol, chloramphenicol)
    - *b* Hepatocellular disease (hepatitis, cirrhosis)*
  - *6* Sepsis

II Predominantly *conjugated* hyperbilirubinemia
- *A* Impaired hepatic excretion (intrahepatic defects)
  - *1* Familial or hereditary disorders
    - *a* Dubin-Johnson syndrome; Rotor syndrome
    - *b* Recurrent (benign) intrahepatic cholestasis
    - *c* Cholestatic jaundice of pregnancy
  - *2* Acquired disorders
    - *a* Hepatocellular disease* (e.g., viral or drug-induced hepatitis)
    - *b* Drug-induced cholestasis (e.g., oral contraceptives, methyltestosterone)
    - *c* Sepsis
- *B* Extrahepatic biliary obstruction (mechanical obstruction, e.g., stones, stricture, tumor of bile duct)

* *In hepatocellular disease (hepatitis and cirrhosis) there is usually interference in the three major steps of bilirubin metabolism—uptake, conjugation, and excretion. However, excretion is the rate-limiting step and is usually impaired to the greatest extent. As a result, conjugated hyperbilirubinemia predominates.*

APPROACH TO THE PATIENT WITH JAUNDICE Once jaundice is recognized clinically or chemically, it is important to determine whether it is predominantly due to unconjugated or conjugated hyperbilirubinemia. *A simple clue in this regard is to determine whether bilirubin is present in the urine.* Its absence in the urine suggests unconjugated hyperbilirubinemia (since this pigment is not filtered by the glomerulus); its presence indicates conjugated hyperbilirubinemia. One can then proceed to the chemical measurement of the bilirubin pigments in the serum. In predominantly unconjugated hyperbilirubinemia, 80 to 85 percent of the total serum bilirubin is measured as unconjugated by the van den Bergh reaction, but more than 96 percent by the more accurate HPLC method. The patient is considered to have predominantly conjugated hyperbilirubinemia when more than 50 percent of the serum bilirubin is of the conjugated type. The serum of such patients will contain both mono- and diglucuronide conjugates.

An approach to the classification of jaundice based on this important distinction is presented in Table 38-2. Derangements of bilirubin metabolism may occur through any of four mechanisms: (1) overproduction, (2) decreased hepatic uptake, (3) decreased hepatic conjugation, and (4) decreased excretion of bilirubin into bile (due to both intrahepatic and extrahepatic factors). Jaundice may also be described on the basis of the pathogenetic mechanisms or disease processes leading to increased bilirubin levels. Thus, the terms *hemolytic jaundice, hepatocellular jaundice,* and *obstructive* (or *cholestatic*) *jaundice* are often used. Though these classifications and terms are helpful, in any one patient more than a single derangement or more than one "type" of jaundice may be present. For example, a patient with cirrhosis may have not only impaired liver cell function (and hence hepatocellular jaundice) but also hemolysis. Furthermore, obstructive jaundice may be due to either *mechanical* obstruction of the biliary radicles or *functional* factors causing impaired hepatic excretion of bilirubin into bile.

In the present chapter a brief description of the major types of jaundice is given. A more detailed discussion of the individual disease entities is found in Chap. 246.

Jaundice with predominantly unconjugated bilirubin in the serum

OVERPRODUCTION OF BILIRUBIN When an increased amount of hemoglobin is released from red blood cells into either the bloodstream or tissues, increased bilirubin production occurs. This is reflected by an increase in unconjugated bilirubin levels in the serum, but with levels rarely exceeding 3 to 4 mg/dL. There may also be a slight increase in conjugated bilirubin, but on a percentage basis the amount is comparable to what is found in normal serum, i.e., 4 percent or less of total bilirubin. For a detailed description of the causes of increased bilirubin production, see Chap. 246.

IMPAIRED HEPATIC UPTAKE OF BILIRUBIN As indicated previously, the uptake of bilirubin by the liver cell involves dissociation of the pigment from albumin, and then binding to ligandin. In some cases of drug-induced jaundice (e.g., due to flavaspidic acid) and possibly in some patients with Gilbert's syndrome, there may be a derangement in this phase of bilirubin metabolism (see Chap. 246).

IMPAIRED GLUCURONIDE CONJUGATION Both acquired and genetic derangements in hepatic glucuronyl transferase occur. In the fetus and at birth, glucuronyl transferase activity is low and appears to account in part for the *neonatal jaundice* normally found between the second and the fifth days of life. *Mild* decreases in glucuronyl transferases occur in Gilbert's syndrome, *moderate* decreases are found in Crigler-Najjar syndrome type II, and the enzyme is totally *absent* in the rare Crigler-Najjar syndrome type I (see Chap. 246).

Acquired defects in bilirubin glucuronyl transferase activity may be produced by drugs (i.e., enzyme inhibition) or intrinsic liver disease. However, with liver cell damage, the excretory capacity of the liver is impaired to a greater extent than is the conjugating capacity. Therefore in most hepatocellular diseases, the hyperbilirubinemia is predominantly of the conjugated type (see Chap. 246).

Jaundice with predominantly conjugated bilirubin in the serum

IMPAIRED EXCRETION OF BILIRUBIN BY THE LIVER The impaired excretion of bilirubin into the biliary canaliculi, whether due to functional or mechanical factors, results in predominantly conjugated hyperbilirubinemia and bilirubinuria. The presence of *bilirubin in the urine is evidence of conjugated hyperbilirubinemia* and is a most important point in the differential diagnosis of jaundice. Such findings are identical to those occurring in complete obstruction of the bile duct, emphasizing that *jaundice due to hepatocellular disease can seldom be differentiated from that due to extrahepatic obstruction solely on the basis of changes in bile pigment metabolism.* Indeed there are often instances when the two conditions are not distinguishable by any biochemical criteria, and liver biopsy or other diagnostic procedures (e.g., ultrasound) are needed for the definitive diagnosis.

When there is interference in the excretion of conjugated bilirubin into bile, by what mechanism does this pigment enter the systemic circulation? Several postulates have been proposed for this "reentry": (1) rupture of the bile canaliculi secondary to the necrosis of the hepatic cells that constitute their walls; (2) occlusion of the canaliculi by inspissated bile or their compression by swollen hepatic cells; (3) obstruction of the terminal intrahepatic bile ducts (cholangioles) by inflammatory cells; (4) altered hepatic cell permeability; and (5) impaired excretion, resulting in accumulation of conjugated bilirubin in the hepatocytes, and secondary diffusion into the plasma. Although some of these postulates are speculative, it is likely that several of these mechanisms occur. For example, occasionally in histologic sections, escape of bile through rents in the walls of canaliculi in areas of necrosis is apparent. Also, microscopic studies of the liver of rats injected with fluorescent dyes have shown reflux of bile from canaliculi into sinusoids. However, no anatomic damage needs to be invoked, because when unconjugated bilirubin is infused into normal subjects at high rates, conjugated hyperbilirubinemia occurs; this is explained most logically by passive diffusion.

EXTRAHEPATIC BILIARY OBSTRUCTION Complete obstruction of the extrahepatic bile ducts leads to jaundice with predominantly conjugated hyperbilirubinemia, bilirubinuria, and clay-colored stools. Failure of bile to reach the intestine results in virtual disappearance of urobilinogen from the stool and urine. The concentration of bilirubin rises progressively but then usually plateaus at a level of 30 to 40 mg/dL. To some extent this plateau may be explained by a balance between renal excretion and diversion of bilirubin to other metabolites. In hepatocellular jaundice, such a plateau tends not to occur, and bilirubin levels in excess of 50 mg/dL may be found, in part due to concomitant hemolysis and renal insufficiency.

Partial obstruction of the extrahepatic bile ducts can also give rise to jaundice but only if the intrabiliary pressure is increased, because the excretion of bilirubin does not diminish until the intraductile pressure approaches the maximal secretory pressure of approximately 250 mmHg bile. Jaundice may occur at much lower pressures if the obstruction is complicated by infection of the ducts or hepatocellular injury. Therefore, jaundice, bilirubinuria, and clay-colored stools are inconstant findings in partial biliary obstruction, and the amount of urobilinogen in urine and stool varies with the degree of occlusion.

The functional reserve of the liver is so great that *occlusion of the intrahepatic bile ducts* does not give rise to jaundice unless the drainage of bile from a large segment of the parenchyma is interrupted. Either of the two major hepatic ducts or a large number of secondary radicles may be occluded without production of jaundice. In experimental animals the ducts draining at least 75 percent of the parenchyma must be occluded before jaundice appears.

Additional points of terminology In clinical practice, a patient may be described as having *obstructive,* or *cholestatic,* jaundice. By this is meant that clinically, and especially biochemically, there is little to suggest hepatocellular damage and that the main features point to interference with, or obstruction in, the flow of bile. Typically one would expect such a patient to show (1) predominantly conjugated hyperbilirubinemia, (2) minimal biochemical changes of parenchymal liver damage, and (3) a moderate to a marked increase in the serum alkaline phosphatase level [usually three or four times normal (or greater than 250 IU per liter)]. As emphasized in Chaps. 244 and 245, an *elevated alkaline phosphatase level* in a patient with jaundice or liver disease, in the absence of other disorders such as bone disease, is most suggestive of interference with bile secretion or an infiltrative process in the liver. However, *laboratory tests alone may not permit differentiation of intrahepatic from extrahepatic cholestasis.*

Some clinicians reserve the term obstructive jaundice for those cases in which anatomic obstruction can be demonstrated and use the term cholestatic jaundice for cases of parenchymal liver disease in which the obstructive phase is on a functional basis. Nevertheless, because these two entities frequently are indistinguishable by clinical and biochemical criteria, the terms obstructive jaundice and cholestatic jaundice are often used interchangeably.

Hepatocellular disorders in which jaundice associated with an obstructive, or cholestatic, phase occurs include (1) occasional cases of viral hepatitis, (2) drug reactions, especially those due to chlorpromazine and methyltestosterone, (3) some cases of alcoholic hepatitis or alcohol-induced fatty liver, (4) jaundice in the last trimester of pregnancy, (5) most cases of Dubin-Johnson or Rotor syndrome, (6) benign recurrent intrahepatic cholestasis, and (7) certain types of postoperative jaundice. These and other conditions are discussed in Chaps. 246 and 247.

In summary, all forms of conjugated hyperbilirubinemia have by definition an impairment in the excretion of bilirubin into bile. In most cases of parenchymal liver disease, a broad derangement is shown by the biochemical tests of liver function. However, when the major detectable alterations of liver function tests include (1) conjugated hyperbilirubinemia and (2) moderate to marked elevation of the serum alkaline phosphatase level, the terms obstructive or cholestatic jaundice may be appropriate. Additional procedures, including operation, are often needed to determine the cause of the cholestasis (see Chaps. 243 and 245).

HEPATOMEGALY

In the supine position, the major part of the liver lies beneath the right rib cage. In some normal persons the liver edge may be palpable 1 to 2 cm below the right costal margin, and a palpable liver edge by itself does not necessarily indicate hepatomegaly. In evaluating liver size by physical examination, two factors other than ability to palpate the liver edge need to be considered, namely, (1) the location of the upper border of liver dullness by percussion, and (2) the body habitus.

Normally, the upper edge of liver dullness on the right side in the midclavicular line is at the level of the fifth rib, but in asthenic habitus it may be lower. The liver edge normally descends 1 to 3 cm with deep inspiration. In hypersthenic subjects, the liver may extend over to the left side of the abdominal wall, with the lower edge high and not palpable; in hyposthenic subjects with a very acute costal angle, the liver may lie in the right half of the abdomen, the edge being palpable by as much as 6 to 8 cm below the right costal margin lateral to the right rectus abdominis muscle. Thus, palpability does not necessarily imply hepatomegaly.

In determining liver enlargement by palpation, one should be certain that the liver is being palpated rather than other right upper quadrant masses such as gallbladder, colonic neoplasm, or fecal material in the colon. Liver enlargement is often confirmed by radiologic studies, including hepatic scintiscans, computerized tomography, and ultrasonography.

In many cases of generalized liver enlargement, the left lobe will be felt in the epigastrium between the xiphoid and umbilicus. The liver should be carefully palpated during deep inspiration to determine whether the edge is tender, regular or irregular, firm or soft, rounded and thickened, or sharp. The edge is tender and often rounded with hepatic inflammation, as in hepatitis, or when the liver is acutely congested, as in cardiac decompensation. Pulsation of the liver may be found with tricuspid valvular incompetence. A carcinomatous liver may be rocklike in hardness; the cirrhotic liver is very firm in consistency. The largest livers are often found with carcinoma (primary or metastatic), marked fatty infiltration, congestive cardiac decompensation, Hodgkin's disease, and amyloidosis. Rapid decrease in liver size may occur with improvement of congestive failure, mobilization of fat from the liver, or massive hepatic necrosis.

In a patient with hepatomegaly, auscultation is sometimes helpful. A friction rub may be audible (and palpable) in the right upper quadrant; it is usually due to a recent biopsy, tumor, or perihepatitis. In portal hypertension a venous hum may be audible between the umbilicus and the xiphoid. An arterial murmur or bruit over the liver may indicate tumor, usually hepatocellular carcinoma.

Some of the causes of a palpable liver and hepatomegaly are given in Table 38-3.

TABLE 38-3 Causes of a palpable liver and hepatomegaly

I Palpable liver without hepatomegaly
- *A* Right diaphragm displaced downward (e.g., emphysema, asthma)
- *B* Subdiaphragmatic lesion (e.g., abscess)
- *C* Aberrant lobe of liver (Riedel's lobe)
- *D* Extremely thin or relaxed abdominal muscles
- *E* Occasionally present in normal persons

II Hepatomegaly
- *A* Vascular congestion (e.g., congestive heart failure, hepatic vein thrombosis)
- *B* Bile duct obstruction (e.g., lesion in common duct leading to hepatomegaly and subsequently to biliary cirrhosis)
- *C* Infiltrative disorders
  - *1* Bone marrow and reticuloendothelial cells
    - *a* Extramedullary hematopoiesis
    - *b* Leukemia
    - *c* Lymphoma
  - *2* Fat
    - *a* Fatty liver (e.g., secondary to alcohol, diabetes, or toxins)
    - *b* Gaucher's disease and some other lipidoses
  - *3* Glycogen (e.g., diabetes, especially after insulin excess)
  - *4* Amyloid
  - *5* Iron (hemochromatosis and hemosiderosis)
  - *6* Granuloma (tuberculosis, sarcoid)
- *D* Inflammatory disorders
  - *1* Hepatitis—due to drugs or infectious agents
  - *2* Cirrhosis—except in late stages when prolonged scarring may lead to a *small,* shrunken liver
- *E* Tumors—primary or metastatic
- *F* Cysts—polycystic disease, congenital hepatic fibrosis

REFERENCES

BERLIN N, BERK P: Quantitative aspects of bilirubin metabolism for hematologists. Blood 57:983, 1981

BLANKAERT N, SCHMID R: Physiology and pathophysiology of bilirubin metabolism, in *Hepatology: A Textbook of Liver Disease,* D Zakim, T Boyer (eds). Saunders, Philadelphia, 1982, pp 246–296

McDONAGH AF et al: Blue light and bilirubin excretion. Science 208:145, 1980

VAN HOOTEGEM P et al: Serum bilirubins in hepatobiliary disease: Comparison with other liver function tests. Hepatology 5:112, 1985

WEISS JS et al: The clinical importance of a protein-bound fraction of serum bilirubin in patients with hyperbilirubinemia. N Engl J Med 309:147, 1983

WOLKOFF AW et al: Hereditary jaundice and disorders of bilirubin metabolism, in *The Metabolic Basis of Inherited Disease,* 5th ed, JB Stanbury et al (eds). New York, McGraw-Hill, 1983, pp 1385–1420

39 ABDOMINAL SWELLING AND ASCITES

ROBERT M. GLICKMAN / KURT J. ISSELBACHER

ABDOMINAL SWELLING Abdominal swelling or distention is a common problem in clinical medicine and may be the initial manifestation of a systemic disease or of otherwise unsuspected abdominal disease. *Subjective* abdominal enlargement, often described as a sensation of fullness or bloating, is usually transient and is often related to a functional gastrointestinal disorder when it is not accompanied by objective physical findings of increased abdominal girth or local swelling. *Obesity* and lumbar lordosis, which may be associated with prominence of the abdomen, may usually be distinguished from true increases in the volume of the peritoneal cavity by history and careful physical examination.

Clinical history Abdominal swelling may first be noticed by the patient because of a progressive increase in belt or clothing size, the appearance of abdominal or inguinal hernias, or the development of a localized swelling. Often, considerable abdominal enlargement has gone unnoticed for weeks or months, either because of coexistent obesity or because the ascites formation has been insidious, without pain or localizing symptoms. Progressive abdominal distention may be associated with a sensation of ''pulling'' or ''stretching'' of the flanks or groins and vague low back pain. Localized *pain* usually results from involvement of an abdominal organ (e.g., a passively congested liver, large spleen, or colonic tumor). Pain is uncommon in cirrhosis with ascites and when it is present, pancreatitis, hepatoma, or peritonitis should be considered. Tense ascites or abdominal tumors may produce increased intraabdominal pressure, resulting in *indigestion* and *heartburn* due to gastroesophageal reflux or *dyspnea, orthopnea,* and *tachypnea* from elevation of the diaphragm. A coexistent pleural effusion, more commonly on the right, presumably due to leakage of ascitic fluid through lymphatic channels in the diaphragm, may also contribute to respiratory embarrassment. The patient with diffuse abdominal swelling should be questioned about increased alcoholic intake, a prior episode of jaundice or hematuria, a change in bowel habits, or a past history of rheumatic heart disease. Such historical information may provide the clues that will lead one to suspect an occult cirrhosis, a colonic tumor with peritoneal seeding, congestive heart failure, or nephrosis.

Physical examination A carefully executed *general physical examination* can yield valuable clues concerning the etiology of abdominal swelling. Thus palmar erythema and spider angiomas suggest an underlying cirrhosis, while supraclavicular adenopathy (Virchow's node) should raise the question of an underlying gastrointestinal malignancy. *Inspection* of the abdomen is an important but often cursorily performed aspect of the abdominal examination. By noting the abdominal contour, one may be able to distinguish localized from generalized swelling. The tensely distended abdomen with tightly stretched skin, bulging flanks, and everted umbilicus is characteristic of ascites. A prominent abdominal venous pattern with the direction of flow away from the umbilicus often is a reflection of portal hypertension; venous collaterals with flow from the lower part of the abdomen toward the umbilicus suggest obstruction of the inferior vena cava; flow downward toward the umbilicus suggests superior vena cava obstruction. "Doming" of the abdomen with visible ridges from underlying intestinal loops is usually due to intestinal obstruction or distention. An epigastric mass, with evident peristalsis proceeding from left to right, usually indicates underlying pyloric obstruction. A liver with metastatic deposits may be visible as a nodular right upper quadrant mass moving with respiration.

Auscultation may reveal the high-pitched, rushing sounds of early intestinal obstruction or a succussion sound due to increased fluid and gas in a dilated hollow viscus. Careful auscultation over an enlarged liver occasionally reveals the harsh bruit of a vascular tumor, especially a hepatoma, or the leathery friction rub of a surface nodule. A venous hum at the umbilicus may signify portal hypertension and an increased collateral blood flow around the liver. A fluid wave and flank dullness which shifts with change in position of the patient are important signs that indicate the presence of peritoneal fluid. In obese patients, small amounts of fluid may be difficult to demonstrate; on occasion the fluid may be detected by abdominal percussion with patients on their hands and knees. Doubt about the presence of peritoneal fluid may be resolved by careful paracentesis with a small-gauge (no. 19 or 20) needle. Careful percussion should serve to distinguish generalized abdominal enlargement from localized swelling due to an enlarged uterus, ovarian cyst, or distended bladder. Percussion can also outline an abnormally small or large liver. Loss of normal liver dullness may result from massive hepatic necrosis; it may also be a clue to free gas in the peritoneal cavity, as from perforation of a hollow viscus.

Palpation is often difficult with massive ascites, and ballottement of overlying fluid may be the only method of palpating the liver or spleen. A slightly enlarged spleen in association with ascites may be the only evidence of an occult cirrhosis. When there is evidence of portal hypertension, a soft liver suggests that obstruction to portal flow is extrahepatic; a firm liver suggests cirrhosis as the likely cause of the portal hypertension. A very hard or nodular liver is a clue that the liver is infiltrated with tumor, and when accompanied by ascites, it suggests that the latter is due to peritoneal seeding. The presence of a hard periumbilical lymph node (Sister Marie Joseph's nodule) suggests metastatic disease from a pelvic or gastrointestinal primary tumor. A pulsatile liver and ascites may be found in tricuspid insufficiency.

An attempt should be made to determine whether a mass is solid or cystic, smooth or irregular, and whether it moves with respiration. The liver, spleen, and gallbladder should descend with respiration unless they are fixed by adhesions or extension of tumor beyond the organ. A fixed mass not descending with respiration may indicate that it is retroperitoneal. Tenderness, especially if localized, may indicate an inflammatory process such as an abscess; it may also be due to stretching of the visceral peritoneum or tumor necrosis. Rectal and pelvic examinations are mandatory; they may reveal otherwise undetected masses due to tumor or infection.

Radiographic and laboratory examinations are essential for confirming or extending the impressions gained on physical examination. Upright and recumbent films of the abdomen may demonstrate the dilated loops of intestine with fluid levels characteristic of intestinal obstruction or the diffuse abdominal haziness and loss of psoas margins suggestive of ascites. Ultrasonography is often of value in detecting ascites, determining the presence of a mass, or evaluating the size of the liver and spleen. Computerized axial tomography (CT scanning) provides similar information. A plain film of the abdomen may reveal the distended colon of otherwise unsuspected ulcerative colitis and give valuable information as to the size of the liver and spleen. An irregular and elevated right side of the diaphragm may be a clue to a liver abscess or hepatoma. Studies of the gastrointestinal tract with barium or other contrast media are usually necessary in the search for a primary tumor.

ASCITES The evaluation of a patient with ascites requires that the *cause* of the ascites be established. In most cases ascites will appear as a part of a well-recognized illness, i.e., cirrhosis, congestive heart failure, nephrosis, or disseminated carcinomatosis. In these situations, the physician should determine that the development of ascites is indeed a consequence of the basic underlying disease and not due to the presence of a separate or related disease process. This distinction is necessary even when the cause of ascites seems obvious. For example, when the patient with compensated cirrhosis and minimal ascites develops progressive ascites that is increasingly difficult to control with sodium restriction or diuretics, the obvious temptation is to attribute the worsening of the clinical picture to progressive liver disease. However, an occult hepatoma, portal vein thrombosis, spontaneous bacterial peritonitis, or even tuberculosis may be responsible for the decompensation. The disappointingly low success in diagnosing tuberculous peritonitis or hepatoma in the patient with cirrhosis and ascites reflects the too-low index of suspicion for the development of such superimposed conditions. Similarly, the patient with congestive heart failure may develop ascites from a disseminated carcinoma with peritoneal seeding. The thorough evaluation of each patient with ascites, even in the presence of an "obvious" cause, will help avoid these errors.

Diagnostic paracentesis (50 to 100 mL) should be part of the routine evaluation of the patient with ascites. The fluid should be examined for its gross appearance, protein content, cell count, and differential cell count, as well as Gram's and acid-fast stains and culture. Cytologic and cell-block examination may disclose an otherwise unsuspected carcinoma. Table 39-1 presents some of the features of ascitic fluid typically found in various disease states. In some disorders, such as cirrhosis, the fluid has the characteristics of a transudate (less than 2.5 g protein per deciliter and a specific gravity less than 1.016); in others, such as peritonitis, the features are those of an exudate. Although there is variability of the ascitic fluid in any given disease state, some features are sufficiently characteristic to suggest certain diagnostic possibilities. For example, blood-stained fluid with more than 2.5 g protein per deciliter is unusual in uncomplicated cirrhosis but is consistent with tuberculous peritonitis or neoplasm. Cloudy fluid with a predominance of polymorphonuclear cells and a positive Gram stain are characteristic of bacterial peritonitis; if most cells are lymphocytes, tuberculosis should be suspected. The complete examination of each fluid is most important, for occasionally only *one* finding may be abnormal. For example, if the fluid is a typical transudate but contains more than 250 white blood cells per cubic millimeter, the finding should be recognized as atypical for cirrhosis, nephrosis, or congestive heart failure and should warrant a search for tumor or infection. This is especially true in the evaluation of cirrhotic ascites where occult peritoneal infection may be present with only minor elevations in the white blood cell count of the peritoneal fluid (300 to 500 cells per cubic millimeter). Since Gram's stain of the fluid may be negative in a high proportion of such cases, careful culture of the peritoneal fluid is mandatory. Direct visualization of the peritoneum (laparoscopy) may disclose peritoneal deposits of tumor, tuberculosis, or metastatic disease of the liver. Biopsies are taken under direct vision often adding to the diagnostic accuracy of the procedure.

Chylous ascites refers to a turbid, milky, or creamy peritoneal fluid due to the presence of thoracic or intestinal lymph. Such a fluid shows Sudan-staining fat globules microscopically and an increased triglyceride content by chemical examination. A turbid fluid due to leukocytes or tumor cells may be confused with chylous fluid (pseudochylous), and it is often helpful to carry out alkalinization and ether extraction of the specimen. Alkali will tend to dissolve cellular proteins and thereby reduce turbidity; ether extraction will lead to clearing if the turbidity of the fluid is due to lipid. Chylous ascites is most often the result of lymphatic obstruction from trauma, tumor, tuberculosis, filariasis (see Chap. 163), or congenital abnormalities. It may also be seen in the nephrotic syndrome.

Rarely, ascitic fluid may be *mucinous* in character, suggesting either pseudomyxoma peritonei (Chap. 242) or rarely a colloid carcinoma of the stomach or colon with peritoneal implants.

TABLE 39-1 Ascitic fluid characteristics in various disease states

Condition	Gross appearance	Specific gravity	Protein, g/dL	Cell count: Red blood cells, >10,000/mm³	Cell count: White blood cells, per mm³	Other tests
Cirrhosis	Straw-colored or bile-stained	<1.016 (95%)*	<2.5 (95%)	1%	<250 (90%);* predominantly mesothelial	
Neoplasm	Straw-colored, hemorrhagic, mucinous, or chylous	Variable, >1.016 (45%)	>2.5 (75%)	20%	>1000 (50%); variable cell types	Cytology, cell block, peritoneal biopsy
Tuberculous peritonitis	Clear, turbid, hemorrhagic, chylous	Variable, >1.016 (50%)	>2.5 (50%)	7%	>1000 (70%); usually >70% lymphocytes	Peritoneal biopsy, stain and culture for acid-fast bacilli
Pyogenic peritonitis	Turbid or purulent	If purulent, >1.016	If purulent, >2.5	Unusual	Predominantly polymorphonuclear leukocytes	+ Gram's stain, culture
Congestive heart failure	Straw-colored	Variable, <1.016 (60%)	Variable, 1.5–5.3	10%	<1000 (90%); usually mesothelial, mononuclear	
Nephrosis	Straw-colored or chylous	<1.016	<2.5 (100%)	Unusual	<250; mesothelial, mononuclear	If chylous, ether extraction, Sudan staining
Pancreatic ascites (pancreatitis, pseudocyst)	Turbid, hemorrhagic, or chylous	Variable, often >1.016	Variable, often >2.5	Variable, may be blood-stained	Variable	Increased amylase in ascitic fluid and serum

* *Since the conditions of examining fluid and selecting patients were not identical in each series, the percentage figures (in the parentheses) should be taken as an indication of the order of magnitude rather than as the precise incidence of any abnormal finding.*

On occasion, ascites may develop as a seemingly isolated finding in the absence of a clinically evident underlying disease. It is then that a careful analysis of ascitic fluid may indicate the direction the evaluation should take. A useful framework for the workup starts with an analysis of whether the fluid is an exudate or transudate. *Transudative ascites* of unclear etiology is most often due to occult cirrhosis, right-sided venous hypertension raising hepatic sinusoidal pressure, or hypoalbuminemic states such as nephrosis or protein-losing enteropathy. Cirrhosis with well-preserved liver function (normal albumin) resulting in ascites invariably is associated with significant portal hypertension (see Chap. 249). Evaluation should include liver function tests, liver spleen scan or other hepatic imaging procedure (i.e., CT or ultrasound) to detect nodular changes in the liver, or a colloid shift of isotope to suggest portal hypertension. On occasion a wedged hepatic venous pressure can be useful to document portal hypertension. Finally, if clinically indicated, a liver biopsy will confirm the diagnosis of cirrhosis and perhaps suggest its etiology. Other etiologies may result in hepatic venous congestion and resultant ascites. Right-sided cardiac valvular disease and particularly constrictive pericarditis should raise a high index of suspicion and may require cardiac imaging and cardiac catheterization for definitive diagnosis. Hepatic vein thrombosis is evaluated by visualizing the hepatic veins using imaging techniques (angiography, CT scans, magnetic resonance imaging) to demonstrate obliteration, thrombosis, or obstruction by tumor. Uncommonly, transudative ascites may be associated with benign tumors of the ovary, particularly fibroma (Meigs's syndrome) with ascites and hydrothorax.

Exudative ascites should initiate an evaluation for primary peritoneal processes, most importantly infection and tumor. Routine bacteriologic culture of ascitic fluid often will yield a specific organism causing infectious peritonitis. Tuberculous peritonitis (Table 39-1) is best diagnosed by peritoneal biopsy, either percutaneously or via laparoscopy. Histologic examination invariably shows granulomata which may contain acid-fast bacilli. Since cultures of peritoneal fluid and biopsies for tuberculosis may require 6 weeks, characteristic histology with appropriate stains allows antituberculosis therapy to be started promptly. Similarly the diagnosis of peritoneal seeding by tumor can be made by cytologic analysis of peritoneal fluid or by peritoneal biopsy. Appropriate diagnostic studies can then be undertaken to determine the nature and site of the primary tumor. Pancreatic ascites (Table 39-1) is invariably associated with an extravasation of pancreatic fluid from the pancreatic ductal system, most commonly from a leaking pseudocyst. Ultrasound or CT examination of the pancreas followed by visualization of the pancreatic duct by direct cannulation (viz. endoscopic retrograde cholangiopancreatography, ERCP) will usually disclose the site of leakage and permit resective surgery to be carried out.

An analysis of the physiologic and metabolic factors involved in the production of ascites (see Chap. 249 for details), coupled with a complete evaluation of the nature of the ascitic fluid, will invariably disclose the etiology of the ascites and permit appropriate therapy to be instituted.

REFERENCES

BAR-MEIR S: Analysis of ascitic fluid in cirrhosis. Dig Dis Sc 24:136, 1979

CATTAN EL JR et al: The accuracy of the physical examination in the diagnosis of suspected ascites. JAMA 247:1146, 1982

CONN HO: Spontaneous bacterial peritonitis: Multiple revisitations. Gastroenterology 70:455, 1976

GARCIA-TSAO G et al: The diagnosis of bacterial peritonitis. Hepatology 5:91, 1985

GRAKE TMS et al: Peritoneoscopy in the diagnosis of tuberculous peritonitis. Gastrointest Endosc 27:66, 1981

RECTOR WG JR, REYNOLDS TB: Superiority of the serum: Ascites albumin difference over the ascites total protein concentration in separation of "transudative" and "exudative" ascites. Am J Med 77:83, 1984

section 6 Alterations in urinary function and electrolytes

40 ALTERATIONS IN URINARY FUNCTION

FREDRIC L. COE

AZOTEMIA, OLIGURIA, AND ANURIA

AZOTEMIA Measurements of urea and creatinine concentrations in serum are often obtained to assess the glomerular filtration rate (GFR). Both substances are produced at a reasonably constant rate, by the liver and muscles, respectively. As discussed in Chap. 218, they undergo complete glomerular filtration and are not reabsorbed extensively by the renal tubules; hence their clearances tend to reflect the GFR. An increase in their serum concentrations, termed *azotemia* (*azo,* "containing nitrogen"), occurs as the GFR falls. Creatinine is a more reliable index of GFR than urea because of the latter's lower back diffusion from tubule lumen to peritubular blood. The GFR may be reduced by a fall in the filtration rates of individual functioning nephrons or by a reduction in the total number of functioning nephrons. (See Table 40-1.)

Reduced single-nephron glomerular filtration rate TUBULAR FUNCTION NORMAL An important response of the normal kidney to a severe sodium-conserving stimulus, such as extracellular fluid volume depletion, is reduction of the single-nephron glomerular filtration rate (SNGFR) and subsequent reabsorption of an increased fraction of the reduced amounts of NaCl and water that enter the tubules. The resulting azotemia is called *prerenal azotemia,* in which urinary Na concentration falls below 20 (often below 1) meq per liter (see Table 40-1). The fractional excretion of Na can be calculated (see Chap. 219) and used as an additional index of prerenal azotemia. Secretion of vasopressin is stimulated by depletion of extracellular fluid volume, and as a consequence, the distal tubules and collecting ducts become fully permeable to water. The concentrating mechanisms in the inner medulla (Chap. 218) are very efficient when flow rates through the loops of Henle and the collecting ducts are low. As a result, the filtrate that escapes reabsorption in the proximal tubule undergoes maximal osmotic concentration, the urine volume becomes small, and it has a high osmolality, above 500 mosmol per kilogram of water. Most of the filtered creatinine escapes tubular reabsorption, and consequently the ratio of the urine-to-plasma (U/P) creatinine concentrations is very high, 40 or more. Because urea can back-diffuse more completely than creatinine, the blood urea nitrogen (BUN) level rises more than the serum creatinine concentration. Normally, the ratio of BUN to serum creatinine concentration is 10:1; with depletion of the extracellular fluid volume this ratio rises. An elevated ratio can also be produced by unrelated factors such as tetracycline administration, adrenocortical steroid therapy, the presence of blood in the gastrointestinal tract, and increased protein turnover due to trauma or burn.

Prerenal azotemia can occur in any edema-forming condition during the phase in which NaCl and water accumulate. Typical examples include the nephrotic syndrome and hepatic cirrhosis with ascites (Chaps. 28 and 223). When a diuretic is being administered to inhibit the tubular reabsorption of NaCl, urine volume and Na concentration may be normal or elevated, even though SNGFR falls

TABLE 40-1 Pathophysiologic mechanisms of azotemia

		Laboratory findings					
Mechanism of reduced GFR	Clinical examples	Oliguria	Urine osm, mosmol/kg	Urine $[Na^+]$, meq/L	$\left(\frac{U}{P}\right)_{creat}$	$\left(\frac{U}{P}\right)_{urea}$	BUN / Serum creat
REDUCED SNGFR							
Tubules normal (prerenal azotemia)	Severe dehydration, edema-forming states, diuretic agents, systemic hypotension, acute glomerular disease,* acute urinary obstruction, incomplete renal vascular obstruction	Nearly always present	>500	<20	>40	>8	>10
Tubules damaged (acute renal failure)	Acute tubular necrosis, nephrotoxic agents, glomerulonephritis with tubule injury	Common	<350	>40	<20	>2	10
REDUCED NEPHRON NUMBER							
Elevated SNGFR	Chronic tubulointerstitial-renal disease Surgical loss of renal tissue	Rare†	[290	>40	3–10	3–10]	10
Normal SNGFR	Diffuse chronic glomerulonephritis Diabetic nephropathy	Rare†	[100–350‡	10–100‡	>10	>3]	>10
Reduced SNGFR	Any of the factors that can reduce SNGFR (listed above) may lower SNGFR in a patient who has a reduced number of functioning nephrons	Common	290	>20	>10	<3	>10

* *Acute obstruction causing reduced SNGFR is called postrenal azotemia.*
† *Occurs only when total GFR is below 5% normal; urine chemistry values are helpful only when oliguria is present and are therefore enclosed in brackets.*
‡ *Varies with diet and with the level of GFR. When GFR is below 20% normal, osmotic concentration of the urine is usually impossible.*
NOTE: = *osm = osmolality; creat = creatinine concentration; U = urine; P = plasma.*

in response to the combination of the underlying edema-forming stimulus and further extracellular fluid volume depletion from the drug. Oliguria may appear upon withdrawal of the drug as the renal tubules resume intense reabsorption of NaCl and water. Prerenal azotemia may also be seen when renal blood flow is reduced by systemic hypotension, incomplete renal arterial or venous occlusion, or other cause (Chap. 127). Acute incomplete obstruction of the ureter and acute glomerular injury may also reduce SNGFR and leave tubule function relatively intact; postrenal azotemia is a term often applied when acute obstruction lowers SNGFR and causes azotemia. Whenever chronic obstruction of any portion of the urinary tract or glomerulonephritis damages nephrons extensively, the high urinary osmolality, U/P ratios for creatinine or urea, and low urinary Na concentrations disappear, and the kidneys behave as they do when nephron number is reduced.

TUBULE FUNCTION IMPAIRED Certain acute renal diseases which produce azotemia lower SNGFR and at the same time damage the tubules sufficiently to reduce or even abolish their reabsorptive function, producing *acute renal failure*. Acute tubular necrosis, exposure to nephrotoxic agents, and all forms of acute tubulointerstitial disease are excellent examples. Azotemia and oliguria appear, but the urinary Na concentration exceeds 20 meq and usually 40 meq per liter; the U/P ratios for urea and creatinine are below 2 and 20, respectively; and urine osmolality is below 350 mosmol per kilogram of water. The ratio of BUN to serum creatinine is not elevated (see Chap. 219).

Reduced nephron number INCREASED SNGFR If one kidney is removed, the other grows larger, its nephrons enlarge, and the SNGFR increases until the total GFR becomes nearly normal for two kidneys. The tubules are overperfused with filtrate, but they appear to cope well with their increased reabsorptive burdens, perhaps in part because they are longer and wider and possess more cells. If more kidney tissue is removed, the remnant nephrons enlarge further, and their SNGFR rises. Extreme overperfusion of the tubules interferes with Na conservation. At the same time, total GFR comes to depend more and more upon expansion of the extracellular fluid volume largely because the increase in SNGFR is due not only to anatomic growth of the glomeruli but also to a relatively high rate of blood flow per glomerulus. Nephron adaptations to reduced nephron number are detailed in Chap. 218.

Azotemia occurs because the total GFR, i.e., the product of the elevated SNGFR and the markedly reduced nephron number, is low. Tubular conservation of filtered H_2O and Na conservation are poor, so fluid and salt intake must be liberal. Clinical states that produce this picture include surgical loss of renal substance secondary to trauma, neoplasm, stone, and destruction of kidneys by bacterial infection or tuberculosis, polycystic and medullary cystic renal diseases, and all the chronic tubulointerstitial nephropathies (Chaps. 226 and 228). In each of these disorders, the nephrons that remain viable are either fully intact or behave as though the SNGFR is better preserved than tubule function.

SNGFR NORMAL The SNGFR does not appear to increase despite a reduction of nephron number in diseases such as glomerulonephritis and diabetic glomerulosclerosis, where the glomerulus is the primary site of damage. In these diseases total GFR falls directly with nephron number and is not supported by elevated SNGFR. Since the tubules are not confronted with an excessive reabsorptive burden, sodium conservation is adequate. In these disorders, superimposed conditions that lower SNGFR, such as depletion of extracellular fluid volume, can cause oliguria with low urine sodium concentration and U/P ratios for creatinine and urea above 20 and 3, respectively. The serum urea to creatinine ratio will rise distinctly.

SNGFR REDUCED In patients with chronic renal disease in whom total GFR has been sufficient to support life only because of a very high SNGFR, inadvertent dehydration or any other factor (Table 40-1 and Chaps. 218 and 219) that lowers the SNGFR can provoke oliguria and severe azotemia. Under these circumstances, urine Na concentration falls, but not below 20 meq per liter, as in the normal person, because SNGFR, though reduced from a previously elevated level, may still be above normal. The U/P ratios for creatinine and urea will be low, usually below 10 and 3, respectively, despite oliguria, and urine osmolality will not rise above the plasma level. The serum urea to creatinine ratio may rise, but not above 20. In less extreme situations, reduction of SNGFR will worsen azotemia and alter urine chemistry in the same directions but to a lesser extent.

OLIGURIA AND ANURIA *Oliguria* refers to a urine volume insufficient to sustain life, usually less than 400 mL per 24 h in an adult of average size. Daily urine volume is difficult to measure when flow rate is low, because small absolute errors of volume measurement, in the range of 50 to 100 mL of urine each day, or of timing of collection, may represent large percentage errors.

Anuria, which is the absence of urine flow, is caused mainly by urinary obstruction, which must be excluded as a first step (Chap. 230). Total renal arterial and venous occlusion is another important cause. Severe renal diseases such as cortical necrosis and rapidly progressive glomerulonephritis produce anuria in the adult, but so rarely that anuria should never be ascribed to a primary renal disease until patency of the urinary tract and major renal blood vessels has been established.

Approach to the patient with azotemia or oliguria A critical issue is whether azotemia has been stable and long-standing (chronic renal failure, Chap. 217) or is recent and increasing (acute renal failure, Chap. 219; pre- and postrenal azotemia). If azotemia is recent, and oliguria present, the most discriminating additional measurements include serum urea and creatinine concentrations, and the Na, urea, and creatinine concentrations and osmolality of a concurrent urine sample. Reduction of SNGFR with well-preserved tubule function is usually present when urine osmolality exceeds 500 mosmol per kilogram of water, Na < 20 meq per liter, the U/P ratios for urea and creatinine > 8 and 40, respectively, the urinalysis is normal, and the BUN is more than 10 times the serum creatinine concentration. The prognosis for recovery of adequate GFR is good, if the cause of reduced SNGFR can be reversed. When urine osmolality is below 350 mosmol per kilogram of water, Na > 40 meq, the U/P values for urea and creatinine < 2 and 20, respectively, and the BUN exceeds the serum creatinine by only tenfold, tubule function has been lost, and some form of acute or chronic renal failure usually is present.

ABNORMAL URINARY CONSTITUENTS

PROTEINURIA Normal adults may excrete up to 150 mg protein daily. Of this, only 10 to 15 mg is albumin; the rest is composed of over 30 different plasma proteins and of glycoproteins that derive from the renal cells. Tamm-Horsfall mucoprotein, the most prevalent of the urine proteins that do not arise from plasma, is produced by the cells of the ascending limb of the loop of Henle and is excreted at the rate of 25 mg per day. Daily excretion of more than 150 mg protein is properly termed *pathologic proteinuria,* but in common usage the word *proteinuria* suffices. Protein excretion above 3.5 g per 24 h is termed *massive* proteinuria and usually occurs when glomeruli have been damaged enough to allow plasma proteins, especially albumin, to enter the urine. Urinary albumin loss lowers serum albumin concentration, and the consequent fall in intracapillary oncotic pressure fosters the accumulation of tissue edema (Chap. 28); serum lipids rise, for reasons detailed in Chap. 223. The combination of *massive proteinuria, hypoalbuminemia, edema,* and *hyperlipidemia* is often called the *nephrotic syndrome;* but this term is becoming synonymous with massive urinary protein loss alone. Hypoalbuminemia, elevated blood lipids, and edema are pathophysiologic consequences of massive proteinuria and occur only when hepatic albumin synthesis, though normal or even increased, fails to compensate for urine albumin losses; these features are not a direct result of renal disease.

Detection of proteinuria Proteinuria is usually detected by urine "dipsticks" that register a trace result in response to as little as 50 mg protein per liter, and a distinct color change of the 1+ level at about 300 mg protein per liter. Since proteinuria can be missed if the urine is very dilute, fasting morning samples that tend to be concentrated are usually studied. Dipsticks respond best to albumin, so that a negative result can occur when large amounts of other protein, or protein fragments such as light chains, are being excreted. Dipstick proteinuria requires additional evaluation by the measurement of 24-h excretion rate. If total protein excretion is abnormal, it is helpful to characterize the proportions of albumin and globulins in the urine by cellulose acetate electrophoresis or other methods. Immunoelectrophoresis is required to identify immunoglobulin fragments, kappa or lambda light chains, when their presence is suggested by a monoclonal peak on routine urine electrophoresis.

Mechanisms of proteinuria TUBULAR PROTEINURIA Normal low-molecular-weight (<40,000) serum proteins, such as beta$_2$ microglobulin (11,600 mol wt), lysozyme (14,000 mol wt), or light chains (22,000 mol wt) are readily filtered by the glomeruli but are reabsorbed so efficiently that only trace amounts enter the urine. Diseases that selectively damage the tubules more than glomeruli (Chap. 226) cause excessive excretion of these small proteins with little or no increase in albumin excretion. The resulting proteinuria is usually between 1 and 3 g per 24 h, and edema and lipid disorders do not occur because albumin losses are small. Bence Jones protein, which is probably a dimer of two light chains, light chains themselves, and myoglobin are examples of proteins whose plasma concentrations may increase as a consequence of disease. If their filtered load rises enough to exceed tubular reabsorptive capacity, "overflow" proteinuria may occur.

GLOMERULAR PROTEINURIA Normal glomeruli filter very little albumin or globulin. Glomerular capillary endothelial cells form a barrier penetrated by pores of about 1000 Å diameter that holds back cells and other particles but offers no impediment to most proteins. The glomerular basement membrane traps molecules about 50 Å in effective radius, above 100,000 daltons molecular mass. The *foot processes (podocytes)* of the visceral epithelial cells (Fig. 40-1) cover the urinary aspect of the glomerular basement membrane and produce a series of narrow channels through which molecules that traverse the basement membrane must pass. Anionic molecules, like albumin, are filtered less freely than are neutral or positively charged molecules of the same size, so little albumin enters the filtrate. This charge selectively appears to be due to anionic glycoproteins that cover the surfaces of the foot processes and contribute to the matrix structure of the basement membrane (Chap. 218). The glycoproteins are anionic because they contain the dicarboxylic amino acids, glutamic and aspartic acid, and sialic acid. At the pH of blood (7.4) or urine (4.5 to 7.5) carboxylic and sialic acid residues are dissociated and, therefore, have a negative charge; albumin also carries an overall negative charge. The negatively charged portions of the glycoproteins repel those of albumin and retard filtration.

Glomerular disease can disrupt any of these filtration barriers. Injury limited to the polyanion glycoproteins would tend to produce selective losses of anionic proteins, such as albumin, that would be filtered more completely by the normal glomerulus but for their charge. Extensive injury that involves the entire basement membrane, not only its polyanion components, may increase losses of very large proteins as well as albumin.

The selectivity of proteinuria varies with the extent of glomerular injury. However, the clinical value of measuring selectivity has not been fully defined. The basis of such measurements is to express the excretion rate of a protein as a fraction of its theoretical maximal filtered load, which is the product of its serum concentration and the GFR. This fraction must reflect the relative filtration efficiency of the protein to that of a completely filtered GFR marker, usually inulin or creatinine, provided that tubular reabsorption and renal production or catabolism are negligible. The slope of a plot of such a clearance ratio against the molecular weight for a variety of serum proteins is one index of filtration selectivity. A more practical version of this test is based upon the ratio of the clearance fractions of two proteins of different molecular weight, such as IgG and transferrin (Chap. 223).

Approach to the patient with proteinuria Given dipstick proteinuria of the 1+ level or more, 24-h urine protein excretion should be measured. If it is above 150 mg, electrophoresis should be carried out to determine the proportions of albumin and other proteins. Excretion mainly of albumin signifies a glomerular lesion. When the total daily protein excretion exceeds 3.5 g, by definition the nephrotic syndrome is considered to be present; milder albuminuria is called an *asymptomatic urinary abnormality*. The initial steps in evaluating proteinuria are outlined in Chap. 217. Subsequent details of differential diagnosis are in Chaps. 223 and 224. Tubular proteinuria usually reflects a hereditary or acquired tubular disorder (Chap. 228) or tubulointerstitial nephropathy (Chap. 226). The presence of large amounts of Bence Jones protein suggests that multiple myeloma may be present (Chap. 258).

HEMATURIA AND CASTS **Isolated hematuria** Bleeding in the urinary tract from the urethra to the renal pelvis produces isolated hematuria, without significant proteinuria, cells, or urinary casts. Total hematuria, which occurs evenly throughout voiding, means that blood has had the opportunity to mix fully with the bladder urine. When bleeding occurs mainly at the beginning or end of micturition, a prostatic or urethral origin is more likely.

FIGURE 40-1 *Top. Diagram showing normal structures separating the capillary lumen and urinary space in the glomerulus. In the process of glomerular filtration, an ultrafiltrate of plasma traverses the glomerular capillary wall through endothelial fenestrae, basement membrane, and slit diaphragms. Macromolecules in the plasma are believed to be restricted from entry into glomerular urine by each of these wall structures. In addition, circulating polyanions (e.g., albumin) are thought to be retarded by negatively charged glycosialoproteins, which, as shown by the shaded area in the upper panel, are distributed throughout the glomerular wall. Bottom. A corresponding electron micrograph of the same structures. (Drawing by NL Gahan from BM Brenner, R Beeuwkes, Hosp Prac, vol 13, no 7, 1978. Reproduced with permission.)*

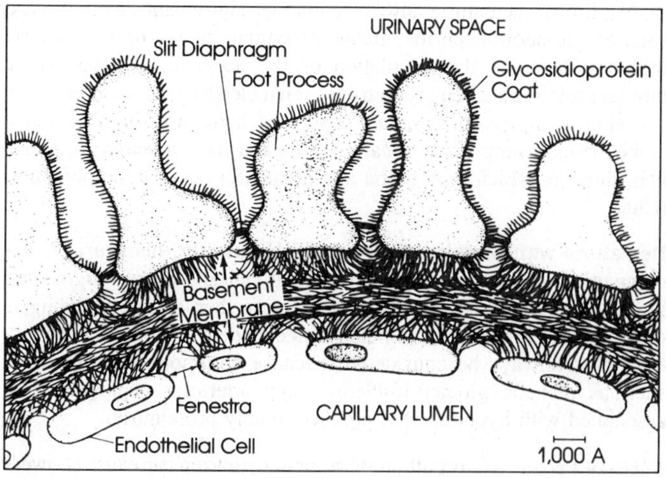

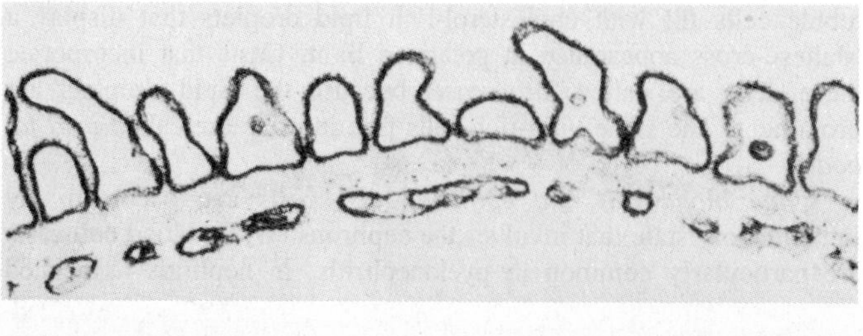

Common causes of *isolated* hematuria are urinary tract stones, benign and malignant neoplasms of the urinary tract, tuberculosis, trauma, and prostatitis; few primary renal diseases cause it. As discussed in Chaps. 217 and 223, *focal glomerulitis,* in the syndrome of benign recurrent hematuria or in Berger's disease, i.e., IgA nephropathy, is usually associated with red blood cell casts. Analgesic nephropathy and sickling states cause isolated hematuria, but modest proteinuria; papillary necrosis or azotemia often is present and suggests a renal origin. Hemoglobin electrophoresis is appropriate whenever a sickling disorder is suspected.

Examination of the prostate and external urethra is the basic first step in the evaluation of isolated hematuria. Intravenous pyelography and renal ultrasonography are the next. If no lesion is found and no obvious cause of bleeding such as renal stone passage is present, cystoscopy and retrograde pyelography may become necessary. At cystoscopy, blood may be found to issue from only one ureter, a helpful clue which indicates a localized lesion rather than a primary renal disease. Disorders of coagulation, and thrombocytopenia, as well as urinary infection, must be excluded. Because infection with tuberculosis and fungi may be difficult to detect, multiple urine samples must be cultured and examined by microscopy. Computerized tomography of the kidney and sometimes renal arteriography may be needed to disclose anatomic lesions such as cysts or tumors.

Hematuria associated with urinary tract infection Bacterial infection of the lower urinary tract or of the kidneys frequently causes hematuria. The presence of associated pyuria suggests the diagnosis of infection, and the demonstration of pathogenic bacteria in concentrations above 10^5 colonies per milliliter of urine establishes it. Acute cystitis or urethritis in women is an especially common cause of gross hematuria; in such symptomatic patients infection is documented by colony counts above 10^2 colonies per milliliter. Urinary tuberculosis can produce isolated hematuria, but pyuria often is present as well.

Hematuria with evidence of renal disease NEPHRONAL HEMATURIA Blood that enters the tubular fluid anywhere along the nephron can be trapped in a cylindrical mold of gelled Tamm-Horsfall protein to produce red blood cell casts. Tamm-Horsfall protein gels when concentrated at a low pH, as occurs during dehydration, or when exposed to myoglobin, hemoglobin, albumin, Bence Jones protein, and pyelographic contrast media. Degenerated red blood cells and clumps of hemoglobin can produce deeply pigmented casts that have the same significance—nephronal hematuria—as red blood cell casts.

Nephronal hematuria always connotes significant renal disease such as glomerulonephritis, tubulointerstitial injury, or a vasculitis that has damaged the circulation of the nephron. Glomerular or tubular proteinuria often accompanies renal bleeding, as a consequence of nephron injury. In general, nephronal hematuria of proteinuria alone arises from primary renal diseases that have a better prognosis than those in which proteinuria and hematuria occur in combination (Chap. 217).

Hematuria with proteinuria or casts Frequently, hematuria is accompanied by proteinuria, but red blood cell and deeply pigmented granular casts are absent. The presumption then is that bleeding is of nephronal origin, but a coincident independent lesion of the urinary tract must always be considered, because common renal diseases, such as diabetic glomerulosclerosis and arteriolar nephrosclerosis associated with hypertension, produce mainly proteinuria.

TYPES OF CASTS Heavy albuminuria or dehydration can cause showers of transparent, refractile "hyaline" casts. During heavy proteinuria, tubule cells fill with cholesterol-rich lipid droplets that display a Maltese-cross appearance in polarized light. Casts that incorporate these cells are called *fatty casts* because the lipid droplets are prominent. The same lipid-rich cells free in urine are called *oval fat bodies.*

White blood cell and epithelial cell casts can occur in any inflammatory state that involves the nephrons. White blood cell casts are particularly common in pyelonephritis, in nephritis associated with systemic lupus erythematosus, and during transplant rejection. When white blood or epithelial cells degenerate, they form granular nonpigmented casts that contain cellular debris and aggregated proteins. So-called *waxy* casts, with few granules and very distinct margins, arise when cell debris has broken down to a fine dispersion so that granules are no longer visible and are most common in chronic and progressive renal diseases.

Broad casts, of unusual width, are thought to arise in the dilated tubules of enlarged nephrons that have undergone compensatory hypertrophy in response to a reduction of functioning renal mass. A urine sample that contains a combination of broad and waxy casts as well as cellular or granular casts or red blood cells indicates a chronic smoldering process and has been termed a *telescoped* urine. This abnormality, first described in polyarteritis nodosa and systemic lupus erythematosus, can also be found in many chronic forms of glomerulonephritis with active glomerulitis.

Approach to the patient with hematuria Many urinalyses should be performed to determine whether the hematuria is isolated or associated with other features of primary renal disease, i.e., cells, casts, or proteinuria. The magnitude and type of associated proteinuria should be determined. As a general rule intravenous pyelography should be performed, if it can be done safely, even when the hematuria is of definite nephronal origin. Not only lesions of the urinary tract, but renal tumors or cysts, discrete areas of papillary necrosis, or signs of renal venous obstruction may be present. The source of isolated hematuria must always be ascertained, and this means a detailed examination of the urinary tract by cystoscopy, retrograde pyelography, and arteriography to disclose tumor, stone, cysts, or other cause. Renal ultrasonography and computer-assisted tomography are particularly helpful in detecting and evaluating renal cysts and tumors and should precede cystoscopy and arteriography. If all the studies disclose normal structures, a nephronal origin of hematuria is likely even if no red blood cell casts are present. The role of renal biopsy in such cases is detailed in Chaps. 223, 224, and 226. Hematuria with infection or overt renal disease usually requires no steps beyond intravenous pyelography. Evaluation of hematuria is detailed further in Chap. 217.

POLYURIA AND NOCTURIA

POLYURIA A reasonable definition of polyuria is a urine volume above 3 liters per day, but this should be qualified to exclude normal individuals who desire a large fluid intake and therefore form large volumes of urine. Patients cannot always distinguish polyuria from urinary frequency, the frequent voiding of small volumes. Since voiding volumes may not be clear from the history, polyuria must be substantiated by 24-h urine collection before one begins an investigation of causes.

Causes Polyuria can arise from inadequate secretion of vasopressin, failure of the renal tubules to respond to vasopressin, solute diuresis, or natriuresis (Table 40-2). It may also occur as a physiologic adaptation to deliberate excessive water drinking. The normal physiology of urine formation and mechanisms responsible for renal water conservation are discussed in Chap. 218.

DIABETES INSIPIDUS (see also Chap. 323) The term *diabetes insipidus* is applied to situations in which inadequate renal water conservation causes polyuria and secondary thirst. Either vasopressin insufficiency (central diabetes insipidus) or renal unresponsiveness to vasopressin (nephrogenic diabetes insipidus) may be responsible. In both, water reabsorption is reduced all along the distal nephron, because passive water movement from tubules into the hypertonic outer and inner medullary interstitium is slow. But even though the rate of water movement out of the collecting ducts is low for a given osmotic difference between the tubule lumen and interstitial fluid, the fluid that enters the collecting ducts is so abnormally dilute and copious in volume that more water enters the inner medulla than under normal circumstances and medullary solutes are washed out into the vasa recta. Wash-out is incomplete and vasopressin administration can lead to formation of an osmotically concentrated urine, but the maximal urine osmolality that can be attained is below normal.

Vasopressin-sensitive (central) diabetes insipidus may be idiopathic or secondary to hypophysectomy or trauma or to neoplastic, inflammatory, vascular, or infectious causes (Table 40-2). Idiopathic diabetes insipidus can be inherited as an autosomal dominant trait; but more commonly it is sporadic and appears in childhood. In both forms there is selective destruction of the neurons that produce vasopressin in the supraoptic nucleus.

Rarely, nephrogenic diabetes insipidus is familial and congenital; but usually it is acquired from renal disease (Table 40-2). Hypercalcemia and hypokalemic nephropathy are important reversible causes of nephrogenic diabetes insipidus. Lithium carbonate, methoxyflurane (1,1-difluoro-2,2-dichloroethyl methyl ether) anesthetic, and demeclocycline, a tetracycline derivative, can also produce nephrogenic diabetes insipidus.

SOLUTE DIURESIS Excessive filtration of a poorly resorbed solute such as glucose, mannitol, or urea can depress reabsorption of NaCl and water in the proximal tubule and cause their loss in the urine, producing polyuria. Urine Na concentration is below that of blood, so that more water than salt is lost from the body and serum hypertonicity can be produced. Glucosuria in diabetes mellitus is a common cause of solute diuresis. Iatrogenic solute diuresis may arise from mannitol infusion, angiographic contrast media, and high-protein gavage feedings, which produce an excessive excretion of urea. Any degree of solute diuresis can cause polyuria, so further evaluation of renal concentrating ability should be postponed until the solute diuresis is corrected.

NATRIURETIC SYNDROMES Excessive chronic Na loss may occur during the course of tubulointerstitial or cystic renal diseases. Polyuria and polydipsia are accompanied by an unusually large daily Na requirement. Examples of this phenomenon include medullary cystic disease, Bartter's syndrome, and the diuretic phase of acute tabular necrosis, in which Na and water losses are very large.

PRIMARY POLYDIPSIA Whether because of habit, predilection, psychiatric disorder, a specific lesion in the brain, or medication (Table 40-2), some people drink enough water every day to produce polyuria. The body and the kidneys rarely if ever are injured by chronic polydipsia, but the condition can be confused with diabetes insipidus, which it resembles closely. During deliberate polydipsia, extracellular fluid volume is normal or high, and vasopressin secretion is reduced to a basal level because serum osmolality tends to be near the lower limits of normal. Reabsorption of water from the end distal convoluted tubule and collecting ducts is reduced so that all the surplus water can be excreted into the urine. The inner medulla loses its urea and NaCl gradients because of wash-out, as in diabetes insipidus. Wash-out may be more severe than in diabetes insipidus because primary polydipsia tends to cause expansion of the extracellular fluid volume, whereas primary renal water loss does the opposite. Volume expansion raises total delivery of NaCl and water to the thick ascending limb of Henle's loop and therefore to the inner medulla, all things being equal. It also raises renal blood flow, and increased flow through the vasa recta reduces their ability to trap solutes in the medulla.

Approach to the patient with polyuria Solute diuresis and natriuretic syndromes usually are apparent from the history, physical examination, urinalysis (glucosuria), clinical setting, blood count, blood glucose, and serum creatinine or the BUN. Diagnostic problems occur mainly when stable, chronic polyuria and polydipsia of uncertain origin are present. Here, one must try to distinguish between vasopressin-sensitive diabetes insipidus, nephrogenic diabetes insipidus, and primary polydipsia; the best-established way to do this is by measuring the response of urine osmolality to water deprivation and the administration of vasopressin.

The patient should have free access to water and receive a normal diet that provides approximately 100 mmol NaCl per day for 3 days; then a total fast is instituted. During the fast, pulse and blood pressure should be measured every 30 min and body weight every hour, using an accurate balance. When 3 percent of the initial body weight has been lost or 14 h have elapsed, urine and serum osmolality are measured. A normal subject will lower urine volume below 0.5 mL/min and raise urine osmolality to above 700 mosmol per kilogram of water. In complete diabetes insipidus, nephrogenic or vasopressin-sensitive, the urine osmolality will remain below 200 mosmol/kg and urine flow will remain above 0.5 mL/min, but some rise in osmolality and fall in flow will occur given incomplete diabetes insipidus. If urine osmolality is below 700 mosmol/kg, by the end of the fasting period, 5 mU/min of aqueous vasopressin is administered by intravenous drip. Patients with complete or partial vasopressin-sensitive diabetes insipidus will raise their urine osmolality above the level achieved by fasting alone by more than 9 percent (see Chap. 323). No increase will occur given complete nephrogenic diabetes insipidus, although incomplete forms of nephrogenic diabetes insipidus will permit some response to vasopressin. Infusion of hypertonic saline (Chap. 323) is useful in defining defects of osmoregulator function.

The response of patients with primary polydipsia is quite different. During fluid restriction the secretion of vasopressin increases, and at the completion of the test the flow rate and osmolality of the urine will reflect a physiologic level of vasopressin acting upon normal tubules that traverse a medullary interstitium whose urea and NaCl concentrations have been reduced by chronic wash-out. In other words, the wash-out will set the upper limit on urine osmolality, and patients with primary polydipsia thus demonstrate a submaximal concentrating ability in spite of intact vasopressin secretion. Exogenous vasopressin can increase urine osmolality very little, <9 percent, because medullary wash-out, not vasopressin insufficiency or insensitivity, is the main limiting factor. Usually the urine osmolality will be above 400 mosmol/kg by the end of the fluid deprivation test, in contrast to the lower values of approximately 200 mosmol/kg encountered in patients with diabetes insipidus; but it may be impossible to distinguish incomplete diabetes insipidus from primary polydipsia, in some cases, by using the fluid deprivation test alone. However, measurement of serum antidiuretic hormone levels by radioimmunoassay may increase diagnostic accuracy.

NOCTURIA Whether an individual sleeps through the night without urinating depends upon a diurnal rhythm in which the volume of urine formed during sleep does not exceed bladder capacity, because of reduced renal osmotic concentration, high sodium excretion, solute diuresis, or low bladder capacity.

All the polyuric states may cause nocturia. Urinary concentrating

TABLE 40-2 Causes of polyuria

I Inadequate renal water conservation
- *A* Diabetes insipidus
  - *1* Vasopressin-sensitive (posthypophysectomy; posttrauma; postpituitary ablation; idiopathic, supra- or intrasellar tumors or cysts; histiocystosis or granuloma; encroachment by aneurysm; Sheehan's syndrome, meningoencephalitis; Guillain-Barré's syndrome; fat embolus; empty sella)
  - *2* Nephrogenic
    - *a* Acquired tubulointerstitial renal disease (pyelonephritis, analgesic nephropathy, multiple myeloma, amyloidosis, obstructive uropathy, sarcoidosis, hypercalcemic or hypokalemic nephropathy, Sjögren's syndrome, sickle cell anemia, renal transplantation)
    - *b* Drugs or toxins (lithium, demeclocycline, methyoxyflurane, ethanol, diphenylhydantoin, propoxyphene, amphotericin)
    - *c* Congenital (hereditary nephrogenic diabetes insipidus, polycystic or medullary cystic disease)
- *B* Solute diuresis (glucosuria, high-protein tube feedings, urea or mannitol infusion, radiographic contrast media, chronic renal failure)
- *C* Natriuretic syndromes (salt-losing nephritis, diuretic phase of acute tubular necrosis, diuretic agents)

II Primary polydipsia
- *A* Psychogenic
- *B* Hypothalamic disease
- *C* Drugs (thioridazine, chlorpromazine, anticholinergic agents)

ability falls in most renal diseases (Chap. 218), often at an early stage. Even though overt polyuria may be absent, overnight urine volume frequently exceeds bladder capacity. Nocturia also occurs in edema-forming states. In congestive heart failure, nephrotic syndrome, and hepatic cirrhosis with ascites, fluid accumulates preferentially in dependent portions of the body during the day. At night, with recumbency, tissue capillary forces change and some edema fluid is mobilized, producing the effect of an intravenous saline infusion. Venous insufficiency may produce dependent edema of the legs that is often also mobilized at night, causing nocturia.

Reduced bladder capacity also causes nocturia. Infection, tumor, or stone can cause inflammation and increased irritability. Chronic partial bladder-outflow obstruction, from prostatic hypertrophy, urethral stricture, or benign or malignant neoplasm or stone, causes a frequent stimulus to void and also a thickening of the muscular wall that reduces its compliance. Frequent small voidings may be a clue to this lower urinary tract cause of nocturia, but in its earlier phases chronic obstruction may lead to only one nocturnal voiding of reasonable volume.

DYSURIA, FREQUENCY AND URGENCY, INCONTINENCE, AND ENURESIS

DYSURIA, FREQUENCY, AND URGENCY *Dysuria* refers to pain or burning during urination. *Urinary frequency* means voiding at abnormally brief intervals, due to a sense of bladder fullness that is due not to a full bladder but to a bladder that is irritable and feels full even when it is not. *Urgency* is an exaggerated sense of needing to urinate, due to an irritable or inflamed bladder.

Mechanisms of dysuria REDUCED BLADDER COMPLIANCE When the bladder has a decreased ability to expand, frequency, nocturia, and urgency usually result. When decreased expansion is due to inflammation of the mucosa (cystitis) from infection, radiation, chemicals, or foreign bodies (catheters, stones), burning usually is more prominent than when it is due to infiltration of the muscle by tumors of the bladder or from adjacent organs (prostate, rectum, uterus).

INFECTION Acute bacterial cystitis, which occurs more frequently in women, usually causes great frequency day and night, burning on urination, and, not infrequently, gross hematuria. Prostatitis or prostatocystitis in men can cause a picture similar to acute cystitis in women. When only the prostate is involved, milder symptoms such as vague pain or discomfort in the lower abdomen, groin, perineum, rectum, testes, or penis occur. The symptoms may be associated with urination but more frequently are noticed at times other than during micturition or ejaculation.

PSYCHOSOMATIC CYSTITIS The functional bladder syndrome and chronic glandular urethrotrigonitis are synonyms for a very common but poorly understood affliction of middle-aged and older women, in which pain is usually vague, aching in nature, and in the lower abdomen or vagina. There is daytime frequency without nocturia; pyuria is absent. A complete urologic evaluation usually becomes necessary because symptoms are chronic and hard to eradicate. The functional bladder syndrome must be distinguished from the effects of a cystocele, which can be repaired surgically. (See also Chap. 225.)

Approach to the patient with dysuria The medical history should focus on past as well as present urinary problems. A pelvic examination in women and prostatic examination in men are necessary components of the physical examination. Microscopic examination of a two-glass urinary sediment in all patients and of the prostatic fluid in men, obtained by prostatic massage, is also necessary. The first 20 mL of a voiding, if collected separately, may contain a higher concentration of leukocytes and bacteria than the remainder of the voided urine, when the urethra is the principal site of inflammation or infection. Normal prostatic fluid, not subjected to centrifugation, contains less than 10 leukocytes per high-power field; excessive leukocytes in the prostatic fluid are an important clue to prostatitis and may, when prostatis is chronic, be the only detectable abnormality. Further diagnostic studies will depend upon such positive findings as a history of chronic or recurrent episodes or associated fever, which are rare in lower urinary tract infections except in acute prostatitis, or an abnormality on physical examination such as a pelvic or rectal mass or tenderness, hematuria or pyuria, or excessive leukocytes and macrophages in the prostatic fluid. Serum acid phosphatase may be elevated when carcinoma of the prostate has extended beyond the boundary of the prostatic capsule.

Additional evaluation of dysuria, when the cause is not evident from clinical examination, may include cultures of urine and prostatic fluid for aerobic and anaerobic bacteria, tubercle bacilli, and mycoplasma; excretory urography; and voiding cystourethrography. If these examinations do not reveal the diagnosis, but symptoms are troublesome, urologic evaluations, including cystoscopy and urethroscopy with endoscopic biopsies of visualized abnormalities, and dynamic urinary tract studies may be useful.

INCONTINENCE *Incontinence* refers to the inability to retain urine in the bladder. It results from neurologic or mechanical disorders of the complicated system that controls normal micturition.

Normal bladder function The detrusor muscle, which provides the propulsive force for emptying the bladder, consists of interlacing fibers of smooth muscle that are under parasympathetic autonomic control through the pelvic nerves from sacral spinal cord segments S2, S3, and S4. The smooth muscle of the trigonal portion of the bladder, between the ureteral orifices and the posterior area of the bladder outlet, is innervated by motor fibers from thoracolumbar segments (T11 to L2) of the sympathetic nervous system, in which alpha receptor sites predominate. This layer of muscle extends into the posterior urethra and acts as an involuntary internal sphincter that helps maintain urinary continence even in the absence of voluntary control. The external urethral sphincter and perineal muscles are under voluntary control via the pudendal nerves.

Sensory tracts of pain, temperature, and distention pass from the bladder via the pelvic nerves to sacral spinal levels S2, S3, and S4, creating a simple spinal voiding reflex between the bladder and the sacral spinal cord. The sensory tracts from the bladder further ascend through sacrobulbar pathways to the medulla of the brain and ultimately to cortical centers, from which impulses arise, pass back down the lateral and ventral reticulospinal tracts, and normally suppress the sacral spinal reflex arc controlling bladder emptying.

The normal adult bladder can accommodate as much as approximately 400 mL fluid without a significant increase in intravesical pressure (<20 cmH_2O). Above this point, sensations of fullness are transmitted to the sacral cord. If not suppressed by cortical control, the sacral cord reflexly discharges motor impulses that cause powerful sustained detrusor contraction. Urination can be prevented by cortical suppression of the reflex arc or by voluntary contraction of the external sphincter and perineal muscles. Infants, and adults with spinal cord damage above S2, urinate spontaneously when the bladder fills sufficiently.

Normal micturition is initiated by voluntary suppression of cortical inhibition of the reflex arc and by relaxation of the muscles of the pelvic floor and the external sphincter. The base of the bladder falls; then the trigone contracts, an action that occludes the ureters as they pass through the bladder wall and helps to prevent vesicoureteral reflux of urine during voiding. Finally, the detrusor contracts and voiding occurs.

Causes of incontinence DETRUSOR INSTABILITY In this condition, the bladder becomes prone to uncontrollable contractions—that cause incontinence—because inhibitory neural pathways are damaged. Among the elderly, detrusor instability causes as much as 70 percent of urinary incontinence, and arises from diseases of the central nervous system such as cerebrovascular accidents, Alzheimer's dementia, neoplasm, and, possibly, normal pressure hydrocephalus. Any lesion that disrupts the lateral and vertical reticulospinal tracts can reduce or abolish descending inhibiting impulses to the sacral spinal reflex and can result in detrusor instability. If the descending tracts are completely destroyed, the bladder will empty automatically. Bladder or pelvic infection or tumor, fecal impaction, uterine prolapse, and prostatic hypertrophy are other causes. Whatever the cause, the usual clinical picture is of unpredictable, involuntary voiding, usually >160 mL each time. Imipramine, 25 mg at bedtime, or calcium channel blockers (such as nifedipine) reduce detrusor contractions, and improve continence. Local infection, tumors, or fecal impaction are treated conventionally.

STRESS INCONTINENCE This condition is common in postmenopausal parous women. The structures of the female urethra atrophy when deprived of estrogen, and many become unable to resist the passage of urine under the stress of increased intraabdominal pressure during coughing, sneezing, climbing stairs, and other physical activity, so small amounts of urine escape. Parturition may damage the pelvic support of the bladder so that the bladder and urethra can slip downward from their normal position above the pelvic diaphragm. As they do, the urethra shortens, and the normal urethrovesical angle, important in closing the urethral sphincter, is lost. In men, stress incontinence usually is secondary to prostatic surgery for benign prostatic hypertrophy or prostatic carcinoma. If the external sphincter has also been damaged during operation, total incontinence may result. Surgical elevation of the urethrovesicle angle is helpful in women. Estrogen replacement therapy may prevent atrophy of the urethral mucosa.

MECHANICAL INCONTINENCE Some congenital anomalies, extrophy of the bladder, patent urachus, and ectopic ureteral openings distal to the vesical neck cause mechanical incontinence. They are all correctable only by surgery. Acquired mechanical incontinence can follow transurethral resection of the prostate in which damage has occurred to both the internal and external sphincter mechanisms. Pelvic surgery or irradiation of the uterus or rectum may cause incontinence because of vesicovaginal, ureterovaginal, vesicoperineal, or ureteroperineal fistulas.

OVERFLOW OR PARADOXICAL INCONTINENCE This form of incontinence arises from large residual volumes of urine secondary to obstruction at the bladder neck or along the urethra (urethral stricture) or from neurologic damage. Benign prostatic hypertrophy afflicts upward of 75 percent of older men. It is manifested by nocturia, reduced size and force of the urinary stream, straining to urinate, and terminal dribbling, all due to outflow obstruction. Functional outflow obstruction can occur because of spinal cord disease; the detrusor and external sphincter contract dyssynergistically, i.e., at the same time. Hypotonic neurogenic bladders may occur in diseases which produce autonomic peripheral neuropathy, such as diabetes mellitus, uremia, hypothyroidism, chronic alcoholism, Guillain-Barré syndrome, collagen vascular diseases, and toxic neuropathies associated with some carcinomas (especially lung and kidney). It also may occur because of prolonged overdistention of the bladder. Hydronephrosis and impaired renal function can occur in patients with chronic overflow incontinence. All causes produce a dilated, palpable bladder. Especially in diabetes, patients can control micturition but lose their sensory awareness of bladder filling. Their incontinence can be avoided by scheduled reminders. Outlet obstruction is treated surgically. If the bladder has become adynamic because of prolonged overfilling, bethanechol chloride, 50 to 100 mg per day, may improve emptying.

PSYCHOGENIC AND FUNCTIONAL INCONTINENCE Children, and even some young adults, draw attention to themselves by feigning incontinence and thereby derive some secondary emotional satisfaction. A complete diagnostic evaluation usually is necessary to rule out organic disease even when psychogenic incontinence is strongly suspected. In elderly people, especially those who have a limited ability to walk or who are confused because of central nervous system disease or drugs, incontinence may be *functional*, i.e., due simply to an inability to reach a toilet in time. Treatment depends upon correcting the individual problem in each case.

ENURESIS *Enuresis* refers to the involuntary passage of urine at night or during sleep—hence, the synonym bed-wetting. Some clinicians reserve the term enuresis for those bed wetters who have no gross urologic abnormalities, but it should be used for bed-wetting in general.

The sacral spinal reflex arc alone controls urination in the infant; therefore, enuretic incontinence is normal under the age of 2 years. As the nervous system matures, cortical control over the spinal reflex arc results in the voluntary control over urination and defecation by the age of 2½ years. Even so, enuresis beyond the age of 3 years occurs to some degree in approximately 10 percent of all otherwise normal children and probably is due to a delay in maturation of bladder control, which may be familial.

Although the majority of bed wetters will be dry by the age of puberty, organic diseases, especially infections of the urinary tract, obstructive lesions with overflow incontinence, neurovesical dysfunction, and polyuric conditions that overload the bladder must be suspected in any child who is enuretic beyond the age of 3 years. Patients with organic disease usually, but not always, are incontinent during the day as well as at night. For the majority, who have no overt lesions, imipramine (75 mg at bedtime) may be useful.

REFERENCES

Azotemia, oliguria, and anuria

ABUELO JG: Proteinuria: Diagnostic principles and procedures. Ann Intern Med 98:186, 1983

BRENNER BM et al: Molecular basis of proteinuria of glomerular origin. N Engl J Med 298:826, 1978

BRIDGES CR et al: Glomerular charge alterations in human minimal charge nephropathy. Kidney Int 22:677, 1982

GLASSOCK RJ et al: Primary glomerular diseases, in *The Kidney*, 3d ed, BM Brenner, FC Rector Jr (eds). Philadelphia, Saunders, 1986, p 929

KURTZMAN NA (ed): *Seminars in Nephrology: Acute Renal Failure*, JP Knochel (guest ed). New York, Grune & Stratton, 1981

——— (ed): *Seminars in Nephrology: Chronic Renal Failure*, G Eknoyan (guest ed). New York, Grune & Stratton, 1981

OKEN DE: On the differential diagnosis of acute renal failure. Am J Med 71:916, 1981

PARDO V et al: Benign primary hematuria: Clinicopathologic study of 65 patients. Am J Med 67:817, 1979

Polyuria and nocturia

BERL T (ed): Disorders of water metabolism, in *Seminars in Nephrology*, vol 4. New York, Grune & Stratton, 1984, p 285

ROBERTSON GL, BERL W: Pathophysiology of water metabolism, in *The Kidney*, 3d ed, BM Brenner, FC Rector Jr (eds). Philadelphia, Saunders, 1986, p 385

SCHRIER RW, BICHET DG: Osmotic and nonosmotic control of vasopressin release and the pathogenesis of impaired water excretion in adrenal, thyroid, and edematous disorders. J Lab Clin Med 98:1, 1981

ZERBE RL, ROBERTSON GL: A comparison of plasma vasopressin measurements with a standard indirect test in the differential diagnosis of polyuria. N Engl J Med 305:1539, 1981

Dysuria, frequency and urgency, incontinence, and enuresis

BRADLEY WE: Diagnosis of urinary bladder dysfunction in diabetes mellitus. Ann Intern Med 92:323, 1980

BRADLEY WE, SCOTT FB: Physiology of the urinary bladder, in *Urology*, 4th ed, JH Harrison et al (eds). Philadelphia, Saunders, 1978, vol 1, p 87

DEGROAT WC, BOOTH AM: Physiology of the urinary bladder and urethra. Ann Intern Med 92:312, 1980

HINDMARSH HR, BYRNE PO: Adult enuresis: A symptomatic and urodynamic assessment. Br J Urol 52:88, 1980

MEARES EM JR: Prostatitis syndromes: New perspectives about old woes. J Urol 123:141, 1980

MIKKELSEN EJ, RAPOPORT JL: Enuresis: Psychopathology, sleep stage, and drug response. Urol Clin North Am 7:361, 1980

PLATT R: Quantitative definition of bacteriuria. Infectious Diseases Symposium, July 28, 1983, p 44, Supplement to Am J Med

TURNER-WARWICK R, WHITESIDE CG (eds): *Symposium on Clinical Urodynamics: The Urologic Clinics of North America*, vol 6. Philadelphia, Saunders, 1979

WILLIAMS ME, PANNELL FC: Urinary incontinence in the elderly. Ann Intern Med 97:895, 1982

41 FLUIDS AND ELECTROLYTES

NORMAN G. LEVINSKY

SODIUM AND WATER

PHYSIOLOGIC CONSIDERATIONS (See also Chap. 218) Both physiologically and clinically, sodium and water metabolism are closely interrelated. The sodium content of the body depends on the balance between dietary intake and renal excretion of sodium. In health, extrarenal losses of sodium are negligible. Renal sodium excretion is closely regulated to match dietary content. Within 2 to 4 days after sodium intake stops, urinary excretion decreases to 5 meq per day or less. If dietary sodium is abruptly increased, sodium excretion promptly rises and equals intake within a few days. Thus, in normal persons the sodium content of the body remains quite constant despite wide variations in sodium intake; over the range of 0 to 400 meq per day, total body sodium varies only by about 10 percent.

Renal sodium excretion is regulated by the interplay of multiple control mechanisms. Sodium loads or deficits tend to produce corresponding changes in the central blood volume. Receptors, apparently located in the atria and central arteries, respond to changes in local pressure or flow which signal the volume/capacity relation of the central circulation (*effective blood volume*). If the effective volume is depleted, salt retention is induced, while expansion triggers multiple factors that favor natriuresis. With volume (salt) depletion, renal blood flow falls, due to decreased cardiac output, increased renal sympathetic nerve activity, and activation of the renin-angiotensin system. Glomerular filtration also tends to fall, which reduces filtered sodium. Tubular reabsorption of sodium is enhanced. Proximal reabsorption is stimulated by changes in Starling forces (e.g., increased plasma protein concentration) in the peritubular circulation and by sympathetic nerves which innervate proximal segments directly. Distal tubular reabsorption is enhanced by aldosterone, which is secreted at an increased rate in response to stimulation of the adrenal gland by angiotensin. Volume expansion leads to the opposite changes in renal hemodynamics and in these various regulators of tubular transport. Moreover, one or more natriuretic hormones are secreted in response to increased extracellular volume. Their nature and role are less well defined than that of aldosterone. Peptides in the cardiac atria can increase sodium excretion acutely by hemodynamic or tubular mechanisms. There is some evidence for another natriuretic hormone which decreases tubular salt transport by inhibiting Na-K adenosine triphosphatase (ATPase). Prostaglandins reduce sodium reabsorption in distal nephron segments.

Undoubtedly, other regulatory mechanisms remain to be defined. The multiplicity of control mechanisms prevents abnormalities of any single mechanism from grossly distorting the regulation of sodium excretion. For example, increased aldosterone secretion leads only to limited and transient sodium retention, because the initial accumulation of sodium stimulates opposing natriuretic factors such as increased glomerular filtration and decreased proximal tubular sodium reabsorption.

All but 2 to 5 percent of the sodium in the body is located in the extracellular fluids. (Approximately 40 percent of total body sodium is located in bone, but this fraction does not participate significantly in most physiologic processes and will not be considered further.) Except for minor differences in concentration due to the Gibbs-Donnan effect of plasma proteins, the electrolyte compositions of plasma and interstitial fluid are essentially equal. Consequently, plasma composition can be considered representative of the entire extracellular compartment. Total extracellular volume approximates 20 percent of body weight. Of this, 5 percent represents plasma volume and 15 percent the volume of interstitial fluids. Thus, in a 70-kg individual with plasma sodium concentration of 140 meq per liter, extracellular sodium content will approximate 2000 meq. The volume of intracellular fluid is approximately twice as great as that of extracellular fluid, i.e., about 40 percent of body weight. However, since intracellular sodium concentration is less than 5 meq per liter, total intracellular sodium content is only about 100 to 150 meq. The asymmetric distribution of sodium across cell membranes is maintained by expenditure of a large fraction of the energy derived from cell metabolism, which is required constantly to pump sodium out of cells against its electrochemical gradient. All the principal electrolytes are asymmetrically distributed across cell membranes. The principal electrolytes of the extracellular fluids are sodium, chloride, and bicarbonate. The major electrolytes of the intracellular fluids are potassium, magnesium, calcium, and organic anions, including proteins.

Since sodium salts account for more than 90 percent of the total osmolality of the extracellular fluid, variations in plasma sodium concentration are almost always reflected in equivalent changes in plasma osmolality. Exceptions due to accumulation of other solutes in plasma are discussed later. Although the electrolyte compositions of intracellular and extracellular fluids differ markedly, they are always in osmotic equilibrium, since water moves rapidly across cellular membranes to dissipate osmotic gradients. Therefore, although sodium is largely confined to extracellular fluids, plasma sodium concentration is an index of not only the relative proportions of sodium and water in those fluids but also the relation between total body solute and total body water. An example is the effect of shift of sodium from extracellular to intracellular fluid without a change in total body solute. Movement of sodium into cells would not cause hyponatremia, since water would shift into cells with the sodium. On the other hand, a primary decrease in the concentration of osmotically active solute within cells would decrease total body solute; although there would be no change in total body sodium or water, hyponatremia would result from the shift of intracellular water into the extracellular compartment.

A very effective mechanism involving the *hypothalamus,* the *neurohypophysis,* and the kidney regulates plasma osmolality. Changes of 2 percent or less in plasma osmolality can be detected by osmoreceptors in the hypothalamus. Small increases in osmolality stimulate the secretion of antidiuretic hormone (ADH) from the neurohypophysis, while small decreases suppress secretion of the hormone. Normal plasma osmolality is approximately 280 to 300 mosmol per kilogram of water; the exact level is determined by the "set" of the hypothalamic osmoreceptors in a given individual. When ADH secretion is maximal, urine volume will be about 500 mL per day, and urine osmolality will be 800 to 1400 mosmol/kg. In the absence of ADH, minimal urine osmolality is 40 to 80 mosmol/kg, and maximum water diuresis can reach 15 to 20 liters per day or more. The capacity of this receptor-effector system is sufficient to maintain plasma osmolality within narrow limits despite large variations in the volume and concentration of dietary fluids. ADH secretion is also regulated by changes in extracellular volume. A reduction of 10 percent or more may trigger ADH release even in the absence of changes in plasma osmolality. If volume contraction is sufficiently severe, volume-mediated stimulation of ADH may override osmotic signals and cause water retention despite progressive dilution of body fluids. Conversely, extracellular volume expansion tends to suppress ADH release even if the body fluids are hypertonic.

The total sodium *content* of the body is determined by the renal sodium regulatory mechanisms described earlier. However, the principal determinant of plasma sodium *concentration* is water metabolism rather than total body sodium content. If excess sodium were to be ingested and retained, hypernatremia would be only transient. Water intake would increase because of thirst, and the fluid ingested would be retained because hypernatremia (hyperosmolality) would stimulate ADH secretion. Expanded extracellular volume, not hypernatremia, would be the end result. Conversely, if the osmoregulatory system is functioning normally, loss of moderate amounts of sodium without water would not result in permanent reduction of plasma sodium concentration. The initial reduction would shut off secretion of ADH, and a water diuresis would ensue. The final outcome would be contraction of extracellular volume, while plasma sodium concentration would be restored to normal. It follows that changes in total sodium content tend to cause changes in extracellular volume. In this sense, the sodium content of the extracellular fluid determines extracellular volume. On the other hand, changes in plasma sodium concentration reflect altered regulation of water excretion, not changes in total body sodium content alone. Clinically, plasma sodium concentration per se gives no information about the amount of sodium present in the body. Total body sodium content is determined by the volume of extracellular fluids as well as by the concentration of sodium in these fluids. Extracellular volume is usually the dominant factor since changes in volume tend to be proportionately greater than changes in sodium concentration. Plasma sodium concentration reflects the relative proportions of sodium and water (or, more exactly, of total body solute and water), not the absolute amount of sodium in the body. Either hyponatremia or hypernatremia may occur when total body sodium content is decreased, normal, or increased.

CLINICAL DISORDERS Deficits and excesses of sodium and water occur in a great variety of clinical circumstances. The manifestations of the underlying illness may overshadow the clinical features of the fluid and electrolyte disorder. Theoretically, disturbances of sodium and water metabolism can be classified into four categories, reflecting a primary excess or deficit of water or sodium. Practically, such isolated disturbances are uncommon. A primary excess of sodium leads to edema; it is not ordinarily considered as an electrolyte disorder but as a feature of underlying disease, such as congestive heart failure, hepatic cirrhosis, or nephrotic syndrome. Primary sodium deficits are nearly always accompanied by water depletion, leading to the clinical syndrome of extracellular volume depletion. Pure or disproportionate water excess leads to hyponatremia, relative or absolute water depletion to hypernatremia. A practical clinical classification of disorders of sodium and water metabolism is given in Table 41-1.

VOLUME DEPLETION Combined sodium and water deficits are far more frequent than isolated deficits of either constituent. Although the term *dehydration* is often used for combined deficits, this usage is confusing. Dehydration should be used to describe relatively pure water depletion leading to hypernatremia; *volume depletion* or some similar term should be used for combined deficits.

Pathogenesis As noted earlier, elimination of sodium from the diet will not by itself lead to sodium depletion in the presence of normal renal function, since urinary sodium excretion will quickly fall to very low levels. Therefore, sodium depletion is always due either to extrarenal losses or to abnormal renal losses.

GASTROINTESTINAL The most common cause of volume depletion is loss of a significant fraction of the 8 to 10 liters of gastrointestinal fluids normally secreted daily. Since the principal secretions contain potassium and hydrogen ion or bicarbonate in large amounts, volume depletion due to gastrointestinal losses is often combined with potassium depletion and acidosis or alkalosis.

Significant volume depletion may be caused by sequestration of secretions within an obstructed gastrointestinal tract or within the peritoneal cavity in peritonitis. Rapid reaccumulation of ascites after paracentesis may cause contraction of the effective circulating blood volume.

SKIN The sodium concentration of sweat varies from 5 to 50 meq per liter; sodium concentration increases with higher rates of sweating and in adrenal insufficiency. Because sweat is always a hypotonic solution, sweating leads to water deficits out of proportion to sodium losses. In burns, capillary damage may lead to sequestration of large amounts of sodium and water in the injured skin.

RENAL Abnormal losses of sodium and water in the urine may occur in both acute and chronic renal diseases. Early in the recovery (diuretic) phase of *acute renal failure,* urinary sodium concentration tends to be high (50 to 100 meq per liter), and substantial deficits of both sodium and water may ensue. With rare exceptions, severe sodium and water wasting does not persist beyond the first few days. It is important to discriminate between increased excretion, which represents elimination of excess retained during the oliguric period, and true tubular sodium and water wasting, which depletes normal extracellular volume. Only the latter requires replacement. Acute salt and water wasting due to tubular damage may also occur immediately after relief of prolonged *obstruction* of the urinary tract. Although such a postobstructive diuresis may be severe, it rarely persists for more than several days as a clinically important phenomenon.

Patients with *chronic renal failure* have limited ability to decrease sodium and water excretion in response to decreased intake. They will become progressively volume-depleted if their intake is restricted by the anorexia, nausea, and vomiting characteristic of uremia or because of their physician's instructions. Large deficits may develop insidiously over many days or weeks. A "self-perpetuating cycle" may result, in that volume depletion will tend further to compromise renal function. Severe sodium-wasting renal disease, i.e., negative sodium balance when dietary sodium is normal, is rare. It occurs in occasional patients with tubulointerstitial diseases of the kidney, especially medullary cystic disease.

Renal sodium wasting in the presence of normal intrinsic renal function occurs in three clinical circumstances. Perhaps the most common is sodium depletion due to continued administration of potent *diuretics* to patients after edema has been relieved or to patients whose edema is sequestered and cannot be mobilized. For example, attempted treatment of cirrhotics with ascites may result in depletion of overall extracellular volume rather than mobilization of ascitic

TABLE 41-1 Disorders of sodium and water metabolism

- *I* Combined sodium and water depletion (volume depletion)
  - *A* Extrarenal losses
    - *1* Gastrointestinal (vomiting, diarrhea, gastrointestinal suction, fistulas)
    - *2* Abdominal sequestration (peritonitis, rapid reaccumulation of ascites)
    - *3* Skin (sweating, burns)
  - *B* Renal losses
    - *1* Renal disease (chronic renal failure, salt-wasting tubular disease, diuretic phase of acute renal failure, postobstructive diuresis)
    - *2* Diuretic excess
    - *3* Osmotic diuresis (diabetic glycosuria)
    - *4* Mineralocorticoid deficiency (Addison's disease, hypoaldosteronism)
- *II* Hyponatremia
  - *A* Associated with extracellular volume depletion (see list of causes above)
  - *B* Associated with extracellular volume excess and edema
  - *C* Associated with normal or modestly expanded extracellular volume (no edema)
    - *1* Acute and chronic renal failure
    - *2* Temporary impairment of water diuresis (pain, drugs, emotion)
    - *3* Syndrome of inappropriate secretion of antidiuretic hormone (SIADH)
    - *4* Severe polydipsia
    - *5* Endocrine (glucocorticoid deficiency, hypothyroidism)
    - *6* Essential ("sick cell syndrome")
  - *D* Without plasma hypoosmolality
    - *1* Osmotic (hyperglycemia, mannitol)
    - *2* Artifactual (hyperlipemia, hyperproteinemia, laboratory error)
- *III* Hypernatremia
  - *A* Due solely to water loss
    - *1* Extrarenal
      - *a* Skin (insensible losses)
      - *b* Lungs
    - *2* Renal
      - *a* Diabetes insipidus (central, nephrogenic)
    - *3* Hypothalamic dysfunction
  - *B* Due to water loss associated with sodium loss
    - *1* Extrarenal
      - *a* Sweat
    - *2* Renal
      - *a* Osmotic diuresis (glycosuria, urea)
  - *C* Due to sodium gain
    - *a* Excessive sodium administration
    - *b* Adrenal hyperfunction (hyperaldosteronism, Cushing's syndrome)

fluid. An obligatory *osmotic diuresis* may also cause renal sodium and water wasting despite normal renal function. Marked glycosuria in uncontrolled diabetes mellitus is the most frequent clinical example. Administration of osmotic diuretics such as mannitol is a common iatrogenic cause. Volume depletion in patients receiving high-protein enteral or parenteral alimentation may be due to an osmotic diuresis of urea formed by protein metabolism. Finally, renal sodium wasting despite normal intrinsic function occurs in Addison's disease and hypoaldosteronism due to a *deficiency* of *mineralocorticoids*.

Clinical features and diagnosis The cause of volume depletion can usually be suspected from a history of inadequate salt and water intake together with vomiting, diarrhea, or excessive sweating; the symptoms of poorly controlled diabetes mellitus or of renal or adrenal disease may be elicited. The key findings on physical examination are those of plasma and extracellular volume depletion. Decreased skin turgor is usually present in patients with significant volume contraction but may be difficult to evaluate in the elderly. It can be estimated clinically by noting the slow rate of return of skin to its original position when it is raised between the examiner's fingers. An area of skin normally free of wrinkles and not subject to wide variations in the thickness of subcutaneous tissue, such as that over the sternum, should be selected for this maneuver. Oral mucous membranes may be dry and axillary sweating decreased; these are less reliable diagnostic features than decreased skin turgor. With moderate volume depletion, blood pressure is usually normal when the patient is recumbent, although resting tachycardia may be present. Postural hypotension, i.e., a drop of at least 5 to 10 mmHg in the sitting or standing position, is often present. With greater degrees of volume depletion, even recumbent blood pressure is reduced, and frank shock may occur. The patient with moderate or severe degrees of volume contraction is often lethargic, weak, confused, or obtunded. Such patients are usually oliguric, even when recumbent blood pressure is normal. However, an osmotic diuresis, as occurs in hyperglycemia, tends to prevent oliguria despite volume contraction.

LABORATORY FINDINGS The hematocrit and plasma protein concentration are increased, but values within the normal range are interpretable only if prior values are known. Plasma sodium concentration may be decreased, normal, or increased, depending upon the proportion between deficits of sodium and of water. Plasma creatinine and urea nitrogen are usually increased, since the glomerular filtration rate is decreased (''prerenal azotemia''). Urinary sodium concentration may be of value in differentiating extrarenal and renal sources of sodium loss if the probable cause is not clear from the history. With extrarenal losses, urinary sodium concentration will be less than 10 meq per liter; the concentration will usually exceed 20 meq per liter if renal or adrenal disorders are at fault. However, urinary sodium may ultimately fall below this level even in patients with renal salt wasting if sodium depletion becomes severe.

Treatment The principal clinical manifestations of extracellular volume depletion are due to reduction of plasma and interstitial fluid volume. Since there is no convenient clinical method for assessing these volumes, the effect of treatment must be determined by following the clinical changes in parameters such as blood pressure, urine output, and skin turgor. Modest deficits of sodium and water can often be corrected by increased oral intake in patients not suffering from gastrointestinal disorders. Severe depletion requires therapy with intravenous solutions. Isotonic saline (0.85%) is the infusion of choice in patients whose serum sodium concentration is approximately normal. The amount to be infused can be estimated from the history of prior losses and from the severity of the physical findings of extracellular volume contraction. Patients with moderate volume contraction usually require replacement with 2 to 3 liters of saline, while patients with severe depletion may require much larger volumes. The need for correction of other concurrent electrolyte abnormalities may alter the composition of the required infusion; e.g., some of the sodium may be given as bicarbonate to patients with volume contraction and metabolic acidosis, or potassium may be added in patients with concurrent potassium depletion. In estimating the total amount to be infused, allowance for ongoing losses must be included. Since the amount to be infused cannot be calculated precisely, patients should be monitored carefully to avoid fluid overload and congestive failure.

HYPONATREMIA **Pathophysiology** Hyponatremia indicates that the body fluids are diluted by an excess of water relative to total solute. Hyponatremia is not equivalent to sodium depletion, which is only one of the clinical states in which it may occur (see Table 41-1). Most types of hyponatremia result from defective urinary dilution. The normal response to dilution of body fluids is a water diuresis, which corrects the hypoosmotic state. Normal water diuresis requires three factors: (1) Secretion of ADH must be suppressed. (2) Sufficient sodium and water must reach the diluting sites of the nephron, in the ascending limb of Henle's loop and the distal convoluted tubule. (3) These nephron segments must function normally, reabsorbing sodium while remaining impermeable to water.

Correspondingly, three types of mechanisms may cause defective water diuresis in patients with hyponatremia. (1) Secretion of ADH may continue ''inappropriately'' despite hypotonicity of extracellular fluid, which normally shuts off secretion of the hormone. This may be due to unregulated release of ADH by neoplasms or to nonosmotic stimuli to ADH secretion. The latter include volume depletion and neural factors such as pain and emotion. (2) Insufficient sodium may reach the diluting segments to permit the formation of an adequate amount of dilute urine. Inadequate delivery of tubular fluid to distal sites may be due to reduced glomerular filtration and/or enhanced proximal tubular reabsorption. Even in the absence of ADH, distal tubular segments are not absolutely impermeable to water; small amounts of water continue to leak from the hypotonic tubular fluid into the isotonic cortical and slightly hypertonic medullary interstitial fluid. The amount of water leaking back in this manner becomes an increasingly larger fraction of the volume of dilute urine formed, as the diluting process is progressively limited by decreasing delivery. Hence, urine osmolality rises progressively. In some instances, this mechanism may even result in excretion of a urine hypertonic to plasma, despite the absence of ADH. (3) Sodium transport in the diluting segments may be defective, or water permeability may be excessive at these sites even in the absence of ADH. One of these three factors can account for most types of hyponatremia, as described below.

Types of hyponatremia (Table 41-1) In patients with extracellular *volume depletion,* delivery of sodium and water to the diluting segments of the nephron is reduced because of decreased glomerular filtration, increased proximal tubular reabsorption, or both. ADH secretion is stimulated by the volume contraction. These changes in renal function and hormone secretion limit water diuresis during extracelluar volume depletion. Hyponatremia per se is usually of little clinical significance in sodium (volume) depletion. The major features are those of extracellular volume contraction, described above. Reduction of plasma sodium concentration by more than 10 to 15 meq per liter is rare in the absence of obvious decreases in skin turgor, postural or recumbent hypotension, and some degree of azotemia. Treatment is directed to correction of the volume deficits. In the occasional symptomatic patient with sodium depletion whose plasma sodium concentration is less than 125 meq per liter, some of the intravenous sodium replacement fluids should be administered as hypertonic saline.

In *edematous states* such as congestive heart failure, cirrhosis, and the nephrotic syndrome, hyponatremia paradoxically appears to result from mechanisms similar to those that cause hyponatremia in patients with volume depletion. Although plasma or extracellular volume is normal or increased in most edematous patients, it is believed that the ''effective'' volume is reduced by decreased cardiac output or sequestration of fluid outside the central circulation. The decrease in ''effective'' volume results in diminished delivery of sodium and water to nephron diluting segments, because of reduced glomerular filtration, increased proximal tubular reabsorption, or both. Volume-mediated secretion of ADH is also triggered in these conditions. In some edematous patients essential hyponatremia may be an additional mechanism (see below). In edematous states, the severity and frequency of hyponatremia correlate to some extent with the magnitude of the edema and the seriousness of the underlying condition. Hyponatremia is usually present in patients with advanced disease unless water intake is restricted. The hyponatremia itself is often of little clinical significance. The principal features are those of the underlying disease. However, symptomatic hyponatremia may occur, most often in connection with vigorous diuretic therapy or excessive oral or parenteral intake of dilute fluids.

Hyponatremia associated with edema responds to effective treatment of the underlying disease. Moderate nonprogressive hyponatremia in edematous patients usually does not cause symptoms. Attempts to correct such hyponatremia by restriction of fluid intake induce thirst and discomfort without improving the clinical picture or longevity. Patients with severe or progressive hyponatremia may require some restriction of water intake, especially during vigorous treatment with diuretics. However, moderate limitation to the range of 1000 to 1500 mL per day will often suffice to avoid symptoms of progressive hyponatremia. More severe restriction should be instituted only if specific clinical or laboratory observations warrant. Since edematous subjects have excess total extracellular sodium, hypertonic saline should not be administered except in rare instances in which clinical manifestations of extreme hyponatremia, such as coma or convulsions, justify emergency measures. Furosemide should be given concurrently in such cases to avoid further expansion of the extracellular space. Dialysis can also be used to correct severe hyponatremia without increasing volume in edematous patients.

Multiple factors contribute to hyponatremia caused by *diuretics*. Salt loss may cause volume depletion, which limits water diuresis by mechanisms already described. Furosemide, ethacrynic acid, and thiazides inhibit salt reabsorption in the diluting segments of the nephron and thereby directly limit water diuresis. Thiazides appear to be the diuretics most commonly associated with hyponatremia, probably because they interfere with elaboration of a hypotonic urine by inhibiting sodium reabsorption in the distal convoluted tubule but, unlike loop diuretics, do not limit urine concentration and water retention by interfering with salt transport in the loop of Henle. In addition, potassium depletion caused by many diuretics contributes to hyponatremia through uncertain mechanisms. Hyponatremia due to diuretic therapy is frequent but usually minor in severity. However, moderate or severe hyponatremia may occur in patients who receive diuretics and who drink large quantities of water or other hypotonic fluids. Progressive hyponatremia is an important complication of diuretic therapy in edematous patients, in whom the underlying disease tends to cause hyponatremia (see above) and to whom large doses of diuretics may be given. The treatment of hyponatremia due to diuretics is water restriction and repletion of potassium deficits.

Hyponatremia may result from *impaired water excretion* not associated with a substantial deficit or excess of salt. In this case, extracellular volume is only modestly expanded. Since excess water is distributed throughout both intracellular and extracellular fluids in proportion to their volumes, only one-third of a water excess will be retained in the extracellular compartment. *Oliguric* patients develop dilutional hyponatremia if the volume of oral and intravenous fluids is not restricted appropriately. The ability to excrete a normal volume of dilute urine is progressively limited in advancing *chronic renal failure*. Regulation of water intake by thirst usually prevents dilutional hyponatremia. However, hyponatremia may be precipitated by increased fluid intake (for example, if the patient is instructed to force fluids). Since the ability to regulate salt excretion is also limited in chronic renal failure, in many patients hyponatremia is associated with edema or salt depletion. In patients with normal renal function, water diuresis may be limited temporarily by ADH secretion induced by various neural stimuli such as pain and narcotics. In the postoperative state, these factors, together with administration of large volumes of hypotonic fluids, may cause hyponatremia. The etiology of hyponatremia is usually evident from the clinical setting and a careful review of fluid intake and output. This type of hyponatremia is treated by water restriction. Only if severe symptoms occur is hypertonic saline infusion required.

Hyponatremia in patients with the *syndrome* of chronic *inappropriate* secretion of *antidiuretic hormone* (SIADH) is principally due to water retention, but continued urinary losses of sodium also contribute to a mild negative sodium balance. Renal sodium wasting is related to modest volume expansion, since it can be eliminated by restricting fluid intake. The mechanisms by which extracellular expansion increases sodium excretion have been discussed above. Clinically, SIADH is defined by a unique group of features: (1) Urine osmolality is not maximally dilute even when marked hyponatremia is induced by water loading. In most cases, urine osmolality exceeds plasma osmolality. (2) Plasma creatinine and urea are normal or low, indicating that the glomerular filtration rate is normal or increased. (The elaboration of hypertonic urine is presumptive evidence of ADH secretion if the glomerular filtration rate is normal.) (3) During fluid loading (even if the fluid is saline), hyponatremia increases due to water retention and urinary sodium wasting. It should be noted that sodium wasting during volume expansion may be minimal or even absent in patients with extreme degrees of hyponatremia. (4) During restriction of fluid intake, hyponatremia and urinary sodium wasting are corrected. This response is helpful in occasional patients in whom it may be difficult to distinguish SIADH from mild volume depletion as the cause of hyponatremia. The plasma uric acid also may be of value in making this distinction. Since uric acid excretion tends to vary with "effective" extracellular volume, hyperuricemia is common in volume depletion while hypouricemia is usual in SIADH.

SIADH has been found frequently in patients with oat cell carcinoma of the lung but has also been described in patients with a variety of other *neoplasms*. In some of these patients the tumor secretes ADH or a substance with analogous biologic activity (see also Chap. 323). The syndrome has also been reported in patients with various disorders of the *central nervous system*, including meningitis, encephalitis, tumors, trauma, stroke, and porphyria. It is assumed that ADH in these patients is secreted in response to direct stimulation of the hypothalamic osmoreceptors. *Pulmonary* diseases associated with SIADH, in addition to tumors, include a wide variety of infections.

Pharmacologic agents that induce SIADH include (1) the oral hypoglycemic agents chlorpropamide and tolbutamide; (2) the antineoplastic and immunosuppressive agents vincristine and cyclophosphamide; (3) psychoactive drugs such as haloperidol, thioridazine, carbamazepine, and amitriptyline; and (4) clofibrate. These agents exert their antidiuretic effect either by potentiating the tubular action of small amounts of ADH or by stimulating inappropriate secretion of ADH.

Hyponatremia due to SIADH responds to limitation of fluid intake; restriction to the range of 1000 to 1200 mL per day is ordinarily adequate. Occasional patients who are symptomatic despite water restriction may be treated by enhancing water excretion. This can be accomplished either by increasing solute excretion (by taking a high-salt, high-protein diet or ingesting urea) or by antagonizing ADH with demeclocycline or lithium. Initial therapy with hypertonic saline infusions may be required in a few patients with marked hyponatremia. Concurrent administration of furosemide may facilitate correction of hyponatremia in those patients who do not respond promptly to hypertonic saline alone.

Hyponatremia may occur in certain endocrine disorders, notably adrenal insufficiency and hypothyroidism. Multiple factors appear to play a role in limiting water diuresis in patients with *adrenal insufficiency*. Deficient secretion of mineralocorticoid hormones may lead to sodium depletion, with consequent reduction of glomerular filtration and enhancement of proximal tubular sodium reabsorption. Moreover, glucocorticoid deficiency directly reduces filtration. Therefore, adrenal insufficiency will tend to decrease delivery of sodium to diluting sites. In addition, glucocorticoid deficiency prevents the maintenance of normal water impermeability in distal diluting segments of the nephron. This appears to be due to inappropriate secretion of ADH, although glucocorticoid deficiency may have a direct effect on water permeability of distal tubular epithelium. Since patients with adrenal insufficiency may have the combination of defective dilution of the urine and sodium wasting, hyponatremia due to Addison's disease can occasionally be confused with SIADH. Usually, other clinical features of adrenal insufficiency such as hyperkalemia, pigmentation, and hypoglycemia suggest the correct diagnosis. However, specific tests of adrenal function are indicated whenever the diagnosis is in doubt. Hyponatremia due to adrenal insufficiency is corrected by appropriate hormonal therapy.

Hyponatremia may develop in moderate or severe *hypothyroidism*. Decreased delivery of tubular fluid to diluting segments and persistent release of ADH both limit water excretion in this condition. The diagnosis of this type of hyponatremia is made by recognizing the clinical features of hypothyroidism and from the response to treatment with thyroid hormone.

The normal kidney can excrete 15 to 20 liters of dilute urine per day. Normal water intake, regulated by thirst and habit, is a small fraction of this maximum excretory capacity. Rarely, *psychogenic polydypsia* may be so severe that the rapid ingestion of huge quantities of fluids may overwhelm normal excretory capacity and produce symptomatic dilutional hyponatremia despite normal renal diluting mechanisms. Hyponatremia of this type is diagnosed from the history of massive fluid intake, most often in patients with other evidence of psychiatric illness. Since water excretory capacity is normal, the urine is maximally dilute in this condition. Hyponatremia due to psychogenic polydypsia responds to water restriction. Rare patients who are symptomatic due to extreme degrees of hyponatremia may require intravenous infusion of hypertonic saline.

Some patients may be hyponatremic in the absence of a defect in water diuresis. The terms *essential hyponatremia* and *sick cell syndrome* have been applied to this category. Osmoreceptor cells in the hypothalamus are thought to be "reset" to maintain a decreased level of body fluid osmolality as though it were normal. Urine becomes dilute or concentrated, respectively, if plasma sodium falls or increases slightly from the new "normal" level for the particular patient. The genesis of such a syndrome is speculative. Changes in cellular metabolism may lead to a primary reduction in cellular osmolality. Another possibility is that essential hyponatremia is a variant of SIADH in which there is a nonosmotic stimulus to ADH secretion. When plasma osmolality is reduced sufficiently, osmotic suppression of ADH secretion overcomes the nonosmotic stimulus.

Essential hyponatremia may occur in a variety of chronic illnesses, such as pulmonary tuberculosis, congestive heart failure, and hepatic cirrhosis. This type of hyponatremia is asymptomatic; skin turgor, blood pressure, and renal function are normal, unless altered by the primary disease. Definitive diagnosis of essential hyponatremia requries the demonstration of normal urinary dilution in response to water loading, normal urinary concentration during dehydration, and normal renal sodium excretory responses to sodium loading and restriction. This type of hyponatremia does not require treatment.

Hyponatremia due to *accumulation* of *osmotically active solutes* in the plasma is the sole exception to the rule that hyponatremia means decreased plasma osmolality. In this type of hyponatremia, plasma osmolality is increased. Plasma sodium is diluted by movement of water out of cells along the osmotic gradient created by the addition of a solute such as glucose or mannitol. (High plasma urea levels in patients with renal failure do not cause hyponatremia because urea concentration is equal across cell membranes.) The diagnosis of hyponatremia due to increased plasma concentrations of osmotically active solutes is usually apparent from the history and clinical features of uncontrolled diabetes. Plasma sodium concentration will decrease by about 1.6 meq per liter with every elevation of 100 mg/dL in plasma glucose above normal. This type of hyponatremia should also be considered whenever there is a history of recent administration of mannitol, especially to oliguric patients unable to excrete it promptly. Since plasma osmolality is increased, clinical manifestations of hypotonicity are absent in this type of hyponatremia.

In patients with severe hyperlipemia or, very rarely, with extreme hyperproteinemia, *artifactual* hyponatremia may be reported by the laboratory. In severe hyperlipemia part of any unit volume of plasma

FIGURE 41-1 *Flow chart for differential diagnosis of causes of hyponatremia. Categories (A, B, C, D) and types (C1–6) are keyed to Table 41-1. Abbreviations: Nl = normal; ECF = extracellular fluid; creat = creatinine; CHF = congestive heart failure; BP = blood pressure; Uosm = urinary osmolality; U_{Na} = urinary Na, meq per liter; ↓ = decreased, ↑ = increased.*

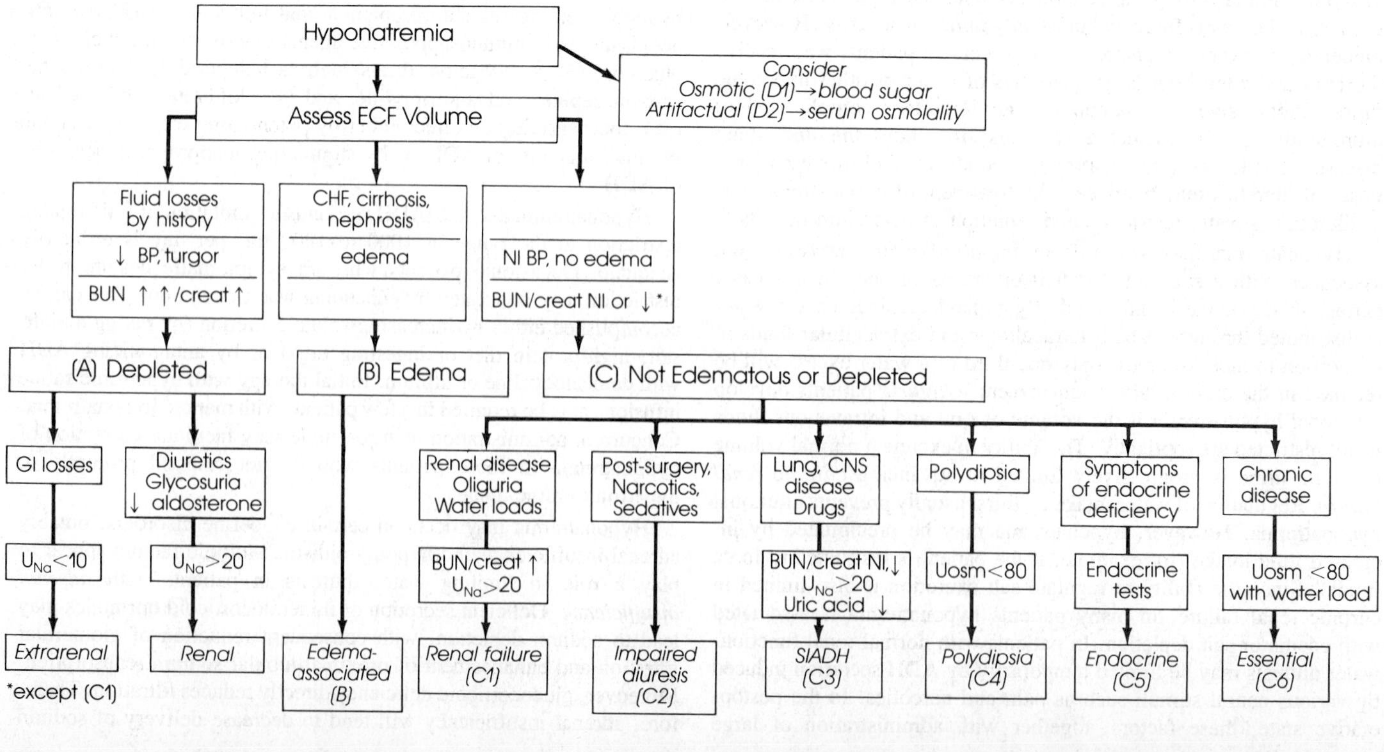

taken for analysis will be lipid, which is sodium-free. This type of hyponatremia rarely occurs unless the plasma is grossly milky. In patients with extreme hyperproteinemia, proteins occupy more than the normal 7 percent of plasma volume, thereby reducing the proportion of aqueous sodium-containing fluid per unit of plasma taken for analysis. In both cases, hyponatremia will be reported by the laboratory because the sodium concentration will be low in milliequivalents per liter of plasma. However, sodium concentration per liter of plasma water and plasma osmolality are normal; hence, this type of hyponatremia has no clinical significance.

Differential diagnosis Although the type of hyponatremia can be defined easily in most patients, precise diagnosis may be difficult in some. More than one type of hyponatremia may occur in a specific disease entity. For example, hyponatremia in patients with hepatic cirrhosis is usually associated with edema or is due to excessive administration of diuretics, but essential hyponatremia may also occur in this condition. Moreover, current categories may prove artificial or inaccurate when the pathophysiology of hyponatremia is more completely understood and specific diagnostic tests such as a radioimmunoassay for ADH are readily available. Despite these limitations, the classification outlined above is a useful framework for diagnosis and treatment.

Figure 41-1 is a flow chart that outlines the major steps in determining the cause of hyponatremia. First, assess extracellular fluid (ECF) volume. The history and physical examination are usually sufficient to determine whether the hyponatremia is associated with a decreased, increased, or normal extracellular volume. In occasional patients, moderate volume depletion may not readily be separable from normovolemia by clinical examination. In that event, measurement of blood urea nitrogen (BUN) and plasma creatinine may be helpful. The plasma creatinine, and especially the BUN, tend to be increased when hyponatremia is associated with volume depletion and normal or decreased when it is associated with a normal or expanded extracellular volume, as in SIADH. The various types of normovolemic hyponatremia can frequently be recognized by a careful review of specific features of the history, such as associated diseases, drug therapy, and fluid intake. However, laboratory tests, such as measurement of serum cortisol, may be needed to confirm a diagnosis.

Measurements of urinary sodium concentration and osmolality are common in the workup. *Urinary sodium concentration* is low (under 10 meq per liter) if hyponatremia is associated with edema or with volume depletion due to extrarenal causes. Urine sodium concentration usually exceeds 20 meq per liter if hyponatremia is due to renal salt losses or to renal failure with water retention. In SIADH, urine sodium concentration usually exceeds 20 meq per liter unless fluid intake has been restricted. Since impaired water diuresis is the mechanism of most types of hyponatremia, measurement of *urinary osmolality* is not usually of value. A maximally dilute urine would be expected only in hyponatremia due to extreme polydipsia or at times in essential hyponatremia. With other causes, urinary osmolality exceeds 150 mosmol per kilogram of water; usually the urine is hypertonic to plasma.

Clinical manifestations Neurologic dysfunction is the principal clinical manifestation of hyponatremia. It is due to intracellular movement of water, leading to swelling of brain cells. The severity of symptoms is related both to the degree of hyponatremia and to the rapidity with which it develops. In chronic hyponatremia, the degree of brain swelling caused by any given reduction in body fluid osmolality is reduced because solute, largely potassium chloride, is lost from the cells. Patients may be lethargic, confused, stuporous, or comatose. If hyponatremia develops rapidly, signs of hyperexcitability such as muscular twitches, irritability, and convulsions may occur. Hyponatremia rarely causes clinical symptoms when plasma sodium is above 125 meq per liter, although occasionally symptoms may occur at higher levels if the decrease in concentration has been rapid.

Treatment Appropriate therapy for the various types of hyponatremia has been outlined. Hyponatremia itself is often of little significance and requires no specific treatment. If severe, symptomatic hyponatremia requires intravenous treatment; the amount of sodium given should be calculated by multiplying the deficit in plasma sodium concentration (milliequivalents per liter) by the total body water (approximately 50 to 60 percent of body weight). Although the administered sodium will remain in the extracellular compartment, the osmotic effect of hypertonic saline will cause water to shift out of cells. The amount needed to raise plasma sodium concentration to the range of 125 to 130 meq per liter should be calculated and infused over several hours. The patient's symptoms and clinical status, especially with respect to circulatory congestion, should be carefully assessed throughout the infusion. Furosemide may be given if fluid overload is present initially or develops during the infusion. Complete correction of hyponatremia, if indicated, is usually best carried out more slowly by water restriction or oral sodium supplementation if possible. Some studies, although controversial, have raised the possibility that rapid, complete correction of hyponatremia may cause neurological damage (central pontine myelinolysis).

HYPERNATREMIA Pathophysiology Hypernatremia is due to a deficit of body water relative to total body solute or sodium content. Without exception, hypernatremia indicates that the body fluids are hypertonic. Normally, minimal increases in tonicity stimulate both thirst and release of ADH. Although renal water retention induced by ADH helps to correct hypernatremia, thirst appears to be the principal defense mechanism. Hypernatremia is usually modest in patients with diabetes insipidus, who lack ADH and may excrete 15 liters or more of urine per day. Thirst stimulates water intake enough to balance even such large water losses. Severe persistent hypernatremia occurs only in patients who cannot respond to thirst by voluntary ingestion of fluid, e.g., infants or mentally obtunded patients. In such individuals, loss of dilute body fluids progressively elevates body fluid osmolality. Initial losses of water are from the extracellular compartment, but water deficits are rapidly equilibrated throughout total body water. The rise in extracellular fluid tonicity causes intracellular water to shift into the extracellular compartment. In effect, approximately two-thirds of pure water deficits are derived from intracellular fluid. Hence, extracellular volume depletion occurs in patients with relatively pure deficits of water only when such deficits are large. The principal clinical features are attributable to decreased intracellular volume, especially dehydration of cells in the central nervous system. Brain cells appear to adapt to chronic hyperosmolality by accumulating increased intracellular solute. When hyperosmolality is rapidly corrected, the increase in total intracellular solute may promote brain swelling even at normal or slightly elevated plasma osmolality. These mechanisms may account for the fact that rapid correction of hypertonicity sometimes causes deterioration of central nervous function. The identity of the excess brain solute is uncertain; electrolyte accumulation accounts for only part of the excess.

Pathogenesis (Table 41-1) For clinical purposes it is useful to classify hypernatremia as due to water loss alone; to water deficits associated with, but proportionately in excess of, sodium deficits; or to retention of sodium. Pure water deficits may be due to extrarenal or renal water losses that are not replaced. Insensible losses of water from the skin or lungs may reach several liters per day, especially in patients with fever, increased respirations, or extensive burns. Renal losses may lead to hypernatremia in diabetes insipidus. Alert patients with diabetes insipidus ordinarily maintain normal or only slightly hypertonic body fluids despite massive renal water wasting by increasing fluid intake appropriately. However, diabetes insipidus may develop acutely after cerebral trauma or neurosurgical procedures. In such patients, careful attention to replacement of urinary losses is mandatory to avoid severe hypernatremia. Defective thirst and ADH regulation occurs in rare patients with hypothalamic disorders, which may be idiopathic ("essential hypernatremia") or due to specific causes such as tumors, granulomas, and cerebrovascular accidents.

Water losses leading to hypernatremia are often associated with sodium deficits. In such cases, the clinical features of extracellular volume depletion and hypernatremia may both be present, and either may predominate. Extrarenal losses of salt and water due to profuse sweating and renal losses due to osmotic diuresis are the major causes of hypernatremia in this category. Since sweat is hypotonic, hypernatremia will develop if profusely sweating patients cannot drink. In an osmotic diuresis, urinary sodium concentration is less than plasma concentration; therefore, hypernatremia tends to occur. Hypernatremia due to a urea diuresis may develop when patients unable to complain of thirst are placed on high-protein feeding. Examples include patients with severe cerebrovascular accidents who are unable to swallow and postoperative neurosurgical patients. In the syndrome of hyperosmolar nonketotic diabetic coma, severe hyperosmolality of the body fluids is due to a combination of hyperglycemia and relative or absolute hypernatremia. The hypernatremia is a consequence of an intense glucose osmotic diuresis in patients who are unable to ingest fluids. Since hyperglycemia itself causes hyponatremia by inducing a shift of water from cells, the presence of hypernatremia in the face of extreme hyperglycemia indicates that total body water is severely depleted.

Infrequently, hypernatremia may result from an absolute excess of sodium rather than from water depletion. Examples are hypernatremia caused by accidental substitution of salt for sugar in infant feeding formulas and administration of excessive amounts of hypertonic sodium chloride or bicarbonate infusions to comatose adults unable to drink. The cause of the common mild hypernatremia in patients with adrenal hyperfunction is uncertain. Presumably, stimulation of renal tubular sodium reabsorption by adrenal steroids initiates the hypernatremia, and the hypervolemia that results resets upward the threshold for ADH release. It is not known why the thirst mechanism fails to maintain normal body fluid osmolality.

Clinical features and diagnosis The principal manifestations of hypernatremia are observed in the central nervous system. Confusion and other evidence of altered mental state; increased neuromuscular irritability, such as twitching and seizures; and obtundation, stupor, or coma may all occur. The magnitude of symptoms depends on the severity of the hyperosmolality. The symptoms are similar whether hyperosmolality is due to hypernatremia or extreme hyperglycemia. The neurologic symptoms appear to be due to dehydration of brain cells. The clinical manifestations of acute hypernatremia are more marked than those of slowly developing hypernatremia. Severe hyperosmolality may cause irreversible neurologic sequelae, apparently due to vascular consequences such as venous sinus thrombosis and hemorrhage from vessels that rupture when the brain shrinks. High mortality rates are associated with extreme hyperosmolality, especially in children and in the elderly.

In patients with pure water deficits, manifestations of extracellular volume depletion are minimal because only one-third of the deficit is derived from extracellular fluid. As noted, combined deficits are common, especially in patients who sweat or experience an osmotic diuresis; in such individuals, the signs and symptoms of volume depletion may overshadow those of hypernatremia.

The cause of hypernatremia can usually be inferred from the history when it is due to extrarenal water loss, an osmotic diuresis, or sodium excess. In these cases, the urine is hypertonic to plasma. The differential diagnosis of pituitary and nephrogenic diabetes insipidus, in which urine concentrating ability is impaired, is discussed in Chap. 323.

Treatment Hypernatremia itself is corrected with water by mouth or by intravenous infusion of 5% dextrose in water. Calculation of water requirements must be based on total body water, since water deficits are drawn from both intracellular and extracellular fluid and both must be repleted. For example, suppose a 70-kg man has a plasma sodium of 160 meq per liter which is to be lowered to 140. Total body water is estimated as 60 percent of 70 kg, which is 42 liters. To reduce plasma sodium, this volume must be increased to (160/140) $\times$ 42 liters, which equals 48 liters. Thus, a positive water balance of 6 liters (48 $-$ 42) is required. Hypernatremia should be corrected slowly; no more than half the water deficit should be replaced in the first 12 to 24 h. As stated above, rapid correction of hypertonicity may cause central nervous function to deteriorate.

In patients with associated sodium deficits, saline solutions should be infused. If the predominant clinical feature is extracellular volume depletion with circulatory insufficiency, treatment should begin with 0.9% saline to replete extracellular volume promptly. If the neurologic effects of hypertonicity predominate, therapy can start with 0.45% saline. In patients with hyperosmolar diabetic coma, sodium deficits are usually large, due to prior glucose osmotic diuresis. Plasma hypertonicity is due to both hyperglycemia and hypernatremia. Treatment consists of isotonic saline (0.9%) to replete extracellular volume and insulin to lower plasma glucose and thereby partly correct hypertonicity. Later, hypotonic saline (0.45%) can replace the remaining water and salt deficits and return plasma sodium to normal.

POTASSIUM

PHYSIOLOGIC CONSIDERATIONS Potassium is the principal intracellular cation. Active transport mediated by Na^+-K^+–stimulated ATPase in cell membranes maintains a cellular concentration of approximately 160 meq per liter, 40 times that in extracellular fluid. All but 2 percent of the 2500 to 3000 meq potassium in the body is within cells. Since potassium is a large fraction of total cellular solute, it is a major determinant of the volume of the cell and the osmolality of the body fluids. Moreover, potassium is an important cofactor in a number of metabolic processes. Extracellular potassium, while a small fraction of the total, greatly influences neuromuscular function. The ratio of intracellular to extracellular potassium concentration is the principal determinant of membrane potential in excitable tissues. Since extracellular potassium concentration is low, small deviations in concentration produce large variations in this ratio; conversely, only large changes in intracellular potassium influence the ratio significantly. These relationships have practical consequences. For example, toxic effects of hyperkalemia can be mitigated by inducing movement of potassium from extracellular fluid into cells.

The relation between plasma and cellular potassium is complex and is influenced by a number of factors, including acid-base balance. Acidosis tends to shift potassium out of cells, and alkalosis favors movement from extracellular fluid into cells. The relation between blood pH and plasma potassium is complex and is influenced by several factors, including the type of acidosis, the duration of the altered acid-base state, and the change in plasma bicarbonate per se. In general, plasma potassium changes less with respiratory acidosis than with metabolic acidosis and less with alkalosis than with acidosis. While the magnitude of the change in plasma potassium cannot be predicted from changes in blood pH alone, a patient with normal total body potassium tends to be hyperkalemic if acidotic and hypokalemic if alkalotic. Hormones also influence the distribution of potassium between extracellular fluid and cells. Insulin, beta-adrenergic catecholamines, and possibly aldosterone promote movement of potassium into cells. These hormones appear to be important parts of the mechanism for moving potassium loads out of plasma. Conversely, alpha-adrenergic agonists impair potassium uptake into cells.

During potassium depletion, plasma potassium initially decreases about 1 meq per liter for each 100 to 200 meq lost. However, plasma potassium falls more slowly after it reaches 2 meq per liter. Thus, a plasma potassium in the range of 2 to 3.5 meq per liter is a reasonably accurate guide to the magnitude of depletion, but plasma potassium concentrations less than 2 meq per liter may reflect a wide range of deficits, from moderate to severe. Plasma concentration increases about 1 meq per liter after acute administration of 100 to 200 meq potassium. Assuming an extracellular volume of 15 liters, 150 meq would be expected to raise plasma potassium by about 10 meq per liter. Thus, the largest fraction of administered potassium rapidly enters cells. Renal excretion also increases promptly. Chronic exposure to high-potassium diets enhances both tissue uptake and renal excretion of the ion; the mechanism of these adaptations is uncertain. Sustained hyperkalemia rarely is caused by excess intake, because these mechanisms normally function so efficiently. Impaired renal excretion and cellular transfer are the usual causes of hyperkalemia.

Of the usual potassium intake of 50 to 150 meq per day, most is excreted in the urine. Normally, stool and sweat contain only about 5 meq per day. As noted, the kidneys respond to acute and chronic changes in potassium intake by corresponding changes in excretion. Excess potassium is excreted promptly; about half of an acute load appears in the urine within 12 h. The renal response to potassium depletion is more sluggish. Excretion does not fall to minimal levels for 7 to 14 days. During this period, a deficit of 200 meq or more may develop in an individual on a potassium-deficient diet. Renal excretory mechanisms for potassium are complex. Potassium in the urine is secreted in the distal convoluted tubule and collecting duct; filtered potassium is nearly quantitatively reabsorbed in more proximal segments. Potassium secretion appears to be determined by the potassium concentration of tubular cells and by an electrochemical gradient favoring diffusion of the ion into tubular fluid. Net excretion is the resultant of secretion and concurrent reabsorption in the distal segments. Among the key influences on this complex system are aldosterone, distal tubular fluid flow rate, acid-base balance, and factors that alter distal tubular electronegativity. Aldosterone stimulates potassium secretion. Thus, hyperkalemia increases potassium excretion by two mechanisms: it stimulates adrenal secretion of aldosterone, and it directly enhances renal secretion, presumably via increased tubular cell potassium. Potassium secretion in the distal tubule is flow-dependent; increased distal delivery of tubular fluid favors potassium excretion. For example, loop diuretics, which enhance distal volume delivery, increase potassium excretion, especially in patients with edema and secondary aldosteronism. Alkalosis enhances and acidosis depresses renal potassium secretion, probably by inducing corresponding changes in tubular cell potassium. If delivery to distal segments of sodium salts of unreabsorbable anions such as excess bicarbonate or carbenicillin is augmented, tubular electronegative potential will increase as sodium is reabsorbed. The enhanced electrical gradient will promote potassium excretion.

POTASSIUM DEPLETION AND HYPOKALEMIA Pathogenesis The principal causes of potassium depletion are listed in Table 41-2. As noted, renal excretion of potassium falls slowly in persons on potassium-deficient diets. During the 10 to 14 days before balance is achieved, significant deficits may occur. Thus, in contrast to sodium, moderate potassium depletion may result from *poor intake* alone. Potassium deficiency is frequent in *gastrointestinal disorders* in which vomiting, diarrhea, or loss of gastrointestinal secretions is prominent. Diarrhea may cause large potassium deficits, since the potassium concentration of liquid stool is 40 to 60 meq per liter. *Loss of gastric secretions* through vomiting or vasogastric suction is also a common cause of potassium depletion. The potassium concentration of gastric fluid is 5 to 10 meq per liter; direct losses contribute only modestly to negative potassium balance. The potassium deficit is primarily due to increased renal excretion. Potassium excretion appears to be stimulated by three mechanisms. Loss of gastric acid leads to *metabolic alkalosis,* which increases tubular cell potassium concentration. The elevated plasma bicarbonate concentration also increases delivery of bicarbonate and fluid to the distal nephron. Finally, secondary hyperaldosteronism due to associated extracellular volume contraction may play a role in maintaining potassium excretion at high levels despite potassium depletion.

All *diuretics* in common use except spironolactone, triamterene, and amiloride promote potassium excretion. In edematous patients with secondary aldosteronism, these agents often cause hypokalemia and potassium depletion. Although hypokalemia also occurs in patients receiving diuretics for treatment of hypertension, potassium depletion is modest if dietary potassium is normal and there are no other factors that stimulate potassium excretion. Potassium excretion is increased during an *osmotic diuresis.* This mechanism leads to potassium depletion in patients with diabetic ketoacidosis, in whom the osmotic diuresis is due to glycosuria and to increased excretion of keto acid anions. However, potassium depletion may be masked by the shift of potassium out of tissues caused by the diabetic acidosis. Failure to recognize potassium depletion may lead to serious cardiotoxicity from sudden hypokalemia when the acidosis is corrected with insulin or alkali. A normal plasma potassium concentration in an acidotic patient strongly suggests potassium depletion.

Urinary potassium loss is often due to *excessive mineralocorticoid activity.* Hypokalemia is characteristic of *primary aldosteronism* but may be minimal in patients with restricted sodium intake. *Secondary aldosteronism* causes renal potassium wasting and hypokalemia in patients with malignant hypertension, Bartter's syndrome, and renin-secreting renal tumors. *Licorice* contains a compound with mineralocorticoid activity; patients who consume huge amounts may become hypokalemic. Excessive levels of *glucocorticoids* stimulate secretion of renal potassium (and hydrogen), leading to hypokalemia and alkalosis in patients with *Cushing's syndrome* and those receiving *therapeutic steroids.*

Renal tubular potassium wasting is a feature of *renal tubular acidosis* (Chap. 228). Some patients with monocytic or myelomonocytic *leukemia* develop hypokalemia. The mechanism is uncertain. Renal potassium wasting in some patients appears to correlate with lysozymuria, and the enzyme may interfere with tubular function. In *Liddle's syndrome,* a rare familial disorder (Chap. 228), renal potassium wasting is an intrinsic tubular abnormality. Certain *antibiotics* may cause hypokalemia by increasing potassium excretion. Carbenicillin in large amounts promotes distal tubular secretion by acting as an unreabsorbed anion; amphotericin B alters distal tubular permeability. Gentamicin has also been reported to cause hypokalemia by unknown mechanisms.

Magnesium depletion can cause potassium depletion, apparently due to increased renal and possibly gastrointestinal losses. Increased aldosterone secretion may play a role in stimulating potassium excretion. Hypokalemia in this condition is associated with hypocalcemia.

Clinical features and diagnosis The most prominent features of hypokalemia and potassium depletion are neuromuscular. Moderate degrees of depletion may be asymptomatic, especially if they develop slowly. Some patients, however, complain of muscle weakness, especially in the lower extremities. With more severe or acute degrees

TABLE 41-2 Causes of potassium depletion and hypokalemia

I Gastrointestinal
- *A* Deficient dietary intake
- *B* Gastrointestinal disorders (vomiting, diarrhea, villous adenoma, fistulas, ureterosigmoidostomy)

II Renal
- *A* Metabolic alkalosis
- *B* Diuretics, osmotic diuresis
- *C* Excessive mineralocorticoid effects
  - *1* Primary aldosteronism
  - *2* Secondary aldosteronism (including malignant hypertension, Bartter's syndrome, juxtaglomerular cell tumor)
  - *3* Licorice ingestion
  - *4* Glucocorticoid excess (Cushing's syndrome, exogenous steroids, ectopic ACTH production)
- *D* Renal tubular diseases
  - *1* Renal tubular acidosis
  - *2* Leukemia
  - *3* Liddle's syndrome
  - *4* Antibiotics
- *E* Magnesium depletion

III Hypokalemia due to shift into cells (no depletion)
- *A* Hypokalemic periodic paralysis
- *B* Insulin effect
- *C* Alkalosis

of hypokalemia and potassium deficiency, marked and generalized weakness of skeletal muscles is prominent. Very severe or abrupt development of hypokalemia may lead to virtually total paralysis, including the respiratory muscles. Rhabdomyolysis may occur. On physical examination, in addition to decreased motor power, the patient may demonstrate decreased or absent tendon reflexes. The smooth muscle of the gastrointestinal tract may be affected, resulting in paralytic ileus.

Abnormalities in the electrocardiogram are common (Chap. 178). The characteristic changes include flattening and inversion of the T wave, increased prominence of the U wave, and sagging of the ST segment. These alterations are not well correlated with the severity of the disturbance in potassium metabolism and cannot be relied on as indexes of the clinical significance of a potassium deficit. Although moderate potassium depletion rarely affects cardiac action, severe or rapid reduction in serum potassium may cause cardiac arrest. Potassium deficiency enhances the cardiac toxicity of digitalis preparations. A variety of atrial and ventricular arrhythmias may occur in hypokalemia, especially in patients receiving digitalis.

Renal tubular function is markedly impaired by potassium depletion (Chap. 226). The most prominent abnormality is decreased concentrating ability, which may cause polyuria and polydipsia. Glomerular filtration rate is normal or slightly reduced; moderate reductions may occur with chronic potassium depletion nephropathy. Renal regulation of potassium excretion remains normal. The urinalysis is benign: protein excretion is normal or minimally increased, and the urinary sediment is normal or demonstrates only a slight increase in hyaline or granular casts.

DIAGNOSIS The cause of hypokalemia and potassium depletion is usually evident from the history. However, patients whose potassium deficiency is caused by chronic abuse of laxatives; psychogenic, self-induced vomiting; or surreptitious use of diuretics rarely volunteer an accurate history. Patients with villous adenomas of the rectum sometimes report that their feces are formed; careful questioning will reveal the elimination of the characteristic mucous secretion of the tumor.

When the history is obscure, *evaluation of urinary potassium excretion* may be helpful in determining the origin of the potassium deficit (Fig. 41-2). If gastrointestinal losses have occurred, urinary excretion is usually less than 20 to 25 meq per liter or per day. Although renal conservation of potassium is slow, excretion falls to these levels by the time that clinically significant deficits of potassium have accumulated. On the other hand, when renal potassium wasting is the cause, urinary concentration usually exceeds 20 meq per liter and excretion is more than 25 meq per day. However, lower concentrations and lower excretion rates may be found in severe depletion, in those patients with excessive mineralocorticoid activity while on low sodium intake, and in patients whose diuretics have been stopped at the time of examination. *Measurement of blood pH* also may help in differential diagnosis. A normal pH or alkalosis is present in most patients who are potassium-depleted. Hypokalemia is associated with acidosis in renal tubular acidosis, diarrhea, and diabetic ketoacidosis, and in patients treated with carbonic anhydrase inhibitors. A third clue to diagnosis is the presence of *hypertension,* which suggests hyperaldosteronism (except Bartter's syndrome) or glucocorticoid excess. Blood pressure is normal in patients whose potassium depletion is due to the other causes listed in Table 41-2. Figure 41-2 is a flow chart which outlines the steps in differential diagnosis of hypokalemia when the cause is not evident from the history.

Treatment When possible, potassium depletion should be corrected by increased dietary intake or supplementation with potassium salts. Potassium chloride is the salt of choice, especially in alkalotic patients. It may be given in the form of an elixir or in tablets in which potassium chloride crystals are imbedded in a wax. Enteric-coated potassium chloride tablets have been responsible for ulceration of the small bowel, due to release of high concentrations of potassium salts. Organic salts such as gluconate or citrate are adequate in patients who are not severely alkalotic and often are used to treat hypokalemia due to renal tubular acidosis. In edematous patients treated with diuretics that cause hypokalemia, potassium deficits should be prevented or treated by increased dietary potassium intake, supplementation with potassium chloride, or addition of "potassium-sparing" diuretics such as spironolactone. More controversial is the need for routine dietary supplements in patients receiving diuretics for treatment of hypertension. Patients with adequate dietary potassium intake usually do not develop significant hypokalemia and probably do not require routine supplements to prevent potassium depletion. However, those who do develop hypokalemia despite adequate diets should probably receive potassium salts, since hypokalemia may be associated with an increased frequency of arrhythmias.

Intravenous treatment is required for patients with gastrointestinal

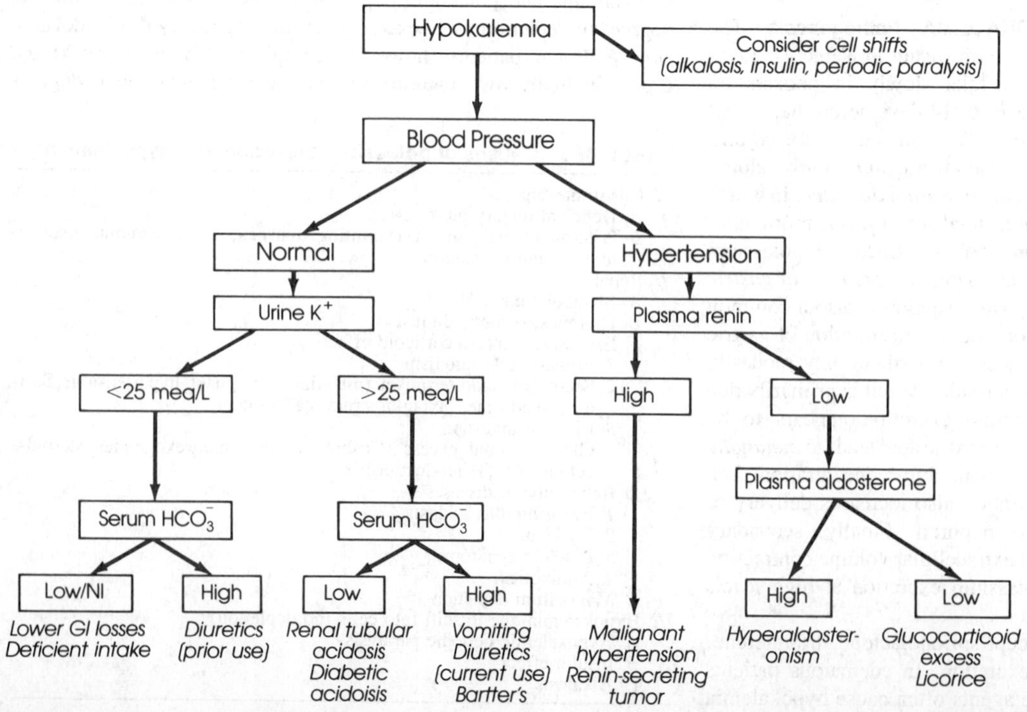

FIGURE 41-2 *Flow chart for differential diagnosis of principal causes of hypokalemia.*

disorders or when the potassium deficiency is severe. It must be emphasized that the potassium *concentration* in commonly available intravenous solutions of potassium chloride is 2000 meq per liter. Concentrations in intravenous infusions should not exceed 40 or at the most 60 meq per liter. The rate of infusion should not exceed 20 meq/h or approximately 200 to 250 meq per day, unless the need for more rapid infusion has been demonstrated in the individual patient by evidence of continuing losses large enough to justify more intensive therapy. The results of treatment are best monitored by repeated determinations of plasma potassium and evaluation of clinical symptoms such as muscular weakness or paralysis. Disappearance of electrocardiographic abnormalities correlates only roughly with improvement in total body potassium content. However, during rapid intravenous administration of potassium, the electrocardiogram should be monitored to avoid cardiac toxicity from inadvertent hyperkalemia.

Hypokalemia and hypocalcemia may occur together, for example, in patients with malabsorption syndrome. The neuromuscular effect of each electrolyte abnormality is masked by the other. Treatment of either disorder alone may precipitate symptoms. Thus, treatment of hypokalemia alone may precipitate tetany, and conversely, treatment of hypocalcemia without correcting the hypokalemia may exacerbate the manifestations of potassium deficiency.

HYPERKALEMIA Pathogenesis The causes of hyperkalemia are shown in Table 41-3. *Inadequate renal excretion* is the most frequent cause (see also Chaps. 220 and 221). When oliguria or anuria is present, as in acute renal failure, progressive hyperkalemia is the rule. Plasma potassium rises by about 0.5 meq per liter per day if there are no abnormal loads. Chronic renal failure does not cause severe or progressive hyperkalemia unless oliguria supervenes. Adaptive changes of unknown etiology increase potassium excretion per residual nephron as chronic renal failure progresses. However, patients with chronic renal failure function at the limits of their excretory capacity. Hence, hyperkalemia may develop rapidly if the potassium load is increased or excretory capacity is limited, e.g., by administration of spironolactone. Selective renal *tubular potassium secretory defects* have been described with renal disease caused by lupus erythematosus, sickle cell disease, rejection of a transplanted kidney, or obstructive uropathy.

Hyperkalemia is a cardinal feature of adrenal insufficiency (Addison's disease) and of selective *hypoaldosteronism*. The common form of the latter disorder in adults is *hyporeninemic hypoaldosteronism* (Chap. 325). Inhibition of the activity of the renin-angiotensin-aldosterone system by beta-adrenergic blockers, nonsteroidal anti-inflammatory drugs, or converting enzyme inhibitors also may induce hyperkalemia.

A kilogram of tissue such as muscle or erythrocytes contains about 80 meq potassium, and damaged cells release potassium into the plasma. Hence hyperkalemia may be seen when there is *muscle-crushing injury, hemolysis,* or *internal hemorrhage*. Acidosis drives potassium out of cells and leads to hyperkalemia. Severe progressive hyperkalemia is not ordinarily a consequence of increased release of potassium from damaged or acidotic tissues alone. However, acidosis and tissue damage often occur together with acute renal insufficiency; under these circumstances, severe hyperkalemia may develop quickly. In contrast to the increase of 0.5 meq per liter per day typical of uncomplicated anuria, plasma potassium in anuric patients with tissue damage may increase 2 to 4 meq per liter per day. Such rapidly progressive hyperkalemia may be an important cause of death in military casualties. In patients with trauma, burns, or neuromuscular diseases such as paraplegia and multiple sclerosis, the muscle relaxant succinylcholine may cause dangerous hyperkalemia. This agent apparently releases potassium from muscle by depolarizing cell membranes. *Arginine hydrochloride,* used to treat metabolic alkalosis, drives potassium out of cells. If potassium excretion is impaired, clinically significant hyperkalemia may occur during arginine infusions. Extreme digitalis poisoning may cause severe hyperkalemia; potassium leaks out of cells because Na^+-K^+-ATPase is inhibited by the drug. *Beta-adrenergic blockers* may induce hyperkalemia by interfering with the action of endogenous beta-catecholamines to enhance movement of potassium into tissues. *Metabolic acidosis* causes hyperkalemia by shifting potassium out of cells. Respiratory acidosis has less striking effects. *Hyperosmolality* also enhances potassium movement from cells. *Insulin deficiency* is conducive to hyperkalemia because the action of insulin to promote potassium movement into cells is diminished. Hyperosmolality or metabolic acidosis may be additional mechanisms of hyperkalemia in insulin-deficient patients. In *hyperkalemic periodic paralysis,* the hyperkalemia is associated with repeated attacks of muscular paralysis. The mechanism of this syndrome is not understood. Ingestion of increased amounts of potassium may precipitate attacks.

The severity of hyperkalemia caused by large oral or intravenous potassium loads is influenced by factors that modulate tissue uptake and renal excretion of potassium. For example, insulin deficiency and treatment with beta-adrenergic blockers tend to augment hyperkalemia by limiting tissue uptake. Volume depletion enhances hyperkalemia by limiting the rate at which the kidney excretes such loads.

Patients with extreme thrombocytosis or, more rarely, extreme leukocytosis in leukemia may demonstrate the phenomenon of pseudohyperkalemia. Platelets or white blood cells release potassium during blood clotting in vitro. While serum potassium may be grossly abnormal, plasma potassium is not increased. Artifactual elevation of plasma potassium may occur if blood is drawn after repeated fist clenching to make veins more prominent during application of a tourniquet. Artifactual hyperkalemia may be suspected when electrocardiographic abnormalities are absent despite apparently marked elevation of serum potassium.

Clinical features and diagnosis The most important toxic effects of hyperkalemia are cardiac arrhythmias. The characteristic sequence of electrocardiographic changes is shown in Fig. 178-15. The earliest manifestation is the development of high-peaked T waves, especially prominent in precordial leads. Hyperkalemia does not prolong the QT interval, unlike other disorders which induce peaking of the T waves. Later changes include prolongation of the PR interval, complete heart block, and atrial asystole. As plasma potassium rises further, ventricular complexes may deteriorate. The QRS complex becomes progressively prolonged and finally tends to merge with the T wave in a sine wave configuration. Terminally, ventricular fibrillation and standstill may occur.

Occasionally moderate or severe hyperkalemia has striking effects on peripheral muscles. Ascending muscular weakness can occur, progressing to flaccid quadriplegia and respiratory paralysis. Cerebral and cranial nerve function are normal, as is sensation.

TABLE 41-3 Causes of hyperkalemia

I Inadequate excretion
- *A* Renal failure
  - *1* Acute renal failure
  - *2* Severe chronic renal failure
  - *3* Tubular disorders
- *B* Adrenal insufficiency
  - *1* Hypoaldosteronism
  - *2* Addison's disease
- *C* Diuretics which inhibit potassium secretion (spironolactone, triamterene, amiloride)

II Shift of potassium from tissues
- *A* Tissue damage (muscle crush, hemolysis, internal bleeding)
- *B* Drugs: succinylcholine, arginine, digitalis poisoning, beta-adrenergic antagonists
- *C* Acidosis
- *D* Hyperosmolality
- *E* Insulin deficiency
- *F* Hyperkalemic periodic paralysis

III Excessive intake

IV Pseudohyperkalemia
- *A* Thrombocytosis
- *B* Leukocytosis
- *C* Poor venipuncture technique
- *D* In vitro hemolysis

Treatment In considering therapy, it is helpful to classify hyperkalemia according to degree of severity. The seriousness of hyperkalemia is best estimated by considering both the plasma potassium and the electrocardiogram. When the plasma potassium is less than 6.5 meq per liter and electrocardiographic changes are limited to peaking of T waves, hyperkalemia is mild. When the plasma potassium is 6.5 to 8 meq per liter and T-wave peaking is the only electrocardiographic abnormality, hyperkalemia is moderate. Severe hyperkalemia is present if the plasma potassium exceeds 8 meq per liter or if electrocardiographic abnormalities include absent P waves, widened QRS complexes, or ventricular arrhythmias. Minimal hyperkalemia can usually be treated by elimination of a cause, such as potassium-sparing diuretics, or by treatment of accompanying acidosis. More severe or progressive hyperkalemia requires vigorous therapy. Severe cardiac toxicity responds most rapidly to infusion of calcium; 10 to 30 mL of 10% calcium gluconate may be infused intravenously within a period of 1 to 5 min under constant electrocardiographic monitoring. While calcium infusions do not alter plasma potassium, they counteract the adverse effects of potassium on neuromuscular membranes. The effect of calcium infusions, while almost immediate, is transient if the hyperkalemia is not treated directly.

In moderately severe hyperkalemia, infusion of hypertonic glucose solutions decreases toxicity by shifting potassium into cells. In the first 30 min, 200 to 500 mL of 10% glucose may be given. An additional 500 to 1000 mL may be infused over the next several hours. Ten units of regular insulin may be given subcutaneously, although this is probably necessary only in insulin-deficient diabetic patients. This treatment may reduce serum potassium by 1 to 2 meq per liter, and effects persist for a number of hours. The infusion of sodium bicarbonate also helps lower serum potassium rapidly by causing potassium to shift into cells; 50 to 150 meq alkali (two to three ampuls) may be added to a liter of glucose. Although this agent is most valuable in acidotic patients, it also is effective in individuals with normal acid-base status. The effect occurs within 1 h and persists for a number of hours. The infusion of hypertonic sodium solutions may also be effective in reversing cardiac toxicity, especially in hyponatremic or volume-depleted patients. In part, the effect depends simply on dilution of plasma potassium, but there may be a direct effect of elevated plasma sodium to antagonize hyperkalemic neuromuscular toxicity as well. Glucose, bicarbonate, and sodium may be combined in a "therapeutic cocktail," formulated by adding an ampul or two of sodium bicarbonate to a liter of 5% dextrose in 0.9% saline.

None of the measures just described removes potassium from the body. Cation exchange resins such as sodium polystyrene sulfonate may be given by retention enema in the treatment of moderate or severe hyperkalemia. Enough potassium may be removed by a single enema to reduce potassium by 0.5 to 2 meq per liter within an hour, and repeated enemas can be given. These resins can also be given repeatedly by mouth to maintain low plasma potassium concentration. Twenty grams is given three or four times a day together with 20 mL of a 70% sorbitol solution, as required to ensure the passage of several loose stools daily. In patients with renal failure, hemodialysis and peritoneal dialysis effectively control hyperkalemia. However, they are relatively slow techniques, and patients with severe hyperkalemia should be treated first with one of the methods previously discussed.

REFERENCES

Sodium and water

BARTTER FC: The syndrome of inappropriate secretion of antidiuretic hormone (SIADH). Dis Month Nov, 1973

BERL T et al: Clinical disorders of water metabolism. Kidney Int 10:117, 1976

MILLER M, MOSES AM: Drug-induced states of impaired water excretion. Kidney Int 10:96, 1976

NARINS RG et al: Diagnostic strategies in disorders of fluid, electrolyte and acid-base homeostasis. Am J Med 72:496, 1982

ROBERTSON GL: Thirst and vasopressin function in normal and disordered states of water balance. J Lab Clin Med 101:351, 1983

———, BERL T: Pathophysiology of water metabolism, in *The Kidney,* 3d ed, BM Brenner, FC Rector Jr (eds). Philadelphia, Saunders, 1986, p 385

WEINER M, EPSTEIN FH: Signs and symptoms of electrolyte disorders. Yale J Biol Med 43:76, 1970

ZERBE R et al: Vasopressin function in the syndrome of inappropriate diuresis. Ann Rev Med 31:315, 1980

Potassium

BIA MJ, DEFRONZO RA: Extrarenal potassium homeostasis. Am J Physiol 240:F257, 1981

HOLLENBERG NK, BROWN RS (eds): Electrolytes and cardiovascular disease. Am J Med 77(5A):1, 1984

KNOCHEL JP: The syndrome of hyporeninemic hypoaldosteronism. Ann Rev Med 30:145, 1979

———: Neuromuscular manifestations of electrolyte disorders. Am J Med 72:521, 1982

RICHARDSON RMA, KUNAU RT JR: Renal regulation of potassium: Abnormal, in *The Kidney: Physiology and Pathophysiology,* 2d ed, DW Seldin, G Giebisch (eds). New York, Raven Press, 1985, p 1251

STERNS RH et al: Internal potassium balance and the control of the plasma potassium concentration. Medicine 60:339, 1981

WRIGHT FS: Sites and mechanisms of potassium transport along the renal tubule. Kidney Int 11:415, 1977

42 ACIDOSIS AND ALKALOSIS

NORMAN G. LEVINSKY

PHYSIOLOGIC CONSIDERATIONS Acids are produced continuously during normal metabolism. Despite the addition of some 20,000 mmol of carbonic acid and 80 mmol of nonvolatile acids to body fluids daily, the free hydrogen ion concentration of these fluids is fixed within a narrow range. The pH of extracellular fluid is normally between 7.35 and 7.45 (hydrogen ion, 45 to 35 nmol per liter). The pH of intracellular fluids cannot be determined with precision, but most methods suggest a mean intracellular pH in the range of 6.9. Intracellular hydrogen ion concentration is not uniform; it varies among intracellular organelles within individual cells. Although the free hydrogen ion concentration of body fluids is low, protons are so reactive that even minute changes in concentration influence enzymatic reactions and physiologic processes. Immediate defense against untoward changes in pH is provided by buffers that can take up or release protons instantaneously in response to changes in acidity of body fluids. Regulation of pH ultimately depends on the lungs and the kidneys.

The principal acid product of metabolism is carbon dioxide, equivalent to potential carbonic acid. The normal concentration of carbon dioxide in body fluids is fixed at 1.2 mmol per liter (P_{CO_2} = 40 mmHg) by the lungs; at this concentration, pulmonary excretion equals metabolic production. Although carbon dioxide reacts with water and body buffers during transport from cells to pulmonary alveoli, no net change in body fluid composition results, since the CO_2 excreted by the lungs is equal to the CO_2 produced by cells. When a nonvolatile acid is produced by metabolism, the protons are removed instantaneously from body fluids by reaction with buffers. In extracellular fluid, bicarbonate is converted to water and carbon dioxide, which is excreted by the lungs. Although this mechanism minimizes changes in acidity, it destroys bicarbonate and uses up cell buffer capacity. The total buffer capacity of the body fluids is about 15 meq per kilogram of body weight. Thus, the normal rate of production of nonvolatile acids would be sufficient to deplete the body buffers completely in 10 to 20 days, were it not for the ability of the kidney to eliminate protons from the body by secretion into the urine, thereby regenerating bicarbonate and cell buffer capacity.

The principal source of nonvolatile acid is metabolism of methionine and cystine in dietary proteins, which produces sulfuric acid. Additional sources include the incomplete combustion of carbohydrates and fats, which produces organic acids; the metabolism of nucleoproteins, which produces uric acid; and the metabolism of organic phosphorus compounds, which releases protons and inorganic phosphates. The diet does not normally contain significant amounts of preformed acid or alkali, but significant amounts of potential acid (e.g., an excess of cationic acids, such as lysine) or alkali (e.g., citrate) may be present.

The principal functions of the kidney in acid-base metabolism can be viewed as retention of existing bicarbonate and generation of new bicarbonate to replace that used to buffer nonvolatile acids. Bicarbonate is reabsorbed in both proximal and distal segments by secretion of protons into tubular fluid. New bicarbonate is generated by secretion of protons onto urinary buffers. Normally, one-third is titrated onto phosphate, converting HPO_4^{2-} to $H_2PO_4^-$, and the remainder onto ammonia. The amount of free acid which can be excreted in the urine is negligible, even at the minimum urine pH of 4.8. However, acidification of the urine is essential for titration of acid onto phosphate and ammonia. Changes in the pH of body fluids lead to regulatory responses by the kidney. Acidosis stimulates renal hydrogen ion secretion. Ammonia production increases, and more protons can be excreted as ammonium. In extreme acidosis, ammonia production may increase tenfold or more above the normal rate of 40 to 50 meq per day. The bicarbonate concentration of extracellular fluid is, in effect, set by the renal rate of proton secretion (bicarbonate reabsorption and generation). If plasma bicarbonate rises without an increase in renal reabsorptive capacity, bicarbonate is excreted rapidly and normal plasma bicarbonate is restored promptly. For example, chronic ingestion of even large amounts of sodium bicarbonate normally produces only minimal sustained elevation of plasma bicarbonate. The rate of proton secretion is influenced by a number of factors, important among them carbon dioxide tension of body fluids, extracellular volume, aldosterone, and body potassium stores. Bicarbonate reabsorption is directly related to carbon dioxide concentration; hypercapnia tends to stimulate, and hypocapnia tends to inhibit, renal bicarbonate retention. Contraction of extracellular volume enhances tubular bicarbonate reabsorption, while volume expansion has the opposite effect. Aldosterone stimulates renal proton secretion; by this effect, hyperaldosteronism promotes metabolic alkalosis, while hypoaldosteronism causes acidosis. In experimental animals, renal bicarbonate reabsorption is inversely related to body potassium stores. In humans, the relation is less clear, but severe potassium depletion has been associated with increased bicarbonate reabsorption and metabolic alkalosis.

The respiratory response to changes in blood pH is almost instantaneous. Acidosis stimulates and alkalosis depresses ventilation. The respiratory center in the medulla appears to respond to a pH intermediate between those of blood and cerebrospinal fluid.

EVALUATION OF ACID-BASE BALANCE In practice, classification of acid-base disorders is based on measurements of changes in the bicarbonate–carbonic acid system, the principal buffer of extracellular fluid. Because intracellular and extracellular buffers are functionally linked, measurement of the plasma bicarbonate system provides useful information about total body buffers. The relationship among the elements of the bicarbonate system is usually described in terms of the Henderson-Hasselbalch equation:

$$\text{pH} = \text{p}K + \log \frac{[\text{HCO}_3^-]}{[\text{H}_2\text{CO}_3]}$$

(The pK of carbonic acid is 6.1. $[H_2CO_3]$ is calculated as αP_{CO_2}; α, the solubility factor for carbon dioxide in body fluids, is 0.031 mmol per liter per mmHg P_{CO_2}. For a normal P_{CO_2} of 40 mmHg, $[H_2CO_3]$ is calculated to be 40 x 0.031 = 1.2 mmol per liter.)

Acidosis is defined as a disturbance which tends to add acid or remove alkali from body fluids, while *alkalosis* is any disturbance which tends to remove acid or add base. Since compensatory processes may minimize or prevent a change in the hydrogen ion concentration of the plasma, some authors prefer to use the terms *acidemia* and *alkalemia* to indicate those situations in which the pH of the plasma is measurably altered. *Respiratory* disorders are those in which the primary change is in the concentration of carbon dioxide (carbonic acid). As can be seen from the Henderson-Hasselbalch equation, a fall in carbon dioxide concentration causes alkalemia, while an increase in carbon dioxide concentration causes acidemia. *Metabolic* disorders are those in which the primary disturbance is in the concentration of bicarbonate. Since bicarbonate appears in the numerator of the buffer salt/acid ratio in the Henderson-Hasselbalch equation, increased bicarbonate concentration causes alkalemia while a decrease in bicarbonate causes acidemia.

A major problem in the assessment of acid-base disorders results from the compensatory responses of the lungs and the kidney. A primary change in carbon dioxide concentration induces a compensatory renal response which alters plasma bicarbonate in the same direction. Conversely, a primary alteration of plasma bicarbonate induces compensatory changes in plasma carbon dioxide. Consider a patient with chronic respiratory insufficiency who has the following set of acid-base parameters: P_{CO_2} = 70 mmHg, $[HCO_3^-]$ = 31 mmol per liter, pH = 7.25. The clinician needs to know whether the elevation of plasma bicarbonate is merely the appropriate renal response to the primary hypercapnia or a metabolic acid-base disorder is superimposed. No calculations or a priori reasoning will provide the answer to this key question. Such information can be derived only from in vivo observations in which the usual compensatory response to a given degree of chronic hypercapnia is determined.

Clinical and experimental observations in humans (and animals) have been made in all common primary acid-base disturbances. They are most readily visualized and used for analysis of clinical acid-base disorders by the "confidence band" technique, as shown in Fig. 42-1. Each band represents the mean ±2 SD, that is, 95 percent of observations, for the compensatory response to each primary disturbance. In the example under discussion, inspection of the confidence band marked *chronic respiratory acidosis* indicates that 95 percent of individuals with chronic elevation of P_{CO_2} to 70 mmHg would have $[HCO_3^-]$ between 34 and 44 meq per liter, due to renal compensation. Thus, the $[HCO_3^-]$ of 31 meq per liter in the example cannot be interpreted as the sole result of an appropriate compensatory response to chronic hypercapnia. A second acid-base disorder, presumably metabolic acidosis, must be superimposed. Obviously, the use of this figure is no panacea, nor does it obviate the need for commonsense clinical evaluation of alternative possibilities. For example, if the patient under discussion had only recently developed

FIGURE 42-1 *Nomogram, showing bands for uncomplicated respiratory or metabolic acid-base disturbances in intact subjects. Each "confidence" band represents the mean ±2 SD for the compensatory response of normal subjects or patients to a given primary disorder. Ac = acute; chr = chronic, resp = respiratory; met = metabolic; acid = acidosis; alk = alkalosis. (Modified from Arbus.)*

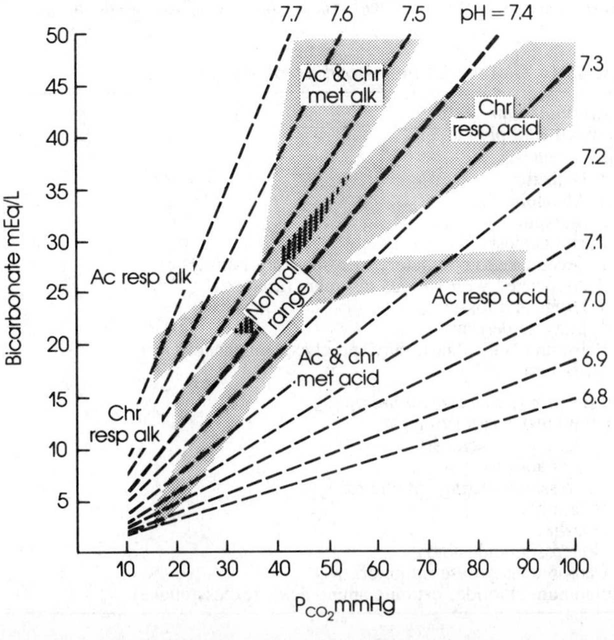

hypercapnia, the [HCO_3^-] of 31 meq per liter would be too high for a purely compensatory response to acute respiratory acidosis and would be interpreted as superimposed metabolic alkalosis. The difference between these two interpretations depends entirely on the clinical recognition of the chronicity of the primary respiratory disorder. The use of Fig. 42-1 in each type of acid-base disturbance is described in the appropriate section of this chapter.[1]

METABOLIC ACIDOSIS

PATHOPHYSIOLOGY Metabolic acidosis is caused by one of three mechanisms (see Table 42-1): (1) increased production of nonvolatile acids, (2) decreased acid excretion by the kidney, (3) loss of alkali. In intracellular fluid excess protons replace potassium, which shifts out of cells, tending to elevate plasma levels. Extracellular bicarbonate is reduced by reaction with hydrogen ions or, in patients wasting alkali, by loss of bicarbonate in urine or stool. The decrease in pH stimulates respiration, and P_{CO_2} is lowered. Inspection of the confidence band for metabolic acidosis (Fig. 42-1) indicates that a decrease in P_{CO_2} of about 1.2 mmHg can be expected for each decrement of 1 mmol per liter in plasma bicarbonate. Complete respiratory compensation for primary metabolic acidosis does not occur. Respiratory compensation for acute acidosis tends to be somewhat greater than for chronic metabolic acidosis. The minimum level of P_{CO_2} which can be attained is approximately 10 mmHg; levels below 15 to 20 mmHg are rarely maintained in chronic metabolic acidosis. When kidney function is normal, net acid excretion increases promptly in response to metabolic acidosis. Most of the initial rise is due to increased titration of urinary phosphate as urine pH falls below 5.2. Over several days, ammonia production by the kidney increases and becomes the most important mechanism for excreting excess protons. Net acid excretion may increase 5 to 10 times above normal, reaching a maximum of several hundred milliequivalents per day.

The most common cause of *acute* metabolic acidosis is increased production of nonvolatile acids. In *diabetic ketoacidosis*, acetoacetic and β-hydroxybutyric acids are produced more rapidly than they can be metabolized (Chap. 327). Severe ketoacidosis may occur in *association* with *acute* and *chronic alcoholism*. Typically patients give a history of prolonged abstention from food, protracted vomiting, and appreciable alcohol intake just before development of the ketoacidosis. β-Hydroxybutyrate, acetoacetate, and lactate accumulate in the plasma. The ketosis may be overlooked because the ratio

[1] *Although the confidence band method does not permit automatic identification of simple or complicated acid-base disorders, it is preferable to techniques such as "buffer base" or "base excess-deficit" for reasons discussed in detail by Schwartz and Relman, N Engl J Med 268:1382, 1963. These terms are not used in this chapter.*

TABLE 42-1 Causes of metabolic acidosis

Increased anion gap
I Increased acid production
A Ketoacidosis
1 Diabetic
2 Alcoholic
3 Starvation
B Lactic acidosis
1 Secondary to circulatory or respiratory failure
2 Associated with various disorders (see text)
3 Drugs and toxins
4 Enzyme defects
C Poisoning (salicylates, ethylene glycol, methanol)
II Renal failure
Normal anion gap (hyperchloremic)
III Renal tubular dysfunction
A Renal tubular acidosis
B Hypoaldosteronism
C "Potassium-sparing" diuretics
IV Loss of alkali
A Diarrhea
B Ureterosigmoidostomy
C Carbonic anhydrase inhibitors
V Ammonium chloride, cationic amino acids (excess intake)

of β-hydroxybutyrate to acetoacetate tends to be high; the nitroprusside test used for clinical detection of plasma ketones responds only to the latter. Blood sugar is usually normal or mildly elevated in these patients. The mechanism of the syndrome is uncertain. *Starvation* may cause mild ketoacidosis because of increased fat metabolism.

Several types of *lactic acidosis* have been recognized (Chap. 328). The most common is *secondary* to severe acute circulatory or respiratory failure, with poor tissue perfusion or arterial oxygen desaturation. The clinical features of shock are usually present. In these patients, lactic acidosis probably is due both to increased production of lactate by hypoxic tissues and to decreased utilization by the liver. Lactic acidosis may also be *associated* with acute hepatic necrosis, leukemia, solid tumors, and uncontrolled diabetes mellitus. The biguanide oral hypoglycemic agents, such as phenformin, were the drugs most often responsible for *drug-induced* lactic acidosis; they are no longer in general use. Certain sugars used for parenteral alimentation, such as fructose, may cause lactic acidosis. Increased lactic acid production contributes to acidosis in *poisoning* by methanol and salicylates. In infants and children, congenital defects in enzymes of carbohydrate metabolism have been identified as causes of lactic acidosis. Primary lactic acidosis in patients without an underlying disease has been reported, but the existence of such a spontaneous disorder is uncertain.

Poisoning and drug toxicity are causes of acute metabolic acidosis. Among the more common agents are salicylates, ethylene glycol, and methyl alcohol (Chap. 171). Salicylates create a metabolic block, which leads to production of a mixture of endogenous organic acids. Methanol and ethylene glycol are converted to acid metabolites, methanol to formic acid and ethylene glycol to glyoxylic and oxalic acids. In addition, these intoxicants create metabolic blocks, which may lead to increased production of endogenous organic acids. Salicylates have the additional effect of stimulating the respiratory center directly. Respiratory alkalosis is the earliest derangement in salicylate intoxication and may be the only acid-base disorder in some patients.

Renal disease is the most common cause of chronic metabolic acidosis. In *chronic renal failure* (Chap. 220), the principal defect is decreased ability to excrete ammonium, but some patients also waste bicarbonate, especially at plasma levels of 18 mmol per liter or above. Acidification of the urine and formation of titratable acidity are usually normal. Plasma bicarbonate tends to fall progressively as renal insufficiency becomes increasingly severe, but plasma bicarbonate usually stabilizes at levels of 12 to 18 mmol per liter; it rarely falls below 10 mmol per liter, even in advanced uremia. The mechanisms of stabilization are thought to be (1) stimulation of acid excretion by advancing acidosis, which occurs to some extent even in the diseased kidney; and (2) buffering of the daily metabolic acid load by carbonate and phosphate in bone. In *acute renal failure* (Chap. 219), plasma bicarbonate decreases by only 1 to 2 mmol per liter per day if reduced renal acid excretion is the only cause of metabolic acidosis. Greater rates of fall suggest the presence, in addition, of some cause of increased acid production.

Chronic metabolic acidosis is the hallmark of *renal tubular acidosis* (Chap. 228), which may be an isolated disorder of tubular acid excretion; part of a Fanconi syndrome, in which other tubular functions are also abnormal; or associated with nonrenal primary disorders (Chap. 307). The acidosis is due to defective renal tubular acidification mechanisms, which limit renal conservation and regeneration of bicarbonate.

Aldosterone stimulates distal tubular acid and potassium secretion. In *hypoaldosteronism*, loss of this effect leads to metabolic acidosis and hyperkalemia. The acidosis is due not only to loss of the direct effect of aldosterone on acid excretion but also to the hyperkalemia, which decreases renal ammonia production. The same factors account for metabolic acidosis caused by the diuretic spironolactone, which blocks the action of aldosterone, and other "potassium-sparing" diuretics such as triamterene and amiloride, which directly inhibit distal tubular secretion of acid and potassium.

Loss of alkali may cause acute or chronic metabolic acidosis. Severe *diarrhea* or intestinal malabsorption usually causes mild to moderate acidosis due to the loss of bicarbonate in liquid stool, in which concentrations of 40 to 60 mmol per liter may be present. Ureterosigmoidostomy, i.e., transplantation of the ureters into the sigmoid colon, leads to metabolic acidosis both because of exchange of chloride for bicarbonate by intestinal epithelium and because renal disease (obstructive uropathy and pyelonephritis) often develops. However, acidosis is not a problem with the more modern technique for urinary diversion, in which a bladder is formed from a small isolated loop of ileum. Carbonic anhydrase inhibitors, such as acetazolamide, cause mild to moderate acidosis by increasing bicarbonate loss in the urine.

Acidosis can be caused by administration of ammonium chloride and lysine or arginine hydrochloride, which form HCl during metabolism. This type of acidosis also may occur during parenteral alimentation with amino acid infusates that contain an excess of the cationic amino acids arginine, lysine, and histidine.

CLINICAL FEATURES AND DIAGNOSIS There are few specific symptoms or signs of metabolic acidosis; diagnosis depends on recognition of the clinical setting and appropriate laboratory studies. In acute metabolic acidosis, hyperventilation is usual and may be intense (Kussmaul respiration). However, it is ordinarily impossible to detect increased respiration by physical examination in patients with chronic metabolic acidosis, despite substantial reduction of P_{CO_2}. Acute, severe acidosis produces a variety of nonspecific symptoms ranging from fatigue through confusion, stupor, and coma. Cardiovascular effects include decreased cardiac contractility and vasodilatation, which may lead to heart failure or hypotension. Chronic metabolic acidosis may produce no symptoms or may be associated with fatigue and anorexia, although it is usually difficult to determine whether these symptoms reflect the acidosis per se or are related to the underlying disease.

The characteristic laboratory features are reduction of plasma bicarbonate and blood pH, together with a compensatory reduction in P_{CO_2} (see Fig. 42-1). Hyperkalemia is often present, due to shift of potassium out of cells. This phenomenon may mask significant potassium depletion (see Chap. 41). Hypokalemia is a clue to conditions in which concomitant potassium depletion is severe, for example, diarrhea or diabetic ketoacidosis, or in which renal potassium-regulating mechanisms are affected, such as renal tubular acidosis or administration of carbonic anhydrase inhibitors.

When the cause of metabolic acidosis is not evident from the history or clinical setting, calculation of unmeasured anions (anion gap) may help in differential diagnosis. Unmeasured anions are calculated by subtracting the sum of plasma bicarbonate and chloride from plasma sodium concentration; the normal value is 8 to 16 mmol per liter. The negative charges on plasma proteins, principally albumin, make up most of the anion gap. Phosphate, sulfate, and organic acid anions normally contribute to unmeasured anions to a lesser degree. When metabolic acidosis is due to increased acid production or renal insufficiency (categories I and II, Table 42-1), the anion gap is usually increased. In acidosis resulting from increased acid production, the increased anion gap is due to accumulation in plasma of the anions of the various acids such as acetoacetate or lactate, which are produced faster than they can be metabolized or excreted. In renal failure, the anion gap increases because sulfate, phosphate, and organic acid anions are not excreted efficiently. In all other types of metabolic acidosis (categories III, IV, V, Table 42-1), the anion gap is normal since there is neither increased production nor decreased excretion of organic acids, sulfate, and phosphate. Plasma chloride concentration is increased approximately as much as plasma bicarbonate is decreased (hyperchloremic acidosis).

In diabetic ketoacidosis a variety of plasma acid-base patterns may develop, depending on the balance between production and renal excretion of ketoacid anions. In most patients there is renal dysfunction, and the anions are retained, leading to an anion-gap acidosis in which the elevation in plasma unmeasured anion is about equal to the reduction in bicarbonate concentration. Patients whose renal function is not impaired may present with a component of hyperchloremic acidosis due to renal excretion of ketone anions and retention of chloride. After therapy that repairs volume depletion and hence renal dysfunction, most patients develop some degree of hyperchloremia, due to the same mechanisms.

TREATMENT The treatment of metabolic acidosis depends on its cause and severity. In *chronic renal failure,* mild or moderate metabolic acidosis does not require treatment. When plasma bicarbonate falls below 15 mmol per liter, it is reasonable to treat patients with oral alkali, such as sodium bicarbonate or sodium citrate. The dose is gradually increased until plasma bicarbonate concentration rises to about 18 to 20 mmol per liter. Some patients appear to benefit symptomatically from elevation of bicarbonate to this level, and fatigue, anorexia, and malaise tend to be alleviated. Caution must be exerted to avoid excessively rapid alkalination of the plasma, which may precipitate tetany; excess sodium given with alkali may aggravate hypertension or edema. Acidosis should be corrected as completely as possible in patients with type 1 (distal) *renal tubular acidosis;* this will avoid hypercalciuria, osteomalacia, nephrocalcinosis, and lithiasis. In type 2 (proximal) renal tubular acidosis, therapy is usually not required (see Chap. 228). Patients with *acute renal failure* also do not ordinarily require specific therapy for acidosis. Dialysis instituted for management of the renal failure should maintain an adequate plasma bicarbonate.

Diabetic *ketoacidosis* responds to insulin, and most patients do not require treatment with alkali (see Chap. 327). However, when acidosis is extreme (pH less than 7.1 or $[HCO_3^-]$ less than 6 to 8 meq per liter), intravenous bicarbonate therapy is justified. The ketoacidosis associated with alcoholism responds rapidly to infusions of glucose and saline. Insulin is not required, nor should alkali be given unless acidosis is extreme. The ketoacidosis of starvation is mild and requires no specific treatment.

Lactic acidosis secondary to acute circulatory or respiratory failure is corrected if treatment of the underlying disorder is successful (see Chap. 328). Since this type of lactic acidosis is usually associated with severe acute circulatory or respiratory failure, the mortality rate is high. Lactic acidosis occurring in other disorders is usually resistant to treatment. Rapid administration of several hundred milliequivalents of alkali may raise plasma bicarbonate in some patients, but in others net production of lactic acid is so rapid that correction of acidosis is difficult. Since vigorous administration of alkali may lead to circulatory overloading, dialysis may be useful. Despite rapid administration of alkali, the mortality rate in these patients is high.

The acidosis due to *diarrhea* or loss of alkaline upper intestinal secretions is usually associated with other volume depletion and potassium deficiency. Treatment of such electrolyte disorders with intravenous infusions appropriate for the patient's specific abnormalities may be required.

Some general points about therapy with alkali are worth emphasis. Oral treatment with sodium bicarbonate should usually begin with 1 g three times daily and be increased to maintain the desired plasma bicarbonate level. Some patients find that sodium bicarbonate leads to upper gastrointestinal discomfort; a 10% sodium citrate solution may be more palatable. In the intravenous treatment of acute metabolic acidosis, sodium bicarbonate is the agent of choice. The amount of bicarbonate to be given depends upon the severity of the acidosis and any associated disorders of serum sodium concentration. Typically, concentrations of bicarbonate between 50 and 150 meq per liter are achieved by adding one to three vials of sodium bicarbonate to a liter of dextrose in water. The concentration of bicarbonate in these vials is 1000 meq per liter (50 meq in 50 mL); these bicarbonate solutions should never be given undiluted in the treatment of acidosis, since rapid infusion may induce serious or even fatal cardiac arrhythmias, especially if given as a bolus through a central venous catheter. The total amount of alkali needed to raise plasma bicarbonate can be estimated from the effects of administration of acid loads. Approximately equal amounts of acid appear to be buffered by extracellular bicarbonate and by intracellular buffers. (In severe acidosis, a greater fraction of the acid load may be buffered within cells.) Therefore, it is appropriate to calculate the amount of alkali needed by assuming that approximately half will accept protons from intracellular buffers and be destroyed; the other half will elevate plasma bicarbonate concentration. Thus, the calculation would be: millimoles of bicarbonate required equals desired increment in plasma concentration (millimoles per liter) times 40 percent of body weight. The 40 percent figure represents twice the extracellular volume. It is rarely desirable to infuse enough alkali to elevate plasma bicarbonate to normal. Possible untoward effects include hypokalemic cardiac toxicity in patients who are substantially potassium-depleted, tetany in patients with renal failure or hypocalcemia, and congestive failure due to excess sodium. Moreover, alkalosis may supervene. Cerebrospinal fluid bicarbonate does not equilibrate rapidly with plasma. Hence the respiratory center, which responds to acidity both of blood and cerebrospinal fluid, maintains some degree of hyperventilation as plasma bicarbonate is increasing. This type of respiratory alkalosis may sometimes persist for several days after correction of metabolic acidosis. In acute acidosis due to overproduction of metabolic acids, successful treatment of the primary disorder will cause rapid metabolic conversion of lactate and ketone bodies to bicarbonate. Thus, excessive administration of bicarbonate early in therapy also may lead to metabolic alkalosis at a later stage of treatment, when endogenous bicarbonate has been reconstituted by improvement in metabolism.

METABOLIC ALKALOSIS

PATHOPHYSIOLOGY Metabolic alkalosis is usually initiated by increased loss of acid from the stomach or the kidney. However, excretion of bicarbonate at high plasma concentrations is normally so rapid that alkalosis will not be sustained unless bicarbonate reabsorption is enhanced or alkali is continuously generated at a great rate. Clinically, maintenance of metabolic alkalosis is most often due to stimulation of bicarbonate reabsorption by a volume (chloride) deficit. During volume depletion, renal conservation of sodium takes precedence over other homeostatic mechanisms, such as correction of alkalosis. Since in alkalosis a large fraction of plasma sodium is paired with bicarbonate, complete reabsorption of filtered sodium requires reabsorption of bicarbonate as well. Alkalosis is sustained until volume depletion is corrected by administration of sodium chloride. This diminishes tubular avidity for sodium and provides chloride as an alternative anion for reabsorption with sodium; excess bicarbonate can then be excreted with sodium.

The other major mechanism which can maintain metabolic alkalosis is hypermineralocorticoidism. Mineralocorticoids stimulate renal hydrogen ion secretion. In patients with excess mineralocorticoid activity, elevation of plasma bicarbonate is initiated by increased urinary loss of protons as ammonium and titratable acidity. Stimulation of tubular acid secretion also enhances bicarbonate reabsorption, thereby sustaining the metabolic alkalosis. Patients with excess mineralocorticoid activity are not volume- or chloride-deficient. Hence, this type of metabolic alkalosis does not respond to sodium chloride administration.

TABLE 42-2 Causes of metabolic alkalosis

I Associated with volume (chloride) depletion
- *A* Vomiting or gastric drainage
- *B* Diuretic therapy
- *C* Posthypercapnic alkalosis

II Associated with hyperadrenocorticism
- *A* Cushing's syndrome
- *B* Primary aldosteronism
- *C* Bartter's syndrome

III Severe potassium depletion

IV Excessive alkali intake
- *A* Acute
- *B* Milk-alkali syndrome

The relation between metabolic alkalosis and potassium is incompletely understood. Alkalosis and hypokalemia often occur together. Alkalosis may cause hypokalemia and potassium depletion through mechanisms discussed in Chap. 41. Conversely, potassium depletion may help to sustain metabolic alkalosis because tubular acid secretion, and hence bicarbonate reabsorption, is stimulated. Whether potassium depletion alone can generate metabolic alkalosis is uncertain; if so, severe potassium depletion is required.

Respiratory compensation for metabolic alkalosis is limited. Alveolar ventilation decreases, and P_{CO_2} is elevated. However, since this response is limited by hypoxia, P_{CO_2} rarely rises above 50 to 55 mmHg.

PATHOGENESIS The principal causes of metabolic alkalosis are outlined in Table 42-2. *Vomiting* and *gastric drainage* usually induce only minimal or moderate alkalosis, but occasional patients, especially those with increased gastric acid secretion, e.g., with acid-peptic disease or the Zollinger-Ellison syndrome, may develop very severe alkalosis. Loss of hydrochloric acid in the gastric fluid initiates the alkalosis. Water and sodium chloride are lost in the vomitus or gastric aspirate. Initially, sodium is lost in the urine as well, coupled to increased bicarbonate excretion (which results from elevation of plasma bicarbonate above the tubular reabsorptive threshold). These losses cause a volume (chloride) deficit, which stimulates tubular reabsorption of bicarbonate and thus maintains the elevated plasma bicarbonate generated by gastric losses of hydrochloric acid.

Alkalosis may be present in patients treated with any *diuretic* except those that specifically inhibit bicarbonate reabsorption, such as acetazolamide, or inhibit distal cation secretion, such as spironolactone and triamterene. The diuretics cause extracellular volume contraction. They inhibit chloride reabsorption in the loop of Henle or distal convoluted tubule, which increases delivery of tubular fluid to more distal nephron segments. The volume deficit and consequent hyperaldosteronism stimulate proton secretion in these segments, generating and maintaining the alkalosis. Alkalosis due to oral treatment with diuretics is usually mild. Acute administration of potent intravenous diuretics such as ethacrynic acid to patients on low-sodium diets may induce more severe alkalosis due to rapid loss of sodium chloride in the urine. Sudden contraction of extracellular volume elevates plasma bicarbonate; renal excretion of excess bicarbonate is prevented by the mechanism discussed above.

Patients with chronic hypercapnia due to respiratory insufficiency maintain high plasma bicarbonate concentrations (see "Respiratory Acidosis," below). If respiration improves, P_{CO_2} falls promptly. However, urinary excretion of excess bicarbonate previously generated by renal compensatory mechanisms takes a number of days. In patients on low-salt diets or diuretics who have a volume (chloride) deficiency, *posthypercapnic* alkalosis of this type may persist indefinitely unless sodium or potassium chloride is added to the diet. The mechanism in this condition is the same as that which causes persistent alkalosis in vomiting, described earlier.

Alkalosis is variable in patients with excess mineralocorticoid activity. Minimal or moderate alkalosis is usually present in patients with *Cushing's syndrome* or *primary aldosteronism*. More marked alkalosis may be seen in patients with extreme adrenal hyperfunction associated with ACTH-secreting tumors, such as bronchogenic carcinoma. Moderate alkalosis is typical of patients with *Bartter's syndrome*.

Although alkalosis and *potassium depletion* are often associated, mild or moderate potassium depletion does not cause sustained metabolic alkalosis. However, extreme degrees of potassium depletion (serum potassium usually 2 meq per liter or less) may cause metabolic alkalosis. This type of alkalosis is not corrected by administration of sodium chloride but does respond to administration of potassium.

For reasons noted earlier, alkalosis due to administration of alkali cannot be sustained unless large amounts are given. When renal function is compromised, alkalosis may be sustained by small exogenous loads. This is apparently the mechanism of alkalosis in the milk-alkali syndrome, in which hypercalcemic nephropathy and alkalosis develop in response to excessive intake of absorbable alkali. The nephropathy limits bicarbonate excretion, thus maintaining the alkalosis.

CLINICAL FEATURES AND DIAGNOSIS There are no specific clinical signs or symptoms. Severe alkalosis may cause apathy, confusion, and stupor. If serum calcium is borderline or low, rapid development of alkalosis may lead to tetany. The diagnosis of metabolic alkalosis depends on recognition of the clinical setting and appropriate laboratory studies. Plasma bicarbonate is increased. P_{CO_2} increases by about 0.6 mmHg for each milliequivalent per liter. Elevation of P_{CO_2} is insufficient to prevent alkalemia (see Fig. 42-1). Plasma potassium concentration is often reduced, and the electrocardiogram may reveal changes in T and U waves typical of hypokalemia (Chap. 178). These changes may be due to alkalosis itself or to associated alterations in potassium metabolism. Despite elevation of plasma bicarbonate, the urine pH is usually less than 7 in patients with sustained metabolic alkalosis. This "paradoxical aciduria" reflects the fact that bicarbonate reabsorption must be increased if metabolic alkalosis is to be sustained.

Differential diagnosis is usually made from clinical features, such as a history of vomiting or the manifestations of Cushing's syndrome. The urinary chloride concentration may be a helpful clue if the diagnosis is not evident. When the alkalosis is associated with volume contraction (category I, Table 42-2), urinary chloride is low, usually less than 10 meq per liter. When the alkalosis is caused by hyperadrenocorticism or severe potassium depletion (categories II and III), urinary chloride is higher, usually 20 meq per liter or more.

TREATMENT Mild or moderate metabolic alkalosis rarely requires specific treatment. In patients with gastric alkalosis, infusion of saline solutions is usually sufficient to enhance renal bicarbonate excretion and to correct alkalosis by mechanisms discussed above. Administration of potassium chloride is also helpful in treating or preventing alkalosis in these patients and those with diuretic-induced alkalosis. In patients with adrenal hyperfunction, alkalosis is corrected by specific treatment of the underlying disease. In Bartter's syndrome hypokalemia, potassium wasting, and alkalosis may be partly corrected by treatment with prostaglandin synthetase inhibitors such as indomethacin. Whenever alkalosis and potassium depletion occur together, potassium depletion should be treated with potassium chloride, not with an organic salt of potassium.

Rarely, with prolonged gastric metabolic alkalosis losses may be severe enough to require intravenous therapy with acidifying agents. Dilute hydrochloric acid or acidifying salts such as ammonium chloride or arginine hydrochloride may be given slowly under such circumstances. In most patients the use of acidifying agents can be avoided by appropriate treatment with saline and potassium chloride. In patients who are volume-expanded or in whom volume loading is inadvisable, therapy with acetazolamide, which enhances renal bicarbonate excretion, may be helpful.

RESPIRATORY ACIDOSIS

PATHOPHYSIOLOGY Failure of ventilation promptly increases P_{CO_2} (carbonic acid) because metabolic production of carbon dioxide is so rapid. Acute respiratory acidosis is modulated to a limited degree by tissue buffers. As can be seen from the curve labeled *acute respiratory acidosis* in Fig. 42-1, immediate tissue buffering elevates plasma bicarbonate only slightly, by about 1 meq per liter for each increase of 10 mmHg in P_{CO_2}. If hypercapnia is sustained, renal acid excretion is enhanced, and bicarbonate reabsorption is stimulated. Over a period of several days, plasma bicarbonate rises approximately 3 meq per liter for each increase of 10 mmHg in P_{CO_2}, thereby minimizing the degree of acidemia. The increment in plasma bicarbonate attributable to renal activity is represented by the difference between the curves marked *chronic respiratory acidosis* and *acute respiratory acidosis*.

PATHOGENESIS (See also Table 215-1) *Acute* respiratory acidosis occurs whenever there is a sudden failure of ventilation. Common causes include depression of the respiratory center by cerebral disease or drugs, neuromuscular disorders, and cardiopulmonary arrest. *Chronic* respiratory acidosis occurs in pulmonary diseases such as chronic emphysema and bronchitis, in which ventilation and perfusion are mismatched and effective alveolar ventilation is decreased. Chronic hypercapnia may also result from primary alveolar hypoventilation or from alveolar hypoventilation related to extreme obesity (Pickwickian syndrome). Acute and chronic diseases characterized principally by interference with alveolar gas exchange, such as chronic pulmonary fibrosis, pneumonia, and pulmonary edema, usually cause hypocapnia rather than hypercapnia. In these conditions, hypoxia stimulates increased ventilation; since carbon dioxide is much more diffusible than oxygen, excretion of carbon dioxide is enhanced despite the barrier to gas exchange. Hypercapnia occurs only with respiratory fatigue or extremely severe disease.

CLINICAL FEATURES AND DIAGNOSIS It is often difficult to separate the manifestations of respiratory acidosis from those of associated hypoxia. Moderate hypercapnia, especially if it develops slowly, probably has no specific clinical features. When P_{CO_2} exceeds 70 mmHg, patients become progressively confused and obtunded. Asterixis may be present. Papilledema may occur, apparently because intracranial pressure is increased by the cerebral vasodilation characteristic of hypercapnia. Dilatation of conjunctival and superficial facial blood vessels may be noted.

The diagnosis of acute respiratory acidosis is usually evident from the clinical situation, especially if respiration is obviously depressed. Proof requires laboratory confirmation that P_{CO_2} is elevated. Acidemia is always present in patients with *acute* hypercapnia. Acidosis in acute cardiopulmonary arrest is usually a combination of a metabolic lactic acidosis and acute respiratory acidosis. Patients with chronic hypercapnia are usually acidemic. However, some individuals with minimal or moderate chronic hypercapnia may have normal or even slightly elevated plasma pH, as may be seen from Fig. 42-1. The mechanism of full compensation or of "overcompensation" in such instances is unknown. However, significant elevation of pH in patients with chronic hypercapnia is almost always due to complicating metabolic alkalosis. Diuretics, low-sodium diets, and posthypercapnic alkalosis are frequent causes of this type of superimposed acid-base disorder.

Because of the differences between plasma bicarbonate in acute hypercapnia and in chronic hypercapnia, proper interpretation of acid-base parameters in respiratory acidosis depends on clinical information.

TREATMENT The only worthwhile approach to treatment of respiratory acidosis is correction of the underlying disorder. Rapid infusion of alkali is justified in cardiopulmonary arrest. In other circumstances, infusions of alkali have no role in practical management of respiratory acidosis.

RESPIRATORY ALKALOSIS

PATHOPHYSIOLOGY Acute reduction in carbon dioxide concentration releases hydrogen ion from tissue buffers, which minimize alkalemia by reducing plasma bicarbonate. Acute alkalosis also enhances glycolysis; increased production of lactic and pyruvic acids lowers serum bicarbonate and raises plasma concentrations of the corresponding anions by a millimole or two. In chronic hypocapnia, plasma bicarbonate is further reduced because the decreased P_{CO_2} inhibits tubular reabsorption and generation of bicarbonate. As in respiratory acidosis, compensation for the chronic state is much more complete than for the acute (Figure 42-1). In acute hypocapnia, plasma bicarbonate falls only about 2 meq per liter for each 10-mm reduction in P_{CO_2}. In chronic hypocapnia, plasma bicarbonate is reduced by 4 to 5 meq per liter for each 10-mm decrease in P_{CO_2}.

The decrement in plasma bicarbonate attributable to renal compensatory activity is shown by the difference between the curves labeled acute and chronic respiratory alkalosis in Fig. 42-1.

PATHOGENESIS Respiratory alkalosis is due to acute or chronic hyperventilation, which lowers P_{CO_2}. The causes of respiratory alkalosis are shown in Table 42-3.

CLINICAL FEATURES AND DIAGNOSIS Depending on its severity and acuteness, hyperventilation may or may not be clinically apparent. In acute respiratory alkalosis, the clinical picture is rather characteristic: patients complain of paresthesias, numbness, and tingling; of light-headedness; and, if alkalosis is sufficiently severe, of manifestations of tetany. Alkalosis directly enhances neuromuscular excitability; this effect, rather than the modest decrease in ionized plasma calcium induced by alkalosis, is probably the major cause of tetany.

TABLE 42-3 Causes of respiratory alkalosis

I Hypoxia
- *A* Acute (e.g., pneumonia, asthma, pulmonary edema)
- *B* Chronic (e.g., pulmonary fibrosis, cyanotic heart disease, high altitudes)

II Respiratory center stimulation
- *A* Anxiety
- *B* Fever
- *C* Salicylate intoxication
- *D* Cerebral disease (tumor, encephalitis, etc.)

III Exercise
IV Gram-negative sepsis
V Hepatic cirrhosis
VI Pregnancy
VII Excessive mechanical ventilation

Severe respiratory alkalosis may cause confusion or loss of consciousness, perhaps due to cerebral vasospasm induced by hypocapnia.

The diagnosis may be suspected from the clinical setting but must be confirmed by analysis of the plasma bicarbonate system. Hypocapnia together with a variable degree of alkalemia is found; plasma bicarbonate is decreased but is rarely below 15 mmol per liter.

TREATMENT The only successful treatment for respiratory alkalosis is elimination of the underlying disorder. In the acute hyperventilation syndrome, sedation, reassurance, and if symptoms are sufficiently severe, rebreathing into a bag will usually terminate the attack.

REFERENCES

ARBUS GS: An in vivo acid-base nomogram for clinical use. Can Med Assoc J 109:291, 1973

BATTLE DC, KURTZMAN NA: Renal regulation of acid-base homeostasis: Integrated response, in *The Kidney: Physiology and Pathophysiology,* 2d ed, DW Seldin, G Giebisch (eds). New York, Raven Press, 1986, p 1539

——— et al: Clinical and pathophysiologic spectrum of acquired distal renal tubular acidosis. Kidney In 20:398, 1981

COGAN MG, RECTOR FC JR: Acid-base disorders, in *The Kidney,* 3d ed, BM Brenner, FC Rector Jr (eds). Philadelphia, Saunders, 1986, p 457

EMMETT M, NARINS RG: Clinical use of the anion gap. Medicine 56:38, 1977

KASSIRER JP, MADIAS NE: Respiratory acid-base disorders. Hosp Practice 15:57, 1980

LEVY LH et al: Ketoacidosis associated with alcoholism in non-diabetic subjects. Ann Intern Med 78:213, 1973

NARINS RG, EMMETT M: Simple and mixed acid-base disorders: A practical approach. Medicine 59:161, 1980

SCHWARTZ WB, RELMAN AS: A critique of the parameters used in the evaluation of acid-base disorders. N Engl J Med 268:1382, 1963

STINEBAUGH BJ et al: Pathogenesis of distal renal tubular acidosis. Kidney Int 19:1, 1981

TANNEN RL: Control of acid excretion by the kidney. Ann Rev Med 31:35, 1980

section 7 Alterations in reproductive and sexual function

43 DISTURBANCES OF MENSTRUATION AND SEXUAL FUNCTION IN WOMEN

BRUCE R. CARR / JEAN D. WILSON

Complaints related to the female reproductive tract can usually be categorized either as disturbances of menstruation, pelvic pain, disturbances in sexual function, or infertility. However, a single disorder, for example leiomyoma of the uterus, can present with symptoms referable to any one or more of these categories. Furthermore, sexual dysfunction can interdigitate with other complaints in several ways. On the one hand, in women who present with complaints related to other reproductive tract functions, the underlying problem may actually be severe sexual dysfunction or marital conflict. Alternatively, women who have severe organic diseases of the pelvis, for example pelvic inflammatory disease, may present with a problem of sexual function such as dyspareunia, which in fact is only a minor manifestation of the underlying disease.

Since normal reproductive function depends on the integrated action of the central nervous system, the endocrine glands, and the reproductive organs, menstrual cycle abnormalities, sexual dysfunction, and infertility may be the result of a variety of systemic and psychological disorders as well as of primary defects in the endocrine and reproductive organs. The endocrine and physiologic changes—normal and abnormal—associated with puberty, reproductive life, and menopause are discussed in Chap. 331. The focus of this chapter is on the initial evaluation of women with disturbances of the reproductive tract.

DISTURBANCES IN MENSTRUATION Disorders of menstruation can be divided into abnormal uterine bleeding and amenorrhea.

Abnormal uterine bleeding The menstrual cycle is defined as the interval between the onset of one bleeding episode and the onset of the next. In normal women of reproductive age the cycle averages 28 ± 3 days, the mean duration of menstrual flow is 4 ± 2 days, and the average blood loss is 40 to 100 mL. Between the menarche and the menopause almost every woman experiences one or more episodes of abnormal uterine bleeding, here defined as any bleeding pattern outside the parameters of frequency, duration, and/or amount of blood loss described above. The decision to evaluate a patient with an abnormal bleeding pattern is based on the severity and frequency of the abnormal bleeding episodes.

When uterine bleeding is suspected, it is essential to establish first that the blood observed by the patient is derived from the uterine endometrium. Rectal, bladder, cervical, or vaginal sources of bleeding must be excluded. Once the bleeding is documented to be uterine in origin, a pregnancy-related disorder (such as threatened or incomplete abortion or ectopic pregnancy) must be excluded by physical examination and appropriate laboratory tests. Abnormal uterine bleeding may also be the initial or principal manifestation of a generalized bleeding diathesis. The remaining causes of abnormal uterine bleeding fall into two general categories: those associated with ovulatory cycles and those associated with anovulatory cycles.

OVULATORY CYCLES Menstrual bleeding with ovulatory cycles is spontaneous, regular in onset, predictable in duration and amount of flow, and frequently associated with discomfort. Uterine bleeding with ovulatory cycles is due to progesterone withdrawal at the end of the luteal phase and requires prior estrogen priming of the endometrium during the follicular phase of the cycle. When deviations from an established pattern of menstrual flow occur but the cycles are still regular, the usual cause is organic disease of the outflow tract. For example, regular, prolonged, excessive bleeding episodes unassociated with a bleeding diathesis are commonly due to abnormalities of the uterus such as submucous leiomyomas, adenomyosis, or endometrial polyps. On the other hand, cyclic, predictable menstruation characterized by spotting or light bleeding is often due to obstruction of the outflow tract as with uterine synechiae or scarring of the cervix. Intermittent bleeding between cyclic ovulatory menses is often due to cervical or endometrial lesions.

ANOVULATORY CYCLES Uterine bleeding that is irregular in occurrence and unpredictable as to amount and duration of flow is called dysfunctional uterine bleeding. Such bleeding is usually painless. Dysfunctional uterine bleeding is the result of a failure of normal follicular maturation with consequent anovulation and may be either transient or chronic. Transient disruption of the synchronous hypothalamic-pituitary-ovarian hormonal patterns necessary for ovulatory cycles occurs most often in the early menarcheal years, during the perimenopausal period, or as the secondary consequence of a variety of stresses and intercurrent illnesses. Persistent dysfunctional uterine bleeding during the reproductive years can occur in several organic diseases that affect ovarian function and is most often due to estrogen breakthrough bleeding. Estrogen breakthrough bleeding occurs when prolonged continuous estrogen stimulation of the endometrium is not interrupted by cyclic progesterone withdrawal. For example, chronic acyclic estrogen production not associated with ovulation can occur in polycystic ovarian disease.

Amenorrhea Amenorrhea is defined as failure of menarche by age 16, regardless of the presence or absence of secondary sexual characteristics, or the absence of menstruation for 6 months in a woman with previous periodic menses. Amenorrhea in a woman who has never menstruated is termed primary; cessation of menses is termed secondary amenorrhea. Because some disorders can cause both primary and secondary amenorrhea, we prefer a functional classification based upon the nature of the underlying defect, namely anatomic defects of the outflow tract (uterus, cervix, or vagina), ovarian failure, and chronic anovulation.

Anatomic defects of the outflow tract include congenital defects of the vagina, imperforate hymen, transverse vaginal septa, cervical stenosis, intrauterine adhesions (synechiae), absence of the vagina or uterus, and uterine maldevelopment. The diagnosis of an anatomic defect is usually made by physical examination and confirmed by demonstrating failure of bleeding following administration of estrogen plus a progestogen for 21 days.

Causes of *ovarian failure* include gonadal dysgenesis, deficiency of 17α-hydroxylase or 17,20-desmolase, resistant ovary syndrome, and premature ovarian failure. Ovarian failure encompasses those disorders in which the ovary is deficient in germ cells and those in which the germ cells are resistant to FSH (follicle-stimulating hormone). The diagnosis of ovarian failure as the cause of amenorrhea is confirmed by a plasma FSH greater than 40 mIU/mL.

Women with *chronic anovulation* fail to ovulate spontaneously but have the capability of ovulating with appropriate therapy. In some patients with chronic anovulation estrogen production is adequate, but estrogen is not secreted in a cyclic fashion. In others estrogen production is deficient.

Women who have adequate estrogen production and demonstrate withdrawal bleeding after progesterone challenge usually have polycystic ovarian disease (see Fig. 331-7). Unusual causes include hormone-secreting ovarian and adrenal tumors. Women with deficient or absent estrogen production, and therefore with absence of withdrawal bleeding after progesterone treatment, usually have hypogonadotropic hypogonadism due either to organic or functional disorders of the pituitary or central nervous system such as brain tumors, pituitary tumors (especially prolactin-secreting adenomas), primary hypopituitarism, or Sheehan's syndrome.

PELVIC PAIN Pelvic pain may originate in the pelvis or be referred from some other region of the body. A pelvic source for such pain is often suggested by the history (for example, dysmenorrhea and dyspareunia) and physical findings, but a high index of suspicion must be entertained for extrapelvic disorders that refer to the pelvis, such as appendicitis, cholecystitis, intestinal obstruction, and urinary tract infections (see Chap. 5).

"Physiologic" pelvic pain PAIN ASSOCIATED WITH OVULATION ("MITTELSCHMERZ") Many women experience low abdominal discomfort with ovulation, typically a dull aching pain at midcycle in one lower quadrant lasting from a few minutes to hours. It is rarely severe or incapacitating. The relationship of the pain to the mechanisms of ovulation is unknown. It may result from peritoneal irritation by follicular fluid released into the peritoneal cavity at the time of ovulation. The onset at midcycle and a short duration of pain are often diagnostic.

PREMENSTRUAL OR MENSTRUAL PAIN In normal ovulatory women somatic symptoms during the few days prior to menses may be insignificant or disabling. Such symptoms include edema, breast engorgement, and abdominal bloating or discomfort. A symptom complex of cyclic irritability, depression, and lethargy is known as the *premenstrual syndrome*. The cause is unknown but may be prostaglandin-mediated.

Severe or incapacitating cramping in women with ovulatory menses but no demonstrable disorders of the pelvis is termed *primary dysmenorrhea*.

Pelvic pain due to organic causes Severe dysmenorrhea associated with disease of the pelvis is termed *secondary dysmenorrhea*. Organic causes of pelvic pain can be classified as (1) uterine, (2) adnexal, (3) vulvar or vaginal, and (4) pregnancy-associated.

UTERINE PAIN Pain of uterine etiology is often chronic and continuous and increases in intensity during menstruation and intercourse. Causes include leiomyomas of the uterus (particularly submucous and degenerating leiomyomas), adenomyosis, and cervical stenosis. Infections of the uterus associated with intrauterine manipulation following dilatation and curettage or with intrauterine devices can also cause significant pelvic pain (see Chap. 331). Pelvic pain due to endometrial or cervical cancer is usually a late manifestation of disseminated disease (see Chap. 331).

ADNEXAL PAIN The most common cause of pain in the adnexae (fallopian tubes and ovaries) is infection (see Chap. 104). Acute salpingo-oophoritis presents as low abdominal pain, fever, and chills, beginning a few days after a menstrual period, and is most often a consequence of chlamydia or of gonococcal disease with or without a superimposed pyogenic infection. Chronic pelvic inflammatory disease results from either a single episode or multiple episodes of infection and may present as infertility associated with chronic pelvic pain that increases in intensity with menses and intercourse. On physical examination the adnexa are tender, and adnexal thickening with or without masses may be present. Pelvic inflammatory disease may become a surgical emergency if peritonitis results from rupture of a tuboovarian abscess. Ovarian cysts or neoplasms may cause pelvic pain that becomes more severe with torsion or rupture of the mass, and ectopic pregnancy must also be considered in the differential diagnosis (see below). Endometriosis involving fallopian tubes, ovaries, or peritoneum may cause both chronic low abdominal pain and infertility; the magnitude of tissue involvement does not always correlate with the severity of symptoms. Endometriosis pain typically increases with menstruation and, if the posterior ligaments of the uterus are involved, with intercourse.

VULVAR OR VAGINAL PAIN Pain in these areas is most often due to infectious vaginitis caused by organisms such as *Monilia, Trichomonas,* or *Gardnerella* and is characteristically associated with vaginal discharge and pruritus. Herpetic vulvitis, condyloma acuminata, and cysts or abscesses of Bartholin's glands may also cause vulvar pain.

PREGNANCY-ASSOCIATED DISORDERS Pregnancy must be considered in the differential diagnosis of pelvic pain in women during the reproductive years. Threatened abortion or incomplete abortion often presents with uterine cramping, bleeding, or passage of tissue following a period of amenorrhea. Ectopic pregnancy may be insidious in presentation and result in severe intraperitoneal hemorrhage and maternal death.

The evaluation of pelvic pain includes a careful history and pelvic examination. This often leads to the correct diagnosis and institution of appropriate treatment. If the pain is severe and the diagnosis is unclear, the workup should follow that outlined for the acute abdomen (Chap. 5). A culdocentesis is indicated if a ruptured ectopic pregnancy is suspected. If there is a question of an adnexal mass such as a tubal pregnancy or if the patient is so obese as to preclude a thorough pelvic examination, sonography may be helpful in the evaluation. Serial human chorionic gonadotropin (hCG) measurements may be helpful in establishing a diagnosis of tubal pregnancy. Finally, diagnostic laparoscopy and laparotomy may be indicated with severe or prolonged pain of undetermined etiology.

SEXUAL DYSFUNCTION Some women with sexual dysfunction describe minor complaints related to the reproductive tract as a means of bringing sexual problems to the attention of the physician. Alternatively, sexual dysfunction may be thought to be the cause of low abdominal discomfort or dyspareunia when the actual etiology is an organic lesion. However, more and more women seek medical advice because of sexual problems that interface in provenance between medicine and sociology.

The normal sexual response begins with sexual arousal which causes genital vasocongestion that results in vaginal lubrication in preparation for intromission. The lubrication is due to the formation of a transudate in the vagina and in conjunction with genital congestion produces the so-called orgasmic platform prior to orgasm. Sexual stimuli (visual, tactile, auditory, and olfactory) as well as healthy vaginal tissue are prerequisites for genital vasocongestion and vaginal lubrication. During the second stage of the sexual response a series of involuntary contractions of the muscles of the pelvis under control of the autonomic nervous system results in a pleasurable cortical sensory phenomenon known as orgasm. Direct or indirect stimulation of the clitoris is important in the production of the female orgasm. In simple terms, sexual dysfunction can be due to interference with the arousal or orgasmic phases of the sexual response. Either disorder can be due to organic or functional cause or both.

Illnesses that impair neurologic function such as diabetes mellitus or multiple sclerosis may prevent normal sexual arousal. Local pelvic diseases such as vaginitis, endometriosis, and salpingo-oophoritis may preclude normal sexual response because of resulting dyspareunia. Debilitating systemic diseases such as cancer and cardiovascular diseases may impair normal sexual response indirectly.

More commonly, failure of a normal sexual response is due to psychological problems that impair sexual arousal. Such problems include misinformation, for example, the perception of sexual satisfaction as bad, or feelings of guilt about previous psychologically traumatic events such as incest, rape, or unwanted pregnancy. In addition, women who have had previous hysterectomy or mastectomy may perceive themselves as "incomplete." Stresses such as anxiety, depression, fatigue, and marital or interpersonal conflicts may lead to failure of the vasocongestive response and prevent normal vaginal lubrication. Women with such experiences may be unable to achieve normal sexual response unless they receive professional counseling by a family physician, psychologist, psychiatrist, or sex therapist. Such problems are approached by attempting to identify and reduce the causative stresses.

Failure to achieve orgasm is a specific form of sexual dysfunction. Many women enjoy sexual encounters to variable degrees without experiencing orgasm because of the pleasure derived from closeness in a cherished relationship particularly with a loving partner. However, for other women sexual relations with rare or absent orgasms are frustrating and unsatisfying. In many instances, failure of orgasm is due to insufficient clitoral stimulation and may be rectified by appropriate counseling and patient education.

A specific entity, "vaginismus," painful, involuntary contractions of the musculature surrounding the entrance to the vagina, is a rare cause of dyspareunia. It is a conditioned response to a previous real or imagined frightening or traumatic sexual experience. Treatment is directed to elimination of the conditioned response by progressive vaginal dilation by the patient in conjunction with marital therapy.

REPRODUCTION Problems of infertility are discussed in detail in Chap. 331. The approach to infertile couples always involves evaluation of both the man and woman. The initial evaluation includes a thorough history and physical examination. The history should elicit information as to the frequency of intercourse, the sexual responses of both, the use of contraceptives or lubricants, previous or past medical illnesses, and all medications taken.

Male-associated factors account for a third of infertility problems. Therefore, one of the first procedures in the workup of infertile couples should be a semen analysis (see Chap. 330). The initial evaluation of the female includes documentation of normal ovulatory cycles. A history of regular, cyclic, predictable, spontaneous menses usually indicates ovulatory cycles, which may be confirmed by basal body temperature graphs, properly timed endometrial biopsies, or plasma progesterone measurements during the luteal phase of the cycle. Also, the diagnosis of luteal-phase dysfunction can be established by these methods. If the woman is anovulatory, attempts to induce ovulation can be undertaken by a variety of methods including clomiphene citrate, human menopausal gonadotropins, bromocryptine mesylate, luteinizing hormone releasing hormone (LHRH) agonists, or wedge resection of the ovaries (Chap. 331).

The most common cause of infertility in women is tubal disease, usually due to infection (pelvic inflammatory disease) or endometriosis. Tubal disease can be evaluated by obtaining a hysterosalpingogram or by diagnostic laparoscopy. The treatment of tubal causes of infertility is primarily surgical.

A cervical factor as a cause of infertility is evaluated by a properly timed postcoital examination. During this examination the sperm motility in cervical mucus is observed. Also, immunologic etiologies for infertility may be present and can be tested for by a variety of laboratory tests. We are unable to account for a cause of infertility in 10 percent of couples.

The desire for fertility control or contraception is also a frequent cause for women to seek medical treatment or evaluation. The most widely used methods for fertility control include (1) rhythm and withdrawal techniques, (2) barrier methods, (3) intrauterine devices, (4) oral steroid contraceptives, (5) sterilization, and (6) abortion. A discussion of these methods and the possible complications of each is found in Chap. 331.

REFERENCES

FORDNEY DS: Dyspareunia and vaginismus. Clin Obstet Gynecol 21:205, 1978

HATCHER RA et al: *Contraceptive Technology 1984–1985*. New York, Irvington, 1984

KASE NG et al: *Principles and Practice of Clinical Gynecology*. New York, Wiley, 1983

MASTERS W, JOHNSON V: *Human Sexual Response*. Boston, Little, Brown, 1966

———, ———: *Human Sexual Inadequacy*. Boston, Little, Brown, 1970

PRITCHARD JH et al: *Williams Obstetrics*, 17th ed. Norwalk Ct., Appleton-Century-Crofts, 1985

SPEROFF L et al: *Clinical Gynecologic Endocrinology and Infertility*, 3d ed. Baltimore, Williams & Wilkins, 1983

44 IMPOTENCE AND INFERTILITY IN MEN

PATRICK C. WALSH / JEAN D. WILSON

A coordinated sequence of physiologic events (psychic, endocrine, vascular, and neurologic) controls normal sexual and reproductive function in men. In this chapter, the discussion is focused on the clinical presentation of sexual disorders in men. (Also see Chaps. 45, "Medical Aspects of Sexuality," and 330, "Disorders of the Testis.")

SEXUAL FUNCTION

NORMAL SEXUAL FUNCTION Simply stated, normal male sexual function can be divided into five events, each of which is under diverse regulation: libido, erection, ejaculation, orgasm, and detumescence.

The first, sexual desire or libido, is regulated by psychic factors and by testicular androgens. Castration produces a decline in libido that can be restored by treatment with testosterone.

The second phase, erection, is primarily a neurologic event that results in modification of the vascular supply to the penis, causing it to become engorged with blood. The neurologic aspect of erection is controlled by both reflex and psychic stimuli. The sensory portion begins with fibers that originate in pacinian corpuscles of the penis and pass via the pudendal nerve to the S2–S4 dorsal root ganglia. The efferent limb begins with parasympathetic preganglionic fibers from S2–S4 which synapse in the perivesicular, prostatic, and cavernous plexuses. From there, postganglionic fibers pass to blood vessels of the corpora cavernosa. Efferent fibers from S3–S4 also travel in the pudendal nerve to the ischiocavernosus and bulbocavernosus muscles. Sympathetic innervation of the male genitalia originates in fibers from the lateral columns of T12 and L1, the so-called thoracolumbar erection center, that synapse in the pelvic and perivesicular plexuses. Postganglionic fibers innervate the smooth muscle of the vas deferens, seminal vesicle, and internal sphincter of the bladder. Sympathetic innervation can act synergistically with the sacral parasympathetics to mediate erection initiated by psychic stimuli but is not mandatory for erection, because most men have normal potency after bilateral complete sympathectomy. The central nervous system modulates erectile response via pathways thought to descend in the lateral columns of the spinal cord. The effect of the central nervous system on erection can either be stimulatory or inhibitory, thus the importance of psychic factors for erection.

While erection is controlled by the parasympathetic nervous system, the transformation of the penis from a flaccid to an erect state is a vascular phenomenon. Blood reaches the penis via terminal branches of the right and left internal pudendal arteries. The erectile tissue of the penis consists of two corpora cavernosa lying side by side on the dorsal aspect of the penis and the corpus spongiosum that surrounds the urethra. This erectile tissue consists of an irregular spongelike system of vascular spaces interspersed between arteries and veins.

Erection is initiated by a decrease in arterial resistance resulting in increased arterial blood flow with a subsequent decrease in venous outflow. The neurotransmitter responsible for these events has not been identified, but vascular or cavernosal smooth muscle relaxation may result from mediation by beta-adrenergic, cholinergic, or vasoactive intestinal polypeptide (VIP) mechanisms. Furthermore, alpha-adrenergic antagonists can cause increased blood flow to the corpus and hence erection.

The third phase, ejaculation, is under control of the sympathetic nervous system and consists of two processes, seminal emission and true ejaculation. Emission results from the contraction of the vas deferens, prostate, and seminal vesicles which causes seminal fluid to enter the urethra. True ejaculation results from contraction of the muscles of the pelvic floor including the bulbocavernosus and ischiocavernosus muscles. Retrograde ejaculation into the bladder is prevented by partial bladder neck closure mediated by the sympathetic nerves.

The fourth phase, orgasm, is a cortical sensory phenomenon in which the rhythmic contraction of the bulbocavernosus and ischiocavernosus muscles is perceived as pleasurable. It is purely psychic. The fact that orgasm can occur without either erection, ejaculation, or bladder neck closure explains why some drugs that prevent erection or ejaculation do not interfere with orgasm.

Detumescence after orgasm and ejaculation may be the result of vasoconstriction of the arterioles supplying blood to the erectile tissue, thus allowing venous drainage to empty the sinuses and the penis to become flaccid. Following orgasm, there is a refractory period that varies with age, physical condition, and psychic factors during which erection and ejaculation are inhibited.

IMPOTENCE Male sexual dysfunction, often termed *impotence*, may be manifested in various ways: loss of desire, inability to obtain or maintain an erection, premature ejaculation, absence of emission, inability to achieve orgasm. Many subjects complain of more than one abnormality simultaneously. These complaints can be secondary to other chronic or debilitating diseases, the consequence of specific disorders of the urogenital or endocrine systems, or the result of psychiatric disturbance. It is mandatory in all instances to exclude organic (and in some instances potentially correctable or treatable) causes.

Loss of desire Because androgens have a major influence on sexual desire in men, a decrease in libido may indicate androgen deficiency arising from either pituitary or testicular disease. This possibility can be tested by the measurement of plasma testosterone and gonadotropins. However, since the level of testosterone required to maintain libido is usually less than the amount necessary for full stimulation of the prostate and seminal vesicles, absence of emission also occurs when the loss of libido is due to hypogonadism. Conversely, if the semen volume is normal, it is unlikely that endocrine factors are responsible for their sexual dysfunction.

Failure of erection The organic causes of erectile impotence can be grouped into endocrine, drug, local, neurologic, and vascular causes (Table 44-1).

Endocrine causes of testicular failure that result in impotence usually cause such profound changes that the disorders are not difficult to recognize (Chap. 330). However, hyperprolactinemia may cause impotence in some patients with pituitary tumors and may not be obvious on physical examination (see Chaps. 321 and 332); hyperprolactinemia suppresses LHRH (luteinizing hormone–releasing hormone) production, resulting in plasma gonadotropins and testosterone values in the low normal range. Bromocriptine mesylate, a dopamine agonist, may lower prolactin levels and reverse impotence in such patients.

Many drugs cause impotence including antihistamines, antihypertensives, anticholinergics, psychogenic agents, and drugs of habituation or addiction. The usual explanation is neurologic blockade, and this may well be the case for those drugs with peripheral parasympatholytic actions such as the tricyclic antidepressants. Others may act by enhancing prolactin secretion. It is not clear whether impotence caused by drugs of addiction such as alcohol, methadone, and heroin is due to reduced testosterone levels or the general condition of the patient.

Penile diseases that cause impotence can almost always be diagnosed by history and physical examination and include previous priapism, penile trauma, and Peyronie's disease.

Many types of neurologic disorders can cause impotence including lesions in the anterior temporal lobe, spinal cord disorders, insufficiency of sensory input such as can occur in diabetic neuropathy and tabes dorsalis, or damage to parasympathetic nerves, for example, following surgical procedures such as total prostatectomy. Transurethral prostatectomy, in contrast, does not cause organic impotence. Furthermore, the nerve supply to the penis (the nervi erigentes) runs through the lateral pedicle of the prostate, and if the nerves are preserved during radical prostate surgery, potency can be preserved in most men. If spinal cord injury is above the thoracolumbar region, reflex erections may occur. Diffuse injury of the spinal cord results in total impotence. Diabetes mellitus deserves special comment. As many as half of diabetic men develop impotence within 6 years of the onset of diabetes, and impotence may be the first clinical manifestation of diabetic neuropathy. However, when a careful neurologic examination is performed including measurement of the cystometrogram, other evidences of neurologic disturbance are usually uncovered. Many of the other polyneuropathies described in Chap. 354 have similar effects.

Vascular insufficiency causes impotence because blood flow into the vascular network of the penis is insufficient to obtain (or maintain) the erect state. The prototype of impaired penile blood supply is the Leriche syndrome. Here impedance to the blood flow into the penis occurs as the result of obstruction of the distal aorta. This usually presents as claudication and impotence; either can occur separately. Likewise, occlusion in smaller vessels supplying the penis can also lead to impotence. Together with neuropathy, vascular insufficiency contributes to the impotence in many men with diabetes mellitus. Decreased blood flow to the penis may be detected using the Doppler technique. By dividing the penile systolic blood pressure by the simultaneously determined supine brachial systolic pressure, the penile/brachial index is obtained. An index of over 0.75 is normal, and one of less than 0.6 is suggestive of vasculogenic impotence. An index of 0.6 to 0.75 is indeterminate. Due to overlap of such abnormal results with those in older potent men it is not possible to be certain that arterial insufficiency is the cause of impotence in a given individual. Normal values exclude arterial insufficiency; abnormal values require confirmatory arteriography.

TABLE 44-1 Some organic causes of erectile impotence in men

I Endocrine causes
- *A* Testicular failure (primary or secondary)
- *B* Hyperprolactinemia

II Drugs
- *A* Antihistamines
  - *1* Cimetidine
  - *2* Diphenhydramine
  - *3* Hydroxyzine
- *B* Antihypertensives
  - *1* Clonidine
  - *2* Methyldopa
  - *3* Propranolol
  - *4* Reserpine
  - *5* Spironolactone
  - *6* Thiazides
- *C* Anticholinergics
- *D* Antidepressants
  - *1* Amitriptyline
  - *2* Doxepin
  - *3* Isocarboxazid
- *E* Antipsychotics
  - *1* Chlorpromazine
  - *2* Haloperidol
  - *3* Thioridazine
- *F* Tranquilizers
  - *1* Diazepam
  - *2* Barbiturates
  - *3* Chlordiazepoxide
- *G* Drugs of habituation or addiction
  - *1* Alcohol
  - *2* Methadone
  - *3* Heroin

III Penile diseases
- *A* Previous priapism
- *B* Penile trauma
- *C* Peyronie's disease

IV Neurologic diseases
- *A* Anterior temporal lobe lesions
- *B* Diseases of the spinal cord
- *C* Loss of sensory input
  - *1* Diabetes mellitus and various polyneuropathies
  - *2* Tabes dorsalis
  - *3* Disease of dorsal root ganglia
- *D* Disease of nervi erigentes
  - *1* Complete prostatectomy
  - *2* Rectosigmoid operations
  - *3* Aortic bypass surgery

V Vascular disease
- *A* Leriche syndrome

Premature ejaculation This disorder seldom has an organic cause. It is usually related to anxiety in the sexual situation, unreasonable expectations about performance, or emotional disorder. A variety of successful therapeutic modalities have been described by Levine.

Absence of emission This symptom may be produced by (1) retrograde ejaculation, (2) sympathetic denervation, (3) androgen deficiency, or (4) drugs. Retrograde ejaculation may occur following surgery on the bladder neck or may develop spontaneously in diabetic men. Demonstration of sperm in a postcoital urine specimen will establish the diagnosis. Following sympathectomy or occasionally after extensive retroperitoneal surgery, the autonomic innervation of the prostate and seminal vesicles is lost, resulting in absence of smooth-muscle contraction at the time of ejaculation. Androgen deficiency results in a decrease in secretions of the prostate and seminal vesicles and in a diminution of the volume of ejaculate. Finally, drugs such as guanethidine, phenoxybenzamine, and phentolamine primarily impair ejaculation rather than erection or libido.

Absence of orgasm If libido and erectile function are normal, the absence of orgasm is almost always due to a psychiatric disorder.

Failure of detumescence Priapism is a persistent painful erection, often unrelated to sexual activity. Priapism is usually idiopathic but can be associated with sickle cell anemia, chronic granulocytic leukemia, or spinal cord injury. The disorder is thought to be secondary to clotting within the penile vascular network. The persistent erection disrupts the network and can lead to fibrosis and subsequent erectile impotence. Early surgical relief of priapism by shunting procedures may prevent subsequent impotence.

Evaluation of impotence The commonest cause of prolonged impotence is an anxiety or depression state. These closely related conditions can be diagnosed by the criteria enunciated in Chap. 11. Other psychological factors such as disinterest in the sexual partner, fear of sexual incompetence, marital discord, deviant sexual attitudes, worry, fatigue, and ill health often operate in various combinations to reduce sexual impulse. The central issue in the evaluation of impotence is to separate those instances due to psychological factors from those due to organic causes (Table 44-1). Usually, the separation can be made on the basis of history. From early childhood through the eighth decade, erections occur during normal sleep. This phenomenon, termed *nocturnal penile tumescence* (NPT), occurs during rapid eye movement sleep, and the total time of NPT averages 100 min per night. Consequently, if the impotent man gives a history of turgid erections under any circumstances (often when awakening in the early morning), the psychic, efferent neurologic, and circulatory systems that mediate erection are intact, and dysfunction is probably due to a psychiatric disorder. In these patients the physical and laboratory examinations should be limited. (Occasional patients with sensory neuropathy may have nocturnal erections.)

If the history of nocturnal erections is questionable, measurements of NPT can be made with the use of a strain gauge attached to a recorder. Alternatively, the penis can be wrapped with gummed, perforated paper; failure to break the perforations on three successive nights suggests absence of nocturnal erections. Although false-negative and false-positive results are possible, these procedures help to differentiate psychogenic and organic impotence. Interestingly, psychogenically impotent men may experience longer and more frequent nocturnal erections than do normal men. Other factors in favor of organic impotence include a similar degree of erectile dysfunction under all circumstances, onset not associated with any particular psychiatric symptomatology, a previous uninterrupted period of normal erectile function, and persistent sexual desire.

Having deduced an organic cause, the fundamental problem is the differential diagnosis of the etiology (Table 44-1). The history should be probed for symptoms of diabetes mellitus, symptoms of peripheral neuropathy or bladder dysfunction, symptoms referable to the vascular system such as intermittent claudication, and symptoms of local disease such as a history of priapism. A thorough drug history should be obtained, and inquiry concerning past operations that may have produced neurologic damage should be made.

Physical examination should include a thorough genital examination to identify abnormalities of the penis. The testes should be palpated for size and abnormal masses; if the length is less than 3.5 cm, hypogonadism should be considered. Evidence of feminization such as gynecomastia and abnormal body hair distribution should be sought. All pulses should be palpated, including the penile pulse, which can be felt by pressing both corpora between the thumb and forefinger and palpating to either side of the midline. However, because only a portion of the superficial dorsal arteries reach the corpus cavernosum, normal dorsal pulse pressures do not exclude the presence of deep cavernous arterial occlusion. If there is an indication from either history or physical examination of a vascular etiology, a Doppler procedure or arteriography may be indicated.

The neurologic exam should measure anal sphincter tone, perineal sensation, and the bulbocavernosus reflex. This reflex is elicited by squeezing the glans penis and noting the degree of anal sphincter constriction. An examination for peripheral neuropathy, including distal muscle weakness, loss of tendon reflexes in the legs, and tests for impairment of vibratory, position, tactile, and pain sensation should also be performed (see Chap. 354). In the absence of a concomitant neurogenic bladder, electromyographic sacral signal tracing of the bulbocavernosus reflex may be a useful ancillary procedure for detection of localized peripheral neuropathy; the methodology involves measurement of bulbocavernosus response latencies following electrical stimulation of the glans. Although this procedure has not been studied exhaustively, improvement by revascularization surgery is unlikely if the test is abnormal.

Laboratory evaluation is probably of minimal value. Measurement of serum testosterone in the absence of evidence of feminization or hypogonadism is seldom helpful.

Treatment of impotence Medical therapy with androgens offers little more than placebo benefit except in hypogonadal men. If a prolactin-secreting pituitary tumor is present, however, either surgical removal or treatment with bromocriptine usually results in return of potency. Surgical therapy may be useful in the treatment of decreased potency related to aortic obstruction; however, potency can be lost rather than improved after aortic operation if the autonomic nerve supply to the penis is damaged. This complication is minimized if an endarterectomy is done or, in a grafting procedure, if the reconstruction of the distal end is performed above the origin of the external iliac arteries.

A useful surgical technique for improvement of potency in refractory patients such as individuals with diabetic neuropathy is the implantation of a penile prosthesis, namely the insertion within the corpora of a small, blunt Silastic rod. The patient must be made aware that full erection is not produced and that the device only prevents buckling during intercourse. Furthermore, the complication rate is high in some series. Alternatively, an inflatable prosthetic device has been devised for implantation on either side of the corpora. A connecting reservoir of material is placed in the perivesicular space and pumps are located in the scrotum. By means of these pumps the penis can be made to become nearly fully erect at the appropriate time and to relax after intercourse. Intracavernous injections of papaverine and/or phentolamine in patients with nonvascular causes for impotence can cause transitory penile tumescence sufficient for coitus. Whether self-injection of these agents will be successful for the management of sexual dysfunction is not clear.

In the larger group of anxiety states and depressive illnesses, measures directed at their alleviation may restore sexual potency, and sexual counseling, education, and psychotherapy are beneficial in alleviating psychogenic factors.

REPRODUCTION

Approximately a tenth of marriages in the United States are barren, and another tenth result in fewer children than desired. The husband is the cause of the infertility in about a third of these marriages.

Infertility can be due to either disorders of the hypothalamic-pituitary system, disorders of the testes, or abnormalities of the ejaculatory system (Table 330-1). When obtaining a history, the physician should collect information about the duration of infertility, fertility in prior marriages of both the husband and wife, the presence of acquired or congenital disease that may lead to infertility, technique and frequency of intercourse, and family history of infertility. To exclude gross abnormalities of the endocrine system, the physical examination should evaluate the distribution of body hair, the presence of gynecomastia, the development of the scrotum and penis, the location of the urethral meatus, and the presence of normal vasa deferentia and epididymides. The size of each testis should be estimated. Because the seminiferous tubules account for more than 75 percent of the testicular mass, a reduction in testicular size (less than 3.5 cm in length) indicates a deficiency in the spermatogenic function of the testis. Finally, with the patient in the upright position, the Valsalva maneuver should be utilized to test for the presence of a varicocele.

The semen analysis provides a semiquantitative estimation of the severity of the dysfunction. The findings are usually considered normal if the semen coagulates and then liquefies, the volume is 2 to 5 mL, the sperm count is greater than 20 million per milliliter, more than 60 percent of the sperm are actively motile, and more than 60 percent have normal morphology. If no sperm are present, the term *azoospermia* is used; if sperm are present but the count is less than 20 million per milliliter, the patient is considered to have *oligospermia*. In the azoospermic man with normal-sized testes, the differential diagnosis includes hyalinization of the seminiferous tubules, Sertoli cell–only syndrome, gonadotropin deficiency, ductal obstruction, and maturation arrest. Plasma testosterone, LH (luteinizing hormone), and FSH (follicle-stimulating hormone) measurements are helpful in separating these conditions. With hyalinization of the seminiferous tubules LH and FSH are elevated, and plasma testosterone is low or borderline normal. Men with Sertoli cell–only syndrome usually have normal LH and testosterone, but elevated FSH levels. In gonadotropin deficiency LH, FSH, and testosterone are low, and in ductal obstruction or maturation arrest all endocrine studies are normal. To differentiate between the last two disorders, a testicular biopsy is necessary. In oligospermic patients, if the history and physical examination are normal, it is unlikely that any further laboratory investigation will be useful in defining the etiology. These patients are usually classified in the large group termed *idiopathic oligospermia*.

REFERENCES

Impotence

Benson GS: Mechanisms of penile erection. Invest Urol 19:65, 1981

Buvat J et al: Comparative investigations in 26 impotent and 26 nonimpotent diabetic patients. J Urol 133:34, 1985

Cole NJ: Drugs that influence sexual expression. Consultant 20:3281, 1980

Davidson JM et al: Effects of androgen on sexual behavior in hypogonadal men. J Clin Endocrinol 48:955, 1979

Ercole JJ et al: Changing surgical concepts in the treatment of priapism. J Urol 125:210, 1981

Fishman JF et al: Experience with inflatable penile prosthesis. Urology 23:86, 1984

Furlow WL (ed): Male sexual dysfunction. Urol Clin North Am 8:1, 1981

Levine SB: Marital sexual dysfunction: Ejaculation disturbances. Ann Intern Med 84:575, 1976

Lue TF et al: Hemodynamics of erection in the monkey. J Urol 130:1237, 1983

MARSHALL PG et al: Nocturnal penile tumescence with stamps: A comparative study under sleep laboratory conditions. J Urol 130:88, 1983
MEYER J: Disorders of sexual function, in *Williams Textbook of Endocrinology*, JD Wilson, DM Foster (eds). Philadelphia, Saunders, 1985, vol 7, pp 476–491
NATH RL et al: The multidisciplinary approach to vasculogenic impotence. Surgery 89:124, 1981
NEWMAN HF et al: Mechanism of human penile erection: An overview. Urology 17:399, 1981
SPARK RF et al: Impotence is not always psychogenic. JAMA 243:750, 1980
VAN ARSDALEN KN et al: Erectile physiology, dysfunction and evaluation: I. Physiology of erection. Monogr Urol 1983, 4:137–156
——— et al: Erectile physiology, dysfunction and evaluation: II. Etiology and evaluation of erectile dysfunction. Monogr Urol 1983, 4:165–185
WALSH PC et al: Impotence following radical prostatectomy: Insight into etiology and prevention. J Urol 128:492, 1982
WINTER CC: Priapism. Urol Surv 28:163, 1978
ZORGNIOTTI AW: Auto-injection of the corpus cavernosum with a vasoactive drug combination for vasculogenic impotence. J Urol 133:39, 1985

Infertility

AMELAR RD et al: *Male Infertility*. Philadelphia, Saunders, 1977, p 153
GREENBERG SH et al: Experience with 425 subfertile male patients. J Urol 119:507, 1970
SHERINS RJ et al: Male infertility, in *Campbell's Urology*, 5th ed, PC Walsh et al (eds). Philadelphia, Saunders, 1985, vol 1, chap 12

45 MEDICAL ASPECTS OF SEXUALITY

PETER REICH

Sexual problems are common in the general population. In one study of healthy, married, middle-aged couples, 40 percent of the men and 63 percent of the women had sexual dysfunctions, primarily impotence and premature ejaculation in men and inability to achieve orgasm in women. In another study 53 percent of outpatients in a general medical group practice described sexual problems when the issue was brought up by the physician during a medical evaluation.

These surveys also showed that patients tend to be reticent about sexual concerns unless they are asked about sexual function by their physicians. Only a fraction of those who were impotent had complained spontaneously of the problem in previous medical contacts. Even those patients who develop erectile dysfunction after taking medications frequently fail to report the problem. Married couples with sexual dysfunctions tend to modify their behavior to compensate for the problem rather than seek medical help.

The reason that many patients find it difficult to discuss sexuality with physicians has not been studied systematically. Some may be inhibited by shyness, embarrassment, guilt, shame, anxiety, or feelings of inadequacy. Old attitudes tend to persist in spite of the current openness about sexuality in general. A common finding in surveys of sexual dysfunction is that patients are often grateful when they are asked about their sexual function and generally perceive the physician as being more competent, thorough, and caring after such questions are asked.

TABLE 45-1 An outline of the sexual history recommended for the initial data base

Introductory question
1 Have you noticed any problems in your ability to have and enjoy sexual relations (sex)?
If positive response, have patient elaborate, then continue with questions.
If negative response, continue with questions.

Men
2 Do you have any problems having or maintaining an erection? If so, in what situations?
3 Do you have any problems having an orgasm (ejaculating) (coming) (too soon, or not soon enough)? If so, in what situations?

Women
2 Do you have any pain during penetration?
3 Do you have any difficulty coming to orgasm? If so, in what situations?

Men and women
4 Are you sexually active?
5 Has your present illness affected your sexual functioning?
6 Do you have any questions or concerns about your sexual functioning?

Clarification of problems
1 How much of a problem is this?
2 How long has this been a problem? When was it better or worse?
3 Do you have any ideas about what causes this problem?
4 Have you ever sought help for this or any other sexual concerns?
5 How do you feel about getting some help now?

SOURCE: *Ende et al.*

The physician in turn may inadvertently discourage the patient from bringing up sexual concerns by subtle indications of discomfort, disapproval, or embarrassment or by failing to ask appropriate and timely questions. Physicians may avoid the subject because of fears of starting an emotionally charged discussion with insufficient time to resolve it. In truth, most physicians can make an initial assessment of sexual symptoms, and a brief inquiry seldom leads to the need for a lengthy discussion.

An objective approach to sexual issues reduces tensions and enables both patient and physician to deal with sensitive material. Often patients harbor fears and misconceptions that may be relieved by open discussion. Sexual symptoms may be the first manifestation of organic disorders, and a change in sexual function at any time of life is an indication for a thorough medical evaluation. Thus, it is the responsibility of the physician to establish an accurate and complete diagnosis including both physiologic and psychological factors and to evaluate the significances of sexual problems in the context of the patient's background and lifestyle. The yield from this aspect of a general medical evaluation can be high in terms of relieving suffering, understanding the patient's medical status, and achieving a good doctor-patient relationship.

THE GENERAL APPROACH TO THE PATIENT More often than in other areas of medicine, the physician needs to take an active role in initiating the discussion of sexual matters. The inclusion of routine screening questions in the review of systems is one way to ensure that the area is not overlooked. Sexuality can be brought up comfortably after questions about menstrual function in women or questions about urinary function in men. Some clinicians prefer linking questions about sexual function to inquiries about relationships and personal satisfactions. To be effective, screening questions should be nonspecific, should not assume that the patient is heterosexual, and should project a nonjudgmental attitude.

Table 45-1 gives an outline of the brief sexual history recommended by Ende et al. for screening purposes. Similar guides can be found in standard texts of psychiatry and of obstetrics and gynecology. It is useful to have such a framework in mind when obtaining a sexual history. A detailed guide to the assessment of sexual function has been published by the Group for Advancement of Psychiatry.

Screening questions vary with the age and the circumstances of the patient. Such questions should be routine or the physician may overlook problems, may return to the subject as an afterthought, or may experience tension or show embarrassment when trying to think of a screening question during the history.

When a sexual complaint is elicited or volunteered, a detailed history of the manifestations and associated symptoms should be obtained. The assessment of a sexual problem is similar to the assessment of a problem involving any other system. The history of a sexual complaint necessarily includes information about relationships with partners; tensions, anxieties, preconceptions, attitudes, and interpersonal factors must be taken into account. A complete history that includes careful attention to multiple determinants, a thorough evaluation of the patient as a person, and a consideration of the context of the symptoms usually yields a working diagnosis that enables the physician either to treat the patient or to make an appropriate referral.

The physician has the special responsibility of initiating a discussion of sexuality when coexisting medical problems are likely to affect sexual function. Patients may fear sexual activity after myocardial infarction or episodes of cardiac arrhythmia or may anticipate loss of sexual function after transurethral prostatectomy, hysterectomy, or other procedures or conditions involving the urogenital tract. Other disorders affect sexuality directly or indirectly through loss of libido or changes in body image (Chaps. 43 and 44). By anticipating sexual problems the physician can help the patient make adjustments and can sometimes prevent disorders that are secondary to fears or misconceptions.

Reassurances about confidentiality may be necessary during the discussion of sexual matters even though such confidentiality is ordinarily assumed in the doctor-patient relationship. The assurance of confidentiality is especially important when the physician also treats other members of the family or when the patient needs to discuss extramarital, deviant, or extralegal behavior.

The dignity of the patient should be kept in mind as the history is taken by observing such simple practices as using scientific words for sexual parts and sexual activities. Vernacular or slang expressions, which are sometimes used in a mistaken effort to put the patient at ease, and jokes or other informal remarks should be avoided even with a patient who uses them. Comments that may seem casual to the physician tend to live on in the patient's mind.

Anticipation of discomfort may lead physicians to choose an evasive route of inquiry while patients might appreciate a direct question. Alternatively, some patients allude to sexual problems indirectly with idiomatic phrases, such as "changing nature" or "problems in relationships"; unless the physician is sensitive to feelings and language the reference may be missed, and the patient may assume that the physician is not interested in further information. Sometimes sexual problems appear indirectly through other complaints relating to the urogenital system.

Two types of patients—the elderly and the homosexual—present special problems in regard to the evaluation of sexual function. The sexuality of elderly patients is often not well understood by physicians. With reasonable health, men retain sexual interest and potency into old age. Impotence at any age is pathologic. Women also retain their sexual response but are more likely to suffer loss of their partner. Physicians may refrain from asking questions because they incorrectly assume that sexual satisfactions can no longer be achieved because of the aging process. Alternatively, patients silently accept a loss of sexual function because of similar misconceptions about the effects of illness or of aging. Depression may be a factor in such instances. Here the questions of the physician, coupled with some reassuring statements about the tendencies of many persons to assume mistakenly they will never be able to enjoy sexual relations again, bring the issue into the open and awaken new hopes in the patient.

Homosexual patients with disorders of sexual function often do not receive sympathetic medical care from heterosexual physicians. In one study of gynecologic care for lesbians a major hindrance in communication was the assumption by physicians that all patients are heterosexual. Homosexual men have similar problems in relating to heterosexual physicians. Some homosexual patients prefer going to homosexual physicians or to clinics run by homophile organizations. Many physicians share with the public at large serious misconceptions about homosexual behavior.

Kinsey and his coworkers showed how common homosexuality is in western societies. In his survey of more than 16,000 American men and women, Kinsey reported that approximately 4 percent of the men and 2 percent of the women are exclusively homosexual throughout their lives, and another 13 percent of the men are predominantly homosexual for at least 3 years of their lives. Occasional or intermittent homosexual contact was common in men and women. Approximately one-third of the men surveyed had had one or more homosexual contacts after puberty. In studies of homosexual men and women no association has been found between homosexuality and family structure, childhood experiences, or parental influences. Early gender nonconformity was the only predictor of homosexual development. Homosexuality was not a conscious choice of the individual but appeared to arise in a predetermined pattern. Homosexuality is also not associated with psychopathology or personality disorder and is compatible with normal productivity in society. In spite of increased acceptance of homosexuality in our culture, gay men and lesbian women often encounter personal rejection and job discrimination. Expectations of rejection may lead patients to conceal homosexuality from their physicians.

With the current epidemic of the acquired immunodeficiency syndrome (AIDS) in homosexual males, it is especially important for the physician to know the sexual orientation of male patients. This information may also provide insight into other disorders to which homosexual men are predisposed, such as hepatitis and proctitis. Homosexual women may also receive better medical care when their sexual orientation is understood. As in other areas of sexuality, a simple direct approach to the issue is generally welcomed by the patient. One experienced clinician advocates asking all patients whether they are homosexual or heterosexual; others simply ask all patients to identify their sexual preference. Whether or not AIDS is a clinical concern, male homosexual patients may be suffering from hidden fears of the disease and would be relieved by an explicit discussion. Even married patients may have covert homosexual activities that have important clinical implications. The parents of homosexual individuals often appeal to physicians for help. They need the reassurance that it is not their fault and that their children can lead satisfying, productive lives while accepting their homosexual orientation. It is important to emphasize that homosexuality is not a disorder and is not associated with psychopathology. It is not a choice taken by the individual and is not amenable to change.

EVALUATION Once a sexual complaint has been elicited, a detailed history of specific behavior should be obtained. Terms for sexual disorders may be misused, exaggerated, or misunderstood by patients. Other sexual complaints reflect misconceptions, ignorance, or fears, and the problems prove to be nonexistent when the behavior is explored in detail. Patients may overestimate or underestimate the extent of a problem, depending upon their psychological orientation. For example, one woman believed herself to be frigid because her sexual partner, for neurotic reasons of his own, compared her in a disparaging way to his previous partners. Much can be learned from the first instance of a sexual problem, from the pattern of behavior after the onset of symptoms, and from inquiring whether the problem is present consistently or varies with the circumstances or nature of the sexual practice.

In every disorder there is a complex interaction between the physical and the emotional, and every sexual symptom needs to be evaluated in the context of the relationships between the patient and the sexual partners and in the context of the sexual practices and attitudes of the patient. A past history, including early experiences, attitudes of parents, and attitudes toward childhood sexuality, development, marriage, and pregnancy may be relevant. Establishing the relationship of sexual function to general health is of fundamental importance, and it is essential to take a complete drug history on every patient, both in regard to drug abuse and to use of prescribed drugs. An understanding of the daily habits of a patient may provide important clues to diagnosis. Fatigue, anxiety, and stress, as well as the timing of the use of alcohol, drugs, and medications, can provide insight into the underlying cause.

A general physical examination with special attention to an examination of the genitalia is essential. At times patients conceal or are unaware of abnormalities of the genitalia. On the other hand, otherwise sophisticated patients may harbor irrational misconceptions or feelings of shame about their bodies and may require concrete reassurance about the adequacy of the genital apparatus. Even if the diagnosis is that of a psychogenic basis for the sexual dysfunction, the patient may disregard assurances that there is no organic basis unless the workup for possible medical causes of the complaint has been thorough.

Appropriate laboratory tests to screen for systemic illnesses together with the specific test for various endocrinopathies, neurologic conditions, and other systemic disorders that may present with sexual problems may be indicated (see Chaps. 43 and 44). Attention to the mental status, including assessment of mood, affect, thought content, judgment, and reality testing, enables the physician to determine whether the sexual symptom is an aspect of a mental disorder. Rarely, sexual problems, especially loss of libido, may be the presenting sign of a disorder of the central nervous system; an examination of mental status can reveal early signs of dementia or of other organic brain conditions.

DIAGNOSTIC CONSIDERATIONS Specific disorders of sexual function are discussed in Chaps. 43 and 44. All of them can vary in severity, from complete loss of function under all circumstances to relatively minor disturbances in specific circumstances or with specific partners. Patients also may vary in their reactions to sexual symptoms, some ignoring or concealing severe disability, others reacting with panic about minor disturbances.

When significant organic factors are present, a useful distinction can be made between sexual symptoms that arise *directly* from organic disorders, such as structural disorders of the urogenital system, neurologic disorders affecting the innervation of the sexual organs, and endocrinopathies that influence sexual physiology, and those that are *secondary* to changes in general health, such as sexual disturbances associated with rheumatoid arthritis, malignancies, renal failure, and other chronic diseases, or those that occur with acute debilitating conditions, such as myocardial infarction, major surgery, and hepatitis. Patients with primary organic disorders may need counseling to help them adjust to permanent losses of sexual function if medical measures cannot reverse the process. Although libido may be affected adversely by a general loss of vitality and by toxic and metabolic factors, the sexual disturbances associated with physical illnesses can also be the expression of hopelessness, depression, or anxiety and may be perpetuated by psychological factors long after the organic problems have disappeared. Persistent sexual dysfunction after a heart attack may reflect fear of sudden death during sexual excitement.

The apparent absence of an organic etiology does not necessarily mean a sexual dysfunction is psychogenic. Subtle vascular or neurologic changes not found on routine evaluations of impotence may underly some instances of erectile dysfunction. The diagnosis of psychogenic impotence should be reserved for cases in which positive evidence of emotional disturbance can be found. Psychological factors that can interfere with the sexual response include fears and conflicts about sex, emotional disturbances that are antithetical to sexual excitement, and anger or dissatisfaction with a partner. Once a sexual failure has occurred for any reason, performance anxiety can develop and lead to further impairment by worry about subsequent encounters. In one study of impotence only 14 percent of cases were diagnosed as psychogenic. In many instances of sexual dysfunction, psychological factors interact with an organic vulnerability to produce overt symptoms.

Primary psychogenic disturbances, those that have been present since puberty, can be distinguished from *secondary* disturbances, those that represent decompensations from previous adequate levels of function. The former often reflect chronic and deep-seated sexual conflicts. When a patient seeks help for a chronic disturbance, the key diagnostic issue may be why help has been sought at this particular time. A secondary decompensation may be the presenting symptom of a psychological defeat or a disturbance in a relationship. Some sexual problems occur in connection with life stresses or transitions, such as retirement, pregnancy, work crises, or bereavement.

Other sexual disorders are manifestations of major mental disorders and respond only to treatment directed at the mental disorders themselves. Diminished sexual responsiveness, impotence, or ejaculatory disturbances may be indications of depression. Bizarre sexual complaints with increased or diminished sexual activity can indicate incipient psychosis. The strange qualities of the symptoms or the intensity of the associated feelings may be the best diagnostic clue to the presence of a psychosis. Hypersexuality can also occur with the onset of mania or as a manifestation of depression, especially in postmenopausal women.

Alcohol may play a significant role in impairment of potency. Often the first episode of secondary impotence is associated with the use of alcohol, and the midlife depressive syndrome that is often related to secondary impotence may be further complicated by alcohol abuse. Barbiturates and opiates also can cause reduced libido and impotence. Antihypertensive agents, tranquilizers, hypnotics, analgesics, and sedatives may also impair sexual function, particularly in the male.

Sexual disturbances may develop after traumatic incidents. For example, impotence can develop after cystoscopic examination or after vasectomy, even though neither procedure has any direct physiologic effect upon sexual function. An automobile accident, assault, pregnancy, contraceptive difficulties, disturbing sexual encounters, and a host of other emotionally significant episodes may cause sudden changes in sexual functioning. In women, either sexual assault or childhood sexual abuse can lead to long-standing sexual inhibition and dysfunctions. Many women are reluctant to share the history of a rape or of an incestuous experience; others may have little memory of traumatic events, especially when they occurred in childhood, although these events may exert a profound effect on adult sexuality.

The diligent physician may inadvertently overdiagnose sexual disturbances. Most patients have self-doubts and sexual dissatisfactions even though they are functioning adequately. It is well to have in mind the concept of a threshold of disturbance to separate the normal vicissitudes from problems that require treatment.

TREATMENT Some sexual problems resolve spontaneously during the evaluation process, especially during an extensive workup. With those problems that persist, the physician must decide whether to treat the patients or to refer them elsewhere. The management of sexual dysfunction due to organic causes is described in Chaps. 43, 44, 330, and 331; sexual problems related to such physical illnesses are appropriately handled by the same physician who treats the physical disorder. Generally, the secondary or reactive psychogenic disorders are most amenable to brief counseling, especially when they occur in response to stress. Patients with more deep-seated problems may best be handled by psychiatrists.

The technique for counseling by the family physician cannot be mapped in a formal way. Sufficient time, a relaxed atmosphere, and genuine interest shown by the physician are necessary. The patient should be encouraged to tell the full story with careful attention to the circumstances surrounding the onset of symptoms, to the attitudes of the patient and partner, to the nature of the patient's relationships, and to factors that might lead to anxiety or depression. Although it may be necessary to review the physical details of the sexual practices, resolution of symptoms may occur with only indirect reference to sexual techniques. Sexual inadequacies often produce anxiety, which in turn leads to further defeats and to inhibition of libido. Without reduction of anxiety and lifting of depression, the process cannot be reversed.

Some physicians choose not to attempt sexual counseling, while others find it a satisfying aspect of practice. In either case, physicians should be familiar with the resources in their communities and understand the capabilities and limitations of various treatments. Physicians who do not undertake sexual counseling themselves usually have referral relationships with gynecologists, urologists, and psychiatrists. In addition, many communities have family services and counseling services. Referral should be tailored to the problems and to the lifestyle and personality of the patient. Some patients prefer to discuss the intimate details of a sexual problem only with a gynecologist or urologist. Others should be directed to a reputable clinic where behavioral approaches to the treatment of sexual dysfunctions are available.

Referral is often a difficult transition for a patient because it implies turning to a stranger after having confided in a physician who has understood the problem. A previously eager patient may lose motivation when referred elsewhere. Some physicians have counselors associated with them in their offices. This system has the advantage of maintaining the personal relationship between counselors and physicians but has the disadvantage of encouraging physicians to rely on counselors for the evaluation of emotional problems rather than carrying through the diagnostic phase themselves. If physicians keep in touch with patients through the process of therapy, it enables them to evaluate the efficacy of the treatment program and to provide support and reassurance.

A few examples will illustrate some of the principles involved in the treatment of patients with sexual disorders.

A.R., a 56-year-old attorney who had recently suffered a myocardial infarct, complained to his physician of loss of libido. He was an energetic, competitive, aggressive self-made man, who enjoyed athletics and was "top man" in his firm. The physician asked him about the details of his daily life and found that the loss of libido was only one of many inhibitions. He avoided arguments, stopped playing handball, reduced his work load, lost weight, and developed insomnia and anorexia. Further questioning revealed fears of sudden death and the fatalistic belief that his days were numbered. He assumed that strict reduction of activity was mandatory. His wife shared his fears and urged him to avoid stress. Together they had decided not to have sexual relations during the period immediately after his heart attack, and he had no desire to resume. In the course of several sessions of counseling the physician reassured him that his fears were exaggerated and that many patients with heart trouble experienced similar feelings, clarified the extent of his disability, and helped him and his wife to plan realistic resumption of many of his previous activities, including sexual relations.

L.D., a 26-year-old woman, consulted a physician because of frigidity. She had left her husband after 6 years of an unfulfilling marriage and had sought satisfaction in a series of brief affairs. The interview revealed a restless, competitive, chronically dissatisfied person who was unhappy in her career and experienced disappointment in close relationships. After careful evaluation of the physical aspects of her sexual difficulties and experiences, the physician decided that her problem reflected long-standing psychological conflicts and referred her to a psychiatrist.

M.B., a 34-year-old salesman, complained to his physician of impotence. He was a nervous, insecure, ineffectual man who worked for his older brother. His wife, an active real estate broker, had become withdrawn and bitter, and his two adolescent children were involved in minor delinquency. The impotence was confined to his relationship with his wife; in a recent extramarital affair he had performed adequately. He said he was unable to satisfy his wife in any way; she was either withdrawn or overly demanding. The physician determined that the impotency had no organic basis and referred the patient to a service agency where the family could be worked with as a unit. Here the wife was found to be depressed and received psychiatric treatment. Later the patient reported that when her depression improved, his potency returned.

C.W., a woman with breast cancer, was asked about her marriage. She reported that her husband had stopped having sexual relations with her when it was discovered that she had metastatic disease. The physician then saw the husband, who confessed to an extramarital affair and the wish to leave his wife. He also described irrational anger directed to his wife and feelings of shame and worthlessness. It emerged that the marriage had been an unusually close one and that he could not bear the anticipation of his wife's death. Sexual contact with her reminded him of his impending loss. His anger and the extramarital affair were responses to grief. The physician met with him for several sessions. By avoiding a moralistic position and by indicating that many spouses of patients with serious diseases have similar feelings and may even find solace in extramarital relationships, the physician helped him to overcome his shame and to share his grief. The process brought dramatic relief, and with occasional contact with the physician he was able to remain with his wife and be helpful to her throughout her terminal illness.

MARITAL COUNSELING BY THE PHYSICIAN The evaluation of sexual problems almost invariably requires some attention to marital or other sexual relationships. Counseling that focuses primarily on these relationships has been designated *marital counseling*. Instead of the usual medical relationship, which emphasizes the individual patient, marital counseling involves both partners, although each may be seen separately at times.

The specific nature of the counseling depends upon the complaints or upon the time of life of the couple. The main requisite is a willingness for physicians to set aside time for this kind of undertaking and to develop an interest in the functional health of patients beyond the specific issues raised by disease. The stresses and transitions in the early years of a marriage should be appreciated as well as the pressures exerted by children. In later years, job problems and conflicts over roles may emerge, followed by development of the "empty nest" syndrome, menopausal and midlife issues, and the male-depressive syndrome as horizons close in and the realities of aging appear.

Most marital problems are not due to sexual difficulties, although sexual problems may be the leading edge, especially in the climate where sexual adjustment is so widely publicized. Sexual satisfaction is dependent on the broader aspects of the relationship between partners and on mental and physical health. The alert physician should probe to these deeper levels during marriage counseling. In this sense, counseling about sexual problems is dependent upon the successful outcome of marriage counseling. Early in the approach the motivation of both partners should be assessed. If one partner is determined to break up the marriage, the counseling may consist of communicating this information to the other partner and perhaps advising legal assistance. On the other hand, apparent determination to seek divorce by either partner needs to be evaluated because it may mask depression, a paranoid reaction, or a hidden problem that is being avoided by flight, such as shame over an affair, fear, illness, or personal failure.

In marital counseling, as with other medical counseling, it is well to avoid giving direct advice about interpersonal relationships. By defining the problem, the physician may enable the patient to arrive at a decision on a course of action. By taking sides in family conflicts or by espousing an ethical position, physicians can inadvertently introduce their own biases or allow themselves to be manipulated by one of the marital partners.

REFERENCES

BELL AP et al: *Sexual Preference: Its Development in Men and Women.* Bloomington, Indiana University Press, 1981

ENDE J et al: The sexual history in general medicine practice. Arch Intern Med 144:558, 1984

FRANK E et al: Frequency of sexual dysfunction in "normal" couples. N Engl J Med 299:111, 1978

GROUP FOR THE ADVANCEMENT OF PSYCHIATRY, COMMITTEE ON MEDICAL EDUCATION: *Assessment of Sexual Function.* New York, Jason Aronson, 1974

KOLODNY RC et al: *Textbook of Sexual Medicine.* Boston, Little, Brown, 1979

LIEF HI et al: *Sexual Problems in Medical Practice.* American Medical Association, 1981

LUDEMAN K: The sexuality of the older person: Review of the literature. Gerontologist 21:203, 1981

MAGGEE MC; Psychogenic impotence: A critical review. Urology 15:435, 1980

MEYER J: Disorders of sexual function, in *Williams' Textbook of Endocrinology,* 7th ed, JD Wilson, DW Foster (eds). Philadelphia, Saunders, 1985, p 312

MUNJACK DJ, OZIER LJ: *Sexual Medicine and Counseling in Office Practice: A Comprehensive Treatment Guide.* Boston, Little, Brown, 1980

SLAGG MF et al: Impotence in medical clinic outpatients. JAMA 249:1736, 1983

46 HIRSUTISM AND VIRILIZATION

WILLIAM J. KOVACS / JEAN D. WILSON

Hirsutism, the growth of hair in women in a pattern characteristic of men, is a common and perplexing problem. The distribution and growth of hair in normal persons is under complex genetic and endocrine control so that there is considerable variability in hair growth in normal men and women. As a consequence, abnormal hair growth is sometimes difficult to define: Some patients may seek medical attention because of what the physician may consider an insignificant cosmetic defect. Others, because of personal or cultural differences, may be undisturbed by surprising degrees of hirsutism. The central issue in dealing with such patients is the separation of those infrequent instances in which hirsutism is a manifestation of an underlying virilizing or defeminizing syndrome from the vast majority of hirsute women in whom excess hair is fundamentally a cosmetic problem.

CONTROL OF NORMAL HAIR GROWTH AND DISTRIBUTION **Endocrine control** Androgens are the major determinants of hair distribution in both sexes. There are three principal circulating androgens in women—dehydroepiandrosterone, derived from the adrenal; androstenedione, which is derived equally from adrenal and ovary; and testosterone, which is both secreted by the ovary and adrenal and formed in peripheral tissue from circulating dehydroepiandrosterone and androstenedione. The production of adrenal androgen is regulated primarily by ACTH, while ovarian androgen secretion is regulated by luteinizing hormone (LH). These various androgens must be converted to testosterone (or dihydrotestosterone) before they can bind to the androgen receptor of target cells and induce an androgenic response. Thus, adrenal androgens virilize only in so far as they serve as precursors for testosterone and dihydrotestosterone.

Several types of relationships can be defined between hair growth and androgens in normal individuals. Eyebrows, eyelashes, and lanugo (fine, downy hair) are not dependent on androgens, while axillary and lower pubic hair are sensitive to the small amounts of androgen secreted by the adrenal. Hair in these regions therefore grows approximately equally in men and women. Hair growth in areas typical of males appears to require the greater androgen levels normally produced by the testes; such areas include the face, upper pubic triangle, chest, and ears. Finally, scalp hair exhibits androgen-mediated regression. The reason different body regions respond differently to the same or similar androgen is unknown. Theoretically, the metabolism of androgens might differ in the various sites, or hormone receptors might vary. The hair follicle, like some other androgen-responsive cells, requires conversion of testosterone to dihydrotestosterone for expression of androgen action, and hair follicles from all regions of the body perform this conversion equally well. Moreover, the same receptor that is essential for androgen action in other cells (Chap. 330) is necessary for the action of dihydrotestosterone in the hair follicle. Genetic disorders with normal testosterone production but absent androgen receptor have deficient or absent axillary, pubic, facial, truncal, and limb hair (Chap. 333). Regional differences in androgen responsiveness of hair in normal individuals may be the consequence of regional differences in the amount of androgen receptor in hair follicles.

Genetic factors Despite similar hormone levels, there is considerable diversity in the distribution of hair between individuals and among different racial groups in regard to facial, truncal, and pubic hair. Dark-haired, darkly pigmented whites of either sex tend to be more hirsute than blond or fair-skinned persons. Orientals, American Indians, and blacks on average are less hirsute than whites. Orientals rarely have facial or body hair except in the pubic and axillary regions, and American Indians, in addition, rarely develop baldness in either sex. Heterogeneity of hair patterns also exists within families.

TABLE 46-1 Clinical signs of defeminization and virilization

Signs of defeminization	Signs of virilization
Amenorrhea	Frontal balding
Decrease in breast size	Increase in size of shoulder girdle muscles
Loss of female body contours	Clitoromegaly
	Coarsening of the voice
	Acne

SOURCE: *After Karp L, Herrmann WL: Diagnosis and treatment of hirsutism in women. Obstet Gynecol 41:283, 1973*

The inheritance of hair patterns is complex and probably polygenic in nature.

Other factors Aging is a prerequisite for the expression of some types of hair development. For example, in men hair on the trunk and extremities frequently increases for several years after maximal levels of plasma androgens have been reached. Conversely, loss of androgen may not result in diminution of normal hair growth in men or reverse hirsutism completely in women. The appearance of pubic hair is frequently the heralding event of puberty in females. Women in the first trimester of pregnancy commonly observe increased hairiness of the face, extremities, and breasts. Menopause is often associated with the loss of hair in the pubic area, axillae, and extremities, whereas growth of hair on the face increases in postmenopausal women. The physiologic basis for these changes is unclear and cannot be explained entirely by changes in androgen levels.

PATHOLOGIC HAIR GROWTH AND DISTRIBUTION In evaluating women for hirsutism the most important feature is whether virilization or defeminization is also present (Table 46-1). In patients with overproduction of androgen defeminizing signs, such as disturbances of menstruation, are more consistent than are the signs of virilization. Virilization should be interpreted with caution for at least two reasons. First, signs of virilization (clitoromegaly, balding, coarsening of the hair, hirsutism) indicate androgen excess at some time in the patient's life but do not necessarily mean that active disease is present at the time of evaluation. It is necessary to measure plasma androgen levels and/or production rates to determine if androgen excess is ongoing. Second, severe overandrogenization may exist in the absence of marked virilization; i.e., at the same level of androgen production clitoromegaly may be present in one patient and not another.

Diagnostic considerations DRUGS Excessive hair growth can be caused by drugs that do not produce other defeminizing or virilizing signs. Such drugs include phenytoin, minoxidil, diazoxide, and hexachlorobenzene. Androgens produce hirsutism as well as virilization. Some synthetic progestogens have androgenic activity.

TUMORS The rapid onset of hair growth with or without accompanying signs of frank virilization suggests a neoplastic source of androgen. Such tumors include androgen-secreting adenomas and carcinomas of the adrenal and ovarian tumors such as arrhenoblastoma, which secrete androgens directly, and Krukenberg tumors of the ovary, which stimulate the surrounding ovarian stromal tissue to produce excess androgen.

POLYCYSTIC OVARIAN DISEASE The most common cause of ovarian hyperandrogenism is polycystic ovarian disease. This disorder has a broad clinical spectrum that ranges from mild hirsutism to complete amenorrhea and virilization. The salient feature for the diagnosis is the pubertal onset of chronic anovulation and hirsutism; enlarged cystic ovaries, obesity, and amenorrhea (i.e., the Stein-Leventhal syndrome) are present in only half or fewer of women with this disorder and need not be present for the diagnosis (see Chap. 331). The fundamental abnormality in polycystic ovarian disease is not fully understood. Elevation of plasma LH concentration causes enhanced androgen secretion by stromal and thecal cells of the ovary.

ATTENUATED FORMS OF ADRENAL HYPERPLASIA The adrenal can also be the source of excess androgen in the absence of tumor. Heritable defects in adrenal steroidogenesis (congenital adrenal hyperplasia) such as 21-hydroxylase deficiency, 11β-hydroxylase deficiency, and 3β-hydroxysteroid dehydrogenase deficiency can produce virilization, and each of these enzyme deficiencies can occur in a "late-onset" form in which hirsutism or virilization and menstrual irregularities appear at the time of expected puberty or in adulthood (see Chap. 333). The clinical presentation in these cases may be indistinguishable from polycystic ovarian disease. Late-onset 21-hydroxylase deficiency is most common and has been most extensively studied; its incidence in the general population of hirsute, oligomenorrheic women is probably on the order of a few percent. The presence of elevated plasma levels of adrenal androgens (such as dehydroepiandrosterone sulfate) or of dexamethasone-suppressible hyperandrogenism does not necessarily imply that the overandrogenization is due to a specific adrenal steroidogenic defect, but these findings may be useful as a guide to therapy.

IDIOPATHIC HIRSUTISM In many women with hirsutism a specific diagnosis cannot be made. The term idiopathic hirsutism applies to those women with evidence of androgen excess but with normal menses, normal-sized ovaries, no evidence of tumors of the adrenal or ovary, and normal adrenal function. Slight elevations of plasma androstenedione and testosterone are commonly present in such women, and testosterone production rates are increased above normal, although to a lesser degree than in patients with polycystic ovarian disease.

Experience with the antiandrogen cyproterone acetate (not available in the United States) indicates that this form of hirsutism is androgen-mediated, since therapy results in improvement. Women with idiopathic hirsutism could constitute the extreme end of a normal continuum of androgen production or represent a true pathologic subset. Some women with the tentative diagnosis of idiopathic hirsutism actually have mild or early polycystic ovarian disease, but in most, hirsutism is not accompanied by or followed by signs of ovarian dysfunction. If such women are merely extremes of the normal range of androgen production, then their hirsutism is fundamentally a cosmetic defect.

DIAGNOSTIC EVALUATION The decision as to when to undertake a complex diagnostic evaluation depends on several factors. Such evaluation is appropriate in all women with hirsutism and virilization; whether it should be performed in women with isolated hirsutism depends upon the severity, distribution, and rate of hair growth. An approach to the diagnostic evaluation of hirsute patients is shown in Fig. 46-1. The clinical history is taken with particular attention to drug ingestion and to the details of pubertal development and menstrual history and their relation to the onset of excessive hair growth. The physical examination is directed to the assessment of sites of growth of androgen-dependent hair (pubic, axillary, facial, truncal, and extremity) and evaluation for signs of virilization, which correlate with higher levels of androgen overproduction and raise the concern of androgen-producing neoplasms. Such signs include laryngeal enlargement (deepening of the voice), temporal balding, clitoromegaly, and increased muscle mass in the limb girdles. Signs of cortisol excess (plethora, centripetal obesity, striae, and cervical and supraclavicular fat pads) should also be sought. Pelvic examination should include a search for palpable ovarian masses. Appropriate laboratory tests include measurement of serum androgens and, when appropriate, radiologic imaging of ovaries and adrenal glands. Basal measurements of dehydroepiandrosterone sulfate greater than 800 ng/dL or of serum testosterone over 200 ng/dL suggest neoplastic sources of androgen excess; plasma testosterone levels in the normal range are more difficult to interpret because total levels in women do not necessarily reflect the free or unbound levels of hormone under conditions when testosterone-binding globulin levels are either increased or decreased. Suspected Cushing's syndrome should be evaluated with standard dexamethasone supression testing if a screening test (such as urinary free cortisol excretion or overnight dexamethasone suppression test) is abnormal. The diagnosis of polycystic ovarian disease is made from the history and clinical features in a woman with chronic anovulation. Women with severe hirsutism associated with cystic acne may be screened for delayed-onset adrenal hyperplasia by the short cosyntropin stimulation test and measurement of plasma 17-hydroxyprogesterone (see Chap. 325).

MANAGEMENT In the case of drug-induced hirsutism and neoplastic disease of the ovary or adrenals treatment is straightforward; administration of the drugs should be stopped, or the tumor should be removed. Adrenal steroidogenic defects are treated with glucocorticoids to suppress excess ACTH and hence inhibit adrenal androgen secretion. In most instances (polycystic ovarian disease as well as idiopathic hirsutism) both cosmetic treatment and suppression of androgen production or antagonism of its action at the receptor level need to be employed.

Cosmetic therapy is directed at the concealment or removal of hair from exposed skin areas. Small amounts of hair can be bleached with hydrogen peroxide. Methods for removal of hair are classified as depilatory (removal of hair from the surface of the skin) or epilatory (removal of the intact hair with the root). Depilatory techniques include shaving and chemical methods. Shaving does not have an adverse effect on hair growth rate or coarseness (although the blunt ends may feel coarse), but shaving of areas other than axillae or legs is unacceptable to most women. Chemical depilatories are effective for limited areas of hair removal and are generally safe if used properly. Most available depilatories are substituted mercaptans, such as thioglycollic acid, which reduce the disulfide bonds in the peptide chains of keratin. The hair fiber swells and softens to a consistency that can be washed from the skin. Care must be taken to avoid skin irritation because of the alkalinity of these preparations. Temporary epilation can be achieved by plucking (useful only for isolated hairs) or wax treatment. The waxes are melted and applied to the skin.

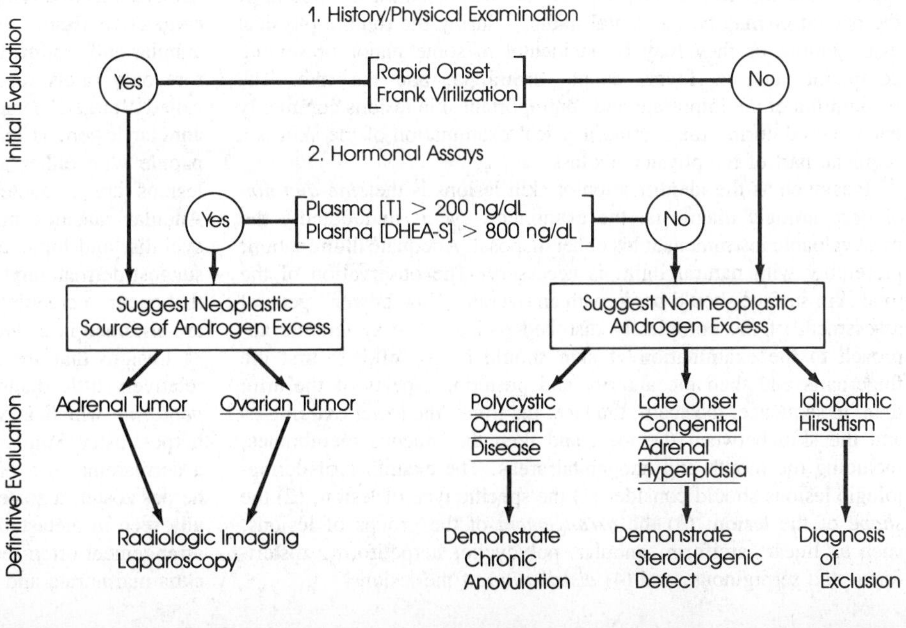

FIGURE 46-1 *Diagnostic approach to the hirsute patient. T = testosterone; DHEA-S = dehydroepiandrosterone sulfate.*

When the wax cools and sets, it is stripped off, removing hair with it. The procedure is uncomfortable, and best results can be obtained by salon treatments. Permanent epilation can be achieved only by electrolysis. The treatments are expensive and time-consuming, and success depends on the skill of the electrologist.

While cosmetic treatment is undertaken, attempts to suppress androgen overproduction may also be appropriate. Treatment with combination oral contraceptives suppresses ovarian androgen secretion when restoration of fertility is not an objective. To minimize side effects the lowest effective dosage of estrogen should be used. Women over 35 years of age, smokers, and those with hypertension, a history of thromboembolic disease, impaired liver function, or suspected estrogen-dependent neoplasm should not be treated with oral contraceptives. Suppression of adrenal androgen overproduction can be achieved with small doses of dexamethasone and is useful in the treatment of women with late-onset 21-hydroxylase deficiency.

Antagonism of the effects of androgens at the hair follicle is the basis for the other main treatment modality, the antiandrogens. Cyproterone acetate has been used with success but is unavailable in the United States. Spironolactone has a dual action of blocking the androgen receptor and of inhibiting androgen production and is a useful alternative therapy. Cimetidine also binds to the androgen receptor and acts as an androgen antagonist, but it is not of general benefit in the treatment of hirsutism.

If pharmacologic therapy is undertaken, the patient should be prepared to make a commitment of 6 months for an adequate trial of efficacy. Even when treatment is long-term, dramatic reversal of established hair growth is unlikely to be achieved by interference with androgen synthesis or action. Such hormonal manipulations can arrest or slow the rate of hair growth, but established hair must be dealt with by use of cosmetic treatment.

REFERENCES

CUMMING DC et al: Treatment of hirsutism with spironolactone. J Am Med Assoc 247:1295, 1982

GIVENS JR: Normal and abnormal androgen metabolism. Clin Obstet Gynecol 21:115, 1978

KIRSCHNER MA et al: Idiopathic hirsutism—an ovarian abnormality. N Engl J Med 294:637, 1976

KUTTENN F et al: Late-onset adrenal hyperplasia in hirsutism. N Engl J Med 313:224, 1985

LUCKY AW et al: Plasma androgens in women with acne vulgaris. J Invest Dermatol 81:70, 1983

RAJ SG et al: Normalization of testosterone levels using a low estrogen-containing oral contraceptive in women with polycystic ovary syndrome. Obstet Gynecol 60:15, 1982

RUBENS R: Androgen levels during cyproterone acetate and ethinyl oestradiol treatment of hirsutism. Clin Endocrinol 20:313, 1984

WILLIAMS GH: Hirsutism, in *Office Practice of Medicine*, WT Branch (ed). Philadelphia, Saunders, 1986, in press

section 8 Alterations in the skin

47 INTERPRETATION OF ALTERATIONS IN THE SKIN

THOMAS B. FITZPATRICK / HARLEY A. HAYNES

CLINICAL EXAMINATION OF THE SKIN

The identification of skin lesions, or alterations, is a problem similar to the recognition of cells in a blood smear: the minute details are of the greatest importance. Lesions may be the presenting complaint of the patient or may be incidental findings during the routine physical examination; or they may be incidental to some major presenting complaint such as fever, cough, arthralgia, and the like. The recognition of the important and nonimportant skin lesions commonly encountered during the routine physical examination of the skin is a requisite part of the physician's task.

Inasmuch as the identification of skin lesions is the *sine qua non* of dermatologic diagnosis, the examiner's eye is undoubtedly the most valuable instrument at his or her disposal. Adequate illumination, preferably with natural light, is necessary. The observation of the total skin surface should begin with an overall, "low-power" general assessment of the completely disrobed patient. The systematic approach to the examination of skin should be as follows: first the fingernails and then the anterior and posterior aspects of the arm; then, in sequence, the scalp, the face, the trunk, the lower extremities and the skin between the toes; and then the mucous membranes, including the mouth and anogenital areas. The examiner of dermatologic lesions should consider (1) the specific *type* of lesion, (2) the *shape* of the lesion, (3) the *arrangement* of the groups of lesions, such as linear, arciform, annular, polycyclic, herpetiform, zosteriform, and serpiginous, and (4) *distribution* of the lesions.

Types of skin lesions can be classified by determining the topographic level of the lesions in relation to the normal skin (Table 47-1). For example, it is possible to distinguish lesions that are in or that protrude from or are superimposed above or below the level of the normal skin. The lesions that are encompassed within the scope of dermatology are listed in Fig. 47-1 and Table 47-1, and the histologic aspects are illustrated in Figs. 47-2 through 47-13.

The *shape* of the individual lesion and the *arrangement* of two or more lesions in relation to each other sometimes constitute important diagnostic clues. A *linear* arrangement of lesions often is indicative of an exogenous cause; also, linear lesions may occur because the pathologic process involves a vein, a lymphatic component, or an arteriole. Linearity can often be seen in various types of cutaneous hamartomas involving epidermal cells or melanocytes or even dermal connective tissue. In contrast, *annular* and *arciform* lesions and annular and arciform arrangements are relatively common and therefore only rarely lead to a specific diagnosis. The *iris* lesion (also called "target" lesion), however, a special and important type of annular lesion, is an erythematous annular or concentric macule or papule with either a purplish papule or vesicle in the center. Iris lesions are characteristic of the erythema multiforme syndrome. Annular macules may be observed in drug eruptions, secondary syphilis, and lupus erythematosus. Annular lesions with scale often suggest dermatophytosis or pityriasis rosea or psoriasis. The wheals that occur in creeping eruptions as well as the nodules in late syphilis are arranged in a *serpiginous* (snake-like) pattern.

Lesions that are contiguous are described as *grouped* and are of relatively little diagnostic value except in the special pattern, *herpetiform,* which is virtually pathognomonic for herpes simplex or herpes zoster. Similarly, the special arrangement, *zosteriform,* follows a dermatome in a bandlike pattern and is characteristically seen in herpes zoster; a zosteriform arrangement of skin nodules is occasionally seen in metastatic carcinoma of the breast. A *reticular* (netlike) arrangement often results from vascular dilatation and is observed in cutis marmorata and livedo reticularis.

The *distribution* of sites of localization of skin eruptions has been greatly overemphasized in dermatologic diagnosis; of far more importance are the type, shape, and arrangement of the lesions. The distribution of eruptions can be classified as *isolated, regional,* or *generalized;* the term *total* (universal) denotes an involvement of all the skin, including the hair and the nails. When the eruption occurs in a bilateral and symmetric distribution, the pathologic stimulus is usually endogenous, i.e., hematogenously disseminated. Bilateral symmetry is characteristic of hypersensitivity and is a common response to a drug. In photosensitivity eruptions, lesions are localized to the parts of the body that are exposed to sunlight. The exposed areas of the face that are usually spared include the fold of skin in the upper eyelids, the skin of the hair-covered scalp, the region below the chin, and the area behind the ears.

TABLE 47-1 Types of skin lesion

Flat lesions (in plane of skin)	Elevated lesions (above plane of skin)	Depressed lesions (below plane of skin)
Macule	Vesicle and bulla	Atrophy*
Infarct†	Pustule	Sclerosis†‡
Sclerosis†‡	Abscess§	Erosion
Telangiectasia‡	Cyst‡	Excoriation
	Papule	Scar‡
	Wheal	Ulcer
	Plaque	Sinus§
	Nodule§	Gangrene*
	Vegetation	
	Keratosis	
	Desquamation (scales)	
	Exudate† (crusts)	
	Lichenification	

* *May also be in the plane of the skin.*
† *May also be below the plane of the skin.*
‡ *May also be above the plane of the skin.*
§ *May also be in or below the plane of the skin.*
SOURCE: *TB Fitzpatrick, in Dermatology in General Medicine, 3d ed, TB Fitzpatrick et al (eds), New York, McGraw-Hill, 1987.*

LABORATORY AND OTHER AIDS IN EXAMINATION OF THE SKIN

There are certain technical, clinical, and laboratory aids and procedures that are indispensable in the clinical examination and interpretation of skin conditions.

VISUAL AIDS **Magnification** Certain diagnostic signs can be revealed only by magnification of the skin lesions, e.g., the follicular plugging indicative of lupus erythematosus, the fine telangiectasia and translucent raised border indicative of basal cell carcinoma, and, if present, the bluish color indicative of early primary malignant melanoma. A pocket magnifier (7×) is necessary for proper identification.

Transillumination Oblique lighting of skin lesions which is done in a darkened room is often required to detect slight degrees of elevation or depression, and is also sometimes useful in estimating the extent of the eruption.

Diascopy Diascopy is an essential technique for the examination of skin because it permits the differentiation of purpura from erythematous macules. Diascopy consists of firmly pressing a microscope slide or a piece of clear plastic over the skin lesion; if the lesion is erythematous, the pressure will reveal compressible capillary dilatation rather than an extravasation of blood, which cannot be blanched. Sarcoidosis, lymphoma, and tuberculosis of the skin are suggested if diascopy of the nodules exhibits either a characteristic hyaline, yellowish-brown, or an "apple-jelly" appearance.

Long-wave ultraviolet light, or Wood's lamp Long-wave ultraviolet light (360 nm), or Wood's lamp, is a necessary source of illumination for complete examination of the skin. Wood's lamp consists of a high-pressure mercury arc lamp with a specially compounded glass filter made of nickel oxide and silica (Wood's filter). This filter permits the passage of a band of radiation of 360 nm, which will reveal fluorescence when light passed through the filter impinges upon certain structures.

FIGURE 47-1 *Common lesions, shown on anterior and posterior views of the patient, encountered during the physical examination of the skin. (From Fitzpatrick et al.)*

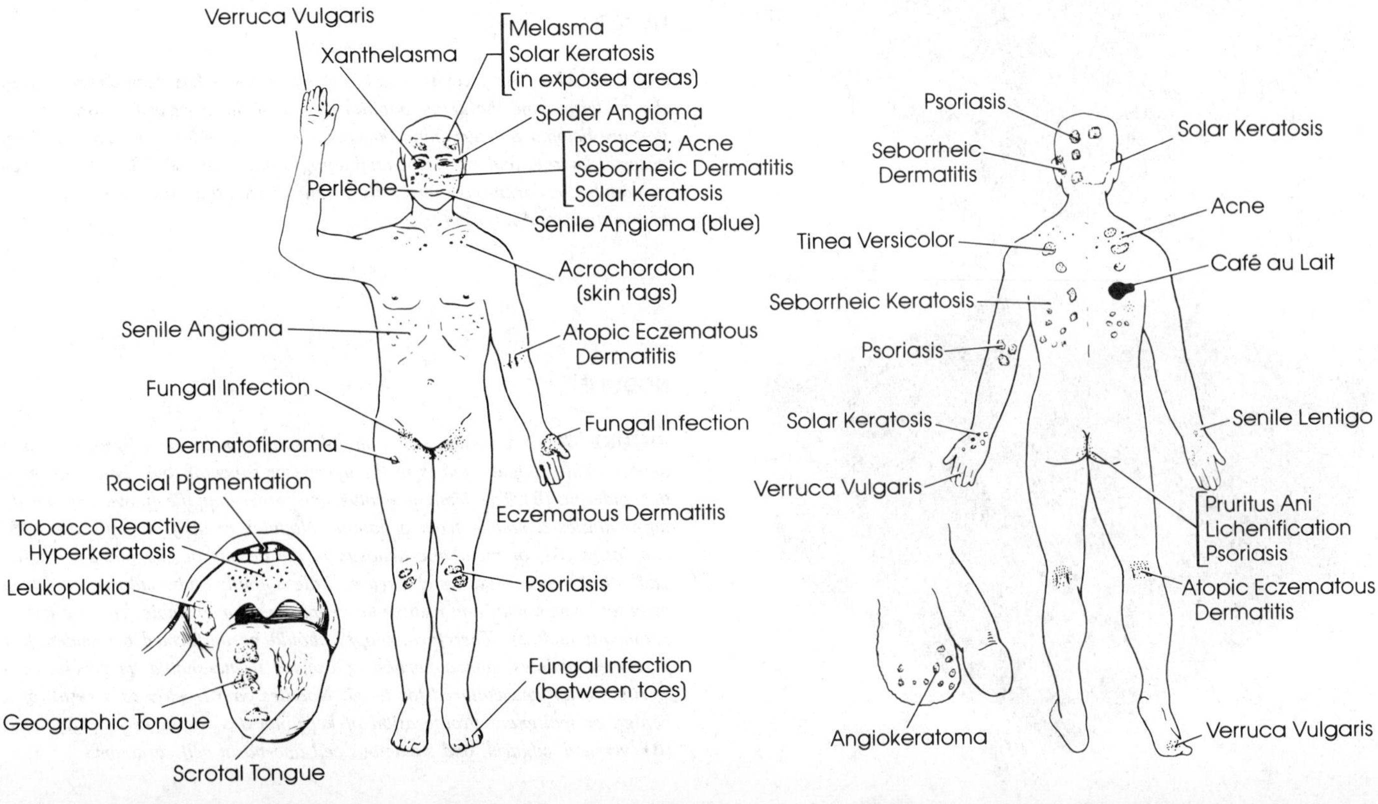

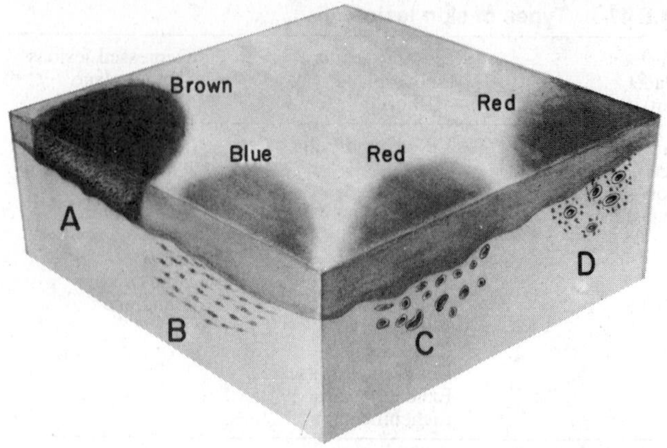

MACULE

FIGURE 47-2 A macule *is a circumscribed area of change in normal skin color without elevation or depression of the surface relative to the surrounding skin. The macules may be of any size and are the result of hypopigmentation (e.g., vitiligo) or hyperpigmentation—melanin (A) or hemosiderin (D)—such as café au lait spots and Mongolian spots (B), or permanent vascular abnormalities of the skin, as in a capillary hemangioma or transient capillary dilation (erythema) (C). Pressure of a glass slide (diascopy) on the border of a red lesion is a simple and reliable method for detecting the extravasation of red blood cells. If the redness remains under the pressure of the slide, the lesion may be purpuric (D); if the redness disappears, the lesion is erythematous and is due to vascular dilation (C).*

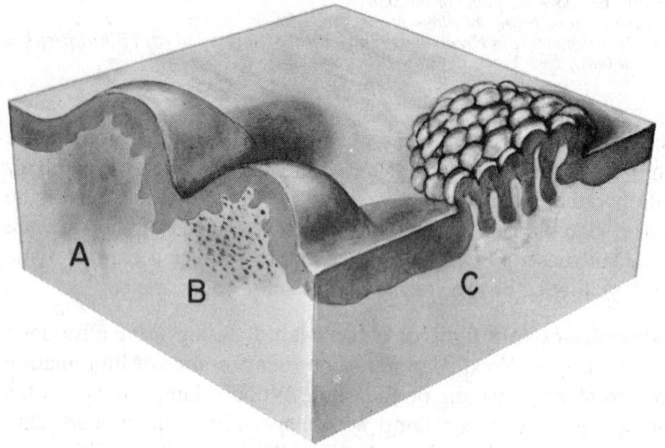

PAPULE

FIGURE 47-3 A papule *is a solid lesion, generally considered as less than 1 cm in diameter. Most of it is elevated above, rather than deep within, the plane of the surrounding skin. The elevation is caused by metabolic deposits (A) in the dermis or by localized infiltrates (B) in the dermis or by localized hyperplasia of cellular elements (C) in the dermis or epidermis. Superficial papules with distinct borders are seen when the lesion is the result of an increase in the number of epidermal cells (C) or melanocytes. Deeper dermal papules resulting from cellular infiltrates have indistinct borders. The topography of a papule or plaque may consist of multiple, small, closely packed, projected elevations that are known as a vegetation (C).*

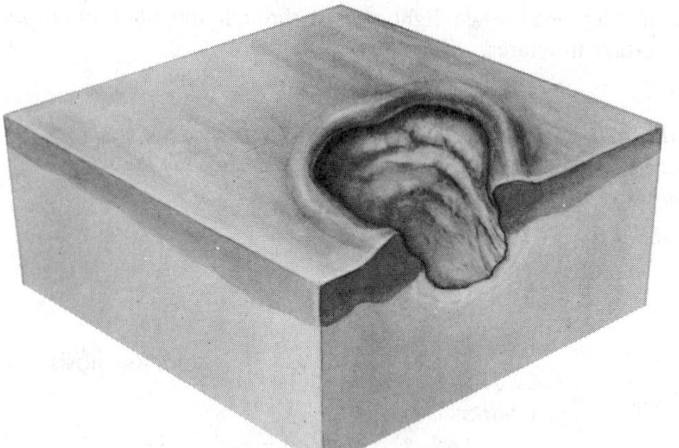

ULCERS

FIGURE 47-4 *An* ulcer *is a lesion in which there has been destruction of the epidermis and the upper papillary layer of the dermis. Certain features that are helpful in determining the cause of ulcers include location, borders, base, discharge, and any associated topographic features of the lesions, such as nodules, excoriations, varicosities, hair distribution, presence or absence of sweating, and adjacent pulses.*

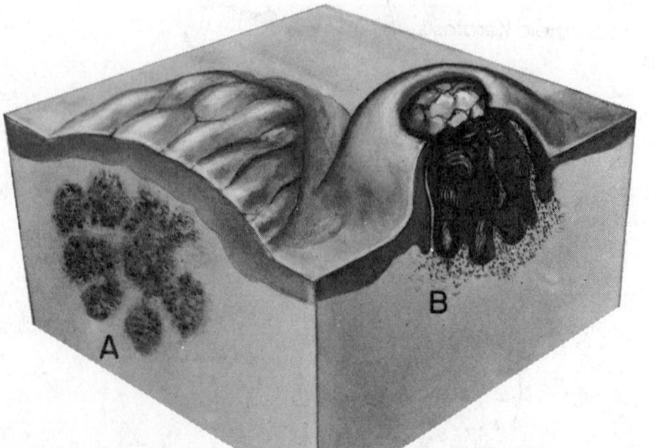

NODULE

FIGURE 47-5 A nodule *is a palpable solid, round, or ellipsoidal lesion deeper than a papule and is in the dermis or subcutaneous tissue (A) or in the epidermis (B). The depth of involvement rather than the diameter primarily differentiates a nodule from a papule. Nodules result from infiltrates (A), neoplasms (B), or metabolic deposits in the dermis or subcutaneous tissue and often indicate systemic disease. Late syphilis, tuberculosis, the deep mycoses, lymphoma, and metastatic neoplasms, for example, can present as cutaneous nodules. Therefore, biopsy should be performed on unidentified persistent nodules, and a portion of excised tissue should be ground in a sterile mortar and cultured for fungi. Nodules can develop as a result of a benign or malignant proliferation of keratinocytes, as in keratoacanthoma (B), verruca vulgaris, and squamous cell and basal cell carcinoma.*

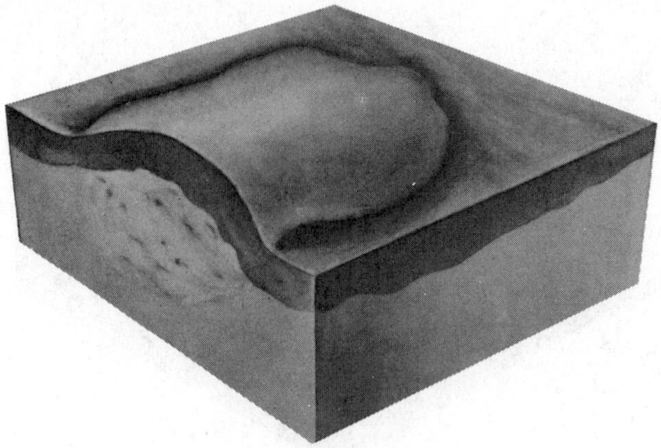

WHEAL

FIGURE 47-6 *A* wheal *is a rounded or flat-topped, pale-red elevation in the skin that is characteristically evanescent, disappearing within hours. Observation of the borders of wheals that have been traced with a skin-marking pencil reveals that the wheals shift relatively rapidly from the involved to the uninvolved adjacent areas. Wheals are the result of edema in the upper layer of the dermis.*

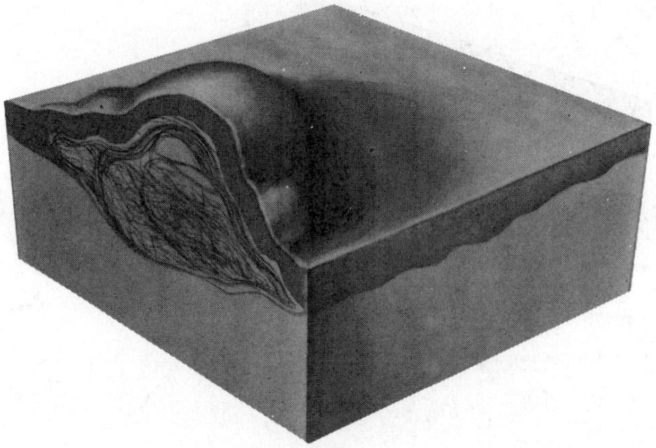

VESICLE

FIGURE 47-7 *A* vesicle *(less than 0.5 cm) or a* bulla *(more than 0.5 cm) is a circumscribed elevated lesion containing fluid. Often the walls are so thin that they are translucent, and the serum, lymph fluid, blood, or extracellular fluid can be seen. Vesicles and bullae arise from a cleavage at various levels of the skin; the cleavage may be within the epidermis (i.e., intraepidermal vesication), or at the epidermal-dermal interface (i.e., subepidermal).*

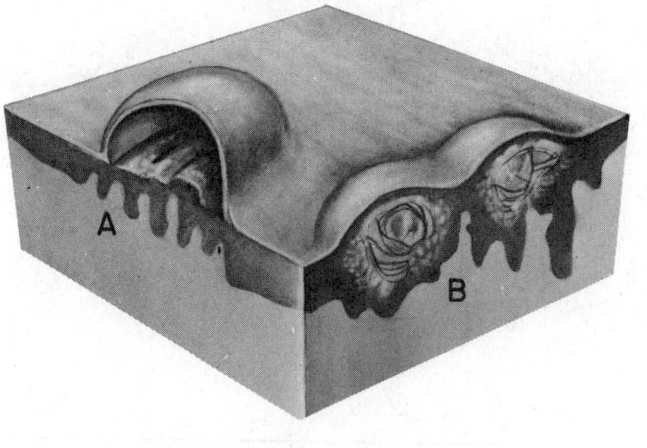

BULLA (A, subcorneal; B, spongiotic)

FIGURE 47-8 *When the cleavage is just beneath the stratum corneum, a* subcorneal vesicle *or* bulla *results (A), as seen in impetigo and subcorneal pustular dermatosis. Intraepidermal vesication may result from intercellular edema, or spongiosis (B), as characteristically seen in delayed hypersensitivity reactions of the epidermis (e.g., in contact eczematous dermatitis), and in dyshidrotic eczema (B).* Spongiotic vesicles *may or may not be seen clinically as vesicles.*

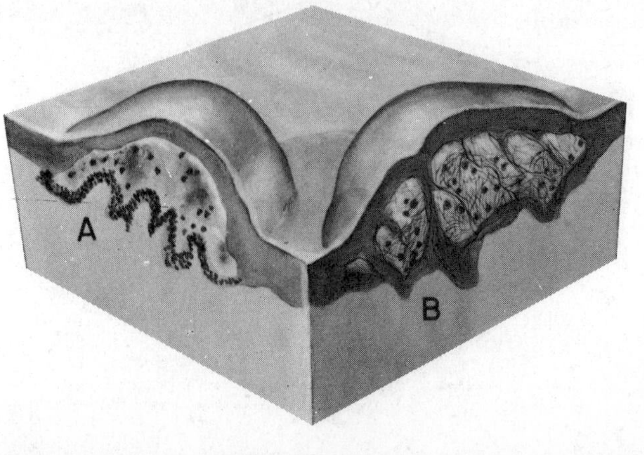

VESICLE (A, acantholytic; B, viral)

FIGURE 47-9 *Loss of intercellular bridges, or desmosomes, is known as acantholysis (A), and this type of intraepidermal vesication is seen in the vesicles or bullae of pemphigus vulgaris; the cleavage is usually just above the basal layer, as in pemphigus vulgaris, but may occur just below the subcorneal layer, as in pemphigus foliaceous. Viruses cause a curious ''ballooning degeneration'' of epidermal cells (B), as in herpes zoster, herpes simplex, variola, and varicella. Viral bullae often have a depressed (''umbilicated'') center.*

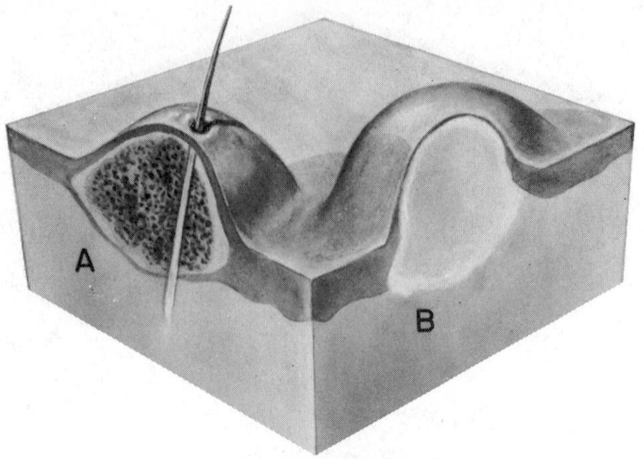

PUSTULE

FIGURE 47-10 *A* pustule *is a circumscribed elevation of the skin that contains a purulent exudate that may be white, yellow, or greenish yellow. This process may arise in a hair follicle (A) or independently (B). Pustules may vary in size and shape; follicular pustules, however, are always conical and usually contain a hair in the center. The vesicular lesions of the viral diseases (varicella, variola, vaccinia, herpes simplex, and herpes zoster) may secondarily become pustular. A Gram's stain and culture should be done on all pustules for identification of intracellular gram positive cocci.*

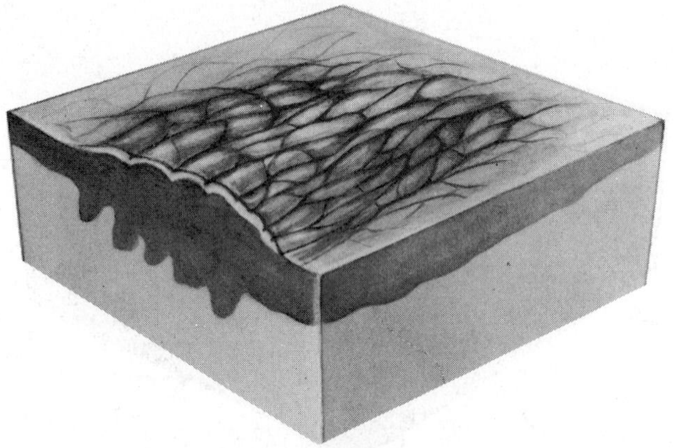

PLAQUE

FIGURE 47-11 *A* plaque *is an elevation above the skin surface that occupies a relatively large suface area in comparison with its height above the skin. Frequently, it is formed by a confluence of papules, as in psoriasis and mycosis fungoides. Lichenification is a proliferation of keratinocytes and stratum corneum forming a plaquelike structure. The skin appears thickened, and the skin markings are accentuated. The process results from repeated rubbing, and frequently develops in persons with atopy. Lichenification occurs in eczematous dermatitis.*

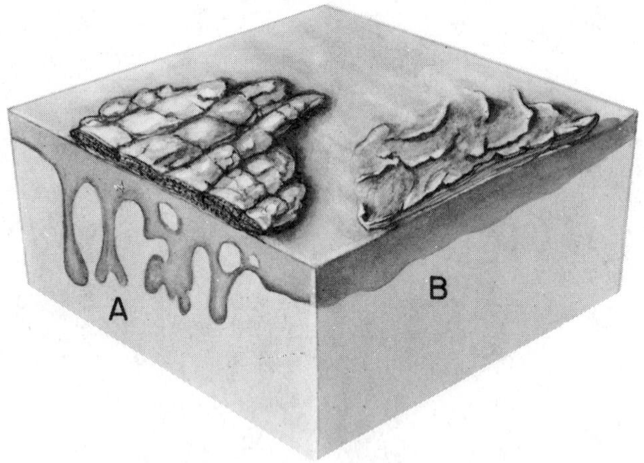

SCALES

FIGURE 47-12 *Epidermal cells are completely replaced every 27 days. The end product of this holocrine process is the stratum corneum. This outermost layer of skin, the stratum corneum, normally does not contain nuclei and is imperceptibly lost. With an increased rate of proliferation of epidermal cells, as in psoriasis, the stratum corneum is not formed normally, and the outermost layers of the skin retain the nuclei. These desquamating layers of skin are seen clinically as* scales. *Densely adherent scales that have a gritty feel (like sandpaper) result from a localized increase in the stratum corneum and are typically seen in solar keratosis (B).*

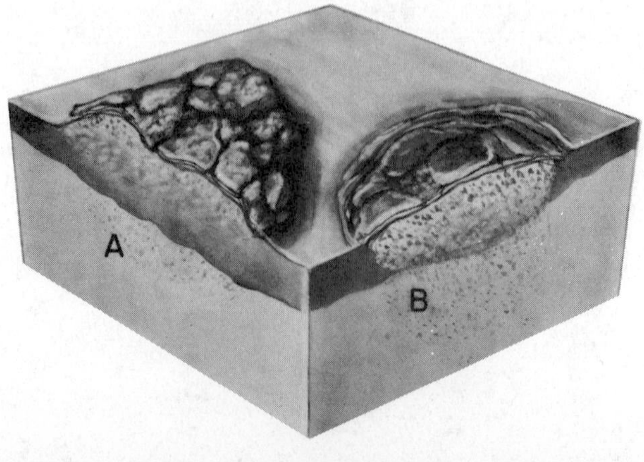

CRUSTS

FIGURE 47-13 Crusts, *resulting when serum, blood, or purulent exudate dries on the skin surface, are the hallmark of pyogenic infection. Crusts may be thin, delicate, and friable (A) or thick and adherent (B). Crusts are yellow when formed from dried serum, green or yellow-green when formed from purulent exudate, or brown or dark red when formed from blood. Superficial crusts occur as honey-colored, delicate, glistening particulates on the surface (A) and are typically seen in impetigo. When the exudate involves the entire epidermis, the crusts may be thick and adherent, and this condition is known as ecthyma (B).*

Wood's lamp is important for the detection of the pinkish-red fluorescence of the urine of patients with porphyria cutanea tarda; the addition of 5% hydrochloric acid greatly intensifies the fluorescence, owing to the oxidation of porphyrin precursors to porphyrins.

Wood's lamp is also a great help in estimating variation in the pigmentation of the skin; it reveals both increased and decreased pigmentation. Inasmuch as melanin is a universal absorber of ultraviolet light, areas of increased melanin will show an increased intensity under Wood's lamp; conversely, areas of decreased melanin will show a decrease in intensity (or an increased reflection) because the ultraviolet light is not absorbed. In this respect, Wood's lamp may be the only means of recognizing the sometimes indistinguishable hypomelanotic macules in tuberous sclerosis, a dominantly inherited trait associated with mental retardation and seizures. The white spots are present at birth and remain throughout life, and therefore represent important markers of this serious genetic disorder. Wood's lamp can be used in mass screening for detection of the fluorescence of dermatophytosis present *in the hair shaft* in ringworm of the scalp.

CLINICAL TESTS **Patch testing** Patch testing is primarily used by dermatologists to detect contact sensitivity. Some contactants are listed in Fisher's monograph on the subject.

Darier's sign One useful clinical response of the skin, Darier's sign, is used as a test for urticaria pigmentosa, and is evoked by the vigorous rubbing of a pigmented macule with the blunt end of a pen. In urticaria pigmentosa (mastocytosis), a palpable red wheal occurs within a few minutes after the physical trauma, owing to the release of histamine by the mast cells in the skin.

LABORATORY PROCEDURES **Examination for bacteria in crusts and biopsy specimens** Gram's stains and bacterial cultures of exudates should be performed on all lesions consisting of crusts and purulent exudates. Ulcers and nodules should be biopsied by removal of a wedge of tissue that extends from the surface down to the subcutaneous fat. The biopsy specimen should be minced in a sterile mortar and cultured for bacteria (including typical and atypical mycobacteria) and fungi.

Examination for mycelia The presence of mycelia may be ascertained by the application of 10% potassium hydroxide to a single tiny portion of scale, which is then gently heated. For fungi and yeasts, scales and hair should be cultured on Sabouraud's medium.

Tzanck test The Tzanck test, or the microscopic examination of cells from the base of vesicles, determines the presence of giant epithelial cells and multinucleated giant cells that occur in herpes simplex, herpes zoster, and varicella. Material taken from the base of a vesicle by gentle curettage with a scalpel is spread gently on a glass slide and prepared with Giemsa's or Wright's stain for the examination.

Dark-field examination of serum for *Treponema pallidum* Dark-field examination of serum from ulcers and erosions on the male and female genitalia is essential for the detection of *Treponema pallidum*. Dark-field examination of material obtained from the oral cavity is not diagnostic because of the presence of nonpathogenic treponemas that are indistinguishable from *T. pallidum*.

BIOPSY Microscopic examination of tissue is particularly applicable in dermatology because biopsies of the lesions can be easily obtained. Although the classic method is an elliptical incision followed by suturing, a satisfactory method for diagnostic purposes is "punch" biopsy. Biopsy of the skin enables correlation of gross and microscopic pathology. For punch biopsy, a small, 3.0- to 4.0-nm, disposable tubular blade is rotated between the thumb and index finger to cut through the entire thickness of the abnormal skin; the resulting cylinder of skin is then lifted out with forceps, and the skin is cut off at its base with a pointed scissors. This simple operation is done under local anesthesia, and the bleeding can be stopped by the use of pressure or absorbable foam; suturing is not usually necessary.

TABLE 47-2 Approach to dermatologic diagnosis

I History
- *A* Duration of lesions: days, weeks, months, years
- *B* Relationship of skin lesions to season, heat, cold, previous treatment, drug ingestion
- *C* Skin symptoms: pruritus, pain, paresthesia
- *D* Constitutional symptoms
  - *1* "Acute illness" syndrome: headache, chills, feverishness, weakness
  - *2* "Chronic illness" syndrome: fatigue, weakness, anorexia, weight loss, malaise
- *E* System review

II Physical examination
- *A* Appearance of patient: uncomfortable, "toxic," well
- *B* Changes in body temperature: elevated
- *C* Normal skin color: white, brown, black
- *D* Skin—four major skin signs: (1) type, (2) shape, (3) arrangement, (4) distribution of lesions
  - *1* Type of lesion

Basic lesions	*Sequential lesions*
Macule	Scale
Papule-plaque	Exudation: dry (crust)
Wheal	wet (weeping)
Nodule	Erosion
Cyst	Scar
Vesicle-bulla	Lichenification
Pustule	
Ulcer (also sequential)	
Hyperkeratosis (also sequential)	
Sclerosis	
Atrophy (also sequential)	
Telangiectasia	
Infarct	
Purpura	

Color of lesions or of skin (if diffuse involvement): "skin color," white, leukoderma, hypomelanosis; red, erythema, pink, violaceous; brown, hypermelanosis, black, blue, gray, orange, yellow. Red purpuric lesions do not blanch with pressure (diascopy).

Palpation
Consistency (soft, firm, hard, fluctuant, boardlike)
Deviation in temperature (hot, cold)
Mobility of lesion or of skin
Presence of tenderness
Estimate of the depth of lesion (i.e., dermal or subcutaneous)

  - *2* *Shape* of individual lesions: round, oval, polygonal, polycyclic, annular (ring-shaped), iris, serpiginous (snake-like), umbilicated
  - *3* *Arrangement* of multiple lesions
    Grouped: herpetiform, zosteriform, arciform, annular, reticulated (netlike), linear, serpiginous (snake-like)
    Disseminated: scattered discrete lesions or diffuse involvement, i.e., without identifiable borders
  - *4* *Distribution* of lesions
    Extent: isolated (single lesion), localized, regional generalized, universal
    Pattern: symmetric, exposed areas, sites of pressure, intertriginous areas, follicular localization, random
    Characteristic patterns: scabies, secondary syphilis, psoriasis, seborrheic dermatitis, lichen planus, pityriasis rosea, dermatitis herpetiformis, atopic dermatitis, vitiligo, acne, erythema multiforme, candidiasis, contact dermatitis, lupus erythematosus, erythrasma, ichthyosis, pemphigus, pemphigoid, porphyria cutanea tarda, xanthoma, necrotizing angiitis (vasculitis)
- *E* Hair and nails
- *F* Mucous membranes
- *G* Miscellaneous physical findings: lymphadenopathy, hepatosplenomegaly, cardiac findings, neurologic findings, ophthalmologic findings

III Laboratory and special examinations
- *A* Dermatopathology
  - *1* Light microscopy: site, process, cell types
  - *2* Immunofluorescence
  - *3* Special techniques: stains, electron microscopy, etc.
- *B* Microbiologic examination of skin material: scales, crusts, or exudate
  - *1* Direct microscopic examination of skin
    For yeast and fungus: 10% potassium hydroxide preparation

For bacteria:	Gram stain
For virus:	Tzanck smear
For spirochetes:	Dark-field examination
For parasites:	Scabies mite from a burrow

  - *2* Culture
    Bacterial: for granulomas, culture
    Mycologic: minced tissue
- *C* General laboratory examinations: blood

  Bacteriologic: culture
  Serologic: ANA, STS

TABLE 47-2 Approach to dermatologic diagnosis *(continued)*

Hematologic: hematocrit or hemoglobin, cells, differential smear, erythrocyte sedimentation rate
Chemistry: Fasting blood sugar, blood urea nitrogen, creatinine

D Wood's light examination

Urine: pink-orange fluorescence in porphyria cutanea tarda (add 5.0% hydrochloric acid)
Hair (in vivo): green fluorescence in tinea capitis (hair shaft)
Skin (in vivo):

	Erythrasma	Coral-red fluorescence
Compared to visible light examination	Hypomelanosis	Decrease in intensity
	Brown hypermelanosis	Increase in intensity
	Blue hypermelanosis	No change in intensity

E Radiographic studies

TABLE 47-3 Clinical classification of skin lesions and syndromes according to the component of the skin primarily involved

I Epidermis (keratinocytes and melanocytes)
- *A* Keratinocytes
  - *1* Scaling macules, papules, or plaques
  - *2* Vesicles and bullae
  - *3* Pustules
  - *4* Exudative (impetiginized) lesions
  - *5* Eczematous dermatitis
  - *6* Erythroderma syndrome (exfoliative dermatitis)*
  - *7* Atrophy, diffuse* or circumscribed
- *B* Melanocytes
  - *1* Hypomelanotic macules
  - *2* Diffuse hypomelanosis*
  - *3* Hypermelanotic (brown) macules
  - *4* Diffuse brown hypermelanosis*

II Dermis (connective tissue and blood vessels)
- *A* Connective tissue component
  - *1* Papules and nodules (with and without inflammation)
  - *2* Ulcers
  - *3* Sclerosis, diffuse* or circumscribed
  - *4* Edema*
  - *5* Atrophy, diffuse* or circumscribed
- *B* Blood vessels
  - *1* Morbilliform and scarlatiniform eruptions
  - *2* Urticarial syndromes
  - *3* Erythema multiforme syndrome
  - *4* Purpura (with and without inflammation)
  - *5* Infarcts
  - *6* Telangiectasia

III Panniculus adiposus (connective tissue and blood vessels)
- *A* Connective tissue component
  - *1* Nodules, noninflammatory, usually nontender
  - *2* Atrophy
- *B* Blood vessels
  - *1* Nodules, inflammatory, usually tender and red
    - *a* Erythema nodosum syndrome

* *Pathologic changes affect large areas of skin, and there are no discrete, circumscribed lesions.*

SOURCE: *TB Fitzpatrick, in Dermatology in General Medicine, 3d ed, TB Fitzpatrick et al (eds), New York, McGraw-Hill, 1987.*

This technique is as harmless and simple as a venipuncture, and supplies enough tissue to permit a definitive histologic diagnosis in most cases.

APPROACH TO DIAGNOSIS In Tables 47-2 and 47-3 an orderly sequence is suggested as a method of establishing a diagnosis in a patient presenting with skin lesions.

REFERENCES

FISHER AA: *Contact Dermatitis*, 2d ed. Philadelphia, Lea & Febiger, 1973

FITZPATRICK TB et al (eds): *Dermatology in General Medicine*, 3d ed. New York, McGraw-Hill, 1987

LAZARUS GS, GOLDSMITH LA: *Diagnosis of Skin Disease*. Philadelphia, Davis, 1980, p 506

ROOK A, WILKINSON DS: The principles of diagnosis, in *Textbook of Dermatology*, A Rook et al (eds). Oxford, Blackwell Scientific, 1979, p 37

48 SKIN LESIONS OF GENERAL MEDICAL SIGNIFICANCE

THOMAS B. FITZPATRICK / JEFFREY D. BERNHARD

The skin is one of the best indicators of serious disease; even an untrained eye can recognize cyanosis, jaundice, or the ashen pallor of shock. The competent physician must be able to detect the subtle skin signs of life-threatening diseases and cutaneous clues to diseases in other organs. Skin lesions are frequently critical in the final resolution of puzzling diagnostic medical problems. Thus, certain cutaneous "marker syndromes," such as erythema nodosum, can be indications of multisystem disease and therefore demand thorough medical evaluation.

The skin (Fig. 48-1) is composed of three layers: (1) the *epidermis,* the outermost part, which consists of two main cell types, keratinocytes and melanocytes; (2) the *dermis,* upon which the epidermis rests, which is composed of a mélange of connective tissue elements, nerves, blood and lymph vessels, glands, appendages, and a few cells (mast cells, fibroblasts, histiocytes); and (3) the *panniculus adiposus* (subcutaneous tissue), which acts as a cushion between the outer layers and the underlying bone. Keratinocytes produce and retain in their cytoplasm the intermediate filament keratin. They constantly turn over, about 27 days are required to complete differentiation and maturation. During maturation the keratinocyte loses its nucleus and retains only the cytoplasm. The latter becomes a highly ordered, two-phase system of keratin filaments embedded in an amorphous matrix, much like the cellulose-lignin system of wood fiber, which is known to be well adapted to withstand shearing and compression forces. The anucleate outermost portion of the epidermis is the *stratum corneum,* which acts as a tough, keratinous membrane. The stratum corneum functions structurally as a "waterproof" wall between the internal fluid milieu and the environment. It is the major barrier of the skin and protects the body against loss of fluids and entrance of toxic agents. It also serves as a passive membrane—some substances move across the skin by passive diffusion in the direction of the concentration gradient.

The skin has a relatively limited number of pathologic responses. If the individual skin lesions are taken to represent the letters of the alphabet, then groups of lesions can be said to form recognizable words or phrases. To the trained eye, these may lead to recognition of a clinically meaningful reaction pattern or diagnosis. The lesions in the majority of patients seen by the general physician can be classified in one of the groups of clinical reaction patterns (see Table 47-3) or types of skin lesion listed in Table 47-1. These skin lesions or clinical reactions may consist of one type of lesion, such as a vesicle or a nodule, or aggregates of various types of lesions, such as papules or vesicles. One or more solitary lesions or one or more groups of lesions may be distributed any place on the body. In some pathologic processes the borders of the lesions may not be defined; this type of diffuse involvement occurs in systemic sclerosis and in pigmentation disorders.

Cutaneous signs of systemic disease not discussed in this chapter include generalized pruritis (Chap. 50), photosensitivity (Chap. 52), and the cutaneous manifestations of internal malignancy (Chap. 300). Cutaneous markers for diseases of other organ systems, such as hyperpigmentation in Addison's disease (Chap. 51) and café au lait macules in neurofibromatosis, are also discussed elsewhere in the text.

In the physician's attempts to identify the specific types of lesions, it is essential to try to estimate the component of the skin that is *primarily* affected, i.e., the epidermis, the dermis, the blood vessels, or the panniculus adiposus. Inasmuch as there are a finite number of disorders that produce pathologic changes in the various individual components, this method of approach will improve the physician's diagnostic acumen. For example, even though erythema multiforme involves the dermis and the epidermis, the *primary component* affected is the blood vessel, and it is this involvement that explains the erythematous macules; the inflammatory process leads subsequently to the development of the cellular infiltrates seen clinically as papules and to destruction of the basement membrane and the development of bullae.

CLASSIFICATION OF LESIONS ACCORDING TO THE COMPONENT OF THE SKIN PRIMARILY AFFECTED

EPIDERMIS Scaling macules, papules, or plaques Generalized scaling macules, papules, or plaques are frequent and important diagnostic problems and are usually a presenting complaint of the patient (see Figs. 47-2, 47-3, and 47-11).

The sudden onset of symmetric, scaling, erythematous macules or papules is often indicative of drug-induced hypersensitivity reactions. Scaling erythematous papules on the scalp and extensor aspects of the arms and legs are suggestive of *psoriasis;* psoriatic lesions often are accentuated on the sites of repeated trauma, such as the elbows and knees. The papules or plaques of psoriasis are often surmounted by a silvery white micaceous scale that is relatively easily removed in layers. In psoriasis, there is a severalfold increase in the normal number of the basal cells of the epidermis. This increase in the basal cell population reduces the turnover time of the epidermis from the normal 27 days to 3 to 4 days. With the consequent shortened interval of epidermal cell migration from the basal layer to the skin surface, the normal events of cell maturation and keratinization do not occur (see A in Fig. 47-12); this failure of maturation is reflected by an array of abnormal morphologic and biochemical changes. In association with the basal cell hyperplasia, there is enhanced metabolism and accelerated synthesis and degradation of nucleoproteins, resulting in an elevated urinary excretion of nucleic acid metabolites such as uric acid. In addition, the subepidermal vasculature proliferates to support the increased rate of cell division. These numerous cytologic, histologic, histochemical, and biochemical alterations are now known to be the result, rather than the cause, of the disease process. The only main fact known at this time about the fundamental cause of psoriasis is that the predisposition to its development is genetically transmitted. An erosive joint disease, *psoriatic arthritis,* is discussed in Chap. 276.

The treatment of psoriasis still remains within the province of the dermatologist. The most effective treatment in the control of *localized psoriasis,* for most patients, is the use of topical corticosteroids, topical coal-tar preparations, and ultraviolet light or sunlight exposures. Corticosteroids can also be injected directly into small, resistant plaques. Systemic corticosteroids are not only ineffective in psoriasis but may cause generalization of the process and are absolutely contraindicated. With certain patients who have generalized psoriasis, it has been necessary to use a variety of systemic chemotherapeutic agents, especially methotrexate; the latter has the capacity to inhibit cell replication without a proportionate inhibition of cell function, i.e., keratinization.

In 1974, a new form of photochemotherapy was introduced which uses oral methoxsalen and a high-intensity, long-wave ultraviolet light source. This approach may replace many of the other forms of therapy. In this so-called PUVA treatment, psoralen (P) is administered by mouth 2 h before total-body irradiation with a special light system that emits predominantly long-wave (320- to 400-nm) ultraviolet light (UV-A). The light alone is ineffective in producing erythema or remission of psoriatic lesions; however, in the presence of one of the psoralens (methoxsalen) the UV-A becomes a potent photoactive agent and produces a remission of psoriatic lesions after multiple exposures. The mechanism of action is probably related in part to the binding of psoralen to DNA by the action of UV-A. Multicenter clinical trials in the United States and Europe involving over 5000 patients have shown that oral methoxsalen photochemotherapy is highly effective in the control of severe psoriasis; in over 80 percent of such patients the psoriasis completely cleared in 3 to 4 weeks of treatment using two or four exposures per week. After clearing, the patients may be given maintenance exposures once per week or less frequently. While methoxsalen photochemotherapy is effective, it requires specialized knowledge and equipment in order to deliver precisely measured amounts of UV-A. PUVA treatment is recommended only for patients with disabling psoriasis because long-term sequelae include premature aging of the skin, skin cancers in certain susceptible patients (i.e., with history of previous exposure to arsenic or ionizing radiation), and cataracts. In extremely disabling and recalcitrant cases, it may be necessary to combine PUVA or UV-B (middle-wave ultraviolet) with other modalities, such as systemic methotrexate, either sequentially or in combination.

The general physician does not always appreciate the impact of psoriasis as a major cause of disability and of disfigurement. Psoriasis affects between 2 and 8 million persons in the United States; about 100,000 are severely affected.

Psoriasiform lesions occurring on the face, lower abdomen, buttocks, groin, perineum, and legs occur in the *glucagonoma syndrome*. The lesions may be almost indistinguishable from subacute psoriasis, but they often have superficial necrosis in the center of the plaques; stomatitis, anemia, and marked weight loss are also present. Hyperglycemia may or may not be present. The eruption disappears rapidly on removal of the glucagon-secreting tumor of the pancreas. Psoriasiform lesions are also seen in Reiter's syndrome (keratoderma blennorrhagicum), mycosis fungoides (cutaneous T-cell lymphoma), nummular eczematous dermatitis, parapsoriasis, certain drug reactions, and dermatophytosis.

Symmetric scaling macules or papules localized on the palms and soles are often seen as the presenting signs of *secondary syphilis;* very frequently generalized lymphadenopathy and oral erosions are present as well.

A relatively common and often baffling generalized scaling eruption is seen in *pityriasis rosea*. In this condition, the scale at the periphery of the lesion is very thin and forms a collarette; the center of the lesion may or may not be scaly. Pityriasis rosea typically has a ''fir-tree'' type of distribution, especially evident on the back. Very

FIGURE 48-1 *Anatomy of the skin. (Copyright 1967 CIBA Pharmaceutical Company, division of CIBA-Geigy Corporation. Reproduced, with permission from the Clinical Symposia, illustrated by Frank H Netter, MD. All rights reserved.)*

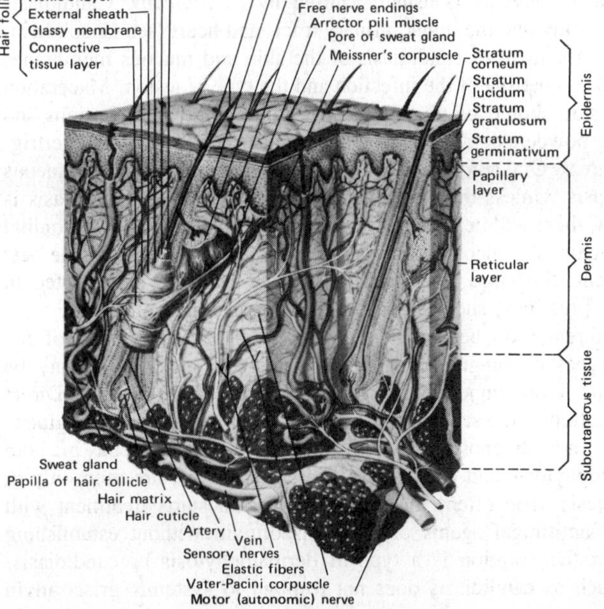

often, but not always, a preceding, single, isolated scaling lesion—the herald patch—is present for several days before generalization of the lesions.

Scaling macules and papules are seen in *dermatophytosis* and *candidiasis,* and it is therefore necessary that some of the scales be examined for the presence of mycelia whenever scaling is present (see "Laboratory Procedures," in Chap. 47).

The various types of *dermatophytosis* (so-called ringworm infections) are confined to the epidermis, hair, toenails, and fingernails, and all (except tinea versicolor) respond to oral griseofulvin. Dermatophytosis is due to three types of fungus: *Microsporum, Epidermophyton,* and *Trichophyton. Microsporum audouini,* a parasite of humans, is the principal pathogen causing epidemic urban fungous infection of the scalp. *Microsporum canis,* which affects the scalp and also the face, where it causes boggy nodules, is a parasite of animals and originates largely from young (usually) farm animals and pets (kittens, puppies, and calves). *Trichophyton rubrum, T. mentagrophytes,* and *E. floccosum,* which also are parasites of humans, are the agents that usually cause dermatophytosis of the feet, the most common site of mycotic infection.

Susceptibility to superficial dermatophyte infection is variable, and appears to depend, at least in part, on individual host responses. The response of dermatophyte infections to oral griseofulvin varies, especially with regard to site of infection. Griseofulvin is effective, even in short courses, in fungous infection of the scalp, trunk, and groin, but even prolonged therapy rarely controls infection of the hands, fingernails, or toenails. Topical treatment with any of the imidazole antifungals is quite effective in infection of the feet, trunk, and groin, but is ineffective for infections of the fingernails or toenails.

The other major category of mycotic infections is represented by candidiasis (monilial infections). These infections do not respond at all to oral griseofulvin and are caused chiefly by *Candida albicans,* and occasionally by *C. tropicalis, C. krusei,* and *C. stellatoidea. C. albicans* can exist as a harmless saprophyte in the gastrointestinal tract and in the vagina. It is more common in females, and is most often present in those who are pregnant or who are taking oral contraceptives or broad-spectrum antibiotics. The association with diabetes mellitus, however, is so common that all patients (regardless of sex) with candidiasis should be screened for this disease.

Despite the fact that *C. albicans* is a normal saprophytic fungus in the vagina and gastrointestinal tract, it is rarely isolated from the exposed surface of the normal skin. *C. albicans* can invade the epidermis when the skin is exposed to high humidity and when the skin becomes macerated; therefore, candidiasis commonly occurs in the intertriginous areas (under the breasts and in the umbilicus, groin, and axillae) and in the oral, as well as the vaginal, mucous membranes. Chronic paronychia is usually caused by *C. albicans.* Candidiasis also may involve the lungs, urinary tract, and heart (see Chap. 147).

The treatment of candidiasis of the skin and mucous membranes depends on the site of the infection and the type of lesion. Maceration of the skin should be treated by air-drying of the area. Lotions and dusting powders containing nystatin are also very useful for intertriginous areas. Oral administration of nystatin is not of value in cutaneous moniliasis. Unless the sexual partner is treated when candidiasis is present, there will be constant retransfer of the infection. For monilial paronychia, 2% alcohol solutions of gentian violet are still the best treatment. Systemic administration of ketoconazole is indicated in certain situations, such as chronic mucocutaneous candidiasis.

Differentiation between dermatophytosis caused by any of the three types of fungus already mentioned and candidiasis may be difficult, if not impossible, without cultures of the fungus. Direct examination of the scales from a scaling eruption in the intertriginous area is not diagnostic because it may reveal mycelia in both dermatophytosis and candidiasis; spores, however, are seen only in candidiasis. Too often, the general physician starts treatment with topical antifungal agents or with griseofulvin without establishing whether the eruption is a type of dermatophytosis or candidiasis. Inasmuch as candidiasis does not respond to systemic griseofulvin and dermatophytes do not respond to nystatin, prescribing these agents for an undiagnosed eruption may result in prolonged disability for the patient. Newer agents such as haloprogin and miconazole are effective against both dermatophytosis and candidiasis.

In the past few years, fungous diseases have assumed a new significance in medicine because of the increased number of patients under treatment with chemotherapeutic agents for leukemia and other neoplasms. Almost all of the saprophytic fungi can invade the tissues of patients who are being treated with chemotherapeutic agents or who have had kidney transplants.

Vesicles and bullae Some diseases may occasionally be associated with vesicles or bullae, such as erythema multiforme or porphyria cutanea tarda, but blisters (vesicles and bullae) are the major feature of a number of disorders: certain bacterial and viral infections; allergic contact dermatitis (such as poison ivy); trauma from mechanical, thermal, or chemical agents; and most important, the bullous diseases of unknown cause (such as pemphigus and pemphigoid).

Grouped vesicles occur in herpes zoster and herpes simplex, whereas scattered, discrete vesicles occur in varicella. A helpful sign in determining the nature of the vesicles is the Tzanck test (see "Laboratory Procedures," in Chap. 47). Epithelial giant cells are present in herpes simplex, herpes zoster, and varicella but are absent in vaccinia and variola. Skin biopsy will also establish the nature of the vesicle or bulla; that is, whether it is intraepidermal (as in virus infections and pemphigus) or subepidermal (as in bullous pemphigoid) (see Figs. 47-7 to 47-9).

Vesicles arranged in linear streaks are characteristic of poison ivy dermatitis. The most reliable clue to the diagnosis of both allergic and primary-irritant contact dermatitis is the localization of vesicles to the skin areas likely to have been exposed to the agent in question. Isolated vesicles and bullae on the dorsal pressure areas of the dorsa of the hands and the face may be the only sign of porphyria cutanea tarda and the variegate porphyria; the diagnosis of the former is immediately confirmed by examination of the urine, using Wood's lamp. These patients do not present with photosensitivity, though the distribution of lesions suggests that sunlight plays a role in their localization.

Scattered, isolated bullae in adults represent a special and serious problem in diagnosis and treatment. *Bullous pemphigoid* and *pemphigus* are chronic and occur primarily in adults; one of them, pemphigus, has serious consequences for the patient. These two disorders need to be distinguished by biopsy of the skin and by immunofluorescence techniques. It is impossible on the basis of clinical diagnosis alone to distinguish between bullous pemphigoid, which is usually a chronic and relatively benign disorder, of limited duration, and *pemphigus vulgaris,* which is a serious disease leading in a relentless course to death, unless treatment with immunosuppressive agents is instituted. Four separate types of pemphigus occur, but pemphigus vulgaris is the most important for the general physician to recognize. Pemphigus vulgaris may begin in the nasal or oral mucous membrane, and the patient may consult the dentist or otolaryngologist first for persistent erosions of the larynx (hoarseness), the mouth, or a bloody nasal discharge. The lesions tend to involve other parts of the body in an unpredictable fashion, but localize chiefly on the umbilicus, scalp, and trunk, although there is no specific distribution pattern. Pemphigus vulgaris affects primarily the middle-aged, particularly between the ages of 40 and 60. It rarely occurs before the age of 17 or after the age of 75. The clinical lesions appear as flaccid bullae from the beginning; they break easily and rarely become very large. The denuded areas (erosions) that form at the site of the ruptured bullae increase in size as the epidermis detaches itself. Occasionally, almost the entire surface may be involved by large, denuded areas; this represents a serious problem in the management of secondary infection and in maintenance of fluid balance—more or less the same problems that occur in a severely burned patient. Oral or nasal mucosal lesions occur in nearly all patients, and more than half have lesions in the mucous membrane of the mouth as the first manifestation of the disease. The disease often starts with only a few lesions in the mouth and may remain limited in extent for several weeks; it then gradually spreads to other parts of the body.

The diagnosis of pemphigus is made on the basis of the light-microscopic examination of the biopsy of an early vesicle and direct immunofluorescence. The earliest change in pemphigus vulgaris consists of intercellular edema followed by disappearance of intercellular bridges in the lower epidermis (see A in Fig. 47-9). This results in loss of cohesion between the epidermal cells (acantholysis) and leads to the formation of clefts and then bullae that are predominantly in suprabasal locations; in other words, the basal cells, although separated from one another, remain attached to the dermis much like a "row of tombstones."

Immunofluorescence allows detection of IgG antibodies specific for an intercellular substance of the skin and mucosa in the serum of patients with pemphigus, and makes possible a differentiation of pemphigus and pemphigoid by the localization of the antibody. The fluorescence is localized precisely to the site of acantholysis in pemphigus; IgG is confined to the intracellular glycocalyx of epidermal cells. In bullous pemphigoid, however, the antibodies react with an antigen in the basement membrane region, and the fluorescence is localized there.

Treatment of pemphigus with systemic corticosteroids, sometimes in combination with azathioprine, is quite successful. Azathioprine alone can control the disease in some patients.

Pustules This skin reaction (see Fig. 47-10) may result from infections or from sterile inflammation. Pustules may arise from preexisting vesicles of any etiology. Infection by pyogenic bacteria, especially staphylococci, as well as by certain fungi and mycobacteria, can produce pustules without a preceding vesicular stage. Noninfectious causes of pustules include acne, pustular psoriasis, and hypersensitivity to drugs, particularly sulfonamides, iodides, or bromides. Purpuric pustules in an acral distribution are characteristic of disseminated gonococcemia, but may also be seen in other forms of bacterial sepsis.

Exudative (impetiginized) lesions Acute infection with gram-positive cocci can occur as a primary process or may be superimposed on eczematous dermatitis or occasionally on any of the vesiculobullous diseases, and is characterized by the presence of crusts (see Fig. 47-13). Such infection on the skin has the same implications as a streptococcal pharyngitis, inasmuch as acute glomerular nephritis develops in a significant percentage of patients with impetiginized dermatitis. Patients with impetiginized dermatitis must be treated with full courses of systemic antibiotics.

Eczematous dermatitis Eczematous dermatitis is not a specific disease entity but a characteristic inflammatory response of the skin due to both endogenous and exogenous agents. Eczematous dermatitis therefore requires a qualifying etiologic term, e.g., *atopic eczematous dermatitis*. Eczematous dermatitis is sufficiently serious to account for the highest incidence of skin disease. Approximately one-third of all patients in the United States seen by dermatologists have eczema. It is responsible for incalculable losses of time and productivity in industry. In Tables 48-1 and 48-2 some of the types of eczematous dermatitis are summarized (see also B in Fig. 47-8 and Fig. 47-11). For the general physician, atopic eczematous dermatitis is the most important disease of this group of disorders. Over 30 percent of atopic patients develop respiratory allergic manifestations (asthma and hay fever). Furthermore, the disease may persist for 15 to 20 years. Cataracts develop in 15 percent of young patients. Finally, patients with atopic eczematous dermatitis are particularly susceptible to infections with herpes simplex and vaccinia. The majority of patients with severe atopic eczematous dermatitis have elevated serum levels of IgE. Control of the intractable pruritus in this disease is difficult, and best results are obtained by judicious use of topical corticosteroids, tar gels, oil baths, lubrication with emollients, and limitation of emotional stress.

Erythroderma syndrome (exfoliative dermatitis) The erythroderma syndrome is an important disorder that may occur as a drug reaction, as a generalized extension of a preexisting dermatitis, such as psoriasis or atopic dermatitis; or in association with lymphoma and leukemia. This syndrome consists of a generalized, erythematous, scaling eruption involving all of the skin surface, and has important implications in general medicine because of the systemic effects occasioned by the massive and continuous exfoliation of the skin. The severity of the metabolic response to exfoliation depends on the duration and

TABLE 48-1 Various types of eczematous dermatitis* of uncertain etiology

Clinical type	Suspected pathogenesis	Diagnostic considerations
Atopic eczematous dermatitis	Hereditary predisposition plus precipitating factors	Eczematous dermatitis, especially localized to the antecubital and popliteal fossae and to the face
Lichen simplex chronicus	Hereditary predisposition plus repeated local trauma	One or more lichenified plaques (see Fig. 47-11), especially on neck
Prurigo nodularis	Repeated local trauma	One or more nodules, especially on extremities
"Neurodermatitis"	Hereditary predisposition plus repeated scratching	Generalized or localized eczematous eruption at sites of repeated trauma
Stasis dermatitis	Chronic venous insufficiency	Signs of venous insufficiency
Nummular eczematous dermatitis	Various precipitating factors (contact irritants, xerosis, emotional stress, etc.)	Discrete coin-shaped patches, usually on extremities and trunk
"Dyshidrotic" eczematous dermatitis	Emotional stress plus other factors‡	Vesicles and bullae on palms and soles
Seborrheic dermatitis	Constitutional diathesis	Greasy scaling patches on scalp, eyebrows, and nasolabial area
Various patterns of eczematous dermatitis	Association with gastrointestinal malabsorption	Eczematous eruption in patient with steatorrhea and abnormal biopsy specimens of the jejunal mucosa
"Eczematous-like eruptions"† with systemic disease: Wiskott-Aldrich syndrome X-linked agammaglobulinemia Phenylketonuria Ahistidinemia Hurler's syndrome Hartnup disease Acrodermatitis enteropathica	Metabolic and immunologic disorders	Related features of clinical syndrome plus immunologic deficiency or biochemical abnormality

* *This term is used by many clinicians for at least four types of eczematous dermatitis that may be exclusively localized to the hands (atopic eczematous dermatitis, allergic contact eczematous dermatitis, nummular eczematous dermatitis, and "dyshidrotic" eczematous dermatitis). Possibly, contact irritants to which the hands are frequently exposed may precipitate or aggravate one of the above-mentioned basic types of eczematous dermatitis.*

† *These eruptions are reported in the literature as eczematous dermatitis, but clear, careful clinical descriptions with cutaneous biopsy specimens are frequently lacking.*

‡ *Such as constitutional diathesis and contact dermatitis.*

TABLE 48-2 Various types of eczematous dermatitis of known etiology

Clinical type	Pathogenesis	Diagnostic considerations
Allergic contact eczematous dermatitis	Chemical allergens (plants, medicaments, cosmetics, metals, fabrics, etc.)	Site and configuration are clues to causal agent; patch tests may confirm diagnosis; avoidance of cause cures eruption
Photoallergic contact eczematous dermatitis	Ultraviolet radiation plus topical chemicals (in soaps, perfumes, citrus fruits, etc.), which then become allergens	Occurs on exposed skin; photopatch tests confirm diagnosis
Polymorphous light-induced eruption—eczematous type	Ultraviolet radiation; sometimes visible light	Occurs on exposed skin; diagnosis implies that all known causes of light-induced eruptions have been eliminated
"Infectious eczematoid dermatitis"	Bacterial products from draining focus (e.g., ear infection)	Occurs near site of infection; responds to treatment of primary infection
Eczematous dermatophytosis	Fungus	Fungi demonstrated in scales or exudate

severity of the process itself. Serious metabolic effects of chronic exfoliative dermatitis occur when the rate of scaling reaches 17 g/m^2 per 24 h. Patients with extensive exfoliative dermatitis may have negative nitrogen balance, edema, hypoalbuminemia, and loss of muscle mass. Another salient feature in these patients is the large extrarenal water loss, due to markedly increased transepidermal water loss across the defective cutaneous barrier. The etiology of exfoliative dermatitis determines its course: the disease eventually clears in patients with psoriasis or atopic dermatitis, whereas the prognosis is relatively poor in patients with lymphoma and leukemia. Approximately 60 percent of patients with exfoliative dermatitis recover within 8 to 10 months, 30 percent die, and 10 percent have a persistent problem unresponsive to therapy.

Atrophy, diffuse or circumscribed Epidermal atrophy is manifested by an almost transparent epidermis and is associated with a decrease in the number of epidermal cells. Atrophic epidermis may or may not retain normal skin markings and is often associated with some alteration in the dermis. Circumscribed epidermal atrophy occurs in discoid lupus erythematosus, in necrobiosis lipoidica diabeticorum, and in striae cutis distensae; diffuse epidermal atrophy occurs with aging and in scleroderma.

The most important atrophic-type disorder is *necrobiosis lipoidica diabeticorum* (NLD) (Plate 5-1). These lesions, which are usually asymptomatic, occur more frequently in women and *on areas subject to trauma* such as the anterior and lateral surfaces of the lower legs. Lesions may also occur on the arms and even on the face. The lesion begins as a small, reddish, elevated nodule with a sharply circumscribed border, gradually enlarges, and becomes flattened and depressed as the skin becomes atrophic. The brownish-yellow–to–orange color is prominent, and blood vessels are readily seen because the atrophic epidermis is smooth, thin, and translucent. The lesions of NLD are often indolent, but shallow ulcerations that are very slow to heal may develop. NLD may apparently occur when diabetes mellitus cannot be detected, but full tests of glucose tolerance, such as the cortisone-glucose tolerance test, have not been done in large numbers of patients who fall into this catgory. NLD is characterized by focal changes in the dermis that present as acellular and intense eosinophilic areas of necrosis bordered by inflammation. Granulomatous inflammation with epithelioid cells, histiocytes, and multinucleated giant cells is a central feature. The blood vessels are always involved, with endothelial proliferation and sometimes even occlusion of arterioles and arteries deep within the dermis; capillary walls are thickened with focal deposits of PAS-positive material. NLD can be controlled with careful intralesional injections of suspensions of triamcinolone acetonide in some patients.

Hypomelanotic macules See Chap. 51.

Diffuse hypomelanosis See Chap. 51.

Hypermelanotic macules See Chap. 51.

Diffuse brown hypermelanosis syndrome See Chap. 51.

DERMIS Papules and nodules (with or without inflammation) Papules and nodules without epidermal change (i.e., scaling) may be either skin color, erythematous, or even slightly pigmented (yellow or brown). Dermal papules and all nodules require a biopsy for definitive diagnosis because they often represent processes that have general medical significance, such as sarcoidosis, or histiocytosis X, tuberculosis, lymphoma, or metastatic carcinoma. Inasmuch as dermal nodules may be present in deep mycotic infections such as coccidioidomycosis, it is necessary to obtain a biopsy not only to rule out malignancy but to culture a portion of the excised tissue for fungi. Cultures of nodules must be made from tissue ground by mortar and pestle. The histologic specimen should be carefully studied for the presence of acid-fast bacilli, since nodules are the presenting feature of leprosy and tuberculosis. Nodules removed from common areas of localization for leishmaniasis (face and arms) should be carefully examined for the presence of parasites.

Papules and nodules with and without inflammation can occur in disorders of the sebaceous glands. Sebaceous glands are distributed largely on the face and scalp, although they can also occur in the labia minora and on the scrotal skin, trunk, nipples, and eyelids. The sebaceous gland is a holocrine gland in which the entire cell is cast off into the excretory stream. Sebum is a complex lipid mixture of squalene (a major product of the steroid pathway), triglycerides, and wax esters. Sebaceous glands are controlled by direct hormonal stimulation by androgens, derived largely from the gonads in both sexes; in the female, but not in the male, adrenal androgens may be important factors in maintaining sebum production. The major disease of the sebaceous gland in humans is *acne vulgaris* which occurs predominantly on the face and, to a lesser degree, on the back, chest, and shoulders. It is characterized by a variety of clinical lesions. These lesions may be either noninflammatory or inflammatory papules and nodules. The noninflammatory papules are called comedones, and these may be either open (blackheads) or closed (whiteheads). Closed comedones are the precursors of papules, pustules, and large inflammatory nodules. In addition, cysts and scars of various sizes may occur; the typical acne scar is a sharply punched-out pit. Pustular and cystic lesions, despite a large amount of purulent exudate that may be recovered following incision, are usually sterile but may contain *Propionibacterium acnes*.

The initial stimulus to the formation of comedones (both the closed and open types) is not precisely known at this time, but the initial histologic event in comedone formation is excessive keratinization within the follicular canal. It is currently believed that lypolysis of triglycerides by *Propionibacterium acnes* releases fatty acids; it is thought that these fatty acids are capable of eliciting an inflammatory process in the follicle wall, which may then rupture. Discharge of the follicular content leads to perifollicular inflammation. The inflammatory infiltrate is lymphocytic, but later, as a result of the presence of keratinous material, gram-positive diphtheroids, and sebum, the infiltrate consists essentially of a foreign-body giant cell reaction.

There should be a careful search of the histologic material, with acid-fast stains, for tubercle and lepra bacilli, for tissue parasites (in leishmaniasis, echinococcus, cysticercosis, schistosomiasis, onchocerciasis, and myiasis), and for fungi (of actinomycosis, blastomycosis, sporotrichosis, coccidioidomycosis, and dermatophytosis). It is necessary to examine tissue sections with the polarizing microscope to detect zirconium and silicon and uric acid crystals. Acne vulgaris is a serious problem, especially common during adolescence, and its therapy is complex and prolonged. Moderate to severe acne vulgaris is best treated by dermatologists who are trained in a number of modalities: topical agents, incision and drainage of cystic lesions, ultraviolet light therapy, and judicious use of systemic antibiotics; x-ray therapy has no place in the treatment of acne vulgaris.

How antibiotics such as tetracycline improve acne is not completely understood, but these drugs are known to suppress the number of propionibacteria and to cause a reduction of free fatty acids on the skin. Because the organisms have been shown to have lipolytic activity in vitro, it is presumed that the antibiotic causes this reduction of free fatty acids. Benzoyl peroxide lotions and gels probably act as antibacterial agents and decrease the bacterial population; these agents are very effective and are widely used by dermatologists.

Estrogens combined with progestins (oral contraceptives) were initially considered to be effective in controlling acne; however, they have been of only limited value in the treatment of acne in females and cannot be given to males. There is no convincing evidence to suggest that particular foods have any effect on the course or severity of acne vulgaris. Acne vulgaris may begin as early as the eighth year or may not appear until the twentieth. It lasts for several years and then subsides spontaneously, usually in the early twenties. In some patients, however, acne vulgaris may continue into the third and fourth decades. Topical antibiotic solutions such as clindamycin or erythromycin are effective new agents for treatment of acne vulgaris. The most dramatically effective new treatment for severe cystic acne is orally administered 13-*cis*-retinoic acid. This drug acts rapidly and is very effective, but it is teratogenic and cannot be used in women of child-bearing age unless effective contraception is guaranteed. Other side effects, such as xerosis and hypertriglyceridemia, and bony spur formation mandate that it be used only in severe cases in which conventional modalities have failed.

Pretibial myxedema (PM) also may cause nodules on the legs and dorsa of the feet. The lesions are usually bilateral and consist of elevated, firm dermal nodules and plaques that are not easily movable. They may be skin color, pink, or, rarely, brown, and, when diascoped, appear yellow and waxy. The epidermis over the nodules may appear normal or may have a marked verrucous (warty) surface. The pathogenesis of pretibial myxedema is not clear. Pretibial myxedema may occur with or without hyperthyroidism (Graves' disease) or before or after treatment of hyperthyroidism, and its development does not parallel the ocular changes (if present). The nodules in pretibial myxedema are accumulations of mucopolysaccharides, which can be demonstrated by special staining of the histopathologic material. LATS (long-acting thyroid stimulator), which is associated in the plasma with immunoglobulin G (7 S gamma globulin), has been implicated in the pathogenesis of pretibial myxedema, exophthalmos, and acropachy; the role of LATS in the pathogenesis of pretibial myxedema has not been established.

Ulcers Ulcers occur as a result of destruction of the epidermis and, at least, the papillary layer of the dermis (see Fig. 47-4). All ulcers of the skin that do not heal within a period of a month must be assumed to be carcinoma until proved otherwise, and it is essential that a biopsy be obtained to rule out malignancy. Ulcers can be divided into two categories: lesions that occur on the legs and feet, and lesions that occur elsewhere on the body. Ulcers not occurring on the legs are rather rare except in primary cancer of the skin or in malignant metastases to the skin. Ulcers arising in nodules with inflammation should be approached in the manner suggested previously for nodules—that is, a biopsy should be obtained, and the tissue examined for bacterial, mycotic, and parasitic diseases. Chancre-like ulcerations and noduloulcerative lesions with regional lymphadenopathy may occur in primary syphilis, primary tuberculosis, and in tularemia, anthrax, glanders, and bubonic plague. Isolated noduloulcerative lesions may be seen in sporotrichosis, coccidioidomycosis, leishmaniasis, cryptococcosis, and tertiary syphilis. Serologic studies are necessary in the diagnosis of syphilis.

The most important etiologic factors in ulceration on the legs and feet are disturbances of circulation. Chronic venous insufficiency leads to ulceration, especially on the medial aspect of the ankle or lower leg, and the ulcers develop in areas of skin with brownish hemosiderin pigmentation and occasionally where there is edema or sclerosis of the area. Hypertensive or ischemic ulcerations tend to start on the lateral aspect of the ankle. Ulceration can also occur as a result of tissue infarction in areas supplied by either large or small blood vessels (arteries, arterioles); infarction may occur as the result of occlusion or constriction due to a variety of etiologic factors, in addition to those already mentioned: emboli, thrombosis, cryoagglutinins, macroglobulinemia, cryoglobulinemia, thrombotic thrombocytopenic purpura, polycythemia, systemic lupus erythematosus, Raynaud's phenomenon, arteriosclerosis obliterans, and thromboangiitis obliterans. Ulceration of the lower extremities also occurs in hemolytic anemia, including sickle cell anemia, thalassemia, and hereditary spherocytosis.

Some ulcers show extensive necrosis of the edges, such as those in *pyoderma gangrenosum,* an indolent ulcer usually on the lower extremities and often associated with ulcerative colitis or regional ileitis. The ulcers in pyoderma gangrenosum have ragged bluish-red overhanging edges and a necrotic base. These lesions often start as pustules or tender red nodules at the site of trauma, and then gradually increase in size until liquefaction necrosis occurs and an irregular ulcer develops. The ulcers are often multiple and may cover large areas of the leg. The histopathologic findings are not specific. The healing of the ulcers usually parallels the activity of the ulcerative colitis, and, inasmuch as the ulceration extends into and involves the reticular layer of the dermis and the subcutis, scarring occurs. Pyoderma gangrenosum and variants of it also occur in association with a number of other conditions such as myeloproliferative disorders and rheumatoid arthritis.

The term *''tropical'' ulcer,* in addition to cutaneous leishmaniasis, now also includes ulceration due to cutaneous diphtheria, treponemal disorders (syphilis, yaws, and bejel), and phagedenic ulcer, a chronic ulcer of the feet and legs caused by mixed bacteria that occurs in persons suffering from starvation and neglect.

Ulcers can be associated with peripheral neuropathy (''neuropathic'' ulcer, or malum perforans) seen in diabetes mellitus, tabes dorsalis, polyneuritis, leprosy, congenital anesthesia, or hereditary sensory radicular neuropathy.

Anal and perianal ulcers are seen in histiocytosis X and in amebiasis. A hanging-drop preparation is necessary to detect *Entamoeba histolytica.*

Ulcers with artificial and bizarre shapes must be suspected of being self-induced by means of destructive agents such as acid and lighted cigarettes. Factitial ulcers are overstudied and, unfortunately, underdiagnosed by most physicians.

Stony-hard, noduloulcerative lesions, particularly around joints (elbows, knees, and fingers) are suggestive of calcinosis cutis or gout; roentgenographic examination enables the detection of calcinosis cutis but shows no opaque bodies in gout.

Sclerosis, diffuse or circumscribed Diffuse sclerosis of the skin is most often seen on the upper extremities, chest, and face in systemic scleroderma (sometimes called progressive systemic sclerosis). Initially, the skin appears yellowish and shows slight nonpitting edema; later, however, it becomes indurated, bound down, and may be markedly hyperpigmented. Calcinosis cutis and Raynaud's phenomenon commonly occur.

Circumscribed sclerosis occurs in *morphea,* which consists of one or more round or oval, firm, reddish plaques up to several centimeters in diameter that become white or yellow centrally, often with a lilac-colored, telangiectatic border. This disorder is not associated with any other organ involvement and is a localized cutaneous form of scleroderma. Another type of localized scleroderma is *linear scleroderma,* in which the morphologic change is the same as that seen in morphea except that the process occurs in bands extending parallel to the long axis of the extremity or along the paramedian line of the forehead and scalp. This form of scleroderma has no relationship to progressive systemic sclerosis.

Edema In addition to the various causes of localized edema and generalized edema, there is a type of edema of the lower extremities that is not often recognized by the physician. This is a bilateral pedal edema which is common in patients with subacute or chronic dermatitis of the lower extremities. This type of edema is most often seen with chronic eczematous dermatitis and psoriasis, but is unrelated to cardiac failure or lymphatic obstruction. It is most probably due to an increased permeability as a result of local capillary damage, which is part of the inflammatory process in the skin. The increased capillary permeability leads to an increased transfer of fluid from the intravascular to the extravascular component of the extracellular fluid space. This type of pitting edema disappears completely when the dermatitis has resolved.

Atrophy, diffuse or circumscribed Dermal atrophy results from a decrease of the papillary or reticular connective tissue and is manifested in the skin as a depression. Circumscribed dermal atrophy may follow trauma, or may occur in association with epidermal atrophy, as in the striae of pregnancy or Cushing's disease.

PANNICULUS ADIPOSUS (SUBCUTIS) Nodules (inflammatory, usually tender, red) Nodules in the subcutis may be recognized by the fact that the skin is usually movable over the nodule; occasionally, however, in inflammatory processes, the nodule may involve both the dermis and panniculus adiposus, and the skin will then not be movable over the nodule. Acute, tender, red nodules on the leg are characteristically found in two disorders: *erythema nodosum syndrome* and *nodular subcutaneous fat necrosis* associated with pancreatitis.

The erythema nodosum syndrome refers to the occurrence of multiple bilateral tender nodules appearing principally on the anterior aspect of the lower extremities and occasionally on the upper extremities and face. The erythema nodosum syndrome is associated with a number of disorders that are unrelated to each other, except for their ability to elicit this distinctive hypersensitivity reaction.

The nodules in erythema nodosum are only slightly elevated, edematous, and sometimes exquisitely tender. Bruising is a characteristic feature of the disease and is due to hemorrhage, leading to the formation of contusions. The lesions never ulcerate or become indurated and very seldom leave any scarring or atrophy. Erythema nodosum is associated with primary tuberculosis and primary coccidioidomycosis, histoplasmosis, *Yersinia* infection, beta-hemolytic streptococcal infections, lymphogranuloma venereum, leprosy, sarcoidosis, ulcerative colitis, Crohn's disease, regional enteritis, drugs (penicillin, sulfonamides, bromides, iodides), and oral contraceptives containing ethynylestradiol and norethynodrel.

Tender, red subcutaneous nodules may also appear on the legs in association with acute pancreatitis and with pancreatic neoplasms and are often erroneously called erythema nodosum. This disorder has been termed *nodular liquefying panniculitis* (NLP). These lesions are distinctive. Their morphologic features are different from those of classic erythema nodosum. The lesions in NLP vary in size from a few millimeters to several centimeters, and, in contrast to the lesions of erythema nodosum, are movable. The lesions of NLP involute in 2 to 3 weeks and may leave a hyperpigmented scar that is slightly depressed. The nodules are often associated with abdominal pain and may also be accompanied by fever and arthralgia. Rarely, lesions may be present on other parts of the body besides the legs. Some of the larger nodules may undergo an abscess-like change, become fluctuant, rupture, and exude a whitish, creamy, or oily viscous material; abscess formation with drainage rarely, if ever, occurs in erythema nodosum. The most common pancreatic neoplasm associated with NLP is an acinous adenocarcinoma of the pancreas. In *Weber-Christian panniculitis,* the subcutaneous nodules, which at first are slightly mobile, become adherent to the overlying skin; then, as the edema subsides in the area of induration, a central depression occurs.

In addition to the above-mentioned entities, various types of vasculitis may also produce tender subcutaneous nodules. Therefore, diagnosis of these lesions often requires an excisional or incisional biopsy.

Nodules (noninflammatory, usually nontender, nonerythematous) Movable, painless, noninflammatory-appearing nodules occur around joints in rheumatic fever, rheumatoid arthritis, and in certain metabolic diseases such as xanthoma, gout, and calcinosis. Metastatic carcinoma or metastatic malignant melanoma may appear as movable, nontender subcutaneous nodules. Sarcoidosis may be manifested in the skin solely as subcutaneous nodules on the lower extremities. Subcutaneous nodules also occur in onchocerciasis and loiasis. *Lipomas,* relatively common causes of subcutaneous nodules, are benign tumors composed of adipose tissue and may be single or multiple and are frequently lobulated; they are often rubbery or compressible and occur most often on the trunk and back of the neck and forearms. Occasionally, subcutaneous lipoma may be painful and associated with marked obesity; this condition, known as *Dercum's disease,* is most common in middle-aged females.

Atrophy, diffuse or circumscribed Atrophy of the panniculus adiposus produces depressions in the skin; these depressions are seen in progressive lipodystrophy, in liquefying panniculitis, and in the localized fat atrophy that occurs at the site of injections of insulin. About 25 percent of diabetics who receive insulin (most often females under the age of 20) have this type of atrophy. The depressed areas of localized fat atrophy show a complete absence of the panniculus, and there is no inflammation. In lipodystrophy, diffuse atrophy of the skin may involve large portions of the body.

BLOOD VESSELS Morbilliform and scarlatiniform eruptions Morbilliform (measles-like) and scarlatiniform eruptions are macular and papular exanthems and can be due to drug hypersensitivities, measles, German measles, erythema infectiosum, other viral exanthems, rickettsial diseases including endemic murine typhus and Rocky Mountain spotted fever, scarlet fever, and secondary syphilis. Many of the diseases manifested by macules or papules and occurring in acutely ill patients with a fever are listed in Table 48-3.

Urticaria Urticaria is characterized by wheals, of which the outstanding feature is their persistence for only a few hours (see Fig. 47-6). This short duration differentiates urticarial wheals from the otherwise almost identical papules of erythema multiforme, which persist for more than 1 or 2 days rather than for a few hours. An acute onset of urticaria is usually related to ingestion of drugs or certain types of foods (shellfish, fresh berries).

Chronic recurrent urticaria is a special problem, and its causes are not easily established. Most patients with this disorder require a careful examination for cryptic diseases such as lymphoma, systemic lupus erythematosus, primary or metastatic carcinoma, intestinal parasites, acute hepatitis, systemic vasculitis, or dermatomyositis. It is especially important, even in chronic urticarias, to carry out a painstaking interrogation of the patient in search of a history of drugs. Aspirin is one of the most common causes of chronic urticaria and can often be missed even in a careful drug history because many patients do not consider aspirin a drug. It is probably true that some patients with chronic urticaria can relate their problem to emotional stress, but this should be considered only after excluding all possible organic causes.

Erythema multiforme syndrome Erythema multiforme syndrome is a characteristic response of the skin and mucous membranes that is related to a number of possible etiologies, including infectious agents (herpesvirus hominis, *Mycoplasma pneumoniae*) and drugs (especially penicillin, antipyretics, barbiturates, hydantoins, and sulfonamides). In 50 percent of patients no etiology is ascertained. The major pathologic change is an acute lymphohistiocytic inflammatory infiltrate around blood vessels and at the dermal-epidermal interface. Degenerative changes in the endothelial cells of the capillaries, marked papillary dermal edema, and keratinocyte necrosis are also seen. There is some evidence for an immune-complex etiology with hypocomplementemic vasculitis.

The lesions occur in a characteristic symmetric distribution and favor the extensor areas of the distal parts of the limbs, the backs of the hands, and the dorsa of the feet; the palms and soles are often involved, even to the exclusion of the dorsal surfaces. Oral lesions, first as blisters and then erosions, occur on the buccal mucous membrane, gums, and tongue, and there is often swelling and crusting of the lips. The syndrome may also include severe toxemia and prostration, high fever, cough, and ''patchy'' inflammation of the lungs. The skin lesions are often characterized by a vivid redness that gradually becomes duller, and they become more indurated, with the development of centers that are pale or may have bullae; these ''target'' or ''iris'' lesions, which are characteristic of erythema multiforme but do not invariably occur, are identified by the clear red area at the periphery that surrounds a pale pink zone and a central livid area, which may contain a bulla. The efficacy of systemic corticosteroids has not been proved, but this therapy is commonly used.

Purpura (with and without inflammation) A purpuric eruption demands immediate exploration for its etiology. Purpura arises in the skin of the vascularized dermis and is almost always confined to the dermis. Purpuric macules gradually disappear after days or weeks, depending on their size. Punctate or tiny purpuric spots are termed *petechiae,* larger (>2.0 cm) macules are spoken of as *suggillations,* and extensive purpuric macules are called *ecchymoses* (see D in Fig. 47-2).

Purpura with inflammation is usually ''palpable,'' i.e., papular, and is seen in systemic vasculitis and in bacteremias such as staphylococcemia, gonococcemia, and meningococcemia. In these bacteremias and in vasculitis, the examination of biopsied skin may establish a diagnosis within 8 h (the time required for processing the tissue). Gentle scraping of the purpuric lesions will produce enough material for a Gram's stain; intracellular gram-negative diplococci are occasionally found in the lesions in acute, but not in chronic, meningococcemia, and are rarely found in acute gonococcemia. The differential diagnosis of palpable purpuric lesions and infarcts occurring in *systemic vasculitis* (necrotizing vasculitis) as compared with those in chronic meningococcemia is not easy. The skin lesions in systemic vasculitis are usually bilateral, and almost symmetric, in their distribution. They tend to be concentrated on the lower extremities, especially on the lower portion and around the ankles and the dorsa of the feet. The lesions in chronic meningococcemia are more randomly distributed, with occurrence on the trunk, lower and upper extremities, and face. Nevertheless, in meningococcemia, lesions can occur in a bilateral distribution, which makes the distinction between chronic meningococcemia and systemic vasculitis difficult, if not impossible, at times. The individual lesions in both chronic meningococcemia and systemic vasculitis may be identical, consisting of a mixture of palpable purpura and urticarial-type papules without purpura. Unfortunately, the histologic findings in biopsy specimens of the lesions in both diseases do not permit a distinction. Therefore, a patient with bilaterally distributed palpable purpuric lesions and fever is best treated with antibiotics before the results of blood cultures are available.

Purpura without inflammation is completely macular, and examination of a blood smear can quickly establish the presence of platelets; if platelets are seen in the smear, thrombocytopenic purpura can be safely ruled out as a possibility.

On the lower legs of older people, a great variety of inflammatory skin diseases, including various types of contact dermatitis, may be associated with purpura; under these circumstances, the purpura does not have the same importance as it does when present on the trunk or upper extremities. Perifollicular purpura, however, on the lower extremities (usually accompanied by follicular hyperkeratosis) is almost pathognomonic of scurvy.

Purpura frequently develops in amyloidosis when the lesions (waxy macules and papules) are pinched. This ''pinch'' purpura, however, may also occur in the normal skin of patients with thrombocytopenic purpura or in the skin of apparently normal elderly persons. (For a full discussion of the classification and differential diagnosis of purpura, see Chaps. 54 and 279.)

Infarcts Infarcts in the skin are usually not pale like those that occur in the kidney but have a variegated dusky red, grayish hue. They are irregularly shaped macules, sometimes slightly depressed below the plane of the skin, and often surrounded by a pink zone of hyperemia. Infarcts are usually slightly tender.

Cutaneous infarctions are important and often diagnostic signs of serious multisystem disease, including both acute and chronic meningococcemia, streptococcal and staphylococcal septicemia, gonococcemia, pseudomonas septicemia, systemic vasculitis, purpura fulminans, systemic lupus erythematosus, and, rarely, dermatomyositis. Degos' disease (malignant atrophic papulosis), in which porcelain-white macules are surrounded by a narrow telangiectatic and erythematous rim, is often associated with similar infarctions in the gastrointestinal and central nervous system.

Telangiectasia Redness of the skin is most freqently caused by transient dilatation of blood vessels (erythema). In contrast to the color produced by fixed blood pigments, as in purpura, the erythema will disappear under the pressure of a glass or plastic slide (see ''Diascopy,'' in Chap. 47). Telangiectasia is the condition in which redness of the skin results from a permanent enlargement in the caliber of small blood vessels (which will be revealed by examination with a hand lens) and an increase in the number of the vessels. Telangiectasia may be composed of fine linear branches of blood vessels appearing distinctly red (i.e., not blue), which are often seen on the nose and face, or of confluent macular areas that appear as a permanent erythema. Erythema in discoid and systemic lupus ery-

TABLE 48-3 Rash and fever in the acutely ill patient: Diagnosis according to type of lesion

DISEASES MANIFESTED BY MACULES OR PAPULES	
Drug hypersensitivities	Rocky Mountain spotted fever (early lesions)*
Scarlet fever	Pityriasis rosea
Erythema infectiosum (fifth disease)	Erythema multiforme
Measles (rubeola)	Erythema marginatum
German measles (rubella)*	Systemic lupus erythematosus*
Enterovirus (echo- and coxsackievirus) infections	Dermatomyositis
Adenovirus infections	''Serum sickness''* (manifested only as wheals)
Typhoid fever	Urticaria, acute (viral hepatitis)
Secondary syphilis	Urticaria, persistent (necrotizing angiitis)
Typhus, murine (endemic)	Lyme disease
DISEASES MANIFESTED BY VESICLES, BULLAE, OR PUSTULES	
Drug hypersensitivities	Variola†
Dermatitis from plants	Enterovirus (echo- and coxsackievirus) infections, including hand-foot-mouth disease
Rickettsialpox	Toxic epidermal necrolysis
Varicella (chickenpox)†	Staphylococcal scaled-skin syndrome
Generalized herpes zoster†	Erythema multiforme bullosum
Disseminated herpes simplex†	
Eczema herpeticum†	
Disseminated vaccinia†	
Eczema vaccinatum†	
DISEASES MANIFESTED BY PURPURIC MACULES, PURPURIC PAPULES, OR PURPURIC VESICLES	
Drug hypersensitivities	Enterovirus (echo- and coxsackievirus) infections
Bacteremia:‡	Rickettsial diseases:
Meningococcemia (acute or chronic)*	Rocky Mountain spotted fever*
Gonococcemia*	Typhus, louse-borne (epidemic)
Staphylococcemia	''Allergic'' vasculitis*‡
Pseudomonas bacteremia	Purpura fulminans‡
Subacute bacterial endocarditis	Acquired immunodeficiency syndrome

* *May have arthralgia or musculoskeletal pain.*
† *One characteristic lesion of these exanthems is an umbilicated papule or vesicle.*
‡ *Often present as infarcts.*
SOURCE: *TB Fitzpatrick, RA Johnson, in Dermatology in General Medicine, 3d ed, TB Fitzpatrick et al (eds), New York, McGraw-Hill, 1987.*

thematosus, dermatomyositis, and psoriasis is caused largely by the presence of telangiectasia.

Telangiectasia may also occur in a scattered, discrete fashion on the upper trunk or on the extremities and is seen characteristically in progressive systemic sclerosis (systemic scleroderma). Telangiectasia occurring around the nail beds, i.e., periungual telangiectasia, is an important diagnostic sign in lupus erythematosus (both discoid and systemic) and in dermatomyositis; these lesions are seen rarely, if at all, in systemic scleroderma or rheumatoid arthritis.

Sharply outlined, red macules or papules 1 to 2 mm in diameter, with an area of radiating telangiectasia, are seen in *hereditary hemorrhagic telangiectasia* (Chap. 281). These occur on the lips, tongue, nasal mucosa, face, and hands.

Generalized telangiectasia occurring in the form of red macules over most of the body surface may be the presenting sign of mastocytosis or urticaria pigmentosa.

Telangiectasia is a prominent and diagnostic feature of *ataxia-telangiectasia,* or Louis-Bar syndrome. Telangiectasia may be present as early as the second year of life but usually develops by the fifth year; it appears first on the bulbar conjunctiva and subsequently involves the ears, the eyelids, the butterfly area of the face, the upper aspect of the chest, and the extremities.

Telangiectasia may occur in a characteristic form known as the *arterial spider,* or spider nevus, spider angioma, or naevus araneus. The main vessel of the spider is an arteriole, and it is usually faintly pulsating, which will show under the diascope. A less common skin lesion usually found with vascular spiders in liver disorders is the telangiectatic *mat* or net, a small red patch composed of intermeshed fine vessels that blanch on pressure. Spider angiomas, usually three or fewer, occur not infrequently in normal children and adults. Numerous spider angiomas often develop during pregnancy or after the ingestion of progestational agents or in rheumatoid arthritis or thyrotoxicosis. Most patients with numerous and prominent vascular spiders, however, have some form of underlying diffuse liver disease, e.g., alcoholic cirrhosis. The progression of subacute hepatitis is often paralleled by the appearance of crops of spiders, and in alcoholic and postnecrotic cirrhosis, almost half the patients have multiple vascular spiders. The mechanism responsible for the development of spider angiomas in liver disease is not known, nor has it been firmly established that the lesions result from disordered metabolism of estrogens by the liver.

REFERENCES

BRAVERMAN I: *Skin Signs of Systemic Disease*. Philadelphia, Saunders, 1981

FARBER EM, COX AJ (eds): *Psoriasis: Proceedings of the Third International Symposium*. New York, Yorke Medical, 1981

FITZPATRICK TB, BERNHARD JD: The structure of skin lesions and fundamentals of diagnosis, in *Dermatology in General Medicine*, 3d ed., TB Fitzpatrick et al (eds). New York, McGraw-Hill, 1987

HENSELER T et al: Oral 8-methoxypsoralen photochemotherapy of psoriasis. Lancet 1:853, 1981

HONIGSMANN H et al: Oral photochemotherapy with psoralens and UVA (PUVA): Principles and practice, in *Dermatology in General Medicine*, 3d ed, TB Fitzpatrick et al (eds). New York, McGraw-Hill, 1987

LEYDEN JJ, KLIGMAN AM: The role of bacteria in acne vulgaris, in *Progress in Diseases of the Skin*, R Fleischmajer (ed). Orlando, Grune & Stratton, 1984, pp 21, 29

PARRISH JA et al: Photochemotherapy of psoriasis with oral methoxsalen and longwave ultraviolet light. N Engl J Med 291:1207, 1974

PECK GL et al: Prolonged remissions of cystic acne with 13-*cis*-retinoic acid. N Engl J Med 300:329, 1979

49 RASH AND FEVER

LAWRENCE COREY / PHILIP KIRBY

Because many infectious and noninfectious diseases produce cutaneous lesions, specific diagnosis of an acutely ill febrile patient with a rash is a clinical skill with important therapeutic implications. Some exanthems are unique to a particular pathogen; others are common to numerous etiologic agents. Classification of exanthematous illness into (1) maculopapular, (2) vesicular, or (3) petechial eruptions is useful in determining the etiology and in understanding the pathogenesis of an exanthem.

PATHOGENESIS Exanthems are cutaneous eruptions due to systemic or contiguous spread of an organism. The pathogenesis of an exanthem may be caused by (1) multiplication of the pathogen in the skin, (2) carriage of the agent in plasma or in infected hematopoietic cells (leukocytes and/or lymphocytes) into integumentary blood vessels, or (3) antigen-antibody or delayed hypersensitivity reactions to antigens derived from the infecting microorganism.

Maculopapular exanthems may be caused by either direct viral or bacterial invasion of the skin or local or systemic immune responses to the microorganism. For example, rubella virus can be recovered from rubella maculopapules as well as from areas of the body not involved by the exanthem. Administration of pooled immune serum globulin after exposure to rubella may not eliminate rubella viremia but does prevent rash. The exanthem of rubeola may be a manifestation of an Arthus reaction produced by the deposition of viral antigen in the endothelium of dermal capillaries. The complex interplay between the host and the pathogen may influence the duration and pattern of a rash. In many viral illnesses, such as enterovirus infections, initial viral replication occurs in the infected mucosal surface and regional lymphatic tissue. A primary viremia then ensues, and ''seeding'' of the virus into target organs, such as liver, muscle, central nervous system, or heart, may occur. Continued viral replication and a secondary viremia with hematogenous spread of the virus to the skin may then follow. The regional multiplication of the virus, primary viremia, and visceral dissemination of virus prior to the development of the exanthem help explain why the initial clinical manifestations of many illnesses occur prior to the development of the rash. Humoral and cellular immune responses which prevent or ameliorate secondary viremia may prevent the development of rash and may explain why exanthems associated with enteroviruses occur more frequently in younger children than in adolescents or adults; young children do not possess cross-reacting antibodies or cannot mount an anamnestic immune response to the infecting agent.

As with maculopapular eruptions, vesicular exanthems can be caused either by direct invasion into the skin by organisms such as herpes simplex virus, varicella-zoster virus, or the coxsackieviruses causing hand-foot-and-mouth disease; by elaboration of a toxin such as in staphylococcal scalded skin syndrome, or by host immune responses such as bullous erythema multiforme or pemphigus.

Petechial eruptions may arise from direct invasion of the cutaneous vasculature by a microorganism, as occurs with septic emboli, or may result from immunologic injury to the vascular endothelium. In Rocky Mountain spotted fever, for example, *Rickettsia rickettsiae* can be demonstrated in the smooth muscle wall of arterioles. Vascular damage, microinfarction, and extravasation of red blood cells produce the characteristic petechial exanthem. Occasionally, a petechial eruption may complicate previous maculopapular or vesicular exanthems, usually coinciding with the development of diffuse intravascular coagulation. In some petechial eruptions, direct evidence of viral or bacterial invasion can be obtained by direct aspiration and culture of the lesion, by demonstration of the agent with Gram's stain, or by immunofluorescent stain to detect microbial agents.

CLINICAL DIAGNOSIS OF MACULOPAPULAR ERUPTIONS Table 49-1 lists the numerous viral, bacterial, rickettsial, and noninfectious agents that may be associated with maculopapular exanthems. One helpful approach to the physical examination of viral maculopapular (not vesicular) rashes is that these eruptions relatively spare the palms and soles in contrast to eruptions associated with drug reactions, bacteria, mycoplasma, and rickettsial and/or immunologic diseases. In the last two entities, a prominent palmar or plantar distribution is often present.

While some exanthematous diseases produce characteristic cutaneous patterns, e.g., measles or erythema infectiosum, overlap in the cutaneous manifestations of viral induced maculopapular exanthems is the rule. Therefore, the presence of associated signs or symptoms as well as the epidemiologic characteristics of the disease, such as the season of the year, the patient's age, and history of exposure and previous immunization, are useful in formulating a diagnostic impression. Because viral maculopapular exanthems are manifestations of the agent's systemic spread, evidence of mucosal viral replication in the form of an enanthem is often a valuable aid in determining the etiology of a viral rash. Koplik's spots in rubeola, ulcerative lesions of the hard and soft palate with herpangina due to coxsackievirus A, and palatal petechiae in early infectious mononucleosis are all helpful clinical signs. Associated clinical findings such as coryza, conjunctivitis, and cough with rubeola; mild fever and posterior auricular lymphadenopathy in rubella; or localized mastitis or furunculosis in staphylococcal scalded skin syndrome should be looked for. Concomitant arthritis, renal disease, and/or heart disease generally suggest entities such as acute rheumatic fever, subacute bacterial endocarditis, serum sickness, or collagen vascular disease.

The distribution of the rash provides important information. Erythema infectiosum presents with a diffuse erythema of the cheeks ("slapped cheeks"). In addition, central clearing of the eruption on the extremities results in a lacelike appearance of the exanthem. Erythema marginatum occurs in 10 percent of patients with acute rheumatic fever and is characterized by a ringed eruption which rapidly spreads to the trunk and extremities. Scarlet fever due to erythrogenic toxin elaborated by a group A streptococcus produces a rash that starts on the neck and spreads to the trunk and extremities within 36 h. The rash consists of numerous punctate papular lesions at the site of hair follicles and feels like rough sandpaper. Circumoral pallor, large red fungiform papillae (strawberry tongue), extension of the rash into body folds including the antecubital fossae, concomitant tonsillitis and cervical lymphadenopathy, and the subsequent desquamation of the rash, especially on the palms and soles, confirm the clinical diagnosis. Erysipelas due to group A (uncommonly group G) streptococci and staphylococci is characterized by an edematous indurated superficial cellulitis. Characteristically, the rash is shiny with a sharply demarcated edge. Occasionally streptococci can be demonstrated on Gram's stain and culture of material aspirated from the advancing edge of the lesion.

Some strains of *Staphylococcus aureus* (phage group 2) can elaborate a toxin which produces a diffuse erythema of the skin (staphylococcal scalded skin syndrome). The development of bullae resulting from the easy separation of the epidermis (Nikolsky's sign) may occur but is not specific for this entity.

Staphylococcal toxic shock syndrome is characterized by the acute onset of fever, hypotension, vomiting, diarrhea, vaginal discharge, and the development of a diffuse scarlatiniform rash with subsequent desquamation (see Chap. 94). This syndrome was reported with increasing frequency in the United States between 1978 and 1980 especially in young menstruating women using tampons. *Staphylococcus aureus*, often in pure culture, was isolated from nearly all of these patients not receiving antimicrobials. Relapses of disease, which are usually milder, are occasionally seen. The staphylococcal strains isolated from these patients appear to elaborate newly described toxin(s).

The course of the eruption is also helpful in differentiating the etiology of viral exanthems. Rubeola usually starts in the hairline area and spreads downward until the involved areas coalesce into a diffuse morbilliform eruption. In contrast, the eruption of

TABLE 49-1 Differential diagnosis of patients with rash and fever

Macules or papules	Vesicles & pustules	Petechiae-purpura
VIRAL		
Rubeola Rubella Enteroviruses Cytomegalovirus Hepatitis B Erythema infectiosum Exanthem subitum Adenoviruses Arboviruses Rhabdovirus group Reoviruses Live virus vaccines (measles, rubella)	Herpes simplex Varicella-zoster Vaccinia Enteroviruses (herpangina) Hand-foot-and-mouth disease (A16) Orf Molluscum contagiosum Vesicular stomatitis virus	Enteroviruses (echovirus) Viral hemorrhagic fevers Dengue Adenoviruses Yellow fever Atypical measles
BACTERIAL		
Group A streptococci: Scarlet fever Erysipelas Erythema marginatum Staphylococcal scalded-skin syndrome Staphylococcal toxic shock syndrome Subacute bacterial endocarditis Secondary syphilis Typhoid fever *Erysipelothrix* *Myobacterium leprae* Rat bite fever Leptospirosis Chronic meningococcemia *Pseudomonas* sepsis Erythema chronicum migrans (Lyme disease)	Staphylococcal scalded-skin syndrome Bullous impetigo	Severe sepsis with diffuse intravascular coagulation Meningococcemia Gonococcemia *Haemophilus influenzae* (type B) *Pseudomonas* sepsis Subacute bacterial endocarditis *Listeria monocytogenes*
RICKETTSIAL		
Rocky Mountain spotted fever (early) Murine typhus	Rickettsialpox	Rocky Mountain spotted fever Epidemic (louse-borne) typhus
FUNGAL		
Candidiasis Sporotrichosis Cryptococcosis Tinea versicolor Pityriasis rosea Tinea corporis		
CHLAMYDIAL		
Psittacosis		
PROTOZOAL		
Toxoplasmosis Trichinosis Scabies		Trichinosis Plasmodia (blackwater fever)
IMMUNOLOGIC		
Erythema multiforme Systemic lupus erythematosis Dermatomyositis Relapsing polychondritis Rheumatoid arthritis Erythema nodosum Urticarial vasculitis Leukemic infiltrate	Erythema multiforme Pustular psoriasis Reiter's syndrome Sweet's syndrome Behçet's syndrome Bowel bypass syndrome Acne fulminans	Immune thrombocytopenic purpura Thrombotic thrombocytopenic purpura Henoch-Schönlein purpura Polyarteritis nodosa Wegener's granulomatosis Cholesterol embolization
UNKNOWN		
Mucocutaneous lymph node syndrome		
DRUGS		
Drug eruptions	Drug eruptions	Drug eruptions

rubella tends to disappear from its original sites of involvement as it spreads.

The rash of Rocky Mountain spotted fever usually starts on the extremities and spreads centripetally to the trunk. In contrast, the rash of roseola subitum starts on the trunk and spreads centrifugally to the arms and legs. Pityriasis rosea is characterized by the development of papular lesions along the lines of cleavage of the trunk (''fir tree'' effect). The development of the earlier appearing ''herald patch'' and the lack of fever characterize this exanthem.

While papular lesions may be a manifestation of viral disease, systemic bacterial and/or fungal disease may also produce these lesions. Chronic meningococcemia may be associated with pale-rose-colored maculopapular lesions that may be mistaken for erythema nodosum when located on the lower extremities. The cutaneous lesions tend to wax and wane with fever. Organisms usually are not demonstrated in Gram's stain or cultures of these lesions. However, blood cultures taken during febrile periods may be positive. The development of discrete papules on the trunk in a patient with a previous history of diarrhea should suggest the possibility of typhoid fever. These ''rose spots'' are 1- to 3-mm papules which disappear in 3 to 4 days. In the untreated patient new lesions will emerge over the next 2 to 3 weeks. *Pseudomonas* bacteremia can also produce small painless papules on the trunk. The papulosquamous lesions of secondary syphilis often involve the trunk, palms, soles, and mucous membranes and may be present for days to several weeks. The serology (VDRL) is invariably positive in secondary syphilis. Erythema chronicum migrans is an exanthem characteristically seen in Lyme disease, an illness caused by the spirochete *Borrelia burgdorferi*. The lesion starts as a small red papule or macule which may gradually expand over a period of days to weeks. Multiple annular or secondary lesions are common. A history of tick bite and associated neurologic, cardiac, and rheumatologic findings are important factors in considering Lyme disease.

Papulonodular lesions can be identified in 10 to 15 percent of patients with disseminated candidiasis. The appearance of these lesions in febrile immunosuppressed patients who fail to respond to antimicrobials should suggest the possibility. Biopsy and culture of the lesions should demonstrate the blastospores and pseudohyphae of *Candida* species.

Noninfectious causes of maculopapular eruptions and fever Drug eruptions are probably the most common noninfectious causes of maculopapular rash and fever. Drug eruptions may be urticarial, bullous, exfoliative, and lichenoid, but the typical drug eruption resembles the exanthem of measles and is often called morbilliform. Drug eruptions begin centrally and extend centrifugally to the extremities, often affecting the palms and soles. They usually begin within one to several weeks after starting a drug, but may be delayed. While most drugs occasionally produce rashes, those most commonly associated with fever and rash include sulfonamides, phenytoin, barbiturates, sulfones, iodides, and bromides. Past and current exposure to the drug is a most important part of the diagnosis.

Several collagen vascular diseases produce distinctive papular rashes and fever. Systemic lupus erythematosus is best known for malar erythema in a ''butterfly'' distribution, but may also include scaly ''discoid'' plaques or bullae. Dermatomyositis is less commonly associated with fever, but has a heliotrope erythema of the periorbital skin and flat violaceous papules over the knuckles (Gottron's papules). Relapsing polychondritis causes episodes of fever and erythema over cartilaginous structures, particularly the superior portion of the ear. Rheumatoid arthritis may present with fever and transient erythematous macules prior to the onset of joint complaints. The diagnosis of collagen vascular diseases usually rests on evidence of specific organ involvement and serologic studies, but recognition and biopsy of skin lesions may be helpful.

Erythema nodosum is a form of panniculitis occurring most commonly in young women. Patients have fever, arthralgias, and exquisitely tender erythematous nodules over the pretibial region bilaterally. Erythema nodosum is often idiopathic, but can be associated with inflammatory bowel disease, streptococcal infection, oral contraceptives, sarcoidosis (Lofgren's syndrome), and many other diseases. Biopsy may be needed for diagnosis and to exclude other forms of panniculitis, such as Weber-Christian syndrome. Erythema multiforme may occur as a papular eruption, but is discussed with vesicular disease. Leukemic or lymphomatous infiltration of the skin may present with fever and adenopathy. Acute monocytic leukemia, myelomonocytic leukemia, chronic lymphocytic leukemia, and non-Hodgkin's lymphoma may all produce nontender plum-colored papules which usually involve the upper body. Biopsy is diagnostic.

CLINICAL DIAGNOSIS OF VESICULAR AND PUSTULAR ERUPTIONS The distribution of the eruption is often helpful in determining a clinical and etiologic diagnosis of a vesicular exanthem. Varicella begins on the trunk, spreads centrifugally, and demonstrates lesions in all stages of healing, i.e., vesicles, ulcers, and crusts. Variola usually begins on the extremities, spreads centripetally, and is characterized by lesions in similar stages of development. The vesicular ulcerative pharyngeal lesions of herpangina are present only on the palate, whereas primary herpes simplex gingivostomatitis also involves the anterior gingival area and/or the lips. Hand-foot-and-mouth disease due to coxsackievirus A16 presents as multiple linear vesicles or pustules on the palms and soles; this is an unusual distribution for either herpes simplex or varicella-zoster virus.

First-episode primary herpes simplex virus (HSV) infection is often accompanied by constitutional symptoms such as fever, malaise, and myalgias; numerous bilaterally distributed lesions; and tender regional lymphadenopathy. In contrast, patients with recurrent HSV are usually afebrile and have only a few clustered unilateral lesions which last from 5 to 12 days. Patients will often complain of a ''prodrome,'' a tingling sensation near or at the eventual site of lesion, from 2 to 48 h prior to the appearance of vesicles. Occasionally, HSV infection will present in a dermatomal distribution that is usually characteristic of herpes zoster. Because cytologic techniques do not differentiate between these two agents, viral cultures or use of specific techniques such as immunofluorescence must be employed in order to differentiate these two viruses.

The appearance of vesicles may be helpful. Herpes simplex and varicella lesions have a surrounding zone of erythema and a thin vesicular roof, and they are tender when irritated. The lesions of molluscum contagiosum are umbilicated, contain an expressible white core, and are usually not tender when scraped gently.

NONINFECTIOUS CAUSES OF VESICULAR AND PUSTULAR ERUPTION Erythema multiforme is a hypersensitivity reaction affecting skin and mucous membranes. The spectrum of erythema multiforme ranges from mild papular reactions to life-threatening bullous diseases referred to as Stevens-Johnson syndrome and toxic epidermal necrolysis. Erythema multiforme has been associated with an extensive list of conditions and often occurs idiopathically, but the most common causes are drugs and infections. Infectious causes include herpes simplex and mycoplasma. Common drug etiologies are phenytoin, sulfonamides, phenobarbital, and penicillins. Recurrent erythema multiforme is usually due to herpes simplex. The classic lesion of erythema multiforme is the target, or iris, lesion with a central dusky papule or vesicle surrounded by concentric rings of erythema and pallor. Lesions are most frequent on the extremities and face, but may be generalized.

Pustular eruptions can be particularly difficult to distinguish from bacterial and viral infections. Culture and biopsy are usually needed to define an etiology. Pustular psoriasis is a rare condition affecting persons both with and without a prior history of psoriasis. The onset is abrupt with disseminated erythematous papules and plaques with superficial pustules and lakes of pus. Annular lesions are common and the oral mucosa is often involved. Progression to erythroderma and death rarely occurs with modern treatment modalities. Reiter's syndrome may produce similar lesions which begin as pustules and become crusted papules called keratoderma blennorrhagicum. The triad of urethritis, arthritis, and conjunctivitis is usually present.

Sweet's syndrome, acute febrile neutrophilic dermatosis, is characterized by fever, leukocytosis, arthralgia, and single or multiple painful erythematous, pustular plaques of the face and upper body. Sweet's syndrome is most frequent in women, may be recurrent, and has been associated with prior upper respiratory infection and myeloproliferative disease. Cultures are negative and biopsy is diagnostic.

Behçet's syndrome is characterized by oral and genital ulceration, uveitis, arthritis, thrombophlebitis, and pustular skin lesions. A characteristic of Behçet's syndrome is formation of pustules at sites of minor trauma such as needle puncture.

Bowel bypass syndrome is believed to be an immune-complex disease due to antigens associated with bacterial overgrowth in an intestinal blind loop. Patients have episodes of fever and sterile pustules of the skin.

Acne fulminans is a rare disease of adolescent males, frequently with no prior history of acne. The onset is sudden, with fever, leukocytosis, arthralgias, and extensive inflammatory cysts of the chest, back, and face. Less common findings include lytic bone lesions and a positive blood culture for *Propionibacterium acnes*.

PETECHIAL ERUPTIONS **Infectious causes** Many hematologic and immunologic entities produce thrombocytopenia as a result of defects in the production, maturation, sequestration, or destruction of platelets. A consequence is the development of petechiae. The physician who is presented with an acutely ill patient with a petechial exanthem must be concerned with systemic, bacterial, or rickettsial disease. The common microorganisms associated with petechial exanthems are listed in Table 49-1. However, any microorganism that is capable of initiating the cascade of hematologic events termed disseminated intravascular coagulation may produce a petechial exanthem.

Petechiae due to septic embolization are characteristic of subacute bacterial endocarditis. Lesions may occur anywhere on the skin and/or mucous membranes but are most common over the upper anterior trunk. Splinter hemorrhages under the nails are difficult to differentiate from traumatic lesions and may be seen in hematologic, malignant, and other infective disorders.

Petechial lesions associated with meningococcemia are small, irregularly shaped, slightly raised, pale-grayish lesions with a vesiculopustular center. The lesions are usually asymmetric and are seen most often on the trunk and extremities, although the conjunctivas and mucous membranes may also be affected. Fulminant meningococcal infection may produce coalescence of the petechiae into grossly ecchymotic areas (purpura fulminans).

Gonococcal infections usually produce lesions on the distal extremities, often over joints. The presence of these pustular, hemorrhagic skin lesions in patients with asymmetric tenosynovitis or polyarthritis, involving the wrists, fingers, knees, or ankles, should suggest the gonococcal arthritis-dermatitis syndrome. The majority of patients with disseminated gonococcal infection do not have symptoms of urogenital, anorectal, or pharyngeal gonococcal disease.

The metastatic lesions of staphylococcal bacteremia include pustules, subcutaneous abscesses, and purulent petechiae. Aspiration of material from the purulent center of the lesion will often reveal gram-positive cocci in clumps. *Pseudomonas* septicemia may produce ecthyma gangrenosum, a round, indurated, painless, necrotic eschar usually located in the anogenital or axillary area. In addition, hemorrhagic lesions with surrounding erythema resembling erythema multiforme may be associated with *Pseudomonas* sepsis.

Rickettsial disease may produce an arteriolar vasculitis that results in a petechial exanthem. The rash of Rocky Mountain spotted fever generally starts as a blanching maculopapular exanthem on the extremities, and after 2 to 4 days petechiae appear in the involved areas. The lesions no longer fade, and increased capillary fragility, manifested by a positive Rumpel-Leede test, is often present. These cutaneous findings in a patient with abrupt onset of fever, chills, headache, myalgias, and arthralgias should suggest this diagnosis. If the patient comes from an endemic area, and a tick bite or tick exposure is present, appropriate therapy should be instituted.

Summer febrile illness due to enteroviruses, especially the echovirus group, may occasionally produce a petechial eruption. While involvement of the face is common, the distribution of the exanthem is usually not distinctive, and because fever, headache, and meningismus may also be present, the clinical differentiation between *Neisseria meningitidis* infection and viral aseptic meningitis may be difficult.

Atypical measles is another viral exanthem that produces a petechial eruption. It begins on the arms and legs and spreads to the trunk and face. The rash differs from typical measles because it has features of raised papules, blisters, and pinpoint hemorrhages into the skin. Koplik's spots are not present, while high fever, cough, bilateral interstitial pulmonary infiltrates, and eosinophils usually are. Patients with this syndrome have a history of previous immunization with inactivated (killed) measles vaccine or of receiving live measles vaccine within 3 months after killed vaccine. The history of previous antigenic exposure to measles virus plus eosinophilia suggests a "hypersensitivity" reaction. A fourfold rise in measles complement fixation antibody titer between acute and convalescent specimens may be demonstrated.

Petechial eruptions and profuse mucosal bleeding are often major manifestations of the viral hemorrhagic fevers. This syndrome is associated with a number of the arenaviruses (Lassa, Junin), arthropod-borne viruses (dengue), and rhabdoviruses (Ebola, Marburg). A history of recent travel to endemic or epidemic areas, involvement of the liver, spleen, heart, kidneys, and lungs, and evidence of diffuse intravascular coagulation are usually present.

Noninfectious causes of petechiae An important differential point in evaluating a patient with a purpuric eruption is between palpable and nonpalpable purpura. Nonpalpable purpura suggests hemorrhage from thrombocytopenia or coagulopathy, but palpable purpura suggests vasculitis. Diseases associated with fever and nonpalpable purpura include immune thrombocytopenic purpura and thrombotic thrombocytopenic purpura. Palpable purpura is usually an indication for skin biopsy for histology and immunofluorescence to confirm and characterize the vasculitis. It is often difficult to distinguish the various types of vasculitis from just the physical examination. Small vessel vasculitis, such as Henoch-Schönlein purpura, serum sickness, and cryoglobulinemia, usually produces symmetric round and oval lesions, located in dependent areas. Larger vessel vasculitis, such as polyarteritis nodosa and Wegener's granulomatosis, produces asymmetric, irregularly shaped lesions which may ulcerate.

Allergic vasculitis (Henoch-Schönlein purpura) is found most frequently in children less than 16 years of age. The presence of symmetric purpuric papules, commonly on the lower extremities, accompanied by abdominal pain, gastrointestinal bleeding, renal involvement (edema, hypoproteinemia, hematuria), and arthralgias characterizes this entity. Cholesterol embolization can mimic polyarteritis nodosa and occurs most commonly as a complication of angiography. Biopsy shows intravascular clefts from cholesterol crystals.

LABORATORY DIAGNOSIS The laboratory studies most useful in determining the etiology of an exanthem in an acutely febrile patient are directed at demonstrating the microorganism at the cutaneous site. Gram's stain and culture of the lesions, dark-field microscopy of spirochetal lesions, and the use of immunofluorescent microscopy of skin scrapings or skin biopsy specimens for the detection of microbial antigens should be employed. Because exanthems are generally manifestations of a systemic illness, blood cultures should be taken prior to antimicrobial therapy. Isolation of the agent from other sites may also be useful, e.g., demonstration of gonococci in throat or urethral smears. Histologic identification of organisms from skin biopsies of lesions may be of great help, especially with slowly growing agents such as fungi or mycobacteria.

Because local viral invasion is characteristic of vesicular exanthems, isolation of the agent from these lesions provides the diagnosis. The development of rapid viral diagnostic testing has been especially useful in the differential diagnosis of vesicular lesions. Biopsies or scrapings of exfoliated cells from vesicular lesions of herpes group viruses (varicella-zoster, herpes simplex virus) contain multinucleated giant cells and/or intranuclear inclusions. However, because the Tzanck smear is only 40 to 70 percent as sensitive as viral isolation, the absence of giant cells does not rule out herpes infection. Herpes simplex and zoster can be differentiated by viral isolation as well as by antigen detection techniques such as fluorescent microscopy or enzyme-linked immunoabsorbent assays (ELISA). Immunofluorescence may also be useful in confirming the diagnosis of immunologically related diseases such as pemphigus vulgaris and vasculitis.

Electron microscopy may be useful for distinguishing the distinct morphology of poxviruses, vaccinia, variola, and molluscum from herpes viruses. In addition, molluscum bodies can be demonstrated by light microscopy with use of a 10% KOH preparation.

In viral exanthems, demonstration of local viral replication in throat secretions or rectal swabs provides presumptive evidence of the etiology of the exanthem; an example is the demonstration of coxsackievirus A16 in throat secretions of patients with hand-foot-and-mouth syndrome. In Behçet's syndrome or in collagen vascular disease, the absence of viruses in an early vesicular or active ulcerative lesion is useful in relating these mucosal lesions to the underlying multisystem illness.

Serologic determinations of acute phase serums are helpful in the diagnosis of syphilis, leptospirosis, streptococcal disease, Epstein-Barr virus infection, hepatitis B, toxoplasmosis, typhoid fever, and occasionally rickettsial disease. Evidence of autoantibody fixation may be useful in diagnosing some collagen vascular diseases. Demonstration of a fourfold or greater rise in antibody titer between acute and convalescent serums will confirm the diagnosis in rubella, rubeola, cytomegalovirus, or rickettsial or chlamydial infection.

MUCOCUTANEOUS LYMPH NODE SYNDROME (KAWASAKI'S DISEASE) Mucocutaneous lymph node syndrome is a multisystem disease of children.

This entity was first described in Japan in the 1960s, but is now frequently recognized in the United States. It affects children from 2 months to 9 years of age, with 50 percent of cases occurring in children under 2 years of age. Occasional cases in young adults have been documented. Characteristically, the patient presents with a fever between 38.3 and 40°C of 1 to 2 weeks' duration which is unresponsive to antimicrobials. Bilateral conjunctivitis; dryness, redness, and fissuring of the lips; diffuse erythema of the oral and pharyngeal mucosa; "strawberry tongue"; and cervical adenopathy may be present. On the third to fifth day of illness, a macular erythematous eruption, usually starting on the extremities, appears. Pronounced reddening of the palms and soles is present, and the child's hands and feet may swell due to an indurative edema. Characteristically during the second week of illness desquamation of the rash starts at the junction of the nails and skin of the fingers and toes. Myocardial involvement is common, with abnormal electrocardiogram findings in over 50 percent of patients. Coronary angiography may reveal aneurysms and pathologic changes in the vessels similar to infantile periarteritis nodosa in 7 to 40 percent of cases. In severe cases, myocardial infarction due to coronary thrombosis may occur. Laboratory abnormalities include an elevated sedimentation rate, normal antistreptolysin O (ASO) titers, elevated C-reactive protein, peripheral leukocytosis, thrombocytosis, high levels of circulating immune complexes, and hypergammaglobulinemia. In the United States, cases have been clustered geographically and temporally. Children of Asian ancestry appear to be at higher risk than white children. The etiology of this entity is unknown. Investigations of outbreaks have revealed no evidence of person-to-person transmission or a common source of exposure. Aspirin in doses (100 mg/kg per day) to produce serum salicylate levels of 15 to 25 mg/dL is used during the acute stage of illness. When fever is controlled, the aspirin may be lowered and given in antithrombotic dosages (10 mg/kg per day). Trials evaluating the use of high-dose intravenous gamma globulin (400 mg/kg) are also underway.

REFERENCES

Centers for Disease Control: Multiple outbreaks of Kawasaki syndrome—United States. Morb Mort Week Rep 34:33, 1985

Cooper PH et al: Acute febrile neutrophilic dermatosis (Sweet's syndrome) and myeloproliferative disorders. Cancer 51:1518, 1983

Furusho K et al: High dose intravenous gammaglobulin for Kawasaki disease. Lancet 2:1055, 1984

Gilchest B, Barden HP: Photodistribution of viral exanthems. Pediatrics 54:136, 1974

Heggin AD: Pathogenesis of rubella exanthems. J Infect Dis 137:74, 1978

Kimura A et al: Measles rash, light and electron microscopic study of measles skin eruptions. Arch Virol 47:295, 1975

Koren MD et al: Probable efficacy of high dose salicylates in reducing coronary involvement in Kawasaki disease. JAMA 254:767, 1985

Melish ME: Kawasaki syndrome: A new infectious disease? J Infect Dis 143:317, 1981

Shands KN: Toxic shock syndrome in menstruating women: Its association with tampon use and *Staphylococcus aureus* and the clinical features of 52 cases. N Engl J Med 303:1436, 1980

Steere AC: The early clinical manifestations of Lyme disease. Ann Intern Med 99:76, 1983

Todd J et al: Toxic shock syndrome associated with phage-group-1 staphylococci. Lancet 2:1116, 1978

Tonneson MG, Soter NA: Erythema multiforme. J Am Acad Dermatol 1:357, 1979

Vanarsdel PP: Allergy and adverse drug reactions. J Am Acad Dermatol 6:833, 1982

50 GENERALIZED PRURITUS

THOMAS B. FITZPATRICK / JEFFREY D. BERNHARD

Generalized pruritus is a frequent and important problem in differential diagnosis for the general physician. Since it may be due to factors as trivial as dryness or as serious as an underlying lymphoma or endocrine abnormality, the evaluation of the patient presenting with pruritus of undetermined origin requires as much clinical judgment as it does knowledge and expertise in examining the skin. For the most part, no particular qualities of pruritus due to an underlying systemic illness permit a specific diagnosis; for example, obstructive biliary disease versus hyperthyroidism or lymphoma. The clinician must rely on the history, physical examination, and laboratory studies to establish the diagnosis.

Itch and pain share common neuroanatomic pathways but are distinct sensory modalities. Free-nerve endings that act as receptors for itch stimuli reside in the papillary layer of the dermis near the dermoepidermal junction, but there are no specific end organs for itching. A variety of diffusable mediators are apparently involved in both peripheral and central aspects of itching. Histamine, trypsin, proteases, and bile salts all cause pruritus when introduced intracutaneously. Prostaglandin E lowers the threshold to itching evoked by both histamine and papain. Prostaglandins are increased in inflamed skin, and may thereby potentiate pruritus in inflammatory dermatoses. Central nervous system opiate peptides and receptors seem to be involved in the perception of itch. The opiate naloxone hydrochloride leads to diminution of itching in several experimental and clinical settings. This may provide a clue as to how opiates relieve pain but exacerbate pruritus.

Patients with pruritus associated with obvious skin lesions, such as vesicles and papules, usually have a primary dermatologic disease. Some of the dermatologic disorders in which pruritus is a common symptom are listed in Table 50-1. Specialized dermatologic approaches, particularly biopsy of the skin, are often required in order to establish the diagnosis.

The itching patient without an apparent skin eruption and with or without the sequelae of chronic scratching (excoriations) and rubbing (lichenification, polished nails) poses a diagnostic challenge. Initially, a search should be undertaken for the primary lesions and subtle evidence of a primarily cutaneous disorder (Table 50-1).

Thorough evaluation of the patient with generalized pruritus in an attempt to discover an underlying systemic disease should include,

TABLE 50-1 Conditions in which pruritus occurs with diagnostic skin lesions

Infestation
Scabies
Pediculosis
Insect bites (especially flea and bedbug)
Inflammatory
Dermatitis herpetiformis
Bullous pemphigoid
Atopic dermatitis
Lichen planus (inconstant)
Miliaria
Urticaria (inconstant)
Dermographism
Aquagenic pruritus
Drug hypersensitivity
Polymorphic light eruption
Infectious
Varicella
Dermatophytosis
Folliculitis
Neoplastic
Mycosis fungoides
Miscellaneous or idiopathic
Xerosis
Anogenital pruritus
Mastocytosis
Sunburn
Exfoliative dermatitis
Lichen sclerosis et atrophicus

SOURCE: *Bernhard.*

in addition to the history and physical examination, the following basic laboratory screening tests: complete blood count; sedimentation rate, urinalysis; blood glucose, liver, thyroid, and renal function tests; chest x-ray; Papanicolaou smear; and stool exam for ova, parasites, and occult blood. Additional tests such as serum protein electrophoresis and radiologic surveys should be performed when indicated. A psychological assessment is helpful. Attributing generalized pruritus of uncertain etiology to a psychological disturbance is unwise until other possibilities have been adequately considered.

Psychogenic pruritus as a reaction to stress occurs but must be considered a diagnosis of exclusion, especially given that the torment of severe itching is stressful in itself. This type of pruritus often affects the skin of the scalp, and may be associated with other sensory complaints such as a bitter taste in the mouth or burning of the tongue. Some patients with psychogenic pruritus are convinced that the itching is caused by some sort of parasite in their skin that cannot be seen by themselves or the physician. Such patients may scratch their skin to the point of ulceration and then assert that the itching has disappeared, owing, they believe, to removal of a parasite or "germ."

Pruritus due to dry skin is a common occurrence in the elderly. On occasion, elderly persons who do not have obviously dry skin experience generalized pruritus that cannot be attributed to emotional stress or to an underlying systemic or cutaneous illness. Such so-called senile pruritus is usually most severe when the patients disrobe to go to bed. It usually begins in one area, particularly the back, and spreads to involve the entire body. Neither psychogenic nor senile pruritus leads to a loss of sleep.

A subtle and important cause of pruritus without a visible rash may be a reaction to drugs, such as aspirin, opiates and their derivatives, and quinidine. Some drugs, such as chlorpromazine, may cause pruritus by inducing cholestasis.

The itching associated with pediculosis corporis may be so intense that it will interfere with sleep. Long linear excoriations along the back are characteristic. The insect can be found in the clothing, particularly along the seams. In scabies, itching is most pronounced at bedtime. The web spaces of the fingers, groin, axillae, and buttocks are most often involved.

For a list of conditions in which generalized pruritus occurs without any evidence of primary skin disease, see Table 50-2.

Generalized pruritus may frequently be the first sign of biliary cirrhosis and may occur many months before the onset of jaundice. It may be the first sign also of lymphoma, and, rarely, of carcinoma. The pruritus may be of sudden onset and may be very severe. It often begins in the palms of the hand and soles of the feet. It is often improved by oral cholestyramine (see Chap. 249).

The treatment of generalized pruritus is unsatisfactory if the primary cause cannot be corrected or eliminated. Exceptions are the excellent response of uremic pruritus to ultraviolet radiation therapy (UV-B) and the response of patients with various forms of cholestasis to oral cholestyramine or activated charcoal. Not one of the systemic medications has been shown to be effective in generalized pruritus. A topical preparation containing 0.5% menthol and 1% phenol in an emollient such as Nivea oil is somewhat helpful in relieving pruritus temporarily. Topical anesthetics containing benzocaine should be avoided because of the high risk of allergic sensitization. When the patient with pruritus also has insomnia, a hypnotic or a sedative should be prescribed. Antihistamines are of little value except in pruritus due to urticaria, but may be of some help in itching due to other causes. It is a general clinical impression that aspirin is helpful in pruritus of any origin, but this has not been proven. The development of drugs that control pruritus remains one of the great challenges of medical research. It is paradoxical that severe pain can be immediately controlled with a variety of agents but there is not yet a single agent so effective for generalized pruritus.

REFERENCES

BERNHARD JD: Clinical aspects of pruritus, in *Dermatology in General Medicine,* 3d ed, TB Fitzpatrick et al (eds). New York, McGraw-Hill, 1987

BERNSTEIN JE: Neuropeptides and the skin, in *Biochemistry and Physiology of the Skin,* LA Goldsmith (ed). New York, Oxford University, 1983, pp 1217–1233

CUNLIFFE WJ: The skin and the nervous system, in *Textbook of Dermatology,* 3d ed, A Rook et al (eds). Oxford, Blackwell, 1979

GILCHREST BA et al: Ultraviolet phototherapy of uremic pruritus. Ann Intern Med 91:17, 1979

GREAVES M: Pathophysiology of pruritus, in *Dermatology in General Medicine,* 3d ed, TB Fitzpatrick et al (eds). New York, McGraw-Hill, 1987

HERNDON, JH, JR: Itching: The pathophysiology of pruritus. Int J Dermatol 14:465, 1975

TABLE 50-2 Conditions in which generalized pruritus may occur without diagnostic skin lesions

Metabolic and endocrine conditions	Malignant neoplasms	Drug ingestion	Infestations	Renal disease	Hematologic disease	Hepatic disease	Psychogenic states	Miscellaneous conditions
Hyperthyroidism Diabetes mellitus Carcinoid syndrome	Lymphoma and leukemia Abdominal cancer CNS tumors Multiple myeloma Mycosis fungoides	Opium derivatives Subclinical drug sensitivities	Pediculosis corporis Scabies* Hookworm (ancylostomiasis) Onchocerciasis Ascariasis Trichinosis Certain zoonoses	Chronic renal failure	Polycythemia vera Paraproteinemia Iron deficiency	Cholestasis (intra- or extrahepatic) Pregnancy (intrahepatic cholestasis)	Transitory: periods of emotional stress Persistent: delusions of parasitosis Psychogenic pruritus Neurotic excoriation	Dry skin (xerosis) "Senile" pruritus† Mastocytosis Pregnancy

* *Diagnostic lesions may be present.*
† *Unexplained intense pruritus in patients over 65 years without obvious "dry skin" and with no apparent emotional stress.*
SOURCE: *Bernhard.*

51 PIGMENTATION OF THE SKIN AND DISORDERS OF MELANIN METABOLISM

THOMAS B. FITZPATRICK / DAVID B. MOSHER

THE MELANOCYTE SYSTEM

DEFINITION OF MELANIN The relative quantities of melanin, oxyhemoglobin, reduced hemoglobin, and carotene account for the wide variations of normal human skin color; melanin is, however, the principal pigment responsible for the color of human skin, hair, and eyes. Melanin is also a density filter that decreases the harmful effects of ultraviolet light on the skin and thereby provides protection against acute sunburn reaction and chronic actinic damage, including skin cancer.

Derived from the Greek word *melas,* "black," melanin is a protein-bound polymer formed by the oxidation of tyrosine by tyrosinase to dihydroxyphenylalanine (dopa) within melanocytes, which are specialized epidermal dendritic cells of neural crest origin. The structure of melanin is unknown because eumelanin is so insoluble that all attempts to degrade it into identifiable fragments have failed. However, all animal melanins are known to contain indoles and are composed basically of indole 5,6-quinone units, in contrast to plant melanins which contain catechols. Pheomelanins are yellow-brown sulfur-containing pigments that, unlike eumelanin, are readily soluble in dilute alkali. Pheomelanins are only present in hair and are the pigments in human red hair.

Skin color is derived from the presence of melanin within the keratinocytes, which are receptor cells for melanocyte-formed mel-

FIGURE 51-1 *Diagram showing the embryonic origin, dispersal, and developmental fate of melanocytes in humans. [By permission from JB Stanbury et al (eds), The Metabolic Basis of Inherited Disease, 5th ed, New York, McGraw-Hill, 1983.]*

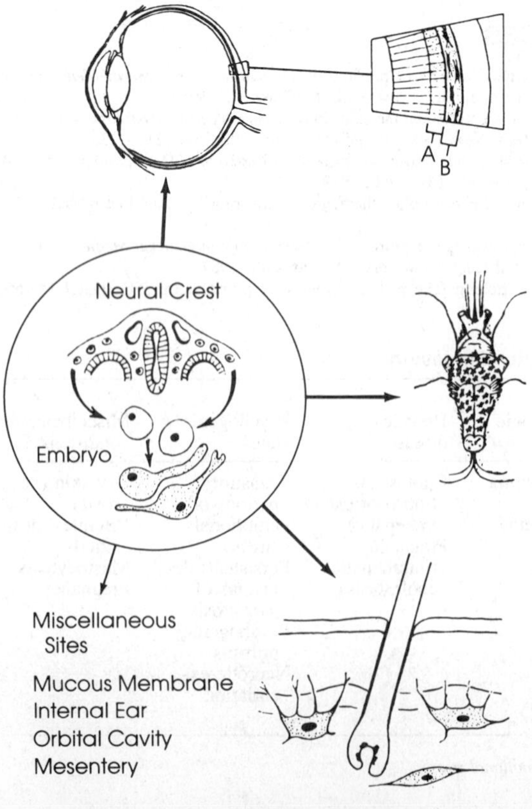

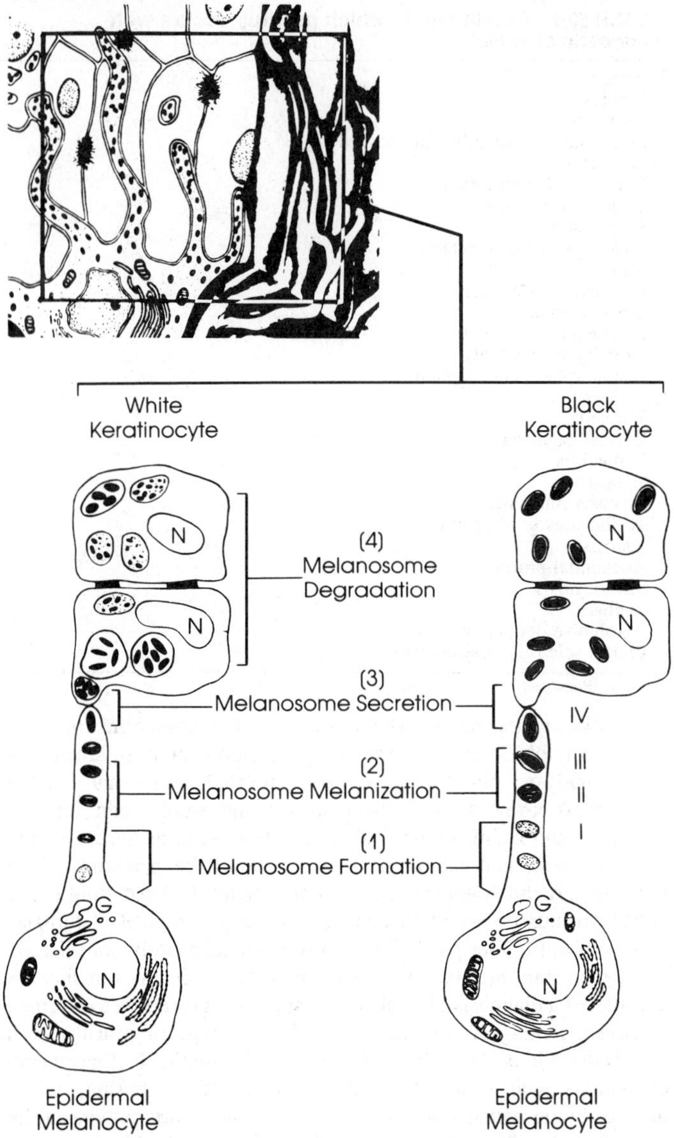

FIGURE 51-2 *Epidermal melanin unit. Four biologic processes in melanin pigmentation underscore the differences in melanosome formation and packaging between blacks and whites: (1) Formation of melanosomes in melanocytes; (2) melanization of melanosomes in melanocytes; (3) secretion of melanocytes by keratinocytes; and (4) transport of melanocytes by keratinocytes, either with degradation of melanosomes within lysosome-like organelles (in whites) or without apparent degradation of melanosomes (in blacks). Note the difference in size between the melanosomes in the black and white epidermal keratinocytes. In the black keratinocytes, the melanosomes are nonaggregated. In the white keratinocytes, groups of several melanosomes are aggregated within membrane-limited lysosome-like organelles, and the melanosomes often appear fragmented (G, Golgi apparatus; N, nucleus; I to IV, the four stages in the development of the melanosome). The epidermal melanin unit is shown at the top. The melanocyte supplies melanosomes to a group of keratinocytes.*

anin-containing organelles called *melanosomes*. Normal skin color is genetic or "constitutive"—that of habitually unexposed skin, as on the buttocks—and "facultative"—that resulting from the sun-induced tanning reaction or from increased pigmentation by pituitary melanocyte-stimulating hormones (MSH).

BIOSYNTHESIS OF MELANIN The melanocyte system is composed of melanocytes found at the dermoepidermal interface, in the hair bulb, uveal tract, retinal pigment epithelium, inner ear, and leptomeninges (Fig. 51-1). The melanocyte system is analogous to, but not known to be related to, the chromaffin system, the cells of which

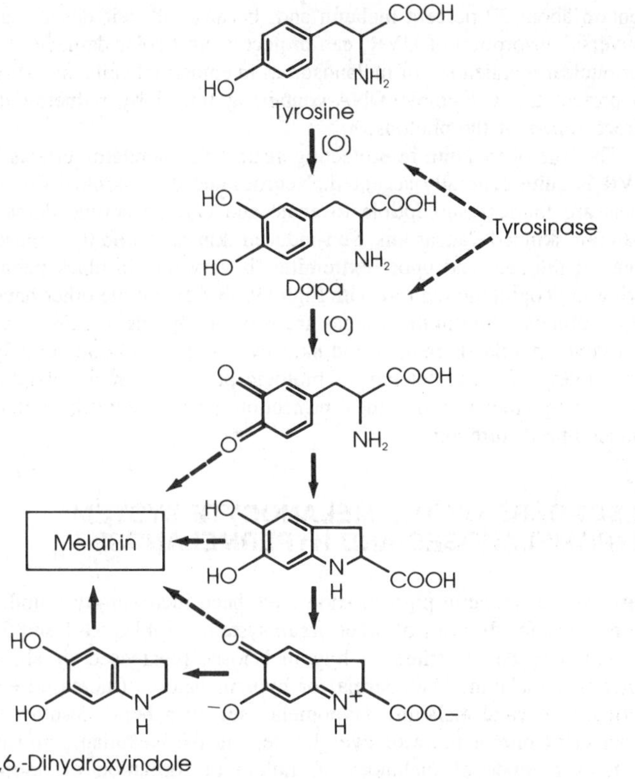

FIGURE 51-3 *Biosynthesis of melanin from tyrosine.*

are also derived from the neural crest and which possess biochemical mechanisms for the hydroxylation of tyrosine to dopa. However, in the latter system the enzyme is not tyrosinase, but tyrosine hydroxylase, and dopa is converted to adrenochrome and not to tyrosine melanin.

Melanocytes within the epidermis at the dermoepidermal interface are dendritic cells that are functionally linked to a number of keratinocytes; each melanocyte and its corresponding associated 36 keratinocytes compose an *epidermal melanin unit* (Fig. 51-2). This functional unit permits organized transfer of specialized tyrosinase-containing, melanin-producing organelles, or melanosomes, to associated keratinocytes. Melanosomes are ellipsoidal organelles which are thought to arise in the area of the endoplasmic reticulum and Golgi apparatus; they are formed as unmelanized spherical structures that darken and become more dense and oval in shape with increasing melanization.

Tyrosinase, the principal enzyme in the pathway of melanin production, is one of a large group of copper-containing aerobic oxidases that catalyze the oxidation of both monohydroxy and *o*-dihydroxy phenols to orthoquinones. In humans and other mammals, this oxidase catalyzes the hydroxylation of the melanin precursor, tyrosine, to dopa and dopa quinone (Fig. 51-3). Tyrosinase is required only for the first step in the biosynthesis of tyrosine melanin, i.e., the orthohydroxylation of tyrosine. It is noteworthy that zinc ions catalyze the conversion of dopachrome to 5,6-dihydroxyindole and that melanosomes have been shown to contain high concentrations of zinc. Recently some new factors have been shown to augment or block the synthesis of melanin *after* the action of tyrosinase.

BIOLOGY OF MELANIN PIGMENTATION Melanin pigmentation (Fig. 51-4), from the clinical point of view, results from the melanin present in the keratinocytes. Inasmuch as the ratio of keratinocytes to melanocytes in the epidermis is 36:1, it is apparent that the amount of melanin present in the keratinocytes must be the predominant factor in the determination of skin color. The relationship of skin color to the location of melanin in the epidermis was studied with the light microscope in American blacks of various hues of brown coloration. In lightly pigmented skin, there was a great variation in both the number and location of melanin particles within the epidermis; only scanty melanin deposits were in the malpighian layer, and no deposits were in the stratum corneum. In fact, in the most lightly pigmented skin, the only melanin particles were in the keratinocytes of the basal layer. In the most heavily pigmented skin, there were melanin particles in the keratinocytes of the basal layer, throughout the malpighian cells, and in the stratum corneum. Based on studies of various skin colors in American blacks and their progeny, it has been estimated that between three to six gene pairs may account for the black-white color gradient. The genetic control of *facultative* color change is not known; it is broadly related to levels of constitutive skin color.

It is apparent from studies of normal skin and of pigmentary disorders, that the intensity of pigmentation, as viewed clinically, depends not only on the rate of melanosome production but also on the number of melanosomes that are transferred to the keratinocytes (Fig. 51-2). Another factor that determines normal and abnormal melanin pigmentation is the degree of melanization of the individual melanosomes. Until recently, three factors—melanosome formation, melanosome melanization, and melanosome secretion—were considered to be the major variables in normal and abnormal melanin pigmentation. In the past few years, however, a fourth variable has been implicated in melanin pigmentation, i.e., the phenomenon of aggregation and degradation of melanosomes that occurs during their transport in the keratinocytes.

Melanosomes are present in melanocytes mainly as nonaggregated (single), membrane-delimited, discrete organelles. In keratinocytes, however, melanosomes occur either as single, or nonaggregated, particles or as aggregates of three or more within a membrane-delimited organelle. These melanosome-containing organelles resemble the melanosome-containing organelles within macrophages that have been identified as lysosomes. In the epidermal keratinocyte, melanosomes appear to undergo a gradual degradation. In heavily pigmented skin, however, intact melanosomes are present in the stratum corneum, indicating that some melanosomes are apparently not degraded with the lysosomes in the epidermis. The regulation of

FIGURE 51-4 *Melanogenesis in human skin, as seen in the light and the electron microscopes and at the molecular level.*

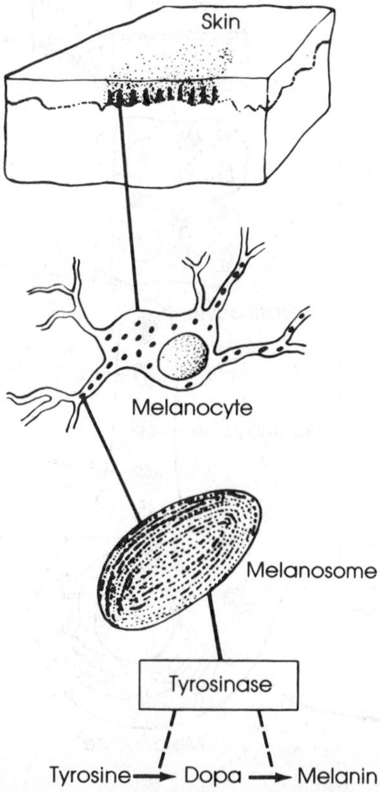

melanogenesis and melanin pigmentation is controlled by three major determinants: genes, hormones, and ultraviolet radiation. These three factors may act independently or in combination. In addition, specific chalones and glycopeptides may markedly affect melanogenesis and melanin pigmentation by exerting negative feedback control and regulating the mitotic activity of melanocytes and keratinocytes. The rate of transfer of melanosomes to keratinocytes may, in fact, regulate the amount of melanosome synthesis. Chalones may also regulate adenylate cyclase activity as well as melanocyte and keratinocyte division. Hormones (MSH) appear to act by a direct effect on adenylate cyclase, which results in increased cyclic AMP leading to increased tyrosinase and melanosome synthesis.

Melanin pigmentation of the skin is related to 10 biologic processes as shown in Fig. 51-5. Aggregation and dispersion of melanosomes probably play little part in the pigmentary anomalies of humans. Such movement has thus far been observed only in specialized effector cells, *melanophores,* present only in vertebrates below mammals in the phylogenetic scale; this movement of melanosomes is under neural and hormonal control in these animals.

In humans, melanocytes by means of their production and transfer of melanin, provide defense against the biologic damage caused by visible and ultraviolet radiation (UVR). Melanin in the uveal tract and in the retinal pigment epithelium protects the eye from visible and longer wavelength (UV-A) radiant energy while UV-B is largely filtered by the cornea. Melanized human epidermis shields the epidermis and dermis by effectively reducing the transmission of UV-B and UV-A radiant energy.

In humans, furthermore, this defense against UVR is highly developed in that exposure of skin to this portion of the electromagnetic spectrum causes the activation of an integrated mechanism (tanning) for the formation of dense organelles containing chromoprotein (melanosomes) and the delivery of these to epidermal cells. Within the epidermal cells, melanosomes scatter and adsorb ultraviolet radiation and remove the damaging free radicals that are generated in the skin after exposure to UVR.

In a heavily pigmented skin, the epidermal cells and the stratum corneum are filled with myriads of melanosomes. Melanosomes contain about 30 percent melanin and, because of their density and universal absorption of UVR, can protect against solar damage. The perinuclear localization of melanosomes in epidermal cells may serve to protect the vulnerable DNA-containing nuclei by reducing the direct impact of the photons.

The role of melanin in protecting against the damaging effects of UVR is quite generally accepted. Negroes and dark-skinned Caucasians are far less susceptible to acute and chronic actinic damage than fair-skinned Caucasians. Sun-induced skin cancer on the exposed areas of the face and upper extremities is very rare in black people living in geographic regions with high UV-B flux; on the other hand, black albinos living in these areas are very susceptible to skin cancer and develop solar keratoses and skin cancer in childhood. Finally, since many of these deleterious biologic processes are involved in skin aging, melanin provides protection against environmentally induced premature aging.

DISORDERS OF THE MELANOCYTE SYSTEM: HYPOMELANOSES AND HYPERMELANOSES

Disorders of melanin pigmentation have been increasingly found to be markers for diseases of other organ systems (Tables 51-1 and 51-2) and may be classified as hypomelanoses (decreased or absent epidermal melanin, leukoderma) or hypermelanoses (increased epidermal or dermal melanin). Hypomelanoses, in general, result from a defect of one or more of over 10 steps in the melanian pathway, such as absence of melanocytes, failure of formation of normal melanosomes, or failure of transfer of melanosomes to keratinocytes. The hypermelanoses are further classified as *epidermal* pigment disorders which present as brown, or as *dermal* pigment disorders which are blue, blue-gray, or gray. Brown hypermelanoses (melanoderma) arise from increased melanin in the epidermis, resulting from increased melanocyte activity, increased numbers of secretory melanocytes, increased numbers of melanosomes, or increased size of melanosomes. The blue-gray hypermelanoses (ceruloderma) represent a virtual ''melanin tattoo''—the presence of melanin in the dermis

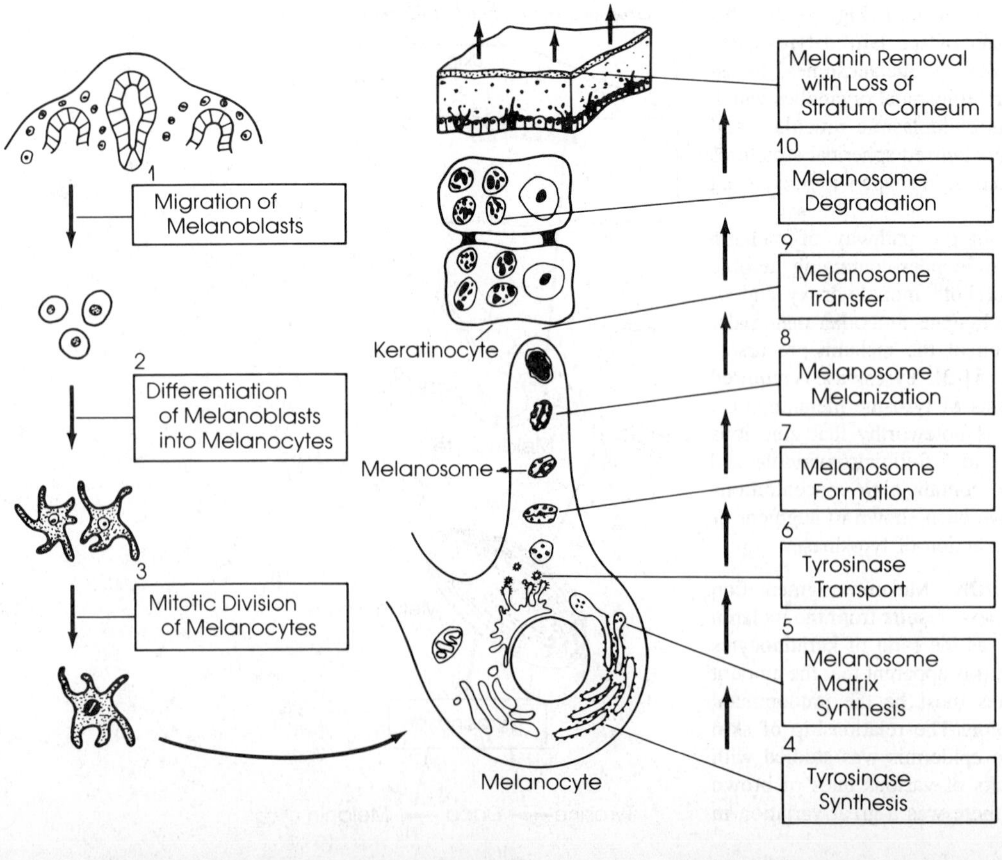

FIGURE 51-5 *Morphologic and metabolic pathway of epidermal melanin pigmentation.*

TABLE 51-1 Pigmentary Changes as Diagnostic Signs in General Medicine

Chief complaint or presenting problem	Pigmentary change	Diseases	Systemic changes
ADDISONIAN BROWN HYPERPIGMENTATION			
"Getting dark"	Generalized diffuse brown hypermelanosis	Addison's disease Hemochromatosis ACTH-producing tumors Systemic scleroderma (early) Porphyria cutanea tarda	Adrenal insufficiency Cirrhosis of liver, diabetes Pituitary tumor, primary; metastatic cancer Dysphagia; pulmonary insufficiency Liver: increased iron stores Diabetes mellitus (25%)
CIRCUMSCRIBED BROWN MACULES			
"Abdominal pain, brown spots on lips, fingers"	Circumscribed, mostly small dark-brown macules (many)	Peutz-Jegher syndrome	Polyposis of small intestine
"Brown spots all over"	Circumscribed small dark-brown macules	"LEOPARD" syndrome	Abnormal ECG Pulmonary stenosis
"Birth mark"; hypertension; precocious puberty	Circumscribed, uniformly brown macules, small or large (café au lait) (few or many)	Von Recklinghausen's neurofibromatosis	Neurofibromatosis of skin and peripheral nervous system; pheochromocytoma; Eye: pigmented hamartoma (Lisch nodules)
		Albright's syndrome	Polyostotic fibrous dysplasia Precocious puberty
		Watson's syndrome	Pulmonary stenosis
"Many dark moles"	Circumscribed dark-brown macules or slightly raised papules with irregular borders and variegation of color (few or many)	Dysplastic nevus syndrome	
CIRCUMSCRIBED WHITE MACULES			
"White spots"	Circumscribed, mostly large white macules (few or many)	Vitiligo Hypothyroidism Thyrotoxicosis Pernicious anemia Adrenal insufficiency Diabetes mellitus	
		Sarcoidosis	Pulmonary findings Uveitis
		Leprosy	Skin (anesthetic white macules) Peripheral neuropathies Hepatosplenomegaly
"Convulsions"; mental retardation	Congenital circumscribed small (1–3 cm) white macules (more than 3)	Tuberous sclerosis	Mental retardation, abnormal EEG Abnormal CT scan Rhabdomyoma of heart
"Eye trouble"; deafness	Circumscribed white macules, poliosis	Vogt-Koyanagi-Harada disease	Uveitis, dysacousia
"Deafness"	White forelock, congenital circumscribed large white macules	Waardenburg's syndrome	Nerve deafness, heterochromia
UNIVERSAL HYPOMELANOSIS			
"Sun sensitivity"; decreased vision	Universal hypomelanosis of skin, hair, and uveal tract	Oculocutaneous albinism, recessive	Decreased visual acuity, iris translucency, nystagmus
"Sun sensitivity"; "Poor tanner"	Type I or type II skin	Oculocutaneous albinoidism, dominant	Iris translucency, normal vision, nystagmus (rare)

in ectopic dermal melanocytes or in dermal macrophages which, because of the Tyndall effect, imparts a characteristic gray, slate, or blue color to the skin. Blue or slate-gray coloration of the skin may also arise from nonmelanin sources—ochronosis, tattoos, pharmacologic agents (chlorpromazine, amiodarone, minocycline), and deposition of other foreign materials in the dermis.

Clinical recognition of circumscribed hypomelanosis ("white spots") and of gray or slate or blue hypermelanosis is usually not difficult. When the degree of hypomelanosis is very slight, when the patient's normal skin color is very light, or when the patient's skin is untanned, the hypomelanotic lesions may be inapparent, and the diagnosis may be facilitated by the use of black light (Wood's lamp; see Chap. 47), which will heighten the contrast between abnormal epidermal pigmentation and normal skin but will not increase the contrast between increased dermal pigmentation and normal skin. Differentiation between abnormal diffuse brown hyperpigmentation (e.g., Addison's disease) normal pigmentation or between diffuse hypomelanosis (e.g., albinism) and normal pigmentation frequently poses a problem because there is such a wide range of skin coloration in normal individuals. Diffuse color changes may be insidious; often patients themselves have been unaware of an unusual or unexplained progressive or gradual deepening of their skin color, such as a summer tan that did not fade. The degree of hypermelanosis that develops is related to the basic skin color of the patient involved. With the onset of Addison's disease, a patient of Mediterranean descent (such as Italian, French, or Spanish) may become intensely pigmented, whereas a light-skinned individual may have only a minimal degree of hypermelanosis. The appearance of pigmentation in mucous membranes and in certain specific areas, such as the axillae and the palmar creases, is usually easier to identify as abnormal than generalized brown hyperpigmentation.

GENETIC MELANIN DISORDERS Patients with pigmentary changes may present with complaints such as "I'm getting dark," "I have many dark moles," "white spots," or "birth spots" (see Table 51-1). Others present with disorders such as deafness, iritis, and seizures,

TABLE 51-2 Disturbances of human melanin pigmentation

Hypomelanosis[a] (Leukoderma) White	Hypermelanosis[a] (Melanoderma) Brown, gray, slate, or blue[b]
GENETIC FACTORS	

Piebaldism[c]
Waardenburg's syndrome[b]
Vitiligo[c,d]
Hypomelanotic macules in tuberous sclerosis[c,e]
Albinism, oculocutaneous:[f,g]
  Tyrosinase-negative
  Tyrosinase-positive
  Yellow mutant
  Brown Rufous
  Hermansky-Pudlak syndrome
  Chédiak-Higashi syndrome
  Cross-McKusick-Green syndrome
Albinism, ocular[c,g,h]
Albinoidism, oculocutaneous[f,g,h]
Pigmentary dilution with immunodeficiency
Phenylketonuria[f,g,h]
Fanconi's syndrome[h]
Homocystinuria[f,h]
Histidinemia[f]
Menkes' kinky hair syndrome[h]
Canities, premature[h]
	Café au lait and freckle-like macules in neurofibromatosis[c]
	Melanotic macules in polyostotic fibrous dysplasia (Albright's syndrome)[c]
	Ephelides (freckles)[c]
	Lentigines[c]
	Lentigines with cardiac arrhythmias[c]
	Becker's nevus
	Neurocutaneous melanosis[c]
	Xeroderma pigmentosum[c]
	Acanthosis nigricans
	Fanconi's syndrome[c]
	Dermal melanocytosis (Mongolian spot)[b,c]
	Incontinentia pigmenti[b,c]

METABOLIC FACTORS	
	Hemochromatosis[f] Hepatolenticular disease (Wilson's disease)[f] Porphyria (congenital erythropoietic, variegata and cutanea tarda)[f] Gaucher's disease[i] Niemann-Pick disease[i] Biliary cirrhosis[i] Chronic renal failure
ENDOCRINE FACTORS	
Hypopituitarism[f] Addison's disease[c] Hyperthyroidism[c]	ACTH-producing and MSH-producing pituitary and other tumors[f] ACTH therapy[f] Pregnancy[i] Addison's disease[f] Melasma[c,j]
NUTRITIONAL FACTORS	

Chronic protein deficiency or loss:[h,k]
  Kwashiorkor
  Nephrosis
  Ulcerative colitis
  Malabsorption
Vitamin B_{12} deficiency[h]
	Pellagra[i]
	Sprue[i]
	Vitamin B_{12} deficiency[i]
	Chronic nutritional insufficiency[c]

CHEMICAL AND PHARMACOLOGIC AGENTS	
Hydroquinone, monobenzylether[c] Hydroquinone[c,e] Miscellaneous catechol and phenol compounds[f] Chloroquine and hydroxychloroquine[h] Arsenical ingestion[c] Corticosteroids, topical and intradermal[c,e]	Arsenical intoxication[f] Busulfan administration[f] Photochemical agents (topical or systemic drugs)[c] 5-Fluorouracil, systemic[f] Cyclophosphamide[f] Nitrogen mustard, topical[c] Bleomycin[c] Fixed (drug) eruption[b,c] Adriamycin BCNU
PHYSICAL AGENTS	
Burns: Thermal, ultraviolet, ionizing radiation[c,l] Trauma[c,l]	Ultraviolet light (suntanning)[c] Thermal radiation[c] Alpha, beta, and gamma ionizing radiation[c] Trauma (e.g., chronic pruritus)[c]
INFLAMMATION AND INFECTION	
Sarcoidosis[c,e] Pinta[c] Yaws[c] Leprosy[c,e] Tinea versicolor[c,e] Post–kala azar[c] Eczematous dermatitis[c,e] Psoriasis[c] Discoid lupus erythematosus[c] Vagabond's leukoderma[c] Miscellaneous postinflammatory hypomelanoses[c,e]	Postinflammation melanoses (exanthems, drug eruptions)[c] Lichen planus[c] Lupus erythematosus, discoid[c] Lichen simplex chronicus[c] Atopic dermatitis[i] Psoriasis[c] Tinea versicolor[c] Pinta in exposed areas[b,c]
NEOPLASMS	
Leukoderma acquisitum centrifugum (including halo nevus)[c] Vitiligo-like hypomelanosis[c,e] associated with melanoma	Malignant melanoma[c,m] Mastocytosis (urticaria pigmentosa)[c] Acanthosis nigricans, with adenocarcinoma and lymphoma[c] Slate-gray dermal pigmentation with metastatic melanoma and melanogenuria[f]
MISCELLANEOUS FACTORS	
Vogt-Koyanagi-Harada syndrome[c] Scleroderma, circumscribed or systemic[c] Canities[h] Alopecia areata[n] Horner's syndrome, congenital and acquired[g] Idiopathic, guttate hypomelanosis[c]	Scleroderma, systemic[f] Chronic hepatic insufficiency[f] Whipple's syndrome[f] Lentigo, senile ("liver spots")[c] Cronkhite-Canada syndrome[c] POEMS syndrome

[a] *Listing includes the pigmentation disorder itself or the condition with which it is associated.*
[b] *Gray, slate, or blue color results from the presence of dermal melanocytes or phagocytized melanin in the dermis.*
[c] *Pigment change is circumscribed.*
[d] *Total loss of pigment in the skin and hair may occur.*
[e] *Loss of pigmentation is usually partial (hypomelanosis); viewed with Wood's lamp, the lesions are not completely devoid of pigment (amelanosis), as in vitiligo.*
[f] *Pigment change is diffuse, not circumscribed, and there are no identifiable borders.*
[g] *Pigment is decreased in the iris.*
[h] *Pigment is decreased in the hair.*
[i] *Pigment change may be diffuse or circumscribed.*
[j] *Idiopathic or due to progestational agents.*
[k] *Hair is gray or reddish.*
[l] *There is a loss of melanocytes.*
[m] *Areas of brown may be admixed with the slate-gray and blue discoloration.*
[n] *Regrown hair is white.*
SOURCE: *Modified from: DB Mosher et al, in Dermatology in General Medicine, 2d ed, TB Fitzpatrick et al (eds), New York, McGraw-Hill, 1979.*

and the pigmentary change is incidental. The following presentation is, however, arranged by etiology rather than by symptoms.

Oculocutaneous albinism is an autosomal recessive trait characterized by congenital, decreased, uniform hypomelanosis of skin and hair; albinism involving the skin alone has not been reported, but ocular albinism with minimal or no cutaneous involvement has been observed. The classic constellation of findings in oculocutaneous albinism includes marked hypomelanosis or amelanosis of skin, white or faintly blondish hair, photophobia, nystagmus, hypopigmented fundus oculi, and translucent irides. Oculocutaneous albinism may be classified according to the presence or absence of tyrosinase in plucked hair follicles of the scalp (the hair bulb incubation test). In normal individuals hair bulbs darken when incubated with tyrosine; in some persons with oculocutaneous albinism the hair follicles darken when incubated in tyrosine, i.e., *tyrosinase-positive,* while in others no such darkening occurs, i.e., *tyrosinase-negative*. These two types of albinism are known to have separate gene loci. In oculocutaneous albinism melanocytes are present, but formation of melanosomes is interrupted in the early stages so that few mature melanosomes are present in albino skin or hair. Whatever tyrosinase is present must be functionally defective and unable to convert enzymatically tyrosine to dopa. Other variants of oculocutaneous albinism include yellow mutant, Hermansky-Pudlak syndrome (hemorrhagic diathesis secondary to storage pool platelet defect), and Chédiak-Higashi syndrome (recurrent infections, hematologic and neurologic abnormalities, and early death from lymphoma). The deficiency of melanin in oculocutaneous albinism has two disturbing consequences for humans: decreased visual acuity and an abnormal degree of intolerance to sunlight. The sensitivity of human albinos to ultraviolet light often leads to the development of carcinoma in exposed areas of the skin. Nearly all albinos in the tropics have actinic keratoses or skin cancers by the third decade. Daily use of effective topical sunscreens and avoidance of unnecessary sun exposure are indicated for all albinos (see Chap. 52).

A syndrome of congenital diffuse pigmentary dilution with immunodeficiency has been described. It is associated with hepatosplenomegaly, neutropenia, thrombocytopenia, and defective helper-T-cell function.

Phenylketonuria is an autosomal recessive disorder of phenylalanine metabolism in which there is a single metabolic block in the conversion of phenylalanine to tyrosine. There is pigmentary dilution of the skin, hair, and irides. The lightening of hair, which is characteristically light blond to dark brown, may be appraised only by comparison with uninvolved siblings. The melanocytes are normal but lack a full complement of melanosomes. Decreased melanin formation results from the fact that excess phenylalanine and its metabolites, present in serum and extracellular fluid, act as competitive inhibitors of tyrosinase and block melanin synthesis.

Vitiligo is an idiopathic, acquired, circumscribed hypomelanosis which is familial in about 30 percent of cases and is characterized by progressively enlarging amelanotic macules (Table 51-3). Vitiligo may be localized, segmental (one or more dermatomes), or generalized. On occasion, vitiligo may become so extensive that all or nearly all the skin becomes white. Characteristic distribution patterns of vitiligo involve extensor surfaces and bony prominences (elbows, knees), the small joints in the hands, and the area around the eyes and mouth. The low back, axillae, and flexor wrists may also be involved. Genitalia, palms and soles, and mucous membranes are often affected. Typically, the vitiligo macules gradually enlarge centrifugally, and new macules appear. In up to 30 percent of cases some minimal and inconsequential spontaneous repigmentation occurs, particularly in sun-exposed areas of skin. White hairs are common in macules of vitiligo, but may also be normally pigmented. Most vitiligo patients are generally healthy, although thyroid disease, diabetes mellitus, Addison's disease, and pernicious anemia occur with increased frequency. Thyroid disease—hyperthyroidism, thyroiditis, hypothyroidism, and nontoxic goiter—may, in fact, be a common coexisting disorder with vitiligo in patients over the age of 50, especially hypothyroidism. Syndromes with multiple endocrinopathies and with hyperthyroidism, hypoparathyroidism, Addison's disease, chronic mucocutaneous candidiasis, and alopecia areata have been described. Iritis may occur in over 10 percent of patients. The pathogenesis of vitiligo is unresolved, but classic hypotheses include destruction of melanocytes by toxic melanin precursors or lymphocytes. Antibodies to normal melanocytes have also been reported.

Electron microscope studies show a total absence of melanocytes in the white vitiligo macules and decreased numbers of melanocytes in "trichrome" areas (macules or margins of vitiligo patches in which a color intermediate between the normal skin color and the vitiligo white is present). Abnormal keratinocytes (with vacuolation) have been observed with transmission electron microscopy in clinically "normal" skin of patients with idiopathic vitiligo. Vitiligo is thus both a marker for multisystem disease and also a tragic social problem for brown and black peoples. The internist should never regard the problem as simply a cosmetic disorder; having ruled out subclinical thyroid disease, Addison's disease, pernicious anemia, and polyglandular endocrinopathy, the brown or black patient should be referred to a dermatologist capable of offering the options for control of the disease. Fair-skinned persons often can learn to "live with their disease" and will not accept treatment.

Options for treatment of vitiligo include sunscreens, cosmetic cover-up, repigmentation, or depigmentation. In over half the patients treated with PUVA photochemotherapy, psoralens, and ultraviolet A [UV-A (sunlight or an artificial UV-A light system; see Chap. 52)] significant repigmentation occurs, particularly on the face and neck, and usually on the trunk, upper arms, and legs. Up to 200 or more treatments may be required, however. In some older patients with extensive areas of depigmentation, irreversible depigmentation of the remaining pigmented skin with topical monobenzylether of hydroquinone cream (Benoquin) is a more practical and feasible approach. These persons look essentially normal but must use sun-protective lotions daily.

Piebaldism is a congenital, autosomal dominant, stable, circumscribed hypomelanosis which resembles vitiligo except that it has a characteristic distribution pattern different from vitiligo and does not usually progress or resolve over time. The hypomelanosis in piebaldism occurs in circumscribed areas on the extremities and anterior surface of the thorax. A white forelock is typical. The eyes are normal, and the patients are otherwise healthy.

Tuberous sclerosis is an autosomal dominant disease which manifests itself by the presence of congenital, circumscribed, white macules in up to 98 percent of cases, and classically by the development (by the fourth year) of seizures, mental retardation, and adenoma sebaceum. The white macules are characteristically located on the trunk or buttocks, are hypomelanotic, number from 3 to 100,

TABLE 51-3 Disorders associated with circumscribed vitiligo-type hypomelanosis

Associated disorder
GENETIC
Vitiligo, with or without:
Hyper/hypothyroidism
Diabetes mellitus
Addison's disease
Pernicious anemia
Hypoparathyroidism
Addison's disease
Chronic mucocutaneous candidiasis syndrome
Piebaldism
Waardenburg's syndrome
Tuberous sclerosis
Ataxia-telangiectasia
CHEMICAL EXPOSURE
Phenolic germicides (O-Syl, Phebocide, etc.)
Hydroquinone, monobenzylether of
Hydroquinone, monomethylether of
NEOPLASTIC
Malignant melanoma (in sites of regression)
Melanocytic nevi (halo nevi)
INFECTIOUS
Leprosy
Pinta
Tinea versicolor
IDIOPATHIC
Vogt-Koyanagi-Harada syndrome
Postinflammation: atopic dermatitis, psoriasis
Sarcoidosis
Scleroderma

and are of typical shape—oval, lance-ovate, or polygonal, like a "thumbprint." The most characteristic, though not the most frequent, is the lance-ovate or American mountain "ash-leaf" macule, which is usually less than 3 cm in its longest dimension and off-white, not pure white, in color. The macules are oriented transversely on the trunk and axially on the extremities. The size and color of these lesions do not change over time. Histologically, these macules contain melanocytes which have decreased numbers of small melanosomes. The presence of three or more circumscribed macules in a patient is strongly suggestive of tuberous sclerosis. Examination with Wood's lamp is often necessary to visualize the lesions.

All persons with unexplained seizures or mental retardation should be screened with a Wood's lamp examination for the presence of white spots to exclude tuberous sclerosis. In addition, examination of parents and siblings with CT scans or magnetic resonance imaging (MRI) is necessary to detect the location, size, and shape of calcifications and intraventricular nodules. MRI may facilitate diagnosis of solid tumors.

Neurofibromatosis (von Recklinghausen's disease) is an autosomal dominant trait characterized by the appearance, usually by the age of 3 and primarily on the trunk and the extremities, of numerous pale yellow-brown macules, or café au lait spots, that vary in diameter from less than 1 cm to more than 15 cm. Spotty generalized pigmentation and axillary freckling may also be present. Often, a few or many soft, rounded, cone-shaped, or pendulous cutaneous tumors covered by normal skin appear by the first or second decade.

The presence in an adult of six or more café au lait spots—which are uniformly hypermelanotic, circumscribed, oval macules with a diameter greater than 1.5 cm (over five greater than 0.5 cm in a child)—is characteristic of neurofibromatosis even in the absence of a positive family history. Lisch nodules (pigmented hamartomas of the iris detected by slit lamp examination) in patients above 6 years are diagnostic of von Recklinghausen's neurofibromatosis; they are not present in Albright's syndrome or in bilateral acoustic neurofibromatosis. In *Albright's syndrome* (polyostotic fibrous dysplasia), however, there are rarely more than three or four such macules, which are usually unilaterally distributed on the buttocks or cervical areas. A single, large, isolated café au lait spot of neurofibromatosis is indistinguishable from the macule of Albright's syndrome. It is possible, however, using light microscopy, to detect melanin macroglobules in whole amounts of epidermis prepared from café au lait macules of neurofibromatosis; these melanin macroglobules are usually not found in the pigmented macules present in Albright's disease or in the café au lait macules observed in 10 percent of the normal population.

Moynahan's syndrome, or "LEOPARD" syndrome, is an autosomal dominant trait in which generalized lentigines (multiple, diffuse, small, dark-brown, circumscribed hypermelanotic macules) have been associated with ECG abnormalities and, in its fully expressed form, with other findings (lentigines, ECG abnormalities, ocular hypertelorism, pulmonary stenosis, abnormal genitalia, retardation of growth, and deafness).

Peutz-Jeghers syndrome is an autosomal dominant disorder in which hyperpigmented, brown to blue macules on the lips and buccal mucosa are associated with similar cutaneous lesions and gastrointestinal polyps. The cutaneous macules, but not the buccal pigmented lesions may fade, by adulthood. This disease is discussed in Chap. 239.

METABOLIC FACTORS Generalized brown hypermelanosis of the skin is a characteristic manifestation of *hemochromatosis, porphyria cutanea tarda,* and *variegate porphyria.* The hyperpigmentation observed in hemochromatosis may be grayish brown or brown and indistinguishable from that of Addison's disease. The diagnosis of hemochromatosis may be established from a skin biopsy which shows hemosiderin deposition in the sweat glands. Melanin deposition is also apparent. Porphyria cutanea tarda may be diagnosed by the clinical presence of vesicles, bullae, atrophic macules, sclerodermoid changes, and milia on the skin of the dorsal hands and face, and in the laboratory by red fluorescence of acidified urine, or the presence of increased urinary uroporphyrin (uroporphyrin to coproporphyrin ratio usually is greater than 3:1). Similar changes may be seen in patients with *variegate porphyria,* which has a distinctive porphyrin profile, especially a high fecal protoporphyrin. The lesions in variegate porphyria are identical to porphyria cutanea tarda and the diseases must be differentiated as they have different responses to treatment and very different associated medical problems (see Chaps. 52 and 312). Primary biliary cirrhosis may be associated with hyperpigmentation in normally sun-exposed areas. Chronic renal failure may also be associated with diffuse hyperpigmentation.

NUTRITIONAL FACTORS In *chronic nutritional deficiency,* in general, macules of dirty-brown hyperpigmentation appear, especially on the trunk. In selective deficiencies, such as protein deficiency in *kwashiorkor,* or when there is protein loss as in *chronic nephrosis, ulcerative colitis,* and *malabsorption syndrome,* there is sometimes dilution of hair color so that the hair becomes a reddish-brown and eventually gray. In other selective deficiencies, such as sprue, there may be a brown hypermelanosis over any area of the body. In *pellagra,* however, the pigmentation is limited to areas of skin exposed to light or to trauma. In *vitamin* B_{12} *deficiency,* there is premature graying of hair and a hypermelanosis most apparent overlying the small joints of the hands.

ENDOCRINE FACTORS Diffuse brown hypermelanosis is a striking feature of primary adrenocortical insufficiency (Addison's disease). There is a marked hyperpigmentation over certain areas, namely, the pressure points (vertebrae, knuckles, elbows, and knees), and in body folds, palmar creases, and gingival mucous membrane. An identifiable type of diffuse hyperpigmentation has also been reported to follow adrenalectomy in patients with Cushing disease. In these patients, there usually are signs and symptoms of pituitary tumors; all tumors recorded have been chromophobe adenomas. A third example of the Addisonian type of melanosis has also been observed in patients with pancreatic and lung tumors. The generalized brown hypermelanosis found in all these conditions results from overproduction of melanocyte-stimulating hormone (MSH) and adrenocorticotropic hormone (ACTH), which share common amino acid sequences. It appears that an excess of α-MSH plays a dominant role in the abnormal pigmentation that occurs in Addison's disease. Both MSH and ACTH are increased in adrenal insufficiency as a result of decreased output of cortisol by the adrenals. Hypermelanosis of the Addisonian type can be produced in adrenalectomized human subjects by the administration of large amounts of homogeneous ACTH and α-MSH. α-MSH is a single-polypeptide chain of 13 amino acid residues and is identical in sequence to the terminal portion of ACTH except for the acetylation of the terminal serine residue. Recent evidence has shown that the polypeptide hormones themselves are produced by cleavage of the larger polypeptides. In mammals, MSH causes a significant darkening of skin as early as 24 h after administration. Mammalian melanocytes have been shown to be uniquely sensitive to α-MSH. Melanocytes appear to possess a unique membrane-bound receptor molecule that is present in the G_2 phase of the cell cycle. Following interaction of this receptor with α-MSH, an enzyme also found within the membrane, adenylate cyclase, is stimulated, leading to an increase in the formation and level of intracellular cyclic AMP. Eight hours following treatment with MSH, tyrosinase activity begins to increase. This effect is followed at 16 h by an increase in melanin formation. Current information suggests that cyclic AMP is the mediator of the MSH effect; this evidence includes the fact that cyclic AMP levels rise soon after exposure to MSH.

Melasma, or the "mask of pregnancy," is found in pregnant women, women on oral contraceptives, and in some otherwise normal women and men. This is a circumscribed brown hypermelanosis of the epidermis, (with a dermal or blue-gray component in some), usually of the forehead, cheeks, upper lip, and chin. MSH levels are normal in these patients. Melasma-like hyperpigmentation has also been observed in patients taking phenytoin or mesantoin. Treatment with topical depigmenting agents in conjunction with opaque covering is effective in about 50 percent of the patients.

CHEMICAL FACTORS Exposure to or use of various chemicals, particularly para-substituted phenol derivatives may cause depigmentation. Topical use of hydroquinone induces a temporary lightening which may be useful in some patients with melasma; monobenzylether of hydroquinone, however, causes a permanent vitiligo-like leukoderma, even remote from the site of application, and is used only to depigment completely the uninvolved pigmented normal skin in patients with extensive vitiligo. Addisonian-like hypermelanosis of the skin follows busulfan therapy, and hypermelanosis may also be seen after use of cyclophosphamide and nitrogen mustard. Inorganic trivalent arsenicals may also produce generalized Addisonian-like hypermelanosis as well as scattered macular hypomelanosis and punctate keratosis of the palms and soles. Blue-gray nonmelanin pigmentation has been observed due to prolonged high doses of chlorpromazine, minocycline, and amiodarone.

PHYSICAL FACTORS Mechanical trauma, as well as burns caused by heat, ultraviolet light, or alpha, beta, and gamma radiation, can lead to hypomelanosis or hypermelanosis. The effects of these physical agents on pigmentation are determined by the intensity and duration of exposure and are limited to the site of injury. Hypomelanosis results from destruction of melanocytes.

INFLAMMATORY AND INFECTIOUS FACTORS Many epidermal proliferative processes resolve and leave aberrations of pigmentation at the sites of involvement; both postinflammatory hypermelanosis (blue-gray, brown, or both) and hypomelanosis may occur following resolution of lupus erythematosus, eczema, psoriasis, lichen planus, drug reactions, pemphigus, viral exanthems, etc. Usually the epidermal hypermelanoses disappear spontaneously within several months, but dermal hypermelanoses are much slower to resolve. White halos surrounding psoriatic plaques are a result of abnormal prostaglandin synthesis and are not an abnormality of melanin biology.

Tinea versicolor, a hypomelanotic, not amelanotic, scaling, circumscribed eruption of the upper anterior and posterior chest in young people, results from the presence in the skin of *Pityrosporum orbiculare* which contains an enzyme that forms azelaic acid, a melanocyte toxin, and results in decreased melanin pigmentation. Sun exposure will result in repigmentation only after appropriate topical antifungal therapy.

Tuberculoid and *lepromatous leprosy* have hypomelanotic macules and papules that are anesthetic. The color, unlike vitiligo, is not pure white, rather, off-white, and the margins of these macules are characteristically indiscrete.

NEOPLASTIC FACTORS Disorders of melanin pigmentation are uncommon features of skin neoplasms. Hypomelanosis has been found around benign nevi (halo nevi) in healthy patients but may also be found in or around malignant melanoma (the primary or metastatic lesion); vitiligo-like hypomelanotic macules remote from the melanoma may also occur. *Leukoderma acquisitum centrifugum* (LAC) refers to the presence of a macule of hypomelanosis surrounding a central pigmented lesion. LAC is most common around nevocellular nevi. Such halo nevi occur in healthy individuals but may also be found in or around melanoma (primary or metastases). The halo is usually eccentrically placed around malignant lesions but concentric around benign ones. *Mycosis fungoides,* which is a cutaneous T-cell lymphoma, may present with vitiligo-like macules. Plaque and systemic lymphoma stages invariably follow after several to many years.

A Vogt-Koyanagi-Harada syndrome has been reported following bacillus Calmette-Guérin (BCG) therapy of melanoma. During terminal stages of malignant melanoma, striking development of blue hypermelanosis may be observed, associated with large amounts of a conjugated derivative of 5,6-dihydroxyindole excreted in the urine (melanogenuria). This intermediate in the metabolic pathway from tyrosine to melanin (Fig. 51-3) can be oxidized to melanin in the absence of tyrosinase; therefore, melanin can be synthesized at almost any site in which oxidation can take place. Diffuse black pigmentation is seen in the peritoneum, liver, heart, muscle, and dermis of patients during the late stages of malignant melanoma. The brown melanin in the dermal phagocytes appears clinically as blue in the skin because of the Tyndall light-scattering phenomenon.

Acanthosis nigricans is characterized by velvety textured hypermelanotic (brown) macules which may be found in the axillae and other areas in patients with various carcinomas, particularly adenocarcinomas of the gastrointestinal tract. Acanthosis nigricans may also be congenital or benign and associated with diabetes mellitus, Cushing's disease, Addison's disease, pituitary adenoma, and other disorders.

Urticaria pigmentosa is characterized by multiple, irregular, round or oval, yellowish brown to reddish brown macules and papules related to the presence of melanin in the epidermis overlying clusters of mast cells. Vigorous rubbing of such lesions results in the development of urticarial wheals (Darier's sign). In children, the skin lesions usually appear in infancy and often spontaneously disappear in several years. The usual course is quite benign, but symptoms of flushing, itching, and urticaria occur in about 30 percent of patients; less than 15 percent experience vomiting, syncope, or shock. The symptoms are presumed to be due to histamine release from mast cells and often coincide with increased urinary excretion of free histamines and metabolites. Urinary levels of 5-hydroxyindoleacetic acid are normal. Antihistamines are of little value. Systemic mastocytosis, in which mast cells infiltrate diffusely into the liver, spleen, gastrointestinal system, and bones, is a rare condition. Mast cell leukemia occasionally develops.

UNKNOWN CAUSES Generalized brown hypermelanosis of the type seen in Addison's disease may be associated with *systemic scleroderma* early in the course of the disorder. Generalized hyperpigmentation occasionally develops in patients with *chronic hepatic insufficiency,* especially that due to portal cirrhosis. The pathogenesis of the pigmentation in both conditions is unknown; MSH levels are not elevated. *Cronkhite-Canada syndrome* is the association of acquired lentigo-like brown macules with gastrointestinal polyposis from the stomach to the rectum. Diarrhea, weight loss, and abdominal pain usually precede the pigmentary changes by several months. Hypopigmented macules with perifollicular hyperpigmented macules are seen in *scleroderma;* such depigmented macules are devoid of melanocytes. Hypomelanotic macules may also be found in a small percentage of patients with *sarcoidosis.* These macules are characteristically not pure white and are circumscribed with indiscrete margins. They may overlie dermal nodules, particularly on the extremities but also at times on the trunk.

REFERENCES

FITZPATRICK TB et al: *Biology and Diseases of Dermal Pigmentation.* Tokyo, University of Tokyo, 1981

KORNER AM, PAWLEK J: Dopachrome conversion, a possible control point in melanin biosynthesis. J Invest Derm 75:192, 1980

MOSHER DB et al: Abnormalities of pigmentation, in *Dermatology in General Medicine,* 3d ed, TB Fitzpatrick et al (eds). New York, McGraw-Hill, 1987

——— et al: Vitiligo: Etiology, pathogenesis, diagnosis and treatment, in *Update: Dermatology in General Medicine,* TB Fitzpatrick (ed). New York, McGraw Hill, 1983

ORTONNE JP et al: *Vitiligo and Other Hypomelanoses of Hair and Skin.* New York, Plenum, 1983

QUEVEDO WC et al: Biology of melanocytes, in *Dermatology in General Medicine,* 3d ed, TB Fitzpatrick et al (eds). New York, McGraw-Hill, 1987

WICK MJ et al: Biochemistry of melanization, in *Dermatology in General Medicine,* 3d ed, TB Fitzpatrick et al (eds). New York, McGraw-Hill, 1987

WITKOP CV et al: Albinism, in *The Metabolic Basis of Inherited Diseases,* 5th ed, JB Stanbury et al (eds). New York, McGraw-Hill, 1983

52 PHOTOSENSITIVITY AND OTHER REACTIONS TO LIGHT

MADHUKAR A. PATHAK / THOMAS B. FITZPATRICK / JOHN A. PARRISH

Humans have evolved in sunlight and depend upon it for much more than an indirect source of food and maintenance of the earth's temperature. Natural light has always been recognized for, and endowed with, health-giving powers. Our skin, eyes, blood vessels, and certain endocrine gland functions respond to radiation from the electromagnetic spectrum of the sun. The formation of vitamin D from sterol precursors in the skin by solar.ultraviolet radiation (UVR) exposure has long been recognized in the management of rickets. Certain of our daily biorhythms are dependent upon the cycles of sunlight. Yet, sunlight can be harmful and damage or kill living cells. Sunlight causes sunburn, damage to deoxyribonucleic acid (DNA), skin cancer, wrinkling and aging changes in the skin, eye inflammation, and possibly cataracts. During the past decade, interest in the reaction of human skin to light has been renewed as a result of

1 The public's obsession with sunbathing, resulting in premature "aging" of the skin (solar elastosis).

2 Demographic data indicating that exposure to sunlight is an important cause of basal cell and squamous cell carcinoma and even melanoma of the sun-exposed parts of the body.

3 The widespread use of certain drugs such as phenothiazines, thiazides and related sulfonamide diuretics, and antibiotics (demethylchlortetracycline), which alter the cutaneous responses to sunlight and cause undesirable photosensitivity reactions.

4 Increased awareness that sunlight is a major cause of discomfort and photosensitivity reactions in patients with certain types of porphyria, especially for those with erythropoietic protoporphyria.

5 The emergence of a new science of photomedicine and photochemotherapy based on the recent advances in molecular photobiology and the availability of high-intensity ultraviolet irradiation systems; this has enabled both researchers and practicing physicians to use UVR and visible radiation with or without the systemic administration of the drug to achieve a striking, therapeutic response in diseases such as psoriasis, polymorphic photodermatitis, mycosis fungoides, lichen planus, vitiligo, uremic pruritus, etc. Visible radiation also has been successfully used in newborn infants in the treatment of neonatal jaundice to prevent bilirubin encephalopathy. Light emitted by certain types of lasers is being increasingly used in the treatment of port-wine stains, telangiectasia, and other vascular lesions.

6 The increased recognition that the exposure of UVR can alter the function and viability of cellular components of the immune system; normal and abnormal immune responses can be altered and can result in local alterations of immune function at the site of exposure or some specific systemic alterations at distant nonexposed sites.

TABLE 52-1 Diseases induced or exacerbated by light

I By light alone
- *A* Genetic: ephelides (freckles)
- *B* Idiopathic
  - *1* Acute solar skin damage (sunburn)
  - *2* Connective tissue degeneration (wrinkling)
  - *3* Telangiectasia
  - *4* Solar keratoses and solar lentigo
  - *5* Basal cell carcinoma
  - *6* Squamous cell carcinoma
  - *7* Malignant melanoma
  - *8* Polymorphous photodermatosis
  - *9* Solar urticaria
  - *10* Actinic reticuloid

II By light plus exogenous agents
- *A* Chemical or drug
  - *1* Phototoxic reactions
  - *2* Phytophotodermatitis
  - *3* Lupus erythematosus (with hydralazine, procainamide)
- *B* Chemical and immunologic: photoallergic reactions

III By light plus metabolite(s)
- *A* Porphyrias
- *B* Porphyria cutanea tarda associated with hexachlorobenzene, estrogens, alcohol

IV By light plus preexisting disease
- *A* Genetic
  - *1* Xeroderma pigmentosum
  - *2* Oculocutaneous albinism
  - *3* Vitiligo
  - *4* Hartnup's syndrome
- *B* Nutritional or metabolic
  - *1* Pellagra
  - *2* Malignant carcinoid
- *C* Viral: herpes simplex
- *D* Unknown: lupus erythematosus (cutaneous, systemic)

There are more than 25 human disorders that are either caused by or aggravated by exposure of the skin to sunlight. These range from degenerative and neoplastic changes to disability and discomfort associated with chemically induced photosensitivity reactions. These abnormal reactions to light in humans are briefly presented in Table 52-1.

This chapter will be concerned with (1) common conditions such as sunburn, the degenerative and neoplastic conditions associated with solar radiation (basal cell carcinoma, squamous cell carcinoma, malignant melanoma, solar keratoses), and chronic sun-induced degeneration; (2) photosensitivity related to drugs and to increased production of photosensitizing porphyrins in patients with all types of porphyrias (except acute intermittent porphyria); (3) certain idiopathic forms of commonly occurring photodermatoses; (4) photochemotherapy; and (5) photoprotection.

The unit of wavelength most commonly used to measure and express nonionizing UVR or visible light is the nanometer (1 nm = 10^{-9} m = 10 Å).

Electromagnetic emanations from the sun comprise a wide range of radiation and include electric waves, radio waves, infrared rays, visible light, UVR, roentgen rays (x-rays), gamma rays, and cosmic rays. The shortest wavelengths that reach the surface of the earth through the atmosphere are about 286 to 290 nm. Wavelengths shorter than 286 nm are principally absorbed by ozone in the stratosphere. In terrestrial sunlight, the UVR region extends from 290 to 400 nm, the visible spectrum from 400 to 760 nm, and the near-infrared and infrared spectrum from wavelengths longer than 760 nm.

The solar spectrum that can affect human skin includes wavelengths of 290 to 760 nm; however, infrared radiation (1.5 to 1000 μm) can produce thermal effects (including burn) and potentiate the photochemical and biologic reactions initiated by UVR or visible radiation. For practical reasons, UVR is often arbitrarily subdivided into three bands designated as (1) UV-A (320 to 400 nm, or long-wave ultraviolet), (2) UV-B (290 to 320 nm, or sunburn spectrum), and (3) UV-C (shorter than 290 nm, or germicidal radiation).

The amount and type of solar radiation, especially UVR, that may reach a given part of the earth at any given time are determined by a great variety of factors, including latitude, time of day, season, altitude, local atmospheric conditions (smog, cloudiness, haze, smoke, dust, fog, humidity, aerosol particles), variations in the thickness of the ozone layer, and height of the sun above the horizon.

Approximately 50 percent of the sun's radiant energy is in the visible portion of the spectrum (400 to 760 nm), about 44 percent in the infrared region, and about 6 percent in the UV region. The damage to skin (sunburn, skin cancer) is evoked by 3 percent of the ultraviolet radiation wavelengths, namely, from 290 to 360 nm.

The transmission of radiant energy varies with wavelength and different areas of the human skin; it may range from 0 to 70 percent. Shorter wavelengths (<285 nm) are mostly absorbed by the dead-cell layer of the stratum corneum; wavelengths that produce sunburn (290 to 315 nm) are also mostly absorbed in the epidermis. About 5 to 15 percent of the impinging UV-B radiation penetrates to the papillary dermis, and the depth of UV-B penetration depends upon the degree of melanin pigmentation of the skin. Longer wavelengths (320 to 760 nm) penetrate more deeply into the dermis. Transmission of different wavelengths depends upon (1) the regional thickness of the epidermis, (2) the degree of hydration, (3) the concentration of UV and visible light-absorbing components such as melanin, proteins (keratin, elastin, collagen), nucleic acid, urocanic acid, carotenoids, and hemoglobin, and (4) the number and spatial arrangement of melanosomes and of blood vessels. In fair-skinned individuals, about 85 to 90 percent of 290- to 315-nm radiation is absorbed by the epidermis and only about 5 to 15 percent can penetrate through the epidermis to reach the dermis. In dark-skinned individuals, nearly 90 to 95 percent of 290- to 315-nm radiation is absorbed by the epidermis. The transmission through the epidermis of long-wave UV radiation (320 to 400 nm) and visible radiation (400 to 760 nm) may range from 20 to 70 percent. The optical properties of hypopigmented epidermis of fair-skinned individuals are such that approximately 2 to 5 percent of 250-nm (germicidal) radiation, about 12 to 15 percent of 300-nm radiation, and about 50 percent of 360-nm radiation can be transmitted to the dermis. Since cutaneous blood flow is about 500 mL/min, the equivalent entire blood volume of an adult person at rest can circulate through the skin every 11 min. Thus, UVR penetrating through the epidermis and impinging on the network of capillaries and small vessels can affect lymphocytes circulating through the skin, and prolonged exposure (over 90 min) may damage a significant portion of the circulating cells. It is now known that UVR induces loss of mononuclear cell viability; they are most sensitive to UV-C (<290 nm) and less sensitive to UV-B and UV-A radiation (sensitivity ratios of 10^4:10:1). UV-induced alterations in immune function appear to be involved in the pathogenesis of experimental photocarcinogenesis in mice. The significance of the alteration of lymphocyte function following exposure to UVR is not well understood, but it is possible that such alterations may play a role in the pathogenesis of UV-induced skin cancer, lupus erythematosus, and some photosensitivity disorders. The alteration of lymphocyte function and immune responses may explain the beneficial effects of phototherapy and photochemotherapy in certain skin diseases.

The most detrimental effect of UVR is cell death. Other effects include mutagenesis, carcinogenesis, interference or inhibition in the synthesis of DNA, RNA, and protein, and also in immune functions. The mutagenic and carcinogenic effects appear to be mediated largely through the action of UV-B radiation on DNA. The most common reactions, such as sunburn, tanning or melanin pigmentation, synthesis of vitamin D, keratosis, and skin aging are also caused by UV-B radiation. Although the longer wavelengths (UV-A, or 320 to 400 nm or 400 to 760 nm) penetrate more deeply and in greater amount into the skin than UV-B, they are much less effective at causing these types of photobiologic phenomena. UV-A radiation is about 800 to 1000 times less effective than UV-B in evoking erythema and other degenerative changes. However, in the presence of certain chemical agents (e.g., drugs that are given orally or endogenous porphyrins in certain porphyrias), these wavelengths become highly damaging and can cause severe skin photosensitization at quite low doses.

Protection against this damage to the "normal" skin has been the subject of much investigation, and many commercially available sunscreens can be recommended in the prevention of sunburn, skin cancer, aging of skin, and in various types of photosensitivity disorders.

SUNBURN AND TANNING

CLINICAL CHANGES Erythema, or sunburn reaction Erythema is caused principally by 290- to 320-nm radiation, maximum solar effectiveness being 300 to 307 nm. UVR emitted by artificial light sources produces erythema maximally at 297 and 254 nm. Radiation greater than 320 nm (320 to 760 nm) is generally considered to be nonerythemogenic, although prolonged exposure to 320- to 400-nm radiation (1.5 to 2 h of midday summer sun in northern latitudes) can produce mild sunburn in normal subjects. The minimal erythema dose (MED) is defined as the lowest UVR dose which produces perceptible redness up to 24 h following exposure to a defined spectral band (either UV-B or UV-A). In fair-skinned individuals, the MED of UV-B is approximately 20 to 50 mJ/cm² (equivalent to approximately 12 to 25 min in northern latitudes during June and July). UV-B doses larger than 3, 6, or 9 times the MED have a short latent period, and the subsequent erythema reaction is more severe; marked erythema, edema, and even bullae may occur. If the total dose is large, pain and systemic symptoms such as fever may occur. The MED of 320 to 400 nm (UV-A) is approximately 25 to 100 J/cm² or about 800 to 1000 times greater than that of UV-B.

Sunburn, suntan, and peeling are experiences familiar to almost the entire fair-skinned population. Individuals vary in their susceptibility to sunburn and suntan. Personal history of sunburning (e.g., easy, moderate, severe, or difficult), peeling, and the ability to acquire tan (minimal, moderate, profuse, etc.) is very helpful to classify people of different ethnic backgrounds into six sun-reactive types as described in Table 52-2.

The sunburn reaction is a complex inflammatory process. The observed histologic changes include the appearance of dyskeratotic cells (containing pyknotic nuclei), spongiosis, vacuolation of keratinocytes, and edema. The dermal changes include an inflammatory infiltrate (mostly lymphocytes), endothelial swelling, and capillary leakage manifested by extravasation of red blood cells. The severity of these changes and the rate at which they evolve depend on the exposure dose, the incident wavelength, and degree of skin pigmentation. Hypopigmented, fair-skinned individuals (e.g., red-haired, freckled individuals such as the Irish or Scottish) are more susceptible to sunburn than pigmented individuals who tan well. The nature of the chromophore that absorbs the light energy which initiates the primary photochemical responses is not well established, although the bulk of evidence suggests that nucleic acids (DNA) are primary targets for the absorption of the 290- to 320-nm radiation. Vasodilatation which accompanies the sunburn reaction appears to result from the activation and release of one or more chemical mediators (e.g., prostaglandins, kinins, serotonin, histamine).

There has been considerable focus on the role of prostaglandins (PG) and related derivatives of arachidonic acid as mediators of the delayed erythema reaction induced by UV-B. Prostaglandins of the PGE and PGF series are low-molecular-weight, oxygenated fatty acid structures synthesized by microsomal enzymes (PG synthase, lipoxygenase, and cyclooxygenase) present in all mammalian cells, including epidermal cells. Increased levels of prostaglandins (PGE series) have been observed in widely different types of cutaneous inflammation reaction, including the UV-induced sunburn reaction. Indomethacin, a nonsteroidal anti-inflammatory agent, when applied topically or given intradermally, can decrease a delayed sunburn response of human skin produced by UV-B radiation. Since indomethacin is known to inhibit prostaglandin synthesis, these findings support the possible role of prostaglandins as mediators of the delayed erythemal response to UV-B radiation. It is of interest to note that prostaglandin levels are increased in skin exposed to an erythemogenic dose of UV-C (germicidal) radiation. However, a PUVA (psoralen + UV-A)–induced phototoxic reaction does not seem to generate elevated levels of prostaglandins, and indomethacin, applied topically

TABLE 52-2 Classification of sun-reactive skin types*

Skin type	History of sunburning and tanning
I	Always burn, never tan, often peel
II	Always burn, tan slightly
III	Always burn, tan moderately (average whites)
IV	Sometimes burn (minimally), always tan (olive skin)
V	Rarely burn, tan easily and substantially (brown skin)
VI	Never burn, tan profusely (blacks)

* *After first exposure to approximately 45 min (3 MED) of summer sun.*

or given intradermally, has no effect in decreasing the intensity of the erythema reaction, suggesting that the mechanism of photosensitization reaction evoked by PUVA is not mediated by PGs. Other mediators including histamine are also believed to be involved in UV-B–induced immediate as well as delayed erythema reaction. Ultraviolet radiation may also have a direct effect on the blood vessels of the upper layer of the dermis (capillaries, venules, and arterioles). The formation of reactive oxygen species such as singlet oxygen, peroxides, superoxide anions, or free radicals appears to play an important role in the damage to cell membranes and lysosomal membranes associated with lipid oxidation. In fair skin, 290- to 320-nm spectrum is known to produce damaging free radicals (molecules with unpaired electrons).

Melanin pigmentation, or tanning Tanning (increase in melanin pigment) that follows exposure of the skin to solar radiation involves two distinct photobiologic processes. The first, *immediate pigment darkening* (IPD), or darkening of preformed pigment in the epidermis, is elicited by wavelengths of 320 to 720 nm. The second, *melanogenesis,* or delayed tanning reaction, is an intricate process that consists of the *erythema response (sunburn)* followed usually in 3 to 4 days by formation of new pigment. Immediate pigment darkening reaction is oxygen-dependent and results from oxidation of melanin through the production of semiquinone-like free radicals in the melanin polymer; transfer of melanosomes from melanocytes and redistribution of already existing melanosomes within the keratinocytes also may occur.

Melanogenesis involves (1) an increase in the number of functional melanocytes, resulting from increased proliferation of melanocytes, and activation of dormant melanocytes; (2) increased arborization of melanocytic dendrites; (3) an increase in the number of melanosomes in proliferating melanocytes; (4) an increase in tyrosinase activity; and (5) an increase in the transfer of melanosomes from melanocytes to keratinocytes. The degree of melanin pigmentation, however, that can be achieved in an individual by exposure to solar radiation is genetically predetermined. People with fair skin who burn easily but do not tan or tan poorly (skin types I and II) cannot with repeated sun exposures achieve that degree of tanning which can be easily achieved by someone genetically able to tan profusely with minimal exposure. Delayed tanning reaction appears to have a protective effect on the skin against subsequent exposures.

CELLULAR AND MOLECULAR CHANGES Hyperplasia Within 72 h after exposure, there is an increase in the number of epidermal cells with a high rate of mitotic activity. The rate of cell proliferation decreases after 7 to 10 days, and the thickness of the epidermis gradually returns to normal within the next 30 to 60 days. In UV-induced hyperplasia the activities of polyamine biosynthetic enzymes, ornithine-decarboxylase (ODC) and *S*-adenosyl-methionine decarboxylase are increased in UV-B irradiated skin, resulting in the elevation of putrescine and spermidine. PUVA and UV-C also induce increased epidermal ODC activity, reflecting the potential role of polyamines in cell growth and hyperplasia.

DNA and RNA changes Damage to DNA by sunburn-producing UV light (290 to 320 nm) may result in mutation or cell death. The principal epidermal DNA photoproducts are pyrimidine dimers (e.g., thymine dimers); these are of the cyclobutane type and are formed between adjacent pyrimidine bases. Cell membranes, DNA, RNA, protein, and other molecules may be altered, and the synthesis of DNA, RNA, and protein may be temporarily inhibited immediately after irradiation. New synthesis is evident by 24 h and is maximal by 60 to 70 h.

Mitosis Inhibition of epidermal mitosis and retardation of basal cell turnover occur within 1 h after irradiation. The epidermal cell cycle is interruped at the S phase of DNA synthesis. Inhibition of mitosis can persist for 7 to 24 h; it is followed by an acceleration of mitotic rate and basal cell turnover that reaches a peak by 48 to 72 h and is associated with epidermal hyperplasia. The mitotic cycle appears to be interrupted in the G_2 stage, in the prophase stage, or in both. The increased mitotic activity and the associated hyperplasia may last for 30 to 60 days. This hyperplasia appears to be due to a combination of the removal of the epidermal mitotic inhibitors (chalones) and stimulation of growth by the action of cyclic adenosine monophosphate (AMP) and guanosine 5′-monophosphate (GMP).

Formation of vitamin D The skin has long been recognized as the site for sun-induced photosynthesis of vitamin D. The action spectrum (290–320 nm) and the photochemical mechanisms involved in the synthesis of vitamin D_3 have been recently elucidated and are described in Chap. 274.

SUN-INDUCED SKIN CANCER

The malignancies and premalignancies unequivocally associated with sun exposure (primarily UV-B radiation) include solar or actinic keratoses, basal cell epitheliomas, squamous cell carcinomas, and keratoacanthomas. Some studies have established that carcinoma of the skin occurs more frequently on the parts of the body habitually exposed to sunlight; thus, the lesions of the head and hands are concentrated on the nose, central portions of the cheeks, eyelids, and dorsum of the hands. In fair-skinned whites who sunburn easily, these cancers are limited almost exclusively to the exposed portions of the face, head, neck, arms, and hands. Black skin, on the other hand, is remarkably resistant to the development of skin cancer on the exposed surfaces, and a similar resistance is seen among the pigmented whites (e.g., East Indians), American Indians, and Asiatics.

Carcinoma of the exposed skin is more prevalent among persons who are outdoors a great deal and is the common cause of cancer in whites in Australia, South Africa, and the southern parts of the United States. The action spectrum for photocarcinogenesis is similar to that of sunburn reaction.

Several studies based on the distribution of local populations in the United States, Australia, and Ireland have emphasized that skin cancer develops earlier and more frequently in people who have light skin and freckles, who burn easily and do not tan on exposure to the sun, and who are of mostly Celtic ancestry (people with skin types I and II). *Australia, with the highest reported incidence of skin cancer* in the world, has a population largely descended from British stock, with about 25 percent claiming Celtic (i.e., Irish, Scottish, and Welsh) extraction. In all three countries surveyed, persons of Celtic ancestry were found to have a disproportionately high incidence of skin cancer. Dark-pigmented races and people who tan well (skin types IV to VI) are least susceptible to skin cancer. Chronically exposed areas of many fair-skinned individuals may develop small hyperkeratotic lesions commonly referred to as *solar keratoses.* These may progress to squamous cell or basal cell carcinomas and may be seen as early as the third decade. Susceptible individuals may exhibit more than one lesion. These can be readily recognized by the use of topical 5-fluorouracil.

All varieties of skin cancer develop in patients with *xeroderma pigmentosum,* an autosomal recessive disorder. This rare defect represents, in the extreme, the basic problem of solar radiation and skin cancer. Patients with this disease have a greatly increased susceptibility to malignant tumors of the skin in the light-exposed areas. The characteristic skin manifestations are atrophy, telangiectasia, hyperpigmented macules, keratoses, and ulcerations, all occurring in sun-exposed areas. Within the first few years of life, basal cell or squamous cell carcinomas or sarcomas or malignant melanomas develop. An inherited enzyme defect may be responsible, at least in part, for the cancer-forming potential in patients with xeroderma pigmentosum. Cultured fibroblasts from patients with xeroderma pigmentosum are incapable of releasing thymine dimers from DNA and, in consequence, are deficient in their ability to repair their UV-damaged DNA. Xeroderma pigmentosum is the most notable human disease in which there is a defect in the excision repair process involving the removal of UV-induced dimers followed by the synthesis and re-forming of new segments of DNA. This enzymatic deficiency may result in a high somatic mutation rate of skin cells after sun exposure and, eventually, in cancer formation. The fact that mutagenesis is largely the result of errors made during the repair of photodamaged DNA and that UVR is known to be mutagenic suggests that the first step toward UV-induced carcinogenesis may be the result of an error made during the repair and replication of the damaged DNA (see Chap. 51 for discussion of sun and melanoma).

SUN-INDUCED DEGENERATIVE CHANGES OF THE SKIN (DERMATOHELIOSIS)

Degenerative skin changes (wrinkling, telangiectasia, keratoses) are more frequent in white-skinned people living in areas where the intensity of UVR is great (e.g., southwestern United States, Australia, South Africa). The term *solar degeneration* or *dermatoheliosis* implies a group of changes in the exposed areas of the skin, including wrinkling, atrophy, hypermelanotic and hypomelanotic macules, telangiectasia, yellow papules and plaques, and keratoses. The furrowed and leathery condition of the skin is seen particularly in persons who have fair skin and poor tanning ability and are constantly exposed to the sun. The most conspicuous and characteristic change may result from biochemical and structural alterations of connective tissue (elastin as well as collagen). The degenerative changes are primarily caused by sunburn-producing (290- to 320-nm) wavelengths and to a limited extent by UV-A (320- to 400-nm) radiation that can penetrate deeply into the dermis. Heat (infrared radiation) may accelerate actinic degeneration.

Chronically light-damaged human epidermis shows shortening or flattening of the rete ridges, thinning of the epidermis (decrease in malpighian cells), and many abnormal cells in disorderly arrangement. There is a progressive degeneration in the papillary and subpapillary zones of the dermis. Other changes include (1) the development of vascular ectasia, (2) accumulation of acid mucopolysaccharides, (3) appearance of abnormal fibrocytes, (4) loss of collagen, (5) degeneration of elastic tissue (''actinic elastosis'') and disorganization of the connective tissue into amorphous masses. In actinically damaged skin the concentration of elastin may be increased and collagen decreased. These changes are mostly irreversible but can be minimized by daily topical application of effective sunscreens.

PHOTOTOXICITY AND PHOTOALLERGY

Sensitivity to sunlight is a common clinical problem. Continuous daily exposure to sun alone may be the major factor responsible for irreversible skin changes (e.g., freckles, telangiectasia, wrinkling, keratoses, atrophy, hypermelanotic and hypomelanotic macules, and carcinomas in the sun-exposed regions). Apart from these chronic changes, human skin can also become hypersensitive to UVR and visible light. The interface between humans and their environment is the skin, and the physical (light) and chemical agents acting directly on it are important etiologic or precipitating factors in photosensitivity disorders.

EFFECT OF DRUGS AND OTHER CHEMICALS IN ASSOCIATION WITH LIGHT EXPOSURE Some chemicals and drugs by themselves may not act as contact irritants and are generally innocuous to skin in the absence of light exposure. However, when the skin is challenged with proper concentrations of the agent and the appropriate light wavelengths, these agents can induce undesirable skin reactions.

Cutaneous photosensitivity is a general term used to refer to the abnormal reaction of the human skin to the stimulus of light. Chemical or drug photosensitivity reactions may be defined clinically as adverse skin responses resulting from the combination of exposure to certain therapeutic or chemical agents and UVR. In most of the drug or chemical photosensitivity reactions, the wavelengths that evoke abnormal reactions are usually but not always in the 320- to 400-nm region. Adverse cutaneous reactions can occur in some individuals who either have ingested certain drugs or have been in contact with certain chemicals (Tables 52-3 and 52-4). These reactions may include an acute, abnormal sunburn response, namely, edema, papules, macules, vesicles, bullae, or acute eczematous or urticarial reactions. There may be desquamation and hyperpigmentation or hypopigmentation. These adverse photosensitivity reactions are classified into two broad categories: (1) phototoxic reactions and (2) photoallergic reactions.

Phototoxic reactions are those reactions exaggerated by UVR in which there is no evidence of participation of the immune system; these reactions usually can be elicited in almost everyone with enough light energy of the appropriate wavelengths and when appropriate concentrations of the agent are either applied topically or given orally. Light plus the offending agent leads to an exaggerated sunburn reaction, with or without painful edema. The reaction can occur within 5 to 18 h after exposure to the sun and is usually maximum at 36 to 72 h. Hyperpigmentation and desquamation can also occur. The reaction is usually confined to the site of exposure. If the applied concentration of the implicated agent is high, bullae or small vesicles may develop. The most common chemicals that induce phototoxicity reactions in humans are (1) anthraquinone dyes; (2) chlorothiazides; (3) chlorpromazines and phenothiazines; (4) coal tars containing anthracene, acridine, phenanthrene, etc.; (5) nalidixic acid; (6) protriptyline; (7) psoralens (8-methoxypsoralen and 4,5',8-trimethylpsoralen); (8) sulfonamides; and (9) tetracycline (demethylchlortetracycline, etc.) (see Table 52-4).

Certain *phototoxic reactions* require the presence of molecular oxygen (e.g., hematoporphyrin, several dyes). The oxygen-dependent reactions are referred to as *photodynamic reactions*. On the other hand, many phototoxic reactions can occur in the absence of oxygen (e.g., psoralen photosensitization). Most reactions have been reported to require UV-A (320- to 400-nm) radiation; however, certain phototoxic reactions can be initiated by the UV-B (290- to 320-nm) as well as by the visible (400- to 700-nm) spectra. The phototoxic reactions in general should be regarded as the undesirable sequelae of augmentation of the primary photochemical reactions that underlie the inflammatory response of skin evoked by UVR. It is believed that a deleterious amount of radiant energy is absorbed by the skin and the photosensitizing agents. This absorbed energy can directly cause cell damage by creating a covalent linking of the sensitizing molecule to the pyrimidines (e.g., thymine) in the cellular DNA. This linkage (the formation of cyclobutane photoadducts of the sensitizer and the pyrimidines) can be lethal to the cell. Photosensitizers like the psoralens selectively intercalate between two base pairs and produce single-strand photoadducts with pyrimidine bases in DNA or interstrand cross-links with epidermal DNA. In addition, the photosensitizing molecule can transfer the absorbed energy and promote formation of free radicals (molecules with unpaired electrons that are highly reactive) and cause damage to the cell membranes and lysosomes. In the presence of certain porphyrins (e.g., hematoporphyrin, protoporphyrin), a reactive singlet form of oxygen can be generated by these photosensitizing molecules. Drug-induced phototoxic reactions may thus involve damage to the DNA, RNA, lysosomes, cell membranes, and other organelles. Certain drugs (chlorpromazine, benoxaprofen) may operate by both photodynamic and photoallergic mechanisms.

Photoallergy to drugs is an acquired and altered capacity of the skin to respond to light in the presence of a photosensitizer, and involves the immune system. Rather than an exaggerated sunburn, the clinical reaction may consist of an eczematous eruption or discrete eruption or discrete papules and plaques. The absorbed light energy may promote a photochemical reaction between the drug and the skin proteins. The drug may act to form a haptenic group and either combines directly with the protein to form a photoantigen or is altered by the absorbed energy; this altered haptenic group then reacts with the proteins to form an antigen. The photoantigen is then processed by macrophages and is believed to come in contact with T cells to

TABLE 52-3 Contact photosensitizers: Chemicals that induce photosensitivity reactions in humans

Name	Use	Reported clinical observations
Halogenated salicylanilides; 3,3′,4′,5-tetrachlorosalicylanilide; 3,4′,5- and 3,3′,5-trichlorosalicylanilide; 3,4′,5- and 3,3′,5-tribromosalicylanilide; 3,5- and 4,5′-dibromosalicylanilide	Deodorant, bacteriostatic agents in soaps	Phototoxic and eczematous photoallergic reactions, burning, itching, cross-photosensitivity reactions
Hexachlorophene	Antimicrobial, antiseptic	Phototoxic reactions
Bithionol or bis(2-hydroxy-3,5-dichlorophenyl) sulfide	Antimicrobial, antiseptic	Photoallergic reactions
Fentichlor (2,2′-dihydroxy-5,5′-dichlorodiphenyl sulfide); multifungin (bromochlorosalicylanilide); Jadit (4-chloro-2-hydroxybenzoic acid *N*-*n*-butylamide)	Antifungal	Phototoxic and photoallergic reactions
5-Flurouracil	Antineoplastic	Acceleration of inflammatory process
p-Aminobenzoic acid (PABA) and esters of PABA	Sunscreen	Photoallergic reactions
4,4′-Bis(3-phenylureido)-2,2′-stilbenedisulfonic acid or blankophor	Fluorescent brightening agent for cellulose, nylon, or wool fibers	Phototoxic and photoallergic reactions
Cadmium sulfide	In tattoos	Erythema
Furocoumarins: psoralen, 8-methoxypsoralen, 5-methoxypsoralen, 4,5′,8-trimethylpsoralen	In vitiligo for increased pigment formation and sun tolerance	Marked erythema, vesicles, bullae, hyperpigmentation
Essential oils: oil of bergamot, oil of lime, oil of cedar, oil of lavender, oil of citron, oil of sandalwood	Cosmetics and beauty aids	Phototoxic reactions and postinflammatory hyperpigmentation
Plants: Umbelliferae, Rutaceae	Used in perfumes or flavorings or as spices	Phytophotodermatitis, hyperpigmentation, vesicles, bullae
6-Methylcoumarin	Used in cosmetics	Photoallergic reactions
Musk ambrette	Used in cosmetics	Photoallergic reactions
Dyes: acriflavine, fluorescein, rose bengal, eosin, erythrocine, trypaflavin, orange red, paraphenylenediamine, methylene blue, toluidine blue, trypan blue, anthraquinone	Cosmetics and dye industry	Erythema, edema, vesicles, pigmentation, phototoxic reaction
Coal tar and coal tar derivatives containing anthracene, phenanthrene, naphthalene, thiophene, and many phenolic agents; pitch, acridine	In therapy for psoriasis and chronic eczema; in hair shampoos	Smarting, exaggerated sunburn, urticarial wheals, tar melanosis

SOURCE: *TB Fitzpatrick et al, in Sunlight and Man: Normal and Abnormal Photobiologic Responses, MA Pathak et al (eds), Tokyo, University of Tokyo Press, 1974.*

manifest any ordinary type of delayed hypersensitivity immunologic response. The complete photoantigen is recognized on subsequent exposure to sensitized T cells in the form of a papulovesicular or an eczematous response.

The clinical manifestations in drug-induced photoallergic reactions may range from acute urticarial lesions, developing within a few minutes after exposure, to eczematous or papular lesions appearing within 24 h or later. The eruption may extend beyond the exposed areas. In recurrent cases, flare-ups of distant, previously uninvolved sites may also occur. Some edema and vasodilatation are common in most of these eruptions. The action spectrum is generally in the long-wave range (320 to 400 nm), and less energy is required than is necessary for the production of phototoxic reactions. In general, photoallergy is much less common than phototoxic reaction, and the light-microscopic examination of a lesional biopsy reveals a characteristic, though not diagnostic, dense perivascular round cell infiltrate.

The various systemic therapeutic agents and their effects on the skin in the presence of light (whether phototoxic or photoallergic reactions) are listed in Table 52-4. The biologic action spectra that induce either the phototoxic or photoallergic reactions are also given.

EFFECT OF PLANTS PLUS LIGHT *Phytophotodermatitis* (phototoxic reactions) can develop as the result of contact with many plants (belonging principally to the families Rutaceae and Umbelliferae, e.g., certain limes, parsley, celery, bishop's weed, figs) and subsequent exposure of the skin to sunlight. The photodermatitis involves a mild-to-severe erythematous reaction with or without vesicles or bullae. Dense postinflammatory hyperpigmentation is visible within 3 to 5 days. Perfumes and colognes containing oil of bergamot are also known to induce hyperpigmentation with or without erythema. The pigmentation in berloque dermatitis occurs in configurations that seem bizarre but actually represent the areas to which the scent was applied; sometimes the hyperpigmentation may be droplike or pendant-like, and has therefore been named accordingly (*berloque* or *berlock*, meaning trinket or pendant). This phytophotodermatitis, as well as that which follows contact with various other plants, is thought to be caused by furocoumarins (e.g., 5-methoxypsoralen, 8-methoxypsoralen, and other psoralens) characteristically present in these plants. The combination of exposure to long-wave UVR (320 to 400 nm) and furocoumarins greatly enhances the erythema and the pigmentation response.

Treatment Therapy of acute phototoxic reactions induced by topical or systemic agents is best achieved by removal of the offending agent and avoidance of exposure to the sun, or both. If necessary, the usual dermatologic procedures for minimizing the discomforts of the inflammatory response should be undertaken. However, in instances in which continued systemic use of the drug is vital, cutaneous photoreactions may be prevented by instructing the patient to remain indoors or by avoiding exposure to sunlight between 10 A.M. and 4 P.M. Generally the problem subsides within a week after discontinuation of the stress (sun and the drug). Sunscreens listed in Table 52-5 also should be prescribed.

EFFECT OF LIGHT PLUS ENDOGENOUS PHOTOSENSITIZERS This category includes several photosensitivity reactions in patients with various types of porphyria (see Chap. 312). The photosensitivity reactions are related to the overproduction in vivo of either proto-, uro-, or coproporphyrins and their precursors. In the porphyrias, endogenously synthesized porphyrin molecules, when exposed to light, cause burning, itching, urticaria, edema, crusting and scarring, vesiculation, atrophy, and many other disabling cutaneous changes. The light-absorbing molecules involved in evoking the cutaneous reactions are a complex of oxidized porphyrins present in abnormal amounts in red blood cells, plasma, skin, liver, stool, and urine. The photodermatitis is optimally produced by a narrow band of light in the region of 400 to 410 nm, which corresponds to one of the absorption peaks of porphyrins. Patients, however, are sensitive to wavelengths from 380 to 600 nm. The most disabling types of photosensitivity reactions are encountered in erythropoietic (congenital) porphyria (Gunther's disease) and in erythropoietic protoporphyria (Chap. 312). Symptoms and signs of sensitivity to sunlight occur in early childhood.

The adverse cutaneous responses to sunlight in patients with erythropoietic protoporphyria (EPP) have been found to be ameliorated by oral ingestion of β-carotene (Chap. 312). Patients who take β-carotene are able to withstand prolonged exposures to sunlight and experience relief from their usual photosensitivity reactions. A recommended treatment is the daily oral ingestion of β-carotene (Solatene) sufficient to maintain blood levels of 600 to 800 μg/dL (usually adults receive a dose of 120 to 180 mg per day; children under 12 years receive 30 to 90 mg per day). Photoprotective effect of β-carotene is observed after 4 to 6 weeks, and the therapy is generally continued throughout the year. In vitro, β-carotene has been found to be an effective quencher for the "singlet" oxygen-generated photoactivated porphyrins. During porphyrin-mediated photosensitivity reactions, peroxide radicals (HO_2^0) are also generated which damage the lipid membranes. It is presumed that β-carotene is preferentially oxidized and that by quenching the "singlet" oxygen, it inhibits lipid peroxide formation.

POLYMORPHOUS LIGHT ERUPTIONS

Polymorphous light eruption (PMLE) is an idiopathic, acquired syndrome characterized by a delayed abnormal response to light and varied morphology. The clinical patterns are pleomorphic or polymorphic in nature. The most common pattern consists of multiple small papules, or papules and vesicles that may become confluent and present at times an eczematous clinical picture. Lichenification due to scratching of the pruritic lesions is not common but certainly occurs. Less frequently, the primary lesion is a large papule that may present an erythema multiforme–like pattern or become confluent to form plaques. This variety is usually, but not exclusively, confined to the face and neck. The only consistent histologic feature in all cases is a dense perivascular infiltrate in the upper and middle dermis. The infiltrate is predominantly lymphocytic and the infiltrating mononuclear cells are mostly T cells. Typically the lesions appear in early spring and after each exposure. The latent period between exposure and the appearance of rash may range from a few hours to 2 days, with the most common interval being 24 to 36 h. Itching is frequent and may occur during sun exposure and even preceding the eruption. Irritating papules may coalesce into plaques, and frequently excoriate and subside within 2 to 5 days if sun exposure is avoided. In the majority of patients, the PMLE condition is seasonal, occurring in the early spring and summer months. Patients tend to improve as the summer progresses. The familial or hereditary form of polymorphous light eruptions has been reported in North American and Latin American Indians.

The sunburn-producing spectrum (UV-B, or 290 to 320 nm) is the most effective waveband for eliciting abnormal PMLE responses. However, in many instances, the action spectrum may extend into the UV-A (320- to 400-nm) region; in some instances it may extend into the visible region. Even alpha particles, x-rays, and germicidal

TABLE 52-4 Systemic photosensitizers: Chemicals that induce photosensitivity reactions in humans

Name	Uses	Clinical observations	Action spectrum, nm
SULFONAMIDES			
Sulfanilamide, sulfathiazole, sulfapyridine, sulfamethazine, sulfaguanidine, sulfisoxazole, monochlorphenamide	Chemotherapy, antibacterial agents	Phototoxic and photoallergic reactions	290–320
SULFONYLUREA			
Carbutamide, tolbutamide (Orinase), chlorpropamide (Diabinese)	Hypoglycemic or antidiabetic drugs	Phototoxic reactions	290–360
CHLORTHIAZIDES			
6-Chloro-7-sulfamyl-3,4-dihydro-1,2,4-thiodiazine 1,1-dioxide (HydroDiuril)	Diuretics, antihypertensive	Papular and edematous eruption, plaques	290–320
Quinethazone (Diuril)	Antihypertensive	Phototoxic and photoallergic reactions	320–400
PHENOTHIAZINES			
Chlorpromazine (Thorazine), promethazine (Phenergan), mepazine, Stelazine, trimeprazine, Compazine, promazine (Sparine)	Tranquilizer, nematode infestation agent, urinary antiseptic, antihistamine	Exaggerated sunburn, maculopapular and urticarial eruptions, gray-blue hyperpigmentation	290–400
ANTIBIOTICS			
Demethylchlortetracycline (Declomycin), chlortetracycline, oxytetracycline, doxycycline	Broad-spectrum antibiotic	Exaggerated sunburn, phototoxic reaction	320–400
Griseofulvin	Antimycotic	Exaggerated sunburn, phototoxic and photoallergic reactions	320–400
Nalidixic acid (NegGram)	Antibacterial	Erythema, bullae	320–400
FUROCOUMARINS: PSORALENS			
4,5′,8-Trimethylpsoralen (trioxsalen), 8-methoxypsoralen (methoxsalen), psoralen	In photochemotherapy of psoriasis and vitiligo; for sun tolerance and increased pigment formation	Erythema, bullae, hyperpigmentation	320–400
ESTROGENS AND PROGESTERONES			
Mestranol and norethynodrel, diethylstilbestrol	Oral contraceptives	Melasma, phototoxic reactions	?290–320
Chlordiazepoxide (Librium)	Tranquilizer, psychotropic	Eczematous eruption	290–360
Triacetyldiphenolisatin	Laxative	Eczematous photoallergic reaction	290–320
Cyclamates, calcium cyclamate, sodium cyclohexylsulfamate	Artificial sweeteners	Phototoxic and photoallergic reactions	290–360

SOURCE: *TB Fitzpatrick et al, in Sunlight and Man: Normal and Abnormal Photobiologic Responses, MA Pathak et al (eds), Tokyo, University of Tokyo Press, 1974.*

TABLE 52-5 Sun protection factors of some brand name sunscreens under indoor or outdoor conditions

Trade name	Ingredients	Type of sunscreen	Sun protection factor (SPF): Indoor solar simulator	Sun protection factor (SPF): Outdoor sunlight	Resistance to: Sweating	Resistance to: Water immersion
PABA sunscreens:						
PreSun-15	5% PABA in 50–70% ethyl alcohol	Clear lotion	15–18	10–12	Excellent	Poor
Pabanol	5% PABA in 50–70% ethyl alcohol	Clear lotion	15–18	6–8	Fair	Poor
Sunbrella	5% PABA in 50–70% ethyl alcohol	Clear lotion	15	6	Fair	Poor
PreSun-15	5% PABA in 50–70% ethyl alcohol	Gel	15	10–12	Good	Fair
PABA ester sunscreens:						
Block out	3.3% isoamyl-*p*-N,N-dimethyl aminobenzoate (padimate A)	Lotion/gel	6–8	6	Good	Fair
PABAFILM	3.3% isoamyl-*p*-N,N-dimethyl aminobenzoate (padimate A)	Lotion/gel	6–8	4–6	Good	Fair
Sundown	3.3% isoamyl-*p*-N,N-dimethyl aminobenzoate (padimate A)	Lotion	8–10	4–6	Good	Fair
Original Eclipse	3.5% padimate A + 3.0% octyldimethyl PABA	Lotion	8–10	4–6	Fair	Fair
Aztec	5.0% homomenthyl salicylate + 2.5% amyl-*p*-dimethyl aminobenzoate	Lotion	6–8	4	Fair	Poor
Sea & Ski	3.3% octyldimethyl PABA	Cream	7–8	4	Fair	Poor
Marbert Sun Creme	Benzyliden-camphor + phenylbenzimidazole-5-sulfonic acid + isopropyl dibenzoyl methane	Cream	15	13–14	Good	Poor
PABA-ester combination sunscreens:						
Coppertone Super Shade-15	7% octyldimethyl PABA + 3% oxybenzone	Milky lotion	15–18	10–12	Excellent	Excellent
Total Eclipse-15*	2.5% glyceryl PABA + 2.5% octyldimethyl PABA + 2.5% oxybenzone	Milky lotion	15–18	10–14	Excellent	Good
MMM-What-A-Tan!	3.0% octyldimethyl PABA + 2.5% benzophenone-3	Milky lotion	15–20	10–12	Excellent	Good
PreSun-15 (water-resistant)	8% padimate O + 3% oxybenzone	Milky lotion	15–20	8–10	Excellent	Good
Clinique-19	Phenyl-benzimidazole-5-sulfonic acid + 2.5% octyldimethyl PABA	Milky lotion	15–19	7–8	Good	Fair
Sundown-15* (sunblock)	7% padimate O + 5% octylsalicylate + 4% oxybenzone	Milky lotion	15–20	10–11	Excellent	Good
Bain de Soleil	7.0% padimate O + 2.5% oxybenzone + 0.5% dioxybenzone	White cream	15–18	9	Excellent	Fair
Elizabeth Arden Suncare Creme-15	Padimate O + oxybenzone	White cream	15–20	14	Good	Excellent
Estee Lauder-15	Phenyl-benzimidazole-5-sulfonic acid + dimethyl PABA	White cream	15–20	9	Good	Fair
Rubenstein Gold Beauty-15	Ethyl-hexyl-*p*-methoxycinnamate + octyldimethyl PABA	Yellow gel	10–12	9	Fair	Poor
Block Out-15	7% octyldimethyl PABA + 3% oxybenzone	Creamy lotion	15	5–8	Good	Good
Shiseido-15	6.5% titanium dioxide + 2.5% octyldimethyl PABA + 0.3% benzophenone-3	Lotion	15–20	8–10	Good	Good
Non-PABA sunscreens:						
Piz Buin-8†	5% ethyl-hexyl-*p*-methoxycinnamate + 3% 2-hydroxy-4-methoxybenzophenone + 4% 2-phenyl-benzimidazole sulfonic acid	Cream	15–20	10–12	Excellent	Good
Piz Bun-8†	5% ethyl-hexyl-*p*-methoxycinnamate + 3% 2-hydroxy-4-methoxybenzophenone	Milky lotion	20–22	10–12	Excellent	Good
TIScreen-15	5% ethyl-hexyl-*p*-methoxycinnamate + 3% 2-hydroxy-4-methoxybenzophenone	Milky lotion	16–20	10–12	Excellent	Good
Piz Buin-4*	4.5% ethyl-hexyl-*p*-methoxycinnamate	Milky lotion	10–12	4–6	Fair	Poor
UVAL	10% 2-hydroxy-4-methoxybenzophenone-5-sulfonic acid	Milky lotion	10–12	4	Poor	Poor
Coppertone	8% homomenthylsalicylate	Lotion	3.5–4	2	Poor	Poor
Ultra Vera-20 (Cheesebrough-Pond's)	Octylmethoxycinnamate + 2-hydroxy-4-methoxybenzophenone	Milky lotion	12–15	6	Fair	Fair
Piz Buin Gletsher Creme-15	Cinnamide + dibenzoylmethane	Yellow lotion	15	12–13	Excellent	Excellent
Piz Buin-12	4.5% octyl-methoxycinnamate + 4.5% zinc oxide + 4.5% talc + 2.2% benzophenone-3	Milky lotion	15–20	12–14	Excellent	Excellent
Physical sunscreens:						
A-Fil	Titanium dioxide + zinc oxide + talc, kaolin, iron oxide, or red veterinary petrolatum	Cream	6–8	4–6	Good	Fair
RV Paque	Titanium dioxide + zinc oxide + talc, kaolin, iron oxide, or red veterinary petrolatum	Cream	10–12	4–6	Good	Fair
Shadow	Titanium dioxide + zinc oxide + talc, kaolin, iron oxide, or red veterinary petrolatum	Cream	4–6	6–8	Good	Fair
Reflecta	Titanium dioxide + zinc oxide + talc, kaolin, iron oxide, or red veterinary petrolatum	Cream	10–12	2–4	Good	Good
Covermark	Titanium dioxide + zinc oxide + talc, kaolin, iron oxide, or red veterinary petrolatum	Cream	10–12	6–8	Good	Fair
Clinique	Titanium dioxide + zinc oxide + talc, kaolin, iron oxide, or red veterinary petrolatum	Cream	10–12	4–6	Good	Fair

KEY: *Excellent = SPF value retained is over 90 to 100% after stress of 45-min swimming; good = SPF value retained is over 75 to 90% after stress of 45-min swimming; fair = SPF value retained is over 50 to 75% after stress of 45-min swimming; poor = SPF value retained is less than 50% after stress of 45-min swimming.*

* *Ingredients may include octyldimethyl PABA + oxybenzone.*

† *Not available in the United States.*

NOTE: *Eyes should always be protected with ultraviolet-opaque goggles or sunglasses while sunbathing or skiing.*

SOURCE: *Pathak et al, in Dermatology in General Medicine, 2d ed, TB Fitzpatrick et al (eds), New York, McGraw-Hill, 1979.*

radiation (290 nm) may produce PMLE. Although the mechanisms underlying these reactions are not known, the evidence suggests a delayed hypersensitivity reaction to an antigen induced by radiation.

TREATMENT Photoprotection with the use of highly effective sunscreens (Table 52-5) or through the avoidance of outdoor activities between 9 A.M. and 5 P.M. during summer months and appropriate long-sleeved clothes may significantly reduce the severity of the clinical response. The synthetic antimalarials are effective in PMLE, but they must be used with great caution to prevent retinopathy and optic nerve atrophy. One of the effective treatments for PMLE is to induce tolerance or hardening of the skin by oral methoxsalen (0.6 mg/kg) photochemotherapy. This tolerance or desensitization by repeated graduated exposures to sunlight or to artificial radiation (UV-A) in combination with psoralens (methoxsalen) is attributed to thickening of epidermis and increased pigmentation and appears to account for the rarity of PMLE in Australia, where the fair-skinned population is exposed to the sun year round. Oral administration of β-carotene (Solatene) has been found to be of limited value.

Several other idiopathic forms of photodermatoses are seen that constitute a rare but large group of light-induced abnormal reactions. *Solar urticaria* following brief exposure to sunlight or artificial radiation is a rare but distinctive condition. The exposed skin reddens, scattered wheals appear and coalesce, and an erythematous flare develops around the wheals with or without urticaria; the cause is unknown. In some patients exposure to UV-B, UV-A, or visible radiation has been followed by the elevation of histamine, degranulation of mast cells, and elevated levels of eosinophil and neutrophil chemotactic factors into the circulation, suggesting that mast cells may play a role. Although antihistamines may benefit some patients, topical broad-spectrum sunscreens and gradual induction of tolerance to natural or artificial radiation by repeated and graded exposures to radiation of appropriate wavelengths have been found to diminish the urticarial reaction.

Actinic reticuloid is another form of chronic, persistent photodermatitis occurring mainly in males who are middle-aged or elderly. It is a most distressing form of persistent photosensitivity characterized by erythematous papular and eczematous eruption; pruritus is generally severe. Lymphomatoid infiltrate is observed histologically with microscopic features implied by the term reticuloid. The patients are severely sensitive to UV-B, UV-A, and even visible radiation. There is a frequent history of eczema present for many years; in some, photosensitivity starts with photocontact dermatitis to a chemical agent. Oral psoralen photochemotherapy appears to help the clearance of photodermatoses.

PHOTOTHERAPY AND PHOTOCHEMOTHERAPY

Phototherapy refers to the therapeutic effectiveness of UVR (usually 290 to 320 nm) or visible radiation without the systemic use of a drug. Photochemotherapy, on the other hand, involves the combination of nonionizing electromagnetic radiation and a systemically administered, photochemically reactive agent. Generally in the doses used, neither the drug alone nor the radiation alone has any therapeutic response; only the combination of the photoactive drug and the radiation, administered at the appropriate time, is therapeutic. Indications for phototherapy include various dermatoses, uremic pruritus, and neonatal hyperbilirubinemia. Phototherapy with blue visible light (430 to 500 nm) causes the photoisomerization of bilirubin, and the resulting water-soluble bilirubin photoproducts are readily excreted in bile and urine. Psoriasis, eczema, and pityriasis rosea may improve with controlled sun exposures. UV-B radiation (290 to 320 nm) is, therefore, a part of the therapeutic regimen for these dermatoses.

The treatment of psoriasis and other proliferative diseases of the skin has involved attempts to inhibit cellular proliferation and DNA synthesis.

The topical application of crude coal-tar products followed by subsequent UV exposure has been a standard treatment for severe generalized psoriasis and was first described by W. H. Goeckerman, M.D., of the Mayo Clinic more than 50 years ago. Although tar-induced phototoxicity affecting DNA synthesis is believed to be responsible for therapeutic effects, it is not yet clear whether the beneficial effects are due to the chemical ingredients of tar alone or the photosensitizing action of UV-A (320 to 400 nm) or UV-B.

ORAL PSORALEN PHOTOCHEMOTHERAPY Psoralens are naturally occurring furocoumarins that are tricyclic compounds, many of which are photochemically reactive [e.g., 8-methoxypsoralen (methoxsalen) and 4,5′,8-trimethylpsoralen (trioxsalen)]. It has been shown that in the presence of psoralens irradiation with UV-A (320 to 400 nm) can result in covalent binding of psoralens to pyrimidine bases in DNA. This photoconjugation may lead to interstrand cross-linking of psoralen between base paired strands of DNA, inhibition of DNA synthesis, and cell death. Psoralens in combination with UV-A (PUVA) are now widely used in treating psoriasis, vitiligo, and mycosis fungoides. Two hours after ingestion of methoxsalen (0.6 mg/kg), patients are exposed to a measured dose of UV-A radiation. The initial dose depends on the patient's skin reactivity to UVR (skin type) and degree of melanin pigmentation of skin. Repeated oral psoralen plus UV-A treatments cause disappearance of psoriatic lesions; a total of 20 treatments given two or three times weekly will usually result in clearance of psoriasis. Maintenance treatments are recommended, once weekly for two months. The scalp and areas to which UV-A does not penetrate do not respond to therapy. Data verifying the efficacy of PUVA have come from several carefully designed, prospective clinical trials involving over 5000 patients at university medical centers throughout the United States and western Europe.

In vitiligo, a disease characterized by amelanotic macules of varying sizes and absence of melanocytes, PUVA treatment can be used in restoring the normal skin color to pigmentless areas of vitiligo macules. Over 70 percent of repigmentation in vitiliginous areas can be achieved. Over 100 to 200 treatments are needed, and this long duration of treatment can often be frustrating, especially when the pigment response is slow, unpredictable, and subject to the presence of functional melanocytes and their proliferation.

The potential long-term concerns of photochemotherapy include premature aging (irreversible changes in connective tissue, blood vessels, and keratinocytes), cataracts, and skin cancer. Oral methoxsalen photochemotherapy using long-wave UVR sources is a new approach. Although over 200,000 patients with psoriasis and thousands of patients with vitiligo have been treated, well-documented examples of actinic keratoses or early squamous cell carcinoma have been infrequently observed in fair skinned patients (skin type I–III) receiving over 80 treatments. Prior history of skin cancer, exposure to ionizing radiation, and arsenic ingestion appear to be predisposing factors for increased incidence of squamous cell carcinoma. However, there is no evidence of cataractogenesis in vitiligo patients treated with psoralens and sunlight over the past 33 years, and adequate eye protection with appropriate UV-A–opaque lenses would largely obviate this risk. Photochemotherapy is an effective treatment which, when compared with other available treatments for generalized psoriasis or vitiligo, appears to have the most acceptable risk/benefit ratio.

Another type of photochemotherapy that appears to be promising is the treatment of tumors with a photosensitizer and visible light. A hematoporphyrin derivative in combination with visible radiation is now being increasingly used for the local treatment of a wide variety of malignant lesions (e.g., metastatic breast carcinoma), including those involving skin. The therapy is based upon the ability of hematoporphyrin to localize in the tumor mass, and its photodynamic efficiency in killing of malignant cells by the photoactivated hepatoporphyrins through the generation of reactive singlet oxygen and subsequent damage to the DNA and other cellular components.

TOPICAL SUNSCREENS IN HEALTH AND DISEASES

Since exposure of skin to UVR is the major cause of skin cancer and actinic aging, the risk can be significantly reduced by decreasing the quantity of harmful radiation reaching the skin with topical application of effective sunscreens. Sunscreens protect viable cells of the skin by absorbing and reflecting the radiation impinging on the skin (see Table 52-5). The majority of sunscreens are designed to protect the user against UV-B (290 to 320 nm). Sunscreens that contain two or more UVR-absorbing chemicals [e.g., benzophenones + cinnamic acid derivatives or benzophenones + PABA ester (padimate O)] appear to filter out both UV-B and UV-A radiation, and at times are referred to as broad-spectrum sunscreens. The effectiveness of a sunscreen is rated on the basis of the sun protection factor (SPF), a term that designates a ratio of MED of the sunscreen-protected skin to the MED of the nonprotected skin; the higher the SPF, the better the skin protection. In counseling people in the prevention of sunburn, skin cancer, aging of the skin, actinic elastosis, and various forms of sun sensitivity, the choice and recommendations of sunscreen depend upon several factors. The most important consideration should be the individual's reactivity to sunlight. People with fair skin, blue eyes, with or without freckles, who burn easily and tan poorly (skin types I and II, Table 52-2) should be given those sunscreens that have an SPF of 10 or greater (Table 52-5). Individuals with skin types III and IV, who burn moderately or minimally but tan well, may be recommended sunscreens with an SPF of 6 to 8. Habitually exposed areas, e.g., face, ears, neck, arms, and hands, should be protected by daily application of a nonoily lotion.

For the greatest protection patients should apply sunscreens with SPF of 10 or more 1 h before exposure. Although many new sunscreens are water-resistant (see Table 52-5), the patient should reapply the sunscreen after swimming or during prolonged sunbathing. In many instances patients may be exquisitely sensitive, irrespective of skin type, and they may require combination therapy with two or more sunscreens (preferably an opaque sunscreen). The drug-induced photosensitization reactions can be minimized or prevented by prescribing topical sunscreens containing benzophenones (Table 52-5). Sunscreens containing PABA or its derivatives should *not* be prescribed for individuals who are photosensitive to certain drugs and manifest phototoxic or cell-mediated delayed hypersensitivity reactions. In patients receiving antihypertensive thiazide diuretics or sulfonamides there may be a cross-reaction with PABA leading to eczematous dermatitis. These patients should be prescribed sunscreens containing benzophenones (see Table 52-5) or opaque sunscreens containing zinc oxide, titanium oxide, and other light-scattering agents such as kaolin.

Individuals with acute sunburn reaction manifesting severe erythema, edema, and painful blistering reaction may be treated with systemic corticosteroids. Oral prednisone, beginning with 40 to 60 mg and tapering over 4 to 8 days, will help to control the severe sunburn reaction.

REFERENCES

HARBER LC, BICKERS DR: *Photosensitivity Diseases: Principles of Diagnosis and Treatment.* Philadelphia, Saunders, 1981

MAGNUS IA: *Dermatological Photobiology.* Oxford, Blackwell, 1976

PARRISH JA: Phototherapy and photochemotherapy of skin diseases. J Invest Dermatol 77:167, 1981

——— et al: Photomedicine, in *Dermatology in General Medicine,* 3d ed, TB Fitzpatrick et al (eds). New York, McGraw-Hill, 1987

PATHAK MA, DUNNICK JK: *Photobiologic, Toxicologic, and Pharmacologic Aspects of Psoralens,* National Cancer Institute Monograph 66, US Department of Health and Human Services, National Cancer Institute, Bethesda, MD, 1984

——— et al: Evaluation of topical agents that prevent sunburn. N Engl J Med 280:1459, 1969

——— et al (eds): *Sunlight and Man: Normal and Abnormal Photobiologic Responses.* Tokyo, University of Tokyo Press, 1974

——— et al: Sunscreens: Topical and systemic approaches for protection of human skin against harmful effects of solar radiation. J Am Acad Dermatol 7:285, 1982

section 9 Hematologic alterations

53 ANEMIA

H. FRANKLIN BUNN

By definition patients with anemia have a significant reduction in red cell mass and a corresponding decrease in the oxygen-carrying capacity of the blood. Normally, blood volume is maintained at a nearly constant level. Therefore, anemia entails a decrease in the concentration of red cells or hemoglobin in peripheral blood.

Under unusual circumstances, the blood values do not accurately reflect alterations in the red cell mass. For example, hemoglobin level and hematocrit are falsely elevated in patients who have sustained an acute reduction in plasma volume owing to hemorrhage, extensive burns, vigorous diuresis, or other types of severe dehydration. In contrast, the blood values may be falsely low in patients who have an expanded blood volume, as in pregnancy or congestive heart failure.

Normal blood values for individuals of various ages are shown in the Appendix. In women in the childbearing age group the blood values are 10 percent lower than in men. At high altitudes, higher values are found, roughly in proportion to the elevation above sea level. Anemia may be defined as a reduction of more than 10 percent below the mean values for the sex. However, since the variations in normal hemoglobin values approach this limit, the documentation of mild anemia may be uncertain.

SIGNS AND SYMPTOMS OF ANEMIA The clinical presentation of the anemic patient depends on the underlying disease as well as on the severity and chronicity of the anemia. The manifestations of anemia per se can be explained by the pathophysiologic principles outlined in this chapter and in Chap. 283. Most of these signs and symptoms represent cardiovascular and ventilatory adjustments which compensate for the decrease in red blood cell mass.

The degree to which symptoms occur in an anemic patient depends on several contributing factors. If the anemia has developed rapidly, there may not be adequate time for compensatory adjustments to take place, and the patient may have more marked symptoms than if an anemia of equivalent severity had developed insidiously. Furthermore, the patient's complaints may depend on the presence of local vascular disease. For example, angina pectoris, intermittent claudication, or transient cerebral ischemia may be unmasked by the development of anemia.

Individuals with mild anemia are often asymptomatic. They may complain of fatigue as well as dyspnea and palpitation, particularly following exercise. Severely anemic patients will often be symptomatic at rest and unable to tolerate significant exertion. When the hemoglobin concentration falls below 7.5 g/dL, resting cardiac output rises significantly with an increase in both heart rate and stroke volume. The patient may be aware of this hyperdynamic state and complain of palpitation or a pounding pulse. Symptoms of cardiac failure may develop if the patient's myocardial reserve is reduced.

The symptoms of severe anemia extend to other organ systems. Patients often complain of dizziness and headache and may experience syncope, tinnitus, or vertigo. Many patients are irritable and have difficulty sleeping or concentrating. Because of decreased blood flow to the skin, patients may become hypersensitive to cold. Gastrointestinal symptoms such as anorexia, indigestion, and even nausea or bowel irregularity are attributable to shunting of blood away from the splanchnic bed. Females commonly develop abnormal menstruation, both amenorrhea and increased bleeding. Males may complain of impotence or loss of libido.

Physical findings *Pallor* is the physical finding most commonly associated with anemia. However, the usefulness of this sign is limited by other factors that affect the color of the skin. The thickness and texture of the skin vary widely among individuals. Furthermore, the blood flow to the skin can undergo wide fluctuations. Normal individuals will appear sallow when blood is shunted away from the skin, whereas anemic patients may appear flushed when overheated or during periods of excitement. The concentration of melanin in the epidermis is another important determinant of skin color. Individuals with a fair complexion may look pale even though they are not anemic. Conversely, pallor is difficult to detect in deeply pigmented individuals. Furthermore, acquired disorders of melanin pigmentation (e.g., Addison's disease, hemochromatosis) or jaundice may interfere with detection of pallor. Nevertheless, even in blacks, the presence of anemia may be suspected by the color of the palms or of noncutaneous tissues such as oral mucous membranes, nail beds, and palpebral conjunctivas. The color of the creases of the palm is a useful sign. When they are as pale as the surrounding skin, the patient usually has a hemoglobin of less than 7 g/dL.

Two factors contribute to the development of pallor in patients with anemia. There is, of course, a decrease in the hemoglobin concentration of blood perfusing the skin and mucous membranes. Also, blood is shunted away from the skin and other peripheral tissues, permitting enhanced blood flow to vital organs. Redistribution of blood flow is an important mode of compensation in anemia.

Other physical findings associated with anemia include tachycardia, wide pulse pressure, and a hyperdynamic precordium. A systolic ejection murmur is often heard over the precordium, particularly at the pulmonic area. In addition, a venous hum may be detected over the neck vessels. These cardiac findings disappear when the anemia is corrected. Patients with hemolytic anemia often have icterus and splenomegaly and occasionally develop superficial skin ulceration over the ankle bones.

APPROACH TO THE PATIENT WITH ANEMIA In evaluating the anemic patient, the physician should proceed in an orderly fashion so that the correct diagnosis can be established with a minimum of laboratory tests and procedures. As in other clinical disciplines, a comprehensive history and meticulous physical examination are of paramount importance in the initial workup of the anemic patient. For example, a family history which reveals a dominant inheritance pattern provides strong support for the diagnosis of hereditary spherocytosis. The discovery of a heart murmur and splenomegaly raises the possibility that the anemic patient may have subacute bacterial endocarditis.

The evaluation of the anemic patient should be based on a firm understanding of the pathophysiologic principles outlined in Chap. 283. As shown in Table 53-1, the clinician must first ask whether the anemia is due to a decreased production of red cells or to enhanced destruction. Moreover, the possibility of blood loss either as the sole etiology or as a contributing factor must always be considered. The examination of the stool for occult blood is an indispensable part of the evaluation of all anemic patients. At this crossroad, laboratory information can be gathered which will establish whether the patient is failing to produce an adequate number of circulating red cells or is undergoing hemolysis.

The *reticulocyte count* is the most useful laboratory test for answering this question. When an appropriate supravital stain is applied to a sample of peripheral blood, the 1- to 2-day-old red cells exhibit a network of purple strands which are aggregates of ribosomes. Reticulocytosis is a reflection of the release of an increased number of young cells from the bone marrow. The degree of increased erythropoiesis can be assessed more quantitatively by determining the reticulocyte index, which uses the hematocrit or packed cell volume (PCV) and is calculated as follows:

$$\text{Reticulocyte index} = \text{reticulocyte \%} \times \frac{\text{patient's PCV}}{\text{normal PCV}}$$

This measure fails to consider the distribution of reticulocytes between the bone marrow and the peripheral blood. When the marrow is greatly stimulated, marrow reticulocytes enter the circulation prematurely. Since the circulation of these "shift reticulocytes" in the peripheral blood is prolonged, the reticulocyte index should be divided by about 2. This factor varies from 1.5 to 3 depending upon the severity of the anemia and the degree of erythropoietin stimulation. This correction should always be made if normoblasts are encountered in the peripheral blood since this finding indicates the premature release of red cell precursors into the circulation. On a routinely prepared smear, "shift reticulocytes" appear larger than average and have a lavender hue, so-called polychromatophilia.

A failure to produce red cells is reflected in an inappropriately low reticulocyte count. In contrast, a significant elevation of reticulocytes is suggestive of hemolysis. Exceptions include (1) the brisk reticulocyte response that is seen in a patient with hemorrhage, (2) reticulocytosis encountered in patients recovering from impaired erythropoiesis (e.g., an individual with pernicious anemia who received an injection of vitamin B_{12} 1 week earlier), and (3) mild to moderate elevations in reticulocytes (3 to 7 percent) encountered in myelophthisic anemia in which the orderly release of cells is affected by alterations of the marrow stroma owing to tumor, fibrosis, or granulomata. These exceptions are often readily appreciated in the initial evaluation of the patient. Furthermore, a number of ancillary laboratory tests described below are useful in determining to what extent hemolysis is occurring. The measurement of unconjugated bilirubin in the serum is a particularly useful guide to the presence of accelerated red blood cell breakdown. Once this information is obtained, the workup can be directed toward the establishment of a specific etiology.

Three additional baseline studies are of critical importance in the initial workup of the patient with anemia: *measurement of red cell indexes, examination of the peripheral blood smear,* and, in many patients, *bone marrow examination.*

Red cell indexes Red cell indexes can be calculated from determinants of hematocrit, hemoglobin concentration, and red blood cell

TABLE 53-1 Initial evaluation of anemia

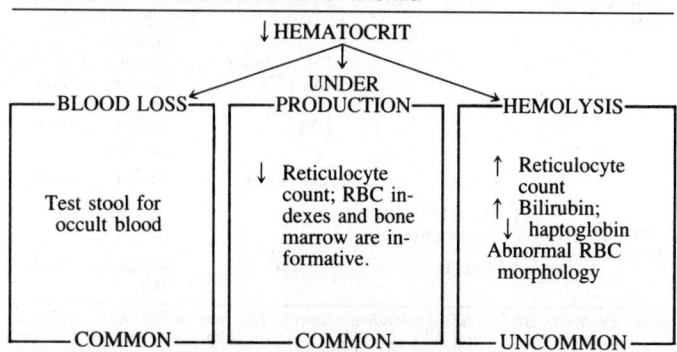

↓ HEMATOCRIT

BLOOD LOSS	UNDER PRODUCTION	HEMOLYSIS
Test stool for occult blood	↓ Reticulocyte count; RBC indexes and bone marrow are informative.	↑ Reticulocyte count ↑ Bilirubin; ↓ haptoglobin Abnormal RBC morphology
COMMON	COMMON	UNCOMMON

count. Measuring the hematocrit or PCV is the simplest and one of the most precise ways to ascertain the concentration of red cells in the blood. Generally, a small sample of anticoagulated blood is drawn into a capillary tube which is sealed at one end and centrifuged. The PCV is the ratio of the volume of packed red cells to the total volume. Alternatively, the concentration of hemoglobin can be determined spectrophotometrically from the absorbance of the cyanmethemoglobin form at a specific wavelength. With the advent of automated red blood cell counting technology, very precise measurements of red blood cell indexes are now readily available in nearly all hospitals and clinical laboratories. The electronic counter makes a direct measurement of the red cell count (RBC/μL) and the mean red cell volume (MCV):

$$\text{MCV (fl)} = \frac{\text{PCV (liters/liters)}}{(\text{RBC}/\mu\text{L}) \times 10^{-9}}$$

This instrument calculates the PCV from the direct measurement of MCV and RBC/μL. In addition, hemoglobin concentration is measured directly on a separate channel. The mean corpuscular hemoglobin concentration (MCHC) is then computed as follows:

$$\text{MCHC (g/dL)} = \frac{\text{Hb (g/dL)}}{\text{PCV (liters/liters)}}$$

A third red blood cell index, the mean corpuscular hemoglobin (MCH), is determined as follows:

$$\text{MCH (pg)} = \frac{\text{Hb (g/dL)}}{(\text{RBC}/\mu\text{L}) \times 10^{-7}}$$

When calculated by an electronic counter, the MCHC is not reliable and is of little use to the clinician. Generally, an automated system provides a printout which includes hemoglobin concentration, red cell count, packed cell volume, and the three red cell indexes (MCV, MCHC, and MCH).

As Table 53-2 shows, the MCV is particularly useful in classifying the anemias due to decreased red cell production. Microcytic anemias have low values for MCV. On microscopic examination, the red cells appear small and often pale. In contrast, in the macrocytic anemias the MCV is elevated and large oval cells (macroovalocytes) are seen on microscopic examination. Unlike the anemias of underproduction, nearly all the hemolytic anemias are normocytic or slightly macrocytic owing to the preponderance of young red cells. Exceptions include the severe forms of thalassemia in which microcytic red cells are accompanied by brisk hemolysis.

TABLE 53-2 Anemias due to decreased red cell production

RBC Indexes	Marrow	Additional lab tests	Diagnosis
Hypochromic, microcytic (↓ MCV)	0 Iron	↓ Fe, ↑ TIBC	Iron deficiency
	+ Iron	↑ Hb A_2, ↑ Hb F	β Thalassemia
	Ring sideroblasts	↓ Hb A_2	Sideroblastic anemia
Macrocytic (↑ MCV)	Megaloblastic	↓ Serum B_{12}, achlorhydria	Vitamin B_{12} deficiency, pernicious anemia
		↓ Serum folate	Folic acid deficiency
Normochromic, normocytic	Normal	↓ Fe, ↓ TIBC	Anemia of chronic inflammation
		↑ Creatinine	Anemia of uremia
		Abn LFT	Anemia of liver disease
		↓ T_4	Anemia of myxedema
	Aplastic	Pancytopenia	Aplastic anemia
Normoblasts, teardrops	Infiltrated: tumor, lymphoma, etc.		Myelophthisic
	Fibrosis	↑ LAP	Myeloid metaplasia

NOTE: *Fe, iron; TIBC, total iron-binding capacity; Hb, hemoglobin; LAP, leukocyte alkaline phosphatase; LFT, liver function tests; Abn, abnormal; MCV, mean corpuscular volume.*

Examination of the blood smear In the evaluation of patients with anemia, the physician should take the time to examine a well-stained peripheral blood film. Figures A5-1 to A5-12 show examples of abnormalities in red cell morphology encountered in various types of anemia. Many subtleties escape the attention of the technologist whose primary purpose in examining the slide is to obtain a white cell differential count. Furthermore, the clinician can approach the specimen with a prepared mind and can scrutinize it for specific abnormalities. As suggested above, the examination can confirm the size and color of red cells as estimated by RBC indexes. Furthermore, while these indexes provide mean statistical values, the microscopic examination can reveal variation in red cell size (anisocytosis) or shape (poikilocytosis), changes which are helpful in the diagnosis of specific anemias. Examination of the blood smear is particularly important in evaluating a patient with hemolysis. Most hemolytic anemias have characteristic morphologic abnormalities. Finally, this practice may yield unexpected dividends. The finding of rouleaux suggests the presence of dysproteinemia as occurs in multiple myeloma. The examination may provide the initial clue that the patient has significant thrombocytopenia.

Bone marrow examination A microscopic examination of the bone marrow is generally indicated in the workup of any *unexplained* anemia. Study of the bone marrow is particularly informative in the anemias of underproduction. The more severe the anemia, the more likely that the procedure will be informative. An assessment of the quantity and quality of red cell precursors may determine whether there is a primary defect in cell production. A marrow biopsy is particularly useful in estimating overall cellularity. The normal differential of nucleated cells in the marrow is shown in the Appendix. The ratio of myeloid (M) to erythroid (E) precursors is normally about 2:1 but may be artifactually increased by the inclusion of circulating leukocytes. The ratio is increased in patients with infection, a leukemoid reaction, or neoplastic proliferation of myeloid cells. Rarely, a high M/E ratio is due to selective aplasia of the red cell precursors. A decreased M/E ratio indicates erythroid hyperplasia (seen in hemolysis or hemorrhage) or ineffective erythropoiesis (e.g., megaloblastic and sideroblastic anemias). The morphology of the precursors may reveal a maturation deficit such as megaloblastic anemia. The bone marrow examination is also important in demonstrating the presence of cellular infiltrates such as those found in leukemia, lymphoma, or multiple myeloma. The demonstration of tumor, fibrosis, or granulomata usually requires a biopsy. A portion of the marrow specimen should be stained with Prussian blue. In addition to providing an assessment of iron stores, the iron stain is required for the identification of sideroblasts.

ANEMIA DUE TO BLOOD LOSS This form of anemia varies considerably in its clinical presentation depending upon the site, severity, and rapidity of the hemorrhage. At opposite extremes are acute fulminant bleeding producing hypovolemic shock and chronic occult blood loss leading to iron-deficiency anemia.

Patients who have sustained an acute hemorrhage generally present with signs and symptoms secondary to hypoxia and hypovolemia. Depending on the severity of the process, the patient will have weakness, fatigue, light-headedness, stupor, or coma and will often appear pale, diaphoretic, and irritable. Vital signs are a reflection of cardiovascular compensation for the acute blood loss (Chap. 29). The patient will have hypotension and tachycardia in proportion to the degree of hemorrhage. Elicitation of postural signs is useful in the initial evaluation of patients with acute blood loss. If the pulse rises 25 percent or more, or the systolic blood pressure falls 20 mmHg or more upon going from a supine to sitting position, the patient is likely to have significant hypovolemia (blood loss >1000 mL) and requires prompt replacement. Acute blood loss in excess of 1500 mL usually leads to cardiovascular collapse.

If the blood loss has been acute and recent, the peripheral blood may not reveal a significant decrease in packed cell volume or hemoglobin, since the red cell mass and plasma volume are contracted in parallel. There often is a moderate leukocytosis and a "shift to the left" in the white cell differential count. Thrombocytosis may be encountered in both acute and chronic blood loss, particularly when the patient is iron-deficient. During the first few days following an acute hemorrhage there is usually an increase in reticulocytes. Occasionally nucleated red cells may appear in the peripheral blood. Since young red cells are larger than old ones, the patient may develop slightly macrocytic red cell indexes (MCV = 95 to 105 fl). As mentioned above, sustained reticulocytosis will be seen if significant blood loss continues, or until iron stores have been exhausted. Internal bleeding may be accompanied by an increase in unconjugated bilirubin. This abnormality is a reflection of an increase in catabolism of heme from extravasated red cells. Patients with acute gastrointestinal blood loss will often have an elevation of blood urea nitrogen owing to impaired renal blood flow and perhaps to the absorption of digested blood protein.

It is of critical importance to assess these patients promptly and institute treatment without delay. A large-bore intravenous line should be placed. While blood is being typed and cross matched, saline, Ringer's lactate, or, preferably, a colloid such as 5% albumin should be infused to correct hypovolemia. Whole blood is then administered as soon as it is available. Monitoring of vital signs and central venous pressure is useful in determining the appropriate amount of volume replacement. During and following these emergency measures, diagnostic studies may reveal the site or sites of bleeding. If the bleeding is unexplained an emergency coagulation profile should be obtained. Demonstration of bleeding from the gastrointestinal tract may require the insertion of a nasogastric tube. Appropriate radiologic studies may be indicated to determine sites of internal bleeding such as retroperitoneal hemorrhage.

Chronic blood loss is usually due to lesions in the gastrointestinal tract or the uterus. The testing of stool specimens for occult blood is an essential, though frequently overlooked, part of the evaluation of anemia. It may be necessary to examine serial specimens over a prolonged period of time since gastrointestinal bleeding is often intermittent. The hematologic manifestations of chronic blood loss are those of iron-deficiency anemia, discussed in detail in Chap. 284.

ANEMIAS DUE TO DECREASED RBC PRODUCTION As shown in Table 53-2, red cell indexes are useful in classifying the anemias due to underproduction of red cells. They can be conveniently grouped into three major categories: microcytic, macrocytic, and normocytic.

The *microcytic* anemias include iron-deficiency anemia (Chap. 284), sideroblastic anemias (Chap. 284), and the thalassemias (Chap. 288). Collectively, they represent a decrease in the availability or synthesis of one of the three major constituents of the hemoglobin molecule: iron, porphyrin, and globin. Since hemoglobin makes up over 90 percent of the protein within the erythrocyte, it is not surprising that these defects in hemoglobin synthesis result in the formation of small, pale red cells. These disorders involve a variable degree of ineffective erythropoiesis (Chap. 283). In addition, the anemias of chronic inflammation and malignancy may be slightly microcytic (Chap. 286). This phenomenon is due to a defect in the availability of iron. However, these disorders are more often normocytic and have been so classified in Table53-2. Measurement of serum iron and iron-binding capacity and evaluation of marrow iron stores are particularly useful in distinguishing between these anemias.

The *macrocytic* anemias generally are associated with megaloblastic morphology in the bone marrow. In most cases, a deficiency of either vitamin B_{12} or folic acid results in an impairment of the replication of DNA, particularly in cells having a high turnover rate. Because nuclear maturation lags behind cytoplasmic development, large red cells tend to be produced in the bone marrow. Megaloblastic anemias are discussed in detail in Chap. 285. Like the microcytic anemias, these disorders are maturation defects associated with ineffective erythropoiesis. Macrocytosis, generally of a lesser degree, may also be encountered in patients with liver disease, hypothyroidism, acute blood loss, hemolytic anemia, aplastic anemia, and alcoholism. However, in these conditions, the red cell precursors in the bone marrow do not appear megaloblastic. The macrocytes in liver disease and hypothyroidism may be related to an increased deposition of lipid in the red cell membrane.

The *normocytic* anemias of underproduction comprise a diverse group of disorders. As shown in Table 53-2, this group can be conveniently subdivided into two categories: those secondary to some other underlying disease and those due to intrinsic pathology within the bone marrow.

The primary disorders of the bone marrow are best approached by microscopic examination of a marrow aspirate and biopsy. This group of anemias is often accompanied by leukopenia and thrombocytopenia. Pancytopenia, usually to a lesser degree, can also be seen in hypersplenism and in the megaloblastic anemias. Aplastic anemia and the myelophthisic anemias are discussed in Chap. 290.

The diagnosis of anemia secondary to some underlying disease is usually quite straightforward. Conversely, the presence of an unexplained normocytic anemia should prompt the search for an underlying disorder such as chronic renal failure, infection, or myxedema. If the presence of such an illness is established, the physician is obliged to investigate whether other factors such as blood loss or a nutritional deficiency contribute to the patient's anemia. Generally, the anemias due to liver disease, chronic inflammation, or an endocrinopathy are of only moderate severity. Unlike the other "secondary" anemias, that due to chronic renal failure can be severe. All these anemias are discussed in more detail in Chap. 286.

HEMOLYTIC ANEMIAS Hemolytic anemias (Table 53-3) are encountered much less frequently than the anemias due to decreased red cell production. Although they are a diverse group, the hemolytic anemias have a number of clinical features in common. Signs and symptoms of patients with hemolysis are briefly mentioned above.

A number of laboratory tests are available to establish the presence of accelerated breakdown of red cells. The reticulocyte count is the single most useful test. Patients with hemolysis nearly always have an elevated reticulocyte count. A variety of serum and urine tests are useful in confirming the presence of hemolysis and assessing its magnitude. Serum haptoglobin and unconjugated bilirubin are particularly useful (Table 53-1). Others are described in detail in Chap. 287 and are summarized in Table 287-2.

Classification of hemolytic anemias Once the presence of hemolysis is established, a large battery of laboratory tests is available for determining the specific diagnosis. Some of these tests are listed in Table 53-3. No other area of internal medicine is better suited to detailed and fruitful diagnostic probing. In the interest of time and

TABLE 53-3 Hemolytic anemias

Blood smear	Additional lab tests	Diagnosis
Schistocytes, helmet cells		Traumatic hemolytic anemia
Spherocytes	+ Coombs' test	Immunohemolytic anemia
	$\uparrow$ Osmotic fragility	Hereditary spherocytosis
Spur cells	Abnormal LFT	Spur cell anemia
	+ Sucrose lysis	Paroxysmal nocturnal hemoglobinuria
Sickle cells	+ Sickle prep	Sickle cell syndromes
Target cells	Abn Hb electrophoresis	Hb C, D, etc.
Heinz bodies	Abn Hb electrophoresis	Congenital Heinz body hemolytic anemia
	$\downarrow$ G6Pd	G6PD deficiency

NOTE: *Hb, hemoglobin; G6PD, glucose 6-phosphate dehydrogenase; LFT, liver function tests; Abn, abnormal.*

money, the clinician should use the available tests in an orderly fashion. This complex group of disorders is easier to approach diagnostically if a concise and workable classification is used. The hemolytic anemias can be grouped in several ways: congenital versus acquired, intracorpuscular versus extracorpuscular, or by anatomic site of the erythrocyte defect. The various kinds of hemolytic anemia are discussed in Chap. 287.

THERAPEUTIC CONSIDERATIONS The effective treatment of anemia, like other disorders, is predicated upon a thorough diagnostic evaluation. There is no reason to administer hematinics such as iron, vitamin B_{12}, or folic acid unless a specific deficiency of these substances has been demonstrated or is anticipated. Although the indiscriminate administration of vitamin B_{12} is not deleterious per se, it lulls both the patient and the physician into false security. In contrast, the inappropriate use of iron preparations over a prolonged period of time can be directly harmful, leading to a state of iron overload. Pyridoxine is indicated only in the treatment of sideroblastic anemias.

Many kinds of anemias can be corrected if a precipitating cause can be uncovered and reversed. If a drug or toxin can be incriminated, its withdrawal may allow full recovery. The outcome of the "secondary" anemias is dependent on whether the underlying condition can be corrected. Anemias due to an endocrinopathy or infection should respond favorably to appropriate treatment. Occasionally, the anemia of malignancy is corrected by the removal of the primary tumor. One of the most dramatic sequelae of a successful renal transplant is the prompt correction of the "anemia of uremia." In chronic disorders such as hepatic cirrhosis or rheumatoid arthritis, the anemia is likely to persist, along with the underlying disease.

Primary disorders of the bone marrow such as aplastic anemia or myelophthisic anemia are often irreversible and are treated with supportive measures. *Androgens* are sometimes employed in this group of anemias, but their efficacy is marginal. Many of these patients require transfusions of red cells and platelets. Because prognosis is so bleak in these disorders, a radical approach to treatment seems justified. As described in Chaps. 290 and 291, bone marrow transplantation and immunosuppressive therapy are now reasonable therapeutic alternatives in selected cases of severe aplastic anemia and acute leukemia.

Several factors should be weighed in determining whether an anemic patient should be transfused. The risks and complications of the administration of blood products are discussed in Chap. 282. Patients with chronic or long-standing anemias are able to compensate in several ways, discussed earlier in this chapter. A considerable reduction in red cell mass can be surprisingly well tolerated, especially if the patient is young or sedentary. Transfusion is seldom indicated in a patient with a chronic anemia whose hemoglobin is 9 g/dL or greater. Those who are expected to respond to the administration of a specific agent such as iron, folic acid, or vitamin B_{12} can usually be spared transfusions. If the anemia has precipitated an episode of congestive heart failure or myocardial ischemia, prompt but cautious administration of packed red cells is indicated. In general, whole blood should be given only if the patient is hypovolemic.

Corticosteroids have only a limited role in the treatment of anemia. These agents are not effective in stimulating erythropoiesis. High doses of a glucocorticoid are indicated in the treatment of immunohemolytic anemia, thrombotic thrombocytopenic purpura, and pure red cell anemia. Otherwise, steroids should be prescribed sparingly unless some coexisting condition dictates their use.

Splenectomy is indicated in the treatment of certain hemolytic anemias. The efficacy of splenectomy correlates with the degree to which the abnormal or defective red cells are sequestered. Splenectomy is virtually curative in hereditary spherocytosis. The operation may be beneficial in selected patients with immunohemolytic anemia, congestive splenomegaly, spur cell anemia, and certain hemoglobinopathies and enzymopathies. Splenectomy has also been recommended early in the treatment of thrombotic thrombocytopenic purpura. The operative morbidity and mortality from elective splenectomy are very low. Occasional patients develop a left subphrenic abscess. Following splenectomy, young children are at risk of developing overwhelming septicemia. This complication is much rarer in adults. Thrombocytosis generally develops promptly following splenectomy. However, in most cases, it is transient. In patients with continued hemolysis or a myeloproliferative disorder (Chap. 289), the thrombocytosis usually persists and may occasionally be associated with thromboembolic phenomena.

REFERENCES

BABIOR BM, STOSSEL TP: *Hematology, A Pathophysiological Approach.* New York, Churchill Livingston, 1984

BECK WS (ed): *Hematology.* Boston, MIT Press, 1985

CROSBY WH: Red cell mass: Its precursors and perturbations. Hosp Prac 15:2, 71, 1980

ERSLEV AJ, GABUZDA TG: *Pathophysiology of Blood.* Philadelphia, Saunders, 1985

HILLMAN RS, FINCH CA: *Red Cell Manual.* Philadelphia, Davis, 1974

WILLIAMS WJ et al (ed): *Hematology,* 2d ed. New York, McGraw-Hill, 1983

WINTROBE MM (ed): *Blood, Pure and Eloquent.* New York, McGraw-Hill, 1980

54 BLEEDING AND THROMBOSIS

ROBERT I. HANDIN

Hemorrhage, intravascular thrombosis, and embolism are common clinical manifestations of many diseases. The hemostatic system usually limits blood loss by precisely regulated interactions between components of the vessel wall, circulating blood platelets, and plasma proteins. However, when disease or trauma damage large arteries and veins, excessive bleeding may occur, despite a normal hemostatic stystem. Less frequently, hemorrhage is caused by an inherited or acquired disorder of the hemostatic machinery itself. A large number of such bleeding disorders have now been identified.

In addition, unregulated activation of the hemostatic system may cause thrombosis and embolism, which can reduce blood flow to critical organs like the brain and myocardium. Although we understand less about the pathophysiology of thrombosis than of hemostatic failure, certain patient groups have been identified that are particularly prone to thrombosis and embolism. These include patients (1) immobilized after surgery, (2) with chronic congestive heart failure, (3) with atherosclerotic vascular disease, (4) with malignancy, or (5) who are pregnant. Most of these "thrombosis-prone" patients have no identifiable hemostatic disorder. However, there are certain patient groups who have inherited or acquired a "hypercoagulable" or "prethrombotic" state which predisposes them to recurrent thrombosis.

The cardinal manifestations of disordered hemostasis which cause bleeding or thrombosis are discussed below, along with the clinical approach to diagnosis and evaluation of these patients. Certain information in the patient's history, such as the mode of onset and sites of bleeding, a family bleeding tendency, and a record of drug ingestion help establish the correct diagnosis. Physical examination can identify bleeding in the skin or joint deformities due to previous hemarthroses. Ultimately, however, bleeding disorders are diagnosed by laboratory tests. General screening tests are utilized first, to document a systemic disorder, and are supplemented by specific tests of coagulation protein or platelet function to arrive at an accurate diagnosis.

The hypercoagulable or prethrombotic patient can also be identified by a careful history. There are three important clues to this diagnosis: (1) repeated episodes of thromboembolism without an obvious predisposing condition; (2) a family history of thrombosis; and (3) well-documented thromboembolism in adolescents and young adults. There are, as yet, no clinically useful screening tests for the prethrombotic state. However, several of the prethrombotic disorders can be diagnosed with specific immunologic and functional assays.

NORMAL HEMOSTASIS

Accurate diagnosis and treatment of patients with either bleeding or thrombosis requires some knowledge of the pathophysiology of hemostasis. The process can be divided into primary and secondary components and is initiated when trauma, surgery, or disease disrupt the vascular endothelial lining and blood is exposed to subendothelial connective tissue. *Primary hemostasis* involves the rapid formation of platelet plugs at sites of injury. This occurs within minutes of injury and is of prime importance in stopping blood loss from capillaries, small arterioles, and venules (see Fig. 54-1). *Secondary hemostasis,* or fibrin formation, results from reactions of the plasma coagulation system and may require a longer time for completion. In this reaction, fibrin strands strengthen the primary hemostatic plug. This is particularly important in larger vessels and prevents secondary bleeding hours or days after the initial injury. Although presented here as separate events, primary and secondary hemostasis are closely linked. For example, activated platelets, accelerated coagulation reactions, products of coagulation, such as thrombin, stimulate platelet aggregation.

Effective primary hemostasis requires three critical events—platelet adhesion, granule release, and platelet aggregation. Within a few seconds of injury, platelets adhere to collagen fibrils in vascular subendothelium. As shown in Fig. 54-2, this interaction is facilitated by the von Willebrand's factor, an adhesive glycoprotein which allows platelets to remain attached to the vessel wall despite the high shear forces generated within the vascular lumen. Von Willebrand's factor accomplishes this task by forming a link between platelet receptor sites and subendothelial collagen fibrils. The adherent platelets then generate and secrete mediators like those depicted in Fig. 54-1.

As in other cells, platelet activation and secretion are regulated by changes in the level of cyclic nucleotides, the influx of calcium, hydrolysis of membrane phospholipids, and phosphorylation of critical intracellular proteins. The relevant pathways are depicted in Figs. 54-3 and 54-4. The binding of agonists such as epinephrine, collagen, or thrombin to platelet surface receptors activates two membrane enzymes—phospholipase C and phospholipase A_2. These enzymes catalyze the release of arachidonic acid from two of the major membrane phospholipids, phosphatidylinositol and phosphatidylcholine. Initially, a small quantity of the released arachidonic acid is converted to thromboxane A_2 (TXA_2), which, in turn, can activate phospholipase C. The formation of TXA_2 from arachidonic acid is mediated by the enzyme cyclooxygenase (see Fig. 54-3). This enzyme is inhibited by aspirin and nonsteroidal anti-inflammatory drugs. Inhibition of TXA_2 synthesis is a common cause of bleeding, as well as the basis for the action of some antithrombotic drugs.

Hydrolysis of the membrane phospholipid, phosphatidylinositol 4,5-biphosphate (PIP_2), produces diacylglycerol (DAG) and inositol triphosphate (IP_3), which play a critical role in platelet metabolism. IP_3 mediates the movement of calcium into the platelet cytosol and stimulates the phosphorylation of myosin light chains. The latter interact with actin to facilitate granule movement and platelet shape change. DAG activates protein kinase C which, in turn, phosphorylates a 47,000-dalton protein that controls platelet granule secretion.

There is a finely balanced mechanism which controls the rate and extent of platelet activation which is illustrated in Fig. 54-3. TXA_2, a platelet product of arachidonic acid, increases phospholipase C activity, which stimulates platelet activation and secretion. In contrast, prostacyclin (PGI_2), an endothelial cell product of arachidonic acid, inhibits phospholipase C activity by raising the intraplatelet cyclic AMP levels which in turn inhibits platelet activation. Similar pathways to regulate activation and secretion occur in other cells.

Following activation, platelets secrete their granule contents into plasma. Endoglycosidases and a heparin cleaving enzyme are released from lysosomes; calcium, serotonin, and adenosine diphosphate (ADP) from the dense granules; and several proteins including von Willebrand's factor, fibronectin, thrombospondin, and a heparin-neutralizing protein (platelet factor 4) from alpha granules. Released ADP modifies the platelet surface so that fibrinogen can attach to a complex formed between membrane glycoproteins IIb and IIIa and link adjacent platelets into a hemostatic plug (Fig. 54-2). Platelet-derived growth factor (PDGF), another alpha granule protein, stimulates the growth and migration of fibroblasts and smooth muscle cells within the vessel wall, which is an important part of the repair process.

As the primary hemostatic plug is being formed, plasma coagulation proteins are activated to initiate secondary hemostasis. An

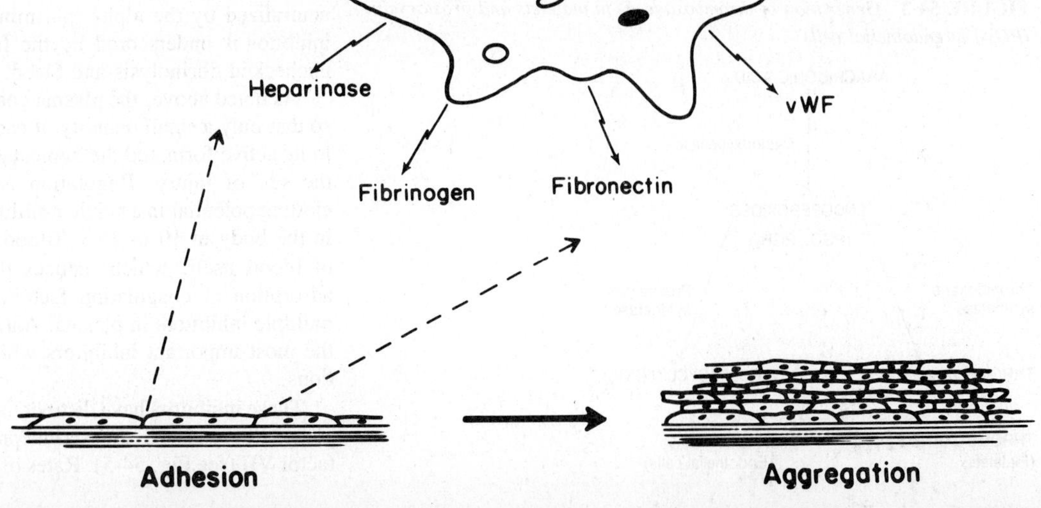

FIGURE 54-1 *Schematic presentation of the major events in primary hemostasis. The first event is platelet adhesion, the interaction of platelets with a nonplatelet surface such as vascular subendothelium. This is followed by platelet activation and secretion. Some of the products secreted by platelets are depicted. Abbreviations—ADP, adenosine diphosphate; PDGF, platelet-derived growth factor, vWF, von Willebrand's factor. The final event is the binding of activated platelets to the adherent monolayer in the process of platelet aggregation.*

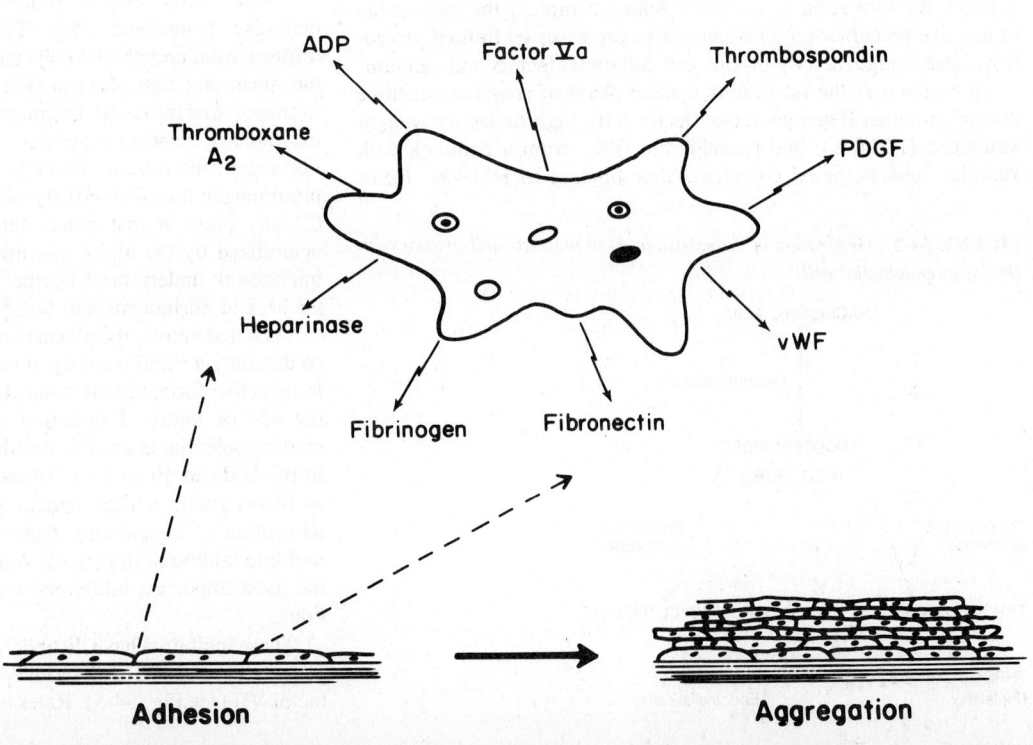

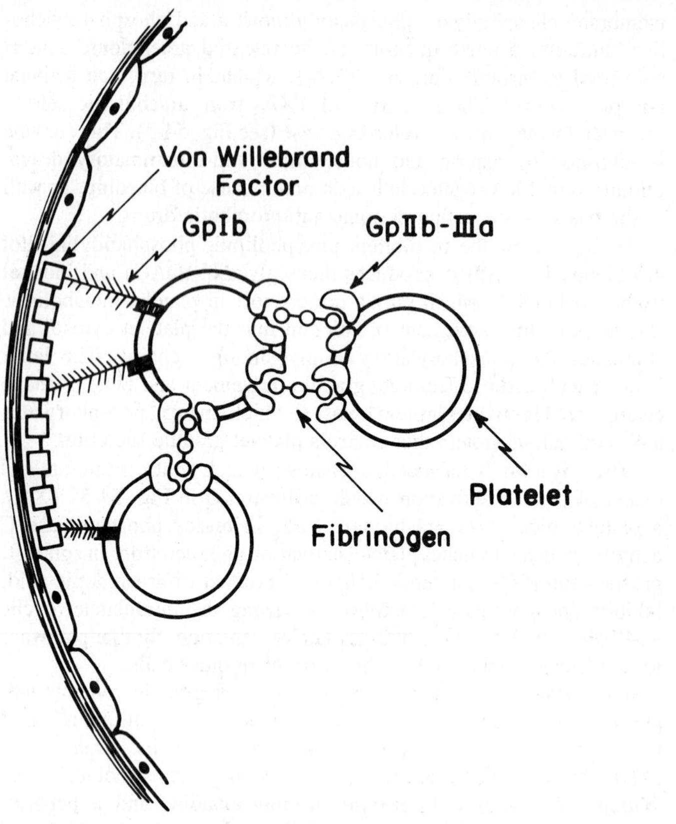

FIGURE 54-2 *The molecular basis of platelet adhesion and aggregation. Adhesion of platelets to vascular subendothelium is facilitated by the von Willebrand's factor which forms a bridge between collagen fibrils in the vessel wall and receptors on platelet glycoprotein Ib (GpIb). In a similar manner, platelet aggregation is mediated by fibrinogen which links adjacent platelets via receptors on the platelet glycoprotein IIb and IIIa complex (GpIIb–IIIa).*

overall picture of the coagulation scheme, including the role of various inhibitors, is shown in Fig. 54-5. The coagulation pathway can be broken down into a series of reactions (outlined in Fig. 54-6) which culminate in the production of sufficient thrombin to convert a small portion of plasma fibrinogen to fibrin. Each of the reactions requires the formation of a surface bound complex, the conversion of inactive precursor proteins into active proteases by limited proteolysis, and is regulated by plasma and cellular cofactors and calcium.

In *reaction 1,* the intrinsic or contact phase of coagulation, three plasma proteins, Hageman factor (factor XII), high-molecular-weight kininogen (HMWK), and prekallikrein (PK), form a complex with vascular subendothelial collagen. After binding to HMWK, factor XII is slowly converted to an active protease (XIIa), which converts both PK to kallikrein and factor XI to its active form (XIa). Kallikrein accelerates XII conversion to XIIa, while XIa participates in subsequent coagulation reactions.

FIGURE 54-3 *Generation of thromboxane A_2 in platelets and prostacyclin (PGI_2) in endothelial cells.*

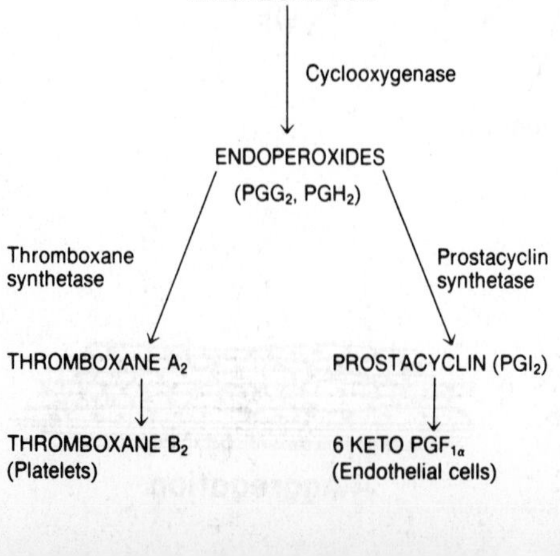

Reaction 2 provides a second pathway to initiate coagulation by converting factor VII to an active protease. In this extrinsic or tissue-factor-dependent pathway, a complex is formed between factor VII, calcium, and tissue factor, a ubiquitous lipoprotein present in cellular membranes which is exposed following cellular injury. Factor VII and three other coagulation proteins—factors II (prothrombin), IX, and X—require calcium and vitamin K for biologic activity. These proteins are synthesized in the liver, where a vitamin K–dependent carboxylase catalyzes a unique posttranslational modification by adding a second carboxyl group to certain glutamic acid residues. Pairs of these di-γ-carboxyglutamic acid (Gla) residues bind calcium, which anchors these proteins to negatively charged phospholipid surfaces. The inhibition of this posttranslational modification by vitamin K antagonists (e.g., warfarin) is the basis of one of the most common forms of anticoagulant therapy.

In *reaction 3,* factor X is activated by the proteases generated in the two previous reactions. In one reaction, a calcium- and lipid-dependent complex is formed between factors VIII, IX, and X. Within this complex, factor IX is first converted to IXa by factor XIa that was generated within the intrinsic pathway (reaction 1). Factor X is then activated by factor IXa in concert with factor VIII. Alternatively, factor X can be activated more directly by factor VIIa generated via the extrinsic pathway (reaction 2). Factor X activation provides an important link between the intrinsic and extrinsic coagulation pathways (see Fig. 54-5).

Reaction 4, the final step, converts prothrombin to thrombin in the presence of factor V, calcium, and phospholipid. Although prothrombin conversion can take place on various natural and artificial phospholipid-rich surfaces, it accelerates several thousand-fold on the surface of activated platelets. Thrombin, the product of this reaction, has multiple functions in hemostasis. Although its principal role in hemostasis is the conversion of fibrinogen to fibrin, it also activates factors V, VIII, and XIII and stimulates platelet aggregation and secretion. Following the release of fibrinopeptides A and B from the alpha and beta chains of fibrinogen, the modified molecule, now called fibrin monomer, polymerizes into an insoluble gel. The fibrin polymer is then stabilized by the cross-linking of individual chains by factor XIIIa, a plasma transglutaminase.

Vessel repair begins immediately after the formation of the definitive hemostatic plug. Tissue plasminogen activator (TPA) diffuses from endothelial cells and converts plasminogen adsorbed to the fibrin clot into plasmin (see Fig. 54-7). Plasmin then degrades fibrin polymer into small fragments which are cleared by the monocyte-macrophage scavenger system. Although plasmin can also degrade fibrinogen, the reaction remains localized because (1) TPA activates plasminogen more effectively when it is adsorbed to fibrin clots, and (2) any plasmin that enters the circulation is rapidly bound and neutralized by the $alpha_2$ plasmin inhibitor. The importance of this inhibitor is underscored by the fact that patients who lack it have unchecked fibrinolysis and bleed.

As noted above, the plasma coagulation system is tightly regulated so that only a small quantity of each coagulation enzyme is converted to its active form and the hemostatic plug does not propagate beyond the site of injury. Regulation is important since there is enough clotting potential in a single milliliter of blood to clot all the fibrinogen in the body in 10 to 15 s. Blood fluidity is maintained by the flow of blood itself, which reduces the concentration of reactants, the adsorption of coagulation factors to surfaces, and the presence of multiple inhibitors in plasma. Antithrombin and proteins C and S are the most important inhibitors which help regulate coagulation reactions.

These inhibitors have distinct modes of action. Antithrombin forms complexes with all the serine protease coagulation factors except factor VII (see Fig. 54-5). Rates of complex formation are accelerated by heparin and heparin-like molecules on the surface of the endothelial cells. This ability of heparin to accelerate the activity of antithrombin is the basis for heparin's action as a potent anticoagulant. Protein C is converted to an active protease by thrombin after it is bound to an endothelial cell protein called thrombomodulin. Activated protein C then inactivates the two plasma cofactors V and VIII to slow down two critical coagulation reactions. Protein C may also stimulate the release of tissue plasminogen activator from endothelial cells. The inhibitory function of protein C is enhanced by protein S. As one might predict, reduced levels of antithrombin, or proteins C and S or dysfunctional forms of the molecule, result in a hypercoagulable or prethrombotic state.

This biochemical description of blood coagulation implies that the process is uniform throughout the body. In fact, the nature of the blood clot varies with the site of injury. In addition, there is little difference between hemostatic plugs, which are a physiologic response to injury, and pathologic thrombi. To underscore the similarity, thrombosis is often described as coagulation occurring in the wrong place or at the wrong time. Hemostatic plugs or thrombi that form in veins where blood flow is slow are richly endowed with fibrin and trapped red blood cells and contain relatively few platelets. They are often called red thrombi due to their appearance in surgical and pathologic specimens. The friable ends of these red thrombi, which often form in leg veins, can break off and embolize to the pulmonary circulation. Conversely, clots that form in arteries under conditions of high flow are predominantly composed of platelets and have little fibrin. These white thrombi may readily dislodge from the arterial wall and embolize to distant sites to cause temporary or permanent ischemia. This is particularly common in the cerebral and retinal circulation and may lead to transient neurologic dysfunction (transient ischemic attacks) including temporary monocular blindness (amaurosis fugax) or strokes. In addition, there is increasing evidence that many episodes of myocardial infarction are due to thrombi which form within atherosclerotic coronary arteries.

CLINICAL EVALUATION

HISTORY Certain elements of the history are particularly useful in determining whether bleeding is due to an underlying hemostatic disorder rather than to a local anatomic defect. One clue is a history of repeated bleeding episodes with common hemostatic stresses such as dental extraction, childbirth, or minor surgery. Bleeding that is sufficiently severe to require a blood transfusion merits special attention. A family history of bleeding and bleeding from multiple sites that cannot be linked to trauma or surgery also suggest a systemic disorder. Since bleeding can be mild, lack of a family history of bleeding does not exclude an inherited hemostatic disorder.

It may be possible to localize the defect to the platelet or plasma coagulation system (Table 54-1). Bleeding from a platelet disorder is usually localized to superficial sites such as the skin and mucous membranes, comes on immediately after trauma or surgery, and is readily controlled by local measures. In contrast, bleeding from

FIGURE 54-4 *The biochemical basis of platelet activation and secretion. Binding of agonists such as thrombin, epinephrine, or collagen sets in motion a chain of events which hydrolyzes membrane phospholipids, inhibits adenylate cyclase, mobilizes intracellular calcium, and phosphorylates critical intracellular proteins. The net result is shape change, movement of granules to the canalicular system, generation of mediators like thromboxane A_2, and granule secretion. Abbreviations—A.C., adenylate cyclase; G, guanine nucleotide binding protein; PIP_2, phosphatidylinositol 4,5-biphosphate; PLC, phospholipase C; DAG, diacylglycerol; PLA_2, phospholipase A_2; PC, phosphatidylcholine; AA, arachidonic acid; CO, cyclooxygenase; AA, arachidonic acid; O_2, oxygen; IP_3, inositol triphosphate; cAMP, cyclic AMP; Ca-CM, calcium calmodulin complex; MLCK, myosin light chain kinase.*

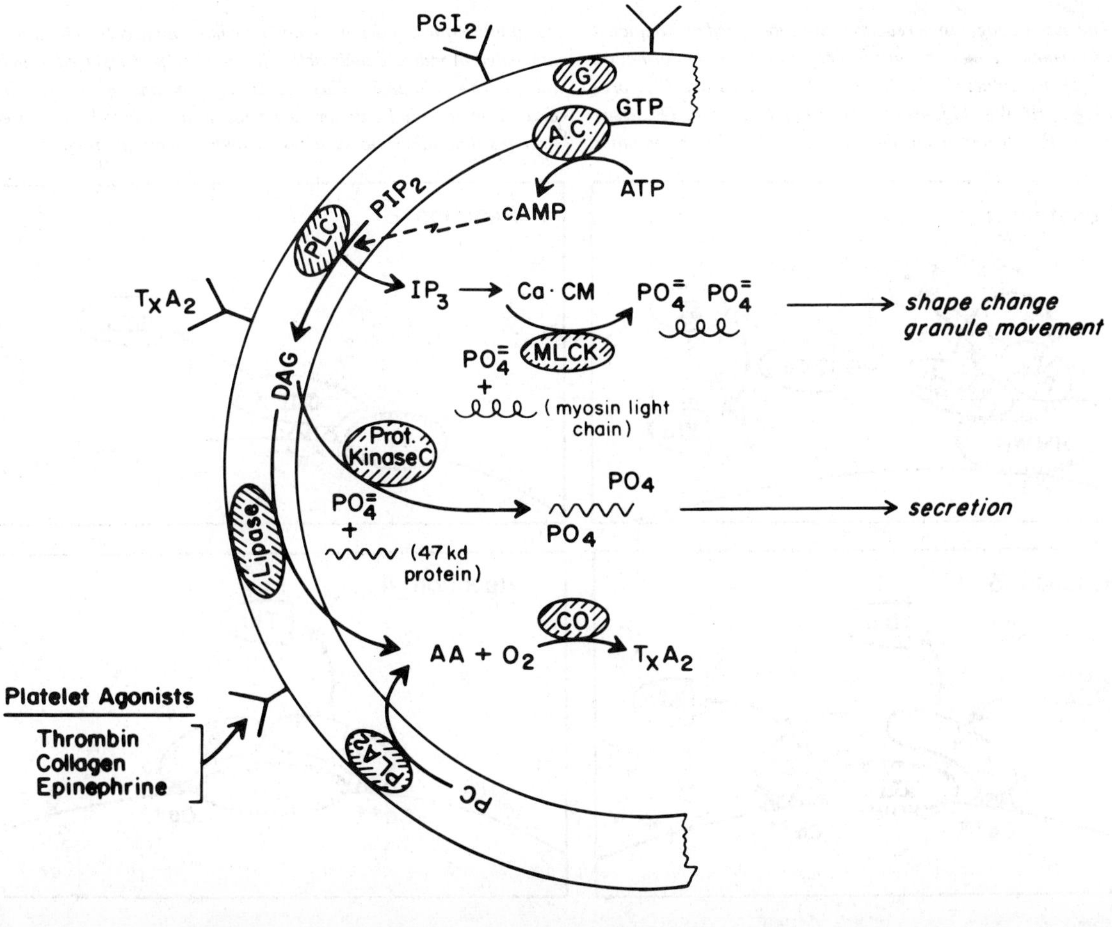

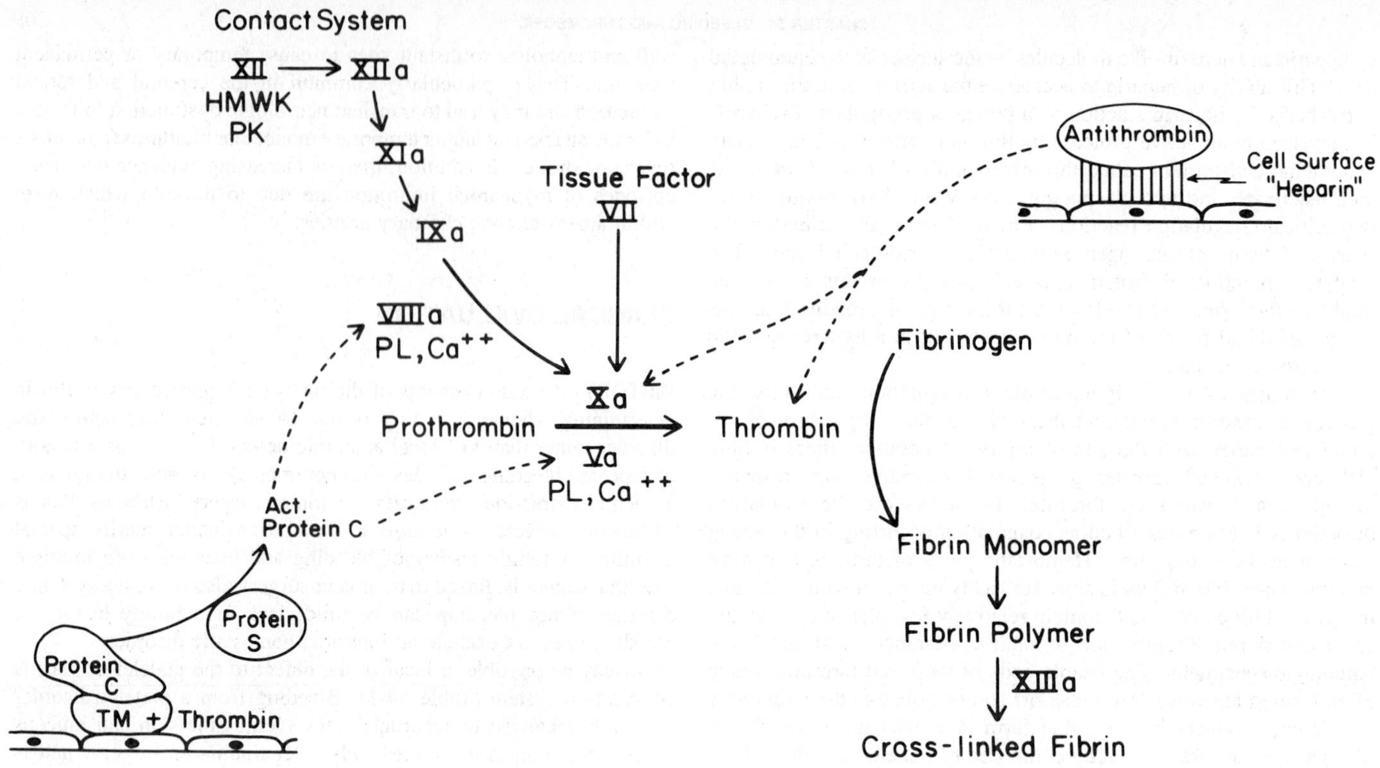

FIGURE 54-5 *A schematic diagram of some of the clinically important coagulation reactions. The unactivated or precursor proteins are indicated by roman numerals, and the active form by the addition of a lower case "a"—a standard convention. Other abbreviations are HMWK, high-molecular-weight kininogen; PK, prekallikrein; PL, phospholipid; TM, thrombomodulin; Ca^{2+}, calcium. There are two independent activation pathways, the contact system and the tissue factor–mediated or extrinsic system. They both merge at the point of factor X activation and lead to the generation of thrombin, which converts fibrinogen into fibrin. These reactions are regulated by antithrombin, which forms complexes with all of the coagulation protein serine proteases except factor VII, and the protein C–protein S system which inactivates factors V and VIII.*

FIGURE 54-6 *The major coagulation reactions are subdivided and depicted in schematic form to emphasize their similarity. They all rely on the formation of surface bound enzyme, cofactor complexes. Abbreviations are PK, prekallikrein; K, kallikrein; HMWK, high-molecular-weight kininogen; TF, tissue factor; Ca^{2+}, calcium; PT, prothrombin; Thr, thrombin. By convention other coagulation factors are indicated by roman numerals, with a lower case "a" appended to indicate their active form. The /\/\/\ is used to indicate the Gla (di-γ-carboxyglutamic acid) containing domains of factors VII, IX, X, Xa, and PT which bind calcium and phospholipid. Hatching is used to indicate proteins that adhere to surfaces by hydrophobic interaction.*

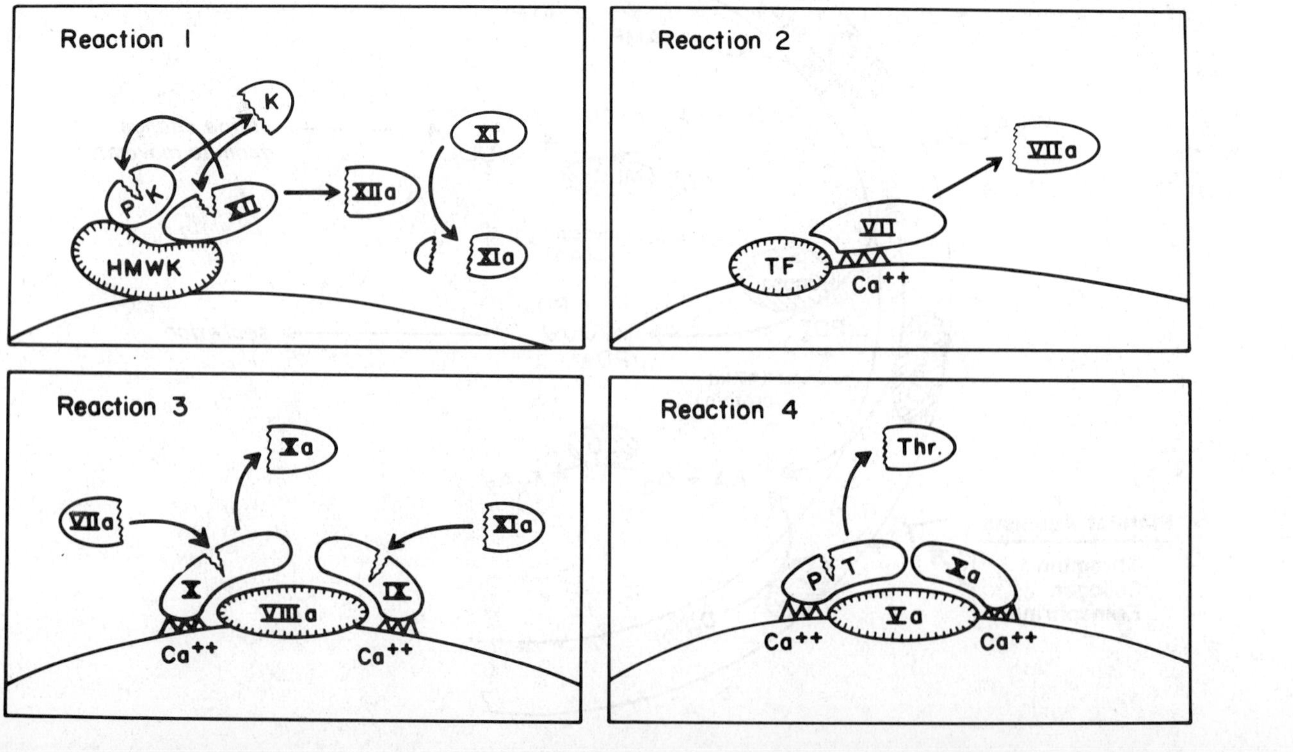

secondary hemostatic or plasma coagulation defects occurs hours or days after injury and is unaffected by local therapy. Such bleeding most often occurs in deep subcutaneous tissues, muscles, joints, or body cavities.

PHYSICAL EXAMINATION In conjunction with a careful history, physical examination can also be of help in evaluating patients with hemostatic disorders. The most common site to observe bleeding is in the skin and mucous membranes. Collections of blood in the skin are called *purpura* and may be subdivided on the basis of the site of bleeding in the skin. Small pinpoint hemorrhages into the dermis due to the leakage of red cells through capillaries are called *petechiae* and are characteristic of platelet disorders—in particular, severe thrombocytopenia. Larger subcutaneous collections of blood due to leakage of blood from small arterioles and venules are *ecchymoses* (common bruises) or, if somewhat deeper and palpable, *hematomas*. They are also common in patients with platelet defects and result from minor trauma. There are other skin and mucous membrane lesions like dilated capillaries or *telangiectasia* that may cause bleeding without any hemostatic defect. In addition, the loss of connective tissue support for capillaries and small veins that accompanies aging increases the fragility of superficial vessels, such as those on the dorsum of the hand, leading to extravasation of blood into subcutaneous tissue—*senile purpura*. Menorrhagia is a serious problem in women with severe thrombocytopenia or platelet dysfunction. In addition, some patients with primary hemostatic defects, especially von Willebrand's disease, may have recurrent gastrointestinal hemorrhage.

As mentioned previously, bleeding into body cavities, retroperitoneum, and joints is a common manifestation of plasma coagulation defects. Repeated joint bleeding may cause synovial thickening, chronic inflammation, and fluid collections and may erode articular cartilage and lead to chronic joint deformity and limited mobility. Such deformities are particularly common in factor VIII and IX deficiency, the two sex-linked coagulation disorders referred to as the hemophilias. For unclear reasons, hemarthroses are much less common in other plasma coagulation defects. Blood collections in various body cavities or soft tissues can cause secondary necrosis of tissues or nerve compression. Retroperitoneal hematomas can cause femoral nerve compression, and large collections of poorly coagulated blood in soft tissues may occasionally mimic malignant growths—the pseudotumor syndrome. Two of the most life-threatening sites of bleeding are in the oropharynx, where bleeding can compromise the airway, and in the central nervous system. Intracerebral hemorrhage is one of the leading causes of death in patients with severe coagulation disorders.

LABORATORY TESTS The most important screening tests of the primary hemostatic system are (1) a *bleeding time* (a sensitive measure of platelet function) and (2) a *platelet count*. The latter is particularly useful as it is readily available and correlates well with the propensity to bleed. The normal platelet count is 150,000 to 450,000 platelets per cubic millimeter of blood. As long as the count

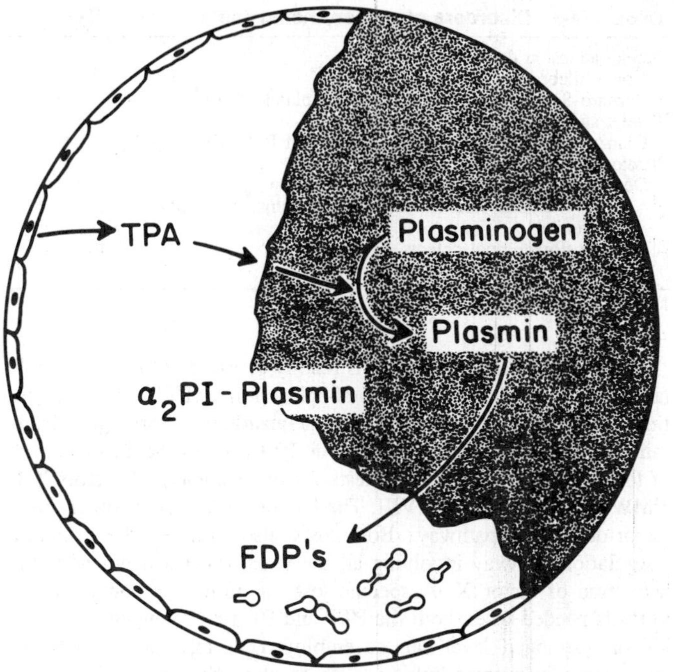

FIGURE 54-7 *A schematic diagram of the fibrinolytic pathway. TPA (tissue plasminogen activator) is released from endothelial cells, enters the fibrin clot, and activates plasminogen to plasmin. Any free plasmin is complexed with a_2 PI (alpha$_2$ plasmin inhibitor). Fibrin is degraded to low-molecular-weight fragments, abbreviated as FDPs, fibrin degradation products.*

is above 100,000 per cubic millimeter, patients are not symptomatic and the bleeding time remains normal. Platelet counts of 50,000 to 100,000 per cubic millimeter cause mild prolongation of the bleeding time so that bleeding occurs only with severe trauma or other stress. Patients with platelet counts less than 50,000 per cubic millimeter have easy bruising, which is manifested by skin purpura with minor trauma and bleeding after mucous membrane surgery. Patients with a platelet count below 20,000 per cubic millimeter have an appreciable incidence of spontaneous bleeding, usually have petechiae, and may have intracranial or other spontaneous internal bleeding. The major causes of thrombocytopenia are outlined in Table 54-2.

Patients with qualitative platelet abnormalities have a normal platelet count and a prolonged bleeding time (Table 54-3). Although any patient with a bleeding time over 10 min has a slightly increased risk of bleeding, the risk does not become great until the bleeding time exceeds 15 or 20 min. When a defect in primary hemostasis is uncovered, specialized testing is needed to determine the cause of the platelet dysfunction (Table 54-3). A precise diagnosis is important since patients with bleeding due to a primary hemostatic disorder may need therapy with platelets, corticosteroids, or plasma fractions, depending on the nature of the disorder.

TABLE 54-1 Differential diagnosis of primary and secondary hemostatic disorders

	Primary hemostasis (platelet defect)	Second hemostasis (plasma proteins)
Onset of bleeding after trauma	Immediate	Delayed—hours or days
Sites of bleeding	Superficial—skin; mucous membranes; nose; gastrointestinal, genetourinary tracts	Deep—joints, muscle, retroperitoneum
Physical findings	Petechiae, ecchymoses	Hematomas, hemarthroses
Family history	Autosomal dominant	Autosomal or X-linked recessive
Response to therapy	Immediate; local measures effective	Requires sustained systemic therapy

TABLE 54-2 Causes of thrombocytopenia

I Decreased marrow production of megakaryocytes
- *A* Marrow infiltration with tumor, fibrosis
- *B* Marrow failure—aplastic, hypoplastic anemias

II Splenic sequestration of circulating platelets
- *A* Splenic hypertrophy—tumor, portal hypertension

III Increased destruction of circulating platelets
- *A* Nonimmune destruction
  - *1* Vascular prostheses, cardiac valves
  - *2* Disseminated intravascular coagulation
  - *3* Sepsis
  - *4* Vasculitis
- *B* Immune destruction
  - *1* Autoantibodies to platelet antigens
  - *2* Drug-associated antibodies
  - *3* Circulating immune complexes—systemic lupus erythematosus, viral agents, bacterial sepsis

TABLE 54-3 Disorders of primary hemostasis

Platelet adhesion defects:
Von Willebrand's disease
Bernard-Soulier syndrome (absence of platelet GpIb)*
Platelet aggregation defects:
Glanzmann's thromboasthenia (absence of BpIIb–IIIa)
Platelet release defects:
Decreased cyclooxygenase activity
Drugs—aspirin, nonsteroidal anti-inflammatory agents
Congenital
Granule storage pool defects
Uremia

* *Gp = glycoprotein.*

Plasma coagulation function is readily assessed with a few simple laboratory tests—the partial thromboplastin time (PTT), prothrombin time (PT), thrombin time (TT), or a quantitative fibrinogen determination (Fig. 54-5, Table 54-4). The PTT screens the intrinsic limb of the coagulation system and tests for the adequacy of factors XII, HMWK, PK, XI, IX, and VIII. The PT screens the extrinsic or tissue factor-dependent pathway. Both tests also evaluate the common coagulation pathway involving all the reactions that occur after the activation of factor X. A specific test for fibrinogen conversion to fibrin is needed when both the PTT and PT are prolonged—either a TT or fibrinogen level can be employed. A test for factor XIII–dependent fibrin cross-linking, such as clot solubility in 5-*M* urea, should be ordered when the PT and PTT are both normal but there is a strong history of bleeding. The fibrinolytic system can be assessed by measuring the rate of clot lysis with the euglobulin lysis or whole blood clot lysis tests and by measuring the level of alpha$_2$ plasmin inhibitor. When abnormalities are noted in any of the screening tests, more specific coagulation factor assays can be ordered to determine the nature of the defect.

There are no clinical tests to screen patients suspected of having hypercoagulable or prethrombotic disorders, although tests are being developed in research laboratories which measure small peptides or enzyme-inhibitor complexes generated during coagulation. For example, radioimmunoassays have been developed for fibrinopeptides A and B, for the thrombin-antithrombin complex, and for prothrombin cleavage fragments. Elevated levels of these products have been reported in patients with prethrombotic disorders and in patients with thromboembolism. At present, patients suspected of having a hypercoagulable state, on the basis of clinical information, should have specific assays to screen for the small number of known defects. Currently available tests can identify 10 to 20 percent of the cases of familial thrombosis and represent only a small fraction of the many patients who present to physicians with thromboembolism.

Inhibitor syndromes or circulating anticoagulants are usually due to antibodies which impair coagulation factor activity. They are an infrequent cause of bleeding which require specialized diagnostic testing. Inhibitors are likely when screening test abnormalities cannot be reversed by adding normal plasma to patient plasma. Antibodies against specific coagulation factors may develop in (1) postpartum females; (2) patients with autoimmune disorders such as systemic lupus erythematosus; (3) patients taking drugs like penicillin and streptomycin; and (4) otherwise healthy elderly individuals. In addition, between 10 and 20 percent of patients with severe hemophilia who have received multiple plasma infusions develop inhibitor antibodies. Some patients, especially those with systemic lupus erythematosus may also have a nonspecific form of anticoagulant antibody which interferes with phospholipid binding of coagulation factors and prolongs the PT and PTT but does not cause clinical bleeding. Occasionally, patients develop inhibitors that are not antibodies. For example, several patients with circulating mucopolysaccharides that have heparin-like actvity have had clinical bleeding.

TABLE 54-4 Relationship between secondary hemostatic disorders and coagulation test abnormalities

Prolonged partial thromboplastin time (PTT):
No clinical bleeding—factors XII, HMWK, PK
Mild or rare bleeding—factor XI
Frequent, severe bleeding—factors VIII and IX
Prolonged prothrombin time (PT):
Factor VII deficiency
Vitamin K deficiency—early
Warfarin anticoagulant ingestion
Prolonged PTT and PT:
Factor II, V, or X deficiency
Vitamin K deficiency—late
Warfarin anticoagulant ingestion
Prolonged thrombin time (TT):
Mild or rare bleeding—afibrinogenemia
Frequent, severe bleeding—dysfibrinogenemia
Heparin-like inhibitors or heparin administration
Clot solubility in 5-*M* urea:
Factor XIII deficiency
Inhibitors or defective cross-linking
Rapid clot lysis
Alpha$_2$ plasmin inhibitor

NOTE: *HMWK = high-molecular-weight kininogen; PK = prekallikrein.*

REFERENCES

BLOOM AL, THOMAS DP (eds): *Haemostasis and Thrombosis*. London, Churchill-Livingstone, 1981

COLMAN RW et al (eds): *Hemostasis and Thrombosis: Basic Principles and Clinical Practice*. Philadelphia, Lippincott, 1982

HANDIN RI: Hemorrhagic Disorders II. Platelets and purpura, in *Hematology*, 4th ed, W Beck (ed). Cambridge, MIT Press, 1985, pp 433–456

ROSENBERG RD: Hemorrhagic disorders I. Protein interactions in the clotting mechanism, in *Hematology*, 4th ed, W Beck (ed). Cambridge, MIT Press, 1985, pp 401–431

55 ENLARGEMENT OF LYMPH NODES AND SPLEEN

BARTON F. HAYNES

Lymph nodes and spleen constitute a major portion of the peripheral immune system, and become enlarged in a wide spectrum of infectious, malignant, autoimmune, and metabolic diseases. Enlargement of lymph nodes (lymphadenopathy) and spleen (splenomegaly) are common clinical findings that can lead to a wide range of diagnostic and therapeutic procedures. The goal of this chapter is to serve as an introduction to these two components of the immune system and to highlight clinical features and diagnostic evaluation of some of the diseases in which lymphadenopathy and splenomegaly occur.

LYMPH NODE STRUCTURE AND FUNCTION Lymph nodes are peripheral lymphoid organs that are connected to the circulation by afferent and efferent lymphatic vessels (Fig. 55-1) and by postcapillary high-endothelial venules. A number of cell types make up the lymph node supportive framework and stroma. Fibroblasts are the predominant cell type in the lymph node capsule and trabeculae. Fibroblast-derived reticular cells are supporting cells found frequently in bone marrow–derived (B) cell areas (follicles and germinal centers) of lymph nodes. Tissue macrophages derived from circulating monocytes are present throughout the normal node. Within cortical areas are interdigitating reticular cells (also called dendritic cells) and Langerhans cells both of which are specialized nonphagocytic, Ia-bearing cells of bone marrow origin that along with macrophages participate in antigen presentation to thymus-derived (T) and B cells (Chap. 62). The outer lymph node cortex contains lymphoid follicles with germinal centers that are the B-cell areas of lymph node (Fig. 55-1). Primary lymphoid follicles are aggregates of IgM- and IgD-bearing B cells and T4$^+$ helper (inducer) T cells prior to antigenic challenge. Secondary lymphoid follicles are the result of antigen stimulation, and contain an outer or mantle layer of IgM- and IgD-bearing B cells and an inner zone (germinal center) of activated B cells, macrophages, reticular cells, and scattered T4$^+$ helper T cells. Between primary and secondary follicle areas (interfollicular zones) and inner lymph node medullary regions are T-cell (paracortical) areas. The majority of T cells in lymph nodes are $T4^+$ helper T cells (approximately 80 percent) while the minority are $T8^+$ suppressor/cytotoxic T cells (approximately 20 percent).

The two most important factors contributing to the composition and distribution of lymphoid cells within lymph node are (1) generation of memory B and T cells de novo from proliferation of antigen-stimulated percursors within lymph nodes, and (2) selective recirculation to and homing of specific types of lymphoid cells to lymph nodes from the circulation. Traffic through lymph nodes is via two general routes (Fig. 55-1). Afferent lymph, containing lymphocytes, macrophages, and antigens, enters the lymph node via the subcapsular space, and drains through paracortical and medullary areas into medullary sinuses that converge to form efferent lymphatic vessels through which lymph exits. B cells from bone marrow and T cells from the thymus enter lymph nodes from the circulation by binding to specific receptors on cells of postcapillary high-endothelial venules. After activation by antigen and clonal expansion, sensitized T and B cells and antibody-secreting plasma cells leave the node in efferent lymph and rejoin the peripheral blood circulation via the thoracic duct.

Lymph nodes function as sites of macrophage, T-cell and B-cell contact with antigen, with a specialized structure that gives rise to optimal T cell, B cell, and macrophage interactions that result under normal conditions in efficient recognition of antigen, activation of the cellular and humoral arms of the immune response, and ultimate elimination of antigen (see Chap. 62).

Lymph node enlargement can be due to (1) an increase in the number of benign lymphocytes and macrophages during response to antigens, (2) infiltration by inflammatory cells in infections involving lymph nodes (lymphadenitis), (3) in situ proliferation of malignant lymphocytes or macrophages, (4) infiltration of nodes by metastatic malignant cells, or (5) by infiltration of lymph nodes by metabolite-laden macrophages in lipid storage diseases.

In normal immune responses, antigen stimulation of macrophages and lymphocytes in lymph nodes exerts profound influences on lymphocyte traffic. One of the earliest effects of antigen is to increase blood flow through the affected node, which during antigen stimulation may reach 10 to 25 times normal levels. Lymphocytes accumulate in antigen-stimulated nodes by increase in traffic through the node, decreased egress of lymphocytes from antigen-stimulated nodes, and by proliferation of responding T and B cells. A lymph node may thus reach 15 times its normal size 5 to 10 days after antigenic stimulation.

DISEASES ASSOCIATED WITH LYMPHADENOPATHY Under normal conditions in adults, the inguinal lymph nodes may be palpable, and are generally 0.5 cm up to 2 cm in size. Elsewhere in the body, smaller lymph nodes due to past infections may be present normally. Enlargement of lymph nodes requires investigation when there are one or more new nodes present equal to or greater than 1 cm in diameter, and not known to arise from a previously recognized cause. However, this is not a rigid criterion and under certain circumstances new multiple or single smaller lymph nodes may warrant investigation as well. Important factors in assessing the significance of enlarged lymph nodes are (1) the patient's age, (2) the physical characteristics of the lymph node, (3) node locations, and (4) the clinical setting associated with lymphadenopathy. Lymphadenopathy reflects significant disease more often in adults than in children because children are more likely to respond to minor stimuli with lymphoid hyperplasia. Lymphadenopathy in patients under 30 years of age is due to benign causes in approximately 80 percent of cases whereas in patients greater than 50 years of age lymphadenopathy is due to benign causes in only 40 percent of cases.

The physical characteristics of peripheral nodes are important. Nodes of lymphomas tend to be rubbery, firm, matted together, and nontender. Nodes involved with metastatic carcinomas are usually hard and fixed to underlying tissue. In acute infections, nodes are tender, asymmetrically enlarged, matted together, and the overlying skin may be erythematous.

The clinical setting is important in assessing lymphadenopathy. In a young college student with fever and recent onset of lymph node enlargement, infectious mononucleosis syndromes are important to consider. In homosexuals, hemophiliacs, and intravenous drug users with systemic lymphadenopathy, the acquired immunodeficiency syndrome (AIDS) or an AIDS-related complex syndrome should be considered (see Chap. 257).

The location of enlarged lymph nodes may suggest important clues to the diagnosis. Enlarged posterior cervical nodes are frequently present in scalp infections, toxoplasmosis, and rubella, whereas anterior auricular nodes suggest infections of the eyelids and conjunctiva. Lymphomas commonly involve cervical lymph nodes and can occasionally involve posterior auricular and occipital nodes as well. Enlarged suppurative cervical nodes are seen in mycobacterial lymphadenitis (scrofula). Unilateral jugular or mandibular lymph node enlargement suggests lymphoma or nonlymphoid head-and-neck malignancy. Supraclavicular and scalene lymph node enlargement is always significant, and frequently results from metastasis from intrathoracic or gastrointestinal malignancies or from lymphomas. Virchow's node is an enlarged left supraclavicular lymph node infiltrated with metastatic tumor usually from the gastrointestinal tract. Unilateral epitrochlear node enlargement is usually due to hand infections; bilateral epitrochlear node enlargement is seen in sarcoidosis, tularemia, and secondary syphilis.

Unilateral axillary adenopathy can be seen with breast carcinoma, lymphomas, infections of the upper extremities, cat-scratch disease, and brucellosis.

Bilateral inguinal adenopathy can be seen in a variety of venereal infections; however, lymphogranuloma venereum and syphilis are associated with unilateral inguinal adenopathy. Progressive inguinal lymph node enlargement without obvious infection suggests malignant disease. Femoral node involvement has been reported to occur in *Pasteurella pestis* infections and lymphomas.

Symptoms that should raise the suspicion of hilar or mediastinal node enlargement are cough or wheezing due to airway compression, recurrent laryngeal nerve compression with hoarseness, paralysis of the diaphragm, dysphagia with esophageal compression, and swelling of the neck, face, or arms due to superior vena cava or subclavian vein compression. Bilateral mediastinal adenopathy is frequently seen in lymphomas, especially the nodular sclerosing type of Hodgkin's disease. Unilateral hilar adenopathy indicates a high likelihood of metastatic carcinoma (usually lung), while bilateral hilar adenopathy is more often benign and is seen in sarcoidosis, tuberculosis, and systemic fungal infections. Bilateral hilar adenopathy in asymptomatic patients or in association with erythema nodosum or uveitis is almost always due to sarcoidosis (Chap. 270). The association of bilateral

FIGURE 55-1 *Schematic lymph node structure. Lymph flows into nodes via afferent lymphatics (A) and leaves nodes via efferent lymphatics (E). B-cell areas are primary and secondary follicles in lymph node cortex while T cells are concentrated in paracortical areas.*

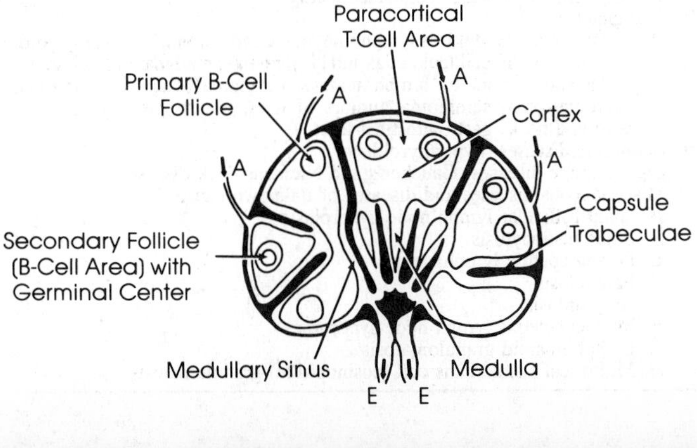

hilar adenopathy with an anterior mediastinal mass, pleural effusion, or pulmonary mass suggests neoplastic disease.

Enlarged retroperitoneal and intraabdominal nodes are not usually inflammatory in origin, but are frequently due to lymphomas or other neoplastic diseases. Tuberculosis can cause mesenteric lymphadenitis with large matted and sometimes calcified nodes.

Some of the diseases associated with lymph node enlargement are listed in Table 55-1 and fall into six general categories: infectious diseases, immunologic diseases, malignant diseases, endocrine diseases, lipid storage diseases, and miscellaneous.

The manifestations of infectious diseases are protean and are best considered according to the type of infectious agent. The most common viral infection associated with systemic lymphadenopathy is Epstein-Barr (EB) virus–associated infectious mononucleosis (see Chap. 138). A variety of other viral diseases including viral hepatitis, cytomegalovirus, rubella, and influenza can cause clinical syndromes similar to those induced by the EB virus. AIDS has recently been shown to be caused by a human retrovirus, human T-cell lymphotropic virus type III (HTLV III), also called lymphadenopathy-associated virus (LAV). In the HTLV III/LAV–associated lymphadenopathy syndrome, cervical, axillary, and occipital nodes are the most commonly involved (see Chap. 257).

Chronic bacterial infections as well as fungal infections may produce considerable lymph node enlargement without signs of local inflammation. Cat-scratch disease is a regional lymphadenitis occurring approximately 2 weeks following a cat scratch or bite. The nodes involved relate to lymph drainage of the wound site with upper extremity adenopathy being the most common, occurring in 50 percent of cases. Fungi associated with primary pulmonary infections (coccidioidomycosis, histoplasmosis) can cause hilar adenopathy. Acute and chronic mycobacterial, parasitic, and spirochetal diseases against which there is a profound cellular and humoral immune response all can result in either systemic or regional enlarged lymph nodes depending on the clinical syndrome in question. Virtually any disease characterized by immune cell activation (systemic lupus erythematosus, rheumatoid arthritis, serum sickness, reactions due to drugs such as diphenylhydantoin, angioimmunoblastic lymphadenopathy) can be associated with regional or systemic adenopathy. Lymph node enlargement associated with malignant disease may be due to direct node involvement by tumor, lymphoid hyperplasia in response to tumor, or both. Generalized lymphoid hyperplasia may occur with hyperthroidism. Patients with lipid storage diseases such as Gaucher's and Niemann-Pick disease can have enlarged lymph nodes, particularly in the abdomen, due to accumulation of lipid-laden macrophages.

TABLE 55-1 Diseases associated with lymph node enlargement

I Infectious diseases
- *A* Viral infections: infectious hepatitis, infectious mononucleosis syndromes (cytomegalovirus, EB virus), AIDS, rubella, varicella–herpes zoster, vaccinia
- *B* Bacterial infections: streptococci, staphylococci, salmonella, brucella, Francisella tularensis, *Listeria monocytogenes, Pasteurella pestis, Hemophilus ducreyi,* cat-scratch disease
- *C* Fungal infections: coccidioidomycosis, histoplasmosis
- *D* Chlamydial infections: Lymphogranuloma venereum, trachoma
- *E* Mycobacterial infections: tuberculosis, leprosy
- *F* Parasitic infections: trypanosomiasis, microfilariasis, toxoplasmosis
- *G* Spirochetal diseases: syphilis, yaws, endemic syphilis (bejel), leptospirosis

II Immunologic diseases
- *A* Rheumatoid arthritis
- *B* Systemic lupus erythematosus
- *C* Dermatomyositis
- *D* Serum sickness
- *E* Drug reactions—diphenylhydantoin, hydralazine, allopurinol
- *F* Angioimmunoblastic lymphadenopathy

III Malignant diseases
- *A* Hematologic: Hodgkin's lymphoma, acute and chronic T-, B-, myeloid, and monocytoid cell leukemias and lymphomas, malignant histiocytosis
- *B* Metastatic tumors to lymph nodes: melanoma, Kaposi's sarcoma, neuroblastoma, seminoma, tumors of lung, breast, prostate, kidney, head and neck, gastrointestinal tract

IV Endocrine diseases: hyperthyroidism

V Lipid storage diseases: Gaucher's and Niemann-Pick diseases

VI Miscellaneous diseases and diseases of unknown cause
- *A* Giant follicular lymph node hyperplasia
- *B* Sinus histiocytosis
- *C* Dermatopathic lymphadenitis
- *D* Sarcoidosis
- *E* Amyloidosis
- *F* Mucocutaneous lymph node syndrome
- *G* Lymphomatoid granulomatosis
- *H* Multifocal Langerhans cell (eosinophilic) granulomatosis

A number of diseases of unknown cause are associated with lymphadenopathy and in many of the diseases in this group, lymphadenopathy is a major manifestation of the disease. Sarcoidosis frequently presents with generalized lymph node enlargement, especially in cervical, inguinal, and epitrochlear areas (Chap. 270). Although giant follicular lymph node hyperplasia can occur in extrathoracic lymph nodes, mediastinal or hilar nodes are involved in 70 percent of cases. In sinus histiocytosis, massive cervical lymph node enlargement often associated with generalized lymphadenopathy occurs and is associated with fever and leukocytosis. Patients with exfoliative dermatitis or other dermatologic syndromes can develop enlarged superficial lymph nodes (called dermatopathic lymphadenitis) which usually regress with resolution of the dermatitis. Lymph node involvement occurs in approximately 30 percent of cases of primary and secondary amyloidosis; only rarely is amyloid lymphadenopathy the major or the only organ involvement. The mechanism of node enlargement in amyloidosis is the accumulation of extracellular masses of amyloid fibrils that compress and eventually obliterate normal lymph node architecture (Chap. 259).

Mucocutaneous lymph node syndrome (Kawasaki's disease) is a systemic lymphadenopathy syndrome, the hallmarks of which are fever, conjunctivitis, erythema of the tongue with protrusion of papillae (strawberry tongue), a truncal exanthem with desquamation of palms and soles, and acute nonsuppurative enlargement of cervical lymph nodes (see Chaps. 49 and 269).

Lymphomatoid granulomatosis is a disease characterized by infiltration of various organs (lungs, skin, central nervous system) with an angiocentric and angioinvasive polymorphic cellular infiltrate consisting of atypical lymphocytes and macrophages. The disease has characteristics of both an inflammatory granulomatous process and a lymphoproliferative disease, with progression to frank lymphoma in up to 50 percent of cases. Lymphadenopathy in the prelymphoma state of lymphomatoid granulomatosis occurs in 40 percent of cases affecting primarily intrathoracic nodes while peripheral adenopathy occurs only rarely (10 percent) (see Chap. 269).

Angioimmunoblastic lymphadenopathy is a disease characterized by fever, generalized lymphadenopathy, hepatosplenomegaly, polyclonal hypergammaglobulinemia, and Coombs-positive hemolytic anemia. Although it is not thought to be a malignant disease, it evolves into B-cell lymphoma in 35 percent of patients, (see Chap. 294).

Diseases characterized by benign and malignant proliferation of tissue macrophages (histiocytes) or of specialized bone marrow–derived cells called Langerhans cells have been termed *histiocytoses* or *histiocytosis X*. In the past, these terms encompassed a number of diseases including unifocal and multifocal eosinophilic granuloma, Hand-Schüller-Christian syndrome, Letterer-Siwe disease, and frank neoplasms of undifferentiated histiocytes. Recently, the identification of the Langerhans cell as the predominant cell in forms of eosinophilic granuloma has prompted reevaluation of these syndromes.

One term currently in use for eosinophilic granuloma syndromes is *Langerhans cell (eosinophilic) granulomatosis,* and this term will be used here. The term histiocytosis X is an outmoded term that refers to a spectrum of diseases encompassing both the benign disorder of Langerhans cell (eosinophilic) granulomatosis and malignant lymphomatous disease.

The classic triad of the *Hand-Schüller-Christian syndrome* (exophthalmus, diabetes insipidus, and destructive bone lesions) occurs with 25 percent of cases of multifocal eosinophilic granuloma but also may occur in malignant lymphoma and carcinoma. *Letterer-Siwe disease* is an acute clinical syndrome of unknown etiology in infants that consists of hepatosplenomegaly, lymphadenopathy, hemorrhagic diathesis, anemia, no familial occurrence, and generalized hyperplasia of tissue macrophages in a variety of organs. It is currently felt that Letterer-Siwe disease represents an unusual form of malignant lymphoma, and is distinct from forms of eosinophilic granuloma.

Histologically, Langerhans cell granulomatosis consists of aggregates of mature eosinophils and Langerhans cells. Langerhans cells are bone marrow–derived cells normally found among epidermal cells of skin and rarely in B-cell areas of lymph node and the medulla of thymus. Langerhans cells contain distinct cytoplasmic granules (Birbeck granules) and contain adenosine triphosphatase and alpha naphthyl acetate esterase. Surface markers of Langerhans cells include class II major histocompatibility complex antigens (Ia-like) and the T6 antigen that is also expressed by the cortical (immature) thymocytes (see Chap. 62).

Unifocal Langerhans cell (eosinophilic) granulomatosis is a benign disease of children and young adults, predominantly in males. Occasionally, it occurs as late as 60 to 70 years of age, and presents as a solitary osteolytic lesion in the femur, skull, vertebrae, ribs, or occasionally the pelvis. Since there are no consistent accompanying laboratory abnormalities, the diagnosis of unifocal Langerhans cell granulomatosis requires biopsy of the lytic bone lesion. Treatment of choice of this condition is excision or curettage of the lesion. Rarely, lesions in inaccessible sites such as cervical vertebrae require moderate doses of irradiation (300 to 600 rads). After initial bone scan and radiographic survey to assess extent of disease, follow-up studies should be performed at 6-month intervals for 3 years. If no additional lesions are present 12 months after diagnosis, development of subsequent lesions is unlikely.

Multifocal Langerhans cell (eosinophilic) granulomatosis also usually presents in childhood, and is characterized by the development of multiple bony lesions at virtually any site—though less commonly in the feet and hands.

Transient or permanent diabetes insipidus due to granulomatous involvement of the hypothalamus occurs in one-third of patients; 20 percent develop hepatomegaly, 30 percent splenomegaly, and one-half of the patients have focal or generalized lymph node involvement. Lesions may also involve the skin, vulva, gingiva, lung, and thymus. Laboratory studies are rarely helpful in the diagnosis of multifocal Langerhans cell granulomatosis, necessitating biopsy of lesions. While generally a benign disease, multifocal Langerhans cell granulomatosis is best treated with low to moderate doses of methotrexate, prednisone, or vinblastine, usually with regression of lesions.

EVALUATION OF THE PATIENT WITH LYMPHADENOPATHY

Good physical examination techniques for palpation and assessment of lymph nodes are essential for providing useful information on which diagnostic and therapeutic decisions can be based. For serial evaluation of nodes, the documentation of each node with regard to size, location, consistency, and mobility at each examination is critical. For cervical nodes the examiner may stand behind or in front of the seated patient to palpate the neck and to examine in sequence the sites of various groups of nodes. Submental nodes are under the chin in the midline and on either side; submandibular nodes are under the jaw near its angle; jugular nodes are along the anterior border of the sternocleidomastoid muscle; supraclavicular nodes are found behind the mid portion of the clavicle. Suboccipital nodes are found in the apex of the posterior cervical triangle, and pre- and postauricular nodes are found in front of and behind the ear pinnae, respectively. Central axillary nodes occur near the middle of the thoracic wall of the axilla; lateral axillary nodes are located near the upper part of the humerus along the axillary vein and are best felt by having the patient's arm elevated. Subscapular nodes can be felt under the anterior edge of the latissimus dorsi muscle, and pectoral nodes are beneath the lateral edge of the pectoralis major muscle. Infraclavicular nodes can be felt under the distal end of the clavicle. Epitrochlear nodes are located approximately 3 cm proximal to the medial humeral epicondyle. Palpation of epitrochlear nodes is best accomplished by palpation across the epitrochlear node area in an anterior to posterior direction. Enlarged abdominal lymph nodes can be difficult to palpate and may only be felt if the patient has a shallow abdominal cavity. Pelvic nodes are best evaluated with deep palpation of the lower abdomen by rolling the extended fingers over the pelvic brim.

The investigation of lymphadenopathy can be organized according to where nodes occur and the type of clinical symptoms present. Enlarged supraclavicular nodes most often result from lymphoma, gastrointestinal, or intrathoracic tumors and should be biopsied. Acute onset of cervical adenopathy in young adults in the absence of head-and-neck infections suggests the diagnosis of infectious mononucleosis syndromes. If localized cervical node enlargement persists and serologic evaluation for EB virus, cytomegalovirus, and toxoplasmosis infections as well as chest x-ray and intermediate-strength PPD skin test are negative, then lymph node biopsy is indicated to seek lymphoma, sarcoidosis, carcinoma, and other diseases listed in Table 55-1.

Unilateral cervical adenopathy warrants a careful ear, nose, and throat examination for malignancy. In the asymptomatic patient with persistent new axillary and/or inguinal adenopathy, a biopsy specimen should be obtained. If fever and constitutional symptoms are present, the cause of infectious mononucleosis–like syndromes should be sought prior to node biopsy.

Generalized lymph node enlargement can be caused by systemic infections, drug reactions, malignancy, or one of the systemic lymphadenopathy syndromes (Table 55-1). History and physical examination can yield clues regarding the possibility of these diagnoses and direct further evaluation (e.g., complete blood count, blood cultures, chest x-ray, serologies, skin tests). If systemic adenopathy persists without an obvious cause being identified, lymph node biopsy is warranted. Once the decision to perform lymph node biopsy has been made, tissue should be processed for culture of appropriate organisms, frozen in liquid nitrogen for lymphocyte typing or other special diagnostic studies for malignant cell types, and processed for routine pathologic evaluation. One can expect information that will lead to a diagnosis in 50 to 60 percent of lymph node biopsies. About 25 percent of patients with nondiagnostic lymph node biopsies will subsequently develop within a year a disease (usually a lymphoma) related to the indication for biopsy. Therefore there should be little hesitation to repeat a nondiagnostic biopsy, especially if enlarged lymph nodes and symptoms persist.

The term *atypical hyperplasia of lymph nodes* refers to neither a clinical nor a pathologic entity, but designates cases in which the pathologist expresses concern about neoplasia and is unable to unequivocally diagnose lymphoma. Since 30 percent of patients whose lymph node biopsies are read as atypical hyperplasia subsequently develop lymphoma, a repeat biopsy is recommended at a later date if node enlargement persists. Needle aspiration biopsy is a safe technique for initial evaluation of superficial adenopathy. While lymph node aspiration can aid in the diagnosis of metastatic tumor and infections, it is rarely helpful in the diagnosis of lymphomas and other hematologic malignancies.

SPLEEN STRUCTURE AND FUNCTION The spleen is a lymphoreticular organ that serves at least four major physiologic functions. First, it is an organ of the immune system and a major site of clearance of microorganisms and particulate antigens from the bloodstream and of generation of humoral or cellular responses to foreign antigens. Second, the spleen is instrumental in sequestration and removal of normal and abnormal blood cells. Third, the vasculature of the spleen plays a role in regulation of portal blood flow. Fourth, while hematopoiesis in the normal adult takes place primarily in the bone marrow, under pathologic conditions when the marrow is replaced or overstimulated to respond, the spleen may become a major site of extramedullary hematopoiesis.

The spleen is arranged into units of areas called red and white pulp (Fig. 55-2). Red pulp contains blood-filled sinuses and pulp

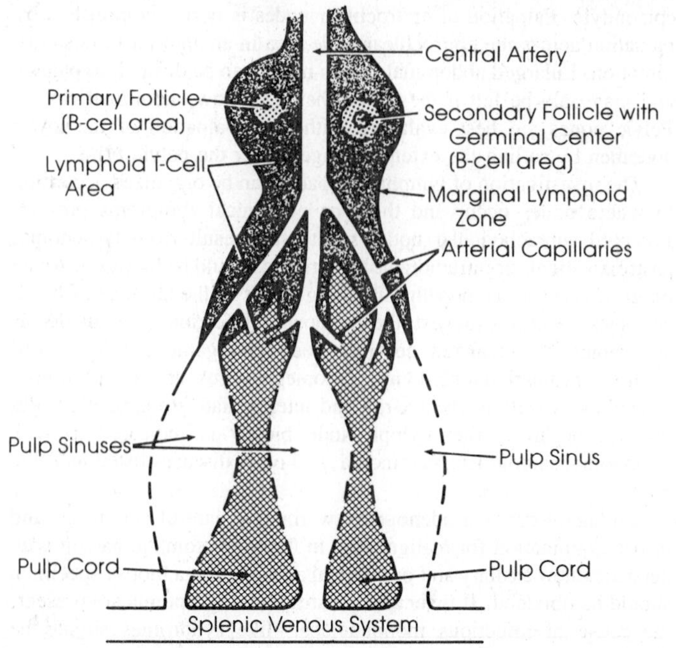

FIGURE 55-2 *Schematic spleen structure. The spleen is made up of multiple units of red and white pulp centered around small branches of the splenic artery called central arteries. White pulp areas of spleen are lymphoid areas while red pulp areas include pulp sinuses and pulp cords. In white pulp, B-cell areas are primary and secondary follicles and the marginal lymphoid zone, while T-cell areas are lymphoid cells around follicles and arterial capillaries. Redrawn with permission from Videbaek et al.*

cords lined by reticuloendothelial cells. White pulp contains centrally located arterioles, surrounded by densely packed small lymphocytes, which are primarily $T4^+$ helper T lymphocytes. Adjacent to the T-cell periarteriolar lymphocyte sheath is the follicular zone of B lymphocytes which also contains germinal centers made up of B cells and macrophages. The outermost portion of white pulp is another B-cell layer called the marginal zone which blends into red pulp areas.

The blood supply and the route of blood flow is unique in the spleen, and splenic anatomy can best be defined in terms of route of blood flow (Fig. 55-2). Blood enters the spleen by the splenic artery. The splenic artery divides into branches which penetrate into the spleen via connective tissue projections called trabeculae and from the trabeculae branch into smaller arteries called central arteries. From central arteries the bloodstream reaches the arterial capillaries. The periarteriolar lymphoid sheaths of T cells surrounding B-cell follicles persist around the arterial vessels until they become small arterioles. Blood in central arterioles empties partly through arterial capillaries directly into splenic venules and then into splenic veins. The central arterioles also empty into macrophage-lined sinuses of red pulp and into the fibrous network of reticuloendothelial cells and tissue macrophages called pulp cords. Blood in red pulp sinuses and pulp cords empties directly into the splenic venous system. During red blood cell passage from central arteries to pulp cords, and finally to spleen sinuses, red cells are concentrated in the macrophage-rich pulp cords. Normally circulating red cells accumulate in pulp cords with subsequent passage through critical small openings of sinus endothelium into red pulp sinuses and on to the splenic venous system. Packing of red cells in pulp cords with subsequent passage through small slits into sinuses is termed *erythrocyte conditioning*. Upon senescence, red cells become less deformable and are unable to pass into sinuses; they are retained in pulp cords and phagocytosed by macrophages—a process termed *culling*. Erythrocyte particulate matter such as nuclear material (Howell-Jolly bodies), denatured hemoglobulin (Heinz bodies), or malaria parasites can be pinched off during passage of red cells from pulp cords into sinuses and retained in the spleen while the rest of the red cell passes back into the circulation—a process termed *pitting*.

Many of the mechanisms of spleen enlargement are exaggerated forms of normal spleen function. While there is a wide variety of diseases associated with enlargement of the spleen, there are six basic pathophysiologic mechanisms of splenic enlargement. (1) Splenic enlargement occurs from reticuloendothelial or immune system hyperplasia in infectious diseases such as bacterial endocarditis or in immune diseases such as Felty's syndrome. Reticuloendothelial hyperplasia also occurs in diseases associated with destruction of abnormal red blood cells such as hereditary spherocytosis, thalassemia, or early in the course of sickle cell disease. (2) Splenic enlargement occurs due to altered splenic blood flow in hepatic cirrhosis or splenic, hepatic, or portal vein thrombosis. (3) Malignant neoplasms can involve the spleen either primarily as with lymphomas or angiosarcomas, or secondarily with leukemias or metastatic solid tumors. (4) Splenic enlargement can occur in situations leading to extramedullary hematopoiesis in the spleen such as in myeloid metaplasia or other myelophthisic syndromes. (5) Infiltration of the spleen with abnormal material in amyloidosis and Gaucher's disease can result in splenomegaly. (6) Splenomegaly can also result from space-occupying lesions such as hemangiomas and cysts.

DISEASES ASSOCIATED WITH SPLENIC ENLARGEMENT A wide variety of diseases lead to an increase in cellularity and vascularity of the spleen (Table 55-2). Increase in cellularity in infections is due to lymphocyte and macrophage proliferation in both red and white pulp areas. Splenomegaly is often present in acute systemic bacterial infections. Infectious granulomas due to mycobacterial and fungal infections occur in both red and white pulp. In diseases associated with disordered immunoregulation such as rheumatoid arthritis and

TABLE 55-2 Diseases associated with enlargement of the spleen

I Infections
- *A* Infectious mononucleosis
- *B* Bacterial septicemias
- *C* Bacterial endocarditis
- *D* Tuberculosis
- *E* Malaria
- *F* Leishmaniasis
- *G* Trypanosomiasis
- *H* Acquired immunodeficiency syndrome
- *I* Viral hepatitis
- *J* Congenital syphilis
- *K* Splenic abscess
- *L* Disseminated histoplasmosis

II Diseases of disordered immunoregulation
- *A* Rheumatoid arthritis (Felty's syndrome)
- *B* Systemic lupus erythematosus
- *C* Immune hemolytic anemias
- *D* Angioimmunoblastic lymphadenopathy
- *E* Drug reactions with serum sickness syndromes
- *F* Immune thrombocytopenias and neutropenias

III Diseases of disordered splenic blood flow
- *A* Laennec's and postnecrotic cirrhosis
- *B* Hepatic vein obstruction
- *C* Hepatic schistosomiasis
- *D* Portal vein obstruction or cavernous sinus transformation
- *E* Splenic vein obstruction
- *F* Chronic congestive heart failure
- *G* Splenic artery aneurysm

IV Diseases associated with abnormal erythrocytes
- *A* Spherocytosis
- *B* Sickle cell disease
- *C* Ovalocytosis
- *D* Thalassemia

V Infiltrative diseases of the spleen
- *A* *Benign*—amyloidosis, Gaucher's disease, Niemann-Pick disease, Hurler's syndrome, Tangier disease, multifocal Langerhans cell (eosinophilic) granulomatosis, extramedullary hematopoiesis, hamartomas, fibromas, hemangiomas, lymphangiomas, splenic cysts
- *B* *Malignant*—leukemias, lymphomas, Hodgkin's lymphoma, primary splenic tumors, angiosarcomas, metastatic tumors, myeloproliferative syndromes

VI Miscellaneous diseases or diseases of unknown cause
- *A* Idiopathic splenomegaly
- *B* Thyrotoxicosis
- *C* Iron-deficiency anemia
- *D* Sarcoidosis
- *E* Berylliosis

systemic lupus erythematosus, splenic enlargement is often due to lymphoid hyperplasia with enlarged lymphoid follicles present in white pulp areas and increased number of plasma cells and macrophages around red pulp arterioles and pulp cords. Splenic enlargement associated with abnormal splenic blood flow is most commonly due to chronic passive congestion from increased portal vein pressure, or from portal vein obstruction. *Banti's syndrome* is *congestive splenomegaly* with hypersplenism associated with cirrhosis and portal hypertension and is manifested histologically by red pulp congestion with accumulation and concentration of erythrocytes in widened pulp cords and sinuses. In congestive splenomegaly, reticuloendothelial hyperplasia occurs with proliferation of cells lining red pulp cords and sinuses. In splenic enlargement in conditions associated with abnormal erythrocytes such as hereditary spherocytosis, there is pooling of abnormal red cells in sinuses and pulp cords because of increased red cell rigidity and therefore decreased ability to traverse the red pulp sinusoidal endothelium.

Myelosclerosis with myeloid metaplasia is characterized by splenic intrasinusoidal extramedullary hematopoiesis involving all three myeloid cell lines associated with dilated and distended pulp sinuses. In cases of secondary extramedullary hematopoiesis such as in myelophthisic syndromes, extramedullary hematopoiesis may only involve one or two cell lineages, particularly red cells. Infiltrative malignant disease can cause focal or generalized increases in white pulp lymphoid cells as in the case of Hodgkin's disease and lymphocytic lymphoma, or infiltration of red pulp areas with malignant cells as in chronic granulocytic leukemia, acute leukemia syndromes, systemic mast cell disease, and metastatic carcinoma. Infiltrative diseases of the spleen such as Gaucher's and Niemann-Pick disease produce splenic enlargement by increase in number of splenic red pulp histocytes. Thyrotoxicosis can be associated with splenomegaly and is due to thyroid hormone–induced lymphoid hyperplasia. Sarcoidosis causes splenic enlargement by the development of areas of granulomatous inflammation in white pulp lymphoid tissue. A splenic artery aneurysm may cause unexplained splenomegaly, cramping, and left upper abdominal pain; a calcified ring in the splenic area may be seen on x-ray.

The degree of splenomegaly varies with the disease entity. Slight or mild enlargement occurs in chronic passive congestion of the liver due to congestive heart failure, acute malaria, typhoid fever, bacterial endocarditis, systemic lupus erythematosus, rheumatoid arthritis, and thalassemia minor. Moderate splenic enlargement occurs in hepatitis, cirrhosis, lymphomas, infectious mononucleosis, hemolytic anemias, splenic abscesses and infarcts, and amyloidosis. Massive enlargement of the spleen occurs in chronic myelocytic leukemia, agnogenic myeloid metaplasia with myelofibrosis, hairy cell leukemia, Gaucher's and Niemann-Pick diseases, sarcoidosis, thalassemia major, chronic malaria, congenital syphilis, leishmaniasis, and in some cases of portal vein obstruction.

DIAGNOSTIC EVALUATION OF THE PATIENT WITH SPLENIC ENLARGEMENT When normal in size and position, the spleen is generally inaccessible to abdominal palpation. A normal-sized spleen is about 12 cm long and 7 cm wide. Because of the oblique orientation of the spleen to the abdominal cavity, its long axis lies behind and parallel to the tenth rib in the midaxillary line, with splenic width located between the ninth and eleventh ribs. Therefore, to percuss for splenic dullness the patient is placed on the right side and the ninth intercostal space is located by finding the tip of the scapula lying in the seventh intercostal space and counting down to the ninth intercostal space. Dullness outside the ninth and eleventh intercostal spaces suggests splenomegaly, although fluid in the stomach and feces in the colon can cause splenic area dullness as well. Palpation of the left upper quadrant is performed with the patient supine or on the right side by the examiner's right hand; the examiner's left hand is placed under the lower thorax grasping the lower ribs posteriorly. Palpation for spleen enlargement is performed with the patient taking deep breaths to permit the examiner to feel the inferior tip of an enlarged spleen. To avoid missing a massively enlarged spleen, palpation of the left upper quadrant should begin in the lower abdominal cavity with gradual movement up to the left upper quadrant.

Demonstration of mild to moderate splenic enlargement by physical examination may be difficult, particularly in obese patients. Other techniques for assessment of spleen size include ^{99}Tc-colloid liver-spleen scan, computerized axial tomography, and ultrasound scanning of the left upper quadrant. These three techniques can be useful in defining splenic defects such as cysts, infarct, or tumors, or in defining accessory splenic tissue that may be due to congenital accessory spleens or residual foci of splenic tissue following splenic rupture (splenosis).

In the evaluation of the patient with splenomegaly, it is helpful to consider splenomegaly with acute or subacute illnesses separately from splenomegaly with chronic illness. Acute left upper quadrant pain with an enlarged tender spleen suggests subcapsular hematoma, splenic rupture, or splenic infarcts. Rupture of the spleen with splenic hematoma most often follows direct or remote trauma but can occur as well in the setting of infectious diseases such as malaria, typhoid fever, and EB virus–induced infectious mononucleosis. Splenic infarcts due either to in situ red cell sickling (in sickle cell disease) or to emboli (from mural thrombus, atrial myxoma, or cardiac valve vegetation) can usually be detected by spleen scan or arteriogram. More unusual disorders presenting acutely are diffuse splenic metastatic disease and hemorrhage into a splenic cyst.

An acute febrile illness associated with splenomegaly may be due to bacterial endocarditis, infectious mononucleosis syndromes, tuberculosis, and histoplasmosis. Fever, peripheral adenopathy, and splenomegaly, with or without a rash or arthralgias should suggest, in addition to infection mononucleosis, sarcoidosis, Hodgkin's lymphoma, a collagen vascular disease such as systemic lupus erythematosus, or a serum sickness syndrome.

An acute illness with splenomegaly associated with the signs and symptoms of anemia, with or without bleeding, suggests autoimmune hemolytic anemia, myeloproliferative syndromes, or acute leukemia.

Splenomegaly with signs and symptoms of chronic illness suggests a wide range of disorders, many of which are listed in Table 55-2. Liver disease with portal hypertension is a common etiology of splenomegaly in this setting. Patients with congestive splenomegaly from liver disease or portal or splenic vein thrombosis are often asymptomatic. With clinical features of rheumatoid arthritis and leukopenia, Felty's syndrome should be considered. The presence of lymphadenopathy should suggest chronic lymphocytic leukemia or lymphoma. Plethora and an elevated hematocrit suggest polycythemia vera or chronic lung disease, with right heart failure and congestive splenomegaly. Weight loss or other signs of chronic illness suggest leukemia or other myeloproliferative syndromes as well as a variety of hemoglobinopathies. Bone marrow aspiration and biopsy can aid in the diagnosis of leukemia and lymphoma, lipid storage diseases, disseminated fungal or mycobacterial diseases, metastatic malignant diseases, and amyloidosis.

Occasionally laparotomy and splenectomy are indicated in the evaluation of splenomegaly. The decision to perform diagnostic laparotomy in a patient with unexplained splenomegaly is difficult and must take into account the patient's age and clinical signs, symptoms, and laboratory abnormalities present. One study has documented palpable spleens in 3 percent of entering college freshman and no increased risk of any disease during the ensuing 6 years. In another study of older subjects (average age 49) who had undergone splenectomy for undiagnosed splenomegaly and had signs and symptoms of chronic illness, a diagnosis of an underlying disorder was obtained in the majority of patients by splenectomy.

HYPERSPLENISM The term hypersplenism applies to any clinical situation in which the spleen removes excessive quantities of erythrocytes, granulocytes, or platelets from the circulation. General mechanisms of removal of formed blood elements include increased sequestration of cells due to hemodynamic abnormalities of splenic blood flow, or by production of anti-red cell, granulocyte, or platelet antibodies, making the cells vulnerable to clearance by splenic macrophages. Situations in which passive congestion of the spleen occurs produce abnormal sludging of blood in sinuses and red pulp cords. Under these conditions there is plasma pooling, producing marked intrasplenic hemoconcentration and hypoxia, making blood cells more vulnerable to the phagocytic action of pulp cord macrophages. Criteria for diagnosis of hypersplenism include (1) splenomegaly, (2) splenic destruction of one or more cell lines in the peripheral blood, (3) normal or hyperplastic cellularity of bone marrow with normal representation of the cell line deficient in the circulation, and (4) variably, evidence of increased cell turnover in the cell lines affected, i.e., reticulocytosis, increased band forms of neutrophils, or circulating immature platelet forms.

Therapy for hypersplenism relates in large part to the underlying disease or the underlying pathophysiologic process. If the underlying disorder responsible for hypersplenism cannot be corrected, splenectomy is an option for cases in which a severe deficit is present (see below for indications for splenectomy).

HYPOSPLENISM The terms hyposplenia or asplenia are used to indicate diminished or absent splenic function. The usual causes of hyposplenism are splenectomy, congenital absence of the spleen, sickle cell anemia in patients older than 5 years (with autosplenectomy due to repeated infarcts), and splenic irradiation. In sickle cell anemia, persistence of a palpable spleen after age 5 suggests coexisting alpha thalassemia. Findings in the peripheral blood that indicate diminished splenic function include the presence of nucleated red cells, erythrocyte Howell-Jolly bodies, erythrocyte Heinz bodies, as well as target and burr forms of red cells.

Splenectomized patients or patients with functional asplenia (such as in sickle cell disease) are prone to bacterial infections, which are frequently overwhelming and life-threatening, particularly with encapsulated organisms such as *Streptococcus pneumoniae, Neisseria meningitidis, Escherichia coli*, and *Haemophilus influenzae*. This is due to a reduction or absence of the filtration function of the spleen for clearance of antibody-coated bacteria as well as to decreased production of IgG and IgM antibodies (opsonins) needed to bind bacteria. Immunization with pneumococcal vaccine is recommended in patients older than 2 years with hyposplenism and prior to elective splenectomy. The presence of peripheral blood manifestations of hyposplenism (Howell-Jolly bodies) in the presence of a normal-sized or enlarged spleen suggests the presence of splenic infiltrative disease such as a primary splenic angiosarcoma.

INDICATIONS FOR SPLENECTOMY Splenic trauma, whether accidental blunt trauma or intraoperative iatrogenic injury, is the most common indication for splenectomy. En bloc removal of the spleen may be indicated either because of tumor involvement or for a splenorectal shunt. Staging laparotomy with splenectomy remains a major diagnostic procedure for many early stage Hodgkin's disease patients being considered for radiation therapy alone. Splenectomy for selected patients with idiopathic splenomegaly is often necessary when other investigations fail to produce a diagnosis; however, the spleen should not be removed simply because it is palpable. Hypersplenism in lymphomas can cause persistent cytopenias and in select cases responds to splenectomy. B-cell hairy cell leukemia frequently presents with hypersplenism, and splenectomy is often beneficial, producing remission in the majority of cases with a 5-year survival of 50 percent.

Felty's syndrome (rheumatoid arthritis and hypersplenism) and Gaucher's disease both require splenectomy when splenomegaly leads to symptomatic neutropenia or other complications of hypersplenism. Immune thrombocytopenic purpura which persists after trials of medical therapy may benefit from splenectomy (see Chap. 279). Of the hemolytic anemias, hereditary spherocytosis, hereditary elliptocytosis, immune hemolytic anemia with warm-reacting IgG antibody, and pyruvate-kinase deficiency have been improved by splenectomy. Splenectomy is usually necessary late in the course of thalassemia major when neutropenia or thrombocytopenia develops, or when transfusion requirements double. Chronic lymphocytic leukemia (CLL), chronic granulocytic leukemia, and agnogenic myeloid metaplasia may be complicated by symptomatic hypersplenism or, in the case of CLL, immune hemolytic anemia and thrombocytopenia, often necessitating splenectomy. (Chaps. 289 and 292.)

REFERENCES

Lymph node enlargement

Butcher E, Weissman I: Lymphoid tissues and organs in *Fundamental Immunology*, WE Paul (ed). New York, Raven, 1984, pp 109–127

Greenfield S, Jordan MC: The clinical investigation of lymphadenopathy, in primary care practice. JAMA 240:1388, 1978

Ioachim HL: *Lymph Node Biopsy*. Philadelphia, Lippincott, 1982

Lennert K, Stein H: The germinal center, in *Morphology, Histochemistry, and Immunohistology in Lymphoproliferative Diseases of Skin*, M Goos, E Christopher (eds). Berlin, Heidelberg, New York, Springer-Verlag, 1982

Lieberman PH et al: A reappraisal of eosinophilic granuloma of bone, Hand-Schüller-Christian syndrome, and Letterer-Siwe syndrome. Medicine 48:375, 1969

Nathwani BN et al: Malignant lymphoma arising in angioimmunoblastic lymphadenopathy. Cancer 41:578, 1978

Poppema S et al: Distribution of T cell subsets in human lymph nodes. J Exp Med 153:30, 1981

Schroer KR, Franssila KO: Atypical hyperplasia of lymph nodes: A follow-up study. Cancer 44:1155, 1979

Sinclair S et al: Biopsy of enlarged, superficial lymph nodes. JAMA 228:602, 1974

Thomas JA et al: Combined immunological and histochemical analysis of skin and lymph node lesions in histiocytosis X. J Clin Pathol 35:327, 1982

Winterbauer RH et al: A clinical interpretation of bilateral hilar adenopathy. Ann Intern Med 78:65, 1973

Yen-Tsu N et al: Lymph node biopsy for diagnosis: A statistical study. J Surg Oncol 14:53, 1980

Splenic enlargement

Butler JJ: Pathology of the spleen in benign and malignant conditions. Histopathology 7:453, 1983

Eichner ER, Whitfield CL: Splenomegaly: An algorithmic approach to diagnosis. JAMA 246:2858, 1981

Enriquez E, Neiman RS (eds): *The Pathology of the Spleen: A Functional Approach*. Chicago, American Society of Clinical Pathologists, 1976

Hermann RE et al: Splenectomy for the diagnosis of splenomegaly. Ann Surg 168:896, 1964

Lewis SM (ed): *Clinics in Haematology*, vol 12: *The Spleen*. London, Saunders, 1983, pp 361–608

McIntyre OR, Ebaugh FG: Palpable spleens in college freshmen. Ann Intern Med 66:301, 1967

Steinberg MH et al: Evidence of hyposplenism in the presence of splenomegaly. Scand J Haematol 31:437, 1983

Videbaek A et al: *The Spleen in Health and Disease*. Chicago, Yearbook, 1982

56 DISORDERS OF PHAGOCYTIC CELLS

JOHN I. GALLIN

Leukocytes are the major cellular components of inflammatory and immune responses and include neutrophils, lymphocytes, monocytes, eosinophils, and basophils. The blood is the most readily obtainable source of leukocytes and serves as the vehicle for their delivery to the various tissues from the bone marrow, where they are produced. Normal blood leukocyte counts in adults range from 4.5 to 11 $\times 10^6$ cells per cubic millimeter; a table of normal values for different ages can be found in the Appendix. The most prevalent cells are neutrophils (54 to 62 percent), followed by lymphocytes (25 to 33 percent), monocytes (3 to 7 percent), eosinophils (1 to 3 percent), and basophils (0 to 0.75 percent). The various leukocytes are thought to derive from a common stem cell in the bone marrow. Three-fourths of the nucleated cells of bone marrow are committed to the production of leukocytes. Leukocyte maturation in the marrow is generally thought to be under the regulatory control of a number of different factors which are incompletely defined. Because an alteration in the number and type of leukocytes is a frequent association with disease processes, a total white blood count (WBC) (cells per cubic millimeter) and differential counts are obtained frequently. The lymphocytes and basophils are discussed elsewhere. This chapter focuses on the neutrophils, monocytes, and eosinophils.

NEUTROPHILS

MATURATION Important events in the neutrophil life are summarized in Fig. 56-1. In normal humans neutrophils are only produced in the bone marrow. Best estimates indicate that the appropriate number of stem cells necessary to support hematopoiesis is between 400 and 500. There is convincing evidence that human blood monocytes and tissue macrophages produce colony-stimulating factors, hormone(s) required for the growth of monocytes and neutrophils in the bone marrow. The hematopoietic system not only produces enough neutrophils (approximately 1.3×10^{11} cells per 80-kg person per day) to carry out physiologic functions but also has a large reserve stored in the marrow which can be mobilized in response to inflammation or infection. An increase in the number of blood neutrophils is called *neutrophilia*, and the presence of immature cells is termed a "shift to the left." A diminution in the number of blood neutrophils is referred to as *neutropenia*.

Neutrophils evolve from pluripotent stem cells. The final stages of hematopoiesis are characterized by the appearance of cells with distinct morphologic features. The myeloblast is the first recognizable precursor cell and is followed by the *promyelocyte*. The promyelocyte evolves when the classic lysosomal granules, called the *primary* or *azurophil granules*, are produced. The primary granules contain hydrolases, elastase, myeloperoxidase, and cationic proteins. The promyelocyte divides to produce the *myelocyte*, a cell responsible for the synthesis of the *specific* or *secondary granules* which contain unique (specific) constituents such as lactoferrin, vitamin B_{12}–binding proteins, and probably cytochrome b, histaminase, and receptors for certain chemoattractants and adherence promoting factors. The secondary granules do not contain acid hydrolases and therefore are not classic lysosomes. They are readily released extracellularly, and their mobilization is probably important in modulating inflammation. During the final stages of maturation there is no cell division and the cell passes through the *metamyelocyte* stage and then to the *band* neutrophil with a sausage-shaped nucleus. As the band cell matures the nucleus assumes a lobulated configuration.

In settings of severe acute bacterial infection, prominent neutrophil cytoplasmic granules called *toxic granulations* are occasionally seen. Toxic granulations are thought to be immature or abnormally staining azurophil granules. Cytoplasmic inclusions (*Doehle bodies*) can also be seen during infection and probably represent fragments of endoplasmic reticulum. Large neutrophil vacuoles are often present in acute bacterial infection and probably represent pinocytosed (internalized) membrane.

Neutrophils have long been thought to be a homogeneous population of cells. However, studies of neutrophil function have suggested they are heterogeneous. Recently monoclonal antibodies have been developed that recognize only a subset of mature neutrophils. The meaning of neutrophil heterogeneity is not known.

MARROW RELEASE AND CIRCULATING COMPARTMENTS Specific signals, including interleukin 1 (endogenous pyrogen) or the complement fragment C3e, mobilize leukocytes from the bone marrow and deliver them to the blood in an unstimulated state. Under normal conditions about 90 percent of the neutrophil pool is in the bone marrow, 2 to 3 percent in the circulation, and the remainder in the tissues. The blood pool exists as two compartments: the marginated pool adherent to endothelial cells and the freely flowing circulating pool. In response to chemotactic stimuli from tissues (e.g., the complement product C5a, the arachidonic acid derivative leukotriene B_4, or the bacterial product *N*-formylmethionylleucylphenylalanine), neutrophil adhesiveness increases and the circulating cells aggregate to each other and adhere to the endothelium. An increased expression of a glycoprotein receptor for C3bi (also called CR3) appears to be intimately involved with the increased adhesion. Receptors for chemoattractants and opsonins are probably also mobilized; the cells orient toward the chemoattractant source in the extravascular space, increase their motile activity (chemokinesis), and migrate with direction (chemotaxis) into tissues. The process of migration into tissues is called *diapedesis* and involves the crawling of neutrophils between postcapillary endothelial cells which open junctions between adjacent cells to permit leukocyte passage. The endothelial responses (increased blood flow secondary to increased vasodilation and permeability) are mediated by anaphylatoxins (e.g., complement products C3a and C5a) as well as vasodilators such as bradykinin and prostaglandins E and I. In the healthy adult most neutrophils leave the body by migration through the mucous membrane of the gastrointestinal tract. Normally neutrophils spend a relatively short time in the circulation with a half-life of 6 to 7 h. Once in the tissues neutrophils release enzymes such as collagenase and elastase, which may help establish abscess cavities. Neutrophils ingest (phagocytose) pathogenic materials that have been properly altered (opsonized) by substances such as immunoglobulin G (IgG) and the complement product C3b. Fibronectin and the tetrapeptide tuftsin facilitate the phagocytic process.

Concomitant with phagocytosis there is a burst of oxygen consumption and activation of the hexosemonophosphate shunt. Nicotinamide-adenine dinucleotide phosphate (NADPH) oxidase is activated, and through a complex enzyme system containing flavoproteins and cytochrome b, toxic oxygen products (e.g., hydrogen peroxide and hydroxyl radical) are generated. Hydrogen peroxide + chloride + neutrophil myeloperoxidase provide a particularly toxic system that generates hypochlorous acid, hypoclorite, and chlorine. These products oxidize and halogenate microorganisms and tumor cells and when uncontrolled, can damage host tissue. Strongly cationic proteins also participate in microbial killing, and other enzymes, such as lysozyme and acid proteases, help digest microbial debris. After 1 to 4 days in tissues neutrophils die. The second wave of inflammation,

FIGURE 56-1 *Schematic diagram of the life cycle of the neutrophil.*

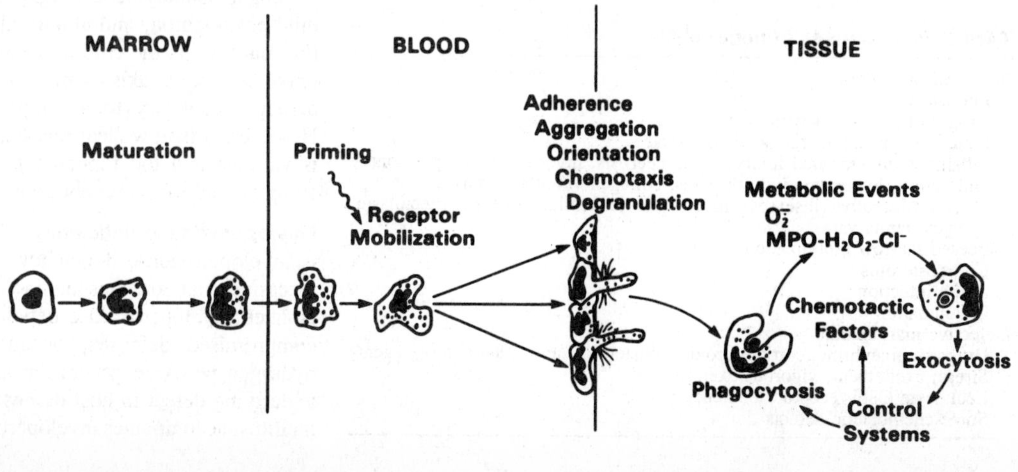

TABLE 56-1 Causes of neutropenia

Decreased production:
- Hematologic diseases—idiopathic, cyclic neutropenia, Chédiak-Higashi syndrome, aplastic anemia, infantile genetic disorders
- Drug-induced—alkylating agents (nitrogen mustard, busulfan, chlorambucil, cyclophosphamide); antimetabolites (methotrexate, 6-mercaptopurine, 5-flurocytosine); noncytotoxic agents [antibiotics (chloramphenicol, penicillins, sulfonamides), phenothiazines, tranquilizers (meprobamate), certain diuretics, anti-inflammatory agents, antithyroid drugs, many others]
- Tumor invasion, myelofibrosis
- Nutritional deficiency—vitamin B_{12}, folate (especially alcoholics)
- Infection—tuberculosis, typhoid fever, brucellosis, tularemia, measles, infectious mononucleosis, malaria, viral hepatitis, leishmaniasis

Peripheral destruction:
- Antineutrophil antibodies and/or splenic trapping:
  - Autoimmune disorders—Felty's syndrome
  - Drugs—aminopyrine, α-methyldopa, phenylbutazone, mecurial diuretics, some phenothiazines

Peripheral pooling:
- Overwhelming bacterial infection
- Hemodialysis
- Cardiopulmonary bypass

monocyte accumulation, occurs within 6 to 12 h of initiation of inflammation. Neutrophils, monocytes, microorganisms in various states of digestion, and altered local tissue cells make up pus, which derives its characteristic green color from myeloperoxidase. Myeloperoxidase and other factors may be important in turning off the inflammatory process by inactivating chemoattractants and immobilizing phagocytic cells.

NEUTROPHIL DYSFUNCTION A defect anywhere in the neutrophil life cycle summarized in Fig. 56-1 can lead to dysfunction and compromised host defenses. The clinical result is often recurrent and severe bacterial and fungal infections creating novel and often difficult management problems.

Neutropenia The consequences of absent neutrophils represent a dramatic demonstration of their importance in host defense. When the neutrophil count is below 1000 per cubic millimeter, there is an increased risk for infection (Chap. 84); when there are fewer than 200 cells per cubic millimeter, the inflammatory process is absent. The causes of neutropenia are multiple and are related to depressed production, peripheral destruction, and peripheral pooling (Table 56-1).

In the newborn severe neutropenia may be seen in the setting of acute bacterial or viral infection and is due to the infant's poor bone marrow reserve. Congenital forms of neutropenia exist and include Kostmann's syndrome (less than 100 neutrophils per cubic millimeter), which is often fatal; more benign chronic idiopathic neutropenia (300 to 1500 neutrophils per cubic millimeter); the hair-cartilage-hypoplasia syndrome; Shwachman syndrome associated with pancreatic insufficiency; and neutropenias associated with other immune defects (X-linked agammaglobulinemia, ataxia-telangiectasia, IgA deficiency). Cyclic neutropenia, an autosomal dominant trait, may occur in infancy. Maternal factors associated with neutropenia in the newborn include transplacental transfer of IgG directed against antigens on fetal neutrophils and drugs (e.g., thiazide) ingested during pregnancy.

The presence of immunoglobulin (IgG) directed toward neutrophils is seen in Felty's syndrome (triad of rheumatoid arthritis, splenomegaly, and neutropenia) (Chap. 263). Patients with Felty's syndrome who respond to splenectomy with an increase in their neutrophil count lower their postoperative serum granulocyte-binding IgG, suggesting that one beneficial effect of splenectomy is reduction in antineutrophil antibody. Drugs that produce neutropenia by increased destruction or sequestration appear to act by serum antibody interaction with drug (antigen) absorbed to the neutrophil. The drugs that cause neutropenia by this mechanism have varying latent periods for their toxicity, although following drug rechallenge neutropenia occurs within hours.

Neutrophilia Neutrophilia results from increased production, marrow release, or defective margination (Table 56-2). Increased production is associated with chronic inflammation or infection and certain myeloproliferative diseases. Increased marrow release is induced by corticosteroids. Release of epinephrine, as with vigorous exercise, excitement, or stress, will demarginate neutrophils and double the neutrophil count. Leukocytosis to 10,000 to 25,000 cells per cubic millimeter occurs in response to infection or other forms of acute inflammation and results from both release of the marginated pool and mobilization of marrow reserves. Persistent neutrophilia of 30,000 to 50,000 cells per cubic millimeter or greater is called a *leukemoid reaction*, a term often used to distinguish this degree of neutrophilia from leukemia. In a leukemoid reaction the circulating neutrophils are usually mature.

ABNORMAL NEUTROPHIL FUNCTION Congenital deficiencies and acquired abnormalities of phagocyte function are described in Table 56-3. The resulting diseases are best considered in terms of the functional defects of adherence, chemotaxis, and microbicidal activity. The distinguishing features of the important congenital lesions are shown in Table 56-4, several of which are discussed below.

C3bi (CR3) receptor deficiency Patients with congenitally (autosomal recessive) abnormal phagocyte adherence lack the plasma membrane receptor for the fragment of the third complement component called C3bi (CR3 by other terminology). Clinically most patients with this syndrome have recurrent bacterial and fungal infections, severe periodontal disease, persistent leukocytosis (15,000 to 20,000 neutrophils per cubic millimeter), and usually a history of delayed separation of the umbilical stump. Neutrophils (and monocytes) from these patients have defective adherence, spreading, aggregation, and chemotaxis.

Hyperimmunoglobulin E–recurrent infection (Job's) syndrome Abnormal neutrophil and monocyte chemotaxis occurs in the hyperimmunoglobulin E–recurrent infection (Job's) syndrome. These patients have recurrent infections with *Staphylococcus aureus* (Chap. 84), and often have characteristically coarse facies, "cold" cutaneous abscesses, dermatitis, markedly elevated levels of plasma IgE including antistaphylococcal IgE, low or absent antistaphylococcal IgA, mild eosinophilia, and abnormal T-suppressor lymphocyte function. For many years the cold abscesses were thought to be a reflection of impaired chemotaxis with too few phagocytes arriving too late, perhaps secondary to a lymphocyte factor inhibiting chemotaxis. However, it is now clear that the chemotactic defect in these patients is variable and the fundamental basis for the impaired defenses is complex and inadequately delineated.

Myeloperoxidase deficiency The most common neutrophil defect is myeloperoxidase deficiency, which is inherited as an autosomal recessive trait and has an incidence of about 1 in 2000 persons. Isolated myeloperoxidase deficiency is not associated with severely compromised defenses, because other defense systems such as hydrogen peroxide generation are accelerated. However, if another underlying defect in host defense, such as poorly controlled diabetes mellitus, accompanies myeloperoxidase deficiency, then host defenses

TABLE 56-2 Causes of neutrophilia

Increased production:
- Idiopathic
- Drug-induced—corticosteroids
- Infection—bacterial, fungal, rarely viral
- Inflammation—thermal injury, tissue necrosis, myocardial and pulmonary infarction, hypersensitivity diseases, collagen vascular diseases
- Myeloproliferative diseases—myelocytic leukemia, myeloid metaplasia, polycythemia vera

Increased marrow mobilization:
- Corticosteroids
- Acute infection
- Inflammation

Defective margination:
- Drugs—epinephrine, corticosteroids, nonsteroidal anti-inflammatory agents
- Stress, excitement, vigorous exercise
- Leukocyte C3bi receptor deficiency
- Some chemotactic defects

TABLE 56-3 Types of neutrophil dysfunction

Function	Drug-induced	Acquired disease	Congenital disorder
Adherence-aggregation	Aspirin; colchicine; alcohol; corticosteriods; ibuprofen; piroxicam	Neonates, hemodialysis	C3bi receptor deficiency
Deformability		Leukemia, neonates, diabetes mellitus, immature neutrophils	
Chemokinesis-chemotaxis	Corticosteroids (high-dose); auranofin; colchicine (weak effect); phenylbutazone, naproxen; indomethacin	Thermal injury; malignancy; malnutrition; periodontal disease; neonates; systemic lupus erythematosus; rheumatoid arthritis; diabetes mellitus; sepsis; influenza virus infection; herpes simplex virus infection; acrodermatitis enteropathica; Down's syndrome; α-Mannosidase deficiency; severe combined immunodeficiency; Wiskott-Aldrich syndrome	Hyper IgE–recurrent infection (Job's) syndrome; Chédiak-Higashi syndrome; specific granule deficiency
Microbicidal activity	Colchicine; cyclophosphamide; corticosteroids (high-dose)	Leukemia; aplastic anemia; certain neutropenias; tuftsin deficiency; thermal injury; sepsis; neonates; diabetes mellitus; malnutrition	Chédiak-Higashi syndrome; specific granule deficiency; chronic granulomatous diseases

are likely to be significantly compromised. An acquired form of myeloperoxidase deficiency occurs in myelomonocytic leukemia and acute myeloblastic leukemia. In acute myelogenous leukemia, pink-staining, apparently aberrant large primary granules, called Auer bodies, are seen.

Chédiak-Higashi syndrome (CHS) CHS is a rare disease with autosomal recessive inheritance characterized clinically by recurrent pyogenic infections (Chap. 84), periodontal disease, partial oculocutaneous albinism, nystagmus, and progressive peripheral neuropathy. About 50 percent of the patients develop a lymphomatous (accelerated) phase of the disease at adolescence. Neutrophils and all cells containing lysosomes from patients with CHS characteristically have large granules. CHS neutrophils and monocytes have impaired chemotaxis and abnormal rates of microbial killing due to slow rates of fusion of the lysosomal granules with phagosomes.

Chronic granulomatous diseases Chronic granulomatous disease (CGD) represents a group of patients with disorders of neutrophil and monocyte oxidative metabolism. Although CGD is rare, occurring in about one in 1 million individuals, it is an important model of defective neutrophil oxidative metabolism. Most often CGD is inherited as an X-linked recessive pattern, although in 15 percent of patients the disease is inherited with an autosomal recessive pattern and an autosomal dominant pattern has been reported in one family. Leukocytes from patients with CGD have severely diminished hydrogen peroxide production. Defects anywhere in the leukocyte's hexose-monophosphate shunt or the NADPH oxidase enzyme system can lead to clinical disease. Patients with CGD characteristically have increased infection with catalase-positive microorganisms (organisms which destroy their own hydrogen peroxide). These patients have an increased propensity to infection with such microorganisms as *Staphylococcus aureus*, *Escherichia coli*, *Serratia marcescens*, *Chromobacterium violaceum*, *Nocardia*, and certain fungi (*Aspergillus* and *Candida albicans*) (Chap. 84). They do not have an increased incidence of infection with catalase-negative microorganisms such as *Streptococcus pneumoniae*. When patients with CGD become infected, they often have extensive inflammatory reactions and lymph node suppuration is common despite the administration of appropriate antibiotics. Aphthous ulcers, gingivitis, and chronic inflammation of the nares are usually present. Granulomas are frequent and can obstruct the gastrointestinal or genitourinary tracts. The excessive inflammatory reactions probably reflect abnormal turnoff of inflammation by failure to degrade chemoattractants and antigens which cause persistent neutrophil accumulation. Impaired killing of intracellular microorganisms by macrophages may lead to persistent cell-mediated immunity and granuloma formation. Surgery is required for thorough drainage of abscesses in the lung, liver, and bones.

TABLE 56-4 Distinguishing features of congenital phagocyte dysfunction syndromes

Disease	Defect	Clinical manifestations
C3bi receptor deficiency	Adherence, aggregation, spreading, chemotaxis, leukemoid reaction	Delayed separation of umbilical stump, depressed inflammation, bacterial infections, gingivitis, periodontal disease
Hyperimmunoglobulin E–recurrent infection (Job's) syndrome	Variable chemotactic defects, very high IgE with anti-*S. aureus* IgE; low anti-*S. aureus* IgA	"Coarse" facies in most patients, "cold" cutaneous abscesses; recurrent pulmonary, bone, upper airway infections with *S. aureus* or *Haemophilus influenza;* mild eosinophilia; mucocutaneous candidiasis
Myeloperoxidase deficiency	Absent myeloperoxidase	Minimal unless another defect, then *Candida albicans* or other fungal infections
Chédiak-Higashi syndrome	Giant lysosomal granules; neutropenia, chemotaxis, degranulation, microbicidal activity, excess O_2 consumption and H_2O_2 production	Recurrent pyogenic infections, especially with *S. aureus;* many patients get lymphomatous-like illness during adolescence; periodontal disease; partial oculocutaneous albinism, nystagmus, progressive peripheral neuropathy
Specific granule deficiency	Absent specific granules; chemotaxis, O_2^- production, bactericidal activity decreased	Recurrent cutaneous, ear, and pulmonary bacterial infections; diminished inflammation
Chronic granulomatous disease	H_2O_2 production absent in neutrophils and monocytes; defective "turn-off" of inflammation	Severe infections of skin, ears, lungs, liver, bone with catalase (+) microorganisms such as *S. aureus, Pseudomonas cepacia, Aspergillus* sp, *Chromobacterium violaceum;* often hard to culture organism; excessive inflammation with granulomas; frequent lymph node suppuration; granulomas can obstruct gastrointestinal or genitourinary tracts; gingivitis, aphthous ulcers

MONONUCLEAR PHAGOCYTES

The mononuclear phagocyte system is defined as a continuum linking monoblasts, promonocytes, and monocytes with the structurally diverse tissue macrophages which make up what was previously referred to as the reticuloendothelial system. Macrophages are long-lived phagocytic cells capable of many of the functions of neutrophils. They are important secretory cells that, through their receptors and secretory products, participate in many complex immunologic and inflammatory processes not attributed to neutrophils. Monocytes leave the circulation by diapedesis more slowly than neutrophils and have a half-life in the blood of 12 to 24 h.

After blood monocytes arrive in the tissues, they differentiate into macrophages with specialized functions suited for specific anatomic locations. Alveolar macrophages, liver Kupffer cells, splenic macrophages, peritoneal macrophages, bone marrow macrophages, lymphatic macrophages, brain microglial cells, and dendritic macrophages all have specialized functions. Macrophage secreted products include lysozyme, neutral proteases, acid hydrolases, arginase, numerous complement components, enzyme inhibitors (plasmin, α_2-macroglobulin), binding proteins (transferrin, fibronectin, transcobalamin II), nucleosides, and interleukin 1 (pyrogen). Interleukin 1 (see Chap. 9) has many important functions including stimulating the hypothalamus to initiate fever, mobilizing leukocytes from the bone marrow, as well as activating lymphocytes and neutrophils. Other macrophage secreted products include reactive oxygen metabolites, bioactive lipids (arachidonate metabolites and platelet activating factors), a neutrophil chemoattractant, factors regulating synthesis of proteins by other cells, bone marrow colony-stimulating factors, factors stimulating fibroblast and microvasculature proliferation as well as factors inhibiting replication of lymphocytes, tumors, viruses, and certain bacteria *(Listeria monocytogenes)*. Macrophages are key effector cells in the elimination of intracellular microorganisms. Their ability to fuse to form giant cells which coalesce into granulomas in response to some inflammatory stimuli is important in the elimination of intracellular microbes and may be under the control of γ-interferon.

Macrophages play an important role in the immune response (see Chap. 62). They process antigen for presentation to lymphocytes, their secreted products modulate lymphocyte function, and macrophages participate in autoimmune phenomena by removing immune complexes and other immunologically active substances from the circulation. Furthermore, they play a role in wound healing, in the disposal of senescent cells, and in the development of atheromas.

DISORDERS OF THE MONONUCLEAR PHAGOCYTE SYSTEM

Many disorders of neutrophils extend to mononuclear phagocytes. Thus drugs which suppress neutrophil production in the bone marrow usually lead to *monocytopenia*. Transient monocytopenia can also be seen after stress or corticosteroid administration. *Monocytosis* is associated with certain infections such as tuberculosis, brucellosis, subacute bacterial endocarditis, Rocky Mountain spotted fever, and malaria. Monocytosis is also seen in kala azar, malignancies, leukemias, myeloproliferative syndromes, hemolytic anemias, chronic idiopathic neutropenias, granulomatous diseases such as sarcoidosis, regional enteritis, and some collagen vascular diseases. Patients with neutrophil C3bi receptor deficiency, the hyperimmunoglobulin E–recurrent infection (Job's) syndrome, Chédiak-Higashi syndrome, and chronic granulomatous diseases all have defects in the mononuclear phagocyte system.

Certain viral infections impair mononuclear phagocyte function. For example, influenza virus infection is associated with abnormal monocyte chemotaxis. Abnormal monocyte chemotaxis and clearance of IgG-coated erythrocytes (discussed below) is also seen in the acquired immunodeficiency syndrome (AIDS), which is caused by a human retrovirus (see Chap. 257). It is likely that the defects of the monocyte-macrophage system in AIDS contribute to the increased susceptibility to opportunistic infection due to intracellular microorganisms such as *Pneumocystic carinii* and *Mycobacterium avium-intracellulare*. T lymphocytes produce a factor, possibly deficient in AIDS, that induces Fc-receptor expression and phagocytosis by mononuclear phagocytes. In other diseases, such as T-cell lymphomas, excessive release of such a T-cell factor is thought to cause erythrophagocytosis by splenic macrophages.

Specific defects of the mononuclear phagocytes have been described in certain autoimmune diseases. Removal of IgG-coated radiolabeled autologous erythrocytes, presumably via the Fc receptor of splenic macrophages, is profoundly abnormal in patients with active systemic lupus erythematosus. Patients with other autoimmune diseases characterized by tissue deposition of immune complexes, as seen in Sjögren's syndrome, mixed cryoglobulinemia, dermatitis herpetiformis, and chronic progressive multiple sclerosis, also have defects in Fc-receptor function as judged by clearance of IgG-coated erythrocytes (see Chap. 261). Clinically, normal subjects with genetic haplotypes commonly associated with autoimmune disease (i.e., HLA-B8/DRw3) also have an increased incidence of defective Fc receptor–specific functional activity, suggesting that this defect may predispose individuals with this genetic profile to immune complex disease.

EOSINOPHILS

Eosinophils and neutrophils share similar morphology, many lysosomal constituents, most chemotactic responses, phagocytic capacity, and oxidative metabolism. However, there are major differences between the two cell types, and little is known about the natural function of eosinophils. Eosinophils are much longer lived than neutrophils and, unlike neutrophils, tissue eosinophils can recirculate. During most infections eosinophils do not appear to have any important function. However, in invasive parasite infections, such as hookworm, schistosomiasis, strongyloidiasis, toxocariasis, trichinosis, filariasis, echinococcosis, and cysticercosis, the eosinophil likely plays a central role in host defense. Eosinophils are also associated with bronchial asthma, cutaneous allergic reactions, and other hypersensitivity states.

The characteristic red-staining eosinophil granules (Wright's stain) contain a number of unique constituents. The distinctive feature of the eosinophil granule is its crystalline core consisting of an arginine-rich protein (major basic protein) with histaminase activity, which is probably important in host defense against parasites. Eosinophil granules also contain a unique eosinophil peroxidase which catalyzes the oxidation of many substances by hydrogen perioxide and may facilitate killing of microorganisms. Eosinophil peroxidase, in the presence of hydrogen perioxide and halide, initiates mast cell secretion in vitro and thereby may contribute to inflammation. Other substances found in eosinophils include cationic proteins, some of which bind to heparin and reduce its anticoagulant activity. Eosinophil cytoplasm contains Charcot-Leyden crystal protein, a hexagonal bipyramidal crystal first described in leukemia and then in sputum from asthma patients, which is a lysophospholipase and may function to restrict the toxicity of certain lysophospholipids. Eosinophils also contain a powerful neurotoxin. Because patients with hypereosinophilic syndrome and cerebral spinal fluid eosinophilia exhibit varied neurologic abnormalities, eosinophil-derived neurotoxin may play an important role in central nervous system disease.

Several factors enhance the eosinophil's function in host defense. For example, T-cell-derived eosinophil stimulation promoter enhances the ability of eosinophils to kill parasites. Mast-cell-derived eosinophil chemotactic factor of anaphylaxis (ECFa) increases the number of eosinophil complement receptors and enhances eosinophil killing of parasites. In addition, eosinophil colony-stimulating factors produced by macrophages may not only increase eosinophil production in the bone marrow but also activate eosinophils to kill parasites.

EOSINOPHILIA More than 500 eosinophils per cubic millimeter of blood is common in many settings besides parasite infection. The most common cause of eosinophilia is probably allergic reactions to drugs such as iodides, aspirin, and sulfonamides. Allergies such as hay fever, asthma, and eczema commonly are associated with eosinophilia. Eosinophilia is also seen in collagen vascular diseases (e.g., rheumatoid arthritis, eosinophilic fasciitis, allergic angiitis, and granulomatosis) and malignancies (e.g., Hodgkin's disease, mycosis fungoides) as well as the hyperimmunoglobulin E–recurrent infection (Job's) syndrome and the chronic granulomatous diseases; the mechanism for the eosinophilia in these diseases is not known. The most dramatic increases in eosinophils occur in hypereosinophilic syndromes incuding Loeffler's syndrome, eosinophilic leukemia, as well as idiopathic hypereosinophilic syndrome (with counts as high as 50,000 to 100,000 eosinophils per cubic millimeter).

The idiopathic hypereosinophilic syndrome represents a heterogeneous group of disorders with the common feature being prolonged eosinophilia of unknown cause and associated organ system dysfunction, including the heart, central nervous system, kidneys, lungs, gastrointestinal tract, and skin. The bone marrow is involved in all subjects, but the most severe complications involve the heart and central nervous system. Eosinophils are found in the involved tissues and are thought to cause tissue damage by local deposition of toxic eosinophil proteins such as eosinophil cationic protein and eosinophil major basic protein. In the heart the pathological changes lead to thrombosis which may result in endocardial fibrosis and restrictive endomyocardiopathy. Similar pathological changes are thought to contribute to the damage of tissues in other organ systems. Although the mechanism for the hypereosinophilia is not known, it has been shown that chemotherapy with corticosteroids usually induces remission. In patients unresponsive to corticosteroids, a cytotoxic agent, such as hydroxyurea, has been used successfully to lower the peripheral blood eosinophil counts and to improve markedly prognosis. Aggressive medical and surgical approaches are also employed when managing patients with cardiovascular complications.

EOSINOPENIA This occurs with stress, such as acute bacterial infection, and following administration of corticosteroids. The mechanism of eosinopenia of acute bacterial infection is unknown but is independent of endogenous corticosteroids since it occurs in animals following total adrenalectomy. There is no known adverse effect of eosinopenia.

DIAGNOSIS AND MANAGEMENT OF PHAGOCYTE DYSFUNCTION

Diagnosis of phagocytic cell disorders is suggested from clinical evaluation. Neutropenia or impaired neutrophil function is frequently associated with depressed inflammation. Aphthous ulcers of the mucous membranes (gray ulcers without pus) are not uncommon. Gingivitis is common and periodontal disease is frequent in some patients. Characteristically, patients with phagocyte defects have recurrent and often severe bacterial or fungal infections which often present as difficult management problems. Patients with congenital defects can have infections within the first few days of life. In some disorders the frequency of infection is variable and patients can go months or even years without major infection. Adults over 30 years of age with congenital defects are unusual, suggesting that patients with such defects die at an early age. However, in recent years, with aggressive management, adults with these diseases are being seen with increasing frequency. Skin, ear, upper and lower respiratory tract and bone infections are common. Sepsis and meningitis are rare.

Initial studies of white blood count and differential and often bone marrow exam are followed by assessment of bone marrow reserves (steroid challenge test), marginated circulating pool of cells (epinephrine challenge test), and marginating ability (endotoxin challenge test). In vivo assessment of inflammation is possible with a Rebuck skin window test, in which the ability of leukocytes to accumulate at a superficial abrasion and adhere to a glass coverslip is tested. In vivo clearance of IgG-coated erythrocytes provides a useful way to monitor the mononuclear-phagocyte (reticuloendothelial) system. In vitro tests of phagocyte aggregation, adherence, chemotaxis, phagocytosis, degranulation, and microbicidal activity (for *Staphylococcus aureus*) help pinpoint cellular or humoral lesions which can then be further characterized at the molecular level. Deficiencies of oxidative metabolism are screened with the nitroblue tetrazolium dye (NBT) test, which is based on the ability of products of oxidative metabolism to reduce yellow, soluble NBT to blue-black formazan, an insoluble material which precipitates intracellularly and can be seen microscopically. Further aspects of neutrophil oxidative metabolism are defined by studies of superoxide and hydrogen perioxide production.

The most important aspect of patient management is to appreciate that patients often have delayed inflammatory responses. Therefore, clinical manifestations may be minimal despite overwhelming infection, and unusual infections must always be suspected in some patients. Early signs of infection demand prompt, aggressive use of antibiotics and surgical drainage of abscesses. Prolonged antibiotics are often required, and in life-threatening infections daily white blood cell transfusions (enriched for neutrophils) are probably beneficial, although their use is still controversial. In patients with the chronic granulomatous diseases, prophylactic antibiotics (trimethoprim-sulfamethoxazole) probably diminish the frequency of life-threatening infections. Rigorous oral hygiene reduces but does not eliminate the discomfort of gingivitis, periodontal disease, and aphthous ulcers; tooth brushing with a hydrogen peroxide–sodium bicarbonate paste helps some patients. Ketoconazole has caused dramatic improvement of mucocutaneous candidiasis in patients with the hyperimmunoglobulin E–recurrent infection (Job's) syndrome. Treatment to restore myelopoiesis in patients with neutropenia due to impaired production has included use of androgens, glucocorticoids, lithium, and immunosuppressive therapy. Cure of some congenital phagocyte defects is theoretically possible by bone marrow transplantation (see Chap. 291). However, complications of bone marrow transplantation are still great, and with rigorous medical care many patients with phagocytic disorders can go for years without a life-threatening infection.

REFERENCES

Adams DO: Macrophage activation and secretion. Fed Proc 41:2193, 1982

Anderson DC et al: The severe and moderate phenotypes of heritable Mac1, LFA-1 deficiency: Their quantitative definition and relation to leukocyte dysfunction and clinical features. J Infect Dis 152:668, 1985

Babior BM: The respiratory burst of phagocytes. J Clin Invest 73:599, 1984

Buescher ES et al: Use of an X-linked human neutrophil marker to estimate timing of Lyonization and size of the dividing stem cell pool. J Clin Invest 76:1581, 1985

Dale DC et al: Chronic neutropenia. Medicine 38:128, 1979

Dinarello, CA: Interleukin 1. Rev Infect Dis 6:51, 1984

Donabedian H, Gallin JI: The hyperimmunoglobulin E–recurrent infection (Job's) syndrome. A review of the NIH experience and the literature. Medicine 62:195, 1983

Dreskin SC et al: Immunoglobulins in the hyperimmunoglobulin E and recurrent infection (Job's) syndrome. Deficiency of anti-*Staphylococcus aureus* immunoglobulin A. J Clin Invest 75:26, 1985

Fauci AS et al: The idiopathic hypereosinophilic syndrome: Clinical, pathophysiologic, and therapeutic considerations. Ann Intern Med 97:78, 1982

Gallin JI: Abnormal phagocyte chemotaxis: Pathophysiology, clinical manifestations, and management of patients. Rev Infect Dis 3:1196, 1981

———: Neutrophil heterogeneity exists, but is it meaningful? Blood 63:977, 1984

———: Neutrophil specific granule deficiency. Ann Rev Med 36:263, 1985

———, Eauci AS (eds): *Advances in Host Defense Mechanisms,* vol. 1: *Phagocytic Cells.* New York, Raven, 1982

——— et al: Recent advances in chronic granulomatous disease. Ann Intern Med 99:657, 1983

Gleich GJ, Loegeung DA: Immunobiology of eosinophils. Ann Rev Immunol 2:429, 1984

Smith PD, et al: Monocyte function in the acquired immune deficiency syndrome. Defective chemotaxis. J Clin Invest 74:2121, 1984

Tauber AI et al: Chronic granulomatous disease: A syndrome of phagocyte oxidase deficiences. Medicine 62:286, 1983

PART TWO BIOLOGIC CONSIDERATIONS IN THE APPROACH TO CLINICAL MEDICINE

section 1 Genetics and human disease

57 GENETIC ASPECTS OF DISEASE

JOSEPH L. GOLDSTEIN / MICHAEL S. BROWN

GENETIC PRINCIPLES

More than one-fifth of the proteins (and hence genes) in each human being exist in a form that differs from the one present in the majority of the population. This remarkable genetic variability, or polymorphism, among "normal" people accounts for much of the normal variation in body traits such as height, intelligence, and blood pressure. These genetic differences also determine the ability of each individual to meet environmental challenges, including those that produce disease. All human diseases can be considered to result from an interaction between an individual's unique genetic makeup and the environment. In certain diseases, the genetic component is so overwhelming that it expresses itself in a predictable manner without a requirement for extraordinary environmental challenges. Such diseases are termed *genetic disorders*.

MOLECULAR BASIS OF GENE EXPRESSION All hereditary information is transmitted from parent to offspring through the inheritance of deoxyribonucleic acid (DNA). DNA is a linear polymer composed of purine and pyrimidine bases whose sequence ultimately determines the sequence of amino acids in every protein made by the body. The four types of bases in DNA are arranged in groups of three, each triplet forming a code word, or codon, that signifies a particular amino acid. A *gene* represents the total sequence of bases in DNA that specifies the amino acid sequence of a single polypeptide chain of a protein molecule.

Genetic information encoded in the DNA of the chromosomes is first transcribed into a *ribonucleic acid* (RNA) copy. During transcription the ribose nucleotides align themselves along the DNA according to base-pairing rules. Thus, adenine of DNA pairs with uridine of RNA, cytosine pairs with guanine, thymine pairs with adenine, and guanine pairs with cytosine. The ribose bases are joined together by RNA polymerase. The resulting *RNA transcript* forms the template for translation into the amino acid sequence of a protein. Figure 57-1 shows the DNA and mRNA code words for each of the amino acids in protein.

Figure 57-2 illustrates a schematic diagram of the genetic control of protein synthesis in higher organisms, including humans. The DNA of most genes is fragmented into discrete coding regions (exons) separated by noncoding regions (introns or intervening sequences). The *coding regions* contain the bases that specify the sequence of amino acids in the polypeptide chain. The *intervening sequences* are

FIGURE 57-1 *The genetic code.*

First nucleotide	Second nucleotide: **A** or *U*			**G** or *C*			**T** or *A*			**C** or *G*			Third nucleotide
A or *U*	**AAA**	*UUU*	Phe	**AGA**	*UCU*	Ser	**ATA**	*UAU*	Tyr	**ACA**	*UGU*	Cys	**A** or *U*
	AAG	*UUC*		**AGG**	*UCC*		**ATG**	*UAC*		**ACG**	*UGC*		**G** or *C*
	AAT	*UUA*	Leu	**AGT**	*UCA*		**ATT**	*UAA*	Stop	**ACT**	*UGA*	Stop	**T** or *A*
	AAC	*UUG*		**AGC**	*UCG*		**ATC**	*UAG*		**ACC**	*UGG*	Trp	**C** or *G*
G or *C*	**GAA**	*CUU*	Leu	**GGA**	*CCU*	Pro	**GTA**	*CAU*	His	**GCA**	*CGU*	Arg	**A** or *U*
	GAG	*CUC*		**GGG**	*CCC*		**GTG**	*CAC*		**GCG**	*CGC*		**G** or *C*
	GAT	*CUA*		**GGT**	*CCA*		**GTT**	*CAA*	Gln	**GCT**	*CGA*		**T** or *A*
	GAC	*CUG*		**GGC**	*CCG*		**GTC**	*CAG*		**GCC**	*CGG*		**C** or *G*
T or *A*	**TAA**	*AUU*	Ile	**TGA**	*ACU*	Thr	**TTA**	*AAU*	Asn	**TCA**	*AGU*	Ser	**A** or *U*
	TAG	*AUC*		**TGG**	*ACC*		**TTG**	*AAC*		**TCG**	*AGC*		**G** or *C*
	TAT	*AUA*		**TGT**	*ACA*		**TTT**	*AAA*	Lys	**TCT**	*AGA*	Arg	**T** or *A*
	TAC	*AUG*	Met	**TGC**	*ACG*		**TTC**	*AAG*		**TCC**	*AGG*		**C** or *G*
C or *G*	**CAA**	*GUU*	Val	**CGA**	*GCU*	Ala	**CTA**	*GAU*	Asp	**CCA**	*GGU*	Gly	**A** or *U*
	CAG	*GUC*		**CGG**	*GCC*		**CTG**	*GAC*		**CCG**	*GGC*		**G** or *C*
	CAT	*GUA*		**CGT**	*GCA*		**CTT**	*GAA*	Glu	**CCT**	*GGA*		**T** or *A*
	CAC	*GUG*		**CGC**	*GCG*		**CTC**	*GAG*		**CCC**	*GGG*		**C** or *G*

Note: The DNA codons appear in boldface type; the complementary RNA codons are in italics. A = adenine, C = cytosine, G = guanine, T = thymine, U = uridine (replaces thymine in RNA). In RNA, adenine is complementary to thymine of DNA; uridine is complementary to adenine of DNA; cytosine is complementary to guanine, and vice versa. "Stop" = termination. The amino acids are abbreviated as follows:

Ala = alanine	*Cys = cysteine*	*His = histidine*	*Met = methionine*	*Thr = threonine*
Arg = arginine	*Gln = glutamine*	*Ile = isoleucine*	*Phe = phenylalanine*	*Trp = tryptophan*
Asn = asparagine	*Glu = glutamic acid*	*Leu = leucine*	*Pro = proline*	*Tyr = tyrosine*
Asp = aspartic acid	*Gly = glycine*	*Lys = lysine*	*Ser = serine*	*Val = valine*

composed of bases that act as spacers between the coding regions; they are not translated into protein. The transcription of DNA produces a faithful copy of the entire gene sequence; thus, the RNA transcript contains altering coding and intervening sequences. The RNA transcript is edited in the nucleus before it passes into the cytoplasm. In the editing process, the intervening sequences are excised, and the coding regions are spliced together to form one continuous gene (Fig. 57-2).

After processing, the edited RNA, which is called *messenger RNA* (mRNA) leaves the nucleus and enters the cytoplasm where it becomes associated with *ribosomes* and thereby serves as a template for the ribosomal synthesis of proteins. Each of the 20 amino acids is attached in the cell cytoplasm to a specific molecule called *transfer RNA* (tRNA). Each tRNA contains a triplet sequence of purine and pyrimidine bases that is "complementary" to a specific codon in the mRNA. These tRNA molecules with their attached amino acids line up along the mRNA molecule in the precise order dictated by the genetic code. Under the action of cytoplasmic enzymes (initiation factors, elongation factors, and termination factors), peptide bonds are formed between the various amino acids, and the completed protein is released from the ribosome. For a more detailed account of the molecular basis of gene expression, see Chap. 58.

MAINTENANCE OF GENETIC DIVERSITY THROUGH TRANSMISSION AND SEGREGATION OF GENES The amount of DNA in the nucleus of each human cell is sufficient to code for more than 50,000 genes and hence to specify more than 50,000 polypeptide chains. The genes are arranged in a linear sequence of DNA that together with certain histone proteins form rod-shaped bodies called *chromosomes*. Each somatic cell contains 46 chromosomes, arranged in 23 pairs, one of each pair derived from each parent. Thus, each individual inherits two copies of each chromosome and hence two copies of each gene. The chromosomal location of the two copies of each gene is termed the *genetic locus*. When a gene occupying a genetic locus exists in two or more different forms, these alternate forms of the gene are referred to as *alleles*.

In humans, a given gene always resides at a specified genetic locus on one particular chromosome. For example, the genetic locus for the Rh blood group is on the short arm of chromosome 1; at this site there are two Rh genes, one on chromosome 1 derived from the mother and the other on chromosome 1 derived from the father. When two genes at the same genetic locus are identical, the individual is a *homozygote*. When the two genes differ (i.e., two different alleles are present at the locus), the individual is a *heterozygote*. Each normal human is heterozygous at approximately 20 percent of genetic loci and homozygous at 80 percent. Figure 57-3 shows a map of human chromosome 1, illustrating the location of a representative sample of genes that have been assigned loci on this chromosome.

The genetic information carried on chromosomes is transmitted to daughter cells under two different sets of circumstances. One of these occurs whenever a somatic cell (i.e., a nongerm cell) divides. This process, called *mitosis*, transmits identical copies of each gene to each daughter cell, thus maintaining a uniform genetic makeup in all cells of a single individual. The other set of circumstances prevails when genetic information must be transmitted from one individual to an offspring. This process, called *meiosis*, produces germ cells (i.e., ova or spermatozoa) that possess only one copy of each parental chromosome, thus allowing for new combinations of chromosomes to occur when ovum and sperm cell fuse during fertilization.

During meiosis, the 46 chromosomes of an immature germ cell arrange themselves in 23 pairs at the center of the nucleus, each pair being composed of one chromosome derived from the mother and its homologous chromosome derived from the father. At a specified point in the meiotic process, the two partner chromosomes separate, only one of each pair going into each daughter cell, or gamete. Thus, meiosis produces gametes with a reduction in the number of chromosomes from 46 to 23, each gamete having received one chromosome from each of the 23 pairs. The assortment of the chromosomes within each pair is random so that each germ cell receives a different combination of maternal and paternal chromosomes. During the process of fertilization, the fusion of ovum and sperm cell, each of which has 23 chromosomes, produces an individual with 46 chromosomes.

The independent assortment of chromosomes into gametes during meiosis produces an enormous diversity among the possible genotypes of the progeny. For each 23 pairs of chromosomes, there are 2^{23} different combinations of chromosomes that could occur in a gamete, and the likelihood that one set of parents will produce two offspring with the identical complement of chromosomes is one in 2^{23} or one in 8.4 million (assuming no monozygotic or identical twins).

RECOMBINATION Adding to the genetic diversity in humans is the phenomenon of *genetic recombination*. During meiosis, when homologous chromosomes are paired, bridges frequently form between corresponding regions of the chromosome pair. These bridges, or *chiasmata*, are regions in which the two chromosomes break at identical points along their length and subsequently rejoin, the distal segments having been switched from one homologous chromosome to another. This process is designated *crossing over*. Although no net change in the amount of genetic material occurs during crossing

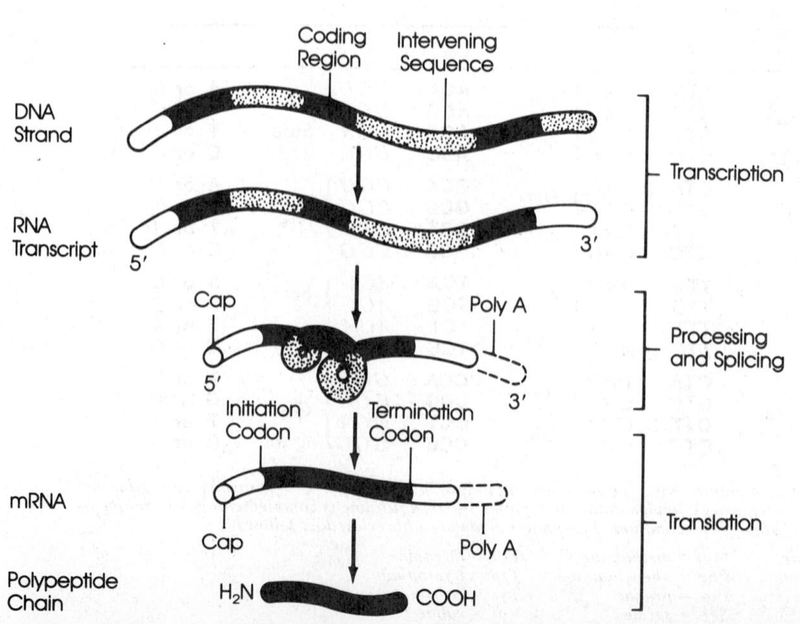

FIGURE 57-2 *A schematic diagram of the genetic control of protein synthesis, illustrating the flow of genetic information from the base sequence of DNA to the RNA transcript (transcription) to mRNA (processing) to the polypeptide chain of a protein molecule (translation). Although DNA exists in a double-stranded form, only one of the two strands is used as a template for transcribing the RNA transcript. Solid sections represent coding regions in DNA, RNA transcript, mRNA, and amino acid sequence in polypeptide chain; dotted sections represent intervening sequences in DNA and RNA transcript.*

over, a recombination of genes does occur. For example, consider a chromosome with two loci, A and B, located at opposite ends of the same chromosome. On this particular chromosome, the A locus has a rare allele *x*, and the B locus also has a rare allele *y*. Without the phenomenon of recombination every offspring that inherited the *x* allele at the A locus would also inherit the *y* allele at the B locus. However, if recombination occurs, the A locus with the *x* allele would then be on the opposite chromosome from the B locus with the *y* allele. In this case any offspring that inherited the *x* allele at the A locus could not inherit the *y* allele at the B locus.

Crossing over occurs with great frequency in every meiosis in humans, and the resultant recombination of genes may occur at any point on a chromosome. The farther apart two genes are on the same chromosome, the greater is the likelihood that a crossing over will occur in the space between them. When two genes are on the opposite ends of a long chromosome, the probability of recombination is so great that their respective alleles are transmitted to offspring almost independently of one another, just as if the two gene loci were on different chromosomes. On the other hand, gene loci that are close together on the same chromosome are said to be *linked* so that there is a great likelihood that offspring will inherit the same combination of alleles that are present on the parental chromosome.

Several examples of *gene linkage* can be seen from the map of human chromosome 1 (Fig. 57-3). For example, the locus for the gene specifying the Rh blood group factor and the locus for the gene producing one form of the dominant trait hereditary elliptocytosis occur in close proximity on this chromosome. Thus, if a subject with hereditary elliptocytosis transmits the disease to an offspring, the offspring will usually inherit the allele that is present at the Rh locus on this chromosome. If the Rh allele happens to be a rare one in the population (such as r'), one can assume that whichever offspring inherits the r' allele at the Rh locus will also inherit the abnormal allele at the elliptocytosis locus. On the other hand, if an offspring does not exhibit the r' allele, he or she will not usually have elliptocytosis. The concept of linkage does not imply an association between any particular set of Rh alleles and the disease state elliptocytosis, rather between the two genetic loci. Thus, in different families the abnormal elliptocytosis allele may be linked to the R^1, R^0, r_2, or any other allele at the Rh locus, depending on the allele that happened to be at that locus when the elliptocytosis mutation occurred. Stated another way, the elliptocytosis locus is linked to the Rh locus in every family, but the particular Rh allele with which it is associated differs from family to family.

MUTATION Broadly defined, a *mutation* is a stable, heritable alteration in DNA. Although the causes of mutation in humans are largely unknown, a variety of environmental agents, such as radiation, viruses, and chemicals, are among the factors that are implicated.

Mutations can involve a visible alteration in the structure of a chromosome, such as a deletion or translocation of a portion of a chromosome, or they can involve a minute change in one of the purine or pyrimidine bases of a single gene. Most commonly, such "point" mutations consist of the substitution of one base for another, changing the meaning of the codon containing that base, hence their designation as *missense mutations*. For example, in the gene coding for the β chain of hemoglobin, the sixth position normally contains the nucleotide triplet CTC, which codes for the amino acid glutamic acid (Fig. 57-1). The mutation that gives rise to hemoglobin C produces a change of the first base of this triplet from cytosine to thymine, changing the triplet to TTC, which codes for lysine. On the other hand, the mutation that gives rise to hemoglobin S produces a change in the second base of the same triplet (from thymine to adenine), producing CAC, which codes for valine. Thus, in the sixth position of the β chain of hemoglobin, the normally occurring glutamic acid may be replaced with either lysine (producing hemoglobin C) or valine (producing hemoglobin S). More than 90 such single-base mutations in the hemoglobin β chain have been identified, and many of these mutations produce distinct clinical syndromes. Of all the mutations so far elucidated in humans, most involve such single-base changes.

Besides producing an amino acid substitution, a single-base substitution can also cause another abnormality in protein synthesis—premature chain termination. Three mRNA code words (UAA, UAG, and UGA) normally do not specify an amino acid but constitute the signal that the message has ended and that the protein chain should be released from the ribosome (Fig. 57-1). If a change occurs in DNA that produces one of these mRNA code words [for example, a switch in an mRNA triplet from UAU (tyrosine) to UAA (termination)], the polypeptide chain would be terminated prematurely when translation had reached that point. Such mutations, called *non-sense mutations,* produce short fragments of proteins that have reduced function.

CELLULAR MECHANISM BY WHICH MUTANT GENES PRODUCE DISEASES Critical to the understanding of heredity is the concept that the only information transmitted from generation to generation is the sequence of bases in DNA and that these sequences in turn specify only the primary structure of RNA and protein molecules. All other chemical reactions—such as the synthesis of complex lipids and carbohydrates, the formation of membranes and other cellular organelles, and the accumulation and partitioning of inorganic ions—occur as a secondary consequence of the action of specific proteins. Many of these proteins are enzymes that catalyze the biochemical conversion of one molecule into another. Others are structural proteins such as collagen and elastin, and still others are regulatory proteins that dictate how much of each enzyme and each structural protein is made.

Since proteins are the cellular molecules whose structures are encoded by genes, mutations in genes exert their deleterious effects by altering the structure of enzymes, structural proteins, or regulatory

FIGURE 57-3 *Gene map of human chromosome 1, illustrating a representative sample of the genes that have been localized to this chromosome. The black bands represent those genetic regions of the chromosome that stain brightly by a fluorescent dye such as quinacrine; the white bands are the negatively staining regions; the hatched area is a variable region that stains differently (i.e., either brightly or negatively) in the chromosomes of different individuals. Each gene is listed opposite its genetic locus on the right. (Data provided by VA McKusick.)*

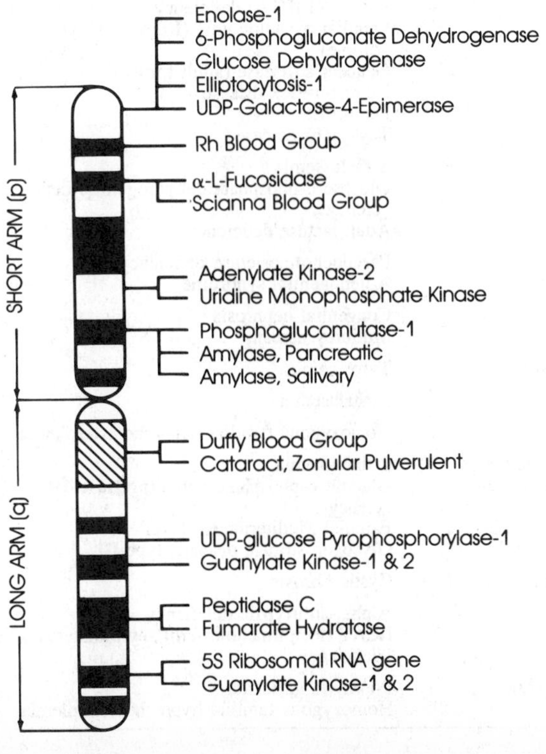

proteins. For example, in a disease such as glycogen storage disease, type I (von Gierke's disease), massive accumulation of glycogen in the liver is due not to a primary structural abnormality in the polysaccharide glycogen but to a structural abnormality in a protein, glucose 6-phosphatase, an enzyme that is required to liberate glucose so as to permit glycogen breakdown. Other examples of the biochemical mechanisms by which mutant genes alter cellular metabolism are discussed below under "Simply Inherited Disorders."

GENETIC HETEROGENEITY When two or more mutations can produce a similar clinical syndrome, genetic heterogeneity is said to exist. Hemophilia is one example of a genetically heterogeneous syndrome. A clinically similar bleeding disorder can be caused by mutations at either of two loci on the X chromosome, one leading to a deficiency of factor VIII (classic hemophilia) and the other causing a deficiency of factor IX (Christmas disease). Most, if not all, hereditary diseases, when carefully analyzed, will probably prove to be genetically heterogeneous.

Genetic heterogeneity may result from the existence of a series of different mutations at a single genetic locus (allelic mutations) or from mutations at different genetic loci (nonallelic mutations). For example, drug-induced hemolysis of red blood cells can occur in patients with several different types of allelic mutations at the glucose 6-phosphate dehydrogenase locus. On the other hand, hemophilia is an example of a syndrome in which nonallelic mutations can produce a similar clinical picture (see above).

In some cases of heterogeneity, both the genetic locus and the mode of inheritance differ. Diseases such as spastic paraplegia, Charcot-Marie-Tooth peroneal muscular atrophy, and retinitis pigmentosa are inherited as autosomal dominant traits in some families, as autosomal recessives in others, and as X-linked recessives in still others. The identification of such genetic heterogeneity in these disorders is of obvious importance for correct genetic counseling.

TABLE 57-1 Examples of simply inherited disorders that occur with increased frequency in specific ethnic groups

Ethnic group	Simply inherited disorder
African blacks	Hemoglobinopathies, especially Hb S, Hb C, persistent Hb F, α and β thalassemias Glucose 6-phosphate dehydrogenase deficiency
Armenians	Familial Mediterranean fever
Ashkenazi Jews	Abetalipoproteinemia Bloom's syndrome Dystonia musculorum deformans (recessive form) Factor XI (PTA) deficiency Familial dysautonomia (Riley-Day syndrome) Gaucher's disease (adult form) Neimann-Pick disease Pentosuria Tay-Sachs disease
Chinese	α thalassemia Glucose 6-phosphate dehydrogenase deficiency Adult lactase deficiency
Eskimos	Pseudocholinesterase deficiency Adrenogenital syndrome
Finns	Congenital nephrosis Mulibrey nanism
French Canadians	Tyrosinemia
Japanese	Acatalasemia
Lebanese	Homozygous familial hypercholesterolemia
Mediterranean peoples (Italians, Greeks, Sephardic Jews)	β thalassemia Glucose 6-phosphate dehydrogenase deficiency Familial Mediterranean fever Glycogen storage disease, type III
Northern Europeans	Cystic fibrosis
Scandinavians	$Alpha_1$-antitrypsin deficiency LCAT (lecithin:cholesterol acyltransferase) deficiency
South African whites	Porphyria variegata Homozygous familial hypercholesterolemia

TAKING THE FAMILY HISTORY

The investigation of a patient with a possible genetic disorder begins with the *family history*. The first step is to obtain certain information on the *proband* or *index case* (i.e., the clinically affected person who has brought the family to attention) and on each of the *first-degree relatives* (i.e., the parents, siblings, and offspring of the proband). This information includes the given name, surname, maiden name, birth date or current age, age at death, cause of death, and name or description of any disease or defect.

The second step is to ask questions designed to survey the family for the presence of disease or defect. (1) Has any relative an identical or similar trait? (2) Has any relative a trait that is absent in the proband but is known to occur in some patients with the same disease? This question requires that the physician have some knowledge about the manifestations of the disease in question. For example, when obtaining the family history from a proband with dissecting aneurysm caused possibly by Marfan's syndrome, one should ask about the occurrence of eye abnormalities, cardiac abnormalities, and skeletal abnormalities in the relatives. (3) Has any relative a trait that is recognized to be genetically determined? The purpose of this question is to ascertain the occurrence of hereditary disease in the family even though the particular patient may not be involved. (4) Has any relative an unusual disease, or has any relative died of a rare condition? The purpose of this question is to identify a condition that might be genetically determined though not recognized as such by the informant. In addition, this question may help to identify conditions in relatives that might be etiologically related to the patient's problem. For example, a patient with pheochromocytoma should be suspected of having von Recklinghausen's disease if he or she has a brother with scoliosis and mental retardation, both of which can be manifestations of the neurofibromatosis (von Recklinghausen's) gene. (5) Is there any consanguinity in the family? This inquiry should be made directly. In addition, one should ask whether common last names appear in the families of husband-wife pairs. Consanguineous marriage may be the source of a rare autosomal recessive syndrome, and sometimes its presence in the family may not be known by the proband. (6) What is the ethnic origin of the family? Persons of various ethnic origins, such as blacks, Jews, and Greeks, have increased chances of specific genetic diseases. Table 57-1 lists examples of simply inherited disorders that are found with increased frequency in various ethnic groups.

CATEGORIES OF GENETIC DISORDERS

Genetic diseases generally fall into one of three categories: (1) *Chromosomal disorders* involve the lack, excess, or abnormal arrangement of one or more chromosomes, producing excessive or deficient genetic material. (2) *Mendelian or simply inherited disorders* are determined primarily by a single mutant gene. These disorders display inheritance patterns which can be classified into autosomal dominant, autosomal recessive, or X-linked types. (3) *Mulifactorial disorders* are caused by an interaction of multiple genes and multiple exogenous or environmental factors. Although many of these multifactorial disorders, such as essential hypertension and cleft lip and palate, are said to run in families, the inheritance pattern is complex and the risk to relatives is less than in the single-gene (mendelian) disorders. Each of these categories presents different problems with respect to causation, prevention, diagnosis, genetic counseling, and treatment.

CHROMOSOMAL DISORDERS The karyotype of an individual (i.e., the number and structure of the chromosomes) can be ascertained from readily accessible body tissues, such as peripheral blood lymphocytes or skin, by growing them in tissue culture until active cell proliferation occurs and then preparing single cells for examination of chromosomes by microscopy. Each individual chromosome can be identified by special staining of DNA sequences, for example, by the affinity of fluorescent dyes (such as quinacrine hydrochloride) for certain chromosomal segments that can be visualized by fluorescence microscopy or by treatment with special dyes (Giemsa) and proteolytic enzymes (trypsin). These techniques produce characteristic *banding patterns* for each chromosome (Fig. 57-4).

The number of chromosomes in normal individuals is 46, of which 44 are the 22 pairs of *autosomes* and the other two are the *sex chromosomes*. Women have two X chromosomes (XX), and men have one X chromosome and one Y chromosome (XY). Each of the 22 pairs of autosomes and the two sex chromosomes can be distinguished on the basis of size, location of the centromere (which divides the chromosome into arms of equal or unequal length), and the unique banding pattern (Fig. 57-4). The relative length of the arms and the position of the centromere are used as further criteria to divide the human chromosomes into seven groups (designated A to G) (Fig. 57-4).

For a complete discussion of the etiology and clinical features of chromosomal abnormalities affecting humans, the reader is referred to Chap. 60.

SIMPLY INHERITED DISORDERS Disorders caused by the transmission of a single mutant gene show one of three simple (or mendelian) patterns of inheritance: (1) autosomal dominant, (2) autosomal recessive, or (3) X-linked. The distinction between "dominant" and "recessive" is one of convenience in pedigree analysis and does not imply a fundamental difference in genetic mechanism. The term *dominant* implies that a mutation is clinically manifest when an individual has a single dose of this mutation (or is *heterozygous* for it), while *recessive* implies that a double dose (or *homozygosity*) is required for clinical detection. Genes are never dominant or recessive; their effects, however, produce clinical patterns that are classified as dominant or recessive. Despite their overall clinical "normality," individuals who are heterozygous for "recessive" genes often have biochemical abnormalities that are demonstrable in the laboratory; on the other hand, those who are homozygous for "dominant" genes are usually more severely affected than are the heterozygotes.

With few exceptions, each of the approximately 1200 mendelian diseases is rare. However, as a group these disorders constitute an important cause of morbidity and death, accounting directly for more than 5 percent of all hospital admissions.

The genes for more than 100 simply inherited diseases have been assigned to specific chromosomes. Disease-producing genes assigned to the X chromosome outnumber those so far assigned to any single autosome. This is because assignment to the X chromosome requires only pedigree studies showing X-linked inheritance (see below). Assignment to an autosome is more complicated, requiring sophisticated techniques of somatic cell hybridization or pedigree studies showing linkage between a disease-producing gene and a "marker" gene that is known to be on a certain chromosome. Table 57-2 shows a partial list of those human genetic diseases that have been mapped to specific chromosomes.

The demonstration that a particular disease or syndrome shows one of the three mendelian patterns of inheritance implies that its pathogenesis, no matter how complex, is due to an abnormality in a single protein molecule. For example, in sickle cell anemia, the entire clinical syndrome, including such seemingly unrelated disturbances as anemia, pain crises, nephropathy, and predisposition to pneumococcal infections, are all the physiologic consequences of having thymine instead of adenine at a specific site in the gene that codes for the β chain of hemoglobin, producing a substitution of a valine for a glutamic acid in the sixth amino acid position in the protein sequence.

In many mendelian disorders, especially in those with dominant inheritance, it is not possible to demonstrate directly the protein that is primarily altered by the mutation. In such cases (e.g., adult polycystic kidney disease and tuberous sclerosis) only the distal physiologic effects of the mutation are recognizable. Nevertheless, it is safe to assume that a single primary defect exists whenever a disease is transmitted by a single gene mechanism and that the various manifestations of the disease all can be related to the mutational event by a more or less complicated "pedigree of causes." Table 57-3 lists the most commonly encountered mendelian disorders affecting adults.

Autosomal dominant disorders Dominant diseases are those manifest in the heterozygous state, that is, when only one abnormal gene (*mutant allele*) is present and the corresponding partner allele on the homologous chromosome is normal. The gene responsible for an autosomal dominant disorder is located on one of the 22 autosomes, and both males and females can be affected. Since alleles segregate independently at meiosis, there is a 1 in 2 chance that the offspring of an affected heterozygote will inherit the mutant allele and, similarly, a 1 in 2 chance of the offspring inheriting the normal allele.

Figure 57-5 shows a typical pedigree involving an autosomal dominant trait. The following features are characteristic: (1) Each affected individual has an affected parent (unless the condition arose by a new mutation or is mildly expressed in the affected parent); (2) an affected individual will bear, on the average, both normal and affected offspring in equal proportions; (3) normal children of an affected individual will have only normal offspring; (4) males and females are affected in equal proportions; (5) each sex is equally likely to transmit the condition to male and female offspring, with male-to-male transmission occurring; and (6) vertical transmission of the condition through successive generations occurs, especially when the trait does not impair reproductive capacity.

While half of the offspring of an individual with an autosomal dominant condition will inherit the disease, it is not necessarily true that each affected person must have an affected parent. In every autosomal dominant disease a certain proportion of affected persons owe their disorder to a new mutation rather than to an inherited mutation. Since the estimated frequency of mutation is 5×10^{-6} mutations per gene per generation and since a dominant trait, by definition, requires a mutation in only one of a pair of alleles, one would expect that about 1 in 100,000 newborn persons would possess a new mutation at any given genetic locus. Many of these mutations

FIGURE 57-4 *The karyotype of a normal male showing the chromosomes of a single somatic cell in the metaphase stage of cell division. The photographic images of the chromosomes have been cut out and arranged according to descending length and varying arm ratio. The chromosomes have been stained by the Giemsa technique, which allows each chromosome pair to be identified by its unique banding pattern. Chromosomes 1 to 22 are the autosomes. The sex chromosomes in this normal male are an X and a Y. The normal female has an identical karyotype except for the absence of the Y chromosome and the presence instead of a second X chromosome. (Courtesy of K Hirschhorn.)*

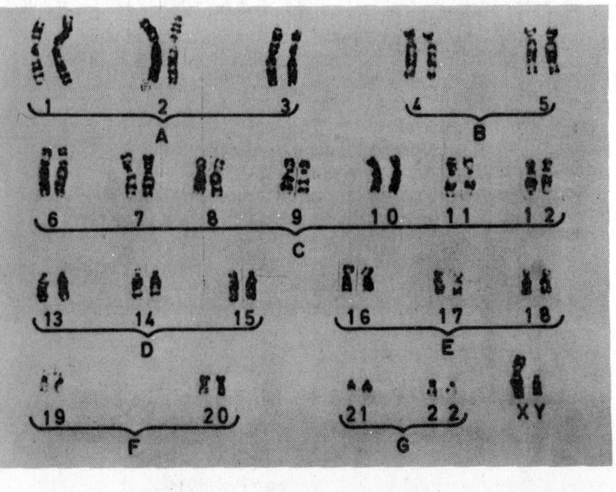

either do not impair the function of the gene product or involve a recessive function so that the mutation is clinically silent. Others, however, cause a defective gene product that gives rise to a dominant trait. The parent in whose germ cells the mutation arose is clinically normal. Likewise, the siblings of the affected individual are normal since the mutation affects only a single germ cell. However, the affected individual transmits the disease to half of his or her children.

The proportion of patients with dominant disorders who represent new mutations is inversely proportional to the effect of the disease in question on biologic fitness. The term *biologic fitness* refers to the ability of an affected individual to produce children who survive to adult life and reproduce. In the extreme case, if a dominant mutation produced absolute infertility, then all observed cases would of necessity represent new mutations, and it would be impossible to prove the genetic transmission of the trait. In less severe disorders, as in tuberous sclerosis, the severe mental retardation reduces biologic fitness to about 20 percent of normal, and the proportion of cases due to new mutations is about 80 percent. Other examples of the relation between biologic fitness and the proportion of new mutations in dominant disorders are shown in Table 57-4.

TABLE 57-2 Partial list of human genetic diseases that have been mapped to specific chromosomes

Chromosome	Disease
1	Elliptocytosis
	RH erythroblastosis
	Gaucher's disease (severe form)
2	Carbamoylphosphate synthetase deficiency
3	Generalized gangliosidosis
	Orotic aciduria
4	Huntington's chorea
	Analbuminemia
5	Sandhoff's disease
	Maroteaux-Lamy's syndrome (mucopolysaccharidosis VI)
6	Complement C2 deficiency
	Complement C4 deficiency
	Hemochromatosis
	Congenital adrenal hyperplasia (21-hydroxylase deficiency)
7	Argininosuccinic aciduria
	Ehlers-Danlos syndrome (one form)
	Osteogenesis imperfecta (one form)
9	Citrullinemia
	Galactosemia
	Nail-patella syndrome
10	Hexokinase deficiency (hemolytic anemia)
	Cholesteryl ester storage disease, Wolman's syndrome
11	Acatalasemia
	Syndrome of Wilms's tumor, aniridia, gonadoblastoma, retardation
	β thalassemia; sickle cell anemia
	Acute intermittent porphyria
12	Phenylketonuria
	Triosephosphate isomerase deficiency (hemolytic anemia)
13	Retinoblastoma
14	Nucleoside phosphorylase deficiency (immunodeficiency)
	Alpha$_1$-antitrypsin deficiency
15	Prader-Willi syndrome
	Tay-Sachs disease
16	α thalassemia
	Gout due to adenine phosphoribosyltransferase deficiency
	LCAT deficiency
17	Growth hormone deficiency (type 1A)
	Glycogen storage disease II (acid maltase deficiency)
19	Familial hypercholesterolemia
	Familial type 3 hyperlipoproteinemia
	Myotonic dystrophy
	Complement C3 deficiency
20	Adenosine deaminase deficiency (immunodeficiency)
22	Metachromatic leukodystrophy
	Hurler's syndrome (mucopolysaccharidosis I)
	Scheie's syndrome (mucopolysaccharidosis V)
X	X-linked ichthyosis due to placental steroid sulfatase deficiency
	Ocular albinism
	Chronic granulomatous disease
	Duchenne muscular dystrophy
	Testicular feminization syndrome
	Phosphoglycerate kinase deficiency (hemolytic anemia)
	Fabry's disease
	Lesch-Nyhan syndrome
	Fragile site associated with X-linked mental retardation
	Color blindness
	Hemophilia A
	Glucose 6-phosphate dehydrogenase (G6PD) deficiency

SOURCE: *McKusick.*

TABLE 57-3 Some relatively frequent mendelian disorders affecting adults

AUTOSOMAL DOMINANT DISORDERS
Familial hypercholesterolemia
Hereditary hemorrhagic telangiectasia
Marfan's syndrome
Hereditary spherocytosis
Adult polycystic kidney disease
Huntington's chorea
Acute intermittent porphyria
Osteogenesis imperfecta tarda
von Willebrand's disease
Myotonic dystrophy
Idiopathic hypertrophic subaortic stenosis (IHSS)
Noonan's syndrome
Neurofibromatosis
Tuberous sclerosis
AUTOSOMAL RECESSIVE DISORDERS
Deafness
Albinism
Wilson's disease
Hemochromatosis
Sickle cell anemia
β thalassemia
Cystic fibrosis
Hereditary emphysema (alpha$_1$-antitrypsin deficiency)
Homocystinuria
Familial Mediterranean fever
Friedreich's ataxia
Phenylketonuria
X-LINKED DISORDERS
Hemophilia A
Glucose 6-phosphate dehydrogenase deficiency
Fabry's disease
Ocular albinism
Testicular feminization
Chronic granulomatous disease
Hypophosphatemic rickets
Color blindness

Many new mutations appear to occur in the germ cells of fathers who are of relatively advanced age. Such a "paternal age effect" is seen, for example, in Marfan's syndrome in which the average age of fathers of sporadic or "new mutation" cases (37 years) is in excess of the mean age of fathers generally (30 years) and also in excess of the age of fathers who transmit Marfan's disease due to an inherited mutation (30 years).

Before one concludes that a dominant disorder in a given patient with unaffected parents is the result of a new mutation, it is important to consider two other possibilities: (1) that the gene may be carried by one parent in whom the disease is of low expressivity (discussed below), and (2) that extramarital paternity may have occurred. The latter is found in about 3 to 5 percent of randomly studied children in the United States.

Most autosomal dominant disorders show two characteristic features that are not usually seen in recessive syndromes: (1) *delayed age of onset* and (2) *variability in clinical expression.* Delayed age of onset is seen in disorders such as Huntington's chorea and adult polycystic kidney disease. These disorders do not manifest clinically

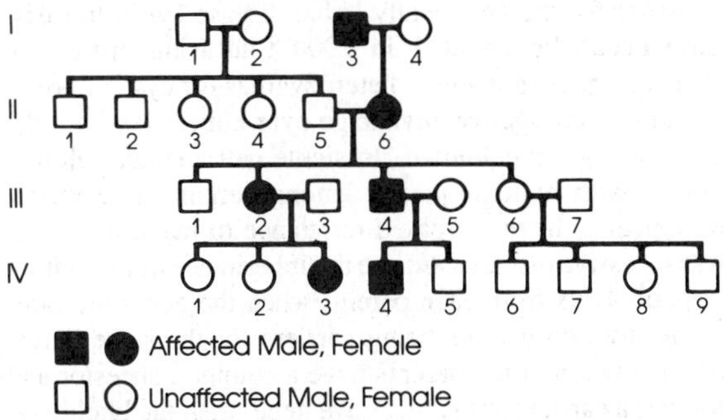

FIGURE 57-5 *Pedigree pattern of an autosomal dominant trait. Note the* vertical *pattern of inheritance.*

until adult life, even though the mutant gene is present from the time of conception. Variability in clinical expression is illustrated dramatically by the multiple endocrine adenoma–peptic ulcer syndrome. Patients in the same family inheriting the same abnormal gene may have hyperplasia or neoplasia of one or more endocrine glands (including the pancreas, parathyroid glands, and pituitary gland), as well as of adipose tissue. The resulting clinical manifestations are diverse; different members of the same family may develop peptic ulcers, hypoglycemia, kidney stones, multiple lipomas of the skin, or bitemporal hemianopsia. The recognition that each family member suffers from the same genetic abnormality can be difficult, as illustrated by the family pedigree in Fig. 57-6.

Dominant mutations involve a type of gene product that produces clinical symptoms when only 50 percent of the gene product is defective. The defective genes usually do not encode enzymes, since a 50 percent deficiency of most enzymes produces no symptoms (see "Recessive Disorders" below). Rather, dominant diseases are likely to involve abnormalities in two classes of proteins: (1) those that regulate complex metabolic pathways, such as membrane receptors and rate-limiting enzymes in pathways under feedback control, and (2) key structural proteins, such as hemoglobin or collagen.

The basic biochemical defects have been identified in only a handful of the approximately 600 autosomal dominant disorders. These include familial hypercholesterolemia (abnormal cell surface receptor that binds plasma low-density lipoprotein and thereby regulates cholesterol metabolism); hereditary methemoglobinemia and several hemolytic anemias due to unstable forms of hemoglobin (abnormal hemoglobin molecule); hereditary angioneurotic edema (abnormal protein inhibitor of an enzyme involved in the serum complement system); acute intermittent porphyria (abnormal enzyme that catalyzes a rate-limiting step in the heme biosynthetic pathway); and pseudohypoparathyroidism, type 1 (abnormal guanine nucleotide-binding regulatory component or *G*-protein of the adenylate cyclase system).

Autosomal recessive disorders Autosomal recessive conditions are clinically apparent only in the homozygous state, that is, when both alleles at a particular genetic locus are mutant. By definition, the gene responsible for an autosomal recessive disorder must be on one of the 22 autosomes; thus, both males and females can be affected.

TABLE 57-4 Approximate proportion of patients affected by new mutations in some autosomal dominant disorders

Disorder	Percentage
Achondroplasia	80
Tuberous sclerosis	80
Neurofibromatosis	40
Marfan's syndrome	30
Myotonic dystrophy	25
Huntington's chorea	4
Adult polycystic kidney disease	1
Familial hypercholesterolemia	Very low

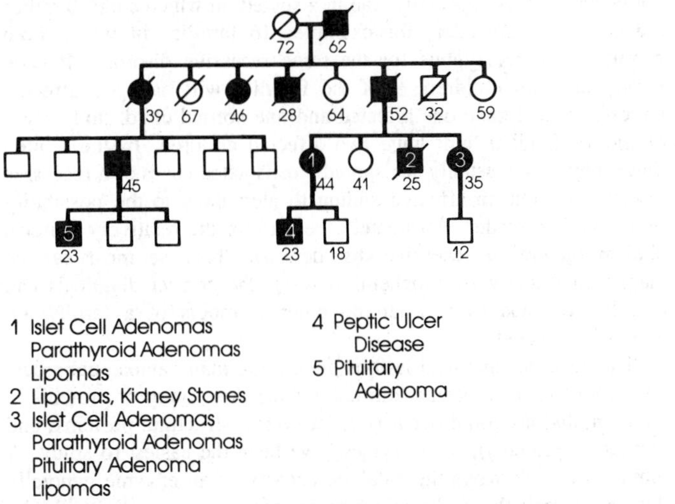

FIGURE 57-6 *Pedigree of a family affected with the multiple endocrine adenoma–peptic ulcer syndrome, a disorder inherited as an autosomal dominant trait. Circles denote females; squares, males. Open circles and squares denote unaffected relatives; closed circles and squares denote affected relatives. Deceased relatives are indicated by the oblique line. The age of each relative is indicated below his or her symbol. Note the marked variation in clinical expression among living affected heterozygotes.*

Figure 57-7 shows a pedigree in which an autosomal recessive trait is present in the family. The following features are characteristic: (1) the parents are clinically normal; (2) only siblings are affected, and vertical transmission does not occur; and (3) males and females are affected in equal proportions.

The relative infrequency of recessive genes in the population and the requirement for two abnormal genes for clinical expression combine to create special conditions for autosomal recessive inheritance: (1) the more infrequent the mutant gene in the population, the stronger the likelihood that affected individuals are the product of consanguineous matings (see below); (2) if a husband and a wife are both carriers for the same autosomal recessive gene, 25 percent of the children will be normal, 50 percent will be heterozygous carriers, and 25 percent will be homozygous and affected with the disease; (3) if an affected individual marries a heterozygote (as may occur with consanguineous marriage), half the children will be affected, and a pedigree simulating dominant inheritance will result; and (4) if two individuals with the same recessive disease marry, all their children will be affected.

The clinical picture in autosomal recessive disorders tends to be more uniform than that of dominant diseases, and the age of onset is often early in life. As a general rule, recessive disorders are more commonly diagnosed in children, while dominant diseases are more frequently encountered in adults.

Since with recessive inheritance only one of four children in a sibship is expected to be affected, multiple cases in a family may

FIGURE 57-7 *Pedigree pattern of an autosomal recessive trait. Note the* horizontal *pattern of inheritance.*

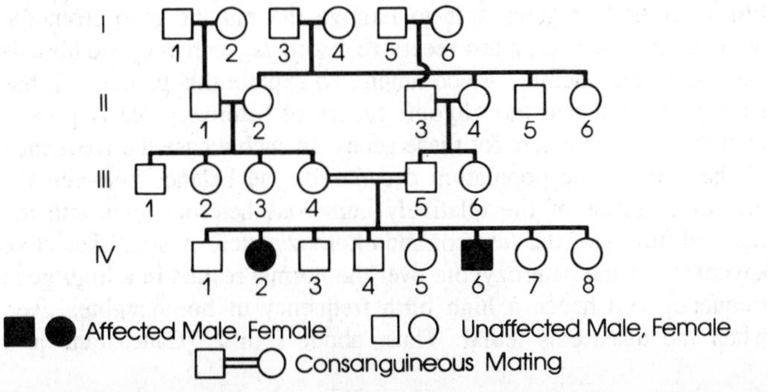

not occur. This is especially true in a society in which small families are common. Consider, for example, 16 families in which both parents are heterozygous for the same recessive disorder. If each family has two children, 9 of the families will have no affected children, 6 will have one affected and one normal child, and only 1 of the 16 families will have two affected children. In the United States physicians usually see sporadic or isolated cases of a recessive disorder without an affected sibling to alert them to the possibility of a genetic disorder. Fortunately, because of the relatively uniform clinical picture of recessive disorders and because most can be diagnosed directly by biochemical tests, the correct diagnosis can usually be made even when no other members of a family are clinically affected.

The basic biochemical lesions underlying many autosomal recessive disorders have been identified. Of the three types of proteins in which mutations could occur (i.e., enzymes, structural proteins, and regulatory proteins), the enzymes have been the easiest to study. A mutation that destroys the catalytic activity of an enzyme generally does not impair the health of a heterozygote (i.e., an individual who has one mutant allele specifying a functionless enzyme and one normal allele on the partner chromosome specifying a normal enzyme). In this situation each cell in the body usually produces about 50 percent of the normal number of active enzyme molecules. However, normal regulatory mechanisms function to avert any clinical consequences of this 50 percent deficiency, and so heterozygotes usually are clinically normal. On the other hand, when an individual inherits functionless alleles at both loci specifying an enzyme, the reduction in enzyme activity is too great for a compensatory mechanism to overcome, and a disease results. For example, heterozygotes for phenylketonuria have half the normal activity of phenylalanine hydroxylase, but they are clinically asymptomatic because the body compensates for the half-normal level of the enzyme by raising the substrate concentration approximately twofold. Under these conditions a normal amount of phenylalanine can be metabolized with no symptoms. On the other hand, the homozygote for phenylketonuria has such a severe reduction in phenylalanine hydroxylase activity that enormous levels of phenylalanine and its derivatives accumulate, causing detrimental brain development. As in the case of phenylketonuria, the majority of enzyme deficiency states produce *simultaneously* both a simple accumulation of one or more metabolites preceding the enzymatic block and a deficient production of other metabolites distal to the block in the metabolic pathway.

Most of the genetic enzyme deficiencies that have been elucidated are not only inherited as recessive traits but also tend to involve enzymes that participate in catabolic pathways. Frequently these enzymes degrade organic molecules that are ingested in the diet, such as galactose (galactosemia), phenylalanine (phenylketonuria), and phytanic acid (Refsum's syndrome). A special class of such catabolic diseases is that in which the deficiency affects an acid hydrolase that occurs within lysosomes. In these *lysosomal storage disorders* the substrate, usually a complex lipid or polysaccharide, accumulates within swollen lysosomes in specific organs, giving the cells a foamy appearance. Examples of such lysosomal diseases include the mucopolysaccharidoses such as Hurler's syndrome (α-iduronidase deficiency) and the lipid storage diseases such as Gaucher's disease (glucocerebrosidase deficiency).

In general, recessive diseases are rare because the reduced biologic fitness of homozygotes acts to remove the mutant gene from the population. However, a few recessive disorders, such as cystic fibrosis and sickle cell anemia, are common. To explain this paradox, it has been postulated that the biologic fitness of heterozygotes is greater than that of noncarriers for these genes. In such a case the frequency of the gene in the population depends on the balance between the increased fitness of the relatively numerous heterozygotes and the reduced fitness of the less common homozygotes. A small selective advantage of the heterozygote over the normal results in a high gene frequency and hence a high birth frequency of homozygotes even when the disease is lethal. Thus, about 1 in 22 Caucasians is a heterozygous carrier for the genetically lethal disease cystic fibrosis, and the disease occurs in about 1 in 2000 Caucasian births. To maintain such a high gene frequency, heterozygotes for cystic fibrosis must have a definite reproductive advantage over noncarriers, but the nature of this advantage is unknown. In sickle cell anemia, another recessive disorder with high frequency among certain populations, heterozygotes appear to have increased resistance to malaria.

Inasmuch as recessive diseases require the inheritance of a mutation at the same genetic locus from each parent, when the genes are rare, the likelihood of any two parents being carriers for the same defect becomes small. However, if the parents have a common ancestor and if that ancestor was a carrier for the recessive gene, then the likelihood that two of the descendants have inherited the gene becomes relatively great. The rarer the recessive gene, the stronger the likelihood that an affected individual will have resulted from such a consanguineous mating. On the other hand, certain recessive genes are so common in the population that the likelihood of two random parents being carriers is great enough to eliminate the need for consanguinity. For common traits such as sickle cell anemia, phenylketonuria, cystic fibrosis, and Tay-Sachs disease, all of which have a high carrier frequency in certain populations, consanguinity in the parents is unusual.

In general, consanguinity is infrequent in families with recessive diseases in the United States. This is because the rate of consanguinity in the general population is low. In most of the United States (as opposed to areas with relative geographic isolation such as northern Norway and Switzerland), a disorder must indeed be rare before it is associated with an important frequency of consanguinity. For example, consanguinity is expected in a large proportion of families having children with very rare disorders such as the Laurence-Moon-Biedl syndrome and abetalipoproteinemia.

Genetic compounds represent a special type of recessively inherited disorder in which the affected individual's two mutant genes, although located at the same genetic locus, are not identical. The mutations in the paternal and maternal alleles presumably involve different alterations in the DNA of the same gene. SC hemoglobinopathy is an example of such a *heteroallelic* compound state in which individuals have a gene for sickle cell hemoglobin on one chromosome and a gene for hemoglobin C on the homologous chromosome.

X-linked disorders The genes responsible for X-linked disorders are located on the X chromosome; therefore, the clinical risk and severity of the disease are different for the two sexes. Since a female has two X chromosomes, she may be either heterozygous or homozygous for a mutant gene, and the trait may therefore demonstrate either recessive or dominant expression. Males, on the other hand, have only one X chromosome, so they can be expected to display the full syndrome whenever they inherit the gene regardless of whether the gene behaves as a recessive or as a dominant trait in the female. Thus, the terms *X-linked dominant* or *X-linked recessive* refer only to the expression of the gene in women.

An important feature of all X-linked inheritance is the absence of male-to-male (i.e., father-to-son) transmission of the trait. This follows because a male must always contribute his Y chromosome to his sons; hence, he can never contribute his X chromosome. On the other hand, a male contributes his one X chromosome to all his daughters.

The pedigree in Fig. 57-8 illustrates the characteristic features of X-linked recessive inheritance. (1) In contrast to the vertical transmission in dominant traits (parents and children affected) and the horizontal transmission in autosomal recessive traits (siblings affected), the pedigree pattern in X-linked recessive traits tends to be oblique because of the occurrence of the trait in the sons of normal carrier sisters of affected males (uncles and nephews affected) (Fig. 57-8*A*); (2) male offspring of carrier women have a 50 percent chance of being affected; (3) all female offspring of affected males are carriers, and affected males do not transmit the disease to their sons (Fig. 57-8*C*); (4) unaffected males do not transmit the trait to any

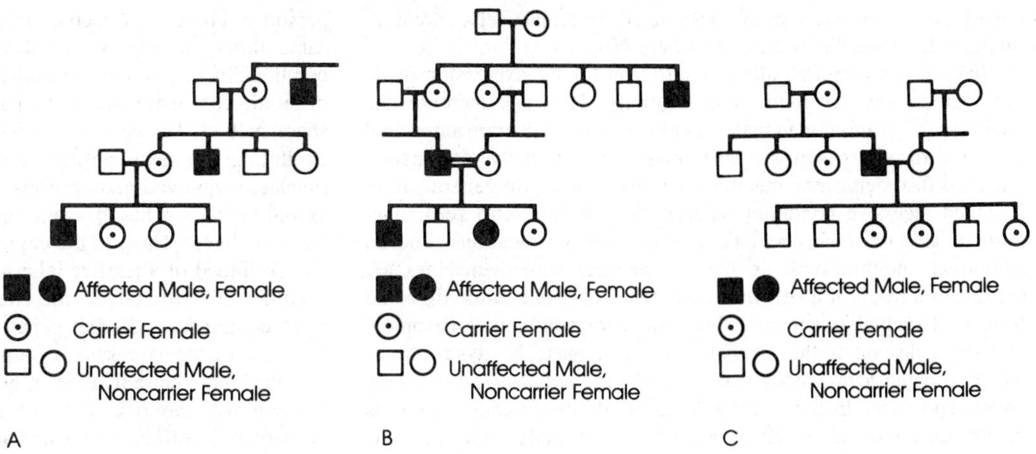

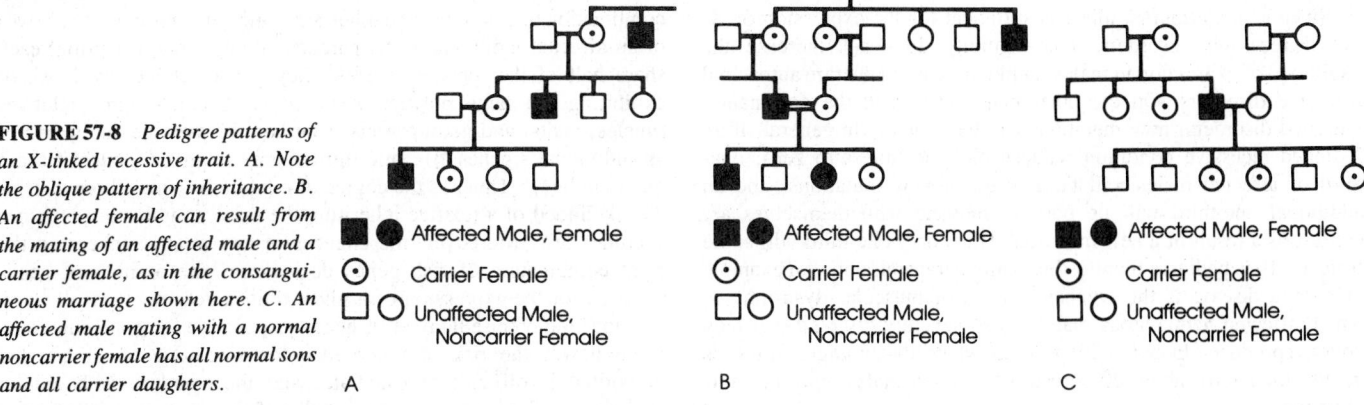

FIGURE 57-8 *Pedigree patterns of an X-linked recessive trait. A. Note the oblique pattern of inheritance. B. An affected female can result from the mating of an affected male and a carrier female, as in the consanguineous marriage shown here. C. An affected male mating with a normal noncarrier female has all normal sons and all carrier daughters.*

offspring; and (5) affected homozygous females occur only when an affected male fathers the child of a carrier female (Fig. 57-8*B*).

Examples of X-linked recessive disorders in humans include hemophilia A, nephrogenic diabetes insipidus, the Lesch-Nyhan syndrome, Duchenne form of muscular dystrophy, glucose 6-phosphate dehydrogenase deficiency, testicular feminization, and Fabry's disease. Color blindness is also inherited as an X-linked recessive trait, but it is sufficiently frequent (occurring in about 8 percent of white males) that the occurrence of homozygous color-blind females is no rarity.

X-linked dominant inheritance is illustrated by the pedigree in Fig. 57-9. Its characteristic features are as follows: (1) Females are affected about twice as often as males; (2) an affected female transmits the disorder to half of her sons and half of her daughters; (3) an affected male transmits the disorder to all his daughters and to none of his sons; and (4) the syndrome is more variable and less severe in heterozygous affected females than in hemizygous affected males. One common trait, the Xg(a+) blood group, is inherited as an X-linked dominant trait, as is vitamin D–resistant rickets (hypophosphatemic rickets).

Some rare conditions may be inherited as X-linked dominant traits in which there is lethality in the hemizygous male. The characteristics of this form of inheritance are illustrated by the pedigree in Fig. 57-10: (1) The disorder occurs only in females who are heterozygous for the mutant gene, (2) an affected mother transmits the trait to half of her daughters, (3) an increased frequency of abortions occurs in affected women, the abortions representing affected male fetuses. Conditions that appear to be transmitted by this mode of inheritance include incontinentia pigmenti, focal dermal hypoplasia, orofaciodigital syndrome, and hyperammonemia due to ornithine transcarbamylase deficiency.

Expression of X-linked traits in females tends to be variable because of the phenomenon of X-chromosome inactivation. Early in embryonic development one of the two X chromosomes in each somatic cell of a female is inactivated. The inactivation process is random, so that for each cell there is an equal probability that the paternally or maternally derived X chromosome will be inactivated. The inactivated X chromosome is rendered permanently nonfunctional, so that all progeny of the initial cell inherit the same active and inactive X chromosomes. Thus, each female is a mosaic; on the average, half of her cells express the X chromosome of the father, and half express the X chromosome of the mother. If a mutation in a gene is carried on one of her X chromosomes, about one-half of the cells in each tissue will be normal and the other half will manifest the mutant phenotype. However, chance or selection of one or the other set of clones of cells may disturb these proportions in any given individual. Depending on the proportions of mutant and normal X chromosomes in each tissue, a genetically heterozygous female may either be clinically normal or have mild or severe manifestations of the disease. To illustrate, mothers of boys with the X-linked recessive Duchenne form of muscular dystrophy may occasionally show mild manifestations of the disease, such as limb girdle weakness or hypertrophied calves.

In each female cell the nonfunctional X chromosome can be visualized by several techniques. By ordinary staining, the inactivated X chromosome in metaphase appears heteropyknotic (condensed in appearance), and it replicates late in the mitotic cycle (''late-labeling'' with tritiated thymidine). In nondividing cells the inactivated X chromosome can be observed as a clump of chromatin at the periphery of the nucleus—the so-called X chromatin or Barr body. In abnormal states with more than two X chromosomes such as 47, XXX, all but

FIGURE 57-9 *Pedigree pattern of an X-linked dominant trait.*

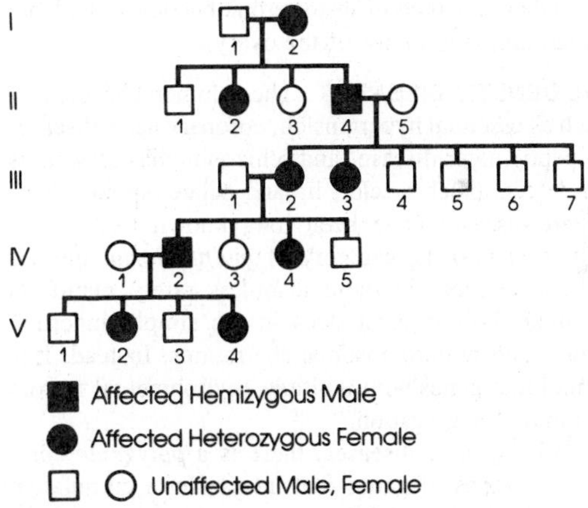

FIGURE 57-10 *Pedigree pattern of an X-linked dominant trait lethal in the hemizygous male.*

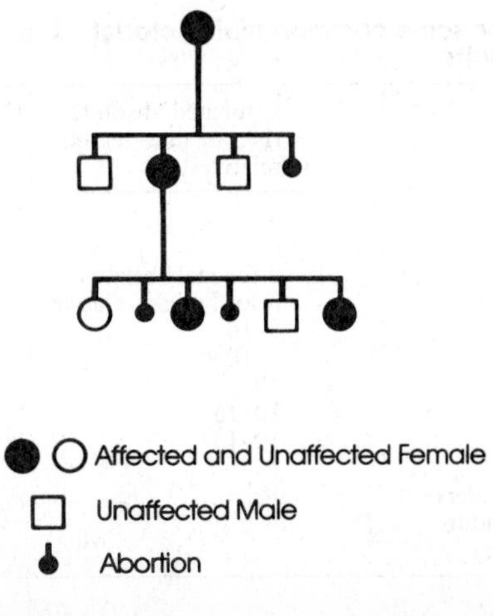

one of the X chromosomes are inactivated, so female cells may have multiple X chromatin bodies (see Chap. 60).

Since a single mutant allele is sufficient for the expression of X-linked recessive disorders, consanguinity does not increase the likelihood of expression in males, unlike the case in the rare autosomal recessive disorders. On the other hand, just as in the dominantly inherited disorders, new mutations can be a factor. In general, if an X-linked recessive condition reduces biologic fitness to zero, one-third of affected males will be a result of new mutations, and an additional one-third will be born to mothers who themselves are carriers as a result of a new mutation. Thus, only one-third will come from a classic pedigree manifesting oblique transmission. An example of such a disease is the Duchenne form of muscular dystrophy in which affected hemizygous males are so severely disabled that they never reproduce. In hemophilia A, in which the biologic fitness is greater than zero, about 20 percent of affected males represent new mutations.

In families in which only one male is affected with an X-linked recessive disease and there is no other family history of the trait, it is essential for proper genetic counseling that the mother undergo biochemical tests or other relevant studies to determine whether she is a carrier. If she is a carrier, half of her daughters will be carriers and half of her sons will be affected. On the other hand, if her affected son represents a new mutation, only his daughters will inherit the gene. At present, biochemical tests can identify female carriers for several X-linked diseases including the Lesch-Nyhan syndrome, Fabry's disease, Hunter's syndrome, hemophilia, and the Duchenne form of muscular dystrophy.

The distinction between X-linked inheritance and *sex-influenced autosomal dominant inheritance* is important. Baldness is probably inherited as an autosomal dominant trait, yet it is manifested mainly in men and rarely in women. Heterozygous females express the baldness gene only when a source of testosterone becomes available as occurs with a masculinizing tumor of the ovary.

MULTIFACTORIAL GENETIC DISEASES The common chronic diseases of adults (such as essential hypertension, coronary heart disease, diabetes mellitus, peptic ulcer disease, and schizophrenia) as well as the common birth defects (such as cleft lip and palate, spina bifida, and congenital heart disease) have been long known to "run in families." They fit best into the category of *multifactorial genetic diseases*. The genetic element in these disorders rarely manifests itself in an all-or-none fashion as it does in the simply inherited (mendelian) disorders and in chromosomal aberrations. Instead, it is the interaction of multiple genes with multiple environmental factors that produces the familial aggregation.

In the multifactorial genetic diseases, there is a *polygenic component* consisting of a series of genes that interact in a cumulative fashion. An individual who inherits the right combination of these genes passes beyond a "threshold of risk," at which point an *environmental component* determines whether and to what extent that person is clinically affected. In order for another individual in the same family to express the same syndrome, the same or similar combination of genes must be inherited. Since the first-degree relatives of an affected individual (i.e., parents, siblings, and offspring) each share half of that person's genes, they are all at increased risk of exhibiting the same polygenic syndrome. Second-degree relatives (uncles, aunts, and grandparents) share on the average one-fourth of an individual's genes $(\frac{1}{2})^2$, and third-degree relatives (cousins) share one-eighth $(\frac{1}{2})^3$. Thus, as the degree of relation becomes more distant, the likelihood of a relative inheriting the same combination of genes becomes less. Moreover, the chances of any relative inheriting the right combination of risk genes decrease as the number of genes required for the expression of a given trait increases.

Since the precise number of genes responsible for polygenic traits is unknown, the risk of inheritance for a relative of an affected individual is difficult to calculate, and the standard is based on empiric risk figures (i.e., a direct tally of the proportion of affected relatives in previously reported families). In contrast to the simply inherited disorders in which 25 or 50 percent of the first-degree relatives of an affected proband are at genetic risk, multifactorial genetic disorders are generally observed empirically to affect no more than 5 to 10 percent of first-degree relatives. Moreover, in contrast to mendelian traits, the recurrence risk of multifactorial conditions varies from family to family, and its estimation is significantly influenced by two factors: (1) the number of affected persons already present in the family, and (2) the severity of the disorder in the index case. The greater the number of affected relatives and the more severe their disease, the higher the risk to other relatives. For example, the risk of cleft lip in the siblings of a child with unilateral cleft lip is about 2.5 percent, but if the lesion in the index case is bilateral, the risk in the siblings rises to 6 percent. Table 57-5 lists the empiric risk figures for the familial recurrence of a number of multifactorial genetic diseases.

The hypothesis of a polygenic component in the inheritance of multifactorial diseases has been given a sound basis in recent years by the demonstration that at least one-third of all gene loci harbor polymorphic alleles that vary among individuals. Such a large degree of variation in normal genes undoubtedly provides the substrate for variations in genetic predisposition with which environmental factors can interact. So far, the genetic loci most strikingly associated with predisposition to specific diseases are those that constitute the HLA system (also called the *major histocompatibility gene complex*) (see Chap. 63). The HLA gene complex is located on the short arm of chromosome 6. It consists of four closely linked but distinct loci (A, B, C, and D). The products of these genes are proteins that are found on the surface of body cells and that enable an individual's immune system to distinguish its own cells from those of someone else. Each HLA locus in the population consists of multiple alleles, each of which produces an immunologically distinct protein. For example, an individual may inherit any 2 of 20 alleles at the HLA-B locus.

An important observation of recent years has been the finding that certain alleles at the HLA loci predispose individuals to certain specific diseases. For example, if the B27 allele at the HLA-B locus is inherited by an individual, that person has a 121-fold greater chance of developing ankylosing spondylitis than an individual who lacks this allele (Table 57-6). Ankylosing spondylitis remains a multifactorial disease, however, because its development clearly requires one or more other factors in addition to the B27 allele. Thus, less than 15 percent of people who inherit this allele develop this disease. Table 57-6 lists some of the diseases associated with alleles at the HLA loci. Several of them are suspected to be of viral etiology, suggesting that the HLA loci may dictate the mode of expression of certain viral diseases. A more detailed discussion of the HLA system is presented in Chap. 63.

Multifactorial disorders are heterogeneous in the sense that the relative contribution of the polygenic factors ("risk genes") and environmental factors to the etiology vary greatly from patient to patient. However, it is important to remember that among common

TABLE 57-5 Empiric risks for some common multifactorial genetic diseases affecting adults

Disorder in index case	Estimated absolute risk for first-degree relatives, %
Cleft lip and/or palate	3
Congenital heart disease	4
Coronary heart disease	8 for male relatives 3 for female relatives
Diabetes mellitus	5–10
Epilepsy	5–10
Hypertension	10
Manic-depressive psychosis	10–15
Psoriasis	10–15
Schizophrenia	15
Thyroid disease (autoimmune disorders including hyperthyroidism, thyroiditis, primary myxedema, simple goiter)	10

phenotypes which are largely multifactorial, often a small proportion will be created by major mutant genes. For example, although coronary heart disease is usually of multifactorial etiology, about 5 percent of subjects with premature myocardial infarctions are heterozygotes for familial hypercholesterolemia, a single-gene disorder that produces atherosclerosis in the absence of any other predisposing factor. Similarly, in a small proportion of patients with other common diseases such as peptic ulcer disease or "essential" hypertension, the condition is not multifactorial but determined by a single gene, as in the multiple endocrine adenoma–peptic ulcer syndrome or the medullary thyroid carcinoma–pheochromocytoma syndrome, respectively.

TABLE 57-6 Alleles at the HLA loci associated with multifactorial genetic diseases

Disease	HLA locus	Specific allele	Relative risk*
Ankylosing spondylitis	B	B27	121
Reiter's syndrome	B	B27	40
Psoriasis with arthritis	B	B27	5
Celiac disease	B	B8	10
Chronic active hepatitis	B	B8	4
Myasthenia gravis	B	B8	4
Diabetes mellitus (insulin-dependent)	DR	DR3/DR4	33
Hyperthyroidism	DR	DR3	4
Addison's disease	B	B8	7
	DR	DR4	10
Multiple sclerosis	DR	DR2	7

* Relative risk *is the probability of the disease developing in an individual with the specific allele, divided by the probability of its development in an individual who does not possess this specific allele.*

INTERACTION BETWEEN SINGLE GENETIC AND ENVIRONMENTAL FACTORS

Many diseases result from an interaction between a specific genotype and a specific environmental factor. In particular, inherited single-gene mutations may produce clinically significant and often life-threatening idiosyncratic responses to certain drugs.

Table 57-7 lists the most important of these *pharmacogenetic disorders,* which encompass all the mendelian modes of inheritance. Perhaps the most common is glucose 6-phosphate dehydrogenase deficiency, an X-linked recessive trait in which a variety of drugs may precipitate a hemolytic anemia. Plasma pseudocholinesterase deficiency and hepatic transacetylase deficiency are examples of autosomal recessive traits which alter drug catabolism so that when the muscle relaxant suxamethonium or the antituberculous drug isoniazid is administered, apnea or peripheral neuropathy, respectively, may ensue. Malignant hyperthermia is an autosomal dominant trait in which acute hyperpyrexia, muscle rigidity, and hyperkalemic cardiac arrest may be induced by administration of any one of several anesthetic agents. Acute intermittent porphyria is another example of a genetic disorder that is exacerbated by drugs, such as barbiturates.

Misinterpretation of adverse drug reactions may result in serious harm to patients. In general, all unusual idiosyncratic reactions should be considered to be genetically determined until proved otherwise. Fortunately, the pharmacogenetic disorders are a group of diseases for which therapy is straightforward: avoidance of the noxious drug by patient and relatives.

In addition to drugs, other factors in the environment may aggravate specific genetic traits. Cigarette smoke may have deleterious effects on persons homozygous and possibly heterozygous for alpha$_1$-antitrypsin deficiency, who are predisposed to the development of emphysema. Patients with xeroderma pigmentosa and anhydrotic ectodermal dysplasia are unusually sensitive to sunlight and high temperatures, respectively. Avoidance of milk at an early age prevents many of the complications ordinarily seen in persons with galactosemia.

Genetic-environmental interactions are particularly important in pregnancy. Women who are affected with phenylketonuria may

TABLE 57-7 Examples of inherited disorders involving an abnormal response to drugs

Disorder	Molecular abnormality	Mode of inheritance	Frequency	Clinical effect	Drugs producing abnormal response
Slow inactivation of isoniazid	Isoniazid acetylase in liver	Autosomal recessive	~50% of U.S. population	Polyneuritis	Isoniazid, sulfamethazine, sulfamaprine, phenelzine, dapsone, hydralazine
Suxamethonium sensitivity	Pseudocholinesterase in plasma	Autosomal recessive	Several mutant alleles; most common affects 1 in 2500	Apnea	Suxamethonium, succinylcholine
Warfarin insensitivity	? Altered receptor or enzyme in liver with increased affinity for vitamin K	Autosomal dominant	Rare	Inability to achieve anticoagulation with usual doses of drug	Warfarin
Glaucoma	Unknown	? Autosomal dominant	Common	Increased intraocular pressure	Corticosteroids
Malignant hyperthermia	Unknown	Autosomal dominant	~1 in 20,000 anesthetized patients	Severe hyperpyrexia, muscle rigidity, death	Such anesthetics as halothane, succinylcholine, methoxyfluorane, ether, cyclopropane
Unstable hemoglobins:					
Hemoglobin Zurich	Arginine substitution for histidine at sixty-third position of β chain of hemoglobin	Autosomal dominant	Rare	Hemolysis	Sulfonamides
Hemoglobin H	Hemoglobin composed of four β chains	Autosomal dominant	Rare	Hemolysis	Sulfisoxazole
Glucose 6-phosphate dehydrogenase deficiency	Glucose 6-phosphate dehydrogenase in erythrocytes	X-linked recessive	~ 1 × 10^8 affected persons in world; common in persons of African, Mediterranean, Asiatic origin; multiple mutant alleles	Hemolysis	Analgesics, sulfonamides, antimalarials, nitrofurantoin, other drugs

SOURCE: *ES Vesell, N Engl J Med 287:904, 1972.*

develop high plasma phenylalanine levels during pregnancy, and thus their offspring may suffer from a variety of phenylalanine-induced birth defects even though the offspring may not themselves have phenylketonuria. Other examples of diseases resulting from an adverse genetic relation between the mother and fetus include erythroblastosis caused by Rh incompatibility and diabetic embryopathy, a term that refers to a series of major birth defects occurring in about 5 percent of the offspring of women who are clinically diabetic during pregnancy.

REFERENCES

HARRIS H: *The Principles of Human Biochemical Genetics*, 3d ed. New York, American Elsevier, 1980

LEWIN B: *Genes*, 2d ed. New York, Wiley, 1985

MCKUSICK VA: *Mendelian Inheritance in Man: Catalogs of Autosomal Dominant, Autosomal Recessive and X-Linked Phenotypes*, 6th ed. Baltimore, Johns Hopkins, 1983

———: The human gene map. *Clin Genet* 27:207, 1985

STANBURY JB et al: *The Metabolic Basis of Inherited Disease*, 5th ed. New York, McGraw-Hill, 1983

VOGEL F, MOTULSKY AG: *Human Genetics: Problems and Approaches*, 2d ed. Berlin, Springer-Verlag, 1986

58 MOLECULAR GENETICS AND MEDICINE

ARTHUR L. BEAUDET

The human genome contains about 3×10^9 (3 billion) base pairs of DNA and encodes 30,000 to 100,000 gene products. The length of DNA frequently is quantitated in thousands of bases (kilobases, kb), e.g., the human genome is 3 million kb in length. Each individual inherits two copies of this genome, and the DNA is packaged as 23 pairs of chromosomes. Each chromosome contains a single linear duplex DNA molecule. Most of the DNA sequences that encode proteins occur as unique (single copy) sequences in the genome. Many gene products show similarities in amino acid sequence and can be viewed as members of large gene families, e.g., the globin gene family. A large amount of DNA in the genome appears not to be functional. Hundreds or thousands of repetitive DNA sequences of uncertain function are present in the genome; some are dispersed, and some are clustered.

If one were to print *one copy* of *one strand* of the human genome, it would fill a text 170 times the size of *Harrison's*. The analogy of the human genome to a large book can be carried further. The book can be envisioned as being bound into 46 separate volumes, each the equivalent of one chromosome. Individuals would inherit one paternal set of 23 volumes and one maternal set of 23 volumes. Sickle cell anemia would be the equivalent of changing a single letter on one page of one volume from each of the sets, while deletion of the alpha-globin gene cluster in alpha thalassemia might represent the equivalent of the loss of one or two pages of text in each set. Digestion of genomic DNA with restriction enzymes, which recognize specific short DNA sequences and cut DNA at these sites, would be the equivalent of cutting the line of text each time a specific word occurred.

The human genome is polymorphic in two ways. One way is by differences in primary DNA sequence, and the second involves the biologic significance of such variations. Beginning at the single nucleotide level, the DNA sequence for the human genome can be variable or relatively constant at a given position. As an example, a DNA base would be highly variable if 50 percent of genes in the population had an A (adenine) nucleotide at the position, 40 percent of genes had a G (guanine) nucleotide there, and 10 percent of genes had a C (cyotosine) nucleotide. Nucleotide positions where more than 1 percent of genes show a nonmajority sequence are designated *polymorphic sites*. Only 1 in 200 to 1 in 500 nucleotide positions qualify as polymorphic. Most nucleotide positions are relatively invariant, the vast majority having the same sequence. The remaining positions have intermediate frequencies of variation. Nucleotide sequence variation is greater in nonfunctional parts of the genome, less in regions of the genome that encode protein sequence or have other important functions. The consequence is that each copy of the human genome varies from every other copy in millions of sequence-specific ways. The nucleotide variations might be envisioned as a multimillion digit serial number embedded within each copy of the human genome. The variability in primary sequence goes beyond single-base changes to include presence or absence of whole segments of DNA. Indeed, considerable length variations occur in the human genome. Inversions of DNA sequence also occur, and translocations between chromosomes also cause DNA variation.

The second type of genetic variation involves phenotypic effect. The alteration of a single nucleotide or single gene may have a dramatic effect. Indeed, certain DNA sequence alterations may be lethal at the stage of the gamete, fertilized egg, or preimplantation embryo. These instances in which a single alteration has a large effect on the phenotype are single-gene disorders; such disorders have been the focus of most efforts to understand human genetic disease up to the present. However, most of the nucleotide differences between human genomes do not cause any significant phenotypic effect. A continuum exists whereby variations in DNA sequence have phenotypic effects ranging from none to minuscule, to small, to moderate, to large, or to overwhelming. In many instances, multiple genetic loci may interact with each other and/or with environmental factors to produce a phenotypic effect. For example, genetic variations in lipoprotein genes, lipoprotein receptor genes, genes that influence intermediary metabolism, and other genes probably interact with diet, smoking, and additional environmental factors to determine susceptibility to atherosclerosis. Together, variations in DNA sequence and in the biologic effect caused by these differences create individuality. Individuals are probably as heterogeneous in susceptibility to hypertension, atherosclerosis, cancer, psychiatric symptoms, and obesity as in their facial appearance and fingerprint patterns.

ANALYSIS OF THE HUMAN GENOME

POWER OF THE RECOMBINANT DNA TECHNIQUES The size, the complexity, and the variability of the human genome constitute barriers to the analysis of individual traits and genes. The feasibility for such analysis was greatly enhanced by the development of recombinant DNA technology. This technology allows for the analysis of one DNA fragment at a time and has provided an index for the human genome and made it possible to locate and isolate individual genes, segments of genes, or nucleotide sequences from the vast DNA library. One of the most powerful of these techniques, so-called cloning of DNA, makes it possible to isolate individual genes or portions of genes, to make an unlimited number of copies of such DNA fragments, and to transcribe and translate the genes so isolated. The various genes and gene products can then be utilized for diverse studies of gene structure and function in normal and disease states. Other recombinant DNA techniques make it possible to analyze genetic variation in individuals directly using clinical samples. Using DNA-hybridization techniques and restriction fragment length polymorphisms (RFLP), to be described below, disease traits can be analyzed both directly and by genetic linkage of polymorphic sites.

The cloning of DNA involves isolation of DNA fragments and insertion of a sequence into the nucleic acid from another biologic source (vector) for manipulation and propagation. The most widely used vectors for this purpose are bacterial plasmids, which have a genome of small, circular, double-stranded DNA. Among other properties, these plasmids can encode resistance to multiple antibiotics, and hence bacteria containing the plasmids can be isolated by virtue of their antibiotic resistance. The plasmids contain a site of origin for DNA replication, and they exist in the bacterial cell as extrachromosomal DNA. Many copies of the plasmid genome can be present in a single bacterium, allowing both high levels of expression of the cloned genes and easy isolation of plasmid DNA.

Another group of vectors are derived from modifications of bacteriophage λ. These bacteriophages can accommodate up to about 15,000 base pairs of inserted DNA and are suitable for preparation of DNA libraries. Cosmid vectors are constructed from fragments of bacteriophages and plasmids; such cosmids can accommodate even larger segments of inserted DNA and combine some technical advantages of λ vectors and of plasmid vectors. Recombinant DNA molecules are grown and manipulated in a host organism such as *Escherichia coli*. Frequently, host strains with impaired genes for recombination are utilized to reduce rearrangements in the cloned foreign DNA.

The development of techniques for the cloning of genes and of other applications of recombinant DNA technology was dependent on the specificity of nucleic acid hybridization and the use of enzymes that cleave DNA at specific sites (restriction endonucleases).

Nucleic acid hybridization Many of the steps in recombinant DNA analysis take advantage of the fact that the complementary nature of nucleic acid interaction is the result of base pairing during the synthesis of DNA and RNA (see Chap. 57). Linear pieces of double-stranded (native) DNA can be treated with heat or alkali to dissociate the two strands to yield single-stranded (denatured) DNA. The denatured DNA can be incubated under conditions that allow for nucleic acid hybridization, i.e., the recognition of two complementary strands and re-formation of double-stranded molecules by base pairing. Nucleic acid hybridization is so sensitive that a single-stranded DNA molecule can be hybridized specifically to a complementary strand of RNA or DNA present at about 1 part in 10,000. Many recombinant DNA studies involve the preparation of one radioactive strand of nucleic acid which is then used as a "probe" in the analysis. It is possible to identify and distinguish both fully homologous sequences and partially homologous sequences. The specificity of nucleic acid hybridization, sometimes in combination with other techniques, allows detection of a single gene among tens of thousands or of a viral sequence in the midst of other nucleic acid sequences.

Restriction endonucleases The discovery in microorganisms of restriction endonucleases, commonly known as restriction enzymes, facilitated recombinant DNA manipulations. The enzymes recognize a specific oligonucleotide sequence in double-stranded DNA and cleave the DNA at this site. Many of these enzymes recognize different DNA sequences (Fig. 58-1). Some enzymes recognize sequences only four nucleotides in length. For example, the enzyme *Hae* III cleaves the sequence 5′-GGCC-3′. Other enzymes recognize sequences six nucleotides in length. The enzyme *Hind* III cleaves the sequence 5′-AAGCTT-3′ (T = thymine). Other enzymes, such as *Mst* II, recognize a seven-base-pair sequence but tolerate any nucleotide pair in the middle position. The sequence specificity of restriction enzymes is a powerful tool in dissection of large genomes. When human DNA is digested with a particular restriction enzyme, hundreds of thousands of DNA fragments are generated with remarkable reproducibility. Such fragments can vary from a few nucleotides to several thousand nucleotides in length, depending on the enzyme used. Restriction enzymes that recognize a sequence only four base pairs long cleave the DNA into smaller fragments than enzymes that recognize a six-base-pair sequence. With the use of multiple restriction enzymes to analyze a particular segment of DNA, it is possible to define a detailed map of restriction endonuclease cleavage sites for the region. Such a map can span a region of from several hundred to tens of thousands of base pairs of DNA. As described below, variations in the sequences of those cleavage sites can be utilized to analyze variations in the human genome. In addition, the sequence specificity of restriction endonucleases has been used

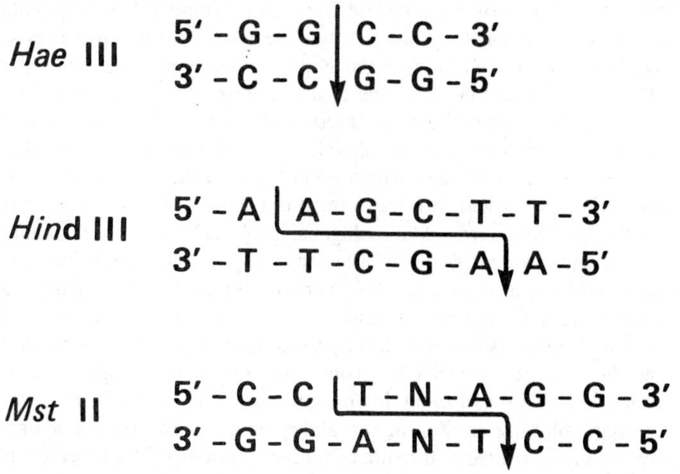

FIGURE 58-1 *DNA sequence specificity and nuclease activity for three restriction endonucleases.* Hae *III leaves a blunt end while the other enzymes leave single-stranded ends.*

to analyze for differences in the sequence of a particular site in the human genome as will be demonstrated below.

Southern blotting Many analyses of the human genome involve a specific application of DNA-DNA hybridization, the blotting procedure developed by E.M. Southern. For clinical analysis, *Southern blotting* (Fig. 58-2) begins with the isolation of genomic DNA from cells such as peripheral leukocytes or amniotic fluid cells. The high-molecular-weight genomic DNA is digested with a restriction enzyme

FIGURE 58-2 *Southern blotting analysis of genomic DNA.*

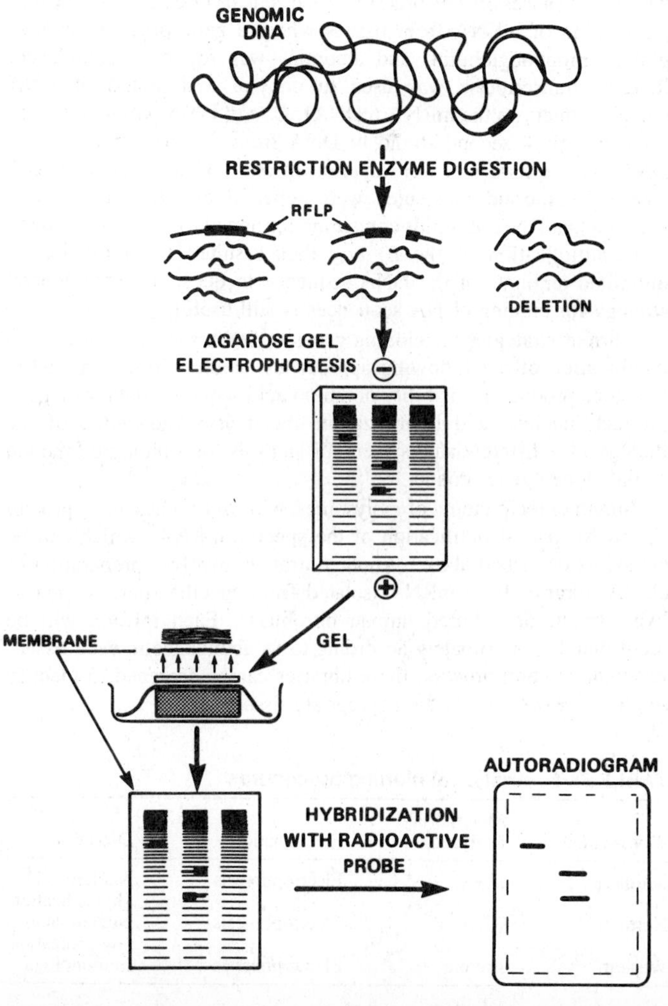

to yield a series of reproducible fragments. These DNA fragments are separated by electrophoresis in agarose gels. After electrophoresis, the DNA is transferred from the gel to a membrane that binds the DNA. The membrane is treated to denature the DNA and is soaked in a solution containing a radioactive single-stranded nucleic acid probe. The probe will form a double-stranded nucleic acid complex at sites on the membrane where homologous DNA is present. The membrane is washed to remove unbound radioactivity, and regions on the membrane where homologous DNA sequences were bound are detected using x-ray film. The sensitivity of Southern blotting is achieved by splitting the DNA into small segments, fractionating the fragments, and applying a sensitive detection method to pick out specific fragments (nucleic acid hybridization). Overall, this method can detect genomic DNA fragments that represent a single gene or about 1 part in 1 million in the genome. The clinical power of Southern blotting resides in the ability it gives to analyze a tiny portion of the primary structure of human genomic DNA taken from an individual.

An analogous procedure starting with RNA for analysis has been termed *northern* (in contrast to Southern) *blotting*. In this procedure, the presence or absence of a particular mRNA as well as its approximate size can be determined. The term *western blotting* describes a derivative procedure designed to analyze protein antigens. Proteins are separated by electrophoresis and transferred to a solid membrane through a blotting procedure. The membrane is analyzed by incubation with antibodies followed by a second step for enzymatic or radioactive detection of bound antibody. Thus, Southern blotting, northern blotting, and western blotting each combines a fractionation and a detection method to provide a sensitive technique for the analysis of DNA, RNA, and protein, respectively (Table 58-1).

Illustrative strategy for DNA cloning Technical aspects of DNA cloning will be described briefly; for details see Watson. Many of the early successful efforts to clone eukaryotic genes involved purification of mRNA from tissues where a gene product, such as globin, immunoglobulin, and albumin, was found in abundance. Reverse transcriptase was used to copy a first strand of DNA complementary to the mRNA (cDNA). *E. coli* DNA polymerase was used to copy a second strand of DNA from the first strand. Insert DNA and vector DNA were hybridized and introduced into *E. coli* where the mosaic molecules were repaired and ligated to yield recombinant DNA plasmids containing foreign cDNA inserts. Growth and multiplication of the *E. coli* then resulted in production of unlimited amounts of the DNA sequence in question. This general strategy for cloning cDNA sequences is still useful.

Current strategies for cloning genes or DNA sequences use some combination of the following approaches: availability of antibodies to a gene product; availability of amino acid sequence data for a gene product; nucleic acid hybridization specificity; knowledge of the biology of a differentiated system; or analysis for a biologic function of the cloned gene product.

Immunoprecipitation of polysomes with antibodies to a protein allows for partial purification of the specific mRNA, which can be cloned as described above. Another strategy involves preparation of cDNA libraries from mRNA isolated from specific sources such as liver, brain, or cultured human fibroblasts. Each mRNA will be represented approximately according to its abundance in each tissue. After the cloning process, these libraries can be screened to identify sequences expressed in the appropriate tissue.

TABLE 58-1 Analytical blotting procedures

Blot method	Material analyzed	Fractionation	Detection
Southern	DNA	Electrophoresis	Nucleic acid hybridization
Northern	RNA	Electrophoresis	Nucleic acid hybridization
Western	Protein	Electrophoresis	Immunologic

Occasionally, functional properties of a gene can facilitate cloning of DNA sequences. Enzymes produced may complement bacterial deficiencies, or products of eukaryotic genes produced by bacteria may have biologic properties that are assayable or can be identified with specific antibodies. If amino acid sequence data are available for a protein, the specificity of the genetic code allows for reverse translation of this sequence into a nucleic acid sequence with limited ambiguity. Single-stranded oligonucleotide probes then can be synthesized and used to screen cloned DNA libraries by hybridization techniques to identify sequences that could encode the protein (see Chap. 57). Using various strategies, more than 300 mammalian genes have been cloned. Isolation of a cloned gene in other mammalian species usually is sufficient to isolate the human equivalent by using the nonhuman clone as a probe to screen human cDNA and genomic DNA libraries using nucleic acid hybridization techniques.

Construction of recombinant DNA libraries is an essential part of strategies for recombinant DNA analysis of human biology, and cDNA libraries are available from most human tissues. Construction of genomic DNA libraries is designed to achieve a series of clones that will include all human sequences without regard to expression. These libraries usually are constructed by restriction enzyme digestion of total human genomic DNA followed by insertion into appropriate recombinant DNA vectors. Genomic DNA libraries have also been prepared from individual human chromosomes that are separated by fluorescence-activated sorting prior to cloning.

For more detailed analysis of genes or DNA, cloned DNA fragments can be sequenced to determine their nucleotide structure. Using these methods, the normal sequence and the mutant sequence for many human genes have been determined.

RFLP MAP OF THE GENOME In 1978, Kan and Dozy demonstrated genetic variation in the size of fragments generated after digestion of normal human DNA with restriction endonucleases. These differences are caused by the DNA sequence polymorphisms discussed above. Restriction enzyme digestion and Southern blotting analysis make it possible to identify these polymorphisms and utilize them as markers for specific sites within the genome. If one of the base pairs in the recognition sequence for a restriction enzyme is variable between individual copies of the genome, or if there is a length variation in the DNA, there will be variation in the size of DNA fragments generated by the restriction enzyme digestion. When the probe for Southern blotting analysis identifies a unique DNA sequence, the pattern of resulting fragments is simple. These restriction fragment length polymorphisms (RFLP) reflect the polymorphisms in normal DNA and are inherited according to mendelian principles. Typical RFLPs are demonstrated in Fig. 58-3. Highly polymorphic sites occur when a sequence is tandemly repeated a variable number of times to give extensive length variation at the site. Although each restriction enzyme detects only a portion of nucleotide variation, the large number of different restriction enzymes available and the extent of genetic heterogeneity allow for detection of almost unlimited numbers of RFLPs.

The ability to analyze primary DNA structure in clinical samples and the availability of gene markers in the form of RFLPs have made it possible to generate a detailed human gene map. Multiple RFLPs detectable in a small region can be linked together to form a series, or haplotype, of tightly clustered DNA markers to enhance the informativeness of such analyses (see "Disorders of globin genes" below). Such haplotypes are equivalent to determination of tiny bits of the unique "serial number" in each copy of the genome. It is also possible to demonstrate linkage of RFLPs to genes for human disease. In the cases of Huntington's disease, cystic fibrosis, and adult polycystic kidney disease the availability of RFLPs made it possible to obtain cloned DNA markers near the disease genes before the identity of the mutant gene or its normal allele was known. "Chromosome walking" (cloning immediate flanking DNA fragments) over short distances is possible, and strategies have been suggested for hopping longer distances to adjacent DNA. It will eventually be possible to clone the gene responsible for any mendelian disorder. A

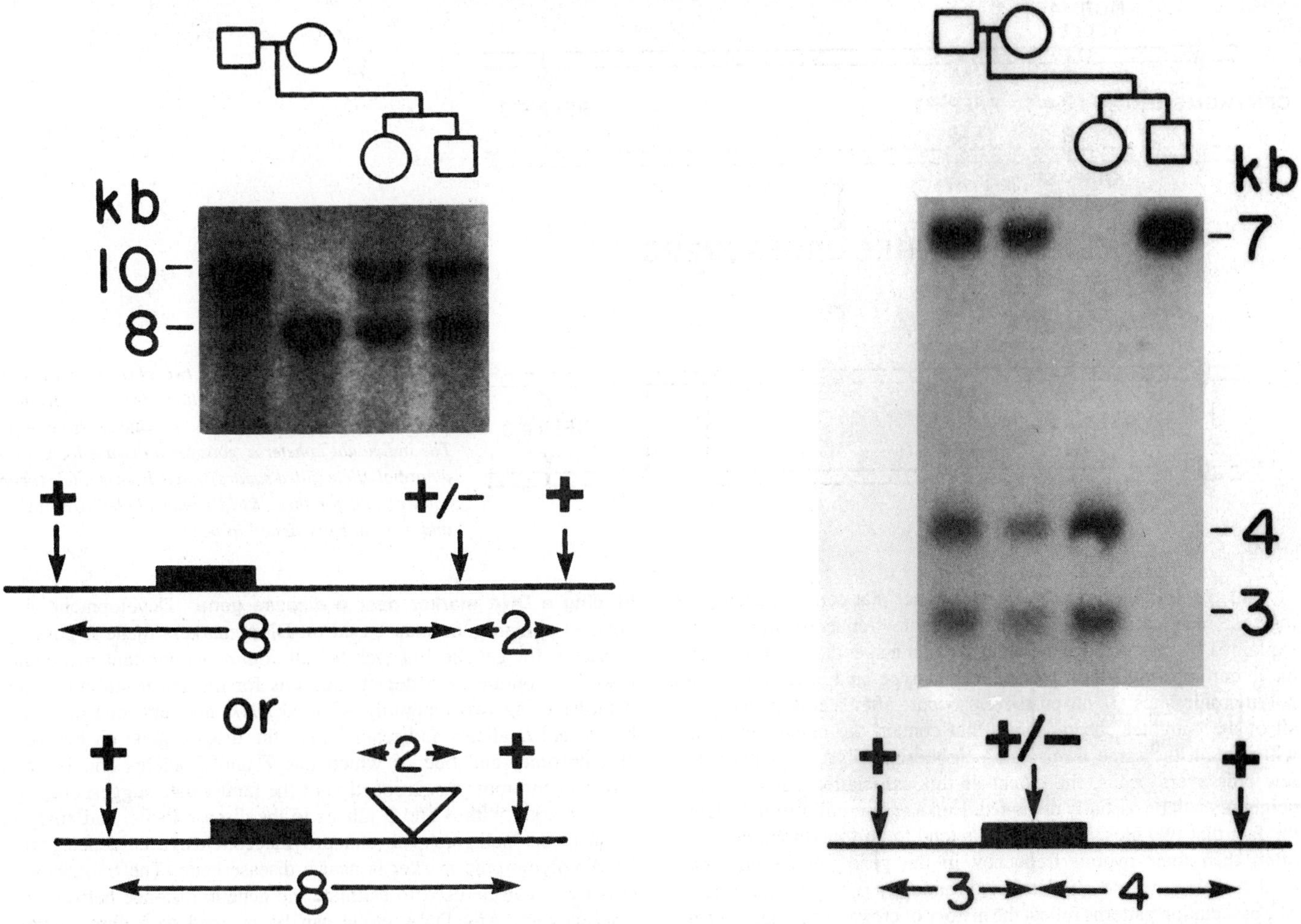

FIGURE 58-3 *Examples of restriction fragment length polymorphisms in human DNA. The solid blocks indicate segments of DNA used as probe. Parents are homozygous and children are heterozygous for the left panel, while the parents are heterozygous and children are homozygous for the right panel. Symbols above the arrows indicating cutting (+) or noncutting (−) by the restriction endonuclease. Numbers indicate DNA length in kilobases.*

detailed human gene map would also make it possible to analyze the role of individual loci in diseases with polygenic or multifactorial etiologies. RFLPs should not be confused with mutant genes. Mutations that cause disease are almost always too rare to be classified as polymorphisms, and only occasionally can they be detected directly with restriction enzymes.

Genetic linkage and linkage disequilibrium The general concepts of genetic recombination and linkage are discussed in Chap. 57. For autosomal genes, each new individual inherits one copy of each chromosome from each parent. Each chromosome is a unique mosaic of polymorphic DNA sequences derived by crossing-over between grandparental chromosomes through the process of meiotic recombination (Fig. 58-4). Genes on different chromosomes are inherited independently, but genes close together on the same chromosome are inherited together unless a meiotic crossover occurs between the two genes. Genes far apart on the same chromosome are inherited as if they were on different chromosomes because of the high likelihood of meiotic crossovers between two distant loci. Genetic distance is expressed in centimorgans (cM) and is a measure of the likelihood of crossover between two loci. The usual clinical concern is whether the disease gene or the normal gene was transmitted from an individual to the next generation. This is true for prenatal diagnosis, presymptomatic diagnosis, and heterozygote detection. If the mutant gene in question can be detected directly by DNA analysis, genetic linkage need not be considered. However, diagnostic analysis frequently relies on a genetic variation near the disease locus for clinical diagnosis. In current terms, this usually means utilization of an RFLP as the nearby genetic marker. If the cloned disease gene is available as a probe, there is negligible likelihood of a crossover between the disease gene and a nearby RFLP (RFLP #1, Fig. 58-4). If the cloned disease gene is not available, it may be possible to use another cloned DNA fragment near the disease gene. In this instance, there will be occasional crossover between the disease locus and the RFLP (RFLP #2, Fig. 58-4). Other RFLPs may be so far from the disease locus that no functional linkage is demonstrable (RFLP #3, Fig. 58-4). There are on average 30 to 35 crossovers during meiosis in males and perhaps twice as many during meiosis in females. The frequency of meiotic crossing-over is not uniform along the length of chromosomes.

For clinical linkage analysis, it is essential that some genetic marker near the disease gene be informative. This means that the individual who is heterozygous for the disease locus must also be heterozygous for a nearby genetic marker. Most analyses can be made informative, since RFLPs are frequent and since it is usually possible to identify useful polymorphisms at important sites. A second requirement is the need to know the *phase* between the two loci for genetic analysis. If an RFLP yields a 10-kb DNA fragment and a 5-kb DNA fragment, it is necessary to know whether the disease gene is linked with the 10-kb fragment and the normal gene with the 5-kb fragment or vice versa. With this knowledge of phase, analysis of which fragment size was transmitted will indicate whether the disease gene or the normal gene was transmitted. The accuracy of such predictions depends upon the proximity of the two genetic loci and the possibility for crossover. Determination of phase usually rests upon previous occurrence of disease within a family or the use of biologic tests to determine the phenotype or genotype. Examples of RFLP analysis in clinical situations will be presented below.

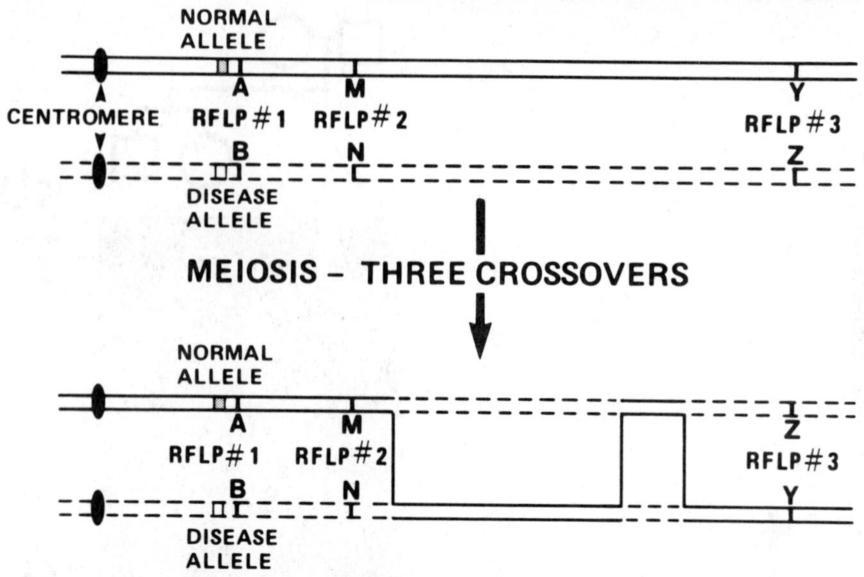

FIGURE 58-4 *Depiction of two chromosomes (one in solid lines and one in dotted lines) from an individual before (above) and after (below) meiotic crossing over. The individual is heterozygous for a disease locus with a normal allele (filled square) and a disease allele (open square) and for three RFLPs with alleles A/B, M/N, and Y/Z. See discussion in text.*

Linkage disequilibrium refers to the fact that certain genes occur together in homogeneous populations more frequently than can be explained by chance. Any new mutation at a specific site must occur on a chromosome of a particular genotype and near preexisting polymorphic sites. If no crossovers occur, after a few generations, all of the daughter chromosomes that contain the mutant gene also will contain the same immediate neighboring DNA sequences. If a few crossovers occur, the extent of this association between close neighbors will be partially disrupted. Linkage disequilibrium describes the fact that two closely linked traits tend to be found together more often than their overall frequency in the gene population would predict if they were each distributed randomly (i.e., in equilibrium). The association patterns reflect the history of crossover events between very close genetic loci. Therefore, a particular RFLP haplotype frequently may be inherited together with a disease gene.

Linkage disequilibrium was demonstrated with the first RFLP described by Kan and colleagues near the beta-globin locus. The enzyme *Hpa* I gives rise to a 13-kb, 7.6-kb, or 7-kb fragment of the beta-globin gene based on a polymorphism in the 3′ flanking region of the gene. The sickle cell mutation is found preferentially with the 13-kb variant in some west African and Mediterranean populations. Linkage disequilibrium affects clinical analyses in two principal ways. First, when developing a haplotype for adjacent RFLPs, extensive linkage disequilibrium is common, so that only a portion of all possible haplotypes (RFLP combinations) are observed. Second, occasional strong linkage disequilibrium between an RFLP haplotype and a disease allele may be of diagnostic value as discussed for alpha$_1$-antitrypsin deficiency below.

Finding a DNA marker near a disease gene Development of a detailed human gene map based on DNA markers made it possible to search for genetic linkages for all common important mendelian disorders. Figure 58-5 depicts analysis for linkage to an autosomal disorder using two randomly selected DNA markers, one of which has *A* and *B* alleles and resides near the disease gene on the same chromosome, and one of which has *Y* and *Z* alleles and is on a different chromosome. Inspection of the family data suggests linkage of the marker with *A* and *B* alleles to the disease locus, and analysis of sufficient pedigree data can provide conclusive evidence that a DNA polymorphic marker is near a disease gene. The frequency of crossovers can be used to estimate the genetic distance between the two markers. Any DNA clone can be mapped to a chromosome. This strategy was used to identify an anonymous (random) DNA segment linked to the Huntington's chorea locus at a distance of 3 to 5 cM on the short arm of chromosome 4. Likewise, a highly polymorphic DNA region near the alpha-globin cluster is linked to the adult polycystic kidney disease locus on chromosome 16. Analogous efforts can be applied to autosomal recessive diseases; for example, the cystic fibrosis gene was mapped to chromosome 7 using this strategy.

CURRENT VIEW OF A TYPICAL GENE A typical gene produces an mRNA that is translated into a protein (Fig. 58-6) (also see Chap. 57). The end of the gene where transcription (RNA synthesis) originates is referred to as the 5′ end, relative to the orientation of the mRNA. The site where transcription begins is referred to as the Cap site. At least some of the DNA sequences required for initiation

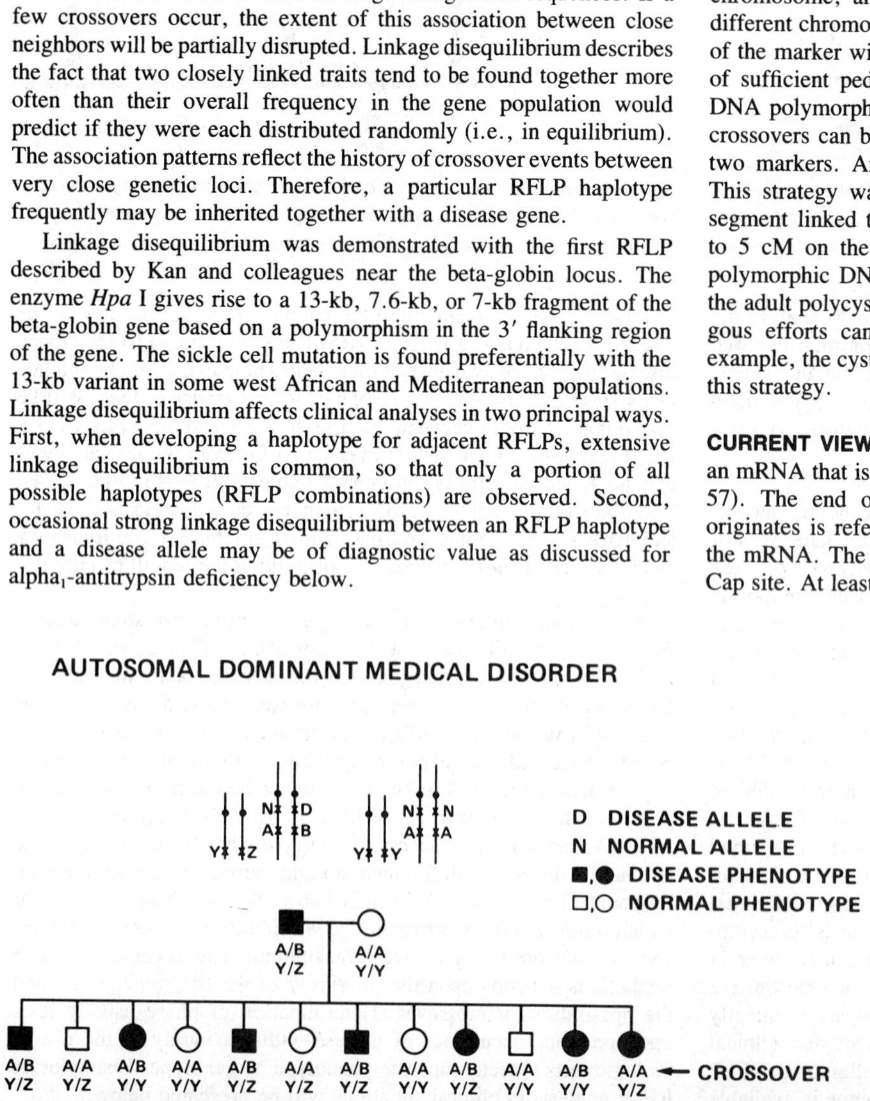

FIGURE 58-5 *Example of a search for linkage of DNA markers to an autosomal dominant disease.* A *and* B *are DNA marker alleles at one site, and* Y *and* Z *are alleles at another site. Two pairs of chromosomes are depicted for each parent. The* B *haplotype and the disease allele are inherited together from the father except for the last-born child in whom a crossover occurred, and the* A *haplotype was inherited with the disease allele.*

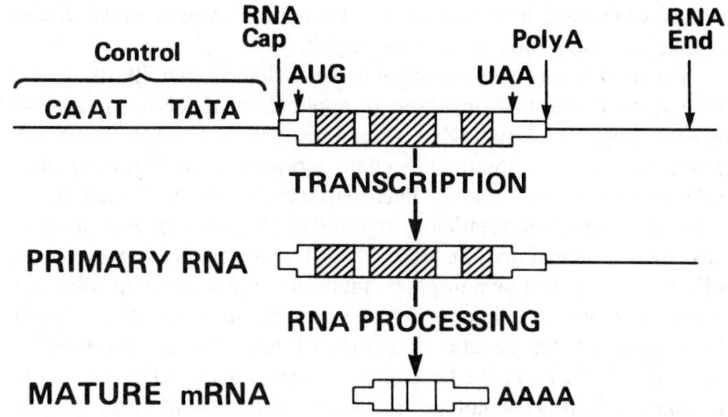

FIGURE 58-6 *A typical gene encoding a protein product. Sequences included in mature mRNA (exons) are represented by open blocks with narrower regions for untranslated sequences. Introns (intervening sequences) are shown as hatched blocks.*

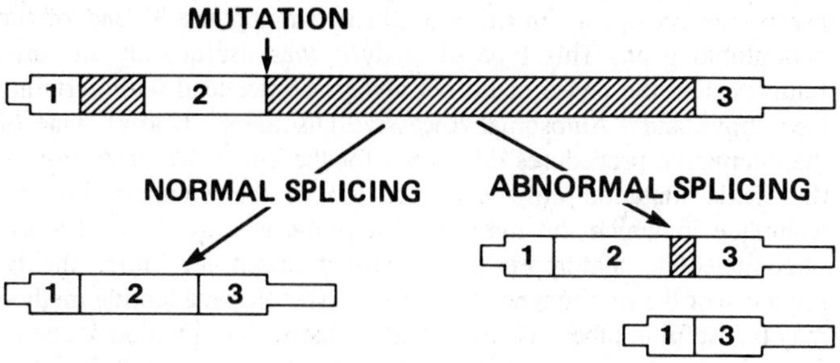

FIGURE 58-7 *A splicing mutation in the beta-globin gene. Exons are numbered and introns are hatched. A mutation in the first nucleotide in the second intron causes the formation of two abnormal mRNA products (right).*

and regulation of transcription are located upstream from this region (opposite from the direction of transcription, to the left in Fig. 58-6). Many upstream regions contain sequences referred to as TATA boxes and CAAT boxes, which are involved in the initiation and control of transcription. Important sequences for gene regulation may also occur even further upstream and downstream from the Cap site. The segments of DNA sequence that are retained in mature processed mRNA are called exons. These exons are separated by segments called intervening sequences (IVS) or introns, which initially are copied into RNA but which are spliced out in the formation of mature mRNA; i.e., the initial transcript contains an RNA copy of both introns and exons, whereas mature mRNA contains copies only of exons. Untranslated RNA sequences are present in mature mRNA and occur upstream from the protein initiator (AUG) codon and downstream from the terminator (UAA, UAG, or UGA) codon. Transcription proceeds beyond the site where mature mRNA will end. The initial RNA transcript is processed by nuclease cleavage at a poly-A recognition site and subsequent addition of A (adenine) nucleotides to the 3′ end of the mRNA.

Many types of mutation are known. The gene can be entirely deleted. The gene can be rearranged by partial deletion, insertion, or inversion of significant segments. Single-base changes in the coding region generate missense or nonsense codons that cause amino acid substitution or premature chain termination. Mutations in the initiator or terminator codon also can cause disease. In addition, mutations can cause abnormalities of mRNA splicing, usually by changing conserved sequences near intron-exon boundaries. These abnormalities of splicing usually generate mRNAs that do not produce a functional product (Fig. 58-7). Mutations also can occur in control regions and in the polyadenylation signal. In addition, disease mutations may occur in parts of the genome that do not encode proteins, although there are few examples of such instances. The diversity of mutations means that detection of mutant genes at a DNA level can be quite complex.

CLINICAL APPLICATIONS OF MOLECULAR DIAGNOSIS

DISORDERS OF GLOBIN GENES The most extensive experience in the molecular analysis of disease involves globin chain abnormalities, and insights applicable to other genes have come from the study of these mutations. For large deletions of major portions of a globin chain cluster, Southern blotting analysis can be used to demonstrate the presence of a homozygous defect (Fig. 58-8). Gene deletion is a common cause for alpha thalassemia, and prenatal diagnosis of these defects is straightforward using either cDNA or genomic DNA probes. Identification of heterozygous deletions requires either careful quantitation or demonstration of abnormal junction fragments from the deleted site. Large deletions are a less frequent cause of mutations in the beta-globin cluster, but such deletions can be demonstrated in hereditary persistence of fetal hemoglobin (Fig. 58-8) and in some forms of delta-beta thalassemia.

By comparison, most single nucleotide changes in the genome are not demonstrated readily by Southern blotting analysis. The first method for molecular diagnosis of sickle cell anemia involved the

FIGURE 58-8 *Depiction of Southern blot analysis of human globin genes. Above, DNA was isolated from a normal individual and from patients with homozygous hereditary persistence of fetal hemoglobin (HPFH) or homozygous alpha thalassemia. DNA was digested with the enzyme* Eco *RI. A mixed DNA probe was prepared by reverse transcription of reticulocyte globin mRNA. Below, arrows indicate* Eco *RI cut sites in the alpha- and beta-globin regions, and numbers indicate DNA fragment sizes in kilobases. (Adapted from YW Kan, AM Dozy, Proc Natl Acad Sci, USA 75:5631, 1978.)*

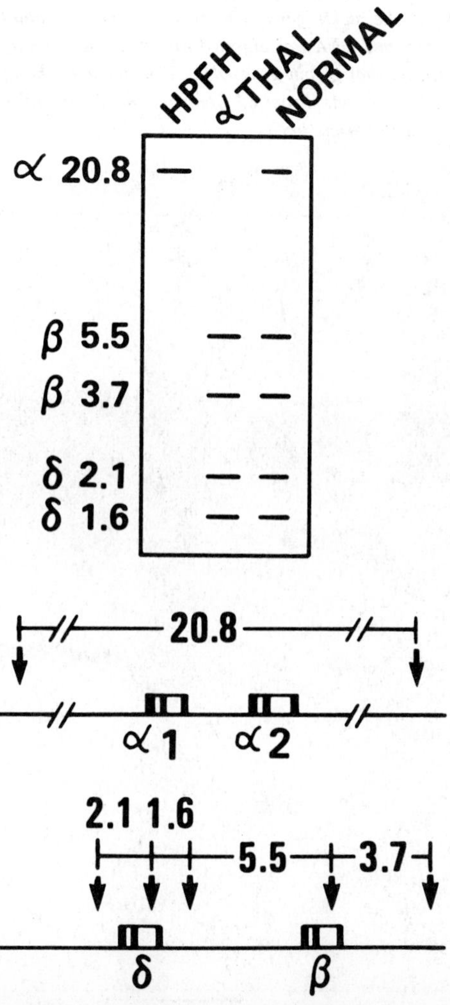

use of the previously mentioned RFLP flanking the 3′ end of the beta-globin gene. This type of analysis was useful only in some families, and the phase could not always be deduced with certainty (see above and "Autosomal Recessive Disorders" below). One of the alternative procedures developed for the direct demonstration of the sickle mutation utilizes a variation of the Southern blotting technique in which the hybridization probe is a synthetic 19-base oligonucleotide that represents a perfect match for either the β^S sequence or the β^A sequence (Fig. 58-9). The oligonucleotide method may be useful in other instances where a particular mutation accounts for a large proportion of disease in the population but has two drawbacks: first, most genetic diseases are heterogeneous at the molecular level, and specific oligonucleotides are required for each mutation; second, the method is so demanding technically as to limit widespread application.

Another method for direct detection of the sickle cell mutation circumvents these technical difficulties. A portion of the nucleotide sequence in the β^A gene is 5′-CCTGAGG-3′, and the corresponding sequence in the sickle gene is 5′CCTG*T*GG-3′. The GAG to GTG change causes the glutamic acid to valine substitution. The restriction enzyme *Mst* II cuts the sequence 5′CCTNAGG-3′ and hence will cut the β^A but not the β^S sequence at this site (Fig. 58-10*A*). Digestion of genomic DNA with the enzyme *Mst* II yields a 1.15-kb fragment for the normal gene and a 1.35-kb fragment for the β^S gene. Southern blotting analysis using *Mst* II and the appropriate beta-globin fragment as a DNA probe allows identification of the AS, AA, and SS genotypes (Fig. 58-10*B*). This is the method of choice for prenatal diagnosis of sickle cell anemia but is not applicable to most other

FIGURE 58-9 *Southern blot analysis using oligonucleotide probes to diagnose sickle cell anemia. The 19 base probes were Hβ19A′ for the normal sequence and Hβ19S for the sickle gene. The genotype for individuals is indicated above each lane, and DNA was digested with a restriction enzyme. HβG1 represents cloned normal globin gene DNA. The smear in the upper region is nonspecific hybridization. (From BJ Conner et al, Proc Natl Acad Sci, USA 80:278, 1983, with permission.)*

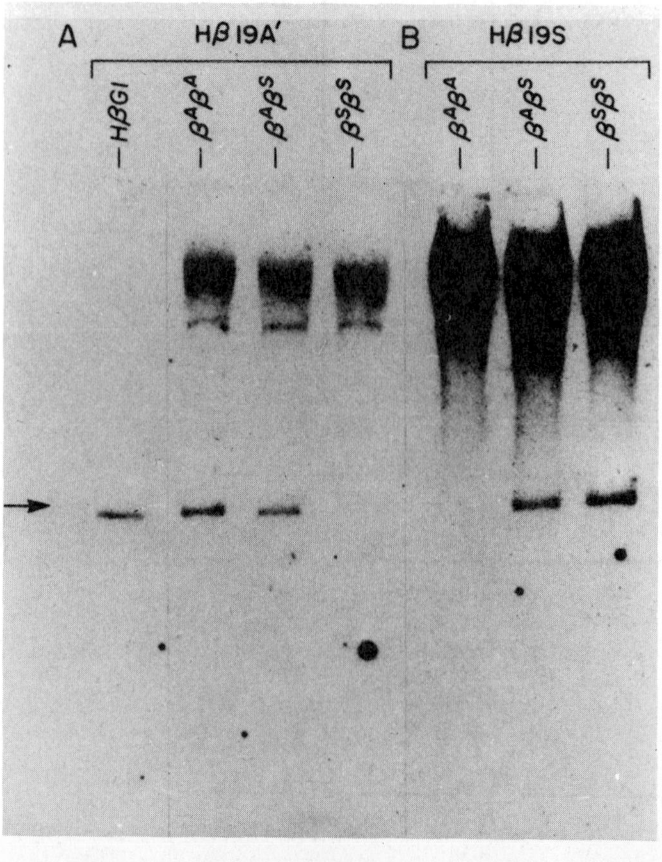

diseases. Indeed, it is unusual for a mutation to both cause disease and be common enough to cause RFLP.

The molecular heterogeneity in beta thalassemia illustrates the magnitude of the task involved in application of DNA analysis for genetic diagnosis. Small DNA alterations, primarily single-nucleotide changes, that cause premature chain termination and splicing aberrations are common among beta-thalassemia alleles. Mutations involving 5′ upstream regulatory regions or the polyadenylation signal also cause thalassemia. Indeed, 17 different splicing mutations, 10 different frameshift or nonsense mutations, and 6 different transcriptional mutations are known for the beta-globin gene (Fig. 58-11). One approach for genetic diagnosis of beta thalassemia involves analysis of RFLPs in the beta-globin cluster. Such variations can be assembled into a haplotype for each chromosome (Fig. 58-12). Assuming that haplotype analysis is informative, prenatal diagnosis can be accomplished in instances where a previous affected child has occurred. In general, each new mutation is associated with a particular haplotype and occurs with limited geographic distribution. In isolated populations, hematologic analysis for heterozygote detection and haplotype analysis can identify carriers and establish a presumed genetic phase for heterozygote screening and prevention of thalassemia. Such analysis becomes much more complicated with admixture of various thalassemia mutations as a consequence of population movements. For example, in Greek or Italian populations in North America, it can be difficult to perform prenatal diagnosis using haplotype analysis if a couple has not had a previous affected child to establish the phase. Direct demonstration of mutant genes using oligonucleotide probes, diagnostic restriction enzyme digestions, or some other method has advantages since requirements for informative markers and determination of phase are eliminated. However, because of the heterogeneity of molecular defects, each family represents a substantial diagnostic project. Comparison of sickle cell anemia, where a single mutation accounts for all of a particular disease phenotype, with beta thalassemia, where extreme molecular heterogeneity is involved in the generation of a particular phenotype, provides important lessons for the study of other loci.

OTHER SINGLE-GENE DISORDERS The term autosomal dominant describes a condition in which heterozygous individuals have a significant disease phenotype. For autosomal recessive disorders, heterozygous individuals are healthy, and only homozygous or compound heterozygous individuals have a disease phenotype (see Chap. 57). These distinctions remain important when considering molecular diagnosis of single-gene disorders.

Autosomal recessive disorders DNA analysis of fetal cells sometimes provides an opportunity for prenatal diagnosis of autosomal recessive disorders such as $alpha_1$-antitrypsin deficiency, phenylketonuria (PKU), and cystic fibrosis. Although these disorders represent a range of disease burden and although few couples at risk may or may not choose prenatal diagnosis, the diseases illustrate the principles involved for autosomal recessive disorders. A hypothetical series of PKU families is illustrated in Fig. 58-13. Phenylalanine hydroxylase is the defective enzyme in PKU, and at least eight RFLPs are detectable using the cloned cDNA for the gene. Each family depicted has a previous child with PKU. For family 1, the analysis is informative, and the phase can be deduced; both parents are heterozygous for an RFLP, and the first affected child indicates that the 5-kb fragment is with the disease gene in both parents. For family 2, the analysis is informative only for the father. For family 3, both parents are heterozygous for the RFLP, but the phase cannot be determined adequately, and the analysis is only partially informative. For family 4, the analysis is uninformative since both parents are homozygous at the RFLP site. For family 5, complete information can be obtained using two RFLPs, since the father is informative for one analysis and the mother is informative for the other analysis. Because more than one RFLP is potentially informative, most families are fully informative, and prenatal diagnosis can be provided to the majority of families with a previously affected child. DNA analysis

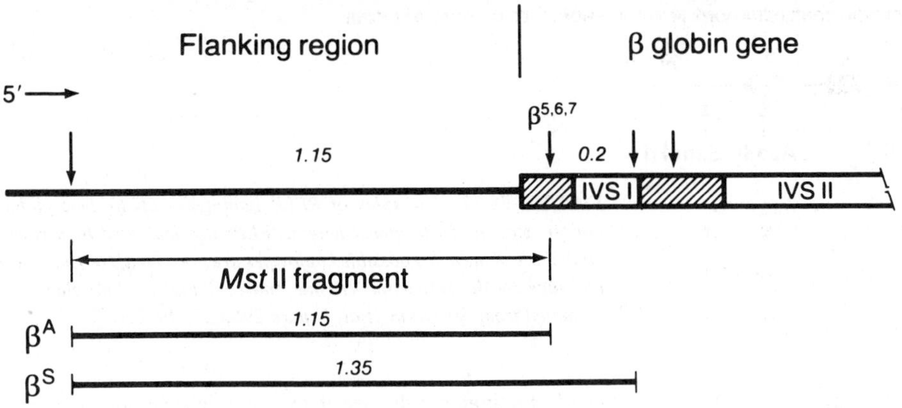

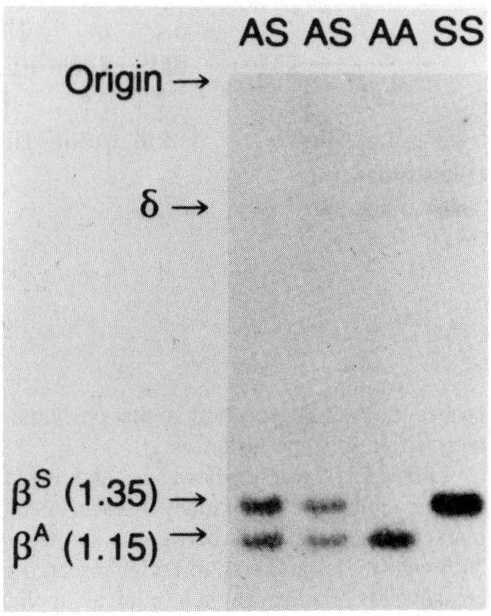

FIGURE 58-10 *Southern blot analysis to diagnose the sickle globin mutation directly. Arrows indicate* Mst *II sites, including the one corresponding to amino acid positions 5, 6, and 7. The* Mst *II fragment of 1.15 kb is the probe; see text. (From JC Chang, YW Kan, N Engl J Med 307:30, 1982; reprinted with permission.)*

may also detect heterozygous relatives such as aunts, uncles, and siblings in families with an affected child.

In the case of alpha$_1$-antitrypsin deficiency, precise genotypic diagnosis and heterozygote detection can be achieved postnatally using protein electrophoresis. A few mutations, primarily the *Z* allele (a single-nucleotide change causing an amino acid substitution), account for most instances of the disease. Prenatal diagnosis can be carried out using oligonucleotide probes to distinguish the transmission of the *Z* allele or the normal allele from each parent to the fetus. In addition, linkage disequilibrium involving an RFLP occurs in the 5′ flanking region of the alpha$_1$-antitrypsin gene, and the presence of a particular RFLP haplotype in this region is virtually diagnostic of the presence of the *Z* allele. This degree of linkage disequilibrium is unusual. Because of the feasibility of population-based identification of specific alleles for alpha$_1$-antitrypsin, it would be possible to offer prenatal diagnosis to couples both of whom have the MZ genotype, even if they have not had a previous affected child.

Diagnosis using linked DNA probes is not in widespread use for autosomal recessive disorders, but the identification of DNA markers near the cystic fibrosis gene should alter this situation. The *met* oncogene and a random DNA marker are closely linked (about 1 cM) to the cystic fibrosis gene on chromosome 7. These DNA markers provide the opportunity for prenatal diagnosis and heterozygote detection in cystic fibrosis families. The principles are similar to those discussed for PKU (Fig. 58-13) except that crossovers between the DNA marker and the cystic fibrosis gene will occur. In attempts to carry out prenatal diagnosis in a family with one previously affected child, there are four opportunities for crossing over, two in the first affected child who is used to determine the phase in the parents and two for the fetus. If a linked DNA marker were 1 cM from the disease gene, there would be a risk of erroneous diagnosis of almost 4 percent. Thus, linkage diagnosis of this type requires RFLP markers that are close to the mutant gene. Such DNA markers allow for heterozygote detection within affected families but not within the general population.

One rare autosomal recessive form of growth hormone deficiency is due to homozygous deletion of the growth hormone gene. This disorder exemplifies the usefulness of molecular analysis. First, DNA analysis can establish the etiology of severe growth failure in such an infant. Second, the analysis has prognostic significance, since such children are more likely to produce antibodies to exogenous growth hormone and may be resistant to growth hormone replacement therapy. Third, the analysis identifies this as a recessive defect with a high risk of recurrence. Fourth, DNA analysis can make prenatal diagnosis possible for such families. DNA analysis also is useful for prenatal diagnosis of recessive disorders, such as carbamyl phosphate synthetase deficiency, in which enzyme activity is not expressed in cultured amniotic cells.

DNA analysis has less to offer when a deficient enzyme can be measured in amniotic cells and the techniques for prenatal diagnosis are well established. Biologic tests such as enzyme assay make it possible to detect defective function without regard to heterogeneity of the molecular defect. For example, prenatal diagnosis and heterozygote detection for lysosomal storage disorders such as Tay-Sachs disease are likely to be uninfluenced by cloning of the mutant genes.

Autosomal dominant disorders Some genes involved in autosomal dominant disorders have been cloned, the low-density lipoprotein (LDL) receptor and antithrombin III being two examples. For the LDL receptor genetic heterogeneity is common; most cases of familial hypercholesterolemia are due to inherited mutant alleles rather than new mutation. At least one RFLP has been identified using gene

FIGURE 58-11 *Location of 30 mutations causing beta thalassemia. Symbols are (△), frameshift and nonsense mutations; (◇), RNA splicing mutants; (●), transcriptional mutants; (○), RNA cleavage mutant. (From SE Antonarakis et al, Hum Genet 69:1, 1985.)*

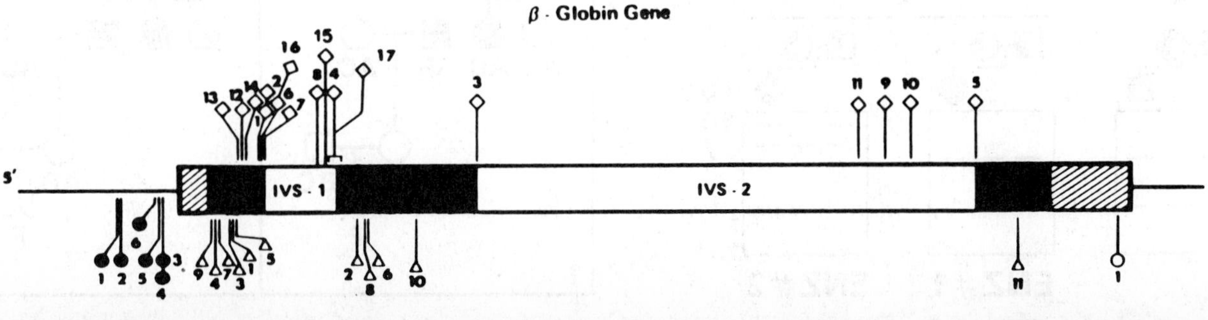

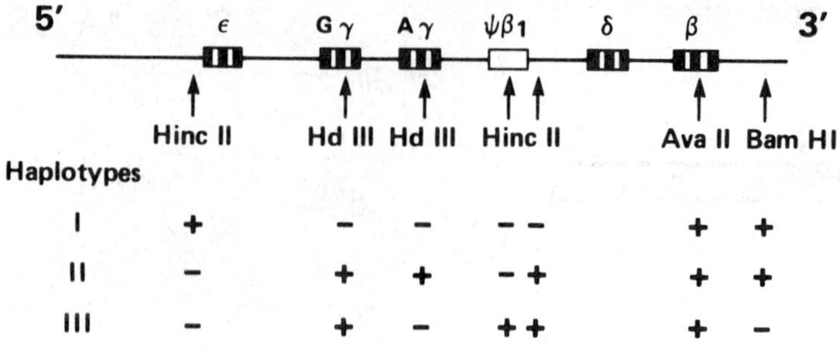

FIGURE 58-12 *Examples of RFLP haplotypes at the beta-globin cluster. Restriction fragment length RFLPs are indicated by arrows. Only three of the many possible haplotypes are presented; (+) indicates cleavage by the restriction enzyme and (−) indicates no cleavage. (Adapted from SH Orkin et al, Nature 296:627, 1982.)*

probes for the LDL receptor so that presymptomatic diagnosis should be possible in some instances.

Linked DNA markers have been identified for Huntington's disease and for adult polycystic kidney disease. As of 1985, the nearest DNA markers are at distances between 2 and 6 cM from the disease loci. Although these markers are major research tools, the occurrence of crossovers complicates their clinical application. Identification of closer DNA markers or the disease genes themselves is needed. For Huntington's disease, presymptomatic diagnosis is not usually warranted because it may lead to an unacceptable psychological burden for affected individuals, but it is possible to make both presymptomatic and prenatal diagnosis of the disorder. Hypothetical examples of Huntington's disease families and haplotype analyses based on RFLPs are presented in Fig. 58-14. For this illustration, it is assumed that the DNA marker is 3 cM away from the disease gene and that the chance of a crossover for meiosis in males or females would be 3 percent. For family 1, the analysis is informative, and the Huntington's disease allele is in phase with the B haplotype. It can be predicted with approximately 97 percent certainty that the pregnant mother has inherited Huntington's disease, and prenatal diagnosis can be offered with about 94 percent accuracy. In family 2 numerous individuals are dead, and presymptomatic diagnosis cannot be offered to the pregnant woman, although one form of prenatal diagnosis can be offered. If the fetus inherits the B (grandpaternal) haplotype from the mother, there is a high risk of Huntington's disease, while there is low risk of Huntington's disease if the fetus inherits the A (grandmaternal) haplotype from the mother. If all pregnancies for this couple with fetal haplotypes BB or BC were terminated, and those with AB or AC were continued, half of all pregnancies would be terminated, but the risk of transmission of Huntington disease would be reduced without clarifying the mother's risk. Using this approach, the terminated pregnancies would likely be affected with Huntington's disease in about half of these families where the parent is affected but would be unaffected in the half of families where the parent is unaffected. Because of the early death of affected individuals, the circumstances in family 2 may be common. The circumstances for adult polycystic kidney disease are similar but differ in that presymptomatic diagnosis using renal ultrasound is generally accurate. A highly polymorphic marker, the result of length variation in tandem repetitive sequences, is closely linked to the adult polycystic kidney disease locus (Fig. 58-15). Availability of linked probes offers the opportunity for prenatal diagnosis of adult polycystic disease, but the acceptability of prenatal testing within affected families is not established.

Certain general features can be recognized for autosomal dominant disorders. In instances such as defects of the LDL receptor where molecular heterogeneity is common, haplotype analysis using RFLPs should be useful. In instances such as Huntington's disease where the great majority of the disease may occur in descendents from one or a few mutations (e.g., molecular heterogeneity would be limited or absent), it would be important to clone the disease gene and identify the molecular defect. Direct identification of the mutation would make presymptomatic and prenatal diagnosis possible in all cases. DNA analysis would be expected to be of limited usefulness in disorders such as achondroplastic dwarfism, where the majority of disease is due to new mutations. There is no opportunity to anticipate the occurrence of new mutations, and molecular prenatal diagnosis is impractical for the new mutation cases since a test must detect all molecular defects and would have to be used in all pregnancies. Thus, cloning the gene for achondroplasia would not provide a

FIGURE 58-13 *Hypothetical families with a child affected with phenylketonuria. Simplified but realistic examples of Southern blot analyses using the phenylalanine hydroxylase cDNA as a probe are depicted. Families are numbered above, and restriction fragment sizes are indicated in kilobases; see text.*

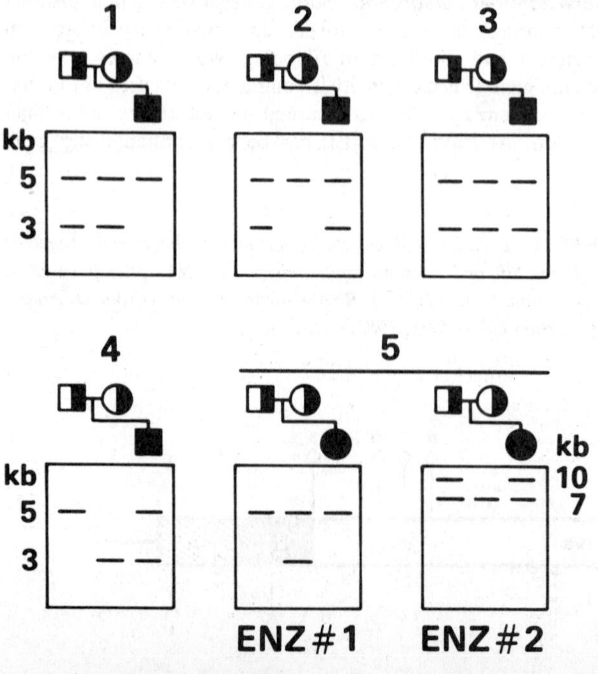

FIGURE 58-14 *Hypothetical families with Huntington's disease. A, B, and C indicate haplotypes for RFLPs detectable with a linked DNA probe. Solid symbols are symptomatic individuals, and P indicates a pregnancy; see text.*

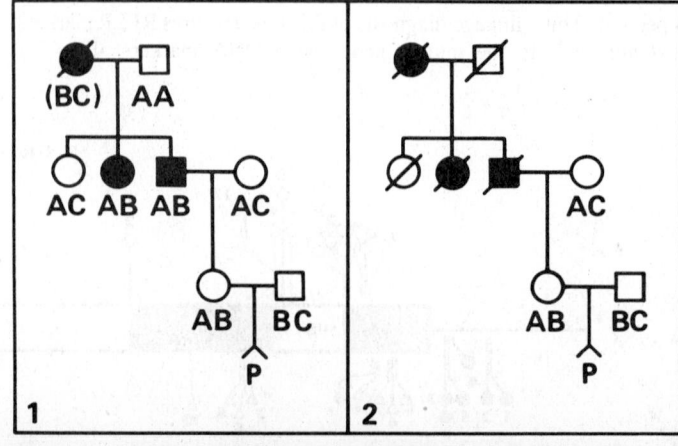

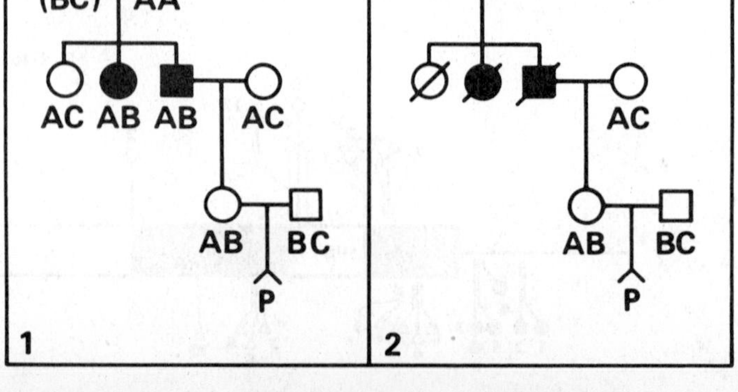

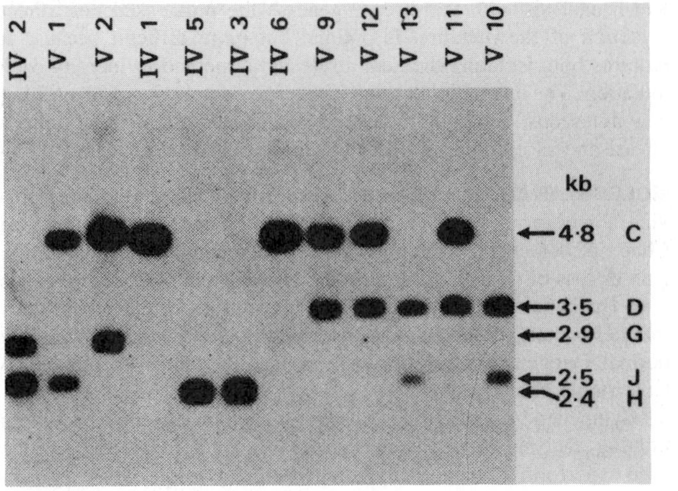

FIGURE 58-15 *Southern blotting analysis of a family affected with adult polycystic kidney disease. Alleles C, D, G, J, and H are detected with a linked, highly polymorphic probe. Designations above each lane refer to pedigree positions, and every person with the C allele also has polycystic disease. (From ST Reeders et al, Nature 317:542, 1985; reprinted with permission.)*

practical option for prenatal detection of most cases. Furthermore, diagnosis by DNA analysis is likely to be handicapped by extensive molecular heterogeneity for disorders such as Marfan's syndrome, tuberous sclerosis, and others, where there are usually few affected individuals in each family. Molecular diagnosis is particularly complicated in disorders involving collagen genes because of the size and complexity of the genes and the degree of molecular heterogeneity (see Chap. 319). Some mutations in a collagen gene cause autosomal dominant disorders, while different mutations in the same gene cause autosomal recessive phenotypes.

X-Linked disorders The same principles apply with modifications for X-linked disorders for which the cloned gene is available, as for factor VIII deficiency (hemophilia A) or factor IX deficiency (hemophilia B). Deletion, gross rearrangement of the gene, or fortuitous mutation within a restriction enzyme site allows for direct detection of the mutation in occasional cases. Alternatively, it may be necessary to rely on linkage analysis using RFLPs detected with the cloned gene as a probe. Analysis of males establishes the phase of linkage between the RFLP and the disease gene, even when the males do not transmit the disease, because males have a single X chromosome. Hypothetical families with hemophilia A are presented in Fig. 58-16, where the cloned factor VIII gene has been used as the DNA probe. In family 1, the analysis is informative, and the phase (hemophilia gene with the B haplotype) can be deduced from analysis of the affected grandson or the unaffected grandfather. Family 2 illustrates the advantages of direct detection of mutations, as compared to RFLP analysis, when it is unclear if the propositus is the result of inherited or new mutation. It is possible to determine if the pregnant woman is a heterozygote only if the mutation can be detected directly and not by RFLP analysis. If the mutation cannot be detected directly, heterozygote testing for this woman depends on analysis of factor VIII activity and antigen. It is possible to offer prenatal diagnosis to family 2 by establishing that if the mother is a carrier, only male fetuses with the B haplotype are at increased risk and that if the mother is a noncarrier, male fetuses are not at risk. In family 3, two brothers, one affected and one normal, inherited the same haplotype. Since the chance of a crossover within the factor VIII gene is low, it is probable that the affected child is the result of new mutation, the mother is not a carrier, and the pregnancy is not at significant risk for a second new mutation. Because random X-inactivation complicates heterozygote detection for X-linked diseases using enzyme

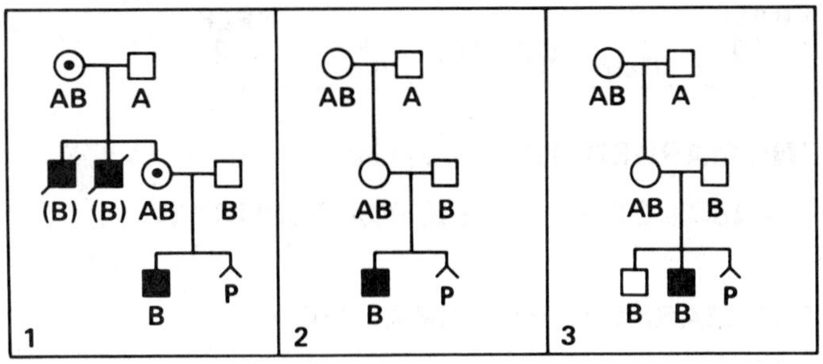

FIGURE 58-16 *Families with hemophilia A. The A and B haplotypes are based on RFLPs detected using the factor VIII gene as a probe. Solid squares indicate affected males, a dot in a circle indicates an obligate carrier female, P = pregnancy; see text.*

assays, DNA analysis when possible is preferable for heterozygote detection.

Some of the complications in the use of linkage analysis for determination of linkage phase are illustrated for a hypothetical X-linked disorder in Fig. 58-17. In each instance the pregnant woman is an obligate carrier, and the DNA marker is 10 cM from the disease locus. In family 1, the probability that the A haplotype is with the disease gene in the mother is .90, based on the findings in the grandson, and prenatal diagnosis in males would be about 81 percent accurate because of the combined uncertainty regarding phase and chance of crossover for the fetus. Family 2 is identical to family 1 except that haplotype information is available for the grandfather, indicating that the disease gene is in phase with the B haplotype in the mother. The affected boy in family 2 must be the result of a crossover, and prenatal diagnosis of males would be about 90 percent accurate. Note that fetuses of haplotype A are predicted to be affected for family 1 and normal for family 2. For family 3, the probability that the phase links the B haplotype with the disease allele is .99, because two affected sons exhibit the same phase (note difference from family 1 with only one affected). The accuracy of prenatal diagnosis in males would be about 90 percent. Similar principles apply in determining phase with autosomal markers.

The advantages of two flanking linked markers are depicted in Fig. 58-18, again using X-linked inheritance as an example. Assuming each marker is 10 cM from the disease locus, prenatal diagnosis can be carried out with 90 percent accuracy if only one marker is informative. If both markers are informative, there will be a 20 percent chance of crossover between the two DNA markers and about a 1 percent chance of a double crossover. Thus, for about one-fifth of families, the analysis will be inconclusive, but such analysis would be 99 percent accurate if the linkage phase were preserved between the two flanking markers.

CLINICAL GUIDELINES Some of the diseases where DNA analysis is helpful are listed in Table 58-2. Molecular studies should be offered to families affected with these diseases as part of prereproductive

FIGURE 58-17 *Issues involved in the determination of phase of linkage using an X-linked example. A and B represent haplotypes based on RFLPs detected using a DNA marker 10 cM from the disease locus; P = pregnancy; see text.*

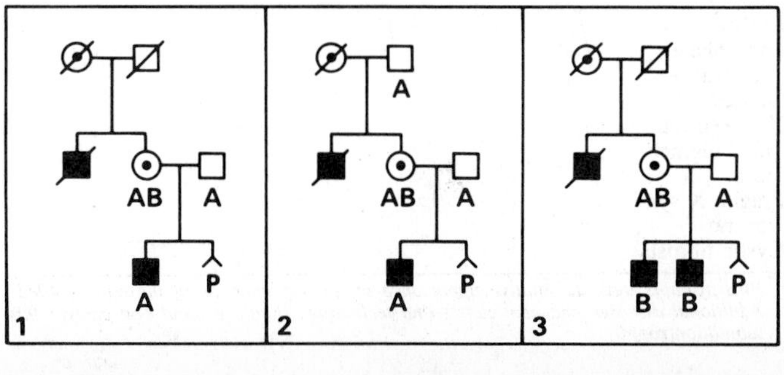

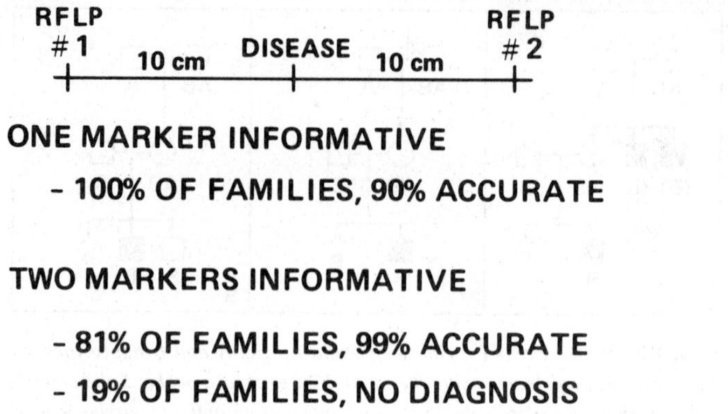

FIGURE 58-18 *Demonstration of the effect of flanking linked genetic markers for an X-linked disease; see text.*

evaluation and counseling. Blood for DNA should be stored from patients affected with Huntington's disease, Duchenne's muscular dystrophy, cystic fibrosis, and polycystic kidney disease. Lack of DNA from affected individuals or from older family members may prevent genetic diagnostic testing for younger family members.

In summary, RFLP analysis with a linked marker is useful, and

TABLE 58-2 Role of molecular analysis for diagnosis of genetic disease

Disease	Detection of mutation*	RFLPs with gene probe	RFLPs with linked marker	Comments
Sickle cell anemia	+ + + +			*Mst* II analysis
Beta thalassemia	+ +	+ +		Very heterogeneous
Alpha thalassemia	+ + +	+		Many deletions
Hemophilia A	+	+ +	+	
Hemophilia B	+	+ +	+	
Phenylketonuria		+ + + +		
Alpha$_1$ antitrypsin *ZZ*	+ +	+ +		
Antithrombin III deficiency	+	+ +		Biologic tests valuable
Familial hypercholesterolemia	+	+ +		Biologic tests valuable
Growth hormone deficiency	+			Rare form
Lesch-Nyhan syndrome	+ +	+ +		Heterozygote detection
Retinoblastoma			+ + +	Inherited form
Huntington's disease			+ + +	Delay over ethical concerns
Myototonic dystrophy			+ +	
Adult polycystic kidney disease			+ + +	
Ornithine transcarbamylase deficiency	+	+ + +		Prenatal and heterozygote
Carbamyl phosphate synthetase deficiency		+ + +		
X-linked retinitis pigmentosa			+ + +	
Fragile X syndrome			+ + +	
Cystic fibrosis			+ + +	

* *Plus symbols indicate relative importance of an approach as of the end of 1985. Additional diseases and new clones and techniques should expand and change this tabulation rapidly.*

RFLP analysis with the disease gene as the probe is better; direct detection of the mutation is optimal but more difficult because it requires both isolating the gene itself and a method to identify each mutation. The examples also emphasize the complexity of identifying new mutations, determining heterozygote status, establishing linkage phase, and ascertaining if a linkage analysis will be informative.

MOLECULAR CYTOGENETICS Recombinant DNA techniques provide a bridge between single-gene disorders and cytogenetics (see Chap. 60). Genetic alterations range from single-base changes to gain or loss of an entire chromosome. As an example, some patients with Duchenne's muscular dystrophy have gross cytogenetic abnormalities, other patients have large deletions of DNA with apparently normal cytogenetic analysis, and presumably others will prove to have single-base changes.

Cytogenetic abnormalities can be studied using either Southern blotting analysis or in situ hybridization. Southern blotting can be used to perform a dosage analysis regarding any unique DNA segment as exemplified in Fig. 58-19. For any chromosomal deletion, duplication, or translocation, it is possible to determine if a particular DNA probe falls within the abnormal region. Indeed, DNA analysis detects heterozygous deletions that are too small to document by conventional cytogenetics. For example, about half of the patients with the Prader-Willi syndrome have deletions or other abnormalities of the proximal portion of the long arm of chromosome 15. Molecular studies of those patients with normal cytogenetic findings might identify deletions too small to detect microscopically. For research purposes, Southern blotting can be applied to the analysis of somatic cell hybrids that contain translocated or rearranged chromosomes separated from their normal homologues. With these techniques, it is possible to determine the location of any DNA marker relative to any cytogenetic breakpoint.

The technique of in situ hybridization involves the use of radioactive DNA probes for direct reannealing to chromosomal DNA in fixed tissue preparations. Such annealing can be detected by autoradiographic techniques over chromosomal regions that contain unique complementary DNA sequences. Clinically, the technique can be used to determine the presence or absence of a DNA segment within an abnormal chromosome and hence to determine whether a segment is deleted or to demonstrate the position of a DNA segment relative to a balanced translocation breakpoint. DNA analysis has also been used to detect Y chromosome–specific sequences in 46 XX males and 46 XX true hermaphrodites (see Chap. 333).

MOLECULAR ONCOLOGY At least three types of molecular changes, all of which alter the expression of the oncogenes, are known to be associated with human tumors (see Chap. 59). These include single-base changes in the coding region of the normal oncogenes, amplification of the copy number, and chromosomal translocations with breakpoints in or adjacent to oncogenes. Each of these alterations can be recognized with Southern blotting. Analysis of tumor DNA for changes in oncogene sequence, for oncogene amplification, and for relevant translocations may ultimately provide diagnostic and therapeutic information for individual patients.

Other tumors are associated with the loss of function of both alleles at specific sites in the genome, for example, at regions of the genome that normally function to suppress tumor formation. If one normal allele for such a gene is inactivated by a first event, loss or alteration of a segment of the other chromosome in this region would cause loss of suppressor function. This was first demonstrated for an association of retinoblastoma with a region of chromosome 13q and subsequently was demonstrated for chromosome 11p in Wilm's tumor. Loss of the second functional gene frequently involves a mechanism that affects adjacent DNA (e.g., cytogenetic deletion). It is possible to compare tumor DNA and uninvolved DNA from the same individual and deduce whether loss of heterozygosity has occurred near the "suppressor" locus. In the case of dominantly inherited retinoblastoma, linkage analysis using DNA markers is useful for genetic counseling, and the heterozygosity analysis of a tumor can be used

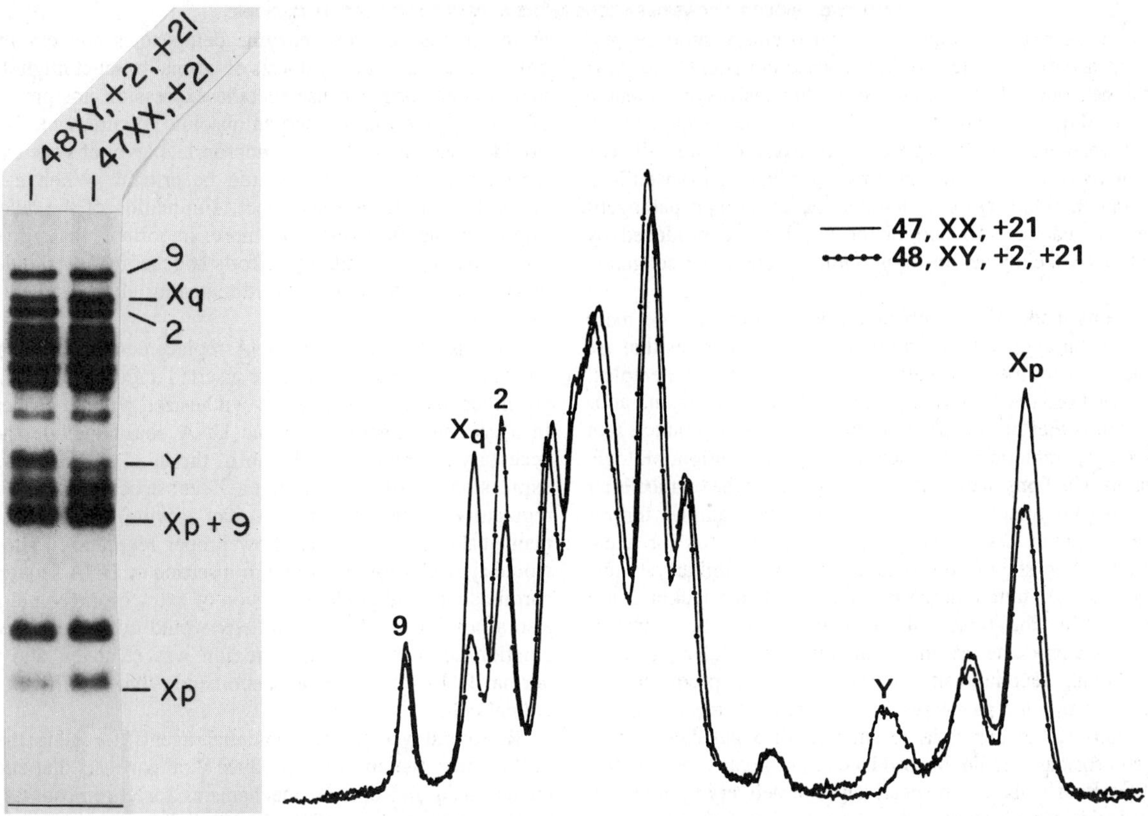

FIGURE 58-19 *Example of dosage analysis using cytogenetically abnormal cell lines. Southern blotting was performed using a cDNA probe which cross-reacts with genomic DNA sequences on 11 different chromosomes including X and Y. Chromosome composition is indicated above the lanes in panel A. Densitometric tracings are presented in panel B with dosage differences for DNA sites on chromosomes 2, Xp, Xq, and Y, but similar dosage for a site on chromosome 9. (From TS Su et al, Am J Hum Genet 36:954, 1984.)*

to determine the phase of linkage, with the retained allele marking the defective chromosome and the lost allele marking the normal constitutional chromosome.

DIAGNOSTIC VIROLOGY AND MICROBIOLOGY Virtually all microorganisms have DNA or RNA genomes that can be detected by nucleic acid hybridization techniques. As discussed above, such hybridization techniques are sensitive and specific, and in human specimens, such as stool, urine, blood, and tissue biopsies, they can be used to detect nucleic acid sequences from microorganisms. These techniques may prove especially suitable for diagnosing cytomegalovirus, rotavirus, Epstein-Barr virus, and other viruses.

MISCELLANEOUS APPLICATIONS DNA fragments that hybridize with multiple, repeated, highly polymorphic sequences in the genome can be used to define polymorphic differences between individuals in a single analysis, even when each variant fragment cannot be readily assigned to a particular chromosomal site. This type of analysis is very useful for quickly detecting nonidentity between individuals. For example, a single Southern blot analysis can distinguish between nonidentical twins and between host cells and donor cells after bone marrow transplantation. These probes offer considerable advantages over conventional genetic markers and may be useful for paternity testing and as a forensic tool to link individuals to semen, blood, and hair root samples. Tissue typing at the HLA loci is also feasible using RFLPs, and such DNA studies may complement or supplant immunologic methods.

CLINICAL PRODUCTS FROM RECOMBINANT DNA

Cloned DNA sequences can be used for the synthesis of proteins and peptides. The major advantages of this strategy are the ability to produce an unlimited amount of a purified product and the avoidance of contamination by pathogens. Production can be carried out in bacteria or in yeast.

Bacteria do not splice eukaryotic messenger RNA properly so that the coding region is usually provided as cDNA clones or as synthetic DNA sequences. The coding region must be linked to bacterial DNA segments that control transcription and initiation of translation. The major difficulties involve the lack of eukaryotic mechanisms for posttranslational processing. Almost all bacterial and eukaryotic proteins undergo proteolytic cleavage at the amino terminus to remove the initiator methionine, and multiple proteolytic cleavages may be involved, as in the production of various hormones from the proopiomelanocortin gene. Other forms of posttranslational modification include carbohydrate addition, phosphorylation, acylation, formation of disulfide bridges, and vitamin K–dependent carboxylation. Improperly or incompletely processed proteins may not function normally and may be antigenic.

These obstacles have been overcome for the synthesis of human insulin. Ordinarily, production of mature insulin involves the formation of three disulfide bridges in a single polypeptide chain followed by proteolytic cleavage to remove the C peptide and leave the α and β chains linked. One strategy was to produce the α and β chains separately from synthetic DNA sequences. Because the mature insulin chains do not contain the amino acids methionine and tryptophan (an unusual and fortuitous circumstance), it was possible to remove the initiator methionine chemically. The chains were then combined, and the proper disulfide bridges formed in vitro.

For the production of growth hormone, bacterial peptidase does not remove the amino terminal methionine from the protein. This results in the production of a growth hormone with an extra methionine residue at the amino terminus. Although the methionyl growth hormone is active in humans, concern regarding immunologic effects delayed release for general use. Growth hormone represents an instance where the natural product was in extremely short supply, and the occurrence of Creutzfeldt-Jakob disease in patients receiving growth hormone isolated from human tissues emphasizes the potential advantages of the recombinant DNA product (see Chap. 322). Production of recombinant DNA products in tissue culture cells can circumvent many or most of the concerns regarding posttranslational processing, but the chances of contamination by human pathogens may be greater. Factor VIII and factor IX that are produced by recombinant DNA techniques in tissue culture cells have coagulant activity.

Some proteins made by recombinant DNA technology are more suitable for clinical applications than others. Those proteins that are present in the circulation are most amenable to replacement therapies. Insulin, growth hormone, clotting factors, alpha$_1$-antitrypsin, antithrombin III, and other plasma proteins are examples of products that could be used for parenteral replacement therapy. In addition, biologic products that have actions in the vascular system or in the extracellular space may have pharmacologic applications. For example, thrombolytic treatment with tissue-type plasminogen activator for acute myocardial infarction shows considerable promise. Similarly, interferon (α, β, and γ), tumor necrosis factor, and interleukin 2 are being evaluated for the treatment of malignancy. The value of recombinant DNA products that must function intracellularly is more tenuous. Although recombinant enzyme could be produced for replacement therapy, the problems of intracellular, tissue-specific targeting remain. For example, large amounts of α-galactosidase A and glucocerebrosidase could be produced for therapy of Fabry's disease and Gaucher's disease, respectively, but delivery systems are unproven. Proteins for which there is no mechanism for endocytosis and proteins required in the central nervous system are unlikely candidates for such replacement therapy. While the majority of recombinant DNA products undergoing trials at present are not completely modified to the mature, posttranslational state, most are biologically active.

Recombinant DNA technology also is useful for the preparation of diagnostic reagents and vaccines. Routine methods for vaccine production involving inactivation of viral particles or development of attenuated live-virus strains carry risks. Occasionally, inactivation of virus is incomplete, or other viruses may contaminate vaccines. Furthermore, preparations of hepatitis B vaccine from human plasma may be contaminated by proteins that cause reactions in allergic individuals. Live attenuated viral strains are subject to change and may cause disease in immunologically compromised recipients. Production of viral proteins by recombinant techniques may provide an acceptable antigen for vaccination. A vaccine for the virus that causes foot-and-mouth disease in cattle is available, and a hepatitis B antigen made in yeast is being tested in humans. An alternative approach to production of new vaccines involves the insertion of one or more DNA sequences encoding antigens into the vaccinia virus genome to produce a polyvalent vaccine. For example, a DNA sequence from influenza virus was recombined with vaccinia to yield a vaccine to protect against vaccinia and influenza.

Diagnostic reagents also can be prepared with recombinant DNA techniques. For example, viral antigens for acquired immune deficiency syndrome (AIDS) and for hepatitis B can be produced for use in radioimmunoassays for viral diagnosis. Various enzymes for diagnostic tests and many of the restriction endonucleases and nucleic acid polymerases used in recombinant DNA diagnosis are produced using the cloned genes for these enzymes.

RESEARCH POTENTIAL

THE PROSPECTS OF GENE REPLACEMENT THERAPY For human genetic disorders in which the mutant gene is identified and the cloned normal gene is available, a number of strategies can be considered for gene replacement therapy (Table 58-3). Gene replacement therapy has a major theoretical advantage over enzyme or factor replacement, since a single treatment could provide permanent correction. If the disease is caused by simple deficiency of the product, as in the case of most enzyme deficiencies and clotting disorders, any restoration of the synthesis of normal product might be beneficial, and neither normal tisuse-specific expression nor precise regulation of gene expression may be an absolute requirement. For other gene products such as globins, an appropriate level of gene expression and tissue-specific expression would be critical. When a mutant gene product has a deleterious effect, elimination of the deleterious gene might be as necessary or more important than provision of a replacement gene. Initially, efforts at gene therapy should be directed at patients with serious life-threatening illness where risk-benefit ratios are acceptable.

At least three types of DNA replacement can be envisioned. In one instance, a cDNA might be inserted under the control of a foreign promoter so that the product is synthesized without proper regulation. In a second strategy, genomic DNA could include the sequences necessary for proper regulation of the level and tissue specificity of expression. Artificial "minigene" constructions that link genomic regulatory regions with cDNA may provide constructions that are of manageable size and that show proper regulation. These strategies would typically involve random insertion of DNA sequences into the chromosome, although expression of extrachromosomal sequences is also a possibility. A third strategy would utilize site-specific recombination so that the mutant region was removed and replaced by normal DNA sequence, a phenomenon that is difficult to effect in animal cells.

Retroviral vectors are potential agents for gene therapy. Such vectors have the ability to produce viral particles that encode foreign nucleic acid and contain mechanisms for chromosomal integration. One current strategy (Fig. 58-20) involves insertion of cDNA or minigene DNA constructions between two viral long terminal repeats (LTRs) in a plasmid vector. These constructions can be introduced into cultured cell lines that provide the viral proteins necessary to package pseudovirus particles that include the gene sequence of interest. For example, bone marrow cells could be removed from a patient with a specific defect, bone marrow stem cells could be infected with these viral particles, and the patient's bone marrow could be repopulated with the altered cells. Delivery to tissues such as liver would be more complex, but can be envisioned.

Alternative strategies might include packaging of DNA in liposomes, development of other viral vectors, and use of vectors that remain in an extrachromosomal state. The risk-benefit ratio for somatic gene replacement therapy must be estimated on an individual basis. Random insertion of DNA sequences into the genome is likely to have some risk for carcinogenesis. However, based on the experience with retroviruses that do not contain oncogenes, this risk might be relatively low if viral progeny are not produced in the recipient. Such risks may be acceptable in patients with life-threatening illness where no reasonable alternative therapy is available. Adenosine deaminase deficiency is a possible candidate disorder for early attempts. Other enzyme deficiencies and clotting factor deficiencies may also be candidate disorders. If proper regulation of globin genes could be achieved, disorders such as sickle cell anemia and thalassemia would constitute important opportunities because of the accessibility of bone marrow for in vitro treatment, because of the frequency of the diseases, and because of their serious nature. Disorders that require careful regulation of gene expression or tissue-specific expression, such as in the central nervous system, are more challenging.

BASIC RESEARCH Over 300 genes have been cloned from human and other mammalian sources. Many of these genes are part of complex functional systems that are only partially understood. A group of genes that control segment differentiation in *Drosophila* have been cloned, and homologous sequences are present in humans and could have functional similarities. Efforts to characterize and clone the genes for Huntington's disease, polycystic kidney disease, cystic fibrosis, and Duchenne's muscular dystrophy should allow for the understanding of the biology of the normal alleles for these genes and could lead to the development of new therapies for some of these disorders.

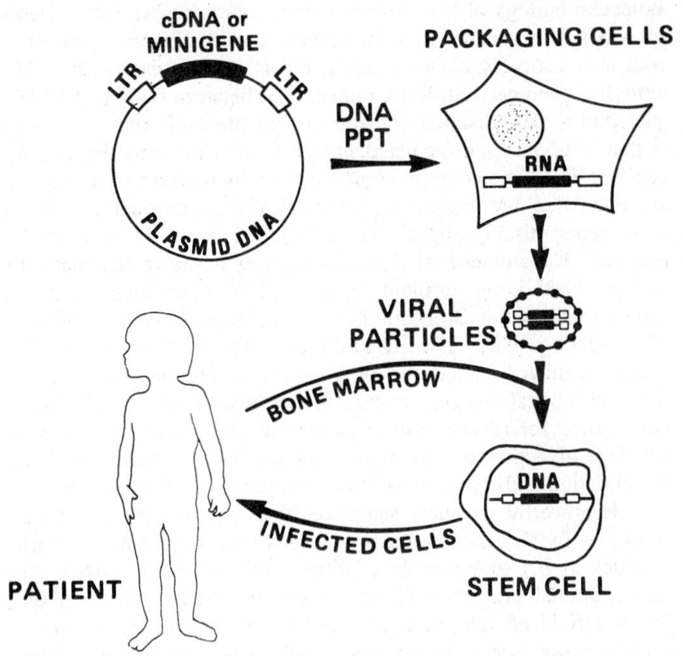

FIGURE 58-20 *One strategy for attempting gene replacement therapy.*

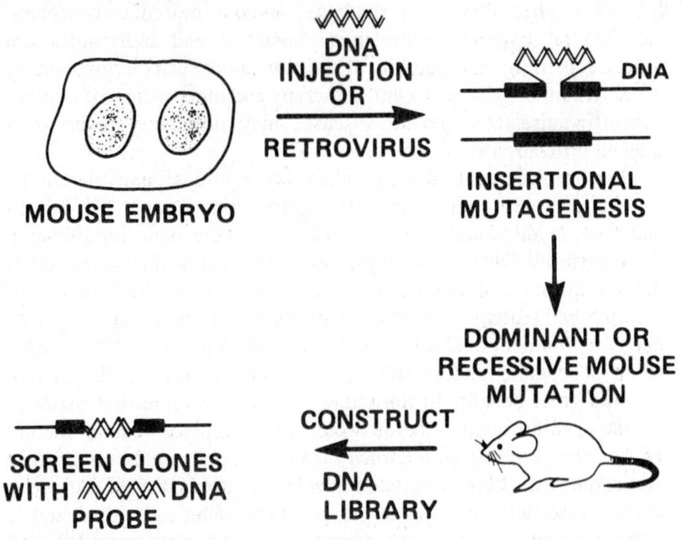

FIGURE 58-21 *Strategy for insertional mutagenesis in mice followed by cloning of the damaged allele.*

Recombinant DNA techniques are likely to be powerful tools for studies of neurobiology and developmental biology. Libraries of cDNA clones can be generated from specific parts of the central nervous system and at specific times in embryogenesis. Another strategy involves the generation of new mutations in mice through insertional mutagenesis (Fig. 58-21). Foreign DNA can be inserted randomly into the genome of early mouse embryos using direct DNA injection or retroviral infection. A functional region of DNA may be interrupted, giving a recessive or dominant phenotype. Phenotypes of biologic interest can be selected such as those causing developmental abnormalities or neurologic dysfunction. The inserted foreign DNA can be used as a probe to clone the damaged region of DNA. Thus, one can generate an informative mutant phenotype and immediately clone the relevant gene. The cloned sequences can be used to search for mRNA sequences to determine the site of tissue-specific expression and the timing of gene expression. If the region encodes a protein, the nucleic acid sequence can be used to deduce the structure of peptides that can then be synthesized and used to generate antibodies. Such antibodies can be used to determine the tissue-specific and cell-specific location of a protein. For example, this insertional mutagenesis strategy was used to identify an embryonic lethal mutation in a type I collagen gene in mice. These tools make it possible to induce informative phenotypes, to explore the molecular basis of the phenotype, and to deduce the related normal biology and physiology.

The availability of a detailed human gene map greatly increases the feasibility of searching for genetic variations associated with predisposition to disease. The fact that there are many known disease associations for the HLA region may be due to a preferential localization of disease susceptibility genes in this region or may reflect the greater opportunity to gather data for highly polymorphic markers. As other parts of the genome become well charted with RFLPs, additional associations may be established between diseases and genetic markers. Such associations may allow identification of genes whose variability predisposes to polygenic or multifactorial diseases.

ETHICAL CONSIDERATIONS Prenatal diagnosis is now possible for diseases with a wide range of burden, such as alpha$_1$-antitrypsin

TABLE 58-3 Human diseases as candidates for gene replacement therapy

Disorders	Burden of disease	Alternative treatment	Disease frequency	Requirement for tissue specificity	Regulation	Relative feasibility*
Hemoglobinopathies	Great	Transfusion, fair to poor	1 in 600 in ethnic groups	Erythroid	Required	+ +
Lesch-Nyhan	Great	Poor	Rare	Brain, ?other	?Not essential	+ +
Adenosine deaminase and nucleoside phosphorylase	Great	Transplant, fair to poor	Very rare	Bone marrow	?Not essential	+ + + +
Phenylketonuria	Small to moderate	Diet, good	1 in 11,000	Liver, ?other	?Not essential	+ +
Urea cycle disorders	Moderate to great	Diet, drug, good to poor	1 in 30,000 for all types	Liver, ?other	?Not essential	+ + +
Alpha$_1$ antitrypsin	Moderate	Poor	1 in 3500	Liver, ?other	?Not essential	+ + +
Hemophilia A & B	Moderate to great	Replacement, fair (AIDS)	1 in 10,000 males	?Any organ, factor VIII	?Not essential	+ + + +
Lysosomal storage diseases	Great	Poor	1 in 1500 for all types	Brain for many	?Not essential	+
Familial hypercholesterolemia	Great	Diet, drug, fair	1 in 500 heterozygotes	Liver, ?other	Some importance	+ +
Cystic fibrosis	Great	Supportive, fair to poor	1 in 2000 whites	?	?	No clone
Duchenne's muscular dystrophy	Great	Poor	1 in 10,000 males	?Muscle	?	No clone
Huntington's disease	Great	Poor	1 in 20,000	?Brain	?	No clone

* *Relative feasibility attempts to take into account requirements for regulation, accessibility of target organ, alternative treatment, and risk-benefit considerations.*

deficiency, phenylketonuria, sickle cell anemia, muscular dystrophy, and familial hypercholesterolemia. Societies and individuals are divided regarding the suitability of abortion under such circumstances. Development of gene replacement therapy and other means of treating presently untreatable genetic diseases may ultimately result in a reduced utilization of abortion.

Gene replacement therapy raises other ethical considerations. Somatic gene replacement therapy requires conventional risk-benefit analyses for individual patients. So long as there is no modification of the germline DNA, few people have serious ethical concerns other than the question of whether such treatment is in the best interest of an individual patient. Experience with cancer chemotherapy suggests that some unintentional low level of damage to germline DNA might be an acceptable undesirable risk of such therapy, if the patient received great benefit. In the future, it is conceivable that methods for site-specific recombination would allow replacement of mutant DNA in the germline with normal material. If one could permanently correct the cystic fibrosis mutation, the Huntington's disease mutation, or the sickle cell mutation in the germline of an individual and if such treatment were safe and effective, would society consider such therapeutic intervention?

REFERENCES

ANTONARAKIS SE et al: DNA polymorphism and molecular pathology of the human globin gene clusters. Hum Genet 69:1, 1985

BEAUDET AL: Bibliography of cloned human and other selected DNAs. Am J Hum Genet 37:386, 1985

BOTSTEIN D et al: Construction of a genetic linkage map in man using restriction fragment length polymorphisms. Am J Hum Genet 32:314, 1980

GILL P et al: Forensic application of DNA "fingerprints." Nature 318:577, 1985

GUSELLA JF et al: DNA markers for nervous system diseases. Science 225:1320, 1984

LAWN RM et al: The molecular genetics of hemophilia: Blood clotting factors VIII and IX. Cell 42:405, 1985

MONACO AP et al: Detection of deletions spanning the Duchenne muscular dystrophy locus using a tightly linked DNA segment. Nature 316:842, 1985

NEWMARK P: Testing for cystic fibrosis. Nature 318:309, 1985

REEDERS ST et al: A highly polymorphic DNA marker linked to adult polycystic kidney disease on chromosome 16. Nature 317:542, 1985

WATSON JD et al: *Recombinant DNA, A Short Course*. Scientific American Books. Distributed by WA Freeman Co. New York, 1983

WILLIAMS DA et al: Introduction of new genetic material into pluripotent haematopoietic stem cells of the mouse. Nature 310:476, 1984

59 ONCOGENES AND NEOPLASTIC DISEASE

PAUL NEIMAN

Upon dividing, cancer cells transmit the neoplastic phenotype to daughter cells. For that reason, it has been generally assumed that the inheritance of the neoplastic phenotype is determined by specific genes. This assumption explains the great appeal of oncogenic viruses for cancer researchers. In spite of their relative genetic simplicity, these agents are capable of inducing all the pathologic and clinical changes associated with neoplastic disease, and in some cases a virus introduces into a normal cell a single gene (oncogene) whose product can initiate and maintain the neoplastic state. These oncogenes represent altered forms of cellular proto-oncogenes, which have important cellular functions in the normal state. Human homologues of some of these oncogenes may play a role in human cancer. This situation prompts a number of questions about the nature of oncogenes, the control of their expression, the biochemical nature of their gene products, and the mechanism of interaction with the metabolism of the host cell.

RETROVIRAL ONCOGENES Interaction of retroviruses with host cells The discovery of oncogenes was a result of the study of the molecular biology of RNA tumor viruses (retroviruses). Retroviruses are widespread in nature, and infection with some of them is associated with neoplastic disease in animals; others are nontumorigenic. The retroviral genome is an RNA molecule of between 8000 and 10,000 nucleotides. The distinctive feature in the life cycle of these agents is that after receptor-mediated entry of the virus into the cell the genomic RNA molecule is copied into DNA (reverse transcription) and integrated into the chromosomal DNA of the host cell (hence the name retroviruses) (Fig. 59-1). This integrated DNA is termed a provirus. The structure of typical proviruses is shown schematically in Fig. 59-2. Long terminal repeats (LTRs) containing sequences copied from both ends of viral genomic RNA are located at each end of the DNA provirus and linked directly to host DNA. These LTRs contain regulatory sequences for the expression of the genes required for viral replication: *gag*, coding for the internal structural protein; *pol*, coding for reverse transcriptase; and *env*, coding for the viral envelope glycoprotein. The regulatory sequences include signals for the initiation and the termination of transcription. They usually also include powerful enhancer sequences that amplify the rate of transcription of viral genes so that proviral RNA transcripts may comprise as much as 0.1 to 1 percent of total cellular messenger RNA. The transcriptional promoter-enhancer sequences usually function only when introduced into particular cell types, accounting for tissue-specific expression of viral genes. In other cases the activity of these enhancer sequences is regulated by steroid hormones. In contrast to many other viruses, retroviruses usually do not kill the host cell when the replicative process is completed; instead their life cycle results in the introduction and expression of exogenous genes and thus in alteration of the phenotype of the host cells.

Acute transforming retroviruses and their oncogenes Infection of animals with retroviruses encoding only the *gag, pol,* and *env* genes results in neoplastic disease after a long latent period. In contrast, acute transforming retroviruses can induce neoplastic disease in vivo in days to weeks and can transform cultured cells in vitro. The prototype of this class of viruses is the Rous sarcoma virus.

The structure of proviruses from these two classes of oncogenic agents is illustrated in Fig. 59-2. Almost all known acute transforming retroviruses are defective, that is, they have lost part of the genes required for replication and hence require co-infection with a standard helper retrovirus for propagation. Such defects result from the replacement of replicative genes of the virus by an oncogene that mediates the direct transforming properties of the virus. (An exception to this general pattern is represented by some strains of Rous sarcoma virus that have both the replicative genes and the viral oncogene.) Although there is variability as to which segment of the viral genome is replaced by the oncogene, the common configuration for acute transforming retroviruses is as depicted in Fig. 59-2. In this case, the oncogene is fused to a 5′ portion of the viral *gag* gene, resulting in the synthesis of a transforming protein that contains *gag* peptides at its amino terminus.

Table 59-1 lists some viral oncogenes (designated by their acronyms), the natural host species, and the types of tumors they induce. In the case of the Rous sarcoma virus, the role of the *src* gene in neoplastic transformation was established by genetic and biochemical means. Mutations that cause reversible inactivation of the *src* gene product at elevated temperature (so-called temperature-sensitive mutations) bring about a reversal of the transformed phenotype to the normal state when infected cells are exposed to elevated temperatures. When the temperature is lowered, the cells again revert to the transformed state. Likewise, deletions of the *src* gene destroy the ability of this virus to induce acute neoplasms. Similar but less complete data exist for other viruses listed in Table 59-1.

Almost all the acute transforming viruses can be detected in vitro by their ability to induce transformation of cultured cells. The standard assay is the formation by infected fibroblasts (or fibroblast-like cell lines) of morphologically altered cells. Some of the leukemia-inducing viruses can transform macrophages and/or hematopoietic cells in vitro.

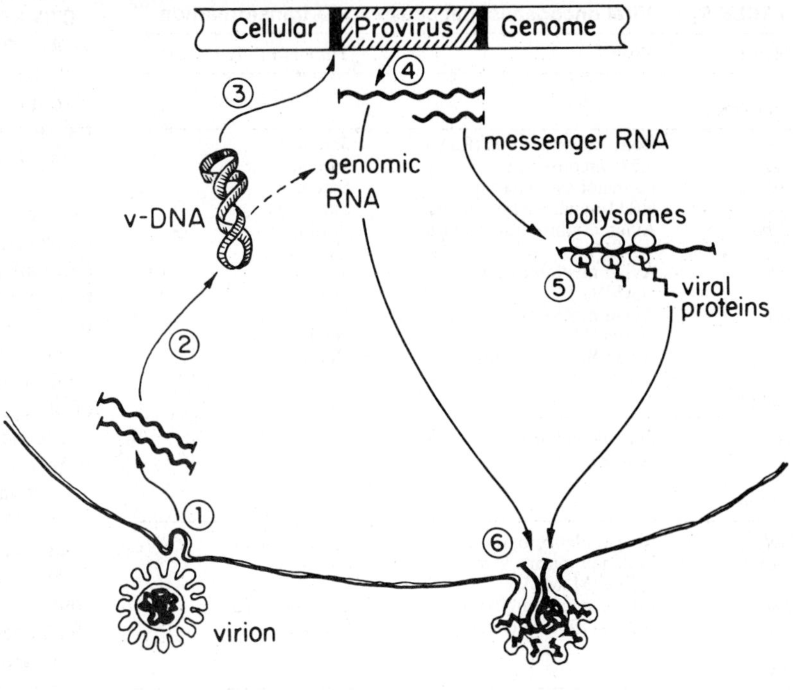

FIGURE 59-1 *Replication of retroviruses. (1) Envelope glycoprotein on the surface of viral particles (virions) recognizes receptors which mediate entry into the cell and release of viral genomic RNA. (2) There are two viral RNA molecules per virion which are copied by reverse transcriptase into circular, supercoiled viral DNA molecules. (3) Some of the circular DNA molecules integrate into host chromosomal DNA at a precise point on the viral DNA molecule and a random, or near random, site on host chromosomes. (4) The integrated viral DNA copy, or provirus, is transcribed into both messenger RNA, which is translated into viral proteins on cellular polysomes (5), and full-length genomic viral RNA, which contains specific sequences serving as packaging signals for virus assembly. (6) Viral RNA and proteins are assembled into particles which bud from the cell surface. The whole process can occur without cytopathic effects on host cells.*

PROTO-ONCOGENES The oncogenes of retroviruses are closely related to normal cellular genes. This relationship was deduced from the discovery of nucleotide sequence homology between the transforming oncogene of Rous sarcoma virus, v-*src* (viral-*src*), and a normal chicken gene, c-*src* (cellular-*src*). Apparently, Rous sarcoma virus originated from a recombination event between c-*src* and an ancestral standard avian retrovirus. This mechanism, recombination between a viral gene and a gene of host origin, is the apparent explanation for the formation of the transforming viruses listed in Table 59-1. The function of the normal genes and their role in nonviral tumor formation is, therefore, a subject of intense interest and investigation.

The normal forms of the oncogenes are highly conserved in nature. There are human homologues of each, and homologues of some are present in all eukaryotic organisms, including invertebrate species and yeasts. This conservation implies that these genes have vital functions in normal cells and suggests that the oncogenic potential of the genes is acquired only after functionally significant alteration (such as occurs from recombination with a retrovirus). Such genes are referred to as *proto-oncogenes* (c-*onc*).

The nucleotide sequences of the protein coding regions of viral oncogenes differ from those of the proto-oncogenes. There are also major differences in the regulation of expression of the viral and cellular genes. For example, the normal cellular form of an oncogene can be expressed without transforming the cell, although usually at a lower level and/or more strictly regulated than with viral oncogenes expressed from proviruses. The relative contributions of overexpression, altered regulation, and structural mutation to the transforming activity of viral oncogenes is not fully resolved. All of these elements may be important to degrees that vary with the individual oncogene and target cell type.

Infection with retroviruses that lack oncogenes can induce neoplastic disease in some animals after a long latent period. A common mechanism for this oncogenic activity is the activation of cellular proto-oncogenes, as illustrated by the induction of lymphomas in the bursa of Fabricius of chickens by avian leukosis virus (ALV). In these neoplasms, a proto-oncogene called c-*myc* is expressed at high levels as a result of the integration fo the promoter-enhancer of the ALV genome near c-*myc*. The fact that these tumors are clonal and that c-*myc* activation occurs only in the tumor cells, coupled with the known oncogenic potential of v-*myc*, supports the idea that c-*myc* plays an important role in these tumors. Table 59-2 lists cellular proto-oncogenes that are known to be activated in retrovirus-induced neoplasms of long latency. Some (*myc* and *erbB*) are homologues of known viral oncogenes. Others (*Int*-1, *Int*-2, *Pim*-1, *Mlvi*-1, and *Mlvi*-2) have not been identified as part of the genomes of acute-transforming viruses. Their oncogenic potential is inferred by analogy.

Human retroviruses Human T-cell leukemia viruses (HTLV) are retroviruses that appear to replicate preferentially in human lymphocytes. Infection with HTLV type I is associated with the development of a specific type of adult T-cell leukemia that occurs with increased frequency in southern Japan and the Caribbean basin. In vitro infection on human T cells by HTLV-I in culture confers a capacity for growth that is independent of exogenous T-cell growth factors (immortali-

FIGURE 59-2 *Comparative structure of the proviruses of standard replication competent and acute transforming retroviruses. In both cases the provirus is bounded by direct long terminal repeat sequences (LTRs) which contain essential regulatory elements including transcriptional promoters and enhancers, signals for the termination of viral RNA transcripts (polyA addition signals), and for integration into the host DNA. Inside the LTRs of standard retroviruses are three genes:* gag *(internal structural proteins),* pol *(reverse transcriptase), and* env *(envelope glycoprotein), which are required for infection and replication. In the acute transforming viruses, all or part of the replicative genes have been replaced by a transforming oncogene which mediates the oncogenic properties of the virus. The most common structure is a fusion of the 5′ portion of the* gag *gene with the oncogene. The standard provirus is transcribed into full-length genomic viral RNA and spliced messenger RNAs for viral proteins. The acute transforming provirus often expresses only one size RNA transcript. It is replication defective and requires co-infection with a standard retroviral "helper" in order to replicate. The* Δgag *symbol indicates that part of the* gag *sequence is missing because it has been deleted.*

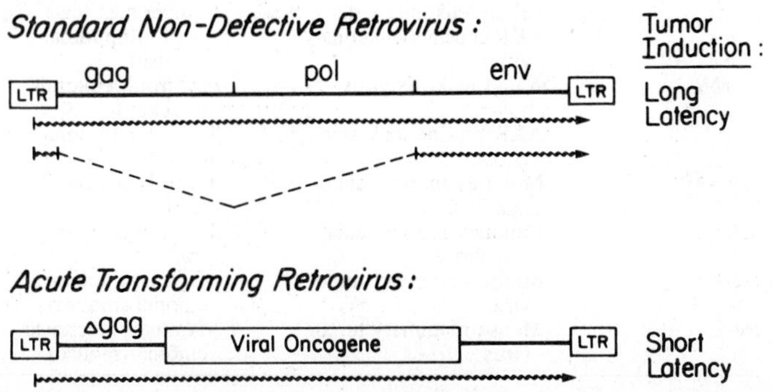

TABLE 59-1 Viral oncogenes that cause acute transformation

Name	Virus	Tumors in vivo
CHICKEN		
src	Rous sarcoma virus (RSV)	Sarcomas
yes	Y73 sarcoma virus	Sarcomas
fps/fes	Fujinami sarcoma virus	Sarcomas
ros	UR11 avian sarcoma virus	Sarcomas
erbB	Avian erythroblastosis virus (AEV)	Erythroid leukemia
myb	Avian myeloblastosis virus (AMV)	Myeloid leukemia
myc	Avian myelocytomatosis virus (MC-29)	Leukemia, endothelioma
ski	Avian SKV770 virus	Unknown
TURKEY		
rel	Reticuloendotheliosis virus (REV)	Lymphomas
MOUSE		
abl	Abelson leukemia virus	B lymphomas
mos	Moloney murine sarcoma virus (MoMSV)	Sarcomas
fos	FBJ osteosarcoma virus	Osteosarcoma
raf	3611 murine sarcoma virus	Sarcomas
RAT		
Ha-*ras*1	Harvey murine sarcoma virus (HaMSV)	Sarcomas, erythroid leukemia
Ki-*ras*2	Kirsten murine sarcoma virus (KiMSV)	Sarcomas, erythroid leukemia
CAT		
fes/fps	Snyder Thielen feline sarcoma virus (ST-FeSV)	Sarcomas
fms	McDonough feline sarcoma virus (SM-FeSV)	Sarcomas
fgr	Gardner-Rasheed feline sarcoma virus (GR-FeSV)	Sarcomas
MONKEY		
sis	Simian sarcoma virus (SSV)	Sarcomas

zation). Infection with a different virus called HTLV-III or lymphadenopathy associated virus (LAV) is associated with the acquired immunodeficiency syndrome. The HTLVs do not appear to contain a host cell–related oncogene. Instead, unique transacting viral regulatory proteins may alter host cell behavior.

Normal human DNA contains structures that appear to be proviruses and that are genetically transmitted in the germline. Their significance is unknown.

TABLE 59-2 Proto-oncogenes and putative proto-oncogenes activated in tumors by nearby integration of retroviral proviruses

Target gene or locus	Virus	Tumor
c-*myc*	Avian leukosis virus	B-cell lymphomas (chicken)
c-*myc*	Feline leukemia virus	Lymphomas (cat)
c-*myc*	AKR-murine leukemia virus	T-cell lymphoma (mouse)
c-*erbB*	Avian leukosis virus	Erythroid leukemia (chicken)
Pim-1	AKR-murine leukemia virus	T-cell lymphoma (mouse)
Mlvi-1	Moloney murine leukemia virus	T-cell lymphoma (rat)
Mlvi-2	Moloney murine leukemia virus	T-cell lymphoma (rat)
Int-1	Mouse mammary tumor virus	Mammary adenocarcinoma (mouse)
Int-2	Mouse mammary tumor virus	Mammary adenocarcinoma (mouse)

ACTIVATED CELLULAR ONCOGENES DETECTED BY TRANSFECTION **The transfection assay for oncogenes** Certain established cell lines have the property of incorporating exogenous DNA into chromosomal DNA with an efficiency that makes experimental gene transfer practical in tissue culture. The transfection technique commonly involves precipitating the DNA onto the surface of the target cells with calcium phosphate followed by the uptake of the DNA into cells by pinocytosis. Some of the ingested DNA molecules are transported to the cell nucleus where they are integrated into the chromosomal DNA. If the transfected DNA contains a gene that can be expressed as a dominant, selectable marker in the recipient cells, transfected cells expressing this trait can be recovered with efficiencies of up to about one in 10^5 possible transfection events. Many of the viral oncogenes in Table 59-1 can induce transformation in this type of assay. Such transformation can be achieved either with pure oncogene DNA or with total chromosomal DNA from cells transformed by retroviruses.

Activated cellular oncogenes can also be detected by this technique in the DNA of tumors not known to be induced by viruses. For example, DNA from chemically transformed animal cells and DNA from a variety of naturally occurring animal and human tumor cells contain transforming genes. Normal high-molecular-weight human DNA does not transform cells, but transforming genes can be activated by fragmentation of normal cellular DNA. These findings support the concept that proto-oncogenes in the normal genome are activated during tumor formation but do not distinguish whether the activation of transforming genes is a cause or an effect of the neoplastic phenotype. Although only a fraction of human tumor DNAs will transform in transfection assays, these observations opened the way for analysis of the molecular genetics of human neoplasia.

The *ras* family of cellular oncogenes Some of the transforming genes detected by transfection of cells with DNA from human tumor cells have been identified (Table 59-3). The most common oncogenes belong to a family of genes called *ras*. The first to be identified was the human homologue of the oncogene of Harvey murine sarcoma virus (Table 59-1) called c-*ras*^{H}, which codes for a protein of 21,000 mol wt called p21 and is activated in a human cell line derived from bladder carcinoma. In cells transformed by Harvey sarcoma virus, p21 is expressed at high levels, and high-level expression of c-*ras*^{H} by experimental linkage of the cellular gene to viral regulatory elements is sufficient to induce cellular transformation. Nevertheless, c-*ras*^{H} is not expressed at high levels in those human tumor cell lines in which it is detectable. Instead, the ability to transform cells appears to be conferred by point mutations that cause amino acid changes either at amino acid position 12 or 61 of the p21 protein. Thus, either altered regulation or mutations of protein structure can activate this proto-oncogene.

A second member of the *ras* family is more frequently activated in human tumors, e.g., the human homologue of the transforming gene of the Kirsten murine sarcoma virus called c-*ras*^{K}. Between 10 and 20 percent of human tumor DNA from diverse neoplasms contains a c-*ras*^{K} gene that transforms cells in transfection assay (Table 59-3). A protein encoded by c-*ras*^{K} is also a p21 molecule, and the transforming activity is due to a structural mutation of this protein similar to that seen for c-*ras*^{H}. This mutation is not present in DNA derived from normal tissues of individuals with carcinomas containing an activated c-*ras*^{K} gene, suggesting that activation is a somatic event which occurs during tumor formation. Finally, in transfection experiments with DNA from some tumors a third member of this family called *ras*^{N} induces transformation. Activation of *ras*^{N} occurs in 10 to 20 percent of human acute myeloid leukemias.

Activation of *ras* is a regular event in some chemically induced epithelial carcinomas in rodents, implying that these genes are activated by chemical carcinogens. However, activated *ras* genes are found only in a fraction of tumors in humans. As yet unidentified alterations of *ras* may occur in human tumors, or alteration of other genes might act in place of altered *ras* genes during tumor development. Neither of these possibilities may be detectable in the standard transfection assays. Alternatively, activation of all oncogenes could be a result of the neoplastic state, rather than an underlying cause. Formal proof for a causative role of activated *ras* genes in the human tumors in which they are found is lacking.

Possible lineage-specific oncogenes In contrast to the *ras* family, which appears to be involved in many types of neoplasms, activation of other oncogenes may be specific to neoplasms of particular cell lineages. The first of these to be identified is called *ChBlym*-1. DNA from chicken lymphomas induced by avian leukosis virus transforms cells in transfection assays, while DNA from normal tissues of the same birds does not have this property. A gene believed to be responsible for this activity, *ChBlym*-1, was obtained from cells transformed by DNA from a bursal lymphoma cell line. It appears to be unrelated to *ras* or the other viral oncogenes described in Table 59-1. As with other oncogenes, nucleotide sequences related to *ChBlym*-1 are conserved in evolution and are present in human DNA.

Human Burkitt's lymphoma resembles the virus-induced lymphomas of chickens in that it is composed of similar B cells at about the same stage of differentiation. The DNA from most Burkitt's lymphoma cell lines can transform cells in transfection assays. This property appears to be due to a gene called *HuBlym*-1, which has about 50 percent homology at the DNA sequence level to *ChBlym*-1. Thus, *Blym* oncogenes are activated in B-cell lymphomas in both chickens and humans but have not been found in other types of tumors. The normal homologues of these transforming genes have not been characterized, so that the cause for activation of the *Blym* oncogenes is not known.

Other B-cell and T-cell neoplasms and adenocarcinomas of the breast contain transforming genes that appear to be distinct for each tumor type. For example, a transforming gene in neoplasms with an intermediate stage of T-cell differentiation, called *Tlym*-1, is distinct from other known oncogenes.

ONCOGENES IMPLICATED IN TUMOR FORMATION BY CHROMOSOMAL TRANSLOCATIONS AND OTHER REARRANGEMENTS A third line of evidence for the activation of oncogenes during tumor formation is derived from the analysis of cytogenetic changes in human neoplasms. Most human tumors are clonal or oligoclonal, that is, composed of cell populations dominated by the progeny of single cells. The dominant cell clones of certain neoplasms are marked by consistent chromosomal abnormalities, such as reciprocal translocations between chromosome 9 and chromosome 22 in chronic myelogenous leukemia (producing the Philadelphia chromosome, Ph′) or between chromosomes 8 and 14 in Burkitt's lymphoma. Indeed, characteristic nonrandom chromosomal changes have been identified in many neoplasms. Genes at or near the site of the DNA rearrangements underlying these cytogenic changes might play a role in the development of the tumors. Advances in in situ hybridization and other techniques of somatic cell genetics have also made it possible to locate the approximate positions of a number of proto-oncogenes on human chromosomes (Table 59-4). Some of these genes are located near the breakpoints of chromosomes that are translocated in particular tumors.

Rearrangement of the c-*myc* locus in Burkitt's lymphoma As noted in Table 59-4, the human c-*myc* gene is located on chromosome 8. This chromosome is invariably involved in a translocation in Burkitt's lymphoma. At the DNA level the translocation involves recombination between the c-*myc* locus on chromosome 8 and an immunoglobulin gene locus, usually near a heavy chain gene on chromosome 14, less often near a light chain gene on chromosomes 2 or 22. This translocation does not appear to affect the structure of the protein coding portion of the c-*myc* locus but instead affects the regulation of its expression. Similar translocations resulting in recombination between c-*myc* and immunoglobulin genes occur in mouse plasmacytomas.

Alteration of c-*abl* expression as a result of chromosomal translocation in chronic myelogenous leukemia The Ph′ chromosome is present both in leukemic cells and in normal marrow cell lineages from most patients with chronic myelogenous leukemia (CML). In this disease, the marrow and peripheral blood are thought to be populated by the progeny of a hematopoietic stem cell that retains its ability to differentiate into red cells, megakaryocytes, and granulocytes. The proliferation of granulocytes, however, is abnormal and excessive, producing the clinical manifestations of CML. Genes whose expression is altered as a consequence of the formation of the Ph′ chromosome are candidates for involvement in the development of CML. The human homologue of the proto-oncogene c-*abl* (Table 59-1) is located near the breakpoint on chromosome 9 for the 9-22 translocation and is transferred to chromosome 22 in the exchange. In the Ph′ chromosome the expression of c-*abl* appears to be both quantitatively and qualitatively altered. The levels of c-*abl* RNA are increased, and both the predominant RNA transcript of the gene and the c-*abl* protein are larger than the c-*abl* RNA and protein molecules in normal cells. The RNA and protein gene products of the c-*abl* focus in CML cells are thought to include a fusion production of the c-*abl* gene and a gene called *bcr* (breakpoint cluster region) at the breakpoint on the recombinant Ph′ chromosome. If this alteration in c-*abl* plays a role in CML, it must be at an early stage of the disease.

Amplified proto-oncogenes in human tumors An increase in gene copy number per cell (gene amplification) can sometimes be manifested at the cytogenetic level by the formation of small chromosome-like structures called double minute chromosomes or by the appearance of homogeneous staining regions (HSRs) on regular chromosomes. HSRs are the result of amplification of segments of DNA within the chromosome to the extent that they are identifiable cytogenetically. As a consequence, the structure contains multiple copies of the gene(s) encoded by the DNA segment. Gene amplification in nontransformed cells can sometimes be induced by growing the cells

TABLE 59-3 **Oncogenes detected in human tumors by transfection of NIH/3T3 cells**

Oncogene	Tumors or tumor-derived cell lines
c-*ras*^{H}	Cell lines derived from EJ/T24 bladder carcinoma, lung carcinoma, and mammary carcinosarcoma
c-*ras*^{K}	Lung, colon, bladder, pancreatic, and ovarian carcinomas; rhabdomyosarcoma
ras^N	Neuroblastoma, fibrosarcoma, promyelocytic and acute myelogenous leukemia, Burkitt's lymphoma, and colon carcinoma
HuBlym-1	Burkitt's lymphoma cell lines (several)
Tlym-1	T-cell lymphoma–derived cell lines*

* *The cloned* Tlym-*1 gene is of mouse origin. A similar transforming gene appears to be activated in human T-cell lymphoma lines as judged by patterns of inactivation by restriction endonucleases.*

TABLE 59-4 **Localization of some proto-oncogenes on human chromosomes.**

Gene	Chromosome	Chromosomal sublocalization, or band*
c-*myc*	8	q24
c-*abl*	9	q34
c-*mos*	8	q22
c-*fes*	15	q24–q25
c-*myb*	6	q22–q24
c-*mil* (raf)	3	p25
N-*ras*	1	cen→p21
c-*ras*^{H}	11	p14.1
c-*ras*^{K}	12	p12.05→ter
c-*ets*	11	q23–q24
c-*erbB*	7	pter→q22
c-*erbA*	17	q21–q22
HuBlym-1	1	p32
c-*fms*	5	q34
c-*fos*	14	q21→q31
c-*ski*	1	NA
c-*sis*	22	q11→ter
c-*src*-1	20	p34–p36
c-*src*-2	1	q12→ter

* *q = long arm, p = short arm, cen = centromere, ter = terminal, NA = not available*

under special conditions. For example, cells containing an amplification of the dihydrofolate reductase gene, which is required for DNA replication, can be selected when cells are grown in the presence of low levels of methotrexate, an inhibitor of dihydrofolate reductase. This increase in gene copy number enhances the amount of enzyme in the cell and overcomes the effects of the inhibitor. Double minute chromosomes and HSRs are present in a variety of tumor cells, suggesting that genes critical to the growth of neoplastic cells may amplify during tumor formation.

The first amplified oncogene recognized in a human tumor cell was the c-*myc* gene which was expressed at a high level in one case of promyelocytic leukemia, both in fresh tumor cells and in a derived cell line. Amplification of c-*myc* appears to be a rare event in this neoplasm and has not been observed in other promyelocytic leukemias. However, double minute chromosomes, amplification of c-*myc* genes, and elevated levels of c-*myc* RNA have been reported in some gastric cancers and small cell carcinomas of the lung, and amplification of the c-*myc* proto-oncogene has been reported in two cell lines derived from human colon carcinoma. Human neuroblastomas are characterized by a high frequency of double minute chromosomes and HSRs. A gene called N-*myc*, which is related to the c-*myc* gene, is amplified and/or expressed at a high level in most neuroblastomas, in cell lines derived from neuroblastomas, and in other neuroendocrine tumors. Considerable heterogeneity occurs within the tumor cell population with respect to the degree of amplification and/or expression of N-*myc*.

FUNCTIONS OF ONCOGENES Studies of the proteins encoded by the viral oncogenes and their normal cellular homologues have provided insight into the functions of these genes. The protein product of the v-*src* gene of Rous sarcoma virus acts as a tyrosine protein kinase, and the oncogenic properties of v-*src* depend upon this enzymatic activity. Five additional viral oncogene proteins (those encoded by *fes/fps, yes, ros, abl,* and *fgr*) are also tyrosine protein kinases. The problem has been to identify the cellular proteins that are modified by these kinases and that are critical for transformation. For example, in cells transformed by Rous sarcoma virus, a number of cellular proteins are modified by the addition of phosphate groups to tyrosine residues, but a role for such changes in oncogenesis has not been established.

Growth factors and receptors An important conceptual advance has come from separate lines of research on oncogene function and growth factor function (Fig. 59-3). The proliferation and differentiation of normal cells are regulated by signals derived from the binding of growth factors to receptors on the cell surface. Two of the better characterized growth factors are platelet-derived growth factor (PDGF), which promotes the growth of connective tissue and smooth muscle cells, and epidermal growth factor (EGF), which is required for optimal growth of epithelial cells in vitro. The receptors for PDGF and EGF possess a tyrosine protein kinase which is activated by binding of PDGF or EGF. Whether the growth factor receptor and oncogene tyrosine protein kinases modify some of the same target proteins inside the cells is not known.

A protein encoded by the viral oncogene of Simian sarcoma virus, *sis,* is closely related to PDGF. The *erbB* oncogene of avian erythroblastosis virus appears to be a truncated form of the receptor molecule for EGF. The *fms* oncogene of a strain of feline sarcoma virus may be related to the receptor of a macrophage growth factor called CSF-1. These observations have led to the postulate that the unregulated growth signal involved in neoplastic transformation might result from changes in growth factors, their receptors, or other elements in the pathway.

***Ras* oncogene proteins** The proteins encoded by *ras* oncogenes are associated with the inner surface of the cell membrane. They share a functional activity, the binding of guanosine triphosphate (GTP), with a family of GTP-binding or G proteins. G proteins are found in association with the adenylate cyclase complex on the inner surface of the cell membrane, and they participate in the transmission of signals from the cell surface that result in changes in intracellular cyclic nucleotide levels (see Chap. 67). In yeast, *ras* genes act through the adenylate cyclase–protein kinase pathway. Thus, transforming *ras* proteins may be a class of altered G proteins that transmit a constitutive growth signal.

Oncogene proteins in the cell nucleus The proteins encoded by three of the oncogenes in Table 59-1, *myb, myc,* and *fos,* are located in the cell nucleus. The normal homologue of *myb* is expressed predominantly in the G1 phase of the cell cycle in some but not all cells. The other two genes appear to be closely tied to the growth factor pathway. When growth-arrested fibroblasts are exposed to PDGF, a specific set of genes (estimated to be between 10 and 30) is expressed, including the proto-oncogenes c-*fos* and c-*myc,* and cellular messenger RNA levels for these genes increase. Expression of c-*myc* is also enhanced in resting B and T lymphocytes after exposure to appropriate mitogens. Once cells enter the growth cycle the expression of c-*myc* remains fairly constant. When cells lose the ability to divide, for example, in postmitotic, differentiated cells, c-*myc* expression ceases. These proto-oncogenes, therefore, may function normally as regulators of cell "activation," growth, and differentiation and may be nuclear targets for growth-factor-derived signals. When altered or deregulated, they may provide a constitutive drive for the uncontrolled cell growth and abnormal differentiation that characterize the neoplastic state. Both the *myc* and *myb* proteins have DNA binding activity, but the mechanism of action of nuclear proteins is not known.

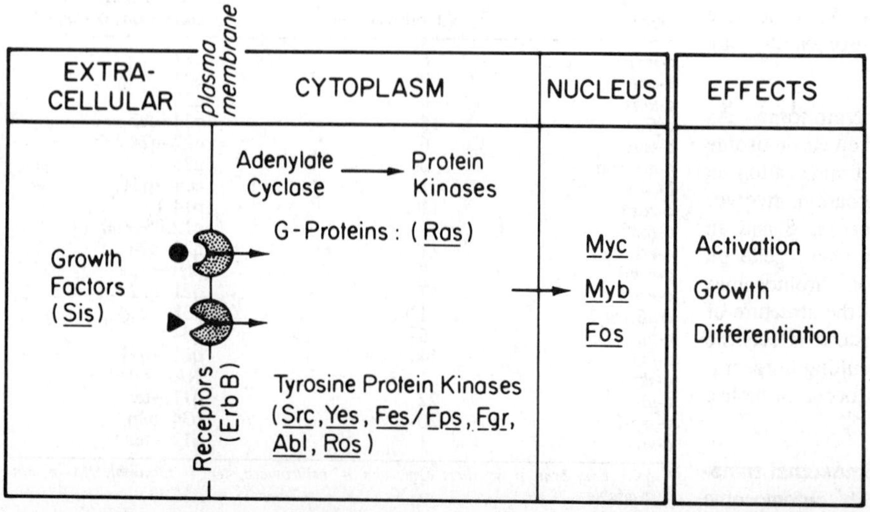

FIGURE 59-3 *Possible relationship of the molecular biology of growth factors to the function of oncogenes. Growth factors are small molecules that signal cell activation, replication, and differentiation by binding to specific receptors on the surface of target cells. As shown, a number of the proteins made by oncogenes fit into the general pathway for growth factor activity. Oncogenes may transform cells by transmitting a constitutive, unregulated signal for cell growth from their particular position in the pathway. For details see text.*

EXPERIMENTAL INTRODUCTION OF ACTIVE ONCOGENES INTO GERM CELLS AND SOMATIC TISSUE STEM CELLS One approach to demonstrating the oncogenic potential of tumor-associated oncogenes is to transfer activated oncogenes into normal cells in vivo and to observe the effects of these genes on development. Several different genes, such as those specifying immunoglobulin and growth hormone, have been introduced by microinjection into fertilized mouse eggs. The injected "trans-genes" become integrated into the genome of progeny mice and, in some cases, are expressed in appropriate cell types (for example, immunoglobulin trans-genes are expressed predominately in B lymphocytes).

The introduction by this technique of a T antigen gene from the DNA tumor virus SV40 into the germline of mice resulted in the formation of choroid plexus papillomas. Likewise, the introduction of altered c-*myc* trans-genes with promoter-enhancer sequences derived from mouse mammary tumor virus into the germline of mice caused the development of mammary tumors in some of the mice. The introduced oncogene appeared to act as a predisposing factor for the acclerated development of mammary carcinomas, but additional events may be required for the full development of mammary tumors in these animals.

Introduction of oncogenes into transplantable stem cells of bone marrow and lymphoid organs is done by infecting stem cells ex vivo with viral vectors containing the genes and then transplanting the cells into appropriately prepared hosts. The introduction of the v-*myc* gene by this technique into the stem cells of the chicken bursa induced pre-neoplastic proliferative lesions that precede the development of B-cell lymphomas. This occurred in the absence of activation of transforming genes like *Blym*-1 that are found in more advanced neoplasms of this type. Consequently, activated *myc* oncogenes may be responsible for the early pre-neoplastic stages of lymphoma formation in this system, while additional events, such as activation of *Blym*-1, may be required for neoplastic progression.

ONCOGENES AND MULTISTAGED TUMORIGENESIS Human cancer and chemically induced neoplasia in animals usually develop as a multistep process in which an abnormal pre-neoplastic cell type evolves into a cell population successively dominated by clones with increasingly malignant characteristics. This evolution of tumor development is thought to be preceded by a latent period, and the whole process may take a significant fraction of the life span of the affected individual. In contrast, acute transforming viruses carrying activated forms of oncogenes that are implicated in nonviral cancer appear to induce neoplasms within days or weeks, i.e., with kinetics that suggest a single-step process. This difference may be due to several factors. First, many of the viral oncogenes encode kinases with multiple cellular targets and may induce abrupt changes that would require several different mutations in more slowly evolving neoplasms. Second, expression of the viral oncogenes is driven by powerful regulatory elements (promoters and enhancers in the proviral LTRs). The transforming potential of the cellular homologues of these same genes can be activated by mechanisms that do not involve such high-level expression, for example, the point mutations at amino acids 12 or 61 of the proteins encoded by the human *ras* tumor-associated oncogenes. In these situations the concerted activity of several genes may be required to induce the same transformed phenotype that can be induced by very high level, unregulated expression of just one of the genes (as occurs with acute transforming retroviruses).

This point is illustrated by transfection experiments suggesting cooperation between oncogenes in inducing transformation of cultured fibroblasts. The activated *ras* genes from human tumor cells can transform immortalized cell lines but cannot induce full morphologic transformation of primary cell cultures. The combination of activated *myc* and *ras* gene clones, however, produces the fully transformed phenotype in primary cell cultures. Thus, in this system *myc* (and other oncogenes that do not alter these cells by themselves) can complement the transforming activating of human *ras* oncogenes. However, when powerful transcriptional enhancer sequences are engineered into the activated *ras* oncogene, this gene can itself transform primary fibroblast cultures, presumably because of a higher level of expression of the oncogene. The requirement for multiple genes in transformation may be conditioned, in part, by the level of oncogene expression, and more than one cellular oncogene may be activated in neoplasms in vivo.

IMPLICATIONS OF ONCOGENE RESEARCH FOR CLINICAL ONCOLOGY The clinical impact of the identification and analysis of human oncogenes and their products may be extensive, indeed revolutionary. For example, efforts to identify and control environmental and nutritional factors that may cause or prevent cancer depend heavily on epidemiologic techniques, animal studies, and clinical trials where disease incidence and mortality are endpoints for measurement. Knowledge of the specific proto-oncogenes that are the targets of environmental carcinogens and of the nature of the changes induced may provide better methods for assessing the actual role of candidate carcinogens and for devising preventive approaches. Delineation of the molecular anatomy of neoplastic change in specific cell lineages should also add new dimensions to diagnosis. An example would be the use of rapid techniques for detecting alteration of the c-*abl* RNA and/or protein for analysis of chronic myelogenous leukemia cells. Knowledge of the molecular mechanisms employed by oncogenes to transform cells may also provide more precise and more specific means for targeting pharmacologic intervention.

REFERENCES

BISHOP JM, VARMUS H: Functions and origins of retroviral transforming genes, in *Molecular Biology of Tumor Viruses; RNA Tumor Viruses,* 2d ed, R Weiss et al (eds). New York, Cold Spring Harbor Laboratory, 1982, pp 999–1108

COHEN S: The epidermal growth factor (EGF). Cancer 51:1787, 1983

COOPER GM, LANE MA: Cellular transforming genes and oncogenes. Biochim Biophys Acta 738:9, 1984

FIALKOW PJ: Clonal origin of human tumors. Ann Rev Med 30:135, 1979

HUNTER T: The proteins of oncogenes. Sci Am 251:70, 1984

LAND H et al: Cellular oncogenes and multistep carcinogens. Science 222:771, 1983

LEDER P et al: Translocations among antibody genes in cancer. Science 222:765, 1983

STILES CD: The molecular biology of platelet-derived growth factor. Cell 33:653, 1983

WEINSTEIN IB: Multistage carcinogenesis involves multiple genes and multiple mechanisms, in *Cancer Cells,* AJ Levine et al (eds). New York, Cold Spring Harbor Laboratory, 1984, pp 229–237

YUNIS JJ: The chromosomal basis of human neoplasia. Science 221:227, 1983

60 CYTOGENETIC ASPECTS OF HUMAN DISEASE

JAMES L. GERMAN III

The chromosome complement of humans, like that of other species, is guarded carefully against change; most chromosome mutations, either structural or numerical, are deleterious. Only rarely is a balanced structural rearrangement (one that results in neither deficiency nor duplication of significant chromosome segments) introduced into the population and transmitted from generation to generation. (Figure 60-1 shows the normal human chromosome complement. In the legend of the figure several terms used in human cytogenetics are defined.) As a rule an abnormal number of autosomes results in early death, except for trisomy of the shortest chromosome. In contrast, an abnormal number of sex chromosomes is often tolerated reasonably well, although infertility or subfertility usually is present. Nevertheless, among human embryos abnormalities in chromosome structure and number are common and are, in fact, the major known cause of embryonic and early fetal wastage. However, not every fetus with an abnormal chromosome complement is aborted, and those that survive constitute the material of medical cytogenetics.

Clinical disorders resulting from chromosome imbalance present varying features including abnormal anatomic development, mental

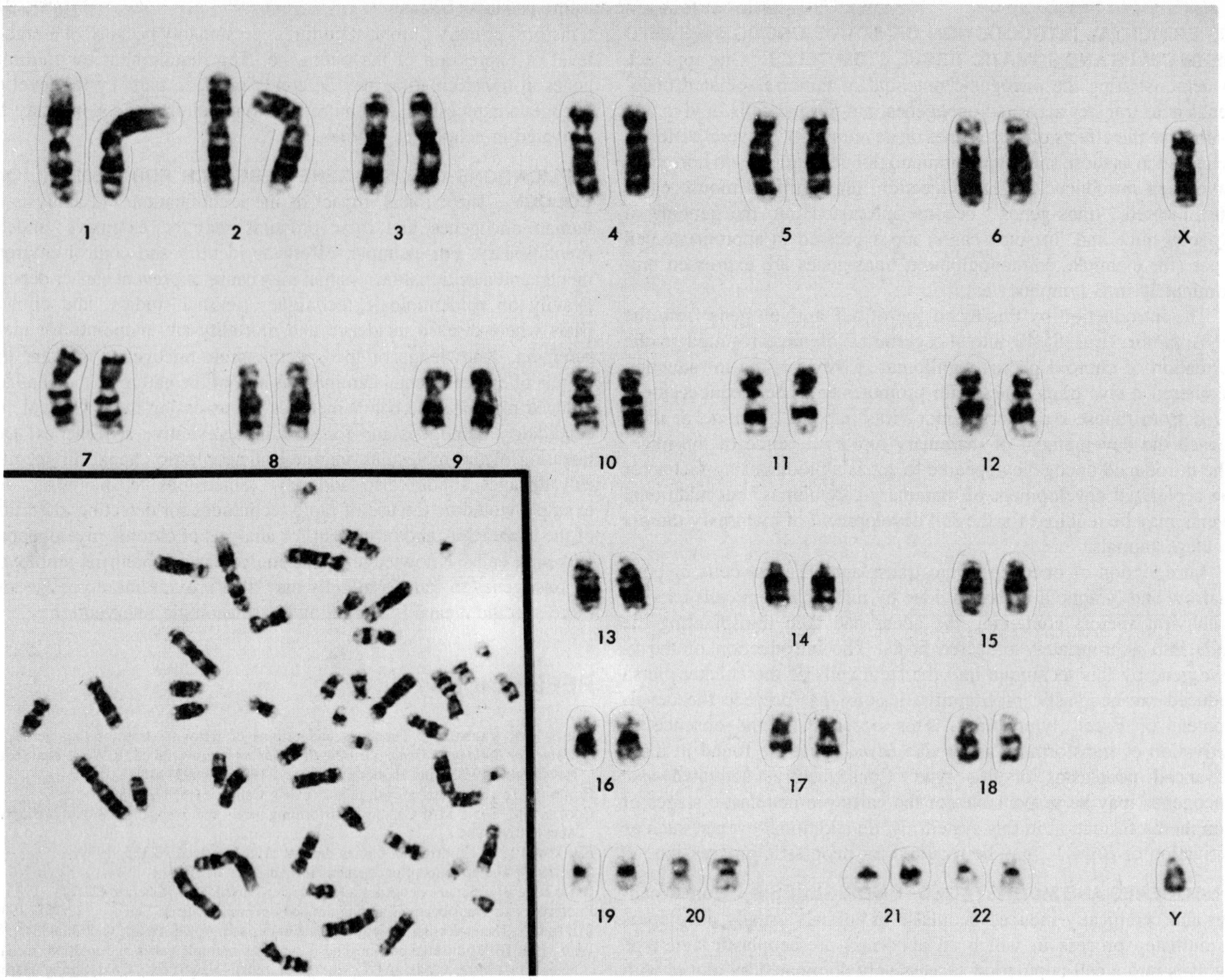

FIGURE 60-1 *Normal human lymphocyte chromosomes arrested in metaphase and stained for G bands (G standing for Giemsa). The inset shows the arrangement of chromosomes in an intact cell, and the remainder of the figure shows their ordered arrangement into a karyotype. By the time mitosis begins, each chromosome consists of two identical parts called sister chromatids and is identified by the relative length, the location of the centromere, and a distinctive sequence of bands of varying lengths and depth of staining. The number of bands visible microscopically varies from cell to cell, depending on the degree of chromosome condensation. The 300 to 400 bands seen in this particular cell can be increased to several times that number if cells with longer chromosomes are chosen for analysis, i.e., many of the bands seen here will resolve into subbands. Normally, the G-band patterns of the two chromosomes of a pair are alike, with the exception of certain polymorphic regions, examples of which are shown in Fig. 60-4.*

The centromere of a chromosome divides it into a short arm (p) and a long arm (q). Numbers 13 to 15, 21, 22, and Y are called acrocentric because of the nearly terminal positions of their centromeres; the minute p of each acrocentric autosome bears a nucleolus-organizing region which often causes a secondary constriction in the metaphase chromosome (the constriction at the centromere being the primary constriction).

By standard nomenclature, this karyotype is described as 46,XY, indicating that its chromosome number is 46, its sex chromosomes are an X and a Y, and the autosomes (those besides the X and Y) number 44. The following examples show the general use of this nomenclature: A normal female karyotype is described as 46,XX. A female cell with an extra chromosome 18 (trisomic for 18) would be described as 47,XX, +18. A cell with only one sex chromosome, an X, and with deletion in the short arm of chromosome 5 would be described as 45,X,5p−. A male cell with a translocation between the long arm of chromosome 2 and the short arm of chromosome 3 would be described as 46,XY,t(2q;3p); exact breakpoints could be indicated by additional characters and symbols.

deficiency, behavioral disorders, and disturbances in growth and sexual development. Sometimes infertility, repeated abortion, or the birth of malformed children is the presenting complaint of persons with abnormal chromosome complements whose own general development is normal.

The disorders just referred to are due to chromosome imbalance that affects tissues throughout the body. In addition, change can occur in the chromosome complement in a single cell of some somatic tissue. Such a mutant cell may have a proliferative advantage over normal cells, in which case a clone bearing the abnormal chromosome complement can develop among otherwise normal cells. Although such mutant clones are in many cases clinically insignificant, much evidence suggests that they are also important in the etiology of cancer.

This chapter is addressed to those aspects of normal chromosome structure and function that constitute the basis for an understanding of the chromosome alterations in human disease. In addition, the chromosome alterations important in adult medicine and their consequences are summarized.

CHROMOSOME STRUCTURE AND FUNCTION The human autosomes are numbered 1 through 22, and the sex chromosomes are denoted X and Y (Fig. 60-1). Each is recognizable microscopically by morphologic features such as relative length and position of the centromere and by staining characteristics (banding pattern). A mammalian chromosome is believed to be composed of one double-stranded chain of deoxyribonucleic acid (DNA) that extends from one end through the centromere to the other end.

Cell-division cycle Chromosomes must duplicate before cell division can occur. This duplication occurs over a period of several hours prior to the onset of mitosis or meiosis in a phase of the cell cycle termed S, for synthesis of DNA (Fig. 60-2). Thus, from the completion of S to the completion of metaphase, each chromosome contains two identical double-stranded helices of DNA, and the nucleus contains four times as much DNA as a spermatozoon or ovum. During mitosis chromosomes are condensed, and the two sister chromatids can be visualized by late prophase or early metaphase (Fig. 60-1). (Metaphase is the stage in the cell-division cycle ordinarily employed for cytogenetic analysis.)

At the onset of anaphase the centromeric regions of each chromosome separate, and the two chromatids move quickly to opposite poles of the mitotic spindle. As soon as each pole receives one full complement of chromatids (now called chromosomes), a nuclear membrane—it had been disassembled late in prophase—is assembled about each cluster to complete formation of the nuclei of the two sister cells that emerge at telophase. The sister cells emerge in what usually is called the G_1 phase of the cell cycle, in which they remain unreplicated unless another division is to be prepared for, whereupon they enter the S phase. Cells engaged in some differentiated function ordinarily remain unreplicated.

Most normal cells in the human body are diploid; i.e., they have twice the haploid number of chromosomes, the number in a gamete (haploid = 23, diploid = 46). In the germ line, which is devoted to gamete formation, cells destined eventually to differentiate into spermatozoa or ova undergo mitotic cell cycles until they enter the two specialized divisions termed *meiosis*. In meiosis, pairing of homologous chromosomes occurs (the paternally derived chromosome 1 with the maternally derived chromosome 1, and so on), and genetic recombination takes place (see Chap. 57). At the first meiotic division homologous chromosomes are segregated, and the diploid chromosome number is reduced to the haploid; i.e., each cell then contains one of each of the 22 (duplicated) autosomes plus one (duplicated) sex chromosome. No S phase takes place between the first and second meiotic divisions (depicted in Fig. 60-2, right), so that at the second division, in which sister chromatids separate, emerging cells maintain the haploid number of chromosomes but are reduced in their content of DNA to half the amount of diploid G_1 cells of somatic tissues. With fertilization of an ovum by a spermatozoon, both the chromosome constitution and the DNA content of the zygote are restored to that of a G_1 somatic cell. An S period in the zygote then permits reinstitution of regular cell-division cycles characteristic of the somatic cells.

Chromosome differentiation A chromosome is differentiated along its length, and some aspects of this differentiation are resolvable in the light microscope. The DNA is complexed with a number of proteins in a highly specific way. The DNA-protein complex together with some associated ribonucleic acid (RNA) is referred to as *chromatin*. The fine structure and the manner in which the DNA is compacted and interacted with proteins are thought to pertain to the control of RNA production and DNA replication, and perhaps to cellular differentiation as well.

The sequences of nucleotide bases in DNA that constitute the genes and that can be transcribed into messenger RNA are distributed throughout the length of the various chromosomes. (These sequences are too short to be resolved microscopically.) Over 400 genes have been mapped to specific chromosomes, in many cases to specific regions of a chromosome. The locations of a few of the many genes of interest in clinical medicine and that have been mapped are shown in Fig. 60-3.

Certain segments of at least 12 chromosomes vary in length among individuals. These segments can be delineated by their staining characteristics (Fig. 60-4). The variable segments consist of nontranscribed, highly repetitive nucleotide sequences of DNA and are transmitted from parent to child in a straightforward mendelian fashion. Techniques of molecular genetics, which are useful as an extension of the microscopic observation of human chromosomes, permit the identification and molecular definition of an even greater number of variable segments of DNA, ones that are submicroscopic. These sometimes are referred to as *restriction fragment-length polymorphisms* (RFLPs). Variations in both the microscopically visible and invisible segments are unassociated with detectable phenotypic effect. However, they can serve as useful cell markers in prenatal diagnosis when they have been shown to lie very close to disease-associated loci (e.g., Duchenne's muscular dystrophy) and in determination of zygosity of twins, paternity, and survival of transplants.

Other microscopically recognizable segments in the short arms of the acrocentric autosomes are devoted to the production of ribosomal RNA and nucleoli. As mitosis progresses, these nucleolus-organizer regions tend to remain relatively uncondensed later than other regions. Consequently, at metaphase they appear understained and thereby demarcate condensed segments of chromatin distal to them on the chromosome arms—*satellites*. (Satellites are examples of the polymorphic segments just mentioned.) Several other regions that remain relatively uncondensed at metaphase and that are seen more often than the remainder of the chromatin to undergo outright disruption ("breakage") are recognizable in a low percentage of cells from some normal individuals and sometimes are called *fragile sites*. In a few cases studied the tendency for such fragile sites to be visible at metaphase is a dominantly transmitted trait. The only such region known to be of significance in relation to a human trait is one located near the distal end (the end away from the centromere) of the long arm of the X chromosome; it segregates in certain families as an X-linked trait in association with a syndrome that features mental defectiveness, a characteristic facies, and macroorchia—the "fragile-X syndrome." (This locus is one of the mapped loci indicated in Fig. 60-3.) Other examples of segmental specialization along the chromosome include *telomeres* and *centromeres*. Telomeres, the distal termini of each arm, have some relationship to the nuclear membrane and probably are important in the maintenance of order in the interphase nucleus; centromeric regions are sites of microtubule attachment at metaphase.

FIGURE 60-2 *Schematic representation of the mitotic and meiotic cell-division cycles, as described in the text. G_1 and G_2 = time gaps before and after S, the period in which DNA replicates. Each of these intervals is several hours in duration; together they constitute interphase. M = mitosis; I and II = the two divisions of meiosis. The DNA content of the cycling cells is indicated on the vertical axis: 1c = the content in a gamete; 2c = that in either an egg immediately postfertilization or a somatic cell emerging from mitosis; 4c = the amount in a cell which has completed chromosome duplication and is ready to enter mitosis or meiosis.*

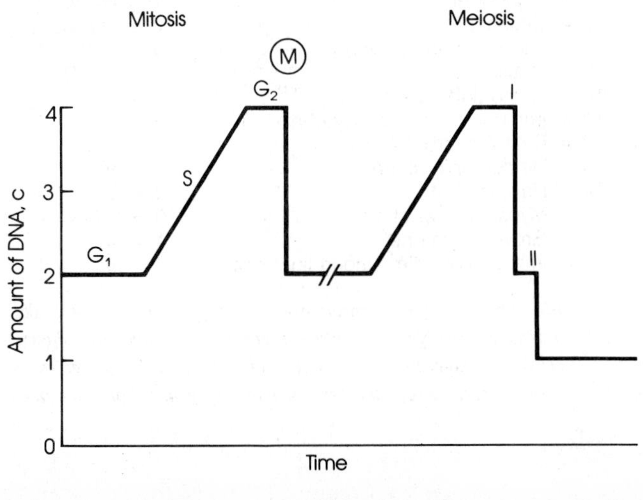

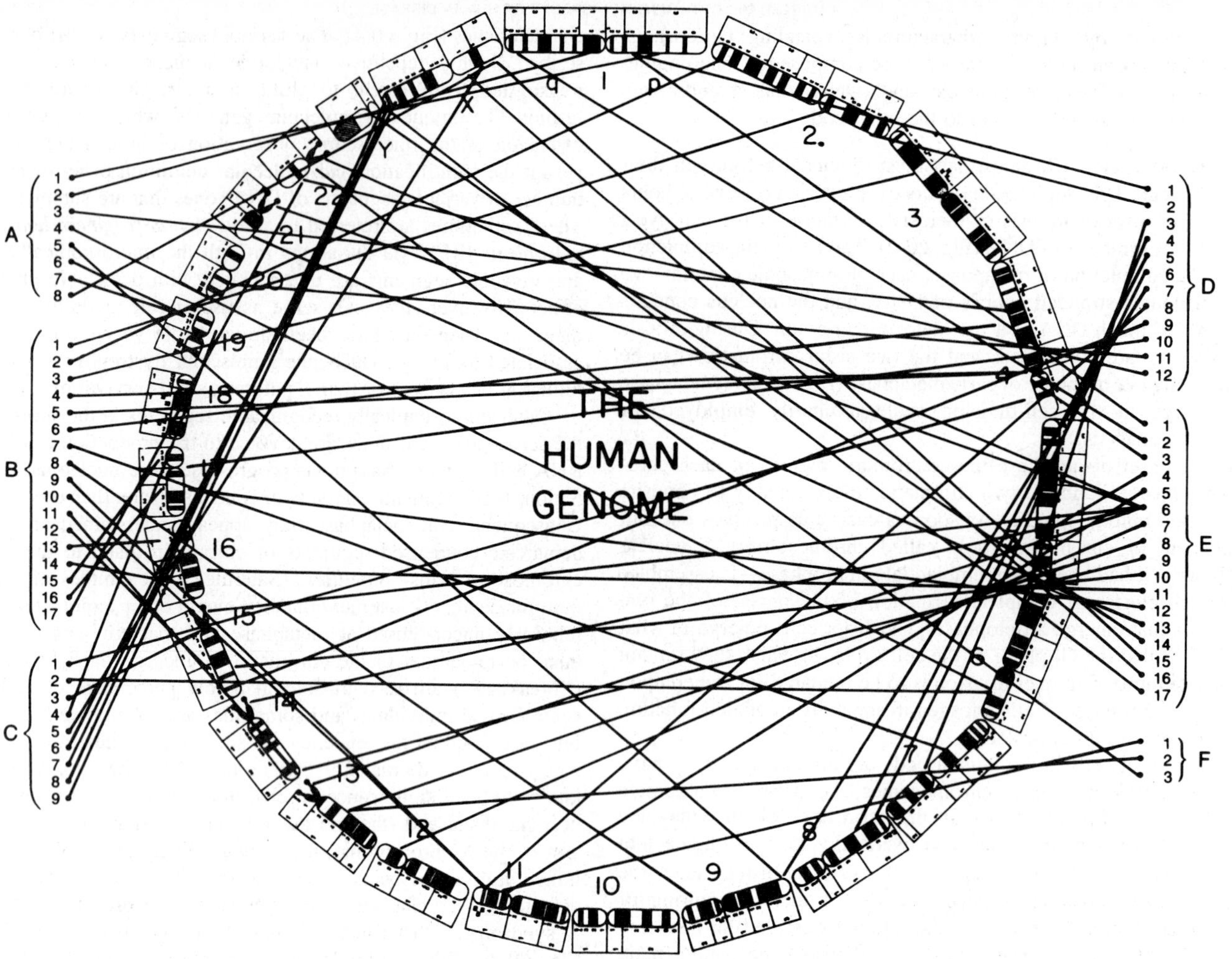

A: CELL SURFACE ANTIGENS
1 = Rhesus
2 = Duffy
3 = MNSs
4 = MHC
5 = ABO
6 = Lewis
7 = Lutheran
8 = Xg

B: DIFFERENTIATED CELL PRODUCTS
1 = Immunoglobulin kappa-light chain
2 = Glucagon
3 = Transferrin
4 = Albumin
5 = Alpha-fetoprotein
6 = Fibrinogen
7 = Collagen I
8 = Interferon (leukocyte)
9 = Insulin
10 = Hemoglobin-beta
11 = Immunoglobulin heavy chain
12 = Beta-2-microglobulin
13 = Hemoglobin-alpha
14 = Haptoglobin
15 = Myosin heavy chain
16 = Growth hormone
17 = Immunoglobulin lambda-light chain

C: GENES FOR DISEASE
1 = Huntington's chorea
2 = Congenital adrenal hyperplasia
3 = Prader-Willi syndrome
4 = Familial hypercholesterolemia (LDL receptor)
5 = Duchenne's muscular dystrophy
6 = Hunter's syndrome
7 = Hemophilia B
8 = Hemophilia A
9 = X-linked mental deficiency

D: CELLULAR ONCOGENES
1 = *N-ras*
2 = *N-myc*
3 = *myb*
4 = *erb B*
5 = *mos*
6 = *myc*
7 = *abl*
8 = *H-ras*
9 = *fes*
10 = *erb A*
11 = *src*
12 = *sis*

E: MISCELLANEOUS
1 = Phosphoglucomutase
2 = 55 ribosomal RNA
3 = Phosphoglucomutase-2
4 = Dihydrofolate reductase
5 = Lactate dehydrogenase A
6 = Ribosomal RNA
7 = Lactate dehydrogenase B
8 = Esterase D
9 = DNA segment D14S1
10 = Hexosaminidase-A
11 = Metallothionein
12 = Thymidine kinase
13 = Superoxide dismutase-1
14 = Testis-determining factor
15 = Steroid sulfatase
16 = DNA segment DXS7
17 = G-6-PD

F: "CANCER GENES"
1 = Wilms's tumor
2 = Retinoblastoma
3 = Meningioma

FIGURE 60-3 *The 24 human chromosomes arrayed in a circle. The distinctive bands demonstrable by several cytogenetic techniques are shown, with the numerical designations that were agreed upon by a series of international conferences. From the several hundred genes that have been mapped to specific chromosome regions, a few of interest in medicine have been selected and their locations indicated. (For a current listing of all known human gene localizations, see McKusick.)*

A further example of chromosome differentiation is the established sequence by which various segments replicate during S; certain segments replicate early, others late. In general, late replication of a chromosome segment correlates with genetic inertness. This correlation is exemplified by one of the two X chromosomes in female cells; the chromosome inactivated by the Lyon effect is almost entirely late-replicating (see Chap. 57 for an explanation of X-chromosome inactivation).

A little-understood type of chromatin is that which long has been referred to as *heterochromatin*. It is tightly condensed, not just at metaphase but throughout interphase. Such condensation of chromatin correlates positively with genetic inactivity and also with late replication. Some regions are condensed and inactive in all cells (constitutive heterochromatin), while others, for example, the X chromosome, may be either condensed and inactive or decondensed and active (facultative heterochromatin). Many chromosome imbalances that permit viability beyond intrauterine life involve chromosome segments that are rich in this apparently inactive, or inactivatable, type of chromatin, e.g., chromosomes that can be trisomic in liveborn individuals or, in the case of X, monosomic. The activity of genes can sometimes be affected, even inactivated, if they are positioned near regions of heterochromatin, as can occur as a result of chromosome breakage and rearrangement.

Therefore, in chromosomal imbalance both the specific genetic loci and the particular types of chromatin deleted or duplicated are important. Also, the significance of a structural rearrangement probably depends on the new and abnormal positioning of structural and regulatory genes in relation to each other and to heterochromatin.

Fortunately for the cytologist, several differentiated features of the chromosome correlate with cytological artifacts that can be produced and visualized in the laboratory. A number of techniques are now in use to display a pattern of bands of various lengths and staining characteristics (Figs. 60-1 and 60-4). These patterns are identical in each chromosome 1, each chromosome 2, etc., varying only in the inert polymorphic regions mentioned above, so that they can be used in clinical cytogenetics to identify chromosomes and to detect and define structural rearrangements.

Sources of error Every aspect of the cell-division cycle is complicated. Doubtless a large number of genetic loci must be active to produce the numerous enzymes and structural proteins required to initiate and complete a cycle. Remarkable precision and accuracy are demanded over and over in matters such as the passage of a cell from G_1 into S, orderly progression of replication, assembly of the mitotic spindle, and spindle function in segregating chromatids during mitosis. An additional battery of loci is activated to permit a cell of the germ line to pass successfully through the complicated stages of meiotic prophase, including pairing of homologous chromosomes, genetic recombination, and then disjoining of chromosomes. Probably all these mechanisms and processes are subject to errors, some spontaneous, others promoted by some unfavorable environmental influence (e.g., Fig. 60-5) or by the presence of deleterious mutations involving one of the many steps just mentioned. Furthermore, the genetic material itself is subject to damage, and certain types of unrepaired or erroneously repaired lesions in DNA theoretically may predispose to chromosome rearrangement. Errors at many of these steps lie behind chromosome imbalance. Errors that occur in germ cells, during fertilization, and in early postfertilization divisions are important in relation to embryonic maldevelopment and infertility; errors in somatic cells are important in relation to neoplasia.

CHROMOSOME ABNORMALITIES Mutations of a single base in a gene and deletions and duplications of chromosome segments involving even hundreds of base pairs are not visible to the cytogeneticist. In fact, for the normal chromosome banding pattern to be detectably disturbed, a lengthy segment of DNA must be deleted, duplicated, or transposed. This means that a chromosome mutation that is microscopically detectable must involve relatively huge amounts of DNA. It is noteworthy, however, that the same environmental agents known to produce point mutations (mutagens in the usual sense) are in general also chromosome-breaking agents, and vice versa. Thus, it seems safe to assume the existence of a spectrum extending from mutations visible to the cytogeneticist all the way down to those that must be defined by nucleotide sequencing. Mutations visible to the cytogeneticist ordinarily exert a more widespread effect on development than do point mutations; ordinary genes—often many of them—as well as other specialized types of chromatin whose function usually is unknown, are involved in cytologically visible mutations.

If an entire chromosome is affected in an imbalance, the genome is said to be either trisomic or monosomic for the chromosome (thus, trisomy 13, monosomy X). Genes and chromatin carried on the affected chromosome then are present in triple or single dose, respectively, rather than the normal double dose. Abnormal dosage affecting less than an entire chromosome, the result of chromosome

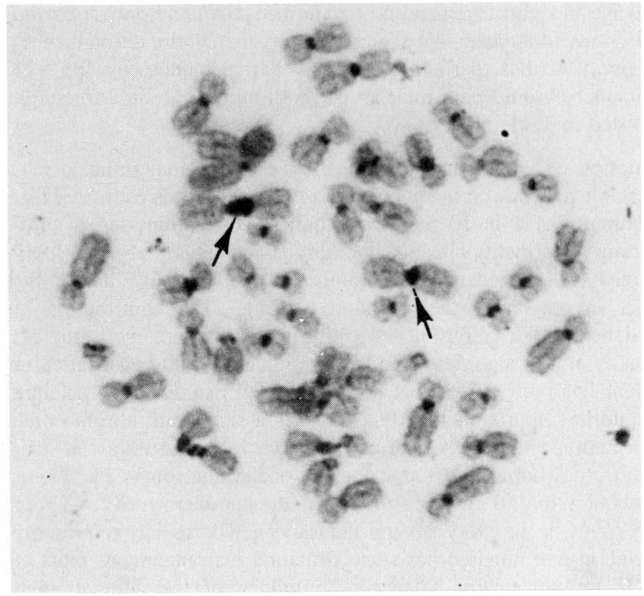

FIGURE 60-4 *Metaphase chromosomes stained for C bands (C standing for centromeric or constitutive heterochromatin), showing inherited variation in lengths of C bands in chromosome 1 (arrows).*

FIGURE 60-5 *Breaks and rearrangements (arrows) in metaphase chromosomes of a blood lymphocyte that received ionizing irradiation before being stimulated by phytohemagglutinin to enter S and divide.*

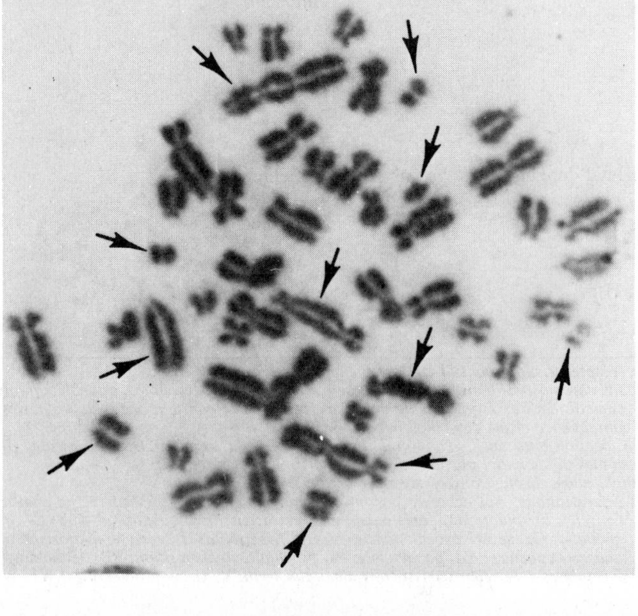

breakage and rearrangement, is often termed *partial trisomy* or *partial monosomy*, to indicate that segments rather than entire chromosomes are involved (thus, partial trisomy 13q, partial monosomy 4p). The commoner chromosome imbalances, both numerical and structural, are listed in Table 60-1.

Incidence The frequency with which chromosomal imbalance is detectable depends on the population investigated. It is estimated that a minimum of 1 in 10 recognized human conceptions has a chromosome abnormality. In human embryos and fetuses aborted spontaneously, the incidence of chromosome imbalance is higher the earlier in pregnancy the sampling is made. The contribution of imbalance to late abortion and stillbirth, though not well studied, probably also is significant. In the more than 65,000 consecutive or random live-born babies that now have been examined in different laboratories, approximately 1 in 200 has a significant chromosome abnormality, either numerical or structural. In such studies, at least 1 in 700 newborns is trisomic for one of the autosomes 21, 18, or 13; about 1 in 350 newborn males has the complement 47,XXY or 47,XYY. One in every several thousand newborns has monosomy X. One in five hundred has some structural rearrangement, most of which are genetically balanced. Samplings of the general adult population reveal an occasional inherited balanced structural rearrangement as well as the expected number of XXY, XYY, and XXX complements; the inherited, apparently innocuous segmental polymorphisms (e.g., Fig. 60-4) and minor structural rearrangements demonstrable by banding techniques are found in abundance.

In populations of individuals with mental deficiency, 10 to 15 percent have a chromosome abnormality, the proportion being greater if the individuals also have anatomic malformations. In some groups of male criminals and in infertile men an increased incidence of individuals with an extra sex chromosome, an X or a Y, is found. Infertile women also include many individuals with extra or missing sex chromosomes and an appreciable number with structural chromosome rearrangement; approximately one-fourth of women with primary amenorrhea have some abnormality of the X chromosome. Among infertile men and women, individuals with genes that interfere with meiosis, so-called meiotic mutants, are also found occasionally.

Numerical abnormalities Trisomy (47 chromosomes) is the most common chromosome imbalance in early spontaneous abortuses, followed by monosomy (45 chromosomes) and triploidy (69 chromosomes). The extra or missing chromosomes can be either paternal or maternal in origin, and the error in segregation of chromosomes

TABLE 60-1 The commoner chromosome imbalances that recur in the human population and that can result in clinically recognizable syndromes*

Imbalance	Chromosomes affected	Karyotypes†	Clinical features‡
	Sex chromosome:		
Monosomy	X	45,X	Turner's syndrome
Segmental deficiency—"partial monosomy"	X	46,XXp-; 46,XXq-; 46,X,r(X); 46,X,iso(Xp); 46,X,iso(Xq);	Turner's syndrome or some features of it
	Y	46,XYp-; 46,XYq-; 46,X,r(Y); 46,X,iso(Yp); 46,X,iso(Yq)	Turner's syndrome, or some features of it; "mixed gonadal dysgenesis" syndrome may result when a 45,X cell line coexists; risk of testicular neoplasia
	Autosome:		
	4	46,XY,4p-	Gr, Cf, Mi, Ey, Sk, Ge, Ht, Co, Me
	5	46,XY,5p-	Cri-du-chat syndrome: Cr, Mi, Cf, Me
	11	46,XY,11p-	WT, Ge, Me
	13	46,XY,13q-	RB, Cf, Me
	15	46,XY,15q-	Prader-Willi syndrome
	18	46,XY,18p-	Gr, Cf, Ea, Te, Po, Sk, Ht, Me
	18	46,XY,18q-	Cf, Hy, Sk, Ey
	21	46,XY,r(21)	Cf, Hp, Ea, Me
	Sex chromosome:		
Trisomy	X	47,XXX	Se, Me (mild), Ps
	X	47,XXY	Klinefelter's syndrome
	Y	47,XYY	Ta, Ac, Su, B; but often normal
	Autosome:		
	8	46,XY/47,XY,8+	Cf, Sk, Me (moderate)
	13	47,XY,13+	Trisomy 13 syndrome: Cp, Ey, Pd, Po, Ht, D, V, Sc, F, Ar, Me
	18	47,XY,18+	Trisomy 18 syndrome: Cf, Ea, V, F, Gr, D, He, Me
	21	47,XY,21+	Trisomy 21 syndrome (Down's syndrome)
Segmental duplication—"partial trisomy"	Sex chromosome: Y	46,X,t(X;Y)§	True hermaphroditism or XX male
	Autosome:		
	9	+9p†	Cf
	22	+22q¶	Gr, Cf, Ea, Cp, He, Hy, Co
Chimerism	Entire complement	46,XY/46,XX	Pseudo- or true hermaphroditism; dimorphism of blood-cell-surface antigens

* *For complete listing, consult DeGrouchy and Turleau.*

† *The sex chromosome constitution might be either XY or XX, but in the example karyotypes given, XY arbitrarily is used.*

‡ *The clinical features given include only some of the more constant ones. Deficiency of one segment often is accompanied by duplication of another, and the phenotypic effect is the consequence of the combined imbalance.*

§ *Translocation onto an X of the minute segment of the Y responsible for testicular differentiation. Random inactivation of either the normal X or the one bearing Y material determines the gonadal phenotype(s)—testis or ovary, respectively.*

¶ *Brought about through any of several rearrangements.*

NOTE: *Abbreviations: Ac, acne; Ar, arrhinencephaly; B, behavior disorder; Cr, characteristically abnormal cry; Cf, characteristic craniofacial dysmorphism; Co, convulsions; Cp, cleft lip–palate; D, early death; Ea, characteristically abnormal ears; Ey, eye anomaly; F, characteristically flared, overlapping fingers; Ge, abnormality of external genitalia; Gr, severe growth deficiency; Hp, hypertonia; Ht, cardiac malformation; Hy, infantile hypotonia; Me, intellectual deficit; Mi, microcephaly; Po, characteristically abnormal posture; Pd, polydactyly; Ps, psychotic predisposition; RB, retinoblastoma; Sc, scalp defect; Se, secondary amenorrhea; Sk, skeletal anomalies; Su, subfertility; Ta, tallness; Te, characteristically abnormal teeth; V, visceral anomalies; WT, Wilms's tumor with aniridia.*

can occur in the germ line, fertilized egg (zygote), or early embryo. Trisomy of every chromosome except the no. 1 has been observed in spontaneous abortions, trisomy 16 most frequently.

Sex chromosomal trisomy (XXY, XYY, and XXX) is compatible with intrauterine survival; in contrast, autosomal trisomy rarely permits survival to term. However, a small proportion of autosomal trisomics is live-born. For practical purposes these are only trisomy 21, 18, and 13, in decreasing frequency. Trisomies 18 and 13 cause death during infancy. Therefore trisomies of significance in adults are trisomy 21, XXY, XXX, and XYY. A few other autosomal trisomies, such as trisomy 8, have occasionally been reported, usually in mosaicism with a normal cellular component. (Mosaicism is the coexistence of multiple, genetically different populations of cells, all derived originally, however, from a single zygote.)

Autosomal monosomy is rare even among abortion material. In contrast, monosomy X (45,X) occurs in approximately 1.5 percent of recognized conceptions. It is common among spontaneously aborted human embryos (approximately 10 percent) and is present in one in every several thousand live-born babies. The reason for the death of 45,X embryos and fetuses is unknown, although developmental abnormalities doubtless contribute; cardiovascular and renal anomalies are common in the few that survive. In monosomy X, the missing sex chromosome can be either a Y or an X and is either paternal or maternal in origin. Often the second sex chromosome is not completely absent but is replaced by a structurally rearranged Y or X. Mosaicism is common in live-borns with monosomy X; here, tissues are populated not only by cells with a 45,X complement but by other cells, perhaps with a normal complement, either 46,XY or 46,XX, or with a complement in which the second sex chromosome is rearranged in some way.

Triploidy is rare in live-born babies and usually leads to early death, even when in a mosaicism with normal cells: 46,XY/69,XXY. The phenotypic effects of the autosomal trisomies, of 47,XXY, and of monosomy X (45,X) are characteristic and well defined so that their diagnosis usually is not difficult (see Chap. 333). The effects of the 47,XYY and 47,XXX constitutions are less striking, and therefore these complements are underdiagnosed. Mosaicism with coexistence of abnormal and normal populations of cells can cause an abnormal phenotype to approach the normal.

The mechanisms responsible for the numerical abnormalities are undefined and may be multiple. A striking but unexplained maternal age effect exists in trisomies 21, 18, 13, XXY, and XXX. In the case of trisomy 21 (at least), the maternal age effect is present regardless of whether the sperm or the egg contributes the extra chromosome at fertilization. Over one-third of babies with trisomy 21 are born to women over 35, whereas only one-tenth of all births occur in this group. The frequency of trisomy 21 rises from 0.5 to 0.7 per 1000 live births between ages 21 and 23 to 3.1 per 1000 at age 35, 10.5 per 1000 at age 40, and 33.6 per 1000 at age 45. (A paternal age effect may also exist in trisomy 21.) Maternal x-ray irradiation in low dosage is also associated with an increased incidence of trisomy 21. After a child with trisomy 21 is born, the risk to the parents of recurrence in future pregnancies is increased to approximately 1 percent. As to the etiology of monosomy X, the frequent association of the 45,X complement in mosaicism with normal complements and with structural rearrangements of the X and Y suggests that the zygote or the preimplantation embryo may often be the target of a chromosome-breaking event.

Structural abnormalities Some structural chromosome rearrangements are inherited, and others represent new mutations. The etiology of the new rearrangements is unknown, although they are assumed to be partly spontaneous and partly the effect of environmental agents such as mutagenic chemicals or ionizing radiation acting on the germ line, zygote, or early embryo (Fig. 60-5). The majority of de novo rearrangements are paternal in origin.

Many of the known chromosome rearrangements have been detected only once or a few times. Others are detected repeatedly, the same one occurring in unrelated individuals and families. For example, the commonest translocation, one that can occur either as a result of de novo mutation or by inheritance, affects one chromosome 13 and one 14 at or near their centromeres. In this translocation, only inert chromatin is lost from the tiny short arms. Also common is a similar translocation affecting chromosomes 14 and 21.

Chromosome complements bearing rearrangements can be genetically balanced or effectively so, thus imparting no unfavorable phenotypic effect to their bearers; about two-thirds of rearrangements detected during surveys of consecutive live-born babies are balanced. Or, the complement can be unbalanced and affect development adversely, the usual case when rearrangements are detected during surveys of spontaneous abortuses or of individuals with multiple anomalies and mental deficiency.

Some balanced rearrangements are transmitted from generation to generation without producing clinical effects. In other cases, however, they are profoundly important to members of the kindred transmitting them, by being responsible for the conception of embryos with unbalanced genomes. For example, bearers of some 13;14 translocations (mentioned above) are at risk of having children with the trisomy 13 syndrome, and inherited translocations involving chromosome 21 predispose to the trisomy 21 syndrome. Approximately 5 percent of live-borns with the trisomy 21 syndrome have a translocation, and in about a fifth of those it is detectable in one of the parents. Because most babies with the trisomy 21 syndrome due to translocation are born to women under 30, a search for a translocation is important when a child with this clinical syndrome is born to young parents.

Different translocations bestow on their carriers different risks of having offspring with unbalanced rearrangements. These risks cannot be predicted on the theoretical basis of the way the translocation might be expected to behave during meiosis. Useful empiric risk figures have been accumulated for common translocations; e.g., the 14;21 translocation bestows a 2 percent risk on a balanced male carrier and more than a 10 percent risk on a female carrier of having a child with the trisomy 21 syndrome. In contrast, the balanced carrier of a 21;21 translocation can expect only unbalanced offspring. Information of this type is indispensable to those undertaking genetic counseling in relation to chromosome disorders.

DISEASE ASSOCIATIONS Various combinations of abnormalities in malformed and defective individuals have been correlated with variations in the chromosome complement. In this way, clinical syndromes due to specific chromosome imbalances have been defined. (Many of the pediatric conditions are of little significance in adult medicine because of their lethality in infancy or early childhood.)

Autosome imbalance Of the three autosomal trisomies found in live-born babies, only trisomy 21 is compatible with survival past infancy. The phenotype produced by the presence of an extra chromosome 21, formerly known as *mongolism* but now termed the *Down syndrome* or *trisomy 21 syndrome,* is characteristic and easily diagnosed from birth: mental deficiency, short stature, muscular hypotonia, brachycephaly, short neck, typical facies (oblique orbital fissures, flat nasal bridge, small simple or folded ears, nystagmus, mouth hanging open), narrow palate, short broad hands with incurving fifth fingers, gaps between the first and second toes, and characteristic dermatoglyphics. Additional findings may include congenital heart disease, blepharitis, and conjunctivitis, Brushfield's spots of the iris, straight pubic hair, abnormal teeth, a protruding furrowed tongue, a high-arched palate, loose skin of the neck, transverse palmar creases, and hyperflexibility of the joints. Cardiac malformations lead to death in infancy in a third of individuals with trisomy 21, and other malformations and infections may also cause early death. However, subjects who survive infancy often reach adulthood, and some even old age. The proneness to develop leukemia in affected infants is not maintained in later life. Females occasionally become pregnant, and, as expected, approximately half their children have trisomy 21.

Mosaicism of trisomy 21 with normal cells (46/47, +21) may occur in individuals with modified features of the trisomy 21 syndrome, and it is probable that many individuals with this mosaicism go undiagnosed. The risk of such persons having trisomic children is increased, but unfortunately their mosaicism is usually detected only after they have had an affected child. Partial trisomy, partial monosomy, or a combination of the two explains many of the instances in both children and adults of multiple developmental defects combined with mental deficiency. Sometimes a balanced autosomal translocation is detected in normally developed adults who have repeated spontaneous abortion or subnormal fertility, with or without abnormal liveborn children.

Although the phenotypic effects of many of the different segmental chromosome imbalances which can occur are varied and nonspecific, the resulting anomalies sometimes compose recognizable clinical syndromes. Two examples are the following: (1) If a rearrangement causes partial trisomy of just the distal band of the long arm of 21, the clinical features composing the full syndrome associated with an extra chromosome 21 develop. (A triple dose of other segments of the long arm of chromosome 21 also produces adverse effects but not the trisomy 21 syndrome.) (2) Partial monosomy of a short segment within the short arm of chromosome 5 causes mental deficiency, a characteristic facies, and a characteristic cry during infancy. This group of signs is known as the *5p−* (five-p-minus) or *cri-du-chat syndrome*.

Because of the large number of karyotype-phenotype correlations made in recent years, additional specific syndromes produced by imbalance of many different segments now are known (Table 60-1), e.g., the 4p−,9p partial trisomy, 13q−, and 18q− syndromes, to name a few. Rearrangements not previously described and their corresponding clinical syndromes are still being recognized. Any of these syndromes may appear as a result either of de novo chromosome rearrangement or through formation of a genetically unbalanced gamete in a person carrying in balanced state a rearrangement affecting the segment involved.

In most individuals with chromosome imbalance, regardless of which segments are affected, a degree of phenotypic similarity is present. These recurring and nonspecific features include mental deficiency, growth deficiency, dysmorphic ears, nose, and mouth, cardiac malformations of standard types, abnormalities of dermal ridges and creases, and dysmorphic digits. (As a rule, autosomal imbalance need not be considered in the etiology of anatomic defects unaccompanied by mental deficiency.) Why similar abnormalities occur with so many different segmental imbalances is unknown, but when several such features are observed in a single individual, they can be a valuable clinical indication for cytogenetic analysis. Imbalance affecting certain segments also causes specific phenotypic changes; an example is the anomalous cry in the 5p− syndrome mentioned above. Other examples of specificity are retinoblastoma, which may develop when one particular band of chromosome 13 is present in single dose, and the Prader-Willi syndrome, which is often associated with a disturbance of a band near the centromere of chromosome 15. Whereas the nonspecific changes serve to call the clinician's attention to the possibility of some chromosome imbalance, the specific features can suggest the exact segment of the genome affected.

Sex chromosome imbalance (see also Chap. 333) In contrast to autosome imbalance, sex chromosome imbalance has relatively mild phenotypic effects. This is because X chromosomes beyond one in the complement of somatic cells are usually almost totally inactivated and because the Y chromosome bears few genes other than the testis determinants. X-linked loci (in contrast to autosomal loci) function normally in single dose: the male is hemizygous for X-linked genes, having only one X chromosome (with the possible exception of a few loci on the Y that may be homologous to a segment on the X); the female is functionally hemizygous through the Lyon effect. The addition of an extra sex chromosome to the normal male or female complement has a phenotypic effect but insufficient to interfere with intrauterine survival. Since major anatomic defects are usually absent, individuals with the complements 47,XXY and 47,XYY, both of whom are males, and 47,XXX, who are females, ordinarily go unrecognized till adolescence or later, often never to be diagnosed at all.

The *Klinefelter syndrome* (Chap. 333), which in classic form consists of small testes, infertility, gynecomastia, and variable degrees of underandrogenization, sometimes with mild mental deficiency, antisocial behavior, or both, is the consequence of the addition of an extra X to the male complement: 47,XXY. The extra X interferes in some way with the survival of germ cells, and atrophy of the spermatogenic tubules and azoospermia are the consequence. Sometimes the phenotypic effects are surprisingly mild, the testicular atrophy being the only noteworthy feature in otherwise healthy and socially well-adjusted men. The mosaicism 46,XY/47,XXY sometimes occurs and may ameliorate the phenotypic effect of the extra X. More extreme phenotypic effects and mental deficiency result when more than one extra sex chromosome is added to the normal male complement: 48,XXXY or 49,XXXXY.

The phenotypic effect of 47,XYY is less well defined; although increased height, behavioral difficulties, and infertility are common, the extra Y is sometimes found in otherwise normal men. The rare complement 48,XXYY results in infertility, probably because of the extra X, as in the 47,XXY Klinefelter's syndrome. The phenotype associated with 47,XXX is also poorly defined, but women with mild mental deficiency, psychosis, and menstrual abnormalities are increased in frequency; this complement is sometimes detected in normal, healthy women. Further clarification is needed concerning the effects on personality and behavior of all three of the complements 47,XXY, 47,XYY, and 47,XXX.

Loss of the Y or of the second X has drastic effects on development. If it does not cause abortion, it may or may not be recognizable at birth. Loose nuchal skin folds and edema of the hands and feet in a newborn girl, with or without renal or cardiovascular anomalies, may point to the diagnosis of the 45,X complement. The *Turner syndrome* (gonadal dysgenesis) is the manifestation in subsequent life (Chap. 333): short stature resistant to all treatment, infantilism of otherwise normal female external and internal genitalia, germ-cell-free gonads referred to as gonadal streaks, and variable renal, cardiovascular, skeletal, and ectodermal anomalies. Without estrogen administration breast development remains infantile and menstruation does not occur. Although mental deficiency is not a feature, a poorly defined emotional immaturity is common.

The Turner syndrome may be the developmental consequence of several chromosome constitutions besides 45,X. Mosaicism as well as structural abnormalities of a second sex chromosome, either a Y or an X, cause a spectrum of disorders at both the clinical and cytogenetic levels. A normal male or normal female cellular component may be present along with the 45,X cellular component, or one component may bear a structurally abnormal chromosome. Common abnormalities of the Y and X are isochromosome formation (one arm deleted and the other duplicated) or deletion of part or all of one arm. In some affected individuals, all cells have 46 chromosomes, with one normal X plus an abnormal Y or X, for example, 46,XXp−, deletion of a segment of the short arm of one of the X chromosomes. In others, a second or third cellular component may be present as well, for example, 45,X/46,XX/46,XXp−. Clinically pure Turner syndrome may be found in association with various combinations of these karyotypes if one of them is either monosomic or partially monosomic for X. However, when Y-bearing cells coexist with the 45,X cells, for example, 45,X/46,XY, genital ambiguity often develops, and gonads may vary from streaks to functional testes (the syndrome of *mixed gonadal dysgenesis*); here the risk of malignant gonadal neoplasia is significant. When 46,XX cells coexist with 45,X, varying degrees of ovarian function may be maintained, including ovulation. Although the phenotype may approach a normal male or female pattern when normal and abnormal cells coexist, the effects of mosaicism are unpredictable. Thus, the clinical syndrome associated with monosomy X and structurally abnormal Ys or Xs ranges from a predominantly male phenotype through Turner syndrome to an almost normal female phenotype.

Two other rare conditions deserve mention—*true hermaphroditism* and the *46,XX male* (see also Chap. 333): true hermaphroditism is present when both testicular and ova- and follicle-containing ovarian tissue exist in the same individual. In most cases 46,XX is the chromosome complement, and it appears normal by banding. Exceptionally, true hermaphrodites have the complement 46,XY; rarely is the chimerism 46,XY/46,XX found, each of the two cellular components having been derived from a different zygote. Second, males occasionally have the complement 46,XX. As in 47,XXY men, the second X interferes with meiosis, and azoospermia results. In both the 46,XX true hermaphrodite and the 46,XX male, the rule that a Y is required for testicular differentiation appears to break down. However, the two conditions may have the same etiologic basis; the most plausible explanation is occult translocation of the testis-determining segment of the Y to another chromosome.

X-linked mental deficiency In the general population more males than females are mentally deficient, and mental deficiency when familial affects males preferentially. In some such kindreds, severe mental deficiency segregates as an X-linked trait.

Although chromosome imbalance is not responsible, one cause, as mentioned above, can be diagnosed by cytogenetic techniques. In a significant proportion of families in which mental deficiency is segregating, the X in the affected males and that same X in their mothers is, or can be made, recognizable cytogenetically by technical manipulations. Near the end of its long arm (Xq) this phenotypically unusual X chromosome, in a variable but usually small proportion of metaphases from affected persons, exhibits an attenuated, and therefore faintly staining, segment. Because this segment usually can be seen to have broken in some of the metaphases, it is sometimes referred to as a fragile site, and the condition the *fragile-X syndrome*. (The "fragile X" is not demonstrable in all families with X-linked mental deficiency.)

Chromosome change in cancer The theory that an alteration in the chromosomal complement may be the cause of cancer was advanced almost seven decades ago, but the matter is still unsettled. Chromosome changes are plentiful in cancer, but this very fact—too many changes—has been a major reason many have rejected them as of etiologic significance. However, support for the idea that chromosome alteration is significant in the etiology of human cancer has come from two observations: (1) the known environmental "causes" of human cancer (carcinogenic chemicals and ionizing radiation) are also chromosome-breaking agents (Fig. 60-5); and (2) three recessively inherited disorders result in increased chromosome breakage and rearrangement in cells in culture, and in each the risk of cancer is increased—Bloom's syndrome, Fanconi's anemia, and ataxia-telangiectasia. Thus, the known environmental and the known genetic causes of increased chromosome mutation all predispose to cancer.

Most human cancers have altered chromosome complements. Table 60-2 lists some of those found with regularity. In the leukemias, lymphomas, and certain myeloproliferative disorders, the alterations are less extensive than in solid tumors and, therefore, easier to define. In certain lymphomas, chromosome 14 is often found to have undergone structural rearrangement, with the breakpoint at one specific segment. In over 95 percent of chronic granulocytic leukemias, a translocation affecting chromosome 22 (usually chromosome 9 is the other chromosome affected) is detected, the so-called Ph^1 chromosome and a no. 22 lacking much of its long arm can be demonstrated in most cases; if the disease progresses into a "blastic" phase, the karyotype often evolves, certain additional chromosome changes being added stepwise in a nonrandom sequence. In this and certain other leukemias, the various chromosome changes have diagnostic value, as well as a limited value in prognosis and choice of therapy.

Solid tumors, which generally are studied later in their course than conditions affecting the bone marrow, show extensive karyotypic changes, both structural and numerical. Different cells from a single tumor have similar numerical changes and structural rearrangements, but in the same type tumor from another person the changes usually seen are different. This apparent lack of specificity is partly due to the complexity of the changes, however, and a few examples of chromosome alterations specific for a solid tumor are known; for example, meningiomas are associated with a deletion of chromosome 22 in almost every case. The cytogenetic findings in both solid tumors and leukemias demonstrate the clonal nature of human cancer.

TECHNICAL CONSIDERATIONS Human metaphase chromosomes can be examined in any tissue in which sufficient cells are cycling. Preparations can therefore be made directly from almost any embryonic tissue and from adult bone marrow, lymphoid tissue, and selected malignant tissues. In searches for mosaicism, the study of multiple tissues is often required. Some tissues unlikely to yield cells in metaphase can be placed in culture, and chromosome preparations can be made from cells that reach mitosis in vitro. Blood T lymphocytes stimulated to enter cell-division cycles by phytohemagglutinin are the standard material for diagnosing constitutional chromosome imbalance. In some myeloproliferative disorders and leukemias, unstimulated circulating blood cells divide spontaneously after a few hours in culture. Long-term cultures of fibroblasts can be derived from minute skin biopsies or from fragments of many other types of tissue, although more elaborate laboratory facilities and a longer period of time are required before cytogenetic preparations can be made. Amniotic fluid is among the sources of cells suitable for culture, and the cells, which are fetal in origin, are widely used in the prenatal diagnosis of chromosome imbalance, particularly in pregnancy in women of advanced age or who already have borne a child with a chromosome imbalance. Metaphase preparations also can be made from chorionic villi biopsied in the first trimester of pregnancy.

Nucleated cells in interphase can be used for the study of sex chromatin. Cells from buccal mucosa and hair follicles are perhaps the most readily obtained, but surgical and autopsy specimens or cells in culture are at times useful also. X chromatin (formerly called the Barr body), a condensed body apposed to the nuclear membrane

TABLE 60-2 Some of the recurring chromosome abnormalities encountered in human neoplasms

Neoplasm	Aberration	Chromosome regions affected
Leukemia:		
Chronic granulocytic	Translocation	9q34 and 22q11
Acute nonlymphocytic:		
M1	Translocation	9q34 and 22q11
M2	Translocation	8q22 and 21q22
Me	Translocation	15q22 and 17q11
Chronic lymphocytic	Trisomy	12
Acute lymphocytic		
L1–L2	Translocation	9q34 and 12q11
L2	Translocation	4q21 and 11q23
L3	Translocation	8q24 and 14q32
Lymphoma:		
Burkitt's	Translocation	8q24 and 14q32
Follicular	Translocation	14q32 and 18q21
Solid tumors:		
Benign:		
Meningioma	Deletion or monosomy	22
Parotid, mixed	Translocation	3p25 and 8q21
Malignant:		
Lung, small cell	Deletion	Bands 3p14 to 3p23
Neuroblastoma	Deletion	Bands 1p31 to 3p36
Ovary, cystadenocarcinoma	Translocation	6q21 and 14q24
Retinoblastoma	Deletion	Band 13q14
Wilms's tumor	Deletion	Band 11p13

NOTE: *The FAB (French-American-British) classification of leukemias is employed above. The chromosome breakpoint and band nomenclature is that of the Paris Conference* (Birth Defects: Original Articles Series VIII *(7):1–46, 1971). The chromosome and chromosome-arm designation (e.g., 9q means the long arm of chromosome no. 9) appears first and is followed by the chromosome region and band on that arm (e.g., 9q34 means the fourth band in the third region of the long arm of chromosome no. 9).*

and present in normal female cells, is composed of the chromatin of one X chromosome. The X responsible for X chromatin in any particular cell is the one genetically inactivated and late-replicating. Therefore, the number of X-chromatin masses is an indication of the number of X chromosomes in excess of 1. Y chromatin, a predominantly genetically inactive segment of the Y chromosome demonstrated by quinacrine staining and fluorescence microscopy, is present in interphase nuclei of Y-bearing cells (for example, 48,XXYY cells contain one X-chromatin and two Y-chromatin masses).

Meiotic chromosome preparations from testicular biopsies are sometimes useful in obscure cases of infertility. Here translocations and genetically determined disturbances in meiotic pairing may be identified.

Recombinant DNA technology has been employed in conjunction with conventional cytogenetic techniques to define chromosome abnormalities in finer detail. As probes for specific loci or chromosome segments have become available, it has been possible to identify segments of chromosomes involved in rearrangements in which banding techniques had lacked the required resolution. In prenatal diagnosis, probes for RFLPs (mentioned earlier) sometimes are used to identify which chromosome has been inherited by the fetus. This can be useful in pregnancies at risk of X-linked disease, determining in male fetuses whether the single X chromosome is the one that bears a particular undesirable locus that one of the parents is known to carry, such as that for Duchenne's muscular dystrophy or hemophilia. Recombinant technology also can be useful in conditions that follow a dominant pattern of inheritance, such as Huntington's chorea, determining whether the undesired mutant gene is present in the complement of the fetus by determining whether an RFLP closely linked to the mutant gene is or is not present. In a few instances, probes for undesirable mutant genes themselves are available. Probes specific for the Y chromosome can define the sex of an embryo or fetus if a few cells can be obtained, for example by chorionic villus biopsy or amniocentesis. They also can be of diagnostic value in obscure cases of intersex in which a Y chromosome, or a segment of the Y, is being sought.

Sometimes, metaphase chromosomes are analyzed to determine whether damage to the genetic material has been induced by some environmental agent (radiation, chemical, virus). Cells that have proliferated in vivo may be used in search of evidence of damage to the genetic material of a given person or of a population. Alternatively, cultured cells can be treated with the agent in question to determine whether the agent is clastogenic (capable of breaking chromosomes) or whether it promotes chromatid exchange and rearrangement. A test system less laborious than metaphase-chromosome analysis, but one capable of showing that chromosome breakage has occurred either in vivo or in vitro, is the determination of the proportion of nondividing cells having micronuclei. A micronucleus is produced when a chromosome fragment lacking a centromere lags at anaphase (as it will be obliged to do) and is encompassed in a separate nuclear at telophase. The micronucleus assay is useful in the survey of populations for clastogen exposure, which is equivalent to mutagen and carcinogen exposure.

REFERENCES

BERG K et al (eds): *Cytogenetics and Cell Genetics*, vol 32: *Human Gene Mapping 6 (1981). Sixth International Workshop.* Basel, Karger, 1982

DE GROUCHY J, TURLEAU C: *Clinical Atlas of Human Chromosomes*, 2d ed. New York, Wiley, 1984

GERMAN JL: Studying human chromosomes today. Am Sci 58:182, 1970

MCKUSICK VA: The human gene map. Clin Genet 27:207, 1985

SCHWARZACHER HG: *Methods in Human Cytogenetics*. New York, Springer-Verlag, 1974

SIMPSON JL: *Disorders of Sexual Differentiation*. New York, Academic, 1976

61 PREVENTION AND TREATMENT OF GENETIC DISORDERS

JOSEPH L. GOLDSTEIN / MICHAEL S. BROWN

APPROACHES TO PREVENTION

The trend for couples to have smaller families has heightened the concern that children should be healthy and free of genetic diseases. Thus, primary-care physicians are called upon to play a more active role in the prevention and treatment of hereditary diseases. In most situations, genetic advice can be given by the primary physician once the relatively simple principles of medical genetics (Chap. 57) and genetic counseling (discussed below) have been mastered.

RETROSPECTIVE GENETIC COUNSELING The prevention of genetic diseases requires the identification of matings that are capable of producing defective genotypes. These may involve matings in which one of the two individuals carries a dominant or X-linked gene mutation or a balanced translocation, or matings in which both individuals are carriers of a deleterious recessive gene at the same locus. Such individuals are usually identified through an affected child or near relative, in which case retrospective genetic counseling can be provided.

When advising family members about the risk of transmitting a disorder that has already affected someone in the family, the counselor's first step is to be certain of the *correct diagnosis*—in particular, to make certain that the problem in question is really of genetic origin. This is especially important in disorders that may have either a genetic or a nongenetic etiology, such as deafness or mental retardation. Second, if the disease has a hereditary element, the possibility of *genetic heterogeneity*, i.e., a situation in which clinically similar genetic disorders show varying patterns of inheritance, must be considered. For example, there are two types of hereditary methemoglobinemia that resemble each other quite closely, but one shows autosomal recessive and the other autosomal dominant inheritance.

To estimate the *recurrence risk*, one must initially determine what is known of the genetic mechanisms controlling the relevant disorder. When more than one genetic mechanism exists, or when environmental factors can cause clinically indistinguishable traits, the *relative probabilities* of the different mechanisms operating in the particular family are computed. For conditions determined by simple mendelian inheritance, there is no difficulty in predicting the probability of an offspring being affected, provided that the genotypes of the parents can be recognized. Identification of the parental genotype is easiest for autosomal recessive and X-linked disorders since the basic lesions in these two forms of mendelian inheritance frequently involve simple enzyme deficiencies for which biochemical tests are now available.

For autosomal dominant disorders, identification of the parental genotype is more difficult since the basic defect is known for only a few of these disorders, and the diagnosis of the heterozygote for a dominant disorder depends almost exclusively on the clinical evaluation and a careful pedigree analysis. In counseling a family in which one relative is affected with a dominant disorder, it is important that appropriate clinical examination of all first-degree relatives and selected distant relatives be carried out. If relatives appear unaffected, the clinical symptoms may be masked by *delayed age of onset* and *variability in expression*, or the possibility of a new dominant mutation must be entertained. Table 61-1 lists the most commonly encountered dominant disorders affecting adults and the methods available for detection of the heterozygote.

When advising families about multifactorial genetic diseases, such as diabetes mellitus, in which the inheritance pattern is not clear-cut, the physician must resort to empiric risk estimates that have been derived from retrospectively assembled data (Table 57-5).

TABLE 61-1 Methods for detection of asymptomatic heterozygotes in frequently encountered dominantly inherited disorders

Disorder	Method of heterozygote detection: Physical findings	Method of heterozygote detection: Laboratory tests	Therapeutic advantage of early diagnosis
GASTROINTESTINAL, LIVER, AND PANCREAS			
Gilbert's disease		Serum bilirubin	Avoid confusion with more serious forms of liver disease
Peutz-Jeghers syndrome	Melanin spots on lips, buccal mucosa, and digits	X-ray of small intestine	Clarify cause of gastrointestinal bleeding
Familial polyposis		X-ray of colon; colonoscopy	Prevent colon carcinoma
Gardner's syndrome	Multiple sebaceous cysts; lipomas; fibromas; osteomas; dental abnormalities; desmoid tumors	X-ray of colon and small intestine; colonoscopy	Prevent colon carcinoma
METABOLIC AND ENDOCRINE			
Medullary thyroid carcinoma-pheochromocytoma syndrome		Serum calcitonin; measurement of blood pressure	Prevent thyroid carcinoma and complications of hypertension
Multiple endocrine adenomatosis	Multiple lipomas	Serum calcium, gastrin, blood sugar; x-rays of sella turcica, stomach, and small intestine	Prevent complication of hyperparathyroidism, hypoglycemia, peptic ulcer, metastatic cancer
Familial hyperparathyroidism		Serum calcium, parathyroid hormone	Prevent renal damage and other complications of hypercalcemia
Familial hypercholesterolemia	Tendon xanthomas, xanthelasma, arcus corneae	Serum cholesterol; low-density lipoprotein receptor activity of cultured fibroblasts	Prevent premature coronary heart disease
HEART AND VASCULAR			
Holt-Oram syndrome	Abnormality of thumb and carpals; murmur of atrial septal defect	X-ray of hands; cardiac evaluation	Prevent complications of atrial septal defect
Noonan's syndrome	Hypertelorism; small chin; low-set ears; ptosis; pectus deformity; cryptorchidism; murmur of pulmonic stenosis	Cardiac evaluation; x-ray of skeleton; intravenous pyelogram (renal anomalies)	Prevent heart failure
Idiopathic hypertropic subaortic stenosis (asymmetric septal hypertrophy)	Presystolic gallop; characteristic carotid arterial pulse	ECG; echocardiogram	Prevent sudden death, syncope, angina, heart failure
Dominantly inherited form of atrial septal defect	Heart murmur	ECG showing first-degree heart block, right bundle branch block, right axis deviation	Prevent complications of atrial septal defect
HEMATOLOGIC			
Hereditary spherocytosis	Splenomegaly; jaundice	Blood smear; reticulocyte count; hemoglobin; osmotic fragility test	Prevent anemia, cholelithiasis
Hereditary hemorrhagic telangiectasia	Telangiectasia of tongue, lips, conjunctiva, ears, fingers; pulmonary AV fistula	X-ray of lungs	Clarify cause of nosebleeds and gastrointestinal bleeding
Von Willebrand's disease		Immunologic and functional assays of plasma antihemophilic globulin levels; bleeding time	Prevent gastrointestinal and urinary bleeding
CONNECTIVE TISSUE AND BONE			
Ehler-Danlos syndromes (types I, II, III)	Loose-jointedness; fragile, stretchable, bruisable skin; subcutaneous calcified spherules		
Marfan's syndrome	Ectopic lens; mitral and aortic murmurs; excessive length of extremities	Slit-lamp examination; metacarpal index by x-ray	Reduce risk of aortic dissection; prevent blindness
Osteogenesis imperfecta	Multiple fractures; loose-jointedness; blue scleras; deafness; aortic regurgitation	X-ray of bones	
RENAL			
Alport's syndrome	Nerve deafness; cataracts, lenticonus, spherophakia	Urinalysis, slit-lamp examination	Prevent uremia
Nail-patella syndrome	Dysplastic nails; absent patellas	X-ray of pelvis (iliac horns); urinalysis	Clarify cause of hematuria and azotemia
Polycystic kidney disease		Urinalysis; intravenous pyelogram; renal arteriogram; measurement of blood pressure	Prevent uremia and complications of hypertension
Renal tubular acidosis		X-ray of kidneys (nephrocalcinosis); urine pH, calcium; serum electrolytes, calcium	Prevent acidosis, osteoporosis, kidney stones

TABLE 61-1 Methods for detection of asymptomatic heterozygotes in frequently encountered dominantly inherited disorders *(continued)*

	Method of heterozygote detection		
Disorder	Physical findings	Laboratory tests	Therapeutic advantage of early diagnosis
RESPIRATORY			
Hereditary angioneurotic edema		Serum level of Cl esterase inhibitor of complement	Reduce risk of sudden death caused by laryngeal edema and clarify cause of acute abdominal pain
DERMATOLOGIC			
Neurofibromatosis	Café au lait spots; neurofibromas; scoliosis		Prevent malignant degeneration of neurofibromas
Waardenburg syndrome	Wide bridge of nose; frontal white blaze of hair; heterochromia iridis; white eyelashes; deafness		Clarify cause of deafness
Basal-cell nevus syndrome	Multiple basal-cell carcinomas; jaw cysts; pits on palms and soles; skeletal defects (ribs, spina bifida, scoliosis)	X-rays of skull (calcification of falx cerebri) and skeleton	Removal of cutaneous cancers; provide cosmetic surgery
NEUROLOGIC			
Charcot-Marie-Tooth disease	Pes cavus; atrophy of anterior tibial and calf muscles (''stork legs''); absence of deep tendon reflexes	Biopsy of muscle and of sural cutaneous nerve	Improve walking by corrective shoes and orthopedic measures
Myotonic dystrophy	Myotonia; muscle wasting of temporal and sternocleidomastoid muscles; cataracts; frontal baldness; signs of hypogonadism	Slit-lamp examination; electromyography; measurement of serum immunoglobulins; electrocardiogram	Anticipate complete heart block
Acute intermittent porphyria		Measurement of uroporphyrinogen synthetase activity in red blood cells	Reduce risk of neuropathic attacks by avoidance of aggravating drugs such as barbiturates
Tuberous sclerosis	Adenoma sebaceium; cutaneous white macules; shagreen patch; periungual fibromas		Prevent seizures
Huntington's chorea	Paranoia, other personality changes; choreic movements; dementia		
Periodic paralysis syndromes (hypo-, hyper-, and normokalemic types)	Cold-induced myotonia	Electromyogram; serum potassium	Reduce frequency of attacks by avoidance of aggravating agents such as high-carbohydrate diet and exposure to cold
PHARMACOGENETIC			
Malignant hyperthermia		Serum creatine phosphokinase	Prevent fatal episode of hyperthermia induced by general anesthesia

Once the parental genotypes are determined, the genetic prognosis is usually presented in terms of probability that a given couple will produce an affected offspring. The physician must make certain that the couple understands not only the meaning of such risk figures, but also the severity of the disease and the variability in clinical expression. In other words, in dealing with a disorder such as neurofibromatosis, it is important for the parents to realize not only that they have a 50 percent risk of producing a child with this disorder but also that a certain proportion of patients with the disorder have severe disease, a certain proportion have mild disease, etc. They should also have an understanding of the potential impact of the disease on their family; a disease that is lethal at birth might be classified as more ''severe'' than one that is lethal at age 16, but the latter is likely to have a more profound impact on the family.

Although different families react in different ways to the same risk, most couples who seek genetic advice take a responsible course of action that is based on the information quoted. Generally, the physician should avoid giving direct advice as to whether a couple ''should'' or ''should not'' have children. For serious genetic disease, with a recurrence risk equal to or greater than 1 in 10, most parents are deterred from planning further children. When the risk is less than 1 in 10, most parents continue with additional pregnancies.

PROSPECTIVE GENETIC COUNSELING In contrast to retrospective genetic counseling in which advice is given after the birth of at least one affected family member, in prospective genetic counseling advice is provided to possible carriers of recessive genes before an affected individual is born. As a first step, this requires the identification of heterozygous individuals by a population-screening procedure. Second, unmarried heterozygotes are instructed about the risk of their having affected children if they marry another heterozygote for the same gene. Finally, if two heterozygotes are already married, there is the possibility of interrupting the birth of affected infants if the disease can be diagnosed in utero by amniocentesis.

Population screening for heterozygote detection is possible for several autosomal recessive disorders (such as sickle cell anemia, thalassemia major, and Tay-Sachs disease) that occur in certain populations with high frequency. For example, 8 percent of the American black population carries the sickling gene, and 4 percent of Ashkenazi Jews are carriers of the Tay-Sachs gene.

Screening programs raise many ethical and social problems. Informing a healthy person that he or she is carrying a specific mutant gene that may cause disease in the children if a certain type of mate is chosen differs from counseling parents who have already had an affected child. Little is known about the social and psychologic effects as well as occupational discrimination that may result from discovering that a person carries a ''bad'' gene.

PRENATAL DIAGNOSIS The use of transabdominal amniocentesis permits diagnosis of certain genetic diseases at a stage early enough

TABLE 61-2 Inborn errors of metabolism for which prenatal diagnosis is feasible (partial list)

DISORDERS OF CARBOHYDRATE METABOLISM
Glycogen storage diseases—Types II, III, and IV
Galactosemia
Galactokinase deficiency
Pyruvate decarboxylase deficiency
DISORDERS OF AMINO ACID METABOLISM
Argininosuccinicaciduria
Citrullinemia
Homocystinuria
Maple syrup urine disease
Methylmalonic aciduria
Isovaleric acidemia
Ketotic hyperglycinemia
DISORDERS OF LIPOPROTEIN AND LIPID METABOLISM
Homozygous familial hypercholesterolemia (receptor-negative type)
Refsum's syndrome
DISORDERS OF LYSOSOMAL ENZYMES
Mucopolysaccharidosis, type I (Hurler's syndrome)
Mucopolysaccharidosis, type II (Hunter's syndrome)
Mucopolysaccharidosis, type III (Sanfillipo's syndrome, types A and B)
Mucopolysaccharidosis, type VI (Maroteaux-Lamy syndrome)
Mucopolysaccharidosis, type VII (β-glucuronidase deficiency)
I-cell disease
Lysosomal acid phosphatase deficiency
Wolman's syndrome and cholesteryl ester storage disease
Fabry's disease
Gaucher's disease
Krabbe's disease (globoid cell leukodystrophy)
Metachromatic leukodystrophy
Niemann-Pick disease
Tay-Sachs disease
Sandhoff's disease
Generalized gangliosidosis
Juvenile gangliosidosis
Fucosidosis
Mannosidosis
Farber's disease (lipogranulomatosis)
DISORDERS OF STEROID METABOLISM
21-Hydroxylase deficiency—congenital adrenal hyperplasia
Steroid sulfatase deficiency (X-linked ichthyosis)
DISORDERS OF PURINE AND PYRIMIDINE METABOLISM
Lesch-Nyhan syndrome
Hereditary orotic aciduria
Xeroderma pigmentosum
Adenosine deaminase deficiency (combined immunodeficiency)
DISORDERS OF METAL METABOLISM
Menkes' syndrome
DISORDERS OF PORPHYRIN AND HEME METABOLISM
Acute intermittent poryphyria
DISORDERS INVOLVING CONNECTIVE TISSUE, MUSCLE, AND BONE
Hypophosphatasia (some types)
DISORDERS OF THE BLOOD AND BLOOD-FORMING TISSUES
Sickle cell anemia
α Thalassemias
β Thalassemias
Glucose 6-phosphate dehydrogenase deficiency
DISORDERS OF TRANSPORT
Cystinosis

to terminate a pregnancy and to prevent the birth of a defective child. This procedure gives high-risk couples the opportunity to have unaffected children provided they are willing for the pregnancy to be terminated in the event that an abnormal fetus is detected. Amniocentesis consists of the transabdominal aspiration of amniotic fluid from the uterus. The procedure is preferably performed between the fourteenth and sixteenth weeks of pregnancy. When performed by a trained gynecologist, the technique is safe for both mother and fetus.

Direct examination of the amniotic fluid itself may be diagnostic. For example, an elevated level of α-fetoprotein is a relatively good indicator of the presence of spina bifida or another neural tube abnormality. More frequently, prenatal diagnosis requires culture of the fetal cells in vitro, a process which usually takes 3 weeks. By this means the karyotype of the fetus can be determined to ascertain fetal sex and to detect chromosomal aberrations. Moreover, many inborn errors of metabolism can be detected by assays of specific enzyme activities or restriction length DNA polymorphisms (Chap. 58) in the cultured fetal cells. Table 61-2 lists those inborn errors for which prenatal diagnosis is currently feasible. More disorders are constantly being added to this list.

A promising new approach to prenatal diagnosis, called chorionic villus sampling, allows the identification of genetic abnormalities between the ninth and twelfth week of gestation. The technique involves passing a catheter through the cervix into the placenta and obtaining a sample of developing chorionic villi, which consists of trophoblastic and mesenchymal cells. A single aspiration typically yields 10 to 25 mg of wet tissue, which is sufficient for studies of chromosomes, enzyme activities, and DNA polymorphisms. Ongoing clinical trials suggest that this is a relatively safe procedure with a miscarriage rate of about 4 percent, a figure that does not exceed the rate in the general population.

Prenatal diagnosis is currently indicated in the following high-risk situations: (1) couples having a previous child with spina bifida or anencephaly, (2) couples having a previous child with a chromosomal aberration such as the trisomy 21 form of Down's syndrome, (3) couples in whom either the husband or wife carries a balanced translocation chromosome for Down's syndrome, (4) couples at high risk for having a child with a detectable inborn error of metabolism, and (5) pregnant women 35 years of age and older. Table 61-3 lists the major indications for prenatal diagnosis, the risks involved, and methods by which the abnormal fetus can be detected.

APPROACHES TO TREATMENT

The goal of treatment for genetic diseases is to modify the natural history of the genetic trait so that an affected person may live a

TABLE 61-3 Major indications for prenatal diagnosis

Clinical situation	Estimated risk to fetus, %	Method of detection of abnormal fetus
Couples having a previous child with spina bifida or anencephaly	5	Measurement of α-fetoprotein in amniotic fluid
Couples having a previous child with a chromosomal disorder such as the trisomy 21 form of Down's syndrome	2	Chromosomal analysis of cultured amniotic fluid cells
Couples in whom either the husband or wife carries a balanced translocation for Down's syndrome	5–20	Chromosomal analysis of cultured amniotic cells
Pregnant women 35 years of age and older whose risk of having a child with Down's syndrome is increased	1–2	Chromosomal analysis of cultured amniotic fluid cells
Couples at risk for having a child with a detectable inborn error of metabolism (see Table 61-2)	25 or 50	Biochemical analysis of cultured amniotic fluid cells

TABLE 61-4 Some treatable hereditary disorders affecting adults

Method of treatment	Disorder
DIETARY RESTRICTION OF SUBSTRATE	
Lactose	Lactase deficiency
Galactose	Galactosemia and galactokinase deficiency
Fructose	Fructose intolerance
Neutral fats	Familial lipoprotein lipase deficiency
Phytanic acid	Refsum's syndrome
Phenylalanine	Phenylketonuria
REPLACEMENT OF DEFICIENT END PRODUCT	
Vitamin D and phosphate	Hypophosphatemic rickets
Cortisol	Adrenogenital syndromes
Thyroxine	Familial goiters
Uridine	Orotic aciduria
DEPLETION OF STORAGE SUBSTANCE	
Sterol removal by bile-acid binding resins heterozygotes	Familial hypercholesterolemia and inhibitors of cholesterol synthesis
Cystine removal by D-penicillamine	Cystinuria
Copper removal by D-penicillamine	Wilson's disease
Iron removal by phlebotomy	Hemochromatosis
Uric acid removal by uricosuric agents	Gout
AMPLIFICATION OF ENZYME ACTIVITY	
Pyridoxine (vitamin B_6)	Homocystinuria
Vitamin B_{12}	Methylmalonic aciduria
Phenobarbital	Crigler-Najjar variant and other forms of unconjugated hyperbilirubinemia
REPLACEMENT OF MUTANT PROTEIN	
Gamma globulin	Agammaglobulinemia
Factor VIII (AHG)	Hemophilia
Infusion of irradiated erythrocytes containing adenosine deaminase	Severe combined immunodeficiency disease
ORGAN TRANSPLANTATION	
Kidney	Fabry's disease, cystinosis, Alport's syndrome, polycystic kidney disease (adult form)
Allogeneic bone marrow	Lymphopenic hypogammaglobulinemia (Swiss type), Wiscott-Aldrich syndrome, severe combined immunodeficiency disease
Liver	Familial hypercholesterolemia (homozygotes)
SURGERY	
Splenectomy	Hereditary spherocytosis
Portacaval shunt	Glycogen storage disease (type I) and homozygous familial hypercholesterolemia
Colectomy	Familial polyposis of the colon
Thyroidectomy	Medullary thyroid carcinoma syndrome

comfortable and healthy life despite a mutant genotype. Such treatment can be achieved for a number of inherited diseases using a variety of approaches, including (1) the exclusion or restriction of toxic foods, (2) metabolic supplementation, (3) removal of toxic products, (4) surgery, and (5) organ transplantation. Table 61-4 lists examples of hereditary diseases affecting adults that can be successfully treated at the present time.

REFERENCES

Emery AEH, Rimoin DL: *Principles and Practice of Medical Genetics,* vols 1 and 2. Edinburgh, Churchill Livingstone, 1983

Epstein CJ et al: Recent developments in the prenatal diagnosis of genetic diseases and birth defects. Ann Rev Genet 17:49, 1983

Jackson, LG: First-trimester diagnosis of fetal genetic disorders. Hosp Pract 20(3):39, 1985

Stanbury JB et al: *The Metabolic Basis of Inherited Disease,* 5th ed. New York, McGraw-Hill, 1983

section 2 Clinical immunology

62 INTRODUCTION TO CLINICAL IMMUNOLOGY

BARTON F. HAYNES / ANTHONY S. FAUCI

Basic research in immunology has resulted in advances in many clinical areas, ranging from allergy and rheumatology to neurology and cardiology. Monoclonal antibody technology has revolutionized the study of cell surface antigens of effector and regulatory immune cells and provided monospecific reagents to essentially any target molecules. The isolation, cloning, and sequencing of genes for antigen receptors on B cells (immunoglobulins) and T cells (α and β chains of T-cell antigen receptor) and of products of the major histocompatibility locus (HLA antigens) have yielded the probes necessary to begin to understand immune effector function. These include diversification of the T- and B-cell antigen repertoire, induction of self-tolerance (self-antigen nonreactivity), and regulation of immune cell growth and differentiation. Molecular biology techniques have likewise provided genetic probes for study and production of large quantities of secreted molecules (products from lymphocytes, *lymphokines;* from monocytes, *monokines*) that regulate immune cell function. Finally, the discovery of the human T-cell lymphotropic virus (HTLV) family of retroviruses (see Chap. 293) that causes forms of leukemia (HTLV type I, adult T-cell leukemia) and immunodeficiency [HTLV III/LAV (lymphadenopathy-associated virus), acquired immunodeficiency syndrome (AIDS)] and analysis of the genetic mechanisms of HTLV alteration of normal T-cell growth has led to understanding of some aspects of normal and abnormal immune cell growth. This knowledge regarding control of immune cell growth and differentiation will lead to new and specific modes of therapy for diseases of disordered immunoregulation such as autoimmune diseases, immunodeficiency diseases, and malignant diseases of the immune system. The aim of this chapter is to provide the essentials of immunology with particular emphasis on those principles relevant to understanding at a basic level the protean clinical and laboratory manifestations of disordered immunity.

PHENOTYPE AND FUNCTION OF IMMUNE CELLS The dual limbs of the immune system are the thymus-derived (T) lymphocyte and the bone marrow–derived or bursa-equivalent (B) lymphocyte, both of which derive from a common stem cell. Other cell types such as the monocyte-macrophage play major roles in the inductive, regulatory, and effector phases of the immune response. The principal effector and regulatory cells of the immune system are T, B, and large granular lymphocytes and monocyte-macrophages. Nonlymphoid cells such as neutrophils, eosinophils, and basophils play roles in the inflammatory response that results from certain immune-mediated reactions and as such must be considered in the scheme of immune cell function (Table 62-1). The proportion and distribution of immunocompetent cells in various tissues reflect cell traffic, homing patterns, and functional capabilities. Bone marrow contains pluripotent stem cells capable of giving rise to all hematopoietic cell types and is the major site of maturation of B cells, monocyte-macrophages, and granulocytes. T-cell precursors also arise from bone marrow stem cells but leave bone marrow while immature and home to thymus for completion of maturation. Mature T lymphocytes, B lymphocytes, and monocytes enter the circulation and home to peripheral lymphoid organs (lymph nodes, spleen) and the gut-associated lymphoid tissue (tonsil, Peyer's patches, and appendix) and await activation via interaction with foreign antigens. Mature myeloid effector cells (neutrophils, eosinophils, basophils) leave the bone marrow and circulate in peripheral blood as well as home to tissues to perform effector functions associated with the response to foreign antigens (Fig. 62-1).

T CELLS T lymphocytes arise from bone marrow precursor cells that migrate to the thymus during fetal and early postnatal life. T lymphocytes differ from other immune effector cell types in that the pool of effector T cells is established in the thymus early in life and is maintained throughout life by antigen-driven expansion of long-lived T cells that reside primarily in peripheral lymph organs and recirculate in blood and lymph. Mature T lymphocytes contribute 70 to 80 percent of normal peripheral blood lymphocytes, 90 percent of thoracic duct lymphocytes, 30 to 40 percent of lymph node cells, and 20 to 30 percent of spleen lymphoid cells. In lymph nodes T cells occupy deep paracortical areas around B-cell germinal centers and in spleen are in periarteriolar areas of white pulp (see Chap. 55). T cells are the primary effectors of cell-mediated immunity with subsets of T cells maturing into cytotoxic cells capable of lysis of viral infected or foreign cells. T cells are also the primary regulator cells of T- and B-lymphocyte and monocyte function via the production of lymphokines and direct cell contact; in addition, T cells regulate erythroid cell maturation in bone marrow.

Human T cells express cell surface proteins that are markers of discrete stages of intrathymic T-cell maturation; many of these molecules mediate or augment specific T-cell functions (Table 62-1). The earliest identifiable cells of T lineage are prothymocytes located in the subcapsular cortical region of thymus (Fig. 62-2), many of which express the sheep-erythrocyte-binding protein, T11, and the pan-T-cell specific protein, 3A1-p40 (stage I). With further maturation, prothymocytes enter the inner thymic cortex, acquire the cortical thymocyte protein T6, and coexpress T-lineage molecules T4 and T8 (stage II). More than 90 percent of stage II thymocytes that arise in the inner cortex die intrathymically, with only a minority of thymocytes achieving phenotypic and functional maturity. Mature T cells located in small foci within the inner cortex and throughout the thymic medulla express the T-cell antigen receptor-associated T3 molecules (20,000 to 25,000 mol wt), p80 molecules thought to be important in T-cell homing to peripheral lymphoid tissues, and high-density cell surface HLA-A, -B, and -C antigens (stage III). With maturity, T-cell expression of the T6 antigen ceases, and T-cell subset antigens T4 and T8 are reciprocally expressed. Mature $T4^+$ cells induce B-cell differentiation, induce $T8^+$ cytotoxic T-cell proliferation, produce various lymphokines, and regulate certain stages of erythropoiesis. A subset of $T4^+$ cells may also function as cytotoxic effector cells, and recognize foreign antigen in the context of major histocompatibility complex (MHC) class II (Ia) antigens. $T8^+$ cells function as suppressor T cells of B-cell antibody synthesis and as cytotoxic effector T cells that recognize foreign antigen associated with class I antigens (see Chap. 63).

TABLE 62-1 Characteristics of human immune and inflammatory effector cells

Cell type	Functional surface molecules	Cellular function mediated via surface molecules
T lymphocyte	T3/T-cell antigen receptor complex	Antigen recognition, T-cell activation.
	Sheep erythrocyte receptor (T11 antigen)	T-cell activation.
	T4 antigen	Marker of inducer-helper T cells, and a subset of cytotoxic T cells. T4 molecule facilitates antigen recognition by $T4^+$ cells, and is a surface recognition molecule via which HTLV III/LAV (AIDS) virus infects this subset.
	T8 antigen	Marker of suppressor and cytotoxic T cells. T8 molecule facilitates $T8^+$ cell recognition of antigen via class I MHC molecules.
	Interleukin 2 (IL-2) receptor	Present on activated T cells, binds IL-2.
B lymphocyte	Surface immunoglobulins (sIg)	Antigen recognition, cell activation.
	IgG Fc receptors	Bind immune complexes.
	C3 receptors	Bind immune complexes.
Large granular lymphocyte (LGL)	IgG Fc receptors	Bind immune complexes.
Monocyte-macrophage	IgG Fc receptors	Bind and phagocytose immune complexes.
	C3 receptors	Bind and phagocytose immune complexes.
	MHC class II (Ia) antigens	Antigen presentation to T and B cells.
	Chemotactic receptors	Cellular polarization and chemotaxis.
Neutrophil	IgG Fc receptors	Bind and phagocytose immune complexes.
	Chemotactic receptors	Cell polarization and chemotaxis.
	C3 receptors	Bind and phagocytose immune complexes.
Eosinophil	IgG Fc receptors	Bind immune complexes.
	C3 receptors	Bind immune complexes.
Basophil–mast cell	IgE Fc receptors C3 receptors	Release of granules containing mediators of immediate hypersensitivity after cross-linking of Fc-bound IgE with allergen (antigen).

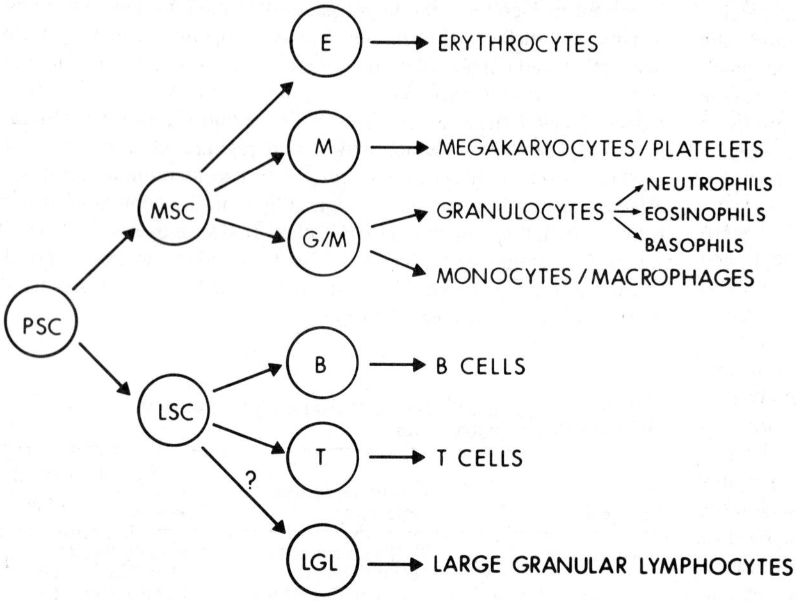

FIGURE 62-1 *Model of hematopoietic stem cell differentiation. Multipotential hematopoietic stem cells (HSC) may give rise to more restricted progenitor cells with self-renewal capacity. Thus, lymphocyte-committed stem cells (LSC) give rise to T and B cells. Another group of hematopoietic cells, for which the immediate progenitor is a more differentiated myeloid stem cell (MSC), includes erythrocytes, megakaryocytes, and platelets as well as the granulocyte, monocyte-macrophage series; the origin of large granular lymphocytes in this schema is hypothetical. (Adapted from MD Cooper et al, with permission.)*

T-cell maturation stages I, II, and III are clinically relevant in that T-cell malignancies can be grouped generally as being derived from one of these stages. T-cell acute lymphoblastic leukemia and lymphomas share phenotypic similarities with stages I or II T cells and thus are malignancies of immature T cells. Forms of cutaneous T-cell lymphoma (mycosis fungoides, Sézary syndrome) and the syndrome of adult T-cell leukemia (associated with HTLV I infection) share the phenotype of stage III T cells and therefore are malignancies of mature T cells.

The structural basis for the association of T-cell functional competence and surface expression of the T3 antigen results from the fact that two of the T3 proteins are bound to the T-cell antigen receptor. The T-cell antigen receptor, called Ti, is a 90,000-mol wt heterodimer composed of one 50,000-mol wt and one 43,000-mol wt B chain. The α and β T-cell antigen receptor molecules possess amino acid sequence homology and structural similarities to immunoglobulin heavy and light chains. The Ti β chain contains four separately encoded regions, namely the V (variable), D (diversity), J (joining), and C (constant) regions, and the Ti α chain consists of at least V, J, and C regions. Thus, the T-cell antigen receptor has constant and variable regions, and the gene for the α and β chains of the T-cell antigen receptor undergo gene rearrangement during T-cell maturation culminating in synthesis of the completed Ti molecule.

FIGURE 62-2 *Model of human intrathymic T-cell maturation. Immature T cells in subcapsular cortex (stage I) and inner cortex (stage II) give rise to mature T cells in small foci in thymic inner cortex and medulla (stage III). Stage III thymocytes migrate to the periphery (peripheral blood, lymph nodes, spleen) and after challenge with antigen, expand into memory-T-effector-cell populations.*

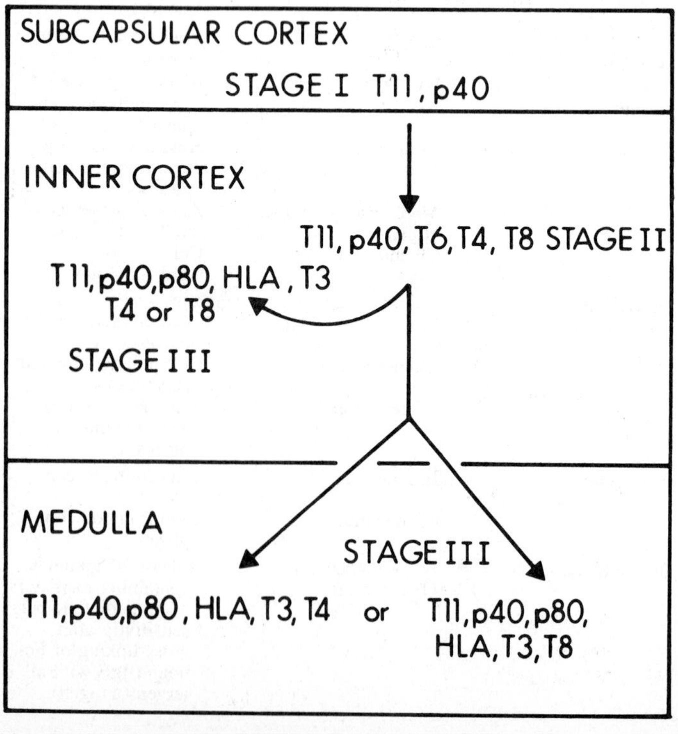

The epithelial component of the thymus is arranged in zones that correspond to those seen in Fig. 62-2 for thymocyte subsets. Thymic epithelial cells containing the thymic hormones thymopoietin, thymulin, and thymosin α_1 are located primarily in the subcapsular cortical and medullary thymic zones. Thymic hormones are thought to play important roles in supporting early stages of T-cell maturation. The specificity of mature T cells is largely determined within the thymus. For example, elimination of T cells capable of reacting against autologous (self) antigens may occur intrathymically, thus preventing autoimmune reactivity. Positive selection likely occurs intrathymically as well. T cells recognize foreign antigens in association with cell surface molecules encoded for by the major histocompatibility complex (MHC) on antigen-presenting cells. Specifically, cytotoxic $T8^+$ T cells recognize antigens in association with class I (HLA-A, -B, and -C) MHC molecules, and $T4^+$ helper and $T4^+$ cytotoxic T cells recognize and respond to foreign antigens in the context of class II (Ia-like) MHC molecules. The association between surface phenotype of T cells and the class of MHC molecules recognized suggests that the T4 and T8 antigens themselves are required to facilitate recognition of, or binding of, T cells to foreign antigens. This ability to corecognize foreign antigen with autologous class I and II MHC antigens on monocyte-macrophages is referred to as *MHC restriction* of immune cell interactions.

B CELLS Mature B cells comprise 10 to 15 percent of human peripheral blood lymphocytes, 50 percent of splenic lymphocytes, and approximately 10 percent of bone marrow lymphocytes and express on their surface intramembrane immunoglobulin molecules that function as B-cell antigen receptors. B cells also express surface receptors for the Fc region of IgG molecules as well as receptors for activated complement components (C3d, C3b). The primary function of B cells is to produce antibodies. Mature B cells are derived from bone marrow precursor cells that arise continuously throughout life (Figs. 62-1 and 62-3). Like myeloid and erythroid cells, B cells are constantly replaced every few days through cell division from marrow precursor cells. However, the maturation of B lymphocytes differs from myeloid and erythroid cell lineages in that B lymphocytes have antigen-dependent and antigen-independent phases of maturation (Fig. 62-3). Pre-B cells arise from precursor cells in bone marrow and are identified by the presence of cytoplasmic immunoglobulin M (cIgM) (initially IgM heavy chain followed by cytoplasmic light chain synthesis). Pre-B cells mature to immature B cells that no longer express cIgM but rather express surface IgM molecules (sIgM). Immature B cells migrate to the periphery and continue antigen-independent maturation, expressing surface IgD, diversifying the B-cell antigen repertoire, and switching the B-cell surface immunoglobulin isotype such that either surface IgM, IgG, IgA, or IgE is expressed along with IgD. Only one Ig heavy and light chain variable region and thus only one antigen specificity is expressed by each B cell. In lymph organs, B cells are the principal cells in lymph node cortical germinal centers and medullary cords and in primary and secondary germinal centers in the white pulp of spleen (see Chap. 55). On contact with antigen, mature B cells in peripheral lymph nodes and spleen either terminally differentiate into antibody-secreting plasma cells or proliferate to form populations of long-lived memory B cells that are capable of interaction with antigen when rechallenged with the same antigen (Fig. 62-3).

LARGE GRANULAR LYMPHOCYTES Large granular lymphocytes (LGL) (previously called "null cells") constitute approximately 5 to 10 percent of peripheral blood lymphocytes, and are nonadherent, nonphagocytic cells with large azurophilic cytoplasmic granules. LGL express surface receptors for the Fc portion of IgG (see Table 62-1), and many LGL express T lineage markers and proliferate in response to interleukin 2 (T-cell growth factor). Functionally LGL share features with both monocyte-macrophages and neutrophils in that subsets of LGL mediate antibody-dependent cellular cytotoxicity (ADCC) and natural killer cell activity. ADCC is the binding of an opsonized (antibody-coated) target cell to an Fc receptor–bearing effector cell via the Fc region of antibody resulting in lysis of the target by the effector cell. Natural killer (NK) cell activity is the nonimmune (i.e., effector cell never having had previous contact with the target), non-antibody-mediated killing of target cells, usually malignant cell types. Thus, LGL that mediate natural killer activity may play an important role in immune surveillance and destruction of cells that spontaneously undergo malignant transformation in vivo.

MONOCYTE-MACROPHAGES Monocytes arise from precursor cells within bone marrow (Fig. 62-1) and circulate with a half-life ranging from 1 to 3 days. Monocytes leave the peripheral circulation by marginating in capillaries and then migrating into a vast extravascular pool. Tissue macrophages arise by migration of monocytes from the circulation and by proliferation of macrophage precursors in tissue. Common locations of tissue macrophages (and some of their specialized names) are lymph node, spleen, bone marrow, perivascular connective tissue, serous cavities such as peritoneum, pleura, synovium, skin connective tissue, lung (alveolar macrophage), liver (Kupffer cell), bone (osteoclast), and central nervous system (microglia).

The monocyte-macrophage system plays a major role in the expression of immune reactivity by mediation of functions such as the presentation of antigen to lymphocytes and the secretion of factors such as interleukin 1 (IL-1) that are central to activation of T lymphocytes. Under certain circumstances monocytes can also mediate immunoregulatory functions such as suppressor cell activity. In addition, monocyte-macrophages mediate effector functions such as destruction of antibody-coated bacteria, tumor cells, or even normal hematopoietic cells in certain types of autoimmune cytopenias. Activated macrophages can also mediate NK-like activity and eliminate cell types such as tumor cells in the absence of antibody. Monocyte-macrophages express surface receptors for a number of molecules, including the Fc region of IgG, activated complement components, and various lymphokines (macrophage inhibitory and activating factors) (Table 62-1). In addition, monocyte-macrophages express cell surface MHC class II (Ia-like) antigens and specific cell surface differentiation antigens. Finally, macrophage secretory products are more diverse than those known for any other cell of the immune system. These secretory products allow the macrophage to exert both pro- and anti-inflammatory effects and to regulate other cell types. Among monocyte-macrophage–secreted products are hydrolytic enzymes, products of oxidative metabolism, and IL-1, also called leukocytic pyrogen and lymphocyte-activating factor, which affects lymphocytes, hepatocytes, fibroblasts, synoviocytes, and cells within the hypothalamus.

NEUTROPHILS, EOSINOPHILS, AND BASOPHILS Granulocytes are a feature of nearly all forms of inflammation and represent a nonspecific amplification and effector component to a specific response. Unchecked accumulation and activation of granulocytes can lead to host tissue damage as seen in neutrophil- and eosinophil-mediated necrotizing vasculitis. Granulocytes are derived from stem cells in bone marrow (Fig. 62-1). Each type of granulocyte (neutrophil, eosinophil, basophil) is derived from a different subclass of progenitor cell which is stimulated to proliferate by proteins tropic for each cell type. During terminal maturation stages of granulocytes, class-specific nuclear morphology, and cytoplasmic granules appear that allow for histologic identification of granulocyte type. Neutrophils express Fc receptors for IgG and activated complement components (C3b, C3d)

FIGURE 62-3 *Model of B-cell differentiation. B cells undergo antigen-independent and antigen-dependent maturation stages that culminate in terminal differentiation into either antibody-secreting plasma cells or memory B cells.*

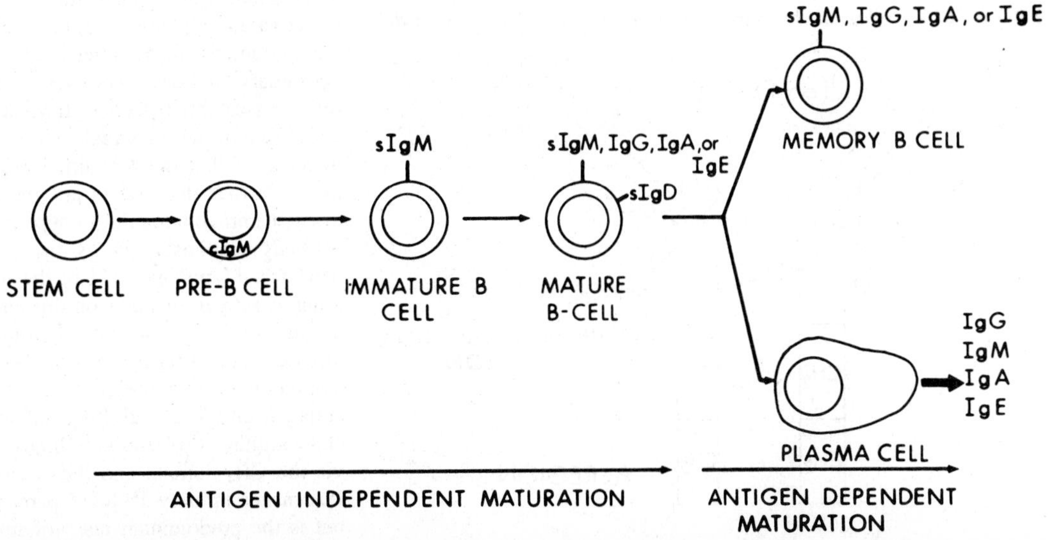

TABLE 62-2 Mediators released from human mast cells and basophils

Mediator	Actions
Histamine	Smooth muscle contraction, increased vascular permeability
Slow reacting substance of anaphylaxis (SRSA) (leukotriene D4)	Smooth muscle contraction
Eosinophil chemotactic factor of anaphylaxis (ECF-A)	Chemotactic attraction of eosinophils
Platelet-activation factor	Activation of platelets to secrete serotonin and other mediators
Neutrophil chemotactic factor (NCF)	Chemotactic attraction of neutrophils
Leukotactic activity (leukotriene B4)	Chemotactic attraction of neutrophils
Heparin	Anticoagulant
Basophil kallikrein of anaphylaxis (BK-A)	Cleavage of kininogen to form bradykinin

(Table 62-1). Upon neutrophil interaction by immune complexes, azurophilic granules (containing myeloperoxidase, lysozyme, elastase, and other enzymes) and specific granules (containing lactoferrin, lysozyme, collagenase, and other enzymes) are released, and microbicidal superoxide radicals (O_2^-) are generated at the neutrophil surface. The generation of superoxide is thought to lead to inflammation by direct injury to tissue and cells and by alteration of macromolecules such as collagen and DNA.

Eosinophils express Fc receptors for IgG and are potent cytotoxic effector cells for various parasitic targets. Intracytoplasmic contents of eosinophils, such as major basic protein, eosinophil cationic protein, and eosinophil-derived neurotoxin, are capable of directly damaging tissues and may be responsible in part for the organ system dysfunction in the hypereosinophilic syndromes (see Chap. 56). Since the eosinophil granule contains anti-inflammatory types of enzymes (histaminase, arylsulfatase, phospholipase D), eosinophils may downregulate or terminate ongoing inflammatory responses in normal homeostasis.

The normal functions of basophils are not known; the capacity of basophil mediators to increase local delivery of antibodies and complement by increasing vascular permeability is hypothetical. Thus, the basophil is identified principally with allergic reactions and some delayed cutaneous hypersensitivity states. Certainly the promotion of increased vascular permeability by basophils is important in the genesis of inflammatory lesions in some vasculitis syndromes (see Chap. 269). Basophils express surface receptors for IgE, and upon cross-linking of basophil-bound IgE by antigen, basophils release their granules containing histamine, eosinophil chemotactic factor of anaphylaxis, heparin, platelet-activating factor, and slow reacting substance of anaphylaxis—all mediators of components of immediate (anaphylaxis) hypersensitivity responses (Table 62-2). In addition basophils express surface receptors for activated complement components (C3a, C5a).

FIGURE 62-4 *Schematic structure of the immunoglobulin G (IgG) molecule.*

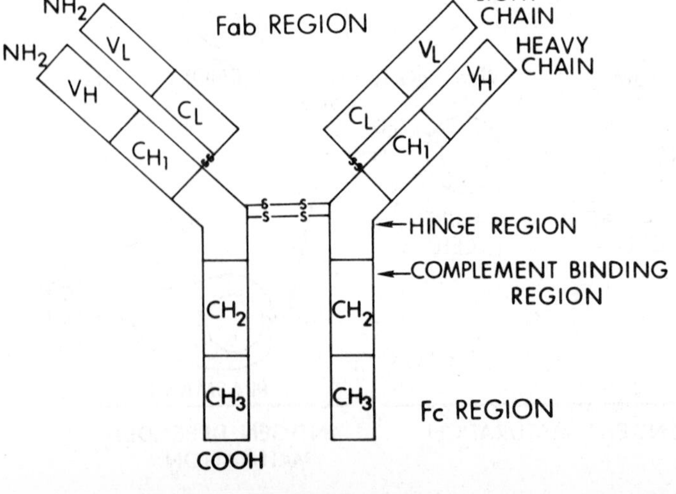

HUMORAL MEDIATORS OF IMMUNITY: IMMUNOGLOBULINS Immunoglobulins are the products of differentiated B cells and mediate the humoral arm of the immune response. Their primary functions are to bind to antigen and bring about the inactivation or removal of the offending toxin, microbe, parasite, or other foreign substance from the body. The structural basis of immunoglobulin molecule function and immunoglobulin gene organization has provided insight into the role of antibody in normal protective immunity and in the mediation of unwanted immune-mediated damage by immune complexes, and autoantibody formation against host determinants.

All immunoglobulins have the basic structure of two heavy and two light chains (Fig. 62-4). Immunoglobulin isotype is determined by the type of heavy and light chain present. IgG and IgA can further be divided into subclasses (IgG1, IgG2, IgG3, IgG4, and IgA1, and IgA2) based on specific antigenic determinants on heavy chains. The characteristics of human immunoglobulins are outlined in Table 62-3. The four chains are covalently linked by disulfide bonds. Each chain is made up of a variable (V) region and constant (C) regions (also called domains) made up of homologous units of 110 amino acids. Light chains have one variable (VL) and one constant (CL) region; heavy chains have one variable region (VH) and three or four constant (CH) regions, depending on isotype. As the name suggests, constant regions are made up of homologous sequences and share the same primary structure as all other chains of the same isotype and subclass. Constant regions are involved in biologic functions of immunoglobulin molecules. The CH_2 domain of IgG and the CH_4 domain of IgM are involved with binding complement components. The CH region at the carboxy terminus end of the IgG molecule, the Fc region (Fig. 62-4), binds to surface Fc receptors of macrophages, LGL, B cells, neutrophils, and eosinophils.

Variable regions (VL and VH) constitute the antibody-binding (Fab) region of the molecule. Within the VL and VH regions are hypervariable regions of extreme sequence variability that constitute the antigen-binding site unique to each immunoglobulin molecule. The idiotype is the specific region of the Fab portion of the immunoglobulin molecule to which antigen binds. Antibodies against the idiotype portion of an antibody molecule are called *anti-idiotype* antibodies. The formation of anti-idiotype antibodies in vivo during a normal B-cell antibody response may generate a negative (or "off") signal to B cells to terminate antibody production (see "Autoimmunity").

IgG makes up approximately 75 percent of the total serum immunoglobulin. The four IgG subclasses are numbered in order of their level in serum, IgG1 is found in greatest amounts and IgG4 the least. IgG subclasses have clinical relevance in their variability in binding macrophage and neutrophil Fc receptors and in their variability to activate complement (Table 62-3). IgG antibodies are frequently the antibodies made after rechallenge of the host with antigen (secondary antibody response). Of the immunoglobulin isotypes only IgG crosses the placenta. IgM antibodies normally circulate as a 950,000-mol wt pentamer with 160,000 monomers joined by a molecule called the J chain, a 15,000-mol wt nonimmunoglobulin molecule that also effects polymerization of IgA molecules. IgM is the first immunoglobulin to appear in the immune response (primary antibody response) and is the initial type of antibody made by neonates. Membrane IgM in the monomeric form also functions as a major antigen receptor on the surface of the mature B cell. IgM is an important component of immune complexes in autoimmune diseases. For instance, IgM antibodies against IgG molecules (*rheumatoid factors*) are present in high titers in rheumatoid arthritis, other collagen diseases, and some infectious diseases (subacute bacterial endocarditis). IgM antibody binds the C1 component of complement via the CH_4 domain and thus is a potent activator of complement. IgA makes up only 10 to 15 percent of total serum immunoglobulin but is the predominant class of immunoglobulin in secretions. IgA

TABLE 62-3 Characteristics of human immunoglobulins

Isotype	Molecular weight	Heavy chain	Light chain	Adult average serum level (mg/dL)	Half-life (days)	Complement activation: Classical pathway	Complement activation: Alternative pathway	Binding to cells via Fc	Other biologic properties
IgG	150,000	γ_1, γ_2, γ_3, γ_4	κ or γ	1250 ± 300	23.0	IgG1, IgG2, IgG3, yes; IgG4 no	IgG1, IgG2, IgG3, no; IgG4 yes	Macrophages, neutrophils, eosinophils large granular lymphocytes	Placental transfer
IgM	190,000 (950,000)*	μ	κ or λ	125 ± 50	5.1	Yes	No	Lymphocytes	Primary antibody response, rheumatoid factor
IgA	160,000 (385,000)†	α_1, α_2	κ or λ	210 ± 50	5.8	No	Yes	Lymphocytes	Antibody in mucous secretions
IgD	175,000	δ	κ or λ	4	2.8	No	Yes	None	Primary lymphocyte surface molecule
IgE	190,000	ε	κ or λ	0.03	2.5	No	Yes	Mast cells, basophils	Mediates anaphylaxis, allergy

* *IgM circulates as a pentameric molecule.*
† *Secretary IgA is a dimer.*
SOURCE: *Adapted with permission from DJ Jeske, JD Capra, Immunoglobulin: Structure and Function, in Fundamental Immunology, WE Paul et al (eds), New York, Raven, 1984.*

in secretions (tears, saliva, nasal secretions, gastrointestinal tract fluid, and human milk) is in the form of secretory IgA (sIgA), a polymer consisting of two IgA monomers, a joining molecule called J chain, and a glycoprotein called the secretory piece.

Of the two IgA subclasses (IgA1 and IgA2), IgA1 is primarily found in serum, whereas IgA2 is more prevalent in secretions. IgA fixes complement via the alternative pathway and has potent antiviral activity in human beings by prevention of virus binding to respiratory and gastrointestinal epithelial cells. IgD is found in minute quantities in serum (Table 62-3) and along with IgM is a major receptor for antigen on the B-cell surface. Present in serum in very low concentrations (Table 62-3), IgE is the major class of immunoglobulin involved in arming mast cells and basophils by binding to these cells via the IgE Fc region. Antigen cross-linking of IgE molecules on basophil and mast cell surfaces results in release of mediators of immediate hypersensitivity responses (Table 62-2).

Similar to the genes for the T-cell antigen receptor, the heavy and light chains of immunoglobulin are each encoded by multiple genetic elements physically separated in germline DNA but brought together to create a single active gene in B cells.

The variable regions of light chains (e.g., κ light chains) are constructed from two genes called VK and JK. These genes, though on the same chromosome, are far apart in the germline but during B-lymphocyte maturation are brought close together with excision of intervening DNA sequences (gene rearrangement). There are approximately 300 VK genes and 5 JK genes resulting in the pairing of VK and JK genes to create 1500 different light chain combinations. The number of distinct κ light chains that can be generated is increased by somatic mutational events within the VK and JK genes, which thus create a large number of specificities from a limited amount of germline genetic information.

Heavy chain immunoglobulin gene rearrangement is more complex than for light chains. The VH domain is created by the joining of three types of germline genes called VH, DH, and JH, thus allowing for even greater diversity in the variable region of heavy chains than in that of light chains.

CELLULAR INTERACTIONS INVOLVED IN REGULATION OF THE NORMAL IMMUNE RESPONSE The net result of activation of the humoral (B-cell) and cellular (T-cell) arms of the immune system by foreign antigen is the elimination of antigen directly by effector cells or in concert with the production of specific antibody. In addition, a series of regulatory cells are activated which modulate T-effector-cell activation and B-cell antibody production. Figure 62-5 is a simplified schematic diagram of the immune system outlining some of these cellular interactions.

MONOCYTE–T CELL INTERACTIONS Many of the activation and regulatory effects of lymphocytes and monocytes occur via soluble mediators. Monocyte-macrophages are required for optimal activation of T cells by antigens or by mitogens (nonspecific activators of lymphocytes). A soluble macrophage product, IL-1, can substitute in some cases for intact macrophages. Upon contact with antigens or mitogens, macrophages secrete IL-1, two effects of which are (1) the induction of receptors for T-cell growth factor or interleukin 2 (IL-2) on T cells and (2) the induction of IL-2 secretion. IL-2 in turn effects activation of T cells resulting in expansion of effector and regulatory T cells that have also been induced to express IL-2 receptors. Effector T cells mediate a variety of functions including the killing of virally infected cells, graft rejection, graft-versus-host reaction, delayed type of hypersensitivity, and the release of lymphokines (Table 62-4).

T CELL–T CELL AND T CELL–B CELL INTERACTIONS The expression of immune cell function is the result of a complex series of phases. Both T and B lymphocytes mediate immune functions, and each of these cell types when given appropriate signals passes through stages, from activation and induction to proliferation, differentiation, and ultimately effector functions. The effector function expressed may be at the end point of a response, such as secretion of antibody by a differentiated plasma cell, or it might serve a regulatory function that modulates other functions such as is seen with inducer or suppressor T lymphocytes which modulate both differentiation of B cells and activation of cytotoxic T cells. As shown schematically in Fig. 62-5, upon activation via IL-1 and IL-2, regulatory T-cell subsets are generated that exert positive and negative forces on effector cells. Thus, for B cells and cytotoxic ($T4^+$ or $T8^+$) T cells, there are $T4^+$ inducer and $T8^+$ suppressor cells that either facilitate or downregulate effector cell function. For B cells, trophic effects are mediated by a variety of cytokines, particularly T cell–derived B-cell growth factor (BCGF) and B-cell differentiating factor (BCDF) which act at sequential stages of B-cell maturation resulting in the induction and propagation of B-cell proliferation, differentiation, and ultimately antibody secretion. For T cells, trophic factors include inducer-T-

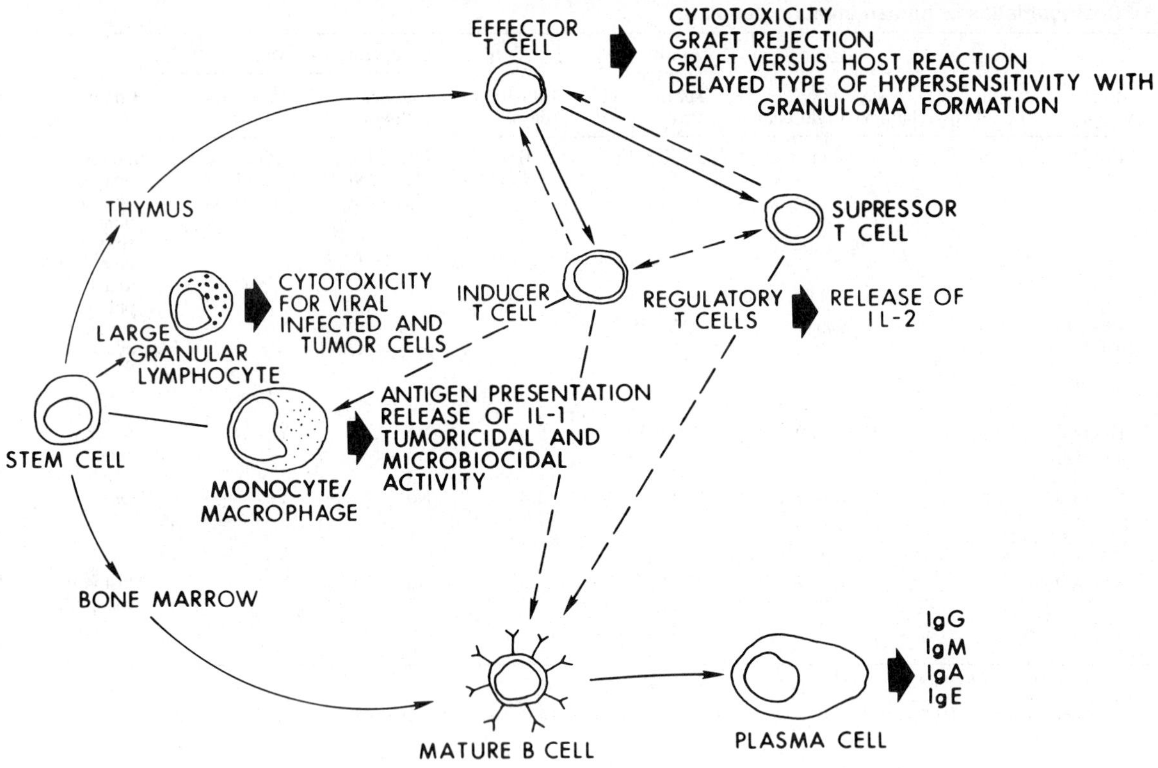

FIGURE 62-5 *Schematic representation of cellular interactions involved in the generation of cell-mediated and humoral immunity. [Adapted with permission from AS Fauci, in WN Kelly et al (eds).]*

cell secretion of IL-2. These complex cellular and humoral interactions involve a delicate balance among positive and negative influences and ultimately result in expression of an appropriate immune response. The slightest imbalance in these immunoregulatory circuits may result in aberrant immune function leading to clinically apparent immune-mediated disease.

THE COMPLEMENT SYSTEM The complement system is a cascading series of enzymes, regulatory proteins, and proteins capable of cell lysis. There are two arms of the complement system (Fig. 62-6). Activation of the classical complement pathway via C1, C4, C2, and activation of the alternative complement pathway via factor D, C3, and factor B lead to cleavage and activation of C3. C3 is a protein whose products are critical for opsonization (antibody and complement coating in preparation for phagocytosis) of bacteria and other foreign antigens. A protein fragment (C3b) results from the activation of C3 and is necessary for activation of the terminal complement components. These components (C5 to C9) when activated form a molecule called the membrane attack complex which inserts into cell membranes resulting in osmotic lysis of the cell. C3b also joins with a cleavage product of factor B (called Bb) to form C3bBb, also known as the alternative pathway C3 convertase. Activation of the classical complement pathway results in cleavage of C4 and C2 with a resulting complex of fragments called C4b2a, also called the classical pathway C3 convertase. Both the classical C3 convertase (C4b2a) and the alternative pathway C3 convertase (C3bBb) function to cleave C3 to form active C3b, thus driving activation of terminal complement components and the C5 to C9 membrane attack complex. The fact that C3b can combine with Bb to form the alternative C3 convertase gives rise to a potent positive feedback loop for production of C3b and thus continued activation of terminal complement components. Activation of the classical complement pathway is by interaction of antigen and antibody-forming immune complexes that bind C1q, a subunit of C1. Immunoglobulin isotypes that bind C1q and activate the classical pathway are IgM, IgG1, IgG2, and IgG3. In contrast, IgA1, IgA2, and IgD activate complement via the alternative pathway. In addition, nephritic factors (IgG autoantibodies against C3bBb, the alternative pathway C3 convertase) are present in serum of some patients with membranoproliferative glomerulonephritis, and binding of nephritic factors to C3bBb results in stabilization of C3bBb enzyme activity and favors positive feedback into the C3b alternative pathway amplification loop. Activation of the complement cascade via the classical pathway by IgG- or IgM-containing immune complexes is rapid, efficient, and leads to activation of terminal complement components. In contrast, activation of the alternative pathway via IgA-containing immune complexes or by bacterial endotoxin is slower and less efficient in terminal component activation. Thus, the immunoglobulin isotype composition of immune complexes is a critical factor in determining complement activation, and therefore in determining efficiency of clearance of immune complexes by Fc receptor–bearing cells within the immune system (see Chap. 261).

In addition to the role of complement in opsonization and cell lysis, several complement component fragments are potent mediators of cell activation. C3a and C5a bind to receptors on mast cells and basophils resulting in release of histamine and other mediators of anaphylaxis. C5a is also a potent chemoattractant for neutrophils and monocyte-macrophages (Table 62-5).

TABLE 62-4 Soluble mediators of the immune response and the targets of their action

Target cells	Factors
Monocyte-macrophage	Migration-inhibitory factor (MIF) Leukotrienes Prostaglandins
Lymphocytes	Lymphocytotoxin (LT) T-cell growth factor, interleukin 2 (IL-2) Gamma interferon B-cell growth factor (BCGF) B-cell differentiation factor (BCDF)
Neutrophils	Leukocyte-inhibitory factor (LIF) Chemotactic factors
Other cell types	Eosinophil chemotactic factor (ECF) Basophil chemotactic factor (BCF) Interferons (IF) Colony-stimulating factor (CSF) Osteoclast-activating factor (OAF)

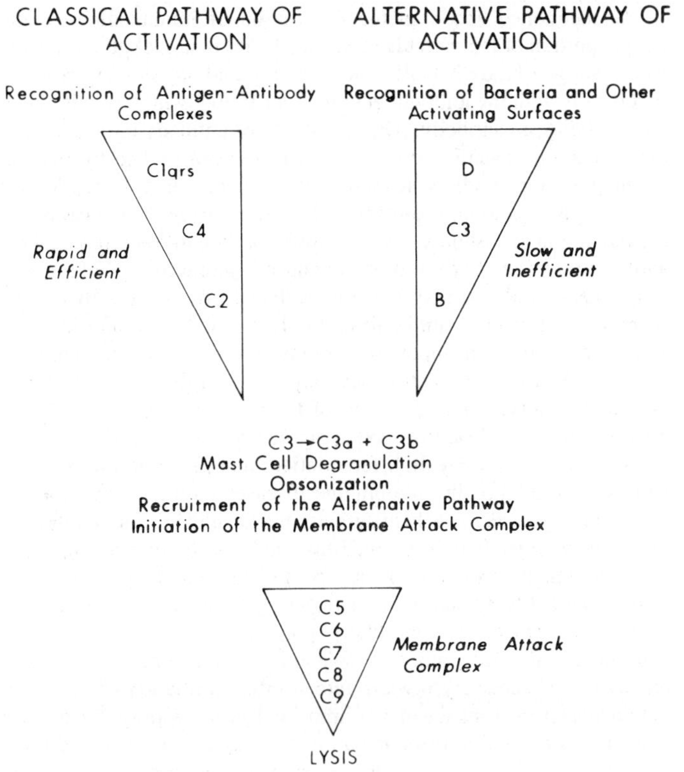

FIGURE 62-6 *Components of the complement system. [Adapted with permission from WE Paul, in WE Paul (ed).]*

MECHANISMS OF IMMUNE DAMAGE Several scenarios of host defense in response to foreign antigen culminate in the rapid and efficient elimination of nonself substances (Table 62-6). These scenarios interface those classic arms of the immune system (T cells, B cells, macrophages) with cells and soluble products that are mediators of inflammatory responses (neutrophils, eosinophils, basophils, kinin and coagulation systems, and complement cascade). Three general phases of host defense involve (1) specific and nonspecific recognition of foreign antigens mediated by T and B lymphocytes, macrophages, and the alternative complement pathway, (2) amplification of the inflammatory response with recruitment of specific and nonspecific effector cells by complement components, lymphokines and monokines, kinins, arachidonic acid metabolites, and mast cell–basophil products, and (3) macrophage, neutrophil, and lymphocyte participation in the phase of antigen destruction and ultimate removal of antigen by phagocytosis of antigen particles (macrophage, neutrophil) or by direct cytotoxic mechanisms (macrophage, neutrophil, lymphocyte). Under normal circumstances, orderly progression of host defenses through these phases results in a well-controlled immune and inflammatory response that protects the host from the offending antigen. However, regulatory dysfunction of any of the systems involved in host defense can damage host tissue and produce clinically apparent disease.

IMMUNE-COMPLEX FORMATION (TYPE III REACTION) Clearance of antigen by immune-complex formation between antigen and antibody is a highly effective mechanism of host defense. However, depending on the level of immune complexes formed and their physicochemical properties, immune complexes may or may not result in host and foreign cell damage. After antigen exposure, certain types of soluble antigen-antibody complexes freely circulate and, if not cleared by the reticuloendothelial system, can be deposited in blood vessel walls and in other tissues such as renal glomeruli. The precise mechanisms whereby immune complexes damage tissues, particularly blood vessels, are discussed in detail in Chaps. 261 and 269.

TABLE 62-5 Biologic activities of some complement components

Component	Activity
C4, C2 kinin	Increases vascular permeability.
C3a	Anaphylatoxin; evokes histamine release from basophils, serotonin from platelets.
C5a	Anaphylatoxin; evokes histamine release from basophils; potent chemoattractant for monocytes and neutrophils.
C3b	Enhancement of phagocytosis by neutrophils and monocytes. Promotes immune-complex binding to cells within monocyte-macrophage system, as well as neutrophils. With Bb forms alternative pathway C3 convertase and amplifies alternative pathway. Promotes solubilization of immune complexes.
C5–C9	Membrane attack complex; forms transmembrane channels leading to cell destruction.

SOURCE: *Adapted with permission from S Ruddy, in WN Kelly et al (eds).*

IGE-MEDIATED ALLERGIC REACTIONS AND ANAPHYLAXIS (TYPE I) Mast cells and basophils have receptors for the Fc portion of IgE, and cell-bound IgE effectively "arms" basophils. Basophil mediator release is triggered by antigen interaction with Fc receptor–bound IgE; the mediators released are responsible for the pathophysiologic changes of allergic disease (Table 62-2). The mediators released from mast cells can be divided into three broad categories of actions:

1 Those that increase vascular permeability and contract smooth muscle (histamine, SRS-A, BK-A)
2 Those that are chemotactic for or activate other inflammatory cells (ECF-A, NCF, leukotriene B4)
3 Those that modulate the release of other mediators (BK-A, platelet-activating factor)

CYTOTOXIC REACTIONS OF ANTIBODY (TYPE II) In this type of immunologic injury, complement-fixing (C1 binding) antibodies against normal or foreign cells or tissues (IgM, IgG1, IgG2, IgG3) bind complement via the classical pathway and initiate a sequence of events similar to those initiated by immune-complex deposition resulting in cell lysis or tissue injury. Examples of type II antibody-mediated cytotoxic reactions include red cell lysis in transfusion reactions, Goodpasture's syndrome with anti-glomerular basement membrane antibody formation, and possibly juvenile-onset diabetes mellitus with anti-islet cell antibody production.

TABLE 62-6 Mechanisms of immunologically mediated inflammation

Mechanism type	Characteristics of inflammatory response	Clinical disease type
I Allergic (IgE-mediated)	Basophil and mast cell products leading to immediate flare-and-wheal.	Atopy, anaphylaxis
II Cytotoxic or tissue-specific antibody (IgM- or IgG-mediated)	Acute inflammation via phagocytic cells and deposition of complement in tissues, lysis or phagocytosis of target cells.	Goodpasture's syndrome, anti-red cell antibodies in transfusion reactions
III Immune complex (IgG-, IgM-, IgA-mediated)	Accumulation of neutrophils, macrophages, complement components.	Systemic necrotizing vasculitis, systemic lupus erythematosus, serum sickness syndromes
IV Delayed hypersensitivity	T cell–induced mononuclear cell accumulation of regulatory and effector T cells and macrophages. Lymphokines and monokines released. Often granuloma formation.	Tuberculosis, sarcoidosis, rheumatoid arthritis, Wegener's granulomatosis

CLASSIC DELAYED HYPERSENSITIVITY REACTIONS (TYPE IV) Inflammatory reactions initiated by mononuclear leukocytes and not by antibody alone have been termed delayed hypersensitivity reactions. The term *delayed* has been used to contrast the secondary cellular response which appears 48 to 72 h after antigen exposure to an ''immediate'' hypersensitivity response generally seen within 12 h of antigen challenge initiated by basophil mediator release or preformed antibody. For example, in an individual previously infected with *Mycobacterium tuberculosis* (TB) organisms, intradermal placement of TB protein purified derivative (PPD) as a skin test challenge results in an indurated area of skin at 48 to 72 h, indicating previous exposure to TB. The cellular events that result in classic delayed hypersensitivity responses are centered around T cells, their soluble products, and macrophages. In the general schema outlined in Fig. 62-5, antigen is processed by macrophages and presented to T cells expressing a cell surface receptor specific for the antigen. Macrophage-secreted IL-1 amplifies antigen-induced T-cell triggering; antigen-specific T cells clonally expand; and lymphokines are secreted to recruit other T cells and macrophages nonspecifically to participate in the inflammatory response. Once recruited, macrophages frequently undergo epithelioid cell transformation and form giant cells. This type of mononuclear cell infiltrate is termed *granulomatous inflammation*. Examples of diseases in which delayed-type hypersensitivity plays a major role are fungal infections (*histoplasmosis*), mycobacterial infections, chlamydial infections (*lymphogranuloma venereum*), helminth infections (*schistosomiasis*), reactions to toxins (*berylliosis*), and hypersensitivity reactions to organic dusts (*hypersensitivity pneumonitis*). In addition, delayed-type hypersensitivity responses may play a role in *rheumatoid arthritis* and Wegener's granulomatosis.

AUTOIMMUNE DISEASE Autoimmune diseases are characterized by production of either antibodies that react with host tissue or immune effector T cells that are autoreactive. Since B-cell responses in human beings generally require inducer T cells, a B-cell autoantibody response directly implies disordered T-cell immunoregulatory control. Examples of clinically relevant autoantibodies are antithyroid antibodies in thyroiditis, and anti-DNA, antierythrocyte, and antiplatelet antibodies in systemic lupus erythematosus.

The clonal selection theory was put forth by Burnet in 1949 to explain autoimmunity. Burnet proposed that the contact of antibody-forming cells with their respective antigens during fetal or early postnatal life lead to their elimination. Thus, in this theory self-reactive clones are avoided unless they arise in later life by somatic mutation of lymphocytes. The progeny of such mutant cells would give rise to self-reacting antibodies. As the study of autoimmunity has progressed, it has become clear that the genesis of autoimmune B and T cells is far more complex than originally thought. Certain drugs (procainamide, phenytoin) and infectious agents (Epstein-Barr virus, *Mycoplasma pneumoniae*) can elicit the production of autoantibodies to a wide array of host antigens in otherwise normal persons. Moreover, normal mice produce autoantibodies when given injections of nonspecific activators of lymphocytes (mitogens). In all of these circumstances, the autoantibodies combine with ubiquitous antigens: DNA, IgG (as the target of an IgM rheumatoid factor), phospholipids (cardiolipins), erythrocytes, lymphocytes, or cytoskeletal components (vimentin, keratins). Thus, production of autoantibodies is an inherent property of the normal immune system. The immune system controls the tendency to produce autoantibodies by a network of feedback controls exerted by T and B cells. It is generally thought that B cells normally are inhibited from terminal differentiation by suppressor T cells, a lack of inducer T cells, or both. In autoimmunity an imbalance between the two types of T cells can perturb the immunoregulatory network; this may be associated with activation of autoreactive B cells. In some instances, autoantibodies may arise by a normal T- and B-cell response activated by foreign organisms or substances that contain antigens, particularly polysaccharides, that cross-react with similar polysaccharides in body tissues.

As mentioned above in the description of immunoglobins, the unique portion of the variable region of the immunoglobulin molecule where antigen binds is called the *idiotype*, and an antibody reactive specifically with the idiotypic region of an antibody molecule is called an *anti-idiotypic* antibody. The specificity of antibody molecules and the regulation of antibody production have been probed by making rabbit anti-human idiotypic antibodies. There are also autologous anti-idiotypes (auto-anti-idiotypes) that arise during the course of the normal immune response. For example, auto-anti-idiotypes against antitetanus antibodies develop during normal immunization of humans to tetanus toxoid and may serve to deliver ''off'' signals to B cells secreting antitetanus antibodies. Idiotypes and auto-anti-idiotype antibodies may be an important component of the immunoregulatory network. Anti-idiotype antibodies may also be relevant to two types of autoimmunity: (1) dysfunction of the idiotype–anti-idiotype antibody system could lead to B-cell hyperreactivity by lack of generation of ''off'' signals for B-cell differentiation, and (2) some anti-receptor antibodies produced in autoimmune diseases (anti-acetylcholine receptor antibodies in myasthenia gravis, anti-insulin receptor antibodies in forms of type I diabetes mellitus, and anti-thyrotropin receptor antibodies in thyrotoxicosis) may be anti-idiotype antibodies made against the antibody combining site (idiotype) of an autoantibody.

Finally, genetic factors likely play a role in the genesis of autoimmune disease, either by selecting for inherent B-cell hyperreactivity and tendency toward autoantibody formation or via other unknown factors. Linkage of autoimmune diseases with known genetic loci such as the major histocompatibility complex has provoked great interest. Myasthenia gravis, thyrotoxicosis, and pernicious anemia are all associated with HLA-B8 (class I) and -DR3 (class II) alloantigen expression (Chap. 63) and are also associated with certain immunoglobulin heavy chain allotypic markers. Genetic marker systems such as HLA types and immunoglobulin heavy chain allotypic antigens may be associated with autoimmunity by making the host susceptible in some way to antiself immune cell activation. Thus, multiple genes and/or events are operative in the ultimate generation of the clinical autoimmune state.

CLINICAL EVALUATION OF IMMUNE FUNCTION Clinical assessment of immunity requires investigation of the four major components of the immune system that participate in host defense and in pathogenesis of autoimmune diseases: humoral immunity (B cells), cell-mediated immunity (T cells, monocytes), phagocytic cells of the reticuloendothelial system (polymorphonuclear cells, macrophages), and complement. Clinical problems that require an evaluation of immunity include chronic infections, recurrent infections, unusual infecting agents, and certain autoimmune syndromes. The type of clinical syndrome under evaluation can provide information regarding possible immune defects. Defects in cellular immunity generally result in viral, mycobacterial, and fungal infections. An extreme example of deficiency in cellular immunity is the acquired immunodeficiency syndrome (see Chap. 257). Antibody deficiencies result in recurrent bacterial infections, frequently with organisms such as *Streptococcus pneumoniae* and *Haemophilus influenzae* (Chap. 256). Disorders of phagocyte function frequently are manifest by recurrent skin infections, often due to *Staphylococcus aureus* (Chap. 56). Finally, deficiencies of early complement components are associated with autoimmune phenomena, and deficiencies of late complement components are associated with recurrent *Neisseria* infections (Table 62-7). Table 62-8 summarizes useful initial screening tests of immune function. For evaluation of antibody-mediated immunity, measurement of total serum immunoglobulin levels, measurement of specific antibody titers to commonly administered antigens (such as tetanus toxoid), and determination of isohemagglutinin titers yield information necessary for institution of appropriate therapy. In certain cases of hypogammaglobulinemia, quantitation of B-cell markers and in vitro B-cell functional assays are of use.

For assessment of cell-mediated immunity, the total lymphocyte count coupled with an appropriately placed battery of intradermal

TABLE 62-7 Clinical syndromes associated with complement deficiencies

Deficient protein	Clinical syndrome*
C1q	Glomerulonephritis and poikiloderma congenitale
C1r	Glomerulonephritis, SLE
C1s	SLE-like syndrome
C1 INH	Hereditary angioedema, SLE
C4	SLE, Sjögren's syndrome
C2	SLE, discoid lupus, polymyositis, common variable hypogammaglobulinemia, Hodgkin's disease, glomerulonephritis
C3	Glomerulonephritis, SLE, *Neisseria* infections
C5	*Neisseria* infections
C6	*Neisseria* infections
C7	SLE, RA, Raynaud's phenomenon, vasculitis, *Neisseria* infections
C8	SLE, *Neisseria* infections
C9	*Neisseria* infections

* *SLE = systemic lupus erythematosus, RA = rheumatoid arthritis.*
SOURCE: *Adapted with permission from S Ruddy, in WN Kelly et al (eds).*

skin tests provides a useful index of T-cell and macrophage response to antigens in vivo.

Anergy is the absence of an appropriate delayed hypersensitivity reaction and can be general anergy with lack of T-cell responses to many types of antigens or specific anergy with lack of T-cell responses to one antigen type. Anergy is determined by absence of reactivity in delayed hypersensitivity skin testing to antigens against which the patient is sensitized. For example, a battery of skin tests including *Candida*, histoplasmin, trichophytin, and *Mycobacterium tuberculosis* are placed intradermally. Most normal adult subjects should react to one of these four antigens. If there is no response on two separate occasions, the subject is said to be *anergic*. The causes for anergy vary in different diseases. Generalized anergy occurs in chronic fungal and TB infections and in sarcoidosis. An example of specific anergy is lack of T-cell responses to *Candida* antigen in mucocutaneous candidiasis.

Quantitation of total T cells and T4 and T8 T-cell subsets can be clinically useful. However, changes in the T4/T8 ratio occur in many clinical conditions and are not specific. In certain situations such as evaluation of a transplant recipient for response to donor antigens, the measurement of lymphocyte activation by determination of the amount of tritiated thymidine incorporated into lymphocyte DNA in response to donor antigens and mitogens is of use.

The evaluation of patients with recurrent cutaneous skin infections such as Job's syndrome and chronic granulomatous disease requires quantitation of neutrophil numbers and tests of neutrophil function. Functional neutrophil tests include nitroblue tetrazolium test, superoxide generation, chemotaxis, and quantitation of the ability of neutrophils to kill bacteria (Chap. 56).

TABLE 62-8 Initial screening tests of immune function

Humoral immunity
Quantitative immunoglobulin levels, IgG, IgM, IgA, IgE
Tests of specific antibody formation (antitetanus toxoid)
Isohemagglutinin titer (anti-A, anti-B): measures IgM response
Cell-mediated immunity
White blood cell count with differential: measures total lymphocytes
Delayed hypersensitivity skin tests: measures specific T-cell and macrophage response to antigens
Phagocytosis
White blood cell count with differential: measures total neutrophils
Nitroblue tetrazolium test (NBT), superoxide production: measures metabolic function
Chemotaxis: measures cell motility
Quantitative measurement of intracellular bacterial killing
Complement
Total hemolytic complement (CH_{50}): quantitates complement activity
Assay of individual complement components: defines complement component deficiencies

SOURCE: *Adapted with permission from AJ Ammann, Immunodeficiency diseases, in Basic and Clinical Immunology 5th ed, DP Stites et al (eds), Los Altos, Lange Medical, 1984.*

The total hemolytic complement (CH_{50}) determination measures the ability of a test sample of serum to lyse 50 percent of a standard suspension of sheep erythrocytes coated with rabbit anti-sheep erythrocyte antibody. This reaction requires the entire classical complement reaction sequence. For the classical activation pathway (C1, C4, C2) or the terminal sequence (C5 to C9) the CH_{50} determination is a reliable screen for homozygous deficiencies. A normal CH_{50}, however, does not exclude heterozygous partial deficiencies of classical complement components. When the CH_{50} level is subnormal, individual component measurements (usually by radioassay) are required to determine specific component deficiency states.

REFERENCES

Acuto O, Reinherz EL: The human T cell receptor: Structure and function. N Engl J Med 311:1019, 1984

Butcher E, Weissman IL: Lymphoid tissues and organs, in *Fundamental Immunology*, WE Paul (ed). New York, Raven, 1984, pp 109–127

Cooper MD et al: Lymphocytes, in *Fundamental Immunology*, WE Paul (ed). New York, Raven, 1984

Fauci AS et al: Activation and regulation of human immune responses: Implications in normal and disease states. Ann Intern Med 99:61, 1983

Haynes BF: The human thymic microenvironment. Adv Immunol 36:87, 1984

Kehrl JH et al: Human B cell activation, proliferation and differentiation. Immunol Rev 78:75, 1984

Kelly WN et al (eds): *Textbook of Rheumatology*, 2d ed. Philadelphia, Saunders, 1985, chaps 2,7,9, and 10

Paul WE: Introduction to the immune system, in *Fundamental Immunology*, WE Paul (ed). New York, Raven, 1984

Plaut M, Lichtenstein LM: Cellular and chemical basis of the allergic inflammatory response, in *Allergy: Principles and Practice*, E Middleton et al (eds). St. Louis, Mosby, 1978, pp 115–138

Romain PL, Schlossman SF: Human T cell subsets: Functional heterogeneity and surface recognition structures. J Clin Invest 74:1559, 1984

Shoenfeld Y, Schwartz RS: Immunologic and genetic factors in autoimmune disease. N Engl J Med 312:100, 1985

Stites DP et al (eds): *Basic and Clinical Immunology*, 5th ed. Los Gatos, Lange Medical, 1984

63 THE MAJOR HISTOCOMPATIBILITY GENE COMPLEX

CHARLES B. CARPENTER

Antigenic differences between members of a species are called *alloantigens*, and when these play a determining role in the rejection of allogeneic tissue grafts they are called *histocompatibility antigens*. Evolution has conserved a single closely linked region of histocompatibility genes, the products of which are prominently displayed on cell surfaces and provide a strong barrier to allotransplantation. The terms *major histocompatibility antigens* and *major histocompatibility gene complex* (MHC) refer to the gene products and genes of this chromosomal region. Many minor histocompatibility antigens, in contrast, are encoded throughout the genome. They represent weaker allotypic differences on molecules that serve a variety of functions. Structures bearing MHC antigens play a major role in immunity and in self-recognition in the differentiation of cells and tissues. Much of the evidence for MHC control of the immune response comes from work in animal models in which immune-response genes have been mapped within the mouse (H-2), rat (RT1), and guinea pig (GPLA) MHC. In humans the MHC is called *HLA*. The individual letters of HLA have various meanings, and by international agreement HLA is the logo for the human MHC.

Several generalizations can be made about the MHCs. *First*, three classes of gene products are encoded within the small [<2 cM (centimorgans)] region of the MHC. Class I molecules, expressed on virtually all cell surfaces, consist of one heavy and one light polypeptide chain and are the products of three reduplicated loci: HLA-A, HLA-B, and HLA-C. Class II molecules, restricted in expression to B lymphocytes, some monocytes, and activated T lymphocytes, consist of two polypeptide chains (α and β) of unequal length and are the products of several closely linked genes, collectively termed the HLA-D region. Class III molecules are the C4, C2, and Bf components of complement. *Second,* class I and class II molecules either form complexes with nominal antigens or the histocompatibility antigens and nominal antigens are conjointly recognized by T lymphocytes having appropriate antigen receptors. Self versus nonself discrimination in the initiation and effector phase of the immune response is thereby intimately directed by class I and II molecules. *Third,* restricted cell-to-cell interactions involving suppressor T lymphocytes are not clearly defined in humans, but HLA genes are important for some suppressor activities. *Fourth,* genes for enzyme systems having no apparent relationship to immunity are located in the region of the MHC, as are genes of importance in skeletal growth and development. The known loci of the HLA region on the short arm of chromosome 6 are shown in Fig. 63-1.

LOCI OF THE HLA SYSTEM Class I aptigens HLA antigens of the class I type are defined serologically by human sera, principally from multiparous females, and to a limited extent by monoclonal antibodies. They are present in varying densities in most body tissues, including B cells, T cells, and platelets but not in mature red blood cells. The number of serologically defined specificities is large, and the HLA system is the most polymorphic genetic system known in humans. Three clearly defined loci are recognized within the HLA complex for class I, serologically defined (SD), HLA antigens. Each class I antigen consists of an 11,500-dalton beta$_2$ microglobulin subunit and a 44,000-dalton heavy chain that carries the antigenic specificities (Fig. 63-2). There are 70 clearly defined A and B specificities, and eight C-locus specificities are known. Antigens of the major complex are prefixed by HLA, but this may be omitted when the context is clear. Antigens tentatively accepted by the World Health Organization have a *w* after the locus designation. The number following the locus designation is the name of the antigen. The HLA antigens of African, Asian, and Oceanic peoples are not well defined

FIGURE 63-1 *Schematic representation of human chromosome 6, showing the location of the HLA region in the 21 region of the short arm. The HLA-A, HLA-B, HLA-C loci encode class I heavy chains (44,000 daltons), while the beta$_2$ microglobulin light chain (11,500 daltons) of the class I molecule is encoded by genes of chromosome 15. HLA-D region (class II) is centromeric to the A, B, C loci, with genes for closely linked complement components C4A, C4B, Bf, and C2 in the B-D region. The order of the complement genes is uncertain. Each D region class II molecule is made up of an α and a β chain. They appear on the cell surface in distinct sets, DP, DQ, and DR. The numbers preceding α or β indicate that there are different genes for the chains of a given set; e.g., for DR, there are three β-chain genes, so that the expressed molecule may be 1βα, 2βα, or 3βα. The antigens DRw52 (MT2) and DRw53 (MT3) are on the 2β chain, while DR is on 1β. DRα is not polymorphic, while molecules bearing the DQ antigens have polymorphism in both α and β chains (2α2β). The other DQ set (1α1β) has limited polymorphism. Polymorphism in DP is confined to the β chains. The overall length of the HLA region is about 3 cM.*

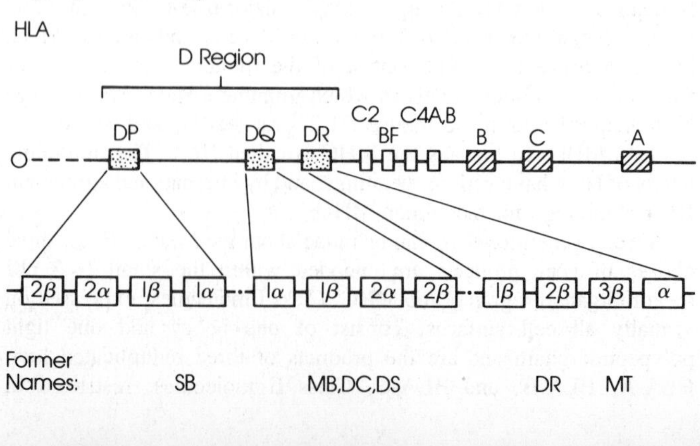

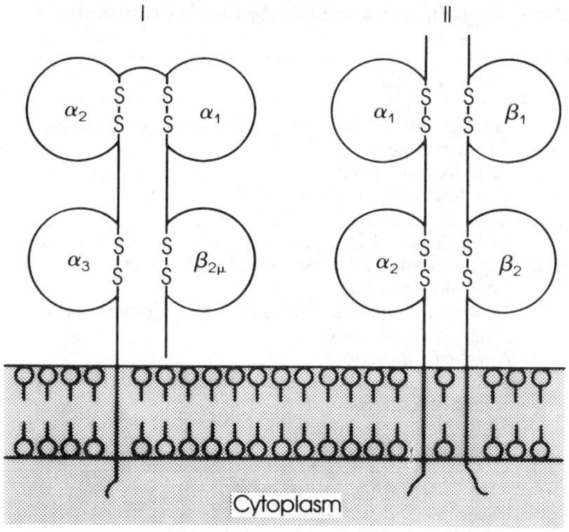

FIGURE 63-2 *Schematic representation of classes I and II molecules on the cell surface. Class I molecules are composed of two polypeptide chains. The 44,000-dalton heavy chain passes through the plasma membrane. Its external portion consists of three domains (α_1, α_2, α_3) formed by disulfide bonding. The beta$_2$-microglobulin ($\beta_{2\mu}$) light chain (11,500 daltons) encoded by chromosome 15 is noncovalently bound to the heavy chain. Amino acid sequence homologies among class I molecules is 80 to 85 percent, falling to 50 percent or less in portions of α_1 and α_2 which most likely represent the sites of alloantigenic polymorphism. Class II molecules consist of two noncovalently associated polypeptide chains, a 34,000-dalton α and a 29,000-dalton β. Each chain has two domains formed by disulfide bridging. [From CB Carpenter and EL Milford, Renal Transplantation: Immunobiology in The Kidney, B Brenner, F Rector (eds), Saunders, New York, 1985, with permission.]*

at present, although they include some of the antigens commonly found in people of West European ancestry. The distribution of HLA antigens is distinctive for certain racial groups and can serve as anthropologic markers in the study of migration patterns and diseases.

Since chromosomes are paired, each individual has six serologically defined HLA-A, HLA-B, and HLA-C antigens, three from each parent. Each of these chromosomal sets is termed a *haplotype,* and by simple mendelian inheritance one-fourth of siblings have identical haplotypes, half share a haplotype, and the remaining one-fourth are completely incompatible (Fig. 63-3). Evidence that this gene complex plays the major role in the transplantation response comes from the fact that haplotype-matched sibling donor-recipient combinations show excellent results in kidney transplantation, in the vicinity of 85 to 90 percent long-term survival (see Chap. 221).

Class II antigens The HLA-D region is adjacent to the class I loci on the short arm of chromosome 6 (Fig. 63-1). This region encodes a series of class II molecules, each consisting of a 29,000-dalton α chain and a 34,000-dalton β chain (Fig. 63-2). Incompatibility for this region, particularly concerning the DR antigens, determines the in vitro proliferative response of lymphocytes to mismatched haplotypes. This mixed lymphocyte response (MLR) is assessed by the degree of proliferation of a *mixed lymphocyte culture* (MLC) and is positive even when HLA-A, HLA-B, and HLA-C antigens are identical (Fig. 63-3). HLA-D antigens are defined by reference-stimulating lymphocytes that are homozygous for HLA-D and are inactivated by x-irradiation or mitomycin C to make the reaction unidirectional. There are 19 such antigens (HLA-Dwl-19) recognized by homozygous typing cells.

Attempts to define HLA-D by serology first established a series of D-related (DR) antigens expressed on class II molecules of B lymphocytes, monocytes, and activated T lymphocytes. Other closely related antigen systems were soon discovered and given various local names (MB, MT, DC, SB). The separate identity of sets of class II

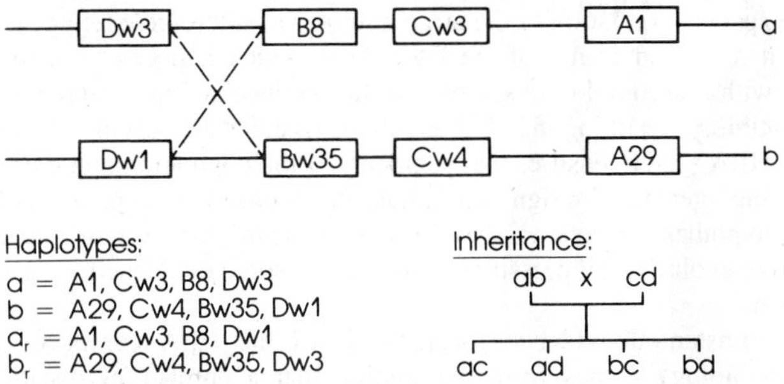

FIGURE 63-3 *HLA region, chromosome 6: inheritance of HLA haplotypes. Each chromosomal segment of linked genes is termed a haplotype, and each individual inherits one haplotype from each parent. The A, B, C, and D antigens of haplotypes a and b are shown for this hypothetical individual in chromosomal order on the diagram, and also below as they would be written in text. If individual ab were to marry cd, their offspring would be of four types only, as far as HLA is concerned. Occasionally (dotted cross) recombination occurs in the germ line (meiosis) of a parent, resulting in an altered haplotype. The frequency of recombinant children is a measure of the map distance (1 percent recombination frequency = 1 cM; see Fig. 63-1). (From CB Carpenter, Kidney International, 14:283, 1978.)*

molecules is now established, and the genes for their respective α and β chains have been isolated and sequenced. The class II gene map shown in Fig. 63-1 describes a minimal number of genes and molecular sets. Although a class II molecule may be composed of a DRα from one parental haplotype and a DRβ from the other parent (transcomplementation), α and β combinatorial possibilities outside of each DP, DQ, DR set rarely, if ever, occur. DR, and to some extent DQ, molecules provide the stimuli for the primary MLR. The secondary MLR is called the *primed lymphocyte test* (PLT) and occurs rapidly over 24 to 36 h instead of 6 to 7 days. DP alloantigens were discovered from their ability to provide PLT stimulation, although they do not produce a primary MLR. While B lymphocytes and activated T lymphocytes express all three sets of class II molecules, DQ antigens are not expressed on 60 to 90 percent of monocytes, which are virtually all DP- and DR-positive.

Molecular genetics Each polypeptide chain of class I and class II molecules bears several polymorphic sites in addition to the "private" antigen defined by alloantisera. In the *cell-mediated lympholysis* (CML) test the specificity of killer T cells (T_c), which arise during the proliferative events in MLR, is determined by testing upon target cells from donors other than those providing the MLR stimulus. Antigen systems defined by this method show a close but imperfect correlation with class I private antigens. Cloning of cytotoxic cells has revealed the presence of a variety of polymorphic target determinants on HLA molecules, some of which are identifiable by alloantisera or monoclonal antibodies derived from immunization of mice with human cells. Some of these reagents can be used to identify private determinants of HLA, while others are directed to more "public" (sometimes called supertypic) determinants. One such system of public HLA-B antigens has two alleles, Bw4 and Bw6. Most HLA-B private antigens are associated with either Bw4 or Bw6. Other systems are restricted to subsets of HLA antigen groups. For example, HLA-B-bearing heavy chains carry additional sites that are common to B7, B27, Bw22, and B40 or to B5, B15, B18, and Bw35. Other types of shared antigenic determinants exist, as exemplified by a monoclonal antibody which reacts with a site shared between HLA-A and HLA-B heavy chains.

The amino acid sequence and peptide maps of several HLA molecules show that the class I hypervariable regions are clustered in outer α_1 domain (Fig. 63-2) and the adjacent portion of α_2. Variability in the sequences of class II molecules differs from locus to locus. Remarkably, the class I α_3 domain, the class II α_2 and β_2 domains, and the portions of the T8 (Leu 2) cell surface molecule which function in T-cell interactions (see Chap. 62) all show significant amino acid sequence homologies with immunoglobulin constant regions. These findings suggest evolutionary elaboration within a family of gene products which have immune recognition functions. When genomic DNA for HLA is examined, typical exon-intron sequences of DNA have been found for class I and class II, exons having been identified for signal peptides (5′), each of the domains, a transmembrane hydrophobic segment, and a cytoplasmic segment (3′). cDNA probes are available for most of the HLA chains, and enzymatic digests have been used to study patterns of *restriction fragment length polymorphisms* (RFLP), many of which correlate with class II serologic and MLR patterns. There are 20 to 30 class I genes, however, making assessment of polymorphism by RFLP difficult. Many of these genes are not expressed (pseudogenes), while some could represent additional class I loci that are expressed only on activated T cells, and are of uncertain function. Development of HLA-A or HLA-B locus specific probes will help to resolve this complexity.

Complement (class III) Structural genes for three complement components, C4, C2, and Bf, are present in the HLA-B-D region (Fig. 63-1). There are two loci for C4, coding for C4A and C4B, formerly recognized as the Rodgers and Chido red blood cell antigens, respectively. These antigens are, in fact, absorbed plasma C4 molecules. Other complement components are not closely linked to HLA. No crossovers have been found between the C2, Bf, and C4 loci. They are all encoded within a 100-kilobase segment between HLA-B and HLA-DR. There are two alleles of C2, four of Bf, seven of C4A, and three of C4B, plus blanks for each locus (QO). The extensive polymorphism of complement types (complotypes) makes them useful for genetic studies. The four most common extended haplotypes found in people of western European ancestry are shown in Table 63-1. MLRs between unrelated individuals who are matched for these extended haplotypes are nonreactive, whereas reactivity is common if unrelated individuals are matched for only HLA-DR and -DQ. Such identical extended haplotypes may be conserved from a common ancestor.

Other sixth-chromosome genes Deficiency of steroid 21-hydroxylase, an autosomal recessive trait, results in the syndrome of congenital adrenal hyperplasia (Chaps. 325 and 333). The gene for the enzyme is localized in the HLA-B-D region. The 21-hydroxylase gene adjacent to C4A is deleted in affected individuals along with C4A (C4AQO), and the HLA-B locus gene may have been altered to convert B13 to the rare Bw47 found only in affected haplotypes. A late-onset variant of 21-hydroxylase deficiency is also linked to HLA, although congenital adrenal hyperplasia due to 11β-hydroxylase deficiency is not HLA-linked. Idiopathic hemochromatosis, an autosomal recessive disorder, is linked to HLA, as has been shown in several family studies (see Chap. 310). Although the pathogenesis of this disease is unknown, the gene that modulates gastrointestinal iron absorption is near HLA-A (Table 63-2).

Immune response genes HLA-D is analogous to the mouse H-2I region as established by studies of in vitro responses to synthetic polypeptide antigens, keyhole limpet hemocyanin, collagen, and tetanus toxoid. Presentation of antigenic fragments on the surfaces of macrophages or other cells bearing class II molecules requires conjoint recognition of a class II + antigen complex by T lymphocytes bearing the appropriate receptor(s) (see Chap. 62). The crux of this "self + X" or "altered self" hypothesis is that in the T-dependent immune response, help from the T helper/inducer cell (T_H) occurs

TABLE 63-1 Common extended HLA haplotypes

HLA-B	HLA-DR	BF	C2	C4A	C4B
8	3	S	C	QO	1
7	2	S	C	3	1
57	7	S	C	6	1
44	7	F	C	3	1

TABLE 63-2 Linkage of genetic defects to HLA

	Gene location	Common haplotype found
C2 deficiency	HLA-B-D	Aw25, B18, BfS, DR2
21-OH deficiency	HLA-B-D	A3, Bw47, BfF, DR7
21-OH deficiency (late onset)	HLA-B-D,	B14, BfS, DR1
Idiopathic hemochromatosis	HLA-A	A3, B14
Paget's disease	HLA-A-D	
Spinocerebellar ataxia	HLA-A-D	
Hodgkins' disease	HLA-A-D	

only if the appropriate class II determinant can be synthesized. The genes for the latter are Ir genes. Since allogeneic class II determinants are perceived as already altered, the allogeneic MLR response represents a model for the immune system in which additional nominal antigen does not need to be added (Fig. 63-4). Effector phases of immunity require recognition of nominal antigen together with a self structure. The latter in humans, as in mice, is the molecule bearing class I histocompatibility antigens. Human cell lines infected with influenza virus are lysed by immune cytotoxic T lymphocytes (T_c) only if an HLA-A- or HLA-B-locus antigen is shared between the attacking and target cells. Again, the allogeneic MLR provides a model for development of class I restricted cytotoxic T lymphocytes (Fig. 63-4). When primed cells are propagated and cloned, an array of restrictions to different class I and II molecules and epitopes can be discerned. At the level of the antigen presenting cell, for example, a given T_H clone recognizes an antigenic fragment conjointly with a specific site on a class II molecule via its receptor (T_i). The restriction elements for some microbial antigens are DR or Dw alleles. Suppression of immune responses (i.e., low responder status) to cedar pollen, streptococcal antigen, and schistosomal antigen is linked to HLA as a dominant trait, suggesting the existence of immune suppressor (Is) genes. Specific allele associations with immune response (e.g., ragweed Ra5 antigen with DR2 and collagen with DR4) have also been demonstrated.

DISEASE ASSOCIATIONS If the major histocompatibility complex serves a critical natural biologic function, what might that be? One hypothesis is that it plays a role in immune surveillance against neoplastic cells that develop in the course of an individual's lifetime. The system could also play an important role in pregnancy because of the histoincompatibility that always exists between the mother and the fetus. The high degree of polymorphism may also ensure survival of the species in relation to the large numbers of microbiologic agents present in the environment. Self-tolerance which happens to cross-react with microbiologic agents would produce a high degree of susceptibility, resulting in lethal infection, whereas the polymorphism in the HLA system ensures that segments of the population recognize offending agents as foreign and initiate the appropriate response. All these hypotheses relate to the survival value of the system under selective evolutionary pressures, and there is some evidence for each of them.

Circumstantial evidence for the role of the HLA complex in immunobiology comes from the finding that a number of disease processes are positively associated with certain HLA antigens within the population. The search for such associations has been stimulated by the discovery of immune response genes linked to the H-2 complex in the mouse. Table 63-3 summarizes the most significant HLA and disease associations.

Most striking is the increased frequency of HLA-B27 in certain rheumatic diseases, particularly ankylosing spondylitis, a condition with a strong familial tendency. B27 is present in about 7 percent of people of West European ancestry, while it appears in 80 to 90 percent of patients with ankylosing spondylitis. Expressed as a relative risk, the antigen B27 confers a susceptibility to the development of ankylosing spondylitis that is 87 times that in the general population. Similarly, acute anterior uveitis, Reiter's syndrome, and reactive arthritis to at least three bacterial infections (yersinia, salmonella, and gonococcus) show a high degree of association with B27. Although the ordinary form of juvenile rheumatoid arthritis (JRA) also shows a similar association with B27, the pauciarticular form of JRA with iritis is DR5-associated. The increased incidence of B27 in psoriatic arthritis is also significant for the central type of the disorder, while Bw38 is associated with both the central and peripheral types. Psoriasis is associated with Cw6. Patients with degenerative arthritis or gout show no alteration in antigen frequencies.

Most other disease associations are with HLA-D region antigens. For example, gluten-sensitive enteropathy (celiac disease, nontropical sprue) in children and adults is associated with DR3 (relative risk = 21). The actual percentage of such patients having this antigen ranges from 63 to 96 percent compared to 22 to 27 percent of controls. The same antigen is also present in increased frequency in patients with chronic active hepatitis and in patients with dermatitis herpetiformis who also have gluten-sensitive enteropathy. Juvenile-onset insulin-dependent diabetes mellitus (type I) is associated with DR4 and DR3 and is negatively associated with DR2. Maturity-onset diabetes is not HLA-associated. A rare allele of Bf (F1) is also found in 17 to 25

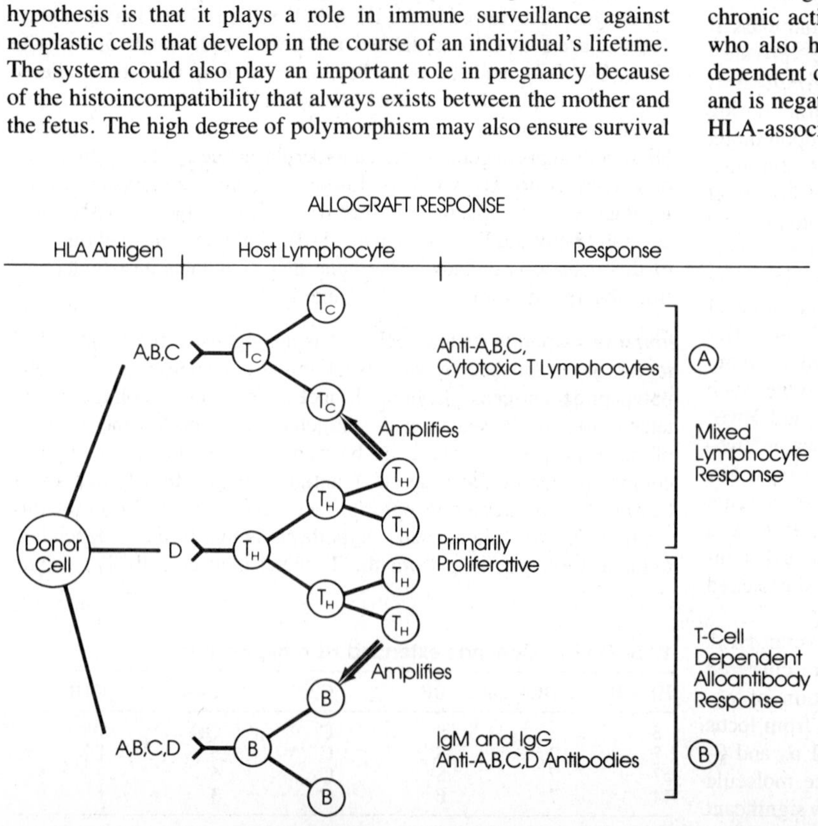

FIGURE 63-4 *Schema of the relative roles of HLA-A, HLA-B, HLA-C, and HLA-D antigens in initiation of the alloimmune response and in the development of effector cells and antibodies. Two main classes of T lymphocytes recognize antigens: T_c, the precursors to the cytotoxic "killer" cells, and T_H, the helper cells for amplification of the cytotoxic response. T_H also provide help to B lymphocytes for production of a fully mature IgG response. Note that T_c generally recognize class I antigens, while the T_H signal is provided principally by HLA-D, which has class II antigens closely associated. (From CB Carpenter, Kidney International, 14:283, 1978.)*

percent of cases of type I diabetes. Hyperthyroidism in the United States is associated with B8, Dw3, while in Japanese populations the association is with Bw35. More extensive studies of healthy and diseased members of various races will help in clarification of which HLA markers are universal. For example, B27 is rare in healthy Japanese but is common in subjects with ankylosing spondylitis. Also, DR4 seems to be the common marker for type I diabetes in all races. Sometimes an HLA marker is clearly associated only with a subgroup within a syndrome. For example, myasthenia gravis without thymoma is more strongly B8, DR3-associated, and the association of DR2 with multiple sclerosis is strong in patients with rapidly progressive deterioration. Goodpasture's syndrome due to autoimmunity to glomerular basement membrane, idiopathic membranous glomerulonephritis, which may be an autoimmune process involving antibodies to an antigen of the glomerulus, and gold-induced membranous nephritis are strongly HLA-DR-associated.

LINKAGE DISEQUILIBRIUM Although the distribution of HLA alleles varies in racial and ethnic populations, the most salient feature of population genetics of HLA antigens is the presence of linkage disequilibria among certain antigens of the A and B, B and C, and B, D, and complement loci. Linkage disequilibrium means that antigens of closely linked loci appear together more frequently than predicted by random association. The classic example is the linkage disequilibrium present between the A-locus antigen, HLA-A1, and B-locus antigen, HLA-B8, in people of western European ancestry. The coincidence of A1 and B8 should be the product of their individual gene frequencies, or 0.17 times 0.11 equals approximately 0.02. The observed frequency of A1 and B8 is 0.08, four times that expected, an increase of 0.06. The latter value is termed Δ (delta), and is a measure of the disequilibrium. Other A- and B-locus haplotype disequilibria have been recognized and include (A3, B7), (A2, B12), (A29, B12), and (A11, Bw35). Furthermore, some D-region determinants are in linkage disequilibrium with B-locus antigens (for example, DR3 and B8), as are some B-locus and C-locus antigens. Serologically defined HLA antigens can serve as markers for the genes of an entire haplotype within a family and as markers for specific genes within a population but only where a linkage disequilibrium exists.

Linkage disequilibrium is of importance because such gene associations may have some bearing on their function. For example, selective pressures during the course of evolution may have been the major factor in the survival of certain gene combinations in a haplotype. Such a theory would suggest, for example, that A1 and B8, along with certain D-region and other determinants, conferred a selective advantage in the face of epidemics such as the plague or smallpox. It would also follow that the descendants of the survivors may display susceptibility to certain diseases because their unique gene complex happens to confer an abnormal response to other environmental agents. The major difficulty with this hypothesis is the assumption that selection must work on several genes simultaneously to account for the observed Δ's; however, the need for complex interactions among the products of the several loci of the major histocompatibility complex is only beginning to be appreciated, and selection might force multiple linkage disequilibria. The conservation of certain extended haplotypes, mentioned above, supports this view.

On the other hand, the selection hypothesis is not necessary to explain linkage disequilibrium. When a population lacking certain antigens is crossed with one in which a high frequency of antigens is in equilibrium, a Δ can develop within a few generations. For example, the increasing Δ value for A1, B8 found in populations from east to west, from India to western Europe, can be explained on the basis of migration and fusion. In smaller groups, consanguinity, founder effects, and gene drift may account for disequilibria. Finally, certain linkage disequilibria could occur as a result of nonrandom crossing over during gametic meiosis, because of chromosomal segments which are either more or less likely to break. Unless there are selective pressures or restrictions in crossing over, linkage

TABLE 63-3 HLA antigens and disease, showing the most highly associated antigens

Disease	Antigen	Relative risk*
RHEUMATIC		
Ankylosing spondylitis	B27	87.0
Reiter's syndrome	B27	37.0
Acute anterior uveitis	B27	10.3
Reactive arthritis (yersinia, salmonella, gonococcus)	B27	18.0
Psoriatic arthritis, central	B27	10.7
	Bw38	9.1
Psoriatic arthritis, peripheral	B27	2.0
	Bw38	6.5
Juvenile rheumatoid arthritis	B27	4.5
	DRw8	3.6
Juvenile arthritis, pauciarticular	DR5	5.2
Rheumatoid arthritis	Dw4/DR4	6.0
Sjögren's syndrome	Dw3	9.7
Systemic lupus erythematosus	DR3	5.8
Systemic lupus erythematosus (hydralazine)	DR4	5.6
GASTROINTESTINAL		
Gluten-sensitive enteropathy	DR3	21.0
Chronic active hepatitis	DR3	6.8
Ulcerative colitis	B5	3.8
HEMATOLOGIC		
Idiopathic hemochromatosis	A3	8.2
	B14	26.7
	A3, B14	90.0
Pernicious anemia	DR5	5.4
SKIN		
Dermatitis herpetiformis	Dw3	15.4
Psoriasis vulgaris	Cw6	4.8
Psoriasis vulgaris (Japanese)	Cw6	10.7
Pemphigus vulgaris (Jews)	DR4	14.4
	A10	5.9
Behçet's disease	B5	6.3
ENDOCRINE		
Type 1 diabetes mellitus	DR4	6.4
	DR3	3.3
	DR2	0.2
	BfF1	15.0
Hyperthyroidism	B8	3.6
	Dw3	3.7
Hyperthyroidism (Japanese)	Bw35	3.9
Adrenal insufficiency	Dw3	10.5
Subacute thyroiditis (de Quervain)	Bw35	13.7
Hashimoto's thyroiditis	DR5	3.2
NEUROLOGIC		
Myasthenia gravis	B8	2.7
	DR3	2.5
Multiple sclerosis	DR2	3.9
Manic-depressive disorder	Bw16	2.3
Schizophrenia	A28	2.3
RENAL		
Idiopathic membranous glomerulonephritis	DR3	12.0
Goodpasture's syndrome (anti-GBM)	DR2	15.9
Minimal change disease (steroid response)	B12	3.5
Polycystic kidney disease	B5	2.6
IgA nephropathy	DR4	4.0
Gold nephropathy	DR3	14.0
INFECTIOUS		
Tuberculoid leprosy (Asians)	B8	6.8
Paralytic polio	Bw16	4.3
Low vs. high response to vaccinia virus	Cw3	12.7
IMMUNODEFICIENCY		
IgA deficiency (blood donors)	DR3	13.0

* *Relative risk* $= \dfrac{(\%\ \text{antigen-positive patients})(\%\ \text{antigen-negative controls})}{(\%\ \text{antigen-negative patients})(\%\ \text{antigen-positive controls})}$.

disequilibria disappear over a period of several generations. A large number of nonrandom associations occur throughout the HLA gene complex, and elucidation of the reasons for their existence may provide insight into the mechanism underlying certain disease susceptibilities.

LINKAGE AND ASSOCIATION The diseases listed in Table 63-2 are examples of HLA linkage wherein the inherited conditions are marked within families by the relevant HLA haplotypes. For C2 deficiency, 21-hydroxylase deficiency, and idiopathic hemochromatosis the mode of inheritance is recessive, with heterozygotes showing partial deficiencies. These genetic defects are also HLA-associated, with an excess of certain HLA alleles in affected unrelated individuals. Also, C2 deficiency is commonly linked to the HLA-Aw25, B18, BS5, D/DR2 haplotype, and idiopathic hemochromatosis exhibits both linkage and strong association with HLA-A3 and B14. The high degree of linkage disequilibria in these HLA-linked diseases may result from mutations in a single founder, and a sufficient period of time may not have passed to bring the gene pool back into equilibrium. In this view, the HLA antigens are simple markers for the linked gene. Alternatively, expression of the defect may require interaction with specific HLA alleles. This latter hypothesis would require a higher mutation rate, with defective gene expression occurring only when linked with certain HLA genes.

Paget's disease and spinocerebellar ataxia are HLA-linked autosomal dominant traits in families having multiple affected members, and Hodgkins disease shows an HLA-linked recessive pattern of inheritance. No HLA associations have been discerned for these disorders, suggesting that there were multiple founders with mutations in linkage with different HLA alleles.

HLA linkage is readily recognized when recessive or dominant inheritance patterns are clear-cut, i.e., when expressivity is high and the process is mostly, if not entirely, determined by a single gene defect. In most of the associations HLA markers represent risk factors involving the operation and modulation of the immune response under the influence of multiple genes. An example of a polygenic immunologic disease is atopic allergy, in which the association to HLA may be evident only in individuals whose genetically controlled (non-HLA) levels of IgE production are low. Another is IgA deficiency (Table 63-3), which is HLA-DR3-associated.

CLINICAL APPLICATIONS The clinical value of HLA typing for diagnosis of disease is limited to B27 and ankylosing spondylitis, where nevertheless there are 10 percent false-positive and false-negative rates. HLA studies are also of value in genetic counseling and early recognition of disease in families with idiopathic hemochromatosis or congenital adrenal hyperplasia due to steroid 21-hydroxylase deficiency, particularly as HLA typing can be performed upon cells obtained by amniocentesis. The high degree of polymorphism of the HLA system also makes it a powerful tool for paternity testing and other medicolegal applications. The implications for diseases such as type I diabetes mellitus and the other diseases showing HLA associations require further study of the components of the HLA system and their role in the pathogenesis of disease.

REFERENCES

Albert E, Mayr W (eds): *Histocompatibility Testing, 1984*. Berlin, Springer-Verlag, 1984

Andersson M et al: Genomic hybridization with class II transplantation antigen cDNA probes as a complementary technique in tissue typing. Hum Immunol 11:57, 1984

Bodmer J, Bodmer W: Histocompatibility, 1984. Immunol Tod 5:251, 1984

Cohen D et al: Clusters of HLA class IIβ restriction fragments describe allelic series. Proc Natl Acad Sci USA 81:7870, 1984

Degos L, Dausset J: Human migrations and linkage disequilibrium of HLA system. Immunogenetics 3:195, 1974

Kaufman JF et al: The class II molecules of the human and murine major histocompatibility complex. Cell 36:1, 1984

Larkhammar D et al: Complete amino acid sequence of an HLA-DR antigen–like beta chain as predicted from the nucleotide sequence: Similarities with immunoglobulins and HLA-A, -B, and -C antigens. Proc Natl Acad Sci USA 79:3687, 1982

Marsh DG et al: Epidemiology and genetics of atopic allergy. N Eng J Med 305:1551, 1981

Möller G (ed): Structure and function of HLA-DR. Immunol Rev 66:1982 (entire volume)

——— (ed): HLA and disease susceptibility. Immunol Rev 70:1983 (entire volume)

Nishimura Y, Sasazuki T: Suppressor T cells control the HLA-linked low responsiveness to streptococcal antigen in man. Nature 302:67, 1983

Qvigstad E et al: Antigen-specific T cell clones restricted by DR, DRw53 (MT), or DP (SB) class II HLA molecules. Inhibition studies with monoclonal HLA-specific antibodies. Hum Immunol 11:207, 1984

Ryder LP et al (eds): *HLA and Disease Registry: Third Report*. Copenhagen, Munksgaard, 1979

White PC et al: HLA-linked congenital adrenal hyperplasia results from a defective gene encoding a cytochrome P-450 specific for steroid 21-hydroxylation. Proc Natl Acad Sci USA 81:7505, 1984

section 3 Clinical pharmacology

64 PRINCIPLES OF DRUG THERAPY

JOHN A. OATES / GRANT R. WILKINSON

QUANTITATIVE DETERMINANTS OF DRUG ACTION

Safe and effective therapy with drugs requires their delivery to target tissues in concentrations within the narrow range that yields efficacy without toxicity. Optimal precision in achieving concentrations of drug within this therapeutic "window" can be achieved with regimens that are based on the kinetics of the drug's availability to target sites. This chapter deals with the principles of drug elimination and distribution that form the basis for loading and maintenance regimens for the average patient and considers instances in which elimination of the drug is impaired (e.g., renal failure). The kinetic basis for optimal utilization of plasma level data is also discussed.

PLASMA LEVELS AFTER A SINGLE DOSE The levels of lidocaine in plasma following intravenous administration decline in two phases as illustrated in Fig. 64-1; such a biphasic decline is typical for many drugs. Immediately following rapid injection, essentially all of the drug is in the plasma compartment, and the high initial plasma level reflects its confinement to this small volume. Subsequently, the drug is transferred into the extravascular compartment, and the period of time during which this occurs is referred to as the *distribution phase*. For lidocaine the distribution phase is virtually complete within 30 min; then a slower rate of fall ensues, referred to as the *equilibrium phase* or *elimination phase*. During this latter phase, the drug levels in plasma and those in the tissues are in pseudoequilibrium.

Distribution phase Pharmacologic events during the distribution phase depend on whether the level of drug at the receptor site is similar to that in the plasma. If this is the case, the pharmacologic effects, whether favorable or adverse, may be inordinately great during this period. For example, following a small bolus dose (50 mg) of lidocaine, antiarrhythmic effects may be evident during the

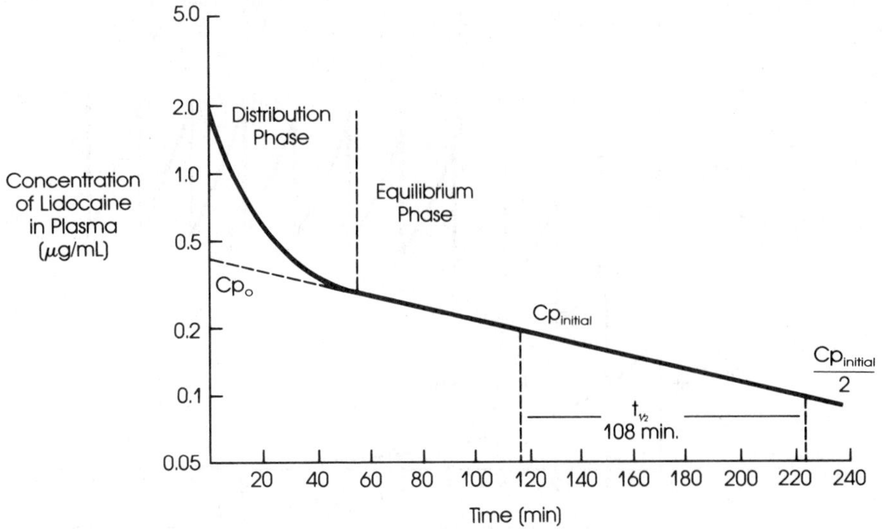

FIGURE 64-1 *Concentrations of lidocaine in plasma following the administration of 50 mg intravenously. The half-life of 108 min is computed as the time required for levels to fall from any given value during the equilibrium phase ($Cp_{initial}$) to one-half that level. Cp_0 is the hypothetical concentration of lidocaine in plasma at time zero if equilibrium had been achieved instantly.*

early distribution phase but disappear as levels fall below those that are minimally effective and even before equilibrium between plasma and tissue is reached. Thus, larger single doses or multiple small doses must be administered to achieve an effect that is sustained into the equilibrium phase. The toxicity of high levels of some drugs during the distribution phase precludes administration of a single intravenous loading dose that will achieve therapeutic levels during the equilibrium phase. For example, the administration of a loading dose of phenytoin as a single intravenous bolus can cause cardiovascular collapse due to the high levels during the distribution phase. If a loading dose of phenytoin is administered intravenously, it must be given in fractions at intervals sufficient to permit substantial distribution of the prior dose before the next is given (for example, 100 mg every 3 to 5 min). For similar reasons, the loading dose of many potent drugs that rapidly equilibrate with their receptors is divided into fractional doses for intravenous administration.

After an oral dose that delivers an equivalent amount of drug into the systemic circulation, plasma levels during the distribution phase do not rise as steeply as after an intravenous bolus dose. Because the drug is not absorbed instantly after oral administration and is delivered into the systemic circulation more slowly, much of the drug is distributed by the time absorption is complete. Thus, procainamide, which is almost totally absorbed after oral administration, can be given as a single 750-mg loading dose with little risk of hypotension; in contrast, loading of the drug by the intravenous route is more safely accomplished by giving the dose in fractions of about 100 mg at 5-min intervals to avoid the hypotension that might ensue during the distribution phase if the entire loading dose were given as a single bolus.

In contrast, other drugs are distributed slowly to their sites of action during the distribution phase. For example, levels of digoxin at the receptor site (and its pharmacologic effect) do not reflect plasma levels during the distribution phase. Digoxin is transported (or bound) to its cardiac receptors more slowly by a process that proceeds throughout distribution. Thus, plasma levels fall during a distribution phase of several hours, while levels at the site of action and pharmacologic effect increase. Only at the end of the distribution phase, when the drug has reached equilibrium with the receptor, does the concentration of digoxin in plasma reflect pharmacologic effect. For this reason, there should be a 6- to 8-h wait after the distribution phase before plasma levels of digoxin are obtained for a guide to therapy.

Equilibrium phase After distribution has proceeded to the point where the concentration of drug in plasma is in equilibrium with that in the tissues outside the vascular compartment, the levels in plasma and tissues fall in parallel as the drug is eliminated from the body. Thus, the *equilibrium phase* is sometimes also referred to as the *elimination phase*.

Most drugs are eliminated as a first-order process. During the equilibrium phase, a characteristic of the first-order process is that the time required for the level of drug in plasma to fall to one-half the original value (the half-life, $t_{1/2}$) is the same regardless of which point on the plasma level curve is chosen as a starting point for the measurement. Another characteristic of the first-order process is that a semilogarithmic plot of the concentrations in plasma versus time during the equilibrium phase is linear. From such a plot (Fig. 64-1) it can be seen that the half-life of lidocaine is 108 min.

One can calculate what amount of the administered dose remains in the body at any multiple of the half-life interval following administration:

Number of half-lives	Amount of dose remaining in the body, %
1	50
2	25
3	12.5
4	6.25
5	3.125

In theory, the elimination process never reaches completion. From a clinical standpoint, however, elimination is essentially complete when it has reached 90 percent. Therefore, for practical purposes, *a first-order elimination process reaches completion after 3 to 4 half-lives.*

DRUG ACCUMULATION—LOADING AND MAINTENANCE DOSES

With repeated administration of a drug, the amount in the body accumulates if the elimination of the first dose is incomplete when the second dose is given, and both the amount of drug in the body and its pharmacologic effect increase with continuing administration until they reach a plateau. The accumulation of digoxin administered in repeated maintenance doses (without a loading dose) is illustrated in Fig. 64-2. As digoxin's half-life is about 1.6 days in a patient with normal renal function, 65 percent of digoxin remains in the body at the end of 1 day. Thus, the second dose will raise the amount of digoxin in the body (and average plasma level) to 165 percent of that following the first dose. Each subsequent dose will result in greater amounts in the body until a plateau is attained. At the plateau, or *steady state,* drug intake per unit of time is the same as the rate of drug elimination. For *all* drugs with first-order kinetics, the time required to achieve steady-state levels can be predicted from the half-life because accumulation also is a first-order process with a half-life identical to that for elimination. Hence, accumulation reaches 90

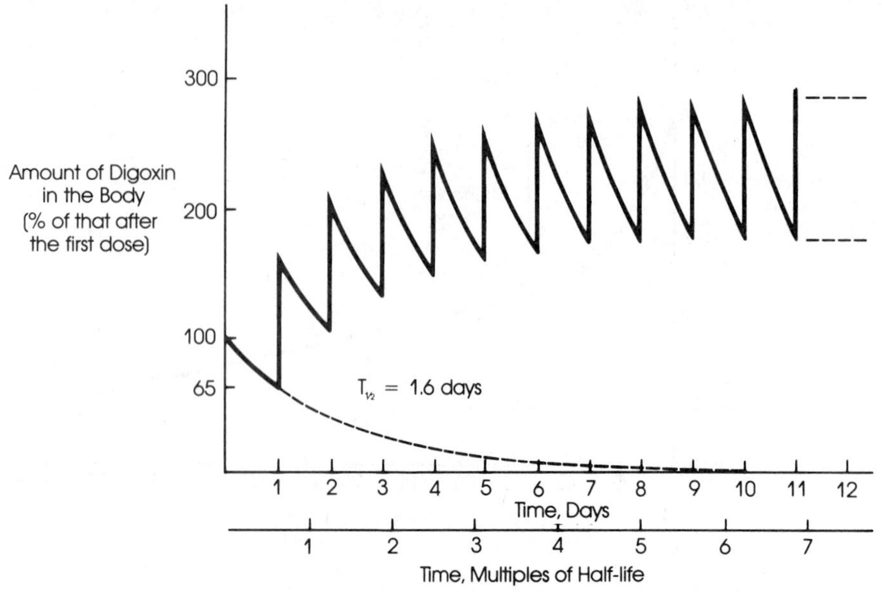

FIGURE 64-2 *The time course of digoxin accumulation when a single daily maintenance dose is given without a loading dose. Note that accumulation is more than 90 percent complete by the end of 4 half-lives.*

percent of steady-state levels at the end of 3 to 4 half-lives. For digoxin, with a half-life of 1.6 days (with normal renal function), accumulation will be practically complete in 5 days. Continuing infusion of a drug at a constant rate also will result in progressive accumulation to a steady state with a time course predictable from the elimination curve for that drug (Fig. 64-3).

When the time required to reach steady-state levels is longer than one wishes to wait, plasma levels may be achieved more rapidly by the administration of a *loading dose*. Loading entails the administration of an amount that will bring the concentration in plasma (at equilibrium) to the level present during steady state. This may be accomplished by the administration of the loading amount as a single dose, or in the case of drugs with low therapeutic indexes (the therapeutic index is the ratio of the toxic dose to the therapeutic dose) the loading amount is administered in a series of fractions of the total loading amount. As the accumulation of procainamide to 90 percent of steady state by infusion would require approximately 10 h (the $t_{1/2}$ is 3 h), a loading regimen is almost always desirable. The load required to suppress an arrhythmia, however, varies among individuals from 300 to 1000 mg, and rapid intravenous administration of the *average loading dose* causes hypotension during the distribution phase in some patients. Therefore, the intravenous loading dose of procainamide is given in fractions (e.g., 100 mg every 5 min) until the arrhythmia is controlled or adverse effects such as hypotension indicate that no further drug should be given. Dividing the loading dose into fractions is appropriate for most drugs that have a low therapeutic index. This permits better individualization of the loading amount and minimizes adverse effects.

The size of loading dose required to achieve the plasma levels at steady state can be determined from the fraction of drug eliminated during the dosage interval and the maintenance dose (in the case of intermittent drug administration). For example, if the fraction of digoxin eliminated daily is 35 percent and the planned maintenance dose is to be 0.25 mg daily, then the loading dose to achieve steady-state levels should be 100/35 times the maintenance dose, or approximately 0.75 mg. Thus,

$$\text{Loading dose} = \frac{100}{\text{\% of drug eliminated per dosage interval}} \times \text{maintenance dose}$$

The fraction of drug eliminated during any dosage interval can be determined from a semilogarithmic graph, in which the total amount in the body at time zero is set at 100 percent and the fraction remaining at the end of 1 half-life is 50 percent.[1] Conversely, if the loading dose is known, the maintenance dose can be similarly calculated.

[1] *Alternatively, the fraction of drug lost from the body during a dosage interval can be determined nongraphically from this equation:*

$$\text{Fraction of drug lost from body} = 1 - e^{-kt}$$

Values for e^{-kt} can be obtained from a table of natural exponential functions or by a calculator, where k (= $0.693/t_{1/2}$) is the fractional elimination constant (described in the next section) and t is the time interval after drug administration.

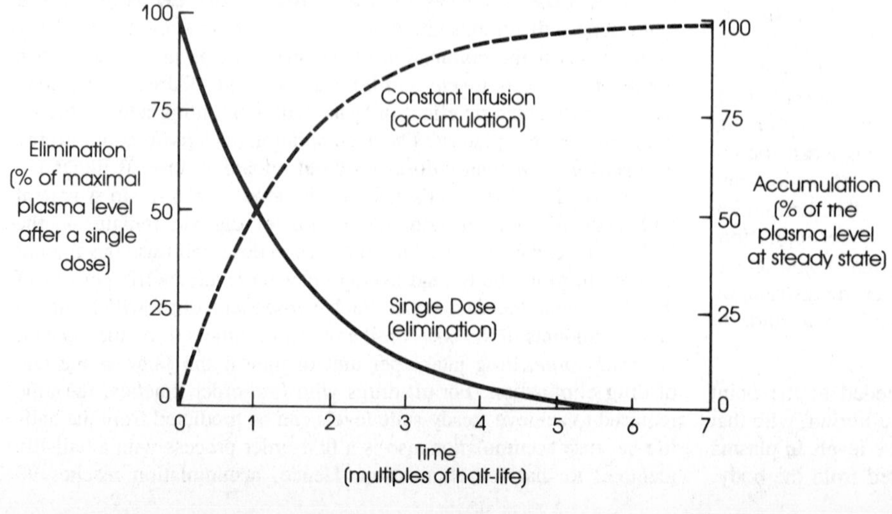

FIGURE 64-3 *The time course of plasma levels of a drug following a single intravenous dose (——) compared with those during a constant intravenous infusion (----). This relationship applies to all drugs that rapidly achieve equilibrium between plasma and tissues.*

Regardless of the size of the loading dose, *after maintenance therapy has been given for 3 to 4 half-lives, the amount of drug in the body is determined by the maintenance dose*. The independence of the plasma levels at steady state from the load is illustrated in Fig. 64-3, which indicates that the elimination of any drug would be practically complete after 3 to 4 half-lives.

DETERMINANTS OF PLASMA LEVELS DURING THE EQUILIBRIUM PHASE An important determinant of the level of drug in plasma during the equilibrium phase after a single dose is the extent to which the drug is distributed outside the plasma compartment. For example, if the distribution of a 3-mg dose of a large macromolecule is confined to a plasma volume of 3 liters, then the concentration in plasma will be 1 mg per liter. However, if a different drug is distributed so that 90 percent of it leaves the plasma compartment, then only 0.3 mg will remain in the 3-liter plasma volume, and the concentration in plasma will be only 0.1 mg per liter. The extent of extravascular distribution at equilibrium can be expressed by the *apparent volume of distribution*, or V_d. V_d expresses the relationship between the amount of drug in the body and the plasma concentration at equilibrium:

$$V_d = \frac{\text{amount of drug in body}}{\text{plasma concentration}}$$

The amount of drug in the body is expressed as mass (e.g., milligrams), and the plasma concentration is expressed as mass per volume (e.g., milligrams per liter). Thus V_d is a hypothetical volume into which a quantity of drug would distribute if its concentration in the entire volume were the same as that in plasma. Although it is not a real volume, it is an important concept because it determines the fraction of total drug in the plasma and therefore the fraction available to the organs of elimination. An approximation of V_d in the equilibrium phase can be obtained by estimating the concentration of drug in plasma at time zero (Cp_0) by back-extrapolation of the equilibrium phase plot to zero time as illustrated in Fig. 64-1. Then, after intravenous administration when the amount in the body at time zero is the dose, we have

$$V_d = \frac{\text{dose}}{Cp_0}$$

For the administration of the large macromolecule mentioned above, the measured Cp_0 of 1 mg per liter after a 3-mg dose indicates a V_d that is a real volume, the plasma volume. This is the exception, however, for the V_d of most drugs is larger than plasma volume; many drugs are so extensively taken up by cells that cellular levels exceed those in plasma. For such drugs, the hypothetical V_d is large, even greater than the volume of body water. For example, Fig. 64-1 indicates that the Cp_0 obtained by extrapolation after administration of 50 mg lidocaine is 0.42 mg per liter, yielding a V_d of 119 liters.

As elimination is performed largely by the kidney and liver, it is useful to consider the elimination of drugs according to the *clearance* concept. For example, in the kidney, regardless of the extent to which removal of drug is determined by filtration, secretion, or reabsorption, the net result is a reduction of the concentration of drug in plasma as it passes through the organ. The extent to which the concentration is reduced is expressed as the *extraction ratio*, or *E*, which is constant as long as first-order elimination occurs.

$$E = \frac{C_a - C_v}{C_a}$$

where C_a = arterial plasma concentration
C_v = venous plasma concentration

If the extraction is complete, $E = 1$. If the total plasma flow to the kidneys is Q (mL/min), the total volume of plasma from which drug is completely removed in a unit time (clearance from the body, Cl) is determined as

$$\text{Cl}_{\text{renal}} = QE$$

If the renal extraction ratio of penicillin is 0.5 and renal plasma flow is 680 mL/min, then penicillin's renal clearance is 340 mL/min. If the extraction ratio is high, as is the case for renal extraction of aminohippurate or hepatic extraction of propranolol, then clearance is a function of organ blood flow.[2]

Clearance from the body is the sum of clearance from all organs of elimination and is the best measure of the efficiency of the elimination processes. If a drug is removed by both the kidney and liver, then

$$\text{Cl} = \text{Cl}_{\text{renal}} + \text{Cl}_{\text{hepatic}}$$

Thus, if penicillin is eliminated by both renal clearance (340 mL/min) and hepatic clearance (36 mL/min) in a normal individual, total clearance is 376 mL/min. If renal clearance is reduced to half, total clearance is 170 + 36 or 206 mL/min. In anuria, total clearance equals hepatic clearance.

Only the drug in the vascular compartment can be cleared during each passage through an organ. To ascertain the effect of a given plasma clearance by one or more organs on the rate of removal of drug from the body, the clearance must be related to the volume of "plasma equivalents" to be cleared, that is, the volume of distribution. If the volume of distribution is 10,000 mL and clearance is 1000 mL/min, then one-tenth of the drug in the body is eliminated per minute. This fraction, Cl/V_d, is known as a *fractional elimination constant* and is designated as *k*:

$$k = \frac{\text{Cl}}{V_d}$$

If the fraction *k* is multiplied by the total amount of drug in the body, the actual rate of elimination at any given time can be determined:

$$\text{Rate of elimination} = k \times \text{amount in body} = \text{Cl}Cp$$

This is the general equation for all first-order processes and expresses the fact that rate is proportional to the declining quantity in a first-order process.

As half-life is a temporal expression of the exponential first-order process, half-life ($t_{1/2}$) can be related to *k* as follows:

$$t_{1/2} = \frac{0.693}{k}$$

$$\text{Because} \quad k = \frac{\text{Cl}}{V_d}$$

$$\text{then} \quad t_{1/2} = \frac{0.693 V_d}{\text{Cl}}$$

As shown in the section on drug dosage in renal failure, the linear relationship of *k* to creatinine clearance makes *k* a useful parameter upon which to estimate changes in drug elimination with reduction in creatinine clearance in renal insufficiency. Half-life is not linearly related to clearance.

The important relationship

$$t_{1/2} = \frac{0.693 V_d}{\text{Cl}}$$

expresses clearly the influence of both clearance and volume of distribution on half-life. Thus, half-life is shortened when phenobarbital induces the enzymes responsible for hepatic clearance of a drug, and half-life is lengthened when a drug's renal clearance is attenuated in renal failure. Also, the half-life of some drugs is shortened when their volume of distribution is reduced. If, as in the case of cardiac failure, the volume of distribution is reduced at the same time that clearance is reduced, there may be little change in drug half-life to reflect the impaired clearance, but plasma levels will be increased,

[2] *When drug is present in the formed elements of blood, then calculation of extraction and clearance from blood is more physiologically meaningful than from the plasma.*

as is the case with lidocaine. In treating patients after an overdose, the effects of hemodialysis on a drug's elimination are dependent on its volume of distribution. When the volume of distribution is large, as with tricyclic antidepressants (V_d of desipramine equals more than 2000 liters), the removal of drug, even with a high-clearance dialyzer, proceeds slowly.

The extent to which a drug is bound to plasma protein also determines the fraction extracted by the organ(s) of elimination. Altered binding changes the extraction ratio significantly, however, only when elimination is limited to the unbound (free) drug in plasma. The extent to which binding influences elimination depends on the relative affinity of the plasma binding versus the affinity of the drug for the extraction process. The high affinity of the renal tubular anion transport system for many drugs leads to extraction of bound and unbound drug, and the efficient process by which the liver removes propranolol extracts most of this highly bound drug from blood.

STEADY STATE With a constant infusion of drug, the infusion rate equals elimination rate at steady state. Therefore,

$$\underset{\text{(amt/unit time)}}{\text{Infusion rate}} = \underset{\text{(amt/vol)}}{Cp} \times \underset{\text{(vol/unit time)}}{\text{Cl}}$$

when the units for amount, volume, and time are consistent.

Thus, if clearance (Cl) is known, the infusion rate to achieve a given plasma level can be calculated. Estimation of drug clearance is discussed in the section on renal disease.

When the dose is given intermittently instead of by infusion, the above relationship between plasma concentration and the dose administered at each dosage interval can be expressed as

$$\text{Dose} = Cp_{\text{av}} \times \text{Cl} \times \text{dosage interval}$$

The average plasma concentration (Cp_{av}) implies, as seen in Fig. 64-2, that levels can be higher and lower than the average during the dosage interval.

When a drug is given orally, only a fraction (F) of the administered dose may reach the systemic circulation. This *bioavailability* may reflect a poorly formulated dosage form that fails to disintegrate or dissolve in the gastrointestinal fluids. Regulatory standards have reduced the extent of this problem. Drug interactions also can impair absorption after oral dosing. Bioavailability may also be reduced due to drug metabolism in the gastrointestinal tract and/or the liver during the absorption process, the *first-pass effect*. This is a particular problem for drugs that are extensively extracted by these organs, and considerable interpatient variability often exists in bioavailability. Lidocaine for the control of arrhythmias is not administered orally because of the first-pass effect. Drugs that are injected intramuscularly may also have low bioavailability, e.g., phenytoin. An unexpected drug response should lead to consideration of bioavailability as a possible factor. Calculation of a dosage regimen should be corrected for bioavailability:

$$\text{Oral dose} = \frac{Cp_{\text{av}} \times \text{Cl} \times \text{dosage interval}}{F}$$

DRUG ELIMINATION THAT IS NOT FIRST-ORDER The elimination of some drugs such as phenytoin, salicylate, and theophylline does not follow first-order kinetics when amounts of drug in the body are in the therapeutic range. For these drugs, the clearance changes as levels in the body fall during elimination or after alterations in dose. This pattern of elimination is said to be *dose-dependent*. Accordingly, the time for the concentration to fall to one-half becomes less as plasma levels fall; this halving time is not truly a half-life, because the term *half-life* applies to first-order kinetics and is a constant. The elimination of phenytoin is dose-dependent, and when very high levels are present (in the toxic range), the halving time may be longer than 72 h, whereas, as the concentration in plasma declines, the clearance increases and the concentration in plasma will halve in 20 to 30 h. When a drug is eliminated by first-order kinetics, the plasma level at steady state is directly related to the amount of the maintenance dose, and a doubling of the dose should lead to doubling of the steady-state plasma level. However, for drugs with dose-dependent kinetics, increases in the dose may be accompanied by disproportionate increases in plasma level. Thus, if the daily dose of phenytoin is increased from 300 to 400 mg, plasma levels rise by more than 33 percent. The extent of increase is not predictable because of the interpatient variability in the extent to which clearance deviates from first order. Salicylates are also eliminated by dose-dependent kinetics at high plasma levels, and in children particular caution must be taken with the administration of high doses. Ethanol metabolism also is dose-dependent, with obvious implications. The mechanisms involved in dose-dependent kinetics may include the saturation of the rate-limiting step in metabolism or a feedback inhibition of the rate-limiting enzyme by a product of the reaction.

INDIVIDUALIZATION OF DRUG THERAPY

Recognition of factors modifying drug action is essential for therapy that provides optimal benefit and minimal risk to each patient.

ALTERATION OF DRUG DOSAGE IN RENAL DISEASE Where urinary excretion is an important route of elimination, renal failure results in decreased drug clearance and therefore slower removal of the drug from the body, so that administration of the usual dosage leads to greater accumulation and an increased likelihood of toxicity. The goal in such cases is to modify the dosage schedule so that the average drug concentration in the plasma of the patient with renal insufficiency is the same and so that the steady state is reached after a similar time interval as in the patient with normal renal function. This is particularly appropriate for drugs with long half-lives and narrow therapeutic indexes (e.g., digoxin).

One approach is to calculate the *fraction of the normal dose* that is to be given at the usual dosage interval. This fraction can be determined from either drug clearance (Cl) or the fractional rate constant (k), based on the fact that both renal clearance and k are proportional to creatinine clearance (Cl_{cr}). Creatinine clearance is best determined directly. However, serum creatinine (C_{cr}) may be used to estimate the value by the following equation which is applicable to men:

$$\text{Cl}_{\text{cr}} = \frac{(140 - \text{age}) \times \text{weight (kg)}}{72 \times C_{\text{cr}}\ (\text{mg/dL})}\ (\text{mL/min})$$

For women, the value should be reduced to 85 percent of that estimated by this equation. This approach to estimation of Cl_{cr} is invalid in severe renal insufficiency ($C_{\text{cr}} > 5$ mg/dL) or with rapidly changing renal function.

The clearance approach Calculation of drug dosage is most accurately based on the clearance of a drug. From data on the clearance of a drug, the dose in renal insufficiency (Dose_{ri}) may be calculated as follows:

$$\text{Dose}_{\text{ri}} = \text{Dose} \times \frac{\text{Cl}_{\text{ri}}}{\text{Cl}}$$

where ri = renal insufficiency
Cl = clearance from the whole body with normal renal function
Cl_{ri} = clearance from the whole body with renal insufficiency
Dose = maintenance dose with normal renal function ($\text{Cl}_{\text{cr}} \sim$ 100 mL/min)

The normal clearance and that in renal impairment can be obtained by employing the data in Table 64-1 in the following equations:

$$\text{Cl} = \text{Cl}_{\text{renal}} + \text{Cl}_{\text{nonrenal}}$$

$$\text{Cl}_{\text{ri}} = \text{Cl}_{\text{renal}} \times \frac{\text{measured Cl}_{\text{cr}}}{100\ \text{mL/min}} + \text{Cl}_{\text{nonrenal}}$$

The Cl_{renal} values in Table 64-1 are those found with $\text{Cl}_{\text{cr}} = 100$ mL/min, and the renal clearance of drug in renal insufficiency is obtained by multiplying Cl_{renal} by the ratio of measured Cl_{cr} (in milliliters per minute) to 100 mL/min.

For gentamicin, with a normal Cl_{renal} of 78 mL/min and $Cl_{nonrenal}$ of 3 mL/min, Cl = 81 mL/min. Therefore, with a Cl_{cr} of 12 mL/min, $Cl_{ri} = 78 \times (12/100) + 3 = 12.4$ mL/min. If the dose of gentamicin for a given infection should be 1.5 mg/kg per 8 h in the presence of normal renal function, then

$$\text{Dose}_{ri} = \frac{1.5 \text{ mg/kg}}{8 \text{ h}} \times \frac{12.4 \text{ mL/min}}{81 \text{ mL/min}} = \frac{0.23 \text{ mg/kg}}{8 \text{ h}}$$

In the patient with renal insufficiency, this computation provides an average plasma level during a dosage interval that is the same as the average plasma level during the dosage interval with normal renal function; the fluctuations between peaks and troughs, however, will be less pronounced.

In some instances it may be desirable to calculate a dose that will yield a certain plasma level at steady state. This approach is most appropriate for constant intravenous infusions where 100 percent of the dose is delivered to the systemic circulation. When clearance of a drug in a patient with renal insufficiency is calculated as above, then

$$\underset{(\text{amt/unit time})}{\text{Dose}_{ri}} = \underset{(\text{vol/unit time})}{Cl_{ri}} \times \underset{(\text{amt/vol})}{Cp}$$

where the time, amount, and volume terms are uniform.

If a plasma concentration of carbenicillin of 100 μg/mL is the therapeutic objective in a patient with a creatinine clearance of 25 mL/min, the infusion rate is calculated as follows. Carbenicillin clearance is

$$Cl_{ri} = 68 \times \frac{25}{100} + 10 = 27 \text{ mL/min}$$

Therefore, carbenicillin should be infused at a rate of 2700 μg/min.

Should the method of calculating dose based on the desired plasma level be applied to intermittent-dose therapy, particular attention should be given to the fact that the calculation is based on an *average* plasma level and that peak plasma levels will be higher. In addition, if an oral drug is not completely absorbed, the computed dose must be divided by the fraction (F) that reaches the systemic circulation (see "Steady State" above).

The fractional rate constant (k) approach For many drugs, clearance data in renal failure are not available. In these cases, the fraction of the normal dose that is required in a patient with renal failure can be approximated from the ratio of the fractional rate constant for elimination from the body in renal failure (k_{ri}) to that with normal renal function (k). This approach requires the assumption that the distribution of the drug (V_d) is not affected by renal disease. The approach is the same as that employed with clearance data:

$$\text{Dose}_{ri} = \text{Dose} \times \frac{k_{ri}}{k}$$

As the ratio k_{ri}/k is the fraction of the usual dose employed in a given degree of renal insufficiency, it is termed the *dose fraction* and may be estimated from the information in Table 64-2 and the nomogram (Fig. 64-4). Table 64-2 gives the fraction of the usual dose of a drug required at a creatinine clearance of zero (dose fraction_0). The nomogram presents the dose fraction as a linear function of creatinine clearance.

To calculate the dose fraction_{ri}, the dose fraction_0 is obtained from Table 64-2, plotted on the left ordinate of the nomogram, and connected by a straight line to the upper right-hand corner of the nomogram. This line describes the dose fraction over a range of creatinine clearances from 0 to 100 mL/min. The point of intersection between the measured creatinine clearance (on the lower abscissa) and this dose fraction line is a coordinate with the dose fraction (on the left ordinate) corresponding with that particular creatinine clearance. For example, if a patient with a creatinine clearance of 20 mL/min requires penicillin G for an infection that would be treated with 10 million units daily in patients with normal renal function, then an appropriate dose would be 2.8 million units daily. This dose is estimated by plotting the dose fraction_0 for penicillin G (0.1) on the left-hand ordinate and connecting it to the top right-hand corner of the nomogram (Fig. 64-4). On this dose fraction line for penicillin G, the coordinate for a creatinine clearance of 20 mL/min corresponds on the left ordinate with a dose fraction of 0.28. Hence, the dose is 0.28 × 10 million units daily.

TABLE 64-1 Clearance of drugs

Drug	Renal clearance,* mL/min	Nonrenal clearance, mL/min
Ampicillin†	340	12
Carbenicillin	68	10
Digoxin†	110	36
Gentamicin	78	3
Kanamycin	60	0
Penicillin G‡	340	36

* *The "normal" renal clearances are those associated with a clearance of creatinine of 100 mL/min.*
† *The fraction of digoxin absorbed after an oral dose (F) is approximately 0.75 and F for ampicillin is 0.5.*
‡ *One microgram of penicillin G = 1.6 units.*

TABLE 64-2 Estimated fraction of usual dose of drug required for a patient with a creatinine clearance of zero (dose fraction_0) and average overall fractional elimination rate constant for a patient with normal renal function (k)

Drug	Dose fraction_0	*k, per hour*
ANTIBIOTICS		
Amikacin	0.01	0.4
Amoxicillin	0.15	0.7
Ampicillin	0.1	0.6
Carbenicillin	0.1	0.6
Cephalexin	0.04	0.7
Cephaloridine	0.08	0.4
Cephalothin	0.02	1.4
Cephazolin	0.06	0.35
Chloramphenicol	0.8	0.3
Clindamycin	0.8	0.2
Cloxacillin	0.25	1.2
Colistimethate	0.3	0.2
Dicloxacillin	0.5	1.2
Doxycycline	0.8	0.03
Erythromycin	0.7	0.5
Gentamicin	0.02	0.3
Isoniazid:		
Fast inactivators	0.8	0.5
Slow inactivators	0.5	0.25
Kanamycin	0.03	0.35
Lincomycin	0.4	0.15
Methicillin	0.12	1.4
Minocycline	0.9	0.06
Nafcillin	0.4	1.2
Oxacillin	0.25	1.4
Oxytetracycline	0.2	0.08
Penicillin G	0.1	1.4
Polymyxin B	0.12	0.15
Rifampin	1.0	0.25
Streptomycin	0.04	0.25
Sulfadiazine	0.45	0.7
Sulfamethoxazole	0.85	0.07
Tetracycline	0.12	0.08
Tobramycin	0.02	0.35
Tricarcillin	0.1	0.6
Trimethoprim	0.45	0.06
Vancomycin	0.03	0.12
MISCELLANEOUS DRUGS		
Chlorpropamide	0.4	0.02
Lidocaine	0.9	0.4
Sulfinpyrazone	0.55	0.3
CARDIAC GLYCOSIDES		
		k, per day
Digitoxin	0.7	0.1
Digoxin	0.3	0.45

The loading dose In addition to adjusting the maintenance dose in renal failure, consideration must also be given to the loading dose. Since this dose is designed to bring the plasma concentration, or more particularly the amount of drug in the body, rapidly to the level at steady state, there is no need to modify the usual loading dose, if one is normally used. The elimination of many drugs is sufficiently rapid that the time required to reach steady state is not significant, and no loading dose is usually used. On the other hand, in renal failure where the half-life may be significantly prolonged, this accumulation period may become unacceptably long. In such a case, a loading dose may be calculated as described in "Drug Accumulation" above for a drug given intermittently. For an infusion, the loading dose may be approximated (when all units are consistent):

$$\text{Loading dose}_{ri} = \frac{\text{infusion rate}_{ri}}{k_{ri}}$$

General considerations for determining dosage in renal insufficiency Because of the differences in volumes of distribution and rates of metabolism, calculations of drug dose in renal failure must be viewed as valuable approximations which prevent the use of doses that are grossly excessive or inadequate for most patients. However, *maintenance dosages are most accurate when plasma level data are employed to enable adjustment of the dose where necessary.*

In all the above calculations, it is assumed that the nonrenal clearance and nonrenal k are constant in renal failure. In fact, when cardiac failure accompanies renal failure, metabolic clearance for many drugs is reduced. Accordingly, when a drug with a narrow therapeutic index, such as digoxin, is used in cardiac failure, an appropriate precaution would be to reduce the value for nonrenal clearance (or k) to about one-half.

Active or toxic metabolites of drugs also may accumulate in renal failure. Meperidine, for example, is cleared largely by metabolism, and its concentration in plasma is little altered by renal insufficiency. However, the plasma concentration of one of its metabolites, normeperidine, is increased when its renal elimination is impaired. As normeperidine has more convulsant activity than meperidine, its accumulation in patients with renal failure probably accounts for the signs of central nervous system excitation such as irritability, twitching, and seizures that result from the administration of multiple doses of meperidine to patients in renal insufficiency.

The metabolite of procainamide, *N*-acetylprocainamide, has similar cardiac effects to those of the parent drug. As *N*-acetylprocainamide is eliminated almost entirely by the kidney, its concentration in plasma is increased by renal failure. Thus, the potential of procainamide to produce toxicity in renal insufficiency cannot be assessed by measuring the plasma concentration of procainamide alone.

FIGURE 64-4 *Nomogram for estimation of the dose fraction (k_{ri}/k) in patients with renal insufficiency. The application of the nomogram is described in the text.*

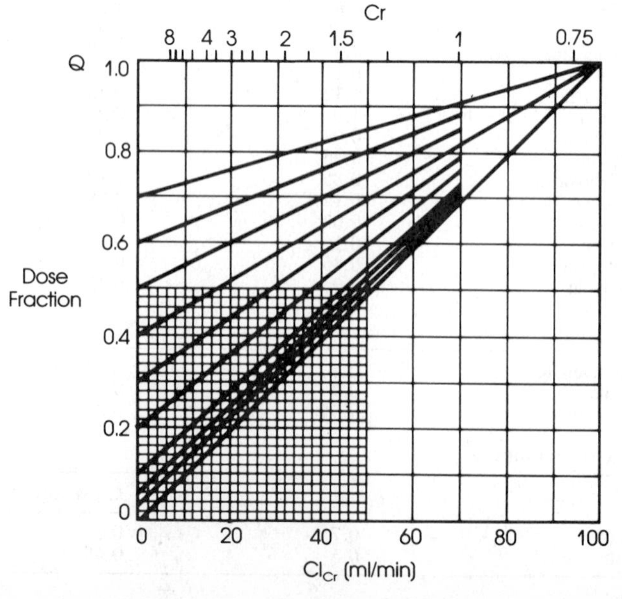

LIVER DISEASE In contrast to the predictable decline in renal clearance of drugs when glomerular filtration is reduced, it is not possible to make a general prediction of the effect of liver disease on hepatic biotransformation of drugs (Chap. 243). Rather, in hepatitis and cirrhosis changes may range from impaired to increased drug clearance. Even in advanced hepatocellular disease, the magnitude of impairment in drug clearance usually is only about two- to fivefold. The extent of such changes, however, cannot be predicted by the common tests of liver function. Consequently, even when it is suspected that drug elimination is altered in liver disease, there is no quantitative base upon which to adjust the dosage regimen other than assessment of clinical response and concentration of drug in plasma.

Portacaval shunting creates a special situation because the effective hepatic blood flow is reduced. This situation has its greatest effect on drugs that normally have a high hepatic extraction ratio so that their clearance is largely a function of blood flow; thus the clearance of such drugs (e.g., propranolol and lidocaine) is remarkably reduced by portacaval shunting. In addition, the fraction of an administered oral dose reaching the systemic circulation is increased, because drug that is shunted around the liver during the absorption process escapes the first-pass metabolism by this organ (e.g., meperidine, pentazocine).

CIRCULATORY INSUFFICIENCY—CARDIAC FAILURE AND SHOCK Under conditions of decreased tissue perfusion, redistribution of the cardiac output occurs to preserve blood flow to the heart and brain at the expense of other tissues (Chap. 29). As a result, the drug is distributed into a smaller volume of distribution, higher drug concentrations are present in the plasma, and the tissues are exposed to these higher concentrations. If either the brain or heart is sensitive to the drug, an alteration in response will occur.

Furthermore, the decreased perfusion of the kidney and liver may impair drug clearance by these organs directly or indirectly. Thus, in severe congestive heart failure, in hemorrhagic shock, and in cardiogenic shock, the response to the usual dose of drug may be excessive, and dosage modification may be necessary. For example, the clearance of lidocaine is reduced by about 50 percent in cardiac failure, and therapeutic plasma levels are achieved at infusion rates of only about half of those usually required. In cardiac failure there also is a significant reduction in lidocaine's volume of distribution which results in the requirement of a smaller loading dose. Similar situations are thought to exist for procainamide, theophylline, and possibly quinidine. Unfortunately, predictors of these types of pharmacokinetic alterations are unavailable. Therefore, loading doses should be conservative, and continued therapy should be monitored closely, following clinical indicators of toxicity and plasma levels.

DISEASE-INDUCED CHANGES IN PLASMA BINDING Many drugs circulate in the plasma partly bound to the plasma proteins. Since only the unbound or free drug can distribute to the site of pharmacologic action, the therapeutic response should be related to the free rather than the total circulating plasma drug concentration. In most cases the degree of binding is fairly constant across the therapeutic concentration range so that significant error is not caused by individualizing therapy on the basis of total drug levels in plasma. However, states such as hypoalbuminemia, liver disease, and renal disease can decrease the extent of drug binding, particularly of acidic and neutral drugs, so that at any total plasma level there is a greater concentration of free drug and a risk of increased response and toxicity. Other conditions, e.g., myocardial infarction, surgery, neoplastic disease, rheumatoid arthritis, and burns, that lead to an increased plasma concentration of the acute-phase reactant alpha$_1$-acid glycoprotein have the opposite effect from basic drugs that are bound to this macromolecule. The drugs for which such changes are important are those that are normally highly bound in the plasma (>90 percent) because a small alteration in the extent of binding produces a large change in the amount of drug in the unbound form.

The consequences of these binding changes, particularly with respect to total drug levels, depend on whether the clearance and distribution are dependent on the unbound or total drug. For many drugs, elimination and distribution are largely restricted to the unbound fraction, and therefore a decrease in binding leads to an increase in the clearance and distribution of the drug. The relative magnitudes of these changes are such that the net effect is to shorten the half-life. The appropriate modification of the dosage regimen in conditions with reduced drug binding is simply to administer the usual daily dose of the drug but in divided doses at more frequent intervals. Individualization of therapy can then be based on either the clinical response or the plasma concentration of unbound drug. It is critical that the patient not be titrated into the usual therapeutic range for concentration of *total* drug in plasma since this will lead to excessive response and toxicity.

In the case of drugs bound to alpha$_1$-acid glycoprotein, the disease-induced increase in binding has the opposite effects of reducing the clearance and distribution of drug. Accordingly, constant rate infusion of lidocaine to control arrhythmias after myocardial infarction leads to an accumulation of drug. However, the clearance of unbound and pharmacologically active drug remains essentially unchanged. Again, it is critical that the patient not be dosed on the basis of total drug concentrations in the plasma since this will be associated with subtherapeutic levels of unbound drug.

INTERACTIONS BETWEEN DRUGS

The effect of some drugs can be altered markedly by the administration of other agents. Such interactions can sabotage therapeutic intent by producing excessive drug action (with adverse effects) or decreasing the action of a drug, rendering it ineffective. Drug interactions must be considered in the differential diagnosis of unexpected responses to drugs, recognizing that patients often come to the physician with a legacy of drugs acquired during previous medical experiences. A meticulous drug history will minimize the unknown elements in the therapeutic milieu; it should include examination of the patient's medications and calls to the pharmacist to identify prescriptions, if necessary.

There are two principal types of interactions between drugs. *Pharmacokinetic interactions* result from alteration in the delivery of drugs to their sites of action. *Pharmacodynamic interactions* are those in which the responsiveness of the target organ or system is modified by other agents.

An index of the drug interactions discussed in this chapter is provided in Table 64-3. Included are interactions which have verified significance in patients and a few of such potential danger that cognizance should be taken of experimental data or case reports suggesting their likely occurrence.

I PHARMACOKINETIC INTERACTIONS CAUSING DIMINISHED DRUG DELIVERY

***A* Impaired gastrointestinal absorption** Cholestyramine, an ionic exchange resin, binds thyroxine, triiodothyronine, and the cardiac glycosides with sufficiently high affinity to impair their absorption from the gastrointestinal tract. This resin probably also interferes with the absorption of other drugs, and it is safest not to give it within 2 h of their administration. Aluminum ions, present in antacids, form insoluble chelates with the tetracyclines, thereby preventing absorption of these drugs. Ferrous ions similarly block tetracycline absorption. Kaolin-pectin suspensions bind digoxin, and when the drugs are administered together, digoxin absorption is reduced by about one-half. However, when kaolin-pectin is administered 2 h after digoxin, there is no effect on absorption of digoxin.

Ketoconazole is a weak base that dissolves well only at acidic pH. Thus, histamine-2 antagonists such as cimetidine, by neutralizing gastric pH, impair the dissolution and subsequent absorption of ketoconazole. Oral administration of aminosalicylate interferes with the absorption of rifampin by an unknown mechanism.

Impaired absorption results in reduction in the total amount of drug absorption, with reduced area under the plasma level curve, reduced peak plasma levels, and lower steady-state concentrations of the drug involved.

***B* Induction of hepatic drug-metabolizing enzymes** When the elimination of the drug is largely by metabolism, an increase in the rate of metabolism reduces its availability to sites of action. The metabolism of most drugs occurs largely in the liver, because of its mass, high blood flow, and concentration of enzymes that metabolize drugs. The initial step in metabolism of many drugs is executed by a group of mixed-function oxidase isoenzymes in the endoplasmic

TABLE 64-3 Drug interaction index

Drug	Section of chapter describing interaction
Acetohexamide	IIB
Allopurinol	IIA
p-Aminosalicylate	IA
Amiodarone	IIC
Amphetamine	IC
Antidepressants, tricyclic (desipramine, nortriptyline, imipramine, doxepin, protriptyline, amitriptyline)	IC
Aspirin	IIB, III
Azathioprine	IIA
Barbiturates (class)	IB
Bethanidine	IC
Carbamazepine	IB
Chloramphenicol	IIA
Chlorpromazine	IC
Cholestyramine	IA
Cimetidine	IA, IIA, IIB
Clofibrate	IIA
Clonidine	IC
Cyclosporine	IB
Dexamethasone	IB
Dicumarol	IIA, IIB
Digitoxin	IA, IB, IIC
Digoxin	IA, IIC
Disulfiram	IIA
Ephedrine	IC
Ethanol	IIA
Guanethidine	IC
Indomethacin	III
Isoniazid	IIA
Kaolin-pectin	IA
Ketoconazole	IA
Lidocaine	IIA
6-Mercaptopurine	IIA
Methadone	IB
Methotrexate	IIB
Metronidazole	IB, IIA
Metyrapone	IB
Nifedipine	IIA
Nonsteroidal anti-inflammatory drugs	III
Oral contraceptive steroids	IB
Phenobarbital	IB
Phenylbutazone	IIA, IIB
Phenytoin (diphenylhydantoin)	IB, IIA
Piroxicam	III
Potassium	III
Prednisone	IB
Probenicid	IIB
Procainamide	IIB
Propranolol	III
Quinidine	IB, IIA, IIC
Ranitidine	IA, IIA
Rifampin	IA, IB
Salicylate	IIB
Spironolactone	III
Tetracycline	IA
Thiazide diuretics	III
Tolbutamide	IIA
Triamterene	III
Verapamil	IIC
Warfarin	IB, IIA, III

reticulum. These enzyme systems containing cytochrome P_{450} oxidize the molecule by a variety of reactions including aromatic hydroxylations, *N*-demethylations, *O*-demethylations, and sulfoxidations. The products of these reactions are usually more polar (and more readily excreted by the kidney).

The biosynthesis of some of the mixed-function oxidase isoenzymes is under regulatory control at the transcriptional level, and their content in the liver can be induced by a number of drugs. Phenobarbital is the prototype of these inducers, and all barbiturates in clinical use increase mixed-function oxidase isoenzymes. Induction with phenobarbital can occur with doses of as little as 60 mg daily. Mixed-function oxidases also are induced by rifampin, carbamazepine, phenytoin, and glutethimide, by occupational exposure to chlorinated insecticides such as DDT, and by chronic alcohol ingestion.

Phenobarbital and other inducers lower plasma levels of many drugs, including warfarin, digitoxin, quinidine, cyclosporine, dexamethasone, prednisolone (the active metabolite of prednisone), oral contraceptive steroids, methadone, metronidazole, and metyrapone. These interactions all have obvious clinical significance. With the coumarin anticoagulants, the patient is placed at major risk when an appropriate level of anticoagulation is achieved while the coumarin drug is coadministered with an inducing agent. Should the inducer then be discontinued, e.g., following discharge from the hospital, plasma levels of the coumarin anticoagulant will rise as the induction effect wears off, leading to excessive anticoagulation. Barbiturates have been shown to lower the plasma levels of phenytoin in some patients, but the clinical effect of reduced phenytoin levels is probably counterbalanced by the anticonvulsant effects of phenobarbital.

There is considerable variation among individuals in the extent to which drug metabolism can be induced. In some patients phenobarbital leads to marked acceleration in the rate of drug metabolism, whereas little induction is seen in others.

In addition to inducing certain of the mixed-function oxidase isoenzymes, phenobarbital has other effects on hepatic function. It increases liver blood flow, bile flow, and the hepatocellular transport of organic anions. The conjugation of drugs and bilirubin may also be enhanced by inducing agents.

C Inhibition of cellular uptake or binding The guanidinium antihypertensives, guanethidine and bethanidine, are transported to their site of action in adrenergic neurons by an energy-requiring membrane transport system for biogenic monoamines. Although the physiologic function of the transport system is reuptake of the adrenergic neurotransmitter, it also transports a variety of ring-substituted bases, including guanethidine and bethanidine, into the adrenergic neuron against a concentration gradient. Inhibitors of norepinephrine uptake prevent the uptake of the guanidinium antihypertensives into adrenergic neurons and thereby block their pharmacologic effects. The tricyclic antidepressants are potent inhibitors of norepinephrine uptake. Consequently, concomitant administration of clinical doses of tricyclic antidepressants including desipramine, protriptyline, nortriptyline, and amitriptyline almost totally abolishes the antihypertensive effects of guanethidine and bethanidine. Although they are less potent inhibitors of norepinephrine uptake, doxepin and chlorpromazine, when given in doses of greater than 100 mg daily, produce dose-related antagonism of the action of the guanidinium antihypertensives. In patients with severe hypertension, the loss of control of blood pressure from these drug interactions can lead to stroke and malignant hypertension.

Amphetamine also antagonizes the antihypertensive effect of guanethidine by displacing it from its site of action within the adrenergic neuron (Chap. 196). Ephedrine, a component of many drug combinations used in asthma, also antagonizes the effect of guanethidine, probably by both inhibition of uptake and displacement from the neuron.

The antihypertensive effect of clonidine is partially antagonized by tricyclic antidepressants. Clonidine lowers arterial pressure by reducing sympathetic outflow from the blood-pressure-regulating centers in the hindbrain (Chap. 196). This central hypotensive action is antagonized by the tricyclic antidepressants.

II PHARMACOKINETIC INTERACTIONS CAUSING INCREASED DRUG DELIVERY

A Inhibition of drug metabolism If the active form of a drug is cleared largely by biotransformation, inhibition of its metabolism leads to a reduced clearance, prolonged half-life, and accumulation of the drug during maintenance therapy. Excessive accumulation due to inhibited metabolism can lead to significant adverse effects.

Cimetidine is a potent inhibitor of the oxidative metabolism of warfarin, quinidine, nifedipine, lidocaine, theophylline, phenytoin, and propranolol. Adverse reactions, many of them severe, have resulted from the administration of these drugs in conjunction with cimetidine. Cimetidine is a more potent inhibitor of mixed-function oxidases than ranitidine, whereas ranitidine is more potent as a histamine-2 antagonist. Thus, ranitidine, when administered in doses of 150 mg twice daily, does not inhibit the oxidative metabolism of most drugs; where reduced drug elimination has been observed, the effects of ranitidine have been less than those of cimetidine and devoid of appreciable pharmacodynamic consequence. Doses of ranitidine higher than 150 mg, however, may produce greater inhibition of drug oxidation.

The metabolism of phenytoin is also inhibited by a number of other drugs. Clofibrate, phenylbutazone, chloramphenicol, dicumarol, and isoniazid can raise the steady-state plasma levels of phenytoin by more than twofold. Impaired metabolism of tolbutamide with severe hypoglycemia has resulted from coadministration of clofibrate, phenylbutazone, and chloramphenicol. Excessive anticoagulation by warfarin may result from inhibition of its metabolism by disulfiram, metronidazole, or phenylbutazone, or by ingestion of ethanol. Warfarin is administered as a racemic mixture, and its *S*(−) isomer has five times the anticoagulant potency of the *R*(+) isomer. Phenylbutazone selectively inhibits the metabolism of the *S*(−) isomer, and only when this isomer is examined specifically can the substantial reduction in its metabolism produced by phenylbutazone be unmasked.

Azathioprine is readily converted in the body to an active metabolite, 6-mercaptopurine, which in turn is oxidized by xanthine oxidase to 6-thiouric acid. When allopurinol, a potent inhibitor of xanthine oxidase, is administered concurrently with standard doses of azathioprine or 6-mercaptopurine, life-threatening toxicity (bone marrow suppression) can result.

B Inhibition of renal elimination A number of drugs are secreted by the renal tubular transport systems for organic anions. Inhibition of this tubular transport system can cause excessive accumulation of a drug. Phenylbutazone, probenecid, salicylates, and dicumarol competitively inhibit this transport system. Salicylate, for example, reduces the renal clearance of methotrexate, an interaction that may lead to methotrexate toxicity. Renal tubular secretion contributes substantially to the elimination of penicillin, which can be inhibited by probenecid.

Inhibition of the tubular cation transport system by cimetidine impedes the renal clearance of procainamide and its active metabolite *N*-acetylprocainamide.

C Inhibition of clearance by multiple mechanisms The concentrations of digoxin and digitoxin in plasma are elevated by quinidine, due largely to inhibition of renal elimination and in part from inhibition of nonrenal clearance as well. An increase in cardiac arrhythmia may occur when quinidine is given in conjunction with a cardiac glycoside.

Amiodarone and verapamil also increase the concentration of digoxin in plasma.

III PHARMACODYNAMIC AND OTHER INTERACTIONS BETWEEN DRUGS Therapeutically useful interactions occur in which the combined effect of two drugs is greater than that of either drug alone.

These favorable drug combinations are described in specific therapeutic sections in this text, and the following is directed toward those interactions that create unwanted effects. Two drugs may act on separate components of a common process and yield effects greater than either alone. For example, small doses of aspirin (less than 1 g daily) do not alter the prothrombin time appreciably in patients who are on warfarin therapy. However, the addition of aspirin to patients anticoagulated with warfarin increases the risk of bleeding because aspirin inhibits platelet aggregation. Thus the combination of impaired functions of platelets and the clotting system increases the potential for hemorrhagic complications in patients receiving warfarin therapy.

Indomethacin, piroxicam, and probably other nonsteroidal anti-inflammatory drugs antagonize the antihypertensive effects of beta-adrenergic receptor blockers, diuretics, converting enzyme inhibitors, and other drugs. The resultant elevation in blood pressure ranges from trivial to severe. Aspirin and sulindac, however, do not elevate the blood pressure in treated hypertensive patients.

The administration of supplemental potassium leads to more frequent and more severe hyperkalemia when potassium elimination is reduced by concurrent treatment with spironolactone or triamterene.

VARIABLE ACTIONS OF DRUGS CAUSED BY GENETIC DIFFERENCES IN THEIR METABOLISM

ACETYLATION Isoniazid, hydralazine, procainamide, and a number of other drugs are metabolized by acetylation of a hydrazino or amino group. This reaction is catalyzed by *N*-acetyl transferase, an enzyme in the liver cytosol that transfers an acetyl group from acetyl coenzyme A to the drug. Individuals differ markedly in the rate at which drugs are acetylated, and there is a bimodal distribution of the population into "rapid acetylators" and "slow acetylators." The rate of acetylation is under genetic control; rapid acetylation is an autosomal dominant trait.

Responses to hydralazine therapy are dependent upon the acetylation phenotype. The hypotensive effect of hydralazine is greater in patients who acetylate the drug slowly, and the lupus erythematosus-like syndrome produced by hydralazine occurs almost exclusively in those with slow acetylation. Thus it may be of value to know the acetylation phenotype as a predictor of which patients with hypertension might benefit from an increase in the dose of hydralazine above the 200 mg daily that can be safely employed in the population at large.

Acetylation phenotype can be determined by measuring the ratio of acetylated to nonacetylated dapsone or sulfamethazine in plasma or urine following administration of a test dose of these acetylation substrates. The ratio of monoacetyldapsone to dapsone in plasma at 6 h after dapsone administration is less than 0.35 for slow acetylators and greater than 0.35 for rapid acetylators. At 6 h following the administration of sulfamethazine, less than 25 percent of the drug in the plasma is in the acetylated form in slow acetylators (rapid acetylators, more than 25 percent); in the urine collected in the 5- to 6-h interval after administration, less than 70 percent of the drug is in the acetylated form in slow acetylators (rapid acetylators, more than 70 percent).

METABOLISM BY MIXED-FUNCTION OXIDASES In healthy individuals taking no other medications, the major determinant of the rate of metabolism of drugs by the hepatic mixed-function oxidases is genetic. Hepatic endoplasmic reticulum contains a family of cytochrome P_{450} isoenzymes with different substrate specificities. Many drugs undergo oxidative metabolism by more than one isoenzyme, and the steady-state concentrations of such drugs in the plasma is a function of the sum of the activities of these and other metabolizing enzymes. When a drug is metabolized by multiple pathways, the catalytic activities of the participating enzymes are regulated by a number of genes so that the frequency of clearance rates and steady-state concentrations of the drug tend to distribute unimodally within the population. The range of activity may differ markedly (tenfold or more) between different individuals, as is the case for chlorpromazine, and there is no way to make a prior prediction of the rate.

For certain metabolic pathways bimodally distributed activity suggests control by a single gene, and several polymorphisms have been identified. As a result, two phenotypic populations are usually present analogous to the situation with *N*-acetylation (see above). A majority of the population are extensive metabolizers (EM), and a smaller group of individuals of the poor metabolizer phenotype (PM) have an impaired, if not an absent, ability to metabolize the drug. For example, about 8 to 10 percent of whites are unable to form the 4-hydroxy metabolite of the test drug debrisoquin, and this trait is inherited in an autosomal recessive fashion. Importantly, the putatively involved cytochrome P_{450} isoenzyme is also involved in the biotransformation of other drugs whose metabolic fate, therefore, cosegregates with the debrisoquin trait. A similar situation occurs with other oxidative polymorphisms that characterize the metabolism of tolbutamide, mephenytoin, and nifedipine. The situation is further complicated by interethnic differences in the frequency of the polymorphisms. For example, impaired hydroxylation of mephenytoin is present in only 3 to 5 percent of whites, but the incidence is about 20 percent in individuals of Japanese descent; likewise, the frequency of the PM phenotype for debrisoquin hydroxylation appears to decrease as one moves from Western (8 to 10 percent) to Eastern (0 to 1 percent) population groups.

Polymorphisms in drug metabolizing ability may be associated with large differences in the disposition of the drug among individuals, especially when the involved pathway is a major contribution to the overall elimination of the drug. For example, the oral clearance of mephenytoin differs 100- to 200-fold between individuals of the EM and PM phenotypes. As a result, peak plasma concentrations and bioavailability after oral administration may be profoundly increased and the rate of drug elimination decreased in PM individuals. This in turn results in drug accumulation and exaggerated pharmacologic responses, including toxicity, when usual drug dosages are administered to patients with the PM phenotype. Effective individualization of drug therapy is even more critical when using drugs exhibiting polymorphic drug metabolism.

CONCENTRATION OF DRUGS IN PLASMA AS A GUIDE TO THERAPY

Optimal individualization of therapy is assisted by measuring the concentration of certain drugs in plasma. Genetic variation in elimination rates, interactions with other drugs, disease-induced alterations in elimination and distribution, and other factors combine to yield a wide range of plasma levels in patients given the same dose. Furthermore, the problem of noncompliance with prescribed regimens during continuing therapy is an endemic and elusive cause of therapeutic failure (see below). Clinical indicators assist the titration of some drugs into the desired range, and no chemical determination is a substitute for careful observations of the response to treatment. However, the therapeutic and adverse effects are not precisely quantifiable for all drugs, and in complex clinical situations estimates of the action of a drug may be misleading. For example, previously existing neurologic disease may obscure the neurologic consequences of intoxication with phenytoin. Because clearance, half-life, accumulation, and steady-state plasma levels are difficult to predict, the measurement of plasma levels is often useful as a guide to the optimal dose. This is particularly so when there is a narrow range between the plasma levels yielding therapeutic and adverse effects. For drugs having such characteristics, e.g., digoxin, theophylline, lidocaine, aminoglycosides, and anticonvulsants, numerous dosing methods have been developed in an attempt to improve the relationship between dosing, plasma drug concentration, and response. Some of these

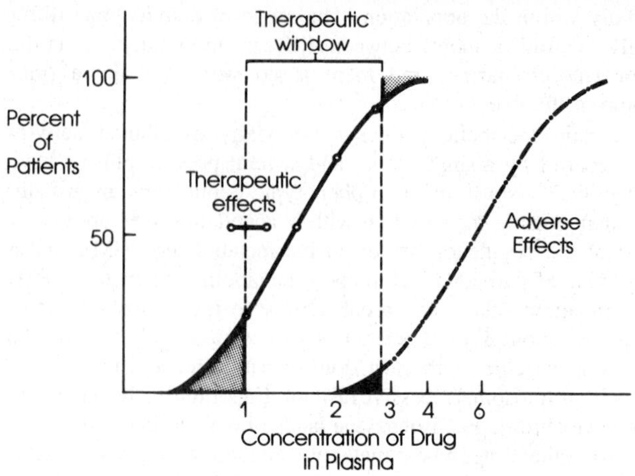

FIGURE 64-5 *The cumulative percentage of patients responding to increasing levels of drug in plasma with both therapeutic and adverse effects. The therapeutic "window" defines the range of concentrations of drug that will achieve therapeutic effects in most patients with adverse effects in only a small percentage.*

methods are accurate and useful, for example, the Bayesian feedback approach, but others are not accurate or have not been sufficiently validated. Further examination of their cost effectiveness is necessary to establish their place in routine patient care.

The variability among individual responses to given plasma levels must be recognized. This is illustrated by a hypothetical population dose-response curve (Fig. 64-5) and its relationship to the therapeutic range or therapeutic "window" of desired plasma levels. The defined therapeutic window should include the levels at which the majority of patients achieve the intended pharmacologic effect. However, a few people are sensitive to the therapeutic effects of most drugs, responding to lower levels, whereas others are sufficiently refractory as to require levels that impose the likelihood of adverse effects as a price for therapeutic benefit. For example, a few patients with strong seizure foci require plasma levels of phenytoin exceeding 20 μg/mL to control seizures. Dosages to achieve this effect may be appropriate.

As also illustrated in Fig. 64-5, some patients are prone to adverse effects at levels that are tolerated by most of the population, and therefore elevation of levels to those with a high probability of therapeutic effect may bring on unwanted actions in the exceptional patient. Table 64-4 presents the concentrations of a number of drugs in plasma that are associated with adverse and therapeutic effects in most patients. Its use within the guidelines discussed should permit more effective and safer therapy for those patients who are not "average."

TABLE 64-4 Concentrations of drugs in plasma: Relation to efficacy and adverse effects

Drug	Efficacy*	Adverse effects†
Amikacin	20 μg/mL	40 μg/mL
Carbenicillin	100 μg/mL‡	300 μg/mL
Carbamazepine	3 μg/mL	10 μg/mL
Digitoxin	12 ng/mL	25–30 ng/mL
Digoxin	0.8 ng/mL	2.0 ng/mL
Ethosuximide	40 μg/mL	100 μg/mL
Gentamicin	4 μg/mL§	12 μg/mL
Lidocaine	1.5 μg/mL	5 μg/mL
Lithium	0.5 meq/liter	1.3 meq/liter
Penicillin G	1–25 μg/mL¶	
Phenytoin (diphenylhydantoin)	10 μg/mL	20 μg/mL
Procainamide	4 μg/mL	8 μg/mL
Quinidine	2.5 μg/mL	6 μg/mL
Theophylline	8 μg/mL	20 μg/mL

* *The therapeutic effect is infrequent or slight at levels below these.*
† *The frequency of adverse effects increases sharply when these levels are exceeded.*
‡ *Minimal inhibitory concentration (MIC) for most strains of Pseudomonas aeruginosa. MIC for other, more sensitive, organisms is less.*
§ *Dependent on the MIC. Higher levels (up to 8 μg/mL) may be desired when host defenses are impaired.*
¶ *There is a wide range of MIC of penicillin for various organisms, and the MIC of all those for which penicillin is used is < 20. "Massive" penicillin therapy with 20 million units daily achieves levels of 20 to 25 μg/mL in patients with clearance of creatinine of 100 mL/min.*

EFFECTIVE PARTICIPATION OF THE PATIENT IN THERAPEUTIC PROGRAMS Measurement of the concentration of a drug in plasma is the most effective approach to determining when patients have failed to take the drug. Such "noncompliance" is a frequent problem in the long-term treatment of diseases such as hypertension and epilepsy, occurring in 25 percent or more of patients in therapeutic environments that lack special efforts to involve patients in the responsibility for their own health. Occasionally, noncompliance can be uncovered by sympathetic, nonincriminating questioning, but more often it is recognized only after determining that the concentration of drug in plasma is nil or is recurrently low. Because other factors can cause plasma levels to be lower than expected, comparison with levels obtained during in-patient treatment may be required to confirm that noncompliance did, in fact, occur. Once the physician is certain of noncompliance, a nonaccusatory discussion of the problem with the patient may elucidate a reason for the noncompliance and serve as a basis for more effective participation of the patient in the care subsequently. Many approaches have been tried to enhance the patients' exercise of responsibility for their own treatment, most based on improved communication regarding the nature of the disease and the expectations of treatment success and treatment failure. This communication includes an opportunity for the patient to relate problems associated with treatment, and it may be improved by involving nurses and other paramedical personnel in the process. Minimizing the complexity of the regimen is helpful, both in terms of the number of drugs and the frequency of administration. Educating patients to assume the principal role in their own health care requires a blend of the art and science of medicine.

REFERENCES

BENET LZ, SHEINER LB: Design and optimization of dosage regimens: Pharmacokinetic data, in *Goodman and Gilman's The Pharmacological Basis of Therapeutics*, 7th ed. AG Gilman et al (eds). New York, Macmillan, 1985, p 1663, Appendix II.

BURTON ME et al: Comparison of drug dosing methods. Clin Pharmacokinet 10:1, 1985

CHENNAVASIN P, BRATER DC: Nomograms for drug use in renal disease. Clin Pharmacokinet 6:193, 1981

DETTLI L: Elimination kinetics and dosage adjustment of drugs in patients with kidney disease. Prog Pharmacol, vol 1, no 4, 1977

SHAND DG et al: Pharmacokinetic drug interactions, in *Handbook of Experimental Pharmacology*, vol 28: *Concepts in Biochemical Pharmacology*, JR Gillette, JR Mitchell (eds). New York, Springer-Verlag, 1975, p 272

SHEINER LB, TOZER TN: Clinical pharmacokinetics: The use of plasma concentrations of drugs, in *Clinical Pharmacology: Basic Principles in Therapeutics*, 2d ed, KL Melmon, HF Morrelli (eds). New York, Macmillan, 1978, p 71

WILKINSON GR, SHAND DG: A physiological approach to hepatic drug clearance. Clin Pharmacol Ther 18:377, 1975

65 ADVERSE REACTIONS TO DRUGS

ALASTAIR J. J. WOOD / JOHN A. OATES

The beneficial effects of drugs are coupled with the inescapable risk that they may also cause untoward effects. The morbidity and mortality that result from these untoward effects often present diagnostic problems, for these drugs can involve every organ and system of the body.

Major advances in the investigation, development, and regulation of drugs ensure in most instances their uniformity, effectiveness, and relative safety, as well as identify their recognized hazards. However, the extremely large number and variety of drugs and drug products available over the counter (OTC) or by prescription from a physician make it impossible for patient or physician to obtain or retain the knowledge necessary to use all these drugs well. It is understandable, therefore, that many OTC drugs are used unwisely by the public and that restricted drugs may be prescribed incorrectly by physicians.

Most physicians use no more than 50 drug products in their practice, gaining familiarity with their effectiveness and safety. Most patients probably use only a limited number of OTC drugs. Nevertheless, many patients receive care and drug prescriptions from more than one physician, and surveys have shown that in any 30-day period patients may consume more than three different OTC drug products containing nine or more different chemical agents.

Twenty-five to fifty percent of patients may make errors in self-administration of prescribed medicines, and this can be responsible for adverse drug effects. Elderly patients are most likely to commit such errors. One-third or more of patients also may not take their prescribed medications. It also seems likely that many patients commit similar errors in taking OTC drugs by not reading or following the directions for use of the medicines provided on the containers. Physicians must recognize that providing directions with prescriptions does not always guarantee their patients' compliance.

Every drug can produce untoward consequences, even when used according to standard or recommended methods of administration. When used incorrectly, the drug's effectiveness may be reduced, or adverse reactions can be expected to occur more frequently. The administration of several drugs during the same period of time also may result in adverse interactions between drugs (see Chap. 64).

In the hospital all the drugs a patient is given should be under the control of a physician, and patient compliance is, in general, ensured. Errors may occur nevertheless, in that the wrong drug or dose may be given, or the drug may be given to the wrong patient, although systems improving drug distribution and administration in hospitals have reduced this problem. On the other hand, there are no means for controlling how ambulatory patients take prescription or OTC drugs.

EPIDEMIOLOGY Epidemiologic studies of adverse drug reactions have been helpful in evaluating the magnitude of the overall problem, in calculating the rate of reactions to individual drugs, and in characterizing some of the determinants of adverse drug effects.

Patients receive on the average 10 different drugs while hospitalized. The sicker the patient, the more drugs are given, and as expected, there is a corresponding increase in the likelihood of adverse drug reactions. When fewer than 6 different drugs are given to hospitalized patients, the probability of an adverse reaction is about 5 percent, but if more than 15 drugs are given, the probability is over 40 percent. Retrospective analysis of ambulatory patients has revealed a history of some adverse drug effects in 20 percent of them.

Thus, the magnitude of the problem posed by drug-induced disease has become exceedingly large. Two to five percent of patients are admitted to the medical and pediatric services of general hospitals because of illnesses attributed to drugs. The case/fatality ratio from drug-induced disease in hospitalized patients varies from 2 to 12 percent. A proportion of fetal or neonatal abnormalities may be due to medicines taken by the mother during pregnancy or parturition.

Women experience twice as many gastrointestinal manifestations of adverse drug effects as do men.

A small group of widely used drugs account for a disproportionate number of reactions. A number of studies have shown that aspirin, digoxin, anticoagulants, diuretics, antimicrobials, steroids, and hypoglycemic agents account for as many as 90 percent of all reactions.

ETIOLOGY Most adverse reactions to drugs may be classified into one of two groups. The most frequent are those that result from the exaggerated but predicted pharmacologic action of the drug. Other adverse reactions ensue from toxic effects on cells that result from mechanisms unrelated to the intended pharmacologic actions. These therefore are often unpredictable, are frequently severe, and result from a number of recognized as well as undiscovered mechanisms. Some of the mechanisms of extrapharmacologic toxicity include direct cytotoxicity, the initiation of abnormal immune responses, and the perturbation of metabolic processes in individuals rendered susceptible by genetic enzymatic defects.

EXAGGERATION OF THE INTENDED PHARMACOLOGIC EFFECT By prior consideration of the known factors that modify drug action, these adverse reactions often are preventable.

Abnormally high drug concentration at the receptor site (site of action) due to the pharmacokinetic variability discussed in Chap. 64 is the usual cause. For example, reduction in the volume of distribution, in the rate of metabolism, or in the rate of excretion will all result in higher than expected concentration of the drug at the receptor site with consequent increase in pharmacologic effect.

Alteration in the dose-response curve due to increased receptor sensitivity will result in an increase in drug effect at the same concentration. An example of this is seen in the excessive response to the anticoagulant warfarin at normal and lower than normal blood levels in the elderly.

The shape of the dose-response curve itself also determines the likelihood of the development of adverse drug reactions. These drugs with a steep dose-response curve are more likely to be associated with dose-related toxicity because of the small increase in dose required to produce a large change in pharmacologic effect. An increase in the dose of drugs which exhibit nonlinear kinetics, such as phenytoin (see previous chapter), may produce a proportionately greater increase in the blood level, resulting in toxicity.

Concomitant drug therapy may affect the pharmacokinetics or pharmacodynamics of other drugs. Pharmacokinetics may be affected by alterations in bioavailability, protein binding, or the rate of metabolism or excretion. Pharmacodynamics may be altered by competition for receptor sites, by prevention of the drug's reaching its site of action, or by antagonism or enhancement of the drug's pharmacologic effect. These subjects are discussed in detail in the previous chapter.

TOXICITY UNRELATED TO A DRUG'S PRIMARY PHARMACOLOGIC ACTIVITY **Cytotoxic reactions** Our understanding of these so-called idiosyncratic reactions has greatly improved recently as it has become clear that many of these reactions are due to irreversible binding of drug or metabolites to tissue macromolecules by shared electron (covalent) bonds. Some chemical carcinogens such as the alkylating agents combine directly with DNA. However, it is more commonly only after metabolic activation to chemically reactive metabolites that covalent binding occurs. This metabolic activation usually occurs in the microsomal mixed-function oxidase system, the hepatic enzyme system which is responsible for the metabolism of many drugs (Chap. 64). During the course of drug metabolism by these pathways, reactive metabolites of some drugs may be produced which covalently bind to tissue macromolecules, causing tissue damage. Because of the highly reactive nature of these metabolites, covalent binding often occurs close to the site of production, such as the liver, but the mixed-function oxidase system is found in other tissues as well.

An example of this type of adverse drug reaction is the hepatotoxicity associated with isoniazid, which is metabolized principally by acetylation (Fig. 65-1) to acetylisoniazid, which is then hydrolyzed to acetylhydralazine. The further metabolism of acetylhydralazine by the mixed-function oxidase system liberates reactive metabolites which covalently bind to hepatic macromolecules, causing hepatic necrosis. The administration of drugs known to increase the activity of the mixed-function oxidase system, such as phenobarbital or rifampin, together with isoniazid, is associated with the production of increased amounts of reactive metabolites, increased covalent binding, and hepatic damage.

The hepatic necrosis produced by overdosage of acetaminophen is caused by the covalent binding of reactive electrophilic metabolites to hepatic macromolecules. Normally these reactive metabolites are detoxified by combining with hepatic glutathione. When glutathione becomes exhausted, the metabolites bind instead to hepatic macromolecules with resultant hepatocyte damage. The hepatic necrosis produced by the ingestion of large quantities of acetaminophen can be prevented, or at least attenuated, by the administration of substances such as *N*-acetylcysteine, which reduce the binding of electrophilic metabolites to hepatic proteins with resultant hepatic necrosis. The risks of hepatic necrosis are increased in patients also receiving drugs such as phenobarbital which increase the rate of drug metabolism and rate of production of toxic metabolite(s).

It is likely, though as yet unproved, that other idiosyncratic reactions are caused by the covalent binding of reactive metabolites to tissue macromolecules, with either direct cytotoxicity or via the initiation of an immunologic response.

Immunologic mechanisms Most pharmacologic agents are poor immunogens since they consist of small molecules with molecular weights less than 2000. Stimulation of antibody synthesis or sensitization of lymphocytes by a drug or one of its metabolites usually requires in vivo activation and covalent linkage to protein, carbohydrate, or nucleic acid.

Drug stimulation of antibody production may mediate tissue injury by one of several mechanisms. The antibody may attack the drug affixed to a cell by covalent linkage and thereby destroy the cell, as occurs in penicillin-induced hemolytic anemia. Complexes of antibody-drug-antigen may be passively adsorbed by a bystander cell which is destroyed by activation of complement; this occurs in quinine- and quinidine-induced thrombocytopenia. Drugs or their reactive metabolites may alter host tissue, rendering it antigenic, and stimulate autoantibodies; for example, hydralazine and procainamide can chemically alter nuclear material, stimulate formation of antinuclear antibodies, and occasionally cause lupus erythematosus. Autoantibodies may be stimulated by drugs which neither interact with the host antigen nor have any chemical similarity to the host tissue; for example, alpha methyldopa frequently stimulates formation of antibodies to host erythrocytes, yet the drug does not itself attach to the erythrocyte or share any chemical similarities with the antigenic determinants on the erythrocyte.

Serum sickness (Chap. 260) results from deposition of circulating drug-antibody complexes on endothelial surfaces. Complement activation occurs, chemotactic factors are generated locally, and an inflammatory response appears at the site of complex entrapment. Arthralgias, lymphadenopathy, glomerulonephritis, or cerebritis may result. Penicillin is the most common cause of serum sickness today. Many drugs, particularly the antimicrobial agents, induce production of IgE, which affixes to mast cell membranes. Contact with a drug antigen initiates a series of biochemical events within the mast cell and results in the release of mediators which may produce urticaria, wheezing, rhinorrhea, and occasionally hypotension characteristic of anaphylaxis.

FIGURE 65-1 *Biotransformation of isoniazid to a hepatotoxic metabolite.*

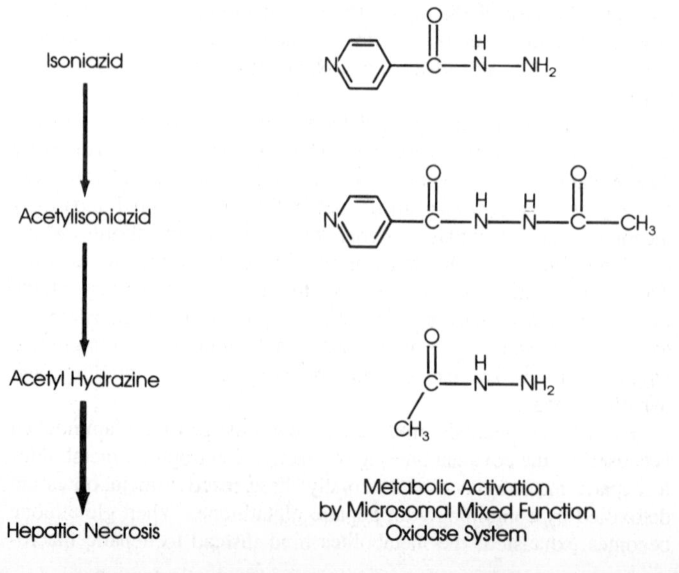

Drugs may also excite cell-mediated immune responses. Topically administered substances may interact with sulfhydryl or amino groups in the skin and react with sensitized lymphocytes to produce the rash characteristic of contact dermatitis. Other types of rashes may also appear from the interaction of serum factors, drugs, and sensitized lymphocytes. The role of drug-activated lymphocytes in the immune mechanisms governing destruction of visceral tissue is unknown.

Toxicity associated with genetically determined enzymatic defects In the porphyrias, drugs which increase the activity of enzymes proximal to the deficient enzyme in the biosynthetic pathway of porphyrins can increase the quantity of porphyrin precursors that accumulate proximal to the deficient enzyme (Chap. 312). These drugs are listed in Table 65-1.

Patients with a deficiency of glucose 6-phosphate dehydrogenase (G6PD) will develop hemolytic anemia on primaquine and a number of other drugs (Table 65-1) which do not cause hemolysis in patients who have adequate quantities of this enzyme (Chap. 287).

Diagnosis The manifestations of drug-induced diseases frequently resemble those associated with other diseases and may be produced by different and dissimilar drugs. Recognition of the role of a drug or drugs responsible for illness is dependent upon appreciation of the possible implication of adverse reactions to drugs in any disease, identification of a temporal relationship between drug administration and development of illness, and familiarity with the manifestations most often caused by particular drugs. Although specific reactions have been described as resulting from the use of particular drugs, there is always a "first," and any drug should be suspected of causing an adverse effect if the clinical setting is appropriate.

Illness related to a drug's pharmacologic action may be more easily recognized than illness attributable to immunologic or other mechanisms. For example, side effects such as cardiac arrhythmias in patients receiving digitalis, hypoglycemia in patients given insulin, and bleeding in patients receiving anticoagulants are more easily related to the prescribed drug than are symptoms like fever or rash, which may be caused by many drugs or by other factors.

Once an adverse reaction is suspected, discontinuance of the suspected drug followed by disappearance of the reaction is presumptive evidence of a drug-induced illness. Reappearance of the reaction upon cautious readministration of the drug may provide confirmatory evidence of the relationship if such confirmation adds useful information to the future management of the patient without entailing undue risk. With concentration-dependent adverse reactions, lowering the dosage may also be followed by disappearance of the reaction, and increasing the dose may cause it to reappear. When the reaction is thought to be allergic, however, readministration of the drug may be hazardous, since anaphylactic shock may develop. Readministration is unwise under these conditions unless alternate drugs are not available and treatment is mandatory.

If the patient is receiving many different drugs when an adverse reaction is suspected, the drugs most likely to be incriminated can usually be identified. All drugs may be discontinued at once, or if this is not practical, then drugs should be discontinued one at a time, starting with the drug under greatest suspicion, and the patient observed for signs of improvement. It must be remembered that the time taken for the disappearance of a concentration-dependent adverse effect will depend on the time taken for the concentration to fall below the range associated with the adverse effect, and this in turn will depend on the initial blood level and on the rate of elimination or metabolism of the drug. Adverse effects of drugs such as phenobarbital which have long half-lives will take a considerable time to disappear.

To assist in the identification of adverse reactions, a table of the drugs recognized as producing a number of reactions appears in this chapter (Table 65-1). This table is not intended to be exhaustive but rather includes well-documented reactions and some less well-

TABLE 65-1 Clinical manifestations of adverse reactions to drugs

- *I Multisystem*
  - *A* Fever
    - Penicillins
    - Novobiocin
    - *p*-Aminosalicylic acid
    - Amphotericin B
    - Antihistamines
    - Cephalosporins
    - Barbiturates
    - Phenytoin
    - Quinidine
    - Sulfonamides
    - Iodides
    - Thiouracil
    - Phenolphthalein
    - Methyldopa
    - Asparaginase
    - Bleomycin
    - Procainamide
  - *B* Drug-induced lupus erythematosus
    - Acebutolol
    - Hydralazine
    - Procainamide
    - Isoniazid
  - *C* Serum sickness
    - Aspirin
    - Penicillins
    - Streptomycin
    - Sulfonamides
    - Propylthiouracil
  - *D* Anaphylaxis
    - Bromsulfophthalein
    - Penicillins
    - Cephalosporins
    - Streptomycin
    - Dextran
    - Iron dextran
    - Procaine
    - Insulin
    - Demeclocycline
    - Iodinated drugs or contrast media
    - Lidocaine
- *II Endocrine*
  - *A* Disorders of thyroid function tests
    - Oral contraceptives
    - Bromsulfophthalein
    - Phenindione
    - Iodides
    - Tolbutamide
    - Chlorpropamide
    - Lithium
    - Acetazolamide
    - Gold salts
    - Dimercaprol
    - Clofibrate
    - Phenothiazines (long-term)
    - Phenylbutazone
    - Sulfonamides
    - Phenytoin
  - *B* Addisonian-like syndrome
    - Busulfan
  - *C* Gynecomastia
    - Estrogens
    - Testosterone
    - Spironolactone
    - Digitalis
    - Reserpine
    - Methyldopa
    - Isoniazid
    - Ethionamide
    - Griseofulvin
  - *D* Galactorrhea (may also cause amenorrhea)
    - Methyldopa
    - Phenothiazines
    - Reserpine
    - Tricyclic antidepressants
    - Dexamphetamine
  - *E* Sexual dysfunction
    - *1* Impaired ejaculation
      - Guanethidine
      - Debrisoquin
      - Bethanidine
      - Thioridazine
    - *2* Decreased libido and impotence
      - Oral contraceptives
      - Sedatives
      - Major tranquilizers
      - Lithium
      - Methyldopa
      - Clonidine
- *III Metabolic*
  - *A* Hyponatremia
    - *1* Dilutional
      - Vincristine
      - Cyclophosphamide
      - Chlorpropamide
      - Diuretics
    - *2* Salt wasting
      - Diuretics
      - Corticosteroid (withdrawal)
      - Enemas
      - Mannitol
  - *B* Hyperkalemia
    - Spironolactone
    - Triamterene
    - Amiloride
    - Cytotoxics
    - Corticosteroid (withdrawal)
    - Succinylcholine
    - Digitalis overdose
    - Potassium salts of drugs
    - Potassium preparations including salt substitute
    - Lithium
  - *C* Hypokalemia
    - Diuretics
    - Laxative abuse
    - Corticosteroids
    - Amphotericin B
    - Alkali-induced alkalosis
    - Insulin
    - Osmotic diuretics
    - Carbenoxolone
    - Gentamicin
    - Degraded tetracycline
    - Vitamin B_{12}
  - *D* Metabolic acidosis
    - Paraldehyde (degraded)
    - Phenformin
    - Acetazolamide
    - Spironolactone
    - Salicylates
  - *E* Hypercalcemia
    - Antacids with absorbable alkali
    - Vitamin D
    - Thiazides
  - *F* Hyperuricemia
    - Thiazides
    - Chlorthalidone
    - Ethacrynic acid
    - Furosemide
    - Aspirin
    - Cytotoxics
    - Hyperalimentation
    - Fructose (IV)
  - *G* Hyperglycemia
    - Corticosteroids
    - Oral contraceptives
    - Chlorthalidone
    - Ethacrynic acid
    - Thiazides
    - Furosemide
    - Diazoxide
    - Growth hormone
  - *H* Porphyria exacerbation
    - Barbiturates
    - Chlordiazepoxide
    - Meprobamate
    - Sulfonamides
    - Estrogens
    - Oral contraceptives
    - Chlorpropamide
    - Phenytoin
    - Glutethimide
    - Griseofulvin
    - Rifampin
  - *I* Hyperbilirubinemia
    - Rifampin
    - Novobiocin
- *IV Dermatologic*
  - *A* Exfoliative dermatitis
    - Penicillins
    - Sulfonamides
    - Barbiturates
    - Phenytoin
    - Phenylbutazone
    - Gold salts
    - Quinidine
  - *B* Toxic epidermal necrolysis (bullous)
    - Barbiturates
    - Phenylbutazone
    - Phenytoin
    - Sulfonamides
    - Phenolphthalein
    - Penicillins
    - Allopurinol
    - Iodides
    - Bromides
    - Nalidixic acid
  - *C* Erythema multiforme or Steven-Johnson syndrome
    - Sulfonamides
    - Barbiturates
    - Phenylbutazone
    - Chlorpropamide
    - Thiazides
    - Sulfones
    - Phenytoin
    - Ethosuximide
    - Salicylates
    - Tetracyclines
    - Codeine
    - Penicillins
  - *D* Erythema nodosum
    - Penicillins
    - Sulfonamides
    - Oral contraceptives
  - *E* Fixed drug eruptions
    - Phenolphthalein
    - Barbiturates
    - Sulfonamides
    - Salicylates
    - Phenylbutazone
    - Quinine
    - Captopril
  - *F* Photodermatitis
    - Tetracyclines, particularly demeclocycline
    - Griseofulvin
    - Sulfonamides
    - Sulfonylureas
    - Thiazides
    - Furosemide
    - Phenothiazines
    - Nalidixic acid
    - Oral contraceptives
    - Chlordiazepoxide
  - *G* Urticaria
    - Aspirin
    - Penicillins
    - Sulfonamides
    - Barbiturates
  - *H* Nonspecific rashes
    - Ampicillin
    - Barbiturates
    - Allopurinol
    - Phenytoin
    - Methyldopa
  - *I* Pigment changes (hyperpigmentation)
    - ACTH
    - Busulfan
    - Phenothiazines
    - Hypervitaminosis A
    - Oral contraceptives
    - Gold salts
    - Chloroquine and other antimalarials
    - Cyclophosphamide
    - Bleomycin
  - *J* Alopecia
    - Cytotoxics
    - Ethionamide
    - Heparin
    - Oral contraceptives (withdrawal)
  - *K* Purpura (see also thrombocytopenia)
    - Corticosteroids
    - Aspirin
  - *L* Lichenoid eruptions
    - Chlorpropamide
    - Gold salts
    - Antimalarials
    - PAS
    - Methyldopa
    - Phenothiazines
  - *M* Eczema (contact dermatitis)
    - Topical antimicrobials
    - Topical local anesthetics
    - Topical antihistamines

- Cream and lotion preservatives
- Lanolin

N Acne
- Anabolic and androgenic steroids
- Corticosteroids
- Bromides
- Iodides
- Oral contraceptives
- Isoniazid
- Troxidone

V Hematologic

A Pancytopenia (aplastic anemia)
- Chloramphenicol
- Phenytoin
- Mephenytoin
- Trimethadione
- Phenylbutazone
- Oxyphenbutazone
- Gold salts
- Mepacrine
- Quinacrine
- Potassium perchlorate
- Sulfonamides
- Cytotoxics

B Agranulocytosis (see also pancytopenia)
- Chloramphenicol
- Sulfonamides
- Phenylbutazone
- Oxyphenbutazone
- Gold salts
- Indomethacin
- Propylthiouracil
- Methimazole
- Carbimazole
- Phenothiazines
- Cytotoxics
- Tolbutamide
- Cotrimoxazole
- Tricyclic antidepressants
- Captopril

C Thrombocytopenia platelet dysfunction (see also pancytopenia)
- Quinidine
- Quinine
- Furosemide
- Chlorthalidone
- Thiazides
- Gold salts
- Cotrimoxazole
- Aspirin
- Indomethacin
- Phenylbutazone
- Oxyphenbutazone
- Chlorpropamide
- Acetazolamine
- Phenytoin and other hydantoins
- Methyldopa
- Carbamazepine
- Digitoxin
- Novobiocin
- Carbenacillin

D Megaloblastic anemia
- Folate antagonists
- Cotrimoxazole
- Phenytoin
- Primidone
- Phenobarbital
- Triamterene
- Trimethoprim
- Oral contraceptives

E Hemolytic anemia
- Methyldopa
- Levodopa
- Mefenamic acid
- Melphalan
- Isoniazid
- Rifampin
- Sulfonamides
- Penicillins
- Cephalosporins
- Insulin
- Quinidine
- Chlorpromazine
- Phenacetin
- *p*-Aminosalicylic acid
- Dapsone
- Procainamide

F Hemolytic anemia (in G6PD deficiency)
- Antimalarials, e.g., primaquine
- Chloramphenicol
- Dapsone
- Nalidixic acid
- Nitrofurantoin
- Sulfonamides
- Aspirin
- Phenacetin
- *p*-Aminosalicylic acid
- Quinidine
- Vitamin C
- Vitamin K
- Cotrimoxazole
- Probenecid
- Procainamide

G Lymphadenopathy
- Phenytoin
- Primidone

H Leukocytosis
- Lithium
- Corticosteroids

I Eosinophilia
- Erythromycin estolate
- Sulfonamides
- Chlorpropamide
- *p*-Aminosalicylic acid
- Imipramine
- Nitrofurantoin
- Procarbazine
- Methotrexate

VI Cardiovascular

A Exacerbation of angina
- Vasopressin
- Oxytocin
- Ergotamine
- Methysergide
- Propranolol withdrawal
- Excessive thyroxin
- Alpha blockers
- Hydralazine

B Cardiomyopathy
- Emetine
- Sympathomimetics
- Phenothiazines
- Lithium
- Sulfonamides
- Daunorubicin
- Adriamycin

C Pericarditis
- Procainamide
- Hydralazine
- Methysergide
- Emetine

D Fluid retention or congestive heart failure
- Estrogens
- Steroids
- Carbenoxolone
- Phenylbutazone
- Indomethacin
- Propranolol
- Mannitol
- Diazoxide
- Minoxidil
- Verapamil

E Arrhythmias
- Sympathomimetics
- Thyroid hormone
- Digitalis
- Quinidine
- Procainamide
- Verapamil
- Atropine
- Propranolol
- Guanethidine
- Emetine
- Propellants in aerosols
- Tricyclic antidepressants
- Phenothiazines, particularly thioridazine
- Lithium
- Anticholinesterases
- Papaverine
- Daunomycin
- Adriamycin
- Lincomycin (intravenous)

F Hypotension (see also arrythmias)
- Nitroglycerin
- Phenothiazines
- Morphine
- Diuretics
- Citrated blood
- Levodopa
- Nifedipine
- Verapamil

G Hypertension
- Oral contraceptives
- Sympathomimetics
- Clonidine withdrawal
- Monoamine oxidase inhibitors with sympathomimetics
- Tricyclic antidepressants with sympathomimetics
- Corticosteroids
- ACTH
- Phenylbutazone

H Thromboembolism
- Oral contraceptives

VII Respiratory

A Nasal congestion
- Reserpine
- Guanethidine
- Isoproterenol
- Oral contraceptives
- Decongestant abuse

B Respiratory depression
- Aminoglycosides
- Polymixins
- Trimethaphan
- Opiates
- Sedatives
- Hypnotics

C Airway obstruction (bronchospasm, asthma; see also anaphylaxis)
- Beta blockers
- Nonsteroidal anti-inflammatory drugs, e.g., aspirin, indomethacin
- Cholinergic drugs
- Tartrazine (drugs with yellow dye)
- Penicillins
- Cephalosporins
- Streptomycin
- Pentazocine

D Pulmonary infiltrates
- Amiodarone
- Nitrofurantoin
- Methysergide
- Bleomycin
- Chlorambucil
- BCNU
- Procarbazine
- Busulfan
- Melphalan
- Cyclophosphamide
- Azothioprine
- Methotrexate
- Mitomycin C
- Sulfonamides

E Pulmonary edema
- Heroin
- Methadone
- Hydrochlorthiazide
- Propoxyphene
- Contrast media

VIII Gastrointestinal

A Dental discoloration
- Tetracycline

B Gingival hyperplasia
- Phenytoin

C Oral ulceration
- Aspirin
- Isoproterenol (sublingual)
- Cytotoxics
- Pancreatin
- Gentian violet

D Taste disturbances
- Penicillamine
- Biguanides
- Griseofulvin
- Metronidazole
- Lithium
- Rifampin
- Captopril

E Dry mouth
- Anticholinergics
- Levodopa
- Tricyclic antidepressants
- Clonidine
- Methyldopa

F Swelling of salivary gland
- Phenylbutazone

TABLE 65-1 Clinical manifestations of adverse reactions to drugs *(continued)*

- Guanethidine
- Bethanidine
- Bretylium
- Clonidine
- Iodides
- *G* Peptic ulceration or hemorrhage
  - Aspirin
  - Phenylbutazone
  - Indomethacin
  - Ethacrynic acid
  - Reserpine (large doses)
- *H* Intestinal ulceration
  - Enteric-coated potassium chloride
- *I* Nausea or vomiting
  - Digitalis
  - Opiates
  - Estrogens
  - Levodopa
  - Potassium chloride
  - Ferrous sulfate
  - Aminophylline
  - Tetracyclines
- *J* Diarrhea or colitis
  - Lincomycin
  - Clindamycin
  - Broad-spectrum antibiotics
  - Magnesium in antacids
  - Guanethidine
  - Debrisoquin
  - Methyldopa
  - Reserpine
  - Digitalis
  - Colchicine
  - Purgatives
  - Lactose excipients
- *K* Constipation or ileus
  - Ganglionic blockers
  - Tricyclic antidepressants
  - Phenothiazines
  - Opiates
  - Aluminum hydroxide
  - Calcium carbonate
  - Barium sulfate
  - Ion exchange resins
  - Ferrous sulfate
- *L* Malabsorption
  - Broad-spectrum antibiotics
  - Neomycin
  - Cholestyramine
  - Colchicine
  - *p*-Aminosalicylic acid
  - Biguanides
  - Phenytoin
  - Primidone
  - Phenobarbital
  - Cytotoxics
- *M* Pancreatitis
  - Corticosteroids
  - Thiazides
  - Azathioprine
  - Oral contraceptives
  - Sulfonamides
  - Opiates
  - Furosemide
  - Ethacrynic acid
- *N* Diffuse hepatocellular damage
  - Halothane
  - Methoxyflurane
  - Methyldopa
  - Isoniazid
  - Rifampin
  - Aminosalicylic acid
  - Ethionamide
  - Phenytoin and other hydantoins
  - Acetaminophen (paracetamol)
  - Salicylates
  - Allopurinol
  - Sulfonamides
  - Tetracyclines
  - Erythromycin estolate
  - Ketoconazole
  - Propylthiouracil
  - Methimazole
  - Oxyphenisatin
  - Methotrexate
  - Pyridium
  - Propoxyphene
  - Monoamine oxidase inhibitors
  - Sodium valproate
  - Nitrofurantoin
  - Aprindine
- *O* Cholestatic jaundice
  - Phenothiazines
  - Androgens
  - Anabolic steroids
  - Oral contraceptives
  - Erythromycin estolate
  - Chlorpropamide
  - Gold salts
  - Methimazole
  - Acetohexamide
  - Nitrofurantoin

IX Renal

- *A* Nephrotic syndrome
  - Penicillamine
  - Gold salts
  - Phenindione
  - Probenecid
  - Captopril
- *B* Tubular necrosis
  - Amphotericin B
  - Aminoglycosides
  - Polymixins
  - Cephaloridine
  - Tetracyclines
  - Colistin
  - Sulfonamides
  - Radioiodinated contrast medium
  - Methoxyflurane
  - Cyclosporin
- *C* Interstitial nephritis
  - Penicillins, particularly methicillin
  - Sulfonamides
  - Phenindione
  - Furosemide
  - Thiazides
  - Allopurinol
- *D* Nephropathies
  - Due to analgesics (e.g., phenacetin)
- *E* Concentrating defect with polyuria (or nephrogenic diabetes insipidus)
  - Vitamin D
  - Lithium
  - Demeclocycline
  - Methoxyflurane
- *F* Renal tubular acidosis
  - Degraded tetracycline
  - Amphotericin B
  - Acetazolamide
- *G* Calculi
  - Acetazolamide
  - Vitamin D
- *H* Obstructive uropathy
  - Intrarenal: cytotoxics
  - Extrarenal: methysergide
- *I* Hemorrhagic cystitis
  - Cyclophosphamide
- *J* Bladder dysfunction
  - Anticholinergics
  - Monoamine oxidase inhibitors
  - Tricyclic antidepressants
  - Disopyramide

X Genital (see also endocrine)

- *A* Vaginal carcinoma
  - Diethylstilbestrol (administered to mother)
- *B* Impairment of spermatogenesis or oogenesis
  - Cytotoxics

XI Neurologic

- *A* Peripheral neuropathy
  - Isoniazid
  - Hydralazine
  - Nitrofurantoin
  - Vincristine
  - Mustine
  - Streptomycin
  - Polymixin, colistan
  - Clioquinol
  - Phenelzine
  - Tricyclic antidepressants
  - Chloramphenicol
  - Procarbazine
  - Ethambutol
  - Ethionamide
  - Glutethimide
  - Demeclocycline
  - Nalidixic acid
  - Tolbutamide
  - Chlorpropamide
  - Methysergide
  - Phenytoin
  - Metronidazole
  - Clofibrate
  - Chloroquine
  - Perhexiline
  - Disopyramide
- *B* Exacerbation of myasthenia
  - Aminoglycosides
  - Polymixins
- *C* Extrapyramidal effects
  - Butyrophenones, e.g., haloperidol
  - Phenothiazines
  - Tricyclic antidepressants
  - Methyldopa
  - Levodopa
  - Reserpine
  - Metoclopramide
  - Oral contraceptives
- *D* Seizures
  - Amphetamines
  - Analeptics
  - Phenothiazines
  - Isoniazid
  - Lidocaine
  - Theophylline
  - Penicillins
  - Nalidixic acid
  - Physostigmine
  - Tricyclic antidepressants
  - Vincristine
  - Lithium
- *E* Stroke
  - Oral contraceptives
- *F* Pseudotumor cerebri (or intracranial hypertension)
  - Corticosteroids
  - Oral contraceptives
  - Tetracyclines
  - Hypervitaminosis A
- *G* Headache
  - Hydralazine
  - Bromides
  - Glyceryl trinitrate
  - Ergotamine (withdrawal)
  - Indomethacin

XII Ocular

- *A* Corneal opacities
  - Vitamin D
  - Mepacrine
  - Chloroquine
  - Indomethacin
- *B* Corneal edema
  - Oral contraceptives
- *C* Cataracts
  - Phenothiazines
  - Corticosteroids
  - Busulfan
  - Chlorambucil
- *D* Glaucoma
  - Mydriatics
  - Sympathomimetics
- *E* Retinopathy
  - Chloroquine
  - Phenothiazines
- *F* Optic neuritis
  - Clioquinol
  - Chloramphenicol
  - Streptomycin
  - Isoniazid
  - Ethambutol
  - Quinine
  - Phenothiazines
  - Penicillamine
  - PAS
  - Phenylbutazone
- *G* Alteration in color vision
  - Troxidone
  - Sulfonamides
  - Streptomycin
  - Methaqualone
  - Barbiturates
  - Digitalis
  - Thiazides

XIII Ear

- *A* Vestibular disorders
  - Aminoglycosides
  - Quinine
  - Mustine

TABLE 65-1 Clinical manifestations of adverse reactions to drugs *(continued)*

B Deafness
- Aminoglycosides
- Ethacrynic acid
- Furosemide
- Quinine
- Bleomycin
- Chloroquine
- Mustine
- Aspirin
- Nortriptyline

XIV Musculoskeletal

A Myopathy or myalgia
- Corticosteroids
- Chloroquine
- Clofibrate
- Oral contraceptives
- Amphotericin B
- Carbenoxolone

B Bone disorders

1 Osteoporosis
- Corticosteroids
- Heparin

2 Osteomalacia
- Anticonvulsants
- Glutethimide
- Aluminum hydroxide

XV Psychiatric disorders

A Schizophrenic-like or paranoid reactions
- Amphetamines
- Lysergic acid
- Levodopa
- Tricyclic antidepressants
- Monoamine oxidase inhibitors
- Bromides
- Corticosteroids

B Depression
- Centrally acting antihypertensives (reserpine, methyldopa, clonidine)
- Propranolol
- Corticosteroids
- Amphetamine withdrawal
- Levodopa

C Hypomania, mania, or excited reactions
- Levodopa
- Sympathomimetics
- Corticosteroids
- MAO inhibitors
- Tricyclic antidepressants

D Hallucinatory states
- Amantadine
- Narcotics
- Pentazocine
- Propranolol
- Levodopa
- Tricyclic antidepressants
- Meperidine

E Delirious or confusional states
- Digitalis
- Anticholinergics
- Bromides
- Sedatives and hypnotics
- Phenothiazines
- Antidepressants
- Corticosteroids
- Isoniazid
- Levodopa
- Amantadine
- Penicillins
- Aminophylline
- Methyldopa

F Sleep disturbances
- Anorexiants
- Levodopa
- Monoamine oxidase inhibitors
- Sympathomimetics

G Drowsiness
- Anxiolytic drugs
- Major tranquilizers
- Tricyclic antidepressants
- Antihistamines
- Methyldopa
- Clonidine
- Reserpine

documented reactions which are sufficiently devastating as to require their consideration. It should be used to suggest the likely causative drug, but the absence of a drug from the table should not be interpreted to mean that it is not responsible for the reaction.

Serum antibody has been demonstrated in some persons with drug allergy involving cellular blood elements, as in agranulocytosis, hemolytic anemia, and thrombocytopenia. For example, both quinine and quinidine can produce platelet agglutination in vitro in the presence of complement and the serum from a patient who has developed thrombocytopenia following this drug.

Eliciting a drug history from patients is important for diagnosis. Attention must be directed to nonprescription, or OTC, as well as to prescription drugs. Each type can be responsible for adverse drug effects, and frequently adverse interactions occur between drugs purchased by patients over the counter and those prescribed by physicians. In addition, it is common for patients to be cared for by several physicians; and duplicative, additive, counteractive, or synergistic drugs may therefore be taken if the physicians are not aware of the patients' drug histories. Every physician should determine what drugs a patient has been taking, at least during the preceding 30 days, before prescribing any medications. A history of previous adverse drug effects in patients is common. Since these patients have a predisposition to other drug-induced illnesses, familiarity with such a history should dictate added caution in prescribing drugs.

Patients with biochemical abnormalities such as erythrocyte G6PD deficiency can be identified; patients with the defect are usually blacks or of Mediterranean descent. Drug-induced hemolytic crisis can be avoided by testing for the enzyme defect before administering these drugs. Similarly, persons with an abnormal serum pseudocholinesterase may have abnormally prolonged apnea when given succinylcholine.

General comments No drug is completely without side effects, and it is important to remember that a side effect in one patient may be the desired pharmacologic effect in another. Recent improvements in drug regulation allow physicians to prescribe drugs with considerable confidence in their purity, bioavailability, and effectiveness. However, while regulatory bodies try to ensure that drugs with serious toxic potential are not marketed, they have to constantly weigh the potential toxicity against the possible benefits. Thus toxicity which would be acceptable for an effective antineoplastic agent would not be permitted in, for example, an oral contraceptive. In addition, because of the necessarily small number of patients treated in premarketing studies, rare adverse reactions cannot be identified, so that the first responsibility for identifying and reporting these effects must rest with the practicing clinician through the use of the various national adverse reaction reporting systems, such as those operated by the Food and Drug Administration in the United States and the Committee on Safety of Medicines in Great Britain. The publication of a newly recognized adverse reaction can in a short time stimulate a very large number of similar such reports which previously had gone unrecognized.

The prevention of adverse drug reactions must first involve a high index of suspicion that the development of a new symptom or sign may be drug-related. Reduction of the dose or discontinuation of the suspected agent will usually clarify the position in concentration-dependent toxic reactions. Physicians should be familiar with the common adverse effects of the drugs they use and, if they are in doubt, should consult the literature.

REFERENCES

Davies DM: *Textbook of Adverse Drug Reactions*, 2d ed. New York, Oxford University Press, 1981

Goldstein RA: Drug allergy: Prevention, diagnosis, and treatment. Ann Intern Med 100:302, 1984

Rossi AC, Knatt D: Discovery of new adverse drug reactions. JAMA 252:1030, 1984

Steel K et al: Iatrogenic illness on a general medical service at a university hospital. N Engl J Med 304:398, 1981

Timbrell JA: Drug hepatotoxicity. Br J Clin Pharmacol 15:3, 1983

66 PHYSIOLOGY AND PHARMACOLOGY OF THE AUTONOMIC NERVOUS SYSTEM

LEWIS LANDSBERG / JAMES B. YOUNG

FUNCTIONAL ORGANIZATION OF THE AUTONOMIC NERVOUS SYSTEM

The autonomic nervous system innervates vascular and visceral smooth muscle, exocrine and endocrine glands, and parenchymal cells throughout the various organ systems. Functioning below the conscious level, the autonomic nervous system responds rapidly and continuously to perturbations that threaten the constancy of the internal environment. The many functions governed by this system include the distribution of blood flow and the maintenance of tissue perfusion, the regulation of blood pressure, the regulation of the volume and composition of the extracellular fluid, the expenditure of metabolic energy and supply of substrate, and the control of visceral smooth muscle and glands.

Autonomic responses, like those of the somatic nervous system, are induced promptly and dissipated quickly, in contrast to the slower, more prolonged effects of circulating hormones. The autonomic nervous system, like the endocrine system, regulates the rate of processes that have intrinsic activities of their own, while the somatic nervous system initiates responses de novo. Although certain autonomic responses are discriminating, many are generalized and influence a variety of effectors in different organs. The interface between the autonomic nervous system and the endocrine system is exemplified by the adrenal medulla. This gland, homologous in many respects with the postganglionic sympathetic neuron, secretes a hormone (epinephrine) into the circulation to interact with adrenergic receptors throughout the body.

ANATOMIC ORGANIZATION The autonomic neurons, located in ganglia outside the central nervous system, give rise to the postganglionic autonomic nerves that innervate organs and tissues throughout the body. The activity of autonomic nerves is regulated by central neurons responsive to diverse afferent inputs. After central integration of afferent information, autonomic outflow is adjusted to permit the functioning of the major organ systems in accordance with the needs of the organism as a whole. Connections between the cerebral cortex and the autonomic centers in the brainstem coordinate autonomic outflow with higher mental functions.

The sympathetic and parasympathetic divisions The preganglionic neurons of the parasympathetic nervous system leave the central nervous system in the third, seventh, ninth, and tenth cranial nerves and in the second and third sacral nerves, while the preganglionic neurons of the sympathetic nervous system exit the spinal cord between the first thoracic and the second lumbar segments. Responses to sympathetic and parasympathetic stimulation are frequently antagonistic, as exemplified by their opposing effects on heart rate and gut motility. This antagonism reflects highly coordinated interactions within the central nervous system; the resultant changes in parasympathetic and sympathetic activity, often reciprocal, provide more precise control of autonomic responses than could be achieved by the modulation of a single system.

Neurotransmitters *Acetylcholine* (ACh) is the preganglionic neurotransmitter for both divisions of the autonomic nervous system, as well as the postganglionic neurotransmitter of the parasympathetic neurons. Nerves that release ACh are said to be cholinergic. *Norepinephrine* (NE) is the neurotransmitter of the postganglionic sympathetic neurons; these nerves are said to be adrenergic. Within the sympathetic outflow postganglionic neurons innervating the eccrine sweat glands (and perhaps some blood vessels supplying skeletal muscle) are of the cholinergic type.

THE SYMPATHETIC NERVOUS SYSTEM AND THE ADRENAL MEDULLA

CATECHOLAMINES All three of the naturally occurring catecholamines, NE, *epinephrine* (E), and *dopamine,* function as neurotransmitters within the central nervous system. NE, the neurotransmitter of postganglionic sympathetic nerve endings, exerts its effects locally, in the immediate vicinity of its release. E, the circulating hormone of the adrenal medulla, influences processes throughout the body. A peripheral dopaminergic system also exists but has not been characterized in detail.

Biosynthesis (Fig. 66-1) Catecholamines are synthesized from the amino acid tyrosine, which is sequentially hydroxylated to form dihydroxyphenylalanine (dopa), decarboxylated to form dopamine, and hydroxylated on the beta position of the side chain to form NE. The initial step, the hydroxylation of tyrosine, is rate-limiting and is regulated so that synthesis of dopa is coupled to norepinephrine release. This regulation is achieved by alterations in both the activity and the amount of tyrosine hydroxylase. In the adrenal medulla and in those central neurons utilizing E as neurotransmitter, NE is *N*-methylated to E by the enzyme phenylethanolamine-*N*-methyltransferase (PNMT). A major portion of the blood perfusing the adrenal medulla is enriched with corticosteroids from the adrenal cortex, and since adrenal PNMT is inducible by glucocorticoids, the capacity of the adrenal medulla to form E may be related to its strategic location within the adrenal cortex.

Catecholamine metabolism (Fig. 66-1) The major metabolic transformations of catecholamines involve *O*-methylation at the metahydroxyl group and oxidative deamination. *O*-methylation is catalyzed by the enzyme catechol-*O*-methyltransferase (COMT), and oxidative deamination is promoted by monoamine oxidase (MAO). COMT in liver and kidney is important in the metabolism of circulating catecholamines. MAO, a mitochondrial enzyme present in most tissues including nerve endings has a lesser role in the metabolism of circulating catecholamines but is important in regulating the catecholamine stores within the peripheral sympathetic nerve endings. The metanephrines and 4-hydroxy-3-methoxymandelic acid (VMA) are the major end products of N and NE metabolism. Homovanillic acid (HVA) is the end product of dopamine metabolism.

STORAGE AND RELEASE OF CATECHOLAMINES Both in the adrenal medulla and sympathetic nerve endings catecholamines are stored in subcellular granules and released by exocytosis. The large stores of catecholamines in these tissues provide an important physiologic reserve that maintains an adequate supply of catecholamines in the face of intense stimulation.

Adrenal medulla The adrenal medullary chromaffin tissue in a pair of normal human adrenal glands weighs about 1 g and contains approximately 6 mg of catecholamines, 85 percent of which is E. Catecholamines are maintained in high concentration within the storage (chromaffin) granule by an active uptake process involving the granule membrane and by an intragranular storage complex that appears to involve ATP, calcium, and a specific granule protein (chromagranin A). Catecholamine secretion, stimulated by ACh from the preganglionic sympathetic nerves, occurs after calcium influx triggers fusion of the chromaffin granule membrane and cell membrane; obliteration of the cell membrane at the point of fusion and extrusion of the entire soluble contents of the granule into the extracellular space complete the process of exocytosis (Fig. 66-1). Approximately 2 to 10 percent of the total adrenal medullary catecholamine store is turned over each day.

Peripheral sympathetic nerve endings The peripheral sympathetic nerve endings form a reticulum or ground plexus that brings the terminal fibers into close contact with effector cells. All the NE in peripheral tissues is in the sympathetic nerve endings, and heavily innervated tissues contain as much as 1 to 2 μg per gram of tissue. NE stored in the nerve endings is in discrete subcellular particles analogous to the adrenal medullary chromaffin granules. MAO in the mitochondria of the nerve endings plays an important role in regulating the local concentration of NE (Fig. 66-1). Amines in storage vesicles are protected from oxidative deamination; amines within the cytoplasm, however, are deaminated to inactive metabolites. Release from the nerve ending occurs in response to action potentials propagated in terminal sympathetic fibers (Fig. 66-1).

THE PERIPHERAL ADRENERGIC NEUROEFFECTOR JUNCTION

Neuronal uptake The peripheral sympathetic nerve endings possess an amine transport system that actively takes up amines from the extracellular fluid. A variety of synthetic and naturally occurring amines are substrates for this process. Neuronal uptake or recapture of locally released NE terminates the action of the transmitter and contributes to the constancy of the NE stores (Fig. 66-1).

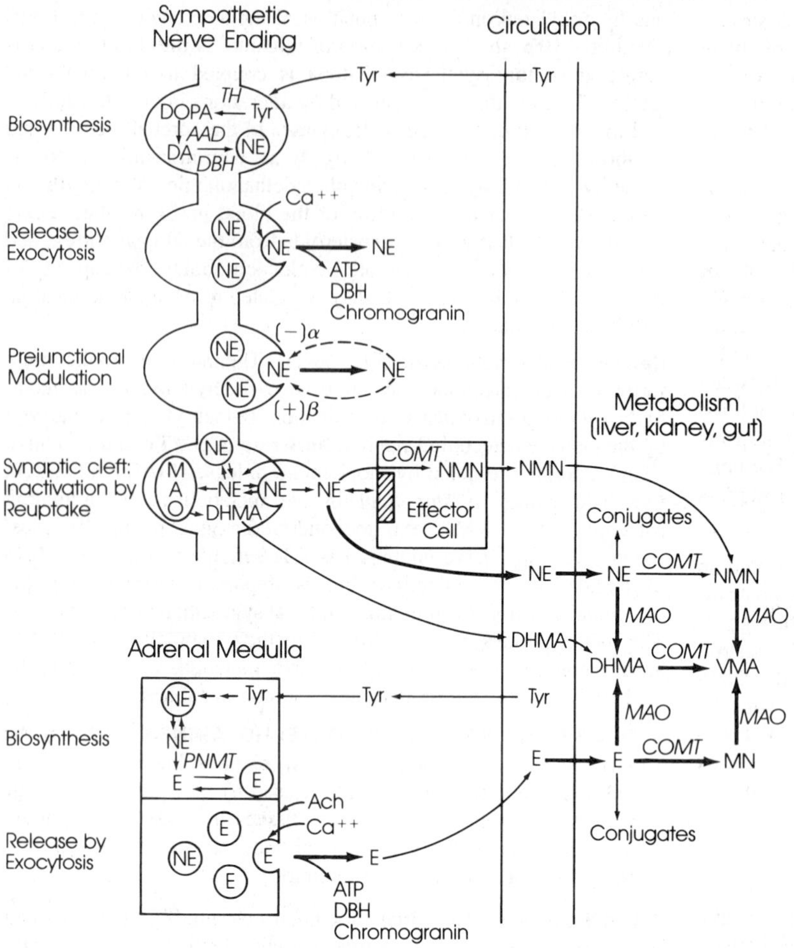

FIGURE 66-1 *Catecholamine biosynthesis, release, and metabolism. Schematic representation of a peripheral sympathetic nerve ending is shown at the top; the bulbous areas on the terminal fiber represent varicosities identified by histochemical fluorescence techniques as areas of high neurotransmitter concentration. The processes of biosynthesis, release, modulation, and reuptake are shown sequentially for demonstration purposes only; in vivo they proceed concurrently. Adrenal medullary chromaffin cells are shown at the bottom of the diagram. (TH = tyrosine hydroxylase, AAD = aromatic-L-amino acid decarboxylase, DA = dopamine, DBH = dopamine-β-hydroxylase, NE = norepinephrine, PNMT = phenylethanolamine-N-methyltransferase, E = epinephrine, COMT = catechol-O-methyltransferase, NMN = normetanephrine, MAO = monoamine oxidase, DHMA = 3,4-dihydroxymandelic acid, VMA = 3-methoxy-4-hydroxymandelic acid.)*

Prejunctional modulation A variety of factors alter the relationship between neuronal impulse traffic and NE release. Diminished temperature and acidosis, for example, both decrease the amount of NE released in response to sympathetic impulses. Several chemical mediators operate at the peripheral sympathetic nerve ending (referred to as prejunctional or presynaptic sites) to modify sympathetic neurotransmission by influencing the amount of NE released in response to nerve impulses. Prejunctional modulation may be either inhibitory or facilitatory. Certain modulators, such as catecholamines and ACh, may either inhibit or facilitate NE release, antagonistic effects that are mediated by different adrenergic or cholinergic receptors, respectively. Those compounds exerting an *inhibitory* effect on NE release at the prejunctional nerve ending include the following: catecholamines (alpha$_2$ receptor), ACh (muscarinic receptor), dopamine (D-2 receptor), histamine (H-2 receptor), serotonin, adenosine, enkephalins, and prostaglandins. *Facilitatory* prejunctional modulators include catecholamines (beta$_2$ receptor), ACh (nicotinic receptor), and angiotensin II. The overall significance of prejunctional modulation, as well as the relative importance of the various mediators, has yet to be established.

PREJUNCTIONAL ADRENERGIC RECEPTORS Catecholamines reduce NE release via prejunctional alpha receptors in a classical negative feedback system. Feedback regulation is complicated by the fact that beta-receptor activation facilitates NE release. Two hypotheses have been advanced to explain how the antagonistic alpha and beta effects on NE release may be integrated physiologically. One hypothesis is that beta-mediated effects occur at lower agonist concentrations than those mediated by the alpha receptor, whereas alpha-mediated responses predominate at higher concentrations of agonist. During low levels of sympathetic stimulation, therefore, when NE concentrations in the synaptic cleft are low, beta-mediated positive feedback may predominate with facilitation of NE release. Conversely, at higher levels of sympathetic stimulation with increased NE concentration in the synaptic cleft, alpha-mediated negative feedback predominates and NE release is inhibited. The other hypothesis is that prejunctional beta receptors are more sensitive to E than NE; circulating levels of E, therefore, might stimulate the prejunctional beta receptors, thereby augmenting NE release and enhancing sympathetic neurotransmission.

PREJUNCTIONAL CHOLINERGIC RECEPTORS Though both inhibitory and facilitatory effects of ACh on NE release have been described, the inhibitory effect of ACh, mediated by the muscarinic cholinergic receptor, occurs at lower ACh concentrations and is probably of greater physiologic significance. This peripheral inhibitory effect of ACh on adrenergic neurotransmission may reinforce the reciprocal changes in central parasympathetic and sympathetic outflow that occur in the regulation of numerous physiologic responses.

CENTRAL REGULATION OF SYMPATHOADRENAL OUTFLOW

Brainstem sympathetic centers Sympathetic outflow is initiated from the reticular formation of the medulla oblongata and pons and from centers in the hypothalamus. Descending fibers originating from these centers synapse in the intermediolateral cell column of the spinal cord with the preganglionic sympathetic neurons. The brainstem sympathetic centers, which have an intrinsic activity of their own, are regulated by many stimuli, including impulses from more rostral areas of the central nervous system (cortex, limbic lobe, hypothalamus); neural afferents that interact at the level of the brainstem centers and at the higher centers; and changes in the physical and chemical properties of the extracellular fluid, including the circulating levels of hormones and substrates. The higher centers, which have connections with the brainstem, coordinate sympathetic outflow with higher mental functions, emotional reactions, and the homeostatic needs of the internal environment. Although the hallmark of intense sympathoadrenal stimulation is a global response (the fight-or-flight reaction of Cannon), discrete changes in sympathetic outflow to different organ systems influence many autonomic functions.

RELATIONSHIP BETWEEN THE SYMPATHETIC NERVOUS SYSTEM AND THE ADRENAL MEDULLA Sympathetic nervous system activity and adrenal medullary secretion are coordinated but not always congruent. During periods of intense sympathetic stimulation, such as cold exposure and exhaustive exercise, the adrenal medulla is progressively recruited, and circulating E reinforces the physiologic effects of sympathetic stimulation. In other situations the sympathetic nervous system and the adrenal medulla are stimulated independently. The response to upright posture, for example, involves predominantly the sympathetic nervous system while hypoglycemia stimulates only the adrenal medulla.

Sympathetic regulation of the cardiovascular system The sympathetic nervous system plays a major role in the regulation of the circulation. Stretch receptors in the systemic and pulmonary arteries and veins continuously monitor intravascular pressures; the resulting afferent impulses, after relay and integration in the brainstem, alter sympathetic activity in defense of blood pressure and blood flow to critical areas (Fig. 66-2).

ARTERIAL BARORECEPTORS An increase in blood pressure stimulates receptors in the carotid sinus and aortic arch. The ensuing afferent impulses, after relay within the nucleus of the solitary tract (NTS) in the brainstem, suppress the brainstem sympathetic centers (Fig. 66-2). This baroreceptor reflex arc forms a negative feedback loop in which a rise in arterial pressure results in the inhibition of central sympathetic outflow. A brainstem noradrenergic pathway interacts with the NTS to participate in suppression of sympathetic outflow. This noradrenergic inhibitory pathway is stimulated by centrally acting alpha-adrenergic agonists and may be involved in the action of certain antihypertensive drugs, such as clonidine, that potentiate the baroreceptor-mediated vasodepressor response (Chap. 196). In the opposite manner, when the blood pressure falls, decreased afferent impulses diminish central inhibition, resulting in an increase in sympathetic outflow and a rise in arterial pressure.

CENTRAL VENOUS PRESSURE Receptors in the walls of the great veins and within the atria are also involved in the regulation of sympathetic outflow. Stimulation of these receptors by high venous pressure suppresses the brainstem sympathetic centers; when central venous pressure is low, sympathetic outflow increases. The central connections are poorly understood, but the afferent impulses are carried in the vagus (Fig. 66-2).

ASSESSMENT OF SYMPATHOADRENAL ACTIVITY The clinical assessment of sympathoadrenal activity involves the measurement of catecholamines in plasma and of catecholamines and catecholamine metabolites in urine. Quantitation of urinary catecholamines and metabolites is useful in the diagnosis of pheochromocytoma (Chap. 326).

Plasma catecholamines Catecholamines in human plasma may be measured by radioenzymatic isotope derivative techniques or by high performance liquid chromotography in conjunction with electrochemical detection. Plasma catecholamine measurements provide an index of sympathetic nervous system and adrenal medullary activity and have been widely used to assess sympathoadrenal activity in clinical investigation in human subjects. The usefulness of plasma catecholamine measurements is, however, compromised by factors that alter the relationship between the plasma concentration of catecholamines and the functional state of the sympathoadrenal system. The clinical usefulness of plasma catecholamine levels is limited to the evaluation of patients with autonomic insufficiency (Chap. 29) and, on occasion, patients with suspected pheochromocytoma (Chap. 326).

Basal plasma NE concentrations are in the range of 150 to 350 pg/mL; basal E levels are about 25 to 50 pg/mL. The half-time of disappearance of NE from the circulation is approximately 2 min. The plasma NE level is markedly affected by a variety of factors, including posture; accordingly, the conditions under which blood is obtained for assay must be controlled. By convention, basal plasma NE levels are those obtained through an indwelling intravenous line after the patient has rested supine in a relaxed environment for 30 min.

PLASMA NE RESPONSE TO UPRIGHT POSTURE The predictable increase in circulating NE concentration during upright posture provides a convenient test of sympathetic nervous system function. Five minutes of quiet standing results in a two- to threefold increase in plasma NE level. A normal response requires an intact afferent system, appropriate central nervous system relays, and an intact peripheral sympathetic nervous system; a defect of any of these components reduces the increment in circulating NE.

Plasma E levels are also dependent on the physical and mental state of the subject. Change in plasma E with upright posture is usually small. Hypoglycemia and various types of mental stress, however, can cause large increments in the plasma E level.

PERIPHERAL DOPAMINERGIC SYSTEM

In addition to its role as neurotransmitter in the central nervous system, dopamine functions as an inhibitory transmitter in the carotid body and the sympathetic ganglia. A distinct peripheral dopaminergic system is also believed to exist. Dopamine elicits a variety of responses not attributable to stimulation of classic adrenergic receptors; it relaxes the lower esophageal sphincter, delays gastric emptying, causes vasodilation in the renal and mesenteric arterial circulation, suppresses aldosterone secretion, and stimulates renal sodium excretion. The mediation of these dopaminergic effects in vivo is poorly understood. Dopamine does not appear to be a circulating hormone. Unequivocal evidence of peripheral autonomic dopaminergic nerves has not been produced, although such nerves may be present in the kidney. The kidney, furthermore, produces much of the dopamine in the urine since the amount excreted each day (approximately 200 μg per 24 h) cannot be accounted for by clearance of plasma dopamine. Decarboxylation of circulating dopa, which is present in high concentration in the plasma (1500 pg/mL) may contribute to urinary dopamine production. Dopamine generated from the decarboxylation

FIGURE 66-2 *Sympathetic regulation of the circulation. Receptors in the venous and arterial circulations are stimulated by stretch, caused by an increase in pressure; afferent impulses from these receptors are carried to the central nervous system by the ninth and tenth cranial nerves. The net result of these afferent impulses, after relay in the brainstem, is to inhibit central sympathetic outflow. The arterial baroreceptor reflex involves a relay in the nucleus of the tractus solitarius (NTS). (+ = stimulation; − = inhibition.)*

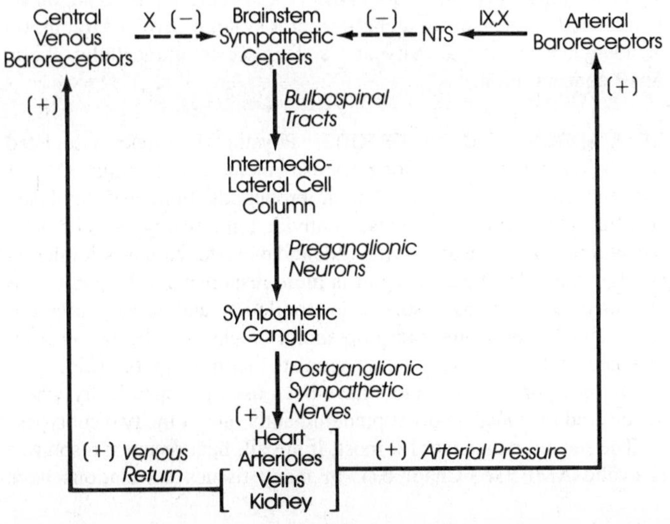

of circulating dopa might also be involved in the mediation of dopaminergic effects in the kidney and other sites. Thus, the nature of the peripheral dopaminergic system is obscure, but the existence of a dopaminergic system in those tissues that respond uniquely to dopamine seems likely.

ADRENERGIC RECEPTORS

Catecholamines influence effector cells by interacting with specific *receptors* on the cell surface. When stimulated by catecholamines, the adrenergic receptor initiates a series of membrane changes followed by a cascade of intracellular events that culminates in a measurable response. Compounds that elicit the response are referred to as *agonists;* those that block the interaction of the agonist with the receptor are referred to as adrenergic *receptor blocking agents* or *antagonists*.

Two major categories of response to catecholamines reflect the activation of two populations of adrenergic receptors, designated *alpha* and *beta*. Selective agonists and antagonists are available, enabling pharmacologic stimulation or blockade of the physiologic effects mediated by one receptor without influencing those mediated by the other. Both alpha and beta receptors have been further divided into subtypes that serve different functions and are susceptible to differential stimulation and blockade.

ALPHA-ADRENERGIC RECEPTORS The alpha-adrenergic receptor mediates vasoconstriction, intestinal relaxation, and pupillary dilatation. E and NE are approximately equipotent as alpha-receptor agonists. Distinct $alpha_1$- and $alpha_2$-receptor subtypes are also recognized. Originally the postsynaptic or postjunctional alpha-adrenergic receptors on effector cells were designated $alpha_1$, while the prejunctional alpha-adrenergic receptors on the sympathetic nerve endings were designated $alpha_2$. Several additional nonneuronal (postsynaptic) processes appear to be mediated by the $alpha_2$ receptor. The $alpha_1$ receptor mediates the classic alpha effects including vasoconstriction; phenylephrine and methoxamine are selective $alpha_1$ agonists, and prazosin is a selective $alpha_1$ antagonist. The second messenger for $alpha_1$-mediated processes has not been identified with certainty but may involve changes in intracellular calcium concentration or in membrane phosphatidylinositol turnover. The $alpha_2$ receptor mediates presynaptic inhibition of NE release from adrenergic nerves and other responses including inhibition of ACh release from cholinergic nerves, inhibition of lipolysis in adipocytes, inhibition of insulin secretion, stimulation of platelet aggregation and, perhaps, initiation of vasoconstriction. Specific $alpha_2$ agonists include clonidine and α-methylnorepinephrine; these agents, the latter derived from α-methyldopa in vivo, exert an antihypertensive effect by interacting with $alpha_2$ receptors within the brainstem sympathetic centers that regulate blood pressure. Yohimbine is a specific $alpha_2$ antagonist. The second messenger for $alpha_2$-receptor systems involves inhibition of adenylate cyclase activity and a decrease in intracellular cyclic AMP concentration.

BETA-ADRENERGIC RECEPTORS Physiologic events associated with beta-adrenergic receptor responses include stimulation of heart rate and contractility, vasodilation, bronchodilation, and lipolysis. Beta-receptor responses can also be divided into two types. The $beta_1$ receptor responds equally to E and NE and mediates cardiac stimulation and lipolysis. The $beta_2$ receptor is more responsive to E than to NE and mediates responses such as vasodilation and bronchodilation. Isoproterenol stimulates and propranolol blocks both $beta_1$ and $beta_2$ receptors. Other agonists and antagonists that have partial selectivity for the $beta_1$ or $beta_2$ receptors have been used therapeutically where the desired response involves predominantly one of the two subtypes.

The second messenger for most, if not all, beta-receptor responses is cyclic AMP (see Chap. 67). In many tissues correlations have been shown between beta-receptor occupancy and stimulation of adenylate cyclase, on the one hand, and between intracellular cyclic AMP accumulation and physiologic response, on the other. While in some systems sequential enzymatic activations involving cyclic AMP–mediated protein phosphorylation couple beta-receptor stimulation and physiologic response, in many tissues the molecular events that mediate beta-adrenergic responses are unknown.

DOPAMINERGIC RECEPTORS Specific dopaminergic receptors, distinct from the classic alpha- and beta-adrenergic receptors, are present in the central and peripheral nervous system and in several nonneural tissues. Two types of dopaminergic receptor serve different functions and have different second messengers. Dopamine is a potent agonist of both types of receptor; the action of dopamine is antagonized by phenothiazines and thioxanthenes. The dopamine-1 receptor mediates vasodilation in the renal, mesenteric, coronary, and cerebral vascular beds. The effects are mediated by a stimulatory effect on adenylate cyclase and an increase in intracellular cyclic AMP. Fenoldopam is an investigational agonist selective for the dopamine-1 receptor. The dopamine-2 receptor inhibits transmission in the sympathetic ganglia, inhibits NE release from sympathetic nerve endings by an effect on the presynaptic membrane (Fig. 66-1), inhibits prolactin release from the pituitary, and causes vomiting. The second messenger for some dopamine-2–mediated processes involves the inhibition of adenylate cyclase. Selective agonists of the dopamine-2 receptor include bromocriptine, lergotrile, and apomorphine, while butyrophenones such as halolperidol (active within the central nervous system) and domperidone (does not cross blood-brain barrier readily) and the benzamide, sulpiride, are relatively selective dopamine-2 antagonists.

REGULATION OF ADRENERGIC RECEPTORS Radiolabeled adrenergic-receptor agonists and antagonists have been utilized as ligands to study adrenergic receptors. In combination with studies of peripheral tissue sensitivity these studies demonstrated that changes in adrenergic receptors occur under a variety of physiologic conditions. Prolonged exposure to alpha- or beta-adrenergic agonists decreases the number of corresponding adrenergic receptors on effector cells. Although the biochemical mechanisms involved are obscure, internalization of the beta-adrenergic receptor within the cell occurs during agonist exposure in some systems, suggesting that internal translocation causes the decrease in receptor number. Alteration in agonist concentration may also affect the affinity of the receptor for the agonist. Adrenergic receptors that utilize adenylate cyclase for the second messenger (beta receptors, $alpha_2$ receptors) exist in high and low affinity states; exposure to agonist diminishes the proportion of receptors in the high affinity state. Such alterations in adrenergic receptors induced by adrenergic agonists are termed homologous regulation. Agonist-induced alterations in adrenergic-receptor density and affinity are believed to contribute to the diminished physiologic response that occurs after prolonged exposure of an effector tissue to adrenergic agonist, a phenomenon known as *tachyphylaxis* or *desensitization*.

Adrenergic receptors are also influenced by factors other than adrenergic agonists, so-called heterologous regulation. Enhanced alpha-adrenergic-receptor affinity, for example, may underlie the potentiation of alpha-adrenergic responses that occur in response to lowered environmental temperatures. Thyroid hormones potentiate beta-receptor responses by alterations in beta-receptor number and in the efficiency of coupling receptor occupancy with physiologic response. Estrogen and progesterone alter the sensitivity of the myometrium to catecholamines by effects on alpha-adrenergic receptors. Glucocorticoids may influence adrenergic function by antagonizing agonist-induced decreases in adrenergic receptors, thereby counteracting tachyphylaxis in response to intense adrenergic stimulation.

Alterations in sensitivity to catecholamines also occur as a consequence of postreceptor changes.

PHYSIOLOGY OF THE SYMPATHOADRENAL SYSTEM

Catecholamines influence all the major organ systems. The effects take place in seconds as compared with the minutes, hours, or days that characterize the actions of the endocrine system and most other control systems that regulate bodily processes. The sympathoadrenal system, moreover, may respond in anticipation of physiologic requirement. An increase in sympathoadrenal activity prior to strenuous exercise, for example, lessens the impact of exercise on the internal environment.

DIRECT EFFECTS OF CATECHOLAMINES **Cardiovascular system** Catecholamines stimulate vasoconstriction in the subcutaneous, mucosal, splanchnic, and renal vascular beds by an alpha-receptor-mediated mechanism. Since vasoconstriction in the coronary and cerebral circulations is minimal, flow to these areas is maintained. The adaptive significance of this priority given the heart and brain is clear; in both of these organs the metabolic requirements relative to blood flow are high, and continuous perfusion is essential for life. Skeletal muscle vasculature contains beta receptors sensitive to low circulating levels of E so that skeletal muscle blood flow is augmented during adrenal medullary activation.

The effects of catecholamines on the heart are mediated by $beta_1$ receptors and include increase in heart rate, enhancement of cardiac contractility, and increase in conduction velocity. The increase in myocardial contractility is illustrated by a leftward and upward shift of the ventricular function curve (Fig. 181-5) that relates cardiac work to ventricular diastolic fiber length; at any initial fiber length catecholamines increase cardiac work. Catecholamines also enhance cardiac output by stimulating venoconstriction, enhancing venous return, and by increasing the force of atrial contraction, thereby augmenting diastolic volume and hence fiber length. The acceleration of conduction in the junctional tissues results in a more synchronous, and hence more effective, ventricular contraction. Cardiac stimulation increases myocardial oxygen consumption, a major factor in the pathogenesis and treatment of myocardial ischemia.

Metabolism Catecholamines increase metabolic rate. The biochemical processes involved and the sites of the increased heat production are not known in humans; in small mammals mitochondrial respiration in brown adipose tissue is uncoupled.

SUBSTRATE MOBILIZATION In a variety of tissues catecholamines stimulate the breakdown of stored fuel with the production of substrate for local consumption; glycogenolysis in the heart, for example, provides substrate for immediate metabolism by the myocardium. Catecholamines also accelerate fuel mobilization in liver, adipose tissue, and skeletal muscle, liberating substrates (glucose, free fatty acids, lactate) into the circulation for use throughout the body. Activation of enzymes involved in fuel breakdown occurs by a beta-receptor ($beta_1$) mechanism for adipose tissue lipolysis and by alpha- and beta-receptor ($beta_2$) mechanisms for hepatic glycogenolysis and gluconeogenesis. In skeletal muscle catecholamines stimulate glycogenolysis (beta receptor) thereby increasing lactate efflux.

Fluids and electrolytes Catecholamines contribute to the regulation of the volume and composition of extracellular fluid. By a direct action on the renal tubule, NE stimulates sodium reabsorption, thereby defending extracellular fluid volume. Dopamine, in contrast, promotes sodium excretion. NE and E also promote cellular uptake of potassium, thereby defending against the development of hyperkalemia. Effects of catecholamines on calcium, magnesium, and phosphate metabolism are complex and depend on a variety of factors.

Viscera Catecholamines affect visceral function by actions on smooth muscle and glandular epithelium. Urinary bladder and intestinal smooth muscle are relaxed while the corresponding sphincters are stimulated. Gallbladder emptying also involves sympathetic mechanisms. Catecholamine-mediated smooth-muscle contraction in the female aids ovulation and ovum transport along the fallopian tubes, and in the male provides propulsive force for the seminal fluid during ejaculation. Inhibitory $alpha_2$ receptors on cholinergic neurons within the gut contribute to intestinal relaxation. Catecholamines induce bronchodilation by a $beta_2$ receptor mechanism.

INDIRECT EFFECTS OF CATECHOLAMINES The ultimate physiologic response induced by catecholamines involves changes in hormone secretion and in blood flow distribution, both of which support and amplify the direct effects of catecholamines.

Endocrine system Catecholamines influence the secretion of renin, insulin, glucagon, calcitonin, parathormone, thyroxine, gastrin, erythropoietin, progesterone, and, possibly, testosterone. Secretion of each of these hormones is governed by complex feedback loops. With the exception of thyroxine and the gonadal steroids, each is a polypeptide not under the direct control of the pituitary gland. Sympathoadrenal input into the secretion of these hormones provides a mechanism for regulation by the central nervous system and ensures a coordinated hormonal response in accord with the homeostatic needs of the organism.

RENIN The juxtaglomerular apparatus of the kidney is heavily innervated. Sympathetic stimulation increases renin release by a direct beta-receptor effect independent of vascular changes within the kidney. The renin response to volume depletion is sympathetically mediated and is initiated by a fall in central venous pressure. Since renin secretion activates the angiotensin-aldosterone system, angiotensin-induced vasoconstriction supports the direct effects of catecholamines on blood vessels, while aldosterone-mediated sodium reabsorption complements the direct increase in sodium reabsorption induced by sympathetic stimulation. Beta-receptor blocking agents suppress renin secretion.

INSULIN AND GLUCAGON The pancreatic islets also receive an extensive sympathetic innervation. Stimulation of pancreatic sympathetic nerves or an elevation in circulating catecholamines suppresses insulin and increases glucagon release. Inhibition of insulin secretion is mediated by the $alpha_2$ receptor, and stimulation of glucagon is mediated by the beta receptor. This combination of effects supports substrate mobilization, reinforcing the direct effects of catecholamines on hepatic glucose output and lipolysis. Although alpha-receptor-mediated suppression of insulin release usually predominates, a beta-receptor mechanism may augment insulin secretion under some circumstances.

SYMPATHOADRENAL FUNCTION IN SELECTED PHYSIOLOGIC AND PATHOPHYSIOLOGIC STATES **Support of the circulation** The sympathetic nervous system functions to maintain an adequate circulation. During upright posture and volume depletion, reduction of afferent venous and arterial baroreceptor impulse traffic diminishes an inhibitory input to the vasomotor center, thereby increasing sympathetic activity (Fig. 66-2) and reducing efferent vagal tone. As a result, heart rate is increased, and cardiac output is diverted from the skin, subcutaneous tissues, mucosa, and viscera. Sympathetic stimulation of the kidney increases sodium reabsorption, and sympathetically mediated venoconstriction enhances venous return. With pronounced hypotension, the adrenal medulla is recruited and E reinforces the effects of the sympathetic nervous system. A similar pattern of sympathetic activation occurs in the postprandial state when blood and extracellular fluid are sequestered in the splanchnic circulation and in the lumen of the gut, respectively.

CONGESTIVE HEART FAILURE The sympathetic nervous system also provides circulatory support during congestive heart failure (Chap. 182). Venoconstriction and sympathetic stimulation of the heart increase cardiac output while peripheral vasoconstriction directs blood flow to the heart and brain. The afferent signals are less clear than in simple volume depletion since the venous pressure is usually elevated. In severe heart failure depletion of cardiac NE may impair the effectiveness of sympathetic circulatory support.

TRAUMA AND SHOCK In acute traumatic injury or shock, adrenal catecholamines support the circulation and mobilize substrates. It is presumed, but unproved, that the sympathetic nervous system is activated as well. In the chronic, reparative phase following injury catecholamines contribute to substrate mobilization and to the elevation in metabolic rate.

EXERCISE Sympathetic activation during exercise increases cardiac output, maintains blood flow, and ensures sufficient substrate to meet the increased needs. Central neural factors, such as anticipation, and circulatory factors, such as fall in venous pressure, trigger the sympathetic response. Mild degrees of exercise stimulate the sympathetic nervous system alone; during more severe exertion the adrenal medulla is activated as well. Conditioning is associated with a decrease in sympathetic nervous system activity both at rest and during exercise.

Hypoglycemia Hypoglycemia causes a marked increase in adrenal medullary E secretion. When glucose concentrations fall below overnight fasting levels, regulatory glucose-sensitive neurons in the central nervous system initiate a prompt increase in adrenal medullary secretion. The increase is especially intense when plasma glucose levels drop below 50 mg/dL when plasma E levels increase 25 to 50 times above baseline, thereby increasing hepatic glucose output, providing alternative substrate in the form of free fatty acids, suppressing endogenous insulin release, and inhibiting insulin-mediated glucose utilization in muscle. Many clinical manifestations of hypoglycemia, such as tachycardia, palpitations, nervousness, tremor, and widened pulse pressure, are secondary to increased E secretion.

Cold exposure The sympathetic nervous system plays a critical role in the maintenance of normal body temperature during exposure to a cold environment. Receptors in the skin and central nervous system respond to a fall in temperature by activating hypothalamic and brainstem centers that increase sympathetic activity. Sympathetic stimulation leads to vasoconstriction in the superficial vascular beds, thereby diminishing heat loss. Heat production is simultaneously increased by shivering, generation of metabolic heat, and substrate mobilization. Acclimatization during chronic cold exposure increases the capacity for metabolic heat production in response to sympathetic stimulation.

Dietary intake Fasting suppresses and overfeeding stimulates the sympathetic nervous system. The reduction in sympathetic activity during fasting or starvation may contribute to the decrease in metabolic rate, bradycardia, and hypotension in these states. Enhanced sympathetic activity during periods of increased caloric intake may contribute to the elevation in metabolic rate associated with a chronic increase in dietary intake.

Hypoxia Chronic hypoxia is associated with stimulation of the sympathoadrenal system, and some of the cardiovascular changes in hypoxia may be dependent upon catecholamines.

PARTICIPATION OF THE SYMPATHETIC NERVOUS SYSTEM IN THE PATHOGENESIS OF SELECTED DISEASE STATES

HYPERTENSION (See also Chaps. 29 and 196) As shown in Fig. 66-3, regulation of arterial pressure by the sympathetic nervous system involves blood vessels, the heart, and the kidneys. The sympathetic nervous system increases peripheral resistance by direct stimulation of the resistance vessels and by activation of the renin-angiotensin system. Increased cardiac output is the result of enhanced cardiac contractility and augmented venous return, the latter a result of venoconstriction and increased renal sodium reabsorption. Stimulation of sodium retention diminishes the capacity of the kidney to compensate for the increase in blood pressure. Antiadrenergic agents lower blood pressure by interacting at many of the sites shown in Fig. 66-3.

The sympathetic nervous system plays at least a permissive role in the maintenance of hypertension (Chap. 29). Despite the elevated blood pressure, sympathetic nervous system activity is not suppressed in hypertensive patients, and reflex control of the circulation is retained, due in part to upward resetting of the baroreceptors. In addition, peripheral sensitivity of the vasculature to NE is either normal or enhanced. The maintenance of sympathetic nervous system activity in patients with hypertension accounts for the hypotensive effects of antiadrenergic agents.

During antihypertensive treatment with vasodilators or diuretics the sympathetic nervous system may be activated in response to decreased pressure in either the venous or arterial circulation (Fig. 66-2). The heightened sympathetic activity that results, in addition to causing tachycardia, may oppose the antihypertensive therapy by activating the various effector systems shown in Fig. 66-3. Antiadrenergic agents, therefore, have a fundamental role in the therapy of most hypertensive patients.

ANGINA PECTORIS (Chap. 189) Sympathetic stimulation of the cardiovascular system increases myocardial oxygen consumption as a consequence of elevated heart rate, enhanced myocardial contractility, and increased myocardial wall tension. Attacks of angina, therefore, are often precipitated by situations associated with sympathetic activation such as exercise, eating, and cold exposure. Beta blockade is beneficial in the treatment of angina (Chap. 29) because

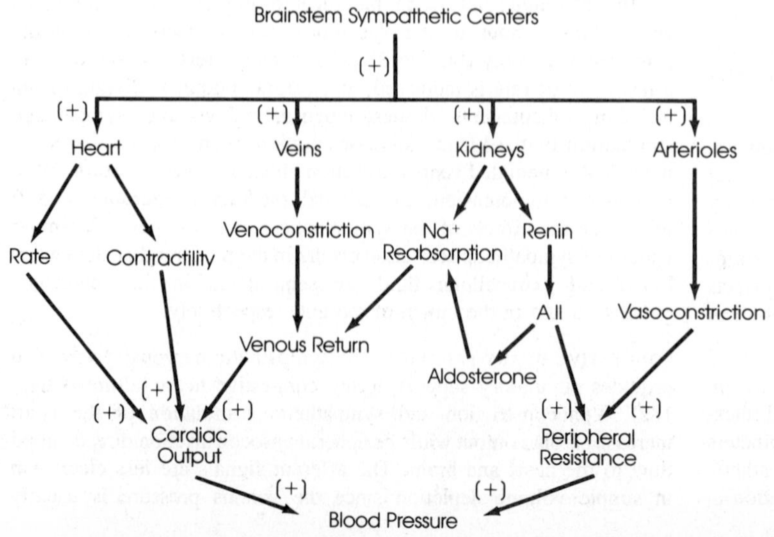

FIGURE 66-3 *Sympathetic nervous system effects on blood pressure. Sympathetic stimulation (+) increases blood pressure by effects on the heart, the veins, the kidneys, and the arterioles. The net result of sympathetic stimulation is an increase in both cardiac output and peripheral resistance. (From JB Young, L Landsberg, in P Sleight et al (eds). Scientific Foundations of Cardiology, London, Heinemann, 1981.)*

of reduction in sympathetic stimulation of the heart. Alpha-adrenergically mediated coronary vasoconstriction may also contribute to coronary spasm.

HYPERTHYROIDISM (Chap. 324) Many of the peripheral manifestations of hyperthyroidism suggest a hyperadrenergic state. Enhancement of beta-receptor responses in hyperthyroidism is due in part to effects on the beta receptor. Thyroid hormone, in some tissues and in some species, increases receptor number; in other tissues, even when beta-receptor number is not increased, coupling of receptor occupancy to the adenylate cyclase cyclic-AMP system is augmented to amplify catecholamine-induced responses. Since thyroid hormone excess does not suppress sympathetic nervous system activity (plasma NE levels are normal in thyrotoxic patients), a "normal" level of sympathetic activity may evoke an exaggerated physiologic response. Many of the adrenergic manifestations of hyperthyroidism are diminished by treatment with beta-receptor blocking agents.

ORTHOSTATIC HYPOTENSION (Chap. 29) The maintenance of arterial pressure during upright posture depends upon an adequate blood volume, an unimpaired venous return, and an intact sympathetic nervous system. Significant postural hypotension, therefore, often reflects extracellular fluid volume depletion or dysfunction of the circulatory reflexes. Diseases of the nervous system, such as tabes dorsalis, syringomyelia, or diabetes mellitus, may disrupt these sympathetic reflexes with resultant orthostatic hypotension. Although any antiadrenergic agent may impair the postural sympathetic response, orthostatic hypotension is most prominent with drugs that block neurotransmission within the ganglia or adrenergic neurons.

The term *idiopathic orthostatic hypotension* refers to a group of degenerative diseases involving either the pre- or postganglionic sympathetic neurons. Involvement of the peripheral sympathetic nervous system is characterized by low basal NE levels, while involvement at the level of the central nervous system or preganglionic sympathetic neurons is associated with normal basal plasma NE levels. In both cases the plasma NE response to upright posture is deficient. Orthostatic hypotension caused by disruption of the preganglionic autonomic neurons within the intermediolateral cell column of the spinal cord often occurs in association with degenerative changes of basal ganglia and other portions of the central nervous system. In the latter situation, known as *multiple systems atrophy*, or the *Shy-Drager* syndrome, orthostatic hypotension occurs along with a variety of neurologic disturbances including Parkinson's disease.

Treatment of orthostatic hypotension is usually unsatisfactory except in the mildest cases. There is no way of reestablishing the normal relationship between fall in venous return and sympathetic neuronal activation. Volume expansion with fludrocortisone and a liberal salt diet in conjunction with fitted stockings to the waist, and elevation of the head of the bed to avoid recumbency, will maintain plasma volume and venous return and frequently provide symptomatic improvement. Rarely a beneficial response may be obtained from treatment with sympathomimetic amines (including clonidine).

PHARMACOLOGY OF THE SYMPATHOADRENAL SYSTEM

A variety of therapeutic agents affect sympathetic nervous system function or interact with adrenergic receptors, making it possible to stimulate or suppress effects mediated by catecholamines with some degree of specificity (Table 66-1).

SYMPATHOMIMETIC AMINES Sympathomimetic amines may directly activate adrenergic receptors (direct acting) or release NE from the sympathetic nerve endings (indirect acting). Many agents have both direct and indirect effects.

Epinephrine and norepinephrine The naturally occurring catecholamines act predominantly by the direct stimulation of adrenergic receptors. NE is employed to support the circulation and elevate the blood pressure in hypotensive states (Chap. 29). Peripheral vasoconstriction is the major effect although cardiac stimulation occurs as well. E, also employed as a pressor, has special usefulness in the treatment of allergic reactions, especially those associated with anaphylaxis. E antagonizes the effects of histamine and other mediators on vascular and visceral smooth muscle and is useful in the treatment of bronchospasm.

Dopamine *Dopamine* is used in treating hypotension, shock (Chap. 29), and certain forms of heart failure (Chap. 182). At low infusion rates it exerts a positive inotropic effect both by a direct action on the cardiac $beta_1$ receptors and by the indirect release of NE from sympathetic nerve endings in the heart. At low doses direct stimulation of dopaminergic receptors in the renal and mesenteric vasculature also results in vasodilation in the gut and kidney and facilitates sodium excretion. At higher infusion rates interaction with alpha-adrenergic receptors results in vasoconstriction, an increase in peripheral resistance, and an elevation of blood pressure.

Beta-receptor agonists *Isoproterenol,* a direct-acting beta-receptor agonist, stimulates the heart, decreases peripheral resistance, and relaxes bronchial smooth muscle. It raises the cardiac output and accelerates atrioventricular conduction while increasing the automaticity of ventricular pacemakers. Isoproterenol is used in the treatment of heart block and bronchoconstriction. *Dobutamine,* a congener of dopamine with relative selectivity for the $beta_1$ receptor and with a greater effect on myocardial contractility than on heart rate, is also used in the treatment of congestive heart failure, often in combination with vasodilators (Chap. 182).

SELECTIVE $BETA_2$-RECEPTOR AGONISTS The cardiac stimulation caused by nonselective beta agonists, such as isoproterenol or epinephrine, is occasionally dangerous when these agents are used in the treatment of bronchoconstriction. Selective $beta_2$ agonists (*metaproterenol, albuterol, terbutaline,* and *isoetharine*) improve the therapeutic ratio by achieving bronchial dilatation with less activation of the cardiovascular system (Chaps. 202 and 208); selectivity is relative, and some cardiac stimulation occurs with these agents, particularly at the higher dose levels. *Ritodrine,* another selective $beta_2$ agonist, is used as a tocolytic agent (as is *terbutaline*) to relax the uterus and antagonize premature labor.

Alpha-adrenergic agonists *Phenylephrine* and *methoxamine* are direct-acting alpha agonists that elevate blood pressure by increasing peripheral vasoconstriction. They are used primarily in the treatment of hypotension and paroxysmal supraventricular tachycardia (Chap. 184), in the latter case by increasing cardiac vagal tone through reflex baroreceptor stimulation. Phenylephrine and a related proprietary compound, *phenylpropanolamine,* are common constituents of decongestant medications (often combined with antihistamines) for the treatment of allergic rhinitis and upper respiratory infections.

Miscellaneous sympathomimetic amines with mixed actions *Ephedrine* has both direct beta-receptor agonist properties and an indirect effect on sympathetic nerve endings, from which it releases NE, and is used primarily as a bronchodilator. *Sudephedrine,* a congener of ephedrine, is less potent at dilating bronchi and serves as a nasal decongestant. *Metaraminol* has both direct and indirect effects on sympathetic nerve endings and is employed in the treatment of hypotensive states.

Dopaminergic agonists The dopamine-2-receptor agonist *bromocriptine* is used to suppress prolactin secretion (Chap. 321). *Apomorphine,* another dopamine-2-receptor agonist, is used to induce emesis.

ANTIADRENERGIC OR SYMPATHOLYTIC AGENTS (See also Chap. 196) **Agents inhibiting central sympathetic outflow** The antihypertensive agents *methyldopa, clonidine,* and *guanabenz* diminish central sympathetic outflow by stimulating a central alpha-adrenergic pathway ($alpha_2$ receptor) that diminishes vasomotor outflow. Central

TABLE 66-1 Some commonly used autonomic drugs[a,b,c]

Agent	Indication	Dose and Route	Comment
ADRENERGIC AGONISTS[d]			
Epinephrine	Anaphylaxis	100–500 μg SC or IM (0.1–0.5 mL of 1/1000 solution of hydrochloride salt); 25–50 micrograms IV (slowly) every 5–15 min; titrate as needed	Nonselective alpha and beta agonist; increases BP, heart rate Bronchodilation
Norepinephrine	Shock Hypotension	2–4 μg of NE base/min IV; titrate as needed	Alpha and $beta_1$ agonist Vasoconstriction predominates Extravasation causes tissue necrosis; infuse through IV cannula
Isoproterenol	Cardiogenic shock Bradyarrhythmias AV block	0.5–5.0 μg/min IV; titrate as needed	Nonselective beta agonist Increases cardiac rate and contractility ($beta_1$) Tachycardia limits usefulness
	Asthma	Inhalation	Dilates bronchi ($beta_2$); cardiac stimulation also occurs
Dobutamine	Refractory CHF Cardiogenic shock	2.5–25 μg/kg/min IV	Selective $beta_1$ agonist with greater effect on contractility than heart rate; a congener of dopamine but not a dopaminergic agonist
Phenylephrine	Hypotension	40–180 μg/min IV	Selective $alpha_1$ agonist; useful in antagonizing hypotension of spinal anesthesia
	Supraventricular tachycardia	150–800 μg slow IV push	Pressor effect induces vagotonic response; do not exceed 160 mm systolic BP
Terbutaline	Asthma	2.5–5.0 mg PO tid; 0.25–0.5 mg SC; inhalation every 4–5 h	Selective $beta_2$ agonist; $beta_1$ (cardiac) effects at higher doses
Albuterol	Asthma	2.0–4.0 mg PO tid or qid; inhalation every 4–6 h	Selective $beta_2$ agonist; $beta_1$ effects (cardiac) at higher doses
Isoetharine	Asthma	inhalation every 2–4 h	Selective $beta_2$ agonist; some $beta_1$ effects
Metaproterenol	Asthma	10–20 mg PO tid or qid; inhalation every 3–4 h	Selective $beta_2$ agonist; some $beta_1$ effects
Ritodrine	Premature labor	100–350 μg/min IV; 10–20 mg every 4–6 h PO	Selective $beta_2$ agonist; hypokalemia. hyperglycemia, hypotension, cardiac stimulation may occur Neonatal hypoglycemia, hypocalcemia reported
DOPAMINERGIC AGONISTS			
Dopamine	Shock	2–5 (μg/kg)/min IV (dopaminergic range) 5–10 (μg/kg)/min IV (dopaminergic and beta range) 10–20 (μg/kg)min IV (beta range) 20–50 (μg/kg)/min IV (alpha range)	Pharmacological effects are dose dependent: renal and mesenteric vasodilation predominate at lower doses; cardiac stimulation and vasoconstriction develop as the dose is increased
Bromocriptine	Amenorrhea-galactorrhea	2.5 mg PO bid or tid	Selective agonist of dopamine-2 receptor; inhibits prolactin secretion
	Acromegaly	5–15 mg PO tid or qid	Lowers growth hormone in a minority of patients with acromegaly
INHIBITORS OF CENTRAL SYMPATHETIC OUTFLOW			
Clonidine	Hypertension	0.1–0.6 mg PO bid	Selective $alpha_2$ agonist; potentiates central baroreceptor depressor reflex Abrupt discontinuation may result in withdrawal syndrome with rebound hypertension
Methyldopa	Hypertension	250–500 mg PO every 6–8 h	Metabolized by decarboxylation and beta-hydroxylation to alpha-methyl-norepinephrine, a centrally active selective $alpha_2$ agonist
ADRENERGIC NEURON BLOCKING AGENTS			
Guanethidine	Hypertension	10–100 mg PO qd	Concentrated in sympathetic nerve endings; blocks release of NE in response to nerve impulses and depletes NE stores; prominent orthostatic hypotension
Bretylium	Ventricular fibrillation and tachycardia	5 mg/kg IV	In addition to blocking NE release, has direct effect on electrical properties of cardiac muscle
BETA BLOCKING AGENTS[e]			
Propranolol	Hypertension	40–160 mg PO bid (or higher)	Lipophilic, nonselective Dosage highly variable
	Angina	10–40 mg PO tid or qid	
	Myocardial infarction	60–80 mg PO tid	Prolongs survival post MI
	Arrhythmias	10–30 mg PO tid or qid; 1–3 mg IV	
	Hypertrophic cardiomyopathy	20–40 mg PO tid or qid	
	Pheochromocytoma	10–20 mg PO tid or qid; 0.5–2.0 mg IV	After alpha blockade initiated
	Essential tremor	20–80 mg PO tid	
	Migraine	20–80 mg PO bid or tid	
	Hyperthyroidism	10–60 mg PO tid or qid	

TABLE 66-1 Some commonly used autonomic drugs[a,b,c] *(continued)*

Agent	Indication	Dose and Route	Comment
Metoprolol	Hypertension Myocardial infarction	50–200 mg PO bid 100 mg PO bid	Selective $beta_1$ (cardiac), lipophilic Prolongs survival post MI
Nadolol	Hypertension Angina	80–320 mg PO qid 80–240 mg PO qid	Hydrophilic, nonselective; lengthen dosage interval with renal failure
Timolol	Hypertension Myocardial infarction	10–30 mg PO bid 10 mg PO bid	Lipophilic, nonselective Prolongs survival post MI
Atenolol	Hypertension	50–100 mg PO qd	Selective $beta_1$, hydrophilic; lengthen dosage interval with renal failure
Pindolol	Hypertension Angina	5–30 mg PO bid 10 mg PO qid	Nonselective, lipophilic with partial agonist activity
ALPHA BLOCKING AGENTS			
Phenoxybenzamine	Pheochromocytoma	10–60 mg PO bid; titrate as needed	Noncompetitive, nonselective alpha blockade
Phentolamine	Pheochromocytoma	5 mg IV (after test dose of 0.5 mg)	Competitive, nonselective alpha blockade
Prazosin	Hypertension CHF	1–5 mg PO bid or tid 2–7 mg PO qid	Competitive, selective $alpha_1$ blockade
COMBINED ALPHA-BETA BLOCKING AGENT			
Labetalol	Hypertension	100–1200 mg PO bid; titrate slowly as needed; 20–80 mg IV (by increments up to 300 mg); 2 mg/min by IV infusion	Competitive alpha and beta antagonist with relatively more activity against beta receptors
DOPAMINERGIC ANTAGONIST[f]			
Metoclopramide	Diabetic gastroparesis	10 mg PO qid	Competitive dopaminergic antagonist with prominent cholinergic agonist activity
	Gastroesophageal reflex Antiemetic (cancer chemotherapy)	10–15 mg PO qid 10 mg IV	
GANGLIONIC BLOCKING AGENT			
Trimethaphan	Hypertensive crisis (aortic dissection)	1–3 mg/min IV	Competitive ganglionic blocker; some direct vasodilating effects; inhibits parasympathetic as well as sympathetic nervous system
CHOLINERGIC AGONIST			
Bethanechol	Urinary retention (nonobstructive)	10–100 mg PO tid or qid; 5 mg SC	M-2 receptor agonist
ANTICHOLINESTERASE AGENTS[g]			
Physostigmine	Central cholinergic blockade	1–2 mg IV (slow)	Tertiary amine; penetrates CNS well; may cause seizures; used to reverse central anticholinergic effects produced by overdose of atropine or tricyclic antidepressants
Edrophonium	Paroxysmal supraventricular tachycardia	5 mg IV (after 1.0 mg test dose)	Induces vagotonic response; rapid onset, short duration of action; effects reversed by atropine
CHOLINERGIC BLOCKING AGENTS[h]			
Atropine	Bradycardia and hypotension	0.4–1.0 mg IV every 1–2 h	Competitive inhibition of M-1 and M-2 receptor; blocks hemodynamic changes associated with increased vagal tone

[a] *Consult complete prescribing information.*
[b] *Doses for children are not given.*
[c] *Only the more common indications and routes of administration are listed.*
[d] *Dopaminergic agonists are listed separately although dopamine, at high doses, is an adrenergic agonist as well.*
[e] *Clinical efficacy of most beta blockers appears similar for major indications. Not all beta blockers are FDA approved for all indications listed in the table.*
[f] *Neuroleptic and antipsychotic agents are also dopaminergic antagonists; these are not included in the table.*
[g] *A major use of cholinesterase inhibitors is in the treatment of myasthenia gravis (Chap 358). These agents, quaternary amines that do not penetrate the CNS, are not included in the table.*
[h] *A wide variety of synthetic atropine derivatives are available for the purpose of (1) diminishing GI tract motility and secretion and (2) increasing urinary bladder capacity. Their usefulness is limited by anticholinergic side effects. Some may be useful as adjuncts in the treatment of peptic ulcer disease.*

nervous system side effects such as sedation are common. When administration of clonidine is stopped abruptly, a withdrawal syndrome characterized by rebound hyperactivity of the sympathetic nervous system can produce a syndrome resembling the crises of patients with pheochromocytoma. *Opiates* may also exert a central sympatholytic effect; the sympathetic excitation of morphine withdrawal responds to clonidine and vice versa. *Propranolol* and *reserpine* may exert some sympatholytic effects at the level of the central nervous system.

Ganglionic blocking agents Ganglionic transmission may be antagonized by drugs that block the (nicotinic) cholinergic synapse between the preganglionic and postganglionic autonomic nerves. These agents inhibit the parasympathetic as well as the sympathetic nervous system. Only *trimethaphan* is in general clinical use; its major application is in the treatment of hypertensive crises, particularly aortic dissection, when controlled hypotension and decreased myocardial contractility are desirable (Chap. 197).

Agents acting at the peripheral sympathetic nerve endings Adrenergic neuron-blocking agents depress the function of the peripheral sympathetic nerves by decreasing the amount of neurotransmitter released. *Guanethidine,* the prototype of this class of drugs, is concentrated in the sympathetic nerve endings by the amine-uptake mechanism. Within the terminal it blocks the release of NE in response to nerve impulses and eventually depletes the nerve of NE by displacing it from the intraneuronal storage granules. The drug is occasionally useful in the management of severe hypertension, although orthostatic hypotension is a limiting side effect. *Bretylium,* an agent whose effects are similar to those of guanethidine, is employed in the treatment of ventricular fibrillation (Chap. 184). Both guanethidine and bretylium are antagonized by agents that affect the amine-uptake transport process such as sympathomimetic amines, tricyclic antidepressants, phenoxybenzamine, and phenothiazines. The antihypertensive action of guanethidine may be rapidly reversed by these drugs.

Reserpine depletes catecholamines from the peripheral sympathetic nerve endings, the brain, and the adrenal medulla. Its antihypertensive effect in humans is usually attributed to depletion of peripheral NE stores within sympathetic nerve endings. The sedation and occasionally morbid depression attending its use result from NE depletion within the central nervous system.

Adrenergic-receptor blocking agents Adrenergic blocking agents antagonize the effects of catecholamines at the level of the peripheral tissue.

ALPHA-ADRENERGIC-RECEPTOR BLOCKING AGENTS *Phenoxybenzamine* and *phentolamine* are utilized principally in treating pheochromocytoma (Chap. 326). Phenoxybenzamine produces prolonged, noncompetitive alpha blockade, while phentolamine leads to reversible, competitive blockade. Because of its rapid action and short duration, phentolamine is commonly used in the treatment of acute hypertensive paroxysms secondary to catecholamine excess, such as occur with pheochromocytoma, with pressor reactions in patients receiving monoamine oxidase inhibitors, and in clonidine withdrawal. Both phentolamine and phenoxybenzamine antagonize $alpha_1$ and $alpha_2$ receptors, although phenoxybenzamine is more potent at the $alpha_1$ receptor site. *Prazosin,* an alpha-adrenergic blocking agent with selectivity for the $alpha_1$ receptor, possesses properties that resemble those of primary vasodilators and is used in the treatment of essential hypertension and as an afterload reducing agent in congestive heart failure. Since none of these agents have much effect on the beta-adrenergic receptor, unopposed beta stimulation may result in tachycardia.

BETA-ADRENERGIC-RECEPTOR BLOCKING AGENTS Beta blocking agents antagonize the cardiovascular effects of catecholamines in angina pectoris, hypertension, and cardiac arrhythmias. The benefit of beta blockade in angina derives from the decrease in myocardial oxygen consumption following reduction in heart rate and myocardial contractility (Chap. 189). The hypotensive effect of beta blockade is not clearly understood (Chap. 196). Diminished cardiac output, decreased NE release at postganglionic sympathetic nerve endings, reduced renin secretion, and suppressed central sympathetic outflow are possible mechanisms. The efficacy of beta blocking agents in the treatment of arrhythmias depends upon reduction of the rate of spontaneous depolarization of pacemaker cells in the sinus node and junctional pacemakers and upon slowing conduction within the atria and atrioventricular node. Beta blockade is also effective in the symptomatic management of hyperthyroidism and the control of tachycardia and arrhythmias in patients with pheochromocytoma. Beta-adrenergic blocking agents are also useful in the treatment of migraine, essential tremor, idiopathic hypertrophic subaortic stenosis, aortic dissection, and possibly in the period following myocardial infarction. Several trials have suggested that beta blocking agents, administered long-term, diminish mortality following acute myocardial infarction. The mechanism may involve antiarrhythmic action, prevention of reinfarction, and reduction in infarct size (Chaps. 184 and 189).

PHARMACOLOGIC PROPERTIES OF BETA-RECEPTOR BLOCKING AGENTS Seven beta blocking agents (atenolol, acebutolol, metoprolol, nadolol, pindolol, propranolol, and timolol) are available for use in the United States. Other agents (alprenolol, bevantolol, oxprenolol, sotalol, etc.,) are in use in other countries and investigational within the United States. The utility of these agents is derived predominantly from blockade of beta-adrenergic receptors. In general, the various agents have similar clinical efficacy.

Although much has been written about other pharmacologic properties including cardioselectivity, membrane stabilizing (local anesthetic) effects, intrinsic sympathomimetic (partial-agonist) activity, and lipid solubility, the clinical significance of these additional properties is small. Local anesthetic properties are most prominent with propranolol; however, membrane stabilization probably does not contribute substantially to the clinical utility. The various beta blockers do differ in their water and lipid solubility. The lipophilic agents (propranolol, metoprolol, oxprenolol) are readily absorbed from the gastrointestinal tract, metabolized by the liver, have large volumes of distribution, and penetrate the central nervous system well; the hydrophilic agents (acebutolol, atenolol, nadolol, sotalol) are less readily absorbed, not extensively metabolized, and have relatively long plasma half-lives. As a consequence, the hydrophilic agents may be administered once per day. Hepatic failure may prolong the plasma half-life of the lipophilic agents, and renal failure prolongs the action of the hydrophilic group. The degree of lipid solubility, therefore, may provide a basis for choice of a particular agent in patients with hepatic or renal insufficiency. Although the hydrophilic agents penetrate the central nervous system less well, central nervous system side effects (sedation, depression, hallucinations) probably occur as frequently with the hydrophilic as with the lipophilic agents.

Some beta-adrenergic blocking agents possess beta-agonist activity. This has been referred to as "intrinsic sympathomimetic activity" or "ISA." Agents with partial agonist activity (pindolol, alprenolol, oxprenolol) cause little or no depression of resting heart rate (partial agonist effect) while blocking the increase in heart rate that occurs in response to exercise or the administration of a beta agonist such as isoproterenol. The presence of partial agonist activity may be useful when bradycardia limits treatment in patients with slow resting heart rates. Although intrinsic sympathomimetic activity may also be useful in patients with depressed left ventricular function and reactive airways, no clear advantage of these agents over beta blockers without partial agonist activity has been demonstrated. Pindolol also produces mild vasodilation, perhaps in part related to peripheral $beta_2$ stimulation. On theoretical grounds intrinsic sympathomimetic activity would be undesirable in the treatment of thyrotoxicosis, idiopathic hypertrophic subaortic stenosis, and aortic dissection.

CARDIOSELECTIVE ($BETA_1$)-ADRENERGIC-RECEPTOR BLOCKING AGENTS Propranolol, the prototype of the nonselective beta-adrenergic blocking agent, induces a competitive blockade of both $beta_1$ and $beta_2$ receptors. Other nonselective beta blocking agents include alprenolol, nadolol, oxprenolol, pindolol, sotalol, and timolol. Metoprolol, acebutolol, and atenolol possess relative selectivity for the $beta_1$ receptor. Although $beta_1$ selective agents have the theoretical advantage of producing less bronchoconstriction and less peripheral vasoconstriction, a clear-cut clinical advantage of the cardioselective agents has not been demonstrated, since the $beta_1$ selectivity is only relative. Bronchoconstriction may occur when $beta_1$ selective agents are administered in full therapeutic doses.

ADVERSE EFFECTS OF BETA BLOCKING AGENTS Aside from the effects on the central nervous system, most adverse reactions to beta blocking agents are consequences of beta-adrenergic blockade. These include the precipitation of heart failure in patients in whom cardiac compensation depends upon enhanced sympathetic drive; the aggravation of bronchospasm in patients with asthma; predisposition to the development of hypoglycemia in insulin-requiring diabetics (blockade of catecholamine-mediated counterregulation and antagonism of the adrenergic warning signs of hypoglycemia); the development of hyperkalemia in diabetic or uremic patients with impaired potassium tolerance; and the enhancement of coronary or peripheral arterial vasospasm.

MISCELLANEOUS ADRENERGIC BLOCKING AGENTS *Labetalol,* approved for use in the United States as an antihypertensive agent, is a competitive antagonist of both alpha- and beta-adrenergic receptors. Although labetalol induces relatively more beta- than alpha-receptor blockade, fall in peripheral resistance may be marked following acute administration of the drug. Vasodilation may be mediated in part by a partial agonist effect on the $beta_2$-adrenergic receptor; labetalol does not possess partial agonist activity for the $beta_1$ (cardiac) receptor.

Metoclopramide is a dopaminergic antagonist with cholinergic agonist properties. It enhances gastric emptying, increases the tone of the lower esophageal sphincter, increases prolactin and aldosterone secretion, and antagonizes emesis induced by apomorphine. It is useful clinically in enhancing gastric emptying (in the absence of organic obstruction such as in diabetic gastroparesis), in antagonizing gastroesophageal reflux, and as an antiemetic during cancer chemotherapy.

THE PARASYMPATHETIC NERVOUS SYSTEM

ACETYLCHOLINE Acetylcholine (ACh) serves as the neurotransmitter at all autonomic ganglia, at the postganglionic parasympathetic nerve endings, and at the postganglionic sympathetic nerve endings innervating the eccrine sweat glands. The enzyme choline acetyltransferase catalyzes the synthesis of ACh from acetyl CoA produced within the nerve ending and from choline, actively taken up from the extracellular fluid. Within the cholinergic nerve endings ACh is stored in discrete synaptic vesicles and released in response to nerve impulses that depolarize the nerve terminals and increase calcium influx.

Cholinergic receptors Different receptors for ACh exist on the postganglionic neurons within the autonomic ganglia and at the postjunctional autonomic effector sites. Those within the autonomic ganglia and adrenal medulla are stimulated predominantly by nicotine (*nicotinic receptors*) and those on autonomic effector cells by the alkaloid muscarine (*muscarinic receptors*). Ganglionic blocking agents antagonize the nicotinic receptors while atropine blocks the muscarinic receptors. The muscarinic (M) receptor, furthermore, has been recently subdivided into two types. The M-1 receptor is localized to the central nervous system and perhaps parasympathetic ganglia; the M-2 receptor is the nonneuronal muscarinic receptor on smooth muscle, cardiac muscle, and glandular epithelium. Bethanechol is a selective agonist of the M-2 receptor; pirenzepine, an investigational agent, is a selective antagonist of the M-1 receptor. This agent markedly reduces gastric acid secretion. The second messengers for muscarinic effects may involve phosphatidylinositol and inhibition of adenylate cyclase activity.

Acetylcholinesterase Hydrolysis of ACh by acetylcholinesterase inactivates the neurotransmitter at cholinergic synapses. This enzyme (also known as specific or true cholinesterase) is present within neurons and is distinct from butyrocholinesterase (serum cholinesterase or pseudocholinesterase). The latter enzyme is present in plasma and nonneuronal tissues and is not primarily involved in the termination of the effects of ACh at autonomic effector sites. The pharmacologic effects of anticholinesterase agents are due to inhibition of neuronal (true) acetylcholinesterase.

PHYSIOLOGY OF THE PARASYMPATHETIC NERVOUS SYSTEM The parasympathetic nervous system participates in the regulation of the cardiovascular system, the gastrointestinal tract, and the genitourinary system. Tissues such as liver, kidney, pancreas, and thyroid also receive parasympathetic innervation, suggesting a role for the parasympathetic nervous system in metabolic regulation as well, although cholinergic effects on metabolism are not well characterized.

Cardiovascular system Parasympathetic effects on the heart are mediated by the vagus nerve. ACh reduces the rate of spontaneous depolarization of the sinoatrial node and decreases heart rate. The heart rate in different physiologic states is the result of coordinated interaction between sympathetic stimulation, parasympathetic inhibition, and the intrinsic activity of the sinoatrial pacemaker. ACh also delays impulse conduction within the atrial musculature while shortening the effective refractory period, a combination of factors which may initiate or perpetuate atrial arrhythmias. At the atrioventricular node ACh reduces conduction velocity, increases the effective refractory period, and thus diminishes the ventricular response during atrial flutter or fibrillation (Chap. 184). The decrease in inotropy induced by ACh is related to a prejunctional inhibitory effect on sympathetic nerve endings as well as to a direct inhibitory effect on the atrial myocardium. The ventricular myocardium is not much affected since innervation by cholinergic fibers is minimal. A direct cholinergic contribution to the regulation of peripheral resistance appears unlikely since parasympathetic innervation of the vasculature is not extensive. The parasympathetic nervous system, however, may influence peripheral resistance indirectly by inhibiting NE release from sympathetic nerves.

Gastrointestinal tract Parasympathetic innervation of the gut is via the vagus nerve and the pelvic sacral nerves. The parasympathetic nervous system increases the tone of gastrointestinal smooth muscle, enhances peristaltic activity, and relaxes the gastrointestinal sphincters. ACh stimulates exocrine secretion from the glandular epithelium and enhances the secretion of gastrin, secretin, and insulin.

Genitourinary and respiratory systems Sacral parasympathetic nerves supply the urinary bladder and genitalia. ACh increases ureteral peristalsis, contracts the urinary detrusor muscle, and relaxes the trigone and sphincter, thereby playing a critical role in the coordination of micturition. The respiratory tract is innervated with parasympathetic fibers derived from the vagus nerve. ACh increases tracheobronchial secretions and stimulates bronchial constriction.

PHARMACOLOGY OF THE PARASYMPATHETIC NERVOUS SYSTEM Cholinergic agonists ACh itself has no therapeutic role because of its widespread effects and short duration of action. Congeners of ACh are less susceptible to hydrolysis by cholinesterase and have a narrower range of physiologic effects. Bethanechol, the only systemic cholinergic agonist in general use, stimulates gastrointestinal and genitourinary smooth muscle with minimal effect on the cardiovascular system. It is used in the treatment of urinary retention in the absence of outflow tract obstruction and, less commonly, in gastrointestinal disorders such as postvagotomy gastric atony. Pilocarpine and carbachol are topical cholinergic agonists used in the treatment of glaucoma.

Acetylcholinesterase inhibitors Cholinesterase inhibitors enhance the effects of parasympathetic stimulation by diminishing the inactivation of ACh. The therapeutic application of reversible cholinesterase inhibitors depends upon the role of ACh as neurotransmitter at the skeletal muscle neuroeffector junction and within the central nervous system, and includes the treatment of myasthenia gravis (Chap. 358), the termination of neuromuscular blockade following general anesthesia, and the reversal of intoxication by agents with a central anticholinergic action. Physostigmine, a tertiary amine, penetrates the central nervous system well, while related quaternary amines (neostigmine, pyridostigmine, ambenonium, and edrophonium) do not. Organophosphorous cholinesterase inhibitors produce irreversible cholinesterase blockade; these agents are used principally as insecticides and are primarily of toxicologic interest. With regard to the autonomic nervous system, cholinesterase inhibitors are of limited use in the treatment of intestinal and bladder smooth-muscle dysfunction such as occurs in paralytic ileus and atonic urinary bladder. Cholinesterase inhibitors induce a vagotonic response in the heart and may be useful in terminating attacks of paroxysmal supraventricular tachycardia (Chap. 184).

Cholinergic-receptor blocking agents *Atropine* blocks muscarinic cholinergic receptors, with little effect on cholinergic transmission at the autonomic ganglia and the neuromuscular junctions. Many of the central nervous system actions of atropine and atropine-like drugs are attributable to blockade of central muscarinic synapses. The related alkaloid, *scopolamine,* is similar to atropine but causes drowsiness, euphoria, and amnesia, effects that make it suitable as a preanesthetic medication.

Atropine increases heart rate and enhances atrioventricular conduction, actions that may be useful in combating the bradycardia or heart block associated with heightened vagal tone. In addition, atropine reverses cholinergically mediated bronchoconstriction and diminishes respiratory tract secretions. These effects contribute to its utility as a preanesthetic medication.

Atropine also decreases gastrointestinal tract motility and secretion. Although various derivatives and congeners of atropine (such as *propantheline, isopropamide,* and *glycopyrrolate*) have been advocated in patients with peptic ulcer or with diarrheal syndromes, the chronic use of such agents is limited by other manifestations of parasympathetic inhibition such as dry mouth and urinary retention. The investigational selective M-1 inhibitor pirenzepine inhibits gastric secretion at doses that have minimal anticholinergic effects at other sites; this agent may be useful in the treatment of peptic ulcer. Atropine and its congener *ipratropium,* when given by inhalation, cause bronchodilation and have been used experimentally in the treatment of asthma.

REFERENCES

FRISHMAN WH: Beta-adrenoceptor antagonists: New drugs and new indications. N Engl J Med 305:500, 1981

———: Pindolol: A new B-adrenoceptor antagonist with partial agonist activity. N Engl J Med 308:940, 1983

INSEL PA: Identification and regulation of adrenergic receptors in target cells. Am J Physiol 247:E53, 1984

LANDSBERG L, YOUNG JB: Catecholamines and the adrenal medulla, in *Williams Textbook of Endocrinology,* 7th ed, JD Wilson, DW Foster (eds). Philadelphia, Saunders, 1985, p 891

———, ———: The influence of diet on the sympathetic nervous system, in *Neuroendocrine Perspective,* vol 4, EE Muller et al (eds). Amsterdam, Elsevier, 1985, p 191

LIMBIRD LE: GTP and Na+ modulate receptor-adenyl cyclase coupling and receptor-mediated function. Am J Physiol 247:E59, 1984

MOSES JW, BORER JS: Beta-adrenergic antagonists in the treatment of patients with heart disease. DM 27:1, 1981

WEINER N, TAYLOR P: Neurohumoral transmission: The autonomic and somatic motor nervous systems, in *The Pharmacologic Basis of Therapeutics,* 7th ed, AG Gilman et al (eds). New York, Macmillan, 1985, p 66

67 THE ADENYLATE CYCLASE SYSTEM

HENRY R. BOURNE

Cyclic 3′,5′-monophosphate (cyclic AMP) acts as an intracellular "second messenger" for a diverse array of peptide hormones and biogenic amines, drugs, and toxins. Consequently, an understanding of the adenylate cyclase system is essential for understanding the pathophysiology and management of many diseases. Investigation of the second messenger role of cyclic AMP advanced our understanding of endocrine, neural, and cardiovascular regulation. Conversely, research aimed at unraveling the biochemical basis of certain diseases has contributed to understanding the molecular mechanisms by which the synthesis of cyclic AMP is regulated.

BIOCHEMISTRY The enzymatic steps involved in the actions of hormones (first messengers) that work via cyclic AMP are depicted in Fig. 67-1, and the hormones that work via this mechanism are listed in Table 67-1. The actions of these hormones are initiated by binding to specific receptors on the external surface of the plasma membrane. The hormone-receptor complex activates the membrane-bound enzyme, adenylate cyclase, which synthesizes cyclic AMP from intracellular ATP. Within the cell cyclic AMP relays the hormonal message by combining with and activating its own receptor, cyclic AMP–dependent protein kinase. The activated protein kinase transfers the terminal phosphate of ATP to specific protein substrates (usually enzymes). Phosphorylation of these enzymes enhances (or in some cases, inhibits) their catalytic activities. Altered activities of these enzymes produce the characteristic effects of the hormone on its target cell.

A second class of hormones acts by binding to membrane receptors that inhibit adenylate cyclase. The action of these hormones, denoted H_i to distinguish them from stimulatory hormones (H_S), is described in more detail below. Figure 67-1 also shows an additional set of biochemical mechanisms that limit the action of cyclic AMP. These mechanisms may also be regulated by hormones. Such regulation allows fine tuning of cell function by additional neural and endocrine pathways.

Biologic role of cyclic AMP Each of the protein molecules involved in the intricate push-pull mechanisms of Fig. 67-1 represents a potential site for regulation of hormonal responsiveness, for therapeutic and toxic actions of drugs, and for pathologic alterations in disease. Specific instances of such interactions are discussed in later sections of this chapter. To set these in context, the general biologic functions of cyclic AMP as a second messenger should be considered. These functions are conveniently illustrated by reference to the regulation of the release of glucose from hepatic glycogen stores (the biochemical system in which cyclic AMP was discovered) by glucagon and other hormones.

TRANSDUCTION OF HORMONAL SIGNALS ACROSS THE PLASMA MEMBRANE The biologic stability and structural complexity of peptide hormones like glucagon make them useful carriers of diverse hormonal messages between cells but impair their ability to penetrate cell membranes. Hormone-sensitive adenylate cyclase allows the information content of the hormonal signal to cross the membrane, although the hormone itself may not.

AMPLIFICATION By binding to a few specific receptors (probably less than 1000 per cell), glucagon stimulates synthesis of a much larger number of cyclic AMP molecules. These cyclic AMP molecules stimulate cyclic AMP–dependent protein kinase, which causes activation of thousands of molecules of hepatic phosphorylase (the enzyme that limits glycogen breakdown) and the subsequent release of millions of glucose molecules from a single cell.

METABOLIC COORDINATION AT THE LEVEL OF A SINGLE CELL In addition to stimulating phosphorylase and causing degradation of glycogen to glucose, cyclic AMP–dependent protein phosphorylation simultaneously deactivates the enzyme that synthesizes glycogen (glycogen synthase) and stimulates enzymes responsible for hepatic gluconeogenesis. Thus, a single chemical signal, glucagon, mobilizes energy reserves via more than one metabolic pathway.

TRANSDUCTION OF DIVERSE MESSAGES INTO A SINGLE METABOLIC PROGRAM Because hepatic adenylate cyclase can be stimulated by epinephrine (acting through beta-adrenergic receptors) as well as glucagon, cyclic AMP allows regulation of hepatic carbohydrate metabolism by two chemically distinct hormones. If the second messenger did not exist, each of the regulatory enzymes involved in hepatic mobilization of carbohydrates would have to be able to recognize both glucagon and epinephrine.

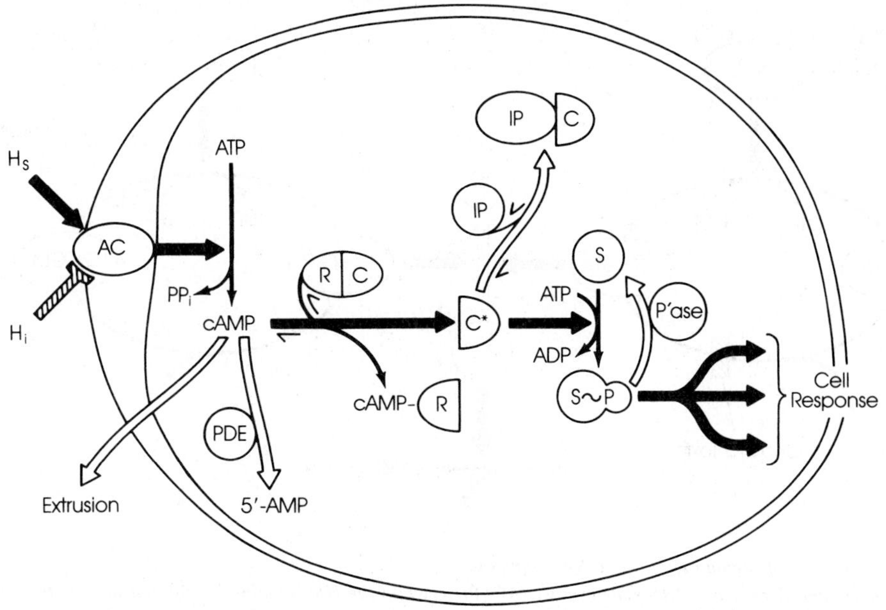

FIGURE 67-1 *Cyclic AMP as an intracellular second messenger for hormones. The diagram depicts an idealized cell containing the protein molecules (enzymes) involved in mediating actions of hormones that work via cyclic AMP. Filled arrows indicate the flow of information from stimulatory hormone (H_s) to cellular response, while open arrows indicate opposing processes that act to modulate or inhibit the flow of information. Extracellular hormones stimulate (H_s) or inhibit (H_i) the membrane enzyme, adenylate cyclase (AC), as described in the text and in Fig. 67-2. AC converts ATP into cyclic AMP (cAMP) and pyrophosphate (PP_i). The intracellular concentration of cyclic AMP depends upon a balance between its rate of synthesis and two processes that remove it from the cell: degradation by cyclic nucleotide phosphodiesterases (PDE), which convert cyclic AMP to 5′-AMP, and extrusion from the cell by an energy-dependent transport system. The intracellular actions of cyclic AMP are mediated or regulated by at least five additional classes of proteins. The first of these, the cyclic AMP–dependent protein kinases (RC), are composed of regulatory (R) and catalytic (C) subunits. In the RC holoenzyme the C subunit is catalytically inactive (inhibited by R). Cyclic AMP acts by binding to the R subunits, freeing C from the cyclic AMP-R complex. Free catalytic subunits (C*) catalyze transfer of the terminal phosphate of ATP to specific protein substrates (S), e.g., phosphorylase kinase. In the phosphorylated state (S~P) these substrate proteins (usually enzymes) initiate the characteristic actions of cyclic AMP within the cell (e.g., activation of glycogen phosphorylase, inhibition of glycogen synthase). The proportion of the kinase substrate proteins in the phosphorylated (S~P) state is regulated by two additional classes of proteins: Kinase inhibitor protein (IP) binds reversibly to C*, rendering it catalytically inactive (IP-C). Phosphatases (P′ase) recycle S~P back to S by removing covalently bound phosphate.*

COORDINATED REGULATION OF DIFFERENT CELLS AND TISSUES BY A FIRST MESSENGER In the classic "fight-or-flight" response to stress, catecholamines bind to beta-adrenergic receptors in heart, adipose tissue, blood vessels, and many other tissues including liver. If cyclic AMP were not available to mediate most of the responses to beta-adrenergic catecholamines (e.g., increased heart rate and contractility, dilatation of vessels supplying skeletal muscle, mobilization of energy from carbohydrate and lipid stores), a huge panoply of distinct enzymes in these tissues would have to possess specific binding sites for regulation by catecholamines.

Similar examples of the biologic functions of cyclic AMP could be adduced from the other first messengers listed in Table 67-1. Cyclic AMP acts as an intracellular mediator for each of these hormones, signifying their presence on the cell surface. Like all good mediators, cyclic AMP provides a simple, economical, and highly specific way of communicating diverse and complex messages.

HORMONE-SENSITIVE ADENYLATE CYCLASE The pivotal enzyme that mediates this system is hormone-sensitive adenylate cyclase. This enzyme is composed of at least five classes of separable proteins, each embedded in the lipid bilayer of the plasma membrane (Fig. 67-2).

Two classes of hormone receptors, R_s and R_i, are exposed on the outer surface of the cell membrane. They contain specific recognition sites for binding hormones that stimulate (H_s) or inhibit (H_i) adenylate cyclase.

The catalytic unit of adenylate cyclase (AC), exposed on the cytoplasmic face of the plasma membrane, converts intracellular ATP to cyclic AMP and pyrophosphate. Two classes of guanine nucleotide–binding regulatory proteins also face the cytoplasm. These proteins, G_s and G_i, mediate the stimulatory and inhibitory effects of R_s and R_i, respectively.

Both the stimulatory and inhibitory coupling functions of the G proteins depend upon their capacity to bind guanosine triphosphate (GTP) (Fig. 67-2). Only the GTP-bound forms of the G proteins

TABLE 67-1 Hormones that utilize cyclic AMP as a second messenger

Hormone	Target organ/tissue	Characteristic effect
Adrenocorticotropic hormone	Adrenal cortex	Cortisol production
Calcitonin	Bone	↓ Serum calcium
Catecholamines (beta-adrenergic)	Heart	↑ Rate, contractility
Chorionic gonadotropin	Ovary, testis	↑ Production of sex steroids
Follicle-stimulating hormone	Ovary, testis	↑ Gametogenesis
Glucagon	Liver	Glycogenolysis, release of glucose
Luteinizing hormone	Ovary, testis	↑ Production of sex steroids
Luteinizing hormone–releasing hormone	Pituitary	↑ Release of luteinizing hormone
Melanocyte-stimulating hormone	Skin (melanocytes)	↑ Pigmentation
Parathyroid hormone	Bone, kidney	↑ Serum calcium, ↓ serum phosphate
Prostacyclin, prostaglandin E_1	Platelets	↓ Platelet aggregation
Thyrotropin	Thyroid	↑ Production and release of T_3, T_4
Thyrotropin-releasing hormone	Pituitary	↑ Release of thyrotropin
Vasopressin	Kidney	↑ Concentration of urine

NOTE: *Only the best-documented cyclic AMP–mediated effects are listed here, although many of these hormones produce multiple effects in several target organs.*

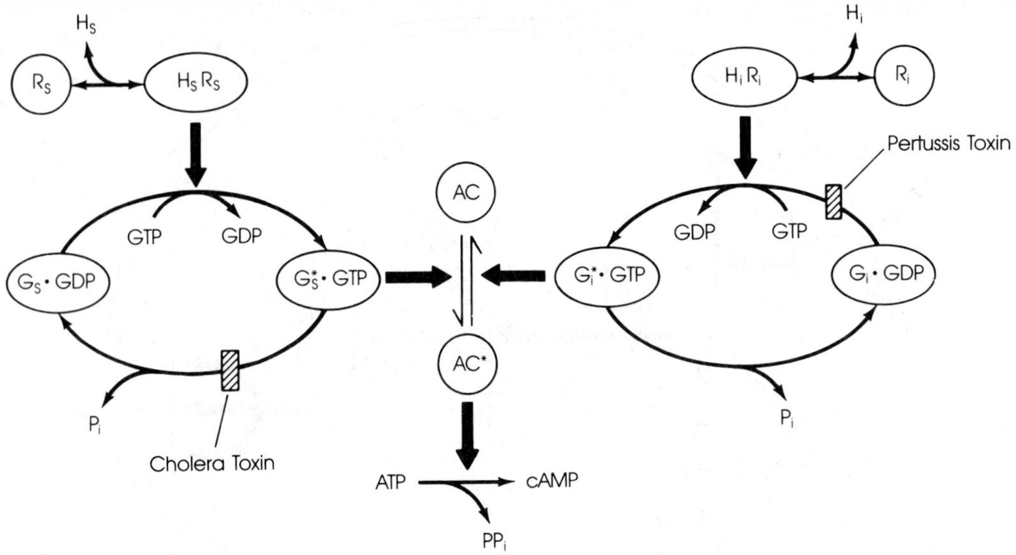

FIGURE 67-2 *Molecular mechanism of regulation of cyclic AMP synthesis by hormones, hormone receptors, and G proteins. Adenylate cyclase (AC) in its active form (AC*) converts ATP to cyclic AMP (cAMP) and pyrophosphate (PP_i). Activation and inhibition of AC are mediated by formally identical systems, shown on the left and right of the diagram. In each system the G protein oscillates between an inactive state, bound to GDP (G-GDP) and an active GTP-bound state (G*-GTP); only the active state of each protein can stimulate (G_s) or inhibit (G_i) AC activity. Each G-GTP complex possesses an intrinsic GTPase activity which converts it to the inactive G-GDP complex. In order to return the G protein to its active state, stimulatory or inhibitory hormone receptor complexes (H_sR_s and H_iR_i, respectively) promote replacement of GDP by GTP at the G protein's guanine nucleotide–binding site. Note that while the HR complex is required to initiate stimulation or inhibition of AC by G_s or G_i, hormone can dissociate from receptor independently of regulation of AC, which instead depends upon the duration of the GTP-bound state of the appropriate G protein, regulated by its intrinsic GTPase. Two bacterial toxins regulate adenylate cyclase activity by catalyzing ADP-ribosylation of the G proteins (see text). ADP-ribosylation of G_s by cholera toxin inhibits its GTPase activity, stabilizing G_s in its active state and thereby increasing cyclic AMP synthesis. In contrast, ADP-ribosylation of G_i by pertussis toxin prevents it from interacting with the H_iR_i complex and stabilizes G_i in the inactive GDP-bound state; as a result, pertussis toxin prevents hormonal inhibition of AC.*

regulate cyclic AMP synthesis. Neither stimulation nor inhibition of AC is permanent; instead, the terminal phosphate of GTP in each G-GTP complex is eventually hydrolyzed, and G_s-GDP or G_i-GDP cannot regulate AC. For this reason, sustained stimulation or inhibition of adenylate cyclase requires continued recycling of G-GDP to G-GTP. In both pathways, hormone-receptor complexes (H_sR_s or H_iR_i) promote the exchange of GDP for GTP. This recycling mechanism temporally and spatially separates the binding of hormones to receptors from the regulation of cyclic AMP synthesis, using the energy stored in the terminal phosphate bond of GTP to amplify the effects of hormone-receptor complexes.

This scheme explains how several different hormones can stimulate or inhibit cyclic AMP synthesis within a single cell. Because receptors are physically distinct from adenylate cyclase, the array of receptors expressed on a cell surface determines the cell's specific pattern of responsiveness to external chemical signals. An individual cell may express three or more different inhibitory receptors and six or more distinct stimulatory receptors. In contrast, all cells appear to contain similar (perhaps identical) G and AC components.

The molecular components of hormone-sensitive adenylate cyclase provide control points for changing the sensitivity of a given tissue to hormonal stimulation. Both R and G components are critical in physiologic regulation of hormonal sensitivity, and alterations of the G proteins are implicated as the primary lesion of four diseases discussed below.

Regulation of sensitivity to hormones (see also Chap. 66) Repeated administration of a hormone or drug often causes gradually increasing resistance to its effects. This phenomenon is variously termed desensitization, refractoriness, tachyphylaxis, or tolerance.

Hormones or neurotransmitters may induce desensitization that is receptor-specific or "homologous." For example, administration of beta-adrenergic catecholamines induces specific refractoriness of heart muscle to readministration of the same amines but not to drugs that do not act via beta-adrenergic receptors. Receptor-specific desensitization involves at least two separate mechanisms. The first, which develops rapidly (within minutes) and is rapidly reversed upon removal of the hormone, functionally "uncouples" receptors from G_s protein and therefore reduces their ability to stimulate adenylate cyclase. The second process involves actual reduction in the number of receptors on the cell membrane, a process termed *receptor down-regulation*. The down-regulation process may require hours to occur and is not readily reversible.

These desensitization processes are part of normal regulation. Removal of normal physiologic stimuli may result in increased sensitivity of a target tissue to pharmacologic stimulation, as in denervation supersensitivity. A potentially important clinical correlate of this increase in receptor number may occur in patients in whom therapy with propranolol, a beta-adrenergic blocking agent, is abruptly withdrawn. Such patients often have transient signs of elevated sympathetic tone (tachycardia, elevation of blood pressure, headaches, tremor, etc.) and may develop symptoms of coronary insufficiency. Peripheral blood leukocytes of subjects receiving propranolol exhibit elevated numbers of beta-adrenergic receptors, and receptor number returns slowly to normal when propranolol is withdrawn. Although the more numerous receptors in leukocytes do not mediate the cardiovascular symptoms and signs of propranolol withdrawal, receptors in myocardium and other tissues likely undergo similar changes.

Sensitivity of cells and tissues to hormones may also be regulated in a "heterologous" fashion—i.e., the sensitivity to one hormone is regulated by a second hormone, acting through a different set of receptors. Regulation of cardiovascular sensitivity to beta-adrenergic amines by thyroid hormones is the most prominent clinical example of heterologous regulation. Thyroid hormones cause an accumulation of an increased number of beta-adrenergic receptors in heart muscle. This increase in receptors partially accounts for the increased cardiac sensitivity of hyperthyroid patients to catecholamines. However, the fact that in experimental animals the increase in number of beta-adrenergic receptors produced by administration of thyroid hormones is not sufficient to account for the increased cardiac sensitivity to catecholamines suggests that thyroid hormones also affect components of the hormone response distal to receptors, possibly including, but not limited to, G_s. Other examples of heterologous regulation include control by estrogen and progesterone of uterine sensitivity to relaxation by beta-adrenergic agonists and the increased responsiveness of many tissues to epinephrine that is produced by glucocorticoids.

A second type of heterologous regulation involves inhibition of hormonal stimulation of adenylate cyclase by agents that act via R_i and G_i, as noted above. Acetylcholine, opiates, and alpha-adrenergic catecholamines act through distinct classes of inhibitory receptors (muscarinic, opioid, and alpha-adrenergic) to decrease the sensitivity of adenylate cyclase in certain tissues to stimulation by other hormones. Although the clinical importance of this type of heterologous regulation is not established, inhibition of cyclic AMP synthesis by morphine and other opiates could account for some aspects of tolerance to opiates. Similarly, relief of such inhibition may be involved in producing the syndrome that follows withdrawal of opiates.

Pseudohypoparathyroidism (see also Chap. 336) A genetic defect involving the G_s component of adenylate cyclase is the molecular basis of pseudohypoparathyroidism type I (PHP-I). This rare inherited disease is characterized by hypocalcemia and hyperphosphatemia, elevated serum parathyroid hormone (PTH), and resistance to the metabolic effects of exogenously administered PTH.

PTH regulates calcium homeostasis at least in part by stimulating adenylate cyclase in kidney and bone. Administration of PTH to normal subjects (and to patients with idiopathic or surgical hypoparathyroidism) causes greatly increased excretion of cyclic AMP in urine. In contrast, PTH causes little or no increase in the urinary cyclic AMP of PHP-I patients. This finding initially raised the possibility that PHP-I is caused by a defect in the PTH receptor, rendering it less capable of stimulating cyclic AMP synthesis.

A defect confined to the PTH receptor, however, could not account for the fact that many PHP-I patients are also partially resistant to other hormones, including thyrotropin (TSH), antidiuretic hormone, glucagon, and gonadotropins. Indeed, some PHP-I patients require replacement therapy for symptomatic hypothyroidism, because of thyroid resistance to TSH. Resistance to the action of the other hormones is for the most part clinically silent and can be detected only with specialized tests.

The fact that these hormones utilize cyclic AMP as a second messenger suggests that PHP-I is caused by a defect distal to hormone receptors, affecting some component common to all cyclic AMP–mediated responses. For many PHP-I patients that component is the G_s protein. Activity of G_s is reduced by about 50 percent in erythrocytes, platelets, and skin fibroblasts of most PHP-I patients. G_s activity was found to be reduced in the kidney of one PHP-I patient and is probably reduced in other endocrine target cells as well, including bone, thyroid, liver, etc.

If G_s deficiency is generalized in PHP-I, why are most of its important clinical consequences related to resistance to a single hormone, PTH? While this question cannot be answered with certainty, it is likely that most hormone responses mediated by cyclic AMP are maintained—in spite of partial G_s deficiency—by a variety of compensatory mechanisms, including elevation of circulating concentrations of the stimulating hormone. Elevated circulating PTH does not suffice to maintain normal calcium homeostasis in PHP-I, however, presumably because the actions of PTH are more critically dependent upon normal activity of G_s. Fortunately, the defect in PTH responsiveness can be bypassed by treatment with vitamin D, which restores serum calcium and phosphate to normal.

Cholera (see also Chap. 115) Elevated cyclic AMP in intestinal mucosal cells causes the massive secretion of water and electrolytes that results in the diarrhea of cholera. Pathogenic *Vibrio cholerae* produce a protein exotoxin that can stimulate cyclic AMP synthesis in virtually all animal cells. The clinical disease is limited to intestinal mucosa because the toxin is not absorbed from the gastrointestinal tract, and other tissues are thus not accessible to the toxin produced by bacteria growing in the intestinal lumen.

Unlike stimulation of adenylate cyclase by hormones, the effect of cholera toxin is slow in onset and does not disappear immediately when the toxin is removed. The reason for this difference is that cholera toxin does not act by reversible binding to a stimulatory receptor but instead acts as an enzyme, producing a stable covalent modification of the G_s protein component of adenylate cyclase. Following binding of the toxin to cells, one of its peptide subunits penetrates the cell membrane, where it catalyzes ADP-ribosylation of G_s, using intracellular nicotinamide adenine dinucleotide (NAD^+) as a substrate:

$$G_s + NAD^+ \xrightarrow{\text{toxin}} G_s\text{-ADP-ribose} + \text{nicotinamide} + H^+$$

ADP-ribosylation of G_s increases cyclic AMP synthesis, apparently by decreasing the rate of hydrolysis of GTP in the G_s-GTP-C complex that synthesizes cyclic AMP (Fig. 67-2).

This biochemical mechanism may explain why the diarrhea of cholera can be produced by a relatively small number of pathogenic organisms and why the diarrhea can persist after the organisms have been eradicated. The first phenomenon stems from the fact that the toxin is an enzyme, so that small numbers of toxin molecules suffice to ADP-ribosylate a substantial fraction of the G_s molecules in a cell. Persistently elevated cyclic AMP synthesis after removal of the toxin, at least in experimental studies, correlates with stability of G_s-ADP-ribose. Most cells apparently lack enzymes capable of removing ADP-ribose from G_s, so that the effect of the toxin disappears only when the G_s-ADP-ribose molecules are replaced by newly synthesized G_s molecules. Recovery from the clinical disease may even require replacement of the mucosal cells themselves. Elucidation of the molecular basis for the action of cholera toxin served as a valuable tool in the discovery and characterization of G_s and advanced our understanding of the biochemical basis of hormone action.

Pertussis (see also Chap. 109) The molecular pathogenesis of pertussis in bronchi closely parallels that of cholera in the gut. Neither organism invades tissues; instead, both cause disease by producing exotoxins that alter cyclic AMP synthesis in host cells. *Bordetella pertussis* secretes two pathogenic exotoxins: The molecular target of one, termed pertussis toxin, is the inhibitory guanine nucleotide–binding protein of adenylate cyclase, G_i. The other toxin is itself an adenylate cyclase molecule.

Like cholera toxin, pertussis toxin catalyzes transfer of ADP-ribose from NAD^+ to a membrane protein; in this case, the protein is G_i. The ADP-ribosylated form of G_i is unable to interact with R_i (Fig. 67-2); as a result, pertussis toxin prevents inhibition of adenylate cyclase by inhibitory ligands such as muscarinic, alpha-adrenergic, and opiate agonists.

The key bronchial target cells for pertussis toxin and the molecular pathways that link ADP-ribosylation of G_i to signs and symptoms of the disease are largely unknown. The ADP-ribosylation reaction does, however, provide an explanation for one puzzle: Antibiotic treatment of pertussis infection does little to limit intensity and duration of disease; indeed, symptoms can persist for 3 weeks or more after organisms have disappeared from the tracheobronchial tree. ADP-ribosylation of G_i (like that of G_s, as described above) is not readily reversible by cellular enzymes. Probably, the disease persists, even in the absence of additional toxin, until the modified G_i proteins or the cells that contain them have been replaced.

The second pathogenic product of *B. pertussis,* adenylate cyclase toxin, remains enzymatically inert until it enters host cells. There it is activated by binding to calmodulin, with a resulting profound elevation of cellular cyclic AMP. Unlike the effect of pertussis toxin, that of the adenylate cyclase toxin rapidly disappears when the source of the toxin is removed; cellular enzymes degrade the bacterial enzyme, and cellular cyclic AMP rapidly returns to normal.

While most of the links between molecular actions of these toxins and the resulting disease are poorly understood, in vitro experiments show that both toxins can interfere with function of human neutrophils—cells that play a crucial role in defense against infection. Cyclic AMP accumulation caused by the adenylate cyclase toxin impairs the neutrophil's ability to kill ingested microorganisms. Pertussis toxin, by ADP-ribosylating G_i or G_i-like molecule, blocks neutrophil responses (chemotaxis, release of lysosomal hydrolases, etc.) to complement and other chemotactic factors. Either or both of these effects could contribute to increased susceptibility to pulmonary infection by other organisms, a frequent complication of pertussis infection.

Aside from their role as tools for exploring transduction of hormonal signals, knowledge of these toxins can produce real clinical dividends. Although the present practice of immunizing with extracts of whole pertussis organisms effectively prevents infection, the immunization itself produces considerable morbidity. Pertussis organisms specifically incapable of producing either of the two toxins are rendered harmless to animal hosts. Accordingly, immunization with purified toxin preparations should prevent disease and may reduce the morbidity of immunization. Results of preliminary clinical trials support both predictions.

Anthrax (see also Chap. 98) Cutaneous infection by *Bacillus anthracis* produces a characteristic lesion, with central necrosis surrounded by prominent subcutaneous edema. While the necrotic lesion appears not to involve the cyclic AMP system, the organism's "edema factor" is in fact adenylate cyclase. Like the adenylate cyclase toxin of pertussis, edema factor gains access to host cells, is activated by cellular calmodulin, and increases intracellular cyclic AMP. Interestingly, there are rare instances of patients who ingest anthrax organisms and develop a watery diarrhea indistinguishable from cholera. Diarrhea in such instances probably results from penetration of edema factor into cells of the intestinal mucosa, with resulting cyclic AMP elevation and secretion of salt and water.

CYCLIC AMP IN CLINICAL MEDICINE A large number of hormones and neurotransmitters act by stimulating adenylate cyclase, and several pharmacologic antagonists act by blocking their binding to specific receptors—e.g., propranolol at beta-adrenergic receptors and cimetidine at H_2-histamine receptors. The therapeutic actions of these agents depend upon elevations or decreases in cyclic AMP content of target cells and tissues in patients. In addition, the methylxanthines (caffeine and theophylline) block cyclic nucleotide phosphodiesterases and may produce some of their therapeutic effects (e.g., bronchodilatation) by elevating cellular cyclic AMP.

In clinical practice, measurements of cyclic AMP in the urine are useful in diagnosing disorders that involve PTH and calcium homeostasis. A substantial fraction of urinary cyclic AMP is made in proximal tubular cells responding to circulating PTH. Thus, urinary cyclic AMP provides a convenient "window" for assessing effects of PTH on the kidney and can reflect elevated PTH (in hyperparathyroidism), decreased PTH (in hypoparathyroidism), or end-organ resistance to PTH (in PHP-I) (see Chap. 336).

At present, however, the real importance of cyclic AMP for medicine is as a tool in understanding normal and pathologic regulation and in developing new drugs. Adenylate cyclase assays are now routinely used to screen new compounds for their ability to stimulate or block adrenergic, histaminergic, and many peptide receptors. Hormone receptors are not the only critical and specific control points in regulation mediated by cyclic AMP; it seems likely that the other proteins depicted in Fig. 67-1 will serve as targets of future therapeutic agents.

OTHER SECOND MESSENGERS Although cyclic AMP is the most thoroughly studied hormonal second messenger, some hormones act by increasing intracellular concentrations of other chemical signals, including calcium ion and cyclic guanosine 3′,5′-monophosphate (cyclic GMP). Certain effects of alpha-adrenergic and cholinergic (muscarinic) agents, for example, appear to be mediated by elevated cytoplasmic concentrations of calcium. Many cell types contain guanylate cyclase, cyclic GMP phosphodiesterases, and protein kinases that are specifically stimulated by cyclic GMP. Nonetheless, the role of this second cyclic nucleotide in normal and pathologic regulation is not well defined.

REFERENCES

Farfel Z et al: Pseudohypoparathyroidism: Inheritance of deficient receptor-cyclase coupling activity. Proc Natl Acad Sci USA 78:3098, 1981

Gilman AG: Guanine nucleotide–binding regulatory proteins and dual control of adenylate cyclase. J Clin Invest 73:1, 1984

Leppla SH et al: Anthrax toxin edema factor: A bacterial adenylate cyclase that increases cyclic AMP concentrations in eukaryotic cells. Proc Natl Acad Sci USA 79:3162, 1982

Weiss AA et al: Pertussis toxin and extra-cytoplasmic adenylate cyclase as virulence factors of *Bordetella pertussis*. J Infect Dis 150:219, 1984

68 ARACHIDONIC ACID METABOLITES RELEVANT TO MEDICINE

R. PAUL ROBERTSON

This chapter focuses on the formation and mechanism of action of the physiologically active metabolites of arachidonic acid and on the biologic phenomena in which these compounds may be involved.

FORMATION OF THE EICOSANOIDS Prostaglandins, the first arachidonic acid metabolites to be recognized, were so named because they were originally identified in seminal fluid and thought to be secreted by the prostate. As other active metabolites were characterized, two major pathways—the cyclooxygenase and the lipoxygenase pathways—became apparent. These synthetic pathways are summarized schematically in Fig. 68-1, and structures of representative metabolites are shown in Fig. 68-2. All products of both the cyclooxygenase and the lipoxygenase pathways are called *eicosanoids*. The products of the cyclooxygenase pathway—the prostaglandins and the thromboxanes—are termed *prostanoids*.

The initial synthetic step for both pathways involves the cleavage of arachidonic acid from phospholipid in the plasma membrane of cells. Free arachidonic acid can then be oxygenated by the cyclooxygenase or lipoxygenase pathway. The first product of the cyclooxygenase pathway is the cyclic endoperoxide prostaglandin G_2 (PGG_2), which is converted to prostaglandin H_2 (PGH_2). PGG_2 and PGH_2 are the key intermediates in the formation of physiologically active prostaglandins (PGD_2, PGE_2, $PGF_{2\alpha}$, and PGI_2) and thromboxane A_2 (TXA_2). The first product of the 5-lipoxygenase pathway is 5-hydroperoxyeicosatetraenoic acid (5-HPETE) which is an intermediate in the formation of 5-hydroxyeicosatetraenoic acid (5-HETE) and the leukotrienes (LTA_4, LTB_4, LTC_4, LTD_4, and LTE_4). Two fatty acids other than arachidonic acid [3,11,14-eicosatrienoic acid (dihomo-γ-linolenic acid) and 5,8,11,14,17-eicosapentaenoic acid] can be converted to metabolites closely related to these eicosanoids. Prostanoid products of the former substrate carry the subscript 1; the leukotriene subscript is 3. Prostanoid products of the latter substrate have the subscript 3 while leukotrienes have the subscript 5. Arachidonic acid forms prostaglandin products with subscripts 2 and leukotrienes with the subscript 4. (The subscripts designate the number of double bonds between carbon atoms in the side chains.)

Virtually all cells have the necessary substrates and enzymes to form some of the metabolites of arachidonic acid, but tissues differ in the enzymes they possess and consequently in the products they form. Eicosanoids are synthesized according to immediate need and are not stored in significant amounts for later release.

The cyclooxygenase products Prostaglandins D_2, E_2, $F_{2\alpha}$, and I_2 are formed from the cyclic endoperoxides PGG_2 and PGH_2. Of these, PGE_2 and PGI_2 exert the broadest physiologic effects. PGE_2 has notable effects in, and is synthesized by, many tissues. PGI_2 (also called prostacyclin) is a dominant product of arachidonic acid in the endothelial and smooth muscle cells of vessel walls and in some nonvascular tissues. PGI_2 is a vasodilator and an inhibitor of platelet

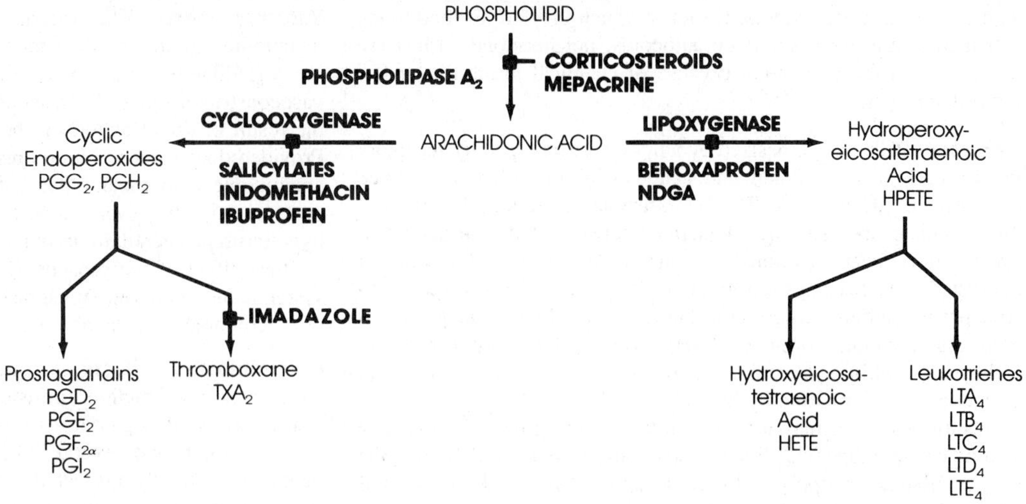

FIGURE 68-1 *The overall scheme of arachidonic acid metabolism. The various drugs act at the various enzymatic steps to inhibit the reactions. The major pathways are the cyclooxygenase and the lipoxygenase pathways. Phospholipase A_2 is inhibited by corticosteroids and mepacrine; cyclooxygenase is inhibited by certain salicylates, indomethacin, and ibuprofen; and lipoxygenase is inhibited by benoxaprofen and nordihydroguaiaretic acid (NDGA). Imidazole prevents TXA_2 synthesis.*

aggregation. PGD_2 is also believed to play a role in platelet aggregation and brain function. $PGF_{2\alpha}$ plays a role in uterine and ovarian function.

Thromboxane synthetase catalyzes the incorporation of an oxygen atom into the ring of the endoperoxide PGH_2 to form the thromboxanes. TXA_2 is synthesized by platelets and enhances platelet aggregation.

The lipoxygenase products The leukotrienes and HETE are the end products of the lipoxygenase pathway. The leukotrienes have histamine-like actions, including induction of increased vascular permeability and of bronchospasm, and appear to have mediator activities for leukocytes. LTC_4, LTD_4, and LTE_4 together have been identified as slow-reacting substance of anaphylaxis (SRS-A). (The pathophysiology of the leukotrienes is discussed in detail in Chap. 202.)

EFFECTS OF DRUGS ON THE SYNTHESIS OF EICOSANOIDS

Many drugs block the synthesis of eicosanoids by inhibiting one or more enzymes in their biosynthetic pathways. Glucocorticoids and antimalarial drugs such as mepacrine interfere with the cleavage of arachidonic acid from phospholipids (Fig. 68-1). Cyclooxygenase is directly inhibited by nonsteroidal anti-inflammatory drugs including salicylates, indomethacin, and ibuprofen. Benoxaprofen, another nonsteroidal anti-inflammatory drug, inhibits the lipoxygenase-mediated conversion of arachidonic acid to HPETE. Tranylcypromine, an antidepressant drug, inhibits the conversion of cyclic endoperoxides to PGI_2, and imidazole inhibits thromboxane synthesis. The fact that a drug inhibits the synthesis of a certain eicosanoid does not mean that a given drug effect is the direct result of a deficiency of that eicosanoid. Most of these drugs inhibit early reactions in the synthetic pathways and therefore block the formation of more than one product. Additionally, some of these drugs have other effects. For example, indomethacin not only inhibits formation of cyclic endoperoxides by cyclooxygenase but may also disrupt calcium flux across membranes, inhibit cyclic adenosine monophosphate (cyclic AMP)–dependent protein kinase and phosphodiesterase, and inhibit one of the enzymes responsible for degradation of PGE_2.

No truly specific synthesis inhibitors nor specific receptor antagonists for individual arachidonic acid metabolites are suitable for human use. The lack of such drugs is a major barrier to elucidating the role of these metabolites in physiologic and pathophysiologic processes.

METABOLISM AND ASSAY OF EICOSANOIDS

Arachidonic acid metabolites are catabolized rapidly in vivo. Prostaglandins of the E and F series, although chemically stable, are almost completely degraded during a single passage through the liver or the lung. Thus, essentially all nonmetabolized PGE_2 measurable in urine is derived from renal and seminal vesicle secretion, whereas PGE_2 metabolites in urine represent total-body PGE_2 synthesis. PGI_2 and TXA_2 are both chemically unstable and also rapidly catabolized. Because PGE_2, PGI_2, and TXA_2 are short-lived in vivo, measurement of their inactive metabolites is commonly used as an index of the rates of their formation. PGE_2 is converted to 15-keto-13,14,-dihydro-PGE_2, PGI_2 is converted to 6-keto-$PGF_{1\alpha}$, and TXA_2 is converted to TXB_2. Five methods are available to measure arachidonic acid metabolites in physiologic fluids: bioassay, radioimmunoassay, chromatography, receptor assay, and mass spectrometry. With each method certain precautions must be taken in handling samples because prostaglandin synthesis may be enhanced during the collection of biologic samples. For example, if blood is allowed to clot or if platelets are not carefully separated from plasma, the generation of large amounts of PGE_2 and TXA_2 during processing can lead to erroneous results. Use of an inhibitor of prostaglandin synthesis in the collection tube minimizes this problem.

PHYSIOLOGY

Prostaglandins and leukotrienes have specific receptor sites on the plasma membranes of cells such as liver, corpus luteum, adrenal gland, adipocytes, thymocytes, uterus, pancreatic islets, platelets, and red blood cells. Most of the binding sites exhibit specificity for eicosanoids of a given type. For example, the liver plasma membrane PGE receptor binds PGE_1 and PGE_2 with high affinity but not prostaglandins of the A, F, and I configurations. The postreceptor mechanisms by which the binding of the prostaglandins alters cell function are poorly understood. The normal physiologic actions of eicosanoids are not mediated via the plasma. Instead, eicosanoids act as local, intercellular, and/or intracellular modulators

FIGURE 68-2 *Structures of representative biologically active eicosanoids.*

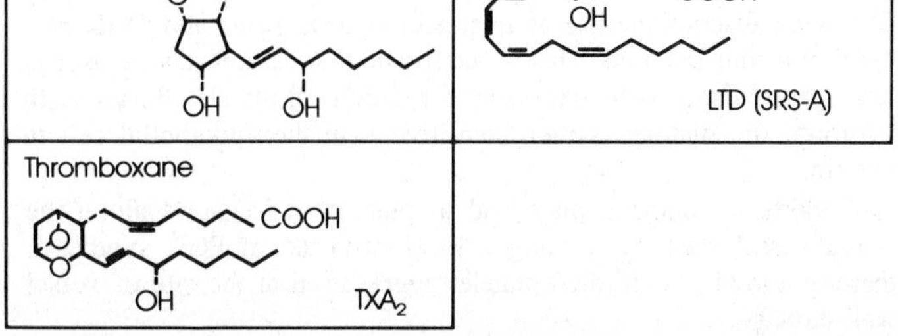

of biochemical activity in the tissues in which they are formed (e.g., a paracrine function). They are autocoids, not hormones. Most are short-lived in the circulation because of chemical instability and/or rapid degradation.

Lipolysis PGE_2 is synthesized by adipocytes, has specific receptors in adipocytes, and is a potent endogenous inhibitor of lipolysis. Since the formation of cyclic AMP is necessary in the action of hormones that stimulate lipolysis, the interactions between PGE and adenylate cyclase have been examined in considerable detail. PGE inhibits lipolysis by decreasing the formation of cyclic AMP in response to epinephrine, adrenocorticotropic hormone (ACTH), glucagon, and thyroid-stimulating hormone (TSH). Thus, PGE may act as an endogenous antilipolytic substance by interfering with the stimulation of cyclic AMP formation by hormones.

Insulin and PGE may act independently during their antilipolytic actions on the adipocyte. For example, insulin but not PGE inhibits the stimulation of lipolysis by exogenous cyclic AMP in isolated adipocytes, but both agents inhibit hormone-stimulated generation of cyclic AMP. This suggests a site of action of insulin distal to the stimulation of adenylate cyclase. In some animals PGE inhibits glucagon-induced lipolysis whereas insulin does not.

Sodium and water balance The renin-angiotensin-aldosterone system is a major regulator of sodium homeostasis, and vasopressin exerts the principal control over water balance. Arachidonic acid metabolites influence both systems. PGE_2 and PGI_2 stimulate renin secretion, and inhibitors of prostaglandin synthesis have the opposite effect. PGI_2 and PGE_2 decrease renal vascular resistance and increase blood flow; this results in redistribution of blood flow from the outer renal cortex to the juxtamedullary region of the kidney. Conversely, inhibitors of prostaglandin synthesis, such as indomethacin and meclofenamate, decrease total renal blood flow and shunt the remaining flow to the outer cortex, which can lead to acute renal venoconstriction and acute renal failure in circumstances such as volume depletion and edematous states. PGE_2 is natriuretic whereas cyclooxygenase inhibitors cause sodium and water retention.

Indomethacin also increases sensitivity to exogenous vasopressin in dogs. Conversely, PGE_2 decreases vasopressin-stimulated water transport. Since this effect of PGE_2 is circumvented by the administration of dibutyryl–cyclic AMP, PGE_2 most likely interferes with the stimulation of adenylate cyclase by vasopressin.

Platelet aggregation Platelets synthesize PGE_2, PGD_2, and TXA_2. Although a physiologic role has not been established for PGE_2 and PGD_2 in platelet function, TXA_2 is a potent stimulator of platelet aggregation; in contrast PGI_2, formed by the endothelial cells of blood vessel walls, is a potent antagonist of platelet aggregation. TXA_2 and PGI_2 may exert their opposing effects by decreasing and increasing, respectively, platelet generation of cyclic AMP.

Inhibitors of endogenous prostaglandin synthesis interfere with platelet aggregation. For example, a single dose of aspirin can suppress normal platelet aggregation for 48 h and longer, presumably by suppressing cyclooxygenase-mediated TXA_2 synthesis. Cyclooxygenase inhibition by a single dose of aspirin is of longer duration in platelets than in other tissues, because the platelet, in contrast to nucleated cells that can synthesize new proteins, does not have the machinery to form new enzyme. Consequently, the effect of aspirin persists until newly formed platelets have been released. Endothelial cells, on the other hand, rapidly recover cyclooxygenase activity following discontinuation of treatment with aspirin, and PGI_2 production is thus restored. This is one reason that patients taking aspirin are not predisposed to excessive formation of platelet thrombi. In addition, the platelet is more sensitive than the endothelial cell to aspirin.

Endothelial damage may lead to platelet aggregation along the blood vessel wall by causing a local decrease in PGI_2 synthesis, thereby allowing unbridled platelet aggregation at the site of vessel wall damage.

Vascular effects The vasoactive properties of arachidonic acid metabolites are among their most impressive actions. PGE_2 and PGI_2 are vasodilators where $PGF_{2\alpha}$, TXA_2, and LTC_4-LTD_4-LTE_4 are vasoconstrictors in most vascular beds. These effects appear to be the result of direct action on the smooth muscle of the vessel wall. Provided that systemic blood pressure is maintained, the vasodilatory arachidonic acid metabolites act to increase blood flow. If blood pressure falls, however, blood flow decreases because with systemic hypotension catecholamine-induced vasoconstriction offsets the vasodilatory effect of the prostaglandins. Thus, significant alterations in systemic blood pressure must be excluded when evaluating the effects of arachidonic acid metabolites on organ blood flow.

Gastrointestinal effects Prostaglandins of the E series influence gastrointestinal function. Infusion of either PGI_2 or PGE_2 into the gastric artery of dogs causes increases in blood flow and inhibition of acid output, and several PGE analogues both inhibit gastric acid output and directly protect the gastrointestinal mucosa when taken orally. In in vitro experiments prostaglandins stimulate gastrointestinal smooth muscle and thereby increase motility, but it is not clear whether these actions are physiologically important.

Neurotransmission PGE inhibits egress of norepinephrine from sympathetic nerve terminals. The effect of PGE on norepinephrine secretion appears to be prejunctional, i.e., at a site on the nerve terminal proximal to the synaptic cleft, and can be reversed by increases in calcium concentration in the perfusing medium. Therefore, PGE_2 may inhibit norepinephrine release by blocking calcium influx. Inhibitors of PGE_2 synthesis can augment norepinephrine release in response to stimulation of adrenergic nerves.

Catecholamines can release PGE_2 from a variety of tissues, probably by an alpha-adrenergic–mediated mechanism. For example, in innervated tissues such as the spleen, nerve stimulation or injection of norepinephrine causes release of PGE_2. This release is blocked after denervation or administration of alpha-adrenergic blockers. Thus, a stimulus that activates the nerve causes release of norepinephrine, which in turn stimulates synthesis and release of PGE_2; PGE_2 then feeds back at the prejunctional level of the nerve terminal to decrease the amount of norepinephrine released.

Pancreatic endocrine function PGE_2 has both stimulatory and inhibitory effects on insulin secretion by the pancreatic beta cell in vitro. In vivo, insulin responses to intravenous glucose in humans are inhibited by PGE_2. This inhibitory effect appears to be specific for glucose because the insulin responses to other secretagogues are not influenced by PGE_2. Studies with inhibitors of prostaglandin synthesis support the concept that endogenous PGE_2 acts in vivo to inhibit insulin secretion. In general, such drugs augment insulin secretion and improve carbohydrate tolerance. An exception is indomethacin, which inhibits glucose-induced insulin secretion and can cause hyperglycemia. The discordant results with indomethacin are likely due to some action other than inhibition of cyclooxygenase. The lipoxygenase pathway appears to play a role in potentiating insulin secretion by participating in stimulus-secretion coupling. In this case a likely active arachidonic acid product may be 12-HPETE.

Luteolysis In the sheep hysterectomy during the luteal phase of the ovarian cycle results in maintenance of the corpus luteum, suggesting that the uterus normally produces a luteolytic substance. A candidate for this substance is $PGF_{2\alpha}$ since it can cause luteal regression.

PATHOPHYSIOLOGY Most postulated roles for arachidonic acid metabolites in disease involve excessive production, but a few disorders may be the result of decreased production. The latter could result from dietary deficiency of arachidonic acid (an essential fatty acid), from damage to a tissue required for prostaglandin synthesis, or from therapy with drugs that inhibit enzymes in the synthetic pathway.

Bone resorption: Hypercalcemia of malignancy (also see Chaps. 303 and 336) Hypercalcemia occurs in association with nonparathyroid malignancies of many different types. Parathyroid hormone excess, as the result either of autonomous production by parathyroid tissue or ectopic formation by the tumor itself, causes a portion of these cases. However, most patients with hypercalcemia of malignancy do not have elevated plasma levels of parathyroid hormone, and the etiology of the hypercalcemia has been the subject of considerable interest.

Prostaglandin E_2 is a potent inducer of bone resorption and of calcium release from bone, and PGE_2 production is elevated in certain hypercalcemic animals with transplantable tumors. Treatment of these animals with inhibitors of PGE_2 synthesis causes reduction of PGE_2 levels and a concomitant decrease in hypercalcemia. Likewise, some patients with hypercalcemia and malignancy have excessive amounts of PGE_2 metabolites in urine, whereas equally elevated levels do not occur in normocalcemic patients with otherwise similar malignancies. Drugs that inhibit prostaglandin synthesis decrease circulating calcium levels in some patients with hypercalcemia of malignancy. Thus, a subset of approximately 5 to 10 percent of patients with hypercalcemia and malignancy have elevated PGE production and can be treated with drugs that inhibit prostaglandin synthesis.

The source of the excess PGE_2 in these patients has not been identified. Increased liver and lung degradation of PGE would be expected to compensate if large amounts of PGE were present in the circulation. It is possible, of course, that such large amounts of PGE_2 are released by a tumor into the circulation that liver and lung degradation cannot handle the load. Alternatively, if lung metastases are present, the venous drainage from the tumors could be delivered into the systemic circulation without passing through lung tissue. A third possible mechanism involves metastatic seeding of bone. Tumor cells synthesize PGE in culture, and metastatic tumor cells in bone could synthesize PGE that acts locally to cause bone resorption. Hypercalcemia of malignancy can occur in the absence of demonstrable bone metastases, but the clinical tools for excluding such metastases, such as radioisotope scans, may not be sensitive enough to detect many small lesions.

Bone resorption: Rheumatoid arthritis and dental cysts (see Chap. 263) Overproduction of PGE_2 has been postulated as a cause of the juxtaarticular osteoporosis and bony erosions in some patients with rheumatoid arthritis. Rheumatoid synovia synthesize PGE_2 in tissue culture, and media from these cultures promote bone resorption; moreover, the inclusion of indomethacin in the culture medium blocks this resorptive capacity. Since indomethacin does not prevent bone resorption due to preformed PGE_2, the PGE_2 produced by the synovia is presumed to be responsible for the resorptive activity.

Cells from benign dental cysts also cause bone resorption and synthesize PGE_2 in tissue culture. Again, bone resorption caused by the culture medium from such cells is decreased if indomethacin is added prior to the incubation. A related problem is that of alveolar bone resorption in patients with periodontal disease, a common inflammatory disease of the gums. PGE_2 levels in inflamed gingiva are greater than in healthy gingival tissue. Thus, it is possible that alveolar resorption might be due, in part at least, to local overproduction of these metabolites.

Bartter's syndrome (see Chap. 228) Bartter's syndrome is characterized by elevated levels of plasma renin, aldosterone, and bradykinin; resistance to the pressor effect of angiotensin; hypokalemic alkalosis; and renal potassium wasting in the presence of normal blood pressure. The basis for the postulated role of prostaglandins in the disorder is that PGE_2 and PGI_2 stimulate the release of renin and that the pressor response to infused angiotensin is blunted by the vasodilator effects of PGE_2 and PGI_2. The increase in renin release leads to increased aldosterone secretion, which in turn can increase urinary kallikrein activity.

In keeping with this postulate, elevated levels of PGE_2 and 6-keto-$PGF_{1\alpha}$ are present in urine of patients with the syndrome. Hyperplasia of renal medullary interstitial cells (which synthesize PGE in culture) has also been demonstrated. These findings led to therapeutic trials of inhibitors of prostaglandin synthesis in the disorder. Indomethacin (and other inhibitors) reverse virtually all the abnormalities except hypokalemia. Thus, a prostaglandin, probably PGE_2 and/or PGI_2, probably mediates some of the manifestations of Bartter's syndrome.

Diabetes mellitus (see Chap. 327) Intravenous administration of large amounts of glucose to normal individuals causes a sudden (first-phase) increase in secretion of insulin into plasma followed by a slower, more prolonged response termed second-phase insulin secretion. Patients with type II (non-insulin-dependent, adult-onset) diabetes mellitus have absent first-phase insulin release in response to glucose and a variable decrease in second-phase insulin secretion. Insulin response to other secretagogues, such as arginine, isoproterenol, glucagon, and secretin, is preserved. Thus, diabetics appear to have a specific defect that interferes with normal perception of glucose signals. Since PGE inhibits glucose-induced insulin secretion in normal individuals, inhibitors of endogenous prostaglandin synthesis have been given to patients with type II diabetes mellitus to ascertain whether insulin secretion can be improved. Both sodium salicylate and aspirin elevate basal plasma insulin levels, partially restore the first-phase insulin response, increase second-phase insulin secretion, and improve glucose tolerance.

Patent ductus arteriosus (see Chap. 185) The ductus arteriosus in sheep is sensitive to the vasodilatory properties of PGE_2, and PGE-like material is present in the ductal wall. Thus, enhanced endogenous PGE_2 might maintain prenatal patency of the ductus. Since inhibitors of prostaglandin synthesis cause constriction of the ductus of fetal lambs, trials with indomethacin were undertaken in premature human infants with isolated patent ductus arteriosus. Such treatment for several days is followed by closure of the vessel in the majority, although some require a second course of therapy, and a minority require surgical ligation. Infants under 35 weeks of gestational age are most likely to respond.

Patients with certain types of congenital heart disease require a patent ductus arteriosus to survive. Ductus-dependent pulmonary blood flow is essential under circumstances in which the ductus is the major channel by which nonoxygenated blood reaches the lungs from the aortic arch, for example, in pulmonary atresia and tricuspid atresia. Since PGE relaxes the smooth muscle in the lamb ductus arteriosus, clinical trials of intravenous PGE were undertaken to attempt to maintain patency of the ductus in such patients as an alternative to emergency surgery. Such PGE infusions for a short time cause a temporary increase in blood flow to the lungs and improve arterial oxygen saturation until the necessary corrective heart surgery can be performed. The large right-to-left shunt in these cardiac malformations allows the intravenously infused PGE_2 to escape pulmonary degradation before arriving at the ductus. In this instance, the disease process itself facilitates delivery of the therapeutic agent.

Peptic ulcer disease (see Chap. 235) Excessive gastric acid secretion in patients with peptic ulcer disease is involved in damaging the mucosa. Various analogues of PGE_2 inhibit gastric acid secretion and are also inherently cytoprotective. These agents are more effective than placebo in relieving pain and decreasing gastric acid secretion in patients with ulcer disease. Moreover, acceleration of the healing of ulcer craters as assessed by endoscopic criteria has been reported in patients receiving PGE analogues as compared with placebo-treated groups.

Dysmenorrhea (see Chap. 331) Dysmenorrhea is usually associated with increased uterine contractions. The fact that some analgesics used to treat this disorder also inhibit prostaglandin synthesis suggests that arachidonic acid metabolites may play a role in the pathogenesis of dysmenorrhea. Prostaglandins of the E and F series are present in human endometrium. Intravenous infusion of either produces uterine contractions, and PGF and PGE levels in menstrual blood are decreased by administration of prostaglandin synthesis inhibitors. Controlled trials comparing prostaglandin synthesis inhibitors with placebo in women with dysmenorrhea suggest that symptomatic improvement is greater following drug therapy.

Asthma (see Chap. 202)

Inflammatory response and immune response (see Chaps. 62 and 260) Drugs such as aspirin have antipyretic, anti-inflammatory, and analgesic effects. Several arguments support a relation between inflammation and the arachidonic acid metabolites: (1) Inflammatory stimuli such as histamine and bradykinin release endogenous prostaglandins in parallel. (2) Leukotriene C_4-D_4-E_4 is more potent than histamine in causing bronchoconstriction. (3) Several arachidonic acid metabolites cause vasodilatation and hyperalgesia. (4) PGE_2 and LTB_4 are present in areas of inflammation. Polymorphonuclear cells release these products during phagocytosis, and they are chemotactic for leukocytes. (5) Some prostaglandins cause increased vascular permeability, a feature of the inflammatory response that gives rise to local edema. (6) Vasodilation induced by PGE is not abolished by atropine, propranolol, methysergide, or antihistamines, known antagonists of other possible mediators of the inflammatory response. Thus, PGE may have a direct inflmmatory effect, and some mediators of inflammation may act by influencing PGE release. (7) Some arachidonic acid metabolites can cause pain in animal models and hyperalgesia or an increased sensitivity to pain in humans. (8) PGE can cause fever after injection into the cerebral ventricles or into the hypothalamus of animals. (9) Pyrogens cause increased concentrations of prostaglandins in cerebrospinal fluid, whereas prostaglandin synthesis inhibitors decrease fever and decrease release of prostaglandins into cerebrospinal fluid.

Arachidonic acid metabolites may also play a role in the immune response. Small amounts of PGE_2 can suppress stimulation of human lymphocytes by mitogens such as phytohemagglutinin, and the inflammatory response is associated with the local release of arachidonic acid metabolites; thus, these substances may act as negative modulators of lymphocyte function. The release of PGE by mitogen-stimulated lymphocytes may constitute a portion of a negative feedback control mechanism by which lymphocyte activity is regulated. Sensitivity of lymphocytes to the inhibiting effects of PGE_2 increases with age, and indomethacin augments lymphocyte responsiveness to mitogens to a greater degree in the elderly. Lymphocytes cultured from patients with Hodgkin's disease release more PGE_2 after the addition of phytohemagglutinin, and lymphocyte responsiveness is enhanced by indomethacin. When suppressor T cells are removed from the cultures, the amount of PGE_2 synthesized is diminished, and the responsiveness of the lymphocytes from the Hodgkin's patients and controls is no longer different. Depressed cellular immunity in patients with Hodgkin's disease may be the result of PGE inhibition of lymphocyte function.

REFERENCES

ROBERTSON RP (ed): Symposium on prostaglandins in health and disease. Med Clin North Am 65:711, 1981

METZ SA et al: Prostaglandins as mediators of paraneoplastic syndromes: Review and update. *Metabolism* 30:299, 1981

GOETZL EJ, SCOTT WA (eds): Regulation of cellular activities by leukotrienes and other lipoxygenase products of arachidonic acid. *J Allergy Clin Immunol* 74:309, 1984

69 THE ENDOGENOUS OPIATE PEPTIDES

MICHAEL ROSENBLATT

The endogenous opiate peptides, the enkephalins and endorphins, are present in the hypothalamus and brain, endocrine glands (pituitary, adrenals, ovaries, and testes), and gastrointestinal tract (including pancreas). These peptides constitute a class of approximately 10 to 15 substances that range in length from 5 to 31 amino acids. Some of them share common biosynthetic and secretory pathways with hormones such as adrenocorticotropin (ACTH), α-melanocyte-stimulating hormone (α-MSH), β-melanocyte-stimulating hormone (β-MSH), and β-lipotropin (β-LPH). They have (1) morphine-like analgesic properties; (2) behavioral effects; and (3) neurotransmitter and neuromodulator functions. Indeed, these peptides may play a role in many functions such as memory, learning, response to stress, reproduction, pain transmission, and regulation of appetite, temperature, and respiration (Table 69-1). In addition, the placebo response, acupuncture-mediated analgesia, stress-induced amenorrhea, and the pathogenesis of shock may be mechanistically linked to the enkephalins and the endorphins. Tranquilization, irritability, agitation, violent behavior, catalepsy, narcolepsy, and catatonia may also be related to the endorphins. Other behavioral phenomena, such as the smoking habit; alcoholism, and drug addiction, may reflect biochemical abnormalities of the system.

The discovery of the enkephalins and endorphins began with opiate receptors, which were identified and characterized before the first endogenous opiate peptides were isolated. The presence of receptors that bind opiate alkaloids such as morphine in the central nervous system and other tissues raised the teleologic issue of the reason for their existence. It seemed unlikely that the receptors were present to interact with exogenously administered drugs; endogenous substances with morphine-like properties were postulated to exist, and efforts were made to identify them.

In 1975, Hughes, Kosterlitz, and colleagues published a report of their discovery of two small (five-amino acid) brain peptides that bind to opiate receptors and are more potent than morphine. They named these substances *enkephalins* (meaning "in the head"). Within months, three more opiate peptides, larger in size than the enkephalins, were isolated from hypothalamic-pituitary extracts and named endorphins (a contraction for "endogenous morphine"). Later dynorphin, α-neoendorphin, and other structures were added to the list. The term *endorphin* is used by some as a general term for all opiate peptides.

STRUCTURE AND BIOSYNTHESIS The structure of several endogenous opiates is provided in Fig. 69-1. Although these substances are chemically unrelated to morphine, molecular modeling studies indicate that the morphine molecule can mimic a predicted conformation of the enkephalins and endorphins that may occur at the instant of interaction with receptor.

Structurally, these substances are identical in the four amino acids at their amino terminus, which constitutes their "active core," although each has different biologic effects. The endorphins as a class bind better to opiate receptors than does morphine itself and are 20 to 700 times more potent than the morphine alkaloids in a variety of in vitro and in vivo bioassays. Rapid lability may cause underestimation of potency in some assays and is the result of enzymatic degradation of the smallest of these substances, the enkephalins.

Although the opiate peptides have common chemical features, they arise via different biosynthetic pathways. In the pituitary β-endorphin, the most abundant endorphin, is synthesized as part of a larger precursor molecule (pro-opiomelanocortin or POMC) that also contains the full sequence of ACTH, α-MSH, β-MSH, and β-LPH (Fig. 69-2). This precursor molecule also has the potential to generate

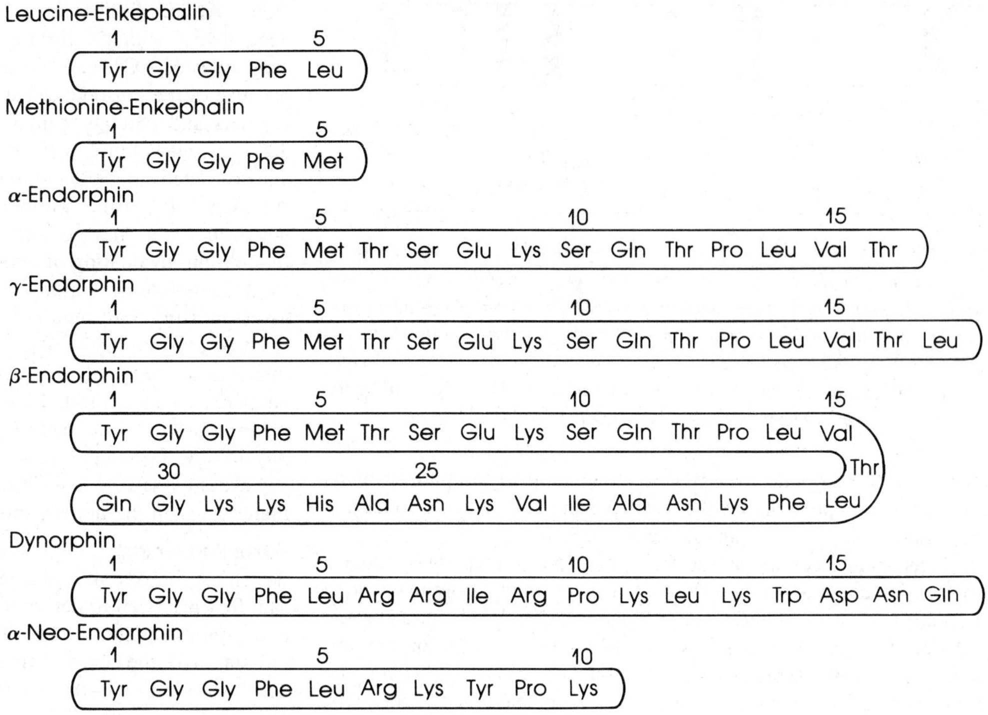

FIGURE 69-1 *Structure of several endogenous opiate peptides. The amino-terminal (leftmost) four amino acids are identical in each peptide. At position 5, a methionine or leucine is found.*

other forms of endorphin, fragments termed α-endorphin and γ-endorphin. "Prohormone-type" cleavage sites exist within POMC and allow the generation of each of the above-mentioned peptides in some anatomic sites. Hence, β-lipotropin is likely a prohormone for β-endorphin. Although β-lipotropin has its own spectrum of biologic properties, its physiologic significance in humans has not been determined. Most importantly, this biosynthetic pathway represents the only means by which the pituitary gland produces ACTH. Therefore, the biosyntheses of ACTH and β-endorphin are inextricably linked in the pituitary by derivation from a single gene that encodes both hormones. Whenever the pituitary secretes ACTH, it also secretes β-endorphin.

Differential processing of POMC occurs within different tissues. Such processing may include metabolic inactivation of peptides generated from the precursor at certain anatomic sites. For instance, although the pituitary gland does not metabolize ACTH to smaller fragments, the hypothalamus converts the precursor molecule to α-MSH. β-MSH is generated in the intermediate lobe of lower species. Humans lack an intermediate lobe as a distinct anatomic entity and hence only produce β-MSH in scattered cells within the pituitary. The cells of the pituitary gland secrete β-endorphin, β-lipotropin, and ACTH. In other cells, the final secretory products are determined by the pattern of cleavage of the large peptide precursor by the enzymatic machinery within that cell. Although several cell types may synthesize the same primary gene product, the final profile of hormone secretion can differ completely.

The enkephalins are derived from different precursors. For example, the adrenal glands biosynthesize enkephalins as part of a large (50,000-mol wt) protein, proenkephalin A, that contains six repeats of the Met-enkephalin sequence and one Leu-enkephalin structure (Fig. 69-3). Again, typical "prohormone-type" cleavage sites delineate the enkephalin structures. Dynorphins and neoendorphins are derived from a third distinct precursor molecule, proenkephalin B.

Additional ("cryptic") peptides are encoded within the structures of these precursor proteins and have the potential to be released by "prohormone-type" cleavages. It is not known whether these cryptic peptides are secreted in vivo, but some have been chemically synthesized and found to have biologic effects.

MECHANISM OF ACTION Like other peptide hormones, the initial step in expression of biologic activity for the opiate peptides is binding to specific receptors on the plasma membrane of target cells.

TABLE 69-1 Biologic effects and possible physiologic roles of endogenous opiates

Analgesia
Catatonic-like state
Seizures
Temperature regulation
Appetite control
Reproductive function (endocrine)
Sexual behavior
Blood pressure decline
Stress response
Release of hypothalamic/pituitary hormones
Memory alteration
Regulation of respiration
Modulation of immune response

At least five functional types of opiate receptors have been characterized: taken together with the multiple forms of endogenous opiate peptides, the complexity of the system is great. The complexity is further increased by variation in response (desensitization, tolerance,

FIGURE 69-2 *Biosynthetic pathway for β-endorphin in the pituitary gland. A single precursor protein, pro-opiomelanocortin (POMC) (molecular weight of approximately 31,000), is initially synthesized from translation of a gene that encodes the structure of adrenocorticotropin (ACTH), β-lipotropin (β-LPH), and β-endorphin. Prohormone-type cleavages can generate other hormones from the same precursor, although this occurs in tissues other than the pituitary. Abbreviations: MSH = melanocyte-stimulating hormone; LPH = lipotropin; CLIP = corticotropin-like intermediate peptide; ACTH = adrenocorticotropin.*

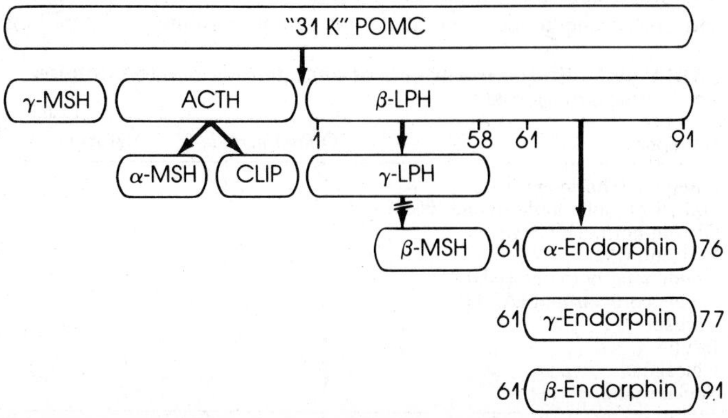

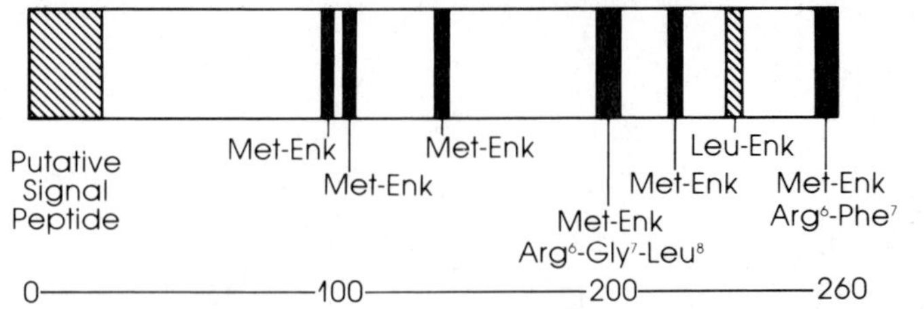

FIGURE 69-3 *Biosynthetic precursor for enkephalins (pre-proenkephalin A) in the adrenal gland. The protein precursor contains 260 amino acids and has a molecular weight of approximately 50,000. Prohormone-type cleavages have the potential to generate six copies of methionine-enkephalin (Met-enk) and one of leucine-enkephalin (Leu-enk) from a single precursor molecule. The signal peptide sequence at the amino terminus (leftmost portion) of the precursor protein is characteristic of secreted proteins.*

etc.) to a given opiate over time or in relation to the pattern of its exposure to receptors and by the fact that a single neuron (or endocrine cell) may secrete more than one neuromediator.

Receptor interaction leads to the formation of a second messenger. For the opiate system in general, receptor interaction leads to a decrease in both basal and stimulated cyclic AMP levels, and chronic exposure to opiate peptides produces a long-term decline in intracellular cyclic AMP levels. As a compensatory response, however, the number of adenylate cyclase units gradually increases with time. This biochemical change may be the physiologic correlate of tolerance and tachyphylaxis, requiring higher doses of opiate to suppress cyclic AMP levels. Sudden withdrawal of opiates at a time when the cell is enriched in adenylate cyclase releases these units from inhibition, resulting in "overshoot" of cyclic AMP levels, and perhaps contributing to development of the opiate withdrawal syndrome.

ENDOCRINOLOGY OF ENDOGENOUS OPIOID PEPTIDES **Endocrine physiology** ACTH, β-endorphin, and β-lipotropin biosynthesis and secretion by the pituitary gland are linked both in normal and in abnormal states. Under normal conditions, β-lipotropin circulates in higher molar concentrations than does β-endorphin, but the radioimmunoassays used clinically recognize both entities. Hence, levels of immunoreactive β-endorphin reflect the combined levels of β-endorphin and β-lipotropin. Such radioimmunoassays provide clinical evidence of the biosynthetic link between ACTH and β-endorphin. For instance, in Addison's disease the plasma levels of both ACTH and immunoreactive β-endorphin are elevated; likewise, glucocorticoid replacement decreases both ACTH and β-endorphin levels. Administration of corticotropin-releasing factor (CRF) stimulates release of both ACTH and immunoreactive β-endorphin in a parallel manner. In Nelson's syndrome (development of a pituitary tumor after bilateral adrenalectomy for Cushing's disease), both plasma ACTH and immunoreactive β-endorphin levels are elevated. Ectopic production of ACTH by tumors is also accompanied by immunoreactive β-endorphin excess. In the latter case, measurement of immunoreactive β-endorphin can be useful as a tumor marker and in some cases serves to monitor treatment.

Cushing's disease Immunoreactive β-endorphin is easily detected and less prone to destruction during sample storage and handling than is ACTH. Furthermore, differentiation of patients with pituitary-dependent Cushing's disease from normal subjects on the basis of a single plasma ACTH and cortisol determination is generally unreliable because of the episodic release and rapid clearance of ACTH in both normals and patients with Cushing's disease (see Chaps. 321 and 325). β-Endorphin and β-lipotropin have a longer half-life in blood and as stated above cross react in most radioimmunoassays. Measurement of plasma immunoreactive β-endorphin, together with plasma cortisol, may be useful for the diagnosis of Cushing's disease. In addition, evaluation of response of the pituitary to maneuvers such as dexamethasone suppression or metyrapone stimulation can be assessed using the β-endorphin radioimmunoassay. Hence, measurement of plasma levels of β-endorphin and β-lipotropin may supplement, if not supplant, those of ACTH in evaluation of the pituitary-adrenal axis in suspected cases of Cushing's disease. Furthermore, patterns of hormonal secretion may be altered in states of abnormal physiology. For example, pituitary tumors responsible for Cushing's disease may secrete a different ratio of β-lipotropin to β-endorphin than occurs in the normal pituitary.

TABLE 69-2 Endocrine effects of endogenous opiate peptides and opiate antagonists

Hormone	Opioid peptide	Naloxone
Luteinizing hormone (LH)	↓	↑
Follicle-stimulating hormone (FSH)	↓	↑
Growth hormone (GH)	↑	↔
Prolactin (Prl)	↑	↔ or ↓
Antidiuretic hormone (ADH)	↓	↑
Adrenocorticotropin (ACTH)	↓	↑
Cortisol	↓	↑
Insulin	↑	↔
Glucagon	↑	↔
Somatostatin	↓	↔

Releasing factors Two general approaches have been employed to determine the role of endorphins in normal physiology (Table 69-2). The first has been to determine the effects of direct administration of endogenous opiate peptides to animals or humans via the systemic circulation or the cerebrospinal fluid. For example, the pharmacologic administration of β-endorphin produces an increase in the secretion of growth hormone (GH), prolactin (Prl), and arginine vasopressin (AVP) and a decrease in the secretion of ACTH, cortisol, luteinizing hormone (LH), and follicle-stimulating hormone (FSH). The effects of β-endorphin on the pituitary gland are not thought to result from direct action on the pituitary but by modulating release of hypothalamic hormones. Hence, they are not direct hypothalamic releasing factors.

An alternate approach to determining the role of the endogenous opiate peptides is to assess the effects of selective antagonists of the opiates, such as naloxone. Such agents block the effects of endogenously secreted opiates, revealing the tonic or physiologic role of opiate peptides. Naloxone administration causes elevations in LH, FSH, and ACTH levels and prevents the stress-mediated rise in prolactin levels. However, naloxone does not cause sustained lowering of GH levels in patients with acromegaly or Prl levels in patients with prolactinomas.

Reproductive endocrinology Administration of opiate antagonists alters the secretory patterns of gonadotropins, suggesting a role for the endorphins in normal reproduction. The effects depend on the sex, age, species, and levels of sex steroids at the time of study. Administration of opiate antagonists causes an increase in the frequency and amplitude of pulsatile secretion of LH, suggesting that gonadotropins are tonically inhibited by endogenous opiate peptides. β-Endorphins are present in hypothalamic portal blood of primates: they are high during the midfollicular and luteal phases of the menstrual cycle but virtually undetectable at the time of menses. Similarly, β-endorphin levels in the hypothalamic portal circulation are low or undetectable in oophorectomized animals, suggesting that ovarian steroids may modulate or play a permissive role in hypothalamic endorphin secretion and that β-endorphin may play a regulatory role in the normal menstrual cycle.

In addition, endorphins may play a role in puberty. Steady increases in plasma β-endorphin levels occur during human puberty, and a decline in the sensitivity of the hypothalamic-pituitary axis to opiate-mediated inhibition of LH secretion occurs in animals as they mature. Thus, "escape" from tonic inhibition may signal the onset of puberty.

Abnormal reproductive function in some women may be linked to alterations in endogenous opiate peptide levels. Extreme stress often produces a delay in the onset of puberty in girls. Similarly, women may develop irregular or absent menses during times of stress, possibly reflecting the effects of stress-increased central endorphin levels and subsequent suppression of pituitary gonadotropin secretion. Female narcotic addicts rarely have normal menses (even prior to marked weight loss), again suggesting a link betwen opiate receptor activation and inhibition of endocrine reproductive function. Finally, peripheral levels of immunoreactive β-endorphin (reflecting pituitary secretion) increase several-fold with intensive and regular exercise, and the development of oligomenorrhea or amenorrhea in women athletes may reflect the effects of exercise-induced β-endorphin on gonadotropin secretion. Hence, under several conditions of "stress," endogenous opiate peptides may serve to suppress ovulation. Finally, in adddition to brain and pituitary, the pro-ACTH/endorphin precursor system is present in the ovaries, testes, and placenta, further suggesting a role for endogenous opiates in reproduction.

Diabetes mellitus Endorphin-containing cells are in close proximity to insulin-containing cells in the endocrine pancreas. β-Endorphin stimulates insulin and glucagon release and inhibits somatostatin secretion, effects that can be reversed by naloxone. Patients with non-insulin-dependent diabetes who receive chlorpropamide develop facial flushing after taking alcohol. This flushing response is blocked by naloxone and reproduced by opiate peptides and is thought to be related to increased sensitivity to endogenous opiates in diabetics. However, a significant role for endorphins in carbohydrate metabolism or a contribution of β-endorphin to the pathophysiology of diabetes has not been established.

NEUROPHYSIOLOGY OF ENDOGENOUS OPIATE PEPTIDES

Anatomic location β-Endorphin is present in the pituitary gland and in the brain. In the human pituitary, ACTH and endorphin-containing cells are found in the anteromedial region of the anterior lobe, at the posterior boundary of the anterior lobe, and in nerve fibers of the posterior lobe. By histochemical criteria, the pituitary is the richest site of endorphin in the body.

The hypothalamus contains neurons that biosynthesize endorphin. These neurons have long projections to other regions of the brain. For example, regions of the brain associated with the limbic system contain substantial quantities of immunoreactive β-endorphin, suggesting a role in memory, learning, and emotions.

Neurons containing the enkephalins are distributed even more widely in the central nervous system. Concentrations are particularly high in the dorsal columns of the spinal cord, a region that contains opiate receptors and that is involved in the transmission of pain (see Chap. 3). Enkephalins are also present in the gastrointestinal tract. Concentrations in the myenteric plexus of the longitudinal muscles of the gut are higher than in the brain. Enkephalins are synthesized in the chromaffin cells of the adrenal medulla and packaged together with the catecholamines in the same secretory granules. Enkephalin is released as part of the sympathetic response to stress together with epinephrine and norepinephrine (Fig. 69-4). Similarly, enkephalin levels in blood are high in pheochromocytoma.

Pain transmission and amelioration The endogenous opiate peptides play a role in regulating pain transmission. In the dorsal horn of the spinal column, enkephalins are released by interneurons that impinge on afferent pain-sensing fibers from the periphery. These pain-transmitting fibers form synapses in the gray matter of the dorsal horn with a second set of neurons, which cross and ascend through the spinal cord as the lateral spinothalamic tract. The release of enkephalins (which may be influenced by descending neuronal input from higher centers) inhibits release of substance P, a neurotransmitter that mediates pain, from afferent fibers entering the dorsal horn (see Chap. 3).

Microinjections of β-endorphin into the central nervous system produce analgesia in animals. Electrical stimulation of regions of the brain involved in pain transmission, such as the periventricular gray area, produces analgesia accompanied by an increase in cerebrospinal fluid levels of endorphins or enkephalins. In the decerebrate cat, localized administration of enkephalin selectively blocks spontaneous firing of neurons involved in pain transmission.

In humans, increased β-endorphin levels have been found in the cerebrospinal fluid of patients with chronic pain from malignancy or causalgia. As in animals, electrical stimulation of periventricular sites produces analgesia accompanied by increased immunoreactive β-endorphin levels, and direct administration of β-endorphin into the cerebrospinal fluid of subjects with terminal malignancies has produced long-lasting analgesia without systemic morphine-like side effects.

Acupuncture and placebo effects The induction of analgesia by acupuncture may be mediated by endogenous opiate peptides. In some studies, the induction of analgesia by acupuncture is accompanied by increased cerebrospinal fluid levels of endorphins whereas coadministration of naloxone (the opiate antagonist) blocks acupuncture-mediated analgesia. Likewise, the effects of placebos may reflect the capacity of an individual to recruit the endogenous opiate peptide system. In studies in which tooth extraction was the pain stimulus, placebo analgesia can be reversed by the administration of naloxone. Similarly, the phenomena of placebo tolerance and dependence are consistent with known properties of the endogenous opioid system.

Behavioral effects Administration of opiate peptides to animals at doses below those required to produce analgesia generates specific and striking behavioral responses. Rats who receive intracerebral β-endorphin display a "catonic-like" behavior, as a consequence of massive hippocampal seizures. Certain stereotyped forms of behavior are also seen, such as the production of "wet-dog shakes." In cats, a rage response is elicited.

Furthermore, it has been suggested that abnormal levels of endogenous opioids or their receptors may play a causal or contributory role in major psychiatric disorders. In one study of schizophrenia, the frequency of auditory hallucinations decreased in patients receiving naloxone. However, other attempts to correlate levels of β-endorphin with states of depression, mania, or other psychiatric disorders have been unsuccessful.

Addictive behavior in humans has also been postulated to be linked to altered levels of endogenous opiate peptides. The susceptibility to chronic abuse of narcotics might be a genetically predetermined disorder of the endogenous opiate system. In addition, certain types of habitual behavior have been described as "addictive." Marathon running and other forms of intensive exercise dramatically increase β-endorphin levels, leading to the hypothesis that such activity creates an internal (central) "self-reward." However, supporting data regarding central nervous system levels of endogenous opiates (perhaps at highly localized anatomic sites) have not been obtained.

OTHER PHYSIOLOGIC AND PATHOPHYSIOLOGIC RESPONSES

Thermogenesis The opiate peptides may play a role in the adaptive response to heat. Chronic exposure of animals to high temperature

FIGURE 69-4 *Hormonal response to stress indicating release of endogenous opiate peptides and other hormones into the systemic circulation and cerebrospinal fluid. Abbreviations: CRF = corticotropin-releasing hormone; EPI = epinephrine; NE = norepinephrine; CNS = central nervous system; ACTH = adrenocorticotropin.*

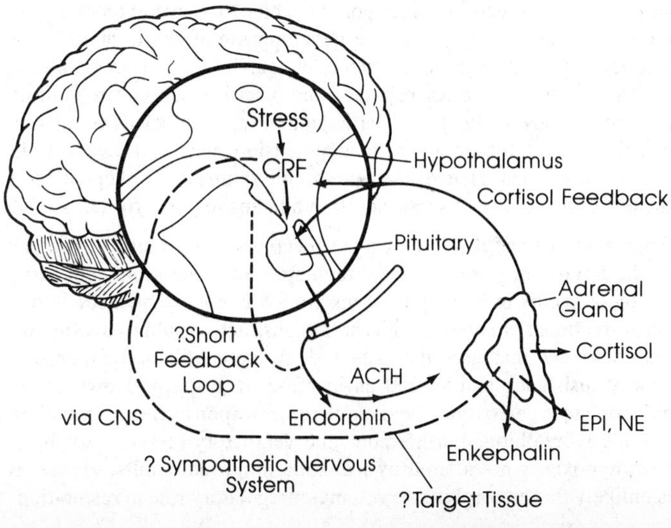

followed by administration of naloxone produces a rapid increase in body temperature. Peptides encoded in the precursor molecule and related to endorphin, such as γ-melanocyte-stimulating hormone (γ-MSH), produce rapid decreases in body temperature.

Stress Increased secretion of β-endorphin and β-lipotropin accompanies the increased ACTH and cortisol levels during stress. Similarly, serum prolactin levels increase in stress. The increase in serum prolactin is blocked by administration of naloxone, suggesting that stress-mediated prolactin release is in part stimulated by endogenous opiates. In certain species, stress-induced eating is blocked by naloxone. The endocrinologic and central role of corticotropin-releasing factor (CRF) as a "stress hormone" links pituitary β-endorphin and β-lipotropin secretion to ACTH and cortisol as part of the stress response, although the target organ(s) for β-endorphin and β-lipotropin action are not known (Fig. 69-4).

Appetite control Endorphins may play a role in normal regulation of appetite and in eating disorders. Genetically obese mice and rats have marked increases in the pituitary content of β-endorphin, β-lipotropin, and ACTH. Injection of β-endorphin into the brain of such animals or injection of morphine subcutaneously produces further increase in food intake. This increase in feeding in genetically obese animals but not in their normal counterparts is blocked by naloxone. Decreased food intake has also been observed in humans given opiate antagonists. The site of action of endorphin in feeding behavior appears to be the hypothalamic paraventricular nucleus. In addition to potential central nervous system sites of endorphin action, opiate receptors are present in the gastrointestinal tract. Furthermore, β-endorphin is synthesized in the pancreas, where it acts (in a paracrine fashion) to stimulate insulin release, perhaps leading to increased food intake and altered glucose utilization.

Blood pressure and shock Severe hypotension or shock stimulates the pituitary release of ACTH, β-lipotropin, and β-endorphin and a subsequent increase in blood cortisol levels. However, a large component of the stress response may not be to the advantage of the organism. In sepsis, immunoreactive β-endorphin levels in blood rise prior to the development of hypotension. Administration of naloxone partially or completely restores blood pressure in experimental hemorrhagic, "neurogenic" or spinal, and septic shock, resulting in decreased mortality in the latter condition. The amount of β-endorphin that is released under these circumstances appears to be regulated (at least in some species); administration of naloxone during endotoxin-mediated shock produces even greater increases in β-endorphin levels, suggesting that β-endorphin secretion is under feedback control. The putative short feedback-inhibitory loop from the pituitary to the hypothalamus could occur via the general circulation since the median eminence of the hypothalamus is one region of the brain which lies outside the blood-brain barrier. Alternatively, one study suggests that pituitary endorphins may ascend to the hypothalamus via the hypothalamic-pituitary portal circulation in what is conventionally regarded as a retrograde direction. It is important to note that several biochemical mediators may contribute to the development of septic shock. For example, platelet-activating factor, arachidonic acid metabolites, kinins, immunoregulatory peptides, and other substances (in addition the endogenous opiates) may participate in septic shock. The relative contribution of these factors to hypotension appears to vary from species to species. Hence, the role of endorphins and enkephalins in the pathophysiology of septic shock in humans requires further study.

Regulation of respiration Opiate receptors are present in regions of the brainstem responsible for regulation of respiration, but a role for these agents in regulation of respiration is not established. In one study treatment of patients with chronic obstructive pulmonary disease with naloxone increased the magnitude of the ventilatory response to airway resistance and caused an increase in dyspnea. However, in another study naloxone did not increase responsiveness to carbon dioxide rebreathing. Furthermore, the ventilatory response to short-term hypoxia is not altered by naloxone in normal adults. Hence, it is unlikely that endorphins serve a major regulatory role in respiration. Rather, they may participate in the fine-tuning of ventilation and may be responsible for variations in respiratory drive among individuals. Alternatively, their effects may be amplified when normal regulatory mechanisms are disturbed.

Immune system interactions The endogenous opiates may provide a biochemical link between the brain, the neuroendocrine system, and the immune system and might provide an explanation for the concept that emotional stress may be associated with compromised immune response, perhaps leading to increased infection and unmasking of malignancy when immune surveillance is nonoptimal.

Opiate receptors are present on human granulocytes, lymphocytes, and monocytes, and there is some evidence that lymphocytes produce a β-endorphin–like substance. Unfortunately, attempts to define a potential regulatory role for opiate peptides in the immune response suggest both suppressive and stimulatory effects, depending on the assay system employed. Opiate peptides stimulate human macrophage chemotaxis, inhibit or increase lymphocyte proliferation, and variably affect natural killer cell activity. The integrated effects of the opiates on immune system responsiveness in vivo remain to be clarified.

CLINICAL IMPLICATIONS Insights gathered from the study of the endogenous opiate peptides hold therapeutic promise in several disorders, particularly in the areas of reproduction, appetite control, and obesity. Elucidation of the pathways and means of transmission of pain has important implications for treatment of pain. Further understanding of the mechanism of action and the cellular responses to the opiate peptides may provide insight into the pathophysiology of addiction, tolerance, and withdrawal from narcotics and into the management of these disorders. Information regarding psychiatric health and disease may also be afforded by study of the endogenous opiates, and naloxone is under investigation as part of the therapeutic regimen for septic shock.

Knowledge of the structure of the endogenous opiates has permitted chemical synthesis of these substances and the design of analogues. Analogues containing any of the following properties might be clinically useful: long duration of action, oral bioavailability, increased potency, selectivity within the spectrum of action of opiates, decreased side effects, and nonaddictive properties.

Many important principles have emerged from the study of the endogenous opiate peptides. The biologic properties of a naturally occurring peptide depend not only on its structure but also on its location and the type of cell with which it interacts. For example, the same chemical substance may act both as a neuromodulator for analgesia and as a hormone that influences gonadotropin secretion.

In addition, study of the opiate peptide system has demonstrated a fundamental pharmacologic principle. Receptors that bind drugs normally interact with endogenous ligands. Such endogenous substances may belong to a chemical class different from the drug (i.e., morphine is an alkaloid, and endorphin is a peptide). Furthermore, the endogenous substances may be more potent and possess fewer side-effects than the currently utilized pharmacologic agent. Exploitation of this principle might uncover endogenous compounds with digoxin-like, tricyclic antidepressant–like, or benzodiazepine-like effects. Isolation of these substances and determination of their structure should provide new biologically active agents.

REFERENCES

Carr DB, Rosenblatt MR: Endorphins in the normal and abnormal pituitary. Proceedings of the International Symposium on Pituitary Tumors, June 1983, in PM Black et al (eds), *Secretory Tumors of the Pituitary Gland (Progress in Endocrine Research and Therapy)*. New York, Raven, 1984, pp 245–261

Hughes J et al: Identification of two related pentapeptides from the brain with potent opiate agonist activity. Nature 258:577, 1975

Martin WR: Pharmacology of opioids. Pharmacol Rev 35:283, 1984

Morley JE: The endocrinology of the opiates and opioid peptides. Metabolism 30:195, 1981

Pert CB et al: Neuropeptides and their receptors: A psychosomatic network. J Immunol 135:820s, 1985

Pfeiffer A, Herz A: Endocrine actions of opioids. Horm Metabol Res 16:386, 1984

Watkins LR, Mayer DJ: Organization of endogenous opiate and nonopiate pain control systems. Science 216:1185, 1982

section 4 Nutrition

70 NUTRITIONAL REQUIREMENTS

DANIEL RUDMAN

ESSENTIAL AND NONESSENTIAL NUTRIENTS AND THEIR THRESHOLDS (REQUIREMENTS, ALLOWANCES, AND TOLERANCES) Over the past few decades diverse factors, including increased personal income, expanded public assistance programs, and vitamin and mineral enrichment of food, have reduced the prevalence of the classic nutritional deficiency diseases. Nevertheless, malnutrition, both overt and subclinical, remains a major problem, especially among the poor, the elderly, alcoholics, the chronically ill, and hospital populations. All too often the patient's nutritional status is ignored during the clinical evaluation, and complete nutritional needs are not met during hospitalization. To approach nutritional care rationally, the physician, understanding how disease affects the two types of nutrient thresholds (requirement and tolerance), must assess the patient's preexisting nutritional status, calculate the needs for maintenance and repletion, and institute the appropriate diet therapy.

The body contains many thousands of species of organic molecules but requires for health the intake of only 24 organic compounds in addition to a source of energy and water: 9 essential amino acids, 2 fatty acids, and 13 vitamins. The vast majority of organic molecules in food, although metabolized or assimilated by the body, are "nonessential" in the sense that their deletion from the diet does not cause illness. The simplicity of the nutritional requirements, compared with the complexity of body composition, is the result of the remarkable capacity for endogenous biosynthesis.

Of the inorganic compounds in food, 15 are believed to be nutritionally essential: calcium, phosphorus, iodine, iron, magnesium, zinc, copper, potassium, sodium, chloride, cobalt, chromium, manganese, molybdenum, and selenium. (It is possible that arsenic, vanadium, and tin may also be essential trace elements.)

The requirement of an essential nutrient is defined as the smallest quantity that maintains normal mass, chemical composition, morphology, and physiologic functions of the body and prevents any clinical or biochemical sign of the corresponding deficiency state. In children, an additional criterion is a normal rate of growth. When the intake of an essential nutrient is limited, the body may conserve that nutrient by increasing absorption (e.g., calcium, iron); by slowing catabolism (e.g., amino acids, calories); by minimizing excretion (e.g., sodium, potassium, magnesium, chloride, phosphate, water); and by mobilizing body reserves (e.g., vitamin A, vitamin B_{12}, essential fatty acids). Only when these homeostatic reactions are inadequate does the nutritional deficiency state appear. The time that elapses, after the intake of an essential nutrient is interrupted (for example, during total parenteral nutrition with an incomplete formula), before a deficiency state develops is proportional to the ratio of body stores divided by daily requirement.

Because requirements vary among individuals due to numerous genetic and environmental circumstances, the recommended dietary allowances (RDA) provide a margin of safety sufficient to meet the needs of 90 to 95 percent of the healthy population (Tables 70-1 and 70-2). RDA is determined as follows:

1 In healthy adults the requirements of protein (or its constituent amino acids) and macrominerals (requirements greater than 100 mg per day) can be assessed by balance techniques. The daily balance of each element equals intake minus output (urinary plus fecal). The requirement of each amino acid or macromineral is the smallest intake that maintains zero balance for nitrogen or for the mineral under study. A negative balance of any essential element, if it persists long enough, leads to illness and death.

2 In the infant or growing child the requirement of energy and essential nutrients is the smallest amount of each that maintains an optimal rate of growth while all others are fed in adequate amounts.

3 For micronutrients (requirement less than 100 mg per day) the requirement is the smallest daily intake that prevents eventual appearance of the nutrient-specific deficiency state.

Table 70-3 lists the amino acids required by infants and adults to illustrate the effect of age on nutrient requirements. Table 70-4 describes the main features of the illness which ensues when each essential nutrient is deficient.

Another nutritional threshold is the maximal tolerance of a nutrient. Just as intake of any essential nutrient below a specific level causes disease, intake above a certain level for many nutrients (either essential or nonessential) disturbs body structure or function. Intakes exceeding tolerance can lead to acute reversible symptoms, acute permanent damage, or progressive systemic impairments (Table 70-5). A physiologic diet provides intakes of each nutrient between the two thresholds of minimal requirement and maximal tolerance. The recognition that tolerance for a nutrient can be exceeded is particularly important during parenteral nutrition, when the gastrointestinal mechanisms (anorexia, emesis, incomplete absorption, diarrhea) that ordinarily help protect the individual from the effects of excessive nutrient intake are bypassed. Although allowance values have been established for the essential nutrients, the actual maximal tolerance levels in many cases are uncertain.

FACTORS ALTERING NUTRITIONAL THRESHOLDS The recommended allowance and the maximal tolerance of each essential nutrient are influenced by many factors: rate of growth, age, exercise, pregnancy and lactation, chemical composition of the diet, diseases, drugs. In addition, the route, rate, and timing of alimentation influence requirements and tolerances. As the "window" between requirement and tolerance narrows, nutritional management becomes more difficult (e.g., protein intake of a cachectic, encephalopathic, cirrhotic patient).

Physiologic factors Growth, exercise, pregnancy, and lactation (Table 70-1) increase the daily requirements per unit of body weight for energy and for most essential nutrients. In the aged person, basal energy requirements per kilogram of lean body mass are the same as those of a younger person; nevertheless, energy requirements decline with age due to the reduced lean body mass and reduced activity. Amino acid and calcium requirements may be higher in old age; optimal nutrient intakes for the elderly are, in general, still uncertain.

Composition of the diet Given diets with identical contents of nitrogen, digestible carbohydrates, fat, vitamins, and minerals, the metabolic availability of the nutrients may vary widely. Thus, all proteins are not equally effective in meeting the daily requirement because of differences in digestibility or in content of essential amino acids (Table 70-6). Gastrointestinal absorption of some minerals is influenced by the presence in the diet of other reactive components; the utilization of vitamins may be influenced by level of intake of organic macronutrients. Examples are given in Table 70-7.

Route, rate, and time (see Chap. 74) The allowances listed in Tables 70-1 to 70-3 apply to enteral nutrition. For some nutrients, different amounts are required for parenteral nutrition. Net gastrointestinal absorption of ingested amino acids, carbohydrates, fats, sodium, chloride, and potassium normally is greater than 90 percent (Table 70-8), and these nutrients have the same RDAs for the intravenous as for the enteral route. For others of the essential minerals, however, net absorption is only 50 percent or less (Table

TABLE 70-1 Recommended daily dietary allowances[a]

					Fat-soluble vitamins		
Age, years	Weight, kg	Height, cm	Energy, kcal	Protein, g	Vitamin A RE[b], μg	Vitamin D, μg[c]	Vitamin E, mg αTE[d]
INFANTS							
0.0–05	6	60	kg × 115	kg × 2.2	420	10	3
0.5–1.0	9	71	kg × 105	kg × 2.0	400	10	4
CHILDREN							
1–3	13	90	1300	23	400	10	5
4–6	20	112	1700	30	500	10	6
7–10	28	132	2400	34	700	10	7
MALES							
11–14	45	157	2700	45	1000	10	8
15–18	66	176	2800	56	1000	10	10
19–22	70	177	2900	56	1000	7.5	10
23–50	70	178	2700	56	1000	5	10
51+	70	178	2400	56	1000	5	10
FEMALES							
11–14	46	157	2200	46	800	10	8
15–18	55	163	2100	46	800	10	8
19–22	55	163	2100	44	800	7.5	8
23–50	55	163	2000	44	800	5	8
51+	55	163	1800	44	800	5	8
PREGNANCY							
			+300	+30	+200	+5	+2
LACTATION							
			+500	+20	+400	+5	+3

[a] *The allowances are intended to provide for individual variations among most normal persons as they live in the United States under usual environmental stresses. Diets should be based on a variety of common foods in order to provide other nutrients for which human requirements have been less well defined.*
[b] *Retinol equivalents; 1 retinol equivalent = 1 μg retinol or 6 μg β-carotene.*
[c] *As cholecalciferol; 10 μg cholecalciferol = 400 IU vitamin D.*
[c] *α-Tocopherol equivalents; 1 mg d-α-tocopherol = 1 αTE.*
[e] *Niacin equivalents; 1 NE = 1 mg niacin or 60 mg dietary tryptophan.*

70-8); consequently the intravenous requirement is only a fraction of the oral one. It is also likely that the requirements of amino acids are not identical by enteral and parenteral routes. After ingestion and absorption into the portal venous system, a portion of the absorbed amino acids is catabolized or transformed during the "first pass" through the liver, where many of the enzymes of amino acid degradation and intermediary metabolism are located. Intravenously infused amino acids, in contrast, partially bypass these catabolic and biosynthetic pathways and reach sites of protein synthesis in muscle and other extrahepatic tissues.

Timing can be important. For example, all of the essential amino acids must be supplied simultaneously to support protein synthesis. If one such essential amino acid, e.g., tryptophan, is administered at a different time than the other amino acids, assimilation of all into protein is curtailed. Similarly, when amino acids, glucose, lipids, and minerals are infused at separate times during the day or week, as often happens in parenteral feeding, assimilation may be impaired. For example, omission of phosphorus or potassium from hyperalimentation solutions impairs retention of the nitrogen furnished by the same fluid.

For these various reasons, the daily requirements of essential nutrients delivered by the parenteral route still remain uncertain.

Disease Nutritional requirements and tolerances may be altered by disease through at least seven mechanisms (see also Table 70-9):

1 Increased utilization of nutrients. Fever, infection, and trauma increase resting metabolic rate and, as a consequence, daily caloric requirements. Folate is utilized more rapidly in patients with hemolysis and increased cell turnover (hemolytic anemia, psoriasis, cancer). Many nutritional requirements are greater during repletion from cachexia than during maintenance of normal nutriture. In this respect, the repletion process in adults resembles growth in children.

TABLE 70-2 Estimated safe and adequate daily dietary intakes of additional selected vitamins and minerals*†

	Vitamins				Trace elements				
	Age, yr	Vitamin K, μg	Biotin, μg	Pantothenic acid, mg	Copper, mg	Manganese, mg	Fluoride, mg	Chromium, mg	Selenium, mg
Infants	0–0.5	12	35	2	0.5–0.7	0.5–0.7	0.1–0.5	0.01–0.04	0.01–0.04
	0.5–1.0	10–20	50	3	0.7–1.0	0.7–1.0	0.2–1.0	0.02–0.06	0.02–0.06
Children and adolescents	1–3	15–30	65	3	1.0–1.5	1.0–1.5	0.5–1.5	0.02–0.08	0.02–0.08
	4–6	20–40	85	3–4	1.5–2.0	1.5–2.0	1.0–2.5	0.03–0.12	0.03–0.12
	7–10	30–60	120	4–5	2.0–2.5	2.0–3.0	1.5–2.5	0.05–0.20	0.05–0.20
	11+	50–100	100–200	4–7	2.0–3.0	2.5–5.0	1.5–2.5	0.05–0.20	0.05–0.20
Adults		70–140	100–200	4–7	2.0–3.0	2.5–5.0	1.5–4.0	0.05–0.20	0.05–0.20

* *Because there is less information on which to base an allowance, these are not given in the main table of dietary allowances but are provided here in the form of ranges of recommended intakes.*
† *Because the toxic levels for many trace elements may be only several times usual intakes, the upper levels for the trace elements given in this table should not be habitually exceeded.*

Water-soluble vitamins							Minerals					
Ascorbic Acid, mg	Thiamin, mg	Riboflavin, mg	Niacin, mg NE[d]	Vitamin B_6, mg	Folacin, μg[f]	Vitamin B_{12}, μg	Calcium, mg	Phosphorus, mg	Magnesium, mg	Iron mg	Zinc, mg	Iodine, μg
35	0.3	0.4	6	0.3	30	0.5	360	240	50	10	3	40
35	0.5	0.6	8	0.6	45	1.5[g]	540	360	70	15	5	50
45	0.7	0.8	9	0.9	100	2.0	800	800	150	15	10	70
45	0.9	1.0	11	1.3	200	2.5	800	800	200	10	10	90
45	1.2	1.4	16	1.6	300	3.0	800	800	250	10	10	120
50	1.4	1.6	18	1.8	400	3.0	1200	1200	350	18	15	150
60	1.4	1.7	18	2.0	400	3.0	1200	1200	400	18	15	150
60	1.5	1.7	19	2.2	400	3.0	800	800	350	10	15	150
60	1.4	1.6	18	2.2	400	3.0	800	800	350	10	15	150
60	1.2	1.4	16	2.2	400	3.0	800	800	350	10	15	150
60	1.1	1.3	15	1.8	400	3.0	1200	1200	300	18	15	150
60	1.1	1.3	14	2.0	400	3.0	1200	1200	300	18	15	150
60	1.1	1.3	14	2.0	400	3.0	800	800	300	18	15	150
60	1.0	1.2	13	2.0	400	3.0	800	800	300	18	15	150
60	1.0	1.2	13	2.0	400	3.0	800	800	300	10	15	150
+20	+0.4	+0.3	+2	+0.6	+400	+1.0	+400	+400	+150	[h]	+5	125
+40	+0.5	+0.5	+5	+0.5	+100	+1.0	+400	+400	+150	[h]	+10	250

[f] *The folacin allowances refer to dietary sources as determined by* Lactobacillus casei *assay after treatment with enzymes ("conjugases") to make polyglutamyl forms of the vitamin available to the test organism.*

[g] *The RDA for vitamin B_{12} in infants is based on average concentration of the vitamin in human milk. The allowances after weaning are based on energy intake (as recommended by the American Academy of Pediatrics) and consideration of other factors such as intestinal absorption.*

[h] *The increased requirement during pregnancy cannot be met by the iron content of habitual U.S. diets nor by the existing iron stores of many women; therefore, the use of 30 to 60 mg of supplemental iron is recommended. Iron needs during lactation are not substantially different from those of nonpregnant women, but continued supplementation of the mother for 2 to 3 months after parturition is advisable in order to replenish stores depleted by pregnancy.*

2 *Malabsorption*. For each nutrient absorbed less efficiently than normal in malabsorption states, the daily requirement is increased correspondingly.

3 *Impaired ability to activate or utilize a nutrient*. The requirement for vitamin D is increased by renal disease that impairs hydroxylation of the vitamin; requirements for folate, thiamin, and pyridoxine in subjects with cirrhosis of the liver may be greater than normal because of impaired hepatic capacity to transform these vitamins into their active forms. Injured or infected patients may utilize glucose and triglyceride less efficiently than healthy individuals.

4 *Abnormally large losses of nutrients*. Impaired conservation of electrolytes or amino acids because of renal disease, burns, blood loss, nasogastric suction, diarrhea, or hemodialysis leads to loss of nutrients. One criterion of normal nutriture for nitrogen and minerals in the adult is zero elemental balance, i.e., enteral or parenteral intake equal to urinary plus fecal output. If output of nitrogen or mineral is increased by abnormal renal or extrarenal loss, then intake must be correspondingly higher to maintain zero balance.

5 *Impaired catabolic or excretory pathways*. Metabolic defects can reduce both requirement and tolerance, because the rate of degradation or excretion of a nutrient is slowed. In children with phenylketonuria or maple syrup urine disease, the requirements for phenylalanine or branched-chain amino acids, respectively, are less than normal. Patients with uremia have a reduced dietary requirement for nonessential amino acids.

6 *Hyperabsorption*. Increased absorption can result in a decrease in both requirement and tolerance. Examples are calcium in hyperabsorptive hypercalciuria, iron in hemochromatosis, and copper in Wilson's disease.

7 *Drugs*. Pharmacologic agents can alter nutritional requirements by

	Electrolytes		
Molybdenum, mg	Sodium, mg	Potassium, mg	Chloride, mg
0.03–0.06	115–350	350–925	275–700
0.04–0.08	250–750	425–1275	400–1200
0.05–0.10	325–975	550–1650	500–1500
0.06–0.15	450–1350	775–2350	700–2100
0.10–0.30	600–1800	1000–3000	925–2775
0.15–0.50	900–2700	1525–4575	1400–4200
0.15–0.50	1100–3300	1875–5625	1700–5100

TABLE 70-3 Recommended daily allowances of the essential amino acids per kilogram of body weight for infants, children, and adult male subjects

Amino acid	Infants*	Children	Adults
L-Threonine	68	28	8
L-Valine	92	25	14
L-Isoleucine	83	28	12
L-Leucine	135	42	16
L-Lysine	99	44	12
L-Tryptophan	21	4	3
L-Methionine-cystine	49	22	10
L-Phenylalanine-tyrosine	141	22	16
L-Histidine	33	?†	?†

* *The preterm infant has additional requirements for arginine, tyrosine, cystine, and taurine.*

† *Essentiality has been established by long-term nitrogen balance and plasma amino acids; however, recommended levels of intake have not been established.*

TABLE 70-4 Symptoms and manifestations of nutrient deficiency

Nutrient	Disorders and symptoms of deficiency	Laboratory tests
Water	Thirst, poor tissue turgor, dry mucous membranes, vascular collapse, altered mental status	Serum electrolytes ↑, serum osmolarity ↑, total body water ↓
Calories (energy)	Weakness and physical inactivity, loss of subcutaneous fat, muscle wasting, bradycardia	Weight loss, MAFA ↓, MAMA ↓, creatinine/height ↓, BMR ↓
Protein	Psychomotor change, dyspigmented, sparse, and easily plucked hair, "flaky-paint" dermatitis, edema, muscle wasting, hepatomegaly, ↓ growth	MAMA ↓, serum albumin, transferrin, retinol binding protein ↓, anemia, creatinine/height ↓, serum nonessential/essential amino acids ↑, urine urea/creatinine ↓
Linoleic acid	Xerosis, desquamation, thickening of skin, hair loss, fatty liver, delayed wound healing	Serum ratio of triene to tetraene fatty acids ↑
Linolenic acid	Visual defect	↓ Serum ω3 fatty acids, thrombocytopenia, abnormal liver function tests
Vitamin A	Xerosis of eye and skin, xerophthalmia, Bitot's spot, follicular hyperkeratosis, hypogeusia, hyposmia	Plasma vitamin A ↓, dark adaptation time ↑
Vitamin D	Rickets and growth failure in children, osteomalacia in adults	Serum alkaline phosphatase concentration ↑, plasma 25-hydroxycholecalciferol ↓, serum Ca^{2+} and P ↓
Vitamin E	Anemia	Plasma α-tocopherol ↓, hemolysis of RBC in dilute H_2O_2
Vitamin K	Bleeding diathesis	Prothrombin time ↑
Vitamin C (ascorbic acid)	Scurvy, petechiae, ecchymoses, perifollicular hemorrhage, spongy and bleeding gums (if not edentulous)	Ascorbic acid concentration in plasma, platelets, whole blood, and white blood cells ↓; urinary ascorbic acid ↓
Thiamin (vitamin B_1)	Beriberi, muscle tenderness and weakness, hyporeflexia, hypesthesia, tachycardia, cardiomegaly, congestive heart failure, encephalopathy	Erythrocyte thiamine pyrophosphate and transketolase activity ↓ and in vitro effect thereon of thiamin pyrophosphate ↑, urinary thiamin ↓, blood pyruvate and α-ketoglutarate levels ↑, lactic acidosis
Riboflavin (vitamin B_2)	Angular stomatitis (or angular scars), cheilosis, magenta tongue, atrophic lingual papillae, corneal vascularization, angular blepharitis, dyssebacia, scrotal (vulvar) dermatosis	EGR activity ↓, and in vitro effect on EGR activity of flavin adenine dinucleotide ↑, pyridoxal phosphate oxidase activity ↓ and in vitro effect thereon of riboflavin ↑, ↓ urinary riboflavin
Niacin	Pellagra, scarlet and raw tongue, atrophic lingual papillae, tongue fissuring, pellagrous dermatosis, diarrhea, dementia	Urinary N^1-methylnicotinamide ↓, urinary 2-pyridone/N^1-methylnicotinamide ratio ↓
Pyridoxine (vitamin B_6)	Nasolabial seborrhea, glossitis, kidney stones, peripheral neuropathy, muscular twitching, convulsions, microcytic anemia	EGOT activity ↓ and in vitro effect of pyridoxal phosphate on EGOT activity ↑, tryptophan load test ↓ (urinary excretion of xanthurenic and quinolinic acids), urinary vitamin B_6 excretion ↓
Folacin	Pallor, glossitis, stomatitis, diarrhea, anemia	Erythrocyte and serum folate concentration ↓, urine formiminoglutamic acid excretion ↑ after histidine load, macrocytic anemia, polymorphonuclear leukocytes hypersegmented, megaloblastic bone marrow
Vitamin B_{12}	Pallor, mild icterus, anorexia, diarrhea, paresthesia, ataxia, optic neuritis, mental changes	Serum vitamin B_{12} ↓, peripheral blood and bone marrow morphology
Biotin	Fatigue, depression, nausea, dermatitis, muscular pains	Urnary biotin ↓, whole blood biotin ↓
Pantothenic acid	Fatigue, sleep disturbances, impaired coordination, nausea	Urinary pantothenic acid ↓
Calcium	Stunted growth, rickets, osteomalacia, convulsions	Osteopenia by x-ray, serum Ca^{2+} ↓
Phosphorus	Weakness, osteomalacia, ↓ phagocytosis, hemolysis, ↓ cardiac function, neurological syndromes, respiratory failure	Osteopenia by x-ray, serum P ↓
Magnesium	Growth failure, behavioral disturbances, weakness, tremor, tetany, seizures, cardiac arrhythmias	Serum, urine, and RBC Mg ↓
Iron	Pallor, weakness, reduced resistance to infection, angular stomatitis, atrophic lingual papillae, koilonychia	Plasma and marrow iron ↓, serum ferritin ↓, microcytic hypochromic anemia
Zinc	Psoriasiform rash, eczematous scaling, growth restriction, hypogonadism, delayed puberty, slow wound healing, hypogeusia, photophobia, anergy	Plasma and 24-h urine zinc ↓
Iodine	Goiter, symptoms of hypothyroidism	TSH ↑, T_4 and T_3 ↓, 24-h urine iodine ↓, RAI uptake ↑
Copper	Pallor	Neutropenia, hypochromic microcytic anemia, hypoferremia, osteopenia, plasma and urine copper ↓, ceruloplasmin ↓
Fluorine	Higher frequency of tooth decay	
Chromium	Glucose intolerance	Serum chromium ↓, urinary chromium ↓
Selenium	Cardiomyopathy, muscle pain	Plasma, RBC selenium ↓, glutathione peroxidose activity ↓
Sodium	Muscle weakness and cramps, confusion, apathy, anorexia, hypotension, oliguria	Serum Na^+ ↓, BUN/creatinine ↑
Potassium	Lassitude, polyuria, ileus, muscular weakness	Serum and urine K^+ ↓, body ^{40}K ↓, abnormal ECG
Chloride	Muscle cramps, apathy, anorexia, alkalosis	Serum Cl^- ↓

NOTES: *BMR = basal metabolism rate; BUN = blood-urea nitrogen; creatinine/height = 24-h urine creatinine/height ratio; ECG = electrocardiogram; EGOT = erythrocyte glutamic-oxaloacetic transaminase; EGR = erythrocyte glutathione reductase; MAFA = midarm fat area; MAMA = midarm muscle area; RAI = radioactive iodine; RBC = red blood cell; T_3 = triiodothyroxine; T_4 = thyroxine; TSH = thyroid-stimulating hormone.*

causing malabsorption or renal loss of a nutrient, by preventing its metabolic utilization, or by accelerating its degradation.

INDIVIDUAL ESSENTIAL NUTRIENTS Water A reasonable allowance is 1 mL/kcal for adults and 150 mL/kg body weight for infants. The minimum requirement, considerably less than the customary allowance, depends on the preformed and potential solutes ingested (largely protein, sodium, chloride, and potassium), the concentrating ability of the kidney, and extrarenal losses. Normally 50 to 100 mL per day is excreted in the feces, 500 to 1000 mL is lost by exhalation and evaporation (insensible loss), and the remainder is excreted in the urine. Water intake must equal these losses to avoid under- or overhydration. Water supply is often inadequate in quantity or quality for impoverished populations in developing nations.

TABLE 70-5 Syndromes that can result from excessive intake or absorption of nutrients by oral route or from excessive infusion by parenteral route

Nutrient	Manifestation of overnutrition
Water	Edema, headache, nausea, hypertension
Calories	Obesity
Proteins	Exacerbation of inborn errors in amino acid catabolism or "nitrogen accumulation diseases, renal damage"
Fat	In predisposed individuals, hyperlipemia
Vitamin A	Headache, vomiting, peeling of skin, anorexia, swelling of long bones, cirrhosis
Vitamin D	Hypercalcemia, nephrolithiasis, impaired renal function
Vitamin K	At high doses may cause jaundice
Ascorbic acid (vitamin C)	Hyperoxaluria
Calcium	Hypercalcemia, mental and renal dysfunction
Magnesium	Diarrhea
Iron	Siderosis, hemochromatosis
Zinc	Fever, nausea, vomiting, diarrhea
Iodine	Depression of thyroid activity, goiter, occasional hyperthyroidism
Copper	Wilson's disease, vomiting
Manganese	Generalized disease of nervous system
Fluorine	Mottling of teeth, increased bone density, neurological disturbances
Sodium chloride	Hypertension, edema, heart failure
Potassium	Muscular weakness, arrhythmia, death

TABLE 70-7 Some essential nutrients for which the daily dietary requirement is influenced by other dietary components

Nutrient	Influence by other dietary component
Protein	Requirement inversely related to calories when the latter are deficient
Essential amino acids	Utilization curtailed if any essential amino acid is deficient
Phenylalanine	Requirement inversely related to tyrosine intake
Methionine	Requirement inversely related to cystine intake
Valine, leucine, isoleucine	Requirement of each is increased by excess of the other branched-chain amino acid(s)
Vitamin E	Requirement proportional to intake of polyunsaturated fat
Thiamin	Requirement proportional to calories
Niacin	Requirement inversely related to tryptophan intake
Vitamin B_6	Requirement increased by protein
Folacin	Requirement increased by alcohol intake
Calcium	Urinary excretion increased by high protein intake
Calcium, magnesium, nonheme iron, zinc	Absorption decreased by phytates
Nonheme iron	Absorption improved by vitamin C or sulfur-containing amino acids
Copper	Absorption decreased by calcium, requirement increased by excess dietary zinc

Maximal tolerance normally is more than 5 liters daily because of the kidney's large capacity for free water clearance. Water requirement and tolerance are increased by factors that cause increased losses in urine, feces, or sweat. The obligatory urinary loss is proportional to the excretion of solutes and the kidney's concentrating capacity; it is increased in proportion to the intake of protein, sodium, potassium, and chloride. Water requirements are increased by deficiency of antidiuretic hormone and decreased when the hormone is secreted inappropriately. Fecal loss of water may increase to over 5 liters per day in severe diarrhea. Nasogastric suction, ileostomy, gastrointestinal fistulas, and burns similarly increase daily water requirements. Water loss is excessive during fever, heavy exercise, or exposure to high environmental temperature. Each degree Celsius of fever causes an obligatory loss of about 200 mL water per day.

Energy To maintain stable weight, energy intake must equal energy output. The output can be divided into basal and activity components. Basal metabolic rate (BMR) is usually measured in the fasting, resting subject immediately after waking (Table 70-10). Values during sleep are about 10 percent less. After each meal, the metabolic rate increases by as much as 30 percent; this thermic effect of food (dietary thermogenesis or specific dynamic action) accounts for about 6 percent of the basal energy expenditure. BMR falls by 20 percent between 30 and 90 years of age; however, this decline disappears when BMR is expressed per kilogram of lean body mass.

Mild, moderate, or severe exercise increases energy expenditure by roughly 30, 50, or 100 (or more) percent, respectively. Energy expenditures in specific types of activity are described in Chap. 317.

The daily energy requirement equals the sum of expenditures incurred by basal metabolism, specific dynamic action, and physical activity. The requirement can be estimated by assessing basal energy expenditure per day from the subject's surface area (Table 70-10), using ideal body weight in this calculation. Subtract 10 percent from basal during the sleeping hours. Add 6 percent to the 24-h basal estimate to cover dietary thermogenesis. From an activity-energy chart, such as is given in Chap. 317, calculate the energy expenditure of the subject's physical activities during a typical day. The daily energy expenditure can be estimated as the sum of basal requirements (minus correction for sleep) plus dietary thermogenesis plus energy requirement for physical activity. Since, on average, 93 percent of energy intake is utilized and 7 percent is lost in feces and urine, the estimated energy requirement for zero balance equals 107 percent of the calculated energy expenditure.

In actual practice, a simpler formula can be used. The Harris-Benedict equations account for sex, weight, height, and age in estimating basal energy expenditure (Table 70-11). To this basal expenditure, 30, 50, or 100 percent is added for sedentary, moderate, or strenuous activity, respectively. Nonstressed hospitalized patients usually require 120 percent of basal energy expenditure, whereas catabolic patients usually require 150 to 200 percent of basal energy expenditure to minimize tissue breakdown or to allow anabolism. Weight is monitored weekly, and if weight increases or decreases in the absence of edema, calories are adjusted accordingly. Short-term changes in weight, however, primarily reflect fluid balance.

Energy expenditure is increased by fever (about 13 percent over basal per degree Celsius), burns (40 to 100 percent), trauma (40 to

TABLE 70-6 Biologic value of food proteins*

Protein source	Biologic value
Milk	93
Egg	93
Beef	76
Peanut meal	74
Potato	69
Oat	65
Rice	65
Corn	50
Soy flour	41
Wheat gluten	40

* *As determined from nitrogen balance studies conducted in the rat, generally at a dietary protein concentration of 5 percent. Tests in the rat at other concentrations, or in other species, give generally similar but not identical biologic values.*

TABLE 70-8 Net absorption of nutrients in normal adults on diets containing mixtures of plant and animal foods

Element	Percent	Element	Percent
Carbohydrate	>90	Manganese	<5
Protein	>90	Fluorine	80–90
Fat	>95	Chromium	1–3
Calcium	5–40	Selenium	>50
Phosphorus	50–60	Molybdenum	40–50
Magnesium	25–50	Cobalt	>50
Iron	5–15	Sodium	>95
Zinc	33	Potassium	80–90
Iodine	>50	Chlorine	>95
Copper	25		

TABLE 70-9 Disorders that alter nutrient requirements by the oral route

Nutrient	Increases dietary requirement	Reduces dietary requirement
Calories	Fever, hyperthyroidism, trauma, malabsorption	Coma, hypothyroidism
Protein	Fever, hyperthyroidism, trauma, azotorrhea	Nitrogen accumulation diseases, inborn errors of urea synthesis
Phenylalanine		Phenylketonuria
Branched-chain amino acids		Maple syrup urine disease
Linoleic acid and fat-soluble vitamins	Malabsorption syndromes	
Folacin	Increased cell turnover	
Calcium	Malabsorption syndromes	Hyperabsorptive hypercalciuria
Phosphorus	Malabsorption syndromes	Renal insufficiency
Magnesium	Malabsorption syndromes	
Iron	Malabsorption syndromes	Hemochromatosis
Zinc	Acrodermatitis enteropathica	
Copper	Malabsorption syndromes	Wilson's disease
Carnitine*	Advanced cirrhosis	

* *No requirement normally.*

100 percent), elective surgery (10 to 20 percent), sepsis (40 to 80 percent), and hyperthyroidism (10 to 100 percent). Hypometabolism, whether due to hypothyroidism, starvation, or other cause, lowers the energy expenditure and, therefore, the energy requirement.

Patients with severe malabsorption may absorb as little as 25 percent of their ingested fat calories and as little as 50 percent of carbohydrate and protein calories, compared with the normal value of over 95 percent. In this situation the oral energy requirement is higher than normal and may prove impossible to achieve if diarrhea is aggravated by increased nutrient intake. In such patients only parenteral nutrition can prevent progressive starvation.

Protein Dietary protein provides a mixture of amino acids for endogenous protein synthesis and is also a metabolic fuel for energy. Healthy adults require nine essential amino acids in amounts varying from 250 to 1100 mg per day. About 7 g of nitrogen as nonessential amino acids is also required for protein synthesis. The requirement and allowance of dietary protein depend on the biologic value of the proteins ingested. Biologic value is defined as the proportion of absorbed protein retained by the body under standard test conditions and is a function of the content of essential amino acids. Nearly optimal ratios of the 9 essential and 11 nonessential amino acids are present in egg and milk proteins, which consequently have the highest biologic values, viz., 90 to 95 (Table 70-6). The biologic value of proteins follows the general order: animal products > legumes > cereals (rice, wheat, corn) > roots. The adult RDA for protein given in Table 70-1, about 50 g per day, assumes a biologic value of about

TABLE 70-10 Basal energy requirements of normal subjects

Age, years	Males, (kcal/m²)/h	Females, (kcal/m²)/h
14–16	46.0	43.0
16–18	43.0	40.0
18–20	41.0	38.0
20–30	39.5	37.0
30–40	39.5	36.5
40–50	38.5	36.0
50–60	37.5	35.0
60–70	36.5	34.0
70–80	35.5	33.0

SOURCE: *EF DuBois, Basal Metabolism in Health and Disease, 3d ed. Philadelphia, Lea & Febiger, 1936, p 151*

TABLE 70-11 Calculation of basal energy expenditure (BEE) by Harris-Benedict equations

WOMEN

$$BEE = 655 + (9.6 \times W) + (1.8 \times H) - (4.7 \times A)$$

MEN

$$BEE = 66 + (13.7 \times W) + (5 \times H) - (6.8 \times A)$$

NOTE: *W = ideal body weight in kilograms, H = height in centimeters, A = age in years*

80, a characteristic value for animal products. The lower the biologic value, the higher the daily protein requirement.

Plant proteins have low biologic value because one or more essential amino acids are usually deficient. Thus for corn (maize), lysine and tryptophan are limiting; for soybeans and green peas, methionine; for rice, lysine and threonine; for wheat, lysine. Therefore, mixtures of vegetable proteins deficient in different essential amino acids have a higher biologic value than either protein separately.

While the usual reason for low biologic value of a particular protein or mixtures of proteins is the limiting content of one or more essential amino acids, a change in the proportion of amino acids or an excess of amino acids can impair the value. For example, when a mixture of amino acids lacking histidine is added to a marginally adequate protein source containing histidine, rats become anorexic and cease growing. This amino acid imbalance is corrected by adding the most limiting amino acid, histidine. An excess of certain amino acids, e.g., methionine and tyrosine, can cause toxic reactions. Requirements for other amino acids can be enhanced by an excess of a structurally similar amino acid, e.g., the branched-chain amino acids, leucine, isoleucine, and valine. These are important considerations in planning the composition of synthetic amino acids for parenteral or enteral feeding, particularly because the anorectic reaction which normally protects against an imbalanced diet is being bypassed.

In other cases essential amino acids may be "spared" by chemically related amino acids. For example cystine and tyrosine, which are synthesized from methionine and phenylalanine, respectively, exert a "sparing" effect in that 80 percent of the methionine requirement and 70 percent of the phenylalanine requirement could be met by giving cystine and tyrosine, respectively.

The daily requirement of a protein, or its constituent amino acids, is influenced by energy intake; the values for protein allowances given in Table 70-1 assume adequate energy intake. When the energy requirement is met by nonprotein calories, a substantial portion of ingested amino acids is utilized for protein synthesis. In contrast, if caloric intake is deficient, some amino acids are diverted from protein synthesis into oxidative metabolism and gluconeogenesis. Under these circumstances, the daily protein requirement is inversely proportional to the energy intake ("protein-sparing effect of nonprotein calories"). Thus, energy undernutrition makes a person more vulnerable to protein starvation, an interaction which accounts for the high prevalence of the combined deficiency state protein-energy undernutrition (see Chap. 72).

The protein-sparing effect of nonprotein calories depends on the source. Carbohydrate spares protein, but in the absence of carbohydrate, fat does not have this action. Protein sparing is maximal when the nonprotein calories include 100 to 150 g carbohydrate per day; the remainder may then be given as fat, carbohydrate, or a mixture of the two.

The daily protein requirement per unit body weight is increased by growth, pregnancy, lactation, fever, infection, trauma, and malabsorption. More protein is required during repletion from cachexia. Protein requirements may be increased in some of the elderly.

To understand how the "nitrogen accumulation diseases," hepatic and renal insufficiency, alter the requirement and tolerance of dietary protein, consider the scheme of amino acid metabolism shown in Fig. 70-1. The daily adult allowance of about 50 g protein serves to maintain protein synthesis (reaction 2) at a rate equal to protein breakdown (reaction 3). Tolerance for protein is normally greater than 250 g per day because of the high capacity of the degradative pathway (reactions 4, 6, 7, and 9). Note that 25 to 40 percent of urea formed in the liver is hydrolyzed by bacteria within the colon and recyles at least once as ammonia (reaction 8). When step 10 is blocked (uremia), the requirement for nonessential nitrogen may be reduced because a small proportion of the ammonia released by urea breakdown is utilized for the synthesis of nonessential amino acids; the carbon skeletons of these acids are readily produced by the intermediary metabolism of glucose. This pathway for endogenous synthesis of nonessential amino acids is the theoretic basis for treating uremics with a diet furnishing a limited amount of protein rich in essential amino acids ("Giovanetti diet"). If to such a diet are added the carbon skeletons (α-keto derivatives) of the essential amino acids, the requirement for the latter nutrients (except for threonine and lysine) is further reduced in part because of the reversibility of transamination (reaction 5 in Fig. 70-1), and in part because the branched-chain keto acids retard the breakdown of proteins in skeletal muscles. Similar considerations apply in the dietary management of cirrhosis of the liver and of hereditary disorders of urea synthesis.

Not only is the daily requirement for protein in some uremics and cirrhotics lower than normal, but the maximal tolerance is curtailed as well. As little as 20 g of protein a day can precipitate or aggravate symptoms of hepatocerebral disease in susceptible patients with liver disease. Intakes of protein customary for healthy subjects in the United States (80 to 100 g per day) can also intensify the uremic syndrome.

One theory to explain the clouded sensorium in liver failure is based on the imbalance of the plasma amino acid profile, namely increased aromatic and decreased branched-chain amino acids. This abnormal ratio, which probably reflects impaired metabolic clearance of aromatic amino acids, might lead to increased synthesis of false neurotransmitters in the brain and subsequent disturbances of neurotransmission. According to this theory, patients with liver failure require a higher ratio of branched-chain to aromatic amino acids in the diet than do individuals with normal liver function.

Reactions 2 and 3 in Fig. 70-1 represent whole-body protein turnover, estimated at about 200 g per day in the 70-kg adult. The major source of amino acids presented for metabolism is from endogenous protein breakdown (reaction 2). Metabolic stress (fever, trauma, infection) increases turnover and reduces efficiency of amino acid reutilization (reaction 3). To achieve nitrogen balance, the protein requirement is increased in the stressed patient by as much as 50 percent.

Fat While the average adult in the United States consumes 40 percent of calories as fat (around 90 g), the dietary requirement is only about 5 percent of total calories as polyunsaturated fatty acids. To minimize the risk of atherosclerosis, the National Institutes of Health have recommended that all Americans (except children under 2 years of age) should reduce total dietary fat intake from the current average level to 30 percent of total calories, reduce saturated fat intake to less than 10 percent of total calories, increase polyunsaturated fat intake but to no more than 10 percent, and reduce daily cholesterol intake to less than 300 mg.

Both the quality and the quantity of the dietary polyunsaturated fatty acids are significant for health. The body contains four classes of unsaturated fatty acids, designated according to the location of the double bond closest to the methyl-terminal, or ω, carbon. Thus, oleic, palmitoleic, linoleic, and linolenic acids, respectively, are 18:1ω9, 16:1ω7, 18:2ω6, and 18:3ω3. Each of these four fatty acids is a precursor for a series of polyunsaturated fatty acids of the same ω class. Only the ω9 and ω7 series can be synthesized by mammals; the ω6 and ω3 compounds are obtained from vegetable and fish or marine animal dietary sources, respectively.

Animals fed a fat-free diet develop a generalized nutritional deficiency syndrome consisting of growth failure, dermatitis, fatty liver, and neurologic and visual abnormalities. Most of these defects are corrected or prevented by the ω6 precursor linoleic acid, but the

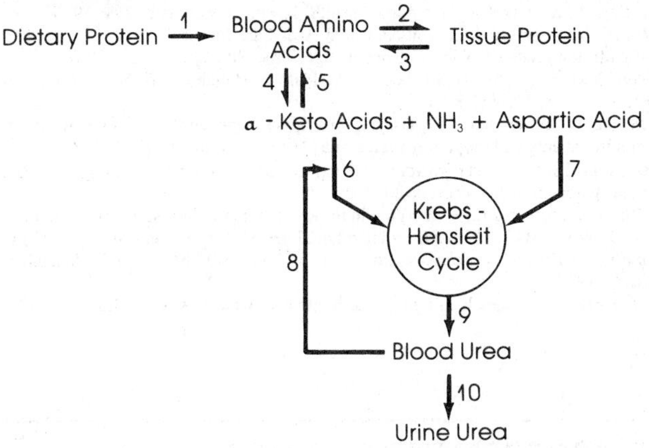

FIGURE 70-1 *Overview of amino acid metabolism.*

neurologic-visual changes reflect depletion of the ω3 class and require linolenic acid for correction. It is now recommended that the human diet contain about 4 percent of calories as linoleic acid and 1 percent as linolenic acid.

Furthermore, the series of 20-carbon-chain eicosanoids (prostaglandins, thromboxanes, prostacyclins, and leukotrienes) derived from each class of polyunsaturated fatty acids has a different profile of bioactivities (see Chap. 68). The ω3 eicosanoids have the unique ability to reduce platelet adhesiveness and lower serum triglycerides. These properties may lower the prevalence of coronary heart disease in populations with a high intake of marine oils.

Naturally occurring animal, fish, and vegetable triglyceride fatty acids are largely 16 or 18 carbons in length. Medium-chain triglycerides (12 to 14 carbons) are clinically useful because they are absorbed through the portal vein, not the splanchnic lymphatics, they are cleared from the circulation more rapidly than long-chain triglycerides, and their fatty acids can be oxidized by carnitine-independent mechanisms in the mitochondria.

Minerals and vitamins The daily allowances and the influence of various conditions on these thresholds are listed in Tables 70-1, 70-2, 70-7, and 70-9. The deficiency syndromes corresponding to each nutrient are listed in Table 70-4, and some clinical effects of exceeding the daily tolerance are given in Table 70-5 (see also Chap. 76). It is important to realize that the mineral and vitamin requirements of the elderly have not been established and that the present recommendations are based on studies of young subjects. Thus, the optimal daily intake of calcium in postmenopausal women is now considered to be 50 percent higher than in youth.

NONESSENTIAL SUBSTANCES Fiber Dietary fiber is a mixture of cellulose, hemicellulose, pectins, algae, polysaccharides, and lignin and contributes 15 to 25 g to the average U.S. diet. The soluble components of these undigestible polymers bind ions, sterols, and bile salts, and the insoluble components add bulk to and accelerate the transit time of the intraluminal contents. Claims have been made for the beneficial effects of dietary fiber on diverticulosis, colon cancer, gallstones, diabetes, and coronary artery disease. Much work is still needed in this area.

Choline, carnitine, inositol These organic compounds have biologic activity, but they have not been considered essential vitamins because several animal species including humans can synthesize them. However, a limited capacity for biosynthesis may be present in immature animals and in certain genetic and acquired disorders; therefore, under these circumstances an exogenous source should be considered.

REFERENCES

Food and Nutrition Board: *Recommended Dietary Allowances*. Washington, D.C. National Academy of Sciences, 1979

GLOMSET JA: Fish, fatty acids and human health. N Engl J Med 312:1253, 1985
MUNRO HN: Nutritional requirements in health. Crit Care Med 8:2, 1980
———: Nutrition-related problems of middle age. Proc Nutr Soc 43:281, 1984
NUTRITIVE VALUE OF AMERICAN FOODS: Agriculture Handbook #456. Agricultural Research Service, USDA, 1975
PHILLIPSON BE et al: Reduction of plasma lipids, lipoproteins, and apoproteins by dietary fish oils in patients with hypertriglyceridemia. N Engl J Med 312:1210, 1985
RECOMMENDED DIETARY ALLOWANCES: National Research Council, Washington, D.C., National Academy of Sciences, 1980
REEDS PJ, GARLICK J: Nutrition and protein turnover in man. Adv Nutr Res 6:93, 1984
RUDMAN D, WILLIAMS PJ: Pathophysiologic principles of nutrition, in *Pathophysiology: The biological principles of disease,* 2d ed, LH Smith Jr, SO Thier (eds). Philadelphia, Saunders, 1985
SANDSTEAD HH: Trace metals in human nutrition. Curr Concepts Nutr 13:37, 1984

71 ASSESSMENT OF NUTRITIONAL STATUS

DANIEL RUDMAN

Undernutrition is a common contributor to morbidity and mortality. As a peculiar discrepancy, however, undernutrition rarely appears in the list of diagnoses or in the progress notes. Consequently, quantitative tests of nutritional status are infrequent in the initial clinical workup, and the progress of the nutritional state is rarely monitored regularly during the course of illness. As a result, undernutrition tends to be recognized late, when it is severe and difficult to treat. This chapter defines feasible methods for identifying and quantifying the deficiency syndromes, for investigating their cause, and for monitoring their course.

MASS AND COMPOSITION OF THE BODY COMPARTMENTS Consideration must first be given to the normal mass and chemical composition of the major body compartments, which are altered by nutritional deficiencies in characteristic ways. The body can be viewed as consisting of four compartments: extracellular fluid, protoplasm (intracellular compartment), bone, and adipose tissue. The first three make up the lean body mass.

The body compartments of a healthy "reference man," 70 kg in weight, 172 cm tall, 35 years old, are summarized in Table 71-1. Typical masses of extracellular fluid, protoplasm, bone, and adipose tissue are 17, 35, 5, and 13 kg, respectively. Chloride is localized almost exclusively in the extracellular fluid, where its average concentration is 96 meq per liter; nitrogen and potassium are largely located in protoplasm, with normal concentrations of 27 g and 150 meq per kilogram of wet weight, respectively; calcium is found primarily in bone, where its concentration averages 260 g per kilogram of wet weight. The adipose tissue contains insignificant levels of these elements.

TABLE 71-1 Approximate mass and major elemental composition of body compartments in a 70-kg healthy "reference man"

	Protoplasm	Extracellular fluid	Bone	Adipose tissue
Mass	35 kg	17 kg	5 kg	13 kg
Body weight	50%	24%	7%	19%
Elemental composition, kg wet wt	27 g N 97 mmol P 150 meq K	140 meq Na 96 meq Cl	260 g Ca 115 g P	

TABLE 71-2 Reifenstein equations for determining change in mass of body compartments

ΔProtoplasm, g	$= 27 \times \Delta N$, g
ΔECF,* g	$= 9.6 \times \Delta Cl$, meq
ΔBone, g	$= 0.1 \times \Delta Ca$, meq
ΔAdipose tissue, g	= ΔBW,† g − [Δ protoplasm, g + ΔECF, g + Δ bone, g]

* *Extracellular fluid.*
† *Body weight.*

DIRECT AND INDIRECT METHODS FOR MEASURING MASS OF BODY COMPARTMENTS If one assumes that the concentrations of chloride, nitrogen, potassium, phosphorus, and calcium remain normal in extracellular fluid, protoplasm, and bone during a period of observation involving expansion or contraction of these compartments, and if one knows the balance (i.e., intake and output) of each element (termed Δ nitrogen, Δ phosphorus, etc.) during this period, then from the equations in Table 71-2 one can calculate the change (Δ) in the mass of each compartment during the period under consideration. The equations are based on the fact that each kilogram of extracellular fluid, protoplasm, or bone gained or lost by the body contains a characteristic amount of chloride, nitrogen, or calcium, respectively.

The urinary excretion of urea nitrogen is accelerated in the patient with trauma, infection or inflammation. A bedside estimate of daily nitrogen balance in grams can be made as follows:

$$\frac{\text{Daily protein intake (g)}}{6.25} - [\text{24-h urine urea nitrogen (g)} + 2.5\text{g}^1]$$

For clinically stable patients, protein intake can be estimated in grams as [24-h urine urea nitrogen (in grams) + 2.5] × 6.25. This approximation is useful in monitoring compliance of patients on low protein diets and in evaluating protein intake of subjects at risk for malnutrition.

Metabolic balance techniques of this type allow estimation of the change in mass of each compartment during the period of observation but provide no information about the absolute mass of the compartment at the beginning and end. Such absolute measurements can be made by several methods: whole-body analysis of potassium (total-body protoplasm), measurement of total-body nitrogen by neutron activation analysis, measurement of extracellular fluid by isotope dilution, measurement of total-body nitrogen by neutron activation analysis, measurement of extracellular fluid by isotope dilution, measurement of total-body water by isotope dilution, calculation of intracellular water (closely related to protoplasmic mass) as total-body water minus extracellular water, measurement of adipose mass by determining whole-body density. These methods are largely restricted to research units. Fortunately, several indirect methods for estimating the mass of body compartments are available to the clinician:

1 In the nonedematous patient, body weight as percent of ideal is a useful indicator of adipose tissue plus lean body mass. Ideal body weight can be estimated from the height/weight tables of the Metropolitan Life Insurance Company or from the following simple formula: in women, 45 kg for the first 152 cm and 0.9 kg for each centimeter over 152; in men, 48 kg for the first 152 cm and 1.1 kg for each centimeter over 152. Reduction of the body weight/ideal body weight ratio to 80 percent in nonedematous patients usually means mild protein-energy undernutrition; a reduction to 70 to 80 percent indicates moderate protein-energy undernutrition; a decline to 70 percent or less indicates severe protein-energy undernutrition.

2 Anthropometric analysis of the midarm requires only a tape measure and caliper. The principle is illustrated in Fig. 71-1; the arm consists of a cylinder of muscle within a sheath of adipose tissue. From the external circumference of the nondominant midarm and the width of the adipose layer (equal to one-half the triceps skin fold), midarm muscle area and midarm fat area can be calculated. The midarm muscle and fat areas are indicators of the body's masses of skeletal muscle and adipose tissue, respectively. Normal average values for adult men and women, respectively, are midarm muscle area, 50.91 and 42.81 cm^2, and midarm fat area, 17.04 and 21.28 cm^2. By taking skinfold measurements at the biceps, subscapular, and suprailiac sites, in addition to the triceps, one

[1] *Two-and-one-half grams is the approximate sum of urinary nonurea nitrogen plus fecal and integumental losses of nitrogen.*

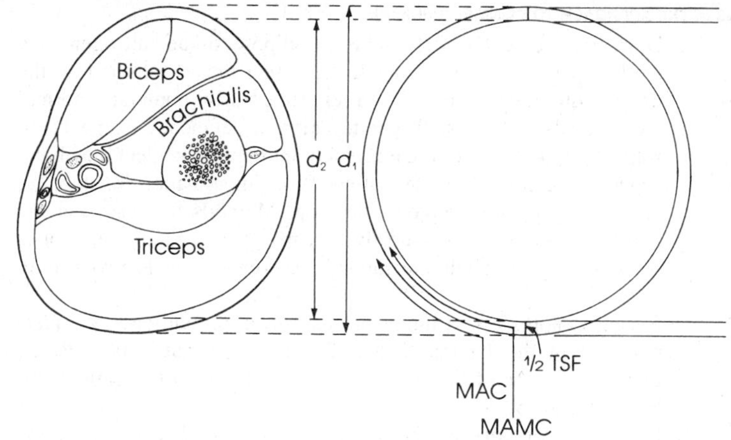

Normal Values (adults)	Male	Female
Triceps skinfold, mm	12.5	16.5
Midarm muscle circumference, cm	25.3	23.2
Midarm fat area, cm^2	17.0	21.3
Midarm muscle area, cm^2	50.9	42.8

Calculation of Mid Upper Arm Muscle Circumference

C_1 = mid upper arm circumference in centimeters

S = triceps skinfold in centimeters

d_1 = arm diameter

d_2 = muscle diameter

Skinfold (S) = 2 X subcutaneous fat = $d_1 - d_2$

Circumference (C_1) = πd_1

Muscle circumference = $C_1 - \pi S$

$$\text{Midarm muscle area} = \frac{(C_1 - \pi S)^2}{4\pi}$$

$$\text{Midarm fat area} = \frac{(S)(C_1)}{2} - \frac{\pi(S^2)}{4}$$

FIGURE 71-1 *Anthropometric measurement of muscle and adipose compartments of the mid-upper arm. Midarm circumference is measured with a tape measure and triceps skinfold with a caliper. (After C Butterworth and C Blackburn, Nutr Today 10:8, 1974.)*

can calculate total adipose mass by the method of Durnin and Womersley. Lean body mass is derived from the difference between fat mass in kilograms and body weight.

3 Urine creatinine is related to lean body mass by the equation:

$$\text{Lean body mass (kg)} = 7.138 + 0.02908 \times (\text{mg creatinine/24 h})$$

The ratio of 24-h creatinine excretion (in grams) to height (in centimeters) is considered a measure of muscle mass and can be used as an index to determine protein depletion. Three qualifying conditions should be considered: (a) diets containing meat influence the quantity of creatinine excreted; (b) impaired renal function results in falsely low creatinine excretion; and (c) creatinine excretion declines with age as a result of smaller muscle mass. In normal men and women the creatinine/height ratio averages 10.5 and 5.8 mg/cm, respectively. In men, ratios in the ranges 8.4 to 9.5, 7.4 to 8.4, and less than 7.4 mg/cm signify mild, moderate, and severe degrees of protein depletion, respectively.

4 Sagittal or horizontal radiograms or computerized tomography (CT) scans of an extremity also provide quantitative information about the mass of representative skeletal muscles but are more expensive.

Skeletal muscle makes up about 30 percent of the lean body mass and atrophies progressively in protein-energy starvation, the most common deficiency state in U.S. hospitals (see Chap. 72). By monitoring the creatinine/height ratio and midarm muscle area, the clinician can identify protein-energy starvation easily and monitor its course.

The visceral compartment, which maintains tissue function, blood protein synthesis, and the immune response, comprises 20 percent of the lean body mass. Under conditions of nutritional inadequacy, protein synthesis declines, metabolic pathways are altered, and the immune system is impaired. Certain blood proteins are sensitive indicators of these events and are used to detect malnutrition and monitor nutritional repletion (Table 71-3). Prealbumin and retinol binding protein have the shortest half-lives (1 to 2 days) and thus

TABLE 71-3 Laboratory tests for the evaluation of nutritional status (adults)

Nutrient evaluation	Test	Deficient (often with clinical manifestations)	Low (usually without clinical manifestations)	Acceptable
Protein	Serum albumin, g/dL	<3.0	3.0–3.5	>3.5
Protein	Serum transferrin, mg/dL	<180–260		180–260
Protein	Serum prealbumin, mg/dL	<20–50		20–50
Protein	Serum retinol binding protein, μg/mL	<30–45		30–45
Protein	Creatinine/height ratio	<90% of Standard	90–95%	>95%
Protein	Nitrogen balance, g	>(−)3	(−)1–3	0–3
Protein, Fe, folacin, vitamin B_{12}	Hemoglobin, g/dL	<12	12–14	>14
Iron	Serum iron, μg/dL	<60		>60
Vitamin A	Plasma retinol, μg/dL	<10	10–20	>20
Vitamin D	Serum Ca × P product, mg/dL	<40		>40
Vitamin D	Alkaline phosphatase, King-Armstrong units/dL	>40	15–40	8–14
Vitamin C	Serum ascorbic acid, mg/dL	<0.20	0.20–0.30	>0.30
Thiamin	Erythrocyte transketolase (% thiamin disphosphate stimulation)	>20	15–20	<15
Riboflavin	Erythrocyte glutathione reductase activity coefficient	>1.40	1.20–1.40	<1.20
Niacin	*N*-Methylnicotinamide excretion, mg/g creatinine	<0.5	0.5–1.59	>1.6
Vitamin B_6	Erythrocyte aminotransferase activity coefficients:			
	Erythrocyte ALT	>1.25		<1.25
	Erythrocyte AST	>1.5		<1.5
Vitamin B_6	Tryptophan load test (xanthurenic acid), mg/day	>50	25–50	<25
Folacin	Serum folate, ng/mL	<3	3.0–6.0	>6.0
Folacin	Erythrocyte folate, ng/mL	<140	140–160	>160
Vitamin B_{12}	Serum vitamin B_{12}, pb/mL	<150	150–200	>200
Ca	24-h urine Ca^{2+}, mg	<50	50–100	>100
P	24-h urine P, mg	<100	100–300	>300
Mg	24-h urine Mg^{2+}, meq	<4	4–8	>8
Na	24-h urine Na^{+}, meq	<20	20–40	>40
K	24-h urine K^{+}, meq	<20	20–40	>40

can be used to monitor patients at high risk of developing protein-energy malnutrition and to evaluate the initial repletion. Presently, these immunoassays are expensive. Transferrin, with a half-life of 8 days, is also useful in monitoring repletion, although concurrent iron-deficiency anemia makes interpretation difficult. Albumin (half-life, 14 days) is the most useful prognostic indicator of protein-energy malnutrition. Albumin synthesis may be impaired in liver disease; nevertheless, in undernourished cirrhotics the albumin level usually rises with nutritional repletion.

SYNDROMES OF UNDERNUTRITION When any of the 39 essential nutrient requirements (Chap. 70) are not met, undernutrition syndromes result. Undernutrition of such micronutrients as nitrogen, sodium, chloride, potassium, calcium, and phosphorus reduces the mass of one or more body compartments, often with associated abnormalities in compartmental chemistry, structure, and function. For example, deficiencies of nitrogen (protein), sodium, and calcium erode protoplasm, extracellular fluid, and bone, respectively. Undernutrition of a micronutrient tends to cause a specific morphologic or functional abnormality in certain tissues without alteration in compartmental mass or elemental composition. While in theory 39 different types of human malnutrition could occur, undernutrition syndromes usually occur in groups rather than in "pure" form.

Deficiency of each essential nutrient can be characterized in terms of symptoms, signs, and chemical and radiographic abnormalities, but deficiency syndromes have several principles in common:

1 Undernutrition can be either primary or secondary in origin. The primary form is due to an inadequate supply of food containing the essential nutrients. In secondary undernutrition an adequate diet is available, but because of illness or medical treatment, nutrients cannot be ingested, absorbed, or metabolized adequately, or the rate of utilization of external losses is excessive. Primary and secondary mechanisms frequently reinforce each other; for example, the hypermetabolism and anorexia of infection precipitate nutritional deficiencies more rapidly in patients who previously subsisted on marginal diets than in well-nourished individuals. To determine whether undernutrition in a particular patient is primary or secondary, the physician must obtain a dietary history, assess personal habits and living conditions, and examine the patient for organic disease.
2 Nutritional deficiency syndromes tend to evolve through three stages. Many essential nutrients are stored in the tissues of the well-nourished subject; for example, iron and vitamins B_{12}, A, and D in liver; essential fatty acids in adipose tissue; nitrogen in a labile reserve in muscle and liver. When intake falls below the daily requirement, these reserves temporarily maintain normal blood levels and forestall manifestation of deficiency (stage 1). In stage 2, blood levels of the nutrient or nutrient-dependent metabolic products decline, but the patient is asymptomatic. In stage 3, clinical signs and symptoms develop. Methods for assessing the nutritional status should ideally be capable of detecting all stages of deficiency. Available techniques, however, usually reveal only stages 2 and 3.
3 Because anorexia is a major mechanism in protein-energy undernutrition in the United States, the intake of nutrients must be measured in one of three ways: by recall, by diary (outpatient), or by observation (inpatient).
4 Change in weight may be ambiguous. In the absence of edema various proportions of weight loss are due to depletion of adipose tissue and lean body mass. In the presence of edema body weight changes are even more difficult to intrepret. Gain in weight can reflect an accumulation of edema, masking erosion of protoplasm; conversely, loss of weight can reflect diuresis with simultaneous expansion of the protoplasmic compartment. An initially obese patient can lose 15 kg because of chronic wasting illness and present with a normal body weight, the still substantial adipose organ masking a shrinkage in the lean body mass. In such instances, direct or indirect estimation of the size of the protoplasmic compartment is essential as described above.
5 The undernourished patient is usually deficient in several nutrients. Common patterns are deficiency of two or more water-soluble vitamins (usually including folate, vitamin C, and/or thiamine) and deficiency of both calcium and magnesium in patients with malabsorption.

TABLE 71-4 Nutritional data base

HISTORY
Previous weight curve
Dietary intake by retrospective recall and prospective diary
Alcohol intake
Socioeconomic and family status, including income
Anorexia, vomiting, diarrhea
Blood loss
Pregnancy, lactation, menses
Vitamin and mineral supplements
Use of drugs that might affect nutrition
PHYSICAL EXAMINATION
General: weight as percent of ideal body weight; triceps skinfold; midarm muscle circumference
Skin: xerosis, follicular hyperkeratosis, pellagrous dermatitis, petechiae, ecchymoses, perifollicular hemorrhages, flaky paint dermatitis, pallor
Hair: dyspigmentation, easy pluckability, thinning, straightening
Head: temporal wasting, parotid enlargement
Eyes: Bitot spots, conjunctival and scleral xerosis, keratomalacia, corneal vascularization, angular palpebritis
Mouth: cheilosis, angular stomatitis, magenta tongue, atrophic lingual papillae, tongue fissuring, glossitis, spongy gums, state of dentition
Heart: cardiomegaly, findings of congestive heart failure
Abdomen: hepatomegaly
Extremities: edema, koilonychia
Neurologic: irritability, weakness, calf tenderness, loss of deep tendon reflexes

The various physical, chemical, and radiographic characteristics of each type of undernutrition are summarized in Table 70-4. The most commonly used chemical indexes of nutrient deficiency are listed in Table 71-3, which gives three average concentration ranges for each test: normal, subnormal without clinical manifestations, and subnormal with clinical signs or symptoms of deficiency. Although these tests are of value in population surveys and in following the response of patients to therapies, coexisting conditions, such as the effect of renal disease on 24-h urinary creatinine, must be taken into consideration.

The clinician must select a reasonable number of historical, physical, and laboratory items to use as a "nutritional data base" for screening for undernutrition. Table 71-4 presents a selection of historical and physical items that reveal most deficiency states in hospital patients. Mullen has shown that a nutritional index based on triceps skin fold, skin reactivity to recall antigens, and serum levels of albumin and transferrin, is a valuable predictor of complications and death after surgery.

Most of the quantitative indexes of nutritional status so far considered are "static" measurements of body composition or of concentrations of nutrients or nutrient-dependent products in body fluids. "Functional" indexes sensitive to nutritional deficiencies include work capacity, dark adaptation, taste acuity, phagocytic activity of leukocytes, cognitive ability, capillary fragility, and reproductive performance. The measurement of such nutrient-dependent physiologic functions is especially important in identifying marginal deficiency syndromes and in documenting the impact of nutritional supplements on the health of populations.

MONITORING THE COURSE OF MALNUTRITION Besides defining the type, severity, and mechanism for the development of undernutrition, it is important to ascertain the rate of progression. This is accomplished by periodic monitoring of body weight, albumin, hematocrit, creatinine excretion, midarm muscle area, midarm fat area, and appropriate blood or urine concentrations of nutrition-dependent variables. An example of the course of progressive protein-energy malnutrition is shown in Fig. 71-2.

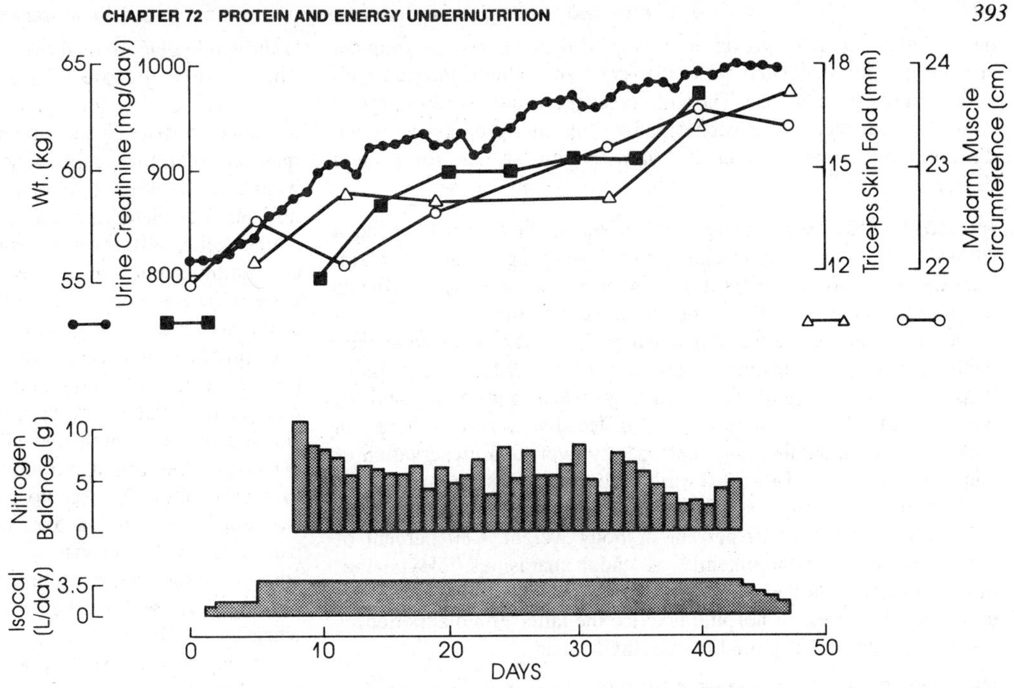

FIGURE 71-2 *The course of a patient with protein-calorie depletion during repletion by nasogastric hyperalimentation.*

REFERENCES

Bistrian BR: A simple technique to estimate severity of stress. Surg Gynecol Obstet 148:675, 1979

Blackburn GL, Thornon PA: Nutritional assessment of the hospitalized patient. Med Clin North Am 63:1103, 1979

Durnin J, Womersley J: Body fat assessed from total body density and its estimation from skinfold thickness: Measurement on 481 men and women from 16 to 72 years. Br J Nutr 32:77, 1974

Forbes GB: Urinary creatinine excretion and lean body mass. Am J Clin Nutr 29:1361, 1976

Herbert V: The five possible causes of all nutrient deficiency: Illustrated by deficiencies of vitamin B_{12} and folic acid. Am J Clin Nutr 26:77, 1973

Maghan KJ et al: The relative proportions of fat, muscle and bone in the normal human forearm as determined by computed tomography. Clin Sci 66:683, 1984

Mullen JL et al: Implications of malnutrition in surgical patients. Arch Surg 114:121, 1979

Phillips LS, Unterman T: Somatomedin activity in disorders of nutrition and metabolism. Clin Endocrinol Metab 13:145, 1984

Reifenstein EC et al: The accumulation, interpretation, and presentation of data pertaining to metabolic balances, notably those of calcium, phosphorus, and nitrogen. J Clin Endocrinol Metab 5:367, 1945

Russell DM, Jeejeebhoy KN: The assessment of the functional consequences of malnutrition. Curr Concepts Nutr 13:113, 1984

Sauberlich HE: Implications of nutritional status on human biochemistry, physiology, and health. Clin Biochem 17:132, 1984

Solomons NW, Allen LH: The functional assessment of nutritional status: Principles, practice and potential. Nutr Rev 41:33, 1983

Sutphen JL: Growth as a measure of nutritional status. J Pediatr Gastroenterol Nutr 4:169, 1985

Vaswani AN et al: Effects of caloric restriction on body composition and total body nitrogen as measured by neutron activation. Metabolism 32:185, 1983

Viteri FE, Alvarado J: The creatinine height index: Its use in the estimation of the degree of protein depletion and repletion in protein calorie malnourished children. Pediatrics 46:696, 1970

72 PROTEIN AND ENERGY UNDERNUTRITION

DANIEL RUDMAN

RELEVANCE TO CONTEMPORARY MEDICINE Protein-energy undernutrition was described in developing nations in the 1930s. The syndrome affects the structure and function of every organ in the body. The causes, manifestations, and treatment have been intensively studied in African and Asian children, in whom the prevalence of the primary form of the disorder is high. The secondary varieties of protein-energy deficiency are common within hospital populations in developed nations. Subacutely or chronically ill patients living longer under the protection of modern therapeutics but handicapped by anorexia, hypermetabolism, or malabsorption may rapidly develop protein-energy malnutrition. A third cause of protein-energy undernutrition in the western world is the syndrome of anorexia nervosa in young women.

DEFINITION AND ETIOLOGY The progressive loss of both lean body mass and adipose tissue results from insufficient consumption of protein and energy, although one or the other may play the dominant role in a given individual. The inadequate intake may be primary or secondary, as discussed in Chap. 71. Synergism between the two mechanisms is common. Patients with scanty reserves of protein and energy develop clinical protein-energy starvation more rapidly than well-nourished subjects when challenged by the hypermetabolism, catabolism, and anorexia of infection or other illnesses.

On a global basis the primary mechanism predominates. Socioeconomic factors that limit the quantity and quality of the diet are paramount. Particularly important is the poor biologic value of many vegetable proteins. The problem is accentuated if energy is inadequate because a large proportion of the dietary amino acids must then be oxidized as fuel instead of used to synthesize tissue and plasma protein. In developed countries, protein-energy malnutrition is often the result of inadequate nutrient intake due to drug or alcohol abuse; to depression and isolation in the aged; or to anorexia, malabsorption, or hypermetabolism in the hospitalized patient.

EPIDEMIOLOGY The prevalence of protein-energy undernutrition can be assessed by measuring percent reduction in midarm fat area, midarm muscle area, 24-h urinary creatinine/height ratio, and serum albumin (see Chap. 71). The rate of growth of the children is a sensitive index of the nutritional state of a population: subnormal height for age ("stunting") usually indicates chronic protein-energy deficiency, and subnormal weight for height ("wasting") manifests recent energy deficit.

Estimates of prevalence of protein-energy depletion in various population groups are given in Table 72-1. In the United States, subclinical protein deficiency is more common in the south than in the north, in blacks and Latin Americans than in whites, and in the poor and the elderly than in the general population. In contrast to developing nations, protein-energy depletion in the general population in the United States tends to be mild and subclinical. In hospitals, on the other hand, severe as well as mild deficiencies are frequent and are usually associated with other types of malnutrition and with underlying organic disease. The widespread prescription of low protein diets to treat hepatic encephalopathy, chronic progressive renal disease, and uremia has created new groups at risk for protein deficiency.

PATHOPHYSIOLOGY Energy and protein deficiencies have been studied most extensively in children of developing nations in whom inadequate or marginal diets, the augmented nutritional requirements of growth, and frequent episodes of infectious disease combine to cause florid manifestations of deficiency. Two syndromes have been distinguished: (1) marasmus, manifested by stunted growth, loss of adipose tissue, and generalized wasting of lean body mass without edema; and (2) kwashiorkor, manifested by growth failure (in children), hypoalbuminemia, edema, fatty liver, and preservation of adipose tissue. Mixed forms (kwashiorkor-marasmus) are common.

In adult secondary protein-energy undernutrition, Bistrian has defined weight loss >10 percent or body weight <80 percent of ideal, without hypoalbuminemia, as "adult marasmus." Hypoalbuminemia alone is termed "adult kwashiorkor." The distinction seems to be useful because in hospital practice the latter group experiences greater morbidity and mortality than the former.

METABOLIC AND ENDOCRINE ASPECTS **Energy deficiency** The events during calorie undernutrition can be viewed as adaptations serving to conserve the lean body mass. The first level of adaptation involves reduction of physical activity and energy expenditure. In early life, if the food intake of balanced diets is reduced to 60 percent of the ad lib intake, growth rate is slowed, puberty is delayed, and adult size is reduced. In rats, mice, and dogs, a moderate degree of underfeeding with a balanced diet (to about 60 percent of ad lib) leads to small, healthy adults. Interestingly, the life span of dogs is increased by a factor of 1.2 to 1.8 compared with ad lib–fed animals; the improved longevity reflects less cancer, better immunity, and preservation of renal function in later life.

Further reduction in caloric intake, or semistarvation, exceeds these adaptations and now leads to adverse effects throughout the body, with increased morbidity, shortened life span, and diminished work capacity. The body responds to semistarvation with an orderly physiologic adaptation, engineered in large part by a reduced secretion of insulin, augmented plasma levels of glucagon and cortisol, curtailed hepatic production of triiodothyronine (T_3) from thyroxine (T_4), and diminished hepatic secretion of somatomedin C despite augmented growth hormone release. The fall in plasma insulin permits free fatty acids and amino acids to be mobilized from adipose tissue and muscle to provide carbon for the continuing oxidative metabolism of the body, while glucose tends to be spared for the central nervous system. The impaired glucose tolerance of starvation sometimes reflects a component of insulin resistance; excessive production of growth hormone, cortisol, catecholamines, free fatty acids, and interleukins may all contribute, especially in the stressed patient. When energy balance is negative, oxidative metabolism claims first priority in the utilization of dietary protein. During starvation, the carbon chains of amino acids also provide substrate for gluconeogenesis, since a continuing supply of glucose is required by the central nervous system. The augmented secretion of ACTH and cortisol contributes to the acceleration of gluconeogenesis. As amino acids are diverted from protein synthesis into oxidative metabolism and gluconeogenesis, protein synthesis is curtailed, particularly in muscle. The low somatomedin level in the underfed child is a probable cause for the slowing of the growth rate. The metabolic rate gradually declines, because of diminished extrathyroidal conversion of T_4 to T_3, decreased synthesis of the T_3 receptor, curtailed production and turnover of catecholamines, and a decrease in dietary thermogenesis. During partial or total deprivation of calories, both lean body mass and adipose tissue contract, but the latter does so more rapidly. In prolonged starvation, the adipose organ may be totally consumed when lean body mass has contracted by only 30 or 40 percent.

During the first week of total starvation, the average patient loses 4 to 5 kg of body weight which consists of about 25 percent adipose tissue, 35 percent extracellular fluid, and 40 percent protoplasm. Losses of nitrogen, potassium, sodium, and chloride represent 3 to 8 percent of the total body content of each element. Negative balances of magnesium, phosphorus, and calcium are also considerable. During ensuing weeks, as further adaptive endocrine and enzymatic adjustments occur, losses of nitrogen and other elements continue but at a slower rate. Ketone bodies now tend to replace glucose as substrate for oxidation in the brain, thereby sparing gluconeogenesis and protein catabolism.

The intracellular compartment does not contract at the same rate in all tissues. The central nervous system does not lose weight. Skeletal muscle atrophies more rapidly than cardiac muscle, and the gastrointestinal tract and liver lose mass more rapidly than kidneys. Mobilization of amino acids from muscle to liver permits the latter to continue to synthesize some albumin and lipoproteins; as a consequence, hypoalbuminemia and fatty liver are not conspicuous. When the loss of muscle mass in protein-energy undernutrition reaches 50 percent, survival is limited; thus, it is unusual to find midarm muscle circumference less than 50 percent of standard in chronically ill adults.

Protein deficiency Frequently the intake of protein is more limited than that of calories. This occurs because dietary protein is more expensive than carbohydrate or fat; because protein of high biologic value (chiefly animal) is more expensive than protein of low biologic value (chiefly vegetable); because high-calorie, low-protein foods (many snack foods, ethanol, starchy root-based vegetables) are in common use in the United States and abroad; and because physicians may administer glucose as the sole organic nutrient in the intravenous feeding of the patient who cannot eat. The deficiency state under these conditions is analogous to kwashiorkor in children. The reduction of insulin secretion, which is a central mechanism in the adaptation to energy starvation, is circumvented. Insulin secreted in response to the dietary or intravenous carbohydrate promotes lipogenesis and retards lipolysis; adipose tissue is preserved, and free fatty acids are not available for oxidation in place of amino acids. The high plasma insulin also impairs mobilization and redistribution of amino acids from skeletal muscle to liver. Plasma amino acids fall, and the total body rate of protein synthesis declines. The synthesis of albumin and transport proteins by the liver is curtailed. Fatty infiltration of the liver is common. Two biochemical mechanisms are probably involved in the steatosis: (1) lack of methionine limits phospholipid synthesis, secondarily impairing lipoprotein formation, and (2) hepatic synthesis of triglycerides from glucose continues. Decreased concentrations of plasma albumin, plasma transferrin, and hemoglobin reflect severe

TABLE 72-1 Prevalence of protein-energy malnutrition in selected groups

Group	Criterion of deficiency	Prevalence of deficiency, %
Children <5 years, 28 developing countries*	Body weight <80% (kwashiorkor) or <60% of standard (marasmus)	25
Pediatric patients, Children's Hospital Medical Center, Boston†	Weight/height <90% of standard; midarm muscle area <15th percentile	37
Cancer patients, Emory University Hospital‡	Creatinine/height <60% std., triceps skin fold <80% std.	50
General surgical patients, Boston City Hospital¶	Midarm muscle circumference, triceps skin fold, serum albumin more than two standard deviations below normal mean	48

* *J Bengou, J Trop Pediatr 13:169, 1967.*
† *R Merritt, Am J Clin Nutr 32:1320, 1979.*
‡ *D Nixon, Am J Med 68:683, 1980.*
¶ *BR Bistrian et al, JAMA 230:858, 1974.*

protein starvation. Edema is characteristic of this stage and results in part from the hypoalbuminemia.

The account above describes the sequence of events in primary protein deficiency. However, variable degrees of energy and protein starvation commonly occur together. A further complication in secondary undernutrition is that the metabolic stress of trauma, infection, fever, or inflammation can cause the release of interleukins that inhibit albumin synthesis. In such patients, the rate of albumin catabolism and its movement from intravascular to extravascular sites are accelerated. Hypoalbuminemia correlates with morbidity and mortality in secondary protein-energy undernutrition, but its pathogenesis is complex.

Mineral metabolism Protein-energy undernutrition is generally associated with a depletion of body minerals. In part this reflects the contraction of protoplasmic and extracellular fluid compartments with their constituent elements (nitrogen, phosphorus, potassium, and magnesium within cells; sodium and chloride in extracellular fluid) being excreted into the urine in the same proportions as in the lean body mass. However, mineral losses are often out of proportion to the contraction of lean body mass. One reason is a shift of potassium and magnesium from muscle to plasma in exchange for sodium. In addition, potassium, magnesium, phosphorus, and calcium intakes may be even less adequate than those of protein and energy (e.g., during prolonged intravenous nutrition with magnesium- or phosphorus-free solutions). Finally, renal and extrarenal losses of these elements may be significant (diuresis, diarrhea, fistulas, etc.).

STRESSED VERSUS NONSTRESSED PROTEIN-ENERGY MALNUTRITION Simple starvation in an otherwise healthy individual, as described above, involves maintenance of glucose production at the expense of muscle tissue. Unchecked protein catabolism would quickly lead to death, but a gradual metabolic adaptation mitigates the effects: the need for gluconeogenesis from amino acids is reduced as the central nervous system adapts to ketone bodies as a fuel source, and basal energy expenditure is reduced.

Protein-energy undernutrition in a patient stressed by trauma, burn, infection, or inflammation proceeds more rapidly. Muscle especially is catabolized at an accelerated rate. The loss of 1.5 to 2 kg of protoplasm in the first week of simple starvation should be compared to the loss of 1.0 to 2.5 kg of protoplasm per day under conditions of severe metabolic stress.

The accelerated pace of protein-energy undernutrition in "stressed semistarvation" has several causes: (1) augmented consumption of glucose because of hypermetabolism and because of the glucose requirement of inflammatory tissues; (2) extra utilization of protein for immune function and wound repair; (3) the exaggerated catecholamine and cortisol responses contributing to hypermetabolism (up to +100 percent), gluconeogenesis, and insulin resistance; (4) production of interleukins. Activated phagocytic cells release one or more metabolically active peptides, variously termed leukocyte pyrogen, leukocyte endogenous mediator, or interleukin 1, which causes prostaglandin E_2 to accumulate in brain, liver, muscle, and adipose tissue, with resultant fever, protein breakdown in muscle, synthesis of acute phase proteins in liver, fat mobilization, insulin resistance, and movement of iron and zinc from the circulation into storage sites in the liver. These features are all prominent in stressed semistarvation.

Studies with heavy isotopes have shed some light on the catabolic response to injury. The rate of turnover of whole-body protein in the normal adult is of the order of 200 g per day. Eighty to ninety percent of the amino acids released by this process are normally reutilized; the remaining 10 to 20 percent are supplied by the diet. The efficiency of the reutilization process depends upon an adequate supply of energy. In unstressed starvation, the rate of protein breakdown remains unchanged, while the rate of protein synthesis declines, with a resultant loss of body protein. In stressed starvation, both protein breakdown and protein synthesis are accelerated, but the former to a greater extent, thereby increasing the loss of body protein. The efficiency of reutilization of the amino acids released by catabolism is reduced in the febrile or injured patient. Branched-chain amino acids may become limiting in the reutilization process, and an increased intake of these building blocks improves muscle protein synthesis in some catabolic patients.

CARDIOVASCULAR-RESPIRATORY AND RENAL RESPONSES The heart and kidneys lose mass progressively during the course of protein-energy starvation. These losses are generally proportional to the erosion of lean body mass, so that ratios of heart mass/lean body mass and kidney mass/lean body mass remain normal. Consequently, a functional insufficiency of these two shrunken organs is not a usual feature of protein-energy depletion. Cardiac output declines in parallel with the falling metabolic rate. Blood pressure is reduced by the fall in cardiac output. The ventilatory response to hypoxia is blunted. Glomerular filtration rate and renal blood flow are lowered. The ability of the kidney to excrete an acid load or to respond to antidiuretic hormone may be impaired. Although these changes in cardiac and renal structure and function are in part appropriate to the reduced lean body mass and hypometabolic state, they may become important handicaps during vigorous nutritional repletion, acute infection, or other circumstances that require rapid increases in cardiac output, metabolic rate, and urinary excretion of solutes. Heart failure and death may occur during the rapid repletion of subjects with severe protein-energy undernutrition.

BLOOD Reduced blood volume, hematocrit, albumin, transferrin, retinol-bending protein, and total lymphocyte count are characteristic in the wasted patient. The anemia of "pure" protein-energy depletion is normocytic and normochromic and usually results from a decreased production of red blood cells, perhaps reflecting the protein requirement for globin synthesis.

In most patients with protein-calorie undernutrition, there are complicating factors such as multiple micronutrient deficiencies; concurrent bacterial, viral, or parasitic infestation; or major underlying disease. In the primary undernutrition in developing nations, iron deficiency is apparent in about 25 percent of patients on admission and becomes evident in 90 percent during recovery. Folate is deficient on admission in 10 to 20 percent. Serum erythropoietin is high. Feeding an adequate diet quickly causes reticulocytosis.

STRUCTURE AND FUNCTION OF GASTROINTESTINAL TRACT AND PANCREAS The gastrointestinal tract and pancreas atrophy. In the small intestine, villous height, mitotic index, and content of disaccharidases and dipeptidases all decline. Exocrine elements of the pancreas atrophy as well, and the production of digestive enzymes is reduced. Bacterial overgrowth may occur in the small intestine. Hypoalbuminemia may lead to edema of the small bowel. These factors combine to produce malabsorption and lactose intolerance. The structural and functional regression of the small intestine results, in part, from decreased oral feeding rather than systemic malnutrition, since patients fully repleted by the parenteral route still exhibit the same lesion.

IMMUNE SYSTEM Lymphatic tissues atrophy. Impaired cell-mediated immunity is evident by all standard tests (blastogenic response of lymphocytes to mitogens, total lymphocyte count, and skin testing with recall antigens). Bactericidal activity of polymorphonuclear leukocytes is decreased. Diminished thymic hormone activity retards the maturation of T cells, and the proportion of circulating T cells of the null variety is increased. Deficiencies of zinc and water-soluble vitamins contribute to the T-cell defects. Plasma B-cell functions (plasma immunoglobin concentrations and humoral responses to antigens) are preserved. Protein-energy-starved patients experience increased morbidity and mortality during common infections and are subject to infection by opportunistic organisms (gram-negative bacteria, *Candida*, herpes simplex). Impaired respiratory function, leading to atelectasis and pneumonia, is a common cause of death. The extent of cutaneous anergy correlates both with the severity of nutritional deficiency and with morbidity and mortality rates.

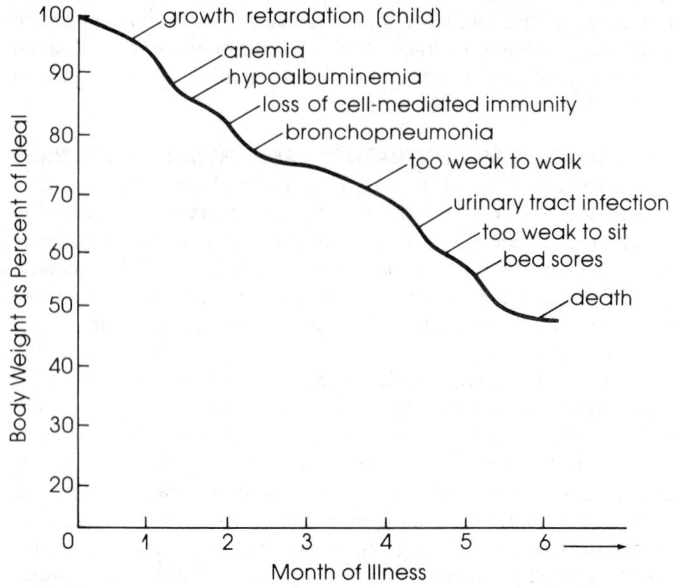

FIGURE 72-1 *Course of a typical case of progressive protein-energy starvation.*

WOUND HEALING The response of fibroblasts to surgical wounds is impaired. Consequently, incisions and enteric anastomoses heal more slowly in undernourished patients; wound dehiscence is common.

TEMPERATURE REGULATION In the absence of fever, basal metabolic rate is reduced. Hypothermia is common. The underlying mechanisms are reduced heat production due to low plasma T_3, possible decreased adrenergic function, loss of thermal insulation when subcutaneous adipose tissue is gone, and resetting of the thermostat in the preoptic nuclei of the hypothalamus. Hypoglycemia may occur (see Chap. 329).

REPRODUCTION Nearly every phase of the reproductive process is impaired in women of child-bearing age. Diminished secretion of luteinizing hormone–releasing hormone (LHRH) by the hypothalamus may cause amenorrhea. Fertility is reduced: if implantation occurs, the risk of early fetal resorption is high. If gestation is completed, the progeny are substandard in weight and length. Lactation is impaired so that postnatal undernutrition is common. Even if postnatal nutrition is adequate, stunted growth in the malnourished infant is in part irreversible, and impairment in learning capacity may be lifelong.

In wasted men, plasma total and free testosterone tend to be low due to various combinations of primary gonadal defect and diminished hypothalamic LHRH production.

CLINICAL MANIFESTATIONS **History** A primary component in the etiology can be uncovered only by reviewing protein and caloric intake and the biologic quality of the dietary protein during the preceding months. Factors that predispose to a secondary etiology include the presence of a known chronic medical problem, prolonged fever, anorexia or other gastrointestinal symptoms, and lack of teeth.

In children failure to gain height and weight is an early sign. In adults weight loss is usual, but a body weight equal to or greater than ideal does not exclude the presence of deficiency of caloric intake, protein, or both. Thus, progressive loss of protoplasm and adipose tissue may be masked by edema; or the patient may have been previously obese, and a substantial loss of lean body mass during the current illness may be masked by a residue of obesity. Listlessness, easy fatigability, sensation of coldness, swollen ankles, and dry, cracked skin are frequent in patients with protein-energy malnutrition.

Physical signs The facies is drawn, temporal regions are concave and fleshless, intercostal spaces are excavated, and the skin hangs in folds on the wasted extremities. ''Flaky paint'' dermatitis and dyspigmentation of skin and hair are common. The patient is pale and may be edematous. Signs of vitamin deficiency may be present. Decubiti and skin ulcers are common in advanced stages.

Vital signs The blood pressure is decreased. The pulse is slow, and the extremities are cool; central temperature may be decreased.

Anthropometrics The midarm fat area and midarm muscle area are reduced in varying ratios dependent on previous nutritional state and relative severity of the energy and protein deficiencies.

Laboratory and x-ray findings The ratio of 24-h urinary creatinine/height is decreased. In the absence of renal disease, this is the most sensitive and practical clinical indicator of protein starvation and should be monitored at monthly intervals in the chronically ill hospital patient. These analyses are valid only in the afebrile state, since urinary excretion of creatinine is increased by fever. Other signs of protein-energy malnutrition include a decrease in serum albumin, serum transferrin, and hematocrit, but these changes are less specific. Nevertheless, protein depletion may be the most common cause of hypoalbuminemia in hospitalized patients, even in patients with hepatic disease. Plasma levels of essential and nonessential amino acid concentrations, and urine urea and creatinine levels are reduced. T-lymphocyte cell function is decreased, as revealed by cutaneous anergy and peripheral lymphopenia (absolute lymphocyte count <1200 cells per cubic millimeter). Glucose tolerance is impaired. Plasma cortisol is often increased (in part because of retarded metabolic clearance), T_3 is decreased, reverse T_3 (rT_3) may be increased, and basal metabolic rate is low. Plasma somatomedin C is low. Heart size is small on chest film. Echocardiography shows a small heart with decreased cardiac output. Sagittal or cross-section x-rays of the arm show a diminished muscle mass.

Course A typical case is illustrated in Fig. 72-1. In children, an early manifestation is slowing of growth. As the protein-energy depletion becomes more severe, pallor, fatigue, and amenorrhea appear. Loss of cell-mediated immunity predisposes to infections. The hypermetabolism and anorexia of intercurrent infection accelerate the progress of cachexia. In advanced undernutrition (midarm fat area <2 cm^2, creatinine/height ratio <60 percent of standard), decubiti, hypothermia, and terminal infection are the rule.

Relation to other deficiency states Usually other nutrients are also depleted. Folic acid, thiamine, riboflavin, nicotinic acid, pyridoxine, ascorbic acid, and vitamin A deficiencies are relatively common in hospital populations in the United States (see Table 72-2). Body content of most minerals is also reduced, but a distinction must be made between absolute and relative decreases. As protoplasmic protein is consumed to supply metabolic fuel and substrate for gluconeogenesis in the underfed patient, the intracellular minerals potassium, phosphorus, and magnesium and some of the microminerals are excreted in parellel with the nitrogen. Such loss is absolute but not relative, since the intracellular and extracellular concentrations of potassium, phosphorus, and magnesium usually remain normal. If the diet is

TABLE 72-2 Undesirable practices affecting the nutritional health of hospital patients

1	Failure to record height and weight on admission
2	Lack of a weight curve in the hospital chart
3	Prolonged use of glucose and saline intravenous feedings
4	Failure to measure patient's food intake
5	Withholding meals because of diagnostic tests
6	Use of tube feedings of inadequate amount and uncertain composition
7	Ignorance of the composition of nutritional products
8	Failure to recognize increased nutritional needs due to injury or illness
9	Delay of nutrition support until the patient is in an advanced state of depletion
10	Limited availability of laboratory tests to assess nutritional status; failure to use those that are available
11	Failure to correct inadequate dentition or the edentulous state

SOURCE: *After Butterworth.*

also deficient in potassium, phosphorus, or magnesium, a further deficiency occurs, and the intracellular, extracellular, and urinary concentrations may become subnormal. Similar considerations apply to the body content of essential fatty acids. Whether the depletion of potassium, phosphorus, magnesium, or essential fatty acids is absolute or relative, repletion with a feeding solution deficient in that nutrient may lead to chemical and clinical manifestations of the corresponding deficiency state within a few days. Life-threatening hypokalemia, hypophosphatemia, or hypomagnesemia can occur. By similar mechanisms, plasma levels of trace minerals decline during hyperalimentation if adequate rations of these nutrients are not provided.

REFERENCES

Alleyne GAO et al: Protein-energy malnutrition. London, Butler & Tanner, 1977

Baracos V et al: Stimulation of degradation of muscle proteins during fever. A mechanism for the increased degradation of muscle proteins during fever. N Engl J Med 308:553, 1983

Becker DJ: The endocrine responses to protein calorie malnutrition. Ann Rev Nutr 3:187, 1983

Beisel WR: Magnitude of the host nutritional responses to infection. Am J Clin Nutr 30:1236, 1977

———: Metabolic effects of infection. Prog Food Nutr Sci 8:43, 1984

Bistrian BR et al: Prevalence of malnutrition in general medical patients. JAMA 235:1567, 1976

——— et al: Protein status of general surgical patients. JAMA 230:858, 1974

Butterworth CE: The skeleton in the hospital closet. Nutr Today 9:4, 1974

Cahill GF: Starvation in man. N Engl J Med 282:668, 1970

Chandra RK: Numerical and functional deficiency in T helper cells in protein energy malnutrition. Clin Exp Immunol 51:126, 1983

Corman LC: The relationship between nutrition, infection and immunity. Med Clin North Am 69:519, 1985

Cuthbertson DP: Post-traumatic metabolism: A multidisciplinary challenge. Surg Clin North Am 58:1045, 1978

Davies L: Nutrition and the elderly: Identifying those at risk. Proc Nutr Soc 43:295, 1984

Dinarello CA: Interleukin 1. Rev Infect Dis 6:51, 1984

Dowd PS, Heatley RV: The influence of undernutrition on immunity. Clin Sci 66:241, 1984

Fernandes G: Nutritional factors: Modulating effects on immune function and aging. Pharmacol Rev 36:123S, 1984

Graham GG: Poverty, hunger, malnutrition, prematurity, and infant mortality in the United States. Pediatrics 75:117, 1985

Grantham-McGregor S: Chronic undernutrition and cognitive abilities. Hum Nutr Clin Nutr 38:83, 1984

Keusch GT: Nutrition as a determinant of host response to infection and the metabolic sequellae of infectious diseases. Seminars in Infectious Disease 2:265, 1979

Leevy CM et al: Incidence and significance of hypovitaminemia in a randomly selected municipal hospital population. Am J Clin Nutr 17:259, 1965

Long CM: Energy balance and carbohydrate metabolism in infection and sepsis. Am J Clin Nutr 30:1301, 1977

Lundholm KG: Nutritional problems in trauma. Acta Chir Scand (suppl) 522:183, 1985

Masoro EJ: Nutrition as a modulator of the aging process. Physiologist 27:98, 1984

Moldawer LL et al: Muscle proteolysis in sepsis and trauma. N Engl J Med 309:494, 1983

Puri S, Chandra RK: Nutritional regulation of host resistance and predictive value of immunologic tests in assessment of outcome. Pediatr Clin North Am 32:499, 1985

Roe DA: *Drug-Induced Nutritional Deficiencies*. Westport, Conn, AVI, 1976

Steffee W: Malnutrition in hospitalized patients. JAMA 244:2630, 1980

Ten-State Nutrition Survey. 1968–1970. US Department of Health, Education and Welfare Publication (HSM) 72, 1972

73 ANOREXIA NERVOSA AND BULIMIA

DANIEL W. FOSTER

Anorexia nervosa and bulimia are eating disorders in young, previously healthy women who develop a paralyzing fear of becoming fat. The population at risk consists largely of white women from middle- and upper-class backgrounds. The disorders rarely occur in black or oriental women, are unusual in the poor, and are almost never seen in men. The driving force is the pursuit of thinness, all other aspects of life being secondary. In the anorexia nervosa syndrome this aim is achieved primarily by radical restriction of caloric intake, the end result being emaciation. In bulimia massive binge eating is followed by vomiting and excessive use of laxatives. Weight loss in bulimic subjects is not great despite the obsession with food. Some authors consider anorexia nervosa and bulimia to be distinct illnesses, while others classify bulimia as a variant of anorexia nervosa. Clearly, overlap syndromes exist since emaciated patients fulfilling the criteria of true anorexia nervosa may exhibit bulimic behavior, while subjects with bulimia often pass through a phase of anorexia. In this chapter it will be assumed that the two disorders represent different clinical expressions of a primary psychologic disturbance focused on an obsession with body weight.

PREVALENCE Estimates of prevalence for anorexia nervosa range from 0.4 to 1.5 per 100,000 population. In adolescent white girls from middle- or upper-class families rates as high as 1 per 100 have been reported. Prevalence is believed to be increasing. Subclinical variants may be present in up to 5 percent of the socioeconomic group at highest risk. The incidence of bulimia is less certain. Vomiting after eating may occur in as many as 18 percent of women college students. The figure for self-induced vomiting in the general population is probably 1 to 2 percent, but the full-blown bulimic syndrome is less frequent.

DIAGNOSIS The diagnosis of both anorexia nervosa and bulimia is made on clinical grounds. No specific diagnostic tests exist. For many years the criteria of Feighner et al. (Table 73-1) were the basis for diagnosis in research studies. Less strict requirements were formulated for the Diagnostic and Statistical Manual of Mental Disorders III (DSM-III) of the American Psychiatric Association:

1 Intense fear of becoming obese, which does not diminish as weight loss progresses
2 Disturbance of body image; e.g., claiming to "feel fat" even when emaciated
3 Weight loss of at least 25 percent of original body weight, or if under 18 years of age, weight loss from original body weight plus weight gain expected from growth charts may be combined to make 25 percent
4 Refusal to maintain body weight over minimal normal weight for age and height

The uniqueness of the disturbance in body image in patients with eating disorders has been questioned, and some authorities have recommended its omission on the grounds that many normal young women demonstrate the same perceptual distortion. Similarly, the 25 percent figure for weight loss may be too restrictive, particularly in children. A presumptive diagnosis of anorexia nervosa is justified if the following elements are elicited: (1) a history of major weight loss; (2) absence of organic disease sufficient to account for weight loss; (3) absence of severe primary psychiatric illness which might account for failure to eat; (4) extreme restriction of food intake with or without intermittent induction of vomiting; (4) ritualized exercise; and (5) denial of hunger, fatigue, or emaciation.

The criteria for the diagnosis of bulimia in DSM-III appear to be less useful. The picture is that of a normal or near normal weight subject whose life is dominated by gorging and regurgitation in the

TABLE 73-1 Criteria for the diagnosis of anorexia nervosa

1 Onset prior to age 25
2 Anorexia with weight loss of at least 25 percent of original body weight
3 Distorted attitude toward eating, food, or weight that overrides hunger, admonitions, reassurances, and threats
4 No known medical illness that could account for the weight loss
5 No other known psychiatric disorder
6 At least two of the following manifestations:
  a Amenorrhea
  b Lanugo hair
  c Bradycardia (persistent resting pulse of 60 beats per minute or less)
  d Periods of overactivity
  e Episodes of bulimia
  f Vomiting (may be self-induced)

SOURCE: *After Feighner et al.*

absence of the physical changes or symptoms of profound weight loss.

ETIOLOGY The cause of anorexia nervosa and bulimia is unknown. Although primary dysfunction of the hypothalamus has been postulated, the associated hypothalamic abnormalities revert to normal with weight gain and thus are secondary rather than causal.

Most investigators favor a psychiatric etiology, but there is disagreement about its nature. One view holds that the disorders begin in response to inadequate or destructive interpersonal relationships in upper middle class families that are goal-oriented and highly achieving. Despite an outward appearance of normality, interpersonal communication among family members tends to be inadequate, frequently following a pattern in which the father seeks success in his work while the mother turns to her children for fulfillment and in the process becomes overdirective. It is often stated that the families are "enmeshed," meaning that generational boundaries are blurred and that parents and children are constantly involved in each other's problems. Psychoanalytic interpretation tends to focus on anorexia as a mechanism whereby the patient reestablishes control of her own life in a way that cannot be controlled by parental direction. It is not clear how this sequence might result in the intense fear of being fat that is the central feature of both classic anorexia and bulimia.

Although the absence of psychiatric disease is one criterion for diagnosis (Table 73-1), it is now widely held that depression plays a significant role in the eating disorders. Abnormalities of neurotransmitter concentrations have been reported in cerebrospinal fluid, but it is not known whether they are primary or secondary. One report claims an increased prevalence of the HLA-Bw16 haplotype in anorexia nervosa, but this antigen may correlate better with depression than with eating disorders per se.

Cultural issues are likely also important in the prevalence of anorexia nervosa. The quest for health and slimness is a powerful force in modern western society and may reinforce the fear of fatness in patients with established anorexia or tip the borderline case into full-blown disease. Occupation may play a role since dancers have a prevalence of anorexia nervosa 10 times that of the general population. Likewise athletes, particularly runners, often seek to decrease body fat to very low levels (5 to 7 percent).

Whatever the mechanism(s) involved, the behavioral response is obsessive and is difficult to treat.

CLINICAL PICTURE While anorexia nervosa and bulimia may coexist in the same patient, the clinical pictures are ordinarily distinct (Table 73-2).

TABLE 73-2 The eating disorders

	Anorexia nervosa	Bulimia
Predominant sex	Female	Female
Method of weight control	Restriction of intake	Vomiting
Binge eating	Uncommon	Invariant
Weight at diagnosis	Markedly decreased	Near normal
Ritualized exercise	Usual	Rare
Amenorrhea	~100%	~50%
Antisocial behavior	Rare	Frequent
Cardiovascular changes (bradycardia, hypotension)	Common	Uncommon
Skin changes (hirsutism, dryness, carotenemia)	Usual	Rare
Hypothermia	Usual	Rare
Edema	+/−	+/−
Medical complications	Hypokalemia, cardiac arrhythmias	Hypokalemia, cardiac arrhythmias, aspiration of gastric contents, esophageal or gastric rupture

NOTE: *These features are characteristic of pure anorexia nervosa and pure bulimia. Overlap syndromes occur, and anorexia may evolve to bulimia (the bulimia → anorexia transformation is rare).*

Anorexia nervosa The anorexia nervosa syndrome usually begins before or shortly after puberty but may appear later (rarely later than the middle twenties). Many patients have been overweight in childhood. Emaciation is equivalent to that seen in the concentration camp victims of World War II. Despite profound weight loss the patients deny hunger, thinness, or fatigue. They are often physically active, and ritualized exercise programs are common. Frenzied calisthenics or running may follow food intake. There is a preoccupation with food, and elaborate meals may be prepared for others. If social circumstances require them to eat more than usual, vomiting is induced as soon as possible, often in a public restroom. As noted, episodic binge eating may occur and is also followed by emesis. Amenorrhea is nearly always present. It usually accompanies or follows weight loss but in a sixth of patients may appear prior to any physical change. Constipation and cold intolerance are common. The latter are presumably due to a defect in regulatory thermogenesis secondary to hypothalamic dysfunction.

In advanced cases bradycardia, hypothermia, and hypotension are present. Body fat is undetectable, and the bones protrude through the skin. Interestingly, breast tissue is often preserved. The skin may be dry and scaly and is often yellow due to carotenemia, (particularly visible in the palms). Body hair is often increased; it is usually of fine, lanugo quality, but frank hirsutism may occur. Parotid glands may be enlarged as in other forms of starvation. Edema in the absence of hypoalbuminemia is thought to be due to failure of extracellular fluid volume to diminish proportionately with body mass during weight loss. Because of edema in the legs and parotid enlargement, which gives a fullness to the face, the true state of emaciation may be masked when the patient is fully dressed.

Laboratory abnormalities include anemia and leukopenia (with hypocellularity of the bone marrow), hypokalemia, and hypoalbuminemia. Serum β-carotene levels tend to be elevated. Prerenal azotemia may occur if vomiting or laxative use are prominent. The blood urea nitrogen may be as high as 60 to 70 mg/dL. Renal concentrating ability is impaired, possibly due to blunted responsiveness to antidiuretic hormone. Release of vasopressin in response to an osmotic stimulus is also abnormal. Plasma cholesterol is occasionally high, but triglyceride levels are not increased despite low activities of hepatic and lipoprotein lipases. Glucose tolerance is abnormal as in other forms of starvation.

Miscellaneous abnormalities include low levels of IgG, IgM, and a variety of proteins in the complement pathways. Despite these findings immune function is generally preserved, and serious infections are rare. Plasma iron and ceruloplasmin are normal, but iron binding capacity is decreased. Serum zinc and copper are decreased, but concentrations of these metals are normal in hair. Serum amylase may be increased in the absence of signs or symptoms of pancreatitis.

A variety of endocrine abnormalities are seen. Basal levels of luteinizing hormone (LH) and follicle-stimulating hormone (FSH) are low when weight loss is severe, and the LH response to luteinizing hormone–releasing hormone (LHRH) is impaired. FSH response to LHRH is normal, although time to peak increase may be delayed. Studies of the 24-h circadian pattern of LH secretion show regression of the maturational stage to the pattern characteristic of prepubertal or early pubertal girls; i.e., episodic LH release is missing or occurs only during sleep. These findings presumably account, at least in part, for the amenorrhea. Menses return with weight gain, although the weight required for reinitiation of menstruation may be somewhat higher (~ 10 percent) than that needed for the original induction of menarche. Ovulatory menses may be induced in subjects with anorexia nervosa by prolonged treatment with LHRH, suggesting that pituitary gonadotropin release is impaired because of hypothalamic dysfunction. Prolactin levels are normal. Plasma estradiol levels are low, and plasma testosterone is in the normal female range. Testosterone concentrations are low in men with anorexia nervosa.

Growth hormone (GH) in the basal state may be normal or elevated. A rise in GH occurs after injection of thyrotropin-releasing hormone (TRH), as in other states with elevated basal levels of GH such as acromegaly, uremia, and protein-calorie malnutrition. Insulin-like growth factor I (somatomedin C) concentrations are low. Plasma cortisol levels are high despite normal production rates; this is due to decreased metabolism of cortisol and prolongation of the plasma half-life. Dexamethasone suppression tests may be abnormal. Norepinephrine concentrations in plasma are depressed.

Thyroxine (T_4) levels tend to be slightly low but free T_4 is normal. Triiodothyronine (T_3) concentrations are reduced while reverse T_3 (rT_3) levels are increased. Basal levels of thyroid-stimulating hormone (TSH) are usually normal, and TSH response to TRH is intact. The primary defect in thyroid hormone metabolism is decreased activity of the 5′-deiodinase that converts T_4 to T_3 and rT_3 to diiodothyronine in nonthyroidal tissues. These changes are characteristic of starvation and wasting diseases and are not specific for anorexia nervosa.

Bone density is decreased in women with anorexia nervosa. The mechanism is thought to be estrogen deficiency rather than an abnormality in vitamin D metabolism.

Bulimia Bulimia, which means "ox-hunger," refers to the episodic ingestion of large amounts of food in a compulsive fashion, coupled with awareness that the eating pattern is abnormal, a fear that eating cannot be stopped voluntarily, and feelings of depression at completion of the act. Bulimics have a morbid fear of becoming fat. While binge eating may occur in several types of emotional disorders, a high percentage of patients give a history of overt or cryptic anorexia nervosa, suggesting that bulimia is commonly a variant of anorexia nervosa. Episodes of binge eating are followed by induced vomiting, with or without the subsequent ingestion of large quantities of laxatives. Initially vomiting is induced by placing a toothbrush or fingers in the throat, but eventually most patients learn to vomit reflexly.

Binge eating generally occurs daily in the active phase; in a series of 40 patients the mean number of episodes per week was 12, ranging from 1 to 46. The duration of the eating period averaged 1.2 h but could last as long as 8 h. The amount of food ingested can be enormous, up to 50,000 calories a day, although the mean number of calories consumed in a single episode is around 3500. High-carbohydrate foods are favored, and more than one food is usually eaten. The order of frequency in one report was: ice cream→bread→candy→donuts→soft drinks. The term "dietary chaos" describes the eating pattern. Because of the high sugar content of the diet, dental caries are frequent.

Other behavioral abnormalities are common. Secrecy about the eating-vomiting sequence is characteristic so that family and friends are often unaware. Stealing is common, and food is the item most often taken. There is a high rate of alcohol and drug abuse. Depression tends to be more severe than in anorexia nervosa, making suicide a definite risk. Hysterical behavior may occur. Families of patients with bulimia have a higher incidence of affective disorders, alcoholism, and illicit drug use than is seen in families of patients with classic anorexia nervosa.

Despite the close relationship with true anorexia nervosa, a number of differences are noted. While many patients with bulimia are thin, weight loss to the point of emaciation is not seen; generally weight is within 15 percent of the normal range as defined by life insurance tables of ideal weight. Fluctuating weight is common, with cyclical gains and losses. Some patients are modestly overweight. In contrast to anorexia nervosa, about half of the patients continue to menstruate, and a number have become pregnant. Persistent menstruation probably reflects the absence of extreme weight loss. Sexual activity is greater in bulimic subjects than in those with anorexia.

The physical findings associated with bulimia are usually minimal, although subjects with more extensive weight loss may manifest some of the changes seen with anorexia nervosa.

The most common laboratory abnormality is hypokalemia with metabolic alkalosis secondary to vomiting and laxative use. Evaluation of the endocrine system has not been systematically carried out.

PROGNOSIS The course of anorexia nervosa is variable. In long-term follow-up about 50 percent of patients achieve normal weight, 20 percent improve but remain underweight, 20 percent continue anorexic, 5 percent become obese, and 6 percent die. Even when weight gain occurs, signs of persistent illness remain since intermittent dieting, binge eating, vomiting, and laxative use persist in up to two-thirds of patients. Death is usually due to starvation (cardiac arrhythmias primarily) or suicide. Poor prognostic signs include older age of onset, longer duration of illness, history of bulimia or vomiting, extreme weight loss, and presence of significant depression.

The prognosis in bulimia is worse than that of anorexia nervosa, probably because the accompanying psychiatric disturbances are more severe. Suicide occurs twice as frequently. Aspiration pneumonia, acute gastric dilatation, gastric or esophageal rupture, and pancreatitis contribute to higher mortality rates.

TREATMENT There is no specific treatment for anorexia nervosa or bulimia. The intense fear of becoming fat coupled with a perceptual disturbance that causes overestimation of body size results in powerful resistance to therapy. The benefits of psychiatric intervention are marginal. The same can be said of behavior modification techniques and for group and family therapy. Supportive care by an understanding physician may accomplish as much as formal psychotherapy. The patient should be seen regularly for a review of weight change, diet, and exercise patterns. It is often useful to establish a mutually agreeable explicit contract; e.g., if the patient weighs 65 pounds and ideal body weight determined from life insurance tables is 115 pounds, a goal of 90 pounds might be set as a first stage. At every visit the patient should be reassured by the physician that "we will not let you get fat." A calm but realistic review of the dangers of starvation, including sudden death, should be given, coupled with statements like "my job is to help you deal with this illness so that you can have a normal life expectancy with reasonable happiness." The physician must be perceived not as an enemy or a parental surrogate but an advisor and partner in the struggle.

A similar approach should also be used with bulimic patients. Even if the gorging-regurgitation cycle cannot be stopped, the lesser goal of limiting the load of food ingested (to minimize the chance of aspiration or gastric rupture) and decreasing the frequency of events may be achieved. Because depression and antisocial behavior are more common in bulimia, psychiatric therapy is usually required.

Drugs such as phenytoin and cyproheptadine are ineffective in the eating disorders. It is now common to use antidepressants in both anorexia nervosa and bulimia. Imipramine and phenelzine may be the best choices. Potassium supplementation may be required for vomiters.

Hospitalization may be a life-saving measure with severe anorexia nervosa. Sudden death may occur at weights more than 35 percent below ideal, particularly if weight loss has been rapid. Hypokalemia, hypotension, and prerenal azotemia due to volume depletion are other indications for hospitalization. If the patient refuses to eat, a nasogastric tube will be required, but it is better to persuade the patient to eat. Supervision of every meal is initially required, ideally by the same person. During the hospitalization the patient should never be allowed to eat alone. Total parenteral nutrition is rarely indicated. Training in nutrition, occupational therapy, group work with the family, and individual psychotherapy should be included in the treatment plan. The "safety" of eating and assurances that obesity will not result should be emphasized repetitively. Some specialists feel that all seriously affected anorexia patients benefit from initial hospitalization, but this is not a universal view. Hospitalization for bulimic subjects is normally only required for medical complications (e.g., aspiration).

Treatment of patients with the anorexia-bulimia syndrome is a long-term proposition, rife with failure, and requires perseverance by the afflicted subject, the family, and the physician.

REFERENCES

FEIGHNER JP et al: Diagnostic criteria for use in psychiatric research. Arch Gen Psychiatry 26:57, 1972

FOSTER DW: Eating disorders: Obesity and anorexia nervosa, in *Williams Textbook of Endocrinology*, 7th ed, JD Wilson, DW Foster (eds). Philadelphia, Saunders, 1985, pp 1081–1107

HARRIS RT: Bulimarexia and related serious eating disorders with medical complications. Ann Intern Med 99:800, 1983

HERZOG DB, COPELAND PM: Eating disorders. N Engl J Med 313:295, 1985

MITCHELL JE et al: Frequency and duration of binge-eating episodes in patients with bulimia. Am J Psychiatry 138:835, 1981

PYLE RL et al: Bulimia: A report of 34 cases. J Clin Psychiatry 42:60, 1981

SCHWABE AD et al: Anorexia nervosa. Ann Intern Med 94:371, 1981

74 DIET THERAPY

DANIEL RUDMAN

Dietary modifications are indicated in many clinical situations. (1) The pathogenesis of certain chronic diseases is influenced by the long-term intake of dietary factors: sodium in hypertension, calcium in osteomalacia, and calories in obesity are examples of such situations. (2) The symptomatic stage of other disorders can be ameliorated or worsened by dietary components, for example, sodium in congestive heart failure, protein in uremia, and gluten in celiac disease. (3) Protein-energy undernutrition, the consequence of numerous subacute or chronic diseases, can often be prevented or corrected with newer techniques of nutritional support. (4) Drug therapy can modify the requirement for certain nutrients; for example, hydantoin anticonvulsants decrease serum levels of folic acid. Conversely, some foods may influence the effectiveness of drugs; for example, calcium-containing foods chelate oral tetracycline and prevent its absorption.

For these reasons, a controlled diet may be a critical aspect of a therapeutic program. The appropriate period of regulation may be temporary or permanent. In some circumstances, the physical composition and even the route of alimentation may need to be changed, with little or no alteration desired in the content of essential or nonessential nutrients. In other circumstances, a specific nutrient may need to be controlled. The physician who wishes to regulate a specific nutrient without causing a deficiency or excess of other nutrients and without the loss of palatability needs to understand the nutrient composition of the common foods.

DISTRIBUTION OF NUTRIENTS AMONG FOOD GROUPS Because nutrients are not evenly distributed, a variety of foods must be eaten to achieve adequate nutrition. The average diet contains nearly 200 different food items. Isocaloric servings of meat and fruit, for example, have totally dissimilar nutrient contents.

Because of this complexity, foods have been arranged into groups of similar nutrient content. Milk-dairy products, meats-legumes, fruits-vegetables, and breads-cereals are the four groups commonly used (Table 74-1). The recommended number of servings from these groups meets the requirements for approximately three-fourths of the essential nutrients. Additional food selections should be made to fulfill the requirements for energy and certain vitamins and minerals.

It is often desirable to control (either increase or reduce) the intake

TABLE 74-1 The nutrient content of the four food groups compared to the recommended dietary allowances (RDAs)*

Food	Recommended servings	Energy, kcal	Protein, g	Fat, g	Carbohydrate, g	Vitamin A, mg RE	Vitamin E, mg	Ascorbic acid, mg	Thiamine, mg	Riboflavin, mg	Niacin, mg	Vitamin B_6, mg	Vitamin B_{12}, μg	Folacin, μg
MILK GROUP														
2% low fat	2 cups	288	20	10	29	117	0.19	5	0.2	1.0	0.5	0.19	1.9	5
MEAT GROUP														
Egg	1	70	6	5	0	156	0.23	0	0.1	0.1	0.1	0.05	1.0	3
Meat, fish, poultry	4 oz	285	31	18	0	26	0.26	0	0.3	0.2	7.3	0.59	1.6	9
VEGETABLE-FRUIT GROUP														
Leafy green and deep yellow	1/4–1/3 cup	12	1	0	2	254	0.47	20	0	0.1	0.3	0.08	0	22
Other vegetables	1/4–1/3 cup	19	1	0	4	35	0.16	7	0	0	0.4	0.05	0	14
Potato	1 medium	113	3	0	26	0	0.05	24	0.1	0	2.0	0.21	0	9
Citrus fruit	1 serving	44	1	0	10	12	0.04	44	0.1	0	0.3	0.03	0	3
Other fruit	1 serving	92	1	0	22	50	0.22	5	0	0	0.4	0.10	0	5
BREAD-CELL GROUP														
Cereal, enriched or whole grain	3/4 cup	135	4	1	29	0	0.22	0	0.1	0	1.3	0.04	0	15
Bread, enriched or whole grain	3 slices	205	7	2	39	0	0.21	0	0.2	0.1	2.0	0.08	0	17
Fortified margarine	4 tsp	144	0	16	0	66	10.0	0	0	0	0	0	0	0
Totals		1300	75	62	161	716	12.0	105	1.9	1.5	14.6	1.42	4.5	102
RECOMMENDED DIETARY ALLOWANCES†														
Women (23–50 yr)		2000	44			800	12	60	1.0	1.2	13	2.0	3.0	400
Men (23–50 yr)		2700	56			1000	15	60	1.4	1.6	18	2.2	3.0	400

* *Values represent the average nutrient content of a food group*
† *Taken from Recommended Dietary Allowances.*
‡ *Because there is less information on which to base an allowance, ranges of recommended intakes are given.*

of a specific food component or nutrient, such as sodium, potassium, lactose, or oxalate. For this purpose, lists have been compiled of foods that are the richest sources of the relevant substances (Table 74-2). In addition, for use in diabetes mellitus, an exchange food-grouping system (Table 74-3) has been adapted for the basic four food groups. This system makes it easy to exchange one food for another within a food group and allows flexibility and variety in planning a diet.

To meet therapeutic goals, food groups or specific foods can be restricted or augmented. However, such a modification may lead to deficiency or excess of other nutrients present in high concentrations in those foods that were removed from, or added to, the diet.

DIET MODIFICATION Consistency The consistency of the diet can be altered from solid to pureed to liquid. *Soft* denotes a general diet altered by method of food preparation to allow easier chewing. Meats, for example, can be ground. *Pureed* signifies a nutritionally adequate, general diet that has been homogenized for edentulous patients or those who have difficulty swallowing solid foods. *Full liquid* diets contain only liquids or foods that liquefy at room temperature and are often used as a step in the reintroduction of foods to patients in whom oral intake has been withheld and in those recovering from oral or facial surgery. However, it is not suitable for prolonged use because it may contain large amounts of lactose and cholesterol and can be inadequate in iron, folic acid, and vitamin B_6. *Clear liquid* means liquids or frozen foods that are clear. Because there is no fiber residue, this diet is used to prepare the bowel for diagnostic workups or surgery and to serve as the initial step in progressing from nothing by mouth to solid foods. A clear liquid diet provides water, sodium, potassium, and small amounts of carbohydrate; therefore, it is usually used for short periods. When clear liquids are desired for a longer period of time, low-residue enteral feedings should be included in the diet. *Liquid formulas* are nutritionally complete and provide adequate nutrition on a prolonged basis either as a supplement to solid food or as complete nutritional support via enteral tube feeding.

Residue or fiber content The residue or fiber content of a diet can be supplemented or restricted. *Dietary fiber* refers to plant material that is not digested. *Residue* signifies the fecal solids, which are made up of undigested and unabsorbed food and metabolic and bacterial products. In the normal bowel, dietary fiber is the main source of fecal residue.

Low-fiber, low-residue diet contains foods with a minimum of fiber and connective tissue. It is used to limit fecal output and prevent the formation of an obstructing bolus in patients with a narrowed intestinal lumen or with an ileostomy. Patients in an acute phase of diverticulitis, ulcerative colitis, or infectious enterocolitis may also benefit from a low-fiber diet. Low-fiber, high-residue foods (milk, prune juice) may also need to be limited.

High fiber signifies a diet with increased amounts of fiber from fruits, vegetables, and grains. Fiber is a natural laxative. It is useful to (1) increase the volume of residue reaching the colon, (2) increase gastrointestinal motility, (3) decrease intraluminal colonic pressure,

Pantothenic acid, mg	Calcium, mg	Phosphorus, mg	Magnesium, mg	Iron, mg	Zinc, mg	Sodium, mg	Potassium, mg	Dietary fiber, g
1.6	698	547	62	0.5	1.9	298	854	0
0.8	24	90	6	1.1	0.5	54	57	0
0.8	14	274	33	3.1	5.4	88	430	0
0.1	34	22	13	0.6	0.3	12	127	2.0
0.1	19	22	13	0.5	0.2	30	105	1.4
0.3	11	79	14	0.8	0.3	5	614	3.5
0.2	19	17	11	0.3	0.1	1	174	0.4
0.2	10	16	13	0.6	0.2	2	176	1.5
0.2	13	75	21	1.1	0.5	303	73	3.8
								6.4
0.4	68	126	38	1.9	0.8	414	143	0
						200		19
0	4	12	0	0	0	1407	4	
4.7	914	1280	224	10.5	10.2		2758	
4–7‡	800	800	300	18	15	1100–	1875–	
4–7‡	800	800	350	10	15	3300‡	5625‡	

TABLE 74-2 Foods containing large amounts of certain nutrients*

SODIUM	
Salt, catsup, mustard	Cheese, buttermilk
Soy sauce, steak-barbeque sauce	Salted nuts, peanut butter
Worcestershire sauce	Self-rising flour, biscuit mixes
Bouillon cubes	Salted crackers, chips, popcorn
Commercially prepared or cured meats, fish	Pickles, olives
	Commercial salad dressings
Canned foods (except fruit)	Instant cooked cereals
POTASSIUM	
Milk	Vegetables: Artichoke, bamboo shoots, beet greens, chard, dried beans, mushrooms, potato, spinach, sweet potato, tomatoes, winter squash
Meat, fish, poultry	
Fruit: Apricots, avocado, banana, cantaloupe, dates, honeydew, orange, prunes, raisins	
OXALATE	
Spinach	Almonds, cashew nuts
Rhubarb	Chocolate, cocoa
Dandelion greens	Tea
LACTOSE	
Milk, milk products	Milk chocolate, chewing gum
Cheese	Some sugar substitutes
Commercial bread and dessert mixes	Foods with these ingredients: Milk, milk solids, dry milk, curd, whey, whey solids, demineralized whey, lactose
Commercial creamed and breaded meats	
Creamed and dehydrated soups	
Creamed, breaded, buttered vegetables	

* *Adapted from Handbook of Chemical Dietetics and Rudman et al.*

TABLE 74-3 Diabetic exchange list

	Serving size	Carbohydrate, g	Protein, g	Fat, g
Milk, skim	8 oz	12	8	0
Meat:	1 oz			
Lean		0	7	3
Medium fat		0	7	5
High fat		0	7	8
Bread-cereal	1 slice or ½ cup	15	2	0
Vegetables	½ cup	5	2	0
Fruit	Per list	10	0	0
Fat	1 tsp	0	0	5

and (4) reduce insulin requirements in some diabetics by delaying absorption of simple sugars. Patients with chronic diverticulitis or irritable bowel syndrome may benefit from a gradual increase in dietary fiber. Increasing fiber by a mixed diet is preferred to the exclusive use of bran, which interferes with the absorption of calcium, zinc, and iron. It has been suggested that people who habitually consume high-fiber diets may receive some protection from colorectal cancer because of more rapid fecal excretion or reduced production of carcinogens formed from bile acids by colonic bacteria.

Omission of foods Certain foods can be omitted because they irritate the patient or interfere with certain diagnostic tests.

Bland diet previously referred to the extensive use of milk and omission of roughage; highly seasoned foods, condiments, and spices; and caffeine. The rationale for avoiding chemical or mechanical irritation has not been supported by medical research. Therefore, the bland diet has been redefined to exclude only those items documented to cause (1) gastric irritation—red and black pepper, chili powder, caffeine, decaffeinated coffee, tea, cocoa, cold beverages, and alcohol; or (2) decreased lower esophageal sphincter pressue—tomatoes, citrus juices, chocolate, caffeine, decaffeinated coffee, peppermint, and excessively fatty foods. Individuals with gastric or duodenal ulcers or esophageal reflux may benefit from this diet and an eating pattern of frequent, small meals.

Elimination diets are useful in identifying food excitants that cause allergies. Milk, eggs, seafood, nuts, seeds, chocolate, oranges, and tomatoes, the most common excitants, are removed from the diet for a few weeks. If symptoms abate, foods are added back singly and at intervals until the offending foods are determined. Diets to control food allergies should be reviewed for nutritional adequacy.

A *serotonin- and 5-hydroxyindoleacetic acid-restricted diet* eliminates foods that lead to a false-positive diagnosis of malignant carcinoid tumors (see Chap. 299). Bananas, plantains, tomatoes, plums, avocados, pineapples, and walnuts should be omitted for 24 h prior to urine collection for such a workup.

Restriction or supplementation of foods PROTEIN MODIFICATION Protein-modified diets comprise low- and high-protein, altered-amino-acid, low-purine, tyramine-free, and gluten-free diets.

Low-protein diets reduce the intake from an average of 80 to 100 g to 0 to 60 g per day by reducing high-protein items such as meat, eggs, milk, and legumes. Symptoms of nitrogen accumulation (as in hepatic encephalopathy, renal insufficiency, and genetic defects in urea synthesis) respond favorably to such restriction. Selection of proteins with high biologic value minimizes the negative nitrogen balance, but prolonged use of a severely restricted diet can lead to protein malnutrition and other nutrient deficiencies.

The original purpose of treating uremic patients with low-protein diets was to minimize azotemia and metabolic acidosis. It was then reported that, in patients so treated, the loss of residual renal function was slower than in their counterparts eating ad lib. Brenner proposed that chronic consumption of excess dietary protein causes sustained increases in renal blood flow and glomerular filtration rate, with resulting intrarenal hypertension and progressive glomerular sclerosis. Clinical trials are now underway testing the theory that reduction of protein intake to the minimum compatible with nitrogen balance will retard the progress of chronic renal disease.

Patients with chronic hepatic or renal disease or with an inborn error of nitrogen metabolism, who are treated with low-protein diets, must be monitored for manifestations of protein deficiency as described in Chap. 72. Compliance with these diets can be determined from the 24-h urine urea content.

High-protein diets, 100 to 120 g, may be prescribed for emaciated or hypermetabolic patients. Generally, high-protein diets also have increased amounts of other nutrients and a higher energy content. When energy intake is adequate, the nitrogen balance in healthy individuals is not enhanced by increasing protein intake above the recommended dietary allowance (RDA). There are, however, two common situations in which a high protein to calorie ratio improves nitrogen balance: the "stressed" patient (infection, trauma, inflammation, or fever) and the protein-starved patient. In addition, high-protein diets also stimulate ventilatory drive, an effect which can be used to expedite weaning of ventilator-dependent patients.

Altered-amino-acid diets are sometimes useful in the treatment of nitrogen accumulation disorders. Synthetic mixtures of amino acids reduce the accumulation of excess plasma amino acids and tend to return the plasma amino acid profile toward normal, sometimes with clinical improvement. However, protein adequacy must be monitored periodically. Examples of such diets include essential-amino-acid mixtures in uremia, altered ratios of branched-chain to aromatic amino acids in hepatic encephalopathy and the catabolic response to injury, and various altered-amino-acid mixtures in genetic errors of nitrogen metabolism.

Low-purine diets contain reduced amounts of uric acid precursors, as an adjunct in the treatment of gout and uric acid calculi. Sweetbreads, anchovies, sardines, shrimp, mackerel, liver, kidney, meat extracts, and dried legumes are excluded from the diet.

A *tyramine-, dopamine-free diet* eliminates foods containing tyramine or dopamine and fermented or aged foods containing bacteria capable of forming amines. Aged cheese and meats, yeast-containing products, alcoholic beverages, and bananas are omitted. This diet prevents amine-mediated hypertensive crises in patients taking monoamine oxidase inhibitors and is useful in preventing false elevations of urinary catecholamine excretion in the workup of suspected pheochromocytomas.

A *gluten-free diet* eliminates wheat, rye, oat, barley, and their derivatives which contain glutens. This diet provides symptomatic control of gluten-induced enteropathy.

CARBOHYDRATE MODIFICATION Carbohydrate-modified diets restrict total carbohydrates, disaccharides, or monosaccharides.

Low total carbohydrate diets reduce carbohydrates from the customary 50 percent to 20 to 30 percent of total calories. A carbohydrate intake of less than 70 g per day is ketogenic and is helpful in certain forms of childhood epilepsy. Postgastrectomy "dumping" may also be responsive to a diet that limits the intake of osmotically active substances. Therefore, a diet containing 140 g or less of carbohydrate with restricted mono- and disaccharides and administered in small, frequent feedings is recommended.

High carbohydrate diets increase CO_2 production, an effect which can cause respiratory distress or failure in patients with compromised pulmonary function, or impede weaning from the ventilator. A diet high in fat and low in calories is used to decrease CO_2 production.

Lactose- or sucrose-restricted diets reduce the lactose content of the diet from 25 to 30 g to 0 to 10 g per day, depending on the severity of the lactase deficiency (Table 74-2); sucrose is reduced to 5 to 15 g per day in subjects with a sucrase-isomaltase deficiency. Lactose restriction requires the omission of milk and dairy products, the primary sources of calcium in the diet, and therefore calcium supplements should be given when the diet is needed on a long-term basis.

A *galactose-free diet* eliminates all sources of galactose (and thereby lactose) for the treatment of individuals with galactosemia (see Chap. 314).

The *300-g carbohydrate diet* has been advocated by some for 3 days prior to a glucose tolerance test. However, a balanced diet providing at least 150 g of carbohydrate results in a valid test. Individuals on hypocaloric or low-carbohydrate diets should receive a balanced or high-carbohydrate diet for 3 days before the test.

FAT MODIFICATION Fat-modified diets may be restricted in total fat (largely triglycerides), in cholesterol, or both, and may be supplemented with medium-chain triglycerides. These diets are used to treat various types of hyperlipemia (see Chap. 315) or malabsorption.

A typical *low-fat, low-cholesterol diet* for hyperlipemic states furnishes 30 to 35 percent of calories as fat, the composition of which is altered to provide more polyunsaturated and less saturated fat and less than 300 mg cholesterol per day. Some types of hyperlipemia also require restrictions of carbohydrate and calories. Increasing the polyunsaturated/saturated fatty acid ratio requires decreasing the intake of beef, pork, lamb, cheese, and egg yolks and increasing the use of chicken, turkey, veal, and fish. Skim milk is used rather than whole milk, and margarines made with polyunsaturated vegetable oils are substituted for butter. Reducing cholesterol to 300 mg per day or less involves restricting egg yolks to three per week as well as limiting fat from animal sources. Such a change in eating habits requires long-term reinforcement.

For the patient with fat malabsorption, severe chylomicronemia, or chylous ascites, long-chain triglycerides should be restricted to 20 to 50 g per day (10 to 25 percent of total calories). When fat intake is severely restricted, medium-chain triglycerides, which are absorbed independently of long-chain fatty acids, should be added to provide sufficient energy. To document fat malabsorption, a diet containing 100 g fat is eaten during a 3-day stool collection. Actual fat intake must be estimated to determine the extent of malabsorption.

ENERGY MODIFICATION Energy-modified diets are designed for weight reduction, weight gain, or weight maintenance. Conditions that benefit from energy-modified diets include obesity, hypertension, diabetes mellitus, hyperlipemia, cachexia, and hypermetabolic states due to trauma, infection, and burns.

Low-kilocalorie diets usually furnish 800 to 1200 kcal for women and 1000 to 1500 kcal for men. Although a weight-reduction diet is designed to include selections from the four food groups, it may be inadequate to meet all of the recommended daily allowances if the caloric content is severely restricted; therefore, vitamin and mineral supplements may be needed.

High-kilocalorie diets (2800 to 4000 kcal per day) usually are designed to provide the estimated basal energy expenditure of the individual plus an additional 100 to 200 percent for repletion or hypermetabolism. If the patient is not able to consume the required caloric intake as solid food, liquid supplements can be used between meals.

Appropriate *diabetic diets* are fundamental to the treatment of diabetes mellitus with the major goals being restrictions of the intake of sucrose and free glucose and achievement of ideal body weight (see Chaps. 317 and 327). Energy requirements are based on the basal energy expenditure (see Chap. 70) plus an additional allowance of 25, 50, or 75 percent for sedentary, moderate, or strenuous activity levels, respectively. The recommended distribution of caloric intake is 50 to 60 percent from carbohydrate, 12 to 20 percent from protein, and 30 to 35 percent from fat. Three meals per day are usually planned for the obese, non-insulin-dependent diabetic. The type of insulin prescribed and the timing of insulin administration determine the meal patterns in the insulin-dependent diabetic. Usually, each of three meals and an evening snack provide three-tenths and one-tenth, respectively, of the allowed carbohydrate and caloric content. Patients receiving intermediate acting insulins such as NPH insulin may require a midafternoon snack to avoid hypoglycemia during the peak activity of the insulin.

ELECTROLYTE AND MINERAL MODIFICATION Electrolyte-mineral–modified diets consist of low-sodium, low- or high-potassium, low- or high-calcium, and low-phosphorus intakes.

Low-sodium diets reduce sodium consumption from an average daily intake of 4 g (176 meq, 10 g NaCl) to 0.5 to 2 g (22 to 88 meq, 1.3 to 5 g NaCl). Patient compliance is often poor if daily intake is restricted to less than 2 g sodium. The 2-g sodium diet eliminates the foods listed in Table 74-2 and controls the use of milk, salted breads and cereals, and salted margarines but does not require the use of salt-free milk, breads, and margarines, which are expensive and have a low palatability. Patients with persistent edema or ascites may require restriction of sodium of 1 g or even 0.5 g a day.

Low-potassium diets reduce intake from an average of 6 g (153 meq) to 2 g (51 meq) for the patient with hyperkalemia. *High-potassium diets* provide an intake greater than 5.8 g (150 meq) and may be indicated when potassium-wasting diuretics are used (Table 74-2). *Low-calcium diets* reduce the calcium intake from an average of 800 mg to 200 to 400 mg and are used to treat hypercalcemia and some types of nephrolithiasis. The long-term consequences of a low-calcium diet on bone are unknown. A *high-calcium diet* indicates a 1000-mg calcium diet, which is used in the evaluation of hypercalciuria, and a 1500-mg calcium diet for women with postmenopausal osteoporosis. A *low-phosphorus diet,* 700 to 800 mg per day, is used to prevent hyperphosphatemia and secondary enhancement of parathyroid hormone secretion in renal disease. A *low-oxalate diet* is designed to eliminate exogenous sources of chronic oxalate and is useful in hyperoxaluria and in calcium oxalate nephrolithiasis.

Alteration of the feeding route The route of delivery can be changed from oral to enteral tube feeding. Technological improvements in nasoenteral tubes, formulas, and infusion pumps have improved the efficacy and safety of tube feedings. The enteral route has three advantages over intravenous feeding. (1) It maintains the integrity of the intestinal mucosa, and nutrients are handled in a more physiologic manner, (2) it causes fewer metabolic and technical complications, and (3) it can be less expensive than intravenous alimentation. Consequently, clinicians should consider enteral tube feeding before resorting to parenteral nutrition (see Chap. 75).

PATIENT SELECTION Oral intake can be inadequate because of anorexia or mechanical obstruction, increased nutrient losses, or hypermetabolism. Wasting disorders in which enteral feedings may be useful include cerebral vascular accidents, head and neck cancer, anorexia nervosa, trauma, and burns. Contraindications to tube feeding include intractable vomiting, upper gastrointestinal bleeding, and intestinal obstruction. Steatorrhea is a handicap but may be surmounted by the use of chemically defined "elemental" formulas or with antidiarrheal drugs.

TUBE PLACEMENT Several enteral tube placements are used: nasogastric, nasoduodenal, nasojejunal, gastrostomy, jejunostomy, or placement of a gastrostomy feeding tube by percutaneous endoscopy. Because the latter three require surgery or endoscopy, the nasogastric or nasoduodenal route is most frequently chosen. Small-bore Silastic or polyurethane tubing minimizes the complications of nasopharyngitis, rhinitis, otitis media, parotitis, and subsequent stricture. Insertion and maintenance of proper placement are facilitated by a removable wire stylet and a mercury-weight tip. A properly irrigated tube may remain in place for months.

Patients who require permanent tube feedings benefit from gastrostomy: the cosmetic problems of the nasogastric tube are avoided, and there is no need to rely on expensive formulas since the large-bore tube allows the use of blended foods.

Jejunal feedings may be desirable when an obstruction or fistula is proximal to the jejunum. An advantage of the jejunostomy is the reduced risk of aspiration from gastric reflux.

SELECTION OF INFUSION METHOD One of the early disadvantages of enteral tube feedings was the lack of control of the infusion rate, and as a consequence patients sensitive to large volumes or hyperosmolar solutions often developed osmotic diarrhea and cramping. Enteral infusion pumps are now available to ensure a constant drip rate. When large volumes (3000 mL) of a hyperosmolar solution (>500 mosmol per liter) are necessary for repletion, either of two approaches can be tried. A full-strength formula can be begun at 50 mL/h for 24 h, and the rate of infusion daily can be increased as tolerated until the desired volume is achieved. Alternately, the formula can be made isotonic by dilution and infused from the start at a rate of 125 mL/h for 24 h; the concentration of the formula can then be gradually increased each day until full strength is reached. Infusion periods of less than 24 h may be preferable when aspiration is a potential problem.

FORMULA SELECTION Over 80 enteral formulas are available in the United States alone to meet nutritional requirements. Choosing from this array is made easier by the knowledge that the products fall into four categories: elemental (''monomeric''), polymeric, modular, and altered amino acids.

Elemental formulas are composed of di- and tripeptides and/or crystalline amino acids, glucose oligosaccharides, and vegetable oil or medium-chain triglycerides. Residue is minimal, and little digestive action is required. An elemental formula may be of use in patients with the short-bowel syndrome, partial bowel obstruction, pancreatic insufficiency, inflammatory bowel disease, radiation enteritis, or bowel fistulas.

Polymeric formulas are composed of complex nutrients, e.g., protein as casein, lactalbumin, or soy protein; carbohydrate as corn syrup solids or maltodextrins; and fat as vegetable oils or milk fat. There is heterogeneity with regard to lactose content, sodium content, caloric density, content of medium-chain triglycerides, and palatability. Most patients with a functional gastrointestinal tract and few specialized nutrient requirements can utilize a formula from the polymeric group. Unless malabsorption is present, polymeric products are preferable to monomeric ones because the hyperosmolarity of the latter may cause gastrointestinal reactions.

Single nutrient modules, available for protein, carbohydrate, and fat, can be combined or added to a monomeric or polymeric formula to create a formula that meets specialized nutrient requirements. The simplest modular formula involves adding a carbohydrate source to a formula to increase caloric value. For example, a cachectic cirrhotic patient with ascites and encephalopathy may benefit from a high-caloric, low-protein, low-sodium formula.

Altered-amino-acid formulas are indicated in patients with genetic errors of nitrogen metabolism: phenylketonuria, maple syrup urine disease, homocystinuria, tyrosinemia, methylmalonic acidemia, and propionic acidemia. In the acquired disorders of nitrogen accumulation (chronic renal failure and cirrhosis), synthetic formulas are designed to either limit or increase the intake of certain amino acids and thereby provide symptomatic improvement. Patients who are catabolic because of injury or infection may show improved nitrogen balance when the branched-chain amino acid content of their nutritional formula is increased.

PATIENT MONITORING Successful enteral tube feeding requires continual, careful monitoring for possible mechanical, gastrointestinal, fluid, and electrolyte complications. Common examples are as follows. Mechanical: clogging of tube by formula, pulmonary aspiration, esophageal erosion, tube dislodgement; gastrointestinal: vomiting, diarrhea; metabolic: hyperglycemia, hyperosmolar coma, edema, hypernatremia, hypercalcemia; cardiovascular: congestive heart failure.

The guidelines given in Chap. 71 for nutritional assessment should be used to evaluate the effectiveness of the nutrition support.

INDICATIONS FOR DIET THERAPY The majority of diseases would probably be benefited by a dietary modification, either in terms of prevention or palliation. Consequently, the clinical indications for dietary modification are too numerous to be listed here. Some examples are given in Table 74-4. For a comprehensive treatment of this subject, see texts on clinical dietetics.

DRUG-NUTRIENT INTERACTIONS Certain foods or meal patterns can alter drug effectiveness, and certain drugs can alter nutrient requirements. Many drugs influence appetite and food intake. Examples of hypophagic drugs are chemotherapeutic agents, narcotics, digitalis, amphetamines, and phenylbiguanides. Some hyperphagic drugs are tranquilizers, insulin, glucocorticoids, metoclopramide, and antihistamines.

The absorption of a drug is generally slower when it is taken with food, an effect that may be important when rapid onset of drug action is desired. Complete inhibition of drug absorption occurs when calcium-containing foods or iron salts chelate tetracycline, making it insoluble. Enhanced drug absorption results when lipid-soluble drugs are given with fat-containing meals or when alcohol is taken with a timed-release medicine that is alcohol-soluble. Gastric irritation by a drug is lessened if it is taken with meals. The optimal timing of each drug with regard to meals should be specified when it is prescribed; pharmacology texts can be consulted for details.

Drugs frequently alter either the gastrointestinal absorption, the utilization, or the urinary excretion of nutrients, with a resulting increase of nutrient requirements. For example, anticonvulsants cause a deficiency of 1,25-dihydroxycholecalciferol, aluminum hydroxide prevents absorption of dietary phosphate and iron, and glucocorticoids reduce absorption of calcium; broad-spectrum antibiotics suppress synthesis of vitamins by the intestinal flora and can cause a deficiency of vitamin K or biotin; isoniazide impairs the utilization of vitamin B_6; and oral contraceptives interfere with the utilization of folic acid; thiazides, furosemide, and penicillamine cause urinary hyperexcretion of potassium, magnesium, zinc, or copper, or several of these. This subject is treated comprehensively in Roe's monograph. In brief, the patient treated with one or more drugs for extended periods is often a risk for a nutritional deficiency. Conversely, the desired action of a drug can be blocked by a nutrient, such as pyridoxine versus levodopa, or vitamin K versus warfarin.

THE PRINCIPLES OF DIET PRESCRIPTION Several considerations are involved in formulating effective diet therapy. The *dietary modifications* appropriate for a given clinical situation must be selected (change in food consistency, removal of specific foods, reduction or increase of specific nutrients, or change in route of nutrient delivery). The appropriate *degree of restriction* or supplementation should be determined, recognizing that the extreme ranges of dietary modifications may cause noncompliance. Does a cardiac patient need a 2- or 0.5-g sodium diet; does a dysphagic patient require a soft or pureed diet; does a patient with wasting febrile illness require a 2000– or 3000-kcal diet? When more than one dietary modification is appropriate, a decision must be made as to which is the most important. Some combinations are virtually incompatible, such as a low-kilocalorie, high potassium diet; a high-calcium, lactose-free diet; or a high-protein, low-fat diet. The *duration* of the diet prescription must be estimated. Diets with severely limited nutrients should be used for as short a time as possible.

By using the type of information shown in Tables 74-1 to 74-3 and in the American Dietetic Association's *Handbook of Clinical Dietetics,* the dietitian implements the prescribed diet and reports how closely the implemented diet conforms to the desired modifications and whether undesired dietary imbalances may have been created by the prescription. Severely altered diets may be deficient or augmented in nutrients not considered in the original diet prescription; for example, a lactose-free diet is also low in calcium and riboflavin. Therefore, further manipulations may be necessary to prevent secondary deficiencies or excesses inherent in the original diet order. Three examples of prescribed diets and their implementations are given below.

Example 1

I Diagnosis: Obesity and hypertension.
II Physician's order: 1200 kcal, 2 g Na, high-potassium diet.
III Dietitian's response: High potassium (>5.8 g, 150 meq) is difficult to achieve when a kilocalorie restriction is ordered. Potassium supplements may be necessary.

	Energy, kcal*	Na, mg*	K, mg*
2 cups milk, skim	180	240	710
6 oz meat, lean	330	150	780
4 servings bread	280	800	180
4 servings vegetables	100	40	1440
3 servings fruit	120	0	1140
4 servings margarine, oil	180	200	40
	1190	1430 (62 meq)	4290 (110 meq)

* *Values represent the average nutrient content of a food group.*

Nutritional analysis: No deficiencies or excesses of essential nutrients.

TABLE 74-4 Examples of clinical disorders that benefit from appropriate diet therapy

Clinical disorder	Recommended diet therapy	Comments
GASTROINTESTINAL DISORDERS		
Dysphagia	Pureed, liquid supplements	
Reflux esophagitis	Bland, frequent small meals	
Gastric ulcers	Frequent small meals	
Posgastrectomy dumping	Low-carbohydrate, frequent small meals	
Fat malabsorption	Low-fat—MCT supplemented	Mg and vitamin A, D, E, and K supplements
Celiac disease	Gluten-free	
Lactose intolerance	Lactose-free	Ca supplement
HEPATIC DISORDERS		
Alcoholic liver disease:		
Alcoholic hepatitis	High-kilocalorie, high-protein	Multivitamin and folate supplements
Cirrhosis	High-kilocalorie, high-protein	Multivitamin and folate supplements
Encephalopathy	Low-protein, low-ammonia	
Ascites	Low-sodium, high-kilocalorie, high-protein	
RENAL DISORDERS		
Acute, chronic renal failure	Protein, phosphorus, sodium, potassium reduced	1,25-$(OH)_2D_3$, Ca supplements
Nephrotic syndrome	Low-sodium	
Renal osteodystrophy	Low-phosphorus	1,25-$(OH)_2D_3$, Ca supplements
Potassium wasting	High-potassium	
Hypercalciuric nephrolithiasis	Low-calcium, oxalate-free	
CARDIOVASCULAR DISORDERS		
Hyperlipemia:		
Type I	Low-fat	No alcohol
Type IIa	Low-cholesterol, low-saturated-fat, increased-polyunsaturated-fat	
Type IIb, III	Carbohydrate-controlled, low-cholesterol, low-saturated-fat	Achieve and maintain ideal body weight
Type IV	Carbohydrate-controlled, low-cholesterol, low-saturated fat	Achieve and maintain ideal body weight
Type V	Low-fat, low-cholesterol	No alcohol, achieve and maintain ideal body weight
Hypertension	Low-sodium	Achieve and maintain ideal body weight
Congestive heart failure	Low-sodium	
PULMONARY DISORDERS		
Sarcoidosis	Low-calcium	If patient is hypercalcemic
ENDOCRINE-METABOLIC DISORDERS		
Diabetes mellitus	Kilocalorie-carbohydrate, fat-controlled	Achieve and maintain ideal body weight
Reactive hypoglycemia	High-protein, low-carbohydrate, frequent small meals	
Obesity	Low-kilocalorie	
Osteoporosis	High-calcium	Vitamin D supplement
Gout, uric acid stones	Low-purine	
Nephrogenic diabetes insipidus	Low-sodium, protein-controlled	
Hypoparathyroidism	High-calcium	1,25-$(OH)_2D_3$ supplement
Hyperparathyroidism	Low-calcium	
Steroid therapy	Low-sodium, high-protein	
GENETIC DISORDERS		
Galactosemia	Galactose-free	
Sucrose-maltose deficiency	Low-sucrose	
Phenylketonuria	Low-phenylalanine, tyrosine supplemented	
Maple syrup urine disease	Low-leucine, -isoleucine, -valine	Thiamine, when responsive
Homocystinuria	Low-methionine, cystine	Pyridoxine, when responsive
Adrenogenital syndrome	High-sodium	
Propionic acidemia	Low-protein	Biotin, when responsive
Methylmalonic acidemia	Low-protein	Vitamin B_{12}, when responsive
Hypophosphatemic rickets		P, 1,25-$(OH)_2D_3$ supplements
Urea cycle disorders	Low-protein	

NOTE: *Note: 1,25(OH)$_2$D$_3$ = 1,25-dihydroxycholecalciferol.*

Example 2

I Diagnosis
- *A* Cirrhosis of the liver
  - *1* Encephalopathy
  - *2* Ascites
- *B* Chronic pancreatitis
- *C* Malnutrition

II Physician's order: 40 g protein, low ammonia, 1 g Na, low-fat diet with increased calories.

III Dietitian's response: **Increased caloric intake (>2500 kcal) is difficult to achieve when protein and long-chain fatty acids can contribute only 610 kcal. Medium-chain triglycerides (MCT) and foods containing largely sucrose will be needed to increase kilocalories.**

	Protein, g*	Na, mg*	Fat, g*	Energy, kcal*
½ cup milk, whole	4	60	4	75
3 oz meat or eggs	21	75	15	220
4 servings bread or cereal	8	800	0	280
4 servings vegetables	8	40	0	100
10 servings fruit	0	0	0	400
5 servings low-protein desserts	0	0	10	460
4 servings salt-free margarine	0	0	20	180
18 servings MCT mayonnaise	0	0	90	810
	41	975 (42 meq)	139	2525

*** *Values represent the average nutrient content of a food group.***

Nutritional analysis: This diet is deficient in calcium, thiamine, riboflavin, and niacin and needs to be supplemented.

Example 3

I Diagnosis: Same patient as in Example 2, with a fourth problem, anorexia.

II Physician's order: 40 g protein, 1 g Na, low fat, enteral tube feeding.

III Dietitian's response: Modular formula.

	Protein, g	Na, mg	Fat, g	Energy, kcal
750 mL Isocal	25	390	33	790
18 g Casec	15	27	0	60
360 mL Polycose	0	220	0	720
105 mL MCT oil	0	0	105	945
250 mL water				
1500 mL	40	637	138	2515

Nutritional analysis: This diet needs to be supplemented with vitamins A, D, and B_6, and folic acid, iodine, iron, and zinc.

ASSESSMENT OF DIETARY COMPLIANCE Assessment of compliance and evaluation of effectiveness are the final steps in successful diet therapy. When a "calorie count" is ordered for a hospitalized patient, the dietitian can estimate the daily intake of protein, carbohydrate, fat, and kilocalories. Some nutrients can be monitored by blood or urine analysis; for example, compliance with a low-sodium diet can be determined by urinary sodium analysis. An outpatient food intake diary is useful in assessing the home compliance. Improvements in symptoms and signs of the disorder also serve as indicators of effective dietary modification.

REFERENCES

AMERICAN DIETETICS ASSOCIATION: *Handbook of Clinical Dietetics.* New Haven, Yale, 1981

BRENNER BM et al: Dietary intake and the progressive nature of kidney disease. N Engl J Med 307:652, 1982

CRAPO PA: Simple versus complex carbohydrate: Use in the diabetic diet. Ann Rev Nutr 5:95, 1985

GOODHART RS, SHILS ME (eds): *Modern Nutrition in Health and Disease,* 6th ed. Philadelphia, Lea & Febiger, 1980

HATHCOCK JG: Metabolic mechanisms of drug-nutrient interactions. Fed Proc 44:124, 1985

KRAUSE MV, MOHER KL: *Food, Nutrition and Diet Therapy: Textbook of Nutritional Care,* 7th ed. Philadelphia, Saunders, 1984

KROMHOUT D et al: The inverse relation between fish consumption and 20-year mortality from coronary heart disease. N Engl J Med 312:1205, 1985

MIZOCK BA: Branched-chain amino acids in sepsis and hepatic failure. Arch Intern Med, 145:1284, 1985

RANDALL HT: Enteral nutrition: Tube feeding in acute and chronic illness. J Parenter Nutr 8:113, 1984

ROBINSON CH, LAWLES MR: *Normal and Therapeutic Nutrition,* 16th ed. New York, Milwaukee Publishing Co, 1982

ROE DA: Nutrient and drug interactions. Nutr Rev 42:141, 1984

SCHNEIDER HA et al: *Nutritional Support of Medical Practice.* Hagerstown, MD, Harper & Row, 1983

WALSER M: Therapeutic aspects of branched-chain amino and keto acids. Clin Sci 66:1, 1984

75 PARENTERAL NUTRITION

KHURSHEED N. JEEJEEBHOY / JEFFREY P. BAKER

Nutritional support is indicated when a normal oral diet cannot be ingested, absorbed, or tolerated for a significant period of time. When possible the route of support should be enteral (see Chap. 74). However, in patients who cannot eat, do not absorb an oral diet efficiently, or deteriorate on oral feeding, partial or complete nourishment by the parenteral route is indicated until they can be fed and can absorb nutrients orally.

INDICATIONS FOR TOTAL PARENTERAL NUTRITION Total parenteral nutrition (TPN) is indicated in the following situations:

1 *In patients who are unable to eat or absorb normally.* The rate of development of malnutrition is based on a number of factors, including previous dietary history and the coexisting illness. The diagnosis of malnutrition is based upon evidence of muscle wasting, hypoalbuminemia, edema, reduced skin fold thickness, and reduced body weight (see Chap. 71). Weight loss alone is not sufficient evidence of malnutrition because edema or previous obesity may mask the degree of nitrogen depletion actually present.

2 *In well-nourished who are temporarily unable to eat.* An estimate has to be made as to the length of time that oral nutrition will not be available. If the period is likely to exceed 7 to 10 days, then total parenteral nutrition should be administered to avoid undue wasting and malnutrition. This is especially important if sepsis or trauma complicate the clinical picture by accelerating catabolism and tissue wasting.

3 *In patients with Crohn's disease, intestinal fistulas, and pancreatitis.* In such patients food ingestion may exacerbate symptoms and high caloric wastage through fistulas, thus preventing healing. When such patients are given nothing by mouth and receive TPN, they may improve by healing fistulas and reducing the size of inflammatory masses while maintaining good nutritional status.

4 *In subjects with prolonged coma* when tube feeding is not possible.

5 *For nutritional support in patients with marked hypercatabolism or protein loss,* as in those with severe trauma and burns, even if some oral intake is possible.

6 *For nutritional support during therapy for malignant disease,* especially when malnutrition has been caused by diminished food intake rather than by uncontrolled tumor growth. Chemotherapy and complications of radiation therapy are particularly prone to cause anorexia and mucosal inflammation that may limit oral intake. TPN given prior to and with chemotherapy results in an improved nutritional status in these patients.

7 *Occasionally, in malnourished patients,* as in patients likely to undergo surgery.

NUTRIENT REQUIREMENTS DURING TPN Energy and fluid requirements The Harris-Benedict equation is an excellent guide to total energy requirements.

For men:

$$\text{Energy (kcal/24h)} = 66.473 + 13.7516 \times \text{wt(kg)} + 5.0033 \times \text{ht(cm)} - 6.7550 \times \text{age (years)}$$

For women:

$$\text{Energy (kcal/24h)} = 655.0955 + 9.5634 \times \text{wt(kg)} + 1.8496 \times \text{ht(cm)} - 4.6756 \times \text{age (years)}$$

In general, the needs for weight maintenance in afebrile patients are those predicted by these equations. For weight increase, an additional 30 percent of calories is required. Similarly, in septic patients basal energy needs should be increased by 30 percent. As a general rule, 32 kcal/kg per day is sufficient for weight maintenance, and 40 kcal/kg per day is adequate for maintenance in septic patients or for weight gain. In burn patients, when the area of burn exceeds 40 percent of the surface area, caloric requirements may increase by as much as 100 percent.

Basal fluid infusion should be about 1 to 1.2 mL/kcal. To this should be added a volume equivalent to losses from diarrhea, stomal output, nasogastric suction, and fistula drainage. In oliguric patients a basal intake of 750 to 1000 mL should be given, plus a volume equal to that of urine and other losses. In patients with cardiac failure, about 40 mL/kg can be infused provided that the sodium intake is restricted to between 20 and 40 meq per day.

Amino acid requirements The efficient functioning of the body requires maintenance of the integrity of the musculoskeletal system and viscera, together with normal levels of enzymes, hormones, and plasma proteins. All are dependent on new protein synthesis to meet the demands of normal turnover; protein synthesis in turn requires that amino acids be available. A major objective of parenteral nutrition is to provide an adequate supply of amino acids for protein synthesis. Although the amount required is influenced by several factors, nitrogen balance and protein synthesis (including albumin formation) are proportional to the amount of amino acid infused within the range of zero to 2 g amino acids per kilogram of body weight per day. In addition, as mentioned above, severe injury, sepsis, and burns increase nitrogen losses, making it necessary to infuse larger amounts of amino acids. The pattern of amino acids infused is important, since unbalanced mixtures do not support protein synthesis. Enrichment of amino acid mixtures with branched chain amino acids and/or branched chain keto acids may aid protein synthesis in septic patients. Requirements are larger if amino acids are the sole energy source than if some caloric demands are met by fat or carbohydrate.

In ordinary starvation the infusion of 100 g of glucose per day reduces urinary nitrogen loss but does not produce positive nitrogen balance. Infusion of amino acids alone also reduces net nitrogen deficits, and in large amounts (~2 g per kilogram of body weight per day) it can induce a slight positive nitrogen balance. However, amino acids are more efficiently utilized when they are infused along with nonprotein energy sufficient to meet calorie requirements. Positive nitrogen balance is achieved in most malnourished patients (who are not suffering abnormal losses) by infusing 0.5 to 1.0 g of amino acids per kilogram of ideal body weight per day, together with optimal nonprotein calories. Unusual losses, as in protein-rich exudates from burns or in upper gastrointestinal tract contents rich in pancreatic secretions, increase requirements to between 1.5 and 2.0 g/kg per day. As the input of nonprotein energy is increased, nitrogen retention is augmented at all levels of amino acid intake. The protein-sparing effect of carbohydrate and fat is most obvious as intake increases from none to an amount approximating the metabolic rate but is also observed to a lesser degree until the intake approximates 55 to 60 kcal per kilogram of ideal body weight. Beyond this point, additional calories in adults do not significantly improve nitrogen retention.

Relation of nitrogen retention to the source of nonprotein energy Both carbohydrates and lipids can be infused with amino acids to provide sufficient nonprotein energy to meet the metabolic requirements. The two types of substrates are equal in efficacy in malnourished and septic patients after an initial 3- to 4-day period for adaptation to the source of the energy. Hence the source of nonprotein energy chosen depends on factors other than its effect on nitrogen retention.

The first factor of importance in choosing the source of nonprotein energy is osmotic pressure. Concentrated glucose solutions are hyperosmolar and cause thrombosis when administered by peripheral vein. TPN regimens using glucose as the primary energy source thus require placement of a catheter in the superior vena cava where rapid blood flow quickly dilutes the hypertonic infusion. A second factor is the metabolic state of the patient. Glucose requires insulin for utilization, and hypertonic glucose solutions are not ideal for diabetic subjects. In such individuals, lipid infusions avoid or diminish the need for additional insulin and for frequent monitoring of blood glucose. Conversely, triglyceride emulsions may be contraindicated in hyperlipiproteinemic states. A third consideration is that infusing glucose as the sole source of calories causes an increase in the metabolic rate and carbon dioxide production and thus may accentuate ventilatory demands. In such patients, giving half the nonprotein calories as fat reduces carbon dioxide excretion.

Glucose infusion mixtures consist of 25 percent dextrose, 2 percent amino acids, vitamins, and minerals. Lipid emulsions are mixtures of triglyceride, phospholipid (as an emulsifying agent), and glycerol (added to maintain isotonicity). Lipid can be infused concurrently with amino acid–dextrose mixtures using a Y connector and can provide 50 to 80 percent of nonprotein calories. Combinations of these nutrients are sometimes supplied in a single bag and are stable under refrigeration for up to 4 days. These concentrations can be given by peripheral vein without fear of thrombosis. Insulin is not required for metabolism of the fat; indeed, plasma insulin levels are low and free fatty acids and ketones are high when lipid is the major source of nonprotein calories. Lipid infusions can also be discontinued abruptly without danger of hypoglycemia because insulin levels are not elevated. This aspect is important in critically ill patients who may require repeated and unpredictable alterations in therapy, especially when surgery may be performed on short notice. Finally, lipid infusions meet essential fatty acid requirements; linoleic acid is present in sufficient quantities if as little as 500 mL of commercially available triglyceride emulsion (Intralipid) is given daily. While essential fatty acid deficiency is ordinarily rare in adults, lipid deficiency may develop in as little as 1 week with TPN and cause abnormal liver function and skin rash.

It is also possible to administer TPN with a ratio of 1:1 (calorie:calorie) of glucose and lipid calories. Substrate and hormone profiles in the blood following infusion of such a mixture are similar to those in the postprandial state.

Recommendations regarding source (type) of nonprotein energy Lipid-free systems are required only in patients with hyperchylomicronemia. Other patients should receive lipid as a part of the regimen for total parenteral nutrition. The 80 percent lipid system can be given by peripheral vein, minimizing the threat of catheter sepsis and other catheter-related complications. However, the authors recommend a 1:1 (calorie:calorie) lipid-glucose solution, given through a central venous line. This regimen simulates the normal diet and causes neither hyperinsulinemia nor hyperglycemia, thus almost eliminating the need for exogenous insulin.

TABLE 75-1 Vitamin input and blood or plasma vitamin levels in six patients on long-term TPN

	Input* provided by:				Plasma/blood vitamin level	
Vitamin	MVI, per 5 mL	Soluzyme + vitamin C, per 10 mL	Consequent average daily input	Daily (oral) recommended requirement	Average level observed in six patients	Normal range
A	5000 IU		2500 IU	5000 IU	41.6	25–70 μg/dL
D	500 IU		250 IU	400 IU	34.4	28–42 ng/mL
E	5 mg		27.5 mg†	30 mg	0.65	0.8–1.2 ng/dL
B_1	22 mg	10 mg	16.0 mg	1.5 mg	226	10–64 ng/mL
B_2	5 mg	10 mg	7.5 mg	2.0 mg		
Niacinamide	50 mg	250 mg	150 mg	20.0 mg	16	3–6 μg/mL
Pantothenate	12 mg	45 mg	28 mg	10.0 mg	689	150–400 ng/mL
Pyridoxine	6 mg	5 mg	5.5 mg	2.5 mg	40	30–80 ng/mL
Ascorbic acid	500 mg	500 mg	500 mg	75 mg	2.0	0.4–1 mg/dL
Folic acid		5 mg	2.5 mg	0.15 mg	48	4–20 ng/dL
B_{12}		25 μg	12.5 μg	1.0 μg	872	100–900 pg/mL
Biotin				300 μg	63	200–500 pg/mL

* *Given on alternate days.*
† *Of the average of 27.5 mg vitamin E per day 25 mg is provided by infusing 500 mL Intralipid per day.*
SOURCE: *After KN Jeejeebhoy, Ann Coll Physicians Surg Can 9:287, 1976.*

TABLE 75-2 Recommended electrolyte intake per day (mmol)

	Na	K	Ca	Mg	P
Basal*	100–120	80–100	7.5–10	10–12	12–16
Cardiac failure	20–50	80–100	10–15	10–12	12–16
Renal failure	20	†	†	†	†

* *To this basal intake, amounts of Na, K, Cl, and HCO_3 are added to meet losses from fistulas, nasogastric tube drainage, diarrhea, and stomal output.*
† *These ions are added as needed, on the basis of initial and continuing measurements of their circulating level and the clinical state of the patient.*

Other requirements VITAMINS Vitamin requirements are given in Table 75-1. Amounts of vitamins sufficient to meet these needs must be added to the basic solution for parenteral feeding. Excessive amounts of fat-soluble vitamins, in particular vitamins A and D, should not be given because of the danger of hypercalcemia and other toxic effects. (See Chap. 76.) A combination of 5 mL Multivitamin Infusion (MVI) with 10 mL Soluzyme plus vitamin C on alternate days meets the requirements for vitamins A and D and for most water-soluble vitamins. These solutions should be supplemented with vitamin K (5 mg) and vitamin B_{12} (200 μg) initially and at intervals of 3 weeks. Folate (5 mg) is given weekly. Biotin deficiency may occur in infants on TPN, as manifested by acidosis, rash, and alopecia.

ELECTROLYTES Electrolytes are an essential component of total parenteral nutrition. Potassium, magnesium, and phosphorus are necessary for optimal nitrogen retention and tissue formation; sodium and chloride are required to maintain osmolality and acid-base balance. Calcium is required to prevent demineralization of bone. Recommended ranges of intake are given in Table 75-2.

TRACE ELEMENTS Trace elements, in particular zinc, copper, and chromium, are needed when parenteral nutrition exceeds 1 to 2 weeks.

Zinc is essential for wound healing, for defense against infection, and as a cofactor for many enzymes. In its absence ageusia, loss of hair, night blindness, and a skin rash occur. The skin rash is often associated with superficial infection due to staphylococci and yeast and responds only to zinc supplementation. Zinc deficiency also interferes with delayed hypersensitivity. In the absence of excessive gastrointestinal losses, 3 mg zinc per day is sufficient to meet needs. For each liter of intestinal fluids lost through fistulas, stomal output, suction, or diarrhea in patients with extensive resection of the small bowel, an additional 12 mg should be added. If the small bowel is intact, zinc losses are greater, and about 17 mg zinc is required per liter of intestinal fluids lost per day.

Copper deficiency causes anemia and neutropenia. The daily requirement is estimated to be between 0.3 and 0.5 mg, with the larger intake to be given in patients with major losses of gastrointestinal fluid. Copper should not be given to patients with obstructive jaundice. *Manganese* requirement is about 0.8 mg per day. This element also should not be given if obstructive jaundice is present. *Chromium* deficiency is associated with glucose intolerance and neuropathy. The chromium requirement is about 20 μg daily. *Selenium* deficiency has been associated with congestive cardiomyopathy and possibly with muscle disease. Selenium requirements are probably somewhat greater than 10 μg per day.

TABLE 75-3 Representative daily protocols for total parenteral nutrition

Component solutions	100% dextrose regimen[a]	50% dextrose–50% lipid regimen[a]	15% dextrose–85% lipid regimen[a]
Amino acid 2.1%, dextrose 25%, mL	3000	—	—
Amino acid 4.2%, dextrose 25%, mL	—	1500	—
Amino acid 5%, dextrose 12.5%,[b] mL	—	—	1500
Lipid 10%,[c,d] mL	—	1000	1500
Electrolyte mix,[e] mL	60	60	60
Trace element mix,[f] mL	5	5	5
Vitamins,[g] mL	10	10	10
Total volume, mL	3075	2575	3075
Total electrolytes[h]			
Na^+, meq	125	125	132.5
K^+, meq	81	80	87
Ca^{2+}, meq	10	10	10
Mg^{2+}, meq	22	22	16
Cl^-, meq	193	192	148
Ac^-, meq	96	95	112.5
P, mg	582	582	693
Total protein, g	60	60	75
Total nonprotein calories, kcal	2550	2375	2286

[a] *All values represent total 24-h amount. Percentage of total calories derived from dextrose and lipid as noted.*
[b] *Obtained by mixing equal volumes of commercially available 10% amino acid and 25% dextrose.*
[c] *The triglyceride and dextrose–amino acid mixture are infused concurrently through a central venous line using a connector for continuous mixing.*
[d] *Intralipid 10% (Cutter Laboratories) or Liposyn 10% (Abbott Laboratories).*
[e] *Electrolyte mix contains 80 meq Na^+, 10 meq Ca^{2+}, 16 meq Mg^{2+}, 42 meq K^+, and 148 meq Cl^- per 60 mL.*
[f] *Trace-element mix contains 1 mL each of (1) 0.5 mg/mL elemental Cu as cupric chloride ($CuCl_2 \cdot 2H_2O$), 20 μg/mL elemental Cr as chromic nitrate [$Cr(NO_3)_3$], and 120 μg/mL of elemental Se as selenious acid (H_2SeO_3); (2) 120 μg/mL elemental I as potassium iodide (KI); (3) 3 mg/mL elemental Zn as zinc sulfate ($ZnSO_4 \cdot 7H_2O$); and (4) 0.7 mg/mL elemental Mn as manganous chloride ($MnCl_2 \cdot 4H_2O$).*
[g] *Vitamins include MVI injection (USV Pharmaceutical Corporation) once weekly and Soluzyme (Upjohn) six times weekly. Vitamin K is given as Synkayvite (Roche) 10 mg weekly.*
[h] *Total electrolytes are calculated on the assumption that the amino acid mixture used contains electrolytes. The total input of electrolytes in this table has been found to be capable of maintaining balance in patients without abnormal losses of gastrointestinal secretions.*

ROUTES OF ADMINISTRATION Central venous catheterization This route allows infusion of fluids irrespective of osmolality and minimizes the need for repeated venipuncture. However, there is a risk of septicemia and thrombosis if the catheter is not properly inserted and cared for during therapy.

Basic principles of catheter insertion and care are as follows:

1 Catheters should be placed and handled using aseptic technique. Face mask and sterile gloves are required.
2 It should be documented radiologically that the catheter is in the superior vena cava prior to commencement of TPN with hypertonic fluids. If the tip is in another central vein (e.g., the internal jugular), thrombosis may occur.
3 Catheters should be introduced via puncture of a large central vein and not via a peripheral vein.
4 The catheter should not be used to withdraw blood or to measure central venous pressure.
5 The skin puncture site should be cleansed weekly with a detergent, painted with a povidone-iodine solution, and occluded with a dressing. An occlusive, transparent plastic dressing is recommended because the insertion site can then be easily inspected for infection, drainage, and bleeding.
6 Barium-impregnated silicone rubber catheters (e.g., Silastic, Extracorporeal Medical Specialities, Inc.) do not traumatize the central veins and are less likely to be surrounded with a fibrin clot.

Peripheral venous infusion This route is safe and not a likely source of sepsis or thrombotic complications. However, the infused fluids must be isotonic or only mildly hypertonic. To achieve these conditions, nonprotein energy must be given mainly as lipid.

REPRESENTATIVE PROTOCOLS FOR ADMINISTRATION OF TOTAL PARENTERAL NUTRITION The sample protocols in Table 75-3 are designed for a 60-kg individual, are intended to be administered over 24 h, and provide 1 g amino acids and 40 nonprotein calories per kilogram of body weight. Proportionate modifications can be made for larger or smaller persons. Nonprotein energy is provided either as (1) glucose, (2) 50 percent glucose and 50 percent lipid, or (3) 85 percent lipid and 15 percent glucose. The latter is suitable for peripheral venous administration. The infusion materials must be prepared with care. In most centers such preparation is done exclusively by specially trained pharmacists.

HOME PARENTERAL NUTRITION (HPN) Home parenteral nutrition has revolutionized the lives of persons who otherwise would require prolonged hospitalization for long-term nutritional support. A permanent silicone rubber catheter is placed in the superior vena cava via a subclavian or jugular vein and brought to the outside through a subcutaneous tunnel. These catheters may be left in place for years without need for replacement. The patient receives periodic supplies of prepackaged nutrients ready for infusion. The nutrients are infused during sleep. A simple pneumatic cuff placed around the plastic bags containing the prepackaged infusion fluids is safe, inexpensive, and less cumbersome than electromechanical delivery systems. The system is disconnected after the overnight infusion, and the catheter is capped and filled with a heparin solution. The patient is then free to carry out normal activities during the day.

PARTIAL PARENTERAL NUTRITION It is debatable whether amino acids should replace glucose and electrolyte solutions in the management of patients unable to eat for short periods (up to 1 week) following surgery, strokes, or other acute illnesses. In 7 days a patient has (on average) a net negative nitrogen balance of 100 to 110 g when receiving only glucose replacement. If amino acids are given at a level of 1 g per kilogram of body weight per day, the nitrogen loss is cut to 35 to 45 g. This difference is equal to about 3 percent of the total nitrogen content of a 60-kg man. Since such a small deficit probably does not make any difference in clinical outcome (the nitrogen content is quickly replenished when food intake is restored) and since amino acid solutions are expensive, amino acid infusion is not recommended for fasts of up to 1 week. Beyond 1 week, full TPN should probably be given.

In some patients oral intake is possible, but the amounts ingested are inadequate for full nutrition. In such cases an estimate is made of the amount taken orally, and the deficiency is made up by parenteral means. When there is a question about how much of the ingested diet is absorbed (e.g., after bowel resection or with intestinal fistulas), the amount of nutrition given parenterally must be determined by trial and error, using weight gain and other signs of clinical improvement as a guide.

COMPLICATIONS **Technical complications** Most technical complications are due to improper central venous catheter placement. These can be minimized by restricting the placement to designated, trained persons. Complications during insertion include injury to lung and pleura causing pneumothorax and hemothorax, embolism due to shearing off the catheter during placement, and brachial plexus injury. The needle used to locate the subclavian vein should be kept anterior, just behind the clavicle. Catheter embolism is caused by attempting to withdraw the catheter while keeping the needle stationary, thus severing the catheter. The needle and catheter should be withdrawn as a unit. Attention to these two simple principles can minimize serious problems.

Technical complications resulting from inappropriate catheter placement include infusion of nutrients into pleura and mediastinum due to a misplaced catheter and thrombosis of jugular and central veins. These can be avoided by infusing only normal saline solution until it has been established radiographically that the catheter is in the lower superior vena cava. High placement or misplacement may result in venous thrombosis if hypertonic solutions are not diluted by a rapid flow of blood; such dilution occurs in the superior vena cava. Late problems can arise from air embolism or catheter clotting. Air embolism can be avoided by using Luer-Lok connections. If catheter thrombosis occurs it can be unblocked by injecting urokinase; it is rarely necessary to remove a blocked catheter.

Septic complications Septic complications may occur because the cutaneous puncture site and catheter tract form a direct route for access of bacteria and fungi to the central veins. The presence in this tract of a foreign body, such as the catheter, aids the process. Hence, catheter sepsis can be avoided by inserting it under strict aseptic conditions after proper skin preparation and by regular cleansing and dressing of the catheter site using strict aseptic technique. Catheter placement and care by specially trained teams can reduce sepsis to below 2 to 3 percent. It should be recognized that fever in a patient with a catheter is often *not* due to catheter sepsis. Hence where fever develops despite good catheter care, it is recommended that the TPN be stopped and electrolyte solutions infused while the cause of fever is investigated. Careful physical examination and history review are performed to identify other causes of fever. Blood cultures are taken from peripheral and central venous catheters, and cultures of sputum, wound, and urine are obtained. If no other cause for sepsis is found and blood cultures are positive, the catheter is removed and the patient is carefully watched. With pure catheter sepsis prompt defervescence should ensue. A new catheter can be inserted 48 hours after the fever has subsided. The common error is to assume that the fever is caused by catheter sepsis and thus to deny TPN to a patient who then becomes more malnourished and even more prone to sepsis.

Metabolic complications In patients with sepsis hyperglycemia may occur owing to insulin resistance and high levels of counterregulatory hormones such as catecholamines and cortisol. The treatment is to replace glucose calories with lipid calories and/or to add insulin. During TPN the blood glucose levels should not be allowed to go below 150 mg/dL because of the danger of hypoglycemia. The unexpected appearance of hyperglycemia may herald a febrile episode caused by sepsis. In contrast, hypoglycemia may occur either owing to the sudden stopping of the hypertonic glucose infusion or rarely in a patient receiving TPN and insulin whose sepsis has been cured.

Hyperammonemia and a picture resembling hepatic encephalopathy may occur in patients who have been infused with a mixture of essential amino acids containing little or no arginine. In such patients, care should be taken to give only minimal nitrogen infusions.

Hypertriglyceridemia may occur with overfeeding. The treatment is to reduce total calorie intake and to discontinue lipid infusions.

Electrolyte disturbances Anabolism is associated with the cellular uptake of potassium, magnesium, and phosphorus. This can result in hypokalemia, hypomagnesemia and hypophosphatemia. The latter can cause disorientation, convulsions, and coma because hypophosphatemia results in low red cell levels of 2,3-diphosphoglycerate (2,3-DPG) and thus reduced oxygen transfer to tissues. These abnormalities should not occur with the use of the mixtures given in Table 75-2 and with proper monitoring.

Acid-base balance The metabolism of the basic amino acids in their chloride forms results in the production of protons and chloride, which, if unbuffered, can accumulate and cause hyperchloremic acidosis. For this reason all current amino acid mixtures contain sodium acetate. The conversion of acetate to bicarbonate serves to buffer the protons produced by the metabolism of basic amino acids. Hence, disturbances of acid-base balance do not occur unless there is loss of bicarbonate from other sources, such as diarrhea, or unless lactic acid acidosis develops.

Liver disease Minimal elevations of serum alkaline phosphatase and aminotransferases are common (70 to 90 percent) during TPN and are usually not associated with jaundice. These abnormalities are as frequent in patients given glucose-electrolyte solutions or those fed by mouth as in those given TPN, which suggest that TPN is only one factor in their development. In occasional patients (1.5 to 2 percent) jaundice and cholestasis develop with minimal hepatocyte injury; hyperbilirubinemia is common in septic patients. Minor abnormalities of liver function are of no consequence, but sepsis should be treated appropriately.

During TPN, "sludge" accumulates in the gall bladder and may lead to obstructive changes in the biliary tract. In some patients cholecystectomy for gall bladder disease has been followed by relief of jaundice despite continuing TPN.

An enlarged, tender, fatty liver may develop if excess calories are given as carbohydrate. The treatment is to reduce caloric intake and replace 50 percent of it with lipid. The pathogenesis appears to be conversion of a portion of the infused carbohydrate to fat. The fat accumulates in the liver as triglyceride. Decreasing or replacing infused carbohydrate reduces the fatty liver.

Hypercalcemia and pancreatitis Pancreatitis associated with hypercalcemia can occur during TPN. This may be relieved by eliminating vitamin D from the infusion.

Metabolic bone disease In some patients receiving home TPN, osteomalacia and osteoporosis have occurred, leading to bone pain and fractures. The mechanism for these changes is not clear.

REFERENCES

ANDERSON GH et al: Design and evaluation by nitrogen balance and blood aminograms of an amino acid mixture for total parenteral nutrition of adults with gastrointestinal disease. J Clin Invest 53:904, 1974

——— et al: Dose-response relationships between amino acid intake and blood levels in newborn infants. Am J Clin Nutr 30:1110, 1977

BAKER JP et al: A randomized trial of total parenteral nutrition in critically ill patients. Gastroenterology 87:53, 1984

BATSTONE GF et al: Metabolic studies in subjects following thermal injury. Intermediary metabolites, hormones and tissue oxygenation. Burns 2:207, 1976

BLACKBURN GL et al: Protein sparing therapy during periods of starvation with sepsis or trauma. Ann Surg 177:588, 1973

CAHILL GF JR et al: Starvation in man. N Engl J Med 282:668, 1970

CRAIG RP et al: Intravenous glucose, amino acids and fat in the postoperative period. Lancet 2:8, 1977

GREENBERG GR et al: Protein-sparing therapy in postoperative patients. Effects of added hypocaloric glucose or lipid. N Engl J Med 294:1411, 1976

IZSAK EH et al: Pancreatitis in association with hypercalcemia in patients receiving total parenteral nutrition. Gastroenterology 79:555, 1980

JEEJEEBHOY KN et al: Metabolic studies in total parenteral nutrition with lipid in man: Comparison with glucose. J Clin Invest 57:125, 1976

——— et al: Total parenteral nutrition at home: Studies in patients surviving 4 months to 5 years. Gastroenterology 71:943, 1976

———: Protein sparing effect of amino acids, in *Clinical Nutrition Update: Amino Acids*, HL Green et al (eds). Chicago, American Medical Association, 1977

———: Role of measuring albumin synthesis as a way of measuring protein body repletion, in ibid.

KORETZ RL, MEYER JH: Elemental diets–Facts and fantasies. Gastroenterology 78:393, 1980

MENG HC, WILMORE DW (eds): *Fat Emulsions in Parenteral Nutrition*. Chicago, American Medical Association, 1976

MESSING B: Does total parenteral nutrition induce gallbladder sludge formation and lithiasis? Gastroenterology 84:1012, 1983

ROULET M et al: A controlled trial of the effect of parenteral nutrition support on patients with respiration failure and sepsis. Clin Nutr 2:97, 1983

RUDMAN D et al: Elemental balances during intravenous hyperalimentation of underweight adult subjects. J Clin Invest 55:94, 1975

SHIKE M et al: A possible role for Vitamin D in the genesis of parenteral-nutrition-induced metabolic bone disease. Ann Int Med 95:560, 1981

76 VITAMIN DEFICIENCY AND EXCESS[1]

JEAN D. WILSON

The role of vitamins in disease has changed within the past few decades. Deficiencies of single vitamins are now rarely endemic, even in developing nations, and instead occur either as a portion of states of malnutrition, as a result of food faddism, as a complication of more widespread disease such as malabsorption, as a complication of complex therapy such as hemodialysis or total parenteral nutrition, or as the result of an inborn error of metabolism. Indeed, disorders of vitamin excess may now be more common than vitamin deficiency.

In considering the pathophysiology of vitamins several points are worth emphasis. (1) The fact that organic compounds cannot be synthesized within the body and are required constituents of the diet is the result of mutations, and the provision of vitamins in the diet is a form of therapy for an inborn error of metabolism. In some instances, such as the limited ability to synthesize thiamine, the requirement is common to many if not all animals, and the mutation must have occurred early in evolution; in others, such as the single-gene defect that prevents ascorbic acid synthesis, humans share the defect with only a few other species, such as the guinea pig. (2) The feature that separates vitamins from other necessary organic constituents in the diet is that small amounts of them are required, in contrast to the relatively large amounts of essential amino acids and essential fatty acids. This is a consequence of the fact that vitamins function not as building blocks of tissue mass or as substrates for energy production but rather as prosthetic groups for quantitatively minor tissue constituents or as catalytic cofactors for biologic reactions; like most catalysts they are required only in small amounts. (3) Deficiency of some vitamins has never been described in humans (e.g., pantothenic acid) implying that these vitamins are either so ubiquitous in food sources or are conserved so efficiently by the body that deficiency can become manifest, if at all, only in the context of a mixed nutritional and vitamin deficiency. (4) Alcoholism is the background upon which many vitamin deficiencies develop in the United States. This is the consequence of several interlocking factors including diminished intake, impairment of absorption and storage of vitamins, and in some cases predisposing genetic factors. In those instances in which alcoholism is not associated with an increased frequency of disease (e.g., pellagra), the etiology of the disorder is more complicated than a simple deficiency state. (5) Biochemical means of proving vitamin deficiency, once suspected, are limited, and the role of vitamin deficiency in disease states is frequently not recognized because nonspecific vitamin therapy is a common part of standard supportive care. As a consequence, understanding the manifestations of vitamin deficiency and a high index of suspicion in the appropriate clinical setting are essential for considering the diagnosis, and demonstration of a response to replacement therapy may be the most accurate way to confirm a diagnosis. (6) The widespread consumption of excessive amounts of vitamins can occur either as the indirect consequence of dietary practice or, more commonly, as the result of deliberate ingestion. The toxicity of the fat-soluble vitamins A and D has long been established, whereas the toxicity syndromes produced by the water-soluble vitamins are inconsistent and less well characterized.

DEFICIENCY STATES

NIACIN (PELLAGRA) Biochemistry *Niacin* is the generic term for nicotinic acid (3-pyridinecarboxylic acid) and derivatives that exhibit the nutritional activity of nicotinic acid (Fig. 76-1). In one sense niacin is not a vitamin since it can be formed from the essential amino acid tryptophan. In the human an average of about 1 mg of niacin is formed from 60 mg of dietary tryptophan. Accordingly, estimates of the adequacy of dietary intake must take into account the tryptophan content of the diet as well as the content of niacin. Many foodstuffs, especially cereals, contain bound forms of niacin from which the vitamin is not nutritionally available.

The absorption, tissue distribution, and metabolism of the vitamin are poorly understood. Approximately one-fifth of the vitamin is decarboxylated, and the remainder is excreted in the urine as methylated products, largely *N*-methylnicotinamide and its derivatives.

Mechanism of action Niacin is an essential component of nicotinamide adenine dinucleotide (NAD) and nicotinamide adenine dinucleotide phosphate (NADP), coenzymes for many oxidation-reduction reactions.

Requirements The requirements and recommended daily allowances for niacin and tryptophan are listed in Tables 70-1 and 70-2. In contrast to most vitamins, the requirement for niacin does not appear to be increased during pregnancy. Requirement is primarily determined by the amino acid composition of the diet.

[1] *For vitamin D, see Chap. 337 and for the hematologic vitamins, see Chap. 285.*

Experimental depletion After the institution of a diet deficient in niacin and tryptophan, the urinary excretion of niacin metabolites reaches minimal values (<1.5 mg per day) after 1 to 2 months and remains constant thereafter. Clinical deficiency develops shortly after excretion becomes stable at a low level and consists of dermatitis, glossitis, stomatitis, diarrhea, proctitis, mental depression, abdominal pain, vaginitis, dysphagia, and amenorrhea, findings similar to those in pellagra.

Clinical deficiency Pellagra was previously an endemic disease in the American south and in many other parts of the world. The endemic disease is usually associated with a high intake of maize (American corn) and can be cured by the administration of niacin; nevertheless, the fact that large populations of people exist on a diet in which maize is the major source of protein but nevertheless are free of endemic pellagra implies that the relation between maize intake and the development of the disease is not straightforward. As a consequence, the concept of the pathogenesis of pellagra has evolved from that of a pure vitamin deficiency or a mixed deficiency of tryptophan and available niacin in the diet to a more complicated etiology. The disorder may be due to an imbalance in dietary amino acids; the niacin equivalent (available niacin and tryptophan) of maize, although low, is no lower than that of some cereals that are unassociated with endemic pellagra. Furthermore, the leucine content of common varieties of maize is high, whereas a hybrid strain of maize, opaque 2, has lower leucine but similar tryptophan and niacin contents. Dogs fed a diet rich in conventional maize or a diet rich in opaque 2 maize supplemented with leucine develop experimental pellagra, whereas dogs fed the opaque 2 maize alone do not. This finding presumably explains why pellagra can result from a diet rich in millet (sorghum, jowar), which has a leucine content similar to that of maize but a niacin and tryptophan content (and availability) equivalent to that of rice. Leucine is believed to inhibit the synthesis of nicotinic acid mononucleotide and consequently the synthesis of NAD and NADP. Thus, development of symptomatic niacin "deficiency" may depend on the amino acid content of the rest of the diet as well as upon the intake of the vitamin and its precursors. The second possibility is that the milling of maize influences the bioavailability of the niacin in the cereal. On the one hand, treatment of maize with alkali in the preparation of foods in Latin America may serve to hydrolyze bound nicotinic acid and to inactivate toxins that may accumulate in stored grain contaminated with molds. On the other hand, degermination of the cereal during the usual milling process in the United States may inhibit the liberation of bound

FIGURE 76-1 *The structure and principal functions of some of the vitamins associated with human disorders.*

Vitamin	Active Derivative or Cofactor Form	Principal Function
Niacin 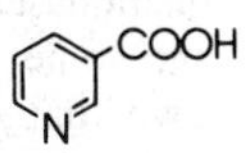	Nicotinamide Adenine Dinucleotide Phosphate (NADP) and Nicotine Adenine Dinucleotide (NAD)	Coenzymes for Oxidations and Reductions
Thiamine 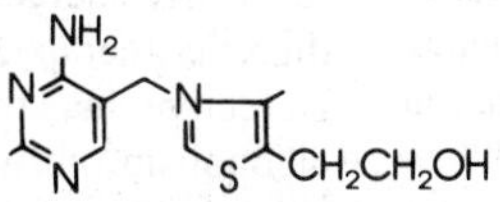	Thiamine Diphosphate	Coenzyme for Cleavage of Carbon-Carbon Bonds
Pyridoxine 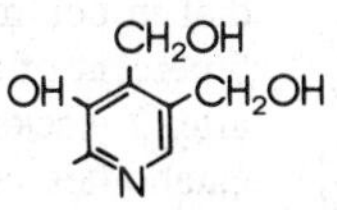	Pyridoxal Phosphate	Cofactor for Enzymes of Amino Acid Metabolism
Riboflavin 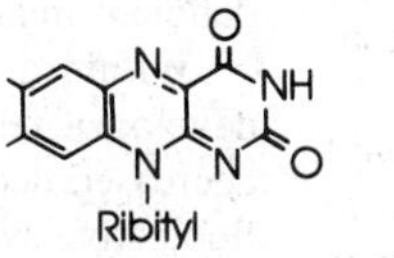	Flavin Mononucleotide (FMN) and Flavin Adenine Dinucleotide (FAD)	Cofactor for Oxidation-Reduction Reactions and Covalently Attached Prosthetic Groups for Some Enzymes
Ascorbic Acid 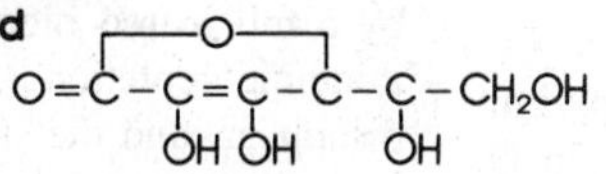	Ascorbic Acid and Dehydroascorbic Acid	Participation as a Redox Ion in Many Biological Oxidation Reactions
Vitamin A 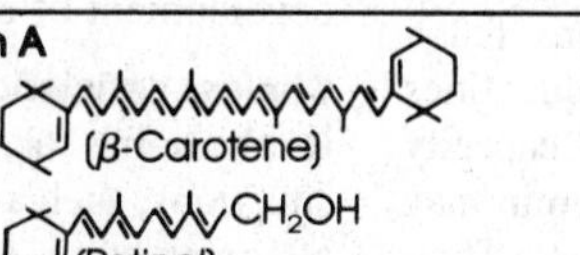	Retinol, Retinal, and Retinoic Acid	Formation of Carotenoid Proteins (Vision) and Glycoproteins (Epithelial Cell Function)
Vitamin E 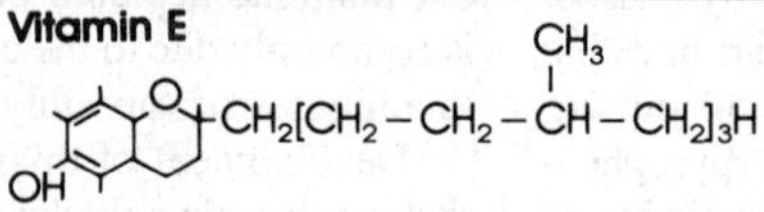	Tocopherol	Antioxidant
Vitamin K 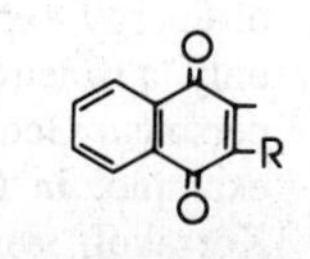	Menaquinone	Cofactor for Post-Translational Carboxylation of Many Proteins Including Essential Clotting Factors

niacin. The effect of these treatments, respectively, would be to prevent or to predispose to the development of pellagra when maize is a major element of the diet.

Whatever the cause, endemic pellagra disappeared coincident with the improvement of nutritional education and with the widespread supplementation of grain cereals with niacin. At present, pellagra is an occasional secondary manifestation of two disorders that profoundly affect tryptophan metabolism, the carcinoid syndrome, in which up to 60 percent of tryptophan is catabolized by what is ordinarily a minor pathway of metabolism (see Chap. 303), and Hartnup disease (see Chap. 307), an inherited disorder in which several amino acids including tryptophan are absorbed poorly from the diet. In both disorders pellagra is due to diminished availability of effective niacin equivalents and can be cured by the administration of large amounts of the vitamin.

Pellagra is a chronic wasting disease typically associated with dermatitis, dementia, and diarrhea. The dermatitis is bilateral, symmetric, and present in sites exposed to sunlight, and is due to photosensitivity. The mental changes are less discrete; fatigue, insomnia, and apathy may precede the development of an encephalopathy characterized by confusion, disorientation, hallucination, loss of memory, and eventually, frank organic psychosis. Paresthesias and polyneuritis may be the result of coexisting deficiencies of other vitamins. Diarrhea, when it occurs, results from widespread inflammation of the mucous surfaces; other mucosal abnormalities include achlorhydria, glossitis, stomatitis, and vaginitis. The course is progressive over a several-year period, and death is usually due to secondary complications.

The relation between the known coenzyme function of NAD and NADP and these various symptoms has not been defined. Levels of NAD and NADP in erythrocytes are lower in patients with pellagra than in normal individuals, but the coenzymes are essential to so many reactions in intermediary metabolism that profound deficiency of the coenzymes is incompatible with life. The mental changes in pellagra may be associated with diminished conversion of tryptophan to serotonin.

No biochemical test is of diagnostic value, and diagnosis must be based upon suspicion and response to replacement therapy. As predicted, excretion in the urine of the metabolites of nicotinic acid and tryptophan is lower than average but not lower than in patients with generalized malnutrition (Table 71-4). Plasma tryptophan and erythrocyte NAD and NADP levels are also low. The skin lesions are characterized by hyperkeratosis, hyperpigmentation, and desquamation.

The administration of small amounts of niacin (10 mg per day) in the face of limiting amounts of dietary tryptophan is sufficient to cure endemic pellagra. Large amounts (40 to 200 mg per day) may be required in Hartnup disease and in the carcinoid syndrome.

THIAMINE (BERIBERI) Biochemistry Thiamine contains pyrimidine and thiazole moieties linked by a methylene bridge (Fig. 76-1). The vitamin is synthesized by a variety of plants and microorganisms but not ordinarily by animals. However, rats and pigeons fed a thiamine-free diet can be protected from deficiency by large quantities of the pyrimidine and thiazole moieties, suggesting a small capacity to couple the subunits together. Limited amounts of the vitamin may be synthesized by microorganisms in the gastrointestinal tract. Thiamine is absorbed both by an active-transport process and by passive diffusion. The capacity to absorb the vitamin in the human intestine is limited to about 5 mg per day. Approximately 25 to 30 mg are stored in the body, 80 percent as thiamine diphosphate (pyrophosphate), 10 percent as thiamine triphosphate, and the remainder as free thiamine monophosphate. Large amounts are present in skeletal muscles (about one-half of body stores), heart, liver, kidneys, and brain. A number of thiaminase enzymes inactivate thiamine by splitting the vitamin into its two component parts. Several metabolites are excreted in the urine, principally thiamine itself (which is secreted by the renal tubules), an acetylated derivative, and end products of thiamine catabolism, mainly derivatives of thiazole acetate and pyrimidine carboxylate.

Mechanism of action Thiamine diphosphate acts as a coenzyme for several reactions that cleave carbon-carbon bonds—the oxidative decarboxylation of α-keto acids (pyruvate and α-ketoglutarate) and keto analogues of leucine, isoleucine, and valine, and the transketolase reaction in the pentose phosphate pathway. Many features of thiamine deficiency are the result of inhibition of these enzymatic reactions and/or the accumulation of the proximal metabolites. Thiamine may also have a specific role in neurons independent of its coenzymatic function in general metabolism; thiamine and its esters are present in axonal membranes, and electrical stimulation of nerves effects the hydrolysis and release of thiamine diphosphate and triphosphate.

Requirements The recommended daily allowances for thiamine are given in Tables 70-1 and 70-2. The vitamin has a widespread distribution in food and is absent only from oils, fats, cassava, and refined sugar. In vegetable products the vitamin is largely in the form of thiamine. The outer layers of cereal grains are especially rich in the vitamin; hence, machine-milled rice is a poor source. In animal tissues thiamine is present largely in the form of phosphate esters. The esters are dephosphorylated by phosphatases in the intestine, and only the free vitamin is absorbed. A substantial loss of the vitamin takes place during cooking above 100°C.

Several factors influence the absorption and metabolism of the vitamin (and hence alter daily requirements). One is the presence of thiaminases in foods including fresh fish, clams, shrimp, mussels, and some raw animal tissues, and in microorganisms in the colon. Two, daily needs decrease when fat forms a large part of the diet and increase as carbohydrate intake increases. Requirements are increased in pregnancy, during lactation, in thyrotoxicosis, and by fever. Accelerated loss of thiamine from the body may occur with diuretic therapy, hemodialysis, peritoneal dialysis, and diarrhea. Defective intestinal absorption can occur in malabsorption states, alcoholism, chronic malnutrition, and folate deficiency.

Experimental depletion Following the institution of a thiamine-free diet in control subjects, thiamine excretion in the urine decreases to 5 percent of the control value after a week and becomes undetectable after 2 weeks. However, the excretion of the pyrimidine and thiazole catabolites of thiamine remains unchanged for as long as a month, indicating that the body pool is slowly utilized during a period of deficient intake.

Within a week after the institution of a deficient diet, subjects develop a resting tachycardia, followed by the onset of weakness, decreased deep tendon reflexes, and (in some) a sensory neuropathy. Subjective symptoms include generalized malaise, headache, nausea, and aching of the muscles. Appearance of these symptoms is paralleled by a fall in red blood cell transketolase activity. Within a week of thiamine repletion (2 mg per day) all abnormal physical findings disappear, and the subjective symptoms clear after 2 weeks. (Experimental depletion in humans has never been carried to the point of development of severe cerebral or cardiovascular symptoms.)

Clinical deficiency In developed nations thiamine deficiency occurs in alcoholics or food faddists or in the context of special clinical situations, such as chronic peritoneal dialysis, hemodialysis, refeeding after starvation, or after the administration of glucose to asymptomatic but thiamine-depleted patients. In developing countries the disorder is commonly due to the consumption of milled rice or foods containing thiaminases or (possibly) other antithiamine factors.

Development of thiamine defeciency in chronic alcoholics is due to low thiamine intake, impaired thiamine absorption and storage, accelerated destruction of thiamine diphosphate, and varying degrees of energy expenditure. However, clinical manifestations develop in only a fraction of alcoholics and other chronically malnourished persons. Genetic factors may be involved in susceptibility. For example, in fibroblasts cultured from patients with the Wernicke-Korsakoff syndrome the thiamine-requiring transketolase binds thiamine diphosphate only one-tenth as avidly as in those of controls. This finding implies that an underlying genetic polymorphism is clinically silent when the diet is adequate but becomes overt if thiamine intake is low or marginal.

The two major manifestations of thiamine deficiency involve the cardiovascular (wet beriberi) and nervous systems (dry beriberi and the Wernicke-Korsakoff syndrome). The typical patient has mixed symptoms involving both the cardiovascular and nervous systems, but pure cardiovascular, pure polyneuritic, and pure cerebral forms also occur. The factors that determine the relative preponderance of these manifestations are related in part to the duration and severity of the deficiency, the degree of physical exertion, and the caloric intake. Severe physical exertion, high carbohydrate intake, and a moderate degree of chronic deficiency favor wet beriberi with little or no peripheral neuritis, whereas an equal deficiency with caloric restriction and relative inactivity favors the development of dry beriberi.

Beriberi heart disease comprises three major physiologic derangements: (1) peripheral vasodilation leading to a high-output state, (2) biventricular myocardial failure, and (3) retention of sodium and water leading to edema. In the chronic form peripheral vasodilatation leads to increased arteriovenous shunting of blood, rapid circulation time, tachycardia, increased cardiac output, and a venous congestive state characterized by elevated peripheral venous pressure, elevated right ventricular end-diastolic pressure, decreased arteriovenous extraction of oxygen, sodium retention, and edema. Disordered blood flow (decreased cerebral and renal blood flow and increased flow to muscles) is common. Cardiac output increases so that notwithstanding the lowered peripheral vascular resistance ventricular work, arterial blood pressure, and pulmonary wedge pressure tend to be elevated. Temporary appearance or worsening of hypertension may occur during thiamine repletion, presumably due to closing of arteriovenous shunts and temporary volume overload.

In acute fulminant cardiovascular (shoshin) beriberi, the myocardial lesion is the central feature of a course in which severe dyspnea, restlessness, and anxiety eventuate in acute cardiovascular collapse and death within hours to days. Physical findings include stocking-glove cyanosis, extreme tachycardia, marked cardiomegaly, hepatomegaly, arterial bruits, and neck vein distention. The venous pressure is high, and the circulation time is rapid. Because of the fulminant course edema may be minimal or absent. Administration of thiamine rapidly restores peripheral vascular resistance, but improvement in the myocardial abnormality may be delayed so that low-output failure supervenes during treatment.

Three types of nervous system involvement occur: peripheral neuropathy, Wernicke's encephalopathy (cerebral beriberi), and the Korsakoff syndrome. The neuropathy may or may not be painful and is characterized by a symmetric impairment of sensory, motor, and reflex function that affects the distal segments of limbs more severely than the proximal ones. The histologic lesion is a noninflammatory degeneration of myelin sheaths. No meaningful distinction can be made between this disorder and so-called alcoholic neuropathy on the basis of either clinical or neurologic criteria.

Wernicke's encephalopathy ordinarily develops in an orderly sequence and consists of vomiting, nystagmus (horizontal more commonly than vertical), palsies of the rectus muscles leading to unilateral or bilateral ophthalmoplegia (and decrease in the nystagmus), fever, ataxia, and progressive mental deterioration that eventuates in a global confusional state and may progress to coma and death. Improvement occurs after thiamine replacement, although Korsakoff's syndrome may supervene. Thus, the eye palsies are corrected, the nystagmus improves in one-half, the ataxia improves or disappears in two-thirds, and the global confusional state disappears to be replaced by Korsakoff's syndrome. The latter consists of retrograde amnesia, impaired ability to learn, and (usually) confabulation. The patient is usually alert and responsive and exhibits no serious defect in behavior. Recovery (complete or partial) from Korsakoff's syndrome can be expected only in one-half.

In summary, Wernicke's encephalopathy and the amnesic psychosis of Korsakoff's syndrome are not separate clinical events; instead, the changing ocular and ataxic signs, the transformation of the global confusional state into the amnesic-confabulatory syndrome, and the development of a nonconfabulatory amnesic state are successive stages in the recovery from a single process. The clinical features, differential diagnosis, course, and pathology of cerebral beriberi are discussed in detail in Chap. 349.

Various biochemical tests to detect thiamine deficiency include the measurement of blood thiamine, pyruvate, α-ketoglutarate, lactate, and glyoxylate; measurement of the urinary excretion of thiamine and thiamine metabolites; a thiamine-loading test; and measurement of urinary methylglyoxal. The most reliable is the measurement of whole-blood or erythrocyte transketolase activity. Any enhancement in enzymatic activity resulting from added thiamine diphosphate (TPP) is referred to as the TPP effect (expressed in percent). If the activity of the enzyme is increased more than 15 percent by the added thiamine diphosphate, then a deficiency state is probably present (Table 71-4). Due to variability in activity, measurement of isolated transketolase levels is not useful, but demonstration of an increase in activity after treatment coupled with a significant stimulation in vitro by added thiamine diphosphate prior to treatment suggests the presence of thiamine deficiency.

Another criterion for the diagnosis is the assessment of clinical response to thiamine administration. Clinical improvement may be dramatic in cardiovascular beriberi, and an increase in blood pressure and decrease in heart rate may be seen within 12 h after start of therapy. Diuresis and reduction in heart size may be apparent within 1 to 2 days.

Prompt administration of thiamine is indicated when beriberi is diagnosed or suspected. Fifty milligrams per day should be given intramuscularly for several days after which 2.5 to 5 mg per day can be administered by mouth. Larger amounts are usually not absorbed. All patients should also receive other water-soluble vitamins in therapeutic quantities.

Thiamine-responsive inborn errors of metabolism A number of thiamine-responsive inborn errors of metabolism have been described in which patients respond to pharmacologic doses of thiamine. These include thiamine-responsive megaloblastic anemia, for which the mechanism is unknown; thiamine-responsive lactic acidosis, which is due to low activity of pyruvate carboxylase in liver; thiamine-responsive branched-chain ketoaciduria, which is due to low activity of a ketoacid dehydrogenase; and intermittent cerebellar ataxia which may result from an abnormal pyruvate dehydrogenase. In addition, the autosomal recessive disorder subacute necrotizing encephalomyelopathy (Leigh's disease) may be related to a diminished amount of thiamine triphosphate in neural tissue; a factor has been isolated from the urine of such patients that inhibits the enzyme that synthesizes thiamine triphosphate. The clinical response of patients with Leigh's disease to pharmacologic doses of the vitamin appears to be minor, however.

PYRIDOXINE (VITAMIN B_6) Biochemistry The biologic activity of the vitamin B_6 group is displayed by pyridoxine, pyridoxal, and pyridoxamine and their 5-phosphate esters (Fig. 76-1). The coenzyme form is pyridoxal 5-phosphate, and the other compounds owe their activity to conversion to pyridoxal 5-phosphate. The vitamin is widely and uniformly distributed in all foods; muscle meats, liver, vegetables, and whole-grain cereals are among the best sources.

Mechanism of action Pyridoxal phosphate acts as a cofactor for many enzymes involved in amino acid metabolism, including transaminases, synthetases, and hydroxylases. In humans the vitamin is of particular importance in the metabolism of tryptophan, glycine, serine, glutamate, and the sulfur-containing amino acids. Pyridoxal phosphate is also required for the synthesis of the heme precursor δ-aminolevulinic acid. A large portion of body stores of pyridoxine is in muscle phosphorylase, where it functions to stabilize the enzyme rather than as a catalyst. It also plays a poorly understood role in neuronal excitability, possibly as a result of its function in transsulfuration reactions or in γ-aminobutyric acid metabolism

Requirements The recommended daily allowances are described in Tables 70-1 and 70-2. Even more than for most vitamins, the requirement is increased in pregnancy and by the ingestion of estrogens. In both conditions abnormal tryptophan metabolites are excreted in urine, and this can be prevented by supplementation with pyridoxine. Estrogens appear to inhibit the role of pyridoxal phosphate in tryptophan metabolism. Pyridoxine requirement may also be increased by high protein intake. The ingestion of ethanol interferes with the metabolism of pyridoxal phosphate, the ethanol metabolite acetaldehyde displacing the coenzyme from proteins and thus enhancing its degradation.

Experimental depletion The feeding of pyridoxine-deficient diets leads to chemical evidence of deficiency (increased xanthurenic acid and decreased pyridoxine in urine) within a week. Electroencephalographic abnormalities are demonstrable within 3 weeks, and some subjects have grand mal seizures. Deficiency induced with the pyridoxine antagonist deoxypyridoxine causes, in addition, seborrheic dermatitis, cheilosis, glossitis, nausea, vomiting, weakness, and dizziness.

Clinical deficiency The widespread occurrence of the vitamin in food is probably the reason that the naturally occurring pure pyridoxine deficiency does not occur except when the pyridoxine content of food is either destroyed or converted to less available protein-bound forms during processing, as has happened in some infant formulas. It is a paradox, therefore, that pyridoxine deficiency is now frequent due to the fact that many commonly used drugs act as pyridoxine antagonists. Hydrazines such as *isoniazid* induce peripheral neuritis that can be prevented by pyridoxine supplementation; these drugs combine with pyridoxal and pyridoxal phosphate to form hydrazones. The hydrazones inhibit enzymes such as pyridoxal kinase, induce convulsions directly, and accelerate pyridoxine loss in the urine and thus induce a vitamin deficiency. *Cycloserine* also causes an increase in the excretion of the vitamin in the urine and produces profound neurologic effects, presumably by forming a complex with pyridoxal phosphate that competes with the cofactor for apoenzymes. *Penicillamine* acts as an antagonist by forming a thiazolidine derivative with pyridoxal phosphate. In each of these instances abnormal tryptophan metabolism and convulsions can be prevented by supplementation with the vitamin.

Estimates of vitamin deficiency have been based upon the correction of clinical signs of deficiency following administration of the vitamin, measurement of the excretion of tryptophan metabolites after tryptophan-loading tests, measurement of various amino acid transferase activities in blood, and measurement of the excretion of pyridoxine or its metabolites or of oxalate in urine (Table 71-4). The most commonly used index is the measurement of urinary tryptophan metabolites, particularly xanthurenic acid, following tryptophan loading. Alternatively, cystathionine can be assayed after administration of a methionine load. In vitro measurement of red blood cell glutamic pyruvic transaminase in the presence and absence of pyridoxal phosphate may be a better indicator of pyridoxine status than either loading test.

The appropriate management is prevention of deficiency. Supplementation of the diet with 30 mg of pyridoxine returns tryptophan metabolism to normal in pregnancy, in users of oral contraceptives, and in patients taking isoniazid. Doses as high as 100 mg per day may be required in subjects taking penicillamine.

Pyridoxine-responsive diseases Several genetic disorders cause abnormalities in vitamin B_6 metabolism. In one group, infants develop convulsions and brain damage and die if not provided with large daily supplements of pyridoxine; these children have an apoenzyme for glutamic acid decarboxylase that has a decreased binding affinity for pyridoxal phosphate. Consequently they do not form normal amounts of γ-aminobutyric acid, a physiologic inhibitor of neurotransmission. Another group of patients has pyridoxine-responsive chronic anemia; pyridoxine supplementation results in prompt hematologic improvement but does not correct the morphologic abnormality in the erythrocytes.

The synthesis of cystathionine from homocystine and serine and its cleavage to cysteine and homoserine are catalyzed by two pyridoxal phosphate enzymes. The changes that occur in deficiency of these two enzymes and in xanthurenic aciduria due to kynureninase deficiency have been reviewed by Mudd. Some patients with vitamin B_6–responsive xanthurenic aciduria or cystathioninuria have a mutant apoenzyme that interacts abnormally with pyridoxal phosphate, a defect that can be largely corrected by elevated concentrations of the cofactor. In contrast, the vitamin B_6 response in patients with homocystinuria due to cystathionine synthetase deficiency is due to an enhancement of the activity of the residual amount of normal enzyme present rather than a restoration of the affected enzyme levels to normal.

RIBOFLAVIN Riboflavin in the form of the coenzymes flavin mononucleotide (FMN) and flavin adenine dinucleotide (FAD) participates in a variety of oxidation-reduction reactions (Fig. 76-1). In addition, covalently attached flavins are essential to the structure of such enzymes as succinate dehydrogenase and monoamine oxidase. The vitamin is absorbed from the gastrointestinal tract either as free riboflavin or the 5′-phosphate by a specific transport process. The requirements and recommended daily allowances are listed in Tables 70-1 and 70-2. Covalently linked vitamin accounts for less than one-tenth of the tissue pool. The vitamin is excreted in urine predominantly in the free form although a small fraction of the daily turnover is the result of catabolism by microorganisms in the gastrointestinal tract.

Riboflavin deficiency can be induced in humans by feeding a riboflavin-deficient diet or by the administration of riboflavin antagonists such as galactoflavin. The deficiency syndrome is characterized by sore throat, hyperemia and edema of the pharyngeal and oral mucous membranes, cheilosis, angular stomatitis, glossitis, seborrheic dermatitis, and normochromic, normocytic anemia due to red cell hypoplasia of the bone marrow. These features can be rapidly and completely reversed by riboflavin administration. Thyroid hormones and adrenal steroids enhance FMN and FAD synthesis; certain psychotropic agents (phenothiazines and tricyclic antidepressants) competitively inhibit flavin coenzyme biosynthesis, but these agents alone do not induce deficiency. Instead, riboflavin deficiency almost invariably occurs in combination with other vitamin deficiencies.

VITAMIN C (SCURVY) Biochemistry In most animals ascorbic acid (vitamin C) can be synthesized from glucose. However, humans, other primates, and the guinea pig are unable to synthesize L-ascorbic acid and require vitamin C in the diet. These species can perform the various reactions required for the biosynthesis of the vitamin from D-glucose except for one step, the conversion of L-gluconogammalactone to L-abscorbic acid. The enzyme that catalyzes this reaction (L-gluconolactone oxidase) is missing because of a mutation; thus the need for vitamin C in the diet is the result of an inborn error in carbohydrate metabolism.

Mechanism of action L-Ascorbic acid readily undergoes reversible oxidation and reduction as follows:

$$\text{L-ascorbic acid} \rightleftharpoons \text{dehydro-L-ascorbic acid} + 2H^+ + 2e$$

This property of the vitamin is the key to understanding its role as a redox agent for biologic oxidation. However, ascorbic acid does not act as a conventional cofactor since its requirement can usually be replaced by other compounds with similar redox properties. The best understood function is in the synthesis of collagen; absence of the vitamin leads to impairment of peptidyl hydroxylation of procollagen and a reduction in collagen formation and secretion by connective tissue. Nonhydroxylated collagen is unstable and cannot form the triple helix required for normal tissue structure. Many features of scurvy result from this defect in collagen synthesis, including the capillary fragility that underlies the hemorrhagic features, the poor healing of wounds, and (in part) the bony abnormalities of children. Collagens that normally have the highest content of hydroxyproline are most severely affected, accounting for the early disruption of the adventitia, media, and basal laminae of blood vessels. Ascorbic acid also functions to prevent oxidation of tetrahydrofolate and thus protect the active folic acid pool and to regulate iron distribution and storage, probably by influencing the valence of stored iron and maintaining a normal ratio of ferritin to hemosiderin. Scorbutic patients excrete incompletely oxidized products of tyrosine metabolism, but the significance is not clear.

Requirements The recommended daily allowances for vitamin C are described in Tables 70-1 and 70-2. The vitamin is present in milk and some meats (kidney, liver, fish) and is widely distributed in fruits and vegetables. A portion is lost after prolonged storage of unprocessed fruits and vegetables (for example, potatoes), but it is partially preserved (half or greater) by most means of food processing (boiling, steaming, pressure cooking, preserving jams and jellies, freezing, dehydration, and canning). As a consequence the recommended daily allowances can be met with even a modest intake of fruits and vegetables. The utilization of the vitamin is increased during pregnancy and lactation and in thyrotoxicosis, and absorption is decreased in diarrheal states and in achlorhydria.

Experimental depletion The total-body pool of vitamin C varies from 1.5 to 3 g. When a deficient diet is instituted, the pool is depleted at a constant rate that may be as high as 4 percent per day. In monkeys the major catabolic pathway involves oxidation of the alcohol at carbon 6 to an aldehyde and then to an acid. Because of differences in initial pool size and rates of turnover, differences in the completeness of deficiency in various experimental diets, and variation among normal subjects at the cellular or enzymatic level, the time required for development of symptoms ranges from 1 to 3 months in different studies. Manifestations of deficiency correlate better with the total pool size than with plasma or blood levels. The first symptoms (petechial hemorrhages and ecchymoses) develop when the pool size is less than 0.5 g; with further depletion (pool size 0.1 to 0.5 g) abnormalities include gum involvement, hyperkeratosis, congested hair follicles, arthralgias, Sjögren's syndrome, coiled hairs, and joint effusions. When depletion is extreme (pool size <0.1 g), dyspnea, edema, oliguria, and neuropathy supervene. Progress of the disease may then be rapid.

Symptoms do not improve until the normal pool is repleted, and the larger the therapeutic dose, the more rapid the repletion. However, with doses as small as 6.5 mg per day the body pool eventually returns to normal, and amelioration of symptoms follows.

Clinical deficiency Clinical scurvy now occurs for the most part in areas of urban poverty. An increased incidence occurs at 6 to 12 months of age in infants whose processed milk formulas are unsupplemented with citrus fruit or vegetables as a result of maternal error or neglect. Another peak occurs in middle and old age; edentulous men who live alone and cook for themselves are particularly prone to develop scurvy. Clinical scurvy is more severe than the experimental disease, doubtlessly because affected individuals usually have deficiencies of other dietary constituents as well and because the groups at risk (infants and the elderly) are especially vulnerable. The disorder has different clinical features in adults and children.

In adults the features include perifollicular hyperkeratotic papules in which hairs become fragmented and buried; perifollicular hemorrhages; purpura beginning on the backs of the lower extremities coalescing to become ecchymoses (Fig. 76-2); hemorrhage into the muscles of the arms and legs with secondary phlebothromboses; hemorrhages into joints; splinter hemorrhages in the nail beds; gum involvement (only in people with teeth) that includes swelling, friability, bleeding, secondary infection, and loosening of the teeth; poor healing of wounds and breakdown of recently healed wounds; petechial hemorrhages in the viscera; and emotional changes. Symptoms resembling those of Sjögren's syndrome may occur. Terminally, icterus, edema, and fever are common, and convulsions, shock, and death may occur abruptly.

In infancy and childhood hemorrhage into the periosteum of long bones causes painful swellings and may result in epiphyseal separation. The sternum may sink inward, leaving a sharp elevation at the rib margins (scorbutic rosary). Purpura and ecchymoses may develop in the skin, and gum lesions occur if the teeth have erupted. Retrobulbar, subarachnoid, and intracerebral hemorrhages rapidly culminate in death if treatment is delayed.

Severe to moderate anemia is common both in children and in adults, is usually normochromic and normocytic, and is due to bleeding into tissues. The anemia may be macrocytic and/or megaloblastic (one-fifth of patients in one series). Many foods that contain vitamin C also contain folate, and diets that cause scurvy may also cause folate deficiency. However, ascorbic acid deficiency also results in an increased oxidation of formyl tetrahydrofolic acid to inactive folate metabolites and may cause a decrease in the active folate pool. Whether changes in iron distribution and storage are involved in the pathogenesis of the anemia is unclear. Whatever the mechanism, the anemia is corrected with refeeding and replenishment of vitamin C and the institution of a balanced diet.

In some hospitals platelet ascorbic acid levels are useful in diagnosing scurvy and are usually less than one-fourth of the normal value (52 ± 22 μg per 10^{10} platelets). Plasma levels of the vitamin correlate less well with the clinical state (Table 71-4). In infants x-ray changes of the bones may be diagnostic. Indirect bilirubin is frequently elevated. Capillary fragility is abnormal. The remainder of the laboratory tests are nondiagnostic.

Scurvy is potentially fatal; if the diagnosis is suspected, blood should be obtained, and ascorbic acid therapy should be instituted

FIGURE 76-2 *Hemorrhages and ecchymoses in a patient with scurvy. (Photograph, courtesy of Dr. Leonard L. Madison.)*

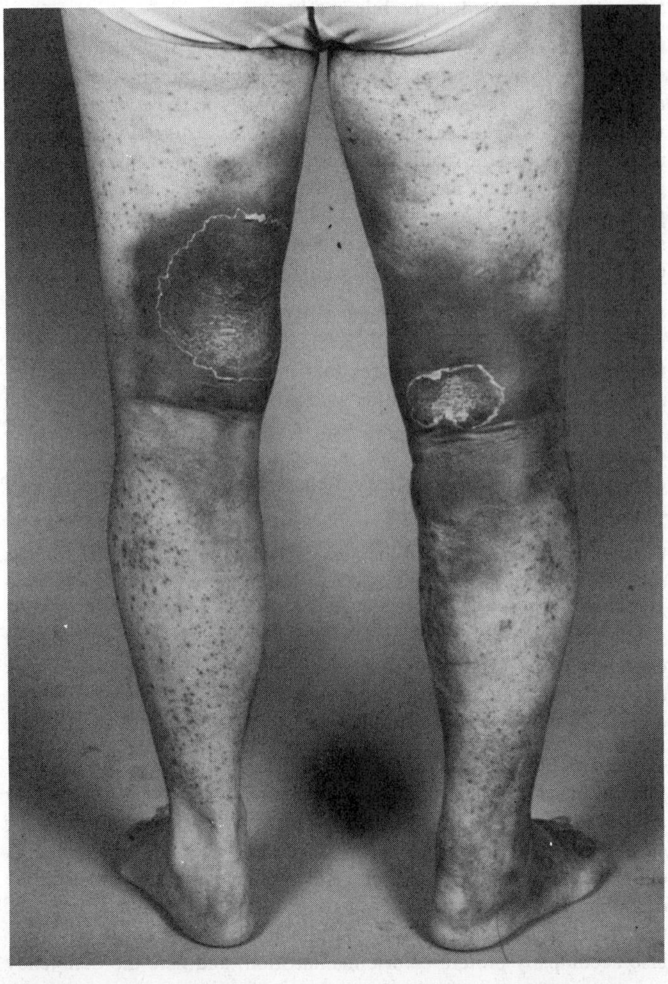

promptly. The usual dose in adults is 100 mg three to five times a day by mouth until 4 g has been administered, then 100 mg per day. In infants and children administration of 10 to 25 mg three times a day is adequate. A diet rich in vitamin C should be initiated simultaneously. Spontaneous bleeding usually ceases within 24 h, muscle and bone pains subside quickly, and the gums begin to heal within 2 to 3 days. Even large ecchymoses and hematomas resolve in 10 to 12 days, although pigmentary changes in areas of extensive hemorrhage may persist for months. Serum bilirubin becomes normal within 3 to 5 days, and the anemia is ordinarily corrected within 2 to 4 weeks.

VITAMIN A Biochemistry Vitamin A (retinol) can either be ingested or synthesized within the body from plant carotenoids (Fig. 76-1). Preformed vitamin A is present in animal tissues, and the best sources are liver, milk, and kidney, where it occurs largely in the form of fatty acid esters. The esters are hydrolyzed during digestion, absorbed in the free form, reesterified with fatty acids within the intestinal mucosa, and enter the circulation in association with lymph chylomicrons. The carotenoid substrates for synthesis of vitamin A, mainly β-carotenes, are widely distributed in plants. β-Carotene can either be absorbed intact or cleaved at the central double bond in the intestinal mucosa (or lumen) to form two molecules or retinaldehyde. Retinaldehyde is subsequently reduced by an aldehyde reductase to retinol. Retinol from whatever source is stored as retinyl esters in the parenchymal cells of the liver. The normal body retinol pool varies from 300 to 900 mg.

Prior to release from the liver retinyl esters are hydrolyzed, and the free alcohol is mobilized bound to a specific transport protein, retinol-binding protein (RBP), for transport to peripheral tissues. In vitamin A deficiency the release of RBP from the liver is inhibited, and the protein accumulates in liver; with repletion RBP is rapidly released from preformed stores. The pathway by which retinol is catabolized and excreted has not been defined; approximately equal amounts are excreted in the bile and urine.

Mechanism of action The best-defined function of vitamin A is its role in vision; in the retina vitamin A constitutes the prosthetic group of a series of carotenoid proteins that provide the molecular basis for visual excitation. In addition, vitamin A is required for growth, reproduction, and the maintenance of life. Retinol-phosphate-mannose glycolipid is present in a variety of cell membranes, and the vitamin plays a primary role in sugar transfer reactions involved in the synthesis of glycoproteins. The importance of glycoprotein to every cell implies that this is an equally important function of the vitamin.

Requirements The recommended daily allowances for vitamin A are listed in Tables 70-1 and 70-2. The assumed utilization efficiency for the conversion of β-carotene to vitamin A in the human is one-sixth (0.167). Other carotenoids with provitamin A activity have, on the average, one-half the activity of β-carotene. Pregnancy and disease states in which there is impaired absorption or storage, excessive utilization, or increased excretion of vitamin A may lead to increased requirements.

Experimental depletion When experimental subjects are fed a diet deficient in both retinol and carotene, plasma levels fall to less than 10 μg/dL, and the body pool shrinks to less than one-half the control value. Deficiency is manifested by follicular hyperkeratosis, impaired dark adaptation, and abnormalities of the electroretinogram. These changes are corrected after supplementation with 150 μg of retinol or 300 μg of β-carotene per day.

Clinical deficiency Endemic results from inadequate amounts of the vitamin and of the carotene provitamins in the diet and probably always occurs in conjunction with deficiency of other nutrients or complicating diseases. In some developing countries vitamin A deficiency is a major cause of blindness in the young as a consequence of failure to incorporate green leafy vegetables or other sources of the provitamin or vitamin into the diet. Vitamin A deficiency may also accompany protein-calorie malnutrition, and here the deficiency is due in part to a defective release mechanism from the liver secondary to inadequate retinol-binding protein. In developed nations vitamin A deficiency is usually due either to intestinal malabsorption (as in sprue or after intestinal bypass surgery), abnormal storage (liver disease), or enhanced destruction or excretion of the vitamin (proteinuria). Vitamin A deficiency has also occurred in patients receiving total parenteral nutrition because of loss of vitamin A after prolonged storage of intravenous fluid.

Night blindness is the earliest symptom of deficiency, followed by degenerative changes in the retina. The bulbar conjunctiva becomes dry (xerosis), and small gray plaques with foamy surfaces develop (Bitôt's spots). These early lesions are reversible with vitamin A. The more serious effects of vitamin A deficiency are ulceration and necrosis of the cornea (keratomalacia), leading to perforation, endophthalmitis, and blindness. Patients may also have dryness and hyperkeratosis of the skin.

Vitamin A levels in plasma are not reliable for the assessment of stores in individual cases. Measurements of dark adaptation, rod scotometry, and electroretinography are reliable indicators of vitamin A stores but require trained personnel and expensive equipment; consequently, the diagnosis is usually based upon a high index of suspicion in malnourished children or in patients with known predisposing factors for its development.

Night blindness and the milder conjunctival changes respond well to 30,000 IU of vitamin A daily for a week. Corneal damage constitutes a therapeutic emergency, and the usual treatment is 20,000 IU per kilogram of body weight per day for 5 days.

VITAMIN E Biochemistry Eight naturally occurring tocopherols possess vitamin E activity. The structure of alphatocopherol, the most widely distributed and most active of the tocopherols, is shown in Fig. 76-1. The vitamin is absorbed from the gastrointestinal tract by a mechanism similar to that for other fat-soluble vitamins and enters the bloodstream via the lymph, associated first with chylomicrons and then with plasma betalipoproteins. Indeed, plasma levels correlate closely with plasma lipid levels. The vitamin is stored in all tissues, and the tissue stores can protect against vitamin deficiency for long periods. Approximately three-fourths of the vitamin is excreted in bile, and the balance is excreted as glucuronides in urine. Metabolites with quinone structures (including one similar to ubiquinone) are present in tissues.

Mechanism of action The vitamin probably acts as an antioxidant rather than as a specific cofactor. In so acting it presumably inhibits oxidation of essential cellular constituents and prevents the formation of toxic oxidation products. Other antioxidants such as selenium, sulfur-containing amino acids, and the ubiquinone group can reverse the symptoms of vitamin E deficiency in animals.

Requirements The estimated daily requirement is 10 to 30 mg per day (Tables 70-1 and 70-2). Diets containing large amounts of polyunsaturated fatty acids increase and diets containing antioxidants decrease the requirement. The vitamin is widely distributed in food, so that a primary deficiency state has never been recognized in otherwise healthy children or adults. Newborn infants have plasma concentrations about one-fifth that of maternal levels, implying poor placental transfer, but human milk (in contrast to cow's milk) has sufficient levels to meet the requirements in infants.

Experimental depletion In long-term studies of vitamin E depletion vitamin E concentrations in plasma declined significantly only after months on a deficient diet. No manifestations of the depletion were detected in normal volunteers, making it difficult to establish that tocopherol is a human vitamin.

Clinical deficiency In the appropriate clinical setting vitamin E deficiency is associated with a discrete syndrome. Intestinal malabsorption can cause deficiency of all fat-soluble vitamins including vitamin E, and children with chronic cholestatic liver disease appear to be particularly susceptible, due to a combination of malabsorption of vitamin E and trapping of the vitamin in plasma by the associated hyperlipemia, so that tissue stores may be depleted despite a normal tocopherol level in serum. Indeed, the ratio of serum vitamin E to total serum lipid is the preferred index for assessing vitamin E status. The manifestations of deficiency include areflexia, gait disturbance, decreased proprioceptive and vibratory sensation, and paresis of gaze and are associated with degeneration of the posterior columns of the spinal cord, selective loss of large-caliber, myelinated axons in peripheral nerves, and appearance of spheroids in the gracile and cuneate nuclei of the brain. Treatment (50 to 100 IU per day by mouth) is most effective when initiated early in the course of the disease.

VITAMIN K Vitamin K consists of a quinone ring attached to a side chain (labeled *R* in Fig. 76-1) that varies depending on the source of the vitamin. Vitamin K_1 (phylloquinone) is present in most edible vegetables, particularly in green leaves, and vitamin K_2 is produced by intestinal bacteria. The many compounds with vitamin K activity are structurally related to the simpler compound, 2-methyl-1,4-naphthoquinone (menadione). Menadione is formed in the gut by the removal of the side chain from the vitamin by intestinal bacteria. After absorption, menadione is converted in the body to the active menaquinone. The vitamin is a component of a specialized microsomal enzyme system that effects the posttranslational γ carboxylation of glutamic acid in proteins of the plasma, bone, kidney, and urine, including the precursor proteins for the clotting factors VII, IX, X, and possibly V. Death from hemorrhage in deficiency states ensues before deficiency of the other carboxylated proteins becomes manifest.

Under ordinary circumstances about 80 percent of vitamin K is absorbed from the small bowel into the intestinal lymph. Because the naturally occurring forms of vitamin K are fat-soluble and are poorly stored in the body, deficiency can occur in association with diseases that interfere with fat absorption. In addition, long-term treatment with antimicrobial drugs may temporarily eliminate intestinal bacterial as a source for vitamin K. The warfarin anticoagulant drugs induce hypoprothrombinemia by inhibiting the γ carboxylation of the precursor protein.

Newborn infants tend to be deficient in vitamin K and have low plasma levels of several coagulation factors in the prothrombin complex. Such deficiencies result from minimal stores of vitamin K at birth, lack of an established intestinal flora, and a limited dietary intake of the vitamin.

Routine determination of prothrombin should be performed prior to surgical procedures or delivery. Subjects with levels below 70 percent of normal should receive therapy with vitamin K. Vitamin K deficiency can be separated from hypoprothrombinemia of liver disease by measurement of the noncarboxylated prothrombin precursor that accumulates in plasma in the vitamin deficiency.

VITAMIN EXCESS

Fat-soluble vitamins are stored to a variable extent in the body and hence are more likely to cause adverse effects when taken in excess; excess states for vitamins D (see Chap. 337) and A are particularly well characterized. Water-soluble vitamins are readily excreted in the urine and stored only to a limited extent. Consequently, toxicity states for these vitamins only occur when large amounts are taken for prolonged periods.

VITAMIN A AND CAROTENES Carotenemia Carotenemia results from excessive intake of vitamin A precursors in foods, principally carrots. Excess carotene is not injurious apart from the cosmetic effect; the fact that carotenemia does not cause hypervitaminosis A indicates that the conversion of carotene to vitamin A must be regulated. Carotenemia is manifested by yellowing of the skin with greatest intensity on the palms and soles and by a corresponding yellowness of serum. The yellowing of the skin can be distinguished from jaundice in that the scleras remain white. Hypothyroid patients are particularly susceptible. The omission of carrots from the diet leads to the rapid disappearance of the pigmentation. Discoloration of the skin can also result from the consumption of excessive amounts of other colored fruits and vegetables.

Vitamin A toxicity Hypervitaminosis A can result from accidental overingestion by hunters or explorers (polar bear liver), as the result of food faddism (usually caused by overly solicitous parents), or as a side effect of inappropriate therapy. Acute toxicity from a single massive dose consists of abdominal pain, nausea, vomiting, headache, dizziness, sluggishness, papilledema, and in infants a bulging fontanel followed within a few days by generalized desquamation of the skin and recovery. Chronic toxicity occurs following ingestion of 40,000 units or more daily for protracted periods and is characterized by bone and joint pain, hyperostoses, hair loss, dryness and fissures of the lips, anorexia, benign intracranial hypertension, low-grade fever, weight loss, and hepatosplenomegaly. The only diagnostic laboratory finding is elevation of the vitamin in serum, chiefly in the form of retinyl esters. The concentration of retinol-binding protein is normal, and the excess vitamin A circulates in association with lipoprotein. Relief is prompt on withdrawal of the vitamin from the diet.

VITAMIN E Relatively large doses of vitamin E have been taken by some for extended periods without causing apparent harm. In others, a variety of nonspecific complaints have been reported including malaise, gastrointestinal complaint, headaches, and possibly hypertension. However, true toxicity appears to occur in two situations—in subjects receiving oral anticoagulants and in premature infants. In large amounts, vitamin E can apparently antagonize vitamin K and inhibit prothrombin time; this phenomenon results in a marked potentiation of oral anticoagulants. Premature infants given parenteral vitamin E are reported to have developed ascites associated with hepatosplenomegaly, cholestatic jaundice, azotemia, and thrombocytopenia.

VITAMIN K Dietary supplements high in vitamin K can block the effects of oral anticoagulants and when given to pregnant women can cause jaundice in the newborn.

PYRIDOXINE Most adults can consume up to 10 times the recommended daily allowance of 2 mg pyridoxine per day without adverse effects. However, severe peripheral neuropathies have developed after ingestion of several grams per day for prolonged periods; symptoms include ataxia, perioral numbness, and clumsiness of the hands and feet, and the findings include loss of position and vibration sense without impairment of reflexes or sensory function. Recovery is slow after ingestion ceases. Lower doses (25 mg per day) can antagonize the effects of levodopa in Parkinson's disease and decrease the anticonvulsant effects of phenytoin.

VITAMIN C Vitamin C is widely used in megavitamin therapy because of the claim that large doses of the vitamin (a gram or greater per day) are effective in preventing or minimizing the symptoms of the common cold. However, in controlled studies, no significant differences in occurrence, severity, or duration have been demonstrated in subjects treated with a placebo compared with the vitamin. Use of the vitamin in this way is unwarranted and probably unwise. The long-term use of ascorbic acid in these doses can interfere with the absorption of vitamin B_{12}, cause uricosuria, and predispose to formation of oxalate kidney stones. In addition, large doses enhance the development of metabolizing enzymes in the fetus and may cause rebound scurvy in the offspring of mothers who have ingested large amounts of the vitamin during pregnancy. However, pharmacologic doses (200 mg daily) may correct leukocyte abnormalities in patients with the Chédiak-Higashi syndrome (see Chap. 56).

NIACIN Large doses of niacin have been used for treatment of hypercholesterolemia and occasionally for other purposes. The vitamin causes release of histamine, which in turn can cause severe flushing, pruritis, and gastrointestinal disturbances and may aggravate asthma. Acanthosis nigricans may occur. In doses of 3 g per day niacin has been reported to cause elevation of serum uric acid and of fasting glucose.

REFERENCES

Niacin deficiency

BOLLET AJ: The conquest of pellagra. Resid Staff Physician 28:31, May 1982

CASTIELLO RJ, LYNCH PJ: Pellagra and the carcinoid syndrome. Arch Dermatol 105:574, 1972

DARBY WJ et al: Niacin. Nutr Rev 33:289, 1977

DE LANGE DJ, JOUBERT CP: Assessment of nicotinic acid status of population groups. Am J Clin Nutr 15:169, 1964

GOLDSMITH GA: Experimental niacin deficiency. J Am Dietetic Assoc 32:312, 1956

GOPALAN C, RAO KSJ: Pellagra and amino acid imbalance, in *Vitamins and Hormones*, PL Munson et al (eds). New York, Academic, 1975, vol 33, p 505

JEPSON JB: Hartnup disease, in *The Metabolic Basis of Inherited Disease*, 4th ed, JB Stanbury et al (eds). New York, McGraw-Hill, 1978, p 1563

SCHOENTAL R: Mouldy grain and aetiology of pellagra: The role of toxic metabolites of *Fusarium*, Biochem Soc Trans 8:147, 1980

Thiamine deficiency

BLASS JP, GIBSON GE: Abnormality of a thiamine-requiring enzyme in patients with Wernicke-Korsakoff syndrome. N Engl J Med 297:1367, 1977

BROWN GM: Biogenesis and metabolism of thiamine, in *Metabolic Pathways*, 3d ed, DM Greenberg (ed). Academic, New York, 1970, p 369

HOYUMPA AM: Mechanisms of thiamine deficiency in chronic alcoholism. Am J Clin Nutr 33:2750, 1980

KAWAI C et al: Reappearance of beriberi heart disease in Japan. Am J Med 69:383, 1980

KOZAM RL et al: Cardiovascular beriberi. Am J Cardiology 30:418, 1972

KURIYAMA M et al: Blood vitamin B_1, transketolase, and thiamine pyrophosphate (TPP) effect in beriberi patients. Clin Chim Acta 108:159, 1980

PINCUS JH et al: Thiamine derivatives in subacute necrotizing encephalomyelopathy. Pediatrics 51:716, 1973

SCRIVER CR: Vitamin-responsive inborn errors of metabolism. Metabolism 22:1319, 1973

VICTOR M et al: *The Wernicke-Korsakoff Syndrome*, Philadelphia, Davis, 1971

ZIPORIN ZZ et al: Excretion of thiamine and its metabolites in the urine of young adult males receiving restricted intakes of the vitamin. J Nutr 85:287, 1965

Pyridoxine deficiency

FRIMPTER GW et al: Vitamin B_6-dependency syndromes: New horizons in nutrition. Am J Clin Nutr 22:794, 1969

GERSHOFF SN: Vitamin B_6, in *Nutrition Reviews' Present Knowledge in Nutrition*, 4th ed, DM Hegsted et al (eds). Washington, DC, The Nutrition Foundation, 1976, p 149

HARRIS JW, HORRIGAN DL: Pyridoxine-responsive anemia-prototype and variations on the theme, in *Vitamins and Hormones*, RS Harris et al (eds). New York, Academic, 1964, vol 22, p 721

JAFFE IA: The antivitamin B_6 effect of penicillamine: Clinical and immunological implications, in *Advances in Biochemical Psychopharmacology*, MS Ebodi et al (eds). New York, Raven, 1972, vol 4

LUHBY AL et al: Vitamin B_6 metabolism in users of oral contraceptive agents: I. Abnormal urinary xanthurenic acid excretion and its correction by pyridoxine. Am J Clin Nutr 24:684, 1971

MUDD SH: Pyridoxine-responsive genetic disease. Fed Proc 30:970, 1971

SAUBERLICH HE et al: Biochemical assessment of the nutritional status of vitamin B_6 in the human. Am J Clin Nutr 25:629, 1972

Riboflavin deficiency

MERRILL AH JR et al: Formation and mode of action of flavoproteins. Ann Rev Nutr 1:281, 1981

PINTO J et al: Inhibition of riboflavin metabolism in rat tissue by chlorpromazine, imipramine, and amitriptyline. J Clin Invest 67:1500, 1981

RIVLIN RS: Hormones, drugs, and riboflavin. Nutr Rev 37:241, 1979

Ascorbic acid deficiency

BAKER EM et al: Ascorbic acid metabolism in man. Am J Clin Nutr 19:371, 1966

BARNES MJ, KODICEK E: Biological hydroxylations and ascorbic acid, in *Vitamins and Hormones*, P Munson et al (eds). New York, Academic, 1972, vol 30, p 1

BARNESS LA: Nutritional aspects of vegetarianism, health foods and fad diets. Nutr Rev 59:153, 1977

BOXER LA et al: Correction of leucocyte function in Chédiak-Higashi syndrome by ascrobate. N Engl J Med 295:1041, 1976

HODGES RE et al: Clinical manifestations of ascorbic acid deficiency in man. Am J Clin Nutr 24:432, 1971

SATO P, UDENFRIEND S: Studies on ascorbic acid related to the genetic basis of scurvy, in *Vitamins and Hormones*, P Munson et al (eds). New York, Academic, 1978, vol 36, p 33

TOLBERT BM et al: New information on synthesis and metabolism of ascorbic acid. Nutr Rev 35:22, 1977

VILTER RW: Effects of ascorbic acid deficiency in man, in *The Vitamins*, WH Sebrell Jr et al (eds). New York, Academic, 1967, vol 1, p 457

WALLERSTEIN RO, WALLERSTEIN RO JR: Scurvy. Sem Hematol 13:211, 1976

Vitamin A deficiency

DELUCA LM: The direct involvement of vitamin A in glycosyl transfer reactions of mammalian membranes, in *Vitamins and Hormones*, PL Munson et al (eds). New York, Academic, 1977, vol 35, p 1

HOWARD L et al: Vitamin A deficiency from long term parenteral nutrition. Ann Intern Med 93:576, 1980

SAUBERLICH HE et al: Vitamin A metabolism and requirements in the human studied with the use of labeled retinol, in *Vitamins and Hormones*, RS Harris et al (eds). New York, Academic, 1974, vol 32

SMITH FR, GOODMAN DS: Vitamin A transport in human vitamin A toxicity. N Engl J Med 294:805, 1976

———, ———: Vitamin A metabolism and transport, in *Present Knowledge in Nutrition*, 4th ed, DM Hegsted et al (eds). Washington, DC, The Nutrition Foundation, 1976

SOMER A et al: Clinical characteristics of vitamin A responsive and nonresponsive Bitot's spots. Am J Ophthalmol 90:160, 1980

SRIKANTIA SG: Human vitamin A deficiency, in *World Review of Nutrition and Dietetics*, GH Bounre (ed). Basel, S Karger, 1975, vol 20, p 185

WALD G: Molecular basis of visual excitation. Science 162:230, 1968

Vitamin E deficiency

GUGGENHEIM MA et al: Progressive neuromuscular disease in children with chronic cholestasis and vitamin E deficiency: Diagnosis and treatment with alpha tocopherol. J Pediatr 100:51, 1982

HORWITT MK: Interrelations between vitamin E and polyunsaturated fatty acids in adult men, in *Vitamins and Hormones*, GF Marrian and KV Thimann (eds). New York, Academic, 1962, vol 20, p 541

ROSENBLUM JL et al: A progressive neurologic syndrome in children with chronic liver disease. N Engl J Med 304:503, 1981

SOKOL RJ et al: Vitamin E deficiency with normal serum vitamin E concentrations in children with chronic cholestasis. N Engl J Med 310:1209, 1984

——— et al Mechanism causing vitamin E deficiency during chronic childhood cholestasis. Gastroenterology 85:1172, 1983

Vitamin K deficiency

BERTINA RM et al: New method for the rapid detection of vitamin K deficiency. Clin Chim Acta 105:93, 1980

DOISY EA JR, MATSCHINER JT: Biochemistry of vitamin K, in *Fat-Soluble Vitamins*, RA Morton (ed). Elmsford, NY, Pergamon, 1970, vol 9, p 293

OLSON RE, SUTTIE JW: Vitamin K and α-carboxyglutamate biosynthesis, in *Vitamins and Hormones*, PL Munson et al (eds). New York, Academic, 1977, vol 35, p 59

SHEARER MJ et al: Studies on the absorption and metabolism of phylloquinone (vitamin K) in man, in *Vitamins and Hormones*, RS Harris et al (eds). New York, Academic, 1974, vol 32, p 513

SUTTIE JW: *Vitamin K Metabolism and Vitamin K-Dependent Proteins*. Baltimore, University Park Press, 1980

Vitamin excess

ALHADEFF L: Toxic effects of water-soluble vitamins. Nutr Rev 42:33, 1984

CHALMERS TC: Effects of ascorbic acid on the common cold. Am J Med 58:532, 1975

CORRIGAN JJ JR: The effect of vitamin E on warfarin-induced vitamin K deficiency. Ann NY Acad Sci 82:361, 1982

HERBERT V: The vitamin craze: Arch Intern Med 140:173, 1980

LORCH V et al: Unusual syndrome with fatalities among premature infants: Association with a new intravenous vitamin E product. Morb Mort Week Rep 33:198, 1984

LOMBAERT A, CARTON H: Benign intracranial hypertension due to A-hypervitaminosis in adults and adolescents. Eur Neurol 14:340, 1976

ROBERTS HJ: Perspective on vitamin E therapy. JAMA 246:129, 1981

SCHAUMBURG H et al: Sensory neuropathy from pyridoxine abuse: A new megavitamin syndrome. N Engl J Med 309:445, 1983

STEIN HB et al: Ascorbic acid–induced uricosuria: A consequence of megavitamin therapy. Ann Intern Med 84:385, 1976

77 DISTURBANCES IN TRACE ELEMENT METABOLISM

KENNETH H. FALCHUK

CLASSIFICATION AND FUNCTIONS The "trace elements" comprise metals in biologic fluids at concentrations below one microgram per gram of wet weight. Most are essential nutrients for human beings (Table 77-1). Others (As, Ni, Sn, V, Si) are essential for some plants and/or vertebrates including mammals and may be required by humans. The functions of trace elements and of other, more abundant metals (Na, K, Ca, Mg) are determined, in part, by their charges, mobilities, and binding constants to biologic ligands. Elements in one group (Na, K) bind weakly to negatively charged ligands and can cross cellular membranes without major impediment. They are used by living systems as charge carriers to conduct electric impulses along nerves, etc. Those in a second group (Mg, Ca) form moderately stable but not tight complexes with enzymes, nucleic

TABLE 77-1 Requirements and functions of trace elements in humans

Element	Requirements, mg/day*	Amount† Total, g per 70 kg body weight	Blood μg/dL	Serum μg/dL	Selected biochemical functions	Enzymes Class	Example
Fe	10–20	4.0	45000	100	Oxygen transport	Oxidoreductases	Cytochrome oxidase
Zn	15–20	3.0	800	100	Nucleic acid and protein synthesis and degradation, alcohol metabolism	Transferases, hydrolases, lyases, isomerases, ligases, oxidoreductases	Carboxypeptidases, alcohol dehydrogenases, alkaline phosphatases
Cu	2–6	0.25	100	100	Hemoglobin synthesis, connective tissue metabolism, bone development	Oxidoreductases	Superoxide dismutase, ferroxidase (ceruloplasmin)
Co	0.0001	1.1	0.02	0.0007	Methionine metabolism	Transferases	Homocysteine methyltransferase
Mn	2–5	0.02	0.09	0.06	Oxidative phosphorylation; fatty acid, mucopolysaccharide, and cholesterol metabolism	Oxidoreductases, hydrolases, ligases	Diamine oxidase, pyruvate carboxylase
Mo	0.15–0.5	0.07	1.5	0.07	Xanthine metabolism	Oxidoreductases	Xanthine oxidase
Se	0.05–0.2	(−)	20	13	Antioxidant	Oxidoreductases, transferases	Glutathione peroxidase
Ni	(−)	(−)	2.5	0.1	?Stabilizing RNA structure	Oxidoreductases, hydrolases	Urease
Cr	0.005–0.2	0.0006	(−)	0.02	?Binding of insulin to cells, glucose metabolism		

* *Requirements may differ for different age groups and physiologic states, e.g., pregnancy.*
† *Reported normal values vary owing to differences in sample preparation, analytical instruments, and small quantities present in biologic materials.*
(−), reported values variable or not available.

acids, and other ligands. They act as biochemical "triggers," altering and/or controlling the functions of these molecules, e.g., Ca affects muscle contraction and relaxation (Chap. 357). Those in a third group (Fe, Zn, Cu, and others) form strong, static complexes with and become integral functional components of enzymes (Table 77-1).

METAL DEFICIENCY OR TOXICITY All metals can cause disease through deficiency, imbalance, or toxicity. Deficiency usually results when dietary intake is inadequate or when intake is adequate but other conditioning factors come into play. Deficiencies can be caused by metal malabsorption in chronic diarrheal diseases, surgical resection of the small intestine, or formation of metal complexes with dietary components that are not readily absorbed, e.g., between phytates and Zn. Deficiency states can also result from increased losses through urine, pancreatic juice, or other exocrine secretions or from metabolic imbalances produced by antagonistic or synergistic interactions between metals. Large amounts of Ca, for example, decrease the absorption of and induce deficiency of Zn. Similarly, Mo and Cu compete with each other; excessive Mo in cattle leads to Cu deficiency characterized by diarrhea and wasting. Proven manifestations of trace element deficiencies in humans, except for iron, were previously rare but have been recognized more frequently with the use of total parenteral nutrition (TPN) (Chap. 75). Clinical criteria for the recognition of deficiency states include decreases in metal content of whole blood, serum, hair and/or other accessible fluids and tissues, changes in the activities of metalloenzymes, and characteristic signs and symptoms (Table 77-2).

Toxic effects are dependent on the chemical form, the amount ingested, the route of entry into the body, the biologic ligands associated with the metal, the tissue distribution, the concentration achieved, and the excretion rate. Mechanisms of toxicity include inhibition of enzyme activity by binding to essential amino acid residues, alterations in nucleic acid function and structure, alteration in protein synthesis, effects on membrane permeability, and inhibition of phosphorylation, among others. Metal toxicity in patients undergoing chronic renal dialysis is important because of the frequency and severity of the resulting problems and because of the number of metals involved, e.g., Al, Zn, Cu, Ni, and Sn (Chap. 221). For example, even when it is present only in trace amounts in dialysis fluids, Al is readily absorbed into blood and accumulates in brain, bone, and erythroid tissues, causing disabling neurologic, skeletal, and hematologic disorders. These include malaise, memory loss, asterixis, dementia, twitches, and other manifestations of metabolic encephalopathy including seizures and death. Osteomalacia unresponsive to vitamin D, fractures, muscular pain, weakness, and anemia may occur. Documentation of increase in plasma Al concentration following deferoxamine administration is diagnostic.

DISORDERS OF METABOLISM OF SPECIFIC METALS **Zinc** Zn absorption in the small intestine is decreased by fibers, phytate, phosphate, Ca, and Cu. In contrast, amino acids, peptides, iodoquinol and other chelating agents increase Zn absorption. Excretion of Zn occurs principally through secretions of the pancreas and intestine. Nearly 99 percent of total-body Zn is inside cells, the remainder is in plasma and extracellular fluids. Serum Zn, approximately 70 percent of which is loosely bound to albumin and other proteins, is the source of metal for cellular needs. Serum Zn content does not normally vary, but it decreases when intake or absorption is reduced (e.g., in regional enteritis) or when urinary losses are increased (e.g., in nephrotic syndrome; in cirrhosis of the liver or other hypoalbuminemic states; during the administration of penicillamine or other chelating agents; in high catabolic states as after trauma, burns, or surgery; and in hemolytic anemias and sickle cell disease). Plasma Zn also decreases in the acute phase of myocardial infarction, infections, malignancies, and hepatitis and other diseases. The decreases may be due to redistribution from plasma to tissues and are probably mediated by ACTH, cortisol, and/or a leukocyte protein (leukocyte endogenous mediator). Clinical deficiency may follow these decreases in serum content. The Zn requirement of the developing fetus, pregnant woman, and growing child or adolescent is higher than that of adult men or nonpregnant women. Therefore, the former groups are more susceptible to Zn depletion. Zn deficiency in pregnant animals can lead to fetal Zn deficiency, which results in high mortality rates or congenital malformations of nearly all organ systems. Zinc deficiency has not been described in pregnant women, but has been reported in adolescents who eat dirt, in patients who receive TPN without supplemental Zn (see Chap. 75), and in patients with the autosomal recessive defect acrodermatitis enteropathica. In the latter disease, deficiency in plasma Zn may be the consequence of a defect in Zn absorption. The onset of symptoms often occurs when an affected infant is weaned from human to cow's milk. Zn may also play a role in the maintenance of normal taste and in wound healing.

Tissues with a high cellular turnover, including skin, gastrointestinal mucosa, chondrocytes, spermatogonia, and thymocytes are characteristically affected (Table 77-2). The dermatologic abnormalities (hyperkeratosis, parakeratosis, acrodermatitis, and alopecia) call attention to the possibility of Zn deficiency. The usual distribution of the keratotic lesions is in areas that are readily traumatized (elbows, knees), but the lesions can develop in other areas as well. The keratotic lesions can become pustular or crusting, red, scaly plaques. Superinfections are common with either fungi or bacteria.

Toxicity follows inhalation of Zn fumes (by welders), oral ingestion, or intravenous administration. Inhalation of high concentrations of zinc oxide fumes leads to an acute illness called *metal-fume fever* or *brass chills,* manifested by fever, chills, excessive salivation, headaches, cough, and leukocytosis. Dialysis fluids can be contaminated with Zn from the adhesive plaster used on the dialysis coils or from galvanized pipes. The toxic syndrome associated with hemodialysis is characterized by anemia, fever, and central nervous system disturbances (Table 77-2). Toxic amounts of Zn decrease chemotaxis, phagocytosis, pinocytosis, and platelet aggregation.

TABLE 77-2 Disorders of metal metabolism in humans

Element	Deficiency	Toxicity*
Fe	Anemia	Hepatic failure, diabetes, testicular atrophy, arthritis, cardiomyopathy, peripheral neuropathy, hyperpigmentation
Zn	Growth retardation, alopecia, dermatitis, diarrhea, immunologic dysfunction, failure to thrive, psychological disturbances, gonadal atrophy, impaired spermatogenesis, congenital malformations.	Gastric ulcer, pancreatitis lethargy, anemia, fever, nausea, vomiting. respiratory distress, pulmonary fibrosis
Cu	Anemia, growth retardation, defective keratinization and pigmentation of hair, hypothermia, degenerative changes in aortic elastin, mental deterioration, scurvy-like changes in skeleton	Hepatitis, cirrhosis, tremor, mental deterioration, Kayser-Fleischer rings, hemolytic anemia, renal dysfunction (Fanconi-like syndrome)
Mn	Bleeding disorder (increased prothrombin time)	Encephalitis-like syndrome, Parkinson-like syndrome, psychosis, pneumoconiosis
Co	Anemia (B_{12} deficiency)	Cardiomyopathy, goiter
Mo	? Esophageal cancer	? Hyperuricemia
Cr	? Impairment of glucose tolerance	Renal failure, dermatitis (occupational), pulmonary cancer
Se	Cardiomyopathy, congestive heart failure, striated muscle degeneration	Alopecia, abnormal nails, emotional lability, lassitude, garlic odor to breath
Ni	?	Dermatitis (occupational), lung and nasal carcinomas, liver necrosis, pulmonary inflammation
Si	? Impaired early bone development	Pulmonary inflammation, granuloma, fibrosis
F	? Impaired bone and dental structure	Motted dental enamel, nausea, abdominal pain, vomiting, diarrhea, tetany, cardiovascular collapse

* *Symptoms are dependent on route of entry and tissue distribution (see text).*

Copper The liver, kidney, heart, and brain contain the highest amounts of Cu. Over 90 percent of plasma Cu is associated with ceruloplasmin, while 60 percent of that in red blood cells is bound to superoxide dismutase. The major excretory pathway is through the bile. The serum Cu concentration is normally constant. Increases occur in patients with acute myocardial infarction, leukemia, solid tumors, infections, portal and biliary cirrhosis, hemochromatosis, thyrotoxicosis, and connective tissue disorders. The consequences of the increases are unknown. Conversely, decreases occur in the nephrotic syndrome, kwashiorkor, the hepatolenticular degeneration of Wilson's disease (see Chap. 311), severe diarrheal diseases with malabsorption, and other conditions associated with increased excretion or decreased synthesis of ceruloplasmin. Premature infants who are fed diets deficient in Cu develop decreased serum ceruloplasmin and Cu levels, anemia, osteopenia, skin and hair depigmentation, and psychomotor retardation. Cu deficiency in subjects receiving TPN causes anemia and neutropenia.

A more complex disorder of Cu metabolism occurs in Menkes' disease, an X-linked recessive disorder. Intestinal Cu uptake is normal, and tissue Cu content varies; that of intestinal, kidney, and skin (fibroblast) cells is normal or high, while that of serum, liver, brain, and (likely) vascular cells is low. Ceruloplasmin content and the activities of some Cu enzymes (e.g., connective tissue amine oxidases) also are decreased. The clinical picture is similar to that of nutritional Cu deficiency in animals except that anemia does not occur (Table 77-2). The patients have kinky hair, and decreased amounts of mature collagen and elastin cause dissecting aneurysms, sudden cardiac rupture, emphysema, and osteoporosis. Death usually occurs in the first 5 years of life.

Excessive oral intake of Cu or hemodialysis with water contaminated with Cu is toxic. The acute symptoms include hemolytic anemia, nausea, vomiting, and diarrhea. The renal and hepatic failure and the central nervous system disorders that eventually develop (Table 77-2) are typical of the Cu toxicity syndrome in hepatolenticular degeneration (Wilson's disease). (See Chap. 311.)

Cobalt Co is a component of vitamin B_{12}, and deficiency syndromes are those associated with deficiency of the vitamin (see Chap. 286). Pharmacologic doses of Co induce erythropoiesis. Chronic administration blocks iodine uptake by the thyroid, resulting in development of goiter.

Cardiomyopathy, congestive heart failure with pericardial effusions, polycythemia, thyroid enlargement, and neurologic abnormalities have been reported as manifestations to Co toxicity in drinkers of beer to which the metal had been added as a foam stabilizer. Co accumulates in the heart, forms a complex with lipoic acid, and interferes with decarboxylation reactions critical to both pyruvate and fatty acid metabolism.

Manganese Mn acts both as an activator of enzymes and as a component of metalloenzymes (Table 77-1). Defects of the skeletal, central nervous, and gonadal systems occur in Mn deficiency in animals. Humans obtain sufficient Mn throughout normal dietary intake so that a deficiency syndrome is rare. In one reported instance an increase in prothrombin time, unresponsive to Vitamin K, was noted. In serum, Mn is bound to transmanganin. Mn is excreted primarily in bile and pancreatic secretions.

Serum Mn increases following myocardial infarction and decreases for unknown reasons in children with convulsive disorders. Miners who inhale large quantities of Mn dust over long periods of time develop asthenia, anorexia, apathy, headache, impotence, leg cramps, speech disturbances, and occasionally even more severe toxic symptoms (Table 77-2).

Selenium Se is a component of glutathione peroxidase and plays a critical role in the control of oxygen metabolism, particularly in catalyzing the breakdown of H_2O_2. The metal is required for the growth of human fibroblasts and other cells in tissue culture. Furthermore, Se cures or prevents Keshan disease, a syndrome that is endemic to Keshan Province in China where the soil may be deficient in the metal. Keshan disease is characterized by multifocal myocardial necrosis and reduced blood and serum Se content. The clinical severity varies from severe arrhythmias and cardiogenic shock to a mild form with cardiac enlargement as the only significant finding. Peripheral myopathies may develop as a consequence of muscle degeneration (Table 77-2). Children and women of child-bearing age are particularly susceptible. Se protects animals from a number of carcinogenic chemicals and viral agents; a role in human cancer prevention is not established. Se binds Cd, Hg, and other metals and mitigates their toxic effects, even though the measurable levels of the metals remain elevated.

Se toxicity occurs in animals, but humans who have consumed vegetables grown in soil containing high selenium content have not become ill. Se poisoning has been reported due to ingestion of water containing large amounts of the metal.

Other trace elements *Silicon* is present in bone and skin and may play a role in the cross-linkage of collagen. Deficiency in animals results in decreased growth, abnormal early bone development, and decreased hexosamine content of epiphyses and epiphyseal plates. No instance of deficiency in humans has been described. Inhalation of fine particles of SiO_2 causes granuloma formation and chronic fibrosis (silicosis) of the lungs (see Chap. 204).

Fluoride is a constituent of teeth and bone. It prevents dental caries, and its use in patients with osteoporosis has resulted in increased mineralized bone (see Chap. 339). Complications of long-term ingestion by such patients include calcification of bony ligaments and tendons. Chronic intake of fluorides also causes fluorosis, a syndrome characterized by weakness, weight loss, anemia, brittle bones, and mottling of teeth (if taken during stages of enamel formation). Acute ingestion of toxic amounts, as found in some insect poisons, causes severe abdominal pain, nausea, vomiting, diarrhea, and hypocalcemia. Eventually, tetany and cardiorespiratory arrest occur.

A deficiency of any one of *arsenic, nickel, tin,* and *vanadium* causes pathologic manifestations in plants and some vertebrates. Their roles in human health are undefined.

REFERENCES

FALCHUK KH: Effect of acute disease and ACTH on serum zinc proteins. N Engl J Med 296:1129, 1977

KARCIOULU ZA, SARPER RM: *Zinc and Copper in Medicine,* Springfield, Ill., Charles C Thomas, 1980

Metabolic and physiological consequences of trace element deficiency in animals and man. Philos Trans R Soc Lond [Biol] 294:1, 1981

MILLINER DS et al: Use of the deferoxamine infusion test in the diagnosis of aluminum-related osteodystrophy. Ann Intern Med 101:775, 1984

PRASAD AS: *Trace Elements in Human Health and Disease.* New York, Academic, 1976, vol II

REINHOLD JG: Trace elements—A selective survey. Clin Chem 21:476, 1975

TING-KAI L, VALLEE BL: The biochemical and nutritional roles of other trace elements, in *Modern Nutrition in Health and Disease,* 6th ed, RS Goodhart and ME Shils (eds). Philadelphia, Lea and Febiger, 1980

UNDERWOOD EJ: *Trace Elements in Human and Animal Nutrition,* 3d ed. New York, Academic, 1971

WILLIAMS RJP: The Tilden lecture. Q Rev Chem Soc (Lond) 24:331, 1970

section 5 Neoplastic diseases

78 PRINCIPLES OF NEOPLASIA

JOHN MENDELSOHN

INTRODUCTION The last few years have witnessed remarkable progress in understanding the biologic and biochemical bases for cancer. This is not to imply that the problem of neoplastic disease is solved. Gains in the treatment of cancer in adults have been gradual and have focused upon those malignancies characterized by unusual sensitivity to radiation and chemotherapy. These include primarily acute myelocytic leukemia, the lymphoproliferative malignancies, testicular cancer, and breast cancer. New treatment modalities involving immunotherapy and agents that promote normal cell maturation remain experimental and are under intensive investigation. Meanwhile, the search has begun for compounds which can interact with oncogene products, gene regulators, and growth factors and their receptors. Research employing modern technology in molecular genetics and immunology promises to provide a new array of anticancer agents which could move rapidly into clinical trials. This is possible because understanding cancer as a pathologic process is buttressed by new knowledge of cancer as an acquired genetic derangement.

This chapter provides an overview of the biology, etiology, and clinical sequelae of the neoplastic process, followed by a description of the general methods for diagnosing cancer and determining its stage, or extent of spread. Cancer treatment is presented in the following chapter, and the details of managing patients with specific types of malignant disease will be found in the chapters devoted to disorders of various specific organs.

Definition The terms cancer, neoplasia, and malignancy are usually used interchangeably in both the technical and popular literature. The disease called cancer is best defined by four characteristics which describe how cancer cells act differently from their normal counterparts.

1 *Clonality:* In most cases, cancer originates from a single stem cell which proliferates to form a clone of malignant cells.
2 *Autonomy:* Growth is not properly regulated by the normal biochemical and physical influences in the environment.
3 *Anaplasia:* There is a lack of normal, coordinated cell differentiation.
4 *Metastasis:* Cancer cells develop the capacity for discontinuous growth and dissemination to other parts of the body.

Properties similar to each of these characteristics *can* be expressed by normal, nonmalignant cells at certain appropriate times—for example, during embryogenesis and wound repair—but in cancer cells the characteristic is inappropriate or excessive. The process by which a normal cell is converted into one which exhibits these characteristic traits is termed *malignant transformation.*

THE CLINICAL PROBLEM One-third of all individuals in the United States will develop cancer. The 5-year relative survival rate for these

TABLE 78-1 Estimated new cases and deaths for major sites of cancer—1984

Site or type	Number of cases	Deaths
Lung	139,000	121,000
Colon-rectum	130,000	59,000
Breast	116,000	38,000
Prostate	76,000	25,000
Uterus	55,000*	10,000
Urinary tract	57,000	19,000
Mouth	27,000	9,000
Pancreas	25,000	23,000
Leukemia	24,000	17,000
Ovary	18,000	12,000
Melanoma	18,000†	7,000

* *Includes cervix. If carcinoma in situ is included, cases total over 99,000.*
† *Estimated new cases of skin cancer (nonmelanoma) = about 400,000.*
NOTE: *Estimates are based on rates from the N.C.I. SEER program 1973–1979.*

patients (the probability of escaping death from cancer for 5 years following diagnosis) has risen to nearly 50 percent as a result of progress in the early diagnosis and the therapy of this disease. However, cancer remains second only to cardiac disease as a cause of death in this country. Twenty percent of Americans die from cancer; this amounted to 450,000 deaths in 1984. Half of the deaths were due to the three most common types of cancer: lung, breast, and colon-rectum. Lung cancer is more prevalent in males, while breast cancer is the commonest form of malignancy in females. Cancer of the colon and rectum is equally common in males and females.

Information is provided yearly by the American Cancer Society, summarizing the incidence and mortality rates for the common types of cancer. Table 78-1 and Fig. 78-1 present just a small portion of the extensive data available. Of particular importance is the clear documentation in Fig. 78-1 that deaths from lung cancer are increasing in the face of stable or falling rates for a number of other types of malignant disease.

Cancer typically presents to the physician as an abnormal growth, or tumor, which causes illness by production of biochemically active molecules, by local expansion, or by invasion into adjacent or distant tissue sites. The symptoms of the illness depend upon the specific molecular products and the location(s) of the tumor. Each type of cancer has a relatively distinctive natural history that describes the likely clinical course of the particular neoplastic process. Designing a proper treatment plan for an individual patient with malignant disease depends upon determining the extent of disease spread, together with a knowledge of the natural history and the available therapeutic alternatives for the particular type of cancer.

TUMOR CELL BIOLOGY AND BIOCHEMISTRY Since all cells in an organism originate from a single fertilized egg (zygote), all carry the identical genetic information. The proliferation and differentiation of this cell into an embryo, and eventually into a mature organism, involve selective and coordinated expression of the genomic repertoire. Control of gene expression is accomplished through incompletely understood molecular interactions which can be modulated, in part, by chemical influences in the environment. The genomic repertoire includes information which permits cells to expand clonally, to function with varying degrees of autonomy, to differentiate and dedifferentiate, and to move from one part of the organism to another in a coordinated way. In the adult, the process of wound healing activates expression of these cellular characteristics in a more "embryo-like" fashion, but under well-coordinated control. In the case of malignancy, the normal control process is subverted or bypassed due to the anomalous activities of a select group of genes (oncogenes) which have central importance to the regulation of cellular activities. A detailed discussion of oncogenes is provided in Chap. 59.

Clonality Careful cytogenetic analysis of metaphase chromosome preparations from cancer cells has yielded a wealth of information about the neoplastic process. It has become clear that virtually all solid tumors and a majority of hematopoietic malignancies display abnormalities in the karyotype which are inherited by the population of tumor cells. These may involve translocations of chromosomal fragments into new locations, as well as additions or deletions of parts of chromosomes or whole chromosomes. A particular karyotypic alteration often occurs in a substantial fraction of all patients with a form of cancer. The first and most well known example of this is the Philadelphia chromosome (Ph^1) observed in 85 percent of patients with chronic myelogenous leukemia (CML), in which the long arm of chromosome 22 is translocated onto the long arm of chromosome 9. This alteration is so characteristic of CML that when analysis of some cases of acute lymphocytic leukemia demonstrated the identical translocation, it was inferred that the disease represented an unusual conversion from CML (which usually progresses to acute myelocytic leukemia). Characteristic chromosomal rearrangements have been described in a number of other human cancers.

The observation of uniform karyotypic abnormalities in all cells within a tumor provides strong evidence for the clonal origin of the

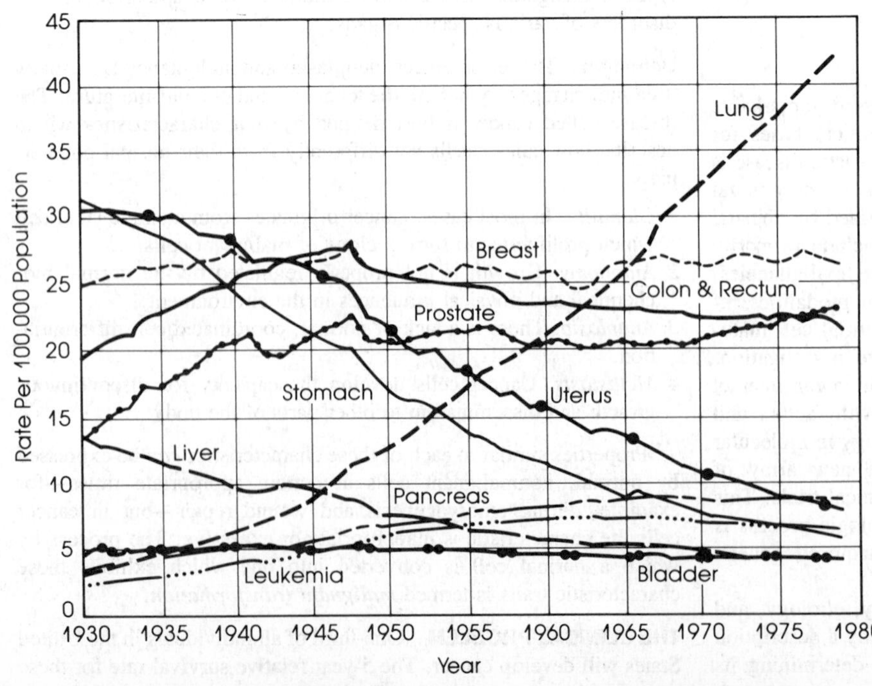

FIGURE 78-1 *Cancer death rates by site in the United States, 1930 to 1979. (Prepared by the American Cancer Society from data provided by the National Center for Health Statistics and the Bureau of the Census.)*

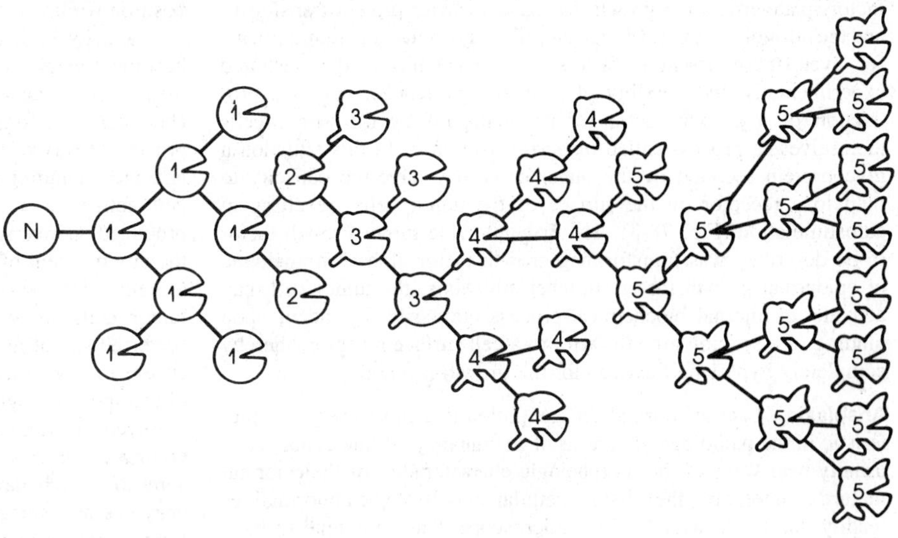

FIGURE 78-2 *A schematic model of clonal progression. The N cell is normal. Five* hypothetical *genetic changes are noted. The first does not result in malignancy but the second does. The third adds invasiveness, the fourth confers the capacity to disseminate and produce metastases, and the fifth provides resistance to chemotherapy. Each may be accompanied by incremental alterations in the karyotype, with an increasing tendency to aneuploidy during further clonal evolution.*

tumor. In turn, the chromosomal abnormalities serve as markers of the presence of a common malignant state in the individual cells.

A remarkable concordance between the chromosome locations of a number of human cellular oncogenes and the break points involved in chromosome translocations in human malignancies has been demonstrated. Furthermore, in many cases, these locations correlate with "fragile" sites in the chromosome. Treatment of cultured cells with agents that inhibit the DNA repair process induces chromosomal breaks far more frequently at many of these loci. A reasonable hypothesis, currently under investigation, links these phenomena and suggests that chromosomal rearrangements may result in activation of cellular oncogenes. For example, in Burkitt's lymphoma, the typical translocation between chromosomes 8 and 14 places the cellular *myc* gene adjacent to the immunoglobulin heavy chain locus, a site of gene activation in the normal lymphocyte.

Studies of the selective expression of the X-linked isoenzymes of glucose 6-phosphate dehydrogenase in heterozygotic patients have provided further evidence for the clonal origin of most cancers from single progenitor cells. Examination of both glucose 6-phosphate dehydrogenase isoenzymes and karyotypes in CML patients has demonstrated clonal abnormalities in erythroid, myeloid, and megakaryocytic cells, as well as B lymphocytes, suggesting that this malignancy originates in a precursor cell common to all of these cell lineages.

While there is convincing evidence for the origin of cancer from genetic alterations in a single cell, further heritable alterations commonly occur, resulting in the presence of a heterogeneous mixture of subclones in a mature tumor cell population which has proliferated enough to be clinically detectable. This heterogeneity can be demonstrated by assaying a variety of characteristics in the subpopulations within a tumor; for example, further abnormalities in the karyotype, varied drug sensitivites and metastatic capacities, differences in growth rates, and the presence or absence of hormone receptors or particular cell surface glycoproteins. With time, therefore, the progressive accumulation of heritable abnormalities in tumor subpopulations typically results in highly significant phenotypic changes which have their clinical counterpart in development of resistance to previously effective therapy or in increased metastatic spread. The appearance of new chromosomal abnormalities in patients with PH^1-positive CML heralds the onset of a rapidly progressive, fatal phase of the disease. A schematic model of this process of clonal progression is shown in Fig. 78-2. It remains to be determined when in the life history of a typical malignancy the process of clonal progression occurs: the sequence of genetic alterations may occur early, with later expansion of selected subpopulations from a heterogeneous mixture of cells as circumstances change; alternatively the genetic alterations may occur close to the time when they are detected by changes in the behavior of the tumor cells.

Following the discovery of cellular oncogenes, evidence rapidly accumulated to show that successive activation of two or more of these genes may be the molecular genetic explanation for clonal progression in tumor cell subpopulations. Activation of cellular oncogenes may be due to a variety of genetic mechanisms in addition to translocation. These mechanisms include gene amplification, or insertion of promoters of transcription adjacent to (*cis*) or in a *trans* relationship to a cellular oncogene, with or without accompanying mutations of specific nucleotides in the oncogene DNA sequence. Many of these changes are undetectable in the karyotype, but can be identified by restriction digest analysis of cellular DNA or by DNA sequencing.

Autonomy Environmental influences which regulate the proliferation of normal cells are circumvented when the process of malignant transformation occurs. This is demonstrable by a variety of experimental assays which document, in different ways, the capacity of the malignant cells to continue to proliferate under normally nonconducive conditions. These assays are listed in Table 78-2.

At least initially, the autonomy of human malignancies is relative rather than absolute. The well-known experiments of Huggins and associates in the 1950s led to a new form of cancer therapy which took advantage of the initial dependence of certain tumors upon the normal influences of sex hormones. The conversion of many prostatic and breast cancers from sensitivity to resistance to hormone therapy vividly demonstrates the further development of autonomy through clonal progression.

Many tumor cell lines can proliferate in culture medium without the usual requirement for serum, provided that a "cocktail" containing three to five essential growth factors and other growth-promoting agents is added. Examples of such factors are epidermal growth

TABLE 78-2 Experimental detection of malignant transformation

Assay	Normal cell	Transformed cell
Capacity of single cells to form colonies in agar suspension	Unsuccessful	Successful
Density-dependent inhibition of cell proliferation in liquid culture	Yes	No
Generations obtained by continuous division in liquid culture	Limited to about 50	Unlimited
Requirements for serum or growth factors	Invariable	Reduced or absent
Capacity to grow as xenografts	Absent	Present

factor, platelet-derived growth factor, the carrier protein transferrin, and the hormone insulin. Malignant cells may obviate the requirements for even these essential factors. One mechanism, demonstrated experimentally and possibly of clinical significance, involves production of a growth factor (or its analogue) by the tumor cells themselves, a process called *autocrine secretion*. In this situation a glycoprotein secreted by the tumor cells may have the capacity to bind to a receptor on the surface of the tumor cells, resulting in autostimulation (Fig. 78-3). The first autocrine tumor growth factor to be described was transforming growth factor alpha, an analogue of epidermal growth factor. In other situations, the tumor cell may activate an internal biochemical process ordinarily dependent upon binding of a specific growth factor to a cell surface receptor, thereby completely bypassing the need for the growth-promoting agent.

Anaplasia Lack of normal differentiation is a most useful characteristic in the pathologic diagnosis of malignancy. While cancer cells usually bear some of the morphologic characteristics of their normal mature counterparts, they display cellular and histologic abnormalities readily detectable with the light microscope. The cells tend to have large nuclei, with more apparent chromatin and prominent nucleoli. There are increased mitoses, as well as abnormal mitoses and giant cells containing multiple nuclei, reflecting aneuploidy and/or a failure of karyokinesis. The degree of morphologic derangement typically correlates with the extent of disease spread or the metastatic potential of the tumor. The histologic appearance of malignancy is one of disarray, with partial or complete loss of normal tissue architecture. Partial formation of structures such as glands or villi may be suggested, even in poorly differentiated malignancies.

Although the term is not used this way, the process of anaplasia may be expressed at a biochemical level as production of hormones or hormone-related peptides, which are either improperly regulated by normal feedback mechanisms (e.g., excessive corticosteroid production by an adrenal carcinoma), or are not appropriate for the particular cell type if it were normally differentiated (e.g., ACTH production by a carcinoma of the lung). In such cases, the genomic repertoire of the malignant cell is expressed inappropriately. Another example is the unregulated production of immunoglobulin (partial or complete chains) by neoplastic derivatives of B lymphocytes.

Histologic features which are abnormal but do not meet the criteria of anaplasia (loss of differentiation) are designated *dysplastic*. Such changes may be seen in "premalignant" situations, for example, in the epithelial lining of the bronchi of cigarette smokers. These abnormalities are often reversible. Cessation of smoking can lead to normalization of the lung epithelium over a period of 5 years.

Metastasis This term encompasses a number of phenotypic traits which together result in the clinical problem which most often leads to death from cancer. The cells lose their adherence and restrained position within an organized tissue, move into adjacent sites, develop the capacity both to invade and to egress from blood vessels, and become capable of proliferating in unnatural locations or environments. These changes in growth patterns are accompanied by biochemical alterations which have the capacity to promote the metastatic process. Invasive tumors may secrete a variety of tissue-degrading enzymes including collagenases and lysosomal hydrolases. Plasminogen activators which lead to promotion of fibrinolysis are also produced. Conversely, procoagulant compounds may be released into the environment of the tumor cells at stages when focal aggregation of cells might be of survival value. In experimental situations where tumor cells show a propensity to select a particular organ as a preferred site of metastasis, surface molecules on the metastatic cells appear to have a high affinity for endothelial cells in the vasculature of the specific target organ. A large number of biochemical steps are involved in the progression of a tumor from a homogeneous proliferating clone to a group of heterogeneous subpopulations of cells, some of which have progressively accumulated the entire array of enzymes and surface molecules required for metastasis. It may be for this reason that the rate of metastasis is low during early tumor growth, in spite of the well-documented fact that malignant cells are often released from a tumor into the circulation continuously and in large numbers. Agents which could block critical steps in the metastatic process would be of great value in the armamentarium of antineoplastic agents.

FIGURE 78-3 *A diagrammatic representation of autocrine, paracrine, and endocrine secretion. Peptide growth factors are shown in latent form within the cell. The thickened, semicircular regions of the cell membrane represent receptor sites. (From MB Sporn, GJ Todaro, N Engl J Med 303:878, 1980.)*

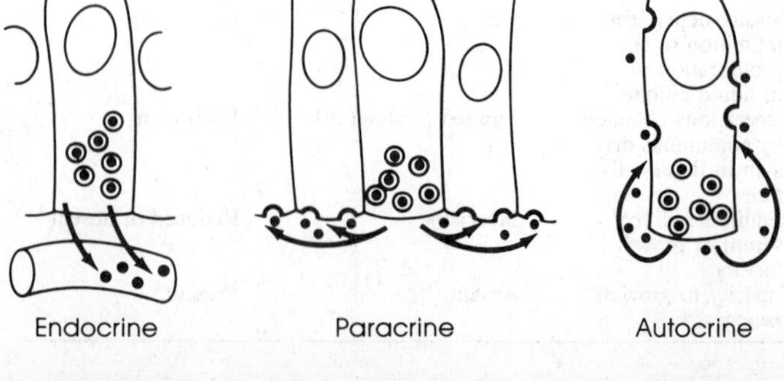

It appears that clonal progression of a tumor generates biochemical or physiologic alterations which confer greater autonomy, greater degrees of anaplasia, and a greater capacity to metastasize. Because there is progressive selection for cells with increased tumorogenic capacity, the process has been called clonal evolution and has been compared to Darwinian evolution, in this case at a cellular level.

ETIOLOGY Patterns of cancer incidence vary with sex, race, and geographic location. In addition, the types of tumors observed vary with age. Hereditary traits and variations in the internal environments around cells explain some of the differences in cancer incidence. It is clear from epidemiologic investigations that variations in diet and exposure to chemical and physical agents in the external environment contribute to the development of neoplasia. The environmental agents which have been linked to the incidence of cancer fall into three broad categories: radiation, a variety of chemicals, and viruses.

Genetic factors For many of the common malignancies, the incidence of cancer is higher among patients with positive family histories than among unselected patients, usually in the range of up to threefold. However, the risk can rise to as high as twenty-five- to thirtyfold in certain groups of patients with a familial history of breast cancer or bowel cancer. In addition, there are a number of uncommon inherited disorders involving either (1) a high risk for the occurrence of a particular neoplasm, or (2) the presence of multiple preneoplastic lesions that can progress to frank malignancy.

The hereditary neoplasms (Table 78-3) may occur as the only manifestation of a gene defect, or as part of a generalized syndrome involving multiple developmental abnormalities. The inheritance patterns in these disorders are generally autosomal dominant, with varying penetrance. Half of the children of patients with these disorders will inherit the gene defect.

The preneoplastic states are grouped into four major categories by Fraumeni (Table 78-3). The hamartomatous syndromes show autosomal dominant inheritance patterns. The most common is neurofibromatosis, occurring in 1 of 3000 live births. The neurofibromas undergo sarcomatous changes in about 10 percent of patients, with development of gliomas in the brain or optic nerve, meningiomas, acoustic neuromas, or pheochromocytomas. The genodermatoses are rare autosomal recessive genetic disorders which conspicuously involve the skin. Chromosome breakage disorders are characterized by the recessive inheritance of chromosomal instability and rearrangements of karyotypes; patients have an increased incidence of acute leukemia. The immune deficiency ataxic telangiectasia is also characterized by chromosomal fragility. Patients with hereditary or acquired immunodeficiency states have an increased incidence of neoplasia, most commonly the lymphoproliferative malignancies.

Race is a genetic factor in the incidence of cancer, but interpretation of epidemiologic data is made difficult by the concurrent effects of environmental and socioeconomic influences. Both the incidence and the death rate from cancer is higher in American blacks than in American whites, with all of the difference being accounted for by the higher cancer rate in black males. It is believed that later detection and less adequate treatment may account for part, but not all, of the difference in survival. The important effect of environmental factors is made clear by documented differences in cancer incidence for Asians living in Hawaii and in California.

Radiation It is estimated that less than 3 percent of cancers result from exposure to radiation. Radiation that can remove electrons from atoms is called ionizing radiation. It includes electromagnetic waves such as x-rays and gamma rays, as well as charged particles such as protons. The unit of radiation dose measures the energy absorbed in matter as a result of exposure to radiation: 1 rad = 100 erg/g; 1 gray = 1 joule/kg = 100 rad.

Information on the capacity of radiation in relatively large doses to induce cancer in humans comes from studies on survivors of atomic bomb blasts, on individuals accidentally exposed to irradiation or radiative fallout, and on patients exposed to radiation for diagnostic purposes or for therapy. It has been learned that nearly all tissues are susceptible to tumor induction by radiation, but with variable sensitivity. The most sensitive tissues are the bone marrow, breast, and thyroid. The latent period is only 2 to 5 years for acute leukemia, and 5 to 10 years for most solid tumors. There is a higher incidence of leukemia in patients who have received radiation therapy for neoplastic diseases and for ankylosing spondylitis, and of thyroid cancer in children irradiated for thymic enlargement.

Solar radiation, resulting from exposure to electromagnetic radiation from the sun, is the primary risk factor in skin cancer. The evidence for this linkage comes from a variety of epidemiologic and experimental observations. Skin cancer is rare in blacks and the deeply pigmented racial groups, whereas it is especially common in fair-complexioned individuals. It occurs primarily on the parts of the body exposed to sunlight and has a higher incidence in outdoor workers. Patients with genetic diseases such as xeroderma pigmentosa and albinism, which are exacerbated by sunlight, have very high risks for the development of skin cancer.

The carcinogenic effect of solar irradiation is greatest in the spectral range of 290 to 320 nm (UV-B radiation), which produces delayed erythema in human skin (sunburn). This range of wavelengths correlates with the action spectrum for UV-induced damage to DNA.

Exposure to solar ultraviolet irradiation is also a risk factor in melanoma. As with skin cancer, there is a higher incidence of melanoma among populations living at a latitude nearer the equator, where exposure to UV irradiation is greatest.

Tobacco Numerous epidemiologic studies have demonstrated that the principal carcinogenic agent in our environment is inhaled tobacco smoke. The incidence of lung cancer is more than tenfold higher in male smokers than in nonsmokers. Furthermore, tobacco smoking is associated with increased rates of cancer of the oral cavity, esophagus, kidney, bladder, and pancreas. Particulate matter in tobacco smoke, known as "tar," contains a long list of chemicals, primarily polycyclic hydrocarbons, which have been shown experimentally to be contact carcinogens. In addition, the metabolic activation of tobacco components, for example, the cyclic *N*-nitrosamines, can produce carcinogens with the capacity to act upon the cells of internal organs. Tobacco-related malignancies account for one-third of all cancer deaths among men in the United States and for 5 to 10 percent of all female cancer deaths. Unfortunately, this figure is rising in females. As a result of increased use of tobacco by women in the period since World War II, the incidence of lung cancer in females is expected to pass that of breast cancer by 1990.

TABLE 78-3 Hereditary cancer syndromes

I Hereditary neoplasms
- Retinoblastoma
- Nevoid basal cell carcinoma syndrome
- Multiple endocrine adenomatosis (Werner's syndrome)
- Pheochromocytoma and medullary thyroid carcinoma (Sipple's syndrome)
- Chemodectomas
- Polyposis coli
- Gardner's syndrome
- Tylosis with esophageal carcinoma

II Preneoplastic states
- *A* Hamartomatous syndromes
  - Neurofibromatosis
  - Tuberous sclerosis
  - von Hippel–Lindau syndrome
  - Multiple exostoses
  - Peutz-Jeghers syndrome
  - Cowden's multiple hamartoma syndrome
- *B* Genodermatoses
  - Xeroderma pigmentosum
  - Albinism
  - Werner's syndrome
  - Epidermodysplasia verruciformis
  - Polydysplastic epidermolysis bullosa
  - Dyskeratosis congenita
- *C* Chromosome breakage disorders
  - Bloom's syndrome
  - Fanconi's syndrome
- *D* Immune deficiency syndromes
  - Ataxia-telangiectasia
  - Wiskott-Aldrich syndrome
  - Late-onset immunologic deficiency
  - X-linked agammaglobulinemia

SOURCE: *From JF Fraumeni, Jr, in JF Holland, E Frei.*

Clearly the single most effective action which could be taken against cancer at the present time involves not an application of molecular genetic research, but cessation of smoking. Fortunately, it appears that smoking cessation results in a gradual decrease in risk, so that after 10 to 15 years, exsmokers have nearly the same risk of lung cancer as nonsmokers. Because the habit of smoking is difficult to break, the physician's role in cessation of smoking is of critical importance. Doctors should deliver a *firm* antismoking message.

Occupational exposure The first report of cancer related to occupational hazards was Percival Pott's observation of an unusually high frequency of scrotal cancer among London chimney sweeps in 1775. It is now known that skin cancer (including scrotal) can be induced by a variety of coal tar products, such as the materials contacted in the London chimneys. Epidemiologic studies also have related lung cancer to exposure to coal by-products. Table 78-4 provides a partial listing of industrial agents which are known to cause cancer.

Air pollution It is clear that lung cancer incidence is increased by tobacco smoking and by certain industrial and occupational exposures (primarily related to coal tar and combustion by-products). Once the risks resulting from exposure to these factors are taken into account, the epidemiologic evidence that links ambient air pollution to lung cancer remains inconclusive. Studies correlating the incidence of lung cancer with increased levels of polycyclic hydrocarbons and benzo(a)pyrene in urban air are complicated by the difficulty of eliminating the contribution of exposure to these compounds through tobacco smoking as well as occupational exposure.

TABLE 78-4 Examples of occupational causes of cancer

Etiology	Site of malignancy
Arsenic (inorganic)	Lung, skin, liver
Asbestos	Mesothelium, lung
Benzene	Leukemia
Benzidine	Bladder
Chromium compounds	Lung
Radiation (mining, dial painting)	Numerous locations
Mustard gas	Lung
Polycyclic hydrocarbons (coal by-products)	Lung, skin
Vinyl chloride	Angiosarcoma of liver

Medications Certain drugs and hormones have been shown to be carcinogenic. The synthetic nonsteroidal estrogen diethylstilbestrol (DES), which was used for a period of time to reduce fetal wastage in pregnant women, caused an increased incidence of vaginal and cervical cancer in daughters who were exposed in utero. Conjugated estrogens have been shown to increase the incidence of endometrial cancer in patients treated for menopausal symptoms. The use of progesterone concomitantly, together with decreased estrogen dose, may obviate this problem.

Alkylating agents have been shown to cause an increased incidence of acute myelocytic leukemia and probably other malignancies. They are used in therapeutic situations in which the poor prognosis of malignancy far outweighs the increased risk of an additional cancer in the future. However, because of this risk, new drug regimens which avoid the use of alkylating agents are being explored in situations where substantial long-term benefits from chemotherapy have been demonstrated, for example, in Hodgkin's disease.

The recipients of organ transplants who are treated with immunosuppressive agents, such as azathioprine and prednisone, have an increased incidence of histiocytic lymphoma as well as a variety of solid tumors. A similar increased incidence is observed in individuals with inherited and acquired immunodeficiency, for example, AIDS. This has been attributed to reduced immune surveillance, but a variety of other explanations are equally likely, such as activation of a latent oncogenic virus or chronic immunostimulation in conjunction with a compromised and malfunctioning immune system.

Diet The role of diet and nutrition in carcinogenesis has been the subject of intensive investigation and equally intensive controversy. There are numerous nutritional hypotheses of carcinogenesis. Some of these have led to unconventional forms of cancer therapy that are based upon no scientific evidence. Unfortunately, these putative dietary therapies are propagated upon a patient population for which proven treatment modalities are often unsuccessful in achieving cure, and at a time when there is a popular emphasis on healthful nutrition.

Epidemiologic analyses of international variations in cancer incidence and comparisons of the types and frequencies of cancer in populations with different dietary habits have yielded a great deal of evidence that cancers of most major sites are influenced by diet. These studies were reviewed in an authoritative publication, *Diet, Nutrition, and Cancer*. Interim dietary guidelines are suggested which are both consistent with good nutritional practices and likely to reduce the risk of cancer: (1) Reduce the intake of fat, saturated and unsaturated, from its present average level (40 percent) to 30 percent of total calories in the diet. (2) Include fruits (especially citrus), vegetables (especially carotene-rich and cruciferous), and whole cereal grain (fiber) in the daily diet; these provide amounts of vitamins A and C as well as fiber adequate to obviate the need for dietary supplements. (3) Minimize consumption of salt-cured or smoked food. (4) Use alcoholic beverages in moderation, since they increase the risk of certain cancers, especially when combined with cigarette smoking.

Experimental data lend support to the inferences from epidemiologic studies, but additional research is necessary to understand how dietary factors influence carcinogenesis. For example, epidemiologic evidence strongly correlates the intake of fat with the occurrence of cancer at several sites, especially the breast and colon. Possible explanations for this observation include increased adiposity, leading to greater conversion of androstenedione to estrone, which could influence carcinogenesis in the breast; and stimulation of increased bile salt excretion which could alter gut flora and thereby augment the production of carcinogenic substances by the bacteria in the colon. Vitamin C may act to prevent cancer by blocking endogenous formation of *N*-nitroso compounds in the gastrointestinal tract, but there are no data showing that taking vitamin C will prevent cancer in human beings. Dietary fiber enhances the rapid transit of potential carcinogens through the colon, which could explain the low incidence of bowel cancer and rectal cancer in tropical Africa.

It is important to stress that the accumulated scientific evidence does not support the anticarcinogenic value of particular vitamins, minerals, or nutritional supplements in amounts greater than provided by a prudent diet. Certainly their use in high doses in the therapy of established malignant disease is not indicated. The physician must be alert to the scientifically unproven dietary treatments which patients with cancer may be urged to undertake. Of course the greatest tragedy occurs when patients whose malignancy could be cured by proven therapeutic modalities are misled into depending upon such dietary manipulations.

Viruses Although there has been extensive research on viral oncogenesis with experimental murine tumors, viruses have been implicated as the cause of only one human cancer, an uncommon malignancy of T lymphocytes. There are a number of situations in which viruses are linked to the occurrence of specific cancers with a high incidence in particular geographic locations, although a causative role has not been established. The Epstein-Barr virus is closely associated with African Burkitt's lymphoma as well as nasopharyngeal carcinoma in Asia. Cofactors in the development of these malignancies might be holoendemic malaria in African Burkitt's lymphoma, and a particular configuration of histocompatibility antigens in the case of nasopharyngeal carcinoma among Chinese. While the Epstein-Barr virus can infect human B lymphocytes (infectious mononucleosis) and transform them in cell culture, evidence is lacking that such a transformation is the cause of clinical malignancy.

Hepatitis B infection is correlated with the incidence of hepatocellular carcinoma, but again there is no evidence for a causal relationship. Chronic hepatocyte infection by the virus might predispose to carcinogenesis in these cells. There may be a variety of contributing factors, including malaria, malnutrition, and exposure to aflatoxin. There also is a statistical correlation between herpes simplex 2 viral infection, which is sexually transmitted, and the incidence of cervical cancer.

Risk of cancer Knowledge of genetic and environmental factors that may contribute to cancer incidence can be utilized by the conscientious physician to identify patients who have an increased risk of malignancy. The presence of certain hereditary diseases in a patient's family may suggest procedures that can lead to early detection and prevention, for example, early surveillance by colonoscopy and prevention by prophylactic colectomy in persons who have familial polyposis of the colon. Environmental factors that increase cancer risks should be identified and avoided. It is evident, however, that changing an individual's life-style in order to avoid exposure to a carcinogen can require an extraordinary level of effort on the part of both the patient and the physician.

CLINICAL SEQUELAE The presence of a malignant lesion may not, in itself, cause symptoms in a patient with cancer. The primary lesion may, for a period of time, be unnoticed and unimportant for the normal maintenance of body functions, in which case its clinical significance is due to its potential for growth and spread. In addition, the presence of metastasis need not result in symptomatic illness. Patients with carcinoma of the bowel, whose disease may have spread beyond the limits of surgical curability, may live for many months or even years with easily detectable metastatic lesions in the lung or abdomen, yet remain free of symptoms until the function of a vital organ is compromised or obstructive problems appear.

Malignancies produce clinical symptoms in three general ways (Table 78-5): by direct effects resulting from invasion or compression of normal tissues; by release of cytokines, hormones, and other biologically active agents into the local and systemic environment; and by secondary psychological effects upon the patient. Each of these factors may contribute profoundly to the degree of illness experienced by the patient. Clinical symptoms resulting from released biologically active agents, as well as systemic problems caused by as yet undetermined mechanisms, are usually grouped under the category of "paraneoplastic syndromes."

TABLE 78-5 Symptoms caused by malignant diseases

I Mass effects
- *A* Ablation by crowding or by invasion
- *B* Obstruction of vessels, tubes, and ducts
- *C* Rupture of blood vessels

II Remote effects (paraneoplastic syndromes)
- *A* Ectopic hormone production
- *B* Neuropathies and CNS abnormalities
- *C* Dermatologic abnormalities
- *D* Metabolic disorders
  - *1* Anorexia, weight loss
  - *2* Fever
  - *3* Chronic inflammation
- *E* Hematologic disorders
- *F* Immunosuppression
- *G* Collagen vascular disorders

III Psychosocial effects
- *A* Loss of control
- *B* Acceptance of personal finitude
- *C* Fear of pain and mutilation
- *D* Separation and loneliness

Mass effects of malignancy In most cases tumors produce clinical problems as a result of local expansion, with obliteration of normal tissues, as the malignant cells proliferate within the confines of the involved organ: marrow replacement by leukemia results in reduced production of the normal cellular elements of the blood; lung cancer compromises oxygen exchange in involved alveoli; primary or metastatic cancer in bone causes weakened trabecular architecture, resulting in pathologic fractures; hepatomas replace normal hepatocytes and interfere with liver function. A second result of local expansion is compression of normal structures, with partial or complete obstruction of tubular organs, blood vessels, and lymphatics: colonic cancer may obstruct the gastrointestinal tract; lung cancer blocks airflow through bronchi and can obstruct pulmonary venous return; hepatic and biliary malignancies produce obstructive jaundice; a variety of intraabdominal neoplasms can encase the ureters, causing renal failure; in the extreme case, penetration of blood vessels can violate the integrity of the vasculature, resulting in hemorrhage. A third result of local expansion is pain, due to pressure on or stretching of nerve fibers. When neoplasia causes increased pressure on nervous tissue within the confines of the skull, the symptoms include headache and vomiting as well as seizure disorders and brain dysfunction.

Paraneoplastic syndromes The malignant process is felt to develop as a result of the unregulated and/or inappropriate expression of certain genes crucial to cell proliferation and differentiation. The aggressiveness of the malignant process is increased by the subsequent uncovering of additional genetic information. In this evolutionary process, abnormal genetic information may be expressed which results in severe physiologic effects upon the patient. As noted above, there may be excessive synthesis of a gene product which is normally found in the particular cell type, or the malignant cell may produce a molecule which does not ordinarily originate from its normal counterpart.

A common type of molecule produced by malignant tumors falls into the category of polypeptide hormones. The synthesis of antidiuretic hormone or ACTH by small cell carcinoma of the lung or parathormone by some squamous cancers are examples. These can produce clinical illness by mediating normal physiologic functions to an excessive degree. Other active molecules have been detected which are homologous with or identical to known growth factors. The potential for autonomous stimulation of proliferation mediated by production of essential growth-promoting agents has been discussed.

From this brief introduction, it can be seen that biologically active agents produced by malignant cells can be clinically important for a number of reasons:

1 They may serve as markers for the presence of a type of tumor. Detection of such markers early in the course of the disease might increase chances for cure. They also may be used to follow the clinical progress of the disease and anticipate recurrence.

2 They may produce symptoms as a result of their intrinsic biologic activity. In some cases these can become the major clinical problems determining survival (e.g., hypercalcemia).

3 They may serve to promote the growth of the tumor directly. In turn, growth-promoting agents of this type may become the focus of new approaches to anticancer treatment.

The paraneoplastic sequelae of cancer which involve ectopic hormone production are described in Chap. 303, and the neurologic manifestations of neoplasia in Chap. 304. Cutaneous manifestations of internal malignancy are discussed in Chap. 300. The association of malignancy with certain metabolic disorders, hematologic abnormalities, and immunosuppression will be further described here.

Metabolic disorders One of the major and most characteristic problems seen with cancer is weight loss, usually associated with anorexia. The extensive wasting which results is known as cachexia. The cause for this commonly observed and often life-limiting disturbance remains to be determined in spite of the fact that many contributing factors have been identified. Abnormalities of taste and smell, physiologic malfunction of the gastrointestinal tract, excessive energy demands made by the tumor, and failure to adapt energy expenditure to the levels of nutrient intake have been implicated as causes of cachexia in patients with cancer. Biochemical abnormalities in energy metabolism have been well-characterized in these patients. Fatty acids are oxidized in preference to glucose, and anaerobic glucose metabolism is increased while oxidative phosphorylation is reduced. This results in an inefficient expenditure of ATP, which might lead to an energy deficit. However, none of these observations is felt to account for the magnitude of the problem.

Typically, the anorectic patient simply cannot ingest food, in spite of a clear understanding of the need for increased nourishment. The chief complaint is unpalatability. An aversion to meat has been clearly documented. While nausea may be a component of the syndrome, emesis occurs rarely. This may be because the patient feels so satiated that no food intake is tolerated.

Provision of alimentation through enteral tubes or by the intravenous route has the potential to provide total parenteral nutrition (TPN) to patients with cancer, and the techniques for performing these procedures have been well described by investigators managing nonmalignant disease. At present there is no indication that the provision of nutritional support at this level can, by itself, affect the course of malignant disease. However, clinical trials have suggested a role for nutritional supplementation, including TPN, in preparing nutritionally deprived cancer patients for potentially beneficial surgical procedures or chemotherapy programs which otherwise might not have been tolerated due to the wasted state of the patient.

A polypeptide produced by macrophages has been isolated and named cachectin. This molecule can mimic the syndrome of cachexia in experimental animals. It may ultimately explain the pathogenesis of this puzzling and vexing syndrome.

Fever is another sign associated with malignancy, and it is usually attributable to infection. Because of the debility which often accompanies cancer, and the depression in circulating granulocytes and mononuclear cells resulting from aggressive therapeutic measures, the types of infection seen may be unusual. Infection by endogenous bacteria, fungi, viruses, and protozoa must be considered when evaluating fever of unknown etiology in patients with malignancy (see Chap. 9). There remain unusual instances when fever can not be explained by infection and must be attributed to a cause intrinsic to the neoplasm itself.

Hematologic abnormalities Anemia is found with increased incidence in advanced stages of malignant disease. The mechanisms accounting for anemia are, in nearly all cases, extrinsic to the tumor, and may be due to several mechanisms. Increased destruction of erythrocytes can result from hypersplenism, microangiopathic hemolysis, and autoantibodies, seen especially in the lymphoproliferative malignancies. Anemia due to occult bleeding is one of the cardinal signs of malignancy in the gastrointestinal tract. Decreased production of erythrocytes may result from iron deficiency related to bleeding, vitamin B_{12} or folate deficiency, erythron depletion due to tumor crowding in the marrow, toxicity secondary to chemotherapy or radiotherapy, and the anemia associated with chronic inflammatory disease.

Granulocytopenia is commonly associated with marrow infiltration by hematologic malignancies, and also results from chemotherapy. The etiologies of thrombocytopenia are comparable to those associated with anemia. Depression in one or all of the circulating hematopoietic elements may result from one of the various forms of marrow failure or aplastic anemia which are known to be preleukemic.

An increase in the formed elements of the blood may also occur. Erythrocytosis resulting from inappropriate production of erythropoietin is observed not only in polycythemia vera, but also in renal cell carcinoma, hepatoma, and cerebellar hemangioma. An elevated granulocyte count may result from marrow infiltration by tumor cells, or an inflammatory response to malignancy, and frank leukemoid reactions may be seen with nonhematopoietic tumors. Thrombocytosis unrelated to primary marrow disease is commonly associated with a systemic malignancy.

A hypercoagulable state is a rare clinical complication of malignancy, although it may be far more prevalent at a subclinical level. Mucin-producing tumors and adenocarcinomas, especially those of the pancreas and stomach, head the list of tumors reported to be associated with clinical disseminated coagulopathy (DIC). This may present as a migratory thrombophlebitis of unknown etiology, which can produce venous thrombosis as well as pulmonary embolism. Hypercoagulation also may be associated with marantic (nonbacterial) endocarditis and resultant thromboembolic episodes, which further complicate the clinical picture. The treatment of the primary malignancy is the only successful therapeutic attack on the problem. Anticoagulation, following the principles for treatment of DIC (Chaps. 54 and 281), may provide short-term benefits in acute situations, but with attendant risks.

Acute promyelocytic leukemia is often associated with abnormalities of hemostasis related to a hypercoagulable state. The malignant immature granulocytes can release procoagulant materials which initiate DIC. In this case, the addition of anticoagulation to the initial phase of antileukemia therapy results in an improved chance for a successful outcome.

Immunosuppression Advanced cancer is accompanied by abnormalities in immune function which can be demonstrated by skin testing against common antigens and by examination of lymphocyte responses to mitogenic stimulation in vitro. Moreover, in general, the extent of malignant disease correlates well with the degree of immune dysfunction. In spite of a vast experimental literature on this subject, the two significant questions concerning immunosuppression in cancer patients continue to be unanswered: (1) What is the mechanism(s) of inhibition? (2) Is the immunosuppression merely secondary to the malignant state, or could it play an etiologic role (failure of "immune surveillance")?

Experimental data have implicated defects in both T- and B-cell function, as well as abnormalities of macrophages, in the etiology of the reduced immune competence in cancer patients. Primary malignancies of lymphocytes are accompanied by abnormalities in the functioning of the particular cell type involved. Some of the lymphoproliferative malignancies are characterized by an increase in autoimmune reactions, most notably in 25 percent of patients with chronic lymphocytic leukemia. In addition, both chemotherapy and radiotherapy can produce long-standing suppression of immune function.

One approach to cancer treatment involves attempts to stimulate an effective immune response with the hope that immune antitumor activity can act alone or in concert with the standard therapeutic modalities to eliminate the malignant cell population. Monoclonal antibodies against antigens present in relatively increased quantities on tumor cells may provide ways to reconstitute or hyperconstitute immune responses to malignancy. Treatment with cytokines such as the interferons has produced some interesting preliminary results, and therapy with high concentrations of interleukin 2 is under active investigation.

Psychosocial effects The diagnosis of cancer immediately raises in the mind of the patient and his or her family a host of questions and fears which require the undivided attention of an empathetic, considerate, and skilled physician. This is especially true when the particular form of cancer has a poor chance for cure, or when malignancy has recurred.

Of the variety of psychosocial problems experienced by patients, two which are particularly difficult to deal with are helplessness and loss of control. These involve both economic control and personal control of one's activity and one's future. Closely tied to these problems and adding to the feeling of helplessness is the difficulty of accepting personal finitude. A third major source of mental anguish is the fear of pain and mutilation. Finally, separation from loved ones, both anticipated and real, creates a void of loneliness and a fear of abandonment.

The reactions to the mental stresses which are produced by these problems can only be dealt with effectively by a professional who has become familiar with the patient's personality and his or her social and intellectual environment. Although one or another emotion may dominate at a particular time, the responses commonly observed include anger, denial, withdrawal, and depression. Added to these problems is the complexity resulting from the response of the patient's family to the illness and to the patient's own response to the illness. In spite of these stresses, some patients with incurable malignancies are able to adapt and reorient their lives in a creative and meaningful way. The intellectual and emotional challenge to the physician is obvious, and careful attention must be given to managing the patient's (and the family's) responses to malignancy in addition to providing specific treatment for the disease.

Does the patient's psychological attitude have a role in the cause or treatment of malignant disease? The question is a complex and controversial one. There is evidence, which is contested, that life stresses can predispose to systemic illness by producing anxiety or depression. One theory postulates that stress leads to a reduction in immunologic function, resulting in inadequate immune surveillance, but this explanation for the pathogenesis of cancer is not adequately supported by available clinical data. There are also claims that correction of emotional difficulties and development of positive attitudes can serve as effective anticancer therapy. In favor of psychological support and counseling is the clear benefit to the quality of life which can be achieved by helping patients with malignancy to develop positive attitudes and to gain some measure of control over *how* they are living. However, scientific evidence does not demonstrate that the patient's psyche can achieve regression or cure of the malignant process. Some of the strongest and most responsible advocates of counseling and attitudinal approaches to cancer patient management also stress the need for concurrent treatment with standard anticancer therapies.

DIAGNOSIS AND STAGING There are four general goals in evaluating a patient for the presence of malignancy. First, information must be gathered leading to biopsy of a candidate lesion, which alone can establish the pathologic diagnosis of neoplasia. The second goal is to determine as precisely as possible the extent of tumor spread, both at the site of origin and as metastases. The process of obtaining this information is known as *staging*. The third goal is to determine the growth rate and time course of the neoplasm in the particular patient undergoing diagnostic evaluation. The dictum that "every person is different" holds for cancers as well. Each malignancy is different, although there is a natural history which broadly characterizes each type of neoplasm. The rate of tumor growth can be determined by sequential assessment, using physical examinations or radiologic techniques, occasionally aided by the measurement of serum markers of tumor activity. The physician's ingenuity and persistence often come into play; an example is determining the existence of past radiologic studies, locating them, and obtaining them for review. The fourth goal in the evaluation is to determine the effects of the malignancy upon the health and performance of the patient. The importance of this in the design of a management plan is obvious, since control of symptoms and proper modification of acitivity levels will improve the well-being of the patient. In addition, it has become increasingly evident that the patient's performance status provides important data in predicting prognosis as well as response to anticancer therapy.

There are two widely used clinical scales of performance status, the Karnofsky scale and a modification developed by the Eastern Cooperative Oncology Group. The influence of performance status upon prognosis is demonstrated by a report correlating performance and median survival in patients with inoperable lung cancer (Table 78-6).

TABLE 78-6 Influence of pretreatment performance status on patients with inoperable lung cancer*

Performance status scale†			Median survival (weeks)	Patients in group (percent)
ECOG	Karnofsky	Definitions		
0	100	Asymptomatic, normal activity	34	2
1	80–90	Symptomatic, but ambulatory	24–27	32
2	60–70	Symptomatic, in bed less than 50% of day, needs minimal assistance	14–21	40
3	40–50	Symptomatic, in bed more than 50% of day, requires considerable assistance	7–9	22
4	20–30	100% bedridden, severely disabled	3–5	5

* *N = 5022 males with inoperable lung cancer of all histologic types entered onto VA Lung Group protocols from 1968–1978.*

† *Eastern Cooperative Oncology Group (ECOG) performance status scale, and DA Karnofsky et al, Cancer 1:634, 1948.*

SOURCE: *Adapted from JD Minna et al, in VT DeVita, Jr et al.*

Pathologic diagnosis The diagnosis of cancer is made by pathologic examination. While there are definite limitations to histologic and cytologic examination of tumor specimens, this procedure is essential in order to exclude inflammatory processes as well as hyperplasia or benign tumors. In addition, the tissue of origin of a malignancy must be known in order to select the appropriate therapy. Specimens for pathologic examination are usually obtained by biopsy of a suspicious lesion. The procedure may involve a surgical operation under general anesthesia, but in many cases tissue specimens can be obtained through local incision (e.g., breast cancer) or by removal of a piece of tissue under direct visualization (bronchoscopy, colonoscopy). When direct visualization is not possible because of the internal location of a suspected lesion, it is often possible to obtain tissue fragments or clumps of cells by fine-needle biopsy aspiration, guided by computerized axial tomography or fluoroscopy. In addition, suitable cytologic preparations can be obtained by washing or scraping surface lesions, as is commonly done to evaluate lesions on the cervix or in bronchi. Finally, in the case of malignancy involving the hematopoietic system or growing in body cavities (e.g., ascites), needle aspiration of tumor cells in suspension can be performed.

To make the diagnosis of cancer the pathologist looks for histologic and cytologic features characteristic of the disease. These include pleomorphism of cellular and nuclear structure, a high rate of mitosis and the presence of large or multiple nuclei, disordered tissue architecture, destruction or invasion of normal tissue boundaries, and the presence of cells in inappropriate locations (metastases). Special stains are useful for identifying chemical components characteristic of particular cell types and tissues. Additional evidence can be brought to bear upon the pathologic diagnosis, using the results of immunohistochemical studies, flow cytometry data on cellular DNA content, karyotype analysis, and electron microscopy. However, in the overwhelming majority of cases, the diagnosis is made with the light microscope, on the basis of morphologic evaluation of the cells individually and as organized into tissue structures.

After the pathologic diagnosis of malignancy is established, the description usually includes three characteristics which classify the neoplasia:

1 The tissue of origin (e.g., adenocarcinoma, epidermoid carcinoma, sarcoma, leukemia)
2 Anatomic origin (e.g., colon, lung, breast)
3 Degree of differentiation (e.g., well-differentiated or poorly differentiated)

Each of these characteristics gives the therapist information relevant to the selection of treatment and to the prognosis. Although this terminology for classification is followed in general, there are many examples of exceptions based upon customary nomenclature involving particular tissues of origin or on the use of eponyms (e.g., Hodgkin's disease, glioblastoma multiforme).

Staging of cancer The staging of a cancer patient involves the detection of the anatomic extent of the tumor, both in its primary location and in metastatic sites. This process is of critical importance in the clinical management for a number of reasons:

1 The optimal treatment plan for an individual patient is selected on the basis of the stage of disease.
2 By determining the presence of early metastatic disease, treatment can often be designed which can increase the chance for cure, or delay the development of symptoms even if cure is not achievable.
3 Staging provides information from which the physician can better evaluate the prognosis.
4 Because half of the cases of cancer cannot be cured by the therapies available today and because rapid advances in the development of anticancer treatment are occurring, management of an individual patient often involves new drugs or experimental procedures which are in the process of being evaluated for toxicity and efficacy. Staging to determine the extent of disease accurately is essential for evaluating factors influencing the results of such new treatments.

The anatomic extent of disease is best described and communicated to other professionals by a standardized nomenclature known as the TNM system. The three elements characterized in this system are the primary *t*umor, the regional lymph *n*odes, and *m*etastases (Table 78-7). The details of classification were decided upon by the International Union against Cancer (UICC) and the American Joint Committee for Cancer Staging (AJCCS). There is a scale of subcategories with designations ranging from 0 to 4 for each of the three tumor characteristics listed in the table. These scales were chosen because they can provide useful predictions of the clinical course. The primary tumor is classified by its size and the extent of local involvement. The involvement of lymph nodes is typically stratified by the spread to locations at a varying distance from the primary lesion and by the number of involved nodes. The most relevant information regarding metastases is their presence or absence. The details of stratification within the TNM system vary for each type of malignancy and are highly individualized. They depend on the characteristic growth patterns and lymphatic drainage patterns of neoplasms of the various

TABLE 78-7 TNM system of anatomic staging

T: Primary tumor	
T0	No evidence of primary tumor
T1–4	Ascending degrees of increase in tumor size and involvement
N: Regional lymph nodes	
N0	No evidence of disease in lymph nodes
N1–4	Ascending degrees of nodal involvement
M: Distant metastasis	
M0	No evidence of metastasis
M1–4	Ascending degrees of metastatic involvement

TABLE 78-8 Tumor (T), node (N), metastasis (M) classification and stage grouping lung cancer*

Occult cancer	TX	N0	M0
Stage Ia	T1,T2	N0	M0
Stage Ib	T1	N1	M0
Stage II	T2	N1	M0
Stage III	T3	N0,N1	M0
	Any T	N2	M0
Stage IV	Any T	Any N	M1

* *TX, positive cytology; T1, less than or equal to 3 cm, no invasion; T2, more than 3 cm, extension to hilar region must be at least 2 cm distal to carina; T3, gross extension, effusion, atelectasis of an entire lung; N1, hilar nodes; N2, mediastinal nodes; M1, distant metastasis.*

SOURCE: *P. Rubin; modified from American Joint Committee.*

organs. There is not always agreement about the definitions of the TNM characteristics, which can create confusion.

The stage of the tumor is typically divided into three or four categories (e.g., I to IV). For each type of malignancy, the various T, N, and M designations are assigned to one of four stages, in order to develop separation into groupings which correlate with data on prognosis and clinical responses to therapy. This is best described by mentioning a specific example. For the neoplasm with the highest mortality rate, non-small cell carcinoma of the lung, the therapy which has the best chance for curing the patient is surgery. The staging system for lung cancer (Table 78-8) is designed in a way which stratifies patients into groups, for which different treatment protocols are indicated. For the stages I and II patients, surgery is the treatment of choice. The extent of the surgical procedure depends on the extent of disease designated by the T and N classification within these two stages. Total excision of all tumor is the therapeutic goal, with 5-year postresection survival rates of 50 percent for stage I and 15 percent for stage II. Only occasional patients with stage III come to surgery, because of the usual nonresectability of the disease at this stage and the lack of survival benefit from removal of the primary tumor in the presence of unresectable metastases.

Clinical evaluation How does the clinician proceed to evaluate a patient for the presence of malignant disease? Early detection depends primarily on awareness of the hereditary and environmental factors contributing to the incidence of cancer, combined with thorough exploration for symptoms and signs which could lead to further diagnostic workup. The seven warning signals widely publicized by the American Cancer Society are useful to remember (Table 78-9) and are usually covered in a review of systems. A careful physical examination is especially useful in detecting early breast cancer, cancer of the colon, skin cancer, and head-and-neck cancers. Three diagnostic screening tests have proved of value in early detection: (1) the exfoliative cytology (''Pap smear'') screen for cervical cancer, (2) fecal occult blood testing, accompanied by periodic sigmoidoscopy, and (3) mammograms.

The prudent guidelines for early cancer detection provided by the American Cancer Society can be summarized as follows. A cancer-related checkup is recommended every 3 years for those 20 to 40 years of age. For breast cancer screening, an examination of patients in this age group by a physician is recommended every 3 years, a self-examination every month, and one baseline breast x-ray between the ages of 35 and 40. For detection of cervical and uterine cancer, a pelvic examination is recommended every 3 years and a Pap test at least every 3 years after two initial negative tests 1 year apart.

In the age group of 40 and over, a yearly cancer checkup is recommended by the American Cancer Society. Women over 40 are advised to have a professional breast examination every year, a self-examination every month, and a breast x-ray every 1 to 2 years for those 40 to 49 years of age, and every year for those 50 and over. For screening of cervical and uterine cancer in this age group, a pelvic examination is recommended every year, a Pap test at least every 3 years after two negative tests a year apart, and an endometrial tissue sample at menopause if the patient has high-risk factors. For colon and rectal cancer, a digital rectal examination is suggested every year after 40, and a stool occult blood test every year after 50 as well as a sigmoidoscopic examination every 3 to 5 years after two initial negative tests 1 year apart.

TABLE 78-9 Cancer's seven warning signals

Change in bowel or bladder habits
A sore that does not heal
Unusual bleeding or discharge
Thickening or lump in breast or elsewhere
Indigestion or difficulty in swallowing
Obvious change in wart or mole
Nagging cough or hoarseness

SOURCE: *American Cancer Society.*

The three most common malignancies involve bowel, lung, and breast, and it is significant that screening tests are suggested for only two of these. Unfortunately, trials of mass screening for lung cancer with chest x-rays and sputum cytology have not resulted in reduced mortality, even when subjects believed to be at high risk were followed. However, the physician who is evaluating a patient in order to attempt to detect cancer early must learn whether or not the patient smokes cigarettes and should attempt to intervene.

The approach to a patient who presents to the physician with a history of symptoms or with abnormal physical findings which could be attributed to cancer involves selection of appropriate diagnostic procedures from a wide variety of available radiologic tests and laboratory studies (Table 78-10). The choice of diagnostic procedures used in the staging of cancer patients is guided by the natural history of the various types of malignancy. For example, knowledge that distant spread of breast cancer most frequently occurs to the lung, liver, bone, brain, and contralateral breast leads to consideration of studies of each of these organs as part of the staging workup. In addition, the diagnostician must know the probability of spread to these various metastatic sites in the presence or absence of abnormal findings in the history, physical examination, and standard blood studies. For the asymptomatic patient with breast cancer who has no abnormal physical findings outside of a small palpable breast lesion, and normal hematologic and blood chemistry values, a chest x-ray and a mammogram are the tests typically performed to stage the patient prior to a decision for definitive therapy. Evaluation of the other organs to which breast cancer commonly metastasizes has not been proven to be worthwhile in this situation. Similar considerations go into planning the diagnostic workup for patients with each of the various forms of malignancy. It is for this reason that a thorough familiarity with the natural history of malignancies of the various organs, as well as the efficacy of a wide variety of diagnostic procedures in detecting these cancers, is essential.

Tumor markers A tumor marker is an abnormality which is specific for a particular type of malignancy. For example, the Ph^1 chromosome abnormality in the karyotype is a marker for chronic myelogenous leukemia, and the exclusive presence of either κ or λ chains on the surface of a population of lymphocytes is a marker of the lymphoproliferative malignancies. Often, the term *marker* is used in a more restrictive sense, referring to molecules which are produced in abnormal amounts or under abnormal circumstances and are released into the circulation. Assays of such markers may be of great help to the clinician in a number of ways: (1) screening of high-risk individuals for the presence of malignancy, (2) diagnosis of malignancy, (3) monitoring of the effectiveness of therapy, (4) early detection of recurrence, and (5) immunodetection of metastatic sites, using radioactive-labeled antibodies against the markers.

The utility of tumor markers depends upon the sensitivity of assays for their presence, and the specificity of the markers for a particular malignant cell type. Data collected from a large number of studies have demonstrated that absolutely specific tumor markers do not exist, except for idiotypic immunoglobulin chains produced by malignant lymphocytes. However, the anaplasia and autonomy of the tumor cells permit production of molecules in greater than normal amounts or at inappropriate times in the life of the organism, and in this sense the abnormalities may become specific.

The tumor marker of greatest use to the clinician is human

chorionic gonadotropin (HCG), which has specificity because of its nearly exclusive production by the trophoblastic epithelium of the placenta under normal circumstances. HCG levels rise during pregnancy. The hormone also may be secreted into the blood by trophoblastic tumors, as well as germ cell neoplasms of the testes and ovaries. Other neoplasms have been reported to be associated with elevated HCG levels, but the serum concentration rarely exceeds 10 ng/mL, whereas trophoblastic tumors can produce concentrations over 100,000 ng/mL. The usefulness of the assay for HCG is markedly enhanced by clinical data which show that changes in the serum HCG concentration in patients with secreting trophoblastic malignancies accurately reflect changes in the tumor burden. Therefore, decisions on the appropriate time to discontinue therapy can be based on the time course of serum levels, and decisions to reinstate therapy for recurrent disease are made on the basis of reappearance of HCG in the serum. The clinical test for HCG utilizes a radioimmunoassay for the beta subunit, to avoid cross reactivity with luteinizing hormone.

Two clinically useful tumor markers are products of genes which are expressed during the normal differentiation of fetal tissue but are partially or completely suppressed in the adult. These markers have been termed oncofetal antigens. Carcinoembryonic antigen (CEA) was originally thought to be specific for bowel cancer, but further studies have shown it to be a nonspecific tumor-associated antigen which also may be elevated in a variety of benign conditions. In the gastrointestinal tract, the molecule, a glycoprotein with a molecular weight of 180,000, is concentrated in the glycocalyx of epithelial cells, from which it is released into the lumen of the bowel. In the presence of malignancy, CEA concentrations may be elevated in the blood and other body fluids. Serum levels of CEA above the normal concentration of 2.5 ng/mL are found in greater than 50 percent of neoplasms involving the colon, pancreas, stomach, lung, and breast. A variety of common nonmalignant conditions are associated with elevation of CEA, but typically not over 10 ng/mL. These include cigarette smoking, chronic pulmonary disease, alcoholic cirrhosis, hepatitis, and inflammatory bowel disease. CEA is not selective for cancer, and measurements of its levels should not be used in screening for the presence of malignant disease. However, serial measurements of CEA levels in patients with secreting malignancies can provide valuable information on the efficacy of treatment and the recurrence of disease. The possibility that early elevation of serum CEA can predict recurrence of bowel cancer soon enough to allow further surgical resection for cure is under study.

The second clinically useful oncofetal antigen is alpha fetoprotein (AFP), which is produced by the liver and gastrointestinal tract epithelium during gestation and which falls to levels less than 20 ng/mL after birth. Serum levels are elevated in 70 percent of patients with hepatocellular cancer, the majority of patients with nonseminomatous testicular cancer, and occasional patients with neoplasms of the gastrointestinal tract. As with CEA, the serum concentration of AFP may be elevated in benign conditions, especially in inflammatory disease of the liver. Its utility is in monitoring tumor activity, especially in the case of testicular tumors.

Elevation of either AFP or HCG is found in 80 to 90 percent of all nonseminomatous germ cell tumors of the testes. However, absence or normal levels of these biochemical markers of malignancy cannot be interpreted as proof that there is no tumor. Some tumors do not produce these marker molecules. Furthermore, because of tumor heterogeneity, it is possible for marker concentrations to fall in the presence of tumor, if a nonproducing subclone begins to grow preferentially. For this reason, recurrence of disease need not be accompanied by recurrence of elevated marker levels.

Other biochemical markers with clinical utility include calcitonin, with which familial medullary carcinoma of the thyroid can be detected in individuals who appear to be normal. Prostatic acid phosphatase levels are useful in determining the extent (stage) of prostatic cancer, and in monitoring the response to therapy.

There are many tumors which, because of increased cellular mass or loss of normal regulation, produce excessive quantities of polypeptides normally secreted into the circulation by the tissue of origin. Examples include the immunoglobulin molecules produced in multiple myeloma, and insulin or gastrin hypersecretion by islet cell tumors. In addition, tumors may secrete molecules which ordinarily are not produced in the tissue from which they are derived. This phenomenon has already been discussed in the description of the paraneoplastic syndromes, because in many cases these marker molecules have biologic activities which can produce clinical illness in the patient. In some cases of malignant disease, cultures of tumor cells have been found to secrete a variety of polypeptide hormones atypical of the tissue of origin. In addition, molecules related to normal hormones or to their precursor forms may be present in the patient's serum, in the absence of any demonstrable clinical effects. These observations provide evidence for the broad scope of genetic deregulation which may accompany the process of oncogene expression and carcinogenesis.

TABLE 78-10 Methods for clinical evaluation

I History
II Physical examination, including examination of oropharynx, Pap test, and proctoscopy
III Radiologic studies
- *A* Roentgenogram
- *B* Ultrasound
- *C* Computerized axial tomography
- *D* Angiography and lymphangiography
- *E* Nuclear medicine
- *F* Magnetic resonance imaging

IV Laboratory studies
- *A* Hematologic evaluation
- *B* Chemical tests of internal organ function
- *C* Tumor markers

V Pathologic examination of tissue

REFERENCES

CALABRESI P et al: *Medical Oncology: Basic Principles and Clinical Management of Cancer*. New York, Macmillan, 1985

DEVITA VT JR et al: *Cancer: Principles and Practices of Oncology*. Philadelphia, Lippincott, 1985

GROBSTEIN C et al: *Diet, Nutrition and Cancer*. Washington DC, National Academy Press, 1982

HOLLAND JF, FREI E: *Cancer Medicine*. Philadelphia, Lea & Febiger, 1982

RUBIN P: *Clinical Oncology for Medical Students and Physicians*. New York, American Cancer Society, 1983

SCHOTTENFELD D, FRAUMENI JF JR: *Cancer Epidemiology and Prevention*. Philadelphia, Saunders, 1982

79 PRINCIPLES OF CANCER THERAPY

VINCENT T. DeVITA, JR.

BIOLOGY OF TUMOR GROWTH

The principles of cancer therapy are based on our knowledge of the biology of tumor growth. The realization, two decades ago, that even small primary cancers shed viable tumor cells into the circulatory system as they grow in their primary site fundamentally altered the thinking about the likelihood of eradicating cancers using methods of local control alone and led to the development of systemic methods of treatment such as chemotherapy and biologic therapy. The cancer phenotype appears to be created by alterations in genetic mechanisms important in developmental biology. A family of highly conserved genes exists in the normal genome as proto-oncogenes, and alteration in their structure, or rearrangement of their location within the genome, appears to be responsible for deregulation of growth by production of abnormal proteins or abnormal quantities of proteins vital to cell growth. Although originally identified in defective oncogenic retroviruses, the existence of proto-oncogenes in normal tissue and oncogenes in many human cancers has been proved by DNA transfection experiments (see Chap. 59). Increased or abnormal expression has been shown in small cell lung cancer, colon and breast cancers, and lymphomas. The malignant phenotype is most likely the end result of the expression of the cascade of these genes. That the products of these genes are important in cell growth is underscored by their partial homology with some growth factors and receptors of growth factors. Experiments in transgenic mice (mice given single copies of oncogenes by insertion into the fertilized eggs) are providing powerful tools for identifying the cascade of genes activated for each histologic type of cancer and approaches for controlling the expression of these genes as a future means of preventing, diagnosing, or treating human cancer. For example, methylphosphonate derivatives of nucleosides complementary to the DNA of known oncogenes that can penetrate cell membranes have been shown to be capable of blocking the translation of messenger RNA and interfering with the function of these genes in vitro.

If proto-oncogenes are important regulatory elements in embryonic growth, it should not be surprising that deregulation could lead to abnormally sustained growth. In addition to uncontrolled growth, cancer cells migrate and kill largely by metastasizing and crowding out other vital organs. Several groups have cloned the genes that appear to regulate the capacity of cells to metastasize suggesting that like regulation of growth, the capacity to metastasize represents the deregulation of genetic mechanisms once responsible for normal cell migration. The capacity to metastasize appears to be related to the ability of a malignant cell to express receptors for the basement membrane protein laminen and of enzymes such as collagenases that are necessary to fix the cell to the basement membrane and to disrupt it, to allow the cell to escape from its primary site. In human studies, breast cancer cells have been shown to express large numbers of laminen receptors with a direct correlation between expression of laminen receptors and involvement of axillary lymph nodes. Developing the capacity to metastasize may be a relatively late step in the genetic cascade leading to clinically relevant cancers, a fact that would account for late metastases associated with some large tumors of certain histologic subtypes. Interfering with the ability of cancer cells to migrate has therapeutic implications. Blocking laminen receptors with laminen fragments in vitro has been shown to interfere with metastatic potential in vivo.

FIGURE 79-1 *The cell cycle. The gap terminology divides the cell cycle into phases M, G_1, S, and G_2. M is the period of cell division. G_1 is the period of normal cell metabolism but without replicative DNA synthesis; cells that stay in G_1 for long periods are often referred to as being in the G_0 phase. The S, or DNA synthetic, phase is the period of doubling of the DNA content; it is followed by the G_2, or tetraploid, phase, which precedes cell division. Normal and cancer cells have similar cycle times, in general: M, 0.5 to 1 h; G_1, 2 h to infinity; S, 6 to 24 h; G_2, 2 to 8 h.*

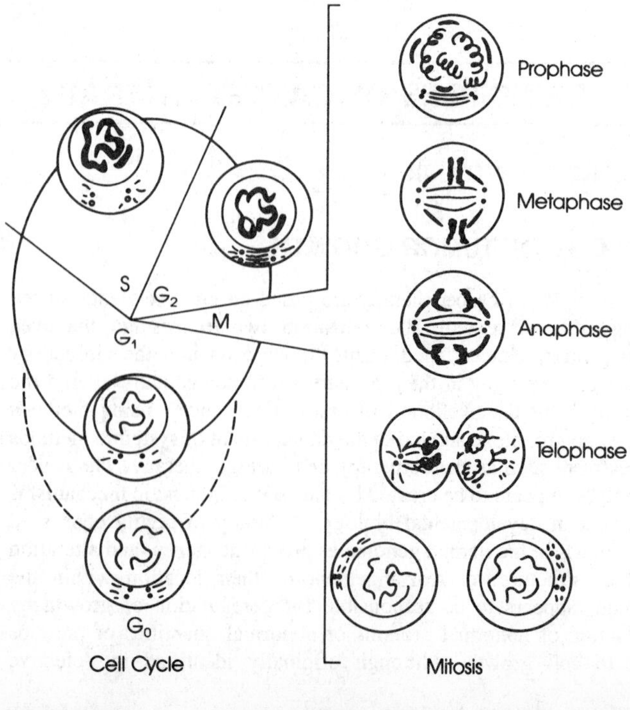

Once cells become malignant, the kinetics of their growth can be easily determined and are similar to the growth of normal tissues. There are three general classes of normal tissue with regard to growth characteristics: renewing (marrow and germ cells), expanding (liver, kidney, and endocrine glands), and static (neurons and striated muscle). For static tissues such as neurons, the cells live for the duration of the life of the host and are normally not replaced if lost. For expanding tissue, mitotic potential becomes apparent in cells only when cell loss takes place (trauma, surgical resection), and then the tissue is replenished. Adult cells of renewing populations have a finite, usually short, life span, and continued replacement from a stem cell pool normally takes place. As long as cell birth does not exceed cell loss, a neoplastic process is not evident even though, in a strict sense, cells of renewing tissue like bone marrow "metastasize." Regardless of the tissue of origin, the kinetics of growing populations of tumor cells resemble those of renewing populations of normal tissue. Growth characteristics of expanding tumor masses are best described as a Gompertzian function. As the mass increases, the growth is matched by exponential retardation of growth. The tumor doubling time (the time required for a given mass to double its volume) is a complex value influenced by the cell cycle time, the fraction of cells in the population undergoing cell division, and the rate of cell loss from the mass. The phases of a cell cycle are illustrated in Fig. 79-1. Cells not in cycle but viable and capable of entering cell division under proper circumstances are said to be in a resting phase (G_0). The fraction of cells in cycle in a given population (proliferative pool, growth fraction) determined by incorporation of tritiated thymidine into DNA (labeling index) markedly influences the growth of the tumor. Although cell cycle times are relatively constant in tumors of a given histologic type, considerable species differences exist in cycle times of normal and tumor tissue. For a given cycle time, a tumor with a high growth fraction will double faster than a tumor with a low growth fraction if cell loss (death, metastasis, shedding) is constant. High rates of cell loss account for long doubling times in tumors known to have high growth fractions. Cell loss begins early in the growth of a tumor. Even small (1 to 2 mm), apparently localized tumors can be assumed to shed cells into surrounding tissue (e.g., shedding from the surface of a colon cancer into the lumen of the bowel) or into lymphatics and/or the bloodstream. Cell loss may be due to departure of cells with active metastatic potential or to shedding of cells unable to produce viable colonies. The fact that some cancers can be cured by local treatment reaffirms the fact that many shed cells are unable to establish metastatic colonies for a variety of reasons, one of which may be that deregulation of the genes controlling migration may not yet have taken place.

CLONAL EVOLUTION OF CANCER The concept that cancer originates from a single transformed cell, or clone, is supported by cytogenetic studies of human neoplasms. The classic example is multiple myeloma, a malignant proliferation of antibody-secreting plasma cells, which is characterized by elevated levels of a single immunoglobulin molecule in blood or urine. In addition, tumor-specific abnormalities in chromosome structure have been demonstrated in more than 95 percent of all tumors. The first example described was the Philadelphia chromosome, which occurs in approximately 95 percent of patients with chronic myelogenous leukemia (CML) (Chap. 289). The abnormal chromosome 22 has been identified in hematopoietic precursor cells, in some cases, several years prior to the onset of overt leukemia. The clonal evolution of this disease is further supported by studies of X-inactivation mosaicism. Each cell of the female determines at the early stage in embryogenesis whether the paternal- or maternal-derived X chromosome will remain active or suppressed. The X-linked enzyme glucose 6-phosphate dehydrogenase (G6PD) has proved a useful marker for such studies of clonal origin because it is polymorphic in the black population. Women who are heterozygous at the G6PD locus for the common gene Gd^B and the variant Gd^A normally have two distinct cell populations reflected in their enzyme electrophoretic pattern. While the nonleukemic G6PD heterozygotes have both the A and B enzyme type in white blood cells, patients with chronic myelogenous leukemia demonstrate only one enzyme type in their leukemic granulocytic series, suggesting that the disorder originated from a single cell. Oncogenes have been located at some translocation sites including loci on chromosome 9 (c-*abl*) and 22 (c-*sis*) in CML and on chromosome 14 (c-*myc*) in Burkitt's lymphoma. In this instance, the c-*myc* gene product appears normal but is constitutively expressed because it has been brought under control of the promoter sequences of the heavy chain immunoglobulin gene on chromosome 14. Cytogenetic abnormalities in malignancies such as acute myelogenous leukemia appear to be predictors of response to treatment and to be characteristic of specific cell types. In patients who relapse after complete remission attained by chemotherapy, the original cytogenetic abnormality usually reappears but may be associated with additional translocations. In follicular lymphomas, biclonal tumors have been identified by examining the rearrangement of their immunoglobulin genes. Two other hereditary tumors, neurofibroma and trichoepithelioma, have demonstrated a double enzyme phenotype, indicating multicellular origin. These exceptions suggest that the somatic mutation theories of oncogenesis may not be valid for all neoplasms.

CHEMOTHERAPEUTIC AGENTS USED FOR THE SYSTEMIC TREATMENT OF CANCER

CYTOTOXIC DRUGS Radiotherapy and surgery offer ways of reducing the tumor mass in specific regions of the body amenable to surgical excision or high doses of radiotherapy. Neither is applicable to the destruction of the widely disseminated or circulating tumor cells characteristically present in most patients with cancer. The stimulus for the development of systemic treatment of cancer can be traced to the success in identifying and using antibiotics for bacterial infections and antiprotozoan drugs for malaria. Drug development for cancer began with the accidental identification of the lympholytic activity of mustard gases used in World Wars I and II. Nitrogen mustard, an antitumor drug, is a derivative of mustard gas and was used to treat lymphomas in the 1940s. Because all of the successfully treated patients subsequently relapsed, the initial success in the treatment of Hodgkin's disease and lymphocytic lymphomas with this drug was followed by an overwhelming disappointment and skepticism that cancer could be successfully treated by drugs. Further excitement was created with the identification of the effectiveness of the antimetabolite methotrexate, first used successfully against acute childhood leukemia and then in the treatment of choriocarcinoma. In that instance, remissions produced by the drug appeared permanent. The need for a standardized approach to the development of anticancer drugs was recognized in the 1950s. Since then, many synthetic drugs, fermentation, and plant products have been identified as possessing antitumor activity against rodent tumors. These compounds have been selected both by rational synthesis and random screening. Six major classes of antitumor agents: alkylating agents, antimetabolites, plant alkaloids, antitumor antibiotics, endocrine agents, and biologicals as well as some miscellaneous drugs are now available either commercially or in investigational clinical studies. These are shown with their acute and delayed toxicity in Tables 79-1 and 79-2. Detailed discussions of the mechanism of action and pharmacology of these agents are found in the references.

THE DEVELOPMENT OF DRUG RESISTANCE Limitations of cancer surgery are related to the tolerable removal of normal tissue. Resistance to radiotherapy is relative to the dose of radiation tolerated by the adjacent normal tissue. While toxicity to normal tissue limits the use of cancer drugs at very large doses, permanent resistance to a cancer drug is an inherent property of the cancer cell itself. Drug resistance can be viewed as either temporary or permanent. Temporary resistance refers to the inability of drugs to kill cancer cells because the cells are in the wrong phase of the cell cycle, are in pharmacologic sanctuaries such as the central nervous system or testis, where drugs may not penetrate in sufficient doses, or are in the center of a poorly vascularized tumor, unreachable by the active moiety of a drug. Permanent resistance refers to ways by which the organism alters a fundamental mechanism of activating, deactivating, or transporting a drug or of repairing damage caused by the agent. Methods of overcoming temporary drug resistance have been quite successful and include treating tumors when the number of cells is small and growing actively, introducing drugs into pharmacologic sanctuaries (such as intrathecal use of methotrexate in leukemia), and reducing tumor mass by surgery or radiotherapy to facilitate drug exposure of individual cells by reducing residual mass size, such as in ovarian cancer, where omentectomy and removal of all resectable tumor masses appears to influence subsequent capacity to respond to chemotherapy. Explanations based on cell kinetics are inadequate to explain the invariably inverse relationship between curability and cell number because in rodent tumors, resistance has been shown to develop over an increase in tumor cell number from 10^3 to 10^8. At these population sizes, cell cycle kinetics have been shown to remain constant. Also, in human adjuvant studies, the use of chemotherapy in the early stages of cancer has only been slightly more effective in curing patients than use of the same drugs in patients with advanced disease in spite of the favorable kinetics in micrometastases.

In 1979, Goldie and Coldman proposed that development of permanent resistance to cancer drugs occurred in a fashion similar to the development of resistance in bacteria to bacteriophage and was a spontaneous genetic effect. They proposed a model by which mutation to drug resistance was related to both the mutation rate and the cell number. There are several important implications of this model. First, because of the sharp relationship to cell number at any given mutation rate, the likelihood of curability decreases rapidly over small increases in tumor mass encompassing as few as six tumor doublings or a 2 log increase in cell number. If the mutation rate is 10^{-6} or greater, the likelihood of a singly or a doubly drug-resistant line appearing in a population of cells of less than 10^9, the usual level of clinically detectable tumor, is almost a certainty. These data suggest that the failure of drugs to cure many patients with advanced cancer is due to the presence of multiple permanently drug-resistant cell lines. If the mutation rate is in the range of 10^{-6}, the *absolute number* of resistant cell lines in a mass should be low enough, however, not to negatively influence the initial response to treatment. Complete remissions should be possible, but cell lines resistant to treatment would regrow and account for relapse in the phase of continued exposure to the effect of chemotherapy (Fig. 79-2). This is consistent with the clinical observations that initially responsive tumors will regrow during continued exposure to drug therapy in some cases. Also, the mutation rate is a stochastic phenomenon in bacteria and probably in the genetically unstable cancer cell. It may be different in tumors of the same type and stage, accounting for the variable responses and cure rates of uniformly staged and treated patients of the same histologic type.

The most persistent chemotherapeutic puzzle has been the unresponsiveness of tumors of visceral origin to chemotherapy when compared to childhood cancers and those of the hematologic system; in many cases, responses to chemotherapy are not observed in some visceral cancers at all. While at first this seemed inconsistent with the Goldie-Coldman hypothesis, there are several ways to account for this observation. First, these tumors may be inherently resistant to drugs as a result of the constant exposure of their normal tissue counterpart to the environment. They may possess detoxification mechanisms developed to protect them from exposure to natural toxins from which many anticancer drugs have been developed. Second, the mutation rate in tumors developed from these tissues

TABLE 79-1 Some commercially available anticancer drugs and hormones (dose-limiting effects are italicized)

Drug	Acute toxicity	Delayed toxicity*
Aminoglutethimide (Cytadren—Ciba)	Drowsiness; nausea; dizziness	Hypothyroidism (rare); bone marrow depression; fever; hypotension; masculinization
Asparaginase (Elspar–Merck)	*Nausea and vomiting; fever;* chills; headache; hypersensitivity, anaphylaxis; abdominal pain; hyperglycemia leading to coma	CNS depression or hyperexcitability; acute hemorrhagic pancreatitis; coagulation defects; thrombosis; renal damage; hepatic damage
Bleomycin (Blenoxane—Bristol)	*Nausea and vomiting; fever;* anaphylaxis and other allergic reactions	*Pneumonitis and pulmonary fibrosis; rash;* stomatitis; alopecia; Raynaud's phenomenon
Busulfan (Myeleran—Burroughs Wellcome)	*Nausea and vomiting;* rare diarrhea	*Bone marrow depression;* pulmonary infiltrates and fibrosis; hyperpigmentation; alopecia; gynecomastia; ovarian failure; azospermia; leukemia; chromosome aberrations; cataracts; Addisonian syndrome
Carmustine (BCNU; BiCNU—Bristol)	*Nausea and vomiting;* local phlebitis	*Delayed leukopenia and thrombocytopenia* (may be prolonged); pulmonary fibrosis (may be irreversible); delayed renal damage; gynecomastia; reversible liver damage
Chlorambucil (Leukeran—Burroughs Wellcome)	Minimal nausea at low doses	*Bone marrow depression;* pulmonary infiltrates and fibrosis; leukemia; hepatic toxicity; hallucinations
Cisplatin (cis-diamine-dichloroplatinum; cis-DDP; Platinol—Bristol)	*Nausea and vomiting;* anaphylactic reactions; fever; hemolytic-uremic syndrome; Raynaud's syndrome	*Renal damage;* bone marrow depression; ototoxicity; hemolysis; hypomagnesemia; peripheral neuropathy; hypocalcemia; hypokalemia; dementia
Cyclophosphamide (Cytoxan—Bristol; Neosar—Adria)	*Nausea and vomiting;* type 1 (anaphylactoid) hypersensitivity; facial burning with IV administration	*Bone marrow depression;* alopecia; hemorrhagic cystitis; sterility (may be temporary); pulmonary infiltrates and fibrosis; hyponatremia; leukemia; bladder cancer
Cytarabine HCl (cytosine arabinoside; Cytosar-U—Upjohn)	*Nausea and vomiting;* diarrhea; anaphylaxis	*Bone marrow depression;* conjunctivitis; megaloblastosis; oral ulceration; hepatic damage; fever; pulmonary edema and encephalopathy with high doses
Dacarbazine (DTIC; DIC; DTIC—Dome-Miles)	*Nausea and vomiting;* diarrhea; anaphylaxis; pain on administration; flulike syndrome	*Bone marrow depression;* alopecia; renal impairment; hepatic necrosis; facial flushing, paresthesia; photosensitivity
Dactinomycin (actinomycin D; Cosmegen—Merck)	*Nausea and vomiting;* diarrhea; local reaction and phlebitis; anaphylactoid reaction	*Stomatitis; oral ulceration; bone marrow depression;* alopecia; folliculitis; dermatitis in previously irradiated areas
Daunorubicin (daunomycin; Cerubidine—Ives)	*Nausea and vomiting;* diarrhea; red urine (not hematuria); severe local tissue damage and necrosis on extravasation; transient (EKG changes); anaphylactoid reaction	*Bone marrow depression; cardiotoxicity* (may be irreversible); alopecia; stomatitis; anorexia; diarrhea; fever and chills
Doxorubicin (Adriamycin—Adria)	*Nausea and vomiting;* red urine (not hematuria); severe local tissue damage and necrosis on extravasation; diarrhea; transient ECG changes; ventricular arrhythmia; anaphylactoid reaction	*Bone marrow depression; cardiotoxicity* (may be irreversible, but may be decreased by weekly schedule); alopecia; stomatitis; anorexia; diarrhea, fever; chills; conjunctivitis
Estramustine phosphate sodium (estracyt; Emcyt—Roche)	*Nausea and vomiting;* diarrhea	Mild gynecomastia; increased frequency of vascular accidents; myelosuppression (uncommon); edema dyspnea; pulmonary infiltrates and fibrosis; leukemia
Etoposide (VP16-213; Vepesid—Bristol)	*Nausea and vomiting;* diarrhea; fever	*Bone marrow depression;* alopecia; peripheral neuropathy; allergic reactions; hepatic damage
Floxuridine (FUDR—Roche)	*Nausea and vomiting*; diarrhea	*Oral and gastrointestinal ulceration; bone marrow depression;* alopecia; dermatitis
Fluorouracil (5-FU; Fluorouracil—Roche; Adrucil—Adria)	*Nausea and vomiting;* diarrhea; hypersensitivity reaction	*Oral and gastrointestinal ulcers; bone marrow depression;* neurologic defects, usually cerebellar; alopecia
Hydroxyurea (Hydrea—Squibb)	*Nausea and vomiting;* allergic reactions to tartrazine dye	*Bone marrow depression;* stomatitis; dysuria; alopecia; rare neurologic disturbances
Lomustine (CCNU; Cee-NU—Bristol)	*Nausea and vomiting*	*Delayed (4 to 6 weeks) leukopenia and thrombocytopenia* (may be prolonged); transient elevation of transaminase activity; neurologic reactions; pulmonary fibrosis
Mechlorethamine (nitrogen mustard; HN2; Mustargen— Merck)	*Nausea and vomiting;* local reaction phlebitis	*Bone marrow depression;* alopecia; diarrhea; oral ulcers; pulmonary infiltrates and fibrosis; leukemia
Melphalan (Allkeran—Burroughs Wellcome)	Mild nausea; hypersensitivity reactions	*Bone marrow depression* (especially platelets); pulmonary infiltrates and fibrosis; leukemia
Mercaptopurine (6-MP; Purinethol—Burroughs Wellcome)	*Nausea and vomiting;* diarrhea	*Bone marrow depression; cholestasis and rarely hepatic necrosis; oral and intestinal ulcers;* pancreatitis; allopurinol may increase overall toxicity
Methotrexate (MTX; Methotrexate—Lederle; Mexate—Bristol; Folex—Adria)	*Nausea and vomiting;* diarrhea; fever; anaphylaxis	*Oral and gastrointestinal ulceration* (perforation may occur); *bone marrow depression;* hepatic toxicity including cirrhosis and acute hepatic necrosis; renal toxicity; pulmonary infiltrates and fibrosis; osteoporosis; chills, fever; alopecia; depigmentation; infertility; menstrual dysfunction; encephalopathy and anaphylactoid reactions with high doses

TABLE 79-1 Some commercially available anticancer drugs and hormones (dose-limiting effects are italicized) *(continued)*

Drug	Acute toxicity	Delayed toxicity*
Mitomycin (Mutamycin—Bristol)	*Nausea and vomiting;* local reaction if extravasation; fever; hemolytic-uremic syndrome	*Bone marrow depression* (cumulative); stomatitis; alopecia; pulmonary fibrosis; hepatotoxicity; renal toxicity
Mitotane (o, p′-DDD; Lysodren—Bristol)	*Nausea and vomiting;* diarrhea	*CNS depression;* rash; visual disturbances; adrenal insufficiency; brain damage with long-term high dosage; hematuria; hemorrhagic cystitis; albuminuria; hypertension; orthostatic hypotension; cataracts
Plicamycin (Mithracin—Miles)	*Nausea and vomiting;* diarrhea; fever	*Hemorrhagic diathesis; bone marrow depression* (thrombocytopenia); coagulation abnormalities; hepatic damage; hypocalcemia and hypokalemia; stomatitis; renal damage
Procarbazine HCl (Matulane—Roche)	*Nausea and vomiting;* CNS depression; Antabuse-like effect with alcohol	*Bone marrow depression;* stomatitis; peripheral neuropathy; pneumonitis; leukemia
Streptozocin (streptozotocin; Zanosar—Upjohn)	*Nausea and vomiting;* local pain; chills and fever	*Renal damage;* hypoglycemia; hyperglycemia; liver damage; diarrhea; bone marrow depression (uncommon); fever; eosinophilia
Tamoxifen citrate (Nolvadex—Stuart)	*Nausea and vomiting*; hot flashes; transient increased bone or tumor pain	Vaginal bleeding and discharge; rash; hypercalcemia; thrombocytopenia; peripheral edema; depression; dizziness; headache; decreased visual acuity; corneal changes; retinopathy
Thioguanine (6-TG; Tabloid Brand Thioguanine—Burroughs Wellcome)	*Occasional nausea and vomiting*	*Bone marrow depression;* hepatic damage; stomatitis
Thiotepa (triethylene-thiophosphoramide; Thiotepa—Lederle)	*Nausea and vomiting;* local pain	*Bone marrow depression;* menstrual dysfunction; interference with spermatogenesis; pulmonary infiltrates and fibrosis; leukemia
Vinblastine sulfate (Velban—Lilly)	*Nausea and vomiting;* local reaction and phlebitis with extravasation	*Bone marrow depression;* alopecia; stomatitis; loss of deep tendon reflexes; jaw pain; muscle pain; paralytic ileus; inappropriate antidiuretic hormone (ADH) secretion
Vincristine sulfate (Oncovin—Lilly)	Local reaction with extravasation	*Peripheral neuropathy;* alopecia; mild bone marrow depression; constipation; paralytic ileus; inappropriate ADH secretion; hepatic damage; jaw pain

* *Cutaneous reactions (sometimes severe), hyperpigmentation, and ocular toxicity have been reported with virtually all nonhormonal anticancer drugs.*
SOURCE: *Adopted from* The Medical Letter *(Feb. 15, 1985), with permission.*

may also be higher due to the exposure to potential carcinogens such as those in cigarette smoke and other chemicals. Third, the impression that tumors of 1 cm in size have gone through 30 doublings to reach 10^9 cells as shown below in Fig. 79-3 is based on the assumption of exponential growth, a rare event in both animal and human tumors. Cell loss approaches 90 percent in some well-studied human visceral malignancies effectively requiring as many as 1200 doublings to reach 10^9 cells. If the likelihood of a mutation to resistance is related to the number of generation cycles, then such tumors could be largely composed of resistant cell lines at the time of diagnosis, at which time they are also unresponsive to multiple chemotherapeutic agents. This is consistent with the clinical data on the doubling times of some highly drug-resistant human cancers, such as colon cancer, which have been reported to be about 2 years.

The clinical implications of the Goldie-Coldman hypothesis are profound. First, it is the only reasonable explanation for the effectiveness of combination chemotherapy and the invariably inverse relationship between cell number and curability. Second, it underscores the need to treat with drugs early in the natural history of the disease. Third, it strongly suggests that delays in treatment as short as a few weeks to a month may markedly alter tumor curability by drugs. Such an effect has been suggested in one human breast cancer adjuvant drug trial where a delay of chemotherapy by 1 month negatively influenced the outcome of the study. It also provides an explanation for the failure of adjuvant chemotherapy to be as effective as initially expected since in most circumstances, the sum total of multiple deposits of micrometastases very likely exceeds 10^9 cells.

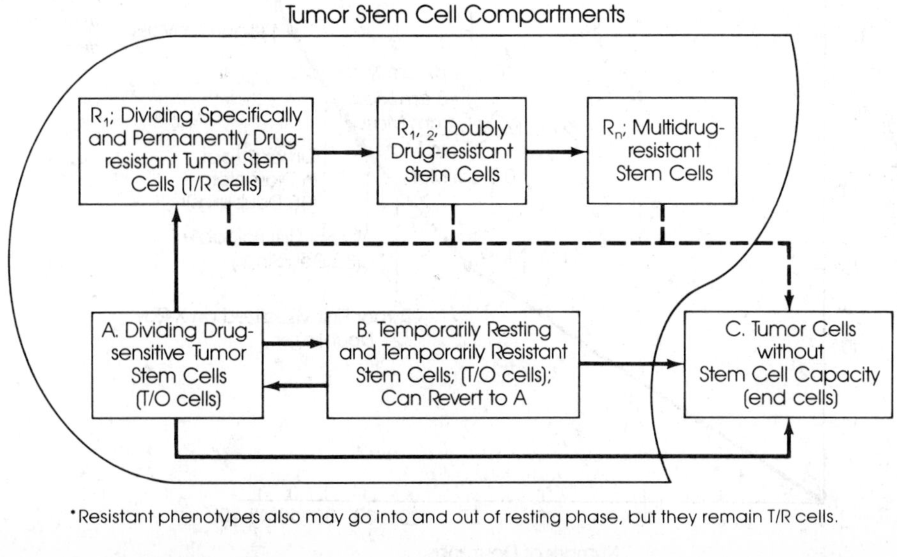

FIGURE 79-2 *Various compartments and flow between compartments in a hypothetical tumor mass.*

TABLE 79-2 Investigational drugs

Drug	Acute toxicity	Delayed toxicity
Amsacrine (AMSA—Bristol, Parke-Davis)	Nausea and vomiting; diarrhea; pain or phlebitis on infusion	Bone marrow depression; hepatic injury; convulsions; stomatitis; ventricular fibrillation; alopecia
Azacitidine (Mylosar—Upjohn)	Nausea and vomiting; diarrhea; fever	Leukopenia (may be prolonged); thrombocytopenia; hepatic damage; muscle pain and weakness; bone marrow depression; possibly cardiotoxicity
Bisantrene (ADC, ADAH—Lederle)	Nausea and vomiting; hypotension; flulike illness; fever; phlebitis	Leukopenia; thrombocytopenia
Deoxycoformycin (DCF)		Nephrotoxicity
Flutamide (Eulexin—Schering)	Nausea	Gynecomastia; impotence
*Hexamethylmelamine (HMM)	Nausea and vomiting	Bone marrow depression; CNS depression; peripheral neuritis; visual hallucinations
Ifosfamide (Ifex—Mead Johnson)	Nausea and vomiting	Bone marrow depression; hemorrhagic cystitis; alopecia; sterility (may be temporary)
Interferon (Roferon-A—Roche; Intron-A—Schering; Wellferon—Burroughs Wellcome)	Fever; chills, myalgias; fatigue; hypotension	Bone marrow depression; anorexia; renal damage; hepatic damage
*Leuprolide (LH-releasing hormone analogue—Lupron-Abbott)	Transient increase in bone pain; hot flashes	Impotence; gynecomastia
Mitobronitol (Myelobromol—Sinclair, UK)	Gastrointestinal disturbances	Bone marrow depression; alopecia
Mitolactol	Mild nausea	Bone marrow depression
*Mitoxantrone HCL (DHAD; Novantrone—Lederle)	Green pigment in urine, green sclera; nausea	Bone marrow depression; cardiotoxicity; alopecia, white hair
Tegafur (ftorafur—Mead Johnson)	Nausea and vomiting; CNS symptoms including dizziness and lethargy	Stomatitis; bone marrow depression; alopecia; dermatitis
*Teniposide (VM-26—Bristol)	Nausea and vomiting; diarrhea; phlebitis; anaphylactoid symptoms	Bone marrow depression; alopecia; peripheral neuropathy
*Vindesine sulfate (Eldisine—Lilly)	Local reaction if extravasation; fever; nausea and vomiting; diarrhea	Bone marrow depression; alopecia; peripheral neuropathy; jaw pain

* *Commercially available in Canada.*
SOURCE: *Adopted from* The Medical Letter *(Feb. 15, 1985), with permission.*

Many mechanisms of specific permanent resistance to available chemotherapeutic agents have been identified, and most occur on a genetic basis demonstrated by gene transfer experiments. These are listed in Table 79-3. Two require special mention. Pleiotropic resistance, development of resistance to multiple different classes of antitumor agents without prior exposure, has been described in rodent and human cancers. In a single step, pleiotropic resistance produces cross-resistance to most of the best and most available anticancer agents, the large complex plant- and microbial-derived products. It is often associated with the appearance of a surface glycoprotein, 170,000 daltons in size, the quantity of which is related to the degree of resistance. The presence of this protein may prove to be a useful way of identifying such lines before therapy is initiated. Pleiotropic resistance appears to be associated with defective drug accumulation due to increased drug efflux. A wide variety of drugs, including many which themselves do not possess any antitumor activity, have been demonstrated in various experimental systems to potentiate cytotoxic effects of certain chemotherapeutic drugs (Table 79-4). The calcium antagonists, calmodulin inhibitors, polyene antibiotics, triparonal analogues, and antiarrhythmic agents all appear to exert their effect, at least in part, by increasing the net accumulation of antineoplastic drugs in resistant tumor cells. Since pleiotropic drug

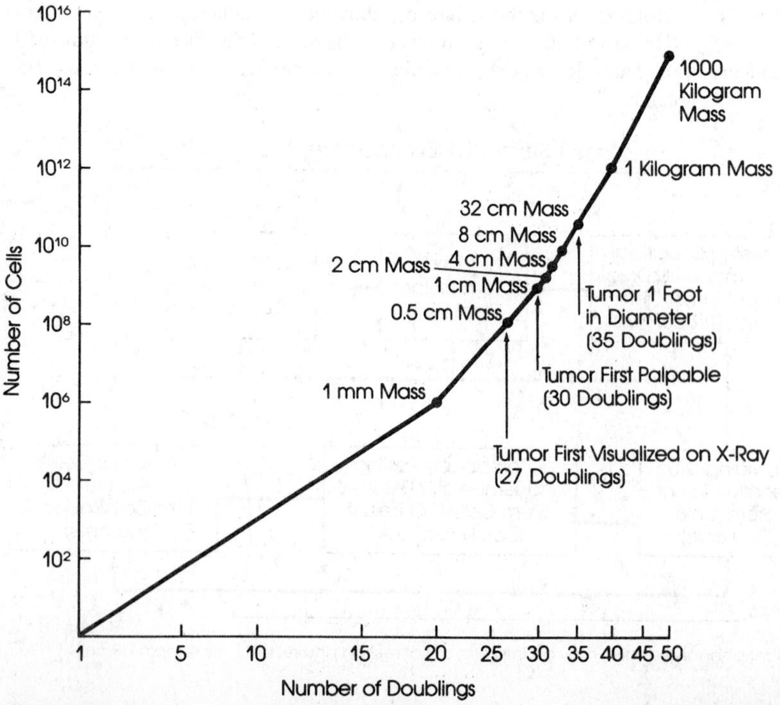

FIGURE 79-3 *A schematic representation of the life cycle of a human tumor. Number of cells present in the body is shown on the ordinate with number of population doublings on the abscissa. Clinical phenomena are related to expected size of tumor mass on plotted line. Most tumors have completed at least two-thirds of their growth (32 doublings) at the time of diagnosis of a 1-cm mass.*

TABLE 79-3 Mechanisms of resistance to cytotoxic drugs

General mechanism	Drug	Specific alteration
Defective transport	Methotrexate Melphalan Mechlorethamine	Decreased carrier-mediated uptake
	Cytarabine	Decreased membrane nucleoside binding sites
Defective metabolism to active species	Cytarabine	Decreased deoxycytidine kinase activity
	5-Azacitidine	Decreased uridine-cytidine kinase activity
	5-Fluorouracil	Decreased uridine kinase activity, decreased orotic acid phosphoribosyltransferase, decreased uridine phosphorylase
	6-Mercaptopurine 6-Thioguanine	Decreased HGPRT activity
	Methotrexate	Defection polyglutamation
	Doxorubicin	Decreased P_{450} or flavin reductase
Increased drug inactivation	6-Mercaptopurine 6-Thioguanine	Increased membrane alkaline phosphatase
	Cytarabine	Increased cytidine deaminase activity
	Alkylators	Increased intracellular glutathione or metallothioneine
Altered DNA repair	Alkylators Cisplatin Doxorubicin	Increased efficiency of excision of damaged bases and/or ligation of excised segment
Gene amplification with increased target protein	Cadmium	Increase in metallothioneine gene copy number
	N-Phosphonacetyl-L-aspartic acid	Increase in aspartate transcarbamylase gene copy number
	Methotrexate	Increase in DHFR gene copy number
	5-Fluorouracil	? Increase in thymidylate synthetase gene copy number
	Pentostatin	? Increase in adenosine deaminase gene copy number
Altered targets	Methotrexate	Altered DHFR
	Vincristine	Altered tubulin
	5-Fluorouracil	Altered thymidylate synthetase
	Hydroxyurea	Altered ribonucleotide reductase
	Steroids	Altered steroid receptor Altered steroid receptor complex binding to DNA
Altered nucleotide pools	Cytarabine 5-Fluorouracil	Increased intracellular CTP and dCTP pools
Salvage pathways	Methotrexate	Increased purine salvage
	5-Fluorouracil	Increased thymidine kinase activity
Pleiotropic drug resistance	Doxorubicin Vinca alkaloids	Defective drug accumulation due to increased energy-dependent efflux
	Dactinomycin Other natural products	? Specific membrane glycoprotein markers

resistance is associated with a decreased accumulation of antineoplastic drugs, the agents which increase cellular drug levels are attractive candidates for clinical trials aimed at reversing primary acquired resistance as well as the broad cross-resistance frequently observed in cancer patients who have relapsed.

Finally, gene amplification has been shown to be associated with drug resistance. This plasticity of the human genome appears to occur as a result of the reduplication of transcription if it is halted or slowed down and can be induced by agents that slow DNA synthesis such as low doses of alkylating agents and x-irradiation. Thus, marginally effective chemotherapeutic agents and/or exposure to radiation therapy may induce resistance to drugs like methotrexate without prior exposure to the drug, a factor which is influencing the design sequence of these cancer treatments. The realization that permanent specific drug resistance is a spontaneous event that can be studied and possibly circumvented is the working hypothesis for a new generation of clinical investigations in cancer therapy which emphasize early chemotherapy, in some cases *prior to* surgery (head and neck, and breast cancers), to determine if the tumor is inherently sensitive, and shorter and more intensive adjuvant chemotherapy courses to maximize the therapeutic effect while minimizing the exposure of surviving cancer cells to chemotherapeutic agents that might increase their mutation rate.

DIFFERENTIATING AGENTS There is increasing evidence that in some cases, cancers such as the leukemias represent an arrest in development. Drugs such as the polar planar compound hexamethylbisacetamide, retinoid derivatives, and biologicals such as interferon have been shown to cause leukemia cells to differentiate in vitro, and in a few reports, the retinoid 13-*cis*-retinoic acid has been shown to cause some differentiation in human acute myelogenous leukemia. Two drugs, dimethylformamide and hexamethylbisacetamide, developed only because of their ability to differentiate cells rather than their cytotoxicity, have reached clinical trials.

ENDOCRINE THERAPY Tumors such as those originating in the prostate and uterine endometrium or lymphoid tissue may respond to hormonal manipulation. The mechanism of interaction of hormones and receptors has been carefully studied. Hormones bind to receptors in the cytoplasm and nucleus and sterically alter the shape of the receptor protein itself, which interacts with DNA and is responsible for initiating specific messenger RNA and protein synthesis. Following this interaction, cytoplasmic receptor concentration is restored and the cycle can be repeated. The adrenal corticosteroids are unique among the steroid hormones because they exert some antitumor effect in tissues not normally considered to be endocrine organs, such as the malignant cells in acute lymphatic leukemia. Receptors for corticosteroids have been identified in the cytosol of leukemic cells which, along with other nonspecific effects of the corticosteroids, probably explains their antitumor action. Receptors also exist for progesterones and androgens.

TABLE 79-4 Modulation of drug resistance

Drugs	Antineoplastic* drugs affected	Proposed mechanism of increased cytotoxicity
Calcium antagonists Verapamil Nifedipine Nitrendipine Caroverine	VCR, DNR, ADR	Increased accumulation by blocking efflux
Calmodulin inhibitors Prenylamine Trifluoroperazine Clomipramine	VCR, DNR ADR	Same as above
Amphotericin Tween 80 Perhexiline maleate	ADR, ACT-D, BCNU ADR ADR	Alterations in lipid composition of plasma membrane leading to increased accumulation
Triparanol analogues Tamoxifen	ADR	Increased drug accumulation
Antiarrhythmic drugs Quinidine	ADR, VCR	Increased drug accumulation
Antihypertensive Reserpine	ADR	Increased drug accumulation
Thiol depleter Buthionine sulfoximine	L-PAM, PLAT, ADR	Drug inactivation, free radical metabolism, protection/repair of DNA

* *Abbreviations: VCR, vincristine; DNR, daunorubicin; ADR, adriamycin; L-PAM, melphalan; PLAT, cisplatin. BCNU, 1,3 bis(2 chloroethyl)1-nitrosourea; ACT-D, actinomycin-D.*

Although prostate and uterine fundal cancers have been shown to possess binding proteins for their respective hormones, the correlation between the frequency and quantity of binding proteins and the response to hormonal therapy has been most carefully studied in breast cancer. While hormones are effective alone, they are being used increasingly with other modalities of therapy either to synchronize tumor cells and increase their vulnerability to cytotoxic drugs (in breast cancer) or as noncytotoxic components of combination drug programs (in leukemias, lymphomas, breast and prostate cancers). Agonists of hypothalamic neuropeptides have been used to down-regulate receptors on hormone-responsive tissues as a new approach to hormone blockade, sometimes in combination with hormone antagonists. In prostate cancer, this has produced impressive early clinical results without the cardiovascular toxicity associated with estrogen use.

BIOLOGICALS AND CANCER THERAPY Since the host's immunologic system may be involved in the control of malignant processes, immunologic approaches to cancer treatment have been under investigation for over two decades. Manipulation of the exquisite information available on the complex network of the immune system holds considerable promise for the development and use of very specific biologicals as an integral part of the systemic approach for the treatment of cancer. Since the development of the hybridoma technique in 1975, large quantities of monoclonal antibodies have become available that react to tumor-associated antigens on tumors such as colon, lung, pancreas, and melanoma, and leukemias and lymphomas. Clinical studies are in progress to evaluate their role used alone when they are complementing fixing antibodies; coupled with toxins, such as a chain of the chemical toxin ricin or *Pseudomonas* toxin; or coupled with radioisotopes, especially alpha particle emitters. Early clinical studies have shown that monoclonal antibodies can produce temporary regressions in leukemias and lymphomas. Recombinant DNA techniques have also led to the cloning of genes for potent lymphokines, and large quantities of purified biologicals once only available in minute amounts for laboratory studies are now available for clinical trials. These include T-cell growth factor (interleukin 2), tumor necrosis factor, and interferon. In experimental systems, biologicals work best when the tumor burden is small, and thus their use after surgery or radiotherapy or after chemotherapy-induced remissions is an important investigational area. Antitumor agents are immunosuppressive, but as patients recover from their effects, their immunologic reactivity may be enhanced temporarily, and this could be the optimal time for biologic therapy.

Purified interleukin 2 (IL 2) has been used to amplify and activate a population of lymphocytes referred to as LAK cells (lymphokine-activated killer cells) which differ from natural killer cells by virtue of their ability to kill fresh autologous tumor cells from both rodents and humans regardless of their immunogenicity. Combinations of IL 2 and LAK cells have produced cures in well-controlled rodent experiments in animals with metastatic tumors. Investigational trials in humans using large doses of recombinant IL 2 and LAK cells concomitantly have produced complete and partial remissions in patients with advanced metastatic melanoma, colon cancer, and renal and lung cancers, and this holds promise as a new form of biologic therapy in adjuvant studies for earlier stages of these diseases.

Local nonspecific immunotherapy is sometimes useful and utilizes delayed hypersensitivity reactions at the site of skin tumors. Bacillus Calmette-Guérin (BCG) injections into skin nodules of patients with recurrent breast cancer or melanoma can be an effective way of controlling local disease although not often used. Delayed hypersensitivity has been produced in patients by cutaneous application of dinitrochlorobenzene. Subsequent application of this substance in superficial epidermoid and basal cell carcinomas has a cure rate equal to topical chemotherapy with 5-fluorouracil. The macrophage plays an important role as a sensor cell in the modulation of the immunologic response to antigenic tumors in rodents. Studies aimed at stimulating macrophages are in progress with levamisole, an antiprotozoan drug that improves depressed lymphocyte function by stimulating macrophages. Coupled with 5-fluorouracil, levamisole has significantly reduced the relapse rate and improved survival in one adjuvant program in colon cancer.

INFLUENCE OF TUMOR MASS ON CURABILITY AND DOSE-RESPONSE RELATIONSHIPS

The growth and size of a tumor are generally measured in order of magnitude or logs. A human tumor, when first diagnosed as, for example, a 1.0-cm mass, contains approximately 1 billion cancer cells, whereas 10^{12} cells has been estimated to represent a lethal body burden for some malignancies. Tumor mass is an important variable for all modalities of treatment.

SURGERY The mass of the primary tumor is directly correlated with the degree of local invasion, and, in turn, the degree of local invasion is a constant predictor of the likelihood of metastases in most malignancies especially in colon and breast cancer and malignant melanoma. Within a given histologic subset of each cancer, tumor mass exerts a profound effect on curability by surgery alone.

DOSE RESPONSE AND RADIATION THERAPY For clinical purposes, a dose-response curve for radiotherapy can be constructed for specific tumors in which local tumor control is plotted as a function of dose. For a specific type of cancer, the larger the mass, the less the likelihood of destroying the tumor without severe damage to normal surrounding tissues. The radiation dose-response curve is illustrated in Fig. 79-4. The fraction of surviving cells is plotted on a log scale against radiation dose. The slope of the exponential portion of the curve, usually referred to as D_0 (mean lethal dose) is a standard reference point. D_0 is the dose required to place one inactivating event in each pertinent biologic entity. The more radiosensitive the cell, the steeper the curve. Owing to the random nature of these energy deposits, some energy will be deposited in a cell which has already been destroyed, while some will escape altogether. According to the Poisson distribution, instead of destroying all the cells, the D_0 destroys only 63 percent of them. Therefore, the dose required to reduce the number of cells in a population to 37 percent of the original number is the D_{37}, which is an index of radiosensitivity. For most cells, this value lies between 0.80 and 2 Gy (80 and 200 rad). The surviving fraction after two mean lethal doses is 37 $\times$ 37 percent or 13.7 percent, and after three mean lethal doses, it is 5.1 percent, etc. In practice, the logarithmic curve is not exactly a straight line. There is a small shoulder to overcome before the curve is exponential. With a strictly exponential curve, $D_0 = D_{37}$. The shoulder on the curve reflects doses below which the cell can repair radiation-induced damage. The dose at which the curve becomes exponential (D_q) is the threshold dose. Repair of radiation-induced damage can take place within 2 h. The identification of D_q, D_0, D_{37} repair time, and mechanisms of repair has important implications in clinical dose fractionation, particularly in studies combining drugs with radiation therapy.

DOSE RESPONSE AND CHEMOTHERAPY When chemotherapy was first developed, it was reserved in the main for advanced cases, after surgery and radiation therapy had failed. Most chemotherapy is able to reduce cell numbers by one to 3 logs; this is capable of producing only minimal palliation in a patient with 10^{12} tumor cells due in part to the relatively large number of cancer cells out of cell cycle less vulnerable to drugs that kill by virtue of interfering with cell growth or division. Total eradication of tumor cells is therefore not possible in advanced metastatic cancer in all but the most drug-sensitive malignancies. The cytotoxic action of anticancer agents is defined by first-order kinetics; they kill a constant fraction of cells rather than a constant number. A course of therapy with a capacity to kill 10^3 tumor cells will reduce a tumor with 10^{10} cells to 10^7, or a neoplasm of 10^5 to 10^2 cells. The majority of single drugs have a limited cell kill potential.

The implication of the fractional killing effect is that to effectively eradicate a drug-sensitive tumor population, it is necessary either to increase the dose of drug(s) within limits tolerable to the host or to begin treatment when the number of cells is sufficiently small to allow tumor destruction at reasonably tolerated doses. The killing effect of cancer chemotherapeutic agents has a definite selectivity for cancer cells over normal cells. The clinical counterpart of animal experiments showing a markedly increased sensitivity to drugs of tumor cells over normal cells can be inferred from the dramatic antitumor effects noted in some patients with drug-sensitive tumors without permanent damage to the patients' bone marrow or gastrointestinal tract.

Conceptually, tumor cells can be divided into three distinct kinetic compartments, each with its particular significance in relation to the effectiveness of chemotherapy (Fig. 79-2). First, there is the fraction of tumor cells sensitive to chemotherapy and actively growing that is most vulnerable to drug treatment. Second, there is a population of cells which are temporarily nondividing but, nevertheless, have the capability of returning to a replicative stage. In terms of cell cycle kinetics, these cells are in an extended G_1 or G_0 phase and are considerably less sensitive to antitumor agents, particularly the cell cycle phase–specific antimetabolites, even though this type of resistance may be temporary. Then there is a compartment of cells that have permanently lost proliferative capacity but which still contribute to the estimated mass of the tumor at the bedside until they die and are absorbed. The dose-response curves for both toxicity and therapeutic effect for cancer drugs are steep. In some rodent experiments, a 20 percent reduction in dose leads to a 50 percent reduction in cure rate. The observation has been extended to doses of single drugs within effective drug combinations. Loss of the curative effect of a combination of drugs is seen with modification of the most effective agent in the combination to accommodate the toxicity of other drugs used with it. Dose rate refers to the administration of a given amount of a drug over a finite time. Since most chemotherapeutic agents are toxic to dividing cells, intervals between treatment cycles are dictated by the recovery of normal renewing tissue pools, most often the bone marrow, which takes approximately 18 to 28 days in humans. Prolonged intervals between cycles of treatment, even if drugs are given at full doses, reduces the dose rate and may allow for both regrowth of tumors and development of permanent resistance. This has been clearly demonstrated in animal models and in the clinic in the treatment of acute myelogenous leukemia, Hodgkin's disease, and small cell lung cancer. Since the effect of most drug treatment programs is reported on the basis of a fixed dose rate, ad hoc alterations of the use of specific treatment regimens in the clinic for purposes of convenience, an all too common event, very likely reduce the reported good effects of the treatment program.

TREATMENT OF LOCALIZED OR REGIONAL TUMOR

SURGICAL THERAPY Surgery is still considered the primary treatment for most early cancers. However, many tumors are operable but not fully resectable, and some that appear resectable (control of the tumor and lymph node compartments) have micrometastatic disease outside the tumor field. This point can best be illustrated using colon and breast carcinoma as examples. Lymph nodes involved in breast cancer (stage II) and colon cancer (Duke's C) serve as indicators of metastatic potential and are associated with low 5-year survivals without further treatment. Increasingly radical surgery in both these cancers has not been demonstrated to provide additional benefit, but minimal surgical procedures, such as lumpectomy with radiotherapy to the breast, give results as good as those attained with radical or modified radical mastectomy. As surgery has become less radical, the complexity of the procedures has sometimes increased, such as in limb-sparing surgery for extremity sarcomas.

LASER SURGERY Laser surgery is another way of excising benign or malignant lesions. The biologic effects of laser surgery in general and the commonly used CO_2 laser surgery in particular are unique. The wavelength of the CO_2 laser is readily absorbed by all biologic structures with very little scatter. When focused appropriately, the incision may be quite fine with minimal damage to adjacent tissue. Combined with an operating microscope, laser surgery is a precise technique. Biologic material is vaporized rather than cauterized. Blood vessels and lymphatics up to 0.5 mm are sealed during treatment. These features minimize trauma, facilitate healing, and shorten hospital stays. The chief drawbacks to laser surgery are the inability to cauterize larger vessels and destroy larger regions of tissue. Carbon dioxide laser surgery is used in cancers of the head and neck region and in the tracheobronchial tube, where its controlled depth of penetration is useful in avoiding perforation. It is under evaluation in the treatment of brain tumors. No claims have been made for improved survival, but significant palliation can be achieved in obstructing tracheobronchial and esophageal lesions treated through a rigid endoscope. It may also be more advantageous than cold knife surgery in patients with blood dyscrasias and in seriously ill patients. Complications are serious heat damage to patients and operating personnel and eye damage from reflected light, both of which can be easily avoided.

Surgeons also perform nontherapeutic procedures in newly diagnosed patients for staging purposes only, such as laparotomy in Hodgkin's disease and other lymphomas (see Chap. 294) and second-look procedures in ovarian and colon cancer. Indications for use of these procedures vary with treatment options, and they should never be performed by the surgeon in vacuo, without prior consultation with the physician, or team of physicians, who will eventually be called upon to provide the definitive treatment.

Indications for more mutilating radical surgical procedures such as hemicorporectomy, pelvic exenteration, and radical head and neck surgery have diminished as methods of combining treatments have proved successful. They are offered to patients with locally advanced primary tumors or locally recurrent tumors for which no other means of controlling the regional tumor or systemic treatment is available. If the patient understands fully the degree of mutilation involved, a careful search reveals no metastases, the risk of recurrent disease is not unreasonably great, and the operation is technically feasible, then the risks of mortality must be weighed against the chance for controlling the tumor. These are very individual decisions shared by the patient, the family, and the physician. Significant advances in reconstructive surgery of the head, neck, and pelvic regions have been made and the greater availability of more acceptable prostheses may make these radical procedures more acceptable.

FIGURE 79-4 *Radiation dose-response curve (see text).*

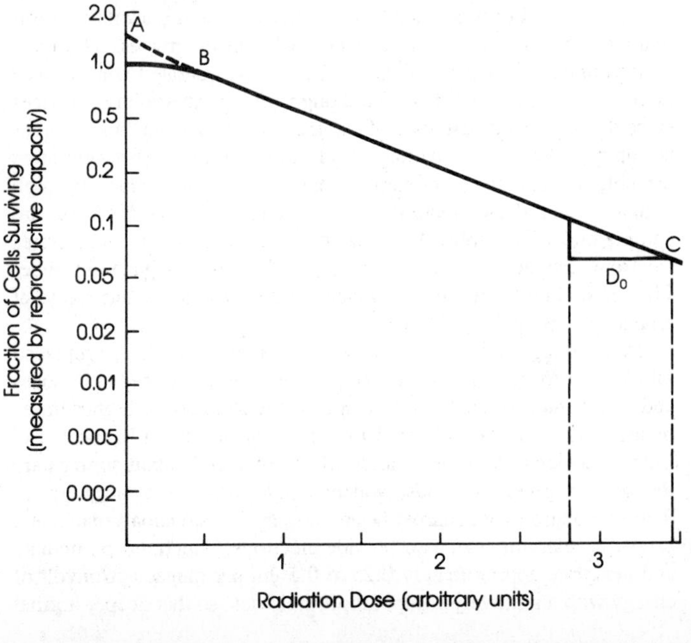

RADIATION THERAPY Radiation therapy is another regional form of treatment used for the control of localized cancers. The ideal in radiation therapy of malignant disease is achieved when the tumor is completely eradicated and the surrounding normal tissues in the treated volume show little or no evidence of structural or functional injury. The important factor in successful treatment is the difference in radiosensitivity of neoplastic and normal cells. The difference depends on the capacity for intracellular repair of normal and neoplastic cells and the ability of normal organs to continue to function well if they are only segmentally damaged. If surrounding tissue can tolerate twice the radiation dose of a given tumor, then the tumor is radiosensitive. On the other hand, tumor which extensively involves both lungs and may be cured by a dose of 30 Gy (3000 rad) cannot be treated effectively with radiation therapy because of the greater radiosensitivity of the surrounding lung tissue. As with normal tissue, however, different tumors have a different range of radiosensitivity, some being responsive to as little as a few hundred rad, and others being incurable with as much as 100 Gy (10,000 rad). This range of sensitivity can exist even within a specific tumor type.

TYPES OF RADIOTHERAPY EQUIPMENT The term *x-ray* or *roentgen ray* is applied to electromagnetic, nonparticulate, ionizing radiations produced by man-made machines, whereas gamma rays emanate from naturally occurring or artificially produced radioactive elements such as radium or cobalt 60. These radiations of very short wavelengths have extremely high penetrating power in materials of low atomic number such as water and tissue, but are stopped effectively in materials of high atomic number such as lead. The ionizing events following irradiation lead to the production of free radicals in the water molecules of the cell microenvironment. Such free radicals and oxidizing agents interact with DNA molecules and produce a large number and variety of DNA breaks and damage. The exact lesion of x-ray irradiation remains undefined, but once alterations in nucleotide sequences occur, a change in transcription, or defective repair, results in cell death. At one time, the best-available apparatus for "deep therapy" operated at 200 to 250 kV, referred to as the *kilovoltage range*. The *supervoltage energy range* is generally taken to be 2 to 10 MeV, and *megavoltage energies* are those above 10 MeV. Radium emits gamma rays from about 1 MeV, while the artificially produced isotope cobalt 60 (^{60}Co) emits gamma rays of about 1.4 MeV. The mere presence in a unit of a quantity of ^{60}Co does not make it a true supervoltage instrument. The great tissue penetration which characterizes the supervoltage range is obtained only when the radiation source is far removed (preferably 70 cm to 1 m) from the surface of the patient. Since the output of the source decreases inversely as the square of its distance from the patient, units containing very large amounts of ^{60}Co (7.4×10^{13} to 11.1×10^{13} Bq, or 2000 to 3000 Ci) are required to produce adequate intensities and reasonably short treatment times at treatment distances of 1 m or greater. The units which contain smaller amounts of ^{60}Co and are operated at a distance of 50 cm or less should not be thought of as supervoltage devices since the physical distribution of gamma ray beams from these sources is comparable with kilovoltage rays. Linear (electron) accelerators are able to generate high-energy radiations without employing high voltages, and those operating in the range of 4 to 10 MeV are commercially available. A similar device, the betatron, accelerates electrons magnetically in a circular path within a vacuum tube. Commercial units presently available produce electrons and x-rays at a peak energy of 18 to 30 MeV.

Megavoltage radiation equipment has almost completely replaced kilovoltage sources in cancer therapy. Because of reduced skin doses and lesser internal scatter with megavoltage irradiation, higher doses of irradiation can be delivered to tumors at any depth in the body. Linear accelerators in the 4- to 35-MeV range and cobalt sources are the photon generators most widely employed. Linear accelerators deliver radiation with sharper beam margins than do cobalt machines. Linear accelerators can also provide electrons, which are particulate and penetrate approximately 0.25 to 0.5 cm per megaelectronvolt of energy with a relatively abrupt falloff in tissues, so that deeper normal tissues are spared from irradiation. The low penetrance of electron beams is proving useful in intraoperative radiotherapy, which seeks to avoid radiation to normal tissues distal to the target organ and those moved aside at surgery.

Other forms of particulate irradiation which are more penetrating than the electron and which have very favorable physical and biologic characteristics for the treatment of cancer are being developed. These include fast neutrons, charged particles such as protons or helium ions, and negative pi mesons. These particles cause a more intense deposition of energy per unit path in the tissue [high linear energy transfer (LET)] than does ordinary photon radiation. They also have the theoretical advantage of greater relative biologic effectiveness (RBE), in part because of lower oxygen-enhancement ratios (OER), which should treat hypoxic fractions of tumors more effectively. Fast neutrons are now being tested in clinical trials using medically dedicated neutron generators. Preliminary results suggest some advantage in patients with head and neck cancers and striking improvements in patients with salivary gland cancers. Attempts to avoid toxicity to normal tissues and improve fractionation techniques include the use of intraoperative radiotherapy for abdominal primaries where normal bowel can be moved outside of the radiation field. Clinical studies in the United States and Japan have shown that dose fractions much larger than conventional fractions can be delivered at the time of surgery and may improve local control in gastric and pancreas cancers; effects on survival have not yet been demonstrated.

Doses of radiation are expressed in units called grays (Gy). One gray equals 100 rad or 1 rad equals 0.01 Gy. These units indicate the amount of absorbed energy per unit volume of tissue. The biologic effects of irradiation are dependent on the time over which the radiation is delivered and the dose per fraction. Usual dose fractionation is about 10 Gy (1000 rad) per week, delivered in 1.5- to 2.5-Gy (150 to 250 rad) fractions. Delivering tumoricidal doses with kilovoltage sources required prolonged periods of time and utilization of many fractions when skin tolerance was the major limiting factor. With megavoltage irradiation this is no longer the case, and shorter and more intense irradiation dose fractionation is being developed and studied.

RADIOSENSITIZERS; CHEMICALS Tumor masses have been shown to contain significant fractions of hypoxic cells due to the inadequacy of the blood supply (as the mass increases) in large tumors. Since the free radical state of molecular oxygen interacts with ionization products created by radiation beams, radiation therapy to such tumors is less effective than to fully oxygenated tumors. In experimental tumor systems, the size of the hypoxic fraction has been shown to be directly proportional to the failure rate of local treatment.

Attempts to improve the cell kill of hypoxic cells have involved the use of hypoxic cell sensitizer drugs. Of the compounds tested as hypoxic cell sensitizers, the 2-nitroimidazoles appear to have the greatest potential because of pharmacologic properties that promote distribution of drug to the central portion of tumors in spite of poor blood supply. Among these, metronidazole and another experimental derivative, misonidazole have been active in animal model systems. These compounds act by mimicking oxygen in fixing DNA damage caused by radiation. They improve radiosensitivity of hypoxic cells as tested both in vitro and in vivo. They do not sensitize normal oxic cells to radiation and therefore exert a selective effect between tumors and normal tissues. The use of hypoxic radiosensitizers has been limited in clinical trials due to neurotoxicity. Newer studies are examining different dosing and fractionation to avoid this side effect, and newer, less lipophilic compounds are in early clinical trials.

There are other compounds that are not hypoxic cell sensitizers that enhance the effect of radiotherapy. One group is the thiol-depleting agents. All cells contain thiols, some of which are nonprotein sulfhydryls that act to protect DNA from radiation damage. Compounds such as *N*-ethylmaleimide or a synthesis blocker like buthionine sulfoximine can render cells radiosensitive. Some chemicals are radioprotectors and theoretically can protect normal tissue from the effects of radiotherapy. So far, only one radioprotector, a sulfhydryl compound—ethiofos— has been developed. In animal studies, it protects normal and tumor tissue equally.

Cytotoxic drugs also act as radiosensitizers to both normal and tumor tissue. Pyrimidine analogues, particularly bromodeoxyuridine and idoxuridine, constitute such a class of radiosensitizers when used in noncytotoxic doses. Radiosensitization occurs when a halogenated pyrimidine is substituted for thymidine in cellular DNA. Sensitization requires prolonged infusion since these compounds are incorporated into the cell only during DNA synthesis. Clinical studies in brain tumors using prolonged intravenous infusions are yielding promising results. In some cases, the use of cancer drugs in cytotoxic doses concurrently with radiotherapy (small cell lung cancer; stage II breast cancer) has improved local control and survival. The toxic effects of drugs like doxorubicin, dactinomycin, and bleomycin are enhanced on normal tissues such as the skin, heart, and lungs when used with radiotherapy.

HYPERTHERMIA Cell sensitivity to heat in the range of 43 to 45°C is increased in the presence of low pH, hypoxia, poor perfusion, and low nutrient supply, conditions found in the interior of many tumors, and tumor cells have been found to be more sensitive to heat than normal cells. Heat tends to kill cells in S phase, the most radioresistant phase of the cell cycle. In animal studies, closely spaced or concurrent use of heating and radiation therapy produces more effective tumor control than either modality alone, and in some cases, allows lower doses of radiation therapy to be used. Experimental data suggest that the antitumor effect of hyperthermia also includes inhibition of radiation damage repair. There are major technical problems, however, with the three chief ways of delivering hyperthermia in the clinics (microwaves, ultrasound, and radio frequency currents) largely related to heat distribution in tumors of varying size and depth and to thermometry techniques to measure heat distribution. Hyperthermia's potential in the treatment of cancer is clear; microwave hyperthermia has received Federal Drug Administration (FDA) approval for use with photon radiotherapy, and several important clinical studies are in progress. Hyperthermia also sensitizes cells to chemotherapy, and clinical trials using whole-body hyperthermia are in progress to evaluate the combination of drugs, heat, and radiotherapy to overcome the limitations of hyperthermia used as a regional treatment.

PHOTODYNAMIC THERAPY A new approach to treatment of cancers limited to geographic regions, photodynamic therapy (PDT), combines exposure to radiated light in the visible range and non-cytotoxic drug therapy. Light-absorbing chemicals such as hematoporphyrin derivatives are selectively retained by cancer cells. The cancer cells are killed when exposed to certain wavelengths of light. Dramatic responses have been reported in rodents and humans with superficial lesions such as skin tumors or in intrabronchial tumors when hematoporphyrin-exposed cells are exposed to laser beams of the appropriate wavelengths through an endoscope. Experiments in rodents with ascites tumors show that complete resolution of ascites is possible since the entire abdominal cavity can be exposed to light. PDT is relatively nontoxic, but its limitations are similar to radiation therapy in that all tumor cells must be exposed to light. Such a circumstance is difficult to achieve with cells in circulation.

CHOICE OF LOCAL MODALITY Treatment with radiotherapy instead of surgery, using more sophisticated equipment, has the advantage of being less mutilating and, where it provides equivalent results, is the preferred approach. This choice will depend in some cases on the expertise in a given institution. For example, in the treatment of stage I carcinoma of the cervix, either modality provides equal survival rates. In localized carcinoma of the vocal cords because radiotherapy has a high cure rate and spares the vocal cords, it is preferred to surgery. In carcinoma of the prostate, with stage A and B, radiotherapy is the preferred approach because it produces survival figures equivalent to those with surgery with far lower risk of impotence. In women with breast tumors less than 4 cm in size, radiotherapy to the breast and axillary nodes is the primary treatment after lumpectomy if the institutional radiotherapist has the necessary technical skills. In carcinoma of the rectum below the peritoneal reflection, radiotherapy alone in small, nonulcerated, and superficial lesions is quite effective in controlling the tumors; radiotherapy can improve survival figures when used in conjunction with surgery and chemotherapy in patients with rectal cancer which is more extensive. In epidermoid cancers of the anal canal, radiotherapy with chemotherapy has replaced abdominoperineal resection and colostomy while producing equivalent survival rates.

In some cases, however, the routine use of radiotherapy as an adjunct to surgery should be avoided. In carcinoma of the breast, routine postmastectomy radiotherapy of the *chest wall* and lymph node areas adds nothing to the results of surgery, does not improve survival, but does cause significant morbidity. Local recurrences are rare in the absence of systemic metastases, and local recurrences can be controlled by radiotherapy or drug treatment when they occur.

In stage IIB carcinoma of the ovary (limited to the pelvis), radiotherapy alone should be discouraged since further drug therapy is usually required. Its use as the primary treatment of stage III ovarian cancer (widespread intraabdominal disease) is also contraindicated. Except in rare instances, routine radiotherapy in lung cancer has been ineffective, although it improves local control and survival when used concurrently with effective drug treatment of small cell carcinoma. In testicular cancer, the routine use of retroperitoneal radiotherapy following lymphadenectomy is no longer used in patients with nonseminomatous tumors. Routine preoperative or postoperative therapy of stage I uterine fundal cancer may not offer additional benefit to surgery.

TREATMENT OF ADVANCED CANCER

CHEMOTHERAPY The most important aspect of cancer chemotherapy trials conducted in the 1960s and realized in the 1970s was the demonstration that drugs could cure patients with some types of advanced cancer. The most important initial goal of the more intensive drug treatment programs is similar to the goal of surgery and radiation therapy for localized tumor—that is, to erase all clinical evidence of disease (complete remission). The length of time the patient remains free of disease after all therapy is discontinued is used as an indication of the magnitude of the reduction of tumor cell number. These indicators of successful treatment have been valid, and survival has improved commensurate with an increase in the rates and duration of complete remission for metastatic cancers when drug combinations have been compared with single agents.

Cancers can generally be grouped into categories according to the effectiveness of systemic treatment. Table 79-5 lists types of cancers for which current chemotherapeutic programs have major activity and are clinically quite useful. In some cases, patients are curable even though the body burden of tumor cells is very high. In most cases maximum benefit is achievable only by drug combinations. In Hodgkin's disease, acute childhood leukemia, diffuse large cell lymphomas, and testicular tumors, disease-free survival after cessation of treatment extends to over 15 years. Considering the tumor volume in most of these patients at the time of treatment ($\pm$ 10^{11} cells), these results are quite remarkable. The break in the survival curve varies for each disease. A 2-year disease-free interval from the end of treatment is sufficient to consider patients cured with such virulent, rapidly growing tumors as choriocarcinoma, Burkitt's lymphoma, and diffuse large cell lymphomas, while 4 or more years are required to evaluate the results of treatment in Hodgkin's disease, acute childhood leukemia, breast cancer, and testicular cancer. Widespread use of these treatment programs has resulted in marked improvement in relative survival rates concomitant with a sharp decrease in national mortality in patients with Hodgkin's disease and other lymphomas, testes cancer, acute leukemia of childhood, other pediatric neoplasms, ovarian carcinoma, and premenopausal women with breast cancer. Chemotherapy has moderate and useful activity in the cancers listed in Table 79-6, although cure is not generally possible once the diseases have metastasized. Adjuvant studies have proved positive in

TABLE 79-5 Diseases in which chemotherapy has major activity

Cancer type	Drugs currently preferred	Alternative drugs
Acute lymphocytic leukemia (ALL)	Induction: vincristine + prednisone ± asparaginase ± doxorubicin	Daunorubicin, cyclophosphamide, cytarabine, thioguanine, vindesine,* teniposide,* mitoxantrone,* etoposide
	CNS prophylaxis: intrathecal methotrexate ± radiotherapy	CNS prophylaxis: high-dose IV methotrexate
	Maintenance: combination chemotherapy with methotrexate + mercaptopurine or other combinations	Maintenance: doxorubicin and/or asparaginase in addition to methotrexate and mercaptopurine
Acute myelocytic leukemia (AML)	Daunorubicin + cytarabine ± thioguanine	Amsacrine,* azacitidine,* high-dose cytarabine, teniposide,* etoposide, mitoxantrone*
Anal cancer	Fluorouracil + mitomycin†	
Brain		
Adult gliomas†	High-dose methotrexate with citrovorum factor rescue; carmustine or lomustine	Procarbazine, doxorubicin, vincristine
Medulloblastoma†	Vincristine + carmustine ± mechlorethamine ± methotrexate Mechlorethamine + vincristine + procarbazine + prednisone (MOPP)	
Breast cancer†	Tamoxifen, progestins; cyclophosphamide + methotrexate + fluorouracil ± prednisone (CMF or CMFP); cyclophosphamide + doxorubicin ± fluorouracil (AC or CAF)	Vincristine, vinblastine, mitomycin, mitolactol,* mitoxantrone,* teniposide,* estrogens, androgens, prednisone, aminoglutethimide
Choriocarcinoma	Methotrexate ± dactinomycin	Vinblastine, chlorambucil, bleomycin, etoposide, cisplatin, 6-mercaptopurine
Embryonal rhabdomyosarcoma†	Vincristine + dactinomycin + cyclophosphamide (VAC) ± doxorubicin	Methotrexate, thiotepa
Ewing's sarcoma†	Cyclophosphamide + doxorubicin + vincristine (CAV)	Dactinomycin
Hairy cell leukemia	Interferon,* deoxycoformycin*	Chlorambucil
Hodgkin's disease	Mechlorethamine + vincristine + procarbazine + prednisone (MOPP) Doxorubicin + bleomycin + vinblastine + dacarbazine (ABVD) MOPP alternated with ABVD	Lomustine, carmustine, etoposide, teniposide,* streptozotocin
Lung		
Small cell (oat cell)	Cyclophosphamide + doxorubicin + vincristine (CAV); cyclophosphamide, methotrexate, lomustine (CMC)	Cyclophosphamide + doxorubicin + vincristine + etoposide (CAVE)
	Etoposide + cisplatin	Procarbazine, mechlorethamine
Lymphocytic lymphoma		
Burkitt's lymphoma	Cyclophosphamide Cyclophosphamide + vincristine + methotrexate	Carmustine, methotrexate, ifosfamide*
Diffuse large cell lymphoma	Prednisone + methotrexate-leucovorin doxorubicin + cyclophosphamide + etoposide—mechlorethamine + vincristine + procarbazine + prednisone (ProMACE-MOPP) Methotrexate, doxorubicin, cyclophosphamide, vincristine, prednisone, bleomycin (MACOP-B) Bleomycin + doxorubicin + cyclophosphamide + vincristine + dexamethasone + methotrexate with leucovorin rescue (M-BACOD) Bleomycin + doxorubicin + cyclophosphamide + vincristine + prednisone + procarbazine (COP-BLAM) Cyclophosphamide + vincristine + methotrexate-leucovorin + cytarabine (COMLA)	Bleomycin, chlorambucil, lomustine, carmustine, cytarabine, etoposide, teniposide,* amsacrine,* asparaginase, methotrexate, high-dose cytarabine, ifosfamide*
Follicular lymphoma	Investigational protocols similar to those used in diffuse large cell lymphomas or observation for low-grade follicular lymphomas; combination chemotherapy for intermediate or high-grade	Cyclophosphamide or chlorambucil or vincristine or prednisone or etoposide (combinations not demonstrably superior to single agents); cytarabine, asparaginase, methotrexate, interferon,* anti-idiotype monoclonal antibody*
Mycosis fungoides	Mechlorethamine (topical in ointment base); combination chemotherapy as in Hodgkin's disease or non-Hodgkin's lymphoma	Vinblastine, methotrexate, psoralen + ultraviolet light (PUVA), interferon,* deoxycoformycin*
Ovary	Melphalan (or cyclophosphamide) ± cisplatin ± doxorubicin (CP, CAP); cyclophosphamide + hexamethylmelamine* + doxorubicin + cisplatin (CHAP); high-dose cisplatin plus cyclophosphamide	Hexamethylmelamines,* fluorouracil, chlorambucil, thiotepa, vincristine, ifosfamide,* megestrol acetate Intraperitoneal: fluorouracil, methotrexate, melphalan, or doxorubicin
Osteogenic sarcoma†	Doxorubicin and/or high-dose methotrexate + leucovorin rescue ± bleomycin ± cyclophosphamide ± dactinomycin anal	Melphalan, mitomycin, cisplatin
Sarcomas† (soft tissue, adults)	Doxorubicin + cyclophosphamide	Vincristine, methotrexate, ifosfamide,* dacarbazine
Testicular	Cisplatin + vinblastine + bleomycin (PVB); ± etoposide for bulky tumor	Vinblastine + dactinomycin + bleomycin + cyclophosphamide + cisplatin (VAB-6)
	Bleomycin + etoposide + cisplatin (BEP)	Etoposide, cyclophosphamide, methotrexate, plicamycin, dactinomycin, melphalan, chlorambucil
Wilms's tumor	Dactinomycin + vincristine for favorable histology; ± doxorubicin for unfavorable prognostic factors	Doxorubicin, cyclophosphamide

* *Available only for investigational use.*
† *Drugs have major activity when combined with surgical resection, radiotherapy, or both (primary multimodal therapy).*
SOURCE: *Modified from* The Medical Letter *(Feb. 15, 1985).*

TABLE 79-6 Diseases in which chemotherapy has moderate activity

Cancer type	Drugs currently preferred	Alternative drugs
Adrenocortical carcinoma	Mitotane	Doxorubicin, aminoglutethimide, cyclophosphamide, cisplatin
Bladder	Cisplatin and/or doxorubin ± methotrexate ± vinblastine; thiotepa or doxorubicin instillation	Mitomycin, fluorouracil, vinblastine, methotrexate, instillation of mitomycin or BCG*
Cervix	Cisplatin + bleomycin ± methotrexate	Cyclophosphamide, vincristine, methotrexate, mitomycin, fluorouracil, doxorubicin, vinblastine
	Bleomycin + mitomycin + vincristine ± cisplatin	
Chronic lymphocytic leukemia	Chlorambucil ± prednisone	Cyclophosphamide, vincristine
Chronic myelocytic leukemia (CML)		
Stable phase	Busulfan; hydroxyurea	Mitobronitol,* mercaptopurine, thioguanine, melphalan
Acute phase	Daunorubicin + cytarabine + vincristine + prednisone ± thioguanine	Amsacrine,* azacitidine,* vincristine
	Vincristine + prednisone for lymphoid variant	
Endometrial	Megestrol acetate or hydroxyprogesterone caproate or medroxyprogesterone	Fluorouracil, tamoxifen, melphalan
	Doxorubicin ± cyclophosphamide	
Gastric	Fluorouracil + doxorubicin + mitomycin (FAM)	Cisplatin
	Fluorouracil + doxorubicin + semustine*	
Head and neck, squamous cell	Bleomycin + cisplatin ± methotrexate; cisplatin + fluorouracil	Vinblastine, cyclophosphamide, mitomycin, doxorubicin
Islet cell carcinoma	Streptozocin ± fluorouracil	Cyclophosphamide, doxorubicin, dacarbazine
Kaposi's sarcoma (epidemic)	Etoposide or interferon*	
Lung cancer		
Non-small cell	Cyclophosphamide + doxorubicin + cisplatin†	Methotrexate, etoposide, lomustine, fluorouracil, ifosfamide,* mitomycin, mitomycin + vinblastine
	Vindesine* + cisplatin	
	Vinblastine + cisplatin	Mitomycin + vinblastine + cisplatin
		Fluorouracil + doxorubicin + mitomycin (FAM)
Myeloma	Melphalan (or cyclophosphamide) + prednisone	Carmustine, vincristine, lomustine, doxorubicin, interferon*
	Melphalan + carmustine + cyclophosphamide + prednisone	
	Dexamethasone + doxorubicin + vincristine	
Neuroblastoma	Doxorubicin + cyclophosphamide + cisplatin + teniposide*	Mechlorethamine, daunorubicin, dacarbazine, vinblastine, prednisone, cisplatin, teniposide,* etoposide
Prostate	Leuprolide* ± flutamide*	Diethylstilbesterol, estramustine, megestrol acetate, fluorouracil, cyproterone,* flutamide ± (antiandrogen), methotrexate; cisplatin ± cyclophosphamide ± doxorubicin
Retinoblastoma	Doxorubicin + cyclophosphamide	

* *Available only for investigational use.*
† *Drugs have major activity only when combined with surgical resection, radiotherapy, or both (adjuvant chemotherapy).*
SOURCE: *Modified from* The Medical Letter *(Feb. 15, 1985).*

non-small cell lung cancer and head and neck cancers that, if confirmed, could change the outlook of these diseases in a major way.

Tumors listed in Table 79-7 are frequently thought of as resistant to treatment, but on occasion significant palliation can be provided for patients by the careful use by an experienced physician of existing chemotherapeutic agents. However, studies using adjuvant 5-fluorouracil plus levamisole have shown a statistically significant improvement in relapse-free and overall survival at 4 years in Duke's B_2 and C colon cancer, and the combination of 5-fluorouracil and radiation therapy has been shown to improve survival in patients with locally unresectable pancreatic cancer. These studies are being reconfirmed in larger-scale clinical trials. Biological therapy with interleukin 2 and activated lymphocytes has produced significant regression of metastases in patients with colon, renal, lung cancer, and malignant melanoma; and preliminary results with specific monoclonal antibodies have shown useful responses in a few patients with colorectal and pancreas cancer and malignant melanoma.

CONTINUOUS INFUSION CHEMOTHERAPY Two advances in technology have reawakened an interest in the methods of delivery of chemotherapy to sites of specific tumor involvement: the availability of improved infusion devices, and sensitive methods for measuring the active moiety of both drugs and their cellular targets within the biologically active range. Organ-directed chemotherapy holds considerable promise as a component of multimodal therapy to deliver drugs at higher concentrations for prolonged periods. This approach can ovecome pharmacokinetic problems in drugs with short half-lives and cell kinetic problems by exposing tumor cells to effective concentrations for periods well in excess of their cell cycle times. In liver perfusions, advantage can be taken of drugs that are metabolically inactivated by the normal liver to avoid systemic toxicity. At the

TABLE 79-7 Diseases in which chemotherapy has minor activity

Cancer type	Drugs currently preferred	Alternative drugs
Colorectal	Fluorouracil;† intraarterial floxuridine	Methotrexate
Esophagus	Cisplatin + vinblastine + bleomycin	5-Fluorouracil, doxorubicin
Liver	Doxorubicin; fluorouracil ± methotrexate	Fluorouracil, floxuridine, amsacrine,* intraarterial floxuridine, vinblastine
Melanoma	Dacarbazine	Dactinomycin, carmustine, procarbazine, vinblastine, interferon*
Pancreatic	Fluorouracil + doxorubicin + mitomycin (FAM); fluorouracil + radiation†	Streptozocin + mitomycin + fluorouracil (SMF); mitomycin, doxorubicin, streptozocin, semustine,* ifosfamide*
Renal	No good choice	Vinblastine, lomustine, interferon*

* *Available only for investigational use.*
† *Clinically useful only in patients with locally unresectable diseases.*
SOURCE: *Modified from* The Medical Letter *(Feb. 15, 1985).*

present time, however, continuous intravenous infusions of anticancer drugs have not shown a clear benefit over pulse or short-term infusions with the possible exception of the continuous intravenous infusion of bromodeoxyuridine or iododeoxyuridine coupled with radiotherapy in the treatment of gliomas. Intraarterial infusion therapy is presently being restudied in patients with metastases from colon cancer limited to the liver. While the results suggest some improvement in terms of increased response rates, most studies are not well enough controlled to recommend the therapy over systemic treatment except under investigational conditions, and because survival has not been improved. The combined use of 5-fluorodeoxyuridine infusions coupled with external radiation therapy to the liver appears to offer some advantage in survival. Attempts are being made to redirect the blood supply away from normal liver to liver metastases by using vasoconstrictors or by trapping drugs in the tumor vasculature temporarily by administration with starch granules which are subsequently dissolved by amylase. Studies are needed to couple infusion therapy with resection of hepatic metastases to focus on minimal residual disease. Intraperitoneal therapy of ovarian cancer using dialysis techniques appears promising and takes advantage of the rapid systemic clearance of many anticancer drugs and the slow diffusion out of the peritoneal cavity of large, non-lipid-soluble molecules. Its use in early-stage disease is still experimental.

Implantable elastomer access ports with self-sealing silicone diaphragms are being used to administer continuous infusions and have reduced the risk of infection associated with tunneled central venous catheters. Extravasation during infusions into the ports remains a problem with drugs such as adriamycin. Several new portable infusion pumps are available as delivery devices. The totally implantable Infusaid pump driven by an internal fluorocarbon energy source is an effective tool in evaluating organ-directed therapy. Implantable access ports and infusion devices are already allowing greater flexibility of scheduling in experimental protocols, with greater comfort to the patient.

THE USE OF SURGERY AND RADIOTHERAPY AS AN ADJUNCT IN PATIENTS WITH ADVANCED CANCER Surgery and radiotherapy, although considered treatment of localized primary cancers, have an increasingly important role in the treatment of patients with advanced metastatic cancer either in an attempt to cure or to palliate. Seemingly solitary brain metastases should be removed surgically, particularly in young people, if at all possible, since the likelihood of rapid demise without such treatment is high, and occasional long-term control is possible. Pulmonary metastases of a variety of sarcomas can be resected even when multiple nodules are present and long-term survival is possible. This has been true particularly in patients whose tumors can be shown to have long doubling times prior to surgery. Removal of metastases to the lungs is important in patients with testicular tumors because of the histologic heterogeneity of this tumor and the likelihood that a metastasis has resulted from growth of a clone of a histologic type resistant to the drugs employed. The resection of apparently localized hepatic metastases of colorectal cancer has resulted in long-term disease-free survival in as many as 25 percent of such patients. These results coupled with the recent information on the biochemistry of metastases have altered the previous universally pessimistic attitude toward patients who develop recurrent tumors. Reducing tumor bulk by resecting major masses of tumor in patients with widespread disease to reduce the body burden of tumor prior to chemotherapy has, however, not proved as useful as anticipated except in ovarian cancer. In one controlled clinical trial, in locally advanced testis tumor, debulking surgery did not improve the ultimate results of chemotherapy.

Surgeons are often asked to provide palliation for patients whose conditions are incurable by any modality. The operative risks are often high and the therapeutic yield, from the surgical point of view, low, but considerations of comfort and ability to return home during the terminal months of illness often make such procedures worthwhile. Palliation should be considered, for example, in intestinal obstruction due to ovarian and pancreatic cancer, in gastrointestinal bleeding, and for urinary diversions; and to relieve pain with neurosurgical procedures. The primary physician often is in the best position to make the judgment regarding the feasibility of such palliative procedures.

In highly radiosensitive tumors, radiotherapy may be used to reduce the areas of prior tumor involvement in patients with advanced metastatic cancers to enhance the cure rate with drugs, as in patients with some types of lymphomas. In diseases that are systemic at diagnosis, such as leukemia and small cell lung cancer, prophylactic use of radiotherapy to treat the brain and meninges before disease is evident has been successful as an ancillary method to drug treatment and has resulted in prolonged disease-free survival. Palliative radiotherapy has many applications in patients with metastatic cancer. In emergency situations, it can be used in conjunction with drugs to provide rapid relief of superior mediastinal obstruction, or to relieve ureteral obstruction in patients with lymphomas or testicular tumors which are drug-resistant. It can provide frequent and useful relief of bone pain and may prevent fractures, if used prophylactically to treat lesions of weight-bearing bones. In these cases, the primary treatment is usually with drugs and the radiation field should be only as large as required to control the lesion in question. For lytic lesions of weight-bearing bones, greater than 2.5 cm in diameter, especially those involving the cortex, prophylactic internal fixation followed by radiation therapy is the treatment of choice. Radiation of the brain and spinal cord are important examples of palliation which, when used early and effectively, can prevent catastrophic neurologic incapacitation in the final months of illness.

MULTIMODAL PRIMARY (ADJUVANT) TREATMENT

A major reduction in national mortality rates from the common visceral cancers appears likely to occur only if current and future systemic treatment programs are applied more effectively in the perioperative period to the treatment of those large numbers of patients who develop recurrences if treated with surgery or radiotherapy alone. Multimodal therapy began by combining the standard surgical and/or radiotherapeutic approaches with newly developed systemic treatment, without alterations, for their use in combination. This approach, while effective in many cases, was often quite toxic. Multimodal primary therapy has now evolved to a process of tailoring each component of the treatment program to maximize the strength of the modality while minimizing the toxicity. This approach has not only improved survival but has markedly altered the methods and morbidity of local control in a significant number of cancers. In cancers in which systemic treatment can cure patients with visible metastases, the effect has been most dramatic. In choriocarcinoma, chemotherapy has replaced hysterectomy; in Hodgkin's disease, chemotherapy alone has become the treatment of choice in stage III, or in combination with radiotherapy, in some patients with stage II disease; in pediatric tumors, in the 60 percent of patients with Wilms's tumor who have favorable histology, surgery and a two-drug combination has replaced the use of surgery, radiotherapy, and a three-drug combination (which included doxorubicin), sparing the patient the growth-retarding effects of radiotherapy and the cardiotoxicity of doxorubicin; in diffuse large cell lymphoma, chemotherapy has proved effective enough in advanced disease that it has replaced radiotherapy as the treatment of choice in stage II disease and in some cases of stage I disease; in nonseminomatous testicular cancer, chemotherapy with the use of sensitive biologic markers has become the primary treatment once orchiectomy is performed; in small cell lung cancer, better local control and improved survival has been achieved if radiotherapy is used concurrently with chemotherapy. In tumors where cure of visible metastatic disease is not yet possible with combination chemotherapy but a major clinical effect is achievable against micrometastases, there has also been an influence on methods of local control which has in some cases resulted in improvement in survival as well. In breast cancer, equivalent local control is achieved with lumpectomy and radiotherapy for women with tumors less than 4 cm; improved survival and decreased mortality is possible when chemotherapy is added in patients with lymph node tumor metastases; in extremity sarcomas a marked improvement in survival is observed with limb-sparing surgery and radiotherapy coupled with combination chemotherapy; and in anorectal cancers equivalent local control and survival without the need for colostomy is attainable with concurrent use of radiotherapy and chemotherapy.

The four most important considerations in the development of drug programs for post- and perioperative use are the following: (1) the identification of populations of patients who, even after optimal surgery or radiotherapy for their primary disease, have a high risk of recurrence and death from their cancer (e.g., stage II breast cancer, Duke's C colon cancer); (2) the availability of a proven systemic form of treatment; (3) the weighing of the potential benefits of treatment against short- and long-term risks of added drug treatment, keeping in mind that a fraction of patients exposed to adjuvant drug treatment would not have developed recurrent tumor; and (4) proper study design. Since measuring the reduction of tumor masses is not a possible end point during adjuvant studies, few can be accepted unless comparisons of treated groups and untreated controls are made, or the risk of recurrence is known to be very high and is spread over so narrow a time frame as to obviate the need for concurrent controls. In the latter case, historical controls may suffice. An example of a tumor requiring controls in adjuvant studies is stage II (T_1,N_1,M_0) melanoma. Sex, site, level of invasion of the primary, and degree of nodal involvement all affect not only the risk but the time of recurrence, which may be spread over periods from a few months to several years.

The most difficult question is the level of effectiveness required of systemic therapy in patients with advanced metastatic tumor before it is feasible to use it in an adjuvant program. Clinical studies have shown that changes in measurements of tumor masses in patients with metastatic disease are sufficiently variable to render partial response rates of 10 percent or less in drug-treated patients the equivalent of "biologic noise." Presently, only single agents, drugs and biologicals, or combinations of both with response rates of 20 percent or higher are considered acceptable for postoperative treatment programs. The attractiveness of a candidate program is enhanced considerably if some fraction of treated patients attain complete rather than partial responses. There is uncertainty as to whether drugs which are apparently inactive against advanced cancer are potentially useful against a small number of cancer cells present in the postoperative period when fewer resistant cell lines are likely to be present and vulnerability to drugs may be different.

The sequencing of chemotherapy and radiation therapy has varied from site to site with the use of radiotherapy before, during, and after chemotherapy. The standard method of using radiotherapy with chemotherapy in the past has been to give radiotherapy first followed by chemotherapy. Numerous clinical trials are now in progress testing the alternative approaches described above. The limit of tolerance for radiotherapy on normal tissue has been the operative guide to therapy rather than the ability to control the tumor and to determine whether combinations of radiation and drugs are additive, synergistic, or inhibitory. There is increasing evidence that the concurrent use of chemotherapy and radiotherapy produces superior results as in brain tumors, breast cancer, extremity sarcomas, anal cancers, and pediatric tumors and lymphomas. These observations are consistent with the Goldie-Coldman hypothesis, which predicts that either concurrent or alternating cycles of chemotherapy and radiotherapy could maximize reduction of resistant cell lines in major tumor masses. Although the concurrent use of radiation therapy and chemotherapy tends to be more toxic, alterations in dosing and fractionation may be possible with less toxicity.

COMPLICATIONS OF THERAPY

Each side effect of treatment must be weighed against the potential benefit to be derived. Patients must be apprised of all the risks involved, both in undergoing therapy and in refusing it. In a disease highly treatable with chemotherapy, it is rare that nausea, vomiting, and temporary hair loss should be of sufficient significance to withhold or reduce treatment. Many treatments are carcinogenic to some degree. The opportunity to identify this risk has come about only following the advent of successful treatment of patients with metastatic cancer, since long disease-free survival provides the follow-up time necessary to bring this to light. Radiation therapy is known to be carcinogenic, but the risk, when it is used alone, is relatively low in a given treatment field. Combinations of drugs and x-rays, however, are associated with a higher risk of second malignancies such as acute myelocytic leukemia and tumors in the irradiated field. This has been noted in long-term survivors of Hodgkin's disease who had received both combination chemotherapy (MOPP) and radiation therapy. In several studies, it is estimated that patients treated with both extensive radiation therapy and MOPP chemotherapy have an incidence of acute myelocytic leukemia between 5 and 10 percent within 10 years. Patients who are long-term survivors of Wilms's tumors treated with both radiation and drug therapy have also had a high incidence of secondary malignancies in the radiation treatment field. In addition, there is some evidence that long-term exposure to alkylating agents in patients with otherwise normal bone marrow may be associated with late marrow dysplasia which may eventuate in acute myelocytic leukemia. These potential risks are particularly germane to the use of these drugs in adjuvant treatment programs although in several large series of studies, the risk of leukemia in drug-treated breast cancer patients was less than 0.5 percent and the benefit far outweighed the risks.

The physician should be familiar with normal tissue tolerance for radiation and its acute and late effects. Acute radiation effects are largely on cell-renewal tissue—skin, oropharyngeal mucosa, small intestine, rectum, bladder mucosa, and vaginal mucosa. Acute radiation effects such as skin reactions, weight loss, nausea and vomiting, mucositis, and blood count depression may appear during or near the end of treatment and are usually reversible. Others, such as pneumonitis, may not appear until several weeks or months following treatment and then resolve. Since the effect on rapid-cell-renewal tissues will be dependent on the balance between cell birth and cell death, it will be crucially affected by the time allowed for repopulation. It will also be dependent upon the cell kill per fraction. Therefore, fraction size will be important. The radiotherapist frequently observing the oral mucosa and seeing an excessive reaction knows that a small decrease in fraction size or a small treatment break may allow rapid resolution of the problem since these changes will permit reconstitution of normal tissue. Late consequences of radiation therapy are its dose-limiting effect, which often progresses with time and is usually irreversible. They include necrosis, fibrosis, fistula formation, nonhealing ulceration, and damage to specific organs such as spinal cord transection or blindness. Normal tissues and organs differ in radiosensitivity. The risk of complications increases with dose and, if delivery is by megavoltage sources in the usual fractions, occurs when the dose exceeds the following: both lungs 15 Gy (1500 rad); both kidneys 24 Gy (2400 rad); liver 30 Gy (3000 rad); heart 35 Gy (3500 rad); spinal cord 40 Gy (4000 rad); intestine 55 Gy (5500 rad); brain 60 Gy (6000 rad); bone 75 Gy (7500 rad). While the mechanisms of late toxicity are not clear, they do not appear to depend primarily on the rapid proliferation of a cell-renewal tissue. Clinically, late effects appear to be much more dependent on the total dose of radiation and the size of the radiation fraction. Only if the same fractionation scheme is used with the same normal tissue end point, the same volume irradiated, and the same treatment technique can acute and late effects be correlated. If any of the treatment parameters is varied, the acute reactions to radiation may be dissociated from eventual late effects. Rather than serve as a guide, these acute reactions will then be misleading. There are a number of examples in radiation therapy in which the total dose has been increased, the fraction size increased or maintained constant, but the time has been extended to minimize acute effects. Such maneuvers have resulted in unacceptable late complications.

There are two hypotheses for the mechanism of late radiation effects. One theory holds that all late effects are due to damage to vascular-connective tissue stroma. A variation on this hypothesis is that damage to the endothelial cells determines late effects. An alternative hypothesis suggests that both the acute and late effects of radiation and cytotoxic chemotherapy are due to depletion of the major target cell-renewal tissues. Acute effects depend on the balance between cell killing and compensatory cellular replication of both the stem and proliferative compartments. The development of late effects requires that stem cells have only a limited proliferative capacity. Compensation for extensive or repeated cell killing may exhaust this capacity, resulting in eventual tissue failure.

Chemical and radiation therapy produce sterilization in both sexes which may be reversible but often is not. If at all reversible, the time necessary for reversal may be several years. Anticancer drugs and radiotherapy are teratogenic. It should never be assumed that chemotherapy and radiotherapy themselves are sufficient methods of contraception. All patients in the childbearing age who are treated with radiation and/or drugs should be fully informed of the risks and be advised of contraceptive measures. When pregnancy occurs during chemotherapy or exposure to radiotherapy, abortion should be considered because of the high risk of teratogenesis if the pregnancy is discovered in the first trimester, even though there are abundant case reports of normal children born to women treated with drugs in the first trimester. Treatment of women who develop tumors while pregnant is best withheld until delivery, which may need to be hastened. Chemotherapy can be used safely in the third trimester, but because of the uncertain long-term effects on the fetus, should not be employed unless the situation is critical.

NUTRITION AND CANCER

A profound state of malnutrition, the cachexia of malignancy, is frequently the most debilitating feature of this disease process. In many instances, it can be attributed to anorexia with an associated distortion of taste sensation or acquired aversion to specific foods, particularly meat. There are, however, patients in whom the extent of weight loss far exceeds the deficit in quantity and quality of calories consumed. In addition to the loss of adipose tissue and protein stores, these patients have a marked degree of insulin resistance with abnormal glucose tolerance. It has been demonstrated that malignancies can cause an augmentation of hepatic and renal gluconeogenesis secondary to enhanced Cori cycle activity, as well as an excessive utilization of fatty acids as metabolic fuel, which can theoretically contribute to a net energy loss by normal tissue. Hyperalimentation with total parenteral nutrition (TPN) with solutions based on 50 percent glucose and mixtures of essential amino acids and vitamins, containing about 3000 calories per day, is used to restore nutritionally depleted patients who have a chance for tumor control by surgery, chemotherapy, and/or radiotherapy. TPN through a catheter placed in the superior vena cava is also indicated in patients with pain on deglutition, fistulas, or intestinal obstruction. When possible, oral hyperalimentation is preferred and effective. TPN in patients who have lost 10 lb or more body weight is associated with an average weight gain of 6 lb in a mean of 24 days, even when chemotheray and radiotherapy are given simultaneously. There is no evidence that TPN preferentially enhances tumor growth. Catheter-related sepsis occurs in about 2 percent of patients. Hyperosmolar, nonketotic coma can be avoided with gradual increases in the concentration of glucose.

HYPERURICEMIA AND OTHER CONSEQUENCES OF RAPID CELL LYSIS

Hyperuricemia is most common in patients with acute leukemia but occasionally occurs in other malignancies. The high serum uric acid levels are due to the increased formation and destruction of tumor cells and accompanying breakdown of nucleoproteins. Chemotherapy and radiotherapy may cause further elevations in serum uric acid and urinary urate excretion. Uric acid is actively secreted by the kidney, and its solubility is highest in alkaline urine. When the concentration exceeds the solubility, uric acid precipitates in the tubules causing obstruction, decreased glomerular filtration, and eventually anuria. Allopurinol prevents the formation of uric acid from xanthine and hypoxanthine. Prophylactic use of this drug in patients with a large volume of tumor prior to treatment, in anticipation of high urate load, should obviate the need to treat uric acid nephropathy. Urate nephropathy can also be prevented by ensuring a water diuresis. Administration of sodium bicarbonate to maintain the urinary pH above 7.0 is helpful. Secondary gout is uncommón except in patients with polycythemia vera. The excessive production of lactate by suboxygenated masses of tumor causes lactic acidosis in patients with leukemia and Burkitt's lymphoma. The lactic acidosis can be reversed by cytotoxic chemotherapy directed against the tumor. The elaboration of large quantities of lactic dehydrogenase (LDH) has been observed in these settings. Cytotoxic therapy in highly drug-sensitive tumors can cause rapid tumor lysis with release of intracellular phosphates and potassium leading to serious hyperkalemia, hypocalcemia, and potentially fatal cardiotoxicity.

REFERENCES

AARONSON SA, TRONICK SR: The role of oncogenes in human neoplasia, in *Important Advances in Oncology*, VT DeVita et al (eds). Philadelphia, Lippincott, 1985, pp 3–15

CHABNER BA (ed): *Pharmacologic Principles of Cancer Treatment*. Philadelphia, Saunders, 1982

———, MYERS CE: Clinical pharmacology of cancer chemotherapy, in *Cancer: Principles and Practice of Oncology*, 2d ed, VT DeVita et al (eds). Philadelphia, Lippincott, 1985, pp 290–328

DEVITA VT et al: The effect of combined modality therapy on local control and survival. Int J Radiat Oncol Biol Phys (in press)

GOLDIE GH, COLDMAN AJ: The genetic origin of drug resistance in neoplasms: Implications for systemic therapy. Cancer Res 44:3643, 1984

LIOTTA LA: The mechanisms of cancer invasion and metastasis, in *Important Advances in Oncology*, VT DeVita et al (eds). Philadelphia, Lippincott, 1985, pp 28–41

section 6 Geriatric medicine

80 THE BIOLOGY OF AGING

WILLIAM R. HAZZARD

The phenomenon of aging has always fascinated mankind. This interest probably derives from the fact that until comparatively recently only a small fraction of people actually lived into old age. The concept of retirement, for example, did not exist until the latter portion of the nineteenth century. However, several forces have brought aging and its consequences into the social and scientific limelight. These forces can best be appreciated by contrasting representative longevity curves of the populations of developing and developed nations (Fig. 80-1). The curves reflect the high birthrates and high infant and childhood mortality rates that are characteristic of developing nations and the correspondingly low rates observed in developed countries. Socioeconomic development results in improved nutrition, housing, education, personal and public hygiene, and eventually in a reduced birthrate. These factors are also responsible for increases in the median age of the population and in expected longevity at birth. However, once maturity has been achieved, extension of longevity is less pronounced. This upper limit of longevity is depicted in Fig. 80-1. Note the similar ages at which the upper ends of longevity curves from populations with disparate degrees of socioeconomic development intersect the abscissa. Survival beyond 120 years of age has not been documented beyond question.

Hence, the change in the modern era is not an increase in the upper limit of the human life span but is an increase in the proportion and number who survive to approach that limit. This trend is the result of a narrowing of the gap between *primary aging*, which is genetically determined and immutable, and *secondary aging*, which is attributable to personal, social, and environmental factors that may be subject to change. When large numbers of individuals age in concert, society itself reflects the aging process. The United States is now experiencing such a redistribution of population toward an older median age. A steady state, with about a fourth of the total population in the ages 1 to 19 years and another fourth in the age group over 55 years, will be reached in another half century (Fig. 81-1). Unless more efficient and effective means are devised for meeting the needs of an aging population, health and social services for the elderly will be overwhelmed.

AGING AT THE CELLULAR LEVEL Clinical and epidemiologic research on aging has lagged behind studies of aging at the cellular level. This has occurred in large part because of the difficulty in separating the primary effects of aging from the secondary effects of the diseases that accompany aging. Only when reduced to the simplest unit of organization, the cell, can aging be studied independently of age-related disease. Even at this level knowledge about aging is primitive, and several theories of aging remain extant. Research in this area was given its major impetus when human skin fibroblasts were found to have a limited potential for replication, about 50 population doublings under the most favorable conditions (the Hayflick phenomenon). This limit is an inherent property of the fibroblasts themselves and not of their environment. A finite and relatively fixed number of doublings is also characteristic of the proliferative potential of certain other cells, such as arterial smooth-muscle cells. Consistent with the suggestion that these cell culture studies may reflect aging in vivo, the actual number of potential doublings of a given fibroblast in vitro is inversely related to the age of its donor. Furthermore, fibroblasts from donors with Werner's syndrome, a single gene defect that causes dramatic acceleration of aging, undergo fewer doublings than cells from age-matched controls.

As a consequence of these findings in cultured cells, several theories have been advanced to attempt to explain senescence on the basis of alteration at the genomic level. One theory, Szilard's mutation hypothesis, holds that as DNA mutations accumulate in somatic cells, chromosomal inactivation and cell death ensue. Related theories suggest that senescence occurs via cumulative errors in formation of RNA or through progressive errors in protein synthesis, resulting in an ''error catastrophe'' (a theory that has receded from favor, as formal tests have failed to document such cumulative errors in aging cells). Such mutations have also been invoked to explain the age-related increase in autoimmunity. However, the effects of mutation need not be permanent. Indeed, the capacity for DNA repair in fibroblasts and the amount of reserve or redundant DNA sequences may correlate with longevity of various species. Finally, it has been proposed that the accumulation of free radicals that occurs with aging (the result of decreased activity of superoxide dismutase) may cause reduced resistance to intra- and extracellular injury.

These theories of ''intrinsic'' aging have been challenged because they are based on in vitro phenomena and hence are far removed from processes occurring in the aging whole organism. In addition, such theories do not explain the marked differences in replicative potential observed among various cell types. For instance, while fibroblasts exhibit senescence in vitro, cells of gastrointestinal and hematopoietic origin appear capable of replication throughout their life span, and kidney and liver cells replicate at all ages in response to unilateral nephrectomy or partial hepatectomy. Still other cells,

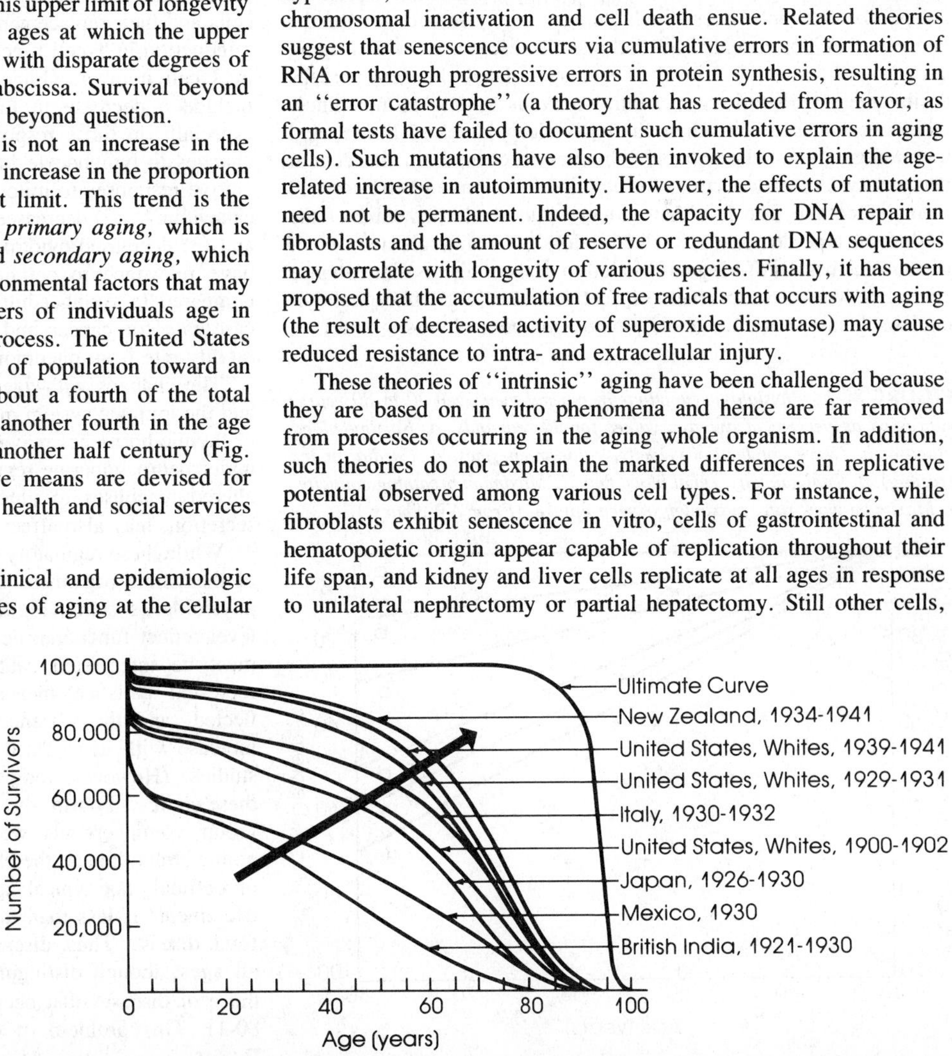

FIGURE 80-1 *Survival curves in different countries varying in degree of socioeconomic development. Diagonal arrow indicates change accompanying such development. (Reprinted by permission from L Hayflick, N Engl J Med 295:1302, 1976.)*

such as those of the central nervous system and striated muscle, do not replicate during adult life. However, regardless of replicative potential, no nonmalignant cell—and this includes all of the hematopoietic cells—survives indefinitely (in contrast to cancer cells). Thus, while considerable variation occurs in generation time and replicative potential of different cell types within a given species and of the same cell type among species, senescence at the cellular level appears to be a universal feature of normal cells.

But do these in vitro phenomena relate to aging in vivo? Even the strongest proponents of the intrinsic school of cellular aging acknowledge that the probability is small that organisms age solely because one or more cell populations lose proliferative capacity. Perhaps, in aging cells, decrements in functional capacities other than proliferative capacity render the organism vulnerable to death. This possibility has been supported in other studies by Hayflick and his colleagues, who have reported that fibroblasts lose the capacity to synthesize and lyse collagen prior to the loss of replicative capacity. Therefore, attention has been focused upon the regulatory processes that control the functions of tissues and whole organisms, specifically the nervous, endocrine, and immune systems.

One school has focused upon the role of central nervous system monoamines, notably dopamine, norepinephrine, and serotonin. These neurotransmitters are altered in certain age-related neurologic diseases. Parkinson's disease, for instance, is associated with major deficiencies of monoamines (e.g., striatal dopamine) and can be partially treated by L-dopa replacement. Furthermore, changes in catecholamine metabolism occur in the normal aging brain, and the elderly are more susceptible to development of parkinsonian symptoms following treatment with phenothiazines. Hence, age-related changes in dopamine uptake and catecholamine metabolism may lower the threshold for induction of parkinsonian symptoms by drugs that deplete or antagonize catecholamines. Such changes may also account for the late onset of postencephalitic Parkinson's disease, in which aging unmasks an earlier viral insult. Other age-related changes, perhaps attributable to alterations in central nervous system monoamines, include changes in circadian rhythms, sleep patterns, libido, and thermoregulation. Alternatively, cholinergic changes in the central nervous system may account for certain alterations in behavior and mental function. The fact that patients with senile dementia of the Alzheimer type demonstrate selective loss of cholinergic neurons of the nucleus basalis of Meynert has led to trials of agents that enhance central nervous system levels of acetylcholine [e.g., phosphatidylcholine (lecithin) and the cholinesterase inhibitor physostigmine].

FIGURE 80-2 *Physiologic functions in normal men aged 30 to 80 years, expressed as percent of average values for 30-year-olds. a. Fasting blood glucose. b. Nerve conduction velocity, cellular enzymes. c. Cardiac index (resting). d. Vital capacity, renal blood flow. e. Maximum breathing capacity. f. Maximum work rate, maximum oxygen uptake. (From NW Shock.)*

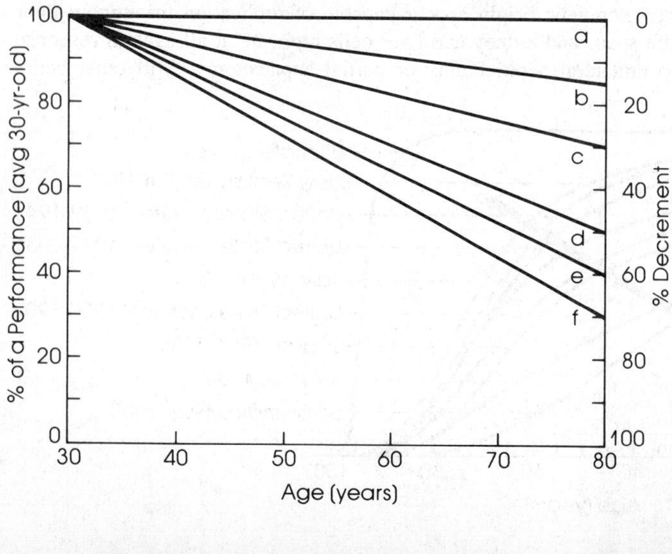

Changes in endocrine function with aging may be related to these neurotransmitter alterations. For example, normal aging is accompanied by a decline in glucose tolerance, and the incidence of diabetes mellitus is increased in the aged. The higher prevalence of nonketotic hyperosmolar coma in the elderly diabetic may be due to the impaired osmoregulation and diminished thirst perception that are common even among the healthy elderly. Clinical and subclinical thyroid deficiency is also more common. Thyroid insufficiency and perhaps the increased incidence of diabetes mellitus may be secondary to age-related increases in autoimmunity. Another age-related change in endocrine function relates to events associated with the menopause in women. It is not established whether the cessation of ovulation is due solely to depletion of primordial follicles within the ovary or whether changes in the neuroendocrine regulation of the ovary that accompany aging are also in part responsible. Whatever the etiology, menopausal endocrine changes, including diminished estradiol secretion, diminished negative feedback control of gonadotropin production at the level of the hypothalamus, compensatory increases in follicle-stimulating hormone (FSH) and luteinizing hormone (LH) secretion, and abnormal thermoregulation, have profound consequences at both psychological and physiologic levels. The endocrine changes in the aging male—though less dramatic—may be of equal import. These include both a decrease in mean plasma testosterone (most evident at the morning peak of the circadian cycle) and an increase in mean plasma estrogens, so that increasing feminization in aging men parallels diminished estrogen production in women.

The immune system may function as the pacemaker of the aging process. The thymus normally reaches maximal size in childhood and begins involution after puberty. Other lymphoid tissues generally reach maximal size soon after puberty and undergo gradual atrophy thereafter. Such atrophy is characterized by a reduction in lymphoid cells and their replacement by connective tissue. In addition there is a reduction in T-cell function that is even greater than the reduction in T-cell number. Other age-related changes in immune function include a decrease in the primary immune response of B cells, especially in those responses requiring T-cell interaction. Specific changes in lymphocyte function include (1) decreases in the proliferative responses to mitogens such as phytohemagglutinin and concanavalin A, (2) decreased suppression of B lymphocytes by T cells, and (3) decreased cytotoxic activity of T cells. These changes may have relevance to certain diseases of the elderly. For example, compared to young adults, the elderly have four to five times the case rate for cancer and tuberculosis and six to seven times the fatality rate from pneumonia.

The changes with age in neurotransmitters, endocrine function, and the immune system may be interlinked. For instance, production of thymic hormones may decrease with age, and this in turn may be under neuroendocrine regulation. Other endocrine changes, such as altered responses to glucocorticoids or changes in glucocorticoid secretion, may also affect the immune response.

While these regulatory systems may be of importance in the aging of the whole organism, age-related decrements occur in nearly all physiologic systems (Fig. 80-2). Such decrements at the organ system level reflect functional decrements at the cellular level. These data must be interpreted cautiously, for several reasons. First, they represent statistical means. Second, individual variation is not reflected, and the variance in physiologic performance appears to increase with age. Third, they were derived from cross-sectional studies. (However, longitudinal follow-up has largely reproduced these curves.) Fourth, the study subjects were all men and of an elite group, volunteers who were highly educated and in upper socioeconomic strata; hence, the changes depicted are perhaps representative of optimal, not typical aging. Nevertheless, the magnitude of the decrements is less than that associated with functional disability or frank disease. Thus, disease, not aging, is a threat to homeostasis at all ages, though distinguishing the primary effects of aging from those of diseases that occur with aging remains a challenge (Table 80-1). This problem of distinguishing between the primary and

TABLE 80-1 Primary vs. secondary aging. Examples of primary age-related changes and age-related disease effects

Organ system	Clinical manifestation	Primary age-related change	Secondary aging factors (disease and time-related factors including drug effects)
Skin	Wrinkling Purpura with minor trauma Susceptibility to pressure sores and slower healing Dry skin/pruritis Hair loss; hair graying	Atrophy (especially subcutaneous), decreased elasticity, increased vascular fragility, decreased sweating and sebaceous gland secretions, decreased hair and hair pigment, diminished cell replication	Sun exposure Chemical exposure
Eyes	Presbyopia, decreased dark adaptation Cataract Glaucoma Macular degeneration	Altered lens elasticity Altered biochemistry and physiology of vitreous and retina	Diabetes ? Cataract ? Glaucoma ? Macular degeneration Drug effects (miosis)
Ears	Decreased hearing, esp. high frequency; decreased sound discrimination	Diminished function of hair cells in the vestibular apparatus	Traumatic hearing loss Ménière's disease Drug toxicities
	Diminished position sense—"dizziness," falls	Diminished vestibular function	"Benign positional vertigo"
Nose and mouth	Decreased taste and food enjoyment Dry mouth	Diminished olfaction Diminished number of taste buds; diminished taste levels and salivation	Zinc deficiency Periodontal disease Drug-induced dry mouth, decreased salivation Diminished social eating cues
Gastrointestinal tract	Dysphagia, gastroesophageal reflux	Diminished esophageal motility and sphincter function	Hiatal hernia
	Hypochlorhydria with bacterial overgrowth	Diminished acid, pepsin, and trypsin secretion	Pernicious anemia
	Constipation	Decreased intestinal motility	Constipation secondary to low-residue diet, laxative abuse
	Altered drug metabolism	Altered hepatic enzymes	Chemical abuse altering drug metabolism (smoking, alcohol)
Respiratory system	Decreased vital capacity, FEV_1, maximum breathing capacity	Diminished lung elasticity	Chronic obstructive pulmonary disease secondary to smoking, pollution
		Diminished respiratory musculature	Diminished respiratory muscle power secondary to lack of exercise
Cardiovascular system	Diminished cardiac reserve, increased pulse pressure, increased vulnerability to hypotension and syncope	Diminished myocardial cell number, increased left ventricular and arterial resistance, diminished chronotropic response, diminished vascular baroreceptor (adrenergic) sensitivity	Atherosclerosis-related ischemia, ventricular dysfunction, arrhythmias, hypertensive heart disease, congestive heart failure
Renal-urinary system	Decreased glomerular filtration rate, tubular reabsorption	Diminished number of nephrons, changes in tubular function	Hypertension-related nephrosclerosis Drug-induced renal disease (aminoglycosides, nonsteroidal anti-inflammatory agents)
	Obstructive uropathy and overflow incontinence Stress incontinence	Decreased bladder tone, decreased bladder capacity, diminished sphincter tone, prostatic hyperplasia (men), diminished tone of pelvic musculature (women)	Urinary tract infections
Endocrine-metabolic system	Menopause (vasomotor symptoms, vaginal atrophy) Diminished male libido, potency, sexual drive	Hypogonadism Relatively abrupt (women) Relatively slow (men)	Surgical hypogonadism (oophorectomy), hypogonadism secondary to alcohol abuse
	Relative glucose intolerance	Diminished insulin response to glucose load, decreased insulin sensitivity (increased adiposity)	Increasing incidence of diabetes mellitus
	Diminished thyroid reserve	Diminished thyroid response	Autoimmune thyroiditis and hypothyroidism; hyperthyroidism (often apathetic)
Musculoskeletal system	Decreased strength	Decreased muscle fiber number and diameter	Disuse atrophy (sedentary lifestyle)
	Increased vulnerability to fracture	Diminished bone mineral content	Gonadal steroid deficiency; diet-, alcohol-, tobacco-, and drug-related osteoporosis
		Diminished bone formation	Osteomalacia secondary to Vitamin D deficiency (deficient diet and lack of sun exposure)
	Joint stiffness and inflammation	Increased stiffness of tendons, connective tissue Diminished joint cartilage	Drug-induced osteoarthritis (fluoride) Traumatic osteoarthritis (occupational, recreational)
Central nervous system	Hypothermia Hyperthermia	Diminished tolerance to temperature variation	Hypothermia from hypothyroidism
	Dehydration	Diminished thirst and drinking	Hyperosmolar, nonketotic coma in diabetes mellitus
	Postural hypotension, "dizziness," syncope, falls	Diminished postural reflexes and autonomic regulation	Drug-induced dehydration Autonomic insensitivity
	Slowness of movement Retarded rate of learning	Neuronal loss in the nucleus basalis, decreased cholinergic neurotransmitters and choline acetyltransferase activity Diminished basal ganglia function	Drug-induced cognitive dysfunction Delirium Drug-induced parkinsonism Alzheimer's disease Parkinson's disease
	Retarded positional correction, falls Altered sleep patterns	Diminished dorsal column function	Drug-induced ataxia, alcoholic cerebellar degeneration
Immune system	Increased susceptibility to infections and malignancy Impaired response to immunization Increased autoantibodies	Diminished cellular immunity (decreased helper cells) Diminished primary antibody response Increased abnormal immunoglobulins and autoimmunity	Nutritional deficiency Autoimmune diseases (thyrotoxicosis, thyroiditis, pernicious anemia)

secondary effects of aging will become more difficult as average longevity increases (death rates are declining most rapidly among the elderly and notably among those over 85), particularly since age-related decrements in functional capacity can pose a threat to the independence of the individual even in the absence of clear-cut disease. Thus age-related decrements may produce morbid symptoms in the elderly, especially under conditions of stress and acute illness. The simultaneous impairment of multiple systems in the elderly patient may explain the cascade of complications that can be initiated by a seemingly trival perturbation as well as the exponential rise in death rate among the very old (e.g., above age 93). The longevity curve of individuals above age 93 suggests that death may occur almost as a random phenomenon.

SUMMARY AND PROJECTION Aging occurs in all cells except those that undergo malignant transformation. While age-related phenomena may be most readily detected in assays of cellular replication in vitro, changes in cell function of a more subtle nature may be more relevant to aging of the whole organism. Such changes are likely to be amplified in systems that regulate metabolism and function of the whole organism, such as the nervous, endocrine, and immune systems. The aging phenomenon in its entirety must represent a mixture of cellular and systemic physiologic changes intrinsic to the species and of environmental insults that interact with the intrinsic processes.

Enhanced survival into old age is predominantly the result of changes in the environment that accompany socioeconomic development. During the twentieth century such changes have resulted in an increased average longevity in developed nations. However, there is little evidence that the upper limit of the human life span, ca. 120 years, has been altered, nor is there a realistic prospect for such a change. Hence, biologic aging in the human, though poorly understood, proceeds inexorably, resulting in a maximal life span that appears to be relatively fixed.

Many physiologic functions decline in an age-related manner, and attempts have been made to estimate physiologic (as contrasted to chronologic) age by application of a battery of tests to presumably healthy individuals of different ages. Although such profiles of performance may permit a gross estimate of biologic age that is useful in predicting a specific outcome in groups of subjects, these tests have no clinical utility in dealing with individuals. Hence, while general awareness of the limited reserve in many systems is of importance in geriatric practice, a careful search for disease-specific causes of decline is imperative in the elevation of patients of all ages.

REFERENCES

ADLER WH et al: Aging and immune function, in *The Biology of Aging*, JA Behnke et al (eds). New York, Plenum, 1978, p 221

GOLDBERG AP et al: Diabetes mellitus in the elderly, in *Principles of Geriatric Medicine*, R Andres et al (eds). New York, McGraw-Hill, 1985, p 750

FINCH CE: The regulation of physiological changes during mammalian aging. Quart Rev Biol 51:49, 1976

FRIES J: Aging, natural death, and the compression of morbidity. N Engl J Med 130:135, 1980

GOLDSTEIN S: The biology of aging. N Engl J Med 285:1120, 1971

HAYFLICK L: Theories of biological aging, in *Principles of Geriatric Medicine*, R Andres et al (eds). New York, McGraw-Hill, 1985, p 9

MARTIN GM et al: Replicative lifespan of cultivated human cells: Effects of donor's age, tissue, and genotype. Lab Invest 23:86, 1970

SHOCK NW: Physiological and chronological age, in *Aging—Its Chemistry*, AA Dietz (ed). Washington, D.C., American Association for Clinical Chemistry, 1980, p 3

81 HEALTH PROBLEMS OF THE ELDERLY

WILLIAM R. HAZZARD / JOHN R. BURTON

Increased concern for the health problems of the elderly is a result of the changing distribution of the population by age that occurs as nations develop socioeconomically (Fig. 81-1), a redistribution that is producing a rise in the proportion of the oldest segments of the American population (Fig. 81-2). This special concern reflects several phenomena: the close association between the aging process and the disease accumulated by the elderly (Table 80-1), the multiple disabilities, both apparent and potential, among those who survive into old age, the chronic and progressive nature of many of these disabilities, the disproportionate per capita consumption of health care resources by the elderly because of their vulnerable health status, and concern about the magnitude of health care expenditures as a proportion of gross national product. The challenge to the system for health and social care is to match the resources of the system to the needs of an aging population so as to improve both efficiency and effectiveness.

The principles of geriatric medicine overlap the principles of internal medicine. Information relevant to the medical care of the elderly is dispersed throughout this text, and a companion volume, *The Principles of Geriatric Medicine*, is available. Accordingly, this chapter is addressed to integrative aspects of geriatric medicine, including comprehensive assessment, preventive medicine, nutrition, and pharmacology of the elderly.

COMPREHENSIVE GERIATRIC ASSESSMENT Comprehensive geriatric assessment is indicated in various circumstances, all having in common a change in social, physical, or health care status. The profile of a typical patient would be one 75 years of age or older (a common threshold to define the younger end of the geriatric age spectrum) (1) whose physician has died or retired, (2) whose physician desires consultation or is not prepared to undertake long-term management of such a problem, (3) whose family perceives a change in health status that may require intervention, (4) whose locale has changed perhaps in response to a deteriorating health status, or (5) who has experienced a new medical problem or social crisis (or any combination of the five). Commonly this assessment is part of the decision-making process about the advisability of admission to a long-term care facility. The purpose of assessment is to review the physical, mental, and social situation with the view toward detecting and treating reversible causes of disease and disability, stabilizing those that may be progressing unnecessarily, introducing rehabilitative strategies to restore function, or adjusting the social or physical environment to provide independence and/or support in a deteriorating situation. The search for a cure for a given disease or even the establishment of a specific diagnosis is less often a primary goal than the formulation of a strategy, often practical in nature, to preserve independence, dignity, and function in a multiply disabled and frail individual. Since hospitalization is itself a risk to the precarious homeostasis of the elderly, this assessment should be carried out in the ambulatory setting wherever possible, the hospital being reserved for the treatment of acute disease.

Dimensions of assessment A comprehensive geriatric assessment includes five dimensions: physical health, mental health, social/economic status, environmental circumstances, and, most important, functional status.

Sometimes patients have undergone multiple previous assessments by generalists or specialists. The physician performing a geriatric assessment therefore may begin with a detailed review of available records so as to avoid redundancy in laboratory or radiologic testing. This aims both at avoiding the risk and cost of unnecessary testing and at identifying any points of uncertainty that remain after previous

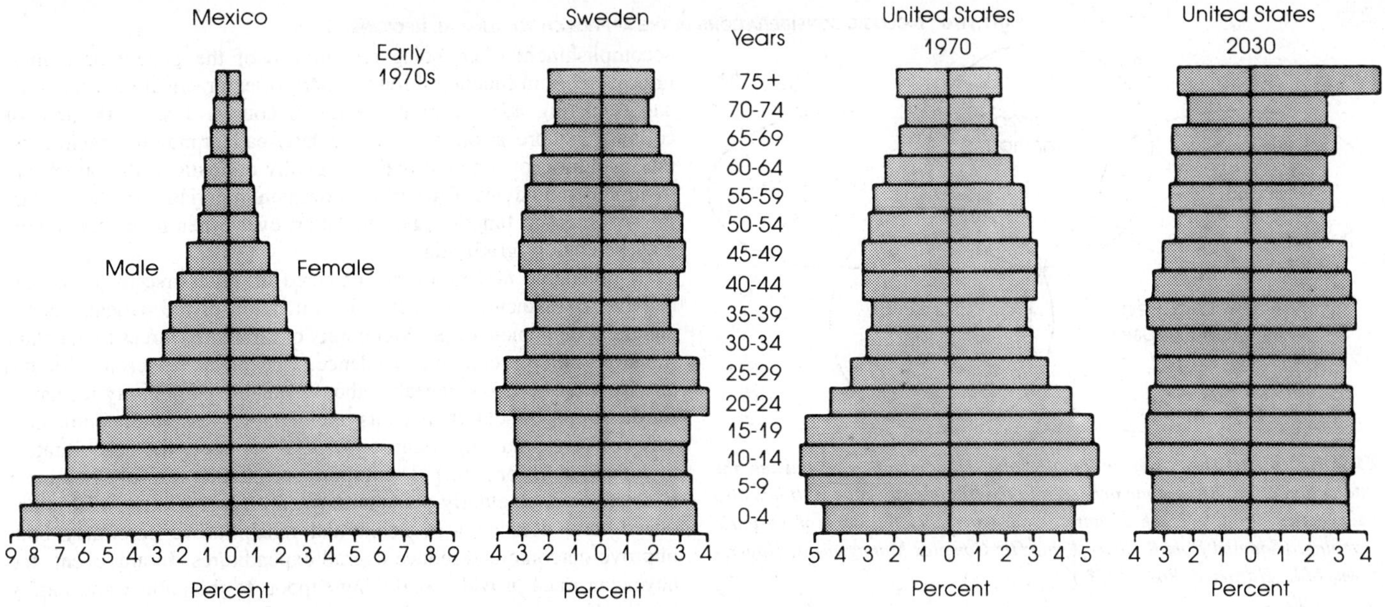

FIGURE 81-1 *Comparative profiles of population age and sex distributions among three nations in the present era and in the United States in 2030 (when a steady state will be approached). From AR Somers, The high cost of health care for the elderly: Diagnosis, prognosis, and some suggestions for therapy, J Health Politics, Policy, and Law 3(2):163, 1978.*

assessments. When geriatric assessment is performed as a consultation, few if any additional laboratory or radiologic examinations may be required. To assist in the systematic collection of requisite clinical and sociologic data, one of the several instruments developed for such assessment may be used, such as the Older American's Resources and Service Group (OARS) assessment form (Duke University Center for the Study of Aging and Human Development, Durham, NC 27710), which takes approximately 1 h to administer. A useful and somewhat shortened version of the OARS instrument, taking approximately half the time to administer, is the Functional Assessment Inventory (FAI) (Suncoast Gerontology Center, University of South Florida Medical Center, Tampa, FL 33612). A general limitation of all such assessment forms is that they have been developed for research use in groups of subjects rather than for the management of an individual patient. They are also less useful in circumstances of rapidly changing physical and mental status (such as in the hospital setting) than in a more stable circumstance over the long term. Therefore, physicians often develop individual approaches to geriatric assessment, commonly relying upon selected portions of the OARS or FAI for the cataloguing of social and economic resources and upon their own assessments of physical and mental health. All mechanisms of assessment, however, should include a systematic analysis of several dimensions.

PHYSICAL HEALTH Physical health should be assessed through the traditional medical history and physical examination, though the evaluation may have to be tailored to the limited physical and mental reserves of the elderly patient; e.g., perhaps conducted over a series of short office visits. Special care must also be taken to compensate for impediments to communication with the elderly patient. For example, the patient may have a problem with mobility, may not understand or be confused by questions, may have difficulty in vision or with hearing, and may become fatigued. Aids for the hearing impaired may be helpful, and the light should be facing the examiner to allow an element of lip-reading by the patient. The physician must be especially careful to evaluate those systems more often the focus of the interest of subspecialists outside the realm of internal medicine: the eyes, the ears, the teeth and mouth, the skin, and the nervous system. Problems such as immobility and incontinence may bridge more than one discipline (Fig. 81-3).

MENTAL HEALTH Depressive illness, delirium, dementia, and other mental disorders are especially debilitating in the elderly: hence, special focus upon cognitive function and mood is required. Systematic evaluation may be enhanced by use of simple scales or standards such as those for measuring depression or mental assessment.

SOCIAL AND ECONOMIC RESOURCES Social circumstances often heavily influence the physical and mental status and represent constraints to problem-solving. Critical areas for social/economic assessment include identification of those who will provide care for the patient in time of need. These "supporters" are critical for the maintenance of the elderly patient in the community and commonly include the spouse, adult children, or perhaps neighbors or landlords. Especially important is identification of those who will provide support of unlimited duration (usually confined to family members). Sources of intermittent or indirect support include church, community, and relevant social agencies. A cardinal rule of geriatric medicine is to "support the supporters," and supporter fatigue may precipitate a geriatric assessment, hospitalization, or long-term institutionalization. Not uncommonly, sickness or death of a prime supporter may be catastrophic for an elderly patient previously living independently in the community. The review of social resources also includes the taking of a financial inventory and establishing the degree to which public or private resources may need to be marshalled in support of the patient.

ENVIRONMENTAL CIRCUMSTANCES The physician should understand the physical environment in which the patient lives: Are there stairs to be climbed? Is the bathroom accessible to the precariously mobile individual? Are there hazards to ambulation in the dwelling (loose

FIGURE 81-2 *Percentage change from 1970 to 1980 in the population of United States residents by age groups. (Adapted from Bureau of Census: General population characteristics, 1980 Census of Population, Washington, DC, US Department of Commerce.)*

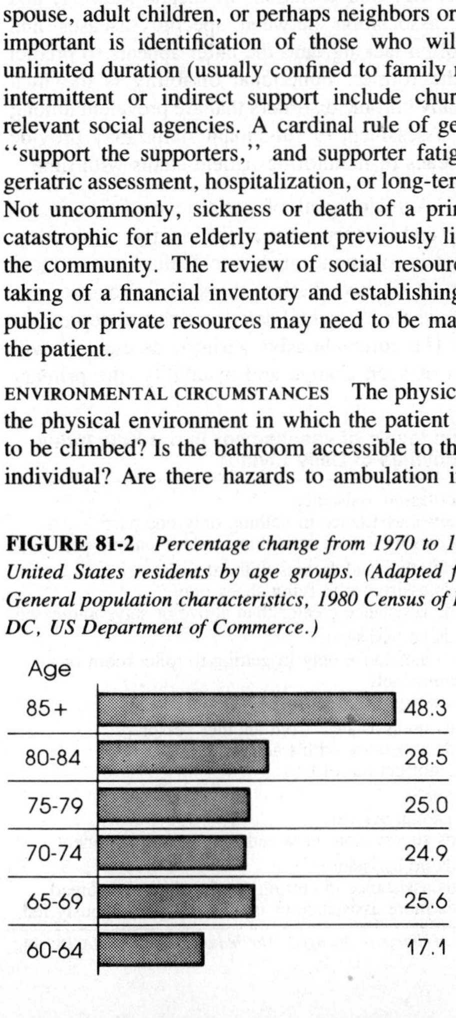

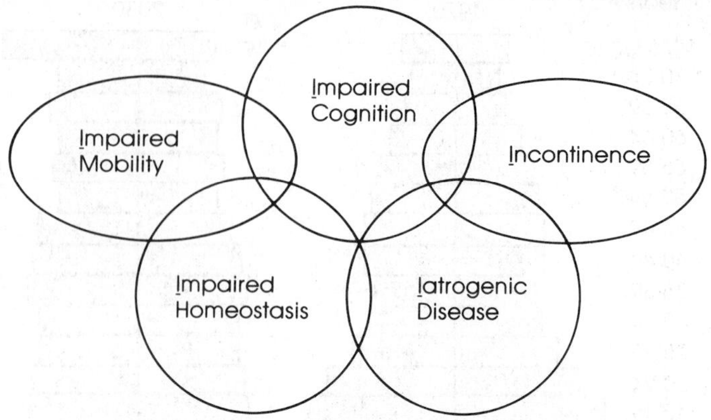

FIGURE 81-3 *The geriatric quintet or "O complex" emphasizes the interaction of problems commonly seen in the frail elderly patient. It has also been called the five Is of geriatrics and represents the core of geriatric teaching. (Adapted from R Cape, Aging: Its Complex Management, Hagerstown, Md., Harper & Row, 1978.)*

cords or rugs, clutter, sharp-edged furniture, etc.)? Are there fire hazards, especially for the cognitively impaired patient (e.g., open-flame stoves)?

FUNCTIONAL STATUS Care provided to the frail elderly patient must conform to the patient's functional ability. Scales of the activities of daily living (ADL) and "instrumental" activities of daily living (IADL) have been developed. Perhaps the most well-known and widely used is the Katz Functional Assessment Scale (Table 81-1). Six basic functions are assessed: bathing, dressing, toileting, transferring, continence, and feeding. More complex activities necessary for independent living include meal preparation, shopping, financial management, housekeeping, transportation, medication taking, and laundering. A strong association between specific diseases and functional capacity is often lacking, and the latter appears to predict outcome better than the former. Functional disability is the final common pathway of many chronic disorders that are prevalent among the elderly, and serial assessment of functional status may provide the most meaningful means of monitoring patient status with time.

Value of assessment A major goal of geriatric medicine is the preservation of function and independence in the elderly. At the time of assessment the patient is commonly in a state of flux: one or more chronic conditions may be in exacerbation, the social circumstances may be changing for the worse, or mental deterioration and depression may have supervened. The comprehensive geriatric assessment will dissect the components of such change and instability, the primary accomplishment often being reassurance of the patient or family, improvement in function through small, often practical interventions, and rendering advice about the future course. Just as the rate of collapse in a precariously situated elderly patient may be precipitous, the restitution of function may be equally dramatic with appropriate treatment and advice. Cure is less common in geriatric medicine than improvement in function, but the latter, even when relatively minor, may be equally gratifying.

If reversible factors are not detected in the course of a comprehensive assessment, the goal is identification of the patient's needs and the arrangement of the community or family resources to maintain function and preserve independence. The physician caring for the elderly must be knowledgeable about available community resources for the support of elderly patients, including professional, nonmedical services (e.g., nursing, dentistry, social services, the rehabilitative therapies, nutrition, etc.). The importance of such careful assessment is clear. Half of elderly persons may be inappropriately institutionalized, and detailed assessment and rehabilitative care may both improve outcome and reduce overall expenditures. In any event, the physician must provide continuing support to the patient and family because few problems are short-term and because needs may change abruptly. Home visits for assessment and intermittent care allow evaluation of the environmental conditions and also allow assessment of interactions of the patient with family and other supporters. Such home visits are especially important for the physician who does not have access to a multidisciplinary assessment team (e.g., social worker, rehabilitation therapists).

TABLE 81-1 Areas and levels of assessment in the Katz Index of Independence in Activities of Daily Living*

Bathing	______	Receives no assistance
	______	Receives assistance in bathing only one part
	______	Receives assistance in bathing more than one part
Dressing	______	Gets clothes and dresses without assistance
	______	Needs assistance in tying shoes only
	______	Needs assistance greater than above or stays undressed
Toileting	______	Needs no assistance
	______	Needs assistance only in getting to toilet room or in cleaning self
	______	Does not go to toilet room
Transferring	______	Needs no assistance from another person
	______	Needs assistance with transferring
	______	Does not get out of bed
Continence	______	Continent
	______	Occasional accident
	______	Needs supervision, uses catheter, or is incontinent
Feeding	______	Needs no assistance
	______	Needs assistance in cutting meat or buttering bread
	______	Needs more assistance or is tube- or intravenously fed

* *From S Katz et al, Studies of illness in the aged: The Index of ADL, JAMA 185:94, 1963.*

PREVENTIVE MEDICINE IN THE ELDERLY Effective intervention to retard or prevent many of the time-related chronic disease processes that pass the clinical threshold in old age must begin long before age 75: hypertension must be treated, dyslipoproteinemia must be diagnosed and managed, bone demineralization must be prevented or retarded, pulmonary function must be preserved by cessation of cigarette smoking, etc. "Preventive gerontology" involves intervention throughout the lifespan. Among the elderly, preventive medicine should focus upon short-term problems and solutions, balancing the risks and costs as well as the potential benefits of intervention (including their estimated duration). Particular attention should focus on the prevention of phenomena that may trigger catastrophic collapse such as immunizations (notably one-time polyvalent pneumococcal vaccination, maintenance of adequate tetanus protection, and annual influenza vaccination), elimination of environmental hazards (classically the scatter rug), and preservation of adequate physical activity, nutrition, and social interactions. Furthermore, even in the frail elderly, systematic exercise programs may improve the sense of well being. This type of preventive medicine is an important part of the periodic health evaluation of the elderly patient with its emphasis upon social, psychological, and functional issues in addition to the usual physical and mental evaluation.

Nutrition and aging A frequent final common pathway of functional decline in the elderly is malnutrition, notably when acute illness is superimposed on chronic disease and disability. Few data have been gathered relative to the prevalence, incidence, and severity of such malnutrition. For example, micro- and macronutrient requirements have not yet been defined for the elderly. By ordinary criteria, significant malnutrition among free-living elderly is common only among the poor and sick. On the other hand, barriers to adequate nutrition are imposed both by primary aging and by the common disease concomitants of the aging process: decline in smell and taste perception causes diminished enjoyment of food; salivation decreases, and mastication is commonly impaired through dental losses and disease; swallowing may be difficult, choking is common, and esophageal motility is diminished; gastric acid and pepsin secretion are diminished, and gastric motility may be reduced (as may that of the small and large intestine, constipation being common); biliary secretion is commonly impaired, and gall bladder disease is common;

perhaps most important, since physical activity is diminished, appetite is also suppressed, and the intake of both macro- and micronutrients may be decreased to the point of marginal deficiency. Social and psychological cues to eating frequently are lacking, and depression is common; for example, death of a spouse may jeopardize intake not only because of the anorexia of the depression associated with bereavement but also by removing the incentive to prepare a tasteful and nutritious meal. The impact of accompanying weight loss and malnutrition is immediately apparent. Weight loss, a cardinal manifestation of disease at all ages, should signal an exhaustive search for its cause in the elderly, for whom it represents a proximate and ominous sign of decline. The cause may be obvious, e.g., malignancy, or cryptic; e.g., tuberculosis or endogenous depression. Just as often the cause cannot be determined, and long-term assessment may be required before the cause of the weight loss can be ascertained. As with geriatric medicine in general, the search for iatrogenic or social causality is of prime importance: e.g., digitalis intoxication; lack of enjoyment through an enforced diet (for example, one that is severely fat- or carbohydrate-restricted); or depression following translocation of a patient from a supportive social environment to one of isolation, as in a retirement community providing no interaction. In any event the prognostic significance of weight loss is nowhere more evident than among the elderly, since malnutrition may represent a serious barrier to recovery from illness and is correlated with the development of pressure sores, infections, muscle wasting, and weakness that prevent ambulation and self care.

Nutritional assessment in the elderly is not unlike that in the nonelderly. Laboratory tests such as serum albumin, lymphocyte count, or transferrin levels appear to add little to the clinical assessment of weight/height (commonly expressed as the Quetelet or body mass index [BMI], weight/height^2), or more valuable, documentation of a change in weight. Measurement of skinfold thickness also adds an objective dimension to evaluation (see Chap. 71), though it is subject to imprecision because of increased skin flaccidity and the lack of adequate standards for the elderly. Calorie counts or reviews of dietary intake may be useful, particularly if food avoidance is suspected. If inadequate intake is documented in the hospitalized patient, intervention is indicated with oral, enteral, or parenteral supplements. Other laboratory measurements are of derivative use only; e.g., folate and/or B_{12} levels if the patient demonstrates a macrocytic anemia.

Nutritional therapy is frequently attempted in the elderly, though success may be elusive and difficult to document. Oral multivitamin and mineral supplements are taken commonly with or without physician advice. The rationale for such supplementation is apparent, however, given the low risk of "one-a-day" vitamin supplementation and the relatively high risk of micronutrient deficiency in the elderly patient whose nutritional status is marginal. Increased calcium intake (1000 to 1500 mg per day) is also recommended in middle-aged and elderly women to prevent or retard osteoporosis. The addition of liquid, calorie-rich supplements in the malnourished patient may be helpful and at times essential (e.g., in the patient with oral pathology or dysphagia for solid foods). However, in the anorectic patient these seldom suffice to overcome antecedent weight loss and may create a false sense of security. Where functional impediments exist (e.g., a swallowing disorder following a stroke), a specific nutritional regimen may be critical in promoting recovery, for example, enteral or parenteral feeding with early consideration of gastrostomy in those requiring chronic enteral alimentation. While many formulations with varying degrees of osmolality, caloric density, and caloric distribution have been introduced for such feeding (see Chap. 74), caloric restitution is of primary importance given adequate protein and micronutrient replacement. Whereas the determinants of disease usually play the dominant role and nutritional supplements only a permissive role in recovery, malnutrition per se can be the cause of depression and even anorexia itself; correction by hyperalimentation may increase activity, positive mood, and eating and permit wound healing and recovery from infection.

Pharmacology in the elderly Iatrogenic disease is one of the major problems of geriatric medicine (Fig. 81-3) and is of primary concern to the physician caring for the elderly. Pharmacologic misadventures are prominent in this concern. Since the elderly commonly have multiple disorders, treatment with multiple medications ("polypharmacy"), both appropriate and inappropriate, is common. While special characteristics of the elderly place them at risk from side effects of drugs, no principle is as important as that multiple drugs enhance the hazard of complications from those drugs.

Approximately 90 percent of the elderly take at least one medication, and the majority take two or more. The most commonly prescribed drugs are those for the treatment of cardiovascular disease, antihypertensives, analgesics, and anti-inflammatory agents. Over-the-counter medications account on average for some 40 percent of the drugs consumed by the elderly; inventory of these agents is important in the search for pharmacologic causes of disease and disability. Patients confined to long-term care facilities commonly take even more medications, psychotropic agents surpassing all others in such institutions (in up to 75 percent of institutionalized as opposed to 25 percent of ambulatory patients). As a consequence of this high prevalence of drug ingestion, adverse drug reactions occur in 6 to 40 percent of those over 60 years of age in various series, are a common cause of hospitalization, and may be difficult to detect. The risk factors for such reactions, in addition to multiple drug usage, include being a woman (perhaps attributable to small body size and failure to adjust dosage accordingly), hepatic or renal insufficiency (leading to drug accumulation), and previous drug reactions. Whether age is a factor independent of its association with disease is not established; what is clear, however, is that the elderly are at particularly high risk to drug misadventures.

Other aspects of drug therapy in the elderly are also relevant. Compliance is of particular concern. In some studies 25 to 50 percent of outpatients fail to take their medications, underscoring the impor-

TABLE 81-2 Summary of factors affecting drug disposition in the geriatric patient

Pharmacokinetic parameter	Age-related physiologic changes	Pathologic conditions	Environmental factors
Absorption	Increased gastric pH Decreased absorptive surface Decreased splanchnic blood flow Decreased gastrointestinal motility	Achlorhydria Diarrhea Gastrectomy Malabsorption syndromes Pancreatitis	Antacids Anticholinergics Cholestyramine Drug interaction Food or meals
Distribution	Decreased total-body water Decreased lean body mass Increased body fat	Dehydration Hepatic failure Malnutrition Renal failure	Protein-binding displacement
Metabolism	Decreased hepatic mass Decreased enzyme activity Decreased hepatic blood flow	Congestive heart failure Fever Hepatic insufficiency Malignancy Malnutrition Thyroid disease Viral infection or immunization	Dietary composition Drug interaction Acceleration of metabolism Inhibition of metabolism Insecticides Tobacco (smoking)
Excretion	Decreased renal blood flow Decreased glomerular filtration rate Decreased tubular secretion	Hypovolemia Renal insufficiency	Drug interactions

SOURCE: *Vestal*

TABLE 81-3 Examples of drugs usually given in reduced dosage in the elderly*

Drug (or drug class)	Possible consequences of standard dosage regimen
Aminoglycosides	Ototoxicity and nephrotoxicity
Benzodiazepines	Unwanted CNS depression—more common with larger doses
Carbamazepine	Drowsiness or ataxia may develop
Chlormethiazole	Confusion possible with larger doses
Digoxin	Digitalis toxicity
Haloperidol	Extrapyramidal reactions
Levodopa	Hypotension common
Meperidine	Respiratory depression
Metoclopramide	Confusion common
Thioridazine	Confusion common
Thyroxine	Myocardial infarction
Vitamin D	Renal toxicity

* *The drugs listed are examples only; this is not intended to be an exhaustive listing*
SOURCE: *From World Health Organization, Health care in the elderly: Report of the technical group on use of medicaments by the elderly, Drugs 22:279, 1981.*

tance of careful review of drug-taking practices at the initial and subsequent assessments in the outpatient setting. In one study 59 percent of ambulatory patients above age 60 made one or more medication errors (26 percent potentially serious ones), and multiple errors are common (especially in patients above 75 years of age). The causes of errors in drug taking include problems in communication and understanding on the part of the patient or supporter, the use of multiple drugs, and the employment of complicated and changing regimens.

Age-related differences also exist in pharmacokinetics (summarized in Table 81-2). In the elderly body water and lean body mass are diminished relative to adipose mass. Hence water-soluble drugs are distributed in a smaller space (i.e., at a higher concentration per dose administered). Alcohol is one such agent that not only has a higher concentration after a given oral dose in the elderly because of a diminished space of distribution but also appears to have an increased effect (producing gait disturbances with smaller amounts ingested, for example). Since renal clearance may decline progressively with age, drugs cleared by the kidney (such as digoxin) must be given in reduced doses. However, some drugs (such as beta-adrenergic blocking agents) are actually of diminished potency in the elderly. Overall, prudence in drug prescription should be exercised both as to the quantity of each agent made available and the number of such agents prescribed (see Table 81-3). The principles for prescribing drugs in the elderly are summarized in Table 81-4.

TABLE 81-4 Principles of drug prescription for geriatric patients

1 Evaluate the need for drug therapy.
- *a* Not all diseases afflicting the elderly require drug treatment.
- *b* Avoid drugs if possible, but do not withhold on account of age drugs that might enhance the quality of life.
- *c* Strive for a diagnosis prior to treatment.

2 Take a careful history of habits and drug use.
- *a* Patients often seek advice and receive prescriptions from several physicians.
- *b* Knowledge of existing therapy, both prescribed and nonprescribed, helps anticipate potential drug interactions.
- *c* Smoking, alcohol, and caffeine may affect drug response.

3 In general, use smaller doses in the elderly.
- *a* Often the standard dose is too large for the elderly patient.
- *b* While the effect of age on drug metabolism by the liver is less predictable, renal excretion of drugs and their active metabolites tends to decline.
- *c* The elderly are particularly sensitive to drugs affecting central nervous system function.

4 Titrate drug dosage with patient response.
- *a* Establish reasonable therapeutic endpoints.
- *b* Adjust dosage until endpoints are reached or unwanted side effects prevent further increases.
- *c* Use an adequate dose, particularly in the treatment of pain associated with malignancy.
- *d* Sometimes combination therapy is appropriate and effective.

5 Simplify the therapeutic regimen and encourage compliance.
- *a* Try to avoid intermittent schedules. Once- or twice-daily dosage is ideal.
- *b* Select a dosage form appropriate for the patient.
- *c* Label drug containers clearly. When appropriate, specify standard containers.
- *d* Give careful instructions to both patient and a relative or friend. Explain why the drug(s) is (are) being prescribed.
- *e* Suggest the use of a medication calendar or diary.
- *f* Encourage the return or destruction of outdated medications.

SOURCE: *Vestal*

REFERENCES

ANDRES R et al: *Principles of Geriatric Medicine*. New York, McGraw-Hill, 1984

BRESLOW L, SOMERS AR: The lifetime health monitoring program: A practical approach to preventive medicine. N Engl J Med 296:601, 1977

HAZZARD WR: Preventive gerontology: Strategies for healthy aging. Post-Graduate Medicine 27(1):22, 1983

KANE RA, KANE RL: *Assessing The Elderly: A Practical Guide to Measurement*, Lexington, MA, Lexington Books, 1981

RUBENSTEIN LZ et al: Effectiveness of a geriatric evaluation unit. N Engl J Med. 31:1664, 1984

VESTAL RE: Clinical pharmacology, in *Principles of Geriatric Medicine*, R Andres et al (eds). New York, McGraw-Hill, 1984

WILLIAM TF et al: Appropriate placement of the chronically ill and aged: A successful approach by evaluation. JAMA 226:1332, 1973

PART THREE DISORDERS CAUSED BY BIOLOGIC AND ENVIRONMENTAL AGENTS

section 1 Important considerations in infectious diseases

82 AN APPROACH TO INFECTIOUS DISEASES

ROBERT G. PETERSDORF / RICHARD K. ROOT

THE SCOPE OF INFECTIOUS DISEASES The vast majority of human and animal diseases of known etiology are produced by biologic agents: viruses, rickettsias, bacteria, mycoplasma, *Chlamydia,* fungi, protozoa, or nematodes. No small part of the past and present importance of infectious diseases in medical practice is attributable to their enormous frequency and the public health implications of their contagiousness. However, developments in sanitary engineering, vector control, immunization, and specific chemotherapy have modified the situation favorably. Although important exceptions remain, infectious diseases as a class are more easily prevented and more easily cured than any other major group of disorders. Despite the elimination of some infectious diseases such as smallpox and the profound reduction in the morbidity and mortality rates of many, humans are by no means free of infection. In fact, the total human load of disease produced by microbial parasites has decreased only modestly, primarily through smallpox and malaria control and better health care in developing countries. As certain specific microbial infections have been controlled, others have emerged as troublesome therapeutic and epidemiologic problems. With the introduction of cytotoxic drugs, massive irradiation in the treatment of malignant diseases, and immunosuppressive agents to control the rejection of transplanted organs, the insertion of prosthetic devices into the bloodstream, and the progressive longevity of people with chronic degenerative diseases, infections due to organisms previously considered saprophytic or commensal have increased. These infections have also been termed *opportunistic*. Worldwide concern has been aroused by the occurrence of infection of T lymphocytes by retroviruses causing either their malignant transformation or cytolysis. The profound immunosuppression characteristic of human lymphotrophic virus III lymphadenopathy-associated virus (HTLV III/LAV) infection and lysis of T helper cells is known as the *acquired immunodeficiency syndrome* (AIDS) (see Chap. 257). Multiple opportunistic infections cause death in the majority of patients with AIDS.

Because of better environmental sanitation and other measures that now prevent contact with many microbial agents, and the development of acquired immunity early in childhood, certain infections have been seen more frequently in adults. For example, as contact with poliomyelitis virus in childhood declined in many countries, paralytic poliomyelitis became more common in young adults. *Haemophilus influenzae* meningitis and pneumonia is being reported more frequently in adults than heretofore, and decreasing infection with the tubercle bacillus raises questions about the status of antituberculous immunity in adults. For reasons that are not clear, hepatitis A is predominantly a disease of young adults, while non-A, non-B hepatitis tends to occur in individuals over 35 years of age.

As antimicrobial agents reduce the mortality associated with certain common infections, other microbes emerge as important causes of human disease. If an infection occurs during or immediately following a course of chemotherapy, it is often caused by a microorganism that is resistant to the drug that was given; such an infection is termed a *superinfection.* While it is relatively unusual nowadays for patients to die of uncomplicated pneumococcal pneumonia, a disease readily handled with available antimicrobials, it is common to see serious disease produced by microorganisms which are much more resistant even though they are often part of the normal microbial flora in humans. These include staphylococci, gram-negative enteric bacilli, and a variety of anaerobes and fungi. One important mechanism by which resistance is conferred on gram-negative enteric bacteria is the action of R factors (see Chap. 85).

Agents not previously known as causes of human disease are being identified rapidly. *Legionella pneumophila* (see Chap. 117) was first described in 1976 and in the ensuing 6 years much of the epidemiology, microbiology, pathogenesis, clinical course, prognosis, and treatment have been worked out. Since the original description of *L. pneumophila* less virulent but related microorganisms that cause pneumonia have been described (see Chap. 117). However, in contrast to *L. pneumophila,* these organisms turned out not to be new pathogens. Rather, they had been described in the past and given different names and the discovery of *L. pneumophila* placed them into the proper taxonomic and clinical framework. A different manifestation of an old organism is the relationship between *Staphylococcus aureus* and the toxic shock syndrome (see Chap. 94). In this situation a well-known organism appears to be elaborating a toxin that causes a severe systemic illness. The precise mechanism whereby this toxin produces disease is not known. Yet another relatively new entity that was presumed to be of infectious etiology, Lyme arthritis (see Chap. 277), has been found to be caused by a spirochete. These brief descriptions of new diseases are cited to illustrate the ever-changing array of infectious diseases.

Particularly striking is the spectrum of infections that are seen in AIDS patients in addition to malignancies such as Kaposi's sarcoma and lymphomas (see Chap. 257). AIDS patients who present with opportunistic infections caused by viruses [cytomegalovirus (CMV), herpes simplex], bacteria (*Mycobacterium avium-intracellulare, M. tuberculosis*), parasites (*Pneumocystis carinii, Toxoplasma gondii, Cryptosporidium*), and fungi (*Cryptococcus neoformans, Histoplasma capsulatum,* and *Candida albicans*) invariably die despite transiently effective antimicrobial therapy, and current attempts at immune reconstitution. This tragic outcome emphasizes the vital role of the cellular immune defenses in protection against these organisms and in surveillance against certain malignancies. No wonder one-quarter of people that seek medical attention, even in developed countries, do so for infections, and the number is much higher in the developing world. It should also come as no surprise that, in the United States, 25 percent of prescriptions that are written are for antibiotics.

In this and the subsequent chapters, principles of host-parasite interaction, the usefulness of diagnostic procedures, important epidemiologic issues, principles of chemotherapy, major infectious syndromes not associated with specific organ systems (which are found under diseases of these organ systems), and approaches to preventing infections are stressed. In subsequent chapters of this section, diseases caused by specific etiologic agents are described. Together, the syndromic as well as etiologic approach provides a thorough compendium to the study of infectious diseases.

THE PARASITE AND THE HOST The interaction between microorganism and humans that results in infection and disease is complex. Much has been learned about the way in which microbes enter the body, the ways in which they produce tissue injury, the influence of specific immunity and "nonspecific" resistance of the host in contributing to the manifestations of both infection and protection, and the mechanisms of recovery. It is not yet possible to transfer in any specific way much of the information that has been acquired to the individual patient with an infection. However, considerable progress is being made. Examples are the sexual transmission of hepatitis A virus; the major role that *Chlamydia* are found to play in the causation of pelvic inflammatory disease (see Chap. 91); the role of Norwalk and rotaviruses in infectious diarrheas (see Chap. 89); and advances in antimicrobial therapy in containing heretofore difficult-to-treat bacteria (see Chap. 88).

INFECTION AND CLINICAL DISEASE Microorganisms of different species or different strains of the same species vary widely in their capacity to produce disease, and human beings are not equally susceptible to the disease caused by a given bacterium or virus. Furthermore, while a specific infectious disease will not occur in the absence of the causative organism, the mere presence of the organism in the body does not lead invariably to clinical illness. Indeed, the production of symptoms in humans by many parasites is the exception rather than the rule, and the *subclinical infection* or the "carrier state" is the usual host-parasite relationship. *Disease* in a clinical sense is not synonymous with the presence of the organism or *infection* in a microbiologic sense. In fact, for most organisms the number of subclinical infections far exceeds that of clinical disease.

MECHANISMS OF INJURY It is customary to refer to bacteria or other microorganisms that are capable of producing disease as *pathogenic*. *Virulence*, the *degree* of pathogenicity, should be distinguished from *invasiveness*, the ability to spread and disseminate in the body. For example, *Clostridium tetani* is pathogenic and, by virtue of its exotoxin, highly virulent, but it is almost completely lacking in invasiveness. Moreover, in certain circumstances and in certain anatomic locations, mildly "pathogenic" organisms can produce fatal disease, or highly "pathogenic" species can multiply without producing any harmful effect.

A few microorganisms produce *toxins* that account for the tissue damage and physiologic alterations of infection. *Hypersensitivity* to components of the organism is demonstrable in several infections to account for the manifestations of disease. For many pathogenic agents, an explanation of their damaging effects upon the host is incomplete or wholly lacking. Generally, therefore, the aim of therapy is to stop multiplication or to kill the microorganisms with appropriate drugs; in diseases caused by toxin-producing organisms, the use of antitoxin (as in tetanus or diphtheria) is the definitive procedure, and chemotherapy is of secondary importance. A relatively new example of a toxin-mediated infection is the toxic shock syndrome, in which the toxin is elaborated by *S. aureus*. In this situation, this ordinarily invasive organism does not usually invade local tissues.

The tendency of certain pathogenic organisms to *localize in certain cells or organs* and to produce disease in a specific anatomic site or evoke a combination of symptoms referable to certain organs often suggests the identity of the causative organism. For example, the pneumococcus usually causes infection in the lung but almost never in the kidney, and *H. influenzae* infections are confined almost solely to the respiratory tract and meninges. Similarly, in the presence of disease known to be caused by a given agent, involvement of other tissues can be anticipated or predicted. Examples include the multiple lung abscesses which are so characteristic of hematogenously disseminated staphylococcal disease and the metastatic skin lesions which complicate *Pseudomonas* bacteremia.

Frequently, the proper management of infectious disease involves the use of techniques completely unrelated to microbiology or chemotherapy, in an effort to support the function of damaged organs. Survival in varicella pneumonia usually depends upon treatment of respiratory failure; in the management of endocarditis, valve replacement is often more difficult than the eradication of the causative organism; in cholera the repletion of the volume deficit and in Weil's disease the treatment of acute renal failure with peritoneal or hemodialysis are the important therapeutic objectives.

RESISTANCE AND SUSCEPTIBILITY Many so-called host factors are known to influence the likelihood that disease will occur if organisms enter the tissues, or to play a determining role in the outcome once the infection has become established. These include the integrity of mucocutaneous barriers, the action of local macrophages, the adequacy of polymorphonuclear leukocyte responses, the function of the complement systems, and the presence or absence of specific antibodies or specific cellular immunity. In the earliest stages of infection, the balance between nonspecific defenses and virulence factors of organisms determines whether or not infection progresses to become clinically apparent.

In experimental animals, sex, microbial strain, age, route of infection, the presence of specific antibody, associated diseases, nutritional state, and the use of such procedures as exposure to ionizing radiation or high environmental temperature, administration of antimetabolites, adrenal steroids, epinephrine, and metabolic analogues can be shown to exert a profound effect on infection by bacteria, viruses, fungi, and other agents.

In humans, these factors are no less important, although controlled studies are lacking for many. Alcoholism; diabetes; deficiency or absence of immunoglobulins (see Chap. 256); defects in cellular immunity (see Chap. 260); malnutrition; chronic administration of steroid hormones; chronic lymphedema; ischemia; the presence of foreign bodies such as bullets, calculi, or bone fragments; obstruction of a bronchus, the urethra, or any hollow tube; agranulocytosis or congenital defects in bactericidal or virucidal activity; various blood dyscrasias, and many other circumstances influence susceptibility to systemic or local infection. Furthermore, in those instances where the extenuating condition is remediable, the probability of recovery is enhanced. An interesting example is provided by the high incidence of tuberculous and fungal infections in patients undergoing jejunoileal bypass for morbid obesity. In some of these patients, the infection could not be reversed until the bypass was reconstructed.

Racial differences in susceptibility, such as the poor resistance of dark-skinned people to tuberculosis and their predilection for developing disseminated coccidioidomycosis, are well established. Resistance to infection may be determined genetically. The relation of sickle cell trait to malaria is one example. The increased frequency and severity of some infections in children, of others in pregnant women, and still others in the aged are familiar. In the elderly, it is important to distinguish between infections complicating age-related diseases (e.g., urinary tract infection in prostatic hypertrophy) versus age-related alterations in specific immunity (e.g., tuberculosis reactivation from suppressed cellular immunity).

Prior contact with an organism or its products, whether by active infection or by artificial immunization, increases resistance to some infections, such as measles, diphtheria, and pertussis, by stimulating antibody production, but seems to have little influence on resistance to others, such as gonorrhea.

Knowledge of all the factors involved in human resistance and susceptibility to infection is incomplete. While various disorders can be shown to alter nonspecific or specific immune mechanisms, the precise contributions of such alterations to clinical manifestations often remain incompletely defined. Given the multiplicity of defenses against microorganisms, profound depression of one or more is usually required to cause repeated or unusually severe infections. For example, unless granulocyte counts fall below 1000 per cubic millimeter (normal >1800 per cubic millimeter), or a major bactericidal mechanism is deleted from all polymorphonuclear leukocytes (e.g., oxygen-forming capacity), as in chronic granulomatous disease (see Chap. 272), life-threatening bacterial or visceral fungal infections are not increased in incidence. Many individuals (~1 in 500) may lack serum or secretory IgA, yet relatively few suffer infectious complications. Similarly, many patients with deficiencies of serum complement components may have no infectious complications or long infection-free intervals. While coexistent infection with CMV, Epstein-Barr virus (EBV), hepatitis, or other sexually transmitted pathogens may serve as promotors for HTLV III/LAV infection in exposed patients, life-threatening opportunistic infections do not occur, as a rule, until the T-helper population is markedly depleted. Not all patients who become colonized with *Haemophilus influenzae* B or *Neisseria meningitidis* develop clinically apparent or severe infection in the absence of specific antibodies. These observations highlight the complex nature of the interactions between microorganisms and the human host which determine the outcome of encounters with infectious agents.

PATHOGENESIS OF INFECTION With relatively minor variations, the development of an infectious disease follows a consistent pattern. The parasites enter the body through the skin, nasopharynx, lung, intestine, urethra, or other portal. A number of microorganisms adhere to their site of primary attack through fimbriae, pili, and surface antigens; the adherence of *Bordetella pertussis* to respiratory epithelium, the gonococcus to urethral epithelium, and possibly some gram-negative urinary pathogens known as "adhesins" to the epithelium of the renal pelvis are some examples. These surface factors couple to specific cellular receptors, the availability, distribution, and turnover of which play a major role in regulating the character of the local microbial flora. Once established in the host, the organisms can multiply and, in so doing, establish a local or primary lesion. From this site, there may be local spread along fascial planes or tubular structures, such as a bronchus or ureter. The next step may be systemic spread of the microorganisms via the circulating blood. Bacteria can enter the bloodstream by direct invasion of vessels, a relatively unusual occurrence, or more commonly by traversing peripheral lymph nodes to enter the thoracic duct lymph and thence the venous system. In the bloodstream, they spread to other tissues and can produce distant or secondary lesions. In infections such as tetanus and diphtheria, distant lesions are produced by toxins elaborated at the primary site without systemic spread of the bacteria. The infectious process may terminate in recovery or death at any stage: the local lesion, systemic spread, or distant lesion.

The apparent inconsistency of this pattern in clinical medicine is attributable to the fact that the infection is recognized as a clinical entity only at the stage when symptoms are most likely to appear. For example, pneumococcal pneumonia is a local lesion, and the distant lesion, pneumococcal meningitis, is referred to clinically as a complication. In meningococcal infections, the local lesion, nasopharyngitis, is rarely symptomatic and has no status as a clinical entity, but the stage of spread, meningococcemia, and the commonest distant lesion, meningitis, are clinical entities. A rarer distant lesion, arthritis, is called a complication. In a patient who has osteomyelitis, a clinical entity, a recent furuncle may be referred to as a predisposing factor. In another patient with extensive furunculosis who develops osteomyelitis, the infection in bone may be regarded as a complication of the superficial infection. The stages mentioned are in no way limited to bacterial diseases; the primary lesion of poliomyelitis is intestinal and is usually asymptomatic, viremia may occur without neurologic involvement, or a distant lesion manifested by symptomatic involvement of the central nervous system may be established.

Because clinical usage and terminology are based upon the symptomatic illness that leads patients to seek medical aid, the consistency of this general sequence in the pathogenesis of infection is often not recognized. However, the concept is useful and offers some basis for systematizing what may otherwise seem to be a miscellaneous collection of unrelated clinical signs and symptoms.

CLINICAL MANIFESTATIONS OF INFECTIONS So varied are the disorders attributable to infection or infestation of humans by lower organisms that generalizations about them are difficult. The clinical manifestations of infection can duplicate those of diseases of any other etiology. However, certain clinical features are highly suggestive of infection, including abrupt onset, fever, chills, myalgia, photophobia, pharyngitis, acute lymphadenopathy and splenomegaly, gastrointestinal upset, and leukocytosis or leukopenia. It is obvious that the presence of one, several, or all of these features does not constitute proof of the microbial origin of illness in a given patient. Conversely, serious, even fatal, infectious disease may exist in the absence of fever or other signs and symptoms.

Although there is no infallible clinical criterion of infection, it is possible to recognize accurately many specific infectious diseases from information obtained by *history, physical examination, blood count, and urinalysis*. The importance of interrogation about past illness, predisposing factors such as alcoholism, familial disease, exposure to ill persons, contact with animals or insects, ingestion of contaminated food, type and order of onset of symptoms, and recent or remote residence in endemic areas is discussed in the subsequent chapters that deal with specific diseases and etiologic agents. Cardinal physical signs are also described for each entity.

The mechanisms that produce most of the signs and symptoms of human infection are incompletely known. The endogenous production of a family of polypeptides known collectively as interleukin 1 (IL-1) appears instrumental in producing many of the clinical manifestations of infection including chills and fever, leukocytosis, myalgias, lassitude, and a negative nitrogen balance (see Chap. 8). The physiologic alterations underlying "malaise," "postinfectious asthenia," "toxicity," and other common complaints are completely mysterious. The factors responsible for leukocytosis or leukopenia are only partially understood (see Chap. 56). Why the rash of typhus begins on the trunk while that of another rickettsiosis, Rocky Mountain spotted fever, begins on the extremities is unanswered. Failure to understand these manifestations does not impair their clinical usefulness, although it is probable that understanding them might lead to more accurate diagnosis and better management.

DIAGNOSTIC PROCEDURES The specific procedures for the diagnosis of infectious disease have become sufficiently complex to warrant separate discussion. This is provided in Chap. 83.

Importance of specific diagnosis in infectious diseases The diagnostic procedures employed for infectious diseases are no more absolute than those in other diseases; they cannot be blindly equated with the science of microbiology. The responsibility for interpreting the facts supplied by the bacteriologist, immunologist, and virologist in the total context of a patient's illness remains that of the physician. A positive tuberculin skin test certainly does not indicate that a patient has active tuberculosis. The finding of *Candida albicans* in a stool culture does not necessarily mean that a patient's diarrhea is caused by intestinal candidiasis. The presence of staphylococci in nasal cultures from a patient with headaches does not establish a diagnosis of staphylococcal sinusitis. A throat culture containing group A beta-hemolytic streptococci does not rule out diphtheria, nor does such a culture establish that a febrile illness in a patient with mitral stenosis is a recurrence of acute rheumatic fever rather than bacterial endocarditis. A positive serologic test for syphilis may indicate a treponematosis other than syphilis, syphilis that is active or inactive, or an unrelated disease such as systemic lupus erythematosus.

The etiologic agent From a practical point of view, two important steps are vital to the correct diagnosis of infection: (1) the organ(s) or organ systems involved must be found, and (2) the etiologic agents causing the infections must be identified precisely. Chapter 83 deals with the diagnostic approaches that are available. Most of the remaining chapters in this part take up the specific bacteria, spirochetes, fungi, rickettsias, viruses, *Mycoplasma,* and protozoa which cause infections. The common syndromes caused by these agents are described either in chapters dealing with specific organisms or in chapters dealing with infections in individual organ systems such as pneumonia (see Chap. 205), bacterial endocarditis (see Chap. 188), urinary tract infections (see Chap. 230), osteomyelitis (see Chap. 340), meningitis (see Chap. 346), and infectious arthritis (see Chap. 277).

When confronted with specific organ involvement, it is important to know the most common pathogens which cause disease in the involved organ. Table 82-1 provides a listing of those pathogens. The disease syndrome may be modified by previous conditions or therapy, thus emphasizing the need for specific diagnostic studies. Used in conjunction with the individual chapters dealing with specific agents and the summary of chemotherapy (see Chap. 88), the table should provide a rational guide to treatment which often must be instituted before the results of cultures and antimicrobial sensitivity tests are available.

ANTIMICROBIAL THERAPY The impact of chemotherapy upon mortality and morbidity from infection and upon epidemic disease is a matter of record. These therapeutic agents, however, have in no way lessened the importance of specific diagnosis; indeed, their availability has increased the need for obtaining exact etiologic information. It requires but a moment's reflection to realize that the substitution of a prescription for a broad-spectrum antibiotic or a quick injection of penicillin for the systematic collection of facts and thoughtful consideration of diagnostic possibilities is a fallacious, unwise, and dangerous practice. Numerous antibiotics with overlapping spectra are now available, dosages for different infections vary widely, the drugs themselves are potentially dangerous, and their administration entails considerable expense. They should never be prescribed as placebos, antipyretics, or substitutes for diagnosis. In the vast majority of instances in which this is done, patients recover just as they would if no "therapy" had been given, and the drugs are wasted. More importantly, an inadequate dosage of a drug or the wrong agent may suppress symptoms temporarily without achieving cure and may make isolation of the etiologic agent difficult, delay recognition of the true nature of an illness, and postpone the institution of curative treatment. Furthermore, antibiotics may select out resistant variants or facilitate the transfer of R factors between pathogenic and commensal enterobacteria. Resistant variants can then replace sensitive strains and pose the additional hazard of spread to others. Finally, to expose a patient to the risk of a drug reaction without proper indication is inexcusable, whether the drug is an antibiotic, a sedative, a laxative, or a narcotic.

EPIDEMIOLOGIC CONSIDERATIONS Just as the decision to administer antibiotics to a patient with a febrile illness of presumed infectious etiology must be made on an individual basis, the selection of cases in which extensive cultural and serologic testing is required is a matter of judgment. The majority of common grippe-like illnesses subside spontaneously, and symptomatic treatment is sufficient. However, because of this tendency toward spontaneous recovery and also because the results of serologic tests may not be available until after recovery has taken place, the effort to determine the specific

TABLE 82-1 The syndromic approach to treatable infections

	Etiologic agents		
Type of infection	Common	Relatively common	Unusual but important
Skin and subcutaneous tissue	*Staphylococcus aureus*	*Streptococcus pyogenes, Candida,* superficial fungi	Gram-negative bacilli (burns, wounds)
Sinusitis	*Streptococcus pneumoniae, Haemophilus influenzae*	*S. pyogenes, H. influenzae, S. aureus*	Mucorales
Pharyngitis	Respiratory viruses, *S. pyogenes*	Gonococcus	*Corynebacterium diphtheriae*
Epiglottitis	*H. influenzae*		
Otitis, mastoiditis	*S. pneumoniae, H. influenzae* (children)	*S. aureus, S. pyogenes*	*Pseudomonas, Proteus*
Pneumonitis	*S. pneumoniae, Mycoplasma pneumoniae, Mycobacterium tuberculosis*	*S. aureus, Klebsiella-Enterobacter,* respiratory viruses, *Legionella pneumophilia*	*S. pyogenes,* gram-negative enteric bacilli, psittacosis, systemic fungi, *Pneumocystis, H. influenzae, Pasteurella multocida*
Empyema and lung abscess	*S. aureus,* anaerobic streptococcus, *Bacteroides, Fusobacterium*	*Klebsiella* (abscess)	
Bacterial endocarditis	*Streptococcus viridans, S. aureus,* enterococcus	*S. pneumoniae,* anaerobic streptococci	*Pseudomonas, Candida, Staphylococcus epidermidis, Listeria monocytogenes*
Gastroenteritis	*Salmonella, Shigella,* enteric viruses, *Campylobacter jejuni, Escherichia coli* (enterotoxic)	*S. aureus,* clostridia, *Giardia*	*Yersinia enterocolitica, Entamoeba histolytica, Vibrio cholerae, V. parahemolyticus*
Peritonitis, cholangitis, intraabdominal abscess	*E. coli,* enterococcus, *Bacteroides,* anaerobic streptococcus, *Fusobacterium*	*Klebsiella-Enterobacter, Proteus* spp.	Clostridia, *S. aureus*
Urinary infection (cystitis, pyelonephritis)	*E. coli, Klebsiella-Enterobacter,* paracolon, *Proteus,* enterococcus	*Pseudomonas*	*S. aureus, S. saprophyticus*
Urethritis	Gonococcus, *Chlamydia trachomatis*	*Treponema pallidum, Mycoplasma*	
Pelvic inflammatory disease	Gonococcus, *E. coli, Bacteroides,* anaerobic streptococci, *Chlamydia trachomatis*	*Klebsiella-Enterobacter,* enterococcus, *Fusobacterium*	Clostridia, *S. aureus*
Bones (osteomyelitis)	*S. aureus*	*Salmonella*	*S. pyogenes*
Joints	*S. aureus,* gonococcus, *S. pneumoniae, H. influenzae*	*S. pyogenes, Neisseria meningitidis*	
Meninges	*S. pneumoniae, H. influenzae, N. meningitidis*	*E. coli, Klebsiella-Enterobacter, Proteus, Pseudomonas*	*S. pyogenes, M. tuberculosis, Cryptococcus, S. aureus, Listeria monocytogenes*

etiology of illness is often considered an impractical, "academic" procedure. If pursued universally such an attitude fails to recognize that in addition to the individual patient, the welfare of the community must be considered. For example, a clinical diagnosis of "virus pneumonia" may turn out, following serologic tests, to be psittacosis. Although the "index" patient may have recovered completely, others in the community may be at risk until the pet parakeet which was the source of the illness has been eliminated. Even more pertinent is the tracing of sexual contacts of patients with sexually transmitted infections. There is no way to eradicate the present-day epidemic of sexually transmitted diseases without this essential "shoe-leather epidemiology." Equally important is the tracing of tuberculosis, particularly in the refugees from southeast Asia who are populating many communities in the United States, and in whom the prevalence of the disease is very high. The physician must be alert to the possibilities of disease transmission or recognize important clustering of cases in caring for patients with infectious diseases.

Pursuing the diagnosis of obscure, often self-limited, illnesses may be academic, but this approach has led to clarification of some important etiologic relations. For example, the syndrome of infectious mononucleosis has been linked with development of antibody to a herpes-like virus, the EB virus (see Chap. 138), which also has a causal relationship to Burkitt's lymphoma and carcinoma of the posterior nasopharynx. Some congenital anomalies have been related to prenatal viral infections; this relationship is well known for rubella (see Chap. 133), but a number of other viruses (CMV, varicella, herpes simplex) have been implicated, although with less certainty. The finding of bacteria-like bodies in the intestinal mucosa of patients with Whipple's disease and the improvement of these patients with tetracycline therapy provides another example of an entity of unknown etiology entering the realm of infectious diseases. The virus etiology of a number of severe fatal demyelinating diseases of the central nervous system has been well established (see Chap. 347). A variety of DNA and retroviruses have now been implicated in the pathogenesis of specific neoplasms in human beings, and their relationship to endogenous "oncogenes" defined.

The recent past has witnessed several striking examples of how careful epidemiologic observations can be wedded to excellent microbiologic and serologic techniques to define the causes of previously mysterious or new diseases. These include the establishment of *Legionella* species in aqueous reserviors as a cause of epidemic pneumonia or grippe-like illness in normal and immunosuppressed hosts, the documentation of a tick-borne *Borrelia* species as the cause of Lyme disease (see Chap. 127), and the isolation of a newly occurring retrovirus infecting T lymphocytes as the agent responsible for AIDS. Not only has the etiology of newly recognized diseases been defined by these approaches, but linkage to other disorders for which the pathogenesis remains obscure has been suggested. For example, host responses to infection with *Borrelia burgdorferii* provide clues to mechanisms involved in chronic arthritis. The infectious and neoplastic complications of AIDS demonstrate the manner in which cellular immunity may both regulate responses to chronic intracellular infections and participate in surveillance against neoplasia. It seems likely that the continued pursuit of the potential role of infectious agents in other disorders of unknown etiology will disclose new pathogenetic relationships.

REFERENCES

Gallin JI, Fauci AS (eds): *Advances in Defense Host Mechanisms*, vol 5, *Acquired Immunodeficiency Syndrome (AIDS)*. New York, Raven, 1985

International Conference on Acquired Immunodeficiency Syndrome. Ann Intern Med 103:653, 1985

Mandell GL et al (eds): *Principles and Practice of Infectious Diseases*, 2d ed. New York, Wiley, 1985

Root RK: Infectious diseases: Pathogenetic mechanisms and host responses, in *Pathophysiology—The Biological Principles of Diseases*, 2d ed, LH Smith Jr, SO Thier (eds). Philadelphia, Saunders, 1985

83 THE DIAGNOSIS OF INFECTIOUS DISEASES

JAMES J. PLORDE

The diagnosis of an infectious disease requires the direct or indirect demonstration of a pathogenic microbe on or within the tissues of the afflicted host. The major ways in which this is accomplished are described in this chapter.

DIRECT MICROSCOPIC EXAMINATION The direct microscopic examination of body fluids, exudates, and tissues is both the simplest and one of the most helpful laboratory procedures available for the diagnosis of infectious diseases. In many situations the examination allows an accurate, highly specific identification of the causative agent. Examples include the recognition of *Borrelia* or *Plasmodium* species in blood smears taken from patients with relapsing fever or malaria. More commonly, only a tentative identification can be made on the basis of microbial morphology. Nevertheless, this is often sufficiently precise to allow the selection of an appropriate chemotherapeutic agent pending the results of more definitive investigations. A variety of techniques are used in direct microscopy. If the agent being sought is sufficiently large or characteristic, the specimen can be prepared as an unstained wet mount and examined by light-field, dark-field, or phase contrast microscopy. More commonly, a dried smear is made; this allows the application of a variety of stains which assists the visualization and identification of the microbe in question.

Wet mounts Dark-field examination of fluid from genital lesions for the spirochete of syphilis is a well-known, but neglected, procedure. More often, wet mounts are used for the diagnosis of fungal and parasitic infections. The examination of hair fragments, skin scrapings, or nail clippings in a drop of 10% KOH is useful in establishing the presence of superficial mycoses. At times, as for tinea versicolor infections, the fungous elements will be sufficiently characteristic to allow the specific identification of the causative agent. Occasionally a presumptive diagnosis of a systemic fungus infection can also be established with this procedure. Two examples are cryptococcal meningitis diagnosed by demonstrating the encapsulated organism in an india ink preparation of cerebrospinal fluid, and coccidioidomycosis identified by finding characteristic spherules in expectorated sputum.

Examination of wet mounts of stool or duodenal drainage is also the initial step in establishing the diagnosis of intestinal protozoal infections such as amebiasis, giardiasis, and cryptosporidiosis. Moreover, it is the definitive procedure diagnosing intestinal helminthic infections including ascariasis, trichuriasis, strongyloidiasis, and hookworm. Finally, filariasis and sleeping sickness can be recognized by demonstrating the characteristic motility of microfilariae and trypanosomes in blood or other body fluids.

Stain-enhanced microscopy Despite many recent technical advances in the field of microbiology, Gram's stain remains, after 90 years of use, the best single technique available for the rapid diagnosis of bacterial infections. It can be applied to virtually all clinical specimens and is of particular value in the examination of exudates, aspirates, and body fluids, including cerebrospinal fluid and urine. Gram's stains are examined first under the lower-power objective to demonstrate the presence of pink-staining inflammatory cells. The paucity of such cells in the presence of many squamous epithelial cells suggests that the specimen was contaminated during the process of collection and may not be representative of the inflammatory process. The smear is then examined for the presence of bacteria using the oil immersion lens; bacteria appear either as dark-blue (gram-positive) or pink (gram-negative) bodies. Their color and morphologic appearance often make possible a presumptive identification of the genus and occasionally the species of the organism. The demonstration of pneumococci in the sputum, Enterobacteriaceae in the urine, staphylococci in localized abscesses, gonococci in urethral exudates, clostridia in foul-smelling discharge, and pneumococci, meningococci, or *Haemophilus influenzae* in stained smears of the cerebrospinal fluid permits the initiation of specific chemotherapy with the assurance that the regimen is the proper one. In some immunosuppressed patients *Candida* blastoconidia and pseudohyphae can be found in blood smears several days before candidemia is demonstrable by culture.

A variety of other stains are available for the demonstration of specific microbes. Mycobacteria have the unique capacity to resist the decolorization by strong mineral acid alcohol solutions once they have been stained with basic carbol-fuchsin or one of the fluorochromes. This allows their immediate recognition in body tissues and fluids. The presence of a large number of acid-fast bacilli in the expectorated sputum establishes the presumptive diagnosis of respiratory tuberculosis and is sufficient evidence for initiating isolation procedures and antituberculosis therapy once additional specimens are collected for culture. Subsequent examination of the sputum with acid-fast stains is an important element in monitoring the success of therapy. The traditional Ziehl-Neelsen and Kinyoun stains are being supplanted by the fluorochromes which allow a much more rapid scanning of smears using relatively low magnification.

Acid-fast smears can also be used to identify *Cryptosporidium* in the stool of patients with diarrhea. If mineral acid rather than acid-alcohol is used for decolorization, pathogenic strains of *Nocardia* may be visualized in body fluids or exudates. When an even weaker decolorizing agent such as organic acid is used, organisms such as *Actinomyces* may also be seen.

Both Giemsa's and iodine stains may be used to diagnose chlamydial infections involving the eye, urethra, or cervix. When epithelial cells obtained by scraping these areas are stained with Giemsa's stain, a typical semilunar dense inclusion body composed of many blue- or purplish-staining particles is seen adjoining the nucleus of the cell. Iodine stains reveal a similar reddish-brown mass in scrapings from the eye but are not useful in cervical specimens.

A number of stains are available for the definitive identification of parasites. *Pneumocystis carinii* can be recognized in transbronchial brush biopsies using a modified Wright's stain, toluidine blue, or methenamine silver. The latter produces a very distinctive black-stained cyst. Blood and tissue protozoa such as plasmodia and *Leishmania* can be demonstrated best with Romanowsky-type mixtures containing methylene blue and eosin. These render the nuclei red to violet and the cytoplasm blue. The identification of intestinal protozoa, on the other hand, requires the use of stains such as iron hematoxylin or trichome to demonstrate the taxonomically important nuclear detail.

Immune microscopy This method combines the specificity of immunologic procedures with the speed of direct microscopy. In the immunofluorescent technique, smears thought to contain viral, bacterial, fungal, or parasitic organisms are stained with specific antibody preparations labeled with fluorescent compounds and examined with a fluorescent microscope. The most useful application of this technique is the examination of brain tissue for herpes simplex or rabies virus; lung tissue, pleural fluid, and sputum for *Legionella* spp.; and cervical, urethral, and conjunctival scrapings for trachoma-inclusion conjunctivitis agent. Direct fluorescent antibody staining of nasal epithelial cells may also be used for the rapid diagnosis of influenza, parainfluenza, and respiratory syncytial virus infections. The direct immunofluorescence technique for detecting antibody-coated bacteria in the urinary sediment has been useful in distinguishing kidney from bladder infection in females.

The accuracy and reliability of immunofluorescent techniques continues to improve as older polyclonal antiserums are replaced with more specific monoclonal reagents. The need for expensive fluorescent microscopes, the poor quality of many of the commercially available conjugated antiserums, and the need for well-trained technologists restrict the routine use of these procedures to reference laboratories.

Enzyme-linked immunosorbent assay (ELISA) tests are similar to the immunofluorescence test except that the antiserum is reacted with an enzyme-labeled antispecies conjugate. After treatment with an appropriate substrate, a color change can be visualized with the ordinary light microscope, obviating the need for expensive equipment.

Electron microscopy The electron microscopic examination has been useful in the identification of certain viruses which do not produce cytopathic effects in cell cultures. It has been particularly valuable in the detection of rotaviruses in the stool specimens of infants and small children suffering from gastroenteritis. The large number and characteristic appearance of these virus particles allow specific identification to be made on morphologic grounds alone. Electron microscopy has also been used in the diagnosis of the so-called winter vomiting disease caused by the Norwalk and Hawaii agents. These agents are morphologically similar to those of the picornavirus group, and specific identification requires aggregation of the virus particles with immune serum. This technique of immune electron microscopy may have wide application in virology and has been used to identify virus-like particles associated with non-A, non-B hepatitis in experimental animals.

DETECTION OF MICROBIAL ANTIGENS, BY-PRODUCTS, AND GENOMES The relative nonspecificity of many direct microscopic methods and the delay inherent in culture procedures have resulted in the introduction of a variety of techniques aimed at the rapid detection of microbial antigens, by-products, or genomes.

Counterimmunoelectrophoresis The most widely used of the antigen detection techniques is counterimmunoelectrophoresis (CIE). In this variation of the agar gel diffusion test, the specimen being tested for antigen is placed in an agar well and specific antiserum in a second apposed well. An electric current is then passed through the agar resulting in rapid confluence of antigen and antibody with the formation of a precipitant within a matter of minutes. CIE has proved most useful for the rapid diagnosis of bacterial meningitis in childhood where the cerebrospinal fluid is checked for the presence of pneumococcal, meningococcal, group B streptococcal, or *H. influenzae* antigens. The technique has approximately the same order of sensitivity as Gram's stain but has the advantage of heightened specificity. CIE has also been used for the detection of the above-mentioned bacterial antigens in serum, pneumococcal capsular antigens in sputum, and the detection of rotavirus and enterovirus in stool.

Particle agglutination These tests have been utilized in many of the same situations as CIE and require less technical skill for their performance. Although greater sensitivity has been claimed for particle agglutination, both latex and coagglutination tests have been plagued by false-positive reactions from heat-labile serum components and rheumatoid factor. Perhaps their greatest usefulness has been in the detection of bacterial antigens in the urine and spinal fluid of children with acute meningitis and cryptococcal antigen in the blood and spinal fluid of patients with chronic meningoencephalitis. Particle agglutination tests have been introduced for the detection of pneumococci in the sputum, group A streptococci in throat swabs, *Candida* antigen in serum, and rotavirus, as well as the enterotoxin of *C. difficile* in stool. The place of these newer tests remains to be determined.

Radioimmunoassay (RIA) The most spectacular application of this technique is in the detection of hepatitis B surface antigen–associated (HBsAg-associated) infection and in the prevention of such infections by the screening of blood and blood products for the presence of the antigen. This procedure is highly sensitive, and results can be obtained within a few hours with commercially available test kits. In this method HBsAg-labeled ^{125}I competes with antigen in a test serum for a specific antibody in the test mixture. Free and bound antigens are separated by washing. The reactivity of the antigen-antibody complex is then analyzed with a gamma counter. Experimental RIA procedures have also been developed for the detection of circulating antigens in disseminated fungal infections.

Enzyme-linked immunosorbent assays The method, as described above under "Direct Microscopic Examination," can be adapted for the visual or spectrophotometric detection of microbial antigens. Increasingly, it is coming to replace radioimmunoassay techniques in the diagnosis of hepatitis A and B infections and is extensively utilized to ascertain the presence of rotavirus in the diarrheal stool of infants. It has been successfully used to detect circulating antigens in candidiasis, aspergillosis, and toxoplasmosis. Enzyme immunoassays may soon play an important role in the diagnosis of *C. trachomatis* and gonococcal cervicitis and urethritis.

Urine screening tests A number of nonmicroscopic bacteriuria screening tests are commercially available. Each is designed to decrease the time and cost involved in the diagnosis of urinary tract infections. Bioluminescence, filtration-colorimetry, or chemical procedures are employed to determine the presence or absence of bacterial and/or leukocytic enzymes in the urine specimen. The tests can be performed reliably by individuals with minimal technical training and require only minutes to complete. Generally, specimens demonstrating a positive screening test are cultured; a negative result is reported as such, and the specimen discarded. The sensitivity, specificity, and reproducibility of these tests do not differ significantly from those obtained with a microscopic examination of a stained urine smear conducted by a competent microbiologist; all reliably detect specimens containing 10^5 or more colony-forming units (CFU) per milliliter of urine, but are insufficiently sensitive at lower colony counts. The considerably higher cost of the screening tests vis-à-vis microscopic examination is partially offset by their technical simplicity. The ultimate role of these screening tests in the detection of bacteriuria remains uncertain.

DNA probes The utilization of recombinant DNA techniques has made it possible to isolate, reproduce, and label single-stranded nucleotide sequences from the genome of specific microorganisms that are unique to that particular strain, species, genus, or group. These labeled DNA fragments, or probes, can be added to body fluids, exudates, or tissues thought to contain the pathogen in question, and the mixture treated with heat or chemicals to separate the microbial DNA into single strands. Following treatment, the DNA strands reanneal. This reassociation, or hybridization, is highly specific occurring only between strands bearing complementary nucleotide sequences. If the specimen contains nucleotide sequences complementary to those of the probe, they will be hybridized and labeled.

The potential advantages of such probes are in their unique specificity, their capacity to detect a single pathogen among a plethora of others, and the capacity to identify microorganisms that are either difficult or impossible to recover by cultural methods. Their most immediate impact will be on the diagnosis of viral, chlamydial, mycobacterial, enteric bacterial, and parasitic infections. Probes have already been developed for a wide variety of agents, including herpes simplex virus I and II, cytomegalovirus, enteroviruses, Epstein-Barr virus, hepatitis B virus, adenovirus, varicella-zoster virus, rotavirus, human T-cell leukemia virus, enterotoxigenic *E. coli, Yersinia enterocolitica, Salmonella* spp., *Shigella* spp., *Campylobacter* spp., *Mycobacteria* spp., *Leishmania mexicana, L. braziliensis,* and *Plasmodium falciparum*. To date, only the *E. coli* probes have undergone large-scale clinical trials.

Ultimately, the utility of DNA probes in clinical medicine will rest on the simplification and commercialization of the hybridization procedure and the development of practical, highly sensitive labels. To date, most probes have utilized radioisotopic markers (usually ^{32}P). These demonstrate a high level of sensitivity but require prolonged processing for autoradiographic detection, have an extremely limited shelf life, and require the storage and disposal of radioactive materials, making them impractical for the clinical laboratory. Colorimetrically detected enzymatic labels have been developed which circumvent these drawbacks; to date, however, all appear to be somewhat less sensitive than the radiometric labels and decidedly less sensitive than most cultural procedures. With the anticipated development of more satisfactory, nonradiometric labels, the DNA probe may well alter the diagnosis and management of infectious diseases in a dramatic and fundamental way. They are unlikely, however, to displace cultural methods for infections in which the recovery, characterization, and susceptibility testing of the pathogenic agent is critical to the management of the sick patient.

Gas chromatography This method involves the direct examination of clinical specimens by gas-liquid chromatography for the detection of characteristic microbial by-products. It has been thought helpful in differentiating aerobic from anaerobic organisms in pus and blood. It has also been used to differentiate staphylococcal, streptococcal, and gonococcal from traumatic arthritis and to detect *Candida* in the blood of patients with fungemia. Although the role of gas chromatography in the identification of anaerobic bacteria is established, its usefulness in the direct analysis of clinical specimens remains to be determined.

CULTURE Despite the time and complexity, the isolation of the etiologic agent by cultivation in artificial media, tissue cultures, or animals is generally the most definitive procedure available.

The diagnostic value of a culture specimen, however, depends to a large extent on the likelihood that it has been collected free of contamination with the resident microbial flora and transported to the laboratory in a fashion that ensures survival of fastidious organisms.

Specimen collection When specimens from deep closed lesions are collected, the site of percutaneous needle aspiration should be cleansed first by using 70% isopropyl or ethyl alcohol and then disinfected with a 2% tincture of iodine or an appropriate iodophor. The iodine is applied in a concentric fashion beginning at the site of aspiration and allowed to act for 1 to 2 min before the aspiration is performed. The area should not be probed or manipulated unless sterile gloves are worn or the involved fingers have also been disinfected. If the initial attempt at collection fails, subsequent efforts should be carried out with a new needle through a freshly disinfected site. At the completion of the procedure the iodine should be removed with alcohol to avoid the danger of sensitization. If the specimen for culture is drawn through an indwelling cannula, the site of withdrawal must be disinfected in the same fashion.

When specimens are to be collected from the uterus or a draining wound or sinus tract, the orifice must be thoroughly cleansed and disinfected as described above, a sterile intravenous catheter or multilumen tube is introduced as deeply as possible through the orifice, and the specimen aspirated into a sterile syringe. Culture from an open lesion may be collected by biopsy, aspiration from the margin, or by swabbing the surface. In the first two situations the wound is prepared as for a deep closed lesion. For swab cultures, the wound surface is cleansed only with sterile saline to remove debris and saprophytic flora.

Transportation All specimens submitted for microbial culture should be transported to the laboratory as rapidly as possible, preferably within 1 h. Delay beyond this time may result in death of fastidious organisms, overgrowth of contaminants, and/or change in the number of bacteria unless special procedures are employed to overcome these problems. Rapid transportation is particularly important when dealing with blood, body fluids, and exudates which may harbor pathogenic *Neisseria* or anaerobes. The container should be clean, sterile (stool specimens excepted), and appropriately labeled. Respiratory secretions, urine, large pieces of tissue, and large volumes of fluid can be safely transmitted in plastic containers with leakproof lids. Aspirates are conveniently and safely transported in the same syringe used in the collection procedure, providing all air is expressed from the syringe and the needle is capped with a sterile holder. Alternatively, such fluid may be injected into a sealed gassed-out vial suitable for transport of anaerobic specimens. If such vials are used, it is important that the indicator in the vial be checked to ascertain whether it is still colorless. A pink or blue color indicates the presence of oxygen and suggests that the vial is no longer adequate for the transport of specimens for anaerobic culture. Small pieces of tissue (less than 1 cm^2) are transported best in sterile rubber-stoppered gassed-out tubes. After the anaerobic indicator is checked, the tube is held upright to minimize the loss of the heavy inert gas, the stopper removed, specimen inserted, and the tube recapped.

Swabs submitted for the culture of group A beta-hemolytic streptococci can be transported in dry sterile test tubes. All other swabs should be submitted in one of several commercially available transport media. These prevent both the desiccation of organisms implanted on the swab and the overgrowth of hardy organisms at the expense of more fastidious ones. Although special anaerobic transport materials are available, use of swab cultures for the recovery of such organisms is not encouraged.

Culture of specific specimens UPPER RESPIRATORY TRACT Because the throat and nasopharynx are normally heavily colonized by both saprophytic and potentially pathogenic bacteria, culture of this area is seldom useful except when a particular bacterial pathogen is being sought, e.g., *Streptococcus pyogenes, Bordetella pertussis, Corynebacterium diphtheriae,* meningococci, or gonococci.

Throat cultures. When throat cultures are submitted to the laboratory without specifying the pathogen being sought, the laboratory will generally report only the presence or absence of *S. pyogenes.* Since a single properly obtained throat swab will detect at least 90 percent of patients with streptococcal pharyngitis, a negative culture is very helpful in excluding the possibility of this disease. Similarly, a heavy or predominant growth of group A beta-hemolytic streptococci in patients presenting with the signs and symptoms of streptococcal pharyngitis is highly predictive of an antibody response to streptococcal antigens and, therefore, presumably disease. It is far more difficult to interpret cultures with a light or nonpredominant growth of *S. pyogenes.* A large proportion of these patients do not mount an appreciable immunologic response, suggesting that bacterial growth represents a carrier state.

Throat cultures may not be indicated in adults presenting with sore throat if they lack fever, cervical lymphadenopathy, or recent exposure to another patient with streptococcal pharyngitis since fewer than 5 percent of this population have positive cultures. Conversely, adults with temperatures of 38°C or higher, tender cervical lymphadenopathy, or pharyngeal exudate are so frequently culture positive that immediate antibiotic therapy is more cost-effective than waiting for the result of culture.

Mouth cultures. Usually massively mixed flora of aerobic and anaerobic bacteria is present in mouth cultures, and they are not clinically useful except when a careful attempt to avoid contamination with indigenous flora has been made. This is particularly true for the isolation of *Actinomyces israelii.* This organism is part of the normal oropharyngeal flora, and the time and effort required for its isolation is not justified unless an uncontaminated specimen can be provided.

LOWER RESPIRATORY TRACT Although culture of expectorated sputum is the most frequently employed technique for the diagnosis of lower respiratory tract infections, both its sensitivity and specificity are open to question. Studies of patients with bacteremic pneumococcal pneumonia have shown the etiologic agent to be present in the sputum in only 50 to 94 percent of cases. Moreover, expectorated sputum is almost always contaminated with oropharyngeal flora including, in many cases, bacterial species commonly associated with pulmonary infections. Even when a potential pathogen is recovered, its role in the causation of a lower respiratory tract infection is uncertain. Attempts to remove saliva and nasal secretions from the sputum by repeated washing or to differentiate upper and lower tract organisms on the basis of quantitative sputum culture have been ineffective or unacceptably tedious. Some confusion can be avoided if the specimen is collected appropriately and screened carefully for both gross and microscopic characteristics prior to inoculation of the culture. Ideally, sputum specimens should be collected early in the morning under direct supervision of a physician or respiratory therapist. If the patient is unable to produce sputum, coughing may be stimulated by lowering the head of the patient's bed for a few minutes or exposing the patient to an aerosol of warm hypertonic saline.

Because sputum is rarely homogeneous, it should be examined carefully for bits of pus and blood. These should then be used to prepare a Gram's stain smear which is examined for the presence of squamous epithelial cells (SEC) and leukocytes under the low-power objective (10×) of the microscope. If there are fewer than 10 SEC and greater than 25 leukocytes per field, the results of the culture are more likely to represent lower tract flora. This is particularly true if a single or clearly predominant bacterial type grows, or, in the case of chronic obstructive pulmonary disease, if both pneumococci and *H. influenzae* are isolated. If squamous epithelial cells number more than 10 per low-power field, the specimen can be considered heavily contaminated with oropharyngeal flora and should be discarded. In most cases a second carefully collected expectorated sputum will yield a satisfactory specimen.

Direct endotracheal or endobronchial aspiration may be employed when a satisfactory expectorated sputum cannot be produced. However, such specimens are subject to contamination by oropharyngeal flora which is introduced during the passage of the aspiration instrument. Fiberoptic bronchoscopy, which allows the direct visualization and aspiration of bronchial secretions, is a relatively inocuous procedure and may result in a somewhat better specimen. When it is accompanied by a brush biopsy performed through an occluded double-lumen tube, the material obtained is unlikely to be diluted with saliva or topical anesthetics and may be utilized for anaerobic cultures. Alternatively, the specimen may be collected by a technique that totally bypasses the oropharynx. The most widely used is transtracheal aspiration. This method entails a definite risk of hemoptysis, subcutaneous and mediastinal emphysema, vagal discharge, or respiratory embarrassment and is contraindicated in the presence of a bleeding diathesis. It should be used only when results from expectorated sputum are unsatisfactory and the infection is severe enough to merit the attendant risks. The technique produces a more reliable sputum specimen than expectoration and is probably the only other satisfactory method for collecting specimens for anaerobic culture. However, some 20 percent of specimens from patients without clinical evidence of pneumonia yield potential respiratory pathogens. These "false-positive" specimens are primarily from patients who have chronic pulmonary disease, who have recently suffered minor bouts of aspiration, or in whom the tip of the catheter was coughed into the hypopharynx during the collection procedure.

Needle aspiration of a pulmonary infiltrate under fluoroscopic control also produces specimens of excellent quality. The percutaneous method gives both a high yield and accurate results but has at least a 5 percent chance of complications, particularly pneumothorax. The morbidity risk is greater than with transtracheal aspiration biopsy, but the diagnostic yield may be superior.

Whatever technique is used to sample the lower respiratory tract, a concomitant blood culture should always be obtained. If a pleural effusion is present, it should also be aspirated and cultured.

In addition to bacterial pathogens, pneumonia can be caused by viruses, *Rickettsia, Chlamydia, Mycoplasma pneumoniae,* and *Legionella* and related agents. Techniques for the recovery of these agents from the sputum are generally not available in a routine clinical microbiology laboratory, and the diagnosis is most frequently made by clinical and/or serologic methods. *L. pneumophila* can be cultured from expectorated sputum, lung tissue, or empyema fluid. In addition, it can be demonstrated by direct fluorescent antibody staining in these specimen types and in transtracheal aspirates. This allows early diagnosis and rapid institution of appropriate therapy. For discussion of the techniques used for the recovery of mycobacteria and fungi from the lower respiratory tract, the chapters devoted to these organisms should be consulted.

URINE CULTURES Voided urine, like expectorated sputum, is usually contaminated with the normal microbial flora, in this case from the urethra and external genitalia. Urine cultures, however, are more reliable than those of expectorated sputum, because the periurethral area can be disinfected and the urethra itself flushed with the first portion of the urine stream before a sample is taken. In addition, quantitation of the bacterial growth is helpful in separating contaminated specimens from true infection. In general, bacterial counts exceeding 100,000 organisms per milliliter of urine indicate true bacteriuria while those less than 1000 organisms per milliliter reflect contamination with perineal or urethral flora. Before a high bacterial count can be accepted as evidence of infection, however, the following factors need to be considered: (1) the adequacy of the disinfection procedures, (2) the sex of the patient, (3) the interval between specimen collection and plating, and (4) the number of bacterial species isolated. Patients must be carefully instructed in the techniques of collecting clean voided specimens or the collection supervised by a trained attendant. In females, the labia must be separated and the periurethral area repeatedly cleansed with an appropriate disinfectant and then rinsed with warm sterile water. Cleansing procedures appear to be unnecessary in males. During the void, the first 20 to 25 mL is discarded, and the specimen is caught directly in a sterile container without interrupting the stream. The cup should be held in a way to avoid contact with the legs or perineal area. When this procedure is followed conscientiously, a single specimen from a male which yields a colony count in excess of 100,000 organisms per milliliter is highly indicative of bacteriuria. In women, the colony count must exceed 100,000 organisms per milliliter in two consecutive urine specimens before infection can be considered to be present. Because urine is a good culture medium, contaminating organisms will multiply to large numbers if the urine is allowed to stand at room temperature for prolonged periods of time. For this reason, specimens which cannot be dispatched to the laboratory within an hour should be refrigerated. They can be held at 4°C for 4 to 6 h without an appreciable change in the bacterial colony count. In most instances, urinary tract infections are caused by a single bacterial species. The isolation of three or more species in a urine culture usually reflects contamination even when the colony count is high. True polymicrobial bacteriuria does occur but is generally restricted to patients with chronic indwelling urethral catheters. In contrast, colony counts of less than 100,000 organisms per milliliter may represent true bacteriuria. For example, $\geq 10^2$ CFU per milliliter in symptomatic dysuric women and $\geq 10^3$ in symptomatic men are significant counts. In fact, up to one-third of urinary tract infections are associated with counts less than 100,000 organisms per milliliter. Patients receiving antimicrobial therapy and specimens obtained by ureteral or urethral catheterization and by suprapubic aspiration also are likely to contain a low number of organisms.

When an adequate clean-voided urine specimen cannot be obtained, or when anaerobic cultures are desired, suprapubic aspiration may be employed. Specimens obtained in this manner are unlikely to be contaminated, and even slight growth may be significant. When an indwelling catheter is in place, a specimen should be collected directly from the catheter by means of a sterile needle and syringe after careful disinfection of the exterior surface or sampling port. Urine should not be taken from the drainage tube or bag, because these are frequently contaminated. Occasionally Foley catheter tips are submitted to the laboratory for culture when a catheterized patient shows signs or symptoms of urinary tract infection. Statistical analysis has shown this practice to be both futile and potentially misleading.

Examination of a Gram's stain smear of uncentrifuged urine is often helpful in the rapid diagnosis of urinary tract infection. The presence of many squamous epithelial cells and mixed bacterial flora indicates contamination and the need for another specimen. In the absence of the epithelial cells, the presence of one or more bacterial cells per 20 oil immersion fields usually indicates true bacteriuria especially when accompanied by one or more leukocytes.

BLOOD CULTURES Cultures should be obtained from all febrile patients who have rigors, are seriously ill, are thought to have endocarditis or intravascular infection, or are immunosuppressed. If viremia, fungemia, brucellosis, tularemia, leptospirosis, or an infection with cell wall–deficient bacteria is suspected, the laboratory should be contacted for special instructions. The sensitivity of most culture techniques is volume-dependent, with yields increasing approximately 2 percent for each milliliter of blood drawn over 5 mL. In general, three blood cultures of 10 to 30 mL taken at intervals of no less than 60 min are adequate to document the presence of bacteremia in an adult. In emergent situations, two cultures taken simultaneously from different anatomic sites will usually suffice. In patients who have received antimicrobial agents within the previous 2 weeks or in whom endocarditis is suspected, a total of six cultures taken over a 2-day period may be useful. If the patient is receiving antimicrobial agents, the cultures should be taken immediately prior to the next dose, and the laboratory should be notified to allow the addition of penicillinase, use of an antibiotic removal device, or extensive dilution of the blood specimen. The collection of specimens over and above the number listed above is seldom helpful in detecting occult bacteremia unless the culture procedures, media, or conditions of incubation are altered to allow detection of fastidious organisms.

Specimens are best collected by percutaneous venipuncture. If possible, aspirations from the femoral vein should be avoided since disinfecting the skin of the groin is often difficult and the concentration of organisms in the venous drainage of the lower extremity is generally less than that found in the venous blood of the arms. The increasingly common practice of drawing blood for culture through an indwelling intravascular cannula often results in a higher level of contamination without substantially improving the detection of bacteremia. Similarly there is no evidence that arterial blood cultures possess any advantage over venous cultures. Bone marrow cultures may reveal the etiologic agent when it cannot be obtained by other means in occasional patients with disseminated salmonellosis, tuberculosis, and deep mycoses.

To minimize the chance of contamination with skin flora, the site of aspiration should be carefully disinfected as described above. Following aspiration, the blood should be inoculated into both aerobic and anaerobic broths immediately. The dilution ratio of blood to broth should be at least 1:5 to minimize the normal bactericidal activity of serum and the activity of any antimicrobial agents that may be present. If direct inoculation into broth is not feasible, the blood may be drawn into a sterile Vacutainer tube containing sodium polyethanol sulfanate (SPS). This anticoagulant is anticomplementary and inactivates leukocytes and certain aminoglycoside and polypeptide antibiotics. Nevertheless, it will not delay bacterial death indefinitely, and Vacutainer specimens should be sent to the laboratory for dilution in broth within 30 min of the time the blood is drawn. If fungemia is suspected, the laboratory should be notified since some of the standard techniques described above are less satisfactory for the isolation of fungi.

Gram's stain examination of buffy coat smears is seldom indicated. Although a number of microorganisms, particularly meningococci and staphylococci, can be detected within granulocytes in approximately 4 percent of submitted blood culture specimens, the procedure is time-consuming and seldom of therapeutic value. It may be justified if fungemia is suspected. The toxicity of amphotericin B therapy precludes initiation of treatment without strong evidence of systemic fungal infection. Because these organisms may require 2 to 5 days to grow, a positive buffy coat smear would be of obvious therapeutic importance.

Approximately two-thirds of blood cultures from bacteremic patients are found to be positive within 24 h and 90 percent within 3 days. Despite strict adherence to disinfectant procedures on the ward and sterile technique in the laboratory, contamination occasionally occurs. The following are characteristics of "false-positive" blood cultures: (1) repeat cultures are seldom positive for the same organism, (2) bacterial growth in broth generally occurs after 2 days of incubation, and (3) the organisms are often identified as diphtheroids, *Bacillus*, or *Staphylococcus epidermidis*. However, any of these species can occasionally be responsible for true bacteremia, particularly in immunosuppressed patients.

CEREBROSPINAL FLUID Examination of the cerebrospinal fluid (CSF) from patients suspected of having meningitis represents one of the major emergency procedures faced by the clinical microbiology laboratory. Bacterial meningitis can be rapidly fatal if treatment is delayed or inadequate, and appropriate therapy often requires specific identification of the etiologic agent. Because of the clinical urgency, CSF specimens should be collected as soon as the diagnosis is considered, and the specimen promptly transported to the laboratory. The laboratory should be notified if the specimen has been collected from an abscess within the central nervous system to ensure that it is cultured both aerobically and anaerobically. If possible, at least 2 mL CSF should be obtained and the specimen sent for glucose, quantitative protein level, and cell count in addition to microbiologic studies. A simultaneous blood sugar also should be drawn for correlation with the CSF glucose level. Fastidious organisms, particularly *Neisseria meningitidis,* may not survive prolonged storage at temperatures below that of the body. If a delay in CSF examination cannot be avoided, specimens should be held at 37°C.

After receipt, the specimen is concentrated by centrifugation or filtration, Gram stained, and cultured. The inflammatory response in the CSF is helpful in distinguishing acute bacterial meningitis from nonbacterial forms of the disease. In bacterial meningitis, polymorphonuclear leukocytes predominate, while in tuberculous, fungal, or protozoal meningitis, the inflammatory cells usually consist of lymphocytes, and the response is less intense. Although polymorphonuclear leukocytes may dominate early in the course of aseptic meningitis, there is usually a clear shift to mononuclear cells within 8 h. Cytologic changes in the CSF may also be seen in patients with brain abscess. However, smears and cultures are generally negative in these cases unless the abscess ruptures into the subarachnoid space or into the ventricles. The Gram's stain smear of the CSF should be examined carefully for stainable organisms, particularly meningococci, pneumococci, *Enterobacteriaceae, Listeria,* and staphylococci in patients with atrioventricular shunts. Stainable, but nonviable, organisms occasionally contaminate sterile plastic containers and may result in a "false-positive" Gram's stain. In addition, in cases of partially treated bacterial meningitis there is a tendency for gram-positive organisms to stain gram-negative.

When a large number of organisms are present and specific antiserums are available, the etiologic agent can often be rapidly identified by the quellung reaction or a precipitin test. Counterimmunoelectrophoresis and particle agglutination tests are even more sensitive and may be positive when the Gram's stain is not. Moreover, detection of microbial antigens in the CSF is often the only method of identification of an infectious agent from a patient with partially treated meningitis. In the presence of a significant number of mononuclear cells without stainable bacteria, encapsulated cryptococci or cryptococcal antigen can be identified with the India ink preparation or latex agglutination tests, respectively.

Regardless of the results of these studies, the CSF must be cultured and any resulting growth identified to the species level. Mycobacterial and fungal cultures should be set up on patients who present with chronic meningitis and a mononuclear inflammatory response in the CSF.

Naegleria fowleri, the cause of amoebic meningoencephalitis, can often be recognized by its amoeboid movements in wet-mount preparations of cerebrospinal fluid. This organism should be looked for in patients who develop hemorrhagic meningoencephalitis during the summer months (see Chap. 153).

GASTROINTESTINAL TRACT Cultures of the mouth, periodontal lesions, or saliva usually yield a mixed flora of aerobic and anaerobic organisms including *A. israelii* and *Candida* spp. The isolation of these organisms is without significance unless the specimen was collected in a way which avoided contamination with indigenous flora. If actinomycosis is suspected, the laboratory should be contacted for special instructions. The diagnosis of oral thrush and Vincent's infection can be made with stained smears from scrapings of the suspected lesion.

Cultures of ileostomy or colostomy stomas, gastrointestinal fistulas, and rectal fissures invariably grow both aerobic and anaerobic intestinal flora. They are seldom helpful, therefore, unless a search is made for specific intestinal pathogens.

Fecal cultures are helpful in determining the etiology of diarrhea and in detecting carrier states. Such specimens are routinely cultured for species of *Salmonella, Shigella,* and *Arizona.* Many laboratories are now also looking for *Vibrio parahemolyticus, Yersinia enterocolitica, Campylobacter jejuni,* and *Clostridium difficile,* the agent of antibiotic-associated pseudomembranous enterocolitis. Cell culture and particle agglutination techniques can be used for the direct detection of *C. difficile* toxin in the stool of diarrheal patients. There is at present no convenient and reliable cultural method of identifying enterotoxogenic strains of *E. coli,* the Norwalk-like viruses, or rotaviruses in the clinical laboratory. The laboratory should be alerted as to whether any of these, or any other unusual infection such as candidiasis, clostridial food poisoning, or cholera, are suspected.

Although rectal swabs are adequate for the diagnosis of bacterial diarrhea, they are less satisfactory for the detection of carrier states. If swabs are used, they should show obvious soiling and be sent to the laboratory in appropriate transport media. Whole stool should be collected free of urine, placed in clean waxed cardboard cartons, and promptly dispatched to the laboratory. If delivery cannot be made within 1 h, the stool should be preserved in phosphate-buffered glycerol to prevent death of fastidious organisms such as *Shigella* spp. It is seldom necessary to submit more than three consecutive daily specimens.

GENITAL TRACT Genital specimens are submitted primarily for the diagnosis of venereal disease including gonorrhea, syphilis, herpes, chancroid, trichomoniasis, and chlamydial infections. Instructions for the collection of specimens should be sought in the sections of the text dealing with these specific diseases. In addition to the venereal pathogens, a number of organisms may infect the endometrium, tuboovarian tissues, and vagina. Endometrial cultures must be collected through a double- or triple-lumen tube inserted through a decontaminated cervical os if contamination with vaginal and cervical flora is to be avoided. The specimens should be delivered to the laboratory in either a gassed-out vial or a sealed syringe to ensure recovery of anaerobic organisms. When a patient presents with vaginitis, a specimen is collected by swabbing the vaginal fornix under direct visualization. If trichomoniasis is suspected, the swab should be placed in a small amount of sterile saline and sent to the laboratory immediately. If the concentration of organisms is large, and if the swab is received within 10 to 15 min, the organism can be identified without difficulty by its characteristic motility in a wet-mount preparation. The use of special culture techniques improves the likelihood of detecting light infections. Cultural examination usually focuses on the recovery of agents thought capable of causing vaginitis such as *Gardnerella vaginalis,* group B beta-hemolytic streptococci, *Mobiluncus* spp., and *Candida albicans.*

EXUDATES AND BODY FLUIDS Pus from undrained abscesses as well as pericardial, pleural, peritoneal, and synovial fluids is best collected by syringe and needle aspiration through disinfected skin. Prior rinsing of the syringe with a sterile anticoagulant such as heparin or SPS will help prevent formation of clots. Because anaerobic organisms are commonly involved in infection of these areas, the syringe should be sealed and sent immediately to the microbiology laboratory. Alternatively, the aspirate may be injected into a gassed-out anaerobic transport vial. The use of swabs is not encouraged since the sample size is small and fastidious organisms including anaerobes are unusually susceptible to desiccation and oxidation. Deep suppurative lesions which communicate with the surface of the body through fistulas or sinus tracts present a difficult problem in specimen collection. The communicating pathway is generally colonized by a wide variety of bacterial flora which contaminate drainage being ejected through the fistula opening. The degree of contamination can be lessened in many instances by carefully disinfecting the orifice and aspirating material via a sterile plastic catheter inserted deep into the sinus. Even when these precautions are taken, however, sinus tract cultures often fail to correlate well with pathogens isolated from operative specimens. For this reason, a bacteriologic diagnosis of draining suppurative lesions should be based on a culture of currettings or biopsy rather than sinus drainage. If actinomycosis is suspected, the draining sinus tract may be covered with gauze which is left in place until it is thoroughly saturated. The gauze is then submitted to the laboratory where it is carefully examined for the presence of granules which can be picked out and then identified.

SKIN, SOFT TISSUE, AND SUPERFICIAL WOUNDS Specimens collected from these areas are usually heavily contaminated with the normal flora of their respective sites. Swab cultures should be obtained only if gross pus is present or if there is need to confirm the presence or absence of only a single bacterial pathogen, such as *C. diphtheriae;* in this case, the wound should first be cleansed mechanically with saline to remove as much exudate as possible. Material from bullae and areas of cellulitis is best obtained with a syringe. Successful aspiration of an area of cellulitis may require several thrusts and withdrawals, care being taken to maintain the tip of the needle beneath the surface of the skin and a significant vacuum in the barrel of the syringe. If sterile saline is injected prior to aspiration, this solution should not contain a preservative which may affect the viability of some bacteria. Alternatively, a punch biopsy may be obtained of the area after appropriate disinfection. Similarly, cultures from open lesions may be obtained by biopsy or by aspirating from the margins of these lesions using a syringe and needle. Semiquantitative cultures of burn eschars are useful in identifying patients at risk of bacteremia.

Intravenous and intraarterial catheter segments are best collected by disinfecting the area of the skin penetrated by the catheter, carefully withdrawing the catheter, and aseptically cutting off the 5-cm section that had been located just under the skin into a sterile container. This is then delivered to the microbiology laboratory where semiquantitative cultures are done. In general, catheters which are contaminated during removal will have only a few colonies on agar plates, while infected catheters will show heavy growth.

SKIN TESTS Exposure to antigens of certain types, by various routes, and under circumstances not completely understood often results in the development of immediate (anaphylactic, atopic) hypersensitivity or delayed (bacterial, tuberculin) hypersensitivity.

Active infection with some, but not all, bacteria and viruses results in delayed hypersensitivity to the infecting agent in some, but not all, individuals. Clinically, this allergic state is detected by intradermal injection of the organism or one of its components; in a sensitive individual, induration and erythema will appear at the local site within 24 to 48 h. If an individual is highly "sensitive" or if the amount of antigen injected is excessive, there may be extensive local inflammation with necrosis, vesicle formation, edema, regional lymphadenopathy, and even malaise and fever. Antigens prepared in concentrations unlikely to provoke severe reactions are generally available for intradermal testing for tuberculosis, leprosy, mumps, lymphogranuloma venereum, cat-scratch disease, chancroid, brucellosis, tularemia, glanders, toxoplasmosis, blastomycosis, histoplasmosis, coccidioidomycosis, and many other infections. The immune reaction to vaccination is also an example of delayed dermal hypersensitivity.

The reliability, specificity, and usefulness of the individual tests differ and are discussed in the chapters on specific infection.

Intradermal injection of antigens derived from sources other than microorganisms usually produces an immediate *wheal-and-erythema* reaction which subsides promptly. The greatest clinical usefulness of this type of reaction is in the detection of allergy to foreign serums, pollens, and animal dander (see Chap. 260). The skin tests for demonstrating infestation with helminths (trichinosis, filariasis) produce reactions of the immediate type in allergic individuals, but many of the antigens employed are so nonspecific that they are of little use in diagnosis.

IMMUNOLOGIC METHODS These diagnostic methods are intended to supply evidence of past or present infection by demonstrating antibodies in serum or other body fluids, or indicating changed reactivity of the host (hypersensitivity, allergy) to products of the organism.

Serologic tests The finding on a single occasion that a patient's serum contains antibody which reacts with a certain antigen merely indicates that the patient has had previous contact with the antigen or a closely related substance. For this reason, with rare exceptions, the clinical interpretation of serologic tests depends on serial determinations. If the antibody titer is found to *rise or fall significantly,* the response likely is a result of recent contact with the antigen. In subsequent chapters, the need for serologic testing of acute phase and convalescent serum is emphasized repeatedly. *In any patient with a puzzling illness, a sterile specimen of serum should be preserved in a frozen state so that it can, if necessary, be studied and compared with serum collected at a later date.*

Prior contact with an antigen may be the result of past immunization with vaccines; interpretation of serum agglutinin titers for typhoid bacilli is often made difficult by prior immunization. The so-called anamnestic reaction, a nonspecific stimulation of antibody formation by an acute illness (e.g., a rise in *Brucella* agglutinins in a patient with acute tularemia), occurs only when the two organisms are antigenically related, and rarely presents a serious problem.

Some mention of "nonspecific" serologic changes may serve to emphasize again that clinical laboratory tests have come into use *only because they have been found to correlate reasonably well with clinical findings.* In several diseases it has been found, often accidentally, that serum antibody develops which will react with antigens derived from sources other than the etiologic agent (which may actually be unknown). Common examples are heterophil agglutinins in infectious mononucleosis, cold agglutinins in mycoplasma pneumonia, and the agglutination of certain strains of *Proteus* bacilli by serum of patients with rickettsial diseases. The VDRL test for syphilis and related flocculation tests are performed with antigens derived from sources completely unrelated to *Treponema pallidum.*

The results of serologic tests must be interpreted in the light of other information about the patient, including such factors as previous immunizations and illnesses, the possibility of exposure to chemically but etiologically unrelated antigens, and the importance of a changing titer in serial tests as opposed to a single isolated observation.

VIROLOGIC SPECIMENS The selection of specimens for the diagnosis of viral illness depends on both the stage of the disease and its clinical presentation. If the patient is seen early in the course of illness, frequently it is possible to demonstrate viral antigen in body tissue or fluids and/or to recover the virus by appropriate culture techniques. If the patient is seen later, during the recovery or convalescent stages, the diagnosis is often best established by serologic means. The type of specimen submitted for culture and the method of specimen transport depend to some extent on the nature of the illness. Throat swabs are helpful in the diagnosis of most viral infections. Because respiratory viruses are extremely labile, the swabs are placed in a buffered, high-protein transport medium containing antibiotic agents. If the specimen is to be transported to another institution, the specimen should be stored at −60°C and shipped on dry ice.

Cerebrospinal fluid from patients presenting with meningitis or encephalitis can also be submitted for culture. As with throat swabs, these specimens should be stored at low temperatures and shipped on dry ice. Stool should be collected in patients with respiratory illnesses, meningitis, or encephalitis, if either adenoviruses or enteroviruses are thought to be involved. Since these organisms are hardy, the feces can be collected in any sterile screw-top bottle and dispatched without refrigeration. Urine cultures are seldom helpful except in the diagnosis of cytomegalovirus and rubella infections. Vesicular fluid is a rich source of virus and viral antigen in patients presenting with exanthems. Pericardial fluid may be of help in patients with myocarditis or pericarditis. Viral blood cultures are seldom useful except in the diagnosis of arboviral infections. Isolation techniques for these viruses are highly specialized and are not available in most virus laboratories. Buffy coat cultures for cytomegalovirus and herpesvirus may be of help in immunosuppressed patients. Brain biopsy is the best single method for diagnosing herpes simplex encephalitis (see Chap. 136). The biopsy specimen should be placed in a sterile screw-top bottle and stored and dispatched in the frozen state.

REFERENCES

EISENBERG HD et al: Collection, handling and processing of specimens, in *Manual of Clinical Microbiology*, 4th ed, EH Lennette et al (eds). Washington, DC, American Society for Microbiology, 1985

ENGLEBERG NC, EISENSTEIN BI: The impact of new cloning techniques on the diagnosis and treatment of infectious diseases. N Engl J Med 311:892, 1984

PLORDE JJ: Newer methods in microbial diagnosis, in *Contemporary Issues in Infectious Diseases*, vol 4: *Septic Shock*, RK Root, MA Sande (eds). New York, Churchill Livingstone, 1985

TODD JK: Nonculture techniques using blood specimens for the diagnosis of infectious disease, in *Proceedings of a Symposium: Body Fluids and Infectious Diseases*, Am J Med, July 28, 1983, vol 75, pp 37–43

WASHINGTON JA II: Bacteria, fungi and parasites, the clinician and microbiology laboratory, in *Principles and Practice of Infectious Diseases*, 2d ed, GL Mandell et al (eds). New York, Wiley, 1985

84 INFECTIONS IN THE COMPROMISED HOST

HENRY MASUR / ANTHONY S. FAUCI

DEFINITION Patients who lack resistance to infection because of a deficiency in any of their multifaceted host defenses are referred to as compromised hosts. Other terminologies such as "abnormal host," "immunosuppressed host," or "immunocompromised patient" are often used, but these terms have different connotations. The latter two terms refer specifically to a subpopulation of compromised hosts whose major deficiency in antimicrobial activity is related to their defective immune response.

An expanding spectrum of diseases can now be controlled or cured by complex and aggressive surgery, implantation of foreign bodies, or powerful cytotoxic or anti-inflammatory drugs. As non-infectious complications such as hemorrhage or uremia or graft rejection are being managed with increasing success, infection is becoming the major threat to the quality and duration of survival in many different patient populations.

HOST DEFENSE MECHANISMS

Antimicrobal defense mechanisms (Table 84-1) consist of complex, interacting systems that protect the host from endogenous and exogenous microbes. The degree to which a patient becomes abnormally susceptible to infection by this microbial environment depends on which mechanisms are compromised, how severe the derangements are, and how these derangements interact. For instance, as isolated abnormalities, total absence of serum IgA or complement component C9 would probably have minor, if any, impact on host susceptibility to infection. Isolated abnormalities such as total absence of circulating neutrophils, serum IgG, or complement component C3 would, in contrast, lead to recurrent and life-threatening infections. Similarly, partial deficiencies in host defense mechanisms can have variable impact on susceptibility to infection depending on the specific mechanism, the degree of deficiency, and the presence of concomitant abnormalities. A modest decrease in circulating neutrophil count to 25 percent of the lower limit of normal or a decrease in serum IgG concentration to 50 percent of the lower limit of normal would probably be managed with only moderate difficulty if either was an isolated and transient abnormality. If such a neutrophil count were present concurrently with a major defect in the skin or mucous membrane for a prolonged period of time, patient survival would far more likely be threatened.

Recognition of which specific and nonspecific host defenses are compromised is important in order to develop effective clinical strategies for predicting the probable onset of infection and the most likely causative organisms; for formulating the appropriate diagnostic approach; and for developing the optimal therapeutic and preventive plan. However, based on an understanding of the mechanisms of host defenses, such an approach must be supplemented by clinical experience with specific patient populations. Because there are complexities of various host defense mechanisms that are not fully understood, it cannot be assumed that all patient populations with the same measured deficiency in antimicrobial defense (as assessed by current laboratory techniques) will behave identically. For example, patients with cytomegalovirus infection (Chap. 137) have immunologic profiles that are similar in certain respects to the profile of patients in the early phases of the acquired immunodeficiency syndrome (AIDS) (Chap. 257). However, the susceptibility of these two populations to life-threatening opportunistic infection is vastly different, with AIDS patients being far more susceptible.

PHYSICAL AND CHEMICAL BARRIERS Physical and chemical barriers (Table 84-1) are part of a complex and interacting system of nonspecific host defense mechanisms that are essential for preventing the introduction and spread of microbial pathogens. These barriers utilize a wide variety of properties to protect the host, including the physical presence of structural barriers (e.g., morphologic integrity of skin or mucous membranes, epiglottis, sphincters); chemical processes (e.g., gastric acidity, pancreatic enzymes, cutaneous fatty acids or lysozyme); physical removal of organisms (e.g., peristalsis, sloughing of squamae, urine flow); and competition from less virulent flora. Interference with any of these mechanisms can increase the host's susceptibility to infection.

INFLAMMATORY RESPONSES Circulating phagocytes (neutrophils, monocytes, eosinophils, and basophils) arise from the bone marrow and upon appropriate signals enter the peripheral circulation and are distributed to local tissues, where they form the cornerstone of the inflammatory response. Recruitment of phagocytes from the bloodstream is a complicated process which involves the phagocytes' aggregation, adherence to the vascular endothelium, passage through endothelial spaces, and migration to local tissue sites (Chap. 56). An effective inflammatory response depends on the ability of the phagocyte to adhere, deform, have random locomotion, and respond to a chemical signal with directed movement. Humoral mediators influence local structures in ways that affect the phagocyte's ability

TABLE 84-1 Mechanisms of host defense

Physical and chemical barriers
Morphologic integrity of skin, mucous membranes
Sphincters
Epiglottis
Normal secretory and excretory flow
Endogenous microbial flora
Gastric acidity
Inflammatory response
Circulating phagocytes
Complement
Other humoral mediators (bradykinins, fibrinolytic systems, arachidonic acid cascade)
Reticuloendothelial system
Tissue phagocytes
Immune response
T lymphocytes and their soluble products
B lymphocytes and immunoglobulins

to reach various loci: an example is the influence the complement cascade (especially C3a and C5a) has on the potential spaces between endothelial cells. Humoral mediators including the complement system, the arachidonic acid cascade, kinin-generating systems, and products of cellular elements (fibroblasts, neutrophils, macrophages, lymphocytes, and microorganisms) also guide directly the locomotion of the phagocytes. Once the phagocyte arrives at a focus of infection, it can adhere to the microorganism, ingest it, and digest it, particularly if the organism has been opsonized by antibodies or complement products. A wide variety of gram-positive and gram-negative bacteria as well as fungi are killed by neutrophils in this manner.

RETICULOENDOTHELIAL SYSTEM Circulating microorganisms are cleared from the bloodstream by tissue phagocytes that are derived from circulating monocytes. These phagocytes include macrophages in the liver (Kupffer cells), spleen, lymph nodes, lung (alveolar macrophages), and brain (microglial nodules). The antimicrobial activities of these monocytes and macrophages are strongly influenced by opsonins such as IgG or C3b which enhance the rate of particle ingestion, and by a large variety of soluble mediators produced primarily by mononuclear leukocytes. The efficacy of the reticuloendothelial system is also influenced by characteristics of specific organisms which often possess adaptive properties allowing the microbes to resist specific steps necessary for microbial activity such as phagocytosis (cryptococci), lysosome-phagosome fusion (toxoplasma), or lysosomal degradation (leishmania).

Immune response The major cellular components of the immune response are T lymphocytes and B lymphocytes (Chap. 62). These cells are distributed throughout the body in the bloodstream and at tissue sites. They interact in a highly complex fashion among themselves and with monocytes, macrophages, immunoglobulins, and the complement cascade. T lymphocytes are the major cellular component of the cell-mediated immune system. They secrete a multitude of soluble products which influence the functional status of other T lymphocytes, B lymphocytes, monocytes, and macrophages. B lymphocytes and plasma cells secrete specific antibodies which have important roles in eradicating certain infections. As noted above, the ability of the monocytes and macrophages to ingest and kill a wide variety of bacteria, fungi, and protozoa is dependent on the ability of the T lymphocyte to activate these cells. Any process which requires opsonization with antibody, such as the process which occurs between neutrophils and many bacteria, can also be profoundly influenced by the regulatory effect of T lymphocytes on B lymphocytes (Chap. 62).

ETIOLOGY AND PATHOGENESIS OF INFECTION

In compromised hosts the occurrence of infectious diseases reflects the impaired interaction of immunologic and nonimmunologic host defense mechanisms with the host's endogenous and exogenous microbial environment. Potentially pathogenic microorganisms may arise from the host's endogenous flora, and factors which change this microbial flora have an important impact on the organisms that are likely to cause disease. Such factors include antimicrobial therapy, nonsterile invasive procedures or trauma, ingestion or inhalation of infected material, and hospitalization itself. Infectious diseases in compromised patients are more often related directly to alterations in host defense mechanisms than to changes in the microbial flora, although both factors are undoubtedly important. Numerous processes can predispose to serious infection by compromising the anatomic and physical barriers of host defense. For example, the skin and mucous membranes can be breached by conditions such as tumor invasion, tumor necrosis, or vascular insufficiency induced by arteritis or atherosclerosis; by injury such as burns, pressure, or trauma; by therapy such as radiation or cytotoxic chemotherapy; by a drug-induced cutaneous slough; and by procedures such as venipuncture or surgery. The respiratory tract can become the site of infection when its anatomic barriers are disrupted: the epiglottis may fail to protect the lower tract when the patient's consciousness is impaired or during intubation or bronchoscopy. The patient's ability to expel organisms may be adversely affected if infection, tumor, or drugs that alter the state of consciousness or prevent coughing; if mucociliary transport is disrupted by a congenital disorder of ciliary subunits (such as Kartagener's syndrome) or by smoke or other inhaled toxins, anesthetic agents, or cytotoxic therapy; or if an airway is obstructed by tumor, a foreign body, or lymph node enlargement. The gastrointestinal tract can become a less effective barrier against entry of organisms if gastric acidity is abolished by a surgical procedure or antacid therapy (infections with *Salmonella* and *Mycobacterium* are particularly important in this regard); or if its mucosa is eroded by tumor or cytotoxic therapy, especially in neutropenic patients. Obstruction of the intestinal or biliary tract by tumor, a stricture, or a stone also allows endogenous or introduced flora to gain access to capillary and lymphatic systems. The genitourinary tract can become a portal of entry for infections if its mucosa is eroded by tumor, irradiation, or cytotoxic therapy. Obstruction of urine flow by tumor, strictures, stones, or prostatic hypertrophy also allows organisms to multiply and gain access to the capillaries and lymphatic systems. Renal failure associated with oliguria or anuria deprives the genitourinary system of the ability to flush out microorganisms and obviates the antimicrobial effects of urine itself. The insertion of foreign bodies into the urethra during catheterization or cystoscopy is an iatrogenic cause for exogenous organisms to be introduced into this system. Any locus in the body can become the site of infection if devitalized tissue or foreign bodies are seeded by bacteria or become infected by direct penetration. Spontaneous or traumatic hematomas, necrotic tissue, infarcts, calcified heart valves, and prosthetic devices (joints, heart valves, or central nervous system appliances) are particularly prone to infection.

Defects in inflammatory and immune function may permit infections that would normally be promptly eradicated to progress and cause clinically important disease. These quantitative or qualitative defects may be related to a congenital disorder, an underlying acquired disease, or drug therapy. Several specific types of defects are associated with particularly frequent or severe infectious complications.

LEUKOCYTE DISORDERS The clinical consequences of leukocyte disorders depend on which subpopulations of leukocytes are numerically or functionally affected, and how prolonged the dysfunction is (Table 84-2) (Chap. 56). Neutropenia (less than 3000 neutrophils per cubic millimeter) is the most commonly encountered defect in inflammatory host defense mechanisms (Chap. 56). As the neutrophil count falls below 1000 cells per cubic millimeter, there is a progressive increase in susceptibility to bacterial and fungal infections and a progressive decrease in the clinical signs and symptoms of inflammation which ordinarily provide clinical clues to the location of the infection. Susceptibility to infection increases dramatically when the peripheral neutrophil count falls below 500 cells per cubic millimeter and increases even more markedly when the count falls below 100 cells per cubic millimeter. The rate of decline and the duration of neutropenia are also important indexes which influence the clinical consequences. Neutropenia can occur because of bone marrow failure, peripheral destruction of cells, or pooling or sequestration of cells. The most common causes of neutropenia are antineoplastic or cytotoxic chemotherapy, neoplastic invasion of the bone marrow, aplastic anemia, and idiosyncratic drug reactions.

Neutrophil dysfunction can also result in a substantial predisposition to serious infection. Dysfunction may be a manifestation of a congenital disorder such as chronic granulomatous disease or Chédiak-Higashi syndrome (Chap. 56). Neutrophil dysfunction can also be a consequence of drug therapy, e.g., corticosteroids. In this regard, certain multiple drug chemotherapeutic regimens may alter both the number and the function of circulating neutrophils.

Lymphopenia in adults is defined as less than 1000 lymphocytes per cubic millimeter. The clinical consequences of lymphopenia

TABLE 84-2 Infections associated with common defects in inflammatory or immunologic response

Host defect	Examples of diseases or therapies associated with defects	Common etiologic agents of infections
INFLAMMATORY RESPONSE		
Neutropenia	Hematologic malignancies Cytotoxic chemotherapy Aplastic anemia	Gram-negative bacilli *Staphylococcus aureus* *Candida* species *Aspergillus* species
Chemotaxis	Chédiak-Higashi syndrome	*Staphylococcus aureus* *Streptococcus pyogenes*
	Job's syndrome	*Staphylococcus aureus* *Haemophilus influenzae*
	Protein-calorie malnutrition	Gram-negative bacilli
Phagocytosis (cellular)	Systemic lupus erythematosus Chronic myelogenous leukemia Megaloblastic anemia	*Streptococcus pneumoniae* *Haemophilus influenzae*
Microbicidal defect	Chronic granulomatous disease	Catalase-positive bacteria and fungi: Staphylococci *Escherichia coli* *Klebsiella* species *Pseudomonas aeruginosa* *Candida* species *Aspergillus* species *Nocardia* species
	Chédiak-Higashi syndrome	*Staphylococcus aureus* *Streptococcus pyogenes*
COMPLEMENT SYSTEM		
C3	Congenital Liver disease	*Staphylococcus aureus* *Streptococcus pneumoniae*
	Systemic lupus erythematosus	*Pseudomonas* species *Proteus* species
C5	Congenital	*Neisseria* species Gram-negative rods
C6, C-7, C-8	Congenital Systemic lupus erythematosus	*Neisseria meningitidis* *Neisseria gonorrhoeae*
Alternate pathway	Sickle cell disease	*Streptococcus pneumoniae*
	Splenectomy	Salmonella species
IMMUNE RESPONSE		
T-lymphocyte deficiency	Thymic aplasia Thymic hypoplasia Hodgkin's disease Sarcoid Lepromatous leprosy	*Listeria monocytogenes* *Mycobacterium* species *Candida* species *Aspergillus* species *Cryptococcus neoformans* *Herpes simplex* *Herpes zoster*
	Acquired immunodeficiency syndrome	*Pneumocystis carinii* Cytomegalovirus *Herpes simplex* *Mycobacterium avium-intracellulare* *Cryptococcus neoformans* *Candida* species
T lymphocyte	Mucocutaneous candidiasis	*Candida* species
	Purine nucleoside phosphorylase deficiency	Fungi Viruses
B-cell deficiency/dysfunction	Bruton's X-linked agammaglobulinemia	*Streptococcus pneumoniae* Other streptococci
	Agammaglobulinemia	*Haemophilus influenzae*
	Chronic lymphocytic leukemia	*Neisseria meningitidis* *Staphylococcus aureus*
	Multiple myeloma	*Streptococcus pneumoniae* *Staphylococcus aureus* *Klebsiella pneumoniae* *Escherichia coli* *Giardia lamblia*
	Dysglobulinemia	*Pneumocystis carinii* Enteroviruses
	Selective IgM deficiency	*Streptococcus pneumoniae* *Haemophilus influenzae* *Escherichia coli*
	Selective IgA deficiency	*Giardia lamblia* Viral hepatitis *Streptococcus pneumoniae* *Haemophilus influenzae*
Mixed T- and B-cell deficiency/dysfunction	Common variable hypogammaglobulinemia	*Pneumocystis carinii* Cytomegalovirus *Streptococcus pneumoniae* *Haemophilus influenzae* Various other bacteria
	Ataxia-telangiectasia	*Streptococcus pneumoniae* *Haemophilus influenzae* *Staphylococcus aureus* Rubella *Giardia lamblia*
	Severe combined immunodeficiency	*Candida albicans* *Pneumocystis carinii* Varicella Rubella Cytomegalovirus
	Wiskott-Aldrich	Infections seen in T- and B-cell abnormalities

depend on which subset(s) is affected; regardless of the total lymphocyte count, severe infections of various types may occur if profound deficiencies of either B lymphocytes or T lymphocytes are present. Substantial reductions in helper T lymphocytes have particularly important consequences in terms of susceptibility to infection. The most common causes of lymphopenia are hematologic malignancies, corticosteroid therapy, antilymphocyte globulins, cytotoxic drugs, and infection with certain viruses such as cytomegalovirus (Chap. 137) and HTLV III (Chap. 257). Congenital lymphopenias can also have severe consequences.

Lymphocyte dysfunction can predispose to life-threatening infection even if lymphocyte number is normal. Lymphocyte dysfunction is most often a consequence of corticosteroids or of cytotoxic antineoplastic or anti-inflammatory therapy.

IMMUNOGLOBULIN DISORDERS Profound decrease in the ability to synthesize functional immunoglobulin, particularly IgG, can cause a marked increase in susceptibility to microbial disease (Chap. 62). Patients with significant reductions in IgG (usually less than 200 to 300 mg/dL) characteristically have recurrent infections due to encapsulated bacteria, particularly *Streptococcus pneumoniae, Hemophilus influenzae,* and *Neisseria meningitidis,* and to certain protozoa (*Pneumocystis carinii* and *Giardia lamblia*). Selective IgA deficiency, when severe, can be associated with similar infections, particularly due to *Giardia lamblia,* as well as severe viral hepatitis. The few documented cases of significant selective IgM deficiency have also been associated with severe infections, particularly those associated with gram-negative organisms such as *Neisseria meningitidis*. Causes of clinically important immunoglobulin deficiency or dysfunction include both congenital and acquired disorders, malignancies (multiple myeloma, chronic lymphocytic leukemia), sickle cell disease, and childhood splenectomy (Table 84-2) (Chap. 256).

COMPLEMENT DISORDERS The consequences of total absence of functional complement proteins depend on which of the specific components are deficient (Table 84-2) (Chap. 62). Deficiencies of the early components (C1, C4, C2) have been associated with pneumococcal infections while deficiencies of C3, C5, C6, C7, or C8 may lead to relapsing *Neisseria meningitidis* or *Neisseria gonorrhoeae* infections. The majority of severe deficiencies are reported with inherited disorders, although there are reports relating significant deficiencies to systemic lupus erythematosus, cirrhosis, and splenectomy.

SPLENECTOMY The spleen is a major site for T cell–independent immune responses, and a large number of B lymphocytes reside there as do monocytes and macrophages. The spleen has an important role in the phagocytosis of circulating opsonized organisms. Following splenectomy young children are at high risk for fulminant infections due to *Streptococcus pneumoniae*, *Haemophilus influenzae*, and *Neisseria meningitidis*. In contrast, when otherwise healthy adults undergo splenectomy, they probably are at only modestly increased risk for these infections, especially during the first 3 years after surgery. However, they may be at risk for developing fulminant infection with intraerythrocytic protozoa such as *Plasmodium malariae* and *Babesia*.

DIAGNOSIS

The diagnosis of infections in compromised patients requires special attention because the clinical manifestations of infection may be atypical. Unusual causative organisms may require special considerations for optimal specimen acquisition and processing, and microbial diseases may become life-threatening with remarkable rapidity. It is important to recognize patients who are at high risk of infection in advance of the onset of their microbial disease so that subtle symptoms and signs can be sought prospectively, especially at those times and in those sites where a particular patient population has been shown to be most susceptible. For instance, fever during the second or third postoperative week following insertion of a prosthetic heart valve or removal of a large traumatic abdominal hematoma should alert the clinician to look for the source even if the temperature elevation is not impressive, as infected prosthetic heart valves or abdominal clots may be fatal rapidly if not treated aggressively. Because of surgical trauma and instrumentations, kidney transplant recipients are known to be at very high risk for bacterial wound and urinary tract infections during the first postoperative month, while opportunistic viral, fungal, or protozoan diseases occur characteristically during the second through sixth months. A patient with a hematologic malignancy needs particular scrutiny when the neutrophil count falls precipitously to 100 cells per cubic millimeter (a time that is usually predictable from the pharmacokinetics of the chemotherapeutic regimen). Similar scrutiny would be appropriate for an adult with recently diagnosed multiple myeloma, an infant who had recently undergone splenectomy, or an AIDS patient whose total helper-T-lymphocyte population had fallen close to zero. Knowledge of these patterns should not substitute for a comprehensive clinical evaluation in any individual patient, but such information does allow the clinician to focus on times, sites, and microorganisms that are highly likely to be causing or soon to be causing clinical disease.

THERAPY

In compromised patients the therapy of infectious complications ideally should include reconstitution of deficient antimicrobial defenses, drainage of localized collections of infected material, and specific antimicrobial therapy. In actively infected patients some antimicrobial defense mechanisms can be augmented and improved. Examples include the infusion of fresh frozen plasma to augment complement components, the administration of immune serum globulin to restore IgG levels, and the tapering of immunosuppresive drugs (such as corticosteroids or cytotoxic agents) to restore cell-mediated immune mechanisms or neutrophil production. Neutropenia is the most common host defense mechanism which predisposes to recurrent life-threatening infections. Augmentation or replacement of neutrophils can be achieved temporarily by white blood cell transfusions or permanently by bone marrow transplantation. However, both of these procedures are expensive, technically difficult, and not always effective.

The administration of antimicrobial chemotherapy to various populations of compromised patients is associated with many critical but unresolved controversies. Should empiric therapy be initiated or should the institution of antimicrobial therapy be postponed until the etiologic agent is identified? Which antimicrobial drugs and which combinations provide optimal empiric or specific therapy? What duration of therapy is optimal considering the etiologic agent and the deficient host defense system?

Empiric therapy is clearly appropriate for some patient populations. Profoundly neutropenic patients who have a spiking fever benefit as a group from prompt empiric therapy using a broad-spectrum regimen directed against the major gram-positive and gram-negative pathogens. In contrast, patients who are compromised because of achlorhydria, a recently resected colon carcinoma, or a bronchoscopic examination usually do not benefit from empiric therapy initiated solely because of a temperature elevation.

INFECTION PREVENTION

In compromised patients certain types of infections can be prevented by avoiding damage to physical barriers, bolstering host defenses, reducing acquisition of new potential pathogens, and suppressing colonizing flora. Damage to physical barriers can be minimized by avoiding invasive procedures such as venipuncture, indwelling vessel catheters, urinary catheterization, or surgery. Bolstering host defenses can be accomplished directly in some patient groups. For example, immune serum globulin can be given prophylactically to hypogammaglobulinemic patients; hyperimmune varicella-zoster immunoglobulin can prevent or reduce the severity of varicella-zoster virus disease after acute exposure; immunization with vaccines against pneumococcal, haemophilus, meningococcal, or other likely pathogens may be helpful for groups with specific susceptibilities such as splenectomized individuals; bolstering nutritional status may also be of benefit in certain patients. Unfortunately, most methods to enhance depressed cell-mediated immunity or to mobilize or supplement low neutrophil counts have been clinically ineffective. Reducing the acquisition of potential pathogens can be faciliated by simple techniques such as having hospital personnel wash their hands before patient contact and by appropriate isolation from specific potentially contagious organisms such as *Herpes zoster*, *Mycobacterium tuberculosis*, or multiply antibiotic-resistant gram-negative bacilli. More stringent measures such as laminar flow isolation or control of the sterility of food and water have not proved to be useful or cost-effective when the survival of most patient populations is assessed, although these measures will decrease the rate of infection for patients with prolonged and profound granulocytopenia. Suppression of endogenous organisms is an important concept since more than 80 percent of organisms causing disease in neutropenic cancer patients can be found in the endogenous flora of the host. From a practical point of view, gut sterilization or prophylactic systemic antibiotics have not been effective consistently in recent studies. However, antimicrobial prophylaxis of certain specific infections that have exceedingly high attack rates in certain defined populations can be quite effective. The impressive protection which trimethoprimsulfamethoxazole provides against *Pneumocystis carinii* pneumonia in children with acute lymphocytic leukemia is a striking example.

REFERENCES

Brown AE, Armstrong DA: Symposium on infectious complications of neoplastic disease. Am J Med 76:413, 631, 1984

Eraklis AJ et al: Hazard of overwhelming infection after splenectomy in childhood. N Engl J Med 276:1255, 1967

Gallin JI, Fauci AS: *Advances in Host Defense Mechanisms*, vol 1: *Phagocytic Cells*. New York, Raven, 1982

———: *Advances in Host Defense Mechanisms*, vol. 2: *Lymphoid Cells*. New York, Raven, 1983

———: *Advances in Host Defense Mechanisms*, vol 3: *Chronic Granulomatous Disease*. New York, Raven, 1983

Kapadia SB: Multiple myeloma: A clinicopathologic study of 62 corresponding autopsy cases. Medicine 5:380, 1980

Lau WK et al: Comparative efficacy and toxicity of amikacin/carbenicillin versus gentamicin/carbenicillin in leukopenic patients. Am J Med 62:959, 1977

Notter DT et al: Infections in patients with Hodgin's disease: A clinicial study of 300 consecutive adult patients. Rev Infect Dis 2:761, 1980

Pizzo PA et al: Empiric antibiotic and antifungal therapy for cancer patients with prolonged fever and granulocytopenia. Am J Med 72:101, 1982

——— et al: Fever in the pediatric and young adult patient with cancer: A prospective study of 1001 episodes. Medicine 61:153, 1982

———, Schimpff SC: Strategies for the prevention of infection in the myelosuppressed or immunosuppressed cancer patient. Cancer Treat Rep 67:223, 1983

Ross SC, Densen P: Complement deficiency states and infection. Epidemiology, pathogenesis and consequences of neisserial and other infections in an immune deficiency. Medicine 63:243, 1984

Rubin RH, Young LS: *The Clinical Approach to Infection in the Immunocompromised Host*. New York, Plenum, 1981

Tramont, EC: General or non-specific host defense mechanisms, in *Principles and Practice of Infectious Diseases*, 2d ed, GL Mandell et al (eds). New York, Wiley, 1985, pp 25–31

85 HOSPITAL-ACQUIRED INFECTIONS

PIERCE GARDNER / PAUL M. ARNOW

DEFINITIONS Hospital-acquired infections (also called nosocomial infections) are significant causes of human morbidity and mortality. They are defined as infections occurring in patients after admission to the hospital that were neither present nor in incubation at the time of admission. Infections acquired in the hospital but not manifest until after the patient is discharged are also included. Although many of these infections can be prevented, some cannot, and the term *hospital-acquired infection* should not be equated with *iatrogenic infection,* which indicates an infection caused by a diagnostic or therapeutic intervention such as the insertion of a urethral or intravenous catheter. *Opportunistic infections* occur in patients with impaired host defenses and are commonly caused by infectious agents that do not ordinarily produce disease in healthy individuals. Many opportunistic infections are caused by organisms in the patient's own flora (*autochthonous infections*) and are often unavoidable because they are related to defects in mucosal barriers or other host defenses rather than preventable environmental risks.

ETIOLOGY AND EPIDEMIOLOGY **Incidence and cost** Hospital-acquired infections occur in from 2 to 10 percent (average, 5 percent) of patients admitted to general hospitals. The highest infection rates are reported from municipal hospitals and tertiary-care centers, while the prevalence of these infections is much lower in community hospitals. These differences in rates appear to be due to the greater severity of underlying disease of patients in municipal and tertiary-care hospitals and may also reflect greater utilization of invasive procedures and diagnostic tests in the management of these patients. On the average, hospital-acquired infections have a mortality rate of 1 percent and contribute to the death of at least an additional 3 percent of cases. Therefore the estimated 2 million hospital-acquired infections which occur annually in the United States result in approximately 20,000 deaths and contribute to the mortality of an additional 60,000 patients. Nosocomial infections add over 7.5 million hospital days and over 1 billion dollars to the national health care costs.

Causative pathogens Gram-negative bacilli lead the list of nosocomial pathogens (Table 85-1). Their statistical importance is due in large part to their role in urinary tract infections, but gram-negative bacilli also are important pathogens at other sites. Many of these organisms, especially pseudomonads and *Klebsiella,* require minimal nutrients and are able to establish reservoirs in the inanimate hospital environment, as well as in patients. In addition, gram-negative bacilli develop resistance to antibiotics more readily than gram-positive cocci. In large part, resistance among gram-negative bacilli is due to the acquisition of plasmids called *resistance factors* (R factors). R-factor plasmids consist of extrachromosomal circular DNA, which mediates antibiotic resistance by coding for enzymes that inactivate the drug or by modifying systems involved in antibiotic uptake. Several properties of plasmids are of major public health concern: (1) Resistance to several antibiotics is often linked on the same R factor; (2) R-factor transfer can occur across species and even genera of gram-negative bacilli; (3) small gene fragments encoding for a single antibiotic-inactivating enzyme have been incorporated into diverse plasmids which are spread among many genera of gram-negative bacilli. Certain gram-negative bacilli (most often *Enterobacter, Pseudomonas,* and *Serratia*) have developed an additional chromosomal mechanism of resistance to penicillin and cephalosporin drugs, i.e., the induction of β-lactamase enzymes. Because production of these enzymes is enhanced by exposure to β-lactam antibiotics (especially the newer cephalosporins), widespread use of these antibiotics in hospitals exerts selective pressure for the emergence of these difficult-to-treat gram-negative bacilli.

Among gram-positive cocci, *Staphylococcus aureus,* the scourge of the 1950s and early 1960s, remains the most important pathogen.

TABLE 85-1 The percentage distribution of the most frequently isolated nosocomial pathogens by site of infection, 1983

Pathogen	Urinary tract	Surgical wound	Lower respiratory tract	Blood-stream	Skin	Other	Total isolates	%
E. coli	31.7	11.4	7.1	9.5	7.7	7.3	5779	18.6
S. aureus	1.6	19.0	12.8	12.8	33.3	16.4	3356	10.8
Enterococci	14.9	11.4	1.6	7.3	9.5	7.3	3308	10.7
P. aeruginosa	12.5	8.1	15.1	6.1	7.2	6.2	3286	10.6
Klebsiella spp.	7.6	4.8	12.8	9.1	4.4	4.0	2288	7.4
Coagulase-negative staphylococci	3.7	8.4	1.1	14.2	9.5	11.1	1892	6.1
Enterobacter spp.	4.4	6.9	10.0	6.9	4.1	4.1	1811	5.8
Proteus spp.	7.3	5.0	4.4	1.7	3.5	3.2	1667	5.4
Candida spp.	5.1	1.4	4.2	5.6	4.5	13.4	1570	5.1
Serratia spp.	1.2	2.0	5.6	2.8	1.8	1.8	691	2.2
All others	10.0	21.6	25.3	24.0	14.5	25.2	5364	17.1
Number of isolates	13,165	6163	4490	2292	1798	3104	31,012	100.0

SOURCE: *Centers for Disease Control, National Nosocomial Infections Study, 1983, Morb Mort Week Rep (Suppl) 33:2SS, 1984.*

Multiply antibiotic-resistant strains of *S. aureus* have appeared in many hospitals in Europe and North America in recent years and have been responsible for epidemics of infections, primarily in critical care units. These strains are generally resistant to all β-lactam agents and often to erythromycin, clindamycin, and the aminoglycosides as well. For serious infections caused by these strains, vancomycin is the drug of choice. There is epidemiologic and laboratory evidence to suggest that resistant *S. epidermidis* strains are an important reservoir of genes mediating multiple resistance and can transfer these genes to *S. aureus*. Bacterial tolerance (organisms are inhibited but not killed by bactericidal drugs) is common among currently isolated strains of *S. aureus*, but the clinical significance of this in vitro observation has not been clearly defined in human infections. The enterococcus (group D streptococcus), long recognized as an important pathogen in nosocomial urinary tract infections, is emerging as a significant wound pathogen particularly in patients who have received broad-spectrum cephalosporins (to which enterococci are uniformly resistant).

The spectrum of microorganisms recognized to be important nosocomial pathogens has expanded considerably. Opportunistic infections caused by low-virulence bacteria (*Staphylococcus epidermidis*, JK diphtheroid) and fungi (*Aspergillus*, *Candida*, and agents causing mucormycosis) have become commonplace. Respiratory viruses, especially respiratory syncytial virus and influenza, have gained increased recognition as causes of significant morbidity when acquired during hospitalization. Other viruses transmissible in blood (hepatitis viruses, HTLV III) are of concern to hospital personnel as well as patients.

Transmission of nosocomial pathogens Contact with hospital personnel remains the principal means of transmission of nosocomial pathogens and hand-washing by hospital personnel remains the principal control measure. Other less important modes of transmission include the airborne route, by which infections such as chickenpox and tuberculosis are spread, and contact with environmental sources. The inanimate hospital environment usually is not the source of infecting pathogens, and improved understanding of the epidemiology of nosocomial infections has generally focused attention on other aspects of infection control. However, environmental reservoirs have proved to be of primary importance in clusters of cases of aspergillosis caused by inhalation of spores from dust or fireproofing material, and in epidemics of Legionnaires' disease linked to contaminated cooling towers or hot tap water in hospitals.

Host factors The age and underlying disease of patients, the integrity of their mucosal and integumentary surfaces, and the status of their immunologic defenses are among the major determinants of both the incidence and outcome of hospital-acquired infections (see Chap. 84).

COMMON HOSPITAL-ACQUIRED INFECTIONS Urinary tract infections These infections account for approximately 40 percent of hospital-acquired infections and are usually a consequence of instrumentation of the urethra, bladder, or kidneys. The most common predisposing factor is the insertion of an indwelling urethral catheter which bypasses the normal anatomic barriers to ascending infection. Hospital surveys show that 10 to 15 percent of all adult patients have indwelling urinary catheters, many of which are unnecessary. Because the urinary tract is the most common site of infection resulting in gram-negative bacteremias, steps to prevent catheter-related infections merit special emphasis and include the following:

1 Restrict the use of indwelling catheters except when required for management of bladder outlet obstruction or for close monitoring of fluid and electrolyte balance in severely ill patients.
2 Rigorously adhere to sterile technique during insertion of the catheter.
3 Maintain a system of closed drainage. Good technique can usually keep the urine sterile for 5 to 7 days. After that, the risk of infection increases with time, 5 to 10 percent for each day of catheterization.
4 Keep the collecting tubing and bag unobstructed and in a dependent position.
5 When urine specimens are required, aspirate the specimen from the sampling port in the collecting tubing by use of a sterile needle and syringe rather than by breaking the closed drainage system.
6 Consider intermittent straight catheterization for patients with anticipated short-term needs for bladder drainage in order to avoid using an indwelling catheter altogether.

Wound infections Most surgical wound infections are caused by organisms introduced directly into the tissues at the time of operative procedures. Most infecting organisms originate from the resident flora of the patient, although personnel in the operating theater may occasionally be the source of infection, especially with group A streptococci or *S. aureus*. The major factors affecting the incidence of wound infection include the type of operation, its duration, the skill of the surgeon, and the basic health of the patient. Operations involving contaminated sites, such as the bowel or vagina, are more likely to be complicated by infection than operations on sites which are sterile prior to surgery. Operations of long duration, or ones in which devitalized tissue, foreign bodies, or hematomas are left behind, are associated with increased rates of wound infection. Other factors predisposing to wound infection include advanced age, poor nutritional status, the presence of distant foci of infection, diabetes mellitus, renal failure, and corticosteroid therapy.

Most wound infections become apparent from 3 to 7 days following surgery. Early postoperative wound infections (those occurring within 24 to 48 h of surgery) are commonly caused by group A *Streptococcus* or *Clostridium* spp. Staphylococcal wound infections characteristically become evident 4 to 6 days after surgery, and those caused by gram-negative bacilli and anaerobic bacteria may not appear for a week or more. If perioperative antibiotics are used, the manifestations of infection may be delayed. Gram-stained smears of wound exudate, together with culture, often provide valuable early clues to the bacterial cause of wound infections.

In addition to emphasis on maintaining sterility in the operating room and insistence on operative techniques that minimize tissue trauma and blood loss, increasing attention is being given to preventing postoperative wound infections with short prophylactic courses of systemic antibiotics during the perioperative period. The principles that should govern the use of antibiotics in this situation include (1) beginning the drug during the immediate preoperative period but not earlier, (2) ensuring adequate tissue levels throughout the surgery, giving intraoperative doses of antibiotics if necessary, and (3) discontinuing antibiotic prophylaxis within 24 to 48 h following surgery. These brief courses of antibiotics do not appear to alter the patient's flora or promote colonization with resistant strains. Prolonged pre- and postoperative courses are unnecessary, expensive, and potentially harmful because of the increased risk of drug toxicity and superinfection. Antibiotic prophylaxis administered according to these principles has reduced infectious morbidity in a wide variety of operative procedures that are traditionally associated with major risk of infection including colon surgery and vaginal hysterectomy.

Nonsurgical wounds that are common sites of nosocomial infection include burns, decubitus ulcers, and cutaneous ulcers resulting from venous or arterial occlusive disease. In general, the offending pathogens are similar to those found in surgical wound infections, except that burn wound infections are frequently caused by *Pseudomonas aeruginosa*, and ulcers of the pelvis and lower extremities usually contain fecal flora. Bacteremic *Pseudomonas* infections may result in bacterial vasculitis and cutaneous infarction manifested by hemorrhagic bullae (ecthyma gangrenosum, see Chap. 105).

Pneumonia Lower respiratory tract infections are the leading cause of mortality among hospital-acquired infections, although they rank third in incidence behind urinary tract infections and wound infections. The major pathogens are the gram-negative bacilli and *S. aureus*, all of which characteristically cause a necrotizing bronchopneumonia. These organisms usually reach the lower respiratory tract by aspiration from the pharynx rather than by hematogenous spread. This is consistent with the observation that the pharyngeal flora of seriously ill patients contains an increased number of gram-negative bacilli. The three settings in which nosocomial pneumonias occur most commonly are in (1) obtunded patients whose gag reflex and cough are ineffective, (2) patients with underlying pulmonary disease or congestive heart failure whose pulmonary clearance mechanisms are impaired, and (3) patients who require respiratory tract instrumentation or ventilatory assistance.

Because antibiotic treatment of nosocomial pneumonia is often ineffective, preventive measures assume special importance. Positioning the patient in a swimmer's or Gatch position is the cornerstone of prevention of aspiration in obtunded patients. Treatment of congestive heart failure will improve the effectiveness of the lung's defenses and will reduce lung edema fluid that serves as an excellent culture medium. Emphasis should be placed on sterile technique when performing tracheal toilet, and the breathing circuits on ventilatory assistance equipment must be properly maintained. The routine use of positive pressure breathing machines in perioperative care is unnecessary and subjects patients to the risk of infection inherent in exposure to ventilatory equipment.

Although patients with pulmonary tuberculosis are now diagnosed and managed in general hospitals, nosocomial spread of the tubercle bacillus is uncommon. Recognition of active cases of pulmonary tuberculosis and prompt institution of respiratory isolation and appropriate chemotherapy are the principal means by which in-hospital spread of the disease can be limited. General hospitals located in communities with an appreciable incidence of tuberculosis should maintain an active surveillance program for their employees.

Hospital transmission of viral respiratory pathogens is common, especially on pediatric services but except for influenza and respiratory syncytial virus, rarely results in severe disease. It is now recognized that hospital personnel often become infected by patients' respiratory viruses and that direct and indirect contact spread of viruses on the hands of personnel is a more important route of transmission than airborne spread. When influenza A is widespread in the community, amantadine prophylaxis, as well as immunization, should be considered for unimmunized hospital patients identified as being at high risk for complications of influenza. Increasing the immunization levels among hospital personnel is likely to reduce the risk of nosocomial transmission of influenza viruses.

Bacteremia Although invasion of the bloodstream can occur in any nosocomial infection, the infected vascular cannula is the most common and also most preventable cause of hospital-acquired primary bacteremia and fungemia. Annually in the United States more than 10 million persons (more than one in four hospitalized patients) receive intravenous therapy, and therefore even a low rate of infection assumes major clinical significance. Infections related to intravenous therapy account for about 5 percent of all nosocomial infections and 10 percent of all positive blood cultures. The most common causative organisms are *S. epidermidis, S. aureus,* gram-negative bacilli, and enterococci; when hyperalimentation fluid is administered through the catheter, *Candida* also is an important pathogen. Although microorganisms can enter a fluid delivery system at any point, contamination most commonly occurs at the site of entry into the skin during cannula insertion or subsequent manipulation and may be followed by migration of organisms along the cannula into the bloodstream. Occasionally hematogenous seeding of the cannula may occur. Intravenous fluids may become contaminated as a result of adding medications, or, rarely, in the process of manufacture. A clue to the possible presence of infusate contamination is unexpected bacteremia caused by one of the few pathogens (*Enterobacter, Klebsiella, Serratia, Pseudomonas cepacia,* or *Citrobacter freundii*) capable of sustained growth in intravenous solutions containing 5% dextrose.

The type of cannula, the choice of insertion site, the adequacy of skin preparation, and the duration of cannula use determine the risk of cannula-related septic complication. Stainless steel needles, especially scalp vein needles, are preferable to plastic cannulas, which carry greater risks of local phlebitis, contamination, and sepsis. Suppurative phlebitis, one of the most feared complications of cannula-related infections, is virtually unknown with steel needles. Arms are better insertion sites than legs owing to lower rates of phlebitis and sepsis. When cannula infection is suspected, semiquantitative microbiologic evaluation of the removed cannula tip by culture or by direct examination of a Gram-stained catheter segment is very useful in identifying patients with heavily colonized cannulas who are at high risk of developing bacteremia or fungemia. Preventive measures designed to reduce the incidence of intravenous-associated infections are listed in Table 85-2. With meticulous care, central venous catheters used for parenteral hyperalimentation can be maintained free of infection for prolonged periods. However, infectious complications, particularly *Candida* sepsis, are not uncommon in this setting. Intravascular catheters used for pressure monitoring pose many of the same risks as those used for infusion therapy; in addition, the presence of an indwelling pulmonary artery catheter during a period of bacteremia may increase the risk of developing endocarditis.

Transient bacteremia following diagnostic or therapeutic manipulations of the mouth or respiratory, gastrointestinal, or genitourinary tract are usually well-tolerated by the normal host. However, the patient with valvular or congenital heart disease or a prosthetic valve may be at risk of developing endocarditis during such episodes and should receive antibiotic prophylaxis when undergoing procedures associated with significant risk of bacteremia. These procedures include dental manipulations, urinary tract instrumentation, abdominal surgery, and other surgery involving infected tissue. For patients with prosthetic heart valves, these recommendations have been extended. Detailed programs of prophylaxis are given in the chapter on infective endocarditis (see Chap. 188).

TABLE 85-2 Guidelines to reduce the risk of infusion-associated infections

1	Limit use of vascular cannulas to specific clinical circumstances when other routes of administration of fluids or drugs are not feasible.
2	Avoid high-risk infection sites, such as the legs.
3	Use stainless steel needles in preferences to plastic catheters when possible.
4	Adequately disinfect skin over the insertion site.
5	Use sterile technique in insertion of cannulas.
6	Securely anchor the cannula to limit to-and-fro motion.
7	Apply sterile dressing over the insertion site (antibiotic ointment optional).
8	Inspect insertion site daily and remove the cannula if inflammation, phlebitis, or cannula malfunction is present.
9	Change peripheral cannulas at frequent (48–72 h) intervals.

NOSOCOMIAL INFECTIONS OF SPECIAL INTEREST Hepatitis B The risk of hospital-acquired hepatitis B is significant not only for patients but also for hospital personnel who work with infected patients or handle their blood specimens. Patients at special risk of hepatitis B virus infection include those who receive blood products or undergo hemodialysis. The widespread practice of screening blood products for the presence of hepatitis B surface antigen (HBsAg) has markedly reduced the incidence of posttransfusion hepatitis B, and most posttransfusion hepatitis is now caused by other hepatitis viruses (non-A, non-B hepatitis). However, transmission of hepatitis B virus remains an endemic problem on many hemodialysis units and oncology services. For poorly understood reasons, hepatitis B virus infections are often more severe in previously healthy personnel than in patients.

Measures to prevent nosocomial hepatitis B infections should include (1) meticulous attention to precautions designed to limit spread of pathogens by needle accidents or direct contact; (2) labeling and careful handling of all blood and tissue specimens from infected patients; (3) encouragement of hepatitis B immunization for hospital personnel whose work places them at high risk of infection, (4) prompt passive-active immunization with hepatitis B immune globulin and hepatitis B vaccine for susceptible personnel or patients who have had a specific hepatitis B risk (i.e., needle-stick from an infectious patient).

Considerable concern has been generated about the infectivity of the approximately 1 percent of physicians and dentists who are asymptomatic carriers of HBsAg. Although several instances of transmission of infection from health care workers to patients have been identified, the great majority of HBsAg-positive health care personnel do not appear to present a hazard to their patients. They should be encouraged to pay particular attention to personal hygiene and hand-washing and should wear gloves during invasive procedures or contact with mucous membranes. If these precautions are observed, their patient-related activities need not be restricted.

Acquired immunodeficiency syndrome (AIDS) Epidemiologic and laboratory evidence indicates that human T-cell lymphotrophic virus III is spread primarily by the same routes (blood and intimate sexual contact) as hepatitis B but is less transmissible. Blood and secretion precautions appear adequate to protect other patients and hospital personnel participating in the care of patients with AIDS. The risk of transmission of opportunistic pathogens from patients with AIDS to other patients also appears to be very low, although in patients with active *Pneumocystis* pneumonia the potential for cross-infection may warrant respiratory precautions.

Legionnaires' disease Nosocomial Legionnaires' disease has been widely reported in the United States and Europe, usually affecting immunocompromised patients. Although contamination of hospital cooling tower water accounts for some cases, sustained epidemic or hyperendemic problems have almost always been traced to heavy contamination of hot tap water by *Legionella* species. Infectious aerosols of tap water can be produced presumably by showers and during operation of some humidifiers and respiratory devices filled with tap water. A causative role of contaminated hospital tap water has been substantiated by the efficacy of hyperchlorination or superheating of hospital tap water in curtailing epidemics.

***Clostridium difficile*, colitis** Bacterial superinfection with *C. difficile* is a consequence of alteration of bowel flora by antimicrobial therapy. Patients with *C. difficile* colitis excrete large numbers of organisms and represent a risk to other patients. Therefore, enteric precautions and thorough cleaning of bathroom areas of patients with *C. difficile* disease should be implemented.

CONTROL MEASURES Infection control team The goals of those concerned with infection control are (1) to reduce the risk of patients acquiring infections in the hospital, (2) to provide adequate care for patients with a potentially communicable infection, and (3) to minimize the infectious risks of employees, visitors, and community contacts. The functions of the infection control team include (1) development of enforceable policies necessary for appropriate management of patients with communicable infections; (2) development of a surveillance system which identifies patients with communicable infections, quantitates the incidence and prevalence of hospital-acquired infection, and investigates problems that are likely to be remediable; (3) feedback to physicians and other staff regarding identified problem areas and surveillance finds, including surgical wound infection rates; (4) liaison with personnel from nursing, central supply, housekeeping, maintenance, pharmacy, and other hospital services to ensure that an appropriate infection control environment is maintained; (5) education of employees in appropriate techniques to prevent the spread of infectious agents within the hospital; (6) communication with employee health services to ensure adequate immunization of hospital employees and to provide care when personnel are exposed to a potentially communicable disease; and (7) monitoring of antibiotic utilization and susceptibility patterns of common nosocomial pathogens. Generally an effective infection control program can reduce nosocomial infection rates by one-third. Most large hospitals employ full-time personnel, nurses and/or physicians, to lead the multidisciplinary team effort that is necessary to carry out these functions.

Prevention The basic principles of hand-washing between patient contacts, appropriate isolation of patients harboring communicable microorganisms, and application of epidemiologic methods to identify and correct potential sources of infection remain the cornerstones of prevention of nosocomial infections.

EMPLOYEE HEALTH SERVICE Preventive medicine applies not only to patients but also to hospital personnel. The employee health service should maintain an employee surveillance program for communicable diseases such as tuberculosis and routinely immunize personnel who are susceptible to measles, mumps, poliomyelitis, diphtheria, or tetanus. In addition, personnel of both sexes who are likely to come into contact with pregnant women should be tested for rubella antibodies, and, if susceptible, immunized before being allowed to work in areas where contact with pregnant women is likely. Personnel whose work will involve frequent handling of blood or direct contact with patients at high risk of having hepatitis B should receive hepatitis B vaccine. Annual influenza immunization should be encouraged both to reduce the risk of nosocomial influenza transmission to patients and to minimize winter absenteeism.

Hospital personnel who develop significant infectious diseases should be removed from patient contact during the period of communicability. The dangers of paronychias and other pustular lesions due to *S. aureus* or group A streptococci are often underestimated by the staff, and it is commonly forgotten that susceptible contacts may develop chickenpox following exposure to persons with herpes zoster.

ADMISSION SCREENING A patient scheduled for elective admission who has, or is thought to be incubating, a communicable disease should not be admitted until the period of communicability has passed. Screening on admission for communicable infections is particularly important for pediatric patients and for patients being admitted to oncology and transplant services where there may be a concentration of immunocompromised patients. Infections usually considered to be of minor importance, such as chickenpox or measles, can be devastating in such patients.

CONTAINMENT Each pathogen has its characteristic mode(s) of spread, and, on the basis of this knowledge, isolation precautions can be tailored to fit the situation. Isolation procedures are time-consuming and expensive and can hinder essential patient care activities if applied too rigidly. They should be used only when necessary and for the shortest period consistent with good medical practice. The following types of isolation and precautions are in common use:

1. Strict isolation, where both airborne and contact transmission of an organism are possible, e.g., varicella pneumonia
2. Respiratory isolation, where the infectious agent is contained in airborne droplet nuclei of respirable size, e.g., tuberculosis
3. Wound skin precautions, where direct or indirect contact with infected skin lesions or dressings may transmit the organism, e.g., a staphylococcal wound infection
4. Enteric precautions, where transmission usually occurs via the fecal-oral route and where contact with articles contaminated by feces is to be avoided, e.g., hepatitis A
5. Protective (reverse) isolation, where the precautions are designed to protect an unusually susceptible patient with impaired host defenses from organisms in the environment, e.g., patients with burns
6. Blood precautions, where transmission is by accidental percutaneous or mucous membrane inoculation with blood or serum, e.g., hepatitis B
7. Resistant-organism precautions, where precautions are designed to reduce the spread of multiply resistant bacteria to other patients and the hospital environment

If preventive measures fail and a communicable infection develops in an inpatient, the following principles of containment should be observed:

1. Prevent further transmission of disease by the index case by either isolating the patient or, if the patient's condition allows, arranging for discharge from the hospital.

2 Identify all contacts of the index case and determine their susceptibility and degree of exposure.
3 If prophylactic measures are available, administer them appropriately to exposed susceptible individuals.
4 Design a plan to prevent the spread of the infectious agent from the exposed susceptibles to other patients and personnel. This plan must recognize the epidemiology of the communicable disease in question, the effectiveness and feasibility of various control measures, and the potential consequences of further disease transmission.

Methods commonly employed to limit the tertiary spread of communicable diseases by exposed susceptibles are (1) early discharge of patients when feasible, (2) arranging assignments of exposed personnel to avoid patient contact during the period of communicability, and (3) cohorting exposed susceptible patients and personnel together and treating them as an epidemiologic unit. Although cohorting is cumbersome, it remains a major measure for control of hospital outbreaks of chickenpox and epidemic diarrhea.

PROGNOSIS Most nosocomial infections are diseases of medical progress, and the ever-increasing orientation of modern medicine to technologically sophisticated procedures, both diagnostic and therapeutic, makes it likely that the risk of patients acquiring infections in the hospital will continue to increase. On the other hand, many of the factors that promote infections in the hospital have been identified, and measures for their control have been developed. Influencing hospital personnel to carry out these control measures, such as handwashing, catheter care, and restraint in the use of antibiotics, remains a major challenge.

REFERENCES

BENNETT JV, BRACHMAN PS (eds): *Nosocomial Infections*. Boston, Little, Brown, 1979

COMMITTEE ON IMMUNIZATIONS: *Guide for Adult Immunization*. Philadelphia, American College of Physicians, 1985

CONTE JE JR et al: Infection control guidelines for patients with the acquired immunodeficiency syndrome (AIDS). N Engl J Med 309:740, 1983

COOPER GL, HOPKINS CC: Rapid diagnosis of intravascular catheter–associated infection by direct gram staining of catheter segments. N Engl J Med 312:1142, 1985

DIXON RE (ed): Symposium on nosocomial infections. Am J Med 70:379, 478, 631, 744, 899, 986, 1981

GARNER JS, SIMMONS BP: CDC guidelines for isolation precautions in hospitals. Infect Contr 4:249, 1983

HALEY RW et al: The efficacy of infection surveillance and control programs in preventing nosocomial infections in US hospitals. Am J Epidemiol 121:182, 1985

KIM K-H et al: Isolation of *Clostridium difficile* from the environment and contacts of patients with antibiotic-associated colitis. J Infect Dis 143:42, 1981

MEYER RD: *Legionella* infections: A review of five years of research. Rev Infect Dis 5:258, 1983

86 SEPTIC SHOCK

DAVID C. DALE / ROBERT G. PETERSDORF

DEFINITION Septic shock is characterized by inadequate tissue perfusion, following bacteremia most frequently with gram-negative enteric bacilli. Hypotension, oliguria, tachycardia, tachypnea, and fever are observed in most patients. The circulatory insufficiency is due to diffuse cell and tissue injury and the pooling of blood in the microcirculation.

ETIOLOGY Septic shock may be associated with gram-positive infections, notably those due to staphylococci, pneumococci, and streptococci, although it is more common following gram-negative bacteremia. The most frequently causative organisms are *Escherichia coli, Klebsiella-Enterobacter, Proteus, Pseudomonas,* and *Serratia*. *Neisseria meningitidis* bacteremia and gram-negative anaerobic bacteremia with *Bacteroides* spp are also important causes of septic shock. In gram-negative bacteremia, the shock syndrome is not due to bloodstream invasion with bacteria per se but is related to toxins from the organisms. Endotoxin, the lipopolysaccharide moiety of the microbial cell wall, is the best-studied of these toxins.

EPIDEMIOLOGY Gram-negative bacteremia and septic shock occur primarily in hospitalized patients who usually have underlying diseases which render them susceptible to bloodstream invasion. Predisposing factors include diabetes mellitus; cirrhosis; leukemia, lymphoma, or disseminated carcinoma; cancer chemotherapy and immunosuppressive drugs; and a variety of surgical procedures and antecedent infections in the urinary, biliary, or gastrointestinal tracts. Particularly at risk are neonates, childbearing women, and elderly men with prostatic obstruction. The incidence of gram-negative bacteremic sepsis is increasing, and it is now as high as 12 cases per 1000 admissions in some large urban hospitals. In addition to the predisposing factors mentioned above, the widespread use of antibiotics, adrenal steroids, intravenous catheters, humidifiers and other hospital equipment, and the increasing longevity of patients with chronic diseases contribute to this serious problem (see Chaps. 84 and 85).

PATHOGENESIS AND PATHOLOGY Most of the bacteria causing gram-negative sepsis are normal commensals in the gastrointestinal tract. From there they may spread to contiguous structures, as in peritonitis after appendiceal perforation, or they may migrate from the perineum into the urethra or bladder. Gram-negative bacteremia follows infection in a primary focus, usually the genitourinary tract; biliary tree; gastrointestinal tract or lungs; and, less commonly, the skin, bones, and joints. In burn patients and in patients with leukemia, the skin or the lungs are often portals of entry. In many instances, notably in patients with debilitating diseases, cirrhosis, and cancer, no primary focus is apparent. When bacteremia is followed by metastatic lesions in distant sites, classic abscess formation occurs. More often, however, the autopsy findings in gram-negative sepsis reflect primarily the infection at the primary locus and show involvement of target organs: pulmonary edema, hemorrhage, and hyaline membrane formation in the lungs; tubular or cortical necrosis in the kidney; patchy necrosis in the myocardium; superficial ulceration in the gastrointestinal tract; and thrombi in the capillaries in many tissues.

PATHOPHYSIOLOGY **Basic mechanisms** Septic shock occurs because bacterial products react with cell membranes and components of the coagulation and complement systems to activate coagulation, injure cells, and alter blood flow, particularly through the microcirculation. Experimental studies conducted by injection of bacteria and endotoxin suggest that many of these responses are stimulated simultaneously; much of the present understanding of the pathophysiology of septic shock depends on studies of the effects of bacterial endotoxin and its toxic component, lipid A.

Endotoxin and other bacterial products activate cell membrane phospholipases to liberate arachidonic acid and initiate synthesis and release of leukotrienes, prostaglandins, and thromboxanes. In cells containing phospholipase A_2 (e.g., neutrophils, monocytes, platelets), platelet activating factor (PAF) is also generated. These inflammatory mediators have major influences on vasomotor tone, microvascular permeability and the aggregation of leukocytes and platelets. For instance, thromboxane A_2 and prostaglandin $F_{2\alpha}$ produce marked pulmonary vasoconstriction, leukotrienes C_4 and D_4 induce microvascular leakage, and leukotriene B_4 and PAF promote neutrophil aggregation and activation. Although the opposing actions and interactions of these substances are complex, their net effect in initiating the shock state appears to be very significant (see Chap. 68, "Prostanoids and Eicosanoids").

Microorganisms activate the classic complement pathway, and endotoxin activates the alternate pathway; both result in generation of C3a and C5a with effects on leukocyte and platelet aggregation and vascular tone. Complement activation, leukotriene generation, and the direct effects of endotoxin on neutrophils lead to accumulation of these inflammatory cells in the lungs, release of their enzymes, and production of toxic oxygen radicals which damage the pulmonary endothelium and initiate the acute respiratory distress syndrome (ARDS). Activation of the coagulation system results in thrombin generation and platelet thrombi formation in the microcirculation in many tissues.

Infusion of gram-negative bacteria or endotoxin stimulates release of catecholamines and glucocorticosteroids by the adrenals, histamine from mast cells, and serotonin from platelets. Opioid secretion in the central nervous system, bradykinin generation from kininogen, and the production of the vasoactive arachidonate derive from many cells simultaneously. Tachycardia, hypotension, and eventual circulatory collapse are attributed to the combined effects of these vasoactive substances. Inhibitors and antagonists of these substances are used experimentally and clinically to alter the course of septic shock. It has been recognized for some time that glucocorticosteroid infusion before administration of endotoxin in experimental animals is protective, an effect attributed to the prevention of arachidonic acid release from cell membranes. If the endotoxin is given first, the effect of glucocorticoids is far less impressive. Opioid secretion, i.e., β-endorphins and enkephalins, may be critical in the development of the shock state. Naloxone, an opiate antagonist, significantly improves cardiovascular function in several experimental situations.

Septic shock results in cell injury and death from the direct effects of endotoxin and other bacterial products, from the indirect effects of endogenous mediators, and from tissue anoxia. The vascular endothelium is particularly exposed; experimental studies demonstrate diffuse injury to and vacuolization and desquamation of these cells. Anoxia and the release of hormones (e.g., catecholamines, glucagon, insulin, glucocorticoids) dramatically shift tissue metabolism from aerobic to anaerobic and cause abnormal lipid metabolism, protein catabolism, hypoglycemia, and lactic acidosis. Many clinical consequences of septic shock are a result of these metabolic changes.

Hemodynamic alterations Early in the development of shock, blood pools in the capillary bed and plasma proteins leak into the interstitial fluid. This, in turn, results in a sharp decrease in effective circulating blood volume, lowered cardiac output, and systemic arterial hypotension. Further sympathetic activity, vasoconstriction, and selective reduction of blood flow to visceral organs and skin follow. If ineffective perfusion of vital organs is permitted to continue, metabolic acidosis and severe parenchymal damage ensue, and shock is then irreversible. In humans, the kidneys and lungs are the organs particularly susceptible to endotoxin; oliguria as well as tachypnea and, in some instances, pulmonary edema develop early. In general, the heart and brain are spared early in shock, and myocardial failure and coma are late and often terminal manifestations of the shock syndrome. There is also experimental evidence that, after the administration of live gram-negative bacteria, significant arteriovenous shunting occurs around the capillary beds of susceptible organs. This intensifies tissue anoxia. In some instances the injured cells seem unable to utilize available oxygen. The net result of defective tissue perfusion is a sharp decrease in arteriovenous (AV) oxygen difference and lactic acidemia.

Early in septic shock, the picture is usually one primarily of vasodilatation with an increase in cardiac output, a decrease in systemic vascular resistance, a decrease in central venous pressure, and an increase in stroke volume. In contrast, later in septic shock, the predominant picture is one of vasoconstriction with an increase in systemic vascular resistance, a decrease in cardiac output, a decrease in central venous pressure, and a decrease in stroke volume. The study of large groups of patients with septic shock has revealed certain patterns of clinical and laboratory abnormalities:

1. Shock characterized by a normal cardiac output, normal blood volume, normal circulation time, normal or high central venous pressure, normal or high pH, and *reduced* peripheral resistance. These patients have warm, dry skin. While hypotension, oliguria, and lactic acidemia are present, the prognosis is generally good. Shock in this group has been attributed to shunting of blood through AV communications, making it unavailable for perfusion of vital organs.
2. Patients with low blood volume, low central venous pressure, high hematocrit, increased peripheral resistance, low cardiac output, hypotension, oliguria, but only a moderate elevation of blood lactate and normal or slightly high pH. These patients may be hypovolemic before bacteremia, and their prognosis is reasonably good, provided intravascular volume is restored, bacteremia is treated with appropriate antibiotics, septic foci are removed or drained, and vasoactive drugs are given.
3. Shock characterized by normal blood volume, high central venous pressure, normal or high cardiac output, reduced peripheral resistance but *marked metabolic acidosis,* oliguria, and very high blood lactate, indicating ineffective tissue perfusion or impaired oxygen utilization. Despite the presence of warm, dry extremities in these patients, the prognosis is unfavorable.
4. Shock characterized by low blood volume, low central venous pressure, low cardiac output, marked decompensated metabolic acidosis, and severe lactic acidemia. In these patients the extremities are cool and cyanotic. The prognosis is extremely poor.

These observations suggest that there are various stages of septic shock, from hyperventilation, respiratory alkalosis, vasodilatation, and high or normal cardiac output in early shock, to perfusion failure characterized by high-grade lactic acidemia, metabolic acidosis, low cardiac output, and small AV oxygen difference in irreversible, late shock. Moreover, in some patients there is little correlation between the outcome and the hemodynamic abnormalities.

COMPLICATIONS Coagulation defects In most patients with septic shock there is a deficiency in several clotting factors, due to consumption of these factors, a syndrome termed *disseminated intravascular coagulation* (DIC). The pathogenesis of this syndrome involves the activation of the intrinsic clotting system by factor XII (Hageman factor) followed by deposition of fibrin-platelet aggregates on the capillary thrombi that have formed as a result of the generalized Shwartzman reaction. The fibrin-platelet aggregates are typical of DIC, which is characterized by a decrease in factors II, V, and VIII, fibrinogen, and platelets. There may be some degree of fibrinolysis, with appearance of split products. These clotting abnormalities are present to some degree in most patients with septic shock, but usually there is no clinical bleeding, although hemorrhagic phenomena due to thrombocytopenia or deficiency in clotting factors occur occasionally. A more important effect of further disseminated intravascular coagulation is development of capillary thrombi, particularly in the lung. Unless there is bleeding, the coagulopathy requires no therapy and disappears spontaneously as shock is treated.

Respiratory failure Respiratory failure is the most important cause of death in patients with shock, particularly after the hemodynamic aberrations have been corrected. This important cause for the acute respiratory distress syndrome (ARDS) is characterized by pulmonary edema, hemorrhage, atelectasis, hyaline membrane formation, and formation of capillary thrombi. The severe pulmonary edema may be a consequence of a marked increase in capillary permeability. It may occur in the absence of heart failure. Respiratory failure may develop and progress even as other abnormalities return to normal. Pulmonary surfactant decreases, and pulmonary compliance becomes progressively compromised.

Renal failure Oliguria occurs early in shock and is probably due to low intravascular volume and inadequate renal perfusion. If renal perfusion remains inadequate, acute tubular necrosis develops. In an occasional patient, renal cortical necrosis, as occurs in the generalized Shwartzman reaction, is seen.

Cardiac failure Many patients with septic shock develop myocardial failure even though they were free of heart disease before development of shock. On the basis of experimental data, heart failure has been attributed to a product of lysosomal enzyme activity in the ischemic splanchnic region. This product has been termed myocardial depressant factor (MDF). Functionally, there is left ventricular failure as indicated by an increase in left ventricular end-diastolic pressure.

Other organs Superficial ulcerations of the gastrointestinal tract manifested by hemorrhage are common, as are abnormalities in liver function, characterized by hypoprothrombinemia, hypoalbuminemia, and mild jaundice.

CLINICAL MANIFESTATIONS Usually gram-negative bacteremia begins abruptly with chills, fever, nausea, vomiting, diarrhea, and prostration. When septic shock develops, there are, in addition, tachycardia; tachypnea; hypotension; cool, pale extremities, often with peripheral cyanosis; mental obtundation; and oliguria. When present in its full-blown form, gram-negative shock is detected readily, but occasionally the findings are quite subtle, particularly in old, debilitated patients or in infants. Unexplained hypotension, increasing confusion, and disorientation or hyperventilation may be the only clues to septic shock. Some patients are hypothermic, and in the absence of fever the diagnosis is often missed. Jaundice occurs occasionally and signifies infection in the biliary tree, intravascular hemolysis, or "toxic" hepatitis. As shock progresses, oliguria persists, and heart failure, respiratory insufficiency, and coma supervene. Death usually occurs from pulmonary edema, generalized anoxemia secondary to respiratory insufficiency, cardiac arrhythmias, disseminated intravascular coagulation with bleeding, cerebral anoxia, or a combination of these factors.

LABORATORY FINDINGS The laboratory data in septic shock vary greatly and depend in many instances on the cause of the shock syndrome and on the stage of shock. The hematocrit is often elevated and falls to below normal as the volume deficit is repaired. There usually is *leukocytosis* with a white blood cell count between 15,000 and 30,000 per cubic millimeter with a shift to the left. However, the white blood cell count may be normal, and some patients have leukopenia. The *platelet count* is usually decreased, and the prothrombin time and partial thromboplastin times may be abnormal, reflecting a consumption of *clotting factors*.

The *urinalysis* shows no specific abnormalities. Initially, the specific gravity is high; as oliguria persists, isosthenuria develops. The *blood urea nitrogen* (BUN) and *creatinine* are elevated, and creatinine clearance is reduced.

Simultaneous measurements of urine and plasma osmolalities are a useful clue to impending renal failure. If the urinary osmolality is greater than 400 mosmol and the ratio of urine to plasma osmolality is greater than 1.5, renal function is preserved and oliguria is probably due to volume depletion. On the other hand, a urine osmolality of less than 400 mosmol and a urine/plasma ratio less than 1.5 signify renal failure. Other useful clues to suggest prerenal azotemia are urine sodium less than 20 meq per liter, a urine creatinine/serum creatinine ratio greater than 40, or a BUN/serum creatinine ratio greater than 20. Electrolyte patterns vary considerably, but there is a tendency to *hyponatremia* and hypochloremia. The serum potassium may be high, low, or normal. The *bicarbonate concentration* is usually low and *blood lactate* is elevated. A low blood pH and high level of blood lactate are the most reliable clues to poor tissue perfusion.

Early in endotoxin shock there is *respiratory alkalosis* manifested by a low P_{CO_2} and high arterial pH, probably because of progressive anoxemia and an attempt to blow off CO_2 to compensate for developing lactic acidemia. As shock progresses, *metabolic acidosis* develops. There often is striking *anoxemia,* and P_{O_2} values below 70 mmHg are common. The *electrocardiogram* generally shows depression of the ST segment, inversion of the T waves, and a variety of arrhythmias, and may mistakenly suggest the diagnosis of myocardial infarction.

In untreated septic shock, the blood cultures should reveal the causative pathogens, but bacteremia may be intermittent and the blood cultures may be negative. Furthermore, many patients will have received antimicrobial agents when they are first seen, masking the bacteriologic diagnosis. *A negative blood culture does not exclude the diagnosis of septic shock.* Culture of the primary septic focus may aid in the diagnosis, but the bacteriology may have been altered by prior chemotherapy. The ability of endotoxin to coagulate the blood of the horseshoe crab *Limulus* is the basis of a test for endotoxemia, but this test is not widely available and is of limited clinical usefulness.

DIAGNOSIS The diagnosis of septic shock is not difficult in the presence of chills, fever, and an overt focus of infection. However, none of the obvious clues may be present. Elderly, debilitated patients, in particular, may have severe infections in the absence of fever. Unexplained confusion and disorientation and hyperventilation without abnormal chest x-rays should call the diagnosis to mind. Pulmonary embolism, myocardial infarction, cardiac tamponade, aortic dissection, and silent hemorrhage are entities often confused with septic shock.

COURSE The rational treatment of septic shock depends upon careful monitoring of patients. A flow sheet for recording clinical data is very helpful. Specifically four basic indexes need to be followed at the bedside:

1 The status of the *pulmonary circulation* and, to a lesser extent, of left ventricular function should be monitored by insertion of a Swan-Ganz catheter. A pulmonary wedge pressure in excess of 15 to 18 cmH_2O signifies fluid overload. When a Swan-Ganz catheter is not available, the *central venous pressure* (CVP) should be measured. Insertion of a catheter into the great veins or right atrium provides an accurate index of the relation between right ventricular competence and effective blood volume and should be used as a guide to fluid replacement therapy. When the CVP exceeds 12 to 14 cmH_2O, there is some danger of overloading the circulation and precipitating pulmonary edema. It is important to be sure that the flow through the catheter is free and that the catheter is not in the right ventricle. Either a Swan-Ganz catheter or a CVP line should be placed in every patient with septic shock.
2 The *pulse pressure* serves as an estimate of stroke volume.
3 *Cutaneous vasoconstriction* provides a clue to peripheral resistance, although it does not reflect accurately blood flow to kidney, brain, or gut.
4 Hourly *urine output* should be used to monitor splanchnic blood flow and visceral perfusion. Usually this requires placement of an indwelling urethral catheter.

By means of these four measurements the patient with shock can be followed carefully and managed intelligently. Indirect arterial blood pressure does not provide an accurate picture of the hemodynamic situation, and perfusion of vital organs may be adequate in patients with hypotension; conversely, some patients with normal blood pressures may have marked pooling and inadequate visceral blood flow. Direct measurement of arterial pressure is helpful but not necessary. Where possible, these patients should be treated in intensive care units in hospitals that have laboratories available for measurement of arterial pH, blood gases, blood lactate, renal function, and electrolytes.

TREATMENT Support of respiration In many patients with septic shock arterial P_{O_2} is markedly depressed. It is essential to establish an airway at the outset and to administer oxygen nasally, or by mask or by endotracheal intubation. Ventilatory support with a respirator should be employed early to avoid acidosis and hypoxia.

Volume replacement With the CVP or pulmonary wedge pressure as a guide, blood volume should be replaced with blood (if anemia is present), plasma, or other colloids, especially human serum albumin, and appropriate electrolyte solutions, primarily dextrose-saline and bicarbonate (which is preferable to lactate for treating the acidosis). Bicarbonate should be given to increase the blood pH to about 7.2 to 7.3 but not higher under most circumstances. The quantity of fluid required may be considerably in excess of "normal" blood volume and may amount to 8 to 12 liters in only a few hours. Large quantities may be required even when the cardiac index is normal. *Oliguria in the presence of hypotension is not a contraindication to continued vigorous fluid therapy*. In order to guard against pulmonary edema, diuresis with furosemide should be attempted when the CVP reaches a level of approximately 10 to 12 cmH_2O and the pulmonary artery pressure 16 to 18 cmH_2O.

Antibiotics Blood cultures and cultures of relevant body fluids or exudates should be taken before instituting antimicrobial therapy. Drugs should be given intravenously, and bactericidal agents used when possible. When the results of blood cultures and sensitivities are known, one of the appropriate drugs recommended in the chapters dealing with the specific infections and discussed in Chap. 88 should be given. Without specific knowledge of the infecting organism, the first principle of initial therapy is that it should be comprehensive, covering all of the pathogens likely to be involved. Clinical clues often guide the initial antimicrobial choices. For example, a young woman with dysuria, chills, and flank pain and septic shock is likely to have *Escherichia coli* bacteremia. Gram-negative sepsis in a burn patient is probably caused by *Pseudomonas*. During an epidemic of influenza, treatment should include coverage for *Staphylococcus aureus* because this is a frequent and serious cause of bacterial superinfection and pneumonia in this setting.

When the cause of septic shock is unknown, therapy should be initiated with both gentamicin (or tobramycin) and a cephalosporin or a penicillinase-resistant penicillin; many physicians add carbenicillin to this regimen. Because of their toxic effect on the vestibular portion of the eighth nerve, gentamicin, tobramycin, and other aminoglycosides must be given cautiously to oliguric patients. If *Bacteroides* is suspected, chloramphenicol, 7-chlorlincomycin (clindamycin), or carbenicillin can be added. As soon as culture results become available, therapy can be adjusted appropriately.

Surgical intervention Many patients with septic shock have an abscess, infarcted or necrotic bowel, inflamed gallbladder, infected uterus, pyonephrosis, or other local situations which lend themselves to surgical drainage or excision. As a rule, successful treatment of shock requires surgical intervention even if the patient is desperately ill. Operations should not be postponed "to get the patient in shape" because these patients' condition will continue to deteriorate unless the septic focus is removed or drained.

Vasoactive drugs Usually, septic shock is accompanied by maximal stimulation of alpha-adrenergic receptors, and pressor agents which act by stimulating these receptors, such as norepinephrine, levarterenol, and metaraminol, are generally not indicated. The two groups of drugs which have been of value in septic shock are beta-receptor stimulants (notably isoproterenol and dopamine) and alpha-receptor blocking agents (phenoxybenzamine and phentolamine).

Dopamine hydrochloride is used widely for treatment of shock. Unlike other vasoactive agents, this drug increases renal blood flow and with it glomerular filtration, sodium excretion, and urine flow. This effect is seen at low doses [1 to 2 (μg/kg)/min]. At a dose of 2 to 10 (μg/kg)/min, the beta receptors in the heart are stimulated with a resulting increase in cardiac output but without increase in heart rate or blood pressure. Between 10 and 20 (μg/kg)/min there is some effect on the alpha receptors with a rise in blood pressure. Above 20 (μg/kg)/min, alpha stimulation predominates, and vasoconstriction may reverse the dopaminergic effects on the renal and splanchnic circulations. Treatment should be started at 2 to 5 (μg/kg)/min and the dose increased until urine flow and blood pressure respond. Most patients respond to doses of 20 (μg/kg)/min or less. Side effects include ectopic rhythms, nausea and vomiting, and occasionally tachyarrhythmias. They usually disappear with reduction in dosage.

Isoproterenol counteracts arteriolar and venous constriction in the microcirculation by its direct vasodilating effect. In addition, the drug exerts a direct inotropic effect on the heart. Cardiac output is increased by stimulation of the myocardium and by reduction of cardiac work as peripheral resistance decreases. The dose of isoproterenol is 2 to 8 μg/min for the average adult. Ventricular arrhythmias may result from this drug, and shock may be made worse if fluid administration does not keep pace with relieved vasoconstriction.

Phenoxybenzamine, an adrenolytic agent, effects a central phlebotomy by reducing resistance and increasing intravascular capacity. Hence there is a redistribution of blood. Blood leaves the lungs, relieving pulmonary edema and enhancing gas exchange. Central venous pressure and left ventricular end-diastolic pressure fall, cardiac output rises, and peripheral venous constriction regresses. The recommended dose is 0.2 to 2.0 mg/kg intravenously. Small doses can be injected instantaneously and large doses over a period of 40 to 60 min. Fluids must be given simultaneously to compensate for the increment in venous capacitance; failure to do so aggravates shock. Phenoxybenzamine[1] is not available for general use, and experience with phentolamine has not been great enough to recommend it.

Diuretics and digitalis It is important to maintain urine flow to try to prevent the development of renal tubular necrosis. Once the volume status of the patient is repaired, a diuretic, preferably furosemide, should be given to keep the hourly urine output up to greater than 30 to 40 mL/h. In patients who remain hypotensive despite an elevated CVP or pulmonary wedge pressure, digoxin may be beneficial but should be given cautiously because of the frequent occurrence of acid-base abnormalities, hyperkalemia, and impaired renal function in shock patients.

Glucocorticosteroids Numerous experimental studies provide a rationale for the use of corticosteroid therapy to ameliorate the effects of endotoxemia and septic shock. Steroids appear to protect cell membranes from endotoxin-mediated injury, to prevent transformation of arachidonic acid to its vasoactive derivatives, to decrease platelet aggregation, and to reduce the extracellular release of leukocyte enzymes. Some studies suggest that steroids also may have a direct effect on reducing peripheral vascular resistance. Because of the complexity of the clinical circumstances surrounding the patient with endotoxic shock, it has been difficult to prove that steroid therapy is clearly helpful. Some controlled studies have demonstrated a benefit for treating patients with methylprednisolone (30 mg/kg) or dexamethasone (3 mg/kg) as soon as shock was recognized. Therapy was repeated in 4 h in the most severely ill patients. These studies and experience in many shock centers support the early use of steroids in high doses for relatively brief periods (24 to 48 h). Late in septic shock, steroids are probably of no benefit. Prolonged steroid therapy substantially increases the problems of hyperglycemia, gastrointestinal bleeding, and other steroid side effects and should be avoided.

Other measures Hemorrhage must be controlled with whole blood, fresh frozen plasma, cryoprecipitate, or platelet transfusion, depending on the clotting abnormality. The use of naloxone, prostaglandin synthesis inhibitors, and prostacyclin is still experimental. Treatment of disseminated intravascular coagulation with heparin remains a controversial and hazardous procedure. Hyperbaric oxygen has been tried in gram-negative bacteremia with indifferent results.

PROGNOSIS The measures described above usually will resuscitate most patients, at least temporarily. Indicators of a favorable response are

1 Improved sensorium and general appearance
2 Decreased peripheral cyanosis
3 Warming of the skin over the extremities
4 Urine output of 40 to 50 mL/h
5 Increased pulse pressure
6 Return of CVP and pulmonary artery pressure to normal
7 Increased blood pressure

The ultimate outcome, however, is dependent upon several other factors:

1 Ability to eliminate the source of infection with surgery or

[1] *This drug has not been approved for this purpose by the Food and Drug Administration at the time of publication.*

antibiotics. The prognosis of urinary tract infections, septic abortions, abdominal abscesses, gastrointestinal or biliary fistulas, and subcutaneous or anorectal abscesses is better than that of primary foci in the skin or lungs. However, extensive abdominal surgery, even if necessary, is associated with a poor prognosis.

2 Previous contact with the organism. Patients with chronic urinary tract infections who develop bacteremia rarely have severe gram-negative shock, perhaps because they have become tolerant to the endotoxin.

3 Underlying disease. Patients with lymphoma or leukemia who develop septic shock while their hematologic disease is out of control rarely recover; conversely, if hematologic remission is achieved, the shock is more likely to respond to therapy. Patients with antecedent heart disease and with diabetes mellitus also have a poor prognosis.

4 Metabolic status. The development of severe metabolic acidosis and lactic acidemia—irrespective of cardiac output—is associated with a poor prognosis.

5 Development of pulmonary insufficiency even after the hemodynamic abnormalities have been corrected is associated with an unfavorable outcome.

The overall mortality rate of septic shock remains 50 percent; however, with better monitoring and more physiologic treatment, the outcome should improve.

PREVENTION The poor results in the treatment of septic shock are not due to lack of potent antibiotics or vasoactive agents. Rather, failure to institute therapy sufficiently early is a major roadblock to success. Septic shock usually is recognized too late, all too often after irreversible changes have taken place. Because 70 percent of patients who are likely to develop septic shock are in the hospital *before* signs and symptoms of shock appear, it is essential to watch patients who are candidates for development of shock assiduously, to treat their infections vigorously and early, and to perform appropriate surgery before catastrophic complications occur. It is particularly important to watch for infected venous and urinary catheters which may act as portals of entry for the organisms that cause gram-negative sepsis and to remove them from all patients as soon as feasible. There is some preliminary evidence that early therapy of septic shock improves the ultimate outcome. Finally, the protective effect of antiserum in experimental animals may, at some time in the future, be applicable to humans.

REFERENCES

BERNTON EW et al: Opioids & neuropeptides: Mechanisms in circulatory shock. Fed Proc 44:290, 1985

BRYAN CS et al: Analysis of 1,186 episodes of gram-negative bacteremia in non-university hospitals: The effects of antimicrobial therapy. Rev Infect Dis 5:629, 1983

HOUSTON MC et al: Shock diagnosis and management. Arch Intern Med 144:1433, 1984

HOUTCHENS BA, WESTENSKOW DR: Oxygen consumption in septic shock: Collective review. Circ Shock 13:361, 1984

KREGER BE et al: Gram-negative bacteremia: III. Reassessment of etiology, epidemiology and ecology in 612 patients. Am J Med 68:332, 1980

———: Gram-negative bacteremia: IV. Re-evaluation of clinical features and treatment in 612 patients. Am J Med 68:344, 1980

MCCABE WR et al: Pathophysiology of bacteremia. Am J Med 75:225, 1983

MIZOCK B: Septic shock—a metabolic perspective. Arch Intern Med 144:579, 1984

PARKER MM, PARRILLO JE: Septic shock: Hemodynamics and pathogenesis. JAMA 250:3324, 1983

ROOT RK, SANDE MM: *Septic Shock*. New York, Churchill Livingstone, 1985

SCHUMER W: Steroids in the treatment of clinical septic shock. Ann Surg 184:333, 1976

SPRUNG CL et al: The effects of high-dose corticosteroids in patients with septic shock. N Engl J Med 311:1137, 1984

87 LOCALIZED INFECTIONS AND ABSCESSES

JAN V. HIRSCHMANN

GENERAL CONSIDERATIONS

While many bacterial diseases are conveniently described by their specific etiologic pathogens, in some their location primarily determines the clinical picture. Examples of such infections include abscesses, soft tissue infections, bacterial endocarditis (see Chap. 188), pyogenic infections of the central nervous system (see Chap. 346), urinary tract infections (see Chap. 225), lung abscess (see Chap. 205), mediastinitis (see Chap. 214), appendicitis and appendiceal abscess (see Chap. 241), diverticulitis (see Chap. 239), osteomyelitis (see Chap. 340), and infections of the pericardium (see Chap. 194). Many pathogens can cause infections in these sites; although their bacteriologic identification may be time-consuming, knowledge of the usual flora causing infection in certain anatomic loci should permit appropriate therapy before the results of cultures are available.

ETIOLOGY Localized pyogenic infection can develop in any region or organ of the body, and may be initiated by *trauma* and secondary bacterial contamination, by some *alteration in local conditions* that renders a tissue susceptible to infection with organisms already present as part of the "normal flora" to which it is ordinarily resistant, by *contiguous spread* from a nearby lesion, or by *metastatic implantation* of microorganisms carried in blood or lymph.

Under appropriate conditions of lowered local host defenses, almost any common bacteria can initiate an infectious process. Cultures from open lesions such as those of the skin or from intraabdominal foci arising from perforations of the gastrointestinal tract frequently contain several bacterial species; as expected, the organisms found most frequently are the "normal flora" of these regions.

Infection in some areas is more likely to be caused by certain organisms, such as staphylococci in the skin and coliform bacteria in the urinary tract, and special features of the tissue reaction produced by some bacterial species make it possible to recognize infection by them with considerable accuracy. The *staphylococci* produce rapid necrosis and early suppuration with large amounts of creamy yellow pus (see Chap. 94). Group A beta-hemolytic streptococcal infections (see Chap. 95) tend to spread rapidly through tissues, causing intense edema and erythema but relatively little necrosis and thin, serumlike exudate; anaerobic bacteria (see Chap. 102) produce necrosis and profuse, brownish, foul-smelling pus.

The identification of infecting organisms is important in the choice of antimicrobial chemotherapy. However, when infection occurs in certain areas, as in paranasal sinuses or cutaneous ulcers, or shows up in sputum, it is unlikely that treatment will render cultured specimens sterile. In these locations, serial cultures during antimicrobial administration are typically unhelpful, and therapy should be guided largely by the clinical response.

PATHOGENESIS Factors predisposing to the initiation and persistence of infection in a tissue include trauma, obstruction of normal drainage (sweat glands, biliary tract, bronchial tree, urinary tract), ischemia (infarction, gangrene), chemical irritation (by gastric contents, bile, or intramuscularly injected drugs), hematoma formation, accumulation of fluid (lymphatic obstruction, cardiac edema), foreign bodies (bullets, splinters, sutures), and others such as the occurrence of stasis or turbulence in the vascular system.

Infection in soft tissue usually begins as a *cellulitis,* a diffuse acute inflammation with hyperemia, edema, and leukocytic infiltration but little or no necrosis and suppuration. With some organisms, this is followed by necrosis, liquefaction, accumulation of leukocytes and debris, suppuration, loculation of the pus, and formation of one or more *abscesses*. Abscess formation is particularly likely to follow infection in a preexisting space or cavity, such as the fallopian tubes or lung cysts.

The local spread of infection generally follows the path of least resistance along fascial planes; proper surgical treatment requires a knowledge of these routes, which will be described for specific infections later in this chapter. Lymphatic spread may lead to lymphangitis, lymphadenitis, or, if the regional nodes suppurate, to the formation of a *bubo*. Involvement of local venules or large veins may cause infective thrombophlebitis with resulting bacteremia, septic embolization, and systemic dissemination of infection. Staphylococci, streptococci, and *Bacteroides* are notorious for frequently producing vascular lesions of this type.

Depending upon the infecting organism and the anatomy of the affected region, a small abscess may subside completely; there may be gradual encapsulation of the accumulated pus and persistence of the focus in a quiescent state; or the lesion may "point" and rupture into adjacent tissues or to the outside surface of the body, as usually happens with furuncles. Spontaneous drainage ordinarily leads to resolution of a superficially situated suppurative focus. However, if the abscess is deeply situated and well encapsulated, persistence of a fistulous tract and the formation of a chronic, draining sinus often occur. *The development of persistent sinuses over an area of suppuration produced by ordinary pyogenic bacteria should always suggest involvement of underlying bone or the presence of a foreign body*. Fistulas that open onto the skin are, of course, soon colonized by microorganisms from the external environment. Ordinary bacterial cultures of drainage fluid almost invariably show a mixed flora and are unreliable for the etiologic diagnosis of the underlying disease. This is particularly important in disorders that characteristically lead to persistent sinus formation, such as tuberculosis and actinomycosis. In these situations, superficial organisms about the opening of the sinus tract may mask the true nature of the lesion by obscuring the real pathogen.

MANIFESTATIONS Secondary infection of wounds and cutaneous ulcers is usually recognizable by inspection. Infections of the skin and subcutaneous tissues almost invariably produce the classic manifestations: *redness, tenderness, heat,* and *swelling*. Reddish streaks extending proximally and associated with tender enlargement of regional lymph nodes indicate lymphangitis. Systemic symptoms may be absent or mild, or there may be fever, malaise, prostration, and leukocytosis.

Infection and suppuration in deeper tissues or in body cavities often cause local pain and tenderness, but locating and determining the exact nature of the lesion may be difficult. Palpating a tender mass is helpful, but muscle spasm and intervening structures often interfere. Abdominal or pelvic examination under anesthesia is sometimes useful in these circumstances.

Auscultation may reveal a friction rub over an abdominal viscus, the pleura, or the pericardium. The rapid development of an effusion in the pericardium, pleura, abdomen, or a joint should suggest infection. Similarly, fluid detected by transillumination of paranasal sinuses or inspection of the tympanic membrane may be the first sign of infection.

Depending on the location of an abscess, symptoms and signs referable to encroachment upon adjacent structures may dominate the picture. Respiratory obstruction may be the first sign of mediastinal abscess; dysphagia often first calls attention to peritonsillar or retropharyngeal abscesses; and tamponade is sometimes the initial clue to pericardial infection. Localizing signs of dysfunction are especially striking and important with brain and spinal cord abscesses, although brain abscesses may be clinically silent (see Chap. 346). In some patients local pain and tenderness or signs of dysfunction are mild or equivocal, and fever, prostration, and weight loss dominate the picture. The fever may be low-grade but is often hectic, with repeated rigors and drenching night sweats. Fatigue and anemia are frequent, and weight loss may be so rapid that emaciation occurs within a few weeks. A patient with these symptoms and signs may have chronic subphrenic, perinephric, or other abscess in the complete absence of any detectable physical sign pointing to the location of a large accumulation of pus. Because of prior antimicrobial therapy, some deep-seated abscesses present the picture of a chronic illness manifested by no more than malaise, easy fatigability, low-grade fever, mild anemia, and an elevated sedimentation rate.

Fluctuation of a mass on palpation is a reliable sign that it contains fluid, perhaps pus, but failure to detect this sign when examining deeper structures does not exclude suppuration as a cause, indicate that the mass is noninfectious, or prove that drainage is unnecessary.

LABORATORY FINDINGS Peripheral polymorphonuclear leukocytosis is frequent with abscesses, and significant unexplained elevation of the white blood cell count in any patient should lead to a search for localized suppuration. Depending on the severity and duration of infection, there may be a chronic normocytic, normochromic anemia. The sedimentation rate is almost always rapid. Mild albuminuria, occasionally noted in febrile patients, has no diagnostic import.

Pus or fluid obtained by needle aspiration or incision of a suspected lesion should *always* be stained and examined directly in addition to being cultured aerobically and anaerobically. Pus is a poor metabolic substrate, and bacteria may fail to grow in cultures from an abscess of long standing. In such instances, the findings on microscopic examination may be the only guide in choosing proper chemotherapy. *Failure to examine exudates with Gram's stain is the single greatest deterrent to appropriate antimicrobial therapy;* the internist as well as the surgeon should be sure that this procedure is performed.

Blood cultures are often positive in intravascular infections such as septic thrombophlebitis and endocarditis and in pyogenic infections in which localized abscesses are metastatic, as in staphylococcal, streptococcal, and *Salmonella* bacteremias. Moreover, manipulation, including surgical incision, of any localized infection may cause transient bacteremia.

Noninvasive techniques are often helpful in the diagnosis of abscess. X-ray examinations may indicate localized collections of pus when they show atypical collections of gas, displacement of organs, and tissue densities in abnormal locations. Radionuclide scans may demonstrate abscesses in brain, liver, spleen, and thyroid. The isotope [^{67}Ga] gallium citrate is selectively concentrated in areas of suppuration, but in noninfectious inflammation and neoplasms as well, and many have found gallium scans of limited value in locating abscesses. Scans using ^{111}In-labeled leukocytes may be more accurate. The technique of diagnostic ultrasound is not only useful in localizing abscess but also may provide clues to the size of the abscess and to the presence of multiple abscesses or loculation. Computerized tomography (CT scan) is very helpful in demonstrating abscesses, especially in the brain and abdominal cavity, including the retroperitoneum.

THERAPEUTIC CONSIDERATIONS Recognition of the striking symptomatic improvement that follows spontaneous evacuation of a suppurative focus led long ago to the adoption of *surgical incision* for the treatment of abscesses. The exact reasons that local and constitutional manifestations improve with adequate drainage of pus are unknown, but clinically the benefits are unequivocal.

Incision of infected tissue before the stage of liquefaction and accumulation of pus is often deleterious, fails to relieve discomfort, and may even at times facilitate spread of infection. For this reason, it is sometimes necessary to wait until an abscess "ripens," i.e., localizes and "comes to a head." The *application of heat* to an area of superficial inflammation will relieve pain and often speed the subsidence of cellulitis without suppuration. If necrosis of tissue is already under way, hot applications appear to facilitate localization of the process and accumulation of pus, making incision and drainage feasible at an earlier time. Another procedure that helps reduce swelling and relieve pain is *elevation of the affected part*.

The availability of specific chemotherapeutic drugs has modified the need for heat, elevation, and incision surprisingly little. The early administration of chemotherapeutics has reduced the incidence of suppurative complications in many disorders, but once suppuration has appeared, antimicrobial drugs become remarkably incapable of eradicating the infecting organisms, although they may mask the classic clinical features of abscess formation.

Some antimicrobials, notably the penicillins, appear to retain their antibacterial activity in the presence of pus, while others, exemplified by the aminoglycosides, are at least partially inactivated. However, inability of the drug to penetrate into an area of suppuration is rarely the reason for therapeutic failure. Although this possibility exists in some infections, such as osteomyelitis, it is usually overcome by increasing dosage. Because direct instillation of the antibiotic into an infected area is not, by itself, a curative procedure, other factors are probably more important than faulty diffusion of the agent into the purulent focus.

An established inflammatory exudate is a relatively poor environment for bacterial multiplication. Because the penicillins and cephalosporins are bactericidal only against multiplying organisms, failure of these antibiotics to eradicate bacteria in an abscess may be related to the organisms' inactive metabolic state. Although the mechanism of their antibacterial action differs from that of the penicillins, bacteriostatic agents such as tetracycline or chloramphenicol also are incapable of eradicating bacteria in the static phase of growth. By definition, these drugs only inhibit multiplication of bacteria and usually exert no direct lethal action; the death of organisms in any infection treated with bacteriostatic agents depends on other mechanisms. For most pyogenic bacteria, phagocytosis is one of the most important of these (although there must be others not so carefully studied), and, in the absence of phagocytes or in circumstances which inhibit their activity, bacteriostatic drugs are relatively ineffective. In fluid-filled cavities, particularly in the metabolically unfavorable milieu of an abscess, phagocytosis is greatly reduced. Consequently, despite inhibition of bacterial multiplication, organisms can remain dormant and survive for long periods of time. It is probably a combination of these two circumstances, decreased multiplication of bacteria and decreased phagocytosis, that makes infection in the heart valves, for example, so relatively resistant to antimicrobial therapy. Large doses of bactericidal drugs for long periods are needed to achieve cure.

Antimicrobial drugs may obviate suppuration if given early or prevent spread of an existing abscess, but usually are no substitute for surgical drainage. Indeed, their use in the face of a lesion requiring evacuation of pus is one of the most common serious errors in treating pyogenic infections.

In empyema, suppurative pericarditis, or pyarthrosis, excellent therapeutic results are sometimes achieved by aspiration of pus and systemic antimicrobial therapy. Success, however, depends as fully on the adequacy of drainage as it does upon the administration of the antibiotic, and if loculation occurs or the exudate becomes too viscid to remove, surgical incision and drainage become mandatory.

In infective thrombophlebitis, surgical interruption of the veins by ligation or, in some cases, by total excision of an infected segment is sometimes indicated to prevent seeding of other organs by infected emboli.

CLINICAL FEATURES OF INFECTIONS IN VARIOUS REGIONS

SUPERFICIAL ABSCESSES Skin and subcutaneous tissues *Impetigo* is a superficial infection caused by group A hemolytic streptococci, sometimes combined with *Staphylococcus aureus*. It is primarily a disease of children, common in warm weather, characterized by multiple erythematous lesions which vesiculate and are intensely pruritic. In adults impetigo is most commonly an infectious complication of a chronic dermatitis. Local spread occurs through scratching and release of infected vesicle fluid. Serious complications are metastatic abscesses and acute glomerulonephritis. Treatment consists of local and general cleansing of the skin, appropriate systemic antibiotics, and therapy of any underlying dermatologic condition present.

Deeper infections of the skin are almost invariably staphylococcal in origin and are described in Chap. 94. Erysipelas, a characteristic dermal lesion produced by group A streptococci, is described in Chap. 95.

Lymphadenitis with or without suppuration may complicate any pyogenic skin lesion and is often striking with superficial streptococcal infections. Specific diseases characterized by suppurative regional lymphadenitis include lymphogranuloma venereum (see Chap. 150), cat-scratch disease (see Chap. 118), tularemia (see Chap. 113), and bubonic plague (see Chap. 114).

Infections of the hand These are almost invariably secondary to trauma. Because of the rapidity with which infection can spread through the complex fascial spaces of the hand, wrist, and forearm, and produce irreparable functional damage, *any deep infection in this area should receive expert surgical attention immediately*. The availability of antibiotics has in no way lessened the importance of such care.

The ordinary *paronychia,* or "run-around," is a superficial infection of the epithelium lateral to a nail, usually a result of tearing a hangnail and most frequently caused by staphylococcus. Hot applications will lead to subsidence of paronychial cellulitis, but often a superficial blister of pus appears. A small incision or simply separation of the nail fold from the nail will promote adequate drainage. If the infection burrows beneath the nail to form a painful *subungual abscess,* incision and drainage with partial or complete removal of the nail are necessary. Recurrence is common, especially in nail biters, and this seemingly trivial infection can cause painful disability. Chronic paronychial inflammation, usually from *Candida,* occurs in those with prolonged or frequent immersion of hands in water.

What appears to be a small furuncle of the webs of the fingers sometimes produces a *collar-button abscess,* consisting of a superficial and deep compartment connected by a narrow tract. Evacuation of the shallow pocket without emptying the deeper abscess can lead to puzzling persistence of infection. Sometimes a foreign-body granuloma forms in the skin of the digital webs. This is most common in barbers, in whom a hair is the core of the foreign-body granuloma, the "barber's interdigital pilonidal sinus."

Infection of the distal phalanx of a finger, usually acquired by pinprick, thorn prick, etc., may lead to the formation of a *felon,* or *whitlow*. This is a suppurative infection in the tightly enclosed fibrous compartments of the finger pulp, the "anterior closed space," which can compromise the distal blood supply by compression of the digital arteries, with consequent necrosis of bone and the development of osteomyelitis. The manifestations are swelling, extreme pain, and tenderness of the palmar surface of the fingertip. The treatment is immediate incision directly over the lesion, sometimes by the use of a trephine, and cutting all the fibrous septa that radiate from the periosteum to the subcutaneous fascia.

Suppurative tenosynovitis, usually a complication of a puncture wound, is an even more serious infection of the hand; early diagnosis and treatment are mandatory to prevent permanent disability from destruction of the tendon or its sheath. The three cardinal manifestations of tenosynovitis are (1) exquisite tenderness limited to the course of the sheath, (2) flexion of the fingers, and (3) excruciating pain, most marked at the base of the digit, on extension of the involved finger. *Immediate incision* of the sheath is indicated, not only to prevent damage to the tendon itself but also to avoid proximal extension of the process into the major fascial spaces of the hand or forearm. Vigorous antibiotic treatment should accompany surgery. The definitive treatment of any serious infection of the hand is a matter for a skilled surgeon, but the early recognition of the need for surgery often falls to other physicians.

Human bites lead to very important hand infections which, if neglected, almost invariably produce a highly destructive, necrotizing lesion contaminated by a mixture of aerobic and anaerobic organisms. A deliberately inflicted bite on the hand or elsewhere is usually recognized as dangerously contaminated, but wounds on the knuckles produced by striking an opponent's teeth with the fists may not be recognized as potentially dangerous. In general, bite wounds should be cleaned thoroughly and not sutured. Patients should be given prophylaxis for tetanus and antibiotics, preferably both a penicillinase-resistant penicillin and ampicillin.

Chronic cutaneous ulcers A partial list of the causes of chronic ulcers of the skin includes circulatory disturbances, such as varicose veins and obliterative arterial disease, extensive injury from frostbite or burns, trophic changes accompanying many neurologic disorders, bedsores or decubiti, systemic diseases such as sickle cell disease, neoplasms, and various infections. No matter what the underlying disease, secondary infection is very likely to occur and to interfere with healing, complicate grafting or other restorative procedures, or produce extension of the process.

The management of secondary bacterial infection in skin ulcers associated with obliterative arterial disease, a common problem in diabetics, is especially important, because infection frequently precipitates spreading gangrene and makes amputation necessary.

The microflora of chronic cutaneous ulcers almost invariably comprises bacteria of many species, including staphylococci, aerobic and anaerobic streptococci, coliform bacilli, and members of the *Proteus* and *Pseudomonas* groups. Depending on the patient's environment and on systemically or locally administered antimicrobial drugs, the predominating bacterial species show great variation in serial cultures. Resistant strains or species commonly replace sensitive organisms during the course of chemotherapy.

Treatment of chronic dermal ulcers should be directed toward the underlying disorder but should also include *local debridement* and *chemotherapy*. Debridement by surgical excision is often needed, but the local application of wet-to-dry dressings or other forms of "medical debridement" frequently suffice. Intensive systemic administration of antibiotics should be carried out only in conjunction with definitive surgical procedures or when infection can be controlled in no other way. The prevention of infection by "prophylactic" administration of antimicrobial drugs is futile because it results in the development of a flora resistant to the drugs being used. The *local application of antibacterial agents* is sometimes highly effective, and in managing chronic mixed infections of this type several potent but toxic antibiotics have great value. An ointment or solution containing neomycin, bacitracin, and polymyxin exerts a bactericidal effect against a wide variety of organisms and will sometimes temporarily sterilize a chronic lesion. Other useful topical medications are furacin and 3% acetic acid, which is especially helpful in *Pseudomonas* infections.

Diphtheritic ulcer of the skin is discussed in Chap. 96.

INFECTIONS OF THE HEAD AND NECK Pustules of the nose and upper lip may be particularly dangerous, because they can extend intracranially through the angular vein to the cavernous sinus. These lesions should be treated conservatively, manipulation or incision should be avoided if possible, and systemic antibiotics should be used if local swelling or redness appears.

Suppurative parotitis Typically, suppurative parotitis occurs in elderly and chronically ill patients who have a dry mouth from decreased oral intake, following general anesthesia and surgery, or from medications with atropine-like effects, such as antihistamines or phenothiazines. In most patients, it is an ascending infection due to *S. aureus,* which normally colonizes the opening to Stensen's duct. Occasionally, there is an obstructing calculus. Its onset, usually sudden, is heralded by unilateral local pain and swelling, frequently with fever and chills. Frank pus can often be expressed from the duct and may show gram-positive cocci in clumps. The gland itself is firm and tender, often with redness and edema of the overlying skin. Treatment consists of systemic antimicrobial therapy with a penicillinase-resistant penicillin or some other agent effective against *S. aureus,* unless another organism is isolated, combined with improved hydration and oral hygiene. Massage of the gland and sialagogues, like lemon drops, help promote drainage through the duct. Surgery is usually unnecessary and should be reserved for patients failing to improve after 4 to 5 days of medical management.

Miscellaneous infections Antibiotics have reduced the incidence of many formerly common suppurative complications of streptococcal pharyngitis. However, as a result of streptococcal sore throat, *Bacteroides* infections of the pharynx, or introduction of infection by trauma to the floor of the mouth or the pharyngeal wall, abscesses of the deep cervical structures still occur. *Suppurative cervical adenitis,* once an all-too-common sequel to streptococcal pharyngitis in children, is now rare. *Peritonsillar abscess* (*quinsy*) is manifested by fever, sore throat, cervical lymphadenopathy, unilateral pain radiating to the ear on swallowing, and enlargement of the tonsil with redness and swelling of the adjacent soft palate. Treatment with penicillin and irrigations of warm saline solution sometimes suffices, but if digital palpation reveals fluctuation, needle aspiration or surgical drainage is indicated. Some recommend tonsillectomy immediately or several weeks later; others reserve it for patients with recurrent tonsillar infections. Organisms associated with peritonsillar abscess include *Streptococcus pyogenes* and oral anaerobic bacteria.

The course of *deep cervical infections* depends upon the anatomic arrangement of fascial planes. Infection in this area is serious and is attended by fever, prostration, and leukocytosis. A tender mass may be palpated, but *surgical evacuation of such an infection should not be delayed because of failure to detect fluctuation,* which is usually absent because of the dense fascial layers.

Infection of the *sublingual* and submandibular spaces, so-called Ludwig's angina, causes brawny induration of the submaxillary region, edema of the floor of the mouth, and elevation of the tongue. It usually originates from apical abscesses of the second and third mandibular molars. There are severe pain, dysphagia, and, within hours, dyspnea from respiratory obstruction. The causative organisms of this and other neck abscesses are mainly streptococci and oral anaerobes. Mortality was formerly about 50 percent. *Treatment* consists of large doses of penicillin and careful observation. With significant airway obstruction, tracheostomy is necessary. Since the infection is largely a cellulitis, incision and drainage are reserved for evidence of fluctuation.

The retropharyngeal space lies between the muscles anterior to the cervical vertebrae and the pharyngeal mucosa. *Retropharyngeal abscess,* formerly common in children, is manifested by dysphagia, progressive stridor, pain, and fever. The bulging mass is easily seen and can completely occlude the airway within hours. Incision and drainage are mandatory; spontaneous rupture may lead to death by aspiration. Esophageal perforation during endoscopy may result in abscess as a late complication. Tuberculous abscess, secondary to spinal disease, occasionally appears in the retropharyngeal space; it is painless, and relief of obstruction follows surgical incision.

Submastoid abscess, or suppuration in the submastoid space, known as *Bezold's abscess,* is usually secondary to otitis and produces nuchal rigidity, which may lead to a mistaken diagnosis of otogenous meningitis. Infection can extend down the carotid sheath to the mediastinum. A suppurative thrombophlebitis of the jugular vein usually accompanies this infection, and the vessel is easily felt as a tender cord. Bacteremia and systemic spread of infection are common, and the involved venous segment may require excision. Spontaneous rupture of the carotid artery with rapid death from exsanguination is a rare complication.

Therapy of head and neck abscesses includes surgical incision and drainage, open treatment of infected wounds, and systemic antibiotics, which should include agents active against anaerobic organisms, particularly if there is foul-smelling pus. Penicillin is usually the drug of choice.

INTRAABDOMINAL ABSCESSES

A useful classification divides intraabdominal abscesses, according to location, into three major types, each with several subdivisions: (1) intraperitoneal, (2) retroperitoneal, and (3) visceral (Table 87-1). The clinical features vary but usually include fever, with no characteristic pattern (ranging from mild to hectic), leukocytosis, and an elevated erythrocyte sedimentation rate. Common, but not universal, are pain near the abscess, anorexia, weight loss, nausea, vomiting, and altered bowel habits. A tender mass may be palpable. Plain abdominal films may suggest an abscess by showing a soft tissue density, displacement of adjacent organs, or extraintestinal gas from a perforated viscus or produced by the infecting organisms within the abscess cavity.

The most useful noninvasive diagnostic techniques are ultrasound and CT examinations. Ultrasound has a diagnostic accuracy of about 80 to 90 percent and is most effective in detecting abscesses in the right upper quadrant, retroperitoneum, and pelvis. It shows a sonolucent mass that may have internal echoes when debris and septations are present. The appearance is usually indistinguishable from other fluid-filled masses, but clinical features and, if necessary, needle aspiration of the mass should discriminate among the possible causes. Since gas blocks the beam, ultrasound is not useful when large amounts of gas are present, as occurs in the stomach and splenic flexure, which makes the left upper quadrant a difficult area to examine. Similarly, loops of gas-filled bowel impair evaluation of the midabdomen. Since the transducer must have good skin contact, wounds, fistulas, stomata, and surgical dressings may make ultrasound examination impossible.

These factors do not affect CT scans, which are therefore especially useful in the postoperative patient, when there are no focal signs or symptoms, or when the area of concern is the left upper quadrant, pancreas, or midabdomen. CT scans are positive in over 90 percent of patients with abscesses, characteristically demonstrating fluid collections with well-defined walls that enhance following intravenous administration of contrast material. Unless gas lies within the mass, however, these findings do not distinguish abscesses from simple cysts, old hematomas, or mucinous metastases. Clinical features or needle aspiration should determine the correct diagnosis.

Effective treatment must include antimicrobial agents active against the responsible organisms. While the infecting flora varies, it commonly comprises bowel organisms, a complex mixture of aerobic and anaerobic bacteria, including *Bacteroides fragilis*. An appropriate therapeutic choice is a combination of an aminoglycoside, such as gentamicin, and an antianaerobic agent such as clindamycin, chloramphenicol, or metronidazole. Cefoxitin alone is an effective alternative, but an aminoglycoside should be added if the infection is hospital-acquired or the patient has received previous antimicrobial therapy.

Antimicrobial therapy alone is often sufficient for some abscesses—appendiceal, renal, and some hepatic—but cure usually also requires drainage of pus, either by surgery or percutaneous catheters, inserted with ultrasonic or CT guidance. Criteria for percutaneous drainage include (1) pus thin enough to be evacuated through the catheter; (2) no more than two abscess cavities or loculations; (3) the absence of a continuing source of contamination, such as a perforated viscus; (4) a drainage route that does not traverse bowel, uncontaminated organs, or sterile pleural or peritoneal spaces. The third criterion excludes appendiceal and diverticular abscesses and the fourth excludes most pelvic and interloop abscesses. Overall, percutaneous drainage is appropriate for less than 50 percent of intraabdominal abscesses. It is also not very successful in pancreatic abscesses. When used appropriately, however, its success rate is about 85 percent, with the catheters typically remaining in place for about 10 to 20 days.

TABLE 87-1 Intraabdominal abscesses

Intraperitoneal:
- Subphrenic:
  - Right suprahepatic
  - Right subhepatic
  - Left subphrenic
  - Lesser sac
- Midabdominal:
  - Right lower quadrant
  - Left lower quadrant
  - Interloop
- Pelvic

Retroperitoneal:
- Anterior retroperitoneal
- Perinephric

Visceral:
- Hepatic
- Splenic
- Pancreatic
- Renal

INTRAPERITONEAL ABSCESS These infections usually arise from a generalized peritonitis caused by perforated abdominal viscera, penetrating trauma, or postoperative infections. Some derive from localized peritonitis when infection extends from a contiguous site. With generalized peritonitis, the effects of gravity, intraabdominal pressure, and respiratory movements favor localization to the subphrenic spaces, the pelvis, and paracolic gutters lateral to the ascending and descending colon.

Subphrenic abscess These abscesses occur in the subphrenic space, arbitrarily defined as lying between the diaphragm and the transverse colon and possessing four subdivisions. The *suprahepatic* and *subhepatic* spaces are located on the right side; on the left there is a single *subphrenic* space plus the *lesser sac,* a space posterior to the stomach and anterior to the pancreas. About 55 percent of subphrenic abscesses are right-sided, 25 percent left-sided, and 20 percent multiple. Over 90 percent are complications of abdominal surgery, especially on the biliary tract, stomach, and duodenum. The contamination causing infection can occur during surgery or afterward, especially from anastomotic leaks. Symptoms typically begin 3 to 6 weeks after surgery, but occasionally develop only months later. Fever, nearly universal, is often mild, rather than dramatic. Abdominal pain is usual, but localized tenderness less common, and a palpable mass rare. By causing diaphragmatic irritation, inflammation that spreads to the pleural cavity, and abdominal distention, subphrenic abscesses often produce thoracic symptoms such as cough, dyspnea, and chest pain. Shoulder discomfort, referred pain from an irritated diaphragm, and hiccups sometimes occur. On chest examination there may be dullness to percussion, diminished breath sounds, basilar crackles, and rarely, a pleural friction rub. Chest roentgenograms, usually abnormal, may demonstrate ipsilateral atelectasis, pleural effusion, elevated hemidiaphragm, and basilar pneumonia.

Midabdominal abscess These abscesses include those in the right and left lower quadrants and between loops of bowel (interloop abscesses). *Right lower quadrant abscesses* usually arise as a complication of acute appendicitis, but occasionally from colonic diverticulitis, Crohn's disease, or upper alimentary tract perforations that drain down into the right paracolic gutter. Most commonly, fever, right lower quadrant pain, and a palpable mass occur following symptoms suggesting acute appendicitis. Occasionally, the abscess causes partial or complete small bowel obstruction. Appendiceal abscesses are usually treatable with antibiotics alone. *Left lower quadrant abscesses* complicate left colonic perforations, usually from diverticulitis, carcinoma, or Crohn's disease, and cause fever, left lower quadrant pain, and a palpable mass. *Interloop abscesses* are collections of pus between the folded surfaces of the small and large intestines and their mesenteries, generally arising from anastomotic disruptions, bowel perforations, or Crohn's disease. The clinical features, which are often very subtle, include mild fever, with or without vague abdominal discomfort. Abdominal tenderness, mechanical bowel obstruction, or a palpable mass occasionally occurs. Plain abdominal roentgenograms may show bowel wall edema, separation of bowel loops, localized ileus, and air-fluid levels on upright films.

Pelvic abscess These are complications of acute appendicitis, colonic diverticulitis, or acute salpingitis. The major symptoms are fever and lower abdominal discomfort. Those adjacent to the colon may cause diarrhea; those next to the bladder may cause urinary frequency and urgency. On abdominal examination tenderness is common, but peritoneal signs, guarding, or a palpable mass are unusual. Rectal or vaginal examination may reveal a mass anterior to the rectum or in the cul-de-sac. Pelvic abscesses usually require surgical drainage, but those arising from acute salpingitis typically resolve with antibiotic therapy alone.

RETROPERITONEAL ABSCESS The retroperitoneum is the space between the posterior peritoneum and the transversalis fascia lining the posterior portion of the abdominal cavity. The *anterior retroperitoneal* space, lying between the posterior peritoneum and the anterior renal fascia, contains the extraperitoneal portion of the alimentary tract: the ascending and descending colon, the duodenal loop, and the pancreas. Abscesses in this space usually develop from pancreatitis or perforations in these extraperitoneal parts of the intestines. The major clinical features are fever, abdominal or flank pain and tenderness, and a palpable mass.

The *perinephric* space, situated between the anterior and posterior layers of the renal (Gerota's) fascia on each side of the body, contains the kidney, adrenal, and ureter. Perinephric abscesses almost always occur from rupture of a renal parenchymal abscess through the renal capsule. Such an abscess may be staphylococcal following hematogenous dissemination from another site, usually the skin, but more commonly it arises from pyelonephritis, especially associated with renal calculus disease. The causative organisms, therefore, are usually *Escherichia coli, Proteus* sp., and *Klebsiella-Enterobacter*. The major symptoms are fever, chills, and unilateral flank pain. Dysuria is frequent, and most patients have unilateral flank or abdominal tenderness, often with a palpable mass. Leukocytosis, pyuria, and a positive urine culture are typical. Blood cultures are positive in 20 to 40 percent of patients. Perinephric abscess usually differs clinically from uncomplicated acute pyelonephritis by the longer duration of symptoms before hospitalization (usually more then 5 days) and the failure of patients to become afebrile within 5 days after receiving antimicrobial therapy. Chest roentgenograms often show ipsilateral pneumonia, atelectasis, pleural effusion, or elevated hemidiaphragm. Findings on excretory urogram include a nonvisualizing or poorly visualizing kidney, distorted calyces, anterior renal displacement, and unilateral fixation of the kidney, best demonstrated by fluoroscopy or inspiration-expiration films. Ultrasound and CT are very effective in detecting these abscesses. Treatment includes appropriate systemic antibiotics, surgical drainage, and relief of any urinary obstruction; occasionally, nephrectomy is necessary.

VISCERAL ABSCESS **Hepatic abscess** These abscesses are usually amebic (see Chap. 153) or bacterial (pyogenic). Bacterial liver abscesses usually develop by one of five mechanisms: (1) portal vein bacteremia arising from an infected intraabdominal site, such as appendicitis, diverticulitis, or perforated bowel; (2) systemic bacteremia originating from a distant site, in which bacteria reach the liver via the hepatic artery; (3) ascending cholangitis in a biliary tract completely or partially obstructed by stone, malignancy, or stricture; (4) direct extension from a contiguous focus of infection outside the biliary tract, such as a subphrenic abscess; or (5) trauma, either penetrating, with direct introduction of organisms into the liver, or blunt, causing a hematoma that becomes secondarily infected. In most cases the cause is apparent, but in some the pathogenesis of the abscess is unexplained ("cryptogenic"). Most abscesses are single; multiple abscesses are typically microscopic and are associated with systemic bacteremia or complete biliary tract obstruction. In these cases, the onset is acute, and the clinical features of the predisposing disease predominate.

Most other cases of hepatic abscess have a subacute onset, and an illness lasting several weeks is the rule. Fever is nearly always present and is accompanied by such nonspecific symptoms as chills, nausea, vomiting, anorexia, weight loss, and weakness. Right upper quadrant abdominal pain or tenderness is present in about one-half of patients, as is hepatomegaly. Some complain of right pleuritic chest pain. Jaundice is usually evident only when there is biliary tract obstruction.

Laboratory findings in most patients include one or more of the following: anemia, leukocytosis, increased erythrocyte sedimentation rate, increased alkaline phosphatase, decreased serum albumin, and usually mildly increased serum bilirubin. The chest roentgenogram is abnormal in about one-half of patients and shows right-sided basilar atelectasis, pneumonia, pleural effusion, or an elevated hemidiaphragm.

The radionuclide liver scan demonstrates filling defects for most abscesses greater than 2 cm in diameter. Ultrasound scans are usually positive and can distinguish fluid-filled from solid masses, helping to discriminate between infectious and neoplastic lesions. Computerized tomography is the most accurate method of demonstrating multiple abscesses.

The bacteriology of liver abscesses depends upon the cause. With systemic bacteremia staphylococci or streptococci are common. Abscesses originating from an intraabdominal infection, however, usually contain aerobic gram-negative rods, especially *E. coli* and *Klebsiella-Enterobacter;* anaerobic bacteria, especially anaerobic gram-positive cocci, *Fusobacterium nucleatum,* and *B. fragilis;* or a mixture of aerobes and anaerobes. Blood cultures are positive in about half of patients but may not grow all the organisms present in the abscess.

Treatment consists of surgical or percutaneous catheter drainage supplemented by appropriate antibiotic therapy. When the bacteriology is unknown, chloramphenicol or a combination of clindamycin and an aminoglycoside should be effective. Antibiotics are usually continued for several weeks following drainage. In uncomplicated pyogenic abscesses, antimicrobial therapy alone may be curative following diagnostic needle aspiration to determine the pathogens.

In correctly diagnosed and treated patients the mortality rate is about 20 to 40 percent, and is higher in those with multiple rather than single abscesses.

In patients with a clinical picture suggesting a liver abscess and an abnormal hepatic radionuclide, CT, or ultrasound scan, it is important to distinguish between a bacterial and an amebic abscess, since the latter rarely requires drainage. Features suggesting an amebic etiology are age under 50; single rather than multiple abscesses; a history of diarrhea, especially if bloody; the presence of *Entamoeba histolytica* in the stool; and the absence of a condition predisposing to bacterial liver abscess. The most helpful differential point is that nearly all patients with amebic liver abscesses have a positive serology for *E. histolytica*.

Splenic abscess Most splenic abscesses are multiple, small, and clinically silent lesions found incidentally at autopsy and occurring as a terminal manifestation of uncontrolled infection elsewhere. Clinically important splenic abscesses are generally solitary and arise from (1) systemic bacteremia originating in another site, such as endocarditis or salmonellosis; (2) infection, probably by the hematogenous route, of a spleen damaged by bland infarction (as occurs in hemoglobinopathies, especially sickle cell trait or sickle cell disease), trauma, penetrating or blunt (with superinfection of a subcapsular hematoma), or other diseases (malaria, hydatid cysts); or (3) extension from a contiguous focus of infection, such as a subphrenic abscess. The most common organisms are staphylococci, streptococci, anaerobes, and aerobic gram-negative rods, including *Salmonella*.

The onset is typically subacute, and the major features are fever and left-sided pain which is often pleuritic and located in the upper abdomen, lower chest, or flank. The pain may radiate to the left shoulder. Left upper quadrant abdominal tenderness and splenomegaly are common, but an audible splenic friction rub is rare. Leukocytosis is usually present.

Radiographic findings may include (1) a left upper quadrant soft tissue abdominal mass, (2) extraintestinal gas from gas-forming organisms in the abscess, (3) displacement of other organs, including the colon, kidney, and stomach, (4) elevation of the left hemidiaphragm, and (5) left pleural effusion. A liver-spleen radionuclide scan is valuable in detecting abscesses larger than 2 or 3 cm, and an ultrasound scan may be positive for macroscopic splenic abscesses, but CT scan is the most reliable diagnostic test.

Treatment consists of appropriate systemic antibiotics and splenectomy. Splenic abscesses should be considered a possible, although rare, cause of continued bacteremia in acute endocarditis despite appropriate chemotherapy, and splenectomy may be necessary to achieve final eradication of the infection.

Pancreatic abscess These abscesses usually occur in a site of pancreatic necrosis following acute pancreatitis. Typically, the patient improves after the attack of pancreatitis, but about 10 to 21 days later fever, abdominal pain and tenderness, nausea, vomiting, and sometimes persistent ileus occur. Less commonly, the abscess develops shortly after the attack begins. In those cases, persistent fever, leukocytosis, and abdominal findings beyond 7 to 10 days should suggest an abscess. A mass is palpable in about half of the cases. The serum amylase is irregularly elevated, but leukocytosis is usually present. The serum alkaline phosphatase may be increased and the albumin decreased.

Chest roentgenograms often show a left pleural effusion, basilar atelectasis or pneumonia, or a raised hemidiaphragm. Ultrasound is very useful in revealing fluid-filled pancreatic masses but may be unable to distinguish infected from uninfected fluid. CT is the most accurate test for abscesses and may show pancreatic gas, peripancreatic fluid collections, or masses, but only pancreatic gas is diagnostic of infection.

Treatment is surgical drainage and appropriate antibiotic therapy. Since the usual organisms are coliforms, staphylococci, streptococci, and anaerobes in varying combinations, chloramphenicol or clindamycin and an aminoglycoside are reasonable choices until culture results return. Even with surgical drainage the mortality rate is about 40 percent, and recurrent abscesses requiring reoperation are common.

Renal abscess Single or multiple abscesses of the renal *cortex* may be the result of metastatic implantation of staphylococci from another focus. There is no relationship to previous renal disease; the infection occurs in younger individuals, is usually unilateral, and occurs on the right side oftener than on the left. Many patients give a history of recent skin infection such as furuncle. Although acute pyelonephritis is a diffuse disease with foci of cellular infiltrates in the interstitium of the renal medulla, these inflammatory foci may coalesce to form single or multiple distinct abscess cavities in the medulla. This situation probably ensues more frequently than is generally appreciated.

The onset of renal abscess is abrupt, with chills and fever, followed by costovertebral pain and tenderness. If the abscess is cortical, the urine contains *no white blood cells;* medullary abscesses are usually accompanied by pyuria. The stained urinary sediment may show myriads of gram-positive cocci in cortical abscesses and gram-negative organisms in medullary abscesses. Transient gross or microscopic hematuria may occur at the onset. The white blood cell count is usually elevated and may exceed 30,000 cells per cubic millimeter. Physical signs are usually localized to the region of the kidney, but abdominal spasm may lead to confusion with appendicitis, cholecystitis, or pancreatitis. Early in the disease, ureteral calculus or acute hydronephrosis may be considered as possible diagnoses. Sudden onset of *fever, leukocytosis, and renal pain in the absence of pyuria* should suggest the diagnosis of a renal cortical abscess, especially in a patient with infection elsewhere. Obstruction of the ureter by pus or cellular debris may also yield a urine sediment sparse in white blood cells and bacteria. Excretory urograms typically reveal an intrarenal mass, and ultrasound and CT scans usually demonstrate the abscess as a fluid-filled defect. *Treatment* consists of appropriate antibiotics, adequate fluids, and relief of pain. An abscess may suddenly discharge into the renal pelvis, with relief of pain and the passage of cloudy urine containing enormous numbers of leukocytes and bacteria. Recovery is ordinarily prompt, and chronic sequelae are rare. Failure to achieve prompt defervescence following treatment suggests an incorrect diagnosis or the necessity of drainage, either by needle aspiration or by surgery.

MISCELLANEOUS ABSCESSES

RETROFASCIAL ABSCESS The retrofascial space, lying between the transversalis and psoas fascias, contains the psoas and quadratus lumborum muscles. Abscesses in this area usually derive from infections in the vertebrae, ilium, and sacroiliac joints. Less frequently, they represent extensions from abscesses in the anterior retroperitoneal space. Sometimes no adjacent source of infection is apparent; these "primary" infections are usually staphylococcal and almost surely have a hematogenous origin. The symptoms of retrofascial abscesses are abdominal pain in the iliac or inguinal region and, particularly with psoas muscle involvement, hip pain and posterior thigh pain and paresthesias. Careful palpation of the lower abdomen or groin often reveals a mass, and rectal or vaginal examination may disclose fullness and tenderness. Pain on hip motion is common, the hip is flexed, and extension or internal rotation of the hip is very painful. Plain abdominal films may demonstrate a mass or loss of the psoas shadow; excretory urograms may show displacement of the kidney or ureter and scoliosis with concavity on the side of infection. Ultrasound usually reveals a soft tissue mass, but CT scans typically provide more precise information, including evaluation of the adjacent bones. Treatment consists of drainage and appropriate antimicrobial therapy.

PROSTATIC ABSCESS These abscesses, typically occurring in middle age, are complications of acute prostatitis, cystitis, urethritis, or epididymitis. Most patients are *afebrile* and have urinary frequency, retention, or dysuria. Less common features are hematuria, perineal pain, and a purulent urethral discharge. Some patients have persistent or recurrent urinary infections despite apparently adequate antimicrobial therapy. Rectal examination may reveal prostatic tenderness or fluctuance, but sometimes there is only prostatic enlargement or even no abnormality at all. Pyuria and positive urine cultures are usual, but not invariably so. Many of these abscesses are unexpected discoveries at prostatic surgery or endoscopy performed for apparent benign prostatic hypertrophy. Treatment is appropriate antibiotics and surgical drainage by transurethral or perineal incision. The usual pathogens are aerobic gram-negative rods and, less frequently, *Staphylococcus aureus.*

RECTAL ABSCESS Most of these infections are superficial and involve the perirectal region, and many are associated with fistulas. Infection in the apocrine glands (hidradenitis) or folliculitis in the perianal region, extension of cryptitis or obstructions in the "anal glands" which open into the crypts of Morgagni, and contamination of submucosal hematomas, sclerosed hemorrhoids, or anal fissures may lead to abscess formation. In most patients, the cause of infection is not apparent. These are usually painful, easily palpable, often visible on inspection. Treatment is incision and drainage. Antibiotics are rarely necessary unless there is extensive perineal cellulitis.

Difficulties in diagnosis are likely to arise with infections higher in the rectum. Most are in the ischiorectal area, but those above the pelvic diaphragm, the so-called supralevator abscess, are particularly elusive. Patients with this type of infection often have fever, malaise, and leukocytosis for several days or even weeks before any symptoms referable to the rectum develop. There is vague pelvic discomfort, relieved by defecation, and constipation punctuated by short episodes of diarrhea is common. In males, the inflammation often involves the base of the bladder, and urinary urgency or retention may occur, falsely centering attention on the urinary tract as the source of fever and malaise. Eventually, the abscess produces severe pain, chills, and fever; palpation and instrumentation will reveal the swelling in the rectal ampulla. Such an abscess may surround the rectum and produce narrowing that is differentiated from neoplasm by the fact that the mucosa remains intact. A useful sign of deep rectal abscess is severe pain with pressure in the region between the anus and the coccyx. The supralevator space is continuous with the ischiorectal space, with both the gluteal and obturator regions, and with the retroperitoneal space. In neglected cases, the abscess may drain through the skin of the perineum, the groin, or the buttock or may extend as high as the perirenal areas. Rectal abscesses are not uncommon in patients with preexisting anorectal disease, diabetes, alcoholism, and neurologic disease; infections in this area are also peculiarly frequent in patients with acute leukemia, especially when neutropenia is present. Because the clinical picture may be that of "fever of unknown origin" for a long period, it is important that thorough digital and endoscopic examination of the rectum be carried out in patients with unexplained fever. Patients with diabetic ketoacidosis should receive a careful rectal examination because a rectal abscess may be the infection responsible for precipitating the ketoacidosis.

A rectal abscess may be a forerunner of both ulcerative colitis and regional enteritis, and may occur months and even years before other overt manifestations of these diseases. For this reason, proctosigmoidoscopy, colonoscopy, barium enema, and, often, upper gastrointestinal roentgenograms are indicated in nonhealing or recurrent rectal lesions.

Treatment of high rectal abscesses consists of incision and drainage, analgesics, and antibiotics directed at *E. coli, Klebsiella-Enterobacter, Bacteroides,* and a variety of streptococci, which constitute the polymicrobial flora of these lesions.

REFERENCES

BARTLETT JG et al: Anaerobic infections of the head and neck. Otolaryngol Clin North Am 9:655, 1976

CHOW AW et al: Orofacial odontogenic infections. Ann Intern Med 88:392, 1978

FEDERLE MP et al: Computed tomography of pancreatic abscesses. Am J Roentgenol 136:879, 1981

GOLIGHER JC: *Surgery of the Anus, Rectum, and Colon,* 5th ed. New York, Macmillan, 1984

HAU T et al: Pathophysiology, diagnosis, and treatment of abdominal abscesses. Curr Probl Surg 21:8, 1984

HOVERMAN IV et al: Intrarenal abscess: Report of 14 cases. Arch Intern Med 140:914, 1980

LINSCHEID RL et al: Common and uncommon infections of the hand. Orthop Clin North Am 6:1063, 1975

MCDONALD MI et al: Single and multiple pyogenic liver abscesses. Medicine 63:291, 1984

SART MG, ZUIDEMA GD: Splenic abscess—Presentation, diagnosis and treatment. Surgery 92:480, 1982

SIMONS GW et al: Retroperitoneal and retrofascial abscesses. J Bone Joint Surg 65-A:1041, 1983

88 CHEMOTHERAPY OF INFECTIONS

HAROLD C. NEU

INTRODUCTION There are many reasons for the plethora of new antimicrobial agents. The most important are changes in the host, the appearance of new pathogens, and the resistance of new and old pathogens to previously available antimicrobial agents. Changes in the host include prolonged survival of critically ill patients due to use of cancer chemotherapy, transplantation, and prosthetic devices. The problem of resistance has been particularly severe due to the worldwide dissemination of plasmids which have the ability to convey resistance to multiple antimicrobial agents simultaneously. Most antimicrobial agents in general use act by inhibiting the growth of the infecting microorganism rather than by enhancing host defense mechanisms. In the past, physicians often were faced with few choices of antimicrobial agents with which to treat an infection. Today that situation has been changed due to the discovery of new agents or the molecular modification of existing compounds. In addition to considerations of efficacy and toxicity which have the major impact on the selection of antimicrobial agents, cost is becoming increasingly important. This chapter deals with some general observations on antimicrobial therapy, and a description of most antibacterial agents. Recommendations for therapy of infections are made in the chapters dealing with individual diseases. Tables 88-1 and 88-2 summarize important information concerning the drugs discussed in this chapter.

FACTORS INFLUENCING SELECTION OF ANTIMICROBIAL AGENTS AND OUTCOME OF THERAPY Several factors bear directly on the selection of an antimicrobial agent. First there must be a knowledge of the infecting microorganism. In many situations this is not the case at the time therapy is initiated. As a consequence, antimicrobial therapy is started empirically in many situations. Even empiric selection of an antimicrobial agent, however, should be based on a knowledge of the likely pathogens and their antimicrobial susceptibility. For example, it is recognized that the most common cause of urinary tract infections is gram-negative bacilli and that *Escherichia coli* is the most common source of outpatient urinary tract infections. Hence, in most instances, therapy should be selected to inhibit this microorganism. However, therapy for treatment of a nosocomial urinary tract infection might be quite different. Bacteria other than *E. coli* are likely to produce this infection, particularly in the presence of an indwelling urethral catheter, and nosocomial pathogens are likely to be resistant to many antibiotics.

The host plays an extremely important role in the selection of an antimicrobial agent, as the antibiotics chosen to treat a febrile, neutropenic patient will be different than those for a healthy individual with a minor infection. Host factors also have an important impact on the route of administration of antimicrobial agents and upon the duration of therapy.

IDENTIFICATION OF THE INFECTING ORGANISMS There are a number of techniques for the rapid identification of the infecting microorganism. A Gram stain is a simple, inexpensive, and rapid method to identify many bacteria and fungi. This technique should be applied to all available body fluids such as urine, wound exudate, synovial fluid, pleural fluid, peritoneal fluid, and cerebrospinal fluid (CSF). Gram stains of sputum, if properly collected, are useful in the diagnosis of the causative organisms involved in bacterial pneumonia. *Campylobacter* can be identified in stains of stool. Another technique which may be useful is antigen detection in body fluids such as CSF (see Chap. 83).

In situations in which material for diagnosis is not available, knowledge of the most likely pathogens will be beneficial in directing the selection of an antimicrobial agent. For example, following an animal bite an organism such as *Pasteurella multocida* should be suspected. Cellulitis in the foot of a diabetic patient should suggest hemolytic streptococci of groups A, B, or G and *Staphylococcus aureus,* as well as mixed infections including anaerobes.

ANTIMICROBIAL SUSCEPTIBILITY OF INFECTING MICROORGANISMS There are a number of different methods for determining the susceptibility of bacteria to antimicrobial agents. Susceptibility of viruses and fungi is in a less well developed state, and very few laboratories have the ability to determine susceptibility of parasites to antiparasitic drugs.

A commonly used method to determine bacterial susceptibility to antibiotics is a disk diffusion method, which is simple, inexpensive, and provides data within 24 h. It is only semiquantitative and is not useful for many slow-growing or fastidious organisms, and has not been adequately standardized for anaerobic bacteria. With the disk

TABLE 88-1 Serum and body fluid levels after oral administration of various antibiotics

Drug	Unit dose* (oral)	Average peak level, µg/mL: Blood†	Urine‡	Bile§	CSF¶	Half-life, h: C_{cl} >80mL	C_{cl} <10mL	Dose adjustment renal failure
Amoxicillin	0.5 g	10	1000	10	NA	1	6	Minor
Ampicillin	0.25 g	1.5	50	5	NA	1	6	Minor
Cephalexin	0.25 g	8	500	3	NA	1	8–20	Major
Cephradine	0.25 g	8	500	85	NA	1	8	Major
Chloramphenicol	1 g	13	100	3	6	2	5	Minor
Ciprofloxacin	0.75 g	4	100–300	8	1	3	5–10	Major
Clindamycin	0.15 g	2	30	20	NA	2	6–10	Minor
Cloxacillin	0.5 g	8	200	—	NA	1	4	Minor
Dicloxacillin	0.5 g	15	200	—	NA	1	2–4	Minor
Doxycycline	100 mg	2.5	100	15	NA	15–20	15–20	No
Erythromycin estolate	0.25 g	1.4	200	800	NA	1.5–2	4–6	No
Indanyl carbenicillin	1 g	15	600	NA	NA	1–2	15	Major
Metronidazole	0.25 g	5	50	5	2	8	8	Minor
Minocycline	100 mg	2.5	100	15	NA	15	15–25	Minor
Norfloxacin	500 mg	4	200	—	NA	3–8	8–20	Major
Oxfloxacin	400 mg	6	100–500	5–15	NA	5–10	10–20	Major
Penicillin V	0.25 g	2	300	4	NA	1	2	No
Rifampin	8 mg/kg	10	50	100	0.5	1.5–5	1.5–5	No
Sulfadiazine	1.0 g	25	100	25	15	10	12–25	Major
Tetracycline	0.25 g	2.2	100	15	NA	6–8	30–50	Major
TMP/SMX	0.16 g TMP + 0.8 g SMX	1 + 30	10 + 100	3 + 30	0.5 + 15	10	25	Major

* *Doses listed are the lowest doses that would normally be employed for adults or children over 32 kg with normal renal function in the treatment of systemic infections.*
† *Blood levels are at 1–2 h after IM or at the end of 20–30 min IV infusion. In most instances considerably higher serum levels are attainable with higher dosages. For example, 2g of ampicillin would yield a peak blood level of 70–90 µg/mL, 2g of cefoxitin a peak blood level of 120–140 µg/mL.*
‡ *Drug concentrations may be significantly lower if the patient is producing a very dilute urine or if creatinine clearance is below 10 mL/min. Concentration based on mean levels for the first 4 h after drug is administered.*
§ *Assuming normal liver function.*
¶ *Meningeal inflammation; in meningitis higher doses than those listed would normally be employed resulting in higher CSF levels.*
NOTE: *NA = not appropriate therapy for meningitis; — = data not available; TMP/SMX = trimethoprim/sulfamethoxazole*

TABLE 88-2 Serum and body fluid levels after parenteral administration of various antibiotics

Drug	Unit dose[a] (parenteral)	Average peak level, µg/mL: Blood[b]	Urine[c]	Bile[d]	CSF[e]	Half-life, h: C_{cl} >80mL	C_{cl} <10mL	Dose adjustment renal failure	Effect of hemodialysis
Amdinocillin	1 g	70	>1000	5–30	1–5[f]	1	4	Minor	Yes
Amikacin	5 mg/kg IM or IV	25	200	5	5	2	30	Major	Yes
Ampicillin	1.0 g IV	35	500	10	3[f]	1	4	Minor	Yes
Azlocillin	3.0 g IV	190	>2000	100	—	1	4	Minor	Yes
Aztreonam	1 g	160	>1000	5–10	1–5[f]	1.5–2	6	Minor	Yes
Carbenicillin	4.0 g IV	250	>1000	50	20	1	15	Major	Yes
Cefamandole	1.0 g IV	70	1000	100	NA	0.7	8	Minor	Yes
Cefazolin	1.0 g IV	110	>1000	50	NA	2	25	Major	Yes
Ceftizoxime	1.0 g IV	80	>1000	30	1–10[f]	1.6	19	Major	Yes
Cefoperazone	2.0 g IV	250	>1000	>100	NA	2	2–4	No	No
Cefotaxime	1.0 g IV	80	>1000	15	10[f]	1	4	Minor	Yes
Cefoxitin	1.0 g IV	70	1000	100	1–5	0.8	10	Major	Yes
Cefuroxime	0.75 g	40	>1000	10–30	1–30[f]	1.5	20	Major	Yes
Ceftazidime	1 g	80	>1000	5–10	1–30[f]	1.8	1.5	Major	Yes
Ceftriaxone	1 g	150	>1000	200	1–30[f]	8	16	No	Yes
Cephalothin	1.0 g IV	70	500	10	0.7	0.5	8	Minor	Yes
Cephapirin	1.0 g IV	70	500	10	NA	0.5	8	Minor	Yes
Chloramphenicol	1.0 g IV	15	100	3	10	1–2	3–5	No	Yes
Ciprofloxacin	200 mg	4	100	5	?	3–4	5–10	Yes	Yes
Clindamycin	0.6 g IV	15	30	40	NA	2	6–10	No	No
Erythromycin	1 g IV	10	20	80	1	1–2	4–6	No	No
Gentamicin	1.5 mg/kg IM or IV	6	50	2	1	1–2	4–6	Major	Yes
Imipenem	0.5 g IV	30	100	10	1	1	6	Major	Yes
Kanamycin	5.0 mg/kg IM or IV	20	200	5	NA	2	35	Major	Yes
Methicillin	2.0 g IV	80	1000	30	5	0.5	4	Minor	Yes
Metronidazole	8.0 mg/kg IM	25	100	20	10	8	8	Minor	Yes
Mezlocillin	3.0 g IV	190	>2000	100	—	1	4	Minor	Yes
Moxalactam	1.0 g IV	100	>1000	60	1–30[f]	2	19	Major	Yes
Nafcillin	1.0 g IV	70	150	40	2	1	2	Minor	No
Oxacillin	1.0 g IV	70	500	2.5	1	1	2	Minor	No
Penicillin G	3 million units IV	115	300	15	6	1	4	Minor	Yes
Piperacillin	3.0 g IV	190	>2000	50	20	1	4	Minor	Yes
Ticarcillin	3.0 g IV	190	>2000	50	20	1	15	Major	Yes
Tobramycin	1.5 mg/kg IM or IV	6	50	2	1	2	35	Major	Yes
Vancomycin	0.5 g IV	30	100	3	3	6	120	Major	No

[a] *Doses listed are the lowest doses that would normally be employed for adults or children over 32 kg with normal renal function in the treatment of systemic infections.*
[b] *Blood levels are at 1–2 h after IM or at the end of 20-30 min IV infusion. In most instances considerably higher serum levels are attainable with higher dosages. For example, 2g of ampicillin would yield a peak blood level of 70–90 µg/mL, 2g of cefoxitin a peak blood level of 120–140 µg/mL.*
[c] *Drug concentrations may be significantly lower if the patient is producing a very dilute urine or if creatinine clearance is below 10 mL/min. Concentration based on mean levels for the first 4 h after drug is administered.*
[d] *Assuming no biliary obstruction.*
[e] *Meningeal inflammation; in meningitis higher doses than those listed would normally be employed resulting in higher CSF levels.*
[f] *Value at higher dose*
NOTE: *NA = not appropriate therapy for meningitis; — = data not available*

method, results are usually given as susceptible, resistant, and intermediate. A *susceptible* zone of inhibition correlates with serum and urine levels that are readily achievable with standard doses of the agent being tested. A *resistant* reading indicates that the zone of inhibition, using regression analysis, is less than that which would correspond to a concentration that could be achieved in blood or serum under normal circumstances. *Intermediate* susceptibility means that the organism falls into a category that is necessary because of the splay in data correlating zone size with minimum inhibitory concentrations (MIC). This is particularly true if the infecting organism is found in a urine specimen in which the concentration of antimicrobial agent would be much higher than in blood or tissues.

Quantitative data on the susceptibility of particular organisms can be determined by micro or macro broth-dilution techniques. These methods detect the lowest concentration of antimicrobial agent that prevents visible growth after an 18- to 24-h incubation period. This is referred to as the minimal inhibitory concentration (MIC). To understand MIC values it is essential to understand the pharmacokinetics of an antimicrobial agent. In general, an organism is considered susceptible when the MIC is no more than one-fourth of the readily obtainable peak serum level of the antimicrobial agent. Using the microdilution method, it is also possible to determine the minimal bactericidal concentration (MBC) or minimal lethal concentration (MLC). This is defined as the concentration of drug that reduces the original inoculum by 99.9 percent as judged by subculture on antibiotic-free medium. MBC determinations are necessary in only a few situations that will be discussed below.

The large number of antimicrobial agents has made it difficult for laboratories to test routinely all antimicrobial agents against an isolate. Many laboratories will use a particular compound as the class representative for a group of compounds. For example, among the first-generation cephalosporins, cephalothin is the representative drug that, either in a disk or in a broth-dilution system, is used to represent susceptibility to cephapirin, cefazolin, cephalexin, and cephradine.

Occasionally, susceptibility tests provide incorrect information. For example, methicillin-resistant *S. aureus* appear susceptible to cephalosporin antibiotics, but are not. Most susceptibility tests do not readily identify a resistant subpopulation.

Some microorganisms have remained susceptible to the same drugs since antibiotics were discovered, and in them development of resistance is exceedingly rare. Examples are group A streptococci which are susceptible to penicillins and cephalosporins. Hence most laboratories do not report susceptibilities of group A streptococci. However, group A streptococci may be resistant to erythromycin, and if the use of this drug is contemplated, susceptibility tests may be necessary. Most strains of *Streptococcus pneumoniae* remain susceptible to penicillin. However, some isolates have intermediate susceptibility; that is, the MICs are between 0.1 and 1.0 mL. Although such penicillin concentrations can readily be achieved in the blood and lung, it may be difficult to achieve cerebrospinal fluid concentrations that are tenfold this level. For this reason, pneumococci isolated from the CSF should be tested for penicillin susceptibility, particularly in patients who do not respond promptly to the drug.

CLINICAL PHARMACOLOGY Knowledge of the clinical pharmacology of antimicrobial agents has become increasingly important in selecting therapeutic programs that are both effective and safe. Antimicrobial agents can be administered by the oral, intramuscular, intravenous, intraperitoneal, or topical routes. After absorption they dissolve in the plasma and are variably bound to plasma proteins. From the plasma they are distributed to various extracellular tissues and fluids in which they may be free or bound. As an antibiotic is distributed into extravascular compartments, there is an initial fall in plasma concentration. Peak concentrations of antimicrobial agents after intravenous infusion occur at the end of the infusion. In contrast, after intramuscular injection, and after oral ingestion, there is an initial slow distribution phase, that is, a combination of absorption and simultaneous excretion or metabolism. Peak serum levels following oral ingestion of antimicrobial agents usually occur at 1 to 2 h. Continued decrease in serum levels of antimicrobial agents is related to renal and biliary excretion and to the hepatic metabolism of some drugs. The amount of drug that reaches the extravascular tissues in which the infection is present depends not only on the concentration gradient from serum to tissue, but also on protein binding in serum and in tissues and the diffusibility of the agent. The diffusibility of antimicrobial agents is a function of their molecular size, dissociation constant, and lipid solubility.

There are several pharmacokinetic indexes that are useful in adjusting dosage of antimicrobial agents. The half-life of a drug is the time required for the plasma concentration to fall by one-half as it is being eliminated from the body. Half-life refers to the drug elimination phase after the absorption of the drug has been completed and the drug has been distributed throughout its entire volume of distribution. The assumption is that the fall in plasma concentration parallels the fall in the total amount of drug in the body. However, direct extrapolation of the frequency of dosing from half-life considerations is not completely appropriate. The MIC of the infecting organism, site of infection, and host defense mechanisms must be considered in determining dose frequency.

Another pharmacokinetic index that may be useful for guiding therapy is the volume of distribution (V_d). This is the volume in which the total amount of drug in the body would have to be uniformly distributed in order to give the observed plasma concentration. Simplistically it is calculated by the formula $V_d = A/C_p$, where A is amount of drug administered and C_p is plasma concentration. The volume of distribution does not correspond to an actual anatomic or physiologic space. It is useful for determining initial or loading doses and in calculating subsequent or maintenance doses to achieve safe, therapeutic plasma concentrations. When a drug dose is given repetitively at regular intervals, the peak concentration and the minimal concentration eventually reach a constant state if there is no change in the rate of drug elimination. With most antimicrobial agents it is not necessary to use an initial loading dose. However, when agents such as the aminoglycosides are used to treat serious infections such as suspected bacteremia or pneumonia, a loading dose which will provide an initial plasma and tissue concentration well above the MIC of the suspected infecting microorganisms is usual.

The half-life distribution data of many antibiotics have been determined in healthy young males. Prolongation of a drug half-life often may result from renal or hepatic dysfunction. Half-life may also be influenced by age and may be shortened in certain disease states. Other drugs administered concomitantly can also either prolong or shorten a drug's half-life.

HOST FACTORS THAT AFFECT ANTIMICROBIAL CHEMOTHERAPY A number of different host factors have a significant influence on the efficacy and toxicity of antimicrobial agents.

Allergic history It is critical to obtain a history of previous adverse reactions to antimicrobial agents since similar reactions may occur to drugs within the same class.

Age Certain antimicrobial agents should not be given to individuals in some age groups. For example, sulfonamides should not be administered to pregnant females or to newborns because sulfonamides bind to serum albumin, displacing bilirubin, which may result in kernicterus. Premature and newborn babies produce an inadequate amount of glucuronyltransferase, the enzyme that inactivates chloramphenicol, and some newborns treated with this drug may develop the "gray baby syndrome," which is characterized by progressive pallor, cyanosis, vasomotor collapse, and death. Tetracyclines should not be administered to pregnant females, newborn infants, or to children below 8 years of age because the drugs bind to developing bone and tooth structure, which may cause brownish discoloration of the teeth.

Renal function The majority of antimicrobial agents are removed from the body by renal excretion. There are several periods in life when renal function has not achieved complete development or has begun to deteriorate. Glomerular and some tubular functions do not develop to adult levels until at least 2 months of age, and drugs administered to premature or newborn infants must be given at different dosage schedules than those used for older children or adults. With advancing age, renal function decreases, and approximately 1 percent of glomerular clearance is lost per year over the age of 30. Antimicrobial agents removed from the body purely by glomerular filtration will accumulate as glomerular filtration declines, resulting in toxicity to other organs or to the kidney itself. Even compounds removed from the body by tubular secretion will accumulate as renal function falls below creatinine clearance of 20 mL/min. Toxic levels of certain penicillins, aminoglycosides, tetracyclines, and quinolones may develop in the presence of markedly reduced renal function. Serum creatinine or blood urea nitrogen may not reflect the true state of renal function in an elderly individual with a small body mass. Hence in calculating the dose of antimicrobial agent it is necessary to consider age, sex, and body weight.

Hepatic function Some antimicrobial agents are metabolized and removed from the body primarily by hepatic mechanisms. These include some of the macrolides, rifamycins, imidazoles, chloramphenicol, and linconoid drugs. Reductions in dose may be necessary to avoid toxic concentrations of these agents. Chloramphenicol is likely to accumulate in patients with impaired hepatic function, while clindamycin and tetracyclines accumulate in patients with severe liver disease. The half-lives of both rifampin and isoniazid are prolonged in patients with extensive hepatic disease. Some drugs which are excreted by biliary mechanisms are excreted by the kidney in the presence of marked elevations of bilirubin. Conversely, some compounds that are normally excreted by the kidney are excreted in the bile in the presence of renal failure. In the presence of combined biliary and hepatic disease, toxic levels may be reached. Examples would be a cephalosporin such as cefoperazone, which is primarily excreted by biliary mechanisms, or carbenicillin and ticarcillin, which are primarily renally excreted; in the presence of combined hepatic and renal failure these drugs accumulate in tissues to a greater extent.

Pregnancy Antimicrobial agents cross the placenta to varying degrees. Most penicillins, cephalosporins, and erythromycins are not teratogenic and are safe in pregnant women. Tetracyclines should not be used in pregnancy not only because of their effect upon fetal dentition but also because they have a propensity to cause fatty necrosis of the liver, pancreatitis, and possible renal damage in pregnant females. If streptomycin is used to treat tuberculosis in pregnancy, it can cause abnormalities of vestibular function and hearing in the child.

Genetic factors A number of different antimicrobial agents will produce hemolysis in patients with glucose 6-phosphate dehydrogenase deficiency. These include sulfonamides, nitrofurantoin, furazoline, chloramphenicol, pyrimethamine, and various sulfones.

The rate at which isoniazid is inactivated by acetylation in the liver is genetically determined. In the United States and North European populations, 50 to 60 percent of individuals are slow inactivators of this drug. Polyneuritis is seen more frequently as a complication of isoniazid therapy in individuals who are slow acetylators.

Site of infection. The site of infection is one of the most important factors in determining the choice of an antimicrobial agent and the dose and route by which the antimicrobial agent is administered. For antimicrobial therapy to be effective, adequate concentrations of a drug must be delivered to the site of the infection. In many situations, if the local concentration of an antimicrobial equals or exceeds the minimum inhibitory concentration of the infecting microorganism, cure will result. This statement is true only for those areas of the body in which there are adequate host defenses such as polymorphonuclear cells, complement, and antibody. In those areas of the body in which these factors are inadequate or absent, such as in the spinal fluid or on the heart valves, concentrations at least fourfold and preferably five- to tenfold above the MIC, or even MBC, are needed to achieve a cure. In some situations, even though concentrations above the MICs of the infecting organisms may not be achieved, there will be a significant effect on the microorganisms that will aid the host's defenses against the infection. Subinhibitory concentrations of antimicrobial agents alter the adherence properties of microorganisms; treated bacteria then do not accumulate to a number adequate to achieve further invasion. Subinhibitory concentrations also alter surface structures, reducing opsonic requirements and enhancing phagocytosis. Subinhibitory concentrations of antibiotics, by binding to the surface of microorganisms, enhance the intracellular killing of bacteria ingested by phagocytic cells. These factors may explain the unusual circumstances in which antimicrobial agents in seemingly inadequate doses result in clinical cure. Nonetheless, the major goal of therapy should be to achieve concentrations above the MIC in all tissues.

In general, antimicrobial agents are widely distributed and achieve adequate concentrations in many infected sites. These include the pleural, pericardial, and infected joint fluids, and infections in muscles or skin structures associated with cutaneous infection. Important exceptions to this statement include vegetations on the heart valves in endocarditis. Although the heart valve is exposed to the circulation, the bacteria often are trapped deep within the fibrin vegetation. The organisms are growing less rapidly making them less susceptible to many antibiotics and there is inadequate phagocytic function in the focal infection on the heart valve. Because of these factors, therapy of bacterial endocarditis requires agents that are bactericidal, that are administered for long periods of time, and that achieve such high concentration in the blood so that diffusion of the antibiotic into the vegetation is facilitated (see Chap. 188).

Meningitis is another disease in which the concentration of antimicrobial agent in the infected space is critical. Many antimicrobial agents cross the blood-brain barrier poorly and do not produce adequate cerebrospinal fluid levels. For example, aminoglycoside antibiotics do not produce effective cerebrospinal fluid levels when given parenterally. Lipid-soluble agents can cross the spinal fluid barrier easily, accounting for the utility of chloramphenicol. This agent has proved highly effective in the therapy of meningitis due to *Streptococcus pneumoniae, Haemophilus influenzae,* and *Neisseria meningitidis* because of the achievable bacteriostatic and bactericidal concentrations it produces in the cerebrospinal fluid. Chloramphenicol is not useful in treating meningitis due to *E. coli* or *Klebsiella penumoniae,* even if the organisms are susceptible in vitro, because the drug is not bactericidal for these organisms, and concentrations eightfold above the MIC cannot be achieved within the cerebrospinal fluid. Fortunately a number of new bactericidal antimicrobials such as cefotaxime, ceftizoxime, ceftriaxone, ceftazidime, and moxalactam all enter the cerebrospinal fluid in concentrations adequate to treat both the common causes of meningitis and the less frequently encountered gram-negative organisms. However, experience with any of these agents is relatively sparse, and it is not clear whether reasonable drug levels are achieved in brain abscesses.

Another infectious site that may be particularly refractory to treatment involves bones in areas of devitalized tissue, as occurs in diabetics and other patients with inadequate blood supply due to vascular insufficiency. Here the penetration of the antimicrobial agents to the site of the infection may be only borderline or inadequate. For this reason antimicrobial agents must be administered in high concentrations for prolonged periods of time to yield adequate concentration within bone. Even with extended periods of therapy, many cases of chronic osteomyelitis are never completely cured since some of the bacteria are in a resting state and do not come into contact with the antimicrobial agent.

Abscesses present a particular problem, and in many instances the surgeon's knife is the only mechanism by which an abscess can be cured. Certain exceptions to this dictum exist, however. For example, lung abscess can be treated without surgical intervention in most situations since the abscess can drain via the bronchi, and the antimicrobial agents kill bacteria in the surrounding inflammatory tissue. However, lung abscesses 8 to 10 cm in diameter frequently do not respond to antimicrobial therapy alone since there is inadequate diffusion of the antimicrobial agent into the cavity and organisms persist. Hence the size of the abscess may influence the ultimate outcome. Other abscesses which respond to antimicrobial therapy alone are those of the ovary, brain, and liver. Ultrasound, computer tomography scanning (CT), and magnetic resonance imaging (MRI) have demonstrated detectable decreases in abscess size. The question that remains unanswered is whether these "imaged abscesses" are equivalent to the abscesses that were in the past diagnosed clinically, and that were remanded to surgery. In general, abscesses in other parts of the abdomen require external drainage, since antimicrobial agents by themselves fail to sterilize the majority of them. Exceptions to this rule have been noted with some anaerobic microorganisms; compounds such as metronidazole diffuse into the abscess and destroy the anaerobic organisms.

Local factors within an abscess can have an important impact upon the activity of certain antimicrobial agents. For example, in the case of a mixed aerobic and anaerobic abscess, the anaerobic organisms may produce β-lactamases that will destroy the β-lactam compound which is being used to inhibit the aerobic gram-negative bacilli. Aminoglycoside antibiotics are significantly less active in an anaerobic abscess since they require an aerobic environment for antimicrobial activity. This class of drugs is also dependent on oxidative phosphorylation to achieve transport across the cell membrane.

Other local circumstances may have a marked impact upon the effectiveness of antimicrobial agents. Aminoglycoside antibiotics are less effective at an acid pH than they are at pH 7.4. Gentamicin or tobramycin might inhibit a *Klebsiella* at 0.1 μg/mL in a Mueller-Hinton broth of pH 7.4, but this condition is not present in the infected lung, where the pH in infected areas is 6.4 to 6.5. Aminoglycosides are ten- to thirtyfold less active at this pH than they are at pH 7.4. Cellular debris from decaying white cells will complex with aminoglycosides and reduce their activity. In a hyperosmolar environment some β-lactam antimicrobial agents may be less effective because they will not produce death of the microorganism but merely change its cell shape. Agents such as methenamine, nitrofurantoin, and chlortetracycline are more active at an acid pH; the activities of erythromycin, clindamycin, and aminoglycosides are greater in an alkaline milieu.

Foreign bodies have an extremely important effect on the response to antimicrobial agents. For example, infections of prosthetic heart valves or joint implants usually are not cured by antimicrobial agents even though the organisms infecting the foreign body are highly susceptible to bactericidal β-lactam or aminoglycoside antibiotics. The reasons for this are complex, but probably involve the development of a glycocalyx which adheres to the foreign material and provides a cover for the microorganisms. A number of studies have revealed that organisms such as *Staphylococcus epidermidis* send projections into small defects in the polypropylene material which is used in catheters and other foreign devices. The methylacrylate used in artificial joints provides a large number of interstices in which microorganisms hide, covered by fibrinous material, and are not exposed to antimicrobial agents. Indwelling urethral catheters are another example of a foreign body which makes it virtually impossible to eradicate infecting microorganisms. Even silicone catheters have a deposit of gelatinous material on the inner aspect of the catheter. Microorganisms persist within this material, and unless the catheter is removed, the organisms will not be eradicated. Other examples of foreign material are suture materials. Even though wire sutures are much less likely to cause infection than braided fiber sutures, sternal wound infections following cardiac surgery usually cannot be completely eradicated as long as the wire sutures remain in place and the infection remains undrained. Calculi, whether in the urinary or biliary tracts, provide a haven for microorganisms. The microorganisms are incorporated into the calculus and will periodically be released as the calculi undergo remodeling. Thorough knowledge of the mechanical, metabolic, and physiologic factors involved in infection is essential in planning therapy to bring about optimal results in infections located in different parts of the body, and different strategies must be applied to infections within the urinary, pulmonary, and central nervous systems.

ANTIMICROBIAL COMBINATIONS Although the majority of infections can be treated with a single antimicrobial agent, there are definite situations in which the combination of antimicrobial agents is necessary. Combination antimicrobial therapy is used much more frequently than necessary. It provides a false sense of security, suggesting that all possible causes have been dealt with and a successful outcome will be more likely. In certain situations inappropriate use of combinations of antimicrobial agents may actually have deleterious results.

The combination of two or three antimicrobial agents may result in one of three different effects. Drugs are said to be *additive* when the activity of the drugs in combination equals the sum of their separate, independent activities. *Synergistic* activity implies that the activity of two or three antimicrobials is greater than the sum of their independent activities. Drugs are considered *antagonistic* when the activity of the combination is less than the sum of the independent effects.

A number of reasons have been advanced for the use of antimicrobial combinations. Preventing the emergence of resistant organisms is one of the most common indications for combination therapy, but this is true only for tuberculosis. The mycobacteria causing tuberculosis consist of a population of organisms of varying susceptibility to antituberculous drugs. In any focus of infection containing a large number of bacilli, particularly in a tuberculous lung cavity, there will be a small percentage of organisms that are intrinsically resistant to the antituberculous agent. In this setting the organisms reach such large numbers that they include a number of drug-resistant mutants which occur naturally and spontaneously at a rate of 1 in 10^{-6} organisms. For this reason, two or three drugs are utilized in the treatment of this disease. The concept of the use of multiple drugs in the treatment of tuberculosis is particularly important when isoniazid-resistant organisms are found in specific patient populations such as those from the far east or the Caribbean.

Another example of preventing the emergence of resistance has been to use rifampin to treat infections other than those caused by mycobacteria. Use of rifampin as a single agent to treat staphylococcal infections rapidly results in the emergence of strains resistant to the antibiotic. However, the combination of a β-lactam antibiotic with rifampin reduces the chance for the emergence of such resistant strains. It has been suggested that the combination of an aminoglycoside with aminothiazolyl cephalosporins (see below) or monobactams (aztreonam) will prevent the emergence of resistance in *Enterobacter* or *Citrobacter* species. Although it is possible to demonstrate this phenomenon in the test tube, there are no clinical studies demonstrating that such a combination is less likely to result in the emergence of resistant organisms. This is particularly true when resistance to gram-negative bacteria is mediated by R factors. These plasmids often code for several enzymes leading to the development of resistance to multiple drugs simultaneously.

A second major reason for combination therapy is to treat polymicrobial infections. Intraperitoneal and pelvic infections are usually due to an aerobic and anaerobic flora. Although some antimicrobial agents inhibit both aerobic and anaerobic species, it may not always be feasible to use these drugs clinically. Combination therapy might include an agent effective against the anaerobic organism and an agent effective against the aerobic gram-negative rod. Another example of this might be the use of an agent such as clindamycin and a third-generation cephalosporin to treat hospital-acquired aspiration pneumonia caused by an anaerobic oral flora, which would be inhibited by the clindamycin and organisms acquired in the hospital such as *Klebsiella* which would be inhibited by the cephalosporin. Brain abscesses are frequently caused by *Bacteroides* and anaerobic or microaerophilic streptococci. Metronidazole penetrates extremely well into the abscess and has excellent activity against the *Bacteroides* species. However, it is not active against streptococcal species. Penicillin will penetrate the brain adequately to kill the streptococcal species but could not be used singly since it would be destroyed in the brain abscess by the β-lactamases frequently elaborated by the *Bacteroides* strains.

A theoretical reason for the use of drug combinations is to lower concentrations of compounds that have toxic potential. Although this is an interesting concept, there is little clinical evidence to substantiate the use of two drugs at lower concentrations than that at which they would normally be utilized. For example, using amphotericin B and 5-fluorocytosine to treat cryptococcal meningitis with lower doses of amphotericin has not decreased nephrotoxicity from the amphotericin. This illustrates that in practice it is difficult to reduce toxicity while continuing therapy with toxic drugs.

One of the major indications for combined antimicrobial therapy is to provide a broad spectrum of coverage for the patient who is neutropenic and has significantly compromised host defenses. It has been the practice to use a broad-spectrum antipseudomonas penicillin combined with an aminoglycoside as an initial therapy for the febrile neutropenic patient. Studies of new highly active β-lactam compounds such as ceftazidime which inhibit the major pathogens causing bacteremia in these patients open this concept to question. Nevertheless, combination therapy will probably continue to be used in such patients since gram-negative organisms continue to be a major cause of infection in neutropenic patients, and it is necessary to provide antimicrobial activity against aerobic gram-negative species, staphylococci, and *Corynebacterium* species until the true pathogen becomes apparent.

Although synergism can be demonstrated in the laboratory with many antimicrobial combinations, in only a few clinical settings has combination therapy proved more effective than single agents. The most widely accepted combination therapy is penicillin G or ampicillin with an aminoglycoside, streptomycin or gentamicin, for the treatment of enterococcal endocarditis. There is clear clinical evidence that this combination is more effective treatment for this infection than a single drug. The penicillin enhances the uptake of the aminoglycosides by the enterococci, which are killed as a result. Similar synergism can be demonstrated between semisynthetic penicillinase-resistant penicillins, such as nafcillin or oxacillin, and gentamicin against *S. aureus*. However, clinical data do not show that this combination has advantages over use of a single drug. Combinations of antipseudomonas penicillins such as carbenicillin, ticarcillin, azlocillin, or piperacillin with gentamicin, tobramycin, or amikacin are synergistic against many strains of *Pseudomonas aeruginosa*. Both animal experiments and clinical trials have demonstrated the superiority of these combinations in neutropenic hosts. However, there are no convincing data that treatment of neutropenic patients infected with organisms such as *E. coli, Klebsiella, Serratia*, or other members of the *Enterobacteriaceae* with two agents will result in a more favorable outcome, despite the demonstration of synergism in vitro.

There are several other examples of synergism in vitro that have clinical application. One of these is the combination of trimethoprim with sulfamethoxazole. These two agents act by inhibiting two critical points in the folic acid cycle which is part of the production pathway of DNA nucleotides. In vitro and animal experiments readily demonstrate that on a milligram basis, the two drugs are more effective than either drug singly. However, the major situation in which such a combination is absolutely necessary is in treatment of *Pneumocystis carinii* infection. In urinary tract infections trimethoprim alone is as effective as the combination of the two agents. Trimethoprim has not been compared to the combination in the treatment of serious infections outside the urinary tract.

Combination of a β-lactam drug with a β-lactamase inhibitor is another example of the synergistic combination of two drugs. Augmentin is a combination of amoxicillin and clavulanate and timentin a combination of ticarcillin and clavulanate. This combination of a β-lactamase-susceptible β-lactam with a β-lactamase inhibitor enhances the antibacterial spectrum of the drug that would normally be destroyed by β-lactamase. Augmentin inhibits *Haemophilus, Branhamella, E. coli, Salmonella*, and *S. aureus* strains which are resistant to amoxicillin. In the case of timentin, the ticarcillin is effective against *Bacteroides* species, *Klebsiella*, and staphylococci which would normally destroy the agent. Sulbactam is another β-lactamase inhibitor which has been combined with ampicillin or cefoperazone to prevent their destruction by β-lactamases.

Another form of synergy has been to use compounds which interfere with cell wall synthesis but inhibit different enzymes. The amdino, amdinocillin, which binds to a specific penicillin-binding protein different from the penicillin-binding proteins to which other penicillins and cephalosporins bind, when combined with various β-lactams has been shown to be synergistic both in vitro and in animal models. Clinical studies have also demonstrated that such synergy is possible. However, it is not clear that this approach is more effective than utilizing a single drug which has activity superior to the two-combination compounds. Combinations of fosfomycin, a cell wall inhibitor, and β-lactams are synergistic in experimental situations, but clinical studies showing the superiority of such combinations are not available.

Disadvantages of antimicrobial combinations There are a number of examples of antagonism of antimicrobial agents. The most impressive historical example was the demonstration that penicillin alone was more effective than a combination of penicillin and chlortetracycline for the treatment of pneumococcal meningitis. There have been other reports that the treatment of meningitis with a combination of ampicillin and chloramphenicol has been associated with a higher mortality than the use of ampicillin alone. One of the most common uses of combination therapy has been in the treatment of meningitis due to β-lactamase-producing *Haemophilus influenzae* or to relatively resistant *Streptococcus pneumoniae*. The effectiveness of cephalosporins such as cefuroxime, cefotaxime, and ceftriaxone for treatment of childhood meningitis make it unnecessary to use combination therapy, although experience with the newer drugs is limited, and to date they are more costly.

There are in vitro examples of antagonism between β-lactams. For example, cefoxitin will induce β-lactamase production in *P. aeruginosa* and *Enterobacter cloacae*. The combination of cefoxitin and an antipseudomonas penicillin can be shown to be antagonistic in vitro. Certain animal experiments have also shown that this combination is antagonistic. Nonetheless, many patients have been treated with the combination of cefoxitin and azlocillin or other antipseudomonas penicillins without evidence of reduced efficacy. In general, however, it seems wise to avoid combined use of a β-lactam that is a good β-lactamase inducer and other β-lactams that might be inactivated by high levels of the enzyme. This is particularly likely to occur during treatment of *Pseudomonas, Enterobacter, Serratia*, and *Citrobacter* infections.

Combination therapy may on occasion result in superinfection with other organisms, particularly fungi, since the combination obliterates the normal protective flora of the oropharynx and the intestine. This problem can be avoided by discontinuing unnecessary empiric combination therapy once the diagnosis has been established.

Another adverse effect of combination therapy may be increased drug reactions or other metabolic side effects. Examples of such toxicity are the combination of cephalothin and gentamicin, resulting in increased nephrotoxicity. There is a slightly increased risk of hepatic toxicity in patients receiving both isoniazid and rifampin, but this is outweighed by the more rapid eradication of tubercle bacilli and the more rapid clinical improvement seen with this combination.

ROUTE OF ADMINISTRATION OF ANTIMICROBIAL AGENTS Having determined the most appropriate agent to treat a given infection, the most appropriate route of administration should be determined. The choice usually lies between the oral and the parenteral route. Oral administration of antimicrobial agents has generally been for infections that are mild and are treated on an outpatient basis. As hospital costs have risen, reevaluation of this concept is necessary. Some serious infections initially may be treated parenterally; then therapy can be completed with an oral antibiotic. Examples would be osteomyelitis, or severe skin infections that have begun to respond to parenteral therapy. When drugs are administered by the oral route, it is important to be certain that the patient takes the drug in a manner that will result in the best serum and tissue levels. The absorption of many antimicrobial agents is markedly decreased by food. Some compounds such as the tetracyclines form a soluble chelate with magnesium, calcium, aluminum, or iron. In a number of infections it may be possible to administer an oral antimicrobial agent twice a day rather than four times a day. This may be an important way to achieve patient compliance.

The parenteral route is generally used for agents that are not absorbed from the gastrointestinal tract, and for serious infections in which a high concentration of the antimicrobial agent is needed immediately. Examples are suspected bacteremia, meningitis, and gram-negative pneumonia. Intravenous administration of most drugs is preferred since it provides for high serum concentration. There are no definitive data that show whether bolus, 3- to 5-min injection, infusion over 15 to 30 min, or continuous administration of a drug by the intravenous route is more effective in curing bacterial infection. Serum concentrations adequate to treat many infections will be achieved after intramuscular administration. With some agents with extremely long half-lives it may be possible to complete therapy of serious infections by administration of the drug intramuscularly once a day. It is rarely necessary to instill antimicrobial agents into infected cavities. There are certain exceptions to this, however. Peritonitis in patients receiving peritoneal dialysis may respond better to administration of the antimicrobial agent in the dialysis solution. Certain forms of meningitis will require intraventricular or intrathecal therapy. This is true for meningitis due to *Coccidioides immitis* and some gram-negative species.

MONITORING PATIENT RESPONSE TO ANTIMICROBIAL THERAPY With some antimicrobial agents it is essential that serum levels of the agent be monitored. This is true for the aminoglycoside antibiotics, for which peak levels should be obtained to determine that effective concentrations are being achieved and trough levels should be measured to determine that the drugs are not accumulating and producing nephrotoxicity or ototoxicity. In most situations, it is not necessary to monitor serum concentrations of β-lactam antibiotics. The one exception to this would be in renal failure, where the drugs may accumulate to toxic levels.

Serum bactericidal titers, defined as the dilution of serum which will kill the infecting pathogen in vitro, have been used extensively to monitor therapy of bacterial endocarditis. There has been wide variation in the performance of serum bactericidal titers, but guidelines for their use have been developed. If a standardized inoculum of organisms is used and standard media and techniques employed, the tests are useful in certain clinical situations. For example, a peak serum bactericidal titer >1:64 correlates with a 98 percent bacteriologic cure of endocarditis. However, clinical cure cannot be predicted since damage to the valve as a result of the endocarditis may result in valvular insufficiency requiring surgery. Most experts feel that a peak serum bactericidal titer greater than 1:8 correlates with a successful outcome in osteomyelitis, bacteremia, septic arthritis, and empyema.

SPECIFIC ANTIMICROBIAL AGENTS

PENICILLINS Penicillins can be conveniently divided into several classes on the basis of antibacterial activity. There are overlaps among the groups, but differences within the groups usually are pharmacologic rather than clinical.

Natural penicillins Penicillin G and penicillin V are the two natural penicillins. Penicillin G is available as an orally, intramuscularly, and intravenously administered compound. Penicillin G is combined with procaine as a 1:1 molar salt which extends the half-life of the drug, and it is combined with benzathine to produce a long-acting repository form of penicillin. Penicillin V is available only for oral use. The antibacterial activity of penicillin G and penicillin V includes *S. pneumoniae,* beta-hemolytic streptococci, viridans group streptococci, and microaerophilic and anaerobic streptococci. Most *S. aureus* and *S. epidermidis* produce β-lactamases which destroy both penicillin G and V. *Neisseria meningitidis* are susceptible to penicillin G as are many *N. gonorrhoeae*. However, in certain parts of the world penicillinase-producing *N. gonorrhoeae* are a significant problem. Penicillin G has excellent activity against clostridial species and also inhibits many of the oral *Bacteroides* species and *Fusobacterium* species. Penicillin V does not have good activity against species such as *Haemophilus* or *Branhamella,* which may be important pathogens causing sinusitis, otitis, and other upper respiratory infections. Infrequently encountered organisms for which penicillin G remains an excellent drug are *Erysipelothrix, Listeria monocytogenes, Pasteurella multocida, Streptobacillus, Spirillum, Fusospirochetes, Treponema pallidum,* and *Actinomyces israelii,* as well as the *Borrelia* which causes Lyme disease.

Penicillin G is not stable in gastric acid and should not be used as an oral preparation. In contrast, penicillin V is 60 percent absorbed when given orally, and food causes only a minor decrease in absorption. Penicillin V is an effective agent in treatment of streptococcal infections and less serious forms of pneumococcal pneumonia. It should not be used, however, to treat syphilis, gonorrhea, or *Haemophilus* infections. Procaine penicillin G remains a useful drug administered twice daily for the therapy of pneumococcal pneumonia, but oral penicillins probably are equally useful. Although procaine penicillin is still used in the treatment of gonorrhea, oral ampicillin or amoxicillin can be used, combined with tetracycline, since the treatment of urethritis usually is directed against both gonorrhea and *Chlamydia* (see Chap. 90). Penicillin G remains the treatment of choice for viridans group streptococcal endocarditis and for pneumococcal and meningococcal meningitis. Since penicillin G has a short half-life due to rapid tubular secretion, it must be administered on a 4- or 6-hourly basis. Only minor dosage adjustments are necessary until the creatinine clearance falls below 30 mL/min. Even in the presence of renal failure, doses of 4,000,000 to 6,000,000 units per day can be administered safely. Benzathine penicillin, which has a half-life of a week, can be used in the treatment of streptococcal pharyngitis, in the therapy of primary and early syphilis, and in the prevention of recurrences of rheumatic fever when administered once monthly.

Aminopenicillins Aminopenicillins are so-called because of the presence of an amino group on the β-acyl side chain of the penicillin nucleus. A number of different compounds are available. They differ microbiologically to a minor degree. Ampicillin was the first aminopenicillin. Subsequently, amoxicillin was produced, and other agents such as bacampicillin, cyclacillin, epicillin, hetacillin, and pivampicillin have been synthesized. Aminopenicillins retain the in vitro activity of penicillin G. In addition, they inhibit *H. influenzae* and are more active against *Streptococcus faecalis,* and *S. faecium* than is penicillin G. Many *E. coli* are inhibited by aminopenicillins, as are *Proteus mirabilis*. In the United States, many *Salmonella* species and *Shigella* species are inhibited by ampicillin, but in developing countries most strains are resistant to aminopenicillins. Aminopenicillins inhibit most mouth organisms, but do not inhibit *Pseudomonas* species, *Klebsiella, Enterobacter,* and the majority of *Bacteroides fragilis* species. In some parts of the United States, 25 percent of *H. influenzae* contain a β-lactamase, making them resistant to the aminopenicillins.

Amoxicillin and bacampicillin are absorbed approximately twice as well as ampicillin. Bacampicillin is an ester of ampicillin that is converted in the intestinal mucosa and in serum to free ampicillin. Administered parenterally, ampicillin is well distributed to body compartments and achieves therapeutic concentrations in the cerebrospinal, pleural, joint, and peritoneal fluids in the presence of inflammation. Urinary levels are high, even in the presence of markedly reduced renal function. Although ampicillin can be administered intramuscularly, orally administered amoxicillin will produce serum levels comparable to those achieved by intramuscular injection of similar amounts of ampicillin. Ampicillin currently is used in the treatment of outpatient urinary tract infections, upper respiratory infections, otitis media, sinusitis, bacterial exacerbations of bronchitis, and community-acquired pneumonia. It is effective therapy for pneumococcal and meningococcal meningitis, and is used in the therapy of enterococcal endocarditis, always in combination with an aminoglycoside. In the oral form, amoxicillin should replace ampicillin due to its better absorption. The one clinical setting in which amoxicillin is inferior to ampicillin is in the treatment of shigellosis. This is probably related to better absorption of the drug so that less of the active compound is present within the intestine. Amoxicillin and bacampicillin can be administered in most situations three times a day, and still achieve adequate blood, tissue, and urinary levels for treatment of susceptible organisms.

Although allergic reactions of the hypersensitivity type to the aminopenicillins occur with the same frequency as with penicillin G or V, there is an increased risk of skin rash with oral ampicillin. It is estimated that 8 to 10 percent of patients receiving oral ampicillin develop a skin rash. As many as 90 percent of patients with infectious mononucleosis receiving ampicillin develop a maculopapular rash beginning approximately 4 days after therapy is instituted. This rash does not represent true penicillin allergy and does not mean that the patient can never receive a penicillin again.

Penicillinase-resistant penicillins A number of different penicillinase-resistant penicillins were developed for the treatment of staphylococcal infections. These agents inhibit *S. aureus* and *S. epidermidis,* as well as *S. pyogenes* and *S. pneumoniae*. None of them has activity against *S. faecalis* (enterococcus) or against aerobic or anaerobic gram-negative bacilli. Methicillin was the first antistaphylococcal β-lactamase-stable penicillin.

S. aureus resistant to all β-lactams are referred to as methicillin-resistant. These isolates have an altered penicillin-binding protein as the basis of their resistance, and hence these *S. aureus* and similar strains of *S. epidermidis* are resistant to all penicillins and to cephalosporins as well. In vitro tests of methicillin-resistant staphylococci against cephalosporins tend to be unreliable, and may show these organisms to be sensitive when, in fact, they are resistant. Methicillin-resistant staphylococci may be inhibited by carbapenems, such as imipenem, or by other penem antibiotics. However, the drug of choice for methicillin-resistant staphylococci is vancomycin.

Methicillin can only be used parenterally since it is not acid-stable, and it has a short half-life, necessitating intravenous administration every 4 h. Since interstitial nephritis is a relatively common side effect, methicillin is rarely used today.

Nafcillin has more intrinsic activity than methicillin against both staphylococci and streptococci. It is excreted primarily by the liver, and to a lesser extent by the kidney. Nafcillin should not be used orally since absorption by this route is erratic, whether the drug is taken fasting or with food. The usual dosage of nafcillin is 4 to 12 g per day, depending upon the severity of the infection, and 100 to 200 mg/kg per day for children. Intravenous nafcillin may result in more severe phlebitis than other antistaphylococcal penicillins, and in high doses may result in more suppression of white cells.

The isoxazolyl penicillins consist of oxacillin, which should be used only parenterally due to poor oral absorption, and the oral preparations cloxacillin and dicloxacillin. In many countries, flucloxacillin is also available as an oral drug and in some countries cloxacillin is available for parenteral use. Although dicloxacillin produces higher blood levels than cloxacillin, it is slightly more protein-bound, 96 vs. 94 percent, than cloxacillin. The active antibiotic levels of the two drugs are actually quite similar. In general, cloxacillin or dicloxacillin are administered in doses of 0.5 or 0.25 g four times a day, respectively.

Although the primary indication for the use of antistaphylococcal penicillins is infection due to penicillinase-producing staphylococci, they are often administered before the etiologic agent is known. Blood levels with the penicillinase-resistant penicillins are adequate to inhibit *S. pneumoniae* and most hemolytic streptococci; therefore, it is not necessary to give both a penicillinase-resistant penicillin and penicillin G simultaneously. However, infections caused by *S. faecalis* (enterococcus) and *Neisseria* do not respond to penicillinase-resistant penicillins, and ampicillin should also be used if these organisms are suspected.

Carboxy penicillins Carbenicillin was the first penicillin with activity against *P. aeruginosa* and certain indole-positive *Proteus* species. Ticarcillin is also a carboxy penicillin, but it is fourfold more active than carbenicillin. Both of these compounds are destroyed by β-lactamases of gram-positive and some gram-negative organisms, but they are less readily destroyed by the β-lactamases of species such as *Pseudomonas, Enterobacter, Morganella,* and *Proteus-Providencia*. Carbenicillin and ticarcillin are less active than ampicillin against *S. pyogenes, S. pneumoniae,* and *Streptococcus faecalis* (enterococcus). However, they have excellent activity against non-β-lactamase-producing *Haemophilus, N. meningitidis,* and *N. gonorrhoeae*. In general, the antibacterial activity of the carboxy penicillins against *E. coli, Proteus, Salmonella,* and *Shigella* species is similar to ampicillin. They are inactive against *Klebsiella* since they are destroyed by the β-lactamase of these organisms.

Ticarcillin and carbenicillin have activity against oral and intestinal *Bacteroides* species, although higher concentrations are required than are needed to inhibit the Enterobacteriaceae. Both carbenicillin and ticarcillin act synergistically with aminoglycosides to inhibit *P. aeruginosa*. The pharmacokinetics of ticarcillin and carbenicillin are virtually identical. Because of the greater in vitro activity of ticarcillin, it has replaced carbenicillin. The drugs are rarely used intramuscularly since peak serum levels are only 20 μg/mL after a 1-g dose. These levels are inadequate for tissue *Pseudomonas* infections, but provide adequate concentrations in the urine. Both agents are administered in dosages of 200 to 300 mg/kg per day, divided into 4- or 6-hourly doses for 24 h. Both carbenicillin and ticarcillin are excreted by the renal tubules and accumulate in the presence of renal dysfunction. Since each drug contains 4.7 meq of sodium, full doses of 12 to 30 g per day may precipitate congestive heart failure. Hypokalemia may also result since the nonreabsorbable portion of the anion is delivered to the distal tubule where it triggers a hydrogen ion exchange, resulting in potassium loss. Carbenicillin and other penicillins bind to ADP receptor sites on platelets, and prevent normal platelet aggregation. Bleeding times are prolonged and clinical bleeding may occur in the presence of high serum levels. Carbenicillin or ticarcillin cannot be administered in the same solution as aminoglycosides since they complex with the aminoglycoside, rendering the aminoglycoside inactive. This does not normally occur in the body, except in the presence of renal failure, when very high concentrations of the antipseudomonas penicillins result in complexing with aminoglycosides. Ticarcillin has proved useful in the therapy of aspiration pneumonia in the hospital setting, in the therapy of the febrile neutropenic patient, in treatment of intraabdominal infection, and in treatment of gynecologic infections.

In the United States, there is only one oral antipseudomonas penicillin, indanyl carbenicillin. This is an alpha-carboxy ester of carbenicillin that has no intrinsic activity of its own, but is acid-stable and moderately well absorbed in the gastrointestinal tract, where it is hydrolyzed to yield free carbenicillin. Indanyl carbenicillin does not provide adequate serum or tissue levels for systemic infection and is useful only for the treatment of urinary tract infections or prostatitis. In the presence of decreased renal function, urine levels may be lower and may be inadequate to treat *Pseudomonas* urinary tract infections.

Ureido penicillins Ureido penicillins, azlocillin, mezlocillin, piperacillin, and apalcillin,[1] in contrast to the carboxy penicillins, are derivatives of ampicillin in which the presence of a side chain linked to the amino group on the alpha carbon provides increased binding to penicillin-binding proteins and more rapid passage through porin channels of gram-negative bacteria. Ureido penicillins are destroyed by β-lactamases of *S. aureus, E. coli, Klebsiella,* and *Bacteroides.* Azlocillin is 8 to 16 times more active than carbenicillin against *P. aeruginosa* and is less active against indole-positive *Proteus* species. It has the same activity as ampicillin against streptococcal species. It is not absorbed orally and must be given by the intravenous route to provide adequate serum levels to treat *Pseudomonas* infections. Since ureido penicillins show nonlinear pharmacokinetics, these drugs should be used in a larger dose administered at intervals of 6 h, rather than the 4-h interval used for carbenicillin. Azlocillin also does not accumulate in the blood in renal failure to the same degree as do carbenicillin and ticarcillin. Its half-life increases to a maximum of only 4 h, even when renal insufficiency is present, necessitating less adjustment in dosage. Azlocillin has been shown to enter the cerebrospinal fluid in the presence of meningeal inflammation, but levels are only 10 percent of serum levels. The drug is used primarily to treat *Pseudomonas* infections; the usual dose is 12 to 18 g per day.

Mezlocillin is a ureido penicillin that differs from carbenicillin and ticarcillin by being more active against streptococci, particularly enterococci. Its activity against streptococci is similar to ampicillin's. It also inhibits approximately 60 percent of *Klebsiella* in a concentration of 16 μg/mL; virtually no *Klebsiella* are inhibited by carbenicillin or ticarcillin. It is also more active against *B. fragilis* and *H. influenzae.* Mezlocillin has activity against *P. aeruginosa* similar to that of ticarcillin. Mezlocillin can be given at 6-hourly intervals, and the dose needs to be reduced only moderately as renal function declines. Mezlocillin is the least likely of the broad-spectrum penicillins to alter bleeding times, but the clinical significance of this is unknown. The drug has been effective in the treatment of respiratory, urinary, gynecologic, and surgical infections. Usual doses are 12 to 18 g per day for adults.

Piperacillin has excellent activity against streptococcal species, *Neisseria, Haemophilus,* and it is the most active penicillin, and probably the drug of choice against *P. aeruginosa.* It also inhibits many *P. cepacia* which are increasingly important organisms in hospital infections. Like the other acyl ureido penicillins, it is destroyed by β-lactamases. It inhibits many community-acquired *Klebsiella* and *Bacteroides* species but will not inhibit Enterobacteriaceae which contain the plasmid β-lactamase. The human pharmacology of piperacillin is similar to the other ureido penicillins. It should be administered in a dose of 12 to 18 g per day, at 6-hourly intervals.

Other penicillins Amdinocillin is penicillin active only against gram-negative species since it does not bind to the penicillin-binding proteins of gram-positive organisms. It has poor activity against *Haemophilus* and *Neisseria,* but is extremely active against *E. coli,* many *Klebsiella, Enterobacter,* and *Citrobacter* species. It has variable activity against *Proteus* species and does not inhibit *Pseudomonas* or *Bacteroides fragilis.* Amdinocillin acts synergistically with other penicillins and has been used in this way. Amdinocillin is not acid-stable and cannot be used orally except as the pivolyl ester which is well absorbed and immediately hydrolyzed, yielding the free compound in serum.

Temocillin[1] is a 6-alpha-methoxy derivative of ticarcillin. This penicillin is not destroyed by plasmid- or chromosomally mediated β-lactamases, but it has markedly reduced activity against gram-positive species and *Pseudomonas.* Temocillin inhibits the majority of *E. coli, Klebsiella, Enterobacter, Proteus, Serratia,* and *Citrobacter* at readily achievable concentrations. *Bacteroides* are resistant. Temocillin has a half-life in humans of 4 to 6 h. It can be administered twice or three times daily. It accumulates in the presence of renal failure and is only partially removed by hemodialysis. Temocillin is not available in the United States, but is currently used in Europe to treat urinary infections and soft tissue infections due to gram-negative bacilli.

Untoward reactions to penicillins The major adverse effects of penicillin are hypersensitivity reactions which range from minor rashes to immediate anaphylaxis. Anaphylactic reactions and accelerated urticarial reactions are due to IgE antibody. Patients who have had such reactions should not receive penicillins. Drug fever is common with all penicillins. Intestinal side effects produced by penicillins are diarrhea or bouts of enterocolitis, some of which are due to overgrowth of *Clostridium difficile.* Neutropenia, platelet dysfunction, and hemolytic anemia have followed the use of all the penicillins. Minor elevations in serum glutamic oxaloacetic transaminase (SGOT) occur most often with oxacillin, nafcillin, or carbenicillin. Neurologic adverse effects in the form of seizures will occur if penicillin G is administered in high doses to patients with decreased renal function. Renal toxicity has varied from allergic angiitis to interstitial nephritis most commonly with methicillin, but this complication can occur with all penicillins.

CEPHALOSPORINS Cephalosporins differ from penicillins by the presence of a dihydrothiazine ring rather than the five-membered thiazolidine ring fused to the four-membered β-lactam ring. Because of their structural configuration, cephalosporins have been modified chemically to produce compounds with different microbiologic and pharmacologic properties. In order to understand their antimicrobial activity, it is useful to divide cephalosporins into so-called generations. In a particular group of cephalosporins, there may be marked differences in microbiologic activity and pharmacologic properties. Like the penicillins, cephalosporins inhibit cell wall biosynthesis and are bactericidal. First-generation cephalosporins include some compounds that can be used only parenterally and some that can be used orally. The parenteral agents are cephalothin, cephapirin, cephaloridine, cefazolin, and cephradine. Oral compounds are cephalexin, cephradine, cefadroxil, and cefaclor.

First-generation cephalosporins First-generation cephalosporins inhibit group A, B, C, and G streptococci and most viridans group streptococci. They are active against *S. pneumoniae, S. aureus,* and *S. epidermidis.* Among the Enterobacteriaceae, *E. coli, P. mirabilis,* and *Klebsiella* species are inhibited. None of these first-generation drugs inhibit *Serratia, Enterobacter,* indole-positive *Proteus, P. aeruginosa,* or *B. fragilis* species. Although a number of the drugs inhibit *H. influenzae,* only cefaclor can be considered therapeutically useful against *Haemophilus.* None of these agents is therapeutic for *Neisseria* species, although all of them have some inhibitory activity against these organisms in vitro.

In some hospitals, 20 to 30 percent of *E. coli* and *Klebsiella* are resistant to first-generation cephalosporins. Nonetheless, one of these agents, cefazolin, has continued to be both useful and heavily used. Cefazolin has a half-life of approximately 2 h and can be administered either by the intramuscular or intravenous routes. It accumulates in the body in the presence of decreased renal function, and dosage adjustments must be made in the presence of renal failure. It is normally administered in doses of 0.5 to 1 g every 6 to 8 h. Cefazolin has proved useful as therapy of respiratory, skin, and urinary tract infections, and as therapy of endocarditis due to viridans streptococci in penicillin-allergic patients. It is also appropriate therapy for osteomyelitis due to staphylococcal species. Cefazolin is useful as a prophylactic antimicrobial agent at the time of orthopedic surgery, prosthetic valve surgery, and upper gastrointestinal operations. Cephalothin and cephapirin have extremely short half-lives, 4 h, and are converted in the body to less active desacetyl derivatives. These drugs should be administered every 4 h, and for this reason they are used much less frequently today.

Both cephalexin and cephradine are well absorbed after oral ingestion, yielding peak blood levels in the range of 15 to 20 μg/mL

[1] *Not available in the United States.*

after a 0.5-g dose. Although these cephalosporins are less active against *S. aureus* than the parenteral first-generation cephalosporins, serum and tissue concentrations are adequate to treat many minor staphylococcal infections in penicillin-allergic patients. Both drugs have a half-life of approximately 1 h and are usually administered three or four times daily. The drugs are totally excreted in the urine, yielding high concentrations inhibitory to common urinary pathogens.

Cefadroxil is a parahydroxy derivative of cephalexin which has a longer half-life, allowing it to be administered twice daily. Otherwise, its antimicrobial activity is identical to that of cephalexin.

Cefaclor has found utility primarily as a therapeutic agent for respiratory infections in children caused by *H. influenzae* or other susceptible organisms. It is poorly β-lactamase stable but the concentrations in ear fluid are adequate to eradicate β-lactamase-producing *H. influenzae*. It should not be used for serious infections caused by β-lactamase-producing strains and is ineffective in urinary tract infections due to β-lactamase-producing *E. coli* and *Klebsiella*.

Second-generation cephalosporins Second-generation cephalosporins probably should not be grouped as a class since the compounds within this class have markedly different antibacterial and pharmacologic properties. All of these agents are administered parenterally and can be used either intramuscularly or intravenously, although they are most frequently used by the intravenous route. Cefamandole has excellent activity against streptococcal and staphylococcal species with the exception of *S. faecalis* (enterococcus). It is more active than first-generation cephalosporins against *E. coli* and *Klebsiella* and has increased activity against *H. influenzae*. It is destroyed by β-lactamases of some gram-negative species, and is not active against *Bacteroides* or *Pseudomonas* species. Although a number of *Enterobacter* and *Citrobacter* strains are inhibited by cefamandole in vitro, clinically it is not useful to treat infections due to these organisms because resistance develops rapidly. Cefamandole has a relatively short half-life, 0.7 h, and it is administered every 4 to 6 h in doses of 1 to 2 g. The drug does not produce adequate concentrations in the cerebrospinal fluid, and it should not be used in patients in whom meningitis is suspected.

Cefuroxime is a β-lactamase-stable cephalosporin that inhibits most streptococcal and staphylococcal species, *H. influenzae*, penicillinase-producing *N. gonorrhoeae*, and β-lactamase-producing Enterobacteriaceae. It is not active against *S. faecalis* (enterococcus), *Bacteroides fragilis*, or *P. aeruginosa*. Cefuroxime has a half-life of approximately 1.5 h, permitting administration at 8-hourly intervals. It enters the cerebrospinal fluid in concentrations adequate to treat meningitis due to *H. influenzae*, *S. pneumoniae*, and *N. meningitidis*. CSF concentrations are inadequate to treat meningitis due to *E. coli* or *Klebsiella* species. Cefuroxime has been used in the therapy of respiratory infections, biliary tract infections, soft tissue infections, osteomyelitis, and urinary tract infections. It can also be used for therapy of meningitis in children and young adults.

Cefonicid is a cephalosporin structurally related to cefamandole. However, substitution of a different moiety at position 3 of the dihydrothiazine ring has provided the compound with a long half-life of approximately 4 to 5 h. Cefonicid activity is similar to that of cefamandole and cefuroxime, with the exception of lower activity against *S. aureus* that may not be clinically important. Cefonicid has been used in a single daily dose administered either intravenously or intramuscularly to treat respiratory, skin, and urinary tract infections due to susceptible organisms. It should not be used to treat meningeal infections.

Ceforanide is similar in structure and antimicrobial activity to cefamandole, but is somewhat less active against *H. influenzae*. Higher serum levels are achieved following intramuscular injection since the drug is highly protein-bound. It has a half-life of approximately $3\frac{1}{2}$ h, and has been used in a single or twice-daily dose to treat susceptible infections.

Cefotiam[1] is a second-generation cephalosporin with activity against streptococci, staphylococci, and most Enterobacteriaceae. It is not β-lactamase-stable and possesses high activity because of its affinity for penicillin-binding proteins. Cefotiam has a short half-life of 0.5 h, similar to many of the first-generation cephalosporins. Therefore, it must be administered every 4 h. Cefotiam is not available in the United States, but is used in Europe and Japan.

Cefoxitin is a cephalosporin which possesses a methoxy group affixed to the β-lactam ring. This provides excellent β-lactamase resistance, but decreases activity against gram-positive organisms such as staphylococci. Cefoxitin inhibits most staphylococci at concentrations of 2 to 4 μg/mL, and *S. pneumoniae* are inhibited at similar concentrations. It possesses no activity against *S. faecalis* (enterococcus). Cefoxitin inhibits *E. coli* and *Klebsiella* species resistant to first-generation and other second-generation cephalosporins. It lacks activity against *Enterobacter* and *Citrobacter* species, and does not inhibit *Pseudomonas*. Cefoxitin has excellent activity against *B. fragilis*, inhibiting the majority of clinical isolates at a concentration between 16 to 32 μg/mL, which is readily achieved in humans. Cefoxitin has a half-life of approximately 0.8 h. It is widely distributed to body sites, but does not yield adequate concentrations within the CSF. The drug accumulates in the presence of decreased renal function, and dose adjustments must be made when renal failure is present. Cefoxitin has been widely used as therapy of mixed aerobic and anaerobic intraabdominal infections and in the treatment of gynecologic infections. In some centers, cefoxitin combined with doxycycline is the therapy of choice for pelvic inflammatory disease. Cefoxitin has also been used as a parenteral prophylactic agent administered at the time of intraabdominal surgery on the colon, particularly in patients in whom oral prophylactic programs are not feasible. Cefoxitin has also proved useful in the therapy of anaerobic pleuropulmonary disease where it is an alternative to penicillin or clindamycin therapy. It is effective for treatment of gonorrhea due to penicillinase-producing *Neisseria*.

Third-generation cephalosporins Third-generation cephalosporins can be grouped into several convenient classes. The first of these are the aminothiazolyl iminomethoxy cephalosporins which consist of cefotaxime, ceftizoxime, cefmenoxime, and ceftriaxone. These agents possess excellent activity against hemolytic streptococci and *S. pneumoniae*, inhibiting these species at concentrations <0.1 μg/mL. They do not inhibit *S. faecalis* (enterococci). The compounds are highly active against *H. influenzae*, *N. meningitidis*, and *N. gonorrhoeae*, including β-lactamase-producing strains. Because of their high affinity for penicillin-binding proteins, these compounds inhibit the majority of the Enterobacteriaceae at concentrations below 4.0 μg/mL, although some *Enterobacter* and *Citrobacter* are resistant. These four agents do not have much activity against *P. aeruginosa* and *Acinetobacter*, and they are much less active than cefoxitin against *B. fragilis*.

Cefotaxime has a half-life of approximately 1 h, and it is converted to a desacetyl derivative which has a half-life of approximately 1.6 h. Although the desacetyl derivative is less active than the parent compound, it is more active than most second-generation cephalosporins and acts synergistically with the parent compound to inhibit some microorganisms. Cefotaxime produces concentrations in the CSF ranging from 1 to 30 μg/mL, depending upon the degree of inflammation and the dose used. It has proved effective as therapy of meningitis due to group B streptococci, *E. coli*, *H. influenzae*, *N. meningitidis*, *S. pneumoniae*, *Klebsiella*, and some infections due to *Enterobacter* and *Serratia*, although failures have occurred with these organisms. Agents that have been employed more frequently (penicillin, ampicillin) should be used unless the patient is allergic to them or the organism is resistant. Although cefotaxime has a relatively short half-life, its high activity and the presence of an active metabolite indicate that it can be administered 8-hourly in most infections, except in febrile neutropenic patients.

Ceftizoxime has a slightly longer half-life than cefotaxime at 1.6 h. It also has proved useful in the therapy of gram-negative meningitis and can be administered every 8 to 12 h in the majority of infections.

Cefmenoxime[1] has a half-life of 1 h. It is normally administered at 6-h intervals. It is not approved at this time for therapy of meningitis.

Ceftriaxone differs from the aforementioned compounds because it has a half-life of approximately 7 h in normal individuals. Sixty percent of ceftriaxone is cleared by the kidney, and the remainder of the drug is cleared through the biliary system. Although ceftriaxone is 95 percent bound to serum proteins, it produces such high serum levels that adequate free drug is available to inhibit the majority of gram-positive and gram-negative bacteria with the exception of *S. faecalis* (enterococci), *Pseudomonas,* and *B. fragilis.* Ceftriaxone enters the CSF and is removed from the CSF extremely slowly. Levels well above the minimum inhibitory concentration for most meningeal pathogens are present 24 h after the administration of a single dose. Ceftriaxone has been administered once and twice daily to treat a variety of infections. It should be used twice daily in the therapy of meningitis, although a successful outcome has been achieved with single daily administration of the drug in some meningeal infections. Ceftriaxone offers the possibility of once-daily intramuscular therapy in the home setting to complete treatment instituted initially within the hospital.

Moxalactam is an oxacephalosporin with oxygen replacing the sulfur in the bicyclic ring structure. Moxalactam has decreased antistreptococcal and antistaphylococcal activity compared to agents such as cefotaxime and ceftizoxime. It has excellent activity against *H. influenzae,* including penicillinase-producing strains, *N. gonorrhoeae,* and the majority of the β-lactamase-producing members of the Enterobacteriaceae. Moxalactam inhibits many strains of *P. aeruginosa* although relatively high concentrations are needed in comparison to its activity against organisms such as *E. coli* and *Klebsiella.* Moxalactam is not hydrolyzed by *Bacteroides* β-lactamases and inhibits *B. fragilis* at concentrations <16 μg/mL. Moxalactam has a serum half-life of approximately 2 h and is excreted primarily in the urine, accumulating in the body in the presence of decreased renal function. The drug possesses an *N*-methylthiotetrazole group at position 3 of the bicyclic structure. This structure has been associated with two adverse reactions. The first is a disulfiram reaction when alcohol is ingested. This is caused by interference with alcohol dehydrogenase and the accumulation of acetaldehyde. A second adverse reaction is hypoprothrombinemia which appears related to two factors; one is the effect of the drug on the intestinal flora, but the second is due to dimer formation of the *N*-methylthiotetrazole which interferes with the production of vitamin K. Moxalactam administered in doses above 4 g per day also will cause platelet dysfunction due to its effect on ADP receptors on the platelets, analogous to the effect produced with high doses of carbenicillin. Because of these factors, patients receiving moxalactam should receive vitamin K at least twice weekly, and platelet function should be assessed by bleeding times. Moxalactam enters the CSF and has proved effective treatment for meningitis caused by *H. influenzae, E. coli, Klebsiella,* and *N. meningitidis.* It is less active against group B streptococci and *S. pneumoniae* and hence should not be used in situations in which these organisms might be the etiologic agent. Concern over bleeding problems associated with moxalactam has limited its use in the United States. When used in mixed infections due to aerobic gram-negative bacilli and anaerobic species, close attention must be paid to bleeding and clotting functions.

Cefotetan is a 7-alpha-methoxy cephalosporin that has in vitro activity similar to cefoxitin against anaerobic microorganisms and activity slightly less than that of the aminothiazolyl cephalosporins against gram-positive cocci and the Enterobacteriaceae. It does not inhibit *Pseudomonas* species. Cefotetan has a half-life of approximately 4 h, and can be administered twice or three times daily. Since it possesses an *N*-methylthiotetrazole group, however, it potentially can cause clotting abnormalities and disulfiram-type reactions.

Cephalosporins with activity against *Pseudomonas aeruginosa* Cefoperazone is a cephalosporin that has activity against the majority of gram-positive microorganisms, Enterobacteriaceae, and will inhibit a significant number of *P. aeruginosa* at concentrations below 32 μg/mL. It is not completely β-lactamase-stable and is destroyed by some β-lactamase-producing *E. coli, Klebsiella,* and *B. fragilis* strains. Cefoperazone is approximately 85 percent protein bound. Following a 2-g dose, peak blood levels of 250 μg/mL are achieved. The half-life of the drug is approximately 2 h. Only 25 percent of cefoperazone is removed from the body by the kidney; the remainder is removed by biliary mechanisms. Cefoperazone is used in a dose of 2 g twice daily to treat gram-positive and gram-negative infections. Higher doses are usually needed to treat serious *Pseudomonas* infections. Since cefoperazone contains an *N*-methylthiotetrazole group, it can produce disulfiram reactions and prolongation of the prothrombin time. It does not, however, alter platelet function.

Ceftazidime is an aminothiazolyl cephalosporin that contains a propyliminocarboxy grouping on the acyl side chain. This provides the compound with excellent activity against *P. aeruginosa* and many strains of *P. cepacia* and *Acinetobacter.* It is slightly less active than cefotaxime against streptococcal species and fourfold to eightfold less active against *S. aureus,* but has similar activity against the Enterobacteriaceae. Ceftazidime has no activity against *B. fragilis* and is inactive against many clostridial species. Ceftazidime is cleared primarily by glomerular filtration and has a half-life of approximately 1.8 h. It enters the CSF in concentrations adequate to inhibit the majority of organisms producing meningitis and has been used successfully to treat a number of patients with meningitis caused by *P. aeruginosa.* Ceftazidime accumulates in the presence of decreased renal function, and dosage adjustments must be made in patients with markedly decreased renal function. Ceftazidime has proved to be a successful drug in a variety of different serious infections, including pneumonia, bacteremia, urosepsis, osteomyelitis, and deep skin structure infections due to Enterobacteriaceae and *P. aeruginosa.* It also has been extremely useful in therapy of suspected infection in the febrile neutropenic patient where it has been used singly or in combination with vancomycin.

Cefsulodin[1] is a unique cephalosporin since it inhibits only *P. aeruginosa.* This compound does not bind to penicillin-binding proteins of the majority of gram-positive species or of the Enterobacteriaceae. Cefsulodin is removed from the body by glomerular filtration and tubular secretion. It has a half-life of approximately 1 h and is administered normally on a 6-hourly dosage program by the intravenous route. Cefsulodin has been used to treat pulmonary infections in cystic fibrosis patients, osteomyelitis, necrotizing otitis, bronchitis, and urinary tract infections due to *P. aeruginosa.*

OTHER β-LACTAM ANTIBIOTICS A number of novel compounds belonging to the β-lactam class have been developed. These agents differ widely in their antibacterial and pharmacologic properties.

Imipenem Imipenem is a prototype of the thienamycin class of compounds. These compounds possess a novel chemical structure that differentiates them from penicillins and cephalosporins. Biochemically, they are carbapenems. Imipenem has excellent in vitro activity against aerobic gram-positive species such as the hemolytic streptococci and *S. pneumoniae;* it inhibits *S. faecalis* at concentrations similar to those of ampicillin and vancomycin. It is also active against *S. aureus* and *S. epidermidis* including β-lactamase-producing strains and inhibits *Listeria monocytogenes.* The majority of the Enterobacteriaceae are inhibited by concentrations <1 μg/mL, as are *H. influenzae* and *N. gonorrhoeae. P. aeruginosa,* including strains resistant to penicillins and to aminoglycosides, are inhibited by concentrations of 1 to 6 μg/mL. *P. cepacia* and *Acinetobacter* are inhibited, but *P. maltophilia* are resistant. Imipenem inhibits the majority of anaerobic species including *B. fragilis,* including isolates resistant to moxalactam and cefoxitin. Imipenem is not absorbed after oral ingestion due to its instability in gastric acid. It is hydrolyzed in the kidney by a peptidase, dehydropeptidase-1, which is located on the brush border of the proximal renal tubular cells. To overcome the problem of destruction of imipenem, a dehydropeptidase inhibitor, cilastatin, is administered with imipenem.

Imipenem has a relatively short half-life of approximately 1 h;

doses of 500 mg to 1 g provide serum, tissue, and urine concentrations sufficient to inhibit the majority of bacteria. Imipenem has been used to treat bacteremia, respiratory infections, intraabdominal infections, bone and joint infections, endocarditis, and urinary tract infections due to organisms that are susceptible to it and that are resistant to other β-lactams and to aminoglycosides. Toxicity has been minimal to date, although leukopenia has been reported, nausea occurs in some patients following too rapid infusion, and, rarely, seizures have occurred.

Monobactams Aztreonam is a monocyclic β-lactam which inhibits only aerobic gram-negative bacteria and does not inhibit gram-positive or anaerobic organisms. Most Enterobacteriaceae, *Haemophilus*, and *Neisseria* species, including β-lactamase-producing strains, are inhibited by <1 μg/mL. Most *P. aeruginosa* are inhibited by 16 μg/mL. Aztreonam is not absorbed following oral ingestion. It has a half-life between 1.5 and 2 h, and following doses of 1 g, serum and urine concentrations above the MICs of most Enterobacteriaceae and *Pseudomonas* are readily achieved. Aztreonam accumulates in the presence of renal failure with an increase in half-life to 6 h. The drug has been used to treat a variety of serious infections due to aerobic gram-negative species including *E. coli, Klebsiella, Serratia*, and *Pseudomonas*. It has been used in combination with clindamycin or antistaphylococcal penicillins in mixed infections where aztreonam has been utilized as a replacement for the aminoglycosides. Aztreonam enters the CSF, but only a small number of patients with meningitis have been treated with it.

β-LACTAMASE INHIBITORS Augmentin is a combination of amoxicillin and clavulanate. Clavulanate is a β-lactamase inhibitor that has minimal antibacterial activity of its own, but inhibits the β-lactamases of *S. aureus*, Enterobacteriaceae, *Bacteroides, Klebsiella*, and *Branhamella* species. Clavulanate produces inhibition of β-lactamases with destruction of the enzyme. Potassium clavulanate is moderately well absorbed from the gastrointestinal tract and peak serum levels occur approximately at the same time as with amoxicillin. The combination of clavulanate and amoxicillin does not significantly alter the pharmacologic properties of either drug. Augmentin can be administered every 8 h and has been used to treat skin infections due to β-lactamase-producing staphylococci, otitis due to *H. influenzae*, and urinary tract infections due to β-lactamase-producing *E. coli* and *Klebsiella*. It has also been used in deep cutaneous infections due to anaerobic microorganisms and in upper respiratory infections in which *Branhamella* has been shown to be an important component.

Timentin is a combination of 3 g ticarcillin and 100 or 200 mg of clavulanate. Timentin increases the activity of ticarcillin to include *S. aureus*, β-lactamase-producing *Haemophilus, Bacteroides* species, *Klebsiella*, and many of the β-lactamase-producing *E. coli* strains. Timentin has been used to treat intraabdominal infections, osteomyelitis, and urinary tract infections and as combination therapy in the febrile neutropenic patient.

Sulbactam[1] is a 6-desamino penicillin sulfone that acts as an inhibitor of plasmid and chromosomally mediated β-lactamases. Sulbactam acts synergistically with penicillins and cephalosporins. It has been combined with ampicillin, and in the presence of concentrations of 8 μg/mL of sulbactam and 16 μg/mL of ampicillin, the majority of staphylococci, *Klebsiella, Haemophilus, E. coli*, and *Bacteroides* is inhibited. Sulbactam has pharmacokinetics in humans similar to ampicillin. It is administered intravenously since, by the oral route, it produces excessive diarrhea. The ampicillin-sulbactam combination has been used successfully to treat urinary tract, intraabdominal, and respiratory infections due to β-lactamase-producing microorganisms.

VANCOMYCIN Vancomycin is a glycopeptide that is active only against gram-positive species. It has assumed increasing importance because of the widespread appearance of methicillin-resistant staphylococci and the recognition of antibiotic-associated colitis caused by *C. difficile*. Vancomycin inhibits cell wall synthesis and is bactericidal. It is active against all hemolytic streptococcal species, *viridans* group streptococci, *S. pneumoniae, L. monocytogenes*, and the *Corynebacterium* species resistant to other β-lactam drugs. Vancomycin can be administered only by the intravenous route. It is eliminated from the body by glomerular filtration and has a half-life of approximately 6 h in individuals with normal renal function. In the presence of anuria, its half-life may be prolonged to between 5 to 9 days, and it may be detected in serum for as long as 21 days after a single 1-g dose. Vancomycin is not absorbed from the gastrointestinal tract. It can be used orally, but not parenterally, to treat enterocolitis, since it is not secreted into the intestine. Following intravenous administration of a 1-g dose, peak levels of 20 to 125 μg/mL are found in serum, and when given orally, concentrations between 100 to 800 μg/mL are found in the stool. Vancomycin enters the CSF poorly. It may be administered once weekly to patients in renal failure as therapy for serious staphylococcal or streptococcal infections. Hemodialysis does not remove vancomycin. Rapid infusion of vancomycin will produce histamine release characterized by fever, chills, and generalized erythema. This reaction can be mitigated by antihistamine drugs, e.g., benadryl. Vancomycin also produces ototoxicity. It is probably minimally nephrotoxic, but when used with an aminoglycoside, nephrotoxicity and ototoxicity may be increased. Vancomycin is the therapy of choice for methicillin-resistant staphylococcal infections and for therapy of *S. faecalis* endocarditis in penicillin-allergic patients. Vancomycin is also useful in the prevention of bacterial endocarditis in patients allergic to penicillin, particularly those who have a prosthetic heart valve (see Chap. 188).

AMINOGLYCOSIDES AND SPECTINOMYCIN Streptomycin was the first aminoglycoside isolated in 1944 from the fungus *Streptomyces griseus*. Some 5 years later, neomycin was discovered. In 1957, kanamycin was isolated and remained the predominant aminoglycoside until the advent of gentamicin. A number of other aminoglycosides have come into clinical use in the last two decades. Aminoglycoside antibiotics are defined by the presence of amino sugars linked by a glycoside bound to an aminocyclitol ring. All aminoglycosides contain amino groups and hydroxyl groups which are important in the antibacterial activity of the compounds, as well as being the sites of enzymatic inactivation by bacterial enzymes. The drugs' ototoxicity and nephrotoxicity is also determined by their structure. Aminoglycosides are bactericidal since they bind irreversibly to proteins in the ribosomes and cause the interruption of the flow of genetic information. Enzymatic modification of the aminoglycosides by enzymes in plasmid-carrying bacteria results in their inactivation since compounds that have been adenylated, phosphorylated, or acetylated do not bind well to ribosomes and fail to induce a protein which facilitates their uptake by bacteria.

A number of generalizations can be made about their antibacterial activity. Most of them inhibit the members of the Enterobacteriaceae, that is, *E. coli, Klebsiella, Serratia, Enterobacter*, etc. Gentamicin, tobramycin, amikacin, sisomicin, and netilmicin all inhibit *S. aeruginosa*, but kanamycin does not. None of the agents are active against anaerobic species such as *Clostridium* or *Bacteroides*. They are not active against a number of gram-positive cocci, including *S. pneumoniae* or hemolytic streptococci. Aminoglycosides act synergistically with penicillins to inhibit *S. faecalis* and with antipseudomonas penicillins to inhibit *Pseudomonas*. They also act synergistically with nafcillin or oxacillin against *S. aureus*.

Aminoglycosides are highly water soluble and stable over a wide pH range, but can be inactivated by β-lactam antibiotics, particularly carbenicillin. They are markedly less active at acid pH, and their activity is decreased in the presence of divalent cations such as calcium and magnesium. An anaerobic environment markedly decreases their effectiveness against both Enterobacteriaceae and staphylococci. They are also inactivated by nucleic acid debris from decaying cells.

A pharmacologic property common to all the aminoglycosides is that they are not normally absorbed from the intestine. However, the small amounts absorbed can be sufficient to produce toxicity in the patient with markedly decreased renal function. This is particularly true when neomycin is administered orally in large amounts. The drugs can be absorbed when applied to burns or after irrigation of ulcers or wounds if excessive amounts are used and will produce oto- and nephrotoxicity following such topical application. Aminoglycosides are well absorbed after intramuscular use. Peak serum levels occur 30 to 90 min after an intramuscular injection, and in normal individuals with creatinine clearances >100 mL, their half-life is approximately 2 h. Aminoglycosides are widely distributed in the extracellular fluid volume and enter pleural, peritoneal, and synovial fluids. They do not penetrate the CSF or the eye. Extremely high concentrations are present in renal cortical tissue and persist there for up to several weeks after a course of therapy. All aminoglycosides are removed from the body by glomerular filtration. The drugs are not metabolized, and biliary excretion is minimal. With all the aminoglycosides, there is marked accumulation in the presence of decreased renal function. The half-life of the drugs in the presence of anuria is 35 to 50 h. Urinary concentrations in normal individuals are 25 to 100 times the plasma concentrations. However, in the presence of decreased renal function, only a small amount of drug is present in the urine.

The pharmacokinetics of aminoglycosides in children and the elderly are markedly different than those in young healthy adults. Although the volume of distribution in the elderly is similar to that in young adults, half-lives are considerably longer due to decreased glomerular function. Glomerular function in the elderly may not necessarily be reflected by a higher serum creatinine because of decreased creatinine production in this group. It is therefore important always to use a calculated creatinine clearance in order to estimate the half-life of an aminoglycoside in the elderly. The equation of Cockroft and Gault by which aminoglycoside concentrations may be calculated is

$$C_{cr}(\text{min}) = \frac{(140 - \text{age}) \times \text{wt (kg)}}{\text{Cr (mg/dL)} \times 72}$$

In obese patients, the volume of distribution of aminoglycosides is approximately 75 percent of that in normal patients. In calculating doses, this must be taken into consideration. Conversely, in a markedly protein-malnourished individual, there will be a larger volume of distribution so that the total body weight should be multiplied by 120 percent compared to that of the normal patient.

In initiating therapy with aminoglycosides, a loading dose should be administered in order to achieve a therapeutic serum level as quickly as possible. Reasonable serum levels, 30 to 60 min after the initial dose, are between 5 and 10 μg/mL for gentamicin, tobramycin, netilmicin, and sisomicin, and between 20 and 40 μg/mL for kanamycin and amikacin. A loading dose of 2 mg/kg for gentamicin, tobramycin, and netilmicin and a loading dose of 8 mg/kg for amikacin are satisfactory. The loading dose is the same whether or not elimination is impaired by renal dysfunction. Since loading doses are sizable, they should be given intravenously over 20 to 30 min to avoid the risk of neuromuscular toxicity. In individuals with creatinine clearances >80 mL/min, a dose of 1.5 to 2 mg/kg of gentamicin, tobramycin, or netilmicin every 8 h, or 5 mg/kg of amikacin every 8 h, provides adequate peak and trough levels. The daily dose of aminoglycosides must be reduced in patients whose renal function is impaired. A simple way of calculating the total daily dose is to calculate the patient's creatinine clearance based on age, sex, weight, and serum creatinine. The clearance of aminoglycosides is linearly related to creatinine clearance. Therefore, the ratio of the patient's creatinine clearance to a normal creatinine clearance approximates the aminoglycoside clearance. An individual with a creatinine clearance of 30 mL/min or 30 percent should receive 30 percent of the usual daily dose. Instead of 4.5 to 6 mg/kg per day, the dose should be reduced to 1.5 to 2 mg/kg per day. This dose can be administered either as a reduced dose at the regular time interval of 8 h, or the total dose can be divided and administered at less frequent intervals. Calculated predictions of aminoglycoside levels provide reasonable approximations, but blood levels should be measured, both at the peak and trough, and dose adjustments should be made accordingly.

Toxicity of aminoglycosides All aminoglycosides share similar toxicity. Hypersensitivity is exceedingly rare, but all of these drugs will produce some degree of nephrotoxicity. The initial renal toxicity is nonoliguric renal failure. There is a loss of concentrating ability, proteinuria, casts in the urine, and renal enzymuria. Subsequently, the serum creatinine and blood urea nitrogen (BUN) will rise. Nephrotoxicity involves the proximal tubular cells. Risk factors for development of toxicity are old age, concomitant hypotension at the onset of aminoglycoside therapy, use of other nephrotoxic agents simultaneously, and, perhaps, concomitant liver disease. Aminoglycoside nephrotoxicity is usually mild and reversible. However, it can result in renal failure and may even require dialysis. For this reason, it is critical to follow aminoglycoside blood levels in patients receiving these drugs. Ototoxicity can be aimed at either the cochlea or the vestibular apparatus. The mechanism of the toxicity is the destruction of hair cells within the organ of Corti or those in the ampullar cristae. Once these cells have been damaged, they cannot regenerate. Detectable toxicity occurs in 3 to 5 percent of patients receiving aminoglycosides. Although tinnitus and a feeling of fullness in the ears may precede hearing loss, it is not a useful guide to hearing damage. Since the high tones outside the conversation range are affected first, ototoxicity may not be recognized initially. Auditory and vestibular toxicity appear to be dose- and duration-related, and probably are due to the development of plasma levels outside the therapeutic range. Less frequent forms of toxicity seen with these drugs are neuromuscular blockade and malabsorption.

Individual aminoglycosides Today streptomycin has several uses, including treatment of selected cases of tuberculosis, for which it is administered twice weekly, tularemia, plague, and brucellosis. Streptomycin is used in the treatment of endocarditis due to *S. faecalis* or viridans streptococci, provided that the strains are susceptible to less than 2000 μg/mL. Neomycin's sole use today is in bowel preparation for intestinal surgery, combined with erythromycin or metronidazole. Kanamycin has been superseded by other aminoglycosides. Gentamicin remains useful as a first-line agent in the treatment of gram-negative infections, particularly because of its low cost. Tobramycin is more active than gentamicin against *P. aeruginosa* and less active against *Serratia* species. Its clinical efficacy is equivalent to that of gentamicin, but there is some evidence that tobramycin is somewhat less nephrotoxic than gentamicin. In general, tobramycin should be used in patients at major risk for nephrotoxicity, in individuals with preexisting decreased renal function, or when *P. aeruginosa* is a pathogen. Amikacin is less likely to be inactivated by plasmid-mediated resistance enzymes. Amikacin should be used particularly in those situations in which it is likely that there is aminoglycoside resistance. Amikacin's use has often been restricted in order to prevent development of resistance to the drug. However, a number of studies have indicated that resistance to aminoglycosides does not increase if amikacin is the drug primarily used. Cost considerations may play a role since gentamicin is much less expensive. Netilmicin is a derivative of gentamicin which is less nephrotoxic and less ototoxic. It is less active against *Pseudomonas* than is gentamicin or tobramycin, but it inhibits a number of strains of *E. coli, Klebsiella,* and *Serratia* resistant to gentamicin and tobramycin. Its precise role compared to older drugs has not been defined. Spectinomycin is an amino cyclitol antibiotic that has been used in a single 2-g intramuscular dose to treat gonorrhea due to penicillinase-producing strains. Its use has been superseded by compounds such as ceftriaxone, which can be administered in 125-to 250-mg intramuscular doses to treat penicillinase-producing gonococcal strains.

TETRACYCLINES Tetracyclines are bacteriostatic agents that have activity against a broad spectrum of microorganisms. They inhibit many gram-positive and gram-negative species and are active against a number of other important organisms which include Rickettsiae, *Chlamydia,* and *Mycoplasma.* They also inhibit *Actinomyces,* but do not inhibit *Nocardia.* Resistance to the tetracyclines has appeared in many species. Some strains of *S. pneumoniae* and *S. pyogenes* are resistant. Many staphylococci are resistant to the tetracyclines as well as many enteric organisms such as *Shigella.* In general, organisms resistant to one tetracycline are resistant to all members of the group. Tetracyclines can be divided into three groups based on pharmacology. The short-acting group consists of tetracycline, chlortetracycline, and oxytetracycline. The intermediate group consists of demeclocycline and methacycline, and the long-acting compounds are doxycycline and minocycline. Tetracyclines are incompletely absorbed from the gastrointestinal tract, and their absorption is increased if they are taken in the fasting state. Their absorption is decreased by milk, milk products, and magnesium-containing antacids and iron. The binding of tetracyclines to plasma proteins varies with the type of drug. They enter the CSF, but concentrations are inadequate for treatment of most cases of meningitis. Since the agents cross the placenta, they cannot be given to pregnant women since they will be sequestered into bone and tooth structures causing abnormalities. High concentrations of the drugs are found in the bile, and there is a significant enterohepatic circulation. Minocycline is excreted in saliva and lacrimal secretions producing antibacterial concentrations in the oropharynx; for this reason it has been used as prophylaxis for meningococcal disease. However, since minocycline can cause vestibular toxicity, it has been supplanted by rifampin. With the exception of doxycycline and chlortetracycline, the tetracyclines are eliminated from the body primarily by glomerular filtration. In the presence of renal failure, the half-life of all tetracyclines, except these two drugs, increases markedly.

The tetracyclines are associated with a number of adverse effects. These include skin rashes, some of which occur in the presence of solar exposure. Gastrointestinal effects include nausea, vomiting, and diarrhea. The diarrhea may be either a direct toxic effect, or due to pseudomembranous colitis. Severe hepatotoxicity has occurred during prolonged therapy with high doses, particularly in pregnant women. In some, often debilitated, patients there may be catabolic effects with protein breakdown, weight loss, and nitrogen retention. Tetracyclines also have been shown to interfere with the production of protein in patients receiving hyperalimentation. Tetracycline's effect on the gut flora may cause prolongation of prothrombin time.

Tetracyclines are rarely the drugs of choice in most common bacterial infections because of the large number of other drugs available. Nonetheless, there are some specific indications for use of these compounds. In rickettsial infections such as Rocky Mountain spotted fever, typhus, or scrub typhus, tetracycline remains the drug of choice. They are drugs of choice in the treatment of sexually transmitted chlamydial infections and are useful in the treatment of *Mycoplasma* infections. Tetracyclines have proved useful in the therapy of Lyme disease in adults, brucellosis, relapsing fever due to *Borrelia,* and, combined with streptomycin, for treatment of complicated plague. They have also proved useful in therapy of infections due to *Actinomyces* and in *Pasteurella multocida* infections in penicillin-allergic patients. Tetracyclines have been used in a number of syndromes such as acne, bacterial exacerbations of bronchitis, malabsorption syndrome, and sinusitis. They are not the drugs of choice for streptococcal or pneumococcal infections or for anaerobic infections in the abdomen.

CHLORAMPHENICOL Chloramphenicol is a broad-spectrum antibiotic that became available in the United States in 1949. It is extremely active against a variety of organisms including aerobic and anaerobic bacteria, *Rickettsia, Chlamydia, Mycoplasma,* and *Spirochaeta.* The organisms most commonly causing meningitis in childhood, *H. influenzae, S. pneumoniae,* and *N. meningitidis,* are highly susceptible to chloramphenicol. Most *B. fragilis* are inhibited by it.

Chloramphenicol is well-absorbed from the gastrointestinal tract. Blood levels following oral ingestion are superior to those achieved after intravenous injection since the inactive chloramphenicol succinate ester which is used in the intravenous preparation is incompletely hydrolyzed within the body. Blood levels following intramuscular injection are probably as good as those following IV administration, but no parenteral route is as effective as oral administration. Chloramphenicol is metabolized in the liver where it is conjugated with glucuronic acid and is excreted in an inactive form by the kidneys. It diffuses well into many tissues and body fluids and produces excellent concentrations in the cerebrospinal fluid and brain tissue. In the presence of renal disease, the half-life of the drug is not significantly increased. In contrast, in patients with hepatic disease, serum levels may increase yielding levels capable of producing bone marrow suppression.

The most important toxic effect of chloramphenicol is its effect upon bone marrow. Approximately 1 in 25,000 patients who receive the drug develop aplastic anemia. This is an unpredictable, idiosyncratic response. There is also a dose-related anemia and leukopenia which is predictable when blood levels are above 25 μg/mL. This toxicity is reversible when the antibiotic is discontinued. Chloramphenicol cannot be given to newborns since they are unable to conjugate the drug and develop toxicity due to excessive levels of free compound.

The precise role for chloramphenicol is not clear. There are a number of different drugs which can be used to treat meningitis since the new cephalosporins enter the CSF and provide concentrations that are effective against the leading pathogens. A number of alternatives, including metronidazole, clindamycin, and cefoxitin, are available to treat severe *B. fragilis* infections. Many strains of *S. typhi* are resistant to chloramphenicol, and other drugs such as trimethoprim-sulfamethoxazole will need to be used instead.

Chloramphenicol undergoes a number of significant drug interactions. It prolongs the half-life of tolbutamide, chlorpropamide, phenytoin, and warfarin by inhibiting hepatic microsomal enzymes.

ERYTHROMYCIN Erythromycin is a macrolide antibiotic that acts primarily in a bacteriostatic fashion. It is effective against a wide range of microorganisms which include *S. pyogenes, S. pneumoniae,* many strains of *Neisseria,* some strains of *H. influenzae, C. diphtheriae, Clostridium, Listeria, Treponema,* and a number of anaerobic cocci and oral *Bacteroides* species. It is effective against *Mycoplasma pneumoniae* and *Legionella pneumophila.*

Erythromycin is used by either the oral or intravenous route. There are a number of different erythromycin preparations available. Esters and salts of erythromycin are more acid-stable. The erythromycin base and ethyl succinate forms are better absorbed when taken in the fasting state. The stearate form is better absorbed when taken with meals. It was originally thought that the estolate produced higher blood levels than other forms, but that appears to be an artifact of the assay system. The estolate salt is associated with more cholestatic hepatitis than are the other forms. The normal half-life of erythromycin is 1.5 h, and appreciable serum levels are maintained for at least 6 h. Therefore, in a number of infections such as streptococcal pharyngitis, the drug can be administered on a twice-daily basis. In anuric patients, reduction in dosage is generally not necessary.

Erythromycin is one of the safest antibiotics, and untoward reactions are extremely uncommon except for cholestatic hepatitis. The main side effect has been epigastric distress and nausea. Hearing loss does occur in association with large doses administered to elderly patients with renal insufficiency. Erythromycin used concomitantly with oral theophylline preparations may cause increased blood levels of theophylline and potential theophylline toxicity. Erythromycin also causes elevation in urinary catecholamines and in 17-hydroxycorticosteroids. The major use of erythromycin is to treat streptococcal pharyngitis in the penicillin-allergic patient, or in the treatment of otitis media, often in combination with sulfonamides. Erythromycin can also be used during pregnancy to treat skin infections or, in high doses, to treat syphilis in pregnancy. Erythromycin in a dose of 0.5 to 1 g every 6 h is the therapy of choice for *Legionella* pneumonia, and it is the drug of choice for *M. pneumoniae* infections.

LINCOMYCIN AND CLINDAMYCIN Lincosamide antibiotics inhibit many of the same organisms as do the erythromycins. Lincomycin is rarely used today and clindamycin is the primary agent in this class. Clindamycin inhibits *S. pneumoniae, S. pyogenes,* and viridans group streptococci. It does not have activity against *S. faecalis* (enterococcus). Many strains of *S. aureus* and *S. epidermidis* are inhibited by clindamycin, and it has excellent activity against most anaerobic species, including *Clostridium* and *Bacteroides*. It also inhibits *Chlamydia*.

Clindamycin is well-absorbed following oral ingestion and can also be administered intramuscularly or intravenously. The serum half-life is approximately 2.5 h, and the drug is metabolized primarily in the liver. Dosage adjustments are minor except in the presence of hepatic failure. Clindamycin produces high concentrations in bone, and has been found to enter white blood cells. Its most significant toxic effect is diarrhea, which has often been associated with pseudomembranous colitis caused by *C. difficile*. If diarrhea develops during clindamycin therapy, the drug should be discontinued. If diarrhea persists, proctoscopy or assay for *C. difficile* toxin should be performed and therapy with oral vancomycin or metronidazole instituted.

The major therapeutic use of clindamycin is for anaerobic infections or as a combination with an aminoglycoside. Clindamycin provides coverage against streptococcal, staphylococcal, and anaerobic species while the aerobic gram-negative organism is attacked by the aminoglycoside. Clindamycin has also been successfully combined with the monobactam aztreonam replacing the aminoglycoside. Clindamycin has proved to be an excellent agent for the therapy of anaerobic pulmonary disease, particularly in patients who have failed to respond to penicillin. Topical solutions of clindamycin are useful in the treatment of severe acne.

RIFAMPIN Rifampin is a macrocyclic antibiotic produced by a *Streptomyces*. Rifampin is available in the United States only for oral use. The drug has been used primarily in the treatment of tuberculosis. However, rifampin has a broad range of activity, inhibiting many microorganisms. It is extremely active against both coagulase-positive and -negative staphylococci. It also inhibits *N. meningitidis, N. gonorrhoeae,* and *H. influenzae*. It is the most active agent known against *L. pneumophila* and is also effective against *L. micdadei*. It inhibits *C. difficile* at concentrations less than 1 μg/mL and inhibits the majority of streptococci and *S. pneumoniae* at concentrations of less than 0.1 μg/mL. Although rifampin inhibits many of the Enterobacteriaceae and some strains of *Pseudomonas,* resistance develops rapidly. The drug inhibits *Chlamydia,* but *Ureaplasma urealyticum* and *Treponema pallidum* usually are resistant.

Rifampin is well-absorbed from the gastrointestinal tract and, following ingestion of 600 mg in an adult or 10 mg/kg in children, peak serum concentrations of approximately 7 μg/mL are reached. Concentrations increase over the first several days that the drug is taken. With repeated doses, drug levels decrease because the drug stimulates the hepatic enzymes responsible for its metabolism. The drug is approximately 75 percent protein-bound. Rifampin is both metabolized and excreted by the liver. The desacetyl derivative is not reabsorbed and is excreted via the stool; only 5 to 30 percent of the dose is excreted in the urine. In general, dosage adjustment is unnecessary in renal failure, but a lower dose should be used in patients with severe hepatic dysfunction. Food will interfere with the absorption of rifampin, lowering and delaying peak blood levels. Rifampin penetrates into all body tissues and enters white cells. High concentrations are found in lacrimal and salivary secretions; the drug penetrates well into bone. Cerebrospinal fluid levels as high as 1.3 μg/mL have been observed during treatment of meningitis.

The adverse effects of rifampin are few. On occasion, it will produce a flulike syndrome in individuals who take the drug intermittently. There have also been reports of interstitial nephritis, thrombocytopenia, and hemolytic anemia. Rifampin alters the metabolism of a number of drugs; it decreases the effect of exogenous steroids and interferes with birth control pills. It artificially lowers the serum concentration of thyroxin; tri-iodothyronine remains normal. Patients should be warned that rifampin will cause red discoloration of urine and can cause permanent staining of soft contact lenses. Rifampin crosses the placenta and has produced teratogenic effects in rodents, but such effects have not been observed in humans. However, the drug should only be used during pregnancy for severe tuberculosis. The major use of rifampin is in short-term (6 to 9 months) treatment of tuberculosis, combined with isoniazid (see Chap. 119). It is also used as prophylaxis for contacts of patients with meningococcal meningitis in a dose of 600 mg for 2 days in adults and 20 mg/kg for 2 days in children. It has also been recommended for prophylaxis of children under 4 years of age who have had close contact with a child with *H. influenzae* type B meningitis. Rifampin, combined with cloxacillin, has proved quite effective in eradicating nasal carriage in individuals with recurrent furunculosis. It may also be used to eradicate methicillin-resistant staphylococci when used in combination with vancomycin or trimethoprim-sulfamethoxazole. Rifampin has been used in the therapy of endocarditis due to tolerant *S. aureus* and for treatment of *Corynebacterium* species endocarditis. It is useful in patients who have failed to respond to erythromycin in Legionnaire's disease. Rifampin also may be useful combined with nafcillin or vancomycin in the treatment of chronic staphylococcal osteomyelitis.

METRONIDAZOLE Metronidazole is a nitroimidazole which is a potent bactericidal agent. It kills organisms within a twofold dilution of the inhibitory concentration: 99 percent of *B. fragilis* are inhibited by 8 μg/mL and 100 percent of *Fusobacterium* by 4 μg/mL. Most clostridial species are inhibited by 4 μg/mL. However, anaerobic gram-positive cocci may be less susceptible, as are *Actinomyces* and *Arachnida*. It is highly active against *C. difficile*. *Proprionibacterium acnes* are resistant, but *Gardnerella vaginalis, Campylobacter fetus,* oral *Spirochaeta,* and *Treponema* are inhibited by metronidazole.

Metronidazole is rapidly and almost completely absorbed when given orally. It can also be absorbed by rectal instillation and is available as an intravenous solution. There is minimal protein binding; the drug has a long half-life of 8 h. Absorption of metronidazole is not affected by food although peak levels are markedly delayed. Metronidazole is metabolized in the liver to a variety of hydroxy and glucuronide derivatives. Both metronidazole and its metabolites are eliminated in the urine and in the feces. Metronidazole dosage does not need to be adjusted in renal failure, but the drug is rapidly removed by hemodialysis. Therefore, additional doses should be given after dialysis. Although metronidazole is usually administered every 6 h, with its prolonged half-life, this frequent dosing is probably unnecessary. The standard dose is 500 mg every 6 h, but 500 mg every 8 h is adequate.

There are a number of adverse effects related to metronidazole. Rare but important reactions are seizures and encephalopathy, peripheral neuropathy, disulfiram-like reaction with alcohol, potentiation of the effects of warfarin, and, extremely rarely, pseudomembranous colitis. Minor problems that are associated with the drug are development of gastrointestinal disturbance, metallic taste, maculopapular rashes, or vaginal burning. Metronidazole is tumorigenic in rats. There is no evidence that this occurs in humans. Nevertheless, the drug should probably not be used in pregnancy.

Metronidazole is effective in treatment of serious anaerobic infections, with some exceptions. It is not useful in actinomycosis, and it has not been very effective in aspiration pneumonia, probably because of the large number of streptococci found in this infection. It is particularly useful in intraabdominal infections since it is able to penetrate abscesses and kill *Bacteroides* within the abscess. It has also been used in other anaerobic infections including bacteremia, osteomyelitis, and head-and-neck infections. Metronidazole can be used in the management of pseudomembranous colitis due to *C. difficile;* it is extremely inexpensive when administered orally. It is the drug of choice if oral vancomycin is not available. Metronidazole is a useful drug in the treatment of *Trichomonas* vaginitis and has also proved useful in the therapy of amebic liver abscess and intestinal amebiasis. It may be useful in *Blastocystis hominis* infections. Metronidazole has been used as prophylaxis for elective colonic surgery and gynecologic surgery or at the time of emergency appendectomy. However, the drug has no activity against gram-positive or gram-negative aerobic organisms.

POLYMYXINS Polymyxins are cyclic basic polypeptides. There are two compounds available, polymyxin B sulfate and polymyxin E, or colistin. Polymyxins are active only against aerobic gram-negative bacteria such as *Pseudomonas* and members of the Enterobacteriaceae. The compounds are not absorbed when given orally and must be administered parenterally. They are rapidly sequestered within the kidney and liver, reducing their clinical value. Both drugs produce very serious neuro- and nephrotoxicity. In view of the large number of other compounds available, there is no reason to use them.

SULFONAMIDES AND TRIMETHOPRIM Sulfonamides are bacteriostatic and act by interfering with folic acid metabolism in bacteria. They are generally classified as short-, medium-, or long-acting sulfonamides, sulfonamides limited to the gastrointestinal tract, and topical sulfonamides. Sulfonamides inhibit a variety of gram-positive bacteria and members of the Enterobacteriaceae, including *E. coli, Klebsiella,* and *Proteus.* They are also active against *Haemophilus,* but do not have activity against *P. aeruginosa.* The major problem with sulfonamides is that bacteria rapidly become resistant on the basis of plasmid-mediated production of altered enzymes. Most sulfonamides are administered orally, although sulfamethoxazole is available for intravenous use. Sulfonamides are absorbed rapidly from the small intestine and stomach. The compounds are distributed throughout the body and enter the CSF, synovial, pleural, and peritoneal fluids in concentrations that approximate 80 percent of serum levels. Sulfonamides are metabolized in the liver by acetylation and glucuronidation. They are excreted via glomerular filtration with partial reabsorption and tubular secretion. Sulfonamides differ widely in their protein binding, plasma half-life, metabolism, and solubility.

One of the major reasons that sulfonamide use has fallen off is that these agents produce a large number of serious side effects. These include a rash that appears in 3 to 5 percent of individuals, fever, jaundice, serum sickness–like syndrome, and acute hemolysis in the G6PD-deficient patient. They also may cause agranulocytosis, thrombocytopenia, and leukopenia. Sulfonamides cannot be administered during the last month of pregnancy since they cross the placenta and displace bilirubin from albumin and increase the risk of kernicterus. Long-acting sulfonamides have been associated with fatal hypersensitivity reactions; this has been noted with the longer-acting sulfonamides used in malarial preparations. By binding to albumin sites, sulfonamides may displace drugs such as warfarin, methotrexate, and hypoglycemic agents such as chlorpropamide. Sulfonamide concentrations are increased by indomethacin, salicylates, and probenecid. Tubular necrosis due to deposition of sulfa crystals within the kidney rarely occurs today.

Sulfadiazine is the most active sulfonamide attaining the highest blood and cerebrospinal fluid levels. However, it tends more often to produce crystalluria; hence sulfisoxazole and sulfamethoxazole are used more frequently. Mixtures of three sulfonamides are also available and can be used in the treatment of toxoplasmosis. Long-acting sulfonamides should be avoided because of the risk of severe erythema multiforme. Topical sulfonamide preparations such as silver-sulfadiazine or mafenide are extremely useful to reduce the number of bacteria in burn eschars.

Trimethoprim is a 2,4-diaminopyrimidine that is a dihydrofolate reductase inhibitor. Trimethoprim is active against most gram-positive cocci and gram-negative rods with the exception of *P. aeruginosa* and *Bacteroides.* It also has relatively poor activity against *Neisseria* species, and against *Chlamydia* and *Nocardia.* Resistance to trimethoprim has been fairly slow to develop. However, in the far east, strains of *Salmonella* and *Shigella* have become resistant, and toxigenic *E. coli* have been isolated in Central America which are resistant to trimethoprim and the combination of trimethoprim and sulfamethoxazole.

Trimethoprim is available as a single agent or a combined agent in a fixed combination of one part trimethoprim to five parts sulfamethoxazole. It is also available as an intravenous combination which contains one part trimethoprim and five parts sulfamethoxazole. Like the sulfonamides, trimethoprim is well-absorbed from the gastrointestinal tract. Most of the drug is excreted in the urine via tubular secretion; it has a serum half-life of 9 to 11 h in normal individuals. Trimethoprim-sulfamethoxazole can usually be given to patients with creatinine clearances greater than 30 mL/min in the usual doses and given in half doses to patients whose creatinine clearances are in the range of 15 to 30 mL/min. Trimethoprim itself may cause fever and rash and depression of white cells and platelets. This problem often can be avoided by the simultaneous administration of folinic acid. Pseudomembranous enterocolitis also can occur following use of trimethoprim-sulfamethoxazole.

Trimethoprim-sulfamethoxazole has been useful in the treatment of urinary tract infections, acute bacterial exacerbations of chronic bronchitis, and gastrointestinal infections due to *Salmonella, Shigella,* and toxigenic *E. coli.* Trimethoprim also is useful in the treatment of gonorrhea. Trimethoprim-sulfamethoxazole is used in high-dose oral or intravenous therapy of *Pneumocystis carinii* infections. Trimethoprim-sulfamethoxazole has also proved useful as prophylaxis in neutropenic children and in chronic granulomatous disease of childhood. The combination has been of particular value in the prevention of recurrent bacteriuria in women with recurrent urinary tract infections.

QUINOLONES Quinolones are synthesized chemically. They include nalidixic acid which inhibits gram-negative bacteria and, to a lesser extent, gram-positive organisms. It has been used primarily for the treatment of urinary tract infections. Nalidixic acid is a naphthyridine derivative while the new quinolones, which are some thousandfold more active than nalidixic acid, are true quinolone compounds. All of these agents bind to an enzyme, DNA gyrase, which is involved in the production of new DNA molecules.

The compounds can be considered in groups; nalidixic acid, oxolinic acid, and cinoxacin are one group. They inhibit the majority of strains of *E. coli, P. mirabilis, Klebsiella,* and *Enterobacter* at concentrations that readily can be achieved in urine. *Pseudomonas* species are resistant as are most gram-positive organisms, *S. aureus, S. pneumoniae,* and *S. faecalis.* Cross-resistance occurs between all three of the compounds. These agents are given by the oral route and are almost completely absorbed from the gastrointestinal tract. They are metabolized in the liver to biologically active and inactive compounds that are excreted by the kidney. The major difficulty with these agents has been the rapid development of resistance to them; hence they have not proved very effective in the treatment of urinary tract infections.

The new carboxyfluoroquinolones such as norfloxacin, enoxacin, pefloxacin, ofloxacin, and ciprofloxacin differ from the previously mentioned drugs because they have an extended antibacterial spectrum. All of these agents inhibit virtually all of the Enterobacteriaceae at concentrations below 1 μg/mL. In addition, they show varying activity against *Pseudomonas,* depending upon the particular compound. For example, ciprofloxacin is extremely active against *P. aeruginosa* and other *Pseudomonas* species, inhibiting isolates resistant to β-lactam and aminoglycoside antibiotics. The agents also inhibit *Haemophilus, Branhamella,* and methicillin-resistant staphylococci. They tend to have less activity against *S. pneumoniae* and generally do not inhibit *Bacteroides* and many clostridial species except at high concentrations.

These agents differ in their oral absorption. Oxfloxacin and enoxacin are more readily absorbed than are norfloxacin and ciprofloxacin. Absorption is markedly reduced in the presence of antacids, but not by H-2-blocking agents. The compounds are widely distributed in the body and are metabolized to both active and inactive products within the liver. The majority of these excretion products leave the body via the urinary tract, and they tend to accumulate in the presence of decreased renal function. The quinolones have been known to enter the CSF at therapeutic concentrations against *H. influenzae*, *N. meningitidis*, and Enterobacteriaceae, but they do not yield adequate concentrations for treatment of *S. pneumoniae* infections. High concentrations are achieved in bone, and studies of experimental osteomyelitis have demonstrated that the agents are superior to aminoglycosides. Several of these agents are available in Europe and Japan, but at present none are available for use in the United States. The compounds have been used in the treatment of urinary tract infections, respiratory tract infections, gastrointestinal disease due to *Salmonella* and *Shigella*, and pathogenic *E. coli* and *Campylobacter*. They have been successfully used in the treatment of osteomyelitis and skin infections. Ciprofloxacin has been extremely effective in therapy of *Pseudomonas* infections, including those occurring in cystic fibrosis patients.

Toxic and adverse reactions to these agents have been fairly rare. Gastrointestinal side effects have included nausea, vomiting, and occasionally diarrhea. Nonspecific rashes and urticaria have occurred. Ophthalmologic side effects have consisted of decreased visual and color perception, both of which have returned to normal with cessation of therapy. Central nervous system symptoms noted with nalidixic acid include headache, vertigo, seizures, and psychosis, but such reactions have not been reported with the 4-quinolones. It is too early to determine the precise role of these compounds in the chemotherapy of infection. However, they appear to be new and exciting agents to treat multiresistant microorganisms.

ANTITUBERCULOSIS DRUGS (See Chap. 119) Isoniazid remains one of the most important drugs for the treatment of tuberculosis. It should be included in any regimen for the treatment of patients with tuberculosis at any site. Isoniazid is well absorbed orally and can also be administered intramuscularly in patients unable to take oral medication. It enters the cerebrospinal fluid in concentrations adequate to treat tuberculous meningitis. The major concern with the use of isoniazid involves its hepatotoxicity. Approximately 15 percent of individuals who receive isoniazid develop elevations in SGOT. Individuals under 20 years of age rarely if ever have significant liver toxicity, but the frequency of hepatotoxicity in adults over 50 approximates 2 to 3 percent. The mechanism of toxicity remains unknown. Peripheral neuropathy may be seen in individuals who receive large doses and is more likely to be seen in individuals with alcoholism, diabetes, or uremia, and in particular those who are slow acetylators of the drug. Pyridoxine will not alter isoniazid's action, but will ameliorate the neuropathy. Isoniazid may also produce fever, skin eruption, and sideroblastic anemia. The most important aspect of monitoring isoniazid use is to follow liver function tests in older individuals.

Ethambutol is a tuberculostatic agent that is administered orally. It is well-absorbed from the gastrointestinal tract and is widely distributed throughout the body, including the cerebrospinal fluid. Resistance to the drug develops readily and hence it must always be used as a second drug to a primary compound such as isoniazid or rifampin. Retrobulbar neuritis occurs if the drug is used in large doses. For this reason, the dose should be kept under 15 mg/kg per day. Although complete blindness has occurred, visual acuity usually returns when the drug is stopped, and eventually patients' visual acuity will gradually return to normal.

Pyrazinamide is an analogue of nicotinamide that is used in short-course therapy for tuberculosis because of its bactericidal action against the tubercle bacillus. It may prove to be an extremely useful agent since it is active at an acid pH which is present in tuberculous cavities. Moreover, the compound appears to enter cells where the pH may be acid. Pyrazinamide is well absorbed orally and distributed throughout the body, including the CSF. It is metabolized in the liver, and its metabolic products are excreted in the urine. It should not be administered to individuals with renal failure. At doses of 20 to 35 mg/kg per day, the drug appears to cause a minimal amount of hepatotoxicity. Liver function tests should be monitored in individuals receiving pyrazinamide, particularly if they are receiving rifampin and isoniazid at the same time. The drug has been reported to cause gout. In certain settings, pyrazinamide can be administered once a week, and it is well tolerated in a twice-weekly program of 50 mg/kg when used in short courses.

There are a number of studies of the use of investigational antituberculous drugs to treat *M. avium-intracellulare* infections, which are a major problem in AIDS patients. One of these, ansamycin, is a rifampin derivative. Another agent is clofazimine, a drug that is ordinarily used in the treatment of leprosy. Results to date are not too encouraging. In vitro, ciprofloxacin, a new quinolone, has proved quite effective against atypical mycobacteria.

ANTIFUNGAL AGENTS See Chap. 146.

ANTIVIRAL AGENTS See Chap. 129.

ANTIPARASITIC AGENTS See Chap. 151 for a general discussion and Chaps. 153 to 168 for treatment of specific diseases.

REASONS FOR FAILURE OF CHEMOTHERAPY

This chapter, as well as the chapters which deal with specific disease entities, has documented that there are few microorganisms with the exception of fungi and viruses that are not susceptible to some antimicrobial agents. Nonetheless, a large number of patients who develop infections continue to die. In these patients, antimicrobial agents have failed. The failure of chemotherapy often is more apparent than real, and may be attributed to a number of different causes.

First, the infection being treated may not be due to a treatable microorganism but to a viral infection that will not respond to the chemotherapeutic agents that are being used. Antibiotics do not prevent bacterial complications of many viral infections.

A second common reason for failure of antimicrobial therapy is that purulent material has not been drained, or that a focus of obstruction or a foreign body has not been removed. Antimicrobial agents do not work well in these situations.

Third, fever may continue, not due to the infection, but as the result of development of hypersensitivity to one of the agents being used to treat the patient. Drug fever is particularly common with many of the antimicrobial agents of the β-lactam and sulfonamide class.

Occasionally, chemotherapy fails because the incorrect drug has been chosen or the culture results have been misinterpreted. This may be particularly true in respiratory infections. One of the most common errors when such a patient is not responding is to add more antimicrobial agents indiscriminately, when the correct course would be to discontinue therapy and observe the patient.

With many of the new antimicrobial agents, failure to provide an adequate dose of antibiotic is less frequently a problem than it was formerly. However, this still may be true in certain infections in which penetration of the antimicrobial agent to the particular area of the body is inadequate unless large doses are utilized.

Perhaps most importantly, the type of patient requiring antimicrobial therapy has shown a marked change in the past decade. More and more, today's patients lack host defenses, and include premature infants, elderly patients with degenerative and debilitating diseases, or patients who have received multiple antimicrobial agents, antineoplastic or immunosuppressive drugs, or who have undergone major surgical procedures. These individuals will tend to have much more difficulty in responding to antimicrobial therapy than normal uncompromised hosts, most of whom remain free of life-threatening infections.

REFERENCES

BARZA M: Imipenem: First of a new class of beta-lactam antibiotics. Ann Intern Med 103:552, 1985

GERDING DN (ed): Role of aminoglycosides as first-line therapy in multiple clinical settings. Am J Med 79(1A):1, 1985

NEU HC (ed): Advances in cephalosporin therapy: Beyond the third generation. Am J Med 79(2A):1, 1985
——— (ed): β-Lactamase inhibition: Therapeutic advances. Am J Med 79(5B):1, 1985
REMINGTON JS (ed): Carbapenems: A new class of antibiotics. Am J Med 78(6A):1, 1985
SCULLY BE, NEU HC: Use of aztreonam in the treatment of serious infections due to multiresistant gram-negative organisms, including *Pseudomonas aeruginosa*. Am J Med 78:251, 1985
SNAVELY SR, HODGES GR: The neurotoxicity of antibacterial agents. Ann Intern Med 101:92, 1984
WINSTON DJ et al: Moxalactam plus piperacillin versus moxalactam plus amikacin in febrile granulocytopenic patients. Am J Med 77:442, 1984

89 ACUTE INFECTIOUS DIARRHEAL DISEASES AND BACTERIAL FOOD POISONING

CHARLES C. J. CARPENTER

Acute diarrheal illnesses caused by bacterial, viral, or protozoal pathogens vary from slightly annoying bowel dysfunction to fulminant, life-threatening diseases. Largely because of the recognition of enterotoxigenic *Escherichia coli* as a major cause of acute diarrheal disease in adults and the identification of rotavirus as a frequent cause in young children, specific etiologic agents have been isolated from 80 to 85 percent of patients with acute diarrheal illnesses. Those illnesses caused by bacterial pathogens are more often life-threatening, at least among adults, and for that reason they will be addressed first. This chapter is aimed at presenting an overview of these diseases; in most instances, the entities are discussed in more detail in the chapters dealing with the specific etiologic agent.

In considering the bacterial diarrheas, it is useful to divide them into two groups, those caused by invasive and those caused by noninvasive microorganisms. The invasive pathogens, of which *Shigella* (see Chap. 108) may be considered the prototype, generally cause abdominal pain, fever, and other systemic symptoms, often including headache and myalgia. Illness caused by the noninvasive pathogens, of which cholera (see Chap. 115) is the prototype, is generally characterized by the absence of fever and few systemic symptoms (except those directly related to intestinal fluid loss). The invasive pathogens characteristically destroy gut mucosal cells, typically involving the terminal ileum and colon, and both leukocytes and erythrocytes are present, to a variable degree, in the stool. Inflammatory cells are generally absent from the stool in acute diarrheal disease caused by noninvasive bacterial pathogens.

NONINVASIVE BACTERIAL PATHOGENS

ENTEROTOXIGENIC *ESCHERICHIA COLI* Etiology and epidemiology Enterotoxin-producing *E. coli* (ETEC), which have the dual capacity to adhere to small-bowel epithelial cells and to produce one or more diarrheagenic toxins, are recognized as a major cause of acute diarrheal disease throughout most of the world and are the most common cause of "traveler's diarrhea." Largely because current techniques for demonstrating toxigenicity remain cumbersome, the epidemiology of ETEC diarrhea is poorly understood. ETEC are responsible for the majority of cases of traveler's diarrhea in visitors to the developing nations in South America, Africa, and Asia. ETEC are also one of the two (with rotavirus) leading causes of acute diarrheal illnesses in children throughout the developing world. ETEC have been implicated as a major cause of fulminant, cholera-like diarrheal disease in adult patients in south and southeast Asia but generally cause milder, self-limited diarrhea in adults in other parts of the developing world. There is no satisfactory explanation for the difference in severity in diarrhea caused by ETEC in different geographic areas. ETEC are rarely incriminated in episodic diarrheal illness in children and adults in the United States.

Pathogenesis The ability to cause diarrheal disease is not restricted to any one *E. coli* serotype but appears to be dependent upon the presence of both a plasmid-mediated colonization factor, which allows the *E. coli* to adhere to small-bowel mucosal cells, and one or more plasmids which code for the production of one or both of the two diarrheagenic toxins which may be produced by *E. coli*. The kinetics and mode of action of one of the toxins, which is heat labile (LT) and of relatively high molecular mass (~83,000 daltons), are similar to those of cholera enterotoxin (see Chap. 115); the diarrheagenic effect results from stimulation of adenylate cyclase in the gut epithelial cells. The other toxin, which is heat stable (ST) and of a lower molecular mass (<2000 daltons), has a more rapid onset of action and probably exerts its effect through stimulation of guanylate cyclase in the gut mucosal cells. Either or both toxins may be produced by ETEC. Most isolates from patients with severe diarrheal disease in Bangladesh produce both LT and ST, whereas isolates from patients in other developing nations have shown widely varying capacities for the production of LT, ST, or both. The wide clinical spectrum may be, in part, related to the predominant production of either LT or ST by the culpable microorganisms. The nutritional status of the host may also be a factor in determining the clinical response to ETEC.

Manifestations Both clinical observations and volunteer studies indicate that the incubation period is generally between 24 and 72 h. The illness which follows is quite variable, ranging from the fulminant, cholera-like disease often seen on the Indian subcontinent to the much milder Mexican "turista," in which the symptoms of mild, watery diarrhea, abdominal cramps, and occasional low-grade fever are more troublesome than life-threatening. Vomiting occurs in fewer than half the adults with *E. coli* diarrhea and is seldom responsible for major fluid losses.

In fulminant cases, the severe diarrhea seldom lasts longer than 24 to 36 h, and the response to either oral or intravenous electrolyte repletion is predictable and dramatic. With milder disease, the symptoms subside more gradually, occasionally persisting for a week or longer.

Laboratory findings As with cholera, no erythrocytes and few, if any, polymorphonuclear leukocytes are seen in a stool preparation stained with Loeffler's methylene blue. Because *E. coli* occurs normally among stool flora, and because its ability to produce enterotoxin is not restricted to any specific serotype, there is no rapid and simple means to make the laboratory diagnosis of enterotoxigenic *E. coli*. Bioassays for LT, based on the ability of *E. coli* isolates to produce fluid in isolated intestinal loops of experimental animals or to stimulate adenylate cyclase in cells in tissue culture, as well as the suckling mouse bioassay for ST, are reliable but of little value in patient management. Newer technology, utilizing DNA probes for rapid identification of the genes responsible for ST and LT production, appears promising and may be adapted for widespread use for epidemiologic purposes in the future.

Treatment The intestinal fluid losses are qualitatively identical to those in cholera. Therefore, in those patients who develop clinically significant saline depletion, the principles of fluid administration are identical to those described for cholera (see Chap. 115). Oral solutions containing electrolytes plus glucose or sucrose are consistently effective in correcting the saline depletion. Antibiotics (tetracycline, 30 mg/kg per day, given orally at 6-h intervals for 48 h; trimethoprim, 200 mg twice daily for 5 days; or trimethoprim, 160 mg, with sulfamethoxazole, 800 mg, twice daily for 5 days) are effective in decreasing the duration of illness but are not essential. Bismuth subsalicylate, 60 mL hourly for four doses, provides symptomatic relief (less frequent stools, less severe abdominal cramps). Both diphenoxylate and loperamide may provide rapid relief of abdominal cramps, but neither drug has been shown to alter the volume of intestinal fluid loss.

Prognosis With even the more fulminant cases of disease caused by ETEC with adequate fluid replacement, the prognosis is excellent.

Prevention Careful hygienic practices, with special attention to ingestion of clean water and adequately cooked foods, provide the most certain protection against enterotoxigenic *E. coli*. Doxycycline, 100 mg per day, is 60 to 90 percent effective as a prophylactic agent, the effectiveness varying with the tetracycline sensitivity of the ETEC in the geographic area. Trimethoprim, 160 mg, with sulfamethoxazole, 800 mg, taken once daily, is also effective in prophylaxis against traveler's diarrhea caused by ETEC.

CHOLERA See Chap. 115.

OTHER ENTEROTOXIGENIC ENTEROBACTERIACEAE Noninvasive strains of *Klebsiella* and *Enterobacter* occasionally have been implicated in acute diarrheal disease in developing areas of the world. The clinical illness produced is indistinguishable from the milder cases of diarrhea caused by enterotoxigenic *E. coli*, and treatment is the same.

CLOSTRIDIUM PERFRINGENS (See Chap. 101) This organism remains a significant cause of diarrheal disease and is implicated in many cases of acute food poisoning in the United States. Both the epidemiologic background and the clinical picture of *C. perfringens* diarrhea differ strikingly from those of *E. coli*. *Clostridium perfringens* diarrhea tends to occur in a microepidemic pattern following ingestion of contaminated meat, poultry products, or legumes. The relatively short incubation period of 6 to 12 h is an important diagnostic clue. Typically, two or more patients who have ingested the same meat dish become ill at roughly the same time. The production of a specific enterotoxin by the actively sporulating microorganisms in the intestinal tract appears to be responsible for all the symptoms. The clinical picture of diarrhea caused by *C. perfringens* is different from that caused by enterotoxigenic *E. coli* in one important respect, because moderately severe cramping abdominal pain, which is usually less prominent with *E. coli*, is a major presenting symptom. Treatment consists of symptomatic therapy with codeine to alleviate the cramping abdominal pain and intravenous fluid therapy in the small proportion of patients in whom there is clinical evidence of saline depletion. The illness is self-limited and rarely lasts for more than 24 h. Because of the relatively short natural course of the illness, antimicrobial therapy is of no value. Because *C. perfringens* normally inhabits mammalian and avian intestinal tracts, prevention is dependent upon adequate cooking and handling of meat and poultry products. The practice of allowing cooked meat products to cool slowly toward room temperature over 12 to 24 h permits germination of contaminating clostridial spores; this practice must be avoided.

STAPHYLOCOCCUS AUREUS (See Chap. 94) Acute staphylococcal diarrhea, classic "food poisoning," is due entirely to ingestion of preformed enterotoxin, and the causative organisms are often absent from the stool during the acute illness. This form of diarrhea often occurs in institutional outbreaks and is characterized by a short incubation period (2 to 6 h), relatively short duration (usually less than 10 h), and very high attack rates (often greater than 75 percent of the population at risk). In addition to its distinctive epidemiologic features, acute staphylococcal diarrhea differs from other noninvasive bacterial diarrheas by the prominence of vomiting, which is an almost constant feature and is apparently mediated by a direct effect of the absorbed toxin on the central nervous system. Treatment is directed toward correction of the saline depletion (intravenous fluids are required in 10 to 20 percent of patients) and, when necessary, toward symptomatic relief of vomiting. Because staphylococcal food poisoning is caused by preformed enterotoxin and is not perpetuated by viable microorganisms, antimicrobials are of no value.

A good example of the explosive nature of staphylococcal food poisoning was provided by an outbreak on a jet liner flying from Anchorage to Copenhagen. In this episode, 57 percent of 343 passengers developed an acute illness characterized by vomiting, diarrhea, and cramping abdominal pain. Of the 200 affected individuals, 30 required intravenous fluids, but none had serious sequelae. The food, contaminated by a pustule on the hand of a food handler, had not been adequately refrigerated aboard the plane, allowing abundant growth of the staphylococcus, with production of enterotoxin. Since staphylococci are ubiquitous, the prevention of massive contamination is dependent largely on control of growth conditions, primarily temperature. *Staphylococcus aureus* can multiply at temperatures from 4 to 46°C, and if contaminated food is allowed to remain at ambient temperatures after cooking, these organisms have ample opportunity to multiply, especially in such items as cream pastries, potato salad, and mayonnaise.

BACILLUS CEREUS *Bacillus cereus* is a cause of acute diarrheal disease which, although uncommon, has been identified with increasing frequency in Europe. The illness results from gross contamination of food with this gram-positive rod, which is capable of producing at least two discrete enterotoxins, one having characteristics similar to those of the labile enterotoxin of *E. coli* and the other having effects similar to that of staphylococcal enterotoxin. *Bacillus cereus* may, therefore, cause two distinct clinical syndromes, a diarrheal form resulting from the *E. coli* LT type of enterotoxin and an emetic form caused by the staphylococcal type of enterotoxin. The diarrheal syndrome caused by *B. cereus* is generally similar to that caused by enterotoxin-producing *E. coli*, with the exceptions that abdominal cramps are more common (75 percent of cases) and both the incubation period (6 to 14 h) and median duration of illness (20 h) are shorter. The emetic syndrome is clinically indistinguishable from that caused by staphylococcal enterotoxin, with a short incubation period (median 2 h), short duration (median 9 h), and prominent vomiting (100 percent compared with less than 25 percent in the diarrheal syndrome). Because both syndromes are self-limited and generally mild, no specific therapy is indicated. When *B. cereus* food poisoning is suspected clinically, the diagnosis can be confirmed by demonstration of 10^5 or more *B. cereus* organisms per gram in epidemiologically incriminated food. *Bacillus cereus* grows readily on simple laboratory media, including blood agar, but will not generally be identified as a pathogen unless such identification is specifically requested. Isolation of *B. cereus* from stool alone does not establish it as the etiologic agent because the organism is frequently found in the fecal flora of normal individuals. Since *B. cereus* is ubiquitous in soil, as well as in many raw, dried, and processed foods, proper food handling is the only practical means of preventing this form of food poisoning. The emetic form of *B. cereus* food poisoning almost invariably has been associated with ingestion of contaminated fried rice. *Bacillus cereus* is commonly present in uncooked rice, and its spores survive boiling and germinate, with production of the enterotoxin, when boiled rice is left unrefrigerated. Brief rewarming before serving is not adequate to destroy the relatively heat-stable toxin. Prompt refrigeration of boiled rice will prevent transmission of the disease.

INVASIVE AND/OR DESTRUCTIVE ENTERIC PATHOGENS

INTRODUCTION Shigellae characteristically invade the colon and terminal ileum, destroy segments of intestinal mucosa, cause extensive inflammatory changes in the lamina propria, and are the prototype of the invasive enteric bacterial pathogens. Other important invasive bacterial enteric pathogens include *Salmonella, Yersinia enterocolitica, Campylobacter jejuni, Vibrio parahemolyticus,* and invasive *E. coli*, which may have the capacity both to damage intestinal mucosa and to produce an enterotoxin. As opposed to the noninvasive pathogens, the invasive enteric organisms frequently cause systemic symptoms, including headache, myalgias, chills, and fever. As a general rule, antiperistaltic agents such as opiates, diphenoxylate, loperamide, and atropine are contraindicated in diarrheal disease caused by invasive enteric pathogens because they clearly worsen the clinical course in human shigellosis, as well as in salmonellosis and shigellosis in animal models.

The major therapeutic challenge in invasive bacterial diarrheas is that of distinguishing between (1) shigellosis and yersiniosis, in which antimicrobial therapy decreases the duration and severity of illness and shortens the period of fecal shedding of the pathogen, and (2) infections caused by *Salmonella,* which are characterized primarily by watery diarrhea and few systemic symptoms and in which antimicrobial therapy does not alter the duration of illness and may cause prolonged excretion of the pathogen.

SHIGELLOSIS See Chap. 108.

SALMONELLOSIS See Chap. 107.

YERSINIA ENTEROCOLITICA See Chap. 114.

CAMPYLOBACTER JEJUNI **Etiology and epidemiology** *Campylobacter jejuni* was first implicated in acute diarrheal disease in humans in 1972; by 1979 *C. jejuni* was second only to *Giardia lamblia* among recognized causes of waterborne diarrheal disease outbreaks in the United States. Attack rates have been highest in adolescents and young adults. *C. jejuni* occurs in the intestinal flora of many wild and domestic animals and poultry, and can be transmitted to humans by milk and water polluted by such animal carriers. The distribution of *C. jejuni* is worldwide, and *C. jejuni* appears to cause from 5 to 10 percent of acute diarrheal illnesses in both the industrialized and the developing areas of the world. Ingestion of raw milk and of water from contaminated mountain streams has been implicated in *Campylobacter enteritis* in North Ameria; in outbreaks associated with ingestion of raw milk, attack rates have reached 60 percent.

Pathogenesis *C. jejuni* causes patchy destruction of mucosa of both the small intestine, especially the distal ileum, and the colon; the stools, therefore, regularly contain pus cells and are occasionally grossly bloody. *C. jejuni* rarely produces transient bacteremia; when it does, it is likely to occur in an immunocompromised host.

Manifestations An incubation period of 2 to 6 days, longer than that of most bacterial enteric pathogens, is followed by fever, cramping abdominal pain, and diarrhea that is initially watery but later contains blood and mucus. The diarrhea, generally mild but occasionally voluminous, usually ceases within 2 to 5 days without specific antimicrobial therapy; on rare occasions the diarrhea may persist for 3 to 4 weeks. In some cases, the abdominal pain may be more prominent than the diarrhea, and the clinical picture may simulate acute appendicitis or, rarely, pancreatitis. (This may also be true in *Yersinia* enterocolitis; see Chap. 114.) In such cases, laparotomy has revealed acutely inflamed mesenteric lymph nodes as well as patchy inflammation of the small bowel. Acute reactive arthritis, similar to that associated with other invasive bacterial diarrheas (*Shigella, Salmonella, Yersinia*) may follow *C. jejuni* enteritis and is often associated wtih the HLA-B27 antigen.

Laboratory findings Diagnosis depends upon isolating *C. jejuni* from stool. Since this curved, motile bacillus does not compete well with other enteric flora on standard enteric media, it will rarely be isolated from stool unless special techniques are utilized. These include incubation at 42°C in a microaerobic atmosphere on blood agar to which a number of antimicrobials have been added. Serologic diagnosis is rarely helpful, as there are many serotypes of *C. jejuni,* and agglutination tests require use of the homologous organism.

Treatment Since *C. jejuni* usually produces a short, self-limited illness, antimicrobial therapy is not essential to management. Erythromycin, 30 mg/kg per day, does, however, significantly decrease the duration of fecal shedding of *C. jejuni* and may shorten the mean duration of illness. In the occasional patient who develops clinical signs of saline depletion, oral and/or intravenous fluids of the same sort used in cholera are uniformly effective (see Chap. 115).

OTHER *CAMPYLOBACTER* INFECTIONS The observation of small, curved, gram-negative rods with characteristic corkscrew-like motility in many stool specimens from which *C. jejuni* cannot be isolated has led to the identification of several additional species of *Campylobacter* which are associated with human disease. All such species, like *C. jejuni,* appear to be epizootic, but precisely which animals are the most common vectors for specific *Campylobacter* species is not known. This discussion will be limited to three species of *Campylobacter,* which represent the spectrum of illness caused by these microorganisms.

Campylobacter coli, although slightly different in biochemical characteristics, is identical to *C. jejuni* in morphology, growth characteristics and epidemiology, as well as in the illness which it produces.

Campylobacter fetus is similar to *C. jejuni* in morphology and growth characteristics but has a marked predilection for patients with chronic renal, hepatic, and neoplastic disease, alcoholism, and compromised immune function. Although the intestinal tract of the compromised host is the presumed site of entry, the intestinal infection may be mild or subclinical, and overshadowed by a bacteremic illness, associated with high fever, which often follows a prolonged or relapsing course and may be complicated by endocarditis, infection of preexisting aortic aneurysms, and/or septic phlebitis. Persistent bacteremia may be enhanced by the relative resistance of *C. fetus* to the bactericidal activity of normal serum.

Although occasional patients have had self-limited *C. fetus* sepsis, *C. fetus* bacteremia is usually fatal unless treated with antimicrobials. Gentamicin is thought to be the drug of choice, although no controlled observations are available. At least 4 weeks of antimicrobial treatment is recommended because of the tropism of *C. fetus* for intravascular sites.

Campylobacter cinaedi sp. n. has been the most frequently isolated of four *Campylobacter*-like organisms (CLOs) which have been associated with proctitis, proctocolitis, and enteritis in homosexual males. Although morphologically similar to *C. jejuni,* the CLOs grow poorly at 42° (and are therefore missed by the standard technique used to isolate *C. jejuni* and *C. fetus*), and prototype CLO strains show little (< 2 percent) DNA homology with *C. jejuni* and *C. fetus.* The CLO organisms grow slowly in a microaerophilic environment on modified brucella agar supplemented with 10% sheep blood.

Despite the differing growth characteristics, the CLOs produce changes which are indistinguishable from those caused by *C. jejuni* on sigmoidoscopic and histologic examination. Although the CLOs are sensitive to erythromycin, no controlled studies of antimicrobial therapy are available.

VIBRIO PARAHEMOLYTICUS **Etiology and epidemiology** *Vibrio parahemolyticus* is a curved, aerobic, nonmotile, gram-negative bacillus. Although present in coastal waters throughout the temperate zone, it has most commonly been associated with acute diarrheal illness in Japan, presumably because of the frequency of ingestion of raw seafood. It is regarded as the prototype of the halophilic vibrios because it grows more rapidly in 6% NaCl solutions than in the isotonic or hypotonic media used to culture most bacterial pathogens. *V. parahemolyticus* is responsible for a relatively small (< 10 percent) proportion of acute diarrheal illnesses in both adults and children in rural Bangladesh, where an association with seafood is less clearly established. It has been implicated in several outbreaks of acute diarrheal disease in the coastal United States, always as a common-source outbreak related to ingestion of inadequately cooked seafood, usually shrimp. Secondary cases caused by person-to-person transmission occur rarely. Several epidemics of *V. parahemolyticus* infections on cruise ships have been reported.

Pathogenesis Although *V. parahemolyticus* produces a toxin capable of causing intestinal fluid accumulation in experimental animals, the role of this toxin in human disease is not certain. *V. parahemolyticus* causes patchy mucosal damage in both distal ileum and colon; stools usually contain numerous polymorphonuclear leukocytes and are occasionally grossly bloody. The volume of fluid lost with *V. parahemolyticus* infection is relatively small, and intravenous fluids are seldom required. The illness is self-limited, with a median duration of just under 24 h.

Manifestations Within 6 to 48 h after ingestion of raw or inadequately cooked seafood, the patient develops an acute diarrheal illness. The volume of fluid lost is not great, moderately severe abdominal cramps may be a prominent feature, and chills and fever are observed in roughly half the cases. Vomiting is generally not prominent and occurs in no more than one-third of patients. The illness is self-limited, and no deaths have been reported in outbreaks involving over a thousand patients in the United States.

Laboratory findings When a common-source outbreak of acute diarrheal disease occurs in a group exposed to fresh or frozen seafood, the index of suspicion should be high and the diagnosis should be confirmed by plating a rectal swab on thiosulfate–citrate–bile salt–sucrose (TCBS) agar, on which typical colonies of *V. parahemolyticus* appear in 24 h. (This organism grows poorly and is therefore easily overlooked on deoxycholate culture plates.) The stool generally has numerous polymorphonuclear leukocytes and a smaller number of erythrocytes, but these findings are less prominent than in shigellosis.

Treatment No therapy is required by the large majority of patients. Antimicrobial therapy shortens neither the course nor the duration of pathogen excretion. Antiperistaltic agents are not of clear-cut benefit. An occasional patient may lose sufficient quantities of intestinal fluid to require oral or intravenous fluid therapy.

Prognosis The outcome is almost always good. Fatal cases, occasionally reported from Japan, have occurred in rare instances in patients with serious underlying disease.

VIBRIO MIMICUS *Vibrio mimicus* has been identified as a pathogen in sporadic outbreaks of acute diarrheal disease, occurring in previously healthy individuals of all age groups who have ingested raw seafood (especially oysters) along the Gulf Coast. The epidemiology of *V. mimicus* infections differs from that caused by *V. parahemolyticus* in that, with the exception of one small outbreak, all isolates have represented single, sporadic cases. Although *V. mimicus,* like *V. cholerae,* is not a halophilic vibrio (it grows more rapidly in 1% NaCl than in higher salt solutions), it does not produce cholera enterotoxin, and it causes an illness in which the presenting features are clinically indistinguishable from those caused by *V. parahemolyticus*.

Fever occurs in at least 40 percent of cases and bloody diarrhea in roughly 15 percent. Since the illness is self-limited, treatment is symptomatic. Antibiotic therapy is of no value.

INVASIVE *ESCHERICHIA COLI* Invasive *E. coli,* which are far less common pathogens than enterotoxigenic *E. coli,* may cause a clinical syndrome quite similar to shigellosis with the exceptions that vomiting seldom occurs with the invasive *E. coli* and the illness is of shorter duration. Diarrhea caused by invasive *E. coli* is rare in the United States but has been a significant cause of short-term disability in eastern Europe and southeast Asia. Since the illness caused by invasive *E. coli* is relatively short-lived, antimicrobial therapy has not been shown to be helpful.

CYTOTOXIC *ESCHERICHIA COLI* A single *E. coli* strain, 0157:H7, has been implicated in widely distributed sporadic cases of hemorrhagic colitis in the United States. Undercooked meat, especially hamburger, has been the most frequently identified mode of transmission. All age groups have been affected, and the clinical illness has been indistinguishable from shigellosis. Colonoscopy has demonstrated inflammation, edema, and/or hemorrhage, primarily in the ascending and proximal transverse colon. The mean duration of illness has been 8 days.

All *E. coli* 0157:H7 isolates tested have been noninvasive (Sereny test negative) but have produced Vero cytotoxin which is immunologically indistinguishable from the Shiga toxin produced by *Shigella dysenteriae* type I. Available data indicate that the hemolytic-uremic syndrome is as frequent following *E. coli* 0157:H7 colitis, as it is following shigellosis caused by *S. dysenteriae* type I.

With the exception of the few individuals who developed the hemolytic-uremic syndrome, the illnesses have been self-limited. Treatment with appropriate antimicrobials has not been shown to alter the duration or severity of the illness, but the sporadic occurrence of cases has prevented controlled studies of antibiotic therapy.

ACUTE VIRAL DIARRHEAS

Acute viral gastroenteritis is discussed in detail in Chap. 139. These illnesses are both more common and more life-threatening in small children than adults. In the United States, rotaviruses account for a large proportion of diarrheal illnesses during the first 2 years of life and usually occur during the winter. They have seldom been implicated in adult illness. In rural Bangladesh, infection with rotavirus accounts for roughly 60 percent of episodes of diarrhea in children from 6 to 24 months of age and for about 5 percent in the 2- to 5-year-old age group; it seldom occurs in adolescents and adults. The illness usually presents with vomiting followed by watery diarrhea and low-grade fever, with little or no associated abdominal pain. Vomiting is a prominent and almost constant early manifestation of rotavirus enteritis but rarely persists beyond the first 24 h. Diarrhea often persists for 4 to 8 days. Although the illness is generally not life-threatening, many patients require fluid and electrolyte repletion. Since the vomiting is usually short-lived, fluid repletion can generally be achieved by the oral route, using the same fluids that are effective in the treatment of cholera (see Chap. 115).

The diagnosis can be confirmed by a variety of tests including demonstration of the virus in stool by electron microscopy, a rise in complement-fixing antibody titers, and radioimmunoassay. The most useful and reliable test for rapid diagnosis under field conditions consists of direct demonstration of the antigen in stool by the enzyme-linked immunosorbent assay (ELISA).

Norwalk and Norwalk-like viruses, now implicated in roughly a third of episodes of epidemic gastroenteritis involving adults in the United States, usually cause relatively mild, short (< 36 h), and self-limited disease, for which neither fluid nor drug therapy is necessary (see Chap. 139).

ACUTE PROTOZOAL DIARRHEAS

Giardia lamblia has emerged as a major cause of acute diarrheal disease (see Chap. 160). Although formerly thought to be a pathogen only in children and later considered to be a significant cause of diarrheal disease only in developing nations, this organism is the pathogen most commonly incriminated in outbreaks of waterborne diarrheal disease in the United States where it occurs most commonly in the Rocky Mountain states and more frequently causes disease in visitors than in the indigenous population. The illness characteristically presents with the sudden onset of watery diarrhea and malabsorption, accompanied by mild to moderate abdominal discomfort, bloating, and flatulence. Symptoms may occasionally persist for weeks unless appropriate antimicrobials are administered. Prolonged disease with malabsorption occurs from time to time in previously normal individuals but is particularly common in patients with IgA deficiency, who tend to have the most severe form of giardiasis.

The attack rate may be quite high (> 50 percent) in individuals exposed to contaminated water sources. In certain groups of North American travelers returning from Leningrad, where the water supply appears to be heavily contaminated with *Giardia* cysts, up to 60 percent of individuals have developed clinical giardiasis. The usual incubation period is 10 to 20 days. The illness, therefore, frequently develops after a traveler returns home, and the travel history is a critical element in suspecting the diagnosis. Occasionally the disease occurs endemically in individuals who have not traveled. The diagnosis can be confirmed in approximately half the cases by examining the stool for cysts; if the stool examination is negative in a patient with characteristic clinical features, duodenal aspirates or biopsies will usually yield the characteristic trophozoites. Treatment with quinacrine, 100 mg tid for 5 to 7 days, is generally curative; metronidazole, 250 mg tid for 7 days, is an equally effective alternative regimen.

TRAVELER'S DIARRHEA

Diarrhea is by far the most common health problem of travelers to developing countries. Of more than 16 million travelers annually from industrialized nations to developing countries, approximately one-third will develop diarrhea. The incidence of traveler's diarrhea (TD) varies markedly by destination.

ETIOLOGY AND EPIDEMIOLOGY Virtually all cases of TD are caused by infectious agents, acquired through ingestion of fecally contaminated food and/or water. Especially risky foods include raw vegetables, raw meats, and raw seafood. Foods sold by street vendors are a common source of enteropathogens. Bacterial pathogens account for the great majority of episodes. Overall, the most common etiologic agents in TD are enterotoxigenic *E. coli* (ETEC), which are responsible for 50 to 75 percent of episodes. The culpable ETEC may produce LT, ST, or both enterotoxins, with considerable geographic variation. Other recognized enteropathogens can be isolated from most of the remainder of cases, but with great regional differences in prevalence. For example, *Shigella* causes up to 10 percent of TD in Mexico but is an unusual etiologic agent in North Africa. *Vibrio parahemolyticus* is a relatively common cause of TD in Japanese travelers in Asia but has not been associated with TD in South America. Viruses (rotavirus, Norwalk-like virus) and protozoa (amoebas, *Giardia*) are collectively responsible for fewer than 10 percent of cases of TD.

PATHOGENESIS The pathogenesis varies with the culpable etiologic organism, but most cases of TD, even when caused by *Shigella,* are self-limited illnesses and have not been associated with serious sequelae in previously healthy individuals.

MANIFESTATIONS Episodes of TD usually begin abruptly, with urgent diarrhea, abdominal cramps, nausea, and often low-grade fever. In the great majority of cases, the fluid loss is not voluminous, and symptoms subside within 3 to 5 days.

TREATMENT For the great majority of patients, fluid losses do not demand specific replacement fluids. Patients want relief from the two specific problems of abdominal cramps and diarrhea. Bismuth subsalicylate, taken as Pepto-Bismol liquid, in a dose of 60 mL qid, can decrease the severity of symptoms. Diphenoxylate and loperamide both provide symptomatic relief, but should not be used in the rare patient with high fever or blood in the stool; the antimotility agents should be discontinued if symptoms persist beyond 48 h. Patients with more severe symptoms (e.g., more than three loose stools within 8 h) may benefit from antimicrobial treatment. Trimethoprim, 160 mg, with sulfamethoxazole, 800 mg, twice daily, or trimethoprim alone, 200 mg twice daily for 3 days, has proved effective in shortening the mean duration of symptoms from 4 to 1.5 days. It is not certain that these antimicrobials will prove equally effective in all parts of the developing world.

PREVENTION The only sure prevention is to avoid ingestion of contaminated water and food, a goal that is not practical for most travelers. Carefully controlled studies have demonstrated that two antimicrobials, doxycycline and trimethoprim-sulfamethoxazole, when taken prophylactically, are consistently effective in reducing the incidence of TD by 50 to 86 percent in various parts of the developing world. Because of the calculable risks of administration of prophylactic antimicrobials to several million travelers annually, balanced against the generally self-limited course of TD, prophylactic antimicrobials are not routinely recommended for prevention of TD. Travelers are advised, however, to obtain therapeutic doses of effective antimicrobial agents (vide supra) prior to travel to high-risk areas, so that the more severe episodes of TD can be treated early, without recourse to potentially dangerous over-the-counter drugs.

REFERENCES

BARKER WH JR et al: *Vibrio parahemolyticus* outbreak in Covington, Louisiana, in August, 1972. Am J Epidemiol 100:316, 1974

BLACKLOW NR, CUKOR G: Viral gastroenteritis. N Engl J Med 304:397, 1981

BLASER MJ et al: *Campylobacter* enteritis in the United States: A multicenter study. Ann Intern Med 98:360, 1983

———, RELLER BL: *Campylobacter* enteritis. N Engl J Med 305:1444, 1981

CARPENTER CCJ, SACK RB: Infectious diarrheal syndromes, in *Update I: Harrison's Principles of Internal Medicine,* KJ Isselbacher et al (eds). New York, McGraw-Hill, 1981, pp 209–229

CONSENSUS CONFERENCE: Traveler's diarrhea. J Am Med Assoc 253:2700, 1985

DUPONT HL et al: Pathogenesis of *Escherichia coli* diarrhea. N Engl J Med 285:1, 1971

——— et al: Symptomatic treatment of diarrhea with bismuth subsalicylate among students attending a Mexican university. Gastroenterology 73:715, 1977

——— et al: Treatment of traveler's diarrhea with trimethoprim/sulfamethoxazole and with trimethoprim alone. N Engl J Med 307:841, 1982

GORBACH SL et al: Traveller's diarrhea and toxigenic *Escherichia coli.* N Engl J Med 292:933, 1975

GRIFFIN MR et al: Foodborne Norwalk virus. Am J Epidemiol 115:178, 1982

GUERRANT RL et al: Role of toxigenic and invasive bacteria in acute diarrhea of childhood. N Engl J Med 293:576, 1974

——— et al: Campylobacteriosis in man: Pathogenic mechanisms and review of 91 bloodstream infections. Am J Med 65:584, 1978

KAPLAN JE et al: Epidemiology of Norwalk gastroenteritis and the role of Norwalk virus in acute nonbacterial gastroenteritis. Ann Intern Med 96:756, 1982

MERSON MH et al: Traveler's diarrhea in Mexico. A prospective study of physicians and family members attending a Congress. N Engl J Med 294:1299, 1976

QUINN TC et al: Infections with *Campylobacter jejuni* and *Campylobacter*-like organisms in homosexual men. Ann Intern Med 101:187, 1984

REMIS RS et al: Sporadic cases of hemorrhagic colitis associated with *Escherichia coli* 0157:H7. Ann Intern Med 101:624, 1984

SACK DA et al: Oral rehydration in rotavirus diarrhea: A double blind comparison of sucrose with glucose electrolyte solution. Lancet 2:280, 1978

——— et al: Prophylactic doxycycline for traveller's diarrhea. N Engl J Med 298:758, 1978

SACK RB et al: Enterotoxigenic *Escherichia coli* isolated from patients with severe cholera-like disease. J Infect Dis 123:378, 1971

——— et al: Human diarrheal disease caused by enterotoxigenic *Escherichia coli.* Annu Rev Microbiol 29:333, 1975

TAYLOR DN et al: *Campylobacter* enteritis from untreated water in the Rocky Mountains. Ann Intern Med 99:38, 1983

TERRANOVA W et al: Current concepts: *Bacillus cereus* food poisoning. N Engl J Med 298:143, 1978

ZEN-YOJI H et al: Epidemiology, enteropathogenicity and classification of *Vibrio parahemolyticus.* J Infect Dis 115:436, 1965

90 SEXUALLY TRANSMITTED DISEASES

KING K. HOLMES / H. HUNTER HANDSFIELD

Venereology encompasses not only the five "venerable" venereal diseases (syphilis, gonorrhea, chancroid, lymphogranuloma venereum, and granuloma inguinale) but also a growing number of other diseases which might be considered the "new generation" of sexually transmitted diseases (STDs). The most recently recognized STD is the acquired immunodeficiency syndrome, caused by the AIDS retrovirus (see Chaps. 257 and 293). Like gonorrhea, many of these newer STDs became epidemic in nearly all countries of the world during the past quarter-century. With increasing interest in these diseases and improved methods for diagnosis has come awareness of the growing consequences of STD on health and society, which extend beyond the traditional sphere of venereology; for example, major impact of the newer STDs has been noted on maternal and infant morbidity and on human infertility and reproduction.

CLASSIFICATION OF SEXUALLY TRANSMITTED DISEASES These diseases can be classified on the basis either of their etiologies or their clinical manifestations. Table 90-1 gives an etiologic classification of STD. Sexual transmission has been implicated as an important factor in the propagation of each of the pathogens listed in this table. There have been sporadic case reports of sexual transmission of many other pathogenic agents, but the diseases caused by these other agents are not generally considered, since sexual transmission seems to be a minor factor in their propagation. For each of the agents listed in Table 90-1, there are one or more diseases or syndromes known to be caused by the agent, and others (indicated by a question mark) for which a causal association is suspected but not proven.

APPROACH TO SEXUALLY TRANSMITTED DISEASE The STDs are viewed throughout the world as a related set of infections for several reasons: knowledge of infectious diseases and dermatology are important for diagnosis and management; skills in the genitourinary examination are required; they are sexually transmitted; and coinfections are common. However, the principal reason for dealing with STDs as a unique set of infections is that no single STD can be regarded as an isolated problem. STDs are not endogenous or transmitted by fomites, food, flies, or casual contact. *An infected partner always exists*. The sexual history and management of sexual partners are therefore of paramount importance. Failure to identify and examine or refer at least one partner represents a failure in management, both at the community level (since sources of spread of infection are not identified) and at the patient level (since reinfection is not prevented). Most persons with genital discharges, lesions, or pain cease sexual activity and seek medical care. Accordingly, those who transmit infection usually are among the minority who are infected but asymptomatic, or who do not understand the implications of their symptoms. Therefore, they do not seek medical attention spontaneously, and physicians must see that they are examined and treated, or referred. In the United States, local health departments will usually identify and treat contacts of some diseases (e.g., syphilis, gonococcal pelvic inflammatory disease), but for most STDs this responsibility is shared by the patient and the physician. With the increasing importance of potentially incurable viral STDs (AIDS retrovirus infection, genital herpes, genital papillomaviruses, hepatitis B virus carriage), the role of counseling to reduce transmission is growing. It is necessary for the clinician to consider the approach to STD syndromes before an etiologic diagnosis is established. Table 90-2 lists some of the most common clinical syndromes and their complications associated with sexually transmitted pathogens. Strategies for the management of some of the common syndromes are outlined below.

MALE URETHRITIS Urethritis in the male is classified as gonococcal or nongonococcal. The incidence of gonococcal urethritis has stabilized in many western countries, while that of nongonococcal urethritis (NGU) continues to rise, suggesting that current measures for control of NGU are relatively ineffective. In general, gonorrhea and NGU are equally common among men seen in STD clinics in the United States, whereas NGU is approximately three times as common as gonorrhea among men seen by physicians in private practice and 10 times as common as gonorrhea among college students.

About 40 percent of NGU is caused by *Chlamydia trachomatis*. Herpes simplex virus and *Trichomonas vaginalis* each cause a small additional proportion of NGU cases in the United States, but about 50 percent of cases cannot be attributed to any of these three pathogens. *Ureaplasma urealyticum* has been implicated in case-control studies as a probable cause of many of the *Chlamydia*-negative cases. A newly described organism, *Mycoplasma genitalium*, is also under investigation as a possible cause of this syndrome. Since facilities for detection of *U. urealyticum* and *M. genitalium* are not widely available, and the role of these agents is not certain, the diagnosis of male urethritis usually does not include cultures for either organism. However, diagnostic testing for *C. trachomatis* is increasingly available, using isolation of the agent in tissue cell culture, or direct immunofluorescent staining of urethral exudate or enzyme-linked immunosorbent assay for detection of chlamydial antigen. The following steps should be taken in evaluating sexually active men with symptoms of urethral discharge and/or dysuria:

1 Establish the presence of urethritis. Commonly in NGU, and less often in gonorrhea, discharge can be demonstrated only by milking the urethra after the patient has not voided for several hours, preferably overnight. If no overt discharge is demonstrable, urethral inflammation can be documented by inserting a small urethrogenital

TABLE 90-1 Twenty-four sexually transmitted pathogens and the diseases they cause

Agent	Disease or syndrome
BACTERIA	
Neisseria gonorrhoeae	Urethritis, epididymitis, proctitis, cervicitis, endometritis, salpingitis, perihepatitis, bartholinitis, pharyngitis, conjunctivitis, prepubertal vaginitis, ?prostatitis, accessory gland infection, amniotic infection syndrome, disseminated gonococcal infection, chorioamnionitis, premature rupture of membranes, and premature delivery
Chlamydia trachomatis	Urethritis, epididymitis, proctitis, cervicitis, endometritis, salpingitis, perihepatitis, bartholinitis, prepubertal vaginitis, otitis media in infants, ?chorioamnionitis, ?premature rupture of membranes, ?premature delivery, inclusion conjunctivitis, infant pneumonia, trachoma, and lymphogranuloma venereum
Mycoplasma hominis	Postpartum fever, ?salpingitis
Ureaplasma urealyticum	?Nongonococcal urethritis, ?chorioamnionitis, ?premature delivery
Treponema pallidum	Syphilis
Gardnerella vaginalis and other vaginal bacteria	Bacterial vaginosis
Haemophilus ducreyi	Chancroid
Calymmatobacterium granulomatis	Donovanosis (granuloma inguinale)
Shigella spp.	Shigellosis in homosexual men
Campylobacter spp.	Enteritis, proctocolitis in homosexual men
Group B streptococcus	Neonatal sepsis, neonatal meningitis
VIRUSES	
AIDS retrovirus (HTLV III/LAV)	Acute mononucleosis-like syndrome, AIDS-related complex (including persistent generalized lymphadenopathy), acquired immunodeficiency syndromes, ?subacute encephalitis and other neurologic syndromes
Herpes simplex virus	Initial and recurrent genital herpes, aseptic meningitis, neonatal herpes, cervical dysplasia and carcinoma, ?carcinoma in situ of the vulva
Hepatitis B virus	Acute hepatitis B, chronic active hepatitis, persistent (unresolved) hepatitis, polyarteritis nodosa, chronic membranous glomerulonephritis, ?mixed cryoglobulinemia, ?polymyalgia rheumatica, hepatocellular carcinoma
Hepatitis A virus	Acute hepatitis A
Cytomegalovirus	Heterophil-negative infectious mononucleosis, congenital infection, gross birth defects and infant mortality, cognitive impairment (e.g., mental retardation, sensorineural deafness), varied manifestations in the immunosuppressed host
Human papilloma virus types 6, 11, 16, 18, 31	Condyloma acuminatum, laryngeal papilloma, cervical dysplasia, Bowen's papulosis, ?squamous cell carcinoma of the cervix, vulva, penis, and anus
Molluscum contagiosum virus	Genital molluscum contagiosum
PROTOZOA	
Trichomonas vaginalis	Trichomonal vaginitis
Entamoeba histolytica	Amebiasis in homosexual men
Giardia lamblia	Giardiasis in homosexual men
FUNGI	
Candida albicans	Vulvovaginitis, balanitis
ECTOPARASITES	
Phthirius pubis	Pubic lice infestation
Sarcoptes scabiei	Scabies

TABLE 90-2 Selected syndromes and complications with corresponding sexually transmitted etiologic agents*

Syndrome	Agent
MEN	
Urethritis	*N. gonorrhoeae, C. trachomatis,* herpes simplex virus, *T. vaginalis U. urealyticum*
Epididymitis	*C. trachomatis, N. gonorrhoeae*
Intestinal infections:	
Proctitis	*N. gonorrhoeae,* herpes simplex virus, *C. trachomatis*
Proctocolitis or enterocolitis	*Campylobacter* spp., *Shigella* spp., *E. histolytica*
Enteritis	*G. lamblia*
Hepatitis	Hepatitis A and B viruses, cytomegalovirus, *T. pallidum*
Acquired immunodeficiency and related syndromes	AIDS retrovirus (HTLV III/LAV)
WOMEN	
Lower genitourinary tract infection:	
Vulvitis	*C. albicans,* herpes simplex virus
Vaginitis	*T. vaginalis, C. albicans, ?G. vaginalis*
Cervicitis	*N. gonorrhoeae, C. trachomatis,* herpes simplex virus
Urethritis	*N. gonorrhoeae, C. trachomatis,* herpes simplex virus
Pelvic inflammatory disease	*N. gonorrhoeae, C. trachomatis, ?Mycoplasma hominis*
Infertility:	
Postsalpingitis, postobstetric, postabortion	*N. gonorrhoeae, C. trachomatis, ?M. hominis*
Pregnancy morbidity: Chorioamnionitis, amniotic fluid infection, prematurity, premature rupture of membranes, postpartum endometritis, ectopic pregnancy	Several STD agents have been implicated in one or more of these conditions
MEN AND WOMEN	
Neoplasia	
Squamous cell epithelial dysplasia and cancer (cervix, vulva, penis, anus)	?Human papillomavirus, ?herpes simplex virus
Hepatocellular carcinoma	Hepatitis B
Kaposi's sarcoma	AIDS retrovirus (?cofactors)
Non-Hodgkin's lymphomas	
Genital ulceration with or without regional lymphadenopathy	Herpes simplex virus, *T. pallidum, H. ducreyi, Cal. granulomatis, C. trachomatis* (LGV strains)
Acute arthritis with urogenital or intestinal infection	*N. gonorrhoeae, C. trachomatis, Shigella* spp., *Campylobacter* spp.
Genital warts, molluscum contagiosum	Human papilloma virus, molluscum contagiosum virus
Ectoparasite infestations	*Sarcoptes scabiei, Phthirius pubis*
Heterophil-negative mononucleosis	Cytomegalovirus, ?Epstein-Barr virus
NEONATES AND INFANTS	
TORCHES syndrome†	Cytomegalovirus, herpes simplex virus, *T. pallidum*
Conjunctivitis	*C. trachomatis, N. gonorrhoeae*
Pneumonia	*C. trachomatis, ?U. urealyticum*
Otitis media	*C. trachomatis*
Sepsis, meningitis	Group B streptococcus
Cognitive impairment, deafness	Cytomegalovirus, herpes simplex virus, *T. pallidum*
AIDS and AIDS-related diseases	AIDS retrovirus

* *For each syndrome, some cases cannot yet be ascribed to any cause and must currently be considered idiopathic.*
† *TORCHES is an acronym for toxoplasmosis, rubella, cytomegalovirus, herpes, and syphilis. The syndrome consists of various combinations of encephalitis, hepatitis, dermatitis, and disseminated intravascular coagulation.*

swab 2 to 3 cm into the urethra and examining the Gram-stained direct smear prepared from this swab for leukocytes. Five or more leukocytes per 1000× field in areas containing cells suggests urethritis. Patients with symptoms who lack objective confirmatory evidence of urethritis on two occasions 1 week apart may have functional problems and generally do not benefit from repeated courses of antibiotics.

2 *Exclude complications or alternative diagnoses.* Epididymitis and systemic complications, such as the gonococcal arthritis-dermatitis syndrome and Reiter's syndrome, should be excluded by brief history and examination. Bacterial prostatitis and cystitis should be excluded by appropriate tests in men with dysuria who lack signs of urethritis. However, digital examination of the prostate gland is seldom informative in patients with urethritis, unless concomitant symptoms such as perineal, suprapubic, or rectal discomfort are present.

3 *Evaluate for gonococcal and chlamydial infection.* The diagnosis of gonorrhea is confirmed by demonstrating typical gram-negative diplococci within neutrophils. The diagnosis of NGU is warranted if gram-negative diplococci are not found. Smears containing only extracellular or atypical gram-negative diplococci are equivocal. In most settings, an attempt should be made to isolate *N. gonorrhoeae* by culture in order to document antimicrobial susceptibility, and also because the predictive value of Gram-stained urethral smears is dependent on the experience of the laboratory. Diagnostic testing for *C. trachomatis* (culture or detection of antigen by immunodiagnosis) should also be performed if resources are available, regardless of the presence or absence of gonorrhea, since coinfection with *N. gonorrhoeae* and *C. trachomatis* is common in men with urethritis. Treatment recommended for gonorrhea includes antimicrobials also effective against *C. trachomatis,* but detection of *Chlamydia* in the male will facilitate management of sexual partners. An approach to the diagnosis of urethritis is illustrated in Fig. 90-1. The treatment of gonorrhea and chlamydial infections is discussed in Chaps. 104 and 150, respectively.

EPIDIDYMITIS Acute epididymitis is almost always unilateral and must be differentiated from testicular torsion, tumor, and trauma. Torsion, a surgical emergency, usually occurs in adolescents and young adults and is suggested by sudden onset of pain, elevation of the testicle within the scrotal sac, and absence of blood flow on Doppler examination or ^{99}Tc scan. In sexually active men under age 35, acute epididymitis is usually caused by *C. trachomatis,* or less commonly by *Neisseria gonorrhoeae,* and is usually associated with overt or subclinical urethritis. Antimicrobial agents are the mainstay of therapy; optimal treatment for epididymitis due to *C. trachomatis* is doxycycline 100 mg twice daily for 10 days. For gonococcal epididymitis, this regimen should be preceded by a single dose of an antibiotic active against both penicillin-sensitive and penicillin-resistant *N. gonorrhoeae,* such as ceftriaxone 125 to 250 mg intramuscularly. Bed rest and scrotal elevation may hasten symptomatic relief.

Acute epididymitis in older men or following urinary tract instrumentation is usually caused by urinary pathogens such as coliform bacteria or *Pseudomonas aeruginosa.* Urethritis is usually absent, but bacteriuria is present. Treatment should be initiated with a broad-spectrum, parenteral antibiotic (e.g., tobramycin) and continued with the appropriate antibiotics as determined by sensitivity tests. An algorithm for diagnosis and management of acute epididymitis in sexually active men is presented in Fig. 90-2.

LOWER GENITOURINARY TRACT INFECTION IN WOMEN Infections of the female urinary tract, cervix, vulva, and vagina produce dysuria, vulvar irritation, dyspareunia, and altered quality or increased quantity of vaginal discharge. Diagnostic confusion may be attributable not only to the symptomatology, which is nonspecific, but also to the lack of consistent application of available laboratory tests, and to the difficulty in differentiating true inflammatory conditions from functional genitourinary complaints. Two steps are required in the evaluation of lower genitourinary symptoms in women: (1) differentiation among cystitis, urethritis, vaginitis, cervicitis, and cervical ectopy, and (2) exclusion of associated upper tract disease (e.g., pyelonephritis, salpingitis).

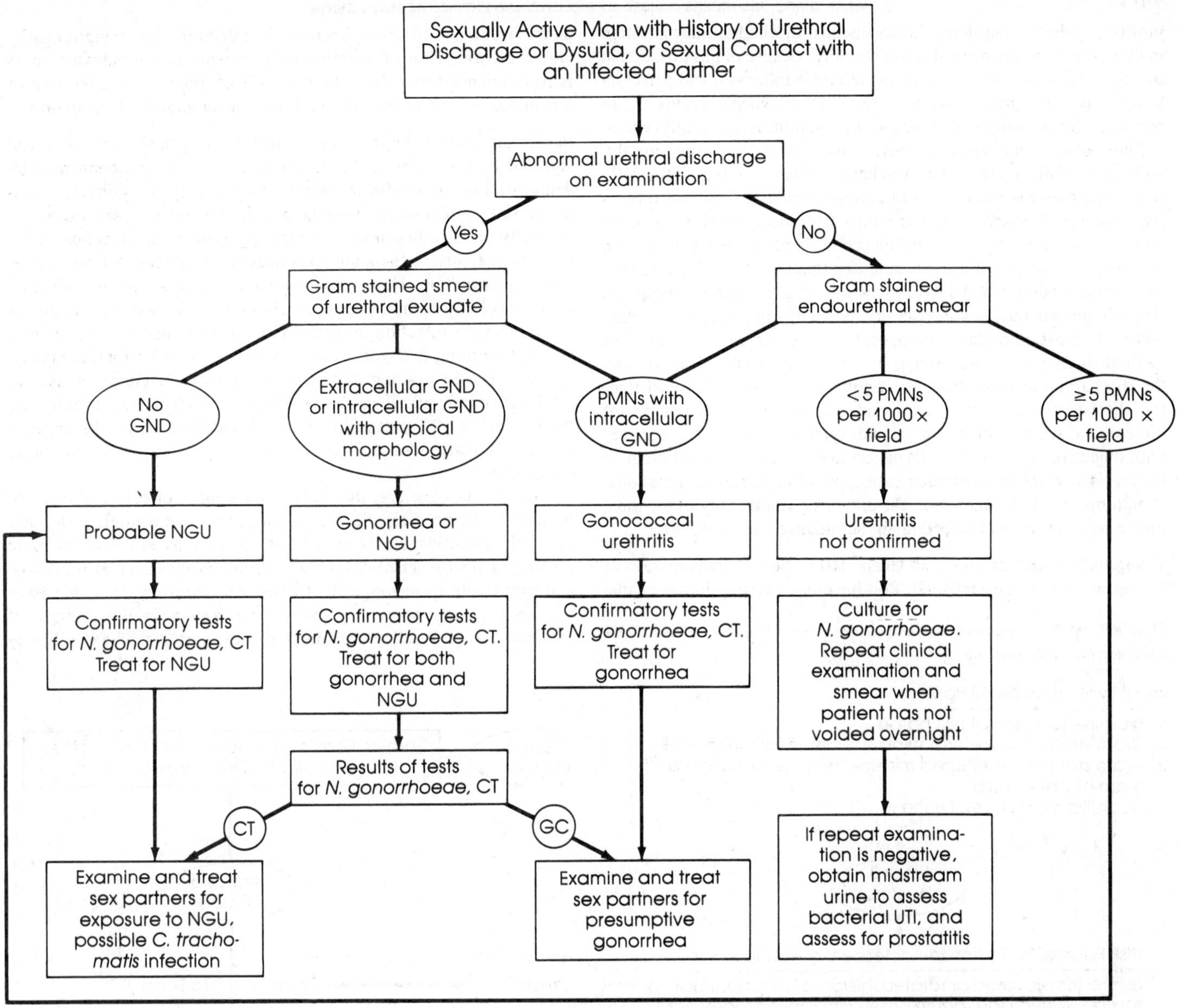

FIGURE 90-1 *Evaluation of sexually active men with suspected urethritis. PMN = polymorphonuclear leukocyte; GND = gram-negative diplococci; NGU = nongonococcal urethritis; UTI = urinary tract infection.*

Cystitis and urethritis Although dysuria is more common in bacterial urinary tract infection (UTI) than in vaginitis, dysuria is often attributable to vaginitis in young women because vaginitis is substantially more common than UTI. Localization of dysuria as "internal" is suggestive of UTI or "urethritis," while "external" dysuria (caused by painful contact of urine with the labia) is associated with vulvovaginitis. In a study of female college students with dysuria, urgency, or frequency without vaginal infection, about half had bacterial cystitis with 10^5 bacteria or more per milliliter of urine, and one-quarter had bacterial cystitis with less than 10^5 bacteria per milliliter (usually between 10^2 and 10^5 per milliliter). About one-quarter had urethral symptoms without bacteriuria—often termed the *urethral syndrome* or *dysuria-frequency syndrome*. In the latter group, about half had pyuria, and most of these were infected with *C. trachomatis*, while most of those without pyuria had no demonstrable infection and improved with placebo therapy. In populations whose risk of gonorrhea is higher than that of college students, *N. gonorrhoeae* is also a common cause of the urethral syndrome.

DIAGNOSIS AND THERAPY As outlined in Fig. 90-3, the first step in the evaluation of dysuria and frequency in sexually active women is the differentiation of cystitis or urethritis from vaginitis by history and examination. Among women without vaginitis, bacterial UTI must then be differentiated from the urethral syndrome. The finding of a single conventional urinary pathogen, such as *Escherichia coli* or *Staphylococcus saprophyticus*, in a concentration of $\geq 10^2$ per milliliter in a properly collected midstream urine specimen from a symptomatic woman with pyuria indicates probable bacterial UTI, whereas pyuria with fewer than 10^2 conventional uropathogens per milliliter of urine ("sterile pyuria") suggests the diagnosis of acute urethral syndrome due to *C. trachomatis* or *N. gonorrhoeae*. Gonorrhea should be excluded by culture of the cervix and urethra. Chlamydial infection should be excluded by culture or specific immunologic tests for chlamydial antigen in urethral and cervical specimens. Treatment with tetracycline (e.g., tetracycline HCl, 500 mg four times daily for 7 days) has been shown to alleviate symptoms in women with "sterile" pyuria and dysuria, but not in women without pyuria or isolation of a pathogen. The sexual partners of such patients should also be examined and considered for treatment.

VAGINITIS In self-referred women attending STD clinics, vaginitis is the most common diagnosis. In most patients, bacterial vaginosis is the most common cause of vulvovaginal symptoms, followed by candidiasis, with trichomoniasis least common.

Vaginal infection, without UTI, is characterized by one or more of the following: increased volume of discharge; abnormal yellow color of discharge caused by increased concentration of polymorphonuclear leukocytes; vulvar itching, irritation, or burning; dyspareunia; and malodor. *Trichomonas vaginalis* characteristically produces a profuse, yellow, purulent, homogeneous discharge that is often malodorous and may be frothy, presumably because of gas production by vaginal bacteria. The vaginal epithelium is inflamed, and petechial lesions may be present on the cervix ("strawberry cervix"). In contrast, the predominant symptom in candidiasis is usually vulvar itching, often with signs of vulvitis as well as vaginitis, usually without a distinct odor. The discharge, often scanty, is typically white and may resemble curds of cottage cheese or adherent thrush-like plaques. *Bacterial vaginosis* formerly was termed *nonspecific vaginitis,* a misnomer since the syndrome is associated with certain microorganisms and is usually noninflammatory. It is characterized by vaginal malodor and increased white or gray vaginal discharge that is homogeneous, low in viscosity, and uniformly coats the vaginal walls. A most important component of the clinical evaluation of vaginal discharge is ascertaining by speculum examination whether the discharge emanates from the vagina or the cervix, and whether the discharge is, in fact, abnormal. Occasionally, symptoms of increased discharge or other vaginal symptoms are not associated with objective signs of vaginitis or cervicitis. Although psychological testing is normal in most such cases, possible causes of functional symptoms should be explored. The diagnosis and therapy of the three major types of vaginal infection are summarized in Table 90-3.

***T. vaginalis* vaginitis** (see also Chap. 161) Sexual transmission of *T. vaginalis* is well established. Routine culture testing indicates that many women and most men with infection are asymptomatic. However, treatment of asymptomatic as well as symptomatic cases is recommended to reduce the reservoir of infection and the risk of transmission, and to prevent the future development of symptoms.

DIAGNOSIS AND THERAPY In women with typical symptoms and signs of trichomoniasis, the diagnosis can usually be confirmed by demonstration of motile trichomonads and polymorphonuclear leukocytes in vaginal secretions mixed with normal saline and examined promptly under a low-power or high dry (400×) microscopic field. In such patients, wet-mount examination is at least 80 percent as sensitive as culture. However, in women without symptoms or signs, culture is often required to detect trichomonal infection. The diagnosis of *T. vaginalis* infection in men is more difficult and requires culture of early morning first-voided urine sediment or of urethral scrapings obtained before voiding. The pH of vaginal secretions is usually ≥5.0 in symptomatic *T. vaginalis* infections. As in bacterial vaginosis, the addition of 10% potassium hydroxide (KOH) to vaginal secretions liberates a fishy odor due to various amines formed by microbial metabolism.

Nitroimidazoles are the only consistently effective drugs for treating trichomoniasis. Several studies show that a single 2.0-g oral dose of metronidazole is at least 90 percent as effective as more prolonged dosage schedules. Other nitroimidazoles such as tinidazole and ornidazole have longer half-lives than metronidazole, but have not been clearly shown to give better results in the therapy of trichomoniasis. Routine treatment of sex partners is advisable to

FIGURE 90-2 *Evaluation and management of patients with unilateral testicular pain and swelling.*

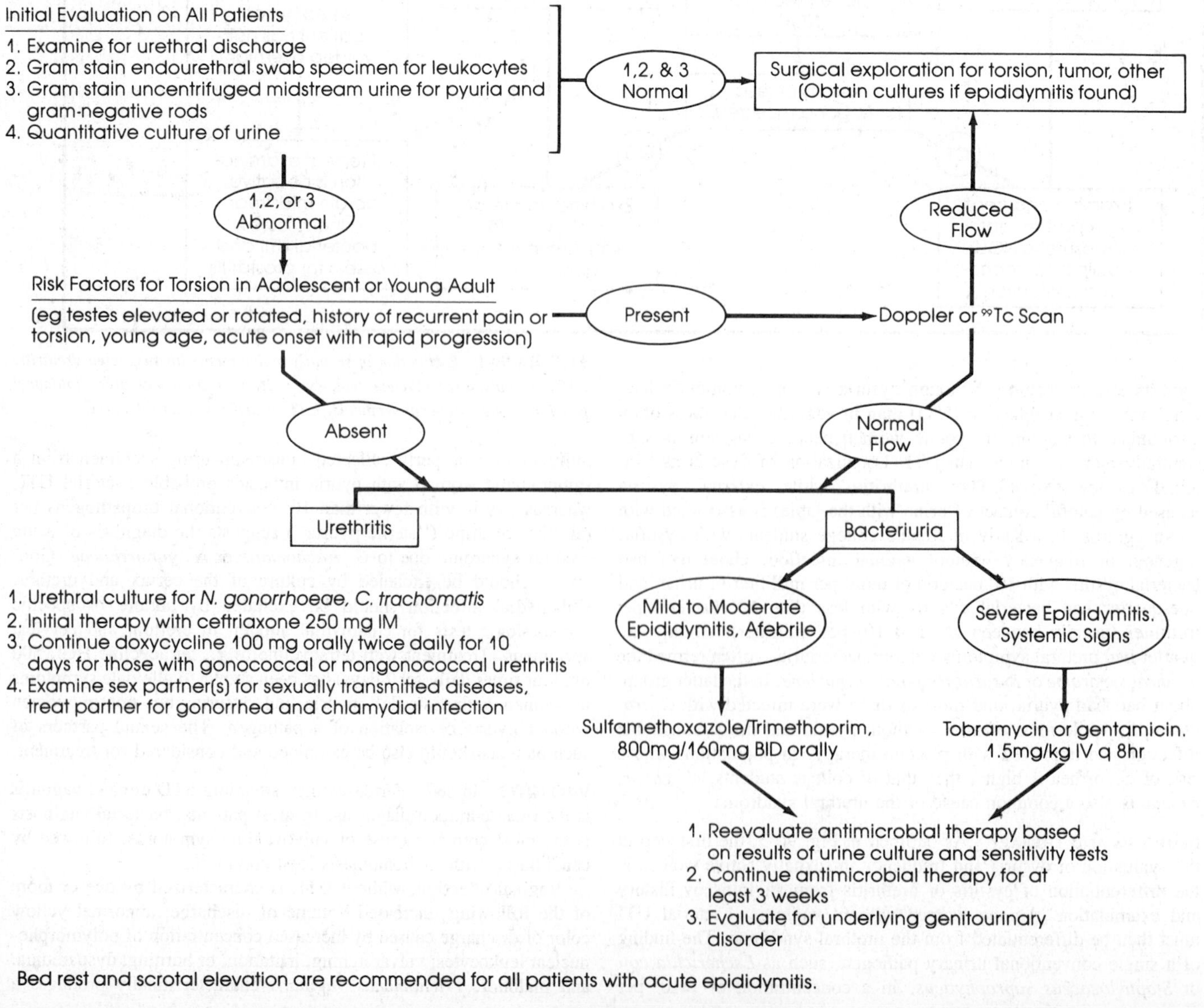

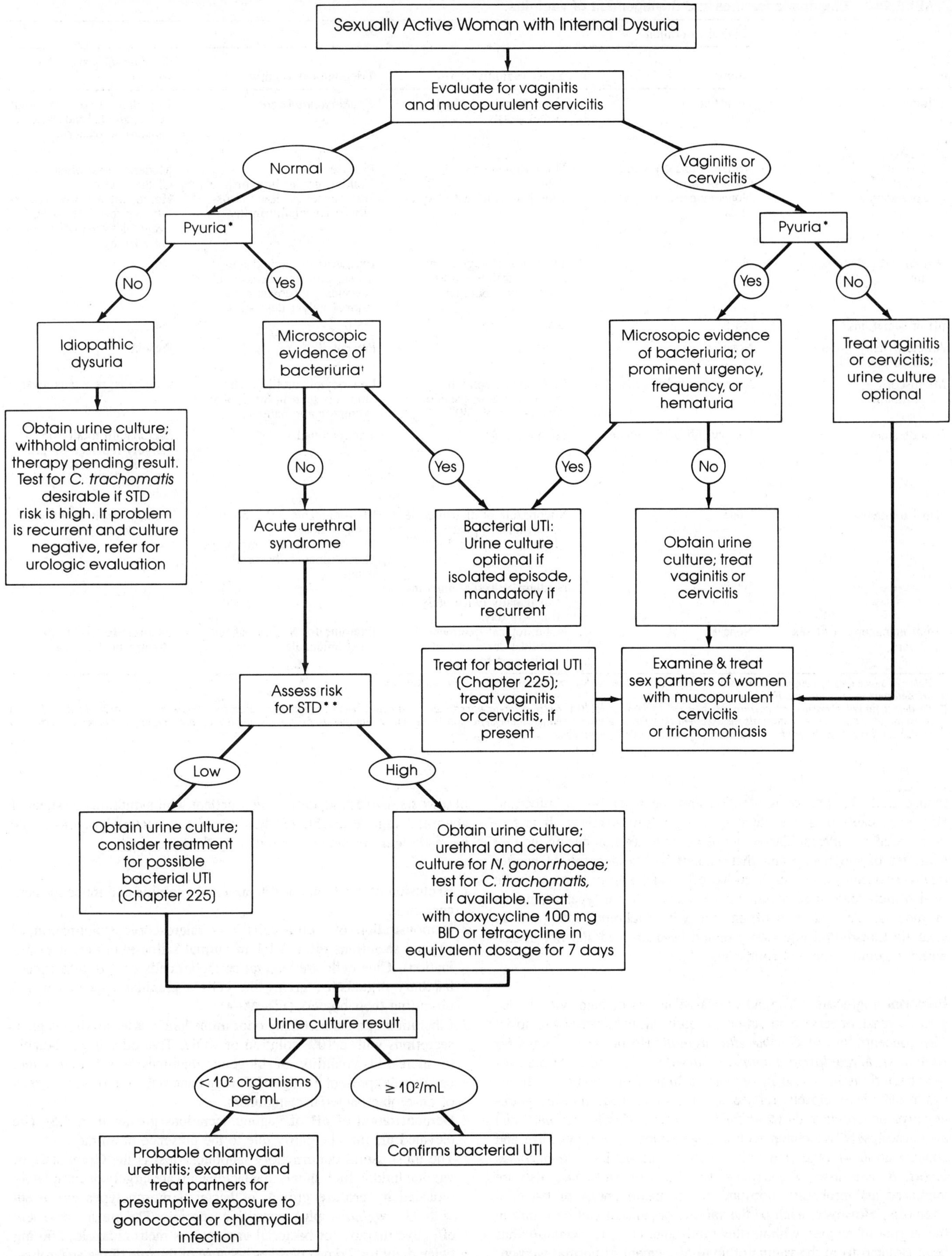

FIGURE 90-3 *Evaluation of sexually active women with "internal" dysuria. *Pyuria is defined as ≥ 20 WBC per 400× microscopic field of a centrifuged midstream urine specimen, or ≥ 1 WBC per 400× field of uncentrifuged urine.*

†Microscopic evidence of bacteriuria is the presence of ≥ 1 bacillus per 400× field of an uncentrifuged midstream specimen of urine.

***Evaluation of STD risk is based on number and nature of sexual partner(s), recent change in partner, marital status, past history of STD, etc.*

TABLE 90-3 Diagnostic features and management of vaginitis

	Clinical Condition			
	Normal	Yeast vaginitis	Trichomonal vaginitis	*Gardnerella*-associated vaginosis
Etiology	Uninfected	*Candida albicans* and other yeasts	*Trichomonas vaginalis*	Uncertain; associated with *G. vaginalis* and various anaerobic bacteria
Discharge:				
Amount	Variable; usually scant	Scant to moderate	Profuse	Moderate to profuse
Color*	Clear or white	White	Yellow, green, brownish	Clear or white
Consistency	Nonhomogeneous, flocculant	Clumped; adherent plaques	Homogeneous, low viscosity; occasionally frothy	Homogeneous, low viscosity, uniformly coating vaginal walls; occasionally frothy
Associated inflammatory signs	None	Erythema of vaginal mucosa, introitus; vulvar dermatitis common	Erythema of vaginal mucosa, introitus; occasional cervical petechiae; occasional vulvar dermatitis	None
pH of secretions†	≤4.5	≤4.5	≥5.0	>4.5
Amine ("fishy") odor with 10% KOH‡	None	None	Present	Present
Microscopy Wet mount	Normal epithelial cells	Leukocytes, epithelial cells; yeasts or pseudomycelia in 50–80%	Leukocytes; motile trichomonads seen in 80–90% of symptomatic patients	Clue cells; few leukocytes
Gram's stain	Lactobacilli predominate	Fungal elements	Trichomonads	Lactobacilli totally or largely replaced by profuse flora consistent with *G. vaginalis* and anaerobes
Usual treatment	None	Miconazole or clotrimazole intravaginally, each 50–100 mg daily for 7 days Nystatin, 100,000 units intravaginally twice daily for 7–14 days	Metronidazole 2.0 g orally (single dose) Metronidazole 250 mg orally three times daily for 10 days	Metronidazole 500 mg orally twice daily for 7 days
Usual management of sex partners	None	None; topical treatment if candidal dermatitis of penis is present	Examine for STD; treat with metronidazole	Examine for STD; no treatment if normal

* *Color of secretions is determined by examining a swab coated with secretions against a white background.*
† *pH determination is not useful if blood is present.*
‡ *To detect fungal elements, secretions are digested by boiling in 10% KOH prior to microscopic examination; to examine for other features, secretions are mixed (1:1) with physiologic saline. Gram's stain also is excellent for detecting yeasts and pseudomycelia and is the only technique useful for distinguishing lactobacilli from other bacteria, but is less sensitive than the saline preparation for detection of* T. vaginalis.

reduce both the risk of reinfection and the reservoir of infection. However, caution is warranted in using nitroimidazoles. It is recommended that metronidazole not be given to women during the first trimester of pregnancy and that alcohol be avoided for 24 h after treatment because of a disulfiram-like effect of the drug. Metronidazole is also mutagenic, and massive doses cause several types of tumors in rodents. The partners of patients with trichomoniasis (and all sexually transmitted infections) should be examined and not treated without examination and counseling.

Bacterial vaginosis Vaginal discharge not associated with *T. vaginalis*, yeast, or cervical infection is usually due to bacterial vaginosis. The concentration of *Gardnerella vaginalis* (formerly *Haemophilus vaginalis*), *Mycoplasma hominis, U. urealyticum,* and certain anaerobic bacteria is increased in vaginal washings from women with this syndrome. Two closely related species of curved, motile, gram-negative anaerobic rods (*Mobiluncus curtisii, Mobiluncus mulieris*) also are closely associated with this syndrome. The prevalence and concentration of other anaerobic bacteria, particularly *Bacteroides bivius, B. capillosis, Peptococcus* spp., and *Eubacterium,* also are increased and probably contribute to the pathogenesis of bacterial vaginosis. However, each of the various organisms can be found in the vagina of women without this syndrome; e.g., *G. vaginalis* has been isolated from the vagina of up to 50 percent of normal women. Metronidazole treatment of the male sex partners of women with bacterial vaginosis does not prevent recurrence of the syndrome in the female.

DIAGNOSIS AND TREATMENT In a patient with symptoms or signs of abnormal vaginal discharge, the diagnosis of bacterial vaginosis can be made with reasonable certainty by the following:

1 Exclusion of candidal and trichomonal vaginitis and mucopurulent cervicitis.
2 Demonstration of "clue cells" by microscopic examination of vaginal secretions diluted 1:1 in normal saline (wet-mount examination). Clue cells are vaginal epithelial cells coated with coccobacillary organisms, giving the cells a granular appearance and obscuring their borders (Fig. 90-4).
3 Liberation of a distinct fishy odor immediately after mixing vaginal secretions with a 10% solution of KOH. This odor is attributable to increased volatility of biogenic diamines (e.g., putrescine, cadaverine) present in vaginal fluid in bacterial vaginosis, the result of anaerobic bacterial metabolism.
4 Demonstration of pH of vaginal secretions greater than 4.5. The elevated pH may be partly due to the presence of amines.
5 The most useful confirmatory laboratory test is the Gram stain of vaginal fluid, which shows that lactobacilli are largely or completely replaced by profuse growth of bacterial morphotypes consistent with *G. vaginalis* plus anaerobic species. The most consistent effective therapy for bacterial vaginosis is metronidazole, 500 mg twice daily for 7 days, perhaps because of the role of the anaerobes, which are highly susceptible to metronidazole in this infection. Ampicillin, 500 mg four times daily for 7 days, has been effective in about 40 to 50 percent of cases of bacterial vaginosis, and is

the primary alternative to metronidazole. Sulfonamide-containing vaginal creams are usually ineffective, probably because sulfonamides are inactive against both *G. vaginalis* and many vaginal anaerobes. Tetracycline therapy also is usually ineffective. Treatment of male partners of women with this syndrome does not affect recurrence rates and is not indicated.

Vulvovaginal candidiasis *Candida albicans* accounts for about 80 percent of yeasts isolated from the vagina, while *Torulopsis glabrata* and other less commonly encountered *Candida* species are found in the remainder. Overt vulvovaginitis is more common among women colonized by *C. albicans* than among those colonized with *T. glabrata* or other species. Most cases of vulvovaginal candidiasis probably result from increased growth of yeasts that previously colonized the vagina, or by spread of organisms from the anus. Some cases of recurrent vulvovaginal candidiasis may be due to sexual transmission from a colonized male.

DIAGNOSIS AND THERAPY The diagnosis of yeast vaginitis involves demonstration of fungal elements by microscopic examination of vaginal secretions in saline or 10% KOH, or by Gram's stain. Demonstration of pseudohyphae strengthens the diagnosis of vaginitis due to *C. albicans*. Microscopic examination is less sensitive than culture, but culture has the disadvantage of detecting asymptomatic carriage in women who may not require therapy. The pH of vaginal secretions is usually less than 4.5, and the vaginal odor is normal. Vulvitis often accompanies vaginitis and may result in superficial erosions that must be differentiated from genital herpes. In most circumstances, therapy for candidal vaginal infection is indicated only if the patient is symptomatic. The usual treatment is intravaginal miconazole or clotrimazole, 100 mg once daily for 7 days; intravaginal nystatin is less effective. Simultaneous therapy with oral nystatin, with the intent of eradicating colonic colonization with *Candida*, does not reduce the risk of recurrent yeast vaginitis. Treatment of the sex partner is not routinely indicated, although this has not been studied rigorously.

MUCOPURULENT CERVICITIS Mucopurulent cervicitis refers to inflammation of the columnar epithelium and subepithelial lesions of the endocervix, and of any contiguous columnar epithelium that lies exposed in an ectopic position on the exocervix. Mucopurulent cervicitis in the female can be regarded as the "silent" partner of urethritis in the male, being equally common and caused by the same agents but more difficult to recognize. It is the most common major STD syndrome in women and can lead to pelvic inflammatory disease, and in pregnant women may lead to obstetrical complications. Improved recognition and treatment of this syndrome would greatly improve the control of STD. Mucopurulent cervicitis usually is caused by *C. trachomatis*, sometimes by *N. gonorrhoeae*. About one-third of cases are associated with neither of these organisms; these have been correlated with *U. urealyticum* infections, but this requires confirmation. The syndrome can usually be differentiated clinically from cervicitis caused by primary or recurrent herpes simplex virus infection, which produces lesions on the stratified squamous epithelium of the exocervix, as well as on the columnar epithelium; and from vaginitis caused by *C. albicans* or *T. vaginalis*.

DIAGNOSIS AND THERAPY The diagnosis is made by demonstrating mucopurulent discharge from the cervical os (analogous to demonstrating abnormal exudate in the male urethra) or by demonstrating increased numbers of polymorphonuclear leukocytes in Gram-stained or Papanicolaou smears of endocervical discharge from women without visible mucus (analogous to criteria now widely used to diagnose urethritis in men without overt urethral discharge). Cervical ectopy (see below) that is edematous and bleeds readily when swabbed is also a common sign of mucopurulent cervicitis due to *C. trachomatis*. Cervical biopsy in such cases shows infiltration of the stroma and epithelium predominantly by lymphocytes, plasma cells, and histiocytes characteristically with lymphoid germinal centers (follicular cervicitis).

A simple way to demonstrate mucopurulent discharge from the cervix, which augments the visual documentation of abnormal exudate, is to observe the color of cervical mucus on a white swab removed from the endocervix; a yellow color indicates the presence of mucopus. After the results of this "swab test" are noted, the cervical mucus should be rolled *thinly* on a slide for Gram staining. An area of the slide should be identified which contains strands of cervical mucus which are not contaminated by vaginal squamous epithelial cells or bacteria. The presence of ≥ 10 polymorphonuclear cells per $1000\times$ microscopic field within strands of cervical mucus suggests cervicitis. In studies in STD clinics and student gynecology clinics, the prevalence of *C. trachomatis* infection has been approximately 50 percent among women with mucopurulent cervicitis by the above criteria and 10 percent among women without it. The presence of a characteristic pattern of inflammatory cells on Papanicolaou smears of endocervical cells is also increasingly being used by cytopathologists to suggest the possibility of chlamydial infection and the need for specific confirmatory testing.

Mucopurulent cervicitis requires antimicrobial therapy. An etiologic diagnosis should always be established to guide management of sexual partners, but therapy should usually be initiated against the most likely causes of this syndrome, while results of diagnostic tests are pending. The diagnosis of gonococcal cervicitis is made by Gram's stain and culture of an endocervical specimen. If a specimen is properly collected from within the endocervix after first wiping the cervix clean to remove vaginal material, then the sensitivity of the Gram's stain showing intracellular gram-negative diplococci (in comparison with culture) is about 50 percent. However, the specificity approaches 100 percent, and observation of intracellular gram-negative diplococci by an experienced microscopist indicates gonococcal

FIGURE 90-4 *A. Vaginal epithelial "clue cells." Note granular appearance due to adherent* G. vaginalis *and indistinct cell margins. 400×. B. Normal vaginal epithelial cells. The cell margins are distinct and lack granularity.*

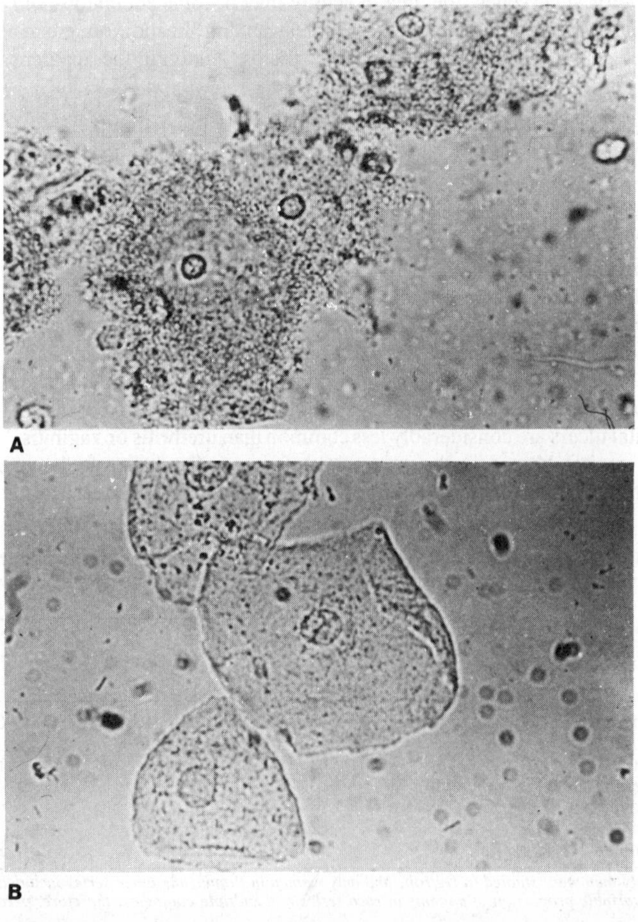

A

B

infection, even if the culture is negative. The sensitivity of a single endocervical culture for *N. gonorrhoeae* is 80 to 90 percent.

Chlamydial infection of the cervix can be confirmed by culture or antigen detection. The sensitivity of a single endocervical culture for *C. trachomatis* is estimated to be 80 percent or more. The sensitivity of antigen detection approaches that of isolation of the organism in cell culture. Antigen detection by direct immunofluorescence is specific in experienced hands, but detection by enzyme immunoassay may be less specific. While diagnostic test results are pending, therapy can be initiated with a single-dose regimen effective for gonorrhea, plus tetracycline hydrochloride, 500 mg four times per day, or doxycycline, 100 mg twice daily, orally for 1 week. For pregnant women, erythromycin base or stearate, in a dose of 500 mg four times daily for 7 to 14 days, can be substituted for the tetracycline-doxycycline treatment. The male sex partners of women with nongonococcal mucopurulent cervicitis should be examined for urethritis and other STD, and treated for exposure to any infection found in the female. If cultures for *C. trachomatis* are not available, the male partners should be treated for presumptive chlamydial infection, regardless of whether urethritis is documented.

Cervical ectopy Cervicitis must be differentiated from cervical ectopy, which is often mislabled "cervical erosion." Ectopy represents the presence of the 1-cell-thick columnar endocervical epithelium in an exposed visible "ectopic" position on the cervix, where it appears redder than the 20-cell-thick stratified squamous vaginal epithelium. When ectopy is present, the cervical os may contain clear or slightly cloudy mucus, but not mucopus. Colposcopy shows that the epithelium is intact and not ulcerated. Ectopy is normally present during early adolescence and gradually recedes as squamous metaplasia replaces the ectopic columnar epithelium. Oral contraceptive usage or pregnancy favors persistence or reappearance of ectopy. The use of cauterizing procedures to eliminate ectopy is controversial. The presence of ectopy may make the cervix more susceptible to infection with *N. gonorrhoeae* or *C. trachomatis* by exposing a larger surface area of susceptible columnar epithelium. When mucopurulent cervicitis supervenes, the area of ectopy may become edematous and fragile, with bleeding induced by gentle swabbing. In addition, edema of the cervix may result in eversion of the os, enlarging the apparent area of ectopy.

ULCERATIVE LESIONS OF THE GENITALIA Genital skin lesions can be classified as ulcerative or nonulcerative. Nonulcerative genital lesions include several sexually transmitted infections such as scabies, genital warts, *Candida* balanitis or vulvitis, or genital molluscum contagiosum, as well as a broad spectrum of nonsexually transmitted dermatologic conditions.

The incidence and etiology of ulcerative lesions of the genitalia vary greatly in different areas of the world (Table 90-4). In Asia and Africa, genital ulcers are seen as frequently as gonorrhea in some STD clinics, and chancroid is the commonest cause, while genital herpes is relatively uncommon. In the industrialized western countries, genital ulcers are considerably less common than urethritis or vaginitis, and genital herpes is the commonest form, with chancroid being relatively uncommon. Syphilis has been the second commonest form of genital ulcer in all areas of the world and must always be excluded. Lymphogranuloma venereum (LGV) and donovanosis (granuloma inguinale) are rare causes of genital ulceration.

DIAGNOSIS AND THERAPY In industrialized countries, the differential diagnosis of genital ulceration, when trauma and excoriated lesions are excluded, usually rests among genital herpes simplex virus (HSV) infection, syphilis, and, rarely, chancroid. Epidemiologic factors that increase the likelihood of chancroid, LGV, or donovanosis include acquisition of infection in a developing country and sexual contact with a prostitute, a homosexual, or an individual of low socioeconomic status. The clinical findings are occasionally definitive (e.g., presence of herpetic vesicles), and clinical findings plus epidemiologic considerations usually help to guide initial therapy pending further studies. Nevertheless, most genital ulcerations cannot be diagnosed confidently on clinical grounds. It is axiomatic to exclude syphilis by appropriate serology in all cases. Dark-field examination should also be performed, by experienced technicians when possible, on lesions suggesting primary or secondary syphilis. Direct immunofluorescence using monoclonal antibodies to *T. pallidum* is at least as sensitive and specific as dark-field microscopy for detection of *T. pallidum* in lesion exudate, and can be performed on specimens sent to a central laboratory. This procedure should become available in the future. Chancroid should not be used as "wastebasket" diagnosis for all ulcerative lesions not attributable to syphilis or genital herpes since few such lesions are confirmed as chancroid, except in developing nations, or in certain local outbreaks (e.g., Manitoba, California, New York City, or Florida in recent years). Selective enrichment media are available for isolation of *Haemophilus ducreyi* from such cases.

The following general guidelines are recommended for management of ulcerative genital lesions (Fig. 90-5):

1 *If typical painful herpetic vesicles or pustules are present:* In this case the clinical diagnosis of herpes is warranted, although a serologic test for syphilis should be performed. If desired, the diagnosis can be confirmed by isolation of HSV in 90 percent and by cytology (Papanicolaou smear) in about two-thirds of patients with intact vesicles or pustules. Immunochemical detection with specific monoclonal antibody is also a promising technique.
2 *If painful nonvesicular ulcer(s) raise the suspicion of herpes or chancroid:* If the lesions(s) or inguinal node(s) is painful or has other features suggestive of herpes or chancroid, attempts to demonstrate HSV or *H. ducreyi* are indicated. All methods of HSV detection are somewhat less sensitive in the ulcerative stage than in the vesicular stage. Syphilis should be excluded by dark-field examination and serologic testing, both of which should be repeated 1 to 2 weeks later if negative initially and if other diagnoses cannot be confirmed.
3 *If painless ulcerative lesions suggest the diagnosis of syphilis:* If lesions are at all suggestive of syphilis, or there are epidemiologic reasons to suspect syphilis, such as recent exposure, then dark-field examination and a rapid serologic test for syphilis should be performed for prompt diagnosis. If these are negative, two more dark-field examinations on successive days are recommended, and

TABLE 90-4 Etiology of genital ulcers in six studies, showing marked difference in populations*

	Percent of patients†					
	Detroit (N=100)	Seattle (N=82)	Nairobi (N=97)	Swaziland (N=155)	Johannesburg/ Soweto (N=102)	Papua (New Guinea) (N=101)
Chancroid	2	1	62	44	61	0
Genital herpes	40	55	5	12	17	0
Syphilis	17	12	11	19	9	50
Lymphogranuloma venereum	0	0	0	12	1	23
Donovanosis	0	0	0	1	1	46
Other	12	12	5	0	4	
Unknown	37	21	24	15	15	15

* *Only men were studied in Detroit, and only women in Papua; the other series included both sexes.*
† *A variable proportion of patients in each series had multiple etiologies; therefore, percentages total >100.*

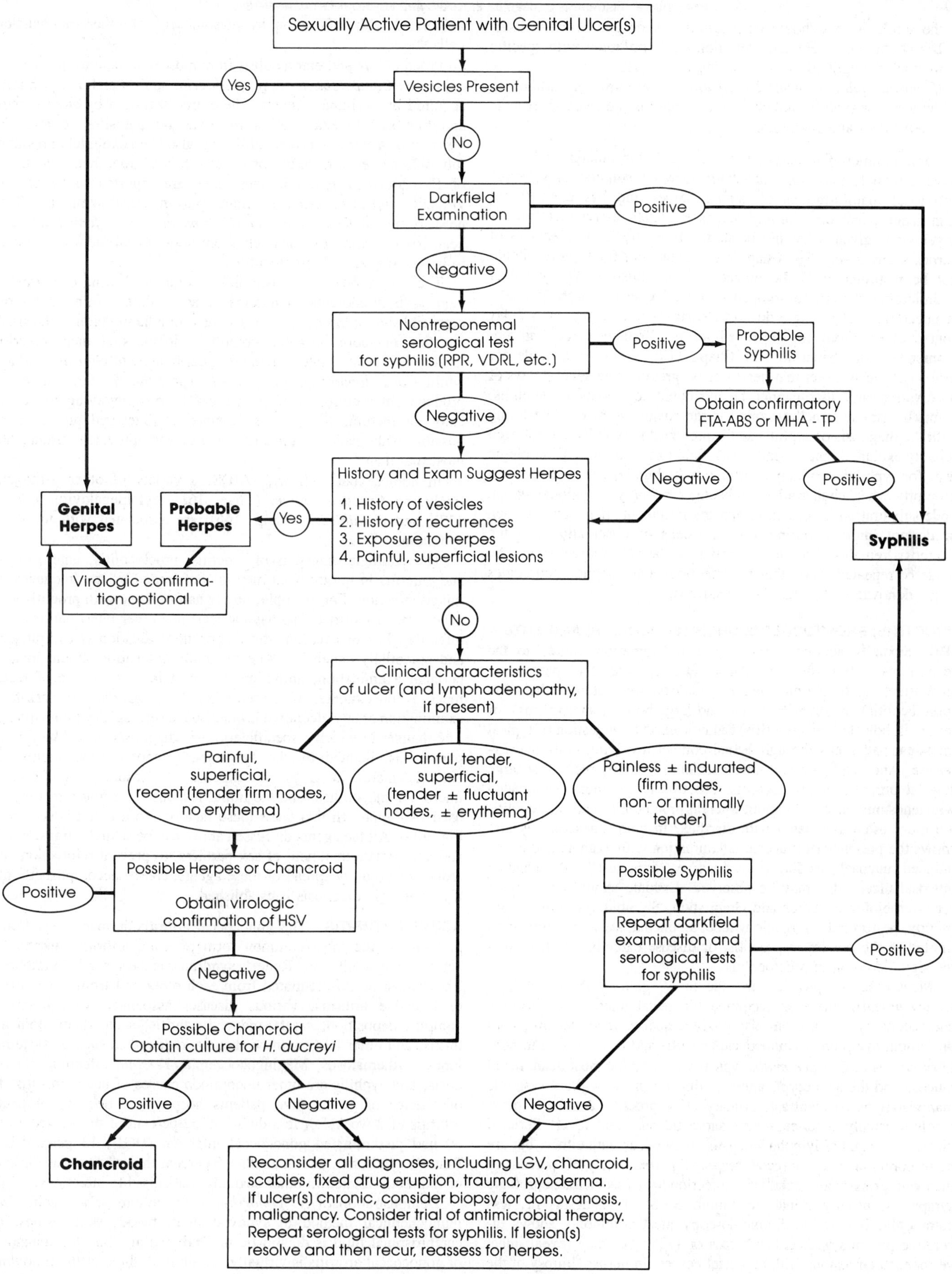

FIGURE 90-5 *Evaluation of sexually active persons with genital ulcer–inguinal lymphadenopathy syndromes.*

the serologic test should be repeated 1 week and 6 weeks later. Direct immunofluorescent detection of *T. pallidum* with specific monoclonal antibody is a promising technique.

4 *If chronic painless genital ulceration progresses:* In addition to the tests for syphilis and chancroid, biopsy is indicated to exclude donovanosis and carcinoma.

Oral antimicrobial therapy is not indicated for undiagnosed ulcerative genital lesions. Oral acyclovir speeds resolution of systemic and local manifestations of genital herpes and has a small but significant effect on recurrent herpes if started early; therefore, if acyclovir is given, it should be started promptly if the diagnosis of herpes seems likely (see Chap. 136). Treatment for syphilis should not be instituted until the diagnosis is established. The value of antimicrobial therapy for idiopathic ulcerative lesions of the genitalia is uncertain, but a single dose of ceftriaxone, 250 mg, or a 7-day course of erythromycin or trimethoprim-sulfamethoxazole, as recommended for chancroid (see Chap. 110), seems reasonable for lesions of recent onset that persist or progress during several days of observation and that cannot be attributed to herpes or syphilis. Trimethoprim-sulfamethoxazole has the advantage of not interfering with the diagnosis of syphilis and is preferred if syphilis has not been reliably excluded, and repeated dark-field examinations and serologic tests for syphilis are planned. Antimicrobial therapy should be given promptly when chancroid is probable, especially if regional lymph node suppuration is present or appears imminent. If patients worsen or do not improve during 1 or 2 weeks of observation and the diagnosis remains obscure, attempts to isolate *H. ducreyi* should be made or repeated, and other noninfectious and infectious etiologies (e.g., donovanosis) should be considered.

PROCTITIS, PROCTOCOLITIS OR ENTEROCOLITIS, AND ENTERITIS Sexually acquired proctitis, or inflammation limited to the rectum, results from direct rectal inoculation of typical STD pathogens. In contrast, inflammation which extends from the rectum to the colon (proctocolitis), involves the small and large bowel (enterocolitis), or the small bowel alone (enteritis) can be caused by ingestion of typical intestinal pathogens through sexual contact involving oral-fecal exposure. Anorectal pain and mucopurulent or bloody rectal discharge suggest proctitis or proctocolitis. Proctitis is commonly associated with tenesmus and constipation, whereas proctocolitis and enterocolitis are more often associated with diarrhea. In both, anoscopy usually shows the presence of mucosal inflammation with exudate and easily induced mucosal bleeding (i.e., positive "wipe test"). Petechial or mucosal ulcers also may be observed. Exudate should be sampled for microbiologic studies and Gram stain. Sigmoidoscopy or colonoscopy, performed if possible without an enema, shows inflammation limited to the rectum in proctitis, or disease extending at least into the sigmoid colon in proctocolitis.

Most cases of proctitis are due to *N. gonorrhoeae,* HSV, or *C. trachomatis;* these are acquired via rectal intercourse. Primary and secondary syphilis can also produce anal or rectal lesions, with or without symptoms. Gonococcal proctitis and proctitis due to non-LGV strains of *C. trachomatis* typically involve the most distal rectal mucosa and the anal crypts and are clinically mild, without systemic manifestations. In contrast, primary HSV proctitis and LGV proctocolitis usually produce severe anorectal pain and fever. Perianal ulcers and inguinal lymphadenopathy may occur with either, but are more common with anorectal herpes. Approximately 50 percent of men with primary anorectal HSV infection have associated neurologic symptoms, usually urinary retention, S5-S5 dysesthesias or, less commonly, impotence. Sigmoidoscopy most commonly shows ulcerative proctitis with either herpes or LGV, but may reveal intact vesicopustular lesions with anorectal herpes. In herpes, biopsy of the rectal mucosa shows microulcerations and may show intranuclear inclusions or perivascular lymphocytic cuffing. In LGV, biopsy typically shows crypt abscesses, granulomas, and giant cells, findings indistinguishable from those of Crohn's disease or idiopathic ulcerative proctocolitis. Syphilis can also produce rectal granulomas, usually associated with infiltration by plasma cells or other mononuclear cells.

Proctocolitis and enterocolitis in homosexual men are most often caused by *Campylobacter* spp. or *Shigella* spp., which are primarily acquired by oral-anal contact. These are diagnosed by stool culture and microscopic examination for ova and parasites. *Entamoeba histolytica,* a cause of proctocolitis, has also been extremely prevalent (up to 25 percent) in studies of selected homosexual men, but strains of *E. histolytica* found in these men are reported to be of low virulence and of uncertain relationship to intestinal symptoms. Two new species of *Campylobacter* (*C. cinaedi* and *C. fennellae*) have been isolated almost exclusively from homosexual men, and appear to be associated with proctocolitis.

The occurrence of diarrhea and abdominal bloating or cramping pain, without anorectal symptoms, in association with normal anoscopy and sigmoidoscopy, is consistent with inflammation of the small intestine or more proximal colon. In homosexual men, enteritis limited to the small intestine is often attributable to *Giardia lamblia,* while *Campylobacter* spp., *Shigella* spp. and *E. histolytica* can produce enterocolitis with or without lesions involving the distal colon or rectum. *Blastocystis hominis,* an intestinal protozoan of possible pathogenic significance, is also very prevalent among homosexual men.

In homosexual men with AIDS, a variety of other pathogens [including *Cryptosporidium* (Chap. 161), cytomegalovirus (Chap. 137), and *C. albicans* (Chap. 146)] are associated with intestinal symptoms.

The etiologic diagnosis of proctitis, proctocolitis, enterocolitis, and enteritis in homosexual men is confounded by the frequency of mixed infection. For example, nearly half of those with proctitis who have rectal gonorrhea also have at least one other intestinal or rectal infection. For this reason, the diagnostic evaluation is complicated and potentially expensive. The minimum evaluation should include perianal examination, anoscopy, Gram stain, and culture of rectal mucosa (or exudate, if present) for *N. gonorrhoeae,* dark-field examination of any ulcerative lesions, and a serologic test for syphilis. The manner in which a specific etiologic diagnosis should be further pursued is dictated by the syndrome (proctitis, proctocolitis, or enteritis/enterocolitis), by the expense, the results of preliminary microbiologic studies, and the initial response to empiric therapy, if used. An approach that takes these factors into account is shown in Fig. 90-6. All the agents discussed above can be sexually transmitted, and appropriate treatment of sex partners, to prevent reinfection and reduce community spread of these agents, can be accomplished only if an etiologic diagnosis is established.

ACUTE ARTHRITIS The gonococcal arthritis-dermatitis syndrome probably is the most common form of acute arthritis in sexually active young adults, and Reiter's syndrome is the second commonest. These must be differentiated from each other and from other forms of infective arthritis, various diseases associated with immune-complex deposition, crystal-induced arthritis, acute rheumatoid arthritis, and other less common rheumatic disorders such as systemic lupus erythematosus. Meningococcemia, *Yersinia* infection, sarcoidosis, and syphilis are other uncommon causes of acute arthritis. In one series of consecutive patients hospitalized because of acute arthritis of 2 weeks' or less duration, 52 percent of those aged 15 to 30 had disseminated gonococcal infection (DGI), 13 percent had Reiter's syndrome, and in another 5 percent the arthritis was directly or indirectly related to other sexually transmissible infections.

Demonstration of *N. gonorrhoeae* by culture or a specific immunochemical method in synovial fluid, blood, skin lesions, or cerebrospinal fluid is diagnostic of DGI. Failing this, the diagnosis of gonococcal arthritis is virtually certain if all three of the following criteria are met: (1) *N. gonorrhoeae* is recovered from a mucosal site of infection or from the patient's sex partner; (2) typical pustular or hemorrhagic skin lesions are distributed primarily on the extremities; and (3) a therapeutic antibiotic trial produces prompt defervesence and improvement of the arthritis. If only two of the above three

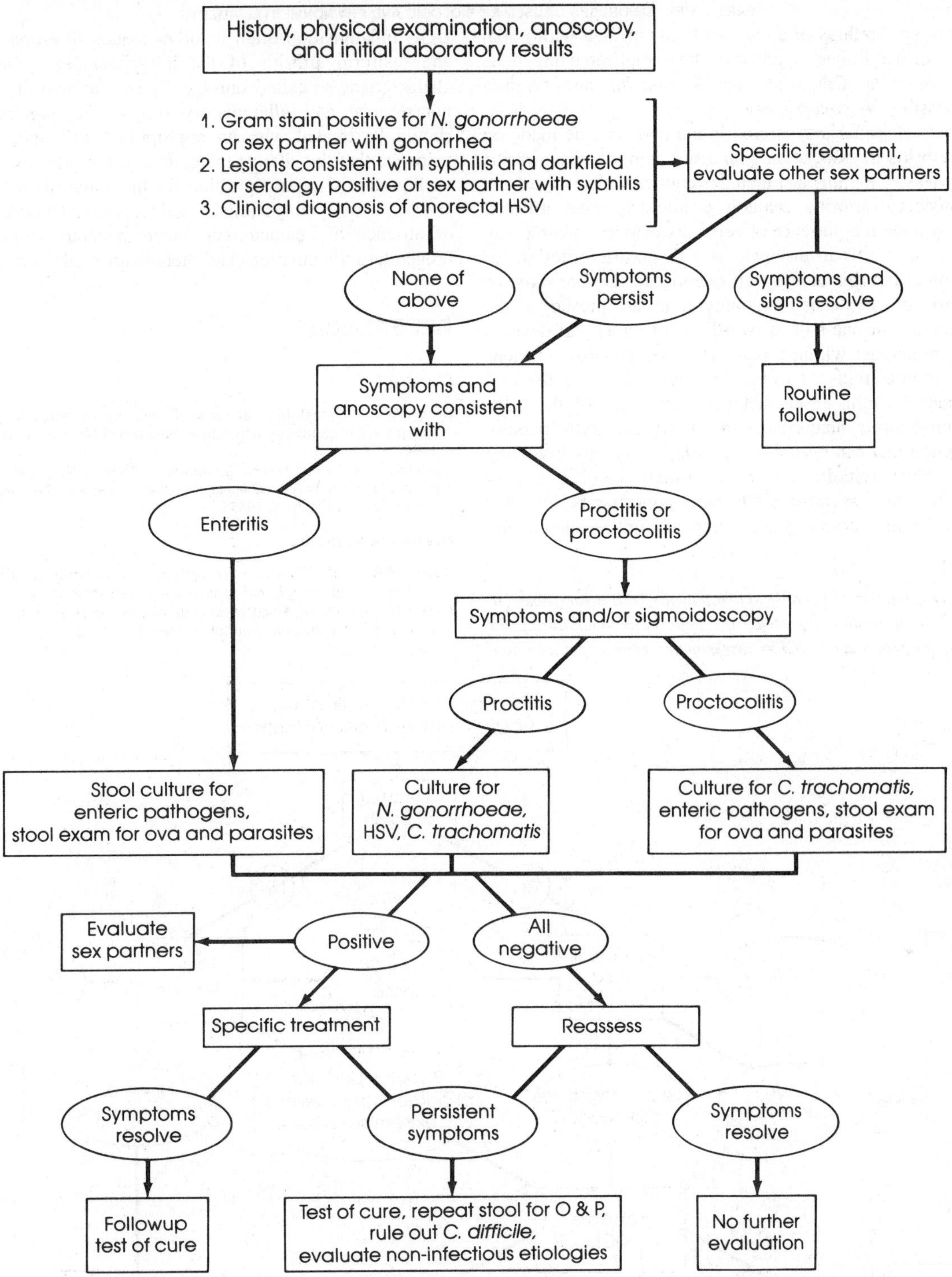

FIGURE 90-6 *Algorithm for management of anorectal and/or intestinal symptoms in homosexually active men. Anoscopy, cultures for* N. gonorrhoeae, *and a serologic test for syphilis should be performed in all cases. Empirical therapy for enteritis or proctitis could be given pending results of microbiologic studies. HSV = herpes simplex virus; O + P = ova and parasites.*

criteria are met, the diagnosis of gonococcal arthritis remains highly probable, especially if the other diagnoses listed above are excluded.

DGI due to penicillinase-negative strains of *N. gonorrhoeae* is best treated with intravenous crystalline penicillin G, 10 million units per day until clear-cut clinical improvement occurs, followed by oral ampicillin 500 mg four times daily to complete 7 to 10 days of antibiotic therapy. Patients who are allergic to penicillin may be given 7- to 10-day courses of cefoxitin or cefotaxime 4 to 6 g daily intravenously, or ceftriaxone 1 to 2 g daily intravenously; mildly ill patients may be given tetracycline 500 mg four times daily for 7 to 10 days. Cefoxitin, cefotaxime, or ceftriaxone should be used for DGI due to penicillinase-producing gonococci. Patients with gonococcal arthritis with highly purulent synovial effusions occasionally have persistent fever and arthritis despite adequate antimicrobial therapy, and they may require repeated closed-joint irrigations with saline before improvement occurs.

Reiter's syndrome occurs in a sporadic (apparently sexually transmitted) form and a postdysenteric form, which sometimes occurs in discrete epidemics. Reiter's syndrome is most commonly diagnosed in men, although some series include many women. Approximately 80 percent of patients have the HLA-B27 haplotype, compared with fewer than 10 percent of the general population. The pathogenesis of Reiter's syndrome is not understood, but it is believed that any of several mucosal infections in a predisposed (e.g., HLA-B27–positive) host triggers an immune response that causes the arthritis and mucocutaneous lesions. *C. trachomatis* is believed to be the most common precipitating infectious agent in the sporadic form and can be isolated from the urethras of up to two-thirds of men with initial episodes of this form of Reiter's syndrome. Other implicated infectious agents include *Shigella, Campylobacter, Salmonella,* and *Yersinia* species, and possibly *N. gonorrhoeae*.

The diagnosis of Reiter's syndrome in the male can be made on the basis of urethritis in association with acute, noninfective arthritis that persists at least 1 month, and includes entities which have been called postgonococcal arthritis, sexually acquired reactive arthritis, and others. In women the presence of cervicitis or sterile pyuria may be equivalent to urethritis in the male as a diagnostic criterion for Reiter's syndrome, but this is less well established. One or more of the characteristic mucocutaneous manifestations are present at the time of presentation in one-half to two-thirds of cases and develop in most of the remainder within a year. The mucocutaneous lesions include acute conjunctivitis or uveitis, painless ulcers of the oral mucosa, circinate balanitis (a characteristic dermatitis of the glans penis), and keratoderma blenorrhagicum (a hyperkeratotic papulosquamous eruption that can resemble psoriasis, commonly involving the palms and soles). Initially, the arthritis usually involves four or fewer joints, distributed asymmetrically. Any joint may be involved and sacroiliac arthritis is common, a differential point compared with DGI. Inflammation often involves tendon insertions (enthesopathy), and fusiform arthritis of the interphalangeal joints produces the characteristic so-called sausage digits. The mainstay of treatment is nonsteroidal anti-inflammatory drugs. The precipitating infection should be treated with an appropriate antibiotic, but there is no evidence that this affects the course of the arthritis.

Figure 90-7 is an algorithm for the diagnosis of acute arthritis in sexually active young adults, based on synovial fluid analysis, presence or absence of characteristic mucocutaneous lesions, evidence of urogenital inflammation, and therapeutic trials with antibiotics.

REFERENCES

General

BERG AO et al: Establishing the cause of genitourinary symptoms in a family practice: Comparison of clinical examination and comprehensive microbiology. JAMA 251:620, 1984

HOLMES KK et al (eds): *Sexually Transmitted Diseases*. New York, McGraw-Hill, 1984

TAYLOR-ROBINSON D (ed): *Clinical Problems in Sexually Transmitted Diseases*. Dordrecht, Martinus Nijhoff, 1985

Urethritis in males

BOWIE WR et al: Etiology of nongonococcal urethritis: Evidence for *Chlamydia trachomatis* and *Ureaplasma urealyticum*. J Clin Invest 59:735, 1977

JACOBS NF, KRAUS SF: Gonococcal and nongonococcal urethritis in men: Clinical and laboratory differentiation. Ann Intern Med 82:7, 1975

FIGURE 90-7 *Evaluation of sexually active patients with acute, nontraumatic arthritis. This algorithm represents the logic used in analyzing the results of the tests or procedures. DGI = disseminated gonococcal infection.*

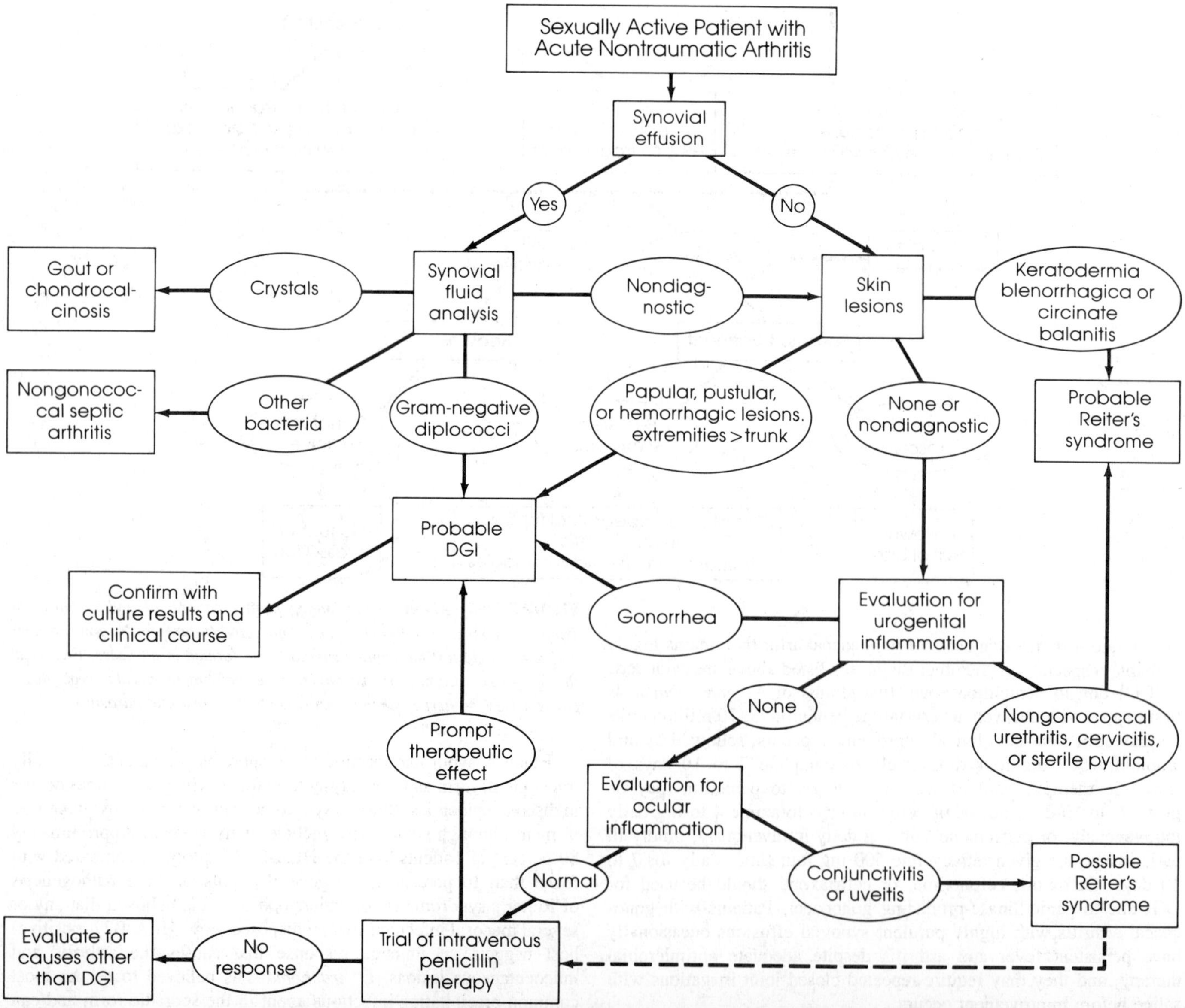

Epididymitis

BERGER RE et al: Etiology, manifestations, and therapy of acute epididymitis: Prospective study of 50 cases. J Urol 121:750, 1979

Urethral syndrome

STAMM WE et al: Causes of the acute urethral syndrome in women. N Engl J Med 303:409, 1980

Vaginitis

HOLMES KK: Lower genital tract infections in women, in *Sexually Transmitted Diseases*, KK Holmes et al (eds). New York, McGraw-Hill, 1984, pp 557–589

KRAUS SF: *Trichomonas vaginalis:* Reevaluation of its clinical presentation and laboratory diagnosis. J Infect Dis 141:137, 1980

MÅRDH PA, TAYLOR-ROBINSON D (eds): *Bacterial Vaginosis*. Stockholm, Almqvist & Wiksell, 1984

ORIEL JD et al: Genital yeast infections. Br Med J 4:761, 1972

SPIEGEL CA et al: Anaerobic bacteria in nonspecific vaginitis. N Engl J Med 303:601, 1980

Cervicitis

BRUNHAM RC et al: Mucopurulent cervicitis—the ignored counterpart in women of urethritis in men. N Engl J Med 311:1, 1984

KIVIAT NB et al: Cytologic manifestations of cervical and vaginal infections: I. Epithelial and inflammatory cellular changes. JAMA 253:989, 1985

Genital ulcers

CHAPEL TA et al: The microbiological flora of penile ulceration. J Infect Dis 137:50, 1978

KRAUS SJ: Genital ulcer adenopathy syndrome, in *Sexually Transmitted Diseases*, KK Holmes et al (eds). New York, McGraw-Hill, 1984, pp 706–714

NSANZE H et al: Genital ulcers in Kenya: Clinical and laboratory study. Br J Vener Dis 57(6):378, 1981

Proctitis, proctocolitis, enterocolitis, enteritis

QUINN TC et al: The polymicrobial etiology of intestinal infections in homosexual men. N Engl J Med 309:576, 1983

Arthritis

HOLMES KK et al: Disseminated gonococcal infection. Ann Intern Med 74:979, 1971

POLLOCK PS, HANDSFIELD HH: Arthritis, in *Sexually Transmitted Diseases*, KK Holmes et al (eds). New York, McGraw-Hill, 1984, pp 745–760

91 PELVIC INFLAMMATORY DISEASE

KING K. HOLMES

DEFINITION The term *pelvic inflammatory disease (PID)* usually refers to ascending infection of the uterus, fallopian tubes, and broad ligaments. Intrauterine infection can be primary (spontaneously occurring and usually sexually transmitted) or secondary to invasive intrauterine surgical procedures (e.g., dilatation and curettage, termination of pregnancy, insertion of an intrauterine device, or hysterosalpingography), or to parturition. Endometritis or endomyometritis is particularly common following delivery by cesarean section.

PID is uncommon during pregnancy itself. The uterotubal junction is closed as early as the seventh week of pregnancy, and the choriamnion becomes approximated to the endocervical os, sealing off the intrauterine cavity, at the twelfth to fifteenth week of gestation. As a consequence, ascending intrauterine infection prior to the twelfth week of gestation may be associated (either as cause or effect) with endometritis and spontaneous abortion, while ascending infection after the twelfth week may be associated with chorioamnionitis. Rarely, infection may extend secondarily to the pelvic organs from adjacent foci of inflammation, such as appendicitis, regional ileitis, or diverticulitis; as a result of hematogenous dissemination, such as tuberculosis; or as a rare complication of certain tropical diseases, such as schistosomiasis. However, the great majority of cases of PID arise spontaneously, without predisposing surgical trauma, obstetrical events, other systemic infection, or adjacent intraabdominal disease.

Spontaneously occurring PID can be divided into chronic and acute types. Chronic PID due to tuberculosis has become uncommon in developing countries; other forms of chronic PID, due to chronic infection with *Chlamydia trachomatis* or secondary to IUD usage, have been described but have not been adequately studied.

The term *PID* is most often used today to refer to cases of acute spontaneously occurring infection ascending from the cervix or vagina. The clinical diagnosis of PID is imprecise. About 10 percent of women with suspected acute PID are found at laparoscopy to have other problems, such as acute appendicitis, endometriosis, ectopic pregnancy, fallopian tube torsion, or corpus luteum bleeding, while another quarter have no laparoscopic evidence of acute disease, and only about 65 percent have laparoscopic evidence of acute salpingitis. Use of endometrial biopsy together with laparoscopy provides evidence of a continuum, progressing from cervicitis alone to endometritis, to salpingitis, to pelvic peritonitis, to generalized peritonitis, to perihepatitis, or to pelvic abscess. In this chapter, the term *PID* is used to refer to the clinical syndrome which includes each of these conditions, and the term *salpingitis* is restricted to patients with visually or histopathologically confirmed inflammation of the fallopian tubes. The distinction between endometritis and salpingitis may be important, because long-term sequelae are common after salpingitis. These sequelae include infertility due to bilateral tubal occlusion, peritubal adhesions, ectopic pregnancy due to tubal damage without occlusion, chronic pelvic pain, and recurrent PID.

ETIOLOGY The etiology of PID has seemed to vary greatly in several studies for reasons related to patient selection as well as methodology. As is summarized in Table 91-1, the agents most often implicated in acute PID include those which are primary causes of cervicitis (*Neisseria gonorrhoeae* and *C. trachomatis*) and those which can be regarded as abnormal components of the vaginal flora.

In the United States, gonococci were isolated from 44 percent of women with acute PID in a multicity cooperative study during the 1970s. From 1980 through 1985 in Seattle, *N. gonorrhoeae* and *C. trachomatis* have each been found in about half of all patients with proven PID: about one-fourth had gonorrhea alone, one-fourth had chlamydial infection alone, and one-fourth had both infections. However, in Scandinavian countries, where gonococcal infection is under better control, endocervical gonococcal infection has been found in less than one-fourth of women with PID during the past decade, while chlamydial infection has been roughly twice as common as gonococcal infection in this group. In general, PID is most often associated with gonorrhea in populations having a high incidence of gonorrhea in developing countries and in indigent, central city urban populations in developed countries. In several studies of women with PID, up to two-thirds with positive endocervical cultures for *N. gonorrhoeae* have had positive endometrial, peritoneal, or tubal cultures for this organism. Similarly, studies of women with proven PID have shown that *C. trachomatis* can be demonstrated by

TABLE 91-1 Cervical and vaginal organisms most often implicated in acute PID

	Vaginal flora		
Cervical pathogens	Anaerobic bacteria	Facultative bacteria	Mycoplasma
N. gonorrhoeae *C. trachomatis*	*Bacteroides* spp. *Peptococci* *Peptostreptococci* *Mobiluncus* spp. *Actinomyces* spp.	Enterobacteriaceae *H. influenzae* *G. vaginalis* *Streptococcus*, groups B, D	*M. hominis* *U. urealyticum*

culture or immunofluorescent staining in the endometrium or tubes of the majority of those who have endocervical chlamydial infection.

Anaerobic and facultative anaerobic organisms (especially *Bacteroides* species, anaerobic gram-positive cocci, *Escherichia coli*, and group B and group D streptococci) and genital mycoplasmas have been isolated from specimens obtained at laparoscopy from the peritoneal fluid or fallopian tubes in a varying proportion—typically one-fourth to one-third—of women with PID studied in the United States. These vaginal organisms can be found in association with chlamydial or gonococcal infection, as well as in women without them, and have been implicated particularly often in women wearing intrauterine contraceptive devices. The importance of vaginal organisms in salpingitis has probably been overestimated in studies based on culture obtained by culdocentesis or endometrial aspiration, procedures in which contamination of the aspirated specimen by vaginal flora could occur. However, as noted above, specimens obtained by laparoscopy have also contained anaerobic and facultative species in some patients with PID.

It should be apparent that it is extremely difficult to determine the exact microbial etiology in the individual patient with PID because of the frequency of mixed infection, the difficulty in sampling the fallopian tube itself, and the complexity of microbiologic techniques required to detect the various fastidious pathogens which most often cause this disorder.

In general, first episodes of acute PID are particularly likely to be caused by *N. gonorrhoeae* and/or *C. trachomatis*. These sexually transmitted pathogens are somewhat less often implicated in recurrent bouts of acute PID, episodes occurring in IUD users, and episodes precipitated by invasive intrauterine diagnostic or therapeutic procedures, which are often associated with ascending infection caused by the more virulent components of the endogenous vaginal flora.

EPIDEMIOLOGY It has been estimated that the annual incidence of PID in the United States during the mid-1970s was about 850,000 cases per year, and the direct and indirect costs of PID and its complications (excluding the cost of fetal death due to ectopic pregnancies) totaled an estimated $1.25 billion per year. These cost estimates do not include the growing costs of tubal microsurgery and in vitro fertilization for women rendered infertile because of salpingitis. PID is not a reportable disease in the United States; survey data from the National Drug and Therapeutic Index and the National Ambulatory Medical Care Survey suggest that the incidence of PID increased from the mid-1960s through the mid-1970s and may have decreased since then. The incidence of one of the major sequelae of salpingitis, ectopic pregnancy, progressively rose each year from 13,200 cases in 1967 to 67,000 cases in 1981. Similar trends in ectopic pregnancies have been seen in Canada and England. There is some evidence that the percentage of involuntary infertility has also increased in the United States during the same period.

Acute PID is almost exclusively a disease of sexually active women. The risk appears to be several times greater in sexually active teenagers who are 15 to 16 years old than among women 20 to 24 years of age. Important risk factors other than young age include a previous history of gonorrhea or of salpingitis, and use of an intrauterine device, particularly the Dalkon shield. In most studies, the relative risk of PID among IUD users was higher in nulliparous women than in parous women. On the other hand, women using oral contraceptives appear to be at decreased risk of PID, particularly gonococcal PID, and for this reason some experts advocate use of oral contraceptives by women at high risk for PID. Barrier methods of contraception prevent PID by reducing the risk of chlamydial and gonococcal infection. Tubal sterilization reduces (but does not completely eliminate) the risk of salpingitis by preventing intraluminal spread of infection into the tubes.

PATHOGENESIS Factors cited as possibly contributing to intracanalicular upward spread of gonococci and *Chlamydia* from the endocervix to the endometrium and endosalpinx include estrogen-dominated (thin) cervical mucus, attachment to sperm which migrate upward into the tubes, use of an intrauterine device, and menstruation. The onset of symptoms of gonorrhea-associated PID and of *Chlamydia*-associated PID often occurs during or just after the menstrual period. In fallopian tube organ cultures in vitro, gonococci attach to the surface of the secretory columnar cells (but not the ciliated cells) of the endosalpinx. Gonococcal pili and perhaps other surface proteins are important in this attachment. Gonococci then are taken into the secretory cells by endocytosis. They pass through the cells, and perhaps between cells, and are extruded through the base of the cell into the submucosal connective tissue. Ciliary motion ceases, and then ciliated cells, although not directly invaded by gonococci, are sloughed from the mucosa during this process—a factor which may render the tubes more susceptible to superinfection by other organisms. It is uncertain whether this loss of ciliated cells is irreversible in vivo. Gonococcal endotoxin and peptidoglycan are at least partly responsible for these cytotoxic effects.

Gonococci associated with PID are significantly more resistant to penicillin and less likely to belong to the Arg-Hyx-Ura- auxotype than are strains causing uncomplicated gonorrhea. Also, gonococci isolated from the fallopian tubes reportedly form transparent colonies, whereas paired isolates from the cervix more often form opaque colonies, reflecting phenotypic changes in the protein composition of the gonococcal outer membrane which may be important in the pathogenesis of PID.

C. trachomatis also infects the columnar cells of the fallopian tube, but produces little damage in tubal organ cultures, perhaps because the host response is more important in the pathogenesis of chlamydial salpingitis. Chlamydial endometritis and salpingitis have been better studied than gonococcal endometritis or salpingitis in vivo, partly because animal models have been developed for chlamydial salpingitis, but not for gonococcal salpingitis. In chlamydial mucopurulent cervicitis (MPC), cervical biopsies show inclusions containing *Chlamydia* within columnar cells, and submucosal and stromal infiltration by mononuclear cells, polymorphonuclear leukocytes, and lymphoid aggregates containing transformed lymphocytes. Routine endometrial biopsies from consecutive women with chlamydial MPC show endometritis in approximately one-half. Although endometritis detected in this way is correlated with uterine tenderness, abnormal menstrual bleeding, and leukocytosis, symptoms of abdominal pain and fever are usually lacking, underscoring the subclinical nature of many cases of upper genital tract chlamydial infection. It is not known what proportion of those with endometritis also have salpingitis, since laparoscopy has not been performed in the absence of more suggestive symptoms and signs of salpingitis. However, among women with chlamydial MPC who do have symptoms and signs suggestive of salpingitis, the great majority who undergo endometrial biopsy and laparoscopy have both endometritis and salpingitis. Chlamydial inclusions are demonstrable by direct immunofluorescence in columnar epithelial cells of the endometrium and endosalpinx. The endometrial biopsies show plasma cells in the superficial endometrial stroma—a finding also seen to a lesser extent in gonococcal endometritis, but never in the uninfected endometrium. In addition, there is dense infiltration of the surface epithelium by acute and chronic inflammatory cells, lymphoid aggregates containing transformed lymphocytes in the stroma, and acute and chronic inflammatory cells in the lumens of the endometrial glands. Experimental inoculation of the fallopian tubes of lower primates produces mild acute salpingitis and ciliary sloughing, which is completely reversible. However, if experimental tubal inoculation is preceded by repeated inoculation of the cervix, a more intense salpingitis results and progresses to peritubular scarring. This suggests that in the female genital tract, as in the eye, it is repeated exposure to *C. trachomatis* which leads to the greatest degree of tissue inflammation and damage.

The pathogenesis of PID attributable to mycoplasmas or other vaginal anaerobic or facultative organisms is less well studied. It is possible that other vaginal organisms implicated in PID cause tubal infection in women whose tubes have already been damaged by a primary sexually transmitted pathogen (i.e., *N. gonorrhoeae* or *C. trachomatis*). Since the anaerobic organisms and mycoplasmas implicated in PID are found in the vagina most often and in greatest concentration in bacterial vaginosis (nonspecific vaginitis), it is possible that bacterial vaginosis itself is a predisposing risk factor for PID (in the same manner that poor oral hygiene is a risk factor in aspiration pneumonia).

Certain other iatrogenic factors, such as dilatation and curettage or cesarean section, are known to pose a greater risk of causing PID in women with endocervical gonococcal or chlamydial infection. It remains to be determined whether such procedures are also a greater risk in women with bacterial vaginosis.

CLINICAL MANIFESTATIONS Tuberculous salpingitis Unlike nontuberculous salpingitis, genital tuberculosis often occurs in older women, and about half are postmenopausal. In a large review of cases in Sweden, 38 percent had had previously diagnosed tuberculosis. The commonest presenting symptoms were abnormal vaginal bleeding (41 percent), pain including dysmenorrhea (25 percent), and infertility (13 percent). Most had normal bimanual pelvic examinations, though about one-quarter had adnexal masses. The most common method of diagnosis was endometrial biopsy, showing tuberculous granulomas, associated with a positive culture in many cases.

Nontuberculous salpingitis The evolution of symptoms classically proceeds from a mucopurulent vaginal discharge caused by cervicitis—possibly associated with dysuria and frequency due to urethritis, or with anorectal pain, tenesmus, rectal discharge, and bleeding due to proctitis—to midline abdominal pain and abnormal vaginal bleeding caused by endometritis, to bilateral lower abdominal and pelvic pain caused by salpingitis, to nausea and vomiting and increased abdominal tenderness caused by peritonitis. Some patients have generalized abdominal pain caused by generalized peritonitis, or pleuritic right upper quadrant pain caused by perihepatitis. The pattern in which symptoms evolve varies from patient to patient and is also related to the etiology of the PID.

The onset of IUD-associated PID is typically gradual, and may be preceded by typical malodorous vaginal discharge characteristic of bacterial vaginosis. The onset of gonococcal PID is typically more acute than that of chlamydial PID, although both are often associated with menses.

The abdominal pain is usually described as dull or aching. In some cases, pain is lacking or is atypical, and active inflammatory changes can be found in the course of an unrelated evaluation or procedure such as a tubal ligation or laparoscopic evaluation for infertility. Metrorrhagia precedes or coincides with the onset of pain in about 40 percent of women with PID, symptoms of urethritis occur in 20 percent, and symptoms of proctitis in 7 percent of patients.

Speculum examination shows evidence of mucopurulent cervicitis in the majority of women with gonococcal or chlamydial PID. Cervical motion tenderness is produced by stretching of the adnexal attachments on the side toward which the cervix is pushed. Bimanual examination reveals uterine fundal tenderness due to endometritis, and abnormal adnexal tenderness due to salpingitis which is usually, but not necessarily, bilateral. Adnexal swelling is palpable in about one-half of women with acute salpingitis, but evaluation of the adnexae in a patient with marked tenderness is not completely reliable, even by an experienced examiner. An initial temperature >38°C is found in only about one-third of patients with acute salpingitis, and fever is not required for the diagnosis.

Laboratory findings include elevation of the erythrocyte sedimentation rate (ESR) in 75 percent and elevation of the peripheral white blood cell count in about 60 percent of patients with salpingitis. C-reactive protein is elevated in most women with acute PID. Microscopic examination of a saline wet-mount preparation of vaginal fluid has revealed more than one polymorphonuclear leukocyte per vaginal epithelial cell in nearly all patients with laparoscopically confirmed salpingitis in Swedish studies, and some experts consider the absence of white blood cells in vaginal fluid or cervical mucus as incompatible with the diagnosis of acute PID.

Certain clinical manifestations of acute PID have been correlated with etiologic findings. For example, the onset of salpingitis is related to menses in women with gonorrhea or chlamydial infection. Women with gonorrhea or chlamydia-associated salpingitis are significantly younger than women with other forms of salpingitis. As is summarized in Table 91-2, women with chlamydia-associated salpingitis tend to have an indolent disease with mild symptoms of significantly longer duration and with less fever when compared to women who have gonorrhea-associated salpingitis, but paradoxically, those with chlamydia-associated salpingitis have had significantly higher erythrocyte sedimentation rates and more severe inflammatory reactions seen in laparoscopy. It is suspected that for all recognized cases of symptomatic *Chlamydia* salpingitis, there is an equal number of unrecognized cases of indolent subclinical *Chlamydia* salpingitis, and that subclinical chronic or recurrent *Chlamydia* salpingitis may be a major cause of infertility in women.

IUD-associated PID also tends to be indolent and is less often associated with fever, but more often with adnexal masses, than is PID not associated with IUD use.

Perihepatitis and periappendicitis Symptoms of perihepatitis, including pleuritic upper abdominal pain and tenderness, usually localized to the right upper quadrant, occur in 5 to 10 percent of women with acute PID. The onset of symptoms of perihepatitis occurs during or after onset of symptoms of PID and may overshadow the lower abdominal symptoms, leading to a mistaken diagnosis of cholecystitis. In up to a quarter of all cases of acute salpingitis in some studies, laparoscopy performed early reveals inflammation ranging from edema and erythema of the liver capsule to exudate with fibrinous adhesions between the visceral and parietal peritoneum. When treatment is delayed, and laparoscopy is performed late, dense "violin-string" adhesions are seen over the liver; these cause chronic exertional or positional right upper quadrant pain when traction is placed on the adhesions. Although perihepatitis, also known as the Fitz-Hugh–Curtis syndrome, was for many years attributed to gonococcal PID, it has been recognized that most cases of perihepatitis have been associated with chlamydial salpingitis. In patients with chlamydial salpingitis, serum microimmunofluorescent antibody titers against *C. trachomatis* are typically much higher when perihepatitis is present than when it is absent, and it has been suggested that repeated chlamydial infections are responsible for perihepatitis.

Physical findings include right upper quadrant tenderness and usually show evidence of adnexal tenderness and cervicitis, even in patients whose symptoms are not suggestive of salpingitis.

Liver function tests are nearly always normal, since inflammation is largely limited to the liver capsule, usually sparing the parenchyma.

TABLE 91-2 Characteristics of laparoscopically verified salpingitis associated with *C. trachomatis* alone, *N. gonorrhoeae* alone, or neither agent (from Svensson et al, 1980)

	Chlamydia-associated, % (*N*=68*)	Gonococcus-associated, % (*N*=19†)	Not gonococcus- or chlamydia-associated, % (*N*=64)
Temperature >38°C	27	74	30
Duration pelvic pain >3 days	85	68	62
ESR >30	65	32	28
Laparoscopic appearance of tubes, moderately severe or severe	78	74	47

* C. trachomatis *isolated from cervix, urethra, rectum, or tubes; or serologic evidence of acute chlamydial infection.*

† N. gonorrhoeae *isolated from cervix, urethra, or tubes; no cultural or serologic evidence of* C. trachomatis *infection.*

SOURCE: *Svensson et al.*

Oral cholecystogram may show nonfunction of the gallbladder, but ultrasonography of the right upper quadrant is normal. The presence of mucopurulent cervicitis and pelvic tenderness in a young woman with subacute pleuritic right upper quadrant pain with normal ultrasonography of the gallbladder points to a diagnosis of perihepatitis.

Periappendicitis (appendiceal serositis which does not involve the intestinal mucosa) has been found in approximately 5 percent of patients undergoing appendectomy for suspected appendicitis, and can occur as a complication of gonococcal or chlamydial salpingitis.

DIAGNOSIS Early diagnosis and initiation of therapy are essential to minimize tubal scarring. Appropriate treatment must not be withheld from patients who have an equivocal diagnosis. Since delay in therapy may lead to progression of tubal scarring, it is better to err on the side of overdiagnosis and overtreatment. On the other hand, it is essential to differentiate between salpingitis and other pelvic pathology, particularly surgical emergencies such as appendicitis and ectopic pregnancy.

No clinical or laboratory finding short of laparoscopy is pathognomonic for salpingitis, and there is reluctance to perform laparoscopy in all cases of suspected salpingitis. The following minimum criteria for the clinical diagnosis of salpingitis are advocated: (1) lower abdominal pain of <3 weeks' duration; (2) pelvic tenderness on bimanual pelvic examination; and (3) evidence of lower genital tract infection (e.g., white blood cells outnumber all other cells in the vaginal fluid). Approximately 60 percent of such patients have salpingitis at laparoscopy.

The presence of additional findings such as a rectal temperature >38°C, a palpable adnexal mass, and elevation of the ESR >15 mm/h also raise the probability of salpingitis, which was found at laparoscopy in 68 percent of patients with one of these additional findings, 90 percent of patients with two or more, and 96 percent of patients with three or more additional findings. However, only 17 percent of all patients with laparoscopy-confirmed salpingitis had three additional findings. The serum C-reactive protein is usually elevated in women with confirmed PID.

Mucopurulent cervicitis is probably responsible for the presence of leukocytes in vaginal fluid in PID, and it is likely that mucopurulent cervicitis would be a useful discriminatory sign in differentiating PID from other causes of lower abdominal pain.

Several clinical features other than the presence of cervicitis favor a diagnosis of salpingitis. These include onset with menses, history of recent abnormal menstrual bleeding, presence of an IUD, history of previous salpingitis, and exposure to a male with urethritis. Detection of polymorphonuclear leukocytes in fluid aspirated by culdocentesis supports a diagnosis of suspected salpingitis. Urethritis or proctitis may occur in chlamydial or gonococcal infection but may also represent a urinary tract infection or an intestinal source for the patient's symptoms. Early onset of nausea and vomiting would favor appendicitis or other disorders of the gut. A missed menstrual period dictates evaluation for ectopic pregnancy. The more sensitive assays for human chorionic gonadotropin which are now available are usually, but not always, positive.

TABLE 91-3 Laparoscopic findings in patients with false-positive or false-negative clinical diagnoses of acute PID

False-positive clinical diagnosis		False-negative clinical diagnosis, unexpected PID at laparoscopy	
Laparoscopic diagnosis	Percent	Clinical diagnosis	Percent
Acute appendicitis	24	Ovarian tumor	20
Endometriosis	16	Acute appendicitis	18
Corpus luteum bleeding	12	Ectopic pregnancy	16
Ectopic pregnancy	11	Chronic salpingitis	6
Pelvic adhesions only	7	Acute peritonitis	6
Benign ovarian tumor	7	Endometriosis	5
Chronic salpingitis	6	Uterine myoma	5
Miscellaneous	15	Atypical pelvic pain	6
		Miscellaneous	6

SOURCE: *Jacobsen and Weström.*

Ultrasonography is sometimes useful to differentiate pelvic abscess from an inflammatory mass involving tubes, ovary, bowel, and omentum, but is not sufficiently sensitive to detect salpingitis.

Laparoscopy is the most specific method for diagnosis of acute salpingitis. Although it may be normal if inflammation is limited to the endosalpinx or endometrium, patients with suspected PID who have normal laparoscopy have a better prognosis, with few if any sequelae, when compared with patients who have abnormal laparoscopic findings. The primary and uncontested value of laparoscopy in women with lower abdominal pain is exclusion of other surgical problems. Table 91-3 clearly shows that the most common and serious problems that may be confused with salpingitis are usually unilateral. Unilateral pain or pelvic mass, though not incompatible with PID, is a strong indication for laparoscopy unless the clinical picture warrants laparotomy instead. Atypical clinical findings such as the absence of lower genital tract infection, a missed menstrual period, or failure to respond to appropriate therapy are other frequent indications for laparoscopy.

Laparoscopic criteria used for the diagnosis of salpingitis include (1) erythema of the fallopian tube; (2) edema of the fallopian tube; and (3) seropurulent exudate or fresh, easily lysed adhesions at the fimbriated end or on the serosal surface of a fallopian tube. Laparoscopic findings are further scored as mild, where the above manifestations are mild and the tubes are freely movable and patent; moderate, when the above manifestations are more marked, tubes are not freely movable, and patency is uncertain; and severe, when findings consist of an inflammatory mass.

Endometrial biopsy showing plasma cell endometritis is relatively sensitive and highly specific for the diagnosis of PID, being found in at least two-thirds or more of women with laparoscopically confirmed salpingitis, and absent in women without PID.

The etiologic diagnosis of PID can be further studied by cultures or specimens obtained by endocervical swab, endometrial aspiration, or culdocentesis, or by laparoscopy or laparotomy. Endocervical swab specimens should be examined by Gram stain for granulocytes and gram-negative diplococci and by culture for *N. gonorrhoeae.* The sensitivity of Gram stain is about 60 percent and specificity >95 percent, compared with culture. The endocervical swab specimen should also be tested for *C. trachomatis* whenever possible. Although isolation of either *N. gonorrhoeae* or *C. trachomatis* from the cervix does not prove that either agent is also present in the upper genital tract, this should strongly support the diagnosis of PID. A 1985 study showed that the clinical diagnosis of PID made by expert gynecologists was confirmed by laparoscopy or endometrial biopsy in only 60 percent of all consecutive patients, but in 90 percent of those who also had positive cultures for *N. gonorrhoeae* or *C. trachomatis.* There is no evidence that isolation of anaerobes or facultative anaerobes from the cervix or vagina correlates with the presence of these organisms in the upper genital tract in acute PID, but this has not been well studied. The value of culture of culdocentesis and endometrial aspirate specimens is disputed because of the risk of contamination of the specimen with vaginal flora. When laparoscopy is performed, material can be obtained directly from the cul-de-sac or the fimbriated opening of the tube, or by tubal aspiration if pyosalpinx is present. Such specimens should be cultured for anaerobic and facultative pathogens, as well as for *N. gonorrhoeae* and *C. trachomatis.*

TREATMENT Hospitalization should be considered in all women with PID. Hospitalization is strongly recommended when (1) the diagnosis is uncertain, (2) surgical emergencies such as appendicitis and ectopic pregnancy must be excluded, (3) a pelvic abscess is suspected, (4) severe illness precludes outpatient management, (5) the patient is pregnant, (6) the patient is assessed as unable to follow or tolerate an outpatient regimen, (7) the patient has failed to respond to outpatient therapy, or (8) clinical follow-up after 48 to 72 h of instituting antibiotic treatment cannot be arranged. The treatment of choice is not established. No single agent is active against the entire spectrum of pathogens (Table 91-4). Several antimicrobial combinations do provide a broad spectrum of activity against the major pathogens in vitro, but many have not been adequately evaluated for clinical efficacy in PID.

Examples of combination regimens with broad activity against major pathogens in PID

1 Doxycycline 100 mg, twice a day, IV, plus cefoxitin 2.0 g, four times a day, IV. These drugs should be continued IV for at least 4 days and at least 48 h after the patient defervesces. Doxycycline should be continued in a dose of 100 mg by mouth, twice a day, after discharge from the hospital to complete 14 days of therapy. This regimen provides excellent coverage for *N. gonorrhoeae,* including penicillinase-producing *N. gonorrhoeae* (PPNG), and *C. trachomatis.*

2 Clindamycin 600 mg, four times a day, IV, plus gentamicin 2.0 mg/kg, IV, followed by 1.5 mg/kg, three times a day, IV, in patients with normal renal function. These drugs should be continued for at least 4 days and at least 48 h after the patient defervesces. Clindamycin should be continued in a dose of 450 mg, by mouth, four times a day, after discharge from the hospital to complete 14 days of therapy. This regimen provides optimal activity against anaerobes and facultative gram-negative rods, and limited data suggest that it is active against *C. trachomatis* and *N. gonorrhoeae* when recommended doses are used.

Patients who are not hospitalized should also receive a combined regimen with broad activity, such as cefoxitin 2.0 g, IM, followed by doxycycline 100 mg, by mouth, twice a day for 14 days. Although a single loading dose of amoxicillin, ampicillin, or procaine penicillin with probenecid, as recommended for uncomplicated gonorrhea (see Chap. 104), could be used in place of cefoxitin, these regimens are not effective against PPNG and have less activity against anaerobes and facultative gram-negative rods. Tetracycline could also be used in a dose of 500 mg, four times a day, in place of doxycycline, but it is less active against certain anaerobes, and requires more frequent dosing; both represent major drawbacks in the treatment of PID.

Management of sexual partners All persons who are sexual partners of patients with PID should be examined for STD and promptly treated with a regimen effective against uncomplicated gonococcal and chlamydial infection.

Follow-up All patients who are treated as outpatients should be clinically reevaluated in 48 to 72 h. Those not responding favorably should be hospitalized. A culture to test whether cure has been achieved should be performed as needed.

Removal of an intrauterine device Although the exact effect of IUD removal on the response of acute salpingitis to antimicrobial therapy and on the risk of recurrent salpingitis is unknown, removal of the IUD is recommended soon after antimicrobial therapy has been initiated. When an IUD is removed, contraceptive counseling is necessary.

Surgery Surgery is necessary only rarely for treatment of salpingitis, except in the face of life-threatening infection such as rupture or threatened rupture of a tuboovarian abscess, or for drainage of an abscess. Ultrasonography is useful for diagnosing and following pelvic abscesses. When surgery is performed, conservative procedures are usually sufficient. Pelvic abscesses can often be drained by posterior colpotomy, and peritoneal lavage can be used if there is generalized peritonitis.

PROGNOSIS Of women treated for PID on an ambulatory basis with IM penicillin followed by a 10-day course of ampicillin, or with a 10-day course of tetracycline alone, in a cooperative trial in the United States, nearly 20 percent treated with either drug were judged to be clinical failures. Among 900 women who underwent long-term follow-up for a mean period of 8 years after successful treatment of the acute episode with various regimens in Sweden, late sequelae included infertility due to bilateral tubal occlusion, ectopic pregnancy due to tubal scarring without occlusion, chronic pelvic pain, and recurrent salpingitis. Chronic pain lasting longer than 6 months was seen in 18 percent of patients and infertility due to tubal occlusion in 17 percent; 4 percent of pregnancies that did occur were ectopic, representing approximately a sixfold increase over the expected rate of ectopic pregnancies.

The rate of infertility after salpingitis was found to be related to age of the patient, etiology of salpingitis, duration of symptoms when treatment was started, severity of salpingitis by laparoscopy at the time of diagnosis, and number of episodes of salpingitis. The rate of infertility due to tubal occlusion among women exposed to a chance of pregnancy was 14 percent for women 15 to 24 years of age and 26 percent for women 25 to 34 years of age; the risk for women of all ages combined was 11 percent after one episode of salpingitis, 23 percent after two episodes, and 54 percent after three or more episodes. The risk was 6 percent after one episode of *N. gonorrhoeae*–associated salpingitis and 21 percent after one episode of nongonococcal salpingitis. Infertility was demonstrated in about 20 percent of women after one episode of *C. trachomatis*–associated salpingitis.

Although the rate of infertility after *C. trachomatis*–associated salpingitis has not been determined in a similar prospective study, a preliminary analysis of such cases suggests about a 10 percent rate of tubal occlusion after therapy. A striking relationship has also been shown in several countries between infertility due to tubal occlusion and the prevalence and titer of antibody to *C. trachomatis.*

Recurrent salpingitis has been seen in approximately 15 to 25 percent of women treated for salpingitis in various studies.

PREVENTION Prevention of PID depends first on the effective use of current methods for control of gonococcal and chlamydial infection. These methods include providing ready access to modern methods of diagnosis and effective treatment, and treatment of sex partners to control further spread. The decline in popularity of the intrauterine device, particularly in nulliparous women, has undoubtedly helped to reduce the incidence of PID. It is possible, but not proven, that increased use of oral contraceptives might reduce the risk of PID,

TABLE 91-4 Approximate activity of the antimicrobial agents most commonly used to treat PID against the pathogens most commonly implicated in PID

			Vaginal anaerobes			
	N. gonorrhoeae	*C. trachomatis*	GPC*	GNR†	Facultative GNR	*M. hominis*
Ampicillin/penicillin G	4+	1+	4+	2+	2+	0
Tetracycline HCl	3+	4+	4+	2+	2+	2+
Doxycycline	3+	4+	4+	3+	2+	2+
Cefoxitin	4+	0	4+	3+	4+	0
Gentamicin/tobramycin	3+	0	1+	0	4+	2+?
Clindamycin	0	2+	4+	4+	0	3+
Metronidazole	0	0	4+	4+	0	0

* *GPC = Gram-positive cocci (peptococci, peptostreptococci).*
† *GNR = Gram-negative rods (anaerobic GNR include* Bacteroides; *facultative GNR include Enterobacteriaceae,* H. influenzae).
NOTE: *No single antimicrobial agent offers optimal activity against all of these pathogens, but certain combinations (e.g., cefoxitin plus doxycycline, gentamicin plus clindamycin) have complimentary activity against these pathogens.*

particularly the risk of recurrent PID among women who have already experienced one episode of PID.

The complications of salpingitis can be minimized by early diagnosis and prompt treatment. It seems logical, but is unproven, that broad-spectrum therapy effective against all of the common causes of PID would offer the best outcome. Similarly, hospitalization to ensure rest and adequate compliance may improve the rather dismal long-term prognosis for tubal function. One placebo-controlled study showed that concurrent anti-inflammatory therapy with prednisolone hastened the reduction of acute inflammatory changes but did not improve the end results as measured by fertility, hysterosalpingographic findings, or chronic pain. However, since the dose of prednisolone used was relatively low, and since the antibiotics used concurrently would not be very effective against chlamydial or anaerobic infection, the potential value of anti-inflammatory therapy has not been adequately evaluated.

REFERENCES

Acute Pelvic Inflammatory Disease (PID): 1985 STD Treatment Guidelines. Morb Mort Week Rep 34(4S):92S, 1985

Eschenbach DA et al: Polymicrobial etiology of acute pelvic inflammatory disease. N Engl J Med 293:166, 1975

Falk V: Treatment of acute nontuberculous salpingitis with antibiotics alone and in combination with glucocorticoids. Acta Obstet Gynecol Scand 44(Suppl):1, 1965

——— et al: Genital tuberculosis in women. Am J Obstet Gynecol 138:974, 1980

Gjønaess H et al: Pelvic inflammatory disease: Etiologic studies with emphasis on chlamydial infection. Obstet Gynecol 59:550, 1982

Henry-Suchet J et al: *Chlamydia trachomatis* associated with chronic inflammation in abdominal specimens from women selected for tuboplasty. Am J Obstet Gynecol 138:1022, 1980

Jacobsen L, Weström L: Objectivized diagnosis of acute pelvic inflammatory disease. Am J Obstet Gynecol 105:1088, 1969

Mårdh PA et al: *Chlamydia trachomatis* infection in patients with acute salpingitis. N Engl J Med 296:1377, 1977

Møller BR et al: Pelvic infection after elective abortion associated with *Chlamydia trachomatis*. Obstet Gynecol 59:210, 1982

Osser S, Persson K: Epidemiologic and serodiagnostic aspects of chlamydial salpingitis. Obstet Gynecol 59:206, 1982

Paavonen J et al: Comparison of endometrial biopsy and peritoneal fluid cytologic testing with laparoscopy in the diagnosis of acute pelvic inflammatory disease. Am J Obstet Gynecol 151:645, 1985

St John RK, Brown ST (eds): International symposium on pelvic inflammatory disease. Am J Obstet Gynecol 138:845, 1980

Svensson L et al: Differences in some clinical and laboratory parameters in acute salpingitis related to culture and serologic findings. Am J Obstet Gynecol 138:1017, 1980

——— et al: Infertility after acute salpingitis—with special reference to *Chlamydia trachomatis*-associated infections. Fertil Steril 40:322, 1983

Thompson SE et al: High failure rates in outpatient treatment of salpingitis with either tetracycline alone or penicillin/ampicillin combination. Am J Obstet Gynecol 152:635, 1985

Wasserheit JN et al: Microbial causes of proven pelvic inflammatory disease and efficacy of clindamycin with tobramycin. Ann Intern Med (in press)

Wølner-Hanssen P et al: Endometrial infection in women with chlamydial salpingitis. Sex Transm Dis 9:84, 1982

92 PREVENTION OF INFECTION: IMMUNIZATION AND ANTIMICROBIAL PROPHYLAXIS

LAWRENCE COREY / ROBERT G. PETERSDORF

There are three major ways to prevent infections: (1) by reducing exposure, (2) by acquiring or inducing immunity, and (3) by using antimicrobial agents to prevent colonization and infection. Exposure can be reduced by diminishing the prevalence of the infecting agent, by community-wide vaccination programs, and by isolating infected patients in cohorts. On an individual basis, however, the most reliable way to prevent infectious disease is to provide effective immunization or chemoprophylaxis against the causative agent. This chapter summarizes current immunization practices and principles of antimicrobial prophylaxis. Additional details are provided in the chapters dealing with individual diseases.

IMMUNIZATION

Immunity may be defined as the ability of the individual to resist or overcome infection; it may be innate or acquired. For many infectious diseases, immunity is acquired during recovery from an infection or induced by the administration of vaccines prepared from inactivated or live microorganisms of modified disease-producing potential, or from specific antigen(s) derived from these organisms. The purpose of immunization, therefore, is to provoke a specific immunologic response to a selected microbial agent or its antigens with the expectation that this will result in humoral, and/or secretory, and/or cell-mediated immunity. While this protection may diminish over time, future exposures to the same stimulus will result in a rapid return of the immune response because of heightened reactivity of antibody-forming, phagocytic, and other cells that mediate immune mechanisms (see Chap. 62).

Certain infectious diseases present special situations that impede the development of vaccines. For example, *Salmonella* organisms and rhinoviruses consist of several hundred antigenically unique strains, making production of a vaccine difficult. Second, the portal of entry of an organism and the role of local immunity are important in determining whether a vaccine given parenterally will offer protection from either infection or disease. Third, even when effective immunizing agents are available, difficulties in delivering them to the susceptible population may preclude their use.

GENERAL PRINCIPLES OF IMMUNIZATION Infections can be prevented or controlled by active and/or passive immunization. Active immunization with live attenuated vaccines generally results in subclinical or mild clinical illness which duplicates, to a limited extent, the disease that is marked for prevention; generally, it provides both local and durable humoral immunity. "Killed" or inactivated vaccines, such as influenza, rabies, typhoid, and cholera vaccines, maintain immunogenicity, without infectivity, but have several disadvantages including the large amount of antigen that must be administered by the parenteral route and the greater time period between administration of the antigen and the appearance of a protective effect. Table 92-1 summarizes active immunizing agents.

The use of any biological substance requires balancing its benefits and risks, and each vaccine must be evaluated accordingly. While some immunizations, such as diphtheria, tetanus, and poliomyelitis, are recommended for all individuals, others should be used only in those who have an increased risk of either acquiring the disease or developing complications. Pneumococcal polysaccharide vaccine, influenza vaccine, hepatitis B vaccine, bacillus Calmette-Guérin (BCG) vaccine, and meningococcal vaccine are some examples.

Inactivated vaccines can be administered simultaneously at separate sites, although vaccines known to be associated with severe side effects should generally be given on separate occasions. Some vaccines contain trace amounts of preservatives or antibiotics to which patients may be sensitive, and, although reactions to them are unusual, reviewing the manufacturers' package insert prior to use of these agents may be helpful. Live virus vaccines prepared by growing viruses in cell culture are usually devoid of potential allergic substances. Many live virus vaccinations can be given simultaneously; measles, mumps, and rubella are some examples. However, when more than one dose of live viral vaccine is required, repeated administration should be separated by at least 1 month. After administration of an immunobiologic, the patient should be given a written record of its receipt and information about the necessity and timing of subsequent doses.

Contraindications to vaccination Virus replication following administration of live attenuated virus vaccines can be accentuated in immune-deficiency diseases and in patients whose immune responses have been suppressed as in leukemia, lymphoma, or generalized malignancy or following therapy with corticosteroids, alkylating drugs, antimetabolites, and radiation. Such patients should not be given live attenuated virus vaccines. Vaccination of persons with severe febrile disease should be deferred to avoid superimposing the adverse effects of the vaccine on the underlying illness. Because of a theoretical risk to the developing fetus, live attenuated virus vaccines generally should not be given to pregnant women. For some vaccines, particularly live attenuated rubella vaccine, pregnancy is an absolute contraindication to vaccination. Passively acquired antibody can interfere with the response to live attenuated virus vaccines; therefore, administration of live vaccine should be postponed until approximately 3 months after passive immunization.

IMMUNIZATION IN ADULTS Most immunization policies have been directed at vaccinating infants and children. A substantial portion of the morbidity and mortality from vaccine-preventable diseases occurs in adolescents and adults. Foreign students, immigrants, and refugees are often at increased risk of vaccine-preventable illnesses. A systematic approach to immunization is needed by all adult health care providers to ensure that their patients are protected against those diseases that can be averted or mitigated by vaccination.

Diphtheria Because of the widespread use of diphtheria toxoid, the incidence of diphtheria in the United States has declined drastically, and only 11 cases were reported between 1980 and 1982. However, 62 percent of adults aged 18 to 39, and over 50 percent of those over 60 lack protective levels of circulating antitoxin to diphtheria. The myocardial and peripheral nervous system involvement associated with *Corynebacterium diphtheriae* is due to elaboration of an exotoxin (see Chap. 96). Diphtheria toxoid is a cell-free preparation of diphtheria toxin treated with formaldehyde. The quantity of toxoid varies among products, and the concentration of diphtheria toxoid in adult preparations is lower than in the pediatric formulation. Adverse reactions are thought to be related to dose and age. Diphtheria immunization is at least 95 percent effective in reducing both the risk of diphtheria and the severity of clinical illness. Diphtheria toxoid provides protection against only the toxin and not the somatic components of *C. diphtheriae,* and local infection, either in the respiratory tract or skin, may occur in immune individuals. Nontoxigenic strains also may cause mild, focal infections.

All children under 7 years should receive routine immunization against diphtheria in the form of absorbed diphtheria and tetanus toxoids and pertussis vaccine (DPT). Absorbed toxoids are produced by the addition of aluminum compounds to the formaldehyde-inactivated toxoid and are more antigenic than the fluid (plain) preparation. Children should receive a primary series of three doses of DPT vaccine before they are a year old, a booster at 18 months, and another when they enter school. A preparation without pertussis vaccine is available for primary immunization of children who are unable to tolerate the pertussis vaccine (DT). Because pertussis is less common and less severe in older children and adults, the preparation recommended for use in adults is a combination of tetanus and diphtheria toxoid in which the diphtheria toxoid is reduced to a maximum of two flocculating units per dose to avoid the febrile reactions that may accompany repeated exposure to diphtheria toxoid. This vaccine (Td) is recommended for primary immunization of adults and children older than 6 years of age and is also routinely used for booster immunization, both for the prevention of tetanus at the time of injury and for diphtheria prophylaxis. For primary immunization in adults, three intramuscular doses of Td should be given, the second dose 1 to 2 months after the first, and the third 6 to 12 months later. Thereafter, boosters at 10-year intervals should be given.

Tetanus (see Chap. 99) The incidence of tetanus has decreased dramatically with the routine use of tetanus toxoid, a formaldehyde-detoxified bacteria-free filtrate of *Clostridium tetanus.* The 75 cases of tetanus that are reported yearly in the United States almost exclusively occur in adults who are unimmunized or inadequately immunized. Two doses of the absorbed toxoid or three doses of fluid toxoid usually result in a protective level of antibody, 0.01 unit per milliliter tetanus antitoxin. Immune pregnant women confer temporary protection to their infant through placental transfer of maternal antibodies. Tetanus toxoid may be used singly or in combination with diphtheria toxoid (DT or Td), or with both diphtheria toxoid and pertussis vaccine (DPT). When used singly, primary immunization with the fluid toxoid is given in three doses at least 1 month apart with a booster 8 to 12 months later. The absorbed form should be given in two doses, 1 month apart. Primary immunization with tetanus toxoid is highly recommended for all children and adults. Clinical tetanus does not necessarily provide immunity against subsequent tetanus. Boosters after wound infection are recommended at 5-year intervals. Routine boosters at 10-year intervals (at mid-decade ages (25, 35, 45) are recommended. Systemic reactions after toxoid (Td) are uncommon. Arthus-like hypersensitivity reactions beginning 2 to 8 h after injection may be seen in persons who have received multiple boosters of tetanus toxoid. A history of a severe hypersensitivity or neurologic reaction from a previous booster constitutes a contraindication to further booster shots. Local side effects do not preclude a booster at 10-year intervals.

Pertussis Endemic pertussis infection is prevalent throughout the world. Complications and mortality of infection are greatest in children, especially those under 6 months. While controversy about the use of pertussis vaccine has occurred, routine use of the vaccine reduces the morbidity and mortality associated with pertussis infection in the neonate. Pertussis infection in adults and older children is usually mild, while systemic and local side effects from vaccination are increased in older children and adults. Pertussis vaccination is routinely recommended for children 1 year of age. Vaccination is *not* recommended for use in adults or children over 6 years of age. In exceptional cases such as persons with chronic pulmonary disease exposed to children with pertussis, or health care personnel exposed during outbreaks of pertussis, a booster dose of adsorbed pertussis vaccine (0.20 to 0.25 mL) may be useful.

Poliomyelitis (see Chap. 139) Routine polio vaccination of adults residing in the United States is not necessary because most are immune and the risk of exposure is small. However, susceptible adults at increased risk by virtue of travel or exposure to wild or vaccine poliovirus should receive primary immunization with either inactivated or wild attenuated polio vaccines. Both a live attenuated oral polio vaccine (OPV) and an inactivated polio vaccine (IPV) are licensed in the United States. A primary vaccination series with either OPV or IPV produces immunity to all three types of poliovirus in over 95 percent of recipients. OPV has been favored over IPV because it is easier to administer, orally versus injection; some studies indicate that it confers more resistance in the alimentary tract to reinfection; and it interferes with simultaneous infection by wild polioviruses. These properties are of special value during epidemics of poliomyelitis. Vaccination with OPV results in shedding of virus contained in the vaccine, and spread of virus to unvaccinated persons occurs. Rarely, recipients of oral vaccine or people in contact with them have contracted paralytic polio. The risk of vaccine-associated polio has been estimated to be one case per 9 million doses distributed to vaccinees and one case per 7 million doses distributed in household contacts. The relative risk of paralytic disease is slightly higher in susceptible adults than in children. Oral trivalent polio vaccine is the principal vaccine used in the United States. IPV is recommended in selective circumstances such as primary immunization of susceptible adults and in persons with immunodeficiencies and their household contacts. Primary immunization with IPV consists of four doses: three at 1- to 2-month intervals and a booster 6 to 12 months after the third. Booster doses at 2- to 3-year intervals either with IPV or with one dose of OPV after primary immunization with IPV will sustain long-lasting immunity.

For infants and children, the primary series of vaccination with

TABLE 92-1 Active immunization in adults *(continued)*

	Type of vaccine	Administration and frequency*	Comments
ALL ADULTS			
Tetanus and diphtheria	Adsorbed toxoid	IM at least every 10 years	Usually administered together as Td vaccine
Poliomyelitis	Live attenuated	Oral polio vaccine (OPV)	Preferred for routine use and during epidemics
	Formalin-inactivated	Inactivated polio vaccine (IPV)	Selective use in unimmunized adults
Measles, mumps, rubella	Live attenuated	SC once	All adults born after 1957 should have measles—see text for specific recommendations re: mumps and rubella vaccine
WOMEN OF CHILDBEARING AGE			
Rubella vaccine	Live attenuated	SC once	Postpartum vaccination of antibody negative persons
POSTPUBERTAL MALES			
Mumps	Live attenuated	SC once	Prevention of orchitis in susceptible seronegative males
PERSONS AT HIGH RISK OF ACQUIRING DISEASE OR DEVELOPING COMPLICATIONS OF DISEASE			
Influenza vaccine	Inactivated	SC yearly	Directed at reducing morbidity and mortality in those at risk of complications of influenza, e.g., chronic heart and lung disease and those over 65 years
Pneumococcal polysaccharide vaccine	Purified polysaccharide vaccine	SC once	Same population as influenza vaccine, functional or surgical asplenia, agammaglobulinemia, cirrhosis, multiple myeloma, and nephrotic syndrome
Hepatitis B vaccine	Inactivated subunit vaccine	3 doses IM at 0, 1, and 6 months	High-risk groups for acquisition of hepatitis B, including household contacts of hepatitis B patients, patients requiring a large volume of clotting factors, illicit drug users, homosexual men, and selected medical and dental personnel
Haemophilus influenzae type B	Purified capsular polysaccharide	SC once	Routine use in children more than 24 months of age; selected populations (day care of children 18–24 months and adults at high risk of getting invasive *H. influenzae* disease, e.g., asplenia, hypogammaglobulinemia)
POPULATIONS EXPOSED TO LOCALIZED OUTBREAKS			
Meningococcal vaccine	Purified capsular polysaccharide	SC once	Control of localized epidemics and adjunct to chemoprophylaxis in household contacts
Measles vaccine	Live attenuated	SC once	Control of outbreaks usually among adolescents or young adults
BCG vaccine	Live attenuated	SC or intradermally, once	Used in groups with excessive risk of new infection with tuberculosis or individuals persistently exposed to sputum-positive tuberculosis
Adenovirus vaccine	Live attenuated bivalent (types 4 and 7)	PO once	Used only for military recruits
Typhoid vaccine	Inactivated bacilli	SC in two doses	Household contact of documented *Salmonella typhi* carrier
Rubella vaccine	Live attenuated	SC once	Control of outbreaks among adolescents and young adults
TRAVELERS TO FOREIGN COUNTRIES			
Smallpox	Live vaccinia virus	Intradermally, every 3–5 years	No indications for smallpox vaccine in civilians
Yellow fever	Live attenuated	SC once per 10 years	Administered at yellow fever vaccination centers
Cholera	Phenol-inactivated suspension of *Vibrio cholerae*	SC approximately every 6 months	Only 50% effective and not effective in decreasing transmission of disease
Typhoid	Inactivated bacilli	SC in half doses 4 weeks apart	70–90% efficacy in ''normal'' exposure

TABLE 92-1 Active immunization in adults *(continued)*

	Type of vaccine	Administration and frequency*	Comments
Plague	Formaldehyde-inactivated *Yersinia pestis*	Primary series = three IM doses. First dose 1 mL; second dose 4 weeks later, 0.2 mL; third dose 5 months later, 0.2 mL	Agricultural workers who reside in plague-endemic areas
Poliomyelitis	Oral or inactivated polio vaccine	See text	Unimmunized adults should receive a complete primary series or at least 2 doses of IPV 1 month apart; if not, then a single dose of OPV is recommended; for high-risk travel in immunized adults, a single dose of OPV or IPV is recommended
Japanese encephalitis	Inactivated, purified mouse-brain vaccine	2 doses IM, 7–10 days apart	Not licensed in U.S.
Hepatitis A	Immune serum globulin	IM every 3 months	See "Passive Immunization" in this chapter

* *PO, orally; SC, subcutaneously; IM, intramuscularly.*

OPV consists of three doses. The first two should be given not less than 6 and preferably 8 weeks apart. The third dose should follow 8 to 12 months after the second dose. A booster dose of trivalent OPV should be given when the child enters kindergarten or first grade. Additional preadolescent immunization (at age 11 to 12) has been recommended to provide additional protection during adulthood. Live attenuated oral polio vaccine is acceptable for adults who have been vaccinated previously or whose circumstances do not allow adequate time for administration of IVP and who are not in a category in which oral vaccine is contraindicated.

Measles (see Chap. 132) While measles vaccine has markedly reduced the incidence of measles in the United States, localized outbreaks, particularly among teenagers and young adults, continue to occur. Measles mortality and encephalitis are greatest in adults, and efforts to eliminate measles in both the child and adult populations is currently underway. Measles vaccine is an attenuated live virus (Schwarz) vaccine derived from passage of the Edmonston strain of measles virus grown in a culture of chick embryo cells. The current vaccine differs from the older live attenuated Edmonston strain vaccine which was administered with human immune globulin.

Vaccination with the Schwarz strain produces life-long immunity in more than 95 percent of recipients. Revaccination of previously immune persons is not associated with significant adverse effects. Measles vaccine is recommended for all persons born after 1957 who lack documentation of prior vaccination on or after their first birthdays or who lack a firm diagnosis of measles. Persons born before 1957 can generally be considered immune. During measles outbreaks, it is recommended that all susceptible children, as well as adolescents and adults at risk, be immunized. Individuals who received measles vaccine before 12 months of age or who received killed measles vaccine followed within 3 months by live vaccine or a measles vaccine of unknown type between 1963 and 1967 should be revaccinated; travelers should be immune to measles before leaving the United States. Repeat vaccination with live measles vaccine poses no increased risk for individuals who have previously had natural measles or who have been vaccinated.

Up to 15 percent of vaccinated children will have fever lasting up to 5 days between the fifth and twelfth days after vaccination. Local induration and edema at the injection site may occur in persons who previously received killed measles vaccine.

IMMUNIZATION IN WOMEN OF CHILDBEARING AGE Rubella (see Chap. 133) The purpose of rubella vaccination is to prevent rubella embryopathy in the fetus. The direct approach to this goal would be to immunize all women before they become pregnant. However, the difficulty is being sure that a woman is not pregnant at the time of vaccination, and the increased risk of joint symptoms associated with vaccination in women has rendered this approach impractical. Because children are a major source of spread of rubella to pregnant females, rubella vaccination has been routinely recommended for all children older than 12 months. When given in combination with measles antigen, rubella vaccine should be administered when a child is about 15 months of age to achieve the maximum rate of measles seroconversion.

Since 1969 when rubella vaccine was first licensed, the incidence of rubella has declined steadily. However, 954 cases of the congenital rubella syndrome have been reported in the United States since the vaccine was introduced. An estimated 10 to 15 percent of young adults are susceptible to rubella, and outbreaks continue to occur at universities and places of employment that entail a higher risk, such as hospitals. Routine premarital rubella antibody determinations would help identify susceptible females before their first pregnancy. Testing for rubella antibody during the perinatal or antepartum period and vaccination of susceptible women in the immediate postpartum period is recommended. Rubella immunization of both male and female medical personnel having frequent contact with pregnant women is also recommended.

Rubella vaccine is prepared in cell cultures and is administered by subcutaneous injection. A single dose induces antibodies in approximately 95 percent of susceptible persons. There is no risk to susceptible contacts of vaccinees. Rubella vaccine virus has been demonstrated to cross the placenta and infect the fetus. Through 1983, 214 susceptible pregnant women who inadvertently received rubella vaccine within 3 months before or after conception and who continued their pregnancies to term have been evaluated. None of these infants had recognizable malformations attributable to rubella. However, fetal infection with vaccine-like rubella virus may produce pathologic changes in developing organs. The risk of teratogenicity is felt to be much lower from the vaccine virus than from the wild virus. If a pregnant woman is inadvertently vaccinated or if she becomes pregnant within 3 months of vaccination, she should be advised of the low (3 percent) risk of congenital infection to the fetus, and the theoretical risk of congenital rubella syndrome.

VACCINATION DURING PREGNANCY When a vaccine or toxoid is to be given during pregnancy, waiting until the second or third trimester to minimize concern about teratogenicity is advisable. Pregnant women not previously vaccinated against tetanus or diphtheria should receive two doses of Td. For those with an incomplete primary series, the completion of the series should be achieved. Booster doses of Td may be given during pregnancy. While live virus vaccines are not usually administered to pregnant women, if immediate protection against poliomyelitis or yellow fever is required, these vaccines may be administered. If yellow fever protection is necessary only for travel, then a waiver letter may be obtained. Indications for the administration of human immune globulin and inactivated vaccine such as hepatitis B, influenza, and rabies are not altered by pregnancy.

VACCINATION OF SUSCEPTIBLE POSTPUBERTAL MALES

Mumps (see Chap. 141) Mumps is primarily a disease of school-aged children; only about 15 percent of the cases occur in adolescents and adults. Most mumps infections are subclinical or self-limited. Meningoencephalitis occurs in up to 15 percent of cases and is usually uncomplicated and benign, although nerve deafness may be seen in 1 in 15,000 cases. Orchitis, usually unilateral, may occur in 20 percent of postpubertal males. The incidence of subsequent sterility is low. Live attenuated mumps vaccine (Jeryl-Lynn strain) grown in chick embryo cell cultures has been available since 1967. Mumps vaccination is recommended for all children older than 1 year and especially in children approaching puberty, adolescents, and adults, particularly males, who have not had mumps or who have no serologic evidence of mumps immunity. Skin testing is not a reliable indication of past infection. Persons with prior mumps or who have received vaccine are not at risk from live mumps vaccine. A single dose is given subcutaneously; continuing protection against infection and protective antibodies have both been shown to persist for at least 12 years after vaccination. Parotitis after vaccination is very rare. Patients with severe febrile illness or hypersensitivity to egg products, with malignancy who are receiving immunosuppressive therapy, or who are pregnant should not be vaccinated. Mumps vaccine virus has been shown to infect the placenta, but virus has not been isolated from fetal tissue.

VACCINATION OF PERSONS WITH CHRONIC HEART, PULMONARY, AND METABOLIC DISEASE

Influenza (see Chap. 130) Influenza occurs every year in the United States but with variation in incidence and geographic distribution. Epidemics occur periodically; more are caused by influenza A viruses than by influenza B. More importantly, influenza A epidemics are notable for causing mortality in excess of what is usually expected. In the 1957 to 1958 Asian influenza epidemic, nearly 70,000 excess deaths were reported in the United States during the 12-week epidemic period. Most nationwide influenza epidemics have resulted in 10,000 to 20,000 excess deaths. Hospitalization rates in high-risk groups will increase two- to fivefold. During influenza epidemics, deaths occur primarily among persons with chronic cardiovascular, pulmonary, renal, metabolic, or immunologic diseases. Surveys indicate that almost 50 percent of elderly persons have high-risk conditions, but only 25 percent of these get vaccinated. Vaccination of high risk populations has been shown to reduce mortality and complications associated with influenza. Vaccination of the entire population has not been considered a reasonable public health policy because protection is of limited duration owing to both the antigenic drift of the virus, as well as the short-lived antibody response to the inactivated vaccine, and the low incidence of serious infections in healthy persons.

Influenza vaccines are inactivated products of the prevalent circulating types of influenza virus. The vaccine usually contains influenza A and influenza B prototype antigens. Two types of vaccines are available, whole virus vaccines and "split-product" or subunit vaccines. Generally, whole virus vaccines are more immunogenic but have a slightly higher reaction rate than split-product vaccines. Studies with both preparations indicate a 60 to 95 percent protection rate, depending upon the population group studied and the relationship between the "epidemic" strain and the vaccine strain. In adults either form of vaccine can be used, but because of the high frequency of febrile reactions, children under 12 should receive two doses of split-product vaccine at approximately 3- to 6-week intervals. Vaccine is generally administered during the fall of the year and is given subcutaneously. While intradermal vaccination may elicit a good humoral antibody response, the clinical efficacy of this route of administration has not been well documented. Because even the zonally centrifuged inactivated influenza vaccines contain trace amounts of egg protein, patients who are allergic to egg or egg protein should not receive this vaccine. Severe adverse reactions to influenza vaccine are uncommon. Among recipients of A/New Jersey/76 swine influenza vaccine, an excess risk of Landry-Guillain-Barré syndrome occurred (10 cases for every million vaccinated), an incidence five to six times higher than in unvaccinated persons, but more recent (nonswine) influenza vaccines have not been associated with an increased risk of the Landry-Guillain-Barré syndrome.

Influenza vaccine is the preferred form of prophylaxis, because of its low cost, efficacy, and slight toxicity. Amantadine hydrochloride has been effective in preventing influenza infection especially during interepidemic intervals. Patients at risk of developing the complications of influenza who failed to receive their annual influenza vaccination should be placed on 100 mg amantadine hydrochloride twice daily during the period in which influenza A virus is identified in the community or until adequate protection after receipt of influenza vaccine has occurred.

Pneumococcal vaccine (see Chap. 93) Despite antibiotic therapy, the morbidity and mortality of pneumococcal disease remains a problem. Bacteremic pneumococcal disease appears to be more common in persons with sickle cell anemia, anatomic or functional asplenia, agammaglobulinemia, multiple myeloma, nephrotic syndrome, cirrhosis, alcoholism, diabetes mellitus, chronic cardiorespiratory disease, and after organ transplantation; in these situations vaccination is generally indicated. Other situations in which pneumococcal vaccine may be of benefit include closed populations in which systemic pneumococcal disease has been identified as an epidemic or endemic problem, or where an antibiotic-resistant strain of pneumococcus has emerged.

The pneumococcal polysaccharide vaccine licensed for use in the United States contains purified capsular material extracted separately from 23 types of *Streptococcus pneumoniae* (Danish types 1, 2, 3, 4, 5, 6F, 7F, 8, 9N, 9V, 10A, 11A, 12F, 14, 15B, 17F, 18C, 19A, 19F, 20, 22F, 23F, and 33F). These 23 types are responsible for about 87 percent of bacteremic pneumococcal disease in the United States. One dose of vaccine contains 25 μg of each polysaccharide. The majority of adults and most children over 2 years of age respond with development of measurable humoral antibody 2 to 3 weeks after vaccination. Immunity exists only against the pneumococcal types contained in the vaccine, although theoretically there may be some degree of cross-protection among immunologically similar types. The duration of protection is unknown, but elevated antibody levels appear to persist 3 to 5 years after immunizations. Booster doses are not recommended because of accentuated local adverse reactions. Persons who received the previous tetradecavalent (14-type) vaccine should not get the newer 23 valent vaccine. Vaccination reduces the likelihood of acquiring the pneumococcal types in the vaccine in the nasopharynx. There has been no evidence of a relative increase in disease caused by other microbial pathogens among vaccine recipients. Vaccination appears to reduce the incidence of pneumococcal pneumonia and bacteremia due to types in the vaccine by about 70 percent. Efficacy may be slightly lower in persons with cirrhosis or renal failure. Two-thirds of persons with serious pneumococcal disease have been hospitalized in the prior 5 years. This suggests that vaccination of high-risk patients who come to hospitals should be performed. Local erythema and pain at the injection site occur in approximately half the patients. Fever and myalgias are reported in fewer than 1 percent of recipients. Serious adverse reactions are rare, about 5 per 1 million doses.

Hepatitis B vaccine Hepatitis B vaccine (HBV) is a subunit, inactivated preparation containing the hepatitis B surface antigen (HBsAg). It is manufactured by concentration purification and inactivation of the hepatitis B virus from human donors with high titers of hepatitis B surface antigen in their plasma. Hepatitis B vaccine contains 20 μg/mL of HBsAg protein. Three 1-mL doses of vaccine given 1 and 6 months apart are recommended; O.5-mL (10 μg) doses are recommended for infants and children from 3 months to 9 years of age. For immunosuppressed patients and patients undergoing hemodialysis three 40-μg doses are recommended. Anti-HBs can be detected in the serum of both adults and children in over 90 percent of recipients after a complete vaccination series. Vaccine should be administered in the deltoid; lower seroconversion rates are seen with buttock injections. The protective efficacy of hepatitis B vaccine for the prevention of clinical hepatitis B has been approximately 95 percent in homosexual men, 90 percent in medical staff of hemodialysis units with endemic hepatitis B, and 75 percent in patients with renal insufficiency undergoing chronic hemodialysis in units with endemic hepatitis B. The duration of vaccine-induced protection and the need for boosters are not known.

Because of the cost and limited availability of vaccine, vaccination strategy is based on selective immunization of high-risk groups. These include susceptible household and sexual contacts of patients with acute and/or chronic hepatitis B, illicit users of injectable drugs, homosexual men, patients requiring blood clotting factor concentrations and large-volume transfusions, residents and staff of institutions and hemodialysis units, infants born to HBsAg-positive women, and closed communities where hepatitis B is endemic. Selective vaccination of health care personnel, including laboratory personnel who handle blood and blood products, nursing staff, and medical and dental personnel having frequent contact with groups with hepatitis B or blood products, is also recommended. These persons should be vaccinated as soon as possible after they begin work in a high-risk environment. The vaccine appears to have no effect on patients who are carriers of hepatitis B surface antigen and has not been associated with either resolution or worsening of chronic hepatitis B infection.

Postexposure immunization with a combination of hepatitis B immune globulin (HBIG) plus hepatitis B vaccine is useful in some clinical situations, such as immunoprophylaxis of infants born to mothers with acute or chronic hepatitis B, sexual contacts of patients with acute or chronic hepatitis B, or needle stick exposure from a known HBsAg carrier. When administered at a different site, HBIG does not appear to alter the subsequent development of anti-HBs after hepatitis B vaccine, and the combination of HBV and HBIG obviates the need for a second dose of HBIG.

***Haemophilus influenzae* vaccine** (see Chap. 109) *H. influenzae* type B infection is largely a disease of children, with peak attack rates between 6 months and 1 year of age. After 5 years of age, *H. influenzae* disease is not usually a significant problem. A polysaccharide vaccine has been newly licensed in the United States for routine use in all children at age 24 months. The vaccine could be used at age 18 months in high-risk groups, such as children attending day-care centers. Insufficient data are available on the efficacy and immunogenicity of vaccine in older children and adults. The vaccine should be used in children with chronic conditions associated with a high risk of type B disease such as hypogammaglobulinemia, asplenia, and Hodgkin's disease.

VACCINES USEFUL IN LOCALIZED OUTBREAKS **Meningococcal vaccine** (see Chap. 103) Meningococcal disease is endemic throughout the world. Occasionally, epidemics occur. In civilians in the United States meningococcal infections occur primarily in single isolated cases; serogroup B cause most of the illnesses, with serogroups C and W-135 accounting for the remainder. Secondary cases occur more frequently in household contacts than in the general population, and appropriate antibiotic prophylaxis has been the principal method of reducing the risk for immediate contacts. Vaccines have been used to curtail outbreaks of groups A and C meningococcal disease, and when epidemic meningococcal disease due to groups A or C occurs, the population at risk should be identified and vaccinated. Vaccination also should be considered as an adjunct to antibiotic prophylaxis for household contacts of cases of meningococcal disease caused by serogroups A, C, Y, or W-135. Because half of the secondary cases in families occur more than 5 days after the primary case, this is enough time to allow potential benefit from vaccination if antibiotic chemoprophylaxis has not been successful.

Two meningococcal polysaccharide vaccines, bivalent A-C, and quadrivalent A, C, Y, and W-135, are licensed for selective use in the United States. These vaccines are chemically defined antigens consisting of purified capsular polysaccharides and induce specific immunity to the serologic groups. The vaccine is administered parenterally as a single dose. Adverse reactions consist principally of localized erythema lasting 1 to 2 days. The vaccine appears effective in all age groups beyond the first year of life, and there is suggestive evidence of efficacy in children as young as 3 months of age. The duration of immunity and the need for booster doses has not been established.

BCG vaccine Efforts to control tuberculosis in the United States are directed toward the early identification and treatment of active cases and preventive therapy with isoniazid. Use of BCG vaccine should be considered for uninfected persons (skin test negative to 5 tuberculin units) who are exposed repeatedly to untreated or inadequately treated individuals or to individuals harboring resistant organisms, or health care workers and others with an annual infection rate of greater than 1 percent despite control measures. The protection from BCG vaccine is relative, and neither permanent nor predictable. BCG recipients should have repeat skin tests 2 to 3 months later; if they are negative, vaccination should be repeated. The World Health Organization (WHO) recommends that BCG vaccine be administered by the intradermal route, but vaccine for percutaneous administration is also available. Severe ulceration at the vaccination site occurs in about 1 percent of vaccinees. BCG should not be given to persons with impaired immune responses, and although no harmful effects of BCG on the fetus have been observed, it is best to avoid vaccination during pregnancy.

Adenovirus vaccine The epidemiologic syndrome of epidemic acute respiratory disease due to adenovirus 4 or 7 is almost exclusively a problem of military recruits. While an effective oral attenuated adenovirus vaccine has been manufactured, clinical illness caused by these adenoviruses has not been associated with significant morbidity or mortality in the civilian population, and hence use of this vaccine outside the military is not recommended.

Typhoid vaccine Routine typhoid vaccination is not recommended in the United States. Selective immunization is indicated for persons who are household contacts of a documented typhoid carrier or travelers to areas where typhoid is endemic. Typhoid vaccine is generally not necessary for persons affected by flooding or other natural disasters or for those in rural summer camps. Typhoid vaccine consists of whole typhoid bacilli that have been killed, concentrated, and preserved by various methods. The vaccine should be given in two doses of 0.5 mL subcutaneously or 0.1 mL intradermally, according to the manufacturers' recommendations. Booster doses at intervals of 3 years or more are recommended. Local reactions such as erythema, induration, and moderate fever for about 24 h may occur. Controlled trials indicate a 70 to 90 percent protection rate from clinical typhoid. Immunity may be overcome by exposure to high inocula of *Salmonella,* and localized gastrointestinal infection accompanied by diarrhea may still occur. A newly developed *oral* typhoid vaccine affords protection and is much easier to administer, particularly in endemic areas.

VACCINATION OF TRAVELERS TO FOREIGN COUNTRIES There are two objectives for immunization of foreign travelers: (1) to satisfy a country's requirements, as modified by international regulations, regarding prevention of the introduction and spread of disease (e.g., yellow fever, cholera, and smallpox), and (2) to protect the traveler.

Smallpox vaccination (see Chap. 134) In May 1980, the WHO declared the world free of smallpox. A smallpox vaccination certificate is not required by any country as a condition of entry for international travel. In May 1983, the distribution of smallpox vaccine for civilian use in the United States was discontinued. In the United States, smallpox vaccination is recommended only for persons who work in high-security laboratories with variola virus. Smallpox vaccine should *not* be used for the treatment of warts or prevention of recurrent herpes simplex virus infections.

Yellow fever vaccine Many countries require a current international certificate of vaccination against yellow fever from persons older than 6 months who have been in the countries reporting yellow fever (South America and the African subcontinent) in the preceding 6 days. Because these requirements change and often vary with the length of stay in the country, all travelers to areas where yellow fever is endemic should seek current information from health departments or international airlines before departing. Yellow fever vaccine must be administered at a designated yellow fever center. Vaccination certificates are valid for a period of 10 years, beginning 10 days after vaccination. The only yellow fever vaccine licensed in the United States is a live attenuated vaccine produced in chick embryos which must be administered subcutaneously in 0.5-mL amounts. Fever and malaise occur in 10 percent of recipients, but major reactions such as encephalitis are very rare. While pregnant females should generally not be vaccinated with live attenuated virus, the risk to the fetus is small, and pregnant women who must travel to areas where the risk of yellow fever is high should be vaccinated. Yellow fever virus vaccine should not be given to patients with severe underlying diseases such as leukemia or those receiving immunosuppressive therapy.

Cholera (see Chap. 115) Travelers to the Middle East, Asia, and Africa may require evidence of cholera vaccination. Ideally, travelers to these countries should be vaccinated 1 month prior to their departure. A single primary series or booster dose of vaccine is generally sufficient. The risk of cholera for travelers who use ordinary tourist accommodations is very slight, and currently available cholera vaccines are only about 50 percent effective in reducing the incidence of clinical illness for a period of only 3 to 6 months. They do not prevent transmission of disease.

Typhoid Travelers going to regions where food and water sanitation is poor may wish to receive typhoid vaccine. However, care in selecting food and water is the best protection.

Japanese encephalitis (see Chap. 143) Cases of Japanese encephalitis have occurred in travelers. An effective inactivated mouse-brain vaccine is available from Japan. While currently not licensed in the United States, the vaccine may be obtained under an investigational permit from the Centers of Disease Control. Candidates for the vaccine are persons who plan a visit of 3 or more weeks during the time of peak encephalitis activity to those areas in which Japanese encephalitis occurs and whose itinerary includes extensive travel to rural areas and intensive exposure to mosquito vectors. Short visits to urban areas are not an indication for vaccination.

Plague (see Chap. 114) Immunization against *Yersinia pestis* is recommended only for laboratory workers and for individuals such as Peace Corps volunteers or agricultural advisors who reside in plague-enzootic or plague-epidemic rural areas where avoidance of rodents and fleas is difficult. Travelers to countries or areas reporting endemic plague do not need to receive vaccine.

UNUSUAL OCCUPATIONAL EXPOSURES In general, vaccination of personnel such as laboratory or field workers whose vocation or avocation puts them at particular risk of developing an immunizable disease should receive preexposure immunization. For example, laboratory workers involved with rabies, *Y. pestis,* smallpox, *Rickettsia prowazekii, R. rickettsii,* yellow fever virus, or Venezuelan or Eastern equine encephalitis viruses, anthrax bacillus, or tularemia should be vaccinated against the appropriate agent. Occupational exposure requiring vaccination includes preexposure immunization against rabies for veterinarians, spelunkers, and other animal handlers exposed to potentially rabid dogs, cats, skunks, foxes, and bats; *Yersinia* vaccination for field workers in endemic areas; and anthrax vaccination for industrial workers who process hides, hair, bone meal, and wool of potentially infected animals.

PASSIVE IMMUNIZATION (Table 92-2) Prophylaxis or therapy of infection can also be accomplished by passive immunization which involves the administration of preformed antibody obtained from humans or other animals who have been actively immunized. Because animal antiserum can induce a hypersensitivity response in the recipient, antiserums from humans are preferable. The duration of immunity provided by passive immunization is brief. Intracellular virus generally is not affected by antibody, and once infection has been initiated, the role of antibody is limited to resisting the spread of the virus.

Hepatitis A (see Chap. 247) Immune serum globulin (ISG) administered before exposure and during the incubation period of hepatitis A is 80 to 90 percent effective in preventing or modifying the disease. The prophylactic effect of ISG is greatest when given early in the incubation period, and the use of ISG more than 2 weeks after exposure or after onset of clinical illness is not indicated. Immune serum globulin is recommended for household contacts of patients with hepatitis A but not for contacts at school, hospital, or work. In institutional settings where periodic epidemics of hepatitis A are common, the administration of ISG to residents and staff may limit the spread of the disease. The dose of ISG for postexposure prophylaxis is 0.02 mL per kilogram of body weight.

The risk of hepatitis A for residents of the United States traveling abroad is small. Travelers to tropical areas or to developing countries who bypass the usual tourist routes should probably be given ISG. For travelers at risk for 2 to 3 months, a single intramuscular dose of 0.02 mL/kg is recommended. Travelers staying in developing countries or in tropical areas longer than 3 months should receive a single injection of ISG, 0.06 mL per kilogram of body weight, every 5 months. Immune globulin modified for intravenous administration may be given as prophylaxis to those for whom intramuscular preparations are contraindicated because of thrombocytopenic or hemorrhagic disorders. The manufacturer's recommendations should be closely followed concerning dose and route of administration.

Hepatitis B (see Chaps. 85 and 247) Hepatitis B immune globulin (HBIG) alone or in combination with hepatitis B vaccine is used for postexposure prophylaxis of hepatitis B. Some controversy exists about the relative efficacy and/or cost benefit of ISG-containing antibody to hepatitis B surface antigen (anti-HBs) or hyperimmune globulin containing a high titer of anti-HBs [hepatitis B immunoglobulin (HBIG)]. HBIG is recommended for susceptible health care personnel who are anti-HBs-negative and who have a percutaneous or mucous membrane exposure to blood from documented HBsAg-positive donors. Ideally, a single dose of HBIG (0.06 mL/kg or 5 mL for adults) should be administered within 48 h of exposure. Because of its lower cost and more likely potential for preventing non-A, non-B hepatitis, ISG may be used in susceptible persons with needle exposures from unknown sources. A series of 3 doses of hepatitis B vaccine should also be initiated within 1 week of exposure. Vaccine and HBIG may be given simultaneously, but in different sites. For those who do not choose to take hepatitis B vaccine, a second dose of HBIG should be given 1 month later. HBIG and hepatitis B vaccine are 90 percent effective in preventing chronic hepatitis B infection in neonates born to mothers with acute or chronic hepatitis B. HBIG should be given to the infant within 24 h of birth (preferably in the delivery room), and hepatitis vaccination should be initiated within the first week of life. For homosexual exposure to an HBsAg-positive male, a single dose of HBIG should be given to susceptible contacts within 14 days of sexual exposure. Hepatitis B vaccine should then be initiated. For heterosexual exposure to persons with acute hepatitis B, a single dose of HBIG is also recommended. If the index case remains HBsAg-positive for 3 months and exposure is continuous, a second dose of HBIG and vaccination should be considered.

Varicella-zoster serum immune globulin (VZIG) If administered within 72 h after exposure, VZIG may prevent or ameliorate varicella-zoster among immunosuppressed susceptible patients. Indications for the use of VZIG are listed in Chap. 135. VZIG is not indicated in established varicella-zoster or in adults with a past history of varicella.

Diphtheria antitoxin (see Chap. 96) Diphtheria antitoxin may be useful in the prophylaxis of asymptomatic unimmunized household

TABLE 92-2 Passive immunization

Disease	Preparation	Route and dose*	Comments
Hepatitis A	ISG, human	IM (0.02–0.06 mL/kg) IV (100 mg/kg)	Household contacts
Hepatitis B	Human hepatitis B immunoglobulin ISG, human	IM (0.06 mL/kg; two doses 4 weeks apart) IM (0.05 mL/kg; two doses 4 weeks apart)	HBIG is preferred prophylaxis for direct parenteral exposure (needle stick) or mucous-membrane contact in susceptibles; if unavailable, ISG should be given. HBIG should be administered to neonates born to mothers with hepatitis B.
Vaccinia immunoglobulin	Human VIG	IM (0.3 mL/kg)	Use in eczema vaccinatum, disseminated vaccinia, vaccinia in pregnancy
Herpes zoster	Human varicella-ZIG	IM (125 units per 10 kg, up to 625 units)	Prevention and amelioration of varicella in susceptible immunosuppressed patients
Diphtheria	Diphtheria antitoxin, horse	IM or IV (10,000–100,000 units)	Dose dependent on extent of membrane and degree of toxicity; may also be used in unimmunized household contacts
Tetanus	Human tetanus immunoglobulin (TIG)	IM (250 units)	When given with tetanus toxoid, use separate syringes and sites
Rabies	Human rabies immunoglobulin Equine antirabies globulin	One-half locally and one-half IM (20 IU/kg) One-half locally and one-half IM (40 IU/kg)	Used for postexposure prophylaxis with rabies vaccine Same as above
Pertussis	Pertussis immunoglobulin, human	IM (1.5 mL, repeat in 5–7 days)	No studies suggest efficacy in susceptible infants
Measles	ISG, human	IM (0.2 mL/kg or 20–30 mL)	Susceptible household contacts less than 1 year old, exposed susceptible pregnant females, or immunodeficient persons
Rubella	ISG, human	IM (20–30 mL)	Exposed susceptible pregnant females who will not consider termination
Botulism (Chap. 100)	Horse serum, trivalent AB	One-half IM and one-half IV (8–32 mL)	Use only therapeutically: greatest efficacy in type E
Snake bite (Chap. 170)	Polyvalent crotaline antivenom (pit vipers)	IV (dose function of severity of bite)	See Chap. 170
Spider bite (Chap. 170)	Equine	IM (2.5 mL)	*Latrodectus* (black widow spider) poisoning

* *IM, intramuscularly; IV, intravenously.*

contacts along with (1) chemoprophylaxis with either oral erythromycin or intramuscular benzathine penicillin or (2) immunization with diphtheria toxoid. The risk of diphtheria among household contacts, which was approximately 20 percent before the antibiotic era but is negligible now, must be weighed against that of serum sickness from equine antiserum before this product is used.

Tetanus immune globulin (TIG) (see Chap. 99) The product of choice when contaminated wounds are present in persons whose history of previous tetanus immunization is uncertain or inadequate is TIG. The current recommended prophylactic dose of TIG is 250 to 1000 units given intramuscularly. TIG does not interfere with the primary immune response to tetanus toxoid given at the same time but at a different site.

Rabies (see Chap. 142) Postexposure prophylaxis for rabies consists of both passive and active immunization. Human rabies immune globulin is the preferred immunizing agent. The dose is 20 IU per kilogram of body weight given half intramuscularly and half intravenously.

Pertussis (see Chap. 109) Hyperimmune pertussis globulin does not appear effective in preventing disease among unvaccinated susceptible neonates.

Measles (see Chap. 132) Immune serum globulin should not be used to control measles outbreaks. Live measles vaccination can usually prevent development of disease if administered within 2 days of exposure. Immune serum globulin should be reserved for susceptible household contacts of measles patients, particularly for those under 1 year of age, exposed pregnant females, or persons in whom measles vaccine is contraindicated, such as immune deficient hosts. The usual dose is 10 to 20 mL intramuscularly.

Rubella (see Chap. 133) After exposure to rubella, ISG will not prevent infection or viremia with rubella virus but may modify or suppress symptoms. The routine use of ISG for postexposure prophylaxis of rubella in early pregnancy is not recommended, and infants with congenital rubella have been born to women who were given ISG shortly after exposure.

CHEMOPROPHYLAXIS OF INFECTION

USE OF A SINGLE DRUG Antibiotics have been used prophylactically to (1) prevent the acquisition of an exogenous organism, (2) prevent a resident organism from infecting a normally sterile site, and (3) prevent a dormant pathogenic organism from causing disease. In general, antimicrobial prophylaxis with a single drug, administered over a moderate period of time and directed at a single pathogen, has been successful. Examples of this type of prophylaxis employing low doses of ''narrow-spectrum'' antimicrobials include the prevention of recurrent episodes of rheumatic fever secondary to group A streptococcal disease with benzathine penicillin, of malaria with chloroquine, and of influenza A with amantadine. Table 92-3 lists some clinical situations where prolonged chemoprophylaxis either to prevent exposure to an exogenous organism or reactivation of a dormant organism in a uniquely susceptible host has been useful.

There are also situations in which the short-term use of antibiotics may prevent bacteremia, as in prophylaxis of bacterial endocarditis in individuals with acquired or congenital heart disease, or may abort localized mucosal infections. Here the use of antibiotics is based on the rationale that brief exposure to an antimicrobial, early in the disease before bacterial multiplication has led to established infection, may prevent full-blown disease. Some examples of short-term prophylaxis are given in Table 92-4.

ANTIBIOTICS PROPHYLAXIS IN SURGERY Controlled evaluations of short courses of prophylactic antimicrobials have indicated that the selective use of antibiotics, particularly in operative procedures

TABLE 92-3 Drugs that may be administered prophylactically for prolonged exposure or for extended periods of time

Disease or organism	Drug
Group A streptococcus (rheumatic fever) (Chap. 186)	Penicillin G, sulfonamide
Influenza A infection* (Chap. 130)	Amantadine
Malaria (Chap. 154)	Chloroquine and/or pyrimethamine, sulfadoxine
Tuberculosis contacts (Chap. 119)	Isoniazid
Recurrent urinary tract infection in females (Chap. 225)	Trimethoprim-sulfamethoxazole, nitrofurantoin
Recurrent otitis media (Chap. 212)	Sulfisoxazole, ampicillin, trimethoprim-sulfamethoxazole
IMMUNOSUPPRESSED PATIENTS	
Pneumocystis carinii in cancer patients receiving cytotoxic agents* (Chap. 158)	Trimethoprim-sulfamethoxazole
Bacterial infections in granulocytopenic patients (Chap. 84)	Trimethoprim-sulfamethoxazole, liquid nonabsorbable antibiotics (vancomycin, gentamycin, nystatin)
Bacterial infection in persons with defective antibody synthesis	Immune serum globulin for intravenous use
Herpes simplex virus infections in patients receiving cytotoxic agents (Chap. 136)	Acyclovir†
Cytomegalovirus infection in renal transplant patients (Chap. 137)	Leukocyte interferon†

* *May require only short courses.*
† *Not licensed by the Food and Drug Administration.*

involving potentially contaminated surgical sites, will lower the rate of postoperative infections. The following principles should be applied in using antimicrobial prophylaxis in surgery (Table 92-5): (1) there must be a high prevalence of postoperative infections that are potentially severe before employing antimicrobial drugs; (2) the prophylactic antimicrobial must be effective against the most frequent postoperative pathogens; (3) the drug should be administered from immediately before and during the operation, and for only a short period thereafter; and (4) where possible, prophylaxis should be carried out with a single drug. In studies of cardiac, colorectal, vaginal, and biliary tract surgery, single-dose antibiotic prophylaxis has been as effective as multiple postoperative administration of antibiotics. Antibiotic prophylaxis is recommended in clean surgical procedures that involve insertion of prostheses where the development of infections can be severe or fatal. Other operations such as those involving clean-contaminated, contaminated, or "dirty" wounds, where the infection rates vary from 10 to 40 percent, also warrant prophylactic antibiotics. This topic is also discussed in Chap. 85. For choice of the appropriate agent, Chap. 88 should be consulted.

TABLE 92-4 Short-term antimicrobial prophylaxis

Disease	Antibiotic
USUALLY EFFECTIVE	
Subacute bacterial endocarditis:	
Streptococcus viridans	Penicillin V or procaine penicillin G plus streptomycin
Enterococcus	Ampicillin or penicillin G or vancomycin plus gentamicin or streptomycin
Neisseria gonorrheae (ophthalmia)	Silver nitrate, penicillin, tetracycline
Neisseria gonorrheae (genital infection)	Tetracycline
Nongonococcal urethritis	Tetracycline
Congenital or incubating syphilis	Penicillin
Toxigenic *Escherichia coli* ("tourista")	Tetracycline, trimethoprim-sulfamethoxazole, bismuth subsalicylate
Enteropathogenic *E. coli* diarrhea	Neomycin or kanamycin
Neisseria meningitidis	Sulfonamides (sensitive strains only), rifampin, minocycline
Corynebacterium diphtheriae	Erythromycin, clindamycin, penicillin, benzathine penicillin
SOMETIMES EFFECTIVE	
Shigellosis	Ampicillin, neomycin
Chronic bronchitis*	Ampicillin, tetracycline
Short-term urethral catheterization (<24 h)	Ampicillin, tetracycline, nitrofurantoin, trimethoprim-sulfamethoxazole

* *Prophylaxis may require prolonged administration.*

ANTIBIOTICS IN SUSCEPTIBLE HOSTS In contrast to short-term antimicrobial prophylaxis with a single drug, which is unlikely to be deleterious, attempts to prevent infection with multiple drugs administered in high doses for relatively prolonged periods are much more likely to be harmful. Adverse effects of "prolonged" antimicrobial prophylaxis include (1) superinfection (defined as an infection with a resistant organism that has developed during antibiotic therapy), (2) increased incidence of toxic or allergic reactions to drugs, (3) increased cost, and last but not least, (4) a sense of false security on the part of attending physicians or surgeons, resulting in less stringent observation of the patient. However, many of the patients who are given antibiotics prophylactically are precisely the ones who are susceptible to complicating infections, and particular care must be taken to watch assiduously for the development of infection and to treat it promptly when it occurs. Such policy is often superior to the use of antimicrobial prophylaxis.

Prophylactic antibiotics have not been useful in preventing bacterial complications of antecedent viral respiratory illness such as influenza

TABLE 92-5 Systemic antimicrobial prophylaxis in surgery

	Antibiotic
PROPHYLAXIS INDICATED	
Obstetric-gynecologic surgery:	
Vaginal and abdominal hysterectomy	A cephalosporin (cefazolin), metronidazole
Caesarean section after prolonged rupture of membranes	A cephalosporin
Colorectal surgery	Neomycin and erythromycin base, doxycycline, cefoxitin, metronidazole, gentamicin plus clindamycin, cefamycin
Appendectomy	Doxycycline, cefoxitin, ampicillin
Cardiac surgery (including coronary artery bypass)	A cephalosporin
Valvular, noncardiac thoracic surgery	A cephalosporin
Orthopedic surgery (joint replacement, prosthesis, compound fractures)	A cephalosporin or penicillinase-resistant penicillin
Peripheral artery surgery with graft replacement	A cephalosporin
Contaminated surgical wounds	A cephalosporin
Prostatectomy with preoperative bacteriuria	Treat according to bacterial sensitivity tests
PROPHYLAXIS OF VALUE IN SELECTED PATIENTS	
Gastroduodenal surgery (obstructing duodenal ulcer, achlorhydria, chronic cimetidine therapy, gastric ulcer, malignancy, bypass for obesity)	A cephalosporin
Biliary tract surgery (elderly, obstructed)	A cephalosporin
Microsurgical craniotomy	A cephalosporin
Extensive ear, nose, or throat surgery	A cephalosporin
PROPHYLAXIS UNLIKELY TO BE OF VALUE	
Clean abdominal surgery	
Gynecologic surgery (other than mentioned above)	
Genitourinary surgery in persons with sterile urine	
Simple lacerations	

TABLE 92-6 Antibiotic prophylaxis in susceptible hosts in whom its use is not indicated

OUTPATIENT USE
Viral respiratory disease
Viral exanthems
Preventing acute exacerbations of asthma
HOSPITALIZED PATIENTS
Preventing pneumonia in comatose patients
Preventing tracheal colonization with pathogenic organisms
Preventing infections in patients with congestive heart failure
Prolonged urethral catheterization (>24 h)
Prolonged intravenous catheterization (>48 h)
High-dose steroid therapy
Prematurity
Shock

or in preventing colonization of pathogenic organisms in intensive care units. Indeed, in these and many other clinical situations the risk of superinfection with resistant, difficult-to-treat organisms outweighs the unlikely effectiveness of prophylactic antibiotics (Table 92-6). However, in some populations, such as victims of severe burns or patients with severe granulocytopenia, antibiotic prophylaxis may be useful. Infections in granulocytopenic patients are often life-threatening. Most infections develop in persons with prolonged (>14 days) and profound (<100 granulocytes per milliliter) granulocytopenia. Mucosal damage by tumor therapy allows invasion of organisms colonizing the alimentary and respiratory tracts and the oral cavity, resulting in pneumonitis, esophagitis, colitis, and perianal infections. Many infections are due to the patient's indigenous flora, and others are due to organisms acquired from the hospital environment. In selected patients, reduction of indigenous flora and prevention of colonization by microbial suppression using oral nonabsorbable antibiotics such as gentamicin, vancomycin, and nystatin (GVN) with or without laminar airflow rooms or selective suppression of alimentary canal microbial flora with trimethoprim-sulfamethoxazole with or without antifungal agents such as ketoconazole have been effective. The necessity of maintaining continuous GVN therapy, the difficulty of patient compliance, the emergence of trimethoprim-sulfamethoxazole–resistant organisms, and the existence of localized outbreaks of unusual organisms indicate that continued evaluation of these prophylactic antibiotic regimens is needed. Among organ transplant patients, the use of systemic acyclovir to prevent endogenous reactivation of herpes simplex virus infections has been demonstrated. Immunobiogens, such as the interferons or immunoglobulins, have been effective in prevention of cytomegalovirus infections in selected instances, and their further evaluation is indicated.

REFERENCES

Adult immunization: Recommendations of the immunization practices advisory committee. Morb Mort Week Rep 33, no. 15, 1984

Broome CV: Pneumococcal disease after pneumococcal vaccination. N Engl J Med 303:549, 1980

Centers for Disease Control: 1985 STD treatment guidelines. Morb Mort Week Rep 34(4S), 1985.

Committee on Immunization, Council of Medical Societies: Guide to adult immunization. Am Coll Phys 1985

DuPont HL: Chemotherapy and chemoprophylaxis of traveler's diarrhea. Ann Intern Med 102:258, 1985

Goldman PG, Petersdorf RG: Prophylactic antibiotics: Controversies give way to guidelines. Drug Ther June 1979, pp 57–77

Hirschmann JV, Inui TS: Antimicrobial prophylaxis: A critique of recent trials. Rev Infect Dis 2:1, 1980

Immunization Practices Advisory Committee, CDC: Poliomyelitis prevention. Ann Intern Med 96:630, 1982

Krugman S: Effect of human immune serum globulin on infectivity of hepatitis A virus. J Infect Dis 34:70, 1975

Levin S: Selected overview of nongynecologic surgical intraabdominal infections: Prophylaxis and therapy. Am J Med 79(suppl 5B):146, 1985

Ruben FL: Antitoxin responses in the elderly to tetanus-diphtheria (Td) immunization. Am J Epidemiol 108:145, 1978

Schimpff SE: Infection prevention during profound granulocytopenia. Ann Intern Med 93:358, 1980

Shapiro ED: Controlled evaluation of the protective efficacy of pneumococcal vaccine for patients at high risk of serious pneumococcal infection. Ann Intern Med 301:325, 1984

Weiss BP: Tetanus and diphtheria immunity in an elderly population in Los Angeles County. Am J Public Health 73:802, 1983

section 2 Diseases caused by gram-positive organisms

93 PNEUMOCOCCAL INFECTIONS

ROBERT AUSTRIAN

ETIOLOGY The pneumococcus *(Streptococcus pneumoniae)* is a gram-positive encapsulated coccus that usually grows in pairs or short chains. In the diplococcal form, the adjacent margins are rounded and the opposite ends slightly pointed, giving the organisms a lancet shape. In stained preparations of exudate, gram-negative forms are sometimes present. Pneumococcal colonies are surrounded by greenish discoloration on or in blood agar and are confused at times with other alpha-hemolytic streptococci to which they are closely related. Their isolation from respiratory secretions may be facilitated by inclusion of 5 μg gentamicin per milliliter in the medium. Pneumococci can be distinguished by their bile solubility and mouse virulence or by serologic typing. Another method with approximately 90 percent specificity, utilizing inhibition of pneumococci by Optochin-impregnated paper disks, is less cumbersome.

The capsular substances are complex polysaccharides and are the basis for dividing pneumococci into serotypes. Organisms exposed to type-specific antiserum show a positive capsular precipitin reaction, the *Neufeld quellung reaction;* by this means, 84 serotypes have been identified. All are pathogenic for human beings, but types or groups 1, 3, 4, 7, 8, 9, and 12 are encountered most frequently in clinical practice. Types or groups 6, 14, 19, and 23 often cause pneumonia and otitis media in children but are less common in adults.

Specific typing of pneumococci remains of great clinical importance if pneumococcus is to be identified with regularity, and recognition of pneumococcus has decreased significantly since the abandonment of capsular typing by most clinical laboratories. The detection of pneumococcal capsular polysaccharides in sputum and in other body fluids by immunologic methods such as counterimmunoelectrophoresis (CIE) or latex agglutination provides an alternative to bacteriologic techniques for the presumptive diagnosis of pneumococcal infection. Because of cross reactions between the polysaccharides of pneumococci and of other bacterial species, immunologic diagnosis is less specific than bacteriologic diagnosis.

PATHOGENESIS The mechanism by which pneumococci damage the mammalian host is obscure, and no toxin elaborated by the organism has been shown to play a major pathogenic role in pneumococcal infection, although components of the cell wall may cause inflammation. The capsular polysaccharides, though nontoxic, are known to be necessary factors in virulence and to protect the organism to a certain extent from phagocytosis.

Although "pneumococcal pharyngitis" is a doubtful entity, invasion of the tissue of the nasopharynx may occur in the infant and occasionally in the nonimmune adult and be followed by spread to the circulation via the cervical lymphatics. At times, secondary infection of serous cavities in the absence of demonstrable focal infection of the upper or lower respiratory tract may occur. The organisms multiply readily in vivo and may produce acute inflammation of the lungs, serous cavities, and endocardium.

The normal human respiratory tract is provided with a variety of mechanisms which guard the lungs from infection. The lower respiratory tract is protected by the glottis and larynx, and material passing these barriers stimulates the expulsive cough reflex. Removal of small particles impinging on the walls of the trachea and bronchi is facilitated by their mucociliary lining; and growth of bacteria reaching normal alveoli is inhibited by their relative dryness and by the phagocytic activity of alveolar macrophages. Any anatomic or physiologic derangement of these coordinated defenses tends to augment the susceptibility of the lungs to infection. Anesthesia, alcoholic intoxication, convulsions, and disturbed innervation of the larynx depress the cough reflex and may permit aspiration of infected material. Alterations in the tracheobronchial tree leading to anatomic changes in the epithelial lining or to localized obstruction increase the vulnerability of the lungs to infection. Pulmonary edema, local or generalized, resulting from viral infection, inhalation of irritant gases, cardiac failure, or contusion of the chest wall, provides a fluid menstruum in the alveoli for the growth of bacteria and their spread to adjacent areas of the lung. Viral infection of the respiratory epithelium with concomitant disruption of its component cells interferes significantly with the clearance of bacteria from the lungs, an observation in accord with the high incidence of pneumococcal pneumonia during epidemics of viral influenza and its frequent clinical association with sporadic viral respiratory infections.

Pneumonia begins usually in the right lower, right middle, or left lower lobe, those areas to which gravity is most likely to carry upper respiratory secretions aspirated during sleep. Bronchial embolization with infected mucinous secretions during the course of an upper respiratory infection appears to be the initiating factor in many cases of pneumococcal pneumonia. Protected initially from phagocytosis by mucinous material, the bacteria multiply and, in infected alveoli, evoke the outpouring of proteinaceous fluid which serves both as a nutrient and as a vehicle for spread to adjacent alveoli. Soon thereafter, polymorphonuclear leukocytes migrate from the pulmonary capillaries to phagocytize a part of the pneumococcal population before the appearance of detectable antibody. Delay in the polymorphonuclear leukocytic response occurs during alcoholic intoxication and certain forms of anesthesia, permitting spread of infection. Glucocorticosteroids may also interfere with leukocyte migration. Later, as the pneumonic lesion evolves, macrophages appear in the exudate and remove the debris of fibrin and cells. It is probable that antibody to the capsular polysaccharide of the invading pneumococcus makes its appearance locally in the lung before being detectable in the circulation. Such antibody increases the efficiency of phagocytosis approximately twofold and causes agglutination of the organisms and their adherence to alveolar walls, thereby slowing their dissemination in the lung. The outcome of infection depends, therefore, on the rate at which bacteria can multiply in the edema fluid and spread, and on the host's ability to immobilize and destroy them by phagocytosis. Individuals with hypogammaglobulinemia and patients with multiple myeloma (see Chap. 258) incapable of producing anticapsular antibody are prone to recurrent attacks of pneumococcal pneumonia. Repeated infection with the same pneumococcal type should always prompt a search for dysgammaglobulinemia.

Failure of local defense mechanisms in the lung results in lymphatic spread of pneumococci to the hilar lymph nodes. In the sinusoids of these organs, a sequence of events not unlike that in the lung ensues. If infection is not checked in this secondary line of defense, organisms find their way into the thoracic duct and then into the circulation. Although transient bacteremia may occur at the onset of many cases of pneumococcal pneumonia, it is detectable in only 20 to 30 percent of cases. Bacteremia, which reflects the body's inability to localize the pulmonary infection, is a poor prognostic sign and carries with it the danger of metastatic infection. The mortality of treated or untreated bacteremic pneumococcal pneumonia is four times that resulting from comparably managed nonbacteremic infections. Metastatic infection secondary to bacteremia may occur in the meninges, joints, or peritoneum or on the endocardium. Direct spread from the infected lung may give rise to empyema or to pericarditis.

Natural recovery from pneumococcal infection coincides usually, but not invariably, with the appearance of detectable type-specific antibody in the circulation and is often accompanied by a dramatic and abrupt fall in temperature, the so-called crisis. Antibody aids recovery by increasing the efficiency of phagocytosis and by limiting dissemination of the organisms. Bacteriostatic drugs, such as sulfonamides, facilitate control of the infection by limiting the size of the pneumococcal population, but the host's defense mechanisms are still required for the elimination of the bacteria. Bactericidal agents, such as penicillin, cause the death of pneumococci in the lung and are effective when some of the host's defense mechanisms are compromised. With the arrest of infection, the alveolar exudate undergoes liquefaction, the inflammatory debris is removed by expectoration and via the lymphatic channels, and the lung is restored to its normal state. Necrosis of pulmonary tissue as a result of pneumococcal infection is distinctly uncommon. Primary pneumococcal lung abscess is a rare clinical entity, although the diagnosis is mistakenly made at times when pneumococcal infection complicates lung abscess of other origins.

In addition to causing pneumonia and its metastatic sequelae, pneumococcus can extend from the nasopharynx to its adjacent structures, giving rise to otitis media, mastoiditis, paranasal sinusitis, or conjunctivitis. Soft tissue abscesses are rare but may occur.

PNEUMOCOCCAL PNEUMONIA

Pneumococcal pneumonia is a disease of considerable uniformity, in contrast to other infections such as typhoid fever and tuberculosis. The diseases produced by different pneumococcal serotypes show little variation in severity or in clinical manifestations. The prognosis in type 3 pneumococcal pneumonia is usually regarded as poor, probably because type 3 infections occur frequently in the aged and in patients with other debilitating diseases, such as diabetes and congestive heart failure. The usual lesion in adults is segmental or lobar in distribution, but in children and the aged, bronchopneumonia, characterized by patchy involvement, is frequent.

MANIFESTATIONS Pneumonia is often preceded for a few days by coryza or some other form of common respiratory disease. The onset is frequently so abrupt that the patient can state the exact hour that illness began. There is a sudden *shaking chill* in more than 80 percent of the cases and a rapid rise in temperature, with corresponding tachycardia and an increase in respiratory rate (tachypnea). Most patients with pneumococcal pneumonia have a single rigor unless antipyretic drugs are administered, and repeated chills should suggest another etiologic agent.

About 75 percent of patients develop severe *pleuritic pain* and *cough,* productive of pinkish or "rusty" mucoid sputum within a few hours. The chest pain is agonizing, and respirations become rapid, shallow, and grunting as the patient tries to splint the affected side. Many patients are mildly cyanotic as a result of hypoxia caused by $\dot{V}/\dot{Q}$ (ventilation perfusion ratio) abnormality or shunt, which accompanies altered respiration, and show dilatation of the alae nasi when first seen. Patients appear acutely ill; but nausea, headache, and malaise are not prominent, and most individuals are alert. Pleuritic pain and dyspnea are the dominant complaints.

In the untreated disease, there are sustained fever of 102.5 to 105°F (39.2 to 40.5°C), continued pleuritic pain, cough, and expectoration; and *abdominal distention* is frequent. *Herpes labialis* is a common complication. After 7 to 10 days, there are diaphoresis, abrupt defervescence, and dramatic improvement in well-being, the "crisis."

In cases which terminate fatally, there is usually extensive pulmonary involvement, and dyspnea, cyanosis, and tachycardia are prominent. Circulatory collapse or a picture resembling adult respiratory distress syndrome has been observed. Death in a few patients is associated with empyema or some other suppurative complication such as meningitis or endocarditis.

Physical examination reveals restricted motion of the affected hemithorax. Tactile fremitus may be decreased during the initial day of illness but is usually increased when consolidation is fully established. Deviation of the trachea away from the affected lung suggests pleural effusion or empyema. The percussion note is dull, and if the lesion is in an upper lobe, impaired motion of the diaphragm can be detected on the affected side. Very early in the course of infection, breath sounds are diminished, but as the lesion evolves, they become tubular or bronchial in quality, and bronchophony and whispered pectoriloquy can be elicited. These findings are accompanied by fine crepitant rales.

EFFECT OF SPECIFIC CHEMOTHERAPY Pneumococcal pneumonia usually improves promptly when an appropriate antimicrobial drug is given. Within 12 to 36 h after initiation of treatment with penicillin, temperature, pulse, and respiration begin to fall and may reach normal values, pleuritic pain subsides, and the spread of the inflammatory process is halted. The temperature of approximately half the patients, however, requires 4 days or longer to become normal, and failure of the patient's temperature to reach normal in 24 to 48 h should not prompt a change in antibacterial therapy in the absence of other indications.

COMPLICATIONS The typical course of pneumococcal pneumonia can be modified by the development of one or more local or distant complications:

In the lung ATELECTASIS Atelectasis of all or part of a lobe may occur during the active stage of pneumonia or after treatment has been instituted. The patient may complain of sudden recurrence of pleuritic pain and show rapid respirations. Small areas of atelectasis are often detected by x-ray in the absence of symptoms. These areas usually clear with coughing and deep breathing, but bronchoscopic aspiration is occasionally necessary. If atelectasis is allowed to persist, the affected area becomes fibrotic and functionless.

DELAYED RESOLUTION Return to normal of physical findings in the lung after pneumococcal pneumonia is usually complete within 2 to 4 weeks. X-ray evidence of residual pulmonary consolidation, however, may persist as long as 8 weeks, and other radiologic manifestations of the infection (volume loss, stranding, and pleural disease) may persist for up to 18 weeks. The process of resolution may require a longer time in those over 50 years of age and in those with chronic obstructive airway disease or alcoholism.

ABSCESS Lung abscess is a rare sequel to pneumococcal infection, although pneumococcal pneumonia is a not uncommon complication of lung abscess of other origins. It is manifested by continued fever and profuse expectoration of purulent sputum. X-ray shows one or more cavities. This complication is exceedingly rare in patients who receive penicillin therapy and is most likely to follow infection with pneumococcus type 3.

In adjacent structures PLEURAL EFFUSION Pleural effusion detectable in lateral decubitus x-rays of the chest occurs in approximately half of patients with pneumococcal pneumonia and is associated with delay in the initiation of therapy and with bacteremia. Usually the effusion is sterile and is absorbed spontaneously within a week or two. At times, however, the effusion is large and requires aspiration or drainage.

EMPYEMA Before the introduction of effective chemotherapy, empyema occurred in 5 to 8 percent of patients with pneumococcal pneumonia; it is now observed in less than 1 percent of treated cases. It is manifested by persistent fever or pleuritic pain, together with signs of pleural effusion. In the early stages, the gross appearance of infected fluid may not differ from that of a sterile pleural effusion; later, there is a profuse outpouring of polymorphonuclear leukocytes and fibrin, resulting in an exudate of thick greenish pus containing large clots of fibrin. The quantity of exudate may become large enough to displace mediastinal structures. In neglected cases, this process leads to extensive pleural scarring, with limitation of thoracic movement. Rupture and drainage through the chest wall *(empyema necessitatis)* occurs, but is rare. Metastatic *brain abscess* is an occasional complication of chronic empyema.

PERICARDITIS A particularly serious complication is spread of infection to the pericardial sac. This lesion is characterized by pain in the precordial region, a friction rub synchronous with the heartbeat, and distention of cervical veins, although one or all of these findings may be absent. The possibility of coexisting purulent pericarditis should be considered whenever a very ill patient with pneumonia develops empyema.

Metastatic infections *Arthritis* occurs more often in children than in adults. The affected joint is swollen, red, and painful, with a purulent effusion. It usually subsides promptly with systemic administration of penicillin, although aspiration and intraarticular injection of penicillin may be necessary in adults.

Acute bacterial endocarditis complicates pneumococcal pneumonia in fewer than 0.5 percent of cases. Its manifestations and treatment are discussed below. *Meningitis,* another complication of pneumococcal pneumonia, is also discussed subsequently.

Paralytic ileus Gaseous abdominal distention is commonly present and in severely ill patients may assume such serious proportions that the term *paralytic ileus* is justified. This complication further impairs respiratory movement by elevation of the diaphragm and constitutes a difficult problem in management. A rarer and more serious gastrointestinal complication is acute gastric dilatation.

Impaired liver function Alterations in hepatic function are common during the course of pneumococcal pneumonia, and mild jaundice is not at all rare. The pathogenesis of the jaundice is not entirely clear, although in some patients it appears to be related to glucose 6-phosphate dehydrogenase deficiency.

LABORATORY FINDINGS *Sputum* should be obtained in the physician's presence before the administration of antimicrobial drugs to ensure its quality. Although resort to transtracheal aspiration or lung puncture may be necessary on occasion to establish the cause of pneumonia, routine use of these invasive techniques is not recommended because of their attendant, albeit infrequent, complications. When stained by Gram's method, the sputum shows polymorphonuclear leukocytes and variable numbers of gram-positive cocci, singly and in pairs. These can be typed directly by the Neufeld quellung technique, and this procedure should be used to facilitate diagnosis whenever possible. The *blood culture* is positive for pneumococci during the first days of untreated illness in 20 to 30 percent of cases. The white blood count usually shows a polymorphonuclear *leukocytosis* ranging from 12,000 to 25,000 cells per cubic millimeter. A normal white count or leukopenia is sometimes observed in patients with overwhelming infection and bacteremia. Occasionally, pneumococci may be seen directly in granulocytes of patients with bacteremia by examining the buffy coat after staining with Wright's stain. These patients often have asplenia. *X-ray of the chest* usually reveals a homogenous density in the affected area of the lung. In well-established cases, the density may occupy one or more entire lobes. Atypical patterns of consolidation may be seen in patients with underlying chronic pulmonary disease.

EXTRAPULMONARY PNEUMOCOCCAL INFECTION

PNEUMOCOCCAL MENINGITIS The pneumococcus is second only to the meningococcus as a cause of purulent meningitis in adults; in children, meningitis caused by *Haemophilus influenzae* is also more frequent than pneumococcal infection.

Pneumococcal meningitis can develop as a "primary" disease without preceding signs of infection elsewhere; as a complication of pneumococcal pneumonia; by extension from otitis, mastoiditis, or sinusitis; or following a skull fracture which creates an opening between the subarachnoid space and the nasal cavity or paranasal sinuses. Patients with pneumococcal endocarditis frequently develop meningeal infection. Patients with multiple myeloma and with sickle cell disease seem to be prone to pneumococcal infection of the meninges, just as they are to pneumonia.

The *manifestations* are of those of any acute pyogenic meningitis (see Chap. 346) and include chills, fever, headache, nuchal rigidity, Kernig's and Brudzinski's signs, delirium, and cranial nerve palsies. Evidence of otitis, sinusitis, or pneumonia should be carefully sought by physical and roentgenographic examination in all patients.

The *spinal fluid* is under increased pressure, appears cloudy, often with a greenish tint, and shows a high protein and low glucose content. Stained smears usually reveal gram-positive diplococci and polymorphonuclear leukocytes; in some patients, the number of cells in the spinal fluid is surprisingly small, and much of the cloudiness is produced by the bacterial content. The diagnosis can be established rapidly by identification of pneumococci in the spinal fluid by Gram's stain. Immunologic tests (CIE or latex agglutination) are positive in approximately 80 percent of culture-positive cases and may provide a presumptive bacterial cause of infection in some patients from whose spinal fluid no organism is recovered.

With appropriate chemotherapy, recovery can be expected in 70 percent of cases; the prognosis is better in children than in infants or in adults. Relapse may occur but is unusual if adequate treatment is carried out. Subarachnoid block, the result of accumulation of large amounts of thick exudate in the meningeal space and at the base of the brain, is an unusual complication.

PNEUMOCOCCAL ENDOCARDITIS Endocarditis is usually a complication of pneumonia or meningitis. The clinical picture is that of acute bacterial endocarditis (see Chap. 188), with remittent fever, splenomegaly, and metastatic infection of the lungs, meninges, joints, eye, and other tissues. Petechiae are uncommon. The infection can attack normal valves and is particularly likely to occur on the aortic valve. The valvular infection is destructive, and loud murmurs and heart failure develop rapidly. Rupture or perforation of cusps or even rupture of the aorta may occur. The blood culture is consistently positive for the pneumococcus in the absence of treatment with antimicrobial drugs; yet at the same time antibodies to the infecting organism may be demonstrable in the blood, a combination of findings seldom observed except in endocarditis or brucellosis. Although the infection is relatively easy to cure with penicillin, damage to valve leaflets, especially to the cusps of the aortic valve, may be followed by rapidly progressive heart failure. Surgical repair or replacement of damaged valvular structures should be carried out early, before heart failure becomes intractable.

PNEUMOCOCCAL PERITONITIS Pneumococcal peritonitis is a rare disease and is probably the sequel to transient pneumococcal bacteremia, although, because of its somewhat greater frequency in young girls, it has been hypothesized that the organism may gain entry to the peritoneum via the vagina and fallopian tubes. Peritonitis was formerly a common complication of the nephrotic syndrome, particularly in children, but it occurs now with a frequency of less than 2 percent. In adults, the disease is seen in association with cirrhosis or with carcinoma of the liver. The diagnosis is made by examination of the ascitic fluid; blood cultures are often positive, and a polymorphonuclear leukocytosis is the rule.

TREATMENT

SPECIFIC ANTIMICROBIAL THERAPY Although resistance of pneumococci to antimicrobial drugs has not been regarded as a significant problem in the past, some strains have been found to be resistant to one or all of the following agents: penicillins, cephalosporins, tetracyclines, chloramphenicol, erythromycin, clindamycin, co-trimoxazole, and aminoglycosides. For this reason sensitivity of the infecting organism to the drug(s) to be used should be determined, particularly in treating extrapulmonary infection. In the absence of resistance or of hypersensitivity to it, penicillin G (benzylpenicillin) is the drug of choice for all manifestations of pneumococcal infection. Strains of pneumococcus manifesting increased resistance to penicillin have been recovered infrequently from humans; and although the level of such resistance does not often preclude treatment with this antibiotic, awareness of the phenomenon is necessary. Although the minimum curative dose for *pneumonia* caused by strains of usual sensitivity to penicillin is less than 60,000 units daily and a dose of 600,000 units daily provides a good margin of safety in treating adults with bacteremic or nonbacteremic infection with such strains in the absence of an extrapulmonary focus, the occurrence of pneumococci showing increased resistance to penicillin makes the initiation of therapy with larger amounts desirable today. Treatment may be started with doses of 600,000 units of aqueous crystalline penicillin G or procaine penicillin administered at 12-h intervals to be continued until the patient has been afebrile for 48 to 72 h. Pneumococcal pneumonia can be treated with an oral penicillin, preferably one resistant to gastric acid (see Chap. 92), in dosage equivalent to 2.4 to 4.8 million units of penicillin G. *Peritonitis* caused by sensitive strains responds usually within 36 to 48 h to 2 to 4 million units of penicillin daily.

Pneumococcal meningitis in adults should be treated with 18 to 24 million units of penicillin G daily intravenously. In some clinics, even larger amounts are used, though care must be taken to avoid neurotoxicity from excessive dosage. Intrathecal administration of penicillin is unnecessary, and supplementation of penicillin with broad-spectrum bacteriostatic drugs such as tetracyclines may exert a deleterious effect. All pneumococcal isolates from cerebrospinal fluid should be tested promptly for their sensitivity to antibacterial drugs. Vancomycin appears currently to be the drug of choice for treatment of meningitis caused by pneumococci resistant to multiple antimicrobial agents.

Moderate doses of penicillin G are used to treat pneumococcal endocarditis—8 to 12 million units daily by intravenous infusion. Rapidly developing heart failure as a result of valvular injury and a tendency to form myocardial abscess, however, often lead to a fatal outcome despite the use of antibiotics. Prompt surgical repair or replacement of damaged heart valves should be considered when cardiac failure develops.

Cephalosporins in parenteral doses of 1 to 2 g daily are effective in pneumococcal pneumonia but must be administered with caution to those hypersensitive to penicillin. Many members of this class of β-lactam drugs cannot be used to treat meningitis because of their poor ability to penetrate the blood–cerebrospinal fluid barrier. Several of the newer cephalosporins, including cefotaxime and ceftriaxone, show promise of efficacy in treating pneumococcal meningitis although experience with each is limited. The tetracyclines in doses of 1 to 2 g daily, erythromycin in doses of 1.6 g daily, or clindamycin in doses of 1.2 g daily are effective treatment for pneumococcal pneumonia if it is caused by a sensitive strain, but they are recommended only for patients who have had untoward reactions to penicillins or cephalosporins. Despite its efficacy, chloramphenicol should not be used to treat pneumococcal infections other than meningitis in patients hypersensitive to penicillin who are infected with a drug-sensitive strain. For patients with illness caused by multiply drug-resistant pneumococci, vancomycin in doses of 2 g daily is the drug of choice. Sulfonamides have little place in the present-day treatment of pneumococcal pneumonia and are useless in endocarditis and meningitis. Aminoglycosides, such as gentamicin, tobramycin, and amikacin, should not be employed to treat pneumococcal infection.

Pneumococcal arthritis responds to systemic penicillin, but aspiration and intraarticular instillation of the drug may be necessary.

Empyema should be detected and treated as early as possible. When an effusion is found, fluid should be removed and examined for bacteria, leukocytes, glucose concentration, and pH. The presence of bacteria, pus, a pH below 7.0, and/or a pleural fluid glucose below 40 mg/dL are indications for institution of closed-chest tube drainage. Failure of early cure of empyema may be followed by pleural fibrosis and necessitate subsequent surgical decortication of the lung to restore pulmonary function.

OTHER MEASURES Oxygen administered through a face mask should be used to treat significant cyanosis, cardiac failure, and delirium. In the presence of adult respiratory distress syndrome, positive end-expiratory pressure may be indicated. Codeine, 32 to 64 mg every 4 h, will usually control pleuritic pain. When pain is severe, it may require intercostal nerve block with 1 to 2% procaine for relief.

PROGNOSIS AND PREVENTION

Although the mortality from pneumococcal pneumonia has diminished significantly since the advent of antimicrobial drugs, available evidence indicates that the incidence of the disease has changed little, if at all. The fatality rate in patients over the age of 12 years with bacteremic pneumococcal pneumonia treated with an antibiotic is 18 percent, and in patients over the age of 50 and in those with underlying systemic illness, it is significantly higher.

Signs of poor prognosis in pneumonia include leukopenia, bacteremia, multilobar involvement, any extrapulmonary focus of pneumococcal infection, presence of preexisting systemic disease, circulatory collapse, and occurrence of the infection in the first year of life or after the age of 55. Infection with pneumococcus type 3 has a higher mortality rate than that caused by other pneumococcal types. Death is most likely to occur in individuals sustaining irreversible physiologic damage early in the course which is unaltered by antimicrobial therapy. Until the nature of the injury produced by pneumococcus is understood and ways are devised to repair it, vaccination will remain the principal means of protecting those at high risk of a fatal outcome.

A 23-valent vaccine containing the capsular polysaccharides of pneumococcal types 1, 2, 3, 4, 5, 6B, 7F, 8, 9N, 9V, 10A, 11A, 12F, 14, 15B, 17F, 18C, 19F, 19A, 20, 22F, 23F, and 33F, which include the serotypes or groups responsible for 90 percent of bacteremic infections in the United States, is recommended for prevention of pneumococcal infection caused by these serotypes in individuals at high risk of a fatal outcome. Those at higher-than-average risk are individuals over the age of 55 and patients with a variety of chronic systemic illnesses including heart disease, chronic bronchopulmonary disease, hepatic disease, renal insufficiency, diabetes, and a variety of malignancies. Persons of all ages with sickle cell disease have an increased risk of developing pneumococcal infection, and the vaccine is recommended for those with this disorder over the age of 2 years. Since anatomic or functional asplenia is associated with fulminant overwhelming pneumococcal septicemia with disseminated intravascular coagulation, giving rise to a clinical picture resembling the Waterhouse-Friderichsen syndrome, such individuals should also be immunized. However, the vaccine does not contain the antigens of all pneumococcal types, and infection caused by antigens not included may occur occasionally in immunized subjects. Reactions to the vaccine are usually absent or mild, although in the occasional individual they may resemble those following immunization with typhoid vaccine: local pain, erythema, and elevation of temperature. The most severe local and systemic reactions to the vaccine appear to be associated with preexisting high levels of antibody to one or more of the antigens in the vaccine. Because of the persistence of pneumococcal antibodies after a single injection of vaccine, reimmunization in less than 5 years after the initial injection is not recommended. The vaccine is 80 to 90 percent effective in immunocompetent adults but may afford little, if any, protection to those with agamma- or dysgammaglobulinemia or to patients who have been subjected recently to intensive antitumor chemotherapy and radiation. In children under 6 years, immunologic responsiveness to different capsular antigens develops at different times as a result of maturational characteristics of the human immune system, and protection may be of shorter duration than in the adults. Further data are needed to define the utility of the vaccine in childhood. If necessary, pneumococcal vaccine may be administered concomitantly with influenza viral vaccine, provided each vaccine is injected from a separate syringe at a separate site.

REFERENCES

AUSTRIAN R, GOLD J: Pneumococcal bacteremia with especial reference to bacteremic pneumococcal pneumonia. Ann Intern Med 60:759, 1964

——— et al: Prevention of pneumococcal pneumonia by vaccination. Trans Assoc Am Phys 89:184, 1976

FRUCHTMAN SM et al: Adult respiratory distress syndrome as a cause of death in pneumococcal pneumonia. Chest 83:598, 1983

GOPAL V, BISNO AL: Fulminant pneumococcal infections in "normal" asplenic hosts. Arch Intern Med 137:1526, 1977

HEFFRON R: *Pneumonia with Special Reference to Pneumococcus Lobar Pneumonia.* Cambridge, Harvard, 1979

KAPLAN SL: Antigen detection in cerebrospinal fluid—pros and cons. Am J Med 75:109, 1983

LIGHT RW et al: Parapneumonic effusions. Am J Med 69:507, 1980

MARINO PL et al: Bacteremic pneumococcal pneumonia and myoglobinuric renal failure. Am J Med 80:521, 1986

ROBBINS JB et al: Considerations for formulating the second-generation pneumococcal capsular polysaccharide vaccine with emphasis on the cross-reactive types within groups. J Infect Dis 148:1136, 1983

SHAPIRO ED, CLEMENS JD: A controlled evaluation of the protective efficacy of pneumococcal vaccine for patients at high risk of serious pneumococcal infections. Ann Intern Med 101:325, 1984

STEPHEN JJ et al: The radiographic resolution of *Streptococcus pneumoniae* pneumonia. N Engl J Med 293:798, 1975

TUOMANEN E et al: The induction of meningeal inflammation by components of the pneumococcal cell wall. J Infect Dis 151:859, 1985

WARD J: Antibiotic-resistant *Streptococcus pneumoniae:* Clinical and epidemiologic aspects. Rev Infect Dis 3:254, 1981

94 STAPHYLOCOCCAL INFECTIONS

RICHARD M. LOCKSLEY

The staphylococci, of which *S. aureus* is the most important human pathogen, are hardy gram-positive bacteria that colonize the skin of most human beings. If the skin or mucous membranes are disrupted by surgery or trauma, staphylococci may gain access to and proliferate in the underlying tissues, giving rise to a typically localized, superficial abscess. Although these cutaneous infections are most commonly harmless and self-limited, the multiplying organisms may invade the lymphatics and the blood, leading to the potentially serious complications of staphylococcal bacteremia. These complications include septic shock, which may be indistinguishable from that caused by gram-negative bacteria, and serious metastatic complications, including endocarditis (see Chap. 188), arthritis (see Chap. 277), osteomyelitis (see Chap. 340), pneumonia (see Chap. 205), and abscesses (see Chap. 87) in virtually any organ in the body. Certain strains of *S. aureus* produce toxins that can cause skin rashes or that mediate multisystem dysfunction, as in toxic shock syndrome. Coagulase-negative staphylococci, particularly *S. epidermidis,* are important nosocomial pathogens, with a particular predilection for infecting vascular catheters and prosthetic devices. *S. saprophyticus* is a common cause of urinary tract infection.

ETIOLOGY AND MICROBIOLOGY Staphylococci are gram-positive, nonmotile, aerobic or facultatively anaerobic, catalase-positive cocci within the family Micrococcaceae. The name derives from the typical clustering of organisms (the Greek *staphyle,* "bunch of grapes") observed microscopically in stained specimens taken from colonies grown on solid media. Pathogenic staphylococci are distinguished from nonpathogenic micrococci by the ability of staphylococci to ferment glucose anaerobically and by their sensitivity to lysostaphin endopeptidase. *S. aureus,* the most important human pathogen in the genus, is named for the golden color of colonies grown aerobically on solid media, the color results from the production of carotenoids. All staphylococcal strains producing coagulase are designated *S. aureus*. In contrast to coagulase-negative staphylococci, *S. aureus* ferments mannitol, produces DNase, and displays greater susceptibility to lysostaphin. *S. aureus* is generally hemolytic when cultured on blood agar. Commercially available kits using specific antibodies linked to latex particles or beads can distinguish *S. aureus* from coagulase-negative staphylococci by particle agglutination. *S. aureus* strains typically exhibit greater expression of biochemical activity (production of coagulase, toxins, hemolysins) than coagulase-negative staphylococci.

There are currently 12 recognized and 2 proposed species of coagulase-negative staphylococci, of which *S. epidermidis* and *S. saprophyticus* are the most important clinically. *S. saprophyticus* can be identified by its resistance to novobiocin and nalidixic acid, although this is reliable only for urinary isolates.

Differentiation among strains of *S. aureus* or *S. epidermidis* has been used to identify a common source during epidemics or intrahospital outbreaks of staphylococcal disease. Strains of *S. aureus* may be distinguished by antimicrobial susceptibility profiles, by patterns of lysis by staphylococcal bacteriophages (phage typing), and by analysis of plasmids within the organism. Of these three tests, antibiotic susceptibility testing has the least and plasmid analysis the most discriminatory ability. Attempts to differentiate strains of *S. epidermidis* using biotyping, antimicrobial susceptibility, or serotyping alone have been generally unsatisfactory. Only 20 to 40 percent of hospital isolates of *S. epidermidis* can be typed by standard phage typing. Plasmid analysis is the most reliable method distinguishing among strains.

EPIDEMIOLOGY The coagulase-negative staphylococci are part of the normal flora of the skin, mucous membranes, and lower bowel; *S. epidermidis* is the commonest species isolated. *S. aureus* transiently colonizes the anterior nares in 70 to 90 percent of persons and may be recovered for relatively prolonged periods of time in 20 to 30 percent of them. Nasal carriage is often accompanied by secondary colonization of the skin. Independent colonization of the perineal area occurs in 5 to 20 percent of persons, and vaginal carriage has been demonstrated in 10 percent of menstruating females. Higher carriage rates of *S. aureus* have been documented in hospital employees (including physicians and nurses), hospitalized patients, and patients whose care requires frequent puncture of the skin, e.g., insulin-dependent diabetic patients, dialysis-dependent renal failure patients, and patients receiving frequent desensitization injections for allergies. Drug abusers who use needles also have enhanced *S. aureus* carriage rates. Presumably, disturbances in the local cutaneous barrier allow *S. aureus* to establish and maintain colonization successfully.

S. saprophyticus demonstrates enhanced adherence to urothelial cells compared to *S. epidermidis*. Approximately 5 percent of healthy males and females have low colony counts of *S. saprophyticus* in the urethral or periurethral areas.

Although staphylococci can survive in the environment for prolonged periods of time, and airborne spread of organisms can be demonstrated, person-to-person transfer via contaminated hands is the most important mechanism for transmission of staphylococci. Hospitalized patients with active staphylococcal infection or those who become heavily colonized, particularly at cutaneous sites (surgical wounds, burns, decubitus ulcers), constitute the greatest reservoir for nosocomially acquired infection. Such patients shed an enormous number of organisms, and the hands of hospital personnel caring for these patients become readily colonized. Failure to use aseptic technique and neglect of hand washing allows transmission of the organisms to the skin of other patients. Strains of both *S. aureus* and *S. epidermidis* may become endemic in areas of the hospital housing patients with large integumental defects, particularly when widespread antimicrobial use favors the acquisition of multiply resistant strains (burn units, intensive care units, bone marrow transplant units). Less frequently, otherwise healthy hospital employees who are nasal carriers have been implicated in nosocomial outbreaks. Upon careful examination, most of these carriers will have active dermatologic infections during the time that effective transmission of staphylococci is documented.

If infections arising from the urinary tract are excluded, *S. aureus* and *S. epidermidis* together have become the most common cause of nosocomial infection in United States hospitals. They are the most frequently isolated pathogens in both primary and secondary bacteremias, and in cutaneous and surgical wound infections.

PATHOGENESIS Infection by staphylococci usually results from a combination of bacterial virulence factors and diminution in host defense. Important microbial factors include the ability of the staphylococcus to survive under harsh conditions, its cell wall constituents, the production of enzymes and toxins that promote tissue invasion, its capacity to persist intracellularly in certain phagocytes, and its potential to acquire resistance to antimicrobials. Important host factors include an intact mucocutaneous barrier, an adequate number of functional neutrophils, and removal of foreign bodies or devitalized tissues.

Microbial factors Cell wall components of *S. aureus* include a large peptidoglycan complex that confers rigidity to the organism and enables it to survive under unfavorable osmotic conditions, a unique teichoic acid linked to peptidoglycan, and protein A, found both attached to peptidoglycan over the outermost parts of the cell and released in soluble form. Both peptidoglycan and teichoic acid are capable of activating the complement cascade via the alternative pathway. Although important for opsonization of organisms for ingestion by phagocytes, complement activation may also play a role in the pathogenesis of shock and disseminated intravascular coagulation. Protein A binds to the Fc portion of certain classes of IgG as well as to the Fc receptor on phagocytes and may serve as a blocking factor preventing neutrophil ingestion of the organisms. Specific receptors for laminin, the major glycoprotein of the vascular basement membrane, may mediate the widespread metastatic potential of *S. aureus*. Some strains of *S. aureus* may be coated by an antiphagocytic capsule that requires specific antibodies for ingestion. The cell wall of certain strains of *S. epidermidis* is also capable of activating complement; shock and disseminated intravascular coagulation during infections by these organisms have been described, although less frequently than with *S. aureus*. The capacity of *S. epidermidis* to adhere to intravascular cannulas and prosthetic devices may explain the propensity of these organisms to cause foreign body infections; the nature of the adherence ligands is unknown.

Certain enzymes produced by *S. aureus* may play a role in virulence. Catalase degrades hydrogen peroxide and may protect the organism during phagocytosis when it must withstand the phagocyte's respiratory burst. This may be important in intracellular persistence of some ingested staphylococci. Coagulase is present in both soluble and cell-bound forms, and causes plasma to clot by formation of thrombinlike material. The high correlation between coagulase production and virulence suggests that this substance is important in the pathogenesis of staphylococcal infections, but its precise role as a determinant of pathogenicity has not been determined. Many strains also produce hyaluronidase, an enzyme that degrades hyaluronic acid in the connective tissue matrix and that may promote spreading of infection. *S. saprophyticus* produces urease, an enzyme capable of breaking down urea to ammonium, alkalinizing the urine, and favoring the formation of struvite stones.

S. aureus may produce numerous extracellular toxins. Toxins may be encoded by chromosomal or plasmid DNA. At least one toxin, enterotoxin A, is encoded by bacteriophage DNA integrated into the bacterial chromosome. Four different red cell hemolysins—designated alpha, beta, gamma, and delta toxins—have been identified. Alpha toxin is also dermonecrotic when injected subcutaneously into animals. Delta toxin inhibits water absorption by elevating cAMP in guinea pig ileum and may play a role in the acute watery diarrhea seen in some cases of staphylococcal infection. Leukocidin lyses granulocyte and macrophage membranes by producing membrane pores permeable to cations.

While the role of the above factors in virulence is incompletely understood, the staphylococcal enterotoxins, exfoliatin toxins A and B, and the toxic shock syndrome toxin—TSST-1—each have been implicated in disease. Five serologically distinct enterotoxins (A through E) have been implicated in food poisoning due to *S. aureus*. The toxins enhance intestinal peristalsis and seem to induce vomiting via a direct effect on the central nervous system. The exfoliatin toxins mediate the dermatologic manifestations of the staphylococcal scalded skin syndrome. The toxins cause intraepidermal cleavage of the skin at the stratum granulosum, leading to bullae formation and denudation. Antibodies to the toxins are protective in both humans and animals. Toxins have been suggested to mediate toxic shock syndrome (TSS) because of the multisystem dysfunction present in the absence of positive blood cultures. TSST-1, so designated because of evidence for additional toxins, is produced by over 90 percent of *S. aureus* recovered from women with menstrual TSS and over 60 percent of nonmenstrual cases. The toxin causes hypotension, conjunctival and cutaneous hyperemia, and fever when injected into rabbits; death may result from multisystem failure and mimics human TSS. TSST-1 induces human monocytes to release interleukin 1 (endogenous pyrogen), which may mediate some of the symptoms of TSS. Interleukin 1 produces fever, neutrophilia, acute phase protein synthesis, and, through its influence on cellular arachidonic acid metabolism, muscle proteolysis, and, potentially, diarrhea and hypotension. Low magnesium ion concentrations enhance the production of TSST-1. The gene encoding TSST-1 has been cloned and seems to be missing or rearranged in toxin-negative strains of *S. aureus*.

Antimicrobial resistance by staphylococci favors their persistence in the hospital environment. Over 90 percent of both hospital and community strains of *S. aureus* causing infection are resistant to penicillin. Resistance is due to the production of β-lactamases, usually by plasmids. Introduction of the penicillinase-resistant antimicrobials was followed shortly by the isolation, initially in Europe and Scandinavia, of the so-called methicillin-resistant *S. aureus* (MRSA). These organisms are resistant to all the β-lactam antimicrobics, as well as to the cephalosporins, despite the fact that standard disk susceptibility testing may indicate sensitivity to cephalosporin drugs. Resistance of MRSA is chromosomally mediated and is not due to enzymatic alteration of the drug. It probably involves alterations of staphylococcal penicillin-binding proteins. Not uncommonly, MRSA has acquired R plasmids mediating some combination of resistance to erythromycin, tetracycline, chloramphenicol, clindamycin, and aminoglycosides. MRSA has become increasingly common worldwide, particularly in tertiary care referral hospitals. In the United States, approximately 5 percent of hospital isolates of *S. aureus* are MRSA; one-third of hospitals surveyed have experienced bacteremias due to MRSA. Despite the theoretic survival advantage of MRSA, the isolation of these organisms has remained relatively constant since 1980. Outbreaks continue to occur periodically in the form of intrahospital epidemics. The community carriage rate of MRSA is low, although selected patient populations, like parenteral drug abusers, may have MRSA at the time of admission to the hospital. These isolates remain susceptible to vancomycin.

Tolerance to β-lactams is an in vitro phenomenon characterized by resistance of the organism to the lethal action of normally cidal antimicrobials. It is characterized by a marked discrepancy between the minimal inhibitory and the minimal bactericidal concentrations of the drug. The mechanism may relate to a defect in the normal activation of autolytic enzymes of the bacteria by cell wall–active antimicrobials. Demonstration of the trait is influenced markedly by physicochemical conditions, and the nature and significance of tolerance remains controversial. Although tolerance has been reported to influence the outcome of severe staphylococcal infection adversely, it has been difficult to incriminate tolerance to β-lactams as a significant cause of antibiotic failure in animal models of infection. This may reflect the in vitro observation that continued treatment with β-lactams will kill tolerant *S. aureus*, although killing proceeds more slowly.

Most instances of *S. epidermidis* infection are nosocomially acquired and typically express greater variability and degrees of antimicrobial resistance than those of *S. aureus*. Virtually all isolates contain R plasmids that produce β-lactamase and are resistant to penicillin. Approximately one-third are resistant to aminoglycosides and two-thirds are resistant to tetracycline, erythromycin, clindamycin, and chloramphenicol. Hospital isolates of *S. epidermidis* containing multiple antimicrobial-resistant plasmids can serve as important reservoirs for the acquisition of resistance by *S. aureus;* transfer of R plasmids from *S. epidermidis* to *S. aureus* via conjugation has been demonstrated both in vitro and on the skin.

Methicillin resistance is common among *S. epidermidis* strains; over 80 percent of isolates from cases with prosthetic valve endocarditis in one study were methicillin-resistant. Methicillin resistance is heterotypic among *S. epidermidis*—only one in 10^4 cells may express resistance under nonselective conditions. Conditions of temperature, pH, osmolality, and the presence of chelating agents and heavy metals all may influence the demonstration of resistance. Methicillin-resistant isolates may appear susceptible by routine susceptibility testing. The most reliable identification of these organisms is by their growth from a large inoculum (10^7 cells) spread on agar containing 20 μg/mL methicillin. Cross-resistance to the other β-lactam antimicrobials and to the cephalosporins is always present, although as with MRSA, these bacteria may appear susceptible to cephalosporins using conventional disk testing. As with *S. aureus, S. epidermidis* strains remain susceptible to vancomycin and usually to rifampin, although resistance to the latter may occur rapidly when the drug is used alone.

Host factors The importance of host factors in resisting staphylococcal infections is demonstrated by the observation that enormous numbers of bacteria are required to establish experimental infections in humans and animals. Areas where skin or mucosal continuity is broken provide portals of entry for staphylococci. More than 50 percent of serious staphylococcal infections of deep tissues arise from cutaneous foci; a smaller number originates from the respiratory, gastrointestinal, or less frequently, genitourinary tract. Direct inoculation of organisms into the blood is an important route of infection in hospitalized patients with intravenous catheters and in drug abusers.

Staphylococci often invade the integument via plugged hair follicles and sebaceous glands, or areas involved by burns, wounds, abrasions, insect bites, or dermatitis. Colonization and invasion of the lungs may occur when the normal mucociliary clearance mechanisms are either bypassed, as occurs with endotracheal intubation, or depressed, as occurs following viral infections of the lung (influenza) or in patients with cystic fibrosis. Mucosal damage to the gastrointestinal tract following cytotoxic chemotherapy or radiotherapy predisposes to invasion from that site.

Once the integument has been breached, local bacterial multiplication is accompanied by inflammation and tissue necrosis at the site of infection. Neutrophils rapidly enter the area and ingest large numbers of staphylococci. Thrombosis of surrounding capillaries occurs; fibrin is deposited about the periphery; later, fibroblasts create a relatively avascular wall about the area. The fully developed staphylococcal abscess consists of a central core of dead and dying leukocytes and bacteria which gradually liquefies to form characteristic thick, creamy pus, surrounded by a fibroblastic wall. When host mechanisms fail to contain the cutaneous or submucosal infection, staphylococci may enter the lymphatics and the bloodstream. Common sites of metastatic seeding include the diaphyseal ends of long bones in children, and the lungs, kidneys, cardiac valves, myocardium, liver, spleen, and brain.

Polymorphonuclear leukocytes capable of normal chemotaxis, ingestion, and killing appear to be the major protective mechanisms against staphylococcal disease. Persons with inherited or acquired defects in any of these leukocyte functions, or with neutropenia itself, are particularly susceptible to staphylococcal infections. A low number of staphylococci is capable of surviving within phagocytes, which may account for the relatively slow response of staphylococcal infections to antimicrobials and the potential for relapse.

Although infections may occur in all age groups, serious staphylococcal infections most commonly afflict the young and the old—particularly those with underlying debilitating diseases. Primary staphylococcal pneumonia is common in infants but rare in adults. Acute staphylococcal osteomyelitis is almost exclusively a disease of children. Superficial staphylococcal pyoderma is more frequent in infants, whereas actual abscess formation occurs more often in adults. While these examples suggest some role for immunity in resistance against staphylococci, there has been no satisfactory demonstration that human staphylococcal disease is followed by effective immunity or that infection can be modified significantly by vaccination. Virtually 100 percent of adults possess antistaphylococcal antibodies in their serum. Except for the neutralizing antibodies to the exfoliatin toxin and the suggestion of a protective effect of antibodies against TSST-1, the role of humoral immunity in modifying or protecting against staphylococcal infection is unclear.

The presence of a foreign body such as a suture or a prosthetic device markedly decreases the inoculum of staphylococci required to produce experimental infection. Once established, such infections are very difficult to cure without removal of the foreign body. Strains of *S. epidermidis* are capable of adhering firmly to and invading plastic catheters, and of secreting a protective glycocalyx covering the adherent colonies. Neutrophil function is also altered in the presence of a foreign body; phagocytosis and killing of *S. aureus* are diminished.

DIAGNOSIS The diagnosis of all staphylococcal infections is made by Gram's stain and culture of purulent material, either aspirated pus or involved tissue, or by culture of normally sterile body fluids. Typical clustering of organisms may not be seen in clinical specimens; individual cocci and even short chains of three or four organisms may be present. Bacteria in the static phase or within leukocytes may appear gram-negative. Abundant neutrophils, many containing intracellular organisms, are usually present, except in severely neutropenic patients.

SPECIFIC DISEASES **Superficial infections** Infection of hair follicles manifested by a minute erythematous nodule without involvement of the surrounding skin or deeper tissues is termed folliculitis. A more extensive and invasive follicular or sebaceous gland infection with some involvement of subcutaneous tissues is termed a furuncle, or boil. Itching and mild pain are followed by progressive local swelling and erythema, and the overlying skin becomes exquisitely painful on pressure or motion. Relief of pain occurs promptly after spontaneous or surgical drainage.

Furuncles occur most commonly in areas subjected to maceration or friction, poor personal hygiene, or involved by acne or dermatitis. The face, neck, axillae, buttocks, and thighs are common sites. Staphylococcal infection may involve the apocrine sweat glands in the axilla or groin (hidradenitis suppurativa). These infections may be deep-seated, slow to localize and drain, and are prone to recurrence and scarring.

Staphylococcal infections within the thick, fibrous, inelastic skin of the back of the neck and upper part of the back lead to formation of a carbuncle. The relative thickness and impermeability of the overlying skin lead to lateral extension and loculation, and a large, indurated, painful lesion with multiple ineffective drainage sites results. Carbuncles produce fever, leukocytosis, extreme pain, and prostration. Bacteremia is common.

Staphylococci frequently colonize impetiginous lesions, but most impetigo is due to group A streptococci. However, staphylococcal impetigo does occur, and while it cannot be clearly differentiated on the basis of its clinical features from streptococcal impetigo, it tends to produce multiple superficial, localized lesions, at different stages of development, has a grayish rather than golden yellow crust, and less often produces high fever.

Treatment of most superficial infections does not require the use of antibiotics. Local moist heat, attention to personal hygiene, and washing with germicidal soaps that leave an inhibitory residue on the skin (hexachlorophene, chlorhexidine, triclosan) are usually sufficient. For more severe or recurrent disease, oral antibiotic therapy with dicloxacillin or cloxacillin (2 g per day in four divided doses) for 7 to 10 days may be effective. Incision and drainage should be utilized selectively. Disease presenting with prominent constitutional symptoms or facial or periorbital infection, should be treated with intravenous doses of appropriate antimicrobials as outlined in the section on bacteremic disease.

Toxin-mediated staphylococcal diseases STAPHYLOCOCCAL SCALDED SKIN SYNDROME (SSSS) SSSS is a generalized exfoliative dermatitis complicating infection by toxin (exfoliatin)-producing strains of *S. aureus*. The disease typically occurs in newborns (Ritter's disease) and in children under the age of 5; it is rare in adults. Strains of *S. aureus* causing SSSS in the United States are frequently phage group II, type 71. The disease begins with a localized cutaneous infection often accompanied by a nonspecific viral-like prodrome. Fever and leukocytosis are mild. A scarlatiniform rash begins in the perioral area, becomes generalized over the trunk and extremities, and finally desquamates. The disease may consist of rash alone (staphylococcal scarlet fever), or large, flaccid bullae develop that may be localized (more common in adults) or generalized. The bullae burst, resulting in red, denuded skin resembling a burn. Friction applied to healthy areas of skin cause the epidermis to wrinkle and separate (Nikolsky's sign). *S. aureus* can usually be recovered from the skin and nasopharynx. Therapy includes antistaphylococcal antibiotics and local skin care. Recovery usually occurs.

In adults, SSSS has been grouped with other severe scalding syndromes such as toxic epidermal necrolysis (Lyell's disease). Drug reactions are the most frequent cause of toxic epidermal necrolysis in adults, and the syndrome may be differentiated from SSSS by skin biopsy. Cleavage of the skin in drug-induced toxic epidermal necrolysis occurs at the basal cell layer resulting in full-thickness denudation, with a greater potential for superinfection and significant fluid and electrolyte loss. In SSSS, cleavage occurs within the epidermis. Kawasaki's disease and toxic shock syndrome should also be considered in the differential diagnosis of SSSS.

TOXIC SHOCK SYNDROME Toxic shock syndrome (TSS) was described in 1978 as a multisystem disease presenting with high fever, a "sunburn" rash that went on to desquamate, and hypotension in children who had group I *S. aureus* isolated from mucosal or sequestered sites. In 1980 TSS became epidemic among young, primarily white, women, with onset during menstruation. A strong correlation was found between TSS and recovery of *S. aureus* from vaginal or cervical cultures of affected patients. The occurrence of a rash, the infrequency of bacteremia, and the association with *S. aureus* suggested a toxin-associated illness. Subsequently a marker toxin, TSST-1, which is produced by most TSS staphylococcal isolates and is believed to mediate the syndrome, was identified. Other undiscovered toxins may mediate TSS among TSST-1–negative isolates. Most *S. aureus* isolates belong to group I.

Epidemiologically, TSS was associated with the introduction of certain brands of hyperabsorbent tampons. Their prolonged intravaginal use, together with the capacity of the materials used in these tampons to bind magnesium, has been associated with increased growth of intravaginal *S. aureus* and enhanced TSST-1 production. Public education and removal of hyperabsorbent tampons from the market have resulted in a marked decrease in the number of reported cases of TSS. Although the majority of cases continue to occur among menstruating females, nonmenstrual TSS now accounts for 25 to 30 percent of TSS cases in the United States.

The diagnosis of TSS is based on clinical criteria that include high fever, a diffuse "sunburn" rash that desquamates on the palms and soles over the subsequent 1 to 2 weeks, hypotension that may be orthostatic, plus evidence of involvement in three or more organ systems. These commonly include gastrointestinal dysfunction (vomiting or diarrhea), renal or hepatic insufficiency, mucous membrane hyperemia, thrombocytopenia, myalgias with elevated creatinine phosphokinase (CK) levels, and disorientation with a normal cerebrospinal fluid examination. Milder forms of the syndrome have been reported.

The onset is acute and typically occurs around the start of menses in a young woman using tampons. The vaginal mucosa is hyperemic, and *S. aureus* can be cultured from the vaginal discharge. Blood cultures are usually negative. Clinical findings are the same in nonmenstrual-associated TSS. Cutaneous infections, postpartum vaginal and cesarean-section wound infections, surgical wound infections, focal tissue infections (abscesses, empyema, osteomyelitis), and rarely primary staphylococcal bacteremia have been associated with TSS. Signs of infection may be minimal among patients with postoperative wound infections where the onset typically occurs on the second day after surgery. The mortality rate of TSS is 3 percent and is most often due to refractory hypotension and the development of the adult respiratory distress syndrome (ARDS) with or without disseminated intravascular coagulation.

Treatment is directed at correcting shock and treating renal failure, pulmonary insufficiency, and disseminated intravascular coagulation when present. Antistaphylococcal antibiotics should be administered parenterally. Focal collections of *S. aureus* must be drained. Up to 30 percent of menstruating women with TSS may have recurrences with subsequent menses, although these are generally milder. The use of antistaphylococcal antibiotics to treat TSS and discontinuation of tampon use significantly decrease the likelihood of recurrences.

The differential diagnosis of TSS includes Rocky Mountain spotted fever, meningococcemia, streptococcal scarlet fever, toxic epidermal necrolysis, and Kawasaki's syndrome.

Staphylococcal food poisoning See Chap. 89.

Invasive staphylococcal infections BACTEREMIA AND ENDOCARDITIS Bacteremia due to *S. aureus* may arise from any local infection, either at extravascular (cutaneous infections, burns, cellulitis, osteomyelitis, arthritis) or intravascular foci (intravenous catheters, dialysis access sites, intravenous drug abuse). Up to one-third of patients do not have an identifiable focus.

Rarely, patients with bacteremia die within 12 to 24 h with high fever, tachycardia, cyanosis, and vascular collapse. Nonencapsulated strains may trigger disseminated intravascular coagulation, producing a disease mimicking meningococcemia. Commonly, the disease progresses more slowly, with hectic fever and metastatic abscess formation in the bones, kidneys, lungs, myocardium, spleen, brain, or other tissues.

A major complication of *S. aureus* bacteremia is endocarditis (see Chap. 188). *S. aureus* is the second most common cause of endocarditis, and the commonest cause among drug addicts. Among nonaddicts, normal valves are involved in 30 to 60 percent of cases, and older, frequently hospitalized, patients with underlying medical disease are most often infected. The mitral, aortic, or both valves may be involved. The disease typically pursues an acute course with high fever, progressive anemia, and frequent embolic and extracardiac septic complications. Progressive valvular insufficiency leads to significant murmurs in 90 percent of patients. Valve ring and myocardial abscesses are common. The mortality rate is 20 to 30 percent. Infection of the aortic valve, the development of uncontrolled congestive heart failure, or evidence of central nervous system involvement are poor prognostic signs; these patients frequently require surgical intervention.

Among addicts, *S. aureus* most frequently involves the tricuspid valve. Evidence for septic pulmonary emboli (chest pain, hemoptysis, nodular infiltrates) is common. Audible murmurs and peripheral stigmata of endocarditis are less common than in nonaddicts. Myalgias and back pain may be the major presenting symptoms and obfuscate the diagnosis. The mortality rate is 2 to 10 percent.

Differentiation of isolated bacteremia from endocarditis may be difficult. Patients with normal heart valves with an identifiable, easily managed or removable primary focus of infection, who receive and respond promptly to appropriate antibiotic therapy, and who do not develop evidence of metastatic complications during the subsequent 2 weeks on therapy, usually can be treated for bacteremia alone. Patients with underlying valvular disorders, with murmurs of valvular regurgitation, with community-acquired disease and no obvious focus, with infection secondary to drug abuse, with evidence for embolic events, or with echocardiographic evidence for vegetations should be treated for endocarditis. The presence of antibodies to the teichoic acid cell-wall component of *S. aureus* after 2 weeks of illness has been used to discriminate between endocarditis or bacteremia with metastatic foci, and uncomplicated bacteremia. Although a negative test supports the diagnosis of simple bacteremia, a positive titer is less specific for complicated disease.

Three carefully collected blood cultures are adequate for the diagnosis in most instances; usually all are positive for *S. aureus*. More cultures may be required if the patient has previously received antibiotics. Purulent skin lesions and urine should also be cultured before starting antibiotic therapy. The urine may be positive in up to a third of cases of staphylococcal bacteremia (with colony counts typically lower than 10^5 per millimeter), and staphylococcal bacteriuria in this setting does not indicate metastatic renal infection.

Intravenous therapy should be initiated with a penicillinase-resistant agent. Nafcillin (1.5 g every 4 h) and oxacillin (2.0 g every 4 h) are preferred to methicillin because of the high incidence of interstitial nephritis with methicillin. Gentamicin (1 mg/kg every 8 h, adjusted for renal function) is frequently added for the first 48 to 72 h because of evidence for synergy with β-lactam antimicrobials against *S. aureus* and the tendency for patients treated with both drugs to defervesce more rapidly and to achieve earlier sterilization of the bloodstream. Rare isolates that do not produce β-lactamase should be treated with intravenous penicillin G (4×10^6 units every 4 h). First-generation cephalosporins (cephalothin, cefazolin) have also been used successfully in infections with both penicillinase-positive and -negative strains of *S. aureus*. Patients with serious penicillin allergy or with infections due to methicillin-resistant *S. aureus* should be treated with vancomycin (0.5 g every 6 h, adjusted by monitoring blood levels).

Cases of uncomplicated *S. aureus* bacteremia can be treated for 2 weeks. These patients should be followed carefully; relapses should be treated as endocarditis. Right-sided endocarditis in drug addicts has been successfully treated with 2 weeks of intravenous therapy followed by 4 weeks of oral dicloxacillin (1 to 1.5 g every 6 h). All other cases of endocarditis should receive 4 to 6 weeks of parenteral antimicrobials. Prosthetic valve endocarditis should be treated with an appropriate penicillin or vancomycin, plus gentamicin, with or without rifampin, for 6 weeks. Most cases will require surgery as well.

The response to antimicrobials in staphylococcal endocarditis may be slow. The fever may not disappear until the second week of therapy. Persistent fever or signs of sepsis should prompt a search for metastatic abscesses that require drainage.

S. epidermidis is the most common isolate in primary nosocomial bacteremias and the most frequent organism infecting intravenous access devices. It has been recognized as a major cause of bacteremia among neutropenic cancer patients, arising either from long-term, indwelling central catheters or from the gastrointestinal tract. Continued fever, progressive sepsis, multiple pulmonary abscesses, and death may result if this complication is left untreated.

Although an uncommon cause of native valve endocarditis, *S. epidermidis* is the commonest cause of prosthetic valve endocarditis (40 percent of cases). Most cases are due to inoculation of organisms at the time of surgery but may not become clinically apparent until 1 year later. Infections frequently involve the valve ring and require surgical intervention. Over 50 percent of patients die.

Because coagulase-negative staphylococci are frequent blood culture contaminants, distinguishing infection from contamination can be difficult. Positive blood cultures demand careful inspection of catheter sites and repeat blood cultures, even in the absence of symptoms, in patients with indwelling catheters, or with prosthetic heart valves or vascular grafts. Speciation of multiple isolates may be useful if isolates can be demonstrated to be the same; plasmid analysis may be required. Catheters should be removed and cultured, although antibiotic therapy alone has been successful for treatment of bacteremic catheter-related infections.

Hospital-acquired *S. epidermidis* infections are usually multiply antibiotic resistant. Methicillin resistance is heterotypic and difficult to exclude. For these reasons, all serious *S. epidermidis* infections should be treated with vancomycin in doses used for *S. aureus*. Prosthetic valve endocarditis should be treated for 6 weeks with vancomycin plus gentamicin, with or without rifampin.

OSTEOMYELITIS *S. aureus* is responsible for the majority of cases of acute osteomyelitis (see Chap. 340). This infection occurs most commonly in children under the age of 12, but adults are also susceptible to acute osteomyelitis, especially of the spine. Approximately 50 percent of patients give a history of a furuncle or superficial staphylococcal infection preceding osteomyelitis. In children, the frequent localization in the diaphyseal end of the long bones is thought to be due to the endarterial circulation of the diaphysis. Many patients give a history of preceding trauma to the involved area. Clavicular osteomyelitis has complicated septic thrombosis of a catheterized subclavian vein.

Once established, infection spreads through the newly formed juxtaepiphyseal bone to the periosteum or along the marrow cavity. If the infection reaches the subperiosteal space, the periosteum is lifted, a subperiosteal abscess forms, and rupture with infection of the subcutaneous tissues may occur. Rarely, the joint capsule is penetrated, producing pyogenic arthritis. There is death of bone, producing a sequestrum, followed by new bone formation, the involucrum. Occasionally indolent staphylococcal infections of bone may persist for years within dense granulation tissue about a central necrotic cavity, a so-called Brodie's abscess.

Osteomyelitis in children may present as an acute process beginning abruptly with chills, high fever, nausea, vomiting, and progressive pain at the site of bony involvement. Muscle spasm about the affected bone is a common early sign, and the child may refuse to move the affected limb. Leukocytosis is common. Blood cultures are positive for *S. aureus* in 50 to 60 percent of cases early in disease. The tissues overlying the involved bone become edematous and warm, and the skin becomes erythematous. Anemia develops during the course of untreated disease.

Staphylococcal vertebral osteomyelitis in the adult differs considerably from acute osteomyelitis in the child. The onset is less abrupt, and there is a greater tendency for bony fusion with obliteration of the disk space. The lumbar spine is most frequently affected.

Osteomyelitis should be suspected in any child with fever, limb pain, and leukocytosis. Similarly, back or neck pain in an adult, when accompanied by fever, should raise the possibility of vertebral osteomyelitis. A history of a preceding cutaneous infection, local tenderness over the bone, and culture of *S. aureus* from the blood are confirmatory. Roentgenograms are usually normal during the first week, but radionuclide scans may be abnormal. Bony rarefaction, local periosteal elevation, and new bone formation can frequently be seen during the second week. Needle aspiration or bone biopsy should be performed if necessary to obtain a specific etiologic diagnosis prior to institution of chemotherapy. In chronic osteomyelitis, sinus tracts are often present, but cultures of the sinus tracts are not reliable in the diagnosis.

Therapy should be initiated parenterally using a penicillinase-resistant semisynthetic penicillin as outlined for bacteremia and endocarditis, and continued for 4 to 6 weeks. Cephalosporins and clindamycin have also been used. Uncomplicated osteomyelitis in children has been managed with 2 weeks of intravenous therapy followed by 2 to 4 weeks of oral therapy. Vancomycin can be used in penicillin-allergic patients and in infections due to methicillin-resistant organisms. Surgery may be required to remove devitalized bone and to drain soft tissue and periosteal abscesses. Neurologic findings due to epidural abscess and cord compression complicating vertebral osteomyelitis demand early surgical intervention. Aggressive treatment of acute osteomyelitis has decreased the incidence of chronic osteomyelitis, with its penchant for recurrent flare-ups and fistula formation. The cure rate for acute staphylococcal osteomyelitis is approximately 90 percent, and death is rare.

PNEUMONIA (See Chap. 205) *S. aureus* causes approximately 1 percent of community-acquired bacterial pneumonias. This disease occurs sporadically except during influenza outbreaks, when staphylococcal pneumonia is relatively more common, although still less frequent than pneumococcal pneumonia.

Primary staphylococcal pneumonia in infants and children frequently presents with high fever and cough. Multiple thin-walled abscesses, or pneumatoceles, are present on the chest roentgenogram. Empyema formation is common. Cough may be nonproductive, and blood cultures are usually negative, frequently necessitating empiric antistaphylococcal therapy. In older children and healthy adults staphylococcal pneumonia is generally preceded by an influenza-like respiratory infection (influenza, measles, or other viruses). Onset of staphylococcal involvement is abrupt, with chills, high fever, progressive dyspnea, cyanosis, cough, and pleural pain. The sputum may be bloody or frankly purulent.

Staphylococci frequently colonize the bronchiectatic airways in children with cystic fibrosis and may cause recurrent episodes of bronchopneumonia. Nosocomial staphylococcal pneumonia typically occurs in intubated patients in intensive care units and in debilitated patients who are prone to aspiration. Residents of nursing homes may have an increased incidence of staphylococcal pneumonia. Infections distal to an obstructing bronchogenic carcinoma may also be caused by *S. aureus*. These infections can begin insidiously, with increasing fever, tachycardia, and tachypnea the only indications of infection. The disease may also be less abrupt when pulmonary involvement occurs during the course of staphylococcal bacteremia, as in patients with right-sided endocarditis. Cavitation, pleural involvement, and empyema are common.

The course of staphylococcal pneumonia may be stormy despite adequate antimicrobial therapy. Gradual defervescence starting 48 to 72 h after the initiation of therapy is typical.

Staphylococcal pneumonia must be differentiated from other pneumonias. The preceding influenza-like illness, rapid onset of pleural pain, cyanosis, and prostration out of proportion to physical findings should suggest primary staphylococcal pneumonia. Sputum

Gram's stain showing masses of neutrophils and gram-positive intraleukocytic cocci provides supportive evidence. Leukocytosis is generally present. When pneumonia develops suddenly or insidiously in debilitated hospitalized patients, staphylococci should be considered in the differential diagnosis.

Parenteral therapy should be initiated with antistaphylococcal antimicrobials as outlined for serious bacteremia and endocarditis. Two weeks of intravenous therapy is usually adequate if complications do not develop. The presence of an empyema usually necessitates chest tube drainage and may be complicated by the formation of loculations or bronchopleural fistulas. Ultrasound or computerized tomography scan may be required to identify loculated collections of pus for drainage.

URINARY TRACT INFECTION *S. saprophyticus* is, after *Escherichia coli,* the most common cause of primary, nonobstructive urinary tract infection in sexually active young women. It is responsible for 10 to 20 percent of infections in healthy outpatients. Symptoms of urgency, frequency, and burning are indistinguishable from urinary infections due to other agents. Fever is absent or low-grade. Although lower tract infection is most common, pyelonephritis has been reported.

The diagnosis is established by examination of the urinary sediment, which characteristically reveals pyuria, microscopic hematuria, and cocci in clumps. The organism may be identified by its resistance to novobiocin and nalidixic acid. *S. saprophyticus* grows readily on blood agar, but less well on MacConkey agar and may be missed by currently available rapid diagnostic methods that depend on nitrate reduction or glucose utilization. The criterion for greater than 10^5 bacteria per milliliter developed for gram-negative urinary tract infection is unreliable.

The organism is susceptible to most antimicrobials used for urinary tract infection, including ampicillin, trimethoprim, sulfonamides, and nitrofurantoin. Relapses after appropriate therapy should raise the consideration of infected renal calculi, which may be formed because of the organism's capacity to produce urease.

Isolation of *S. aureus* from a well-collected urine specimen should prompt consideration of staphylococcal bacteremia, which may have been complicated by renal, perinephric, or prostatic abscesses.

Miscellaneous infections *S. epidermidis* and *S. aureus* rank first and second among pathogens infecting prosthetic devices and intravascular grafts. *S. epidermidis* infections tend to be more insiduous and frequently pursue a prolonged course with high morbidity due in part to the temptation to regard positive cultures as contaminants. Subtle clinical findings are common—prosthetic hip infections may present with pain and loosening of the prosthesis, and cerebrospinal fluid shunt infections may present as hypocomplementemic glomerulonephritis due to circulating immune complexes.

S. aureus is a frequent cause of mastitis in nursing mothers; the infant is usually colonized. Although *Clostridium difficile* is the most common cause of postantibiotic colitis, overgrowth of *S. aureus* in the ileum and cecum may be responsible occasionally. *S. epidermidis* is a common cause of endophthalmitis complicating ocular surgery.

CONTROL OF INTRAHOSPITAL OUTBREAKS OF STAPHYLOCOCCAL DISEASE (See Chap. 85) Hospital outbreaks of staphylococcal disease may develop rapidly in burn units, intensive care units, or neonatal care units—areas housing debilitated patients under continuous antibiotic pressure. The index case is frequently a patient recently discharged or transferred from another hospital where the organism is endemic. The implicated strains of *S. aureus* are frequently methicillin-resistant (MRSA).

Control demands the rapid identification of the patient reservoir in the affected care units by cultures of wounds, nares, and perineum; urine cultures should be obtained from patients with indwelling urinary catheters. Isolation of culture-positive patients together with reinforcement of the need for proper aseptic technique and hand washing by hospital personnel decreases transmission. Housekeeping antisepsis using phenolic cleaning agents should be carried out in the rooms of colonized patients. Early discharge of colonized patients should be encouraged. Charts should be labeled and patients returned to strict isolation upon readmission to the hospital until shown to be culture-negative.

Although nasal carriers among hospital personnel may transmit the organism, efficient dissemination occurs by persons with cutaneous diseases (eczema, atopic dermatitis) that have become colonized with *S. aureus*. Such personnel should be removed from clinical duties until they become culture-negative either spontaneously or following therapy.

Decolonization of the skin and nares in patients and personnel has been accomplished by whole-body washing with antiseptic soaps that leave an inhibitory residue on the skin—hexachlorophene, chlorhexidine, or triclosan. Topical antibiotics are ineffective. Oral antibiotics may be required to abolish the carrier state. Rifampin (600 mg every day for 5 days) has been used successfully alone or, depending on the sensitivity of the staphylococcal isolate, combined with trimethoprim-sulfamethoxazole, doxycycline, or dicloxacillin to prevent the emergence of rifampin resistance.

REFERENCES

ARCHER GL: *Staphylococcus epidermidis* and other coagulase-negative staphylococci, in *Principles and Practice of Infectious Diseases,* GC Mandell et al (eds). New York, Wiley Medical, 1985, pp 1117–1123

CHAMBERS HF et al: *Staphylococcus aureus* endocarditis: Clinical manifestations in addicts and nonaddicts. Medicine 62:170, 1983

GARBE PL et al: *Staphylococcus aureus* isolates from patients with nonmenstrual toxic shock syndrome. Evidence for additional toxins. JAMA 253:2538, 1985

HOVELIUS B, MARDH P-A: *Staphylococcus saprophyticus* as a common cause of urinary tract infections. Rev Infect Dis 6:328, 1984

LOWY FD, HAMMER SM: *Staphylococcus epidermidis* infections. Ann Intern Med 99:834, 1983

SHEAGREN JN: *Staphylococcus aureus.* The persistent pathogen. New Engl J Med 310:1368, 1437, 1984

WALDVOGEL FA: *Staphylococcus aureus* (including toxic shock syndrome) in *Principles and Practice of Infectious Diseases,* GC Mandell et al (eds). New York, Wiley Medical, 1985, pp 1097–1117

95 STREPTOCOCCAL INFECTIONS

ALAN B. BISNO

Streptococci are among the commonest bacterial pathogens of humans. They are responsible for a diverse spectrum of diseases including pharyngitis and tonsillitis, scarlet fever, erysipelas, impetigo, lymphangitis, and perinatal infections of mother and child. Certain representatives of this genus are prominent causes of endocarditis and urinary tract infections. In addition to their role in causing acute pyogenic infections, strains of *Streptococcus pyogenes* are capable of giving rise to the delayed nonsuppurative sequels of acute rheumatic fever and acute glomerulonephritis.

ETIOLOGY AND CLASSIFICATION Streptococci are spherical or ovoid bacterial cells which grow in pairs or chains of varying lengths. Most are facultative anaerobes, although some taxonomists include certain strict anaerobes in the genus. The organisms are gram-positive, usually nonmotile, non-spore-forming, and catalase-negative. No single system of classification suffices to differentiate this heterogeneous group of organisms. Instead, classification depends upon a combination of features, including patterns of hemolysis observed on blood agar plates, antigenic composition, growth characteristics, and biochemical reactions.

When cultivated on blood agar plates, streptococci may produce one of three different patterns of hemolysis. Alpha-hemolytic colonies are surrounded by a zone of partial hemolysis; in addition, such organisms usually produce a greenish discoloration in the medium due to the presence of an unidentified reductant of hemoglobin. This greening reaction gives rise to the designation "viridans" streptococcus, which is often applied to alpha-hemolytic strains. Strains of *S. pneumoniae* are alpha-hemolytic, as are many other streptococci which normally inhabit the upper respiratory and gastrointestinal tracts. Beta-hemolytic colonies are surrounded by clear colorless zones within which the red blood cells in the medium have been completely lysed. This pattern of complete hemolysis is shown by *S. pyogenes* and many of the other streptococci pathogenic for humans. Gamma streptococci fail to produce hemolysis upon blood agar plates.

Although classification of streptococci on the basis of hemolytic reactions is quite useful in certain clinical situations, more precise identification of streptococci is accomplished by differentiation into serogroups, as originally described by Lancefield, on the basis of antigenic differences in cell wall carbohydrates or teichoic acids. These antigens are readily extracted from streptococcal cell walls and identified by precipitin reactions using specific antiserums. The majority of beta-hemolytic streptococci isolated from human infections belong to groups A to D and G. Certain alpha-hemolytic and nonhemolytic strains also contain group-specific antigens. The most important of these are the group D streptococci, including the so-called enterococci, among which many strains fail to show beta hemolysis. There are 21 recognized species of streptococci. Species designation is based upon growth characteristics under varying conditions of temperature, pH, and media composition. Five species do not possess group antigens, and, conversely, a number of serogroups do not encompass any of the recognized species.

Anaerobic streptococci include members of the family Peptococceae, genus *Peptostreptococcus*; five species are recognized. Hemolytic reactions of these organisms are variable, and no satisfactory method of classifying them has been devised.

GROUP A STREPTOCOCCAL INFECTIONS

Streptococci of Lancefield's group A (*S. pyogenes*) are uniquely important because of the frequency with which they cause human infections and their role as precursors of rheumatic fever and glomerulonephritis.

ETIOLOGY The *group-specific carbohydrate* of group A streptococci is a polymer of rhamnose and *N*-acetylglucosamine. There are approximately 80 recognized and provisional group A serotypes. The typing system is based upon antigenic differences in a cell wall constituent known as *M protein,* which is the principal virulence factor of group A organisms. Strains rich in M protein are highly resistant to phagocytosis by polymorphonuclear leukocytes in vitro and are capable of initiating disease in humans and experimental animals. Strains lacking M protein are avirulent. The antiphagocytic effect of M protein is due, at least in part, to its ability to prevent opsonization of the organism by the complement system. Acquired human immunity to streptococcal infection is based upon development of opsonic antibodies directed against the antiphagocytic moiety of M protein. This immunity is type-specific and lasts for many years, perhaps indefinitely. M proteins of certain types share antigenic determinants with human heart tissue.

T protein serves as the basis of a subsidiary typing system which has been useful in classifying strains not typeable by the M systems; unlike M protein, the T antigen plays no role in virulence. *Lipoteichoic acid,* a substance which has a marked affinity for biological membranes, has been found to play a crucial role in colonization by binding group A streptococci to fibronectin and to specific receptor sites on human epithelial cells. The streptococcal *cell membrane* contains a number of antigenic structures, certain of which have been reported to share determinants with constituents of human heart and with basement membrane of the renal glomerulus. During the early logarithmic phase of replication, streptococci are enveloped in a slimy *hyaluronic acid capsule* which serves to retard phagocytosis and, therefore, represents an accessory virulence factor. Streptococcal hyaluronate is nonantigenic in humans, presumably because it is identical to that found in human connective tissue.

As streptococci grow in vitro or in vivo, they elaborate a number of extracellular products. *Erythrogenic toxin (pyrogenic exotoxin),* which is induced by lysogeny with a temperate bacteriophage, is responsible for the rash of scarlet fever. There are four serologically distinct toxins, the effects of which may be neutralized by antibody. Two distinct hemolysins are elaborated. *Streptolysin O* is reversibly inhibited by oxygen (hence exerting its effect primarily on subsurface colonies) and irreversibly inhibited by cholesterol. It is produced by almost all group A strains as well as by many group C and G organisms. Titration of antistreptolysin O (ASO) antibodies in human serums is the most widely used serologic procedure to detect group A streptococcal infection in clinical practice. Hemolysis on the surface of blood agar plates is due primarily to the action of *streptolysin S.* Although streptolysin S differs from streptolysin O in being oxygen-stable and nonantigenic, both hemolysins possess the capacity to damage membranes of polymorphonuclear leukocytes, platelets, and subcellular organelles. A number of other extracellular products exert effects which might serve to facilitate the organisms' survival in vivo by liquefying pus [streptokinase and deoxyribonucleases (DNases) A to D] or by allowing spread through tissue planes (*hyaluronidase* and *proteinase*). The role of these substances in streptococcal virulence remains unproved.

The two most frequent types of group A streptococcal infection are pharyngitis and pyoderma. They differ markedly in their epidemiologic, clinical, and bacteriologic characteristics.

STREPTOCOCCAL PHARYNGITIS Epidemiology The incidence of this ubiquitous infection is highest in children aged 5 to 15 years; males and females are affected equally. The great majority of such infections are due to group A streptococci, but strains of other serogroups, particularly group C or G, are involved occasionally. The organism is ordinarily transmitted directly from person to person, most likely by droplet spread, and crowding markedly facilitates interpersonal transmission. This may account for the increased incidence of streptococcal pharyngitis in northern latitudes during the colder months of the year, as well as for the explosive outbreaks which occur in military recruit camps and other crowded institutional settings. Common-source epidemics of streptococcal sore throat with high attack rates occasionally occur following contamination of a food item with beta-hemolytic streptococci.

Patients with acute streptococcal pharyngitis harbor large numbers of organisms in the anterior nares and throat. If antibiotics are not administered, the organisms may persist in the upper respiratory tract for weeks to months after symptoms have subsided. However, as the length of the carrier state increases, the organisms decrease in number, disappear from the anterior nasal secretions, and lose detectable M protein. Therefore, convalescent carriers are less likely than acutely ill patients to transmit group A streptococci to exposed individuals. Group A pharyngeal carriage rates vary with geographic location, season of the year, and age group. Among school-age children, rates of 15 to 20 percent have been reported; the carriage rate among adults is considerably lower.

Symptoms The usual incubation period of streptococcal pharyngitis is between 2 and 4 days. The classic syndrome, as observed in older children and adults, is ushered in by the rather abrupt onset of sore throat, particularly by pain on swallowing. Associated symptoms include headache, malaise, feverishness, and anorexia. Chilliness is a frequent symptom, but true rigors are rare. Nausea, vomiting, and abdominal pain are common in children.

Physical signs The patient appears moderately ill with tachycardia and fever which frequently exceeds 38.3°C (101°F). There is diffuse erythema, edema, and lymphoid hyperplasia of the posterior pharynx. The uvula is edematous. The tonsils, if present, are enlarged, reddened, and covered by a punctate or coalescent exudate which may be yellow, gray, or white. Discrete areas of pinhead-size exudate may be present on the hypertrophied lymphoid follicles of the posterior pharynx. On the soft palate, small, red, raised follicular lesions with yellowish centers (''doughnut lesions'') are occasionally seen. The anterior cervical lymph nodes at the angles of the jaw are enlarged and tender. Cough and hoarseness, if present, are mild and, in the absence of the signs and symptoms indicated above, do not suggest the diagnosis of streptococcal pharyngitis. Laryngeal involvement with loss of voice is not a feature of streptococcal infection.

The full-blown clinical syndrome of acute exudative tonsillopharyngitis is seen frequently during explosive epidemics of streptococcal disease, particularly those occurring in institutional settings such as military recruit camps. In endemically occurring infections among civilian populations, however, the illness is frequently much milder. Indeed, in such circumstances, only about half the children with sore throats and positive cultures for group A streptococci will have tonsillar exudate, and a third or less may have fever greater than 38.3°C (101°F) or marked leukocytosis. Patients who have undergone tonsillectomy tend to experience a milder clinical syndrome. In infants, streptococcal upper respiratory infections tend to be less sharply localized to the lymphoid tissue of the faucial and posterior pharyngeal areas. Infections at this age are characterized by rhinorrhea with excoriation of the nares, low-grade fever, anorexia, and a protracted clinical course. Exudative pharyngitis in children under 3 is rarely streptococcal in etiology.

Course The course of streptococcal pharyngitis is usually brief and self-limited. Fever abates within a week, usually within 3 to 5 days. Constitutional symptoms and sore throat disappear with defervescence or shortly thereafter. Several weeks may be required, however, for the tonsils and lymph nodes to return to normal size.

SCARLET FEVER When streptococcal pharyngitis is due to a lysogenic strain producing erythrogenic toxin, and when the host does not possess neutralizing antibody to the toxin, scarlet fever ensues. The situation may be more complex than was previously thought, because a preexisting state of hypersensitivity to streptococcal products may predispose to the development of scarlet fever.

The rash usually appears within 2 days after onset of sore throat, involves first the neck, upper chest, and back, then spreads over the remainder of the trunk and the extremities, and spares the palms and soles. The rash may be difficult to appreciate in black patients. It consists of a diffuse erythema, which blanches on pressure, with numerous 1- to 2-mm punctate elevations that impart a ''sandpaper'' texture to the skin. Discrete lesions are absent from the face, but there is a generalized facial flush which contrasts with the prominent circumoral pallor. The rash is more intense along skin folds, such as those of the antecubital fossae and axillary folds, and in these locations often produces linear striations of confluent petechiae known as *Pastia's lines,* which are due to increased capillary fragility.

The exanthem of scarlet fever is accompanied by an enanthem, consisting of punctate erythema and petechiae on the soft palate. Early in the disease, the tongue is covered with a white coat through which hypertrophied papillae protrude as islands of red (white strawberry tongue). By the fourth or fifth day the coating is gone and the entire tongue appears beefy red (red strawberry or raspberry tongue). In rare cases, scarlet fever may be complicated by jaundice, pleural effusion, and arthralgia.

The rash usually lasts 4 to 5 days and is followed by extensive desquamation which begins as early as a few days or as late as 3 to 4 weeks after onset of the disease and is often a striking feature of the convalescent phase of scarlet fever.

Although scarlet fever usually follows upper respiratory infection due to group A streptococci, rarely erythrogenic toxins are produced by streptococci of other groups and by certain strains of staphylococci. Moreover, scarlet fever may follow streptococcal impetigo or secondary streptococcal infection of superficial wounds or surgical incisions. The disease must be differentiated from various of the childhood exanthems (e.g., rubeola, rubella, exanthem subitum), toxic shock syndrome, Kawasaki disease, infectious mononucleosis when the latter is associated with rash, miliaria, and drug eruptions. The management of scarlet fever consists of adequate treatment of the causative infection.

Complications Streptococcal pharyngitis may give rise to suppurative complications, among which acute otitis media and acute sinusitis are the most frequent. Suppurative cervical lymphadenitis may also occur. Inflammation of the faucial area induced by streptococcal infection may give rise to peritonsillar cellulitis, peritonsillar abscess, or retropharyngeal abscess. The abscesses themselves, however, usually contain a variety of oropharyngeal flora, including anaerobic bacteria, with or without group A streptococci. A variety of other complications, common in the past, are almost never seen in the antibiotic era: (1) extension up the cribriform plate of the ethmoid or via the mastoid, giving rise to meningitis, brain abscess, or thrombosis of cerebral venous sinuses; and (2) bacteremia with metastatic foci of infection such as suppurative arthritis, endocarditis, osteomyelitis, or liver abscess. Streptococcal pharyngitis is associated with two delayed nonsuppurative sequels: acute rheumatic fever (ARF) and acute glomerulonephritis (AGN). These are discussed in Chaps. 186 and 223, respectively.

Diagnosis Sore throat due to group A streptococci must be differentiated from that caused by a number of other agents. *Diphtheria* is rare in immunized populations. It is characterized by the presence of an extensive diphtheritic membrane, and in severe cases by respiratory embarrassment due to laryngeal involvement, as well as by myocarditis and cranial nerve palsies. Cultures on Loeffler's medium will be positive for *Corynebacterium diphtheriae*. Gonococcal tonsillopharyngitis should be suggested by a history of homosexuality or fellatio and confirmed by appropriate cultures. *Vincent's angina* is characterized by sore throat and tonsillopharyngeal exudate. Unlike streptococcal sore throat, however, there is an insidious onset without constitutional symptoms, pharyngeal ulcerations are frequent, and the disease is usually unilateral.

The major differential diagnostic confusion is with viral upper respiratory infections, which occur more frequently than streptococcal infections. In many cases, the viral etiology may be suspected because of the more prominent catarrhal, ''common cold–like'' quality of these viral infections. *Adenoviruses* may cause an exudative pharyngitis which is indistinguishable clinically from that due to group A streptococci. *Infectious mononucleosis* also produces severe exudative pharyngitis with fever and toxicity and at times is accompanied by a rash which may be confused with scarlet fever. The generalized lymphadenopathy, splenomegaly, prolonged fever, and presence of abnormal lymphocytes and heterophile antibodies in the peripheral blood serve to differentiate this entity. Pharyngitis due to group A coxsackieviruses (*herpangina*) or to primary infection with *herpes simplex* is characterized by formation of vesicles, which rupture and leave shallow ulcers. *Influenza* virus infections frequently occur in epidemics; they are accompanied by severe myalgias, bronchitis is a frequent clinical feature, and all age groups are affected. *Mycoplasma pneumoniae* infections may cause pharyngitis that at times may be exudative. Bullous myringitis, if present, should suggest this diagnosis.

Although use of algorithms incorporating combinations of epidemiologic data, symptoms, and signs may enhance diagnostic accuracy, in many instances it is impossible to differentiate streptococcal from nonstreptococcal sore throat on clinical grounds alone. For this reason, precise diagnosis requires identification of the infecting organism in the pharynx. This is achieved most reliably by a throat culture. In obtaining the culture, it is important to rub the cotton swab over both tonsils or tonsillar fossae, the oropharynx, and the nasopharynx posterior to the uvula. The swab should be inoculated onto a sheep blood agar plate to allow evaluation of patterns of hemolysis after overnight incubation. If beta-hemolytic streptococci are isolated, they may be identified presumptively as group A if growth is inhibited around a low-potency (0.04-unit) bacitracin disk. Definitive identification may be accomplished by fluorescent antibody, agglutination, or precipitin techniques. A number of the positive cultures obtained, particularly those with relatively few organisms on the culture plate, will represent streptococcal carriers rather than cases of acute infection. It is not possible to differentiate cases from carriers confidently on the basis of culture results, but culture does serve to exclude from antimicrobial therapy the bulk of patients with sore throat (approximately 70 percent) who have negative cultures for beta-hemolytic streptococci. A number of commercial kits are available which allow detection of group A antigen directly from throat swabs by immunologic means. These kits provide results within less than an hour, some within a few minutes. The direct antigen tests are highly specific, and the physician may proceed confidently on the basis of a positive result. Although the immunologic tests are in general quite sensitive, they fail to identify reliably patients with very weakly positive cultures. Many such patients are, however, asymptomatic carriers. The precise role of group A antigen tests, which provide rapid results at the expense of somewhat reduced sensitivity compared to throat culture, has not been established.

In selecting patients for throat culture or antigen testing, it should be borne in mind that group A streptococcal pharyngitis and acute rheumatic fever are extremely rare in children under 3 in the United States. Likewise, first attacks of rheumatic fever are rare in older adults. Routine use of streptococcal diagnostic procedures is less cost-effective in these groups.

Assays of serum antibodies to streptococcal extracellular products (e.g., ASO) provide confirmatory evidence of recent streptococcal infection in patients suspected of having ARF or AGN, but such tests are of no value in the diagnosis of acute streptococcal infection.

Treatment Therapy of streptococcal pharyngitis is directed primarily toward prevention of ARF and of suppurative sequelae. It is unclear whether treatment of the antecedent streptococcal infection will prevent development of AGN. Prevention of ARF depends upon eradication of the infecting organism from the pharynx, and attainment of this objective requires prolonged antibiotic treatment. Penicillin is the drug of choice. It is inexpensive and nontoxic and all group A streptococci have remained exquisitely sensitive to it. A single intramuscular injection of benzathine penicillin G, 600,000 units for children weighing 27 kg (60 lb) or less and 1.2 million units for all others, ensures a prolonged penicillinemia and is the most effective form of therapy. Given the current low risk of ARF in most areas of the United States, many physicians now choose oral therapy for compliant patients. This is an attractive alternative because the risk of severe allergic reactions is presumed to be less with oral than with intramuscular penicillin. A full 10 days of therapy is required, however, and this is often difficult to achieve, because patients are usually asymptomatic well before the 10 days have elapsed. If oral therapy is elected, penicillin V, 125 to 250 mg, three to four times daily, is the treatment of choice.

Penicillin-allergic individuals may be treated with oral erythromycin. Prescribing information for the various formulations should be consulted for the precise dosage. For most preparations, the dose is 40 mg per kilogram of body weight per day, to be administered in two to four equally divided portions. The total daily dose should not exceed 1 g.

Nearly all group A streptococci in the United States have remained susceptible to erythromycin, but extensive resistance has been reported in certain areas of the world such as Japan. On the other hand, tetracycline-resistant strains are encountered with some frequency in the United States, and this drug is not recommended. Sulfonamides are ineffective in eradication of established streptococcal infection, although they are useful prophylactically in preventing new pharyngeal acquisitions of group A streptococci and in preventing recurrences of ARF (see Chap. 186).

Because of the very low incidence of ARF and because a high proportion of "treatment failures" occur in streptococcal carriers rather than in acutely infected patients, routine follow-up cultures are not needed in asymptomatic individuals. Exceptions should be made, however, if there is a history of ARF in the patient or family contacts.

Appropriate antibiotic therapy is effective in preventing ARF, even when initiated as long as 9 days after the onset of acute pharyngitis. Therefore, in the patient seen early in the course of illness, the delay in initiating therapy occasioned by processing a throat culture is not ordinarily a matter of concern. Although treatment also speeds resolution of fever, sore throat, and systemic symptoms associated with streptococcal pharyngitis, the effect of antibiotics is in most cases not dramatic. Indeed, given the self-limited course of the illness, it is difficult to demonstrate clinical improvement in antibiotic-treated vs. placebo-treated patients if therapy is initiated more than 24 h after onset of symptoms. Unless patients have high fever, severe systemic toxicity, or evidence of suppurative complications, initiation of antimicrobial therapy can await the results of throat culture.

In patients judged to be more severely ill, therapy may be initiated at the time of the initial visit after a throat culture has been obtained. If oral antibiotic therapy is elected, the throat culture serves as a guide to the necessity of completing a full 10-day course or, alternatively, of recalling the patient for definitive therapy with an injection of benzathine penicillin G.

Patients with more severe suppurative complications, such as mastoiditis or ethmoiditis, require larger doses of penicillin than those used for treatment of uncomplicated sore throat. When streptococcal upper respiratory infection is complicated by the development of abscesses associated with suppurative cervical adenitis or in the peritonsillar or retropharyngeal soft tissues, incision and drainage are usually required.

The role of tonsillectomy, if any, in the management of patients with frequent recurrences of acute pharyngitis or in the prevention of ARF remains undefined. Clinical episodes of pharyngitis occur less frequently and tend to be milder following tonsillectomy, but this may possibly make detection and appropriate treatment of immunologically significant streptococcal infections more difficult.

Family contacts of patients with streptococcal sore throat frequently develop symptomatic infections or become asymptomatic pharyngeal carriers. Symptomatic secondary cases in families should be treated appropriately. Asymptomatic family contacts should also be cultured in high-risk circumstances. These include the presence of a rheumatic subject in the family or of known cases of ARF occurring in the general area. In situations where the risk is lower, cultures of asymptomatic family contacts need not be performed routinely.

STREPTOCOCCAL SKIN INFECTIONS Erysipelas Also known as Saint Anthony's fire, erysipelas is an acute infection of the skin, with marked involvement of cutaneous lymphatic vessels, caused by group A streptococci. Other streptococci and *Staphylococcus aureus* have been implicated on rare occasions. The disease most frequently affects infants, young children, and elderly individuals. The commonest site of involvement is the face, where cutaneous infection originates from an upper respiratory source, presumably by way of small or inapparent breaks in the skin. Erysipelas may also result from streptococcal infection of wounds, surgical incisions, or even areas of dermatophytosis, in which case any portion of the body may be involved.

The onset is usually abrupt; initial symptoms include malaise, chilliness, feverishness, headache, and vomiting. The skin lesion may begin with itching and mild discomfort at the site of infection and is followed shortly thereafter by a small area of erythema which enlarges during the ensuing hours. The lesion spreads rapidly, reaching its maximum extent in 3 to 6 days. It is warm, pink to deep red in color, and has an advancing elevated margin which protrudes irregularly into the surrounding areas of normal skin. Vesicles and bullae may appear; these rupture leaving crusts on the surface. While the advancing margin remains inflamed, central clearing may be evident with a return of the skin to normal appearance or with residual pigmentation. The eruption may be less well demarcated in areas where the skin is loose, but edema and erythema are constant features. Facial erysipelas commonly involves the bridge of the nose and one or more cheeks in a "butterfly" distribution (Fig. 95-1).

The disease process may be accompanied by high fever and bacteremia. Recovery is usually apparent by the end of a week, but

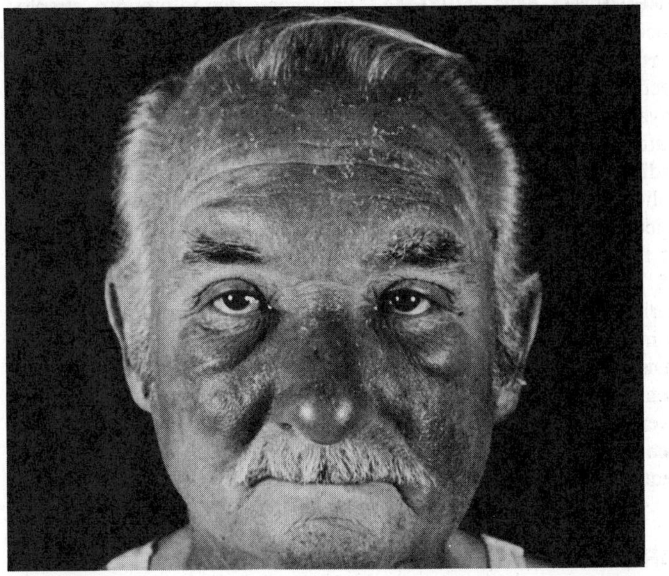

FIGURE 95-1 *This patient with facial erysipelas exhibits the characteristic "butterfly" distribution of the lesion. The picture was obtained after 48 h of penicillin therapy when the acute inflammation and systemic toxicity had abated slightly.*

this varies with the severity of the infection. The substantial mortality attending bacteremic cases of erysipelas in the preantibiotic era has been markedly reduced by penicillin. Fatalities still occur among children within the first few months of life and elderly, debilitated, immunosuppressed individuals. The disease is noted for its propensity to recur, especially in areas of chronic lymphatic obstruction.

The diagnosis of erysipelas is primarily clinical. Group A streptococci may at times be isolated from the respiratory tract or the bloodstream. Culture of edema fluid or of saline injected intracutaneously and then withdrawn from the advancing margin may yield streptococci, but this maneuver is rarely successful.

Pyoderma This term is used collectively to denote localized purulent streptococcal skin infections. Some pyoderma lesions represent obvious secondary infections of wounds or burns. For the most part, however, the term is used synonymously with streptococcal impetigo or impetigo contagiosa and refers to discrete purulent lesions which appear to be primary infections of the skin. Streptococcal impetigo differs from streptococcal pharyngitis in a number of particulars (Table 95-1). Epidemiologically, impetigo is more prevalent among underprivileged children residing in warm, humid climates such as the southeastern United States or the tropics. However, the disease may also occur during the summer in northern settings, such as the American Indian reservations of Minnesota. The peak incidence is in young children (2 to 6 years), and there is no definite sex or racial predisposition.

The mode of spread of streptococcal pyoderma is unknown, but personal contact and insect vectors such as *Hippelates* flies are probably both important. "Skin strains" of group A streptococci (i.e., strains of M and T types usually associated with pyoderma) are capable of contaminating unbroken skin, from where they may be inoculated intradermally by local scratches, abrasions, or insect bites. Nasal and pharyngeal carriage of skin strains is frequent in children with impetigo, but such carriage does not ordinarily occur until after establishment of cutaneous carriage or overt infection.

The pattern of immunologic responses to streptococcal impetigo differs from that associated with upper respiratory infection. In particular, the ASO response to impetigo is weak, perhaps because streptolysin O is inactivated by lipids present in the skin. Brisk antibody responses to anti-DNAse B and anti-hyaluronidase, as well as to the Streptozyme slide hemagglutination reagent, are observed, however. Type-specific anti-M responses are variable, depending in part upon the antigenicity of the infecting strain, but in general such responses are weaker than in pharyngeal infections. The role of type-specific antibodies in protection against reinfection in pyoderma has not been adequately studied.

Streptococcal impetigo occurs on exposed areas of the body, most frequently on the lower extremities. The lesions remain well-localized but are frequently multiple. They begin as papules but rapidly evolve into vesicles surrounded by an area of erythema. The vesicular lesions are rarely recognized clinically; they give rise to pustules which gradually enlarge, then break down over 4 to 6 days to form characteristic thick crusts. The lesions heal slowly, leaving depigmented areas. A deeply ulcerated form of impetigo is known as *ecthyma*. Although regional lymphadenitis often occurs, systemic symptoms are not ordinarily present.

In addition to the indolent, impetiginous skin infections of young children, a more severe and extensive form of pyoderma has been observed in combat troops serving in hot, wet environments such as the jungles of southeast Asia. During the Vietnam conflict, such "jungle sores" became a major medical problem among infantry personnel. In their most common form, they consist of multiple ecthymatous ulcers located on the ankle or dorsum of the foot. The ulcers are usually circular, punched-out lesions 0.5 to 3.0 cm in diameter, have borders, and are surrounded by a zone of erythema. They are filled with purulent material and covered with grayish-yellow adherent crusts. Secondary cellulitis or lymphadenitis may be present.

The diagnosis of streptococcal pyoderma is made by culture. Adequate cultures require removal of the surface crusts in order to obtain specimens from the base of the lesions. Although both *S. pyogenes* and *Staphylococcus aureus* may be isolated from the lesions, the former is the major pathogen. Morphologically characteristic lesions respond well to penicillin therapy, even when penicillinase-resistant staphylococci are recovered. These lesions contrast with bullous impetigo, which is ordinarily due to *S. aureus* and not to streptococci. Antibiotic regimens are the same as those for pharyngitis, and benzathine penicillin G, oral penicillin V, or oral erythromycin all result in cure rates in excess of 95 percent. Topical antiseptics and antibiotics are of little or no value. Prevention of pyoderma depends primarily upon adherence to good personal hygiene, with special attention to frequent scrubbing with soap and water.

Streptococcal pyoderma does not give rise to ARF. This observation remains unexplained, but may indicate a requirement for infection at the pharyngeal site, with its rich endowment of lymphoid tissue, in order to initiate the immunologic events leading to ARF. On the other hand, studies of populations in which ARF and AGN occur simultaneously indicate that the streptococcal strains responsible for each sequela are distinct and suggest that "pyoderma strains" of

TABLE 95-1 Comparative features of pharyngitis and pyoderma due to group A streptococci

	Pharyngitis	Pyoderma
Predominant geographic distribution	Ubiquitous	Subtropic-tropic
Season (temperate zone)	Winter-spring	Summer-fall
Peak age group	5–15 years	2–5 years
Mode of spread	Direct contact (droplet)	Unknown (?insects)
Clinical illness	Acute	Indolent
Streptococcal types	Generally lower-numbered M types	Generally higher-numbered M types
ASO responses	Good	Weak
Type-specific antibody responses	Generally good	Variable, often poor
Nonsuppurative sequelae	Acute rheumatic fever, acute glomerulonephritis	Acute glomerulonephritis

SOURCE: *Modified from Wannamaker LW, N Engl J Med 282:23, 1970* group A streptococci may be nonrheumatogenic. When pyoderma is due to a nephritogenic strain of group A streptococcus, AGN may ensue. Indeed, pyoderma is by far the commonest antecedent of poststreptococcal glomerulonephritis in subtropical and tropical regions of the world. Strains of a number of M types (49, 55, 57, and others) have been associated with both sporadic cases and large epidemics of pyoderma-associated nephritis in diverse geographic areas. There are no conclusive data to indicate that treatment of an individual case of pyoderma will prevent the subsequent occurrence of AGN in that patient. Such treatment is important, however, in eradicating nephritogenic streptococci from the environment in epidemiologic settings in which these strains are prevalent.

Cellulitis Streptococcal cellulitis may occur in areas of tissue damage due to trauma, operative wounds, or stasis ulceration. Although such infections are frequently due to group A organisms, beta hemolytic streptococci of groups G, B, or C may be responsible. Cellulitis is an acute inflammation of the skin and subcutaneous tissues marked by pain, tenderness, erythema, fever, and often regional lymphadenopathy. In contrast to erysipelas, the margins of the lesions are neither elevated nor sharply demarcated from the surrounding uninvolved tissue. Rarely such lesions may progress to frank gangrene. Certain patients who have undergone saphenous venectomy for coronary bypass surgery experience recurrent bouts of acute streptococcal cellulitis in the months to years after surgery. The cellulitis always involves the saphenous donor extremity. Frequently the patients suffer from tinea pedis, and uncontrolled observations suggest that eradication of the superficial fungal infection, which may serve as a nidus for streptococcal colonization, may result in abolition of the recurrent attacks.

Cellulitis of the perianal area may be manifested by painful defecation or by pruritus; asymptomatic anal colonization has been the source of several outbreaks of hospital-acquired streptococcal infection. Vaginal colonization by group A streptococci has a number of features in common with perianal involvement. In both instances there is a close epidemiologic association with streptococcal upper respiratory infection. Anal and vaginal streptococcal infection may be either symptomatic or asymptomatic. At least one outbreak of nosocomial streptococcal infection has been attributed to an asymptomatic vaginal carrier.

LYMPHANGITIS AND PUERPERAL SEPSIS Local trauma, whether or not complicated by frank cellulitis, may give rise to *acute lymphangitis*. This entity is characterized by the appearance of red linear streaks extending from the portal of entry to the draining regional lymph nodes, which are enlarged and tender. Systemic symptoms, including chills, fever, malaise, and headache, are prominent, and the process may be accompanied by demonstrable bacteremia.

Streptococcal bacteremia, from whatever cause, may give rise to metastatic foci of infection, such as suppurative arthritis, osteomyelitis, peritonitis, endocarditis, meningitis, or visceral abscesses. Streptococcal bacteremia may complicate parenteral drug abuse; such infections are often associated with local abscesses at the injection site and/or infective endocarditis (see Chap. 94). The clinical course of streptococcal bacteremia may be fulminant and lead rapidly to prostration, shock, purpura fulminans, disseminated intravascular coagulation, and death.

Puerperal sepsis follows abortion or childbirth when streptococci invade the endometrium and surrounding structures and then the lymphatics and bloodstream. The process may be further complicated by pelvic cellulitis, septic pelvic thrombophlebitis, peritonitis, or pelvic abscess. The causative organism may be transmitted to the pregnant woman directly by medical personnel or attendants, as was demonstrated by Semmelweiss in the mid-nineteenth century. Group B streptococci have supplanted other organisms as the most frequent cause of perinatal streptococcal infections of mother and child (see below). Anaerobic streptococci, along with other anaerobic organisms, have also been implicated.

PNEUMONIA AND EMPYEMA Pneumonia due to group A streptococci is uncommon and usually occurs following influenza, measles, pertussis, or varicella. The illness occurs in epidemic form in military recruit camps and is characterized by abrupt onset of fever, chills, myalgia, dyspnea, cough, pleuritic chest pain, and hemoptysis. Patients are severely ill and often cyanotic. Pathologically and radiologically, this is usually a bronchopneumonia, and lobar consolidation is uncommon. A characteristic feature of streptococcal pneumonia is the early and rapid accumulation of copious amounts of thin, serosanguinous empyema fluid. Bacteremia occurs in 10 to 15 percent of cases. Extension of the pneumonic process to the pericardium may give rise to a purulent pericarditis. Other potential complications include mediastinitis, pneumothorax, and bronchiectasis. Therapy consists of at least 4 to 6 million units of parenteral penicillin daily in the form of aqueous procaine penicillin G, given every 6 to 12 h intramuscularly, or intravenous aqueous crystalline penicillin G, and adequate drainage of empyema fluid, which usually requires insertion of a chest tube.

GROUP B STREPTOCOCCAL INFECTIONS

Streptococci belonging to serogroup B have been of interest to veterinarians because of their association with bovine mastitis, an association which led to their species designation as *S. agalactiae*. The organisms are beta-hemolytic and usually, but not uniformly, resistant to bacitracin. In addition to the presence of group B carbohydrate in their cell walls, *S. agalactiae* may be identified by biochemical means, including their production of hippuricase and so-called CAMP factor and their failure to hydrolyze bile esculin agar. Group B streptococci may be subdivided by means of surface polysaccharides and protein antigens into five serotypes: Ia, Ib, Ic, II, and III.

Human strains of group B streptococci, which appear to be biologically distinct from bovine strains, frequently colonize the female genital tract as well as the throat and rectum. Asymptomatic vaginal carriage rates in postpubertal women generally have ranged between 6 and 25 percent, depending on the bacteriologic methods employed and on the socioeconomic status and geographic residence of the women sampled. The majority of serious group B infections occur as perinatal events. Maternal infections include chorioamnionitis, septic abortion, and puerperal sepsis. *Streptococcus agalactiae* now ranks with *Escherichia coli* as one of the two most frequent causes of neonatal sepsis and meningitis. Neonatal disease takes one of two forms. Early-onset disease, occurring within the first 10 days of life, is usually due to organisms acquired from the maternal genital tract. It involves primarily the lungs, probably as a result of aspiration of infected amniotic fluid, but the organism can be cultured from the blood, nasopharynx, skin, and myocardium. Early-onset group B streptococcal infection occurs in approximately two of every thousand live births (the incidence is higher following prolonged or complicated delivery) and is attended by a high mortality rate. Late-onset disease occurs in infants over 10 days old, may be due to nosocomial transmission of group B streptococci, is manifested primarily by meningitis and bacteremia, and has a lower mortality rate than early-onset disease. Although the serotypes involved in early-onset illness are variable, type III organisms predominate as the cause of late-onset meningeal infection. Transplacentally acquired antibodies to type III organisms may protect against late-onset disease: they are reported to be present in serums of most women delivering healthy babies but are usually lacking in serums of mothers whose offspring develop late-onset meningitis due to type III group B streptococci.

Group B streptococci also cause a group of adult infections not associated with the puerperium. These include urinary tract infections in both sexes; the infections in men often occur in elderly individuals, perhaps due to associated prostatism. A second syndrome occurs in patients with adult-onset insulin-dependent diabetes mellitus, peripheral vascular insufficiency, and suppurative gangrenous lesions, infected with *S. agalactiae*. Bacteremia may accompany this syndrome. Other adult infections due to group B organisms include endocarditis, pyogenic arthritis, pneumonia, empyema, meningitis, peritonitis, and terminal bacteremia in patients with malignancy. Although recovered from a small proportion of throat cultures, group B streptococci are rarely, if ever, the cause of clinically significant pharyngitis. All strains are susceptible to penicillin, which is the drug of choice, although group B organisms have higher minimal inhibitory concentrations for penicillin than do group A strains. Life-threatening group B infections in neonates are often treated initially with aminoglycosides in addition to high doses of penicillin, because this combination is synergistic in vitro and because of occasional reports of penicillin tolerance in group B strains. Only occasional strains are resistant to erythromycin. Tetracyclines should not be used without prior susceptibility testing because resistance to them is quite common.

OTHER STREPTOCOCCAL INFECTIONS

Although streptococci of groups C and G are human commensals, both are capable of causing pharyngitis, and epidemics of upper respiratory disease due to these organisms have been reported, particularly following ingestion of contaminated foods. Strains of both serogroups produce streptolysin O, and pharyngeal infections with groups C and G elicit rises in ASO titer. Streptococci of groups C and G are highly susceptible to penicillin.

Most human infections with group C are due to *S. equisimilis*. There have, however, been several reports of outbreaks of human disease due to *S. zooepidemicus*, in which the vehicle was unpasteurized or inadequately pasteurized milk or cheese. Clinical manifestations have included pharyngitis, cervical adenitis, and disseminated deep tissue infections. In two outbreaks, cases of poststreptococcal glomerulonephritis ensued.

Group G streptococcal bacteremia often arises from cutaneous foci such as localized cellulitis or decubitus ulcers, and chronic lymphatic obstruction and venous insufficiency are important predisposing factors. The patients involved frequently have underlying conditions such as malignancy, alcoholism, or parenteral drug abuse. Bacteremia may lead to severe or even life-threatening complications such as endocarditis, meningitis, or septic arthritis.

Lancefield's group D streptococci consist of enterococcal species (*S. faecalis, S. faecium, S. durans*) and nonenterococci (*S. bovis, S. equinus*). Group D streptococci are frequent causes of urinary tract infection in patients with structural abnormalities of the urinary tract and are responsible for 10 percent or more of cases of bacterial endocarditis. They are isolated from infected decubitis ulcers and intraabdominal abscesses, usually in combination with other bacteria. These microorganisms are ordinarily alpha-hemolytic or nonhemolytic but may be beta-hemolytic. The treatment of severe enterococcal infections, particularly bacterial endocarditis, is complicated by the fact that the organisms are resistant to many antibiotics and are relatively resistant to the penicillins. In the therapy of enterococcal endocarditis, a combination of intravenous penicillin G or ampicillin in high doses plus an aminoglycoside antibiotic should be used, because this combination exerts a synergistic effect in the killing of enterococci (see Chap. 188). Formerly, streptomycin was the aminoglycoside of choice, but high-level resistance (>2000 μg/mL) to streptomycin and kanamycin has been found in a significant number of enterococcal isolates and synergy is not observed in the presence of such high-level resistance. Gentamicin is the drug of choice along with penicillin or ampicillin in treatment of serious enterococcal infections due to organisms which are highly resistant to streptomycin. The combination of penicillin and tobramycin is not lethal in vitro for strains of *S. faecium*.

Certain enterococcal strains have developed resistance by a variety of mechanisms to many of the aminoglycoside antibiotics. Fortunately, gentamicin remains an effective synergistic agent for treatment of most deep tissue enterococcal infections encountered in the United States. In treatment of individual cases, however, it is advisable to rule out the presence of high-level gentamicin resistance by in vitro testing. Treatment of life-threatening enterococcal infections in patients who cannot tolerate penicillin is difficult. Cephalothin and clindamycin are of no value, but vancomycin, in combintion with gentamicin, is likely to be effective.

Nonenterococcal group D streptococci, of which *S. bovis* is the major pathogen, remain extremely sensitive to penicillin and are amenable to therapy with this agent alone. Bacteremia or endocarditis due to *S. bovis* has been associated with carcinoma of the colon. Laboratory differentiation of *S. bovis* from enterococci is sometimes difficult. Likewise, *S. mutans*, a penicillin-sensitive viridans streptococcus which is normally found in the mouth and occasionally causes endocarditis, may be confused with group D streptococci. A series of precise biochemical tests is required to identify the various species correctly. In particular, enterococci grow in 6.5% sodium chloride, while *S. bovis* and *S. mutans* do not.

Streptococci of most groups have been isolated at least occasionally from infected heart valves, soft tissues, or visceral abscesses. Such infections may occur as "opportunists" following surgical manipulation or in patients with malignant disease. Danish and Dutch investigators have reported a number of instances of meningitis and bacteremia in humans due to streptococci of serogroup R, a group of organisms well-known as pathogens of swine. In nearly all human cases there had been a history of contact with pigs.

Viridans streptococci are normal inhabitants of the oropharynx and gastrointestinal tract. They remain the most frequent causative agents of subacute bacterial endocarditis (see Chap. 186). The taxonomy of these organisms is confused, but one classification scheme recognizes five species (in addition to *S. pneumoniae*): *salivarius, mitior, milleri, sanguis,* and *mutans*. Although viridans streptococci are not usually considered to be highly invasive, *S. milleri* is capable of causing serious pyogenic infections such as liver and brain abscesses, peritonitis, and empyema. Cases of endocarditis due to *S. milleri* are more likely to be complicated by abscess formation in peripheral tissues than are similar infections due to other species of viridans streptococci. *Streptococcus milleri* is usually considered "microaerophilic," and its clinical behavior is similar to that of the anaerobic streptococci. All the viridans species, including *S. milleri*, are susceptible to penicillin. Modest increases in the minimal inhibitory concentrations of oral streptococci to penicillin occur following prolonged oral therapy or high-dose intravenous therapy with this antibiotic.

Anaerobic streptococci (see Chap. 102) abound in the mouth, intestinal tract, and vagina. They may be found, often in combination with other anaerobic and aerobic microorganisms, in abscess cavities throughout the body. In the head and neck, anaerobic streptococci may be found in infected paranasal sinuses, brain abscess, dental abscess, infections of the retropharyngeal or lateral pharyngeal spaces, and in cases of Ludwig's angina. In the chest, these organisms occur in lung abscesses and empyema fluids. Abscesses of the liver and other intraabdominal viscera, as well as perirectal abscesses and pelvic abscesses in women, may be due in part to peptostreptococci. These organisms may also thrive in dead or devitalized muscle, skin, or subcutaneous tissue. *Streptococcal myositis* is characterized by marked edema, crepitant myositis, pain, and the presence of chains of gram-positive cocci in a seropurulent exudate. *Hemolytic streptococcal gangrene* may occur after trauma or surgery or without an obvious portal of entry. It is characterized by necrosis of subcutaneous and dermal tissues with spread along fascial planes. *Progressive synergistic gangrene* usually develops about a surgical incision and consists of an ulcerated lesion surrounded by gangrenous skin. The infection is associated particularly with the use of through-and-through sutures after abdominal surgery, and is thought most often to be due to the synergistic action of *S. aureus* and microaerophilic streptococci. *Chronic burrowing ulcer* is a deep soft tissue infection caused by microaerophilic streptococci which erodes through subcutaneous tissue to emerge as an ulcer at a distant site. Management of anaerobic streptococcal infections consists of drainage of abscesses, debridement of devitalized tissues, and high-dose intravenous penicillin therapy.

REFERENCES

AMERICAN HEART ASSOCIATION, COMMITTEE ON RHEUMATIC FEVER AND BACTERIAL ENDOCARDITIS: Prevention of rheumatic fever. Circulation 70:1118A, 1984

AUCKENTHALER R et al: Group G streptococcal bacteremia: Clinical study and review of the literaure. Rev Infect Dis 5:196, 1983

BADDOUR LM, BISNO AL: Recurrent cellulitis after coronary bypass surgery: Association with superficial fungal infection in saphenous venectomy limbs. JAMA 251:1049, 1984

———: Non-group A beta-hemolytic streptococcal cellulitis. Am J Med 79:155, 1985

BREESE BB, HALL CB: *Beta Hemolytic Streptococcal Diseases.* Boston, Houghton Mifflin, 1978

BRENNAN RO, DURACK DT: The viridans streptococci in perspective, in *Current Clinical Topics in Infectious Diseases,* JS Remington, MN Swartz (eds). New York, McGraw-Hill, 1984

EDWARDS MS, BAKER CJ: *Streptococcus agalactiae* (group B streptococcus), in *Principles and Practice of Infectious Diseases,* 2d ed, GL Mandell et al (eds). New York, Wiley, 1985

GALLAGHER PG, WATANAKUNAKORN C: Group B streptococcal bacteremia in a community teaching hospital. Am J Med 78:795, 1985

LAM K, BAYER AS: Serious infections due to group G streptococci. Am J Med 75:561, 1983

SCHWARTZ RH et al: Penicillin V for group A streptococcal pharyngotonsillitis: A randomized trial of seven vs ten days' therapy. JAMA 246:1790, 1981

SHULMAN ST: *Pharyngitis: Management in an Era of Declining Rheumatic Fever.* New York, Praeger, 1984

STOLLERMAN GH: *Rheumatic Fever and Streptococcal Infection.* New York, Grune & Stratton, 1975

96 DIPHTHERIA

JAMES P. HARNISCH

DEFINITION Diphtheria is an acute infectious disease produced by *Corynebacterium diphtheriae*. It is characterized by a local inflammatory lesion, usually in the upper part of the respiratory tract, and a toxic reaction involving primarily the heart and peripheral nerves.

ETIOLOGY *Corynebacterium diphtheriae* is a gram-positive, nonsporulating, nonmotile rod. There is a characteristic swelling at one end of the bacillus, which gives it a club shape. A Chinese-letter configuration is usually seen in stained smears owing to the alignment of the bacilli at sharp angles with each other. Diphtheria bacilli have been classified into *mitis, gravis,* and *intermedius* groups on the basis of colonial morphology, appearance on tellurite medium, fermentation reactions, and ability to produce hemolysis. European workers have suggested that there is a significant difference in the clinical manifestations and in the severity of disease related to the strain; gravis and intermedius infections are thought to be accompanied by more severe toxic manifestations and a higher death rate. In the United States, the gravis strain is comparatively uncommon, and less significance is attached to the relationship of the type of organism and the clinical form of the disease.

Corynebacterium diphtheriae produces a protein exotoxin which is responsible for many of the clinical manifestations; as little as 0.0001 mg is lethal for guinea pigs. Strains of diphtheria bacilli which elaborate exotoxin are lysogenic with the temperate β-converting phage. Absence of lysogeny generally is associated with lack of toxin formation and virulence. However, symptomatic diphtheria may also follow invasion by strains of *C. diphtheriae* that cannot be shown to produce toxin.

EPIDEMIOLOGY Diphtheria occurs primarily in the temperate zone and is still very common in some parts of the world. Since 1966, there has been an irregular increase in the number of cases of diphtheria in the United States. Two outbreaks in Texas early in the 1970s accounted for most of the cases. However, since 1973, more than 75 percent of the cases were reported from the Pacific northwest and the southwest. The western provinces of Canada experienced a similar increase in diphtheria. Until this geographic trend was recognized, the highest frequency had been in children between 1 and 9 years of age. The attack rate for unimmunized children was 70 times higher than the rate for children who had received primary immunization. Within the United States since 1980, few cases have been reported annually, and 70 percent have occurred in adults. In the Pacific northwest, isolates have been obtained predominantly from indigent adults with symptomatic skin lesions. A high incidence is observed among native Americans both in urban centers and on tribal lands. Another striking change has been a decrease in the incidence of laryngeal involvement. In general, diphtheria is acquired by droplet transmission from active cases or carriers, but fomites may play a role in the spread of cutaneous infection. Each diphtheria infection must be classifed as either a case or a carrier. A *case* is an individual who is colonized in the respiratory tract with *C. diphtheriae* and is symptomatic. The concomitant presence of other organisms, such as beta-hemolytic streptococci, does not change the definition or prognosis of a diphtheria case. A *carrier* is colonized with *C. diphtheriae* but lacks symptoms. No attempt should be made to classify an instance of cutaneous diphtheria as a case or a carrier.

PATHOGENESIS AND PATHOLOGY The commonest portal of entry for the diphtheria bacillus is the upper respiratory tract. The skin, genitalia, eye, and middle ear may also be sites of invasion. Growth of the organism is superficial in most cases, and there is little tendency to invade the lymphatics or bloodstream except in the terminal stages. The exotoxin elaborated in the local lesion is absorbed and carried by the blood to all parts of the body. The intensity of the toxic effects is greatest when the primary lesion is in the pharynx, less when it is in the larynx, and least when it is on the nasal mucosa or skin. Simultaneous involvement of the pharynx, larynx, trachea, and bronchial tree is associated with most severe intoxication.

The *membrane,* the primary lesion of diphtheria, is thick, leathery, and blue-white and is composed of bacteria, necrotic epithelium, phagocytes, and fibrin. It is surrounded by a narrow zone of inflammation and is firmly adherent to the underlying tissues; bleeding follows its forcible removal. Ulceration is not a regular feature. Regional lymphadenitis is frequent.

The *toxic manifestations* involve primarily the heart, kidneys, and peripheral nerves. The brain is rarely affected. Cardiac enlargement is frequent; this appears to be related to myocarditis rather than hypertrophy. The kidneys may be enlarged and reveal cloudy swelling and interstitial changes. Bronchopneumonia due to *C. diphtheriae* or to secondary invading organisms occurs in some patients, especially those with laryngeal involvement. Membrane is present throughout the bronchial tree when the diphtheria bacillus is responsible for the pulmonary infection. The peripheral nerves may reveal fatty degeneration, disintegration of the medullary sheaths, and involvement of the axis cylinder. Both motor and sensory fibers are affected, but the main impact is on the motor innervation. The anterior horn cells and the posterior columns of the spinal cord may be damaged. Other central nervous system involvement includes cerebral hemorrhage, meningitis, and encephalitis. Petechial and purpuric lesions are occasionally present in the kidneys, skin, or adrenals. Endocarditis due to *C. diphtheriae* is rare.

Death results from respiratory obstruction by membrane or edema, or from the effects of toxin on the heart, nervous system, or other organs.

IMMUNITY Susceptibility to the complications of diphtheria is related to the presence or absence of circulating antibody to exotoxin. The Schick test yields a rough estimate of the quantity of antitoxin in the circulation. This test is carried out in the following manner: 0.1 mL purified diphtheria toxin (one-fiftieth the minimum lethal dose) dissolved in buffered human serum albumin is injected intradermally on the volar surface of the forearm; 0.1 mL purified diphtheria toxoid is injected into the other arm as a control. These areas are examined at 24 and 48 h and between the fourth and seventh days and interpreted in the following way:

1 *Positive reaction.* The site of injection of toxin begins to redden in 24 h; the reddening increases and reaches a maximum in about a week, at which time the lesion may be as large as 3 cm in diameter and moderately swollen and tender. There is usually a small (1 to 1.5 cm) dark-red central zone which gradually turns brown, desquamates, and leaves a pigmented area. The area of toxoid injection shows no reaction. A positive test indicates little or no circulating antitoxin and no immunity.
2 *Negative reaction.* There is no reaction at the site of injection of either toxoid or toxin. This is consistent with a blood antitoxin level of 1/30 to 1/100 unit and immunity to ordinary exposure.
3 *Pseudoreaction.* Inflammation at both sites of injection within 12 to 14 h, which reaches a maximum in 48 to 72 h and then fades. This usually indicates immunity plus hypersensitivity to the toxin or other materials in the solution.
4 *Combined reaction.* This begins like the pseudoreaction, but the inflammatory response at the toxin site persists after that in the area of toxoid injection has faded. It indicates delayed sensitivity to toxin or other proteins and either low levels or no antitoxin. The incidence of combined reactions increases with age and is highest in unimmunized groups living in areas where diphtheria is prevalent.

Individuals with negative Schick tests occasionally contract diphtheria, and some persons with positive Schick reactions do not develop the disease after exposure. In some parts of the United States fewer than 50 percent of adults have ''protective'' levels of circulating antitoxin. The Schick test is not used routinely in the United States, and the lack of ability to perform it should not delay the treatment of asymptomatic contacts of diphtheria.

Second attacks of respiratory diphtheria are rare despite the fact that about 10 percent of patients who have had the disease remain Schick-positive. This suggests that factors other than antitoxin may play a role in protection against infection. Recidivism with cutaneous diphtheria has been observed during large outbreaks. Underlying chronic dermatoses constitute a common feature of this phenomenon. In general, immunized patients have a milder illness than unimmunized ones when the initial clinical picture and level of circulating antitoxin are the same. Early therapy of diphtheria with antibiotics may lead to recurrence of the disease if exposure to fresh infections occurs shortly after discontinuation of treatment, suggesting that the development of antitoxic immunity is suppressed in these cases. Full immunization with diphtheria toxoid does not prevent nasopharyngeal carriage of the organism but significantly reduces the case fatality ratio. It also ameliorates the symptoms of active disease.

CLINICAL MANIFESTATIONS The incubation period of diphtheria is 1 to 7 days. The local symptoms vary with the site of the primary lesion. A membrane is not always present. The constitutional reaction usually is of only minor to moderate severity in uncomplicated disease. Fever is usually low [37.8 to 38.3°C (100 to 101°F)], unless infection with another organism (often group A *Streptococcus pyogenes*) supervenes. When toxic manifestations are absent, patients feel well except for varying degrees of discomfort at the site of the local lesion. Pallor, listlessness, tachycardia, and weakness are common in more severe cases. Nausea or vomiting is more frequent in young children. Peripheral vascular collapse often develops in the terminal stages of the disease.

Nasal diphtheria Diphtheria is occasionally restricted to the nasal mucosa. It is usually localized to the septum or turbinates in the anterior portion of one side of the nose, does not extend, and may persist for a long time. A foreign body is frequently present. A unilateral serosanguineous discharge is characteristic. When the disease is located in the posterior nasal areas, it commonly extends to the pharynx, from which toxin is absorbed.

Pharyngeal diphtheria The early diphtheritic membrane in the pharynx consists of small areas of soft exudate which wipe off easily and leave no bleeding points. As the disease progresses, the discrete exudate coalesces to form an easily removable thin sheet which spreads to cover tonsils or pharynx, or both. Later, it becomes thicker, bluish white, gray, or black, depending on the degree of hemorrhage, and is so firmly attached to the underlying tissues that attempts to remove it result in bleeding. If infection with group A *Streptococcus pyogenes* is superimposed, the pharynx is diffusely red and edematous. Sore throat is the most common complaint. Pain on swallowing may occur in over 25 percent of the cases and in some patients may be severe. There is a moderate leukocytosis with 15,000 or fewer white blood cells per cubic millimeter.

Local spread of the pharyngeal membrane may occur, and the throat, tonsils, and soft and hard palates become completely covered. Patients with severe disease may develop so-called malignant diphtheria, characterized by marked edema of the submandibular areas and the anterior neck, giving the characteristic ''bullneck'' appearance. Respiration is noisy, the tongue protrudes, the breath is foul, and the speech thick. The pharyngeal tissues are red and edematous, and the cervical lymph nodes are enlarged. The skin is pale and cool. The patient complains of overwhelming weakness. Purpuric eruptions of the skin, particularly on the neck and anterior chest wall, may appear occasionally. Drowsiness and delirium are common.

Laryngeal diphtheria Involvement of the larynx is usually the result of extension of the diphtheritic membrane from the pharynx. The infection may rarely be limited to the larynx or trachea. This possibility must be considered in the differential diagnosis of all cases of ''croup''; it can be ruled out only by direct examination of the airway. The clinical features of this type of disease are described below.

Cutaneous diphtheria Until recently, diphtheria of the skin was a problem primarily in tropical areas where it is responsible for some cases of ''jungle sore.'' However, since 1972, there has been a significant increase in skin diphtheria in the Pacific northwest and the southwest. A high attack rate has occurred in native Americans and in indigent males living in ''skid row'' areas where crowding and poor personal and community hygiene abound. *Corynebacterium diphtheriae*, being unable to penetrate unbroken skin, invades wounds, burns, or abrasions. Coagulase-positive *Staphylococcus aureus* and/or beta-hemolytic streptococci frequently are recovered concomitantly. Although the lesions develop most often on the extremities, they may appear at any site including the perianal area. In tropical zones, the typical lesion appears as a round, deep, ''punched-out'' ulcer, 0.5 cm to several centimeters in diameter. In the early stages, it is covered by a gray-yellow or gray-brown membrane which strips off easily to reveal a clean hemorrhagic base that dries quickly and becomes covered by a thin, leathery, dark-brown or black, adherent membrane. In the untreated case, this separates spontaneously 1 to 3 weeks after infection. The margin of the fully developed ulcer is usually slightly undermined, purple, rolled, and sharply defined. When lesions are infected with a toxigenic strain, anesthesia over the lesion develops within a few weeks. In temperate climates, the lesions are not sufficiently specific to permit visual diagnosis. Cutaneous diphtheria should be suspected in any adult with skin lesions, particularly in the proper epidemiologic setting. Antibiotic therapy will change the character of the skin lesions. Twenty percent of patients with cutaneous diphtheria also have infections in the nasopharynx with the same biotype. Myocarditis or neuropathy occurs in about 3 percent of patients with cutaneous diphtheria. The Landry-Guillain-Barré syndrome develops occasionally.

Diphtheritic lesions in other areas Diphtheria may involve the uterine cervix, vagina, vulva, bladder, urethra, or penis (after circumcision). Toxic manifestations are common. The tongue, buccal mucous membrane, gums, and esophagus may also be affected. Infection of the conjunctiva occurs rarely. Otitis media may occur as an isolated syndrome or secondary to diphtheria in the upper part of the respiratory tract; the aural infection may become chronic; virulent organisms may be isolated from the discharge for many months.

COMPLICATIONS OF DIPHTHERIA The complications of diphtheria are of two types: (1) those that result from spread of the membrane in the respiratory tract, and (2) those due to the effects of the toxin.

Extension and spread of membrane The membrane of diphtheria may spread from the fauces over the posterior pharyngeal wall into the larynx, trachea, and, uncommonly, the bronchial tree, leading to severe illness and a high incidence of toxic manifestations. Occlusion of the airway is manifested by tachypnea and, as obstruction increases, restlessness, use of accessory muscles of respiration, cyanosis, and finally death. In some cases, the membrane extends diffusely into the bronchial tree and produces clinical manifestations of pneumonia. Hoarseness and a crouplike cough are seen with laryngeal involvement. Bronchopulmonary diphtheria is very serious, not only because of obstruction but also because of the large surface from which toxin can be absorbed; the death rate is very high. When the pulmonary lesion regresses, pieces of membrane may break off and produce sudden occlusion of the airway; a cast of the bronchial tree may be coughed up. Occasionally, pharyngeal membrane has extended into the esophagus and cardia of the stomach.

Toxic complications of diphtheria Diphtheria toxin is produced only by isolates of *C. diphtheriae* lysogenic for corynephages that carry the tox structural gene. Nontoxigenic strains can be converted to toxin-producing organisms through transference of this phage. The bacterial host regulates expression of the tox structural gene. The toxin is a single polypeptide chain composed of two fragments. Fragment B recognizes specific surface receptors on sensitive cell membranes, and fragment A crosses the plasma membrane. In the cytoplasm, protein synthesis is inhibited by fragment A through the inactivation of the eukaryotic translocating enzyme, elongation factor 2. A cofactor, nicotinamide adenine dinucleotide, is required for activity of the toxin. The effects of the toxin on the myocardium are thought to result from its ability to decrease the rate of oxidation of long-chain fatty acids by interfering with the metabolism of carnitine. Because of this action, triglycerides accumulate in the myocardium and cause fatty degeneration of muscle.

Myocarditis develops in about two-thirds of patients with diphtheria. However, it is clinically evident in only about 10 percent of cases; alterations in the intensity of the heart sounds, systolic murmurs, bundle branch block, incomplete or complete heart block, atrial fibrillation, and ventricular premature beats or tachycardia, or both, are common. Ventricular fibrillation is a constant threat and is frequently responsible for sudden death. Ninety percent of patients with atrial fibrillation, ventricular tachycardia, or complete heart block die. Overt congestive cardiac failure is uncommon. Evidence of decompensation of the right side of the heart usually develops first; the most common symptom is pain in the right upper quadrant of the abdomen due to rapid engorgement of the liver. Failure of the left side of the heart may appear later. Diphtheritic heart disease is not necessarily "benign" in survivors of the disease; permanent cardiac damage may occur. Fibrosis of the myocardium has been observed in patients who have expired several weeks after "mild" myocarditis was detected electrocardiographically. The degree and extent of fibrotic change have often been greater than could have been predicted on the basis of the type of abnormality present in the ECG.

Peripheral neuritis may occur in the course of diphtheria. Paralysis of the soft palate and posterior pharyngeal wall occasionally appears very early in the disease (2 to 3 days). A more common neuritis (10 percent of cases) usually develops 2 to 6 weeks after onset of the disease. It is characterized by cranial nerve dysfunction; the IIId, VIth, VIIth, IXth, and Xth cranial nerves are most commonly involved. Loss of accommodation, nasal voice, and difficulty in swallowing are the most frequent manifestations. However, any of the peripheral nerves may be affected, with resulting paralysis of the extremities, diaphragm, or intercostal muscles; death may occur from failure of respiration. The peripheral neuritides which appear in the second to the sixth weeks of the disease are characterized primarily by motor loss; sensory changes are uncommon and, when present, are minor. Demyelination is the usual pathologic change. Nerve conduction studies show a marked dissociation between the time course of clinical features and electrophysiologic abnormalities: peripheral nerve conduction velocities are minimally affected early in the disease despite profound weakness. During clinical recovery the electrophysiologic abnormalities are most apparent. Peripheral neuritis may not appear until 2 to 3 months after the onset of diphtheria. In these cases, the clinical picture and course resemble infectious polyneuritis. The outstanding findings are loss of sensation in the "glove-and-stocking" distribution and albuminocytologic dissociation in the cerebrospinal fluid identical with that observed in the Landry-Guillain-Barré syndrome. Motor weakness and areflexia may develop with progression of involvement. Facial diplegia may accompany the other neurologic manifestations. A fatal, rapidly ascending paralysis of the Landry type may develop rarely. Complete recovery is the rule in this late peripheral neuritis, although it may require as long as a year. Encephalitis is a rare toxic complication of diphtheria.

Shock, which develops suddenly and without warning, is an occasional cause of sudden death in this disease. In some instances, this may be a consequence of myocarditis; in others, no cause can be discovered.

Other complications Cerebral infarction with hemiplegia occurs rarely; it is probably due to embolization from atrial thrombi in patients with myocarditis and cardiac dilatation. Superinfection of the lungs is a risk in all patients with diphtheria who are given antimicrobial agents. Purpuric skin eruptions may be seen in severe, malignant cases; thrombocytopenia occurs rarely. A mild morbilliform rash may be present during the early stage of diphtheria. Secondary invasion of the pharynx by group A *S. pyogenes* may take place in patients who have not received an antibiotic. Serum sickness occasionally follows the use of antitoxin. Relapses of diphtheria may occur when patients given antimicrobial agents are exposed to fresh cases soon after therapy has been discontinued. Bacteremia, endocarditis, and meningitis are rare complications.

COURSE AND PROGNOSIS The diphtheritic membrane may be present for only 3 to 4 days in mild cases, even when no antitoxin is given; it usually lasts for about a week in cases of moderate severity. Commonly, the pharyngeal lesion increases in extent and thickness during the first 24 h after the administration of antitoxin. As the disease begins to recede, the exudate softens, wipes off easily, leaving no bleeding areas, becomes patchy so that it resembles the picture of "follicular" tonsillitis, and finally disappears, leaving normal underlying mucous membrane.

The fatality rate of diphtheria prior to the use of specific antitoxin was about 35 percent in average cases and 90 percent in those with laryngeal involvement. Since specific serotherapy has been employed, this rate has been reduced to a range of 3.5 to 22 percent, but it is still highest when the larynx is affected. The overall death rate in the United States is about 10 percent. Death is most frequent in the very young and the old. Immunization is a factor of great importance in prognosis. The fatality rate in immunized individuals is one-tenth that in the unimmunized population. Paralysis is 5 times and "malignant" disease 15 times less common in immune than in nonimmune individuals. As a rule, the longer the delay in the administration of antitoxin, the greater the incidence of complications and death. However, antitoxin is ineffective in reducing risks of complications and death if it is given much later than 48 h after diphtheria begins.

A white blood cell count higher than 25,000 per cubic millimeter is associated with a higher risk of complications and death.

DIAGNOSIS The clinical features of the fully developed diphtheritic membrane, especially in the pharynx, are sufficiently characteristic to suggest the possibility of the disease in most instances. However, the appearance of the pharyngeal exudate alone does not clinch the diagnosis. There are a number of other infections in which pseudomembranes resembling those of diphtheria are present; among those are infectious mononucleosis, streptococcal pharyngitis, viral exudative pharyngitis, fusospirochetal infection, and acute pharyngeal candidiasis.

The specific diagnosis of diphtheria depends completely on demonstration of the organism in stained smears and their recovery by culture. Methylene blue–stained preparations are positive, in experienced hands, in 75 to 85 percent of cases. Diphtheria bacilli can be recovered by culture on Loeffler's medium in 8 to 12 h if patients have not been receiving antimicrobial agents. *Corynebacterium diphtheriae* also multiplies, but more slowly, on ordinary blood agar. If an antibiotic, especially penicillin or erythromycin, has been administered prior to obtaining cultures, the organisms may not grow for as long as 5 days or may fail to grow at all.

Staining of suspected material with fluorescein-labeled diphtheria antitoxin may allow rapid diagnosis. Toxigenicity of *C. diphtheriae* isolates should be determined by passive agar diffusion (Elek plate method), guinea pig inoculation, or counterimmunoelectrophoresis. Biotype determination will help characterize the epidemiology of an outbreak. Restriction endonuclease digests of *C. diphtheriae* DNA may prove useful in the study of isolates recovered during an occurrence of diphtheria. Comparison of electrophoretic gel patterns of restriction enzyme digests can help identify newly introduced strains from the preexistent resident organisms. Phage typing is too difficult to be of immediate epidemiologic assistance during an outbreak.

TREATMENT Patients with diphtheria should be isolated and kept at strict bed rest; physical effort should be reduced during the early convalescent stages. Local therapy of the diphtheritic pharyngeal lesion is useless. The only specific treatment for diphtheria is antitoxin. Antiserum must never be given until the patient's sensitivity to horse serum, using the eye and skin tests, has been determined. There are several regimens for the administration of antitoxin, and the amount given is often based on an empiric decision. In general, the more severe the disease or the more extensive the membrane formation, the greater the amount of antitoxin required. Mildly symptomatic cases may be treated with 10,000 to 20,000 units. Moderately severe cases, such as those with a pharyngeal membrane, should be given 20,000 to 40,000 units. Severe diphtheria, as with laryngeal involvement, requires 50,000 to 100,000 units. The total dose should be given at one time rather than in split doses over a long period. For doses less than 20,000 units, the intramuscular route is convenient. When this method is used, only one-half the dose should be given intramuscularly and the remainder intravenously in order to expedite delivery of the antitoxin. Alternatively, after appropriate testing for sensitivity, the entire amount of antitoxin may be given intravenously in 100 to 200 mL isotonic saline over a 30-min period. Desensitization should be attempted if the initial skin or eye test is positive. A rare patient may be sensitive to such a high degree that the antiserum cannot be administered without the risk of death.

Antitoxin should be given as early in the course of diphtheria as possible. It is capable of binding or inactivating only the toxin present in blood or extracellular fluid. Once the toxin has entered the cell, the effect cannot be reversed or prevented. Antitoxin must be given when diphtheria is suspected clinically; laboratory confirmation prior to administration of the antitoxin is not necessary. Since mortality increases directly with delay in use of antitoxin, it is better to treat clinically suspect but culture-negative cases than to withhold specific therapy.

A history of military service is not reliable proof of adequate immunization. From World War II until 1956, immunization for diphtheria in the United States military was inconsistent. Since 1957, all branches of the armed forces have routinely immunized their pesonnel. When the immunization history is not clear, it is best to provide antitoxin promptly. Antimicrobial agents do not alter the course, incidence of complications, or outcome of diphtheria.

Patients with laryngeal obstruction should be watched very carefully. In mild cases, inhalation of warm or cool steam may be beneficial. If advancing signs of airway obstruction develop, intubation or tracheostomy is indicated. These procedures must never be delayed until cyanosis appears, because, at this point, stimulation of the pharynx or trachea may produce cardiac standstill and death. Sedative or hypnotic agents should never be given because they may obscure increasing respiratory difficulty.

The pulse and blood pressure should be measured frequently. Little can be done to alter the course of the myocarditis. Quinidine has been tried to prevent and treat arrhythmias but appears to be of no value; there is some suspicion that it may produce deleterious effect. The use of procainamide when ventricular premature beats or tachycardia supervene has been suggested, but no documented observations of its effect have been recorded. The administration of digitalis for cardiac failure in diphtheria is controversial. Some consider this drug to be completely contraindicated; others feel, however, that, used carefully, digitalis may be given safely and with beneficial effects. Shock should be treated according to its etiology (see Chaps. 29 and 139). There is no evidence that corticosteroids and corticotropin are of any value in the treatment of diphtheria or any of its complications. Antibiotics should be used to treat symptomatic cases only after antitoxin is administered. Circulating exotoxin is not affected by antibiotics, and their prompt use may give a sense of false assurance. Patients with diphtheria should be quarantined until two successive cultures of the nose, throat, or other infected areas, taken at 24-h intervals, are negative. If antibiotics have been given, cultures should not be taken until at least 24 h after cessation of therapy.

Treatment of carriers *Corynebacterium diphtheriae* usually disappears from the upper part of the respiratory tract after 2 to 4 weeks in patients who do not receive antimicrobial drugs; in a small number of individuals the organism may persist for a long time or even permanently. The most effective treatment of the acute and chronic carrier state is erythromycin. A dose of 2 g per day orally in divided doses for 7 days appears to be adequate. The enteric-coated base, estolate, and ethyl succinate forms of erythromycin are preferred to ensure adequate serum concentrations without regard to food intake. Alternative antimicrobials include procaine penicillin G, 600,000 units intramuscularly every 12 h for 10 days; clindamycin, 150 mg four times a day orally for 7 days; and rifampin, 600 mg as a single oral dose for 7 days. Tetracyclines, semisynthetic penicillins, aminoglycosides, and oral cephalosporins are inadequate for the eradication of *C. diphtheriae*. Parenteral cephalosporins such as cephalothin or cefamandole are effective. In two areas of North America endemic for cutaneous diphtheria, resistance of *C. diphtheriae* to erythromycin has been recognized. The origin of the plasmid in erythromycin-resistant strains is not clear; fortunately such isolates are uncommon. Initial observations indicate that plasmids are not usually detectable in respiratory isolates of *C. diphtheriae* and are rare in skin isolates. Re-treatment is indicated for carriers whose organisms do not disappear on the first trial. This is preferable to tonsillectomy, which may be considered a last resort should the carrier state persist despite repeated courses of antibiotic. Persistence of the organism after appropriate antimicrobial therapy may represent a lack of compliance rather than drug resistance.

PREVENTION Diphtheria is, for the most part, a preventable disease. Immunization at the age of 3 months should be routine. Diphtheria toxoid is best given together with tetanus toxoid and pertussis vaccine (DPT), because antibody titers are higher with combined immunization than with either agent alone. Booster doses should be administered at the age of 1 year and again just before a child goes to school. Although it has been suggested that Schick testing is not necessary in those who have been immunized, some physicians still carry this out to determine the status of antitoxic immunity. A Schick test acts as a booster. A negative reaction does not indicate absolute protection. The development of highly purified toxoid has made it possible to protect adults with little or no risk of untoward sequelae. In this situation, a combination of adult tetanus-diphtheria (Td) toxoid containing 1 to 2 flocculation (Lf) units per milliliter should be used. With this preparation, severe reactions can be avoided. The Moloney test need not be carried out. Adults should receive booster doses at least every 10 years. Unfortunately, reimmunized adults are the exception, and many elderly patients have low and nonprotective levels of circulating antitoxin. They constitute a high-risk group during any diphtheria outbreak.

Treatment of unimmunized persons exposed to an active case of diphtheria remains controversial. One approach has been to administer 3000 units of equine antitoxin intramuscularly, after appropriate skin and eye tests. In some countries (not in the United States) human diphtheria antitoxin is available. The concentration achieved with this product is sufficient only for passive protection of the asymptomatic, unimmunized contact but is not high enough for treatment of symptomatic disease. If human diphtheria immunoglobulin is used, active immunization must be delayed for 6 weeks. Alternatively, cultures of *C. diphtheriae* can be taken, and a primary series of immunizations initiated. The exposed individual then can be observed closely for signs of active disease. If symptoms occur, antitoxin can be given immediately. In those who have been previously immunized, a booster dose of toxoid is usually sufficient. Cultures from the nasopharynx or open wounds should be obtained from close contacts or family members of a diphtheria case or carrier.

REFERENCES

Belsey MA, LeBlanc DR: Skin infections and the epidemiology of diphtheria; acquisition and persistence of *C. diphtheriae* infections. Am J Epidemiol 102:179, 1975

Brooks GR et al: Diphtheria in the United States 1959–1970. J Infect Dis 129:172, 1974

Good I: Myocardial changes in fatal diphtheria: A summary of observations in 221 cases. Am J Med Sci 219:257, 1948

Goor RS, Pappenheimer AM Jr: Studies on the mode of action of diphtheria toxin. J Exp Med 126:899, 913, 923, 1967

Harnisch JP et al: A decade of diphtheria among urban adults: The epidemiology of diphtheria in modern Americans. Ann Intern Med (in press)

Ipsen J: Circulating antitoxin at the onset of diphtheria in 425 patients. J Immunol 54:325, 1946

———: Immunization of adults against diphtheria and tetanus. N Engl J Med 251:459, 1954

Kurdi A, Abdul-Kader M: Clinical and electrophysiological studies of diphtheritic neuritis in Jordan. J Neurol Sci 42:243, 1979

McCloskey RV et al: The 1970 epidemic of diphtheria in San Antonio. Ann Intern Med 75:495, 1971

Naiditch MJ, Bower AG: Diphtheria: A study of 1,433 cases observed during a ten-year period at the Los Angeles County Hospital. Am J Med 17:229, 1954

Pappenheimer AM Jr: Diphtheria toxin. Annu Rev Biochem 46:69, 1977

———, Murphy JR: Studies on the molecular epidemiology of diphtheria. Lancet 2:923, 1983

Scheid W: Diphtherial paralysis: An analysis of 2,292 cases of diphtheria in adults which include 174 cases of polyneuritis. J Nerv Ment Dis 116:1095, 1952

Schiller J et al: Plasmids in *Corynebacterium diphtheriae* and diphtheroids mediating erythromycin resistance. Antimicrob Agents Chemother 18:814, 1980

Thompson NL, Ellner PD: Rapid determination of *Corynebacterium diphtheriae* toxigenicity by counterimmunoelectrophoresis. J Clin Microbiol 7:493, 1978

Wittels B, Bressler R: Biochemical lesion of diphtheria toxin on the heart. J Clin Invest 43:630, 1964

97 INFECTIONS CAUSED BY *LISTERIA MONOCYTOGENES* AND *ERYSIPELOTHRIX RHUSIOPATHIAE*

PAUL D. HOEPRICH

LISTERIA MONOCYTOGENES INFECTIONS

DEFINITION Listeriosis, a disease caused by *L. monocytogenes*, consists of many clinical syndromes. Perinatal infection, acquired either transplacentally or during parturition, is the most nearly unique form of listeriosis.

ETIOLOGY *Listeria monocytogenes* are gram-positive, non-acid-fast, microaerophilic, motile bacilli that form smooth colonies but do not produce either capsules or spores. Several serotypes have been defined on the basis of O and H antigens. The epidemiologically essential aid of typing is available from the Centers for Disease Control in Atlanta, Georgia. Types 4b, 1b, and 1a account for more than 90 percent of the cases worldwide. Weakly hemolytic gram-positive bacilli are presumed to be *L. monocytogenes* if they are motile (when grown at 20 to 25°C), reduce 2,3,5-triphenyltetrazolium chloride, hydrolyze esculin, and display characteristic animal pathogenicity: (1) The Anton test—3 to 5 days after inoculation into the conjunctival sac of a rabbit or a guinea pig, *L. monocytogenes* cause a keratoconjunctivitis; (2) general listeriosis (intravenous or intraperitoneal inoculation) typically provokes a monocytosis in rabbits, and focal hepatic necrosis in mice.

EPIDEMIOLOGY AND PATHOGENESIS Found on every continent save the Antarctic, *L. monocytogenes* are distinct from the nonhemolytic, nonpathogenic, bacilli (found mainly in soil, decaying matter, and feces) that are designated *L. innocua* or assigned to the new genus *Murraya*. *Listeria ivanovii* and *L. seeligeri* have rarely been associated with disease in humans, whereas *L. welshimeri* has not; all three are differentiable from *L. monocytogenes* by biochemical and augmentation hemolysis (CAMP) tests. Although typical *L. monocytogenes* have been isolated from silage, other vegetative sources, and 1 to 5 percent of specimens of human feces, listeriosis is uncommon and occurs sporadically with a frequency of two to three cases per million population per year. Listeriosis is actually more common in urban than rural dwellers, occurring most frequently in July and August (northern hemisphere). The reservoir from which human beings become infected is frequently occult and the mode of transmission often obscure. However, outbreaks associated with the ingestion of coleslaw made from contaminated cabbage, pasteurized milk, and fresh Mexican-style cheese document the importance of food-borne transmission. Transmission from the infected pregnant female to her offspring is well established as a route of infection.

Transplacental perinatal infection results in disseminated fetal listeriosis. The fetus is usually stillborn or is prematurely ejected, virtually always with lethal listeriosis. Fetal listeriosis acquired during delivery is typically not clinically evident for 1 or 2 weeks postpartum and usually presents as a meningitis.

Listeriosis is preponderantly a disease of persons under 1 year and over 55 years of age.

Persons in apparent good health may develop listeriosis. However, other diseases, particularly those with diminished cell-mediated immunity (listerias are cytophilic), facilitate the occurrence of listeriosis: for example, neoplasms (especially of the lymphoreticular system) and any conditions requiring treatment with pharmacologic doses of glucosteroids, irradiation, or cytotoxic agents; alcoholism; cardiovascular disease; diabetes mellitus; and tuberculosis.

MANIFESTATIONS *Listeriosis of the newborn,* the most nearly unique clinical form of listeriosis, ranges from meningitis that is clinically apparent within 1 month postpartum to diffuse disseminated disease in aborted, premature, stillborn infants, and neonates, who die within minutes to days after birth. If clinical disease is delayed to 1 to 4 weeks postpartum, it is generally localized to the central nervous system, as is the rule when children 1 month to 6 years of age are afflicted.

Infants born alive with listeriosis may or may not have fever; yet these babies are critically ill, with cardiorespiratory distress, vomiting, and diarrhea. Dark-red skin papules are frequent, particularly on the lower extremities. Hepatosplenomegaly may be present. This form of listeriosis is also known as septic or miliary granulomatosis. The findings at necropsy are characteristic and mimic those seen in listeriosis of rodents: widely disseminated abscesses varying in size from grossly visible to microscopic, involving, in order of decreasing frequency, liver, spleen, adrenal glands, lungs, pharynx, gastrointestinal tract, central nervous system, and skin. Typically, the lesions are abscesses, but classic granulomas may be seen, depending principally on the duration of infection before death. Microscopic examination of a Gram-stained smear of meconium from the normal newborn infant does not disclose bacteria; fetal listeriosis results in meconium laden with gram-positive bacilli. For this reason, examination of meconium by Gram's stain and by culture should be carried out whenever there is gross soiling of the amniotic liquid with meconium, prematurity, or unexplained fever in the mother before or at the onset of labor. This is particularly important because listeriosis in the pregnant woman may be asymptomatic or may cause a nonspecific illness. A week to a month prepartum, there may have been malaise, a chill, diarrhea, pain in the back or flanks, and itching. Even when symptomatic, the disease is benign and self-limited in the mother; however, as symptoms subside, a decrease or cessation of fetal movement may be noted. Infection of the fetus may occur as early as the fifth month of gestation but occurs most often in the third trimester. Following delivery of infants with proved fetal listeriosis, cervical cultures are, or soon become, negative for *L. monocytogenes;* subsequent conception, gestation, and delivery of normal offspring are usual.

Meningitis accounts for about three-fourths of the cases verified by culture and is the predominant clinical form of listeriosis. Meningitis caused by *L. monocytogenes* cannot be distinguished on clinical grounds from meningitis caused by other kinds of bacteria.

Nonmeningeal listeriosis of the central nervous system is associated with fever, nausea and vomiting, headache, and listeremia; the cerebrospinal fluid is normal. Localizing neurologic signs may develop (especially if abscess forms), or the picture may be that of an encephalitis.

Listeremia that has no identifiable source and is associated with high fever, and severe prostrating illness (typhoidal listeriosis) occurs most often in patients with cancers and immunosuppression. However, primary listeremia may also develop in patients with cirrhosis, alcoholism, pregnancy, and no discernible underlying disease.

Listerial endocarditis is generally a chronic process without singular manifestations. About half of the patients have no known predisposing cardiac disease.

Other rare forms of listeriosis include ocular infections, dermatitis, infections of serous cavities, and abscesses in various organs.

LABORATORY FINDINGS Although *L. monocytogenes* grow well on the usual culture media, etiologic diagnosis by isolation and identification may be hampered by failure of differentiation from *Corynebacterium* spp., *Erysipelothrix rhusiopathiae,* and *Streptococcus* spp. Recognition of listerial colonies in a mixed culture, as may result with vaginal or cervical specimens, is difficult and may be aided by using selective media and/or enrichment procedures.

Serodiagnosis by assay for agglutinins has not been useful because of the common finding of so-called natural antibodies. Such nonspecific reactions may reflect the known antigenic relationship between *Staphylococcus aureus* and several listerial serotypes. The humoral antibody response to listeriosis in humans is almost exclusively IgM throughout the disease, whereas staphylococci elicit IgG as well as IgM; i.e., treatment of serums with 2-mercaptoethanol may not eliminate nonspecific reactivity.

Monocytosis is not common in human listeriosis. Leukocytosis with neutrophilia, as in any acute bacterial infection, is seen in listerial meningitis, nonmeningeal infection of the central nervous system, primary listeremia, listerial endocarditis, and abscesses in hosts capable of mounting a granulocytic response. In most patients with listerial meningitis, the findings in the cerebrospinal fluid do not differ from those found in other bacterial meningitides, but occasional patients may have a relative increase in mononuclear cells.

DIFFERENTIAL DIAGNOSIS Abortion, premature delivery, stillbirth, and neonatal death are more often due to causes other than listeriosis: Rh incompatibility, syphilis, or toxoplasmosis.

In patients with leptomeningitis, conjunctivitis, endocarditis, bacteremia, or polyserositis, reports of isolation of "diphtheroids" or "nonpathogens" must always be challenged. A statement that *L. monocytogenes* has been excluded should be required.

TREATMENT *Listeria monocytogenes* are susceptible to several antimicrobials in vitro, including penicillin G, ampicillin, erythromycin, rifampin, streptomycin, gentamicin, co-trimoxazole, tobramycin, and the tetracyclines. Tolerance, i.e., inhibition at low concentrations with much higher concentrations needed for killing, is characteristic with the penicillins, erythromycin, rifampin, co-trimoxazole, and streptomycin. Accordingly, combination therapy is necessary for maximally listericidal therapy, e.g., penicillin G [150 to 200 mg (240,000 to 320,000 units) per kilogram of body weight per day, intravenously, as six equal portions every 4 h] plus tobramycin (5 to 6 mg per kilogram of body weight per day, intravenously, as three equal portions every 8 h). Ampicillin and gentamicin (same dosages) may be substituted but offer no advantage. Such treatment is appropriate for listeriosis of the newborn (2 weeks), listeremia in pregnancy (2 weeks), primary listeremia (4 weeks), listerial endocarditis (4 to 6 weeks), and any form of listeriosis outside the central nervous system in immunosuppressed patients (4 to 6 weeks).

As gentamicin and tobramycin do not enter the central nervous system reliably, high-dosage therapy with penicillin G [200 to 300 mg (320,000 to 480,000 units) per kilogram of body weight per day, intravenously, as six equal portions every 4 h] is the primary treatment. Ampicillin may be substituted in the same dose, but the cephalosporins, including the newer derivatives, should not be used. Optimal treatment of patients who are allergic to the penicillins is uncertain; candidate antimicrobials include erythromycin (40 to 50 mg per kilogram of body weight per day, intravenously, as four equal portions every 6 h); doxycycline (3 mg per kilogram of body weight, intravenously as a loading dose, and 1.5 mg per kilogram of body weight per day, intravenously, as two equal portions every 12 h for maintenance); co-trimoxazole (15 and 75 mg per kilogram of body weight, respectively, per day, intravenously, as 3 equal portions every 8 h). Treatment should be continued in full dosage by intravenous injection for 14 to 21 days after defervescence.

PROGNOSIS Prompt, vigorous antimicrobial treatment of the acute forms of listeriosis, excepting fetal listeriosis, is usually curative. On the basis of agglutinin titers, specific antibody disappears during the months following cure. However, reinfection has not been reported.

ERYSIPELOTHRIX RHUSIOPATHIAE INFECTIONS

DEFINITION Erysipeloid is the commonest and most nearly unique form of infection in humans caused by *Erysipelothrix rhusiopathiae.* Infective endocarditis and arthritis are rare forms of erysipelothricosis in human beings.

ETIOLOGY As gram-positive, microaerophilic bacilli, *E. rhusiopathiae* may be confused with nontoxinogenic *Corynebacterium* spp. and *Listeria monocytogenes.* However, *E. rhusiopathiae* is nonmotile and fails to grow on media selective for *Corynebacterium* spp. Also, unlike *L. monocytogenes, E. rhusiopathiae* only rarely causes conjunctivitis, following conjunctival inoculation, or monocytosis, after intravenous inoculation, in the rabbit. Because alpha hemolysis is commonly evident after 48 h of incubation of *E. rhusiopathiae,* confusion with streptococci may also occur. Isolates of *E. rhusiopathiae* appear to be serologically homogeneous. Although serodifferentiation from other gram-positive bacilli is possible, few laboratories are capable of definitive serodiagnosis.

EPIDEMIOLOGY AND PATHOGENESIS Primarily a saprophyte, *E. rhusiopathiae* is worldwide in distribution. Human beings are virtually always infected by traumatic dermal inoculation; erysipeloid is the usual result. The disease is almost wholly restricted to persons who in their occupations handle edible or nonedible dead animal products. If the bacilli are not successfully confined to the skin, bacteremia may result and may lead to infective endocarditis; in about two-thirds of the reported cases, there was no evidence of preexisting valvular heart disease.

The seasonal incidence of erysipeloid parallels that of swine erysipelas, being highest in summer and early fall. Yet persons who tend pigs, even pigs ill with porcine erysipelas, do not commonly develop erysipeloid.

MANIFESTATIONS Erysipeloid begins 2 to 7 days after injury, often after the initial lesion has healed. An itching, burning, painful irritation may precede and always accompanies the appearance of the maculopapular, nonvesiculated, sharply defined, raised, purplish-red zone surrounding the site of entry. There is local swelling, and when, as is usual, a finger or the hand is involved, nearby joints may become stiff and painful. Centrifugal spread from the site of inoculation is apparent in a day or so. Movement is slow, 1 to 2 cm per 24 h maximally, and more rapid proximally than distally; involvement of the terminal phalanx of a finger is rare, while spread to other fingers and the hand distal to the wrist is common. With extension, the original center subsides without desquamation or suppuration. There are usually no systemic signs or symptoms; regional lymphangitis and lymphadenitis are rare. Untreated, the disease heals within 3 weeks in most patients, although relapse has been observed.

The manifestations of erysipelothrical endocarditis may be either acute or chronic, depending on the virulence of the infecting strain and on the state of resistance of the host. Usually, there are no classic erysipeloid skin lesions to suggest the disease at the time that endocarditis is clinically evident. However, a history of recent erysipeloid may be helpful.

Erysipelothrical arthritis is not clinically characteristic but usually can be related to erysipeloid or erysipelothrical bacteremia. Isolation of *E. rhusiopathiae* from synovial fluid has not been reported.

LABORATORY FINDINGS The usual culture media are adequate for the growth of *E. rhusiopathiae*. However, differentiation from diphtheroids, listerias, and streptococci depends primarily on the clinician's alerting the laboratory to the possibility of erysipelothricosis.

In erysipeloid, *E. rhusiopathiae* are best recovered by incubating, in broth containing glucose, a full-thickness biopsy of skin removed from the advancing edge of a lesion. Culture of an aspirate obtained after injection of sterile, bacteriostat-free 0.9% NaCl solution into the periphery of a lesion is less likely to yield *E. rhusiopathiae*.

With endocarditis and arthritis, the findings are in keeping with the respective clinical syndromes and are in no way characteristic for *E. rhusiopathiae*.

DIFFERENTIAL DIAGNOSIS The appearance and location of erysipeloid, its slow and limited spread, the lack of constitutional reaction, the history of occupation and injury, all serve to identify this disease. The afflicted skin in *erysipelas* is very erythematous, and the face and scalp are affected; there are regional lymphangitis and lymphadenitis, leukocytosis, fever, and malaise. Eczematous lesions may itch, but they display vesicles and little abnormal color. The various erythemas have a different location and do not usually itch or burn; they are more apt to be chronic and nonmigratory.

TREATMENT The penicillins, the cephalosporins, erythromycin, clindamycin, the tetracyclines, and chloramphenicol inhibit *E. rhusiopathiae* in vitro at concentrations practical in therapy. Penicillin G is the agent of choice. Erysipeloid is adequately treated by injection of 1.2 million units of benzathine penicillin G. Erythromycin (15 mg/kg per day in four equal portions taken orally for 5 to 7 days) is an alternative. Cure of erysipelothrical endocarditis has been effected by the daily injection of 2 to 20 million units of penicillin per day for 4 to 6 weeks; the dose should be monitored by determination of the bactericidal activity of serum from the patient against the infecting strain. Intractable cardiac failure may oblige surgical excision of an infected valve and insertion of a prosthesis.

PROGNOSIS Penicillin therapy is highly effective in curing erysipelothrical infections. As with infective endocarditis from any cause, the prognosis is primarily a function of the severity of the valvular damage. Of cases reported since penicillin became available, about 25 percent were fatal; earlier diagnosis, and, perhaps, earlier resort to surgical excision and replacement of infected valves, may improve the outcome.

REFERENCES

BOJSEN-MOLLER J: Human listeriosis. Diagnostic, epidemiological and clinical studies. Acta Pathol Microbiol Scand B 229:13, 1972

FLEMING DW et al: Pasteurized milk as a vehicle of infection in an outbreak of listeriosis. N Engl J Med 312:404, 1985

HALLIDAY HL, HIRATA T: Perinatal listeriosis—a review of twelve patients. Am J Obstet Gynecol 133:405, 1979

HOEPRICH PD: Listeriosis, in *Infectious Diseases*, 3d ed, PD Hoeprich (ed). Philadelphia, Lippincott-Harper, 1982, chap 51

———: Erysipeloid, in *Infectious Diseases*, 3d ed, PD Hoeprich (ed). Philadelphia, Lippincott-Harper, 1982, chap 103

Listeriosis outbreak associated with Mexican-style cheese—California. Morb Mort Week Rep 34:357, 1985

NELSON E: Five hundred cases of erysipeloid. Rocky Mount Med J 52:40, 1955

ROCOURT J, GRIMONT PAD: *Listeria welshimeri* sp. nov. and *Listeria seeligeri* sp. nov. Int J Syst Bacteriol 33:866, 1983

SCHLECH WF III et al: Epidemic listeriosis—evidence for transmission by food. N Engl J Med 308:203, 1983

SEELIGER HPR: *Listeriosis*. Basel, Karger, 1961

98 ANTHRAX

DONALD KAYE / ROBERT G. PETERSDORF

DEFINITION Anthrax is a disease of wild and domesticated animals that is transmitted to humans by contact with infected animals or their products, by insect vectors which act as mechanical carriers of the etiologic organism, or, rarely, in some developing parts of the world by direct contact, such as use of common household articles. The characteristic lesion of human anthrax is a necrotic cutaneous ulcer. Occasionally, inhalation can produce a severe infection with mediastinitis and pulmonary manifestations. Rarely, ingestion can cause gastrointestinal or oropharyngeal infection. Meningitis and other forms of dissemination may result from anthrax bacteremia.

ETIOLOGY *Bacillus anthracis* is a large, encapsulated, gram-positive, nonmotile, aerobic, spore-forming microorganism that grows well in most nutrient media. On agar, it produces grayish-white colonies with comma-shaped projections ("Medusa's head"). The colonies are sticky and tend to stand up in stalagmite fashion when lifted with a loop. Microscopic examination of *B. anthracis* from artificial media or in tissue reveals parallel chains of bacilli which resemble boxcars. The pathogenicity of *B. anthracis* for laboratory animals, including mice and guinea pigs, differentiates it from *B. subtilis* and *B. cereus,* which it closely resembles. The spores are killed by boiling for 10 min but can survive for up to 20 years in soil and animal products, an important factor in the persistence and spread of the disease. Uncultivated soil is more favorable to sporulation, and dry climates also favor the persistence of organisms. The anthrax bacillus possesses a capsule of glutamyl polypeptide, which interferes with phagocytosis of the microorganism. In addition, it contains an anticomplementary substance and elaborates a toxin which is probably of importance in determining virulence.

EPIDEMIOLOGY Anthrax is worldwide; repeated outbreaks have occurred in southern Europe, notably Greece and Turkey, the Middle East (particularly Iran), Africa (Zimbabwe and Gambia), Australia and New Zealand, and on both American continents. From 1975 to 1976, under 2000 cases of anthrax were reported to the World Health Organization. This is very likely an underestimate. In the United States, immunization programs for high-risk occupational groups, better industrial protective measures, and decreased contact with contaminated animal products have markedly reduced the number of reported cases of anthrax. No cases were reported in 1981 to 1983, and one case was reported in 1984.

Cattle, horses, sheep, goats, and swine are most commonly infected. There have been outbreaks of anthrax among animals in the United States, centering mostly in South Dakota, Nebraska, Arkansas, Mississippi, Louisiana, Texas, Washington, and California. The disease tends to occur in animals in late summer and early fall. An outbreak of anthrax, acquired from goatskin bongo drum heads and goatskin rugs, occurred in Haiti and was imported into the United States.

The disease in humans is acquired by butchering, skinning, or dissecting infected carcasses or by handling contaminated hides, wool, hair, or other materials. The majority of cases of human anthrax involve workers handling imported and unprocessed wool, hair, or hides, or bone meal used as fertilizer. Gardeners have been infected accidentally by inhaling bone meal fertilizers, and inhalation anthrax has been reported following exposure to exhausts of a tanning plant. The disease usually follows inoculation of bacilli or spores into the skin, often through a wound or abrasion. Intestinal infection has followed ingestion of contaminated meat. In Africa outbreaks of anthrax have been attributed to flies which carry the organism from infected carcasses or to biting flies which may carry the bacillus in their blood. This may account for the absence of lesions on the fingers and hands. In Gambia, under crowded conditions, human-to-human transmission has been implicated through the use of common palm-brushes (loofahs).

PATHOGENESIS Germination of spores occurs within hours of inoculation. The spores germinate, form capsules, and release toxin that causes brawny edema and necrosis. The malignant pustule which follows cutaneous inoculation of anthrax organisms is characterized by vesiculation, neutrophilic infiltration, gelatinous edema, and necrosis. Suppuration is rare in the absence of secondary pyogenic infection; hence, the term *malignant pustule,* which is often used to describe cutaneous anthrax, is inappropriate. Spread of the bacilli to the regional lymph nodes may be followed by systemic dissemination. Examination of tissues from fatal human cases reveals masses of the bacteria in blood vessels, lymph nodes, and the parenchyma of various organs. There is scanty or no cellular exudation at these foci, but hemorrhage and edema are widespread.

In inhalation anthrax the spores are phagocytosed by alveolar macrophages, and germination occurs in mediastinal lymph nodes. There is necrosis of tissue in the nodes and mediastinum resulting in hemorrhagic mediastinitis with associated bacteremia. Respiratory failure may occur either from a hemorrhagic pneumonia secondary to bacteremia or from a direct effect of *B. anthracis* toxin on pulmonary capillaries.

Meningeal anthrax results from bacteremia following a primary cutaneous lesion or from inhalational infection.

Intestinal anthrax occurs by ingestion of infected, poorly cooked animal meat. Spores enter the submucosa and regional lymph nodes where they germinate and cause hemorrhage and necrosis with associated bacteremia. In oropharyngeal anthrax the bacilli damage cervical or submandibular lymph nodes.

B. anthracis toxin has three components: edema factor, lethal factor, and protective antigen. Toxin is important in the pathogenesis of some of the manifestations of the disease. Its persistence may explain delayed response after onset of antimicrobial therapy. Immunity to subsequent infection seems to follow anthrax.

MANIFESTATIONS In the past in the United States, 95 percent of cases were cutaneous and 5 percent were acquired from inhalation. Meningitis occurred in less than 5 percent of cases. Gastrointestinal and oropharyngeal forms of anthrax were extremely rare.

Cutaneous anthrax Human anthrax usually begins on an exposed body surface (such as the upper extremity or face) as a painless pruritic, erythematous papule which vesiculates and ulcerates to form a black eschar. Tiny satellite vesicles are frequent. The ulcer may be surrounded by extensive edematous swelling which is nontender, nonpitting, and so characteristic of anthrax that it is a valuable diagnostic sign. After about 5 days the ulcer begins to subside, but edema may persist for several weeks. Mild tenderness and enlargement of regional lymph nodes are frequently present. Constitutional symptoms are often absent despite extensive local changes, but there may be mild fever, headache, and malaise. Conditions that may resemble cutaneous anthrax are staphylococcal skin infections, plague, tularemia, and orf.

In 10 to 20 percent of untreated cutaneous anthrax, the infection spreads from the hemorrhagic regional lymph nodes to the bloodstream. There is high fever, prostration, and a rapidly fatal course. These cases usually involve the meninges.

Inhalation anthrax Also termed *woolsorter's disease,* this is a highly fatal disseminated infection characterized by cyanosis, dyspnea, mediastinitis, and hemoptysis and is probably dependent on the entry of spores into the lungs. The illness is biphasic and initially consists of an insidious onset of mild fever, malaise, fatigue, myalgia, nonproductive cough, and a feeling of substernal oppression. This phase lasts several days, and there may be some improvement before the acute onset of a second stage consisting of dyspnea, cyanosis, stridor, and shock. Pleural effusions and mediastinal widening on chest x-ray are characteristic. Most patients die within 24 h despite treatment. It has been postulated that underlying lung disease, such as sarcoid, may predispose to inhalation anthrax.

Meningeal anthrax This is an acute fulminant infection. The cerebrospinal fluid is hemorrhagic, purulent, or both.

Intestinal anthrax There is fever, nausea, vomiting, and abdominal pain. Hematemesis, bloody diarrhea, and ascites may develop. Clinically, it may resemble an acute abdomen. The disease usually has been fatal, although a few patients have been cured by resection of the involved bowel.

Oropharyngeal anthrax Patients have fever and cervical or submandibular lymphadenopathy with edema.

LABORATORY DIAGNOSIS The fluid from the cutaneous lesion frequently contains many bacilli, demonstrable by Gram's stain and culture, but when patients have been given topical or systemic antibiotics, cultures and smears may be unreliable. Blood cultures are usually positive in disseminated anthrax, but only 10 percent of patients with cutaneous ulcers have bacteremia. The blood leukocyte count is normal in mild cases, but there is polymorphonuclear leukocytosis in most patients with disseminated disease. Patients with meningeal involvement show bloody spinal fluid, in which the organisms are easily found by direct examination or culture.

A 24-h culture on blood agar shows characteristic colonies. Inoculation of a suspected colony of *B. anthracis* will kill guinea pigs in 24 h, and the organism can be recovered from the left ventricle.

The indirect microhemagglutination test (IMH test) has detected antibodies in 93 percent of patients, 98 percent of vaccinees, and none of the controls. It is useful in confirming the diagnosis.

TREATMENT For cutaneous anthrax, 600,000 units of aqueous procaine penicillin should be given every 6 h until the local edema subsides. Then oral therapy can be continued for a total of 7 to 10 days. In penicillin-allergic patients, erythromycin or tetracycline may be used in doses of 500 mg every 6 h for 7 to 10 days. The eschar goes through its natural evolution in spite of treatment, and lymph node enlargement may persist for several days. *Bacillus anthracis* cannot be recovered from the skin lesion after 24 to 48 h of penicillin. For inhalation anthrax, 20 million units of penicillin should be given intravenously, but it is doubtful that the drug acts sufficiently rapidly to reverse the process. In meningeal anthrax, similar large doses of penicillin plus 300 to 400 mg hydrocortisone should be given. It is not clear whether the addition of steroids affects the outcome favorably.

PREVENTION The potential for infection of personnel in industrial plants where contaminated animal products are handled exists. An outbreak of inhalation anthrax with a high mortality rate was reported in a goat hair processing mill in the United States in the late 1950s. Sterilization of all raw wool, mohair, etc., would probably remove the hazard but has had only limited use. A vaccine prepared from the "protective" antigen of *B. anthracis* is available and is effective in reducing the incidence of infection in an exposed population. Spore vaccines of various types are used with good effect in domestic animals in endemic areas but are not suitable for use in humans. Animals dying with anthrax should be disposed of safely.

PROGNOSIS The cutaneous disease was fatal in 20 percent of cases before antimicrobial drugs were available. The mortality rate of cutaneous anthrax now is less than 1 percent with proper treatment. In the rare cases of inhalational, meningeal, and intestinal anthrax the prognosis is poor despite antibiotic therapy.

REFERENCES

BRACHMAN PS: Inhalation anthrax. Ann NY Acad Sci 353:83, 1980

———: Anthrax, in *Bacterial Infections of Humans: Epidemiology and Control*, A Evans, H Feldman (eds). New York, Ms Hilary Evans Publishing, 1982, pp 63–74

FEELEY JC, PATTON CM: *Bacillus*, in *Manual of Clinical Microbiology, 3*, EH Lennette et al (eds). Washington, DC, American Society of Microbiology, 1980, p 145

LAFORCE FM: Woolsorters' disease in England. Bull NY Acad Med 54:956, 1978

NALIN DR et al: Survival of a patient with intestinal anthrax. Am J Med 62:130, 1977

SIRISANTHANA T et al: Outbreak of oral-oropharyngeal anthrax: An unusual manifestation of human infection with *Bacillus anthracis*. Am J Trop Med Hyg 33:144, 1984

99 TETANUS

HARRY N. BEATY

DEFINITION Tetanus is an acute, often fatal, disease caused by an exotoxin produced in a wound by *Clostridium tetani*. It is characterized by generalized increased rigidity and convulsive spasms of skeletal muscles.

ETIOLOGY *C. tetani* is a strictly anaerobic, gram-positive rod which is motile and readily forms a single, spheric, terminal endospore that swells the end of the organism and produces a characteristic "clubbed" appearance.

The organism grows well on blood agar at 37°C under anaerobic conditions. *C. tetani* is relatively inert biochemically, with no proteolytic activity and no fermentation of carbohydrates. Vegetative forms are no more resistant to adverse conditions than other bacteria are, but spores are highly resistant to antiseptics and moderately resistant to heat.

Ten types of *C. tetani* can be distinguished on the basis of flagellar antigens. All these types have one or more common somatic antigens and are capable of producing at least two exotoxins. One, a hemolysin, is relatively unimportant clinically. The other, tetanospasmin, generally referred to as tetanus toxin, is a protein with a molecular weight of approximately 145,000 in its dimer form and is responsible for the clinical manifestations of tetanus. The tetanospasmins produced by the various types of *C. tetani* are nearly identical antigenically. For this reason, one antitoxin is needed to neutralize the tetanus toxins produced by all strains.

EPIDEMIOLOGY The tetanus bacillus is found in the superficial layers of soil and as a saprophyte in the intestinal tract of humans and certain animals. It is most frequently encountered in densely populated regions in hot, damp climates and in soil rich in organic matter. Urbanization, mechanization of agriculture, and socioeconomic factors such as poverty and lack of availability of health services also significantly influence the occurrence of this disease.

Worldwide, there are probably 300,000 to 500,000 cases of tetanus each year, with a mortality rate of roughly 45 percent. There is no racial predilection, but the male-to-female ratio is 2.5:1, even among neonates, in which the exposure is presumably equal. In the United States, there are about 100 reported cases each year, which occur almost exclusively in nonimmunized or only partially immunized individuals. The incidence of disease is high among nonwhites in the southern states, and in the last decade, about two-thirds of patients have been 50 or older. However, spores of *C. tetani* are distributed widely throughout urban and rural areas of the entire country, and are found commonly on clothing and in house dust, placing the nonimmune individual at risk after relatively minor household injuries. Tetanus has been known to follow surgery and innocuous procedures such as skin testing or intramuscular injection of medication. The disease is inordinately common in narcotic addicts, perhaps because heroin is frequently "cut" with quinine, which drastically lowers the redox potential at the site of injection and favors the growth of *C. tetani*.

Tetanus neonatorum is a major cause of infant mortality in developing countries and is directly related to poor obstetric conditions and lack of maternal immunization programs.

PATHOGENESIS AND PATHOLOGY *C. tetani* is a noninvasive organism. Therefore, tetanus can occur only after spores or vegetative bacteria gain access to tissues and produce toxin locally. The usual mode of entry is through a puncture wound or laceration on an extremity. However, tetanus may follow elective surgery, burn wounds, chronic skin ulcers, otitis media, dental infection, abortion, and pregnancy. Neonatal tetanus usually follows infection of the umbilical stump. Tetanus not infrequently follows trivial injuries not seen by a physician, and in 10 to 20 percent of cases there is neither a history of injury nor a detectable lesion.

Wounds undoubtedly are contaminated frequently with spores of *C. tetani*, but tetanus develops rarely because germination of spores occurs only when the oxygen tension is much lower than that of normal tissue. Spores may survive in the body for months to years and finally produce disease at some later date after minor trauma that alters local conditions. Toxin production in wounds is favored by necrotic tissue, foreign bodies, calcium salts, and associated infections that establish low oxidation-reduction potentials. Infection caused by the tetanus bacillus remains strictly localized, but the toxin produced is transported to the central nervous system via neural pathways. Toxin entering the circulation persists for days, and probably must enter peripheral nerves to spread centrally and cause disease.

The typical clinical manifestations of tetanus are caused by the effect of tetanospasmin on the central nervous system. The toxin attacks synaptic functions to produce disinhibition of both the alpha and gamma motor systems. Generalized muscle rigidity arises from uninhibited afferent stimuli entering the central nervous system from the periphery. When the stimuli become more vigorous, spasms occur. Emotional and, to a lesser extent, visual stimuli can also cause muscle spasm. Tetanus toxin also has other effects. Peripherally it produces neuromuscular blockade similar to that of botulinum toxin, and it acts directly on muscle to produce contraction which is unaccompanied by an action potential in nerves. Certain clinical manifestations suggest that tetanus toxin also has an effect on the sympathetic nervous system.

All the effects of tetanus toxin appear to be self-limited and completely reversible, because patients who recover from the disease have no residual defect. Although there are no distinguishable pathologic changes that are characteristic of tetanus, brainstem lesions have been reported in patients dying from tetanus, and toxic myocarditis has been recognized.

CLINICAL MANIFESTATIONS The *incubation period* of tetanus, i.e., the time between injury and the appearance of unmistakable symptoms, ranges from 2 to 56 days. However, over 80 percent of patients become symptomatic within 14 days. A short incubation period indicates severe disease.

Nonspecific premonitory symptoms such as restlessness, irritability, and headache are encountered occasionally, but the commonest presenting complaints are pain and stiffness in the jaw, abdomen, or back and difficulty swallowing. As the disease progresses, stiffness gives way to rigidity, and patients often complain of difficulty in opening their mouths. In fact, trismus is the commonest manifestation of tetanus and is responsible for the familiar descriptive name of *lockjaw*. As more muscles are involved, rigidity becomes generalized, and sustained contractions of facial muscles produce a characteristic expression called *risus sardonicus*. The intensity and sequence of muscle involvement is quite variable. In a small proportion of patients, only local signs and symptoms develop in the region of the injury. In the vast majority, however, most muscles are involved to some degree, and the signs and symptoms encountered depend upon the major muscle groups affected.

Reflex spasms usually occur within 24 to 72 h of the first symptoms, an interval referred to as the *onset time*. A short onset time is associated with a poor prognosis. Spasms are caused by sudden intensification of afferent stimuli arising in the periphery and may be both painful and dangerous. As the disease progresses, more intense and longer-lasting spasms occur with increasing frequency. Respiration may be impaired by laryngospasm or tonic contraction of respiratory muscles, which prevents adequate ventilation. Hypoxia then may lead to irreversible central nervous system damage and death.

Patients are almost invariably conscious and mentally alert at the time of admission. Low-grade fever, profuse sweating, and tachycardia are common. Deep tendon reflexes are hyperactive, and there may be labile hypertension. The physical examination should be undertaken with care, because reflex convulsive spasms may be precipitated easily. Physical examination should include evaluation of wounds and determination of the extent of rigidity; the severity of trismus; the presence or absence of dysphagia and respiratory embarrassment; the frequency, intensity, and duration of convulsive spasms; and the presence of complications such as respiratory infection.

Characteristically, the manifestations of tetanus increase in severity for about 3 days and then remain stable for the next 5 to 7 days. After about 10 days, spasms begin to occur less frequently, and by the end of 2 weeks, they disappear altogether. Although residual stiffness may persist for a prolonged period, most survivors recover completely in 4 weeks.

Tetanus neonatorum is a severe form of the disease that usually occurs within 10 days of birth. Early signs include difficulty sucking, irritability, and excessive crying, associated with peculiar grimacing. Intense rigidity characteristically produces opisthotonus, flexion of the arms, clenched fists, extension of the legs, and plantar flexion of the toes. Typical spasms occur with minimal stimuli.

Complications Complications contribute significantly to the morbidity and mortality of tetanus. Some result from overly vigorous therapy and prolonged bed rest, while others are attributed to the action of tetanus toxin. Inadequate ventilation is a constant threat. In addition to hypoxia, atelectasis is a common consequence of impaired respiration. Difficulty in swallowing leads to aspiration of secretions, which may also cause atelectasis and initiate pulmonary infection. Thrombophlebitis is occasionally encountered, but bland venous thrombosis is more common and may lead to pulmonary embolization. Cardiovascular complications thought to be due to hyperactivity of the sympathetic nervous system include vasomotor instability, hypertension, tachycardia, arrhythmias, and severe vasoconstriction. Pulmonary edema and hypotension may occur as a consequence of myocarditis. High fever usually signifies secondary infection. Pneumonia is a common late complication of tetanus; other sites of secondary infections include the original wound, decubitus ulcers, and the urinary tract of patients with indwelling bladder catheters. Fractures of midthoracic vertebrae are probably due to severe spasms and are particularly common among children and adolescents. Gastrointestinal complications include acute peptic ulceration, paralytic ileus, and constipation. Hemolysis is seen in a small proportion of patients.

Pneumonia is a major cause of death. Other autopsy findings include congestion of viscera and, occasionally, intracranial hemorrhage or thrombosis. In about 20 percent of cases, no obvious pathology is identified, and death is attributed to the direct effects of tetanus toxin.

LABORATORY FINDINGS There are no laboratory findings characteristic of tetanus. Granulocytosis is seen in about one-third of patients, but anemia is rare. Blood chemistries are almost always normal initially, but various fluid and electrolyte disturbances may arise in the course of the disease. The electrocardiogram usually shows only sinus tachycardia, but occasionally T-wave inversion is seen. Roentgenograms are not helpful except in the evaluation of complications.

The diagnosis of tetanus is entirely clinical and does not depend upon bacteriologic confirmation. *C. tetani* is recovered from the wound in only 30 percent of cases, and not infrequently it is isolated from patients who do not have tetanus. Laboratory identification depends on cultural and morphologic characteristics and demonstration of toxin production in mice.

DIFFERENTIAL DIAGNOSIS No disease resembles fully developed tetanus. However, strychnine poisoning and dystonic reactions due to phenothiazines and metoclopramide produce a syndrome that has been referred to as pseudotetanus. These rare reactions usually follow brief exposure to drugs and subside 24 to 48 h after their administration is discontinued. Early in the course of true tetanus, exclusion of local causes of jaw pain may be difficult, and the combination of neck stiffness and fever may suggest meningitis. However, this can be excluded by lumbar puncture, because in tetanus the spinal fluid is normal. When there is doubt about the diagnosis, clinical observation usually settles the issue within a matter of hours.

TREATMENT In order to formulate a rational plan of therapy, it is useful to assess the severity of tetanus. Because of the poor prognosis of tetanus in older individuals, the disease should be considered moderate to severe in all patients over 50.

General measures Patients must be hospitalized. After initial evaluation, necrotic tissue and foreign bodies should be removed from the infected wound, and abscesses should be drained. Patients should be placed in a quiet room and observed closely for development of complications or unexpected changes in the course of the disease. While it is a good general principle to disturb patients as little as possible, vital signs must be monitored and aspiration must be averted by positioning the patient carefully and by aspirating nasopharyngeal secretions frequently. Care must be taken to prevent development of decubitus ulcers or contractures, but many routine nursing procedures should be omitted because they may precipitate uncomfortable or dangerous spasms. Initially, nutrition is not a major consideration, and fluid and electrolyte balance should be maintained over the first several days by administration of appropriate solutions intravenously, accompanied by careful recording of intake and output. Patients with severe tetanus are in an intense catabolic state, and may have tremendous fluid losses. Early consideration should be given to intravenous hyperalimentation as a means of meeting the nutritional requirements of these patients.

Antiserum Antiserum does not neutralize tetanus toxin fixed in the central nervous system and does little to ameliorate symptoms already present at the time of admission. However, the case/fatality ratio in mild to moderately severe disease is reduced significantly when antiserum is administered early. Human tetanus immune globulin (TIG) is generally available in the United States, and is far superior to equine antiserum. Because its half-life is about 25 days, only one dose of 3000 to 10,000 units intramuscularly is recommended, even though as little as 500 units may be equally effective. Local infiltration at the site of the wound is of no proven value. Hypersensitivity reactions do not occur with TIG, obviating the need for pretreatment testing.

If human antitoxin is not available, a single dose of equine antiserum should be given after the patient has been tested for hypersensitivity to horse serum. Although the dosage of heterologous antitoxin often recommended for adults is 100,000 to 200,000 units, 10,000 units is probably optimal. Anaphylaxis can occur despite negative sensitivity tests, and patients must be observed carefully to institute treatment at the first sign of an anaphylactic reaction. Up to 25 percent of patients develop delayed reactions including serum sickness after equine antitoxin. Occasionally, serious neurologic complications accompany other manifestations of serum sickness.

Active immunization of patients with tetanus is necessary, because the disease does not confer natural immunity. However, there is no need to begin primary immunization until the patient has recovered.

Management of muscle spasms Muscle relaxation is the key to therapy, but mild sedation is desirable also because it reduces the effect of sensory stimuli. Ideally, this should be accomplished without significantly affecting respiration. Although a variety of agents have been used in the treatment of tetanus, none has achieved universal acceptance. Among the barbiturates, phenobarbital, in adult doses of 50 to 100 mg every 3 to 6 h, produces adequate sedation and may suffice in the management of mild tetanus. When rapid action is required, amylbarbital or pentobarbital, 50 to 200 mg intravenously, may be used. Frequent and severe spasms cannot be managed with barbiturates alone, because the dosage required for control leads to unconsciousness and suppressed respiration. For this reason, muscle relaxants usually are used, either alone or in combination with barbiturates, in the treatment of moderate or severe tetanus. Electromyographic studies have shown that the phenothiazines effectively produce relaxation while sparing the sensorium and respirations. Chlorpromazine, in doses of 200 to 300 mg a day, minimizes rigidity and decreases the frequency of spasms. Diazepam, in adult doses of 40 to 120 mg a day, is very effective in the treatment of tetanus; it acts quickly, relieves rigidity, and has significant sedative effect without depressing respiration. Given alone to patients with moderately severe disease, diazepam has been shown to lower oxygen consumption from levels that are three to five times normal to near normal. In combination with other drugs, diazepam may significantly reduce mortality in nonneonates with severe tetanus. Other drugs which have been employed extensively include dantrolene, mephenesin, meprobamate, paraldehyde, and chloral hydrate.

Another approach to the management of muscle spasms involves the use of neuromuscular blocking agents such as tubocurare or pancuronium. This method can be used only where facilities and personnel are available to provide controlled mechanical ventilation for the paralyzed patient. It should be reserved for treatment of severe tetanus that is not adequately controlled by other measures. In centers with a team experienced in handling these patients, this approach, in conjunction with meticulous attention to other details of care, has produced encouraging results.

Tracheostomy Tracheostomy has an important role in the management of tetanus. It protects against suffocation due to laryngospasm, reduces the risk of aspiration, and facilitates mechanical assistance of ventilation. While most patients with mild tetanus and some with more severe disease can be managed without it, all patients should be considered candidates for tracheostomy, and the necessary equipment should be at the bedside. Where secretions are copious or respiration has been compromised, the need for tracheostomy should be recognized early, and whenever possible it should be performed electively rather than as an emergency.

Other measures Although antibiotics are frequently prescribed to treat the infected wound and prevent toxin production, there is no indication that they influence the disease favorably. If antibiotics are used, penicillin G is the drug of choice because it is highly effective against the tetanus bacillus, and its limited spectrum is less likely to predispose patients to superinfections. Appropriate cultures to detect complicating infections should be obtained periodically throughout the course of the disease, and specific antibiotics prescribed when indicated. Adrenocortical steroids have been used empirically in the treatment of tetanus, but there is limited clinical evidence to support their effectiveness. Likewise, beneficial results have been claimed for hyperbaric oxygen, but insufficient information is available to evaluate its potential. Adrenergic blockade may control some of the cardiovascular manifestations of tetanus.

PREVENTION *C. tetani* is so ubiquitous in nature that the only hope for prevention of tetanus lies in massive immunization programs. Effective active immunization is possible, and if applied universally, according to recommendations, tetanus could be virtually eliminated. Even tetanus neonatorum could be prevented, because infants are protected by antibody that passes the placental barrier. Two types of tetanus toxoids are available for immunization, a fluid and an adsorbed form. The adsorbed toxoid is preferred because it produces higher antitoxin titers and longer-lasting immunity. Immunization failures are exceedingly rare.

According to current recommendations, children 2 months to 6 years of age should be immunized with diphtheria and tetanus toxoids and pertussis vaccine (DPT). Ideally, the first dose should be administered within 2 or 3 months of birth, the second and third should follow at 4- to 8-week intervals, and the fourth dose should be given 1 year after the third. Schoolchildren and adults should be immunized with three doses of adult-type tetanus and diphtheria toxoids (Td). The second dose should be given 4 to 8 weeks after the first, and the third 6 months to 1 year after the second. A booster of DPT is recommended for children 4 to 6 years of age. Thereafter and for everyone else who has received a primary immunization series, routine boosters of Td should be given every 10 years. Side effects are uncommon after the primary series, but occur more frequently in persons who have received an excessive number of booster injections. Reactions usually take the form of local swelling, erythema, lymphadenopathy, and fever, but on rare occasions more severe hypersensitivity reactions occur.

In the management of wounds, the question of prophylaxis against tetanus frequently arises. Because active immunization is so effective, a reliable immunization history can greatly simplify the problem. If a patient has received three or more doses of toxoid, antiserum need not be given, and a toxoid booster is required only if more than 5 to 10 years has elapsed since the last dose. The shorter interval pertains for all but clean, minor wounds. In all other instances, the decision must be made on an individual basis, taking into consideration the characteristics of the wound, the conditions under which it was incurred, its age, and the patient's previous active immunization

TABLE 99-1 Guidelines for tetanus prophylaxis

Active immunization	Toxoid	Antitoxin	
		Minor wound*	Other wounds
Uncertain	Yes	No	Yes
None	Yes	No	Yes
< 3 doses	Yes	No	Yes‡
≥ 3 doses	No†	No	No

* *Fresh, clean, minor wounds incurred in a setting unlikely to cause tetanus.*
† *Unless more than 10 years since last dose; 5 years if the wound is other than minor.*
‡ *Except in patients who have received at least two previous doses of toxoid and have fresh non-tetanus-prone wounds.*

against tetanus. Table 99-1 provides guidelines that may be useful in making appropriate decisions about tetanus prophylaxis. For patients who have received fewer than two doses of toxoid, the primary immunization series should be completed in the succeeding weeks to months.

When passive immunization is contemplated, TIG is preferred to horse serum because it offers longer protection and freedom from serious reactions. The recommended prophylactic dose for adults is 250 units intramuscularly, which ensures a protective level of antitoxin in the plasma (> 0.01 unit per milliliter) for as long as 4 weeks. If TIG is not available, equine antitoxin in doses of 3000 to 6000 units should be administered after careful screening for sensitivity to horse serum. When both toxoid and antitoxin are indicated, they can be given simultaneously, but separate syringes and separate injection sites should be used. The adsorbed toxin is the preparation of choice in this situation.

Prompt and adequate care of wounds is also important in preventing tetanus. They should be cleaned carefully, and foreign bodies or necrotic, devitalized tissue should be removed. Administration of tetracycline or penicillin is advocated by some to prevent multiplication of *C. tetani,* but tetanus may occur in spite of prophylactic antibiotics, and their role in the prevention of tetanus has not been established. However, severe wounds should be examined regularly and treated promptly with antimicrobials if infection develops.

PROGNOSIS The overall case fatality ratio of tetanus in the United States ranges between 40 and 60 percent. This reflects the fact that the incidence of tetanus is 8 to 10 times greater among people over 60 compared with people 10 to 20 years of age, and the mortality rate is 25 to 50 times greater in the elderly. Neonatal tetanus is uncommon in this country but is fatal in more than 60 percent of cases. The shorter the incubation period and onset time, the poorer the prognosis. Three-fourths of the deaths occur within the first week, primarily from pulmonary infection, aspiration, or pulmonary embolization. Survivors recover completely, but remain susceptible to the disease unless actively immunized with tetanus toxoid.

REFERENCES

BRAND DA et al: Adequacy of antitetanus prophylaxis in six hospital emergency rooms. N Engl J Med 309:636, 1983

CENTERS FOR DISEASE CONTROL: Diphtheria, tetanus, and pertussis: Guidelines for vaccine prophylaxis and preventive measures. Morb Mort Week Rep 30:392, 1981

NEWTON-JOHN HF: Tetanus in Victoria, 1957–1980. Med J Aust 140:194, 1984

O'KEEFE SJD et al: The metabolic response and problems with nutritional support in acute tetanus. Metabolism 33:482, 1984

SCHER KS et al: Inadequate tetanus protection among the rural elderly. South Med J 78:153, 1985

SIMONSEN O et al: Immunity against tetanus and effect of revaccination 25–30 years after primary vaccination. Lancet 2:1240, 1984

TIDYMAN M et al: Adjunctive use of dantrolene in severe tetanus. Anesth Analg 64:538, 1985

100 BOTULISM

HARRY N. BEATY

DEFINITION Botulism is an acute form of poisoning that results from ingestion of a toxin produced by *Clostridium botulinum.* The illness is characterized by progressive descending muscle paralysis and may be fatal.

EPIDEMIOLOGY The disease was first recognized over 200 years ago by German physicians. Botulism was rare in the United States before World War I. Subsequent growth of commercial and home canning led to a great increase in cases. Knowledge of the habitat of *C. botulinum,* the foods often incriminated, and the conditions necessary for the destruction of *C. botulinum* spores led to the virtual elimination of botulism from the commercial canning industry, and most cases of clinical botulism now follow consumption of improperly canned, home-preserved foods. However, the need for constant surveillance is emphasized by periodic outbreaks of botulism caused by commercially processed foods. Two of the largest outbreaks ever reported in the United States occurred in the late 1970s and contrast sharply with the usual situation in which fewer than three individuals are affected after eating home-canned or improperly handled fresh foods.

ETIOLOGY *C. botulinum* is a strictly anaerobic, spore-forming, gram-positive rod that elaborates a potent exotoxin during growth and autolysis. Morphologically and culturally similar strains are differentiated into types A through G on the basis of antigenic characteristics of the toxin each produces. In the past two decades, food-borne outbreaks of human disease have been caused most frequently by type A toxin followed in frequency by types B and E. Type F is implicated rarely, and in about 15 percent of outbreaks, the type of toxin involved is not determined. Types C and D produce disease almost exclusively in animals, including wild waterfowl, cattle, horses, and mink. Type G had been isolated from soil infrequently, but in 1977 and 1978 the organism and its toxin were recovered at autopsy from five patients in Switzerland who died suddenly and unexpectedly.

Spores of organisms producing type A or B toxins are widely distributed in soil throughout the world. Producers of type A toxin are most common in the United States, especially along the Pacific Coast and the Rocky Mountain states. Type B toxin-producers have been found more frequently in the eastern states and in Europe. Type E toxin is found in organisms from lakeshore mud, coastal sand, and sea-bottom silt in northern latitudes, which accounts for the high incidence of type E strains in fish-borne botulism. Organisms that produce the type F toxin have been found in marine sediments collected off the coast of California and Oregon and in salmon taken from the Columbia River.

Botulinus toxins are the most potent poisons known. They have been purified and identified as simple proteins. Although they differ in terms of antigenicity, molecular size, electrophoretic mobility, and amino acid content, they appear to have a similar effect on neuromuscular transmission. Biologic differences are manifested by the variable susceptibility of specific animal species to the different toxins.

Spores of *C. botulinum* can withstand 100°C for several hours. Moist heat at 120°C for 30 min will destroy spores of all types, but the toxins are considerably more heat-labile. All varieties of toxin are destroyed by boiling for 10 min, or by temperatures of 80°C for 30 min.

PATHOGENESIS For years, botulism was considered a disease that occurred almost exclusively after ingestion of preformed toxin. With the recognition that infant botulism may follow ingestion of *C. botulinum* spores which germinate, proliferate, and produce toxin in the intestinal tract, this concept has been modified. The Centers for Disease Control now report human cases of botulism in four categories: food-borne botulism, infant botulism, wound botulism, and unclassified. The latter includes a small number of adult cases each year for which no ingestion of contaminated food can be documented.

Botulinus toxins exert their major effect by blocking neuromuscular transmission in cholinergic nerve fibers. They either inhibit the release of acetylcholine or bind with it at or near its site of release within presynaptic clefts. Muscle reactivity to acetylcholine applied directly to the motor end plate is unimpaired. Central nervous system cholinergic pathways do not appear to be affected significantly in humans.

Food-borne botulism Food-borne botulism can occur when the following conditions are met: (1) a food product is contaminated with viable *C. botulinum* bacilli or spores; (2) proper conditions for germination of the spores exist; (3) time and conditions permit production of toxin before eating; (4) the food is not heated or is heated insufficiently to destroy botulinus toxin; and (5) the toxin-containing food is ingested by a susceptible host. Though a relatively anaerobic environment and temperatures above 30°C (86°F) are optimal for toxin production, strict anaerobic conditions are not necessary, and toxin production by some type E strains has been observed at temperatures as low as 3°C (38°F).

Although a variety of home-processed foods have been sources of botulism in the United States, certain foods seem to be safer than others. This may be because low pH (acidity) inhibits germination of spores and, therefore, toxin production. Commercially processed foods and improperly handled fresh foods have been implicated in outbreaks of botulism. Contaminated foods may appear putrefied, but frequently look and taste perfectly normal, regardless of toxin type.

Botulinus toxins are absorbed primarily in the stomach and upper part of the small intestine. They are large protein molecules which are absorbed after they have been reduced in size by proteolytic enzymes that do not destroy their activity. Either absorption is incomplete or toxins are inactivated partially by digestion, because the amount of toxin that appears in the bloodstream is variable, and in animals the lethal dose orally is 1000 times greater than the lethal dose intravenously. Toxin that reaches the lower part of the small intestine and colon may be absorbed slowly, which probably accounts for the delayed onset and the prolonged symptoms in many patients.

Infantile botulism It is not clear why botulism occurs in some babies who ingest *C. botulinum* spores and not in others. Age is an important factor; 90 percent of recognized cases have occurred in children under 6 months, and in certain animal models the syndrome can only be reproduced during a few days of early life. The intestinal tract of infants with botulism is colonized with *C. botulinum,* and it is assumed that the manifestations of the syndrome are slowly progressive because toxin is absorbed as it is produced rather than all at once, as is the case in food-borne botulism. Studies comparing the fecal flora of infants who have botulism with that of controls suggest that colonization of the intestine with *C. botulinum* may occur because of a delay in establishment of the normal fecal flora, the presence of organisms that promote or inhibit *C. botulinum* colonization, or a change in intestinal function that favors germination and growth of ingested spores. Diet is an important factor in the development of infant botulism. Honey has been the source of *C. botulinum* spores in a number of cases, and the current recommendation is that honey not be fed to children under 12 months. Honey has not been shown to contain botulinus toxin, so it is a safe food for older children and adults. Breast-feeding may provide relative protection against infant botulism. Supplementary iron may increase a baby's susceptibility to the fulminant form of the disease. Spores can be ingested from a variety of environmental sources, but for the majority of cases no source of *C. botulinum* is identified.

Wound botulism In contrast to food-borne botulism, wound botulism results from toxin produced by *C. botulinum* infecting a wound that is typically traumatic and contaminated with soil. The wound often seems clinically insignificant. From 1982 to 1983, six cases of this rare syndrome were reported in chronic drug abusers, five of whom abused drugs intravenously, and four of whom had superficial skin infections.

CLINICAL MANIFESTATIONS Botulism may vary from a mild illness for which patients seek no medical advice to a fulminant disease which ends in death within 24 h. Symptoms usually begin 12 to 36 h after ingestion of toxin, although the extremes of 3 h to 14 days are recorded. In general, the earlier symptoms appear, the more serious the disease.

The commonest symptoms are diplopia, blurred vision, and bulbar weakness manifested by dysphonia, dysarthria, dysphagia, and dry mouth. Symmetric paralysis of the extremities appears and may progress rapidly in a descending or ascending manner. Weakness of the respiratory muscles may occur early, but may be asymptomatic until function is moderately impaired.

Impairment of cholinergic autonomic transmission may result in constipation, urinary retention, and reduced salivation and lacrimation. Nausea and vomiting are early symptoms in half the patients, but the absence of these symptoms does not rule out botulism.

On examination, patients are usually alert, oriented, and afebrile, even with severe disease. Ocular signs include ptosis, weakness of extraocular motion, and in some patients failure of accommodation. The pupils are normal in many patients, but in some cases may react sluggishly or may be dilated and unreactive to light. Widespread neuromuscular block results in symmetric flaccid weakness of the palate, tongue, larynx, respiratory muscles, and extremities. Severe paralytic ileus and bladder distention may be present. Deep-tendon reflexes are intact in milder cases, but if significant paralysis is present they are reduced or absent. No pathologic reflexes are detectable. Findings on sensory examination are always entirely normal. Some patients have apparent gait disturbances and incoordination, but this is due to generalized weakness.

Once symptoms are noted, the disease may progress rapidly over several days, with significant changes in status occurring at hourly intervals. A period of stabilization is then followed by gradual recovery over days to months, depending on the severity of intoxication. The mechanism of recovery is not well understood. In wound botulism the patient may be febrile, but the clinical manifestations are otherwise similar. A 10- to 14-day incubation period is common from the time of infection to the onset of toxic symptoms. The clinical spectrum of infant botulism ranges from asymptomatic carriage of *C. botulinum* to a fatal illness indistinguishable from the sudden infant death syndrome. Constipation, poor feeding, and "failure to thrive," alone or in combination, may be the only signs of the illness, but these manifestations may be followed by progressive weakness of skeletal muscles, cranial nerve palsies, "floppiness" of the head, and impaired respiration.

LABORATORY FINDINGS Routine laboratory studies do not aid in diagnosing botulism. When botulism is suspected, public health authorities should be consulted to assist in special studies to confirm the diagnosis. Specimens of blood, feces, and gastric contents, as well as suspected foods and their containers, should be obtained. Because of the extreme potency of botulinus toxin, careful collection and laboratory precautions should be used. The food, stool, and serum should be studied for the presence of toxin by the mouse bioassay technique and submitted for special anaerobic culture. This battery of tests will result in an overall case recognition rate of about 85 percent. Immunofluorescent techniques are useful for the early recognition of the organisms. If wound botulism is suspected, the exudate should be submitted for culture and toxin analysis.

The spinal fluid is usually normal, although mild elevations in protein concentration may occur. Electrocardiographic abnormalities, including minor disturbances in conduction, nonspecific T-wave and ST-segment changes, and various disorders of rhythm, have been described. Electrodiagnostic studies have been shown to be of value in differentiating botulism from other paralytic diseases. The evoked motor action potential may be of low voltage but will facilitate with tetanic stimulation in a manner similar to the myasthenic syndrome (Eaton-Lambert syndrome). Electromyography may show small, short-duration, overly abundant motor units. In severe cases, denervation can occur, resulting in fibrillation activity after several weeks.

DIFFERENTIAL DIAGNOSIS Botulism must be differentiated from other conditions that produce generalized paralysis. In the Guillain-Barré syndrome, mild sensory abnormalities are nearly always present, and the spinal fluid protein is often elevated. The variant of the Guillain-Barré syndrome with ophthalmoplegia, areflexia, and ataxia (Fisher's syndrome) may prove particularly confusing. The course of myasthenia gravis is seldom so acute, and the deep tendon reflexes and pupils are normal. Some patients with botulism may show mild improvement after injection of edrophonium (Tensilon), but this improvement is not of the magnitude seen in myasthenia gravis. In tick paralysis the weakness is generally of an ascending pattern, patients may have paresthesias, and a tick is found. In diphtheria, palatal weakness is frequently the first symptom, and a history of prior pharyngitis may be obtained. Cutaneous diphtheria can be differentiated from wound botulism by appropriate cultures. In poliomyelitis the spinal fluid is abnormal and the weakness is often asymmetric and spares the ocular muscles. Vascular accidents of the brainstem can be recognized by associated neurologic signs. Belladonna poisoning presents with markedly dilated pupils and delirium. In organophosphate poisoning the pupils are markedly miotic. Shellfish poisoning, aminoglycoside antibiotic paralysis, and familial periodic paralysis might also prove confusing.

Patients with marked dry mouth may develop a picture simulating pharyngitis. Patients with gastrointestinal complaints and ileus may appear to have other forms of food poisoning or intestinal obstruction.

TREATMENT The most immediate threat to the survival of patients with botulism is respiratory failure. Patients with symptoms or known exposure should be hospitalized. Close observation is essential, and vital capacity should be measured frequently. If respiratory insufficiency develops, the patient may require assisted ventilation. Respiratory difficulties may develop rapidly; intubation or tracheostomy should be performed before onset of respiratory failure, and may be needed to manage secretions even if ventilation is otherwise adequate.

If there is no ileus, cathartics and enemas should be given to remove unabsorbed toxin from the intestine, but magnesium citrate and magnesium sulfate should not be given, as the magnesium may potentiate the neuromuscular block produced by botulinus toxin. Nasogastric suction and intravenous hyperalimentation may be needed if ileus is severe. If the bladder is atonic, a catheter will be required. Meticulous nursing care and physical therapy are essential.

As soon as the diagnosis of botulism is suspected, the patient should be tested for hypersensitivity to horse serum and treated with trivalent ABE antitoxin (Connaught), which is available from public health authorities. Type-specific antitoxin has been of benefit in several outbreaks of type E intoxication, but the value in type A and B outbreaks is less certain, particularly when paralysis has already occurred. Nonfatal hypersensitivity reactions occur in 15 to 20 percent of patients receiving the equine antitoxin, and those that react to a test dose must be desensitized prior to further treatment. Antibiotics should be reserved for specific infectious complications. In infant botulism, where multiplication of ingested organisms may be a factor, antibiotics have been ineffective in eradicating the organism, though this eventually may occur spontaneously. The value of antibiotic therapy in wound botulism has not been determined. It is essential that public health officials be notified so that toxin-containing foods can be confiscated and persons with possible exposure can be notified.

A number of reports have described the use of guanidine hydrochloride in the treatment of botulism. About two-thirds of the reported cases have shown some improvement with oral doses of 15 to 50 mg/kg per day, but the drug seems ineffective in patients with severe respiratory impairment, and probably has no effect on mortality rate. Dose-related side effects include gastrointestinal upset, paresthesias, and fasciculations. Idiosyncratic reactions include cardiac arrhythmias and blood dyscrasias.

PROGNOSIS The current mortality rate of food-borne botulism in the United States is about 10 percent, with type A outbreaks having somewhat higher mortality than types B and E. The case/fatality ratio of hospitalized cases of infant botulism is about 2 percent. Death from botulism is due to complications such as respiratory failure and pneumonia. With rapid diagnosis and aggressive supportive care, even severely involved patients can recover fully. Some patients may have mild residual weakness due to denervation atrophy. Artificial respiratory support may be required for many months, and clinical weakness and autonomic symptoms may be noted for as long as 1 year after the onset of disease.

REFERENCES

ARNON SS: Infant botulism. Annu Rev Med 31:541, 1980

DOWELL VR et al: Botulism and tetanus: Selected epidemiologic and microbiologic aspects. Rev Infect Dis 6(suppl 1):S202, 1985

HUGHES JM et al: Clinical features of types A and B food-borne botulism. Ann Intern Med 95:442, 1981

LONG SS et al: Clinical, laboratory, and environmental features of infant botulism in southeastern Pennsylvania. Pediatrics 75:935, 1985

McDONALD KL et al: Botulism and botulism-like illness in chronic drug abusers. Ann Intern Med 102:616, 1985

SELLIN LC: Botulism—an update. Milit Med 149:12, 1984

TACKET CO: Equine antitoxin use and other factors that predict outcome in type A food-borne botulism. Am J Med 76:794, 1984

101 OTHER CLOSTRIDIAL INFECTIONS

DENNIS L. KASPER

DEFINITION Bacteria of the genus *Clostridium* are gram-positive, spore-forming, obligate anaerobes which are ubiquitous in nature. There are over 60 recognized species of clostridia, many of which generally are considered saprophytic. Some of these species are pathogenic for humans and animals, particularly under conditions of lowered oxidation-reduction potential. Infections associated with these organisms range from localized wound contamination to overwhelming systemic disease. The three major disease categories for which clostridia are responsible include intestinal disorders, skin and soft tissue infections, and bacteremias. Toxins play a major role in some of these syndromes.

ETIOLOGY In humans, clostridia normally reside in the gastrointestinal tract and in the female genital tract, although they occasionally can be isolated from the skin or the mouth. As with other pathogenic anaerobic bacteria, clostridia are quite aerotolerant. Of the known species of the genus *Clostridium,* at least 30 have been isolated from human infections. Clostridia characteristically produce abundant gas in artificial media and form subterminal endospores. *C. perfringens,* the most important of the species discussed in this chapter, is encapsulated, nonmotile, and rarely sporulates in artificial media; the spores usually can be destroyed by boiling. *C. tetani* and *C. botulinum* are discussed in Chaps. 99 and 100, respectively.

Clostridia are present in the normal intestinal flora in concentrations of 10^9 to 10^{10} per gram. Of the 30 or more species which normally colonize humans, *C. ramosum* is the most common, followed by *C. perfringens.* These organisms universally are present in soil in concentrations of up to 10^4 per gram. Although clostridia morphologically are typical gram-positive organisms, many species appear to be gram-negative in clinical material or in stationary phase cultures. Therefore, Gram stains of cultures or clinical material should be interpreted with great care.

C. perfringens is the most common of the clostridial species isolated from tissue infections and bacteremias, followed in frequency by *C. novyi* and *C. septicum*. In the category of enteric infections, *C. difficile* is an important cause of antibiotic-associated colitis, and *C. perfringens* is associated with food poisoning and enteritis necroticans.

PATHOGENESIS Severe infections due to clostridial species are relatively uncommon despite the fact that clostridia can be cultured from most severe, traumatic wounds. Essential to the development of severe disease appears to be the presence of tissue necrosis and a low oxidation-reduction potential. *C. perfringens* requires about 14 amino acids and 6 or 7 additional growth factors for optimum growth. These nutrients are not found in appreciable concentrations in normal body fluids but are present in necrotic tissue. When *C. perfringens* grows in necrotic tissue, a zone of tissue damage due to the toxins elaborated by the organism allows for progressive growth. In contrast, when only a few bacteria leak into the bloodstream from a small defect in the intestinal wall, the organisms do not have the opportunity to multiply rapidly because blood as medium for growth is relatively deficient in certain amino acids and growth factors.

C. perfringens possesses 17 possible virulence factors, including 12 active tissue toxins and enterotoxins. *C. perfringens* has been divided into five types (A through E) on the basis of four major toxins: alpha, beta, epsilon, and iota. The alpha toxin is a phospholipase C (lecithinase) that splits lecithin into phosphorylcholine and diglyceride. This alpha toxin has been associated with gas gangrene and is known to be hemolytic, destroy platelets, and cause widespread capillary damage. When injected intravenously, it causes massive intravascular hemolysis and damages liver mitochondria. Alpha toxin may be important in the initiation of muscle infections which may progress to gas gangrene. Experimentally, the higher the concentration of alpha toxin present in the culture fluid, the smaller the infecting dose of *C. perfringens* required to produce infection. The protective effect of antiserum is directly proportional to its content of alpha antitoxin. Beta, epsilon, and iota toxins are also known to increase capillary permeability.

C. difficile produces a cytotoxin and an enterotoxin. The cytotoxin is potent in tissue culture assays and is a relatively sensitive and specific marker for *C. difficile*–induced enteric disease. The enterotoxin, designated toxin A, appears to be substantially more potent in biologic assays using animal models. Therefore, this toxin may play an important role in the expression of clinical disease.

CLINICAL MANIFESTATIONS **Intestinal disorders** FOOD POISONING *C. perfringens* is the second or third most common cause of food poisoning in the United States. Outbreaks generally have resulted from problems in the cooling and storage of foods cooked in bulk. The food sources primarily involved are meat, meat products, and poultry. Generally, the implicated meats have been cooked, allowed to cool, and then recooked the following day, often in a stew or hash. Strains of *C. perfringens* that contaminate meat manage to survive initial cooking. During reheating, the organisms sporulate and germinate. The disease is associated with an attack rate often as high as 70 percent. Symptoms of food poisoning from type A strains develop 8 to 24 h after ingestion of foods heavily contaminated with the organism. The primary symptoms include epigastric pain, nausea, and watery diarrhea lasting 12 to 24 h. Fever and vomiting are uncommon. Symptoms usually last less than 24 h. Diarrhea appears to be caused by a heat-labile protein enterotoxin. The enterotoxin inhibits glucose transport, damages the intestinal epithelium, and causes protein loss into the intestinal lumen, with minimal activity in the ileum.

ENTERITIS NECROTICANS Enteritis necroticans (*pigbel*), caused by type C strains of *C. perfringens,* has been the cause of necrotizing enteritis and death, occurring after a feast, in children and adults in New Guinea. A similar disease, *darmbrand,* was epidemic in Germany after World War II. It has been proposed that the highlanders of Papua, New Guinea, are susceptible to enteritis necroticans because their intestinal lumen contains low levels of digestive proteases, as a result of a low-protein diet, and the presence of a heat-stable trypsin inhibitor in sweet potato, their staple food. The low level of intestinal proteolytic activity is thought inadequate to destroy the lethal beta toxin produced by *C. perfringens* type C. Clinical features include acute abdominal pain, bloody diarrhea, vomiting, shock, and peritonitis; death occurs in 40 percent of patients. Pathologically, there is an acute ulcerative process of the bowel restricted to the small intestine. The mucosa is lifted off the submucosa, forming large denuded areas. Pseudomembranes composed of sloughed epithelium are common, and gas may dissect into the submucosa. The source of the organisms may be the patient's own intestinal flora, because cultures of ingested pig have failed to yield the organism. In clinical trials, antitoxin against the beta toxin of *C. perfringens* has been of considerable benefit in changing the course of established disease. In a large-scale trial, children immunized with *C. perfringens* beta toxoid were protected from disease.

ANTIBIOTIC-ASSOCIATED COLITIS Strains of *C. difficile,* which produce toxins detectable in the stool, have been identified as the major cause of colitis in patients with antibiotic-associated diarrhea.

In order to diagnose this type of colitis, there should be no other identifiable cause of diarrhea and the onset of symptoms must occur either during antimicrobial administration or within 4 weeks after the implicated agent has been discontinued. The drugs implicated most commonly in *C. difficile* enterocolitis are clindamycin, ampicillin, cephalosporins, and the aminoglycosides. With the possible exceptions of vancomycin and streptomycin, nearly all antibiotics have been associated with this syndrome. Antibiotic-associated diarrhea is associated with 6.6 to 26 percent of clindamycin usage, and with 5 to 9 percent of ampicillin usage.

Antimicrobial-associated diarrhea can be divided into four anatomic categories: (1) normal colonic mucosa, (2) mild erythema with some edema, (3) granular, friable, or hemorrhagic mucosa, and (4) pseudomembrane formation.

Most commonly, patients with antibiotic-associated diarrhea have a normal, minimally erythematous colonic mucosa with some edema. Occasionally colitis is more severe and characterized by granular, friable, or hemorrhagic mucosa. Stool examination in these patients may reveal large numbers of red blood cells and some leukocytes. Biopsy shows subepithelial edema with round cell infiltration of the lamina propria and focal extravasation of erythrocytes. *C. difficile* toxin has been found in 15 to 46 percent of stools from patients in these first three categories, suggesting that other factors exist in the pathogenesis of antibiotic-associated diarrhea. The most characteristic form of antibiotic-associated colitis caused by *C. difficile* is pseudomembranous colitis (PMC). More than 95 percent of patients with documented PMC have positive stool toxin assays. Close inspection of pseudomembranes reveals exudative punctate raised plaques with skip areas or edematous hyperemic mucosa. These plaques can enlarge and coalesce over large segments of intestine in the later stages of disease. The clinical spectrum of antibiotic-associated PMC is diverse. Diarrhea is the common feature and is usually watery, voluminous, and without gross blood or mucus. Most patients have abdominal cramps and tenderness, fever, and leukocytosis. However, the symptoms may vary considerably. At one end of the spectrum are patients with annoying diarrhea but no systemic signs or symptoms, while at the other end there is severe systemic toxicity, fever to 104 or 105°F, and peripheral white blood cell counts of up to 50,000 per cubic millimeter. Fecal examination frequently reveals leukocytes. Without specific therapy, the course is highly variable. Some patients have prompt resolution of symptoms with discontinuation of the drug, while others have protracted diarrhea with large stool volumes for up to 8 weeks, with resultant hypoalbuminemia and electrolyte imbalance. Severely ill patients with toxic megacolon and colonic perforation have been reported. In those who are severely ill, mortality rates may be as high as 30 percent, while most patients with minimal symptoms have resolution of disease with discontinuation of antibiotics. In the majority of patients, symptoms begin 4 to 10 days after antibiotic therapy is initiated. However, about 25 percent of patients do not have symptoms until the implicated antimicrobial agent has been discontinued, in some cases as long as 4 weeks afterward. A few cases have been reported within hours after initiation of antibiotic therapy.

Diagnostic evaluation of patients with PMC should include examination of the stool for the presence of *C. difficile* cytotoxin. Although several assays are available, the tissue culture assay is the most practical and sensitive. The assay is performed by incubating stool filtrates with tissue culture cells and monitoring for a cytopathic effect which can be neutralized by antitoxin to either *C. sordellii* (which is cross-reactive with *C. difficile,* but does not cause PMC) or C. *difficile*. Endoscopy, although useful in establishing the presence of PMC, does not establish the etiology and should be reserved for more serious disease manifestations to exclude alternative diagnoses. Isolation of *C. difficile* from stool cultures is difficult.

Skin and soft tissue infections Originally, three categories of traumatic wound infections due to clostridia were described: simple contamination, anaerobic cellulitis, and anaerobic myonecrosis. With the availability of better anaerobic bacteriologic techniques, it has been necessary to expand this classification to encompass other entities in which clostridia are isolated, usually mixed with other bacteria. These infections are frequently suppurative, and the patients may have systemic symptoms. The classification of clostridial soft tissue disease also includes diffuse spreading cellulitis and fasciitis with systemic toxic manifestations.

SIMPLE CONTAMINATION Clostridia are cultured most often from wounds in the absence of clinical signs of sepsis. As many as 30 percent of battle wounds can be contaminated by clostridia without signs of suppuration, and 16 percent of penetrating abdominal wounds yield clostridia on culture despite treatment with cephalothin and kanamycin. In cases of trauma clostridia are isolated with equal frequency from suppurative and well-healing wounds. Based on these findings, the diagnosis of clostridial infection should be clinical rather than bacteriologic.

SUPPURATIVE INFECTION IN TISSUE Clostridia are recovered frequently from various suppurative conditions in conjunction with other anaerobic and aerobic bacteria. These conditions exist with severe local inflammation, but without systemic signs induced by clostridial toxins. These infections include intraabdominal sepsis, empyema, pelvic abscess, subcutaneous abscess, frostbite with gas gangrene, infected stumps in amputees, brain abcess, prostatic abscess, perianal abscess, conjunctivitis, and infected aortic grafts.

Clostridia are isolated in approximately two-thirds of patients with intraabdominal infections resulting from intestinal perforation. *C. ramosum, C. perfringens,* and *C. bifermentans* are the most commonly isolated species. The clinical presentation does not differ from that of other patients with similar infections in which clostridia are not cultured (Chap. 102).

An interesting association has been made between malignancy and the isolation of *C. septicum* in the absence of grossly contaminated deep traumatic wounds. A major site for these malignancies is the gastrointestinal tract, particularly the colon. An association with leukemia or other solid tumors also has been noted. Some of these patients present with *C. septicum* bacteremia and have a fulminant clinical course; others develop localized suppurative infection in the abdomen or the abdominal wall without bacteremia. Presumably this infection arises from a silent perforation that leads to intraabdominal abscess formation.

Clostridia have been isolated from suppurative infections of the female genital tract, particularly tuboovarian and pelvic abscess. The major species involved here has been *C. perfringens.* Most of these are mild suppurative infections without evidence of uterine gangrene. Isolation of *C. perfringens* has been reported in as many as 20 percent of diseased gallbladders at surgery. One clinical syndrome, emphysematous cholecystitis, is caused by clostridial species at least 50 percent of the time. In this syndrome there is gas formation in the biliary radicles and the wall of the gallbladder. It is seen most often in diabetic patients. Although the mortality rate in this entity is higher than in more common forms of cholecystitis, there is no evidence of myonecrosis.

Clostridia are among the many organisms found in empyema fluids or isolated by transtracheal aspiration from patients with lung abscesses. There is no clinical clue to the presence of clostridia (as opposed to other organisms) in these infections. *C. perfringens* has been reported as a cause of empyema arising from aspiration pneumonia, pulmonary emboli, and infarction. However, the majority of cases of clostridial empyema are secondary to trauma.

LOCALIZED INFECTION OF THE SKIN AND SOFT TISSUE WITHOUT SYSTEMIC SIGNS This condition was originally referred to as anaerobic cellulitis. It is a localized infection involving the skin and soft tissue due to clostridia in pure or mixed culture. There are no systemic signs of toxicity, although the infection may invade locally, producing necrosis. These infections tend to be relatively indolent, spreading slowly to contiguous areas. Localized infections tend to be relatively free of pain and edema. Perhaps because of the lack of edema, gas that is limited to the wound and the immediately surrounding tissue may be more evident than in gas gangrene. In these localized infections gas is never found intramuscularly. Cellulitis, perirectal abscesses, and diabetic foot ulcers are typical infections from which clostridial species can be isolated. If inadequately treated, these localized infections advance by extension through subcutaneous tissue and fascial planes into muscle and may produce severe systemic disease, with signs of toxemia.

An interesting localized form of suppurative myositis has been described in heroin addicts. These patients develop local pain and tenderness in discrete areas (particularly the thigh and forearm) with the subsequent appearance of fluctuance and crepitance that require surgical drainage. The unusual aspect of these infections is that they remain localized without systemic signs of toxicity. Moreover these local areas are not necessarily sites of trauma or heroin injection. Pathologically there are subcutaneous abscesses, purulent myositis, and fasciitis, from which clostridia are recovered in pure culture; though, on occasion mixed infections involving aerobes and anaerobes are found.

SPREADING CELLULITIS This condition is best described as diffuse spreading cellulitis and fasciitis, but myonecrosis is absent, and only mild inflammation is seen in muscle. These patients present with the abrupt onset of a syndrome which progresses rapidly through the fascial planes within hours. Patients demonstrate suppuration and gas in soft tissues as well as overwhelming toxemia. This infection is rapidly fatal. On physical examination there is subcutaneous crepitance, but little localized pain. Surgery is of no proven value because there are no discretely involved tissues amenable to resection, as may be the case in myonecrosis.

However, incision of the affected area should be performed, because in rapidly advancing fasciitis, it is still the cornerstone of therapy. The initial local lesion may be quite inocuous and arises from an area involved by tumor or other infection and not from injury. The systemic toxic effects include hemolysis and injury of capillary membranes. Usually, this infection is uniformly fatal within 48 h, despite intensive therapy involving antitoxin and exchange transfusion. This syndrome is seen most commonly in patients with carcinoma, especially of the sigmoid or the cecum. Presumably, the tumor invades the fascia, and tumoral contents leak into the abdominal wall. These patients present with extreme toxicity and occasionally with total-body crepitance. The syndrome differs from necrotizing fasciitis caused by other organisms in three respects: (1) the extreme rapidity of death with clostridia, (2) the rapidity with which the organism moves through tissue, and (3) the systemic effects of the toxin typified by massive hemolysis.

CLOSTRIDIAL MYONECROSIS (GAS GANGRENE) Clostridial myonecrosis occurs when bacteria invade healthy muscle from adjacent traumatized muscle or soft tissue. The infection originates in a wound contaminated with clostridia. Despite the fact that more than 30 percent of deep wounds are infected with clostridia, the incidence of clostridial myonecrosis is quite low. These infections occur in military or civilian settings. In wartime situations, an essential factor in the genesis of gas gangrene appears to be trauma, particularly involving deep lacerated wounds of muscle. The entity of clostridial myonecrosis is relatively uncommon after simple, through-and-through bullet wounds without shattering of bone, and relatively common following shrapnel fragmentation wounds, particularly when deep muscle is involved. In civilian cases, gas gangrene can occur after trauma or surgery. The trauma need not be severe; however, the wound must be deep, necrotic, and without communication to the surface, conditions which favor anaerobic infection.

The incubation period of gas gangrene is usually short: almost always less than 3 days, and frequently less than 24 h. Eighty percent of cases are caused by *C. perfringens,* while *C. novyi, C. septicum,* and *C. histolyticum* cause most of the other cases. Typically, gas gangrene begins with the sudden appearance of pain in the region of the wound, a point that helps to differentiate it from spreading cellulitis. Once established, the pain steadily increases in severity, but remains localized to the infected area and only spreads if the infection spreads. Soon after pain develops, local swelling and edema, accompanied by a thin, often hemorrhagic exudate appear. These patients frequently develop marked tachycardia, but elevation in temperature may be only minimal. Gas frequently is not obvious at this early stage and may be absent completely. Frothiness of the wound exudate may be noted. The skin is tense, white, often marbled with blue, and cooler than normal. The symptoms rapidly progress; swelling, edema, and toxemia increase and a profuse serous discharge appears. The discharge can have a peculiar sweetish smell. Gram stain of the wound exudate shows many gram-positive rods with relatively few inflammatory cells.

The diagnosis hinges on surgery to demonstrate and define the extent of muscle involvement. At surgery, the muscle is characteristically pale, edematous, and does not contract when probed with the scalpel. As the surgeon dissects further, the muscle appears beefy red and nonviable and can progress to become black, friable, and gangrenous. It is important to establish a diagnosis early, and frozen section biopsy of muscle has been proposed as a diagnostic modality.

Patients with myonecrosis are reported to have peculiar changes in mental status. Despite hypotension, renal failure, and often body crepitance, they have a heightened awareness of their surroundings. This increased mental acuity persists until just before death, when they lapse into toxic delirium and coma. They have a complete appreciation of the gravity of the circumstances, and a most profound and distressing terror of impending death. In untreated cases, as the local wounds progress, the skin becomes bronzed; bullae appear, become filled with dark red fluid, and are accompanied by dark patches of cutaneous gangrene. Gas appears in later phases but may not be as obvious as in anaerobic cellulitis. Jaundice is rarely seen in wound gas gangrene (in contrast to uterine infections), and when it does appear, is almost invariably associated with hemoglobinuria, hemoglobinemia, and septicemia. There have been reports of cases of clostridial myonecrosis without a history of trauma. These patients have bullous lesions and crepitance of the skin; they present with a rapidly worsening course which includes myonecrosis, especially of the extremities.

CLOSTRIDIAL SEPTICEMIA Clostridial septicemia is an uncommon but almost invariably fatal illness occurring after clostridial infection primarily of the uterus, colon, or biliary tract. This entity must be differentiated from transient clostridial bacteremia which is much more common than septicemia. Bacteremia is not necessarily associated with a poor outcome. *C. perfringens* causes the majority of septicemic infections, as well as the majority of cases of transient bacteremia. *C. septicum,* which is more common in patients with malignant disease, and *C. sordellii* and *C. novyi* account for most of the remainder of cases. Clostridia account for 1 to 2.5 percent of all positive blood cultures in major hospital centers. The majority of these isolates represent transient bacteremia and only rarely true septicemia. In transient bacteremias clostridia are isolated frequently from the blood with other aerobes or anaerobes. Clinically, primary sites of infection can be identified in fewer than half the cases, with pelvic, biliary, or bowel sources the most common.

The majority of cases of clostridial septicemia originate from the female genital tract following septic abortion. In these cases when a foreign body or solution is introduced into the cervix, clostridia are introduced from the foreign object itself or from the perineum or vagina. In the uterus there may be residual necrotic fetal and placental tissues and traumatized endometrium that allow the growth of clostridia. Only a small fraction of cases of septic abortion are followed by serious septicemic illness. Approximately 1 percent of all women hospitalized after septic abortion have clostridial sepsis.

In these patients, sepsis, fever, and chills begin from 1 to 3 days after the attempted abortion. The initial signs are malaise, headache, severe myalgias, abdominal pain, nausea, vomiting, and occasionally diarrhea. Frequently a bloody or brown vaginal discharge is noted. Patients may rapidly develop oliguria, hypotension, jaundice, and hemoglobinuria. The hemolysis, which is secondary to *C. perfringens* alpha toxin, causes a characteristic bronzing of the skin. As in myonecrosis, the mental status of severely ill patients is characterized by increased alertness and apprehension. Local examination of the pelvis reveals foul cervical discharge, occasionally with gas. Frequently laceration marks around the cervix or perforation of the cervical segment are evident. If the infection involves the myometrium or has spread to the adnexa, extreme tenderness, guarding, and an adnexal mass may be found.

Laboratory studies in septicemic patients reveal an elevated white count and may show pink, hemoglobin-tinged plasma. Anemia is proportional to the degree of hemolysis, and the hematocrit may be extremely low. Platelets may be reduced, and there is often evidence of disseminated intravascular coagulation. Oliguria or anuria, increasingly refractory hypotension, and hemorrhage and bruising may develop.

Clostridia may enter the bloodstream from the gastrointestinal or biliary tract. This occurrence is associated with ulcerative lesions or obstruction of the small or large intestine, necrotic or infiltrating malignancy, bowel surgery, or various abdominal catastrophes. The patient may present with an acute febrile illness with chills and fever, but no other signs of localized infection. Intravascular hemolysis occurs in as many as half the cases. Biliary or gastrointestinal symptoms, if present, may be the only clue to the etiology. Positive blood cultures provide the definitive clue for the diagnosis in these patients.

Patients with malignant disease also can develop rapidly fatal clostridial sepsis, particularly from a gastrointestinal focus. The most common species in this setting is *C. septicum.* Characteristic signs and symptoms include fever, tachycardia, hypotension, abdominal pain or tenderness, nausea, vomiting, and preterminally, coma. The tachycardia may be out of proportion to the fever. Only about 20 to 30 percent of patients will develop hemolysis. A striking feature of this syndrome is the rapidity of death, which frequently occurs in less than 12 h.

The relatively common entity of transient bacteremia due to clostridia can arise in any hospitalized patient but is most common with a predisposing focus in the gastrointestinal tract, biliary tract, or uterus. Fever frequently resolves within 24 to 48 h without therapy. Despite the finding of clostridial bacteremia following septic abortions and the frequent isolation of clostridia from the lochia, most of these patients do not have evidence of septicemia. In one series of 60 patients with clostridial bacteremia, half of the cases could be associated with an infected site, while the other half had a totally unrelated illness, such as tuberculous pneumonia, meningitis, or benign gastroenteritis. Frequently, by the time the blood culture reports return, the patients are completely well and sometimes have been discharged. Therefore, when a blood culture report is positive for clostridia, the patient must be assessed clinically rather than simply treated for the positive blood culture alone.

DIAGNOSIS The diagnosis of clostridial disease must be based primarily on clinical findings. Because of the presence of clostridia in many wounds, their mere isolation from any site including the blood does not necessarily indicate severe disease. Smears of wound exudates, uterine scrapings, or cervical discharge may show abundant large gram-positive rods as well as other organisms. Cultures should be placed in selective media and incubated anaerobically for identification of clostridia.

The urine of patients with severe clostridial sepsis may contain protein and casts, and the patients may develop severe uremia. Profound alterations of circulating erythrocytes are seen in such severely toxemic patients. Patients have a hemolytic anemia, which develops extremely rapidly, along with hemoglobinemia, hemoglobinuria, and elevated levels of serum bilirubin. Spherocytosis, increased osmotic and mechanical red blood cell fragility, erythrophagocytosis, and methemoglobinemia have been described. Disseminated intravascular coagulation may be seen in patients with severe infection. In patients with severe septicemia, a Wright or Gram stain smear of peripheral blood or buffy coat may demonstrate clostridia.

X-ray examination sometimes provides an important clue to the diagnosis by revealing gas in muscles, subcutaneous tissue, or the uterus. However, the finding of gas is not pathognomonic for clostridial infection. Other bacteria, particularly anaerobes, mixed with aerobic organisms may produce gas.

The diagnosis of clostridial myonecrosis can be established by frozen section biopsy of muscle. The diagnosis of *C. difficile*–associated colitis is made by the identification of *C. difficile* toxin in stool.

TREATMENT The treatment of choice for clostridial infection is penicillin G, 20,000,000 units a day. In cases of penicillin sensitivity or allergy, other antibiotics should be considered, but all should be tested for in vitro efficacy because of the occasional isolation of resistant strains. Chloramphenicol, 4 g per day, usually is an effective alternative. Clostridia are generally, but not universally, susceptible in vitro to cefoxitin, carbenicillin, clindamycin, metronidazole, doxycycline, minocycline, tetracycline, and vancomycin. The actual choice of antimicrobial agent should be tailored to the specific conditions.

Simple contamination of a wound with clostridia should not be treated with antibiotics.

Localized skin and soft tissue infection can be managed by debridement rather than with systemic antibiotics. Drugs are required when the process extends into adjacent tissue, or when fever and systemic signs of sepsis are present.

Suppurative infections should be treated with antibiotics. Frequently, broad-spectrum antibiotics must be used because of mixed flora in these infections. Aminoglycosides can be used for the aerobic gram-negative bacteria and mixed infections.

The use of a polyvalent gas gangrene antitoxin is still recommended by some authorities. At present the antitoxin is not produced in the United States, and most centers have discontinued its use in management of patients with suspected gas gangrene or clostridial postabortion sepsis because of questionable efficacy and the substantial risk of hypersentitivity to horse serum.

The use of hyperbaric oxygen in the treatment of gas gangrene is also controversial. Studies in humans are not well designed to answer questions on efficacy, but several knowledgeable authors believe that hyperbaric oxygen therapy has contributed to dramatic clinical improvement. It may, however, be associated with untoward effects due to oxygen toxicity and high atmospheric pressure. Some centers without hyperbaric chambers have reported acceptable mortality rates, indicating that expert surgical and medical management and control of complications are probably the most important factors in treating gas gangrene.

Treatment of *C. difficile* enterocolitis The treatment of *C. difficile*–associated colitis requires discontinuation of the offending antimicrobial agent. In some patients symptoms will resolve over a period of 2 weeks. However, specific therapy has been beneficial. The most widely used agent in the treatment of antibiotic-associated diarrhea ascribed to *C. difficile* is oral vancomycin. Most strains of *C. difficile* are susceptible to achievable concentrations of vancomycin. This antibiotic is poorly absorbed after oral administration and high levels appear in the stool. Dosing should begin with 125 mg orally four times a day for 7 to 10 days, but the dose may be increased to 500 mg orally four times a day. It has been reported that oral metronidazole at a dose of 500 mg three times a day for 7 to 10 days is also effective. A few cases of *C. difficile* colitis have developed after oral metronidazole therapy for other infections. Because response to the two treatment regimens is comparable and metronidazole is less costly, it is reasonable to initiate treatment with metronidazole. However, if diarrhea persists, then therapy should be changed to oral vancomycin. Therapy with oral cholestyramine was initially reported to provide dramatic improvement in patients with pseudomembranous colitis (PMC). Subsequent studies have shown that cholestyramine, as well as other anionic resins, bind the cytotoxin produced by *C. difficile*. However, comparative trials in animals have shown that cholestyramine is distinctly inferior to oral vancomycin. Combination therapy with oral vancomycin and cholestyramine in refractory cases has been successful. Although not adequately tested, bacitracin may be promising in the therapy of PMC. This drug is poorly absorbed when administered orally, resulting in high levels in the colonic lumen. Toxin production in PMC persists in 5 to 10 percent of treated patients. Relapses are reported in up to 20 percent of patients, but patients usually respond to a second course of oral vancomycin.

REFERENCES

BARTLETT JG et al: Antibiotic-associated pseudomembranous colitis due to toxin-producing clostridia. N Engl J Med 298:531, 1978

———, TAYLOR NS: Antibiotic-associated colitis, in *Medical Microbiology*, CSF Easman, J Jeljaszewicz (eds). London, Academic Press, 1982, pp 1–48

BORNSTEIN DL: Clostridial myonecrosis, in *Medical Microbiology and Infectious Diseases*, A Braude (ed). Philadelphia, Saunders, 1981, Chap. 239

DORNBUSCH K et al: Antibiotic susceptibility of *Clostridium* species isolated from human infections. Scand J Infect Dis 7:127, 1975

FINEGOLD SM: *Anaerobic Bacteria in Human Disease*. New York, Academic, 1977

GORBACH SL: Other *Clostridium* species (including gas gangrene), in *Principles and Practice of Infectious Diseases*, GL Mandell et al (eds). New York, Wiley, 1985

———, THADEPALLI H: Isolation of *Clostridium* in human infections: Evaluation of 114 cases. J Infect Dis 131:S81, 1975

JENDRZEJEWSKI JW et al: Nontraumatic clostridial myonecrosis. Am J Med 65:542, 1978

KORANSKY JR et al: *Clostridium septicum* bacteremia. Am J Med 66:63, 1979

LAWRENCE G et al: Prevention of necrotizing enteritis in Papua, New Guinea by active immunization. Lancet 1:227, 1979

PRITCHARD JA, WHALLEY PJ: Abortion complicated by *Clostridium perfringens* infection. Am J Gynecol 111:484, 1971

SMITH LDS: Virulence factors of *Clostridium perfringens*. Rev Infect Dis 1:254, 1979

SUTTER VL, FINEGOLD SM: Susceptibility of anaerobic bacteria to 23 antimicrobial agents. Antimicrob Agents Chemother 10:736, 1976

TEASLEY DG et al: Prospective randomized trial of metronidazole versus vancomycin for *Clostridium difficile*–associated diarrhea and colitis. Lancet 2:1043, 1983

THADEPALLI H et al: Abdominal trauma, anaerobes, and antibiotics. Surg Gynecol Obstet 137:270, 1973

102 INFECTIONS DUE TO MIXED ANAEROBIC ORGANISMS

DENNIS L. KASPER

DEFINITIONS Anaerobic bacteria are organisms that require reduced oxygen tension for growth, failing to grow on the surface of solid media in 10% CO_2 in air. Microaerophilic bacteria can grow in 10% CO_2 in air or under anaerobic or aerobic conditions. Facultative bacteria can grow in the presence or absence of air. This chapter addresses infections caused by nonsporulating anaerobic bacteria. In general, anaerobes associated with human infections are relatively aerotolerant. They can survive for as long as 72 h in the presence of oxygen, although generally they will not multiply in this environment. Less pathogenic anaerobic bacteria, which are also part of the normal flora, die after brief contact with oxygen, even in low concentrations.

The nonsporulating anaerobic bacteria exist as normal flora on the mucosal surfaces of humans and animals. The major reservoirs of these bacteria are the mouth, gastrointestinal tract, skin, and the female genital tract. Of the oral flora, anaerobes are the predominant commensal organisms, ranging in concentrations from 10^9 per milliliter in saliva to 10^{12} in gingival scrapings. In the oral cavity the relative concentration of anaerobic to aerobic bacteria ranges from 1:1 on the surface of the tooth to 100 to 1000:1 in the gingival crevice. Anaerobic bacteria are not found in the normal intestine until the distal ileum. In the colon, the proportion of anaerobes increases significantly, as does the overall bacterial count. For example, in the colon there are 10^{11} to 10^{12} organisms per gram of stool, with a ratio of anaerobes to aerobes of approximately 1000:1. In the female genital tract there are approximately 10^9 organisms per milliliter of secretions, with a ratio of anaerobes to aerobes of approximately 10:1. Hundreds of species of anaerobic bacteria have been identified as part of the normal flora of humans. Identification of as many as 500 different anaerobic species in fecal specimens reflects the diversity of the anaerobic flora. Despite the complex array of bacteria which exist in the normal flora, relatively few species are isolated commonly from human infection.

Anaerobic infections occur when the harmonious relationship between the host and bacteria is disrupted. Any site in the body is susceptible to infection with these indigenous organisms when the mucosal barriers or skin are compromised by surgery, trauma, tumor, or situations, such as ischemia or necrosis, which reduce local tissue redox potentials. Because the sites that are colonized by anaerobic bacteria contain many species of bacteria, disruption of anatomic barriers allows penetration of many organisms, resulting frequently in mixed infections involving multiple species of these anaerobes combined with facultative or microaerophilic organisms. Such mixed infections are seen in the head and neck (chronic sinusitis, chronic otitis media, Ludwig's angina, and periodontal abscesses). Brain abscesses and subdural empyema are the most frequent anaerobic infections of the central nervous system. Anaerobes are responsible for pleuropulmonary diseases such as aspiration pneumonia, necrotizing pneumonia, abscesses, or empyema. Similarly, anaerobes play an important role in various intraabdominal infections such as peritonitis, intraabdominal abscesses, and liver abscesses. They are isolated frequently in female genital tract infections such as salpingitis, pelvic peritonitis, tuboovarian abscess, vulvovaginal abscesses, septic abortions, and endometritis. Anaerobic bacteria also are frequently found in infections of the skin, soft tissue, bones, and as a cause of bacteremia.

ETIOLOGY It is useful to consider the classification of these organisms based on Gram-staining characteristics. The major anaerobic gram-positive cocci producing disease are peptostreptococci. The principal anaerobic gram-negative bacilli are the *Bacteroides* family, which includes the *Bacteroides fragilis* group, fusobacteria, and the pigmented *Bacteroides*. The *B. fragilis* group contains the anaerobic pathogens most frequently isolated from clinical infections. Members of this group are part of the normal bowel flora. Several distinct species comprise the group, including *B. fragilis, B. thetaiotaomicron, B. distasonis, B. vulgaris,* and *B. ovatis*. Of this group *B. fragilis* is the most important clinical isolate. However, in the normal fecal flora, the frequency with which *B. fragilis* is isolated is low compared to other *Bacteroides* species. A second major group of *Bacteroides* are part of the indigenous oral flora. These are primarily pigment-producing bacteria which were previously classified under the species *B. melaninogenicus*. Current terminology of this group has changed so that several distinct species are recognized, including *B. gingivalis, B. asaccharolyticus,* as well as *B. melaninogenicus*. Fusobacteria are also isolated from clinical infections, including necrotizing pneumonia and abscesses.

Infections due to anaerobic bacteria most frequently are mixed infections with more than one organism. Infections may be due to one or several anaerobic species, or a combination of anaerobic organisms and aerobic bacteria acting synergistically. The concept of mixed infections requires a restatement of Koch's postulates since the idea of one organism, one disease, which applies to many infections, does not apply to infections caused by multiple strains of bacteria behaving in a cooperative fashion.

APPROACH TO THE PATIENT WITH ANAEROBIC BACTERIAL INFECTIONS There are seven important features to remember when approaching the patient with presumptive infection due to anaerobic bacteria. (1) Most of these organisms are harmless commensals, and very few cause disease. (2) In order for these organisms to cause infection, they must spread beyond the normal mucosal barriers. (3) Conditions favoring the propagation of these bacteria, particularly a lowered oxidation-reduction potential, are necessary. Therefore, these infections arise in sites of trauma, tissue destruction, compromised vascular supply, or as complications of preexisting infections that produce necrosis. (4) A characteristic of anaerobic infections is the complex array of infecting flora. For example, as many as 12 different types of organisms can be isolated from suppurative sites. (5) Anaerobic organisms tend to be found in abscess cavities or in necrotic tissue. The detection of an abscess in a patient which fails to yield organisms on routine culture should alert the physician that this abscess is likely to contain anaerobic bacteria. However, often smears of this "sterile pus" are teeming with bacteria on Gram stain. The malodorous nature of the pus is also an important clue to anaerobe infections. Although some facultative organisms, such as *Staphylococcus aureus,* also are capable of causing abscesses, abscesses in organs or within deeper body tissues should call to mind anaerobic infection. (6) Treatment need not be directed at all of the organisms in the infectious site. However, some species in particular require specific therapy. The best example of this principle is the need to treat *B. fragilis*. Many of these synergistic infections can be cured with antibiotics directed at some, but not all, of the organisms. The hypothesis is that antibiotic therapy, combined with drainage, disrupts the interdependent relationship among the bacteria and that species which are resistant to the antibiotic do not survive without the co-infective organisms. (7) Manifestations of disseminated intravascular coagulation are unusual in patients with infection due to these bacteria.

EPIDEMIOLOGY Difficulties in obtaining appropriate cultures, contamination of cultures by aerobic bacteria or normal flora, and the lack of readily available reliable culture techniques have made accurate incidence or prevalence data on anaerobic infections unavailable. It can be stated, however, that these infections are encountered frequently in hospitals with active surgical, trauma, and obstetric and gynecologic services. In several centers anaerobic bacteria account for approximately 8 to 10 percent of positive blood cultures. In these situations *B. fragilis* predominates. Also, anaerobes have been isolated in up to 50 percent of clinical cultures from other sites.

PATHOGENESIS Because of the specific growth requirements of these organisms and their presence as commensals on mucosal surfaces, conditions must arise which allow these organisms to penetrate mucosal barriers and enter tissue with a lowered oxidation-reduction potential. Therefore, tissue ischemia, trauma, surgery, perforated viscus, shock, or aspiration provide environments conducive to the proliferation of anaerobes. Highly fastidious anaerobes lack the enzyme superoxide dismutase (SOD) that in other organisms reduces toxic superoxide radicals, thereby lessening the potentially lethal effects of superoxide. A general correlation exists between the intracellular concentration of SOD and the oxygen tolerance of anaerobic bacteria; organisms that contain SOD have a selective advantage after exposure to aerobic environments. For example, in the case of a perforated viscus, hundreds of species of anaerobic bacteria are spilled into the peritoneal cavity, but many of these organisms are unable to survive because the highly vascularized tissue provides an adequate oxygen supply. The entry of oxygen into the environment results in selection of aerotolerant organisms.

Anaerobic bacteria produce a number of exoenzymes which are capable of enhancing their virulence. These enzymes include a heparinase elaborated by *B. fragilis* which may contribute to intravascular clotting and lead to a requirement for increased doses of heparin in patients on heparin therapy. Collagenase, produced by *B. melaninogenicus,* may enhance tissue destruction. Both *B. fragilis* and *B. melaninogenicus* possess lipopolysaccharides (endotoxins) which lack the biologic potency characteristic of endotoxins associated with aerobic gram-negative bacteria. The biologic inactivity of the endotoxin may account for the rarity of shock, disseminated intravascular coagulation, and purpura in *Bacteroides* bacteremia compared to facultative and aerobic gram-negative rod bacteremia.

B. fragilis is unique among the various pathogenic anaerobic species in its ability to form abscesses as a sole pathogen. *B. fragilis* has capsular polysaccharides which are a virulence factor, and these polysaccharides stimulate directly the formation of abscesses in experimental models of intraabdominal sepsis. Other anaerobic species require the presence of synergistic facultative species to induce abscesses.

CLINICAL MANIFESTATIONS **Anaerobic infections of the head and neck** Infections of the mouth can be divided into those infections that arise from the supragingival or subgingival dental plaque. Supragingival plaque formation begins with the adherence of gram-positive bacteria to the tooth surface. This form of plaque is influenced by salivary and dietary components, oral hygiene, and local host factors. Once established, the acquisition of pathogenic bacteria as well as an increase in the amount of plaque is responsible for the ultimate development of gingivitis. Early bacteriologic changes in the supragingival plaque initiate an inflammatory response in the gingiva. These changes include edema, swelling, and increase in gingival fluid and are responsible for the development of caries and endodontic (pulp) infections. Also, these changes are responsible partially for the subsequent pathogenic alteration in the subgingival plaque which arise from poor or inadequate oral hygiene. Subgingival plaque is associated with periodontal disease and disseminated infection arising from the oral cavity. Bacteria that colonize the subgingival area are primarily anaerobic. The black-pigmented gram-negative anaerobic bacilli belonging to the *Bacteroides* group, principally *B. gingivalis* and *B. melaninogenicus,* are the most important. Infections in this area are frequently mixed and involve both anaerobic and aerobic bacteria. After establishment of local infection either in root canals or in the periodontal area, infection may extend into the mandible, causing osteomyelitis; to the maxillary sinuses; or to local tissues in the submandibular or submental spaces, depending upon which teeth are involved. Periodontitis also may result in spreading infection that can involve adjacent bone or soft tissues. This form of infection may be due either to oral *Bacteroides* or to *Fusobacterium.*

GINGIVITIS Gingivitis may become a necrotizing infection (trench mouth, Vincent's stomatitis). The onset of disease is usually sudden and is associated with tender bleeding gums, foul breath, and a bad taste. The gingival mucosa, especially the papillae between the teeth, become ulcerated and may be covered by a gray exudate which is removable with gentle pressure. These patients may become systemically ill, developing fever, cervical lymphadenopathy, and leukocytosis. Occasionally, ulcerative gingivitis can spread to the buccal mucosa, the teeth, and the mandible or maxilla, resulting in widespread destruction of bone and soft tissue. This infection is termed *acute necrotizing ulcerative mucositis* (cancrum oris, noma). This infection destroys tissue rapidly, causing the teeth to fall out and large areas of bone, even the whole mandible, to be sloughed. A strong putrid odor frequently is present, although the lesions are not painful. The gangrenous lesions eventually heal, leaving large disfiguring defects. This infection is seen most commonly following a debilitating illness, or in severely malnourished children in underdeveloped areas of the world. It has been known to complicate leukemia or to develop in individuals with a genetic deficiency of catalase.

ACUTE NECROTIZING INFECTIONS OF THE PHARYNX These occur in association with ulcerative gingivitis, although they also may occur alone. The major complaints are an extremely sore throat, foul breath, and a bad taste in the mouth, accompanied by a sensation of choking and fever. Examination of the pharynx demonstrates that the tonsillar pillars are swollen, red, and ulcerated and covered with a grayish membrane that peels easily. Lymphadenopathy and leukocytosis are common. The disease may last for only a few days or may persist for weeks if not treated. Lesions begin unilaterally but may spread to the other side of the pharynx or the larynx. Aspiration of the infected material by the patient can result in lung abscesses. Soft tissue infection of the oral-facial area may or may not be odontogenic in origin. *Ludwig's angina,* a periodontal infection usually arising from the third molar, may produce submandibular cellulitis that results in marked local swelling of tissues with pain, trismus, and superior and posterior displacement of the tongue. Submandibular swelling of the neck develops, which can result in the inability to swallow and respiratory obstruction. In some cases tracheostomy may be life-saving. Both mixed anaerobic and aerobic infection originating from the oral flora have been implicated in the etiology of this syndrome.

FASCIAL INFECTIONS These arise from the spread of organisms originating in the upper airways to potential spaces formed by the fascial planes of the head and neck. Although there are few well-documented reports on the microbiology of these syndromes, anaerobes from the oral flora have been implicated in many cases studied with adequate bacteriology. *Staphylococcus aureus* and *Streptococcus pyogenes* have been implicated in space infections related to overlying skin infections, such as boils or impetigo, whereas anaerobes are associated with space infections arising from diseases of the mucous membranes, dental manipulations, or occurring spontaneously.

SINUSITIS AND OTITIS While there are a few reports of the role of anaerobic bacteria in acute sinusitis, it is likely that these reports underestimate the frequency with which anaerobes are involved in these infections because of improper collection of specimens. Material for culture is obtained by aspiration at the inferior nasal meatus without decontamination of the nasal mucous membranes. In contrast, no conflict exists concerning the importance of anaerobes in chronic sinusitis. Anaerobic bacteria were found in 52 percent of specimens collected during external frontoethmoidotomy or radical antrotomy via the canine fossa. These methods avoid nasal mucosal bacterial contamination. Similarly, anaerobic bacteria are much more easily implicated in chronic suppurative otitis media than in acute otitis media. Purulent exudate from chronically draining ears has been found to contain anaerobes in up to 50 percent of patients. A variety of anaerobes have been isolated from these chronic infections, particularly *Bacteroides* species. In contrast to other infections of the head and neck, *B. fragilis* has been isolated from up to 28 percent of patients with chronic otitis media.

COMPLICATIONS OF ANAEROBIC HEAD AND NECK INFECTIONS Contiguous spread of these infections craniad may result in osteomyelitis of the skull or mandible, or in intracranial infections such as brain abscesses or subdural empyema. Caudad spread can produce mediastinitis or pleuropulmonary infections. Hematogenous complications also may result from anaerobic infections of the head and neck. Bacteremia, which can occasionally be polymicrobial, has been reported and can lead to endocarditis or other distant infections. When infections spread to produce suppurative thrombophlebitis of the internal jugular vein, a destructive syndrome with prolonged fever, bacteremia, septic emboli to both the lung and brain, and multiple metastatic foci of suppurative infection may develop. This syndrome has been reported with septicemia from species of *Fusobacterium* following exudative pharyngitis. This entity (Lameer's postanginal septicemia) is uncommon in this era of antimicrobial agents.

Central nervous system infections Of the many infections of the central nervous system, brain abscesses most frequently are associated with anaerobic bacteria. If optimal bacteriologic techniques are employed, as many as 85 percent of brain abscesses yield anaerobic bacteria. The anaerobic bacteria found most often in these infections are anaerobic gram-positive cocci, followed in frequency by fusobacteria and *Bacteroides* species. Frequently, facultative or microaerophilic streptococci and coliforms are involved in brain abscesses as mixed infections. Brain abscesses arise from either direct extension of suppurative infection involving the sinuses, mastoids, or middle ear, or from hematogenous dissemination from infection elsewhere, particularly the lungs. Brain abscess is discussed in greater detail in Chap. 346.

Pleuropulmonary infections Anaerobic pleuropulmonary infections result from the aspiration of oropharyngeal contents, which is associated commonly with an altered state of consciousness or absent gag reflex. There are four clinical syndromes associated with anaerobic pleuropulmonary infection produced by aspiration: simple aspiration pneumonia, necrotizing pneumonia, lung abscess, and empyema.

ANAEROBIC ASPIRATION PNEUMONITIS Anaerobic aspiration pneumonitis must be distinguished from two other types of aspiration pneumonitis, neither of which are bacterial diseases. One aspiration syndrome results from aspiration of solids, usually food. Obstruction of major airways with resulting atelectasis is typical. Moderate nonspecific inflammation occurs. Therapy consists of removal of the foreign body.

A second aspiration syndrome is more easily confused with bacterial aspiration. This is the so-called Mendelson's syndrome, resulting from regurgitation of stomach contents and aspiration of chemical material, usually gastric juices. Pulmonary inflammation including destruction of alveolar lining with transudation of fluid into the alveolar space occurs with remarkable rapidity. Typically this syndrome develops within hours often following anesthesia when the gag reflex is depressed. The patient becomes tachypneic, hypoxic, and febrile. The leukocyte count may rise, and the chest x-ray may evolve suddenly from normal to a complete whiteout bilaterally within 8 to 24 h. Minimal sputum production occurs. The pulmonary signs and symptoms can resolve quickly with symptomatic therapy or result in respiratory failure with subsequent development of bacterial superinfection over a period of days. Antibiotic therapy is not indicated unless bacterial infection supervenes. The signs of bacterial infection include sputum, persistent fever, leukocytosis, and clinical evidence of sepsis.

In contrast to these syndromes, bacterial aspiration pneumonia develops more slowly. It is seen in patients who are hospitalized and have a depressed gag reflex, elderly patients, or those with transient impaired consciousness such as can result from seizures or alcoholic blackouts. Patients who enter the hospital with this syndrome typically have been ill for several days, generally complain of low-grade fever, malaise, and sputum production. Usually the history reveals a predisposition for aspiration, such as alcohol overdose or residence in a nursing home. Sputum characteristically is not malodorous unless the process has been present for at least a week. Mixed bacterial flora with many polymorphonuclear leukocytes are present on Gram stain; reliable cultures can be obtained only by avoiding contamination with normal oral flora, i.e., by transtracheal aspiration. Chest x-rays show consolidation in dependent pulmonary segments. These dependent areas are the basilar segments of the lower lobes if the patient aspirated while upright or sitting, as is noted commonly in nursing home patients, or in the posterior segment of the upper lobe, usually on the right side, or the superior segment of the lower lobe if aspiration has occurred in the supine position. Organisms isolated reflect the pharyngeal flora; *B. melaninogenicus, Fusobacterium* species, and anaerobic cocci are the most frequent isolates. The patient who aspirates in a hospital setting also may have mixed infection involving facultative bacteria, including enteric gram-negative rods.

NECROTIZING PNEUMONITIS This is a form of anaerobic pneumonitis characterized by numerous but small abscesses which spread to involve several pulmonary segments. The process can be indolent or fulminating. This syndrome is observed less commonly than either aspiration pneumonia or lung abscess, and includes features of both types of infection.

ANAEROBIC LUNG ABSCESSES These result from subacute anaerobic pulmonary infection. The clinical syndrome typically involves a history of constitutional symptoms including malaise, weight loss, fever, chills, and foul-smelling sputum which may occur over a period of weeks. Patients who develop lung abscesses characteristically have dental infection and periodontitis, but there are reports of lung abscesses in patients who are edentulous. Abscess cavities may be single or multiple, and generally occur in dependent pulmonary segments. Anaerobic abscesses must be distinguished from tuberculosis, neoplasia, and other causes of lung abscess, despite the fact that the clinical syndrome is usually typical. Oral anaerobes predominate, although *B. fragilis* is isolated in up to 10 percent of cases. *Staph. aureus* may be found as well. Although in vitro resistance by *B. fragilis* to penicillin is common, this antibiotic generally is successful in treatment when combined with vigorous pulmonary toilet, perhaps because of the synergistic nature of the infection. Bronchoscopy is indicated only to rule out the presence of airway obstruction but should be delayed until the antimicrobial has begun to affect the disease process so that it does not spread the infection. Bronchoscopy has no role in enhancing drainage. Surgery is almost never indicated and can be hazardous because of spillage of abscess contents into the lungs.

Empyema Empyema is a manifestation of long-standing anaerobic pulmonary infection. The clinical presentation resembles other anaerobic pulmonary infections including the presence of foul-smelling sputum. Patients may complain of pleuritic chest pain and marked chest wall tenderness.

Empyema may be masked by overlying pneumonitis and should be considered especially in cases of persistent fever in a patient receiving therapy. Diligent physical examination and the use of ultrasound to localize a loculated empyema are important diagnostic tools. The presence of a foul-smelling exudate obtained by thoracentesis is typical. Drainage is required. Defervescence, a return to a feeling of well-being, and resolution of the process may require several months of therapy for empyema as well as lung abscesses.

Extension from a subdiaphragmatic infection also may result in an anaerobic empyema. Septic pulmonary emboli may originate from intraabdominal or female genital tract infections and can produce anaerobic pneumonia.

Intraabdominal infections Because anaerobic bacteria outnumber aerobic bacteria in normal bowel flora by 100 to 1000:1, it is not surprising that disruption of the bowel wall will result in peritonitis with a preponderance of anaerobic bacteria. Colonic perforation releases large numbers of these bacteria and therefore entails a high risk of intraabdominal sepsis. Following peritonitis, abscesses may develop in any part of the peritoneal cavity and retroperitoneal spaces. The peritoneum reacts with a marked inflammatory response and effectively walls off the infection in a very short time. If an intraperitoneal abscess is localized, typical signs and symptoms appear (Chap. 87). For example, *subphrenic abscess* may cause an ipsilateral sympathetic pleural effusion, and the patient may have pleuritic type pain and splinting of the hemidiaphragm on the affected side. Constitutional symptoms include fever, chills, and malaise. There is a history of abdominal surgery, trauma, or other conditions that predispose to disruption of the bowel wall. In contrast, more subtle clinical signs must be sought when an intraabdominal abscess is not readily localized. Peritonitis and abscess formation are closely related processes. Often following surgery to repair a bowel perforation, a patient may be febrile without localizing abdominal signs or general clinical deterioration. Persistent leukocytosis may be related to the operative procedure and/or resolving peritonitis. Attention should be directed to the presence and character of wound drainage which if profuse, cloudy, or foul-smelling suggests the possibility of purulent anaerobic infection. Gram stain revealing a mixed fecal flora is frequently helpful. *B. fragilis* is isolated from approximately 70 percent of surgical wounds after trauma involving perforation of the lower gut, and a similar percentage of isolates follows elective colonic surgery. Antibiotics effective against *B. fragilis,* as well as facultative bacteria, are important in therapy, although they are not a replacement for surgical or percutaneous drainage. Appendicitis with perforation and abscess formation is the most common intraabdominal anaerobic infection. Diverticulitis involves nonsporulating anaerobes and can result in perforation followed by generalized peritonitis, but generally results in small walled-off infections that do not require surgical drainage. Abdominal ultrasound, gallium- or indium-labeled neutrophil scans, computerized tomography (CT) scans, or combined liver-spleen and lung scans may be helpful in localizing intraabdominal abscesses. Surgical exploration, however, may be necessary to establish the site of such an infection.

Among visceral abdominal infections involving nonsporulating anaerobes, the most common is *liver abscess;* nonsporulating anaerobes are isolated from approximately 50 percent of liver abscesses. Liver abscess results from both bacteremic spread (sometimes following blunt trauma with localized infarction of hepatic tissue) and from contiguous infection, especially within the peritoneal cavity. Infection may spread from the biliary tract or from the portal venous system (suppurative pyelophlebitis) which results from direct extension of pelvic or intraabdominal sepsis. Symptoms and signs often suggest infection that can be readily localized, but nonspecific symptoms of fever, chills, weight loss, nausea, and vomiting are also seen in many patients. Only half the patients have hepatomegaly, right upper quadrant abdominal tenderness, and jaundice. The diagnosis can be confirmed by ultrasound, CT scan, or radioisotopic scanning. Occasionally more than one diagnostic procedure may have to be utilized. More than 90 percent of patients with liver abscesses have a leukocytosis and elevation of the serum alkaline phosphatase and aspartyl transaminase. Fifty percent have associated anemia, hypoalbuminemia, and elevated serum bilirubin. A basilar pulmonary infiltrate, pleural effusion, or elevated hemidiaphragm can be seen on chest x-ray. One-third of these patients have bacteremia. Open surgical drainage is indicated when an abscess is associated with other lesions requiring surgical drainage. Otherwise, percutaneous drainage using ultrasonography or CT scan to guide the catheter may be combined with antimicrobial therapy. If a liver abscess arises from contiguous gallbladder infection, cholecystectomy is essential.

Pelvic infections The vagina of a healthy woman is one of the major reservoirs of both anaerobic and aerobic bacteria. In the normal flora of the female genital tract, anaerobes outnumber aerobes by a ratio of approximately 10:1. These anaerobes include anaerobic gram-positive cocci and *Bacteroides* species. Serious infections of the upper female tract contain organisms found in the normal vaginal flora. Anaerobes are isolated from the majority of such patients. The major pathogens consist of *B. fragilis, B. melaninogenicus,* anaerobic cocci, and clostridial species. Anaerobes frequently are encountered in tuboovarian abscess, septic abortion, pelvic abscess, endometritis, and postoperative wound infection, particularly following hysterectomy. Although these infections are frequently mixed, involving both anaerobes and coliforms, pure anaerobic infections without coliform or other facultative bacterial species occur more often in pelvic infections than intraabdominal infections. These infections are characterized by drainage of foul-smelling pus or blood from the uterus, generalized uterine or local pelvic tenderness, and continued fever and chills. Suppurative thrombophlebitis of the pelvic veins may complicate the infections and lead to repeated episodes of septic pulmonary emboli.

Skin and soft tissue infections Injury to skin, bone, or soft tissue by trauma, ischemia, or surgery creates a suitable environment for anaerobic infections. These infections are most frequently found when the site is prone to contamination with feces or upper airway secretions. Examples include wounds associated with intestinal surgery, decubitus ulcers, or human bites. Anaerobic bacteria can be isolated in cases of crepitant cellulitis, synergistic cellulitis, or gangrene and necrotizing fasciitis. Furthermore, these organisms have been isolated from cutaneous abscesses, rectal abscesses, and axillary sweat gland infections (hydradenitis suppurativa). Anaerobes frequently have been isolated from foot ulcers in diabetic patients. These types of soft tissue or skin infections usually represent processes with mixed flora. A mean of 4.8 bacterial species can be isolated with a roughly 3:2 ratio of anaerobes to aerobes. The most frequently isolated organisms include *Bacteroides* species, anaerobic streptococci, group D streptococci, clostridial species, and *Proteus* species. The presence of anaerobes in these types of infections is associated with a higher frequency of fever, foul-smelling lesions, or a visible foot ulcer.

Anaerobic bacterial *synergistic gangrene* (Meleney's) typically occurs several days postoperatively. This lesion is characterized by the development of a wound infection which is exquisitely painful, red, and swollen, followed by induration. Erythema surrounds a central zone of necrosis. A granulating ulcer which may heal forms at the original center as necrosis and erythema extends outward. Symptoms are limited to pain. Fever is not typical. These infections most usually involve a combination of anaerobic cocci and *Staph. aureus.* Treatment includes surgical removal of necrotic tissue and antimicrobial therapy.

NECROTIZING FASCIITIS This is a rapidly spreading destructive disease of the fascia, usually attributed to group A streptococci, but it can be caused by anaerobic bacteria including *Peptostreptococcus* and *Bacteroides* species. Similarly, myonecrosis can be associated with mixed anaerobic infection. Fournier's gangrene is an anaerobic cellulitis involving the scrotum, perineum, and anterior abdominal wall in which mixed anaerobic organisms spread along deep external fascial planes and cause extensive loss of skin.

Bone and joint infections Although *actinomycosis* (Chap. 147) accounts on a worldwide basis for the majority of anaerobic infections in bone, other organisms are frequently isolated in such infections. In particular, anaerobic or microaerophilic cocci, *Bacteroides* species, *Fusobacterium,* and *Clostridium* species can be found. These infections frequently arise in the setting of soft tissue infections in adjacent soft tissues. Hematogenous seeding of bone is uncommon. Oral *Bacteroides* are seen in infections involving the maxilla and mandible, whereas *Clostridium* species have been reported as common anaerobic pathogens in cases of osteomyelitis of the long bones, following fracture or trauma. Fusobacteria have been isolated in pure culture from osteomyelitis adjacent to the perinasal sinuses, and, in the preantibiotic era caused fatal mastoid infections. Anaerobic and microaerophilic cocci have been reported as significant pathogens in infections involving the skull or mastoid.

In cases of anaerobic septic arthritis, the most common isolates are the *Fusobacterium* species. Most of these patients have uncontrolled peritonsillar infections progressing to septic cervical venous thrombophlebitis and resulting in hematogenous dissemination which shows a predilection for the joints. Most of these infections occurred in the preantibiotic era. Following the introduction of antibiotics, the isolation of *Fusobacterium* species from joints has been less common. Unlike anaerobic osteomyelitis, most cases of pyoarthritis caused by anaerobes are not polymicrobial and may be acquired hematogenously. Anaerobes are important pathogens in infections involving prosthetic joints; in these infections the causative organisms are part of the normal skin flora, such as the anaerobic gram-positive cocci and *P. acnes.*

In patients with osteomyelitis, the most reliable source of culture is a bone biopsy obtained free from normal uninfected skin and subcutaneous tissue. If mixed flora is isolated from a bone biopsy, all isolates should be treated. When an anaerobic isolate is recognized as a major or sole pathogen involving a joint, the treatment regimen should be similar to treatment of arthritis caused by aerobic bacteria. Therapy includes management of underlying disease states, appropriate antimicrobial therapy, temporary joint immobilization, percutaneous drainage of effusions, and usually removal of infected prostheses or internal fixation devices. Surgical drainage and debridement such as sequestrectomy are essential for removal of necrotic tissue that would sustain anaerobic infections.

Bacteremia Transient bacteremia is a well-known event that occurs in healthy people when the anatomic mucosal barriers are injured (e.g., toothbrushing). These bacteremic episodes, which are often due to anaerobes, have no pathologic consequences. However, anaerobic bacteria compose nearly 10 to 15 percent of bacterial blood isolates from clinically ill patients when proper culture techniques are used. *B. fragilis* is the single most frequent anaerobic isolate. The portal of entry can usually be deduced along with the likely underlying problem that led to seeding of the bloodstream, by identification of the organism and understanding its place of normal residence. For example, mixed anaerobic bacteremia including *B. fragilis* implies colonic pathology with mucosal disruption from neoplasia, diverticulitis, or some other inflammatory lesion. The initial manifestations are determined by the portal of entry and reflect the localized condition. However, when bloodstream invasion occurs, patients can become extremely ill with rigors and hectic fevers ranging up to 105°F. The clinical picture may be quite similar to that seen in sepsis with aerobic gram-negative bacilli. Although other complications of anaerobic bacteremia such as septic thrombophlebitis and septic shock have been reported, the incidence of these complications in association with anaerobic bacteremia is low. Anaerobic bacteremia is potentially fatal and requires rapid diagnosis and appropriate therapy. The source of bacteremia must be identified and managed appropriately. The choice of antimicrobial therapy depends on the identification of the infecting organism.

ENDOCARDITIS (Chap. 188) Endocarditis due to anaerobes is uncommon. However, anaerobic streptococci, which are often classified incorrectly, are responsible for this disease more frequently than is appreciated, although general incidence data are unavailable. Gram-negative anaerobes are unusual causes of endocarditis.

DIAGNOSIS Because of the time and difficulty involved in the isolation of anaerobic bacteria, diagnosis of these infections must frequently be made on presumptive evidence. Infections caused by these nonsporulating anaerobic bacteria have unique characteristics that serve as useful clues in aiding diagnosis. Certain clinical settings such as avascular, necrotic tissues with lowered oxidation-reduction potential favor the diagnosis of an anaerobic infection. When infections occur in proximity to mucosal surfaces normally harboring anaerobic flora, such as the gastrointestinal tract, female genital tract, or oropharynx, anaerobes should be considered as potential etiologic agents. A foul odor often is present since anaerobes produce certain organic acids as they proliferate in necrotic tissue. Although the presence of these odors is pathognomonic for anaerobic infection, the absence of odor does not exclude these organisms as potential etiologic agents. Fifty percent of documented anaerobic infections lack a characteristic foul odor. Because anaerobes often coexist with other bacteria to form a mixed or synergistic infection, Gram-stained exudate frequently reveals numerous pleomorphic cocci and bacilli suggestive of anaerobes. Sometimes these organisms will have morphologic characteristics associated with specific species.

The presence of gas in tissues is highly suggestive, but not diagnostic, of anaerobes. Culture reports from obviously infected sites which yield no growth or only streptococci or a single aerobic species such as *E. coli*, when a Gram stain reveals mixed flora, imply that the anaerobic microorganisms failed to grow because of inadequate transport and/or culture techniques. Failure of a patient to respond to antibiotics that are not active against anaerobes, for example, aminoglycosides, and, in some circumstances, penicillin, cephalosporins, or tetracyclines, suggests the possibility of anaerobic infection.

There are three critical steps to diagnose anaerobic infection: (1) proper specimen collection, (2) rapid transportation of these specimens to the microbiologic laboratory, preferably in anaerobic transport media, and (3) proper handling of these specimens by the laboratory. Collection of specimens must be performed by meticulously sampling infected sites avoiding contamination with normal flora. When there is a likely contamination of a specimen with normal flora, the specimen is unacceptable for processing by the bacteriology laboratory. Examples of unacceptable specimens for anaerobic culture include: (1) sputum collected by expectoration, or nasal tracheal suction, (2) bronchoscopy specimens, (3) direct collections through the vaginal vault, (4) collections of urine by voided specimen, and (5) feces. Specimens which can be cultured for anaerobes include blood, pleural fluid, transtracheal aspirates, pus obtained by direct aspiration from an abscess cavity, fluid obtained by culdocentesis, suprapubic bladder aspirates, cerebrospinal fluid, and lung puncture specimens.

Because even brief exposure to oxygen may kill these organisms and result in failure to isolate them in the laboratory, abscess cavities which are aspirated with a syringe should have the air expelled and the needle capped with a sterile rubber stopper. Specimens can be injected into transport bottles containing a reduced medium or brought immediately in syringes to the laboratory for direct culture on anaerobic media. In general, swabs should not be used. However, if a swab must be used, it should be placed in a reduced semisolid carrying medium before transport to the laboratory. It is important to remember that delays in transportation may lead to failure to isolate anaerobes due to exposure to oxygen, or overgrowth of facultative organisms which may eliminate or obscure the anaerobes that are present. All clinical specimens from suspected anaerobic infections should be Gram-stained and examined for organisms with characteristic morphology. It is not unusual for organisms to be observed on Gram stain but not isolated in culture. If purulent materials are found to be sterile, or organisms are seen on Gram stain, but do not grow in the culture, suspicion should be raised that anaerobes are involved and that improper transportation or handling of the specimen in the laboratory has occurred.

TREATMENT Successful therapy of anaerobic infections involves a combination of appropriate antibiotics, surgical resection, and drainage. Although the operative approach ultimately may be decisive, surgical intervention alone may be inadequate. Drainage of abscess cavities should be carried out as soon as fluctuation or localization occurs. Perforations must be closed promptly, devitalized tissues or foreign bodies removed, closed spaces drained, tissue compartments decompressed, and adequate blood supply established. Appropriate antibiotics should be employed because anaerobic sepsis can continue postoperatively with intermittent symptoms and insidious extension of the process. Frequently it is necessary to begin antimicrobial therapy of anaerobic infections on a presumptive basis before culture and susceptibility data are available. The selection of initial antibiotic therapy should be based on knowledge of the pathogens likely to be present in a specific clinical setting, in combination with the Gram stain findings which should suggest the likelihood of certain species of organisms. Because many anaerobic infections tend to be mixed with coliforms and other facultative organisms, it is advisable, in general, to use drugs active against both anaerobic and aerobic components. In general, if anaerobes are suspected, the choice of antibiotics can be made reliably since patterns of antimicrobial susceptibility are quite predictable. Because *B. fragilis* is resistant to penicillin, a major decision concerns the likelihood of the presence of this organism. *B. fragilis*, in general, does not play a significant role in infections above the diaphragm, including head and neck infections, pleuropulmonary infections, and central nervous system infections. However, septic processes originating below the diaphragm, including in the pelvic and abdominal cavity, frequently contain *B. fragilis*, and specific antimicrobial therapy directed at these organisms should be employed.

In infections arising from sources above the diaphragm, because *B. fragilis* is isolated rarely or is of dubious pathogenic significance, penicillin G is the most widely used antibiotic for treatment. Depending on the site of infection and the severity, the dose of penicillin G recommended is variable. For the treatment of lung abscesses, a dose of 6 to 12 million units per day for at least 4 weeks is recommended (Chap. 205). Infrequently, infections arising from oral organisms will fail to respond to penicillin. In such cases these patients should be treated with drugs effective against penicillin-resistant anaerobes such as clindamycin, chloramphenicol, or cefoxitin. Reports of increasing resistance of *B. melaninogenicus* to penicillin may account for some of these treatment failures.

Infections arising from a colonic source are likely to contain *B. fragilis* and present a different problem. Many therapeutic failures have been noted in patients with documented *B. fragilis* infection who were treated with penicillin or first-generation cephalosporins. In major studies of intraabdominal sepsis, the use of antibiotics effective against anaerobes has clearly reduced the incidence of postoperative infection and serious infectious complications. Based on such data, it is clear that in suspected *Bacteroides* infection, appropriate antimicrobial therapy must be initiated. Although the number of antimicrobial agents effective against *B. fragilis* is somewhat limited, there currently are several choices which are useful; no single regimen has demonstrated clear superiority over another. In general, greater than 80 percent cure rates can be achieved in patients with *B. fragilis* infection when treated with appropriate antimicrobial therapy.

Of the currently available drugs for the treatment of *B. fragilis* infections, several can be considered as potentially useful primary agents. These include clindamycin, metronidazole, and cefoxitin. Although chloramphenicol has produced some good results in studies of intraabdominal and female pelvic infections, there have been case reports of therapeutic failures, including cases of persistent *B. fragilis* bacteremia in the face of adequate treatment. Cefamandole, cefoperazone, cefotaxime, and moxalactam have all had generally higher minimum inhibitory concentrations (MICs) against this organism than the other antibiotics mentioned above.

Regimens for therapy of specific infections must be tailored to the initial infecting site and the clinical situation. For example, intraabdominal sepsis should be treated with either clindamycin, 600 mg intravenously every 8 h, or metronidazole, 7.5 mg/kg every 8 h. An aminoglycoside such as gentamicin or tobramycin should be included in the regimen to treat facultative gram-negative bacilli. Cefoxitin has compared favorably to the regimen of clindamycin and an aminoglycoside in treating serious mixed infections of the abdomen or skin, which frequently include *B. fragilis* among the causative pathogens. However, an aminoglycoside should be added to cefoxitin in patients who have either received prior antibiotic therapy, or who have acquired their infections in the hospital. Such patients are at high risk for infection involving cefoxitin-resistant organisms such as *Enterobacter, Pseudomonas,* or *Serratia*.

Chloramphenicol can be used in patients with intraabdominal or central nervous system infections at a dose of 30 to 60 mg/kg per day, depending on the severity of illness. Chloramphenicol has been used successfully in the treatment of central nervous system infections due to anaerobic bacteria. Penicillin G and metronidazole also cross the blood-brain barrier and are bactericidal for the organisms which cause brain abscess. In patients who have meningitis or endocarditis due to anaerobic bacteria, a bactericidal agent is preferred.

Although other semisynthetic penicillinase-resistant penicillins are not active against anaerobes, carbenicillin, ticarcillin, or piperacillin combine the antimicrobial spectrum of penicillin G with increased activity against *B. fragilis* based on the higher dose of drug administered. This group of antibiotics, although not recommended as first-line therapy of anaerobic infection, has been used successfully in some cases.

Nearly all drugs mentioned above have certain significant, toxic side effects. Chloramphenicol produces fatal aplastic anemia in 1:40,000 to 100,000 patients who receive the drug. Clindamycin, the cephalosporins, the penicillins, and even, rarely, metronidazole have been associated with the development of pseudomembranous colitis due to *Clostridium difficile*. Since diarrhea may precede frank development of pseudomembranes, the administration of these drugs should be discontinued if diarrhea develops during therapy.

Due to widespread resistance, tetracycline and doxycycline are not reliable for the therapy of anaerobic infections. Erythromycin and vancomycin have some activity against gram-positive anaerobes but are not recommended for the therapy of serious infection.

Anaerobic infections which have failed to respond to treatment or relapse after initial response should be recultured. The need for surgical drainage or debridement should be reassessed. Superinfection should be considered, potentially due to resistant gram-negative facultative or aerobic bacteria. Drug resistance also must be entertained, particularly if chloramphenicol was the antibiotic used. Repeated cultures should then yield the initial organism.

Other supportive measures in the management of anaerobic infections include careful attention to fluid and electrolyte balance, since extensive local edema formation may lead to hypovolemia; hemodynamic support for septic shock; immobilization of infected extremities; maintenance of adequate nutrition during chronic infections by enteral or parenteral hyperalimentation if oral intake is inadequate; relief of pain; and anticoagulation with heparin for thrombophlebitis. Hyperbaric oxygen therapy is of no value.

REFERENCES

Balows A et al: *Anaerobic Bacteria: Role in Disease*. Springfield, Thomas, 1974

Bartlett JG, Finegold SM: Anaerobic infections of the lung and pleural space. Am Rev Resp Dis 110:56, 1974

Finegold SM: *Anaerobic Bacteria in Human Disease*. New York, Academic, 1977

Gorbach SC: Anaerobic bacteria, in *Principles and Practices of Infectious Diseases*, GL Mandell et al (eds). New York, Wiley, 1985

———, Bartlett JG: Anaerobic infections. N Engl J Med 290:1177, 1974

Harding GKM et al: Prospective randomized comparative study of clindamycin, chloramphenicol and ticarcillin, each in combination with gentamicin in therapy for intraabdominal and female tract sepsis. J Infect Dis 142:384, 1980

Kasper DL et al: Virulence factors of anaerobic bacteria. Rev Infect Dis 1:246, 1979

——— et al: Capsular polysaccharides and lipopolysaccharides from two strains of *Bacteroides fragilis*. Rev Infect Dis 6:525, 1984

Ledger WJ: *Infection in the Female*. Philadelphia, Lea and Febiger, 1977

Mansheim BJ, Kasper DL: Infections produced by non-sporulating anaerobic bacteria, in *Seminars in Infectious Diseases VII*, L Weinstein, BJ Fields (eds). New York, Grune & Stratton, 1979

Mathisen GE et al: Brain abscess and cerebritis. Rev Infect Dis 6:5101, 1984

Nakata MN, Lewis RP: Anaerobic bacteria in bone and joint infections. Rev Infect Dis 6:5165, 1984

Newman MG: Anaerobic oral and dental infections. Rev Infect Dis 6:5107, 1984

Onderden K et al: Use of a model of intraabdominal sepsis for studies of the pathogenicity of *Bacteroides fragilis*. Rev Infect Dis 6:5191, 1984

Perera MR et al: Presentation, diagnosis and management of liver abscess. Lancet 2:629, 1980

Sutter VL et al: *Wadsworth Anaerobic Bacteriology Manual*, 3d ed. St Louis, Mosby, 1980

section 3 Diseases caused by gram-negative organisms

103 MENINGOCOCCAL INFECTIONS

HARRY N. BEATY

DEFINITION *Neisseria meningitidis* causes a variety of infections, most notably, meningitis and bacteremia.

ETIOLOGY In stained smears, meningococci are gram-negative single cocci or diplococci with flattened adjacent sides. They grow well on solid or semisolid media containing blood, serum, or ascitic fluid, and thrive best at temperatures between 35 and 37°C in an atmosphere reduced in oxygen and containing 5 to 10 percent CO_2. The organism is recovered readily from biologic fluids when fresh specimens are inoculated on warm chocolate agar plates that are incubated 18 to 24 h in a candle jar or in a more sophisticated apparatus that provides a suitable environment.

The biochemical reactions of the *Neisseria* are relatively limited, but they contain cytochrome oxidase, which is responsible for the positive "oxidase" test; the clinically significant species usually are differentiated by their ability to produce acid in glucose, maltose, or sucrose. Typically, the meningococcus ferments both glucose and maltose, but on occasion maltose-negative strains have been isolated.

Meningococci can be divided into serologic groups on the basis of agglutination reactions with immune serum. The present classification includes groups A through Z. Clinically significant new groups encompass Y and W135. The major groups are remarkably heterogeneous, but subclassification with additional serologic markers has been possible. Noncapsular antigens have provided the basis for dividing strains of groups into distinct types.

EPIDEMIOLOGY The natural habitat of meningococci is the nasopharynx of humans, and no other reservoir or vector has been recognized. Transmission from person to person is through inhalation of droplets of infected nasopharyngeal secretions. It is unlikely that the disease is spread by contact with contaminated fomites. Meningococci cause either epidemic or sporadic disease, and historically, there has been a cyclic variation in the prevalence of meningococcal infection with peaks of increased frequency occurring every 8 to 12 years and lasting 4 to 6 years. The last, quite minor, peak occurred in 1965. Subsequently, the incidence has declined to a fairly constant rate of about 1 case per 100,000 population per year. The prevalence of meningococcal infection is also subject to seasonal influences; the lowest attack rate occurs in midsummer and the highest in winter and early spring.

The attack rate of meningococcal disease is highest for children between 6 months and 1 year. The lowest attack rate occurs in individuals over 20. There is no clear-cut reason for sexual predominance, but males develop meningitis and meningococcemia more frequently than females. The attack rate in household contacts of sporadic cases of meningococcal disease is up to 1000 times the overall endemic rate; in epidemic periods, the attack rate among household contacts may be as much as 15,000 times that of the general population. Experience with group A outbreaks in Alaska and the northwestern part of the United States indicates that alcoholics and Alaska natives are at increased risk of infection, as are patients with deficiency in one or more components of complement. Military recruits also are particularly susceptible to meningococcal disease, although outbreaks among this population have disappeared coincident with the routine use of vaccines during the past 10 years.

In the first half of this century, most epidemics of meningococcal disease in the United States were caused by group A organisms. In the past two decades, first group B then group C meningococci were responsible for outbreaks in both the military and civilian populations. Currently, group B is responsible for 50 to 55 percent of reported cases. The proportion of isolates that are groups C, W135, and Y are 20 to 25, 15, and 10 percent, respectively. Only 1 to 2 percent of isolates are group A, but in Alaska and the Pacific Northwest 30 to 60 percent of patients with meningococcal disease are infected with this serogroup.

Studies of meningococci isolated from patients with meningococcal disease show that a very small proportion of strains in the environment cause disease. Common membrane antigens, closely related restriction endonuclease patterns, and the ability to form pili and release endotoxin have been correlated with "virulence."

Coincident with shifts in the predominant serogroup causing disease, there has been a waxing and waning of the proportion of isolates that are resistant to sulfadiazine. In the early 1960s, the majority of group B meningococci were resistant to sulfadiazine; in 1982 over 90 percent were sensitive. Similarly, when group C emerged as the predominant serogroup, sulfadiazine resistance was the rule. While sulfadiazine resistance has been recognized among isolates of all major serogroups, it is now uncommon in all but group B strains, 30 percent of which are resistant.

The potential for the meningococcus to produce serious outbreaks of disease has been reemphasized by epidemics in Brazil, Finland, and parts of Africa. Massive immunization programs curtailed two of these major epidemics.

Carriers Between epidemics, 2 to 15 percent of the individuals in urban centers harbor meningococci in the nasopharynx. When sporadic cases of meningococcal disease occur, the carrier rate in close contacts may rise to 40 percent, and in closed populations or during epidemics, may approach 100 percent. Although some individuals harbor meningococci for years, nasopharyngeal infection is usually transient, and in 75 percent of carriers the organism disappears within a few weeks to a few months. Case-to-case transmission of infection is documented rarely, and carriers, not patients, are the foci from which disease is spread. Even so, the prevalence of meningococcal disease can be attributed to the prevailing carrier rate only in a general way, and the occurrence of clinical disease is most dependent on the immunologic status of the host, other factors that lead to spread of infection beyond the nasopharynx, and strain virulence.

Immunity The fact that meningococcal meningitis is primarily a disease of childhood has suggested that natural immunity develops in most individuals within the first two decades of life. There is a correlation between susceptibility to meningococcal disease and absence of bactericidal antibody in the serum, and most adults have antibodies to pathogenic strains of meningococci. Natural immunization appears to result from asymptomatic carriage of meningococci in the nasopharynx. Not only does the carrier state produce antibodies to the infecting strain, but cross-reacting antibodies may develop, even after colonization with nongroupable organisms. The immunity conferred by meningococcal meningitis or meningococcemia is usually group-specific, and second episodes of meningococcal disease have been encountered. Deficiency of complement components C6, C7, or C8 is a significant risk factor for repeated episodes of bacteremia with the pathogenic *Neisseria*, and is seen more frequently in patients with initial infections than in the general population.

PATHOGENESIS The primary focus of meningococcal infection is the nasopharynx. In most instances, this infection is subclinical, but occasionally localized inflammation occurs and mild symptoms develop. Dissemination of meningococci from the nasopharynx occurs via the bloodstream, and generally is followed by clinical manifestations of meningococcal disease. *Purulent meningitis* is a form of metastatic infection and is either associated with signs and symptoms of meningococcemia or constitutes the predominant clinical expression of illness. Rarely, more extensive inflammation causes an acute diffuse encephalitis.

Although the mechanisms that produce tissue injury are unknown, in laboratory animals, an endotoxin that is biochemically and biologically similar to endotoxins of enteric bacilli appears to be involved. It may be responsible for hypotension and vascular collapse observed in fulminant meningococcemia and may also play a role in the pathogenesis of the purpura and visceral hemorrhages associated with meningococcal bacteremia. Thrombosis of dermal venules, adrenal sinusoids, and renal glomerular capillaries is most commonly seen in patients who die of fulminant meningococcemia and is strikingly similar to the pathologic changes observed in the experimental Shwartzman reaction induced by endotoxin.

CLINICAL MANIFESTATIONS Ninety to ninety-five percent of patients with meningococcal disease have meningococcemia and/or meningitis.

Meningococcemia Thirty to fifty percent of patients who develop overt disease have meningococcemia without meningitis. The onset of clinical illness may be abrupt, but patients usually have nonspecific prodromal symptoms of cough, headache, and sore throat followed by the sudden development of spiking fever, chills, arthralgia, and muscle pains that may be particularly severe in the lower extremities and back. Patients usually appear acutely ill with an inordinate degree of prostration. In addition to high fever, tachycardia, and tachypnea, mild hypotension may be present. However, clinical shock does not occur unless fulminant meningococcemia supervenes. In the course of meningococcal bacteremia, about three-fourths of the patients develop a characteristic petechial rash. Lesions are frequently sparse, and the axillae, flanks, wrists, and ankles are most commonly involved. Often petechiae are located in the center of lighter-colored macules, and they may become nodular as the disease progresses. The diagnosis of meningococcemia occasionally can be established by demonstrating gram-negative diplococci in scrapings from these nodular lesions. In severe cases, purpuric spots or large ecchymoses develop, and a widespread petechial or purpuric eruption suggests fulminating disease. However, the absence of rash does not necessarily indicate that the illness will be mild.

Fulminant meningococcemia, or the Waterhouse-Friderichsen syndrome, is meningococcemia associated with vasomotor collapse and shock. It occurs in 10 to 20 percent of patients with generalized meningococcal infection, and is associated with a high fatality rate. The onset is abrupt, and profound prostration frequently occurs within a few hours. Petechiae and purpuric lesions enlarge rapidly, and hemorrhage into the skin may be extensive. Early in the preshock stage, there is generalized vasoconstriction; patients are alert and pale, with circumoral cyanosis and cold extremities. Upon entering the shock stage, however, coma develops, the cardiac output decreases, and the blood pressure drops. Unless incipient shock is recognized and appropriate therapy is instituted early, death from cardiac and/or respiratory failure almost invariably occurs. Patients who recover may have extensive sloughing of skin lesions or loss of digits because of gangrene.

Chronic meningococcemia is a rare form of meningococcal infection that lasts for weeks or months and is characterized by fever, rash, and arthritis or arthralgia. Typically, the fever is intermittent, and during afebrile periods, which may last several days, patients appear remarkably well. The usual rash is a maculopapular or polymorphous eruption that waxes and wanes with the fever, but petechial or nodular lesions may be seen. Joint involvement is present in two-thirds of the patients, and splenomegaly is detected in about 20 percent. If the diagnosis is not suspected or treatment is otherwise delayed, complications such as meningitis, carditis, or nephritis may occur.

Meningitis Meningitis is a common form of meningococcal disease that occurs primarily in children from 6 months to 10 years. Fever, vomiting, headache, and confusion or lethargy are the commonest symptoms; in about one-fourth of the patients, symptoms begin abruptly and rapidly increase in severity. The more typical patient, however, has symptoms of an upper respiratory tract infection followed by an illness that progresses over several days. Twenty to forty percent of patients have meningitis without clinical evidence of meningococcemia, and the diagnosis depends upon bacteriologic examination of the cerebrospinal fluid. However, when meningitis occurs in association with a petechial or purpuric rash, a presumptive diagnosis of meningococcal disease is warranted, because this pattern of illness is seen only rarely in other infections.

Rarer manifestations The meningococcus is a rare cause of purulent conjunctivitis or sinusitis. Primary pneumonia previously was considered a rare manifestation of meningococcal infection, but increasing numbers of cases are being reported. In one study of military recruits, 68 cases of clinical pneumonia due to group Y meningococci were reported. Bacterial endocarditis, primary pericarditis, arthritis, and osteomyelitis have also been reported. On rare occasion, meningococci have produced genital infections clinically indistinguishable from gonococcal disease. *N. meningitidis* has been isolated with increasing frequency from the genitourinary tract and anal canal of symptomatic and asymptomatic patients of both sexes.

LABORATORY FINDINGS Aside from bacteriologic data, laboratory studies are of little value in establishing the diagnosis of meningococcal infection. Polymorphonuclear leukocyte counts usually range from 12,000 to 40,000 cells per cubic millimeter, but in meningococcemia, normal or low leukocyte counts may be encountered. Anemia is uncommon, and levels of serum electrolytes and blood urea nitrogen are normal unless shock develops. Patients with prominent hemorrhagic manifestations may have low platelet counts and decreased levels of circulating clotting factors as a result of disseminated intravascular coagulation. In meningitis, the cerebrospinal fluid pressure is increased, and the fluid usually contains from 100 to 40,000 polymorphonuclear leukocytes per cubic millimeter. The protein content is increased, and the concentration of glucose is almost always less than 35 mg/dL and often is between 0 and 10 mg/dL.

Meningococci often can be recovered from cultures of blood or spinal fluid, and, on occasion, material aspirated from skin lesions or joints yields the organism. In addition, gram-negative diplococci may be seen in stains of nodular petechiae or the buffy coat of blood from patients with meningococcemia. In meningococcal meningitis, a smear of the spinal fluid is diagnostic in about half the patients but often shows only a few intracellular bacteria which are located with difficulty.

COMPLICATIONS Herpes labialis occurs in 5 to 20 percent of patients with meningococcal disease. Other complications, which result from neurologic damage or secondary foci of infection, are uncommon following appropriate treatment and are often transient. Seizures or deafness occur in 10 to 20 percent of patients during the acute stages of meningitis, but postmeningitic epilepsy is rare, and the frequency of permanent eighth nerve damage is probably less than 5 percent. Peripheral neuropathy, cranial nerve palsies, and hemiplegia are seen occasionally, but usually clear completely within 2 to 4 months. Hydrocephalus and thrombosis of venous sinuses, once frequent sequelae of meningococcal meningitis, are encountered rarely. A number of patients complain of recurrent headache, emotional lability, insomnia, backache, memory loss, and difficulty in concentrating for months after an episode of meningitis. The organic basis for these symptoms is obscure, but they usually disappear a year or two after the infection.

Arthritis is a common metastatic complication of meningococcemia and occurs in 2 to 10 percent of patients. As a rule, multiple joints are involved, and signs and symptoms may not appear until after treatment of meningitis or meningococcemia has been instituted. Joint fluid usually contains many granulocytes, but meningococci are recovered infrequently. Arthritis may be immunologically mediated in those instances when cultures are sterile. Permanent joint changes are rare.

Other purulent complications have become extremely uncommon since antibiotics have gained widespread use. Pneumonia occurs occasionally, but it is uncertain whether it is caused by the meningococcus or coincidental infection with other bacteria. Bacterial endocarditis is quite rare, but a high proportion of patients who die of meningococcal infection have myocarditis. The etiology of these myocardial changes is uncertain, but cardiac failure may be an important factor in the pathogenesis of the shock syndrome in meningococcemia. A pericardial friction rub or electrocardiographic change of pericarditis is seen in about 5 percent of patients, and rarely purulent pericarditis may develop.

DIAGNOSIS The diagnosis of meningococcal disease depends upon recovering *N. meningitidis* from cultures of blood, spinal fluid, or petechial scrapings from patients with a typical clinical picture. Detection of antigen in spinal fluid by latex agglutination or counterimmunoelectrophoresis is valuable in diagnosing meningococcal meningitis. These techniques do not detect antigens of group B organisms, however. Recovery of meningococci from the nasopharynx does not, in itself, establish the diagnosis of meningococcal disease.

Few diseases need to be considered seriously in the differential diagnosis of meningococcal disease. If meningococcal meningitis is not accompanied by manifestations of bacteremia, it is indistinguishable from meningitis caused by other common pathogens. Occasionally, the common viral exanthems, mycoplasma infection, Rocky Mountain spotted fever (see Chap. 148), and vascular purpuras may be confused with meningococcemia.

TREATMENT Antimicrobial therapy of suspected or documented meningococcal disease should be instituted as early as possible. Penicillin G is the drug of choice, and should be administered intravenously. The dosage for treatment of meningitis in adults is 12 to 24 million units per day, and in the pediatric age group, 16 million units/m^2 per day. Meningococcemia alone can be treated with 5 to 10 million units per day, because it is not necessary to achieve high levels of antibiotic in the spinal fluid. If treatment with these doses is continued for a minimum of 7 days, or 4 to 5 days after the patient becomes afebrile, relapse is extremely rare. Meningococci are susceptible to chloramphenicol, but it should not be used unless a patient is allergic to penicillin. Then chloramphenicol hemisuccinate 4.0 to 6.0 g per day in divided doses (in adults) is an acceptable alternative. Some of the "third-generation" cephalosporins (see Chap. 88) have been used to treat small numbers of patients with meningococcal meningitis, but they should not be employed routinely until more extensive clinical research documents their efficacy. *Because a significant proportion of meningococci isolated are resistant to sulfonamides, these drugs should not be used alone in the treatment of meningococcal infections,* and their use in combination with penicillin offers no advantage.

Patients with meningococcal infections require supportive treatment as well as antimicrobial therapy. Maintenance of fluid and electrolyte balance and prevention of respiratory complications in comatose patients are of primary concern. When shock occurs, visceral perfusion must be improved by maintenance of an adequate intravascular volume, treatment of heart failure, and support of the blood pressure. Vasoactive drugs should be employed according to the pathophysiologic derangement in each individual case. These derangements can be determined best by carefully monitoring the blood pressure, pulse, arterial blood gases, cardiac output, peripheral resistance, pulmonary artery wedge pressures, and arteriovenous oxygen differences. When blood pressure must be raised immediately, norepinephrine may be indicated. However, if improved tissue perfusion is the primary goal, an agent such as dopamine is likely to be more effective. When heart failure is present, diuretics and digitalis should be given. When disseminated intravascular coagulation is recognized, treatment with heparin, whole blood, or fibrinogen can be tried, but dramatic results should not be expected. Massive doses of adrenal cortical steroids as used in the treatment of septic shock (see Chap. 86) may be helpful, but lower "replacement" doses are of uncertain value.

PREVENTION With the widespread emergence of sulfonamide-resistant meningococci, alternate methods of preventing meningococcal disease in closed populations were sought. High-molecular-weight polysaccharide antigens from organisms of serogroups A, C, Y, and W135 have been shown to induce a group-specific bactericidal antibody response after subcutaneous injection. Currently, a quadrivalent vaccine containing these antigens is available for use in control of outbreaks. Routine immunization is recommended only for particular high-risk groups. An effective group B vaccine has not yet been developed.

For intimate contacts of sporadic cases of meningococcal disease, chemoprophylaxis should be administered. If the organism isolated from the patient is sensitive to sulfonamides, 2 days of prophylaxis with one of these drugs is recommended. When sensitivities are not known or the organism is resistant to sulfonamides, rifampin in dosage of 600 mg every 12 h for 2 days for adults and 5 to 10 mg/kg every 12 h for children can be expected to eradicate the carrier state temporarily and minimize spread of meningococci.

With increased availability of an effective vaccine, its use as an adjunct to chemoprophylaxis for household or other intimate contacts of sporadic cases of meningococcal disease has been recommended.

PROGNOSIS Before the introduction of antibiotics, meningococcal meningitis and meningococcemia were almost invariably fatal. With prompt and appropriate chemotherapy, the mortality rate of meningitis without fulminant meningococcemia has dropped to less than 10 percent in the United States, and neurologic sequelae are rare. The mortality of fulminant infection remains high primarily because patients are often in irreversible shock when treatment is instituted. Most deaths occur within 24 to 48 h of admission, and the capacity of the meningococcus to kill a perfectly healthy individual within a few hours remains one of the most awesome characteristics of this disease.

REFERENCES

Band JD et al: Trends in meningococcal disease in the United States, 1975–1980. J Infect Dis 148:754, 1983

Black JR et al: Neisserial antigen H.8 is immunogenic in patients with disseminated gonococcal and meningococcal infections. J Infect Dis 151:650, 1985

Buchan H et al: An outbreak of meningococcal disease: Implications for community medicine. NZ Med J 97:860, 1984

Centers for Disease Control: Meningococcal vaccines. Morb Mort Week Rep 34:255, 1985

Ross SC et al: Complement deficiency states and infection: Epidemiology, pathogenesis and consequences of neisserial and other infections in an immune deficiency. Medicine 63:243, 1984

104 GONOCOCCAL INFECTIONS

KING K. HOLMES

DEFINITION Gonorrhea, an infection of columnar and transitional epithelium caused by *Neisseria gonorrhoeae,* is the most common reportable communicable disease in the United States. Anatomic sites which can be infected directly by the gonococcus include the urethra, rectum, conjunctivas, pharynx, and endocervix. Local complications include endometritis, salpingitis, peritonitis, and bartholinitis in the female, and periurethral abscess and epididymitis in the male. Systemic manifestations of gonococcemia include arthritis, dermatitis, endocarditis, and meningitis as well as myopericarditis and hepatitis.

ETIOLOGY *Neisseria gonorrhoeae* is a gram-negative coccus usually found in pairs with flattened adjacent sides. It forms oxidase-positive colonies and is differentiated from other *Neisseria* by its ability to utilize glucose but not maltose, sucrose, or lactose, and by specific immunologic reactions.

Colonies examined within 20 h of inoculation from clinical specimens contain organisms covered by fimbria (pili). As the colonies grow older, their appearance changes, reflecting the loss of pili. Piliated organisms cause infection and urethritis after inoculation into the urethras of male volunteers, whereas nonpiliated organisms do not. Pili mediate attachment to various epithelial cells, and interfere with neutrophil phagocytosis. The process by which piliated gonococci throw off nonpiliated variants, and vice versa, is termed *phase variation,* and is mediated by chromosomal rearrangement. Each pilus is composed of repeating peptide subunits (pilin) which have a molecular weight of about 20,000. The pilin subunits consist of conserved and variable regions. The variable regions are prone to rapid antigenic variation in vitro and in vivo. Antigenic variation of pilin may allow gonococci to adapt rapidly to attachment onto different types of epithelial surfaces, and to evade the host's antibody response to pilin.

The trilaminar outer membrane of the gonococcus contains several classes of proteins, including proteins I, II, and III, and lipopolysaccharide (Fig. 104-1). Like pili, protein II also is thought to function as a ligand, mediating the attachment of gonococci to various types of human cells. As in the case with pili, individual strains of gonococci may or may not choose to express protein II, and several antigenic variants of protein II may be expressed at different times by the same strain. The presence or absence of protein II also influences colony morphology, and protein II may be responsible for the clumping of gonococci which is so evident on Gram-stained smears of urethral exudate.

Opaque colonies contain organisms which express protein II, and predominate in isolates from the male urethra, and in cervical isolates obtained from women in midcycle. Transparent colonies lack protein II, and predominate in isolates from women during menses, and in isolates from blood, synovial fluid, or fallopian tubes.

Protein I (32,000 to 36,000 mol wt) is quantitatively the major outer membrane protein, present as a trimer aggregated with protein III. Protein I molecules act as porins, forming transmembrane channels that permit exchange of hydrophilic molecules through the outer membrane. Protein I molecules have been shown to move rapidly from gonococcal outer membranes to the more fluid cytoplasmic membrane of human cells. This process may initiate endocytosis of the gonococcus, representing the first step in gonococcal invasion of the epithelium.

The lipopolysaccharide of the gonococcus contains lipid A and core oligosaccharide, but no repeating polysaccharide side chain. No capsular polysaccharide has yet been isolated, but high-molecular-weight surface polyphosphates have been demonstrated which may have functions similar to those of capsular polysaccharides in other organisms.

Gonococcal typing Gonococcal strains now can be typed on the basis of nutritional requirements (auxotyping) or surface antigenic variation of protein I. Unlike pili and protein II, the protein I expressed by any single strain of gonococcus is antigenically stable, although there is considerable antigenic heterogeneity of protein I between strains. There are two different kinds of protein I, known as IA and IB, and individual strains contain either protein IA or protein IB, but not both. Monoclonal antibodies against different epitopes of protein IA and protein IB can be used to classify gonococci into a large number of serovariants known as serovars IA1 to IA18, and IB1 to IB28.

EPIDEMIOLOGY The only natural hosts for *N. gonorrhoeae* are humans. In the United States the annual age-specific incidence rates tripled from 1963 to 1978, when over 1 million cases were reported and an equal number probably went unreported. During this period of epidemic gonorrhea, the incidence increased fastest in young white females. After 1978, the incidence of gonorrhea fell steadily every year through 1984, when 879,000 cases were reported. In 1985, the incidence again rose unexpectedly by 5 percent. The current increase has been limited to heterosexuals; gonorrhea (and syphilis) in homosexual men has continued to decline rapidly because of fear of AIDS and a decline in homosexual promiscuity. The resurgence of gonorrhea in heterosexuals is unexplained, but could be related to

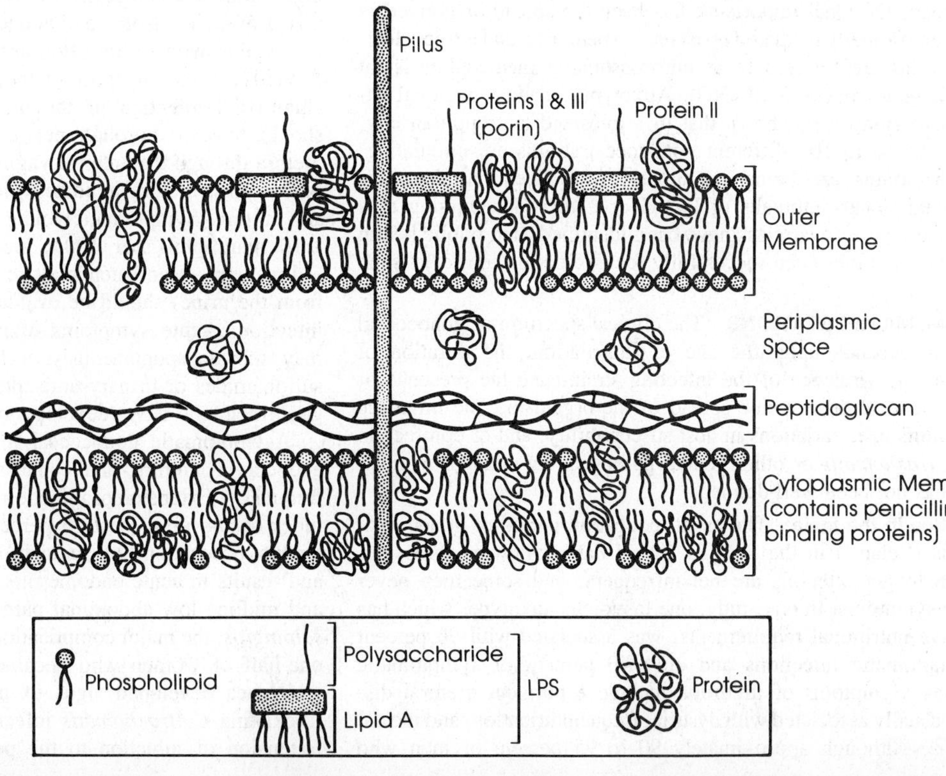

FIGURE 104–1 *Diagram of the envelope of* N. gonorrhoeae, *showing structures thought to influence pathogenesis, antimicrobial susceptibility, and antigenicity.*

reallocation of public health efforts from gonorrhea control toward control of other sexually transmitted diseases such as AIDS.

Gonorrhea incidence and prevalence rates are known to be related to age, sex, sex preference, race, socioeconomic status, marital status, urban residence, and level of education—risk factors which influence sexual behavior, illness behavior, and accessibility of health care. Among sexually active individuals, the highest rates occur in teenagers, in non-whites, in the poor and poorly educated, in large cities, and in unmarried persons—particularly those who live alone. Such individuals comprise a "core group" of "efficient transmitters" who play a disproportionate role in the spread of gonorrhea. The incidence is highest in men, while the prevalence is highest in women. The prevalence rate is so high among women in the United States that routine endocervical cultures have been advocated for gonorrhea case detection in asymptomatic women age 30 or under who are considered to be at high risk because of sexual behavior or demographic factors cited above. However, greater reliance should be placed upon contact tracing, which is far more efficient for control of gonorrhea, than upon routine endocervical culturing, which is expensive and does not focus on those most likely to transmit the infection. The single most important axiom about the epidemiology of this disease is that *gonorrhea is usually spread by carriers who have no symptoms or have ignored symptoms.* Symptomatic patients, male or female, have usually been recently infected by such carriers, who must in turn be traced and treated to prevent reinfection. *Men and women with symptomatic gonorrhea should always be interviewed to identify their recent sex contacts, who should be examined and treated if infected.*

There are interesting regional differences in the antibiotic resistance of *N. gonorrhoeae*. In 1976, penicillinase-producing strains of *N. gonorrhoeae* (PPNG), completely resistant to penicillin and ampicillin, appeared almost simultaneously in two areas of the world: in England, where they had probably been imported from west Africa, and in the United States, where they had been imported from the Philippines. The β-lactamase enzymes produced by these strains are encoded on small plasmids identical to plasmids found in *Haemophilus influenzae*. PPNG first became established and then spread in areas of the world where prostitution is exceptionally common and where access to subcurative antimicrobial therapy is unrestricted. PPNG now comprise 50 percent or more of all gonococci in many areas of Africa and Asia, and have by now become well established in many regions of the United States (e.g., Miami, New York, Los Angeles) and Europe. Of equal importance has been the spread of gonococci with chromosomally mediated resistance to penicillin and tetracycline. These strains are referred to as chromosomally mediated resistant *Neisseria gonorrhoeae* (CMRNG). Auxotyping and monoclonal antibody serotyping have shown that in a midsized metropolitan city, as many as 60 to 100 different gonococcal strains are circulating, and new strains are being continously introduced. Against this background, local outbreaks of PPNG or CMRNG belonging to a single auxotype-serovar class have been identified, and public health efforts have at times been successfully focused on the control of such strains.

CLINICAL MANIFESTATIONS The clinical spectrum of gonococcal infections depends upon the site of inoculation, the duration of infection, the virulence of the infecting strain, and the presence or absence of local or systemic spread of the organism. The influence of inoculum size, variations in host susceptibility, and of coinfection with *C. trachomatis* or other genital pathogens on clinical manifestations has not been well-defined.

Gonorrhea in the male The usual incubation period of gonococcal urethritis ("clap") in the male is 2 to 7 days following exposure, although longer intervals are not infrequent, and some men never develop symptoms. In one study, one fastidious auxotype, which has distinctive nutritional requirements, was associated with 96 percent of asymptomatic infections and only 40 percent of symptomatic infections. Symptoms of urethritis include a purulent urethral discharge, usually associated with dysuria, frequent urination, and meatal erythema. Although approximately 90 to 95 percent of men who acquire urethral gonococcal infection develop urethral discharge, most symptomatic men seek treatment and are removed from the infectious pool. The remaining men who never develop symptoms or who ignore their symptoms constitute about two-thirds of the infected men at any point in time, and they serve as the main source of spread of infection to women. Before antibiotic treatment became available, symptoms of urethritis persisted for an average of 8 weeks, and unilateral epididymitis occurred in 5 to 10 percent of untreated men. Epididymitis is now an uncommon complication (see below), and gonococcal prostatitis occurs rarely, if at all. Other local complications of gonococcal urethritis which are now unusual include inguinal lymphadenitis, edema of the penis due to dorsal lymphangitis or thrombophlebitis, submucous inflammatory "soft" infiltration of the urethral wall, periurethral abscess or fistula, unilateral inflammation or abscess of Cowper's gland (which lies between the thumb and forefinger when the forefinger is in the anal canal and the thumb is positioned anteriorly on the perineum), and, rarely, seminal vesiculitis.

In homosexual men, rectal and pharyngeal gonococcal infection are common. Gonococcal isolates from homosexual men tend to be more resistant to antimicrobials than are isolates from heterosexuals. This may be due to the fact that certain highly susceptible types are rapidly killed by bile salts and fatty acids in feces and rarely occur in homosexual men, while gonococci possessing a gene for multidrug resistance (*mtr*) are resistant to bile salts and fatty acids and occur with increased frequency in homosexual men. Rectal infection may be asymptomatic from the outset or may produce anorectal pain, pruritus, tenesmus, and a bloody, mucopurulent rectal discharge. Proctoscopy and appropriate laboratory studies are essential to exclude several other conditions which cause similar symptoms (see Chap. 90). These symptoms may subside without treatment, leaving a chronic asymptomatic carrier state. Pharyngeal gonococcal infection occurs in approximately 20 percent of homosexual men or heterosexual women who engage in fellatio with men who have urethral infection, and in a smaller proportion of heterosexual men. Pharyngeal infection may produce exudative tonsillitis but frequently is asymptomatic; asymptomatic pharyngeal gonococcal infection usually clears spontaneously over several weeks, even without therapy.

Gonorrhea in the female Acute uncomplicated gonorrhea in the female often causes dysuria, frequent urination, increased vaginal discharge due to exudative endocervicitis, abnormal menstrual bleeding, and anorectal discomfort. While dysuria and frequency in young men arouse the suspicion of gonococcal urethritis, the same symptoms in a young woman are often automatically attributed to "cystitis." Actually, some of those without bacteriuria have gonococcal or chlamydial infection of the urethra. Young women with dysuria should have a thorough pelvic examination. Compression of the urethra through the anterior vaginal wall against the symphysis pubis may express urethral exudate which can be examined by Gram's stain and culture. Symptomatic young women with "sterile pyuria" (i.e., ≥ 10 neutrophils per $100\times$ microscopic field in the centrifuged sediment of clean-catch midstream urine; no uropathogens isolated from the urine) should be evaluated for gonococcal and chlamydial infection. Acute symptoms of gonococcal urethritis in the female may subside spontaneously or following subcurative therapy with sulfonamides or urinary antiseptics. The proportion of women with gonorrhea who never develop symptoms is undefined.

Asymptomatic gonococcal infection in the female involves the endocervix, urethra, anal canal, and pharynx, in decreasing order of frequency. Extension of infection from the endocervix to the fallopian tubes occurs in at least 15 percent of women with gonorrhea. This tends to occur soon after acquisition of infection or during menstruation and results in acute endometritis, with abnormal menstrual bleeding and midline low abdominal pain and tenderness, followed by *acute salpingitis,* the major complication of gonorrhea. One study suggested one-half of women who became infected after recent exposure to gonorrhea developed signs of pelvic inflammatory disease (PID). Coexisting *C. trachomatis* infection may increase the rate of PID. Extension of infection to the pelvis may produce signs of pelvic peritonitis, accompanied by nausea and vomiting, and may lead to pelvic abscess. Early antibiotic treatment, before development of adnexal masses, restores normal tubal function and fertility in nearly all cases of gonococcal salpingitis. However, if prominent adnexal swelling has occurred before treatment is begun, bilateral tubal damage occurs in 15 to 25 percent.

Spread of gonococci or chlamydia into the upper abdomen may cause *perihepatitis* (Fitz-Hugh–Curtis syndrome) manifested by right upper quadrant or bilateral upper abdominal pain and tenderness, and occasionally by a hepatic friction rub.

Acute inflammation of Bartholin's gland is usually unilateral and frequently is due to gonococcal infection. The acutely infected duct is surrounded by a red halo and exudes pus at the posterior third of the labium majus. Occlusion of the duct results in formation of a Bartholin's abscess. Chronic Bartholin cysts are rarely caused by active gonococcal infection.

There is suggestive evidence that endocervical gonococcal infection is associated with prematurity and premature rupture of membranes.

Gonorrhea in children During childbirth, the gonococcus may infect the conjunctivas, pharynx, respiratory tract, or anal canal of the newborn. The risk of contamination increases with prolonged rupture of membranes. Prevention of gonococcal ophthalmia by prophylactic use of 1% silver nitrate eyedrops has led to the emergence of inclusion conjunctivitis caused by *Chlamydia* as a more common form of ophthalmia neonatorum. Since neonates and young infants lack bactericidal IgM antibody against *N. gonorrhoeae,* they may be at increased risk for gonococcal bacteremia. During the first year of life, infection of the infant usually results from accidental contamination of the eye or vagina by an adult. Between 1 year of age and puberty, many cases of gonorrhea involve vulvovaginitis in females who have been molested by a relative, and medicolegal considerations necessitate a complete bacteriologic diagnosis and child welfare consultation. Auxotyping and serotyping of isolates from the sexual assault victim and accused assailant have been used as evidence in court.

Disseminated gonococcal infection The incidence of disseminated gonococcal infection (DGI) varies with time and place, in relation to the local incidence of infection with strains of gonococci that have a propensity to produce bacteremia. Approximately two-thirds of patients with DGI are women, and symptoms of bacteremia often begin during menses. The majority of men and women with gonococcemia do not have symptoms of urogenital, anorectal, or pharyngeal gonococcal infection. As noted below, serum complement-mediated bactericidal activity appears essential for protection against gonococcal bacteremia.

Patients typically present either with symptoms and signs of gonococcemia, or with purulent arthritis affecting one or two joints. The onset of gonococcemia is characterized by fever, polyarthralgias, and papular, petechial, pustular, hemorrhagic, or necrotic skin lesions. Approximately 3 to 20 such lesions appear, usually on the distal extremities. Gonococci are demonstrable by immunofluorescent staining in about two-thirds of gonococcal skin lesions. The initial joint involvement is characteristically limited to tenosynovitis involving several joints asymmetrically. The wrists, fingers, knees, and ankles are most often involved. Circulating immune complexes have been demonstrated at this stage of infection in some but not all studies. Serum complement levels are normal (except in those with complement deficiency), and the role of immune complexes, if any, is uncertain. Without treatment, the duration of gonococcemia is variable; the systemic manifestations of bacteremia may subside spontaneously within a week. Alternatively, septic arthritis ensues, often without prior symptoms of fever, polyarthralgias, or skin lesions. Pain and swelling then increase in one or, very occasionally, more joints, with accumulation of purulent synovial fluid, leading to progressive destruction of the joint if treatment is delayed.

IgM antibody to gonococcal lipopolysaccharide, present in normal human serum, is bactericidal for most strains of gonococci in the presence of complement. Gonococci isolated from patients with DGI have stable resistance to normal human serum. These strains usually contain protein IA, and are highly susceptible to penicillin. They often require arginine, hypoxanthine, and uracil for growth, and are referred to as belonging to the AHU auxotype. Patients deficient in complement components C5, C6, C7, and C8 are uniquely susceptible to gonococcemia and meningococcemia because they cannot mount a serum bactericidal response to gonococci or meningococci. Gonococci isolated from patients with tenosynovitis and skin lesions are even more resistant to pooled normal human serum than are isolates from patients with purulent arthritis, suggesting that the two different DGI syndromes may be determined by characteristics of the causative organism.

The probability of positive blood cultures decreases after 48 h of illness, and the probability of recovery of gonococci from synovial fluid increases with increasing duration of illness. Gonococci are infrequently recovered from early effusions containing less than 20,000 leukocytes per cubic millimeter, but are usually recovered from effusions containing more than 80,000 leukocytes per cubic millimeter. In the individual patient, gonococci are seldom recovered from blood and synovial fluid simultaneously.

Other common manifestations of disseminated gonococcal infection include mild myopericarditis and "toxic" hepatitis. Endocarditis and meningitis are infrequent but severe complications. Endocarditis is suggested by pathologic or changing heart murmurs, major embolic phenomena, severe myocarditis, deterioration of renal function, or an unusually large number of skin lesions.

PATHOGENESIS Understanding of the pathogenesis of gonorrhea has developed rapidly. Epidemiologic data suggest that only about one-third of men become infected after a single exposure to gonorrhea, and under experimental conditions an inoculum of 10^3 organisms appears necessary to establish urethral infection in 50 percent of male volunteers. Factors which may confer resistance to infection are undefined. Components of the urethral or vaginal flora, such as *Candida albicans, Staphylococcus epidermidis,* and certain types of lactobacilli, can inhibit *N. gonorrhoeae* in vitro and may provide some natural resistance in vivo. Lactoferrin is present at mucosal surfaces, where it presumably competes with gonococci for iron, which is required for growth of the organism. AHU strains of gonococci compete poorly with lactoferrin, which could explain the tendency of such strains to cause asymptomatic mucosal infections. Gonococci infect mucus-secreting epithelial surfaces, and mucus could be a physical barrier or competitive inhibitor between the gonococcus and its target cell receptors.

Attachment of gonococci to mucosal cells is mediated in part by pili and by protein II. Local antibody to pili can partially block attachment. Pili also impede phagocytosis of gonococci by neutrophils, and antibody to pili is opsonic. An enzyme produced by the pathogenic *Neisseria,* IgA1 protease, which inactivates sIgA1, may interfere with IgA-mediated antiadherence activity, resulting in increased attachment.

Following attachment to columnar or transitional epithelium, gonococci penetrate through or between cells to reach the subepithelial connective tissue. Transfer of gonococcal protein I into the host cell may initiate endocytosis by the epithelial cell. Gonococcal lipopolysaccharide (LPS) and peptidoglycan are toxic for fallopian tube organ cultures. Gonococci also produce proteases, phospholipases, and elastases which may play a role in pathogenesis. In subepithelial tissue, and in blood, gonococci presumably interact with serum antibody, including natural IgM antibody directed against LPS antigens, with generation of the chemotactic factor C5a and formation of the bactericidal C5b-C9 attack complex. Insertion of the attack complex into the outer membrane of serum-sensitive gonococci results in gonococcal cell lysis. Although an attack complex is also formed when serum interacts with gonococci characterized by stable serum resistance, the insertion of the complex into the outer membrane of the organism has an abnormal configuration which does not result in rapid cell lysis. Furthermore, human serum also appears to contain IgG antibody directed against protein III which blocks the bactericidal action of IgM antibody for strains of gonococci with stable serum resistance. Following phagocytosis by neutrophils, the susceptibility of gonococci to intracellular killing is controversial. During in vivo growth, gonococci apparently develop phenotypic serum resistance and resistance to neutrophil-mediated killing. The mechanisms responsible for these phenotypic changes are largely undefined.

Spread of gonococci from the cervix to the endometrium and salpinges may be enhanced in women using an intrauterine device and impeded by oral contraceptive usage. Menstruation further increases the risk of intraluminal ascent from the cervix and evidently also predisposes to gonococcal bacteremia. Therefore, susceptibility to gonorrhea, to ascending gonococcal PID, and to gonococcemia depends upon a complex interplay of host factors and virulence properties of the organism.

DIFFERENTIAL DIAGNOSIS Gonococcal infection produces several common clinical syndromes which have multiple etiologies or which mimic other conditions. In particular, the epidemiology and clinical manifestations of *Chlamydia trachomatis* infections closely resemble those of gonococcal infections. The differential diagnosis of urethritis, epididymitis, and proctitis in men, vaginitis and cervicitis in women, and of acute arthritis in young adults is discussed in Chap. 90. The differential diagnosis of pelvic inflammatory disease is discussed in Chap. 91.

LABORATORY DIAGNOSIS The Gram's stain of urethral or endocervical exudate is considered diagnostic of gonorrhea when typical gram-negative diplococci are seen within leukocytes, is equivocal if only extracellular or atypical gram-negative diplococci are seen, and is negative if no gram-negative diplococci are seen. When these criteria are employed by experienced microbiologists, the sensitivity and specificity of Gram's stain of the urethral exudate approach 100 percent. Even so, in areas where resistant gonococci are seen, culture should be performed to allow testing of isolates for antimicrobial resistance. The specificity of Gram's stain of purulent cervical exudate also is high, but the sensitivity is only about 50 percent. Thayer-Martin (TM) medium, which contains antibiotics to inhibit most other organisms selectively, is most useful for recovering the gonococcus from the endocervix, rectum, and pharynx, which are colonized by a mixed bacterial flora. The concentration of vancomycin should not exceed 3 μg/mL, and even this concentration may inhibit a small proportion of gonococci. After inoculation, the medium should be placed in an atmosphere containing 3 to 10 percent carbon dioxide to permit growth of the gonococcus. This can be accomplished in a candle jar, by generation of carbon dioxide chemically within packets which are sealed after inoculation, or within special CO_2 incubators. Inoculated media should be incubated at 36°C for 48 h, and putative gonococcal colonies should be confirmed by oxidase reaction, Gram's stain, and sugar utilization tests or agglutination reactions using antiserums which are specific for *N. gonorrhoeae*. The latter two of these tests are especially important for isolates from the pharynx and rectum and for cultures obtained from populations which have a low prevalence of gonorrhea, such as prenatal patients.

In men with incubating or chronic asymptomatic urethral infection without exudate, or as a test of cure following treatment, a very thin swab should be inserted 2 cm into the anterior urethra and used to inoculate TM medium. Cultures of the pharynx and rectum should be obtained from homosexual men with suspected gonorrhea.

The most efficient test for gonorrhea in women is the endocervical culture, which is positive on a single examination in approximately 80 to 90 percent of those with gonorrhea. This diagnostic yield can be increased by performing a second endocervical culture and by performing cultures of the rectum, urethra, and pharynx.

Standard blood culture broth medium containing 3 to 10 percent carbon dioxide should be used in culturing blood and is also recommended for culturing synovial fluid. In pus from skin lesions, *N. gonorrhoeae* is more often demonstrable by immunofluorescent staining than by culture. Techniques designed to detect gonococcal infection by testing of a single serum have been limited by inability to differentiate antibody due to past gonorrhea from antibody due to current infection, and by false-positive tests caused by cross-reactive antibody to *N. meningitidis*. For these reasons, serologic tests for gonorrhea have had a very low predictive value, and they are not used in clinical practice.

Another diagnostic approach is the detection of gonococcal antigen in urethral or cervical secretion by enzyme-linked immunosorbent assay (ELISA). In men with urethritis, the Gram stain is just as accurate, quicker, and cheaper. In women, these tests may be an acceptable alternative to culture for diagnosis of endocervical gonococcal infection in settings where culture is not at all feasible. However, the positive predictive value of the currently available test requires further study in populations with a low prevalence of gonorrhea; the medical-legal and psychosocial implications of a false-positive diagnosis of gonorrhea can be troublesome.

TREATMENT The preferred drugs for gonococcal infection for several years have been penicillin G, ampicillin, or amoxicillin, tetracycline hydrochloride, and spectinomycin. Although long-acting forms of penicillin (such as benzathine penicillin G) are effective in syphilotherapy, they have *no place* in the treatment of gonorrhea. Penicillin V and the isoxazolyl penicillins are not recommended for the treatment of gonococcal infection. Similarly, first-generation cephalosporins are not used for gonorrhea. In 1985, the Centers for Disease Control issued new treatment guidelines for gonorrhea because of several new developments. The incidence of infections due to penicillinase-producing *N. gonorrhoeae* has increased, and outbreaks have occurred with CMRNG. A high frequency of coexistent chlamydial infection in heterosexual patients with gonococcal infections has been demonstrated, and the importance of serious complications related to chlamydial infections has been established. Several new and more expensive β-lactam antibiotics which are effective in gonococcal infection (especially ceftriaxone) have come onto the market. Spectinomycin resistance has been noted frequently in England, Korea, and occasionally elsewhere. The following guidelines for gonococcal infections attempt to consider these new developments, but they do not represent a comprehensive list of all possible treatment regimens. These guidelines are adapted from recommendations made by a CDC advisory committee in 1985. As is shown in Table 104-1, a regimen combining a single oral dose of amoxicillin or ampicillin plus probenecid, or IM ceftriaxone without probenecid, together with a 7-day course of tetracycline or doxycycline, is recommended for uncomplicated gonococcal infections in heterosexual adults. These combination regimens can be expected to provide adequate therapy for gonorrhea at any site, including the pharynx, and eliminate coexisting *C. trachomatis* infections. In patients who can not tolerate tetracycline, the single-dose oral ampicillin or amoxicillin/probenecid regimen can be followed by erythromycin base or stearate, 500 mg by mouth four times daily for 7 days, or by erythromycin ethylsuccinate, 800 mg by mouth four times daily for 7 days. All tetracyclines are ineffective as single-dose therapy, and even a 7-day course of tetracycline has been ineffective in a small but growing proportion of patients, especially females, with gonorrhea.

Homosexual men with uncomplicated gonococcal infection should be treated with ceftriaxone, 250 mg IM; or with 4.8 million units of aqueous procaine penicillin G, plus 1.0 g of probenecid. Men allergic to penicillin should receive spectinomycin, 2.0 g, in one intramuscular injection. Any of these regimens provides adequate treatment for urethral and anorectal gonorrhea, but spectinomycin is not effective for pharyngeal gonorrhea. Coexisting chlamydial infection is less common in homosexual men with gonorrhea than in heterosexual men with gonorrhea, and therefore the 7-day course of tetracycline is often omitted in treating homosexual males. With parenteral penicillin G, the risk of anaphylaxis in patients who deny previous penicillin allergy has been about 0.04 percent. The risk of procaine reaction due to transient neurotoxic serum concentrations of procaine is probably between 0.1 and 1 percent with the currently recommended dosage.

All patients with gonorrhea should have a serologic test for syphilis at the time of diagnosis. Patients with incubating seronegative syphilis, without clinical signs of syphilis, are likely to be cured by any of the recommended regimens (except spectinomycin) and need not have later follow-up tests for syphilis. However, patients with gonorrhea who also have syphilis or who are established contacts of someone with syphilis should be given additional treatment appropriate to the stage of syphilis. As a test of cure of gonorrhea, follow-up cervical, rectal, and other appropriate cultures should be obtained from women, and urethral and other appropriate cultures from men, 3 to 7 days after completion of therapy.

The patient in whom gonorrhea persists after treatment with one of the nonspectinomycin regimens above should be treated with 250 mg of ceftriaxone intramuscularly or with 2.0 g of spectinomycin intramuscularly (except in areas where spectinomycin resistance is a problem). Most recurrent gonococcal infections after treatment with the recommended schedules are due to reinfection and indicate a need for improved contact tracing and patient education. Since infection by PPNG is a cause of treatment failure, posttreatment isolates should be tested for pencillinase production.

Patients with proven infection by PPNG or CMRNG, or who are likely to have acquired gonorrhea in areas where such strains are common (Africa, Asia, and currently certain metropolitan areas such as Miami), and their sexual partners should receive ceftriaxone, 250 mg, or spectinomycin, 2.0 g, intramuscularly in a single injection. Tetracycline or doxycycline may be added to treat coexistent chlamydial infection. Other newer β-lactam antibiotics (cefotaxime, cefuroxime), and certain new oxyquinolones are also very effective for resistant gonorrhea, but the long half-life of ceftriaxone, together with its in vitro activity, make it the optimal drug for single-dose therapy of resistant gonorrhea at present. Cefoxitin is also effective for PPNG infection in a dose of 2.0 g intramuscularly, together with 1.0 g of probenecid by mouth. Cefoxitin is widely used for PID (with doxycycline) because of its activity against other organisms often implicated in PID, as well as against *N. gonorrhoeae*.

Postgonococcal urethritis (PGU) usually becomes apparent about 2 to 3 weeks after treatment of gonorrhea with a penicillin or a cephalosporin. PGU often is caused by *C. trachomatis* which may have been acquired at the same time as gonorrhea but did not become clinically apparent until later because of the longer incubation period of chlamydial infection. When PGU occurs, it can be managed, like nongonococcal urethritis, with tetracycline, 0.5 g four times a day for at least 7 days. Similarly, mucopurulent cervicitis in women often persists or appears after treatment of gonorrhea with a penicillin, is often caused by *C. trachomatis*, and can be treated like PGU with tetracycline 0.5 g four times a day for 7 days. Men and women exposed to gonorrhea should be examined, cultured, and treated with one of the recommended treatment schedules.

All pregnant women should have endocervical cultures for gonococci at the time of the first visit as an integral part of the prenatal care. A second culture late in the third trimester should be obtained from women at high risk of gonococcal infection.

Drug regimens of choice in pregnancy are ampicillin or amoxicillin, each with probenecid as described above, or ceftriaxone. Women allergic to penicillin, cephalosporins, or probenecid can be treated with spectinomycin, 2.0 g intramuscularly. Erythromycin in the dosage recommended above for chlamydial infection can be added to treat coexistent chlamydial infection. Tetracycline should not be used in pregnant women because of potential toxic effects for mother and fetus.

The management of pelvic inflammatory disease is discussed in Chap. 91. Hospitalization of women with PID is recommended whenever practical. Adequate treatment of women with acute PID must include examination and appropriate treatment of sex partners because of their high prevalence of nonsymptomatic urethral, gonococcal, or chlamydial infection. Failure to treat sex partners may lead to recurrent salpingitis.

Treatment of gonococcal arthritis can be accomplished satisfactorily with several regimens. Gonococci recovered from patients with gonococcal arthritis have been significantly less resistant to penicillin or tetracycline than isolates from patients with uncomplicated gonorrhea. However, because of the threat of endocarditis, meningitis, and joint sepsis, all patients with disseminated infection should preferably be hospitalized and treated with aqueous crystalline penicillin G intravenously, 10 million units per day for at least 3 days, and until clinical improvement occurs. Treatment can then be completed on an outpatient basis with ampicillin or amoxicillin, 2 g per day orally, to complete a 7- to 10-day course of therapy. Treatment with ampicillin, 3.5 g daily orally with 1 g probenecid, followed by 0.5 g four times a day for 7 days, also probably represents adequate therapy for disseminated gonococcal infection. Failure to improve with one of these regimens strongly suggests a diagnosis other than disseminated gonococcal infection. Repeated joint aspiration or closed irrigation of the joint with sterile saline may be required to reduce inflammation in patients with high synovial fluid leukocyte counts. Open drainage is seldom, if ever, required for gonococcal arthritis, except in infants with hip infection. Temporary immobilization of the joint may reduce discomfort for the patient and may be useful during initial ambulation in patients with persistent effusions of the

TABLE 104-1 Recommended treatment for gonococcal infection

Diagnosis	Treatment of choice
Uncomplicated gonococcal infection in adults	Amoxicillin 3.0 g or ampicillin 3.5 g single oral dose, or ceftriaxone 250 mg intramuscularly. Amoxicillin and ampicillin (but not ceftriaxone) to be accompanied by 1.0 g probenecid by mouth. Complete therapy with tetracycline 0.5 g by mouth four times a day or with doxycycline 100 mg by mouth twice daily for 7 days (if penicillin-allergic, give the 7-day tetracycline or doxycycline regimen alone).
Uncomplicated gonococcal infection in homosexual men	Aqueous procaine penicillin G (APPG), 4.8 million units total dose given intramuscularly at two sites, with 1.0 g probenecid by mouth (if penicillin-allergic, give spectinomycin 2.0 g in one intramuscular injection*).
Treatment failures, penicillinase-producing *N. gonorrhoeae*, or chromosomally mediated resistant *N. gonorrhoeae*	Spectinomycin 2.0 g single intramuscular dose* *or* ceftriaxone 250 mg single intramuscular dose.
Gonorrhea in pregnancy	Same as for uncomplicated gonococcal infection in adults, except that erythromycin should be substituted for tetracycline for coexisting chlamydial infection (see text) (if penicillin-allergic, give spectinomycin 2.0 g single intramuscular dose).
Disseminated gonococcal infection	Hospitalization is recommended. Aqueous crystalline penicillin G, 10 million units intravenously per day for at least 3 days (longer if meningitis or endocarditis occur), followed by ampicillin or amoxicillin, 0.5 g by mouth four times daily to complete 7 days of antibiotic treatment.
Gonococcal PID	Hospitalization is recommended; see Chap. 91 for suggested antimicrobial therapy.
Gonococcal epididymitis	See Chap. 90 for recommended therapy.
Pediatric gonococcal infection	Children who weigh 100 lb (45 kg) should receive adult regimens; for those who weigh less than 100 lb, see discussion in text.

* *Not effective for pharyngeal gonococcal infection (see text).*

knee or ankle. Antibiotics should not be injected directly into the joint. Once the diagnosis of gonococcal arthritis is proven, then occasional patients may benefit from use of anti-inflammatory agents along with antimicrobial therapy. However, if the diagnosis is suspected, but not proven, then early use of anti-inflammatory drugs will prevent monitoring the response to antimicrobial therapy, which is usually rapid and often of diagnostic importance in gonococcal arthritis.

Meningitis and endocarditis caused by the gonococcus require high-dose intravenous penicillin therapy, typically for 10 to 14 days for meningitis and 1 month for endocarditis. In penicillin-allergic patients with disseminated gonococcal infection, ceftriaxone, 1.0 g IV once daily, or cefotaxime, 500 mg IV four times daily for 14 days may be used. Similar doses are acceptable for arthritis, and higher doses may be effective for meningitis and endocarditis, although experience so far is negligible, and cross-allergenicity with penicillin may occur.

Gonococcal conjunctivitis in the adult or newborn should be managed as a medical emergency by irrigation of the conjunctiva with saline, together with penicillin G or ceftriaxone given intravenously.

Pediatric gonococcal infection The infant born to a mother with gonorrhea is at high risk of infection and requires treatment with a single intravenous or intramuscular injection of aqueous crystalline penicillin G, 50,000 units to the full-term infant or 20,000 units to the low-birth-weight infant. Topical prophylaxis for neonatal ophthalmia is not adequate treatment for infections at other sites. Clinical illness requires additional treatment.

Neonates with gonococcal ophthalmia should be hospitalized and isolated for 24 h after initiation of treatment. Aqueous crystalline penicillin G, 100,000 units per kilogram per day, in four divided daily doses intravenously should be administered for 7 days. Irrigation of the eyes with saline or buffered ophthalmic solutions should be performed immediately and then repeated as often as necessary to eliminate discharge. Topical antibiotic preparations alone are not sufficient or required when appropriate systemic antibiotic therapy is given. Both of the parents of a newborn with gonococcal ophthalmia must be treated for gonorrhea.

Neonates with arthritis and bacteremia should be hospitalized and treated with aqueous crystalline penicillin G, 100,000 units per kilogram per day, intravenously in four divided doses for 7 days (at least 10 days for meningitis).

Uncomplicated gonococcal vulvovaginitis, urethritis, proctitis, or pharyngitis in older children can be treated at a single visit with amoxicillin, 50 mg/kg, orally with probenecid, 25 mg/kg (maximum 1.0 g), or with ceftriaxone, 125 mg IM. This regimen is recommended for proctitis and pharyngitis. Patients should be evaluated for coinfection by chlamydia.

Topical and/or systemic estrogen therapy is of no benefit in gonococcal vulvovaginitis. All children should have follow-up cultures, and the source of infection should be identified, examined, and treated. Child abuse should be carefully considered and evaluated.

Children who are allergic to penicillins can be treated with spectinomycin, 40 mg/kg, intramuscularly. Children older than 8 years may be treated with tetracycline, 40 mg/kg per day, by mouth, in four divided doses for 5 days. For treatment of complicated disease, the alternative regimens recommended for adults may be used in appropriate pediatric dosages.

PPNG infection in neonates should be treated with ceftriaxone, 125 mg intramuscularly, but experience is limited.

Treatment of gonorrhea in developing countries Ironically, the proportion of gonococcal infections caused by PPNG or CMRNG is highest in developing countries, which can least afford spectinomycin, ceftriaxone, or other new antimicrobials effective against these strains. Inexpensive alternatives to penicillin G and tetracycline, the traditional mainstays of gonorrhea therapy, have been generally disappointing. For example, a sulfonamide-trimethoprim combination which initially cured over 95 percent of cases of gonorrhea in African countries, fell to less than 75 percent efficacy within 2 years after it became a popular regimen in Kenya. One innovative approach has been the use of 4.8 million units of procaine penicillin G intramuscularly plus 1.0 g probenecid orally (a standard regimen for non-PPNG infections) together with 125 mg of clavulanic acid (in the form of one capsule of amoxicillin-clavulanate) to inhibit gonococcal β-lactamase. This inexpensive regimen has been effective in small trials in Kenya, even against PPNG infections. Gentamicin, in a 280-mg single intramuscular dose, has also been used effectively in this setting. Use of newer cephalosporins in lower than recommended doses, to reduce cost, should be discouraged.

PREVENTION AND CONTROL There is probably no more striking illustration than gonorrhea of the failure of a specific treatment alone to eradicate a communicable disease. Vaccination is not available. A field trial of a purified gonococcal pili vaccine in U.S. soldiers in Korea showed that the vaccine was not effective. Use of the condom can prevent transmission, and the extensive use of condoms for contraception may be responsible for the low rates of gonorrhea in some countries (e.g., Japan). Spermicidal preparations used with a diaphragm probably offer some protection against gonorrhea and chlamydial infection, though this has not been proved convincingly. Prophylactic antibiotics (e.g., 200 mg minocycline or doxycycline taken soon after sexual exposure) reduce the risk of infection, but are not recommended for general use or for individuals with known exposure to gonorrhea, who should receive one of the regimens recommended for established gonorrhea.

To contain the increasing spread of antimicrobial-resistant gonococci, several measures are important: (1) routine use of diagnosis by cultures and testing of isolates for antimicrobial resistance or β-lactamase production; (2) routine use of spectinomycin or ceftriaxone for gonorrhea treatment failures; (3) rapid epidemiologic tracing of contacts of patients with gonorrhea, particularly treatment failures of those known to be infected with resistant gonococci; and (4) routine use of spectinomycin or ceftriaxone in areas where PPNG exceeds a certain threshold proportion (e.g., >5 percent) of all gonococcal isolates. The most effective public health measure now available for control of gonorrhea is tracing sexual contacts of infected patients. Experienced interviewers are able to identify and bring to treatment an average of one additional case for every patient interviewed.

REFERENCES

Britigan BE, Sparling PF: Gonococcal infection: A model of molecular pathogenesis. N Engl J Med 312:1683, 1985

Centers for Disease Control: 1985 STD treatment guidelines. Morb Mort Week Rep 34(4S):75S, 1985

Curran JW et al: Female gonorrhea. Its relations to abnormal uterine bleeding, urinary tract symptoms and cervicitis. Obstet Gynecol 45:195, 1975

Easmon CSF et al: Emergence of resistance after spectinomycin treatment for gonorrhoea due to beta-lactamase–producing strain of *Neisseria gonorrhoeae*. Br Med J 284:1604, 1982

Handsfield HH et al: Asymptomatic gonorrhea in men. Diagnosis, natural course, prevalence and significance. N Engl J Med 290:117, 1974

——— et al: Treatment of the gonococcal arthritis-dermatitis syndrome. Ann Intern Med 84:661, 1976

——— et al: Epidemiology of penicillinase-producing *Neisseria gonorrhoeae* infections: Analysis by auxotyping and serogrouping. N Engl J Med 306:950, 1982

Holmes KK et al: Disseminated gonococcal infection. Ann Intern Med 74:979, 1971

Hook EH III, Holmes KK: Gonococcal infections. Ann Intern Med 102:229, 1985

Knapp JS et al: Serologic classification of *Neisseria gonorrhoeae* using monoclonal antibodies directed against outer membrane protein I. J Infect Dis 150:44, 1985

Panikabutra K et al: Randomized comparative study of ceftriaxone and spectinomycin in gonorrhea. Genitourin Med 61:106, 1985

Petersen BH et al: *Neisseria meningitidis* and *Neisseria gonorrhoeae* bacteremia associated with C6, C7, or C8 deficiency. Ann Intern Med 90:917, 1979

Roberts M et al: Molecular characterization of two beta-lactamase specifying plasmids isolated from *Neisseria gonorrhoeae*. J Bacteriol 131:557, 1977

Roberts RB: *The Gonococcus*. New York, Wiley, 1977

Schoolnik GK et al (eds): *The Pathogenic Neisseria*. Washington, DC, American Society for Microbiology, 1985

105 DISEASES CAUSED BY GRAM-NEGATIVE ENTERIC BACILLI

DENNIS R. SCHABERG / MARVIN TURCK

INTRODUCTION The Enterobacteriaceae are a group of gram-negative nonsporing rods which are aerobic but can grow under anaerobic conditions, and which are commonly found in the gastrointestinal tract. They are characterized biochemically by their ability to ferment glucose, their ability to reduce nitrates to nitrites, and the fact that they are oxidase-negative. The diverse genera in this family, including *Escherichia, Salmonella, Shigella, Klebsiella, Serratia, Enterobacter, Proteus, Morganella, Yersinia, Providencia,* and other less common genera, are differentiated by serologic tests and computerized analysis of biochemical reactions. It is important to make this differentiation, not only taxonomically but also because of epidemiologic and therapeutic implications.

Other gram-negative bacilli which are not members of the family Enterobacteriaceae may also be causes of infection. Important genera include *Pseudomonas, Acinetobacter,* and *Eikenella.*

ESCHERICHIA COLI INFECTIONS

ETIOLOGY *Escherichia coli*, of the family Enterobacteriaceae, is a commensal in the gastrointestinal tract. It may spread from the tract to infect contiguous structures if normal anatomic barriers are interrupted, as occurs in appendiceal perforation. It is believed that the urinary tract is infected from without via urethral contamination, but direct hematogenous spread may also account for renal infection. Once infection has occurred in a primary focus, further spread to distant organs may occur via the bloodstream. A consequence of bacteremia that occurs potentially with all gram-negative bacilli is endotoxin shock (Chap. 86). In more than 50 percent of *E. coli* infections, the urinary tract is the portal of entry; infections emanating from the hepatobiliary tree, peritoneal cavity, skin, and lung are also common. Some patients with *E. coli* bacteremia have no demonstrable portal of entry; they often have neoplastic and hematologic diseases. There may be other defects in host resistance, including diabetes mellitus, cirrhosis, and sickle cell anemia or recent administration of irradiation, cytotoxic drugs, adrenal steroids, or antibiotics. There is also epidemiologic evidence that *E. coli* and other Enterobacteriaceae tend to colonize the skin and mucous membranes of debilitated patients, possibly accounting for the increased frequency of these infections in patients with advanced illness. There is a common misconception that *E. coli* bacterial infections are characterized by a foul-smelling, feculent exudate. Such an odor is caused by anaerobic streptococci or *Bacteroides* species, which are often associated with coliform bacteria in mixed infections.

EPIDEMIOLOGY Strains of *E. coli* are characterized by their somatic (O), flagellar (H), and capsular (K) antigens, and there are hundreds of different serologic varieties. Any of the strains is capable of causing disease. Clinical and epidemiologic studies have demonstrated that certain specific *E. coli* serotypes are more frequently incriminated in diarrheal disease of the infant and newborn as well as in outbreaks of enteric disease in adults. Strains incriminated in infantile diarrhea probably are disseminated within nurseries by symptomatic or asymptomatic infant carriers, mothers, and staff. Although fecal contamination is the usual mode of spread, airborne contamination and fomite spread may also occur.

Some epidemiologic studies have suggested that *E. coli* 04, 06, and 075 are responsible for most *E. coli* infections other than infantile diarrhea. It is unclear whether these strains actually are more virulent or merely are more prevalent than other somatic types.

Strains of *E. coli* with K1 antigen are recovered from an inordinate number of neonates with meningitis. These K antigens have been implicated in promoting adherence to host cells and in resisting phagocytosis.

MANIFESTATIONS **Urinary tract infections** *Escherichia coli* accounts for over 75 percent of urinary tract infections, including cystitis, pyelitis, pyelonephritis, and asymptomatic bacteriuria (see Chap. 225). Strains cultured from patients with acute uncomplicated urinary tract infections are almost invariably *E. coli,* whereas other Enterobacteriaceae and strains of *Pseudomonas* become prevalent among patients with chronic infection.

Peritoneal and biliary infections *Escherichia coli* can usually be cultured from a perforated or inflamed appendix or from abscesses secondary to perforated diverticula, peptic ulcers, subphrenic or lesser sac abscesses, or mesenteric infarction. Often, other organisms, including anaerobic streptococci, clostridia, and *Bacteroides,* are found along with *E. coli.* Acute cholecystitis with gangrene and perforation is often associated with *E. coli* infection. An air-fluid level associated with stones or a circumferential layer of gas in the wall of the gallbladder may be detectable by x-ray and is characteristic of acute emphysematous cholecystitis. From the gallbladder, infection may ascend via the biliary tree to produce cholangitis and multiple liver abscesses. More rarely, *E. coli* infection in the peritoneal cavity may produce a septic thrombophlebitis of the portal vein (pylephlebitis), which in turn is followed by liver abscesses.

Bacteremia Invasion of the bloodstream is the most serious manifestation of *E. coli* infection; it is characterized usually by the sudden onset of fever and chills but sometimes only by mental confusion, dyspnea, or unexplained hypotension. It is most common in patients with urinary tract infection and biliary or intraperitoneal sepsis. In some patients no portal of entry is evident. Most cases occur in elderly males, presumably because of the high incidence of urethral instrumentation and catheterization in this group. Hyperventilation may be an early sign. Hypotension may be present from the onset but usually occurs within 12 to 16 h after bacteremia; if it is persistent, it is accompanied by oliguria and often by mental confusion, stupor, and coma, a syndrome known as *gram-negative* or *endotoxin shock* (see Chap. 86). Occasionally, *E. coli* bacteremia develops in patients with cirrhosis without an overt portal of entry. This has been attributed to portosystemic shunts both in and around the liver, impaired reticuloendothelial function, and diminution in humoral and cellular defense mechanisms. Persistence or reappearance of bacteremia with *E. coli* or other members of the Enterobacteriaceae on therapy, so-called breakthrough bacteremia, has a poor prognosis and suggests an intraabdominal focus for infection or undrained pus.

Other manifestations *Escherichia coli* may produce abscesses anywhere in the body. Subcutaneous infections are found at the site of insulin administration in diabetics, in ischemic extremities, and in surgical wounds. Perirectal phlegmons are not uncommon in patients with leukemia. Subcutaneous abscesses, especially among diabetics, are often characterized by formation of gas in tissue, which may be detected by crepitation or by x-ray and which must be differentiated from clostridial infection. This is most rapidly accomplished by Gram's stain. *Escherichia coli* may cause pneumonia de novo; also, *E. coli* are often cultured from sputum in pulmonary superinfections.

Neonatal infection Neonates, particularly premature infants, often develop *E. coli* bacteremia associated with meningitis and bloodborne pyelonephritis. Fecal soiling and absence of maternal gamma-globulin (IgM) antibody are two of the factors which render this group particularly susceptible to *E. coli* infections.

Gastroenteritis Children under 2 years of age develop gastroenteritis typified by nausea, vomiting, and diarrhea. Most outbreaks have occurred in nurseries and have been due to specific strains of enteropathogenic *E. coli* (EPEC). These strains can produce toxins, one of which is heat labile (LT) and similar to the toxin elaborated by *Vibrio cholerae,* while the other is heat stable (ST) (see also Chaps. 89 and 115). Fluorescent antibody techniques have been useful in the rapid identification of organisms with serotypes frequently implicated in this syndrome. Although theoretically any *E. coli* strain might be cultured, since the genetic information coding for toxin production is found on a plasmid and can be transferred between *E. coli* strains, the number of different serotypes involved remains restricted. Although diarrhea is usually mediated through production of enterotoxins, occasionally *E. coli* may be enteroinvasive, involving the mucosa and causing disease akin to *Shigella* dysentery. The rapid dehydration, with its attendant high mortality, demands prompt recognition of this condition, isolation of the infants, and treatment of both patients and contacts. *Escherichia coli* is also recognized as a cause of acute diarrheal disease in adults, especially in travelers abroad.

LABORATORY FINDINGS There are no characteristic laboratory abnormalities. The white blood cell count is usually elevated, and there is a preponderance of granulocytes. At times, however, the white count is normal or low. When *E. coli* infection occurs in previously healthy individuals, anemia is absent, but more commonly there is anemia which is usually related to underlying disease. *Escherichia coli* grows readily in a variety of bacteriologic media and should be cultured from appropriate secretions and blood. In the presence of bacteremia there can be metabolic derangements, including azotemia, metabolic acidosis, hypokalemia, and hyperkalemia as well as a variety of coagulation defects.

DIAGNOSIS *Escherichia coli* cannot be differentiated from most other gram-negative bacteria on Gram's stain, and culture followed by appropriate biochemical characterization is necessary to identify the organism precisely. Serologic typing of *E. coli* may be useful in individual patients with recurrent urinary tract infections in order to help differentiate between relapse and reinfection.

TREATMENT As with other infections, drainage of pus and removal of foreign bodies are essential. If *E. coli* is suspected as the etiologic agent in a particular infection, choice of an appropriate antimicrobial will depend upon the site and type of infection as well as upon its severity; outcome is often related to underlying disease. For example, in acute, uncomplicated urinary tract infection in females, the disease is frequently self-limited even without antimicrobial therapy, and there is no evidence that antibiotics are superior to sulfonamides. Conversely, *E. coli* bacteremia in a patient with leukemia may not respond to antimicrobials unless a hematologic remission is achieved simultaneously.

In most situations, antibiotics should be selected on the basis of in vitro susceptibility tests. Although no drug is uniformly active against all strains of *E. coli,* a number of agents are effective against the majority of clinical isolates. Although resistant strains can be encountered, especially in hospital-acquired *E. coli,* ampicillin remains an effective drug when given in doses of 2 to 4 g per day intravenously, intramuscularly, or orally. For severe infections the dose of ampicillin can be raised to 12 g per day, usually given intravenously. The cephalosporins are also effective against *E. coli;* compounds such as cefazolin and cephapirin provide effective therapy. Newer so-called third generation cephalosporins have lower minimal inhibitory concentrations (MICs) for *E. coli*; this increased activity coupled with slightly enhanced CNS penetration make them useful for the therapy of meningitis due to *E. coli* (see Chap. 346). Gentamicin and tobramycin have been employed effectively in the initial treatment of severe *E. coli* infections in doses of 5 mg/kg per day in divided doses every 8 h. Amikacin is very active against isolates which are resistant to the other aminoglycosides in doses of 15 mg/kg per day, divided to be administered every 8 to 12 h. Tetracyclines and chloramphenicol are still used in the treatment of *E. coli* infection, but better drugs are now available. Although combinations of antimicrobials have been recommended there is little need to employ more than one agent in most situations. Nitrofurantoin (400 mg) and nalidixic acid (2 to 4 g) are reserved for treating patients with *E. coli* bacteriuria, and should not be employed when infection is suspected outside the urinary tract. Trimethoprim/sulfamethoxazole is also useful in urinary tract infections.

PREVENTION Isolation and antimicrobial therapy of infants and contacts are essential to abort epidemic infantile diarrhea. In adults, many *E. coli* infections are hospital-associated, and their incidence can be reduced by limiting use of indwelling urinary and intravenous catheters, by careful surgical aseptic technique, by appropriate isolation of infection-prone patients, and by judicious use of antibiotics, glucocorticosteroids, and cytotoxic agents.

KLEBSIELLA-ENTEROBACTER-SERRATIA INFECTIONS

ETIOLOGY Next to *E. coli,* strains of *Klebsiella, Enterobacter,* and *Serratia* are the most important enteric organisms infecting humans. These are also of the family Enterobacteriaceae. In many laboratories *Klebsiella* are more resistant to antibiotics than are *E. coli,* and their isolation from blood, purulent exudates, and urine is of more serious epidemiologic and prognostic significance. The Friedlander bacilli (*K. pneumoniae*) are encapsulated gram-negative bacilli found among the normal flora of the mouth and intestinal tracts. *Klebsiella* are closely related to the genera *Enterobacter* and *Serratia* and may be differentiated only by certain amino acid decarboxylase tests. In addition to differentiation by these biochemical tests, which identify the *Klebsiella, Enterobacter,* and *Serratia* groups, strains of *Klebsiella* usually are nonmotile and form large mucoid colonies on solid media, whereas the other species are typically motile. Strains of *Klebsiella* can be further distinguished on the basis of type-specific capsular antigens; more than 75 known capsular types have been identified. There is little evidence that certain types are more virulent than others, and the main role of capsular typing of *Klebsiella* is an epidemiologic tool in nosocomial outbreaks of infection.

Klebsiella rhinoscleromatis is probably the causative agent of rhinoscleroma, and *K. ozenae* has been isolated occasionally from the noses of patients with ozena, a chronic severe rhinitis associated with turbinate atrophy and progressive anosmia. *Klebsiella oxytoca* is the new designation for indole-positive strains of *K. pneumoniae*.

PATHOGENESIS *Klebsiella, Enterobacter,* and *Serratia* are all capable of causing disease in diverse anatomic sites. However, results of clinical and epidemiologic studies suggest that differences in pathogenicity may exist among these genera and that precise taxonomic identification is of value. Although infections of the respiratory tract with *K. pneumoniae* have been emphasized most in the past, the urinary tract presently accounts for the majority of clinical isolates. In this site clinical manifestations and pathogenesis are similar to those of infections produced by *E. coli,* but *Klebsiella* is more frequently found in patients with complicated and obstructive urinary tract disease. Infections of the biliary tract, peritoneal cavity, middle ear, mastoids, paranasal sinuses, and meninges also are not uncommon. In these locations, *Klebsiella* is more frequent than either *Enterobacter* or *Serratia* and is more likely to produce an illness of greater severity. The apparent increased frequency of infection by *Serratia* represents an increase primarily due to nosocomial spread of this organism. *Enterobacter* species have been incriminated frequently in outbreaks of in-hospital bacteremia attributed to contaminated intravenous solutions.

MANIFESTATIONS Symptoms and signs of common infections caused by *Klebsiella*—namely, those involving the urinary tract, biliary tree, and peritoneal cavity—are indistinguishable from those caused by *E. coli.* These infections commonly occur in diabetics and in the form of superinfections in patients who have received antimicrobials to which these organisms are resistant. *Klebsiella* infection is also an important etiologic factor in septic shock. *Serratia* and *Enterobacter* are almost exclusively nosocomial pathogens. These organisms have been implicated as pathogens in a wide variety of infections, most frequently pneumonia, urinary tract infections, and bacteremia.

Pneumonia *Klebsiella* is well recognized as a pulmonary pathogen but probably accounts for less than 1 percent of all cases of bacterial pneumonia. The disease is most common in men over 40 years of age and is most frequently found in alcoholics. Other factors associated with increased susceptibility include diabetes mellitus and chronic bronchopulmonary disease. Aspiration of oropharyngeal secretions containing *Klebsiella* organisms is the likely inciting factor among alcoholic patients. The clinical manifestations are indistinguishable from those of pneumococcal pneumonia (see Chap. 93), with sudden onset of chills, fever, productive cough, and severe pleuritic chest pain. Patients are frequently delirious and prostrated, but this may also occur with pneumococcal infection. The pulmonary lesion is most frequent in the right upper lobe but often rapidly progresses and, if untreated, may spread from lobe to lobe. Cyanosis and dyspnea develop rapidly, and jaundice, vomiting, and diarrhea may be present. Physical findings consist primarily of consolidation, unless pleural effusion or necrotizing pneumonitis with rapid cavitation has intervened. The blood leukocyte count may be elevated but is often low, which probably is a reflection of severe infection in an alcoholic patient with poor bone marrow reserve and folate deficiency. Lung abscess and empyema are much more frequent than they are in pneumococcal pneumonia; they are related to the destructive capabilities of this organism. So-called characteristic radiographic features such as bulging fissures and loss of lung volume occur only occasionally; they also may be found in pneumococcal infection as well as in necrotizing pneumonia caused by other gram-negative species.

Klebsiella, Serratia, and *Enterobacter* are frequently seen in nosocomial pneumonia. Older patients become colonized with gram-negative bacilli in the oropharynx, and these organisms can then gain access to the respiratory tract and cause pneumonia or purulent bronchitis. Common-source outbreaks, with contamination of a variety of respiratory therapy devices, have been implicated in infections with these pathogens, especially *Serratia.* As a general rule, the most drug-resistant strains of *Serratia* are nonpigmented and account for the majority of nosocomial isolates. However, pigmented and multiply sensitive *Serratia* isolates are also seen in device-related infections. Rarely, infection with *Klebsiella* may progress, often in indolent fashion, to a chronic necrotizing pneumonitis resembling tuberculosis. The principal symptoms are productive cough, weakness, and anemia.

DIAGNOSIS Diagnosis of community-acquired pneumonia is established by an awareness of the clinical setting in which *Klebsiella* infections occur and by isolation of the organism. A presumptive diagnosis of *Klebsiella* pneumonia should be made on the basis of a Gram's stain of the sputum which shows a predominance of short, plump, gram-negative bacilli, frequently surrounded by a clear space because of the capsule. Often these gram-negative organisms occur together with gram-positive cocci, and because the gram-positives are easier to see, the gram-negative bacteria may be ignored and the diagnosis may be missed. This, in turn, may lead to potentially serious delays in instituting therapy. Additional proof of *Klebsiella* infection in the lung is the isolation of the organisms from blood and pleural exudate. In extrapulmonary infections, the organisms are readily seen in, or cultured from, pus or secretions of involved organs.

The diagnosis of nosocomial respiratory infection with these organisms may be more difficult, mainly because colonization has to be distinguished from infection. Careful evaluation of the clinical course is necessary in establishing a diagnosis. Transtracheal aspiration of sputum for culture and Gram's stain may be useful in difficult cases.

TREATMENT *Klebsiella, Enterobacter,* and *Serratia* have variable susceptibility to antimicrobial drugs, and cultures of these organisms need to be tested in vitro. Frequently, antimicrobial therapy needs to be begun before results of antibiotic susceptibility tests are available. In general, most strains of *Klebsiella* are susceptible to the aminoglycosides and the newer third generation cephalosporins. *Klebsiella* isolates do not respond to most penicillin analogues, although many isolates are inhibited by newer ureidopenicillins, e.g., mezlocillin. *Serratia* isolates are frequently resistant to many antimicrobials, and resistance to gentamicin and tobramycin is being encountered with increasing frequency. Amikacin has been used effectively in these drug-resistant infections. The antimicrobial regimen of choice in the treatment of *Klebsiella, Enterobacter,* and *Serratia* infection will vary from one institution to another depending on the resistance patterns as well as upon the degree of clinical severity of infection. In severely ill patients, the combination of an aminoglycoside such as tobramycin or gentamicin (3 to 5 mg/kg per day) or amikacin (15 mg/kg per day) with cephalothin, cephapirin, or cefazolin (4 to 12 g per day) is usually preferred. The new cephalosporins and/or cephamycins, i.e., cefoxitin, or third generation compounds also may be active against *Klebsiella, Enterobacter,* and *Serratia.* Occasionally, one or all of these compounds may be more active than the older cephalosporins, and in vitro susceptibility tests will be required to select the most appropriate agent. Because of the relatively poor blood and tissue levels obtained with the polymyxins, they should not be employed as first-line agents in the treatment of severe *Klebsiella* infections despite apparent in vitro susceptibility. Regardless of the antimicrobial regimen employed, treatment should be continued for a minimum of 10 to 14 days and prolonged if there is extensive cavitation. Pleural effusions must be drained; antibiotic therapy alone is not sufficient treatment for closed-space infections of the pleural cavity. At times, rib resection with open drainage may be necessary and should be considered if effusions recur.

PROGNOSIS Before the introduction of antimicrobials, the fatality rate from these infections varied from 50 to 80 percent, and death within 48 h was not infrequent. Even with antimicrobial treatment the course of these infections is quite variable and the prognosis must be guarded. For the most part, the prognosis reflects the age group involved and the frequent association of *Klebsiella* infections with alcoholism, malnutrition, and severe underlying disease.

PROTEUS, MORGANELLA, AND *PROVIDENCIA* INFECTIONS

ETIOLOGY The genus *Proteus* of the family Enterobacteriaceae consists of gram-negative bacilli which do not ferment lactose and are characterized by their active motility and spreading growth on solid media. Organisms once thought to be related and once classified as *Proteus* have recently been renamed based on detailed DNA studies. *Proteus morganii* has been reclassified as *Morganella morganii,* while some biogroups of *Proteus rettgeri* have been reclassified as *Providencia stuartii* and *Providencia rettgeri. Proteus mirabilis* and *Proteus vulgaris* retain their nomenclature; *Proteus mirabilis* causes 75 to 90 percent of human infections. It is distinguishable from the other organisms mentioned by its inability to form indole. All four split urea, with production of ammonia. Some strains of *Proteus vulgaris* share a common antigen with certain rickettsia, which accounts for the appearance of antibodies against *Proteus* organisms (Weil-Felix reaction) in typhus, scrub typhus, and Rocky Mountain spotted fever. The *Providencia* group of organisms resembles those of the genus *Proteus* closely except for some differences in biochemical tests.

EPIDEMIOLOGY AND PATHOGENESIS These organisms are normally found in soil, water, and sewage and are part of the normal fecal flora. Occasionally, they have been implicated as a cause of epidemic diarrhea in infants, but the evidence for this is inconclusive. They are frequently cultured from superficial wounds, draining ears, and sputum, particularly in patients who have received antibiotics; they replace the more susceptible flora eradicated by these drugs.

MANIFESTATIONS These organisms are rarely primary invaders but produce disease in locations previously infected by other pathogens. These locations include skin, ears and mastoid, sinuses, eyes, peritoneal cavity, bone, urinary tract, meninges, lung, and bloodstream.

Cutaneous infections These organisms can be isolated from surgical wounds, particularly after antimicrobial therapy, but they do not interfere with normal wound healing provided that the tissues are viable and foreign bodies are not present. Burns, varicose ulcers, and decubitus ulcers may become contaminated with these organisms, often in company with other gram-negative bacilli or staphylococci.

Infections of the ears and mastoid sinuses Otitis media and mastoiditis, especially with *Proteus mirabilis,* can result in extensive destruction of the middle ear and mastoid sinuses. Fetid otorrhea, cholesteatoma, and granulation tissue constitute a chronic focus of infection in the middle and inner ears and mastoid, and deafness ensues. Paralysis of the facial nerve is an occasional complication. The great danger of these infections lies in intracranial extension, leading to thrombosis of the lateral sinus, meningitis, brain abscess, and bacteremia.

Ocular infections These pathogens may cause corneal ulcers, usually following trauma to the eye, which occasionally terminate in panophthalmitis and destruction of the eyeball.

Peritonitis Because they are part of the normal intestinal flora, these organisms may be isolated from the peritoneal cavity following perforation of viscera or mesenteric infarction.

Urinary tract infections These organisms are a common cause of urinary tract infections, usually in patients with chronic bacteriuria, many of whom have had obstructive uropathy, a history of bladder instrumentation, and repeated courses of chemotherapy. They are often recovered from bacteriuric patients with renal or bladder calculi. This may be related to the urease activity which renders the urine alkaline and provides a fertile medium for formation of ammonium-magnesium-phosphate stones.

Bacteremia Bloodstream invasion is the most serious manifestation of infection with this organism. In 75 percent of cases, the urinary tract serves as the portal of entry; in the remainder, the biliary tree, gastrointestinal tract, ears and sinuses, and skin are the primary foci. Bacteremia is frequently preceded by cystoscopy, urethral catheterization, transurethral prostatic resection, or other operative procedures. Clinically, the signs, symptoms, and laboratory findings of sepsis—high fever, chills, shock, metastatic abscess, leukocytosis, and rarely thrombocytopenia—are indistinguishable from those of bloodstream infections with *E. coli, Klebsiella,* or other gram-negative bacteria.

DIAGNOSIS The diagnosis of *Proteus, Morganella,* or *Providencia* infection depends on culture of the organism from blood, urine, or exudate and its identification by appropriate biochemical tests. It is especially important to separate *Proteus mirabilis,* the indole-negative species, from organisms that are indole-positive, because only *P. mirabilis* is susceptible to the action of penicillin and many other antibiotics. *Proteus* organisms are often present in mixed infections with other pathogens. Particular care should be exercised in the isolation of other organisms growing in the same medium with *Proteus mirabilis* or *Proteus vulgaris* lest they be masked by spreading growth. The spreading character of these bacteria also may make antibiotic sensitivity tests difficult to interpret.

TREATMENT Most strains of *Proteus mirabilis* are sensitive to penicillin in high concentration (10 units per milliliter or greater), ampicillin, carbenicillin, gentamicin, tobramycin, or amikacin, and the cephalosporin antibiotics. *Proteus mirabilis* bacteriuria can be readily eradicated with any of these drugs during treatment; ampicillin in dosage of 0.5 gm every 4 to 6 h is highly effective. In severe infection, therapy should be parenteral: 6 to 12 g ampicillin or 20 million units of penicillin G plus tobramycin or gentamicin in divided doses of 5 mg/kg per day, if renal function is adequate. There is some evidence that an aminoglycoside is synergistic with ampicillin and penicillin G in *P. mirabilis* infections. In view of the numerous more effective agents, there is no reason to use chloramphenicol in *P. mirabilis* infections. In general, all strains of *P. mirabilis* are resistant to tetracycline. Most strains other than *P. mirabilis* are predictably sensitive only to aminoglycosides and the third generation cephalosporins. Carbenicillin, ticarcillin, and the new ureidopenicillins are effective against many isolates. Ideally, therapy should be based on in vitro susceptibility, or lacking this, an awareness of local resistance patterns. As with all other gram-negative infections, appropriate attention must be given to drainage of pus, maintenance of fluid and electrolyte status, and, if endotoxin shock is present, treatment of circulatory collapse.

PSEUDOMONAS INFECTIONS

ETIOLOGY *Pseudomonas aeruginosa* is a motile gram-negative rod which generally is not encapsulated and forms no spores. It grows readily in all ordinary culture media, and on agar it forms irregular, soft, iridescent colonies which usually have a fluorescent yellow-green color because of diffusion into the medium of two pigments, pyocyanin and fluorescin. *Pseudomonas* produces acid but no gas in glucose, and it is proteolytic. It is oxidase-positive and produces ammonia from arginine. A number of different strains have been identified by immunofluorescent techniques or bacteriophage typing. There is no evidence that these strains vary in their virulence for humans. Other *Pseudomonas* species (*P. maltophilia, P. cepacia, P. fluorescens, P. testosteroni,* and *P. putida*) also may cause infection in human beings. For the most part, these organisms have been associated with common-source nosocomial outbreaks; in addition, they have been incriminated in bacteremia, endocarditis, and osteomyelitis in narcotic addicts.

EPIDEMIOLOGY *Pseudomonas* organisms are present on the skin of some normal persons, particularly in the axilla and anogenital regions. They are uncommon in the stools of adults not receiving antibiotics. In the majority of instances, *Pseudomonas* organisms are cultured as avirulent secondary contaminants in superficial wounds or from the sputum of patients treated with antibiotics. Ordinarily this is of little consequence because the organisms merely fill the bacteriologic vacuum left by the elimination of more sensitive bacteria. Occasionally, however, infections with *Pseudomonas* organisms occur in the ear, lung, skin, or urinary tract of patients, often after the primary pathogen has been eradicated by antibiotics. Serious infections are almost invariably associated with damage to local tissue or with diminished host resistance. Despite the many potential virulence factors shared by strains of *Pseudomonas,* the organism rarely causes disease in healthy persons. Patients compromised by cystic fibrosis and those with neutropenia appear at particular risk to severe infection with *P. aeruginosa.* Premature infants; children with congenital anomalies and patients with leukemia (who are usually receiving antibiotics, adrenal glucocorticosteroids or antineoplastic drugs); patients with burns; and geriatric patients with debilitating diseases are likely to develop *Pseudomonas* infections. Most often these infections occur in the hospital environment, and they generally are exogenous infections with the organism acquired from sources other than the patient's normal flora. In hospitals, the organisms have been cultured from a variety of sources that share in common an aqueous environment, including such items as sinks, antiseptic solutions, and aqueous medications. The organism is prevalent in urine receptacles and on catheters, and on the hands of hospital staff. In several outbreaks, *Pseudomonas* urinary tract infections appear to have been transmitted from patient to patient by human carriers. Similar epidemics have been reported in nurseries among premature infants, and cross infection on burn wards is common. Although *P. aeruginosa* is found in the gastrointestinal tract of only approximately 5 percent of normal adults, carriage rates increase in hospitalized patients.

PATHOGENESIS The portal of entry of *Pseudomonas* organisms varies with the patient's age and underlying disease. In infancy and childhood, the skin, umbilical cord, and gastrointestinal tract predominate; in old age, the urinary tract is more often the primary focus. Often the infections remain localized to the skin or subcutaneous tissues. In burns, the region below the eschar may become massively infiltrated with bacteria and inflammatory cells and usually serves as the focus for bacteremia, the single most lethal complication. Hematogenous dissemination is characterized by hemorrhagic nodules in many areas, including the skin, heart, lungs, kidneys, and meninges. The histologic picture is one of necrosis and hemorrhage. Typically the walls of arterioles are heavily infiltrated with bacteria, and the vessels are partially or wholly thrombosed.

Most strains of *P. aeruginosa* produce a layer of slime which is rich in carbohydrate and shares heat stable somatic antigenicity with the cell wall. Antibody against the specific serologic type of slime antigen affords protection to experimental challenge. Most isolates also produce a number of exotoxins. Exotoxin A, which shares many properties with diphtheria toxin, is the most potent toxin produced by *P. aeruginosa*. In life-threatening infection with *P. aeruginosa*, high antibody titers against exotoxin A correlate with increased survival.

MANIFESTATIONS *Pseudomonas* infections occur in many locations, including the skin, subcutaneous tissues, bone and joints, eyes, ears, mastoid and paranasal sinuses, meninges, and heart valves. Bacteremia without a detectable primary focus may also occur and should raise the question of contaminated intravenous medications, intravenous solutions, or antiseptics used for preparing an intravenous site, especially when *Pseudomonas* species other than *P. aeruginosa* are isolated.

Infections of the skin and subcutaneous tissues *Pseudomonas* organisms are frequently cultured from surgical wounds, varicose and decubitus ulcers, and burns, particularly following antibiotic therapy. Draining tuberculous or osteomyelitic sinuses may become secondarily infected. The mere presence of *Pseudomonas* in these sites is of little significance provided that bacterial multiplication deep in subcutaneous tissues does not occur and bacteremia does not ensue. Cutaneous infections usually heal after removal or slough of devitalized tissue. *Pseudomonas* organisms may be responsible for green nails in persons whose hands are excessively exposed to water, soap, and detergents, who have onychomycosis, or whose hands are subject to mechanical trauma. The organism can usually be cultured from the nail plate. *Pseudomonas* has been incriminated in whirlpool-associated dermatitis. The disease is benign and resolves spontaneously.

Osteomyelitis Osteomyelitis is unusual with *Pseudomonas* except as a complication of bacteremia, intravenous drug abuse, or puncture wounds. If a puncture wound, especially a nail puncture of the foot in a child, fails to respond to standard therapy within 3 to 4 days, complicating *Pseudomonas* osteomyelitis must be considered.

Infections of the ear, mastoid, and paranasal sinuses Otitis externa is the most common form of *Pseudomonas* infection which involves the ear. It is particularly troublesome in tropical climates and is characterized by chronic serosanguineous and purulent drainage from the external auditory canal. A rapidly progressive, severe infection due to *Pseudomonas* involving the ear, referred to as malignant otitis externa, can develop, especially in diabetics. In contrast to the usual otitis externa, this infection requires aggressive management including surgical debridement and parenteral antimicrobial therapy. Otitis media or mastoiditis usually occurs as a superinfection following eradication of gram-positive organisms by antimicrobial agents.

Infections of the eye Corneal ulceration is the most severe form of ocular *Pseudomonas* infection. It usually follows a traumatic abrasion and may terminate in panophthalmitis and destruction of the globe. Purulent conjunctivitis occurs as a manifestation of *Pseudomonas* infection in premature infants. Contamination of contact lenses or lens fluid may be an important means of infecting the eyes with *Pseudomonas*.

Urinary tract infections *Pseudomonas* organisms are common pathogens in the urinary tract and are usually found in patients with obstructive uropathy who have been subjected to repeated urethral manipulations or to urologic surgery. *Pseudomonas* bacteriuria is in no way unique and cannot be distinguished from infection with other organisms on clinical grounds.

Gastrointestinal tract *Pseudomonas* organisms have been implicated as a cause of epidemic diarrhea of infancy. In addition, a number of infants dying from neonatal sepsis have the classic necrotic, avascular ulcers of *Pseudomonas* bacteremia in the bowel at autopsy. A "typhoidal" form of *Pseudomonas* infection characterized by fever, myalgia, and diarrhea occurs predominantly in the tropics. This illness, also called 13-day fever or Shanghai fever, is self-limited, and the prognosis is good.

Respiratory tract Primary *Pseudomonas* pneumonia is infrequent and culture of this organism from the sputum usually is indicative of aspiration of oropharyngeal contents with secondary infection following eradication of a more sensitive flora with antibiotics. The normal oropharyngeal flora of hospitalized patients is frequently replaced by gram-negative rods, including *Pseudomonas*, early in hospitalization. A variety of nosocomial events, most notably administration of sedative medications, endotracheal intubation, and intermittent positive pressure breathing treatments, can predispose to respiratory infection with *Pseudomonas*. Pulmonary infection is often associated with microabscesses. The organism is often isolated from the sputum of patients with bronchiectasis, chronic bronchitis, or cystic fibrosis who have lingering infections punctuated by multiple courses of chemotherapy, and it is recovered frequently from the stomata of tracheostomy sites. *Pseudomonas* bronchitis and bronchiolitis may be the terminal event in cystic fibrosis, and sputum isolates from these patients often have a characteristic mucoid colonial morphology when cultured on agar.

Meningitis Spontaneous *Pseudomonas* meningitis is unusual, but the bacilli may be introduced into the subarachnoid space by lumbar puncture, spinal anesthesia, intrathecal medication, or head trauma. Shunts performed for hydrocephalus may become contaminated with *Pseudomonas*, and revision or removal of the shunt offers the best hope of cure.

Bacteremia Bloodstream invasion tends to occur in debilitated patients, premature infants, children with congenital defects, patients with lymphomas, leukemias, or other malignant tumors, and elderly patients who have undergone surgery or instrumentation of the biliary or urinary tract. *Pseudomonas* bacteremia is an important cause of death in patients with severe burns. In adults, *Pseudomonas* bacteremia is indistinguishable from bloodstream infection with other bacterial species except for two findings: (1) ecthyma gangrenosum, the classic skin lesion, often located in the anogenital or axillary region as a round, indurated, purple-black area about 1 cm in diameter with an ulcerated center and a surrounding zone of erythema; and (2) rarely, the passage of green urine, presumably due to the hemoglobin pigment verdoglobin. Organisms usually can be cultured from cutaneous lesions and may provide an early clue to the diagnosis.

Bacterial endocarditis A number of cases of *Pseudomonas* subacute bacterial endocarditis have followed open-heart surgery. Usually the organisms become implanted on a silk suture or a synthetic patch employed for closure of septal defects. Reoperation with removal of the vegetation and foreign bodies offers the best hope of cure. *Pseudomonas* endocarditis has been found on normal heart valves in patients with burns and in drug addicts. Metastatic abscesses in bone, joint, brain, adrenal glands, and lungs are frequent consequences of *Pseudomonas* endocarditis.

TREATMENT Localized *Pseudomonas* infection can be treated by irrigation with 1% acetic acid or topical therapy with colistin or polymyxin B. Debridement and drainage of purulent material is essential when deeper tissues are involved. For deep-seated tissue infections and life-threatening infection, such as pneumonia or bacteremia, parenteral therapy must be employed. The aminoglycoside antibiotics, tobramycin and gentamicin, inhibit most strains of *Pseudomonas*. In patients with normal renal function, 5 mg/kg per day in divided doses will provide inhibitory levels. Amikacin is also active against *Pseudomonas* and is especially useful against strains which have developed enzyme-mediated drug resistance to tobramycin and gentamicin. It should be given in doses of 15 mg/kg per day in divided doses. Ticarcillin and mezlocillin are active against most strains of *Pseudomonas* in doses of 16 to 20 g per day. Piperacillin and azlocillin are active in vitro against some isolates not inhibited by ticarcillin. These isolates are usually nosocomial in origin. The combination of an aminoglycoside active against *Pseudomonas* plus an antipseudomonal penicillin is frequently employed to delay emergence of resistance during therapy and provides enhanced activity, especially in granulocytopenic patients with *Pseudomonas* infection. Asymptomatic bacteriuria, particularly when confined to the bladder, should be treated with the least toxic agent, which at times may be a sulfonamide or tetracycline. The antimicrobial susceptibility of *Pseudomonas,* except for *P. aeruginosa,* is variable, and some of these isolates may be resistant to aminoglycoside antibiotics. Some of the newer cephalosporins like cefoperazone and ceftazidime are also active in vitro against many isolates of *Pseudomonas*.

PROPHYLAXIS *Pseudomonas* cross infections in hospitals can be reduced by careful attention to aseptic techniques and good infection control practices (see Chap. 85). Systemic antibiotic prophylaxis aimed at preventing colonization and infection with *Pseudomonas* organisms has been notoriously unsuccessful and should be interdicted. A polyvalent vaccine for *Pseudomonas* has been developed, as well as hyperimmune gamma globulin, but it has not been used widely.

PROGNOSIS The mortality rate in *Pseudomonas* bacteremia is 75 percent and is highest in patients with shock or severe associated disease such as massive third-degree burns, leukemia, or prematurity. When bacteremia originates in the urinary tract and is not accompanied by shock, the prognosis is considerably better. Localized *Pseudomonas* infections do not present a threat to life unless hematogenous dissemination occurs.

ACINETOBACTER INFECTIONS

DEFINITION Organisms of the genus *Acinetobacter* are pleomorphic, gram-negative bacilli which are easily confused with members of the genus *Neisseria*. Severe infections with these organisms, including meningitis, bacterial endocarditis, pneumonia, and bacteremia, have been described with increasing frequency.

ETIOLOGY *Acinetobacter calcoaceticus* var. *lwoffi* was described by DeBord as *Mima polymorpha* in 1939. It is one of two well-characterized varieties of *Acinetobacter,* the other being *Acinetobacter calcoaceticus* var. *anitratus,* formerly called *Herellea vaginicola*. Organisms described as *Bacterium anitratum* and B5W are synonymous with *Acinetobacter*. These organisms are pleomorphic, gram-negative, encapsulated, and nonmotile. They grow well on ordinary media, forming white, convex, smooth colonies. Diplococcal forms predominate in colonies grown on solid media; rods and filamentous forms are more common in liquid media. The species can be differentiated from the Enterobacteriaceae by their negative nitrate reaction and from members of the genus *Neisseria,* which they may resemble morphologically, by their simple growth requirements, their bacillary form in liquid media, and their usually negative oxidase reaction.

EPIDEMIOLOGY AND PATHOGENESIS *Acinetobacter* organisms are ubiquitous. Twenty-five percent of normal subjects are skin carriers of *Acinetobacter*. The striking association of *Acinetobacter* bacteremia with cutdowns or indwelling intravenous catheters favors the skin as a major portal of entry in human beings. The increasing incidence of *Acinetobacter* pneumonia, both as a primary infection and as a superinfection, also points to the respiratory tract as an important portal of entry. It appears that *Acinetobacter* organisms are normal human commensals of relatively low virulence which produce colonization much more frequently than infection. Infections seem to occur in patients subjected to the same epidemiologic pressures encountered with nosocomial, gram-negative bacilli; serious infections are produced under conditions of decreased host resistance, or in the presence of instrumentation, or with prior broad-spectrum antimicrobial therapy. An unexplained predominance of *Acinetobacter* pulmonary infections occurring in late summer has been noted. The role of these organisms as a cause of conjunctivitis, vaginitis, and urethritis requires further documentation.

MANIFESTATIONS Serious infections caused by *Acinetobacter* include (1) meningitis, (2) subacute and acute bacterial endocarditis, (3) pneumonia, (4) urinary tract infections, and (5) bacteremia. Usually, the signs and symptoms associated with infections in these sites are no different from those produced by other pathogens. Occasionally, *Acinetobacter* may be the cause of a fulminating bacteremia, with high fever, vascular collapse, petechiae, and ecchymoses, which is indistinguishable from fulminant meningococcemia. More often, however, bacteremia is associated with an overt portal of entry, such as infected cutdowns or indwelling intravenous catheters, surgical wounds, or burns; it may follow urethral or other surgical instrumentation. The clinical picture presented by these patients is dominated by endotoxemia, and the prognosis is poor.

DIAGNOSIS The diagnosis of *Acinetobacter* infection can be missed, either because the clinical bacteriology laboratory is unfamiliar with these organisms and reports them incorrectly or because they are considered contaminants. The confusion attending the taxonomic classification of these organisms has not simplified matters. For practical purposes, isolation of *Acinetobacter* from blood, spinal fluid, sputum, urine, or pus should be considered significant unless there is no evidence of infection on clinical grounds. Since *Acinetobacter* isolates are resistant to penicillin and members of the genus *Neisseria* are sensitive, differentiation of these organisms is of obvious importance.

TREATMENT Antibiotic sensitivities of *Acinetobacter* strains vary, but most strains are inhibited by gentamicin, tobramycin, amikacin, and the ureidopenicillins such as piperacillin. Sensitivity to the tetracyclines is unpredictable, and most strains are resistant to penicillin, ampicillin, the cephalosporins, erythromycin, and chloramphenicol. For serious systemic infections, the appropriate antibiotic, generally an aminoglycoside, should be administered, and since these organisms may produce localized abscesses, surgical drainage may be necessary.

EIKENELLA INFECTIONS

ETIOLOGY *Eikenella corrodens* is a facultatively anaerobic or capnophilic gram-negative rod which is oxidase-positive. As colonies develop on blood agar, characteristic "pitting" or "corroding" of the agar is seen with many strains and generally requires 48 to 72 h of growth to develop.

EPIDEMIOLOGY *Eikenella corrodens* is an inhabitant of the mouth, upper respiratory tract, and gastrointestinal tract of humans. Infections frequently involve bowel or oral contamination. A striking association between *Eikenella* infections and methylphenidate abuse has been noted, perhaps related to the low redox potential created by "skin popping" of this agent as well as a tendency for needles to become contaminated with oral secretions through needle licking.

MANIFESTATIONS The most common infection caused by *Eikenella* is that of skin or soft tissue. Endocarditis, pneumonia, osteomyelitis, and meningitis are reported but are rare. *Eikenella* infections frequently mimic infections caused by strict anaerobes such as *Bacteroides* *fragilis* or *Peptostreptococcus*. The infections are indolent and frequently mixed with aerobic gram-positive cocci, and drainage is often foul-smelling. Abscess formation is common.

TREATMENT *Eikenella corrodens* is susceptible to penicillin, ampicillin, carbenicillin, and tetracycline. Adequate drainage of purulent material is essential in the management of these infections. Ampicillin or penicillin coupled with surgical drainage generally provides a good response. Of note is the marked resistance of *Eikenella* to clindamycin, making the differentiation between *Eikenella* infections and those caused by mixed anaerobes even more important.

REFERENCES

Enterobacteriaceae: General

KREGER BE et al: Gram negative bacteremia. Am J Med 68:332, 1980

MAKI DG: Nosocomial bacteremia: An epidemiologic overview. Am J Med 70:719, 1981

MOORE RD et al: Association of aminoglycoside plasma levels with therapeutic outcome in gram-negative pneumonia. Am J Med 77:657, 1984

SCHABERG DR et al: Epidemics of nosocomial urinary tract infection caused by multiply-resistant gram-negative bacilli: Epidemiology and control. J Infect Dis 133:363, 1976

TANCREDE CH, ANDREMONT AO: Bacterial translocation and gram-negative bacteremia in patients with hematological malignancies. J Infect Dis 152:99, 1985

Escherichia coli infections

BERK SL, MCCABE WR: Meningitis caused by gram-negative bacilli. Ann Int Med 93:253, 1980

CONN HO, FESSEL JM: Spontaneous bacterial peritonitis in cirrhosis. Medicine 50:161, 1971

GERACI JE et al: Endocarditis due to gram-negative bacteria. Mayo Clin Proc 57:145, 1982

Klebsiella-Enterobacter-Serratia infections

COOPER R, MILLS J: *Serratia* endocarditis. Arch Intern Med 140:199, 1980

MELTZ DJ, GRIECO MH: Characteristics of *Serratia marcescens* pneumonia. Arch Intern Med 132:359, 1973

RENNIE RP, DUNCAN IBR: Emergence of gentamicin resistant *Klebsiella* in a general hospital. Antimicrob Agents Chemother 11:179, 1978

Proteus infections

IANNINI PB et al: Multidrug resistant *P. rettgeri*. Ann Intern Med 55:161, 1976

LEWIS J, FEKETY FR: *Proteus* bacteremia. Johns Hopkins Med J 124:151, 1969

MUSCHER DM et al: Role of urease in pyelonephritis resulting from urinary tract infections with *Proteus*. J Infect Dis 131:177, 1975

Pseudomonas infections

BAGEL J, GROSSMAN ME: Subcutaneous nodules in *Pseudomonas* sepsis. Am J Med 80:528, 1986

BODEY GP et al: Infections caused by *Pseudomonas aeruginosa*. Rev Infect Dis 5:279, 1983

COLLINI FJ et al: Ecthyma gangrenosum in a kidney transplant recipient with *Pseudomonas* septicemia. Am J Med 80:729, 1986

DOGGETT RG (ed): *Pseudomonas aeruginosa: Clinical manifestations of infection and current therapy*. New York, Academic, 1979

FLICK MR, CLUFF LE: *Pseudomonas* bacteremia. Review of 108 cases. Am J Med 60:501, 1976

POLLACK M: The role of exotoxin A in *Pseudomonas* disease and immunity. Rev Infect Dis 5(suppl):S979, 1983

Acinetobacter infections

BUXTON AE et al: Nosocomial respiratory tract infection and colonization with *Acinetobacter calcoaceticus*. Am J Med 65:507, 1978

GLEW RH et al: Infections with *Acinetobacter calcoaceticus:* Clinical and laboratory studies. Medicine 56:79, 1977

RETAILLIAU FH et al: *Acinetobacter calcoaceticus:* A nosocomial pathogen with unusual seasonal pattern. J Infect Dis 139:371, 1979

Eikenella infections

BROOKS GF et al: *Eikenella corrodens*, a recently recognized pathogen. Medicine 53:325, 1974

GOLDSTEIN FJC et al: Isolation of *Eikenella corrodens* from pulmonary infections. Am Rev Resp Dis 119:55, 1979

106 MELIOIDOSIS AND GLANDERS

JAY P. SANFORD

MELIOIDOSIS Definition Melioidosis is an infection of humans and animals with a protean clinical spectrum. Melioidosis, which means "a resemblance to distemper of asses," bears a striking resemblance to glanders both clinically and pathologically, but is epidemiologically dissimilar.

Etiology Melioidosis is caused by a gram-negative motile bacillus, *Pseudomonas pseudomallei,* which can be differentiated from *P. mallei* by bacteriologic and serologic means. *P. pseudomallei* (also known as Whitmore's bacillus) is a small, gram-negative, motile, aerobic bacillus. When it is stained with methylene blue, Wayson's, or Wright's stain, marked irregularities with a bipolar "safety pin" pattern are observed. It grows well on standard bacteriologic media, with a characteristic wrinkling of colony surfaces after 48 to 72 h of incubation. Two antigenic types have been distinguished, type I (Asian), found widely, including in Australia, and type II (Australian), found mainly in Australia. Both types are equally pathogenic.

Epidemiology The disease is endemic in Southeast Asia where human and animal cases occur commonly. Disease in humans has been reported from adjacent areas including India, Borneo, the Philippines, Guam, Indonesia, Sri Lanka, New Guinea, and Australia (north Queensland, Northern Territory). Cases in humans or animals have been reported from Madagascar, Chad, Kenya, Central West Africa (Niger, Upper Volta), Iran, and Turkey. In 1976, *P. pseudomallei* was isolated from animals in the Paris zoo just behind Notre Dame. In Madrid, horses kept for serum died from melioidosis. Human melioidosis has been described only rarely in the western hemisphere (Panama, Ecuador)—a neonatal case in Hawaii, a case in Georgia, and a possible case in Oklahoma. With these exceptions, confirmed melioidosis has occurred in United States or European residents only when they have traveled in endemic areas. As of January 1973, when all American forces had been withdrawn from Vietnam, there had been 343 cases with 36 deaths reported in United States Army personnel who were or had been in Vietnam.

Pseudomonas pseudomallei is a saprophyte which can be isolated from soil, stagnant streams, ponds, rice paddies, and market produce in endemic areas. Its ubiquitous nature is illustrated by its isolation as a laboratory contaminant. *Pseudomonas pseudomallei* is capable of causing disease in epizootic form among sheep, goats, swine, and horses. Outbreaks have occurred in dolphins in oceanariums in Paris and Hong Kong. Occasional isolates have also been reported from cows, rodents, dogs, cats, wallabies, and birds. Although animals are susceptible to the disease, they apparently do not represent a reservoir for human disease. Attempts to culture *P. pseudomallei* from the urine and feces of a large variety of healthy animals have been unsuccessful. Arthropod-borne infection does not occur naturally. Humans contract melioidosis by soil contamination of skin abrasions. Ingestion, nasal instillation, and inhalation are other probable methods of spread. In contrast to glanders, infections have been uncommon, but can occur, in laboratory workers. *P. pseudomallei* has been recovered from urine specimens from two patients, both diabetic, who had urethral catheters, while hospitalized in an endemic area. Person-to-person transmission of melioidosis is rare. Venereal transmission from a patient with chronic prostatitis with *P. pseudomallei* isolated from prostatic secretions to his wife, who had never been in an endemic area and who had a hemagglutination titer of 1:10,240, has been recorded. Also, the development of melioidosis in a 2-day-old newborn in Hawaii and demonstration of a significant antibody titer in a nurse who had never been in an endemic area but who had worked on wards with melioidosis patients raise the question of spread from person-to-person within a hospital.

Pathology In acute infections, the majority of lesions occur in the lungs, with occasional abscesses in other organs. In subacute infections, lung abscesses tend to be more extensive, and lesions are found throughout the body, in the skin, subcutaneous tissue, meninges, brain, eye, heart, liver, kidney, spleen, bone, prostate, synovial membranes, and lymph nodes. The acute abscesses are characterized by an outer border of hemorrhage, a medial zone heavily infiltrated with polymorphonuclear leukocytes, and an inner core of necrotic debris containing large histiocytes with two or three nuclei that have been termed giant cells. A striking histologic feature has been the marked karyorrhexis. In chronic infections, the lesion consists of a central area of caseation necrosis, mononuclear and plasma cells, and granulation tissue. Calcification does not occur.

Melioidosis is associated with impaired cellular immunity; total lymphocyte counts are usually less than 1000 per cubic millimeter; the percentage of total T cells is less than 50 percent due to a decrease in T helper cells; and skin tests with dinitrochlorobenzene are negative. The number of T suppressor cells is normal, as is the number of B cells.

Clinical manifestations The clinical manifestations of melioidosis are variable. The illness can present as an acute, subacute, or chronic process. The incubation period has not been defined; however, judging by the lapse of time between injury and the development of infection, it may be as short as 2 days. Following a laboratory accident, an incubation period of 3 days ensued. Clinically inapparent infections may remain latent for a number of years after an individual leaves an endemic area, with an interval of 26 years reported in one patient. Men are more often affected than women, a finding which is thought to represent occupational exposure. Melioidosis may be recognized as inapparent infection, asymptomatic pulmonary infiltration, acute localized suppurative infection, acute pulmonary infection, acute septicemic infection, or chronic suppurative infection.

INAPPARENT INFECTION In Thailand, Vietnam, and Malaysia, 6 to 8 percent of healthy adult men have significant antibody titers against *P. pseudomallei,* with the prevalence reaching 20 percent in a group of Army recruits from the rice-growing states of western Malaysia. Only 1 percent of Thai women had positive reactions. None of the serums from a control group from the United States was positive. The prevalence of significant antibody titers has been reported as 2 percent for Europeans living in Vietnam and 1 to 9 percent in unselected patients in United States Army hospitals and in a group of normal uninjured soldiers who had served in Vietnam. Occasionally, asymptomatic infections have been discovered by routine chest x-ray. In northern Queensland, the prevalence of positive indirect hemagglutination titers (1:40 or higher) is as high as 10.6 percent, averages 5.7 percent, and is equal in men and women. Ten percent of serums from inhabitants of a village in Upper Volta were positive, yet melioidosis had never been recognized.

ACUTE LOCALIZED SUPPURATIVE INFECTION Infection by inoculation of a break in the skin usually results in a nodule with an area of acute lymphangitis and regional lymphadenitis. There are usually fever and generalized malaise. This form of infection may rapidly progress to the acute septicemic form.

ACUTE PULMONARY INFECTION The most common form of the disease has been pulmonary infection, which may represent a primary pneumonitis or hematogenous spread. The acute pulmonary infection can vary in severity from a mild bronchitis to overwhelming necrotizing pneumonia. The onset may be abrupt without prodromal symptoms or more gradual, with headache, anorexia, and generalized myalgia. Fever occurs in almost all patients, is often in excess of 38.9°C (102°F), and may be associated with rigors. Dull or pleuritic chest pain is common. Cough, with or without sputum, occurs. There may be mild pharyngitis. Tachypnea may be out of proportion to the fever and findings on physical or x-ray examination. Chest findings may be minimal but usually consist of rales in the area of pneumonitis. In the absence of dissemination, the spleen and liver are not palpable. Laboratory findings include total leukocyte counts ranging from normal to 20,000 cells per cubic millimeter. Mild normochromic, normocytic anemia may appear during the illness. The pneumonia usually involves the upper lobes with the radiographic appearance of consolidation. Thin-walled cavities, usually 2 to 7 cm in diameter, frequently occur. Without specific therapy, the temperature may become normal within a few days; however, the upper lobe cavitation persists, resulting in a radiographic appearance of tuberculosis. While uncommon, pleural effusions, a pleural mass, and bilateral hilar adenopathy have been reported. Progressive pulmonary spread or hematogenous dissemination with the development of septicemic manifestations may ensue.

ACUTE SEPTICEMIC INFECTION This is the form originally described primarily among narcotic addicts. Subsequent reports, however, have shown a predilection for debilitated patients with diabetes mellitus and alcoholism. The onset may be abrupt, with the dominant symptoms depending upon site of major involvement. In individuals with bacteremia complicating pneumonitis, symptoms may include disorientation, extreme dyspnea, severe headache, pharyngitis, watery diarrhea, and development of cutaneous pustular lesions on the head, trunk, or extremities. There is high fever, extreme tachypnea, a flushed skin, and cyanosis. Muscle tenderness may be striking. On examination of the chest, signs may be absent, or rales, rhonchi, and pleural rubs may be heard. The liver and spleen may be palpable. Signs of arthritis or meningitis may appear. Patients with the septicemic form usually have a rapidly progressive fatal course, which in many instances may be too fulminant to be altered by therapy. The leukocyte count may be normal or slightly increased. Chest radiographs most commonly show irregular nodular densities 4 to 10 mm in diameter disseminated throughout the lungs. These enlarge, coalesce, and often undergo cavitation as the disease progresses. Pleural effusion is rare. Other radiographic patterns include unilateral irregular mottled densities which become confluent.

CHRONIC SUPPURATIVE INFECTION In some patients secondary abscesses develop which dominate the clinical picture. Organs involved include skin, brain, lung, myocardium, liver, spleen, prostate, bones, joints, lymph nodes, and even the eye. These patients may be afebrile.

RECRUDESCENT INFECTION Activation of inapparent or quiescent infection may present as acute localized suppurative, acute pulmonary, acute septicemic, or chronic suppurative disease remote from the probable time of exposure (up to 26 years having been reported). Surgery, trauma, intercurrent illness such as severe influenzal pneumonia, diabetic ketoacidosis, alcoholic debauches, or radiation therapy appeared to act as triggering events. Since *P. pseudomallei* is an intracellular parasite and is associated with suppression of T helper lymphocytes, it is only a matter of time before melioidosis will be added to the list of infections which occur in individuals with HTLV-III virus infections and the acquired immunodeficiency syndrome (AIDS), especially in areas where *P. pseudomallei* is endemic.

Diagnosis Melioidosis should be considered in the differential diagnosis of any febrile illness in an individual who has been in an endemic area, especially if the presenting features are those of fulminant respiratory failure, if multiple pustular or necrotic skin or subcutaneous lesions develop, or if there is a radiographic pattern of tuberculosis in a patient from whom tubercle bacilli cannot be isolated.

Microscopic examination of exudates will reveal poorly staining, small, gram-negative bacilli which show the characteristic staining irregularities and "safety pin" bipolar staining with methylene blue. *Pseudomonas pseudomallei* will grow on most laboratory media, including eosin methylene blue agar (EMB) or MacConkey's agar, in 24 to 48 h. The organisms can be differentiated from *P. mallei* and *P. aeruginosa* by standard bacteriologic procedures, although isolates may pose problems in identification with some commercial medium kits. The characteristic wrinkling of the colonies may require 72 h or longer. The hemagglutination, direct agglutination test, and complement fixation test are aids in diagnosis if a fourfold or greater rise in titer is demonstrated in paired serums. Single low titers are difficult to interpret because of nonspecific responses. The complement fixation test is said to be specific with titers above 1:8 during the acute illness, but may cross-react with *P. mallei*. A negative complement fixation test does not exclude disease. The hemagglutination and agglutination tests show more cross-reactions. Titers of 1:40 or more suggest infection. In one-third of patients, with both fulminating and subacute disease, the serology has been negative at the time the culture became positive.

Treatment The treatment regimen should vary with the form of the disease. Individuals with low-titer positive serologic tests but with no clinical evidence of infection do not require therapy. The choice of antibiotics in active infection should be based upon sensitivity studies, and therapy should be given for a minimum of 30 days. *Pseudomonas pseudomallei* is usually sensitive in vitro to the tetracyclines, chloramphenicol, novobiocin, kanamycin, amikacin, sulfadiazine or sulfisoxazole, trimethoprim-sulfamethoxazole, and the third-generation antipseudomonal cephalosporins, especially ceftazidime, and in most instances is resistant to penicillin G, ampicillin, carbenicillin, dicloxacillin, streptomycin, gentamicin, tobramycin, first- and second-generation cephalosporins, vancomycin, clindamycin, and rifampin. In patients with pneumonitis who are not too ill, effective therapy has included tetracycline, 2 to 3 g daily (40 mg/kg); chloramphenicol, 3 g daily (40 mg/kg); or trimethoprim-sulfamethoxazole (4 mg/kg trimethoprim, 20 mg/kg sulfamethoxazole) for 60 to 150 days. Ceftazidime, 6 g daily (100 mg/kg), has been reported to be effective. If the patient is severely ill, two of these antimicrobials in combination should be given for 30 days followed by another 30 to 120 days of trimethoprim-sulfamethoxazole alone. The mean interval for sputum cultures to become negative has been 6 weeks. If sputum cultures remain positive for 6 months, surgery with lobectomy should be considered. In patients with extrapulmonary suppurative lesions, therapy should be continued for 6 months to 1 year. The usual principles of surgical drainage should be followed. In desperately ill patients with severe pneumonitis or the septicemic form, multiple antibiotics should be administered by the parenteral route. Current recommendations for antibiotics in the septicemic form of melioidosis are tetracycline, 4 to 6 g per day (80 mg/kg); chloramphenicol, 4 to 6 g per day (80 mg/kg); and one of the following: trimethoprim-sulfamethoxazole (9 mg/kg trimethoprim, 45 mg/kg sulfamethoxazole), kanamycin (30 mg/kg), or novobiocin (60 mg/kg). In vitro studies have revealed antagonism between the following pairs of drugs: chloramphenicol-kanamycin, tetracycline-kanamycin, and sulfadiazine-chloramphenicol. Though the significance of such antagonism in clinical therapy has not been assessed, the data favor selection of trimethoprim-sulfamethoxazole or novobiocin as the third drug. The dosage should be tapered rapidly as clinical improvement occurs. Experience with the third-generation antipseudomonal cephalosporins is extremely limited; however, a combination of ceftazidime (in a dose of 100 mg/kg or 6 g daily) and trimethoprim-sulfamethoxazole is likely to emerge as the recommendation of choice. Levamisole[1] (150 mg twice per week) has been used as an adjunct to antibiotic therapy in several patients with results that suggest it may be beneficial in the treatment of relapses.

Prognosis Prior to antimicrobials, the mortality rate of apparent infection was 95 percent. With better diagnosis and more prolonged appropriate therapy, the mortality rate in all except the septicemic form is low. Even with vigorous appropriate antibiotics and supportive therapy, the mortality rate in patients with melioidosis septicemia is greater than 50 percent. Very few patients have had long-term follow-up, and the incidence of late relapses is approximately 20 percent.

Prevention There is no means of active immunization. In endemic areas, vigorous cleansing of abrasions and lacerations is recommended.

[1] *This drug has not been approved for this purpose by the Food and Drug Administration at the time of publication.*

GLANDERS Definition Glanders is a serious infection of equine animals caused by *P. mallei*, which is transmitted occasionally to other domestic animals and to human beings.

Etiology *Pseudomonas mallei* is a small, slender, nonmotile, gram-negative bacillus. When it is stained with methylene blue, marked irregularities in staining are observed. Organisms grow on most common meat infusion media but require glycerol for optimum growth.

Epidemiology Glanders was at one time widespread throughout Europe, but owing to the introduction of control measures, its incidence has decreased steadily in most countries. The disease still occurs in Asia, Africa, and South America, but not in the United States and western Europe. Glanders has never been common in humans; the occasional infection, however, may be very serious. There have been no naturally acquired infections in the United States since 1938.

Glanders is primarily a disease of horses, mules, and donkeys, although goats, sheep, cats, and dogs sometimes naturally contract the disease. Infection of lions at a safari park in Italy attributed to feeding imported horse meat has been reported. Pigs and cattle are resistant. In horses, the disease may be systemic, with prominent pulmonary involvement (*glanders*) or may be characterized by subcutaneous ulcerative lesions, and lymphatic thickening with nodules (*farcy*). Inhalation, ingestion, and inoculation through breaks in the skin have been suggested as routes of infection in animals. In humans, the disease occurs primarily in individuals with close contact with horses, mules, or donkeys through inoculation of or a break in the skin or by exposing the nasal mucosa to contaminated discharges. A number of instances of airborne infection have been reported in laboratory workers.

Pathology The acute lesion is characterized by nodules consisting of polymorphonuclear leukocytes surrounded by a zone of congestion. A characteristic histologic feature is a peculiar nuclear degeneration known as chromatotexis which occurs early and is extensive. Small foci of deeply staining detritus within the abscess result from this degeneration. In older nodules, the reaction is characterized by epithelioid cells surrounding an area of central necrosis. Giant cells may be present. Virtually any organ may be involved.

Clinical manifestations The manifestations which frequently overlap may be categorized as (1) acute localized suppurative infection, (2) acute pulmonary infection, (3) acute septicemic infection, and (4) chronic suppurative infection. Nearly 60 percent of patients have been between the ages of 20 and 40 years. The disease has been rare in women, probably because there is opportunity for contact.

Infection acquired by inoculation through an abrasion in the skin usually results in a nodule with an area of acute lymphangitis. The incubation period is probably 1 to 5 days. In all types of acute glanders, there are usually fever, generalized malaise, and prostration.

Infection of the mucous membranes may result in a mucopurulent discharge involving the eye, nose, or lips followed by extensive ulcerating granulomatous lesions which may or may not be associated with systemic reactions. With systemic invasion, a generalized papular eruption which may become pustular is frequent. This septicemic form of disease is usually fatal in 7 to 10 days.

Infection by inhalation is followed by an incubation period of 10 to 14 days. The more common symptoms include fever, occasionally associated with rigors, generalized myalgia, fatigue, headache, and pleuritic chest pain. Other symptoms consist of photophobia, lacrimation, and diarrhea. Findings on physical examination are usually normal except for fever and occasional lymphadenopathy, especially in the cervical chain, and splenomegaly. Laboratory findings include mild leukocytosis with 60 to 80 percent neutrophilic leukocytes, but leukopenia with relative lymphocytosis has been recorded. In the acute pulmonary form, chest radiographs characteristically reveal circumscribed densities which suggest early lung abscesses. Other findings may include lobar or bronchopneumonia. In the chronic suppurative form of the disease, the most frequent finding consists of multiple subcutaneous and intramuscular abscesses which most often involve the arms or legs. Approximately one-half the patients will have associated fever, lymphadenopathy, and nasal discharge or ulceration. Visceral involvement including pulmonary or pleural, ocular, skeletal, hepatic, splenic, and meningeal or intracranial involvement occurs in some patients.

Diagnosis Microscopic examination of exudates may reveal small gram-negative bacilli which stain irregularly with methylene blue; however, organisms generally are very scanty. *Pseudomonas mallei* and *P. pseudomallei* cannot be distinguished morphologically. Culturing is often avoided because of the hazard to laboratory personnel; however, if cultures are made, growth occurs on most meat infusion nutrient media. The material is often contaminated with other microorganisms, and incubation with penicillin G (1000 units per milliliter) prior to culturing may be helpful. Subcutaneous inoculation of material into a guinea pig or hamster affords an alternative means of isolation. Blood cultures are usually negative except in the terminal stages of disease. Serologic tests show a rapidly rising agglutination titer, which reaches levels of 1:640 within 2 weeks. Serum from normal persons has been reported to show agglutination titers in dilutions up to 1:320. The complement fixation test is less sensitive but more specific and usually becomes positive during the third week; it is considered positive in dilutions of 1:20 or greater.

Treatment The limited number of recent infections in human beings has precluded evaluation of most of the antibiotic agents. Sulfadiazine has been found to be an effective agent in experimental animals and in humans. The dosage utilized has been approximately 100 mg/kg administered in divided doses. In experimental infections, 3 weeks of therapy gave better results than 1 week. Penicillin is ineffective. Tetracycline, chloramphenicol, the antipseudomonal aminoglycosides, carbenicillin, the third-generation antipseudomonal cephalosporins, and trimethoprim-sulfamethoxazole have not been evaluated. In the absence of clinical experience and pending in vitro susceptibility studies, it would seem most reasonable to utilize the regimens appropriate for patients with melioidosis. In the acute infections, appropriate supportive measures are essential, and in chronic suppurative infections, the usual principles of surgical drainage should be followed.

Prognosis The prognosis depends upon the type of infection. The acute septicemic form has been uniformly fatal. The localized or chronic forms have a much better prognosis.

Prevention Next to acquisition from diseased horses, the commonest source of natural disease in human beings has been contact with human glanders. Isolation is indicated.

REFERENCES

ASHDOWN LR, GUARD RW: Prevalence of human melioidosis in northern Queensland. Am J Trop Med Hyg 33:474, 1984

DODIN A, FERRY R: Recherche epidemiologique du bacille de Whitmore en Afrique. Bull Soc Pathol Exot 67:121, 1974

———, GALIMAND M: Whitmore's bacillus. Rec Med Vet 152:323, 1976

EICKHOFF TC et al: *Pseudomonas pseudomallei:* Susceptibility to chemotherapeutic agents. J Infect Dis 121:95, 1970

EVERETT ED, NELSON R: Pulmonary melioidosis, observations in 39 cases. Am Rev Resp Dis 112:331, 1975

GUARD LR et al: Melioidosis in far north Queensland. Am J Trop Med Hyg 33:467, 1984

HOWE C, MILLER WR: Human glanders: Report of six cases. Ann Intern Med 26:93, 1947

JACKSON AE et al: Recrudescent melioidosis associated with diabetic ketoacidosis. Arch Intern Med 130:268, 1972

MCCORMICK JB et al: Human-to-human transmission of *Pseudomonas pseudomallei*. Ann Intern Med 83:512, 1975

MAYS EE, RICKETS EA: Melioidosis: Recrudescence associated with bronchogenic carcinoma twenty-six years following initial geographic exposure. Chest 68:261, 1975

SANFORD JP: Melioidosis: Another great imitator, in *Infectious Diseases: Current Topics in Diagnosis and Treatment*, DN Gilbert, JP Sanford (eds). New York, Grune & Stratton, 1978

SCHLECH WF III et al: Laboratory-acquired infection with *Pseudomonas pseudomallei* (melioidosis). N Engl J Med 305:1133, 1981

TANPHAICHITRA D, SRIMUANG S: Cellular immunity in tuberculosis, melioidosis, pasteurellosis, penicilliosis and role of levamisole and isoprinosine. Dev Biol Stand 57:117, 1984

WALL RA et al: A case of melioidosis in West Africa. J Infect Dis 152:424, 1985

WILKINSON L: Glanders: Medicine and veterinary medicine in common pursuit of a contagious disease. Med Hist 25:363, 1981

ZAJTCHUK R et al: Surgical treatment of melioidosis. J Thorac Cardiovasc Surg 66:838, 1973

107 *SALMONELLA* INFECTIONS

RICHARD L. GUERRANT

The genus *Salmonella* consists of three species which include more than 2000 different serologic types. Striking variation in pathogenicity of serotypes occurs, but almost all are pathogenic for animals and humans. Specific host preferences characterize certain serotypes, such as *S. typhi,* which under natural conditions of transmission produces disease only in humans. *Salmonella* infections in humans present a spectrum of clinical syndromes, which sometimes overlap. The syndromes are (1) enteric fever (typhoid or paratyphoid fever), (2) acute gastroenteritis, (3) bacteremia, and (4) localized infection which may occur at almost any site. In addition, *asymptomatic intestinal infections* and *transient convalescent intestinal carrier* states are common. Occasionally, a focus of infection persists in the gallbladder or urinary tract to produce a *chronic carrier* state.

ETIOLOGY Salmonellae are motile gram-negative bacilli that ferment glucose but do not ferment lactose or sucrose. *S. typhi* and *S. cholerae-suis* can usually be distinguished from most other serotypes by biochemical means. *S. typhi* does not produce gas and is ornithine-negative, which distinguishes it from almost all other *Salmonella* serotypes. *S. cholerae-suis* is almost uniquely trehalose-negative and is often dulcitol-negative. The many serotypes are identified by highly specific O (somatic) and H (flagellar) antigens. A given serotype will contain a specific combination of multiple O and H antigens. Identification by serotype is accomplished routinely only in major salmonella typing centers, which have the necessary collection of antiserums required for such work. Salmonellae are also divided into groups on the basis of O antigen composition. Most isolates from natural sources fall into five groups, A to E.

The species *S. typhi* and *S. cholerae-suis* consist of only one serotype each (in groups D and C, respectively). Considerable overlap in antigenic composition is responsible for the cross-reactivity which is commonly seen in serologic tests with salmonellae.

While *S. typhi* infections in the United States have declined to around 500 isolations per year (most of which are imported from abroad), non-*typhi Salmonella* infections appear to be increasing steadily, especially in patients who are immunocompromised or who are taking antibiotics.

Despite its passive, laboratory-based system of reporting, the Centers for Disease Control report a steady increase from less than 20,000 isolations of salmonellae annually from humans in the United States in 1968 to nearly 40,000 in 1983. This near doubling in frequency contrasts with the infrequency of *Salmonella* infections in developing countries and suggests, with increasing resistance to antimicrobial agents, that human salmonellosis is increasing, perhaps in association with agricultural practices in industrialized countries. It is estimated that over 2 million cases of human *Salmonella* infections occur each year in the United States.

In descending order, the most frequently isolated serotypes in 1983 were *S. typhimurium, S. heidelberg, S. enteritidis, S. newport, S. agona, S. infantis, S. saint-paul, S. montevideo, S. oranienburg,* and *S. typhi*. The 10 most frequently isolated serotypes account for over 70 percent of the total isolates from humans. *Salmonella typhimurium* perennially accounts for 25 to 35 percent of the isolates. *S. agona,* an organism apparently introduced indirectly via animals fed Peruvian fish meal in 1971, continues to increase. There is increasing appreciation of the association of *Salmonella* infections with raw milk consumption (especially *S. dublin*), and with antibiotic use in humans.

Typhoid fever, the classic example of enteric fever, is considered separately from other *Salmonella* infections because of its historical importance, the host specificity of *S. typhi,* and the extensive clinical experience with the disease.

TYPHOID FEVER

DEFINITION Typhoid fever is an acute systemic disease resulting from infection with *S. typhi*. The disease is unique to humans. It is characterized by malaise, fever, abdominal discomfort, transient rash, splenomegaly, and leukopenia. The most prominent major complications are intestinal hemorrhage and perforation. The disease is the classic example of enteric fever caused by salmonellae. However, enteric fever, similar to typhoid, can also be caused by other *Salmonella* serotypes and is termed *paratyphoid fever*.

EPIDEMIOLOGY *Salmonella typhi* gains access to the body by the oral route in almost all cases as a consequence of the ingestion of contaminated food, water, or milk. Humans are the only true reservoir of *S. typhi* in nature, and persons with typhoid fever, or convalescent or chronic carriers, always serve as the ultimate source of infection. Infected individuals can excrete millions of viable typhoid bacilli in the feces, which are the usual source of contamination of food or drink. Patients with active disease also occasionally have organisms in respiratory secretions, vomitus, or other body fluids. Flies or other insects can carry organisms from feces or other infected material to food or drink and have been implicated in a few outbreaks. The fact that *S. typhi* may survive freezing or drying enhances the possibility of spread by contaminated ice, dust, foods, and sewage. Oysters or other shellfish are contaminated at times in polluted waters and occasionally serve as sources of typhoid.

The incidence of typhoid fever has steadily decreased in the United States during the past century to the present relatively low level of less than 600 cases per year. The decrease in incidence has been coincident with improvement in socioeconomic conditions and is specifically related to development of pure water supplies, effective sewage disposal, pasteurization of milk, and methods to detect and control spread of organisms from persons with active disease or from carriers. Typhoid continues to occur on a large scale in countries where sanitation is suboptimal. Over 60 percent of the patients with typhoid fever in the United States have acquired their infections in areas where the disease is endemic, with 65 percent of these being from Mexico and India. However, fatalities are more common with domestically acquired cases, probably because the diagnosis is not suspected early. About 4 percent of cases in the United States are laboratory-acquired.

Typhoid can be eradicated ultimately because the infection is confined to humans and both the disease and the carrier state can be controlled with appropriate drugs. The importance of sewage disposal, a pure water supply, and control of carriers is highlighted repeatedly by the occurrence of outbreaks which develop when defects in sanitation occur such as failure of adequate water chlorination or during natural disasters such as flood.

The sex distribution of patients with typhoid fever in the United States shows no significant predilection. In recent years, about 75 percent of cases have occurred in persons less than 30 years of age. In contrast, the chronic carrier state is much more common in females than males (the female/male ratio is 3:1) and in older individuals (88 percent are over 50 years of age).

There is no seasonal variation in incidence of typhoid fever in the United States. However, in areas of the world where the disease is endemic, the incidence increases in the summer months.

PATHOGENESIS The outcome of the interaction between the typhoid bacillus and humans is determined during the early hours after ingestion of the organisms. Typhoid bacilli reach the small intestine shortly after ingestion and may multiply there. The organisms may then penetrate the mucosa with minimal epithelial destruction and enter intestinal lymphatics, perhaps via Peyer's patches, to be carried to the bloodstream. This initial early bacteremia apparently occurs within 24 to 72 h after ingestion of organisms and is rarely detected in natural infections because patients are usually asymptomatic at this early stage. The bacteremia is transient and is rapidly terminated as bacilli are phagocytized by cells of the reticuloendothelial system. Nevertheless, viable bacilli are disseminated throughout the body and apparently persist within reticuloendothelial cells. After intracellular multiplication takes place, organisms reenter the bloodstream, producing a continuous bacteremia for days or weeks. The reappearance of bacteremia corresponds with the onset of manifestations of the disease. The intracellular organisms are eventually destroyed as manifestations of disease subside and recovery ensues. Enhanced intracellular killing and recovery appear to be related to the onset of delayed hypersensitivity. Recovery is unrelated to the appearance, even in high titer, of agglutinins against the somatic, flagellar, or Vi antigens of the typhoid bacillus.

The number of organisms ingested is an important determinant of whether typhoid fever results from exposure to *S. typhi.* Studies in volunteers have shown that about 10^7 typhoid bacilli of the Quailes strain must be taken orally to produce typhoid fever in 50 percent of normal volunteers. The number of organisms ingested also influences the incubation period, and short incubation periods, in general, correspond to large doses of organisms. The volunteer studies have also demonstrated that different strains of typhoid bacilli vary considerably in their capacity to produce disease in humans.

The normal flora of the upper intestinal tract is an important protective mechanism against invasion by *S. typhi.* Volunteer studies have demonstrated that antimicrobial therapy a day or so before oral challenge with *S. typhi* markedly decreases the number of viable bacilli required to produce disease. It is possible that certain factors known to be associated with typhoid outbreaks, such as malnutrition, enhance susceptibility to typhoid infection by alterations in the intestinal flora or other host defenses.

During the phase of persistent bacteremia, all organs are repeatedly exposed to typhoid bacilli. Abscess formation may occur but is unusual. However, localization does occur in the gallbladder in almost all cases. Organisms multiply in the bile to high titer, usually without manifestations of cholecystitis, and are excreted with bile into the intestinal tract. Stool cultures, which are usually negative for *S. typhi* during the incubation period and early phases of the disease, become positive in a large proportion of cases during the third or fourth week of the disease, when excretion of organisms in the bile reaches a peak.

The factors responsible for the fever, leukopenia, and other manifestations of typhoid fever have been inadequately defined. Typhoid bacilli contain biologically active lipopolysaccharides or endotoxins which produce fever, leukopenia, thrombocytopenia, and hyperplasia of reticuloendothelial cells when injected into animals or humans. It is assumed that endotoxins play an important role in the pathogenesis of the signs and symptoms of typhoid fever. However, the evidence regarding the role of endotoxin in causing the manifestations of typhoid is inconclusive. For example, tolerance to the pyrogenic effects of endotoxins can be demonstrated during convalescence from typhoid fever, which suggests release of endotoxins during infection. While laboratory evidence for low-grade, subclinical disseminated intravascular coagulation can often be demonstrated in patients with typhoid fever, endotoxemia is usually not detectable. Other studies show that typhoid fever follows a normal course in volunteers rendered tolerant to endotoxins prior to challenge, indicating that more complex mechanisms than endotoxemia alone are responsible for the sustained fever and toxemia. It has been suggested that endogenous pyrogens released by local inflammatory effects of *S. typhi* endotoxin may sustain the pyrexia in typhoid fever.

PATHOLOGY The most prominent microscopic lesion in typhoid fever is proliferation of large mononuclear cells in many different tissues. Mononuclear hyperplasia leads to lymphadenopathy, splenomegaly, and impressive enlargement of lymphoid tissues in the intestines, especially in the terminal ileum (Peyer's patches). Proliferating mononuclear cells may also be observed in bone marrow, liver, and lung. Studies in volunteers using ^{131}I-tagged aggregated albumin have shown increased phagocytic activity of the reticuloendothelial system by the third to fifth day after onset of symptoms. Necrosis in hyperplastic Peyer's patches may be associated with erosion of blood vessels in the lesions in the intestinal tract, which leads to oozing of blood or massive hemorrhage. Lesions may extend deep into the intestinal wall and cause perforation, usually in the distal ileum, an event which characteristically occurs late in the disease, most often in the third febrile week.

The gallbladder and bile ducts are routinely infected during the disease. As a rule, this biliary infection is asymptomatic, although acute cholecystitis may occur occasionally. Biliary infection terminates spontaneously during convalescence in the vast majority of patients within 12 months, but about 3 percent of adults continue to harbor organisms in the gallbladder and become chronic carriers of the typhoid bacillus.

MANIFESTATIONS The incubation period averages about 10 days but may vary from extremes of 3 to 60 days depending on the infecting dose.

The clinical manifestations and duration of illness vary markedly from one patient to another. Mild forms of the disease, characterized primarily by fever, may last only a week, or illness may be prolonged, lasting 8 weeks or more if untreated.

In a typical patient not treated with antimicrobials, the illness lasts about 4 weeks. The onset is insidious with headache, malaise, anorexia, and fever. Headache may be the first manifestation of disease and is usually generalized and severe. Chilly sensations are common, and frank chills may be observed. The fever is remittent, frequently increasing in a steplike manner from day to day as the illness develops. Abdominal discomfort, bloating, and constipation are common during the early phase of illness. A dry cough is observed in about two-thirds of the patients and occasionally may be so prominent as to direct attention away from the generalized nature of the infection. Nosebleeds may occur during the early phase of illness.

The temperature gradually increases for 5 to 7 days and then plateaus as a continuous or mildly remittent fever in the range of 39 to 40°C. The temperature may be sustained at these levels with little variation for 2 or 3 weeks. A relative bradycardia occurs in 30 to 40 percent of the patients. The prolonged persistent fever leads to general debility; patients are weak and anorectic. Mental dullness is common and delirium may occur. Abdominal pain and marked distention are usual. Constipation during the early phase of illness may give way to diarrhea later in the course of the disease.

The characteristic rash (rose spots) is most often observed during the second week of the disease. The lesions are small, 2- to 4-mm, erythematous macules which occur in small numbers on the upper abdomen and anterior thorax. The lesions blanch on pressure and last only 2 to 3 days. Some reports describe rose spots in as many as 90 percent of patients, whereas other reports indicate a frequency of only 10 percent or even less. The evanescent nature of the rash and the difficulties encountered in detecting lesions in highly pigmented individuals probably account for the marked variation in incidence reported in the literature.

The liver and spleen are frequently enlarged and palpable after the first week of illness. The spleen is palpable in about three-quarters of the patients. The liver may be tender, and occasionally a friction rub is audible over the spleen.

Abdominal tenderness is frequent and distention occurs in the majority of cases. Marked abdominal pain with signs of peritonitis should call attention to the possibility of perforation of the bowel.

After the third week, the symptoms slowly abate, and the temperature returns to normal over a period of days.

Jaundice secondary to extensive mononuclear cell infiltration in the liver and hepatic cell necrosis is a rare complication of typhoid. Acute renal failure also is observed rarely; the pathogenesis of this so-called typhoid nephritis has not been adequately defined. Disseminated intravascular coagulation may develop in severe typhoid and lead to additional clinical manifestations secondary to thrombosis or hemorrhage.

Complications Prior to the introduction of chloramphenicol, the prolonged febrile course of typhoid often led to profound debility, weight loss, and multiple nutritional deficiencies. Intestinal hemorrhage and bowel perforation, the most feared complications, were common causes of death in 12 to 32 percent of cases. The frequency of complications in typhoid fever has been reduced to 2 percent or less since the advent of effective chemotherapy.

INTESTINAL HEMORRHAGE Erosion of blood vessels in hyperplastic and necrotic Peyer's patches or in other mononuclear cell accumulations in the wall of the intestine leads to bleeding into the intestinal tract. Occult blood in feces is quite common during the course of the disease, occurring in 20 percent or more of patients. Gross blood is present in feces in about 10 percent of patients, and massive hemorrhage occurs occasionally. Major hemorrhage is usually a late complication, occurring most often during the second or third week of disease. A sudden drop in blood pressure or temperature may be the first manifestation of hemorrhage.

INTESTINAL PERFORATION The pathologic process in the lymphoid tissues of the intestine may also involve the muscular and serosal layers of the bowel and lead to perforation. Prior to the advent of chloramphenicol, perforation occurred in about 3 percent of patients with typhoid. The incidence has been reduced by antimicrobial therapy to about 1 percent. Perforation is most common in the distal 60 cm of ileum and is observed most frequently during the third week of the disease. The onset of perforation may be quite unexpected during an otherwise uncomplicated convalescence. Pain in the right lower quadrant of the abdomen is the most frequent initial manifestation, but signs of localized or generalized peritonitis develop rapidly.

OTHER COMPLICATIONS Typhoid bacilli may localize in any tissue in the body with the production of localized suppurative infection. Meningitis, chondritis, periostitis, osteomyelitis, arthritis, and pyelonephritis are examples of localized infections that may be observed occasionally. Pneumonia is not unusual and may be caused by the typhoid bacillus or by a secondary bacterial invader, such as the pneumococcus. Severe deep thrombophlebitis may occur during the febrile period. Late complications also include peripheral neuritis, deafness, and alopecia. Hemolytic anemia may be observed, especially in infected individuals deficient in glucose 6-phosphate dehydrogenase.

Relapse After illness has subsided for a variable period, usually about 2 weeks, all the manifestations which characterized the initial infection may recur. Blood cultures, negative during convalescence, may become positive again. Although relapse may be severe, it is usually milder and of shorter duration than the original illness. The incidence of relapse was about 5 to 10 percent prior to the introduction of effective chemotherapy. Chloramphenicol has not decreased the frequency of relapse; in fact, the relapse rate in chloramphenicol-treated patients is higher than in patients not receiving the drug. Periods of antimicrobial therapy longer than 2 weeks do not seem to alter the incidence of relapse. Relapse cannot be correlated with the titer of agglutinins against the flagellar, somatic, or Vi antigens of the typhoid bacillus.

Chronic carriers Although the vast majority of patients with typhoid fever eradicate the site of infection in the gallbladder during convalescence, about 3 percent of adults do not, and these individuals become chronic typhoid carriers who continue to excrete organisms in feces for years, usually for life. A chronic carrier is defined as a person documented to have been excreting typhoid bacilli in the stool for a period of at least 1 year. In the United States, almost all chronic carriers have a persistent site of infection in the gallbladder from which organisms reach the intestinal tract in bile. Chronic carriers may be detected by follow-up of patients with typhoid fever, but many carriers give no history of typhoid. In these patients, it is assumed that the initial illness was so mild as to go unrecognized or undiagnosed. Once organisms have been demonstrated in the stools for as long as a year, it is unlikely that the focus of infection in the gallbladder will terminate spontaneously. The chronic carrier state is rare in children and occurs more commonly with increasing age and is about three times more common in women than men. It is possible that these age and sex characteristics are related to the greater prevalence of gallbladder disease in older women, a factor which would favor persistence of organisms in the biliary tract.

The chronic biliary carrier is usually asymptomatic. Despite millions of organisms entering the intestine in each milliliter of bile, patients show no systemic manifestations. Gallstones and dysfunction of the gallbladder on cholecystogram can be demonstrated in a large proportion of chronic carriers, and carriers occasionally develop acute cholecystitis.

In areas of the world where *Schistosoma haematobium* infections are common, a chronic urinary carrier state results from localization of typhoid bacilli or other *Salmonella* serotypes in the obstructed urinary tract or adjacent lesions resulting from the schistosomiasis. These chronic urinary carriers not only excrete *Salmonella* in the urine but also may have intermittent bacteremic episodes which are not necessarily accompanied by fever.

LABORATORY FINDINGS Leukopenia of 3000 to 4000 cells per cubic millimeter is characteristic of the febrile phase of typhoid fever. A sudden increase in leukocyte count to 10,000 cells per cubic millimeter or higher should suggest the possibility of intestinal perforation, hemorrhage, or a pyogenic complication, but these complications may occur in the absence of leukocytosis. A normocytic normochromic anemia develops during the course of the disease and may be aggravated by blood loss from intestinal lesions. Occult blood and a mononuclear leukocytosis in feces is common from the second week of disease. Urine is usually normal except for transient albuminuria during the febrile period.

The most dependable way to establish a definitive diagnosis of typhoid fever is by blood culture. Organisms can be recovered by culture of blood in 70 to 90 percent of patients during the first week of disease. Bacteremia is continuous and prolonged. Positive blood cultures are obtained in as many as 30 or 40 percent of patients during the third week of disease, but the incidence of bacteremia rapidly decreases after this time. Blood cultures frequently are positive during relapse. Recent evidence in partially treated cases suggests that culture of bone marrow may yield the organism when other cultures are negative, especially after antibiotics have been given.

Only about 10 to 15 percent of patients have positive stool cultures during the first week of disease. However, the frequency of positive stool cultures increases as the disease progresses, reaching a maximum of about 75 percent during the third or fourth week of illness. The frequency of positive cultures then begins to decline so that only about 10 percent of patients have positive stool cultures 8 weeks after onset of illness. Most of these patients' cultures become negative over the next several weeks or months, but about 3 percent of adults continue to excrete organisms even after 1 year. Persistent excretion in these chronic carriers is secondary to infection in the gallbladder and biliary tract.

The incidence of positive urine cultures varies markedly during the course of typhoid fever and parallels the frequency of positive stool cultures. At least some of the positive cultures represent contamination of urine with feces harboring typhoid bacilli.

The majority of patients, but certainly not all, develop a fourfold or greater rise in serum agglutinins against the somatic or O antigens of the typhoid bacillus during the course of the disease. Detection of *S. typhi* Vi, D, or d antigens in the urine of patients with typhoid fever may be even more sensitive. A fourfold or greater increase in serum titer in the absence of recent typhoid immunization is compatible with infection with *S. typhi* but is by no means specific. All the group D organisms, one of which is *S. typhi,* as well as organisms in groups A and B, have certain common antigens which can evoke the formation of antibodies reactive with the O antigen used in the Widal test. Agglutinins against flagellar or H antigens also appear, frequently in higher titer than agglutinins against the O antigens. However, the H agglutinins are even more subject to nonspecific variation than O agglutinins and are of no value in diagnosis. Agglutinins begin to appear after about 1 week of illness and reach a peak titer during the fifth or sixth week. Early antimicrobial therapy may dampen the immunologic response in patients with typhoid fever. Relapse bears no relation to agglutinin titer. Rheumatoid factor activity in high titer can be detected in a large proportion of patients with typhoid or paratyphoid fever.

DIFFERENTIAL DIAGNOSIS The clinical features of typhoid fever, while characteristic and suggestive of the diagnosis, are certainly not pathognomonic. Many other diseases give a clinical picture which may be confused with typhoid; these include the rickettsioses, brucellosis, tularemia, leptospirosis, psittacosis, infectious hepatitis, infectious mononucleosis, primary atypical pneumonia, miliary tuberculosis, malaria, lymphoma, and rheumatic fever. Typhoid should be considered in any patient with unexplained fever, especially if there is a history of recent foreign travel to endemic areas.

TREATMENT Antimicrobial therapy Chloramphenicol is the antibiotic of choice for the treatment of typhoid fever caused by sensitive organisms. Despite the fact that a number of antimicrobial agents show excellent in vitro activity against *S. typhi,* chloramphenicol has consistently been shown to be more effective in terminating the febrile toxic course of the disease in the greatest proportion of patients in the shortest period of time. Nevertheless, the response to chloramphenicol is not dramatic or rapid. Subjective improvement usually occurs within about 48 h after beginning therapy, but the temperature usually does not return to normal for 2 to 5 days after initiating treatment. Bacteremia usually clears within hours after therapy is instituted, but occasionally organisms can be recovered from the blood 24 to 48 h after beginning treatment. The dose of chloramphenicol should be 50 mg per kilogram of body weight per day divided into three or four equal doses given orally at intervals of 6 to 8 h. After the patient has become afebrile, the dose may be reduced to 30 mg/kg per day. Therapy should be continued for 2 weeks. If chloramphenicol cannot be given by the oral route, comparable doses should be given parenterally.

Ampicillin in doses of 80 mg/kg per day or 6 g per day for adults divided into four or six doses given parenterally or a combination of trimethoprim and sulfamethoxazole is effective in the treatment of typhoid, but the response is not as predictable or as prompt as with chloramphenicol. If there is a contraindication to therapy with chloramphenicol, ampicillin, amoxicillin, or trimethoprim-sulfamethoxazole is recommended.

Occasional patients with typhoid without evidence of suppurative complications do not respond clinically even after 4 or 5 days of antimicrobial therapy, even though blood cultures become negative. Delayed responses of this type occur in only about 1 percent of patients treated with chloramphenicol, in contrast to 5 or 10 percent of patients treated with ampicillin.

Chloramphenicol-resistant strains have been reported since 1972 from many areas of the world, predominantly Mexico, southeast Asia, and India. Resistance is due to a transferable R factor which also codes for resistance to sulfonamides, tetracycline, and streptomycin. *Salmonella typhi* resistant to both chloramphenicol and ampicillin have been isolated from a few patients, and the in vivo acquisition of resistance to chloramphenicol, and sulfonamide/trimethoprim, in a patient treated with these drugs, has been reported. If chloramphenicol resistance is encountered, then ampicillin, amoxicillin, or trimethoprim-sulfamethoxazole should be used.

Adrenal hormones The administration of dexamethasone, prednisone, or steroids with similar activity can terminate within a matter of hours the severe febrile toxemic state seen in some patients. Because of the lag in time between institution of antimicrobial therapy and evidence of response, patients with life-threatening toxemia, hypotension, or clouded sensorium should be treated with a brief course of corticosteroids in addition to chloramphenicol. While 300 mg of cortisone (or 60 mg prednisone) have been effective, very high doses of dexamethasone (3 mg/kg) have been shown to reduce mortality in very severe typhoid fever. In any case, steroids should be rapidly tapered over 24 to 48 h. Hypothermia and hypotension occasionally occur within hours after initiation of steroids.

Supportive treatment Nursing care and attention to nutritional requirements are important. Laxatives and enemas should be avoided despite constipation because of the danger of precipitating hemorrhage or perforation. Salicylates should not be used, because in addition to their effects on blood platelets and irritating action on the bowel, these compounds can induce wide swings in temperature with very uncomfortable chills and sweats. Hypothermia and hypotension occur in some patients after administration of salicylates.

Hemorrhage and perforation Patients should be observed carefully to detect these complications at an early stage. Typing and cross matching should be carried out at the time of initial diagnosis of typhoid, and transfusion is indicated in the event of significant hemorrhage. Patients with typhoid are poor surgical risks. If perforation is suspected, emphasis should be placed on efforts to combat shock and decompress the bowel. Additional antimicrobials may have to be added to control peritonitis. Small perforations may localize and can be managed without surgical intervention. However, if evidence of localization does not develop, prompt surgical intervention may be required.

Relapse The therapy of relapse is identical to that for the primary episode.

Chronic carriers Chronic carriers should be investigated for the presence of gallstones or a nonfunctioning gallbladder. Carriers without evidence of gallstones or gallbladder disease on cholecystogram or with ultrasound usually can be cured with a prolonged course of ampicillin. One program which has been found to be effective consists of 6 g ampicillin divided into four equal oral doses each day with probenecid for a period of 6 weeks. If gallstones or a nonfunctioning gallbladder are demonstrated, antimicrobial therapy is unlikely to be effective in terminating the carrier state. These patients should have cholecystectomy, which cures the chronic carrier state in about 85 percent of patients. Ampicillin may be used in conjunction with cholecystectomy. Therapy should be started a few days prior to the procedure and continued for 2 or 3 weeks. One study has reported success of sulfamethoxazole-trimethoprim and rifampin in the treatment of chronic *Salmonella* carriers.

PREVENTION AND CONTROL Control of typhoid fever involves improved sanitation, sewage control, and water supplies, and identification and cure or control of chronic carriers. Although immunization with typhoid vaccine affords significant protection against typhoid infection, the degree of immunity is not great and can be readily overcome with a large dose of organisms. Nevertheless, immunization is recommended for individuals living or traveling in areas where the disease is endemic and for persons working with the organism in laboratories. Adults should receive 0.5 mL vaccine on two occasions separated by a period of 1 or 2 weeks. A booster is recommended every 3 years to maintain immunity. Immunization with typhoid vaccine causes a transient elevation for several months in titer of agglutinins against typhoid O antigens and a persistently elevated titer for H antigens. A live, attenuated vaccine is being developed that shows promising efficacy in initial field trials.

All typhoid patients should be reported to local health authorities, and stool specimens should be cultured during convalescence. Three consecutively negative stool cultures obtained at weekly intervals indicate that a carrier state has not developed.

Caution should be observed to prevent spread of infection from persons with active disease or from carriers. Chronic or convalescent carriers should not be allowed to prepare food until clear documentation shows that at least three or more stool cultures are negative for typhoid bacilli. Carriers should be cautioned regarding routine sanitary techniques.

PROGNOSIS The mortality rate from typhoid fever prior to the introduction of chloramphenicol was about 12 percent. Death was associated with toxemia, inanition, pneumonia, bowel perforation, and intestinal hemorrhage. The mortality rate is still about 2 percent; deaths are observed primarily in infants, the aged, or individuals with malnutrition or other underlying diseases, or in those in whom the diagnosis is not suspected early.

SALMONELLA INFECTIONS OTHER THAN TYPHOID FEVER

DEFINITION Bacteria of the genus *Salmonella* may produce asymptomatic infection of the intestinal tract in humans or several different clinical syndromes including acute gastroenteritis (or enterocolitis), bacteremia, paratyphoid fever, or localized infections ranging from osteomyelitis to endocarditis. The clinical syndromes resulting from infection with *Salmonella* cannot always be sharply differentiated and sometimes overlap.

Salmonella infections are among the most prevalent recognized communicable diseases caused by bacteria in the United States today. These infections are transmitted in the vast majority of cases from animals to humans and occasionally from person to person and, in normal hosts, are usually brief, self-limited, and mild.

EPIDEMIOLOGY Salmonellae can be isolated from the intestinal tracts of humans and many lower animals. The prevalence of asymptomatic excretors of these organisms in the general population has been estimated to be about 0.2 percent (with probably over 2 million cases annually in the United States), but the most important reservoir of salmonellae is in domestic and wild animal species in which infection rates vary from less than 1 to more than 20 percent. An incomplete list of animals from which *Salmonella* species have been isolated includes chickens, turkeys, ducks, pigs, cows, dogs, cats, rats, parakeets, as well as certain cold-blooded animals and insects. Animals sold as pets, especially baby chicks, ducks, and turtles, may also harbor *Salmonella* and serve as sources of infection.

Salmonella infection is almost always acquired by the oral route, usually by ingestion of contaminated food or drink. Rare exceptions are *Salmonella* infections acquired by intravenous platelet transfusions or contaminated fiberoptic instruments. Any food product is a potential source of human infection. The source of contamination of food or drink may be asymptomatic human carriers or persons with active clinical disease, but the greatest single source of human infection in the United States is the vast reservoir of *Salmonella* in lower animals. The high incidence of infection in domestic animals used as a source of food for humans and present methods of processing foods and food products in bulk result in the availability of foods for human consumption with a potentially high incidence of contamination with *Salmonella*. For example, a significant proportion varying from 1 to more than 50 percent of raw meats purchased in retail markets is contaminated with *Salmonella*. Meat is contaminated by many routes, but the most common are natural infection of the animal used as a source of meat and contamination of the carcass during slaughter and processing. Eggs or egg products, including dried or frozen eggs, are also common sources of *Salmonella* infection. Of the various animal species, domestic fowl, including chickens, turkeys, ducks, and eggs and egg products, constitute the single largest reservoir of infection and the source most often responsible for infection of humans. Adequate cooking of food prior to human consumption serves to decrease the possibility of infection. However, salmonellae may survive cooking at low temperature, or food may be recontaminated after cooking by organisms from kitchen equipment or personnel. Raw or inadequately pasteurized milk is increasingly recognized as a potential vehicle of *Salmonella* infections, especially with *S. dublin,* that may cause more severe or bloodstream infections.

Food or drink may also be contaminated by rats, mice, insects, or other vermin harboring these organisms. Cross infection occurs occasionally by the airborne route from dried foods such as egg whites or dust which contain viable *Salmonella*. *Salmonella* contamination of a large variety of processed foods has also been documented. Some of these foods contain ingredients of animal origin such as eggs, whereas others contain contaminated products of vegetable origin such as coconut or yeast. A variety of pharmaceutical products of animal origin have been shown to be responsible for *Salmonella* infections of humans; these products include carmine dye, pancreatin, bile salts, and extracts of various organs such as thyroid, adrenal, and stomach.

Pet turtles are an important source of *Salmonella* infection in humans, especially in children, accounting for perhaps as many as 10 to 20 percent of reported *Salmonella* infections in certain areas. Turtles are infected on breeding farms and continue to excrete organisms in feces into tank water for long periods of time. Although knowledge of the manner of transmission to humans is incomplete, it is likely that turtle feces or tank water harboring salmonellae contaminates the hands of handlers, from which organisms are passed to the mouth or to food or drink.

Salmonella species may also be transmitted directly or via fomites from humans to humans or from animals to humans without the intervention of contaminated food or drink, but this method of spread is not common. However, cross infection of this type has been shown to be responsible for a number of outbreaks of salmonellosis among patients in nurseries and hospitals. Nosocomial salmonellosis poses a particular threat to newborns, immunosuppressed patients, patients in burn units, and those receiving multiple broad-spectrum antibiotics, who may be infected by relatively few organisms. Multiply drug-resistant salmonellae are often found in this setting. Nursery outbreaks have been traced to newborn infants from mothers with recent *Salmonella* infections.

Fish meal, meat meal, bone meal, and other by-products of the meat-packing industry are often contaminated with *Salmonella* organisms. These products are incorporated in animal and poultry feeds and apparently play an important role in the perpetuation of infection among domestic animals that can be spread to humans.

The true incidence of *Salmonella* infection is difficult to determine. The reported isolations of salmonellae from humans in the United States represent about 10 cases per 100,000 population per year. However, reported cases represent only a small proportion of the actual number because bacteriologic studies are usually performed only on patients with severe or protracted diarrhea, and many outbreaks are not investigated. It is estimated that over 2 million cases probably occur each year, affecting nearly 1 percent of the population in the United States. Although *Salmonella* infection occurs throughout the year, the Salmonella Surveillance Unit of the National Communicable Disease Centers has observed a distinct seasonal pattern with the greatest number of isolations reported from July through November for each year.

A close correlation exists between the *Salmonella* serotypes most often responsible for human infection and those isolated from animals in any specific geographic area. The similarities document the importance of nonhuman reservoirs of *Salmonella* in the epidemiology of *Salmonella* infection in humans.

PATHOGENESIS The course of events after salmonellae have gained access to the gastrointestinal tract is determined by the dose, serotype, and invasive potential of the organism, and by the resistance of the host. Different *Salmonella* serotypes show marked variation in invasive potential and capacity to produce disease in humans. For example, *S. anatum* characteristically produces asymptomatic intestinal infection and rarely invades the bloodstream. In contrast, *S. cholerae-suis*, the most invasive serotype, frequently produces bacteremia and metastatic infection. Bloodstream invasion may occur as a complication of gastroenteritis but usually develops without preceding intestinal symptoms. Bacteremia with any serotype may be transient or prolonged, and may be accompanied by recurrent chills and fever or manifestations of paratyphoid fever. Bloodborne bacteria may localize at any site and lead to suppuration in bone, joints, meninges, pleura, or other tissues.

Multiplication of ingested organisms in the intestinal tract may be followed by symptoms of gastroenteritis. The intestinal irritation and inflammation are produced by a true infection deep in the mucosa as evidenced by polymorphonuclear leukocytes typically found in the diarrheal stool. However, studies in animals have shown that mucosal invasion alone is not sufficient to account for the intestinal fluid observed in experimental infections. The secretory effects of certain strains of *S. typhimurium* can be abolished in animals by indomethacin without altering the invasive process. This has led to the hypothesis of a possible enterotoxin-like effect on upper intestinal transport. An enterotoxin-like effect has also been shown with culture filtrates of *Salmonella* in animals and tissue culture models used to study *Escherichia coli* and cholera enterotoxins.

Studies in human volunteers indicate that large numbers of viable organisms must be ingested to produce clinically apparent disease. However, a transient carrier state can be produced with doses 10 or 100 times smaller than those required to evoke symptoms of infection. The minimal infectious dose varies markedly among different serotypes.

Many host factors influence the frequency and nature of *Salmonella* infections. The minimal infectious dose varies considerably among different individual hosts and can be reduced by antacids, antimotility drugs, or antimicrobial agents in experimental animals. Some have reported the precipitation of severe systemic disease following antimotility therapy for mild gastroenteritis.

The bacterial flora of the intestine is important in determining the fate of ingested salmonellae. Increasingly impressive epidemiologic and experimental data show that antibiotics increase the susceptibility to *Salmonella* infections. Symptomatic infections in outbreaks are often associated with recent antibiotic consumption. Administration of certain antibiotics by the oral route to mice results in a 10,000-fold increase in susceptibility to infection with *S. enteritidis*. In experimental typhoid fever in volunteers, the dose of *S. typhi* required to initiate infection by the oral route in humans can also be reduced sharply by giving certain antimicrobials orally prior to challenge. Epidemiologic studies have also shown that prior antimicrobial therapy alters the capacity of the human intestinal tract to eradicate *Salmonella* acquired naturally. The effect of antibiotic therapy may be related to a marked diminution in the number of *Bacteroides* or other organisms which produce substances such as short-chain fatty acids that inhibit the growth of *Salmonella*. Alteration in intestinal flora also has been suggested as a mechanism of the increased susceptibility of patients with previous major gastric surgery, especially gastrectomy and gastroenterostomy, to intestinal infection with salmonellae. However, reduced acidity or rapid emptying time consequent to gastric surgery may also play a role by increasing the number of viable organisms reaching the small intestine.

Cell-mediated immune mechanisms are also important in host resistance to infection with salmonellae. About one-third of patients who are hospitalized because of salmonellosis have some type of major underlying disease, such as leukemia, lymphoma, lupus erythematosus, or aplastic anemia. Several reports describe an increased frequency of persisting or recurring *Salmonella* infections in patients with the acquired immunodeficiency syndrome (AIDS). In a few other diseases there is evidence to indicate a particular predisposition to infection by salmonellae that exceeds susceptibility to other bacterial species. Patients with sickle cell anemia and other hemolytic processes are unusually susceptible to bloodstream invasion by salmonellae. In patients with sickle hemoglobinopathies there is a strong tendency for localization in bone, and salmonellae, not staphylococci, are the most common cause of osteomyelitis in patients with sickle cell diseases. *Salmonella* bacteremia is also an unusually frequent complication of the acute hemolytic phase of bartonellosis (see Chap. 116).

Infants are more susceptible to *Salmonella* infection and remain convalescent carriers for a longer period of time than adults. The mortality rate from the disease is also higher in infants and in the elderly than in young adults.

CLINICAL MANIFESTATIONS Gastroenteritis Although gastroenteritis often occurs in large epidemics among individuals who have eaten the same contaminated food, family outbreaks and sporadic cases are even more common. After an incubation period of 8 to 48 h, there is sudden onset of colicky abdominal pain and loose, watery diarrhea, occasionally with mucus or blood. Nausea and vomiting are frequent but are rarely severe or protracted. Fever of 38 to 39°C is common, and there may be an initial chill. Patients usually have mild to moderate abdominal tenderness on palpation, but severe tenderness, even with rebound, occurs in occasional patients. Peristalsis is usually hyperactive. Abdominal findings may be prominent in some patients and lead to confusion with certain intraabdominal emergencies, such as acute appendicitis or acute cholecystitis. Colonic involvement with tenesmus and with mucosal friability and crypt abscess may also occur. Symptoms usually subside promptly within 2 to 5 days and recovery is uneventful. However, the illness is occasionally more protracted, with persistence of diarrhea and low-grade fever for 10 to 14 days. Fatalities rarely exceed 1 percent of the affected population and are limited almost entirely to infants, the aged, and debilitated patients.

The causative organism can often be isolated from the suspected food and from feces during the acute illness. Stool cultures usually become negative for salmonellae within 1 to 4 weeks, but occasional patients continue to excrete organisms for months. Organisms tend to persist in the stools of infants and young children for longer periods than in older children or adults. The blood leukocyte count is usually normal. The blood culture is usually negative.

Enteric or paratyphoid fever Certain species can produce an illness clinically indistinguishable from typhoid fever, with prolonged fever, rose spots, splenomegaly, leukopenia, gastrointestinal symptoms, and positive blood and stool cultures. The organisms most likely to produce this picture are *S. cholerae-suis* and *S. enteritidis*, serotypes *paratyphi A* and *paratyphi B*. Occasionally a typical attack of food poisoning is followed in a few days by manifestations of paratyphoid fever. Generally, paratyphoid fevers tend to be milder than *S. typhi* infections, but differentiation on clinical grounds is not possible in the individual case. Recovery may be followed by continued excretion of the causative organism in the stools for several months, but the chronic carrier state is less frequent than in typhoid fever.

Bacteremia *Salmonella* species may produce a syndrome characterized primarily by prolonged fever and positive blood cultures. Although symptoms of gastroenteritis can precede bacteremia, they are usually lacking, and most cases arise sporadically. In many instances, the only manifestations are prolonged fever, which is usually spiking and is accompanied by repeated rigors, sweats, aching, anorexia, and weight loss. The characteristic features of typhoid and paratyphoid fever, such as rose spots, persistent leukopenia, and sustained fever, are absent. Stool cultures are usually negative. In contrast to the constant bacteremia of typhoid fever, discharge of organisms into the bloodstream is intermittent, and repeated blood cultures may be required to demonstrate the causative organism. At some time in the course of the illness, localizing signs of infection appear in about one-fourth of the cases. Pulmonary infection in the form of bronchopneumonia or abscess, pleurisy, empyema, pericarditis, endocarditis, pyelonephritis, meningitis, osteomyelitis, and arthritis is relatively common. The blood leukocyte count is usually normal, but with the development of focal lesions, polymorphonuclear leukocytosis as high as 20,000 to 25,000 cells per cubic millimeter occurs. *Salmonella* bacteremia can be a very puzzling disorder, especially before localization takes place, and should be considered in cases of fever of unknown origin.

A prolonged febrile illness lasting weeks or months and characterized by weight loss, marked anemia, hepatosplenomegaly, and bacteremia with *Salmonella* has been described in Brazil and other areas of the world in patients with hepatosplenic schistosomiasis due to *Schistosoma mansoni*. Intermittent bacteremia with *Salmonella* also occurs in patients with *Schistosoma haematobium* infection who are also urinary carriers of *Salmonella*.

Local pyogenic infections *Salmonella* organisms can produce abscesses in almost any anatomic site, and these can occur independently of previous symptoms of gastroenteritis or other systemic illness, or as complications of bacteremias. There is nothing characteristic about the suppurative lesions, and the correct etiologic diagnosis is rarely made on the basis of clinical findings alone. There is a strong tendency for salmonellae to localize in tissues that are the site of preexisting disease. Localization has been described in aneurysms, bone adjacent to aortic aneurysms, hematomas, and many different tumors, including hypernephroma, ovarian cyst, and pheochromocytoma. Meningeal localization of infection is common in newborns and infants, and occasional small outbreaks of *Salmonella* infection in nurseries have consisted almost entirely of meningitis. In addition to suppurative joint disease, a chronic aseptic polyarthritis has been described.

DIAGNOSIS Febrile gastroenteritis produced by presumed viral agents, *Campylobacter jejuni* or *Shigella* sp., can be distinguished from *Salmonella* gastroenteritis only by appropriate stool cultures, especially in sporadic cases. Polymorphonuclear fecal leukocytes are frequently present in *Salmonella* gastroenteritis and in bacillary dysentery (shigellosis), but not in viral, giardial, or enterotoxin-induced gastroenteritis. Staphylococcal food poisoning usually is not associated with fever, and vomiting is a more prominent feature than in most *Salmonella* infections. Systemic manifestations are usually much less striking in patients with gastroenteritis caused by enterotoxigenic *E. coli* and *Clostridium perfringens*. Many toxic agents and drugs can produce diarrhea, nausea, and abdominal pain, but fever is rarely a feature of these disorders, and the diagnosis depends upon a history of exposure or ingestion. The diagnosis of paratyphoid fever or *Salmonella* bacteremia depends upon isolation of the causative organism. Agglutination tests with acute and convalescent serums as performed in the usual clinical laboratory are not very helpful. The possibility of an underlying disease should be considered in every patient with a severe *Salmonella* infection.

TREATMENT The treatment of *Salmonella* gastroenteritis is supportive. Dehydration should be corrected by parenteral administration of fluids and electrolytes. Abdominal cramps and diarrhea often are much improved if the patient takes nothing by mouth for 8 to 12 h. Antimicrobial therapy does not shorten the clinical course of *Salmonella* gastroenteritis, but actually prolongs the duration of excretion of organisms in the stool and may increase the clinical relapse rate. Unless there is documented bacteremia or a protracted febrile course suggesting the diagnosis of enteric fever, antibiotics are *not* indicated in uncomplicated *Salmonella* gastroenteritis. Because of the predilection of *Salmonella* bacteremia to colonize endovascular foci, it has been suggested that patients over 50 years old, especially those with atherosclerotic arterial aneurysms, prosthetic vascular prostheses or valves, or even underlying valvular or coronary disease, who develop febrile *Salmonella* enteritis and suspected bacteremia should be considered for early antimicrobial therapy. Certainly, persons with documented bacteremia or those who relapse with these actual or potential intravascular foci should receive effective antimicrobial therapy.

There has been a steady increase in the frequency of antimicrobial resistance due to transferable resistance factors among *Salmonella* isolates from humans. This may be due in part to the widespread use of antibiotics in animals and in humans.

Chloramphenicol in doses of 3 g daily in adults is the antibiotic of choice in systemic infections including *Salmonella* bacteremia, metastatic infection, and paratyphoid fever. The response is characteristically slow, and the temperature rarely returns to normal until 3 to 4 days after beginning therapy. Therapy should be continued for at least 2 weeks, but in certain infections, such as osteomyelitis or meningitis, the duration may have to be extended. As resistance to multiple antibiotics is increasing, antibiotic sensitivity of the organism should be tested in cases of bacteremia, metastatic infection, or enteric fever.

Because of the hematologic toxicity of chloramphenicol, some prefer ampicillin to treat systemic infections caused by sensitive *Salmonella* strains, and ampicillin is preferred over chloramphenicol for suspected intravascular infection as noted above. However, a significant proportion of *Salmonella* strains are highly resistant to ampicillin in vitro. For this reason, ampicillin should not be used in therapy of serious infections unless it is known that the causative organism is sensitive. As in cases of typhoid fever, the combination of trimethoprim and sulfamethoxazole holds promise in the therapy of *Salmonella* infection when the organism is resistant to chloramphenicol and ampicillin. The tetracycline derivatives have sometimes appeared to exert a beneficial effect, but streptomycin, polymyxin, neomycin, kanamycin, and the sulfonamides are generally ineffective.

Antimicrobial therapy is usually not indicated in convalescent or asymptomatic transient carriers of *Salmonella* species. The carrier state will cease spontaneously in 1 to 3 months in the vast majority of individuals.

The chronic carrier state with localization of infection in the gallbladder and positive stool cultures for a period of time exceeding 1 year is rarely caused by *Salmonella* serotypes other than *S. typhi* and *S. paratyphi* A and B. Its treatment has been discussed. Surgically accessible suppurative lesions should be drained.

PREVENTION AND CONTROL Continuous surveillance and careful reporting of all *Salmonella* isolates improve awareness of new strains, common sources, antibiotic resistance, and the carrier state. Because of the great number of specific serotypes, surveillance and serotyping have occasionally brought attention to widespread occurrence of relatively rare serotypes traced to single sources. Adequate cooking of meat and egg products and careful surveillance of poultry products and persons who handle food have been only moderately successful in controlling salmonellosis. Probably most important, besides food surveillance, is personal hygiene, including handwashing. Transient or permanent carriers should be warned to take these precautions and, as much as possible, to avoid food preparation. Minimizing the time that foods are allowed to stand at room temperature (as between cooking and refrigeration) should reduce the chances of bacterial growth to infectious inocula.

Careful obstetrical histories for any diarrheal illness at the time a woman enters for delivery should always be obtained, and mothers and infants so affected should be isolated until cultures rule out *Salmonella* carriage. Finally, because of the increasing antibiotic resistance, the indiscriminate use of unnecessary or "prophylactic" antimicrobial agents should be avoided.

REFERENCES

ALVAREZ-ELCORO S et al: *Salmonella* bacteremia in patients with prosthetic heart valves. Am J Med 77:61, 1984

BAINE WB et al: Institutional salmonellosis. J Infect Dis 128:357, 1973

BLASER MJ et al: *Salmonella typhi:* The laboratory as a reservoir of infection. J Infect Dis 142:934, 1980

BUTLER T et al: Typhoid fever: Studies of blood coagulation, bacteremia and endotoxemia. Arch Intern Med 138:407, 1978

COHEN PS et al: The risk of endothelial infection in adults with *Salmonella* bacteremia. Ann Intern Med 89:931, 1978

FREERKSEN E et al: Treatment of chronic salmonella carriers. Chemotherapy 23:192, 1977

HOFFMAN SL et al: Reduction of mortality in chloramphenicol-treated severe typhoid fever by high-dose dexamethasone. N Engl J Med 310:82, 1981

HOLMBERG SD et al: Drug-resistant *Salmonella* from animals fed antimicrobials. N Engl J Med 311:617, 1984

HOOK EW: Typhoid fever today. N Engl J Med 310:82, 1981

HORNICK RB, GRIESMAN S: On the pathogenesis of typhoid fever. Arch Intern Med 138:357, 1978

Human *Salmonella* isolates—United States, 1980. Morb Mort Week Rep 30:377, 1981

JACOBS JL et al: *Salmonella* infections in patients with the acquired immunodeficiency syndrome. Ann Intern Med 102:186, 1985

KAYE D et al: Treatment of chronic enteric carriers of *Salmonella typhosa* with ampicillin. Ann NY Acad Sci 145:429, 1967

LEVY SB: Playing antibiotic pool: Time totally the score. N Engl J Med 311:617, 1984

MANDAL BK: Typhoid and paratyphoid fever. Clin Gastroent 8:715, 1979

POTTER ME et al: Unpasteurized milk. The hazards of a health fetish. JAMA 252:2048, 1984

QUE JU, HENTGES DJ: Effect of streptomycin administration on colonization resistance to *Salmonella typhimurium* in mice. Infect Immun 48:169, 1985

RYDER RW et al: Increase in antibiotic resistance among isolates of *Salmonella* in the U.S. J Infect Dis. 142:485, 1980

TAUXE RV et al: Turtle-associated salmonellosis in Puerto Rico. JAMA 254:237, 1985

TAYLOR DN et al: Typhoid in the United States and the risk to the international traveler. J Infect Dis 148:599, 1983

TURNBULL PCB: Food poisoning with special reference to *Salmonella*—Its epidemiology, pathogenesis and control. Clin Gastroent 8:663, 1979

108 SHIGELLOSIS

RICHARD D. PEARSON / RICHARD L. GUERRANT

DEFINITION Shigellosis refers to an acute bacillary infection of the intestinal tract produced by one of four *Shigella* species. The spectrum of disease ranges from mild, watery diarrhea to severe dysentery characterized by crampy abdominal pain, tenesmus, fever, and signs of systemic toxicity.

ETIOLOGY The genus *Shigella* of the family Enterobacteriaceae is composed of a group of closely related species which are nonmotile, nonencapsulated, nonsporulating, gram-negative rods. They are aerobes or facultative anaerobes and grow best at 37°C. The species differ in their ability to ferment carbohydrates. All strains produce acid, but not gas, from glucose and either fail to ferment lactose or do so slowly. The four species are further subdivided into a total of approximately 40 serotypes. Four species or groups are separated on the basis of major somatic (O) antigens and fermentation patterns: *S. dysenteriae* (group A), *S. flexneri* (group B), *S. boydii* (group C), and *S. sonnei* (group D). In developing countries, *S. dysenteriae* type 1 and *S. flexneri* are the most common isolates. They predominated in the United States and Europe prior to 1940, but *S. sonnei* has been the most frequent isolate since that time.

Shigella species have lipopolysaccharide endotoxin which is chemically and biologically similar to the endotoxins of other Enterobacteriaceae. *Shigella dysenteriae* type 1 (Shiga bacillus) also produces an exotoxin. The exotoxin has since been shown to have enterotoxin activity which may cause intestinal secretion as well as cytotoxic properties directed against intestinal epithelial cells. It may also account for the neurotoxicity observed in children with shigellosis. *S. flexneri* and *S. sonnei* produce a similar exotoxin although in smaller amounts.

EPIDEMIOLOGY Shigellosis is worldwide in distribution and remains a major problem in countries which lack effective sanitation and where malnutrition is common. In 1983, approximately 15,000 cases of shigellosis were reported in the United States; *S. sonnei* was responsible for 66 percent. Children under 10 years of age accounted for the greatest number of cases. In the United States, shigellosis is particularly common among children in day-care centers and among male homosexuals. In emerging nations, *S. flexneri* and *S. dysenteriae* type 1 remain the most important pathogens.

Humans and other primates are the only known reservoirs of *Shigella* species. The portal of entry is the gastrointestinal tract. Shigellosis is one of the most communicable of the bacterial diarrheal diseases; ingestion of fewer than 100 organisms can produce disease among healthy volunteers. Spread of *Shigella* is primarily person-to-person through contaminated hands or objects or by consumption of contaminated food or water. Poor sanitation, low standards of personal hygiene, crowded conditions, and a high proportion of children in the population favor spread of infection in the developing world. Outbreaks of shigellosis in the United States have tended to occur in confined populations where there are poor sanitary conditions or hygiene such as day-care centers, cruise ships, Indian reservations, mental institutions, geriatric wards, or other custodial care centers. Secondary transmission in industrialized countries frequently follows acquisition of shigellosis by children in day-care centers. Fecal-oral transmission of *Shigella* among male homosexuals has been increasingly recognized. *Shigella* species have caused traveler's diarrhea in visitors to Russia and other areas of the world. Laboratory-acquired cases are also well-documented.

Common source outbreaks have involved food contaminated by careless handlers who are *Shigella* carriers. Outbreaks associated with drinking water have occurred, and swimming in contaminated water has led to infection. However, food- and waterborne transmission appear to be less important in shigellosis than in cholera or typhoid fever, in which larger inocula are usually necessary to produce disease.

In developing countries where spread of disease is primarily person-to-person, carriers may be the important reservoir. In patients who receive no antibiotic treatment, fecal excretion of *Shigella* usually lasts 1 to 4 weeks, but in a small percentage of cases shedding persists for much longer periods. Prolonged carriage seems to be more common among the malnourished.

PATHOGENESIS AND PATHOLOGY After ingestion, the organism is thought to colonize and multiply in the upper small bowel where it may cause secretion early in illness. The colon rapidly becomes the principal site of pathology in *Shigella* dysentery. *Shigella* penetrate epithelial cells, multiply intracellularly, and spread laterally to cause cell death. Superficial microulcers and inflammation result.

The multiple factors which contribute to the virulence of *Shigella* are under polygenic control. There is a strong correlation between invasiveness and gastrointestinal virulence. Virulent *Shigella* produce an exotoxin that has cytotoxic, enterotoxic, and neurotoxic properties. It is composed of active and binding subunits, binds to a glycoprotein membrane receptor on epithelial cells, is transported into the cell by an energy-dependent mechanism, and inhibits protein synthesis by catalytic inactivation of the 60S ribosomal subunit. Roles for enterotoxin activity in causing secretion, cytotoxin activity in causing cell damage, and neurotoxin activity in producing the neurologic manifestations of shigellosis have been postulated but not proven. A 120–140 Mcal plasmid encoding translucent colony morphology, smooth lipopolysaccharide, and antigenic peptides is necessary, but not sufficient for invasiveness. Necessary chromosomal traits include somatic antigens, intestinal survival, invasiveness as assessed by the Serény test, and possibly exotoxin production.

Innate and acquired host defenses against *Shigella* are not completely understood. Gastric acidity and bile do not appear to provide effective barriers. Increased intestinal motility during infection may contribute to clearance of the organism. Normal intestinal flora may impede the growth of *Shigella*. Humoral immunity is thought to be important in acquired host defense against *Shigella*, protection deriving mainly from coproantibodies (IgA). After natural infection, serotype-specific antibodies and enterotoxin-neutralizing antibodies are identified in serum within 1 to 2 weeks. Serotype-specific vaccine efficacy has also been demonstrated. Breast-feeding appears to be protective in newborns. This may be mediated by maternal antibodies against *Shigella* or nonspecific factors. Cellular immune responses during or following shigellosis in humans have not been thoroughly characterized, but in vitro studies indicate that Fc receptor–bearing lymphocytes, monocytes, and granulocytes can kill *Shigella* in the presence of anti-*Shigella* antisera.

CLINICAL MANIFESTATIONS The spectrum of shigellosis ranges from mild diarrhea to severe dysentery with crampy abdominal pain, tenesmus, fever, and systemic toxicity. Symptoms usually begin abruptly 1 to 7 days after exposure. Patients initially have watery stools accompanied by fever (as high as 41°C), diffuse abdominal pain, nausea, and vomiting. Other symptoms include myalgias, chills, backache, and headache. Dysentery develops after the first few days of illness and is associated with tenesmus and frequent, small, bloody, mucoid stools. Fever subsequently decreases, and abdominal pain may localize to the lower quadrants. Diarrhea peaks at about 7 days. Bloody dysentery is more common and appears earlier in infection with *S. dysenteriae* type 1 than with other serotypes. Neonatal infection, which is uncommon even in endemic areas, may present with weight loss, poor feeding, diarrhea, and occasionally jaundice.

The physical examination is normal in mild cases, or there may be signs of severe dehydration. Diffuse or localized lower abdominal tenderness is often present, but there is seldom evidence of peritoneal irritation. Bowel sounds are usually hyperactive. Diffuse mucosal edema, hyperemia, and superficial ulceration are seen on proctosigmoidoscopy.

Shigellosis is generally a self-limited disease, but in certain patients, particularly infants and the elderly, severe dehydration or even malnutrition may be precipitated by fluid and electrolyte loss, anorexia, and fever. In normal hosts who do not receive antibiotics, fever usually resolves after 3 or 4 days, but diarrhea and abdominal cramps may continue for 1 to 2 weeks. The overall mortality rate associated with shigellosis in the United States is less than 0.1 percent, but the illness is often more severe and the prognosis poorer among children and the elderly. *S. dysenteriae* type 1 produces more severe infection than other *Shigella* species, and mortality rates in epidemics in the developing world have been high, particularly in malnourished children.

Extraintestinal complications of *Shigella* infection are uncommon. In addition to headache, meningismus or seizures may occur. Seizures are most common in children under 5 years of age and are not always associated with marked temperature elevation. The cerebrospinal fluid is usually normal. Transient peripheral neuropathy has followed *S. dysenteriae* type 1 infection, and the Guillain-Barré syndrome has followed by 1 week an outbreak of *S. boydii* gastroenteritis. *Shigella* species are infrequently recovered from the bloodstream, possibly because *Shigella* are susceptible to complement-mediated lysis in serum. Hematogenous dissemination is relatively infrequent except in malnourished infants, and *Shigella* abscesses and meningitis have been reported. Respiratory symptoms are rare. Cough, chest pain, pulmonary infiltrates, and pleural effusions may occur, but *Shigella* species are seldom isolated from sputum. As with other types of inflammatory colitis, Reiter's syndrome with arthritis, sterile conjunctivitis, and urethritis may follow shigellosis, usually within 1 to 4 weeks after the onset of diarrhea in patients with HLA-B27 histocompatibility antigens (see Chap. 268). Some *Shigella* isolates have antigens that immunologically cross-react with the B27 locus. Isolated, nonsuppurative monoarticular or oligoarticular arthritis may also follow shigellosis. This condition is usually self-limited and resolves within several months without deformity. Urinary tract infections due to *Shigella* species have been reported but are rare. A hemolytic-uremic syndrome has been observed with shigellosis in children. It tends to occur in association with leukemoid reactions, severe colitis, and circulating endotoxin but usually without demonstrable bacteremia. Culture-positive, purulent keratoconjunctivitis occasionally results from direct autoinoculation of the eye by contaminated fingers.

DIAGNOSIS AND LABORATORY FINDINGS Shigellosis should be considered in every febrile illness associated with diarrhea. The stool is usually watery and contains variable amounts of mucus, blood, or pus. There is no consistent alteration in the peripheral blood white count during shigellosis. Occasionally a leukemoid reaction with 50,000 or more polymorphonuclear cells per cubic millimeter is encountered. An increase in band forms is frequent. Anemia is uncommon. Serum electrolyte abnormalities may result from vomiting and diarrhea.

The finding of fecal leukocytes and erythrocytes in a fresh stool specimen indicates inflammatory enteritis. A definitive diagnosis is established when a *Shigella* species is isolated from stool culture. The organisms are relatively fastidious and easily destroyed in fecal specimens which have been allowed to stand or dry. Cultures should be immediately plated from freshly passed stool or a rectal swab, or if that is not possible, placed into transport media. An enteric agar medium (MacConkey or *Shigella-Salmonella,* SS), a moderately selective agar (xylose-lysine-desoxycholate, XLD), and an enrichment broth (gram-negative or selenite broth) should be used. The stool culture is usually positive during acute shigellosis. During the postacute phase, multiple stool cultures may be necessary to isolate the organism. Antibodies develop in the serum of the majority of patients with positive cultures, but are not detectable until after the patient has recovered. Although not useful in the acutely ill patient, serology may be helpful in identifying endemic serotypes or in documenting the occurrence of an epidemic.

The differential diagnosis of inflammatory colitis characterized by fever, gross or microscopic blood in the stool, and fecal leukocytes includes infection with *Shigella* species, *Campylobacter jejuni, Salmonella* species, enteroinvasive *Escherichia coli, Yersinia* species, *Vibrio parahemolyticus,* cytotoxigenic *Clostridium difficile,* and *Entamoeba histolytica* (see Chap. 89). These pathogens cannot be clearly distinguished on clinical grounds. The onset of amebic colitis is often more gradual than that of shigellosis, the diarrhea less voluminous, and fecal leukocytes are pyknotic or absent. In viral gastroenteritis, fever is uncommon and the stool does not usually contain blood or pus. The bacterial causes of inflammatory colitis can be differentiated with certainty only be microbiologic studies. Shigellosis occasionally causes more prolonged, intermittent diarrhea resulting in a clinical picture that mimics ulcerative colitis. The extraintestinal manifestations of shigellosis may initially suggest acute meningitis, infectious arthritis, or other diseases.

TREATMENT Correction of fluid and electrolyte loss is a mainstay of therapy and can be accomplished with an oral glucose-electrolyte solution and ad libitum fluids if the patient is mild to moderately dehydrated, not vomiting, and able to drink. Otherwise, intravenous fluids may be necessary. The clinical state of hydration must be monitored especially closely in infants and the elderly. Once appetite returns, regular food or breast-feeding of infants should be offered to replace the acute protein-calorie deficit.

Although shigellosis is usually a self-limited disease, chemotherapy is effective in reducing the duration of fever and in shortening the period of *Shigella* carriage. Stool cultures become negative within 48 h after initiation of antibiotic treatment for susceptible strains, and clinical relapses after therapy are rare. Emergence of antibiotic resistance has been an important problem throughout the world. Resistance is usually mediated by R factors. In the United States, 90 percent of *Shigella* isolates are resistant to sulfonamides, and many are now resistant to ampicillin.

The treatment of choice for shigellosis when susceptibility is unknown or when ampicillin/tetracycline–resistant strains are encountered, is trimethoprim-sulfamethoxazole (trimethoprim 160 mg plus sulfamethoxazole 800 mg) every 12 h orally for 5 to 6 days. Ampicillin 50 mg/kg per day in four equally divided doses for 5 days is considered the treatment of choice for sensitive strains. Clinical failures have been observed with amoxicillin, and it should not be used. A single dose of 2.5 g of oral tetracycline has been used successfully in some adult patients. Tetracycline should be avoided in children under 10 years of age because of its deposition in growing teeth and bone. Other antibiotics which are active against *Shigella* in vitro have not been effective in vivo. These include cefamandole, cephalexin, cefaclor, and kanamycin. Experience in widely scattered areas around the world indicates that trimethoprim-sulfamethoxazole resistance is now emerging among *Shigella* species. Newer drugs such as bicozamycin or quinoline compounds including nalidixic acid or ciprofloxacin may be necessary to treat infections with these strains. Antimotility drugs such as paregoric, loperamide, and diphenoxylate hydrochloride with atropine (Lomotil) are contraindicated because they may worsen the clinical illness and prolong excretion of *Shigella.*

PREVENTION Preventive measures should be aimed both at the individual and the community. Good personal hygiene with hand washing after defecation is important. Infected patients should not prepare food, and toilets should be adequately disinfected. In the future, immunologic control may become possible given the relatively limited number of serotypes of *Shigella* which cause disease. Serotype-specific protection has been shown with orally administered live, attenuated *Shigella* vaccines in humans, but a completely stable, nonreverting vaccine strain capable of producing long-lasting immunity is not available.

Community measures include the development of adequate sewage disposal systems and safe water supplies. Hospitalized patients should be placed on stool isolation precautions, not allowed to contact others, and have their linen and clothing isolated. Attending personnel must wash their hands and instruments after patient contact. Patients who have recovered from shigellosis should not prepare food until their stool culture is negative.

REFERENCES

BARRETT-CONNOR E, CONNOR JD: Extraintestinal manifestations of shigellosis. Am J Gastroenterol 53:234, 1970

DRITZ SK et al: Patterns of sexually transmitted enteric diseases in a city. Lancet 2:3, 1977

DUPONT HC: *Shigella* species (bacillary dysentery), in *Principles and Practice of Infectious Diseases 2,* GL Mandell et al (eds). New York, Wiley, 1985, pp 1269–1273

KEUSCH GT: The epidemiology and pathophysiology of invasive bacterial diarrheas with a note on biological considerations in control strategies, in *Diarrhea and Malnutrition: Interactions, Mechanisms and Interventions,* LC Chen, NS Scrimshaw (eds). New York, Plenum, 1983, pp 45–72

PICKERING LK et al: Diarrhea caused by *Shigella,* rotavirus, and *Giardia* in day-care centers: Prospective study. J Pediatr 99:51, 1981

SANSONETTI PJ et al: Genetics of virulence in enteroinvasive *Escherichia coli,* in *Microbiology—1985,* L Leive et al (eds). Am Soc Microbiol, 1985, pp 74–77

SHIGELLOSIS— United States, 1983. Morb Mort Week Rep 33:616, 1984

STRUELENS MJ et al: *Shigella* septicemia: Prevalence, presentation, risk factors, and outcome. J Infect Dis 152:784, 1985

TACKETT CO, COHEN ML: Shigellosis in day care centers: Use of plasmid analysis to assess control measures. Pediatr Infect Dis 2:127, 1983

109 *HAEMOPHILUS* INFECTIONS

RALPH D. FEIGIN / FREDERICK M. MURPHY[1]

Haemophilus influenzae was isolated by Pfeiffer in 1892 from the sputum of individuals afflicted during an influenza pandemic. The requirement of blood for in vitro growth and its presumptive role in the pandemic prompted the designation. Other species have since been classified as members of the *Haemophilus* genus on the basis of morphology and physiology: small, pleomorphic, aerobic or

[1] *The editors wish to acknowledge the contribution of David H. Smith, M.D. It is on his chapter in the tenth edition of* Principles of Internal Medicine *that this revision is based.*

facultatively anaerobic, nonmotile, non-spore-forming, gram-negative bacilli that require enriched media containing blood or certain preformed growth factors present in blood.

There are 16 species belonging to the genus *Haemophilus*. The single most important member is *H. influenzae*. Other important pathogenic species include *H. aegypticus, H. ducreyi, H. parainfluenzae, H. aphrophilus,* and *H. paraphrophilus*. Previously included in the genus *Haemophilus* were *H. vaginalis* and *H. pertussis*. Neither of these two species has a strict requirement for either growth factor X or V; therefore, they are excluded from this genus. *H. vaginalis* is now classified as *Gardnerella vaginalis* and is considered in Chap. 143. *H. pertussis* is now classified as *Bordetella pertussis* and is included in this chapter.

HAEMOPHILUS INFLUENZAE **Etiology** *H. influenzae* is distinguished by its growth requirement of a heat-labile V factor and a heat-stable X factor found in erythrocytes and its inability to hemolyze erythrocytes during growth. V factor can be replaced by coenzyme I (DPN), coenzyme II (TPN), or nicotinamide nucleoside, and X factor by hematin. X factor is not required for anaerobic growth. Fermentation reactions and tests of other metabolic activities are variable and not useful in identification but may help in "biotyping" individual isolates. Based upon indole production and ornithine decarboxylase and urease activities, seven biotypes (I to VII) have been described.

Optimal growth of *H. influenzae* is realized with media in which erythrocytes are disrupted to release the growth factors, e.g., chocolate or Levinthal agar. "Satellism," growth around colonies of hemolytic *Staphylococcus aureus* which release growth factors, is often used to identify *H. influenzae*. Some strains grow best in 5 to 10% carbon dioxide; many laboratories therefore incubate specimens suspected of containing *H. influenzae* in a candle jar or an incubator purged with carbon dioxide. Since viability of this bacterium is lost rapidly on drying or heating, clinical specimens should be inoculated without delay.

The organism exists with or without a polysaccharide capsule. Colonies of nonencapsulated isolates are usually 0.5 to 1.5 mm in diameter and appear granular after overnight incubation on solid agar; those of encapsulated isolates are usually 3 to 4 mm in diameter and initially appear mucoid or glistening. *H. influenzae* grown on enriched media appear microscopically as relatively uniform, small coccobacilli (1×0.3 μm); under less than optimal growth conditions, long filaments or short chains are common. Because *H. influenzae* in clinical specimens often have variable morphology and do not always react with safranin dye, gram-stained smears of infected material are frequently misdiagnosed.

The outer membrane of *H. influenzae,* like that of other gram-negative bacilli, is composed of a lipopolysaccharide (endotoxin)-containing cell wall and a number of proteins, some of which are common to all isolates. Determination of the composition of *H. influenzae* outer membrane proteins has been useful for epidemiologic studies. The antigenic activity of *H. influenzae* endotoxin and these outer membrane proteins has not been defined. Only a small percentage of isolates recovered from the respiratory tract are encapsulated. Six antigenically distinguishable capsular types, designated a to f, have been identified. Each is a complex carbohydrate. Type a, b, and c capsules share antigenic determinants with those of certain pneumococci. In addition, type b capsule, polyribose ribitol phosphate (PRP), cross-reacts immunologically with the capsules or cell walls of several species of gram-positive bacteria and enteric bacilli.

Strains with decreased or absent capsular antigen arise spontaneously from encapsulated strains. This variation proceeds M (fully encapsulated) → S (partially encapsulated) → R (nonencapsulated). The genetic basis of this variation and the natural existence of its converse, i.e., R→S→M, remain undescribed. DNA purified from an M strain can transform an R strain to the serotype of the donor M strain. Transformation of *H. influenzae* in the host has not been studied, but the demonstration of pneumococcal transformation in experimentally infected mice supports the possibility that this occurs. Transformation between *H. aegypticus* and *H. influenzae* and between *H. influenzae* and *H. parainfluenzae* demonstrates the close genetic relation of these species.

The physiologic release by *H. influenzae* b of its capsular antigen (PRP) during growth in vitro and in the host provides the basis for clinically useful immunologic detection systems, e.g., countercurrent immunoelectrophoresis or agglutination of latex particles to which antibody is absorbed.

H. influenzae was previously susceptible to many antibiotics, but a significant percentage of strains is now resistant to ampicillin, and resistance to tetracycline has been increasing. Ampicillin-resistant strains are widely but variably distributed and are as pathogenic and transmissible as antibiotic-sensitive strains. Ampicillin resistance, which is plasmid-mediated, occurs in 25 percent of isolated strains of *H. influenzae* type b, and higher resistance rates have been reported. Chloramphenicol-resistant and multiple-resistant (chloramphenicol, tetracycline, and/or ampicillin) strains have been isolated with increasing frequency.

Epidemiology *H. influenzae* infects only humans and primarily in the upper respiratory tract. It can be recovered from the nasopharynx of up to 90 percent of healthy individuals with the frequency of infection related inversely to age. The colonization rate of type b organisms averages 5 percent. Asymptomatic nasopharyngeal infection lasts days to a few months, is not eradicated by systemic antibody, and often is not eliminated by antibiotic therapy adequate to cure type b meningitis.

H. influenzae diseases occur worldwide and for the most part are endemic. Systemic *H. influenzae* diseases have a marked age relationship: children of 6 to 48 months are highly susceptible; newborns, older children, and adults are uncommonly affected. Systemic type b diseases occur at an attack rate up to 6000 times normal among children of susceptible ages who have intimate contact with primary cases and among persons with certain diseases that increase their susceptibility, e.g., sickle cell disease, splenectomy, agammaglobulinemia, and treated Hodgkin's disease. Alcoholic adults appear to be at modestly increased risk of *H. influenzae* pneumonia. Increased risk also is noted among blacks, the poor, urban dwellers, and members of large families. In temperate climates, systemic *H. influenzae* diseases occur most commonly during the late winter and spring.

The incidence of systemic *H. influenzae* b diseases has increased fourfold during the past 3 to 4½ decades, and more adults are being affected. The basis for this increased attack rate is not understood, but improved diagnostic laboratories and diminution in the prevalence of type-specific immunity due to excessive use of antibiotics have been suggested as possible mechanisms. Changes in antigenic composition and/or virulence of the organism and the prevalence of cross-reactive antibodies also may be responsible for this change.

Pathogenicity The relatively common asymptomatic nasopharyngeal infection occasionally develops into symptomatic disease which may spread contiguously to involve the sinuses, middle ear, or bronchi, or may invade local tissues, causing epiglottitis, pneumonia, or pericarditis. The frequent bacteremia associated with local invasion may lead to metastatic disease such as facial cellulitis, meningitis, or septic arthritis. Nonencapsulated strains produce luminal diseases, while systemic diseases are caused almost entirely by encapsulated *H. influenzae,* of which at least 95 percent are type b.

The pathogenicity of invasive strains is related directly to the inhibition of phagocytosis by the capsule. The basis for the disproportionate virulence of type b strains is under study, as is the role of outer membrane proteins and other constituents. Animal studies indicate that, unlike other bacteria, piliated strains have no apparent advantages over nonpiliated *H. influenzae* for colonization or invasion. Synergy between *H. influenzae* and certain respiratory viruses has been demonstrated in studies of human disease and experimental models.

Immunity Susceptibility to *H. influenzae* is correlated inversely with age and with anticapsular antibody titer. Antibodies to the PRP capsule of *H. influenzae* b promote phagocytosis and bacteriolysis in vitro, protect animals from lethal concentrations of *H. influenzae* b, and are responsible for the efficacy of the anti–*H. influenzae* b serum used in the preantibiotic era. The genesis of naturally occurring anti-PRP antibody is not known but may result from nasopharyngeal carriage of *H. influenzae* b or from infection with cross-reacting bacteria such as *E. coli* K100, which also has a capsule composed of PRP. Antibodies to strain-specific, noncapsular protein antigens also protect against lethal inocula of *H. influenzae* b in animals, increase the clearance rate of bacteria administered intravenously, and may be protective in humans. Immunity may result from a composite effect of anticapsular and antisomatic antibodies as well as from cellular immunity.

Studies of patients recovering from systemic *H. influenzae* b disease and those immunized with PRP have revealed that infants respond infrequently and poorly, younger children have intermediate reactivity, while older children and adults develop marked, non-boostable responses. A few children fail to produce anti-PRP antibody (measured by radioimmunoassay) following systemic disease and subsequently develop a second distinct episode of invasive type b disease. Although these children appear to have been "immunologically nonreactive" for periods up to months, all subsequently raised anti-PRP antibody activity. These observations indicate the need for further study and close follow-up of young children recuperating from invasive *H. influenzae* b disease. Likewise, survivors of intensive therapy for Hodgkin's disease—chemotherapy, splenectomy, and/or radiation—produce transient, infantlike anti-PRP antibody responses, even following systemic *H. influenzae* b disease.

Clinical manifestations *H. influenzae* can cause local respiratory tract or invasive diseases. Surveys of hospitalized children indicate that *H. influenzae* b is now the most common cause of bacteremic disease and that about one-half of children with *H. influenzae* disease have meningitis, one-sixth pneumonia, about 10 percent bacteremia without a primary focus, facial cellulitis, or epiglottitis, and 1 percent pyarthrosis. Adults may develop *H. influenzae* bacteremia, meningitis, and, less commonly, epiglottitis; however, bronchitis, due to non-encapsulated strains, and pneumonia are more common.

H. influenzae diseases are generally acute with symptoms reflecting the pyogenic process; however, the clinical course of certain of these diseases may be surprisingly prolonged.

MENINGITIS *H. influenzae* is the most common cause of bacterial meningitis, primarily affecting children 9 months to 4 years of age. The signs and symptoms depend on the patient's age and the time in the course of the disease when medical care is sought. Young children and those early in the disease generally have a nonspecific clinical picture: preceding upper respiratory tract symptoms, fever, anorexia, lethargy, vomiting, and, with older children and adults, headache. A history of stiff neck or back may be elicited. Mental confusion, paresis of cranial nerves, coma, convulsions, opisthotonus, and shock occur with more prolonged and serious disease. The clinical findings are identical to those of other bacterial causes. Age and certain types of concurrent disease, e.g., cellulitis, pyarthrosis, or epiglottitis, suggest *H. influenzae,* but the diagnosis depends on bacteriologic studies. Demonstration of PRP in cerebral spinal fluid by latex agglutination or CIE (counterimmunoelectrophoresis) permits rapid diagnosis.

PNEUMONIA *H. influenzae* may cause either a broncho- or lobar pneumonia. Up to 75 percent of the children with lobar pneumonia have an associated empyema. Purulent pericarditis may develop in up to 5 percent of cases. Concomitant otitis media due to *H. influenzae* is frequent. Lobar disease, particularly with pleural involvement, is most often confused with pneumococcal or *S. aureus* pneumonia, but the course can be prolonged enough to suggest tuberculosis. Elderly patients, particularly those with primary lung disease and/or alcoholism, are being infected increasingly by *H. influenzae*.

BACTEREMIA WITHOUT LOCALIZED DISEASE Children, particularly those 6 to 24 months of age, may develop bacteremia without evidence of localized disease. This condition most often occurs in those with a temperature greater than 102°F and an elevated circulating neutrophil count. Persons with sickle cell disease, previous splenectomy, or chemotherapy for Hodgkin's disease are at increased risk of bacteremia without localized disease. Although pneumococci are the most common cause of this syndrome, *H. influenzae* b is the second most common etiologic agent. Fever, chills, anxiety, anorexia, and lethargy dominate the clinical picture. Among highly susceptible persons, this disease can progress to shock and death within a few hours.

CELLULITIS *H. influenzae* causes a cellulitis, particularly among children 6 to 24 months of age. It is characterized as a raised, warm, tender area of distinctive reddish-blue hue, usually located on one cheek or, less commonly, the periorbital area. The child is moderately febrile and toxic and has a history of preceding rhinorrhea, fever, and, at times, ipsilateral otitis media. The cellulitis develops and spreads within a few hours. *H. influenzae* cellulitis on the limbs or hands is seen rarely and usually in older children. The distinctive color, location, and clinical course suggest the etiology. Bacteremia is almost always present, and a secondary focus is present in 10 percent of cases.

EPIGLOTTITIS *H. influenzae* b is the leading cause of this potentially lethal disease. The mean age in children is 4 years with males outnumbering females. Caucasians predominate. Bacteremia is detected in 90 percent of cases, but extraepiglottic foci are rare. The disease is characterized by the rapid onset of fever, dysphagia, toxicity, anxiety, stridor, retractions, and drooling. Patients assume a typical position of sitting forward with protrusion of the mandible and hyperextension of the neck to maximize airway diameter. The dramatic clinical presentation is usually sufficient to justify direct laryngoscopy and, if epiglottitis is present, endotracheal intubation. This should be performed in a setting where emergency tracheostomy can be performed if attempted intubation is unsuccessful. Lateral neck radiographs can be helpful if the diagnosis is not obvious and the patient is stable. Examination of the oropharynx utilizing a tongue depressor may precipitate complete airway obstruction and respiratory arrest and probably should not be attempted.

Acute epiglottitis in adults most often has a viral etiology and a more indolent clinical course of dysphagia and sore throat and less often requires intubation or tracheostomy. When due to *H. influenzae,* the clinical course approximates that in children but is less severe.

PYARTHROSIS *H. influenzae* b joint disease occurs during a septic invasion with or without other systemic disease usually in children under 2 years of age. Single, large, weight-bearing joints are usually involved, and concomitant osteomyelitis is present in up to 22 percent of cases. Response to systemic antibiotics without surgical drainage is dramatic and curative, but long-term follow-up reveals some joint dysfunction in a significant number of children.

PERICARDITIS *H. influenzae* b causes purulent pericarditis usually associated with pneumonia. The clinical signs and symptoms are generally similar to those caused by other pyogenic bacteria, but the course is often more prolonged.

OTHER RESPIRATORY TRACT DISEASE *H. influenzae* is the second leading cause of childhood otitis media and often causes sinusitis. Nearly all the etiologic strains are nonencapsulated. These diseases cannot be distinguished clinically from those produced by other microbial agents, nor can the disease caused by encapsulated or nonencapsulated *H. influenzae* be differentiated clinically. Fever, local pain, irritability, and, in sinusitis, foul breath, postnasal drip, and cough predominate. Chronic bronchitis, particularly among adults and those with agammaglobulinemia, is often caused by nonencapsulated *H. influenzae* or mixed bacterial species among which *H. influenzae* predominates. Cough productive of purulent sputum, dyspnea with prolonged expiration, and anorexia dominate the clinical picture, which is aggravated by smoking and by inhalation of respiratory pollutants.

OTHER DISEASES *H. influenzae* can cause endocarditis and brain abscess, but such cases are rare and are usually associated with a primary underlying disease. *H. influenzae* endophthalmitis, pyelonephritis, and osteomyelitis have been reported. Pharyngitis is only rarely caused by *H. influenzae,* and this organism plays no role in bronchiolitis.

Diagnosis The etiology of many *H. influenzae* diseases, especially facial cellulitis and epiglottitis, can generally be suspected on the basis of the history and clinical findings. Chemical analysis of infected fluids is consistent with any pyogenic etiology. Leukocytosis is common, and children often have a significant anemia. Gram stains of infected body fluids correlate with culture results in 70 percent of cases. Among the remainder of culture-positive specimens, 15 percent have negative smears, while another 15 percent have misinterpreted smears. Staining such specimens with methylene blue generally does not improve these results. Quellung reactions are even less accurate.

PRP can be detected in the serum, CSF, or concentrated urine of up to 95 percent of patients with meningitis by countercurrent electrophoresis, the enzyme-linked immunosorbent assay (ELISA) technique, latex agglutination, or coagglutination. Several studies have compared these various techniques. CIE is the least sensitive, and the ELISA technique requires too much time to be clinically practical. Despite the apparent widespread distribution of immunologically cross-reactive antigens among bacteria in nature, false-positive reactions are unusual. PRP is generally detected in infected pericardial fluid or joint fluid but is found infrequently in the serum of children with epiglottitis, presumably due to the fulminant course of this disease and the time required for antigen release from invasive bacteria. Detection of antigen in the supernatant of liquid cultures can expedite laboratory diagnosis. Since antigen often persists after antibiotic therapy, its detection is helpful in the diagnosis of patients with systemic *H. influenzae* diseases who have received antibiotics.

Positive nasopharyngeal cultures are not meaningful because of the high carriage rate of *H. influenzae* by healthy individuals. Needle aspiration of the edge of the site of cellulitis or of diseased lung markedly increases the rate of bacterial isolation and is recommended, particularly in patients who are critically ill or who have a complicated course. Cultures of empyema, pericardial and joint fluid, and an inflamed epiglottis are diagnostic. Blood cultures are positive in up to 80 percent of patients with *H. influenzae* septic arthritis, facial cellulitis, epiglottitis, and meningitis prior to the onset of antibiotic therapy. Even if antibiotic therapy has been initiated, the yield is sufficiently great to recommend that blood cultures be taken. It has been suggested that *H. influenzae* pneumonia, in which 30 percent of persons have a positive blood culture, is underdiagnosed. The role of PRP detection in this diagnosis deserves further evaluation.

Treatment Without treatment, systemic *H. influenzae* disease, particularly meningitis and epiglottitis, has a very high, if not uniform, mortality. Chloramphenicol therapy yields very high concentrations of antibiotic in joint and cerebrospinal fluid relative to serum and produces excellent clinical results. The potential toxicity of chloramphenicol and the excellent results obtained with ampicillin made this agent the antibiotic of choice for *H. influenzae* diseases for many years. However, the current prevalence of ampicillin-resistant strains requires that all systemic diseases that might be due to *H. influenzae* be treated with chloramphenicol, 100 mg/kg per day for children, 4 g per day for adults, given intravenously in divided doses at 6-h intervals until the etiologic agent is proved to be sensitive to ampicillin. Some, including the American Academy of Pediatrics, recommend that ampicillin also be added to the initial chloramphenicol therapy. If the etiologic strain is sensitive, ampicillin is given intravenously in doses of 200 to 400 mg/kg per day for children and 6 g per day for adults, divided into six infusions given at 4-h intervals.

Chloramphenicol given orally yields higher serum levels of the antibiotic than identical doses given intravenously; administration of chloramphenicol by intramuscular injection yields variable and unpredictable blood levels and is contraindicated. Routine sensitivity testing of *H. influenzae* in invasive disease has become increasingly important, and the increasing frequency of ampicillin- and chloramphenicol-resistant strains of *H. influenzae* has stimulated a search for new antimicrobial agents for the treatment of meningitis.

In one excellent prospective randomized study moxalactam was shown to be as effective and safe as ampicillin or chloramphenicol in the treatment of meningitis. Other agents that have been employed successfully for the treatment of multiply resistant *H. influenzae* diseases in a small number of patients include ceftriaxone, ceftazidime, cefotaxime, and cefuroxime.

Amoxicillin is recommended for outpatient therapy of disease caused by *H. influenzae*. Alternative antibiotics when the organism is resistant to ampicillin or the patient is allergic to penicillin include cefaclor, trimethoprim-sulfamethoxazole, erythromycin-sulfasoxazole, cefaclor plus a sulfonamide, or chloramphenicol. Although chloramphenicol is an excellent antibiotic for oral therapy of serious *H. influenzae* infections, its routine use on an outpatient basis is not recommended because of its hematologic toxicities and the potential for accelerating the emergence of chloramphenicol resistance. Tetracycline can be used in adults to treat bronchitis and other respiratory diseases caused by sensitive strains.

The duration of chemotherapy for *H. influenzae* disease depends on the disease and the status of the individual patient. All systemic diseases should be treated with intravenous drugs at least until cultures of the infected area are sterile and the patient is afebrile and without clinical and laboratory evidence of active infection for 3 to 5 days. Patients with meningitis are therefore usually treated for 10 to 14 days. Occasionally, ampicillin does not clear the bacteria from the CSF, and relapses follow the cessation of therapy. Most therapeutic failures with ampicillin have been associated with antibiotic courses that are too brief, employ too low a dose, or are given otherwise than by the intravenous route; some result from localized disease that was not completely eradicated with standard treatment. In treatment failures, re-treatment according to the above guidelines should be undertaken, usually with chloramphenicol.

Patients with endocarditis or pericarditis should receive 3 to 6 weeks of intravenous therapy. Ampicillin and chloramphenicol diffuse well into inflamed joint spaces, and there is no indication for local instillation of antibiotics. Children with otitis media may be treated orally with amoxicillin in dosage of 50 mg/kg per day (adults 2 g per day in four divided doses) until their symptoms are alleviated plus 3 to 4 days; hence, the usually total course is 7 to 10 days. Sinusitis requires therapy of 3 or more weeks; therapy of bronchitis may need to be prolonged even longer.

Antibiotic therapy is only one facet of the management of the patient with a systemic *H. influenzae* disease. Careful evaluation of the airway, consideration of oxygen therapy and transfusion, vigorous treatment of shock and disseminated intravascular coagulation, conservative fluid replacement, anticonvulsant therapy, and medical management of cerebral edema are often critical. Repeated aspirations of an infected joint or empyema may be needed, but installation of a surgical drain is rarely required. The creation of a pericardial ''window'' for drainage in patients with pericarditis is preferable to repeated aspirations.

Prevention A large, prospective study coordinated by the Centers for Disease Control has shown that secondary cases of invasive *H. influenzae* diseases occur at significantly increased rates among young, household contacts. Specifically, the risk in household contacts was as follows: for those less than 6 years of age, 0.5 percent; less than 4 years, 2.1 percent; and less than 1 year, 6 percent. Several studies have shown that attack rates in day care center contacts less than 4 years of age range from 0 to 1 percent.

Several antibiotic regimens were studied between 1978 and 1984 to determine their efficacy in eradicating *H. influenzae* b from the nasopharynx. The only reliably effective regimen proved to be rifampin in a 20 mg/kg dose (maximum 600 mg per day) provided once daily for 4 days. This regimen is not only effective in eliminating nasopharyngeal carriage of *H. influenzae,* but also appears to be efficacious in preventing secondary cases of disease among household contacts.

The American Academy of Pediatrics currently recommends that rifampin be given orally once each day for 4 days in a 20 mg/kg dose (maximum 600 mg per day) to all household contacts (including adults) in households where there are children other than the index case younger than 4 years of age. Prophylaxis of contacts should begin as soon as possible after the diagnosis is established in the index case. Prophylaxis of day-care center or nursery school contacts is no longer recommended unless two or more cases of invasive disease have occurred among attendees within a 60-day period. It is also important to provide the same prophylactic regimen for all children with invasive disease prior to discharge from the hospital since they may still harbor the organism in their nasopharynx despite appropriate antibiotic therapy.

The increased attack rate and the constant mortality (5 to 10 percent) and neurologic morbidity (30 percent) during the past two decades for *H. influenzae* meningitis in children and the prevalence of ampicillin-resistant strains have stimulated an attempt to produce a vaccine to prevent *H. influenzae* diseases. Because of the primacy of the type b capsule in pathogenicity and the efficacy of anticapsular serum, attention was focused initially on a vaccine composed of purified capsular PRP. Such a vaccine has been found to be nontoxic and immunogenic for older children and adults. A single dose protects children older than 18 months from septic diseases for at least 4 years; however, the vaccine is not immunogenic or protective for children less than 18 months of age. This PRP vaccine is now licensed, and it is recommended for children 2 to 5 years of age and is suggested beginning at 18 months of age for those at high risk of invasive disease, such as the Alaskan Inuit, Navajo Indians, sickle cell disease patients, and day-care center attendees. Efforts have been made to investigate the immunogenicity of several vaccines in which PRP has been linked to a protein carrier such as pertussis, tetanus toxoid, or diphtheria. Such combinations have improved immunogenicity in infants compared to PRP alone (particularly the PRP-diphtheria vaccine), but further studies are needed to establish their efficacy.

Oral ingestion of nonpathogenic species of *Escherichia coli* which have an immunologically cross-reactive capsule may elevate systemic anti-PRP antibody activity. However, the observation in one center of an unusually high incidence of intestinal carriage of such *E. coli* among children with *H. influenzae* b meningitis has precluded further studies. Other studies are evaluating the role of *H. influenzae* outer membrane proteins either as a primary vaccine or a polysaccharide carrier, with the hope that such a vaccine might be protective against diseases caused by nonencapsulated as well as encapsulated *H. influenzae.*

HAEMOPHILUS AEGYPTICUS *H. aegypticus,* also known as the Koch-Weeks bacillus, causes conjunctivitis in humans. Morphologically and biochemically, this organism closely resembles an unencapsulated *H. influenzae.* Moreover, *H. aegypticus* and *H. influenzae* share certain antigens and can be transformed by DNA of the other species.

The conjunctivitis, which primarily affects children, occurs worldwide, often in epidemics, and in some areas seasonally. It must be distinguished from trachoma-inclusion conjunctivitis (TRIC) agents, adenoviruses, and other bacterial agents such as pneumococcus, *S. aureus,* and *Neisseria gonorrhoeae.* Therapy consists of local instillation of antibiotic drops or ointment, such as sulfonamide, polymyxin B, or gentamicin five or six times daily, and moist soaks to keep the eyelids clean.

HAEMOPHILUS APHROPHILUS *H. aphrophilus* is a small, nonmotile, aerobic, gram-negative coccobacillus which requires factor X (but not V) and high concentrations of CO_2 (5 percent is optimal) for growth. It is part of the normal oral flora, and although uncommon, is being recognized increasingly as a cause of many types of infection, particularly bacteremia, endocarditis, and brain abscess. Other reported infections due to *H. aphrophilus* include acute and chronic sinusitis, pneumonia, empyema, osteomyelitis, septic arthritis, otitis media, peritonitis, cholecystitis, periapical dental abscess, meningitis, deep tissue abscess, wound infection, and necrotizing fasciitis.

H. aphrophilus by itself can cause disease in otherwise normal individuals, but most cases are associated with predisposing conditions such as malignancy, immunosuppression, rheumatic or congenital heart disease, recurrent otitis media, and asthma.

Most strains are sensitive to the majority of commonly used antibiotics including penicillin, cephalosporins, aminoglycosides, tetracycline, and chloramphenicol.

HAEMOPHILUS DUCREYI *H. ducreyi* causes a localized venereal disease, chancroid (see Chap. 110). This disease is uncommon in the United States, but is endemic throughout the tropics, and accounts for 50 percent of genital ulcers in Kenya. The organism requires X but not V factor for growth. In clinical specimens and colonies grown on solid medium, the organism appears as small ovoid rods arranged in pairs, groups, or parallel chains. The disease is characterized by painful, nonindurated ulceration of the genitalia with enlarged, and often suppurative, regional lymph nodes. Chancroid must be distinguished from primary syphilis; not infrequently the two diseases occur simultaneously. Isolation on special selective media is successful in only 50 to 70 percent of cases, even in the best equipped laboratories. Because of the increasing incidence of sulfa and tetracycline resistance, which is usually plasmid-mediated, the recommended therapy is now trimethoprim-sulfamethoxazole or erythromycin.

HAEMOPHILUS PARAINFLUENZAE This species differs from *H. influenzae* by requiring V but not X factor for growth. Since *H. influenzae* does not require X factor for anaerobic growth, diagnostic confusion can arise, especially in stabbed cultures. This phenomenon may have played a role in certain systemic infections allegedly caused by *H. parainfluenzae* which, on further testing, were found to be due to *H. influenzae.*

Acute upper respiratory disease, e.g., otitis media, and less commonly meningitis, pneumonia, and brain abscess have been ascribed to *H. parainfluenzae.* Rarely, in less than 1 percent of cases, it is the infecting agent in endocarditis, and its isolation in this disease is often delayed (mean of 6 to 8 days) due to fastidious growth requirements and need for blind subculturing onto chocolate agar. *H. parainfluenzae* may be confused with *H. paraphrophilus,* which causes clinically identical endocarditis and from which it is very difficult to differentiate biochemically. A small but significant percentage of *H. parainfluenzae* carries plasmids mediating β-lactamase production and ampicillin resistance.

BORDETELLA PERTUSSIS *Bordetella pertussis* causes an acute infection of the respiratory tract that is most serious in infants and young children and is characterized by a repetitious, paroxysmal cough and prolonged, inspiratory stridor. The word *pertussis* means intensive cough, and this designation is preferable to "whooping cough" since not all patients with pertussis whoop.

Etiology The vast majority of cases of pertussis syndrome are caused by *B. pertussis;* however, *B. parapertussis, B. bronchiseptica,* and several adenoviruses can produce an identical illness.

B. pertussis is a minute, nonmotile, non-spore-forming, aerobic, gram-negative coccobacillus with extremely fastidious growth requirements. This organism is inhibited by many factors present in routine bacteriologic media. The classic medium for the primary isolation of *B. pertussis* (Bordet-Gengou) contains blood and starch. Addition of penicillin inhibits the growth of other organisms. The absence of an antigenic relation and with it the ability to transform *B. pertussis* with *H. influenzae* DNA or vice versa suggests that these species are not closely related. *B. pertussis* does not require X or V factors for growth; therefore, it cannot be included in the genus *Haemophilus. B. pertussis* is related closely, however, to *B. para-*

pertussis, which can cause a milder, similar disease in humans, and *B. bronchiseptica,* which causes respiratory disease in animals but rarely in humans. They have similar growth requirements and morphologic appearance and can be distinguished from each other by specific agglutination reactions.

Freshly isolated *B. pertussis* is in phase I, the virulent, morphologically uniform, encapsulated, and piliated form. Passage in culture may induce nonvirulent forms (phase II, III, or IV). Phase I organisms are required for transmission of disease and for the production of vaccine.

Epidemiology *B. pertussis* exists worldwide and naturally affects only humans, although nonhuman primates and mice can be infected experimentally. Pertussis is one of the most contagious infectious diseases because it is transmitted by aerosolized droplets. (The infectivity of respiratory secretions and contact transmission is not well studied.) Up to 90 (and in some reports 100) percent of exposed, susceptible persons develop the disease. Asymptomatic infection is rare. Although pertussis occurs endemically, it produces epidemics in a susceptible population. There is little seasonal variation in the incidence of pertussis. Females are affected more frequently than males, and this difference is accentuated with increasing age.

More than 50 percent of *B. pertussis* disease occurs in infants, presumably owing to deficient maternal immunity and possibly the lack of transplacental transfer of a protective bacteriologic antibody. Although adults were thought to be resistant to pertussis, neither the disease nor active immunization provides lifelong immunity; in fact, pertussis is not an uncommon cause of bronchitis in adults. More than 5 percent of cases now occur in individuals 15 years of age or older. Hospital personnel also are at increased risk, as evidenced by reports of epidemics involving hospital staff and patients.

About 3000 cases of pertussis are reported each year in the United States, but most observers think this number is falsely low because of the difficulty in bacteriologic confirmation. Reported cases probably represent 15 to 25 percent of the number of actual cases. Prior to widespread active immunization initiated in the 1940s, pertussis was a major cause of morbidity and mortality with the vast majority of deaths occurring in children less than 1 year of age. Since 1944, the pertussis mortality rate has decreased over 85-fold, although it has remained relatively constant since 1974. Pertussis remains a very significant health problem in developing countries, particularly in areas of poor nutrition and immunization. The limitation in the rate of immunization to pertussis in Great Britain to 30 percent of children has been accompanied by an epidemic affecting as many persons as in the prevaccine era. Certain adenoviruses can cause a clinical picture identical to that of pertussis, but there can be little doubt that *B. pertussis* is a primary pathogen.

Pathogenesis Inhaled phase I *B. pertussis* organisms attach to the ciliated respiratory epithelium by pili; the organisms multiply on the surface of the airways, but do not invade the bloodstream. Acute inflammation results: epithelial cell ciliary action is inhibited and mucous secretions are stimulated. The subsequent necrosis results in patchy ulceration of respiratory epithelium. The bronchi and bronchioles are primarily affected; the trachea, larynx, and nasopharynx may be involved, but less severely. The mucopurulent exudate can compromise the diminutive airway of the infant or small child. Focal atelectasis and emphysema and peribronchial infiltration by inflammatory cells, particularly lymphocytes, are common, and bronchopneumonia may develop.

Pertussis is mediated by a surface protein toxin which is composed of histamine-sensitizing factor (HSF), lymphocytosis-promoting factor (LPF), islet-activating protein (IAP), beta-adrenergic blockadelike effect, adjuvant effect, and mitogenicity. A heat-stable lipopolysaccharide endotoxin is also present on the surface of the organism but probably is not important in the pathogenesis of the disease. Additional biologically active components include a cytoplasmic heat-labile toxin (HLT), a tracheal cytotoxin (TCT), an intracellular adenylate cyclase, cell surface filamentous hemagglutinin (FHA), and surface agglutinogens. The capsule of *B. pertussis* is antiphagocytic. Antibody against capsular antigen is not protective.

Antipertussis secretory IgA is protective and specifically inhibits bacterial adherence to cilia. Antitoxin antibodies also are protective and either inhibit fixation of toxin to receptor cells or neutralize toxin. The role played by cell-mediated immunity in pertussis remains unclear.

Clinical manifestations Following an incubation period of 6 to 20 days (mean 7 days), sneezing, mild fever, rhinorrhea, anorexia, and a mild cough become evident (catarrhal period) and last 1 to 2 weeks, after which the cough increases in frequency and intensity. Paroxysms of cough are followed, particularly in infants, by a prolonged, often distressing, inspiratory gasp (the whoop). The cough occurs at variable intervals, often every few minutes, for 2 to 4 weeks (paroxysmal period). The disease is much more severe in the infant. The cough inhibits oral intake, and swallowed mucus may provoke vomiting, resulting in significant dehydration and weight loss. The cough can provoke venous congestion with hemoptysis, epistaxis, and small blood vessel hemorrhage. Hypoxia is more common and severe than is usually appreciated clinically and may be responsible for seizures, hypoxic encephalopathy, or coma. The contribution of toxin to neurologic complications is unclear. Adults and older children are less ill and have symptoms of a severe, prolonged bronchitis. The paroxysmal period is followed by a recovery period that lasts 1 to 6 weeks, during which the cough decreases in frequency and intensity. Spasms can be provoked during recovery, however, particularly by smoke or irritating inhalants.

Pneumonia, either caused by *B. pertussis* itself or more likely by secondary bacterial pathogens, is the most frequent complication of pertussis and is responsible for more than 90 percent of deaths in children under 3 years of age. Mucous plugging may result in atelectasis. Apnea is frequent. Other complications include activation of latent tuberculosis, otitis media (frequently due to *Streptococcus pneumoniae*), subarachnoid or intraventricular hemorrhage, severe alkalosis secondary to persistent vomiting, epistaxis, subdural hematomas, rupture of the diaphragm, umbilical or inguinal hernia, rectal prolapse, and meningoencephalitis.

Diagnosis The clinical diagnosis is suggested by a history of contact, the classic cough, and a marked absolute lymphocytosis. The diagnosis depends on the identification of *B. pertussis* in respiratory secretions. Success of isolation is favored by the immediate culture of a deep nasopharyngeal (NP) specimen in a freshly prepared selective medium. Because the characteristic pearllike colonies cannot be appreciated for 4 to 6 days, inhibitors of normal NP flora, e.g., methicillin, are added to the medium to prevent overgrowth of *B. pertussis*. The recovery rate on "cough plates" is too low to recommend this technique. *B. pertussis* can be isolated from as many as 90 percent of patients during the catarrhal stage of the disease but from no greater than 50 percent during the paroxysmal stage. Fluorescent-labeled antibody can detect *B. pertussis* in NP smears, but false-positive results may be obtained with up to 40 percent of specimens and false-negative tests in 10 to 20 percent. Serologic studies are of little value. Blood cultures are sterile and are not recommended; chest radiographs may show peribronchial thickening, atelectasis, or emphysema, but are not diagnostic. Dual infection with adenoviruses occurs, and positive viral cultures do not exclude *B. pertussis* as an etiologic agent.

An enzyme-linked immunosorbent assay (ELISA) can be used to detect IgM, IgA, and IgG antibodies in serum and may be useful in patients with negative cultures. The ELISA technique also can be used to detect IgA against *B. pertussis* in nasopharyngeal secretions beginning in the second or third week of illness up to at least 3 months. This antibody is induced by infection but not by vaccination. Pertussis may be distinguished from viral, mycoplasmal, and other bacterial causes of tracheobronchitis by a history of contact, the character and duration of symptoms, and the laboratory findings. The results of cultures are definitive.

Spasmodic coughing also may be associated with bronchiolitis; bacterial, mycoplasmal, and viral pneumonia; tuberculosis; cystic fibrosis; foreign bodies; and disease causing airway compression such as malignancy or chronic obstructive pulmonary disease. These diseases can be distinguished by their clinical and laboratory findings and by the course of the illness.

Treatment General supportive care is critical: careful nursing, avoidance of stimuli that provoke paroxysms, oxygen, suctioning of respiratory secretions, and attention to caloric needs and fluid and electrolyte balance. A single controlled study reporting beneficial effects of steroids in severely ill infants deserves attention.

B. pertussis is sensitive to many antibiotics in vitro. Antibiotics can eliminate infection and, if given in the catarrhal phase, prevent disease. Since the pathologic process is well-developed by the time paroxysms occur, antibiotic therapy given thereafter does not affect the clinical course. Erythromycin is preferred and should be used to prevent interpersonal transmission. Tetracycline and chloramphenicol are almost as effective as erythromycin but are not recommended because of potential toxicity, particularly for infants. Ampicillin appears to be relatively ineffective in eradicating nasopharyngeal infection. Antibiotic therapy may reduce the frequency and morbidity of secondary bacterial infection. Hyperimmune, antibacterial rabbit serum has no effect on bacterial shedding or clinical manifestations and is not recommended.

Prevention Patients suspected of having pertussis should be isolated until the diagnosis is disproved or the infection is eradicated by antibiotics. Exposed susceptibles should be vaccinated to prevent disease (see below) and treated with erythromycin to prevent infection and retransmission.

Prior to the availability of a vaccine, pertussis caused as many deaths in the United States as all other contagious diseases of children *combined*. In order to prevent the disease, a vaccine composed of a chemical extract of bacterial cells was developed. Because of the risk of pertussis to infants, the proposal was made to start immunization as early in life as possible. Unfortunately, pertussis immunization at 7 days of age produced a limited antibody response in only a small percentage of infants and resulted in reduced booster responses at 1 year. This vaccine is now mixed with diphtheria and tetanus toxoids, for convenience and because pertussis enhances the antibody responses to the toxoids, and is given five times during the first 6 years of life, with three doses being given at 2-month intervals starting at 8 weeks of age.

Although the vaccine was 70 to 80 percent effective in preventing disease among intimately exposed children, its effectiveness and toxicity have been questioned. Completely immunized children may develop pertussis, although the disease is milder than among the unimmunized. Furthermore, the protection provided by the vaccine is transient, with minimal resistance being evident a decade or later following the last immunization. Indeed, improved housing, hygiene, and nutrition are cited by some as responsible for the dramatic decline in pertussis during the past several decades. However, available data indicate that the rate of decline in the attack rate of pertussis in the United States has been positively affected by the vaccine. The association of an epidemic of pertussis in Great Britain with a decline in pertussis immunization also strongly supports the efficacy of the vaccine.

Pertussis vaccine provokes local reactions in up to 50 percent of recipients; neurologic complications, including uncontrollable screaming fits, convulsions, and encephalopathy, are a rare but real risk. However, the efficacy of the vaccine far outweighs the risk of significant neurologic complications. Convulsions, alteration of consciousness, shock, persistent screaming for 3 h or more, high-pitched cry, focal neurologic signs, temperature of 40.5°C or greater, and anaphylaxis following pertussis vaccination are contraindications to further doses. Immunization of infants residing in the United States should be deferred if they previously have had a seizure. Such individuals may be more prone to experience a convulsion after receipt of pertussis vaccine. There is no convincing evidence that isolated seizures either produce permanent neurologic disease or aggravate existing neurologic conditions. Children with neurologic disorders such as inherited defects that may be associated with seizures could be at increased risk of seizures following receipt of pertussis vaccine. Immunization of these children may be deferred, but such deferral is suggested on a case-by-case basis; the situation should be reevaluated at each visit to a physician.

Prematurity is not believed to increase the likelihood of seizures following pertussis immunization. Children with developmental delay or cerebral palsy who are not otherwise predisposed to seizures generally are not considered to be at increased risk of seizures following pertussis immunization. Because toxic reactions are more common in older persons, the vaccine is rarely given to those over 6 years of age. However, older persons with chronic pulmonary disease and exposed hospital personnel may be candidates for an absorbed pertussis vaccine (0.1 to 0.25 mL).

REFERENCES

Haemophilus aphrophilus

BIEGER RC et al: *Haemophilus aphrophilus:* A microbiologic and clinical review and report of 42 cases. Medicine 57:345, 1978

ELSTER SK et al: *Hemophilus aphrophilus* endocarditis: A review of 23 cases. Am J Cardiol 35:72, 1975

Haemophilus influenzae

BAND JD et al: Prevention of *Haemophilus influenzae* type b disease. JAMA 251:2381, 1984

FLEMING DW et al: Secondary *Haemophilus influenzae* type b in day-care facilities. Risk factors and prevention. JAMA 254:509, 1985

KAPLAN SL et al: Prospective comparative trial of moxalactam versus ampicillin or chloramphenicol for treatment of *Haemophilus influenzae* type b meningitis in children. J Pediatr 104:447, 1984

LEVIN DC et al: Bacteremic *Haemophilus influenzae* pneumonia in adults: Report of 24 cases and review of the literature. Am J Med 62:219, 1977

MUSTOE T, STROME M: Adult epiglottitis. Am J Otolaryngol 4:393, 1983

PELTDA H et al: *Haemophilus influenzae* type b capsular polysaccharide vaccine in children: A double-blind field study of 100,000 vaccines 3 months to 5 years of age in Finland. Pediatrics 60:730, 1977

ROTBART HA, GOLDE MP: *Haemophilus influenzae* type b septic arthritis in children: Report of 23 cases. Pediatrics 75:254, 1985

SMITH AL: Antibiotic resistance in *Haemophilus influenzae*. Pediatr Infect Dis 2:352, 1983

SMITH DH et al: Responses of children immunized with the capsular polysaccharide of *Haemophilus influenzae* type B. Pediatrics 52:637, 1973

TODD JK, BRUHN FW: Severe *Haemophilus influenzae* infections. Am J Dis Child 129:607, 1975

Update: *Haemophilus influenzae* b polysaccharide vaccine: Morb Mort Week Rep 35:144, 1986

WARD JI et al: *Haemophilus influenzae* meningitis: A national study of secondary spread in household contacts. N Engl J Med 301:122, 1979

Haemophilus parainfluenzae

CHUNN CJ et al: *Haemophilus parainfluenzae* infective endocarditis. Medicine 56:99, 1977

FRAZIER JP: Meningitis due to *Haemophilus parainfluenzae:* Report of three cases and review of the literature. Pediatr Infect Dis 1:119, 1983

Haemophilus aegipticus

ALBRITTON WL: Infections due to *Haemophilus* species other than *H. influenzae*. Ann Rev Microbiol 36:199, 1982

Haemophilus ducreyi

PLUMMER FA et al: Antimicrobial therapy of chancroid: Effectiveness of erythromycin. J Infect Dis 148:726, 1983

Bordetella pertussis

AMERICAN ACADEMY OF PEDIATRICS COMMITTEE ON INFECTIOUS DISEASES: Pertussis vaccine. Pediatrics 74:303, 1984

BASS JW et al: Antimicrobial treatment of pertussis. J Pediatr 75:768, 1969

BUCHANAN RD, GIBBONS NE (eds): *Bergey's Manual of Determinative Bacteriology*, 9th ed. Baltimore, Williams & Wilkins, 1984

CHERRY JD: The epidemiology of pertussis and pertussis immunization in the United Kingdom and the United States: A comparative study. Curr Probl Pediatr 14(2):1, 1984

DONALDSON P, WHITACKER J: Diagnoses of pertussis by fluorescent antibody staining of nasopharyngeal smears. Am J Dis Child 99:423, 1960

KOPLAN JP et al: Pertussis vaccine—An analysis of benefits, risks and costs. N Engl J Med 301:906, 1979

NELSON JD: The changing epidemiology of pertussis in young infants: The role of adults as reservoirs of infection. Am J Dis Child 132:371, 1978

110 CHANCROID

ALLAN R. RONALD / FRANCIS A. PLUMMER

DEFINITION Chancroid, or soft chancre (ulcer molle), is an acute sexually transmitted infection characterized by painful genital ulcerations often associated with inflammatory inguinal adenopathy which may progress to suppuration. The diagnosis is established by isolation of *Haemophilus ducreyi* from the lesion or a suppurative node and by exclusion of syphilis, genital herpes, and other specific causes of genital ulceration.

ETIOLOGY The isolation of *H. ducreyi* from ulcers proves the microbial etiology of chancroid. Gram-positive cocci and anaerobic gram-negative rods are often also present. However, there is no evidence that these organisms are independent pathogens or require specific therapy, and the clinical response to antimicrobial therapy parallels the susceptibility of *H. ducreyi*. In areas where chancroid is common, *H. ducreyi* can be isolated from up to 90 percent of ulcers that clinically appear to be chancroid. The organism is a gram-negative facultative aerobe which requires hemin (X factor) but not nicotinamide adenine dinucleotide (V factor) for growth. Many strains also require serum. Although no unique biochemical or immunologic features are known, the colonial morphology of *H. ducreyi* is distinct in that the yellow-gray colonies can be moved intact across the agar surface. Some strains demonstrate a typical streptobacillary "chaining" appearance on Gram stain, but this feature is variable and cannot be used as a taxonomic criterion.

EPIDEMIOLOGY The incidence of chancroid is unknown, owing to inaccurate diagnosis and incomplete reporting. It is common in southeast Asia and Africa, and is more prevalent than syphilis in many countries. Less than 1000 cases are reported annually in the United States. However, localized outbreaks do occur; for example, hundreds of cases involving predominantly migrant workers occurred in southern California in 1981 and 1982. The sex ratio of reported cases in the United States is five males to one female. Uncircumcised males are more susceptible to the disease. Prostitution plays a major role in transmission, and among merchant seamen and military troops whose sexual contacts are prostitutes, chancroid is more common than syphilis. The role of cervical carriage in the transmission of *H. ducreyi* is uncertain. Over one-half of the secondary sex partners of men with chancroid develop clinical chancroid. Asymptomatic carriage without disease has not been proven to occur.

FIGURE 110-1 *The classic chancroid.*

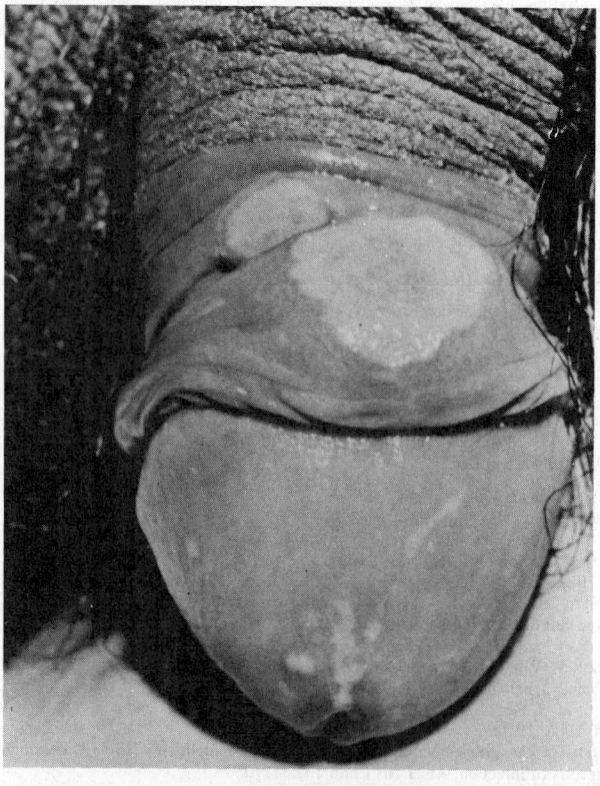

CLINICAL MANIFESTATIONS After an incubation period of 3 to 10 days, a small inflammatory papule appears which ulcerates within 2 to 3 days. The classic chancroidal ulcer (Fig. 110-1) is superficial, ranging in size from a few millimeters to several centimeters in diameter. The edge is ragged and undermined. The ulcer base is covered by a necrotic exudate. The ulcers are often multiple and may merge to form giant or serpiginous ulcers. Occasionally, the lesions remain pustular and resemble folliculitis or pyogenic infection. In contrast to syphilis, the chancroidal ulcer in males is painful and not indurated. The most frequent areas of localization are the preputial orifice, the internal surface of the prepuce, and the frenulum in men, and the labia, fourchette, and perianal region in women. The lesions in females tend to be more superficial and less painful. Extragenital ulcers are rare.

Acute, painful, tender inflammatory inguinal adenopathy occurs in almost 50 percent of patients and is frequently unilateral. If the patient is untreated, the involved nodes become matted, forming a unilocular suppurative bubo. The overlying skin becomes erythematous and tense and finally ruptures, forming a deep single ulcer.

DIAGNOSIS The morphologic diagnosis of genital lesions is fraught with error, and many lesions diagnosed as chancroid are actually genital herpes or syphilis. In the United States, one study of 100 consecutive men with penile ulceration disclosed genital herpes in 22, syphilis in 17, and traumatic lesions in 8. Classic chancroidal ulcers were noted in 12, only 2 of whom had ulcers that yielded *H. ducreyi*. In another study, two patients with suspected granuloma inguinale had positive cultures for *H. ducreyi*. These lesions have been termed *pseudogranuloma inguinale chancroid*. In contrast, in Kenya, of 97 consecutive men with penile ulceration, 60 were infected with *H. ducreyi*, 11 had syphilis, and only 4 had genital herpes.

Primary genital infection with herpes simplex virus produces tender inguinal adenopathy, but can be distinguished by the history of onset with vesicular lesions or of recent exposure to herpes and the presence of systemic symptoms such as fever and myalgia. Chancroid rarely causes systemic symptoms.

The chancre of primary syphilis is indurated, and the associated adenopathy is bilateral, nontender, and nonsuppurative. To exclude syphilis, all patients with genital ulcers should have two dark-field examinations performed on separate days, together with monthly serologic tests for syphilis for 3 months.

Lymphogranuloma venereum (LGV) differs from chancroid in that the adenopathy develops after the ulcer is healed. It is indolent, often bilateral and nontender, and develops multilocular suppuration and fistulas.

The diagnosis of chancroid is confirmed by the isolation of *H. ducreyi* from an ulcer or bubo. Exudate should be directly plated onto chocolate agar enriched with 1% Isovitalex and 5% sheep serum, plus 3 μg/mL of vancomycin. Colonies usually appear within 48 h of incubation in 5% CO_2 with 100% humidity but may require 4 to 5 days. No serologic tests are available for the diagnosis of chancroid.

TREATMENT Untreated chancroidal ulcers persist for long periods of time and often progress. Small lesions may heal within 2 to 4 weeks. Although sulfonamides and tetracyclines have been considered effective for chancroid, the emergence of multiresistant strains has resulted in many failures with both agents. Many isolates of *H. ducreyi* possess plasmids which mediate resistance to sulfonamides, tetracyclines, chloramphenicol, ampicillin, and kanamycin. Trimethoprim/sulfamethoxazole 320/1600 mg daily or erythromycin 2 g daily, each for 1 week are the regimens recommended by the Centers for

Disease Control. Trimethoprim/sulfamethoxazole will not interfere with the dark-field examination for *Treponema pallidum* or with the development of a positive serologic test for syphilis. The usual time to healing after onset of therapy is about 9 days. Several single-dose regimens including trimethoprim 640 mg/sulfonamide 3200 mg, spectinomycin 2 g IM, and ceftriaxone 250 mg IM have proved very effective for chancroid in Kenya. Fluctuant buboes should be aspirated to prevent rupture. Lymph node suppuration may progress despite otherwise effective therapy. Buboes larger than 5 cm in diameter almost always require aspiration.

Sexual contacts of patients with chancroid should be examined for ulcers, and treatment of contacts is recommended. Although the epidemiology of chancroid suggests that effective control measures, specifically designed for limited target populations such as prostitutes and known sexual contacts, could halt the spread of this disease, further prospective epidemiologic studies to demonstrate this are required.

REFERENCES

BLACKMORE CA et al: An outbreak of chancroid in Orange County, California: Descriptive epidemiology and disease-control measures. J Infect Dis 151:840, 1985

CHAPEL T et al: How reliable is the morphologic diagnosis of penile ulcers? Sex Trans Dis 4:150, 1977

FAST M et al: Treatment of chancroid by clavulanic acid with amoxicillin in patients with beta-lactamase-positive *Haemophilus ducreyi* infection. Lancet 2:509, 1982

HAMMOND GW et al: Comparison of specimen collection and laboratory techniques for isolation of *Haemophilus ducreyi*. J Clin Microbiol 7:39, 1978

——— et al: Epidemiologic, clinical, laboratory and therapeutic features of an urban outbreak of chancroid in North America. Rev Infect Dis 2:867, 1980

HANDSFIELD HH et al: Molecular epidemiology of *Haemophilus ducreyi* infection. Ann Intern Med 95:315, 1981

KRAUS SJ et al: Pseudogranuloma inguinale caused by *Haemophilus ducreyi*. Arch Dermatol 118:494, 1982

MCNICOL PJ et al: The plasmids of *Haemophilus ducreyi*. J Antimicrob Chemother 14:561, 1984

NSANZE H et al: Genital ulcers in Kenya: A clinical and laboratory study of 97 patients. Br J Vener Dis 57:378, 1981

PLUMMER FA et al: Short course of single-dose antimicrobial therapy of chancroid in Kenya: Reports of studies with rifampin-trimethoprim and rifampin alone. Rev Infect Dis 5:S565, 1983

——— et al: Single-dose therapy of chancroid with trimethoprim-sulfametrole. N Engl J Med 309:67, 1983

——— et al: Epidemiology of chancroid and *Haemophilus ducreyi* in Nairobi. Lancet 2:1293, 1983

RONALD AR et al: Chancroid and *Haemophilus ducreyi*, in *Sexually Transmitted Diseases*, KK Holmes et al (eds). New York, McGraw-Hill, 1984

———, PLUMMER FA. Chancroid and *Haemophilus ducreyi*. Ann Intern Med 102:705, 1985

111 DONOVANOSIS (GRANULOMA INGUINALE)

KING K. HOLMES

DEFINITION Donovanosis (granuloma inguinale) is a mildly contagious, chronic, indolent, progressive, autoinoculable, ulcerative disease involving the skin and lymphatics of the genital or perianal areas. The disease may be sexually transmitted and is associated with the presence in affected tissues of an intracellular microorganism, identified morphologically as the Donovan body.

ETIOLOGY Donovanosis was described by McLeod in India in 1882, and in 1905 Donovan described the intracellular bodies which are thought to cause the disease. Encapsulated bacteria resembling Donovan bodies have been recovered from lesions and pseudobuboes of granuloma inguinale by inoculation of chick embryo yolk sacs or yolk-agar medium. These bacteria, which are known as *Calymmatobacterium granulomatis,* measure 1.5 by 0.7 μm. They are antigenically related to *Klebsiella* species but do not reproduce the disease when inoculated intradermally in humans. It is uncertain whether these isolates are responsible for the disease. Electron microscopic studies of Donovan bodies confirm their morphologic resemblance to gram-negative bacteria.

EPIDEMIOLOGY Donovanosis is endemic in the tropics, particularly in New Guinea and among Hindus in India, and in parts of the Caribbean and Africa. In the United States the disease is rare. Most cases occur in the southeastern states and involve homosexual men. In reported cases the sex ratio of males to females is nearly 10:1. The disease is uncommon in Caucasians. The reported frequency of donovanosis in conjugal partners of chronically infected patients ranges from 1 to 64 percent. Evidence for sexual transmission includes the age-specific incidence, which corresponds to that of other sexually transmitted diseases, the frequent concomitant presence of syphilis, and the predilection for genital involvement in heterosexuals and for anorectal infection in homosexually active men.

CLINICAL MANIFESTATIONS The incubation period ranges from 8 days to 12 weeks, but most lesions appear within 30 days after sexual exposure.

Donovanosis begins as a papule, which ulcerates and develops into a painless elevated zone of clean, beefy-red, friable granulation tissue. The edges are irregular and spread by continuity or by autoinoculation of approximated skin surfaces. Secondary anaerobic infection may produce pain and a foul-smelling exudate. Less common complications of the disease include deep ulcerations, chronic cicatricial lesions, phimosis, lymphedema, and exuberant epithelial proliferation which grossly resembles carcinoma. In men, the lesions are usually located on the glans, prepuce, or shaft of the penis (Fig. 111-1*A*) or the perianal area, while infection of the labia is most common in women. Lesions in women often arise at the fourchette and progress anteriorly in a V shape along the vulva. Extragenital lesions may occur, involving the face, neck, mouth, and other sites. The chronicity of the disease is of diagnostic importance, since several months often elapse before patients seek treatment. Extension to the inguinal region by autoinoculation, by continuity, or via the lymphatics results in diffuse intradermal and subcutaneous swelling or suppuration, known as "pseudobubo," because involvement of the underlying lymph nodes is minimal. Locally destructive lesions and secondary infection may produce severe morbidity or death. Fatal disseminated disease, involving the bones, joints, or liver, has been reported after several years of chronic local infection. The relationship of donovanosis to subsequent carcinoma of the genitalia is uncertain.

DIAGNOSIS Early donovanosis may be mistaken for the primary chancre or condyloma latum of syphilis. Epithelial proliferation resembling carcinoma in the genital or perianal region in a young individual should always raise the suspicion of donovanosis if unnecessary destructive surgery is to be avoided. Chronic ulcerative or cicatricial changes may resemble lymphogranuloma venereum.

Amebiasis can produce penile lesions resembling donovanosis. In the United States, *Haemophilus ducreyi* has frequently been isolated from lesions resembling donovanosis; this has been termed *pseudogranuloma inguinale–chancroid.* Histologic studies in donovanosis reveal marked acanthosis and pseudoepitheliomatous hyperplasia. The dermis contains an inflammatory infiltrate consisting mainly of plasma cells and histiocytes. Because Donovan bodies are seldom detectable in sections stained with hematoxylin and eosin, these changes may lead to an erroneous diagnosis of carcinoma and to unnecessary destructive surgery. Although silver impregnation techniques are useful for demonstration of Donovan bodies in sections, the diagnosis is best made by examination of impression smears prepared from specimens obtained by punch biopsy of granulation tissue from the periphery of a lesion; the deep portion of the specimen is removed, crushed between two slides which are air-dried and fixed in methanol, and stained with Wright-Giemsa stain. With this method, Donovan bodies appear as very rounded coccobacilli, 1 by 2 μm in size, which lie within cystic spaces in the cytoplasm of large mononuclear cells (Fig. 111-2). The capsule stains as a dense acidophilic zone surrounding the bacterium, which resembles a closed

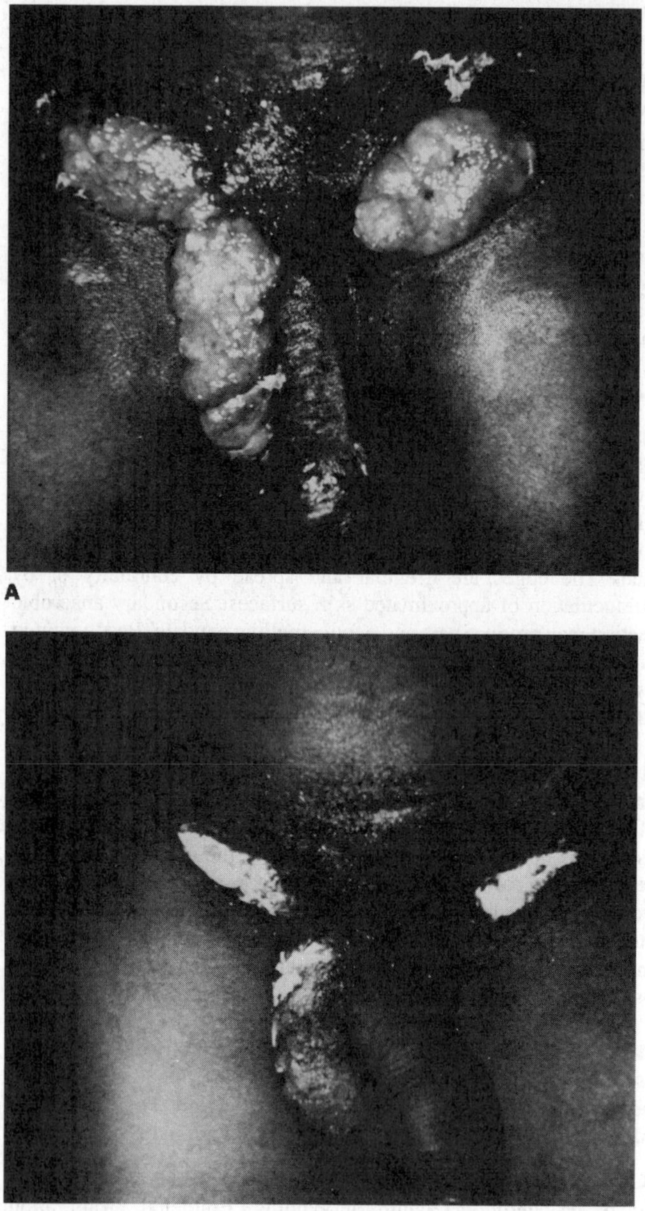

A

B

FIGURE 111-1 *A. Extensive granuloma inguinale, extending along the scrotum and involving both inguinal areas, with elevated, clean, exuberant granulation tissue. B. Same patient, following treatment. (Courtesy of A Brathwaite.)*

safety pin because of bipolar condensation of chromatin. The pathognomonic mononuclear cell is 25 to 90 μm in diameter and has many cystic areas containing Donovan bodies.

Perianal donovanosis may resemble condylomata lata of secondary syphilis. Other venereal diseases, particularly syphilis, very frequently coexist with donovanosis. Repeated dark-field examinations of lesions before treatment and a serologic test for syphilis should therefore be performed. In countries where donovanosis is endemic, the persistence of suspected condylomata lata after appropriate penicillin therapy for syphilis is highly suggestive of donovanosis.

TREATMENT The treatment of choice is tetracycline, 2 g daily, for at least 10 days. The risk of relapse is reduced if treatment is continued until healing is complete. Healing is usually apparent within 3 weeks, as the lesions become pale and flatter and develop peripheral reepithelialization (Fig. 111-1*B*). Donovan bodies disappear from lesions within a few days after onset of therapy. If tetracycline cannot be given, streptomycin may be used in a dose of 1 g intramuscularly every 12 h for 10 to 15 days. In New Guinea, chloramphenicol, 500 mg every 8 h orally, or gentamicin, 1 mg/kg twice daily, is used for cases which appear resistant to tetracycline. Co-trimoxazole (trimethoprim 160 mg, sulfamethoxazole 800 mg) twice daily for 10 days is also reported to be effective. In pregnant women, erythromycin, 500 mg every 6 h, may be effective. Treatment is reviewed in more detail in the chapter by Hart (1984).

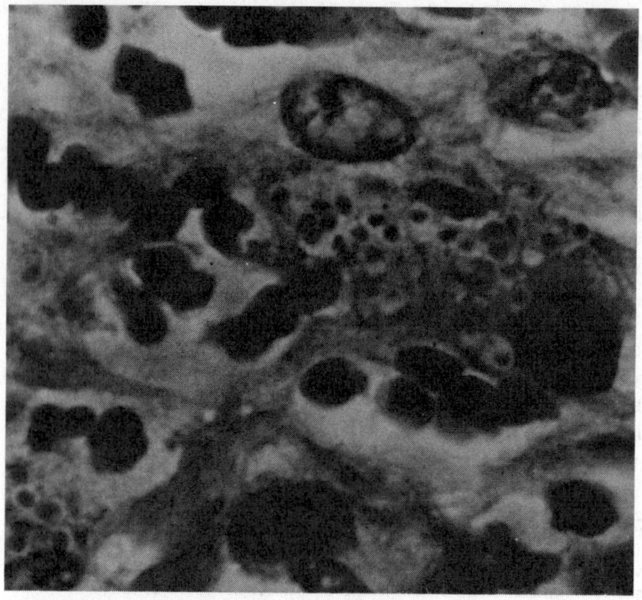

FIGURE 111-2 *Biopsy from granuloma inguinale ulcer, showing mononuclear cells containing Donovan bodies. Wright-Giemsa stain.*

REFERENCES

Davis CM: Granuloma inguinale. A clinical, histological, and ultrastructural study. JAMA 211:632, 1970

Dodson RF et al: Donovanosis: A morphologic study. J Invest Dermatol 62:611, 1974

Garg BR et al: Efficacy of cotrimoxazole in donovanosis. Br J Vener Dis 54:348, 1978

Hart G: Chancroid, donovanosis, lymphogranuloma venerum. US Department of Health, Education, and Welfare Publication (CDC) 75-8302, 1975

———: Donovanosis, in *Sexually Transmitted Diseases,* KK Holmes et al (eds). New York, McGraw-Hill, 1984, pp 393–397

Jofre ME et al: Granuloma inguinale simulating advanced pelvic cancer. Med J Aust 2:869, 1976

Kraus SJ et al: Pseudogranuloma inguinale caused by *Haemophilus ducreyi*. Arch Dermatol 118:494, 1982

Kuberski T: Granuloma inguinale (donovanosis). Sex Transm Dis 7:29, 1980

——— et al: Ultrastructure of *Calymmatobacterium granulomatis* in lesions of granuloma inguinale. J Infect Dis 142:744, 1980

Lal S, Nicholas C: Epidemiological and clinical features in 165 cases of granuloma inguinale. Br J Vener Dis 46:461, 1970

Sowmini CN: Donovanosis, in *International Perspectives on Neglected Sexually Transmitted Diseases: Impact on Venereology, Infertility, and Maternal and Infant Health,* KK Holmes, PA Mardh (eds). Washington, DC, Hemisphere Publishing, 1982, pp 205–217

112 BRUCELLOSIS

DONALD KAYE / ROBERT G. PETERSDORF

DEFINITION Brucellosis (undulant fever, Malta fever, Mediterranean fever) is an infection caused by microorganisms of the genus *Brucella,* which are usually transmitted to humans from domestic animals. The illness is characterized by fever, sweats, weakness, malaise, and weight loss, often without localized findings.

ETIOLOGY Human brucellosis is an infection caused by one of four species: *B. melitensis* (goats), *B. suis* (hogs), *B. abortus* (cattle), and *B. canis* (dogs). Relatively few cases of *B. canis* infection have been reported, but it is probably much more prevalent than is recognized. Although infections are usually confined to the major animal host, infections of swine with *B. abortus* or of cattle with *B. suis* may occur, and *Brucella* infection has been reported in other animals. The species of *Brucella* are separated from one another by biochemical and serologic reactions. The organisms are small, nonmotile, non-spore-forming, gram-negative coccobacilli which grow best at 37°C in trypticase soy broth or tryptose phosphate broth with a pH of 6.6 to 6.8 under increased CO_2 tension.

EPIDEMIOLOGY The natural reservoir of brucellosis is in domestic animals, particularly cattle, swine, goats, and sheep. Brucellosis in the natural host is very contagious. However, spread may occur to secondary hosts such as human beings. Person-to-person spread is rare. Animal-to-animal transmission is usually venereal or by ingestion of infected tissue or milk. Human infection most commonly results from ingestion of infected animal tissues or milk products, or directly through abraded skin.

On the average, approximately 200 cases of brucellosis are reported in the United States every year. However, it has been estimated that only about 4 percent of cases are recognized and reported. On a worldwide basis, the prevalence of the disease correlates closely with the extent of animal brucellosis in a given country. Brucellosis has nearly been eradicated in several European countries, where the incidence of animal brucellosis is also very low. In the United States, areas in which cattle-raising is an important industry generally have a higher incidence of brucellosis.

Brucellosis most frequently occurs in individuals who are exposed to *Brucella*-infected tissues and milk or milk products, including slaughterhouse workers, butchers, farmers, livestock producers, veterinarians, and individuals who ingest unpasteurized milk products. In most of the instances in which brucellosis has been acquired from unpasteurized dairy products, these products were purchased in other countries, particularly in Mexico, the Mediterranean basin, the Far East, and South America. In the United States, brucellosis occurs mainly in males of working age, more than half of them slaughterhouse workers. Fortunately, isolation of *Brucella* from infected meat decreases following refrigeration, but the high rates of accidental cuts and exposure to blood and lymph of freshly killed animals make abattoir workers particularly susceptible to this infection. In Alaska, a number of cases have been transmitted via raw meat from caribou and moose.

In the United States, *B. abortus* is the most frequent cause of brucellosis followed by *B. suis*. *B. melitensis* and *B. canis* are rare causes. Approximately 2 to 3 percent of cases acquired in this country occur in laboratories, often in veterinarians who are accidentally inoculated (via needle or the conjunctival or airborne routes) with live vaccine. The vaccine-induced disease is usually mild.

PATHOGENESIS AND PATHOLOGY *Brucella* invade the body through abraded skin and, less commonly, through the oropharynx, conjunctivae, or respiratory passages. They interact with polymorphonuclear leukocytes (PMN) and tissue macrophages. Many organisms are phagocytized, but if the inoculum is sufficiently large, they spread via the lymphatics to the regional lymph nodes, most commonly in the axillary, cervical, and supraclavicular regions. If localization does not occur there, the organisms spread via the bloodstream to other reticuloendothelial tissues such as the bone marrow, liver, and spleen, but visceral organs such as kidneys, bones, testes, and endocardium are involved as well. *Brucella* can multiply within PMN, tissue macrophages, and cells of the reticuloendothelial system and destroy them. In their intracellular location, *Brucella* are protected both from antibody and from many antibiotics.

The characteristic but nonspecific reaction of tissues to *Brucella* is the appearance of epithelioid cells, giant cells of the foreign body and Langhans' types, and lymphocytes and plasma cells with formation of granulomas. Although many *Brucella* are killed by PMNs, the macrophage is the ultimate cell that destroys *Brucella*. *B. abortus* causes mild disease with noncaseating granulomas in liver and other reticuloendothelial organs. *B. suis* causes more severe disease with local suppurative complications and granulomas that may caseate. *B. melitensis* causes the most severe acute disease with symptoms that may be disabling. *B. canis* causes mild disease similar to that seen with *B. abortus*. Granulomas in brucellosis eventually heal with fibrosis and often calcification.

Although brucellosis is a common cause of abortion in cattle, swine, and goats, there is no evidence that human abortions occur any more frequently with this disease than with other bacteremias.

MANIFESTATIONS Brucellosis may be asymptomatic with only serological evidence of infection. The manifestations of symptomatic brucellosis may be divided into acute brucellosis, localized disease, and chronic brucellosis.

Acute brucellosis The incubation period of acute brucellosis usually varies between 7 and 21 days, but may be months. The onset may be acute with a toxic course, especially when caused by *B. melitensis*. However, the onset is often insidious. Patients frequently have a low-grade fever with no localizing complaints but only malaise, fatigue, headache, weakness, sweats, chills, backache, and myalgias. Most patients are anorectic and lose weight. Some have cough or arthralgias.

Typically there are a multitude of complaints but a paucity of physical findings. When physical findings occur, the major manifestations are splenomegaly (which occurs in 10 to 20 percent of patients), lymphadenopathy (15 percent of patients), and hepatomegaly (less than 10 percent).

Localized brucellosis Localized disease may occur at almost any anatomic location, but osteomyelitis, splenic abscess, genitourinary tract localization, pulmonary involvement, and endocarditis are among the more common sites of involvement. Osteomyelitis usually occurs in the vertebrae, with the lumbosacral area as the most frequent site. There is a disc space infection with involvement of both adjacent vertebrae. Bone scans are positive early, followed by roentgenographic evidence of osteoporosis, anterior vertebral plate erosion, and formation of "parrot-beaked" osteophytes. Arthritis, which is much less common than osteomyelitis, most often involves the knee. Splenic abscesses may occur and result in areas of calcification. Epididymoorchitis and less often clinically apparent prostatic or renal infection may be observed. Meningoencephalitis, myelitis, radiculitis, or neuropathy are the neurologic complications. Pleural effusion and pneumonia are occasional manifestations.

Bacterial endocarditis is the most common cause of death among patients with brucellosis. It has been reported predominantly in males, follows an indolent course, is accompanied by a high rate of congestive heart failure and arterial embolization, and has required both valve replacement and antibiotic therapy to achieve cure.

Chronic brucellosis Chronic brucellosis is defined as ill health for more than 1 year following onset of brucellosis. Included in this group have been patients with relapsing illness with no localized infection, those with localization of infection in one or more organs, and those who have no objective signs of infection (e.g., no fever) and no evidence of active brucellosis (i.e., by serologic methods or by culture). It is doubtful that this last group has active brucellosis; it is more likely their complaints, fatigue and weakness, are psychoneurotic in nature.

An unusual complication that occurs in veterinarians removing placentas from infected animals consists of an erythematous macular, papular, or pustular rash on the hand and arms which is presumed to be a hypersensitivity reaction to *Brucella* antigens.

DIAGNOSIS Brucellosis is a relatively rare disease, and there are many common illnesses that mimic it. Among them are influenza, infectious mononucleosis, toxoplasmosis, viral hepatitis, disseminated gonococcal infection, rheumatic fever, systemic lupus erythematosus, tuberculosis, leptospirosis, and typhoid fever. The clinical suspicion that the patient has brucellosis should be higher in farmers, abattoir workers, and others exposed to infected tissues or animal products.

The definitive evidence of *Brucella* infection consists of isolating the *Brucella* organisms from the patient. However, culturing *Brucella* organisms may be dangerous to laboratory personnel. *All cultures should be clearly marked "possible brucellosis" and should be processed employing sterile techniques in a biohazard hood certified for handling class III infectious agents.* It is recommended that laboratories not having these facilities not undertake *Brucella* cultures.

Cultures Up to half the patients whose blood is submitted for culture early in the course of infection, and who have not received antibiotics, will have *Brucella* organisms in the blood when a culture is grown in trypticase soy broth for 1 to 3 weeks in the presence of 5 to 10% CO_2. However, many laboratories discard blood cultures after 10 days' incubation. This is another reason for the clinician to communicate any suspicion of brucellosis to the laboratory and to urge the laboratory to hold these cultures for at least 4 weeks. Sometimes, bone marrow cultures may be positive in acute brucellosis when blood cultures are not. Later in the course of illness, bacteremia is less frequent and organisms may then be isolated from infected lymph nodes or granulomas involving the spleen, liver, and bone. Altogether, only 15 to 20 percent of cases of brucellosis are confirmed by culture. In localized brucellosis, biopsy and isolation of *Brucella* may be necessary for diagnosis. In the majority of cases of brucellosis, the diagnosis is made serologically.

Serology IgM antibody titers rise early (usually in the first week of infection), peak at about 3 months, and then fall over a period of months. Titers may persist for several years. IgG antibodies appear 2 to 3 weeks after onset of illness, rise to peak titers in about 8 weeks, and persist as long as the infection is active. Therefore, the persistence of IgG antibody indicates continuing active infection. With treatment, IgG antibody titers decrease rapidly and usually disappear within 1 year. With relapse, both IgM and IgG titers increase. The most reliable serologic test is the standard tube *Brucella* agglutination test (STA) which measures antibodies directed primarily at *Brucella* lipopolysaccharide antigens. A fourfold or greater rise in titer of serum specimens drawn 1 to 4 weeks apart is indicative of recent exposure to *Brucella* or *Brucella*-like antigens. The specimen should be tested on the same day, in the same laboratory, under identical conditions. Using this test, most patients develop a rise in titer to *Brucella* antigens within 1 to 2 weeks of illness, and within 3 weeks virtually all patients will show seroconversion. False-positive tests may be due to *Brucella* skin tests, cholera vaccination, and infection with *Vibrio cholerae, Francisella tularensis,* or *Yersinia enterocolitica.* These cross-reactive causes of seroconversion are usually readily eliminated.

Significance of serologic findings A single STA titer of 160 or higher indicates past or present exposure to *Brucella* organisms or antigens that cross-react with *Brucella* species. If there is strong clinical suspicion of brucellosis, dilutions as high as 1:1280 should be made, because false-negative tests due to blocking antibodies have been reported in titers as high as 1:640. Virtually all patients with brucellosis have STA titers $\geq$ 1:160. Lower titers are of no diagnostic significance.

IgG-agglutinating antibodies can be recognized in the STA by extraction with 2-mercaptoethanol (2-ME). This procedure destroys the agglutinating activity of IgM antibodies and allows recognition of only the IgG-agglutinating antibody. Existence of a single elevated titer ($\geq$ 1:160) in the 2-ME *Brucella* agglutination test is good objective evidence of either current or recent infection and the need for treatment. Many patients maintain elevated IgM-agglutinating antibodies for several years, even after presumed complete cure of their infection. For this reason, a 2-ME *Brucella* agglutination test that measures only IgG-agglutinating antibodies is the most useful indicator of whether the patient has been cured.

Other serologic tests are of no additional value. The *Brucella* skin test is of no more significance than a positive tuberculin test in patients suspected of having tuberculosis. Moreover, the test may interfere with interpretation of serologic tests by causing a rise in titer. For this reason, a skin test should not be performed.

Standard agglutination tests for antibodies to *Brucella* use *B. abortus* antigens. Antibodies to *B. melitensis* and *B. suis* cross-react with *B. abortus* but not with *B. canis*. To test for *B. canis* the antigen must be prepared from *B. canis*; these tests are not routinely available.

Other laboratory tests An occasional patient will develop anemia. The white blood cell count is normal or low, and the erythrocyte sedimentation rate may be normal or high.

TREATMENT It is generally accepted that the combination of tetracycline 500 mg orally four times daily for 3 to 6 weeks plus streptomycin 1 g every 12 h intramuscularly for the first 2 weeks will result in cure of brucellosis. This regimen has produced lower relapse rates than has treatment with tetracycline alone. With this program, relapses have occurred in only 2 percent of patients, and these have responded to retreatment. Tetracycline should not be used in pregnant women or children below the age of 8 because of the danger of staining developing teeth. Streptomycin may cause ototoxicity, and the dose must be decreased in patients with renal insufficiency.

A variety of other drugs, including gentamicin in lieu of streptomycin, doxycycline instead of tetracycline, or trimethoprim-sulfa or rifampin have been tried, but none has been found clearly superior to the tetracycline-streptomycin combination. When tetracycline plus streptomycin cannot be used, trimethoprim/sulfamethoxazole (480/2400 mg per day) for 4 weeks is a reasonable substitute. Addition of rifampin (900 mg per day) to the basic tetracycline-streptomycin or trimethoprim-sulfamethoxazole regimen may improve results when response is poor. Despite apparent in vitro activity against strains of *Brucella,* the role of the third-generation cephalosporins, if any, in brucellosis remains to be determined.

Abscesses should be drained when indicated. Splenectomy has been performed in some patients with splenomegaly and multiple relapses and has apparently been successful in preventing further relapses.

Febrile patients with either acute or subacute brucellosis characterized by severe anorexia, depression, and generalized debilitation may be given a short course of steroids. Prednisone in an oral dose of 60 mg a day tapered rapidly over a 5- to 7-day period can be administered and may be helpful. However, it is not necessary in most patients.

Therapeutic use of *Brucella* vaccine is of questionable value and is not recommended. Headache, backache, and generalized aches and pains should be treated with analgesics.

PROGNOSIS Even before antimicrobial treatment, the mortality rate of brucellosis was low, and only 15 percent of patients had an illness exceeding 3 months in duration. With chemotherapy, long illnesses have become quite rare, as have complications. When the morbidity exceeds 1 to 2 months, other causes of illness, previously unsuspected underlying disease, or a complication of brucellosis should be considered. The mortality rate of acute brucellosis is less than 2 percent.

The diagnosis of chronic brucellosis, continued active brucellosis, or a complication of brucellosis can best be made by demonstrating a titer of 1:160 or greater in the 2-ME agglutination test. If the titer is less than 1:40 on this test, it is highly unlikely that persistent illness or relapse is due to brucellosis.

Most patients who develop brucellosis in the course of their work can be permitted to return to their place of work. Immunity to reinfection appears to follow the first *Brucella* infection in most cases, but reinfection can occur.

PREVENTION The elimination of human brucellosis depends upon the eradication of the disease in animals, where the disease can be prevented by the administration of live attenuated *Brucella* vaccine. Such a vaccine is not available for human use in the United States. The risk of brucellosis can be mitigated by consumption of pasteurized milk and pasteurized milk products, by guarding against exposure to freshly killed tissue from potentially infected animals, and by protecting potential portals of entry in high risk individuals (veterinarians, meat inspectors, slaughterhouse workers) with appropriate protective bandages or by the use of gloves or goggles.

REFERENCES

BUCHANAN TM et al: Brucellosis in the United States, 1960–1972: An abattoir-associated disease: I. Clinical features and therapy; II. Diagnostic aspects; III. Epidemiologic evidence for acquired immunity. Medicine 53:403, 415, 427, 1974

———, FABER LC: 2-Mercaptoethanol *Brucella* agglutination test: Usefulness for predicting recovery from brucellosis. J Clin Microbiol 11:691, 1980

CERVANTES F et al: Liver disease in brucellosis: A clinical and pathological study of 40 cases. Postgrad Med J 58:346, 1982

COHEN PS et al: Infective endocarditis caused by gram-negative bacteria. Prog Cardiovasc Dis 22:205, 1980

HEIBIG J et al: *Brucella* aortic endocarditis corrected by prosthetic valve replacement. Am Heart J 106:594, 1983

HEWITT WG, PAYNE DJ: Estimation of IgG and IgM *Brucella* antibodies in infected and non-infected persons by a radioimmune technique. J Clin Pathol 37:692, 1984

LARBRISSEAU A et al: The neurological complications of brucellosis. Can J Neurol Sci 5:369, 1978

LLORENS-TEROL J, BUSQUETS RM: Brucellosis treated with rifampicin. Arch Dis Child 55(6):486, 1980

POLT SS et al: Human brucellosis caused by *Brucella canis:* Clinical features and immune response. Ann Intern Med 97:717, 1982

SPINK WW: *The Nature of Brucellosis.* Minneapolis, University of Minnesota Press, 1956

YOUNG EJ: Human brucellosis. Rev Infect Dis 5:821, 1983

113 TULAREMIA

DONALD KAYE

DEFINITION Tularemia (rabbit fever, deer fly fever) is an infection caused by *Francisella tularensis. F. tularensis* is found in many animals and is transmitted to human beings by direct contact or via an insect vector. The illness is characterized by an ulcerative lesion at the site of inoculation with regional lymphadenopathy, by pneumonia, or by fever without localizing findings.

ETIOLOGY *F. tularensis* is a small, nonmotile, pleomorphic, gram-negative aerobic coccobacillus. It grows poorly in many media but will grow well in glucose-cysteine blood agar, thioglycolate broth, and other media supplemented with cysteine. *F. tularensis* is found only in the northern hemisphere. There are two types of *F. tularensis*. Jellison type A is distributed solely in North America, is virulent for humans and rabbits, produces citrulline ureidase, and ferments glycerol. Type B is found in North America, Europe, and Asia, causes no or mild disease in humans and rabbits, does not produce citrulline ureidase, and does not ferment glycerol. *F. tularensis* cross-reacts serologically with *Brucella* species and *Yersinia pestis.* It contains an endotoxin similar to endotoxins of other gram-negative bacilli.

EPIDEMIOLOGY *F. tularensis* has been found in many mammals including rabbits, squirrels, muskrats, beavers, deer, cattle, and sheep, in birds, in amphibians, and in fish. Tularemia can result from skin contact with any of these species. Tularemia has also been transmitted by cat bite. Ticks, deer flies, and mosquitoes can transmit the bacterium. Ticks transmit *F. tularensis* to their offspring through transovarian passage. In the United States the disease can be carried by *Dermacentor andersoni* (Rocky Mountain wood tick), *Dermacentor variabilis* (American dog tick), *Dermacentor occidentalis* (Pacific Coast dog tick), and *Amblyomma americanum* (Lone Star tick). *F. tularensis* has also been recovered from streams.

In the United States most cases of tularemia result from skin contact with infected wild rabbits (especially cottontail rabbits) or the bite of a tick or deer fly. Infection occasionally results from ingestion or inhalation of infected material. The highest risk groups are hunters and trappers. Therefore, tularemia is most likely to occur in adult males. Person-to-person transmission rarely, if ever, occurs.

Tularemia has been reported from all parts of the United States, but mostly from Arkansas, Missouri, Oklahoma, Texas, and Utah. About 300 cases are reported each year in the United States. Arthropod-borne disease occurs mainly in the spring and summer, and rabbit-produced infection mainly in the winter.

PATHOGENESIS AND PATHOLOGY In human infection, the most common portal of entry is through the skin or mucous membranes. This may be direct through inapparent abrasions or via the bite of a tick or other arthropod. Inhalation or ingestion of *F. tularensis* can also result in infection. Fewer than 50 organisms will result in infection when injected into the skin or inhaled, whereas more than 10^8 are usually required to produce infection via the oral route.

Following inoculation into the skin, the bacteria multiply locally and after 2 to 5 days (occasionally 1 to 10 days) produce an erythematous, tender, or pruritic papule. The papule rapidly enlarges and forms an ulcer with a black base. The bacteria spread to regional lymph nodes producing lymphadenopathy, and further spread with bacteremia may occur. With bacteremia, organisms are cleared from the blood by phagocytic cells of the reticuloendothelial system (mainly in the liver and spleen) and may survive intracellularly for long periods of time.

Affected organs (liver, spleen, lymph nodes) demonstrate areas of focal necrosis initially surrounded mainly by polymorphonuclear leukocytes. Subsequently granulomas form with epithelioid cells and lymphocytes and sometimes multinucleated giant cells surrounding the areas of necrosis which may resemble caseation necrosis. Coalescence of granulomas can lead to formation of abscesses. Nodes may occasionally become fluctuant and even rupture. Healing occurs with fibrosis and calcification of the granulomas.

Contamination of the conjunctiva can result in infection of the eye with regional lymph node enlargement. Aerosolization of *F. tularensis* with inhalation can result in pneumonia. Pneumonia can also occur via the hematogenous route. There is an inflammatory reaction with foci of alveolar necrosis and initially polymorphonuclear leukocytic and later mononuclear cell infiltration with granuloma formation. Chest roentgenograms usually reveal bilateral patchy infiltrates rather than large areas of consolidation. Mediastinal or other regional lymphadenopathy may occur.

Pharyngitis with cervical lymphadenopathy or gastrointestinal tularemia with mesenteric lymphadenopathy may follow ingestion of large numbers of *F. tularensis.* The portal of entry is unknown in typhoidal tularemia, an uncommon form, but may be the skin, lung, or gastrointestinal system. There is fever with no localizing symptoms.

CLINICAL MANIFESTATIONS Tularemia usually has an incubation period of 2 to 5 days after which there is onset of one of a number of syndromes (listed below), all of which are usually associated with fever and chills. Headache, myalgias, and malaise are also often present. Hepatosplenomegaly, which may be tender, is a common finding. About 20 percent of patients develop a generalized maculopapular rash which may occasionally become pustular.

Ulceroglandular tularemia Most patients with tularemia (75 to 85 percent) develop infection secondary to inoculation of the skin. In cases related to rabbits the portal of entry is usually on the finger or hand. In tick-related cases, the site of inoculation is usually on the lower extremities, inguinal or axillary areas, scalp, abdomen, or chest.

At time of onset of illness there is usually an erythematous papule that may be tender or pruritic, or there is already an ulcer present at the portal of entry of the organism. If there is a papule, it evolves over a period of several days to form a punched out ulcer with sharply dermarcated edges and a yellow exudate. The ulcer gradually develops a black base. There is very tender, large regional lymphadenopathy (usually axillary or epitrochlear with tularemia from rabbits, and inguinal or femoral lymphadenopathy with tick-borne disease). The nodes may become fluctuant and may drain spontaneously. In 5 to 10 percent of cases of tularemia, the skin lesion may be inapparent and the lymphadenopathy the only physical finding. This has been called "glandular tularemia."

Oculoglandular tularemia In a small percent of patients (about 1 percent), the conjunctiva serves as the portal of entry for the organism. There is purulent conjunctivitis with regional lymphadenopathy (preauricular, submandibular, or cervical). Corneal perforation may occur.

Oropharyngeal tularemia A rare form of tularemia (less than 1 percent of cases) which may occur after ingestion of *F. tularensis* (usually in undercooked meat) is acute exudative or membranous pharyngitis associated with cervical lymphadenopathy.

Gastrointestinal tularemia Rarely following ingestion of *F. tularensis* there may be ulcerative intestinal lesions with associated mesenteric lymphadenopathy. In addition to fever, the patient has diarrhea, abdominal pain, nausea and vomiting, and gastrointestinal bleeding.

Pulmonary tularemia Involvement of the lung can result from inhalation of *F. tularensis* or as a part of the bacteremia caused by tularemia at another site. Inhalation pulmonary disease occurs most often in laboratory workers and is a serious infection with high mortality. Pulmonary involvement occurs in 10 to 15 percent of patients with ulceroglandular tularemia and in about half of the patients with typhoidal tularemia. There is cough, which is usually nonproductive, and there may be dyspnea or pleuritic chest pain. The physical examination is usually normal. Roentgenograms of the chest usually reveal bilateral patchy infiltrates which have been described as "ovoid densities." Lobar pneumonia may occur, and pleural effusion(s) may be present.

Typhoidal tularemia In about 10 percent of cases of tularemia there is fever without apparent skin lesion or lymphadenopathy. In the absence of a history of possible contact with a vector of the disease, diagnosis is extremely difficult.

Other manifestations Meningitis, pericarditis, peritonitis, endocarditis, and osteomyelitis have all been reported. The meningitis causes a lymphocytic response in the spinal fluid.

DIAGNOSIS Differential diagnosis In patients with fever and large, tender lymphadenopathy the possibility of tularemia should be strongly considered, and an attempt should be made to determine if there was an appropriate animal or arthropod vector contact. The suspicion of tularemia should be especially high in hunters, trappers, game wardens, veterinarians, and laboratory workers. However, in up to 40 percent of patients with tularemia, no history of epidemiologic contact with an animal or arthropod vector can be elicited.

Ulceroglandular tularemia is often so characteristic that it does not present a problem in differential diagnosis, but on occasion it must be differentiated from other diseases. The skin lesion may resemble those seen in sporotrichosis, skin infection with coagulase-positive staphylococci or group A streptococci, syphilis, anthrax, rat bite fever (caused by *Spirillum minor*), rickettsial infections (such as scrub typhus) and *Mycobacterium marinum* infection. However, the regional lymphadenopathy in these diseases is usually not as impressive as in tularemia.

The lymphadenopathy of tularemia must be differentiated from that of plague (Chap. 114), lymphogranuloma venereum (Chap. 150), and cat scratch fever (Chap. 118). However, in these infections there is usually no local lesion resembling the ulcer of tularemia.

Typhoidal tularemia may resemble typhoid fever, other *Salmonella* bacteremias, rickettsial infections (such as Rocky Mountain spotted fever), brucellosis, infectious mononucleosis, toxoplasmosis, miliary tuberculosis, sarcoid, or hematologic malignancies. Tularemia pneumonia may resemble pneumonias caused by other bacteria as well as viral or *Mycoplasma* pneumonia.

Laboratory diagnosis The diagnosis of tularemia is usually made serologically by agglutination methods. A significant rise in titer (i.e., fourfold or greater) in paired serum specimens over a 2- to 3-week period is diagnostic. Agglutinating antibody appears after 1 to 2 weeks of illness. Fifty percent of patients have antibody in the second week, and the rest develop antibody later in the course. Titers peak at 4 to 8 weeks and may remain elevated for years. A single agglutinating titer of $\geq$ 1:160 in a patient who has been ill for at least 2 weeks is highly suggestive of tularemia but may only indicate old infection. Antibodies to *F. tularensis* may cross-react with *Brucella,* but the titers to *Brucella* are usually much lower than the titers to *F. tularensis*.

F. tularensis is rarely observed on Gram stains of skin lesions, sputum, or aspirates of nodes. While cultures of these materials or blood may be positive if processed on appropriate media, there is a major risk of infection in laboratory personnel. Cultivation of *F. tularensis* should only be attempted in laboratories with adequate isolation techniques and experienced personnel.

Isolation of *F. tularensis* can be achieved by inoculation intraperitoneally into guinea pigs, which will die within 10 days, and by direct plating onto glucose-cysteine blood agar. Agents such as cycloheximide, polymyxin B, and penicillin are frequently added to media to suppress other organisms in specimens that may overgrow *F. tularensis*.

A delayed-type skin test (similar to the tuberculin test) with *F. tularensis* antigen or killed whole bacilli has been used. It turns positive during the first week of illness, prior to the appearance of agglutinating antibody, and persists for years. A positive skin test may be helpful in early diagnosis, but the skin test antigen is not available commercially. The skin test can boost titers of agglutinating antibodies.

There are no other helpful laboratory tests in the diagnosis of tularemia. The white blood cell count is usually normal, and the erythrocyte sedimentation rate may be normal as well.

TREATMENT Streptomycin, in a dose of 7.5 to 10 mg/kg every 12 h intramuscularly, is considered the drug of choice in treatment of tularemia. In severe infections, 15 mg/kg every 12 h may be used for the first 48 to 72 h. Therapy is continued for 7 to 10 days. Gentamicin, in a dose of 1.7 mg/kg, intramuscularly or intravenously, every 8 h, is also effective. Virtually all strains are susceptible to streptomycin and gentamicin. Temperature response occurs within 2 days, but skin lesions and lymph nodes may take 1 to 2 weeks to heal. When therapy is not initiated until several weeks of illness have elapsed, the temperature response may be delayed. Relapses are very uncommon with streptomycin therapy.

Tetracycline or chloramphenicol, 30 mg/kg per day in four divided doses for 14 days, has also been used to treat tularemia. While response to these agents is good, the relapse rate is unacceptably high, occurring in up to 20 percent of patients.

If fluctuant nodes require aspiration or drainage, at least several days of antibiotic therapy should be given first to avoid exposure of medical personnel to aerosolization of infected material.

PREVENTION Prevention of tularemia is based on avoidance of exposure and vaccination of high-risk populations. Avoidance of skinning wild mammals, especially rabbits, will decrease the frequency of transmission. Wearing gloves while handling rabbit carcasses will decrease the risk of transmission. Use of insect repellents and prompt removal of ticks will help prevent transmission by ticks in tick-infested areas.

A multiple-puncture intradermal vaccine (used in a fashion similar to vaccinia) made from live attenuated *F. tularensis* and available from the Centers for Disease Control, Atlanta, Georgia, is effective in decreasing the frequency and severity of disease, but will not totally prevent tularemia. Protection is long-lasting. The vaccine induces agglutinins to *F. tularensis* and skin test reactivity. It is effective by stimulating cellular immunity, as circulating antibodies do not seem to be protective.

Veterinarians, hunters, trappers, game wardens, and others who are likely to come in contact with infected wild mammals are candidates for immunization. Laboratory workers who handle specimens containing *F. tularensis* should be immunized.

Prophylactic treatment with streptomycin will prevent development of clinical disease in patients who are incubating *F. tularensis*.

PROGNOSIS If untreated, symptoms of tularemia usually last 1 to 4 weeks but may continue for months. The mortality of severe untreated infection (which includes all tularemia pneumonia) can be as high as 30 percent. However, the overall mortality rate for untreated tularemia is less than 8 percent. Mortality is rare with appropriate therapy. Following tularemia there is usually lifelong immunity.

REFERENCES

BUCHANAN TM et al: The tularemia skin test. 325 skin tests in 210 persons: Serologic correlation and review of the literature. Ann Intern Med 74:336, 1971

KOSKELA P, HERVA E: Cell-mediated and humoral immunity induced by a live *Francisella tularensis* vaccine. Infect Immunol 36:983, 1982

MASON WL et al: Treatment of tularemia, including pulmonary tularemia, with gentamicin. Ann Rev Resp Dis 121:39, 1980

SANDSTROM G et al: Antigen from *Francisella tularensis:* Nonidentity between determinants participating in cell-mediated and humoral reactions. Infect Immunol 45:101, 1984

SANFORD JP: Landmark perspective: Tularemia. JAMA 250:3225, 1983

SCHMID GP: Clinically mild tularemia associated with tick-borne *Francisella tularensis*. J Infect Dis 148:63, 1983

Tularemia. Morb Mort Week Rep 31:39, 1982

YOUNG LS et al: Tularemia epidemic: Vermont 1968. Forty-seven cases linked to contact with muskrats. N Engl J Med 280:1253, 1969

114 PLAGUE AND OTHER *YERSINIA* INFECTIONS

DARWIN L. PALMER

DEFINITION Plague is an acute infectious illness of human beings, wild rodents, and their ectoparasites which is caused by the gram-negative bacillus *Yersinia pestis*. The disease persists because of its firm entrenchment in sylvatic rodent-flea ecosystems throughout the world. Wild rodent contact leads to sporadic human disease; the historically explosive urban epidemics resulted from transmission of disease into rats. Human bubonic plague follows bites by rodent fleas; after several days painful local adenopathy (the bubo) and sepsis spread to other organ systems, and death occurs. Primary plague pneumonia is transmitted between humans by cough-generated aerosols, has a fulminant course, and is almost universally fatal if untreated.

EPIDEMIOLOGY Sylvatic plague involves more than 200 species of wild rodents and is concentrated in the southwestern United States, the southern Soviet Union, India, Indochina, and South Africa. In the United States, ground squirrels, mice, voles, marmots, wood rats, prairie dogs, and chipmunks are potential carriers. Rodent disease is characterized by occurrence in the spring and summer, year-to-year variations in disease activity, chronicity in the populations involved, slow regional spread, and rare geographic regression. The disease dies off in some populations in cyclical fashion, leaving both resistant survivors and infected fleas seeking another host. Disease also persists in natural foci because of latent infection during animal hibernation, by prolonged viability of *Y. pestis* in soil of rodent burrows, by survival of infected fleas, and by persistent infection in relatively resistant rodents. Rodent predators may also spread plague; felines, such as domestic cats, generally die when infected with *Y. pestis,* while canines, such as foxes, coyotes, and dogs, often recover and may serve as serologic sentinels of wild rodent disease. Human disease can be readily acquired from domestic pets when the pets catch and return plague-infected rodents or their fleas to rural homes. Hares and rabbits are occasional nonrodent sources of the disease in humans, especially during the winter hunting season.

Rodent fleas are critical to the natural plague cycle and are implicated in about 85 percent of human cases. After infection, fleas develop obstruction of the foregut, causing regurgitation of plague bacilli during the next blood meal. The rat flea, *Xenopsylla cheopsis,* is an especially efficient plague vector both between rats and between rodents and humans. Transmission without fleas may occur by ingestion of infected carcasses by predators, possibly by contact with infected tissue through an open wound, or by inhalation of infected aerosols. Human body lice as well as ticks are also capable of inter-human or person-to-person transmission.

In the last three decades there has been a rising incidence of sporadic human plague originating in the western United States, with a death rate of 15 percent. This rate, double that seen in large outbreaks, reflects delay in the diagnosis or incorrect therapy due to travel during the incubation period out of plague endemic areas, or failure to elicit a history of animal exposure. Sporadic human plague occurs most frequently in the spring and summer, especially in children or youths under 20 and in adult males, reflecting their increased risk of wild rodent contact. While urban rat–related human outbreaks are now rare, they represent a continued threat; spread from sylvatic rodents into urban rats was documented as recently as 1983 in Los Angeles. Primary plague pneumonia arises as a secondary infection during bubonic/septicemic disease, with subsequent person-to-person spread via infectious aerosols. In closed quarters it is rapidly transmitted. A primary pneumonic plague outbreak in the United States last occurred in 1919, when 13 cases with 12 deaths (including two physicians and one nurse) developed before the disease was recognized and halted by case isolation. Cases of primary human pneumonic plague have also been acquired from domestic cats dying of plague pneumonia.

ETIOLOGY *Yersinia pestis* is a member of the family Enterobacteriaceae. It is a pleomorphic, gram-negative, nonmotile, aerobic bacillus which grows optimally at 28°C. The organism grows readily but slowly on routine media, and cultures should not be discarded before 72 h. Although weakly gram-negative, *Y. pestis* stains best with Giemsa's or Wayson's stains, with which it shows prominent bipolar "safety pin" microscopic morphology. The organism is a facultative intracellular parasite which maintains its virulence by the production of V and W antigens, enabling the organism to resist phagocytic intracellular killing, while production of capsular fraction 1 antigen partially protects the organism from phagocytosis by polymorphonuclear leukocytes. Other virulence factors include pesticin, fibrinolysin, coagulase, and a lipopolysaccharide endotoxin. The production of V and W antigens is plasmid-mediated, dependent on calcium, and may reflect the response of *Y. pestis* to its frequent intracellular location. No separate serotypes are recognized, but biotypes *antigua, orientalis,* and *mediaevalis* have geographic distributions which presumably mark previous epidemic spread. The organism is relatively resistant to drying and may maintain its viability in cool, moist conditions, such as the soil of an animal burrow, for many months. Antibiotic resistance can be developed in the laboratory, and both streptomycin- and tetracycline-resistant strains have been isolated from clinical specimens.

PATHOGENESIS After *Y. pestis* is inoculated into the skin by a flea bite, bacteria migrate to local lymph nodes, where they are taken up but not killed by mononuclear cells. Intracellular multiplication results in development of capsular envelopes containing fraction 1 protein; other toxins are elaborated. An acute inflammatory response is provoked in the lymph node in 2 to 6 days. At this stage the organisms are relatively resistant to phagocytosis by polymorphonuclear leukocytes because of the protection by capsules containing fraction 1 antigen and the lack of specific opsonic antibody. Characteristically, hemorrhagic necrosis of lymph nodes next occurs from which large numbers of bacteria gain access to the bloodstream and other organs. Extension along lymphatics involves both superficial nodes at the site of inoculation, the spleen, and nodes in the abdomen, mediastinum, or perihilar areas. The lung is secondarily infected in 10 to 20 percent, generally as a rapidly progressive, multilobar pneumonia, often with pleural exudate. The early acute inflammatory reaction is followed by lobar consolidation and hemorrhagic necrosis, and if death does not intervene, may progress to abscess formation. Fibrin thrombi may be extensive in the pulmonary vessels as well as in glomeruli and vessels of skin and other organs. Secondarily, the adult respiratory distress syndrome or a rise in pulmonary artery pressure may be seen. Pericarditis with a small amount of seropurulent exudate is frequent, and meningitis may occur late in untreated bacteremic plague. In 5 to 15 percent, the skin, predominantly of the extremities, is involved early on with petechiae and hemorrhages due to thrombocytopenia and vasculitis. Late in the disease, buboes may become fluctuant and occasionally may become superinfected with other bacteria. Endotoxemia can be detected during plague sepsis. It may result in both endotoxin shock and disseminated intravascular coagulation.

MANIFESTATIONS Bubonic plague has an incubation period of 2 to 7 days from flea bite to onset of illness. Although many patients do not remember an insect contact, a small eschar may be found at the bite site. Patients present with a painful bubo and fever accompanied by headache, prostration, and abdominal distress. The bubo, a tender enlarged lymph node or nodes, ranges in size from 1 to 10 cm and is found in the groin in 70 percent; alternatively, buboes may develop in axillary or cervical nodes or in several lymphatic chains simultaneously. Buboes are extremely tender, not fixed to skin or underlying structures, and the overlying skin is often erythematous. Fever and rigors are prominent and occasionally precede appearance of a bubo by 1 to 3 days. Gastrointestinal symptoms are present in more than half the patients, with abdominal pain often extending from the groin bubo and accompanied by anorexia, nausea, vomiting, and diarrhea, which may be bloody. Cutaneous petechiae and hemorrhages occur in 5 to 50 percent, and may be extensive late in the disease. Disseminated intravascular coagulation occurs in subclinical form in as many as 86 percent of patients, 5 to 10 percent of whom have clinical manifestations, including gangrene of the skin, fingers, toes, and penis. If untreated, bubonic disease may proceed without other organ system involvement to generalized sepsis, prostration, hypotension, and death within the next 2 to 10 days. Some patients have very prominent signs of sepsis with no demonstrable bubo. This represents a form of bubonic plague in which lymphatic involvement is limited to deep structures or where the buboes are so small as to be overlooked in the presence of overwhelming signs of infection. Septicemic disease may progress rapidly with chills, fever, rapid pulse, severe headache, nausea, vomiting, delirium, and death within 48 h. In such fulminant sepsis, bacteremia is so prominent that blood buffy coat may readily show *Y. pestis* on Gram stain.

Other than the lymphatics, the lung is the organ most commonly involved, with development of secondary pneumonia in 10 to 20 percent of all patients. Cough, fever, and tachypnea appear on days 2 to 3 of illness, accompanied by minimal pulmonary infiltrates. Later, or less commonly from the start, symptoms worsen rapidly with marked dyspnea, bloody sputum, and evidence of respiratory failure. There may be multilobar involvement, with variable degrees of consolidation, and the sputum may teem with *Y. pestis* and is highly contagious when disseminated by cough-generated aerosols. Primary plague pneumonia is a fulminant illness; time from the initial contact to death ranges from 2 to 6 days. The adult respiratory distress syndrome (ARDS), characterized by noncardiac pulmonary edema, anoxia, and respiratory failure, also occurs as a manifestation of plague sepsis and may be indistinguishable from plague pneumonia except for the absence of bacteria in respiratory secretions. Both *Y. pestis* pneumonia and the ARDS form of illness have a mortality in excess of 75 percent, despite appropriate antimicrobial and supportive therapy. Less commonly, marked perihilar adenopathy may present alone or accompany pneumonia.

Plague meningitis, as a late complication in fewer than 5 percent of untreated patients, is characterized by nuchal rigidity, headache, confusion, and coma, and is often preceded or accompanied by bacteremia.

Rarely, patients with plague have a very mild illness manifested chiefly by low-grade fever and adenopathy. In this group are patients with tonsillar plague, who have positive throat cultures, serologic conversion, and minimal illness. Other less common late complications include persistent hectic fever despite appropriate therapy; fluctuance and spontaneous drainage from buboes; and pulmonary cavitation with abscess formation.

LABORATORY FINDINGS With the exception of definitive microbiologic studies, laboratory tests are of little diagnostic help. A polymorphonuclear leukocytosis of 15,000 to 20,000 cells per cubic millimeter is common, and the white cells may show toxic changes. Rarely, a marked leukemoid reaction with more than 100,000 white cells is seen. Modest elevations of serum glutamic oxaloacetic transaminase are common, but otherwise liver function studies are normal. Evidence of disseminated intravascular coagulation with low platelet counts, prolonged partial thromboplastin times, and positive fibrin degradation products is common. The electrocardiogram is usually normal but may show right axis deviation and peaked P waves indicative of acute cor pulmonale. The chest x-ray will show infiltrates, often with pleural effusion, in secondary or primary plague pneumonia or show evidence of pulmonary edema in patients with the adult respiratory distress syndrome. In meningitis, examination of cerebrospinal fluid demonstrates polymorphonuclear pleocytosis, low sugar, elevated protein, and gram-negative coccobacillary organisms, although culture may demonstrate *Y. pestis* more reliably.

Confirmation of the clinical suspicion of bubonic plague may be obtained by needle-aspiration of a bubo with direct staining of the aspirated material. With either Wayson's or Giemsa's stain, the characteristic bipolar-staining, "safety pin" forms are seen. By fluorescent antibody staining, a presumptive diagnosis may be specifically confirmed in about 80 percent of cases. Cultures of aspirated material, as well as sputum, pleural fluid, and blood, will be positive in a high percentage of patients. Microscopic examination of buffy coat smear may show *Y. pestis* in septicemic cases. A serologic response with a fourfold or greater rise is detected in the second week of illness by complement fixation, hemagglutination or indirect immunofluorescent antibody.

DIAGNOSIS Bubonic plague must be suspected in any febrile patient with painful adenopathy who has a history of wild animal exposure in a plague endemic area, but may be confused with other illnesses. Presentation with fever and a painful groin bubo can mimic granuloma venereum or syphilis or, when more severe, an acute abdominal crisis such as incarcerated inguinal hernia, appendicitis, or a ruptured viscus. Abdominal pain and bloody diarrhea can be mistaken for shigellosis or other acute diarrheal processes. With an axillary or cervical bubo, acute streptococcal or staphylococcal lymphadenitis, tularemia, cat-scratch fever, granuloma venereum, or syphilis may be considered. Bubonic/septicemic disease with an absent or minimal bubo, suggests typhoid fever or bacteremia due to other causes. Primary or secondary pneumonic plague may mimic bacterial pneumonia from any cause.

When plague is suspected, diagnostic maneuvers must include aspiration of buboes with appropriate stains and cultures, as well as blood cultures and cultures from other sources. Cultures should not be discarded early because the organism grows slowly and may only appear in 48 to 72 h. A serologic rise by passive hemagglutination is evident by day 5 and peaks by day 14. Newer serologic methods such as enzyme-linked immunosorbent assay compare well in sensitivity to standard passive hemagglutination tests and are more rapid.

TREATMENT If plague is strongly suspected on clinical and/or epidemiologic grounds, therapy must be started immediately, prior to completion of diagnostic studies. Antibiotic and supportive treatment should reduce the 40 to 100 percent mortality of untreated bubonic or pneumonic plague to 5 to 10 percent. Effective antibiotics include streptomycin, tetracycline, and chloramphenicol. Streptomycin should be given initially at a dosage of 7.5 to 15 mg/kg every 12 h intramuscularly; tetracycline, given intravenously at 5 to 10 mg/kg every 6 h, may be started concurrently and streptomycin discontinued when the patient becomes afebrile. Larger doses, even in those with severe illness, offer no benefit. Tetracycline should be continued for a total of 3 to 4 days after the fever has disappeared. In less severely ill patients, tetracycline alone at 5 to 10 mg/kg every 6 h may be given either by mouth or intravenously. Chloramphenicol in a dose of 12.5 to 25 mg/kg given intravenously every 6 h should be substituted for tetracycline in patients with meningitis due to its better central nervous system penetration. While antibiotic-resistant organisms have appeared only rarely, gentamicin is as effective as streptomycin. Tetracycline or trimethoprim-sulfamethoxazole are effective for the prophylaxis of case contacts and should be given orally for 5 days. Local treatment of the bubo is not indicated unless fluctuance or spontaneous drainage occurs, when cultures should be obtained to detect staphylococci. Ventilatory support for patients with plague pneumonia or adult respiratory distress syndrome may be necessary and lifesaving.

PREVENTION AND CONTROL Individuals working in high-risk occupations in plague endemic areas or conducting laboratory work with *Y. pestis* should consider use of the formalin-killed whole-bacteria vaccine; however, the vaccine must be readministered every 6 months due to rapidly waning immunity. Alternatively, individuals briefly visiting a plague endemic area may take tetracycline or trimethoprim-sulfamethoxazole prophylaxis. Following the presumptive diagnosis of pneumonic plague, patients should be placed in respiratory isolation; simple hand-washing precautions suffice for bubonic cases. Contacts of a patient with plague pneumonia should be given oral tetracycline prophylaxis, at 250 mg four times daily by mouth, and should be advised to seek medical attention upon the development of respiratory symptoms or fever. Possibly due to such precautions, transmission of primary plague pneumonia has not occurred in this country for many years.

The potential for spread of plague into urban rat populations from sylvatic rodent sources is an ever-present risk. Prevention depends on control of urban rat populations and their exclusion from dwellings as well as surveillance of sylvatic rodents and of their local predators. Picnickers, hikers, and others traveling into plague endemic regions during the spring-summer season should be warned that plague is a potential danger. They should avoid touching carcasses or sick rodents and should restrain and treat pets with flea-repellent powders. No practical measures exist for eliminating plague from wild rodent sources. Reducing rodent harborage around rural homes in endemic regions is important. Killing rodents around rural dwellings with rodenticides should be preceded by insect control to prevent displaced rodent fleas from seeking humans or domestic pets.

OTHER *YERSINIA* INFECTIONS (*Y. PSEUDOTUBERCULOSIS* AND *Y. ENTEROCOLITICA*)

ETIOLOGY *Y. enterocolitica* and *Y. pseudotuberculosis* are both non-lactose-fermenting, gram-negative, aerobic bacilli related to one another and to *Y. pestis* and are members of the Enterobacteriaceae. Both organisms grow slowly on media used for the detection of other enteric bacteria, and their detection can be enhanced by cold enrichment incubation at 20 to 25°C. Cold enrichment, however, requires refrigeration for several weeks and is of little use in diagnosis of any one patient. Strains can be distinguished from one another and from *Y. pestis* on the basis of serologic and biochemical reactions as well as by antibiotic sensitivities. As in *Y. pestis,* both organisms elaborate W and V virulence factors and, with *Y. pseudotuberculosis,* virulence is also related to its ability to survive intracellularly. Both organisms produce an endotoxin and *Y. enterocolitica* elaborates a heat-stable enterotoxin which may be of significance in foodborne illness. A large number of serotypes of both organisms exist causing disease in many animal species, but most human infections are caused by a limited number of strains.

MANIFESTATIONS Although recognized most commonly in northern Europe and North America, *Y. enterocolitica* causes enteric infection worldwide and accounts for approximatley 1 to 3 percent of all cases of acute bacterial enteritis. Although the origin of the disease is often unclear, outbreaks traced to both food and water have been reported; person-to-person as well as animal-to-person transmission is common. Manifestations of the disease vary with age. In infants and young children the predominant symptom is acute watery diarrhea lasting 3 to 14 days; 5 percent of children have blood in the stool. In older children and young adults, a syndrome of right lower quadrant pain accompanied by fever and moderate leukocytosis indistinguishable from acute appendicitis occurs. In adults, especially in women over age 40, erythema nodosum often follows enteritis by 1 to 2 weeks. Adults may develop a monoarticular arthritis of the knee, foot, or hand with or without preceding enteritis. Rarely, a severe, disabling suppurative arthritis is seen. Among patients with arthritis, 65 percent have histocompatibility group HLA-B27. *Y. enterocolitica* also causes bacteremia, mostly in individuals with underlying illness such as diabetes mellitus, severe anemia, cirrhosis, or malignancy. Septicemic patients complain of headache, fever, and abdominal pain with or without diarrhea and frequently develop abscesses in multiple organs. Exudative pharyngitis with *Y. enterocolitica* was found in adult patients during the course of an outbreak of milkborne yersiniosis.

Pseudotuberculosis is a rare illness acquired from humans or domestic and wild animals, presumably by fecal-oral contact. Most cases are sporadic and occur in the young, with males more commonly affected than females and with a peak in the winter months corresponding to the peak occurrence in animals. After ingestion, the organisms apparently penetrate the ileal mucosa, localize in the ileocecal lymph nodes, and produce an acute mesenteric adenitis, which is generally accompanied by vomiting, abdominal pain, and diarrhea. Fever is usually high and leukocytosis common. At laparotomy the appendix appears normal, but enlarged mesenteric lymph nodes and inflammation of the terminal ileum may be seen. Complications appear in adults less commonly than with *Y. enterocolitica* but include arthritis, erythema nodosum, and septicemia.

DIAGNOSIS *Y. enterocolitica* and *Y. pseudotuberculosis* cause similar signs and symptoms but may have different reservoirs; the first is characterized primarily by diarrhea and the second by mesenteric adenitis. Therefore *Y. enterocolitica* causes disease similar to other bacterial diarrheas and must be distinguished from them by microbiologic means. Laboratory detection of the organism depends on special cultural techniques. The diagnosis is made best by isolation of the organism from stool in patients with enteritis, or atypical cases of appendicitis, erythema nodosum, or reactive arthritis. Cultures of the pharyngeal exudate, peritoneal fluid, and other body fluids should be obtained where clinically indicated. Hemagglutination titers peak in 8 to 10 days and remain elevated for 18 months after infection. Cross-reactivity with some *Brucella, Salmonella,* and *Vibrio cholerae* antigens occurs. The diagnosis of *Y. pseudotuberculosis* is also made by culture of stool and mesenteric lymph nodes.

THERAPY AND PREVENTION *Y. enterocolitica* organisms are susceptible in vitro to aminoglycosides, chloramphenicol, tetracycline, trimethoprim-sulfamethoxazole, and the third-generation cephalosporins but are generally resistant to the penicillins and first-generation cephalosporins. However, the value of antimicrobial therapy is unclear, because most cases of enteritis are self-limited. Patients with very severe illness or septicemia should be treated, because treatment may shorten both the duration of disease and the shedding of organisms. *Y. pseudotuberculosis* is usually sensitive to ampicillin, tetracycline, choramphenicol, and cephalosporins. No controlled clinical trials demonstrate efficacy of treatment, although patients with septicemic disease should receive ampicillin or tetracycline, because severe infection has a high mortality. Prevention depends on hygienic measures such as careful food handling, availability of clean drinking water, and hand washing to prevent spread within families or other human contacts.

PASTEURELLA MULTOCIDA INFECTION

Pasteurella multocida is a small, aerobic, gram-negative, bipolar-staining coccobacillus, distantly related to *Yersinia* species but differing from them in microbiologic characteristics and clinical disease patterns. Three related species (*P. haemolytica, P. pneumotropica,* and *P. ureae*) cause occasional disease in human beings. All grow well on routine media (but not MacConkey's agar), possess endotoxin, and are sensitive to penicillins, late-generation cephalosporins, tetracyclines, and chloramphenicol, but are variably resistant to aminoglycosides and erythromycin. *P. multocida* is a member of the normal flora of the digestive and respiratory tract of many wild and domestic mammals and birds; carriage in dogs and cats ranges from 50 to 90 percent.

The organism causes septicemia and pneumonia in domestic animals and most frequently results in human infections following animal bites or scratches, especially of cats and dogs. Skin wound infections typically develop rapidly (1 to 2 days) with severe pain, fever, suppuration, and surrounding cellulitis and adenitis. Complications include abscess formation, tendonitis, osteomyelitis, and septic arthritis. Pulmonary infections are next most common, and consist of pneumonia, acute and chronic bronchitis, and sinusitis. Infections occur in those with underlying respiratory disease and may not be associated with animal contact. Bacteremia may accompany pulmonary infection but may also originate from or accompany abdominal abscesses, meningitis, endocarditis, and genitourinary infection.

The diagnosis should be suspected following animal bites. Neither wound nor other organ site infections are clinically unique, often resembling infection due to staphylococci, streptococci, or cat-scratch fever. The diagnosis should be confirmed by laboratory identification of *Pasteurella* species. Therapy of infection with parenteral penicillin or tetracycline is usually effective, but the value of prophylaxis of bite wounds has not been proved.

REFERENCES

Plague

BARNES AM, POLAND JD: Plague in the United States, 1983, Centers for Disease Control Surveillance Summaries, Publication 33 (no 1SS), 1984

BUTLER T: A clinical study of bubonic plague: Observations on the 1970 Vietnam epidemic with emphasis on coagulation studies, skin histology, and electrocardiograms. Am J Med 53:268, 1972

KAUFMAN AF et al: Public health implications of plague in domestic cats. Am J Vet Assoc 179:875, 1981

REED WP et al: Bubonic plague in the Southwestern United States—A review of recent experience. Medicine 49:465, 1970

TOMICH PQ et al: Evidence for the extinction of plague in Hawaii. Am J Epidemiol 119: 261, 1984

P. multocida

WEBER DJ et al: *Pasteurella multocida* infections. Report of 34 cases and review of the literature. Medicine 63:133, 1984

Yersinia

BOYCE JM: *Yersinia* species, in *Principles and Practice of Infectious Diseases,* 2d ed, GL Mandell, et al (eds). New York, Wiley, 1985, pp 1296–1301

BRUBAKER RR: The Vwa$^+$ virulence factor of yersiniae: The molecular basis of the attendant nutritional requirement for Ca^{++}. Rev Infect Dis 5(Suppl 4):S748, 1983

TACKET CO et al: *Yersinia enterocolitica* pharyngitis. Ann Intern Med 99:40, 1983

TERTTI R et al: An outbreak of *Yersinia pseudotuberculosis* infection. J Infect Dis 149:245, 1984

115 CHOLERA

CHARLES C. J. CARPENTER

DEFINITION Cholera is an acute illness which results from colonization of the small intestine by *Vibrio cholerae.* The disease is characterized by its epidemic occurrence and the production in the more severe cases of massive diarrhea with rapid depletion of extracellular fluid and electrolytes.

ETIOLOGY AND EPIDEMIOLOGY *Vibrio cholerae* is a curved, aerobic, gram-negative bacillus with a single polar flagellum. It is rapidly motile and possesses both O and H antigens. Serologic identification is based on differences in the polysaccharide O antigens.

Cholera has been endemic for a century and a half in the Gangetic Delta of West Bengal and Bangladesh and is often epidemic throughout south and southeast Asia. The seventh and most recent pandemic spread of this disease, from 1961 to 1981, extended from the Celebes northward to Korea and westward to the whole of Africa and southern Europe. The last major epidemic of cholera in the western hemisphere occurred from 1866 to 1867. However, since 1978, over 40 persons have developed cholera, serotype Inaba, in coastal Texas or Louisiana. Sporadic cases have occurred after ingestion of inadequately cooked seafood caught in lakes or coastal Gulf waters of Louisiana, and one large (14 cases) common-source outbreak resulted from contamination of drinking water on a Gulf Coast oil rig. Only one other documented case of cholera has been acquired in any other western hemisphere country since 1900.

The majority of epidemics have clearly been waterborne, but direct contamination of food by infected feces also contributes to spread within affected households. Poor sanitation is primarily responsible for the continuing presence of cholera, but host factors, such as relative or absolute achlorhydria, also play an important role in the susceptibility of the individual to infection. In endemic areas, cholera is predominantly a disease of children; in rural Bangladesh, attack rates are 10 times greater in the 1- to 5-year-old age group than in those above 14 years of age. However, when the disease spreads to previously uninvolved areas, the attack rates are initially at least as high in adults as in children.

A chronic gallbladder carrier state has been observed in a small percentage of elderly convalescent cholera patients. The basis for the annual cholera epidemics throughout the Gangetic Delta, for the periodic outbreaks throughout the remainder of south and southeast Asia, and for the occasional global pandemics is, however, not known.

PATHOGENESIS *Vibrio cholerae* produce a protein enterotoxin which is responsible for all known pathophysiologic aberrations in cholera. This enterotoxin, which has a molecular weight of 84,000, stimulates adenylate cyclase in the intestine epithelial cells, and the resultant increase in intracellular cyclic adenosine 3′,5′-monophosphate leads to secretion of isotonic fluid by all segments of the small intestine. The enterotoxin-induced electrolyte secretion occurs in the absence of any demonstrable damage to intestine epithelial cells or to the capillary endothelial cells of the lamina propria. The stool of the adult cholera patient is nearly isotonic, with sodium and chloride concentrations slightly less than those of plasma, a bicarbonate concentration approximately twice that of plasma, and a potassium concentration three to five times that of plasma. The pathophysiologic defect in cholera is extracellular fluid depletion with resultant hypovolemic shock, base-deficit acidosis, and progressive potassium depletion. *Vibrio cholerae* does not invade the gut wall, nor has the enterotoxin been shown, in human disease, to have any direct effect on any organ other than the small intestine.

MANIFESTATIONS The incubation period generally lasts from 12 to 48 h. This is followed by the abrupt onset of watery, generally painless diarrhea. In the more severe cases, the initial diarrheal stool may be in excess of 1000 mL, and several liters of isotonic fluid may be lost within hours, leading rapidly to profound shock. Vomiting generally follows, but occasionally precedes, the onset of diarrhea; the vomiting is characteristically effortless and not preceded by nausea. As saline depletion progresses, severe muscle cramps, commonly involving the calves, occur.

When first seen, the typical severely ill cholera patient is cyanotic, with pinched facies, scaphoid abdomen, poor skin turgor, and thready or absent peripheral pulses. The voice is faint, high-pitched, and often inaudible, and there are tachycardia, hypotension, and varying degrees of tachypnea. In all epidemics there are many subclinical or mild cases in which gastrointestinal fluid loss is not severe enough to require hospitalization. With the *el tor* strain of *V. cholerae,* which has been responsible for the most recent pandemic, the ratio of subclinical infections to clinical cholera cases is greater than 10:1.

The disease runs its course in 2 to 7 days, and subsequent manifestations depend on the adequacy of electrolyte repletion therapy. With prompt fluid and electrolyte repletion, physiologic recovery is remarkably rapid, and mortality exceptionally rare. The important causes of death, in inadequately treated patients, are hypovolemic shock, metabolic acidosis, and uremia resulting from acute tubular necrosis.

LABORATORY FINDINGS In epidemics or in endemic areas, the clinical picture should arouse strong suspicion immediately. The most reliable technique for identification of *V. cholerae* consists of direct plating of a sample of cholera stool on bile salt, gelatin-tellurite-taurocholate (GTT), or thiosulfate–citrate–bile salt–sucrose (TCBS) agar. On bile salt or GTT agar the organisms appear as typical translucent colonies within 24 h. On TCBS agar, *V. cholerae* appear at 24 h as distinct, large, flat yellow colonies. Further classification requires agglutination with type-specific antiserums. In mild or convalescent cases, recovery of vibrios may be enhanced by initial enrichment for 6 h in alkaline peptone water followed by subculture on bile salt, GTT, or TCBS agar. Rapid presumptive diagnosis is possible either by directly observing immobilization of vibrios by type-specific antiserums, by using dark-field or phase microscopy, or by identifying the organisms with immunofluorescent methods.

TREATMENT Successful therapy requires only prompt and adequate replacement of gastrointestinal losses of saline and alkali. A uniformly satisfactory solution for intravenous fluid therapy can be simply prepared by the addition of 5 g sodium chloride, 4 g sodium bicarbonate, and 1 g potassium chloride to 1 liter of pyrogen-free distilled water. If commercially prepared fluids are available, lactated Ringer's solution is generally satisfactory. The intravenous fluids are initially infused at 50 to 100 mL/min, until a strong pulse has been restored. The same fluids should subsequently be infused in quantities equal to the gastrointestinal losses. If losses cannot be measured accurately, intravenous fluids should be given at a rate sufficient to maintain a normal radial pulse and normal skin turgor. Overhydration can be avoided by careful observation of neck venous filling and auscultation of the lungs. Close observation is mandatory during the acute phase of the illness, because the cholera patient can lose as much as 1 liter of isotonic fluid per hour during the first 24 h of the disease. Inadequate or delayed restoration of fecal fluid losses may result in a high incidence of acute renal failure. Serious hypokalemic symptoms are rare in adults, and potassium repletion can be carried out orally if potassium-containing intravenous fluids are not available. Hypokalemia may contribute significantly, however, to the morbidity in inadequately treated pediatric patients, and potassium, 10 to 13 meq per liter, should be included in the intravenous fluids administered to children.

Although adequate intravenous saline and alkali repletion alone results in rapid recovery of virtually all cholera patients, a dramatic reduction in the duration and volume of the diarrhea and early eradication of vibrios from the stool may be effected by antibiotic therapy. Oral tetracycline, 500 mg every 6 h for the first 48 h of treatment, has been most successful. Other antibiotics, including chloramphenicol and furazolidone, are also of value, but both appear to be slightly less effective than tetracycline.

Oral therapy Since the cholera enterotoxin does not alter glucose-facilitated sodium absorption, fluid repletion can be effected by the oral administration of glucose-containing electrolyte solutions. Since the limiting factor in treatment of cholera in both epidemic and endemic situations is often the lack of adequate quantities of intravenous fluids, the availability of an oral treatment regimen has greatly reduced the mortality from cholera outbreaks during the most recent pandemic. An oral rehydration solution (ORS) containing glucose 20 g per liter (or sucrose 40 g per liter), sodium bicarbonate 2.5 g per liter, sodium chloride 3.5 g per liter, and potassium chloride 1.5 g per liter can be readily prepared and should be satisfactory for treatment of all age groups. Roughly, 41 million packets of the salts contained in ORS were distributed by the World Health Organization to a total of 87 countries in 1981 and 1982. ORS, administered orally at a rate equal to the stool losses, can be given to patients with milder cholera throughout the course of illness and is also satisfactory in the more severe cases, once the hypovolemic shock has been corrected by intravenous fluid therapy. Oral therapy does not decrease the rate of intestinal fluid loss but provides an electrolyte solution which can be absorbed at a rate sufficient, in most cases, to counterbalance the continuing fluid losses. Therefore, successful management of the cholera patient with oral therapy requires just as close supervision, with careful monitoring of pulse volume, skin turgor, and neck veins, as does management with intravenous solutions. Supplemental intravenous fluids must be administered whenever clinical signs of saline depletion recur.

PROGNOSIS Under ideal conditions and with prompt and adequate fluid replacement, mortality approaches zero, and significant sequelae are rare. Unfortunately, death rates as high as 60 percent still occur, especially during the initial phases of outbreaks. This high mortality reflects lack of pyrogen-free intravenous fluids in remote areas, the difficulties of initiating treatment promptly when large numbers of cases are occurring in poverty-striken populations, and the compromises which may have to be made under emergency conditions.

PREVENTION Immunization by standard commercial vaccine, containing 10 billion killed organisms per milliliter, provides only limited (40 to 60 percent) protection for a relatively short (4- to 6-month) period in endemic areas. Vaccination, therefore, is not recommended for Americans who are traveling abroad. Careful hygiene provides the only sure protection against cholera.

REFERENCES

CARPENTER CCJ et al: Clinical studies in Asiatic cholera, I–VI. Bull Johns Hopkins Hosp 118:165, 1966

FISHMAN PH: Mechanism of action of cholera toxin: Events on the cell surface, in *Secretory Diarrhea,* M Field *et al* (eds). Bethesda, American Physiological Society, 1980, pp 85–106

GANGAROSA EF et al: The nature of the gastrointestinal lesion in Asiatic cholera and its relation to pathogenesis: A biopsy study. Am J Trop Med Hyg 9:125, 1960

HIRSCHHORN N et al: The treatment of cholera, in *Cholera,* D Barua, W Burrows (eds). Philadelphia, Saunders, 1974, p 235

JOHNSON JM et al: Cholera on a Gulf Coast oil rig. N Engl J Med 309:523, 1983

MAHALANOBIS D et al: Oral fluid therapy of cholera among Bangladesh refugees. Johns Hopkins Med J 132:197, 1973

MORRIS JG JR et al: Non-O group 1 *Vibrio cholerae* gastroenteritis in the United States: Clinical, epidemiologic, and laboratory characteristics of sporadic cases. Ann Intern Med 94:656, 1981

116 BARTONELLOSIS

JAMES J. PLORDE

DEFINITION Bartonellosis (Carrión's disease) is an infection with *Bartonella bacilliformis*. Two well-defined clinical stages occur: an acute febrile anemia of rapid onset and high mortality, designated *Oroya fever,* and a benign eruptive form with chronic cutaneous lesions, called *verruga peruana*. Either of these types may be mild, and asymptomatic cases constitute the greatest epidemiologic hazard.

ETIOLOGY *Bartonella bacilliformis* is a small, motile, aerobic, pleomorphic, gram-negative coccobacillus which stains reddish violet with Giemsa's stain. It can be cultured on enriched media and does not produce a hemolysin. The organisms are sensitive to several antibiotics in vitro.

EPIDEMIOLOGY The disease is limited to certain valleys in the Andes Mountains comprising parts of Peru, Ecuador, and Colombia. It occurs in regions between the altitudes of 2400 and 8000 ft where the phlebotomine sandfly vector, *Lutzomyia,* propagates. Although *L. verrucarum* is the principal vector of the disease, other species are involved in Colombia as well. Asymptomatic cases and convalescent carriers are the only known reservoir of infection. A low-grade bacteremia may persist for years following resolution of symptoms, and *B. bacilliformis* can be recovered from the blood of 5 to 10 percent of the apparently normal population in an endemic area. Epidemics often coincide with immigration of workers from uninfected areas.

PATHOLOGY AND PATHOGENESIS The manifestations of the disease are thought to reflect the immune status of the host. In nonimmune individuals Oroya fever develops. Large numbers of the *Bartonella* bacteria enter the bloodstream, adhere to erythrocytes, and invade the endothelial cells of the capillaries and lymphatics where they multiply. Subsequent invasion and multiplication within erythrocytes results in their phagocytosis and destruction by the liver and spleen. The red blood cell life span is greatly shortened, and anemia develops. This is accentuated by a defective erythropoietic response early in the course of infection. The pathogenesis of the hemolytic anemia remains unknown. Agglutinins and hemolysins have not been found, and tests for mechanical fragility of red blood cells have given variable results. Invasion and swelling of capillary endothelial cells may lead to vascular occlusion and tissue infarcts. It is possible that an impairment of reticuloendothelial function secondary to massive phagocytosis of red blood cells is responsible for the frequency with which *Salmonella* and other coliform bacteremias are seen in Oroya fever.

With developing immunity, the bacteria nearly disappear from the peripheral blood and capillary endothelium. After a latent period they reappear in the skin and subcutaneous tissue where they are apparently responsible for the development of the hemangioid lesions of verruga peruana. Second attacks of Carrión's disease are unusual. When they occur, they almost invariably present as verruga.

CLINICAL MANIFESTATIONS The incubation period is approximately 3 weeks but may be longer. The initial symptoms are fever and pains in the bones, joints, and muscles. At this point the disease often resembles influenza or malaria, but blood cultures are positive. After these prodromes, the patient usually develops one of the two classic forms of the infection.

Oroya fever This form is characterized by sudden onset of high fever, extreme pallor, weakness, and a precipitous drop in the number of red blood cells. The count may fall from normal to 1 million per cubic millimeter within 4 or 5 days. The anemia is characterized by normochromic macrocytes in the peripheral blood, striking polychromasia and polychromatophilia, nucleated red blood cells, Howell-Jolly bodies, Cabot rings, and basophilic stippling. There may also be a mild leukocytosis with a shift to the left. Organisms are numerous in the blood, and stained smears may show 90 percent of the erythrocytes heavily invaded. Salmonellosis, malaria, amebiasis, tuberculosis, and other intercurrent infections may occur and are an important factor in fatal cases.

Muscle and joint pain and headache are severe, and insomnia, delirium, and coma are the terminal manifestations. In untreated patients, the mortality rate may exceed 50 percent; death occurs within 10 days to 4 weeks. With treatment, or sometimes spontaneously, recovery results if the organisms decrease and fever abates. The red blood cell count stabilizes and approaches normal values in about 6 weeks, when convalescence begins.

Verruga peruana This form of the disease, characterized by a profuse skin eruption, may follow the anemic form or may occur in patients without previous symptoms. The verrugas vary in color from red to purple. They may be miliary, nodular, or eroding, and they range in size from 2 to 10 mm up to 3 or 4 cm in diameter. The three types of verruga may occur together; since eruption takes place in successive crops, verrugas of all types and in all stages of development may be found on the same patient. The chief sites involved are the limbs and face, and less frequently the genitalia, scalp, and mucosa of the mouth and pharynx. They may persist for 1 month to 2 years. The eruption is accompanied by pain, fever, and moderate anemia. Bartonellas may be demonstrated in the lesions and cultured from the blood.

DIAGNOSIS A clinical diagnosis of verruga peruana can be made with accuracy in endemic areas. It is confirmed by demonstrating the Giemsa-stained organism in biopsy specimens from representative lesions. During Oroya fever the organism is easily seen on peripheral blood smears. It may be recovered from blood cultures in all stages of the disease.

TREATMENT Oroya fever responds dramatically to a number of antibiotics including tetracycline and chloramphenicol. The latter in a dose of 2 g per day for 7 days is often preferred because of the frequency with which *Salmonella* infections complicate this disease. Fever disappears within 48 h, and the patient recovers rapidly. Transfusions may be required when the anemia is severe. Antibiotic therapy of the verrugal stage may hasten the involution of these lesions. The use of DDT in both the interior and exterior of human dwellings is highly effective in controlling the night-biting sandflies. Insect repellents and bed netting afford personal protection.

REFERENCES

CAUDRA MC: Salmonellosis complication in human bartonellosis. Tex Rep Biol Med 14:97, 1956

DOOLEY JR: Haemotropic bacteria in man. Lancet 2:1237, 1980

KAYE D et al: Factors influencing host resistance to *Salmonella* infections: The effects of hemolysis and erythrophagocytosis. Am J Med Sci 254:205, 1967

RICKETTS WE: Clinical manifestations of Carrión's disease. AMA Arch Intern Med 84:751, 1949

SCHULTZ MG: Daniel Carrión's experiment. N Engl J Med 278:1323, 1968

117 *LEGIONELLA* INFECTIONS

HARRY N. BEATY / A. WILLIAM PASCULLE

DEFINITION *Legionella* infections are acute respiratory infections caused by species of bacteria within the genus *Legionella*. The type species of the genus is *L. pneumophila,* and Legionnaires' disease, the common name for pneumonia caused by this bacterium, is still the prototype for infections with this group of organisms. Collectively, these infections often are referred to as legionellosis. While the various species within the genus *Legionella* are quite distinctive microbiologically, multiple characteristics of the various forms of legionellosis differ inconsequentially from those of Legionnaires' disease and other clinical expressions of *L. pneumophila* infection. Therefore, much of what is known concerning legionellosis is derived, sometimes by inference, from what has been learned about Legionnaires' disease.

HISTORY In July of 1976, an explosive outbreak of severe respiratory illness occurred in Philadelphia—chiefly among delegates of an American Legion Convention. Initial investigation failed to document a familiar infective or toxic etiology, and so a comprehensive, coordinated effort was undertaken to define the epidemiology and cause of the outbreak. As the ensuing saga unfolded, it became apparent that at least 220 cases of pneumonia—34 of which were fatal—resulted from a common source of airborne infection that was present for several days inside and in the immediate vicinity outside one of the convention hotels. The infective agent was proved to be a previously unknown gram-negative bacterium that ultimately was named *Legionella pneumophila*.

Using serologic techniques, it has been shown that the same organism, or antigenically related species, has caused other outbreaks of respiratory illness. One of these occurred among attendees at a convention of Oddfellows, which took place in 1974 at the same Philadelphia hotel that was involved in the outbreak of Legionnaires' disease. The organism also was found to be responsible for nosocomial infections when an outbreak of pneumonia that occurred in 1965 in a psychiatric hospital in Washington, D.C., and involved 81 patients with 14 fatalities was retrospectively attributed to *L. pneumophila* infection. The earliest outbreak of Legionnaires' disease that has been identified occurred in 1957 among employees of a meat packing plant in Austin, Minnesota. Seventy-eight persons were infected, and there were two fatalities.

A second form of disease due to *L. pneumophila* was recognized when it was shown that a brisk epidemic of nonpneumonic, influenza-like illness that occurred in 1968 among employees and visitors of the county health department building in Pontiac, Michigan, had been caused by *L. pneumophila*.

The use of techniques developed for the isolation and characterization of *L. pneumophila* resulted in the subsequent recognition of several closely related organisms, some of which caused human disease. In 1978 and 1979 two outbreaks of nosocomial pneumonia among patients in hospitals in Pittsburgh, Pennsylvania, and Charlottesville, Virginia, were attributed to an organism that was isolated initially by the Pittsburgh workers from the lung tissue of one patient. This "Pittsburgh pneumonia agent," as it was first called, ultimately was shown to be phenotypically similar to but genetically distinct from *L. pneumophila* and was named *Legionella micdadei* in honor of Joseph McDade who first isolated *L. pneumophila*.

Subsequently, a linkage was established between a group of rickettsia-like bacteria first isolated decades ago and the newly recognized genus, *Legionella*. Many of these isolates resembled *L. pneumophila* phenotypically, but were "atypical" antigenically and genetically. Initially these organisms were referred to as "atypical *Legionella*-like organisms" (ALLO), but all are now recognized species in the genus. Currently there are 22 distinct species of *Legionella* consisting of 35 antigenically different organisms (Table 117-1).

ETIOLOGY The legionellae are gram-negative aerobic rods that do not grow on commonly used bacteriologic media. In clinical specimens, the bacteria appear as 0.5-μm rods while organisms from artificial media may be highly pleomorphic and even include filamentous forms many times longer. Most species are motile and contain one or two polar flagella that appear to be antigenically identical among all the species.

Legionellae have complex growth and pH requirements. The medium of choice for their isolation from clinical specimens is buffered charcoal yeast extract agar supplemented with alpha-ketoglutarate (BCYE-alpha). BCYE agar is a very rich culture medium and is in no way selective for legionellae. Many common bacterial species, including *Francisella tularensis,* are capable of growth on this medium as are many fungi, such as *Coccidioides immitis*. The addition of cefamandole, polymyxin, and anisomycin to BCYE-alpha results in a semiselective medium which can be used for the isolation of at least some *Legionella* species from normally contaminated clinical specimens such as sputum. Biochemically, the legionellae do not appear highly diverse and cannot be identified by metabolic testing. When only a few species were known, the legionellae could be rapidly classified by serologic testing with antibody conjugates prepared against the known species. Serologic cross reactions among the first ten species identified were very minor and did not interfere with the production of relatively specific reagents. Several of the recently recognized species, however, cross-react significantly with other species, and specific antisera are not yet available for serologic identification of all *Legionella* species.

At the present time, the definitive identification of an isolate at the species level requires DNA homology studies. It is on the basis of these determinations that the legionellae have been divided into the 22 currently recognized species. Their classification in the genus *Legionella* is based upon their phenotypic similarity.

ECOLOGY AND EPIDEMIOLOGY Legionellosis occurs worldwide, and the legionellae are ubiquitous microorganisms that appear to be part of the natural microbial community of many natural and artificial aquatic ecosystems. They have been isolated from a variety of moist habitats ranging from alpine lakes to the hot springs of Yellowstone National Park.

The ecologic niche of these organisms that has the most direct clinical importance is the warm moist areas of the mechanical systems of large buildings, particularly hotels and hospitals. Legionellae have been found in the evaporative coolers of large air conditioning systems, and aerosols from these cooling towers can carry the organisms significant distances before they are inhaled by a susceptible host. The outbreak of Legionnaires' disease in Philadelphia and of Pontiac fever in Michigan almost certainly arose from contaminated air conditioning systems. Air handling equipment also has been incriminated as a source of nosocomial outbreaks of Legionnaires' disease in Burlington, Vermont, and Memphis, Tennessee, to name only a few.

Potable water distribution systems are a frequent source of these bacteria, particularly in association with nosocomial legionellosis. Overwhelming evidence indicates that the legionellae can thrive in

TABLE 117-1 Recognized species and serotypes of *Legionella*

Organism	Number of serotypes	Human isolation	Environmental isolation
L. pneumophila	10	Yes	Yes
L. micdadei	1	Yes	Yes
L. bozemanii	2	Yes	Yes
L. dumoffii	1	Yes	Yes
L. gormanii	1	Yes	Yes
L. feeleii	2	Yes	Yes
L. longbeacheae	2	Yes	Yes
L. jordanis	1	Yes	Yes
L. oakridgensis	1	Yes	Yes
L. wadsworthii	1	Yes	Yes
L. hackeliae	1	Yes	No
L. maceachernii	2	Yes	Yes
L. sainthelensi	1	No	Yes
L. spiritensis	1	No	Yes
L. jamestownensis	1	No	Yes
L. santicrucis	1	No	Yes
L. anisa	1	No	Yes
L. cherrii	1	No	Yes
L. steigerwaltii	1	No	Yes
L. paresiensis	1	No	Yes
L. rubrilucens	1	No	Yes
L. erythra	1	No	Yes

the hot water distribution system of some buildings. Organisms live and multiply in the sludge of hot water tanks in association with other bacterial species. From there, the organisms can be disseminated throughout the plumbing systems in hospitals, hotels, and even a small number of private homes. Water passing through contaminated fixtures such as shower heads and faucet valves produces an effective aerosol of bacteria.

Medical devices utilizing unsterilized tap water also can become contaminated with legionellae. For example, *L. micdadei* has been isolated from an ultrasonic nebulizer and from room humidifiers. Outbreaks also have been linked to contaminated whirlpools and hot tubs.

The mere presence of legionellae in a water distribution system does not always predict the presence of disease among those potentially exposed. The reasons for this are not yet understood, but one intriguing hypothesis is that not all *Legionella* strains are equally virulent. Virulence, in turn, may be related to the presence of a plasmid.

Infection appears to be acquired by the respiratory route. In the case of Legionnaires' disease, the usual incubation period is 2 to 10 days. While organisms have been identified in the sputum of patients with Legionnaires' disease, person-to-person spread has not been documented. Common-source outbreaks have received the greatest public attention, but hundreds of sporadic cases of legionellosis occur each year. Incidence may increase in the summer and early fall, but these infections occur year-round.

Although Legionnaires' disease has been reported in children, most patients with legionellosis are middle-aged or older. Cigarette smokers and individuals with serious underlying diseases such as chronic renal failure, malignancy, and immunosuppression have increased susceptibility to infection. The mortality rate of Legionnaires' pneumonia that is serious enough to require hospitalization is around 15 percent; among immunocompromised patients it may exceed 50 percent.

Serologic surveys using the indirect fluorescent-antibody technique have shown that less than 5 percent of healthy individuals from around the United States have reciprocal antibody titers to *L. pneumophila* of 128 or higher. However, some more geographically restricted surveys have shown that 15 to 25 percent of the population has similar serologic evidence of significant exposure to *L. pneumophila* or antigenically related organisms. This suggests that the infection may be endemic in some regions.

PATHOLOGY AND PATHOGENESIS Most pathologic features ascribable directly to infection with legionellae are limited to the lungs. Those associated with Legionnaires' disease have been studied most extensively and are representative of changes seen in infections with other organisms in the genus. Apparent lobar involvement almost always represents confluent bronchopneumonia. Prominent microscopic features include extensive exudation of proteinaceous fluid and inflammatory cells into the alveoli. In most cases, the cellular component of the exudate is a mixture of polymorphonuclear neutrophils and macrophages. Extensive lysis of inflammatory cells, with accumulations of nuclear debris and fibrin, is a distinctive feature of this pneumonia. Alveolar septa usually are edematous and infiltrated with inflammatory cells; hyaline membranes are seen in about half the cases. Terminal bronchioles are routinely involved, but larger bronchioles and bronchi are unaffected. None of these changes is unique to pulmonary infection with legionellae, but the histopathologic alterations are sufficiently distinctive to suggest the diagnosis.

Bacteria usually can be demonstrated in the inflammatory exudate with the Dieterle stain or by using direct fluorescent-antibody conjugates. Other stains are less reliable although *L. micdadei* may be demonstrated by acid-fast stains of tissue. Many bacilli appear to be intracellular, and an increase in the number of organisms is associated with lysis of inflammatory cells.

Little is known about the pathogenesis of legionellosis. The fact that cigarette smokers are more susceptible to infection than nonsmokers suggests that the defective alveolar macrophage function plays a role in the development of disease. Experimental evidence indicates that legionellae can survive and proliferate in normal macrophages and other cells, a characteristic that has important pathogenetic implications. The extensive lysis of inflammatory cells and the edema of the interstitium raise the possibility that a toxin is produced by the infecting organism. Such a toxin might be responsible for some of the clinical features seen with this infection.

CLINICAL MANIFESTATIONS The total spectrum of clinical manifestations of legionellosis is not known. Mild respiratory illness has been recognized, but asymptomatic infection has not been excluded as a possible explanation for elevated antibody titers among healthy individuals. The outbreak in Pontiac, Michigan, was characterized by the acute onset and short duration of a moderately severe influenza-like syndrome of fever, myalgia, and headache. Legionellosis with this presentation is referred to as "Pontiac fever" and until an outbreak associated with *L. feeleii* was described, was thought to be caused exclusively by *L. pneumophila* infection.

The more typical patient with legionellosis has pneumonia that is severe enough to require hospitalization. No clinical features distinguish between infections caused by the different species of *Legionella* or between legionellosis and other forms of pneumonia. The most characteristic patients with Legionnaires' disease have malaise and a slight headache, which precedes a rapidly rising fever by less than a day. Within 24 to 48 h, temperatures reach 40°C in about half the patients, and shaking chills are common. A modest, nonproductive cough frequently is present early; it progresses in severity over the first few days of illness and usually becomes productive of variable amounts of mucoid to mucopurulent sputum. Minimal hemoptysis is seen in about 20 percent of patients. Additional symptoms that occur less frequently include dyspnea, pleuritic chest pain, and myalgia. About 25 percent of patients have various combinations of gastrointestinal symptoms which include nausea and vomiting, diarrhea, and abdominal pain. In a few patients, these manifestations predominate despite the presence of pneumonia. In some individuals, the onset of legionellosis is more protracted and the clinical expression less distinctive. These cases are likely to be missed unless the epidemiologic setting or subtle clinical clues stimulate physicians to suspect the diagnosis. The findings on physical examination are not specific for legionellosis, and they are affected by patients' associated diseases. High fever, tachypnea, and tachycardia are common. Patients frequently are flushed, mildly diaphoretic, and appear moderately to severely prostrated. Examination of the chest shows moist rales, but signs of consolidation usually are absent. Chest roentgenograms characteristically show more involvement of the lungs than is suspected on clinical grounds.

During the first 4 to 6 days, the disease becomes progressively worse. An additional 4 to 5 days may pass before dramatic clinical improvement begins, even though appropriate antimicrobial therapy is given. The average duration of fever in one large series was 13 days. Clearing of pulmonary infiltrates lags significantly behind improvement of other manifestations of infection, and minor residual scarring is not uncommon. Many patients experience weakness and easy fatigability for weeks after the acute stages of the illness.

The major complication of legionellosis is respiratory failure. Twenty to thirty percent of patients sick enough to require hospitalization have hyperventilation and hypoxemia. In about half of these patients, progression of disease leads to intubation and mechanical ventilation. The mortality rate among patients with respiratory failure is high. Hypotension and shock, with secondary acute renal failure, are additional complications that may be encountered.

LABORATORY FINDINGS Most patients have a modest granulocytosis, or even neutropenia, but about 20 percent have leukocyte counts in excess of 20,000 per cubic millimeter. The erythrocyte sedimentation rate is elevated, and there is moderate proteinuria. Reversible renal insufficiency and mild changes in liver function have been reported, but it is not always possible to attribute these abnormalities to the infection.

Chest roentgenograms show unilateral pulmonary parenchymal infiltrates in about 65 percent of cases early in the illness. By the time of maximal involvement, the pneumonia has progressed to involve both sides in most cases. Nonspecific poorly marginated rounded opacities or diffuse patchy lobar shadows predominate. Small pleural effusions are seen in about a third of cases.

Routine bacteriologic studies including blood and sputum cultures are negative. Lower respiratory tract secretions obtained by transtracheal aspiration or other suitable techniques show many granulocytes and alveolar macrophages but may show no organisms on Gram's stain and are sterile on routine culture media.

DIAGNOSIS The diagnosis of legionellosis is most firmly established by the demonstration of legionellae in the respiratory secretions of patients by either culture or immunofluorescent staining. Since colonization with these organisms is not known to occur, their demonstration in sputum is confirmation of their role in the infection. Culture of respiratory secretions is somewhat more sensitive than immunofluorescent staining for the detection of these organisms. The highest yields have been achieved when samples of respiratory secretions have been collected without contamination by oral flora. Such specimens include transtracheal aspirates, percutaneous fine-needle aspirates, and bronchoalveolar lavages. The sensitivity of culture for these specimens approaches 90 percent because of the lack of interference from contaminating flora.

When expectorated sputum is employed, two factors reduce the sensitivity of cultural techniques. The first is that contaminating microorganisms may inhibit the growth of the legionellae on nonselective media. In addition, selective media contain antimicrobial agents to which several species are sensitive. For instance, *L. micdadei* does not grow well on these media because it is susceptible to cefamandole, and cultures from patients with this infection may be falsely negative.

Immunofluorescent staining is less sensitive than culture. The antigenic diversity of the genus contributes to the difficulty in making diagnoses by immunofluorescent staining because antibody conjugates are routinely available only for *L. pneumophila, L. micdadei, L. bozemanii, L. dumoffii, L. gormanii,* and *L. longbeacheae*. While it is true that the great majority of cases of legionellosis are caused by *L. pneumophila,* the possibility that a particular patient's disease may be due to a known but undetected species must be kept in mind when evaluating a negative direct fluorescent antibody (DFA) test. Patients with Legionnaires' disease have been shown to shed antigens of the organism in urine. This antigen(s) is detectable in the urine within the first 3 days of illness, which makes the test potentially useful for rapid diagnosis. This test suffers from the same limitation as other serologic tests that might be used to diagnose all forms of legionellosis, in that a large number of reagents will be required to detect all species and serotypes.

Because of the plethora of antigens that must be employed and the vagaries of the immune response to the legionellae, serologic testing is more of epidemiologic than clinical value.

TREATMENT AND PREVENTION Although in vitro sensitivity tests indicate that a number of antibiotics might be effective in the treatment of Legionnaires' disease, clinical experience has shown that the lowest case-fatality ratio is achieved with erythromycin in a dose of 0.5 to 1 g every 6 h for adults and 15 mg/kg every 6 h for children. Tetracycline is less effective. Rifampin has shown promise in laboratory testing, but its propensity to induce resistance may limit its potential usefulness. Certainly, it should not be used alone. With increasing frequency, the combination of rifampin and erythromycin is being used for critically ill patients. It has not been documented, however, that this combination is more effective than erythromycin alone.

Although the case-fatality ratio of patients treated with erythromycin is low, response to treatment frequently is not dramatic. If therapy is continued for at least 14 days, relapses are uncommon. When they occur, they usually respond to a second course of erythromycin. Because Legionnaires' disease can cause pneumonia in patients not sick enough to be hospitalized and who are assumed to have either *Mycoplasma* infection or early pneumococcal infection, erythromycin should be considered the drug of choice for the treatment of pneumonia in an ambulatory care setting.

There is more to treatment of Legionnaires' disease than administration of antibiotics. High fever, diaphoresis, and tachypnea produce excessive fluid loss, and volume replacement with intravenous fluids may be needed. Hypoxic patients should receive supplemental oxygen.

Prevention of legionellosis depends upon identifying contaminated environmental reservoirs and eradicating the organisms from them. These organisms are so ubiquitous, however, that routine surveillance of the environment is of limited value in the absence of disease. A more productive activity for hospitals is active surveillance, involving both the laboratory and infection control personnel, for *Legionella* infections. Attempts should be made to determine if nosocomial cases cluster in time and space so that environmental samples for culture are collected rationally. All possible contacts, such as respiratory therapy equipment and potable water, must be evaluated epidemiologically to determine their relative contribution to patients' risk of developing nosocomial legionellosis.

PROGNOSIS The overall mortality rate of legionellosis is unknown. Among patients with pneumonia who are sick enough to require hospitalization, the mortality rate is around 15 percent. The presence of complicating associated illnesses may raise that figure two- or threefold. Individuals who recover from pulmonary infection with legionellae usually have no significant residua. It is not known whether they are immune to reinfection with the same or related organisms.

REFERENCES

Bernardini DL et al: Neurogenic bladder. New clinical finding in Legionnaires' disease. Am J Med 78:1045, 1985

Brenner DJ et al: Ten new species of *Legionella*. Int J Sys Bacteriol 35:50, 1985

Garbe PL et al: Nosocomial Legionnaires' disease. Epidemiologic demonstration of cooling towers as a source. JAMA 254:521, 1985

Herwaldt LA et al: A new *Legionella* species, *Legionella feeleii* species nova, causes Pontiac fever in an automobile plant. Ann Intern Med 100:333, 1984

Meyer RD: *Legionella* infections: A review of five years of research. Rev Infect Dis 5:258, 1983

Rudin JE, Wing EJ: A comparative study of *Legionella micdadei* and other nosocomial acquired pneumonia. Chest 86:675, 1984

Thornsberry C et al (eds): *Legionella, Proceedings of the 2d International Symposium.* Washington, American Society for Microbiology, 1984

Winn WC Jr et al: The pathology of the *Legionella* pneumonias. Human Pathol 12:401, 1981

118 CAT-SCRATCH DISEASE

LAWRENCE COREY

DEFINITION Cat-scratch disease is an infection characterized by indolent, occasionally suppurative, regional lymphadenitis usually occurring following a scratch or a close contact with a cat. A cutaneous lesion at the site of inoculation is often present, and 90 percent of patients report cat scratches or close contact with cats.

ETIOLOGY The etiology of cat-scratch disease remains undefined. Agents incriminated in the past included atypical acid-fast bacteria, *Chlamydia*-like organisms, and viruses. The current candidate is a small, pleomorphic, presumably gram-negative bacillus identified by Warthin-Starry silver impregnation stain in lymph nodes of 25 of 34 patients who fulfilled the clinical and histologic criteria for cat-scratch disease. The organism was identified most frequently in capillary walls and macrophages lining the sinuses or germinal centers, and rarely from areas of suppuration or microabscess formation. The organism has also been identified in biopsies of cutaneous lesions from patients with the disease. A second group of workers isolated a similarly sized organism from a lymph node of a patient with cat-scratch disease. The putative pathogen is pleomorphic and gram-variable on Gram's stain and may be related to the *Rothia* genus of bacteria. This genus commonly is part of the oropharyngeal flora. The organism is sensitive in vitro to penicillin, erythromycin, cotrimoxazole, cephalosporins, and clindamycin. Koch's postulates have not been fulfilled for this organism.

EPIDEMIOLOGY The disease has been reported in numerous geographic areas; it is most common in fall and winter, and 75 percent of cases occur in children. Reactivity to the skin test antigen is seen in 3 to 20 percent of the population. Persons who have frequent contact with cats, such as veterinarians and family contacts of index cases, have a higher prevalence of past infection as detected by a positive reaction to the skin test antigen. Cats appear to act only as vectors of the disease. The animals are usually not ill and have negative skin tests. Familial occurrence of several infections interspersed by months or years suggests that cats are intermittent or long-term carriers. A compatible syndrome has been described following monkey scratches and injuries due to inanimate objects.

PATHOLOGY The histopathologic appearance of lymph nodes is not specific. Three stages have been described: (1) early lesions show reticulum-cell hyperplasia; (2) intermediate lesions show granuloma formation; and (3) late lesions show microabscesses. These histologic changes are similar to those seen with atypical mycobacterial infections, lymphogranuloma venereum, toxoplasmosis, sarcoidosis, brucellosis, tularemia, and even Hodgkin's disease.

MANIFESTATIONS The incubation period ranges from 3 days to several weeks, usually 3 to 10 days. In a typical case, a primary lesion consisting of a raised, slightly tender, nonpruritic papule. The papule may progress through a small vesicle or eschar over a 2- to 3-day period. Multiple primary lesions have been described. The lesion is often felt to be an insect bite and usually does not cause the patient to present to the physician. In about 40 percent of cases no primary lesion is present, and in some patients no history of inciting trauma is elicited.

Regional lymphadenopathy becomes evident in a few days or as long as 6 weeks after infection. Adenopathy is usually confined to a single region and is usually unilateral and asymmetric; in most instances only one node is involved. The axillary, cervical, preauricular, submandibular, inguinal, femoral, or epitrochlear nodes (in decreasing order of frequency) on one side become visibly swollen and tender, often with redness of the overlying skin. The nodes occasionally suppurate, soften, and drain spontaneously; fistulas heal completely with only slight scarring. Usually the tenderness subsides gradually, and nontender, firm, enlarged nodes remain palpable for some weeks or even months. With rare exceptions, there is no generalized glandular enlargement, and the spleen is not palpable.

Systemic symptoms are usually mild and consist of headache, fever, and malaise, which subside within a few days. Shaking chills and fever with temperatures as high as 104°F can occur but are unusual. Many patients are entirely symptom-free. During the early stages of illness a transient macular or vesicular rash which subsides within 48 h may occur. Erythema nodosum and multiforme and thrombocytopenic purpura have also been reported.

Other clinical forms of this disease include: (1) encephalitis characterized by fever, convulsions, alterations in consciousness, mild cerebrospinal fluid pleocytosis, and elevation in protein (this usually resolves with complete recovery); (2) Parinaud's oculoglandular syndrome characterized by granulomatous conjunctivitis and enlargement of the homolateral preauricular node; (3) mesenteric lymphadenitis; (4) osteolytic bone lesions, which subside spontaneously; and (5) thrombocytopenic and nonthrombocytopenic purpura. In all these syndromes the diagnostic criteria for cat-scratch disease must be present before the illness can be ascribed to this disease.

DIAGNOSIS The following criteria should be fulfilled before a diagnosis of cat-scratch disease is established: (1) history of contact with cats, (2) presence of a primary lesion, (3) regional lymphadenopathy, (4) positive intradermal skin test, (5) biopsy of lymph node with demonstration of histopathologic changes consistent with cat-scratch disease (this may not be necessary if the skin test is positive), (6) demonstration of the presumptive causative bacillus from the primary lesion or lymph node, and (7) failure to demonstrate other causative agents.

The specific diagnosis is made by means of a skin test. In the United States standardized skin test antigen is not commercially available. Antigen for skin tests is prepared by mixing one part pus aspirated from infected lymph nodes with three parts saline solution and inactivating the mixture by heating or by irradiation. A positive reaction is of the delayed tuberculin type, consisting of 5 mm induration and 10 mm erythema, that appears in 24 to 48 h. Although batches of antigen vary in potency, in general patients reacting to one batch react to another. Skin test material can be preserved by freezing. The test becomes positive within 30 days after infection and may persist for many years. Each batch of antigen must be tested against patients known to have had the disease. False-negative reactions have been reported. Approximately 5 percent of normal individuals will have positive reactions.

Other laboratory abnormalities include mild leukocytosis (up to 15,000 cells per cubic millimeter), occasional mild eosinophilia, and an elevated sedimentation rate.

Cat-scratch disease is a benign illness, and the prognosis is uniformly good. Its main clinical importance lies in its possible confusion with other, more serious diseases of the lymphatics. Diseases to be considered are tularemia, lymphatic tuberculosis, sporotrichosis, histoplasmosis, coccidioidomycosis, toxoplasmosis, and bacterial adenitis. Because of the indolent character of the adenopathy, Hodgkin's disease or other lymphomas may be suspected. Cat-scratch disease must be differentiated from tularemia, which occasionally can be transmitted by cats. Neck masses may be confused with thyroglossal duct cysts, cleft cysts, dermoids, cystic hygromas, thryoid and parathyroid adenomas, salivary gland tumors, carotid body tumors, aneurysms, pharyngeal or esophageal diverticula, and mesodermal tumors, as well as lymphomas. Appropriate serologic and cultural tests serve to rule out other infections; biopsy may be needed to exclude tumor. A positive skin test with cat-scratch antigen may obviate the necessity for biopsy.

TREATMENT The disease is self-limited and symptoms resolve spontaneously in 1 to 2 months. Occasionally aspiration of suppurative nodes affords relief of pain. Antibiotics and steroids are ineffective.

REFERENCES

Carithers HA et al: Cat-scratch disease; its natural history. An overview based on a study of 1200 patients. Am J Dis Child 135:1124, 1985

———: Cat-scratch skin test antigen: Purification by heating. Pediatrics 60:928, 1977

Elliot DL et al: Pet-associated illness. N Engl J Med 313:985, 1985

Gerber MA et al: The aetiological agent of cat-scratch disease. Lancet 1:1236, 1985

Lyon LW: Neurologic manifestations of cat-scratch disease. Arch Neurol 25:23, 1971

Margileth AM: Cat-scratch disease: Bacteria in skin at the primary inoculation site. JAMA 252:928, 1984

———, Marcy SM: Cat-scratch disease: Safety of cat-scratch skin test material. Pediatr Infect Dis 3:281, 1984

Wear DJ et al: Cat-scratch disease: A bacterial infection. Science 221:1403, 1983

section 4 Mycobacterial diseases

119 TUBERCULOSIS

THOMAS M. DANIEL

DEFINITION Tuberculosis is a chronic bacterial infection caused by *Mycobacterium tuberculosis* and characterized by the formation of granulomas in infected tissues and by florid cell-mediated hypersensitivity. The usual site of disease is the lungs, but other organs may be involved. In the absence of effective treatment, a chronic wasting course is usual and death ultimately supervenes in most cases.

ETIOLOGY *Mycobacterium tuberculosis,* the tubercle bacillus, is one of more than 30 well-characterized and many unclassified members of the genus *Mycobacterium*. Along with the closely related *M. bovis,* it causes tuberculosis. *M. leprae* is the etiologic agent of leprosy (Chap. 120), and a number of other mycobacterial species produce less common human diseases (Chap. 121). Most mycobacteria are not pathogenic for human beings, and many are readily isolated from environmental sources.

Mycobacteria are distinguished by their surface lipids which render them acid-fast. That is, these organisms cannot be decolorized with acid alcohol after staining. Because of this lipid, heat or detergents are usually necessary to accomplish primary staining.

Important to understanding the pathogenesis of tuberculosis is recognition that *M. tuberculosis* contains many immunoreactive substances. Surface lipids of mycobacteria and water-soluble components of cell wall peptidoglycan are important adjuvants that may exert their effects through their primary actions on host macrophages. *M. tuberculosis* survives the intracellular milieu of macrophages, and this intracellular persistence may be facilitated by cell wall lipids which inhibit phagosome-lysosome fusion. Mycobacteria contain an array of protein and polysaccharide antigens, some probably species-specific but others clearly sharing their antigenicity broadly throughout the genus. Tuberculous infection results in the presentation of antigens to the host in the presence of adjuvants; cell-mediated hypersensitivity is characteristic of tuberculosis and is an important determinant of the disease's pathogenesis.

EPIDEMIOLOGY There is little doubt that tuberculous disease was widely prevalent in ancient times. Tuberculosis was portrayed by European physicians and lay writers of the eighteenth and nineteenth centuries, and early public health data indicate that as many as one-quarter to one-third of all deaths in European cities in the mid-nineteenth century may have been due to tuberculosis. Today tuberculosis is disappearing rapidly from Europe and North America, but in the rest of the world it continues as an important cause of death.

In 1984, a total of 22,255 cases of tuberculosis were reported in the United States, a new case rate of 9.4 per 100,000 per year. In recent years this case rate has been falling at a rate of 5 to 6 percent per year. In 1982, there were 1,807 deaths due to tuberculosis in the United States. It is estimated that 10,000,000 Americans have a positive tuberculin test but that fewer than 1 percent of American children are tuberculin reactors. Tuberculosis in North America tends to be a disease of the elderly urban poor and of minority groups. At all ages case rates among nonwhites tend to be twice those in whites. Hispanic, Haitian, and southeast Asian immigrants may have case rates as high as those of the countries from which they come, and in these individuals the frequency of disease among younger persons reflects its occurrence in those countries. Increasingly, tuberculosis in the United States is being seen in microepidemics, often centered in families.

In the United States tuberculosis has become a disease of the elderly. It is frequently seen in nursing homes. Although transmission of infection can occur at any age, most disease in older persons represents a legacy of previous times. The elderly of today were children when transmission of tubercle bacilli occurred much more frequently. Of those who were infected, many developed disease in young adulthood. Some, especially males, did not and are only now developing reactivation disease in their late years. However, an increasing portion of elderly persons has never been infected, and nosocomial new infection has been recognized as a problem in nursing homes.

Worldwide, tuberculosis case rates are decreasing, but this decrease is not as rapid as the increase in population, so that the number of new cases is rising and will continue to rise. In much of the world transmission of tuberculous infection is declining, but in many impoverished nations this is not true. In some countries estimated new case rates are as high as 400 per 100,000 per year. As in North America and Europe, poverty and tuberculosis go hand in hand. In high-prevalence areas, tuberculosis is seen with equal prevalence in rural and urban settings, and this disease afflicts chiefly young adults. A reasonable estimate of the magnitude of tuberculosis in the world is that half of the population of the world is infected with *M. tuberculosis,* that there are 30 million cases of active tuberculosis in the world, that 10 million new cases occur annually, and that 3 million die of tuberculosis each year. Tuberculosis probably causes 6 percent of all deaths worldwide.

TRANSMISSION *M. tuberculosis* is transmitted from person to person via the aerial route. Although other routes of transmission are possible and have been documented on occasion, none is of major importance. Tubercle bacilli in respiratory secretions form nuclei for water droplets expelled during coughing, sneezing, and vocalizing. Small droplets evaporate within a short distance from the mouth, and thereafter desiccated bacilli remain airborne for long periods. Infection of a susceptible host occurs when a few of these bacilli are inhaled. The number of bacilli excreted by most infected persons is not large; typically, household contact of many months is required for transmission. However, patients with laryngeal tuberculosis, endobronchial disease, recent transbronchial spread of tuberculosis, and extensive cavitary pulmonary disease are often highly contagious. Infectiousness correlates with number of organisms in the expectorated sputum, extent of pulmonary disease, and frequency of cough. Mycobacteria are susceptible to ultraviolet irradiation, and transmission of infection rarely occurs out-of-doors in daylight. Adequate ventilation is the most important measure which can be employed to reduce the infectiousness of the environment. Fomites are not important in the transmission of tuberculosis. Most patients become noninfectious within 2 weeks after the institution of appropriate chemotherapy because of decrease in the number of organisms excreted and decrease in cough.

Transmission of infection with *M. bovis* has long been associated with the consumption of contaminated cow's milk. This organism is no longer a major cause of human disease in much of the world.

PATHOGENESIS The initial entry of tubercle bacilli into the lungs or other site of a previously uninfected individual elicits a nonspecific acute inflammatory response which is rarely noted and is usually accompanied by few or no symptoms. The usual infecting inoculum is no more than one to three organisms which reach the pulmonary alveoli directly via the airborne route. They are then ingested by macrophages and transported to the regional lymph nodes. If spread of the organism is not contained at the level of regional lymph nodes, then tubercle bacilli reach the blood stream and widespread dissemination ensues. Most lesions of disseminated tuberculosis heal, as do most primary pulmonary lesions, although they remain potential foci of later reactivation. Dissemination may result in miliary or meningeal tuberculosis—illnesses with potential for major morbidity and mortality, especially in infants and young children.

During the 2 to 8 weeks after primary infection, while bacilli continue to multiply in their intracellular environment, cell-mediated hypersensitivity develops in the infected host. Immunologically competent lymphocytes enter areas of infection. They elaborate chemotactic factors, interleukins, and lymphokines. In response, monocytes enter the area and undergo transformation into macrophages and subsequently into specialized histiocytic cells which are organized into granulomas. Mycobacteria may persist within macrophages despite increased lysozyme production within these cells, but their further multiplication and spread is usually confined. Healing then occurs, often with late calcification of the granulomas, which sometimes but not always leaves a residual lesion visible on chest radiograph. The combination of a calcified peripheral lung lesion and calcified hilar lymph node is known as a Ghon complex.

In the United States, 95 percent of individuals undergo complete healing of their primary tuberculous lesions with no subsequent evidence of disease. In other populations, where infective inocula may be higher and where nutritional status and other host factors may be less propitious, failure of complete healing may occur in more than 5 percent of individuals. Famine and many intercurrent diseases adversely affect healing and threaten the stability of healed tuberculous lesions.

Tuberculosis—the clinical disease—develops in the minority who do not successfully contain their primary infections. In some individuals tuberculosis develops within weeks after primary infection; in most, organisms lie dormant for many years before entering a phase of logarithmic multiplication leading to disease. Among many factors, age can be identified as a significant factor determining the course of tuberculosis. In infants tuberculous infection frequently progresses rapidly to disease, and the risk of disseminated disease including meningitis and miliary tuberculosis is high. In children older than 1 or 2 years up to about the age of puberty, primary tuberculous lesions almost always heal; most of those destined to develop tuberculosis do so during adolescence or young adulthood. Individuals infected in adulthood are at greatest risk of developing tuberculosis within approximately 3 years following infection. Tuberculous disease is more common in young adult women, whereas it is more common in men later in life.

IMMUNOLOGY Immunity Human beings display native immunity to tuberculosis, with substantial individual variation. Twin studies have demonstrated that tuberculosis is more likely to occur in both members of monozygotic sibships than in dizygotic sibships or other family relationships. Attempts to link susceptibility to tuberculosis to HLA phenotype have produced conflicting data. Although susceptibility to tuberculosis has been associated with race, the evidence is largely anecdotal and is not convincing. As noted, age is an important determinant of native immunity to tuberculosis. Although specific data on nutrition and tuberculosis immunity are lacking, the association of tuberculosis with famine is clear.

Acquired immunity follows primary tuberculous infection. Disease due to exogenous reinfection is probably rare in North America and Europe; it may be more frequent in populations of high prevalence where risk of repeated exposure is great. It is useful to recall that *immunity* in the classic use of the word refers to resistance to infection, whereas *hypersensitivity* describes a state of altered host reactivity. In this sense, immunity may also result from infection with other species of mycobacteria, whether through bacillus Calmette-Guérin (BCG) vaccination or by naturally acquired infection with environmental species of mycobacteria. Studies with BCG in mice have provided substantial evidence that nonspecific immunity extends across generic lines. As an example, BCG protects animals against infection with *Listeria* and *Salmonella,* which are nonrelated intracellular murine pathogens. This nonspecific acquired immunity may reflect primarily macrophage activation.

Antigen-specific immunity is T-lymphocyte-dependent and can be transferred adoptively with lymphocytes. It closely parallels delayed hypersensitivity in its development. It may be an independent phenomenon but is most usefully considered as a functional expression of cellular hypersensitivity.

Tuberculin hypersensitivity Tuberculin hypersensitivity is antigen-specific in nature and follows primary infection. It is chiefly or perhaps entirely directed against protein antigens. It is mediated by T lymphocytes through secretion of lymphokines which act upon effector monocytes.

Mycobacterial antigens have been subjected to extensive immunochemical study. It is clear that there is no single dominant antigen, and that infected and artificially sensitized hosts develop hypersensitivity to an array of mycobacterial proteins. Tuberculin purified protein derivative (PPD), the antigen preparation most frequently employed clinically and epidemiologically to demonstrate tuberculin hypersensitivity, is a crude mixture of largely denatured antigens and is a poor representative of native antigens. Nevertheless, its use has yielded much information.

Mycobacteria are rich in adjuvants. Trehalose dimycolate is the principal adjuvant of chloroform-methanol lipid extracts, wax D, and cord factor. Cell wall arabinogalactan complexed to the underlying peptide constitutes a potent water-soluble adjuvant. Muramyl dipeptide, which lies between the structural polysaccharide arabinogalactan and the cytoplasmic membrane in the cell wall, is a small, soluble, and potent adjuvant. In infection the protein antigens of mycobacteria are always presented to the host in the company of this battery of adjuvants. Purified arabinogalactan has been shown in in vitro studies to be a potent immunosuppressive agent.

Antigen recognition by the sensitized host follows processing by macrophages and depends upon expression by the macrophage at its surface of antigen-specific epitopes in association with Ia antigen, a gene product of the major histocompatability locus. This complex is recognized by specific T lymphocytes. Macrophage synthesis and secretion of interleukin 1 is also necessary for T lymphocyte response to the presented antigen.

Following antigen presentation, T-lymphocyte clonal expansion occurs. Specific subsets of T lymphocytes develop which have antigen-specific immunoregulatory functions and which modulate the immune response. These functions are associated with surface expression of lymphocyte antigens recognizable with monoclonal antibody reagents. Reactivity with monoclonal antibody OKT4 is characteristic of T lymphocytes with helper function, and reactivity with monoclonal antibody OKT8 is characteristic of suppressor T lymphocytes.

Immunoreactive lymphocytes secrete mediators, and in response macrophages become activated and serve as the principal effector cells of tuberculin hypersensitivity. Peripheral blood monocytes from tuberculous patients have been shown to have several features characteristic of activated macrophages, including increased hexose monophosphate shunt activity, augmented surface adhesiveness, expression of characteristic membrane structures, and increased bactericidal activity. Animal studies have demonstrated that these features are T-lymphocyte-dependent. Activated monocytes/macrophages are important immunoregulatory cells possessing suppressor functions.

In tuberculosis, aberrations of this carefully modulated state of hypersensitivity occur with some frequency and are recognizable in 15 percent of acutely ill patients. This has given rise to the suggestion that tuberculosis may present with an immunologic spectrum similar to that seen in leprosy but more subtly expressed. At one pole are patients with chronic cavitary disease, relatively chronic courses, and florid expression of tuberculin hypersensitivity. At the other pole are the less frequently seen patients with cutaneous anergy, a few of whom have absence of granuloma formation and all other manifestations of cellular hypersensitivity and have pancytopenia, widely disseminated disease, and a progressive downhill course. Although the delayed tuberculin skin reaction is the best known manifestation of tuberculin hypersensitivity (see below), granuloma formation is probably its central and most important expression. Granuloma formation is important in containing the spread of infection. Studies with tuberculin antigens on the surface of bentonite or agarose particles have shown that granuloma formation in response to antigen presented in particulate fashion has all of the characteristics of an immunologic hypersensitivity response.

B-lymphocyte-mediated production of antibodies to protein and polysaccharide antigens of mycobacteria is readily demonstrated in tuberculosis. There is no evidence that these antibodies play any role in immunity, hypersensitivity, or pathogenesis of tuberculosis.

CLINICAL MANIFESTATIONS **Primary tuberculosis** Primary tuberculous infection is usually asymptomatic. A nonspecific pneumonitis typically occurs in the lower or midlung zones. Hilar lymph node enlargement is usual and in children is sometimes sufficient to produce bronchial obstruction. In low-prevalence areas primary infection now occurs frequently in adults. It may progress directly to clinical disease which has the pathologic features of reactivation disease. In these persons such perplexing presentations as subapical pneumonias are common.

Reactivation tuberculosis Reactivation tuberculosis is a chronic wasting disease, and constitutional manifestations are often more prominent than respiratory symptoms in patients with pulmonary tuberculosis. Weight loss and low-grade fever are common. Many patients present with typical drenching night sweats over the upper half of the body several times a week.

Pulmonary tuberculosis Pulmonary tuberculosis has a predilection for the apical posterior segments of the upper lobes and the superior segments of the lower lobes of the lungs. The location has been attributed both to posture and to higher intraalveolar oxygen concentration in the uppermost portions of the lung. The extent of disease varies from minimal infiltrates that produce no clinical illness and that are barely discernible on chest radiograph to massive involvement with extensive cavitation and debilitating constitutional and respiratory symptoms. In the absence of effective therapy, pulmonary tuberculosis pursues a chronic and progressive course. There are often periods of long stability and relative well-being, but in most patients these give way to episodes of disease progression with involvement of more and more lung parenchyma.

The onset of pulmonary tuberculosis is usually insidious, and illness may not be noted by the patient for some time. However, it is incorrect to view this onset as one of slow progression. In fact, pulmonary tuberculosis usually reaches its full extent within a few weeks. About one-third of patients will live long lives with chronic illness interspersed with periods of relative well-being. However, the overall death rate of untreated pulmonary tuberculosis probably approaches 60 percent, and the median course to death is about $2\frac{1}{2}$ years.

As pulmonary lesions progress, central necrosis occurs with development of caseation, so named because of the cheesy nature of necrotic material which only partly liquifies in the absence of proteolytic enzymes common in other forms of suppuration. Satellite lesions grow concomitantly. They can usually be recognized on chest radiograph and are often helpful in distinguishing tuberculosis from pulmonary neoplasms. Necrotic material may empty into bronchi resulting in cavitation of the nodular disease. Other parts of the lung may be seeded transbronchially with the development of exudative lesions. In some patients tuberculous pneumonia develops in a lobar or segmental pulmonary distribution. Occasionally transbronchial spread following rupture of a tuberculous peribronchial lymph node into a bronchus leads to tuberculous pneumonia in the absence of other obvious disease. With the progression of pulmonary tuberculosis, the normal pulmonary architecture is lost. Fibrosis, volume loss, and upward contraction are typical. However, recently diseased areas may heal with relatively little destruction when effective chemotherapy is administered.

Pulmonary cavities may persist even though effective chemotherapy has resulted in apparent cure. In the absence of therapy, persistence of cavities is to be expected. Cavities may be a source of major hemoptysis, especially in the presence of continued active disease. Rasmussen's aneurysm consists of a persistent terminal pulmonary artery within such a cavity and may be a source of bleeding. An important cause of bleeding is the presence of an aspergilloma in a chronic tuberculous cavity, and bleeding in this instance may occur without persisting tuberculous disease. Rupture of a tuberculous cavity into the pleural space may lead to tuberculous empyema and bronchopleural fistula.

Chronic cough is the principal respiratory symptom. Sputum is usually scant and nonpurulent. Hemoptysis is frequent and is usually limited to blood streaking of the sputum. Massive, life-threatening hemoptysis is rare.

Findings on physical examination of the lung in patients with pulmonary tuberculosis are typically few and generally can be appreciated only in the presence of extensive disease. Rales which are accentuated or heard only posttussively are characteristic of apical disease. With extensive cavitation, amphoric breath sounds may be present. Dullness to percussion may sometimes be recognized in Krönig's isthmus and at the clavicles, reflecting extensive apical disease.

Contemporary classification of tuberculosis in the United States is based primarily on bacteriologic status, reflecting concern with infectivity. Previously, pulmonary tuberculosis was classified by the extent of disease that was apparent on the posteroantero chest radiograph. *Minimal lesions* are those which are noncavitary and do not exceed in total extent the area of one lung above the second chondrosternal junction and the spine of the fourth or body of the fifth vertebra. *Moderately advanced* disease is that which does not exceed the area of one lung and which has total cavitation diameter of less than 4 cm. Greater extensiveness of disease is termed *far advanced.*

Extrapulmonary tuberculosis PLEURISY WITH EFFUSION Pleurisy with effusion results when the pleural space is seeded with *M. tuberculosis.* Following a peripheral primary infection, the pleural space may be contaminated by organisms that are transported lymphogenously to the pleura and hence across the surface of the lung to the hilum. Pleural effusion occurs, sometimes massively, usually with substantial pleuritic pain. The onset of symptoms is often abrupt. The effusion is most frequently, but not invariably, unilateral. Classically, tuberculous pleurisy with effusion occurs in younger individuals in the absence of pulmonary tuberculosis. However, in current North American experience this disease presents in many individuals past the age of 35 and simultaneous pulmonary tuberculosis is present in about one-third of patients with tuberculous pleurisy. The effusion is exudative in nature, and a protein concentration greater than 3.0 g/dL is the most characteristic feature of the pleural fluid. Lymphocytes usually, but not invariably, predominate among the pleural fluid cells. Mesothelial cells are rare. Needle biopsy of the parietal pleura may reveal granulomas, and such a finding confirms the diagnosis of tuberculous pleurisy. The tuberculin skin test is negative in one-third of patients, sometimes because the disease presents early before tuberculin reactivity develops, and sometimes because this form of tuberculosis is particularly prone to aberrations of immunoregulation. Untreated, tuberculous pleurisy usually remits, but active pulmonary tuberculosis develops within 5 years in two-thirds of cases. Response to chemotherapy is good. Complete removal of pleural fluid is not necessary. There is rarely a need for surgical decortication.

Bronchopleural fistula and tuberculous empyema are catastrophic complications of untreated tuberculosis resulting from rupture of a pulmonary lesion into the pleural space. The diagnosis is usually not difficult, and acid-fast bacilli are usually readily demonstrated in the pleural exudate. Treatment consists of adequate surgical drainage and chemotherapy.

TUBERCULOUS PERICARDITIS AND PERITONITIS The pericardium and peritoneum are serosal surfaces which are not infrequently the sites of tuberculosis. Pericarditis sometimes occurs in association with pleurisy and may represent an extension of that process. More commonly the pericardium is seeded by drainage from an infected lymph node. Exudative effusion occurs and patients present with fever and pericardial pain. A friction rub may be present. Cardiac tamponade occasionally occurs. Chronic constrictive pericarditis is a late sequel. The diagnosis of tuberculous pericarditis is often difficult and sometimes requires thoracotomy for pericardial biopsy.

Tuberculous peritonitis results from hematogenous seeding of the peritoneum or entry of bacilli from an abdominal lymphatic or genitourinary organ source. As with other serositis, an exudative effusion occurs. The onset is usually insidious, and the disease is often mistaken for hepatic cirrhosis in alcoholic patients. As with tuberculous pericarditis, the diagnosis is often difficult, and recovery of the organism from paracentesis fluid is possible only in a minority of cases. Surgical biopsy may be necessary for diagnosis.

LARYNGEAL AND ENDOBRONCHIAL TUBERCULOSIS Tuberculosis of the larynx is usually seen in association with far-advanced pulmonary disease. Occasionally it occurs with only minimal pulmonary involvement. It results from seeding of the mucosal surface during expectoration. The disease progresses from a superficial laryngitis to ulceration and granuloma formation. The epiglottis and hypopharynx are occasionally involved. Hoarseness is the principal symptom of tuberculous laryngitis. In a similar fashion the bronchial mucosa may be seeded, causing tuberculous bronchitis. Indeed, localized bronchitis in segmental bronchi leading to diseased portions of lung is common. Cough and minor hemoptysis are the chief clinical manifestations. Patients with tuberculous laryngitis and extensive bronchitis are usually highly infectious. These forms of disease respond rapidly to chemotherapy and have a favorable prognosis with treatment.

TUBERCULOUS ADENITIS Scrofula is chronic tuberculous lymphadenitis of the cervical lymph nodes. Any of the cervical nodes may be involved, but those high in the neck just below the mandible are the most frequent site of disease. Tuberculous nodes are usually rubbery to palpation and not tender. With progression, they become harder and matted. Chronic draining fistulas may develop, but these are rare, and the course of this form of tuberculosis is usually indolent. The diagnosis is commonly established by surgical biopsy. Lymph node biopsy specimens obtained for this purpose should always be submitted for culture as well as histologic examination, and chemotherapy should be instituted at or before the time of surgery to avoid postoperative fistulas in the surgical wound site. Lymph nodes other than those in the cervical regions are less commonly involved in tuberculosis and account for about 35 percent of tuberculous adenitis. When it was an important cause of disease, *M. bovis* had a predilection for causing scrofula.

In children, *M. scrofulaceum* and *M. intracellulare* are frequently the cause of scrofula. The onset of this disease is usually before 5 years of age. As with tuberculosis, lymph nodes high in the neck are most frequently involved. A single enlarged node is commonly the presenting manifestation. Constitutional symptoms are absent, and the adenitis is usually not tender. Progression is common, with necrosis of the node and the development of fistulous sinus tracts. The organisms involved are usually not susceptible to drugs, and treatment, if necessary, is surgical excision. Spontaneous resolution is usual after puberty.

SKELETAL TUBERCULOSIS Bone and joint disease is a not infrequent manifestation of tuberculosis. Pott's disease, tuberculosis of the spine, usually involves the midthoracic spine. Tubercle bacilli reach the spine hematogenously or through lymphatic channels from the pleural space to paravertebral lymph nodes. Anterior erosion of vertebral bodies leads to collapse. The result is a sharply angulated kyphosis without scoliosis (gibbus deformity). Paraplegia may result. If there is no neurologic compromise, Pott's disease can be treated with chemotherapy. If the spine is unstable, surgical stabilization may be necessary. In the face of new paraparesis, immediate orthopedic consultation should be obtained. Paravertebral "cold abcesses" are a frequent concomitant of tuberculous spondylitis. They usually do not need to be drained, if adequate chemotherapy is given, unless they are very large. They may extend along fascial planes and point in the inguinal region or in other remote sites.

Tuberculosis of joints most frequently affects large weight-bearing joints such as the hips and knees. It responds well to immobilization and chemotherapy. Tuberculous synovitis may occur alone or in association with tuberculous arthritis. In prior years bone and joint tuberculosis was frequently caused by *M. bovis,* an organism that is now rare.

GENITOURINARY TUBERCULOSIS Genitourinary tuberculosis may involve any part of either the male or female genitourinary system. Renal tuberculosis usually presents initially as microscopic pyuria and hematuria with a sterile urine culture. The diagnosis may be established by finding tubercle bacilli on culture of the urine. As the disease progresses, cavitation of the renal parenchyma occurs. In the past, nephrectomy was often performed for renal tuberculosis. However, with adequate chemotherapy surgical removal of a kidney is almost never necessary. The ureters and bladder may be infected by tubular spread of the organism, and ureteral stricture may result.

Tuberculous salpingitis often results in female sterility. Genital tuberculosis in the male most commonly involves the prostate, seminal vesicles, and epididymis. Prostatic and epididymal tuberculosis are characterized by nontender nodular induration detectable by physical examination. The presentation of genital tuberculosis in both males and females is insidious, with chronic or subacute symptoms. The diagnosis is usually made by culture of acid-fast bacilli.

MENINGEAL TUBERCULOSIS The leptomeninges are relatively frequently seeded by organisms which disseminate during primary infection. In young children, tuberculous meningitis may develop at this time. This chronic infection is manifested not only by meningeal signs but also by frequent cranial nerve signs, reflecting a tendency for basilar distribution of the infection. High protein content, low glucose, and lymphocytosis are characteristic of the cerebrospinal fluid. Prior to the advent of effective chemotherapy, this disease was almost always fatal. Chemotherapy with isoniazid, rifampin, and ethambutol is effective. Intrathecal drug administration is not necessary. Late reactivation of meningeal tuberculous foci may produce disease in adults who have no evidence of pulmonary tuberculosis. Tuberculomas of the meninges or brain may become evident in adult life many years after primary infection, and seizures are often their major clinical manifestation.

OCULAR TUBERCULOSIS Tuberculosis may involve almost any part of the eye. Chorioretinitis and uveitis are the most common manifestations. The diagnosis of tuberculosis of the eye is extremely difficult to establish, and most diagnoses are presumptive. The manifestations cannot be distinguished clinically from sarcoidosis or systemic mycoses, but phlyctenular keratitis strongly suggest tuberculosis. Phlyctenular lesions are thought to represent manifestations of tuberculin hypersensitivity rather than bacterial infection. Choroid tubercles are often present in patients with miliary tuberculosis, and their recognition may be helpful in the diagnosis of miliary tuberculosis. Ocular tuberculosis responds well to standard chemotherapeutic agents.

GASTROINTESTINAL TUBERCULOSIS The stomach is extremely resistant to tuberculous infection, and a large number of virulent tubercle bacilli can be swallowed without establishing an infection. Rarely, usually concomitantly with extensive cavitary pulmonary disease and severe debility, swallowed organisms reach the terminal ileum and cecum and tuberculous ileitis develops. Chronic diarrhea and fistula development are the principal manifestations, and the disease is difficult to distinguish from Crohn's disease. Tuberculosis of the liver can occur as an isolated event, but it is usually a manifestation of miliary tuberculosis.

ADRENAL TUBERCULOSIS Hematogenous seeding of the adrenal gland is probably fairly common, but disease due to this infection is rare and usually seen only in association with long-standing and extensive pulmonary tuberculosis. The cortex is most frequently involved. It may lead to adrenal insufficiency. In contrast, carcinomatous involvement of the adrenal cortex, even though very extensive, rarely produces clinical adrenal insufficiency.

CUTANEOUS TUBERCULOSIS Tuberculous infection of the skin is rare in the absence of long-standing, untreated disease elsewhere. Lupus vulgaris is a granulomatous disease of the skin, and it responds well to treatment. Diagnosis is made by skin biopsy. Tuberculin hypersensitivity manifestations are common. Erythema nodosum may be present, although it much more commonly results from other granulomatous diseases including sarcoidosis and systemic mycoses. Tuberculids are poorly understood papular lesions of tuberculin hypersensitivity.

MILIARY TUBERCULOSIS Miliary tuberculosis results from widespread hematogenous dissemination. It often presents as a perplexing fever, sometimes with a double quotidian curve, often accompanied by anemia and splenomegaly, in a patient with a relatively preserved sense of well-being. Miliary tuberculosis is apt to be more fulminating in children than in adults.

Classically, miliary tuberculosis develops following hematogenous dissemination at the time of primary infection, and patients present no antecedent history of tuberculosis. Lesions develop synchronously throughout the body. The appearance of these lesions suggested millet seeds; hence the name miliary tuberculosis. Patients become ill before radiographic changes appear on the chest radiograph; these take 4 to 6 weeks to become recognizable. The typical radiologic findings are soft, uniformly distributed, fine nodules throughout both lung fields. They often can be recognized first on a lateral chest film or an underpenetrated posteroantero radiograph. The diagnosis is difficult, and expectorated sputum rarely contains organisms. Transbronchial biopsy and liver biopsy are usually but not invariably positive. Bone marrow biopsy is positive in approximately two-thirds of patients.

When hematogenous dissemination occurs in a previously diseased individual, a much more fulminant course results. Prostration is common. Diffuse but ragged nodular infiltrates develop within a few weeks, and the sputum is often positive. The diagnosis is rarely difficult.

The subacute form and the rare chronic form of miliary tuberculosis often present major problems in diagnosis. This type of disease is usually attributed to repeated seeding of the blood stream from a tuberculous focus. A very rare form of disseminated tuberculosis occurs with widespread dissemination of disease, a massive number of bacteria in tissues, complete absence of granuloma formation, and pancytopenia. It is termed disseminated nonreactive tuberculosis. It has a poor prognosis, even with chemotherapy.

Tuberculin anergy is common in miliary tuberculosis, and a negative skin test should not be a deterrent to the consideration of this diagnosis. Anergy may extend to other delayed hypersensitivity antigens as well, but it does not always do so. In vitro cultured leukocyte studies also demonstrate hyporesponsiveness, and they suggest that this anergy is mediated by monocytes with suppressor function. With treatment and stabilization of patients with miliary tuberculosis, tuberculin hypersensitivity is restored.

Without treatment, the prognosis for miliary tuberculosis is grave. This disease responds well to chemotherapy, however, and can be treated with the same drug regimens employed for other forms of tuberculosis.

SILICOTUBERCULOSIS Tuberculosis occurs with increased frequency in patients with silicosis and possibly in patients with some other pneumoconioses. The diagnosis is often difficult because of confounding radiographic changes due to the underlying pneumoconiosis. Even with therapy, the prognosis is less favorable than in other patients. Experimental animal work has shown that silica exposure increases susceptibility to infection, and work in both animals and humans has demonstrated that silica impairs macrophage function. Patients with silicotuberculosis should be treated for longer than customary periods. Patients with silicosis who are tuberculin-positive should be considered for isoniazid prophylaxis even when they do not meet other criteria for this form of therapy. It is likely that isoniazid prophylaxis is somewhat less effective in persons with silicosis.

DIAGNOSIS Bacteriology The diagnosis of tuberculosis is established when tubercle bacilli are identified in the sputum, urine, body fluids, or tissues of the patient. For the majority of patients who have pulmonary tuberculosis, the diagnosis can be most readily established by sputum examination. The staining characteristics of *M. tuberculosis* allow its ready identification in clinical specimens, although it is usually present in small numbers so that prolonged study of stained slides is necessary. A slender (less than 0.5 μm diameter), curved, often polychromatically beaded rod, it frequently presents in clinical specimens as pairs or clumps of a few organisms lying side by side. When stained with fluorescent auramine-rhodamine, tubercle bacilli can be seen under usual high-dry (100×) microscope magnification, but the morphology of organisms is often indistinct with this stain and at this magnification. A more definitive stain is accomplished using carbol fuchsin, and this stain requires meticulous scanning with oil immersion (1000×) microscopy. Sputum culture adds to the diagnostic yield and also permits the specific identification of acid-fast bacilli and the study of drug susceptibility of the organisms. However, the generation time of mycobacteria is 20 to 24 h. Primary isolation from clinical specimens usually requires 4 to 8 weeks on classical media. Radiometric techniques using highly selective media allow cultivation in 1 or 2 weeks, but confirmation of the identity of an isolated organism may require additional time. Mycobacteria are aerobes. Modern culture techniques are excellent, and there is no longer reason to inoculate guinea pigs for primary isolation. Niacin production characterizes *M. tuberculosis* and helps to distinguish it from other species.

If expectorated sputum is not readily available for examination, expectoration may be induced or samples obtained by nasotracheal aspiration. Early morning gastric aspiration provides excellent material for culture and for smear examination. Although nonpathogenic mycobacteria are occasionally found in gastric aspirates, their number is so small as to preclude their appearance in smears of gastric aspirates. Bronchoscopy has a high yield in the diagnosis of tuberculosis, but in the absence of other considerations it should not be undertaken unless multiple attempts by simpler means have failed and the diagnosis remains obscure.

The diagnostic yield of sputum smear and culture is directly related to the extent of pulmonary disease. Overall, about two-thirds of patients in whom a positive culture can be obtained will have a positive direct sputum smear. However, only about one-third of patients with minimal pulmonary tuberculosis will have a positive sputum smear, even after multiple examinations. If there is no lesion visible on the chest radiograph, then there is usually little reason to obtain sputum examinations for tubercle bacilli. Conversely, if a patient with extensive cavitary disease or an exudative pneumonic process has a negative sputum smear, diagnoses other than tuberculosis should be sought. If an initial sputum smear is negative, repeated smears should be obtained on separate days. There is rarely indication for obtaining more than five sputum examinations.

It is clear that both the sensitivity and specificity of sputum examinations for tubercle bacilli depend on the experience of those performing the examination. False-positive and false-negative sputum smears occur with distressing frequency in laboratories in which cases of tuberculosis are rarely encountered, and sputum smears performed by medical students and house officers in teaching hospitals are often unreliable. False-positive sputum cultures also have been well documented. Laboratory identification of mycobacteria poses difficult problems for many clinical laboratories, and use of reference laboratories is desirable to confirm speciation.

Serology Serologic tests for the diagnosis of tuberculosis remain experimental and are not routinely available. The most specific serologic tests have used highly purified antigens. Enzyme-linked immunosorbent assay (ELISA) techniques offer the potential for readily applied serologic tests for tuberculosis, and should have great value in the diagnosis of tuberculosis in children and in extrapulmonary disease where sputum examination is not available.

Radiology The chest radiograph is an important tool for both the diagnosis and evaluation of tuberculosis. Healed primary lesions may leave a small peripheral nodule which may calcify with the passing of years. When calcified and present together with a calcified hilar lymph node, this is known as a Ghon complex. Similar lesions result from histoplasmosis, and it is not possible to distinguish between healed primary lesions of these two diseases radiologically. Calcification of right paratracheal lymph nodes is more commonly seen in histoplasmosis.

Multinodular infiltration in the apical posterior segments of the upper lobes and superior segments of the lower lobes is the most typical lesion of pulmonary tuberculosis. Cavitation is frequently present and is usually accompanied by substantial amounts of infiltration in the same pulmonary segments. Laminagrams are often helpful in recognizing satellite nodular lesions, which are characteristic of tuberculosis and not usually seen in carcinoma. Lordotic views may be of help in evaluating disease obscured by the intersection of the third or fourth posterior rib, second anterior rib, and clavicle. They are of little use in evaluating disease located elsewhere. As tuberculosis becomes inactive or heals, fibrotic scarring becomes apparent on the chest radiograph. There is frequently volume loss in the involved upper lobes, and upward and medial retraction of hilar markings is common. Fibrotic lesions may develop calcifications. The activity of tuberculosis may be judged from serial films. It is never wise to judge tuberculosis to be inactive on the basis of a single radiographic examination.

Clinical pathology Other than bacteriologic examinations, clinical laboratory tests contribute relatively little to the diagnosis of tuberculosis. Peripheral blood monocytosis in the range of 8 to 12 percent is common. The erythrocyte sedimentation rate is usually elevated.

Tuberculin test The intracutaneous tuberculin skin test is a reliable means of recognizing prior mycobacterial infection. Its correct interpretation requires some thought and knowledge. The preferred antigen is tuberculin purified protein derivative (PPD). For all routine use the intermediate-strength dose should be used. In North America this is 5 tuberculin units of material which is standardized by bioassay (bioequivalent) against reference antigen designated PPD-S. In other parts of the world, PPD lot RT-23, prepared in Denmark and widely distributed by the World Health Organization, is available. A gravimetric unit has been assigned to this material, and 2 units of this PPD are equivalent to 5 units of PPD-S. Diluents for PPD should contain polysorbate 80, which decreases loss of potency due to adsorption onto glass and plastic surfaces. Multiple puncture devices offer much convenience, but do so at the cost of decreased specificity. They can be recommended only as screening tests, and positive tests should be repeated using intracutaneous PPD.

The tuberculin test is usually applied on the forearm. Reactions should be read by measuring the transverse diameter of induration as detected by gentle palpation at 48 to 72 h. Patients with tuberculosis have normally distributed reaction sizes with the mean and mode at 17 mm. Infected but healthy, nondiseased individuals have similarly distributed reactions. Hence, a reaction to PPD is presumptive evidence of prior mycobacterial infection.

Tuberculin hypersensitivity may result from contact with nonpathogenic, environmental mycobacteria, and this nonspecific reactivity may seriously confound the interpretation of tuberculin tests. The magnitude of this problem varies substantially geographically. Nonspecific tuberculin reactivity is rarely found in northern climates, and in such areas all reactivity to PPD can be considered to reflect infection with *M. tuberculosis*. In many warm and humid climatic zones, including all of the coastal areas of the southeastern United States, nonspecific tuberculin reactivity is common. In such regions it is customary to consider reactions smaller than 10 mm as not significant and attribute them to cross reactivity with environmental mycobacterial antigens. However, considering smaller reactions as not significant always incurs the cost of missing some reactions which bespeak infection with *M. tuberculosis*.

Repeated skin testing may boost reaction size, whether the primary reactivity was directed to *M. tuberculosis* or was nonspecific. Caution must be used in attributing a small increase in reactivity to new infection. It is well-established, however, that repeated skin testing with PPD does not lead to positive reactions in uninfected persons. Positive reactions do not occur as a result of allergy to components of the diluent. Tuberculin reactivity wanes with advancing age, and the booster phenomenon may be useful in this situation. For example, if an older person fails to react to initial testing, repeat testing with intermediate strength PPD may be done after 7 to 10 days. A reaction at this time should be accepted as significant.

PPD is also available in a second strength which contains 50 times the amount of PPD in intermediate-strength material. Except as a test for anergy, this product has little use. Because PPD at this strength so readily elicits nonspecific reactivity, a positive reaction to second-strength PPD is much more apt to give misinformation than to contribute to the correct diagnosis. A first-strength PPD is also available. It contains one-fifth the amount of PPD of intermediate PPD. It has not been adequately standardized for clinical use.

Anergy is the paradoxical absence of dermal tuberculin reactivity in infected persons. It occurs in association with a number of disease states and in immuosuppressed individuals. It also occurs in as many as 15 percent of tuberculous patients with newly active pulmonary disease. In these persons tuberculin reactivity reappears with stabilization of the disease process. One-half of patients with miliary tuberculosis and one-third of patients with newly diagnosed tuberculous pleurisy have negative tuberculin tests. It has become common practice in many medical centers to use a battery of delayed hypersensitivity antigens to serve as controls for tuberculin tests in demonstrating anergy. However, antigens standardized for this purpose are not available, and tuberculin anergy may be antigen-specific. False-negative tuberculin tests may result from technical errors including subcutaneous injection, use of outdated PPD, and permitting PPD to stand in syringes before use. Such errors should not be mistaken for anergy.

TREATMENT The modern treatment of tuberculosis is based on the administration of effective drugs. In the presence of adequate chemotherapy, hospitalization, rest, and improved diet do not contribute to achieving cures. In order to prevent the emergence of drug-resistant mutants which are present initially in very small numbers, two effective drugs are always required. Because of the slow generation time of mycobacteria and because these organisms can be metabolically inactive for long periods of time, prolonged courses of drug therapy are always necessary. Treatment regimens do not differ for pulmonary and extrapulmonary tuberculosis.

Table 119-1 presents dosage and toxicity information on drugs currently in use for the treatment of tuberculosis. Table 119-2 describes several effective treatment regimens. Daily therapy with isoniazid and rifampin for 9 to 12 months represents the most effective regimen available and is capable of achieving a favorable outcome in 99 percent of patients. At this level of success, it probably will be impossible ever to mount a controlled clinical trial sufficiently large to demonstrate that any other regimen is significantly better. Certainly, the addition of a third drug does not offer anything to a patient with drug-sensitive organisms. However, many experts add ethambutol initially until the results of sensitivity tests become available. Daily therapy with isoniazid and ethambutol for 18 months is 90 to 95 percent effective, and it is probably the equal of isoniazid and rifampin in patients with minimal disease. In developing countries where drug costs are a limiting factor, the extremely low cost combination of isoniazid and thioacetazone for 12 to 18 months provides a regimen which can achieve 80 to 90 percent cure rates.

General acceptance has been given to a hypothesis which states that tubercle bacilli exist in tuberculous patients in three pools—a metabolically active extracellular pool and relatively metabolically inactive intracellular and necrotic caseum pools. Only rifampin is thought to be bactericidal for all of these pools, and hence it may not be necessary to continue rifampin-containing regimens for as long as other regimens which rely upon organisms entering the metabolically active pool to achieve sterilization. Isoniazid and streptomycin are both bactericidal against extracellular, metabolically active organisms. Against intracellular organisms, isoniazid and pyrazinamide are bactericidal and streptomycin is inactive. In clinical trials, pyrazinamide has been found to be particularly useful during the first 2 months of treatment. Ethambutol is only bacteriostatic.

The major problem in tuberculosis treatment programs today is patient default. It is unusual for any tuberculosis clinic to achieve a default rate of less than 15 percent, and default rates of 40 to 60 percent are common. Unfortunately, these rates tend to be highest in those parts of the world where high tuberculosis prevalence is coupled with limited resources. Default not only leads to treatment failure but also leads to the emergence and transmission of drug-resistant organisms. This situation has led to an emphasis on short-course therapeutic regimens. However, since most patient defaults occur within the first 6 months of the treatment program, short-course therapy is likely to have a meaningful impact only if the resources conserved by shortening treatment are used to strengthen those components of the program responsible for maintaining patient compliance. Completely supervised regimens are successful for noncompliant patients, but their widespread use is costly. Twice weekly drug administration is effective and facilitates patient supervision.

Short-course treatment programs are best considered as consisting of two phases. An initial 2-month intensive phase of daily therapy should include isoniazid, rifampin, pyrazinamide, and either streptomycin or ethambutol. A consolidation phase of daily therapy with isoniazid and one other drug should be given for at least 4 months, with a 6-month course duration perhaps being superior. In the United States, success has been achieved with a regimen of isoniazid 300 mg and rifampin 600 mg daily for 1 month, followed by isoniazid 900 mg and rifampin 600 mg twice weekly for 8 months.

Relapses after successful therapy should be fewer than 1 percent. Since these few relapses usually present with symptoms and are almost never found by routine x-rays, patients may be discharged from follow-up at the completion of therapy. Relapses are more frequent after short-course therapy, usually occurring within the first year, and follow-up for such patients for 1 or 2 years is justified.

The physician following a patient being treated for tuberculosis should expect symptomatic improvement within the first 2 to 3 weeks in most patients. Clearing of infiltrates on the chest radiograph may not occur within the first month but usually is readily recognized between the second and fourth months. Most patients reach a point of radiologic stability between 4 and 6 months. Although it has become customary to continue drug therapy for arbitrary periods, there is logic in continuing therapy for 6 months after this point of stability is reached, even if this means prolonging the planned period of treatment. Sputum conversion occurs in most patients within the first 2 months. The fact that an individual patient responds more slowly than the norm should not necessarily be a cause for concern, provided the patient is taking effective drugs.

Since there are alternative effective drug regimens, toxicity becomes a factor in choice of therapy. Major individual drug toxicities are listed in Table 119-1; the toxicity of greatest concern is hepatitis. Toxicity sufficient to require change in regimen occurs in 3 to 5 percent of patients taking isoniazid and rifampin and in about 1.5 percent of patients taking isoniazid and ethambutol. The toxicity of isoniazid and thioacetazone appears to vary with racial characteristics of the patient population. It reaches about 30 percent in oriental groups but is only 2 to 5 percent in other populations. Routine monitoring of serum enzymes or other blood test values reflecting liver disease is of little use and is not recommended. Normal values

TABLE 119-1 Drugs used in the treatment of tuberculosis

Drug	Usual daily adult dose	Major toxicity
Isoniazid	300 mg	Hepatitis, peripheral neuropathy, drug fever
Rifampin	600 mg	Hepatitis, influenza-like syndrome, thrombocytopenia (rare)
Streptomycin	0.75–1 g	Deafness, loss of vestibular function, loss of renal function
Pyrazinamide	1.5–2 g	Hepatitis, hyperuricemia
Ethambutol	15 mg/kg	Optic neuritis (extremely rare at this dose)
p-Aminosalicylic acid	12 g	Diarrhea, hepatitis, hypersensitivity reactions
Ethionamide	1 g	Hepatitis
Cycloserine	1 g	Depression, personality changes, psychosis, convulsions
Thioacetazone	150 mg	Exfoliative dermatitis, hepatitis
Kanamycin	1 g	Deafness, loss of renal function, loss of vestibular function (rare)
Capreomycin	1 g	Deafness, loss of vestibular function, loss of renal function
Viomycin	1 g	Deafness, loss of vestibular function, loss of renal function

TABLE 119-2 Effective drug regimens for the treatment of tuberculosis

Regimen (adult drug dose)	Comment
Isoniazid (300 mg) and rifampin (600 mg) daily for 9–12 months	The usual regimen for initial treatment of all patients unless drug resistance is suspected, in which case ethambutol 15 mg/kg should be added.
Isoniazid (300 mg) and ethambutol (15 mg/kg) daily for 12–18 months	The least toxic effective regimen. Suitable for patients with minimal disease. The regimen of choice in pregnant women.
Isoniazid (300 mg) and thioacetazone (150 mg) daily for 12–18 months	The least expensive effective regimen. Streptomycin (0.75–1 g) may be added daily for the first 8 weeks to increase effectiveness, but this doubles both cost and toxicity.
Isoniazid (300 mg), rifampin (600 mg), pyrazinamide (2 g), and streptomycin (1 g) or ethambutol (15 mg/kg) daily for 2 months followed by one of the following:	Initial intensive phase for short course regimens. Short course regimens have only been demonstrated to be effective under conditions of close patient supervision.
a Isoniazid (300 mg) and rifampin (600 gm) daily for 4 months	
b Isoniazid (300 mg) and thioacetazone (150 mg) daily for 6 months	Inexpensive.
c Isoniazid (300 mg), rifampin (600 mg), and streptomycin (1 g) twice weekly for 6 months	Suitable for fully supervised therapy.
Isoniazid (300 mg) and rifampin (600 mg) daily for 1 month followed by isoniazid (900 mg) and rifampin (600 mg) twice weekly for 8 months	Effectiveness demonstrated in ambulatory treatment programs in Arkansas. Has not been compared with other regimens in clinical trials.

do not predict absence of toxicity, and serum enzymes in patients taking isoniazid may rise transiently to three times normal values without the subsequent development of hepatitis. A well-educated patient and an alert treatment supervisor are the principal available safeguards against drug hepatitis. If medication is discontinued during the prodromal phase or promptly with the onset of jaundice, drug hepatitis can be expected to resolve without untoward incident. Isoniazid toxicity is probably due to toxic metabolites of acetyl isoniazid. Induction of cytochrome P-450 enzymes by alcohol or long-acting barbiturates predisposes to isoniazid hepatitis. Isoniazid also causes a peripheral neuropathy which is preventable and reversible by the administration of pyridoxine. Patients with such predisposing factors as old age, diabetes, alcoholism, and malnutrition should be given pyridoxine concomitantly with isoniazid; the usual dose is 50 mg/day.

Isoniazid is known to be safe in pregnant patients. Data are less complete for other drugs but suggest that ethambutol is the companion drug of choice. Rifampin should be used if the tuberculosis is disseminated or very extensive. Streptomycin should not be used in pregnancy because of the risk of fetal ototoxicity. Tuberculosis often pursues an unfavorable course during and just after pregnancy, and treatment of a pregnant woman should never be deferred. It is reasonable to postpone isoniazid prophylaxis until just after delivery.

Patients with chronic renal failure also present special treatment problems, and these patients have tuberculosis case rates approximately 10 times those of the general population. Isoniazid is acetylated to an inactive form by the liver and then excreted by the kidney. Acetyl isoniazid is the precursor of hydrazines which are probably hepatotoxic. Both isoniazid and acetyl isoniazid are not bound by plasma proteins and are dialyzable. The usual daily dose of isoniazid should be given to patients with renal failure at intervals of two or three times weekly. Patients on dialysis should receive the drug following each dialysis. Ethambutol behaves like isoniazid, except that it is excreted by the kidney as the active drug. As with isoniazid, the usual daily dose should be given at longer intervals, and administration should follow dialysis. Optic nerve toxicity of ethambutol appears to be related not to intermittent high drug levels but to sustained high drug levels. Patients with renal failure who are receiving ethambutol should have their color vision and visual acuity monitored regularly. Rifampin is protein-bound, nondialyzable, and excreted in the bile by the liver. No change in dose or interval is necessary in the presence of renal failure. Caution should be exercised in using rifampin in patients with hepatic failure.

Faced with relapse in a previously treated patient, a major concern should be the possibility of drug resistance, and resistance studies of the organism should be obtained in a competent reference laboratory. In fact, in one-third of patients who relapse after adequate drug therapy taken regularly, the relapse is caused by drug-resistant organisms. If, however, the patient took the drug sporadically or the previous regimen was inadequate, then the likelihood of drug resistance having developed is about two chances in three. Therapy for presumed drug-resistant tuberculosis should be instituted with two drugs which the patient has not taken previously, provided that one of these two new drugs is isoniazid or rifampin. Otherwise, four drugs should be used, including as many new drugs as possible. When resistance studies become available, the regimen should be modified appropriately. Data from studies conducted before rifampin became available suggest that it is beneficial to continue isoniazid even when laboratory studies indicate drug resistance. In general, all re-treatment regimens should be closely supervised and directed by physicians with special experience with this problem.

Primary drug resistance should be suspected in patients who appear to have contracted their infection from patients with known drug resistance or with known noncompliance and in patients who come from areas where drug resistance is common. This group includes immigrants from Haiti, southeast Asia, and many areas of Latin America. While laboratory resistance studies are pending, drug therapy should be dictated by the prior treatment of the suspected index case. In immigrant populations, most of the drug resistance of concern is to isoniazid. In this circumstance, therapy should be initiated with isoniazid, rifampin, and ethambutol. One of these drugs may be discontinued when resistance studies become available.

PREVENTION Chemoprophylaxis In one of the largest controlled clinical trials ever conducted, 1 year of isoniazid has been shown to be effective in reducing the incidence of tuberculosis in tuberculin-positive individuals presumed to have been infected with *M. tuberculosis*. The benefit of isoniazid prophylaxis has been demonstrated so clearly that the question of its use now hinges primarily on the risk of drug toxicity, chiefly hepatitis.

In administering isoniazid prophylaxis, highest priority should be assigned to treating household contacts of persons with active tuberculosis and to persons known to have become infected within the preceding year. The risks of developing tuberculosis in these two groups are, respectively, 0.5 percent per year and 3 percent during the first year. Particular attention should be given to treating children in these categories. Prophylaxis of childhood household contacts with isoniazid should be started immediately. After 3 months of therapy, the child should be skin-tested with intermediate-strength PPD. If the skin test is negative at that time, isoniazid may be discontinued. If it is positive, 12 months of prophylaxis should be completed.

In general, younger individuals benefit most from isoniazid prophylaxis because the drug is most effective when the infection is recent and because older individuals have often already outlived a substantial part of their risk. The risk of hepatitis rises with age, reaching approximately 2 percent by the seventh decade. Cost-benefit analyses with large data bases have shown that there is a 1:1 ratio of cases of tuberculosis prevented and hepatitis caused at age 45 when individuals without added risks are considered. Based on this calculation, there is a general consensus that all persons younger than age 35 with a positive tuberculin reaction should receive isoniazid 300 mg per day for 1 year.

It is also possible to develop criteria for the prophylactic use of isoniazid in older persons with remote tuberculosis, either known historically or evident radiographically, who have never received adequate chemotherapy. The annual risk of tuberculosis in such persons is at least 0.5 percent, and isoniazid prophylaxis will prevent 70 percent of the cases. Assuming an isoniazid hepatitis risk of 2 percent, a 1:1 ratio of tuberculosis prevented and hepatitis caused is reached in 5.7 years. Isoniazid 300 mg per day should be given for 1 year to all persons in this category who have a life expectancy greater than 10 years. Other individuals at high risk for the development of tuberculosis include tuberculin-positive persons who have such diseases as the acquired immunodeficiency syndrome (AIDS) and Hodgkin's disease, which alter T-lymphocyte-mediated immunity; patients with silicosis, which alters macrophage function; patients who are receiving adrenocortical steroids chronically; patients with renal failure; and patients receiving immunosuppressive agents. One year of isoniazid prophylaxis should be given to tuberculin-positive persons in these categories regardless of age. As with therapy for active tuberculosis, monitoring serum enzymes is not useful in patients receiving isoniazid prophylaxis.

BCG vaccination Baccillus Calmette-Guérin (BCG) is an attenuated strain of *M. bovis* which has been given to hundreds of millions of persons as a vaccine against tuberculosis. It is clearly safe, but its efficacy is in some dispute. In controlled studies in North America and Britain, it was found to offer greater than 80 percent protection. In well-designed studies in Georgia and Puerto Rico, it offered little or no protection. In a large study carried out in south India, no protection was observed. There may be unusual aspects to the host-parasite relationship in that population that make it hazardous to extrapolate the results from south India to other populations. Even in those studies where no protection was observed, the disseminated forms of tuberculosis which have such high mortalities among children were virtually eliminated. While final judgment on the efficacy of

BCG is reserved, its continued use in high-prevalence areas appears justified.

BCG vaccination induces tuberculin hypersensitivity. However, the dermal reaction to PPD is usually not as large as that which follows natural infection, usually does not persist as long, and varies from strain to strain of vaccine. Individuals with large PPD reactions persisting for many years after vaccination should be viewed as infected and considered for isoniazid prophylaxis.

CONTROL PROGRAMS Tuberculosis control programs must be mounted in varying situations. In most low-prevalence areas, such as those which exist in North America, resources are relatively abundant and disease occurrence is mostly sporadic. Increasingly, tuberculosis is being seen in microepidemics, often centered in family groups. High-risk groups can be identified, immigrant groups and residents and employees of nursing homes being among the most important. Central to any program is an efficient case-reporting and registry system. Contact investigation must be carried out effectively and is especially important when index cases occur in children. The major effective tool for decreasing the spread of infection is chemotherapy for all infectious patients. Chemoprophylaxis also has an important role.

At the other end of the spectrum are high-prevalence areas with few or no resources for tuberculosis control. The single, most effective measure in this situation is the establishment of a network of ambulatory tuberculosis treatment centers providing diagnosis by direct sputum smear and standardized drug therapy. Hospital beds, chest radiographs, sputum cultures, and individualized treatment regimens are all luxuries until basic treatment is available to all. Success has only followed the assumption of responsibility for providing treatment, and this usually means treatment at no cost to the patient. Tuberculosis diagnostic and treatment programs should be integrated into national health programs, but categoric and expert supervision is always necessary. Treatment records should be maintained, but complex registries are of little value.

In high-prevalence areas, BCG vaccine should be offered to every individual under 15 or 20 without prior tuberculin testing. Older individuals can be assumed to have been infected already. Before a mass BCG campaign is initiated, planning should begin for continuing vaccination of newborns or young school children. Community-wide isoniazid prophylaxis programs have not proved to be successful.

REFERENCES

AMERICAN THORACIC SOCIETY: Diagnostic standards and classification of tuberculosis and other mycobacterial diseases (14th ed). Am Rev Respir Dis 123:343, 1981

———: Treatment of tuberculosis and other mycobacterial diseases. Am Rev Respir Dis 128:336, 1983

COMSTOCK GW, EDWARDS PQ: The competing risks of tuberculosis and hepatitis for adult tuberculin reactors. Am Rev Respir Dis 111:573, 1975

——— et al: The tuberculin skin test. Am Rev Respir Dis 124:356, 1981

———: Epidemiology of tuberculosis. Am Rev Respir Dis 125(suppl):8, 1982

DUTT AK et al: Short-course chemotherapy for extrapulmonary tuberculosis. Ann Intern Med 104:7, 1986

EDWARDS LB et al: An atlas of sensitivity to tuberculin, PPD-B, and histoplasmin in the United States. Am Rev Respir Dis 99(suppl):1, 1969

FOX W: The chemotherapy of pulmonary tuberculosis: A review. Chest 76(suppl):785, 1979

GLASSROTH J et al: Tuberculosis in the 1980s. N Engl J Med 302:1441, 1980

GOREN MB: Immunoreactive substances of mycobacteria. Am Rev Respir Dis 125(suppl):50, 1982

GROSSET J: Bacteriologic basis of short-course chemotherapy for tuberculosis. Clin Chest Med 1:231, 1980

GRZYBOWSKI S, ENARSON DA: The fate of cases of pulmonary tuberculosis under various treatment programmes. Bull Int Union Tuberc 53:70, 1978

SNIDER DE, JR: The tuberculin skin test. Am Rev Respir Dis 125(suppl):108, 1982

STEAD WW et al: Tuberculosis as an endemic and nosocomial infection among the elderly in nursing homes. N Engl J Med 312:1483, 1985

TENDAM HG et al: Present knowledge of immunization against tuberculosis. Bull WHO 54:255, 1976

120 LEPROSY (HANSEN'S DISEASE)

RICHARD A. MILLER[1]

DEFINITION Leprosy (Hansen's disease) is a chronic granulomatous infection of humans which attacks superficial tissues, especially the skin and peripheral nerves. Accounts of leprosy extend back to the earliest historical records and document a stigmatization of leprosy patients which transcends cultural and religious boundaries. The clinical and immunologic manifestations of disease form a continuum extending from polar *tuberculoid* leprosy to polar *lepromatous* leprosy. The borderline portion of the spectrum lies between these two extremes, and is usually subdivided into *borderline tuberculoid, borderline*, and *borderline lepromatous* classes. In addition, an early indeterminate form is seen, which may spontaneously remit or develop into overt leprosy.

ETIOLOGY *Mycobacterium leprae,* or Hansen's bacillus, is the causal agent of leprosy. It is an acid-fast rod assigned to the family Mycobacteriaceae on the basis of morphologic, biochemical, antigenic, and genetic similarities to other mycobacteria. Although it has not been cultivated in artificial media or tissue culture, it can be consistently propagated in the foot pads of mice. Systemic infections with manifestations similar to those of human disease can be induced in armadillos and mangabey monkeys. The bacillus multiplies exceedingly slowly, with an estimated optimal doubling time of 11 to 13 days during logarithmic growth in mouse foot pads. The mouse model has been used extensively for the study of antileprosy drugs, and the high bacterial yield from armadillos has been crucial for immunologic studies.

Lepromin is a suspension of killed *M. leprae* prepared from heavily infected human or armadillo tissue. Intradermal injection elicits, somewhat variably, a tuberculin-like reaction at 48 h (Fernandez's reaction) and more consistently, a papular reaction at 3 to 4 weeks (Mitsuda's reaction). The Mitsuda reaction is usually positive in tuberculoid patients and is always negative in lepromatous patients. However, because it is also positive in nearly all normal adults, even those residing in areas free of endemic leprosy, it has no diagnostic value. Lepromin is not commercially available.

EPIDEMIOLOGY There are probably 10 to 20 million persons affected with leprosy in the world. The disease is more common in tropical countries, in many of which the prevalence rate is 1 to 2 percent of the population. A warm environment is not critical for transmission, as leprosy also occurs in certain regions with cooler climates, such as Korea and central Mexico. Distribution of infected individuals within countries is very nonhomogeneous, and districts in which 20 percent of the population is affected can be found. The distribution of cases across the spectrum of leprosy also varies between countries, with lepromatous disease predominating in some countries, such as Mexico, and tuberculoid disease in other areas, including India. Ninety percent of the approximately 270 cases per year diagnosed in the United States have occurred in immigrants from leprosy-endemic countries. Indigenous transmission occurs primarily in Hawaii, the Pacific Island territories, and sporadically along the Gulf coast.

Leprosy can present at any age, although cases in infants less than 1 year of age are extremely rare. The age-specific incidence peaks during childhood in most developing countries, with up to 20 percent of cases occurring in children under 10. Since leprosy is most prevalent in poorer socioeconomic groups, this may simply reflect the age distribution of the high-risk population. The sex ratio of leprosy presenting during childhood is essentially 1:1, but males predominate by a 2:1 ratio in adult cases.

[1] *Dr. Charles C. Shepard (deceased) contributed significantly to the text on which this revision was based.*

Direct human-to-human transmission is believed responsible for most cases of leprosy. Animal reservoirs exist among feral armadillos and possibly among nonhuman primates, but there is little evidence that they have an important role in the epidemiology of human disease. Familial spread is facilitated by the indolence of the clinical illness and the potential for transmission prior to the development of symptoms. Among close family contacts (spouse-spouse or spouse-child) of untreated lepromatous patients the risk of disease is increased approximately eightfold, and the attack rate can be as high as 10 percent. Development of clinical disease in contacts of tuberculoid patients is less common, although sensitive immunologic tests suggest that most of these contacts have been sensitized to *M. leprae*. The site of entry remains a matter of conjecture, but is probably either the skin or the mucosa of the upper respiratory tract. The chief portal of exit is thought to be the nasal mucosa of untreated lepromatous patients. Transmission is theoretically possible from infected breast milk or via hematophagous arthropod vectors, but the importance of these alternative modalities appears to be minor.

The incubation period is frequently 3 to 5 years, but has been reported to range from 6 months to several decades.

PATHOGENESIS The early events following the entry of *M. leprae* into the body have not been described in humans. The bacilli are surrounded by a dense, nearly inert lipid capsule, produce no exotoxins, and engender little inflammatory response. The factors which determine the nature and efficacy of the host response to *M. leprae* are unknown. Immunologic and epidemiologic studies suggest that only a small fraction, possibly 10 to 20 percent, of those exposed to viable bacilli will develop signs of indeterminate leprosy and that only about 50 percent of those with indeterminate disease will progress to full-blown clinical leprosy.

The intensity of the specific cell-mediated immune response to *M. leprae* correlates with the clinical and histologic disease class. Individuals with polar tuberculoid disease have an intense cellular response to *M. leprae* and a low bacillary load, whereas patients with lepromatous leprosy have no detectable cellular immunity to the leprosy bacillus. There is evidence from sibling studies that specific HLA-associated genes may be linked to different classes of disease. HLA-DR3 was inherited preferentially by children with polar tuberculoid disease, whereas HLA-MT1 was associated with polar lepromatous disease. The effect of the HLA-associated genes was limited to influencing the type of leprosy which developed. There was no association between HLA haplotypes and overall susceptibility to leprosy. These findings are analogous to those made in mice infected with *Mycobacterium lepraemurium* or *Leishmania donovani*. In the mouse, innate susceptibility or resistance to these intracellular pathogens is controlled by non-H-2 genes (the H-2 locus in mice is the analogue of the human HLA system), but H-2-linked genes subsequently influence the severity of infection which develops in susceptible mice.

The defect in cell-mediated immunity in lepromatous patients is extremely specific. They do not suffer increased morbidity following infection by pathogens such as viruses or parasites for which cellular immunity is important, and they do not have an increased risk of neoplasia. Tuberculin reactivity may be suppressed in untreated lepromatous disease, but usually returns with treatment, unlike the lepromin response, which remains negative. Patients with lepromatous leprosy have been shown to have an increased number of circulating OKT8 (''suppressor'') lymphocytes which can be specifically activated by *M. leprae* antigens, and the lymphocytes present in their cutaneous granulomas are almost exclusively OKT8-positive. In contrast, OKT4-positive (''helper'') cells predominate among the T cells in the cutaneous lesions of tuberculoid patients. In lepromatous leprosy, cells of the monocyte-macrophage family become engorged with *M. leprae* and are unable to kill or digest the organisms. However, when studied in vitro, monocytes from these patients respond normally to lymphokines and display normal phagocytic and microbicidal activity. These results suggest that an underlying defect in regulation of T-lymphocyte subpopulations is responsible for the immunologic tolerance characteristic of lepromatous leprosy.

Intense bacillemia is very common in lepromatous leprosy, and organisms can often be seen in stained smears of peripheral blood or buffy coats, but high fever and signs of systemic toxicity are absent. Even in the most advanced cases, destructive lesions are limited to the skin, peripheral nerves, anterior portions of the eyes, upper respiratory passages above the larynx, testes, and structures of the hands and feet. The trophism of *M. leprae* for these tissues may be due to the fact that they are all usually several degrees cooler than 37°C. Two sites of preferential involvement are the ulnar nerves near the elbow and the peroneal nerves where they pass around the head of the fibula; above and below these areas where these nerves take deeper courses, they are much less severely involved. In patients with lepromatous leprosy, collections of bacilli are also found in the liver, spleen, and bone marrow. No visceral organ system dysfunction has been associated with the presence of these bacilli, and it is unclear whether they are capable of reproduction at core body temperatures.

CLINICOPATHOLOGIC CLASSIFICATION As is true of other chronic infections, such as syphilis and tuberculosis, the manifestations of leprosy are many and variable. The classification in general use is based on clinical and histopathologic findings.

Lepromatous leprosy is one of the polar forms. The cutaneous involvement is extensive, diffuse, and bilaterally symmetric. Even apparently normal skin will usually contain bacilli demonstrable by staining. Peripheral nerves are heavily infected but often better preserved than in the tuberculoid form. Histologically, there is a diffuse granulomatous reaction with macrophages, large foam (Virchow's) cells, and many intracellular bacilli, frequently in spheroidal masses (globi). Epithelioid cells and giant cells are not found.

Tuberculoid leprosy is the other polar type. Skin lesions are single or few and are sharply demarcated. Neurologic involvement is relatively pronounced and may occur in the absence of cutaneous lesions (pure neural leprosy). The histologic picture consists of lymphocytes, epithelioid cells, and perhaps giant cells; bacilli are frequently absent or difficult to demonstrate.

Classification within the borderline region of the spectrum is less precise. Lesions tend to increase in number and heterogeneity, but decrease in individual size as the lepromatous pole is approached. The histopathology of the granulomas also changes from an epithelioid cell predominance to a macrophage predominance. The presence and number of lymphocytes is variable and correlates poorly with the disease class. Bacilli are present in large numbers in the skin granulomas of borderline and borderline lepromatous patients. For this reason, these groups, together with polar lepromatous leprosy, are referred to as ''multibacillary leprosy.'' Borderline tuberculoid, polar tuberculoid, and indeterminate classes are grouped together as ''paucibacillary leprosy.'' The borderline disease states are unstable and may shift toward the lepromatous form in the untreated patient or toward the tuberculoid pole during treatment. Slight discrepancies between the clinical appearance and histopathologic findings are also common. Change of either polar type to the other is exceedingly rare.

In all forms of leprosy peripheral nerve involvement is a constant feature. In any histologic section involvement of nerves will tend to be more severe than involvement of other tissues. Much of the neural destruction appears to result from the granulomatous reaction of the host, rather than from an innate neurotoxic property of the bacillus.

CLINICAL MANIFESTATIONS Early leprosy The first signs of leprosy are usually cutaneous. One or more hypopigmented or hyperpigmented macules or plaques may be seen. Often an anesthetic or paresthetic patch is the first symptom noted by the patient, but on careful examination skin involvement can also be found. When contacts are examined, a single skin lesion is often noted, especially in children; usually, this is a hypesthetic macule that may clear spontaneously in a year or two, but specific treatment is usually recommended. Sensation is often preserved in early lesions, particularly those on the face.

Tuberculoid leprosy Early tuberculoid leprosy is frequently manifested by a hypopigmented macule, sharply demarcated and hypesthetic. Later the lesions are larger, and the margins are elevated and circinate or gyrate. There is peripheral spread and central healing. Fully developed lesions are densely anesthetic and have lost the normal skin organs (sweat glands and hair follicles). The lesions appear singly or are few in number and are not symmetric. Nerve involvement occurs early, and the superficial nerves leading from the lesions may be enlarged. The larger peripheral nerves (especially the ulnar, peroneal, and greater auricular nerves) may be palpably and visibly enlarged, particularly those closest to the skin lesion. There may be severe neuritic pain. Neural involvement leads to muscle atrophy, especially of the small muscles of the hand. Contractures of the hand and foot are frequent. Trauma, especially from burns and splinters and from excessive pressure, leads to secondary infection of the hands and to plantar ulcers. Later, resorption and loss of phalanges may supervene. When the facial nerves are involved, there may be lagophthalmos, exposure keratitis, and corneal ulceration leading to blindness.

Lepromatous leprosy The skin lesions are macules, nodules, plaques, or papules. The macules are often hypopigmented. The borders of the lesions are ill defined and the centers of raised lesions are indurated and convex (rather than concave as in tuberculoid disease). There is also diffuse infiltration between the lesions. The sites of predilection are the face (cheeks, nose, brows), ears, wrists, elbows, buttocks, and knees. Involvement with infiltration and little or no nodulation may progress so subtly that the disease goes unnoticed. Loss of the eyebrows, especially the lateral portions, is common. Much later the skin of the face and forehead becomes thickened and corrugated (leonine facies), and the earlobes become pendulous.

Nasal symptoms (nasal "stuffiness," epistaxis, and obstructed breathing) are common early symptoms. Complete nasal obstruction, laryngitis, and hoarseness are also frequent. Septal perforation and nasal collapse lead to saddlenose. Invasion of the anterior portion of the eye leads to keratitis and iridocyclitis. Painless inguinal and axillary lymphadenopathy occurs. In adult males infiltration and scarring of the testes lead to sterility. Gynecomastia is common.

Involvement of major nerve trunks is less prominent in the lepromatous form, but diffuse hypesthesia involving the peripheral portions of the extremities is common in advanced disease.

Borderline leprosy The skin lesions of borderline tuberculoid leprosy generally resemble those of tuberculoid disease, but are greater in number and have more poorly defined borders. Involvement of multiple peripheral nerve trunks is more common than in polar tuberculoid disease. Increasing variability in the appearance of the skin lesions is characteristic of borderline leprosy (sometimes referred to as "dimorphic" leprosy). Papules and plaques may coexist with macular lesions. Anesthesia is less prominent than in tuberculoid disease. Borderline lepromatous disease is characterized by very heterogeneous and relatively symmetric skin lesions. The earlobes may be slightly thickened, but the eyebrows and nasal regions are spared.

REACTIONAL STATES The general course of leprosy is indolent, but it may be interrupted by two types of reaction. Both forms of reactions can occur in untreated patients, but more often emerge as complications of chemotherapy.

Erythema nodosum leprosum Erythema nodosum leprosum (ENL), or type 2 lepra reaction, occurs in lepromatous and borderline lepromatous patients, most frequently in the latter half of the initial year of treatment. Tender, inflamed subcutaneous nodules develop, usually in crops. Each nodule lasts a week or two, but new crops may appear. ENL may last only a week or two, or it may continue for long periods. Low-grade fever, lymphadenopathy, and arthralgias can accompany severe ENL. Histologically, ENL is characterized by polymorphonuclear infiltration and deposits of IgG and complement; hence, it resembles an Arthus reaction.

Reversal reaction Reversal reaction, or type 1 lepra reaction, can complicate all three borderline categories. Existing skin lesions develop erythema and swelling, and new lesions may appear. An early influx of lymphocytes into existing lesions is followed by edema and a shift toward tuberculoid histology. Cellular immunity increases. Reversal reactions can be differentiated from disease progression or relapse by mouse inoculations to test bacillary viability and by histologic studies. Downgrading reactions, which clinically mimic reversal reactions, are most common in untreated patients and in women during the third trimester of pregnancy. Skin biopsies reveal a shift toward lepromatous histology and reflect a decrease in cellular immunity.

COMPLICATIONS Leprosy is probably the most frequent cause of crippling of the hand in the world. Trauma and secondary chronic infections can lead to loss of digits or distal extremities. Blindness is also common.

The *Lucio phenomenon* is limited to patients with a diffuse, infiltrative, nonnodular lepromatous disease; it is seen most often in Mexico and central America. Arteritis leads to ulceration of the skin in a characteristic angular pattern, and subsequently to angular thin scars. Severe cases clinically resemble other forms of necrotizing vasculitis and are associated with a high mortality rate.

Amyloidosis is a complication of severe lepromatous disease, especially when complicated by chronic ENL.

DIAGNOSIS The demonstration of acid-fast bacilli in skin smears made by the scraped-incision method is strong evidence for leprosy, but in tuberculoid disease bacilli may not be demonstrable. Wherever possible, a skin biopsy specimen from the affected area should be sent to a pathologist knowledgeable in leprosy. The histologic involvement of peripheral nerves is pathognomonic, even in the absence of bacilli.

The lepromin test has no diagnostic value. Hematologic and blood chemistry tests are likewise of little help. Lepromatous patients frequently have mild anemia, elevated erythrocyte sedimentation rate, and hyperglobulinemia. Between 10 and 40 percent of lepromatous patients have false-positive serologic tests for syphilis or autoantibodies directed against nuclear or cellular antigens.

Major advances in the search for a specific serodiagnostic test for leprosy have been made. A surface glycolipid antigen unique to *M. leprae,* referred to as phenolic glycolipid I, has been purified and its chemical structure determined. Assay systems to detect antibody directed against this antigen have been developed and have a sensitivity of over 95 percent in polar lepromatous disease and about 50 percent in polar tuberculoid cases. The specificity is excellent, even when testing serums from patients with tuberculosis or other mycobacterial diseases. When perfected, these assays may be useful for confirming the diagnosis of leprosy, for monitoring the response to therapy, and for screening contacts of leprosy patients for subclinical disease.

The differential diagnosis includes conditions such as lupus erythematosus, lupus vulgaris, sarcoidosis, yaws, dermal leishmaniasis, and a host of banal skin diseases. The skin lesions of leprosy, especially of turberculoid disease, are characterized by hypesthesia, and peripheral nerve involvement can always be demonstrated. Peripheral neuropathy from other causes and syringomyelia may be confused with leprosy, although skin involvement is not a feature of other diseases causing peripheral neuropathy. The combination of a chronic skin disease and peripheral nerve involvement should always lead to the consideration of leprosy.

TREATMENT The management of leprosy involves a broad, multidisciplinary approach, including consultative services such as orthopedic surgery, ophthalmology, and physical therapy in addition to antimicrobial chemotherapy.

Specific chemotherapy *Dapsone* (4,4′-diaminodiphenylsulfone, DDS, diphenylsulfone), a folate antagonist, is the mainstay of therapy. The daily dosage is 50 to 100 mg in adults. Dapsone is very inexpensive, safe in pregnancy, and has a long serum half-life of about 24 h, allowing once daily administration. Major side effects are relatively uncommon, but include hemolysis, agranulocytosis, hepatitis, and potentially fatal exfoliative dermatitis. In lepromatous disease enough bacilli are killed during the first 10 to 12 weeks of dapsone monotherapy to render mouse foot pad inoculations negative. However, in this form of the disease nonviable bacilli disappear slowly and may be found in the tissues for 5 to 10 years. Moreover, a few viable bacilli (persisters) may survive in the tissues for many years and cause a relapse if treatment is discontinued.

Dapsone resistance is a problem of increasing concern. Secondary resistance is most common in lepromatous patients and presents as a clinical and bacteriologic relapse after several years of apparently successful, regular therapy. Sulfone resistance can be demonstrated by mouse foot pad inoculation. The frequency of this secondary resistance has been 2 to 30 percent in different countries, depending on the sulfone used and the regularity of its administration. Primary dapsone resistance in as many as 30 percent of previously untreated patients has complicated empiric therapy in many parts of the world, but has remained uncommon in newly diagnosed patients in the United States. Because of the problems of dapsone-resistant bacilli and of persister bacilli, multiple drug therapy is now recommended for all multibacillary disease.

Rifampin is the most rapidly mycobactericidal drug known for *M. leprae*. The viability of skin bacilli falls to undetectable levels within 5 days following a single 1500-mg dose of oral rifampin. The usual dosage is 600 mg per day. The high cost of rifampin has limited its use in the developing world, and has led to regimens in which it is given at a dosage of 600 or 900 mg once per month. These intermittent regimens are based on animal studies but have not been extensively evaluated in human disease. Until more clinical experience has been accumulated, many leprologists prefer to treat with daily or twice weekly rifampin. Rare cases of rifampin-resistant *M. leprae* have been reported. Rifampin has not been approved for this purpose by the Food and Drug Administration.

Clofazimine is a compound derived from a phenazine dye. It is highly lipophilic and accumulates in the skin, the gastrointestinal tract, and in macrophages and monocytes. Its pharmacokinetics are poorly understood, but it is usually given in a dosage of 50 to 200 mg per day and has an apparent half-life of over 70 days. Major toxicity is restricted to the skin and the intestinal tract. The reddish skin pigmentation, often accompanied by ichthyosis, is unacceptable to many light-skinned patients, and can lead to poor compliance. The intestinal toxicity is also dose-related and is reflected in diarrhea and cramping abdominal pain. Clofazimine has not been shown to be safe for use during pregnancy. Clofazimine is an investigational drug in the United States and is available for protocol use through the National Hansen's Disease Center, Carville, Louisiana.

Several other agents, including ethionamide, prothionamide, thiambutosine, and amithiozone, have limited activity against *M. leprae* and may be of value in multiple drug regimens. None of these drugs have been approved for this purpose by the Food and Drug Administration.

Therapy for multibacillary disease should consist of three drugs, usually dapsone, rifampin, and clofazimine. If the organism is known to be dapsone-sensitive, the combination of dapsone and rifampin may be adequate for borderline and borderline lepromatous cases, but the likelihood of secondary dapsone resistance makes the addition of a third drug advisable in lepromatous disease. Objective measures of response to therapy, including skin scrapings and biopsies, should be monitored and therapy continued at least until they are consistently negative. The optimal duration of therapy is unknown, but a minimum of 2 years is recommended. Indefinite therapy may be required for lepromatous disease.

Therapeutic regimens containing two drugs, usually dapsone and rifampin, are adequate for paucibacillary leprosy. The World Health Organization recommends a 6-month course, which can be repeated if relapse occurs. Standard practice in the United States is to treat with dapsone and rifampin for the first 6 to 12 months (depending on the clinical response), followed by dapsone alone to complete a total of 24 months of therapy.

Objective evidence of clinical improvement should be visible by the second or third month of treatment. The clinical response to adequate therapy may be confused by intercurrent reactional states, but the disease stops progressing and the skin lesions gradually improve. Recovery from neurologic impairment is limited.

Treatment of reactional states Mild ENL is managed with antipyretics and analgesics. Severe cases can be rapidly controlled with high dosages of prednisone (60 to 120 mg per day). Antimicrobial therapy should be continued as corticosteroid therapy promotes the viability of *M. leprae* in mice not given antileprosy drugs. Rifampin enhances the metabolism of corticosteroids by the liver, necessitating administration of larger doses to achieve a given therapeutic effect. Thalidomide is the most effective drug for ENL. The usual initial dosage is 200 mg twice a day, which can be gradually tapered to a maintenance dosage of 50 to 100 mg per day for patients with chronic ENL. Thalidomide is absolutely contraindicated in women of childbearing age because of its teratogenicity, but has proved relatively free of major side effects in other leprosy patients. This drug has not been approved by the Food and Drug Administration but is available through the National Hansen's Disease Center as an investigational agent. Clofazimine has anti-inflammatory properties as well as antimycobacterial activity and can be valuable in the treatment of chronic ENL, but requires at least 3 to 4 weeks to reach effective levels, making it of little use in acute attacks. Other classes of anti-inflammatory agents including antimalarials such as chloroquine and cytotoxic drugs have been used in difficult cases; in general these unusual situations should be managed in consultation with a leprosy specialist.

Reversal reactions are often acute and can lead to rapid and irreversible neurologic damage. Corticosteroids are indicated for severe reversal reactions. Clofazimine is of some use in chronic situations, but it is generally necessary to continue corticosteroids as well. Reversal reactions do not respond to thalidomide.

Other measures Many of the deformities and disabilities of leprosy are preventable. Plantar ulcers, which are very common, may be prevented by rigid-soled footwear or walking plaster casts, and contractures of the hand may be prevented by physical therapy and application of casts. Reconstructive surgery is sometimes helpful. Nerve and tendon transplants and release of contractures can give patients more functional ability. Vocational retraining is often necessary for those with permanent disability. Plastic repair of facial deformities assists acceptance of patients in society. The psychological trauma which resulted from prolonged segregation is now minimized by home therapy in virtually all cases.

Control Case finding and chemotherapy form the present basis of control because infectiousness is quickly suppressed, as is the development of deformity. Early detection of cases is especially important. In endemic countries this means the establishment of clinics or traveling teams. Family and other close contacts need regular examinations for leprosy. In the United States patients are eligible for treatment by the Public Health Service, and special clinics are located in several major cities, as well as an inpatient facility at the National Hansen's Disease Center in Carville, Louisiana. Risk of transmission is very low, even in untreated patients, and no unusual infection control precautions are required when patients are hospitalized. Chemoprophylaxis with lowered dosages of dapsone is effective, but contact screening by yearly physical examinations is preferred to empiric therapy in most situations. Field trials of bacillus Calmette-Guérin (BCG) vaccination in endemic areas have given conflicting results, but even the most optimistic reports have shown only modest efficacy. A vaccine which combines viable BCG and heat-killed *M. leprae* has shown promise in pilot studies and is now undergoing field trials.

REFERENCES

BLOOM BR, GODAL T: Selective primary health care: Strategies for control of disease in the developing world. V. Leprosy. Rev Infect Dis 5:765, 1983

BULLOCK WE: Rifampin in the treatment of leprosy. Rev Infect Dis 5:S606, 1983

———: *Mycobacterium leprae* (leprosy), in *Principles and Practice of Infectious Diseases,* 2 ed, GL Mandell et al (eds). New York, Wiley, 1985, pp 1406–1413

DUNCAN ME et al: Pregnancy and leprosy: The consequences of alterations of cell-mediated and humoral immunity during pregnancy and lactation. Int J Lepr 50:425, 1982

NEILL MA et al: Leprosy in the United States, 1971–1981. J Infect Dis 152:1064, 1985

RIDLEY DS, JOPING WH: Classification of leprosy according to immunity: A five-group system. Int J Lepr 34:255, 1966

SANSONETTI P, LAGRANGE PH: The immunology of leprosy: Speculations on the leprosy spectrum. Rev Infect Dis 3:422, 1981

VAN EDEN W et al: HLA-linked control of predisposition to lepromatous leprosy. J Infect Dis 151:9, 1985

VAN VOORHIS WC et al: The cutaneous infiltrates of leprosy: Cellular characteristics and the predominant T-cell phenotypes. N Engl J Med 307:1593, 1983

WHO STUDY GROUP: Chemotherapy of leprosy for control programs. WHO Tech Rep Ser 675:7, 1982

YOUNG DB, BUCHANAN TM: A serological test for leprosy with a glycolipid specific for *Mycobacterium leprae*. Science 221:1057, 1983

121 OTHER MYCOBACTERIAL INFECTIONS

STANLEY D. FREEDMAN[1]

INTRODUCTION Myobacteria other than the tubercle bacilli were shown to be agents of human disease in the 1950s. A classification of these organisms based upon colonial morphology and growth characteristics was provided by Runyon. These bacteria are widely distributed in nature as saprophytes, primarily in soil and water. Animals can be infected and serve as reservoirs for infection of humans. Person-to-person transmission has not been documented. Epidemiologic studies using tuberculins from the various species demonstrated the extent of infection in the United States and other countries, as well as notable geographic differences. These organisms have been referred to as atypical mycobacteria or anonymous mycobacteria. Although the organisms are not always anonymous, the frequency with which they are found in the environment demands repeated isolation from a diseased area before they can be accepted as the etiologic agent. With the steady improvement of laboratory techniques including radiometric cultures, species designations are now increasingly familiar and preferred in the study of these pathogens (Table 121-1). With increasing sophistication of medical practice and the emergence of newly recognized diseases, additional syndromes associated with different species have emerged and have assumed major importance.

MYCOBACTERIUM ULCERANS *M. ulcerans* is the etiologic agent of the Buruli or Bairnsdale ulcer. It grows only at 30 to 33°C. Colonies require 7 weeks to appear; isolation is enhanced by inoculation of mouse foot pads. A disease of the tropics, it is concentrated in Australia and Africa. The first sign of infection with *M. ulcerans* is a small painless nodule developing into an extensive granulomatous ulceration usually affecting the extensor surfaces of the extremities. Characteristically, the ulcer is deep with a necrotic base and undermined edges. Wide surgical excision with skin grafting is curative; there are no clear data regarding chemotherapy.

MYCOBACTERIUM MARINUM This organism, previously called *M. balnei,* is a psychrophilic (30°C) photochromogen which inhabits fresh and salt water and causes disease in fish. Human infections are usually associated with some aquatic activity, like working in aquaria and swimming. The organism enters abraded skin and either forms a nodule, which can spread along lymphatics suggesting sporotrichosis, causes verrucous lesions, or, less commonly, ulcerates. The pathology consists of a granulomatous lesion usually without caseation—the so-called swimming pool or fishtank granuloma. Infection is frequently associated with a positive tuberculin test reflecting shared antigens with *M. tuberculosis*. Because the differential diagnosis includes sporotrichosis as well as other mycobacterial infections, appropriate cultures (30 to 32°C incubation) are critical. Infections of tendon sheaths and synovia have been described in association with penetrating injuries. Ulcerations similar to those caused by *M. ulcerans,* as well as disseminated skin lesions, have been reported in immunocompromised patients. Minor lesions can resolve spontaneously. The organism is often sensitive in vitro to rifampin and ethambutol, and these drugs have been curative. Tetracycline, especially minocycline, and trimethoprim/sulfamethoxazole have also been used with favorable results.

MYCOBACTERIUM KANSASII *M. kansasii* produces pigment upon exposure to light, grows at 37°C, and is a long, thick, acid-fast organism with prominent transverse banding. Infections are more common in the central United States, Texas, England, and Wales. The reasons for these geographic variations are unknown, but likely relate to subtle ecologic properties of these organisms. Person-to-person spread is not recognized. Reported cases reflect a preponderance of white adult men.

Pulmonary disease is the commonest expression of this organism, and the clinical picture closely resembles pulmonary tuberculosis although signs and symptoms are milder. Pneumoconiosis and chronic obstructive pulmonary disease (COPD) are considered predisposing conditions. Thin-walled cavities with minimal inflammatory reaction are characteristic. The usual situation, without treatment, is slow progression.

Disseminated disease is now recognized as an important manifestation of *M. kansasii* infections. Such hematogenous spread is associated with pancytopenia, hairy cell leukemia, malignancies, and

[1] *Dr. Charles C. Shepard (deceased) contributed significantly to the text on which this revision was based.*

TABLE 121-1 Human mycobacterial pathogens other than *M. tuberculosis* and *M. leprae*

Mycobacterium	Pigmentation of culture*	Usual site of disease	Usual source of infection	Response to drugs
M. marinum	P	Skin	Swimming pools, aquaria, fish	Good
M. ulcerans	N	Skin	Tropical environment	Variable
M. avium-intracellulare	N	Lungs	Environment, animals?	Poor
M. kansasii	P	Lungs	Environment?	Good
M. xenopi	S	Lungs	Water, animals?	Variable
M. szulgai	S†	Lungs	?	Good
M. scrofulaceum	S	Lungs, lymph nodes	Water, soil	Poor
M. fortuitum	N	Skin (abscesses), lungs	Soil, dirt, water	Poor
M. chelonei	N	Skin (abscesses), lungs	Soil, dirt, water	Poor

* *P = photochromogenic (develops yellow-orange pigment only when exposed to light); N = nonpigmented; S = scotochromogenic (develops yellow-orange pigment in the dark).*
† *Scotochromogenic at 37°C, photochromogenic at 25°C.*

bone marrow and renal transplantations. Fever, anemia, and signs and symptoms referrable to multiple organ system involvement occur. The diagnosis is confirmed by appropriate cultures of involved tissues. Skin and soft tissue involvement is seen and may mimic *M. marinum* infections. Tenosynovitis, osteomyelitis, lymphadenitis, pericarditis, and genitourinary tract infections have been reported.

Diseases due to *M. kansasii* respond well to treatment. Rifampin appears to be the most effective drug and should be used in all initial regimens. Ethambutol and isoniazid are usually the other drugs administered. Over 95 percent of patients respond to this combined regimen. Retreatment programs should be guided by in vitro sensitivity testing, and rifampin used if the organism is sensitive.

MYCOBACTERIUM SCROFULACEUM This scotochromogenic bacillus is a major cause of lymphadenitis in children. Cervical nodes are usually involved, and associated systemic symptoms are rare. Definitive diagnosis requires culture, and definitive therapy requires total excision of the node and sinus tract, if present. There are a few reports of pulmonary disease and osseous and soft tissue infections; dissemination usually is associated with serious underlying conditions. Sensitivity patterns vary, and multiple-drug regimens have been used.

MYCOBACTERIUM SZULGAI At 37°C this organism is scotochromogenic and can be confused with more common tap water contaminants. It was initially recognized as an uncommon pulmonary pathogen; there are also reports of bursitis, lymphadenitis, and tenosynovitis. Most isolates are sensitive to rifampin and ethambutol.

MYCOBACTERIUM XENOPI *M. xenopi* is a slow-growing scotochromogen which infrequently causes tuberculosis-like pulmonary disease in humans. However, reports of disseminated disease are becoming more common and include an association with the acquired immunodeficiency syndrome (see below). Unlike a number of nontuberculous mycobacteria it is sensitive to most of the antituberculous drugs.

MYCOBACTERIUM AVIUM-INTRACELLULARE Although seroagglutination, thin-layer chromatography, and enzyme-linked immunoabsorbent assays can distinguish *M. avium* from *M. intracellulare,* distinction is difficult and they are considered as a complex (MAI). These ubiquitous organisms are particularly prevalent in the southeastern United States and, overall, are the most commonly isolated mycobacteria other than *M. tuberculosis*. Colonization and inapparent infection are common; knowledge of transmission is limited. The lungs are most commonly involved, and the clinical picture is similar to pulmonary tuberculosis. Underlying pulmonary disease, a possible genetic predilection, and age are risk factors. Solitary pulmonary nodules are not uncommon. It is important to be certain of the etiology and the pathogenic role of the organism isolated, because chemotherapy is often associated with morbidity.

Skin involvement and musculoskeletal infections including vertebral osteomyelitis resembling Pott's disease have been described. MAI is a major cause of lymphadenitis in children. Disseminated disease is also recognized in children, and in adults in association with severe underlying diseases. Fever, anemia, leukocytosis, hypergammaglobulinemia, and hepatosplenomegaly are prominent features.

These organisms have been added to the list of opportunistic infections complicating the acquired immunodeficiency syndrome (AIDS). They represent one of the most common life-threatening infections in this syndrome. The manifestations are unique and basically reflect overwhelming infection in these hosts with impaired cellular immunity. There is mycobacteremia, and organisms abound in most organs and body secretions. There is a minimal cellular response, granulomatous or otherwise. Profound diarrhea with intestinal pathology that strikingly resembles Whipple's disease, due to macrophages packed with MAI, is recognized. In other organs these macrophages resemble lepra cells.

Treatment is difficult and unsatisfactory. The organisms are usually resistant to most of the antimycobacterial agents. Yet multiple-drug therapy is recommended with some demonstrable benefit possibly reflecting synergy which is difficult to prove in vitro. Drugs chosen should include those antimicrobials to which the organism is sensitive. Three to six drugs are used concurrently, chosen from among isoniazid, ethambutol, rifampin, ethionamide, pyrazinamide, cycloserine, streptomycin, kanamycin, and capreomycin. Of these, ethambutol, ethionamide, and cycloserine appear more effective. Surgical excision is the treatment of choice for lymphadenitis and is a reasonable alternative for a few other localized infections. The experimental drugs clofazimine and rifabutine have been used along with immunomodulators in patients with MAI infections complicating AIDS (see Chap. 257).

MYCOBACTERIUM FORTUITUM* AND *CHELONEI The unique feature of these acid-fast bacteria is their rapid growth; initial growth may take 1 to 5 weeks, but subsequent subcultures grow within 5 days. Reflecting their meager nutritional requirements, they are readily cultured on most media. These two species account for virtually all the reported infections due to rapid growers. *M. fortuitum* is more frequently associated with posttraumatic and postsurgical skin and soft tissue infection. *M. chelonei* is a more common cause of pulmonary infections and disseminated disease. Subspeciation is not necessary for clinical purposes. Widespread in nature and in hospital environments, and highly resistant to drugs, antiseptics, and disinfectants, rapid growers are important nosocomial pathogens.

Most human infections are associated with interruption of the integument and injury or alteration of the soft tissues. Inhalational pulmonary disease complicates underlying lung disease. Although a chronic granulomatous reaction with caseation may occur, the distinguishing feature is a suppurative process with microabscesses, and diphtheroid-like organisms on Gram stain. Infections have followed cardiothoracic surgery, augmentation mammoplasty, arthroplasty, injections, ocular surgery, and dialysis. Clinical manifestations include lymphadenitis, keratitis, osteomyelitis, meningitis, and endocarditis involving porcine, prosthetic, and natural valves. Hematogenous dissemination is uncommon, and affects those with impaired host defenses.

Adequate debridement and drainage with removal of foreign bodies is indicated whenever possible. Many of these organisms are highly resistant to all antimicrobial agents. However, reflecting their growth characteristics, antimicrobial sensitivity testing is more reliable in determining appropriate chemotherapy. Amikacin is most often effective, but other drugs of proven value include gentamicin, cefoxitin, doxycycline, erythromycin, sulfonamides, rifampin, and ethambutol. Sulfonamides are more active against *M. fortuitum,* and erythromycin inhibits some *M. chelonei.* Because of the emergence of resistant organisms, two or three drugs may be preferable to one.

OTHER MYCOBACTERIA *M. haemophilum* has emerged as a skin pathogen. It is psychrophilic, but requires iron supplements for growth. Virtually all reported cases have been in immunosuppressed patients. Ulcerating skin lesions with acid-fast bacilli that could not be grown have been described in individuals living in Minnesota and the adjacent Canadian border. The disease is self-limited. Unclassified mycobacterial species are being sought as etiologic agents in inflammatory bowel disease; these might be similar to *M. paratuberculosis,* the agent of Johne's disease, an intestinal disease of ruminants.

With increasing laboratory and clinical sophistication, the list of diseases caused by nontuberculous mycobacteria may lengthen.

REFERENCES

Collins CH, Grange JM: *Mycobacterium marinum* infections in man. J Hyg Camb 94:135, 1985

Greene JB, Sidhu GS: *Mycobacterium avium-intracellulare:* A cause of disseminated life-threatening infection in homosexuals and drug abusers. Ann Intern Med 97:539, 1982

LICHTENSTEIN IH, MACGREGOR RR: Mycobacterial infections in renal transplant recipients: Report of five cases and review of the literature. Rev Infect Dis 5:216, 1983

ROTH RI, OWEN RL: Intestinal infection with *Mycobacterium avium* in acquired immune deficiency syndrome (AIDS). Dig Dis Sci 30:497, 1985

RUNYON EH: Anonymous mycobacteria in pulmonary disease. Med Clin North Am 43:273, 1959

SANDERS WE: Other *Mycobacterium* species, in *Principles and Practice of Infectious Diseases*, 2d ed, GL Mandel et al. (eds). New York, Wiley, 1985

WALLACE RJ, SWENSON JM: Spectrum of disease due to rapidly growing mycobacteria. Rev Infect Dis 5:657, 1983

———: Treatment of nonpulmonary infections due to *Mycobacterium fortuitum* and *Mycobacterium chelonei* on the basis of in vitro susceptibilities. J Infect Dis 152:500, 1985

WEINBERG JR, GERTNER D: Disseminated *Mycobacterium xenopi* infection. Lancet 1:1033, 1985

WOLINSKY E: Nontuberculous mycobacteria and associated diseases. Am Rev Resp Dis 119:107, 1979

WONG B, EDWARDS FF: Continuous high-grade *Mycobacterium avium-intracellulare* bacteremia in patients with the acquired immune deficiency syndrome. Am J Med 78:35, 1985

section 5 Spirochetal diseases

122 SYPHILIS

KING K. HOLMES / SHEILA A. LUKEHART

DEFINITION Syphilis is a chronic systemic infection caused by *Treponema pallidum* subspecies *pallidum,* is usually sexually transmitted, and is characterized by an incubation period averaging 3 weeks, followed by a primary lesion associated with regional lymphadenopathy; a secondary bacteremic stage associated with generalized mucocutaneous lesions and generalized lymphadenopathy; a latent period of subclinical infection lasting many years; and, in about one-third of untreated cases, a tertiary stage characterized by progressive destructive mucocutaneous musculoskeletal or parenchymal lesions, aortitis, or central nervous system disease.

ETIOLOGY The discovery of *Treponema pallidum* in syphilitic material was made by Schaudinn and Hoffman in 1905. *Treponema pallidum* is one of the many spiral-shaped microorganisms which propel themselves by spinning around their longitudinal axis. The Spirochaetales include three genera which are pathogenic for humans and for a variety of other animals: the *Leptospira,* which cause human leptospirosis; the *Borrelia,* including *B. recurrentis* and *B. vincentii,* which cause relapsing fever and Vincent's angina, respectively, as well as *B. burgdorferi,* the causative agent of Lyme disease; and the *Treponema,* responsible for the diseases known as treponematoses. The *Treponema* include *T. pallidum* subspecies *pallidum* (hereafter called *T. pallidum*) which causes syphilis; *T. pallidum* subspecies *pertenue, T. pallidum* subspecies *endemicum,* and *T. carateum,* the organisms which cause yaws, endemic syphilis, and pinta (see Chap. 123); and *T. paraluiscuniculi,* the cause of rabbit syphilis. Other treponema include nonpathogenic species found in the human mouth and several species of anaerobic saprophytic genital treponemes of low pathogenicity which often coexist with anaerobic gram-negative rods in ulcerative genital lesions (so-called fusospirochetal infections). These can also be confused with *T. pallidum* on dark-field examination.

Treponema pallidum is a thin, delicate organism with 6 to 14 spirals and tapered ends, measuring 6 to 15 μm in total length and 0.2 μm in width. The cytoplasm is surrounded by a trilaminar cytoplasmic membrane, which in turn is surrounded by a delicate inner mucopeptide layer, the periplast, thought to be composed of alternating molecules of *N*-acetyl glucosamine and *N*-acetyl muramic acid, and which provides some structural rigidity, while an outer lipoprotein membrane is selectively permeable and osmotically sensitive. The spiral structure of *T. pallidum* is maintained by six fibrils, three arising at each end of the organism, which wind around the cell body in a space between the inner cell wall and the outer cell membrane, and may be the contractile elements responsible for motility. None of the four pathogenic treponemes has yet been cultured in vitro in quantities sufficient to permit detailed comparisons of the organisms, and no convincing morphologic, serologic, or metabolic differences between them have been discerned. They are distinguished primarily according to the clinical syndrome they produce. Limited animal inoculation studies also indicate some differences in host range and virulence, even among different strains of *T. pallidum.* The only known natural host for *T. pallidum* is the human. Many mammals can be infected with *T. pallidum,* but only humans, higher apes, and a few laboratory animals regularly develop syphilitic lesions. Virulent strains of *T. pallidum* are maintained in rabbits.

HISTORY The first clear descriptions of syphilis were recorded at the end of the fifteenth century, when a pandemic known as the great pox, as distinguished from smallpox, swept over Europe and Asia. Severe morbidity or death often occurred during the secondary stage, indicating an unexplained virulence then which is almost unknown today, except in congenital syphilis. The sexual mode of transmission of syphilis was recognized early during the European pandemic, and description of the primary and secondary stages of the disease followed. The major cardiovascular and neurologic complications of late syphilis were recognized during the eighteenth and nineteenth centuries. Gummas were not recognized as being syphilitic in origin until this century.

A rapid series of important advances began in 1903 with the successful inoculation of syphilis into primates. The discovery of *Treponema pallidum* in serum from secondary lesions was made in 1905. In 1910, the complement fixation test for the diagnosis of syphilis and an arsenic derivative, arsphenamine (Compound 606, Salvarsan), which was effective in treatment, were introduced.

EPIDEMIOLOGY Nearly all cases of syphilis are acquired by sexual contact with infectious lesions (i.e., the chancre, mucous patch, skin rash, or condyloma latum). Less common modes of transmission include nonsexual personal contact and infection in utero or following blood transfusions.

In the United States, infant deaths due to syphilis, and new admissions of patients with syphilitic psychoses, have fallen by 99 percent since 1940. The total reported number of cases of late and late latent syphilis has fallen almost every year since 1943. The 7.4 cases per 100,000 population reported in 1983 represent a decrease of over 98 percent since 1943. Only 239 cases of congenital syphilis were reported in 1983, a decrease of 98 percent since 1941; however, 321 cases were reported in 1984, an increase of 34 percent over the previous year. The number of new cases of infectious syphilis reached a peak in 1947, then fell steadily to about 6000 in 1957, but then began to increase again in the late 1970s. In 1984, there were 28,559 cases of primary and secondary syphilis and 23,117 cases of early latent syphilis reported; the number of unreported cases was estimated to be greater.

The peak incidence of syphilis occurs in the age group 15 to 34. In the United States, the male/female ratio of reported early cases (<1 year) increased from 0.8:1 in 1950 to 3.2:1 in 1980, and dropped to 2.6:1 in 1983. The high male/female ratio results from the disproportionate representation of syphilis in male homosexuals. Of all men with primary, secondary, or early latent syphilis interviewed in the United States during 1980, one-half were homosexual or bisexual. It has been speculated that the AIDS epidemic has caused a decrease in new sexual exposure in the homosexual population and that this change is largely responsible for the decreasing overall incidence of sexually transmitted diseases, including syphilis, observed since 1983. There are few data to support this hypothesis for syphilis, however. Although there was a 12.7 percent decrease in the total number of reported cases of primary and secondary syphilis from 1983 to 1984, the number of reported cases of primary and secondary syphilis in women also decreased by 12.2 percent during that same period, indicating that the incidence in homosexual men was not decreasing more rapidly than in heterosexuals.

Although the reported incidence of syphilis appears higher in nonwhites than in whites, and is higher in urban than in rural areas, these differences partly reflect the fact that urban racial groups are treated at public clinics, where case reporting is complete. The case rates of early syphilis are highest in the south and southwest, and in those states with large urban populations.

Of patients with reported early syphilis in 1983, 52 percent were self-referred, 24 percent were contact referrals, and 23 percent were identified by serologic screening. Interviews of patients with early syphilis disclose an average of 1.98 sexual contacts at risk per patient. Approximately one of two individuals named as contacts of infectious syphilis becomes infected. Many contacts will have already developed manifestations of syphilis when they are first seen, and about 30 percent of apparently uninfected contacts of infectious syphilis who are examined within 30 days of exposure will actually be in the incubation stage and will themselves develop infectious syphilis if not treated. Because of this, the identification and "epidemiologic" treatment of all recently exposed contacts has become an important aspect of syphilis control. Also important is the identification of syphilitics by serologic testing of pregnant women, hospital admissions, military inductees, and persons undergoing examination in physicians' offices. Of 45 million blood specimens examined during 1980 in the United States, 1.4 million tests were reactive, representing untreated syphilis, previously treated syphilis, or false-positive tests. Of all reported early syphilis cases of less than 1 year's duration in 1983, 47 percent were detected as a direct result of either contact tracing or serologic testing. More controversial are laws and regulations requiring routine premarital serologic testing for syphilis. Of 3.8 million premarital serologies performed in 1978, only 1 in 8461 was positive for infectious syphilis; the number positive for latent syphilis requiring treatment is probably larger, though national data are not available. Each state should review its own data on the yield of premarital testing; in general, the yield is currently highest in certain southern states, Texas, and the District of Columbia.

NATURAL COURSE AND PATHOGENESIS OF UNTREATED SYPHILIS *Treponema pallidum* can rapidly penetrate intact mucous membranes or abraded skin and within a few hours enters the lymphatics and blood to produce systemic infection and metastatic foci long before and after the appearance of a primary lesion. Blood from a patient with incubating syphilis is infectious. The generation time of *T. pallidum* in vivo is estimated to be 30 to 33 h, and the incubation period of syphilis is inversely proportional to the number of organisms inoculated. The concentration of treponemes generally reaches at least 10^7 per gram of tissue before the appearance of a clinical lesion. In experimental infection in rabbits or humans, very low numbers of treponemes can initiate infection which leads to a discernible lesion only after several weeks, although histopathologic changes are evident earlier; intradermal injection of 10^6 organisms usually produces a lesion within 72 h. The number of organisms required for production of symptomatic infection in humans was determined by intradermal injection of three graded doses of *T. pallidum* simultaneously at separate inoculation sites into each of eight volunteers. While lesions developed at all sites infected with 10^3 organisms, chancres appeared at 63 and 38 percent of sites inoculated with 10^2 and 10 *T. pallidum*, respectively, with incubation periods ranging from 20 to 42 days for the lowest dose. Based upon these results, the infectious dose 50 (ID_{50}) was calculated to be 57 organisms. The median incubation period in humans is about 21 days, suggesting an average inoculum of 500 to 1000 infectious organisms for naturally acquired disease. Although the incubation period is traditionally stated as ranging from 9 to 90 days, experimental inoculations of humans and rabbits show that the period from inoculation until the primary lesion is discernible rarely exceeds 6 weeks. Subcurative therapy during the incubation period may delay the onset of the primary lesion, but it is not certain that this reduces the probability of ultimate development of symptomatic disease.

The primary lesion appears at the site of inoculation, usually persists for 2 to 6 weeks, and then heals spontaneously. Histopathology of primary lesions shows perivascular infiltration, chiefly by lymphocytes, plasma cells, and histiocytes, with capillary endothelial proliferation, and subsequent obliteration of small blood vessels. At this time *T. pallidum* is demonstrable in the chancre in spaces between epithelial cells as well as within invaginations or phagosomes of epithelial cells, fibroblasts, plasma cells, and the endothelial cells of small capillaries, within lymphatic channels, and in the regional lymph nodes. Macrophages can be seen taking up treponemes into phagocytic vacuoles where the organisms are destroyed.

The generalized parenchymal, constitutional, and mucocutaneous manifestations of secondary syphilis usually appear about 6 to 8 weeks after healing of the chancre, although 15 percent of patients with secondary syphilis have persisting or healing chancres. In other patients, secondary lesions may appear only several months after the chancre has healed, and some patients may enter the latent stage without ever developing secondary lesions. Secondary maculopapular skin lesions show histopathologic features of hyperkeratosis of the epidermis, capillary proliferation with endothelial swelling in the superficial corium, and dermal papillae with transmigration of polymorphonuclear leukocytes, and in the deeper corium, perivascular infiltration by monocytes, plasma cells, and lymphocytes. Treponemes are found in many tissues including the aqueous humor of the eye and the cerebrospinal fluid. Cerebrospinal fluid abnormalities are detected in as many as 40 percent of patients during the secondary stage. Hepatitis and immune complex–induced glomerulonephritis are relatively rare but recognized manifestations of early syphilis. Generalized lymphadenopathy is present in 85 percent of patients with secondary syphilis, and is characterized by marked follicular hyperplasia, with histiocytic infiltration and lymphocyte depletion of the paracortical areas, where treponema are present in greatest numbers. The reason for the paradoxical appearance of secondary manifestations in the face of high titers of humoral antibody (including immobilizing antibody) to *T. pallidum* is unknown. The secondary lesions subside within 2 to 6 weeks, and the patient enters the latent stage, which is detectable only by serologic testing. In the preantibiotic era, up to 25 percent of untreated patients experienced one or more subsequent generalized or localized mucocutaneous relapses at some time during the first 2 to 4 years after infection. Since 90 percent of such infectious relapses occur during the first year, identification and examination of sexual contacts are most important for patients with syphilis of less than 1 year's duration.

The World Health Organization now arbitrarily divides latent syphilis into early latent (less than 1 year's duration) and late latent (over 1 year's duration) stages. However, because infectious relapse can occur during the first 2 years, and because the risk of congenital syphilis continues to be high during the first 2 years after acquisition of infection, the International Classification of Diseases defines early latent syphilis as less than 2 years' duration and late latent as over 2 years' duration. In the preantibiotic period, about one-third of patients with untreated latent syphilis developed clinically apparent tertiary disease; today, in medically advanced societies, specific and coincidental therapy of early and latent syphilis have greatly reduced the incidence of tertiary disease. In the past, the most common type of tertiary disease was the gumma, a usually benign granulomatous lesion. Today, gummas are very uncommon, perhaps because they respond to very low doses of antitreponemal drugs. The remaining tertiary lesions are caused by obliterative small vessel endarteritis which usually involves the vasa vasorum of the ascending aorta and, less often, the central nervous system. Factors which determine development of tertiary disease are unknown.

The course of untreated syphilis has been studied retrospectively in a group of nearly 2000 patients with primary or secondary syphilis diagnosed clinically, before the dark-field and Wasserman tests came into use (the Oslo Study, 1891–1951); prospectively in 431 black men with seropositive latent syphilis of 3 or more years' duration (the Tuskegee Study, 1932–1972); and retrospectively in a review of 198 autopsies of patients with untreated syphilis.

In the Oslo Study, 24 percent of the patients developed relapsing secondary lesions within 4 years, and 28 percent eventually developed one or more manifestations of late syphilis. Cardiovascular syphilis, including aortitis, was detected in 10 percent, with no cases occurring in those infected before age 15; symptomatic neurosyphilis occurred in 7 percent, and 16 percent developed benign tertiary syphilis (gumma of the skin, mucous membranes, and skeleton). Syphilis was the primary cause of death in 15 percent of males and 8 percent of the females. However, many patients alive when the Oslo Study was completed remained at risk for developing complications, while tuberculosis and other infections prematurely eliminated others before complications of syphilis occurred, so the Oslo figures probably represent minimum estimates of the risk of late complications. Cardiovascular syphilis was found in 35 percent of men and 22 percent of women who eventually underwent autopsy. In general, serious late complications were nearly twice as common in men as in women.

The Tuskegee Study showed that the death rate of untreated syphilitic black men, 25 to 50 years of age, was 17 percent greater than in nonsyphilitics, and 30 percent of all deaths were attributable to cardiovascular or central nervous system syphilis. The ethical issues raised by this study, begun in the preantibiotic era but continuing into the early 1970s, had a major influence on development of current guidelines for human medical experimentation. By far the most important factor in increased mortality was cardiovascular syphilis. Anatomic evidence of aortitis was found in 40 to 60 percent of autopsied syphilitics (versus 15 percent of controls), while central nervous system lues was found in only 4 percent. Hypertension was also increased in the syphilitics. The incidence of cardiovascular syphilis was higher and central nervous system syphilis lower in the prospective Tuskegee Study than in the Oslo Study. These studies each show that about one-third of patients with untreated syphilis develop clinical or pathologic evidence of tertiary syphilis; about one-fourth die as a direct result of tertiary syphilis; and additional excess mortality not directly attributable to tertiary syphilis is also seen. Untreated syphilis may make people more susceptible to other diseases, or individuals who get syphilis coincidentally may be more susceptible to other diseases, perhaps because of socioeconomic factors.

MANIFESTATIONS Primary syphilis The typical primary chancre usually begins as a single painless papule which rapidly becomes eroded and usually, but not always, is indurated, with a characteristic cartilaginous consistency on palpation of the edge and base of the ulcer (Fig. 122-1). Histologic examination of the ulcer shows mononuclear and histiocytic infiltrates with obliterative endarteritis and periarteritis of small vessels. *Treponema pallidum* is seen by electron microscopy to lie in interstitial perivascular spaces and within invaginations or phagosomes of macrophages, neutrophils, endothelial cells, and plasma cells.

In heterosexual men, the chancre is usually located on the penis. In homosexual men, the chancre is often found in the anal canal or rectum, within the mouth, or on the external genitalia. It may occur on any site of the body. In women, common primary sites are the cervix and labia. Primary syphilis is often overlooked in women or in homosexual men. For example, during 1974 in the United States, 42 percent of cases of early syphilis in heterosexual men were detected in the primary stages, whereas only 23 percent of early cases in homosexual men and 11 percent of early cases in women were detected in the primary stages. Anorectal chancres account for only 15 percent of primary syphilis among homosexuals in the United States, suggesting that anorectal chancres are most often asymptomatic or are not sought by clinicians evaluating men with suspected syphilis, or that the clinician fails to consider syphilis in the evaluation of anal lesions in men.

Regional lymphadenopathy accompanies the primary lesion, appearing within 1 week of the onset of the lesion. The nodes are firm, nonsuppurative, and painless. Inguinal lymphadenopathy is bilateral and may occur with anal as well as with genital chancres, since lymphatic drainage of the anus involves inguinal nodes. The chancre heals within 4 to 6 weeks (range 2 to 12 weeks), but the lymphadenopathy may persist for months.

Atypical primary lesions are common. The clinical appearance depends upon the number of treponemes inoculated and upon the preinfection immune status of the patient. A large inoculum produces a dark-field–positive ulcerative lesion in nonimmune human volunteers, but in individuals with a previous history of syphilis may produce either a small dark-field–negative papule, an asymptomatic but seropositive latent infection, or no response at all. A small inoculum usually produces only a papular lesion, even in nonimmune humans. Therefore, syphilis should be considered even in the evaluation of trivial or atypical, dark-field–negative, genital lesions. The most common genital lesions which must be differentiated from primary syphilis include traumatic superinfected lesions, genital herpes simplex virus infection (see Chap. 136), and chancroid (see Chap. 110). *Primary genital herpes* may produce inguinal adenopathy, but the nodes are tender and associated with multiple painful vesicles which later ulcerate, and with systemic symptoms including fever; *recurrent genital herpes* typically begins with a cluster of painful vesicles, usually without associated adenopathy. *Chancroid* produces painful, superficial exudative, nonindurated, more often multiple ulcers; adenopathy is either unilateral or bilateral, is tender, and may suppurate.

FIGURE 122-1 *Primary chancre on the penis. (Reprinted, with permission, from Sexually Transmitted Diseases, Prof. Dr. E. Stolz, Rotterdam, ©Boehringer Ingelheim International, 1977.)*

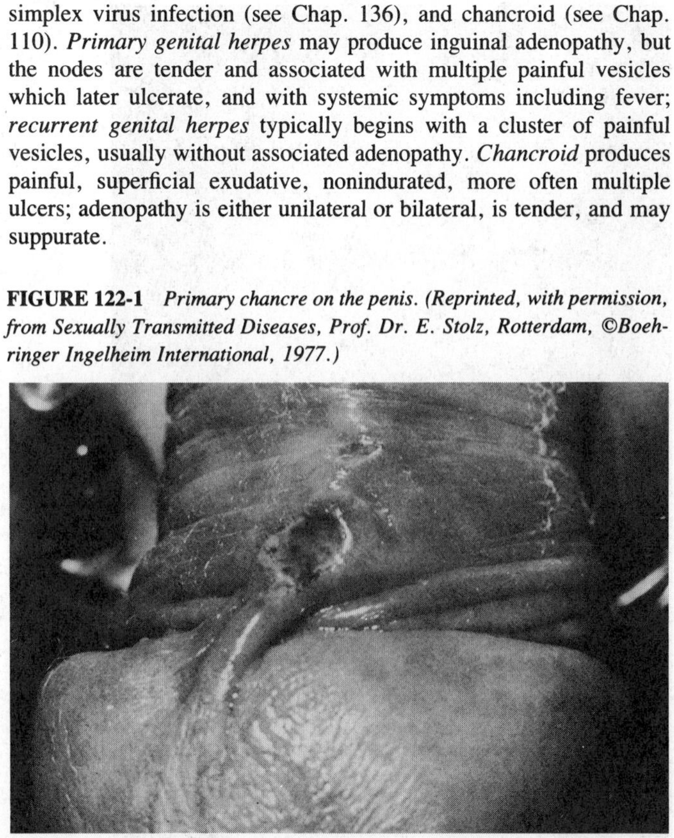

Secondary syphilis The manifestations of the secondary stage are protean but usually include localized or diffuse symmetric mucocutaneous lesions and generalized nontender lymphadenopathy. The healing primary chancre is still present in 15 percent of cases. The skin rash consists of macular, papular, papulosquamous, and occasionally pustular syphilides, often with one or more forms present simultaneously. The eruption may be very subtle, and approximately 25 percent of patients with a discernible rash of secondary syphilis may be unaware that they have dermatologic manifestations. Initial lesions are bilaterally symmetric, pale red or pink, nonpruritic, discrete, round macules, 5 to 10 mm in diameter, distributed on the trunk and proximal extremities (Fig. 122-2). After 1 to 2 months, red, papular lesions 3 to 10 mm in diameter also appear. These may progress to necrotic lesions (resembling pustules) in association with increasing endarteritis and perivascular mononuclear infiltration. These lesions are distributed widely and may occur on the palms, soles (Fig. 122-3), face, and scalp. Tiny papular *follicular syphilides* involving hair follicles may result in patchy alopecia (alopecia areata) and loss of scalp hair, eyebrows, or beard. Nonpatchy hair loss (telogen effluvium) also occurs in secondary syphilis, as in other systemic diseases. Progressive endarteritis obliterans and ischemia result in superficial scaling of papules (*papulosquamous syphilides*) and eventually may lead to central necrosis (*pustular syphilide*). In warm, moist, intertriginous areas, including the perianal area, vulva, scrotum, and inner thighs, axillae, and the skin under pendulous breasts, papules enlarge and become eroded, to produce broad, moist, pink or gray-white highly infectious lesions called *condylomata lata*, which are seen in 10 percent of patients with secondary syphilis. Superficial mucosal erosions, called *mucous patches*, occur in up to one-third of patients and may involve lips, oral mucosa, tongue (Fig. 122-4), palate, pharynx, vulva and vagina, glans penis, or inner prepuce. The typical mucous patch is a silver-gray erosion surrounded by a red periphery and is usually painless.

FIGURE 122-2 *Maculopapular rash of secondary syphilis. (Reprinted, with permission, from Sexually Transmitted Diseases, Prof. Dr. E. Stolz, Rotterdam, ©Boehringer Ingelheim International, 1977.)*

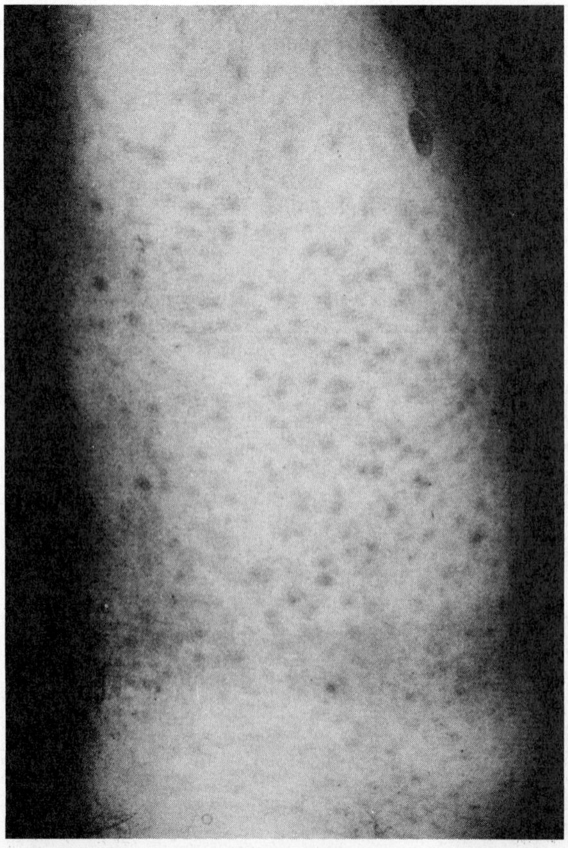

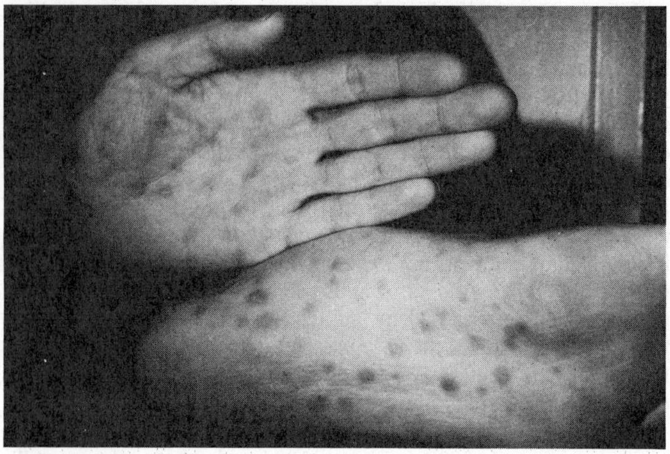

FIGURE 122-3 *Secondary rash on palms and soles. (From Ronald Roddy; reprinted, with permission, from Gynecology and Obstetrics, JW Sciarra (ed), New York, Harper & Row, 1985.)*

During relapses of secondary syphilis, condylomata lata are particularly common, and skin lesions tend to be asymmetrically distributed and more infiltrated, resembling skin lesions of late syphilis, perhaps reflecting increasing cellular immunity.

Constitutional symptoms which may accompany or precede secondary syphilis include sore throat (15 to 30 percent), fever (5 to 8 percent), weight loss (2 to 20 percent), malaise (25 percent), anorexia, headache (10 percent), and meningismus (5 percent). *Acute meningitis* occurs in only 1 to 2 percent of patients, but increased cells and protein have been found in the cerebrospinal fluid in 30 percent or more. *Treponema pallidum* has also been recovered by rabbit inoculation from cerebrospinal fluid during secondary syphilis in up to 40 percent of patients; this is often correlated with other cerebrospinal fluid (CSF) abnormalities, but may also be seen in patients with normal CSF.

Gastrointestinal involvement can be found with surprising frequency during secondary syphilis and may include hypertrophic syphilitic gastritis suggestive of linitis plastica or lymphosarcoma of the stomach, patchy proctitis, or an ulcerative or mass lesion resembling a rectosigmoid neoplasm.

Other less common complications of secondary syphilis include hepatitis, nephropathy, arthritis and periostitis, and iridocyclitis. Ocular findings which suggest secondary syphilis include otherwise unexplained pupillary abnormalities, optic neuritis, and a retinitis pigmentosa syndrome, as well as the classic iritis (especially granu-

FIGURE 122-4 *Mucous patches on the tongue. (From Ronald Roddy; reprinted, with permission, from Sexually Transmitted Diseases, KK Holmes et al (eds), New York, McGraw-Hill, 1984.)*

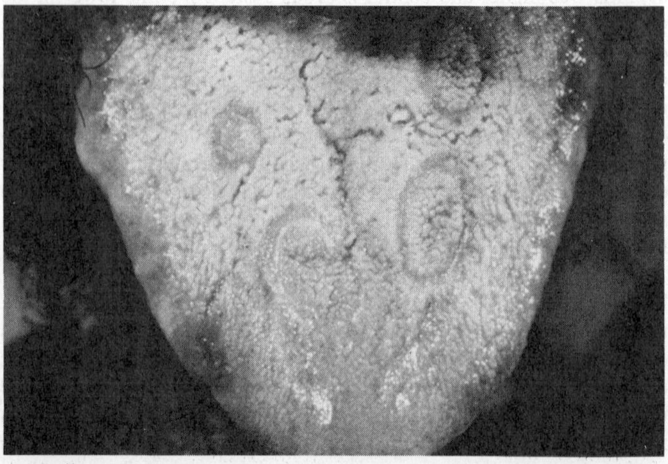

lomatous iritis) or uveitis. The diagnosis of secondary syphilis is often considered only after failure to respond to steroid therapy. *Syphilitic hepatitis* is distinguished by an unusually high serum alkaline phosphatase and by a nonspecific histologic appearance which is unlike viral hepatitis and includes moderate inflammation with polymorphonuclear leukocytes and lymphocytes, some hepatocellular damage, and no cholestasis. The *renal involvement* is associated with proteinuria, an acute nephrotic syndrome, or rarely with hemorrhagic glomerulonephritis and is characterized by subepithelial electron-dense deposits and glomerular immune complexes, suggesting that this complication is a form of immune complex glomerulonephritis. Anterior uveitis has been reported in 5 to 10 percent of patients with secondary syphilis, and *T. pallidum* has been demonstrated in the aqueous humor in such cases.

Latent syphilis A diagnosis of latent syphilis is established by the finding of a positive specific treponemal antibody test for syphilis, together with a normal cerebrospinal fluid examination, the absence of clinical manifestations of syphilis on physical examination and chest films, and a history of primary or secondary lesions, history of exposure to syphilis, or delivery of an infant with congenital syphilis. *Early latent* syphilis encompasses the first year after infection, while *late latent* syphilis, beginning 1 year after infection, in the untreated patient, is associated with relative immunity to infectious relapse and with increasing resistance to reinfection. *Treponema pallidum* may still intermittently seed the bloodstream during this stage, pregnant women with latent syphilis may infect the fetus in utero, and transfusion syphilis has been transmitted from patients with latent syphilis of many years' duration. Until recently, it was thought that untreated late latent syphilis had three possible outcomes; (1) it could persist throughout the life of the infected individual; (2) it could end in development of late syphilis; or (3) it could end with spontaneous cure of infection, with reversion of serologic tests to negative. It is now apparent, however, that the more sensitive treponemal antibody tests rarely if ever become negative. Fifty to seventy percent of untreated patients with latent syphilis never develop clinically evident late syphilis, but the occurrence of spontaneous cure is in doubt.

Late syphilis The onset of slowly progressive inflammatory disease of the aorta or central nervous system begins early during the pathogenesis of syphilis. Evidence of early syphilitic aortitis is present soon after the secondary lesions subside, and it is patients who develop CSF abnormalities during the early stages of syphilis who appear to be at risk of late neurologic complications.

ASYMPTOMATIC NEUROSYPHILIS In patients with untreated latent syphilis, if the CSF is normal 2 years or more after infection, there is probably no future risk of subsequent development of neurosyphilis, except for the purely vascular type. The diagnosis of asymptomatic neurosyphilis is made in patients with no clinical manifestations of neurosyphilis who have cerebrospinal fluid abnormalities, including pleocytosis, elevated protein, or positive cerebrospinal fluid Wasserman or Venereal Disease Research Laboratory (VDRL) tests. One or more of these findings are present in 20 to 30 percent of patients with untreated syphilis after 2 years, and spontaneous regression to normal is rare. The risk of progression to symptomatic neurosyphilis is two or three times greater in whites than in blacks and is twice as common in men as in women. The risk of parenchymal neurosyphilis (tabes dorsalis or general paresis) is five times greater in men than in women. In patients with untreated asymptomatic neurosyphilis, the overall cumulative probability of progression to clinical neurosyphilis is about 20 percent in the first 10 years, but increases with passing time, and is highest in those who show the greatest degree of pleocytosis or protein elevation. The evaluation of CSF for treponemal antibody is controversial and complex and is discussed below under "Laboratory Diagnosis."

SYMPTOMATIC NEUROSYPHILIS Although mixed features are common, the major clinical categories of symptomatic neurosyphilis include meningovascular and parenchymatous syphilis. The latter category includes general paresis and tabes dorsalis. The interval from infection to onset of symptoms is a few months to 12 years (average 7 years) for meningovascular syphilis, 20 years for general paresis, and 25 to 30 years for tabes dorsalis. However, many patients with symptomatic neurosyphilis, particularly in the antibiotic era, do not present a classic picture, but have mixed and subtle or incomplete syndromes. *Meningovascular syphilis* is associated with diffuse inflammation of the pia and arachnoid, together with evidence of focal or widespread arterial involvement of small, medium, or large vessels. The most common presentation is a stroke syndrome in a relatively young adult, involving the middle cerebral artery; however, unlike the usual thrombotic or embolic stroke syndrome of sudden onset, meningovascular syphilis often presents after a subacute encephalitic prodrome with headaches, vertigo, insomnia, and psychologic abnormalities followed by a gradually progressive vascular syndrome. The manifestations of *general paresis* reflect widespread parenchymal damage and include abnormalities corresponding to the mnemonic *paresis* [*p*ersonality, *a*ffect, *r*eflexes (hyperactive), *e*ye (e.g., Argyll Robertson pupils), *s*ensorium (illusions, delusions, hallucinations), *i*ntellect (decreased recent memory orientation, calculations, judgment, insight), and *s*peech]. *Tabes dorsalis* presents symptoms and signs of demyelinization of the posterior column, dorsal roots, and dorsal root ganglia. Symptoms include ataxic, wide-based gait and footslap, paresthesias, bladder disturbances, impotence, areflexia, and loss of position, deep pain, and temperature sensation. Trophic joint degeneration (Charcot's joints) and perforating ulceration of the feet can result from loss of pain sensation. The Argyll Robertson pupil, seen in both tabes dorsalis and paresis, is a small, irregular pupil which reacts to accommodation but not to light. *Optic atrophy* also occurs frequently in association with tabes.

CARDIOVASCULAR SYPHILIS Cardiovascular manifestations are limited to the large vessels in which the blood supply is provided by vasa vasorum. Endarteritis obliterans of the vasa vasorum produces medial necrosis with destruction of elastic tissue, particularly in the ascending and transverse segments of the aortic arch, resulting in uncomplicated aortitis, aortic regurgitation, saccular aneurysm, or coronary ostial stenosis. Until recently, these complications had not been described following congenital syphilis or syphilis acquired before age 14, suggesting some unexplained resistance of the large blood vessels in youth to invasion by *T. pallidum*. The onset of symptoms occurs from 10 to 40 years after infection. Cardiovascular complications are more common and occur at an earlier age in men than in women, and in blacks than in whites. The incidence of symptomatic cardiovascular complications in late untreated syphilis is approximately 10 percent, with aortic regurgitation being two to four times as common as aneurysm. However, syphilitic aortitis can be demonstrated at autopsy in about one-half of black males with untreated syphilis.

Asymptomatic syphilitic aortitis may be suspected in life if linear calcification of the ascending aorta is demonstrated on chest x-ray films, since arteriosclerotic disease seldom produces this sign. Aortic dilatation and a tambour quality of the sound of aortic closure are unreliable signs of aortitis. Syphilitic aneurysms are usually saccular, occasionally fusiform, and do not lead to dissection. Approximately 1 in 10 aortic aneurysms of syphilitic origin may involve the abdominal aorta, but tend to occur above the renal arteries, whereas arteriosclerotic abdominal aneurysms usually are found below the renal arteries. With increasing age, the nervous system is also affected in up to 40 percent of patients with cardiovascular syphilis.

LATE LESIONS OF THE EYES Iritis associated with pain, photophobia, and dimness of vision or chorioretinitis occurs not only during secondary syphilis, but also as a relatively common manifestation of late syphilis. Adhesions of the iris to the anterior lens may produce a fixed pupil, not to be confused with Argyll Robertson pupil.

LATE BENIGN SYPHILIS (GUMMA) Gummas may be multiple or diffuse, but are usually solitary lesions which range from microscopic size to several centimeters in diameter, and histologically consist of granulomatous inflammation with central necrosis surrounded by mononuclear, epithelioid, and fibroblastic cells, occasional giant cells, and perivasculitis. Although *T. pallidum* is rarely demonstrated microscopically, it has reportedly been recovered from the lesions by rabbit inoculation. The most commonly involved sites are the skin and skeletal systems, mouth and upper respiratory tract, larynx, liver, and stomach. Virtually any organ may be involved. Gummas of skin produce painless nodular, papulosquamous, or ulcerative lesions, which are indurated, and form characteristic circles or arcs, with peripheral hyperpigmentation. The lesions are usually indolent, and may heal spontaneously with scarring, but may also be explosive in onset and are often destructive. These lesions may resemble many other chronic granulomatous conditions, including tuberculosis and sarcoidosis, leprosy, and deep fungal infections. Skeletal gummas involve long bones of the legs with greatest frequency, although any bone may be affected. Trauma may predispose to involvement of a specific site. Presenting symptoms usually include focal pain and tenderness. When sufficiently advanced to produce radiographic abnormalities, the findings may include periostitis or destructive or sclerosing osteitis. Gummas of the upper respiratory tract can lead to perforation of the nasal septum or palate. Gummatous hepatitis may produce epigastric pain and tenderness and low-grade fever, and may be associated with splenomegaly and anemia.

The histopathology and extensive tissue necrosis associated with gummas suggest that delayed hypersensitivity to *T. pallidum* produces these lesions. Certain individuals appear to develop an exaggerated delayed hypersensitivity response to *T. pallidum,* presumably mediated by sensitized T lymphocytes and macrophages. In areas where syphilis is endemic in childhood, reinfection may result in gummas; when one member of a household acquires a fresh infection, other members of the household who then become reinfected develop gummas. Experimental inoculation of *T. pallidum* into individuals with latent or late syphilis also sometimes results in gumma formation at the site of inoculation.

Since the histologic changes may be suggestive but are nonspecific, the diagnosis of late benign syphilis is confirmed by serologic testing and by therapeutic trial. Treatment with penicillin results in rapid healing of active gummatous lesions.

Congenital syphilis Transmission of *T. pallidum* from a syphilitic mother to her fetus across the placenta may occur at any stage of pregnancy, but the lesions of congenital syphilis develop only after the fourth month of gestation, when immunologic competence begins to develop. This suggests that the pathogenesis of congenital syphilis may depend upon the immune response of the host rather than upon a direct toxic effect of *T. pallidum.* The risk of infection of the fetus during untreated early maternal syphilis is estimated to be 75 to 95 percent, decreasing to about 35 percent for maternal syphilis of longer than 2 years' duration, with the risk of fetal infection apparently continuing during late latent maternal syphilis. Adequate treatment of the mother before the sixteenth week of pregnancy should prevent fetal damage. During the past decade, the number of reported cases of congenital syphilis in infants less than 1 year of age in the United States has remained steady at about 2 cases per 100 reported cases of primary and secondary syphilis in women. However, the dramatic rise in the number of reported cases of primary and secondary syphilis in women between 1978 and 1983, from 5331 to 9082 cases, was consequently accompanied by a striking 48 percent increase in reported congenital syphilis in infants, from 107 to 158 cases. In 1984, 240 infants with congenital syphilis were reported, a 120 percent increase over the 1978 low figure. A study of 50 cases reported in 1982 showed that 56 percent of the mothers of infected children had not sought prenatal examination, but had reactive serologic tests at delivery, 14 percent had negative or no serologic test performed during prenatal care, and 14 percent were serologically nonreactive at delivery and were presumably infected late in pregnancy. Laboratory error and physicians' delay in therapy only contributed to 2 and 6 percent, respectively, of the cases, and 8 percent represented treatment failure. Syphilis acquired during pregnancy may remain subclinical in the mother while nearly always causing serious fetal infection. Untreated maternal infection may result in up to 40 percent fetal loss (stillbirth is more common than abortion, because of the late onset of fetal pathology), prematurity, neonatal death, or nonfatal congenital syphilis. Of mothers with untreated syphilis of <2 years' duration, 21 percent aborted or had a stillbirth, 13 percent had infants who died within 2 months, 43 percent had infants with syphilis alive at 2 months, and 23 percent had nonsyphilitic infants. Therefore, routine serologic testing in early pregnancy as well as at delivery and repeat serologic testing of "high-risk" pregnant women in the third trimester are fully justified.

Only fulminant cases of congenital syphilis are clinically apparent in live infants at birth, and these babies have a very poor prognosis. The most common clinical problem is the healthy appearing baby born to a mother who has a positive serologic test.

The manifestations of congenital syphilis can be divided into (1) early manifestations, which appear within the first 2 years of life, often between 2 and 10 weeks of age, are infectious, and resemble severe secondary syphilis in the adult; (2) late manifestations, which appear after 2 years, and are noninfectious; and (3) the residual stigmata of congenital syphilis. During 1984, 75 percent of reported cases of congenital syphilis were diagnosed during the first year of life.

The earliest sign of congenital syphilis is usually rhinitis ("snuffles") soon followed by other mucocutaneous lesions. These may include bullae (syphilitic pemphigus), vesicles, superficial desquamation, petechiae, and later, papulosquamous lesions, mucous patches, and condylomata lata. The most common early manifestations are osteochondritis and osteitis, particularly involving the metaphyses of long bones, progressing in severity during the first 6 months of life, then spontaneously subsiding; and periostitis, which continues to progress after the first 6 months. Hepatosplenomegaly, lymphadenopathy, anemia, jaundice, thrombocytopenia, and leukocytosis are common. The anemia is usually hypoproliferative but may be hemolytic (paroxysmal cold hemoglobinuria). The nephrotic syndrome in early congenital syphilis, as in adult secondary syphilis, represents an immune complex–induced glomerulonephritis.

Neonatal congenital syphilis must be differentiated from other generalized congenital infections, including rubella, cytomegalovirus or herpes simplex virus infection, and toxoplasmosis, and also from erythroblastosis fetalis. Neonatal death is usually due to pulmonary hemorrhage, secondary bacterial infection, or severe hepatitis. Pathologic findings include interstitial and perivascular inflammation followed by variable fibroblastic proliferation, involving skin, bones, liver, kidneys, pancreas, spleen, lungs, and intestines, and by extramedullary hematopoiesis.

Late congenital syphilis is defined as congenital syphilis which remains untreated after 2 years of age. In perhaps 60 percent of cases, the infection remains latent, while the clinical spectrum in the remainder differs in certain respects from that of acquired late syphilis in the adult. For example, cardiovascular syphilis rarely develops in late congenital syphilis, whereas interstitial keratitis is much more common and occurs between ages 5 and 25. The onset is acute with photophobia, pain, and circumcorneal injection, followed by superficial and deep vascularization of the cornea, which progresses despite antibiotic therapy, and eventually becomes bilateral. The symptoms and signs may be suppressed with corticosteroid therapy. Although treponemes have occasionally been demonstrated in aqueous humor in interstitial keratitis, the pathogenesis is obscure and is ascribed to "hypersensitivity." Other manifestations associated with interstitial keratitis are eighth-nerve deafness and recurrent arthropathy. Bilateral knee effusions are known as *Clutton's joints.* Examination of CSF discloses asymptomatic neurosyphilis in about one-third of untreated patients without other late clinical manifestations, and clinical neurosyphilis occurs in a quarter of untreated individuals with congenital syphilis over 6 years of age. The clinical manifestations of congenital neurosyphilis correspond to those seen in adult neurosyphilis. Gummatous periostitis occurs between ages 5 and 20 and, as in nonvenereal endemic childhood syphilis, tends to cause destructive lesions of the palate and nasal septum.

Characteristic stigmata include Hutchinson's teeth, the centrally notched, widely spaced, peg-shaped upper central incisors, and "mulberry" molars, sixth-year molars which have multiple, poorly developed cusps, rather than the usual four. The abnormal facies, which includes frontal bossing, saddlenose, and poorly developed maxilla, may also be seen in congenital ectodermal dysplasia. Saber shins, or anterior tibial bowing, are rare but were probably more common in the past when syphilitic periostitis of the anterior tibia was associated with vitamin D deficiency. *Rhagades* are linear scars at the angles of the mouth and nose caused by secondary bacterial infection of the early facial eruption. Other stigmata include unexplained nerve deafness, old chorioretinitis, optic atrophy, and corneal opacities due to past interstitial keratitis.

LABORATORY EXAMINATIONS Dark-field examination technique Dark-field examination is essential in evaluating cutaneous lesions, such as the chancre of primary syphilis, or condylomata lata of secondary syphilis. Although it is often difficult to demonstrate *T. pallidum* in dry maculopapular lesions in secondary syphilis by dark-field examination, the organism may be demonstrated by saline aspiration of lymph nodes during this stage. The surface of the suspected ulcerated lesion should be cleaned with saline and gauze, then gently abraded further with dry gauze, without production of bleeding. The lesion is then squeezed to express a serous transudate, and a drop of the transudate is picked up on the surface of a glass slide. A drop of saline (without bacteriostatic additives) may be mixed with the transudate if necessary, and this is then covered with a coverslip and examined immediately for *T. pallidum* with a dark-field or phase contrast microscope by an experienced individual. A single negative examination does not exclude syphilis, since at least 10^4 treponemes per milliliter transudate must be present to be detected, and prior use of topical antiseptic or cleansing by the patient may obfuscate the examination. Cleansing or use of topical medication should, therefore, be avoided, and the dark-field examination should be repeated on three successive days before being considered negative.

Direct immunofluorescence Most syphilis is diagnosed in private physicians' offices where dark-field microscopy is not available, and alternative methods for the identification of *T. pallidum* in exudate are needed. The direct fluorescent antibody *T. pallidum* (DFA-TP) test, available at central laboratories, uses fluorescein-conjugated polyclonal antitreponemal antibody for detection of *T. pallidum* in fixed smears prepared from suspect lesions. Because of cross-reactive antibodies which will also stain commensal nonpathogenic spirochetes, the antiserum is extensively absorbed with cultured treponemes in an effort to produce a specific reagent.

A refinement of this technique using a monoclonal antibody which is specific for only the pathogenic treponemes has been developed. It has been shown in clinical trials to be as sensitive and specific as dark-field microscopy for examination of suspicious lesions.

Demonstration of *T. pallidum* in tissue It is often necessary to demonstrate *T. pallidum* in tissue when clinical or histopathologic features suggest the diagnosis of syphilis. Although the organism can be found in tissue by appropriate silver stains, these should be interpreted with caution, because artifacts resembling *T. pallidum* are often seen. Treponemes can be demonstrated more reliably in tissue by immunofluorescence, using specific monoclonal or polyclonal antibodies against *T. pallidum*.

Serologic tests for syphilis The profusion of serologic tests for syphilis causes much unnecessary confusion. Syphilitic infection produces two types of antibodies, the nonspecific *reaginic* antibody and specific antitreponemal antibody, which are measured by the nontreponemal and treponemal tests, respectively (Table 122-1). The treponemal tests, as well as the nontreponemal tests, are reactive in persons with any treponemal infection, including yaws, pinta, and endemic syphilis.

The nontreponemal antibodies produced in syphilis contain both IgG and IgM immunoglobulins directed against a lipoidal antigen that results from the interaction of *T. pallidum* with host tissues, and possibly against a lipoidal antigen of *T. pallidum* itself. The term *reagin* is unfortunate, since the unrelated IgE antibody involved in certain allergic phenomena is also known as reagin.

The most widely used nontreponemal or reagin antibody tests are the rapid plasma reagin (RPR) test, which can be automated (ART), and the VDRL slide test. Other less frequently used nontreponemal tests include the unheated serum reagin (USR) and the reagin screen test (RST). In these tests, antibody is detected by the microscopic (VDRL, USR) or macroscopic (RPR, RST) flocculation of the antigen suspension (Table 122-1).

The RPR is often more expensive than the VDRL test but is easier to perform and uses unheated serum; it is the test of choice for rapid serologic diagnosis in a clinic or office setting. The VDRL reagents are less expensive, but must be prepared fresh daily. Although the development of the simpler macroscopic tests has resulted in the replacement of the VDRL by the RPR for examination of serum in many laboratories, the VDRL test remains the standard test for use with cerebrospinal fluid.

RPR and VDRL tests are equally sensitive and may be used for initial screening or for quantitation of serum reagin antibody titer. The reagin titer reflects the activity of the disease: a fourfold or greater rise in titer may be seen during the evolution of primary syphilis; VDRL titers usually reach 1:32 or higher in secondary syphilis; a persistent fall in titer following treatment of early syphilis provides essential evidence of an adequate response to therapy. VDRL titers do not correspond directly to RPR titers, and sequential quantitative testing (as for response to therapy) must employ a single test.

There are three standard treponemal tests: the fluorescent treponemal antibody-absorption (FTA-ABS), the microhemagglutination assay for antibodies to *T. pallidum* (MHA-TP), and the hemagglutination treponemal test for syphilis (HATTS). A third hemagglutination test, the TPHA, is widely used in Canada and Europe, but is not available in the United States.

For the FTA-ABS test, the patient's serum is first diluted with a substance containing nonpathogenic treponemal antigens (sorbent) to bind group-specific antibodies which may be produced against saprophytic oral and genital treponemes. The patient's absorbed serum is then placed on a slide which contains fixed *T. pallidum*. If specific antibody to *T. pallidum* is present in the patient's serum, it is bound to the dried treponemes, and then is detected by the addition of fluorescein-labeled antihuman gamma globulin and subsequent examination of the slide by fluorescence microscopy. The *T. pallidum* hemagglutination tests (MHA-TP, HATTS, and TPHA) also use a sorbent-like diluent for binding treponemal group antibodies. *T. pallidum*–specific antibody is detected by agglutination of *T. pallidum*–coated sheep or turkey erythrocytes. The *T. pallidum* immobilization (TPI) test, in which immobilization of live *T. pallidum* is produced by immune serum plus complement, is the most specific treponemal test, but is more laborious, and in the United States is available only

TABLE 122-1 Common serologic tests for syphilis

NONTREPONEMAL (REAGIN) TESTS
Microscopic flocculation: Venereal Disease Research Laboratory (VDRL)
Macroscopic flocculation: rapid plasma reagin (RPR)
TREPONEMAL TESTS
Immunofluorescence: fluorescent treponemal antibody-absorption (FTA-ABS)
Hemagglutination: *T. pallidum* hemagglutination assay (MHA-TP, HATTS, TPHA)
Immobilization: *Treponema pallidum* immobilization (TPI)

in research laboratories. Both the hemagglutination and FTA-ABS tests are very specific and, when used for confirmation of positive reaginic antibody tests, have a very high positive predictive value for the diagnosis of syphilis. However, even these tests give false-positive rates as high as 1 to 2 percent when used for screening normal populations.

The relative sensitivities of the VDRL, FTA-ABS, and MHA-TP tests in the various stages of syphilis are shown in Table 122-2. The nontreponemal tests are nonreactive in nearly one-third of patients with primary or late syphilis. In early primary syphilis, the detection of antibody can be maximized either by performing an FTA-ABS test or simply by repeating a VDRL test after 1 to 2 weeks if the initial VDRL was negative. However, obtaining a reagin antibody test alone is not sufficient in evaluating late symptomatic syphilis; the more sensitive FTA-ABS test should be obtained routinely in suspected late syphilis. The hemagglutination tests are even less sensitive than the reagin tests in primary syphilis, but are as sensitive as the FTA-ABS in other stages. All treponemal and nontreponemal tests are reactive during secondary syphilis, and a nonreactive result virtually excludes syphilis in a patient with otherwise compatible mucocutaneous lesions. (An estimated 1 to 2 percent of patients with secondary syphilis have a nonreactive or weakly reactive VDRL test with undiluted serum which becomes positive in higher dilutions—the *prozone* phenomenon.)

False-positive serologic tests for syphilis Because the antigen used in the nontreponemal tests is found in other tissues, the tests may be reactive in persons without treponemal infection, although rarely in titers exceeding 1:8. Of all reactive reagin tests, an estimated 20 to 40 percent are false-positive, but the percentages vary widely depending upon the population being examined. In a population which has been selected for screening because of clinical suspicion, history of exposure, or increased risk for sexually transmitted infections, the percentage of reactive tests which are falsely positive is much lower. False-positive reagin tests are classified as acute if they become negative within 6 months. Acute false-positive reagin tests occur during a variety of acute infections, such as viral diseases, mycoplasma pneumonia, and malaria, and following certain immunizations. Chronic reactions, which persist 6 months or longer, occur in addiction, autoimmune diseases, and aging. False-positive reagin tests occur in 25 percent of narcotics addicts, and in 10 to 20 percent of patients with active systemic lupus erythematosus. The autoimmune nature of the false-positive reagin test is suggested by the occurrence of systemic lupus erythematosus or other connective tissue diseases in 15 to 45 percent of chronic false-positive reactors. Other antibodies which have been found with great frequency in serums from chronic false-positive reactors include antinuclear, antithyroid, and antimitochondrial antibodies, as well as rheumatoid factor and cryoglobulins. The Donath-Landsteiner antibody responsible for paroxysmal cold hemoglobinuria is a hemolysin which appears in syphilis. The prevalence of false-positive reagin tests increases with advancing age, and 10 percent of people over 70 years of age have false-positive reactions. Other diseases associated with hyperglobulinemia, such as leprosy, may also produce chronic false-positive reactions.

In the patient with a false-positive reagin test, syphilis is excluded by obtaining a nonreactive treponemal test. The results of the FTA-ABS test are reported as negative, borderline, or reactive. *Borderline* results are more common in patients who are pregnant or have diseases associated with abnormal or increased globulins, and are frequently not associated with either clinical, historical, or other serologic evidence of syphilis. Borderline results should, therefore, always be repeated in questionable cases and interpreted with caution. A typical *reactive* FTA-ABS occurs infrequently in conditions other than syphilis. Although false-positive FTA-ABS tests have been reported in 15 percent of patients with active systemic lupus erythematosus, the fluorescent staining is "borderline" or has an atypical "beaded" appearance in most cases (thought to be due to attachment of antinuclear antibody to treponemal DNA or nucleoprotein leaked through breaks in the outer treponemal membranes). However, because of the occasional occurrence of false-positive FTA-ABS tests, only a positive TPI provides conclusive proof of past or present treponemal infection.

For practical purposes, most clinicians need to be familiar with the three uses of serologic tests for syphilis: (1) for testing large numbers of serums for screening or diagnostic purposes (e.g., RPR or VDRL); (2) for quantitative measurement of reaginic antibody titer in order to assess the clinical activity of syphilis, or to follow the reagin titer in response to therapy (e.g., VDRL or RPR); and (3) for confirmation of the diagnosis of syphilis in a patient with a positive reagin antibody test or with a suspected clinical diagnosis of syphilis (e.g., FTA-ABS, MHA-TP, HATTS).

Evaluation for asymptomatic neurosyphilis Asymptomatic involvement of the central nervous system is detected by examination of cerebrospinal fluid (CSF). CSF abnormalities are very infrequent in the primary stage, but pleocytosis or elevated protein can be demonstrated in CSF from up to 40 percent of patients with secondary or latent syphilis. *T. pallidum* has been recovered by rabbit inoculation from up to 40 percent of those with secondary syphilis, but rarely from those with latent syphilis. The demonstration of *T. pallidum* in CSF is often associated with other CSF abnormalities; however, organisms can be recovered from patients without pleocytosis or elevated protein. In the prepenicillin era, the risk of developing clinical neurosyphilis was roughly proportional to the intensity of spinal fluid changes in early syphilis. CSF examination is essential in any seropositive patient with neurologic signs and symptoms and is recommended in all patients with untreated syphilis of unknown duration or of greater than 1 year's duration. The possibility that asymptomatic neurosyphilis is present in some patients with secondary and early latent disease is not addressed by these recommendations. Because standard therapy for early syphilis fails to achieve treponemicidal levels in the CSF, some experts currently advise lumbar puncture in secondary and early latent syphilis, with follow-up examinations for patients with abnormalities.

CSF is examined for pleocytosis, increased protein concentration, and VDRL reactivity. The CSF-VDRL is very specific if the fluid is not contaminated with blood. The CSF-VDRL is relatively insensitive, however, and may be nonreactive even in progressive symptomatic neurosyphilis. The unabsorbed FTA test on cerebrospinal fluid is reactive far more often than the VDRL test in all stages of syphilis, but may reflect passive transfer of serum antibody into the CSF. Most specialists do not recommend performing an FTA test on spinal fluid. Similarly, the finding of a reactive CSF-FTA-ABS test without other cerebrospinal fluid abnormalities in a patient with nonspecific neurologic findings does not prove a diagnosis of "atypical" neurosyphilis. However, even in the absence of confirmatory CSF examination, a therapeutic trial of penicillin in doses adequate for neurosyphilis is warranted in any patient with a positive serum treponemal antibody test who also has neurologic findings consistent with neurosyphilis.

Attempts to identify a more sensitive and specific marker for neurosyphilis have included CSF oligoclonal banding and measurement of intrathecal production of antitreponemal IgM and IgG. CSF

TABLE 122-2 Reactivity of serodiagnostic tests in untreated syphilis

Test	Stage of disease, % positive*			
	Primary	Secondary	Latent	Tertiary
VDRL	59–87	100	73–91	37–94
FTA-ABS	86–100	99–100	96–99	96–100
MHA-TP	64–87	96–100	96–100	94–100

* *Percentage figures provided should not be interpreted as absolute values because there are small numbers in certain categories and test results vary from study to study.*

SOURCE: *Modified (with permission) from H Jaffe, Management of the reactive serology, in Sexually Transmitted Diseases, KK Holmes et al (eds), New York, McGraw-Hill, 1984.*

from 80 percent of patients with multiple sclerosis and approximately 40 percent of patients with other inflammatory CNS diseases (including neurosyphilis, bacterial meningitis, viral encephalitis, subacute sclerosing panencephalitis) have discrete oligoclonal immunoglobulin bands in the gamma globulin region following agarose gel electrophoresis of CSF. These antibodies are thought to be intrathecally produced and have specificity for the etiologic agent (e.g., *T. pallidum* in syphilis and measles virus in subacute sclerosing panencephalitis); however, an oligoclonal banding pattern per se is not specific for neurosyphilis in a seropositive patient. The intrathecal production of specific anti-*T. pallidum* IgG and IgM antibodies has been estimated by several techniques which are still investigational.

TREATMENT OF ACQUIRED SYPHILIS Penicillin G is the drug of choice for all stages of syphilis. *Treponema pallidum* is killed by very low concentrations of penicillin G, although a long period of exposure to penicillin is required for treatment because of the unusually slow rate of multiplication of the organism. The efficacy of penicillin for syphilis remains undiminished after 40 years of use. Other antibiotics which are effective in syphilis include the tetracyclines, erythromycin, and the cephalosporins. Aminoglycosides inhibit *T. pallidum* only in very large doses, and the sulfonamides are inactive. The optimal dose and duration of therapy have not been established for any antimicrobial for any stage of syphilis. The U.S. Public Health Service recommendations are based on limited therapeutic trials and should be interpreted in light of the considerations noted below.

Recurrence rates for a given regimen increase as infection progresses from incubating syphilis to seronegative primary to seropositive primary to secondary to late syphilis. Therefore it is probable, but unproved, that a longer duration of therapy is required to effect cure as the infection progresses. For these reasons some authorities use more prolonged penicillin therapy than that recommended by the U.S. Public Health Service when treating secondary, latent, or late syphilis.

The optimal dose and duration of therapy have not been carefully evaluated in well-controlled studies. A variety of data suggests that it is necessary to achieve serum levels of penicillin G of 0.03 μg/mL or more for at least 7 days to cure early syphilis. Other tentative conclusions which can be gleaned from published studies include the following: (1) extending therapy with aqueous procaine penicillin G beyond 2 weeks does not improve cure rates for primary or secondary syphilis; (2) studies of experimental syphilis show that *T. pallidum* begin to regenerate if penicillinemia is allowed to fall to subinhibitory levels for periods of 18 to 24 h; (3) in human beings, increases in the dosage of crystalline penicillin G administered over 9 h from 0.03 to 0.6 mg/kg progressively increased the rate of disappearance of *T. pallidum* from chancres, but further increases in dosage did not further speed the disappearance of treponemes; and (4) the serum concentration of penicillin G achieved after one injection of 2.4 million units of benzathine penicillin G probably does not kill *T. pallidum* at the maximum rate.

The treatment regimens currently recommended for syphilis by the Centers for Disease Control are summarized in Table 122-3 and described below.

Early syphilis In very early incubating syphilis, treatment of concurrently acquired gonorrhea with 4.8 million units of procaine penicillin G (plus 1.0 g probenecid) aborts the syphilis. The ampicillin-probenecid and tetracycline regimens recommended for gonorrhea are probably also effective against incubating syphilis, although proof is not available. Follow-up serologic testing for syphilis is considered unnecessary in patients treated for gonorrhea with the recommended dose of procaine penicillin G, ampicillin, or tetracycline. Preventive (abortive, "epidemiologic") treatment is recommended for seronegative individuals without signs of syphilis who were exposed to infectious syphilis within the previous 6 weeks. Before treatment is given, every effort should be made to establish a diagnosis by examination and serologic testing. *The regimens recommended for preventive treatment are the same as those recommended for early syphilis.*

Benzathine penicillin G is the most widely used form of treatment for early syphilis, including primary, secondary, and early latent syphilis, although it is more painful on injection than procaine penicillin G. A single dose of 2.4 million units cures over 95 percent of cases of primary syphilis. Because efficacy for secondary syphilis may be slightly lower, some physicians administer a second dose of 2.4 million units 1 week after the initial dose for secondary syphilis.

TABLE 122-3 Recommended therapy for syphilis

Stage of syphilis	Patients without penicillin allergy	Patients with penicillin allergy
Primary, secondary, or early latent	Benzathine penicillin G, 2.4 million units single dose IM (1.2 million units in each hip).	Tetracycline hydrochloride, 2 g daily for 15 days.
Late latent or latent of uncertain duration	Lumbar Puncture *CSF normal:* Benzathine penicillin G, 2.4 million units IM weekly for 3 weeks. *CSF abnormal:* Treat as neurosyphilis.	Lumbar Puncture *CSF normal:* Treat as neurosyphilis. *CSF abnormal:* Treat as neurosyphilis.
Neurosyphilis* (asymptomatic or symptomatic)	Aqueous procaine penicillin G, 2.4 million units IM daily plus probenecid 500 mg, by mouth, 4 times a day, both for 10 days, followed by benzathine penicillin G, 2.4 million units IM weekly for 3 doses. *Or* aqueous penicillin G, 12 to 24 million units per day IV for at least 10 days, followed by benzathine penicillin G, 2.4 million units IM weekly for 3 doses.	Tetracycline hydrochloride, 2 g daily for 30 days.
Late cardiovascular or benign tertiary	Benzathine penicillin G, 2.4 million units IM weekly for 3 weeks.	Treat as for neurosyphilis.
Congenital (see text)	Aqueous procaine penicillin G, 50,000 units/kg, IM daily for at least 10 days. *Or* aqueous crystalline penicillin G, 50,000 units/kg per day, IM or IV, in two divided daily doses for at least 10 days. *Or, only if CSF normal:* benzathine penicillin G, 50,000 units/kg, IM, in a single dose.	Antibiotics other than penicillin should not be used.
Syphilis in pregnancy	According to stage.	See text.

* *Benzathine penicillin G has given inferior results for treatment of symptomatic neurosyphilis. Although tetracycline was recommended by the CDC Syphilis Therapy Advisory Committee for CNS Syphilis in penicillin-allergic patients, there is minimal experience with this drug (which does not achieve high CSF levels) in CNS syphilis. Doxycycline has higher theoretical efficacy than tetracycline hydrochloride for neurosyphilis because of better CSF penetration, although controlled studies have not been performed. Many patients who give a history of penicillin allergy prove negative when skin-tested for immediate hypersensitivity to penicillin and could be given aqueous crystalline penicillin G for CNS syphilis under close supervision in the hospital. Certain third-generation cephalosporins (e.g., ceftriaxone, cefotaxime) have some promise for penicillin-allergic patients with CNS syphilis but require further evaluation.*

SOURCE: *Sexually transmitted diseases treatment guidelines 1985. Morb Mort Week Rep Suppl 34(4S), 1985*

Late latent and late syphilis Recommended treatment for late latent syphilis with normal CSF, for cardiovascular syphilis, and for late benign syphilis (gumma) is benzathine penicillin G, 2.4 million units intramuscularly once a week for 3 successive weeks (7.2 million units total). Lumbar puncture should be performed in the evaluation of latent syphilis of more than 1 year's duration, in suspected neurosyphilis, and also in late complications other than symptomatic neurosyphilis, since asymptomatic neurosyphilis may coexist with other late complications. Abnormal cerebrospinal fluid findings can then be followed serially as a guide to therapy. No studies of benzathine penicillin G for cardiovascular syphilis have been reported, and the efficacy of penicillin therapy in any form for cardiovascular syphilis has not been proved. The response of cardiovascular syphilis to penicillin is seldom dramatic because aortic aneurysm and aortic regurgitation cannot be reversed by antibiotic treatment, although further progression of these lesions may be arrested.

In contrast, the response of benign tertiary syphilis and of meningovascular syphilis to penicillin G is usually impressive. The response of parenchymal neurosyphilis has been variable. In a cooperative study of the treatment of 1086 general paretics with penicillin, the frequency of clinical improvement or termination of progression ranged from 38 percent of those with severe involvement to 81 percent of those with mild involvement. All patients who relapsed following initial improvement in cerebrospinal fluid pleocytosis had received less than 6 million units of penicillin, and all had improvement of CSF pleocytosis with subsequent therapy. Tabes dorsalis or optic atrophy responds less often. In general, treatment of inactive neurosyphilis in which neurologic damage has already occurred may not produce any clinical change, and retreatment of such cases is not warranted. However, persistence of cerebrospinal fluid pleocytosis, or recurrence of pleocytosis following initial response to treatment, indicates continuing active infection, which should respond to additional treatment. The optimal dose and duration of penicillin for neurosyphilis has not been determined, but administration of 600,000 to 900,000 units of procaine penicillin G daily for 10 days has been about 90 percent effective. The 1985 Centers for Disease Control treatment guidelines for neurosyphilis are presented in Table 122-3. Since benzathine penicillin G given in single doses of 2.4 million units to adults or 50,000 units per kilogram to infants does not produce detectable concentrations of penicillin G in cerebrospinal fluid, this form of penicillin is unreliable for the treatment of neurosyphilis in the adult or infant, and asymptomatic neurosyphilis has been found to relapse in up to one-quarter of patients treated with 2.4 million units of benzathine penicillin. Many authorities therefore do not advocate use of benzathine penicillin alone for treatment of neurosyphilis. On the other hand, administration of intravenous penicillin G in doses of 12 million units or more per day for 10 days or longer ensures treponemicidal concentrations of penicillin G in cerebrospinal fluid, and occasionally cures patients who failed to respond to conventional therapy. There are no data to support the use of antibiotics other than penicillin G for the treatment of neurosyphilis; however, some of the third-generation cephalosporins (e.g., ceftriaxone, cefotaxime) may deserve further evaluation.

Management of syphilis in pregnancy Every pregnant woman should be tested with a nontreponemal test at her first prenatal visit, and women who are at high risk for acquiring sexually transmitted diseases should have a repeat test in the third trimester. In the pregnant patient with presumed syphilis, evidenced by a reactive serology, with or without clinical manifestations, and with no history of treatment for syphilis, expeditious evaluation and initiation of treatment is essential. Therapy should be administered according to stage of the disease, as for nonpregnant patients. Because of the risk of Jarisch-Herxheimer reaction, some experts advise that women with syphilis who are several months pregnant be hospitalized for treatment, to permit early administration of tocolytic therapy if premature labor should occur during the reaction.

If the patient has well-documented penicillin allergy, and this is confirmed by demonstration of an immediate wheal-and-flare response to skin testing with penicilloyl polylysine or penicillin G minor determinant mixture, no satisfactory and proven alternative to penicillin therapy is available. Erythromycin, the commonly recommended alternative in penicillin-allergic pregnant patients, crosses the placenta poorly, with fetal blood levels varying from 0 to 20 percent of maternal levels. The birth of infected infants has been reported following therapy for syphilis in several women treated during pregnancy with recommended doses of erythromycin. Erythromycin estolate is often associated with liver toxicity in pregnancy. Doxycycline, 100 mg twice daily for 15 days, or certain cephalosporins (e.g., ceftriaxone) may be preferable alternatives, although doxycycline has potential toxicity in pregnancy and cephalosporins may produce allergic reactions in some penicillin-allergic patients. After treatment, a quantitative reagin test should be repeated monthly throughout pregnancy, and if a fourfold rise in titer occurs, treatment should be repeated. Treated women who do not show a fourfold decrease in titer in a 3-month period should also be retreated.

Evaluation and management of congenital syphilis Newborn infants of mothers with reactive VDRL or FTA-ABS tests will themselves have reactive tests, whether or not they have become infected, because of transplacental transfer of maternal IgG antibody. Neonatal IgM antibody can be detected in cord or neonatal serums in a modified FTA-ABS test, employing fluorescein-labeled antihuman IgM to detect antitreponemal IgM antibody. However, the specificity of this test is questionable because of evidence that infants with a variety of congenital infections may produce IgM antibody to maternal allotypes of IgG (rheumatoid factor). IgM antibody detected in the IgM-FTA-ABS test may then be directed against maternal IgG antibody bound specifically to *T. pallidum,* rather than against *T. pallidum* itself. Because of the questionable sensitivity and specificity of this test, the IgM-FTA-ABS is not currently recommended. Instead, monthly quantitative reagin tests are performed on asymptomatic infants born to women who were treated adequately with penicillin during pregnancy. Rising or persistent titers indicate infection, and the infant should be treated. If the seropositive mother received inadequate penicillin treatment or treatment other than penicillin, or her treatment status is unknown, or if the infant may be difficult to follow, the infant should be treated at birth. It is unwise to require proof of diagnosis before treatment in such cases. The CSF should be examined as a baseline before treatment of such infants. The calculation of penicillin dosage for treatment of late congenital syphilis is the same as for that used in the infant, until dosage based upon body weight reaches that used for adult neurosyphilis.

Jarisch-Herxheimer reaction A dramatic reaction consisting of fever (average temperature elevation, 1.5°C), chills, myalgias, headache, tachycardia, increased respiratory rate, increased circulating neutrophil count (average total white blood cell count, 12,500 per cubic millimeter), and vasodilatation with mild hypotension, may occur following initiation of treatment of syphilis. This reaction occurs in approximately 50 percent of patients with primary syphilis, 90 percent with secondary, and 25 percent with early latent syphilis. The onset occurs within 2 h of treatment, the peak temperature occurs at about 7 h, and defervescence takes place within 12 to 24 h. The reaction is more delayed in neurosyphilis, with peak fever occurring after 12 to 14 h. In patients with secondary syphilis, an increase in erythema and edema of the mucocutaneous lesions occurs; occasionally subclinical or early mucocutaneous lesions may first become apparent during the reaction. The pathogenesis of this reaction is controversial. Patients should be warned to expect such symptoms, which can be managed by bed rest and aspirin. The Jarisch-Herxheimer reaction in neurosyphilis or cardiovascular syphilis has, on very rare occasions, been associated with acute progression of irreversible organ damage.

Follow-up evaluation of responses to therapy for all stages of syphilis The response of early syphilis to treatment should be determined by following the quantitative VDRL titer 1, 3, 6, and 12 months after treatment. Because the FTA-ABS and hemagglutination tests remain positive in nearly all patients treated for seropositive early syphilis, these tests are not useful in following the response to therapy. After successful treatment of seropositive primary or secondary syphilis, the VDRL titer progressively declines, becoming negative within 3 to 12 months in about 75 percent of seropositive primary cases and 40 percent of secondary cases. Two years after treatment for primary syphilis, nearly all patients have a negative VDRL, although 25 percent of secondary cases and a higher proportion of those treated for early latent syphilis maintain low reagin titers. If the VDRL becomes negative or reaches a fixed low titer within 1 or 2 years, performing a lumbar puncture is unnecessary at that time, since the spinal fluid examination is almost invariably normal and there is little risk of subsequent neurosyphilis. However, if a VDRL titer of 1:8 or more fails to fall at least fourfold within 12 months, if the VDRL titer rises fourfold, or if clinical symptoms persist or recur, retreatment is indicated. Every effort should be made to differentiate treatment failure from reinfection, and the CSF should be examined. Suspected treatment failures, especially those with abnormal CSF, should be treated as described for neurosyphilis. If the patient remains seropositive but asymptomatic after such retreatment, no further therapy is necessary. Patients treated for late latent syphilis frequently have a low-titered VDRL prior to therapy and may not demonstrate a fourfold drop following therapy with penicillin; 56 percent of these patients remain seropositive in low titer for years following therapy. Retreatment is not warranted unless the titer rises or signs and symptoms of syphilis recur.

The activity of neurosyphilis correlates best with the degree of cerebrospinal fluid pleocytosis. Changes in the cerebrospinal fluid cell count, and to a lesser extent, in cerebrospinal fluid protein concentration, provide the most sensitive index of response to treatment. Spinal fluid examination should be performed every 3 to 6 months for 3 years after treatment of asymptomatic neurosyphilis. An elevated cerebrospinal fluid cell count falls to 10 or less per cubic millimeter within 3 to 12 months in 95 percent of adequately treated cases, and becomes normal in all cases within 2 to 4 years. Elevated levels of cerebrospinal fluid protein fall more slowly, and the CSF reagin titer declines slowly over a period of several years.

Persistence of treponemal forms The persistence of *T. pallidum* in the aqueous humor, cerebrospinal fluid, lymph nodes, brain, inflamed temporal arteries, and other tissues following "adequate" penicillin treatment of latent or late syphilis has been suggested by dark-field microscopy and by immunofluorescent antibody and silver staining techniques. It is not surprising that *T. pallidum* might persist in the aqueous humor or cerebrospinal fluid despite penicillin treatment, because of poor penetration of the antibiotic, but peristence in lymph nodes and other sites remains unexplained. Limited evidence indicates no increase in resistance to penicillin of such persistent treponemes. Since the data on persisting treponemes are scanty, no modification of the treatment recommendations for latent or late syphilis seems warranted.

IMMUNITY AND PREVENTION OF SYPHILIS Only about 50 percent of the named contacts of primary and secondary syphilis become infected. The actual risk of infection from a single exposure is probably much lower. The relative importance of variations in sexual and hygienic practices, inoculum size, body and environmental temperature, and other local and systemic factors affecting transmissibility of syphilis remains undefined. There is some interest in the possible efficacy of intravaginal contraceptive gels as prophylactics against venereal diseases including syphilis, since many available preparations have bacteriostatic as well as spermicidal properties. Humans have no natural resistance to infection by pathogenic treponemes. The rate of development of acquired resistance to *T. pallidum* following natural or experimental infection is quantitatively related to the amount of the antigenic stimulus, which depends upon both the size of the infecting inoculum and the duration of infection prior to treatment. Resistance of human beings to reinfection by intradermal inoculation of *T. pallidum* was studied in volunteers. Those who had previously been treated for *early* syphilis developed a primary lesion and a serologic response, while the majority of those who had previously been treated for *late latent* syphilis and all those with *untreated latent* syphilis developed neither primary lesions nor serologic response following inoculation. Two patients treated for late latent or late congenital syphilis developed gummas at the site of inoculation.

The role of serum antibody in conferring immunity to syphilis remains controversial. Reagin antibody is not protective. Passively administered antibody from rabbits recovering from experimental syphilis prevents or delays appearance of clinical manifestations of syphilis; it does not prevent infection. Evidence for the importance of cellular immunity includes histopathologic studies in experimental rabbit syphilis, which demonstrates clearance of treponemes from primary lesions soon after peak infiltration of the lesion by T lymphocytes and macrophages. The histopathology of gummas suggests that the cellular immune response is involved in the pathogenesis of these lesions.

Inability to cultivate pathogenic treponemes in vitro has hindered analysis, purification, and concentration of treponemal antigens, and attempts to induce immunity to syphilis by vaccination have shown limited promise. However, repeated injection of rabbits with gamma-irradiated motile strains has conferred immunity to a rechallenge with 10^5 organisms. Currently, the prevention of syphilis depends upon use of mechanical or antiseptic prophylactic agents, and upon detection and treatment of infectious cases.

REFERENCES

Bryceson ADM: Clinical pathology of the Jarisch-Herxheimer reaction. J Infect Dis 133:696, 1976

Campisi D, Whitcomb C: Liver disease in early syphilis. Arch Intern Med 139:365, 1979

Chapel T: The signs and symptoms of secondary syphilis. Sex Trans Dis 7:161, 1980

Clark EG, Danbolt N: The Oslo study of the natural course of untreated syphilis. Med Clin North Am 48:613, 1964

Fischer A et al: Tertiary syphilis in Denmark 1961–1970, a description of 105 cases not previously diagnosed or specifically treated. Acta Derm Venereol 56:485, 1976

Fiumara NJ: Treatment of primary and secondary syphilis: Serologic response. JAMA 243:2500, 1980

Greene BM et al: Failure of penicillin G benzathine in the treatment of neurosyphilis. Arch Intern Med 140:1117, 1980

Hook EW III et al: Detection of *Treponema pallidum* in lesion exudate with a pathogen-specific monoclonal antibody. J Clin Microbiol 22:241, 1985

Hotson JR: Modern neurosyphilis: A partially treated chronic meningitis. West J Med 135:191, 1981

Idsoe O et al: Penicillin in the treatment of syphilis. Bull WHO 47(Suppl):1, 1972

Jaffe HW: The laboratory diagnosis of syphilis: New concepts. Ann Intern Med 83:846, 1975

Johnson RC (ed): *The Biology of the Parasitic Spirochetes*. New York, Academic, 1976

Luger A et al: Diagnosis of neurosyphilis by examination of the cerebrospinal fluid. Br J Vener Dis 57:232, 1981

Lukehart SA et al: Characterization of lymphocyte responsiveness in early experimental syphilis: II. Nature of cellular infiltration and *Treponema pallidum* distribution in testicular infection. J Immunol 124:461, 1980

Magnuson HJ et al: Inoculation studies in human volunteers. Medicine 35:33, 1956

Mascola L et al: Congenital syphilis. Why is it still occurring? JAMA 252:17, 1984

Mohr JA et al: Neurosyphilis and penicillin levels in cerebrospinal fluid. JAMA 236:2208, 1976

Moore JE, Hopkins HH: Asymptomatic neurosyphilis. VI. The prognosis of early and late asymptomatic neurosyphilis. JAMA 95:1637, 1930

Muller F, Moskophidis M: Estimation of the local production of antibodies to *Treponema pallidum* in the central nervous system of patients with neurosyphilis. Br J Vener Dis 59:80, 1983

Paley SS: Syphilis in pregnancy. NY State J Med 37:585, 1937

Quinn TC et al: Rectal mass caused by *Treponema pallidum:* Confirmation by immunofluorescent staining. Gastroenterology 82:135, 1982

Reimer CB et al: The specificity of fetal IgM: Antibody or anti-antibody? NY Acad Sci 254:77, 1975

Rosahn PD: *Autopsy Studies in Syphilis*. CDC Publication 433, US Department of Health, Education, and Welfare, 1960

Ross WH, Sutton HFS: Acquired syphilitic uveitis. Arch Ophthalmol 98:496, 1980

Sexually transmitted diseases treatment guidelines 1985. Morb Mort Week Rep Suppl 34(4S), 1985

Simon RP: Neurosyphilis. Arch Neurol 42:606, 1985

Turner DR, Wright DJM: Lymphadenopathy in early syphilis. J Pathol 110:305, 1973

Zoller M et al: Detection of syphilitic hearing loss. Arch Otolaryngol 104:63, 1978

123 NONVENEREAL TREPONEMATOSES: YAWS, PINTA, AND ENDEMIC SYPHILIS

PETER L. PERINE

GENERAL CONSIDERATIONS Nonvenereal treponematoses occur in remote, impoverished areas of the world. Yaws, pinta, and endemic syphilis are distinguished from venereal syphilis solely by clinical and epidemiologic features. Yaws and pinta are caused by treponemes which are conventionally designated as unique species (*Treponema pertenue* causes yaws, and *T. carateum* pinta), but no convincing morphologic or antigenic differences have yet been demonstrated among *T. pertenue, T. carateum,* and *T. pallidum.* The etiologic agent of endemic syphilis is generally held to be identical with *T. pallidum* and is sometimes designated as *T. pallidum endemicum.* Pinta involves the skin alone; yaws affects skin and bones; and endemic syphilis involves the skin, bone, and mucous membranes. Each disease tends to progress by stages, but these are neither as distinct nor as predictable as in syphilis. Congenital infections and cardiovascular and central nervous system involvement occur rarely, if ever, in the nonvenereal treponematoses but are common in syphilis. It is unclear whether the clinical and epidemiologic differences among yaws, pinta, endemic syphilis, and venereal syphilis are solely determined by environmental and host factors or are attributable to undefined biologic differences among the causal treponemes. The relationship of the treponematoses is summarized in Table 123-1.

EPIDEMIOLOGY Treponemal antibodies are demonstrable in some proportion of nonhuman primates in regions of Africa where human yaws and endemic syphilis are common, and pathogenic treponemes have been found in skin lesions and lymph nodes of seropositive animals. These treponemes have produced yaws-like lesions in susceptible monkeys and hamsters.

Yaws and endemic syphilis are diseases of young children. Yaws occurs throughout the world between the tropics of Cancer and Capricorn, in humid, warm environments. Transmission of yaws among children is favored by scanty clothing, poor hygiene, and frequent skin trauma. Spread occurs by direct contact with infected lesions and perhaps by passive transfer of treponemes by insects. Endemic syphilis occurs in arid subtropical or temperate climates in Africa, the eastern Mediterranean, the Arabian peninsula, and central Asia. It is not observed in the western hemisphere. Skin-to-skin transmission is less important than in yaws; instead, infection of mucous membranes results from direct mouth-to-mouth contact or from contaminated fomites, such as shared drinking or eating utensils. Venereal syphilis can spread by nonvenereal contact among children and cause household outbreaks in modern cities when crowding and poverty favor transmission of *T. pallidum.*

Although cutaneous pigmentary changes resembling late stages of pinta occur in yaws or endemic syphilis, pinta is a separate, more benign disease which occurs only in the western hemisphere. The onset is typically later than in yaws or endemic syphilis, usually when the person is between 10 and 20 years of age. Pinta is not very contagious, and its mode of transmission is not well defined.

The WHO/UNICEF-assisted mass campaign for eradication of endemic nonvenereal treponematosis from 1948 to 1969 was an unusually successful public health campaign. Over 160 million people were examined in 46 countries, and approximately 50 million cases, contacts, and latent infections were treated. The impact of this program was remarkable. The prevalence of active yaws lesions was reduced from over 20 percent to less than 1 percent in many rural areas. In Bosnia, Yugoslavia, endemic syphilis was eradicated—the only example of eradication of an endemic treponematosis.

Relaxation of active surveillance activities after the mass campaigns has led to a resurgence of yaws, particularly in Africa. Yaws has not been eradicated in any large area. The Ivory Coast, Ghana, Togo, and Benin have large reservoirs of yaws and account for over 90 percent of cases reported to WHO since 1982. North of these countries, the Sahelian nations of Mali, Niger, Burkina Faso, and Senegal have prevalence rates in some areas of 10 to 15 percent for endemic syphilis. These rates exceed those reported before the mass treatment campaigns. Seroactivity and late manifestations of endemic syphilis continue to occur among nomads in Saudi Arabia. The resurgence of yaws and endemic syphilis has led to a new yaws campaign in Ghana in 1980, and other national campaigns are planned to control resurgent yaws and endemic syphilis in Africa.

Antitreponemal and reaginic seroreactivity has been detected in a small percentage of children without clinical disease born after the mass campaigns in some areas (e.g., Nigeria, New Guinea, and Bosnia). This may represent attenuated or asymptomatic infection, or may simply reflect the decreased predictive value of serologic tests (probability that disease is present if the test is positive) when the prevalence of disease is sharply reduced.

In the Americas, foci of yaws persist in Haiti; Dominica, St. Lucia, and St. Vincent; Peru, Colombia, and Ecuador; a few areas of Brazil; and Guyana and Surinam. Pinta is confined to Central America and northern South America, where it appears to have regressed to remote Indian villages. Its prevalence today is probably less than 1 percent of that found 20 years ago.

BIOLOGIC RELATIONSHIPS Specific humoral antibodies to *T. pallidum* are produced in individuals with yaws, pinta, or endemic syphilis, but the time of appearance of antibodies after onset of infections is variable. The fluorescent treponemal antibody absorption (FTA-ABS) test, the *T. pallidum* hemagglutination test (TPHA), and

TABLE 123-1 Etiology, epidemiology, and clinical manifestations of the treponematoses

	Venereal syphilis	Endemic syphilis	Yaws	Pinta
Organism	*T. pallidum*	*T. pallidum endemicum*	*T. pertenue*	*T. carateum*
Transmission	Sexual, transplacental*	Household contacts: mouth-to-mouth or via drinking, eating utensils	Skin-to-skin ? Insect vector	Skin-to-skin ? Insect vector
Usual age	Adult	Early childhood	Early childhood	Adolescent
Primary lesion	Cutaneous ulcer (chancre)	Rarely seen	Framboise (raspberry), or "mother yaw"	Nonulcerating papule with satellites
Secondary lesion	Mucocutaneous; occasional periostitis	Florid mucocutaneous lesions (mucous patch, split papule, condyloma latum); osteoperiostitis	Cutaneous papulosquamous lesions; osteoperiostitis	Pintides
Tertiary	Gumma, cardiovascular, and CNS lues	Destructive cutaneous osteoarticular gummas	Destructive cutaneous osteoarticular gummas	Dyschromic, achromic macules

* *Since the nonvenereal treponematoses are usually acquired in childhood and treponemal bacteremia ceases with time, only in adult-onset venereal syphilis is there any likelihood of a mother giving birth to an infected child.*

the *T. pallidum* immobilization (TPI) test cannot differentiate among the treponematoses.

In addition to the clinical and epidemiologic differences among the treponematoses in humans, the range of susceptible animal hosts and some manifestations of experimental infection are also different. In particular, *T. carateum* has produced an infection in chimpanzees which resembles pinta, but attempts to infect other experimental animals have been unsuccessful. Differences between *T. pallidum* and *T. pertenue* have been reported for infections produced in the rabbit and golden hamster, and experimental rabbit infection with one species conferred greater immunity to reinfection with the homologous species than with the heterologous species. However, these interspecies differences in superinfection immunity are no greater than intraspecies differences among different strains of *T. pallidum*. Individuals who have had yaws or pinta are considered relatively immune to syphilis, and persons with active pinta or syphilis cannot be superinfected with *T. pertenue* by experimental inoculation.

CLINICAL MANIFESTATIONS **Yaws** Also known as pian, framboesia, or bubas, yaws is a chronic infectious disease of childhood caused by *T. pertenue*. The disease is characterized by an initial skin lesion(s) followed by relapsing, nondestructive, secondary lesions of skin and bone. In the late stages, destructive lesions of skin, bone, and joints occur.

The incubation period following experimental inoculation of susceptible human beings is 3 to 4 weeks. Disruption of the skin by insect bites, abrasions, or injuries promotes acquisition of natural infection from infected contacts, most likely by fingers contaminated directly or indirectly with material from early yaws lesions. The initial early lesion is a single papule which is usually located on a leg. The lesion enlarges and becomes papillomatous. This lesion is known as a framboesioma (raspberry) or "mother yaw." It becomes superficially eroded and covered by a thin yellow crust of serous exudate containing *T. pertenue*. Erythema and induration do not occur. The lesion is mildly pruritic, and regional lymphadenopathy occurs. The initial lesion usually heals in 6 months. As a result of treponemal bacteremia and autoinoculation, a generalized secondary eruption of similar lesions appears either before or after the initial lesion has healed and is most extensive on the exposed surfaces of the body. These early cutaneous lesions of yaws have a variety of forms, including desquamative macular and papular as well as papillomatous types (Fig. 123-1). Painful papillomata on the soles of the feet result in a crablike gait referred to as *crab yaws*. Early lesions are infectious and heal slowly; they may result in scarring, hyperpigmentation, or depigmentation, resembling the pigmentary changes seen in pinta. Histologic findings are mononuclear-cell infiltration, acanthosis (Fig. 123-2), hyperkeratosis, and the presence of many treponemes. Other manifestations of early yaws include lymphadenopathy and nocturnal bone pain and polydactylitis due to periostitis. Fever and other constitutional symptoms are rare, however, unless lesions become secondarily infected. Infectious cutaneous relapses are characteristic during the first 5 years after infection. Late yaws lesions occur in about 10 percent of cases, starting 5 years or more after infection, and differ histologically from early lesions in showing endarteritis. Late lesions include gummas of the skin and long bones, particularly of the legs, hyperkeratoses of the soles and palms, osteitis, periostitis, juxtaarticular fibromatous nodes, and hydrarthrosis.

Late lesions of yaws are characteristically extensive and usually destructive. Destruction of the nose, maxilla, palate, and pharynx, termed *gangosa*, or *rhinopharyngitis mutilans*, occurs in late yaws, as well as in leprosy and leishmaniasis. Hypertrophic paranasal maxillary osteitis produces distinctive facies known as *goundou*.

The clinical features of yaws have become less reliable for diagnosis

FIGURE 123-1 *Recrudescent yaws lesions of the left arm with subcutaneous juxtaarticular nodules.*

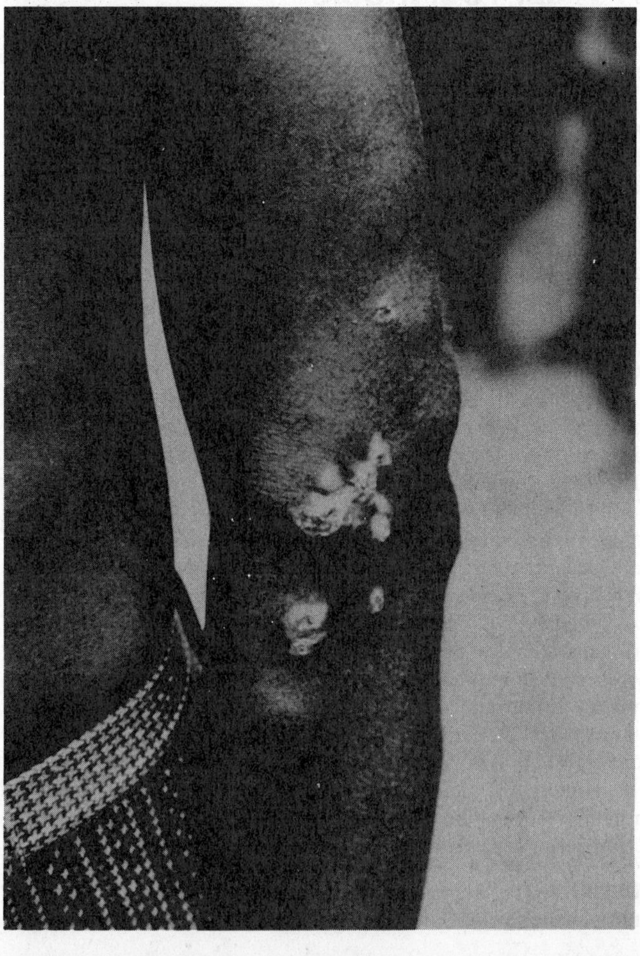

FIGURE 123-2 *Secondary yaws ulceropapillomata on the right leg.*

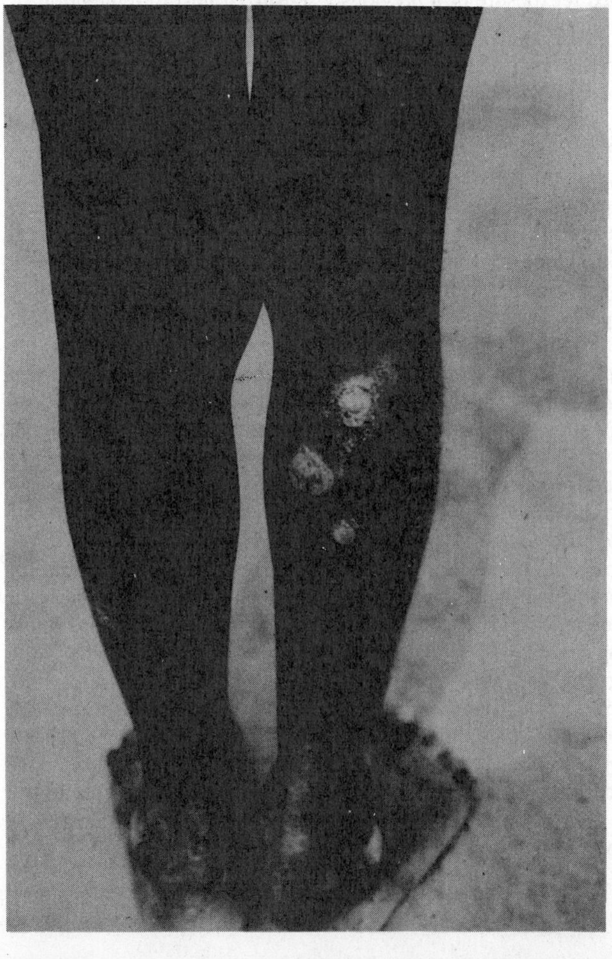

as the prevalence of yaws has decreased, necessitating the use of easily performed serologic tests, such as the rapid plasma reagin (RPR) card test, by paramedical field workers engaged in the consolidation phase of yaws surveillance.

T. pertenue can be demonstrated by dark-field examination in early cutaneous lesions but should not be confused with other spirochetes found in tropical ulcers. The serum reagin antibody tests become positive after 1 month, and the FTA-ABS test is also positive.

Endemic syphilis Synonyms for endemic syphilis are Bejel, Siti, Dichuchwa, Njovera, Belesh, and Skerljevo. It is a chronic nonvenereal, treponemal infection of childhood, characterized by early mucous membrane or mucocutaneous lesions, a latent period of indeterminate duration, and late complications including gummas of bone and skin. The causative organism is indistinguishable from *T. pallidum*. Endemic syphilis differs from congenital syphilis in that dental changes, interstitial keratitis, and neurosyphilis rarely, if ever, occur. Cardiovascular complications are considered rare in both endemic and congenital syphilis.

Primary cutaneous lesions are infrequent and when present are extragenital. The earliest manifestation of endemic syphilis is usually an intraoral mucous patch or mucocutaneous lesion resembling the split papules or condylomata of secondary syphilis. Periostitis is common. Regional lymphadenopathy occurs, but generalized lymphadenopathy is unusual. Treponemes are abundant in the moist early lesions and in aspirates from regional lymph nodes. After a variable latent period, late lesions may develop and are the most frequent clinical manifestations. These resemble the lesions of late benign syphilis and include osseous or cutaneous gummas. Destructive gummas, osteitis, and periostitis of nasopharyngeal structures are more common than in late yaws. Gummas occur on the nipples of mothers who have themselves previously had endemic syphilis who breastfeed infants with oral lesions. Both early and late forms of endemic syphilis thus may coexist in the same family. The tertiary lesions of endemic syphilis sometimes may be a consequence of repeated reexposure of a previously sensitized host to reinfection.

Pinta Also known as mal del pinto, carate, azul, or purupuru, pinta is an infectious disease of the skin caused by *T. carateum*. This disease has three cutaneous stages characterized by marked changes in the skin color, does not involve osseous tissue or viscera, and causes no disability other than that associated with cosmetic disfigurement.

The initial lesion is a small papule which appears 7 to 30 days after exposure and is located most often on the extremities, face, neck, or buttocks. It increases in size slowly by peripheral extension and by coalescing with smaller satellite papules. Regional lymphadenopathy occurs. A secondary eruption not associated with generalized lymphadenopathy appears 1 month to 1 year after the appearance of the initial lesion. The secondary lesions are termed *pintides*, may be numerous, and evolve into a psoriatic or circinate configuration. Pintides are initially red but become deeply pigmented, reaching a slate-blue color after a period of time which is related to exposure to sun. Pigmentation occurs most rapidly on the exposed parts of the body. These pigmented lesions are known as dyschromic macules and contain treponemes which are located principally in the epidermis in older lesions. Histologically there is deposition of pigment in the dermis with decreased melanin pigment in the basal cell layer. Within 3 months to a year, most of the pintides show varying degrees of depigmentation, becoming brown and finally white and giving the skin a mottled appearance. The porcelain-white achromic lesions represent the "late" stage of the disease in which the epidermis is atrophic, and melanocytes and melanin are absent. *T. carateum* can be demonstrated in transudates from initial, early secondary, or dyschromic lesions. Serologic reaginic and antitreponemal antibody tests are positive, but may take four times longer to become positive in pinta than in venereal syphilis.

TREATMENT Treatment is similar for all the endemic treponematoses. Intramuscular injection of 1.2 million units of benzathine penicillin G in adults and half this dose in children results in rapid resolution of lesions and prevents recurrence. Procaine penicillin G in oil and 2% aluminum monostearate (PAM) has been used extensively. In persons who are allergic to penicillin, tetracycline hydrochloride in a dose similar to that used for infectious syphilis (see Chap. 122) is effective. In areas where less than 5 percent of the population has active disease, cases are managed on an individual basis, and all contacts of infected persons are treated with antibiotics.

PREVENTION Although the nonvenereal treponematoses are less amenable to eradication than smallpox, the resurgence of yaws has led some authorities to suggest that the application of *selective epidemiologic control* as used in smallpox eradication be applied to yaws control. This strategy would emphasize ongoing active surveillance, investigation of outbreaks, and treatment of active cases and their contacts rather than mass treatment.

REFERENCES

BURKE JP et al (eds): International symposium on yaws and other endemic treponematoses. Rev Infect Dis 7:S217, 1985

Editorial: Yaws again. Br Med J 2:1090, 1980

GRIN EI, GUTHE T: Evaluation of a previous mass campaign against endemic syphilis in Bosnia and Herzogovina. Br J Vener Dis 49:1, 1973

GUTHE T: Clinical, serological and epidemiological features of framboesia tropica (yaws) and its control in rural communities. Acta Derm Venereol 49:343, 1969

HOPKINS DR: Yaws in the Americas, 1950–1975. J Infect Dis 136:548, 1977

PERINE PL et al: *Handbook of Endemic Treponematoses*. WHO, Geneva, 1984

Treponematoses Research: Report of a WHO Scientific Group, WHO Technical Report Series 455, 1970

WORLD HEALTH ORGANIZATION: Endemic treponematoses. Week Epidem Rec 56:241, 1981

124 LEPTOSPIROSIS

JAY P. SANFORD

DEFINITION *Leptospirosis* is a term applied to disease caused by all leptospiras regardless of specific serotype. Correlation of clinical syndromes with infection by differing serotypes leads to the conclusion that a single serotype of *Leptospira* may be responsible for a variety of clinical features; conversely, a single syndrome, e.g., aseptic meningitis, may be caused by multiple serotypes. Hence there is a preference for the general term leptospirosis rather than the synonyms such as Weil's disease and canicola fever.

ETIOLOGY The genus *Leptospira* contains only one species, *L. interrogans*, which may be subdivided into two complexes, interrogans and biflexa. The interrogans complex includes the pathogenic strains, while the biflexa complex includes saprophytic strains. Within each complex the organisms show antigenic variations that are stable and allow them to be classed as serotypes (serovars). Serotypes with common antigens are arranged in serogroups (varieties). Despite contrary common usage, an example of the correct designation of *Leptospira* is as follows: Pomona serogroup of *L. interrogans* or *L. interrogans* var. pomona, not *L. pomona*. The interrogans complex now contains about 170 serotypes arranged in 18 serogroups (the number in parentheses refers to number of serotypes within the serogroup): Icterohemorrhagiae (18), Hebdomadis (30), Autumnalis (17), Canicola (12), Australis (12), Tarassovi (17), Pyrogenes (12), Bataviae (10), Javanica (8), Pomona (8), Ballum (3), Cynopteri (3), Celledoni (3), Grippotyphosa (5), Panama (2), Shermani (1), Ranarum (2), and Bufonis (1). At least 27 serotypes of *Leptospira* occur naturally in the United States.

EPIDEMIOLOGY Leptospirosis is thought to be the most widespread zoonosis in the world. Cases are regularly reported from all continents except Antarctica and are especially prevalent in the tropics. Although leptospirosis is not a common disease, it has been reported from all regions of the United States including arid areas such as Arizona. Between 1974 and 1983, 61 to 110 cases were reported annually. Infection in humans is an incidental occurrence and is not essential to the maintenance of leptospirosis. The disease occurs in a wide range of domestic and wild animal hosts, including poikilothermic vertebrates. In many species, such as opossums, skunks, raccoons, and foxes, infectivity ratios in the range of 10 to 50 percent are not unusual. Interspecies spread of specific serotypes of leptospiras between animal hosts is frequent, e.g., Pomona, a serotype principally associated with livestock, has been demonstrated in dogs. Infection in animals may vary from inapparent illness to severe fatal disease. Even asymptomatic animals may carry high numbers ($>10^{10}$ organisms per gram) in their kidneys. The carrier state, in which the host may shed leptospiras in its urine for months to years, may develop in many animals. Immunization of dogs may not prevent the carrier, or shedder, state.

Survival of pathogenic leptospiras in nature is governed by factors including pH of the urine of the host, pH of soil or water into which they are shed, and ambient temperature. Leptospiras in most "urine spots" in soil retain infectivity for 6 to 48 h. Acid urine permits only limited survival; however, if the urine is neutral or alkaline and is shed into a similar moist environment which has low salinity, is not badly polluted with microorganisms or detergents, and has a temperature above 22°C, leptospiras may survive for several weeks. Human infections can occur either by direct contact with urine or tissue of an infected animal or indirectly through contaminated water, soil, or vegetation. The usual portals of entry in humans are abraded skin, particularly about the feet, and exposed conjunctival, nasal, and oral mucous membranes. The previously held concept that organisms could penetrate intact skin has been questioned. While leptospiras have been isolated from ticks, these arthropods appear to be unimportant in transmission.

With the ubiquitous infection of animals, leptospirosis in human beings can occur in all age groups, at all seasons, and in both sexes. However, it is primarily a disease of teenage children and young adults (about one-half of patients are between the ages of 10 and 39), occurs predominantly in males (80 percent), and develops most frequently in hot weather (in the United States one-half of infections occur from July to October). The wide spectrum of animal hosts results in both urban and rural human disease. Leptospirosis has been considered an occupational disease; however, improved methods of rat control and better standards of hygiene have reduced the incidence among occupational groups such as coal miners and people who work in sewers. The epidemiologic pattern has changed; in the United States and the United Kingdom, water-associated and cattle-associated leptospirosis is most common. Currently less than 20 percent of patients have had direct contact with animals; they are mostly farmers, trappers, or abattoir workers. In the majority of patients exposure is incidental; two-thirds of cases occur in children, students, or housewives. Swimming or partial immersion in contaminated water, e.g., riding motorcycles through contaminated pools of water, has been implicated in one-fifth of patients and has accounted for most of the recognized common-source outbreaks. In Hawaii, one-fourth of cases have been associated with aquaculture industries, while in Italy leptospirosis remains common in the rice-growing areas of the Po River Valley.

PATHOLOGY In patients who have died with hepatorenal involvement (Weil's syndrome), the significant gross changes include hemorrhages and bile staining of tissues. The hemorrhages, which vary from petechial to ecchymotic, are widespread and are most prominent in skeletal muscle, kidneys, adrenals, liver, stomach, spleen, and lungs.

In skeletal muscle, focal, necrotic, and necrobiotic changes typical of leptospirosis occur. Biopsies early in the illness demonstrate swelling and vacuolation. Leptospiral antigen has been demonstrated in these lesions by the fluorescent antibody technique. Healing ensues by the formation of new myofibrils with minimal fibrosis. The renal lesions in the acute phase involve predominantly the tubules and vary from simple dilatation of distal convoluted tubules to degeneration, necrosis, and basement membrane rupture. Interstitial edema and cellular infiltrates consisting of lymphocytes, neutrophilic leukocytes, histiocytes, and plasma cells are uniformly present. Glomerular lesions either are absent or consist of mesangial hyperplasia and focal foot process fusion which are interpreted as representing nonspecific changes associated with acute inflammation and protein filtration. Microscopic alterations in the liver are not diagnostic and correlate poorly with the degree of functional impairment. The changes include cloudy swelling of parenchymal cells, disruption of liver cords, enlargement of Kupffer cells, and bile stasis in biliary canaliculi. The changes in the brain and meninges are also minimal and are not diagnostic. Microscopic evidence of myocarditis has been recorded. Pulmonary findings consist of a patchy, localized hemorrhagic pneumonitis. Special staining techniques utilizing silver impregnation methods have demonstrated organisms in the lumina of renal tubules but rarely in other organs.

CLINICAL MANIFESTATIONS General features The incubation period following immersion or accidental laboratory exposure has shown extremes of 2 to 26 days, the usual range being 7 to 13 days and the average 10 days.

Leptospirosis is a typically biphasic illness. *During the leptospiremic* or *first phase,* leptospiras are present in the blood and cerebrospinal fluid. The onset is typically abrupt, and initial symptoms include headache, which is usually frontal, less often retroorbital, but occasionally may be bitemporal or occipital. Severe muscle aching occurs in most patients, the muscles of the thighs and lumbar areas being most prominently involved, and often is accompanied by severe pain on palpation. The myalgia may be accompanied by extreme cutaneous hyperesthesia (causalgia). Chills followed by a rapidly rising temperature are prominent. Following the abrupt onset, the leptospiremic phase typically lasts 4 to 9 days. Features during this interval include recurrent chills, high spiking temperatures [usually 38.9°C (102°F) or greater], headache, and continued severe myalgia. Anorexia, nausea, and vomiting are encountered in one-half or more of the patients. Occasional patients have diarrhea. Pulmonary manifestations, usually either cough or chest pain, have varied in frequency of occurrence from less than 25 percent to 86 percent. Hemoptysis occurs but is rare. Adult respiratory distress syndrome has been reported. Examination during this phase reveals an acutely ill, febrile patient, with a relative bradycardia and normal blood pressure. Disturbances in sensorium may be encountered in up to 25 percent of patients. Transient cerebral ischemic attacks in children associated with leptospiral arteritis have been reported from China.

The most characteristic physical sign is conjunctival suffusion, which usually first appears on the third or fourth day. It may be lacking in some patients but more often is overlooked. It may be associated with photophobia, but serous or purulent secretion is unusual. Less common findings may include pharyngeal injection, cutaneous hemorrhages, and skin rashes that are usually macular, maculopapular, or urticarial and usually occur on the trunk. Uncommon findings are splenomegaly, hepatomegaly, lymphadenopathy, or jaundice. The first phase terminates after 4 to 9 days, usually with defervescence and improvement in symptoms. This coincides with the disappearance of leptospiras from the blood and cerebrospinal fluid.

The second phase has been characterized as the "immune" phase and correlates with the appearance of circulating IgM antibodies. The concentration of C3 in serum has remained within normal range during this phase. The clinical manifestations of this phase show greater variability than those during the first phase. After a relatively asymptomatic period of 1 to 3 days, the fever and earlier symptoms recur and meningismus may develop. The fever rarely exceeds 38.9°C (102°F) and is usually of 1 to 3 days' duration. It is not uncommon for fever to be absent or quite transient. Even when symptoms or signs of meningeal irritation are absent, routine examination of cerebrospinal fluid after the seventh day has revealed pleocytosis in 50 to 90 percent of patients. Less common features include iridocyclitis, optic neuritis, and other nervous system manifestations, including encephalitis, myelitis, and peripheral neuropathy.

Some clinicians recognize a third or convalescent phase, usually between the second and fourth weeks, when both fever and aching may recur. The pathogenesis of this stage is not understood.

Leptospirosis during pregnancy may be associated with an increased risk of fetal loss.

Specific features WEIL'S SYNDROME Weil's syndrome, which may be due to serotypes other than Icterohemorrhagiae, is defined as severe leptospirosis with jaundice, usually accompanied by azotemia, hemorrhages, anemia, disturbances in consciousness, and continued fever. There is uncertainty as to the pathogenesis of the syndrome, i.e., whether it represents direct toxic damage due to leptospiras or whether it is the consequence of immune response to leptospiral antigens. The consensus favors toxic damage.

The onset and first stage are identical with the less severe forms of leptospirosis. The distinctive features of Weil's syndrome appear from the third to the sixth days but do not reach their peak until well into the second stage. As in milder forms of leptospirosis, there is a tendency for defervescence about the seventh day; however, with recurrence, fever is marked and may persist for several weeks. Either renal or hepatic manifestations may predominate. Hepatic disturbances include tenderness in the right upper quadrant and hepatic enlargement, both of which are common when jaundice is present. Serum glutamic oxaloacetic transaminase (SGOT) values are rarely increased more than fivefold regardless of the degree of hyperbilirubinemia, which is predominantly conjugated (direct): e.g., serum bilirubin, 40 mg/dL; SGOT, 170 IU. The predominant mechanism appears to be an intracellular block to bilirubin excretion.

Renal manifestations consist primarily of proteinuria, pyuria, hematuria, and azotemia. Dysuria is rare. Serious renal damage usually occurs in the form of acute tubular necrosis associated with oliguria. The peak elevation of blood urea nitrogen usually is seen on the fifth to seventh day. Hemorrhagic manifestations are most prevalent in this group of patients and include epistaxis, hemoptysis, gastrointestinal bleeding, hemorrhage into the adrenal glands, hemorrhagic pneumonitis, and subarachnoid hemorrhage. These have been explained on the basis of diffuse vasculitis with capillary injury. In addition, in some patients hypoprothrombinemia and thrombocytopenia have been observed.

ASEPTIC MENINGITIS A leptospiral etiology has been incriminated in 5 to 13 percent of sporadic cases of aseptic meningitis. The pleocytosis is not present before the immune phase, when it develops rapidly. There are usually tens to hundreds of leukocytes, occasionally 1000, per cubic milliliter, among which neutrophils or mononuclear cells may predominate. The cerebrospinal fluid glucose concentration is almost always normal, but occasional instances of lowered glucose levels (hypoglycorrhachia) have been recorded. In contrast to the observations with many viral causes of aseptic meningitis, with leptospirosis the cerebrospinal fluid protein may exceed 100 mg/dL early in the course. Xanthochromic cerebrospinal fluid has been observed in the presence of jaundice. Each of the serotypes of leptospiras that are pathogenic for humans is probably capable of causing aseptic meningitis. The most prevalent serotypes have been Canicola, Icterohemorrhagiae, and Pomona.

PRETIBIAL (FORT BRAGG) FEVER An illness was observed in the summer of 1942 that had an onset identical with that of the first phase of leptospirosis. The most distinctive feature was the development on about the fourth day of a rash, characterized by 2- to 5-cm, slightly raised, erythematous lesions that were usually symmetrically distributed over the pretibial areas. In contrast to other leptospiral syndromes, splenomegaly occurred in 95 percent of these patients. This outbreak was shown to be due to the Autumnalis serogroup. Subsequently, Pomona has been observed in association with rashes, which are usually truncal but which have also been pretibial.

MYOCARDITIS Cardiac arrhythmias including paroxysmal atrial fibrillation, atrial flutter, ventricular tachycardia, and premature ventricular contractions have been described but are usually of little clinical significance. However, on rare occasions definite cardiac dilatation with acute left ventricular failure has been observed. Associated manifestations have included jaundice, pulmonary infiltrates, arthritis, and skin rashes. The serotypes thus far incriminated have included Icterohemorrhagiae, Pomona, and Grippotyphosa.

CHILDREN Several clinical features which are not seen or are very rare in adults occur in children: hypertension, acalculous cholecystitis (five of nine children in one series), pancreatitis, abdominal causalgia, and peripheral desquamation of a rash which may be associated with gangrene and cardiopulmonary arrest. The features of desquamation, myocardial involvement, and hydrops of the gallbladder suggest Kawasaki syndrome [mucocutaneous lymph node syndrome (see Chap. 49)].

LABORATORY FEATURES Leukocyte counts vary from leukopenic levels to mild elevations in the anicteric patients. In patients with jaundice, leukocytosis as high as 70,000 cells per cubic millimeter may be present. However, regardless of the total leukocyte count, neutrophilia of greater than 70 percent is very frequently encountered during the first stage.

Hemolytic substances have been demonstrated in cultures of pathogenic leptospiras. In contrast to many hemolysins of bacterial origin which are not hemolytic in vivo, the leptospiral hemolysins appear to be active in vivo. In patients with jaundice, anemia may be severe and is most characteristically due to intravascular hemolysis. Other mechanisms of anemia include azotemia and blood loss secondary to hemorrhage. Anemia due to leptospirosis is unusual in anicteric patients.

Thrombocytopenia sufficient to be associated with bleeding (less than 30,000 platelets per cubic millimeter) may be encountered. Additional hematologic abnormalities include elevation of the erythrocyte sedimentation rate in over one-half of patients, but it is usually less than 50 mm/h.

Urinalysis during the leptospiremic phase reveals mild proteinuria, casts, and an increase in cellular elements. In anicteric infections, these abnormalities rapidly disappear after the first week. Proteinuria and abnormalities in the urine sediment usually are not associated with elevations in blood urea nitrogen. Since the anicteric form of the disease often has gone undiagnosed, estimates of the frequency of azotemia and jaundice are probably high. Azotemia has been reported in approximately one-fourth of patients. In three-fourths of these patients, the blood urea nitrogen is less than 100 mg/dL. Azotemia is usually associated with jaundice. The serum bilirubin levels may reach 65 mg/dL; however, in two-thirds of patients the levels are less than 20 mg/dL. During the first phase, one-half of the patients have increased serum creatine phosphokinase (CK) levels, with mean values of five times normal. Such increases are not seen in viral hepatitis, and a slight increase in transaminase with a definite increase in CK suggests leptospirosis rather than viral hepatitis.

DIAGNOSIS Diagnosis is based upon culture of the organism or serologic proof of its existence. The most common initial diagnostic impressions in patients with leptospirosis are meningitis, hepatitis, nephritis, fever of undetermined origin (FUO), influenza, Kawasaki syndrome, toxic shock syndrome, and Legionnaires' disease. Leptospiras may be isolated quite readily during the first phase from blood and cerebrospinal fluid or during the second phase from the urine. Leptospiras may be excreted in the urine for up to 11 months after the onset of illness and may persist despite antimicrobial therapy. Whole blood should be inoculated immediately into tubes containing semisolid medium, such as Fletcher's or EMJH medium. If culture medium is not available, leptospiras reportedly will remain viable up to 11 days in blood to which anticoagulants, preferably sodium oxalate, have been added. Animal inoculation (preferably either suckling hamsters or guinea pigs) may be used and is of particular value if specimens are contaminated. Direct examination of blood or urine by dark-field methods has been employed; *however, this method so frequently results in failure or misdiagnosis that it should not be employed.* Serologic methods are applicable during the second phase; antibodies appear from the sixth to the twelfth days of illness. Two serologic methods are commonly used: a macroscopic or slide agglutination test which is easy to perform but lacks specificity and sensitivity, and hence is suitable for screening only, and the microscopic agglutination test which is more complicated but also more specific. Serologic criteria for diagnosis include a fourfold or greater rise in titer during the course of illness. Cross-agglutination reactions between various serotypes commonly occur so that the infection serotype often cannot be determined with certainty without isolation of leptospiras.

PROGNOSIS The prognosis is dependent upon both the virulence of the organism and the general condition of the patient. Between 1974 and 1981 the mortality rate in reported cases in the United States varied annually between 2.5 and 16.4 percent, averaging 7.1 percent. Age is the most significant host factor related to increased mortality. In a representative series, the mortality rate rose from 10 percent in men less than 50 years of age to 56 percent in those over 51 years of age. The virulence of the infecting leptospiras correlates best with the development of jaundice. In anicteric patients, mortality is extremely rare, but with the development of jaundice, the mortality rate in various series has ranged from 15 to 48 percent. The long-term prognosis following the acute renal lesion of leptospirosis is good. Glomerular filtration rates have returned to normal, usually within 2 months; however, a few patients show residual tubular dysfunction such as a defect in concentrating capacity.

TREATMENT A variety of antimicrobial drugs, including penicillin, streptomycin, the tetracycline congeners, chloramphenicol, and erythromycin, have been effective in vitro and in experimental leptospiral infections. Data concerning the efficacy of antibiotics in human beings have been conflicting. If antimicrobial drugs are to have any beneficial effect, they must be administered within 4 days of the onset of illness. Within 4 to 6 h after initiation of penicillin G therapy, a Jarisch-Herxheimer type of reaction, which suggests antileptospiral activity, may occur. Prospective double-blind studies have demonstrated that doxycycline (200 mg orally taken once per week) is highly effective prophylaxis. Further, doxycycline (100 mg orally taken twice daily for 7 days) when started within 4 days of onset of symptoms significantly shortened the duration of fever and most other symptoms and decreased the frequency of leptospiruria. Both studies were based upon disease acquired in Panama. The epidemiologic conditions and clinical illnesses were typical of leptospirosis generally. It is reasonable to assume that the conclusions are applicable to other areas and would probably apply to other tetracyclines, provided appropriate dosage adjustments were made. There is general agreement that antimicrobials administered after the fifth day of illness have no beneficial effect. There exists the clinical impression that early bed rest may minimize subsequent morbidity. Azotemia and jaundice require meticulous attention to fluid and electrolyte therapy. Since the renal damage is reversible, patients with azotemia should be considered for peritoneal dialysis or hemodialysis. From case reports exchange transfusion has been suggested to be beneficial in the management of patients with extreme hyperbilirubinemia.

REFERENCES

ALSTON JM, BROOM JC: *Leptospirosis in Man and Animals.* Edinburgh, E & S Livingstone, 1958

DAMUDE DF et al: The problem of human leptospirosis in Barbados. Trans R Soc Trop Med Hyg 73:169, 1979

EDWARDS GA, DOMM M: Human leptospirosis. Medicine 39:117, 1960

FEIGIN RD, ANDERSON DC: Human leptospirosis. CRC Crit Rev Clin Lab Sci 5:413, 1975

JOHNSON RC: *The Biology of Parasitic Spirochetes.* New York, Academic, 1976

JOHNSON WD JR et al: Serum creatine phosphokinase in leptospirosis. JAMA 233:981, 1975

MCCLAIN JB et al: Doxycycline therapy for leptospirosis. Ann Intern Med 100:696, 1984

PUBLIC HEALTH LABORATORY SERVICE: Update on leptospirosis. Br Med J 290:1502, 1985

TAKAFUJI ET et al: An efficacy trial of doxycycline chemoprophylaxis against leptospirosis. N Engl J Med 310:497, 1984

WINEARLS CG et al: Acute renal failure due to leptospirosis: Clinical features and outcome in six cases. Q J Med 53:487, 1984

WONG ML et al: Leptospirosis: A childhood disease. J Pediatr 90:532, 1977

125 RAT-BITE FEVER (*STREPTOBACILLUS MONILIFORMIS* AND *SPIRILLUM MINUS* INFECTIONS)

JAN V. HIRSCHMANN

DEFINITION *Rat-bite fever* refers to infection by either *Streptobacillus moniliformis* or *Spirillum minus.* The latter infection is also known by its Japanese name *sodoku.*

ETIOLOGY AND EPIDEMIOLOGY *Streptobacillus moniliformis* is an aerobic nonmotile gram-negative bacterium that may grow in chains of fusiform bacilli. In blood cultures the typical puffball colonies generally appear in 2 to 7 days. Stable L forms frequently develop spontaneously.

The nasopharynx of rats is the natural reservoir of *S. moniliformis,* which grows from as many as half those studied. Human infection usually follows bites from wild rats, but bites from laboratory rats, which can have a high nasopharyngeal carriage rate of the organism, and occasionally other rodents have caused disease. Infection may also occur from ingestion of contaminated food. An epidemic in Haverhill, Massachusetts, in 1926 involving 86 people and caused by contaminated milk or ice cream has led to the term *Haverhill fever* when infection is foodborne.

Spirillum minus is a short, thick spiral gram-negative organism of 2 to 5 μm with two to five curves and terminal flagellae that increase its total length to 6 to 10 μm. On dark-field microscopy the organism has characteristic spasmodic motions of the body and darting movements of the flagella. Although it may be visible on Wright's stains of blood from infected patients or animals, it does not grow on artificial media and requires animal inoculation for isolation from patients.

Carrier rates in wild rats, the natural reservoir, are as high as 25 percent in some locations. In them it may cause interstitial keratitis and conjunctivitis. Human infections with *S. minus* almost always follow rat bites.

CLINICAL MANIFESTATIONS Although up to 22 days may elapse, the incubation period for *S. moniliformis* infection is generally short, typically less than 10 days, usually 1 to 3 days. The onset is sudden, with fever, chills, headache, and myalgias the initial symptoms. The bite site is usually unimpressive; occasionally swelling, ulceration, and regional lymphadenopathy are present. A macular rash develops in about 75 percent of cases, usually 1 to 3 days after the onset of symptoms, and is most prominent on the extremities, where it may involve the palms and soles. Sometimes it may be generalized, petechial, purpuric, or pustular. Arthralgias or arthritis occurs in about half the cases within the first week, usually with multiple, asymmetric large joint involvement. Without treatment the course of disease may be prolonged for several weeks with persistent or recurrent fever and arthritis. Complications of *S. moniliformis* infection include endocarditis and localized abscesses in soft tissues or brain.

In *Spirillum minus* infections the incubation period is typically longer, usually 1 to 4 weeks, with a range of 1 to 36 days. Usually the bite site, after initial prompt healing, becomes swollen, painful, and red at the onset of fever and chills. Lymphangitis and regional lymphadenopathy are often present. The fever is usually relapsing, with febrile periods of 2 to 4 days alternating with afebrile periods of about the same duration. During the fever, headache, photophobia, nausea, and vomiting may occur. Joint complaints are rare. A rash, present in more than half the patients, is usually macular and reddish-brown or purple-red and typically occurs on the extremities. When untreated, this relapsing illness may persist for months. Rarely, bacterial endocarditis develops.

LABORATORY FINDINGS In *S. moniliformis* infections the leukocyte count is typically elevated, with neutrophilia and increased immature forms. The organism can be isolated from blood, joint fluid, or pus. Serologic response can be demonstrated during the second week by agglutination tests.

In *Spirillum minus* infections the leukocyte count may be normal or elevated. The organism may be visible on Wright's stained smears or dark-field examination of the patient's blood. In suspected cases the blood should be injected into the peritoneum of mice or guinea pigs; 5 to 15 days later the organism will be visible on dark-field examination of the animals' blood or peritoneal fluid. In about one-half of patients there are biologic false-positive tests for syphilis.

DIFFERENTIAL DIAGNOSIS With a history of a rat bite, the major clinical features distinguishing *S. moniliformis* from *S. minus* infection are the differences in the incubation period, the condition of the bite site, the nature of the fever, and the presence or absence of joint symptoms.

TREATMENT AND PROGNOSIS Before effective chemotherapy was available, the mortality rate from *S. moniliformis* infections was about 10 percent; for *Spirillum minus* it was about 6 percent. The treatment of choice is the same for both organisms: 7 to 10 days of procaine penicillin, 600,000 units twice daily intramuscularly, or oral penicillin V, 2 g daily in four divided doses. For penicillin-allergic patients oral erythromycin or tetracycline, 2 g daily in four divided doses, is an alternative. Patients with endocarditis should receive a 4-week course of intravenous penicillin G in a daily dose of 12 to 16 million units.

REFERENCES

COLE JS et al: Rat-bite fever. Ann Intern Med 71:979, 1969

MCCORMACK RC et al: Endocarditis due to *Streptobacillus moniliformis*. JAMA 200:77, 1967

Rat-bite fever in a college student—California. Morb Mort Week Rep, June 8, 1984

ROUGHGARDEN JW: Antimicrobial therapy of rat-bite fever: A review. Arch Intern Med 116:39, 1965

126 RELAPSING FEVER

PETER L. PERINE

DEFINITION Relapsing fevers are a group of acute infections characterized by recurrent cycles of pyrexia which are separated by asymptomatic intervals of apparent recovery. They are caused by spirochetes of the genus *Borrelia* and occur in two epidemiologic varieties—louse-borne and tick-borne.

ETIOLOGY Borreliae are slender, helical-shaped, motile organisms measuring 7 to 20 μm long and 0.7 μm in diameter. Unlike other spirochetes, they are readily stained by aniline dyes. They are microaerophilic, and tick-borne strains grow well in Kelly's medium. Tick-borne *Borrelia* strains are more antigenically diverse and widespread in nature than is louse-borne *B. recurrentis*. They are named after their tick vectors, which in the United States include *B. hermsi*, *B. parkeri*, and *B. turicate*.

EPIDEMIOLOGY Louse-borne relapsing fever is transmitted from person to person solely by human body lice, which ingest blood infected with *B. recurrentis*. The spirochetes penetrate the wall of the intestine of the louse and multiply in its body cavity. Infection occurs when the louse is crushed against the bite site or an abrasion is caused by scratching. There is no known animal reservoir. The disease is endemic in remote areas of central and east Africa, the Peruvian Andes, and China, where poverty and crowding promote louse infestation, especially in times of famine and war. Several pandemics have occurred in this century in Africa, the Middle East, and Europe, with 50 million cases and over 5 million deaths. Like typhus, it is now present among the famine refugees in Ethiopia and Sudan. An occasional case of louse-borne relapsing fever has been imported into Europe and North America.

The tick vectors of relapsing fever belong to several species of the genus *Ornithodorus*. These long-lived, soft-shelled (argasid) ticks are reclusive, nocturnal biters which usually feed on ground squirrels and other small rodents. Their bite is painless and lasts for less than an hour. A small pruritic eschar may appear for a few days at the bite site. Ticks of both sexes are potentially infectious, and the spirochetes are transmitted by the female to her progeny. A rodent-tick reservoir of relapsing fever can persist near human dwellings or habitats for decades. Transmission to human beings occurs if the infected tick's saliva or coxial fluid contaminates its feeding site. Most cases in the United States occur during the spring and summer when ticks and rodents are active, particularly in western mountain states, from Texas in the south to Colorado, Washington, Montana, and Idaho in the northwest. Clusters of cases have often been linked to a tick-infested dwelling visited by travelers from different parts of the country.

PATHOGENESIS AND PATHOLOGY Once inoculated into a human, the borreliae reach the bloodstream, producing spirochetemia. Although most organs and tissues are invaded, the organisms remain and multiply primarily in the vascular system. Fever, the first manifestation of the disease, appears 3 to 12 days after infection. The severity of the fever and tissue injury is roughly correlated with the number of circulating spirochetes, which in severe cases can be more than 100,000 per cubic millimeter of blood. Endothelial injury by borreliae is widespread, and subacute disseminated intravascular coagulation with thrombocytopenia and extravasation of blood into serosal membranes and skin is common. Immobilizing (opsonizing) antibodies appear after 3 to 5 days, and the organisms are rapidly cleared from the bloodstream by leukocyte phagocytosis, inducing a febrile crisis of short duration. The precise mechanisms causing the fever and crisis are unknown, but borrelial endotoxin-like substances and/or nonendotoxin particulate pyrogens have been implicated. Fever resolves, but a small number of a new antigenic variant of the spirochete survive in the blood or are sequestered in tissues. A new variant occurs spontaneously by genetic mutation with a frequency of once every 10^3 to 10^4 spirochetes and possesses surface proteins that are different from the infecting or preceding serotypes. They multiply and are detectable in the peripheral blood after a latent period of approximately 1 week, causing a second paroxysm of fever. The number of relapses is fewer in louse-borne than in tick-borne infections and is probably limited by the production of host antibodies directed against common, integral proteins possessed by each new variant.

At autopsy, splenic microabscesses, serosal petechiae, intracranial hemorrhage, diffuse histiocytic myocarditis, and hepatitis with focal necrosis may be seen. The spirochetes can also cross the placenta and cause abortion or relapsing fever in the newborn.

MANIFESTATIONS Symptoms and signs are usually of greater severity in louse-borne relapsing fever and may vary in tick-borne infections depending on the particular species. After an incubation period of 3 to 18 days, the disease begins abruptly with the onset of high fever (39 to 40°C) which remains until the time of crisis. Patients appear acutely distressed, with some alteration in mental status. They complain of headache, muscle and joint pains, weakness, and anorexia. Nausea, vomiting, upper abdominal pain, and nonproductive cough are common. The pulse is increased in proportion to fever, and premature ventricular beats are frequent in louse-borne disease. Cardiac enlargement and heart failure are rare. Meningismus occurs in about 40 percent of patients. The liver and spleen are tender and enlarged in the majority of patients, especially in those with louse-borne disease. Jaundice, secondary to hepatocellular injury, occurs in between 10 and 80 percent of cases, appears late in the course of infection, and is more common in louse-borne disease.

Bleeding is common in both types of relapsing fever. In 10 to 60 percent of cases, a petechial or ecchymotic rash is present. Later, with the development of hepatitis, severe and prolonged epistaxis occurs in 25 percent of patients with louse-borne disease. Less common are hemoptysis, hematuria, and subconjunctival and retinal hemorrhages. Cerebral and gastrointestinal hemorrhage may occur as terminal events in fatal cases. Transient focal neurologic signs may be present without intracranial bleeding. Photophobia is common, and iritis or iridocyclitis leading to permanent visual impairment may develop in patients with tick-borne disease after several relapses.

Three to six days after the onset of symptoms, the attack resolves by crisis. It begins with a brief period of shaking chills which is followed by a transient but pronounced rise in temperature, heart rate, respiratory rate, and systolic blood pressure. This, in turn, is followed by reductions in temperature and peripheral vascular resistance, producing a hypotensive episode of several hours' duration. Acute myocardial failure and fatal cardiac arrhythmias may occur during the hypotensive phase, but most patients recover with return of vital signs to normal within 24 h, leaving the patient weak but comfortable. An identical crisis—the Jarisch-Herxheimer-like reaction—is precipitated by antibiotic therapy. The mediators of the crisis have not been identified, but phagocytosis of opsonized or antibiotically damaged spirochetes is the initiating event. An afebrile period of apparent recovery lasting 5 to 7 days ensues before the patient relapses with fever. In relapse, the symptoms are milder, shorter, and the crisis less severe than in the first attack. While only one or two relapses occur in louse-borne disease, multiple relapses over a period of several weeks are characteristic of tick-borne disease.

LABORATORY FINDINGS A moderate anemia is common. The leukocyte count is usually normal except for leukopenia at the peak of the crisis. The erythrocyte sedimentation rate is elevated. Thrombocytopenia with platelet counts below 150,000 per cubic millimeter and a prolonged bleeding time are seen regularly. Elevated serum aminotransferases, bilirubin, and prolonged prothrombin and partial thromboplastin times are common. Azotemia unrelated to extracellular fluid volume occurs in most patients with louse-borne disease. Electrocardiogram abnormalities include a prolonged QTc interval. The majority of patients with louse-borne and about 30 percent of those with tick-borne relapsing fever develop agglutinins to *Proteus* OXK antigens.

The definitive diagnosis is made by demonstrating borreliae in peripheral blood during a febrile episode by examining blood films stained with Giemsa's or Wright's stains. Repeated examinations may be required. Motile spirochetes can be visualized in wet mounts of freshly drawn blood by dark-field or phase-contrast microscopy. If direct methods are negative and tick-borne disease is suspected, blood may be injected into mice or rats and their blood examined frequently for the presence of spirochetes.

DIFFERENTIAL DIAGNOSIS Many acute febrile illnesses, including Lyme disease, rat-bite fever, salmonellosis, typhus, and Weil's disease, must be considered. Practically, there is seldom confusion if the travel history of the patient is considered and if blood films are examined carefully.

TREATMENT The peripheral blood is quickly cleared of spirochetes by treatment with penicillin, tetracyclines, erythromycin, or chloramphenicol. The first dose of any of these antimicrobial drugs usually provokes a Jarisch-Herxheimer-like reaction beginning 1 to 2 h after treatment is initiated. The severity of the reaction is greater and more predictable in louse-borne than in tick-borne relapsing fever, where it is potentially fatal. Treatment should be given in a hospital where supportive care can be given and vital signs can be monitored carefully. Bed rest is essential for the first 24 h to prevent postural hypotension and precipitation of potentially fatal cardiac arrhythmias. The hyperpyrexia can be treated with acetaminophen and tepid sponging. Most patients are hypovolemic and require 4 or more liters of isotonic saline during the first 24 h. Those with bleeding and jaundice should be given vitamin K; heparin is not effective in controlling the coagulopathy and should not be given.

The treatment of choice in louse-borne relapsing fever is tetracycline, chloramphenicol, or erythromycin stearate, 500 mg in a single oral or intravenous dose. Children under 12 years of age should be given one-half of the adult dose. Meptazinol, in a dose of 100 mg given by slow intravenous injection at the same time as tetracycline, diminishes the Jarisch-Herxheimer-like reaction in louse-borne relapsing fever.

Tetracycline hydrochloride, 500 mg orally every 6 h for 10 days, is the recommended treatment for tick-borne relapsing fever. Doxycycline, 100 mg twice daily, is also effective. The dosage is halved for children under 12 years of age. Erythromycin stearate or chloramphenicol, 500 mg orally every 6 h for 10 days, can be given to patients who are allergic to tetracycline.

PROGNOSIS The untreated mortality rate in epidemics of louse-borne disease is between 30 to 70 percent. Appropriate treatment lowers mortality to less than 1 percent. Adverse signs are deep jaundice, delirium or coma, uncontrolled bleeding, and a marked prolongation of the QTc interval.

Typhus, malaria, and enteric fever may occur simultaneously with louse-borne relapsing fever, and they probably contribute to the mortality rate, particularly during epidemics.

REFERENCES

HORTON JM, BLASER MJ: The spectrum of relapsing fever in the Rocky Mountains. Arch Intern Med 145:871, 1985

JUDGE DM et al: Louse-borne relapsing fever in man. Arch Pathol 97:136, 1974

PERINE PL, TEKLU B: Antibiotic treatment of relapsing fever in Ethiopia: A report of 377 cases. Am J Trop Med Hyg 32:1096, 1983

SOUTHERN PM, SANFORD JP: Relapsing fever: A clinical and microbiological review. Medicine 48:129, 1969

TEKLU B et al: Meptazinol diminishes the Jarisch-Herxheimer reaction of relapsing fever. Lancet 1:835, 1983

WARRELL DM et al: Pathophysiology and immunology of the Jarisch-Herxheimer-like reaction in louse-borne relapsing fever: Comparison of tetracycline and slow release penicillin. J Infect Dis 147:898, 1983

127 LYME DISEASE

ALLEN C. STEERE

DEFINITION Lyme disease, a tick-transmitted spirochetal illness, usually begins with a characteristic expanding skin lesion accompanied by "flulike" or "meningitis-like" symptoms (stage 1). This phase of the disorder may be followed by frank meningitis, cranial or peripheral neuritis, carditis, or migratory musculoskeletal pain (stage 2), or by intermittent or chronic arthritis or chronic neurologic or skin abnormalities (stage 3). Certain aspects of the disease were first recognized in Europe and given different names. The initial skin lesion is known as *erythema chronicum migrans* (ECM), and the neurologic abnormalities are called Bannwarth's syndrome, chronic lymphocytic meningitis, or tick-borne meningopolyneuritis. Two additional dermatologic entities—lymphocytoma and acrodermatitis chronica atrophicans—have also been linked to the disease complex in Europe. Although the frequency of certain manifestations seems to be different in America and Europe, the basic outlines of the illness are similar in both locations.

ETIOLOGY The causative agent of the disease was originally called the Lyme disease spirochete or the *Ixodes dammini* or *I. ricinus* spirochete. All of the isolates tested to date, including those from the United States and Europe, have been shown to be a single species, and the organism has been named *Borrelia burgdorferi.* Lyme spirochetes are 11 to 25 μm long; they have 7 to 11 flagella; and their cytosine/guanine ratio is 27.3 to 30.5 percent. Like other *Borrelia,* they grow in modified Kelly's medium.

EPIDEMIOLOGY Lyme disease has a worldwide distribution that correlates primarily with the geographic ranges of certain ixodid ticks—*I. dammini, I. pacificus,* and *I. ricinus.* The lone star tick, *Amblyomma americanum,* has also been implicated, and other currently unrecognized vectors probably exist.

I. dammini is the principal vector in the northeastern United States from Massachusetts to Maryland and in the midwest in Wisconsin and Minnesota. In surveys of *I. dammini* in these states, 20 percent or more of the ticks have been infected with *B. burgdorferi,* and most of the cases of Lyme disease in the United States have occurred in these areas. *I. pacificus* is the vector in California, Oregon, Nevada, Utah, and Montana. However, surveys have shown that 1 percent or less of these ticks are infected, and accordingly, fewer people have acquired the disease there. Sporadic cases, perhaps related to other vectors, have been reported in the southeast in Virginia, North Carolina, Georgia, and Florida, and in Indiana, Kentucky, Tennessee, Arkansas, and Texas. The disease may be acquired throughout Europe—from Great Britain to Scandinavia to Russia—where *I. ricinus* is the vector, and in Australia. The ticks have different reservoirs; for *I. dammini,* the white-footed mouse is the preferred reservoir of the immature tick, and the white-tailed deer of the mature tick.

Most new cases have onsets during the summer months. Cases have occurred in association with hiking, camping, or hunting trips or among people living in wooded or rural areas. Patients of any age and both sexes are affected. The first known case in the United States occurred in 1962, but more than 1000 people now acquire the infection each summer.

CLINICAL MANIFESTATIONS As with other spirochetal illnesses, Lyme disease occurs in stages, with remissions and exacerbations and different clinical manifestations at each stage. Stage 1 generally lasts for several weeks, stage 2 occurs during the following several months, and stage 3 occurs months to years after the onset of infection. Marked variation is possible in the clinical expression of the disease. Some patients have only ECM. At the opposite end of the spectrum, an occasional patient will have severe involvement of skin, nerves, heart, and joints at the same time. Some patients without ECM have the nonspecific symptoms associated with stage 1. In other patients, neurologic, cardiac, or joint involvement is the presenting sign of the illness.

Stage 1 After an incubation period of 3 to 32 days, ECM, which occurs at the site of the tick bite, usually begins as a red macule or papule that expands to form a large annular lesion, usually with a bright red outer border and partial central clearing. Because of the small size of ixodid ticks, most patients do not remember the preceding tick bite. The center of the lesion sometimes becomes intensely erythematous and indurated, vesicular, or necrotic. In other instances, the expanding lesion remains an even intense red, several red rings are found within the outside one, or the central area turns blue before it clears. Although the lesion can be located anywhere, the thigh, groin, and axilla are particularly common sites. The lesion is warm, but not often painful. Skin biopsies show perivascular infiltrates of lymphocytes and histiocytes, and immune complexes are prominent. In some patients, the Lyme spirochete remains localized to this skin lesion and to regional lymph nodes and is sometimes accompanied by minor constitutional symptoms. In others, the organism spreads hematogenously to many different sites. Within days after the onset of ECM, such patients often develop secondary annular skin lesions, which are similar in appearance to the initial lesion. Additional dermatologic manifestations include malar rash, diffuse erythema, urticaria, or evanescent lesions. Skin involvement is frequently accompanied by severe headache, mild neck stiffness, fever, chills, migratory musculoskeletal pain, arthralgias, and profound malaise and fatigue. Less common manifestations include generalized lymphadenopathy or splenomegaly, hepatitis, sore throat, nonproductive cough, conjunctivitis, iritis, or testicular swelling.

Except for fatigue and lethargy, which are often constant, the early signs and symptoms of Lyme disease are typically intermittent and changing. Even in untreated patients, the early symptoms usually improve or disappear within several weeks. However, fatigue and lethargy and sometimes vague musculoskeletal pain may last for months after the skin lesions have disappeared.

Stage 2 Symptoms suggestive of meningeal irritation may occur early in Lyme disease when ECM is present but are usually not associated with a spinal fluid pleocytosis or objective neurologic deficit. After several weeks to months, about 15 percent of patients develop frank neurologic abnormalities, including meningitis, subtle encephalitic signs, cranial neuritis (including bilateral facial palsy), motor or sensory radiculoneuritis, mononeuritis multiplex, chorea, or myelitis, alone or in various combinations. The usual pattern consists of fluctuating symptoms of meningitis accompanied by facial palsy and peripheral radiculoneuropathy. Cerebrospinal fluid shows a lymphocytic pleocytosis (about 100 cells per cubic millimeter), often with elevated protein, and normal or slightly low glucose. Neurologic abnormalities usually resolve completely within months, but chronic neurologic disease may occur later.

Within several weeks after the onset of illness, about 8 percent of patients develop cardiac involvement. The most common abnormality is fluctuating degrees of atrioventricular block (first-degree, Wenckebach, or complete heart block). Some patients have more diffuse cardiac involvement, including electrocardiographic changes of acute myopericarditis, left ventricular dysfunction on radionuclide scans, or, rarely, cardiomegaly or pancarditis. Cardiac involvement usually lasts only a few weeks but may recur.

During this stage, musculoskeletal pain is common. The typical pattern is migratory pain in joints, tendons, bursae, muscle, or bone, usually without joint swelling.

Stage 3 Within weeks to 2 years after the onset of infection, about 60 percent of patients develop frank arthritis. If arthritis occurs early in the illness, joint swelling is typically mild and transient; marked joint swelling does not usually begin until months later. The typical pattern is intermittent attacks of oligoarticular arthritis in large joints, especially knees. However, both large and small joints may be affected, and a few patients have developed symmetric polyarthritis. Individual attacks of arthritis generally last for a few weeks to months, but most patients have recurrent attacks for at least several years. In a small percentage of patients, involvement in large joints becomes chronic, with erosion of cartilage and bone. By the time arthritis is present, the disease usually seems localized to joints. At this point systemic symptoms are unusual except for fatigue.

Joint fluid white cell counts range from 500 to 110,000 cells per cubic millimeter (average: 25,000 cells per cubic millimeter), mostly polymorphonuclear leukocytes. Tests for rheumatoid factor or antinuclear antibodies are usually negative. Synovial biopsies show fibrin deposits, villous hypertrophy, vascular proliferation, microangiopathic lesions, and a heavy infiltration of lymphocytes and plasma cells.

Although much less common, chronic neurologic or skin involvement (acrodermatitis chronica atrophicans) may also occur years after the onset of infection.

PATHOGENESIS After injection into the skin, the Lyme spirochete may migrate outward in the skin producing ECM and may spread hematogenously to other organs. *B. burgdorferi* has been cultured from blood, skin (ECM), and cerebrospinal fluid and has been seen in skin, myocardial, retinal, and synovial lesions. These findings and the response of all stages of the disease to antibiotic therapy suggest that the organism invades and persists in affected tissues throughout the illness.

Initially, the immune response seems to be suppressed. The mononuclear cells of patients respond minimally to Lyme spirochetal antigens and less than normal to mitogens. Suppressor cell activity is greater than normal. After the first several weeks of infection, mononuclear cells generally have heightened responsiveness to Lyme spirochetal antigens and to mitogens, less suppressor cell activity than normal, and evidence of B-cell hyperactivity—elevated total serum IgM levels, cryoprecipitates, and circulating immune complexes. Specific IgM antibody titers to *B. burgdorferi* peak between the third and sixth week after disease onset; specific IgG antibody titers rise slowly and are generally highest months later when arthritis is present. By that time, antigen-reactive mononuclear cells are concentrated in joint fluid, and immune complexes, which correlate with the total granulocyte count, are always found in the fluid. However, evidence of B-cell hyperactivity is usually not found systemically late in the illness. Patients with neurologic or joint involvement have an increased frequency of the B-cell alloantigen, DR2.

LABORATORY FINDINGS Culture of the Lyme disease spirochete from patients permits definitive diagnosis but is a low-yield procedure. Similarly, spirochetes are rarely seen by direct examination of patient specimens. Therefore, determination of antibody titers is generally the most helpful diagnostic test. Early in the illness, only half of patients have elevated IgM or IgG antibody titers to *B. burgdorferi*. However, after the first several weeks of infection, IgG antibody titers are almost always diagnostic. Antibody to *B. burgdorferi* cross-reacts with other spirochetes, including *Treponema pallidum,* but patients with Lyme disease do not have a positive VDRL test. The most common nonspecific laboratory abnormalities, particularly early in the illness, are a high erythrocyte sedimentation rate, an elevated total serum IgM level, or an increased serum glutamic oxaloacetic transaminase (SGOT) level.

TREATMENT For early Lyme disease, tetracycline, 250 mg four times a day, is the drug of choice in adults. Phenoxymethylpenicillin, 500 mg four times a day, or erythromycin, 250 mg four times a day, are acceptable alternatives. Therapy should be given for at least 10 days, and for up to 20 days, if symptoms persist or recur. In children, phenoxymethylpenicillin is effective (50 mg/kg per day, but not more than 2 g per day) in divided doses for the same duration, or, in cases of penicillin allergy, erythromycin, 30 mg/kg per day, in divided doses for 15 to 20 days, should be used. Approximately 15 percent of patients experience a Jarisch-Herxheimer-like reaction during the first 24 h of therapy.

Later in the illness, parenteral penicillin therapy is usually necessary. In patients with frank meningitis and cranial or peripheral neuropathies, intravenous penicillin G, 20 million units per day in divided doses for 10 days, is effective. In patients with high-degree atrioventricular block or a PR interval of greater than 0.3 s, intravenous penicillin, 10 to 20 million units per day for at least 10 days, and cardiac monitoring are recommended. In patients with complete heart block or congestive heart failure, corticosteroids may be of benefit if the patient does not improve on antimicrobial therapy alone within 24 h. Finally, for established arthritis, benzathine penicillin, 2.4 million units weekly for 3 weeks (total dose: 7.2 million units), or intravenous penicillin G, 20 million units per day in divided doses for 10 to 20 days, seems to be curative in approximately half of patients. In patients who do not respond to antimicrobial therapy, synovectomy may be successful.

PROGNOSIS In stage 1 disease, irrespective of the antibiotic given, nearly half the patients with Lyme disease have minor recurrences of headaches, musculoskeletal pain, or lethargy. These recrudescences correlate significantly with the severity of the initial illness. Eventually, complete recovery ensues.

REFERENCES

Pachner AR, Steere AC: The triad of neurologic manifestations of Lyme disease: Meningitis, cranial neuritis, and radiculoneuritis. Neurology 35:47, 1985

Steere AC, Malawista SE: Lyme disease, in *Principles and Practice of Infectious Diseases,* 2d ed, GL Mandell et al (eds). New York, Wiley, 1985, pp 1343–1349

——— et al: Lyme carditis: Cardiac abnormalities of Lyme disease. Ann Intern Med 93:8, 1980

——— et al: The spirochetal etiology of Lyme disease. N Engl J Med 308:733, 1983

——— et al: The early clinical manifestations of Lyme disease. Ann Intern Med 99:76, 1983

——— et al: Treatment of the early manifestations of Lyme disease. Ann Intern Med 99:22, 1983

——— et al: Neurologic abnormalities of Lyme disease: Successful treatment with high-dose intravenous penicillin. Ann Intern Med 99:767, 1983

——— et al: Successful parenteral penicillin therapy of established Lyme arthritis. N Engl J Med 312:869, 1985

section 6 Viral diseases

128 PRINCIPLES OF VIROLOGY

KENNETH L. TYLER / BERNARD N. FIELDS

STRUCTURE AND CLASSIFICATION OF VIRUSES A typical virus particle (*virion*) contains a core of nucleic acid of either DNA or RNA. There is considerable variability in the structure and size of viral nucleic acids (Table 128-1). The smallest molecular weight genomes, such as those of the parvoviridae, encode three or four proteins, whereas the larger genomes, such as those of the poxviridae, encode more than 50 structural proteins and enzymes. The number of proteins encoded by a viral genome may be greater than predicted from the genome's molecular weight because of the presence of multiple open reading frames and/or the presence of overlapping regions of nucleic acid that can be transcribed into several distinct mRNAs. Extensive nucleotide sequence data are available for part or all of the genomes of many viruses.

The viral nucleic acid is surrounded by either a single or double protein shell (*capsid*). The viral nucleic acid plus the capsid are referred to as the *nucleocapsid*. The viral capsids are composed of smaller repetitive subunits (*capsomeres*) arranged in symmetric constructions. The repeating subunits facilitate assembly of viral proteins into mature virions and reduce the amount of genomic information required to encode structural proteins. Capsids are formed by self-assembly of their structural subunits.

The two fundamental patterns of capsid structural symmetry are icosahedral and helical. Some of the largest viruses, such as the poxviruses, have more complex structural patterns. The retroviruses appear to have icosahedral capsid symmetry and helical core symmetry. Viruses with icosahedral capsid symmetry generally follow principles of physical organization that specify the total allowable number of structural subunits. The nucleic acid in icosahedral viruses is usually in a condensed form and is geometrically independent of the surrounding capsid structure.

Animal viruses with helical symmetry have RNA genomes. A general feature of animal viruses is the binding of protein subunits of the capsid in a regular, periodic fashion along the viral RNA. This close interaction between the capsid proteins and nucleic acid is in sharp contrast to the loose interactions in viruses with icosahedral symmetry and imposes different constraints for viral assembly.

Many viruses have an envelope surrounding the nucleocapsid. The viral envelope is composed of viral-specific proteins and of lipids and carbohydrates derived from host cell membranes. The host cell components are added as the virus buds through the host cell nuclear membrane, endoplasmic reticulum, Golgi apparatus, or cytoplasmic membrane. Different viruses utilize distinctive types of host cell membranes for budding. The factors that determine this specificity are incompletely understood. In some cases viral-specific envelope proteins may include a matrix protein (*M protein*) which lines the inner side of the envelope and is in contact with the nucleocapsid. Viral-specific glycoproteins protrude from the outer surface of the envelope (e.g., as "spikes") and may in some cases contain hydrophobic domains, which span the lipid bilayer of the envelope, as well as internal domains which may contact the M proteins.

Viral proteins, referred to as *structural* or *virion proteins*, can form the viral capsid, can be a major component of viral envelopes, or can be associated with the viral nucleic acid (*core proteins*). A number of viruses contain surface glycoproteins that agglutinate red blood cells (*hemagglutinins*) by binding to receptors on the red cell surface. The orthomyxoviruses and some paramyxoviruses contain the enzyme neuraminidase which may either be identical to (e.g., paramyxovirus) or distinct from (e.g., orthomyxovirus) the hemagglutinin.

Many viruses contain proteins with enzymatic activity. In many cases these enzymes are required for the synthesis of messenger RNA (mRNA) of the appropriate (+) polarity for translation into protein or for replication of the viral genome. An RNA-dependent RNA polymerase activity is found in all (−) polarity RNA viruses. Poxviruses contain a DNA-dependent RNA polymerase. Retroviruses contain an RNA-dependent DNA polymerase commonly referred to as *reverse transcriptase*. Some viruses, including the poxviruses, reoviruses, paramyxoviruses and rhabdoviruses, have RNA "capping enzymes" which modify viral mRNAs at their 5′ end by adding a 7-methylguanosine cap in 5′-5′-triphosphate linkage. Enzymes which polyadenylate the 3′ end of viral mRNAs may also be virally encoded. Additional virally encoded enzymes include protein kinases, nucleoside triphosphate phosphohydrolases, endonucleases, and RNAses.

The earliest classifications of viruses were based solely on their ability to pass through filters with small pore sizes. Subsequent classifications stressed pathogenic properties, specific organ tropisms (e.g., enteroviruses), or epidemiologic characteristics (e.g., arboviruses). Current classifications of viruses are based on a combination of genetic, physicochemical, and biologic factors. These include the type and structure of the viral nucleic acid, the nature of virion ultrastructure including size, type of capsid symmetry, capsid composition, and the presence or absence of an envelope, as well as the strategy used by the virus for genome replication. The reliance on morphologic criteria often means that electron-micrographic studies provide sufficient information to identify both the family and the genus to which a virus belongs. Subdivisions within major viral taxonomic groups may be based on immunologic, cytopathologic, pathogenetic, or epidemiologic features. The application of recombinant DNA techniques will require revision of these classifications based on degrees of genetic relatedness.

REPLICATION Replication refers to the process by which viruses infect susceptible cells, reproduce their genomic material and proteins, and assemble and release infectious progeny. The diversity among viruses in terms of structure and type of genomic material is reflected by the large number of replicative strategies.

The first stage of viral infection of target cells begins with adsorption of the virus particles and ends with the onset of formation of infectious progeny virus. This stage is often referred to as the *eclipse period* and varies from 1 to 5 h (e.g., picornaviruses, togaviruses, rhabdoviruses, orthomyxoviruses, herpesviruses) to 8 to 14 h (adenoviruses, papovaviruses). During this period there is a

TABLE 128-1 Structure of viral nucleic acid

Viral family	Type and form of viral nucleic acid	Approximate mol wt of nucleic acid	Envelope	Capsid symmetry
Parvoviridae	Linear ss(+) or (−)DNA	$1.5–2.0 \times 10^6$	No	I
Adenoviridae	Linear dsDNA	$20–25 \times 10^6$	No	I
Herpetoviridae		$80–150 \times 10^6$	Yes	I
Poxviridae		$85–240 \times 10^6$	Yes	C
Papovaviridae	Supercoiled circular dsDNA	$3–5 \times 10^6$	No	I
(Hepadnaviridae)*	Circular DNA (ds + ss portions)	$1–2 \times 10^6$	Yes	—
Picornaviridae	Linear ss(+)RNA	$2–3 \times 10^6$	No	I
Caliciviridae		$2.6–2.8 \times 10^6$	No	I
Togaviridae		4×10^6	Yes	I
Coronaviridae		$5.5–8 \times 10^6$	Yes	H
Rhabdoviridae	Linear ss(−)RNA	$3.5–4.5 \times 10^6$	Yes	H
Paramyxoviridae		$5–8 \times 10^6$	Yes	H
(Filoviridae)†		$4–5 \times 10^6$	Yes	H
Retroviridae	ss(+)RNA (2 identical copies)	6×10^6	Yes	I,H+
Orthomyxoviridae	Segmented ss(−)RNA (8 segments)	5×10^6	Yes	H
Arenaviridae	Linear ss(−)RNA‡ (2 segments)	$3–5 \times 10^6$	Yes	H
Bunyaviridae	Linear ss(−)RNA‡ (3 segments)	$4.5–7 \times 10^6$	Yes	H
Reoviridae	Segmented linear dsRNA (10–12 segments)	$12–20 \times 10^6$	No	I

* *Proposed name, includes hepatitis B virus.*
† *Proposed name, includes Marburg and Ebola virus.*
‡ *Cohesive ends, noncovalently linked by inverted complementary sequences at the 5′ and 3′ ends.*
NOTE: *ds = double-stranded; ss = single-stranded; + = message sense polarity (RNA can be transcribed directly into protein); − = antimessage sense; i = icosahedral; H = helical; C = complex; I,H+ = icosahedral capsid, helical nucleocapsid.*

dramatic drop in the amount of infectious virus that can be recovered from disrupted cells.

Adsorption appears to be a process that is initially reversible, resulting from random collisions between viruses and target cells. It has been estimated that only one in 10^3 to 10^4 such collisions leads to tighter binding (*attachment*). Attachment is facilitated by the appropriate ionic and pH conditions but is largely temperature-independent and does not require energy. Adsorption of virus to a target cell may involve specific binding of viral proteins to receptors on the cell surface (also called attachment). The virion structure mediating cell attachment has been identified for a number of viruses. For enveloped viruses the viral attachment protein is typically one of the "spikes" inserted on the outer surface of the viral envelope such as the hemagglutinin (HA) of influenza viruses. Some enveloped viruses, such as the herpesviruses and vaccinia, may have more than one type of cell attachment protein. In nonenveloped viruses, surface polypeptides, such as the fiber protein of adenovirus and the hemagglutinin (σ1) protein of reovirus, often function as the viral attachment proteins.

The exact nature of the cellular receptors for animal viruses is known in only a few specific cases. Even when the specific receptor is still unknown, it has been possible to identify "families" or classes of viral receptors using competition binding studies. Viruses of the same species, but different serotypes, may compete for the same receptor class (e.g., poliovirus serotypes 1, 2, 3) or for different receptor classes (e.g., human rhinovirus 2 and 14). Viruses from different families (e.g., coxsackievirus B3 and adenovirus 2) may also compete for the same class of receptor. These types of binding studies suggest that there are generally 10^4 to 10^6 viral binding sites (receptors) per cell.

Once attachment has occurred, the entire virion or a substructure containing the viral genome and any virion polymerases required for its initial transcription must be translocated across the plasma membrane of the cell. The rate of penetration varies depending on the nature of the virus, the type of cells being infected, and environmental factors such as temperature. Some nonenveloped viruses such as poliovirus and reovirus undergo a process of receptor-mediated endocytosis (*viropexis*) and appear in the cytoplasm inside endocytotic vesicles. Other nonenveloped viruses may be able to cross the plasma membrane directly and appear free in the cytoplasm without entering endocytotic vesicles.

Enveloped viruses also utilize at least two strategies for penetration. The first is exemplified by Semliki Forest virus (SFV). SFV, a togavirus, binds to specific cell surface receptors, which then aggregate at distinct sites on the plasma membrane (*coated pits*) and are internalized by receptor-mediated endocytosis. They subsequently appear inside clathrin-coated vesicles within the cell cytoplasm. Fusion between the viral envelope and the endosomal membrane causes release of the viral nucleocapsid into the cytoplasm. A second mechanism for penetration of enveloped viruses occurs with paramyxoviruses (e.g., Sendai). The viral envelope fuses directly with the cell plasma membrane, and the viral nucleocapsid is discharged free into the cytoplasm.

Uncoating is the process of removing or disaggregating part or all of the viral protein capsid in preparation for transcription and translation of the viral genome. In many cases penetration and uncoating are part of a single process. Some picornaviruses, for example, seem to undergo an alteration in capsid structure and integrity and loss of an internal protein as they are translocated across the plasma membrane. The structural alterations associated with loss of the protein may facilitate entry of the viral RNA into the cytoplasm.

Nonenveloped viruses which enter endosomes, such as adenovirus, may induce fusion of lysosomes with the endosome and have their capsid removed by lysosomal enzymes. In the case of reoviruses, intraendosomal proteases sequentially remove the three outer capsid proteins to produce a "subviral particle," a process which leads to activation of the viral transcriptase. Uncoating of poxviruses, such as vaccinia, first involves degradation of the outer protein coat by intraendosomal enzymes and then of the remaining "core," liberating the viral DNA. This step appears to require the synthesis of a virus-specified "uncoating protein."

A number of strategies have evolved for *transcription* of viral genomes into mRNA and *translation* of mRNA into protein. In general, eukaryotic cells require that mRNAs contain only a single initiation site for protein translation (i.e., be monocistronic). One approach is for viruses to contain mRNA that is translated into a large precursor polyprotein, which is then cleaved to produce the various virion proteins. This approach is exemplified by viruses such as the picornaviruses and togaviruses in which the nucleic acid is in the form of (+) polarity, single-stranded RNA (ssRNA) and serves as mRNA. It binds to large polyribosomes and is fully translated ($5' \rightarrow 3'$) to produce a single large polyprotein, which is then cleaved in a series of steps to produce the nonstructural, core, and capsid proteins.

In the case of the togaviruses, the virion RNA also functions as mRNA, yielding a polyprotein that is cleaved to form the nonstructural proteins required for RNA replication. The virion RNA is then transcribed into a (−)RNA template of genomic length, from which two major types of (+)RNA are copied. Major differences exist between the alphaviruses and flaviviruses of the togavirus group. For example, flavivirus mRNA is genomic in length, whereas alphavirus mRNAs of subgenomic size are produced. Also, genes for the structural proteins of the flaviviruses are located at the 5′ end of the viral genome, whereas the structural protein genes of alphaviruses are located at the 3′ end of the viral genome.

In the case of both the picornaviruses and the togaviruses a virally encoded RNA polymerase synthesizes a complementary RNA using the genomic RNA as template. The newly synthesized RNA in turn serves as template for the synthesis of more genomic RNA. The new genomic RNAs may serve as mRNAs or as precursor RNA for progeny virions.

Viruses which contain linear or segmented RNA produce unique mRNAs for each viral protein rather than a single large mRNA molecule. A transcriptase enzyme contained in the virion (the virion polymerase) is required to produce mRNAs from the genomic RNA. The presence of multiple mRNAs allows regulation of the amount of each protein synthesized. A single region of genomic RNA may have multiple reading frames, each of which is transcribed into unique mRNAs, which are in turn translated into distinct proteins. Genomic (−)ssRNA is replicated via a (+)ssRNA intermediate, which then serves as template to synthesize more (−)ss genomic RNA.

Reoviruses contain a RNA-dependent RNA polymerase that transcribes (+)ssRNAs from the (−) strand of each double-stranded (ds) RNA segment. These (+)ssRNAs are extruded from the viral core through channels in the core spike, and serve as monocistronic mRNAs for translation into viral proteins. The viral RNA polymerase also synthesizes (+)ssRNAs, which in turn serve as templates for the complementary (−) strand during replication of the viral genome.

The retroviruses utilize a unique replicative strategy. Viral (+)ssRNA serves as a template for the virion RNA-dependent DNA polymerase (reverse transcriptase) and primer transfer RNAs (tRNAs). A ssDNA copy is produced which is initially hydrogen bonded to its complementary (+)ssRNA. A virally encoded ribonuclease digests the ssRNA, and a complementary DNA strand is synthesized. Then dsDNA is integrated into chromosomal DNA in the host cell nucleus. Transcription of this integrated viral DNA is under the control of the host cell transcriptases.

DNA-containing viruses are capable of using strategies similar to those in eukaryotic cells for replication during lytic infection. Papovaviruses, adenoviruses, and herpesviruses use replicative strategies in which transcription of viral DNA into mRNA occurs in the nucleus of the host cell and depends on host cell enzymes. In the case of papovaviruses (e.g., SV40), the initial proteins produced after infection are the *T antigens* (tumor antigens or *early proteins*). Some of the T-antigen proteins appear to interact with the viral genomic dsDNA by binding near the site of initiation of DNA replication. This binding facilitates DNA replication. Subsequently, mRNAs encoding the capsid polypeptides are transcribed (*late proteins*). The early mRNAs are all derived from only one of the two viral DNA strands (referred to as the E or *E*arly strand), and the late mRNAs from the other (the L or *L*ate strand). Adenoviruses also have early and late genes, but they are intermixed along both strands of the viral DNA rather than on separate strands.

In the replication of both papovaviruses and adenoviruses, early proteins appear to be primarily regulatory in nature and often pleiotropic in function. Late proteins include structural proteins. The individual mRNAs for both early and late proteins are often complementary to dispersed segments of the viral DNA, indicating that extensive splicing, with removal of intervening regions, has occurred. In many cases mRNAs are synthesized from overlapping regions of the viral DNA. This type of redundancy reduces the amount of viral DNA needed to encode viral proteins.

The technique utilized for replication of the viral DNA differs somewhat between the papovaviruses and adenoviruses. In both cases host-derived DNA polymerases are required. DNA replication in the papovaviruses begins at a single fixed origin and then proceeds bidirectionally around the circular dsDNA until two replicative forks meet. The DNA synthesis does not proceed continuously, and small, newly synthesized DNA fragments are later joined together on at least one of the two DNA strands. Replication of the dsDNA in the adenoviridae is simplified by its linear rather than circular arrangement. Replication of each complementary DNA strand occurs independently, and the newly synthesized strands can then initiate another round of replication.

In the case of the herpesviruses, the viral DNA is initially transported to the cell nucleus where transcription and replication occur. The earliest proteins serve a regulatory function, the next proteins to appear are involved in viral DNA synthesis, and the final proteins are primarily structural in nature.

Poxviruses are the most complicated of the known animal viruses, and their replicative cycle is correspondingly complex. All the initial steps of transcription and translation appear to occur in the host cell cytoplasm, which requires that the virus contain its own DNA-dependent RNA polymerase to initiate transcription. One of the virus-encoded early proteins is responsible for the second stage of uncoating which makes the viral DNA fully accessible for transcription and replication. Replication, transcription, and later viral assembly all occur in virus-initiated "factories" within the host cell cytoplasm. Sequential groups of virus-specified proteins can be detected in infected cells. Early proteins include a number of enzymes (e.g., a DNA polymerase and a thymidine kinase), as well as some structural proteins. As infection proceeds, DNA replication begins, the synthesis of the early nonstructural proteins ceases, and the synthesis of late proteins begins. Many of the late proteins are structural proteins; other late proteins include enzymes and proteins that may play a role in viral assembly.

Once replication of the viral genome and synthesis of the viral proteins have been completed, intact virions must then be assembled and released from the host cells. Assembly of the nonenveloped viruses and the nucleocapsid of enveloped viruses often appears to proceed in a crystallization-like fashion which depends on the self-assembly of viral capsomers.

In most cases nonenveloped virions accumulate within the infected cell and are released together when the cell lyses. The events leading to cell disruption include inhibition of the synthesis of host cell protein, lipid, and nucleic acids, disorganization of the host cell cytoskeleton, and alteration of host cell membrane structure. Membrane disruption may result in increased cell permeability and in the release of proteolytic enzymes from lysosomes. The failure to replenish energy-rich substrate molecules inhibits the function of ion transport pumps and disturbs transport of essential nutrients and cellular waste products.

Enveloped viruses are typically released from infected cells by budding. This process may be lethal to the cell. In all cases virus-specified proteins are inserted into host cell membranes in a fashion that restructures the membrane by displacing some of its normal protein components. Viral capsids may then bind to virus-specified matrix proteins which line the cytoplasmic side of these altered patches of membrane. In the case of the smallest enveloped viruses, the togaviruses, the capsids bind to the intracytoplasmic domains of viral proteins inserted in the host cell membrane rather than to matrix proteins.

PATHOGENESIS The signs and symptoms of disease are the result of the culmination of a series of interactions between the virus and the host. A virus must first be able to enter the host, then undergo a period of primary replication, followed by spread to its final target tissue. Once a virus reaches its target organs, it must then infect and successfully replicate in a susceptible population of host cells. The outcome of this last step may be a productive infection with or without cell injury, latent infection, or persistent infection. To transmit infectious virus to the next host the virus must successfully avoid or overcome the host immune response and a wide variety of other host defense mechanisms. A great deal of viral replication can occur before any signs or symptoms of clinical illness are detectable. This "incubation period" can vary from a few days (e.g., influenza), to weeks (e.g., measles, varicella), to months (rabies, hepatitis), to years (slow viruses).

Most viral diseases result from exposure to exogenous virus. However, in some cases disease results from the reactivation of endogenous virus, which has been latent within specific host cells. Examples of infections caused by reactivated endogenous viruses include shingles (herpes zoster), progressive multifocal leukoencephalopathy (JC or BK papovaviruses), recurrent labial and genital herpes (herpes simplex), and some types of cytomegalovirus (CMV) infections.

In the majority of cases, transmission of viral illnesses occurs between members of a susceptible host population (*horizontal spread*). *Vertical spread* of infection occurs when the fetus becomes infected in utero through virus carried in the germ cell line, virus infecting the placenta, or virus in the maternal birth canal. Rubella virus, CMV, herpes simplex virus, varicella-zoster virus, and hepatitis B virus can all produce vertically transmitted congenital infections.

The age and genetic background of the host can have important implications for the outcome of viral infections. Newborns, for example, are particularly susceptible to severe, disseminated herpes simplex virus infections. In contrast, many of the exanthematous illnesses, poliovirus infection, and Epstein-Barr virus (EBV) infection are typically more severe in older individuals than in children. In mice specific genes help determine susceptibility to certain viral infections. These genes may act through effects on the immune system, interferon production, or viral receptors. Inadequate host nutritional status may increase susceptibility to infections such as measles, perhaps by depressing cell-mediated immunity. The host can also influence viral infections in ways that are still poorly understood. Stress may trigger recurrent herpes labialis. Strenuous exercise may have an adverse effect on the course of polio.

Viral infection begins with *entry* into the host, which may occur via a number of routes. The stratum corneum of the skin provides both a physical barrier and a biologic barrier against the entry of viruses. Some viruses overcome the skin barrier by being directly inoculated via insect or animal bites or mechanical devices such as needles. The arthropod-borne viruses are directly inoculated into the bloodstream when an infected tick or mosquito takes a blood meal. Rabies virus and herpesvirus simiae (monkey B virus) enter tissues after an animal bite. Iatrogenic inoculation allows entry of a large number of viruses. Hepatitis B virus, CMV, and human T-cell leukemia/lymphadenopathy-associated (HTLV III/LAV) virus may all be present in contaminated blood products used for transfusion. Infected corneal transplants, infected instruments used in neurosurgical procedures, and infected pituitary tissues used to prepare growth hormone have been implicated as causes of Creutzfeldt-Jakob disease.

Parenteral vaccination using live attenuated virus represents another category of iatrogenic inoculation.

A large number of viruses enter the host by crossing mucosal barriers in the respiratory and gastrointestinal tracts. Respiratory infection can be either by means of aerosol droplets, nasal secretions, or saliva. Entry via either the respiratory or enteric routes requires that the virus overcome a formidable series of host defenses. In the lung, immunologic defenses include secretory IgA, natural killer (NK) cells, and macrophages. Nonspecific glycoprotein viral inhibitors are present in tracheobronchial mucus. Ciliated respiratory epithelial cells continually move mucus away from the lower respiratory tract. The harsh acidic environment of the stomach inactivates acid-labile viruses such as rhinoviruses. Bile salts, present in the lumen of the small intestine, can destroy the lipid envelope of many viruses and may account for the fact that entry via the gastrointestinal route is limited largely to nonenveloped viruses. Proteolytic enzymes and secretory IgA contribute to host antiviral defenses in the gastrointestinal tract. Specific viral capsid proteins may allow some viruses to withstand proteolytic digestion in the gut.

For some enteric viruses, passage across the mucosal barrier of the gut is mediated by a specific population of cells overlying Peyer's patches known as microfold (M) cells. These cells, and perhaps their analogues in bronchial lymphoid tissue, seem to facilitate transport of some viruses, including reoviruses and possibly enteroviruses, to the abluminal surface of the small intestine.

Venereal transmission with entry across the genitourinary or rectal mucosa appears to be important for herpes simplex virus type 2, CMV, hepatitis B virus, and presumably HTLV III/LAV.

For some viruses, the processes of entry, primary replication, and tissue tropism all occur at the same anatomic site. Examples of this type of viral illness include the upper and lower respiratory infections caused by the rhinoviruses, ortho- and paramyxoviruses; the enteritis caused by rotaviruses; and the dermatologic lesions induced by human papillomavirus (warts) and paravaccinia virus (milker's nodules). In other cases a virus enters at one site and must subsequently spread to a distant area, such as the central nervous system (CNS), to produce disease. Enteroviruses enter via the gastrointestinal tract but must spread to the CNS to produce meningitis, encephalitis, and poliomyelitis. Measles virus and varicella virus enter the body through the respiratory tract but then spread to produce skin disease (exanthem) and often generalized organ involvement.

Neural, hematogenous, and lymphatic pathways are all utilized by viruses to spread to target tissues. Rabies virus, herpes simplex virus, herpesvirus simiae (monkey B), varicella-zoster virus, and the scrapie agent spread via nerves. Herpes simplex virus appears to enter nerves via receptors located primarily near synaptic endings rather than on the nerve cell body. Rabies virus accumulates at the motor end plate of the neuromuscular junction (NMJ) and may utilize the acetylcholine receptor (AChR) or a closely related structure to enter the distal axons of motor neurons. Other viruses including La Crosse Bunyavirus and the togavirus Sindbis also accumulate at the NMJ, although their receptor molecules have not been identified. Rabies virus also infects muscle spindles and spreads via sensory nerves to the dorsal root ganglia and spinal cord. The kinetics of neural spread for rabies, herpes simplex, and polio strongly suggest that these agents utilize intraneuronal mechanisms involved with fast axonal transport. The scrapie agent, which appears to spread slowly along neural pathways, may be an example of movement via slow axonal transport. Infection of Schwann cells may provide another "neural" pathway to the CNS. Neural spread may be important not only as a pathway to the CNS but also for spread within the CNS and from the CNS to the periphery.

The olfactory pathway represents a special category of neural spread. The rod processes of olfactory receptor cells lie exposed in the olfactory mucosa. These cells synapse directly with the mitral cells in the olfactory bulb within the CNS. Under experimental conditions, intranasal or aerosol inoculations of rabies virus, herpes simplex virus, poliovirus, and some togaviruses can lead to CNS infection via the olfactory route. This route may provide a naturally occurring pathway to the CNS in humans for rabies and possibly other viruses where high-titer viral aerosols are present, such as in caves occupied by large numbers of rabid bats or in accidental laboratory-acquired infections. An olfactory route of spread might be one explanation for the localization of herpes simplex virus to the orbitofrontal and medial temporal cortex in cases of herpes simplex encephalitis.

Hematogenous spread is important for many viruses. A period of primary replication usually precedes the initial viremia and can be asymptomatic or result in prodromal symptoms. For enteric viruses, primary replication occurs in Peyer's patches and peritonsilar lymphatic tissue. Primary replication of respiratory viruses occurs in epithelial or alveolar cells and for many enteroviruses and togaviruses in skeletal muscle. In some cases virus travels from the site of initial multiplication via lymphatics to regional lymph nodes before entering the bloodstream. The initial (*primary*) viremia often disseminates virus to tissues such as the spleen and liver where continued multiplication in parenchymal cells leads to an amplified secondary viremia. Growth in endothelial cells may help sustain the viremic phase in some togavirus infections. Sustained secondary amplification of the viremia is required if a virus is to overcome clearance by reticuloendothelial cells.

Blood-borne virus can travel free or in association with cellular elements. Hepatitis B virus, picornaviruses, and toga viruses all travel free within plasma; Colorado tick fever virus and Rift valley fever virus are associated with red blood cells; EBV, CMV, rubella, and HTLV III/LAV are lymphocyte-associated.

In some cases viruses use different pathways of spread at different stages in the infectious cycle. Varicella-zoster virus disseminates to the skin by the hematogenous routes to produce "chickenpox." The virus then spreads centripetally along nerves from the skin to neurons in the dorsal root ganglion where it remains latent. Reactivation results in centrifugal spread of virus down sensory nerves to their skin dermatome and the production of "shingles" (zoster). Neural spread of virus presumably accounts for recurrent episodes of oral and genital infection caused by herpes simplex virus. Poliovirus represents an example of a virus capable of spreading by both hematogenous and neural routes. The hematogenous route is generally accepted as the primary pathway to the CNS, although the virus may spread to the CNS via autonomic nerves in the gut. Axonal transport may play a role in the spread of poliovirus within the CNS.

Once a virus has spread from its site of primary replication to a target organ, it must infect a population of susceptible cells. This requires the interaction between specific viral structures (*viral attachment proteins*) and viral receptors on cells. The exact nature of some of these viral receptors is slowly becoming known. Virus-encoded tissue-specific enhancers may in part mediate viral injury to specific cell populations. Lytic infection also requires that all of the subsequent steps in the viral replicative cycle be successfully completed.

HOST FACTORS The antibody response Most viruses make good antigens for stimulating the immune response because they contain a large number of foreign proteins, each of which may contain multiple antigenic sites. In addition, although the amount of viral antigenic material may initially be quite small, there is amplification in its quantity due to viral replication. Few of the antibodies play a significant role in protecting the host against infection, and in some cases they may themselves be implicated in disease pathogenesis.

The immunogenicity of viruses depends on the nature of the virus itself and on a variety of host factors. The slow virus agents responsible for kuru and Creutzfeldt-Jakob disease do not appear to provoke any detectable immune response in the host. The route of viral infection may also play a role in immunity. In experimental influenza infections, intravenous inoculation is more immunogenic than intraperitoneal inoculation, which in turn exceeds the subcutaneous route.

Antibodies which protect the host by destroying the infectivity of virus are referred to as neutralizing antibodies (Nab). The binding of Nab to virus is generally a reversible reaction. Viral infectivity may be reduced because Nab inhibits attachment, penetration, or uncoating of virus; produces aggregation of virions; accelerates viral degradation in vesicles, or enhances viral opsonization and subsequent phagocytosis. In the case of poliovirus, Nab binding appears to induce a conformational rearrangement of the viral outer capsid which blocks viral uncoating but not attachment.

Complement Viruses can trigger activation of both the alternate and classic pathways of complement activation in the absence of an antibody response. Activated complement components (e.g., C3b) may act as opsonins that enhance phagocytosis of viruses. Activation of the alternate complement pathway, in combination with antibody, may produce lysis of enveloped viruses or virus-infected cells. Although the complement system plays a role in the protection against viral infection in animals, human complement deficiency states are not typically associated with an increase in the frequency or severity of viral illnesses.

Cell-mediated immunity Virus-infected cells can be lysed by lymphocytes and other cells through both antibody-dependent and antibody-independent pathways. NK cells are large granular lymphocytes that bind to infected target cells and then secrete cytotoxic molecules contained in azurophilic granular vesicles. NK activity is increased by interferons and possibly by some viral glycoproteins, and does not require antibody. NK cytotoxicity provides one of the earliest host defenses against viral infection (peak activity at 2 to 3 days) and precedes the appearance of antibody (7 days), cytotoxic T lymphocytes (CTL), and delayed type hypersensitivity (DTH). Activated NK cells have been identified in human viral infections caused by CMV, EBV, measles, and mumps virus.

Antibody-dependent lysis of infected cells can occur via antibody-dependent cell-mediated cytotoxicity (ADCC) or via antibody-independent CTLs. In ADCC reactions, virus-specific antibody bound to antigens on an infected cell interacts with Fc receptors for IgG on the surface of specialized lymphocytoid cells [''killer'' (K) cells]. The binding of IgG to the Fc receptor activates the K cell and results in target cell killing. Macrophages, lymphocytes, and PMNs also have Fc receptors and may also participate in ADCC.

Lysis of infected cells mediated by CTLs is class I histocompatibility antigen restricted. CTLs must be activated by antigen presented by macrophages or other antigen-presenting cells (APCs). Activation of CTLs is virus specific and may be specific even for individual strains of the same virus. CTLs from mice infected with lymphocytic choriomeningitis (LCM) only kill LCM-infected target cells from H2 histocompatible mice. The magnitude of the CTL response in mice is controlled by immune response (Ir) genes, and similar regulation may occur in humans.

Interferons Leukocytes produce more than a dozen [alpha (α-)] (''leukocyte'') interferons that share about 70 percent amino acid sequence homology. Beta (β-) (''fibroblast'') interferon is produced by fibroblasts and epithelial cells and has 30 percent homology to α-interferons. Both α- and β-interferons are acid-stable (pH = 2) and relatively heat resistant. ''Immune'' (γ-) interferon is produced by both sensitized and unsensitized T lymphocytes, has different physicochemical properties and different inducers, and uses a different cellular receptor from α- and β-interferons. Genes encoding interferons are located on human chromosomes 9(α and β), 2(β), 5(β), and 12(γ).

Interferons can be induced by both active and inactivated viruses, by double-stranded RNA, and by a number of other compounds. The amount of interferon produced may vary with different viruses. All the interferons have extremely high specific activity and are generally most active in cells of the species in which they are induced (''species-specific''), presumably because of variation in the nature of the interferon receptor. Interferon production appears to involve a derepression of cellular genes induced by the presence of viral nucleic acid in the host cell cytoplasm. This results in the rapid production of mRNAs for interferon and subsequent interferon synthesis.

Newly produced interferon is released into extracellular fluid and then binds to a specific receptor on adjacent cells. The gene encoding the glycoprotein receptor for α- and β-interferon appears to be on human chromosome 21. Binding of interferon to this receptor results in a complex variety of subsequent events. A protein kinase is synthesized which phosphorylates a protein synthesis initiation factor, resulting in inhibition of initiation complex formation and hence of viral protein synthesis. An induced 2,5-oligoisoadenylate synthetase produces 2,5-oligoadenylates, which in turn activate a cellular endonuclease (RNase L) which degrades viral mRNA. Methyltransferase reactions are inhibited which decreases methylation of mRNAs and thereby interferes with viral protein synthesis. In addition to these actions there are changes in target cell surface antigens, resulting in enhanced expression of both class I and class II histocompatability antigens. Interferons also increase the activity of NK cells, CTLs, and cells involved in ADCC reactions. The relative importance of each of these activities in creating the interferon-induced antiviral state is not established.

Virus-induced immunopathology Viruses can combine with virus-specific antibodies to produce circulating immune complexes which may be involved in immunopathogenesis. Virus stimulation of B lymphocytes may result in the production of polyclonal antibodies to antigens unrelated to the inciting virus. Viruses can also induce cross-reacting antibodies to normal host structures which contain antigenic regions similar to those of the virus (*molecular mimicry*). These types of autoantibodies may also lead to immune complex formation. Immune complexes can become trapped in basement membranes at a variety of sites including the skin, the kidney, the choroid plexus, and the walls of blood vessels. These immune complexes result in tissue injury by attracting and activating a variety of inflammatory mediators.

Autoantibodies produced by virus infection may also result in direct tissue injury. Autoantibodies to lymphocytes, platelets, smooth muscle, intermediate filaments, immunoglobulins and myelin basic protein are usually transient and of low titer. These autoantibodies could result from a variety of mechanisms including (1) incorporation of host antigens into viral structures or virus-induced alteration of host antigens, (2) virus-induced alterations in immunoregulatory systems, (3) cross-reactivity between virus antigens and normal host cell structures (molecular mimicry), and (4) eliciting anti-idiotypic antibodies which stimulate host cell receptors.

EPIDEMIOLOGY Viral epidemiology includes the study of the causes, distribution, frequency, modes of transmission, and spread of viral diseases. Accurate enumeration of the incidence and prevalence of viral diseases is an important aspect of epidemiology. Incidence can be defined as the number of *new* cases of a particular disease that appear during a defined period of time, and prevalence as the *total* number of cases. It is often useful to refer to incidence and prevalence *rates,* which are obtained by dividing incidence or prevalence numbers by the size of the total population at risk. Terms such as ''epidemic'' and ''outbreak'' are arbitrary and simply indicate that a greater than expected number of cases of a particular disease has occurred in a specific population, geographic location, or time period.

The appearance of an acute viral disease indicates that an infected host has come into contact with a susceptible individual under conditions that permit the transmission of a particular viral agent. The time interval between exposure to a virus and the development of signs and symptoms of disease is referred to as the ''incubation period'' and can vary from a few days (e.g., influenza) to years (slow virus diseases). Viral infection does not always lead to overt clinical disease. The percentage of those infected who develop overt disease ranges from 100 percent (e.g., rabies, measles) to 0 percent

(BK, JC papovaviruses). In most cases symptomatic disease is less common in children than in adults (e.g., EBV mononucleosis, paralytic poliomyelitis, hepatitis A virus).

Transmission of a virus from an infected host to a susceptible individual can take a variety of forms. Human-to-human transmission can occur from an acutely ill individual, from a chronic carrier, or from mother to fetus. The method of spread can involve respiratory aerosols, fecal-oral contamination, sexual contact, or direct inoculation via infected needles or blood products.

Respiratory aerosolization usually occurs via coughing or sneezing. A sneeze may generate up to 2 million aerosol particles and a cough up to 90,000. The fate of these particles depends both on ambient environmental conditions (e.g., humidity, wind currents) and particle size. Small particles remain airborne longer and can escape the filtering action of the nose, which traps particles larger than 6 μ in diameter. The number of viral particles aerosolized may vary for different strains of the same virus.

For most viruses it is unclear how many viral particles are required to initiate a respiratory infection. For influenza A, adenovirus, or coxsackie A21, as few as 10 particles may be sufficient. Aerosolization is not the only possible route of respiratory transmission. EBV is typically spread by saliva during kissing. A critical pathway of spread for rhinoviruses, which cause the common cold, is from hands to eyes, nose, or mouth—a cycle which can be interrupted by hand washing.

Gastrointestinal transmission occurs when virus shed in feces contaminates food or water and is then ingested by a susceptible individual (''fecal-oral spread''). Stool-tainted hands, resulting from poor personal hygiene, provide another vehicle of spread for enteric viruses. The high incidence of enteric virus infections in infant day-care centers and institutions for the mentally retarded reflect the difficulty of maintaining hygiene in these settings.

In many types of viral disease the vector is an insect or infected animal. In dengue fever there is a continuing cycle between humans and infected mosquitoes. Dengue virus multiplies in the gut of the *Aedes aegypti* mosquito, spreads to its salivary glands, and is injected into a human during the mosquito's blood meal. The infected person develops a high-titer viremia which is sufficient to transmit virus to an uninfected mosquito during biting. In other arbovirus infections the human being is a ''dead-end host'' because the degree of viremia in infected individuals is insufficient to transmit infection to a new group of insect vectors. Examples of this type of cycle are provided by togaviruses, such as eastern, western, and St. Louis encephalitis viruses. The normal animal reservoirs for arboviruses include small birds and mammals. The horse, like humans, is usually a dead-end host, although in Venezuelan equine encephalitis, horses may be a reservoir of virus.

Some arthropod-borne infections do not require a viremic vertebrate intermediate host. Virus can be passed in transovarian fashion to the progeny of an infected tick or mosquito or by venereal transmission between male and female mosquitoes. Transovarian transmission may allow survival of arthropod viruses through the winter months.

Zoonotic infections illustrate another mechanism of disease transmission. In the case of rabies, transmission results from the bite of an infected animal. Many human infections occur when humans are exposed to the excreta (feces, urine, saliva) of infected rodents. Examples include arenavirus infections and the hemorrhagic fevers with renal disease caused by the Bunyaviruses.

Defective agents, such as the adeno-associated human parvoviruses (AAHP) and the delta hepatitis virus (hepatitis D), require coinfection with a ''helper'' virus. Infection with the delta virus is dependent on coincident infection with hepatitis B virus (HBV) and does not occur in its absence. Many details of the epidemiology of these viruses remain to be established. The defective adeno-associated human parvoviruses do not appear to alter significantly the disease produced by the helper adenovirus alone. Conversely, coinfection with HBV and the delta antigen frequently results in fulminant hepatitis.

DIAGNOSIS OF VIRAL DISEASES A reasonably accurate diagnosis of some viral illnesses, such as measles, can be made on clinical grounds alone. In other cases the best that can be done clinically is to identify a group of viruses that are likely pathogens for specific categories of illness. More definitive diagnosis is often necessary because of availability of antiviral agents with activity limited only to certain types of viruses. Definitive diagnosis requires isolation of the virus in animals or in tissue culture, identification of the virus or detection of virus-specified antigens or viral nucleic acids in tissues or body fluids, or documentation of specific serologic responses. The physician must ensure that the appropriate specimens are obtained for diagnostic studies during a suitable phase of the illness, that they are rapidly transported, and that adequate clinical information is provided to the diagnostic laboratories.

In the case of diarrheal or gastrointestinal illness where a viral etiology is suspected, a fresh stool sample is the specimen of choice for virus isolation. In diseases of the respiratory system, including pharyngitis, croup, bronchiolitis, and pneumonia, nasopharyngeal or tracheal *aspirates* provide the best specimens. Nasopharyngeal and throat *swabs* are less satisfactory. When a vesicular rash is present, a needle aspirate of vesicular fluid provides the optimum specimen. When the rash is petechial or maculopapular, both nasopharyngeal aspirates and a stool sample should be obtained. In patients with CNS diseases of suspected viral etiology including meningitis, encephalitis, myelitis, and Guillain-Barré syndrome, a nasopharyngeal aspirate and stool and cerebrospinal fluid specimens should be obtained. A urine sample may be helpful when infection due to CMV, measles, mumps, or papovaviruses is suspected. Blood specimens may be useful for the detection of some arboviruses, herpesviruses, and LCM. Saliva has been used for the detection of rabies and mumps viruses. A brain biopsy specimen is required for the diagnosis of herpes simplex encephalitis, progressive multifocal leukoencephalopathy, subacute sclerosing panencephalitis (SSPE), progressive rubella panencephalitis, and slow virus diseases such as Creutzfeldt-Jakob disease.

Nasopharyngeal or rectal swab specimens should be placed in an appropriate transport medium. In general this consists of a few milliliters of a neutral isotonic salt solution to which a small amount of protein or animal serum has been added. Antibiotics should be added to inhibit bacterial contaminants. Specimens can be placed in a thermos flask filled with crushed ice if any delay in transport is anticipated. Ideally, specimens should be inoculated into the appropriate culture systems on arrival in the virology laboratory. Storage up to 48 h can often be safely done at refrigerator temperature (4°C), and longer storage should be at −70°C. Many viruses quickly lose infectivity if repeatedly frozen and thawed.

Isolation of virus from clinical specimens is done in cell cultures, embryonated eggs, and animals such as suckling mice. Cell culture techniques involve the use of primary cultures of cells prepared from organs of freshly killed animals (e.g., monkey kidney cells); human diploid cell lines such as WI-38 embryo fibroblasts; and continuous (heterodiploid) cell lines such as HeLa, HEp-2, BHK-21, and Vero. Some viruses grow better on certain cell lines than others. Inoculation into the amniotic cavity or the allantoic cavity of embryonated chicken eggs is useful in the isolation of influenza virus. Intraperitoneal and intracerebral inoculation into neonatal mice may be necessary for isolation of coxsackie A viruses and may help in the isolation of many arboviruses, rabies virus, arenaviruses, and orbiviruses. Adult mice or guinea pigs can be used to isolate LCM virus. Identification of the agent responsible for slow virus diseases such as kuru and Creutzfeldt-Jakob disease may require intracerebral inoculation of higher primates such as chimpanzees. Special isolation techniques using brain tissue explants are required to identify measles virus in cases of SSPE, or rubella virus in patients with progressive rubella panencephalitis.

Once cell culture inoculation has been performed, the specimens are examined for distinctive patterns of cytopathic effect (CPE).

Viruses such as HSV and many enteroviruses produce early CPE, whereas cultures may need to be followed for weeks and even subcultured to detect CPE due to CMV, rubella, and some adenoviruses. Cultured cells are examined for cell lysis and vacuolization. The presence of syncytia suggests HSV, RSV, measles, or mumps virus. Cytomegaly is seen with HSV, varicella-zoster virus (VZV), and CMV. Detection of inclusion bodies is aided by the use of Giemsa or other stains. Immunocytochemical staining of cell cultures to detect viral antigens using fluorescein or enzyme-conjugated specific antiviral antibodies can aid in the detection and identification of many viruses. Some viruses produce minimal or no detectable CPE. Ortho- and paramyxoviruses (influenza, parainfluenza, measles, mumps) can be detected by the ability of infected cultures to adsorb certain red blood cells (*hemadsorption*). Infection with rubella can be detected by the ability of infected cultures to block the CPE produced by infection with a second challenge virus (*interference*).

Identification of virus particles or antigens in tissue specimens provides another important method of viral diagnosis. Skin scrapings from the base of vesicles can be stained with Wright or Giemsa stain according to the Tzanck method to help identify HSV or VZV. Similar techniques may help identify CMV-infected cells in urine sediment or measles-infected cells in scrapings from Koplik spots. In some cases, examination of appropriately prepared specimens by electron microscopy (EM) is of diagnostic value; high concentrations ($>10^{67}$ particles per milliliter) of virus must be present. A special technique which concentrates virus in specimens by adsorbing excess fluid and salts on an agarose surface may enable detection of as few as 10^4 particles per milliliter (pseudoreplica technique). EM easily distinguishes between vaccinia and varicella-zoster viruses in vesicular fluid negatively stained with phosphotungstic acid, and may be extremely useful in identifying skin viruses such as human papilloma virus, orf virus, and molluscum contagiosum. The use of specific antisera to aggregate virus in prepared stool specimens facilitates EM detection of rotaviruses, hepatitis A virus, and the Norwalk agent. EM examination of brain biopsy specimens may allow identification of herpes simplex encephalitis, PML, and SSPE.

Detection of virus-specific antigens is facilitated by immunofluorescence and immunocytochemical techniques. These procedures are particularly valuable in diagnosing rabies, herpes infection, PML, and SSPE in brain biopsy specimens; herpes keratitis from corneal scrapings; HSV, VZV, and vaccinia infections from vesicle scrapings; parainfluenza, influenza, and RSV infections from nasopharyngeal aspirates; hepatitis B infections in liver biopsy specimens; and Colorado tick fever virus infection from blood clots. Viral antigens can be detected in these tissue specimens using virus-specific antibodies directly or indirectly coupled with fluorescein isothiocyanate (FITC), or enzymes including horseradish peroxidase (HRP), alkaline phosphatase (AP), and glucose oxidase (GO). Enzyme-linked antibody techniques offer the advantage of increased sensitivity, preservability of stained specimens, and detectability with conventional light microscopy. Coupling a biotin-linked antibody with avidin-linked FITC or enzymes promises to improve immunocytochemical techniques. Radioimmunoassays and immunoassays in which viral antibody coupled to a solid support (ELISA) is used to detect viral antigens have proved useful in the diagnosis of hepatitis A and B virus, rotavirus, and adenovirus infections.

The detection of a fourfold or greater increase in antibody titer to a specific viral agent in a patient's acute and convalescent (3 to 4 weeks later) sera can usually be considered diagnostic of acute infection. A single serum specimen is only occasionally useful in viral diagnosis. A high antibody titer against a rare agent in a typical clinical setting, or a distinct pattern of antibody titers to viral antigens of specific types, may provide presumptive evidence of acute infection. Blood for serology should be collected in anticoagulant- and preservative-free glass tubes, and allowed to clot. Serum should be separated out and stored frozen. A number of different types of antibodies including neutralizing (N), complement-fixing (CF), and hemagglutination-inhibiting (HI) antibodies are routinely assayed. The time course of these antibody responses and their sensitivity and specificity differ greatly.

Restriction enzyme analysis of the genomes of DNA viruses (e.g., HSV, VZV, CMV) and oligonucleotide fingerprinting of ribonuclease T_1 cleaved genomes of RNA viruses (e.g., influenza, dengue enteroviruses) are valuable in epidemiologic studies and in establishing the origin of certain types of viral isolates. In situ hybridization has been utilized for detecting the genomes of viruses in tissue samples. Detection of viral nucleic acids in samples of tissue and body fluid, using cloned virus-specific nucleic acid probes, provides another method for the direct identification of viral pathogens.

PREVENTION OF VIRAL ILLNESS **Vaccines** Currently available vaccines utilize inactivated virus, attenuated virus, or virus subunits to induce active immunization. Formalin– or β-propiolactone–inactivated vaccines are available for rabies, influenza, and polio. Strains used in the inactivated influenza whole-virus vaccine are specified yearly by the FDA. The vaccine is composed of formalin-inactivated natural isolates of influenza virus and laboratory-designed reassortant strains containing the hemagglutinin and neuraminidase genes of the influenza viruses that are currently circulating. As many as 60 to 80 percent of those immunized show a reduction in the frequency or severity of influenzal illness. Guillain-Barré syndrome occurred in 1 in 100,000 individuals vaccinated with the swine influenza vaccine in 1976 to 1977 but has not been associated with subsequent influenza vaccine preparations. Killed polio vaccine is used in Sweden, Finland, and the Netherlands, and in combination with live vaccine in Denmark, but has been supplanted by the Sabin live oral vaccine in the United States, except for use in immunodeficient individuals.

Inactivated virus vaccines have advantages and disadvantages compared to live vaccines. The absence of live virus results in immunization without active infection. Since there is no live virus present, reversion to virulence does not occur, although improperly prepared vaccines can contain virulent virus or adventitious viral contaminants (e.g., SV40, avian leukosis virus). Effective local immunity does not develop, so vaccinated individuals may still transmit virus to the community. In rare cases (measles, RSV), inactivated vaccines have resulted in atypical immunologic responses which potentiated rather than prevented subsequent natural infections.

The attenuated virus vaccines in current use have been developed from either naturally occurring attenuated viruses (e.g., poliovirus type 2 strain 712) or from viruses after serial passage in tissue culture cells or embryonated eggs. These passage-selected viruses have mutations when compared to their wild type parents. For example, the vaccine strain of poliovirus type 1 differs in 21 amino acids from the original parent virus. On some vaccine viruses, the largest number of mutations are located in genes coding for viral surface proteins such as VP1 (polio) or V3 (yellow fever). However, in the case of the type 1 polio vaccine strain mutations responsible for attenuation appear to be distributed throughout the viral genome. In other cases (e.g., mumps) a clear marker for the vaccine virus strain has not been identified.

Following immunization with the oral Sabin polio vaccine, the vaccinated person excretes virus which can infect other individuals in the community. In rare cases, the excreted virus appears to be more virulent than the vaccine strain, and may account for some of the rare cases of paralytic polio in close contacts of vaccinees. Reversion to virulence by the vaccine strain of virus may also cause paralytic polio in vaccinees. Approximately 1 in 10 million vaccinated individuals develops paralytic polio, and there are 3 cases of paralytic polio per 10 million household and community contacts of recent vaccinees. These risks are small and are probably overestimates which include coincidental as well as causal associations. In rare settings, where exposure to polio occurs at a very young age, a combined program using both inactivated (killed) and attenuated vaccines may be of benefit.

Live attenuated measles, mumps, and rubella vaccines can be administered together (MMR) without any loss in immunizing capacity

(>90 percent). Of individuals who receive the measles vaccine alone (Schwarz strain), 10 to 30 percent have mild clinical reactions, and there are rare cases of encephalitis. It is not at all clear that the very rare cases of encephalitis in recipients of measles vaccine are related to the vaccine virus. On the contrary, by preventing natural measles, measles vaccine has been associated with a dramatic reduction in the incidence of SSPE. The attenuated Jeryl Lynn B strain is used in the live mumps virus vaccine. Attenuation took place via serial passage in embryonated eggs followed by chick embryo cell cultures. Adverse effects are rare and include allergic reactions as well as CNS complications. The most commonly used rubella vaccine strain (RA 27/3) was attenuated by multiple passages through the WI-38 line of cultured human diploid fibroblasts. The most notable complications are transient arthralgia and rare cases of arthritis.

A live attenuated vaccine for yellow fever has been prepared using virus derived from passage through chicken embryos. Of those vaccinated intradermally, 95 percent develop an immune response. Serious adverse reactions occur in fewer than 1 in 1 million cases.

A novel approach to vaccination is illustrated by the adenovirus vaccine. In this case the live vaccine virus strains (4, 7) are not attenuated, but the route of administration results in an asymptomatic infection with subsequent immunity. Immunization is via oral ingestion of an enteric coated tablet. Ingested virus does not reach the respiratory tract, but produces an intestinal infection that stimulates an immune response that protects against subsequent adenovirus-induced respiratory infections.

Two vaccines utilize virus subunits rather than whole virus to induce immunity. The influenza subunit vaccine is composed of purified envelope glycoproteins. It appears to be less toxic than live whole virus vaccine but also less antigenic. The hepatitis B vaccine uses a formalin-treated antigen as an immunogen. Purified proteins from cloned viral DNA will be available for use in hepatitis B vaccine and possibly in a herpes vaccine. Synthetic polypeptides analogous to major antigenic sites on viral structural proteins may be of value either as vaccines or as primers that induce a primary immune response that requires a subsequent boost. Nonpathogenic animal viruses which are related to the human rotavirus also show promise as potential vaccines.

ANTIVIRAL THERAPY **Immune globulins** The role in antiviral therapy of immunoglobulins extracted from pooled lots of adult plasma is limited. Antibody titers to specific viruses in different pooled lots of gamma globulin vary over a 10-fold range. Intramuscular administration of immune globulin at the time of exposure to hepatitis A virus can prevent infection or decrease the severity of subsequent illness. A similar beneficial effect has been reported for measles infection and possibly for hepatitis B infection.

Specific immune globulins are made from plasma with high antibody titer against specific viruses. When given within 72 h of exposure to varicella-zoster virus, varicella-zoster immune globulin can prevent or modify subsequent infection. Such therapy is of value in exposed immunocompromised individuals, pregnant women, young infants of mothers who develop chicken pox, and newborns of nonimmune mothers exposed to chicken pox. Hepatitis B immune globulin is useful in preventing infection of individuals exposed to HBsAg-positive material (e.g., a needle stick) or of infants exposed to hepatitis B–infected mothers. Rabies immune globulin is an integral part of postexposure prophylaxis of rabies. Other immune globulins are available but are not widely used.

Antiviral chemotherapy Antiviral chemotherapy depends on the fact that specific stages in the viral replicative cycle or specific viral enzymes and their functions can be selectively inhibited without seriously compromising normal cellular activities. Most currently available antiviral agents have several possible sites of action. Amantadine, rimantadine, and arildone appear to act on an early stage in viral replication, probably penetration-uncoating. Amantadine and rimantadine are given orally. Prophylactic administration of either drug results in a 50 to 90 percent decrease in the incidence of influenza A infections. If either drug is administered therapeutically within 24 to 48 h of the onset of symptoms of influenza A infection, the subsequent illness is milder. Side effects occur in <10 percent and include drowsiness, dizziness, and decreased mental concentration. Arildone appears to inhibit the uncoating of certain viruses including polio and herpes simplex. Initial studies with topical preparations of this drug in the treatment of cutaneous herpes simplex virus infections appear promising.

Iododeoxyuridine (IDU), trifluorothymidine (TFT), vidarabine (ARA-A), and acyclovir appear to exert their antiviral activity by inhibiting viral DNA synthesis by susceptible herpesviruses. Due to their extreme toxicity, IDU and TFT are currently only used as topical preparations. Both drugs are efficacious in the treatment of superficial dendritic keratitis caused by herpes simplex. While acyclovir is extremely effective in herpetic keratitis, no ophthalmic preparation is available. IDU, TFT, and vidarabine are all used effectively in herpes simplex keratitis.

Vidarabine is available both as a 3% ointment for topical use and as an intravenous preparation. The drug is phosphorylated by host cell enzymes to form a triphosphate derivative which acts to inhibit the herpes simplex virus DNA polymerase and may also cause premature termination of elongating viral DNA chains. The drug is mutagenic in vitro and teratogenic for some animal species. The majority of administered drug is converted by the enzyme adenosine deaminase to arabinosyl hypoxanthine, which is largely excreted in the urine. Acute toxicity involves the gastrointestinal, hematologic, and central nervous systems. Poor water solubility results in the need to administer the drug in volumes of fluid which can cause increased intracranial pressure in patients with encephalitis.

Vidarabine 3% ointment is beneficial in the treatment of herpes dendritic keratitis. There are fewer treatment failures and fewer recurrences than with either IDU or TFT. Acyclovir appears to offer the same benefits with less toxicity. Vidarabine is also effective in the treatment of herpes simplex encephalitis. The mortality (at 30 days) in treated biopsy-proven cases is 28 to 33 percent versus 70 percent in placebo-treated cases. Approximately half the vidarabine-treated survivors have normal neurologic function or only mild disability. Younger patients (<30 years) who are treated before they become comatose have a better prognosis than older, comatose patients. Two controlled clinical studies have shown intravenous acyclovir to be significantly more effective than vidarabine. Vidarabine is also effective in the treatment of disseminated herpes simplex infection and in localized CNS infection in neonates. The mortality of disseminated disease was reduced from 85 to 57 percent, and that of localized CNS disease from 50 to 10 percent in treated patients. However, many survivors have severe neurologic sequelae. Both varicella and zoster infections respond to early (<72 h) initiation of vidarabine therapy. In immunocompromised individuals with varicella, treatment with vidarabine decreases the duration of new lesion formation and reduces the risk of visceral complications. Immunocompromised individuals who develop zoster have accelerated healing of skin lesions and decreased cutaneous and visceral dissemination if treated with vidarabine. Unfortunately, the drug does not appear to reduce the incidence of postherpetic neuralgia, although it does seem to reduce its duration.

Acyclovir is the most promising of the currently licensed antiviral drugs with efficacy against herpes simplex virus and varicella-zoster virus. The drug is monophosphorylated by a herpes simplex virus–induced deoxypyrimidine kinase and then di- and triphosphorylated by host cell enzymes. The triphosphate derivative competitively inhibits viral DNA polymerase to a far greater extent than host cell αDNA polymerase. The triphosphate derivative may contribute to the antiviral action of the drug by becoming incorporated into the viral DNA, resulting in premature DNA chain termination and noncompetitive inhibition of the viral DNA polymerase. Selectivity of drug action is based on the initial requirement for phosphorylation by a virus-induced enzyme and the greater degree of inhibition of viral DNA polymerase.

Acyclovir is not teratogenic or carcinogenic in animals, but it does cause mutagenesis in some assays. Acute complications of therapy include reversible alterations in renal function (<10 percent) and encephalopathy (<1 percent). The renal function abnormalities are due to crystallization of the drug in the renal tubules and can be avoided by slow infusion of drug, adequate patient hydration, and dose adjustments for preexisting subnormal renal function.

The 3% topical acyclovir ointment is the drug of choice for herpes simplex dendritic keratitis. Use of the 5% topical ointment results in accelerated clearing and decreased shedding of virus in primary genital herpes. Oral tablets have become available, and oral therapy does result in decreased viral shedding, decreased formation of new lesions, and accelerated healing and shorter duration of symptoms in the initial attacks of genital herpes. Chronic therapy may be of value in suppressing recurrent attacks of genital herpes, but neither treatment of primary or recurrent genital herpes nor suppression prevents the establishment of neuronal latency or abolishes latent infection once it has been established.

Intravenous acyclovir decreases the incidence of visceral dissemination in immunocompromised patients with varicella or zoster. Decreased acute pain and accelerated healing after acyclovir treatment are also seen in immunologically normal individuals with zoster.

Preliminary results from a national cooperative trial of the treatment of herpes simplex encephalitis with acyclovir indicate that the drug is less toxic and significantly more efficacious than vidarabine. Acyclovir is the drug of choice for treatment of herpes simplex encephalitis.

Ribavirin appears to be efficacious, when inhaled as an aerosol, in the treatment of both influenza A and RSV infections. Phosphorylated derivatives of the drug may exert antiviral activity by inhibiting inosine monophosphate dehydrogenase, an enzyme involved in the synthesis of GTP or by inhibiting the guanyltransferase enzyme involved in capping viral mRNAs.

Interferon Preparations of interferon with high specific activity (10^8 units per milligram of protein) have been derived from recombinant DNA expressed in *Escherichia coli* and from Sendai virus stimulation of the Namalwa line of cloned lymphoblasts. These preparations have replaced earlier preparations which were of low specific activity and contained mixtures of various interferon types.

Interferons have been used as topical agents (drops, sprays, gels) and administered by a variety of parenteral routes. Intravenous administration has been associated with severe systemic reactions including shock. Administration by other routes commonly produces fever, fatigue, myalgia, and headache. Laboratory abnormalities include elevated serum transaminases, leukopenia, and thrombocytopenia.

The indications for clinical use of interferon are not established. Intranasal aerosolized α-interferon protects against rhinovirus infection, and α-and β-interferon are also effective in the treatment of virus-associated papillomas and warts. Interferon appears to act synergistically with antiviral chemotherapeutic agents in promoting healing of herpes keratitis and is beneficial in immunocompromised patients with varicella-zoster infections. Prophylactic administration of α-interferon to patients undergoing manipulation of the Vth nerve for intractable trigeminal neuralgia results in a reduced incidence of reactivated herpes labialis infection postsurgery. Interferon (both α and β) decreases the titer of HBsAg, the number of circulating Dane particles, and the level of viral DNA polymerase activity in the serum of hepatitis B virus carriers, but its utility in this setting must await further clinical studies.

REFERENCES

EVANS AS (ed): *Viral Infections of Humans: Epidemiology and Control,* 2d ed. New York, Plenum, 1984

FIELDS BN et al (eds): *Virology.* New York, Raven, 1985

GALASSO GJ et al (eds): *Antiviral Agents and Chemotherapy,* 2d ed. New York, Raven, 1984

JOHNSON RT: *Viral Infections of the Nervous System.* New York, Raven, 1982

NOTKINS AL, OLDSTONE MBA (eds): *Concepts in Viral Pathogenesis.* New York, Springer-Verlag, 1984

129 PRINCIPLES OF ANTIVIRAL CHEMOTHERAPY

RAPHAEL DOLIN

INTRODUCTION The use of antiviral compounds for chemotherapy and chemoprophylaxis of viral diseases is a relatively new development in the field of infectious diseases, particularly when compared to the more than 40 years of experience with antibacterial antibiotics. The principles which underlie the use of antiviral compounds have been modeled after those successfully employed in the treatment of bacterial infections, as outlined in Chap. 88. However, application of these principles to antiviral chemotherapy and chemoprophylaxis presents a number of unique problems.

First, antiviral compounds must possess a high degree of selectivity because of the biologic properties of viruses. Bacteria can replicate extracellularly and have evolved metabolic and structural features which differ considerably from those of mammalian cells. However, viruses must replicate intracellularly and often employ host cell enzymes, macromolecules, and organelles for the synthesis of virus particles. Therefore, safe and effective antiviral compounds must be able to discriminate with a high degree of efficiency between cellular and virus-specific functions. Inhibitors of virus replication which lack this selectivity are likely to be too toxic for clinical use.

Second, because of the nature of virus replication, evaluation of the in vitro sensitivity of virus isolates to antiviral compounds must be carried out in a complex culture system consisting of living cells (e.g., tissue culture). The results from such assay systems vary widely according to the type of tissue culture cells which are employed and the conditions of assay. Furthermore, the precise relationship between the in vitro sensitivity of an isolate and the outcome of antiviral therapy is not well worked out.

Third, information regarding the pharmacokinetics of antiviral compounds, particularly in diverse clinical settings, is limited, particularly when compared to that available for antibacterial antibiotics. For compounds such as acyclovir, considerable detailed pharmacokinetic data are available, while for others such as rimantadine, relatively little information exists. Assays to determine concentrations of antivirals, particularly of active moieties within cells, are not widely available. There are few guidelines with which to adjust dosage levels to maximize antiviral activity and to minimize toxicity. Therefore, clinical use of antiviral compounds must be accompanied by particular vigilance for unanticipated side effects or toxicities.

Fourth, it is clear that highly complex host defense systems play critical roles in the course of viral infections. The presence or absence of preexisting immunity, and the ability to mount humoral and/or cell-mediated immune responses, are especially important determinants in the outcome of viral infections. For example, profound "immunosuppression" may result in infections in which prolonged viral replication is present, and inhibition of such replication by antiviral compounds may be particularly useful. On the other hand, if host defenses are severely depressed, as in bone marrow transplants, antiviral therapy may be relatively ineffective. The state of host defenses and their interactions with antiviral compounds need to be considered when antivirals are utilized or evaluated.

Finally, as with antibacterial antibiotics, the optimal use of antiviral compounds requires that a specific and timely diagnosis be made. For some viral infections, such as herpes zoster, the clinical manifestations are so characteristic that a diagnosis can be made on clinical grounds alone. For other viral infections, such as influenza A, epidemiologic information (i.e., community-wide outbreaks) can be utilized to make a presumptive diagnosis with a high degree of accuracy. However, for most other viral infections, including herpes simplex encephalitis, cytomegalovirus infections, and acute viral gastroenteritis, diagnosis on clinical grounds alone cannot be accomplished with certainty. For such infections, rapid, noninvasive viral diagnostic techniques are sorely needed, and considerable effort is being expended to develop such tests.

Despite the above complexities, the efficacy of several antiviral compounds has been clearly established in rigorously conducted and controlled studies. The compounds which are currently available or likely to be made available in the immediate future for clinical use are discussed below and summarized in Table 129-1.

AMANTADINE AND RIMANTADINE Amantadine (1-adamantanamine hydrochloride) and the closely related compound rimantadine (α-methyl-1-adamantanemethylamine hydrochloride) are primary symmetric amines with antiviral activity limited to influenza A viruses. They inhibit influenza A virus replication at an as yet unspecified step after virus attachment to the cell, either by interference with uncoating of the virus, or with primary transcription of viral RNA. In several experimental systems, rimantadine is two to four times more active than amantadine against isolates of influenza A.

Amantadine and rimantadine have been demonstrated to be effective in the prophylaxis of influenza A in large-scale studies in young adults, and to a lesser extent in children and in elderly subjects. In such studies, efficacy rates of 55 to 80 percent in prevention of influenza-like illness were noted, and even higher rates were reported when virus-specific attack rates were calculated. Amantadine and rimantadine have also been demonstrated to be effective in the treatment of influenza A infection, in studies carried out predominantly in young adults and to a lesser extent in children. Administration of these compounds within 24 to 72 h after the onset of illness has resulted in a reduction of duration of signs and symptoms by approximately 50 percent when compared to a placebo-treated group. The effect on signs and symptoms of illness has been demonstrated to be superior to that of commonly used antipyretic-analgesics. Only anecdotal reports are available concerning the efficacy of amantadine or rimantadine in the prevention or treatment of complications of influenza (e.g., pneumonia).

Amantadine and rimantadine are available only in oral formulations and are ordinarily administered in a dose of 200 mg per day for adults, given once or twice daily. Despite their structural similarities, the pharmacokinetics of the two compounds are different. Amantadine is not metabolized and is excreted almost entirely by the kidney, with a half-life of 12 to 17 h and peak plasma concentrations of 0.4 μg/mL. Rimantadine is extensively metabolized to hydroxylated derivatives and has a half-life of 30 h. Only 30 percent of an orally administered dose is recovered in the urine. The peak plasma levels of rimantadine are approximately one-half those of amantadine, but rimantadine is concentrated in respiratory secretions to a greater extent than amantadine. For prophylaxis, the compounds must be administered daily for the period at risk (i.e., the duration of the outbreak). For therapy, amantadine or rimantadine is generally administered for 5 to 7 days.

Although these compounds are generally well tolerated, 5 to 10 percent of amantadine recipients experience mild central nervous system (CNS) side effects, consisting primarily of dizziness, anxiety, insomnia, and difficulty in concentrating. These side effects are rapidly reversible upon cessation of the drug. In a dose of 200 mg per day, rimantadine is better tolerated than amantadine, and in a large-scale study in young adults, side effects were no more frequent in rimantadine recipients than in placebo recipients. Seizures and worsening of congestive heart failure have also been reported in patients treated with amantadine, although a causal relationship has not been established.

Amantadine is licensed for the prophylaxis and therapy of influenza A in the United States, while rimantadine is experimental as of March 1986. Because of its effectiveness and lack of toxicity, rimantadine may be particularly advantageous for long-term prophylaxis, or for therapy of influenza in subjects at particular risk for development of CNS toxicity, such as elderly individuals. When amantadine is employed in the latter group, the USPHS recommends reduction in dosage to 100 mg per day.

RIBAVIRIN Ribavirin is a synthetic nucleoside analogue which inhibits a wide range of RNA and DNA viruses. The mechanism of action of ribavirin is not completely defined and may be different for different groups of viruses. Ribavirin 5′-monophosphate blocks the conversion of inosine 5′-monophosphate to xanthosine 5′-monophosphate, and interferes with the synthesis of guanine nucleotides and both RNA and DNA synthesis. Ribavirin 5′-monophosphate also inhibits capping of virus-specific RNA in certain viral systems. In studies demonstrating the effectiveness of ribavirin, the compound has been administered as a small-particle aerosol. It has been utilized to treat respiratory syncytial virus (RSV) infection in infants, and to a lesser extent, influenza A and B infection in young adults. In RSV infection in infants, ribavirin administered by continuous aerosol for 3 to 6 days resulted in more rapid resolution of illness, lower respiratory tract signs, and arterial oxygen desaturation when compared to placebo-treated groups. Orally administered ribavirin has not been effective in the treatment of influenza A infections. Ribavirin is currently being evaluated in the therapy of adenovirus and arenavirus infections, including Lassa fever, and in patients with acquired immunodeficiency syndrome.

Large doses of ribavirin administered orally (800 to 1000 mg per day) have been associated with reversible hematopoietic toxicity, but this has not been observed with aerosolized ribavirin, apparently because little drug is absorbed systemically. Aerosolized administration of ribavirin has been approved for treatment of respiratory syncytial virus infection in infants. Because of the need for aerosolized administration, the drug can only be given for this indication under close supervision.

ACYCLOVIR Acyclovir 9-[(2-hydroxyethoxy)methyl]guanine is a highly potent and selective inhibitor of replication of certain herpesviruses, including herpes simplex 1 (HSV-1), herpes simplex 2 (HSV-2), varicella-zoster virus (VZV), and Epstein-Barr virus (EBV). It is relatively ineffective in human cytomegalovirus (CMV) infections.

The high degree of selectivity of acyclovir is related to its mechanism of action, which requires that the compound first be phosphorylated to acyclovir monophosphate. This phosphorylation occurs efficiently in herpesvirus-infected cells by means of a virus-coded thymidine kinase. In uninfected mammalian cells, little phosphorylation of acyclovir occurs, and therefore, the drug is concentrated in herpesvirus-infected cells. Acyclovir monophosphate is subsequently converted by host cell kinases to a triphosphate which is a potent inhibitor of virus-induced DNA polymerase but has relatively little effect on host cell DNA polymerase. Acyclovir triphosphate can also be incorporated into viral DNA, with early chain termination.

Acyclovir is available in intravenous, oral, and topically administered forms. Intravenous acyclovir has been demonstrated to be markedly effective in the therapy of mucocutaneous HSV infections in immunocompromised hosts, reducing time to healing, duration of pain, and virus shedding. When administered prophylactically during periods of intense immunosuppression such as chemotherapy for leukemia or transplantation, but before lesions are present, intravenous acyclovir has also reduced the frequency of HSV-associated disease. After prophylaxis was discontinued, recurrent HSV lesions developed. Intravenous acyclovir has also been demonstrated to be effective in the treatment of HSV encephalitis, and two comparative trials have indicated that acyclovir is more effective than vidarabine for treatment of the latter infection (see below). In immunocompromised patients with herpes zoster, intravenous acyclovir reduced the frequency of

TABLE 129-1 **Antiviral chemotherapy and chemoprophylaxis**

Infection	Antiviral drug	Administration	Dosage	Comment
Influenza A (prophylaxis)	Amantadine	Oral	Adults: 200 mg per day for period at risk Children ≤9 yrs: 4.4–8.8 mg/kg per day not to exceed 150 mg per day	Needs to be administered for the duration of the outbreak. Dosage should be reduced in renal failure and in the elderly. Can be administered along with vaccine.
	or			
	rimantadine	Oral	As above	Not yet licensed by FDA. May be better tolerated than amantadine.
Influenza A (therapy)	Amantadine	Oral	As above for 5–7 days	Both amantadine and rimantadine are effective in uncomplicated influenza. Neither drug has been demonstrated to be effective in complicated influenza (e.g., pneumonia).
	or			
	rimantadine	Oral	As above for 5–7 days	Under study for treatment of complicated influenza in placebo-controlled trials.
Respiratory syncytial virus	Ribavirin	Aerosol	Administered continuously by small-particle aerosol from a reservoir containing 20 mg/mL for 3–6 days	Utilized for treatment of infants and young children hospitalized with RSV pneumonia and bronchiolitis.
Herpes simplex encephalitis	Acyclovir	IV	10 mg/kg every 8 h for 10 days	Acyclovir is the drug of choice for this infection on the basis of comparative trials vs. vidarabine. Optimal results are obtained when therapy is initiated early in illness.
	or			
	vidarabine	IV	15 mg/kg per day as a continous infusion for 12 h for 10 days	
Neonatal herpes simplex	Vidarabine	IV	30 mg/kg per day given as a continuous infusion over 12 h per day for 10 days	Vidarabine reduces mortality, but severe morbidity is frequent. Currently being compared with acyclovir in a clinical trial.
	or			
	acyclovir	IV	10 mg/kg every 8 h for 10 days	
Genital herpes simplex: primary infection	Acyclovir	IV	5 mg/kg every 8 h for 5–10 days	IV route is preferred if infection is of sufficient severity to warrant hospitalization, or if neurologic complications are present.
		Oral	200 mg 5 times per day for 10 days	Preferred route of administration for patients who do not warrant hospitalization. Adequate hydration should be maintained.
		Topical	5% ointment; 4–6 applications per day for 7–10 days	Largely supplanted by oral therapy. May be of use in pregnant women in order to avoid systemic therapy. Systemic symptoms and untreated areas are not affected.
Genital herpes simplex: recurrent infections (therapy)	Acyclovir	Oral	200 mg 5 times per day for 5 days	Clinical effect is modest and is enhanced if therapy is initiated early. No effect on subsequent recurrence rates.

cutaneous dissemination and visceral complications and was more effective than vidarabine in one comparative trial.

The most widespread use of acyclovir is in the therapy of genital herpes simplex virus infections. Both intravenous and oral formulations have shortened the duration of symptoms, reduced virus shedding, and accelerated healing when employed for the treatment of primary genital HSV infections. Oral acyclovir also had a modest effect in the therapy of recurrent genital HSV infections. However, treatment of either primary or recurrent disease did not reduce the frequency of subsequent recurrences, indicating that acyclovir was ineffective in elimination of latent infection. Chronically administered oral acyclovir (for 4 to 6 months) has been shown to reduce the frequency of recurrences markedly while on therapy, although once the drug was discontinued, lesions recurred. Studies are currently underway to examine the effect of acyclovir on the course of recurrent genital herpes simplex infection for longer periods of time.

With the availability of the oral and intravenous forms, there are few indications for topical acyclovir, although treatment with this formulation has shown modest beneficial effects in the therapy of primary genital herpes infections and of mucocutaneous HSV infections in immunocompromised hosts.

Overall, acyclovir is remarkably well tolerated and generally free of toxicity. The most frequently encountered toxicity has been occasional renal dysfunction, particularly after rapid intravenous administration or when patients have been inadequately hydrated. Central nervous system changes, including lethargy and tremors, occasionally have been reported, primarily in immunosuppressed patients. However, whether these changes are related to acyclovir, to concurrent administration of other therapy, or to underlying infection remains unclear. Acyclovir is excreted primarily unmetabolized by the kidney, both by glomerular filtration and tubular secretion. Approximately 15 percent of a dose of acyclovir is metabolized to 9-[(carboxymethoxy)methyl]guanine or other minor metabolites. Reduction in dosage is indicated in patients with creatinine clearances less than 50 mL/min per 1.73 m^2. The half-life of acyclovir is approximately 3 h in normal adults, and peak plasma concentrations after a 1-h infusion employing a 5 mg/kg dose are 9.8 μg/mL. Approximately 22 percent of acyclovir administered orally is absorbed, and peak plasma concentrations of 0.3 to 0.9 μg/mL are attained after administration of a 200-mg dose. Acyclovir penetrates relatively well into the cerebrospinal fluid, with CSF concentrations approaching one-half of those found in plasma.

An analogue of acyclovir, DHPG 9-[(1,3-dihydroxy-2-propoxy)methyl]guanine, has markedly increased activity against CMV, and appears to be the most promising antiviral agent currently available against CMV in humans. DHPG is now undergoing extensive clinical trials in CMV infections.

VIDARABINE Vidarabine (9-β-D-arabinofuranosyladenine) is a purine nucleoside analogue with activity against HSV-1, HSV-2, VZV,

TABLE 129-1 Antiviral chemotherapy and chemoprophylaxis *(continued)*

Infection	Antiviral drug	Administration	Dosage	Comment
Genital herpes simplex: recurrent infections (suppression)	Acyclovir	Oral	200 mg 3–5 times per day for up to 6 months	Suppressive therapy is recommended only for patients with frequent recurrences, at least 6 to 10 per year, for up to 6 months. Occasional "breakthrough" may occur, and asymptomatic shedding of virus occurs. Studies of longer courses of suppression are underway.
Mucocutaneous herpes simplex in immunocompromised patients (treatment)	Acyclovir	IV	250 mg/m² every 8 h for 7 days	Choice of intravenous or oral route will depend on severity of infection and whether patient can take oral medication. Oral or IV administration has supplanted topical therapy except for small, easily accessible lesions.
		Oral	200 mg PO 5 times per day for 10 days	
	or	Topical	5% ointment; 4–6 applications per day for 7 days or until healed	
	vidarabine	IV	10 mg/kg per day for 7 days given as a 12-h infusion	Efficacy has been demonstrated in HSV-1 infections and in patients who were older than 40. Appears to be less useful than acyclovir in this setting.
Mucocutaneous herpes simplex in immunocompromised patients (prevention of recurrences during periods of intense immunosuppression)	Acyclovir	Oral	200 mg 4 times per day	Acyclovir is administered during periods when intense immunosuppression is expected, e.g., antitumor chemotherapy, after transplantation. After therapy is discontinued, lesions recur.
		IV	5 mg/kg every 12 h	
Herpes simplex keratitis	Trifluorothymidine	Topical	One drop of 0.1% ophthalmic solution every 2 h while awake (maximum 9 drops per day)	Therapy should be undertaken in consultation with an ophthalmologist.
	or			
	vidarabine	Topical	0.5-in ribbon of 0.5% ophthalmic ointment 5 times per day	As above.
Varicella in immunocompromised patients	Acyclovir	IV	500 mg/m² every 8 h for 7 days	Studies comparing acyclovir with vidarabine in the treatment of varicella have not been performed. Limited placebo-controlled studies suggest the effects of both drugs on varicella are similar.
	vidarabine	IV	10 mg/kg per day in a 12-h infusion for 5 days	
Herpes zoster in immunocompromised patients	Acyclovir	IV	500 mg/m² every 8 h for 7 days	Efficacy of acyclovir and vidarabine are established for localized zoster, particularly when treated early and acyclovir appears to be more effective. Studies of the effect on disseminated zoster of the two drugs are underway. Oral acyclovir is under study in herpes zoster in immunosuppressed patients and in "normal" hosts.
	or			
	vidarabine	IV	10 mg/kg per day in a 12-h infusion for 5 days	

and EBV. Vidarabine inhibits viral DNA synthesis through its 5′-triphosphorylated metabolite, although the precise molecular mechanisms of action are not completely understood. In the therapy of herpes zoster in immunosuppressed patients, vidarabine, administered in a dose of 10 mg/kg per day for 5 days, resulted in reduction of rates of cutaneous and visceral dissemination, and of postherpetic neuralgia but was less effective than acyclovir in a comparative trial. Beneficial effects have also been observed in the treatment of varicella in immunosuppressed patients. Vidarabine administered in a higher dose (15 mg/kg per day for 10 days) was demonstrated to be effective in the therapy of herpes simplex encephalitis in a placebo-controlled study in which mortality was reduced from 70 to 40 percent in vidarabine recipients at 6 months after therapy. However, comparative studies indicate that acyclovir (30 mg/kg per day) is more effective than vidarabine in the therapy of herpes simplex encephalitis, and acyclovir has supplanted vidarabine as the treatment of choice for that infection. The above studies also indicated that the success of therapy was closely related to administration of the drug early in the illness.

Vidarabine treatment has also reduced the mortality of neonatal herpes simplex infection from 74 percent in placebo recipients to 38 percent, although the majority of survivors have severely impaired central nervous system function. Vidarabine has also been found to be effective in the treatment of HSV mucocutaneous infections in immunosuppressed patients, although the effects observed were limited to patients who had HSV-1 infections and were older than 40. Topically administered vidarabine has been generally ineffective in the treatment of mucocutaneous genital or orofacial HSV infections, but is effective in the treatment of HSV keratitis.

For systemic administration, vidarabine is available only as an intravenous preparation with poor solubility, so that no more than 450 mg of vidarabine can be dissolved in 1 liter of fluid. The dose is administered as a constant 12-h infusion, and substantial fluid loads can result which may be a significant problem in central nervous system infections. In humans, vidarabine is rapidly deaminated by a serum adenosine deaminase to its hypoxanthine derivative, ara-Hx, which has tenfold less antiviral activity than the parent compound, but is the major antiviral moiety in the plasma. When 10 mg/kg of vidarabine is administered, peak levels of ara-Hx are 3 to 6 μg/mL. Cerebrospinal fluid concentrations of ara-Hx are approximately 35 percent of plasma values in adults, although higher ratios have been found in infants. Under these conditions, the serum half-life of ara-Hx is estimated to be approximately 3.5 h, and the primary route of elimination is renal.

Large-scale controlled trials of vidarabine at doses of 10 to 15 mg/kg per day have not been attended by significant toxicity. At somewhat higher doses (20 mg/kg per day), vidarabine has been associated with hematopoietic side effects, including anemia, leukopenia, and thrombocytopenia. Neurotoxicities have also been reported, particularly with high dosages, in patients with hepatic or renal insufficiency, and possibly with concurrent interferon or allopurinol administration. The neurotoxic effects have included tremor, alterations in mentation, rarely coma or seizures, and unusual pain syndromes in the extremities, which have lasted up to 6 months after cessation of therapy.

TOPICAL ANTIVIRALS IUdR (5′-iodo-2′-deoxyuridine) is an inhibitor of DNA virus replication, including herpesviruses and poxviruses. It was formerly used systemically to treat herpesvirus infections, including HSV encephalitis, but because of associated toxicity and lack of demonstrated efficacy, its systemic use has largely been abandoned. However, topical IUdR is effective in the treatment of HSV keratitis, particularly in superficial epithelial infections. Local toxicity in the form of inflammation, pruritus, and allergic manifestations has been reported. In currently available topical formulations, IUdR has not been demonstrated to be effective in the treatment of mucocutaneous HSV infections.

Trifluorothymidine (TFT) is an analogue of deoxythymidine, which is also effective against herpesvirus infections. Because of bone marrow suppression, its use is restricted to topical application in the eye, where it appears to be somewhat more effective and better tolerated than IUdR, and at least as effective as vidarabine. TFT has also been effective in some patients who had not responded clinically to topical IUdR or vidarabine.

INTERFERONS From its earliest descriptions, considerable interest has existed in the application of interferon to the prophylaxis and/or therapy of viral infections. Early studies with human leukocyte interferon demonstrated an effect in the prophylaxis of experimentally induced rhinovirus infections in humans, and in the treatment of varicella-zoster infections in immunosuppressed patients. DNA recombinant technology has made available highly purified alpha, beta, and gamma interferons, which are now being evaluated in a wide variety of viral infections. Results available from such trials have confirmed the effectiveness of interferon in the prophylaxis of rhinovirus infections, and have suggested an effect on certain papillomavirus infections, chronic hepatitis B infections, and cytomegalovirus infections. Definition of the precise role of interferon in the treatment of these and other viral infections awaits the results of ongoing clinical trials.

REFERENCES

DOLIN R: Antiviral chemotherapy and chemoprophylaxis (review). Science 227:1296, 1985

——— et al: A controlled trial of amantadine and rimantadine in the prophylaxis of influenza A infection. N Engl J Med 307:580, 1982

DOUGLAS JM et al: A double-blind study of oral acyclovir for suppression of recurrences of genital herpes simplex virus infection. N Engl J Med 310:1551, 1984

GALASSO G et al (eds): *Antiviral Agents and Viral Diseases of Man*, 2d ed. New York, Raven, 1984

HALL CB et al: Aerosolized ribavirin treatment of infants with respiratory syncytial viral infection: A randomized double blind study. N Engl J Med 308:1443, 1983

REICHMAN RC et al: Treatment of recurrent genital herpes simplex with acyclovir. A controlled trial. JAMA 251:2103, 1984

WHITLEY RJ et al and the NIAID Collaborative Antiviral Study Group: Herpes simplex encephalitis: Adenine arabinoside versus acyclovir therapies. N Engl J Med 314:144, 1986

130 INFLUENZA

RAPHAEL DOLIN

DEFINITION Influenza is an acute respiratory illness caused by infection with influenza viruses. The illness affects the upper and/or lower respiratory tracts, and is often accompanied by systemic signs and symptoms such as fever, headache, myalgia, and weakness. Outbreaks of illness of variable extent and severity occur nearly every winter. Such outbreaks result in significant morbidity in the general population and in increased mortality rates in certain "high-risk" patients, predominantly as a result of pulmonary complications of acute illness.

ETIOLOGY Influenza viruses are members of the Orthomyxoviridae family. Influenza A and B viruses constitute one genus, and influenza C is the other genus. The designation of influenza viruses as types A, B, or C is based on antigenic characteristics of the nucleoprotein (NP) and matrix (M) protein antigens. Influenza A viruses are further subdivided (subtyped) on the basis of the surface hemagglutinin (H) and neuraminidase (N) antigens (see below). Individual strains are also designated according to the site of origin, isolate number, year of isolation, and subtype (e.g., influenza A/Victoria/3/79 H3N2). Influenza B and C viruses are similarly designated, but H and N antigens from those viruses do not receive subtype designations, since intratypic variations in H and N antigens of influenza B and C viruses are less extensive.

Most of the information regarding the molecular biology of influenza viruses has been generated from studies of influenza A viruses, and less is known about the replicative cycle of influenza B and C viruses. Morphologically, influenza viruses A, B, and C are similar. The virions are irregularly shaped spherical particles, 80 to 120 nm in diameter, and contain a lipid envelope from whose surface the hemagglutinin and neuraminidase glycoproteins project. The hemagglutinin serves as the site by which virus binds to cell receptors, while the neuraminidase degrades the receptor and probably plays a role in release of virus from infected cells after replication has taken place. Antibodies directed against the H antigen are the major determinants of immunity against influenza virus, while antineuraminidase antibodies limit viral spread and contribute to reduction of the extent of infection. The inner surface of the lipid envelope contains the matrix protein (M), whose function is incompletely understood but which may be involved in virus assembly and stabilization of the lipid envelope. The virion also contains the nucleoprotein (NP) with which the genome of the virus is associated, as well as three polymerase (P) proteins which are essential for transcription and synthesis of viral RNA. In addition, three nonstructural (NS) proteins of unknown function are also present in infected cells.

The genome of influenza A virus consists of 8 single-stranded segments of viral RNA, which code for the structural and nonstructural proteins. Because the genome is segmented, the opportunity for reassortment of genes during infection is high, and reassortment has been noted to occur frequently during infection of cells with more than one influenza A virus.

EPIDEMIOLOGY Influenza outbreaks occur virtually every year, although the extent and severity of such outbreaks vary widely. Localized outbreaks occur at variable intervals, usually every 1 to 3 years. Global epidemics or pandemics have occurred approximately every 10 to 15 years since the 1918–1919 pandemic (Table 130-1).

The most extensive and severe outbreaks are caused by influenza A viruses. In part, this is a result of the remarkable propensity of the hemagglutinin and neuraminidase antigens of influenza A virus

TABLE 130-1 Emergence of antigenic subtypes of influenza A associated with pandemic or epidemic disease

Year	Subtype of influenza A	Extent of outbreak
1889–90	H2N8*	Severe pandemic
1900–03	H3N8*	?Moderate epidemic
1918–19	H1N1† (formerly HswN1)	Severe pandemic
1933–35	H1N1† (formerly H0N1)	Mild epidemic
1946–47	H1N1	Mild epidemic
1957–58	H2N2	Severe pandemic
1968–69	H3N2	Moderate pandemic
1977–78	H1N1	Mild pandemic

* *As determined by retrospective serologic survey of individuals alive during those years ("seroarcheology").*

† *Hemagglutinins formerly designated as Hsw and H0 are now classified as variants of H1.*

to undergo periodic antigenic variation. Major antigenic variations are referred to as "antigenic shifts," which most likely occur from reassortment of genome segments between viral strains. Antigenic shifts may be associated with pandemics and are restricted to influenza A viruses. Minor variations are called "antigenic drifts" and likely arise from point mutations. These antigenic changes may involve the hemagglutinin alone, or both the hemagglutinin and the neuraminidase. In human infections, three major antigenic subtypes of hemagglutinins (H1, H2, and H3) and two neuraminidases (N1, N2) have been recognized. The hemagglutinins formerly designated as H0 and Hsw1 are now classified as variants of H1. An example of an antigenic shift which involved both the hemagglutinin and neuraminidase occurred in 1957, when the predominant influenza A virus subtype shifted from H1N1 to H2N2, and resulted in a severe pandemic, with an estimated 70,000 excess deaths in the United States alone. In 1968, an antigenic shift occurred which involved only the hemagglutinin (H2N2 to H3N2), and the subsequent pandemic was less severe than that seen in 1957. In 1977, an A/H1N1 virus emerged which caused a pandemic that primarily affected younger individuals, i.e., those born after 1957. As can be seen in Table 130-1, H1N1 viruses circulated from 1918 to 1956, so that individuals born prior to 1957 would be expected to possess some degree of immunity to H1N1 viruses. During most outbreaks of influenza A, a single subtype has circulated at a time. However, since 1977 both A/H1N1 and A/H3N2 viruses have circulated simultaneously resulting in outbreaks of varying severity.

The origin of pandemic strains is unknown. Because of the marked differences between the primary structures of the hemagglutinins of different subtypes of influenza A viruses (H1, H2, or H3), it is believed unlikely that antigenic shifts result from spontaneous mutations in the hemagglutinin gene. Because the segmented genome of influenza viruses may result in high rates of reassortment, it has been suggested that pandemic strains may emerge by reassortment of genes between human and animal influenza viruses. Influenza B viruses do not have an animal reservoir and do not undergo antigenic shift.

Although pandemics provide the most dramatic evidence of the impact of influenza, illnesses that occur in between pandemics account for an even greater total in mortality and morbidity, albeit over a longer period of time. Since 1957, interpandemic illness has been associated with 10,000 or more "excess deaths" on 15 occasions in the United States, resulting in an accumulated mortality of more than 450,000 over that period of time. Influenza A viruses that circulate in between pandemics demonstrate antigenic drifts in the hemagglutinin antigen. These antigenic drifts apparently result from point mutations which involve the RNA segment which codes for the hemagglutinin. Amino acid analysis of "drifted" hemagglutinins indicates that changes in a single amino acid have little effect on the antigenic properties of the hemagglutinin. Epidemiologically significant strains, i.e., those which have potential for causing widespread outbreaks, have changes in at least two of the four major antigenic sites in the HA molecule. Since two-point mutations are unlikely to occur simultaneously, it is believed that antigenic drifts result from point mutations which occur sequentially during the spread of virus from person to person. Antigenic drifts have occurred nearly annually since 1977 for A/H1N1 viruses, and since 1968 for A/H3N2 viruses.

Influenza A epidemics begin abruptly, reach a peak over a 2- to 3-week period, generally last for 2 to 3 months, and often subside almost as rapidly as they began. The first indication of influenza activity in a community is an increase in the number of children with febrile respiratory illnesses who present for medical attention. This is followed by increases in influenza-like illnesses among adults, and eventually by an increase in hospital admissions for patients with pneumonia, worsening of congestive heart failure, and exacerbations of chronic pulmonary disease. Rises in industrial and school absenteeism also occur at this time. An increase in the number of deaths caused by pneumonia and influenza ("excess mortality") is generally a late observation in an outbreak. Attack rates have been highly variable from outbreak to outbreak but most commonly are in the range of 10 to 20 percent of the general population. During the pandemic of 1957, it was estimated that the attack rate of clinical influenza exceeded 50 percent in urban populations, and that an additional 25 percent or more may have been subclinically infected with influenza A virus. Among institutionalized populations and in semiclosed settings where a large number of susceptible individuals is present, even higher attack rates have been reported.

Epidemics of influenza occur almost exclusively during the winter months in the northern and southern hemispheres. It is highly unusual to detect influenza A virus at times other than those in which an outbreak occurs, although rarely serologic rises have been noted at other times of the year. Where or how influenza A virus persists in between outbreaks is unknown. A possible explanation is that influenza A viruses are maintained in the human population on a worldwide basis by person-to-person transmission, and that large population clusters might be able to support a low level of interepidemic transmission. Alternatively, human strains may persist in animal reservoirs, but convincing evidence to support either explanation is not available. In the modern era, rapid modes of transportation may contribute to the transmission of viruses from widespread geographic locales.

The factors which result in the inception and termination of outbreaks of influenza are also incompletely understood. A major determinant of the extent and severity of an outbreak is the level of immunity present in the population at risk. When an antigenically novel influenza virus emerges to which little or no antibody is present in a community, extensive outbreaks may occur. When the absence of antibody is worldwide, epidemic disease may spread around the globe, resulting in a pandemic. Such pandemic waves can occur for several years, until immunity in the population reaches a high level. In the years following pandemic influenza, antigenic drifts among influenza viruses result in outbreaks of variable severity in populations that have high levels of immunity to the pandemic strain which circulated earlier. This situation persists until another antigenically novel pandemic strain emerges. On the other hand, outbreaks may also terminate despite the persistence of a large pool of susceptible individuals in the population. Occasionally, the emergence of a significantly different antigenic variant will result only in a localized outbreak. The "swine influenza outbreak" of 1976 in the United States may be considered to be an example of this, although this outbreak may simply represent the introduction of a swine influenza virus into a crowded human population without spread beyond that setting. It has also been suggested that certain viruses, such as recently circulating A/H1N1 strains, may be intrinsically less virulent and cause less severe disease, even in immunologically virgin subjects, suggesting that other undefined factors besides the level of preexisting immunity play a role in the epidemiology of influenza.

Influenza B causes outbreaks which are generally less extensive and are associated with less severe disease than those caused by influenza A virus. The hemagglutinin and neuraminidase of influenza B virus undergo less frequent and less extensive variation than is seen in influenza A viruses, which may account, in part, for the observation of less extensive disease. Influenza B outbreaks are seen most frequently in schools and military camps, although occasional outbreaks in older individuals have also been noted. The most serious complication of influenza B virus infection is Reye's syndrome (see below). Influenza C has been infrequently associated with human disease, although infection with influenza C virus is widespread.

The morbidity and mortality of influenza outbreaks continue to be substantial. Mortality occurs primarily in certain individuals with underlying diseases who have been characterized as being at "high risk" for complications of influenza. Excess hospitalizations for adults with "high risk" medical conditions have reached rates of 800 per 100,000 during recent outbreaks of influenza. These high-risk conditions are primarily chronic cardiac and pulmonary diseases, as well as increased age, particularly over 65. Increased mortality rates have also been observed among individuals with chronic metabolic, renal, and immunosuppressive diseases, although to a lesser extent than among those with chronic cardiopulmonary diseases.

In addition to the excess mortality, the morbidity of influenza in the general population is also extensive. For each of three outbreaks in the United States that were studied during the 1960s, it has been estimated that direct and indirect economic costs ranged from 1.5 to 3.5 billion dollars, and that today, such costs would be much greater.

PATHOGENESIS The initial event in influenza is infection of the respiratory epithelium with influenza virus, which is acquired from respiratory secretions of acutely infected individuals. In all likelihood, this occurs via aerosols generated by coughs and sneezes, although hand-to-hand, other personal contact, and even fomite transmission may occur. Experimental evidence suggests that infection by small-particle aerosol (less than 10-μm in diameter) is more efficient than that produced by larger droplets. Initially, viral infection involves the ciliated columnar epithelial cells, but it may also involve other respiratory tract cells, including alveolar cells, mucous gland cells, and macrophages. In infected cells, virus replication takes place within 4 to 6 h, after which infectious virus is released to infect adjacent or nearby cells. This results in spread of infection from a few foci to a large number of respiratory cells over several hours. In experimentally induced infection, the incubation period of illness has ranged from 18 to 72 h, depending on the size of the virus inoculum. Histopathologically, degenerative changes can be seen in infected ciliated cells, including granulation, vacuolization, swelling, and pyknotic nuclei. The cells eventually become necrotic and desquamate, and in some areas, previously columnar epithelium is replaced by flattened and metaplastic epithelial cells. The severity of illness is correlated with the quantity of virus shed in secretions, suggesting that the degree of viral replication itself may be an important mechanism in the pathogenesis of illness. Despite the frequent presence of systemic signs and symptoms such as fever, headache, and myalgias, influenza virus has only rarely been detected in extrapulmonary sites, including the bloodstream, and the pathogenesis of systemic symptoms in influenza remains unknown.

The host response to influenza infections involves a complex interplay of humoral antibody, local antibody, cell-mediated immune responses, interferon, and other host defenses. Serum antibody responses may be measured by a variety of techniques and can be detected by the second week after primary infection with influenza virus. Such antibodies may be measured by hemagglutination inhibition (HAI), complement fixation (CF), neutralization, enzyme immunosorbent assays (ELISA), and antineuraminidase antibody assays. Antibodies directed against the hemagglutinin appear to be the most important mediators of immunity, and in several studies, HAI titers of 40 or greater have been associated with protection from infection. Secretory antibodies produced in the respiratory tract are predominantly of the IgA class, and also play a major role in protection against infection. Secretory antibody neutralization titers of 4 or higher have also been associated with protection. A variety of cell-mediated immune responses, both antigen-specific and non-antigen-specific, can be detected early after infection, depending upon prior immunity of the host. These responses include T-cell proliferative, T-cell cytotoxic, and natural killer cell activity. Interferons have been detected in respiratory secretions shortly after shedding of virus has begun, and rises in interferon titers coincide with decreases in virus shedding.

The host defense factors responsible for cessation of virus shedding and resolution of illness have not been specifically defined. Virus shedding generally stops within 2 to 5 days after symptoms first appear, at a time when serum and local antibody responses are often not detectable by conventional techniques, although antibody rises may be detected earlier by use of highly sensitive techniques, particularly in individuals with previous immunity to the virus. It has been suggested that interferon, cell-mediated immune responses, or nonspecific inflammatory responses may be important in the resolution of illness.

MANIFESTATIONS Influenza has been most frequently described as the abrupt onset of systemic symptoms such as headache, feverishness, chilliness, myalgia, or malaise, accompanied by respiratory illness, most frequently manifested by cough and sore throat. In many cases, the onset is so abrupt that patients can recall the precise time of the onset of illness. A typical case of naturally occurring influenza is depicted in Fig. 130-1. However, a wide spectrum of clinical

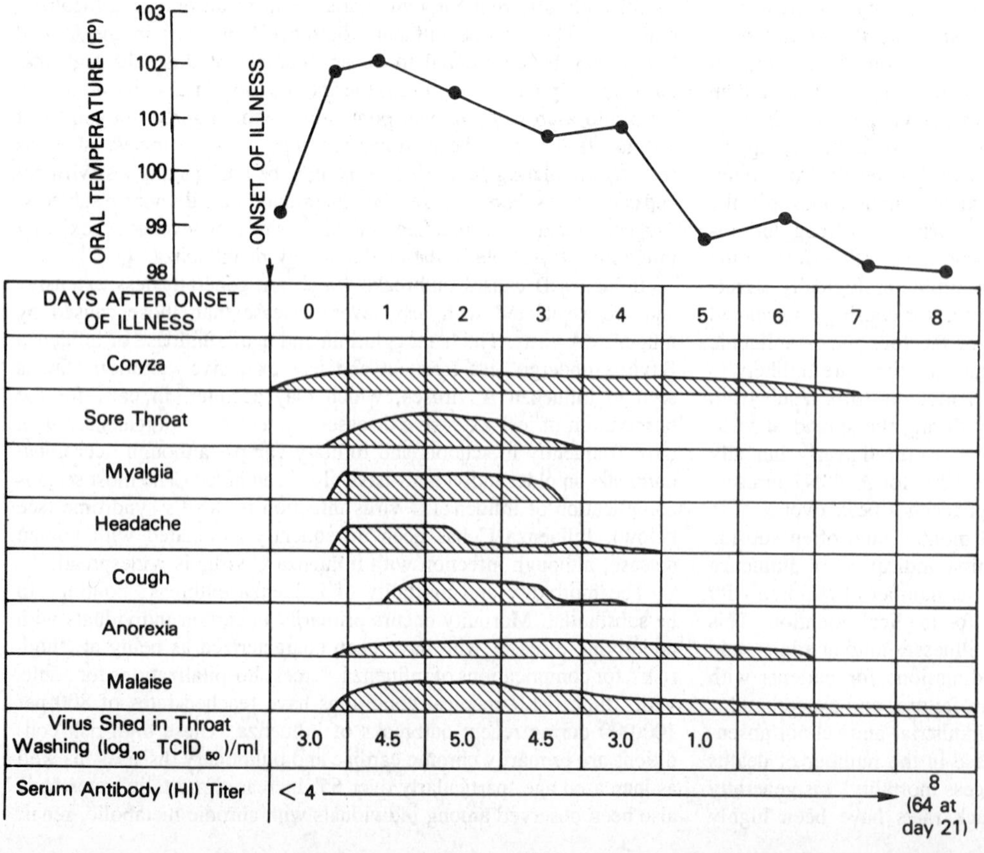

FIGURE 130-1 *Clinical characteristics of a naturally occurring case of influenza A in an otherwise healthy 28-year-old male. (From R Dolin, Am Fam Phys 14:74, 1976.)*

presentations may occur. These can range from mild, afebrile respiratory illnesses similar to the common cold, with either gradual or abrupt onset, to illnesses in which severe prostration with relatively few respiratory signs and symptoms may be present. In the majority of cases which come to a physician's attention, fever is present and can range from 38°C to as high as 41°C. The temperature rises rapidly within the first 24 h of illness, and is generally followed by a gradual defervescence over a 2- to 3-day period, although, on occasion, fever may last for as long as a week. Patients complain of feverish feeling and chilliness, but true rigors are rare. Headache, either generalized or frontal, is often a particularly troublesome complaint. Myalgias may involve any part of the body, but are most common in the legs and lumbosacral area. Arthralgias may also be present.

Respiratory complaints often become more prominent as systemic symptoms subside. Many patients complain of a sore throat or persistent cough which may last for a week or more, and which is often accompanied by substernal discomfort. Ocular signs and symptoms include pain on motion of the eyes, photophobia, and burning of the eyes.

Physical findings are usually minimal in cases of uncomplicated influenza. Early in the illness, the patient appears flushed and the skin is hot and dry, although diaphoresis and mottled extremities, particularly in older patients, may occur. Examination of the pharynx may be surprisingly unremarkable despite a severe sore throat, but injection of the mucous membranes and postnasal discharge can be present. Mild cervical lymphadenopathy may be noted, particularly in younger individuals. Chest examination is largely negative in uncomplicated influenza, although rhonchi, wheezes, and scattered rales have been reported with variable frequency in different outbreaks. Frank dyspnea, hyperpnea, cyanosis, diffuse rales, or signs of consolidation should alert the physician to the presence of pulmonary complications. Patients with apparently uncomplicated influenza have been reported to have a variety of mild ventilatory defects and increased alveolar-capillary diffusion gradients, indicating that subclinical pulmonary involvement may be more frequent than is appreciated.

In uncomplicated influenza, the acute illness generally resolves over a 2- to 5-day period, and most patients have largely recovered in 1 week. In a significant minority, however, symptoms of weakness or lassitude ("postinfluenzal asthenia") may persist for several weeks, particularly in the elderly, and may prove troublesome for those who wish to return to full activity promptly. The pathogenetic basis for this "asthenia" is unknown, although pulmonary function abnormalities may persist for several weeks after uncomplicated influenza.

COMPLICATIONS OF INFLUENZA The most common complication of influenza is pneumonia, which may occur either as "primary" influenza viral pneumonia, secondary bacterial pneumonia, or mixed viral and bacterial pneumonia. Primary influenza viral pneumonia is the least common but most severe of the pneumonic complications. It presents as acute influenza which does not resolve, but instead relentlessly progresses with persistent fever, dyspnea, and eventual cyanosis. Sputum production is generally scanty but can contain blood, and few physical signs may be present early in the illness. In more advanced cases, diffuse rales may be noted, and chest x-ray findings consistent with diffuse interstitial infiltrates and/or acute respiratory distress syndrome may be present. In such cases arterial blood gases show marked hypoxia. Viral cultures, particularly if taken early in illness, show high titers of virus shed in respiratory secretions and in the lung parenchyma. Histopathology of fatal cases of primary viral pneumonia shows a marked inflammatory reaction in the alveolar septa, with edema and infiltration with lymphocytes, macrophages, occasional plasma cells, and variable numbers of neutrophils. Fibrin thrombi in alveolar capillaries, along with necrosis and hemorrhage, have also been noted. Eosinophilic hyaline membranes can also be found lining alveoli and alveolar ducts.

Primary influenza viral pneumonia has a predilection for individuals with cardiac disease, particularly those with mitral stenosis, but has also been reported in otherwise healthy young adults, as well as in older individuals with chronic pulmonary disorders. In some epidemics of influenza (notably 1918 and 1957), pregnancy increased the risk of the development of primary influenza pneumonia.

Secondary bacterial pneumonia is a complication in which bacterial infection develops following a case of acute influenza. With this illness, patients experience a period of improvement for 2 to 3 days after acute influenza, followed by a reappearance of fever, along with clinical signs and symptoms of bacterial pneumonia. These include cough, purulent sputum production, and physical and x-ray signs of consolidation. The most common bacterial pathogens in this setting are *Streptococcus pneumoniae, Staphylococcus aureus,* or *Haemophilus influenzae,* organisms that can colonize the nasopharynx and that cause infection in the wake of changes in bronchopulmonary defenses. The etiology can often be determined by Gram strain and culture of an appropriately obtained sputum specimen. Secondary bacterial pneumonia occurs most frequently in high-risk individuals with chronic pulmonary and cardiac disease and in elderly individuals. Patients with secondary bacterial pneumonias will often respond to antibiotic therapy when it is instituted promptly.

Perhaps the most common of the pneumonic complications that occur during outbreaks of influenza are mixed viral and bacterial pneumonias. The clinical course of this complication contains features of both primary and secondary pneumonias described above. Patients may have a gradual progression of their acute illness, or may show a transient improvement followed by a clinical worsening, with eventual manifestion of the clinical features of a bacterial pneumonia. Sputum cultures may contain both influenza A virus and one of the bacterial pathogens described above. Patchy infiltrates or areas of consolidation may be noted by physical examination and chest x-ray. Patients with mixed viral and bacterial pneumonias generally have less widespread involvement of the lung than those with primary viral pneumonia, and their bacterial infections may respond to appropriate antibiotics. Mixed viral and bacterial pneumonias occur primarily in patients with chronic cardiovascular and pulmonary diseases.

In addition to the pulmonary complications of influenza, a number of extrapulmonary complications may occur. *Reye's syndrome* is a serious complication of influenza B, and to a lesser extent of influenza A virus infection, as well as of varicella-zoster virus infection. It occurs in children most commonly between the ages of 2 and 16, and follows several days after a generally unremarkable viral illness. Reye's syndrome is marked by the onset of nausea and vomiting for 1 to 2 days, after which central nervous system symptoms appear. These are most frequently changes in mental status, ranging from lethargy to coma, and can include delirium and seizures. Hepatomegaly is noted, along with a marked elevation of SGOT, SGPT, and LDH levels. Bilirubin values are only moderately elevated, so that the children are not jaundiced, but blood ammonia levels are elevated in virtually all patients. Hypoglycemia can occur, especially after varicella-zoster virus infection or after viral gastrointestinal illnesses. Children are usually afebrile, and while lumbar puncture generally shows an elevated pressure, the cerebrospinal fluid is quite unremarkable, indicating that an encephalopathy rather than a meningoencephalitis is present. The mortality of the syndrome is related to the state of consciousness on admission and has decreased from more than 40 percent, when the syndrome was originally described, to approximately 10 percent, reflecting earlier recognition and improved management of cerebral edema and hypoglycemia. Histopathology demonstrates little in the way of inflammatory changes in either the liver or the central nervous system. Liver biopsy shows diffuse fatty infiltration of hepatocytes, and swelling and pleomorphism in mitochondria. Cerebral edema and anoxic changes in neurons are the only pathologic changes detected in the central nervous system. The pathogenesis of Reye's syndrome is unknown, but the virus is almost never found in the affected liver and brain. An epidemiologic association with aspirin therapy for the antecedent viral infection has been noted.

Myositis, rhabdomyolysis, and myoglobinuria have also been reported as occasional complications of influenza infection. Although myalgias are exceedingly common in influenza, true myositis is rare. Patients with acute myositis have exquisite tenderness of the affected muscles, most commonly in the legs, and may not be able to tolerate even the slightest pressure, such as the touch of bed sheets. In the most severe cases, there is frank swelling and bogginess of muscles. Markedly elevated serum creatine phosphokinase and aldolase levels are present, and an occasional patient has developed renal failure from myoglobinuria. The pathogenesis of influenza-associated myositis is also unclear, although the presence of influenza virus in affected muscles has been reported.

Myocarditis and pericarditis in association with influenza virus infection was reported during the 1918–1919 pandemic, based largely on histopathologic findings, and has been infrequently documented since that time. ECG changes during acute influenza are commonly noted in patients who have cardiac disease but these have been most often ascribed to exacerbations of the underlying cardiac disease rather than to direct involvement of the myocardium with influenza virus.

Central nervous system (CNS) disease has also been reported during influenza, including encephalitis, transverse myelitis, and Guillain-Barré syndrome. The etiologic relationship of influenza virus to such CNS illnesses remains unestablished.

In addition to complications involving the specific organ systems described above, every influenza outbreak includes a number of elderly and other high-risk individuals who develop influenza, and who subsequently experience a gradual deterioration of underlying cardiovascular, pulmonary, or renal function, occasionally leading to irreversible changes and death. These fatalities contribute to the overall toll of excess mortality associated with influenza A outbreaks.

LABORATORY FINDINGS Laboratory diagnosis is accomplished during the acute illness by isolation of virus from throat swabs, nasopharyngeal washes, or sputum. Virus is usually detected in tissue culture or less commonly in the amniotic cavity of chick embryos within 48 to 72 h after inoculation. Viral antigens may be detected somewhat earlier by use of immunofluorescence techniques in tissue culture, or directly in exfoliated nasopharyngeal cells obtained by washings. The type of influenza virus (A or B) may be identified by either immunofluorescence or hemagglutination inhibition techniques, and the hemagglutinin subtype of influenza A virus (H1, H2, or H3) may be identified by hemagglutination inhibition using subtype-specific antisera. Serologic methods for diagnosis require comparison of antibody titers in sera obtained during the acute illness with those obtained 10 to 14 days after the onset of illness, and are useful primarily in retrospect. Fourfold or greater rises as detected by hemagglutination inhibition, complement fixation, or significant rises by ELISA techniques are diagnostic of acute infection. Complement fixation tests are generally less sensitive than other serologic techniques, but since they detect type-specific antigens, they may be particularly useful when subtype-specific reagents are not available.

The remainder of other laboratory tests are generally not helpful in making a specific diagnosis of influenza virus infection. Leukocyte counts are variable during illness, being frequently low early in illness, and normal or slightly elevated later. Severe leukopenia has been described in overwhelming viral or bacterial infection, while leukocytosis with counts of greater than 15,000 cells per cubic millimeter should raise the suspicion that secondary bacterial infection is present.

DIFFERENTIAL DIAGNOSIS On clinical grounds alone, an individual case of influenza may be difficult to differentiate from an acute respiratory illness caused by a variety of respiratory viruses or by *Mycoplasma pneumoniae*. Severe streptococcal pharyngitis or early bacterial pneumonia may mimic acute influenza, although bacterial pneumonias generally do not run a self-limited course. The presence of purulent sputum in which a bacterial pathogen can be detected by Gram stain is an important diagnostic feature in bacterial pneumonia. The fact that influenza occurs in characteristic outbreaks during the winter months may be very helpful in making a clinical diagnosis. When local health authorities indicate that influenza activity is present in the community, the etiology of an acute febrile respiratory illness can be attributed to influenza with a high degree of certainty, particularly if the typical features of abrupt onset and systemic symptoms are present.

TREATMENT In uncomplicated cases of influenza, symptomatic therapy for headache, myalgia, and fever may be considered, employing either acetaminophen or salicylates, but salicylates should be avoided in children below 16 years of age because of the possible association of salicylates with Reye's syndrome. Since cough is ordinarily self-limited, treatment with cough suppressants is generally not indicated, although codeine-containing compounds may be employed if the cough is particularly troublesome. Patients should be advised to rest and maintain hydration during acute illness, and should return to full activity only gradually after the illness has resolved, particularly if illness has been severe.

The only specific antiviral therapy available for influenza is amantadine. Amantadine is active only against influenza A viruses and has been licensed for the prophylaxis and therapy of influenza A virus infections in the United States. If begun within 48 h of the onset of illness, amantadine reduces the duration of systemic and respiratory symptoms of influenza by approximately 50 percent, and in one study, was superior to aspirin. From 5 to 10 percent of individuals who receive amantadine will experience mild CNS side effects, primarily jitteriness, anxiety, insomnia, or difficulty in concentrating. These side effects disappear promptly upon cessation of the drug. The dose of amantadine for adults is 200 mg per day for 3 to 5 days or up to 48 h after illness has resolved. Because amantadine is excreted almost entirely by the kidneys, the dose should be reduced in individuals with renal insufficiency. Rimantadine, an experimental drug which is a closely related analogue of amantadine, appears to be equally efficacious, and is associated with less frequent CNS side effects than is amantadine. Recently, ribavirin, a nucleoside analogue with activity against a variety of viral agents, has been reported to be effective against both influenza A and B virus infections when administered as an aerosol, although relatively ineffective when administered orally.

Studies demonstrating the therapeutic efficacy of antiviral compounds in influenza have been carried out almost exclusively in uncomplicated disease in young adults, and it is not known whether such compounds are effective in the treatment of complications such as influenza pneumonia. Therapy for primary influenza pneumonia is directed at maintaining oxygenation and is most appropriately managed in an intensive care unit, with aggressive respiratory and hemodynamic support as needed. Bypass membrane oxygenators have been employed in this setting with variable results. When an acute respiratory distress syndrome develops, fluids must be administered cautiously, with close monitoring of blood gases and hemodynamic function.

Antibacterial drugs should be reserved for the therapy of bacterial complications of acute influenza such as secondary bacterial pneumonia. The choice of antibiotics should be guided by Gram stain and culture of appropriate specimens of respiratory secretions, such as sputum or transtracheal aspirates. If the etiology of a bacterial pneumonia is unclear from examination of respiratory secretions, empiric antibiotics should be selected which are effective against the most common bacterial pathogens in this setting, namely, *S. pneumoniae*, *S. aureus*, and *H. influenzae*.

PROPHYLAXIS The major public health measure for prevention of influenza has been the use of inactivated influenza vaccines. Currently, these vaccines are derived from influenza A and B viruses which circulated during the previous influenza season. If the vaccine and currently circulating viruses are closely related, such vaccines would be expected to provide 50 to 80 percent protection against influenza. Currently available vaccines have been highly purified and are associated with few reactions. Up to 5 percent of individuals will experience low-grade fever and mild systemic symptoms 8 to 24 h after vaccination, and up to one-third may have mild redness or tenderness at the vaccination site. Since the vaccine is produced in eggs, individuals with true hypersensitivity to egg products should either be desensitized or should not receive vaccine. Although the 1976 swine influenza vaccine appears to have been associated with an increased frequency of Guillain-Barré syndrome, influenza vaccines administered since 1976 have not been associated with Guillain-Barré syndrome. Live attenuated (''cold-adapted'') influenza A vaccines have also been developed and are currently under evaluation. Such vaccines are administered intranasally and stimulate local antibody production more efficiently than conventional inactivated vaccines.

The U.S. Public Health Service recommends influenza vaccination for individuals with chronic cardiovascular or pulmonary disorders severe enough to have required medical attention during the preceding year, and for residents of nursing homes and other chronic care facilities. The next priority of recommendations is for vaccination of medical personnel who come in contact with high-risk patients. Other populations for whom the vaccine is recommended include otherwise healthy individuals over 65 years of age, individuals with chronic metabolic diseases, including diabetes mellitus, renal dysfunction, anemia, immunosuppression, or asthma. Since commercially available vaccines are inactivated (''killed''), they may be safely administered to immunocompromised patients. Influenza vaccination is also not associated with exacerbations of chronic nervous system diseases such as multiple sclerosis. Vaccination should be administered early in the autumn before influenza outbreaks occur, and should be administered on an annual basis to maintain immunity against the most current influenza virus strains.

Amantadine and rimantadine have also been demonstrated to be effective in the prophylaxis of influenza A. Studies have demonstrated 70 to 90 percent effectiveness of these drugs in preventing illness associated with influenza A virus infection. The major use for prophylaxis with amantadine or rimantadine is likely to be for high-risk individuals who have not received influenza vaccine, or when the vaccines previously administered are relatively ineffective because of antigenic changes in the circulating virus. If vaccination is performed during an outbreak, amantadine can be administered simultaneously with inactivated vaccine, since it will not interfere with an immune response to the vaccine. In addition, there is evidence that the protective effects of amantadine and vaccine may be additive. Amantadine has also been employed to control nosocomial outbreaks of influenza A. For prophylaxis, amantadine, or rimantadine should be instituted promptly when influenza A activity is detected and must be administered daily for the duration of the outbreak. The dosage most frequently employed has been 200 mg per day for adults, but the dose of amantadine should be reduced in patients with renal insufficiency and in the elderly.

REFERENCES

CENTERS FOR DISEASE CONTROL: Prevention and control of influenza. Morb Mort Week Rep 34:261, 1985

———: Prevention and control of influenza. Ann Intern Med 103:560, 1985

DOLIN R et al: A controlled trial of amantadine and rimantadine in the prophylaxis of influenza A infection. N Engl J Med 307:580, 1982

GLEZEN WP: Serious morbidity and mortality associated with influenza epidemics. Epidemiol Rev 4:25, 1982

LAMONTAGNE JR et al: Summary of clinical trials of inactivated influenza vaccines, 1978. Rev Infect Dis 5:723, 1983

MURPHY BR, WEBSTER RG: Influenza viruses, in *Virology*, BN Fields (ed). New York, Raven, 1985, pp 1179–1240

131 COMMON VIRAL RESPIRATORY INFECTIONS

RAPHAEL DOLIN

GENERAL CONSIDERATIONS Acute viral respiratory illnesses are among the most common of human diseases, accounting for one-half or more of all acute illnesses. The incidence of acute respiratory disease in the United States is from 3 to 5.6 cases per person per year. The highest rates occur in children under 1 (6.1 to 8.3 cases per year) and remain high until age 6, when a progressive decrease is noted. Adults in the general population have three to four illnesses per person per year. Morbidity from acute respiratory illnesses accounts for 30 to 50 percent of time lost from work by adults and from 60 to 80 percent of time lost from school by children.

It has been estimated that two-thirds to three-fourths of cases of acute respiratory illnesses are caused by viruses. More than 200 antigenically distinct viruses from 8 different genera have been reported to cause acute respiratory illness, and it is likely that additional agents will be described in the future. The vast majority of these viral infections involve the upper respiratory tract, but lower respiratory tract disease can also occur, particularly in younger age groups and in certain epidemiologic settings.

The illnesses caused by respiratory viruses traditionally have been divided into multiple distinct syndromes, such as the ''common cold,'' pharyngitis, croup (laryngotracheobronchitis), tracheitis, bronchiolitis, bronchitis, and pneumonia. These general categories of illnesses have a certain epidemiologic and clinical utility, e.g., croup occurs exclusively in very young children and has a characteristic clinical course. In addition, some types of respiratory illnesses are more likely to be associated with certain viruses, e.g., the ''common cold'' with rhinoviruses, while others occupy characteristic epidemiologic niches, such as adenoviruses in military recruits. The syndromes most commonly associated with infection with the major respiratory virus groups are summarized in Table 131-1. Despite these associations, it is clear that most respiratory viruses have the potential to cause more than one type of respiratory illness, and frequently features of several types of illness may be present in the same patient. Moreover, the clinical illnesses induced by these viruses are rarely sufficiently distinctive to enable an etiologic diagnosis to be made on clinical grounds alone, although the epidemiologic setting increases the likelihood that one group of viruses rather than another may be involved. In general, laboratory methods must be relied upon to establish a specific viral diagnosis.

This chapter will review viral infections caused by five of the major groups of respiratory viruses: rhinoviruses, coronaviruses, respiratory syncytial virus, parainfluenza viruses, and adenoviruses. Influenza viruses, which are a major cause of mortality as well as morbidity, are reviewed in Chap. 130. Herpesviruses, which occasionally cause pharyngitis and which also cause lower respiratory tract disease in immunosuppressed patients, are reviewed in Chap. 136. Enteroviruses, which account for occasional respiratory illnesses during the summer months, are reviewed in Chap. 139.

RHINOVIRUS INFECTIONS

ETIOLOGY Rhinoviruses are members of the Picornaviridae family, which are small (15 to 30 nm), nonenveloped viruses which contain a single-stranded RNA genome. In contrast to other members of the picornavirus family, such as enteroviruses, rhinoviruses are acid-labile and are almost completely inactivated at pH 3 or lower. Rhinoviruses grow preferentially at 33 to 34°C, which is the temperature of nasal passages in humans, rather than the higher temperature (37°C) of the lower respiratory tract. Currently, there are 113 distinct serotypes among rhinoviruses; additional serotypes are likely to be described in the future.

EPIDEMIOLOGY Rhinoviruses are a major cause of the common cold and have been isolated from 15 to 40 percent of adults with common cold-like illnesses. Infection rates are higher among infants and young children and decrease with increasing age. Rhinovirus infections occur throughout the year, but seasonal peaks occur in early fall and spring in temperate climates. Rhinovirus infections are most often introduced into families by preschool or grade school children below 6 years of age. Between 25 and 50 percent of initial illnesses in family settings are followed by secondary cases, with the highest attack rates occurring in the youngest siblings at home. Attack rates also increase with increasing size of families.

The spread of rhinoviruses appears to be by direct contact with infected secretions, usually respiratory droplets. In volunteer studies, transmission was most efficient by hand-to-hand contact, with subsequent self-inoculation of the conjunctival or nasal mucosa. Transmission appears to be much less efficient following exposure to large or small aerosolized particles. Virus can also be recovered from plastic surfaces inoculated 1 to 3 h previously, suggesting that environmental surfaces may also contribute to transmission. In studies conducted in married couples in which serum antibody was not present in either partner, transmission was associated with prolonged contact (122 h or more) during a 7-day period. Transmission was infrequent unless virus was recoverable from the donor's hands and nasal mucosa, unless at least 1000 $TCID_{50}$ of virus was present in nasal washes of the donor, and unless the donor was at least moderately symptomatic with the "cold." Despite anecdotal observations, exposure to cold temperatures, fatigue, or sleep deprivation has not been associated with increased rates of rhinovirus-induced illness in human volunteer studies.

Infection with rhinoviruses is worldwide in distribution, and by the time they reach adulthood, nearly all individuals have neutralizing antibodies to multiple serotypes, although the prevalence of antibody to any one serotype varies widely. Multiple serotypes circulate simultaneously, and generally no single serotype or group of serotypes has emerged as being more prevalent than others.

PATHOGENESIS Relatively limited information is available on the histopathology and pathogenesis of acute rhinovirus infections in humans. Biopsies performed in experimentally induced and in naturally occurring illness indicate that the nasal mucosa is edematous, often hyperemic, and during acute illness, is covered by a mucoid discharge. There is a mild infiltrate of the mucosa with inflammatory cells, including neutrophils, lymphocytes, plasma cells, and eosinophils. Mucous secreting glands in the submucosa appear hyperactive; the nasal turbinates are engorged, which may lead to obstruction of nearby openings of sinus cavities.

The incubation period for rhinovirus illness is short, and generally ranges from 1 to 2 days. Virus shedding coincides with the onset of illness or may begin shortly before symptoms develop. The mechanisms of immunity to rhinovirus are not well worked out. In some studies, the presence of homotypic antibody significantly reduced the rates of subsequent infection and illness, but conflicting data exist as to the relative importance of serum and local antibody in protection from rhinovirus infection.

CLINICAL MANIFESTATIONS The most common clinical manifestations of rhinovirus infections are those of the common cold. Initially, illness begins with rhinorrhea and sneezing, accompanied by nasal congestion. Sore throat is frequently present and in some cases may be the initial complaint. Systemic signs and symptoms, such as malaise and headache, are mild or absent, and fever is unusual. Illness generally lasts for 4 to 9 days, and resolves spontaneously without sequelae. In children, lower respiratory tract involvement may be seen, including bronchitis, bronchiolitis, and on occasion bronchopneumonia. Rhinoviruses may also cause exacerbations of asthma and chronic pulmonary disease in adults. The vast majority of rhinovirus infections resolve without sequelae, but complications related to obstruction of the eustachian tubes or sinus ostia, including otitis media or acute sinusitis, can occur.

DIAGNOSIS Although rhinoviruses are the most frequently recognized cause of the common cold, similar illnesses may be caused by a variety of other viruses, and the etiologic diagnosis cannot be made on clinical grounds alone. The diagnosis of rhinovirus infection is made by isolation of virus from nasal washes or nasal secretions in tissue culture. In practice, this procedure is rarely carried out because of the benign, self-limited nature of the illness. Because of the large number of serotypes of rhinovirus, diagnosis of rhinovirus infections by serum antibody tests is currently not practical. Common laboratory tests such as white cell count and sedimentation rate are not helpful in the diagnosis of rhinovirus infection.

TREATMENT AND PREVENTION Rhinovirus infections are generally mild and self-limited so that treatment is not necessary. Some patients may benefit from the use of analgesics and nasal decongestants, and reduction of activity is prudent if significant discomfort or fatigability is present. Specific antiviral therapy is not available, although intranasally administered interferon has been effective in the prophylaxis of experimentally induced rhinovirus infections and is currently being evaluated in naturally occurring disease. Experimental vaccines to certain rhinovirus serotypes have been prepared but their utility is questionable, particularly because of the existence of the large number of serotypes and the uncertainty regarding the important mechanisms of immunity. Thorough hand washing or barrier protection against autoinoculation may help to reduce transmission of infection.

TABLE 131-1 Illnesses associated with respiratory viruses

Frequency of respiratory syndromes associated with virus groups

Virus	Most frequent	Occasional	Infrequent
Rhinoviruses	Common cold	Exacerbation of chronic bronchitis and asthma	Pneumonia (children)
Coronaviruses	Common cold	Exacerbation of chronic bronchitis and asthma	Pneumonia and bronchiolitis
Respiratory syncytial virus	Pneumonia and bronchiolitis in young children	Common cold in adults	Pneumonia in elderly
Parainfluenza viruses	Croup and lower respiratory tract disease in young children	Pharyngitis and common cold	Tracheobronchitis in adults
Adenoviruses	Common cold and pharyngitis in children	Outbreaks of acute respiratory disease (ARD)* in military recruits	Pneumonia in children and immunosuppressed patients
Influenza A viruses	"Influenza-like illness"†	Pneumonia and excess mortality in "high-risk" patients	Pneumonia in healthy individuals
Influenza B viruses	"Influenza-like illness"†	Rhinitis and pharyngitis alone	Pneumonia
Enteroviruses	Acute undifferentiated febrile illnesses‡	Rhinitis and pharyngitis	Pneumonia
Herpes simplex viruses	Gingivostomatitis‡ (children) Pharyngotonsillitis (adults)	Tracheitis and pneumonia in immunocompromised patients	Disseminated infection in immunocompromised patients

* *Serotypes 4 and 7.*
† *Fever, cough, myalgia, malaise.*
‡ *May or may not have a respiratory component.*

CORONAVIRUS INFECTIONS

ETIOLOGY Coronaviruses are pleomorphic, single-stranded RNA viruses, 80 to 160 nm in diameter, with clublike projections emanating from the virus envelope, resulting in an appearance which resembles that of the solar "corona" from which their name is derived. Three distinct coronavirus serotypes, designated B814, 229E, and OC43, have been isolated from humans. Coronaviruses are fastidious and are difficult to culture in vitro. Some strains will grow only in human tracheal organ cultures rather than in tissue culture.

EPIDEMIOLOGY Only limited seroepidemiologic studies have been carried out in coronavirus infections. Seroprevalence studies of two of the serotypes, 229E and OC43, have yielded variable rates of serum antibodies, ranging from 12 to 80 percent in various populations. Overall, coronaviruses account for 10 to 20 percent of common colds. Coronavirus infections appear to be particularly prevalent in late fall, winter, and early spring, at a time when rhinovirus infections are less common. Depending on the serotype, a cyclical pattern for outbreaks of coronavirus infection has been suggested, which ranges from every 2 years for OC43, to every 2 to 4 years with 229E.

CLINICAL FEATURES The clinical features of illness caused by coronaviruses are similar to those caused by rhinoviruses. In volunteer studies, the mean incubation period of illness induced by coronaviruses (3 days) is somewhat longer than that caused by rhinoviruses, and the duration of illness is somewhat shorter, with a mean of 6 to 7 days. In some studies, the amount of nasal discharge was somewhat greater in colds induced by coronaviruses compared to those induced by rhinoviruses. Coronaviruses have also been recovered from infants with pneumonia and from military recruits with lower respiratory tract disease, and have also been associated with worsening of chronic bronchitis. However, the overall significance of coronaviruses in lower respiratory tract disease in humans is unclear.

TREATMENT AND PREVENTION The approach to the treatment of common colds caused by coronaviruses is similar to that discussed above for rhinovirus-induced illnesses. Because of the uncertainty regarding the number and relative importance of coronavirus serotypes and the mechanisms of immunity, vaccines against coronaviruses have not been developed.

RESPIRATORY SYNCYTIAL VIRUS INFECTIONS

ETIOLOGY Respiratory syncytial virus (RSV) is a member of the Paramyxoviridae family and comprises the genus *Pneumovirus*. RSV is an enveloped virus approximately 150 to 300 nm in size, so named because virus replication leads to fusion of neighboring cells into large multinucleated syncytia. The single-stranded RNA genome codes for 10 virus-specific proteins. Viral RNA is contained in a helical nucleocapsid surrounded by a lipid envelope bearing two glycoproteins, one of which is the fusion protein which facilitates entry of virus into the cell by fusing host and viral membranes. Respiratory syncytial viruses are of a single antigenic type, although minor antigenic strain variations of uncertain significance have been noted.

EPIDEMIOLOGY RSV is the major respiratory pathogen of young children and is the major cause of lower respiratory disease in infants. Infection with RSV is seen throughout the world, in annual epidemics which occur in either late fall, winter, or spring, and can last up to 5 months. The virus is rarely encountered during the summer. The highest rates of illness occur in infants between 1 and 6 months of age, with peak rates occurring between 2 and 3 months of age. The attack rates among susceptibles are extraordinarily high, approaching 100 percent in settings such as day-care centers where large numbers of susceptible infants are present. RSV accounts for 20 to 25 percent of hospital admissions for pneumonia of young infants and children, and up to 75 percent of cases of bronchiolitis in this age group. It has been estimated that more than half of infants who are at risk will become infected during an RSV epidemic.

In older children and adults, reinfection with RSV is frequent, but disease is milder than in infancy. A "common cold-like syndrome" is the illness most commonly associated with RSV infection in adults. RSV is also an important nosocomial pathogen and can infect up to 25 to 50 percent of the staff on pediatric wards during an RSV outbreak. The spread of virus among families is also efficient, and up to 40 percent of older siblings may become infected when RSV is introduced into the family setting.

RSV is transmitted primarily by close contact with contaminated fingers or fomites, and by self-inoculation of the conjunctiva or anterior nares. Virus may also be spread by coarse aerosols produced by coughing or sneezing but is inefficiently spread by fine-particle aerosols. The incubation period of illness is approximately 4 to 6 days, and virus shedding may last for 2 weeks or longer in children, and for shorter periods of time in adults.

PATHOGENESIS The characteristics of the immune response to RSV are not well elucidated. Because reinfection occurs frequently and is often associated with illness, the immunity that develops after single episodes of infection is not complete or long-lasting. However, the cumulative effect of multiple reinfections ameliorates subsequent disease and provides some temporary measure of protection against infection. Studies of experimentally induced disease in normal volunteers indicate that the presence of nasal IgA neutralizing antibody correlates more closely with protection than does the presence of serum antibody. Studies in infants, however, suggest that maternally acquired antibody provides some protection from lower respiratory tract disease, although severe illness may also occur in infants who have moderate levels of maternally derived serum antibody.

CLINICAL MANIFESTATIONS RSV infection leads to a wide spectrum of respiratory illnesses. In infants, 25 to 40 percent of infections result in lower respiratory tract involvement, including pneumonia, bronchiolitis, and tracheobronchitis. In infants, illness begins most frequently with rhinorrhea, low-grade fever, and mild systemic symptoms, often accompanied by cough and wheezing. Most patients gradually recover in 1 to 2 weeks. In more severe illness, tachypnea and dyspnea develop, and eventually frank hypoxia, cyanosis, and apnea can ensue. Physical examination may reveal diffuse wheezing, rhonchi, and rales. Chest x-ray shows hyperexpansion, peribronchial thickening, and variable infiltrates ranging from diffuse interstitial infiltrates to segmental or lobar consolidation. Illness may be particularly severe in children with congenital cardiac disease, bronchopulmonary dysplasia, or immunosuppression. One study documented a 37-percent mortality rate for infants with RSV pneumonia and congenital cardiac disease.

In adults, the most common symptoms of RSV infection are those of the common cold, with rhinorrhea, sore throat, and cough. Illness may occasionally be associated with moderate systemic symptoms such as malaise, headache, and fever. RSV has also been reported to cause febrile lower respiratory tract disease in adults, including severe pneumonia in the elderly.

LABORATORY FINDINGS AND DIAGNOSIS The diagnosis of RSV infection can be suspected on the basis of the epidemiologic setting, i.e., severe illness in infants during an outbreak of RSV in the community. Infections in older children and adults cannot be differentiated with certainty from those caused by other respiratory viruses. The specific diagnosis is established by isolation of RSV from respiratory secretions, including sputum, throat swabs, or nasopharyngeal washes. Virus is detected in tissue culture and identified specifically by immunologic reactions, employing immunofluorescence, enzyme-linked immunosorbent assay (ELISA), or other techniques. Immunofluorescence microscopy of nasal scrapings or washings provides a rapid diagnostic method that is in use in many diagnostic virology laboratories. Serologic tests which depend on fourfold or greater rises in complement fixing or neutralizing antibody titers are useful for diagnosis in older children and adults but are less sensitive in children under 4 months of age. Compared to complement fixation or neutralization tests, ELISA detects serum antibody rises in infants with more sensitivity. As with other serologic tests, diagnosis requires comparison of acute and convalescent serum specimens and is therefore not useful during the acute illness.

TREATMENT AND PREVENTION Treatment of upper respiratory tract RSV infection consists primarily of symptomatic therapy similar to that for other upper respiratory tract viral infections. For lower respiratory tract infections, treatment includes respiratory therapy, including hydration, suctioning of secretions, administration of humidified oxygen, and antibronchospastic agents as needed. If severe hypoxia is present, intubation and ventilatory assistance may be required. Controlled studies of the treatment of infants hospitalized with RSV infection with aerosolized ribavirin, a nucleoside analogue which is active in vitro against RSV, have demonstrated a beneficial effect on the resolution of lower respiratory tract illness, including improvement of blood gases.

Considerable interest exists in the development of an effective vaccine against RSV. Inactivated virus vaccines have been either ineffective or, in one study, potentiated the disease in infants. Other approaches to vaccine development include immunization with purified, cloned viral glycoproteins of RSV, or generation of stable, live attenuated virus vaccines. In the settings where high rates of transmission occur, such as pediatric wards, barrier methods of protection of hands and conjunctiva may be useful in reducing the spread of virus.

PARAINFLUENZA VIRUS INFECTIONS

ETIOLOGY Parainfluenza viruses are members of the Paramyxoviridae family and comprise the genus *Paramyxovirus*. Parainfluenza viruses are 150 to 250 nm in diameter, enveloped, and contain a single-stranded RNA genome. The envelope is studded with two glycoproteins, one of which possesses both hemagglutinin and neuraminidase activity, while the other glycoprotein contains the fusion activity. The viral RNA genome is enclosed in a helical nucleocapsid and codes for seven virus-specific proteins. There are four distinct serotypes of parainfluenza viruses, all of whom share certain common antigens with other members of the Paramyxoviridae family, including mumps and Newcastle disease virus.

EPIDEMIOLOGY Parainfluenza viruses are distributed throughout the world, although type 4 has been reported less widely, probably because it is more difficult to grow in tissue culture. Infection occurs in early childhood so that by 8 years of age, most children show antibodies to serotypes 1, 2, and 3. Parainfluenza types 1 and 2 cause epidemics during the fall, primarily in odd-numbered years. Type 3 infection has been detected during all seasons of the year, with occasional increases in activity at variable times during the fall, winter, or spring. In recent years, epidemics of type 3 virus have occurred annually in the spring.

The overall contribution of parainfluenza infections to respiratory disease are variable according to both the location and year. In studies carried out in the United States, parainfluenza virus infections accounted for 4.3 to 22 percent of respiratory illnesses in children. In adults, parainfluenza infections are generally mild and account for less than 5 percent of respiratory illnesses. The major importance of parainfluenza viruses is as a cause of respiratory illness in young children, where they are second only to RSV as causes of lower respiratory tract illness. Like RSV, but unlike parainfluenza types 1 and 2, parainfluenza type 3 frequently causes illness during the first month of life, while passively acquired maternal antibody is still present. In contrast, parainfluenza type 1 is the most frequent cause of croup (laryngotracheobronchitis) in children, while serotype 2 causes similar, although generally less severe, disease. Parainfluenza type 3 is an important cause of bronchiolitis and pneumonia in infants, while illnesses associated with parainfluenza type 4 have been generally mild. Parainfluenza viruses are spread through infected respiratory secretions, primarily by person-to-person contact and/or by large droplets. In experimental studies, the incubation period has varied from 3 to 6 days but may be somewhat shorter in naturally occurring disease in children.

PATHOGENESIS Immunity to parainfluenza viruses is incompletely understood, but there is suggestive evidence that immunity to types 1 and 2 infections is mediated by local IgA antibodies in the respiratory tract. Passively acquired serum-neutralizing antibodies also confer some protection against infection with parainfluenza viruses types 1, 2, and, to a lesser degree, type 3.

CLINICAL MANIFESTATIONS Parainfluenza virus infections occur most frequently in children, in whom initial infection with serotypes 1, 2, and 3 is associated with an acute febrile illness in 50 to 80 percent of cases. Children may present with coryza, sore throat, hoarseness, and cough, which may or may not be croupy. In severe croup, fever persists, with worsening coryza and sore throat. A brassy or barking cough may be noted and may progress to frank stridor. In most children, recovery will occur over the next 1 to 2 days, although progressive airway obstruction and hypoxia may ensue occasionally. If bronchiolitis or pneumonia develops, progressive cough accompanied by wheezing, tachypnea, and intercostal retractions may be present. In this setting, a moderate increase in sputum production can be seen. Physical examination shows nasopharyngeal discharge and oropharyngeal injection, along with rhonchi, wheezes, or coarse breath sounds. Chest x-rays can show air trapping and, occasionally, interstitial infiltrates.

In older children and adults, parainfluenza infections tend to be milder, presenting most frequently as the common cold or hoarseness, with or without cough. Lower respiratory tract involvement in older children and adults is uncommon, but tracheobronchitis in adults has been reported.

LABORATORY FINDINGS AND DIAGNOSIS As with other respiratory viral diseases, the clinical syndromes caused by parainfluenza viruses are not sufficiently distinctive to permit a diagnosis to be made on clinical grounds alone, with the possible exception of croup in young children. A specific diagnosis is established by detection of virus in respiratory tract secretions, throat swabs; or nasopharyngeal washings. Virus is detected by growth in tissue culture, either by hemagglutination or by cytopathic effect, or by immunofluorescence of viral antigens in exfoliated cells from the respiratory tract. Serologic diagnosis can be made by fourfold or greater rises in acute and convalescent serum specimens as detected by hemagglutination inhibition, complement fixation, or neutralization tests. However, frequent heterotypic responses occur among the parainfluenza serotypes, so that identification of the serotype which causes the illness often cannot be made by serologic techniques alone.

Acute epiglottitis caused by *Haemophilus influenza,* type B (bacterial croup), must be differentiated from viral epiglottitis. Influenza A virus is a common cause of croup during epidemic periods.

TREATMENT AND PREVENTION For upper respiratory tract illness, symptomatic therapy can be employed as discussed above for other viral respiratory tract illnesses. If complications such as sinusitis, otitis, or superimposed bacterial bronchitis develop, appropriate antibiotics should be administered. Mild cases of croup should be treated with bed rest and moist air as generated by vaporizers. More severe cases require hospitalization and close observation for the development of respiratory distress. If acute respiratory distress develops, humidified oxygen and bronchodilators should be employed. There is no specific antiviral therapy available, although aerosolized ribavirin is currently being evaluated. Effective vaccines against parainfluenza viruses have not been developed.

ADENOVIRUS INFECTIONS

ETIOLOGY Adenoviruses are complex DNA viruses which are 70 to 80 nm in diameter. Human adenoviruses belong to the genus *Mastadenovirus,* of which 41 serotypes are currently recognized. Adenoviruses have a characteristic morphology consisting of an icosahedral shell comprised of 20 equilateral triangular faces and 12 vertices. The protein coat (''capsid'') consists of hexon subunits with group-specific and type-specific antigenic determinants, and penton subunits at each vertex primarily containing group-specific antigens. From each penton, a fiber with a knob at the end projects, which contains type-specific and some group-specific antigens. Adenoviruses have been divided into six or seven subgroups based on the homology of DNA genomes. The adenovirus genome is a linear double-stranded DNA which codes for structural and nonstructural polypeptides. The replicative cycle of adenovirus may result in either lytic infection of cells, or in the establishment of a latent infection (primarily involving lymphoid cells). Some adenovirus types can induce oncogenic transformation, and tumor formation has been observed in rodents, but despite intensive investigation, adenoviruses have not been associated with tumors in humans.

EPIDEMIOLOGY Adenovirus infections occur most frequently in infants and children. Infections occur throughout the year but are most commonly noted from fall to spring. Large-scale surveys have shown that adenoviruses account for 3 to 5 percent of acute respiratory infections in children. Infections are less frequent in adults and account for less than 2 percent of respiratory illness in civilians. Nearly 100 percent of adults have serum antibody against multiple serotypes, indicating that infection is common in childhood. Types 1, 2, 3, and 5 are the most frequent isolates obtained from children. Certain adenovirus serotypes, particularly 4 and 7, but also 3, 14, and 21, are associated with outbreaks of acute respiratory disease (ARD) in military recruits which occur in winter and spring. Transmission of adenovirus infection can occur by inhalation of aerosolized virus, by inoculation of virus in conjunctival sacs, and probably occurs by the fecal-oral route as well. Type-specific antibody generally develops after infection and is associated with protection against infection with the same serotype.

CLINICAL MANIFESTATIONS In children, adenoviruses cause a variety of clinical syndromes. The most common is an acute upper respiratory tract infection, with prominent rhinitis. On occasion, lower respiratory tract disease, including bronchiolitis and pneumonia, can also be seen. Adenoviruses, particularly types 3 and 7, cause pharyngoconjunctival fever, a characteristic acute febrile illness of children which occurs in outbreaks, most often in summer camps. The syndrome is marked by bilateral conjunctivitis in which the bulbar and palpebral conjunctiva have a granular appearance. Low-grade fever is frequently present, along with rhinitis, sore throat, and cervical adenopathy. The illness generally lasts for 1 to 2 weeks and resolves spontaneously. Febrile pharyngitis without conjunctivitis has also been associated with adenovirus infection. Adenoviruses have also been isolated from cases of whooping cough with or without *Bordetella pertussis;* the significance of adenovirus in that disease is unknown.

In adults, the most frequently reported illness has been acute respiratory disease (ARD) in military recruits caused by adenovirus types 4 and 7. This illness is marked by a prominent sore throat and the gradual onset of fever, often reaching 39°C on the second or third day of illness. Cough is almost always present, and coryza and regional lymphadenopathy are also frequently seen. Physical examination may show pharyngeal edema, injection, and tonsillar enlargement with little or no exudate. If pneumonia is present, auscultation of the chest and x-ray may indicate areas of patchy infiltration.

Adenoviruses have also been associated with a number of nonrespiratory tract diseases, including acute diarrheal illness in young children caused by adenovirus types 40 and 41, and hemorrhagic cystitis caused by adenoviruses 11 and 21. Epidemic keratoconjunctivitis, caused most frequently by adenovirus types 8, 19, and 37, has been associated with contaminated common sources such as ophthalmic solutions and roller towels. Adenoviruses have also been associated with disseminated disease and pneumonia in immunosuppressed patients, including patients with acquired immunodeficiency syndrome (AIDS).

LABORATORY FINDINGS AND DIAGNOSIS Adenovirus infection should be suspected in the epidemiologic setting of ARD and in certain of the clinical syndromes such as pharyngoconjunctival fever or epidemic keratoconjunctivitis in which outbreaks of characteristic illnesses occur. In the majority of cases, however, illnesses caused by adenovirus infection cannot be differentiated from those caused by a number of other viral respiratory agents and *Mycoplasma pneumoniae*. A definitive diagnosis of adenovirus infection is established by culture of virus from sites such as the conjunctiva and oropharynx or from sputum, urine, or stool. Virus may be detected in tissue culture by cytopathic changes, and specifically identified by immunofluorescence or other immunologic techniques. Serum antibody rises can be demonstrated by complement fixation, neutralization, ELISA, or radioimmunoassays. Hemagglutination inhibition tests may also be done for those adenoviruses which hemagglutinate red cells.

TREATMENT AND PREVENTION Only symptomatic and supportive therapy is available for adenovirus infections, and no clinically useful antiviral compounds have emerged. Live vaccines have been developed against adenovirus types 4 and 7 and are widely utilized to control this illness in military recruits. These vaccines consist of live, unattenuated virus which is administered in enteric coated capsules. Infection of the gastrointestinal tract with types 4 and 7 does not cause disease but stimulates local and systemic antibodies which protect against subsequent ARD with those serotypes. Vaccines prepared from purified subunits of adenovirus are currently under development.

REFERENCES

Rhinoviruses

D'ALESSIO DJ et al: Short-duration exposure and the transmission of rhinoviral colds. J Infect Dis 150:189, 1984

GWALTNEY JM: Rhinoviruses, in *Viral Infections of Humans*, AS Evans (ed). New York, Plenum, 1982, pp 491–517

MONTO AS, CAVALLARO JJ: The Tecumseh study of respiratory illness. II. Patterns of occurrence of infection with respiratory pathogens, 1965–1969. Am J Epidemiol 94:280, 1971

Coronaviruses

LARSON HE et al: Isolation of rhinoviruses and coronaviruses from 38 colds in adults. J Med Virol 5:221, 1980

MCINTOSH K: Coronaviruses, in *Virology*, BN Fields (ed). New York, Raven, 1985, pp 1327–1330

Respiratory syncytial virus

GLEZEN WP et al: Risk of respiratory syncytial virus infection for infants from low income families in relationship to age, sex, ethnic group and maternal antibody level. J Pediatr 98:708, 1981

HALL CB et al: Aerosolized ribavirin treatment of infants with respiratory syncytial viral infection: A randomized double blind study. N Engl J Med 308:1443, 1983

HENDERSON FW et al: Respiratory syncytial virus infections, reinfections and immunity. N Engl J Med 300:530, 1979

Parainfluenza viruses

CHANOCK RM et al: Myxoviruses. Parainfluenza. Am Rev Respir Dis 88:152, 1963

DENNY FW et al: Croup: An 11 year study in a pediatric practice. Pediatrics 71:871, 1983

TYERYAR FJ: Report of a workshop on respiratory syncytial virus and parainfluenza viruses. J Infect Dis 148:528, 1983

Adenoviruses

BAUM SG: Adenoviruses, in *Principles and Practice of Infectious Diseases*, 2d ed, J Bennett et al (eds). New York, Wiley, 1985, pp 988–994

FOX JP et al: The Seattle virus watch. VII. Observations of adenovirus infections. Am J Epidemiol 105:362, 1977

ZAHRADNIK JM et al: Adenovirus infection in the immunosuppressed patient. Am J Med 68:725, 1980

132 MEASLES (RUBEOLA)

C. GEORGE RAY

DEFINITION Measles, or rubeola, is an acute febrile eruption which has been one of the most common diseases of civilization. Despite the development of effective prophylactic measures it remains a worldwide health problem.

ETIOLOGY The measles virion is composed of a central core of ribonucleic acid with a helically arranged protein coat surrounded by a lipoprotein envelope with small, spikelike structures. The virion is 120 to 200 nm in diameter and is classified as a paramyxovirus.

EPIDEMIOLOGY Measles occurs naturally only in human beings, although infection with the virus can be demonstrated in laboratory colonies of monkeys exposed to infected individuals. Before active immunization was available, epidemics of measles occurred in 2- to 3-year cycles, usually during the spring months, and about 95 percent of urban dwellers developed the disease before the age of 15 years. The virus is transmitted by transfer of nasopharyngeal secretions, either directly or in airborne droplets, to the respiratory mucous membranes or conjunctivas of susceptible individuals. Persons infected with the virus may transmit the disease during a period which extends from 5 days after exposure until 5 days after skin lesions have appeared. The virus is highly contagious, with secondary attack rates among susceptible household contacts usually exceeding 90 percent; asymptomatic primary infections are rare. Measles is typically a disease of childhood in populous areas, but may occur at any age in remote isolated communities if the disease is introduced. In the United States, there has been a distinct shift in age-specific attack rates, with outbreaks most usually occurring among teenagers and young adults. Infants are uncommonly affected under the age of 6 to 8 months, presumably because of the persistence of maternal antibody acquired by transplacental transmission. With increasingly effective attempts at control, the incidence of measles in the United States fell to the lowest level ever recorded in 1983. However, this trend was sharply reversed in 1984 to 1985, with increasing reports of outbreaks primarily among high school and college students.

PATHOGENESIS AND PATHOLOGY It is probable that, after infection, measles virus multiplies in the epithelium of the respiratory tract and is disseminated by way of the blood to distant sites. For a few days before the rash appears, and for 1 or 2 days after, the virus can be isolated from blood or washed white blood cells, conjunctiva, lymphoid tissue, and respiratory mucous membranes and secretions. The virus can be obtained from urine for as long as 4 days after the onset of the eruptions.

The mucous membrane lesions (Koplik's spots) consist of vesicle formation and epithelial necrosis. Histology of the Koplik's spots reveals cytoplasmic and intranuclear inclusions, giant cells, and intercellular edema. Electron microscopy of the Koplik's spots and skin lesions has demonstrated microtubular aggregates which are thought to be the measles virus, and suggests that both the exanthem and enanthem are associated with local viral replication. Large multinucleated epithelial giant cells can be found during the prodrome and acute stages of illness in the buccal mucosa, pharynx, tracheobronchial mucosa, and occasionally in the urine. In addition, reticuloendothelial giant cells (Warthin-Finkeldey cells) are found in hyperplastic lymphoid tissues, including lymph nodes, tonsils, spleen, and thymus. An unusually high number of white blood cells from patients with the disease contain broken chromosomes. The epithelium of the respiratory passages may become necrotic and slough, leading to secondary bacterial infection; in addition, interstitial pneumonia with giant cell infiltration may be observed. Changes in the brain of patients with encephalitis resemble those seen in other postviral encephalitides and consist of focal hemorrhage, congestion, and perivenous demyelination. The pathogenesis is probably similar to experimental allergic encephalomyelitis.

MANIFESTATIONS The time from exposure to the development of the first symptoms of measles infection is usually 9 to 11 days, and from exposure to the appearance of rash is about 2 weeks. The initial manifestations of the disease are malaise, irritability, fever as high as 105°F, conjunctivitis with excessive lacrimation, edema of the eyelids and photophobia, moderately severe hacking cough, and nasal discharge. The prodromal period usually lasts 3 to 4 days, with a range of 1 to 8 days before the onset of a rash. Koplik's spots—small, red, irregular lesions with blue-white centers—appear 1 or 2 days before the onset of the rash on the mucous membranes of the mouth and occasionally on the conjunctiva or intestinal mucosa. The findings of the prodromal illness subside or disappear within 1 or 2 days after the appearance of skin lesions, although the cough may persist throughout the course of the disease.

The red maculopapular rash of measles breaks out first on the forehead, spreads downward over the face, neck, and trunk, and appears on the feet on the third day. The density of lesions is greatest on the forehead, face, and shoulders, where coalescence of individual spots usually occurs. The lesions in each area persist for about 3 days and disappear in the same order in which they appeared, resulting in total duration of rash of about 6 days. As the maculopapules fade, a brown discoloration of the skin may be noticed, and finely granular desquamation may occur. In adults the duration of fever may be longer, the rash more prominent, and the incidence of complications higher.

The course of measles can be altered by the administration of gamma globulin soon after exposure. The incubation period may be prolonged for as long as 20 days. The prodromal period of the modified disease may be shorter, the fever, respiratory symptoms, and conjunctivitis milder, and the rash less marked; Koplik's spots may not be present. An atypical, severe form of measles is seen in some persons who received inactivated measles vaccine several years before exposure. The prodromal period with prominent fever, headache, myalgias, and abdominal pain lasts for 1 or 2 days and is followed by an eruption which may be urticarial, maculopapular, hemorrhagic, and/or vesicular. In contrast to natural measles, the rash begins on the hands and feet and progresses toward the head. The rash is especially prominent on the legs and in the body creases. Peripheral edema and pneumonia have been prevalent in this form of atypical measles. The pneumonia is lobar or segmental; hilar lymphadenopathy and pleural effusion are frequent. Ill-defined nodular shadows may persist at the periphery of the lung for as long as 1 to 2 years.

COMPLICATIONS Measles, usually a benign self-limited disease, may be associated with a number of complicating illnesses. Viral involvement of the respiratory tract may lead to croup, bronchitis, bronchiolitis, or rarely to *interstitial giant cell pneumonia,* which is seen most often in children suffering from severe systemic disease such as leukemia, congenital immunodeficiency, or severe malnutrition, and which is characterized by severe respiratory symptoms, pulmonary infiltrations, and the presence in the lungs of multinucleated giant cells. It may occur in the absence of the typical measles exanthem. *Conjunctivitis,* which is seen regularly in the course of uncomplicated measles, may occasionally progress to corneal ulceration, keratitis, and blindness. *Myocarditis,* characterized by transient changes in the electrocardiogram, occurs in about 20 percent of patients with measles, but clinical evidence of cardiac dysfunction is rare. Viral involvement of the mesenteric lymph nodes and appendix may result in abdominal pain and signs of peritoneal inflammation so severe that surgical exploration is considered. The situation is especially confusing if the evidence of appendiceal involvement becomes manifest during the preeruptive phase of the disease. *Hepatitis,* usually without clinical signs, also frequently occurs. It is usually detected by the presence of a transient elevation of SGOT or SGPT values during the acute phase of illness. *Acute glomerulone-*

phritis has also been transiently observed during the acute phase of illness. Measles infection of pregnant women results in death of the fetus in about 20 percent of the cases; however, a teratogenic effect such as that observed in rubella has not been demonstrated.

Superimposed bacterial pneumonia caused by streptococci, pneumococci, staphylococci, or *Haemophilus influenzae* is considerably more common than giant cell pneumonia and occasionally may progress to formation of empyema or lung abscess. Bacterial otitis media is a frequent sequel of measles infection in children. In tropical areas, stomatitis, probably of bacterial origin, progressing to cancrum oris may be encountered during the course of the disease.

Clinically apparent *encephalomyelitis* occurs in 1 of 1000 patients with measles. It usually begins 4 to 7 days after the appearance of the eruption, but may precede the rash by 10 days or follow it by 24 days. It is characterized by high fever, headache, drowsiness, and coma, and in some patients by focal brain or spinal cord involvement. Death occurs in about 10 percent of affected individuals, and persistent signs of central nervous system damage, including mental changes, epilepsy, and paralysis, are encountered. Electroencephalographic abnormalities without other signs of central nervous system dysfunction may be demonstrated in 50 percent of patients with otherwise uncomplicated measles. A progressive, fatal encephalitis has been described in children with lymphatic malignancies treated with immunosuppressive drugs, with onset 1 to 6 months after an episode of measles. Other, more unusual neurologic complications include transverse myelitis and ascending myelitis. An extremely rare condition, *subacute sclerosing panencephalitis* (see Chap. 347), is probably a late complication of measles. *Thrombocytopenia* may occur 3 to 15 days after the onset of symptoms and results in purpura as well as bleeding from mouth, intestine, and genitourinary tract. Measles is also associated with transient suppression of delayed hypersensitivity to tuberculin, exacerbation of existing tuberculosis, and an increased incidence of new tuberculous infections.

LABORATORY FINDINGS Leukopenia is frequent in the prodromal phase of measles, and the appearance of leukocytosis suggests bacterial superinfection or another complication. Extreme lymphopenia (less than 2000 lymphocytes per cubic millimeter) is considered to be a poor prognostic sign. During the prodrome and in the early eruptive phase, multinucleated giant cells can be identified in stained preparations of sputum, nasal secretions, or urine, and the measles virus can be isolated by inoculation of the same materials onto appropriate cell cultures. Measles antigen can often be detected quickly by fluorescent antibody staining of infected respiratory or urinary epithelial cells. Complement fixation, enzyme immunoassay, immunofluorescent, and hemagglutination inhibition tests are available for serologic confirmation of measles. Spinal fluid protein of patients with encephalomyelitis ranges from 48 to 240 mg/dL, and lymphocyte counts are usually in a range of 5 to 99 per cubic millimeter, although counts as high as 1000 per cubic millimeter have been reported. Bacterial infection can be identified by appropriate cultures.

DIFFERENTIAL DIAGNOSIS Measles, with its prodrome, Koplik's spots, and characteristic rash, is infrequently confused with other diseases. Rubella is a milder disease of shorter duration with mild respiratory complaints or none at all. Infectious mononucleosis and toxoplasmosis can be identified by the presence of atypical lymphocytes and by serologic tests. Secondary syphilis may show skin lesions similar to the measles rash. Other infections which can sometimes mimic measles include those caused by adenoviruses, enteroviruses, *Mycoplasma pneumoniae*, and *Streptococcus pyogenes*, e.g., scarlet fever. Drug reactions, particularly those associated with ampicillin and phenytoin, can also produce a morbilliform rash. The atypical form of measles in patients previously immunized with inactivated vaccine may suggest Rocky Mountain spotted fever, varicella, scarlet fever, or meningococcemia.

PROPHYLAXIS Measles can be prevented by the administration of 0.25 mL/kg gamma globulin within 5 days of exposure. Passive immunization should be considered for any susceptible person exposed to the disease, but is especially important for children under 3 years of age, for pregnant women, for patients with tuberculosis, and for those patients in whom immune mechanisms are impaired. In this instance, a dose of 0.5 mL/kg gamma globulin (maximum of 15 mL) may be necessary. A modified, less severe form of the disease which results in some degree of active immunity may be observed if 0.04 mL/kg gamma globulin is given within 5 days of exposure (see "Manifestations" above). Prophylactic administration of antibiotics does not decrease the frequency or severity of bacterial superinfections.

Active immunity can be induced by the use of live, attenuated measles virus without spread to contacts of vaccinated individuals. Attenuated vaccine (Schwarz, Attenuvax) is associated with few local or systemic reactions. Vaccination induces antibody formation in more than 95 percent of susceptible individuals inoculated at age 15 months or older. The vaccine can induce protection if given before, or within 2 days after, exposure. After this time, active immunization is less predictable in its ability to confer protection to the already exposed individual, although no ill effects have been noted when vaccination followed exposure by more than 2 days. Vaccination results in protection for at least 15 years, but the total duration of immunity is not known. Live measles vaccine should not be given to pregnant women, to patients with untreated tuberculosis, to patients with leukemia or lymphoma, or to those whose immune responsiveness is depressed. Hypersensitivity reactions have not been associated with the vaccine even among egg-sensitive individuals; however, the vaccine should not be given to persons known to be hypersensitive to vaccine components, such as trace amounts of antibiotics. Except in unusual circumstances, vaccination should not be given in the first 13 months of life. However, if epidemiologic circumstances suggest a risk to infants in the 6- to 13-month age group, the vaccine may be used, and a second dose administered at 15 to 18 months of age to ensure adequate seroconversion. The vaccine seems equally effective when administered alone or simultaneously in combination with rubella and mumps vaccines. Measles vaccination has been very effective in decreasing the incidence of measles in the United States without producing serious side effects. Measles occurs most commonly among the unvaccinated, who, for the most part, are members of low socioeconomic groups. The disease rarely occurs in those who have been vaccinated, although there have been vaccine failures. These failures are related, in part, to early vaccination of infants who still have maternal neutralizing antibody or to the use of improperly stored vaccine.

There is no indication for the use of *inactivated* vaccine because of severe atypical measles which has been observed in persons immunized with it (see "Manifestations" above).

TREATMENT No therapy is indicated for uncomplicated measles. Gamma globulin, although effective in prophylaxis, is of no value once symptoms are evident. Patients should be monitored for the development of bacterial superinfections, which should be treated with appropriate antibiotics on the basis of clinical and bacteriologic findings.

REFERENCES

AICARDI J et al: Acute measles encephalitis in children with immunosuppression. Pediatrics 59:232, 1977

BLOCH AB et al: Measles outbreak in a pediatric practice: Airborne transmission in an office setting. Pediatrics 75:676, 1985

COOVADIA HM et al: Immunoparesis and outcome in measles. Lancet 1:619, 1977

FRANK JA JR et al: Major impediments to measles elimination. Am J Dis Child 139:881, 1985

FULGINITI VA, HELFER RE: Atypical measles in adolescent siblings 16 years after killed measles virus vaccine. JAMA 244:804, 1980

GAVISH D et al: Hepatitis and jaundice associated with measles in young adults. Arch Intern Med 143:674, 1983

JOHNSON RT et al: Measles encephalomyelitis—clinical and immunologic studies. N Engl J Med 310:137, 1984

KRAUSE PH et al: Epidemic measles in young adults. Ann Intern Med 90:873, 1979

LAMPE RM et al: Measles reimmunization in children immunized before 1 year of age. Am J Dis Child 139:33, 1985

LIN C, HSU H: Measles and acute glomerulonephritis. Pediatrics 71:398, 1983

133 RUBELLA ("GERMAN MEASLES") AND OTHER VIRAL EXANTHEMS

C. GEORGE RAY

RUBELLA

DEFINITION Rubella ("German measles," "3-day measles") is usually a benign febrile exanthem, but when it occurs in pregnant women, it may lead to serious chronic fetal infection and malformations.

ETIOLOGY In the late 1930s and 1940s rubella was transmitted to humans and monkeys, and in 1962 a viral agent was recovered in cell cultures inoculated with nasopharyngeal secretions of infected persons. The rubella virion, 60 to 70 nm in diameter, is a somewhat spheroidal RNA virus which has been classified in the togavirus family.

PATHOGENESIS AND PATHOLOGY Rubella can be induced in susceptible persons by the instillation of virus into the nasopharynx, and natural infection is probably induced in the same way. Virus is present in blood, throat washings, and occasionally feces for several days before the exanthem becomes apparent. It can be detected in blood for 1 to 2 days, and in throat washings for as long as 7 days before appearance of rash, to 2 weeks after onset. Lymph nodes show edema and hyperplasia.

Congenital rubella results from transplacental transmission of virus to the fetus from an infected mother, and may be associated with growth retardation, infiltration of liver and spleen by hematopoietic tissue, interstitial pneumonia, a decreased number of megakaryocytes in the bone marrow, and various structural malformations of the cardiovascular and central nervous systems. The virus can persist in the fetus during intrauterine life and may be excreted for 6 to 31 months after birth.

EPIDEMIOLOGY Rubella is not as contagious as measles, and immunity to the disease is not so widespread. Estimates of susceptibility to rubella among unimmunized women of childbearing age range from 10 to 25 percent. Before the routine introduction of vaccine in 1969, epidemics occurred at 6- to 9-year intervals; however, this cyclical pattern is no longer seen. In 1964 more than 1.8 million cases of rubella were reported in the United States; in 1984, only 745 cases, an all-time low, were reported. Rubella was once most frequent among children 5 to 9 years of age, but with the advent of immunization programs often directed primarily at this age group as well as at preschoolers, a greater proportion of cases is now being reported among older schoolchildren (15 to 19 years) and young adults (20 to 24 years).

MANIFESTATIONS The time from exposure to the appearance of the rash of rubella is 14 to 21 days, usually about 18 days. In adults there may be a prodromal illness preceding the exanthem by 1 to 7 days. The prodrome consists of malaise, headache, fever, mild conjunctivitis, and lymphadenopathy. In children the rash may be the first manifestation of disease. It is apparent from serologic studies that 25 to 50 percent of infections are subclinical, or may result in only lymph node enlargement without skin lesions; however, rash without lymphadenopathy is uncommon. Respiratory symptoms are mild or absent. Small, red lesions (Forchheimer's spots) occasionally may be seen on the soft palate but are not pathognomonic of the disease.

The rash begins on the forehead and face and spreads downward to the trunk and extremities. The small maculopapular lesions, of lighter hue than those of measles, are usually discrete but may coalesce to form a diffuse erythema suggestive of scarlet fever. The rash may last from 1 to 5 days, but is most commonly present for 3 days. Enlarged, tender lymph nodes appear before the rash, are most impressive during the early eruptive phase, and may persist several days after the rash has disappeared. Splenomegaly or generalized lymphadenopathy may occur, but the postauricular and suboccipital nodes are most strikingly involved. Arthralgias and slight joint swellings may be a complication of rubella, especially in young women. The pain and swelling, involving wrists, fingers, and knees, are most marked during the period of rash and may persist for 1 to 14 days after other manifestations of rubella have disappeared. Recurring joint symptoms for a year or more have also been reported. Purpura with or without thrombocytopenia may occur and may be associated with hemorrhage. Encephalomyelitis following rubella resembles other postinfectious encephalitides and is much less common than encephalitis following measles. Testicular pain is also occasionally reported in young adults.

Congenital rubella The syndrome of congenital rubella has conventionally been thought to consist of heart malformations—patent ductus arteriosus, interventricular septal defect, or pulmonic stenosis; eye lesions—corneal clouding, cataracts, chorioretinitis, and microphthalmia; microcephaly; mental retardation; and deafness. In the American epidemic of 1964, thrombocytopenic purpura, hepatosplenomegaly, intrauterine growth retardation, interstitial pneumonia, myocarditis or myocardial necrosis, and metaphyseal bone lesions were encountered frequently in association with the previously recognized manifestations, leading to the term *expanded rubella syndrome*. Some infants have also been found to have significant humoral and/or cellular immunodeficiency, which generally resolves as chronic viral excretion diminishes and eventually ceases. Any combination of lesions may be seen in an individual infant, and the severity is highly variable.

Later complications include an apparent higher risk of subsequent development of diabetes mellitus. In addition, there are reports of patients with congenital rubella who develop a progressive, subacute panencephalitis, with onset in the second decade of life. This is characterized by intellectual deterioration, ataxia, seizures, and spasticity.

Congenital rubella is usually the result of maternal infection during the first trimester of pregnancy, although well-documented cases have resulted from infection several days before conception; deafness may occur as a result of infection in the fourth month. Serologically identified, asymptomatic maternal rubella can also result in severe fetal disease. It is therefore desirable to ascertain the immune status of every woman, either before conception or as early in the pregnancy as possible, by history of previous immunization or by serologic testing. If rubella antibodies are present before or within 10 days after exposure, the patient is considered immune, and the risk of fetal damage is virtually nil. If antibodies are not detectable and exposure has occurred, acute and convalescent antibody titers should be determined simultaneously on serums obtained 2 to 4 weeks apart, depending upon the time after exposure when the acute sample was drawn.

DIAGNOSIS Rubella is frequently confused with other diseases associated with maculopapular exanthems such as those described in Chap. 49 and with infectious mononucleosis (Chap. 138), as well as with drug eruptions and scarlet fever. *A certain diagnosis of rubella can be made only by virus isolation and identification, or by changes in antibody titers.* Rubella hemagglutination-inhibiting antibodies may be present by the second day of rash and increase in quantity over the next 10 to 21 days. Other serologic tests which are used for diagnosis or determination of immunity include complement fixation (CF), enzyme-linked immunoassay (ELISA), fluorescence immunoassay (FIA), radioimmunoassay (RIA), and a variety of IgM-specific antibody tests. In addition, there are several economic and rapid semiquantitative screening tests to determine immunity: latex agglutination, passive hemagglutination (PHA), and single radial hemolysis. Antibodies detected by ELISA, FIA, and RIA tend to parallel the hemagglutination-inhibiting antibodies, while the appearance of CF antibody lags behind the others by a period of 3 to 7 days and often does not disappear until 1 or 2 years after infection. The PHA antibody first appears even later (14 to 21 days after rash onset), but persists thereafter. The presence of IgM-specific antibodies suggests recent rubella infection (within 2 months); however, they have been known to persist as long as 1 year in some cases. There are no other laboratory findings helpful in the diagnosis of rubella, although lymphocytosis with atypical lymphocytes may occur.

Patients with the congenital rubella syndrome may lose hemagglutination-inhibiting antibodies at age 3 or 4 years. Therefore a negative serologic test in a child over 3 years does not exclude the possibility of congenital rubella. Congenital rubella should be differentiated by appropriate serologic tests from congenital syphilis (see Chap. 122), toxoplasmosis (see Chap. 157), and cytomegalic inclusion virus disease (see Chap. 137). IgM-specific antibodies are often found early in the first year of life in infants with congenital rubella, but virus isolation is the most reliable way to confirm the diagnosis.

PREVENTION In adults and children rubella is usually a mild disease with infrequent complications. However, the severity of congenital infection has prompted efforts to prevent the disease. Administration of gamma globulin to exposed persons can abort the clinical disease, but seroconversion and transmission of the disease from mother to fetus may occur despite the administration of large amounts of gamma globulin soon after exposure.

Active immunization with live attenuated rubella vaccines has been practiced in this country since 1969, especially among young children. The aim has been to decrease the frequency of the infection in the population and to decrease the chance that susceptible pregnant women will be exposed. Because of concern for a possibly enlarging pool of susceptible adolescents and adults, there has been increasing enthusiasm for serologic screening of pubertal females with no history of immunization, followed by selective immunization of those who are seronegative. Such immunization must of course be done with appropriate precautions, as noted below. Persons working in hospitals or clinics who might contract rubella from infected patients or who, if infected, might transmit the infection to pregnant patients should all be required to have proof of immunity (either documented immunization or presence of serum antibody).

The attenuated virus can be detected in the respiratory secretions of vaccinees for as long as 4 weeks after immunization, but transmission to other susceptible individuals rarely, if ever, occurs, even in households where susceptible pregnant women are in contact with children who are being vaccinated. The vaccine induces detectable antibodies in about 95 percent of recipients, but the degree and duration of protection are still being evaluated. After heavy exposure in closed populations, vaccinated individuals sometimes develop subclinical infections (diagnosed by antibody rises and virus isolation). However, viremia has not been demonstrated in immunized persons, which suggests that previously vaccinated pregnant women will not infect their fetuses even if they acquire subclinical rubella.

Side effects of fever, rash, lymphadenopathy, polyneuropathy, or arthralgias occur very seldom in vaccinated children, but joint pain and swelling or paresthesias were seen in more than 25 percent of women who were immunized with the earlier vaccines. This risk has been reduced to less than 2 percent with the advent of vaccines prepared in human embryonic fibroblast cell cultures (RA 27/3 vaccine). The joint symptoms usually begin 2 to 10 weeks after vaccination, and they may be confused with other forms of arthritis. *Rubella vaccine must never be given to pregnant women or to those who may become pregnant within 3 months of immunization.* Although no infant with the congenital rubella syndrome has been reported to have been born to a woman inadvertently vaccinated during pregnancy, the theoretical risk of vaccine virus–induced fetal damage remains. In addition, vaccine is contraindicated in patients with immune-deficiency diseases or who are taking immunosuppressive drugs.

OTHER VIRAL EXANTHEMS

In addition to the diseases such as measles, rubella, and chickenpox which historically have been associated with prominent skin lesions there are other virus infections in which skin manifestations may occur. Table 133-1 lists the other most commonly recognized causes of maculopapular eruptions. Some of them, particularly the enteroviruses, can also occasionally cause papulovesicular or petechial rashes; others are capable of provoking erythema multiforme–like eruptions. One helpful aspect of the physical examination is the observation that viral-caused maculopapular (not vesicular) exanthems usually *relatively* spare the palms and soles. This is in contrast to eruptions associated with drug reactions, bacteria, *Mycoplasma,* and *Rickettsia,* in which a prominent palmar or plantar eruption is often noted.

EXANTHEM SUBITUM (ROSEOLA INFANTUM) Exanthem subitum is a benign disease of infants 6 to 24 months of age that is characterized by a high fever and rash. The disease can be transmitted to humans and monkeys by the transfer of blood obtained from a patient during the first few days of illness. The infectious agent is probably a virus, although it has not been isolated. The first manifestations of disease, after an estimated incubation period of 5 to 15 days, are the abrupt onset of irritability and fever, which last for 3 to 5 days; the temperature may be as high as 105°F. There may be mild pharyngitis and slight lymph node enlargement; convulsions may occur during the height of the fever. On the fourth to fifth day of illness, there is a sudden drop in temperature to normal or below normal; several hours before or after defervescence the rash suddenly and surprisingly appears. It is characterized by faint 2- to 3-mm macules or maculopapules over the neck and trunk and may extend to the thighs and buttocks; it may last for only a few hours or may be present for a day or two. Leukopenia is frequently noted later in the febrile period. The disease is benign and not associated with complications, although rarely an infant may show sequelae as a result of febrile convulsions. In the early, preeruptive phase, the disease may be difficult to differentiate from an acute bacteremia, particularly from one associated with *Streptococcus pneumoniae.* Though a leukocytosis with an increase in band forms is often seen in bacteremias presenting in this fashion, blood cultures are necessary to make the diagnosis.

ERYTHEMA INFECTIOSUM (FIFTH DISEASE) Erythema infectiosum is a mild febrile exanthematous disease with little or no prodrome. The mean incubation period is estimated as approximately 4 to 12 days (median 7 days). The first manifestations are low-grade fever with varying degrees of conjunctivitis, upper respiratory complaints, cough, myalgia, itching, nausea, and diarrhea, followed in many cases by the appearance of indurated, confluent erythema over the cheeks, giving a "slapped face" appearance. A day or so later, a bilaterally symmetric eruption is seen on the arms, legs, and trunk, but rarely on the palms or soles. The lesions are maculopapular and tend to be confluent, forming slightly raised blotchy areas and reticular or lacy patterns. When it occurs, the rash usually lasts about a week, and during this time it may disappear, only to reappear in the same areas a few hours later. The waxing and waning eruption may

TABLE 133-1 Causes of maculopapular eruptions

Viral	Other
Measles	*Mycoplasma pneumoniae*
Rubella	Syphilis
Exanthem subitum	Typhoid fever
Erythema infectiosum	Bacterial toxins: streptococci and staphylococci
Enteroviruses: coxsackievirus, echovirus	Rat-bite fever
Infectious mononucleosis	*Rickettsia*
Adenoviruses	Live-virus vaccines
Reoviruses	Drug eruptions
Arboviruses	Mucocutaneous lymph node syndrome

occasionally persist for several weeks, and can be brought on by fever, heat, exercise, sunlight exposure, or emotional stress. Mild joint pain and swelling have been observed in a large proportion of adults with the disease, and some have had symptoms lasting from a few months to over 4 years. Erythema infectiosum affects all ages but is most common in children of school age and may occur in epidemic form. The etiologic agent has now been identified as a human parvovirus (B19) which also is considered to be the primary cause of aplastic crises in patients with chronic hemolytic anemias such as sickle cell disease and hereditary spherocytosis. The route of transmission of the natural disease is probably respiratory. Subclinical infection is common. Antibody to the virus has been demonstrated in 30 to 50 percent of healthy adults. Specific diagnosis is accomplished by detection of the virus particles in early acute-phase serum by electron microscopy, by demonstration of specific viral DNA in serum or pharyngeal secretions, or more commonly by detection of IgM-specific antibodies in serums collected in the acute or early convalescent phase of illness. However, these methods are not yet routinely available in the United States. A clinical diagnosis of this disease must sometimes be made with caution, since rubella and some enteroviruses have also been shown at times to cause a nearly identical syndrome.

ENTEROVIRAL EXANTHEMS Many individual enteroviruses have been associated with rash. Of these, polioviruses are rarely implicated. More commonly, echovirus serotypes 1 through 7, 9, 11, 12, 14, 16, 18, 19, 20, 25, and 30, coxsackievirus serotypes A4, A5, A6, A9, A10, A16, and B2, B3, and B5 have all been implicated. With the exception of hand-foot-and-mouth disease, usually associated with coxsackievirus A16 or enterovirus 71 infection (see Chap. 139), there is no set of clinical or epidemiologic features that aids in differentiating the specific enteroviral agent involved in a specific case. All are capable of producing maculopapular rashes which vary in intensity and duration, and can also occasionally produce petechial or papulovesicular exanthems and enanthems. In community and household outbreaks, younger children and infants are usually more likely to have exanthems, while other features of enteroviral infection, such as fever, myalgia, and aseptic meningitis, are more prominent among older children and young adults. Two enterovirus infections which have been frequently associated with rashes and have been studied extensively are described as examples of epidemic enteroviral infections.

Boston exanthem (infections with echovirus 16) Echovirus 16 infection was described first and most extensively during an epidemic in Boston in 1951. Children who were infected usually had a disease characterized by exanthem and low-grade fever, while adult family contacts often developed high fever, prostration, and signs of aseptic meningitis with absent or fleeting rash. The first manifestation of the disease in children was fever of 101 to 102°F, lasting for a day or two, pharyngitis with small ulcerated lesions resembling herpangina, and slight enlargement of the cervical and postauricular lymph nodes. The rash appeared during fever or after defervescence and consisted of small pink maculopapules on the face, upper part of the chest, and occasionally on the whole body, including the palms and soles. The rash lasted for 1 to 5 days, and there were no important complications or sequelae. The disease resembled exanthem subitum but occurred in children of all ages and in adults.

Infection with echovirus 9 Infection with this virus in children and adults has been characterized by a febrile illness with a high incidence of aseptic meningitis. The incubation period is 5 to 8 days. About 30 percent of patients have a rash, which may occur with or without meningitis. It is usually maculopapular, developing at the onset of fever. The exanthem appears first on the face and neck, spreads to the trunk and extremities, may involve the palms and soles, although slightly, and persists for 3 to 5 days. Petechiae with or without maculopapules have been recognized; when they are seen in association with meningitis, there may be confusion with meningococcal meningitis. This can be a point of some concern, since concurrent outbreaks of echovirus 9 and meningococcal disease have been observed. A vesicular eruption with crusting lesions has been seen occasionally. An exanthem on the buccal mucosa and soft palate occurs in about 30 percent of patients and consists of small red areas with white centers which resemble Koplik's spots. The disease is usually benign but rarely has been associated with permanent central nervous system damage. Acute rhabdomyolysis with myoglobinuria has also been associated with echovirus 9 infection, and can be severe.

REFERENCES

ANDERSON MJ et al: Experimental parvoviral infection in humans. J Infect Dis 152:257, 1985

CHONMAITREE T et al: Enterovirus 71 infection: Report of an outbreak with two cases of paralysis and a review of the literature. Pediatrics 67:489, 1981

CLARKE WL et al: Autoimmunity in congenital rubella syndrome. J Pediatr 104:370, 1984

Current trends: Rubella and congenital rubella syndrome—United States, 1984–1985. Morb Mort Week Rep 35:129, 1986

HALL CB et al: The return of Boston exanthem. Echovirus 16 infections in 1974. Am J Dis Child 131:323, 1977

HERRMANN KL: Available rubella serologic tests. Rev Infect Dis 7:S108, 1985

HILL HR, RAY CG: The differential diagnosis of viral exanthems and enanthems, in *Infections in Children*, RJ Wedgwood et al (eds). Philadelphia, Harper & Row, 1982, p 235

IMMUNIZATION PRACTICES ADVISORY COMMITTEE: Rubella prevention. Ann Intern Med 101:505, 1984

JOSSELSON J et al: Acute rhabdomyolysis associated with an echovirus 9 infection. Arch Intern Med 140:1671, 1980

NEVA FA et al: Clinical epidemiological features of an unusual epidemic exanthem. JAMA 155:544, 1954

ORENSTEIN WA et al: The opportunity and obligation to eliminate rubella from the United States. JAMA 251:1988, 1984

PLUMMER FA et al: An erythema infectiosum-like illness caused by human parvovirus infection. N Engl J Med 313:74, 1985

PREBLUD SR: Some current issues relating to rubella vaccine. JAMA 254:253, 1985

REID DM et al: Human parvovirus-associated arthritis: A clinical and laboratory description. Lancet 1:422, 1985

SEVER JL et al: Rubella epidemic, 1964: Effect on 6,000 pregnancies. Am J Dis Child 110:395, 1965

TINGLE AJ et al: Failed rubella immunization in adults: Association with immunologic and virological abnormalities. J Infect Dis 151:330, 1985

TOWNSEND JJ et al: Progressive rubella panencephalitis: Late onset after congenital rubella. N Engl J Med 292:990, 1975

WHITE DG et al: Human parvovirus arthropathy. Lancet 1:419, 1985

134 SMALLPOX, VACCINIA, AND OTHER POXVIRUSES

C. GEORGE RAY

Poxviruses are a group of large (200 to 320 nm), brick-shaped, DNA-containing viruses that have a predilection for skin. Many of the poxviruses, such as myxoma and fowl pox agents, cause disease mainly in lower animals. Smallpox (variola major), alastrim (variola minor), vaccinia, and cowpox agents are closely related members of the poxvirus group that cause human disease.

SMALLPOX (VARIOLA)

DEFINITION Smallpox is a severe, contagious, febrile disease characterized by a vesicular and pustular eruption. Alastrim is a similar but milder illness, with a lower mortality rate. Though the difference in severity between these diseases is apparent, the agents of variola major and variola minor are biologically and immunologically indistinguishable from each other in the laboratory.

Smallpox (both variola major and variola minor) is considered to no longer exist in nature. In 1967, the World Health Organization launched an ambitious program aimed at total eradication of smallpox.

Two important epidemiologic factors which suggested that this was possible were the absence of nonhuman reservoirs of the virus and the apparent nonexistence of completely asymptomatic human carriers. As a result of this astonishing effort, the last recorded case of naturally acquired smallpox occurred in Somalia in 1977. After 2 more years of worldwide surveillance with no further infections, global eradication of smallpox was confirmed in 1979 and accepted by the World Health Organization in May 1980. This was followed by destruction of laboratory stocks of virus, with the exception of two laboratories: one in Atlanta, the other in Moscow. Surveillance continues, including studies of poxviruses of animals which are antigenically somewhat similar to smallpox. Some virologists remain legitimately concerned that an animal poxvirus (e.g., monkeypox, whitepox) could undergo mutation and become virulent for humans, although the chance of such an occurrence seems remote. Also, the possibility of ''escape'' of virus from a laboratory, although unlikely, must be considered.

Because the disease appears to be eradicated, the following description may be more of historical than practical interest. However, the disease might reappear unexpectedly, and a discussion of its features and prevention is still warranted.

PATHOGENESIS AND PATHOLOGY The virus gains access to the body by the respiratory tract and multiplies in unidentified sites, probably in lymph nodes or liver. After several days, during which there is no evidence of infection, viremia ensues, with swelling of the endothelium of blood vessels in the corium and perivascular inflammation. Loculated vesicles are the result of cellular destruction and exudation of serum. The infected epithelial cells are swollen and contain intracytoplasmic inclusions surrounded by a halo (Guarnieri bodies). The extent of skin involvement is greater in smallpox than in chickenpox and reaches into the corium. Pitting, most commonly seen on the face, is said to result from destruction of sebaceous glands, which are abundant in this area. The liver, spleen, and lymph nodes may be enlarged and may show focal accumulations of large mononuclear cells.

EPIDEMIOLOGY Smallpox is not as contagious as measles or influenza, and ordinarily face-to-face contact with an infected person is required to transmit the disease; however, airborne dissemination from contaminated fomites has also been shown to occur. A patient with smallpox is infectious from a day before the rash appears until all lesions have healed and the scabs have fallen off. During the early phase of the illness, the virus is transmitted in nasopharyngeal secretions; when the eruption is fully formed, the lesions themselves are a major source of infectious material. Variola virus may contaminate clothing, bedding, dust, or other inanimate objects and remain infectious for months, necessitating disinfection of articles in the patient's environment.

MANIFESTATIONS The incubation period of smallpox, from the time of exposure to the onset of the prodrome, is about 12 days, with extremes of 4 to 17 days. The disease can be divided into a prodrome, an early eruptive phase, and a period of vesiculation and pustule formation. The prodrome is characterized by a temperature of 102 to 106°F, headache, myalgia especially in the back, abdominal pain, vomiting, and in some patients by a transient, blotchy, erythematous eruption. After 3 or 4 days the fever subsides, the symptoms decrease, and the patient seems to recover. It is at this time, when the patient is afebrile, that the focal eruption begins. Early manifestations are painful ulcers on the buccal mucosa and macules which appear first on the face and forearms, and rapidly become firm, shotty papules. The papules increase in number and spread from the face and distal extremities to involve the trunk. The individual lesions may remain discrete and scattered, or they may become confluent and involve most of the body. They are most concentrated on the face and distal extremities, including the palms and soles, and are relatively sparse in the axilla. On the third or fourth day after the appearance of the focal rash, the papules progress to vesicles containing clear fluid, which, over the next few days, becomes cloudy because of infiltration by pus cells and desquamated epithelial cells; hemorrhage into the vesicles and surrounding skin may also be seen. During the course of smallpox, the lesions at any one time, in one area, are all at the same stage of evolution. At the time the vesicles become pustular, there is recurrence of fever, which may persist until healing occurs. The pustules umbilicate and form crusts and scabs which usually fall off 3 weeks after the beginning of illness, leaving small scars or deep pits.

The above description applies to disease of moderate severity. A milder illness may occur in previously immunized persons or in some who have no history of vaccination. It is characterized by the usual incubation period and prodrome, but is followed either by focal eruption of fewer than 100 papules, or by a rash resembling chickenpox. Smallpox with prodrome but with no eruption of any kind has been recognized (variola sine eruptione). The disease may also occur in a rapidly fulminating form (''sledgehammer'' smallpox). After the usual incubation period, the patient develops an initial illness characterized by severe prostration, fever, bone marrow depression, hemorrhagic skin lesions, and bleeding. The disease progresses from inception to death within 3 or 4 days without evidence of the typical focal skin lesions.

Alastrim is similar to mild and moderate forms of variola major in that it has the same incubation period and prodromal illness, but the skin eruption is less extensive, and fatalities are rare.

COMPLICATIONS Bacterial superinfections of the lesions, usually with *Staphylococcus aureus,* may occur in the late pustular stage. Bacterial pneumonia and sepsis may be seen in severe forms of smallpox. Mild conjunctivitis is quite common, and iritis and keratitis have been recognized. Encephalomyelitis may occur in the late stage of the disease and is similar to other postinfectious encephalitides. Osteomyelitis and joint effusions may complicate the disease, and orchitis has also been reported.

LABORATORY FINDINGS Leukopenia is present during the prodromal illness, and there is usually leukocytosis during the pustular stage. Rapid diagnosis of poxvirus infection can be made by the finding of characteristic brick-shaped particles in preparations of vesicle fluid examined by electron microscopy. Specific precipitation in agar by use of antigen prepared from lesions and antivariola or antivaccinia immune serum may also allow detection of poxvirus within a few hours. For definitive identification the virus must be grown in cell culture or on the chorioallantoic membrane and neutralized with specific antiserum.

DIFFERENTIAL DIAGNOSIS The major problem in differential diagnosis is in distinguishing smallpox from chickenpox. Smallpox is preceded by a longer prodrome than chickenpox, and the eruption vesiculates over a period of days instead of hours. The smallpox lesions are all characteristically in the same stage of development, whereas those of chickenpox may, in one area, display all stages of evolution. Electron microscopy and agar precipitation techniques (see above) are especially useful in distinguishing between smallpox and chickenpox. Cytologic examination of scrapings of the base of a vesicle can also be helpful in the differential diagnosis. The presence of multinucleated giant cells and/or intranuclear inclusions strongly suggests a herpes group infection (varicella-zoster or herpes simplex); such findings are not seen with poxvirus infections.

Other conditions which are sometimes confused with smallpox include eczema vaccinatum, eczema herpeticum, rickettsialpox, drug eruptions, some cases of contact dermatitis, and Stevens-Johnson syndrome. The fulminant, hemorrhagic smallpox may closely resemble meningococcemia, typhus, and hemorrhagic fevers.

PREVENTION Smallpox may be prevented among the patient's contacts by vaccination. Because this procedure is most successful if carried out during the early part of the incubation period, all exposed persons, regardless of previous immunization, should be vaccinated immediately upon recognition of exposure. Large, controlled, clinical trials have demonstrated that oral administration of *N*-methylisatin 3-thiosemicarbazone (methisazone), a drug which interferes with poxvirus multiplication, can prevent smallpox and alastrim in patients exposed to the diseases. The use of a drug together with prompt vaccination results in greater chance of protection than either measure alone. A drawback to the use of methisazone is its tendency to induce vomiting. The combined use of vaccination and parenteral administration of vaccinia immune globulin early in the incubation period is also effective in the prevention of smallpox in exposed individuals.

TREATMENT There is no specific therapy for smallpox. Thiosemicarbazone, although effective in prophylaxis, has not been shown to be of value in the treatment of established cases. Fluid deficits should be replaced by the administration of appropriate solutions. During the vesicular and pustular phases of the disease, an attempt should be made to prevent bacterial infection by the use of sterile sheets and aseptic nursing procedures. Antihistamines may be helpful in decreasing pruritus. Application of lotions or ointment should be avoided. Later in the course of the illness, when desquamation has begun, showers or baths may be helpful in removing desquamating tissue. If bacterial infection develops, an antibiotic active against the infecting organism should be given by the parenteral route. Topical antibiotics should be avoided.

VACCINIA

Vaccinia is a virus disease of the skin which is induced by inoculation for the prevention of smallpox. The exact origin of the vaccinia virus is obscure. The material first used by Jenner in 1796 was propagated for many years by successive passage from person to person through use of exudate from fresh skin lesions.

VACCINATION Use of vaccinia virus is now indicated *only* for a few laboratory workers directly involved with smallpox or closely related animal poxviruses, such as monkeypox. A few countries in Asia and Africa still require an up-to-date certification of smallpox vaccination as a condition of entry, even though there is no medical reason to do so. It has been suggested that travelers to these areas obtain smallpox vaccination–waiver letters indicating that vaccination is contraindicated for health reasons, rather than undergo the risk of complications from the vaccine. Many United States military personnel are still routinely vaccinated, representing a continued source for complications and spread of the virus to civilian contacts.

In the past, vaccinia virus has also been occasionally used for the treatment of diseases such as recurrent herpes simplex infection or warts. There is *no* evidence of therapeutic efficacy in these situations, and the use of the virus for these purposes is strictly contraindicated. Live, lyophilized vaccinia virus prepared from vesicle fluid of infected calves maintains potency for 18 months at 46°F. It is dissolved in a diluent solution just prior to use. The usual method for vaccination is to apply a small drop of vaccine to the skin over the deltoid muscle and to press a sterile needle through the vaccine several times in such a way that only the superficial layer of skin is entered, or by simultaneous puncture utilizing a plastic tine device. Vaccination should always induce some form of skin reaction; complete absence of any kind of lesion indicates that the vaccine was not viable or was not administered properly. The reaction which occurs in nonimmune individuals is characterized by a red papule at the site of inoculation 3 to 5 days after vaccination. The papule becomes vesicular on about the fifth or sixth day and pustular by the ninth or eleventh day after inoculation. The vesicle and pustule may be surrounded by a large area of erythema. About 2 weeks after vaccination, the pustule dries and develops a crust which falls off by the end of the third week, leaving a scar. Fever, malaise, and irritability are common in children during the vesicular and pustular phases, and axillary lymphadenopathy may develop and persist for several months. In the partially immune person, a modified reaction develops without fever or constitutional symptoms. A papule appears on the skin within 3 days, vesiculates in 5 to 7 days, and heals without much scarring. The so-called immune reaction described by some, where a papule and/or erythema appears in a few days, then recedes without vesiculation, is an "equivocal" reaction, and may simply represent allergy to the components of an inadvertently inactivated vaccine. A successful vaccination is defined as the presence of a Jennerian vesicle (vesicular, pustular, or crusted) 7 days after inoculation. If the criterion is not met, the patient should be revaccinated, preferably with vaccine from a different lot.

Revaccination every 3 years is required to ensure protection. *Absolute contraindications* to vaccination include individuals with congenital or acquired immune deficiencies, lymphoma, leukemia or other blood dyscrasias, patients being treated with steroids, antimetabolites, alkylating agents, irradiation, and individuals with a history of vaccinia encephalitis. *Relative contraindications* include patients or household contacts with eczema or a history of eczema, severe acne, or other similar dermatologic problems, pregnancy, and infants under 12 months of age. If the necessity to vaccinate any individual in this latter group is great, simultaneous administration of vaccinia immune globulin (VIG), 0.3 mL/kg, is suggested, to be given at a separate site intramuscularly at the time of immunization.

COMPLICATIONS Healing of the primary vaccinal lesion may not occur, and some patients go on to develop slowly progressive necrosis with destruction of large areas of skin, subcutaneous tissue, and underlying structures *(vaccinia gangrenosum).* In addition to the local destruction, there may be metastatic lesions on other parts of the skin surface and in bone and viscera. Vaccinia gangrenosum occurs most frequently in persons with disorders of immunity and, if untreated, is nearly always fatal. *Eczema vaccinatum* is a serious complication that is seen in persons with eczema or other types of chronic skin conditions. Widespread infection in the previously affected areas, as well as in normal skin, may result from direct vaccination of an eczematous patient or from exposure to a recently vaccinated individual. *Generalized vaccinia* in patients without preexisting skin disease is characterized by a few satellite lesions surrounding the inoculation site or by widely disseminated pox resembling the primary vaccination lesion. This condition is usually mild with generally complete recovery. Vaccinia virus may be transferred from the primary inoculation site to the eye or other sites by scratching. *Postvaccinal encephalomyelitis* appears from 2 to 25 days after vaccination. The patient suddenly becomes severely ill with nuchal rigidity, drowsiness, vomiting, convulsions, coma, and signs suggesting disease of the spinal cord. The period of coma lasts for a few days, and in those who recover there are usually no permanent sequelae. Death occurs in about 30 to 40 percent of the patients with encephalomyelitis. *Erythema multiforme bullosum,* or *diffuse blotchy erythema,* may occur in vaccinated patients 7 to 10 days after vaccination, and is thought to be an allergic reaction to the virus or other components of the vaccine.

The rates of adverse effects per million primarily vaccinated persons were vaccinia gangrenosum, 0.9; eczema vaccinatum, 10.4; generalized vaccinia, 23.4; vaccinal lesions resulting from accidental implantation of virus, 25.4; postvaccinal encephalitis, 2.9; other complications, 11.8; the death rate was 1 per million.

Active treatment of vaccinia complications, aside from control of bacterial superinfection and treatment of any underlying defects, is limited. VIG is of possible value in accidental inoculation into secondary sites such as the eye, vaccinia gangrenosum, eczema vaccinatum, and generalized vaccinia. Dosage is usually 0.6 mL/kg intramuscularly, although much larger doses are sometimes used in severe cases. VIG is of no use in erythema multiforme or postvaccinal encephalitis. Thiosemicarbazone has been used in some cases of progressive vaccinia gangrenosum, and 5-Iodo-2′-deoxyuridine is suggested for topical treatment of vaccinial keratitis and conjunctivitis; however, the evidence supporting their efficacy is equivocal.

COWPOX

Cowpox is primarily a disease of the teats and udders of cows. Humans are almost always infected by milking, but occasional spread to contacts may occur from an infected person. The human disease is characterized by low-grade fever and by small papules on the fingers and hand, which go through vesicular and pustular stages resembling the course of vaccinia infection. The lesions may be ruptured by trauma and spread to immediately adjacent areas on the hand and continue to ulcerate for several weeks. Edema, lymphangitis, and axillary lymph node enlargement are common. Very rare cases of post-cowpox encephalitis and serious infections of eczematous persons have been reported. In general, the disease is benign, heals without scarring, and is uncomplicated.

PARAVACCINIA (MILKERS' NODULES)

Paravaccinia is a poxvirus which is antigenically unrelated to cowpox, but produces similar lesions in humans. It is primarily a disease of calves and milk cows, producing lesions on the teats of the cows and oral lesions in the suckling calf. Humans acquire infection through the skin by direct contact. The lesion is usually solitary, beginning as a macule on the finger, hand, or wrist, and progressing to a firm nodule, 1 to 2 cm in diameter, in 10 days. It then crusts and heals without scarring in 2 to 3 weeks. Occasionally, there is associated lymphadenitis. The lesion and its evolution are closely similar to ecthyma contagiosum (orf), a poxvirus of sheep, or bovine papular stomatitis which can also infect humans by direct inoculation.

MOLLUSCUM CONTAGIOSUM

Molluscum contagiosum is spread by direct contact with infected cells. In children, the lesions are commonly seen on the face, trunk, and limbs as a result of skin-to-skin or fomites-to-skin spread. The adult form most commonly occurs in the genital, lower abdomen, and inner thigh areas as a result of sexual contact.

After an incubation period of 2 to 8 weeks, pale, firm, pearllike nodules 2 to 10 mm in diameter develop in the epidermis. The lesions are painless, umbilicated, and not associated with systemic symptoms. A cheesy material can often be expressed from the pore at the center of each. Local spread can occur if the lesions and surrounding skin are traumatized. Pathologic findings include epidermal hyperplasia, ballooning degeneration, and acanthosis. The diagnosis is usually made on clinical grounds, but can be confirmed by demonstration of large, eosinophilic cytoplasmic inclusions (molluscum bodies) in the affected epithelial cells.

If left alone, the lesions disappear in 2 to 12 months. Specific treatment, if desired, is often by curettage or careful removal of the central core by expression with forceps.

REFERENCES

BOWMAN KF et al: Cutaneous form of bovine papular stomatitis in man. JAMA 246:2813, 1981

BREMAN JG, ARITA I: The confirmation and maintenance of smallpox eradication. N Engl J Med 303:1263, 1980

DIXON CW: *Smallpox*. London, Churchill, 1962

GOLDSTEIN JA et al: Smallpox vaccination reactions, prophylaxis, and therapy of complications. Pediatrics 55:342, 1975

MOORE RM: Human orf in the United States, 1972. J Infect Dis 127:731, 1973

NAKANO JH: Poxviruses, in *Manual of Clinical Microbiology*, 4th ed, EH Lennette et al (eds). Washington, DC, American Society for Microbiology, 1985, p 733

ROCKOFF AS: Molluscum dermatitis. J Pediatr 92:945, 1978

WHITE PJ, SHACKELFORD PG: Edward Jenner MD, and the scourge that was. AM J Dis Child 137:864, 1983

135 VARICELLA-ZOSTER VIRUS INFECTIONS

RICHARD J. WHITLEY

DEFINITION Varicella-zoster virus (VZV) causes two distinct clinical entities: varicella, or chickenpox, and herpes zoster, or shingles. Chickenpox, a ubiquitous and extremely contagious infection, is usually a benign illness of childhood characterized by an exanthematous, vesicular rash. With reactivation of latent VZV, more common after the sixth decade of life, the disease presents as a dermatomal, vesicular rash which is usually associated with severe pain.

ETIOLOGY A clinical association between varicella and herpes zoster has been recognized for nearly 100 years. Early in the twentieth century, similarities in the histopathologic findings of skin lesions resulting from varicella and herpes zoster were demonstrated. Isolation of VZV in 1952 permitted a definition of the biology of this virus. Viral isolates from patients with chickenpox and herpes zoster demonstrated similar alterations in tissue culture, specifically the appearance of eosinophilic intranuclear inclusions and multinucleated giant cells, suggesting that the viruses were biologically similar. Later studies proved their identity by rigorous biochemical methods. Restriction endonuclease analysis of viral DNA from a patient with chickenpox who subsequently developed herpes zoster verified the molecular identity of the two viruses responsible for these differing clinical presentations. Varicella-zoster virus is a member of the herpesvirus family, sharing such similar structural characteristics as a lipid envelope, surrounding a nucleocapsid with icosahedral symmetry, a total size of approximately 150 to 200 nm, and centrally located double-stranded DNA with a molecular weight of approximately 80 million. Only enveloped virions are infectious; this may, in part, account for the lability of VZV.

PATHOGENESIS AND PATHOLOGY Primary infection The pathogenesis of chickenpox may evolve in a fashion similar to that proposed by Fenner for mousepox. Transmission is likely by the respiratory route, followed by localized replication at an undefined site, and leading to seeding of the reticuloendothelial system with, ultimately, viremia. The occurrence of viremia in patients with chickenpox is supported by the diffuse and scattered nature of the skin lesions and can be verified in selected cases by the recovery of virus from the blood. Vesicles involve the corium and dermis with degenerative changes characterized by ballooning, multinucleated giant cells, and eosinophilic intranuclear inclusions. Infection may involve localized blood vessels of the skin, resulting in necrosis and epidermal hemorrhage. With disease evolution, vesicular fluid becomes cloudy with the recruitment of polymorphonuclear leukocytes, degenerated cells, and fibrin. Ultimately, the vesicles rupture and release their fluid contents which include infectious virus or are gradually reabsorbed.

Recurrent infection The mechanism of reactivation of VZV that results in herpes zoster is unknown. It is presumed that virus infects the dorsal root ganglia during chickenpox where it remains latent until reactivated. Histopathologic examination of the representative dorsal root ganglia during active herpes zoster demonstrates hemorrhage, edema, and lymphocytic infiltration.

Involvement with active VZV replication in other organs, such as the lung or brain, can occur during either chickenpox or herpes zoster but is uncommon in the immune-competent host. Lung involvement is characterized by interstitial pneumonitis, multinucleated giant cell formation, intranuclear inclusions, and pulmonary hemorrhage. Central nervous system (CNS) infection leads to histopathologic evidence of perivascular cuffing similar to that encountered with measles and other viral encephalitides. Focal hemorrhagic necrosis of the brain, characteristic of herpes simplex virus encephalitis, is uncommon with VZV infection.

EPIDEMIOLOGY AND CLINICAL PRESENTATION Chickenpox Humans are the only known reservoir for VZV. Chickenpox is highly contagious with an attack rate of at least 90 percent among susceptible or seronegative individuals. Both sexes and individuals of all races are infected equally. The virus is endemic in the population at large; however, it becomes epidemic among susceptible individuals during seasonal periods, namely, late winter and early spring in the temperate zone. Children between the ages of 5 and 9 are most commonly affected and account for 50 percent of all cases. Most other cases occur between the ages of 1 to 4 and 10 to 14. Over the age of 15, approximately 10 percent of the population of the United States is susceptible to infection.

The incubation period of chickenpox ranges between 10 and 21 days but is usually between 14 and 17 days. Secondary attack rates in susceptible siblings within a household are defined as between 70 and 90 percent. Patients are infectious approximately 48 h prior to the onset of the vesicular rash, during the period of vesicle formation, generally 4 to 5 days, and until all vesicles are crusted.

Clinically, chickenpox presents with a rash, low-grade fever, and malaise, although a few patients will develop a prodrome 1 to 2 days prior to the onset of the exanthem. In the immune-competent child, this is usually a benign illness that is associated with lassitude and fever from 100 to 103°F of 3 to 5 days' duration. The skin manifestations, the hallmark of the infection, consist of maculopapules, vesicles, and scabs in varying stages of evolution. The evolution of lesions from maculopapules to vesicles occurs over a matter of hours to days. The lesions appear on the trunk and face and rapidly involve other areas of the body. Most lesions are small and have an erythematous base with a diameter of 5 to 10 mm. Successive crops of lesions appear over a 2- to 4-day period. Lesions can also be found on the mucosa of the pharynx or the vagina. The severity of skin lesions varies from individual to individual. Some individuals have very few lesions, while others can have as many as 2000. Younger children tend to have fewer vesicles compared to older individuals. Immunocompromised children, particularly those with leukemia, have more numerous lesions, often with a hemorrhagic base. Healing takes nearly three times longer in this population. These children are at greater risk for visceral complications, which occur in 30 to 50 percent of cases and which are fatal in 15 percent of cases.

The most common infectious complication of varicella is secondary bacterial superinfection of the skin, which is usually caused by *Streptococcus pyogenes* or *Staphylococcus aureus*. This may result from excoriation of skin lesions following scratching. Gram's stain of skin lesions should help clarify the etiology of unusually erythematous and pustulated lesions.

The most common extracutaneous site of involvement in children is the central nervous system and consists of acute cerebellar ataxia. Cerebellar ataxia generally appears approximately 21 days after the onset of the rash and rarely occurs in the preeruptive phase. The most prominent clinical finding is ataxia and meningeal irritation. The cerebrospinal fluid contains lymphocytes and elevated levels of protein. This is a benign complication of VZV infection in children and does not generally require hospitalization. In addition, aseptic meningitis, encephalitis, transverse myelitis, and Reye's syndrome can also occur. Encephalitis is reported in 0.1 to 0.2 percent of children with chickenpox. No specific therapy is available at this time for patients with central nervous system involvement caused by VZV.

Varicella pneumonitis is the most serious complication following chickenpox, occurring more commonly in adults (up to 20 percent) than in children. It usually appears 3 to 5 days into the course of illness and is associated with tachypnea, cough, dyspnea, and fever. Cyanosis, pleuritic chest pain, and hemoptysis are frequent physical findings. Roentgenographic evidence of disease consists of nodular infiltrates and an interstitial pneumonitis. Resolution of pneumonitis parallels improvement of skin rash; however, patients may have persistent fever and compromised pulmonary function for weeks.

Other complications of chickenpox include myocarditis, corneal lesions, nephritis, arthritis, bleeding diatheses, acute glomerulonephritis, and hepatitis. Hepatic involvement, distinct from Reye's syndrome, is extremely common in chickenpox and is usually characterized by an elevation of liver enzymes, particularly serum glutamic oxaloacetic transaminase (SGOT) and serum glutamic pyruvic transaminase (SGPT). Hepatic involvement is usually asymptomatic, although a few patients report nausea and vomiting.

Perinatal varicella is associated with a high mortality rate when maternal disease develops within 5 days before delivery or 48 h post partum. Because the newborn does not receive protective transplacental antibodies and has an immature immune system, illness may be exaggerated. The mortality rate has been reported as high as 30 percent in this group. Congenital varicella with clinical manifestations at birth is extremely uncommon. It is characterized by skin scarring, hypoplastic extremities, eye abnormalities, and usually evidence of central nervous system impairment.

Herpes zoster Herpes zoster, a sporadic disease, is the consequence of reactivation of latent virus from the dorsal root ganglia. It is a disease which occurs at all ages but mainly among the elderly. Most patients who develop herpes zoster have no history of exposure to other individuals with VZV infection at that time. The highest incidence of disease ranges between 5 and 10 cases per 1000 persons for individuals in the sixth through the eighth decades of life. Approximately 2 percent of herpes zoster patients who do not receive immunosuppressive therapy will develop a second episode of infection. This figure is at least fivefold higher in immunocompromised individuals.

Herpes zoster, or "shingles," is characterized by a unilateral vesicular eruption within a dermatome, often associated with severe pain. The dermatomes from T3 to L3 are frequently involved. Unique complications are encountered if the ophthalmic branch of the trigeminal nerve is involved, resulting in zoster ophthalmicus. The factors responsible for reactivation of virus are not known. In the child, reactivation is usually benign, whereas in the adult, acute neuritis and postherpetic neuralgia can be particularly debilitating. The onset of disease is heralded by pain within the dermatome that may precede lesions by 48 to 72 h, followed by an erythematous maculopapular rash which evolves rapidly to vesicular lesions. In the normal host, these lesions may remain few in number and continue to form only for a period of 3 to 5 days. The total duration of disease is generally between 7 and 10 days; however, it may take as long as 2 to 4 weeks before the skin returns to normal. In a very few patients, characteristic localization of pain to a dermatome with serologic evidence of herpes zoster has been reported without skin lesions ever appearing. When branches of the trigeminal nerve are involved, lesions may appear on the face, in the mouth, in the eye, or on the tongue. The ear canal and tongue may be involved as part of the involvement of the sensory branch of the facial nerve (Ramsay Hunt syndrome).

The most debilitating complication of herpes zoster, both in the normal and in the immunocompromised host, is pain associated with acute neuritis and postherpetic neuralgia. Postherpetic neuralgia is extremely uncommon in young individuals; however, at least 50 percent of patients over age 50 with zoster will report pain in the involved dermatome months after resolution of cutaneous disease. Changes in sensation within the dermatome, resulting in either hypo- or hyperesthesia, have been reported.

Central nervous system involvement following localized herpes zoster may be more common than has been reported. Many patients without signs of meningeal irritation will have cerebrospinal fluid (CSF) pleocytosis and moderately elevated levels of CSF protein. Symptomatic meningoencephalitis is characterized by headache, fever, photophobia, meningitis, and vomiting. A rare manifestation of CNS involvement by herpes zoster is granulomatous angiitis with contralateral hemiplegia, which can be diagnosed by cerebral arteriography. Other neurologic manifestations include transverse myelitis with or without motor paralysis.

As with chickenpox, herpes zoster in the immunocompromised host is more severe than in the normal individual. Lesion formation continues for over a week, and total scabbing does not develop in the majority of patients until 3 weeks into the disease's course. Therefore, the natural history of the disease is extended approximately twofold. Patients with Hodgkin's disease and non-Hodgkin's lymphoma are at greatest risk for progressive herpes zoster because cutaneous dissemination develops in about 40 percent of these patients. Among patients with cutaneous dissemination, there is a 5 to 10 percent increased risk of pneumonitis, meningoencephalitis, hepatitis, and other serious complications. However, even in immunocompromised patients disseminated zoster is rarely fatal.

DIFFERENTIAL DIAGNOSIS Chickenpox is a clinical diagnosis which is certainly less confusing now than 20 to 30 years ago when smallpox or disseminated vaccinia could easily be confused with varicella. The characteristic rash of chickenpox and the epidemiologic history of recent exposure should lead to prompt diagnosis. Other viral infections which can mimic chickenpox include disseminated herpes simplex virus infection in patients with atopic dermatitis, and the disseminated vesiculopapular lesions sometimes associated with coxsackievirus, echovirus, or atypical measles infections. These rashes are more commonly morbilliform with a hemorrhagic component rather than vesicular or vesiculopustular. Rickettsialpox can be confused with chickenpox; however, it can be easily distinguished by finding the "herald spot" at the site of the mite bite and a more pronounced headache. The serologic test is also useful in differentiating rickettsialpox from varicella.

Unilateral vesicular lesions in a dermatomal pattern should lead rapidly to the diagnosis of herpes zoster. Both herpes simplex virus infections and coxsackievirus infections can be a cause of dermatomal vesicular lesions. In such situations, a Tzanck smear with supportive diagnostic virology will be helpful in assuring the proper diagnosis. In the prodromal stage of herpes zoster, the diagnosis can be exceedingly difficult and may only be achieved once lesions have appeared, or by retrospective serologic assessment.

LABORATORY FINDINGS The diagnosis of chickenpox or shingles can often be made by history and physical examination. Unequivocal confirmation of the diagnosis is possible only through the isolation of virus in susceptible tissue culture cell lines or by the demonstration of seroconversion or a fourfold or greater antibody rise when comparing acute and convalescent specimens. A rapid impression can be obtained by a Tzanck smear, performed by scraping the base of the lesions in an attempt to demonstrate multinucleated giant cells. Direct immunofluorescent staining of cells from the skin base or detection of viral antigens by other assays (immunoperoxidase) can also be utilized, although such tests are not yet commercially available. The most frequently employed serologic tools for assessing host response are immunofluorescent detection of antibodies to VZV membrane antigens, fluorescent antibody to membrane antigen (FAMA) test, immune adherence hemagglutination, or enzyme-linked immunoabsorbent assay (ELISA). The FAMA and ELISA tests appear to be the most sensitive.

PROPHYLAXIS In the normal host, prophylaxis and treatment of chickenpox are of little relevance since the disease is usually benign. However, because the immunocompromised child is at significant risk for developing progressive varicella, modalities of prevention include passive immunization or experimental administration of a live attenuated vaccine. Immune prophylaxis can be accomplished by the administration of specific zoster immune globulin (ZIG), derived from patients with herpes zoster, varicella-zoster immune globulin (VZIG), or the intravenous formulation of zoster immune plasma (ZIP). Both ZIG and VZIG should be given within 96 h, but preferably within 72 h, of exposure in order to be effective. It is likely that ZIP can be given somewhat later. Indications for the administration of ZIG or VZIG are summarized in Table 135-1. VZIG should be administered to immunodeficient patients under 15 who have a negative or unknown history of chickenpox, who have not been vaccinated against VZV, and who have had a contact in a household, with a playmate for more than 1 h indoors, or in a shared hospital room. It should also be administered to the newborn whose mother had an onset of chickenpox less than 5 days before delivery or 48 h post partum. The use of VZIG for susceptible individuals over 15 must be evaluated on an individual basis. There is no evidence that VZIG is useful for adults with chickenpox, including pregnant women.

An alternative approach to prophylaxis evolved from the development of a live attenuated vaccine for administration to high-risk and normal individuals. Clinical trials performed in Japan and the United States demonstrated efficacy both in normal individuals and in the immunocompromised host. A live attenuated VZV vaccine may be licensed in the United States in the near future, particularly for use in the immunocompromised child.

TREATMENT Medical management of chickenpox in the normal host is directed toward preventing avoidable complications. Obviously, good hygiene including daily bathing, astringent soaks, and closely cropped fingernails are the key to avoiding this complication. Secondary bacterial infection of the skin can be avoided by meticulous skin care, particularly with close cropping of fingernails. Pruritus can be decreased with topical dressings or the administration of antipruritic drugs. Tepid water baths and wet compresses are better than drying lotions for the relief of itching. Domeboro soaks for the management of herpes zoster can be both soothing and cleansing. Administration of antipyretics should be approached with care, especially for the child suffering from chickenpox because of the recent association between aspirin derivatives and the development of Reye's syndrome.

Patients with varicella pneumonia will require excellent supportive nursing care including removal of bronchial secretions and ventilatory support, as needed. Zoster ophthalmicus should be referred promptly and immediately to an ophthalmologist. Therapy consists of administration of analgesics for severe pain and the use of atropine. The role of parenteral administration of antivirals for the management of zoster ophthalmicus remains unknown at this time, although both acyclovir and vidarabine have been utilized.

The treatment of both chickenpox and herpes zoster in the immunocompromised host can be successfully accomplished with intravenous administration of vidarabine or acyclovir. When the former drug is administered to patients with either disease, healing of skin lesions is accelerated and visceral complications are likely to be decreased. For patients with herpes zoster, intravenous vidarabine therapy will also accelerate resolution of acute neuritis and decrease both the duration of postherpetic neuralgia and the frequency of

TABLE 135-1 Recommendations for VZIG utilization

I Exposure:
- *A* Both exposure to person with chickenpox or zoster as:
  - *1* Continuous household contact
  - *2* Playmate of >1-h duration indoors
  - *3* Hospital contact (same room or prolonged face-to-face)
  - *4* Newborn exposure whereby mother had onset of chickenpox <5 days before delivery or 48 h post partum
- *B* And time elapsed ≤96 h (preferably sooner)

II Candidates should:
- *A* Have significant exposure (see *I* above)
- *B* Be susceptible to VZV infection
- *C* Be <15 years of age (older immunocompromised patients require individual decision)
- *D* Have one of the following conditions:
  - *1* Leukemia or lymphoma
  - *2* Congenital or acquired immune deficiency
  - *3* Immunosuppressive treatment
  - *4* Newborn defined above (see *IA4*)

cutaneous dissemination. The dosage is 15 mg/kg per day once daily intravenously over 12 h at a concentration of 0.5 mg of standard intravenous fluids. Acyclovir is not yet approved for this indication by the Food and Drug Administration. The administration of intravenous acyclovir leads to the decreased occurrence of visceral complications but with no effect, demonstrable at this time, on healing of skin lesions or pain. While high-dose intramuscular human leukocyte interferon has been beneficial in a limited number of immunocompromised patients, the more readily available and genetically produced recombinant interferons have not been shown to be effective for treating either varicella or herpes zoster. Concomitant with the administration of an intravenous antiviral to the immunosuppressed host, it is desirable to attempt to wean patients from immunosuppressive treatment.

Management of acute neuritis and/or postherpetic neuralgia can be particularly difficult. In addition to the judicious use of analgesics, ranging from nonnarcotic to narcotic derivatives, supplementation with such drugs as amitriptyline hydrochloride and fluphenazine hydrochloride has been reported to be beneficial for pain relief. Corticosteroids have been reported in some studies to be useful when administered early in the course for prevention of postherpetic neuralgia. Large-scale controlled studies remain to be performed to address the utility and potential complications of such an approach.

Over the next decade, it is likely that significant advances will be achieved in the area of prevention and treatment of varicella-zoster virus infections both in the normal and the immunocompromised host, both with drugs and vaccines.

REFERENCES

Brunell PA et al: Prevention of varicella by zoster immune globulin. N Engl J Med 280:1191, 1969

Gershon AA et al: Live attenuated varicella vaccine. JAMA 252:355, 1984

Hope-Simpson RE: The nature of herpes zoster: A long-term study and a new hypothesis. Proc R Soc Med 58:9, 1965

Prober CG et al: Acyclovir therapy of chickenpox in immunosuppressed children—a collaborative study. J Pediatr 101:622, 1982

Ross HA: Modification of chickenpox in family contacts by administration of gamma globulin. N Engl J Med 267:369, 1962

Weibel RE et al: Live attenuated varicella versus vaccine: Efficacy trial in healthy children. N Engl J Med 310:1409, 1984

Weller TH: Varicella and herpes zoster: Changing concepts of the natural history, control, and importance of a not-so-benign virus. N Engl J Med 309:1362, 1434, 1983

Whitley RJ et al: Early vidarabine therapy to control the complications of herpes zoster in immunosuppressed patients. N Engl J Med 307:971, 1982

———: Vidarabine therapy of varicella in immunosuppressed patients. J Pediatr 1:125, 1982

———: Varicella-zoster virus infections, in *Antiviral Agents and Viral Diseases of Man 2*, GJ Galasso et al (eds). New York, Raven Press, 1984, pp 517–542

Zaia JA et al: Evaluation of varicella-zoster immune globulin: Protection of immunosuppressed children after household exposure to varicella. J Infect Dis 147:737, 1983

136 HERPES SIMPLEX VIRUSES

LAWRENCE COREY

DEFINITION Herpes simplex viruses (HSV-1, HSV-2) (*Herpesvirus hominis*) produce a variety of infections involving mucocutaneous surfaces, the central nervous system, and occasionally visceral organs. The advent of effective antiviral chemotherapy for HSV infections has made prompt recognition of these syndromes of clinical importance.

HISTORY The word *herpes* from the Greek "to creep" was utilized to describe fever blisters by Herodotus in 100 A.D. In the early 1960s it was demonstrated that HSV could be divided by neutralization tests into two antigenic types (HSV-1 and HSV-2) and that there was an association between the antigenic type and the site of viral recovery.

ETIOLOGY The genome of herpes simplex virus is a linear, double-stranded DNA molecule (about 100×10^6 in molecular weight) large enough to encode in excess of 60 to 70 gene products. The structure of the genome is unusual among DNA viruses because two unique nucleotide sequences are flanked by inverted repeated sequences. The two components can invert relative to each other, so that DNA isolated from the virus consists of four isomers differing in their orientation of the two components. About 50 percent of the HSV-1 and HSV-2 genomes are homologous. The homologous sequences are distributed over the entire genome map, and most (if not all) of the polypeptides specified by one viral type are antigenically related to polypeptides of the other viral type. Restriction endonuclease analysis of viral DNA can be utilized to distinguish between the two subtypes and among strains of the two subtypes. The variability of nucleotide sequences from clinical strains of HSV-1 and HSV-2 are such that for practical purposes HSV isolates obtained from two individuals can be differentiated by restriction enzyme patterns unless the isolates are from epidemiologically related sources such as sexual partners, mother-infant pairs, or common source outbreaks.

The viral genome is packaged within a regular icosahedral protein shell (capsid) composed of 162 capsomers. The outer covering of the virus is a lipid-containing membrane (envelope) derived from modified cell membrane, acquired as the DNA-containing capsid buds through the inner nuclear membrane of the host cell. Between the capsid and lipid bilayer of the envelope is the tegument, composed of a number of viral proteins whose properties and functions are largely unknown. Viral replication has both nuclear and cytoplasmic phases. The initial steps of replication include attachment, fusion between the viral envelope and a cell membrane to liberate the nucleocapsid into the cytoplasm of the cell, and disassembly of the nucleocapsid to release the viral DNA. Three classes of HSV genes have been defined. The genes designated α are expressed earliest in infection without any requirement for prior viral protein synthesis. The second class of HSV genes, designated β, require prior synthesis of an α protein but not viral DNA replication. The β proteins include regulatory proteins and enzymes required for DNA replication. Most current antiviral drugs interrupt β proteins such as the viral DNA polymerase enzyme. The third class of HSV genes, designated γ, require viral DNA replication for expression, and most of the structural proteins specified by the virus are γ proteins.

Following replication of the viral genome and synthesis of structural proteins, nucleocapsids are assembled in the nucleus of the cell. Envelopment occurs as the nucleocapsids bud through the inner nuclear membrane into the perinuclear space. In some cells, viral replication within the nucleus forms two types of inclusion bodies, type A basophilic Feulgen-positive bodies that contain viral DNA, and an eosinophilic inclusion body which is devoid of viral nucleic acid or protein, representing a "scar" of viral infection. Virions are then transported via the endoplasmic reticulum and the Golgi apparatus to the cell surface.

HSV infection of certain cells (neurons in particular) does not result in virus replication and cell death. Instead, viral genomes are maintained by the cell in a repressed or largely repressed state compatible with survival and normal activities of the cell, a process called *latency*. Subsequently, activation of the viral genome may occur resulting in viral replication and, in some cases, the redevelopment of herpetic lesions, a process termed *reactivation*. Whereas infectious virus rarely can be recovered from sensory or autonomic nervous system ganglia dissected from cadavers, maintenance and growth of the neural cells in tissue culture results in production of infectious virions, a process called explantation, and subsequent permissive infection of susceptible cells, a process called *cocultivation*. Virus replication was first detected in neurons during reactivation in vitro suggesting that the neuron harbors the latent virus in vivo. Subsequently, viral DNA has been found in neural tissue at times when infectious virus cannot be isolated. HSV DNA extracted from latently infected neural tissue differs from HSV DNA in cells actively replicating virus. Current data suggest that the HSV DNA in latently infected cells may exist in circular or concatameric form.

PATHOGENESIS Exposure to virus at mucosal surfaces or abraded skin permits entry of virus and initiation of replication in cells of the epidermis and dermis. Whether or not clinically apparent lesions develop, sufficient viral replication to permit infection of either sensory or autonomic nerve endings may occur. Whether latency always results from peripheral mucosal infection is unclear. Virus, or more likely, nucleocapsid, is then thought to be transported intraaxonally to the nerve cell bodies in ganglia. In humans, the time from inoculation of virus in peripheral tissue to spread to the ganglia is unknown. During the initial phase of infection, viral replication occurs in ganglia and contiguous neural tissue. Virus then spreads to other mucosal skin surfaces through centrifugal migration of infectious virions via peripheral sensory nerves. This centrifugal spread of virus to the skin from peripheral sensory nerves helps explain the large surface area, and the high frequency of new lesions distant from the initial crop of vesicles which are characteristic in patients with primary genital or oral-labial HSV and the recovery of virus from neural tissue distant from neurons innervating the inoculation site. Contiguous spread of locally inoculated virus may also occur and allow further mucosal extension of disease.

Following resolution of primary disease, infectious virus can no longer be recovered in the ganglia, and the surface viral proteins are not expressed in detectable amounts. The mechanisms by which latency is maintained and by which various stimuli cause reactivation of HSV infection are unknown. Ultraviolet light, immunosuppression, and trauma to the skin or ganglia are associated with reactivation.

Analysis of the HSV DNA from sequentially isolated strains of HSV or from multiple infected ganglia from any one individual has revealed identical restriction endonuclease patterns in most persons. Occasionally, and more frequently in immunocompromised persons, multiple strains of the same viral subtype can be detected in the same person, suggesting that exogenous infection with different strains of the same subtype is possible.

IMMUNITY Host responses to infection influence the acquisition of disease, severity of infection, resistance to development of latency, maintenance of latency, and frequency of HSV recurrences. Both antibody-mediated and cell-mediated reactions are clinically important. Immunocompromised patients with defects in cell-mediated immunity experience more severe and extensive HSV infections than those with deficits in humoral immunity such as agammaglobulinemia. In mice experimental ablation of lymphocytes indicates that T cells play a major role in preventing lethal disseminated disease, although antibodies help reduce virus titers in neural tissue. Some aspects of the pathogenesis of disease may also be related to the host immune response, e.g., stromal opacities associated with recurrent herpetic keratitis. The surface viral glycoproteins have been shown to be antigens recognized by antibodies mediating neutralization and immune-mediated cytolysis (antibody-dependent cell-mediated cytotoxicity, ADCC). Monoclonal antibodies specific for each of the known viral glycoproteins have, in experimental infections, conferred protection against subsequent neurologic disease or ganglionic latency. Multiple cell populations including natural killer (NK) cells, macrophages, a variety of T-lymphocyte populations, and lymphokines generated by these cells play a role in host defenses to HSV infections. In animals passive transfer of primed lymphocytes confers protection from subsequent challenge. Maximum protection usually requires the activation of multiple T-cell subpopulations. Both class I MHC-restricted and class II MHC-restricted responses appear important. Effector cells involved in containing virus include cytotoxic T cells and T cells responsible for delayed hypersensitivity. The latter cells may confer protection by the antigen-stimulated release of lymphokines (e.g., interferons) which may have a direct antiviral effect or activate other nonspecific effector cells.

EPIDEMIOLOGY HSV infections are found worldwide. Standard complement fixation (CF) antibody assays do not distinguish between HSV-1 and HSV-2 infection. However, several serologic assays such as neutralization, indirect immunofluorescence (IFA), passive hemagglutination (PHA), radioimmunoassay (RIA), and enzyme-linked immunosorbent assay (ELISA) can measure the relative selectivity of serum antibodies to the two subtypes. Much of the humoral immune response to HSV is to type common antigenic determinants, making it difficult to detect HSV-2 antibody in persons with prior HSV-1 infection and HSV-1 infection in those with prior HSV-2.

Seroepidemiologic studies performed in the 1940s and 1950s demonstrated that in almost all populations studied, over 90 percent of persons had antibodies to HSV by the fourth decade. In developing countries, similar patterns still prevail. In many western industrialized middle-class populations, however, the age-specific prevalence rates of HSV-1 infection appear to be decreasing, and serosurveys of middle-class populations in the United States indicate only 40 percent of persons between 25 and 29 possessed antibodies to HSV with antibody prevalence increasing by about 1.5 percent per year.

Antibodies to HSV-2 are not routinely detected until puberty, and antibody prevalence rates correlate with past sexual activity. HSV-2 antibodies have been detected in 80 percent of female prostitutes, up to 60 percent of adults of lower, and 20 to 40 percent of middle to higher socioeconomic status, and 0 to 3 percent of nuns. Only about one-third of persons who possess HSV-2 antibody give a history of a prior or current genital ulceration. Consultations with private practitioners for genital herpes increased ninefold in the United States between 1966 and 1981.

HSV infections occur throughout the year. The incubation period ranges from 1 to 26 days (median 6 to 8 days). Contact with active ulcerative lesions or asymptomatically excreting patients can result in transmission. Asymptomatic salivary excretion of HSV-1 has been reported in 2 to 9 percent of adults and 5 to 8 percent of children. HSV-2 has been isolated from the genital tract of from 0.3 to 5.4 percent of males and 1.6 to 8 percent of females attending sexually transmitted disease clinics. The titer of HSV in cultures from lesions is 100 to 1000 times higher than from salivary or genital tract secretions from asymptomatically excreting persons. The efficiency of transmission is likely to be greater during symptomatic versus asymptomatic periods of viral excretion.

CLINICAL SPECTRUM HSV has been isolated from nearly all visceral or mucocutaneous sites. The clinical manifestations and course of HSV depend on the anatomic site of the infection, the age and immune status of the host, and the antigenic type of the virus. First episodes of HSV disease, especially primary infection (that is, first infections with either HSV-1 or HSV-2 in which the host lacks HSV antibodies in acute phase serums), are frequently accompanied by systemic signs and symptoms, involve both mucosal and extramucosal sites, have a longer duration of symptoms, a longer time from which virus is isolated from lesions, and a higher rate of complications than recurrent episodes of disease. Both viral subtypes can cause genital and oral-facial infections, and these infections are clinically indistinguishable. However, the frequency of future reactivations of infection is influenced by the anatomic site and virus type. Genital HSV-2 infection is twice as likely to reactivate and will recur 8 to 10 times more frequently than genital HSV-1 infection. Conversely oral-labial HSV-1 infections will recur more frequently than oral-labial HSV-2 infections.

Oral-facial HSV infections Gingivostomatitis and pharyngitis are the most frequent clinical manifestations of first-episode HSV-1 infection, while recurrent herpes labialis is the most frequent clinical manifestation of reactivation HSV infection. HSV pharyngitis and gingivostomatitis usually result from primary infection and are most commonly seen in children and young adults. Clinical symptoms and signs include fever, malaise, myalgias, inability to eat, irritability, and cervical adenopathy, which may last from 3 to 14 days. Lesions may involve the hard and soft palate, gingiva, tongue, lip, and facial area. HSV-1 or HSV-2 infection of the pharynx usually results in exudative or ulcerative lesions of the posterior pharynx and/or tonsillar pillars. Concomitant lesions of the tongue, buccal mucosa, or gingiva may occur later in the course in one-third of cases. Fever lasting from 2 to 7 days and cervical adenopathy are common. The clinical differentiation of HSV pharyngitis from bacterial pharyngitis, *Mycoplasma pneumoniae* infections, and noninfectious causes of pharyngeal ulcerations such as Stevens-Johnson syndrome may be difficult. No substantial evidence suggests that reactivation oral-labial HSV infection is associated with symptomatic recurrent pharyngitis.

Reactivation of HSV from the trigeminal ganglia may be associated with asymptomatic excretion in the saliva, development of intraoral mucosal ulcerations, or herpetic ulcerations on the vermillion border of the lip or external facial skin. About 50 to 70 percent of seropositive patients undergoing trigeminal nerve root decompression and 10 to 15 percent of those undergoing dental extraction will develop oral-labial HSV infection a median of 3 days after these procedures.

In immunosuppressed patients extension of the infection into mucosal and deep cutaneous layers may occur. Friability, necrosis, bleeding, severe pain, and inability to eat or drink may result. HSV mucositis is clinically similar to mucosal lesions due to cytotoxic drug therapy, trauma, or fungal or bacterial infections. Concomitant HSV and *Candida* infection may also occur commonly. Systemic acyclovir therapy speeds the rate of healing and relieves the pain of mucosal HSV infections in immunosuppressed patients. Patients with atopic eczema may also develop severe oral-facial HSV infections (eczema herpeticum) which may rapidly involve extensive areas of skin and occasionally disseminate to visceral organs. Prompt resolution of extensive eczema herpeticum has been achieved with the administration of intravenous acyclovir. Erythema multiforme (EM) may also be associated with HSV infections, and some evidence suggests that it is the precipitating event in about 75 percent of cases of cutaneous EM. HSV antigen has been demonstrated in both circulatory immune complexes and in skin lesion biopsy of these patients. Patients with severe HSV-associated erythema multiforme may be candidates for chronic suppressive oral acyclovir therapy.

Genital HSV infections First-episode primary genital herpes is characterized by fever, headache, malaise, and myalgias. Pain, itching, dysuria, vaginal and urethral discharge, and tender inguinal adenopathy are the predominant local symptoms. Characteristically widely spaced bilateral distributed lesions of the external genitalia are seen. Lesions may be present in varying stages including vesicles, pustules, or painful erythematous ulcers. Involvement of the cervix and urethra are seen in over 80 percent of women with first-episode infections. First episodes of genital herpes in patients who have had prior HSV-1 infection are associated with less frequent systemic symptoms and faster healing than primary genital herpes. The clinical courses of acute first-episode genital herpes among patients with HSV-1 and HSV-2 infections are similar. However, the recurrence rates of genital disease differ. Over 80 percent of patients with first-episode HSV-2 infection will have a recurrence within 12 months (median number of recurrences, four) compared to 55 percent of those with primary HSV-1 infections (median number of recurrences, less than one). Recurrence rates of genital HSV-2 infections vary greatly between individuals and over time within the same individual. HSV has been isolated from the urethra and urine from men and women without concomitant external genital lesions. A clear mucoid discharge and dysuria are characteristic of symptomatic HSV urethritis. HSV has been isolated from the urethra of 5 percent of women with the dysuria-frequency syndrome. Occasionally, genital tract disease manifested by HSV endometritis and salpingitis in women and HSV prostatitis in men may occur.

Rectal and perianal HSV infections due to HSV-1 and HSV-2 may be seen, especially among homosexual men and/or heterosexual women who engage in anorectal intercourse. Symptoms of HSV proctitis include anorectal pain, anorectal discharge, tenesmus, and constipation. Sigmoidoscopy reveals ulcerative lesions of the distal 10 cm of the rectal mucosa. Rectal biopsies show mucosal ulceration, necrosis, polymorphonuclear and lymphocytic infiltration of the lamina propria, and occasionally multinucleated intranuclear inclusion–bearing cells. Autonomic nervous system dysfunction manifested by burning sacral paresthesias, impotence, and urinary retention may also accompany symptomatic HSV proctitis. Perianal herpetic lesions are also seen in immunosuppressed patients receiving cytotoxic therapy. HSV-1 strains, usually identical to those found in the oropharynx, are obtained from these lesions, suggesting the mode of spread is autoinoculation of the perianal area from HSV-infected saliva and/or finger lesions. Extensive perianal herpetic lesions and/or HSV proctitis may occur in patients with the acquired immunodeficiency syndrome (AIDS). Anecdotal observations suggest healing of these lesions can be achieved with the use of systemic acyclovir.

Herpetic whitlow Herpetic whitlow, HSV infection of the finger, is most often seen in medical practitioners, although it may occur as a complication of primary oral or genital herpes by inoculation of virus via a break in the epidermal surface. Clinical signs and symptoms include the abrupt onset of edema, erythema, and localized tenderness of the infected finger. Vesicular or pustular lesions of the fingertip indistinguishable from pyogenic bacterial infection are seen. Fever, lymphadenitis, and epitrochlear and axillary lymphadenopathy are common. Recurrences may occur. Prompt diagnosis to avoid unnecessary and potentially exacerbating surgical therapy and/or transmission to patients is necessary.

Herpetic eye infections HSV infection of the eye is the most frequent cause of corneal blindness in the United States. HSV keratitis presents with acute onset of pain, blurring of vision, chemosis, conjunctivitis, and characteristic dendritic lesions of the cornea. Use of topical corticosteroids may exacerbate symptoms and lead to involvement of deep structures of the eye. Debridement, topical antiviral, and/or interferon therapy hasten healing. However, recurrences are common and immunopathologic injury of the deeper structures of the eye may occur. Chorioretinitis, usually as a manifestation of disseminated HSV infection, may occur in neonates or those with AIDS. Acute necrotizing retinitis due to HSV is also an uncommon but severe manifestation of HSV infection.

Central and peripheral nervous system infections with HSV-1 and HSV-2 HSV encephalitis is the most common identified cause of acute, sporadic viral encephalitis in the United States, comprising 10 to 20 percent of all cases. The estimated incidence is about 2.3 cases per million persons per year. Cases are distributed throughout the year, and the age distribution appears biphasic with peaks at between 5 and 30 and greater-than-50 years of age. HSV-1 accounts for more than 95 percent of cases. The pathogenesis of HSV encephalitis is varied. In children and young adults primary HSV infection may result in encephalitis; presumably exogenously acquired virus enters the CNS by neurotropic spread from the periphery via the olfactory bulb. However, most adults with HSV encephalitis have clinical or serologic evidence of mucocutaneous HSV-1 infection prior to the onset of the CNS symptoms. In about 25 percent of the cases examined, the HSV-1 strains from the oropharynx and brain tissue from the same patient differ, suggesting that some cases may result from reinfection with another strain of HSV-1 that reached the CNS. Two theories have been proposed to explain the development of actively replicating HSV in localized areas of the CNS in persons from whom the ganglionic and CNS isolates are similar. Reactivation of latent trigeminal or autonomic nerve root HSV-1 infection may be associated with extension of virus into the CNS via nerves innervating the middle cranial fossa. HSV DNA has been demonstrated by DNA hybridization in human autopsy brain tissue. As such, reactivation of long-standing latent CNS infection may be another potential mechanism for the development of HSV encephalitis.

The clinical hallmark of HSV encephalitis has been the acute onset of fever and focal neurologic, especially temporal lobe, symptoms. To date no reliable noninvasive radiologic or virologic technique has been developed to diagnose HSV encephalitis during its early clinical stages, and differentiation of HSV encephalitis from other viral encephalitides and other focal infections and noninfectious processes is difficult. An increase in CSF and serum antibodies to HSV does occur with most cases of HSV encephalitis. However, these antibody rises rarely are present prior to 10 days into the illness and, while useful retrospectively, are not helpful in establishing the clinical diagnosis early in the course of disease. Brain biopsy because of its high sensitivity, low complication rate, and ability to establish alternative potentially treatable diagnoses has been felt by many to be the most expeditious method to diagnose HSV encephalitis. Antiviral chemotherapy reduces the mortality of HSV encephalitis, and intravenous acyclovir appears to be more effective than vidarabine. Even with therapy, however, neurologic sequelae are frequent.

HSV has been isolated from the cerebrospinal fluid from 0.5 to 3 percent of patients presenting to the hospital with aseptic meningitis. HSV meningitis is usually seen in association with primary genital HSV infection. HSV meningitis is an acute self-limited disease manifested by headache, fever, and mild photophobia, which lasts from 2 to 7 days. A lymphocytic pleocytosis in the CSF is characteristic. Neurologic sequelae are rare. Recurrent bouts of aseptic meningitis related to reactivation of HSV have been reported.

Autonomic nervous system (ANS) dysfunction, especially of the sacral region, has been reported in association with both HSV and varicella-zoster infections. Numbness, tingling of the buttock or perineal areas, urinary retention, constipation, cerebrospinal fluid pleocytosis, and impotence in males may occur. Symptoms appear to resolve slowly over a period of days to weeks. Occasionally hypesthesia and/or weakness of the lower extremities may persist for many months. Rarely transverse myelitis manifested by a rapidly progressive symmetric paralysis of the lower extremities or a Guillain-Barré syndrome may occur after HSV infection. Similarly, peripheral nervous system involvement [idiopathic facial paralysis (Bell's palsy)] or cranial polyneuritis may also be related to reactivation of HSV-1 infection. Transitory hypesthesia of the area of skin innervated by the trigeminal nerve and vestibular system dysfunction as measured by electronystagmography are the predominant signs of disease. Studies to determine if antiviral chemotherapy may abort or alleviate the frequency and severity of these signs are unavailable.

Visceral infections HSV infection of visceral organs usually results from viremia, and multiple organ involvement is common. Occasionally, however, the clinical manifestations of HSV infections may involve only the esophagus, lung, or liver. HSV esophagitis may result from direct extension of oral-pharyngeal HSV infection into the esophagus or may occur de novo by reactivation of HSV and spread of virus to the esophageal mucosa via the vagus nerve. The predominant symptoms of HSV esophagitis are odynophagia, dysphagia, substernal pain, and weight loss. Endoscopically there are multiple oval ulcerations on an erythematous base with or without a patchy white pseudomembrane. The distal esophagus is most commonly involved, but with extensive disease diffuse friability of the entire esophagus may ensue. Neither endoscopic nor barium examination can differentiate HSV from *Candida* esophagitis, or from esophageal ulcerations due to thermal injury, radiation, and corrosives. Endoscopically obtained secretions for cytologic examination and culture provide the most accurate material for diagnosis. While controlled trials have not been conducted, anecdotal observations suggest resolution of the symptoms of HSV esophagitis with systemic antiviral chemotherapy.

HSV pneumonitis is uncommon except in severely immunosuppressed patients. Among bone marrow transplant recipients HSV pneumonitis appears to account for approximately 6 to 8 percent of cases of biopsy- or autopsy-proven interstitial pneumonia. HSV-1 infection of the lower respiratory tract may occur from extension of herpetic tracheobronchitis into lung parenchyma. Focal necrotizing pneumonitis usually results. Hematogenous dissemination of virus from oral or genital mucocutaneous disease may also occur, and produce a bilateral interstitial pneumonitis. Concomitant bacterial, fungal, and parasitic pathogens are common in HSV pneumonitis. As the mortality of HSV pneumonia in immunosuppressed patients is high (>80 percent), these patients should be candidates for antiviral chemotherapy. HSV has also been isolated from the lower respiratory tract of persons with acute respiratory distress syndrome (ARDS). However, the relationship between isolation of HSV and the pathogenesis of the respiratory distress syndrome is unclear.

HSV is an uncommon cause of hepatitis in immunocompetent patients. HSV infection of the liver is associated with fever, abrupt elevations of the bilirubin and serum transaminases, and leukopenia (white blood cells <4000 per cubic millimeter). Disseminated intravascular coagulation may also be present.

Other isolated but reported complications of HSV include monoarticular arthritis, adrenal necrosis, idiopathic thrombocytopenia, and glomerulonephritis. Disseminated HSV infection in the immunocompetent patient is rare. In immunocompromised, burn, or malnourished patients, dissemination of HSV to other visceral organs such as adrenal glands, pancreas, small and large intestine, and bone marrow may occur occasionally. Rarely, primary HSV infection in pregnancy may disseminate and may be associated with mortality in both mother and fetus. This, however, is an uncommon event and is usually associated with acquisition of primary infection in the third trimester.

NEONATAL HSV INFECTION Neonates (<6 to 7 weeks of age) appear to have the highest frequency of visceral and/or CNS infection of any HSV-infected patient population. Untreated, over 70 percent of neonatal herpes cases will disseminate or develop CNS infection. Without therapy, the overall mortality of neonatal herpes is 65 percent, and less than 10 percent of neonates with CNS infection experience normal development. While skin lesions are the most commonly recognized features of disease, many infants do not develop lesions until well into the course of disease. In most series 70 percent of neonatal HSV cases are related to HSV-2 infection, almost all of which result from contact via infected genital secretions at the time of delivery. However, congenitally infected infants have been reported, usually from mothers who acquired primary HSV infection during pregnancy. Neonatal HSV-1 infections are usually acquired postnatally through contact with immediate family members with symptomatic or asymptomatic oral-labial HSV-1 infection or from nosocomial transmission within the hospital. Antiviral chemotherapy has reduced the mortality of neonatal herpes to 25 percent. However, the morbidity, especially in infants with CNS involvement, is still very high.

DIAGNOSIS Both clinical and laboratory criteria are useful for establishing the diagnosis of HSV infections. Clinical diagnosis can be made accurately where characteristic multiple vesicular lesions on an erythematous base are present. Scrapings of the base of the lesions and subsequent staining with Wright, Giemsa (Tzanck preparation), or Papanicolaou's stain will demonstrate characteristic giant cells or intranuclear inclusions of a herpesvirus infection. These cytologic techniques are often useful as a quick office procedure to confirm the diagnosis. Limitations of this method are that it does not differentiate between HSV and varicella-zoster infections and is only about 60 percent as sensitive as viral isolation. The laboratory confirmation of HSV infection is best performed by isolation of virus in tissue culture. HSV causes a discernible cytopathic effect in a variety of cell culture systems, and most specimens can be identified within 48 to 96 h after inoculation. The sensitivity of viral isolation varies with the stage of lesions (higher in vesicular than in ulcerative lesions), whether the patient has a first or recurrent episode of the disease (higher in first episodes), and whether the sample is from an immunosuppressed or immunocompetent patient (more antigen in immunosuppressed). Immunofluorescent assays using monoclonal antibodies and some DNA hybridization procedures have approached the sensitivity of viral isolation for detecting HSV from genital or oral-labial lesions but appear only about 50 percent as sensitive as viral isolation for the detection of asymptomatic HSV in cervical or salivary secretions. Laboratory confirmation allows for subtyping the virus, which may be useful epidemiologically as well as in helping to predict the frequency of reactivation after first-episode oral-labial or genital HSV infection. Restriction endonuclease analysis of viral DNA can also be used to differentiate between HSV-1 and HSV-2 as well as to differentiate between strains within the same subtypes, information which may be very useful in identifying common source outbreaks of HSV.

Acute and convalescent serum can be useful in documenting seroconversion during primary HSV-1 or HSV-2 infection. However, only 5 percent of patients with recurrent mucocutaneous HSV infections show a fourfold or greater rise in anti-HSV antibodies between acute and convalescent serums. As such, serologic assays have little utility in diagnosing acute mucocutaneous HSV infection, and are best used to identify persons with past infection.

THERAPY Many aspects of mucocutaneous and visceral HSV infections are amenable to treatment with antiviral chemotherapy. For mucocutaneous infections acyclovir has been the mainstay of therapy. Several antivirals are available for topical use in HSV eye infections: idoxuridine, trifluorothymidine, and topical vidarabine. For HSV encephalitis, intravenous acyclovir is the treatment of choice. For neonatal HSV infections both intravenous vidarabine and acyclovir are effective.

Acyclovir has been shown to be effective in shortening symptoms and the duration of lesions of mucocutaneous HSV infections in immunocompromised patients and first-episode genital herpes in immunocompetent patients (Table 136-1). Intravenous and oral acyclovir will also prevent reactivation of HSV in seropositive immunocompromised patients who are undergoing induction chemotherapy for acute leukemia or in the immediate posttransplant period.

Oral acyclovir tablets have also been shown to speed the healing and resolution of symptoms of first and recurrent episodes of genital HSV-1 and HSV-2 infections. The benefit of treating acute episodes of recurrent genital disease with oral acyclovir is modest, and as such, routine use for recurrent episodes of disease, especially for mild episodes, is not recommended. Chronic daily suppressive therapy may be useful in reducing the frequency of reactivation disease among patients with very frequent genital herpes. However, while daily administration of two to five tablets of oral acyclovir for 4 to 6 months appears safe, selective use of the drug must be advocated until there is better understanding of possible long-term toxicity, the frequency with which resistant strains emerge, and the effects of chronic therapy on the transmission of the disease. Chronic suppressive oral acyclovir does not eliminate ganglionic latency, and reactivation of disease occurs after discontinuing therapy. No data are available on the use of oral acyclovir in the treatment of primary or recurrent gingivostomatitis.

Both intravenous vidarabine 15 mg/kg per day over 12 h daily and intravenous acyclovir 30 mg/kg per day given as 10 mg/kg infusion over 1 h at 8-hourly intervals have been shown to be effective in reducing the mortality of HSV encephalitis. Primary determinants of outcome include young age and early therapy. Comparative trials of the two drugs for the treatment of HSV encephalitis have indicated a lower mortality rate and fewer neurologic sequelae with intravenous acyclovir. The major side effect associated with intravenous acyclovir is transient renal insufficiency usually due to crystallization of the compound in the renal parenchyma. This can be avoided if the medication is given slowly over 1 h and the patient is well-hydrated. As CSF levels of acyclovir average only 30 to 50 percent of plasma levels, the dosage of acyclovir used for treatment of CNS infection (30 mg/kg per day) is double that used for treatment of mucocutaneous or visceral disease (15 mg/kg per day). Vidarabine at doses of 15 mg/kg per day tends to produce more hematopoietic and hepatic toxicity than acyclovir, but this is usually not a limiting problem in treating severe neonatal or CNS infections.

TABLE 136-1 Current status of antiviral chemotherapy of HSV infection*

I Mucocutaneous HSV infections
- *A* Immunosuppressed patients
  - *1* Acute symptomatic first or recurrent episodes: IV acyclovir (5 mg/kg every 8 h) or oral acyclovir (200 mg PO 5 times per day for 7 to 10 days) relieves pain and speeds healing. With localized external lesions 5% topical acyclovir ointment applied 4 to 6 times daily may be beneficial.
  - *2* Suppression of reactivation disease: IV (5 mg/kg every 8 h) or oral acyclovir (400 mg PO 4 to 5 times per day) will when taken daily prevent recurrences during high-risk period, e.g., immediate post-transplantation period.
- *B* Immunocompetent patients
  - *1* Genital herpes
    - *a* First episodes: Oral acyclovir (200 mg PO 5 times per day for 10 to 14 days) is the treatment of choice. IV acyclovir (5 mg/kg every 8 h for 5 days) is given for severe disease or neurologic complications such as aseptic meningitis. Topical 5% ointment or cream applied 4 to 6 times daily for 7 to 10 days may be beneficial in patients without cervical, urethral, or pharyngeal involvement.
    - *b* Symptomatic recurrent genital herpes: Oral acyclovir (200 mg PO 5 times per day for 5 days) has modest benefit in shortening lesions and viral excretion time. Routine use for all episodes not recommended.
    - *c* Suppression of recurrent genital herpes: Daily oral acyclovir 200-mg capsules, 2 to 3 times daily will prevent reactivation of symptomatic recurrences; use at present limited to 6-month course in frequent recurrers.
  - *2* Oral-labial HSV
    - *a* First episode: Oral acyclovir has not been studied yet.
    - *b* Recurrent episodes: Topical acyclovir ointment is of no clinical benefit. Oral acyclovir is not routinely recommended.
  - *3* Herpetic whitlow: Studies of antiviral chemotherapy have not yet been performed.
  - *4* HSV proctitis: Oral acyclovir (400 mg PO 5 times per day) is useful in shortening course of infection. In immunosuppressed patients or in severe infection, IV acyclovir 5 mg/kg every 8 h may be useful.
- *C* Herpetic eye infections
  - *1* Acute keratitis: Topical trifluorothymidine, vidarabine, idoxuridine, acyclovir, and interferon are all beneficial. Debridement may be required; topical steroids may worsen disease.

II CNS HSV infection
- *A* HSV encephalitis: Intravenous acyclovir 10 mg/kg every 8 h (30 mg/kg per day) for 10 days or vidarabine (15 mg/kg per day) decrease mortality; acyclovir is the preferred agent.
- *B* HSV aseptic meningitis: No studies of systemic antiviral chemotherapy. If therapy is to be given IV, acyclovir at 15 to 30 mg/kg per day should be utilized.
- *C* Autonomic radiculopathy: No studies are available.

III Neonatal HSV infection: Intravenous vidarabine (30 mg/kg per day) or acyclovir (30 mg/kg per day). Neonates appear to tolerate this high dose of vidarabine.

IV Visceral HSV infections
- *A* HSV esophagitis: Systemic acyclovir (15 mg/kg per day) or vidarabine (15 mg/kg per day) should be considered.
- *B* HSV pneumonitis: No controlled studies: systemic acyclovir (15 mg/kg per day) or vidarabine (15 mg/kg per day) should be considered.

V Disseminated HSV: No controlled studies, intravenous acyclovir or vidarabine should be attempted. No definite evidence that therapy will decrease mortality.

VI Erythema multiforme associated with HSV: Anecdotal observations suggest oral acyclovir capsules 2 to 3 times daily will suppress EM.

* *IV = intravenous; PO = by mouth.*

PREVENTION The large reservoir of persons with asymptomatic HSV-1 and HSV-2 infections indicates that control of HSV disease through suppressive antiviral chemotherapy and/or educational programs will be limited. Control of HSV infection will require prevention of infection, a goal most likely achievable by vaccination. Effective HSV vaccines are not currently available in the United States. Many heterologous vaccines such as smallpox, bacillus Calmette-Guérin, influenza, and polio vaccines have been used as therapies for genital HSV infection. All have been ineffective. In particular, smallpox vaccine is ineffective in reducing the recurrence rate of herpes. Deaths from disseminated vaccinia infection have occurred, and this potentially dangerous form of therapy should be actively discouraged.

Currently no proven effective means of prophylaxis of HSV has been established. Barrier forms of contraception, especially condoms, may decrease transmission of disease especially during periods of asymptomatic viral excretion. Transmission of disease when lesions were present despite the use of a condom may still occur, and patients should be instructed to avoid sexual activity when genital lesions are present.

REFERENCES

COREY L et al: A trial of topical acyclovir in genital herpes simplex infections. N Engl J Med 306:1313, 1982

———: Genital herpes simplex virus infection: Clinical manifestations, course and complications. Ann Intern Med 98:958, 1983

———, SPEAR P: Infections with herpes simplex viruses. N Engl J Med 314:686, 749, 1986

DOUGLAS JM et al: A double-blind study of oral acyclovir for suppression of recurrences of genital herpes simplex virus infection. N Engl J Med 310:1551, 1984

HILL TJ: Herpes simplex virus latency, in *The Herpesviruses*, 3, B Roizman (ed). New York, Plenum, 1984, pp 175–240

HIRSCH MS, SCHOOLEY RT: Drug therapy: Treatment of herpesvirus infections. N Engl J Med 309(16):963 and 309(17):1035, 1983

MERTZ GJ et al: Double-blind placebo-controlled trial of oral acyclovir in first episode genital herpes simplex virus infection. JAMA 242:1147, 1984

RAMSEY PG et al: Herpes simplex virus pneumonia. Ann Intern Med 97:812, 1982

SHEPP DH et al: Oral acyclovir therapy for mucocutaneous herpes simplex virus infections in immunocompromised marrow transplant recipients. Ann Intern Med 102:783, 1985

STRAUSS SE et al: Acyclovir for chronic mucocutaneous herpes simplex virus infection in immunosuppressed patients. Ann Intern Med 96(3):270, 1982

——— et al: Herpes simplex virus infection: Biology, treatment and prevention. Ann Intern Med 103:404, 1985

WADE JC et al: Intravenous acyclovir to treat mucocutaneous herpes simplex virus infection after marrow transplantation. Ann Intern Med 96:265, 1982

WHITLEY RJ et al: Vidarabine therapy of neonatal herpes simplex virus infection. Pediatrics 66:495, 1980

——— et al: Vidarabine versus acyclovir therapy in herpes simplex encephalitis. N Engl J Med 314:144, 1986

137 CYTOMEGALOVIRUS INFECTION

MARTIN S. HIRSCH

DEFINITION Cytomegalovirus (CMV), which was initially isolated from patients with congenital cytomegalic inclusion disease, is now recognized as an important pathogen in all age groups. In addition to inducing severe birth defects, CMV causes a wide spectrum of disorders in older children and adults, ranging from an asymptomatic, subclinical infection to a mononucleosis syndrome in healthy individuals to disseminated disease in the immunocompromised. Human CMV is one of several related species-specific viruses that cause similar diseases in various animals. All are associated with the production of characteristic enlarged cells; hence the name cytomegalovirus.

ETIOLOGY CMV is a member of the herpesvirus group and thus contains double-stranded DNA, a protein capsid, and a lipoprotein envelope. Like other members of the herpesvirus group, CMV demonstrates icosahedral symmetry, replicates in the cell nucleus, and can cause either a lytic and productive or a latent infection. CMV can be distinguished from other herpesviruses by certain biologic properties such as host range and the type of cytopathology induced. Virus replication is associated with the production of large intranuclear inclusions and smaller cytoplasmic inclusions. The virus appears to replicate in a variety of cell types in vivo; in tissue culture it grows preferentially in fibroblasts. It is unclear whether CMV is oncogenic in vivo. However, the virus can rarely transform fibroblasts and genomic transforming fragments have been identified.

EPIDEMIOLOGY CMV has a worldwide distribution. Approximately 1 percent of newborns in the United States are infected with CMV, and the percentage is higher in many less-developed countries. Communal living and poor personal hygiene facilitate early spread. Perinatal and early childhood infections are common. Virus may be present in milk, saliva, feces, and urine. Transmission of CMV has been identified among young children in day-care centers.

The virus is not readily spread by casual contact but requires repeated or prolonged intimate exposure for transmission. In late adolescence and young adulthood, CMV is often transmitted venereally, and asymptomatic viral carriage in semen or cervical secretions is common. CMV antibody titers approach 100 percent in female prostitutes and in sexually active homosexual men. Transfusion of whole blood or certain blood products containing viable leukocytes may also transmit CMV with a frequency of 2 to 10 percent per unit transfused.

Once infected, an individual probably carries the virus for life. Most commonly these infections remain latent. However, with compromise of T-lymphocyte-mediated immunity, as occurs following organ transplantation or in association with lymphoid neoplasms and certain acquired immunodeficiencies, CMV reactivation syndromes develop frequently.

PATHOGENESIS Congenital CMV infection can follow either primary or reactivation infection of the mother. However, clinical disease in the fetus or newborn is almost exclusively limited to primary maternal infections. Factors determining the severity of congenital infection are unknown; a deficient capacity to produce precipitating antibodies and to mount T-cell responses to CMV are associated with more severe disease.

Primary infection in late childhood or adulthood is often associated with a vigorous T-lymphocyte response that may contribute to the development of a mononucleosis syndrome similar to that observed following Epstein-Barr virus infection (see Chap. 138). The hallmarks of such infections are the appearance of atypical lymphocytes in the peripheral blood; these cells are predominantly activated T lymphocytes of cytotoxic-suppressor phenotype. Polyclonal activation of B cells by the virus contributes to the development of rheumatoid factors and other autoantibodies during CMV mononucleosis.

Once acquired during symptomatic or asymptomatic primary infection, CMV persists indefinitely in tissues of the host. The sites of persistent or latent infection are unclear, but probably involve multiple cell types and various organs. Transmission following blood transfusion or organ transplantation points to silent infections in these tissues. Autopsy studies suggest that lungs, salivary glands, and bowel may also be areas of latent infection.

If T-cell responses of the host become compromised by disease or by iatrogenic immunosuppression, latent virus can be reactivated to cause a variety of syndromes. Chronic antigenic stimulation, as occurs following tissue transplantation, in the presence of immunosuppression, appears to be an ideal setting for CMV activation and CMV-induced disease. Certain particularly potent suppressants of T-cell immunity such as antithymocyte globulin are associated with a high rate of clinical CMV syndromes which may follow either primary or reactivation infection. CMV may itself contribute to further T-lymphocyte hyporesponsiveness which often precedes superinfection with other opportunistic pathogens, such as *Pneumocystis carinii*. CMV and pneumocystis are frequently found together in immunosuppressed patients with severe interstitial pneumonia.

PATHOLOGY Cytomegalic cells in vivo are presumed to be infected epithelial cells. They are two to four times larger than surrounding cells and often contain an 8- to 10-μm intranuclear inclusion that is eccentrically placed and surrounded by a clear halo, resulting in an "owl's eye" appearance. Smaller granular cytoplasmic inclusions may also be demonstrated occasionally. Cytomegalic cells are found in a wide variety of organs including salivary glands, lung, liver, kidney, intestines, pancreas, adrenal glands, and the central nervous system.

The cellular inflammatory response to infection consists of plasma cells, lymphocytes, and monocyte-macrophages. Granulomatous reactions are occasionally observed, particularly in the liver. Immunopathologic reactions may contribute to CMV disease. Immune complexes have been described in infected infants, sometimes associated with CMV-related glomerulopathies. Immune complex glomerulopathy has been observed in some CMV-infected patients following renal transplantation.

CLINICAL MANIFESTATIONS **Congenital CMV infection** Fetal infections range from inapparent to severe and disseminated. Cytomegalic inclusion disease develops in approximately 5 percent of infected fetuses and is seen almost exclusively in infants born to mothers who develop primary infections during pregnancy. Petechiae, hepatosplenomegaly, and jaundice are the most common presenting features (60 to 80 percent). Microcephaly with or without cerebral calcifications, intrauterine growth retardation, and prematurity are noted in 30 to 50 percent of patients. Inguinal hernias and chorioretinitis are observed less commonly. Laboratory abnormalities in decreasing order of frequency include increased serum IgM (>20 mg/dL), atypical lymphocytosis, elevated liver transaminases, thrombocytopenia, hyperbilirubinemia, and increased cerebrospinal fluid protein (>20 mg/dL). Prognosis among severely infected infants is poor with mortality rates of 20 to 30 percent; few patients escape intellectual or hearing difficulties in later years. Differential diagnoses of cytomegalic inclusion disease in infants include syphilis, rubella, toxoplasmosis, herpes simplex or enterovirus infection, and bacterial sepsis.

Most congenital CMV infections are clinically inapparent at birth. Between 5 to 25 percent of asymptomatically infected infants develop significant psychomotor, hearing, ocular, or dental abnormalities over the next several years.

Perinatal CMV infection The newborn may acquire CMV at the time of delivery by passage through an infected birth canal or by postnatal contact with maternal milk or other secretions. Approximately 40 to 60 percent of infants who are breast-fed for over 1 month by seropositive mothers will become infected. Iatrogenic transmission can also result from neonatal blood transfusion. Screening of blood products prior to transfusion to eliminate CMV-positive blood will decrease the risk of infection. The great majority of infants infected at or after delivery will remain asymptomatic. However, protracted interstitial pneumonitis has been associated with perinatally acquired CMV infection, particularly in premature infants, occasionally associated with *Chlamydia trachomatis, P. carinii,* or *Ureaplasma urealyticum* infections. Poor weight gain, adenopathy, rash, hepatitis, anemia, and atypical lymphocytosis may also be present, and CMV excretion often persists for months to years.

CMV mononucleosis The most common clinical manifestation of CMV infection in normal hosts beyond the neonatal period is a heterophil-antibody negative mononucleosis syndrome. This may occur spontaneously or following the transfusion of leukocyte-containing blood products. Although the syndrome occurs at all ages, sexually active young adults are most often involved. Incubation periods range from 20 to 60 days, and the illness generally lasts 2 to 6 weeks. Prolonged high fevers, sometimes accompanied by chills, profound fatigue, and malaise characterize this disorder. Myalgias, headache, and splenomegaly are frequent, but exudative pharyngitis and cervical lymphadenopathy are rare, in contrast to infectious mononucleosis caused by Epstein-Barr virus. Occasional patients will develop rubelliform rashes, often after exposure to ampicillin. Less commonly observed are interstitial or segmental pneumonia, myocarditis, pleuritis, arthritis, or encephalitis. Rarely, Guillain-Barré syndrome may complicate CMV mononucleosis. The characteristic laboratory abnormality is a peripheral blood relative lymphocytosis with greater than 10 percent atypical lymphocytes. Total leukocyte counts may be low, normal, or markedly elevated. Although significant jaundice is uncommon, moderately elevated serum transaminase and alkaline phosphatase levels are often present. Heterophil antibodies are absent; however, transient immunologic abnormalities are common. These may include the presence of cryoglobulins, rheumatoid factors, cold agglutinins, and antinuclear antibodies. Rarely, hemolytic anemia, thrombocytopenia, and granulocytopenia complicate recovery.

Most patients recover without sequelae, although postviral asthenia may persist for months. CMV excretion in urine, genital secretions, or saliva often continues for months to years. Rare patients have recurrent episodes of fever and malaise, sometimes associated with autonomic nervous system dysfunction, e.g., attacks of sweating or flushing.

CMV infection in the immunocompromised host CMV appears to be the most frequent and important viral pathogen complicating organ transplantation. In renal, cardiac, and liver transplant recipients, CMV induces a variety of syndromes including fever and leukopenia, hepatitis, pneumonitis, colitis, and retinitis. The maximal period of risk appears between 1 to 4 months after transplantation, although retinitis is often a later complication. The relative risk of disease appears greater following primary infection than after reactivation. However, reactivation infection is much more common since the population of seronegative recipients of organs from seropositive donors is relatively small. Therefore, the overall morbidity rate from reactivation infection may be equally as high as that after primary infection. Clinical disease is related to the degree of immunosuppression; patients receiving certain immunosuppressive agents, such as antithymocyte globulin, appear more likely to have severe infections than those receiving other agents, such as cyclosporin A.

CMV pneumonia occurs in nearly 20 percent of bone marrow transplant recipients, with a case fatality rate of 88 percent. The risk is greatest between 5 to 13 weeks after transplant, and several risk factors have been identified. These include degree of immunosuppression, acute graft-versus-host disease, older age, seropositivity before transplantation, and granulocyte transfusions.

CMV has become recognized as an important pathogen in patients with the acquired immunodeficiency sydrome (AIDS). CMV infection is nearly ubiquitous in this disorder and often causes disseminated disease, contributing to death. CMV-induced immunosuppression probably also contributes to the T-lymphocyte deficiency initiated by the etiologic retrovirus.

CMV syndromes in the immunocompromised host often begin with prolonged fever, malaise, anorexia, fatigue, night sweats, and arthralgias or myalgias. Liver function abnormalities, leukopenia, thrombocytopenia, and atypical lymphocytosis may be observed during these episodes. The development of tachypnea, hypoxia, and unproductive cough signals respiratory involvement. Radiologic examination of the lung often demonstrates bilateral interstitial or reticulonodular infiltrates, beginning in the periphery of the lower lobes and spreading centrally and superiorly; localized segmental, nodular, or alveolar patterns are less commonly observed. Diagnosis requires lung biopsy, since neither peripheral virus excretion nor high antibody titers provides sufficient information to prove etiology. The differential diagnoses include *P. carinii,* other viral, bacterial, or fungal pathogens, pulmonary hemorrhage, and injury secondary to radiation or cytotoxic drugs.

Gastrointestinal CMV involvement may be localized or extensive and occurs almost exclusively in compromised hosts. Ulcers of the esophagus, stomach, small intestine, or colon may result in bleeding or perforation. CMV infection may lead to exacerbations of underlying ulcerative colitis. Hepatitis frequently occurs, and CMV-associated acalculous cholecystitis has been described.

CMV rarely causes meningoencephalitis in otherwise healthy individuals. However, in patients with AIDS, it has been associated with chronic encephalitis and with subacute encephalopathy which presents as lethargy and social withdrawal and progresses to dementia over weeks to months. Although CMV inclusions have been observed in patients dying of AIDS-encephalopathy, the role of CMV in this disorder is unclear (see Chap. 257).

CMV retinitis is an important cause of blindness in immunocompromised patients, including patients with AIDS and organ transplant recipients. Early lesions consist of small, opaque, white areas of granular retinal necrosis that spread in a centrifugal manner and are later accompanied by hemorrhages, vessel sheathing, and retinal edema (see Fig. A4-14). CMV must be distinguished from other causes of retinopathy including toxoplasmosis, candidiasis, and herpes simplex virus.

Fatal infections are often associated with persistent viremia and multiple organ system involvement. Progressive pulmonary infiltrates, pancytopenia, hyperamylasemia, and hypotension are characteristic, often with a terminal bacterial, fungal, or protozoan superinfection. Extensive adrenal necrosis with CMV inclusions is present at autopsy, as well as CMV involvement of many other organs.

In the renal transplant recipient, CMV also contributes to graft dysfunction by mechanisms other than direct viral cytopathic effects. An immune complex glomerulopathy may accompany CMV infection and should be differentiated from true graft rejection, since the former does not respond well to increased immunosuppression. Kidney biopsy is often necessary to distinguish the two, although CMV viremia and abnormal inverted ratios of T-lymphocyte subsets strongly suggest CMV glomerulopathy.

DIAGNOSIS The diagnosis of CMV infection cannot be made reliably on clinical grounds alone. Virus isolation from appropriate clinical specimens, together with demonstration of a fourfold or greater antibody rise or persistently elevated antibody titers, are the preferred diagnostic approaches. Virus excretion or viremia is readily detected by culture of appropriate specimens on human fibroblast monolayers. If virus titers are high, as is frequently the case in congenital disseminated infection or in patients with AIDS, characteristic cytopathic effects may be detected within a few days. However, in some situations, e.g., CMV mononucleosis, virus titers are low and cytopathic effects may take several weeks to appear. Virus isolation from urine or saliva by itself does not necessarily imply acute infection since excretion from these sites may continue for months to years following illness. Detection of CMV viremia is a better predictor of acute infection.

Advances in molecular biology have allowed DNA-DNA hybridization techniques to be used for rapid detection of CMV in urine and buffy coat specimens with a sensitivity and specificity of approximately 90 percent. To date, these techniques are experimental and require the use of ^{32}P-labeled probes. The use of nonradioactive stable probes will allow this promising technique to become more generally available. Another rapid technique that will be employed increasingly is detection of CMV antigens in specimens by immunofluorescence of immunoperoxidation using monoclonal antibodies directed against CMV-specific antigens.

A variety of serologic assays (complement fixation, immunofluorescence, indirect hemagglutination, enzyme-linked immunosorbent assay) are available to detect antibody rises to CMV antigens. Antibody rises may not be detectable for up to 4 weeks after primary infection, and titers often remain high for years after infection. For this reason, single-sample antibody determinations are of no value in assessing the acuteness of infection. Detection of CMV-specific IgM is sometimes useful in the early diagnosis of infection, particularly in infants with congenital infection; circulating rheumatoid factors may result in occasional false-positive IgM tests.

PREVENTION AND TREATMENT Although no specific therapy is available for CMV infections, prophylactic measures may be useful in certain situations. The use of blood from seronegative donors or blood that was frozen, thawed, and deglycerolized greatly decreases transfusion-associated transmission of CMV. Similarly, matching of kidney transplants by CMV serology, using only organs from seronegative donors for seronegative recipients, reduces primary infections following transplantation. CMV immune globulin has been reported to be useful in certain seronegative bone marrow transplant recipients and is under study in kidney transplant patients. A live, attenuated CMV vaccine is undergoing trial among renal transplant patients. Prophylactic interferon alpha has been demonstrated to prevent reactivation CMV syndromes and to delay CMV excretion in high-risk kidney transplant recipients, i.e., those receiving cadaver organs and antithymocyte globulin. Its use in transplant recipients susceptible to primary infection is under investigation.

Treatment of ongoing CMV syndromes has been largely unsuccessful to date in transplant recipients and in patients with AIDS. Interferons, vidarabine, and acyclovir have failed, whether used alone or in combination. Newer nucleoside derivatives, such as 9-(1,3-dihydroxy-2-propoxymethyl)guanine (DHPG), show considerable activity against CMV in vitro. DHPG also shows promise in early clinical trials against CMV retinitis, colitis, and pneumonitis.

REFERENCES

ADLER S: Transfusion-associated cytomegalovirus infections. Rev Infect Dis 5:977, 1983

BRADY MT et al: Use of deglycerolized red blood cells to prevent posttransfusion infection with cytomegalovirus in neonates. J Infect Dis 150:334, 1984

CHOU S, MERIGAN TC: Rapid detection and quantitation of human cytomegalovirus in urine through DNA hybridization. N Engl J Med 308:921, 1983

GLENN J: Cytomegalovirus infections following renal transplantation. Rev Infect Dis 3:1151, 1981

COHEN JI, COREY GR: Cytomegalovirus infection in the normal host. Medicine 64:100, 1985

FELSENSTEIN D et al: Treatment of cytomegalovirus retinitis with 9-[2-hydroxy-1-(hydroxymethyl)ethoxymethyl] guanine (BWB759U). Ann Intern Med 103:377, 1985

HANDSFIELD HH et al: Cytomegalovirus infection in sex partners: Evidence for sexual transmission. J Infect Dis 151:344, 1985

HIRSCH MS et al: Effects of interferon-alpha on cytomegalovirus reactivation syndromes in renal-transplant recipients. N Engl J Med 308:1489, 1983

HO M: *Cytomegalovirus: Biology and Infection:* New York, Plenum, 1982

JORDAN MC et al: Spontaneous cytomegalovirus mononucleosis: Clinical and laboratory observations in nine cases. Ann Intern Med 79:153, 1973

KLEMOLA E et al: Cytomegalovirus mononucleosis in previously healthy adults. Ann Intern Med 71:11, 1969

MEYERS JD et al: Nonbacterial pneumonia after allogeneic marrow transplantation: review of ten years' experience. Rev Infect Dis 4:1119, 1982

——— et al: Prevention of cytomegalovirus infection by cytomegalovirus immune globulin after marrow transplantation. Ann Intern Med 98:442, 1983

ONORATO IM et al: Epidemiology of cytomegaloviral infections: Recommendations for prevention and control. Rev Infect Dis 7:479, 1985

PASS RF et al: Cytomegalovirus infection in a day-care center. N Engl J Med 307:477, 1982

PLOTKIN S et al (eds): CMV: *Pathogenesis and Prevention of Human Infection.* New York, Alan R Liss, 1984.

SCHOOLEY RE et al: Association of herpesvirus infections with T-lymphocyte subset alterations, glomerulopathy, and opportunistic infections after renal transplantation. N Engl J Med 308:307, 1983

SPECTOR SA et al: Detection of human cytomegalovirus in clinical specimens by DNA-DNA hybridization. J Infect Dis 150:121, 1984

VOLPI A et al: Rapid diagnosis of pneumonia due to cytomegalovirus with specific monoclonal antibodies. J Infect Dis 147:1119, 1983

138 EPSTEIN-BARR VIRUS INFECTIONS, INCLUDING INFECTIOUS MONONUCLEOSIS

ROBERT T. SCHOOLEY

DEFINITION Epstein-Barr virus (EBV) is a B lymphotropic human herpesgroup virus which is worldwide in distribution. Primary infection with EBV during childhood is usually subclinical. Between 25 and 70 percent of adolescents and adults who undergo a primary EBV infection develop the clinical syndrome of infectious mononucleosis. Infectious mononucleosis is defined by the clinical triad of fever, lymphadenopathy, and pharyngitis combined with the transient appearance of heterophil antibodies and an atypical lymphocytosis. EBV is also associated with nasopharyngeal carcinoma and certain B-cell lymphomas.

EPIDEMIOLOGY OF EBV INFECTIONS EBV is a ubiquitous agent that has been found in all population groups surveyed to date. The virus was initially described by Epstein, Achong, and Barr who noted, by electron microscopy, the presence of particles similar in morphology to herpes simplex virus in continuous cell lines which had arisen from tumor tissue obtained from patients with Burkitt's lymphoma. The perceptive observation by the Henles that antibodies to this agent developed in conjunction with infectious mononucleosis in one of their laboratory personnel was followed quickly by large-scale serologic surveys at Yale which confirmed EBV as the etiologic agent for infectious mononucleosis.

EBV is transmitted primarily in saliva, although infections can also be transmitted by blood transfusion. Primary infection tends to occur at an earlier age among lower socioeconomic groups and in developing countries. In industrialized countries approximately 50 percent of individuals have experienced a primary EBV infection by adolescence. These early infections are usually mild and non-specific or clinically inapparent. A second wave of seroconversions to EBV occurs with the onset of the social activity associated with adolescence and young adulthood. Primary EBV infection among this age group accounts for most cases of infectious mononucleosis. The peak incidence of infectious mononucleosis occurs between 14 and 16 years of age for girls, and between 16 and 18 years of age for boys. By adulthood most individuals are EBV-seropositive.

EBV is shed from the oropharynx for up to 18 months following primary infection; thereafter it is shed intermittently by all EBV-seropositive individuals in the absence of a clinical illness. EBV can be isolated from the oropharyngeal washings of 15 to 25 percent of healthy EBV-seropositive individuals on any given day. Immunosuppressed individuals shed the virus more frequently. EBV can be isolated from 25 to 50 percent of the oropharyngeal washings obtained from renal allograft recipients and from virtually all patients with the acquired immunodeficiency syndrome (AIDS). Asymptomatic shedding of EBV by healthy individuals accounts for most of the spread to uninfected members of the population despite the fact that it is not highly contagious. Transmission is largely dependent on salivary contact (e.g., kissing). It is not likely to be transmitted by aerosol or fomites. Thus, isolation restrictions on patients with mononucleosis or individuals likely to be shedding EBV are not appropriate. EBV infection can also be transmitted by blood transfusion.

ETIOLOGY AND PATHOGENESIS OF INFECTIOUS MONONUCLEOSIS By electron microscopy the EB virus appears as an icosahedral nucleocapsid surrounded by a complex envelope and is indistinguishable from other members of the human herpesvirus group. The double-stranded EBV DNA has a molecular weight of approximately 101 $\times 10^6$ and encodes for at least 30 polypeptides. At present, there is no convincing evidence that there are strain differences among EBV isolates which account for the wide range of clinical conditions associated with EBV infection.

When EBV is transmitted by saliva, the initial site of replication is the oropharynx. B lymphocytes support a productive infection by EBV and are the only cells known to have surface receptors for the virus. However, recent studies have documented the presence of the virus within oropharyngeal epithelial cells of patients with infectious mononucleosis. During the acute phase of the illness, EBV antigens can be demonstrated within the nuclei of up to 20 percent of circulating B lymphocytes. After the infection subsides, the virus can be isolated from a small number of B lymphocytes of EBV-seropositive individuals and may also reside within nasopharyngeal epithelial cells.

Virus-host interactions EBV infection has both direct and indirect effects on the cellular and humoral immune responses. Understanding the interactions between EBV and the host provides an insight into the clinical manifestations and complications of EBV infection. Within 18 to 24 h after entry of EBV into B lymphocytes by means of the C3d receptor, Epstein-Barr nuclear antigens (EBNA) are detectable within the nucleus of the infected cell. Expression of EBNA corresponds to the acquisition of the transformed or immortalized phenotype. EBV-infected B lymphocytes also express lymphocyte-determined membrane antigens (LYDMA) which serve as the putative target for the cellular immune response to virus-infected B lymphocytes. Immortalized B lymphocytes can be propagated continuously in vitro and are polyclonally stimulated by EBV to produce immunoglobulin. Antibodies reactive with sheep red blood cells (heterophil) and antibodies with several other specificities are the in vivo correlate of the polyclonal immunoglobulin production demonstrable in vitro and may mediate several of the complications of infectious mononucleosis. A minority of EBV-infected B lymphocytes enter the lytic cycle (production of mature, progeny virus and death of the host cell) and produce EBV antigens that are detected during virus replication. These are divided into the early antigen complex (EA) and viral capsid antigens (VCA). The early antigen complex consists of two groups of antigens; (1) diffuse (EA-D), which are detectable in both the cytoplasm and the nucleus of cells in the lytic cycle, and (2) restricted (EA-R), which are demonstrable only in the cytoplasm. EBV-induced membrane antigens are also produced during productive infection. These antigens serve as markers of infection at the cellular level; the pattern of the antibody response to these antigens is useful diagnostically in the identification of EBV-associated disease states (Table 138-1). After the appearance of VCA the host cell dies and whole virions are released, which can infect and transform additional B lymphocytes.

TABLE 138-1 EBV-specific antibodies

Antibody specificity	Time of appearance in IM	Persistence	Percent of IM patients with antibody	Comments
VCA:				
IgM	At clinical presentation	1–2 months	100	Best indicator of primary infection; not present with reactivation; technically difficult to perform
IgG	At clinical presentation	Lifelong	100	Standard "EBV titer" reported by most commercial and state labs; major utility is as a marker for prior or current infection in epidemiologic studies
EA:				
EA-D	Peaks 3–4 weeks after onset	3–6 months	70	Presence correlates with more severe disease in patients with IM; present in nasopharyngeal carcinoma; IgA anti-EA-D antibodies useful for prediction of NPC in high-risk populations
EA-R	Several weeks after onset	Months to years		Present in high titer in African Burkitt's lymphoma; may be useful as an indicator of reactivation of EBV in immunosuppressed patients
EBNA	3–6 weeks after onset	Lifelong	100	Late appearance of anti-EBNA antibodies in IM makes seroconversion a useful marker for primary infection if IgM anti-VCA antibody studies are not available

NOTE: *IM = infectious mononucleosis; VCA = viral capsid antigen; EA = early antigens; EA-D = diffuse early antigens; EA-R = restricted early antigens; EBNA = Epstein-Barr nucelar antigens; NPC = nasopharyngeal carcinoma.*

An effective immune response to EBV involves humoral and cellular components. Neutralizing antibodies which inactivate cell-free virus and antibodies to VCA and EBNA appear during primary infection in all patients; antibodies to EA-D appear in most patients. The cellular immune response is largely responsible for controlling B-cell proliferation and polyclonal immunoglobulin production triggered by EBV and is composed primarily of T lymphocytes having functional and surface phenotypic characteristics of activated, suppressor-cytotoxic T lymphocytes ($T8^+$, Ia^+). As the illness progresses, memory T lymphocytes capable of limiting proliferation of autologous EBV-infected B lymphocytes are demonstrable. These memory T lymphocytes persist for life. However, latent EBV remains in a small proportion of B lymphocytes and perhaps also in epithelial cells in the oropharynx.

During the primary immune response to EBV, global cellular immune hyporesponsiveness is readily demonstrable. This resolves after resolution of the illness, but reactivation of EBV is facilitated by conditions which interfere with the cellular immune response (immunosuppressive drugs, especially cyclosporin A, and disorders associated with cellular immunodeficiency, e.g., AIDS). EBV and cytomegalovirus (CMV) reactivation in immunosuppressed patients are frequently associated with a return of the immunoregulatory abnormalities characteristic of the primary immune response to these viruses. In the case of CMV, particularly, this hyporesponsiveness may contribute to many of the superinfections which frequently accompany CMV infections in immunocompromised hosts. The cellular hyporesponsiveness associated with EBV reactivation is generally less intense and less prolonged than that associated with CMV but may also contribute to morbidity in immunocompromised individuals.

CLINICAL MANIFESTATIONS **Symptoms and signs** After an incubation period of 4–8 weeks, prodromal symptoms of malaise, anorexia, and chills frequently precede the onset of pharyngitis, fever, and lymphadenopathy by several days. Severe pharyngitis is the symptom which most frequently prompts patients to seek medical attention. Occasionally patients will note only fever or lymphadenopathy or will present with one of the complications of infectious mononucleosis discussed below. Most patients also complain of headache and malaise. Abdominal pain is infrequent in the absence of splenic rupture.

Physical examination Fever is present in 90 percent of patients with infectious mononucleosis and is generally higher in the late afternoon, and may reach 39 to 40°C. Periorbital edema was frequently noted in early series of cases of mononucleosis but has been commented upon less frequently recently. The pharyngitis is usually diffuse; an exudate is observed in one-third of the cases. Palatine petechiae may also be observed. Posterior and/or anterior cervical adenopathy is noted in 90 percent of patients with infectious mononucleosis. Individual nodes are rarely painful and may be moderately tender to palpation. Hepatomegaly is infrequently noted, although mild hepatic tenderness is present in up to half the patients. Approximately half of all patients will have splenomegaly, which is usually maximal in the second or third week of illness. In 5 percent of patients a macular, petechial, scarlatiniform, urticarial, or erythema multiforme-like rash may appear. Administration of ampicillin results in a pruritic, maculopapular eruption in 90 to 100 percent of patients.

Clinical course Infectious mononucelosis is a self-limiting illness in the vast majority of cases. The pharyngitis is maximal for 5 to 7 days and then resolves over the subsequent 7 to 10 days. Fever usually persists for 7 to 14 days, but occasionally may continue somewhat longer. The course of the lymphadenopathy is variable, but rarely exceeds 3 weeks. The most persistent symptom is malaise. Most patients are well enough to return to work or school within 3 to 4 weeks, but occasional patients remain exhausted, have difficulty concentrating, and are unable to return to full activities for months. This subgroup is often found among those who present with a more subacute onset without severe pharyngitis and high fever.

Occasional patients have been reported in which recurrent pharyngitis and fever is accompanied by persistent or resurgent heterophil antibodies. More recently a group of patients has been described with nonspecific symptoms which may include malaise, fatigue, pharyngitis, fever, lymphadenopathy, and difficulty with higher cognitive function. These patients are usually heterophil-negative. The demonstration that some of these patients have anti-VCA and EA-R titers which are higher, and anti-EBNA titers which are lower, than median titers for the general population has led to the speculation that this symptom complex may be a manifestation of ongoing replication of EBV. However, healthy members of the general population not infrequently have antibodies to EA-R antigens, and one should be cautious about applying the diagnosis of chronic active EBV infection to patients with these nonspecific symptoms simply on the basis of the presence of anti-EA-R antibodies. At present, no specific therapy is available for these patients.

Complications Complications of infectious mononucleosis occur infrequently but may be so dramatic as to be the predominant manifestation of the illness (Table 138-2). Hematologic complications include autoimmune hemolytic anemia, which may be mediated by IgM antibodies with anti-i specificity. Hemolytic anemia usually subsides over a 1- to 2-month period. Mild thrombocytopenia occurs in up to 50 percent of cases; profound thrombocytopenia is a rare, but well-recognized, complication and is frequently antibody-mediated. Mild granulocytopenia is frequently observed in uncomplicated infectious mononucleosis, and severe granulocytopenia associated with infection or death has been reported. Antibodies which react with granulocytes have been detected in up to 80 percent of patients and may contribute to the profound granulocytopenia which is occasionally observed. Both the thrombocytopenia and the granulocytopenia are usually self-limited and resolve over 3 to 6 weeks. Corticosteroids have been advocated for treatment of both hemolytic anemia and thrombocytopenia associated with infectious mononucleosis, but efficacy has not been proved in controlled studies. Splenic rupture is an infrequent complication of infectious mononucleosis, often accompanied by the insidious or abrupt onset of abdominal pain, and is usually observed during the second or third week of illness. Surgery, which usually includes splenectomy, is the only effective management.

Neurologic complications of infectious mononucleosis may be the presenting or sole manifestation of the illness. Heterophil antibodies may be absent, and atypical lymphocytes may not be present at the onset of the neurologic event. The most frequent neurologic complications are cranial nerve palsies and encephalitis which may initially present with cerebellar findings. The onset of the encephalitis is usually abrupt. Cerebrospinal fluid findings are not diagnostic, and localization by noninvasive neurodiagnostic studies may suggest

TABLE 138-2 Complications of infectious mononucleosis

Hematologic complications:
- Autoimmune hemolytic anemia
- Thrombocytopenia
- Granulocytopenia

Splenic rupture

Neurologic complications:
- Encephalitis
- Cranial nerve palsies, especially Bell's palsy
- Meningoencephalitis
- Guillain-Barré syndrome
- Seizures
- Mononeuritis multiplex
- Transverse myelitis
- Psychosis

Hepatic complications:
- Hepatitis

Cardiac complications:
- Pericarditis
- Myocarditis

Pulmonary complications:
- Airway obstruction
- Interstitial pneumonitis

herpes simplex encephalitis. Eighty-five percent of patients with EBV-associated neurologic findings recover spontaneously.

Hepatitis is a common component of infectious mononucleosis. Almost 90 percent of patients have mild elevation of hepatic transaminases. Although more serious hepatic sequellae have been reported, severe or permanent hepatic dysfunction is exceedingly rare.

Cardiac abnormalities are uncommon but may include pericarditis, myocarditis, coronary artery spasm, or electrocardiographic abnormalities.

Airway obstruction from pharyngeal or paratracheal adenopathy can occur. This may require surgical intervention but is usually quite sensitive to corticosteroid therapy. Pulmonary parenchymal abnormalities such as interstitial infiltrates are noted infrequently and appear to be more common among children.

Infectious mononucleosis is rarely fatal. Neurologic complications, airway obstruction, and splenic rupture are the most frequent causes of death in previously healthy individuals with primary EBV infection. Sporadic or X-linked cases of overwhelming EBV infection accompanied by lymphoproliferation and hepatic dysfunction have been reported. The X-linked condition, known as X-linked lymphoproliferative (XLP) or Duncan's syndrome, results in the death of 40 percent of affected males during primary EBV infection. In addition to overwhelming lymphoproliferation, XLP patients may manifest severe immunologic or hematologic sequellae such as agammaglobulinemia, aplastic anemia, or lymphocytic lymphoma. The pathophysiology of the XLP syndrome has not yet been completely elucidated, but an X-linked defect in the immune response to EBV may result in failure to control EBV replication or in disordered immunoregulation which leads to the other immunologic sequellae observed in this syndrome.

LABORATORY MANIFESTATIONS Heterophil antibodies Antibodies to sheep erythrocytes which can be removed by prior absorption with beef red blood cells, but not with guinea pig kidney, are termed heterophil antibodies. Heterophil antibodies are demonstrated in 50 percent of children and 90 to 95 percent of adolescents and adults with mononucleosis. Although the classic tube heterophil titer is still performed in many laboratories, the "monospot" test using a commerical kit is a sensitive, specific, easily performed substitute. The frequency of heterophil positivity associated with infectious mononucleosis depends upon the test used, the age of the patient population, and the time during the illness at which the test is performed. Monospot tests may be slightly more sensitive than heterophil titers. Ten to fifteen percent of patients with mononucleosis may be heterophil-negative if tested only during the first week of the illness. If the clinical suspicion of mononucleosis is high enough, retesting for heterophil antibodies during the second or third week of illness is warranted. Heterophil antibodies decline in titer after the acute illness is resolved but may be detectable for up to 9 months after the onset of the illness.

Atypical lymphocytosis A relative and absolute lymphocytosis is present in about 75 percent of cases of infectious mononucleosis. The lymphocytosis usually peaks in the second or third week of illness and is characterized by cells with atypical morphology. These atypical lymphocytes, which are primarily activated T lymphocytes, are larger than mature lymphocytes and often contain eccentrically placed lobulated nuclei with nucleoli, and vacuolated cytoplasm with rolled up edges. As noted above, mild neutropenia and thrombocytopenia are frequently observed. Other laboratory abnormalities include a mild polyclonal increase in immunoglobulins of the IgM, IgG, and IgA classes, and mild elevations of hepatocellular enzymes.

EBV-specific antibody response Antibodies to several EBV-specific antigens arise during primary EBV infection (Table 138-1) Proper utilization of EBV-specific antibody studies may facilitate the diagnosis of primary EBV infection in clinically atypical or heterophil-negative cases. IgM antibodies to the VCA are diagnostic of a primary EBV infection. Unfortunately this study is technically difficult to perform and available only in certain reference laboratories. IgG anti-VCA antibodies are present at clinical presentation in almost all patients and remain detectable for life. IgG anti-VCA antibodies are, thus, useful mainly as a test for susceptibility to EBV and are not useful for the diagnosis of primary infection. Approximately 70 percent of patients with infectious mononucleosis make antibodies to EA-D. Anti-EA-D antibodies usually peak 3 to 4 weeks after the onset of illness and usually disappear after recovery. Antibodies to EBNA appear 6 to 8 weeks into the illness and persist for life. The presence of IgM anti-VCA antibodies, and seroconversion to EBNA is diagnostic of a primary EBV infection. Patients with defects in cellular immunity may fail to make antibodies to EBNA.

DIAGNOSIS The diagnosis of infectious mononucleosis is not difficult in the vast majority of cases. The constellation of fever, pharyngitis, and lymphadenopathy coupled with an atypical lymphocytosis and heterophil antibodies is virtually always due to primary EBV infection and requires no further laboratory studies. Certain patients with EBV-induced mononucleosis, particularly preadolescents, or those with neurologic complications may be heterophil-negative or may lack an atypical lymphocytosis. Primary EBV infection can be diagnosed with certainty in these patients with the proper use of EBV-specific serologic studies (see above). Culturing EBV from oropharyngeal washings or peripheral blood mononuclear cells is laborious, and because of the ubiquity of the virus among EBV-seropositive individuals, it is not diagnostic of primary EBV infection.

Primary CMV infection is the illness most frequently confused with EBV-induced infectious mononucleosis. About two-thirds of adults with heterophil-negative mononucleosis have CMV-induced mononucleosis. Patients with CMV mononucleosis are, on the average, slightly older than those with EBV-induced infectious mononucleosis and usually manifest an illness characterized predominantly by fever and malaise. Pharyngitis and lymphadenopathy are less common than with infectious mononucleosis. CMV-induced mononucleosis is usually more insidious in onset and slower to resolve than EBV-induced mononucleosis. The diagnosis can be made by the isolation of CMV from the peripheral blood, and the demonstration of seroconversion or a fourfold or greater rise in antibody titer to CMV. Although CMV is also shed in saliva and urine by patients with CMV mononucleosis, demonstration of the agent in the blood is a more specific, but less sensitive, indicator of CMV-induced morbidity.

Severe pharyngitis may also be caused by another virus (e.g., herpes simplex) or by group A beta-hemolytic streptococci. Since group A beta-hemolytic streptococci can be isolated from the throat of up to 30 percent of patients with infectious mononucleosis, isolation of this organism does not rule out the diagnosis of infectious mononucleosis. Atypical lymphocytes may also be observed in a number of other conditions including rubella, hepatitis, toxoplasmosis, mumps, and drug reactions. These conditions rarely pose major differential diagnostic problems when careful attention is paid to the other clinical and laboratory features of these illnesses.

MANAGEMENT Infectious mononucleosis usually requires only supportive management. Although patients should be advised to obtain adequate rest, there is no evidence that forced bed rest hastens recovery. Fever and pharyngitis are usually ameliorated by acetaminophen. Because of the infrequent complication of splenic rupture, patients should be advised to avoid contact sports for 6 to 8 weeks after the onset of illness. The timing of return to school or work is determined solely by symptomatology. Patients with mild illness may not require any major changes in routine. Occasional patients with protracted illness may not return to a full school or work schedule for several months. It is important to emphasize to patients that recovery from mononucleosis is often gradual and that the malaise may wax and wane for some time.

Although corticosteroids may hasten defervescence and the resolution of pharyngitis, they are indicated only for certain specific complications of mononucleosis; airway obstruction usually responds dramatically to parenteral corticosteroids. Corticosteroids may also hasten the recovery of patients with severe hemolytic anemia or thrombocytopenia. There is no evidence that corticosteroids are beneficial for the neurologic complications of the illness. Occasional selected patients with protracted illness may benefit from a short course of prednisone, but corticosteroids should be avoided in the majority of patients with infectious mononucleosis.

Acyclovir, interferon alpha, and 9-[2-hydroxy-1-(hydroxymethyl)ethoxy]methyl guanine are active inhibitors of EBV replication in vitro. Their role in the management of EBV infections is currently under evaluation. Interferon alpha has antiviral activity and can decrease shedding of EBV by renal allograft recipients treated with antithymocyte globulin.

EBV-ASSOCIATED MALIGNANCY Since the initial description of EBV in patients with African Burkitt's lymphoma, the virus has been detected in association with several other malignancies. Its role in the pathogenesis of these malignancies remains the subject of intense discussion. EBV DNA sequences have been detected in tumor tissue from more than 90 percent of patients with African Burkitt's lymphomas. American Burkitt's lymphoma, which often affects older children, and more often presents as an intraabdominal tumor, is EBV-associated in only 15 percent of cases. Anaplastic nasopharyngeal carcinoma, a common neoplasm in southeast China, is highly associated with EBV; virtually all adequately studied patients with this malignancy have evidence of EBV in tumor tissue.

There is increasing evidence that implicates EBV in the pathogenesis of certain cases of lymphocytic lymphoma in the immunoincompetent host. B-cell lymphoma is greatly overrepresented among malignancies developing in immunosuppressed individuals such as organ allograft recipients, patients with ataxia telangiectasia, and patients with AIDS. Immunologically privileged areas such as the central nervous system also appear to be particularly susceptible to B-cell lymphomas. Cardiac allograft recipients treated with cyclosporin A appear to be particularly susceptible to B-cell lymphoma. EBV sequences are detectable in up to half of the B-cell malignancies encountered in immunosuppressed individuals. Controversy exists as to whether the B-cell lymphoproliferation, which is initially polyclonal and may be driven by EBV reactivated in the setting of cellular immunodeficiency, is the first step in the development of these malignancies. The process, which is thought to be polyclonal initially, becomes oligoclonal or monoclonal with a second-step chromosomal translocation made more likely by the increased number of proliferating B lymphocytes. The biologic behavior of these tumors does not always correlate with clonality as defined by conventional techniques. Patients have been described who have succumbed to lymphoproliferative processes which appear to be polyclonal by surface immunoglobulin studies. More sensitive techniques of defining clonality, such as that utilizing immunoglobulin gene rearrangement, may reveal that a larger proportion of the polyclonal lymphomas are in fact oligo- or monoclonal. The response of these B-cell lymphomas to conventional chemotherapy is often disappointing. Some have advocated acyclovir therapy; others feel many of these lymphoproliferative syndromes are reversible if the immunosuppression is decreased. Studies of larger numbers of these patients for the presence of EBV sequences and for the progression from a polyclonal to an oligoclonal or monoclonal disorder will shed more light on the role of EBV in oncogenesis in both immunoincompetent and immunologically normal hosts.

REFERENCES

ANDIMAN W et al: Use of cloned probes to detect Epstein-Barr viral DNA in tissues of patients with neoplastic and lymphoproliferative diseases. J Infect Dis 148:967, 1983

EPSTEIN MS et al: Virus particles in cultured lymphoblasts from Burkitt's lymphoma. Lancet 1:702, 1964

GROSE C et al: Primary Epstein-Barr virus infections in acute neurologic diseases. N Engl J Med 292:392, 1975

HANTO DW et al: Epstein-Barr virus induced B-cell lymphoma after renal transplantation. Acyclovir therapy and transition from polyclonal to monoclonal B-cell proliferation. N Engl J Med 306:913, 1982

HAYNES BF et al: Emergence of suppressor cells of immunoglobulin synthesis during acute Epstein-Barr virus-induced infectious mononucleosis. J Immunol 123:2095, 1979

HENLE G et al: Immunofluorescence in cells derived from Burkitt lymphoma. J Bacteriol 91:1248, 1966

HENLE W et al: Epstein-Barr virus specific diagnostic tests in infectious mononucleosis. Hum Pathol 5:551, 1974

HOAGLAND RJ: Infectious mononucleosis. Am J Med 13:158, 1952

JONES JF et al: Evidence for active Epstein-Barr virus infection in patients with persistent, unexplained illnesses: Elevated anti-early antigen antibodies. Ann Intern Med 102:1, 1985

PURTILO DT et al: Epstein-Barr virus infections in the X-linked recessive lymphoproliferative syndrome. Lancet 1:798, 1978

REINHERZ EL et al: The cellular basis for viral-induced immunodeficiency: Analysis by monoclonal antibodies. J Immunol 125:1269, 1980

SCHOOLEY RT et al: Antineutrophil antibodies in infectious mononucleosis. Am J Med 76:85, 1984

SIXBEY JW et al: Epstein-Barr virus replication in oropharyngeal epithelial cells. N Engl J Med 310:1225, 1984

THORLEY-LAWSON DA et al: Suppression of in vitro Epstein-Barr virus infection: A new role for the adult human T lymphocyte. J Exp Med 146:495, 1977

139 ENTEROVIRUSES AND REOVIRUSES

C. GEORGE RAY

GENERAL CONSIDERATIONS

Enteroviruses consist of a major subgroup of picornaviruses that include the polioviruses, coxsackieviruses, echoviruses, and more recently discovered agents that are simply designated enteroviruses. The number of serotypes that infect humans is nearly 70, and more are likely to be found in the future. Their name is derived from their ability to infect intestinal tract epithelial and lymphoid tissues and to be shed into the feces.

Enteroviruses can cause paralytic disease, encephalitis and acute aseptic meningitis syndromes, pleurodynia, exanthems, pericarditis, myocarditis, nonspecific febrile illness, and occasional fulminant disease in the newborn. The spectrum of disease may be even broader. Some infections can lead to permanent damage, and others may trigger chronic, active disease processes.

Since these viruses have many features in common, they will first be considered as a group. Some of the special features of important serotypes will be discussed in detail later in this chapter.

CHARACTERISTICS OF ENTEROVIRUSES As a group, the picornaviruses are extremely small (17 to 28 nm in diameter), single-stranded RNA viruses with icosahedral symmetry. In contrast to the rhinoviruses, the enterovirus subgroup is resistant to ether, acid pH (4.0), and bile. Another feature is cationic stability; in the presence of magnesium sulfate, the viruses become more resistant to thermal inactivation. They can survive for prolonged periods in sewage and even in chlorinated water if sufficient organic debris is present. Although some of the enterovirus serotypes share antigens, there are no significant serologic relationships between the major classes listed in Table 139-1. Definitive identification of isolates usually requires neutralization tests.

Most of these agents can be isolated in primate (human or simian) cell cultures; however, some strains, such as several coxsackievirus group A serotypes, are grown with difficulty in cell cultures, and inoculation of newborn mice may be necessary for detection. Inoculation of newborn mice was one basis for the original classification of group A and B coxsackieviruses. After the mice have been inoculated, at 24 h of age or less, and observed for 2 to 12 days, group A viruses primarily have a widespread, inflammatory, necrotic effect on skeletal muscle, leading to flaccid paralysis and usually death; similar inoculation of group B viruses causes encephalitis, resulting in spasticity and occasionally convulsions. Other organs are variably affected, and histopathologic examination is sometimes helpful in distinguishing the two. Echoviruses and polioviruses rarely have an adverse effect on mice, unless special adaptation procedures are employed. The higher-numbered enteroviruses (types 68 to 72), which have overlapping growth and host characteristics, have been classified separately. Hepatitis A virus has been classified as enterovirus 72 and is discussed in Chap. 247.

Humans are the major natural host for the polioviruses, coxsackieviruses, and echoviruses. There are enteroviruses of other animals with a limited host range that does not appear to extend to humans. Conversely, viruses thought to be identical or related to human enteroviruses have been isolated from dogs and cats. Whether these agents cause disease in these animals is debatable, and there is no evidence of spread from animals to humans.

EPIDEMIOLOGY The enteroviruses have a worldwide distribution, and asymptomatic infection is common. The proportion of infected individuals who will develop illness varies from 2 to 100 percent, depending upon the serotype or strain involved, prior immune status, and the age of the patient. Secondary infections in households are common and range as high as 40 to 70 percent, depending upon factors such as family size, crowding, and sanitary conditions.

There is a seasonal predilection; epidemics are usually observed during the summer and fall. In subtropical and tropical climates, the duration of greatest transmission sometimes extends into the winter. In some years, certain serotypes emerge as dominant strains; they then may wane, only to reappear in epidemics years later. The emergence of dominant serotypes is unpredictable from year to year.

Direct or indirect fecal-oral transmission is considered the most common mode of spread. After infection, the virus persists in the oropharynx for 1 to 4 weeks, and it can be shed in the feces for 1 to 18 weeks. Sewage-contaminated water, contaminated foods, or insect vectors (flies, cockroaches) may occasionally be the source of infection. More commonly, however, spread is directly from person to person. Approximately two-thirds of all isolates are from children 9 years of age or younger.

Incubation periods vary, but relatively short intervals (2 to 10 days) are the rule. Illness is often seen concurrently in more than one family member, and the clinical features may vary within the household.

PATHOGENESIS AND PATHOLOGY After primary replication in the epithelial cells and lymphoid tissues in the upper respiratory and gastrointestinal tracts, viremic spread to other sites can occur. Potential target organs vary according to the virus strain and its tropism, but may include the central nervous system, heart, vascular endothelium, liver, pancreas, gonads, lungs, skeletal muscles, synovial tissues, skin, and mucous membranes. Histopathologic findings include cell necrosis and mononuclear cell inflammatory infiltrates; in the central nervous system, the inflammatory cells are localized most prominently in perivascular sites. The initial tissue damage is thought to result from the lytic cycle of virus replication. Viremia is usually undetectable by the time symptoms appear, and termination of virus replication commences with the appearance of circulating interferon, neutralizing antibody, and mononuclear cell infiltrations of infected tissue. The early antibody response is mediated by immunoglobulin M, which usually wanes 6 to 12 weeks after onset to be replaced by IgG-specific antibodies. The important role of antibodies in the termination of infection is supported by the observation of persistent enterovirus replication in patients with antibody-deficiency diseases.

Although initial acute tissue damage may be caused by the lytic effects of the virus on the cell, many of the secondary sequelae appear to be immunologically mediated. Enterovirus-caused poliomyelitis, disseminated disease of the newborn, aseptic meningitis, encephalitis, exanthems, and acute respiratory illnesses, thought to represent primary lytic infections, can usually be identified through routine methods of virus isolation and determination of specific antibody titer changes. On the other hand, syndromes such as myopericarditis, nephritis, and myositis have been associated with enteroviruses primarily by serologic and epidemiologic evidence. In many of these cases, viral isolation is the exception. The pathogenesis of these infections is not clear; however, it seems likely that the acute phase of the infection may be mild or subclinical and often subsides by the time the clinical illness becomes evident. Illness probably represents a host immunologic response to tissue injury by the virus or to viral or virus-induced antigens that persist in the affected tissues. Experiments with coxsackieviruses in murine models tend to support this hypothesis.

Infection by a specific serotype in an immunologically normal host is followed by a humoral antibody response, which can often be detected by neutralization methods for many years thereafter. There is relative immunity to reinfection by the same serotype; however, reinfection has been reported, usually resulting in subclinical infection or mild illness. Although there is some antigenic sharing between serotypes in some of the enterovirus classes (for example, group B coxsackieviruses), there is no evidence of significant heterotypic immunity to infection by different serotypes.

LABORATORY DIAGNOSIS In acute enteroviral infections, the diagnosis is most readily established by virus isolation from throat swabs, stool or rectal swabs, body fluids, and occasionally tissues. Except in young infants, viremia is usually undetectable by the time symptoms appear. When there is central nervous system involvement, cerebrospinal fluid cultures taken during the acute phase of the disease may be positive in 10 to 85 percent of cases (except in poliovirus infections, in which virus recovery from this site is rare), depending upon the stage of illness and the serotype involved. Direct isolation of virus from affected tissues or body fluids in enclosed spaces (for example, pleural, pericardial, or cerebrospinal fluid) usually confirms the diagnosis. Isolation of an enterovirus from the throat is suggestive of an etiologic association, as the virus is usually detectable at this site for only 2 days to 2 weeks after infection; isolation of virus from fecal specimens only must be interpreted more cautiously, as asymptomatic shedding from the bowel may persist for as long as 4 months.

The diagnosis may be further supported by fourfold or greater neutralizing antibody titer changes between paired acute and convalescent serum samples. This method is expensive and cumbersome, requiring careful selection of serotypes for use as antigens. Serodiagnosis is generally reserved for critical situations in which the etiology is questionable, such as isolation of a virus only from a peripheral source such as the feces, or in illnesses such as myopericarditis, in which the yield on routine culture is low and the number of serotypes that might be expected to be involved is limited. Quantitative interpretations of antibody titers on single serum samples are rarely helpful because of the high prevalence and wide range of titers to different serotypes that can be found in groups of healthy individuals. In acute poliovirus infections, complement-fixing antibody titer determinations on acute and convalescent sera can aid in diagnosis.

White blood cell counts and the erythrocyte sedimentation rates are usually only mildly elevated. If there is necrosis (e.g., liver, lung), a neutrophilic reaction may be noted. Hyperbilirubinemia and elevated transaminase and alkaline phosphatase levels may be seen

TABLE 139-1 Enteroviruses that infect humans

Class	Number of serotypes
Poliovirus	3
Coxsackievirus	
Group A	23*
Group B	6
Echovirus	31
Enterovirus	Types 68–72†

* *Includes several subtypes; coxsackievirus A23 is the same as echovirus 9.*
† The classification of the more recently described enteroviruses is based on overlapping biologic characteristics. These are identified numerically. Enterovirus 72 is hepatitis A virus.

in patients with hepatitis. Albuminuria often occurs transiently, but hematuria is rare.

PROPHYLAXIS AND TREATMENT Vaccines, which are available only for the prevention of poliovirus infections, will be discussed in detail below. Although proper disposal of feces and careful personal hygiene are recommended, the usual quarantine or isolation measures are relatively ineffective in controlling the spread of enteroviruses in the family or community.

None of the currently available antiviral agents or immune serum globulins has been shown effective in treatment or prophylaxis of enterovirus infections. The only exception to this may be the use of high-titered immunoglobulin in the treatment of chronic enteroviral encephalitis in antibody-deficient patients. Otherwise, treatment is entirely symptomatic and supportive. Glucocorticosteroids are usually considered contraindicated; they are sometimes employed, however, in the management of severe myocarditis, but only as a last resort.

POLIOVIRUS INFECTIONS

The most important enteroviruses are the three poliovirus serotypes (types 1, 2, and 3). They first emerged as important causes of disease in developed temperate-zone countries during the latter part of the nineteenth century, and they continue to be a serious public health problem in developing countries.

The particular tropism of polioviruses for the central nervous system (CNS), which they usually reach by passage across the blood-CNS barrier, is perhaps favored by reflex dilatation of capillaries supplying the affected motor centers of the anterior horn of the brainstem or spinal cord. An alternate pathway is via the axons or perineural sheaths of peripheral nerves. Motor neurons are particularly vulnerable to infection and variable degrees of destruction. The histopathologic findings in the brainstem and spinal cord include necrosis of neuronal cells and perivascular "cuffing" by infiltration with mononuclear cells, primarily lymphocytes.

CLINICAL MANIFESTATIONS Most infections (perhaps 90 percent) are either subclinical or extremely mild. When disease does result, the incubation period can be from 4 to 35 days, but is usually between 7 and 14 days. The disease falls into three classes: The first, abortive poliomyelitis, is a nonspecific febrile illness of 2- to 3-day duration with no signs of CNS localization. A second group of patients will additionally develop aseptic meningitis. Recovery is rapid and complete, usually within a few days. The third class, paralytic poliomyelitis, is the major possible outcome of infection and is often preceded by a period of fever and "minor illness." Classically, after several days, symptoms disappear. In 5 to 10 days fever recurs, and signs of meningeal irritation and asymmetric flaccid paralysis ensue. Cramping muscle pain and spasm as well as coarse twitching in affected parts follows. The maximum extent of involvement is apparent within a few days after first paralysis. In children younger than 5 years, paralysis of one leg is most common. In patients 5 to 15 years of age, weakness of one arm or paraplegia is frequent, while in adults quadriplegia is more likely to occur. Urinary bladder and respiratory muscle dysfunction are also frequent in adults. Inoculations of vaccines are associated with involvement of the muscles around the site of injection.

Tendon reflexes are diminished or absent. Sensation is intact, separating poliomyelitis from the usually symmetric paralysis of the Guillain-Barré syndrome. Paralysis due to heavy metal poisoning may also be difficult to distinguish clinically from poliomyelitis.

Among paralytic cases, 6 to 25 percent may be bulbar. Myocarditis, hypertension, pulmonary edema, shock, nosocomial gram-negative or staphylococcal pneumonias, urinary tract infections, and emotional problems are among the complications of severe paralytic disease. Treatment is supportive. About 2 to 5 percent of children and 15 to 30 percent of adults with paralyzing infection die. As temporarily damaged neurons regain their function, recovery begins and may continue for as long as 6 months. Paralysis persisting beyond that time is permanent, and may be associated with complaints of severe pain in the affected areas which sometimes recur years after the illness.

PREVENTION Two types of poliovirus vaccines are currently licensed in the United States: inactivated polio vaccine and live, oral, attenuated virus vaccine. Each contains the three serotypes of poliomyelitis virus.

Inactivated polio vaccine (IPV) was introduced in 1955; it remains the only vaccine used in some countries, notably Sweden, Finland, and the Netherlands, and its efficacy has been excellent. Primary vaccination with four doses (three doses 4 to 8 weeks apart and the fourth 6 to 12 months later) produces antibody responses in more than 95 percent of recipients. The current product is considered safe, with no significant deleterious side effects.

Oral polio vaccine (OPV) is composed of live, attenuated viruses. It was first licensed in the United States in 1963. The vaccine is given as a primary series of three doses (the first two doses usually 6 to 8 weeks apart, and the third 8 to 12 months later) and produces antibodies to all three serotypes in more than 95 percent of recipients. As with IPV, recall boosters are recommended to maintain adequate antibody levels. Like wild poliovirus, OPV viruses infect and replicate in the oropharynx and intestinal tract, and may be shed into the feces for 6 weeks or longer.

One disadvantage of OPV is the remote risk of vaccine-associated paralytic disease in some recipients, such as immunocompromised persons; susceptible adults are at a slightly higher risk than children. There is speculation that some instances of vaccine-associated paralytic disease may also be related to reversion of attenuated virus to more virulent characteristics in vivo after passage from person to person. The incidence of vaccine-associated paralytic poliomyelitis is estimated at approximately 1 per 3.7 million doses distributed. Of the 76 cases reported in the United States during 1969 to 1978, 18 were in otherwise healthy vaccine recipients, 47 in healthy close contacts of vaccine recipients, and 11 in persons with immune-deficiency conditions.

The major advantages of OPV include ease of administration and secondary immunization of nonimmune contacts through shedding of vaccine virus into the intestinal tract, resulting in more widespread immunity in the population. It is also theorized that during outbreaks, transient vaccine virus colonization results in the induction of mucosal immunity (primarily through secretory IgA), which may interfere with subsequent acquisition and spread of wild poliovirus.

The choice between IPV and OPV for routine primary immunization is widely debated; however, it is clear that both are highly effective vaccines, and that routine immunization with one or the other is important in the prevention of disease. Ideally, immunization should commence in infancy. A susceptible adult at risk of exposure to infection because of travel to an endemic area should receive complete immunization. Persons with immunodeficiency or altered immune status should not be exposed to OPV, either directly or by household contact, because of the increased risk of vaccine-associated paralysis.

Although there are no currently recognized areas of wild poliovirus prevalence in the United States, importation of these strains can readily occur from endemic areas in contiguous countries as well as from developing nations abroad. Once introduced into a community, the virus can spread rapidly among susceptible individuals. For this reason, continuing immunization programs are of utmost importance in preventing spread of this disease.

COXSACKIEVIRUSES AND ECHOVIRUSES

The coxsackieviruses and echoviruses are widespread throughout the world. The basic features of their epidemiology and pathogenesis appear to be the same as those of the polioviruses. Unlike polioviruses, they have a greater tendency to affect the meninges and occasionally the cerebrum, and only rarely do they affect anterior horn cells.

The consequences of infection with these agents are highly variable and related only in part to virus subgroup and serotype. Up to 60 percent of infections are subclinical. The main interest in these agents stems from their ability to cause more serious illness, which becomes most evident during epidemics.

Inapparent infection is common, but varies with the infecting strain and the host involved. The manifestations of illness range from mild to lethal and from acute to chronic. Table 139-2 lists the major syndromes and serotypes commonly associated with each. Considerable overlap occurs, however, and it is not surprising to find an enteroviral serotype associated with a specific syndrome which differs from that most often encountered. The group B coxsackieviruses generally appear to have the greatest latitude with regard to tissue tropism.

ASEPTIC MENINGITIS (See Chap. 347) In terms of relative frequency, aseptic meningitis is the most important illness associated with enterovirus infections. This syndrome can be mild and self-limiting; however, it is occasionally accompanied by encephalitis, which can lead to permanent sequelae, particularly in infants. Overall, enteroviruses cause the majority of all nonbacterial CNS infections now observed in the United States.

There may be a mild prodromal malaise, but major illness usually begins with fever, headache, and stiff neck. Kernig's and Brudzinski's signs may be present. Localizing sensory or motor deficits are unusual. Confusion and delirium are common. These acute findings may persist for 4 to 7 days. Cerebrospinal pleocytosis is usually less than 500 cells per cubic millimeter. Early, there may be as many as 90 percent polymorphonuclear leukocytes, but within 48 h the cellular response becomes completely mononuclear. Persistence of polymorphonuclear leukocytes in the cerebrospinal fluid suggests pyogenic meningitis or intracerebral, subdural, or epidural abscess. Gram's stain and appropriate spinal fluid cultures must be done to exclude bacterial meningitis, tuberculosis, or mycotic meningitis. Protein concentration in the cerebrospinal fluid is moderately elevated, but glucose is usually normal. Early in the illness enteroviruses may be isolated from spinal fluid, even in the absence of significant pleocytosis. It usually takes several weeks before the cerebrospinal fluid reverts to normal. An occasional patient may develop a transient syndrome of inappropriate secretion of antidiuretic hormone. In hypo- or agammaglobulinemic syndromes echoviruses have persisted in CSF for months to years, producing a progressive encephalitis.

For attempts at virus isolation, throat, stool, and cerebrospinal fluid specimens should be collected as early in the course as possible. Acute and convalescent serums can also be studied for rises in type-specific neutralizing antibodies in patients in whom viral isolation results are negative or equivocal.

It is not possible to distinguish clinically between aseptic meningitis due to various enteroviruses, arboviruses, Epstein-Barr virus, and mumps. Localizing findings, hemiplegia, oculogyric crises, coma, and bloody spinal fluid favor the diagnosis of type 1 herpes simplex virus encephalitis (see Chap. 136). Although enterovirus aseptic meningitis most often is self-limited and recovery in persons afflicted after the first year of life is usually complete, about 10 percent of patients have more serious involvement of the central nervous system. Minor muscle weakness with reflex changes may persist for weeks to months, but over 90 percent of patients recover completely within a year. Occasionally, choreiform movements, ataxia, nystagmus, transverse myelitis, Guillain-Barré syndrome, poliomyelitis-like symptoms, coma, bulbar involvement, and death result.

OTHER ENTEROVIRAL ILLNESSES *Generalized disease of the newborn* is a highly lethal expression of enteroviral infection, in which the infant may be overwhelmed by simultaneous virus infection of the heart, liver, adrenals, brain, and other organs.

Acute myocarditis and/or pericarditis can be caused by a variety of viral agents; however, it is estimated that as many as 50 percent of cases are associated with infection by coxsackie B viruses. Such infections are usually self-limited, but can lead to a fatal outcome (arrhythmia or heart failure) or cause chronic heart disease (see Chaps. 192 and 194).

The exanthems may or may not be associated with CNS inflammation (see Chap. 133). The observed rashes usually resemble rubella, roseola infantum, or adenovirus macular or maculopapular exanthems, but may also appear as vesicular or hemangioma-like lesions. Hand-foot-and-mouth disease usually affects children and is characterized by a vesicular eruption over the extremities and the anterior oral cavity. Coxsackievirus A16 is the specific agent most frequently implicated, but others, such as enterovirus 71, can cause a similar illness.

Herpangina is an enanthematous (mucous membrane) disease characterized by the acute onset of fever and sore throat. Characteristic small vesicles or white papules (lymphonodules) surrounded by a red halo are seen over the posterior half of the palate, pharynx, and tonsillar areas. This mild, self-limiting (1 to 2 weeks) illness has usually been associated with infection by several different group A coxsackievirus serotypes.

Epidemic myalgia (pleurodynia, or Bornholm disease) is characterized by fever and sudden onset of intense upper abdominal or lower thoracic pain, often accompanied by a frontal headache. The pain may be aggravated by movement, such as breathing or coughing, and usually persists for 3 to 14 days. Coxsackie B viruses are most frequently implicated.

A variety of other illnesses may also result from infections by this subgroup. Epidemic acute hemorrhagic keratoconjunctivitis associated with enterovirus 70 has been reported in Asia and the United States, and disease resembling paralytic poliomyelitis caused by enterovirus 71 infection has occurred in Bulgaria and the United States. In addition, there is some evidence that certain enteroviruses may participate in the pathogenesis of at least some cases of insulin-dependent diabetes mellitus, acute arthritis, polymyositis, hemolytic-

TABLE 139-2 Clinical syndromes reported to be commonly associated with enterovirus serotypes

Syndrome	Coxsackievirus Group A	Coxsackievirus Group B	Echovirus and enterovirus (E)
Aseptic meningitis, encephalitis	2,4,7,9,10	1,2,3,4,5	4,6,9,11,16,30;E70,E71
Muscle weakness and paralysis (poliomyelitis-like disease)	7,9	2,3,4,5	2,4,6,9,11,30;E71
Cerebellar ataxia	2,4,9	3,4	4,6,9
Generalized disease (infants)	—	1,2,3,4,5	3,6,9,11,14,17,19
Exanthems and enanthems	4,5,6,9,10,16	2,3,4,5	2,4,5,6,9,11,16,18,25;E71
Pericarditis, myocarditis	4,16	2,3,4,5	1,6,8,9,19
Epidemic myalgia (pleurodynia), orchitis	9	1,2,3,4,5	1,6,9
Respiratory symptoms	9,16,21,24	1,3,4,5	4,9,11,20,25
Conjunctivitis	24	1,5	7;E70

uremic syndrome, and idiopathic acute nephritis. However, the associations between these viruses and the diseases mentioned have not been clearly elucidated.

REOVIRUS INFECTIONS

The reoviruses (respiratory enteric orphans) are naked virions that contain double-stranded RNA. They are extremely ubiquitous and have been found in humans, simians, cattle, rodents, and a variety of other hosts. Three serotypes are known to infect humans; however, their role and relative importance in human disease remains uncertain. Sporadic cases of febrile upper respiratory infections, exanthems, pneumonia, hepatitis, encephalitis, and gastroenteritis have all been reported to be associated with these viruses. Reovirus type 3 has also been implicated as a possible cause of biliary atresia and neonatal hepatitis. Asymptomatic shedding of reoviruses also occurs, which makes it difficult to prove association with disease. Reoviruses have been used as models in the laboratory for the study and understanding of viral pathogenesis.

Reoviruses can be isolated in cell cultures, particularly primary monkey kidney or human kidney monolayers.

REFERENCES

BARRETT-CONNOR E: Is insulin-dependent diabetes mellitus caused by coxsackievirus B infection? A review of the epidemiologic evidence. Rev Infect Dis 7:207, 1985

BOWEN GS et al: Epidemic of meningitis and febrile illness in neonates caused by ECHO type 11 virus in Philadelphia. Pediatr Infect Dis 2:359, 1983

CHEMTOB S et al: Syndrome of inappropriate secretion of antidiuretic hormone in enteroviral meningitis. Am J Dis Child 139:292, 1985

ERLENDSSON K et al: Successful reversal of echovirus encephalitis in X-linked hypogammaglobulinemia by intraventricular administration of immunoglobulin. N Engl J Med 312:351, 1985

GLASER JH et al: Role of reovirus type 3 in persistent infantile cholestasis. J Pediatr 105:912, 1984

HORSTMANN DM: Control of poliomyelitis: A continuing paradox. J Infect Dis 146:540, 1982

JEHN UW, FINK MK: Myositis, myoglobinemia, and myoglobinuria associated with enterovirus echo 9 infection. Arch Neurol 37:457, 1980

JENISTA JA et al: Epidemiology of neonatal enterovirus infection. J Pediatr 104:685, 1984

JOSSELSON J et al: Acute rhabdomyolysis associated with an echovirus infection. Arch Intern Med 140:1671, 1980

KAPLAN MH et al: Group B coxsackievirus infections in infants younger than three months of age: A serious childhood illness. Rev Infect Dis 5:1019, 1983

KEREIAKES DJ, PARMLEY WW: Myocarditis and cardiomyopathy. Am Heart J 108:1318, 1984

SHARPE AH, FIELDS BN: Pathogenesis of viral infections: Basic concepts derived from the reovirus model. N Engl J Med 312:486, 1985

WOLFE JL et al: Intestinal M cells: A pathway for entry of reovirus into the host. Science 212:471, 1981

140 VIRAL GASTROENTERITIS

HARRY B. GREENBERG

INTRODUCTION In less developed countries, acute infectious diarrheal disease is a leading cause of morbidity in all age groups, and of mortality in infants and young children. In developed countries, acute diarrheal illness remains an important cause of morbidity among both children and adults. Two distinct groups of viruses—the rotaviruses and the Norwalk viruses (Fig. 140-1)—as well as a variety of bacterial pathogens (see Chap. 89) have emerged as important etiologic agents of gastroenteritis. The rotaviruses are primarily pathogens of young children. The Norwalk and related small round viruses affect predominantly older children and adults.

ROTAVIRUS Classification and characterization Rotaviruses are members of the Reoviridae family. The rotavirus virion consists of a 70-nm double-shelled icosahedral capsid which surrounds a genome composed of 11 segments of double-stranded RNA. The virus has two surface proteins which are both involved with viral neutralization. Because rotaviruses have a segmented genome, they are capable of undergoing gene reassortment at very high frequency. The role of gene reassortment in generating rotavirus antigenic diversity is not known. In humans, rotavirus infection is characterized by replication that is localized exclusively in the small intestinal epithelial cells.

Epidemiology Rotavirus infection occurs worldwide. By the age of 3, virtually every individual has been infected by rotaviruses at least once. In areas with a temperate climate, rotavirus infection is seasonal, occurring in the cooler winter months. In tropical areas rotavirus infection tends to occur throughout the year, with some increase in incidence during the cooler rainy season. Rotaviruses are the single most important cause of severe dehydrating diarrhea in infants and young children under 3 in both developed and less developed countries, and account for between 30 and 50 percent of all cases of diarrhea requiring hospitalization or intensive rehydration therapy. Although rotavirus infections are primarily confined to infants and small children, they are frequently associated with diarrhea in adults, particularly family members of affected infants, geriatric patients, and immunocompromised hosts. They account for up to 25 percent of traveler's diarrhea (see Chap. 89). Subclinical infections or mild gastrointestinal illnesses which do not require hospitalization account for the majority of rotavirus infections. Subclinical infections have also been documented in neonates; these infections were shown to protect against severe rotavirus gastroenteritis for up to 3 years. At least four distinct serotypes of human rotavirus have been described. The relationship of the frequency of infection with these serotypes to host immune status is unclear. A large variety of other mammals and avian species can be infected by rotavirus, but it does not appear that these animal rotavirus strains cause disease in humans under natural conditions. Rotaviruses are shed in very large numbers (up to 10^{10} particles per gram of feces) in the stool; it is presumed that transmission occurs via fecal-oral spread.

Pathophysiology Rotavirus infects and kills the mature villus tip cells of the small intestine. The mature epithelial cells are replaced by immature absorptive cells that cannot absorb carbohydrate or other nutrients efficiently. Rotavirus infection leads to an osmotic diarrhea due to nutrient malabsorption. Changes in intracellular cyclic adenosine monophosphate or guanosine monophosphate are not involved in the etiology of rotavirus diarrhea.

Manifestations These range from subclinical infections to mild diarrhea to severe, occasionally fatal, illness. Most information concerning the signs and symptoms of rotavirus infection has been derived from studies of hospitalized young children. The onset of illness is usually abrupt. Vomiting, followed by diarrhea, occurs in over 80 percent of affected children. About one-third of hospitalized children will have a temperature greater than 39°C. Gastrointestinal symptoms usually last between 2 and 6 days. Mucus is commonly found in the stool but white blood cells and red blood cells are present in less than 15 percent of cases. Rotavirus infection frequently occurs in conjunction with respiratory tract symptoms, but there is little evidence to indicate that rotavirus replicates in the repiratory tract. Rotavirus infection has been observed in association with a wide variety of other clinical syndromes, including sudden infant death syndrome, Reye's syndrome, encephalitis, aseptic meningitis, pneumonia, exanthem subitum, Kawasaki's syndrome, necrotizing enterocolitis, gastroenteritis, which may be accompanied by hemorrhage, intussusception, Henoch-Schönlein purpura, hemolytic uremic syndrome, disseminated intravascular coagulation, and Crohn's disease. The etiologic relationship between these clinical syndromes and rotavirus infection is probably coincidental rather than causal. Rotavirus infection may be especially severe, and even fatal, in immunocompromised children.

Clinical immunity Relative immunity to rotavirus illness is acquired following infection early in childhood. Immunity is not complete, and adults with low levels of antibody can be symptomatically infected. Local immunity appears to be the critical determinant in protection.

Diagnosis Because rotavirus is shed in large amounts in the stool, detection is relatively easy. A variety of specific commercial immunoassays are available to detect rotavirus antigen in fecal specimens. There are no pathognomonic signs or symptoms of rotavirus infection, but rotavirus infection is more frequently associated with severe dehydration than other enteric bacterial or viral pathogens.

Treatment and prevention Despite the fact that rotavirus diarrhea is caused by intestinal epithelial cell lysis and death, it can be adequately treated by standard oral rehydration therapy. Only rarely is intravenous rehydration required. Since rotavirus infections have persisted in developed countries with advanced sanitation facilities and widely available clean water, it is unlikely that the viral infection will be preventable by hygienic measures alone. Progress with a number of candidate live attenuated vaccines suggests that prevention through vaccination may be feasible in the next decade.

NORWALK AND RELATED SMALL ROUND VIRUSES **Classification and characterization** A variety of round 27- to 32-nm particles, most of which have a poorly defined ultrastructure, have been identified in the stools of individuals with acute nonbacterial gastroenteritis. These agents have not been definitely classified because they are shed in the stool in small amounts for only a few days, and they have not been adapted to cell culture or to animal models. The Norwalk virus represents the most extensively studied and best characterized member of this group of agents, which also includes such serologically distinct viruses as the Hawaii agent, the Snow Mountain agent, the W-Ditchling agent, the Marin agent, and a number of agents described as either astrovirus-like or calicivirus-like. The Norwalk virus and the Snow Mountain virus appear to have a protein structure similar to typical caliciviruses, and it is likely that most of these 27-nm gastroenteritis agents will prove to be plus-stranded RNA viruses.

Epidemiology Norwalk infection occurs year round, not seasonally. Infection with Norwalk virus is common. From 58 to 70 percent of adults in both developed and less developed countries have antibodies to this virus. Norwalk antibody acquisition occurs at a considerably younger age in children in less developed countries than in those in developed areas, consistent with the presumption that Norwalk virus is spread by the fecal-oral route. In developed countries, Norwalk virus is responsible for approximately one-third of all epidemics of nonbacterial gastroenteritis. Norwalk virus has been incriminated in a variety of food-borne epidemics, and transmission vehicles have included oysters, green salad, and chocolate icing. The virus is a common cause of water-borne epidemics of gastroenteritis and has been shown to be the etiologic agent in nursing home, cruise ship, and institutional (summer camps and schools) outbreaks.

In less developed countries, the role of Norwalk virus infection in the etiology of diarrhea has not been thoroughly investigated.

FIGURE 140-1 *A. A group of Norwalk virus particles observed in the stool of a volunteer. (From AZ Kapikian et al, J Virol 10:1075, 1972.) B. Human rotavirus particle observed in a stool filtrate. (Reprinted with permission from AZ Kapikian et al. Copyright 1974 by the AAAS.) Bars = 100 nm.*

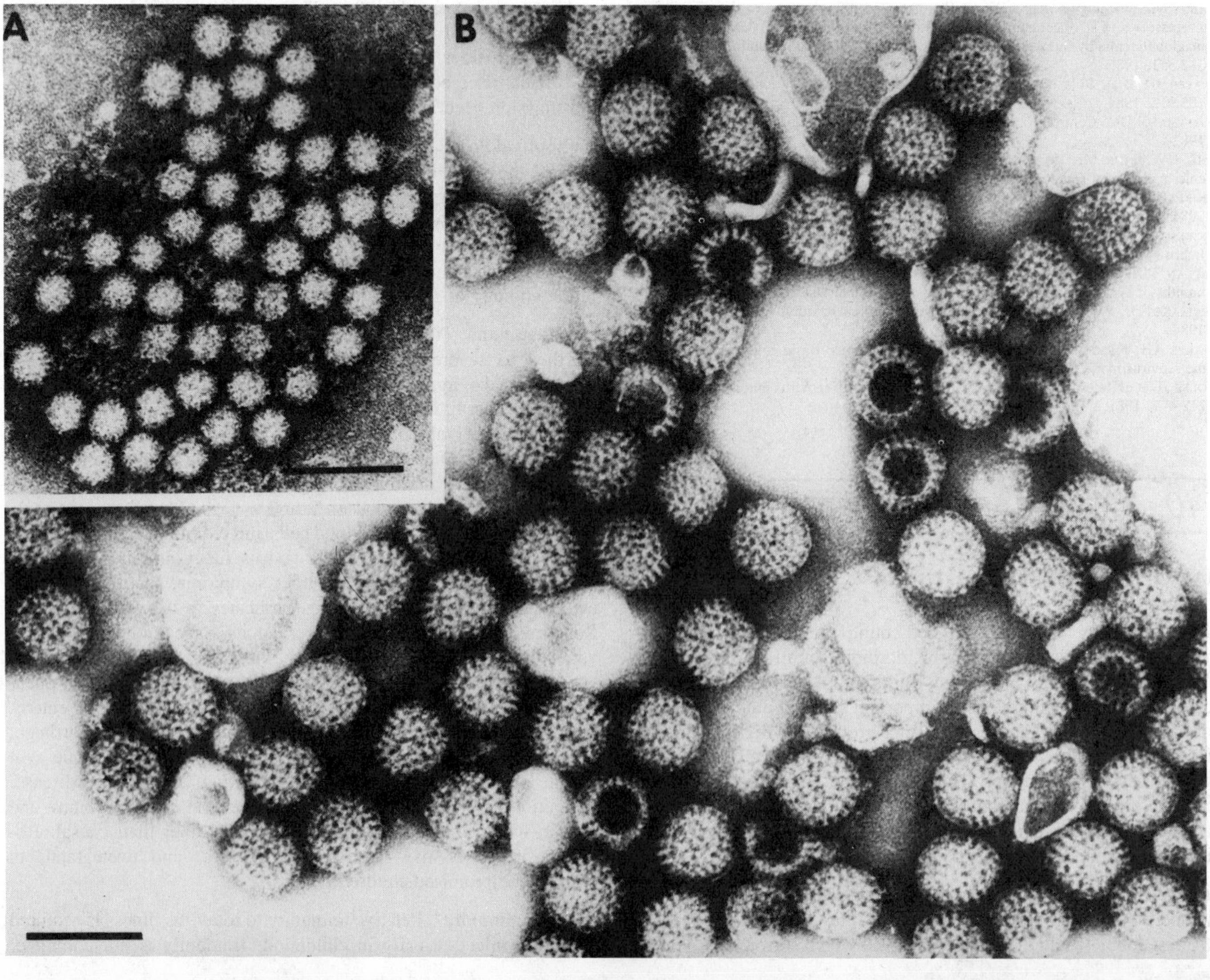

Preliminary studies indicate that Norwalk virus can cause mild diarrhea in young children, but it does not appear to cause severe illness in infants in either developed or less developed countries. The other serologically distinct small round gastroenteritis viruses must be studied in more detail before their epidemiology can be distinguished from Norwalk infection.

Pathophysiology Following infection with Norwalk or Hawaii viruses, the proximal small intestinal architecture is altered with villus shortening, crypt hyperplasia, and lamina propria infiltration by polymorphonuclear and mononuclear cells. Changes are not observed in the stomach or colon. The cells in which viral replication occurs have not been identified. The histologic alterations are accompanied by mild steatorrhea, carbohydrate malabsorption, and decreased levels of some brush border enzymes. Changes in adenylate cyclase activity have not been observed.

Manifestations Norwalk illness has an incubation period of between 18 and 72 h. Disease is characterized by the abrupt onset of nausea and abdominal cramps followed by vomiting and/or diarrhea. Vomiting occurs more frequently in children than adults. Low-grade fever (above 37.5°C) is seen in about half of affected individuals. Headache, myalgias, and abdominal pain are common. The white blood cell count is normal; rarely there is leukocytosis with a relative lymphopenia. Red and white cells are not found in the stool. The illness is usually mild and self-limited, lasting 24 to 48 h.

Clinical immunity For most people long-term (2 years or greater) resistance to Norwalk reinfection does not occur. In volunteers, there is a paradoxical relationship between the level of antibody to Norwalk virus and susceptibility to illness. Low levels of Norwalk antibody in the serum and intestine are associated with clinical resistance to illness. It appears, therefore, that immune mechanisms are not the primary determinants of protection from Norwalk virus.

Diagnosis, treatment, and prevention Radioimmunoassays and ELISA have been developed for Norwalk virus and several other 27- to 30-nm gastroenteritis agents. These tests are not yet available commercially. Norwalk illness is acute and self-limited; treatment is not usually required. In the rare case of severe vomiting or diarrhea, oral or intravenous rehydration is indicated. Because long-term immunity to Norwalk illness does not usually follow natural infection, it seems unlikely that a vaccine will be developed.

MISCELLANEOUS ENTERIC VIRAL PATHOGENS Enteric adenoviruses are a minor (~10 percent) cause of diarrheal illness in infants and children. These viruses differ from other adenovirus strains in a variety of ways including neutralization serotype, restriction endonuclease digestion pattern, and their ability to grow in tissue culture. The role of enteric adenovirus illness in adults or in less developed countries is not known.

Several strains of antigenically distinct rotaviruses, presently called "atypical rotaviruses" (or pararotaviruses) have been identified as the cause of occasional episodes of diarrhea in humans and animals. One strain of atypical rotavirus caused a very large water-borne outbreak of diarrheal disease in adults in China. From the scanty data available, it can be concluded that the atypical rotaviruses are not frequent causes of diarrheal illness in humans.

Corona viruses are frequent causes of diarrheal disease in a variety of animals. Several investigators, using electron microscopy, have identified putative corona virus–like particles in the stools of patients with diarrhea. In most cases, however, these particles do not have the typical morphologic features of corona viruses and may represent bacterial breakdown products or cellular fragments. A serologically distinct corona virus has been shown to cause necrotizing enterocolitis in newborn infants.

REFERENCES

Black RE et al: A two-year study of bacterial, viral and parasitic agents associated with diarrhea in rural Bangladesh. J Infect Dis 142:660, 1980

Brandt CD et al: Pediatric viral gastroenteritis during eight years of study. J Clin Microbiol 18:71, 1983

Estes MK et al: Rotaviruses: A review, in *Current Topics in Microbiology and Immunology*, M Cooper et al (eds). New York, Springer-Verlag, 1983, p 123

Greenberg HB et al: Proteins of Norwalk virus. J Virol 37:994, 1981

Kapikian AZ et al: Visualization by immune electron microscopy of a 27-nm particle associated with acute infectious non-bacterial gastroenteritis. J Virol 10:1075, 1972

——— et al: Reovirus-like agent in stools: Association with infantile diarrhea and development of a serologic test. Science 185:1049, 1974

Kaplan JE et al: Epidemiology of Norwalk gastroenteritis and the role of Norwalk virus in outbreaks of acute non-bacterial gastroenteritis. Ann Intern Med 96:756, 1982

Morse DL et al: Widespread outbreaks of clam- and oyster-associated gastroenteritis. Role of Norwalk virus. N Engl J Med 314:678, 1986

Resta S et al: Isolation and propagation of a human enteric coronavirus. Science 229:978, 1985

Tyrell DA, Kapikian AZ (eds): *Virus Infections of the Gastrointestinal Tract*. New York, Dekker, 1982

Vesikari T et al: Protection of infants against rotavirus diarrhea by RIT 4237 attenuated bovine rotavirus strain vaccine. Lancet 1:977, 1984

141 MUMPS

C. GEORGE RAY

DEFINITION Mumps is an acute communicable disease of viral origin characterized by painful enlargement of the salivary glands and sometimes by involvement of the gonads, meninges, pancreas, and other organs.

ETIOLOGY The causative agent of mumps is a paramyxovirus of intermediate size (120 to 200 nm in diameter). It has a tight helical inner core (RNA) enclosed in an outer envelope of lipid and protein. The virus of mumps has two components capable of fixing complement. These are the soluble, or S, antigens derived from the nucleocapsid, and the V antigen derived from the surface hemagglutinin. The virus can be cultivated in chick embryos and in a variety of mammalian cell cultures.

EPIDEMIOLOGY Human beings are the only natural host for mumps. The disease is worldwide and is endemic in urban communities. Epidemics are relatively infrequent and are confined to closely associated groups who live in orphanages, army camps, or schools. The disease is most frequent in the spring, particularly during April and May. Although mumps is generally considered less "contagious" than measles and chickenpox, this difference may be more apparent than real because many mumps infections (at least 25 percent) tend to be inapparent clinically. In some surveys, 80 to 90 percent of an adult population had serologic evidence of previous infection with mumps. The incidence of mumps in the United States has reached its lowest point since reporting began in 1922.

Infections are rare before the age of 2 years and then increase in frequency, reaching a peak at ages 5 to 9. Clinical mumps may be more common in males than in females. The virus is transmitted in infected salivary secretions, although its isolation from urine suggests that the virus may also spread via this route. Mumps virus is rarely isolated from stools. The saliva is infectious for approximately 6 days prior to the onset of parotitis, and virus has been recovered from this site for as long as 2 weeks after onset of parotid swelling. Viruria also persists for 2 to 3 weeks in some patients. Despite this prolonged secretion of virus, the peak of infectivity occurs a day or two before onset of parotitis and subsides rapidly after the appearance of glandular enlargement.

One attack of clinical or subclinical mumps confers lasting immunity, and second attacks are most unusual. Unilateral parotitis affords protection just as effectively as does bilateral disease.

PATHOGENESIS The virus enters via the respiratory route; during the incubation period of 15 to 21 days it presumably replicates in the upper respiratory tract and cervical lymph nodes, from which it is disseminated via the bloodstream to other organs, including the meninges, gonads, pancreas, breasts, thyroid, heart, liver, kidneys, and cranial nerves. The salivary adenitis is thought by many to be secondary to viremia, but primary spread from the respiratory tract has not been ruled out as an alternative mechanism.

MANIFESTATIONS **Salivary adenitis** The onset of typical parotitis is usually sudden, although it may be preceded by a prodromal period of malaise, anorexia, chilly sensations, feverishness, sore throat, and tenderness at the angle of the jaw. In many cases, however, parotid swelling is the first indication of illness. The glands enlarge progressively over a period of 1 to 3 days, and the swelling resolves within a week after maximal enlargement. The swollen gland extends from the ear to the lower portion of the mandibular ramus and to the inferior portion of the zygomatic arch, often displacing the ear upward and outward. The skin over the gland is usually not warm or erythematous, in contrast to what happens in bacterial parotitis. There may be reddening and pouting of the orifice of Stensen's duct. Usually, pain and tenderness are marked, although at times they are absent. The edema of mumps has been described as "gelatinous," and when the involved gland is tweaked, it rolls like jelly. Swelling may involve only the submaxillary and sublingual glands and may extend over the anterior part of the chest, producing *presternal edema*. Involvement of submaxillary glands alone can cause difficulty in distinguishing mumps from acute cervical adenitis. Swelling of the glottis occurs rarely but may require tracheostomy. Parotitis is bilateral in two-thirds of cases and remains confined to one side in the remainder. The second gland tends to swell as the first is subsiding, usually 4 to 5 days after onset. In general, parotitis is accompanied by a temperature of 100 to 103°F, malaise, headache, and anorexia, but systemic symptoms may be virtually absent, particularly in children. In most patients, the chief complaints refer to difficulty in eating, swallowing, and talking.

Epididymoorchitis Mumps is complicated by orchitis in 20 to 35 percent of postpubertal males. Testicular involvement usually appears 7 to 10 days after onset of parotitis, although it may precede it or appear simultaneously. Occasionally, orchitis occurs in the absence of parotitis. Gonadal involvement is bilateral in 3 to 17 percent of patients. Orchitis is heralded by recrudescence of malaise and appearance of chilly sensations, headache, nausea, and vomiting. Shaking chills and high fevers, with temperatures between 103 and 106°F, are frequent. The testicle becomes greatly swollen and acutely painful. The epididymis is often palpable as a swollen tender cord. Occasionally there may be epididymitis without orchitis. Swelling, pain, and tenderness persist for 3 to 7 days and gradually subside; lysis of fever usually parallels abatement of swelling. Occasionally, the temperature falls by crisis. Mumps orchitis is followed by progressive atrophy of the testicle in one-half the cases. Even after bilateral orchitis, sterility is unusual, provided no significant atrophy has taken place. However, if bilateral testicular atrophy occurs after mumps, sterility or subnormal sperm counts are quite common. Plasma testosterone levels are depressed during acute orchitis but return to normal with recovery. *Pulmonary infarction* has been noted to follow mumps orchitis. This may be the result of thrombosis of the veins in the prostatic and pelvic plexuses in association with the testicular inflammation. Priapism is a rare but painful complication of mumps orchitis.

Pancreatitis Pancreatic involvement is a potentially serious manifestation of mumps, which may rarely be complicated by shock or pseudocyst formation. It should be suspected in patients with abdominal pain and tenderness together with clinical or epidemiologic evidence of mumps. It is difficult to document, since hyperamylasemia, the hallmark of pancreatitis, is also often present in parotitis. Many times the symptoms resemble those of gastroenteritis. Although diabetes or pancreatic insufficiency rarely follows mumps pancreatitis, several children have developed "brittle" diabetes a few weeks after mumps.

Central nervous system involvement Nearly half the patients with mumps have an increased number of cells, usually lymphocytes, in the cerebrospinal fluid (CSF), although symptoms of meningitis, stiff neck, headache, and drowsiness are less common. In typical cases, the onset of overt central nervous system signs and symptoms occurs 3 to 10 days after the onset of parotitis; however, the onset has also been noted to develop prior to the parotitis or 2 to 3 weeks later. In approximately 30 to 40 percent of laboratory-proven cases, there is *no* associated salivary gland involvement at any time in the course of illness. The CSF protein is moderately elevated, and CSF glucose tends to be normal, although in as many as 10 percent of patients low CSF glucose concentrations, in the range of 20 to 50 mg/dL, may be seen. True encephalitis is unusual, although it is responsible for most of the central nervous system sequelae, including behavioral disturbances, headaches, seizures, deafness (usually unilateral), and visual disturbances. At least seven cases of aqueductal stenosis and hydrocephalus have been reported as possible late sequelae to mumps encephalitis, but the association remains unproven. Mumps should also be recognized as capable of presenting a picture of mild paralytic poliomyelitis; definition of the cause depends on isolation of virus or serologic confirmation of mumps in the absence of changing antibody titers to poliomyelitis viruses. Rarely, mumps may produce a transverse myelitis, cerebellar ataxia, or the Guillain-Barré syndrome. Mumps meningitis, without clinical encephalitis, is generally thought to be benign.

Other manifestations Mumps virus tends to involve glandular tissues; inflammation of the lacrimal glands, thymus, thyroid, breasts, and ovaries occurs occasionally. *Oophoritis* may be recognized by persistence of pain in the lower part of the abdomen and fever. It does not result in sterility. Mumps virus has been implicated in the causation of subacute thyroiditis; the diagnosis can be made serologically, and occasionally the virus can be isolated from the thyroid gland. Myxedema following mumps thyroiditis has been reported. Ocular manifestations of mumps include dacryoadenitis, optic neuritis, keratitis, iritis, conjunctivitis, and episcleritis. Although these conditions may transiently interfere with vision, complete resolution is the rule. Mumps *myocarditis*, evidenced primarily by transient abnormalities in the electrocardiogram, is relatively common. On rare occasions it can be fatal but it does not usually produce symptomatic disease or impair cardiac function. Similarly, *hepatic* involvement may be manifested by mild abnormalities in liver function, but icterus and other clinical signs of hepatic damage are extremely rare. *Thrombocytopenic purpura* as a complication of mumps has been described, and an occasional patient has a leukemoid reaction involving predominantly lymphocytes. Tracheobronchitis and interstitial pneumonia have also been associated with mumps infection, particularly among young children.

A rare but interesting manifestation of mumps is *polyarthritis* which is often migratory. It is most common in males between the ages of 20 and 30. Joint symptoms begin 1 to 2 weeks after subsidence of parotitis; usually the large joints are involved. The illness lasts 1 to 6 weeks, and complete recovery is the rule. It is not clear whether arthritis is due to viremia or whether it is a "hypersensitivity reaction."

Acute hemorrhagic glomerulonephritis in the absence of streptococcosis has been reported after mumps. The relationship of these two diseases is not clear.

Late complications With the exception of the rare central nervous system complications, and occasional patients who become sterile following bilateral testicular involvement, mumps leaves no sequelae. There is no firm evidence that stillbirths and offspring with congenital defects are more common among mothers who have mumps during pregnancy. Likewise, the causal relationship between intrauterine mumps infection and endocardial fibroelastosis has not been clearly established.

LABORATORY FINDINGS In uncomplicated parotitis, the blood leukocyte count is normal, although there may be mild leukopenia with relative lymphocytosis. Patients with mumps orchitis, however, may have a marked leukocytosis with a shift to the left. In meningoencephalitis, the white blood cell count is usually within normal limits. The erythrocyte sedimentation rate is usually normal but may rise with testicular or pancreatic involvement. The serum amylase level is elevated both in pancreatitis and in salivary adenitis. It may also be elevated in some patients in whom the sole evidence of mumps is meningoencephalitis, and probably reflects subclinical involvement of the salivary glands. In contrast to the amylase, the serum lipase level is elevated only in pancreatitis, in which hyperglycemia and glucosuria also may occur. The cerebrospinal fluid contains 0 to 2000 cells per cubic millimeter, almost all mononuclear, although occasionally polymorphonuclear cells will predominate in the early stages. The pleocytosis in mumps meningitis tends to be greater than in aseptic meningitides caused by the polio-, coxsackie-, and echoviruses. There is no relationship between the cell count and the severity of central nervous system involvement. Transient hematuria and mild reversible abnormalities in renal function, including inability to concentrate the urine maximally and to clear creatinine, occur in association with the viruria of mumps.

DIAGNOSIS The definitive diagnosis of mumps depends on isolation of the virus from blood, throat swabs, secretions from Stensen's duct, cerebrospinal fluid, or urine. Immunofluorescence methods can detect positive cell cultures in 2 to 3 days rather than the 6 days required with standard methods. In addition, immunofluorescence can be utilized to rapidly detect the viral antigen directly in oropharyngeal cells. Serologic determination of acute infection or susceptibility can be done by a variety of methods. The usual test of choice is the enzyme-linked immunosorbent assay (ELISA). Immunofluorescent assays are also commonly available, and can be used for identification of IgM- and IgG-specific antibody responses. The complement fixation test can also be employed to quantitate antibody responses to the S and V antigenic components for the diagnosis of acute or recent mumps infection. Antibodies to the S antigen develop rather rapidly, often reaching a peak within 1 week after the onset of symptoms, and usually disappear in 6 to 12 months. Complement-fixing antibodies to the V antigen follow a more typical pattern, reaching a peak titer within 2 to 3 weeks after onset, remaining elevated for at least 6 weeks, and then persisting at lower levels for years afterward. Paired serums obtained 2 to 3 weeks apart are recommended. A fourfold increase in titer by any standard assay confirms recent infection. In cases where an acute serum is not obtained until later in the course of illness, an elevation of antibodies to the S antigen which exceeds the V antibody titer or the presence of IgM-specific antibody suggests recent infection. The *skin test* consists of intradermal injection of killed mumps virus; previous exposure will result in a delayed reaction of the tuberculin type and an anamnestic antibody titer rise to mumps. The skin test is unreliable when used alone in determining the immune status of an individual, is useless in the diagnosis of acute mumps, and is no longer commercially available in the United States.

The diagnosis of mumps during an epidemic is usually obvious. Sporadic cases, however, must be distinguished from other causes of parotid enlargement. Parotitis may be caused by other viruses, notably parainfluenza, influenza, and coxsackieviruses. *Bacterial parotitis* usually occurs in debilitated patients with severe underlying diseases, such as uncontrolled diabetes mellitus, cerebrovascular accidents, or uremia. It may also follow surgical operations. The parotid glands are swollen, warm, and tender, and pus can be expressed from the orifices of Stensen's ducts. Marked polymorphonuclear leukocytosis is present. The disease is usually acquired in the hospital, and *Staphylococcus aureus* is the usual causative organism. Dehydration followed by inspissation of secretions in the salivary ducts is an important predisposing factor. *Calculus* in a salivary duct is usually detectable by palpation or by injection of radiopaque media into Stensen's duct. *Drug reactions* may produce tender swelling of the parotid and other salivary glands. "Iodine mumps" is the commonest type; it may follow such procedures as intravenous urography. Mercurialism and the antihypertensive agent guanethidine may also cause parotid enlargement and tenderness. A careful history usually serves to clarify the cause of these reactions. *Cervical adenitis* caused by streptococci, "bullneck" diphtheria, infectious mononucleosis, cat-scratch disease, sublingual cellulitis (Ludwig's angina), and cellulitis of the external auditory canal are usually easy to distinguish from mumps by careful examination. Parotid tumors and chronic infections such as actinomycosis tend to follow a more indolent course, with slowly progressive swelling. The common "mixed tumor" of the parotid is well-circumscribed, nontender, and very firm, almost cartilaginous on palpation. Parotid swelling and fever, often accompanied by lacrimal adenitis and uveitis (Mikulicz's syndrome), may occur in tuberculosis, leukemia, Hodgkin's disease, and lupus erythematosus. The onset may be sudden, but the process is usually painless and of long duration. "Uveoparotid fever" of similar type may be the first manifestation of sarcoidosis; in this disease parotid swelling is frequently accompanied by single or multiple palsies of cranial nerves, particularly the facial nerve, and is referred to as Heerfordt's syndrome. Presternal edema may also be a manifestation of malignant lymphoma involving retrosternal lymph nodes. Bilateral painless parotid swelling unassociated with fever is found in patients with Laennec's cirrhosis, chronic alcoholism, malnutrition, diabetes mellitus, pregnancy and lactation, and hypertriglyceridemia.

Sjögren's syndrome (see Chap. 266) is a chronic inflammation of the parotid and other salivary glands which is often associated with atrophy of the lacrimal glands and occurs most commonly in women past the menopause. With cessation of lacrimal and salivary function, there may be striking dryness of the conjunctiva and the cornea (keratoconjunctivitis sicca) and of the mouth (xerostomia). These patients may also have a variety of systemic manifestations, including arthritis of the rheumatoid type, splenomegaly, leukopenia, and hemolytic anemia. The chronicity of the process and its occurrence in elderly women make confusion with mumps unlikely. Finally, benign hypertrophy of both masseter muscles, presumably due to habitual clenching and grinding of teeth, may be confused with painless parotid swelling.

The causes of aseptic meningitis are discussed in Chap. 347.

Orchitis occurring in the absence of parotitis is likely to remain undiagnosed. Serologic testing may later confirm the diagnosis of mumps. Orchitis may occur in association with acute bacterial prostatitis and seminal vesiculitis. It is a rare complication of gonorrhea. Occasionally testicular inflammation accompanies pleurodynia, leptospirosis, melioidosis, tuberculosis, relapsing fever, chickenpox, brucellosis, and lymphocytic choriomeningitis.

TREATMENT There is no specific treatment for infections with the mumps virus. Patients with parotitis should receive mouth care, analgesics, and a bland diet. Bed rest is advisable only as long as the patient is febrile; contrary to popular belief, physical activity has no influence on the development of orchitis or other complications. Patients with epididymoorchitis may be acutely ill and in great pain. Many forms of treatment, including surgical decompression of the testicle, infiltration of the spermatic cord with local anesthetics, estrogens, convalescent serum, and broad-spectrum antibiotics, have not been regularly effective. Despite failure to document their effectiveness in controlled studies, adrenal steroids have been of considerable benefit in diminishing fever, as well as testicular pain and swelling, and in restoring the sense of well-being in a number of patients. It is important to give a large initial daily dose corresponding to 300 mg cortisone or 60 mg prednisone. Subsequently, administration of the hormone can be tapered off over 7 to 10 days. Adrenal steroids have not exerted an adverse effect on concomitant pancreatitis or meningitis, although they have not benefited patients with meningeal involvement, and their withdrawal has usually been accompanied by a recrudescence of symptoms. Adrenal steroids have not prevented the appearance of parotid involvement on the contralateral side. Mumps arthritis is usually mild and requires no treatment. Mumps thyroiditis may subside spontaneously, but excellent relief has been obtained with adrenal hormones.

PREVENTION A live attenuated mumps virus vaccine (Jeryl Lynn strain) has been highly effective in producing significant rises in mumps antibody in individuals who are seronegative prior to vaccination, and has afforded 75 to 95 percent protection to individuals subsequently exposed to mumps. The vaccine also has boosted antibody levels in vaccinated individuals who are seropositive. The vaccine produces an inapparent, noncommunicable infection. Parotitis after vaccination has been reported only rarely, and central nervous system dysfunction has not been proved to be a complication. It has conferred excellent protection for at least 12 years and has not interfered with vaccines against measles, rubella, and poliomyelitis or with smallpox vaccination given simultaneously. Protection has been demonstrated in both children and adults.

Live mumps vaccine can be administered at any time after 1 year of age, and should be particularly considered for children approaching puberty, adolescents, and adult males who have not had clinical mumps or live mumps vaccine in the past. Individuals living in groups or in institutions should be vaccinated, particularly because it has been shown that physical isolation of mumps patients does not effectively prevent transmission of the infection.

Vaccination is contraindicated in babies under the age of 1 year because of the interfering effect of maternal antibody; in individuals with a history of hypersensitivity to vaccine components; in patients with febrile illnesses, leukemia, lymphoma, or generalized malignancies; in those receiving steroids, alkylating drugs, antimetabolites, or irradiation; and during pregnancy.

It is not known whether the vaccine will prevent infection when administered after exposure, but no contraindication to its use in this situation exists. Neither mumps immune globulin nor ordinary gamma globulin has been shown to be efficacious in postexposure prophylaxis, and therefore neither is recommended.

REFERENCES

BEARD CM et al: The incidence and outcome of mumps orchitis in Rochester Minnesota 1935 to 1974. Mayo Clin Proc 52:3, 1977

GORDON SC, LAUTER CB: Mumps arthritis: Unusual presentation as adult Still's disease. Ann Intern Med 97:45, 1982

IMMUNIZATION PRACTICES ADVISORY COMMITTEE: Mumps vaccine. Ann Intern Med 98:192, 1983

KOPLAN JP, PREBLUD SR: A benefit-cost analysis of mumps vaccine. Am J Dis Child 136:362, 1982

KOSKINIEMI M et al: Clinical appearance and outcome in mumps encephalitis in children. Acta Paediatr Scand 72:603, 1983

LEVITT LP et al: Central nervous system mumps: A review of 64 cases. Neurology 20:829, 1970

SHEHAB ZM et al: Epidemiological standardization of a test for susceptibility to mumps. J Infect Dis 149:810, 1984

142 RABIES AND OTHER RHABDOVIRUSES

LAWRENCE COREY

RABIES

DEFINITION Rabies is an acute viral disease of the central nervous system that affects all mammals and that is transmitted by infected secretions, usually saliva. Most exposures to rabies are through the bite of an infected animal, but on occasion a virus aerosol or the ingestion or transplantation of infected tissues may initiate the disease process.

ETIOLOGY The rabies virus is a bullet-shaped, enveloped, single-stranded ribonucleic acid (RNA) virus of 75 to 80 nm diameter belonging to the rhabdovirus group. Glycoprotein excrescenses, 6 to 7 nm long, each with a knoblike structure at the distal end, cover the surface of the virion. The viral glycoproteins are capable of binding to acetylcholine receptors and contribute to the neurovirulence of rabies virus. These surface structures elicit neutralizing and hemagglutination-inhibiting antibodies, while a nucleocapsid antigen induces a complement-fixing antibody. Neutralizing antibodies to the surface glycoproteins appear to be protective. Antirabies antibodies used in diagnostic immunofluorescent assays are generally directed against the nucleocapsid antigens. Isolates of rabies virus from different animal species and locales have different biologic properties. Antigenic variations in strains have also been documented and may account for differences in virulence and lack of response to some types of rabies vaccination regimens. Interferon is induced by rabies virus, particularly in those tissues with high virus concentrations, and may play some role in retarding progressive infection.

EPIDEMIOLOGY Rabies exists in two epidemiologic forms: *urban,* propagated chiefly by unimmunized domestic dogs and/or cats, and *sylvatic,* propagated by skunks, foxes, raccoons, mongooses, wolves, and bats. Infection in domestic animals usually represents a "spill-over" from sylvatic reservoirs of infection, and human beings can be infected by either. Hence, human infection tends to occur in locales where rabies is enzootic or epizootic, where there is a large population of unimmunized domestic animals, and where human contact with the outdoors is common. While only about 800 rabies deaths are reported to the World Health Organization (WHO) each year, the worldwide incidence of rabies is approximated at 15,000 cases per year. Southeast Asia, the Philippines, Africa, and the Indian subcontinent are areas where the disease is especially common. Increased spread of terrestrial rabies and increased travel to countries where urban rabies is present has made recognition of clinical rabies and its prevention of increasing importance. In the United States human rabies is still exceedingly rare, and 0 to 5 cases are reported yearly.

In most areas of the world, the dog is the important vector of rabies virus for humans. However, the wolf (eastern Europe, arctic regions), the mongoose (South Africa, the Caribbean), the fox (western Europe), and the vampire bat (Latin America) may also be prominent vectors of the disease. Rodents and lagomorphs are rarely infected with rabies. In the United States the most important sources of human disease have been skunks, bats, and raccoons. In the United States, rabies in wildlife accounts for about 85 percent of the reported animal rabies, with dogs and cats comprising only about 2 and 3 percent, respectively. However, most of the reported cases of postexposure prophylaxis are associated with dog bites. Many human cases of rabies in U.S. citizens have resulted from domestic animal bites that occurred outside the country.

Several cases of human-to-human transmission of rabies through corneal transplantation have been documented.

PATHOGENESIS The first event is the introduction of live virus through the epidermis or onto a mucous membrane. Initial viral replication appears to occur within striated muscle cells at the site of inoculation. The peripheral nervous system is exposed at the neuromuscular and/or neurotendinal spindles. The virus then spreads centripetally up the nerve to the central nervous system, probably via peripheral nerve axoplasm. Experimentally, viremia has been shown to occur, but is not thought to play a role in naturally acquired disease. Once the virus reaches the central nervous system, it replicates almost exclusively within the gray matter and then passes centrifugally along autonomic nerves to reach other tissue—the salivary glands, adrenal medulla, kidney, lung, liver, skeletal muscle, skin, and heart. Passage into the salivary glands facilitates further transmission of the disease via infected saliva. The incubation period of rabies is exceedingly variable, ranging from 10 days to over 1 year (mean 1 to 2 months). The time period appears to depend upon the amount of virus introduced, the amount of tissue involved, host defense mechanisms, and the actual distance that the virus has to travel from the site of inoculation to the central nervous system. Studies in animals have shown that host immune responses and viral strains may also influence disease expression. Attenuated strains of rabies virus produce high cytotoxic responses compared with wild "street virus." Animals which develop paralytic rabies (dumb rabies) appear to have a more marked immune response to infection than those which develop fulminant encephalitis.

The neuropathology of rabies resembles other viral diseases of the central nervous system: hyperemia, varying degrees of chromatolysis, nuclear pyknosis, and neuronophagia of the nerve cells; infiltration by lymphocytes and plasma cells of the Virchow-Robin space; microglial infiltration, and parenchymal areas of nerve cell destruction. The pathognomonic lesion of rabies is the Negri body. This eosinophilic mass, approximately 10 nm in size, is made up of a finely fibrillar matrix and rabies virus particles. Negri bodies are distributed throughout the brain, particularly in Ammon's horn, the cerebral cortex, the brainstem, the Purkinje cells of the cerebellum, and the dorsal spinal ganglia. Negri bodies are not demonstrated in at least 20 percent of rabies, and their absence in brain material does not rule out the diagnosis.

MANIFESTATIONS The clinical manifestations of rabies can be divided into four stages: (1) a nonspecific prodrome, (2) an acute encephalitis similar to other viral encephalitides, (3) a profound dysfunction of brainstem centers which produces the classic features of rabies encephalitis, and (4) rarely, recovery.

The prodromal period usually persists for 1 to 4 days and is marked by fever, headache, malaise, myalgias, increased fatigability, anorexia, nausea and vomiting, sore throat, and a nonproductive cough. The prodromal symptom suggestive of rabies is the complaint of paresthesias and/or fasciculations at or about the site of inoculation of virus. This symptom is present in 50 to 80 percent of patients.

The encephalitic phase is usually ushered in by periods of excessive motor activity, excitation, and agitation. Quickly, confusion, hallucinations, combativeness, bizarre aberrations of thought, muscle spasms, meningismus, opisthotonic posturing, seizures, and focal paralysis appear. Characteristically, the periods of mental aberration are interspersed with completely lucid periods, but as the disease progresses, the lucid periods get shorter until the patient lapses into coma. Hyperesthesia, with excessive sensitivity to bright light, loud noise, touch, and even gentle breezes, is very common. On physical examination the temperature may be found to be as high as 40.6°C (105°F). Abnormalities of the autonomic nervous system include dilated, irregular pupils, increased lacrimation, salivation, perspiration, and postural hypotension. Evidence of upper motor neuron paralysis with weakness, increased deep tendon reflexes, and extensor plantar responses is the rule. Paralysis of the vocal cords is common.

The manifestations of brainstem dysfunction begin shortly after the onset of the encephalitic phase. Cranial nerve involvement causes diplopia, facial palsies, optic neuritis, and the characteristic difficulty with deglutition. The combination of excessive salivation and difficulty in swallowing produces the traditional picture of "foaming at the mouth." Hydrophobia, the painful, violent involuntary contraction of the diaphragm, accessory respiratory, pharyngeal, and laryngeal muscles initiated by swallowing liquids, is seen in about 50 percent of cases. Involvement of the amygdaloid nucleus may result in priapism and spontaneous ejaculation. The patient lapses into coma, and involvement of the respiratory center produces an apneic death. The prominence of early brainstem dysfunction distinguishes rabies from other viral encephalitides and accounts for the rapid downhill course. The median survival after the onset of symptoms is 4 days, with a maximum of 20, unless artificial supporting measures are instituted.

If intensive respiratory support is used, a number of late complications may appear and include inappropriate secretion of antidiuretic hormone, diabetes insipidus, cardiac arrythmias, vascular instability, adult respiratory distress syndrome, gastrointestinal bleeding, thrombocytopenia, and paralytic ileus. Recovery is very rare and when it occurs has been gradual. There have been only three well-documented nonfatal cases of rabies in humans. Two of these survivors received partial postexposure prophylaxis and the third, a case of laboratory-associated rabies, probably from an aerosol exposure, had received preexposure prophylaxis.

Occasionally, rabies may present as an ascending paralysis resembling the Landry-Guillain-Barré syndrome (dumb rabies, *rage tranquile*). This clinical pattern occurs most frequently in those bitten by vampire bats or who have received postexposure rabies prophylaxis.

The difficulty of suspecting rabies when it is associated with ascending paralysis is illustrated by the documentation of person-to-person transmission of the virus by tissue transplantation. Corneal transplants from donors who died of presumed Landry-Guillain-Barré syndrome have produced clinical rabies and death in the recipient. Retrospective pathologic examinations of the brains of both patients demonstrated Negri bodies, and rabies virus was subsequently isolated from each donor's frozen eye.

LABORATORY FINDINGS Early in the disease the hemoglobin and routine blood chemistries are normal, but abnormalities occur as hypothalamic dysfunction, gastrointestinal bleeding, and other complications ensue. The peripheral white blood cell count is usually slightly elevated (12,000 to 17,000 per cubic millimeter) but may be normal or as high as 30,000 per cubic millimeter.

As in any viral infection, the specific diagnosis of rabies depends upon (1) the isolation of virus from infected secretions [saliva, rarely cerebrospinal fluid (CSF), or tissue (brain)], (2) the serologic demonstration of acute infection, or (3) the demonstration of viral antigen in infected tissue, e.g., corneal impression smears, skin biopsies, or brain. Samples of brain obtained either on postmortem examination or from brain biopsy should be subjected to (1) mouse inoculation studies for virus isolation, (2) fluorescent-antibody (FA) staining for viral antigen, and (3) histologic and/or electron microscopic examination for Negri bodies. While the mouse inoculation studies for virus isolation and direct FA staining for viral antigen are quite reliable and sensitive, if the patient's life has been prolonged and high levels of neutralizing antibody are present in serum and CSF, "autosterilization" may occur, and these tests may be negative. The use of FA staining of skin biopsies, corneal impression smears, and saliva for evidence of rabies antigen has been helpful in diagnosing rabies during life. Confirmation of these findings either serologically or by demonstration of virus in brain should be sought.

If the patient has not received antirabies immunization, then a fourfold rise in neutralizing antibody to rabies virus in serial serum samples is diagnostic. If the patient has received rabies vaccination, then a clue to the diagnosis may be obtained from the absolute titers of serum-neutralizing antibody and the presence of neutralizing antibody to rabies in CSF. Postexposure rabies prophylaxis rarely produces CSF-neutralizing antibody to rabies. If present, it is usually in low titer, e.g., less than 1:64, whereas CSF titers in human rabies may vary from 1:200 to 1:160,000.

DIFFERENTIAL DIAGNOSIS There is little to distinguish rabies from other viral encephalitides, and the most helpful point in diagnosis is the history of exposure. Other problems to be considered include hysterical reactions to animal bites (pseudohydrophobia), Landry-Guillain-Barré syndrome, poliomyelitis, and allergic encephalomyelitis to rabies vaccine. The latter occurs most commonly after use of nerve tissue–derived vaccine and usually begins 1 to 4 weeks after vaccination.

PREVENTION AND TREATMENT Each year more than 1 million Americans are bitten by animals. In each instance, a decision must be made whether to initiate postexposure rabies prophylaxis. When deciding whether to institute rabies prophylaxis, the following considerations apply: (1) whether the individual came into physical contact with saliva or another substance likely to contain rabies virus; (2) whether rabies is known or suspected in the species and area associated with the exposure (e.g., all persons within the continental United States bitten by a bat that then escapes should receive postexposure prophylaxis); (3) the circumstances surrounding the exposure; and (4) the treatment alternative and complications. A guide for postexposure rabies prophylaxis is illustrated in Fig. 142-1.

If rabies is known to be present or suspected to be present in the animal species involved in a human exposure, the animal should be captured, if possible. Captured wild animals or any ill, unvaccinated, or stray domestic animal involved in a rabies exposure, particularly any animal involved in an unprovoked bite, exhibiting abnormal behavior, or suspected of being rabid, should be captured and killed, and the head should be sent immediately to an appropriate laboratory for rabies FA examination. If examination of the brain by the FA technique is negative for rabies, it can be assumed that the saliva contains no virus, and the exposed person need not be treated. Persons exposed to escaped wild animals capable of carrying rabies (bats, skunks, coyotes, foxes, raccoons, etc.) in an area where rabies is known or suspected to be present should receive both passive and active immunization against rabies.

If a healthy dog or cat bites a person, the animal should be captured, confined, and observed for 10 days. If any illness or abnormal behavior develops in the animal during the observation period, it should be killed for FA examination.

Postexposure prophylaxis Once a decision regarding the necessity to initiate postexposure rabies prophylaxis has been made, the general principle of postexposure therapy is to minimize the amount of virus at the site of inoculation with local treatment of the wound and to establish an early and long-lasting neutralizing antibody titer to rabies virus. In most instances, this includes administration of globulin and vaccines. The following therapeutic regimen is recommended:

1 Local wound therapy with generous scrubbing with soap and then flushing the wound with water is recommended. Both mechanical and chemical cleansing are important. Quaternary ammonium compounds such as 1 to 4% benzalkonium chloride or 1% cetrimonium bromide are also useful. However, 0.1% benzalkonium solutions are less effective than 20% soap solutions. Usually tetanus toxoid and antibiotics (generally penicillin) should be administered.

2 Passive immunization with antirabies antiserum of either equine or human origin. Human rabies immune globulin (RIG) is preferred because of the high incidence of serum sickness (20 to 40 percent) with the equine product. Fifty percent of the total dose of 20 units per kilogram for RIG and 40 units per kilogram for the equine antiserum is given by local infiltration of the wound, and the rest is administered intramuscularly.

3 Active immunization with antirabies vaccine. Human diploid cell vaccine (HDCV) is now the only available antirabies vaccine in the United States. HDCV is an inactivated vaccine prepared from a laboratory strain of rabies virus grown in human diploid cell cultures. The vaccine developed in Europe (Merieux Institute) is a whole-virus preparation. The HDCV developed in the United States is a subunit vaccine dissolved with tri-*n*-butyl phosphate and then inactivated with β-propiolactone. The Merieux product appears more immunogenic, and the Wyeth vaccine was recalled from the U.S. market in February 1985.

Severe reactions to HDCV are uncommon. Immediate hypersensitivity responses such as urticaria have been reported in approximately 1 in 650 recipients. Systemic reactions such as fever, headache, and nausea are generally mild and are reported in 1 to 4 percent of recipients. Local reactions such as swelling, erythema, and induration at the injection site occur in 15 to 20 percent of vaccinees.

Five 1-mL doses of HDCV are given intramuscularly (IM) as soon as possible after exposure. The first dose (day 0) should also be accompanied by antirabies serum (RIG) given in the opposite arm. Subsequent doses of HDCV are given on days 3, 7, 14, and 28. The WHO also recommends a 21- and 90-day dose.

To date, follow-up evaluation of over 575 persons with bites from confirmed rabid animals has shown that no person who has received HDCV in combination with RIG has developed rabies. All persons

FIGURE 142-1 *Postexposure rabies prophylaxis algorithm.*

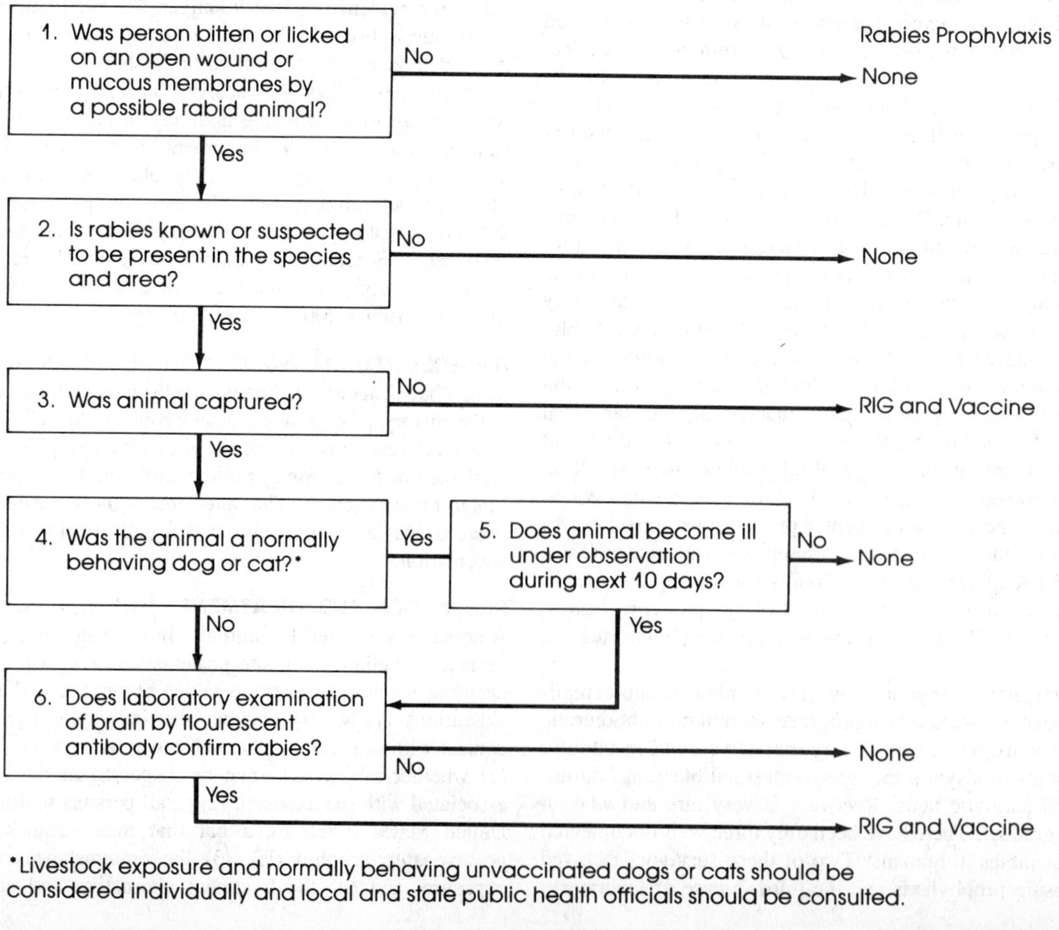

treated with RIG and five 1.0-mL IM doses of HDCV have developed an adequate titer (≥1:5 by the rapid fluorescent focus inhibition test). The combination of RIG plus 0.1-mL intradermal doses at eight sites on day 0, four sites on day 7, and one site on days 28 and 91 also produces good antibody responses.

Preexposure prophylaxis Individuals with a high risk of contact with rabies virus—veterinarians, spelunkers, laboratory workers, and animal handlers—should have preexposure prophylaxis with rabies vaccine. HDCV is the preferred vaccine for preexposure prophylaxis; three IM injections on days 0, 7, and 21 to 28 should be administered. Alternatively, three 0.1-mL doses intradermally in the skin overlying the deltoid region can be administered on the same days. A neutralizing antibody titer should be checked after vaccination. Booster doses may be administered either as a single 1-mL IM or 0.1-mL intradermal injection. Postexposure prophylaxis in individuals previously given preexposure therapy consists of HDCV vaccine alone (two IM doses of HDCV on days 0 and 3 are usually adequate).

Routine booster doses of vaccine at 2-year intervals have been recommended, but up to 6 percent of persons receiving IM booster doses of HDCV have developed an immune complex–like reaction characterized by urticaria, arthritis, nausea, vomiting, and, occasionally, angioedema. While these reactions have been self-limited in patients who develop them, consideration should be given to periodic measurement of antibodies. Booster doses are still recommended for those with low antibody titers who are at continued risk of exposure.

MARBURG VIRUS DISEASE

DEFINITION Marburg virus causes an acute systemic febrile illness characterized by the abrupt onset of headache, myalgias, pharyngitis, rash, and hemorrhagic manifestations. It was recognized first in 1967 when it caused simultaneous outbreaks in the Federal Republic of Germany and Yugoslavia among laboratory workers exposed to imported African green monkeys (*Cercopithecus aethiops*). More recent outbreaks have been reported from Kenya. The clinical manifestations are similar to other hemorrhagic fevers of the arenavirus class or flavivirus group (Argentina and Bolivian hemorrhagic fever, Chap. 144). The high case fatality rate and demonstrated ability for nosocomial spread has made recognition of this rare agent an important worldwide public health concern.

ETIOLOGY The Marburg virus has been isolated in guinea pig and various cell culture systems such as vervet monkey kidney. The virus particle contains lipid and RNA, and under the electron microscope the virus appears as an 80- to 100-nm elongated filamentous particle with occasional "blister-like excrescences." The Marburg virus exhibits some morphologic relationship to other members of the rhabdoviruses, e.g., rabies and Mokola viruses. However, physicochemical studies indicate that the Marburg and Ebola agents (see below) appear unique. A proposal has been made to include them in a new family of agents (Filoviridae).

EPIDEMIOLOGY The initial outbreaks affected 31 patients in Marburg and Frankfurt, Germany, and Belgrade, Yugoslavia, and was epidemiologically linked to monkeys imported from the same source in Uganda. Virus was isolated from the blood and tissue of these monkeys. Of the 25 primary infections, there were seven deaths. Six secondary cases, involving two physicians, one nurse, a postmortem attendant, and the wife of a veterinarian, occurred. Person-to-person transmission was felt to take place via accidental needle sticks or abrasions, although respiratory and conjunctival infection could not be ruled out. The wife of one patient developed Marburg virus disease. Marburg virus was demonstrated in semen of the original patient, despite the presence of circulating antibody, and this secondary case is believed to have been acquired through sexual intercourse. The natural reservoir of Marburg virus is unknown. Serologic examination of a large number of primates in Uganda suggests that monkeys appear to be susceptible but incidental hosts.

PATHOLOGY Marburg virus appears "pantropic" and produces lesions in almost all organs including lymphoid tissue, liver, spleen, pancreas, adrenals, thyroid, kidney, testes, skin, and brain. In lymphoid tissue focal necrosis with degeneration of lymphoid tissue is apparent. In the liver, eosinophilic cytoplasmic bodies resembling the Councilman bodies of yellow fever have been noted. The lungs may show interstitial pneumonitis, as well as vascular lesions in small arterioles indicative of endarteritis. Neuropathologic changes consist of multiple small hemorrhagic infarcts with glial proliferation.

CLINICAL MANIFESTATIONS After an incubation period of 3 to 9 days, patients develop the abrupt onset of frontal and temporal headache, malaise, myalgias, especially in the lumbar area, nausea, and vomiting. Fever of 39.4 to 40°C (103 to 104°F) is characteristic, and about half the patients have conjunctivitis. Between 1 and 3 days after onset, watery diarrhea, which is often severe, lethargy, and a change in mentation are noted. An enanthem of the palate and tonsils, and cervical lymphadenopathy may also be noted during the first week of illness. The most reliable clinical feature is the appearance of nonpruritic maculopapular rash which begins on the fifth to seventh day on the face and neck and spreads centrifugally to involve the extremities. A fine desquamation of the affected skin, especially the palms and soles, appears 4 to 5 days later. Hemorrhagic manifestations, including gastrointestinal, renal, vaginal, and/or conjunctival hemorrhages, generally develop between days 5 and 7 of disease.

During the first week, the temperature continues in the vicinity of 40°C (104°F), falling by lysis during the second week, to increase again between the twelfth and fourteenth days. Other clinical signs apparent in the second week of disease include splenomegaly, hepatomegaly, facial edema, and scrotal or labial reddening. Complications include orchitis, which may lead to testicular atrophy, myocarditis with irregular pulse and electrocardiographic abnormalities, and pancreatitis. The overall case fatality rate has been about 25 percent, with death usually occurring during the eighth to sixteenth days of illness. Recovery is often protracted over a 3- to 4-week period, and during this period loss of hair, intermittent abdominal pain, poor appetite, and prolonged psychotic disturbances have been noted. Late sequelae including transverse myelitis and uveitis have been reported. Marburg virus has been isolated from the anterior eye chamber and semen nearly 3 months after onset of disease.

LABORATORY FINDINGS Abnormalities in granulocyte function are found, and leukopenia is detected as early as the first day, with leukocyte counts as low as 1000 per cubic millimeter, and a neutrophilia by the fourth day. Subsequently, atypical lymphocytes, as well as neutrophils exhibiting the characteristic of the Pelger-Huet anomaly, may appear. Thrombocytopenia appears early and is most marked, often less than 10,000 cells per cubic millimeter, between the sixth and twelfth days. In fatal cases, evidence of disseminated intravascular coagulation can be demonstrated. Hypoproteinemia, proteinuria, and azotemia may occur. Elevations in serum glutamic oxaloacetic transaminase (SGOT) and alanine aminotransferase (SGPT) are usual. Lumbar puncture may be normal or reveal a minimal pleocytosis. The erythrocyte sedimentation rate is usually low.

DIAGNOSIS The characteristic clinical course and epidemiologic features are the basis of the diagnosis. Specific diagnosis requires isolation of the virus or serologic evidence of infection in paired serum samples. Viremia coincides with the febrile state of disease, and virus has been isolated from tissue as well as urine, semen, throat, and rectal swabs. Attempts to isolate virus must be carried out only in *specialized high-security laboratories*. All patients should be kept in strict isolation, and all specimens should be handled and shipped according to World Health Organization guidelines.

TREATMENT Patients have received a multiplicity of drugs without apparent influence on the course of the illness. Convalescent serum was administered to four patients, whose subsequent disease followed a mild course. However, similarly benign outcomes were observed in patients who did not receive serum.

EBOLA VIRUS

Between July and November 1976 simultaneous outbreaks of an acute febrile hemorrhagic disease occurred in southern Sudan and northern Zaire. "Secondary and tertiary" spread of infection, particularly among hospital staff, was noted. In the Sudan over 300 cases with 151 deaths and in Zaire 237 cases with 211 fatalities were reported. The virus isolated from these patients was morphologically similar to but antigenically distinct from the Marburg agent. The name Ebola virus, after the river in Zaire located near the epidemic, has been proposed. Biologic and antigenic differences between strains of Ebola viruses isolated in Zaire and Sudan may account for the differences in mortality between the two outbreaks. Sporadic cases of disease also appear to occur, and a serosurvey revealed a prevalence rate of 7 percent for antibodies to Ebola virus in endemic areas. As with other hemorrhagic fevers, neutrophil leukocytosis, hypofibrinoginemia, thrombocytopenia, and microangiopathic hemolytic anemia are features of the illness.

Ebola virus has been propagated in tissue culture (Vero cells) and in suckling mice and guinea pigs. The source of the outbreak in both the Sudan and Zaire is unknown; however, as with other viral hemorrhagic fevers, peridomestic rodents are suspected as being a reservoir of the infection, and serologic evidence of Ebola virus infection was detected in a domestic guinea pig trapped in Zaire. Once established, nosocomial as well as community-acquired cases occur, especially among those with close and prolonged contact. Parenteral exposure to the virus through disinfected rather than sterilized needles may have played a role in transmission. Barrier nursing and strict isolation precautions using protective clothing appeared to decrease the number of nosocomial cases.

CLINICAL MANIFESTATIONS Clinically, the disease is similar to Marburg virus disease. The incubation period ranges from 4 to 6 days (mean is 7 days). Patients usually present on the fifth day of illness with a history of abrupt onset of headache, malaise, myalgias, high fever, diarrhea, abdominal pain, dehydration, and lethargy. Pleuritic chest pain, a dry hacking cough, and a pronounced pharyngitis were also noted. A maculopapular eruption develops between days 5 to 7 of illness. On black skins the rash is often faint and not recognized until desquamation occurs. Hematemesis, melena, and bleeding from the nose, gums, and vagina are common. Abortion and massive metrorrhagia was a frequent complication among pregnant women. Death usually occurs in the second week of illness and is preceded by severe blood loss and shock.

TREATMENT Patients should be isolated until virologic studies indicate they are free of virus, usually 21 days from onset of illness. Malaria parasites were frequently found in blood films of patients with Ebola virus infection in the Sudan indicating that the presence of parasitemia does not rule out concomitant viral illness. Treatment with plasma containing Ebola virus–specific antibodies has resulted in diminished levels of viremia; however, further tests are required to establish the effectiveness of this form of therapy. Requests for viral isolation as well as convalescent plasma should be addressed to WHO Regional Centers in Atlanta or Geneva.

MOKOLA VIRUS

Mokola virus was first isolated from wild shrews captured in Nigeria and subsequently was shown to be related morphologically and serologically to rabies. However, neither of the two reported cases of human disease (both children) demonstrated classic clinical features of rabies. One patient had a nonfatal illness characterized by fever, pharyngitis, and convulsions. Mokola virus was recovered from her cerebrospinal fluid. The second patient initially had fever, cough, and vomiting, followed in several days by drowsiness, confusion, and generalized flaccid weakness. Her cerebrospinal fluid was normal. She progressed to deep coma and died within 10 days of onset. Mokola virus was isolated from her brain, and histopathologic sections revealed finely granular cytoplasmic inclusions that were distinguishable from Negri bodies in many neurons.

VESICULAR STOMATITIS VIRUS

Vesicular stomatitis is a viral illness of animals which can occasionally infect humans. It presents as an acute self-limited influenza-like disease. The disease in animals is found in the United States and South America and affects chiefly domestic cattle, horses, swine, and wild deer, raccoons, skunks, and bobcats.

In animals, vesicular stomatitis is characterized by the development of vesicles on the oral mucosa, particularly the tongue, udders, and heels. The mode of spread is probably by direct contact; however, epidemics tend to occur in warm weather, and the virus has been isolated from *Phlebotumus* sandflies in Panama and *Äedes* species in New Mexico, suggesting these as possible vectors. Two distinct serotypes, New Jersey and Indiana, have been recognized, and most of the outbreaks in North America have been attributed to the New Jersey strain. The disease is most common in laboratory workers, and in one report three-fourths of laboratory personnel handling experimentally infected animals or manipulating the virus developed neutralizing antibodies. The disease is transmissible, however, under natural conditions among workers having direct contact with infected animals, especially cattle. The incubation period ranges from 1 to 6 days. This is followed by the sudden onset of fever, up to 40°C (104°F), chills, profuse sweating, myalgias, malaise, headache, and pain on ocular movement. One-third to one-half of patients have sore throat and cervical and/or submandibular adenopathy. Small raised vesicular lesions may appear on the buccal mucosa. Conjunctivitis and coryza are present in about 20 percent of cases. Occasionally, small subcorneal, intraepithelial vesicles may appear on the fingers, usually associated with direct inoculation of the virus. Symptoms generally last 3 to 4 days, but occasionally a diphasic course may occur. Inapparent infection is common, and among laboratory workers with serologic evidence of infection, only about one-half reported clinical symptoms. In some areas of Panama, 17 to 35 percent of the population have neutralizing antibodies against vesicular stomatitis virus.

The differential diagnosis includes hand-foot-and-mouth disease, herpangina, primary herpetic pharyngitis and other mucocutaneous syndromes, and influenza. Viral isolation from patients is not common; however, a rise in complement fixation and/or neutralizing antibodies to vesicular stomatitis virus between acute and convalescent serums will help to confirm the diagnosis. Treatment is nonspecific.

REFERENCES

Marburg virus

GEAR JSS et al: Outbreak of Marburg virus disease in Johannesburg. Br Med J 4:489, 1975

SIMPSON DIH: Marburg and ebola virus infections: A guide for their diagnosis, management and control. WHO Offset Publication no 36, Geneva, 1977

SMITH DH et al: Marburg-virus disease in Kenya. Lancet 1:816, 1982

Mokola virus

FAMILUSI JB: Fatal human infection with Mokola virus. Am J Trop Med Hyg 21:959, 1972

Rabies

ANDERSON LJ: Human rabies in the United States, 1960 to 1979. Epidemiology, diagnosis and prevention. Ann Intern Med 100:728, 1984

BAER GM: *The Natural History of Rabies*. New York, Academic, 1975

BAHMANYAR M: Successful protection of humans exposed to rabies: Post exposure treatment with the new human diploid cell rabies vaccine and antirabies serum. JAMA 236:2751, 1976

Compendium of Animal Rabies Vaccines, 1986. Morb Mort Week Rep 34:770, 1986

HATTWICK MA et al: Recovery from rabies: A case report. Ann Intern Med 76:931, 1972

HOUGH SA et al: Human-to-human transmission of rabies virus by a corneal transplant. N Engl J Med 300:603, 1979

PLOTKIN SA: Rabies vaccine prepared in human cell culture: Progress and perspectives. Rev Infect Dis 2:433, 1980
Rabies Prevention, United States, 1984. Morb Mort Week Rep 33:393, 1984
WARRELL MJ et al: Economical multiple site intradermal immunization with human diploid-cell-strain vaccine. Lancet 1:1059, 1985

Ebola virus

MCCORMICK JB et al: Biologic differences between strains of Ebola virus from Zaire and Sudan. J Infect Dis 147:264, 1983
STANSFIELD SK: Antibody to Ebola virus in guinea pigs: Tandala, Zaire. J Infect Dis 146:483, 1982

143 ARBOVIRUS INFECTIONS

JAY P. SANFORD

Most viral infections in humans are either asymptomatic or present as undifferentiated illnesses characterized by fever, malaise, headache, and generalized myalgia. The similarities in clinical features between infections caused by viruses as dissimilar as the myxoviruses (e.g., influenza), the enteroviruses (e.g., poliovirus, coxsackievirus, echovirus), some of the herpesviruses (e.g., cytomegalovirus), and the arboviruses usually preclude an etiologic diagnosis based entirely on clinical manifestations without ancillary information regarding epidemiologic features and serologic findings. The purpose of this chapter is to direct attention to the ever-expanding list of viruses which produce febrile disease in humans. Because the number of agents is large, mention will be made of those which have been best documented, have demonstrated unusual features, or seem to be of greatest potential public health importance.

DEFINITION AND CLASSIFICATION The earliest efforts to classify viruses were based on common pathogenic properties (e.g., hepatitis viruses), common tropisms (e.g., respiratory viruses), or common ecologic characteristics (e.g., arboviruses). The definition of an arthropod-borne virus (arbovirus) was published in 1967 by the World Health Organization:

Arboviruses are viruses which are maintained in nature principally, or to an important extent, through biological transmission between susceptible vertebrate hosts by hematophagous arthropods; they multiply and produce viremia in the vertebrates, multiply in the tissues of arthropods, and are passed on to new vertebrates by the bites of arthropods after a period of extrinsic incubation.

From this definition it can be appreciated that the term *arbovirus* is used in the ecologic sense. Transmission by vectors is not correlated with virus architecture. Current approaches to taxonomy are based upon viral morphology, structure, and function. As a result, for taxonomic purposes, the term *arbovirus* has been eliminated.

The more than 250 antigenically distinct "arboviruses" are now grouped into five families (Table 143-1). The majority of agents contain single-stranded RNA, although some, such as the Reoviridae contain double-stranded RNA.

"Arboviruses" are of importance in both temperate and tropical zones. Representative viruses have been isolated in almost every geographic area outside the polar regions.

"Arbovirus" infection of vertebrates is usually asymptomatic. The viremia stimulates an immune response which sharply limits the duration of the viremia. In "arbovirus" infections other than urban yellow fever, phlebotomus fever, chikungunya, o'nyong-nyong, mayaro, oropouche, dengue, and possibly Ross River virus, infection of humans represents an incidental occurrence which is tangential to the basic maintenance cycle of the virus. Hence, the isolation of virus from arthropod vectors or the detection of infection in the natural vertebrate host may provide a means for early detection and enable control of epizootic infection before significant spread to humans occurs.

TABLE 143-1 Virus taxonomy and arboviruses-arenaviruses*

Family	Genus	Virus "English vernacular name"†
Reoviridae	Orbivirus	Colorado tick fever‡
		Orongo
		Kemerovo
Togaviridae	Alphavirus (group A)	Eastern equine encephalitis‡
		Venezuelan encephalitis‡
		Western equine encephalitis‡
		Sindbis
		Semliki Forest complex
		Chikungunya‡
		O'nyong-nyong
		Ross River‡
		Mayaro
	Flavivirus (group B)	*Associated with encephalitis*
		St. Louis encephalitis‡
		Japanese encephalitis‡
		Murray Valley encephalitis‡
		Tick-borne encephalitis complex‡
		Russian spring-summer encephalitis
		Central European encephalitis
		Negishi
		Powassan‡
		Louping-ill
		Rocio
		Associated with fever-arthralgia-rash
		Dengue fever‡
		West Nile fever‡
		Nine other agents–not of major public health importance
		Associated with hemorrhagic fever
		Yellow fever‡
		Dengue fever‡
		Omsk hemorrhagic fever
		Kyasanur Forest disease
Rhabdoviridae	Vesiculovirus	Vesicular stomatitis Indiana‡
		Vesicular stomatitis New Jersey‡
		Cocal
		Chandipura
		Piry
		Isfahan
	Lyssavirus	Rabies‡
		Mokola
		Duvenhage
Filoviridae		Marburg‡
		Ebola‡
Bunyaviridae	Bunyavirus (16 serogroups)	Twenty-four agents may cause fever, fever-rash. None cause death. None in United States.
		California serogroup
		LaCrosse‡
		Snowshoe hare
		Jamestown Canyon
		California encephalitis
		Tahyna
		Inkoo
	Phlebovirus	Thirty-seven phleboviruses isolated from human beings; none cause death except Rift Valley fever virus.
		Sandfly fever–Naples‡
		Sandfly fever–Sicilian‡
		Rift Valley fever‡
	Nairovirus	Crimean-Congo hemorrhagic fever‡
	Not yet established	Hantaan‡
		Puumala‡
		Prospect Hill‡
		Tchoupitoulas‡
Arenaviridae	Arenavirus	Lymphocytic choriomeningitis‡
		Lassa‡
		Machupo‡
		Junin‡

* *Only agents which have been shown to naturally infect humans are tabulated.*
† *Virus species have not yet been designated formally. The International Committee on Taxonomy of Viruses lists species under the term "English vernacular name."*
‡ *Viruses found in the United States and/or of major public health importance.*

Most human "arbovirus" infections are asymptomatic. When disease is produced, the spectrum of clinical illness is varied both in predominant features and in severity. Most commonly, disease is self-limited with symptoms of fever, headache, malaise, and myalgia. Associated lymphadenopathy may be a feature. "Arboviruses" which may cause three major clinical syndromes—arthralgia-arthritis, encephalitis–aseptic meningitis, or hemorrhagic disease—are tabulated in Table 143-2.

TABLE 143-2 Major clinical syndromes, associated arboviruses-arenaviruses, and major geographic distribution

Clinical syndrome*	Virus	Geographic distribution
Fever, arthralgia, rash	Chikungunya	Africa, southeast Asia
	O'nyong-nyong	East Africa
	Ross River	Australia, Fiji, Samoa, Cook Islands, New Guinea
	Sindbis	Africa, U.S.S.R., Finland, Sweden
	Mayaro	South and Central America
	Dengue fever	Tropical Asia, Oceania, Africa, Australia, Americas
	West Nile fever	Africa, Middle East, U.S.S.R., France, India, Indonesia
	Lymphocytic choriomeningitis	United States, Germany, Hungary, Argentina
Encephalitis/aseptic meningitis	Kemerovo	Central Europe
	Eastern equine encephalitis	Atlantic, Gulf coasts, United States, upper New York, Caribbean, western Michigan
	Venezuelan equine encephalitis	Northern South America, Central America, Mexico, Florida
	Western equine encephalitis	United States, Canada, Central and South America
	Semliki Forest	Africa
	St. Louis encephalitis	United States, Caribbean
	Japanese encephalitis	Japan, Korea, China, India, Philippines, southeast Asia, eastern U.S.S.R.
	Murray Valley encephalitis	Australia
	Rocio	Brazil
	Omsk hemorrhagic fever	U.S.S.R.
	Kyasanur Forest disease complex	India
	Negishi	Japan
	Powassan	New York, eastern Canada
	Louping ill	United Kingdom, Ireland
	Russian spring-summer encephalitis	U.S.S.R.
	Central European encephalitis	Eastern Europe, Scandinavia, France, Switzerland
	California group	North America
	Tahyna	Europe
	Inkoo	Europe
	Phlebotomus fever	Mediterranean basin, Balkans Near and Middle East, east Africa, central Asia, Pakistan, parts of India, southern China, Panama, Brazil
	Rift Valley fever	South and east Africa
	Lymphocytic choriomeningitis	United States, Germany, Hungary, Argentina
Hemorrhagic fever	Yellow fever	South America, Africa
	Dengue	Caribbean, southeast Asia
	Chikungunya	Southeast Asia
	Kyasanur Forest disease	India
	Omsk hemorrhagic fever	U.S.S.R.
	Crimean-Congo hemorrhagic fever	Africa, eastern Europe, Middle East, Asia
	Hantaan	Korea, Japan, Scandinavia, U.S.S.R., central Europe
	Marburg	Uganda, Kenya, Zimbabwe
	Ebola	Zaire, Sudan
	Lassa fever	West Africa
	Machupo	Bolivia
	Junin	Argentina

* *Most agents are more often associated with undifferentiated febrile illness than with the specific syndromes. See text for exceptions.*

"ARBOVIRUS" INFECTIONS PRESENTING CHIEFLY WITH FEVER, MALAISE, HEADACHE, AND MYALGIA Phlebotomus fever Phlebotomus (sandfly, pappataci, or 3-day) fever is an acute, relatively mild, self-limited infection caused by at least five immunologically distinct phleboviruses (Naples, Sicilian, Punta Toro, Chagres, and Candiru). Serologic evidence of human infection has been demonstrated for four additional agents (Bujaru, Cacao, Karimabad, and Salehabad). Humans, the only known host, probably serve as a dead-end host. Voles are suspected of being an endemic host in the Middle East.

PREVALENCE The disease occurs throughout the Mediterranean basin, the Balkans, the Near and Middle East, the eastern part of Africa, the Soviet republics of central Asia, Pakistan, parts of India, and possibly certain parts of southern China. Recently, sandfly fever has been recognized in Panama and Brazil. In the Middle East and central Asia native populations acquire the disease at an early age and develop and maintain high levels of immunity. Cases in Panama and Brazil are sporadic, occurring mainly in persons entering the forest. The apparent absence of phlebotomus fever in indigenous adult populations residing in areas where sandflies are abundant may present a deceptive picture of the actual risk to susceptible persons.

EPIDEMIOLOGY In the Middle East and central Asia, the disease occurs during the hot, dry season (summer or autumn months) and is transmitted to human beings by the bite of infected sandflies (*Phlebotomus papatasii*), which are small (2- to 3-mm) urban flies that can penetrate ordinary house screens. Only the female bites and usually does so during the night. In persons who are not sensitive, there is neither pain nor local irritation after the bite; hence only about 1 percent of patients will remember having been bitten. In contrast, most of the human-biting sandflies (*Lutzomyia* sp.) of tropical America are sylvan in their habits. Transovarial and transstadial transmission of the virus has been demonstrated and in view of the low-titered and transient viremia in humans suggests the phlebotomine fly is both vector and reservoir. In humans, the incubation period averages 3 to 5 days. Viremia is present for at least 24 h before the onset of fever, but is not detectable for more than 2 days after the onset of illness.

CLINICAL MANIFESTATIONS The onset of symptoms is abrupt in over 90 percent of patients, with the temperature rapidly rising to its highest point, which may vary from 37.8 to 40.1°C (100 to 105°F). Headache is nearly always present and often is accompanied by pain on moving the eyes and by retroorbital pain. Myalgia is common and may be localized to the chest, resembling pleurodynia, or to the abdomen. Other symptoms may include vomiting, photophobia, giddiness, neck stiffness, alteration or loss of taste, and arthralgia. Conjunctival injection is present in approximately one-third of patients. Small vesicles may be seen on the palate, and macular or urticarial rashes occur. The spleen is rarely palpable, and lymphadenopathy is absent. The pulse rate may be elevated in proportion to the temperature on the first day; thereafter bradycardia is often present. The fever persists 3 days in most patients, with gradual defervescence. Giddiness, weakness, and feelings of depression are frequently encountered during convalescence. Second attacks 2 to 12 weeks after the first occur in 15 percent of cases.

In common with other "arbovirus" infections, phlebotomus fever may be associated with *aseptic meningitis*. In one series, 12 percent of patients had symptoms and signs sufficient to warrant a lumbar puncture. Findings in these patients included pleocytosis, with an average cell count of 90 per cubic millimeter and a predominance of either polymorphonuclear or mononuclear leukocytes. Spinal fluid protein concentration ranged from 20 to 130 mg/dL. In another series mild papilledema was observed in a few patients with severe illness.

LABORATORY FINDINGS The changes in leukocyte count constitute the only positive laboratory findings. Total leukocyte counts of less than 5000 per cubic millimeter are observed in 90 percent of patients if daily counts are done during the febrile period and convalescence.

The leukopenia may not appear until the last day of fever or even after defervescence. The differential leukocyte count will reveal an absolute decrease in lymphocytes on the first day, accompanied by an increase in nonsegmented neutrophils. During the second or third day, the number of lymphocytes begins to return to normal and may constitute 40 to 65 percent of the total count. Concurrently, there is a reversal in proportion of segmented and band neutrophils. The differential count usually returns to normal within 5 to 8 days after defervescence. Erythrocyte values and urinalyses are usually normal.

DIAGNOSIS In the absence of a specific serologic test, the diagnosis must be made on clinical and epidemiologic grounds.

TREATMENT The disease is self-limited, and no specific therapy is available. Symptomatic care, including bed rest, adequate fluid intake, and analgesia with aspirin, is recommended. Convalescence may require a week or longer.

PROGNOSIS No fatalities have been recorded among the tens of thousands of cases.

Colorado tick fever Colorado tick fever is one of the two tick-transmitted virus diseases of human beings recognized in the United States and Canada, Powassan virus being the other. Though "mountain fever" had been described ever since the advent of immigrants to the Rocky Mountain region, it must be differentiated from mild Rocky Mountain spotted fever. Once the clinical picture of disease had been established, it was renamed Colorado tick fever. A second serotype of the Colorado tick fever serogroup (Eyach virus) was isolated from *Ixodes ricinus* ticks near the village of Eyach in West Germany.

ETIOLOGY Colorado tick fever virus is grouped as an "arbovirus" because it replicates in ticks. It is a double-stranded RNA virus belonging to the orbivirus genus of the Reoviridae family (see Table 143-1).

PREVALENCE The disease has been contracted in Colorado, Idaho, Nevada, Wyoming, Montana, Utah, the eastern portions of Oregon, Washington, California, and northern portions of Arizona and New Mexico, and Alberta and British Columbia. The virus of Colorado tick fever has been isolated from the dog tick, *Dermacentor variabilis*, obtained from Long Island. This observation has not been confirmed, but suggests the possibility that Colorado tick fever may occur over a wider geographic area. Mild and clinically inapparent forms of the disease occur. Up to 15 percent of perennial campers have neutralizing antibodies. The number of cases of Colorado tick fever reported in Colorado is 20 times greater than that of Rocky Mountain spotted fever. In fact, almost one-half of the patients diagnosed as having Rocky Mountain spotted fever in Utah were subsequently shown to have Colorado tick fever.

EPIDEMIOLOGY Colorado tick fever is transmitted to humans by the adult hard-shelled wood tick, *Dermacentor andersoni*. The virus has been found in as many as 14 percent of this species of ticks collected in endemic areas. Transovarial transmission of the virus in the tick has been established. Illness occurs from late March through September, mostly in May and June. Virus can be recovered from blood for 2 weeks in most patients, for at least 1 month in nearly one-half, and from spinal fluid during the acute illness. The virus persists within erythrocytes of convalescent patients for as long as 120 days. Virus can be readily isolated from washed erythrocytes 100 days following infection. Transfusion-associated Colorado tick fever has been reported.

CLINICAL MANIFESTATIONS The incubation period is usually 3 to 6 days, and in 90 percent a history of tick contact within 10 days of onset of illness can be obtained. Failure to obtain such a history militates against the diagnosis. Persons affected usually are those whose occupational or recreational activities bring them in contact with ticks. The disease may occur at any age, although 40 percent in one series were 20 to 29 years of age. The clinical picture is characterized by the sudden onset of severe aching of the muscles of the back and legs, chilliness without true rigors, a rapid increase in temperature, which usually reaches 38.9 to 40°C (102 to 104°F), headache with pain on ocular movement, retroorbital pain, and photophobia. Abdominal pain and vomiting occur in one-fourth of patients; diarrhea is rare. The physical findings are not specific. Tachycardia in proportion to the temperature, flushed facies, and variable conjunctival injection may be present. Occasionally the spleen is palpable. Rash occurs in only 5 percent of patients, but on occasion a petechial rash involving primarily the arms and legs or a maculopapular rash over the entire body may occur. Rarely, punched-out ulcers may form at the site of tick bite. The fever with the associated symptoms lasts about 2 days, then abruptly lyses to normal or subnormal, leaving the patient very weak. After an afebrile period of about 2 days, the fever recurs, may be higher than in the first phase, and may last as long as 3 days. One-half of patients show this saddleback pattern of temperature. Rarely there may be three febrile phases. Convalescence of more than 3 weeks is reported in 70 percent of patients over age 30, while symptoms last less than 1 week in 60 percent of patients under 20. Prolonged convalescence has no relationship to persistent viremia.

Evidence of central nervous system involvement has been recorded in a few patients. The findings are those of either an aseptic meningitis with stiffness of the neck or encephalitis with clouding of the sensorium, delirium, and coma. Single instances of reported complications include epididymoorchitis and patchy pneumonitis.

The clinical manifestations of Eyach virus infection have not been elucidated. Antibodies to Eyach virus were found in patients with various neuropathies.

LABORATORY FINDINGS The most important laboratory feature is moderate to marked leukopenia, although in one-third of confirmed cases leukocyte counts remain about 4500 per cubic millimeter. On the first day of illness, the total leukocyte count may be at normal levels, but usually by the fifth or sixth day there has been a decrease to 2000 to 3000 per cubic millimeter. Characteristically there is a proportionate decrease in lymphocytes and granulocytes. Toxic changes in neutrophils are often conspicuous, and "virocyte" types of lymphocytes are frequently observed. Bone marrow examination reveals "maturation arrest" in the granulocytic series. Erythrocyte values remain normal. Thrombocytopenia has been recorded in an isolated case report. The blood picture returns to normal within a week after the fever subsides.

DIAGNOSIS The diagnosis of Colorado tick fever is suspected on the basis of the epidemiologic history and clinical findings. Because of the infrequency of rash, patients who develop fever and rash after tick bites should be suspected of having Rocky Mountain spotted fever. The usual methods for confirming Colorado tick fever are mouse inoculation and fluorescent antibody (FA) staining of patients' erythrocytes; a combination of the two is best. Special handling of blood is not necessary for the FA test which remains positive for several weeks after clinical illness.

TREATMENT Treatment is entirely symptomatic.

PROGNOSIS The prognosis is excellent.

PREVENTION Only one patient has been reported as having the disease twice. Active immunity with an attenuated virus has been produced, but the immunization itself frequently produced mild disease. Colorado tick fever is best prevented by avoiding contact with the wood tick. Convalescent individuals should be excluded as blood donors for at least 6 months.

Venezuelan equine encephalitis Venezuelan equine encephalitis (VEE) was first noted in equines in Colombia in 1935.

ETIOLOGY Like other alphaviruses, the causative agent of VEE is a 40- to 45-nm, single-stranded RNA virus. Based on serologic tests and oligonucleotide fingerprints a complex of Venezuelan encephalitis viruses has been established: VE subtypes IA to IE, II (Everglades),

III (Mucambo), and IV (Pixuna). IA was the original epidemic strain which occurred in Venezuela, and IB, which was recognized in Ecuador in 1963, spread through Central America into Mexico and was responsible for the epidemic in Mexico in 1971 which spread into southern Texas, with the occurrence of at least 76 laboratory-confirmed human cases. In early 1973, almost 4000 cases occurred in Peru.

EPIDEMIOLOGY VEE has been primarily a disease of equines and other mammals, although occasionally the agent has infected humans. Evidence of human infection (virus isolation or specific neutralizing antibodies) has been found in Colombia, Ecuador, Panama, Surinam, Guyana, French Guiana, Mexico, Brazil, Curaçao, Trinidad, Argentina, Peru, Florida, and Texas. Each subtype of VE virus is unique to its enzootic vector and does not replicate well in other vectors. Most common is an enzootic cycle between *Culex* mosquitoes and forest rodents. Enzootic VEE infects people who enter the rain forest or swamps, rubber tappers, forestry workers, and military personnel on jungle maneuvers. During an epizootic, many species of mosquitoes can transmit virus, especially *Aëdes, Mansonia,* and *Psorophora.* The virus has a wide host range in wild mammals, with at least 20 genera, including capuchin monkeys, rats, mice, opossum, jackrabbit, fox, and bats, being naturally infected. Domestic animals other than equines which have been shown to be infected include cattle and pigs in Mexico and goats and sheep in Venezuela. VEE appears to multiply well in mammals with high titers of virus in the blood; e.g., infected horses may have titers of up to $10^{7.5}$ mouse intraperitoneal lethal doses per milliliter of blood. Though 29 species of wild birds have been shown to be naturally infected with VEE (20 percent of which are colonial nestling herons and related species), whether the VEE-viremia levels in birds are high enough to infect vector mosquitoes is not known. During the initial 3 days of illness, viremia has been detected in approximately two-thirds of patients. The levels of viremia are sufficiently high that humans could serve as a reservoir. VEE virus also has been isolated by pharyngeal swab in a few patients, suggesting the potential for person-to-person transmission. The available observations make it reasonable to consider that the natural vector is a mosquito, with the primary reservoir being either wild or domestic terrestrial mammals. However, natural infection can probably take place without an arthropod vector. Laboratory infections have occurred and are probably due to inhalation of aerosols.

CLINICAL MANIFESTATIONS In humans, infection with VEE virus usually results in a mild acute febrile illness without neurologic complications. No age is spared, and there is no sex preponderance. The incubation period is 2 to 5 days, followed by the abrupt onset of headache, fever often associated with rigors, malaise, and myalgia. Other common symptoms may include nausea, vomiting, diarrhea, and sore throat. Uncommon features include photophobia, seizures, mental confusion, coma, tremors, and diplopia. Lymphadenopathy occurs in one-third of patients. On laboratory examination initial leukocyte counts are normal with 80 percent neutrophils. By the third day leukopenia occurs in two-thirds of patients. The cerebrospinal fluid may reveal pleocytosis with modest increases in protein concentration and normal glucose concentration. Virus may be isolated both from blood and from cerebrospinal fluid. The symptoms usually last 3 to 5 days in mild cases and up to 8 days in more severe cases, although one patient reported from Florida was febrile for 3 weeks. A biphasic course of illness may be encountered, with recrudescence of symptoms at the sixth to the ninth day. In one case report, palatine petechiae were noted and the patient vomited "coffee-grounds" material. In an epidemic in Venezuela in 1962, almost 16,000 cases of acute disease were evaluated; 38 percent were classified as encephalitis, but only 3 to 4 percent had severe neurologic abnormalities: convulsions, nystagmus, drowsiness, delirium, or meningitis. The mortality rate was estimated to be less than 0.5 percent, and nearly all deaths occurred in young children.

Rift Valley fever Rift Valley fever is an acute disease principally of livestock, sheep, goats, cattle, and camels which is widespread throughout east and South Africa. It was first described in humans during an extensive epizootic of hepatitis in sheep in the Rift Valley in Kenya. During an epizootic in South Africa in 1950–1951, an estimated 20,000 humans became infected. Fatal human disease, four cases of hemorrhagic illness and hepatitis, was first reported during an epizootic in South Africa in 1975. In 1977 Rift Valley fever jumped the Sahara to Egypt with a major outbreak. Cases occurred in subsequent years until 1980; an estimated 200,000 cases with 598 reported deaths occurred in 1977. At least one case has been reported in a Canadian tourist.

Virus has been found in several species of mosquitoes: *Culex pipiens, Eretmapodites chrysogaster, Aëdes caballus, Aëdes circumluteolus,* and *Culex theileri. Culex pipiens* has been suggested as the vector in Egypt. While antibodies to Rift Valley fever have been found in wild field rats in Uganda, the reservoir is unknown. It has been suggested that the virus may be maintained by transovarial transmission in floodwater *Aëdes.* Although humans presumably can be infected by arthropods, many infections occur as a result of handling infected animal tissues. In addition, laboratory-acquired infections have been common, suggesting a respiratory route of transmission.

The incubation period is usually 3 to 6 days. The onset is abrupt, with malaise, chilly sensation or rigors, headache, retroorbital pain, and generalized aching and backache. The temperature rises rapidly to 38.3 to 40°C (101 to 104°F). Later complaints include anorexia, loss of taste, epigastric pain, and photophobia. Findings on examination are usually unremarkable except for flushing of the face and conjunctival injection. The temperature curve is often saddleback in type, with an initial elevation lasting 2 to 3 days, followed by a remission and second febrile period. Convalescence is typically rapid. Prior to the outbreak in Egypt, Rift Valley fever was a benign illness with almost no fatalities. In Egypt, approximately 1 percent of patients developed severe complications, such as encephalitis, retinopathy, or hemorrhagic manifestations. Encephalitis appeared as the acute infection waned and was severe with serious residua in some survivors. Hemorrhagic manifestations appeared as the disease evolved with generalized hemorrhages and icterus. Deaths from massive hepatic necrosis occurred 7 to 10 days after onset of illness. The fatality rate in severely ill patients may exceed 50 percent. Visual loss, including light perception, occurred 2 to 7 days after the onset of fever. Macular edema, hemorrhage, vasculitis, retinitis, and vascular occlusion were noted. One-half of patients had some permanent loss of visual acuity. A characteristic finding is an initial normal total leukocyte count followed by leukopenia with a decrease in neutrophils associated with an increase in band forms. The diagnosis is made by isolating the virus from the blood by inoculation of mice. Three-fourths of patients are viremic (up to 10^8 mouse intraperitoneal lethal doses per milliliter blood) when first seen. Neutralizing antibodies have been demonstrated as early as 4 days after onset. There is no specific treatment. A killed vaccine which had been stockpiled in the United States is being utilized.

Zika virus Zika virus was first isolated from a captive rhesus monkey in Uganda and subsequently from wild mosquitoes. Serologic surveys reveal a prevalence of human infection up to 50 percent in central Africa and parts of Asia (Indonesia), but human disease is rarely reported. During investigation in eastern Nigeria of an outbreak of jaundice that was suspected of being yellow fever, physicians isolated Zika virus from one patient and noted that two others had a rise in neutralizing antibodies. The symptoms in these patients included fever, arthralgia, and headache with retroorbital pain. Jaundice was present in one, and bile was demonstrated in the urine of another. Albuminuria was noted in one patient. Prothrombin times were normal. The clinical syndrome appears to simulate mild yellow fever.

Bunyaviruses The family Bunyaviridae consists almost entirely of viruses transmitted to vertebrate animals by arthropods. There are more than 200 viruses in the family, classified into five genera: Bunyavirus (formerly the Bunyamwera supergroup), Uukuvirus, Nairovirus, phlebovirus, Hantaan virus (Table 143-1). The majority of Bunyaviruses were isolated in exploratory surveys of tropical ecosystems in South America, southeast Asia, and Africa. Most Bunyaviruses have not been associated with human infection or disease. Currently, 24 Bunyaviruses have been associated with febrile human disease which may or may not be associated with rashes. This includes the C group, Bunyamwera and Oropouche. The geographic distribution of C-group viruses includes Brazil, Trinidad, and Panama. Isolates have been obtained mostly from forest workers and laboratory technicians. Epidemics have not been recognized. The disease begins with headache, fever [with temperature up to 40.6°C (105°F)], and myalgia. Additional symptoms include malaise, photophobia, vertigo, and nausea. Illness is generally mild, lasting 2 to 4 days, and is occasionally followed by a relapse. No fatalities have been reported. Occasionally a prolonged period of convalescence ensues. Leukopenia, with total leukocyte counts as low as 2600 per cubic millimeter, is a common finding. Diagnosis has been established mainly by virus isolation.

Representative viruses of the Bunyamwera group are found in all inhabited continents except Australia. Only five viruses of the group—Bunyamwera itself, Germiston, Ilesha, Guaroa, and Wycomyia—have been associated with clinical disease. Serologic surveys give evidence of a high prevalence of inapparent infection in some areas. Clinical illness is characterized by low-grade fever, headache, and myalgia which last several days, and may be followed by weakness during convalescence. Infection due to Bunyamwera virus is associated often with arthralgia and sometimes with a rash. Since 1962 seven epidemics of Oropouche disease involving thousands of persons in Brazil, in the populated regions south of the Amazon River, have occurred. Outbreaks occurred during the rainy season. The epidemic vector is the midge of *Culicoides paraensis*. The incubation period is 4 to 8 days. Clinical features include abrupt onset of fever, usually to 39 to 40°C (102 to 104°F), with rigors. Symptoms, which include headache, photophobia, dizziness, myalgia, anorexia, nausea, and vomiting, last 2 to 5 days. Lymphadenopathy, splenomegaly, or rash have not been features. Laboratory findings include leukopenia with relative lymphocytosis. Urinalyses are normal. Mild elevations of transaminase may occur. Fatalities have not been reported.

"ARBOVIRUS" INFECTIONS PRESENTING CHIEFLY WITH FEVER, MALAISE, ARTHRALGIA, AND RASH **Chikungunya** In 1952 an epidemic of a disease occurred in Tanzania, which was given the name *chikungunya* ("that which bends up") because of the sudden onset of joint pains. An alphavirus of the Semliki Forest complex was isolated in 1956 both from serum of patients ill with the disease and from a pool of *A. aegypti* mosquitoes.

Chikungunya virus is responsible for a dengue-like illness in Africa, India, southeast Asia, New Guinea, and Guam, as well as for a rather mild form of hemorrhagic fever in Asiatic children. Outbreaks have been associated with high attack rates, with as many as 80 percent of inhabitants in some settlements becoming ill. In large epidemics, *Aëdes aegypti* is the vector. In Africa, virus is transmitted among monkeys and baboons by forest *Aëdes* mosquitoes, *A. africanus*. The cycle in southeast Asia has not been clearly defined, but humans may be the host.

After an incubation period of 3 to 12 days, the onset is typically abrupt, with a rapid rise in temperature to 38.9 to 40.6°C (102 to 105°F), often associated with a rigor and headache. Pain in large joints occurs early, incapacitating some individuals within a few minutes of onset. The arthralgia is often associated with objective arthritis. Sites of involvement include knees, ankles, shoulders, wrists, or proximal interphalangeal joints. Myalgia, especially backache, and malaise occur frequently. In 60 to 80 percent of patients a maculopapular eruption, which may appear at any time during the febrile course, is noted on the trunk or on the extensor surfaces of the extremities. Mild lymphadenopathy, predominantly in the axillary or inguinal areas, may be evident. Pharyngitis and conjunctival suffusion may be observed in a few patients. Fever continues for 1 to 10 days, and in some patients an afebrile interval of 1 to 3 days is followed by a secondary rise in temperature. The joint pains may continue after the temperature has returned to normal. In a few individuals joint pains have persisted for up to 4 months. Hematocrit values remain normal. Total leukocyte counts may be less than 5000 per cubic millimeter in some patients, while in others they remain normal. Urinalyses are normal. There is no specific antiviral treatment. Anti-inflammatory agents such as aspirin or indomethacin have been utilized. No second attacks have been recognized, and in the absence of the hemorrhagic fever syndrome, no deaths have been described.

Mayaro virus disease Outbreaks involving a number of persons have occurred in Brazil and Bolivia. Survey for antibodies in serums obtained from residents in Rio de Janeiro showed that almost one-third were positive. Mayaro virus has been isolated from a wild mosquito, *Mansonia venezuelansis,* and can be maintained serially in *A. aegypti* and *Anopheles quadrimaculatus*.

The incubation period has not been clearly defined but is about 1 week. Ages of patients have ranged from 2 to 62 years, with both sexes involved. Illness begins abruptly with fever, chills, severe frontal headache, myalgia, and dizziness. Temperatures usually exceed 40°C (104°F). Arthralgia occurs uniformly and is very prominent, occasionally incapacitating, and in some patients precedes the fever by a few hours. Involvement of the wrists, fingers, ankles, and toes predominates. Other initial symptoms (in less than one-third of patients) include nausea, vomiting, and diarrhea. Initial examination reveals inguinal lymphadenopathy (one-half of cases), swelling of affected joints (one-quarter of cases), and occasional conjunctival congestion. The initial clinical features last 3 to 5 days except the arthralgia, which may persist for 2 months. On about the fifth day a maculopapular rash develops over the chest, back, arms, and legs. Rash appeared in 90 percent of children and in one-half of adults and lasted about 3 days.

Laboratory findings include leukopenia with leukocyte counts as low as 2500 per cubic milliliter during the first week. Urinalysis revealed albuminuria (2+) in one-fourth of patients. Some patients showed slight elevations in serum glutamic oxaloacetic transaminase levels.

In Brazil, no relapses were observed and no deaths have been recognized. In Bolivia, more severe illness and several fatalities have been reported.

O'nyong-nyong fever O'nyong-nyong fever was first noted as an epidemic illness characterized by joint pains, rash, and lymphadenopathy in the northern province of Uganda in 1959. The agent is an alphavirus which shows close antigenic relationships with chikungunya viruses. The original outbreak was associated with an explosive epidemic which spread to Tanzania and other areas in east Africa. By 1961, 2 million cases were recorded. In some areas, 91 percent of the population had either clinical disease or inapparent infection. Local outbreaks extended over the entire year. All age groups were affected. The most likely vector is *Anopheles funestus*. The clinical features are similar to those of chikungunya virus infection. The disease disappeared in 1962. While the virus was isolated from *A. funestus* in Kenya in 1978, no further outbreaks have been recognized.

Sindbis virus Sindbis virus, once thought rarely to present as clinical disease, has been recognized in Africa (Uganda, Republic of South Africa), Australia, and Europe (U.S.S.R., Finland, and Sweden). In the U.S.S.R. it is known as Karelian fever, in Sweden as Okelbo disease, and in Finland as Pogosta disease. Clinically, fever is low-grade and accompanied by malaise, myalgia, and arthralgia involving joints and tendons. The most striking feature is a maculopapular rash appearing on the trunk and extremities but usually sparing the face. Unlike the rash of chikungunya or o'nyong-nyong, the rash often becomes vesicular, especially on the feet and hands.

Ross River virus Epidemics of polyarthritis associated with rashes have been observed in Australia since 1928. Outbreaks occur almost entirely in the period December to June. Ross River virus infection was limited to Australia, New Guinea, and the Solomon Islands until 1979 when a major outbreak occurred in Fiji which spread to the Samoan, Cook, and some Melanesian Islands. In the Fiji outbreak in 1979, infection rates were equal at all ages and in both sexes, but clinical attack rates were 4 percent in patients under 20 years of age and 42 percent in adults, and the clinical attack rate of males to females was 1:1.7. The onset is characterized by headache, mild catarrh, and occasionally tenderness of the palms and soles. Initially fever may be absent or minimal [highest 38°C (100.4°F)]. In about one-half of patients, arthritis, involving mainly the small joints, wrists, and ankles and sometimes associated with swelling, and paresthesias precede a rash by 1 to 15 days. In the other half, the rash precedes the arthralgia. The rash, which lasts 2 to 10 days, is usually maculopapular, appears on the cheeks and forehead, occasionally spreads to the trunk, or may be restricted to the limbs. The rash may be pruritic. Vesicles occur rarely. Tender lymphadenopathy occurs in one-fifth of the patients. Joint symptoms persist for 3 weeks to 3 months. The presence of antibody early in the clinical course suggests an immunopathogenesis. Infection has not been associated with fetal loss or congenital anomalies in children. The virus has been isolated from *Culex annulirostris* and *Aëdes vigilax*. Animals may serve as reservoir hosts in Australia. In the Pacific, person-mosquito-person transmission seems likely.

Other "arboviruses" Bunyamwera viruses occasionally have been associated with the syndrome of rash and arthralgia.

"ARBOVIRUS" INFECTIONS PRESENTING CHIEFLY WITH FEVER, MALAISE, LYMPHADENOPATHY, AND RASH **Dengue fever** Dengue is endemic over large areas of the tropics and subtropics, southeast Asia, the South Pacific, and Africa. Outbreaks of dengue have occurred in the Caribbean including Puerto Rico and the U.S. Virgin Islands since 1969. Approximately 3000 cases were reported in Mexico in 1979. Indigenous infection occurred in the United States for the first time in 35 years in the fall of 1980. Eleven cases have been recognized in residents of the Rio Grande valley of Texas. In the summer of 1981, 79,000 cases of dengue-like illness with 31 deaths were reported from Cuba. *Aëdes aegypti,* the vector, has reappeared along the U.S. Gulf Coast; hence, the threat of dengue along the Gulf Coast is real.

ETIOLOGY There are four distinct serogroups of dengue viruses, types 1, 2, 3, and 4, all of which are flaviviruses. In the Caribbean, type 1 was associated with the 1977–1978 outbreak, type 2 in 1968–1969, type 3 in 1963–1964, and type 4 was documented in the western hemisphere for the first time in 1981.

EPIDEMIOLOGY Dengue infections in nature involve primarily human beings and *Aëdes* mosquitoes. Dengue transmission involving monkeys and forest *Aëdes* spp. has been documented in Malaysia and West Africa. *Aëdes aegypti* is the most important worldwide vector species. This species, as well as the less common vector species, is peridomestic, biting humans readily or even preferentially and breeding in small collections of water such as cisterns and backyard litter. Surveys in Texas have revealed containers with water in which *A. aegypti* were breeding in up to 25 percent of premises. They fly during the day. Humans appear to be uniformly susceptible, and susceptibility is not influenced by age, sex, or race. During outbreaks, attack rates may be very high; in Puerto Rico and the U.S. Virgin Islands, the overall rate of clinical illness was 20 percent, with infection rates as determined by serologic survey as high as 79 per 100.

CLINICAL MANIFESTATIONS Dengue viruses frequently produce inapparent infections in humans. When symptoms develop, three broad clinical patterns may be encountered: classic dengue, hemorrhagic fever (see below), and a mild atypical form. Classic dengue (breakbone fever) occurs primarily in nonimmune individuals, specifically nonindigenous adults and children. The usual incubation period is 5 to 8 days. Prodromal symptoms such as mild conjunctivitis or coryza may occur, followed in hours by the abrupt onset of a severe splitting headache, retroorbital pain, backache, especially in the lumbar area, and leg and joint pains. The headache is aggravated by movement. At least three-fourths of patients have ocular soreness, with pain on moving the eyes. A few have mild photophobia. Though true rigors are common during the course, they are usually not present at the onset. Additional symptoms include insomnia, anorexia with loss of taste or bitter taste, and weakness. Mild transient rhinopharyngitis occurs in as many as one-quarter of the individuals. Cough is almost never seen. Epistaxis has been observed. Examination reveals scleral injection (90 percent), tenderness upon pressure on the ocular globe, and nontender posterior cervical, epitrochlear, and inguinal lymphadenopathy. Over one-half of patients have an enanthem characterized initially by pinpoint-sized vesicles over the posterior half of the soft palate. The tongue is often coated. Skin rashes, varying from diffuse flushing to scarlatiniform and morbilliform, are frequently present over the thorax and inner aspects of the arms. These are transient and fade, only to be followed by a more definite maculopapular rash which appears on the trunk on the third to the fifth day and spreads peripherally. The rash may be pruritic and generally terminates with desquamation. Extreme bradycardia is not observed. Within 2 to 3 days after the onset, the temperature may decrease to nearly normal and other symptoms disappear. The remission typically lasts 2 days and is followed by return of fever and the other symptoms, although they are generally less severe than during the initial phase. This "saddleback" diphasic febrile course is considered characteristic, but often is not encountered. The febrile illness usually lasts 5 to 6 days and terminates abruptly. Complaints of fatigue for several weeks after infection are common.

In addition to this "classic" syndrome, an atypically mild illness may occur. Symptoms include fever, anorexia, headache, and myalgia. On examination, evanescent rashes may be seen, but lymphadenopathy is usually absent. The course is usually less than 72 h in duration.

At the onset both in classic and in mild dengue, the leukocyte counts may be low or normal; however, by the third to the fifth day, leukopenia, usually with counts of less than 5000 leukocytes per cubic millimeter, and neutropenia are usually seen. Occasionally albuminuria of moderate degree occurs.

DIAGNOSIS Inoculation of blood obtained within the first 3 to 5 days onto mosquito tissue cell cultures or inoculation into mosquitoes is used for primary viral isolation. Diagnosis can be made by serologic tests employing paired serums for hemagglutination inhibition tests and complement fixation tests. IgM antibodies are produced in primary dengue infections. Specific serologic diagnosis is complicated by cross-reactions with other flavivirus antibodies such as those following immunization with yellow fever vaccine.

TREATMENT Treatment is entirely symptomatic.

PROGNOSIS In the absence of the dengue hemorrhagic fever or dengue shock syndrome, mortality is nil.

PREVENTION An attenuated vaccine for dengue type 2 is undergoing early experimental evaluation. Control depends upon mosquito abatement.

West Nile fever West Nile virus is distributed throughout Africa, the Middle East, parts of Europe (Camargue, France), U.S.S.R., India, and Indonesia. It produces a clinical picture closely resembling dengue. Outbreaks of disease involving several hundred patients occurred in Israel in 1950 to 1952. In one outbreak, over 60 percent of the population developed overt disease.

EPIDEMIOLOGY The disease is highly endemic in Egypt but goes largely unrecognized. Presumably most of the adult population is immune, and the infection in childhood is an undifferentiated mild febrile illness, whereas in Israel it mainly affects adults. The infection occurs in the summer both in Israel and in Egypt. The transmission cycle in the Middle East is bird-to-mosquito-to-bird, with *Culex univittatus* and *Culex pipiens molestus* being the principal vectors. *Culex tritaeniorhynchus* is an important vector in Asia. Although humans and a variety of other vertebrates are infected by the virus, their involvement is tangential.

CLINICAL MANIFESTATIONS The incubation period is 1 to 6 days. Most of the patients in Israel have been young adults, with neither sex predominating. The onset is usually abrupt and without prodromal symptoms. The temperature quickly rises to 38.3 to 40°C (101 to 104°F), with chills occurring in one-third of patients. Symptoms include drowsiness, severe frontal headache, ocular pain, and pain in the abdomen and back. A small number of patients have anorexia, nausea, and dryness of the throat. Cough is uncommon. Signs observed include flushing of the face, conjunctival injection, and coating of the tongue. The prominent finding is general enlargement of lymph nodes, which are of moderate size but are not hard and are only slightly tender. Occipital, axillary, and inguinal nodes are usually involved. The spleen and liver are slightly enlarged in a small proportion of patients. In one-half the patients a rash may appear from the second to the fifth day of illness and may persist for several hours or until defervescence. The rash occurs predominantly over the trunk and consists of pale roseolar maculopapular lesions. The illness is self-limited and lasts 3 to 5 days in 80 percent of patients.

In a few patients, transitory meningeal involvement may be encountered. Spinal fluid examinations may reveal a pleocytosis and some increase in protein concentration.

Leukopenia occurs in the majority of patients, and total leukocyte counts are lower than 4000 per cubic millimeter in one-third. Differential counts vary from a moderate shift to the left to a slight lymphocytosis.

Convalescence is often prolonged, lasting 1 to 2 weeks, with prominent symptoms of fatigue. Enlargement of lymph nodes subsides over several months. Only rarely have complications, sequelae, or fatalities been seen in natural infections, although in one outbreak in a group of elderly patients a high proportion of patients developed meningoencephalitis, and four fatalities ensued.

Accurate diagnosis rests on virus isolation, which can be accomplished because viremia persists for as long as 6 days, or the demonstration of a rising specific antibody titer.

The treatment is symptomatic.

"ARBOVIRUS" INFECTIONS PRESENTING CHIEFLY WITH CENTRAL NERVOUS SYSTEM INVOLVEMENT Four "arboviruses" are presently recognized as numerically important causes of central nervous system disease in the United States: St. Louis encephalitis virus (SLE), eastern equine encephalitis virus (EEE), western equine encephalitis virus (WEE), and the California serogroup (CE) viruses. The spectrum of infection caused by these agents includes inapparent infection, fever with headache, aseptic meningitis, and encephalitis. Some 1500 to 2000 cases of encephalitis are reported in the United States each year. In the absence of epidemics, 5 to 10 percent of these (75 to 200 cases) are confirmed as "arboviral" in etiology. In nonepidemic years, California serogroup viruses (predominantly LaCrosse virus) represent two-thirds to three-fourths of the cases. Because of epidemics of St. Louis and western equine encephalitis, which contribute larger numbers of cases, the overall distribution in the 30 years between 1955 and 1984 has been: SLE 65 percent, CE 20 percent, WEE 13 percent, and EEE 2 percent.

ETIOLOGY Despite the diversity of specific viral etiologies (see Table 143-2), in individual patients the clinical manifestations of aseptic meningitis and encephalitis are very similar, and preclude an etiologic diagnosis without ancillary information regarding epidemiologic and serologic features (see Table 143-3). The clinical features of aseptic meningitis due to "arboviruses" are indistinguishable from those due to the more prevalent enteroviruses. Since transmission to humans in the United States and Canada involves arthropods, specifically mosquitoes, except for Powassan and Colorado tick fever, indigenously acquired disease occurs at times when mosquitoes are prevalent, such as late spring through early fall. The broad clinical picture of "arbovirus" encephalitis will be discussed; then the specific epidemiologic and prognostic features which characterize the major types will be presented.

CLINICAL MANIFESTATIONS The clinical features of "arbovirus" encephalitis differ among age groups. In infants under 1 year of age, the only consistently noted symptoms are sudden onset of fever, which is often accompanied by convulsions. Convulsions may be either generalized or focal. Typically the fever ranges between 38.9 and 40°C (102 and 104°F). Other physical findings may include bulging of the fontanelle, rigidity of the extremities, and abnormalities in reflexes.

In children between 5 and 14 years of age, subjective symptoms are more easily elicited. Headache, fever, and drowsiness of 2 to 3 days' duration before medical attention is sought are common. The symptoms may then subside or become more intense and may be associated with nausea, vomiting, muscular pain, photophobia, and, less frequently, convulsions (less than 10 percent except in California encephalitis). On examination, the child is found to be acutely ill, febrile, and lethargic. Nuchal rigidity and intention tremors are often present, and on occasion muscular weakness can be demonstrated.

In adults, the initial symptoms commonly include the fairly abrupt onset of fever, nausea with vomiting, and severe headache. The headache is most often frontal but may be occipital or diffuse in location. Mental aberrations, represented by confusion and disorientation, usually appear within the subsequent 24 h. Other symptoms may include diffuse myalgia and photophobia. The abnormalities found on physical examination predominantly relate to the neurologic examination, although conjunctival suffusion is frequently seen and skin rashes may occur. Disturbances in mentation are among the most outstanding clinical features. These range from coma through severe disorientation to subtle abnormalities detected only by cerebral function tests such as the subtraction of serial 7s. A small proportion

TABLE 143-3 Features of arboviral encephalitides common in the United States

Etiology	Geographic predominance in the United States	Urban/ rural	Age, years	Sex	Unique clinical features	Mortality, %	Residua
California encephalitis	Midwest	Rural	5–10	M	Seizures	2	Seizures (one-fourth who had them in acute phase), behavioral problems (15%)
Eastern equine encephalitis	Eastern seaboard	Both	<5 >55	=	CSF may have >1000 WBC/ mm^3	50	Children <10 years have emotional lability, retardation, convulsions
St. Louis encephalitis	Eastern and midwest	Both	>35	=	Dysuria	2–12	Ataxia, speech difficulties (5%)
Western equine encephalitis	Entire	Both	<1 >55	=	None	3	Children <3 months have behavioral problems, convulsions

of patients show only lethargy, lying quietly, apparently asleep unless stimulated. Tremor is common and is observed more frequently in individuals over 40 years of age. The tremors vary in location and may be continuous or intention in type. Cranial nerve abnormalities resulting in oculomotor muscle paresis and nystagmus, facial weakness, and difficulty in deglutition may occur and are usually present within the initial several days. Objective sensory changes are unusual. Hemiparesis or monoparesis may occur. Reflex abnormalities are also common; these include exaggerated palmomental reflexes, and suck and snout reflexes. Superficial abdominal and cremasteric reflexes are usually absent. Changes in the tendon reflexes are variable and inconstant. The plantar response may be extensor and fluctuates almost hourly. Dysdiadochokinesia often exists.

The duration of the fever and neurologic symptoms and signs varies from several days to a month but usually ranges from 4 to 14 days. Clinical improvement generally follows the subsidence of the fever within several days unless irreversible anatomic changes have occurred.

LABORATORY FINDINGS Erythrocytes are usually normal. Total leukocyte counts often reveal both a slight to moderate leukocytosis (occasionally greater than 20,000 leukocytes per cubic millimeter) and neutrophilia. Examination of the cerebrospinal fluid usually reveals several hundred cells per cubic millimeter, but on occasion cloudy cerebrospinal fluid with cells in excess of 1000 per cubic millimeter may be seen. Within the first several days of illness, polymorphonuclear neutrophils may predominate. The initial cerebrospinal fluid protein is usually only slightly elevated but on occasion may exceed 100 mg/dL. The level of spinal fluid sugar is normal; a significant decrease should raise serious consideration of an alternative diagnosis. As the illness progresses, mononuclear cells in the cerebrospinal fluid tend to increase so that they predominate and the protein concentration may increase. Other laboratory studies have been performed only sporadically, but abnormalities may include hyponatremia, often due to the inappropriate secretion of antidiuretic hormone, and elevations in serum creatine phosphokinase.

DIAGNOSIS Specific diagnosis requires the isolation of the virus or detection of antibodies with a rising titer between the acute phase of disease and convalescence. Antibodies can be detected by hemagglutination inhibition, complement fixation, or virus neutralization techniques.

TREATMENT Treatment is entirely supportive and requires meticulous attention in the comatose patient.

LaCrosse encephalitis A previously undescribed virus was isolated in 1943 from mosquitoes in Kern County, California. Since 1963, a large number of agents now designated as the California group of viruses have been isolated (Table 143-1). LaCrosse, snowshoe hare, Jamestown Canyon, and California encephalitis viruses cause human encephalitis in North America. Tahyna and Inkoo viruses are associated with febrile and, rarely, encephalitic disease in Europe.

Since 1966 in the midwest United States, LaCrosse virus (California) encephalitis has been incriminated in 5 to 6 percent of cases of acute central nervous system disease, ranking above all agents except the enteroviruses.

EPIDEMIOLOGY LaCrosse virus infection occurs in the north central states, New York, in wooded areas of eastern Texas and Louisiana, and along the eastern seaboard. The virus is maintained by transovarial transmission in woodland mosquitoes, *Aëdes triseratus,* which breed in tree holes in hardwood forests and have adapted to discarded tires. The virus is present in seminal fluid of male mosquitoes and transmitted to the female. The virus overwinters in eggs of *A. triseratus.* Chipmunks and gray squirrels serve as amplifier hosts. LaCrosse virus (California) encephalitis occurs during the summer months (June to October), most often involving boys (60 percent) 5 to 10 years of age (60 percent) who live in rural areas.

CLINICAL MANIFESTATIONS Two clinical patterns of LaCrosse virus disease have been defined. One is a mild form with a 2- to 3-day prodrome of fever, headache, malaise, and gastrointestinal symptoms. About the third day the temperature increases to 40°C (104°F), and the patient becomes lethargic and develops meningeal signs. These findings abate gradually over a 7- to 8-day period without overt sequelae. The second pattern, a severe form which occurs in at least one-half of the patients, begins abruptly with fever, headache, and vomiting, followed shortly by lethargy and disorientation. During the first 2 to 4 days the course is rapidly progressive with the occurrence of seizures (50 to 60 percent), focal neurologic signs (20 percent), pathologic reflexes (10 percent), and coma (10 percent). Focal neurologic signs may include asymmetric flaccid paralysis. Uncommon findings have included arthralgia and rash. Clinical laboratory features include peripheral leukocyte counts ranging from 7000 to 30,000 per cubic millimeter (median 16,000 per cubic millimeter) with neutrophilia. Cerebrospinal fluid examination reveals 10 to 500 cells per cubic millimeter, usually with a predominance of mononuclear cells, protein concentrations of less than 100 mg/dL, and normal sugar concentrations. Electroencephalograms (EEGs) are abnormal in at least 80 percent of patients, revealing slow deltawave activity. In one-half of the patients the abnormality is asymmetric, suggesting focal destructive lesions. Brain scans using [^{99}Tc]pertechnetate and computerized tomography (CT) also may be abnormal, and temporal lobe localization has been observed. Beginning about the fourth day and proceeding over the next 3 to 7 days, there is progressive improvement, with almost all patients becoming afebrile, seizure-free, and ready for discharge from the hospital within 2 weeks after onset.

DIAGNOSIS Serum and CSF should be tested for LaCrosse virus IgM antibodies. Serum capture IgM ELISA tests detected 83 percent on admission in LaCrosse encephalitis. Early specific diagnosis eliminates the need for brain biopsy to exclude herpes encephalitis which is suggested by the temporal lobe localization.

TREATMENT Initial seizure activity is frequently prolonged and difficult to control. The most effective anticonvulsant medication has been parenteral diazepam. Patients with the severe form of disease should be discharged on anticonvulsants such as phenobarbital for 6 to 12 months.

PROGNOSIS The case fatality ratio is low (2 percent or less); however, one-third of patients may have abnormal neurologic findings at the time of discharge. During the early convalescent period, emotional lability and irritability are common. In one series, recurrent seizures occurred in one-quarter of the patients who had seizures during the acute phase. In this same series EEGs were abnormal in one-third of patients evaluated 1 to 8 years after their acute illness. In another series, 15 percent had sequelae, predominantly personality or behavioral problems.

Other California group encephalitides Jamestown Canyon encephalitis is uncommon, but in contrast to LaCrosse encephalitis usually occurs in adults. Snowshoe hare virus has been isolated from mosquitoes throughout Canada and from Alaska. Encephalitis has been reported from the eastern provinces. Clinical features of Tahyna virus disease, which has been seen in children in Europe, include fever, pharyngitis, pneumonitis, gastrointestinal symptoms, and aseptic meningitis. Neither mortality nor sequelae are reported.

Eastern equine encephalitis Eastern equine encephalitis (EEE), an alphavirus, was first isolated in 1933 from the brain tissue of horses during an outbreak of equine illness in New Jersey. The first recognized human outbreak occurred in Massachusetts in 1938.

EPIDEMIOLOGY The virus is distributed along the eastern coast of the Americas from northeastern United States to Argentina. Foci have been found in the Syracuse region of New York, Ontario, Canada, western Michigan, and South Dakota. Viral isolations also have been reported in the Philippines, Thailand, Czechoslovakia, Poland, and the U.S.S.R., but the question of type specificity has not been resolved. In the northeastern United States, epidemics occur in the late summer and early fall. Epizootics in horses precede the occurrence of human cases by 1 to 2 weeks. The disease affects mainly infants, children, and adults over 55 years of age. There is no sex preponderance. Inapparent infection occurs in all age groups, suggesting that the decreased likelihood of developing overt infection in the 15- to 54-year age group is not the result of decreased exposure. The ratio of inapparent infection to overt encephalitis approximates 25:1.

The transmission of EEE involves *Culiseta melanura* mosquitoes and swamp-dwelling birds, e.g., red-winged blackbirds, sparrows, pheasants. Transmission by pecking has been shown in domestic pheasant flocks. *C. melanura* rarely feed on horses or humans, and other mosquitoes, especially *Aëdes sollicitans,* a salt-marsh mosquito which is an avid human feeder, have been postulated as the epidemic vector. The epidemiology of overwintering and maintenance between outbreaks remains unknown. Equine animals and human beings are "dead ends" in the transmission cycle, and infection in them is accidental.

CLINICAL MANIFESTATIONS Though human infections have been thought usually to result in serious, if not fatal, central nervous system involvement, the detection of inapparent infection as well as relatively mild disease establishes the occurrence of milder forms. In many patients, the cerebrospinal fluid is cloudy and contains in excess of 1000 cells per cubic millimeter.

DIAGNOSIS Enzyme-linked immunosorbent assay (ELISA) tests for the detection of specific IgM antibodies in CSF or serum enable early diagnosis, although absence of IgM does not exclude infection. Confirmation can be obtained by a fourfold or more rise or fall in complement fixation (CF), hemagglutination inhibition, or virus neutralization tests.

PROGNOSIS The mortality rate in clinical infection exceeds 50 percent. In the most severe cases, death occurs between the third and fifth days. Children under 10 years of age have a greater likelihood of surviving the acute illness, but they also have a greater likelihood of developing severe disabling residuals: mental retardation, convulsions, emotional lability, blindness, deafness, speech disorders, and hemiplegia.

St. Louis encephalitis St. Louis encephalitis (SLE) was first recognized as an entity during a major outbreak in St. Louis, Missouri, and the surrounding area in 1933. Subsequently, sporadic, unpredictable outbreaks have occurred, for example, in Houston, 1964, Dallas, 1966, Memphis, 1974, northern Mississippi and Illinois, 1975. The attack rate in Greenville, Mississippi, in 1975 was the highest which has been encountered, 10 per 10,000 population.

EPIDEMIOLOGY In the United States, epidemics of SLE fall into two epidemiologic patterns. One pattern is found in the west, where mixed outbreaks of western equine encephalitis and SLE have occurred primarily in irrigated rural areas. The vector has been *Culex tarsalis.* The second pattern occurred in the original St. Louis outbreak and the numerous subsequent epidemics in the midwest, Texas, New Jersey, and Florida. These outbreaks have been more urban in location and are characterized by occurrence of encephalitis in older persons. In such urban-suburban epidemics, the epidemic vectors have been mosquitoes of the *Culex pipiens-quinquefasciatus* complex with the exception of the Florida epidemic, in which *Culex nigripalpus* was incriminated. The presence of SLE virus outside the United States has been proved by isolations in Trinidad, Panama, Jamaica, Brazil, and Argentina. However, except for Jamaica, SLE has not been reported outside the United States. The basic transmission cycle is that of wild bird–mosquito–wild bird. The virus survives the winter in female mosquitoes which ingest a blood meal from a viremic bird before overwintering. The disease in humans usually appears in midsummer to early fall. In urban epidemics, there is no sex predominance while among sporadic cases in the west, men predominate 2:1 due to greater occupational exposure. The human represents an accidental host and plays no role in the basic transmission cycle. Serologic studies following most urban epidemics indicate that infection rates are similar in all age groups, and that the increasing age-specific attack rate for clinical encephalitis which is typical of urban St. Louis encephalitis is probably due to age differences in host susceptibility to overt disease rather than to a higher rate of infection.

CLINICAL MANIFESTATIONS Infection with SLE virus most commonly results in an inapparent infection. Of the patients with confirmed disease, approximately three-fourths have clinical encephalitis; the remainder present with aseptic meningitis, febrile headaches, or nonspecific illness. Virtually all patients over 40 years of age have encephalitic manifestations. Urinary frequency and dysuria have been symptoms in approximately 20 percent of patients despite sterile routine aerobic urine cultures. SLE virus antigen has been demonstrated in urine; this may account for the occurrence of urinary tract symptoms.

DIAGNOSIS The occurrence of either encephalitis or aseptic meningitis as manifested by febrile illness with cerebrospinal fluid pleocytosis in the months of June through September in an adult, especially over 35 years of age, should raise the suspicion of St. Louis encephalitis. Because approximately 40 percent of patients with SLE have antibodies detectable by hemagglutination inhibition at the onset of illness, acute serum for serologic studies should be submitted promptly to a competent laboratory. ELISA tests for the detection of specific IgM antibodies in CSF or serum provide a means of early specific diagnosis.

PROGNOSIS The case fatality ratio in the original St. Louis epidemic was 20 percent. In most subsequent outbreaks the mortality rate has varied from 2 to 12 percent. Subjective nervous complaints, including nervousness, headaches, and easy fatigability and excitability, appear to be the most common residuals. Late organic defects such as speech defects, difficulty in walking, and disturbances in vision were demonstrated in approximately 5 percent of patients 3 years following infection.

Western equine encephalitis Western equine encephalitis (WEE) virus is an alphavirus which was isolated in 1930 in California from horses with encephalitis. In 1938 it was recovered from a fatal human infection.

EPIDEMIOLOGY WEE virus has been isolated in the United States, Canada, Brazil, Guyana, and Argentina. Human disease has been diagnosed in the United States, Canada, and Brazil. In the United States, the virus is found in virtually all geographic areas. The central valley of California represents an important endemic area. The disease occurs mainly in early summer and midsummer. Wild birds, which develop viremia of sufficiently high titer to be able to infect mosquitoes that feed on them, are the basic reservoir. *Culex tarsalis* is the principal vector in the western United States. In areas east of the Appalachian Mountains, another vector must be operative. The virus has been repeatedly isolated from *Culiseta melanura;* however, the importance of this species has been questioned, since it is not primarily a human-biting mosquito. The overwintering mechanism is not known. The ratio of inapparent infection to disease, as evidenced by serologic survey studies, varies from 58:1 in children to 1150:1 in adults. Approximately one-fourth of patients are less than 1 year of age. The highest attack rates occur in persons 55 years or older.

PROGNOSIS The fatality rate approximates 3 percent in laboratory-confirmed cases. The incidence and severity of sequelae are related to age. Sequelae among very young infants are frequent (appearing in 61 percent of a group of patients less than 3 months old) and severe; they consist of upper motor neuron impairment, involving the pyramidal tracts, extrapyramidal structures, and cerebellum, and result in behavioral problems and convulsions. Both the incidence and severity of sequelae diminish rapidly after 1 year of age. Adults may complain of nervousness, irritability, easy fatigability, and tremulousness for 6 months or longer after the acute illness. Probably not more than 5 percent of adults have sequelae which are sufficiently severe to be of practical significance. Postencephalitic seizures are rare.

Japanese encephalitis The name Japanese B encephalitis was employed during an epidemic which occurred in 1924 to distinguish it from von Economo's disease, which was designated as type A encephalitis. The designation as Japanese B no longer seems useful, and the term Japanese encephalitis (JE) will be employed.

EPIDEMIOLOGY Japanese encephalitis virus infection is known to occur in eastern Siberia, China, Korea, Taiwan, Japan, Malaya, Vietnam, Thailand, Singapore, Guam, and India. Since the late 1960s JE has declined in Japan and China. JE remains a major problem in northern Thailand. In temperate climates, the disease shows a late-summer early-fall seasonal incidence. In tropical climates there is no seasonal variation. The mosquito *Culex tritaeniorhynchus* is the major vector species. It is a rural mosquito which breeds in rice fields and preferentially bites large domestic animals, such as pigs, but also feeds on birds and humans. The human is an accidental host in the transmission cycle. In endemic areas, children ages 3 to 15 are primarily affected. Epidemics in nonendemic areas have affected all age groups, but young children and older adults predominate. The ratio of inapparent infection, as evidenced by a serologic survey study of Australian troops in Vietnam, was 210:1.

CLINICAL MANIFESTATIONS The incubation period is 5 to 15 days. As with SLE, illness may present as encephalitis, aseptic meningitis, or febrile headache. The occurrence of severe rigors at the onset has been noted in almost 90 percent of patients. On admission, most patients are alert, but deterioration of mental status occurs in about three-fourths of patients within 3 to 4 days. Localized paresis is found more often than with other "arboviral" encephalitides, e.g., in 31 percent of cases, with predominantly upper extremity involvement; however, it resolves rapidly with defervescence. Convulsions are frequent in children, but occur in less than 10 percent of adults. Severe hyperthermia may occur and require treatment. A peripheral leukocytosis with 50 to 90 percent neutrophils is common. Weight loss has been very striking. The failure of the temperature to lyse, appearance of diaphoresis, tachypnea, and the accumulation of bronchial secretions are grave prognostic signs.

PROGNOSIS The immediate mortality rate has varied from 7 to 33 percent or higher. The rate of occurrence of sequelae varies inversely with the fatality rate; in those series with high fatality rates (33 percent), sequelae occurred in 3 to 14 percent. In another series with a fatality rate of 7.4 percent, the rate of adverse sequelae was 32 percent. Individuals who had neurologic abnormalities during the acute phase but survived have no more than an 80 percent chance for complete recovery. Sequelae consist of seizures, persistent paralysis, ataxia, mental retardation, and behavioral disorders.

Other "arboviruses" with central nervous system involvement A large group of additional "arboviruses" have been associated with encephalitis or aseptic meningitis. Some of these agents are listed in Table 143-2. Though the epidemiologic picture of each of these agents is unique, the general features are sufficiently similar to require laboratory support for their differentiation.

"ARBOVIRUS" DISEASES PRESENTING CHIEFLY WITH HEMORRHAGIC MANIFESTATIONS For 300 years, yellow fever was the only epidemic viral disease known to be accompanied by grave hemorrhagic manifestations. Since the 1930s diverse viral etiologies of the hemorrhagic fever syndrome have been recognized (Table 143-2). Additional agents include members of several families and genera: flavivirus, Filoviridae, phlebovirus, Nairovirus, the Hantaan group of viruses, and arenavirus (Chap. 144). Despite diverse etiologies, there are many similar clinical manifestations. The onset is usually sudden, with headache, backache, generalized myalgia, conjunctivitis, and prostration. From approximately the third day, the initial stage is followed by hypotension, and hemorrhagic manifestations may occur; these are characterized by bleeding gums, epistaxis, hemoptysis, hematemesis, melena, petechiae, ecchymoses, and hemorrhages into most visceral organs. Mild leukopenia develops early, but with the appearance of hemorrhagic manifestations, leukocytosis may occur. The pathophysiology of the cardinal signs is attributable to hematopoietic and capillary damage, with variable localization of lesions. On the basis of limited confirmatory observations, variable degrees of disseminated intravascular coagulation may be in part responsible for the pathophysiology of the hemorrhagic fever syndromes. Death usually occurs in the second week of disease, at which time a high titer of antibody has developed and the patient may have become afebrile. Death is usually associated with coma, which is due not to encephalitis but to an encephalopathy. The pathologic changes may be similar despite diverse viral etiologies, with midzonal hepatic necrosis and acidophilic cytoplasmic inclusions similar to the Councilman bodies of yellow fever.

Yellow fever Yellow fever is an acute infectious disease of short duration and extremely variable severity; it is caused by a flavivirus and is followed by lifelong immunity. The classic triad of symptoms—jaundice, hemorrhages, and intense albuminuria—is present only in severe infections, which make up only a small proportion of the total.

PREVALENCE For more than 200 years, after the first identifiable outbreak occurred in Yucatan in 1648, yellow fever was one of the great plagues of the world. As late as 1905, New Orleans and other southern United States ports experienced at least 5000 cases and 1000 deaths. Because of the existence of the sylvatic form of the disease, protective measures must be maintained against human disease, as demonstrated by outbreaks in Central America from 1948 to 1957. In southern Ethiopia from 1962 to 1964 there were over 100,000 cases with some 30,000 deaths. From 1978 to 1980 there have been outbreaks in Bolivia, Brazil, Colombia, Ecuador, Peru, and Venezuela. In 1979, yellow fever reappeared in Trinidad. During the same time period extensive epidemics were seen in Nigeria, Ghana, Senegal, and Gambia. In Gambia the attack rate was 2.6 to 4.4 percent with a case fatality rate of 19 percent. In 1983, epidemics occurred in Burkino Faso (formerly Upper Volta) and Ghana.

EPIDEMIOLOGY Human infection results from two basically different cycles of virus transmission, urban and sylvatic. The urban cycle is human-mosquito-human, i.e., *Aëdes aegypti*–transmitted yellow fever. After a 2-week extrinsic incubation period, mosquitoes can transmit infection. Sylvan yellow fever differs under various ecologic circumstances. In the rain forests of South and Central America, species of treetop *Haemagogus* or *Sabethes* mosquitoes maintain transmission in wild primates. Once infected, the mosquito vector remains infectious for life; hence it may serve as a reservoir as well as a vector. When humans come into proximity with the forest-canopy mosquitoes, sporadic cases or focal outbreaks may occur. With sylvan yellow fever, males predominate. Focal outbreaks may be quite extensive; in Brazil in 1973 at least 21,000 persons out of 1.5 million (1.4 percent) were infected. In east Africa, the mosquito-primate cycle is maintained by the forest-canopy mosquito, *A. africanus,* which seldom feeds on humans. The peridomestic mosquito *A. simpsoni* feeds upon primates entering the village gardens and can then in turn transmit the virus to humans. Once yellow fever is reintroduced into urban areas, the urban cycle can be reinitiated, with the potential for epidemic disease. Why yellow fever has never invaded Asia despite widespread distribution of human-biting *A. aegypti* mosquitoes has never been satisfactorily explained.

CLINICAL MANIFESTATIONS The incubation period is usually 3 to 6 days. In accidental laboratory- or hospital-acquired infections longer incubation periods (10 to 13 days) have been reported. In considering the clinical features, it is advantageous to classify the illness as to severity: inapparent, mild, moderately severe, and malignant. In mild yellow fever the only symptoms may be the abrupt onset of fever and headache. Additional symptoms may include nausea, epistaxis, relative bradycardia known as Faget's sign [e.g., with a temperature of 38.9°C (102°F) the pulse may be only 48 to 52 beats per minute], and slight albuminuria. The mild illness lasts only 1 to 3 days and resembles influenza except that coryzal symptoms are lacking.

Moderately severe and malignant attacks of yellow fever are characterized by three distinct clinical periods: the period of infection, the period of remission, and the period of intoxication. Prodromal symptoms are usually absent. The onset is characteristically sudden, with headache, dizziness, and temperature elevations to 40°C (104°F) without a relative bradycardia. Young children may have febrile convulsions. The headache is followed quickly by pains in the neck, back, and legs. Often there is nausea with vomiting and retching. Examination reveals a flushed face and injection of the conjunctivae. The congestion of the eyes persists until the third day. The tongue characteristically shows bright-red margins and tip and a white furred center. Faget's sign appears by the second day. Epistaxis and gingival bleeding are common. On the third day of illness, the fever may fall by crisis and the patient enters remission, or, in the malignant form, copious hemorrhages, anuria, or delirium may occur. The stage of remission lasts from several hours to several days. In the third stage, the "classic" symptoms develop; the fever returns but the pulse remains slow. Jaundice becomes detectable about the third day; however, jaundice often is not prominent even in fatal illnesses. Increased epistaxis, melena, and uterine hemorrhages are common, but gross hematuria is rare. Of the classic signs, "black vomit" is more characteristic than is jaundice. Hematemesis usually does not occur before the fourth day and is often associated with a fatal outcome. Albuminuria, which rarely develops before the third day, occurs in 90 percent of patients and may be quite marked (3 to 20 g albumin per liter). In spite of this massive albuminuria, edema or ascites has not been reported. In malignant infections, coma frequently occurs 2 to 3 days before death. Shortly before death, which usually occurs between the fourth and the sixth days, the patient commonly becomes delirious and wildly agitated. Though the duration of fever in the third stage is usually 5 to 7 days, the period of intoxication is the most variable of the stages and may last up to 2 weeks. Clinical yellow fever is relatively free from complications, suppurative parotitis being the most striking of those which do occur. Clinical relapses are not characteristic of yellow fever.

LABORATORY FINDINGS Early in the disease, progressive leukopenia may occur. By the fifth day, total leukocyte counts of 1500 to 2500 per cubic millimeter often are found, the decrease being due mostly to a decrease in neutrophils. Total leukocyte counts return to normal by the tenth day, and in fatal cases there may be a marked terminal leukocytosis. Hemoglobin values remain normal except terminally, when hemoconcentration or bleeding may occur. Platelet counts are normal or decreased. Prolongation of clotting, prothrombin, and partial thromboplastin times is marked in patients with jaundice. Increases in total and conjugated bilirubin occur. In icteric patients, marked elevations of serum glutamic oxaloacetic transaminase occur. Hypoglycemia has been seen in patients with severe hepatic damage. Electrocardiograms may show T-wave changes. Clinical examinations of cerebrospinal fluid have not revealed abnormalities.

DIAGNOSIS Inoculation onto mosquito cell cultures or intrathoracically into mosquitoes are methods of choice for virus isolation from blood. Isolation is most likely from specimens obtained during the first 3 days of illness. Serologic methods include plaque reduction neutralization tests on paired serums and detection of yellow fever IgM antibodies, and antigen usually by ELISA methods. The ELISA method enables confirmation in the field within 3 h.

TREATMENT The management has been symptomatic and supportive and should be based upon assessment and correction of the circulatory abnormalities. If evidence of disseminated intravascular coagulation is present, the administration of heparin should be considered. Close attention to fluids and electrolytes is essential.

PROGNOSIS The overall fatality rate in yellow fever is between 5 and 10 percent of clinical cases; it may be even less since many infections are mild or inapparent.

PREVENTION Effective control measures are available. Immunization has been effective in the prevention of outbreaks. With the occurrence of sylvatic outbreaks, work in the area of epizootic activity should be discontinued and intensive mosquito abatement measures should be instituted. These measures may provide the time necessary for a mass immunization program.

Dengue hemorrhagic fever All four dengue virus serotypes can cause dengue hemorrhagic fever (DHF) and dengue shock syndrome (DSS). Infection with dengue 1, 3, or 4 followed within a few years by dengue 2 may be especially important in the pathogenesis. There is consensus that DHF is an immunologically mediated disease. Enhanced growth of dengue 2 virus occurs in peripheral blood mononuclear phagocytes obtained from dengue immune donors or in cells from normal donors in the presence of subneutralizing concentrations of dengue or cross-reacting heterotypic flavivirus antibodies. Infectious virus-antibody complexes attach and enter mononuclear phagocytes by way of Fc receptors. Increased replication of virus in these cells may be followed by a secondary set of reactions: complement activation, mast cell degranulation, and activation of the kinin system.

PREVALENCE The reasons for the apparent sudden "appearance" of the syndrome in the past 30 years are completely obscure. However, during the 1922 epidemic of dengue fever in Louisiana, hemorrhagic manifestations, including epistaxis, bleeding gums, melena, menorrhagia, and even "black vomit," were observed. DHF is now a leading cause of morbidity and mortality in tropical Asia. During the past 5 years, over 500,000 cases of DHF have been officially reported with major epidemics in the People's Republic of China, Vietnam, Indonesia, Thailand, and Cuba. In the Cuban outbreak in 1981, almost 350,000 persons developed dengue, approximately 10,000 had hemorrhagic manifestations, and 158 died (1.6 percent mortality). DHF in Asia is a disease of childhood with one peak observed in children under 1 year, and a second in children ages 3 to 5. The disease in infants is associated with primary infection in the presence of maternal antibody. Studies in Thailand have estimated the frequency of DSS as 11 cases per 1000 secondary dengue infections. DSS occurs more frequently in girls than boys. Dengue hemorrhagic fever occurs almost exclusively in indigenous populations; it has been observed only rarely in whites of European descent despite the frequent occurrence of classic dengue in this group.

CLINICAL MANIFESTATIONS Illness begins abruptly with a minor stage characterized by fever, cough, pharyngitis, headache, anorexia, nausea, vomiting, and abdominal pain which is often severe. This continues for 2 to 4 days. In contrast to classic dengue, myalgia, arthralgia, and bone pain are unusual. Physical signs include fever varying from 38.3 to 40.6°C (101 to 105°F), injection of the tonsils and pharynx, and palpable lymph nodes and liver. The initial state is followed by abrupt deterioration, with the rapid onset of lassitude and weakness (Table 143-4). On examination the child is found to

TABLE 143-4 World Health Organization's clinical classification of dengue hemorrhagic fever

	Grade	Clinical features	Laboratory findings
DHF*	I	Fever, constitutional symptoms, positive tourniquet test	Hemoconcentration Thrombocytopenia
DHF*	II	Grade I plus spontaneous bleeding (e.g., skin, gums, gastrointestinal tract)	Hemoconcentration Thrombocytopenia
DHF*, DSS*	III	Grade II plus circulatory failure, agitation	Hemoconcentration Thrombocytopenia
DHF*, DSS*	IV	Grade II plus profound shock (blood pressure = 0)	Hemoconcentration Thrombocytopenia

* *DHF, dengue hemorrhagic fever; DSS, dengue shock syndrome.*

be restless and to have cold clammy extremities with a warm trunk and a pallid face with circumoral cyanosis. Petechiae, most frequently located on the forehead and distal extremities, are seen in half the cases. Occasionally there may be a macular or maculopapular rash. The extremities are frequently cyanotic. Hypotension, with narrowing of the pulse pressure, and tachycardia occur. Pathologic reflexes may be observed. Most fatalities occur in the fourth or fifth day of illness, melena, hematemesis, coma, or unresponsive shock being poor prognostic signs. Cyanosis, dyspnea, and convulsions are terminal manifestations. Following this critical period, survivors show steady and quite rapid improvement.

LABORATORY FINDINGS In one study, hemoconcentration was found in one-fifth of the children. The majority had leukocyte counts between 5000 and 10,000 per cubic millimeter, with one-third showing a leukocytosis. Only 10 percent of children had a true leukopenia. The most characteristic findings were thrombocytopenia, rarely with blood platelets under 75,000 per cubic millimeter, positive tourniquet test, and prolonged bleeding time. Prothrombin time and partial thromboplastin times were usually near normal values. Depression of clotting factors V, VII, IX, and X may be present. Bone marrow examination may reveal maturation arrest of megakaryocytes. In Manila or Bangkok, hematuria has been infrequent even with other serious bleeding manifestations; however, in Tahiti, gross hematuria was common. Cerebrospinal fluid examinations are usually normal. Other abnormal laboratory findings may include hyponatremia, acidosis, elevated blood urea nitrogen levels, elevation in serum glutamic oxalacetic transaminase levels, mild hyperbilirubinemia, and hypoproteinemia. Electrocardiograms may reveal diffuse myocardial abnormalities. Two-thirds of patients have radiologic evidence of bronchopneumonia, with many showing pleural effusions.

DIAGNOSIS The World Health Organization (WHO) has established criteria for the diagnosis of DHF: fever—acute onset, high, continuous, and lasting for 2 to 7 days; hemorrhagic manifestations including at least a positive tourniquet test and any of the following: petechiae, purpura, ecchymoses, epistaxis, bleeding gums, hematemesis, or melena; enlargement of the liver; thrombocytopenia, ≤100,000 per cubic millimeter; hemoconcentration, hematocrit increased by ≥20 percent. Criteria for DSS are a rapid, weak pulse with narrowing of the pulse pressure (≤20 mmHg) or hypotension with cold, clammy skin and restlessness. The WHO classification includes a grading of severity (Table 143-4). Minor hemorrhagic manifestations may be seen during the course of classic dengue fever without meeting WHO criteria for DHF. These cases should be termed dengue fever with hemorrhage, not DHF. For specific viral diagnosis, see "Dengue Fever."

TREATMENT The mainstay is correction of circulatory collapse while avoiding fluid overload. Administration of 5% glucose in 0.5 *N* saline at a rate of 40 mL/kg restored blood pressure within 1 to 2 h in one-half of patients. When stable, the rate of administration of intravenous fluids was slowed to 10 (mL/kg)/h. If improvement did not occur, plasma or a plasma expander (20 mL/kg) was administered. Transfusion of whole blood is not recommended. Oxygen should be administered. Glucocorticosteroids have been used, but doses of 25 mg/kg have not resulted in significant improvement. Since the evidence for severe disseminated intravascular coagulation is questionable, use of heparin is not clear-cut, although in a group of Filipino children with type 3 dengue virus, administration of heparin (1 mg sodium heparin per kilogram) was associated with a dramatic rise in number of platelets and level of plasma fibrinogen. Antibiotics are not indicated; sympathomimetic amines and salicylates are contraindicated. Recovery from vascular collapse usually occurs within 24 to 48 h, at which time diuretics and digitalis may be necessary. An uncontrolled trial of interferon was conducted during the 1981 epidemic in Cuba with some indication of efficacy.

PROGNOSIS Mortality has varied from 1 to 23 percent. Deaths have been most common in infants under 1 year of age.

PREVENTION At present, vector control is the only method available to prevent hemorrhagic fever.

Tick-borne hemorrhagic fevers CRIMEAN-CONGO HEMORRHAGIC FEVER At the close of World War II, a new disease entity was recognized in the Crimea region of the U.S.S.R. Retrospective studies demonstrated that an almost identical syndrome had been recognized in the south central Asian republics of the U.S.S.R. for many years. Soviet workers repeatedly isolated virus strains during 1967 to 1969.

The virus of Crimean hemorrhagic fever (CHF) is antigenically identical with Congo virus, which was isolated from patients, cattle, and ticks in Africa (Kenya, Uganda, Congo, and Nigeria). Crimean-Congo hemorrhagic fever (CCHF) virus is now known from South Africa, throughout most of subSaharan Africa, eastern Europe, the Middle East, and Asia as far as the Xinjiang province of China. CCHF occurs where *Hyalomma* ticks are found.

Approximately 30 cases of CCHF have been recorded annually in each of the known areas of occurrence in the U.S.S.R. The cases occur between April and September. The sex distribution of CCHF is equal, and 80 percent of the cases occur in the 20- to 60-year age group, with the majority occurring in dairy and agricultural workers. The major arthropod vectors for transmission to humans are ticks which belong to the genus *Hyalomma*. Cattle and wild hares appear to be important reservoirs, and rooks and other birds have been implicated. Once a case of human CCHF occurs, person-to-person transmission is possible. Nosocomial outbreaks have occurred in the U.S.S.R., Pakistan, India, and Iraq. Transmission is presumed to occur through direct contact with infected blood. There are no data to suggest airborne transmission.

After an incubation period of 3 to 6 days, the onset is abrupt, with temperatures to 40°C (104°F), dizziness, headache, and diffuse myalgia. The course of fever is occasionally biphasic, with an average duration of 8 days. Physical signs include flushing of the face, conjunctival injection, vomiting, and, on occasion, epigastric pain. Hepatomegaly is found in half the patients. Splenomegaly has been reported in 2 to 25 percent of patients. Respiratory symptoms or signs are unusual. Hemorrhagic manifestations generally begin on the fourth day with petechiae on the oral mucosa and skin, epistaxis, gingival bleeding, hematemesis, and melena. Neurologic abnormalities, seen in 10 to 25 percent of patients, include nuchal rigidity, excitation, and coma. Laboratory findings show leukopenia, with the number of white blood cells falling as low as 1000 per cubic millimeter, and thrombocytopenia, which is often severe. Proteinuria and microscopic hematuria are common, but azotemia and oliguria are not. Convalescence may be prolonged. Death is usually attributed to shock or intercurrent infection. Sequelae include transient alopecia and mono- or polyneuritis.

The major approach to therapy has been supportive. Convalescent immune serum has shown promise if administered during the first 3 days of illness. Patients should be isolated with contact restricted to hospital staff and immediate family. Masks and gowns should be worn, and blood and body fluids handled as infectious. The reported mortality rate has shown variation between 9 and 50 percent.

OMSK HEMORRHAGIC FEVER Omsk hemorrhagic fever (OHF) is an acute febrile disease which occurs in the Omsk and Novosibirsk oblasts in the U.S.S.R. and is caused by a flavivirus. The seasonal occurrence of OHF shows a biphasic pattern with peaks in May and August. The transmission cycle is uncertain. OHF is transmitted to humans either by the bite of infected ticks, *Ixodes apronophorus*, or by the handling of infected muskrats. The natural reservoir includes muskrats, other rodents, especially water voles, and ticks. Epidemics occurred from 1945 to 1948, but recently the disease has been less prevalent.

Following an incubation interval of 3 to 8 days, illness begins abruptly with fever, headache, and hemorrhagic manifestations, which include epistaxis and gastrointestinal and uterine bleeding. Rarely, neurologic abnormalities may occur. Laboratory features include leukopenia. In contrast to many of the other hemorrhagic fevers, OHF has a low case fatality rate (0.5 to 3.0 percent).

KYASANUR FOREST DISEASE Kyasanur Forest disease was first recognized in south India in 1957 as a discrete clinical entity shown to be due to a flavivirus. Kyasanur Forest disease occurs following occupational exposure to *Haemaphysalis spinigera* ticks in the tropical forests of western Mysore in southern India. The silent reservoir cycle which infects the primate- and bird-feeding *Haemaphysalis* ticks is now believed to be *Ixodes* ticks transmitted among small forest mammals, especially the shrew. Laboratory-associated infections have been common.

The major symptoms include abrupt onset of fever, headache, fatigue, myalgia (especially of the lumbar area and calf muscles), and retroorbital pain. Cough and abdominal pain occur in half the patients. Additional symptoms may include photophobia and polyarthralgia. Epistaxis and hematemesis are observed in some patients. On examination, findings include relative bradycardia, conjunctival injection, and generalized lymphadenopathy. Fine and coarse rales are frequently heard. Hepatosplenomegaly has been encountered occasionally. During the initial phase, generalized hyperesthesia of the skin occurs occasionally. The fever usually lasts from 6 to 11 days. After an afebrile period of 9 to 21 days, approximately half the patients may develop a second phase, which lasts from 2 to 12 days. This is manifested by recurrence of fever, severe headache, neck stiffness, mental disturbance, coarse tremors, giddiness, and abnormalities in reflexes, as well as by recurrence of many of the initial symptoms. No sequelae have been observed, but convalescence is often prolonged.

Only limited laboratory studies have been performed. During the initial phase, leukopenia is a constant feature, with a total leukocyte count of fewer than 3000 per cubic millimeter by the fourth to sixth day. The leukopenia is associated with neutropenia. During the second phase there is a mild leukocytosis. Lumbar puncture during the second phase has shown a pattern of aseptic meningitis. Diagnosis is based upon virus isolation from blood; this is readily accomplished, since viremia is prolonged. Serologic tests of paired serums also can be performed. The management is supportive. The mortality rate is approximately 5 percent.

HEMORRHAGIC FEVER WITH RENAL SYNDROME Synonyms for this disease (HFRS) include Korean hemorrhagic fever, far eastern hemorrhagic fever, endemic or epidemic nephrosonephritis, Manchurian epidemic hemorrhagic fever, Songo fever, and Churilov's disease. A similar but milder disease in Scandinavia has been called nephropathica epidemica or epidemic nephritis (EN).

In 1932, the Russians first observed HFRS in southeastern Siberia. In April 1951, a previously unknown illness, subsequently recognized as HFRS, broke out among the United Nations forces in Korea.

Etiology In 1976, the antigen of HFRS was reported in the lungs of the rodent *Apodemus agrarius coreae*. Diagnostic increases in immunofluorescent antibodies were demonstrated in 113 of 116 cases of severe HFRS. The agent designated Hantaan virus is a single-stranded RNA virus belonging to the family Bunyaviridae. It has been proposed as a separate genus (Table 143-1). The Hantaan group consists of at least four agents: Hantaan virus (Korean hemorrhagic fever), Puumala virus (nephropathica epidemica), and two viruses from the United States (Prospect Hill virus and Tchoupitoulas virus) which have not been associated with disease.

Prevalence In Korea between April 1951 and January 1953, 2070 cases of EHF were reported among United Nations personnel. The disease usually occurs as an isolated event; hence, overall attack rates have relatively less meaning. With this reservation, attack rates in two United States Army divisions stationed in Korea varied between 1.9 and 2.9 cases per 1000 persons per epidemic season. Approximately 800 cases per year have continued to occur; however, most cases are now seen in Korean civilians and military with less than 10 cases per year in U.S. military personnel. During the past decade the disease has increased in prevalence in Korea, urban Japan, and in China. The People's Republic of China reported 30,000 hospitalized cases in 1980 and 42,000 in 1981. Hundreds of cases of nephropathica epidemica have occurred annually in Finland and other Scandinavian countries since the 1930s. In 1953 a severe form of HFRS was recognized in the Balkan countries, and in 1982 in Greece and France. Antibody studies indicate worldwide distribution. Antibodies in human serums have been found in Argentina, Brazil, Colombia, Belgium, Canada, the United States, including Hawaii and Alaska, southeast Asia, Egypt, and central Africa.

Epidemiology The majority of cases occur in May to June and in October to November. These peaks coincide with rodent density population. Hantaan virus is present in rodent urine, feces, and saliva in high titer. Transmission from rodent to rodent is primarily respiratory, with transmission to people through inhalation of virus-containing dried excreta. There is no evidence for person-to-person transmission. The urban reservoir appears to be the house rat. Laboratory outbreaks have occurred in the U.S.S.R., Korea, Japan, France, and Belgium with Wistar rats implicated in Korea and Japan.

Clinical manifestations There are two forms of disease, a mild illness characteristically diagnosed in Scandinavia as nephropathica epidemica (NE) and the more severe far eastern form (EHF).

Nephropathica epidemica (NE) is characterized by sudden onset of high fever, backache, headache, and abdominal pain. On the third or fourth day, hemorrhagic manifestations may occur and conjunctival hemorrhages, palatine petechiae, and a petechial rash appear on the trunk. About one patient in five is "toxic" and mentally obtunded. Oliguria and azotemia develop. Urinalysis reveals proteinuria, hematuria, and leukocyturia. After about 3 days the rash subsides, the patient develops polyuria, and recovers over several weeks.

EPIDEMIC HEMORRHAGIC FEVER The incubation period in epidemic hemorrhagic fever (EHF) is usually 10 to 25 days, with possible extremes of 7 and 36 days. Visitors who contract the disease in an endemic area may not develop illness until after their return home.

The clinical course of EHF may be divided into phases on the basis of the underlying physiologic aberrations: febrile, hypotensive, oliguric, diuretic, and convalescent. There is considerable variation among patients in the severity of the illness. In one study two-thirds of the 264 cases studied were classified as mild, while 14 percent were termed severe. The illness in most patients was of comparable severity in each phase.

Febrile (invasive) phase From 10 to 20 percent of patients describe vague prodromal symptoms resembling mild upper respiratory infections. The onset is then usually abrupt, often initiated by a chill and accompanied by fever, headache, backache, abdominal pain, and generalized myalgia. Anorexia and thirst are almost universal, while nausea and vomiting are common although not constant symptoms. The headache is most commonly frontal or retroorbital. Eye symptoms, especially mild photophobia and pain on movement of the eyes, are characteristic. Diarrhea is not a feature. Fever is present in almost all patients; the temperature ranges from 37.8 to 41.1°C (100 to 106°F), reaches a peak on the third or fourth day after onset, and falls by lysis on the fourth to seventh day. There is a relative bradycardia. Initially the blood pressure is normal. One of the most typical early findings is a diffuse reddening of the skin, most marked over the face and V area of the neck that may resemble a severe sunburn. The erythema blanches on pressure. Dermographism can be demonstrated in over 90 percent of patients at the same time as the flush. Slight edema of the upper eyelids causes a bleary-eyed appearance. Bulbar and palpebral conjunctivas show injection. Conjunctival petechiae may develop by the third or fifth day of illness. Subconjunctival hemorrhages may be striking. Intense pharyngeal reddening without significant sore throat is typical. The first location for petechiae is usually the palate, where they occur in half the patients. Within 12 to 24 h, petechiae appear at pressure areas such as the axillary folds, lateral chest wall, belt line, hips, and thighs.

Retinal hemorrhages occur rarely. Cervical, axillary, and inguinal nodes are moderately enlarged but nontender. Abdominal and costovertebral tenderness is almost a constant finding. Splenomegaly is unusual and in Korea was generally attributable to malaria with which EHF coexisted in about 1 percent of patients. The degree of flush, fever, and conjunctival injection and the number of petechiae correlate quite well with the overall severity of illness.

Laboratory studies during this phase are often not striking. Initial hemoglobin and hematocrit values are usually normal. Prior to the fourth day, leukocyte counts range from 3600 to 6000 per cubic millimeter but are associated with neutrophilia. Early in the course urine specific gravity may be high. Albuminuria, which is an almost universal finding, appears, often abruptly, between the second and fifth days of illness. The urinary sediment reveals microscopic hematuria and hyaline, granular, red blood cell casts, and/or white blood cell casts. Erythrocyte sedimentation rates are normal during the first week. Capillary fragility tests are usually positive at the time of admission and become most abnormal by the ninth day. Electrocardiographic abnormalities may be seen in 15 to 30 percent of patients; these include sinus bradycardia and low or inverted T waves. Lumbar punctures may reveal gross blood in the spinal fluid.

Hypotensive phase On about the fifth day of illness, during the last 24 to 48 h of the febrile phase, hypotension or shock may occur. In mild cases, only a transient fall in blood pressure occurs; among moderately and severely ill patients shock may persist for 1 to 3 days. In 828 patients, 16.5 percent had clinical shock, and another 14 percent had hypotension without shock. Headache often diminishes, but thirst persists. In the beginning of the hypotensive phase, most patients have warm, dry skin and extremities. As the hypotensive phase progresses and the systolic blood pressure decreases and pulse pressure narrows, the skin becomes cool and moist. Tachycardia replaces the relative bradycardia.

At this stage, an increase in hematocrit with no change in total serum protein level is found. This is thought to reflect a loss of plasma through damaged capillaries. On about the fifth day, all patients develop marked proteinuria. The previously normal urine specific gravity begins to fall and in 2 to 3 days is usually around 1.010. Blood urea nitrogen concentrations begin to increase. Other laboratory findings include leukocytosis with white blood cell counts of 10,000 to 56,000 per cubic millimeter with neutrophilia and toxic granulation. The number of platelets often decreases to less than 70,000 per cubic millimeter.

Oliguric phase (*hemorrhagic or toxic phase*) About the eighth day of illness, blood pressure returns to the normal range and in some instances increases to hypertensive levels. While oliguria may have appeared during the shock phase, it now becomes a prominent feature. Oliguria develops even though hypotension was not recognized. Symptomatically patients continue to feel weak and thirsty and have more severe backache. Protracted vomiting and hiccups may ensue.

Blood urea nitrogen levels increase rapidly and are associated with hyperkalemia, hyperphosphatemia, and hypocalcemia. Metabolic acidosis is rarely severe. Although platelets begin to return to normal, hemorrhagic manifestations become more prominent and include petechiae, hematemesis (analogous to "black vomit" in yellow fever), melena, hemoptysis, gross hematuria, and hemorrhages into the central nervous system. The enlarged lymph nodes may now become tender.

With the onset of diuresis on about the seventh day in moderately ill patients and the ninth to eleventh day in severely ill patients, symptoms of fluid and electrolyte abnormalities and central nervous system or pulmonary complications may appear. Central nervous system symptoms include disorientation, extreme restlessness, lethargy, paranoid delusions, and hallucinations. Grand mal seizures, pulmonary edema, and pulmonary infection occur in some patients.

Diuretic phase With the onset of diuresis, progressive improvement is the rule. Most patients begin to eat and regain their strength. In fatal cases the diuretic phase is associated with a daily urine output of less than 4 liters and often less than 2 liters, in contrast to larger volumes in surviving patients.

Convalescent phase The convalescent phase lasts 3 to 6 weeks. Weight is regained slowly. Complaints include muscular weakness, intention tremor, and lack of stamina. Hyposthenuria and polyuria are present; however, within 2 months most patients are able to concentrate their urine to a specific gravity of 1.023 or greater after a 12-h period of water deprivation.

Diagnosis Diagnosis is based on demonstration of specific IgM antibodies by ELISA or a fourfold change in immune adherence hemagglutination titers in paired serums.

Treatment Clinical management primarily revolves around meticulous supportive care. Trials with a variety of agents including antibiotics, adrenocortical steroid hormones, antihistamines, and convalescent serum were without significant beneficial effect during the Korean epidemics.

Prognosis The Soviet experience indicates a mortality rate of 3 to 32 percent; in China, the case fatality ratio was 7 to 15 percent. Between April 1951 and December 1976 the overall case fatality ratio in Korea was 6.6 percent.

Residua are uncommon. Of 783 surviving patients cared for at the Hemorrhagic Fever Center in Korea between April and December 1952, only 16 were unable to return to duty within a period of 4 months. Fifteen of these individuals still had hyposthenuria. Follow-up studies on former EHF patients 3 to 5 years later showed that they had many more subsequent hospital admissions for urologic problems than did a control group and that the relative frequency correlated with the severity of the acute episode of EHF. Asymptomatic residual renal tubular dysfunction may be more common than has been appreciated.

REFERENCES

"Arboviruses": Definition and classification

FIELDS BN et al (eds): *Virology*. New York, Raven, 1985

"Arbovirus" infections characterized by fever, malaise, headaches, and myalgia

BECKER FE: Tick-borne infections in Colorado. Col Med 27:36, 1930

BOWEN GS et al: Clinical aspects of human Venezuelan equine encephalitis in Texas, 1971. Bull Pan Am Health Org 10:46, 1976

BRICENO ROSSIE AL: Rural epidemic encephalitis in Venezuela caused by a group A arbovirus (VEE). Prog Med Virol 9:176, 1967

CALISHER CH et al: Rio Grande—a new phlebotomus fever group virus from south Texas. Am J Trop Med Hyg 26:997, 1977

DIETZ WH JR et al: Ten clinical cases of human infection with Venezuelan equine encephalomyelitis virus, subtype I-D. Am J Trop Med Hyg 28:329, 1979

FLEMING J et al: Sandfly fever. Review of 664 cases. Lancet 1:443, 1947

GOODPASTURE HC et al: Colorado tick fever: Clinical, epidemiologic and laboratory aspects of 228 cases in Colorado in 1973–1974. Ann Intern Med 88:303, 1978

HUGHES LE et al: Persistence of Colorado tick fever virus in red blood cells. Am J Trop Med Hyg 23:530, 1974

LAUGHLIN LW et al: Epidemic Rift Valley fever in Egypt: Observations of the spectrum of human illness. Trans R Soc Trop Med Hyg 73:630, 1979

LENNETTE EH, KOPROWSKI H: Human infection with Venezuelan equine encephalomyelitis virus. JAMA 123:1088, 1943

SCHERER WF et al: Ecologic studies of Venezuelan encephalitis virus in Southeastern Mexico: VII. Infection of man. Am J Trop Med 21:79, 1972

SIAM AL et al: Rift Valley fever ocular manifestations: Observations during 1977 epidemic in Egypt. Br J Ophthalmol 64:366, 1980

SPRUANCE SL, BAILEY A: Colorado tick fever. A review of 115 laboratory confirmed cases. Arch Intern Med 131:288, 1973

VAN VELDEN et al: Rift Valley fever affecting humans in South Africa: A clinicopathologic study. S Afr Med J 29:867, 1977

"Arbovirus" infections presenting chiefly with fever, malaise, arthralgia, and rash

AASKOV JG et al: An epidemic of Ross River virus infection in Fiji, 1979. Am J Trop Med Hyg 30:1053, 1981

CLARK JA et al: Annually recurrent epidemic polyarthritis and Ross River virus activity in a coastal area of New South Wales. I. Occurrence of the disease. Am J Trop Med Hyg 22:543, 1973

DELLER JJ JR, RUSSELL PK: Chikungunya disease. Am J Trop Med 17:107, 1968
MALHERBE H et al: Sindbis virus infection in man. Report of a case with recovery of virus from skin lesions. S Afr Med J 37:547, 1963
PINHEIRO FP et al: An outbreak of Mayaro virus disease in Belterra, Brazil: I. Clinical and virological findings. Am J Trop Med Hyg 30:674, 1981
ROBINSON MC: An epidemic of virus disease in Southern Province, Tanganyika territory in 1952–53: I. Clinical features. Trans R Soc Trop Med Hyg 49:28, 1955
SHORE H: O'nyong-nyong fever: An epidemic virus disease in East Africa: III. Some clinical and epidemiological observations in the Northern Province of Uganda. Trans R Soc Trop Med Hyg 55:361, 1961

"Arbovirus" infections presenting chiefly with fever, malaise, lymphadenopathy, and rash

ALVAREZ MD, RAMÍREZ-RONDA CH: Dengue and hepatic failure. Am J Med 79:670, 1985
CENTERS FOR DISEASE CONTROL: Dengue in the United States, 1983–1984. CDC Surveillance Summaries 34(255):555, 1985
MARBERG K et al: The natural history of West Nile fever: I. Clinical observations during an epidemic in Israel. Am J Hyg 64:259, 1956
MICKS DW, MOON WB: *Aëdes aegypti* in a Texas coastal county as an index of dengue fever receptivity and control. Am J Trop Med Hyg 29:1382, 1980
PERELMAN A, STERN J: Acute pancreatitis in West Nile fever. Am J Trop Med Hyg 23:1150, 1974
TAYLOR RM et al: A study of the ecology of West Nile virus in Egypt. Am J Trop Med 5:579, 1956

"Arbovirus" infections presenting chiefly with central nervous system involvement

BALFOUR HH JR et al: California arbovirus (LaCrosse) infections. Pediatrics 52:680, 1973
CENTERS FOR DISEASE CONTROL: Arboviral infections of the central nervous system—United States, 1984. Morb Mort Week Rep 34:283, 1985
DICKERSON RB et al: Diagnosis and immediate prognosis of Japanese B encephalitis. Observations based on more than 200 patients with detailed analysis of 65 serologically confirmed cases. Am J Med 12:277, 1952
EDELMAN R, PARYANONDA A: Human immunoglobulin M antibody in the serodiagnosis of Japanese encephalitis virus infections. Am J Epidemiol 98:29, 1973
FINLEY KH et al: Western equine and St. Louis encephalitis. Preliminary report of a clinical follow-up study in California. Neurology 5:223, 1955
GRABOW JD et al: The electroencephalogram and clinical sequelae of California arbovirus encephalitis. Neurology 19:394, 1969
HILTY MD et al: California encephalitis in children. Am J Dis Child 124:530, 1972
KETEL WB, OGNIBENE AJ: Japanese B encephalitis in Vietnam. Am J Med Sci 261:271, 1971
LUBY JP et al: The epidemiology of St. Louis encephalitis (SLE): A review. Ann Rev Med 20:329, 1969
———: Antigenemia in St. Louis encephalitis. Am J Trop Med Hyg 29:265, 1980
SCHNEIDER RJ et al: Clinical sequelae after Japanese encephalitis: One year follow-up study in Thailand. Southeast Asian J Trop Med Public Health 5:560, 1974
WEAVER OM et al: Japanese encephalitis: Sequelae. Neurology 8:887, 1958

"Arbovirus" diseases presenting primarily with hemorrhagic manifestations

BURNEY MI et al: Nosocomial outbreak of viral hemorrhagic fever caused by Crimean hemorrhagic fever—Congo virus in Pakistan, January 1976. Am J Trop Med Hyg 29:941, 1980
CASALS J et al: A current appraisal of hemorrhagic fevers in the USSR. Am J Trop Med 15:751, 1966
CENTERS FOR DISEASE CONTROL: Viral hemorrhagic fever. Initial management of suspected and confirmed cases. Ann Intern Med 101:73, 1984
DENNIS LH et al: The original hemorrhagic fever: Yellow fever. Blood 30:858, 1967
HALSTEAD SB, O'ROURKE EF: Dengue viruses and mononuclear phagocytes: I. Infection enhancement by non-neutralizing antibody. J Exp Med 146:201, 1977
———: Dengue hemorrhagic fever—a public health problem and a field for research. Bull WHO 58:1, 1980
———: The pathogenesis of dengue: Molecular epidemiology in infectious disease. Am J Epidemiol 114:632, 1981
KIRK R: An epidemic of yellow fever in the Nuba Mountains, Anglo-Egyptian Sudan. Ann Trop Med Parasitol 35:67, 1941
LEE HW et al: Isolation of the etiologic agent of Korean hemorrhagic fever. J Infect Dis 137:298, 1978
MONATH TP et al: Yellow fever in the Gambia, 1978–1979: Epidemiologic aspects with observations on the occurrence of Orongo virus infections. Am J Trop Med Hyg 29:912, 1980
———: Pathophysiologic correlations in a monkey model of yellow fever with special observations on the acute necrosis of B cell areas of lymphoid tissues. Am J Trop Med Hyg 30:431, 1981
NELSON ER: Hemorrhagic fever in children in Thailand: Report of 69 cases. J Pediatr 56:101, 1960
PINHEIRO FP et al: An epidemic of yellow fever in Central Brazil 1972–1973: I. Epidemiological studies. Am J Trop Med Hyg 27:125, 1978
Technical guide for diagnosis, treatment, surveillance, prevention and control of dengue hemorrhagic fever. Geneva, World Health Organization, 1982
WORLD HEALTH ORGANIZATION: Hemorrhagic fever with renal syndrome: Memorandum from a WHO meeting. Bull WHO 61:269, 1983

144 ARENAVIRUS INFECTIONS

JAY P. SANFORD

DEFINITION AND CLASSIFICATION The term *arenavirus* is the proposed designation for a group of RNA viruses which have unique morphology. The virions are round, oval, or pleomorphic, with diameters between 60 and 350 nm, and contain an electron-dense membrane with projections and 2 to 10 inclusion-like dense particles (resembling ribosomes) that give the virion an appearance of having been sprinkled with sand (Latin *arenaceus*, "sandy"). Eleven distinct arenaviruses have been described (Table 144-1). All except Tacaribe are parasites of rodents, and most are unique to tropical America. A special property of arenaviruses that cause disease in humans, especially Machupo and lymphocytic choriomeningitis, is their capacity to induce persistent infection in their reservoir hosts with no ill effects and in the absence of an immune response.

LYMPHOCYTIC CHORIOMENINGITIS The first-recognized arenavirus was lymphocytic choriomeningitis (LCM) virus. It was recognized early that LCM was carried by apparently healthy laboratory mice. Clinically LCM has been considered primarily in the context of aseptic meningitis; however, it is associated with at least two clinical syndromes in humans: central nervous system and influenza-like illness which may be associated with rash, arthritis, or orchitis. LCM virus has provided a valuable model for the study of chronic, persistent, and generally symptomless viral infections in laboratory animals.

Prevalence In the United States human infection with LCM virus is rare; however, seroepidemiologic studies on specimens obtained in 1935 to 1940 from persons with no history of central nervous system disease from all parts of the United States revealed neutralizing antibodies in 10 to 28 percent. In recent years, the prevalence of infection seems to have decreased markedly.

Epidemiology The virus of LCM is worldwide in distribution. Foci of LCM virus have been defined in Germany, Hungary, and elsewhere in Europe. Scandinavia appears to be LCM virus–free as are most of the Americas except Argentina. Although infection can be induced

TABLE 144-1 Classification of arenaviruses

Virus	Clinical disease	Reservoir	Known geographic range
Lymphocytic choriomeningitis	Aseptic meningitis, meningoencephalitis, influenzal syndrome, orchitis, arthritis	Mice, hamsters	Worldwide except Australia
Tacaribe		Bats	Trinidad
Junin	Argentinian hemorrhagic fever	*Calomys musculinus*	Argentina
Machupo	Bolivian hemorrhagic fever	*Calomys callosus*	Northeast Bolivia
Amapari			Brazil
Latino			Bolivia
Parana			Paraguay
Pichinde			Colombia
Tamiami			Florida
Lassa	Lassa fever	*Mastomys natalensis*	Nigeria, Liberia, Sierra Leone, Republic of Guinea, Central African Republic
Flexal		*Orzomys* sp.	Brazil

in a variety of animals, mice are the major natural reservoir as well as the primary host in which latent, asymptomatic infection occurs. The latency of infection in the mouse depends upon immunologic tolerance. Animals infected in utero or shortly after birth excrete LCM virus for life without overt disease. Human infections are secondary to contact with an infected rodent. The mode of transmission is thought to be via airborne spread or contact with excrement from infected animals. In the past, most cases have arisen in persons living in rodent-infested houses, but lately outbreaks of LCM virus disease in humans have been reported from Germany and from the United States in which the source of infection was traced to laboratory animals and household pets, specifically hamsters which, like mice, can shed LCM virus in urine and stool. LCM occurs throughout the year but has been more frequent in the colder months when "the mice come in from the fields." Person-to-person transmission has not been demonstrated.

Pathogenesis In natural infection, the portal of entry of the LCM virus is probably through the respiratory tract. Virus multiplication occurs initially in the respiratory epithelium, and an influenza-like illness develops. Dissemination of virus to extrapulmonary sites, presumably to reticuloendothelial cells with multiplication, and viremia occur. LCM virus crosses the blood-brain barrier. In mice, the resulting meningitis is attributed to a cell-mediated immune reaction. Support for this hypothesis derives from observations that disease but not infection can be prevented in experimental animals by neonatal thymectomy, irradiation, or immunodepressant drugs such as cyclophosphamide. Similar pathogenetic mechanisms may operate in humans, although isolation of LCM virus from the CSF of patients with aseptic meningitis is quite common.

Clinical manifestations The exact incubation period is not known. Following experimental inoculation of LCM virus into volunteers, fever occurred in $1\frac{1}{2}$ to 3 days, while an influenza-like constellation of symptoms developed 5 to 10 days after exposure. An influenza-like illness is the commonest clinical pattern. In some patients, up to one-half in some series, the illness may be biphasic with subsequent aseptic meningitis or encephalomyelitis. Fever, usually from 38.3 to 40°C (101 to 104°F), associated with rigors, is uniformly noted. Other symptoms which are encountered in over one-half of patients include malaise, weakness, myalgia (especially lumbar aching), retroorbital headache, photophobia, anorexia, nausea, and light-headedness. Other prominent symptoms which occur in one-fourth to one-half of patients include sore throat, vomiting, and dysesthesias. Later arthralgias, especially in the hands, occur. Less common complaints (up to one-quarter of patients) include aching pain in the chest, associated with pneumonitis; increased hair loss progressing to generalized alopecia, 2 or 3 weeks after the onset of illness; testicular pain or frank orchitis, usually unilateral, again 1 to 3 weeks after onset; and parotid pain, which may lead to a misdiagnosis of mumps. Physical findings in the first week of illness are few. Patients often have a relative bradycardia. Pharyngeal injection without exudate is commonly seen (60 percent). Mild nontender cervical or axillary lymphadenopathy may occur. The initial phase lasts from 5 days to 3 weeks followed by improvement. After a remission of 1 to 2 days many patients relapse with recurrent fever and more prominent headache. Physical signs may include skin rashes, swelling of metacarpophalangeal and proximal interphalangeal joints, meningeal signs, orchitis, parotitis, and alopecia. Convalescence generally is of 1 to 4 weeks' duration, characterized by easy fatigability, an excessive need for sleep, dysesthesias, and occasional dizziness. Patients with aseptic meningitis almost always recover without sequelae. With encephalitis, 25 to 30 percent of patients have neurologic residua.

Laboratory findings Leukopenia and thrombocytopenia are almost uniform during the first week of illness. Although leukocyte counts usually vary between 2000 and 3000 per cubic millimeter, counts as low as 600 per cubic millimeter have been recorded. Differential counts generally show slight relative lymphocytosis. Platelet counts are usually between 50,000 and 100,000 per cubic millimeter. Anemia is not encountered. The erythrocyte sedimentation rate often is normal. Mild elevations of serum glutamic oxaloacetic transaminase (SGOT) and lactic dehydrogenase (LDH) may occur. Chest radiographs may suggest basilar pneumonias. In patients with meningeal signs examination of the cerebrospinal fluid usually reveals several hundred cells per cubic millimeter, although cell counts in excess of 1000 per cubic millimeter are reported in half the patients in some series. Lymphocytes predominate (greater than 80 percent) even early. The initial cerebrospinal fluid protein is usually slightly elevated, but on occasion levels may exceed 150 mg/dL. Although a normal cerebrospinal fluid glucose level is considered the hallmark of viral meningitides, hypoglycorrhachia has been observed in up to 27 percent of patients with LCM, glucose values as low as 15 mg/dL with normal simultaneous blood sugar levels having been reported.

Diagnosis The diagnosis of LCM can be established with certainty by recovery of the virus from blood or spinal fluid. Complement-fixing antibodies are usually detectable 1 to 2 weeks after the onset of infection, peak at 5 to 8 weeks, and are gone by 6 months. Neutralizing antibodies appear after 6 to 8 weeks, increase in titer slowly, and remain high for years. Immunofluorescent studies have detected antibody to LCM virus earlier in the course of illness, and its appearance seems to parallel the development of the neurologic phase. The clinical manifestations of LCM cannot be differentiated from those produced by numerous other viruses.

Treatment There is no specific treatment.

ARGENTINIAN AND BOLIVIAN HEMORRHAGIC FEVERS The first cases of a new American hemorrhagic disease were seen near the Argentinian town of Junin near Buenos Aires in 1953. A virus was isolated from patients' blood and from local rodents and their mites. In 1959, cases of a disease thought to resemble severe epidemic typhus were noted among rural workers in northeastern Bolivia. The similarity between these syndromes was recognized. In 1963, the causal virus was isolated from patients and rodents and named the Machupo virus. Machupo virus is serologically related to but distinct from Junin virus.

Prevalence Junin virus infections have occurred in epidemic form since 1958 with between 100 and 3500 cases reported annually. The hemorrhagic disease in Bolivia has been particularly severe. Of a total population of 4000 to 6000 in the endemic area, 750 persons were affected between 1959 and 1963.

Epidemiology Argentinian hemorrhagic fever (AHF) occurs in sharply endemic seasonal form (February to August), mostly among male rural workers, especially those exposed to fields at the time of the maize harvest. Virus is transmitted in the urine of rodents with chronic infection and viruria. Humans acquire the virus through contact with items or foodstuffs which have been contaminated with infected rodent urine. The main reservior is two species of cricetidae, *Calomys laucha* and *C. musculinus*.

Bolivian hemorrhagic fever (BHF) is similarly transmitted by the urine of *C. callosus* (a mouselike rodent) chronically infected with Machupo virus. Direct person-to-person transmission is possible and may have occurred in the outbreak in Cochabamba. Disease has not occurred in medical personnel attending infected patients.

Clinical features Argentinian hemorrhagic fever presents manifestations of renal, cardiovascular, and hematologic involvement. Inapparent infections are rare. The incubation period is estimated to be 7 to 16 days, followed by a gradual onset of chills, fever, headache, malaise, myalgia, anorexia, nausea, and vomiting. The temperature reaches 38.9 to 40°C (102 to 104°F), facial flushing may be prominent, and there is a painless enanthem of the pharynx. Lymphadenopathy and splenomegaly are not present. From 3 to 5 days after the onset, the signs and symptoms worsen, with the appearance of signs of dehydration, hypotension to 50 to 100 mmHg, oliguria, and relative bradycardia. In the more severe cases, hemorrhagic manifestations, including bleeding from the gums, hematemesis, hematuria, and melena, occur. Progressive oliguria and tremor of the tongue and extremities may develop. Some patients develop psychic manifestations, with agitation, delirium, or stupor. Progressive shock, hypothermia, gallop rhythm, or gastrointestinal bleeding may occur from the seventh to tenth days. In fatal cases, pulmonary edema usually is the cause of death. During convalescence temporary alopecia has been noted. Erythrocyte counts are normal or elevated. The total leukocyte count drops to 1200 to 3400 blood cells per cubic millimeter. Thrombocytopenia may occur. Disseminated intravascular coagulation does not seem to be the mechanism responsible for the hemorrhagic manifestations. Complement components C2, C3, and C5 are decreased. The urine is dark and may approach the color of mahogany, with intense albuminuria. Blood urea nitrogen levels rise rapidly.

The clinical picture of Bolivian hemorrhagic fever is similar to Argentinian, although epistaxis and hematemesis at the onset is more common.

Diagnosis Antibody responses, including IgM antibodies, do not occur before 10 to 20 days.

Treatment Treatment consists of supportive measures, including peritoneal dialysis or hemodialysis-filtration to correct both the azotemia and the pulmonary edema. In AHF, a double-blind trial of administration of immune plasma reduced mortality from 16 to 1 percent. However, fever and cerebellar signs occurred in patients treated with immune plasma. Preliminary studies suggest that ribavirin may be effective in experimental BHF in rhesus monkeys.

Prognosis The mortality rate among patients with Argentinian hemorrhagic fever is usually 3 to 15 percent, while that in Bolivian hemorrhagic fever is 5 to 30 percent.

Prevention In Bolivia, rodent control measures directed primarily against *C. callosus* populations in the houses has resulted in a prompt and dramatic cessation of human cases. In Argentina, the wide dispersal of infected hosts renders rodent control measures futile.

LASSA FEVER A virus disease which is both highly contagious and virulent occurred in a missionary nurse in Lassa, a town in northeast Nigeria, in 1969.

Epidemiology Since the initial outbreak at Lassa in 1969, during which one of the patients was transferred to New York City, there have been other outbreaks near Jos in northern Nigeria in 1970 (32 suspected cases with 10 deaths), in Zorzor, Liberia, in 1972 (11 cases with 4 deaths), and in the eastern province of Sierra Leone with 63 suspected cases admitted to two hospitals between 1970 and 1972. Lassa fever occurs as an endemic disease in eastern Sierra Leone. Population surveys showed more than one-half of older adults had antibodies. Other countries in west Africa having clinical or serologic evidence of Lassa fever include Senegal, Gambia, Guinea, Ghana, Burkina Faso (formerly Upper Volta), Mali, and Ivory Coast. Lassa-related viruses (Mopeia, Mobala) have been isolated from rodents in Mozambique, Zimbabwe, and the Central African Republic; however, they have not yet been associated with human illness. In Jos and Zorzor, outbreaks apparently resulted from person-to-person nosocomial spread from the index case to hospital workers or other patients. In Sierra Leone, the great majority of cases were acquired outside the hospital, although hospital workers were at risk. *Mastomys natalensis,* a multimammate rat widespread in Africa, is the animal reservoir, and primary human cases result from contamination of foodstuffs with rodent urine. Human-to-human transmission may occur through contact with urine, feces, vomitus, or saliva through droplets, and particularly through wounds contaminated with blood. Intrafamilial outbreaks have occurred around several cases. There are a number of cases which have been acquired through accidental autoinoculation with needles while starting intravenous fluids. At least one laboratory-acquired infection has occurred. In Sierra Leone 6 percent of the population surveyed had complement-fixing antibody against Lassa virus, while only 0.2 percent had recognized disease, suggesting mild disease or inapparent infection. In Liberia 10 percent of hospital personnel had antibodies.

Clinical features The incubation period is 1 to 24 days, and was 10 days following accidental inoculation. Patients have ranged from 5 months to 46 years of age; approximately two-thirds are women. Three of eight women in one series were 22 to 28 weeks pregnant during their illness. The apparent predilection for women may relate to exposure to contaminated food or work in hospitals rather than to differences in susceptibility. The onset of illness was described by most patients as insidious. The most frequent initial symptoms were fever (100 percent), chilliness and true rigors, headache (50 percent), malaise (100 percent), and myalgia (50 percent). Most patients did not seek medical attention for 4 to 9 days after onset. Symptoms of a systemic viral illness then developed with anorexia, nausea, vomiting, myalgia, and pain in the chest, epigastrium, and lumbar area. Headache was usually present. Early examination revealed fever and flushing of the face and V area of the neck. Pharyngitis developed early and became progressively more severe during the first week; examination in some cases revealed raised patches of whitish exudate occurring on the palatine arches which occasionally coalesced into a pseudomembrane. Oral ulcerations have been noted in up to one-half of cases. Generalized nontender lymphadenopathy occurred in one-half of patients. During the second week severe lower abdominal pain and intractable vomiting were common, and facial and neck swelling with conjunctival edema and infection frequently developed. Occasionally patients had tinnitus, epistaxis, bleeding from the gums and venipuncture sites, maculopapular rashes, cough, and dizziness. During the acute stage, systolic blood pressures of less than 90 mmHg, with pulse pressures less than 20 mmHg, occurred in 60 to 80 percent of patients. Initially, relative bradycardia was common. During the second week, the patients who recovered defervesced, while the patients who died often developed signs of shock, clouding of the sensorium, rales, signs of pleural effusion, agitation and, on occasion, grand mal seizures. The duration of illness in surviving patients ranged from 7 to 31 days (average 15 days), while that in fatal cases was 7 to 26 days (average 12 days). The mortality rates in Jos and Zorzor were 52 percent and 36 percent, respectively, while in Sierra Leone the rate was 8 percent. During convalescence occasional flurries of rapid involuntary eye movements (oculogyric crises) occurred. Late sequelae include deafness in a number of patients (two of six in one series) and alopecia in one patient.

Laboratory features The hematologic findings include relatively normal hematocrit values and early leukopenia (less than 4000 cells per cubic millimeter in 36 percent) with a relative neutrophilia and immature forms of leukocytes. In two cases in which it was recorded, the erythrocyte sedimentation rate was normal. Urinalyses revealed proteinuria, which was often massive. Chest radiographs may suggest basilar pneumonitis and pleural effusions. Electrocardiographic abnormalities compatible with diffuse myocardial disease have been encountered. Levels of serum enzymes, SGOT, creatinine phosphokinase (CPK), and LDH have been elevated. Lassa virus has been recovered from cerebrospinal fluid in two patients.

Diagnosis Diagnosis can be made by demonstrating a fourfold rise in antibody titer to Lassa virus between acute phase and convalescent phase serum specimens with the indirect fluorescent antibody technique or with Lassa IgM antibodies. The diagnosis is unlikely if IgM antibodies are absent by the fourteenth day of illness.

Treatment The management has been supportive. Infusion of immune plasma from convalescent patients resulted in a dramatic effect in three of four patients. Because of the self-limited nature of the disease, these results cannot be assessed easily. In a study of the antiviral agent ribavirin, 19 of 20 patients treated intravenously within 6 days of onset with a 2.0-g loading dose, followed by 1.0 g every 6 h for 4 days, then 0.5 g every 8 h for another 6 days, survived, whereas 11 of 18 who received no therapy, and 10 of 16 who received convalescent plasma died. In view of the hospital association and the presence of virus in pharyngeal secretions and urine, respiratory and enteric isolation and blood precautions are required. With reasonable isolation practices, nosocomial spread need not be as feared as previously.

OTHER HEMORRHAGIC FEVERS Ebola hemorrhagic fever and Marburg virus disease are caused by members of the family Filoviridae and are discussed in Chap. 142 and summarized in Table 143-1.

REFERENCES

BAUM SG et al: Epidemic non-meningitic lymphocytic-choriomeningitis virus infection. N Engl J Med 274:934, 1966

CASALS J: Arenaviruses. Yale J Biol Med 48:115, 1975

CENTERS FOR DISEASE CONTROL: Viral hemorrhagic fever. Initial management of suspected and confirmed cases. Ann Intern Med 101:73, 1984

FARMER TW, JANEWAY CA: Infections with the virus of lymphocytic choriomeningitis. Medicine 21:1, 1942

FIELDS BN et al (eds): *Virology*. New York, Raven, 1985

FRAME JD et al: Lassa fever, a new virus disease of man from West Africa: I. Clinical description and pathological findings. Am J Trop Med Hyg 19:670, 1970

JOHNSON KM et al: Hemorrhagic fever of Southeast Asia and South America. A comparative approach. Prog Med Virol 9:105, 1967

MCCORMICK JB et al: Lassa fever: Effective therapy with ribavirin. N Engl J Med 314:20, 1986

MACKENZIE RB et al: Epidemic hemorrhagic fever in Bolivia: 1. A preliminary report of the epidemiologic and clinical findings in a new epidemic area in South America. Am J Trop Med Hyg 13:620, 1964

MAIZTEGUI JI et al: Efficacy of immune plasma in treatment of Argentine hemorrhagic fever and association between treatment and a late neurological syndrome. Lancet 2:1216, 1979

MERTENS PE et al: Clinical presentation of Lassa fever cases during the hospital epidemic at Zorzor, Liberia, March–April 1972. Am J Trop Med Hyg 22:780, 1973

MONATH TP et al: Lassa fever in the Eastern Province of Sierra Leone, 1970–1972: II. Clinical observations and virological studies on selected hospital cases. Am J Trop Med Hyg 23:1140, 1974

VANZEE BE et al: Lymphocytic choriomeningitis in University hospital personnel. Clinical features. Am J Med 58:803, 1975

145 VIRAL WARTS

RICHARD C. REICHMAN

DEFINITION Warts are epithelial tumors that result from papillomavirus (PV) infection of skin or mucous membranes.

ETIOLOGY PV, members of the A genus of the family Papovaviridae, are nonenveloped viruses, 50 to 55 nm in diameter, with icosahedral capsids composed of 72 capsomeres. They contain a double-stranded, circular DNA genome of about 8000 base pairs. PV appear to be species specific, and human papillomaviruses (HPV) have not been propagated in tissue culture or in experimental animals. Significant quantities of virus are difficult to obtain, and HPV are incompletely characterized. Suitable HPV antigens have not been available and work on the epidemiology, pathogenesis, immunology, and treatment of HPV-induced disease has been difficult to carry out. Structural viral proteins make up 88 percent of the mass of PV virions. A major capsid protein with a molecular weight of 55,000 and as many as 10 additional polypeptides have been identified by sodium dodecyl sulfate polyacrylamide gel electrophoresis. Four cellular histones are associated with the viral DNA. Type-specific antigenic determinants appear to be located on the virion surface and genus-specific determinants internally. Antisera produced by immunization of experimental animals with disrupted PV virions are broadly cross-reactive.

The genomic organization of all PV is similar. Types and subtypes are defined by degree of polynucleotide sequence homology under stringent conditions. DNA of a distinct PV type has a maximum of 50 percent homology with that of other classified viruses. Viruses with greater than 50 percent but less than 100 percent homology constitute subtypes. More than 40 types of HPV are recognized. Individual types are associated with specific kinds of warts (Table 145-1).

TABLE 145-1 Correlation of human papillomavirus (HPV) type with disease

Virus type	Disease
1	Plantar and palmar warts
2	Common warts
3, 10, 28, 29	Flat warts
4	Plantar and common warts
5, 8, 9, 12, 14, 15, 17, 19–25, 36, 39, 40	Epidermodysplasia verruciformis
6,11	Condyloma acuminatum, respiratory papillomatosis
7	Common warts in meat and animal handlers
13, 32	Focal epithelial hyperplasia (Heck's disease)
16, 18, 31, 33, 35	Genital dysplasias and carcinomas
26, 27	Warts in immunosuppressed patients
30, 34, 37, 38	Isolated cases of benign and malignant neoplasms

EPIDEMIOLOGY Seroepidemiologic studies of HPV infections have been hampered severely by lack of appropriate antigens, and there are few good studies of the incidence or prevalence of human warts in well-defined populations. Common warts are found in as many as 25 percent of some groups, and are most prevalent among young children. Plantar warts are also widely prevalent and occur most commonly among adolescents and young adults. The incidence of venereal warts (condylomata acuminata) has risen dramatically in the last 10 to 15 years, and condyloma acuminatum is one of the most common sexually transmitted diseases in the United States.

CLINICAL MANIFESTATIONS Until the mid-1970s, it was generally believed that there was only one HPV and that clinical and pathologic differences among warts were a function of the nature of the squamous epithelium at the site of infection. With the discovery of multiple HPVs, it has become clear that the specific HPV is an important determinant of the nature of the lesion. Thus, clinical manifestations of HPV infection depend upon location of lesions and virus type. Common warts (verrucae vulgaris) usually occur on the hands, and are flesh-colored to brown, exophytic, hyperkeratotic papules. Plantar warts (verrucae plantaris) differ from most other warts by growing inward. They may be quite painful, and can be differentiated from callus by paring the surface to reveal thrombosed capillaries that bleed easily. Flat warts (verrucae plana) are most common among children and occur on the face, neck, chest, and flexor surfaces of forearms and legs.

Anogenital warts (condylomata acuminata, or venereal warts) occur on skin and mucosal surfaces of external genitalia and perianal areas. The differential diagnosis of anogenital warts includes condylomata lata of secondary syphilis, molluscum contagiosum, pearly penile papules, fibroepitheliomas, and a variety of mucocutaneous malignancies. Anogenital warts are sexually transmitted, and have an incubation period of 1 to 6 months. In men, condylomata are found most frequently at the frenum or coronal sulcus, but they may affect any part of the penis. They occur commonly at the urethral meatus, and may extend proximally. Perianal warts are common among homosexual men, but appear in heterosexual men as well. In women, warts appear first at the posterior introitus and adjacent labia. They then spread to other parts of the vulva and commonly involve the perineum and anus. Condylomata frequently involve the vagina and cervix. These lesions may be present in the absence of external warts. Laryngeal papillomatosis is uncommon, occurs predominantly in preschool children, and may result from acquisition of virus at the time of delivery through an infected birth canal. These lesions are typically multiple and may produce life-threatening airway obstruction. Disease in adults may be acquired by orogenital sexual contact.

Immunosuppressed patients, particularly those undergoing organ transplantation, often develop pityriasis rosea–like lesions from which DNA of several HPV types has been extracted. Occasionally, such lesions appear to undergo malignant transformation.

Epidermodysplasia verruciformis is a rare, autosomal recessive disease characterized by the inability to terminate HPV infection and later development of cutaneous squamous cell malignancies. Lesions resemble flat warts or macules similar to those of pityriasis rosea.

Complications of warts include itching and occasionally bleeding. Rarely, they may become secondarily infected with bacteria or fungi. Large masses of warts may produce mechanical problems such as obstruction of the birth canal. Epidemiologic, cytopathologic and histologic data suggest an association of HPV infection with dysplasia and carcinoma of the uterine cervix. HPV nucleic acid sequences have been detected in cervical scrapings and biopsy specimens from patients with these pathologic findings. Sequences homologous to HPV types 16 and 18 have been found in 70 to 80 percent of specimens of cervical cancer tissue from patients in certain geographic areas. Other genital tract malignancies have also been associated with these viruses.

PATHOGENESIS HPV infection is transmitted by close personal contact and is facilitated by minor trauma at the site of inoculation. It may result from direct contact with another individual, by autoinoculation, or via fomites. All types of squamous epithelium may be infected by HPV, and gross and histologic appearances of individual lesions vary with site of infection and virus type. Exophytic warts are characterized by papillomatosis, hyperkeratosis, and elongation of dermal papillae. Acanthosis, an increase in cellularity, occurs in the prickle cell layer in association with viral DNA synthesis. Late gene expression, manifested by appearance of structural proteins and assembled virions, is evident within nuclei of cells in the granular layer, where koilocytosis develops. Koilocytes are large round cells with pyknotic nuclei and large areas of perinuclear vacuolization surrounded by a ring of dense amphophilic cytoplasm.

Host defense responses to HPV infection are poorly understood. Most immunologic studies are difficult to interpret because crude and poorly characterized preparations have been employed as antigens. The potential importance of type-specific responses has not been adequately evaluated because the recognition that there are multiple HPV types is new, and appropriate antigenic materials are not widely available. Virus-specific IgM and IgG antibodies have been demonstrated in patients with and without clinical evidence of active infection. Cell-mediated immune responses to HPV antigens have also been measured, and patients with defects in cell-mediated immunity appear to be more susceptible than normals to HPV infections. Such patients occasionally develop extensive HPV disease.

DIAGNOSIS Most warts that are visible to the naked eye can be diagnosed correctly by history and physical examination alone. Colposcopy is invaluable in assessing vaginal and cervical lesions, and may prove to be helpful in the diagnosis of oral and cutaneous HPV disease as well. Papanicolaou smears prepared from cervical scrapings often show cytologic evidence of HPV infection. Persistent or atypical lesions should be biopsied and examined by routine histologic methods. In addition, the genus-specific capsid antigen can be identified in tissue sections using immunologic techniques, and virus type can be determined by restriction endonuclease analysis of DNA extracted from infected tissues and by hybridization with nucleic acid probes.

TREATMENT Therapy should be initiated with the knowledge that no treatment of proven safety and efficacy is currently available, and that many warts resolve spontaneously. Frequently used therapies include application of caustic agents, cryosurgery, electrodesiccation, surgical excision, and ablation with laser. Topical antimetabolites such as 5-fluorouracil have been used also. Failure as well as recurrence have been well-documented following all these methods of treatment. The high frequency of recurrence may be explained by the presence of HPV DNA in normal-appearing tissue adjacent to lesions, and in previously involved areas during periods of remission. For many years, topically applied podophyllum preparations have been used in treatment of condyloma acuminatum. However, use of these compounds is associated with resolution rates of less than 50 percent, and initial treatment of venereal warts with cryosurgery may be preferable. Promising preliminary results have been observed in the treatment of laryngeal papillomatosis and condyloma acuminatum with different interferon preparations.

At the present time, no effective methods of prevention are available for warts other than avoiding contact with infectious lesions. Barrier methods of contraception may be helpful in preventing transmission of condyloma acuminatum.

REFERENCES

CRUM CP et al: Human papillomavirus type 16 and early cervical neoplasia. N Engl J Med 310:880, 1984

DURST M et al: A papillomavirus DNA from a cervical carcinoma and its prevalence in cancer biopsy samples from different geographic regions. Proc Natl Acad Sci USA 80:3812, 1983

FERENCZY A et al: Latent papillomavirus and recurring genital warts. N Engl J Med 313:784, 1985

JENSON AB et al: Human papillomaviruses, in *Textbook of Human Virology*, RB Belshe (ed). Littleton, Mass, Wright-PSG Publishing, 1984, pp 951–968

LUTZNER MA et al: Clinical observations, virologic studies, and treatment trials in patients with epidermodysplasia verruciformis, a disease induced by specific human pipillomaviruses. J Invest Dermatol 83:18s, 1984

ORIEL JD: Genital warts, in *Sexually Transmitted Diseases*, KK Holmes et al (eds). New York, McGraw-Hill, 1984, chap 46

PFISTER H: Biology and biochemistry of papillomaviruses, in *Reviews of Physiology, Biochemistry and Pharmacology*, vol 99, RH Adrian et al (eds). New York, Springer-Verlag, 1984, pp 111–210

SHAH KV: Papovaviruses, in *Virology*, BN Fields et al (eds). New York, Raven, 1985

STEINBERG BM et al: Laryngeal papillomavirus infection during clinical remission. N Engl J Med 308:1261, 1983

VANCE JC et al: Intralesional recombinant alpha-2 interferon for the treatment of patients with condyloma acuminatum or verruca plantaris. Arch Dermatol (in press)

section 7 Infections caused by higher bacteria and fungi

146 FUNGAL INFECTIONS

JOHN E. BENNETT

INTRODUCTION Actinomycetes and fungi are considered together in this section, but this should not obscure profound differences between these two groups of organisms. The agents of actinomycosis, nocardiosis, and actinomycetoma are actinomycetes. These organisms are gram-positive higher bacteria which branch but have the diameter, antibiotic susceptibility, and ability to induce a neutrophilic inflammatory response in common with other bacteria. Actinomycetes resemble fungi in causing infections which may be extremely chronic and which are poorly transmissible from person to person. Few other similarities exist between fungi and actinomycetes. This introductory section will concern mycoses.

The diagnosis of a mycosis requires demonstration of the pathogenic fungus in appropriate patient specimens. Visualization of the fungus by smear or histology is a less precise and less sensitive diagnostic method than culture but is more rapid. Culture allows definitive identification of the pathogen and can detect a small number of organisms. False-positives occur with both methods. Artifacts may be mistaken for fungi in smears or histologic sections. *Candida albicans* can be isolated from the mouth, vagina, sputum, urine, or stool in the absence of candidiasis. *Aspergillus* and, occasionally, *Cryptococcus neoformans* appear in sputum of patients without a mycosis. Histology has the uniquely valuable potential of demonstrating the fungus within the area of inflammation. Only this method can show whether *Aspergillus* in the lung or paranasal sinus tissue exists as a pathogen or merely as a saprophyte growing in pooled secretions. Demonstration of fungi in tissue section usually requires special stains, such as methenamine silver.

Skin testing with fungal antigens has little diagnostic value in active infection. Serologic testing is very helpful in diagnosing coccidioidomycosis and cryptococcosis, as well as in following response to therapy of these mycoses. In histoplasmosis, and paracoccidioidomycosis, serologic tests are useful in adding some support to the clinical diagnosis. A positive serology may provide the impetus for more aggressive diagnostic maneuvers. Serologic results differ enough between laboratories that the physician must know the individual laboratory's experience and expertise.

Topical therapy of a mycosis can be very effective if the fungus is confined to the epidermis or squamous mucosa. Ringworm of the glabrous skin, tinea versicolor, and candidiasis of the skin and mucosa often respond to topical therapy, whereas infection of the skin's deeper layers, such as occurs in sporotrichosis, chromomycosis, mycetoma, and blastomycosis, fails to improve with topical drugs. Allergic bronchopulmonary aspergillosis is presented in Chap. 203.

ANTIFUNGAL AGENTS

TOPICAL AGENTS Imidazoles and triazoles These synthetic compounds act by inhibiting ergosterol synthesis in the fungal cell wall and also probably by direct damage to the cytoplasmic membrane. Drug resistance rarely arises in the previously sensitive strains. Agents of this class include three topical drugs already on the market in the United States: miconazole, clotrimazole, and econazole. Ketoconazole cream will soon be on the market. Compounds currently available elsewhere or undergoing trial include tioconazole, bifonazole, terconazole, isoconazole, and sulconazole. Miconazole is available without prescription. As yet, no substantial difference in efficacy or local intolerance between these agents has appeared. All are effective in treatment of cutaneous candidiasis, tinea versicolor, and mild to moderately severe ringworm of the glabrous skin. Vaginal formulations are effective in vulvovaginal candidiasis. Clotrimazole is poorly absorbed from the gastrointestinal tract, but the oral troche is useful as a topical treatment for oral and esophageal candidiasis.

Polyene macrolide antibiotics These broad-spectrum antifungal agents combine with sterol in the fungal cytoplasmic membrane, increasing membrane permeability. Topically they are not active against ringworm but are effective against candidiasis of the skin and mucous membranes. Nystatin suspension is effective in oral thrush, and vaginal troches are effective in vulvovaginal candidiasis. Both nystatin and amphotericin B are available in topical preparations for cutaneous candidiasis. Natamycin ophthalmic suspension is marketed in some countries for mycotic keratitis and conjunctivitis.

Other topical antifungals Ciclopirox olamine and haloprogin have the same clinical spectrum among the cutaneous mycoses as the imidazoles. Tolnaftate and undecylenic acid are effective against ringworm but not candidiasis. Keratolytic agents, such as salicyclic acid, are helpful as accessory drugs for some hyperkeratotic skin lesions. Many other topical antifungal preparations are available.

SYSTEMIC ANTIFUNGALS Griseofulvin Griseofulvin is a useful drug in treating certain kinds of ringworm; however, it is ineffective in treating candidiasis. The microcrystalline and ultramicrocrystalline preparations differ in dose but not in efficacy. Absorption of both is enhanced when drug is ingested with fat-containing foods. Griseofulvin metabolism interacts with phenobarbital and coumarin-type anticoagulants.

Imidazoles and triazoles Ketoconazole is the only systemically absorbed oral drug of this class that is currently available, though similar drugs are now undergoing clinical trial. Absorption of ketoconazole is variable between individuals, not affected by food, and poor in patients taking cimetidine or ranitidine. Simultaneous administration of antacids can also impair absorption. Metabolism is chiefly hepatic, although substantial liver disease has minimal effect on blood ketoconazole concentrations. Ketoconazole blood levels are decreased in patients takin rifampin and also possibly isoniazid. Ketoconazole administration can elevate cyclosporin blood levels and, occasionally, can enhance the anticoagulant effect of warfarin. Neither renal disease nor hemodialysis affects the metabolism of ketoconazole. The most common toxicity of ketoconazole is dose-related nausea, anorexia and, occasionally, vomiting. Hepatotoxicity is idiosyncratic and usually mild. Serious hepatotoxicity is rare but can be fatal. Several dose-related, temporary endocrine effects have been observed: decreased adrenal reserve; gynecomastia; decreased serum testosterone, libido, and potency in males; and menstrual irregularity in females. Pruritus or rash may also occur. Ketoconazole is effective in blastomycosis, histoplasmosis, paracoccidioidomycosis, chronic mucocutaneous candidiasis, esophageal candidiasis, and some forms of disseminated coccidioidomycosis and pseudallescheriasis. Partial improvement may be seen in cutaneous sporotrichosis and chromomycosis. Although vulvovaginal candidiasis, ringworm, and tinea versicolor are responsive to the drug, the toxicity of oral ketoconazole makes topical imidazoles or other drugs preferable for these indications. Miconazole is available as both a topical and an intravenous preparation. The latter is rarely indicated.

Amphotericin B A colloidal preparation of this drug is available for intravenous or intrathecal administration. The drug cannot be given intramuscularly and is not absorbed orally. Sodium or potassium salts must not be added to the infusion solutions because the colloidal drug will precipitate out of solution. In-line filters with 0.22-μm pore diameter may trap some of the colloid. Within the bloodstream, the drug binds first to plasma lipoproteins and then transfers to tissues throughout the body. The tissue-bound drug slowly elutes back into the blood. Catabolism is extremely slow and is not influenced by renal failure, hepatic failure, or hemodialysis. Penetration into cerebrospinal fluid and vitreous humor is poor; however, concentrations in pleural, peritoneal, and articular exudates are adequate for many mycoses. Histoplasmosis, blastomycosis, paracoccidioidomycosis, candidiasis, and cryptococcosis are the most responsive mycoses. Coccidioidomycosis, extraarticular sporotrichosis, aspergillosis, and mucormycosis are less responsive; chromomycosis, mycetoma, and pseudallescheriasis show little if any response. The usual course is 8 to 10 weeks of 0.4 to 0.6 mg/kg daily. Infusions are generally given in 5% dextrose over 2 to 4 h. Severe febrile reactions to initial doses generally prompt use of an initial test dose with 1 mg, followed by escalating doses based upon the gravity of the patient's infection and tolerance of the drug. Essentially all patients show substantial toxic reactions that are related to the dose and duration of therapy. These side effects include azotemia, anemia, hypokalemia, nausea, anorexia, weight loss, phlebitis and, occasionally, hypomagnesemia. Intrathecal amphotericin B is indicated in coccidioidal meningitis and refractory cryptococcal meningitis, though this therapy is associated with formidable toxicity. Doses of 0.1 to 0.5 mg are given three times per week initially, then with decreasing frequency.

Flucytosine Flucytosine (5-fluorocytosine) is a synthetic oral drug useful in cryptococcosis, candidiasis, and chromomycosis. Within the fungal cell, flucytosine is converted to the antimetabolite 5-fluorouracil. Drug resistance appears rather rapidly when flucytosine is used alone. For this reason the drug is used frequently in combination with amphotericin B, permitting a lower dose of the latter. The usual regimen is amphotericin B 0.3 mg/kg daily and flucytosine 37.5 mg/kg every 6 h. Flucytosine is well absorbed from the gastrointestinal tract, even in the presence of food. The drug penetrates well into the cerebrospinal fluid and is excreted unchanged in the urine. Hemodialysis results in significant drug removal. Even modest reductions in renal function may elevate flucytosine blood levels into the toxic range, meaning more than 100 or 125 μg/mL. Elevated levels are associated with a significant incidence of neutropenia and thrombocytopenia. Elevated flucytosine blood levels also seem to predispose to colitis, the other major toxicity of this drug. Hepatotoxicity is idiosyncratic and uncommon. An allergic rash may also occur.

THE DEEP MYCOSES

CRYPTOCOCCOSIS Etiology Cryptococcosis is an infection caused by the yeastlike fungus *Cryptococcus neoformans. C. neoformans* reproduces by budding and forms round, yeastlike cells 4 to 6 μm in diameter. Within the host and on certain culture media, a large polysaccharide capsule surrounds each yeast cell. The fungus grows well as smooth, creamy white colonies on Sabouraud's or other simple media at 20 to 37°C. Certain culture media for ringworm contain cycloheximide, which inhibits *C. neoformans*. Identification is based on gross and microscopic appearance, biochemical tests, and growth at 37°C. The fungus has four capsular serotypes, designated A, B, C, and D, and a perfect state called *Filobasidiella neoformans.*

Pathogenesis and pathology Infection is thought to be acquired by inhalation of fungus into the lungs. Pulmonary infection has a tendency toward spontaneous resolution and is frequently asymptomatic. Silent hematogenous spread to the brain leads to clusters of cryptococci in the perivascular areas of cortical gray matter, basal ganglia, and, to a lesser extent, other areas of the central nervous system. Inflammatory response around these foci is usually scant. In the more chronic cases, a dense basilar arachnoiditis occurs. Lung lesions show an intense granulomatous inflammation. Cryptococci are best seen in tissue by staining with methenamine silver or periodic acid Schiff. A strongly positive mucicarmine stain of the organism in tissue is diagnostic, but staining varies from intense to absent.

Cryptococcus neoformans has been isolated from several sites in nature, particularly weathered pigeon droppings. Patients are usually unaware of any unusual exposure to pigeon droppings. No significant case clustering, highly endemic areas, or racial or occupational predisposition is known. Infection before puberty is uncommon. The male/female ratio is about 2:1. Approximately half the patients have a predisposing condition, such as lymphoma or sarcoidosis, or are receiving supraphysiological doses of adrenal corticosteroids. Patients with the acquired immunodeficiency syndrome (AIDS) are prone to develop rapidly progressive cryptococcosis that is difficult to cure. Neither neutropenia nor hypogammaglobulinemia seems to increase susceptibility to cryptococcosis. Cryptococcosis occurs in animals, especially the cat family. Transmission from animals to humans or from person to person has not been documented.

Clinical manifestations The majority of patients have *meningoencephalitis* at the time of diagnosis. This form of the infection is invariably fatal without appropriate therapy, and death occurs anywhere from 2 weeks to several years from onset of symptoms. Early manifestations include headache, nausea, staggering gait, dementia, irritability, confusion, and blurred vision. Both fever and nuchal rigidity are often mild or absent. Papilledema is present in one-third of the patients at the time of diagnosis. Cranial nerve palsies, typically asymmetric, occur in about one-fourth of the patients. Other lateralizing signs are rare. With progression of the infection, deepening coma and signs of brainstem compression appear. Autopsy often reveals cerebral edema in the more acute cases or hydrocephalus in more chronic cases.

Pulmonary cryptococcosis causes chest pain in about 40 percent of patients and cough in 20 percent. Chest x-ray shows one or more dense infiltrates, which are often well circumscribed. Cavitation, pleural effusions, or hilar adenopathy are infrequent. Calcification is not present, and fibrotic stranding is rarely noticeable.

Skin lesions are present in 10 percent of patients with cryptococcosis. These appear to be hematogenously disseminated because the vast majority of patients will be found to have disseminated infection. One or a few asymptomatic tiny papular lesions appear, slowly enlarge, and tend to show central softening leading to ulceration. Osteolytic bone lesions occur in 4 percent of patients and usually present as a cold abscess. Rare manifestations of cryptococcosis include prostatitis, endophthalmitis, hepatitis, pericarditis, endocarditis, and renal abscess.

Diagnosis Cryptococcal meningoencephalitis must be distinguished from tuberculosis, neoplasm, coccidioidomycosis, histoplasmosis, candidiasis, viral meningitis, and sarcoidosis. Focal lesions are virtually never demonstrable in cryptococcosis by technetium brain scan, cerebral angiography, or electroencephalogram. Computerized tomography (CT) scan will occasionally show one or two areas of decreased density with contrast-enhancing margins. Lumbar puncture is the single most useful test. An india ink smear of centrifuged spinal fluid sediment reveals encapsulated yeast in one-half the cases, but artifacts resembling cryptococci may cause confusion. Cerebrospinal fluid glucose is reduced in half the cases, protein concentration is usually increased, and 20 to 600 leukocytes per cubic millimeter are typically present and consist predominantly of lymphocytes. Approximately 90 percent of patients with cryptococcal meningoencephalitis, including all those with a positive cerebrospinal fluid smear, will have capsular antigen detectable in cerebrospinal fluid or serum by latex agglutination. False-positive tests occur occasionally, making culture the definitive diagnostic test. *C. neoformans* is often present in urine in patients with meningoencephalitis. Fungemia occurs in 10 percent of patients.

Pulmonary cryptococcosis mimics malignancy by x-ray and symptoms. Sputum culture is positive in only 10 percent, and serum antigen tests are positive in only a third. Occasionally, *C. neoformans* appears in one or multiple sputum specimens as an endobronchial saprophyte. Biopsy is usually required for diagnosis of pulmonary cryptococcosis. Cutaneous cryptococcosis may be mistaken for a comedo, basal-cell carcinoma, or sarcoidosis. Biopsy reveals a myriad of cryptococci. Osseous cryptococcosis resembles tuberculosis.

Treatment Cryptococcal meningoencephalitis may be treated either with amphotericin B alone or in combination with flucytosine. Amphotericin B is given as 0.5 to 0.6 mg/kg per day when used alone or as 0.3 mg/kg per day in combination therapy. With either regimen, double-dose therapy on alternate days may be employed. Flucytosine is given as 150 mg/kg per day divided into four doses, 6 h apart. Reduction of the dose is required in patients with compromised renal function. Lesser nephrotoxicity and more rapid culture conversion with the combination have led to its general acceptance. With either regimen, approximately 50 to 70 percent of patients can be cured. Treatment with either regimen is continued for at least 6 weeks and until at least four weekly cultures of 2 to 4 mL cerebrospinal fluid are sterile. Intrathecal amphotericin B is usually reserved for treatment of patients refractory to conventional therapy. Permanent sequelae include dementia, personality change, hydrocephalus, and blindness.

Patients with extraneural cryptococcosis most often require intravenous amphotericin B, with or without flucytosine. Observation or excision of lesions may suffice for some patients who are previously normal, who have a single focus in lung, skin, or bone, and who have no cryptococci in the cerebrospinal fluid, urine, or blood. All too often, however, patients who present with a presumed single focus of extracranial cryptococcosis are discovered to have early asymptomatic meningoencephalitis or dissemination to other organs.

BLASTOMYCOSIS Etiology *Blastomyces dermatitidis* is a dimorphic fungus, growing at room temperature as a white or tan mold but growing within the host or at 37°C as budding, round yeastlike cells. The fungus is identified by its appearance, its dimorphism, and the appearance of small spores borne on hyphae of the mold form. When isolates of the two opposite mating types are grown closely together on specialized culture media, sporulating structures appear which characterize the perfect form, *Ajellomyces dermatitidis*.

Pathogenesis and pathology The infection is restricted by geography and age. Blastomycosis is uncommon in any locality, but the majority of cases occur in the southeast, central, and midatlantic areas of the United States, with occasional cases in other localities in the United States and Canada. Cases have also been encountered in Africa, Mexico, Central America, and, rarely, South America. Most patients are between 20 and 69 years old. The male/female ratio is about 10:1. There is no occupational predisposition.

Infection appears to be acquired by inhalation of the fungus from nature, but the reservoir remains unknown. The fungus has been isolated only rarely from sources other than infected humans or animals. No carrier state or transmission from animal to human or from person to person has been observed. The initial pulmonary infection may heal spontaneously or become chronic. Spread to other portions of the lung, cavitation, or endobronchial lesions may appear in chronic cases. Whether or not the lung lesion resolves spontaneously, infection commonly spreads hematogenously to skin, subcutaneous tissue, bone, prostate, epididymis, or mucosa of the nose, mouth, or larynx. Less commonly, infection spreads to the brain, meninges, liver, lymph nodes, or spleen. Dissemination may not be evident for weeks or years after the appearance of the lung lesion. Progressive infection is only rarely attributable to an underlying disease or immunosuppressive treatment. The inflammatory response includes lymphocytes, giant cells, and neutrophils. Pseudoepitheliomatous hyperplasia may be striking and lead to a mistaken diagnosis of squamous-cell carcinoma.

Clinical manifestations A small number of patients have an acute, self-limited pneumonia. Fever, productive cough, myalgia, and malaise usually have resolved within a month. Pulmonary infiltrates have cleared slowly as *B. dermatitidis* disappeared from the sputum. Laboratory exposure or case clusters in certain geographic sites have suggested the diagnosis in many of these cases. In one such case cluster, the incubation period appeared to be 4 weeks. In none of these case clusters has the exact activity leading to exposure been identified.

The vast majority of patients with blastomycosis have an indolent onset and a chronically progressive course. Fever, cough, weight loss, lassitude, skin lesions, and chest ache are common symptoms. Skin lesions favor exposed areas and enlarge over many weeks from a pimple to a well-circumscribed, verrucous, crusted, or ulcerated lesion. Pain and regional lymphadenopathy are minimal. Large chronic lesions may show central healing with scarring and contracture. Mucous membrane lesions resemble squamous-cell carcinoma. Chest x-ray is abnormal in two-thirds of cases, with one or more pneumonic or nodular infiltrates. Calcification, hilar adenopathy, and large pleural effusions are rare. Osteolytic lesions may occur in nearly any bone and present as cold abscess or a draining sinus. Extension to a contiguous joint may cause indolent swelling, pain, and restricted motion. Prostatic and epididymal lesions resemble tuberculosis clinically.

Diagnosis The diagnosis is made by demonstrating the fungus in culture of sputum, pus, or urine. In experienced hands, diagnosis by appearance of the organism in wet smear or histopathologic section is adequate. The fungus may be visible in a sputum cytology smear but is easily overlooked. Skin tests and serologic tests lack sufficient sensitivity and specificity to be useful.

Treatment A few patients have been observed with transitory lung lesions, but no guidelines are known to distinguish these patients from those who will progress locally or disseminate. Therefore, every patient should receive treatment. Intravenous amphotericin B is the most established drug and is the drug of choice for patients with rapidly progressive infections, severe illness, or meningitis. Skin and noncavitary lung lesions should be treated for about 8 to 10 weeks. The recommended total dose for an adult is about 2.0 g. Cavitary lung disease or infection beyond the lung and skin should be treated for about 10 to 12 weeks with 2.5 g or more. Ketoconazole is an effective drug in patients with indolent nonmeningeal blastomycosis of mild to moderate severity and who take the drug reliably. The initial adult dose is 400 mg once daily, raised after a month to 600 or 800 mg daily if improvement is suboptimal. Therapy is continued for 6 to 12 months. Iodide therapy is ineffective. The mortality rate in appropriately treated cases is 15 percent or less.

HISTOPLASMOSIS Etiology *Histoplasma capsulatum* is a dimorphic fungus that grows in nature or on Sabouraud's agar at room temperature as a mold. Hyphae bear both large and small spores that are used for identification. *H. capsulatum* grows as a small budding yeast in host tissue and on enriched agar, such as blood cysteine glucose, at 37°C. Despite the name, the fungus is unencapsulated. When two isolates of the opposite mating type, both in mold form, are grown closely together on an appropriate culture medium, specialized spore-bearing structures are formed which characterize the perfect state, *Emmonsiella capsulata*.

Pathogenesis and pathology Infection with *H. capsulatum* has been encountered in many areas of the world but is much more frequent in certain areas. Within the United States infection is most common in the southeastern, midatlantic, and central states. Endemic areas are probably determined by the availability of proper conditions in nature for growth of the fungus. *H. capsulatum* prefers moist surface soil, particularly when it is enriched by droppings of certain birds and bats. The fungus has not only been isolated repeatedly from such sites but many case clusters have occurred 5 to 18 days after groups were exposed to such dust, for example, by raking, cleaning dirt-floored chicken coops, bulldozing, or cave exploring. In many endemic areas, 80 percent or more of residents over age 16 have been exposed, judging by skin test reactivity.

Microconidia, or small spores, of *H. capsulatum* are small enough to reach the alveoli on inhalation and are transformed to budding forms. With time, an intense granulomatous reaction occurs. Caseation necrosis or calcification may mimic tuberculosis. The primary infection in children usually heals completely but may leave spotty calcification in the hilar nodes or lung. Transient dissemination may leave calcified granulomas in the spleen. In adults, a rounded mass of scar tissue, with or without central calcification, may remain in the lung. This has been called a *histoplasmoma.* Previous exposure is thought to confer some protection against reinfection, but infection of persons with prior positive skin tests clearly has occurred.

In a small proportion of patients, histoplasmosis becomes a progressive, potentially fatal infection. The disease occurs either as chronic fibrocavitary pneumonia or, less commonly, as disseminated infection. Patients with either form lack a history of acute primary pulmonary histoplasmosis. Chronic pulmonary infection favors otherwise healthy males over the age of 40. A history of cigarette use can be elicited from nearly all patients with chronic progressive pulmonary histoplasmosis. An acute, rapidly fatal course is most likely to be encountered in young children and immunosuppressed patients, including those with AIDS. A more chronic but equally lethal disseminated infection is more common in previously healthy adults.

Clinical manifestations The vast majority of infections are either asymptomatic or mild, and the diagnosis is elusive. Cough, fever, malaise, and chest x-ray findings of hilar adenopathy with or without one or more areas of pneumonitis occur. Erythema nodosum and erythema multiforme have been reported in a few outbreaks. Hilar adenopathy may cause temporary compression of the right middle lobe bronchus in children and young adults. Subacute pericarditis may occur, probably by extension from contiguous lymph nodes. Rarely, hilar nodes undergo a caseous, granulomatous reaction with perinodal fibrosis. Mediastinal structures become encased by progressive fibrosis, and, over many years, compression of the pulmonary veins, superior vena cava, pulmonary arteries, and esophagus may occur. Late in mediastinal disease only rare nonviable histoplasma can be found in caseous residua of lymph nodes.

Patients with *chronic pulmonary histoplasmosis* have a gradual onset over weeks or months of increasing productive cough, weight loss, and sometimes night sweats. Chest x-ray reveals uni- or bilateral fibronodular apical infiltrates. Approximately one-third of cases will stabilize or improve spontaneously early in the course. The remainder have insidious progression. Retraction and cavitation of the upper lobes occur with spread to the apex of the lower lobes and other areas of the lung. Emphysema and bullae formation further compromise pulmonary function. Death from cor pulmonale, bacterial pneumonia, or histoplasmosis occurs after months or years.

Acute disseminated histoplasmosis may be mistaken for miliary tuberculosis (see Chap. 119). Common findings include fever, emaciation, hepatosplenomegaly, lymphadenopathy, jaundice, anemia, leukopenia, and thrombocytopenia. All these features may occur in chronic dissemination as well, but the disease tends to be more localized. Indurated ulcers of the mouth, tongue, nose, or larynx occur in about a fourth of patients. Other focal findings include granulomatous hepatitis, Addison's disease, gastrointestinal ulceration, endocarditis, and chronic meningitis. Chest x-ray abnormalities occur in half the cases and show discrete nodules or a miliary pattern.

The presumed *ocular histoplasmosis* syndrome is a distinct clinical form of uveitis. Although a positive histoplasmin skin test is a requisite for diagnosis, none of these patients has had active histoplasmosis.

Diagnosis Histoplasmosis may be suspected by serologic tests and clinical manifestations, but definitive diagnosis requires demonstration of the organism by culture or histology. Serologic tests are performed with either a culture filtrate called histoplasmin or with whole yeast form cells. The results are interchangeable. Complement fixation is quantifiable and is the best test. Agar gel diffusion with histoplasmin is a useful but not quantifiable test. An H band on agar gel testing is more diagnostic of active histoplasmosis than an M band. Frequent false-negatives and false-positives limit all current serologic tests. Serologic conversion is helpful but occurs rarely except in acute pulmonary histoplasmosis. Higher complement fixation titers, such as 1:32 or greater, are most suggestive of the diagnosis, but no titer is diagnostic. Cross-reactions with serologic tests for blastomycosis are very common. A 5-mm or more diameter area of induration 24 to 48 h after skin testing with histoplasmin has been very helpful in identifying prior exposure to *Histoplasma,* but false-negatives and false-positives are so frequent that skin testing has little value in the study of ill patients. Further, approximately one-fifth of normal volunteers with a positive skin test will convert their histoplasmin serology from negative to positive after skin testing.

Culture of *H. capsulatum* from sputum is difficult but is the procedure of choice in chronic pulmonary histoplasmosis. Digestion by proteolytic enzymes and centrifugation of sputum are helpful. In disseminated histoplasmosis, cultures of bone marrow, blood, centrifuged urine sediment, and biopsy specimens are most often positive. Cultures should be performed on agar surfaces of enriched media at room temperature. Growth occurs in 2 to 6 weeks. Histologic sections of bone marrow, liver, lymph node, lung, and mucosal lesions may yield the diagnosis.

Treatment Acute pulmonary histoplasmosis requires no therapy. Mediastinal fibrosis may benefit by surgery, but the ultimate prognosis is poor. All patients with disseminated or chronic fibronodular pulmonary histoplasmosis should receive chemotherapy. The indications for using ketoconazole, as well as the treatment regimen, are the same as those given in the section on "Blastomycosis." Amphotericin B is given as 0.4 to 0.5 mg/kg per day or double that on alternate days, continued for at least 10 weeks. In chronic pulmonary histoplasmosis, chest x-ray abnormalities improve somewhat, but pulmonary function improves very little. Successful therapy prevents progression. Addisonian crisis is a preventable cause of death in disseminated histoplasmosis.

African histoplasmosis Patients have been encountered in Africa who seem to be infected with *H. capsulatum* except that the yeast form is larger. Clinical manifestations resemble blastomycosis more than histoplasmosis because skin and bone lesions are very common.

COCCIDIOIDOMYCOSIS Etiology *Coccidioides immitis* has two forms, growing as a white fluffy mold on most culture media but as a nonbudding spherical form, a spherule, in host tissue or under specialized conditions. Reproduction in the host tissue is by formation of small endospores within mature spherules. After rupture of the spherule, the released endospores enlarge, become spherules, and repeat the cycle. The fungus is identified by its appearance and by formation of thick-walled, barrel-shaped spores, called *arthrospores,* in the hyphae of the mold form.

Pathogenesis and pathology *C. immitis* is a soil saprophyte in certain arid regions of the United States, Mexico, Central America, and South America. Within the United States, most cases are acquired in California, Arizona, West Texas, and New Mexico. A few cases are acquired in bordering areas and by exposure to fomites from endemic areas, such as cotton bales.

Infection in humans and animals results from inhalation of windborne arthrospores arising from soil sites. This primary pulmonary infection is symptomatic in only 40 percent of individuals, with symptoms ranging from a mild, influenza-like illness to severe pneumonia. Mild, self-limited infections may come to medical attention because of case clusters or hypersensitivity reactions:

erythema nodosum, erythema multiforme, toxic erythema, arthralgia, arthritis, conjunctivitis, or episcleritis. Case clusters occur 10 to 14 days after a group of susceptible individuals is exposed to dust in an endemic area through such activities as unearthing Indian relics, rock hunting, military maneuvers, or construction. Wind storms can carry spores to adjacent nonendemic areas and cause case clusters. The usual course of primary pulmonary infection is complete healing, though an area of pneumonitis on x-ray may heal by forming a coinlike lesion, or coccidioidoma. Less commonly, a single thin-walled cavity remains as a chronic sequela in the area of consolidation. Also, the consolidation may persist as a chronic pneumonia or progress to fibronodular, cavitary disease.

Pleural effusion may be the only manifestation of primary infection. Self-healing of this form is common.

An uncommon but dreaded complication of coccidioidomycosis is dissemination beyond the lung and hilar lymph nodes. Dissemination is more frequent in blacks, Filipinos, Native Americans, Mexican-Americans, and pregnant or immunosuppressed patients, including those with AIDS.

C. immitis incites a chronic granulomatous reaction in host tissue, often with caseation necrosis. Lung and hilar node lesions may show calcification. Both IgM and IgG antibodies against *C. immitis* are induced by infection but neither appears protective. The amount of specific IgG antibody is a rough measure of the antigenic mass, i.e., of the amount of infection, making a high titer a poor prognostic sign. Appearance of delayed hypersensitivity to antigens of *C. immitis* is most common in those clinical forms of disease with a good prognosis, such as self-limited primary pulmonary disease. Negative skin tests to *Coccidioides* antigens occur in roughly half the patients with disseminated disease and portend a poor prognosis.

Clinical manifestations Symptomatic primary pulmonary infection is manifested by fever, cough, chest pain, malaise, and sometimes hypersensitivity reactions. Chest x-ray may show an infiltrate, hilar adenopathy, or pleural effusion. Peripheral blood may show a mild eosinophilia. Spontaneous improvement begins after several days to 2 weeks of illness and usually culminates in complete recovery.

The symptoms of a chronic thin-walled cavity include cough or hemoptysis in half the cases; the other patients are asymptomatic. Chronic progressive pulmonary coccidioidomycosis produces cough, sputum, variable degrees of fever, and weight loss. The first indications of dissemination usually appear during the primary infection. Reactivation with dissemination in later years occurs occasionally, especially if Hodgkin's disease, non-Hodgkin's lymphoma, renal transplantation, or other immunosuppression has supervened. Dissemination should be suspected when fever, malaise, hilar or paratracheal lymphadenopathy, and elevated sedimentation rate show abnormal persistence in patients with primary pulmonary coccidioidomycosis. High complement fixation titers support this concern. With time, lesions appear in the bone, skin, subcutaneous tissue, meninges, joints, and other sites. Without therapy, dissemination may progress rapidly to death or wax and wane for years.

Diagnosis When coccidioidomycosis is suspected, sputum, urine, and pus should be examined for *C. immitis* by wet smear and culture. *The laboratory request should indicate clearly that coccidioidomycosis is suspected because the mold form must be handled with extreme care to prevent infection of laboratory personnel.* On biopsy, smaller spherules must be distinguished from nonbudding forms of *Blastomyces* and *Cryptococcus,* but appearance of the mature spherule is diagnostic.

Serologic tests are very helpful in coccidioidomycosis. Latex agglutination and agar gel diffusion tests are useful in screening serums for antibody to *Coccidioides.* The complement fixation test is used on cerebrospinal fluid and to confirm and quantitate serum antibody detected by screening tests. The number of cases with a positive complement fixation test will depend upon the severity of disease and upon the laboratory performing the test. Positive tests are least common in patients with solitary pulmonary cavities or primary pulmonary infection, while serums from patients with multiorgan disseminated disease are nearly all positive. Seroconversion is helpful in primary pulmonary coccidioidomycosis but may not occur for up to 8 weeks after onset. A positive complement fixation test in unconcentrated cerebrospinal fluid is diagnostic of meningitis. Rarely, a parameningeal focus will cause a positive CSF serology.

Conversion of the skin test from negative to positive ($\geq$5 mm induration at 24 or 48 h) with either coccidioidin or spherulin, the two commercially available antigens, may be observed between the third and twenty-first days of symptoms in primary pulmonary coccidioidomycosis. Skin testing can also be helpful in epidemiologic studies, such as investigation of case clusters or definition of endemic areas. The utility of skin testing as a diagnostic tool is limited by the presence of persistent positive tests resulting from remote exposures to *Coccidioides* and by the frequency of negative skin tests in many patients with either thin-walled cavities or disseminated coccidioidomycosis.

Treatment Primary pulmonary coccidioidomycosis usually resolves spontaneously. Some physicians give a few weeks of intravenous amphotericin B when patients show an unusually severe or protracted primary infection, hoping to abort disseminated or chronic pulmonary disease. There is no solid evidence to support this practice, but the stronger the suspicion of dissemination becomes in any given patient, the more logical this approach appears. Once evidence for dissemination becomes incontrovertible, amphotericin B may be palliative rather than curative. Incomplete recovery and relapse after apparent cure with amphotericin B have been distressingly common in both disseminated and chronic progressive pulmonary infection. The low toxicity and possibility of long-term oral therapy with ketoconazole have encouraged study of this drug in nonmeningeal coccidioidomycosis. Doses of 200 to 400 mg per day have improved some patients with skin, bone, and lung coccidioidomycosis. Patients failing to respond to this dose should have the dose escalated gradually in the 10 to 20 mg/kg per day range to assess clinical response and toxicity. Treatment is continued 12 months or more. A seriously ill or rapidly deteriorating patient should not be treated with this drug. Such patients are given intravenous amphotericin B 0.5 to 0.7 mg/kg daily or a double dose on alternate days until infection appears relatively quiescent, often 10 or 12 weeks. More prolonged courses may be changed to 1.0 mg/kg three times a week. Surgical debridement of bone lesions and drainage of abscesses contribute to cure. Resection of chronic progressive pulmonary lesions is a helpful adjunct to chemotherapy when infection is confined to the lung and in one lobe. A single thin-walled cavity tends to close spontaneously, and ordinarily is not resected. Such a cavity responds poorly to chemotherapy. Coccidioidal meningitis is treated with long-term intrathecal amphotericin B. Hydrocephalus, a frequent complication, renders this therapy less effective. The prognosis in all forms of chronic progressive coccidioidomycosis must be guarded.

THE OPPORTUNISTIC DEEP MYCOSES

CANDIDIASIS Etiology *Candida albicans* is the most common cause of candidiasis, but *C. tropicalis, C. parapsilosis, C. guilliermondii, C. krusei,* and a few other species can cause candidiasis and may even be fatal. *C. parapsilosis* is particularly notable for its ability to cause endocarditis. All *Candida* species pathogenic for humans are also encountered as commensals of humans, particularly in the mouth, stool, and vagina. These species grow rapidly at 25 to 37°C on simple media as oval budding cells. In specialized culture media, hyphae or elongated branching structures called *pseudohyphae* are formed. *C. albicans* can be identified presumptively by its ability to form germ tubes in serum or by the formation of thick-walled large spores, called *chlamydospores.* Final identification of all species requires biochemical tests.

Pathogenesis and pathology Either local or systemic factors may lead to tissue invasion by *Candida*. Chronic maceration predisposes to cutaneous candidiasis, as in diaper rash, intertrigo in obese patients, or paronychia in bartenders or cannery workers. Age is important because neonatal colonization often leads to oral candidiasis (thrush). Women in the third trimester of pregnancy are prone to vulvovaginal thrush. Patients with diabetes mellitus, AIDS, or hematologic malignancy, or who are receiving broad-spectrum antibiotics or high doses of adrenal corticosteroids, are especially susceptible to candidiasis. Breaks in the integrity of the skin or mucous membranes may provide access to deeper tissues. Examples include perforation of the gastrointestinal tract by trauma, surgery, and peptic ulceration; indwelling catheters for intravenous alimentation, peritoneal dialysis, and urinary tract drainage; severe burns; and intravenous drug abuse.

Candida grows within tissues in both yeast and pseudohyphal forms. Rarely, only one form is present. Visceral lesions are characterized by necrosis and a neutrophilic inflammatory response. Neutrophils kill *Candida* yeast cells and damage segments of pseudohyphae in vitro, suggesting a major role for the neutrophil in host defense against this fungus. Visceral lesions show a preference for kidney, brain, spleen, heart, and liver.

Clinical manifestations *Oral thrush* presents as discrete and confluent adherent white plaques on the oral and pharyngeal mucosa, particularly in the mouth and tongue. These lesions are usually painless, but fissuring at the corners of the mouth can be painful. *Cutaneous candidiasis* presents as red, macerated intertriginous areas, paronychia, balanitis, or pruritus ani. Candidiasis of the perineal and scrotal skin may be accompanied by discrete pustular lesions on the inner aspects of the thighs. *Chronic mucocutaneous candidiasis* or *Candida* granuloma typically presents as circumscribed hyperkeratotic skin lesions, crumbling dystrophic nails, partial alopecia in areas of scalp lesions, and both oral and vaginal thrush. Systemic infection is very rare, but disfigurement of the face and hands can be severe. Other findings may include chronic epidermophytosis, dental dysplasia, and hypofunction of the parathyroid, adrenal, or thyroid glands. A variety of defects in T-cell function have been described in these patients. Vulvovaginal thrush causes pruritus, discharge, and sometimes pain on intercourse or urination. Speculum examination reveals an inflamed mucosa and a thin exudate, often with white curds.

From one to multiple small shallow ulcerations due to *Candida* may appear in the esophagus or gastrointestinal tract. Esophageal lesions favor the distal third and may cause dysphagia or substernal pain. Other such lesions tend to be asymptomatic but assume importance in the leukemic patient as a portal for disseminated candidiasis. Within the urinary tract, the most common lesions are either hematogenous renal abscesses, which can cause azotemia, or bladder thrush. Bladder invasion usually follows catheterization or instrumentation of a patient with diabetes mellitus or who is receiving broad-spectrum antibiotics. This lesion generally is asymptomatic and benign. Rarely, retrograde invasion of the renal pelvis leads to renal papillary necrosis.

Hematogenous dissemination of Candida presents with fever and toxicity but with few localizing findings. One or more retinal abscesses may appear and extend slowly into the vitreous humor. The patient may note orbital pain, blurred vision, scotoma, or opacities floating across the visual field. Pulmonary candidiasis is almost always hematogenous and is visible on chest x-ray only when the abscesses are numerous enough to cause a diffuse, vaguely nodular infiltrate. Candidiasis of the endocardium or around intracardiac prostheses resembles bacterial infection of these sites. Chronic *Candida* meningitis or arthritis may occur, from either disseminated disease or insertion of a prosthesis in the case of arthritis. Rare focal manifestations of disseminated disease include osteomyelitis, pustular skin lesions, myositis, and brain abscess.

Diagnosis Demonstration of pseudohyphae on wet smear with confirmation by culture is the procedure of choice for diagnosing superficial candidiasis. Scrapings for the smear may be obtained from skin, nails, and oral and vaginal mucosa. Culture alone is not diagnostic.

Deeper lesions of *Candida* may be diagnosed by histologic section of biopsy specimens or by culture of cerebrospinal fluid, blood, joint fluid, or surgical specimens. Blood cultures in vented bottles or concentrated by lysis-centrifugation are very useful in *Candida* endocarditis and intravenous catheter-induced sepsis but are positive less often in other forms of disseminated disease. The utility of serodiagnosis remains controversial.

Treatment Cutaneous candidiasis of macerated areas responds to measures which reduce moisture and chafing plus a topically applied antifungal agent in a nonocclusive base. Nystatin, ciclopirox, and the imidazole creams such as clotrimazole and miconazole appear roughly equivalent. Nystatin and some imidazoles are available also for vaginal application. Oral candidiasis should be treated with clotrimazole troches or a nystatin suspension. Swallowing nystatin suspension, sucking on clotrimazole troches, or taking ketoconazole, 200 to 400 mg per day, may improve symptoms of esophageal candidiasis. When esophageal symptoms are pronounced, a 5- to 10-day course of intravenous amphotericin B, 0.3 mg/kg per day, may be beneficial. Bladder thrush responds to bladder irrigations with amphotericin B, 50 μg/mL for 5 days. In all forms of skin and mucosal candidiasis, relapse after successful treatment is common.

Intravenous amphotericin B is the drug of choice in disseminated candidiasis. The drug is usually given as 0.4 to 0.5 mg/kg every day or as a double dose on alternate days for several weeks. In patients with no contraindication to the use of flucytosine, administration of that drug in dosage of 100 to 150 mg/kg per day plus amphotericin B, 0.3 mg/kg per day, is an effective alternative. Ketoconazole in an adult dose of 200 mg daily is probably the drug of choice for chronic mucocutaneous candidiasis.

Candida isolated from a properly obtained blood culture should be considered significant, for true false-positives are rare. Whether a patient with candidiasis should receive antifungal therapy will depend on the degree of illness and the likelihood of spontaneous recovery. For example, a febrile, severely immunosuppressed patient with one positive blood culture should receive prompt therapy because a rapidly fatal course is common. A nonimmunosuppressed patient acquiring candidiasis from an indwelling intravenous plastic catheter may recover spontaneously if the catheter is removed promptly. The species of *Candida* is irrelevant to this decision. Patients with candidiasis in whom antifungal therapy is withheld should be observed carefully for the development of endophthalmitis, endocarditis, arthritis, osteomyelitis, or other visceral lesions that require therapy.

ASPERGILLOSIS **Etiology** *Aspergillus fumigatus* is the most common pathogen, but *A. flavus, A. niger,* and several other species can cause disease. *Aspergillus* is a mold with septate hyphae about 2 to 4 μm in diameter. Sporulating structures, called *conidial heads,* may be seen when the fungus is growing in nature, on an artificial medium, or within air-containing spaces of the body. The appearance of the colonies and of conidial heads is used for identification.

Pathogenesis and pathology All the common species of *Aspergillus* which cause disease in humans are ubiquitous in the environment, growing on dead leaves, stored grain, compost piles, hay, and other decaying vegetation. Inhalation of *Aspergillus* spores must be extremely common, but disease is rare. Invasion of lung tissue is almost entirely confined to immunosuppressed patients. Roughly 90 percent will have two of these three conditions: less than 500 granulocytes per cubic millimeter of peripheral blood, supraphysiologic doses of adrenal corticosteroids, and a history of cytotoxic drugs such as azathioprine. Infection in such patients is characterized by hyphal invasion of blood vessels, thrombosis, necrosis, and hemorrhagic infarction. Chronic granulomatous disease of childhood also predisposes to invasive pulmonary aspergillosis, but here the inflammatory response is granulomatous. Blood vessel invasion is rare.

Massive inhalation of *Aspergillus* spores by normal persons can lead to an acute, diffuse, self-limited pneumonitis. Epithelioid granulomas with giant cells and central pyogenic areas containing hyphae are seen. Spontaneous recovery taking several weeks is the usual course.

Aspergillus can colonize the damaged bronchial tree, pulmonary cysts, or cavities of patients with underlying lung disease. Balls of hyphae within cysts or cavities may reach several centimeters in diameter and be visible on chest x-ray. Tissue invasion does not occur. The term *allergic bronchial aspergillosis* denotes the condition of patients with preexisting asthma who have eosinophilia, IgE antibody to *Aspergillus,* and fleeting pulmonary infiltrates from bronchial plugging (see Chap. 203).

Clinical manifestations *Endobronchial pulmonary aspergillosis* presents as chronic productive cough and often hemoptysis in a patient with prior chronic lung disease, such as tuberculosis, sarcoidosis, bronchiectasis, or histoplasmosis. *Aspergilloma* refers to a ball of hyphae within a lung cyst or cavity, usually in the upper lobe. *Aspergillus* may be spread from its endocavitary or endobronchial site to the pleura during the course of bacterial lung abscess or surgery.

Invasive aspergillosis in the immunosuppressed host presents as an acute pneumonia. Infection progresses by hematogenous spread as well as extension to surrounding lung and other contiguous structures. Occasionally the portal of infection in the immunosuppressed host is the paranasal sinus, gastrointestinal tract, skin, or palate.

Aspergillus sinusitis in nonimmunosuppressed patients may take two forms. A ball of hyphae may form in a chronically obstructed paranasal sinus, without tissue invasion. Much less commonly, a chronic, fibrosing granulomatous inflammation with *Aspergillus* hyphae within tissue may begin in the sinus and spread slowly to the orbit and brain.

Growth of *Aspergillus* on cerumen and detritus within the external auditory canal is termed *otomycosis.* Trauma to the cornea may cause chronic *Aspergillus* keratitis. Endophthalmitis follows introduction of *Aspergillus* into the globe by trauma or surgery. *Aspergillus* may infect intracardiac or intravascular prostheses.

Diagnosis Repeated isolation of *Aspergillus* from sputum or demonstration of hyphae in sputum or bronchial brushing specimens suggests endobronchial colonization or infection. Fungus ball of the lung is usually detectable by chest x-ray. Antibody of the IgG class to *Aspergillus* antigens is demonstrable in the serum of many colonized patients and of virtually all patients with fungus ball.

Biopsy is usually required to diagnose invasive aspergillosis of the lung, paranasal sinus, or sites of dissemination. Blood cultures are rarely positive, even in patients with infected cardiac prosthetic valves. *Aspergillus* hyphae can be identified presumptively by histology, but culture is required for confirmation and determination of species. Serologic and skin tests have not proved helpful in invasive aspergillosis.

Treatment Patients with severe hemoptysis due to fungus ball of the lung may benefit by lobectomy. Poor pulmonary function in residual lung and dense pleural adhesions around the lesion can complicate the resection. Systemic chemotherapy is of no value in endobronchial or endocavitary aspergillosis.

Intravenous amphotericin B has resulted in arrest or cure of invasive aspergillosis when immunosuppression is not severe. Combined flucytosine–amphotericin B may be useful in nonneutropenic patients with invasive aspergillosis.

MUCORMYCOSIS (ZYGOMYCOSIS, PHYCOMYCOSIS) Etiology *Rhizopus* and *Mucor* species are the principal pathogens, though *Cunninghamella* and *Absidia* species are occasionally encountered. These molds have broad, rarely septate hyphae of uneven diameter, ranging from 6 to 50 μm. The fungus is inexplicably difficult to grow from infected tissue. When it occurs, growth is rapid and profuse on most media at room temperature. Identification is based upon gross and microscopic appearance of the mold.

Pathogenesis and pathology *Rhizopus* and *Mucor* species are ubiquitous, appearing on decaying vegetation, dung, and foods of high sugar content. Infection is uncommon and largely confined to patients with serious preexisting diseases. Mucormycosis originating in the paranasal sinuses and nose occurs predominantly in patients with poorly controlled diabetes mellitus. Mucormycosis in patients with hematologic malignancy or organ transplantation more often originates in the lung than in the nose and paranasal sinuses. Gastrointestinal mucormycosis occurs in a variety of conditions, including uremia, severe malnutrition, and diarrheal diseases. Infection is acquired from nature, with no person-to-person spread. Elastic bandages contaminated with *Rhizopus* species have caused several postoperative skin and subcutaneous infections.

In all forms of mucormycosis, vascular invasion by hyphae is prominent. Ischemic or hemorrhagic necrosis is the predominant histologic finding.

Clinical manifestations Mucormycosis originating in the nose and paranasal sinuses produces a characteristic clinical picture. Low-grade fever, dull sinus pain, and sometimes nasal congestion or a thin, bloody nasal discharge are followed in a few days by double vision, increasing fever, and obtundation. Examination reveals a unilateral generalized reduction of ocular motion, chemosis, and proptosis. The nasal turbinates on the involved side may be dusky red or necrotic. A sharply delineated area of necrosis, strictly respecting the midline, may appear in the hard palate. The skin of the cheek may become inflamed. Fungal invasion of the globe or ophthalmic artery leads to blindness. Opacification of one or more sinuses is found on x-ray. Carotid arteriogram may show invasion or obstruction of the carotid siphon. Coma is due to direct invasion of the frontal lobe. Early symptoms mimic bacterial sinusitis. Clouding of the sensorium may be attributed to diabetic acidosis. Cavernous sinus thrombosis may be considered when orbital invasion occurs. Without treatment, death may occur in a few days to a few weeks.

Pulmonary mucormycosis is a progressive severe pneumonia, accompanied by high fever and toxicity. The necrotic center of large infiltrates may cavitate. Hematogenous spread to other areas of the lung, as well as to brain and other organs, is common. Survival beyond 2 weeks is unusual. Gastrointestinal invasion presents as one or more ulcers which tend to perforate. Hematogenous dissemination can originate from the gastrointestinal tract, lung, or paranasal sinuses. Sometimes no portal of entry can be found.

Diagnosis Lesions of the lung and craniofacial structures are best diagnosed by biopsy and histologic section. Cultural confirmation should be attempted. Wet smear of crushed tissue can provide rapid diagnosis. Cultures of blood and cerebrospinal fluid are negative. Smear and culture of sputum may be positive during cavitation of a lung lesion. Serologic tests are of little assistance.

Treatment Regulation of diabetes mellitus and decreasing immunosuppressive drugs aid in the treatment. Extensive debridement of craniofacial lesions appears to be very important. Orbital exenteration may be required. Intravenous amphotericin B is clearly of value in craniofacial mucormycosis and should be employed in the other forms of mucormycosis as well. Maximum tolerated doses are given until progression is halted. The drug is continued for a total of 10 to 12 weeks. Appropriate management results in cure of about half of the craniofacial infections. Survival of patients with pulmonary, gastrointestinal, or disseminated mucormycosis is rare.

SPOROTRICHOSIS Etiology *Sporothrix schenckii* lives as a saprophyte on plants in many areas of the world. In nature and on culture at room temperature the fungus grows as a mold, but within host tissue or at 37°C on enriched media it grows as a budding yeast. Identification is by appearance of the fungus in mold and yeast forms. Small spores with a hairlike attachment to hyphae give the fungus the name *Sporothrix.*

Pathogenesis and pathology Infection results when minor trauma inoculates the fungus into subcutaneous tissue. Nursery workers, florists, and gardeners acquire the illness from roses, sphagnum moss, and other plants. Infection may be limited to the site of inoculation (plaque sporotrichosis) or extend along proximal lymphatic channels (lymphangitic sporotrichosis). Spread on an extremity, the usual site, even as far as inguinal or axillary nodes is rare, and hematogenous dissemination from the skin remains unproven. The portal for osteoarticular, pulmonary, and other extracutaneous forms of sporotrichosis is unknown but is likely the lung.

Untreated sporotrichosis shows little evidence of self-healing and is capable of extreme chronicity. The inflammatory response contains both clusters of neutrophils and a marked granulomatous response with epithelioid cells and giant cells.

Clinical manifestations Lymphangitic sporotrichosis, by far the most common manifestation, forms a nearly painless red papule at the site of inoculation. Over the next several weeks, similar nodules form along proximal lymphatic channels. Nodules intermittently discharge small amounts of pus. Ulceration may occur. The proximal extension of these lesions, often with skip areas, is quite distinctive but may be mimicked by lesions of *Nocardia brasiliensis, Mycobacterium marinum,* or, on rare occasions, by *Leishmania brasiliensis* or *M. kansasii.*

Plaque sporotrichosis is a nontender red maculopapular granuloma confined to the site of inoculation. Osteoarticular sporotrichosis presents as mono- or polyarticular arthritis of indolent onset and progression over months or years, involving the elbows, knees, wrists, ankles, and, rarely, smaller joints of the extremities. Periarticular bone gradually appears "moth-eaten," and draining sinuses may appear over joints and bursas. Hematogenous spread to the skin may be observed during polyarticular disease, but none of the skin lesions shows lymphangitic spread. Immunosuppression predisposes to such spread. Pulmonary sporotrichosis usually presents as a single chronic cavitary upper-lobe lung lesion.

Diagnosis Culture of pus, joint fluid, sputum, or skin biopsy specimen is the preferred method of diagnosis. Appearance of *S. schenckii* in tissue is quite variable. In skin lesions, organisms are hard to find.

Treatment Cutaneous sporotrichosis can be cured with oral administration of a saturated solution of potassium iodide, given in increasing divided daily doses up to 4.5 to 9 mL per day for adults, as tolerated. Gastrointestinal disturbance or acneform rash over the cape area and face are common, but therapy should be continued for 1 month after resolution of all lesions. Patients with serious allergic reactions to iodides may respond to local heat, particularly when plaque sporotrichosis is the only form of disease. Extracutaneous sporotrichosis rarely responds to iodides, but cures have been obtained in over half such patients with prolonged courses of intravenous amphotericin B.

RARER DEEP MYCOSES

PARACOCCIDIOIDOMYCOSIS Etiology Formerly called *South American blastomycosis,* this is the mycosis caused by *Paracoccidioides brasiliensis.* A dimorphic fungus, *P. brasiliensis* grows as a budding yeast but may be grown as either yeast or mold on a culture medium. Identification is by gross and microscopic appearance. A superficial resemblance to *Blastomyces dermatitidis* may cause misdiagnosis.

Pathogenesis and pathology Infection is thought to be acquired by inhalation of spores from environmental sources, but the reservoir in nature remains obscure. Pulmonary infection produces few symptoms initially. Hematogenous spread to the mucous membranes of the mouth and nose, the lymph nodes, and other sites brings the patient to medical attention. Fatal cases show spread to the adrenal, the gastrointestinal tract, and many other viscera.

Clinical manifestations Common symptoms include indurated ulcers of the mouth, oropharynx, larynx, and nose, enlarged and draining lymph nodes, lesions of the skin and genitalia, productive cough, weight loss, dyspnea, and sometimes fever. Acquisition of infection is restricted to South America, Central America, and Mexico, but the extreme indolence of this infection may lead to recognition many years after the patient has left the endemic area. Chest x-ray most often shows a bilateral patchy pneumonia.

Diagnosis Cultures of sputum, pus, and mucosal lesions are often diagnostic. The diagnosis can be made by smear or histologic section, though confirmation by culture is preferable. Serologic tests are useful in suggesting the diagnosis and monitoring therapy.

Treatment Milder cases may be cured by one year's treatment with oral ketoconazole, 200 to 400 mg daily. More advanced cases are given intravenous amphotericin B, followed by ketoconazole.

PSEUDALLESCHERIASIS Etiology Also called *Petriellidium boydii, Pseudallescheria boydii* is a mold frequently found in soil. When the fungus is isolated in the imperfect state, it is called *Seedosporium apiospermum.*

Pathogenesis and pathology Wind-borne spores of *P. boydii,* arising in soil, are the presumed source of infection. The fungus grows as a mold within tissue, causing necrosis and abscess formation.

Clinical manifestations *P. boydii* resembles *Aspergillus* in its ability to colonize the endobronchial tree, to form fungus balls in the lung or paranasal sinuses, to invade the cornea or globe following trauma or surgery, and by its propensity to invade the immunosuppressed host. Hyphae of *P. boydii* in tissue may be difficult to distinguish from *Aspergillus.* Infection with *P. boydii* is much less common than with *Aspergillus. P. boydii* is the single most common cause in the United States of mycetoma. Intravascular hyphae, a hallmark of invasive aspergillosis, also can be found in pseudallescheriasis. Occasional normal patients have developed necrotizing pneumonia or abscesses in brain or other organs due to *P. boydii.*

Diagnosis Demonstration of hyphae in tissue and culture confirmation are required for diagnosis.

Treatment Intravenous miconazole or ketoconazole is recommended, but therapeutic response to all drugs has been poor.

TORULOPSOSIS Etiology *Torulopsis glabrata (Candida glabrata)* is a small yeast-like fungus, the same size as the yeast form of *Histoplasma capsulatum. T. glabrata* does not form hyphae or pseudohyphae. Identification is by biochemical tests.

Pathogenesis and pathology *T. glabrata* is a normal inhabitant of the human gastrointestinal tract and vagina. Within tissue, *T. glabrata* causes abscess formation with a neutrophilic inflammatory response. In immunosuppressed patients, a scanty or mononuclear inflammatory response may be seen.

Clinical manifestations Torulopsosis mimics many of the manifestations of candidiasis, but infection is less common and often less severe. Clinical entities include intravenous catheter–induced sepsis or endocarditis, gastrointestinal and disseminated infection in immunosuppressed patients, and retrograde infection of the urinary tract.

Diagnosis *Torulopsis* may be difficult to distinguish from yeast cells of *Candida* in histologic section. Culture is the most reliable diagnostic tool.

Treatment Therapeutic measures used in candidiasis appear appropriate for torulopsosis.

MYCETOMA Etiology *Actinomycetoma* refers to infection by actinomycetes of the genera *Nocardia, Streptomyces,* and *Actinomadura. Eumycetoma* is caused by true fungi of many different genera. The most common agent varies with the locality.

Pathogenesis and pathology The pathogens live in the soil and enter the skin through minor trauma. The most common site of infection is the foot. Infection runs a relentless course over many years, with destruction of contiguous bone and fascia. Grains are found in purulent foci, surrounded by fibrosis and a mononuclear cell inflammatory response.

Clinical manifestations *Mycetoma* is a chronic suppurative infection originating in subcutaneous tissue and characterized by the presence of grains, which are tightly clumped colonies of the causative agent. The infected site shows painless swelling, woody induration, and sinus tracts which discharge pus intermittently. Systemic symptoms and spread to distant sites in the body are not seen.

Diagnosis The clinical picture is characteristic, but confusion with chronic osteomyelitis or botryomycosis may occur. The diagnosis requires demonstration of grains in pus from the draining sinus or in biopsy sections. Many histologic sections may need to be examined to locate a grain.

Treatment Actinomycetoma may respond to prolonged therapy with sulfonamides, trimethoprim-sulfamethoxazole, or other antibacterial agents. Eumycetoma does not respond reliably to any drug. Amputation may be required.

CHROMOMYCOSIS Etiology The five species of fungi currently recognized as causing this syndrome have received a bewildering number of different names. Using Emmons' classification, these fungi are called *Phialophora verrucosa, P. pedrosoi, P. compacta, P. dermatitidis,* and *Cladosporium carrionii.*

Pathogenesis and pathology Infection occurs in tropical and subtropical areas where workers acquire many small puncture wounds from thorns or splinters. Histopathologic section of the skin lesion shows pseudoepitheliomatous hyperplasia and a granulomatous dermal infiltrate. Microabscesses with neutrophils also occur. Clumps of the pathogenic organism are found in these abscesses or elsewhere in the dermis as rounded, thick-walled brown cells. The epidermis and superficial crusts may contain branching brown hyphae.

Clinical manifestations *Chromomycosis* is characterized by chronic verrucoid, ulcerated, or crusted skin lesions. The site of the lesion depends upon the area of trauma but is usually the foot or leg. The lesion begins as a pimple, pustule, or ulcer with slow progression over many years. Lesions may remain flat or become pedunculated. Pain is minimal, but itching is common. Infection usually remains confined to the same extremity, but a few cases have spread hematogenously to cause brain abscess.

Diagnosis Demonstration of the characteristic organisms in histologic sections of skin biopsy is the best diagnostic method. Positive cultures are obtained readily, but accurate identification may require the service of a reference laboratory.

Treatment Prolonged therapy with oral flucytosine appears helpful. Relapse with secondary drug resistance has been encountered with sufficient frequency to make flucytosine plus low-dose intravenous amphotericin B appear preferable for large lesions.

DERMATOPHYTOSIS

Definition Dermatophytosis, also known as ringworm or tinea, is a chronic fungal infection of the skin, hair, or nails.

Etiology Species of *Trichophyton, Microsporum,* and *Epidermophyton* are called *dermatophytes.* They grow in and remain confined to the keratinous structures of the body. Other mycoses can show fungal invasion of keratinous structures, such as candidiasis, pityriasis versicolor, and tinea nigra, but are traditionally not termed *dermatophytoses.*

Pathology and pathogenesis Dermatophyte species are called anthropophilic, zoophilic, or geophilic, depending on whether their usual reservoir within nature appears to be humans, animals, or soil. Infectivity of all those sources is low, and group outbreaks are largely confined to an occasional case clustering of scalp infections in children. Acquisition of a dermatophytosis appears to be favored by minor trauma, maceration, and poor hygiene of the skin. Infection does not seem to confer solid immunity. Repeated infection with the same species is commonplace, particularly with anthropophilic species. Infrequency of scalp infection in adults has been attributed to local factors rather than immunity.

Invasion of the stratum corneum by dermatophytes may cause little inflammation, or, particularly with zoophilic fungi, inflammation can be intense. Shedding of the stratum corneum is increased by inflammation. To the extent that fungal growth cannot keep up with shedding, inflammation may help terminate infection. Conversely, infection is probably favored when shedding is reduced by corticosteroids and cytotoxic drugs. Antifungal drugs interfere with the ability of fungal growth to keep up with shedding.

Clinical manifestations The disease varies with the site of infection and fungal species. Foot infection (athlete's foot, tinea pedis) may present as fissuring of the toe webs, scaling of the plantar surfaces, or vesicles around the toe webs and soles. Interdigital lesions may be pruritic or, when bacterial superinfection occurs, may be painful. Hand infection is less common but resembles foot infection. Scalp dermatophytosis (tinea capitis) is characterized by areas of alopecia and scaling. In so-called endothrix infection, the hair shaft breaks off at the skin surface, leaving the hairs visible as black dots in the scalp. With some forms of scalp infection an intense boggy suppuration occurs, called a *kerion.* Dermatophytosis of the glabrous skin (tinea corporis) presents as circumscribed lesions with a wide variety of appearances. Scales, vesicles, or pustules may appear. Inflammation may be minimal or intense. Central healing of less inflamed lesions may be seen. The serpiginous border of inflammation is the source of the name *ringworm.* Dermatophytosis of the bearded area (tinea barbae) appears as a pustular folliculitis. Onychomycosis (tinea unguium) presents as white discolored nails or thickened, chalky crumbling nails. Peeling and fissuring of the perinychia or keratotic debris under the nail edge may also be seen.

Diagnosis Discolored hairs, scales, and keratotic debris under infected nails should be collected for KOH smear and culture. In the scraping of skin lesions, a drop of water on the skin site may keep the removed scales from flying off and aid in their collection. Culture is important in distinguishing dermatophytes from *Candida* and fungal saprophytes growing in keratinaceous debris.

Treatment Mild or moderately severe lesions of the trunk, groin, and feet often respond to topical therapy with an imidazole or one of the other agents mentioned earlier in this chapter. Hyperkeratotic lesions of the palms and soles respond less well. Ringworm that is moderately severe or severe, that is unresponsive to topical therapy, or that involves the scalp, nails, or bearded area should be treated systemically. The drug of choice is griseofulvin. Either 500 mg of the microcrystalline form or 375 mg of the ultramicrocrystalline form is given once daily or divided into two doses, given with meals. Double this amount has been recommended for refractory infections. Treatment must be continued until all infected keratin is gone. Cutting of infected hair, epilating nails, and cleansing interdigital webs can expedite cure. Secondary bacterial infection of the foot may require soaks or antibacterial agents. Relapse of dermatophyte foot infections may be decreased by measures to keep the feet clean and dry. Griseofulvin-resistant cases may respond to oral ketoconazole, 200 to 400 mg daily.

REFERENCES

Therapy

AMA Department of Drugs: Antifungal agents for systemic mycoses, in *AMA Drug Evaluations,* 5th ed. Chicago, American Medical Association, 1983, pp 1779–1788

BENNETT JE: Treatment of cryptococcal, candidal and coccidioidal meningitis, in *Current Clinical Topics in Infectious Diseases,* JS Remington, M Swartz (eds). New York, McGraw-Hill, 1980, vol 2, pp 54–67
Drugs for treatment of systemic fungal infections. The Medical Letter 24:35, 1982
EMMONS CW: *Medical Mycology.* Philadelphia, Lea & Febiger, 1977
HEIDEMANN HT et al: Amphotericin B nephrotoxicity in humans decreased by salt repletion. Am J Med 75:476, 1983
KERRIDGE D: Present status of antimycotics. Microbiol Sci 2:83, 1985
MEDOFF G, KOBAYASHI GS: Strategies in the treatment of systemic fungal infections. N Engl J Med 302:145, 1980
NIAID MYCOSES STUDY GROUP. Treatment of blastomycosis and histoplasmosis with ketoconazole. Ann Intern Med 103:861, 1986
RIPPON JW: *Medical Mycology. The Pathogenic Fungi and the Pathogenic Actinomycetes.* Philadelphia, Saunders, 1982

Cryptococcosis

BENNETT JE et al: A comparison of amphotericin B alone and combined with flucytosine in treatment of cryptococcal meningitis. N Engl J Med 301:126, 1979
KHOURY MB et al: Thoracic cryptococcosis: Immunologic competence and radiologic appearance. Am J Radiol 141:893, 1984
PERFECT JR et al: Cryptococcemia. Medicine 62:98, 1983

Blastomycosis

EDSON RS, KEYS TF: Treatment of primary pulmonary blastomycosis. Results of long term follow-up. Mayo Clin Proc 56:683, 1981
HABTE-GABR E, SMITH IM: North American blastomycosis in Iowa. Review of 34 cases. J Chronic Dis 26:523, 1973
HALVORSEN RA et al: Pulmonary blastomycosis: Radiologic manifestations. Radiology 150:1, 1984
KLEIN BS et al: Isolation of *Blastomyces dermatitidis* in soil associated with a large outbreak of blastomycosis in Wisconsin. N Engl J Med 314:529, 1986
SAROSI GA, DAVIES SF: Blastomycosis. Am Rev Respir Dis 120:911, 1979

Histoplasmosis

GOODWIN RA et al: Histoplasmosis in normal hosts. Medicine 60:231, 1981
WHEAT LJ et al: Cavitary histoplasmosis occurring during two large urban outbreaks. Analysis of clinical, epidemiologic, roentgenographic, and laboratory features. Medicine 63:201, 1984
——— et al: Histoplasmosis in the acquired immune deficiency syndrome. Am J Med 78:203, 1985

Coccidioidomycosis

BOUZA E et al: Coccidioidal meningitis. An analysis of thirty-one cases and review of the literature. Medicine 60:139, 1980
DRUTZ DJ, CATANZARO A: Coccidioidomycosis. Am Rev Respir Dis 117:559, 727, 1978
———: Amphotericin B in the treatment of coccidioidomycosis. Drugs 26:337, 1983
EINSTEIN HE (ed): Proceedings of the 4th International Conference on Coccidioidomycosis. Washington, DC, National Foundation for Infectious Diseases, 1984
SALOMON NW et al: Surgical manifestations and results of treatment of pulmonary coccidioidomycosis. Ann Thorac Surg 30:433, 1980

Candidiasis

DUPONT B, ROUHET E: Cutaneous, ocular, and osteoarticular candidiasis in heroin addicts: New clinical and therapeutic aspects in 38 patients. J Infec Dis 152:577, 1985
LEVINE MS et al: *Candida* esophagitis; accuracy of radiographic diagnosis. Radiology 154:581, 1985
LEWIS JH et al: The spectrum of hepatic candidiasis. Hepatology 2:479, 1982
ROSE HD, SHETH NK: Pulmonary candidiasis. A clinical and pathological correlation. Arch Intern Med 138:964, 1978
SOLOMKIN JS et al: The role of *Candida* in intraperitoneal infections. Surgery 88:524, 1980

Aspergillosis

FAULKNER SL et al: Hemoptysis and pulmonary aspergilloma: Operative versus non-operative treatment. Ann Thorac Surg 25:389, 1978
RINALDI MG: Invasive aspergillosis. Rev Infect Dis 5:1061, 1983
WEILAND D et al: Aspergillosis in 25 renal transplant patients. Epidemiology, clinical presentation, diagnosis and management. Ann Surg 198:622, 1983
YOUNG RC et al: Aspergillosis: Spectrum of the disease in 98 patients. Medicine 49:149, 1970

Mucormycosis

BARTRUM RJ et al: Roentgenographic findings in pulmonary mucormycosis. Am J Roentgenol 117:810, 1973
LEHRER RI et al: Mucormycosis. Ann Intern Med 93:93, 1980
MANIGLIA AL et al: Cephalic phycomycosis: A report of eight cases. Laryngoscope 92:755, 1982
MEYERS BR et al: Rhinocerebral mucormycosis. Premortem diagnosis and therapy. Arch Intern Med 139:557, 1979

Sporotrichosis

BULLPITT P, WEEDON D: Sporotrichosis: A review of 39 cases. Pathology 10:249, 1978
CROUT JE et al: Sporotrichosis arthritis. Clinical features of seven patients. Ann Intern Med 86:294, 1977
ENGLAND DM, HOCHHOLZER L: Primary pulmonary sporotrichosis. Am J Surg Path 9:193, 1985
FRIEDMAN SJ, DOYLE JA: Extracutaneous sporotrichosis. Int J Dermatol 22:171, 1983
LYNCH PJ et al: Systemic sporotrichosis. Ann Intern Med 73:23, 1970

Paracoccidioidomycosis

CASTANEDA OJ et al: *Paracoccidioides brasiliensis* arthritis. Report of a case and review of the literature. J Rheumatol 12:356, 1985
LONDERO AT, SEVERO LC: The gamut of progressive pulmonary paracoccidioidomycosis. Mycopathologia 75:65, 1981
RESTREPO A et al: The gamut of paracoccidioidomycosis. Am J Med 61:33, 1976
——— et al: Ketoconazole in paracoccidioidomycosis: Efficacy of prolonged therapy. Mycopathologia 72:35, 1980
SUGAR AM et al: Paracoccidioidomycosis in the immunosuppressed host: Report of a case and review of the literature. Am Rev Respir Dis 129:340, 1984

Pseudallescheriasis

BAKERSPIGEL A, SCHAUS D: Petrielliodiosis (pseudallescheriasis) in southwestern Ontario, Canada. Sabouraudia 22:247, 1984
GALGIANI JN et al: *Pseudallescheria boydii* infections treated with ketoconazole. Chest 86:219, 1984
TRAVIS LB et al: Clinical significance of *Pseudallescheria boydii:* A review of 10 years' experience. Mayo Clin Proc 60:531, 1985
WINSTON DJ et al: *Allescheria boydii* infections in the immunosuppressed host. Am J Med 63:830, 1977

Torulopsosis

KAUFFMAN CA, TAN JS: *Torulopsis glabrata* renal infection. Am J Med 57:217, 1974
VALDIVIESO M et al: Fungemia due to *Torulopsis glabrata* in the compromised host. Cancer 38:1750, 1976

Mycetoma

GREEN WO, ADAMS TE: Mycetoma in the United States. Am J Clin Pathol 42:75, 1964
MAHGOUB ES: Medical management of mycetoma. Bull WHO 54:303, 1976
TARALAKSHMI VV et al: Mycetomas caused by *Streptomyces pelletieri* in Madras, India. Arch Dermatol 114:204, 1978

Chromomycosis

LONDERO AT, RAMOS DC: Chromomycosis: A clinical and mycologic study of thirty-five cases observed in the hinterland of Rio Grande Do Sul, Brazil. Am J Trop Med Hyg 25:132, 1976
LOPES CF: Recent developments in the therapy of chromoblastomycosis. Bull Pan Am Health Organ 15:58, 1981

Dermatophytosis

COX FW et al: Oral ketoconazole for dermatophyte infections. Am Acad Dermatol 6:445, 1982
ROBERTSON MH et al: Ketoconazole in griseofulvin-resistant dermatophytosis. J Am Acad Dermatol 6:224, 1982

147 ACTINOMYCOSIS AND NOCARDIOSIS

JOHN E. BENNETT

ACTINOMYCOSIS

DEFINITION Actinomycosis is an indolent suppurative infection caused by certain anaerobic actinomycetes. The microorganisms grow within the tissue as grossly visible tightly knit clusters, called *grains.*

ETIOLOGY *Actinomyces israelii* is the usual pathogen, with occasional cases due to other species of *Actinomyces* (*A. naeslundii, A. viscosus, A. odontolyticus, A. meyeri*) or *Arachnia propionica.* All can form branching gram-positive hyphae, are the same width as bacteria, and grow best in an atmosphere which is either anaerobic or contains 6 to 10% CO_2. Isolation of the causal agent is rendered difficult by the usual presence of mixed flora in actinomycotic abscesses.

PATHOLOGY AND PATHOGENESIS All agents of actinomycosis are commensals in the mouth and gastrointestinal tract of humans. The portal of entry appears to be either a break in the integrity of the mucosa or aspiration into the lung. Poor dental hygiene and dental abscess predispose to cervicofacial lesions. Within the gastrointestinal tract, the appendiceal area is the most common site. Infection presents as a chronic suppurative inflammation, usually in the cervicofacial, thoracic, or abdominal area. In histopathologic section, each grain is typically surrounded by polymorphonuclear neutrophils. The adjacent tissue shows subacute or chronic inflammation with extensive fibrosis and formation of sinus tracts. Giant cells are infrequent. The grain stains variably with hematoxylin and eosin, and may have an eosinophilic coating composed of human proteins. Hyphal filaments cannot be seen on hematoxylin and eosin stain but may be demonstrated in the periphery of the grain by tissue Gram stain (such as Brown and Brenn) or by a heavily stained Gomori methenamine silver. These stains may be useful if there is chance for confusion with the grains of eumycetoma or staphylococcal botryomycosis. The grains are a few millimeters in diameter, making them difficult to miss if they are present in the histologic section being examined. Several sections may have to be searched to find a grain. Grains may be observed grossly in pus or on bandages covering draining sinuses. These pale yellow, cheeselike particles can be crushed on a microscope slide, and the gram-positive branching filaments demonstrated on Gram stain.

Infection spreads by direct extension and hematogenously. Direct extension through the skin causes one or more chronic draining sinuses to appear in the abdomen, chest, or cervicofacial area. Hematogenous foci may appear in bone, brain, liver, or other organs.

CLINICAL MANIFESTATIONS *Cervicofacial actinomycosis* presents as a red or purplish firmly indurated subcutaneous mass, typically in the submandibular area or in the anterior cervical triangle near the angle of the mandible. One or more draining sinuses may be present. Tenderness is slight or absent. Lethargy, weight loss, variable low-grade fever, anemia, and leukocytosis are infrequent in cervicofacial actinomycosis but common in *thoracic* and *abdominal actinomycosis*. Localizing findings in the latter forms include draining sinuses and, in thoracic actinomycosis, cough and purulent sputum. Pulmonic lesions may extend through the chest wall and present as an indolent subcutaneous abscess. Pain or a palpable mass may appear in abdominal actinomycosis. *Pelvic actinomycosis,* once rare, is now being seen in women with intrauterine devices. The indolent onset, variable low-grade fever, abdominal pain, and adnexal mass may lead to an erroneous diagnosis of pelvic inflammatory disease or tumor. In all forms of actinomycosis, disease typically has been present for weeks or months at time of diagnosis.

Chest x-ray may reveal an area of dense pneumonitis. Fibrosis, empyema, or cavitation may be seen. Periappendiceal abscess may appear as an extrinsic mass on barium enema.

DIAGNOSIS Laboratory tests other than culture or histologic section are not helpful. Blood cultures are rarely positive. Isolation of *Actinomyces* or *Arachnia* species from the mouth, sputum, stool, or feculent draining sinuses is not diagnostic. Demonstration of a grain in pus or deep tissue is diagnostic, if botryomycosis and mycetoma can be excluded. Nocardiosis can be distinguished by the absence of grains, identification of the organism in culture, and, usually, by the weak acid-fast staining of *Nocardia.*

TREATMENT Milder cases of actinomycosis, including most cervicofacial infections, respond well to oral tetracycline or penicillin V, an adult dose being 500 mg qid of either drug. Oral erythromycin would be second choice. More severe cases, including most thoracic and abdominal infections, should receive parenteral penicillin G for roughly 6 weeks (in adults 2 to 6 million units per day) followed by prolonged therapy with oral penicillin V or tetracycline. The likelihood of relapse is reduced if the total duration of therapy is 2 to 4 months in mild cases and up to 6 to 12 months in severe forms. Drug resistance has not been encountered in relapses. Curettage of bone lesions, surgical resection of necrotic tissue, and drainage of empyema, brain abscess, or other large collections of pus facilitate recovery but are usually not curative by themselves.

It is common in actinomycosis to isolate microbes other than actinomycetes from pus. In general, the antibiotic susceptibility of these secondary organisms does not have to be considered in the selection of therapeutic agents.

NOCARDIOSIS

DEFINITION Nocardiosis is an acute, subacute, or chronic infection, most often beginning in the lung.

ETIOLOGY *Nocardia asteroides, N. brasiliensis,* and *N. caviae* are the etiologic agents of two different diseases, nocardiosis and mycetoma. In the latter infection, the organism enters the skin by trauma, forms grains within tissue, and spreads slowly to contiguous tissue (see Chap. 146). While nocardiosis can result from local trauma, the organism usually enters via the lung, does not form grains, and is prone to hematogenous spread. Even though the etiologic agents of these diseases do overlap, *N. asteroides* causes most cases of nocardiosis and *N. brasiliensis* is the species usually isolated from mycetoma. *Nocardia caviae* is a rare cause of either disease. *Nocardia brasiliensis* can also cause a lymphocutaneous disease closely resembling sporotrichosis; this infection differs from mycetoma by its lymphangitic spread and by the absence of grains.

Nocardia species are aerobic actinomycetes with branching hyphae the same width as bacteria. Hyphae are weakly gram-positive and weakly acid-fast. Growth appears in 2 to 5 days on blood agar, Sabouraud's agar, or other simple media. Incorporation of antibiotics into the media to inhibit bacterial growth usually inhibits *Nocardia* as well. Colonies become rough and chalky with an orange or yellow hue. Identification of *Nocardia* species, including distinction between *Streptomyces, Actinomadura,* and *Nocardia,* is difficult and best assigned to a reference laboratory.

PATHOGENESIS AND PATHOLOGY *Nocardia* is a soil saprophyte widely distributed throughout the world. Infection is acquired from sites in nature, never from infected persons or animals. Males are infected two to three times more commonly than females. No age or exposure is known to predispose to nocardiosis. Many patients have serious preexisting conditions, such as adrenal corticosteroid therapy, cancer, pulmonary alveolar proteinosis, or chronic granulomatous disease of childhood.

Lesions of nocardiosis show suppuration, necrosis, and abscess formation. Neutrophils are the predominant inflammatory cell. Hyphae are scattered throughout the lesion without formation of grains. Tissue Gram stain or overstained methenamine silver demonstrates the hyphae best. A modified Fite-Faraco stain of histologic sections can be used to demonstrate acid-fastness.

CLINICAL MANIFESTATIONS *Nocardia* pneumonia presents with fever and productive cough of several days' or up to several months' duration. The initial illness may resemble a bacterial pneumonia, but slow radiologic progression continues despite antibiotic therapy, often with cavitation of radiodense central areas. Hematogenous dissemination to brain and subcutaneous tissue is frequent in nocardiosis. A pulmonary portal is usually but not always detectable clinically. Brain lesions are typically multiple abscesses. Purulent meningitis may result from rupture of an abscess into the ventricle. The subcutaneous lesion typically consists of one or a few indolent abscesses. Hematogenous dissemination to other organs occurs but is rarely detectable clinically.

DIAGNOSIS *Nocardia* is difficult enough to detect in sputum culture on Gram stain or in histologic section so that the diagnosis is readily missed. A progressive pneumonia with purulent sputum should suggest the diagnosis, particularly if cavitation or spread to brain or subcutaneous tissue occurs. Sputum, pus, bronchial brushing, or bronchial washing specimens should be examined by Gram stain and modified acid-fast stain. On Gram stain the hyphae are usually branching, beaded, and refractile. They are not strongly gram-positive but take the red counterstain even less well. Conventional acid-fast staining procedures such as Ziehl-Neelsen or a fluorochrome often do not stain *Nocardia*. Identification of branching, weakly acid-fast organisms in histologic section or smear of pus or sputum, is sufficient to establish the diagnosis of nocardiosis. Cultural confirmation is highly desirable, but isolation of *Nocardia* from heavily contaminated specimens is difficult. Isolation of *Nocardia* from otherwise sterile pus is readily accomplished. *Nocardia* is rarely isolated from blood, but diphasic culture media are said to facilitate isolation.

When *Nocardia* is isolated from sputum, the diagnosis of nocardiosis should be suspected, but occasionally no disease can be detected. Rarely, *Nocardia* is an airborne contaminant.

TREATMENT Surgical drainage of empyema and abscesses in brain or subcutaneous tissue is helpful but not sufficient to achieve cure. Virtually all patients should receive prolonged chemotherapy. The treatment of choice is sulfisoxazole or trimethoprim-sulfamethoxazole. Sulfadiazine had been regarded as the drug of choice because of favorable clinical experience and excellent penetration into the cerebrospinal fluid. The poor availability of intravenous solutions and the danger of oliguria with crystalluria has restricted the use of sulfadiazine. Sulfisoxazole therapy is begun orally or intravenously at 100 mg/kg per day in four divided doses. The dose is then adjusted downward to achieve a peak blood concentration of 10 to 15 mg/dL (100 to 150 μg/mL). Alternatively, trimethoprim-sulfamethoxazole can be given orally or intravenously as 50 mg/kg per day of the sulfamethoxazole component, divided into two doses per day. With either regimen, therapy is continued for 6 to 12 months, depending on the severity of the infection and the presence of immunosuppression. Addition of other antibiotics to sulfa drugs may be indicated in patients who show continued deterioration. Ampicillin 150 mg/kg per day is preferred. High doses of minocycline or erythromycin also have been advocated. Parsimonious use of other drugs during sulfa therapy of nocardiosis minimizes the probability that a drug allergy will necessitate discontinuance of sulfa.

Survival has been reported in 92 percent of cases with isolated pulmonary nocardiosis compared to 52 percent in cases with brain abscess. Concomitant use of immunosuppressive therapy seems to impair therapeutic response in nocardiosis.

REFERENCES

Actinomycosis

BARTELS LJ, VRABEC DP: Cervicofacial actinomycosis—A variable disorder. Arch Otolaryngol 104:705, 1978

BENHOF DF: Actinomycosis: Diagnostic and therapeutic considerations and a review of 32 cases. Laryngoscope 94:1198, 1984

DAVIES M, KEDDIE NC: Abdominal actinomycosis. Br J Surg 60:18, 1973

DUGUID HL et al: *Actinomyces*-like organisms in cervical smears from women using intrauterine contraceptive devices. Br Med J 23:534, 1980

FRADIS M et al: Actinomycosis of the face and neck. Arch Otolaryngol 102:87, 1976

LUDMERER KM et al: Draining inguinal ulcer in a middle-aged woman. Am J Med 77:537, 1984

WEESE WC, SMITH IM: A study of 57 cases of actinomycosis over a 36-year period. Arch Intern Med 135:1562, 1975

Nocardiosis

CURRY WA: Human nocardiosis. Arch Intern Med 140:818, 1980

DEWSNUP DH, WRIGHT CN: In vitro susceptibility of *Nocardia asteroides* to 25 antimicrobial agents. Antimicrob Agents Chemother 25:165, 1984

GALLIS HA: The clinical spectrum of *Nocardia brasiliensis* infection in the United States. Rev Infect Dis 6:164, 1984

GEISELER PJ, ANDERSEN BR: Results of therapy in nocardiosis. Am J Med Sci 278:188, 1979

SMEGO RA et al: Trimethoprim-sulfamethoxazole therapy for *Nocardia* infections. Arch Intern Med 143:711, 1983

section 8 Rickettsia, *Mycoplasma*, and *Chlamydia*

148 RICKETTSIAL DISEASES

THEODORE E. WOODWARD

Introduction The rickettsial diseases of humans consist of a variety of clinical entities caused by microorganisms of the family Rickettsiaceae. The rickettsias are obligate intracellular parasites about the size of bacteria and are usually seen microscopically as pleomorphic coccobacilli. Each of the rickettsias pathogenic for humans is capable of multiplying in one or more species of arthropod as well as in animals and humans. Indeed, the majority of the rickettsias are maintained in nature by a cycle which involves an insect vector and an animal reservoir, and infection of humans is unimportant in the cycle. Epidemic typhus presents a number of points of dissimilarity to most of the other rickettsioses. Until recently, the natural cycle of infection was thought to involve only humans and lice. The finding of a sylvatic reservoir in flying squirrels associated with a human illness which resembles classic typhus emphasizes that there are other mechanisms.

A compendium of information of the rickettsial diseases is given in Table 148-1. Because each of the rickettsioses responds therapeutically to tetracyclines or chloramphenicol, the table mentions no therapy. Procedures for diagnostic isolation of the rickettsias are omitted because they generally are less useful than serologic methods, and the techniques which they require are highly specialized and hazardous. Information on isolation may be found in textbooks devoted to viral and rickettsial diseases.

Of all the afflictions of the human race the rickettsial diseases, particularly epidemic typhus, rank among the foremost as a cause of suffering and death. The record of deaths from epidemic typhus in this century in the Balkan countries and in Poland and Russia reached astounding figures. Typhus ravaged Russia and eastern Poland from 1915 to 1922, infecting 30 million of the inhabitants and causing an estimated 3 million deaths.

The past two decades have seen the development of excellent methods for the prevention and treatment of rickettsioses. In fact, these measures have been so successful that the rickettsioses have become of minor importance in the United States and in many other countries. Although conquered, the rickettsioses have not been eliminated, and they could again become rampant if the will to control them, the present high standards of sanitation, and the necessary industrial capacities for production of effective insecticides and therapeutic agents should be decreased through war or disaster.

Pathogenesis Rickettsial diseases develop after infection through the skin or the respiratory tract. Agents of the typhus and spotted fever group are introduced through the bite of the infected arthropod vector. Ticks and mites, which transmit the agents of spotted fever and scrub typhus, inoculate the rickettsias directly into the dermis during feeding. The louse and flea, which transmit epidemic and murine typhus, respectively, deposit infected feces on the skin; infection occurs when organisms are rubbed into the puncture wound made by the arthropod. The rickettsias of Q fever gain entry through the respiratory tract when infected dust is inhaled; moreover, the respiratory route is occasionally implicated in epidemic typhus when infection results from inhalation of dried infected louse feces.

Although organisms probably multiply at the original site of entry in all instances, local lesions appear with regularity only in certain diseases, namely, the initial cutaneous lesions of scrub typhus, rickettsialpox, and boutonneuse fever, and the pneumonitis which develops in about half the persons infected with Q fever.

Volunteers infected with either scrub typhus or Q fever develop rickettsemia late in the incubation period, often some hours before the onset of fever. Similar events probably occur in all the rickettsial diseases; circulating rickettsias can be detected during the early febrile period in practically all patients. Little is known about the pathogenesis of infection during the midportion of the incubation period. However, it is reasonable to assume that during this time, in patients with typhus or spotted fever, a transient low-grade rickettsemia results from release of organisms multiplying at the initial site of infection and that this seeds infection in the endothelial cells of the vascular tree. Vascular lesions developing at such sites account for the pathologic changes, including the rash.

Rickettsias apparently invade and proliferate in the endothelial cells of small blood vessels. Endothelial cell destruction occurs from the proliferation of organisms and eventual disruption. Rickettsias may exert a cytotoxic effect on endothelial cells; in mice the rickettsial toxin causes remarkable increase in capillary permeability, independent of proliferation. The anatomic localization of multiple microscopic-sized lesions and the numerous foci of rickettsial vascular changes with rickettsias present coincide well for organs carefully examined such as the kidney, lung, heart, and liver. Current observations along these lines confirm Wolbach's original conclusion that "the lesions of the blood vessel are due to the presence of the parasite." Absence of inflammatory cell reactions in fulminant Rocky Mountain spotted fever tends to exclude several host-mediated pathogenic mechanisms. A delayed type of hypersensitivity does occur during infection. The entire process, however, is not explainable by immunopathologic mechanisms.

The underlying cause of the toxic-febrile state which characterizes the rickettsial diseases remains unknown. Several rickettsial species contain type-specific toxins which are lethal for mice; these may play a role.

Pathologic physiology Peripheral vascular collapse results in death in fulminating cases during the first week, with capillary dilatation and pooling of blood without increased capillary permeability or loss of fluid into extravascular spaces. As proliferative and thrombotic lesions develop in small vessels, anoxia occurs in the areas supplied, resulting in necrosis and increased capillary permeability, with loss of water, electrolytes, proteins, and erythrocytes. This in turn results in a decrease in blood volume, together with an increase in the

TABLE 148-1 Rickettsial diseases

Disease: Type	Agent	Geographic distribution	Natural cycle: Arthropod	Natural cycle: Mammal	Principal means of transmission to humans	Serologic diagnosis: Weil-Felix reaction	Serologic diagnosis: CF, MA, and IFA reactions*
SPOTTED FEVER GROUP							
Rocky Mountain spotted fever	*R. rickettsii*	Western hemisphere	Ticks	Wild rodents, dogs	Tick bite	Positive OX-19 OX-2	Positive group- and type-specific
Boutonneuse fever	*R. conorii*	Africa, Europe, Middle East, India	↓	↓	↓	↓	↓
Queensland tick typhus	*R. australis*	Australia	↓	Marsupials, wild rodents	↓	↓	↓
North Asian tick-borne rickettsiosis	*R. sibirica*	Siberia, Mongolia	↓	Wild rodents	↓	↓	↓
Rickettsialpox	*R. akari*	United States, Russia, Africa(?)	Blood-sucking mite	House mouse, other rodents	Mite bite	Negative	↓
TYPHUS GROUP							
Endemic (murine)	*R. typhi*	Worldwide	Flea	Small rodents	Infected flea feces into broken skin	Positive OX-19	Positive group- and type-specific
Epidemic	*R. prowazekii*	Worldwide	Body louse	Humans Flying squirrels	Infected louse feces into broken skin	Positive OX-19	↓
	R. Canada	North America	Ticks			Positive OX-19	↓
Brill-Zinsser disease	*R. prowazekii*	Worldwide	Recurrence years after original attack of epidemic typhus			Usually negative	↓
Scrub	*R. tsutsugamushi*	Asia, Australia, Pacific islands	Trombiculid mites	Wild rodents	Mite bite	Positive OX-K	Positive in about 50% of patients
OTHER RICKETTSIAL DISEASES							
Q fever	*R. burnetii*	Worldwide	Ticks	Small mammals, cattle, sheep, goats	Inhalation of dried infected material	Negative	Positive
Trench fever	*R. quintana*†	Europe, Africa, North America	Body louse	Humans	Infected louse feces into broken skin	Negative	None available

* *CF = complement fixation; MA = microscopic agglutination; IFA = immunofluorescent antibody.*
† *Some authorities no longer place the agent in the genus Rickettsia because it can be cultured on artificial media.*

extravascular space and clinical edema. Edema, anoxia of the myocardium, and histologic evidence of myocarditis are disclosed by electrocardiographic abnormalities, including serious arrhythmias. Liver function is impaired. The azotemia which develops in seriously ill patients appears to be prerenal. Clinical manifestations resulting from the peripheral vascular collapse are oliguria and anuria, azotemia, anemia, hypoproteinemia, hyponatremia, edema, and coma. In spotted fever and typhus patients with hemorrhagic skin lesions, consumptive coagulopathy is present. All these alterations are absent or minimal in mild cases or in those who are given specific treatment early.

Pathology The basic changes in the spotted and typhus fever groups are vascular, with resultant widespread lesions in adjacent parenchymatous tissues throughout the body. They are most common in the skin, muscles, heart, lung, and brain. The most conspicuous and diverse are found in Rocky Mountain spotted fever. Here swelling, proliferation, and degeneration of the endothelial cells occur, frequently with thrombus formation which partially or completely occludes the lumen. The muscle cells of the arterioles undergo swelling and fibrinoid changes. The adventitial tissues are infiltrated with mononuclear leukocytes, lymphocytes, and plasma cells. The vascular damage is scattered along the arteries, veins, and capillaries, with normal architecture prevailing throughout most of the vascular bed. The changes in murine, epidemic, and scrub typhus fevers resemble those in Rocky Mountain spotted fever, but thrombosis is uncommon and involvement of the musculature is rare.

Interstitial myocarditis occurs in each of these diseases but is usually most extensive in Rocky Mountain spotted fever and in scrub typhus. In the brain glial nodules are found in all members of the group, but microinfarcts in the brain tissue or in the myocardium are most often observed in spotted fever.

A rickettsial pneumonitis occurs, at least to some extent, in many patients with spotted or typhus fever and is the characteristic pathologic change in patients with Q fever. The process is patchy and consists microscopically of areas of congestion and edema. Within the consolidated areas the alveoli are filled with compact fibrinocellular exudate containing lymphocytes, plasma cells, large mononuclear cells, and erythrocytes, but few, if any, polymorphonuclear leukocytes.

Rickettsias can occasionally be observed microscopically in sections of tissue. Failure to demonstrate them is of no diagnostic significance. They are readily identifiable by the immunofluorescent technique.

Laboratory diagnosis Diagnostic procedures which depend on isolation of the etiologic agent from blood or other clinical material are expensive, time-consuming, and hazardous to laboratory personnel. Primary isolation of rickettsias by inoculation in the yolk sac of the chick embryo or tissue cells usually fails because of the small number of organisms in the patient's blood. Rickettsias have been identified in stained cultured monocytes of infected monkeys and by direct or indirect immunofluorescence of tissues of animals infected with *R. rickettsii*. Except in unusual circumstances, however, currently available serologic tests are adequate for laboratory confirmation of the clinical diagnosis in each of the rickettsial diseases. The demonstration of a rise in titer of specific antibody during convalescence is of prime importance in establishing the laboratory confirmation. Table 148-2 summarizes the serologic results usually encountered in persons who have rickettsial diseases in the United States. The Weil-Felix test employing *Proteus* strains OX-19 and OX-2 gives positive results in patients with spotted fever and murine typhus and negative results in those with rickettsialpox and Q fever. It is useful as a screening procedure but cannot be relied upon to differentiate spotted fever from murine typhus. In patients with Brill-Zinsser disease the *Proteus* OX-19 reaction is usually negative or low in titer.

Serologic tests employing group-specific rickettsial antigens provide data which clearly differentiate the most common infections, i.e., epidemic typhus, murine typhus, Rocky Mountain spotted fever, and Q fever. Moreover, if type-specific rickettsial antigens are employed, it is generally possible to distinguish rickettsialpox from spotted fever and Brill-Zinsser disease from murine typhus.

Utilizing better antigens, other serologic procedures for rickettsial diseases not only distinguish between specific rickettsioses but help to determine the type of immunoglobulin in acute (IgM) and late or recurrent (IgG) illness, such as in recrudescent typhus (Brill-Zinsser disease). The Weil-Felix and complement fixation tests are useful for routine diagnosis; microscopic agglutination, immunofluorescent antibody, and hemagglutination reactions are valuable for specific identification.

Specific antibiotic therapy has little effect on the time of appearance of antibodies or on their ultimate titer, provided treatment is instituted some days after onset of the illness. However, if the illness is cut short by early and vigorous treatment, antibody production may be delayed for a week or so, and also the maximal titers attained may be below those illustrated in Table 148-2. Under these circumstances a sample of blood taken 4 to 6 weeks after onset of illness should also be tested.

The immunofluorescent antibody test is a very useful procedure for detecting rickettsia in the tissues of patients with the typhus group of rickettsioses, the spotted fevers, and Q fever. Identifiable rickettsias have been visualized in skin lesions of patients with Rocky Mountain spotted fever as early as the fourth day of illness and as late as the tenth day. Rickettsias may be visualized in human tissues several days after administration of chloramphenicol or tetracycline. The technique also visualizes rickettsias in ticks and the tissues of animals. This test is useful with paraffin-fixed tissues.

Normochromic anemia occurs in patients severely ill with rick-

TABLE 148-2 Serologic diagnosis of rickettsial diseases in the United States

		Weil-Felix reaction				Complement fixation tests with type-specific antigen				
			Illustrative titer				Illustrative titer			
Group	Disease	Proteus	10th day	20th day	Cases with diagnostic titer	Rickettsial antigen	10th day	20th day	30th day	Cases with diagnostic titer
Spotted fever	Rocky Mountain spotted fever	OX-19 OX-2	40 20	320 160	Most	*R. rickettsii*	20	160	80	Most
	Rickettsialpox	OX-19 OX-2	0 0	0 0	None	*R. akari*	0	64	128	Most
Typhus	Murine typhus	OX-19 OX-2	160 10	640 40	Most	*R. typhi*	0	160	160	Most
	Epidemic typhus squirrel related	OX-19 OX-2	160 10	640 40	Most	*R. prowazekii*	0	160	160	Most
	Brill-Zinsser disease	OX-19 OX-2	160 0	20 0	Infrequent	*R. prowazekii*	1280	640	320	Most
	Q fever	OX-19 OX-2	0 0	0 0	None	*R. burnetii*	10	80	160	Most

ettsial diseases. The white blood cell count in Rocky Mountain spotted fever, rickettsialpox, murine and epidemic typhus, Brill-Zinsser disease, Q fever, and other rickettsial diseases is usually within the normal range; 6000 to 10,000 cells per cubic millimeter. Leukopenia is occasionally observed, and in the presence of complications, such as superimposed infections and extensive vascular lesions, moderate leukocytosis occurs. The differential blood cell count is usually normal.

Thrombocytopenia occurs in severely ill spotted and scrub typhus fever patients with extensive vascular lesions; hypofibrinogenemia, prolonged prothrombin and partial thromboplastin times, and other clotting abnormalities occur.

Treatment Certain physiochemical changes occurring in the patient seriously ill with one of the diseases of the typhus–spotted fever group should be understood before a therapeutic regimen is outlined. These changes are circulatory collapse, coma, oliguria and anuria, azotemia, anemia, hypoproteinemia, hypochloremia and hyponatremia, and edema. These alterations are often absent in the mildly ill, and in them management is much less complicated. The therapeutic principles necessary for treatment of all rickettsioses are (1) specific chemotherapy and (2) supportive care. Attention to both is mandatory for the seriously ill patient first recognized late in the disease. During the first week in the moderately ill patient, supportive therapy may need to be less energetic, because specific chemotherapy usually suffices. The early mild case may be successfully treated at home; more severely ill patients should receive hospital care.

Therapeutic measures advisable for all the rickettsioses will be described in detail. Variations of this regimen which apply to the individual rickettsioses are described in subsections covering those diseases.

SPECIFIC THERAPY Specific therapy is most effective when initiated during the early stages of disease coincident with the appearance of the rash. When therapy is delayed until the rash has become hemorrhagic and widespread, the response is less dramatic. The antibiotics of choice are chloramphenicol and the tetracyclines, which are effective because of their rickettsiostatic properties. They are not rickettsiocidal.

The following antibiotic regimen is considered optimal: for chloramphenicol, an initial dose of 50 mg per kilogram of body weight, and for tetracycline, 25 mg/kg. Subsequent daily doses are the same as the initial loading dose, with the requirement divided equally and given at 6- to 8-h intervals. Antibiotic treatment is continued until the patient has improved and has been afebrile approximately 24 h. In patients too ill to take oral medication, an intravenous preparation of one of the antimicrobials should be employed.

Adrenal cortical hormones may be needed for their antitoxemic effects in patients first observed late in the course of severe illness. Large doses for brief periods of about 3 days, in combination with specific antibiotics, are recommended in critically ill patients.

Therapy with antibiotics is continued until the toxemia has abated, the general condition has markedly improved, and the temperature has remained at normal levels for 24 h. In uncomplicated cases of spotted fever, there is symptomatic improvement within 24 h and the temperature becomes normal in 60 to 72 h.

SUPPORTIVE CARE Frequent turning of the patient relieves pressure from prominent bony parts and also militates against the development of aspiration pneumonia. Proper mouth care, with frequent swabbing of the oral cavity, may avert the development of parotitis and gingivitis. Sucking of the juice of a lemon or the oral use of glycerin or mineral oil is helpful.

A generous intake of protein should be provided by frequent feedings as soon as the disease is suspected, in order to avoid subsequent protein deficiency. Usually food is well tolerated by patients with rickettsial disease, and the daily diet should provide 1 to 2 g protein per kilogram of normal body weight, with adequate carbohydrate and fat to make it palatable. When the patient is uncooperative, the diet may be supplemented by hourly liquid protein feedings via stomach tube, provided that there is no abdominal distention.

At the critical stage, when hypoproteinemia is present and changes in capillary permeability lead to edema and vascular embarrassment, careful attention must be given to parenteral hyperalimentation with high concentration of glucose and amino acids. When indicated by hematologic studies, whole-blood transfusions given slowly are helpful. The judicious administration of one of the plasma expanders at this stage may have a definite favorable effect upon impending circulatory collapse. If the patient is anuric and azotemia is pronounced, overloading the circulation with fluids should be governed by clinical judgment and very careful laboratory studies. Frequent determinations of hemoglobin, hematocrit, electrolytes, and protein, sometimes at intervals of a few hours during crucial periods, are necessary in order to ascertain abnormalities and to permit institution of corrective measures. Dialysis is indicated when there is clear-cut evidence of acute renal failure.

ROCKY MOUNTAIN SPOTTED FEVER **Definition** Rocky Mountain spotted fever is an acute febrile illness caused by *Rickettsia rickettsii*. It is transmitted to humans by ticks. The disease is characterized by sudden onset with headache and chills and by fever which persists for 2 to 3 weeks. A characteristic exanthem appears on the extremities and trunk about the fourth day of illness. Delirium, shock, and renal failure occur in severely ill patients.

Etiology and epidemiology The causative microbe, *R. rickettsii*, is the prototype for the rickettsial group of agents. The minute organisms are purple when stained by Giemsa's method or red by Macchiavello's technique; most of them are gram-negative. These organisms often occur in pairs and possess a cell wall similar in structure and chemical composition to that of gram-negative bacteria; there are a cell membrane, cytoplasmic granules corresponding to ribosomes, and prokaryotic organization of nuclear material. The cell membrane is selectively permeable; the cell wall is the focus of important antigens and an endotoxin-like substance.

The rickettsias grow in the nucleus and the cytoplasm of infected cells of ticks, mammals, and embryonated eggs; the intranuclear situation of the organisms is shared by the other members of the spotted fever group, but not by rickettsias of the typhus group. *Rickettsia rickettsii* is readily distinguishable from the agents of the typhus fevers by cross-immunity tests in guinea pigs and by complement fixation tests employing antigens prepared from infected yolk sac tissues. The differentiation of *R. rickettsii* from closely related members of the spotted fever group frequently requires elaborate procedures. Strains of the agent of Rocky Mountain spotted fever vary considerably in their virulence for humans and animals.

The first reports of spotted fever in Idaho and Montana during the final decade of the last century led to the name Rocky Mountain spotted fever. However, the disease has been reported from all states (except Maine, Alaska, and Hawaii), as well as from Canada, Mexico, Colombia, and Brazil. Although related diseases are found on other continents, this particular infection is limited to the western hemisphere. In the years 1981, 1982, 1983, and 1984 there were 1176, 976, 1126, and 848 cases reported, respectively. The mortality rate was about 20 percent in the days before specific therapy but has decreased to about 7 percent. More than half the cases occur in the south Atlantic and south central states, with the greatest number of these in North Carolina, Virginia, Georgia, Maryland, Tennessee, and Oklahoma.

A number of species of ticks are found infected with *R. rickettsii* in nature, but only two are important in transmitting spotted fever to humans. These are *Dermacentor andersoni*, the wood tick, which is the principal vector in the west, and *D. variabilis*, the dog tick, which assumes this role in the east. *Amblyomma americanum*, the lone star tick, and *D. variabilis* are the common vectors in the west south central states. Infected female ticks transmit the agent transovariably to at least some of their offspring. Ticks which become infected, either through the egg or at one of the stages during their development cycle by feeding on an infected mammal, harbor the rickettsias throughout their lifetime, which may be several years, making the tick a reservoir as well as a vector. Small wild mammals are suspected of playing an important role in spreading the rickettsias in nature by infecting ticks which feed on them during rickettsemia.

Disease in humans is generally acquired from the bite of an infected tick. Transmission is unlikely unless the tick remains attached for a number of hours. Infection may also be acquired through abrasions in the skin which become contaminated with infected tick feces or tissue juices; hence, the hazard associated with crushing ticks between the fingers when removing them from persons or animals. The agent of Rocky Mountain spotted fever has been transmitted accidentally to humans by transfusion of blood taken from a donor just before onset of illness.

There are seasonal variations in the incidence of cases of spotted fever, as well as differences in age and sex distribution of cases. In each instance these differences are related to exposure to ticks. Most cases are seen during the period of maximal tick activity, i.e., April to September, and 60 percent of cases occur in individuals under 20 years of age. This age distribution is undoubtedly influenced by propinquity to the wood and dog ticks. The mortality rate increases with the age of the patient.

Rocky Mountain spotted fever has been acquired by laboratory workers via aerosol transmission, and special precautions are necessary when the agent is handled in the laboratory.

Clinical manifestations INCUBATION PERIOD AND PRODROMATA A history of tick bite is elicited in approximately 80 percent of patients. The incubation period varies between 3 and 12 days with a mean of 7 days. A short incubation period usually indicates a more serious infection.

ONSET In nonvaccinated persons, the onset is usually abrupt, with severe headache, a sudden shaking rigor, prostration, generalized myalgia, especially in the back and leg muscles, nausea with occasional vomiting, and fever which reaches 103 to 104°F within the first 2 days. Pain in the abdominal muscles may be severe, and arthralgia is not uncommon. Deep muscle palpation often elicits tenderness. Occasionally the debut of illness in children and adults is mild, accompanied by lethargy, anorexia, headache, and low-grade fever. These symptoms are similar to those of many acute infectious diseases, making specific diagnosis difficult during the first few days.

PYREXIA Fever continues for approximately 15 to 20 days in untreated cases. The febrile course in children may be shorter. Hyperthermia of 105°F or greater is of unfavorable prognostic significance, although fatalities may occur when the patient is hypothermic, with concurrent vasomotor collapse. Fever generally terminates by lysis over a period of several days, but rarely does so by crisis. Recurrent fever is uncommon except in the presence of secondary pyogenic complications.

The *headache* is generalized and excruciating, and frequently most intense over the frontal area. It persists throughout the first and second weeks of illness in untreated cases. Occasionally headache is mild. Malaise continues for the first week; irritability is notable, and the patient shuns distractions such as questioning and examination.

CUTANEOUS MANIFESTATIONS The rash which is present in practically all cases is the most characteristic and helpful diagnostic sign. It usually appears on the fourth febrile day; the range is 2 to 6 days. Faint-pink macules which fade on pressure have been noted on the first febrile day. The initial lesions are on the wrists, ankles, palms, soles, and forearms. The first lesions are macular, nonfixed, pink, irregularly defined, and measure 2 to 6 mm. A warm compress applied to the extremity accentuates the rash in the early stages. The exanthem is most prominent when the temperature is elevated. After 6 to 12 h, the rash extends centripetally to the axilla, buttocks, trunk, neck, and face. (This is in contrast to the eruption of typhus fever, which begins on the trunk and spreads centrifugally, rarely involving the face, palms, or soles.) The rash becomes maculopapular after 2 to 3 days (it may be felt by light palpation) and assumes a deeper red hue. By about the fourth day it is petechial and fails to fade on pressure. Not uncommonly, the hemorrhagic lesions coalesce to form large ecchymotic blemishes; these lesions tend to form over bony prominences and may ultimately slough to form indolent, slow-healing ulcers. Patients who have had the typical rash show brownish discolorations at the site for several weeks during convalescence. In milder cases, the rash does not become purpuric and may disappear within a few days. Antibiotic therapy may abort the early exanthem; the later fixed lesion fades less rapidly with specific therapy. Occasionally, a rash does not occur or is unnoticed, particularly in dark-skinned patients.

The application of tourniquets for several minutes, or the occasional taking of the blood pressure may provoke additional petechiae (Rumpel-Leede phenomenon), further evidence of capillary abnormalities.

CARDIOVASCULAR AND RESPIRATORY FEATURES During the early stages, the pulse is full and regular and is accelerated in proportion to the height of the temperature, and the blood pressure is well sustained. During the peak of illness in seriously ill patients, the pulse is rapid and feeble, and hypotension of 90 mmHg or less is common. If circulatory failure is sustained, the resultant hypoxia and shock lead to agitation and delirium and contribute to the formation of ecchymoses and gangrene of fingers, toes, genitalia, buttocks, earlobes, and nose. Cyanosis of the peripheral parts of the body is common. Venous pressure determinations show no elevation. A reduction of the total blood volume is occasionally found. The ECG shows low voltage of ventricular complexes, minor ST-segment deflections, and occasionally delay in atrioventricular conduction. These changes are transient and nonspecific. Severely ill patients have a puffy appearance of the face, hands, ankles, feet, and lower parts of the sacrum. Occasionally a severe arrhythmia associated with myocarditis results in sudden death.

Respirations are either normal or slightly accelerated. Cough may be harassing and nonproductive, and localized pneumonitis may occur, but pulmonary consolidation is extremely rare. Pulmonary edema may develop after injudicious use of intravenous fluids.

HEPATIC AND RENAL MANIFESTATIONS In the majority of patients, there is little alteration in renal or hepatic function. The liver may be enlarged, but jaundice is unusual. Oliguria commonly occurs in the seriously ill, and anuria may mark the critically ill patient. Azotemia is common; when marked, it is a very unfavorable sign. Abnormalities in liver function include hypoproteinemia, with reduction in the albumin fraction.

NEUROLOGIC MANIFESTATIONS The principal neurologic manifestations are headache, restlessness, and varying degrees of insomnia. Stiffness of the back is common. The cerebrospinal fluid (CSF) is clear, with normal dynamics and normal chemical constituents. Occasionally, the CSF pressure is elevated; there may be a slight increase in mononuclear cells. Coma and muscular rigidity may occur. Athetoid movements, convulsive seizures, and hemiplegia are grave manifestations. Deafness during the active stages of the disease is not uncommon. As a rule, all neurologic signs abate without residua. Findings based upon follow-up examinations and electroencephalograms may be interpreted as indicative of minor residual brain damage for a year or more following recovery of certain patients from Rocky Mountain spotted fever.

OTHER PHYSICAL MANIFESTATIONS Patients become dehydrated, with extreme dryness of lips, gums, tongue, and pharynx. The skin is hot and dry, the conjunctivas are frequently injected, and the eyes suffused. Photophobia is common in the early stages of illness. Petechial hemorrhages may be noted in the conjunctivas or in the retina. The spleen is enlarged in approximately one-half the cases and is firm and nontender. Abdominal distention is frequent, and occasionally some degree of intestinal ileus is observed. Constipation is usual.

Course In patients with mild and moderately severe cases who are given no specific antibiotic therapy, the disease abates within 2 weeks, and convalescence is rapid. In fatal cases death usually occurs during the latter part of the second week as a result of toxemia, vasomotor collapse and shock, or renal failure. In a few patients, the course is fulminant with death occurring as early as the sixth day of illness.

In vaccinated individuals who contract the disease, the illness is mild, with a short febrile course and an atypical rash.

Prognosis If the serious manifestations of spotted fever mentioned above are regarded as intrinsic parts of the disease, then complications are uncommon and consist mainly of secondary bacterial infections, namely, bronchopneumonia, otitis media, and parotitis. Thrombosis of major blood vessels may result in gangrene of a portion of an extremity. Hemiplegia and peripheral neuritis are rare sequelae.

The overall mortality rate for spotted fever was formerly about 20 percent. Death occurred in more than half of persons over 40 years of age, but the mortality rate was much lower in children and young adults. Since the introduction of the broad-spectrum antibiotics and the development of more precise knowledge regarding correction of the physiologic abnormalities which develop during the disease, fewer deaths occur. Some of the fatalities can be attributed to failure to consider spotted fever in the differential diagnosis and resultant delay in instituting appropriate treatment.

Differential diagnosis During the early stages of infection before the rash has appeared, differentiation from other acute infections is difficult. History of tick bite while living or traveling in wooded or bushy sites known to be in a highly endemic area is helpful. The rash of meningococcemia (see Chap. 103) resembles Rocky Mountain spotted fever in certain aspects, because it is macular, maculopapular, or petechial in the chronic form, and petechial, confluent, or ecchymotic in the fulminant type. The meningococcal skin lesion is tender and develops with extreme rapidity in the fulminant form, whereas the rickettsial rash occurs on about the fourth day of disease and gradually becomes petechial. *Spotted fever is often confused with measles.* The exanthem of rubeola rapidly becomes confluent, while that of rubella *usually remains discrete.*

Murine typhus is a milder disease than Rocky Mountain spotted fever; the rash is less extensive, nonpurpuric, and nonconfluent, and renal and vascular complications are uncommon. Not infrequently differentiation of these two rickettsial infections must await the results of specific serologic tests. Epidemic typhus fever is capable of causing all the pronounced clinical, physiologic, and anatomic alterations seen in patients with Rocky Mountain spotted fever, i.e., hypotension, peripheral vascular collapse, cyanosis, skin necrosis and gangrene of digits, renal failure and azotemia, and neurologic manifestations. However, the rash of classic typhus is noted initially in the axillary folds of the trunk and later extends peripherally, rarely involving the palms, soles, or face. The serologic patterns in these two diseases are distinctive when specific rickettsial antigens are employed. Moreover, louse-borne typhus is now recognized in the United States as a flying squirrel–related illness which occurs sporadically and as Brill-Zinsser disease (recrudescent typhus fever). Rickettsialpox, although caused by a member of the spotted fever group is usually readily differentiated from Rocky Mountain spotted fever by the initial lesion, the relative mildness of the illness, and the early vesiculation of the maculopapular rash. The Weil-Felix reaction is positive in Rocky Mountain spotted fever and in murine and epidemic typhus, but is negative in rickettsialpox. Agglutinins against *Proteus* OX-19 and OX-2 appear in the serum of patients with spotted fever, but only those against OX-19 are generally found in murine and epidemic typhus.

Complications *Pyogenic complications,* including otitis media and parotitis, are encountered in patients severely ill with Rocky Mountain spotted fever and other rickettsioses. These localized infections respond to therapy with appropriate antibiotics combined with surgical measures.

Pneumonitis usually develops as a result of specific rickettsial action. The sputum is scant but should be examined to determine whether superimposed bacterial infection is present. Specific therapy is guided by the results of these laboratory studies. The pneumonitis generally responds to the antibiotic therapy the patient is receiving, but if staphylococcal pneumonia is suspected, a penicillinase-resistant penicillin should be added to the broad-spectrum drug.

Circulatory failure of peripheral or central origin is combated by careful administration of plasma expanders and fluids. Heart failure may develop from the disease or as a result of overzealous intravenous therapy and is recognized by rapid pulse, gallop rhythm, and increase in venous pressure. When the clinical signs reveal unmistakable evidence of cardiac failure, digitalis and diuretics should be employed. Oxygen therapy improves the cardiac and circulatory status and is helpful in hypoxemic patients with involvement of the central nervous system.

Prevention Prevention is attained primarily by avoidance of tick-infested areas. When this is impractical, prophylactic measures include (1) spraying the ground with dieldrin or chlordane for area control of ticks (though there are environmental objections to the use of residual insecticides in area control of ticks, under special conditions such procedures may be warranted); (2) application of repellents such as diethyltoluamide or dimethylphthalate to clothing and exposed parts of the body, or in very heavily infested areas the wearing of clothing which interferes with the attachment of ticks, i.e., boots and a one-piece outer garment, preferably impregnated with repellent; and (3) daily inspection of the entire body, including the hairy parts, to detect and remove attached ticks. In removing attached ticks great care should be taken to avoid crushing the arthropod with resultant contamination of the bite wound; touching the tick with gasoline or whisky encourages detachment but gentle traction with tweezers applied close to the mouth parts may be necessary; the skin area should be disinfected with soap and water or other antiseptics. Similarly, precautions should be employed in removing engorged ticks from dogs and other animals, because infection through minor abrasions on the hands is possible. Improved vaccines containing inactivated *R. rickettsii* are under development and when available commercially should be used for those at great risk, namely, persons frequenting highly endemic areas and laboratory workers exposed to the agent. Because the broad-spectrum antibiotics are such excellent therapeutic agents in spotted fever, there has been less impetus for vaccination of persons who run only a minor risk of infection.

After tick bite in a known endemic area an exposed person should be observed for signs of fever, headache, prostration, and rash; therapy is very effective early in the infection.

MURINE (ENDEMIC) TYPHUS FEVER Definition Murine typhus fever is an acute febrile disease caused by *Rickettsia typhi (mooseri)* and transmitted to humans by fleas. The clinical illness is characterized by fever of 9 to 14 days, headache, a maculopapular rash appearing on the third to fifth day, and myalgia.

Etiology and epidemiology *R. typhi* resembles other rickettsias in morphologic properties, staining characteristics, and intracellular parasitism. Under the electron microscope *R. typhi* is seen to contain dense masses of nuclear material in a less dense homogeneous protoplasmic substance, the whole of which is surrounded by a limiting membrane. It differs from *R. rickettsii* in that it always multiplies within the cytoplasm of cells, in contrast to the intranuclear and cytoplasmic positions of spotted fever rickettsias.

Invasion of the body by *R. typhi* provokes specific and nonspecific immunologic responses. Utilizing highly purified antigens, specific antibodies may be demonstrated readily by complement fixation, microscopic agglutination, and immunofluorescent antibody reactions. The positive Weil-Felix reaction which occurs in this disease is nonspecific, because it is attributable to the presence of a common carbohydrate antigen in *Proteus* OX-19 and *R. typhi* and because the reaction is also positive in epidemic typhus and spotted fever. Group-specific rickettsial antigens are common to both *R. typhi* and *R. prowazekii*.

The common vector of *R. typhi* for rats and humans is the rat flea (*Xenopsylla cheopis*). In nature, the rat louse (*Polypax spinulosis*) may transmit the agent among rodents. Customarily, rat fleas become infected on ingestion of blood from diseased rats; the rickettsias multiply within the intestinal cells of the arthropod and are excreted in the feces. Infection in humans occurs after the flea bite and contamination of the broken skin by rickettsia-laden feces. Dried flea feces may also infect via the conjunctivas or the upper part of the respiratory tract.

Rats and mice are naturally infected with murine typhus, and although the rodent disease is nonfatal, viable rickettsias persist in the brain for variable periods.

Murine typhus is one of the most benign and widespread of the rickettsioses in the United States. Prevalent in the southeastern and Gulf Coast states, it has been identified in most of the other states and in harbor centers throughout the world wherever rats and fleas abound. In the early 1940s, 2000 to 5000 cases of murine typhus were reported annually. This contrasts to 61 and 58 cases reported in the United States in 1981 and 1982, respectively. This sharp reduction was achieved by control of rats and their fleas in known areas of high prevalence. In urban areas the disease is more prevalent during the summer and fall months and occurs predominantly among persons working in proximity to granaries or food depots. There has been an extension to certain rural areas when changing agricultural practices have provided rats with ready access to adequate food supplies. A small cluster of five cases occurred in late 1982 in a rural area in north central Texas. Conceivably, use of rat poison several weeks before the illness forced infected fleas to seek an alternative human host. All five patients recovered; four were treated with tetracycline. Endemic typhus has been reported in laboratory workers. This emphasizes the importance of taking special precautions when working with rickettsial organisms in the laboratory.

Clinical manifestations INCUBATION PERIOD AND PRODROMATA The incubation period ranges from 8 to 16 days, with a mean of 10 days. Common prodromata are headache, backache, arthralgia, and chilly sensations. Nausea, malaise, and transient temperature rises may precede the true onset of disease.

ONSET AND GENERAL SYMPTOMS A frank shaking chill and repeated rigors are present at the onset, associated with a severe frontal headache and fever. This triad of headache, chill, and pyrexia is usually followed within a few hours by nausea and vomiting. Prostration, malaise, and weakness are sufficient to enforce cessation of activity in adults, in contrast to children, whose illness is less severe. Occasionally, mild symptoms make it difficult to define the actual onset.

PYREXIA The usual febrile course in murine typhus lasts for about 12 days in adults; the temperature ranges from 102 to 104°F but may reach 105 to 106°F in children. The temperature may reach high levels abruptly after onset or ascend in a stepwise manner during the first few days. With the appearance of the rash, fever is usually sustained, with partial daily remissions which occasionally reach normal levels in the morning. Defervescence is generally by lysis over several days but sometimes occurs by crisis. Transient mild fever of 100°F is not uncommon during early convalescence. A few patients experience only low-grade fever throughout, but this does not necessarily connote a mild illness.

CUTANEOUS MANIFESTATIONS The early lesions, which are sparse and discrete, are hidden in the axillae and inner surface of the arm. Most patients then develop with surprising suddenness a generalized, dull-red macular rash of the upper part of the abdomen, shoulders, chest, arms, and thighs. The individual lesions are discrete and pea size, with an ill-defined border, and fade on pressure during the first 24 h. They later become maculopapular, in contrast to the exanthem of epidemic typhus, which is persistently macular. The distribution over the trunk with sparse involvement of the extremities, palms, soles, and face differs from the peripheral distribution and facial involvement of Rocky Mountain spotted fever. The murine rash generally appears initially on the fifth febrile day, but rarely it is seen concurrently with the onset of fever or develops as late as the seventh day.

Eighty percent of patients develop a rash which persists for 4 to 8 days and fades before defervescence. The cutaneous manifestations vary greatly in intensity and duration and may be fleeting. They are readily overlooked in dark-skinned patients, in whom they should be sought by light palpation and indirect lighting.

CARDIOVASCULAR AND RESPIRATORY FEATURES An irritating, nonproductive cough is frequent and is occasionally associated with moderate hemoptysis. Early in the second week, rales may be detected in the basilar lung areas. These changes are generally rickettsial rather than bacterial in origin and respond to the broad-spectrum antibiotics. Pulmonary congestion occurs in extremely ill and elderly patients.

Accelerated pulse, hypotension, and general circulatory weakness occur, although less frequently than in patients with epidemic typhus or Rocky Mountain spotted fever.

NEUROLOGIC MANIFESTATIONS Headache is the most common neurologic manifestation of murine typhus and may dominate the clinical picture. It is frontal and continues into the second week of illness. Stupor and prostration may occur in the second week, and in severe cases, there may be delirium, extreme agitation, or coma. Coma in elderly patients after 2 weeks of illness presages death. Nuchal rigidity and general spasticity often suggest meningitis, although the spinal fluid is normal except for slight increases in pressure and lymphocytes (5 to 30 per cubic millimeter). Transient partial deafness occurs occasionally, but rarely is there localized neuritis or hemiplegia. Neurologic sequelae are unusual. Children experience minimal neurologic changes.

OTHER PHYSICAL MANIFESTATIONS During the first 2 days of illness the patient may be nauseated and vomit, but vomiting later in the illness should arouse suspicion of an intercurrent complication. Abdominal pain is bothersome; when associated with diarrhea, it responds to intravenous alimentation. Hepatomegaly and jaundice are unusual. There is splenomegaly in approximately 25 percent of patients.

Photophobia, retroocular pain, and suffusion of the conjunctivas are common but are less severe than in the other typhus and spotted fevers.

Renal function is usually unaltered except in elderly patients with prolonged hypotension. Under these circumstances, azotemia may develop to the degree observed in epidemic typhus. In severe murine typhus, as in the epidemic typhus, hyponatremia and hypoalbuminemia are encountered.

Course After defervescence, murine typhus patients recover rapidly. Fatalities occur between the ninth and twelfth days in elderly or debilitated patients, usually as a result of circulatory and renal failure or intercurrent bacterial infection.

Prognosis The mortality rate in murine typhus was low even before the introduction of modern specific therapy. Only one death occurred in 114 cases studied by Maxcy and none in the 180 reported by Stuart and Pullen.

Differential diagnosis Because murine typhus and Rocky Mountain spotted fever occur in many of the same states, the problem of differential diagnosis often arises. Flea-borne murine typhus, which is predominantly an urban disease, is more likely to occur in late summer and autumn. In contrast, spotted fever is a rural and suburban disease in which exposure to ticks is important. Most cases occur in the spring and summer.

Treatment and prevention Both chloramphenicol and the tetracycline antibiotics have controlled the disease (see above).

Prevention of murine typhus in humans is attained by reducing the natural reservoir and vector by applying measures for eliminating rodents and employing appropriate insecticides in rat-infested areas to control fleas. Spraying of rat burrows with DDT effectively reduces the population of the vector.

EPIDEMIC (LOUSE-BORNE) TYPHUS FEVER Definition The classic epidemic form of typhus is a severe, febrile disease caused by *R. prowazekii* and transmitted to humans by the body louse. Intense headache, continuous pyrexia of about 2 weeks, a macular skin eruption appearing on about the fifth febrile day, malaise, and vascular and neurologic disturbances represent the principal clinical features. Confirmation of the diagnosis is made by demonstration of *Proteus* OX-19 agglutinins and of specific complement-fixing antibodies in convalescence. The broad-spectrum antibiotics are specific therapeutic agents.

Etiology and epidemiology The causative microbe, *R. prowazekii,* is closely related to *R. typhi,* which causes murine typhus; indeed, the two have a number of common antigens.

Human beings generally are infected when rickettsia-laden louse feces are rubbed into the broken skin; scratching the louse bite facilitates this process. *Pediculus humanus corporis,* which is peculiarly adapted to humans, is the only important vector of epidemic typhus. It dies of its infection and fails to transmit rickettsias to its offspring. *R. prowazekii* has been isolated from flying squirrels, and the organism probably infests their ectoparasites. Generally, however, the organism is maintained by a cycle involving human-louse-human. New epidemics apparently originate from patients with Brill-Zinsser disease (recurrent epidemic typhus). Flying squirrels can serve as a potential host to initiate an outbreak of epidemic typhus provided an avid human vector, such as the body louse, is prevalent. Pathogenic rickettsias reside for long periods in patients with epidemic typhus as well as Rocky Mountain spotted fever and scrub typhus. Lice readily become infected when fed on patients with recurrent typhus. Inhalation of dust containing dried louse feces may cause infection. An established nonhuman reservoir such as flying squirrels poses a serious threat.

If uncontrolled, epidemic typhus behaves as a cyclic disease in a susceptible population, extending over a 3-year period. During the first year there is a gradual seeding of cases throughout the group; during the second there is epidemic spread; and during the third the epidemic tapers off, because the majority of persons have become immune. Outbreaks of epidemic typhus last occurred in the United States in the nineteenth century, and its presence is now recognized in the form of Brill-Zinsser disease and flying squirrel–related typhus.

Clinical manifestations Epidemic typhus resembles murine typhus but is more severe. After an incubation period of about 7 days an abrupt onset of headache, chill, and rapidly mounting fever ushers in the illness. Headache, malaise, and prostration continue unabated until the rash appears on the fifth febrile day. It is initially macular in the axillary folds but ultimately invades the trunk and extremities as a pink, irregular macular lesion, which becomes fixed, petechial, and confluent in the later stages.

Neurologic features range from headache and general spasticity to extreme agitation, stupor, and coma. Circulatory disturbances consisting of tachycardia, hypotension, and cyanosis are more profound than those observed in murine typhus and are almost as severe as in Rocky Mountain spotted fever. Ultimately, in untreated cases azotemia often reaches high levels as a result of vascular and renal failure, and death occurs late in the second week of illness. Furthermore, thrombosis of major blood vessels and cutaneous gangrene develop in a manner similar to that seen in the virulent form of Rocky Mountain spotted fever.

The complications and sequelae of epidemic typhus are more severe than those in murine typhus, but not as severe as those in Rocky Mountain spotted fever. However, during certain outbreaks, epidemic typhus was fatal in 60 percent of those infected, and convalescence in survivors was prolonged. Broad-spectrum antibiotics have almost eradicated mortality in this dread disease, provided therapy is instituted before irreversible changes have been established in the tissues.

Differential diagnosis Differentiation of epidemic typhus from the various rickettsioses and other diseases with which it may be confused was described above. The disease is not known to occur in epidemic form in the absence of lousiness in the general population. Under the conditions in which typhus epidemics are likely to occur, other diseases which may cause confusion include malaria, relapsing fever, pneumonia, and tuberculosis. Classic typhus contracted by a previously vaccinated person is usually mild and may be clinically indistinguishable from murine typhus except by serologic methods. An illness simulating Rocky Mountain spotted fever is caused by *R. canada,* a member of the typhus group.

Treatment and prevention Both chloramphenicol and the tetracycline antibiotics have been found to be highly efficient therapeutic agents in epidemic typhus. Usually the patient becomes afebrile after 2 days of treatment. Under field conditions, 100 mg doxycycline in a single oral dose resulted in abatement of clinical manifestations and defervescence in epidemic typhus.

The most effective measures for controlling epidemic typhus are those which eliminate lousiness. DDT or lindane powder when dusted into clothing is suitable for this purpose. If resistant lice are found, malathion or carbaryl may prove effective.

A commercially available vaccine prepared from formalin-treated suspensions of infected yolk sac tissue is an effective immunizing agent. A viable vaccine utilizing an attenuated strain of *R. prowazekii* is effective but is not available commercially.

BRILL-ZINSSER DISEASE (RECRUDESCENT TYPHUS) Brill-Zinsser disease is a recrudescent episode of epidemic typhus fever which occurs years after the initial attack, in persons who had recovered from the epidemic disease acquired while residing in countries where it was prevalent. *R. prowazekii* have been isolated from lice fed on patients during the active stages of illness.

The clinical entity, not always mild, resembles epidemic typhus in the character of the rash, circulatory disturbances, and hepatic, renal, and nervous system changes. Recovery is the rule. The Weil-Felix reaction with the various *Proteus* antigens is usually negative, or positive in very low titer. The specific complement fixation, microscopic agglutination, and immunofluorescent antibody reactions are valuable in establishing the diagnosis. In Brill-Zinsser disease the specific complement-fixing antibodies appear as early as the fourth day after the onset of illness; antibodies are of the IgG class, and the peak response is attained by the eighth to tenth days. Specific antibody titers in the primary attack of epidemic typhus begin later, about the eighth to twelfth day, with maximum titers on about the sixteenth day after onset. Treatment is the same as for other rickettsial infections.

SCRUB TYPHUS Definition Scrub typhus is limited to eastern and southeastern Asia, India, northern Australia, and the adjacent islands. It is caused by *R. tsutsugamushi* and is characterized by a primary lesion at the site of the bite of an infected mite, a fever of about 2 weeks' duration, a cutaneous rash which develops about the fifth day, and the appearance late in the second week of agglutinins against the OX-K strain of *Proteus* bacillus. The broad-spectrum antibiotics are specific therapeutic agents.

Etiology The agent of scrub typhus resembles other rickettsias in its physical properties but differs from them in antigenic structure, vector, and reservoir. The disease is transmitted by larvae of several species of mites, especially *Leptotrombidium* (*Trombicula*) *akamushi* and *L. deliense*. These tiny chiggers attach themselves to the skin and during the process of obtaining a meal of tissue juice may acquire infection from the host or transmit rickettsias to the vertebrate. The infection is maintained in nature by a cycle involving mites and small rodents and by transovarial transmission in mites; human infection represents an accident attributable to propinquity.

Clinical manifestations About 10 to 12 days after infection, illness begins abruptly with chilliness, severe headache, fever, conjunctival injection, and moderate generalized lymphadenopathy, which is most prominent in the nodes draining the area of the primary lesion. The initial lesion at the beginning of fever is evidenced by an erythematous indurated area 1 cm in diameter, surmounted by a multiloculated vesicle; within a few days the vesicle ulcerates and becomes covered with a black crust.

Fever increases progressively during the first week, generally reaching 104 to 105°F, but the pulse remains relatively slow, 70 to 100 beats per minute. The red macular rash, which begins on the trunk about the fifth day and spreads to the extremities, sometimes becomes maculopapular but usually fades in a few days. The course of the disease and the complications resemble those of endemic and epidemic typhus; however, interstitial myocarditis is more prominent than in the other typhus fevers.

Prognosis Before the introduction of the broad-spectrum antibiotics the mortality rate varied from 1 to 60 percent, depending on the geographic area and the virulence of the local strains of *R. tsutsugamushi,* and convalescence was prolonged. With modern therapeutic methods, deaths are rare and convalescence is short.

Differential diagnosis Scrub typhus is to be differentiated from the other members of the typhus and the spotted fever group of diseases as well as from measles, typhoid fever, and the meningococcal infections. The geographic localization of scrub typhus, the primary lesion, and the occurrence of OX-K agglutinins are especially useful in establishing the diagnosis.

Treatment and prevention Chloramphenicol and the tetracycline antibiotics are extremely effective in scrub typhus. Scrub typhus is more amenable to drugs than are the other rickettsial infections, and patients with this disease regularly become afebrile and are decidedly improved within 24 to 36 h after beginning treatment, irrespective of the stage of disease. Antibiotic treatment may be discontinued after several afebrile days.

Relapse of clinical illness is unusual unless specific treatment is initiated early, such as before the fifth febrile day. Under these circumstances, recrudescence is obviated by giving the antibiotic for several days and resuming treatment about 5 days after cessation of the initial course of therapy.

Prevention of disease in the individual is accomplished by the application of miticidal chemicals (dibutyl phthalate, benzyl benzoate, diethyltoluamide, and others) to clothing and the skin. There is no satisfactory vaccine. Chemoprophylactic studies conducted in highly endemic infested areas of scrub typhus showed that single oral doses of chloramphenicol or tetracycline given every 5 days for a total of 35 days (seven doses with 5-day nontreatment intervals) prevents scrub typhus and results in active immunity. This procedure is recommended under special circumstances. A long-acting tetracycline (doxycycline) serves the same purpose.

TRENCH FEVER Definition Trench fever is a febrile disease transmitted between humans by the body louse, *Pediculus humanus corporis*. It is characterized by a sudden onset with headache and severe pain in the muscles, bones, and joints. In most cases, the fever and other symptoms assume a relapsing character. Fatalities are rare. The disease is also known as shin bone fever, Volhynia fever, His-Werner disease, and quintan fever.

Etiology and epidemiology *R. quintana,* the etiologic agent, grows extracellularly in the louse gut, in contrast to other pathogenic rickettsias which can multiply only within cells. A European strain of *R. quintana* has been cultivated on blood agar, and typical trench fever has been induced in volunteers.

Humans are the only known reservoir of infection. The louse does not transmit the organism transovarially but acquires its infection by ingesting the blood of a person with rickettsemia. The organisms multiply extracellularly in the louse gut, without injury to this host, and are excreted in large numbers with the feces. Humans become infected by the inoculation of the contaminated feces into abraded skin or conjunctivas. *R. quintana* may be recovered periodically from human blood for several years after convalescence from an acute attack. Trench fever is known to exist in Mexico, Tunisia, Eritrea, Poland, the U.S.S.R., and possibly China, and there is serologic evidence for its occurrence in Bolivia, Burundi, and Ethiopia.

Pathology Since there have been no recorded fatalities, histologic examination has been confined to excised macules of the skin, which have shown nonspecific perivascular infiltrates without the involvement of the vessel walls that is seen in typhus fever.

Clinical manifestations Clinical manifestations range from a mild afebrile disease to a debilitating illness with a protracted clinical course involving numerous relapses. Following an incubation period of 10 to 30 days the onset may be insidious or dramatically abrupt. The acute disease is characterized by malaise, headache, fever, and bone and body pain, especially severe in the shins. In some cases only one fever peak occurs; in others the fever continues for 5 to 7 days; and in others there is an initial febrile episode lasting 1 to 3 days followed by relapses which characteristically occur at 4- to 5-day intervals. In some cases the fever and symptoms are continuous for 2 or 3 weeks. Enlargement of the spleen and a red macular rash occur in 70 to 80 percent of the cases. Pain and soreness in the muscles usually recur with each febrile relapse.

The disease is marked by a persistent rickettsemia, which is present during the initial attack and which continues during the relapses, throughout the asymptomatic periods between relapses, and for months or even years after cessation of physical symptoms. A relapse has been reported 10 years after the original attack.

Prognosis The disease causes no known deaths, but its duration is variable. About 85 percent of patients are able to return to work within 2 months of onset, but about 5 percent of all cases become chronic. Recovery is even more delayed in the aged and debilitated.

Differential diagnosis During epidemics, typical cases are easily diagnosed on the basis of symptoms. The disease may be differentiated from influenza, typhoid, typhus, dengue, and relapsing fever by the specific laboratory tests available for the diagnosis of each of these diseases.

Treatment and prevention *R. quintana* is highly sensitive in vitro to the broad-spectrum antibiotics, but no reliable information has been obtained about the value of these drugs in treating trench fever. The treatment is symptomatic. Aspirin is used to control pain and discomfort, but codeine may be necessary. Patients should remain in bed for a week or more after complete cessation of subjective and objective evidence of infection. They should be kept under observation for several months.

The methods employed to control epidemic typhus should be equally efficacious in controlling trench fever. These are based on the elimination of lousiness and the improvement of living conditions with provision for frequent bathing and washing of clothing. DDT or lindane powder should be applied by hand or power duster at appropriate intervals to clothes and persons living under conditions favoring lousiness. If resistant lice are found, malathion or other effective lousicides may be substituted as a dusting powder.

RICKETTSIALPOX Definition Rickettsialpox is a mild, nonfatal, self-limited, febrile illness caused by *R. akari,* which is transmitted from mouse to humans by mites. It is characterized by an initial skin lesion at the site of the mite bite, a week's febrile course, and a papulovesicular rash.

Etiology and epidemiology Rickettsialpox was first recognized in New York City in 1946, and about 180 cases were reported annually for several years thereafter. It has been diagnosed in several other areas of the United States, and outbreaks have been reported in European Russia. The vector is a small, colorless mite, *Allodermanyssus sanguineus* (Hirst), which infests small mice and rodents. House mice serve as the reservoir of infection.

R. akari is morphologically and biologically similar to other rickettsias and is antigenically related to, but distinct from, *R. rickettsii*, the cause of Rocky Mountain spotted fever.

Clinical manifestations The initial skin lesion appears about 7 to 10 days after the mite bite as a firm red papule 1 to 1.5 cm in diameter. In a few days, the center vesiculates, and the papule is surrounded by an area of erythema. The regional lymph glands are moderately enlarged. The primary lesion, which is never painful, becomes covered with a black scab; it heals slowly, and a small scar is visible on separation of the crust.

The febrile phase begins 3 to 7 days after the initial lesion, and an exanthem may accompany the fever or begin several days later. The onset of fever is sudden, with chilly sensations or frank chills, headache, sweats, myalgia, anorexia, and photophobia. The pyrexia ranges from 103 to 104°F and continues for about a week, occasionally with morning remissions.

The exanthem is maculopapular-vesicular, generalized in distribution, and may be abundant or scant. The lesions may involve the oral cavity but not the palms or soles. In a week, the vesicles dry and form scabs which eventually scale but leave no scar.

The constitutional symptoms are generally mild, and the course of illness is uncomplicated. No fatal cases have been reported.

The disease may be confused with chickenpox, which is different because it occurs usually in childhood and has no initial lesion and the papular cutaneous lesion is entirely transformed into a vesicle. Variola (smallpox) is accompanied by a more severe constitutional reaction, and the vesicles become pustules. The skin lesions of the other rickettsioses differ in their lack of vesiculation. The Weil-Felix reaction is usually negative in this rickettsial disease, but specific complement fixation, microscopic agglutination, and immunofluorescent antibody reactions are useful diagnostic aids even though there is considerable antigenic crossing with materials from Rocky Mountain spotted fever.

Treatment and prevention Chloramphenicol and the tetracycline antibiotics are all effective for treating patients with rickettsialpox. The temperature reaches normal levels in about 2 days, and recovery is rapid.

Control measures should be directed toward elimination of house mice and the vector mites responsible for transmitting the disease.

OTHER TICK-BORNE RICKETTSIAL DISEASES Definition Boutonneuse fever, North Asian tick-borne rickettsiosis, and Queensland tick typhus, three diseases occurring in the eastern hemisphere, are caused by rickettsias closely related to one another and to the agent of Rocky Mountain spotted fever. Each is transmitted by the bite of an ixodid tick. These mild to moderately severe illnesses are characterized by an initial lesion (called *tache noire* in boutonneuse fever), a fever of several days to 2 weeks, and a generalized maculopapular erythematous rash which appears on about the fifth day and usually involves the palms and soles. Specific complement-fixing antibodies appear in the patients' serums during convalescence, but agglutinins to *Proteus* OX-19 (Weil-Felix reaction) are frequently found only in low titer.

Etiology and epidemiology The etiologic agents of these three diseases are all members of the spotted fever group of rickettsias. Together with *R. rickettsii* and *R. akari* they possess common group antigens which are readily demonstrated by agglutination, complement fixation, microscopic agglutination, and immunofluorescent antibody reactions.

Boutonneuse fever, which may be regarded as the prototype of the three, is caused by *R. conorii*. Modern serologic methods employing specific rickettsial antigens have shown this rickettsia to be the causative agent for a single widely disseminated disease known by various local names. Information on the distribution and etiology of the various tick-borne rickettsial diseases is contained in Table 148-1.

In general, the epidemiology of these tick-borne rickettsioses resembles that of spotted fever in the western hemisphere. Ixodid ticks and small wild animals maintain the rickettsias in nature; if humans intrude accidentally into the cycle, they become a dead end in the transmission chain. In certain areas, the cycle of boutonneuse fever involves domiciliary environments, with the brown dog tick *Rhipicephalus sanguineus* as the dominant vector.

Clinical manifestations These three tick-borne rickettsioses, which occur in different parts of the eastern hemisphere, resemble one another closely. The clinical course is usually milder than that of spotted fever, with a shorter febrile period and fewer severe complications; fatalities are rare and generally limited to the aged and debilitated. The initial lesion, which is present in most cases at the onset of fever, heals slowly; the regional lymph nodes are enlarged. The rash usually remains papular and only in severe cases becomes hemorrhagic.

The clinical picture (including the primary lesion), the geographic location, and epidemiologic considerations are helpful in establishing the diagnosis. The typhus fevers, meningococcal infections, leptospirosis, and measles must be considered in the differential diagnosis; the serologic reactions, i.e., Weil-Felix and complement fixation tests, are of value here.

Treatment and prevention Chloramphenicol and the tetracyclines are effective therapeutic agents for boutonneuse fever. Patients generally become afebrile after 2 to 3 days of treatment, and recovery is rapid. Presumably these measures are also applicable to North Asian tick-borne rickettsiosis and Queensland tick typhus.

The major effective methods of control are concerned with avoidance of tick bites; these include application of new repellents and prompt removal of attached ticks. Effective vaccines are not available commercially.

Q FEVER Definition Q fever is an acute infectious disease caused by *Coxiella burnetii* and characterized by a sudden onset of fever, malaise, headache, weakness, anorexia, and interstitial pneumonitis. Rickettsemia occurs during the febrile period, and specific complement-fixing antibodies are present during convalescence. In contrast to the other rickettsioses, the disease is not associated with a cutaneous exanthem or agglutinins for the *Proteus* bacteria (Weil-Felix reaction).

Etiology and epidemiology *C. burnetii* possesses the general properties of other rickettsias but is somewhat more resistant to inactivation in unfavorable environments and more pleomorphic than the others. Its infectivity after drying under natural conditions is of importance in the spread of infection to humans. *C. burnetii* has a wide host range in nature, but guinea pigs and embryonated eggs are the common laboratory hosts employed for its propagation.

Human cases of Q fever are contracted by inhalation of infected dusts, by handling infected materials, possibly by drinking milk contaminated with *C. burnetii* and, in one instance, by blood transfusion. The disease in Australia is enzootic in animals, especially bandicoots, and is transmitted in nature by ticks. Rickettsia-laden tick feces may contaminate cattle hides, and inhalation of this material has caused infection in humans. In the United States, a number of species of ticks are naturally infected, among them *Dermacentor andersoni* and *Amblyomma americanum,* and in North Africa transovarial transmission of the agent in indigenous ticks has been demonstrated. Sheep, goats, and cows have been found to be naturally infected in North America and in Europe, and *C. burnetii* has been recovered from the milk of such animals. Milk, as well as infected excretions from livestock, probably accounts for certain outbreaks of human disease following inhalation by cows of infected dust from barns and pens. The airborne route of dried contaminated material is the most likely method of spread. A number of epidemics have occurred among laboratory workers engaged in studies on *C. burnetii.* The disease is not transmitted between humans.

Clinical manifestations After incubation of approximately 19 days (the range is 14 to 26 days), the disease begins with headache, chilly sensations, fever, malaise, myalgia, and anorexia. For several days, the temperature ranges from 101 to 104°F; the entire course rarely exceeds 2 weeks and usually ranges from 3 to 6 days. There may be wide fluctuations in the fever. Respiratory and gastrointestinal symptoms are not conspicuous in the early stages. Headache and fever predominate. A dry cough and chest pain occur after about 5 days, when rales are usually audible. Roentgenographic findings indistinguishable from those of primary atypical pneumonia are present usually by the third to fourth day of disease, first as patchy areas of consolidation involving a portion of one lobe, giving a homogeneous ground-glass appearance. Occasionally, a homogeneous localized infiltration may resemble a tumor mass. These manifestations persist beyond the febrile period and may appear in patients who are unaware of pulmonary involvement. Complications are rare, and coincident with defervescence the appetite begins to return. Convalescence progresses slowly for several weeks, during which time the principal disability is weakness. It is not uncommon for patients to lose 7 to 9 kg during the active stages of disease. The disease may be protracted in approximately 20 percent of cases, with fever persisting for longer than 4 weeks, particularly in elderly patients. Occasionally relapse occurs, especially in patients treated with antibiotics during the first several days of disease.

Hepatitis, with the development of clinically detectable icterus, occurs in approximately one-third of patients with the protracted form. This form of Q fever is characterized by fever, malaise, absence of headache or respiratory signs, and hepatomegaly with right upper quadrant pain. Liver biopsy specimens show diffuse granulomatous changes with multinucleated giant cells and scattered infiltrations of polymorphonuclear leukocytes, lymphocytes, and macrophages. *C. burnetii* may be demonstrated in such specimens with the fluorescent antibody technique. Therefore, Q fever must be included in the differential diagnosis of patients with hepatitis and those with hepatic granulomas such as tuberculosis, sarcoidosis, histoplasmosis, brucellosis, tularemia, syphilis, and others.

Endocarditis also has been reported, and *C. burnetii* has been identified by smear and isolation in vegetations on the heart valves obtained at operation or autopsy. The aortic valve is most commonly involved, often with large vegetations. It is important, therefore, to suspect the possibility of Q fever in cases of apparent subacute bacterial endocarditis with persistently negative blood cultures. Operative intervention with replacement of damaged valves is usually necessary for recovery because the available antibiotics are not rickettsicidal. In some selected instances long-term antibiotic therapy has been successful.

A high complement-fixing antibody titer to phase I antigen is present in patients with endocarditis and granulomatous hepatitis.

Prognosis Few fatalities have been recorded and, except for the patient with protracted illness and hepatic involvement or endocarditis, the course of disease is generally uncomplicated and benign.

Treatment and control The tetracycline antibiotics and chloramphenicol are effective in the treatment of patients with Q fever. Most patients, when treated early in the course of disease, respond promptly and recover without relapses. The therapeutic procedures are comparable to those used in spotted fever.

Control of Q fever depends primarily on immunization of susceptible persons with specific vaccines. Vaccines made from phase I rickettsias are potent and afford considerable protection to slaughterhouse and dairy workers, herders, rendering-plant workers, woolsorters, tanners, laboratory workers, and others at risk. Measures should be taken to avoid exposure to infected aerosols; milk from infected domestic livestock must be pasteurized or boiled.

REFERENCES

Andrew R et al: Tick typhus in North Queensland. Med J Aust 2:253, 1946

Bozeman FM et al: Serologic evidence of *Rickettsia canada* infection in man. J Infect Dis 121:367, 1970

——— et al: Epidemic typhus rickettsiae isolated from flying squirrels. Nature 255:545, 1975

Centers for Disease Control: Epidemic typhus—Georgia. Morb Mort Week Rep 33:618, 1984

Derrick EH: The epidemiology of Q fever: A review. Med J Aust 1:245, 1953

DeShazo RD et al: Early diagnosis of Rocky Mountain spotted fever. Use of primary monocyte culture technique. JAMA 235:1353, 1976

Ferguson IC et al: Clinical, virological and pathological findings in a fatal case of Q fever endocarditis. Br J Clin Pathol 15:235, 1962

Gambrill MR, Wisseman CL Jr: Mechanisms of immunity in typhus infections. Infect Immun 8:519, 1973

Harrell GT: Rickettsial involvement of the nervous system. Med Clin North Am 37:395, 1953

Hattwick MAW et al: Rocky Mountain spotted fever: Epidemiology of an increasing problem. Ann Intern Med 84:732, 1976

Hazard GW et al: Rocky Mountain spotted fever in the Eastern United States. N Engl J Med 280:57, 1969

Koster FT et al: Cellular immunity in Q fever: Specific lymphocyte unresponsiveness in Q fever endocarditis. J Infect Dis 152:1283, 1985

Moulton FR (ed): *The Rickettsial Diseases of Man.* Washington, DC, American Association for the Advancement of Science, 1948

Murray ES et al: Brill's disease: I. Clinical and laboratory diagnosis. JAMA 142:1059, 1950

———, Snyder JC: Brill's disease: II. Etiology. Am J Hyg 53:22, 1951

Ormsbee RA et al: The influence of phase on the protective potency of Q fever vaccine. J Immunol 92:404, 1964

——— et al: Serologic diagnosis of epidemic typhus fever. Am J Epidemiol 105:261, 1977

Oster CN et al: Laboratory acquired Rocky Mountain spotted fever: The hazard of aerosol transmission. N Engl J Med 297:859, 1977

Pedersen CE et al: Demonstration of *Rickettsia rickettsii* in Rhesus monkeys by immune fluorescence microscopy. J Clin Microbiol 2:121, 1975

Philip RN et al: A comparison of serologic methods for diagnosis of Rocky Mountain spotted fever. Am J Epidemiol 105:56, 1977

Rocky Mountain spotted fever—United States, 1985. Morb Mort Week Rep 35:247, 1986

Rose HM: The clinical manifestations and laboratory diagnosis of rickettsialpox. Ann Intern Med 31:871, 1949

Smadel JE: Influence of antibiotics on immunologic responses in scrub typhus. Am J Med 17:246, 1954

——— (ed): *Symposium on Q Fever,* Medical Science Publication 6. Washington, DC, Walter Reed Army Institute of Research, 1959

———, Jackson EB: Rickettsial infections, in *Diagnostic Procedures of Viral and Rickettsial Diseases,* 3d ed. New York, American Public Health Association, 1964, p 743

Somenshine DE et al: Epizootiology of epidemic typhus (*Rickettsia prowazekii*) in flying squirrels. Am J Trop Med Hyg 27:339, 1978

Vinson JW: Etiology of trench fever in Mexico, in *Industry and Tropical Health,* vol V. Boston, Harvard School of Public Health, 1964, p 109

Walker DH, Cain BG: A method for specific diagnosis of Rocky Mountain spotted fever on fixed, paraffin-embedded tissue by immunofluorescence. J Infect Dis 137:206, 1978

———, Bradford WD: Rocky Mountain spotted fever in childhood, in *Perspectives in Pediatric Pathology,* vol 6, HS Rosenberg, J Bernstein (eds). New York, Masson Publishing, 1981, pp 35–61

Wolbach SB: Studies on Rocky Mountain spotted fever. J Med Res 41:1, 1919

Woodward TE: Rickettsial diseases in the United States. Med Clin North Am 43:1507, 1959

———: A historical account of the rickettsial diseases with a discussion of unsolved problems. J Infect Dis 127:583, 1973

———: Identification of *Rickettsia* in skin tissues. J Infect Dis 134:297, 1976

149 *MYCOPLASMA* INFECTIONS

WALLACE A. CLYDE, JR.[1]

The mycoplasmas, formerly called pleuropneumonia-like organisms (PPLO) after the organism that causes a highly contagious form of bovine pneumonia and pleurisy, are now designated class Mollicutes, with three families and four genera.

The mycoplasma of chief importance in human disease is *M. pneumoniae,* a respiratory pathogen. Others include *M. hominis* and *Ureaplasma urealyticum,* which involve the genitourinary tract.

[1] *The editors wish to acknowledge the contribution of Vernon Knight. It is on his chapter in the 10th edition of* Principles of Internal Medicine *that this revision is based.*

M. pneumoniae grows on peptone-enriched beef-heart infusion as small round colonies partially buried in the agar without the "fried egg" periphery characteristic of growth of *M. hominis* and many mycoplasmas. *Ureaplasma urealyticum* requires anaerobic incubation and special media of acid pH.

Mycoplasmas are resistant to penicillin and antibiotics known to interfere with polymerization of cell wall precursors, and they do not retain the dye-iodine complex of Gram stain. They are inhibited by tetracyclines and, in selected instances, erythromycin. Like bacteria, they grow outside the cell, possess ribonucleic and deoxyribonucleic acids, and reproduce by fission.

MYCOPLASMA PNEUMONIAE

DEFINITION Pneumonia caused by *M. pneumoniae* is characterized by fever, pharyngitis, cough, and pulmonary infiltration, in which roentgenographic signs are more extensive than indicated by physical examination. Synonyms are primary atypical pneumonia, Eaton agent pneumonia, and cold agglutinin–positive pneumonia. This organism also commonly causes upper respiratory illness without pneumonia and asymptomatic infection.

ETIOLOGY *M. pneumoniae* is distinguished from other mycoplasmas by rapid hemolysis of sheep or guinea pig erythrocytes and utilization of glucose and other sugars. It may be identified serologically by fluorescent antibody, complement fixation, growth inhibition, and indirect hemagglutination tests, all of which are useful for serologic diagnosis of human infection.

EPIDEMIOLOGY In the general population *M. pneumoniae* infection is characterized by intrafamilial spread. In most cases the infection is introduced into the family by a schoolchild. Once it is introduced, most family members become infected. In family outbreaks, pneumonia occurs with greatest frequency among school-age children, with a predominance in males. The disease is less common above age 40. *M. pneumoniae* pneumonia occurs throughout the year, although prolonged wintertime outbreaks may occur in college groups or communities. The total incidence of *M. pneumoniae* pneumonia in a study in Seattle was 1.3 per 1000 per year, which constituted about 15 to 20 percent of pneumonia from all causes. At intervals of several years, epidemics of *M. pneumoniae* pneumonia may occur with about double the usual incidence of disease.

Certain populations are at high risk for acquisition of *M. pneumoniae* infections. This mycoplasma is the leading cause of pneumonia among college students, accounting for 50 percent of all cases. Another group having a high incidence of infections is military recruits; 20 to 50 percent of pneumonia in this setting is caused by *M. pneumoniae*.

M. pneumoniae is probably spread by means of infected respiratory secretions. The organisms can be cultured from sputum of naturally occurring cases and from volunteers infected artificially. In volunteers naturally acquired antibody is associated with a high degree of resistance to infection. However, this immunity is not permanent since second episodes of pneumonia have been documented within 4 to 10 years.

CLINICAL MANIFESTATIONS The incubation period is from 9 to 12 days in experimental infections, but the interval between cases in families is approximately 3 weeks. Illness usually begins with symptoms of upper respiratory infection, which in some patients progresses to bronchitis and pneumonia. Four syndromes of respiratory disease have been identified: pneumonia, tracheobronchitis, pharyngitis, and bullous myringitis. About one-third of cases in family members will develop pneumonia, up to one-half will have tracheobronchitis, 10 percent exhibit only pharyngitis, and 10 percent will be asymptomatic. Children 5 to 10 years old have the greatest incidence of disease. Ear involvement and nondescript skin rashes are common in children, while sinusitis is present in half of adults. Cough is almost universal in pneumonia and is frequent in cases without pulmonary involvement. Blood-flecked sputum may occur in the more severe cases, but gross hemoptysis is rare. A variety of other respiratory and systemic complaints may occur. Fever, nasal congestion, and sore throat are common. In pneumonia, harsh or diminished sounds are frequent but bronchial breathing is uncommon. Fine inspiratory rales are found in most patients but are not impressive. Pleural rubs and pleural effusion are infrequent. Studies on the distribution of pneumonia in one large series showed that more than one-half of cases were multilobular and slightly less than one-half were bilateral. Lower-lobe pneumonia was appreciably more frequent than upper-lobe pneumonia. Pulmonary infiltrates may occur as an isolated area in the lung periphery but more often spread from the hilum.

The disease is variable in severity, but high fever may persist for 1 to 2 weeks in untreated cases. X-ray changes last for as long as 3 weeks in untreated cases, but for 7 to 10 days in treated cases. Even in untreated cases, complications are rare and consist of occasional purulent sinusitis, persistent cough, and, rarely, pleurisy. Prolonged weakness and malaise follow the untreated illness in adults.

Rare complications include meningoencephalitis, polyneuritis, monoarticular arthritis, Stevens-Johnson syndrome, pericarditis, myocarditis, hepatitis, diffuse intravascular coagulation, noncardiogenic pulmonary edema, and hemolytic anemia.

LABORATORY FINDINGS During acute illness leukocytosis in the range of 10,000 to 15,000 leukocytes per cubic millimeter occurs in about 25 percent of cases. Increase in sedimentation rate above 40 mm/h occurs in at least two-thirds of cases. Urinalysis, electrocardiograms, and fluid and electrolyte and liver function studies show no characteristic changes. The complement fixation, fluorescent antibody, indirect hemagglutination, and growth inhibition tests yield specific diagnostic information. The simplicity of the complement fixation test recommends it for general use, although it is less sensitive and specific than the other tests. Fourfold rises in titer often occur within 2 weeks, and maximum rise is achieved in 4 weeks. A nonspecific test for *M. pneumoniae* infection in use for many years is the detection of cold agglutinins. The end point is the dilution of the patient's serum which agglutinates human type O red blood cells at 4°C. The test depends on the presence of a macroglobulin antibody to the I antigen of red blood cells. In *M. pneumoniae* infection, cold agglutinins appear at the end of the first week of illness and can serve as a rapid diagnostic test; they disappear in 2 to 6 weeks. The test is positive in about half the patients, more commonly in those who are severely ill. The cold agglutinin reaction occurs with other red blood cell antigens in infectious mononucleosis, lymphoproliferative diseases, and in several respiratory infections, particularly in children younger than 5 years.

New information about perturbations of host immune response in *M. pneumoniae* infections dictates caution in interpreting serologic data. Due to polyclonal B-cell activation "nonspecific" antibody rises to diverse agents can occur; coupled with T-lymphocyte suppression, this also may explain the appearance of various host tissue autoantibodies and transient anergy. Since other infectious agents, including cytomegalovirus, Epstein-Barr virus, and measles, produce similar effects, diagnostic confusion can result. *M. pneumoniae* serologic tests never should be included in panels of studies for illness of unknown cause.

DIFFERENTIAL DIAGNOSIS Pneumonia due to *M. pneumoniae* needs to be distinguished from pneumonia of all other types. It is usually less severe, is associated with less dense pulmonary infiltration than pneumococcal and other bacterial pneumonias, and occurs throughout the year. Pulmonary infiltrates in the absence of symptoms or physical signs may initially suggest acute pulmonary tuberculosis. In military populations adenoviral pneumonia must be excluded. Pneumonic involvement as a direct result of influenza viral infection or its complication by pneumococcal, streptococcal, staphylococcal, or *Haemophilus influenzae* infection may cause difficulty in diagnosis.

Q fever, psittacosis, and tularemia are less frequent causes of pneumonia that may be difficult to distinguish from *M. pneumoniae* infection. In children, especially young infants, pneumonia due to respiratory syncytial, parainfluenza, adenovirus, and influenza viruses may resemble *M. pneumoniae* infection. Legionnaires' disease (see Chap. 117) resembles severe cases of *M. pneumoniae* pneumonia.

TREATMENT Erythromycin and tetracycline derivatives are effective in treating *M. pneumoniae* disease. For adults, erythromycin (0.5 g every 8 h orally) or tetracycline (250 mg every 6 h orally) for 10 to 14 days usually is prescribed. In severe illnesses the dose may be increased and given for 21 days; intravenous erythromycin at times is useful, but tetracycline is not recommended by this route. For children below age 8, erythromycin is the primary antibiotic at doses of 30 to 50 mg/kg per day orally for 10 to 14 days. Tetracycline is an effective alternative in older patients.

Treatment temporarily reduces the frequency of positive cultures from the respiratory tract, but shedding may continue for several weeks after treatment, a finding similar to that in psittacosis pneumonia. Relapse of *M. pneumoniae* pneumonia occurs occasionally, but such cases respond to re-treatment. In cases in which there is doubt between the diagnosis of *M. pneumoniae* and *Legionella* or pneumococcal infection, erythromycin should be used in preference to a tetracycline. No vaccines are available.

OTHER *MYCOPLASMA* INFECTIONS

A growing body of literature documents evidence of other human *Mycoplasma* infections, particularly in the perinatal period, and a variety of genitourinary syndromes in both sexes. *Mycoplasma* should be suspected in suppurative processes that are bacteriologically sterile, such as urethritis, salpingitis, amnionitis, neonatal meningitis, and pneumonia and pyelonephritis. *Mycoplasma* abscesses and arthritis may occur in immunocompromised hosts. Sexually transmitted *Mycoplasma* diseases are considered elsewhere (see Chap. 91).

Mycoplasmas most commonly encountered are *M. hominis* and *U. urealyticum*. *M. hominis* hydrolyzes arginine in liquid media, producing ammonia which results in an alkaline pH shift. Ureaplasmas are so-named because they cleave urea, again producing ammonia. Selective, differential media have been described which allow demonstration of the unique urease activity on primary isolation within 24 to 48 h.

Very few diagnostic microbiology laboratories perform *Mycoplasma* cultures, and serodiagnosis remains a research tool for species other than *M. pneumoniae*. Specimens should be transported on wet ice (within 24 h or less) or dry ice (greater than 24 h) to reference laboratories for assistance. Generally, *M. hominis* is sensitive to tetracycline and clindamycin but not erythromycin, while ureaplasmas are sensitive to tetracyclines and erythromycin. Since antibiotic sensitivity patterns of these species vary widely, laboratory guidance may be required for effective therapy.

REFERENCES

CASSELL GH, COLE BC: Mycoplasmas as agents of human disease. N Engl J Med 304:80, 1981

CHERRY JD et al: *Mycoplasma pneumoniae* infections and exanthems. J Pediatr 87:369, 1975

CLYDE WA, FERNALD GW: Mycoplasmas: The pathogens' pathogen. Cell Immunol 82:88, 1983

COUCH RB: *Mycoplasma pneumoniae*, in *Principles and Practice of Infectious Diseases*, G Mandell et al (eds). New York, Wiley, 1985, pp 1065–1076

FOY HM et al: Viral and mycoplasmal pneumonia in a prepaid medical care group during an eight year period. Am J Epidemiol 97:93, 1973

KALB RE et al: Stevens-Johnson syndrome due to *Mycoplasma pneumoniae* in an adult. Am J Med 79:541, 1985

MCDADE JE et al: Legionnaires' disease. Isolation of a bacterium and demonstration of its role in other respiratory disease. N Engl J Med 297:1197, 1978

ROIFMAN CM et al: Increased susceptibility to *Mycoplasma* infection in patients with hypogammaglobulinemia. Am J Med 80:590, 1986

150 CHLAMYDIAL INFECTIONS

WALTER E. STAMM / KING K. HOLMES

The genus *Chlamydia* contains two species, *C. psittaci* and *C. trachomatis*. *C. psittaci* is widely distributed in nature, producing genital, conjunctival, intestinal, or respiratory infections in many mammalian and avian species. Genital infections with *C. psittaci* have been well characterized in several species and cause complications such as abortion and infertility. Although mammalian strains of *C. psittaci* are not known to infect humans, avian strains do occasionally infect humans, causing pneumonia.

C. trachomatis is exclusively a human pathogen and was first recognized as the cause of trachoma in the 1940s. Since then, *C. trachomatis* has been recognized as a major sexually transmitted and perinatal infection. Chlamydiae are obligate, intracellular parasites that were originally considered large viruses. However, they possess both DNA and RNA, have a cell wall and ribosomes similar to those of gram-negative bacteria, and can be inhibited by antibiotics such as tetracycline. Therefore, chlamydiae are now classified as bacteria belonging to their own order (Chlamydiales) and genus (*Chlamydia*).

A unique feature of all chlamydia is their complex reproductive cycle. Two forms of the microorganism—the extracellular elementary body and the intracellular reticulate body—participate in this cycle. The elementary body is adapted for extracellular survival and is the infective form transmitted from one person to another. Elementary bodies attach to susceptible target cells (usually columnar or transitional epithelial cells) via specific receptors and enter the cell within a phagosome. Within 8 h, the elementary bodies reorganize into reticulate bodies. These forms are adapted to intracellular survival and multiplication. They undergo binary fission, eventually producing numerous replicates contained within the membrane-bound "inclusion body" which occupies much of the infected host cell. Chlamydial inclusions resist lysosomal fusion until late in the developmental cycle. After 24 h, the reticulate bodies condense and form elementary bodies still contained within the inclusion. The inclusion then ruptures, releasing elementary bodies from the cell to initiate infection of adjacent cells.

C. psittaci and *C. trachomatis* share a genus-specific or group antigen. Antibody against this antigen is measured in the complement-fixation serologic test available in most state health departments. *C. trachomatis* strains can be further characterized serologically on the basis of antibody produced against their major outer membrane protein. These antigens serve as the basis for the serovar classification of Wang and Grayston. Using this system, strains associated with trachoma have generally been those of the A, B, Ba, and C serovars, while serovars D through K have been largely associated with sexually transmitted and perinatally acquired infections. Serovars L_1, L_2, and L_3 produce lymphogranuloma venereum (LGV) and hemorrhagic proctocolitis. These strains demonstrate unique biologic behavior in that they are more invasive than the other serovars, produce disease in lymphatic tissue, grow readily in cell culture systems and macrophages, and are fatal when inoculated intracerebrally in mice and monkeys. Non-LGV strains of *C. trachomatis* characteristically produce superficial infections involving the columnar epithelium of the eye, genitalia, and respiratory tract.

C. psittaci and *C. trachomatis* can be differentiated in the laboratory by inclusion type and sensitivity to sulfonamide. While *C. trachomatis* is sensitive to sulfa, *C. psittaci* is resistant. *C. trachomatis* inclusions contain glycogen and stain with iodine, while *C. psittaci* inclusions do not.

SEXUALLY TRANSMITTED AND PERINATAL *C. TRACHOMATIS* INFECTIONS

SPECTRUM OF *C. TRACHOMATIS* GENITAL INFECTIONS Genital infections caused by *C. trachomatis* are now recognized as the most common sexually transmitted disease (STD) in the United States. An estimated 3 to 4 million cases occur each year. In adults the clinical spectrum of sexually transmitted *C. trachomatis* infections is easily understood because it parallels closely the spectrum of gonococcal infections (Table 150-1). Both agents have been associated with urethritis in both sexes, with epididymitis, mucopurulent cervicitis, acute salpingitis, bartholinitis, proctitis, and the Fitz-Hugh–Curtis syndrome (perihepatitis), and both can be associated with systemic complications, particularly with arthritis. Simultaneous infection with *C. trachomatis* occurs in 30 to 50 percent of women with cervical gonococcal infection and in 25 percent of heterosexual men with gonococcal urethritis.

EPIDEMIOLOGY Genital infections other than LGV are caused by *C. trachomatis* serovars D through K. Although data are lacking, the incidence of genital *C. trachomatis* infection is probably increasing, because the incidence of nongonococcal urethritis (NGU) has risen dramatically over the last two decades, and *C. trachomatis* has consistently been isolated from 30 to 50 percent of men with NGU. The peak age incidence of genital *C. trachomatis* infections is in the late teens and early twenties, resembling other sexually transmitted infections. Further evidence for sexual transmission is the rising prevalence of serum antibody to *C. trachomatis* in proportion to an increasing number of sex partners. The prevalence of chlamydial urethral infection in young men ranges from 3 to 5 percent of men seen in general medical settings, to over 10 percent of asymptomatic soldiers undergoing routine physical examination, to 15 to 20 percent of men seen in STD clinics. Among homosexual men, urethral infection appears less common (4 to 5 percent of homosexual men in STD clinics) than in heterosexual men, but rectal infections occur with a prevalence of 4 to 7 percent in homosexual male STD clinic patients. Cervical infection in women has ranged from 5 percent or more of asymptomatic college students or prenatal patients in the United States, to over 10 percent of women seen in family planning clinics, to over 20 percent of women seen in STD clinics. In the United States, the prevalence of *C. trachomatis* in the cervix of pregnant women is 5 to 10 times higher than that of *N. gonorrhoeae*. The prevalence of genital infection with either agent is highest in individuals who are single, nonwhite, unmarried, and between ages 18 and 24. The ratio of chlamydial to gonococcal urethritis is highest for heterosexual men and those with high socioeconomic status, and lowest for homosexual men and indigent populations. The proportion of infections that are asymptomatic appears to be higher for *C. trachomatis* than for *N. gonorrhoeae*, and symptomatic *C. trachomatis* infections are clinically less severe. It is suspected that mild or asymptomatic chlamydial infections of the fallopian tubes may nonetheless cause ongoing tubal damage and infertility. Furthermore, because the total number of *C. trachomatis* infections exceeds that of *N. gonorrhoeae* infections in industrialized countries, the total morbidity caused by *C. trachomatis* genital infections is comparable with that caused by *N. gonorrhoeae*. The prevalence of *C. trachomatis* is higher than that of *N. gonorrhoeae* in industrialized countries, in part because measures such as treatment of sex partners and routine cultures for case detection in asymptomatic individuals are being applied much more effectively for gonorrhea than for control of *C. trachomatis* infection.

TABLE 150-1 Clinical parallels between sexually transmitted infections due to *Neisseria gonorrhoeae* and *Chlamydia trachomatis*

	Resulting clinical syndrome	
Site of infection	*N. gonorrhoeae*	*C. trachomatis*
MEN		
Urethra	Urethritis	NGU, PGU
Epididymis	Epididymitis	Epididymitis
Rectum	Proctitis	Proctitis
Conjunctiva	Conjunctivitis	Conjunctivitis
Systemic	Disseminated gonococcal infection (DGI)	Reiter's syndrome
WOMEN		
Urethra	Acute urethral syndrome	Acute urethral syndrome
Bartholin's gland	Bartholinitis	Bartholinitis
Cervix	Cervicitis	Cervicitis
Endometrium	Endometritis	Endometritis
Fallopian tube	Salpingitis	Salpingitis
Conjunctiva	Conjunctivitis	Conjunctivitis
Liver capsule	Perihepatitis	Perihepatitis
Systemic	DGI	Reiter's syndrome

CLINICAL MANIFESTATIONS Nongonococcal and postgonococcal urethritis Nongonococcal urethritis is a diagnosis of exclusion that is applied to men with symptoms and/or signs of urethritis who do not have gonorrhea. Postgonococcal urethritis (PGU) refers to nongonococcal urethritis which develops 2 to 3 weeks after treatment of gonococcal urethritis in men. *C. trachomatis* causes 30 to 50 percent of the cases of NGU and PGU in heterosexual men but is less commonly isolated from homosexual men with these syndromes. The cause of the remainder is uncertain, although considerable evidence suggests that *Ureaplasma urealyticum* causes some of these infections.

In current practice, NGU is diagnosed by documentation of a leukocytic urethral exudate and by exclusion of gonorrhea by Gram's stain or culture. *C. trachomatis* urethritis is generally less severe than gonococcal urethritis, although in an individual patient these two forms of urethritis cannot be differentiated solely on clinical grounds. Symptoms include urethral discharge, dysuria (often whitish and mucoid rather than frankly purulent), and urethral itching. The examination may show meatal erythema and tenderness and a urethral exudate which is often demonstrable only by stripping the urethra. About one-third of male STD patients who have *C. trachomatis* urethral infection have no demonstrable signs or symptoms of urethritis. Such patients frequently have first-glass pyuria (15 leukocytes per 400× microscopic field in the sediment of first-voided urine) or an increased number of leukocytes on gram-stained smear prepared from a urogenital swab inserted 1 to 2 cm into the anterior urethra. The smear is first scanned at low power to identify areas of the slide containing the highest concentration of leukocytes. These areas are then examined under oil immersion (1000×). An average of four or more leukocytes in five 1000× (oil immersion) fields is indicative of urethritis and correlates with recovery of *C. trachomatis*. To differentiate between true urethritis and functional symptoms among symptomatic patients, or to make a presumptive diagnosis of *C. trachomatis* infection in asymptomatic men (e.g., male patients in STD clinics, sex partners of women with nongonococcal salpingitis or mucopurulent cervicitis, fathers of children with inclusion conjunctivitis), the examination of an endourethral specimen for increased leukocytes is useful if specific diagnostic tests are not available.

Epididymitis *C. trachomatis* is the major cause of epididymitis in sexually active males. In one study, *C. trachomatis* infection was found by cultures of the urethra, urine, semen, or epididymal aspirate or by serology in 17 of 34 men under 35 years of age who presented with epididymitis, while 7 had gonorrhea; of 16 men over 35 with epididymitis, only 1 had chlamydial infection, and none had gonorrhea. Coliform bacteria and *Pseudomonas aeruginosa* are the most common causes of epididymitis in men over 35. The presence of a urethral discharge or a history of recent urethritis in association with unilateral scrotal pain, swelling, and tenderness suggests the diagnosis of chlamydial or gonococcal epididymitis. However, the presence of midstream pyuria and bacteriuria in an older patient without urethral discharge, but with a history of genitourinary instrumentation or bacterial urinary tract or prostatic infection, suggests coliform or *Pseudomonas* infection. Testicular torsion should be promptly excluded by radionuclide scan, Doppler flow study, or surgical exploration in a teenager or young adult who presents with acute unilateral testicular pain without urethritis. Testicular tumor or chronic infection (e.g., tuberculosis) should be excluded in the patient with unilateral intrascrotal pain and swelling who does not respond to appropriate antimicrobial therapy.

Reiter's syndrome *C. trachomatis* has been recovered from the urethra of up to 70 percent of men with untreated nondiarrheal Reiter's syndrome and associated urethritis. The syndrome consists of conjunctivitis, urethritis, arthritis, and characteristic skin lesions (see Chap. 268). In the absence of overt urethritis, it is important to exclude subclinical urethritis as discussed above.

Proctitis *C. trachomatis* of either the genital immunotypes D through K or the LGV immunotype L_2 causes proctitis in homosexual men and heterosexual women who practice anal intercourse. Either asymptomatic infection or mild proctitis not unlike gonococcal proctitis results from infection with immunotypes D through K. Clinically, these patients present with mild rectal pain, mucus discharge, tenesmus, and, occasionally, bleeding. Nearly all have polymorphonuclear leukocytes in their rectal Gram stain. Sigmoidoscopy in these non-LGV cases of chlamydial proctitis reveals mild, patchy mucosal friability and the disease process is limited to the distal rectum. LGV strains produce a more severe ulcerative proctitis or proctocolitis which histologically resembles Crohn's disease in that giant-cell formation and granulomas are seen (see Chap. 238). The differential diagnosis of proctitis limited to the distal rectum in homosexual men includes gonococcal or herpes simplex virus infection, in addition to *C. trachomatis* infection.

Mucopurulent cervicitis *C. trachomatis* has been isolated from the cervix of 30 to 60 percent of women with gonorrhea or a history of contact with gonorrhea, from 30 to 70 percent of women whose male partners have nongonococcal urethritis, and from 10 to 20 percent of women attending STD clinics who do not have a history of contact with a partner with urethritis. Women who have cervical ectopy or who use oral contraceptives appear to have an increased prevalence of cervical infection with *C. trachomatis*.

Although some women with *C. trachomatis* infection of the cervix have no symptoms or signs, careful speculum examination shows that many have mucopurulent cervicitis. As discussed more fully in Chap. 91, mucopurulent cervicitis is associated with yellow mucopurulent discharge from the endocervical columnar epithelium, and with $\geq$10 polymorphonuclear (PMN) leukocytes per 1000× microscopic field within strands of cervical mucus on a thinly smeared, Gram-stained preparation of endocervical exudate. Pap smear also shows increased PMN leukocytes, as well as a characteristic pattern of mononuclear inflammatory cells, including plasma cells, transformed lymphocytes, and histiocytes. Cervical biopsy shows predominantly a mononuclear infiltrate, often with a follicular cervicitis (i.e., lymphoid aggregates with germinal centers containing transformed lymphocytes.)

Pelvic inflammatory disease (PID) *C. trachomatis* plays an important causative role in salpingitis. *C. trachomatis* infection has been demonstrated in laparoscopically verified salpingitis, recovered from the fallopian tubes in the absence of other pathogens, and serologic evidence of *C. trachomatis* infection has been adduced in women with PID. In the United States *C. trachomatis* has been identified in the fallopian tubes or endometrium in up to 50 percent of women with PID, and its role as an important etiologic agent in this syndrome is now well accepted. The ability of *C. trachomatis* to cause salpingitis has been confirmed in animal models.

Pelvic inflammatory disease occurs via ascending intraluminal spread of *C. trachomatis* from the lower genital tract, and mucopurulent cervicitis is followed by endometritis, endosalpingitis, and finally pelvic peritonitis. Evidence of mucopurulent cervicitis is usually present in women with laparoscopically verified salpingitis. Similarly, endometritis, demonstrated by endometrial biopsy showing plasma cell infiltration of the endometrial epithelium, is present in nearly all women with laparoscopically verified chlamydial (or gonococcal) salpingitis. Chlamydial endometritis also occurs in the absence of clinical evidence of salpingitis: approximately 40 percent of women with mucopurulent cervicitis were found to have plasma cell endometritis in one study. Histologic evidence of endometritis was correlated with an "endometritis syndrome," consisting of vaginal bleeding, lower abdominal pain, and uterine tenderness in the absence of adnexal tenderness, and with peripheral blood leukocytosis. Since laparoscopy was not performed in these patients, it is not known what proportion of those with chlamydial endometritis without adnexal tenderness nonetheless had salpingitis. However, chlamydial salpingitis apparently produces milder symptoms then does gonococcal salpingitis and is associated with less marked adnexal tenderness. The presence of mild adnexal or uterine tenderness in sexually active women with cervicitis should suggest PID.

Infertility associated with fallopian tube scarring has been strongly linked to antecedent *C. trachomatis* infection in serologic studies. Since not all infertile women with tubal scarring and antichlamydial antibody in these studies gave a history of prior PID, subclinical tubal infection may produce scarring. Ectopic pregnancy, which occurs in over 60,000 women in the United States annually, is also thought to be related to chlamydia-induced tubal scarring in many cases.

Perihepatitis, or the Fitz-Hugh–Curtis syndrome, was originally described as a complication of gonococcal PID. However, cultural and/or serologic evidence of *C. trachomatis* infection in most women with this syndrome has come to light. *C. trachomatis* has also been cultured from exudate on the hepatic capsule in laparoscopically verified cases. This syndrome should be suspected whenever a young, sexually active woman presents with an illness resembling cholecystitis (fever and right upper quadrant pain of subacute or acute onset). Symptoms and signs of salpingitis may be minimal.

Urethral syndrome in women *C. trachomatis* has been found to be the most common pathogen isolated from college women with acute dysuria, frequency, and pyuria, together with the absence of uropathogens such as coliforms or *Staphylococcus saprophyticus* in *any* concentration in a clean-catch midstream urine specimen (see Chap. 225). *Chlamydia* can also be isolated from the urethra of women without symptoms of urethritis, and up to 25 percent of female STD clinic patients have had positive *C. trachomatis* cultures from the urethra only.

***C. trachomatis* infection in pregnancy** *C. trachomatis* in pregnancy has been associated in some studies (but not in others) with premature delivery and with postpartum endometritis. Whether these complications are in part attributable to *C. trachomatis* requires further investigation.

PERINATAL INFECTIONS: INCLUSION CONJUNCTIVITIS AND PNEUMONIA

EPIDEMIOLOGY Studies in the United States have demonstrated that 5 to 25 percent of pregnant women have *C. trachomatis* infections of the cervix. In these studies, approximately one-half to two-thirds of the children who were exposed during birth eventually showed laboratory evidence of *C. trachomatis* infection. Roughly half of the infants who developed laboratory evidence of infection (or 25 percent of the group exposed) developed clinical inclusion conjunctivitis. In addition to eye infection, *C. trachomatis* was isolated frequently and persistently from the nasopharynx and the rectum. Pneumonia occurs in about 10 percent of children infected perinatally, and otitis media may in some cases result from perinatally acquired chlamydial infection.

INCLUSION CONJUNCTIVITIS OF THE NEWBORN (NEONATAL CHLAMYDIAL CONJUNCTIVITIS) In the newborn, chlamydial conjunctivitis generally has a longer incubation period than gonococcal conjunctivitis (usually 5 to 14 days vs. 1 to 3 days), but this is not reliable in the individual patient. The other common causes of conjunctivitis in newborns include *Staphylococcus aureus, Haemophilus influenzae, Streptococcus pneumoniae,* and herpes simplex virus. Neonatal chlamydial conjunctivitis has an acute onset and often produces a profuse mucopurulent discharge. However, it is impossible to differentiate *Chlamydia* conjunctivitis from other forms of neonatal bacterial conjunctivitis clinically, and laboratory diagnosis is required. Inclusions within epithelial cells often can be demonstrated in Giemsa-stained conjunctival smears, but these smears are less sensitive than cultures or antigen detection tests. Similarly, Gram-stained smears may show gonococci, or occasional small gram-negative coccobacilli in *Haemophilus* conjunctivitis, but smears should be accompanied by cultures for these agents. Very rarely a trachoma-like eye disease with chlamydial infection occurs in children living in areas that do not have endemic trachoma. This probably is the late result of neonatally acquired infection. If neonatal chlamydial conjunctivitis is not treated appropriately with oral antimicrobials, it may be followed by chlamydial pneumonia.

INFANT PNEUMONIA There is a distinctive pneumonia syndrome in infants infected with *C. trachomatis* which occurs in two to six cases per 1000 live births. The diagnosis of *C. trachomatis* pneumonia has been confirmed by isolation of the organism from lung biopsy and by development of high titers of specific IgM antibody to *C. trachomatis*. This pneumonia has been found in infants from 1 to 4 months of age. The onset is gradual and the course protracted, but the child is usually afebrile. Radiographically, there is diffuse interstitial involvement of the lungs. Most of the infants have a distinctive cough (a series of closely spaced staccato coughs, each separated by a brief inspiration), tachypnea, rales, hyperinflation, slight eosinophilia, and elevated serum immunoglobulins. Clinical illness lasts several weeks, while inspiratory rales and radiologic signs may persist for months. About half of the infants with pneumonia also have conjunctivitis. While many infants with pneumonia have recovered without therapy, a few in whom the illness has been associated with apnea have been severely ill.

LYMPHOGRANULOMA VENEREUM

DEFINITION Lymphogranuloma venereum (LGV) is a sexually transmitted infection caused by *C. trachomatis* strains of the L_1, L_2, or L_3 serovars. Most cases are caused by L_2 infections. The acute disease in heterosexual men is characterized by a transient primary genital lesion followed by multilocular suppurative regional lymphadenopathy. Women, homosexual men, and, occasionally, heterosexual men may develop hemorrhagic proctitis with regional lymphadenitis. Acute LGV is almost always associated with systemic symptoms such as fever and leukocytosis and rarely with systemic complications such as meningoencephalitis. After a latent period of years, late complications include genital elephantiasis, strictures, and fistulas of the penis, urethra, and rectum.

FIGURE 150-1 *Lymphogranuloma venereum. Bilateral inguinal buboes, with the "sign of the groove," caused by adenopathy above and below Poupart's ligament. (Courtesy of A Brathwaite.)*

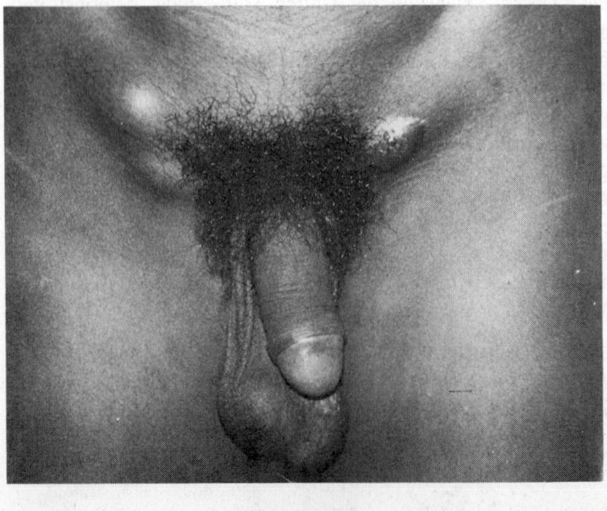

EPIDEMIOLOGY LGV is usually sexually transmitted, but occasional transmission by nonsexual personal contact, fomites, or laboratory accidents has been documented. Laboratory work involving creation of aerosols of this organism (e.g., sonication, homogenization) must be conducted with appropriate biologic containment.

The peak incidence of LGV corresponds to the age of greatest sexual activity, the second and third decades of life. The worldwide incidence of LGV is falling, but the disease is still endemic and a major cause of morbidity in Asia, Africa, and South America. Only 235 cases were reported in the United States in 1982.

The frequency of infection following exposure is believed to be much less than that associated with gonorrhea and syphilis. Early manifestations are recognized far more often in men than in women, who usually present with late complications. In the United States, where the reported sex ratio is 3.4 males to 1 female, most cases involve homosexually active men; travelers, seamen, and military personnel returning from abroad; and individuals of low socioeconomic status living in areas of low endemicity in the southeast. The main reservoir of infection is presumed to be asymptomatically infected individuals, although this has not been directly demonstrated.

CLINICAL MANIFESTATIONS In heterosexuals, a *primary genital lesion* occurs from 3 days to 3 weeks after exposure. It is a small, painless vesicle or nonindurated ulcer or papule located on the penis in men or on the labia, posterior vagina, or fourchette in women. The primary lesion is noticed by less than one-third of men with LGV and only rarely by women. It heals in a few days without scarring and even when noticed is usually not recognized as LGV except in retrospect. LGV strains of *C. trachomatis* have occasionally been recovered from genital ulcers, and also from the urethra of men and the endocervix of women who present with inguinal adenopathy, suggesting that these areas may be the primary site of infection in some cases.

In women and homosexual men, *primary anal or rectal infection* occurs following rectal intercourse. In women, rectal infection with LGV (or non-LGV) strains of *C. trachomatis* presumably can also arise either via contiguous spread of infected secretions along the perineum (as with rectal gonococcal infection in women) or perhaps by spread to the rectum via the pelvic lymphatics. From the site of the primary urethral, genital, anal, or rectal infection, the organism spreads via the regional lymphatics. Penile, vulvar, and anal infection can lead to inguinal and femoral lymphadenitis. Rectal infection produces hypogastric and deep iliac lymphadenitis. Upper vaginal or cervical infection results in enlargement of the obturator and iliac nodes. The most common presenting picture in heterosexual men is the *inguinal syndrome,* which is characterized by painful inguinal lymphadenopathy beginning 2 to 6 weeks after presumed exposure; rarely the onset occurs after a few months. The inguinal adenopathy is unilateral in two-thirds of cases, and palpable enlargement of the iliac and femoral nodes is often present on the same side as the enlarged inguinal nodes. The nodes are initially discrete, but progressive periadenitis results in a matted mass of nodes which become fluctuant and suppurative. The overlying skin becomes fixed, inflamed, and thinned and finally develops multiple draining fistulas. Extensive enlargement of chains of inguinal nodes above and below the inguinal ligament ("the sign of the groove") is common but is not specific, and is present in only a minority of cases (Fig. 150-1). Histologically, infected nodes initially show characteristic small stellate abscesses surrounded by histiocytes. These abscesses coalesce to cause large, necrotic, suppurative foci. Spontaneous healing usually occurs after several months, leaving inguinal scars or granulomatous masses of varying size which persist for life. Massive pelvic lymphadenopathy in women or homosexual men may lead to exploratory laparotomy.

As cultures and serology for *C. trachomatis* are being used more often, increasing numbers of cases of LGV proctitis are being recognized in homosexual men. Such patients present with anorectal pain and mucopurulent, bloody rectal discharge. Although patients may complain of diarrhea, this usually represents frequent, painful unsuccessful attempts at defecation (tenesmus). Sigmoidoscopy reveals ulcerative proctitis or proctocolitis, with purulent exudate and mucosal bleeding. Since the LGV agent is an obligate intracellular pathogen, the histopathologic findings in the rectal mucosa include granulomas with giant cells, along with crypt abscesses and extensive inflammation. These clinical, sigmoidoscopic, and histopathologic findings may closely resemble Crohn's disease of the rectum (Fig. 150-2).

Constitutional symptoms are common during the state of regional lymphadenopathy and, in the presence of proctitis, may include fever, chills, headache, meningismus, anorexia, myalgias, and arthralgias. These findings in the presence of lymphadenopathy are sometimes mistaken for malignant lymphoma. Other systemic complications are infrequent but include arthritis with sterile effusion, aseptic meningitis, meningoencephalitis, conjunctivitis, hepatitis, and erythema nodosum. Chlamydiae have been recovered from the cerebrospinal fluid, and in one case from the blood in a patient with severe constitutional symptoms, indicating the occurrence of disseminated infection. Laboratory infections due to suspected inhalation of aerosols have been associated with mediastinal lymphadenitis, pneumonitis, and pleural effusion.

Associated laboratory findings during the acute stage of infection include leukocytosis and slight elevation of the sedimentation rate. Abnormal liver function tests, hyperglobulinemia, mixed cryoglobulinemia, rheumatoid factor activity, and elevated IgG, IgA, and IgM have been reported in subacute and chronic LGV. False-positive serologic tests for syphilis are rare, and syphilis should be suspected if these tests are positive, as is often the case.

Complications of untreated anorectal infection include perirectal abscess, fistula in ano, and rectovaginal, rectovesical, and ischiorectal fistulas. Secondary bacterial infection probably contributes to these complications. Rectal stricture is a late complication of anorectal infection and usually occurs 2 to 6 cm from the anal orifice, within reach on digital rectal examination. The stricture may extend proximally for several centimeters, leading to a mistaken clinical and radiographic diagnosis of carcinoma.

A small percentage of cases of LGV in men presents with chronic progressive infiltrative, ulcerative, or fistular lesions of the penis, urethra, or scrotum. Urethral stricture may occur and usually involves the posterior urethra, causing incontinence or difficulty with micturition.

An uncommon late complication of LGV is *genital elephantiasis,* a chronic induration and edema of the penis or vulva caused by lymphatic obstruction. Polypoid swelling of the skin and large stellate hyperplastic keloidal scars of the genitalia may be associated with vulvar induration or lymphedema and are difficult to distinguish clinically from granuloma inguinale and genital tuberculosis. Chronic ulcerations of the vulva (esthiomene) and smooth pedunculated perianal growths (lymphorrhoids) also occur. The significance of reports of malignant changes associated with chronic anorectal or genital LGV is uncertain.

DIAGNOSIS Although LGV is uncommon, it frequently enters the differential diagnosis of common conditions such as inguinal lymphadenopathy; vesicular, papular, or ulcerative genital lesions; and perirectal abscess, fistula in ano, or proctitis.

The most reliable method of diagnosis is isolation of an LGV strain of *Chlamydia* from aspirated bubo pus, from the rectum, or from the urethra, endocervix, or other infected tissue. Isolation has been possible from bubo pus in about 30 percent of cases with inguinal lymphadenopathy and from the rectum in most homosexual men who have proctitis. The most widely used immunodiagnostic tests in the past have been the LGV complement fixation (CF) test and the Frei skin tests. An LGV CF titer $\geq$1:64 is suggestive of LGV and can be found in most patients after the bubo has appeared. The titer may not increase in paired serums since most patients have already been infected for several weeks when first seen. The LGV CF test can also become positive during infections with non-LGV strains of *C. trachomatis,* and high titers of CF antibody can be seen in patients who have had severe infections with such non-LGV strains. The Frei skin test is less sensitive than the LGV complement fixation test and is no longer available.

The microimmunofluorescent antibody test detects antibody to *C. trachomatis* in nearly all patients with culture-proven LGV. Serum microimmunofluorescent antibody titers from patients with LGV are usually $\geq$1:512, exceeding the highest titers that occur in chlamydial NGU and can usually be shown to have a characteristic broad pattern of reactivity against many immunotypes of *C. trachomatis.* The histopathology of excised nodes or of rectal biopsy specimens is seldom definitive, but suggestive findings (e.g., stellate abscesses in lymph nodes or granulomas on rectal biopsy) may raise the question of LGV and lead to more specific tests. Fluorescein-conjugated monoclonal antibodies against *C. trachomatis,* and against the L_2 strain of *C. trachomatis,* may prove useful for identification of the agent in properly fixed specimens from lymph nodes or other tissue, and monoclonal antibody to L_2 can be used for rapid identification of L_2 strains isolated in tissue cell culture.

TREATMENT The LGV and non-LGV strains of *C. trachomatis* have similar antimicrobial susceptibilities. Antimicrobial therapy does not have a dramatic effect on the duration and healing of inguinal buboes, but acute constitutional symptoms are often terminated abruptly, and LGV proctitis improves rapidly after antimicrobial therapy has been instituted. Antibiotics are usually not helpful in improving late complications such as rectal stricture or genital elephantiasis unless secondary infection is also present. Genital

FIGURE 150-2 *Histopathologic findings in LGV proctitis in a homosexually active man. Note granulomatous changes, with giant cells, and crypt abscess with adjacent giant cell (insert). These changes resemble those seen in Crohn's disease of the rectum. (From TC Quinn et al, N Engl J Med 305:195, 1981.)*

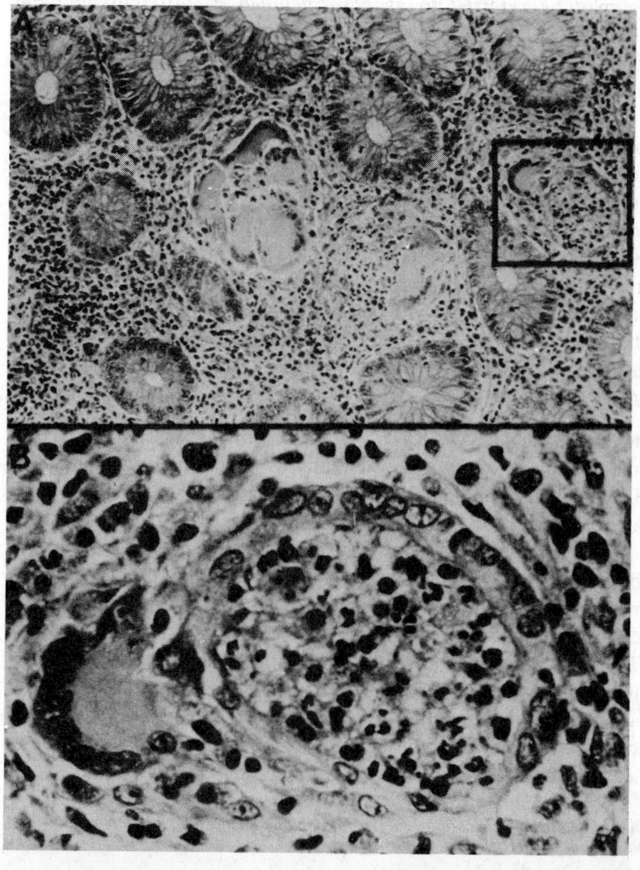

elephantiasis and rectal, penile, and urethral strictures and fistulas usually require surgical correction, although sometimes urethral and even rectal strictures can be managed by repeated mechanical dilation.

The recommended treatment regimen is tetracycline hydrochloride, 0.5 g four times a day for 3 weeks. A sulfonamide preparation, 4 g per day for 3 weeks, can also be used, but occasional isolates have been resistant to sulfonamides in vitro. Fluctuant buboes should be aspirated through normal skin with a syringe and 18-gauge needle as often as necessary to prevent spontaneous rupture. It is not unusual for buboes to increase in size or to develop at another site after initiation of treatment. Although these seldom progress to fistula formation, they should be aspirated if fluctuant. A fourfold or greater fall in CF titer or microimmunofluorescent antibody titer eventually occurs over several months in most treated patients, and LGV *Chlamydia* cannot be isolated from lesions after the initiation of antibiotic treatment.

TRACHOMA AND ADULT INCLUSION CONJUNCTIVITIS[1]

DEFINITION Trachoma is a chronic conjunctivitis associated with infection by *C. trachomatis* serovars A, B, and C. It has produced an estimated 20 million cases of blindness throughout the world and remains an important preventable cause of blindness. Inclusion conjunctivitis is an acute ocular infection caused by sexually transmitted *C. trachomatis* strains (usually serovars D through K) in adults exposed to infected genital secretions and in their newborn offspring.

EPIDEMIOLOGY Epidemiologically, two types of eye disease are caused by *C. trachomatis*. In trachoma-endemic areas where the classic eye disease is seen, transmission is from eye to eye, via hands, towels, flies, and other fomites, and usually involves serovars A, B, or C. In nonendemic areas, organisms of serovars D through K can be transmitted from the genital tract to the eye, usually causing only the inclusion conjunctivitis syndrome with or without keratitis. Rarely the eye disease acquired in this way progresses with the development of pannus and scars similar to endemic trachoma. These cases may be referred to as *paratrachoma* to differentiate them epidemiologically from eye-to-eye transmitted endemic trachoma.

The worldwide incidence and severity of trachoma have decreased dramatically during the past 30 years in areas with improving hygienic and economic conditions. Endemic trachoma is still the major cause of preventable blindness in north Africa, sub-Saharan Africa, the Middle East, and parts of Asia. Transmission of the endemic disease occurs primarily through close personal contact, particularly among young children in rural communities. In endemic areas, trachoma is associated with repeated exposure, but the infection can also be latent. In the United States a mild form of endemic trachoma still occurs in Mexican Americans as well as in immigrants from areas where trachoma is endemic. Acute relapse of old trachoma may be seen occasionally following treatment with cortisone eye ointment or in very old persons exposed in their youth.

CLINICAL MANIFESTATIONS Both endemic trachoma and adult inclusion conjunctivitis present initially as a conjunctivitis characterized by small lymphoid follicles in the conjunctiva. In regions with hyperendemic classic blinding trachoma, the disease usually starts insidiously before the age of 2 years. Reinfection is common and probably contributes to the pathogenesis of trachoma. In experimental primate models, repeated reinfection of the eye at regular intervals produces trachoma-like scarring.

The cornea becomes involved with inflammatory leukocytic infiltration and superficial vascularization (pannus formation). As the inflammation continues, there is conjunctival scarring that eventually distorts the eyelids, causing them to turn inward so that the inturned lashes constantly abrade the eyeball (trichiasis and entropion); eventually the corneal epithelium is abraded and may then develop a bacterial corneal ulcer with subsequent corneal scarring and blindness. Destruction of the conjunctival goblet cells, lacrimal ducts, and lacrimal gland may produce a "dry-eye" syndrome with resultant corneal opacity due to drying (xerosis) or secondary bacterial corneal ulcers.

Communities with blinding trachoma often experience seasonal epidemics of bacterial conjunctivitis with *Haemophilus influenzae* (biotype III or the Koch-Weeks bacillus), which contribute to the intensity of the inflammatory process. In such areas the active infectious process usually resolves spontaneously in affected persons between 10 and 15 years of age, but the conjunctival scars continue to shrink, producing trichiasis and entropion and subsequent corneal scarring in adult life. In areas with milder and less prevalent disease the process may be much slower, with active disease continuing into adulthood; blindness is rare in these cases.

Eye infection with genital *C. trachomatis* strains, usually in sexually active young adults, presents with acute onset of unilateral follicular conjunctivitis and preauricular lymphadenopathy similar to acute adenovirus or herpes virus conjunctivitis. If untreated, the disease may persist for 6 weeks to 2 years. It is frequently associated with corneal inflammation in the form of discrete opacities ("infiltrates"), punctate epithelial erosions, and minor degrees of superficial corneal vascularization. Very rarely conjunctival scarring and eyelid distortion occur, particularly in patients treated for many months with topical corticosteroids. Recurrent eye infections occur most often in patients whose sexual consorts are not treated with antimicrobials.

DIAGNOSIS The clinical diagnosis of classic trachoma can be made if two of the following signs are present:

1 Lymphoid follicles on the upper tarsal conjunctiva
2 Typical conjunctival scarring
3 Vascular pannus
4 Limbal follicles or their sequelae, Herbert's pits

The clinical diagnosis of endemic trachoma should be confirmed by laboratory tests in children with more marked degrees of inflammation. Intracytoplasmic chlamydial inclusions occur in 10 to 60 percent of Giemsa-stained conjunctival smears in such populations, but isolation in cell cultures is more sensitive. Follicular conjunctivitis in adult Europeans or Americans living in trachomatous regions is rarely trachoma.

Sporadic cases of adult inclusion conjunctivitis must be differentiated from adenovirus and herpes simplex virus keratoconjunctivitis during the first 15 days after onset, and later from other forms of chronic follicular conjunctivitis. Demonstration of chlamydial infection by Giemsa- or immunofluorescent-stained smears or by isolation in cell cultures constitutes definitive evidence of infection. Serum antibody does not constitute evidence of chlamydial eye infection since many sexually active adults have serum antibody. A practical diagnostic procedure in cases with chronic follicular conjunctivitis is treatment for 6 days with an oral tetracycline or erythromycin; a marked symptomatic response within 3 to 4 days is highly suggestive of inclusion conjunctivitis, and treatment should be continued for at least 3 weeks.

DIFFERENTIAL DIAGNOSIS The eye and its adnexa may be infected during the course of many cutaneous and systemic viral diseases. Sometimes these ocular infections produce minor manifestations, such as the transient loss of accommodation of dengue and the milder forms of conjunctivitis in systemic adenovirus infections. Other virus infections, however, such as herpes simplex (see Chap. 136), herpes zoster (see Chap. 135), measles (see Chap. 132), and vaccinia (see Chap. 134), occasionally produce serious and permanent visual loss. In addition, congenital viral infections are an important cause of blindness, particularly rubella, which leads to cataracts, microphthalmus, and cytomegalic inclusion disease with retinal involvement.

Among the viral infections limited to the outer eye and manifested as a follicular conjunctivitis are epidemic keratoconjunctivitis (EKC),

[1] *Much of this section is based on the separate chapter on this topic by Doctors Grayston and Dawson in the previous (tenth) edition of this book.*

herpes simplex keratoconjunctivitis, Newcastle disease virus (NDV) conjunctivitis, and acute hemorrhagic conjunctivitis. Adenovirus types 8 and 19 are the usual cause of epidemics of EKC, although milder cases may be associated with other adenovirus types. The most common method for transmission of adenovirus type 8 is through manipulation of the eye by medical personnel, e.g., for foreign-body removal or during an ophthalmologic examination. The virus, which is unusually resistant to inactivation, is transmitted on the fingers, by instruments, or in solutions. One of the rarer causes of EKC, adenovirus type 19, appears to be transmitted person-to-person during small community outbreaks.

Following an incubation period of 5 to 12 days, EKC presents a moderate to very severe follicular conjunctivitis with preauricular lymphadenopathy that is usually unilateral at onset. Severe cases may have subconjunctival hemorrhages and conjunctival membrane formation with subsequent conjunctival scarring. In adults, the associated systemic manifestations are minimal with little if any fever, headache, or malaise, but in children adenovirus type 8 infections may present as febrile upper respiratory disease, or otitis media, with only a minor conjunctivitis; such children may be a source of infection for adults. In EKC, the usual onset of focal corneal involvement is 7 days after onset of conjunctivitis when there is a severe foreign-body sensation, photophobia, and lacrimation. As the conjunctivitis subsides during the second week of the disease, subepithelial corneal opacities 1 to 2 mm in diameter appear, and these opacities may persist for 2 years or longer.

Occasionally herpes simplex virus produces an acute follicular conjunctivitis that is usually accompanied by one or multiple herpetic skin vesicles on the eyelids. In children this may be the primary herpetic infection, but in adults the conjunctivitis is often a recurrent herpetic infection at a new site. The skin lesions may be inconspicuous, misdiagnosed as a sty, or even not present, so that the disease is indistinguishable from early EKC. The cornea may have focal epithelial lesions, a typical linear, branching (dendritic) ulcer, or no involvement at all. The conjunctivitis usually resolves in 2 weeks.

Human infection with Newcastle disease virus, which is related to influenza, occurs mainly in poultry workers, veterinarians, and virologists. In humans, accidental introduction of contaminated material from naturally infected animals or from live virus (e.g., vaccines) is followed in 24 to 72 h by conjunctivitis, edema of the lids, and tearing. Systemic symptoms occur very rarely, and recovery is complete in 10 to 14 days. The diagnosis may be confirmed by virus isolation in embryonated eggs.

Acute hemorrhagic conjunctivitis (AHC) presents as an acute conjunctivitis with numerous punctate hemorrhages on the bulbar conjunctiva which become confluent within 24 h. There is also minor involvement of the cornea. The inflammation subsides in 4 to 5 days, but the hemorrhages do not resolve for 7 to 10 days. The only reported complication has been the rare occurrence of lumbar radiculomyelitis with resultant flaccid paralysis like poliomyelitis. Enterovirus 70 (a member of the picornavirus group) has been identified as the etiologic agent in most epidemics, but some outbreaks have been caused by coxsackievirus A24, another picornavirus. Epidemics of AHC have occurred in the crowded urban populations of developing countries, affecting all age groups and social classes. Occasional outbreaks in Europe have been centered around eye clinics. Community-wide epidemics of AHC have occurred in the United States and Central America.

TREATMENT *C. trachomatis* strains are susceptible to the tetracyclines, erythromycin, and the sulfonamides. Public health control programs for endemic trachoma have consisted of the mass application of tetracycline or erythromycin ointment to the eyes of all children in affected communities for 21 to 60 days or on an intermittent schedule. These programs also include surgical correction of inturned eyelids by a mobile surgical team that visits each locality. Oral erythromycin, but not oral tetracyclines, offers a useful alternative method of mass antibiotic treatment for trachoma of young children and pregnant women.

Adult inclusion conjunctivitis responds well to treatment with full doses of systemic tetracycline or erythromycin for 3 weeks. Treating all sexual consorts of the patient simultaneously is also necessary to prevent ocular reinfection and to avoid the genital diseases due to chlamydial infection. Topical antibiotic treatment is not required in patients treated with systemic antibiotics.

PREVENTION Efforts to develop a practical trachoma vaccine have not been successful. General hygienic measures associated with improved living standards are effective in the elimination of endemic trachoma. Adequate water supply for personal cleanliness may be a key factor. In some areas the reduction of flies in the household is important.

OTHER INFECTIONS CAUSED BY *C. TRACHOMATIS* IN ADULTS *C. trachomatis* has been reported as an infrequent cause of subacute endocarditis and may cause respiratory infections in older children and adults. Serologic evidence supporting a role for *Chlamydia* in community-acquired pneumonia and in acute pharyngitis has been gathered, but the agent has not been isolated from such cases. Immunosuppressed patients with pneumonia have had, in some cases, either serologic or cultural evidence of *C. trachomatis* infection, but more data are necessary to define the role of *Chlamydia* in these patients. Many infections caused by *C. trachomatis* produce few or no symptoms, or symptoms that are nonspecific and thus not diagnostic of *C. trachomatis* infection. These considerations, plus the limited availability and high cost of culture tests for chlamydial infection have markedly hampered confirmation of infection in individual patients and have limited public health control efforts.

PSITTACOSIS

DEFINITION Psittacosis is primarily an infectious disease of birds caused by *Chlamydia psittaci*. Transmission of infection from birds to humans results in a febrile illness characterized by pneumonitis and systemic manifestations. Inapparent infections or mild influenza-like illnesses may also occur. The term *ornithosis* is sometimes applied to infections contracted from birds other than parrots or parakeets, but *psittacosis* is the preferred generic term for all forms of the disease. A previously unrecognized *C. psittaci* strain, the TWAR strain, has been serologically linked with human respiratory illness. This strain appears to cause a mild pneumonitis and/or upper respiratory tract infection in young adults.

EPIDEMIOLOGY Almost any avian species can harbor *C. psittaci*. Psittacine birds (parrots, parakeets, budgerigars) are most commonly infected, but human cases have been traced to contact with pigeons, ducks, turkeys, chickens, and many other birds. Psittacosis may be considered an occupational disease of pet-shop owners, poultry raisers, pigeon fanciers, taxidermists, and zoo attendants. The incidence of human infection in the United States rose steadily from 1930, owing in large measure to the increasing popularity of parrots and parakeets as pets and, as subsequently recognized, transmission of infection by barnyard fowl and pigeons. The number of reported cases reached a peak in 1956 and gradually declined thereafter. By 1963, with acceptance of control measures such as incorporation of tetracyclines in poultry feed, the disease had again become relatively uncommon. However, since 1973, there has been a steady increase in incidence, with cases occurring primarily among employees of poultry processing plants. In 1983, about 150 cases of psittacosis were reported to the Centers for Disease Control. It is suspected that many cases are undiagnosed and not reported. The disease appears to be more common in England, where budgerigars are popular household pets and where restrictions on the importation of these birds have been eased.

The agent is present in nasal secretions, excreta, tissues, and feathers of infected birds. Although the disease can be fatal, infected birds frequently show only minor evidence of illness, such as ruffled feathers, lethargy, and anorexia. Asymptomatic avian carriers are common, and complete recovery may be followed by continued shedding of the organism for many months.

Psittacosis is almost always transmitted to humans by the respiratory route. On rare occasions the disease may be acquired from the bite of a pet bird. Prolonged contact is not essential for transmission of the disease; a few minutes spent in an environment previously occupied by an infected bird has resulted in human infection. The severity of the disease in humans bears no apparent relationship to closeness or duration of contact, although sick birds are more likely to transmit infection than healthy ones. Transmission of a psittacosis-like agent between humans has occurred among hospital personnel, with severe and sometimes fatal infections. There is evidence that these "human" strains are more virulent than native avian organisms. There is no record of infection acquired by eating poultry products.

PATHOGENESIS The psittacosis agent gains entrance to the body through the upper part of the respiratory tract, spreads via the bloodstream, and eventually localizes in the pulmonary alveoli and in the reticuloendothelial cells of the spleen and liver. Invasion of the lung probably takes place by way of the bloodstream rather than by direct extension from the upper air passages. A lymphocytic inflammatory response occurs on both the interstitial and respiratory surfaces of the alveoli as well as in the perivascular spaces. The alveolar walls and interstitial tissues of the lung are thickened, edematous, necrotic, and occasionally hemorrhagic. Histologically, the affected areas show alveolar spaces filled with fluid, erythrocytes, and lymphocytes. The picture is not pathognomonic of psittacosis unless macrophages containing characteristic cytoplasmic inclusion bodies (LCL bodies) can be identified. The respiratory epithelium of the bronchi and bronchioles usually remains intact.

CLINICAL MANIFESTATIONS The clinical manifestations and course of psittacosis are extremely variable. After an incubation period of 7 to 14 days or longer, the disease may start abruptly with shaking chills and fever ranging as high as 40.5°C (105°F), but the onset is often gradual with increasing fever over a 3- to 4-day period. Headache is almost always a prominent symptom; it is usually diffuse and excruciating and often the patient's chief complaint.

Many patients present with a dry hacking cough which is usually nonproductive, but small amounts of mucoid or bloody sputum may be raised as the disease progresses. Cough may appear early in the course of the disease or as late as 5 days after the onset of fever. Chest pain, pleurisy with effusion, or a friction rub may all occur but are rare. Pericarditis and myocarditis have been reported. Most patients have a normal or slightly increased respiratory rate; marked dyspnea with cyanosis occurs only in severe psittacosis with extensive pulmonary involvement. In psittacosis, as in most nonbacterial pneumonias, the physical signs of pneumonitis tend to be less prominent than symptoms and x-ray findings would suggest. The initial examination may reveal fine, sibilant rales, or clinical evidence of pneumonia may be completely lacking. Rales usually become audible and more numerous as the illness progresses. Signs of frank pulmonary consolidation are usually absent. Symptoms of upper respiratory tract infection are not prominent, although mild sore throat, pharyngeal infection, and cervical adenopathy are often present; on occasion they may be the only manifestations of illness. Epistaxis is encountered early in the course of nearly one-fourth of the cases. Photophobia is also a common complaint.

There is commonly a complaint of generalized myalgia, and spasm and stiffness of the muscles of the back and neck may lead to an erroneous diagnosis of meningitis. Lethargy, mental depression, agitation, insomnia, and disorientation have been prominent features of the illness in some epidemics, but not in others; delirium and stupor occur near the end of the first week in severe cases. Occasional patients are comatose when first seen, and the diagnosis of psittacosis may be missed. Gastrointestinal complaints such as abdominal pain, nausea, vomiting, or diarrhea are present in some cases; constipation and abdominal distention sometimes occur as late complications. Icterus, the result of severe hepatic involvement, is a rare and ominous finding. A faint, macular rash (Horder's spots) simulating the rose spots of typhoid fever has been described.

Patients without cough or other clinical evidence of respiratory involvement come to the physician with fever of unknown origin. The pulse rate is slow in relation to the fever. When splenomegaly is present in a patient with acute pneumonitis, psittacosis should be considered; the reported incidence of splenomegaly ranges from 10 to 70 percent. Nontender hepatic enlargement also occurs, but jaundice is rare. Thrombophlebitis is not unusual during convalescence; indeed, pulmonary infarction is sometimes a late complication and may be fatal.

In untreated cases of psittacosis, sustained or mildly remittent fever persists for 10 days to 3 weeks, or occasionally as long as 3 months. Over this period, the respiratory manifestations gradually abate. Psittacosis contracted from parrots or parakeets is more likely to be a severe, prolonged illness than infections acquired from pigeons or barnyard fowl. Relapses occur but are rare. Occasional patients develop endocarditis, and *C. psittaci* infection should be considered in cases of culture-negative endocarditis. Secondary bacterial infections are uncommon. Immunity to reinfection is probably permanent.

LABORATORY FINDINGS The chest x-ray in psittacosis mimics that in a great variety of pulmonary diseases. The pneumonic lesions are usually patchy in appearance but can be hazy, diffuse, homogeneous, lobar, atelectatic, wedge-shaped, nodular, or miliary. The white blood cell count is normal or moderately decreased in the acute phase of the disease but may rise in convalescence. The erythrocyte sedimentation rate is frequently not elevated. Transient proteinuria is common. The cerebrospinal fluid sometimes contains a few mononuclear cells but is otherwise normal. Despite hepatomegaly, liver function tests are generally normal.

The diagnosis can be confirmed only by isolation of the causative microorganism or by serologic studies. The agent is present in the blood during the acute phase of the disease and in the bronchial secretions for weeks or sometimes years after infection, but it is difficult to isolate. Psittacosis is most readily diagnosed by the demonstration of a rising titer of complement-fixing antibody in serum. An acute and convalescent specimen should always be tested. Even a low titer of antibody during the acute febrile phase constitutes presumptive evidence of psittacosis. The prompt initiation of treatment with tetracycline has been shown to delay antibody rise in convalescence for several weeks or months. Interpretation of a single complement fixation test may sometimes be difficult because of the antigenic cross reaction between *C. psittaci* and *C. trachomatis*.

DIFFERENTIAL DIAGNOSIS A history of exposure to birds may be the only clinical basis for differentiating psittacosis from a great variety of infectious and noninfectious febrile disorders. A partial list of pneumonic disease that may be confused with psittacosis includes *Mycoplasma* pneumonia, Q fever, coccidioidomycosis, tuberculosis, enteroviral infection, carcinoma of the lung with bronchial obstruction, and bacterial pneumonias. In the early stages, before pneumonitis appears, psittacosis may be mistaken for influenza, typhoid fever, miliary tuberculosis, infectious mononucleosis, and Legionnaires' disease.

TREATMENT The tetracyclines are consistently effective in the treatment of psittacosis. Defervescence and alleviation of symptoms usually occur in 24 to 48 h after instituting therapy with 2 g daily in four divided doses. To avoid relapse, treatment should probably be continued for at least 7 days after defervescence. In severe cases, oxygen and other supportive measures are indicated.

APPROACH TO THE DIAGNOSIS AND TREATMENT OF *C. TRACHOMATIS* INFECTIONS

Traditionally, three types of laboratory procedures have been used to confirm *C. trachomatis* infection. These include direct microscopic examination of tissue scrapings for typical intracytoplasmic inclusions, isolation of the organism, and detection of antibody in the serum or in local secretions. Direct microscopic examination of Giemsa-stained cell scrapings has an unacceptably low sensitivity, and false-positive interpretations by inexperienced observers are common. Cell culture techniques have replaced the yolk sac of embryonated eggs for isolation of *C. trachomatis*. The cell cultures are much more convenient and sensitive, particularly for strains from the genital tract. While LGV strains grow well in many cell lines, the other *C. trachomatis* strains are much more difficult to culture. The most common cell lines used are McCoy cells and HeLa 229 cells. Both cell lines require special pretreatment and centrifugation of the inoculum onto the monolayer for efficient isolation of genital or ocular trachoma strains. Positive cultures are identified by visualizing typical intracytoplasmic inclusions stained by Giemsa stain, by iodine stain, or by using fluorescein-conjugated monoclonal antibodies.

Although culture remains the "gold standard" for diagnosis of chlamydial infection, it is expensive, technically demanding, and not widely available. Therefore, antigen detection methods have been developed that can be used instead of cultures. In the immunofluorescent slide test, potentially infected genital or ocular secretions are smeared on a slide, fixed, and stained with fluorescein-conjugated monoclonal antibody. When viewing the slide using a fluorescence microscope, the presence of fluorescing elementary bodies confirms the diagnosis. Compared with culture, this test is 85 to 90 percent sensitive and quite specific when used for confirmation of urethral, cervical, or ocular infection in high-risk patients with suspected *C. trachomatis* infection. Its value as a screening test has not been widely assessed. An enzyme-linked immunosorbent assay (ELISA) technique for chlamydial antigen detection has also been developed and provides another alternative to culture. Reported sensitivity and specificity of this test for genital infections has been 67 to 95 percent and 92 to 97 percent in populations studied to date.

Serologic tests have limited usefulness in chlamydial diagnosis. A complement fixation (CF) test with the heat-stable group-reactive antigen has been used to diagnose psittacosis and LGV with some success. It is insensitive in non-LGV *C. trachomatis* infections. The microimmunofluorescence (micro-IF) test with *C. trachomatis* antigens is more sensitive but remains available only in research laboratories. The test measures antibodies by serovar specificity and by immunoglobulin class (IgM, IgG, IgA, secretory IgA) in both serum and local secretions. Serologic diagnosis using the micro-IF test may be useful in several specific instances. In infant pneumonia, a high antibody titer is nearly always present and, since a definite clinical syndrome may bring the infant to the physician early in the course of disease, high-titer IgM antibody and/or fourfold titer rises can often be demonstrated. For similar reasons, serodiagnosis has been used in a research setting in women with chlamydial salpingitis, especially with Fitz-Hugh–Curtis syndrome. In LGV the micro-IF antibody titer against *C. trachomatis* is high (≥1:512) and usually has a characteristic pattern of broad reactivity against all immunotypes of *C. trachomatis* (since LGV strains induce broadly reactive antibody).

Table 150-2 summarizes the diagnostic tests of choice for patients with suspected chlamydial infection. With few exceptions, the most

TABLE 150-2 Diagnostic tests in *C. trachomatis* infection

Infection	Suggestive signs/symptoms	Presumptive diagnosis*	Confirmatory test of choice
ADULT MALES			
Nongonococcal urethritis, postgonococcal urethritis	Discharge, dysuria	Gram stain with more than four polymorphonuclear (PMN) leukocytes per oil immersion field, no gonococci	Urethral culture or antigen detection test for *C. trachomatis*
Epididymitis	Unilateral intrascrotal swelling, pain, tenderness; fever; nongonococcal urethritis	Gram stain with more than four PMN leukocytes per oil immersion field, no gonococci	Urethral culture or antigen detection test for *C. trachomatis*
ADULT FEMALES			
Cervicitis	Mucopurulent cervical discharge, cervical edema, ectopy, bleeding	Cervical Gram stain with ≥10 PMNs per oil immersion field in cervical mucus	Cervical culture or antigen detection test for *C. trachomatis*
Salpingitis	Evidence of pelvic inflammatory disease on examination	*C. trachomatis* should always be suspected in salpingitis	Cervical culture or antigen detection test for *C. trachomatis*
Urethritis	Dysuria and frequency without urgency or hematuria	Mucopurulent cervicitis, sterile pyuria, negative routine urine culture	Urethral and cervical cultures or antigen detection test for *C. trachomatis*
ADULTS OF EITHER SEX			
Proctitis	Rectal pain, discharge, diarrhea, blood; homosexual patient	Negative gonococcal culture and Gram stain; ≥1 PMN leukocytes in rectal Gram stain	Rectal culture or direct immunofluorescence test for *C. trachomatis*
Reiter's syndrome	Nongonococcal urethritis, arthritis, conjunctivitis, typical skin lesions	Gram stain with more than four PMN leukocytes per oil immersion field, no gonococci	Urethral culture or antigen detection test for *C. trachomatis*
LGV	Regional adenopathy, primary lesion, proctitis, systemic symptoms	None	Isolation of LGV strain from node, rectum, occasionally from urethra or cervix; LGV CF-titer ≥1:64; micro-IF titer ≥1:512
NEONATES			
Conjunctivitis	Purulent conjunctival discharge 6 to 18 days postdelivery	Negative cultures and gram stains for gonococci, *Haemophilus* sp., pneumococci, staphylococci	Conjunctival culture or antigen detection test for *C. trachomatis;* Giemsa-stained scraping of conjunctival material can provide more rapid diagnosis but is less sensitive
Infant pneumonia	Afebrile, staccato cough, diffuse rales, bilateral hyperinflation, interstitial infiltrates	None	Chlamydial culture of sputum, pharynx, eye, rectum; micro-IF antibody to *C. trachomatis*—fourfold change in IgG or IgM antibody

* *Although a presumptive diagnosis of chlamydial infection is often made in the syndromes listed when gonococci are not found, a positive test for* Neisseria gonorrhoeae *does not exclude* C. trachomatis, *which is very often also present in patients with gonorrhea.*

suitable method for diagnosis is demonstration of the agent in tissue-cell culture or by antigen detection methods. Selection of the most appropriate of these tests depends upon local availability and expertise. Since *C. trachomatis* is an intracellular pathogen, adequate specimens for chlamydial culture must include epithelial cells. Cultures of pus result in fewer isolations of the organism. In urethritis, a thin-shafted urogenital swab should be inserted at least 2 cm into the urethra to obtain an appropriate specimen. When a cervical culture is taken, the external os should first be cleaned of debris and purulent material, and a plastic-shafted swab then inserted into the cervix, rotated slowly several times, and withdrawn. When conjunctival specimens are sought, the epithelium should be swabbed to remove cells, rather than simply purulent material. All specimens for chlamydial culture should be placed immediately into a transport medium and then either refrigerated if they will reach the laboratory within 12 to 18 h or frozen at −70°C if longer storage is anticipated. A major advantage of antigen detection techniques is their less rigid transport requirements.

From a public health viewpoint, the most effective use of chlamydia diagnostic testing has not been established and will vary depending upon clinical population, local resources, and laboratory expertise. The Centers for Disease Control have recommended empiric treatment (without diagnostic testing if resources are not available for testing) of selected high-risk groups. These include men with NGU or sexually transmitted epididymitis; women with mucopurulent cervicitis (MPC) or PID; asymptomatic sexual partners of patients with these syndromes; women and heterosexual men with gonorrhea (because of the high proportion of these patients who will also have *C. trachomatis* infection); and contacts of men or women with gonorrhea. Where funds for diagnostic testing are limited (e.g., in public clinics serving indigent patients), it is rationalized that these groups will receive empiric therapy in any event, and hence diagnostic testing is not absolutely essential. However, where available, diagnostic testing has several potential benefits in these patients, including confirmation of infection (especially in women with MPC and PID), enhancement of sex partner referral, determination of prognosis, and education of physicians (ability to correlate signs and symptoms with culture results). Where diagnostic testing must be rationed because of limited resources, highest priority should be given to screening asymptomatic high-risk women, especially those seen in high-risk settings (i.e., STD clinics, abortion clinics, family planning clinics), or individuals with a high-risk profile (young, multiple sexual partners, lower socioeconomic status).

ANTIMICROBIAL SUSCEPTIBILITY In laboratory tests, death of inoculated mice and chick embryos, as well as growth in cell cultures, is prevented or inhibited by tetracyclines, erythromycin, and rifampin; sulfonamides and cycloserine are active against *C. trachomatis* but not *C. psittaci;* bacitracin and polymyxin B are less effective; penicillin and ampicillin suppress *Chlamydia* multiplication but do not eradicate the organism in vitro. The cephalosporins also appear relatively ineffective against *C. trachomatis*. Streptomycin, gentamicin, neomycin, kanamycin, vancomycin, ristocetin, spectinomycin, and nystatin are not effective at concentrations inhibitory for most bacteria and fungi. For treatment of human infection, the tetracyclines, erythromycin, and sulfonamides are most useful.

TREATMENT In general, chlamydial infections cannot be eradicated by single-dose or short-term antimicrobial regimens. In most situations, at least 7 days and sometimes 2 to 3 weeks of antibiotic should be given. Treatment failure after treatment of genital infections with a tetracycline usually indicates inadequate therapy, poor compliance, or reinfection. Tetracycline-resistant strains of *C. trachomatis* have not been described.

Therapy of *C. trachomatis* urethritis is more effective than therapy of other forms of NGU. *C. trachomatis* is eradicated from the urethra by treatment with tetracycline hydrochloride, 500 mg four times daily for 7 days, or doxycycline, 100 mg by mouth bid for 7 days. An effective alternative regimen is erythromycin, 500 mg four times daily for 7 days.

Eradication of *C. trachomatis* from the cervix has been demonstrated with similar doses and durations of tetracycline, doxycycline, and erythromycin. Erythromycin base, 500 mg four times daily for 10 to 14 days, is the regimen of choice for pregnant women with *C. trachomatis* infection. Tetracycline hydrochloride, 500 mg four times daily for 14 days, produces clinical and microbiologic cure of epididymitis associated with *C. trachomatis* infection. Treatment of PID is discussed in Chap. 91. Treatment of gonorrhea should include an effective antichlamydial drug (see Chap. 104).

Treatment of sex partners Genital *C. trachomatis* infections have continued to increase in incidence from the mid-1970s to the mid-1980s, whereas gonococcal infections have steadily fallen in incidence over the same period. The increase in chlamydial infection probably is due to the inability of clinicians to diagnose asymptomatic infection and also failure to diagnose and treat *C. trachomatis* infections in symptomatic patients or their sexual partners. Cases of NGU, epididymitis, Reiter's syndrome, and mucopurulent endocervicitis are sometimes not treated with antimicrobials, and sex partners are treated even less often. *C. trachomatis* urethral or cervical infection has been well documented in a high proportion of the sex partners of patients with NGU, epididymitis, Reiter's syndrome, salpingitis, or endocervicitis. This is analogous to the problem of asymptomatic gonococcal infection in sex partners of patients with gonorrhea. Confirmatory laboratory tests for *Chlamydia* should be obtained if possible, but antigen detection tests may be less sensitive in asymptomatic carriers. Even those without evidence of clinical disease who have been recently exposed to proven or possible chlamydial infection (for example, NGU) should be offered therapy.

In neonates with conjunctivitis or infants with pneumonia, erythromycin ethylsuccinate or estolate can be given orally in a dose of 50 mg/kg per day, preferably as 12.5 mg/kg four times daily, for 2 weeks. Careful attention must be given to compliance with therapy—a frequent problem. Relapses of eye infection are common following treatment with topical erythromycin or tetracycline ophthalmic ointment and may occur after oral erythromycin therapy also, so that follow-up cultures should be obtained after treatment. Both parents should be examined for *C. trachomatis* infection and, if diagnostic tests are not readily available, should also be treated with a tetracycline.

REFERENCES

ALEXANDER ER, HARRISON ER: Role of *Chlamydia trachomatis* in perinatal infection. Rev Infect Dis 5:713, 1983

BRUNHAM RC et al: Mucopurulent cervicitis—the ignored counterpart in women of urethritis in men. N Engl J Med 311:1, 1984

CENTERS FOR DISEASE CONTROL: Morb Mort Week Rep 31:65, 1983

———: Morb Mort Week Rep 32:27SS, 1984

COUTTS II et al: Clinical and radiographic features of psittacosis infection. Thorax 40:530, 1985

JONES RB et al: *Chlamydia trachomatis* in the pharynx and rectum of heterosexual patients at risk for genital infection. Ann Intern Med 102:757, 1985

MÅRDH PA et al: *Chlamydial Infections*. Amsterdam: Elsevier Biomedical Press, 1982

SCHACHTER J: Chlamydial infection. N Engl J Med 298:428, 490, 540, 1973

——— et al: Experience with the routine use of erythromycin for chlamydial infections in pregnancy. N Engl J Med 314:276, 1986

STAMM WE et al: Causes of the acute urethral syndrome in women. N Engl J Med 303:309, 1980

———: Use of antigen detection methods for the diagnosis *Neisseria gonorrhoeae* and *Chlamydia trachomatis* infections. Diagn Micro Infect Dis, in press

THOMPSON SE, WASHINGTON AE: Epidemiology of sexually transmitted *C. trachomatis* infections. Epidemiol Rev 5:96, 1983

WORLD HEALTH ORGANIZATION: *Guide to the Laboratory Diagnosis of Trachoma*. Geneva, WHO, 1975

section 9 Protozoal and helminthic infections

151 THE DIAGNOSIS AND THERAPY OF PARASITIC INFECTIONS

JAMES J. PLORDE

Parasitic diseases such as malaria, trypanosomiasis, leishmaniasis, schistosomiasis, and filariasis remain among the major causes of human sickness and death in the world today. A number of technical, social, economic, and political phenomena have combined to produce a dramatic increase in the prevalence of some of these illnesses. This has been most devastating in the case of malaria. Growing resistance of the mosquito vector to insecticides, development of drug-resistant strains of *Plasmodium falciparum,* and cutbacks in many malaria control programs have led to a worldwide resurgence of this disease. At present, over 1 billion people reside in endemic areas; between 125 and 200 million of these are infected at any given time. In Africa, where the intensity of parasite transmission defies current control measures, malaria kills over 1 million children annually. The resurgence of malaria together with an increase in international travel has resulted in an upsurge in the number of infected patients who enter the United States. From 1969 to 1980 civilian malaria cases reported annually to the Centers for Disease Control have increased from 151 to 1864; in the four subsequent years, the number has averaged 1000 cases annually. Over the same 15-year period, the number of infections involving U.S. citizens has climbed steadily from 90 to 360.

In Africa, from the Sahara in the north to the Kalahari Desert in the south, human strains of *Trypanosoma brucei* cause one of the most lethal of all human diseases, sleeping sickness. Animal strains of this species limit food supply in the same area through their impact on animal husbandry. In South America, a related organism, *T. cruzi,* infects several million people, leaving many with severe heart and gastrointestinal lesions (Chagas' disease).

Leishmaniasis is found in parts of Europe, Asia, Africa, and South and Central America where it may present as a chronic, highly lethal infection of the reticuloendothelial system (kala azar), a mutilating mucocutaneous infection (espundia), or a self-limiting skin ulcer (oriental sore).

Schistosomiasis is the most serious of the helminthic infections, affecting an estimated 200 million individuals living between the tropics of Cancer and Capricorn. In many it produces bladder, intestinal, and/or liver disease which can eventually result in death. In many countries irrigation schemes have resulted in the dissemination of the disease to previously uninvolved areas, mitigating the economic gains of these development projects. Although not transmitted in the continental United States, exogenously acquired schistosomiasis involves nearly a half million people now residing in this country.

Wuchereria bancrofti and *Brugia malayi,* two closely related filarial worms, obstruct lymphatic circulation and produce grotesque swellings of the legs, arms, and genitals in tropical populations. Onchocerciasis, another filarial infection, affects millions of people in Africa, leaving thousands blind.

Toxoplasmosis, pneumocystosis, giardiasis, and trichomoniasis are four cosmopolitan protozoan infections well known in the United States. The first infects perhaps one-third of the world's population. Although it is usually asymptomatic, congenital toxoplasmosis may result in abortion, stillbirth, prematurity, or severe neurologic defects. Even when there are no obvious signs at birth, chorioretinitis with visual impairment may occur years later. Asymptomatic toxoplasma and pneumocystis infections can both result in fatal illness later in life during periods of immunosuppression.

In contrast, giardiasis and trichomoniasis seldom result in severe disability; nevertheless their morbidity can be attested to by millions of otherwise healthy individuals. Both appear to be increasing in incidence, apparently the result of changing American lifestyles. Giardiasis is particularly frequent among day-care center attendees, hikers and campers in our western states, and male homosexuals who practice anilingus, while the incidence of trichomoniasis is closely tied to the level of promiscuous heterosexual activity.

DIAGNOSIS Although some of the diseases mentioned above are uncommon in the United States, the continuous arrival of travelers and immigrants from endemic areas of the world makes it necessary to consider them in the differential diagnosis of many illnesses. Typically, neither the clinical manifestations nor the general laboratory findings observed in patients suffering from parasitic infections are sufficiently unique to raise this possibility in the mind of the clinician. Although eosinophilia has long been recognized as a clue to the presence of a hidden parasite, this phenomenon is characteristic only of helminthic infections. Even here its absence does not preclude this diagnosis. The eosinophilia presumably reflects an immunologic response to the complex foreign proteins of the worm and is most marked during the early stages of tissue migration and invasion. Once migration ceases and the worm matures to adulthood, eosinophilia may diminish or disappear.

Unless a careful travel, transfusion, and socioeconomic history is taken, the correct diagnosis may never be entertained. Once considered, however, the presence of a parasitic disease is easily confirmed. Most commonly, this is accomplished by the recovery and morphologic identification of the parasite in the stool, urine, sputum, blood, or tissues of the patient.

In intestinal infections, examination of a wet-mount and/or stained smear of the stool is usually adequate. Because many parasites are passed intermittently or in fluctuating numbers, the examination of a single stool specimen may detect only one-third to one-half of involved patients. The testing of three such specimens collected at intervals of 2 or 3 days will improve this yield substantially. Alternatively, a saline cathartic may be administered to evacuate the cecal area where many protozoa are concentrated, and the entire purge examined. The stool must be free of interfering substances such as antidiarrheal or contrast agents, antacids, and antibiotics. If the appropriate specimens cannot be obtained prior to administration of such substances, testing should be performed 1 week or, in the case of antimicrobial agents, 3 weeks after their discontinuation. Occasionally, specimens other than stool must be examined. In small-bowel infections such as giardiasis and strongyloidiasis, the diagnosis, at times, can be established only by sampling the duodenal contents or by performing a jejunal biopsy. Similarly, eggs of *Enterobius* (pinworm) and *Taenia* (tapeworm) are frequently found on the perianal skin when absent from the feces. Recovery of large-bowel parasites such as *Entamoeba histolytica* and *Schistosoma mansoni* may require colonic intubation with aspiration or biopsy of suspect lesions. Whenever intestinal aspirates or soft to watery fecal specimens are collected, they should be immediately placed in a preservative such as polyvinyl alcohol (PVA) to prevent rapid disintegration of fragile protozoan trophozoites and allow the preparation of permanently stained smears. Protozoan cysts and helminthic ova found in formed stool will survive for 1 to 2 days at room temperature and indefinitely if placed in 5% formaldehyde.

Direct examination of the blood is useful for the detection of malaria parasites, leishmania, trypanosomes, and microfilaria. Preferably, fresh capillary blood should be used to prepare thin and thick blood smears and, when appropriate, wet mounts. Only specially prepared glass slides should be used as traces of soda lime or potash on uncleaned slides may alter the pH of the stain, making recognition of parasites difficult. If an experienced technologist is not available to assist in the bedside preparation of smears, it is preferable to collect venous blood in an EDTA Vacutainer and send it to the laboratory. As in the case of intestinal parasites, organisms in the peripheral blood may fluctuate, requiring the collection of multiple specimens over a period of several days.

Parasites dwelling within the tissues of the host are more difficult to identify. Some discharge their offspring into the sputum (lung flukes) where they can be found with appropriate concentration procedures. In others, larvae can be recovered with skin (*Onchocerca volvulus*) or muscle (*Trichinella spiralis*) biopsies. In some diseases, however, parasite recovery is uncommon. Reliable immunodiagnostic tests have been developed for a few of these. Unfortunately, serologic tests for parasites often lack the sensitivity and specificity of those developed for viral and bacterial agents. This is particularly true for helminths which are broadly cross-reactive with one another. With the use of molecular technologies, more highly specific antigens are being developed. Table 151-1 lists the serologic tests available through the Centers for Disease Control (CDC). In Table 151-2 the diagnostic titer, sensitivity, and specificity of the most frequently requested CDC procedures are given.

Soluble antigens have been detected in the blood, body fluids, tissues, and excreta of a number of protozoan and helminthic diseases, including amebiasis, primary amebic meningoencephalitis, giardiasis, malaria, toxoplasmosis, filariasis, trichinosis, and schistosomiasis. The diagnostic usefulness of such procedures is being explored; at present none are commercially available. Similarly, diagnostic DNA probes have been described for falciparum malaria and cutaneous leishmaniasis. Highly sensitive and specific, these tests may revolutionize the diagnosis of parasitic diseases in the near future, but are not currently commercially available.

TREATMENT Over the past decade, a number of new chemotherapeutic agents have been introduced for the treatment of parasitic diseases. A few, such as praziquantel and nifurtimox, represent the first effective agents available for the treatment of previously refractory diseases (i.e., clonorchiasis, Chagas' disease). Others, such as mebendazole, possess activity against a broad spectrum of helminths, allowing single-drug therapy of multiple intestinal infections. Many of the new agents are better tolerated than the ones they are destined to replace, permitting them to be used in mass therapy programs.

Despite these gains, however, treatment of parasitic diseases remains unsatisfactory. For a number of infections, including cryptosporidiosis, cysticercosis, echinococciasis, and trichinosis, satisfactory anthelmintics are not available. Drug resistance, a phenomenon so common to bacterial pathogens, also threatens the usefulness of some antiparasitic agents. This is particularly serious among the antimalarials. Chloroquine-resistant *P. falciparum,* long present in southeast Asia and Latin America, has now spread to Africa, the continent most devastated by this disease. Some Asian strains of this same organism have now developed resistance to the pyrimethamine-sulfadoxine regimen that has been used so successfully to suppress chloroquine-resistant infections.

Yet another problem relates to the availability of antiparasitic agents in the United States. Many of the drugs recommended in the following chapters have not been approved by the U.S. Food and Drug Administration either for use in this country or for the particular disease indicated. Those available as investigational agents through the Centers for Disease Control are listed in Table 151-3. Others, such as DL-α-difluoromethylornithine (DFMO), must be obtained

TABLE 151-1 Parasitic diseases for which serology is available

	Diagnostic usefulness	
Taxonomic group	High	Marginal
Protozoan	Amebiasis* Babesiosis* Chagas' disease* Leishmaniasis* Toxoplasmosis*	Malaria* Giardiasis Pneumocystosis
Helminthic	Cysticercosis* Echinococcosis* Paragonimiasis* Toxocariasis* Trichinosis*	Ascariasis Clonorchiasis* Dracunculiasis* Filariasis* Schistosomiasis* Strongyloidiasis

** Available at the Centers for Disease Control, Atlanta, Ga.*

TABLE 151-2 Interpretation of tests frequently performed at the Centers for Disease Control

Disease	Test*	Diagnostic titer	Sensitivity %†	Specificity %†	Comments
Invasive amebiasis	IHA	≥:256	70[1], 95[2]	90[3]	*1* Intestinal. *2* Extra-intestinal. *3* Titers may persist for years.
Cysticercosis	ELISA	≥1:32	50[1], 70[2], 95[3]	83–95[4]	*1* Intracranial calcifications, seizures. *2* Meningitis. *3* ↑ Intracranial pressure. *4* Cross-reacts with echinococcosis.
Echinococcosis	IHA	≥1:256	10[1], 88[2]	90–95[3,4]	*1* Lung or calcified cyst. *2* Liver or peritoneal. *3* Cross-reacts with cysticercosis. *4* Titer may persist for years.
	IEP	Arc 5	Very high	—[5]	*5* Arc 5 indicates echinococcosis.
Toxocariasis					
Visceral	ELISA	≥1:32	78	92[1,2]	*1* Cross-reacts with ascariasis but eliminated by preabsorption. *2* In children.
Ocular	ELISA	≥1:8	90	91[3]	*3* Patients with ocular disease.
Trichinosis	BFT	≥1:5	97[1]	90[2]	*1* Detected after third week of illness. *2* Titers may persist for years.

** IHA = indirect hemagglutination; ELISA = enzyme-linked immunosorbent assay; BFT = bentonite flocculation; IEP = immunoelectrophoresis.*
† Superscript numbers refer to comments at right.
SOURCE: *Adapted from data provided by Kenneth W. Walls, Ph.D., December 1985.*

TABLE 151-3 Agents available through the parasitic diseases division, CDC*

Infection	Therapeutic agent
Amebiasis	Dehydroemetine Diloxanide furoate
Chagas' disease (*Trypanosoma cruzi*)	Nifurtimox
Dracunculosis	Niridazole
Fascioliasis	Bithionol
Leishmaniasis	Sodium antimony gluconate (stibogluconate sodium)
Malaria	Parenteral chloroquine hydrochloride Parenteral quinine dihydrochloride
Onchocerciasis	Suramin
Paragonimiasis	Bithionol
Schistosomiasis	Metrifonate Niridazole
Sleeping sickness (*Trypanosoma brucei*)	Melarsoprol Suramin

* *Parasitic Diseases Division, Centers for Disease Control, Atlanta, GA 30333. Day telephone: (404) 329-3670.*

TABLE 151-4 Fecal egg counts associated with illness

Worm	Approximate egg output per female worm per day	Minimum egg output usually associated with illness
Necator americanus	25,000	>2000/mL
Trichuris trichiura	7500	>3000/g
Schistosoma mansoni	60–300	>200/g

SOURCE: *After DP Stevens, Clin Gastroenterol 7:236, 1978.*

directly from the manufacturer. When a clinician prescribes such an agent, the patient should be informed of the drug's investigational status and potential side effects.

Finally, the toxicity of many agents is such that the benefit of treatment must be carefully weighed against its potential side effects. This is particularly true in helminthic infections. Since most worms do not multiply within the body and because disability is usually related to the intensity of infection, treatment is directed primarily at reducing the worm burden of moderately to heavily infected patients. Total eradication is often unnecessary and may be unwise considering the toxicity of many anthelmintics. Light infections should be treated only when (1) small numbers of worms may be dangerous as in the case of strongyloidiasis, (2) the chance of reinfection is slight, and/or (3) the anthelmintic agent in question is without serious side effects. The intensity of many intestinal infections can be determined by enumerating the eggs found in stool (Table 151-4). Multiplying the total seen on direct smear by 750 provides a rough estimate of the number present per gram of feces. The Stoll dilution and the various modifications of the Kato thick-smear technique provide more precise results.

REFERENCES

Drugs for parasitic infections. Med Lett 26:27, 1984

Health Information for International Travel 1981. US Department of Health, Education, and Welfare Publication (CDC) 81-8280. Morb Mort Week Rep 1981;30 (August Suppl)

PLORDE JJ: Introduction to pathogenic parasites, in *Medical Microbiology: An Introduction to Infectious Diseases,* JC Sherris (ed). New York, Elsevier North-Holland, 1982

SMITH JW, BARTLETT MS: Diagnostic parasitology: Introduction and methods, in *Manual of Clinical Microbiology,* 4th ed, EH Lennette et al (eds). Washington, Am Soc Microbiol, 1985, pp 595–611

WALLS KW: Serodiagnosis of parasitic diseases, in *Manual of Clinical Microbiology,* 4th ed, EH Lennette et al (eds). Washington, Am Soc Microbiol, 1985, chap 97, pp 945–984

152 THE IMMUNOLOGY OF PARASITES

JOHN R. DAVID

During the past decade interest in parasitic diseases of humans and in new approaches to their control has increased steadily. One reason for this is the enormous scope of the problem. Over a billion people in the world are affected by parasitic diseases. Although accurate statistics are difficult to obtain, it is estimated that over 200 million people have malaria, the most serious protozoan disease of humans, and that more than a million children die of malaria each year in Africa alone. Schistosomiasis, a disease caused by helminths that are transmitted by snails, affects 200 to 300 million persons. Filarial parasites affect an equal number of people, and one of these, *Onchocerca volvulus,* is the second major cause of blindness in the world. *Trypanosoma cruzi,* another protozoan, is the major cause of heart disease in South America, and hookworm infects over 800 million persons.

With the modernization of developing countries, many of these diseases are becoming more prevalent. For example, the pressure to provide energy for industrialization leads to building dams which have brought about profound changes in the local environment; the lake behind the Volta Dam has increased the coastline by 4000 miles, and the snails on its banks infected with schistosomes have increased the prevalence of schistosomiasis in people living on the lake's borders from a few percent to almost 100 percent. Improvement schemes for agriculture often involve extension of irrigation as is necessary for the cultivation of rice. Some of these projects have been associated with increases in transmission of malaria by mosquitoes, which breed in the irrigation ditches. Another example of the unanticipated effects of progress can be seen in the Amazon basin, where the clearing of the forests in order to reclaim the land for industry and agriculture has greatly increased human contact with sandflies which live in these areas and transmit leishmaniasis.

Another reason for the increasing focus on these diseases by scientists and physicians is that the classic control measures are less than adequate. The most telling example of this is malaria. After World War II, there was great optimism that this disease could be eradicated by spraying homes with DDT and by treating the disease in humans with chloroquine. After an extensive eradication program was instituted in the early 1960s in Sri Lanka, only 18 cases of malaria were reported in that country. However, 5 years later there were over a half million cases. The failure of malaria eradication was due to at least three factors: (1) the surveillance stage of the eradication effort was not maintained; (2) mosquitoes became resistant to DDT; and (3) the parasite became resistant to chloroquine. Moreover, the cost of these control measures proved to be enormous.

The large number of people affected by parasitic diseases, the increasing environmental changes in the developing world, and the failure of classic control programs have stimulated the search for new approaches for the control of these disorders. One of these approaches is immunologic. Currently, immunologists are studying several aspects of parasites' interaction with the host. They are trying to delineate the mechanisms that parasites have evolved to evade the immune response of the host, to define which immune mechanisms they do not escape, and to learn which immune responses are the basis for the pathologic lesions. Immunology is also providing diagnostic tests and ultimately, it is hoped, will provide effective vaccines for some of these diseases. At present, there is not a single vaccine available to protect humans against parasites, despite the availability of several effective vaccines against animal parasitic diseases. For the purposes of this discussion, the most useful way to present the problems of vaccine development in these complex diseases is to give a relatively detailed description of what is being done in one disease, malaria, rather than a cursory summary of many.

MALARIA VACCINE Although investigators are trying to produce vaccines to many parasites, especially intensive work is under way on vaccines for *Plasmodium falciparum*, the most malignant malaria parasite. In order to understand the various approaches that are being pursued, it is necessary to review briefly the life cycle of the malaria parasite (see Chap. 154). When an infected mosquito bites a human, it injects the motile sporozoite, which is in the salivary gland. In less than half an hour, the sporozoite leaves the blood and invades the liver. It then goes through the exoerythrocytic cycle, undergoing asexual division by schizogeny and producing many merozoites. These burst out of the liver cells into the blood and invade erythrocytes. Here, they differentiate into trophozoites, undergo division by schizogony, and burst, liberating more merozoites which reinvade erythrocytes and continue the cycle. Some of the merozoites develop into the sexual stages, the gametocytes. When a mosquito bites an infected person, the gametocytes are taken up in the blood meal and rapidly come out of the erythrocytes. The male microgametes then fertilize the female macrogametes, forming the ookinete and then the oocyst. Further division within the oocyst leads to the infective stage, the sporozoite. Several of these stages can be targeted for immunologic attack by a vaccine.

Sporozoite vaccine Persons can become immune to *P. falciparum* via the sporozoite stage. This has been shown by allowing irradiated infected mosquitoes (containing irradiated sporozoites which cannot divide) to bite humans. Investigations have resulted in the characterization of a single sporozoite antigen. Monoclonal antibodies to this antigen can passively transfer resistance to malaria in rodents and monkeys. Using recombinant DNA technology, the gene coding for the protective sporozoite antigen of *P. falciparum* has been cloned. The protective epitope is made up of four amino acids repeated 23 times. This repeated sequence can be synthesized for the development of a vaccine. The advantages of a sporozoite vaccine are that it might be effective without an adjuvant and that it may protect against different strains of *P. falciparum*. The disadvantage is that immunity is an all-or-none phenomenon; if a few sporozoites evade the immune response, the person will get malaria.

Merozoite vaccine The host encounters merozoites for short periods, as they leave one erythrocyte and invade another. Erythrocytes infected by parasites develop new antigens, probably of parasite origin, on their surface. Both the merozoite and the infected erythrocyte could be targets for a vaccine. Monoclonal antibodies to merozoites and infected erythrocytes of rodent malaria transferred passively can confer partial protection. These monoclonal antibodies have been used to isolate antigens which can induce protective immunity. This vaccine would have the advantage of acting against stages of the parasite that interact with the host for a longer time period than the sporozoites. The disadvantages are that adjuvants are required for effective protection and that the vaccine may be strain-specific.

Gamete vaccine If an animal is made immune to gametes, a state that does not usually occur in nature because the gamete is isolated from the immune apparatus by the erythrocyte membrane, the antigamete antibodies, when taken up with the gametes in the mosquitoes' blood meal, will neutralize the gametes when they leave the erythrocyte. It appears as if at least two antigens are involved in this process because neutralization will occur when two different monoclonal antigamete antibodies act in concert but not when they act alone. A vaccine aimed at gametes would not protect the vaccinated individual from malaria but might be effective in reducing its transmission. It could be useful, therefore, if it were incorporated into a multivalent vaccine.

TABLE 152-1 Some mechanisms of immune evasion

Parasite	Mechanism
Trypanosoma brucei	Antigenic variation
Toxoplasma	Lysosome-phagosome fusion prevented
Malaria, *Babesia*	Escape into host cells
Schistosomes	Host molecule acquisition
	Loss of surface antigens
	Intrinsic membrane changes
	Immune complex blockade
Filaria, *Leishmania*	Specific T-cell suppression
Taenia, amoeba	Inactivation of mediators of inflammation

IMMUNE EVASION BY PARASITES Parasites have developed a variety of ingenious ways of evading the immune response of the host. Some of these are listed in Table 152-1. The most fascinating mechanism is that of antigenic variation by African trypanosomes, the flagellated protozoa transmitted by the tsetse fly that is the cause of sleeping sickness. The trypanosome has a thick surface coat, which is made up of many molecules of a single antigenic glycoprotein. When cloned organisms, all having the same surface antigen, are injected into certain animals, successive waves of parasitemia ensue similar to those seen when a human is bitten by an infected tsetse fly. Each peak consists of organisms expressing a single variant surface glycoprotein antigen (VSG), and this VSG is different from all other VSGs expressed by organisms in previous peaks of parasitemia in the same animal. A cloned organism can produce waves of parasites with over 100 different VSGs! Each peak of parasitemia induces soluble antibody directed at the major VSG. Presumably the antibody eliminates the organism with that specific VSG, but trypanosomes which can switch to another VSG escape. Analysis of the amino acid sequence of a number of VSGs indicates that they do not differ by only a few substitutions which could be explained by point mutations; on the contrary, the amino acid sequence of each VSG is quite different.

Studies on the genes encoding the VSGs have shown that each VSG is encoded by a distinct gene. Every trypanosome, regardless of the VSG it is expressing, contains a copy of each VSG gene. Trypanosomes have several mechanisms for expressing a VSG. For example, the organism expressing a particular VSG gene may have an additional, duplicate copy of that gene; this is referred to as the expression-linked copy. Studies using restriction enzymes indicate that the expression-linked copy is moved to a new site in the trypanosome that is gene-specific for expression. If each gene is visualized as a tape cassette in a library, to express the VSG the cassette is duplicated, the duplicate is removed from the library and inserted into a genetic tape deck, and expressed.

Although it was thought initially that the driving force for antigenic variation was antibody to that antigen, it has been shown that antigenic variation can be triggered in the absence of antibody both in vitro and in vivo.

Some organisms have developed multiple ways of evading the immune response. Schistosomes, for instance, can lose surface antigens after they enter the host, can take up host antigens and masquerade as host tissue, can develop certain intrinsic membrane changes making them resistant to attack even when surface antigens are present, and can shed antigens which may block effector cells and antibodies. A number of parasites, *Toxoplasma* being one example, when engulfed by a macrophage, prevent the fusion of the phagosome with the lysosomes. Others, such as *Leishmania*, do not prevent fusion when engulfed but are resistant to toxic substances in the lysosomes of the macrophage. And still others, such as *Trypanosoma cruzi*, escape from the lysosomes into the cytoplasm.

A number of parasites such as filaria, *Leishmania*, and *Plasmodium* induce strong suppressor mechanisms, including T suppressor cells, which dampen or eliminate the host's effective immune response. Some parasites can destroy mediators of inflammation involved in an effective immune response. For example, *Taenia* destroys complement components, and amoebae produce factors which neutralize chemotactic factors for macrophages. Other parasites such as *Ascaris* appear to have a surface coat that is antigenic and can induce an immune response but is, nevertheless, resistant to its effect. Against these parasites, there is no effective protective immune response.

Although some parasites can evade the immune response, they can induce an effective protective immune response to a subsequent infection by the same species. This is called *concomitant immunity* or *premunition*.

EFFECTOR MECHANISMS AGAINST PARASITES Mechanisms that may be effective against parasites include the following: antibodies, cells including cytotoxic T cells, T-cell–induced activated macrophages, natural killer cells, and a variety of cells that mediate antibody-dependent cell-mediated cytotoxicity. Amplifiers of the immune system such as lymphokines and complement are also involved.

Immunity against several parasites such as malaria, schistosomes, and *Trypanosoma cruzi* can be transferred by antibodies. Nevertheless, evidence obtained in a number of animal models suggests that cell-mediated immunity is also involved against these and other parasites, including the organisms causing malaria, leishmaniasis, toxoplasmosis, schistosomiasis, filariasis, and trichinosis. It is less clear whether protective immunity develops against amoebae, African trypanosomes, or hookworm. There appears to be no naturally acquired immunity to *Ascaris,* guinea worm, or pinworm.

Two immune mechanisms have been described which appear to be unique for helminths. These involve eosinophils in one case and IgE in the other.

EOSINOPHILS AND ANTIBODY-DEPENDENT CELL-MEDIATED CYTOTOXICITY (ADCC) It has been known for over 100 years that eosinophils are associated with helminth infections, but only in the past few years has it become known that these cells can function as killer cells. Specifically, highly purified preparations of eosinophils, when mixed with antibody-coated schistosomula of *Schistosoma mansoni* in vitro, killed the larvae. The antibody formed is of the IgG class, and the eosinophils attach to the Fc portion of the IgG by the cells' Fc receptor. Immune complexes or staphylococcal protein A which can interfere with the binding of esosinophils to the Fc portion of the antibody inhibit the reaction. Incubation at 37°C makes the interaction between eosinophils and antibody-coated schistosomula become irreversible. This is associated with degranulation and the release of major basic protein (MBP), the most abundant protein in the eosinophil granule and eosinophil cationic protein (ECP) over the surface of the schistosomula. MBP and ECP, in turn, are toxic to the larvae. Eosinophils can also kill other helminths such as *Trichinella spiralis,* presumably by a similar mechanism.

Eosinophils from patients with eosinophilia exhibit an enhanced ability to kill antibody-coated schistosomula in vitro; they act as if they were activated. Moreover, a number of soluble substances can enhance the killing capacity of eosinophils in vitro. These include eosinophil stimulator promoter (ESP), ECF-A, a soluble substance similar or identical to eosinophil colony stimulating factor, and a soluble mediator produced by blood monocytes and lymphocytes in culture.

PROTECTIVE ROLE FOR IgE The observation that IgE levels are elevated in some persons in the tropics, notably those infected with helminths, suggests that IgE may act to protect the host against parasites. The mediators released by triggered mast cells could affect the parasites directly or, by increasing vascular permeability and releasing eosinophil chemotactic factors, they could lead to the accumulation of necessary antibodies (IgG) and cells to attack the parasite. IgE-immune complexes can induce macrophage-mediated cytotoxicity to schistosomula. Rats made specifically IgE-deficient by the repeated injection of antiepsilon chain antibodies show markedly impaired resistance to *Trichinella* infection.

IMMUNOPATHOLOGY Immune mechanisms play a major role in the pathology induced by many parasites. Such mechanisms are the cause of the granulomatous reaction to eggs of *S. mansoni* which is the basis of the immunopathology of this disease; immune complex renal disease in malaria and visceral leishmaniasis; heart disease due to *T. cruzi;* the obstructive and ocular disease in filariasis and onchocerciasis; the muscle pathology in trichinosis; the allergic reactions to ruptured hydatic cyst fluid; and the pulmonary complications to migrating nematode larvae. Just as suppressor mechanisms are involved in damping protective immunity, they are also involved in modulating the immunopathology. An example of this is the modulation of *S. mansoni* granulomas by T suppressor cells.

MONOCLONAL AND ANTI-IDIOTYPIC ANTIBODIES Monoclonal antibodies to various stages of malaria parasites have been used to detect antigens that can induce protective immunity. In addition, passive protection has been demonstrated with monoclonal antibodies to the promastigote stage of *Leishmania mexicana* and to schistosomula of *S. mansoni*. Because of their spec·ficity, monoclonal antibodies can also be used for diagnosis because they can be selected not to show the multiple cross-reactions with other parasites that are frequently found with serums from infected animals. For example, species-specific monoclonal antibodies have been developed which can distinguish between five different species of South American *Leishmania* without cross-reacting with *T. cruzi*. Antibodies in the serum of an infected patient will usually cross-react with all these parasites. Diagnostic tests using these antibodies are being developed.

An antibody to an antigen has a specific antigen unique to itself on the immunoglobulin. This antigen is called the *idiotype,* which is the unique amino acid sequence and configuration of the antigen-binding site of that antibody. For instance, it is possible to make an antibody to a particular monoclonal antibody; that antibody will then recognize the idiotype and is called an *anti-idiotypic antibody*. The monoclonal antibody will bind to the anti-idiotype or to the original antigen. If a monoclonal antibody to a parasite were used to induce an anti-idiotypic antibody, it should be possible to induce protective immunity with this anti-idiotype instead of using the antigen. This would have the advantage of bypassing the need to purify antigens and then to produce them in large quantities. This novel strategy for the production of a vaccine is under study.

The rapidly accelerating pace of discovery and definition of the regulatory systems of the immune response, together with the revolution in technology, may soon make it possible to induce stronger protective immunity artificially than that which is acquired naturally, and the prediction that vaccines can be produced against the diseases caused by a number of parasites is based on this assumption.

REFERENCES

BLOOM BR: Games parasites play: How parasites evade immune surveillance. Nature 279:21, 1979

COHEN S, WARREN K (eds): *Immunology of Parasitic Infections*, 2d ed. London, Blackwell Scientific, 1982

———, CROSS GAM (eds): Towards the immunological control of human protozoal diseases: A symposium. Phil Trans Roy Soc London B 307:1, 1984

DONELSON JE, TURNER MJ: How the trypanosome changes its coat. Sci Am 252(2):44, 1985

HOMMELL M: Antigenic variation in malaria parasites. Immunology Today 6:28, 1985

MAHMOUD AF, AUSTEN KF (eds): *The Eosinophil in Health and Disease*. New York, Grune & Stratton, 1981

MARCHALONIS JJ (ed): *Contemporary Topics in Immunobiology*, vol 12: *Immunobiology of Parasites and Parasitic Infections*. New York, Plenum Press, 1984

MOLLER G (ed): *Immunoparasitology*. Immunological Reviews 161. Copenhagen, Munksgaard, 1982, pp 5–269

153 AMEBIASIS

JAMES J. PLORDE

DEFINITION Amebiasis is an infection of the large intestine produced by *Entamoeba histolytica*. It is an asymptomatic carrier state in most individuals, but diseases ranging from chronic, mild diarrhea to fulminant dysentery may occur. Among extraintestinal complications, the commonest is hepatic abscess, which may rupture into peritoneum, pleura, lung, or pericardium.

ETIOLOGY There are seven species of ameba that naturally parasitize the human mouth and intestine, but of these only *E. histolytica* causes disease. *Entamoeba coli* and *E. hartmanni* are the two species with which it is most likely to be confused in examination of stools.

Entamoeba histolytica exists in two forms: the motile trophozoite and the cyst. The trophozoite is the parasitic form and dwells in the lumen and/or wall of the colon, divides by binary fission, grows best under anaerobic conditions, and requires the presence of either bacteria or tissue substrates to satisfy its nutritional requirements. When diarrhea occurs, the trophozoites are passed unchanged in the liquid stool, where they can be distinguished by their size (10 to 20 μm in diameter), directional motility, sharply demarcated clear ectoplasm with slender finger-like pseudopodia, and finely granular endoplasm. In dysentery, the trophozoites are larger (up to 50 μm in diameter), and often contain ingested erythrocytes. In the absence of diarrhea, the trophozoites usually encyst before leaving the gut. The cysts have a chitinous wall which renders them highly resistant to environmental changes, chlorine concentrations found in water purification systems, and gastric acid. With rare exception they are responsible for transmission of disease. Young cysts have a single nucleus, a glycogen vacuole, and sausage-shaped collections of ribosomes known as chromatoid bodies. As the cyst matures, it absorbs its cytoplasmic inclusions and becomes quadrinucleate. The cysts of *E. histolytica* can be distinguished from those of *E. hartmanni* by their larger diameter (10-μm) and from those of *Entamoeba coli* by the presence of one to four nuclei with small centric karyosomes and fine peripheral chromatin and by their thick chromatoid bodies with round ends.

The electrophoretic mobility patterns of four enzymes found in trophozoites have been used to define 22 *E. histolytica* zymodemes. Amebas recovered from patients with invasive disease belong to just 9; all are characterized by the presence of advanced, paired hexokinase bands and/or a beta phosphoglucomutase without an accompanying alpha-phosphoglucomutase band. The zymodemes are highly stable, and transitions between the invasive and commensal isoenzyme patterns have not been observed. Further studies will be required to determine whether the biologic differences between the two groups of organisms are sufficient to warrant the division of *E. histolytica* into separate pathogenic and nonpathogenic species.

Entamoeba histolytica can be cultivated in artificial media, a procedure that is essential for the determination of isoenzyme patterns and preparation of the purified antigens used in serologic testing. Its diagnostic value remains uncertain.

EPIDEMIOLOGY Although *E. histolytica* can sometimes infect rats, cats, dogs, and primates, humans are the principal hosts and reservoir. Because trophozoites die rapidly after leaving the intestine, the asymptomatic cyst passer is the source of new infections; a chronic carrier may excrete several million organisms daily. The infective dose usually exceeds 10^3, but infection has followed the ingestion of a single cyst. These structures are transmitted by the fecal-oral route, usually through direct person-to-person contact. Poverty, ignorance, mental retardation, and other factors which impair personal hygiene facilitate the spread of the parasite. Oral-anal sexual contact produces high infection rates in male homosexuals. Food- and waterborne transmission occur in poorly sanitated areas of the world, including certain southern rural communities, Indian reservations, and migrant farm camps in the United States. Occasionally this results in common source outbreaks; these epidemics, however, are never as explosive as those produced by pathogenic intestinal bacteria. Symptomatic amebiasis is unusual below the age of 10 years in temperate climates, and both intestinal and hepatic lesions predominate in adult males to an extent that is not readily explainable on the basis of different rates of exposure to infection.

It has been estimated that 50 percent of inhabitants of some less well-developed nations, 10 percent of the world's population as a whole, and 1 percent of Americans are infected with *E. histolytica*. Invasive amebiasis, which produces an estimated 30,000 deaths annually, is concentrated in comparatively few parts of the world, most notably Mexico, western South America, south Asia, and west and southeastern Africa. This is presumably related to the concurrent presence in these geographic areas of virulent strains of *E. histolytica* and the hygienic and sanitary conditions necessary for their transmission. Even in areas endemic for invasive disease, however, only 10 percent of infected patients harbor virulent zymodemes of *E. histolytica*. A minority of these experience clinical disease. In the United States the incidence of invasive amebiasis dropped sharply in the four decades preceding the 1970s. Between 1971 and 1974, an average of 3500 cases were reported annually to the Centers for Disease Control; since then the numbers have steadily increased. Isoenzyme studies of *E. histolytica* strains isolated from male homosexuals and inmates of mental hospitals in Great Britain indicate the overwhelming majority belong to nonpathogenic zymodemes, suggesting that virulent strains are now uncommon in the developed nations. Although patients with dysentery and liver abscess can still be found in the impoverished segments of the American population, the bulk of the invasive disease diagnosied in the United States is now acquired outside the country.

IMMUNITY There are both animal and human data suggesting the presence of protective immunity. However, repeated infections are common, and there is no correlation between the presence of circulating antibodies and immunity to infection. It is likely that immunity is incomplete, serves to limit rather than prevent disease, and is cell mediated.

PATHOGENESIS AND PATHOLOGY After ingestion, cysts undergo further nuclear division. In the small intestine, the cyst wall disintegrates, and trophozoites are released. The immature amebas are carried to the large intestine, where they live in the lumen of the gut feeding on bacteria and debris. Experimental and epidemiologic evidence indicates that organisms belonging to nonpathogenic zymodemes, although capable of inducing transient, focal epithelial damage, are seldom responsible for sustained tissue invasion and destruction. In contrast, the almost universal presence of specific humoral antibodies in carriers of pathogenic zymodemes suggests that tissue invasion by these strains is the rule. Only in the minority, however, is this sufficiently extensive to produce symptoms. The factors modulating invasion are not completely understood, but the state of the host and the virulence of the infecting organism both play roles. High iron and carbohydrate intake, corticosteroids, protein malnutrition, and pregnancy all render the host more susceptible. Trophozoite virulence is enhanced by rapid animal passage; presumably, a similar phenomenon occurs in epidemiologic settings conducive to rapid spread of the protozoan from human to human. Direct association with certain strains of bacteria may also enhance the virulence of pathogenic strains, possibly by protecting the ameba from oxidant stress or through the exchange of genetic material.

The precise pathogenic mechanisms responsible for tissue invasion are not fully understood. The invasiveness of a strain correlates well with its phagocytic prowess, production of collagenase and an immunogenic cytotoxic protein, resistance to the host's inflammatory response, and, perhaps most importantly, its capacity to induce histolysis following direct cell-to-cell contact with host tissue. The latter phenomenon is initiated by a lectin-mediated adherence of the trophozoite to a target cell. Cytolysis, which appears to require both intact microfilament function and amebic phospholipase A enzymes, rapidly follows.

Amebic ulceration of the intestinal wall is characteristic. A small mucosal defect overlies a larger, burrowing area of necrosis in the submucosa and muscularis, producing a bottle-shaped lesion. There is little acute inflammatory response, and in contrast to the picture in bacillary dysentery, the mucosa between ulcers is normal. The sites of involvement in order of frequency are cecum and ascending colon, rectum, sigmoid, appendix, and terminal ileum. In the cecum and sigmoid, chronic infection may lead to the formation of large masses of granulation tissue or *amebomas*. Amebas can enter the portal circulation and lodge in venules; liquefaction necrosis of liver tissue leads to the formation of an abscess cavity. Rarely, embolization results in lung, brain, or splenic abscess.

CLINICAL MANIFESTATIONS **Asymptomatic cyst passer** In the majority of patients with this common form of amebiasis, *E. histolytica* probably lives as a commensal in the bowel lumen. Individuals infected in temperate climates are unlikely to harbor virulent strains. However, as invasion can occasionally occur, treatment of all cyst passers is warranted.

Symptomatic intestinal amebiasis In some patients there is intermittent diarrhea consisting of one to four foul-smelling loose or watery stools daily. The stools sometimes contain mucus and blood. Loose stools alternate with periods of relative normality and may persist for months or years. Flatulence and abnormal cramping are frequent. The only physical findings are occasional tender hepatomegaly and slight pain when the cecum and ascending colon are palpated. Sigmoidoscopy sometimes reveals typical ulcerations with areas of normal mucosa interspersed. The diagnosis depends upon finding the organism in the feces or in ulcers.

Fulminating attacks of amebic dysentery are less common. Waterborne outbreaks may occur, but fulminating dysentery is more likely to occur spontaneously in debilitated individuals. Attacks may be precipitated by pregnancy or corticosteroids. The onset in half the cases is abrupt with high fever, between 40 and 40.6°C (104 and 105°F), severe abdominal cramps, and profuse, bloody diarrhea with tenesmus. There is diffuse abdominal tenderness, often so severe that peritonitis is suspected. Hepatomegaly is very frequent, and sigmoidoscopy almost always demonstrates extensive rectosigmoid ulceration. Trophozoites are numerous in stools and in material obtained directly from the ulcers.

In some cases there may be extensive destruction of the colonic mucosa and submucosa, massive hemorrhage or perforation of the bowel wall, with resultant peritonitis. Repeated severe attacks of intestinal amebiasis can lead to an ulcerative postdysenteric colitis. Amebas can usually not be demonstrated in this condition, but serologic tests are strongly positive. Invasion of the appendix may lead to a clinical picture of *appendicitis*. Penetration of trophozoites through the muscle wall of the bowel may result in the development of large masses of granulation tissue. When the entire circumference of the intestine is involved, there may then be partial obstruction, and a movable, tender, sausage-shaped mass is often palpable. This lesion or ameboma is most frequently seen in the cecum where a palpable mass and radiologic demonstration of a ragged encroachment of the lumen may lead to a mistaken diagnosis of adenocarcinoma.

Hepatic amebiasis The term *amebic hepatitis* is used for a syndrome of tender hepatomegaly, right upper quadrant pain, fever, and leukocytosis in patients with amebic colitis. Hepatic biopsy reveals nonspecific periportal inflammation. The absence of ameba within the areas of inflammation, the rarity with which the syndrome is followed by an amebic liver abscess, and the resolution of the liver signs following treatment of the intestinal disease with luminal amebicides indicate that these manifestations are not secondary to spread of trophozoites from the intestine, but are rather a nonspecific accompaniment of amebic colitis. As such, the syndrome does not merit the appellation of "amebic hepatitis."

Hepatic abscess may develop insidiously, with fever, sweats, weight loss, and no local signs other than painless or slightly tender hepatomegaly. In immunologically naive patients, there is more often an abrupt onset, with chills, fever to 40.6°C (105°F), nausea, vomiting, severe upper abdominal pain, and polymorphonuclear leukocytosis. Initially, cholecystitis, perforated ulcer, or acute pancreatitis may be suspected. Over 80 percent of patients with an insidious onset and half of those presenting with acute manifestations have a single abscess. Most commonly, this is localized in the posterior portion of the right lobe of the liver, because this lobe receives most of the blood draining the right colon through the "streaming" effect in portal vein flow. This location is responsible for several features that aid in diagnosis. *Point tenderness* in the posterolateral portion of a lower right intercostal space is frequent even in the absence of diffuse liver pain. Most abscesses enlarge upward, producing a bulge in the diaphragmatic dome, obliteration of the costophrenic gutter, small hydrothorax, basilar atelectasis, and pain referred to the right shoulder.

Liver function tests may be mildly to moderately disturbed and provide little diagnostic aid; the level of the serum glutamic oxaloacetic transaminase (SGOT), however, is of clinical value as it directly reflects the severity of disease. Jaundice is uncommon, and when present implies a grave prognosis. Radiologically, unruptured abscesses do not show a fluid level, and calcification of the liver parenchyma is very rare. Isotope liver scan utilizing two, or preferably three, projections is invaluable in confirming the presence and location of a liver abscess. It becomes positive within the first days of illness, often prior to other imaging techniques. Presumably these early changes reflect either a focal decrease in blood supply or injury to the Kupffer cells rather than liquefaction necrosis. Ultrasonic scanning and computerized tomography, although becoming positive slightly later in the course of the disease, are ultimately as sensitive as isotopic scanning and provide confirmation of the cystic nature of the lesion. The defect seen on imaging commonly persists for several months after the complete recovery of the patient. Serologic tests are positive in over 90 percent of cases.

Needle puncture results in the withdrawal of "pus" which consists of liquefied, necrotic liver. Typically, it is thick and odorless, resembling "chocolate syrup" or "anchovy paste." It may, however, be thin in consistency and yellow or green in color. The pus contains no polymorphonuclear leukocytes (barring secondary bacterial infection) and, usually, no amebas. The parasites are localized in the cyst wall and may be demonstrated in the terminal portion of the aspirate or, at times, by a Vim-Silverman needle biopsy of the cyst wall following aspiration of the abscess.

Hepatic abscess complicates asymptomatic infection of the colon more often than symptomatic intestinal disease, another factor making recognition difficult. Trophozoites or cysts are demonstrable in the feces of only about one-third of patients with abscess, and fewer than one-half can recall significant diarrheal illness.

Pleuropulmonary amebiasis The right pleural cavity and lung are involved by direct extension from the liver in 10 to 20 percent of patients with liver abscess. Rarely, amebic lung abscess has resulted from embolization rather than direct extension.

Manifestations are those of a consolidating pneumonia or lung abscess. If perforation into a bronchus occurs, patients expectorate large amounts of the typical exudate, some patients even commenting that the sputum "tastes like liver." Cough, pleural pain, fever, and leukocytosis are the rule, and secondary bacterial infection is frequent. Rupture into the free pleural space results in a massive pleural effusion; aspiration of "chocolate" fluid is diagnostic.

Other extraintestinal lesions Extension of an abscess from the left lobe of the liver to the pericardium is the most dangerous complication of hepatic abscess. It may be mistaken for tuberculous pericarditis or congestive cardiomyopathy. Less frequently, rapid cardiac tamponade occurs with ensuing dyspnea, shock, and death. *Peritonitis* is a result of perforation of colonic ulcer or rupture of liver abscess. Painful ulcers or condylomata of the genitalia, perianal skin, or abdominal wall (draining sinuses) are unusual complications which may be mistaken for syphilitic, tuberculous, or neoplastic lesions. They usually result from direct extension of intestinal disease; some are thought to result from sexual transmission. Metastatic brain abscess is rare, and an etiologic diagnosis is seldom made clinically. Splenic abscess has been reported but is very unusual.

DIFFERENTIAL DIAGNOSIS **Intestinal amebiasis** Patients with nondysenteric amebiasis are often misdiagnosed as having irritable bowel syndrome, diverticulitis, or regional enteritis. Ameboma may mimic colonic carcinoma or granulomatous disease, while the clinical spectrum of amebic dysentery overlaps those of shigellosis, salmonellosis, ulcerative colitis, and, in endemic areas, schistosomiasis. The invasive bacterial infections are usually more acute, severe, and self-limited than amebiasis. Stools from patients with shigellosis, salmonellosis, and ulcerative colitis contain large numbers of polymorphonuclear leukocytes, while those in amebic infection do not. Nevertheless, amebiasis may closely resemble any of the above diseases both clinically and radiologically and must be considered in the differential diagnosis of any chronic diarrhea or dysentery.

The identification of *E. histolytica* in the stool, however, does not eliminate other diagnostic possibilities. Amebic infection is often superimposed on or exacerbated by other colonic disease including schistosomiasis and cecal carcinoma. For this reason, patients with intestinal amebiasis and abdominal complaints still require stool culture, sigmoidoscopy, and a barium enema.

Hepatic abscess Once a filling defect has been demonstrated by isotope liver scanning, the differential diagnosis includes hepatic neoplasm, hydatid cyst, and pyogenic abscess. Neoplasms can usually be differentiated on the basis of their ultrasonic scanning characteristics, while the lack of constitutional manifestations and presence of an appropriate epidemiologic history is helpful in recognizing echinococcosis. The most difficult problem lies in the exclusion of a pyogenic abscess. An insidious onset in an adult male, a history of chronic diarrhea, significant pleuritic chest pain, and a single right lobe lesion favors the diagnosis of amebiasis. High fever, hyperbilirubinemia, multiple hepatic filling defects, and foul-smelling hepatic aspirate are more suggestive of pyogenic disease. Ultimately, the separation of the two diseases rests upon laboratory procedures.

LABORATORY DIAGNOSIS The diagnosis of intestinal amebiasis depends upon *identification of the organism in the stool or tissues*. Formed stools are microscopically examined initially in saline and iodine mounts for amebic cysts; concentration methods such as the formalin-ether technique increase the yield two- to threefold. Liquid or semiformed stools should be examined immediately in saline solution for the presence of motile hematophagous trophozoites. The addition of a supravital stain such as buffered methylene blue to the saline enhances nuclear detail and minimizes the possibility of confusing fecal leukocytes with amebic trophozoites. If there is any delay in examination of the stool, a portion of the specimen may be refrigerated for a few hours at 4°C, or placed in polyvinyl alcohol and 10% formalin. Definitive identification of *E. histolytica* requires the examination of permanently stained slides prepared from the material preserved with polyvinyl alcohol. An ocular micrometer is necessary to separate *E. hartmanni* from its larger relative. Four to six stool specimens may be required for diagnosis. If possible, the stool should be examined before the administration of antimicrobial, antidiarrheal, or antacid preparations, because all these agents may interfere with the recovery of amebas. Likewise, enemas and radiographic procedures utilizing barium sulfate are best postponed until after a thorough search for *E. histolytica* has been made. A simple, sensitive, and specific enzyme-linked immunosorbent assay has been developed for the detection of *E. histolytica* antigen in the stool. If commercially developed, it could provide a useful alternative to microscopic examination.

Sigmoidoscopy is of value in symptomatic cases. The mucosal lesions should be aspirated and the material examined for trophozoites as described above. Biopsy material obtained from such lesions and stained with periodic acid Schiff solution also will frequently reveal trophozoites.

The diagnosis of extraintestinal amebiasis is difficult. The parasite usually cannot be recovered from stool or tissue. Cultivation of amebas from feces or pus is possible but is not practical in most laboratories. *Serologic tests* employing purified antigens are positive in nearly all patients with proven amebic liver abscess and in a great majority of those with acute amebic dysentery. They are generally negative in asymptomatic cyst passers, suggesting that tissue invasion is required for antibody production. The persistence of significant antibody titers for months to years after complete cure makes serology, particularly in endemic areas, of more value in excluding the diagnosis than in confirming it. Some authors recommend the routine screening of all patients thought to have inflammatory bowel disease for serologic evidence of amebiasis. Steroid therapy could then be withheld in patients with positive tests pending the outcome of parasitological examination. Of the available tests, the indirect hemagglutination and enzyme-linked immunosorbent assays appear to be the most sensitive; average time to positivity is 3 and 2 weeks, respectively. Indirect immunofluorescence, countercurrent electrophoresis, and agar gel diffusion are also highly reliable. A number of these testing procedures are now available as commercial kits, making serologic testing feasible for most laboratories.

TREATMENT Treatment should be aimed at relief of symptoms, replacement of fluid, electrolyte, and blood losses, and eradication of the organism. Amebas may be found in the lumen of the bowel, in the intestinal wall, or extraintestinally. Most amebicides are not effective at all sites or when used alone, and a combination of drugs is often necessary to achieve cure. The available drugs based on their site of action fall into two categories.

Luminal amebicides These oral agents act by direct contact with trophozoites dwelling in the bowel lumen but are ineffective against amebas in tissue. Of the large number of available drugs, diloxanide furoate is one of the most effective and well tolerated but is presently available in the United States only through the Centers for Disease Control. A response rate of 80 to 85 percent has been noted; flatulence appears to be the only major side effect.

Iodoquinol has been effective in 60 to 70 percent of cases. As with its analogue iodochlorhydroxyquin, myelooptic neuropathy has been reported after long-term use. However, no such case has been noted when the dosage was limited to that given in Table 153-1. The drug should not be used in patients with thyroid disease or preexisting optic neuropathy.

Tissue amebicides *Chloroquine phosphate* is a systemic amebicide which is useful in hepatic disease because of its high concentration in the liver. It has little activity elsewhere.

Emetine is an alkaloid derivative of ipecac. When given intramuscularly, it is highly effective in destroying trophozoites in tissue including those in the wall of the intestine. It is ineffective against luminal amebas. Emetine is relatively toxic and may produce vomiting, diarrhea, abdominal cramping, weakness, muscle pain, tachycardia, hypotension, precordial pain, and electrocardiographic abnormalities. The common ECG changes include T-wave inversion and prolongation of the QTc interval. Rarely arrhythmias and prolongation of the QRS complex are seen. A synthetic derivative, dehydroemetine, is thought to be less toxic by virtue of its more rapid excretion and lower concentration in myocardial tissue. It is not free of toxicity, however, and patients treated with either drug should be at bed rest with ECG monitoring. Neither drug should be used in patients with renal, cardiac, or muscle disease, during pregnancy, or in children, unless other drugs fail.

Metronidazole is unique because it is effective against trophozoites at all sites, intestinally and extraintestinally. For intestinal amebiasis it is given in dosage of 750 mg three times daily for 5 to 10 days. Smaller doses are effective in hepatic amebiasis. Metronidazole has an Antabuse-like action, and alcohol should be avoided during its administration. The evidence that this drug is carcinogenic and possibly teratogenic in animals when given in large doses is disturbing. The potential risk in human beings must be weighed against the severity of the disease; it should not be given in the first trimester of pregnancy.

Specific antiprotozoal therapy is outlined in Table 153-1.

In extraintestinal amebiasis including hepatic abscess, metronidazole is the drug of choice. In cases of relapse, impending rupture of an abscess, or in situations where the patient is unable to take oral medication, therapy with dehydroemetine or emetine should be instituted, and oral chloroquine added as soon as possible. Diagnostic trials should employ the chloroquine-emetine regimen because pyogenic liver abscesses may temporarily respond to metronidazole. Most authors prefer to add luminal amebicides to both the metronidazole and chloroquine-emetine programs. Treatment failures have been reported for both emetine-chloroquine and metronidazole. They appear to be unrelated to the organism's resistance.

There is debate over the value of routine aspiration of amebic liver abscesses. Certainly, if there is localized swelling over the liver, marked elevation of the diaphragm, severe localized liver tenderness, and failure to respond to systemic amebicides within 72 h, it should be done. Adequate drainage can usually be accomplished by needle alone, and surgical drainage is rarely necessary. The greatest hazard in needling an abscess is secondary bacterial infection.

PROGNOSIS Intestinal amebiasis usually responds readily and completely to appropriate drugs. Parasitologic relapses sometimes occur, and posttreatment stools should be checked monthly for 6 months. Repeated relapses, however, are usually a manifestation of reinfection, complicating illness, inadequate therapy, or incorrect diagnosis. The fatality rate is less than 5 percent.

Hepatic and pulmonary amebiasis are still accompanied by an appreciable mortality, but no reliable figures are available.

PREVENTION For the individual, avoidance of contaminated food and water, scalding of vegetables, and the use of iodine-releasing tablets in drinking water (chlorine, in the form of halazone, is ineffective) are important measures. Globaline tablets, containing tetraglycine hydroperiodide, are convenient and effective.

Improvements in general sanitation and the detection of cyst passers and their removal from food-handling duties are general measures in prophylaxis, but such segregation of carriers is rarely practiced. Community control of amebic disease by periodic mass treatment with metronidazole and diloxanide furoate has been successful in some areas. Personal chemoprophylaxis for travelers is not recommended.

TABLE 153-1 Drug therapy of amebiasis

	Dosage
ASYMPTOMATIC INTESTINAL CARRIER	
Iodoquinol*	650 mg tid for 20 days
or diloxanide furoate†	500 mg tid for 10 days
MILD TO MODERATE INTESTINAL DISEASE	
Metronidazole	750 mg tid for 5–10 days
plus iodoquinol	As above
or diloxanide furoate	As above
or tetracycline	500 mg qid for 5 days
SEVERE INTESTINAL DISEASE	
Above regimen	
plus dehydroemetine†	1.0–1.5 mg/kg IM per day (maximum 90 mg per day) for up to 5 days
or emetine	1 mg/kg IM per day (maximum 60 mg per day) for up to 5 days
EXTRAINTESTINAL DISEASE	
Metronidazole	As above
plus iodoquinol	
or chloroquine phosphate	1 g per day for 2 days, then 500 mg per day for 4 weeks
plus dehydroemetine†	As above for 10 days
or emetine	As above for 10 days

* *Glenwood Laboratories, Inc., 83 North Summit St., Tenafly, NJ 07670.*
† *Investigational drug available through the Parasitic Drug Service, Centers for Disease Control, Atlanta, Ga., (404) 633-3311, nights and weekends 633-2176.*

PRIMARY AMEBIC MENINGOENCEPHALITIS

Primary amebic meningoencephalitis is caused by free-living amebas of the genus *Naegleria* or *Acanthamoeba.* The former most often affects children and young adults, appears to be acquired by swimming in fresh, warm water, and is almost invariably fatal. *Acanthamoeba* infections involve older immunocompromised individuals, and spontaneous recovery is sometimes seen.

Free-living amebas are ubiquitous in nature where they are commonly found in soil and water. Although generally considered harmless, some varieties are clearly pathogenic for the central nervous system of mammals. In those instances of human meningoencephalitis where the responsible organism has been isolated and cultured, it has, with few exceptions, been identified as an amoeboflagellate, *Naegleria fowleri.*

Over 100 *Naegleria* cases have been reported from different parts of the world including Australia, Belgium, Brazil, Czechoslovakia, Great Britain, Ireland, New Zealand, Zambia, and the United States. Serologic studies suggest that inapparent infections are much more common. Most of the 50 cases recognized in the United States have occurred in the southeastern states, particularly Florida, Georgia, and Virginia. Characteristically the patients have fallen ill during the summer months approximately 1 week after swimming in fresh or brackish water. The 16 Czechoslovakian cases followed swimming in an indoor pool with chlorinated water maintained at 24°C, and 6 cases have been acquired apparently after bathing in hot mineral water. In sub-Saharan Africa, cases appear to follow inhalation of airborne cysts during the dry, windy harmattan season. Histologic evidence suggests that the amebas reach the central nervous system directly via the nasal mucosa at the level of the cribriform plate. Clinically, the illness is rapid in onset, brief in duration, and inexorable in course. The initial symptom is a severe, persistent, frontal headache followed by nausea, vomiting, fever, and nuchal rigidity. Unusual tastes or smells may be noted. Later, drowsiness, confusion, convulsions, and coma appear. Focal neurologic findings may occur late in the course of the illness.

A more benign, chronic form of meningoencephalitis is produced by organisms of the genus *Acanthamoeba.* They appear to be disseminated to the brain and other organs from the skin or respiratory tract. Patients with this clinical syndrome are frequently older, are immunocompromised, lack a history of freshwater swimming, and may recover spontaneously. Pathologically, the disease can be distinguished from *Naegleria* infections by the granulomatous nature of the inflammatory reaction and the presence of both trophozoites and cysts in the tissues. Unfortunately, the identification of the responsible organisms remains in some doubt as they have seldom been recovered by culture. It is possible that the free-living amebas of several species are involved. Approximately a dozen cases of *Acanthamoeba* keratitis have been reported.

A careful examination of the cerebrospinal fluid is the single most helpful diagnostic procedure. In *Naegleria* infections the fluid is usually bloody or sanguinopurulent and demonstrates an intense neutrophilic response. The protein is elevated and the glucose diminished. No organisms are demonstrated on Gram's stain or routine culture. Early examination of a wet preparation of unspun spinal fluid will usually reveal viable trophozoites. They are 10 to 20 μm in diameter, possess a granular cytoplasm, a distinct ectoplasm, and bulbous pseudopodia. If the specimen is allowed to cool, the trophozoites may become immobile and more difficult to recognize. The diagnosis is confirmed with direct fluorescent antibody (DFA) stains. Although the amebas may be easily grown on ordinary culture media which have been seeded with coliform bacteria, this is not helpful in clinical management, so rapidly progressive is the disease. In contrast, the spinal fluid in *Acanthamoeba* infections usually demonstrates a mononuclear response. Trophozoites have been neither cultured nor seen on wet mounts. A positive DFA stain has been seen in a few cases. Treatment with standard antiprotozoal agents seems completely ineffective. *Naegleria,* however, is highly sensitive to amphotericin B, miconazole, tetracycline, and rifampin. To date only four patients have survived a *Naegleria* infection. All were diagnosed early and treated, three with amphotericin B and the other with amphotericin B, miconazole, and rifampin. Intracisternal, as well as intravenous, administration of amphotericin is probably essential to rapidly obtain effective levels in the cerebrospinal fluid. The intraventricular dose is 0.5 to 1 mg for the first few days. The intravenous dose is similar to that for cryptococcal meningitis (see Chap. 146). *Acanthamoeba* are sensitive to sulfanilamides, clotrimazole, 5-FC, and polymyxin B, but no clinical studies have been done.

If the source of the infection can be determined, further *Naegleria* cases might be prevented by closing the area to bathing.

REFERENCES

Amebiasis

ADAMS EB, MACLEOD IN: Invasive amebiasis. Medicine 56:315, 1977

BARBOUR GL, JUNIPER K JR: A clinical comparison of amebic and pyogenic abscess of the liver in sixty-six patients. Am J Med 53:323, 1972

JACKSON TFHG, GATHIRAM V: Seroepidemiological study of antibody responses to the zymodemes of *Entamoeba histolytica*. Lancet 1:716, 1985

KATZENSTEIN D et al: New concepts of amebic liver abscess derived from hepatic imaging, serodiagnosis, and hepatic enzymes in 67 consecutive cases in San Diego. Medicine 61:237, 1982

KNOBLOCH J, MANNWEILER E: Development and persistence of antibodies to *Entamoeba histolytica* in patients with amebic liver abscess: Analysis of 216 cases. Am J Trop Med Hyg 32:727, 1983

MARTINEZ-PALOMO A, MARTINEZ-BAEZ M: Selective primary health care: Strategies for control of disease in the developing world. X. Amebiasis. Rev Infect Dis 5:1093, 1983

MCGOWAN K et al: *Entamoeba histolytica* cytotoxin: Purification, characterization, strain virulence, and protease activity. J Infect Dis 146:616, 1982

RAVDIN JI, GUERRANT RL: A review of the parasite cellular mechanisms involved in the pathogenesis of amebiasis. Rev Infect Dis 4:1185, 1982

THOMPSON JE et al: Amebic liver abscess: A therapeutic approach. Rev Infect Dis 7:171, 1985

TRISSL D: Immunology of *Entamoeba histolytica* in human and animal hosts. Rev Infect Dis 4:1154, 1982

UNGER BLP et al: Use of a monoclonal antibody in an enzyme immunoassay for the detection of *Entamoeba histolytica* in fecal specimens. Am J Trop Med Hyg 34:465, 1985

Primary amebic meningoencephalitis

JOHN DT: Primary amebic meningoencephalitis and the biology of *Naegleria fowleri*. Ann Rev Microbiol 36:101, 1982

MA PE et al: A case of keratitis due to *Acanthamoeba* in New York, New York, and features of 10 cases. J Infect Dis 143:662, 1981

SEIDEL JS et al: Successful treatment of primary amebic meningoencephalitis. N Engl J Med 306:346, 1982

154 MALARIA

JAMES J. PLORDE / NICHOLAS J. WHITE

DEFINITION Malaria is a protozoan disease transmitted to humans by the bite of *Anopheles* mosquitoes. It is characterized by *fever, rigors, splenomegaly, anemia,* and a *chronic relapsing course*. Despite the impressive results of the World Health Organization–sponsored malaria eradication program initiated in 1956, technical and socioeconomic difficulties have led to a resurgence of the disease in many areas of the world. Consequently, malaria remains today, as it has been for centuries, one of the most serious infectious disease problems in the world. In the United States and Europe, several thousand imported cases are seen annually in travelers from endemic areas.

ETIOLOGY *The causative organisms are protozoa of the genus Plasmodium.* The four species known to infect human beings are *P. vivax, P. ovale, P. malariae,* and *P. falciparum*. Human infection begins when a female anopheline inoculates plasmodial *sporozoites* into the lymphohematogenous system while feeding. After a brief passage in the peripheral blood, these organisms invade hepatocytes where they initiate the preclinical hepatic (exoerythrocytic) phase of disease. By a process of asexual multiplication referred to as *schizogony,* a single sporozoite eventually produces 2000 to 40,000 hepatic *merozoites*. In most cases, these daughter cells rupture back into the circulatory system within 1 to 6 weeks. In infections produced by some northern strains of *P. vivax,* release of hepatic merozoites occurs some 10 months after initial infection, a time which coincides with the short mosquito breeding period of the following year. In *P. falciparum* and *P. malariae* infections, the hepatic phase terminates at this point. In the other species, liver forms (*hypnozoites*) persist and produce new episodes of bloodstream invasion months to years later.

The erythrocytic or clinical phase of malaria starts with the attachment of a released merozoite to a specific receptor site on the red blood cell surface. This site appears to differ for each species of malaria; in the case of *P. vivax,* it is related to the Duffy blood group antigens (Fy^a or Fy^b). Duffy-negative (FyFy) individuals, who include the majority of people of West African extraction, are resistant to vivax malaria, presumably for this reason. Glycophorin, a red blood cell membrane sialoglycoprotein, has been implicated as the attachment site for the *P. falciparum*. Following attachment, the merozoite invaginates the cell surface and is slowly interiorized. The intracellular parasite first appears as a ring-shaped trophozoite which later enlarges and assumes an irregular or ameboid shape. Its nucleus then divides into several portions to form a multinucleated *schizont*. Eventually, cytoplasm condenses around each daughter nucleus to form a new generation of merozoites. Forty-eight hours after its original invasion (72 h in the case of *P. malariae*) the erythrocyte ruptures, releasing 6 to 24 merozoites, each of which is capable of initiating a new red blood cell cycle. With repetition of this cycle, some of the red blood cells become filled with morphologically distinct *sexual forms* (gametocytes); these do not induce cell lysis and are unable to undergo further development unless ingested by an appropriate mosquito during a blood meal. In the gut of the mosquito fertilization occurs, and the resulting *zygote* encysts on the outer surface of the gut and releases myriads of *sporozoites*. These migrate to the salivary glands and are inoculated into a human subject at the next feeding.

EPIDEMIOLOGY Malaria survives only in areas of the world where both the anopheline and infected human population remain above certain *critical densities* required for the sustained transmission of disease. Control measures are directed toward reducing both populations to levels that are too low for the infection to survive. Important procedures include drainage or filling of breeding areas, use of residual insecticide sprays, screening, use of skin repellents, effective treatment of cases, and large-scale suppressive drug programs in some human populations.

An active international cooperative program aimed at the eradication of malaria resulted in a significant decline in the incidence of the disease between 1956 and 1968. In over three-quarters of the original malarial areas of the world, the disease was eradicated, or active eradication programs were instituted. Presently, however, malaria still infects between 250 and 300 million inhabitants of 104 countries throughout Africa, Latin America, South America, Asia, and Oceania. Tropical Africa alone harbors 200 million of these afflicted individuals and contributes most of the estimated 1 million deaths that occur annually from this terrible disease. The presence of mobile populations, outdoor-biting mosquitoes, and high levels of disease transmission make successful eradication in these remaining areas unlikely. Furthermore, the emergence of insecticide-resistant mosquitoes as well as a variety of administrative and socioeconomic problems has produced serious setbacks to several previously successful eradication programs. Added to these difficulties has been the continuing spread of drug-resistant *P. falciparum* throughout southern Asia, the western Pacific, Central America, and South America. Resistant strains have been discovered in east and central Africa and the Indian subcontinent, areas previously free of this problem.

Endemic malaria did not disappear from the United States until the 1950s. Imported cases and occasional outbreaks of malaria acquired by mosquito transmission from imported infections (*introduced malaria*) have continued to occur, but until 1966 the total never exceeded 200 cases a year. This number rapidly increased with the return of infected military personnel from southeast Asia, reaching a peak of over 4000 in 1970. Associated with this wave of imported malaria was a smaller increase in the number of infections induced by blood transfusion and intravenous heroin use. Although this epidemic has waned, the incidence of malaria in the civilian population has not (Fig. 154-1). From 1970 to 1979, the number of cases reported annually among tourists, businesspeople, teachers, students, and other civilians rose from 151 to 825; in 1984 and 1985, approximately 1000 cases of malaria diagnosed in this country were reported annually. With rare exceptions, malaria was acquired abroad: approximately 40 percent in Asia, 30 percent in Africa, and 20 percent in the Caribbean or Latin America. Forty percent of the recent infections have involved U.S. citizens; over half of these had been acquired in Africa. Most infections involving foreign civilians occurred in émigrés from southeast Asia. Surveillance studies suggest that 2 to 5 percent of this population are infected at the time of entry to this country. Clinical manifestations usually develop within 6 months of arrival in the United States, but in one-third of the vivax cases they are delayed beyond that point. In 1983, one-fourth of the cases and all three of the deaths were caused by the virulent *P. falciparum*. Most of these cases could have been prevented with appropriate chemoprophylaxis. Until travelers are more fully informed of dangers inherent in traveling unprotected to malarious areas, the number of cases seen in this country each year will continue to increase.

PATHOGENESIS AND PATHOLOGY The invasion, alteration, and destruction of red blood cells by malaria parasites, local and systemic circulatory changes, and the related metabolic abnormalities are all important in the pathophysiology of malaria.

Red blood cell changes Malaria species differ significantly in their ability to invade red blood cells. *Plasmodium vivax* and *P. ovale* attack only immature erythrocytes; *P. malariae*, only senescent ones. During infection with these species, therefore, no more than 1 or 2 percent of cells are involved at any one time. *Plasmodium falciparum*, although preferring younger erythrocytes, invades red blood cells of all ages and may cause extremely high levels of parasitemia, a factor contributing to the lethality of this disease. The presence of certain erythrocytic abnormalities, however, appears capable of limiting the intensity of the parasitemia and its attendant morbidity and mortality. This has been most convincingly demonstrated in patients with sickle cell trait. Parasite growth is retarded in AS cells exposed to conditions of reduced oxygen tension such as that present in the visceral capillary bed. The tactoids formed during sickling of AS cells may also directly damage the parasite and render the deformed erythrocyte more susceptible to phagocytosis. Although not well documented, a similar protective effect may be exerted in thalassemia and in glucose 6-phosphate (G6PD) or pyridoxal-kinase deficiency, since these abnormalities are found more commonly in malarious areas. The protection, if present, may be related in part to the increased susceptibility of such erythrocytes to oxidant damage. In thalassemia and related hemoglobinopathies, the persistent production of fetal hemoglobin may also contribute since maturation of *P. falciparum* is retarded in cells containing hemoglobin F. In subjects with melanesian ovalocytosis, protection is afforded by the rigidity of the erythrocytic wall which prevents merozoite penetration.

Once parasitized, the cells undergo a number of changes. Up to 75 percent of the hemoglobin content is ingested and metabolized by the plasmodia as they begin to grow. In falciparum infections, electron-dense "knobs" form on the eyrthrocytic membrane where it overlays accumulations of parasitic antigen. These structures appear to mediate the attachment of the involved cells to the capillary and postcapillary venous endothelium of the deep tissues, resulting in intravascular agglutination and sludging. Infection with any of the four plasmodium species renders the red blood cell less deformable and hence susceptible to removal by the spleen. With the stimulation of the immune system, circulation of erythrocytes through the splenic cords increases, splenic trapping is enhanced, and parasitized erythrocytes are forced into intimate contact with activated macrophages. Here the intracellular parasite is damaged or destroyed by macrophage-secreted cytotoxins, and/or the erythrocyte itself is phagocytosed. Parasitized cells escaping splenic removal are destroyed at the time of sporulation, a process which elicits fever in the host. The specific mechanism responsible remains obscure, but is presumably related to the release of an intracellular pyrogen.

The severity of the anemia in acute malaria often exceeds that which would be predicted from the loss of parasitized cells alone. Several factors account for this discrepancy; sequestration results in

FIGURE 154-1 *Cases of malaria in civilians and foreigners in the United States (including Puerto Rico, the Virgin Islands, and Guam), 1970–1983. (From Malaria Surveillance: Annual Summary, 1984, Atlanta, GA., Centers for Disease Control, 1985.)*

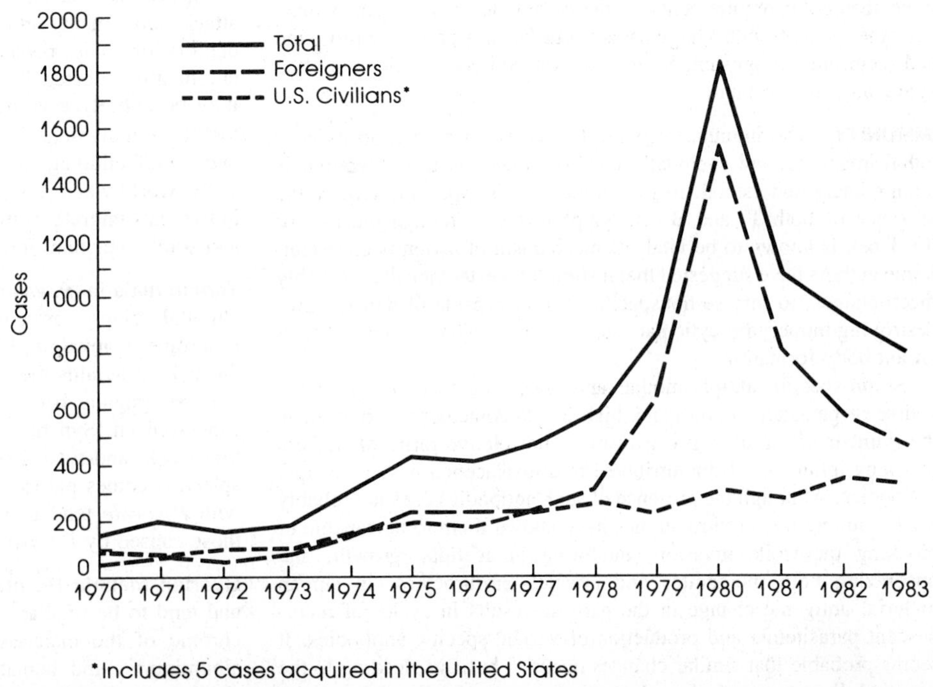

an underestimation of the total number of infected erythrocytes, erythropoiesis is dampened, and nonparasitized as well as parasitized cells are removed from the circulation. The most unusual and profound example of this process is blackwater fever, in which there is massive intravascular hemolysis. More commonly, the red blood cells are destroyed in the reticuloendothelial system of the liver and spleen. The Coombs test is occasionally positive. These phenomena are reflected in other blood components as well. Thrombocytopenia, the result of both splenic pooling and a shortened platelet life span, is common. Disseminated intravascular coagulation occurs in severe falciparum malaria, but is clinically significant in less than 5 percent of cases. The leukocyte and differential white blood cell counts are generally normal.

Circulatory changes Except for the periods of cutaneous vasoconstriction that accompany malarial rigor, the febrile patient is usually warm and well-perfused with low or normal blood pressure and a rapid pulse. In severe falciparum malaria, this vasodilatory state may be exaggerated with hypotension and a decreased central venous pressure. An increase in the radioiodinated serum albumin space and the secretion of aldosterone and antidiuretic hormone suggests a decrease in effective circulating blood volume due to enhanced vascular capacitance. Myocardial function remains surprisingly good despite sequestration of parasitized erythrocytes in the small vessels of the heart. Fluid replacement must be carefully managed if the twin dangers of acute tubular necrosis and pulmonary edema are to be avoided. Occasionally severe shock develops without apparent cause; this has been called *algid malaria* and may be secondary to spontaneous gram-negative rod bacteremia.

Almost all deaths in malaria result from the occlusion of the visceral microcirculation with *P. falciparum*–infected erythrocytes, a reflection of that organism's ability to invade a large proportion of the nonimmune patient's red blood cells and the selective adhesion of these cells to the vascular endothelium of capillaries and postcapillary venules. Although the process involves all deep tissues, it is most intense in the brain. Infants, children, pregnant women, travelers to endemic regions, and other nonimmune or immunocompromised subjects in whom the parasitemia rate may exceed 100,000 per cubic millimeter are most commonly involved.

Metabolic changes Local tissue hypoxia in the regions of abnormal microcirculatory flow is presumed to mediate most pathologic events seen in severe falciparum malaria. Lactic acidosis resulting from anaerobic glycolysis in both host and parasite may be lethal. The large metabolic requirements of the plasmodia in pregnant women and other patients with a large parasite burden may produce a profound and recurrent hypoglycemia; quinine-induced hyperinsulinemia often aggravates this problem.

IMMUNITY The immune response to malaria, which controls nonlethal infections and eventually confers protection to reinfection, is incompletely understood. In simian malaria, it appears to require the presence of both T- and B-cell lymphocytes. Although the role of the T cell is known to be vital, its mechanism of action is uncertain. Some authors have suggested that it stimulates effector cells, probably macrophages, to release nonspecific factors capable of damaging or destroying intraerythrocytic parasites; it may also have a helper effect on antibody formation.

Strain-specific antiplasmodial antibodies do occur early in the course of parasitemia and reach high levels coincident with a fall in the number of circulating organisms. The relative rarity of malaria in young infants has been attributed to transplacental passage of IgG antibodies. Although the presence of such antibodies does not reliably predict immunity, in vitro studies have shown them to be capable of blocking merozoite invasion, inhibiting intracellular growth, and opsonizing both merozoites and infected erythrocytes. In simian malaria, antigenic change in the parasite results in cycles of recrudescent parasitemia and production of variant-specific antibodies. It seems probable that similar changes occur in humans, leading to the eventual disappearance of erythrocytic forms. In falciparum malaria, this results in cure. In vivax and ovale infections, the intracellular hepatic forms escape the humoral immune defenses and may later discharge fresh merozoites into the bloodstream to maintain the infection for a period of 3 to 5 years. *Plasmodium malariae* produces chronic disease of extremely long duration, up to 53 years in one case, despite the lack of a persistent exoerythrocytic focus. This effect is presumably due to long-term survival of circulating parasites in concentrations too low to be detected on routine blood films. How these parasites escape immunologic destruction is unknown. In a closely related simian malaria, however, splenectomy rapidly leads to termination of infection, suggesting that suppressor T cells in the spleen may play a protective role.

MANIFESTATIONS General The incubation period between the bite of the mosquito and onset of symptoms is usually 10 to 14 days in vivax and falciparum malaria and 18 days to 6 weeks in malariae infections. This period may be prolonged in certain vivax infections acquired in temperate climates and in persons who have taken antimalarial suppressants. In the United States, the interval between entry into the country and onset of disease exceeds 6 months in one-quarter of the patients developing vivax infections; it exceeds 1 month in a similar proportion of falciparum cases. There is some variation in clinical manifestations produced by the different plasmodia in nonimmune hosts, but in all, chills, fever, headache, muscle pains, splenomegaly, and anemia are common. Herpes labialis is frequent and usually appears after the infection is well established. Hepatomegaly, mild icterus, and edema are often observed, especially in falciparum infections. Urticaria is common in patients with chronic malaria.

The hallmark of the disease is the malarial *paroxysm,* which recurs regularly in all but falciparum infections. The typical paroxysm begins with a rigor that lasts 20 to 60 min—the "cold stage"—followed by a "hot stage" of 3 to 8 h with temperature of 40 to 41.7°C (104 to 107°F). The "wet stage" consists of defervescence with profuse diaphoresis and leaves the patient exhausted.

First attacks are often severe, and, if untreated, may persist for weeks. The paroxysms eventually become more irregular and less frequent and finally, with the disappearance of parasites from the blood, cease altogether, marking the end of the primary attack. Relapses occur when hypnozoites persisting in the liver reinvade the bloodstream. In hyper- and holoendemic areas (e.g., West Africa), where parasite transmission is intense and constant, individuals first acquire malaria at approximately 6 months of age following the decline of maternal antibody. If the infected child survives the primary attack, subsequent reinfections become progressively milder, although debilitation may persist and become progressive; by adulthood chronically infected individuals are usually afebrile and, at times, may be entirely asymptomatic. This hard-won immunity is readily lost. If an individual leaves an endemic area and returns several years later, reinfection again results in symptomatic disease. In those areas of the world where transmission is intermittent, or when nonimmune individuals migrate from nonendemic to endemic areas, symptomatic and sometimes fatal infections develop in adult life.

Tertian malaria (*P. vivax* or *P. ovale*) This infection is rarely fatal, although relapses are common, and it is the most difficult to cure. A prodrome of myalgia, headache, chilliness, and low-grade fever for 48 to 72 h heralds the onset of the acute illness. Initially, the fever may be irregular because the maturation cycle of the parasite is not synchronized. Synchronization usually occurs toward the end of the first week, and typical paroxysms then occur on alternate days. The spleen becomes palpable at the end of the second week. Infections with *P. ovale* tend to be milder, and primary attacks shorter than those caused by *P. vivax*.

Quartan malaria (*P. malariae*) Paroxysms occur every third day and tend to be regular. The disease is usually the mildest and most chronic of the malarias but responds well to treatment. Edema, albuminuria, and hematuria (*not* hemoglobinuria), a clinical state similar to acute hemorrhagic nephritis, occasionally appear during the course. This complication should not be confused with *blackwater fever*. Chronic *P. malariae* infection may be associated with a clinically and histologically unique nephrosis. Granular deposits of IgG, IgM, C3 component of complement, and *P. malariae* antigens have been noted along the glomerular basement membrane, establishing this as an immune-complex nephropathy. The prolonged duration of asymptomatic parasitemia characteristic of the species helps to explain the frequency with which it is implicated in transfusion-induced malaria. There appears to be positive association between *P. falciparum* and *P. malariae* parasitemias in Africa. Within a given individual, the former is more frequent during the dry season and the latter during the wet season.

Falciparum malaria (*P. falciparum*) Because of an asynchronous cycle of multiplication, the onset may be insidious and fever continuous, remittent, or irregular. Typical paroxysms occur in a minority of patients. Splenomegaly appears rapidly, and headache, mental confusion, postural hypotension, edema, and gastrointestinal symptoms are common. If the acute attack is treated rapidly, the disease is usually mild and recovery uneventful. If left untreated in a nonimmune individual, sequestration of infected red blood cells in the deep tissues can give rise to serious complications. This should be anticipated if the intensity of parasitemia exceeds 100,000 organisms per cubic millimeter. Clinical warning signs include severe anemia, jaundice, hyperventilation, and evidence of central nervous system dysfunction such as delirium, stupor, or coma. Depending upon the organ system involved, one or more of the following *pernicious syndromes* may develop:

Cerebral malaria, the most important complication of falciparum malaria, is a symmetric encephalopathy that presents as unarousable coma in a patient without focal neurologic findings. Convulsions occur in half of all adults and the majority of children. Disturbances in conjugate gaze, alterations in tone, and extensor plantar responses are common; abdominal reflexes are invariably absent. Abnormal posturing may occur. Retinal hemorrhages are found in 13 percent of adults. The cerebrospinal fluid is usually under normal pressure and papilledema is rare. The mortality rate in adults is 20 percent. Most deaths occur within 3 days of admission and are associated with multiorgan dysfunction. Poor prognostic signs include deep coma, infection of more than 5 percent of all red blood cells, a total white blood cell count over 10,000 per cubic millimeter, and evidence of renal impairment. The major differential diagnoses include viral and bacterial meningoencephalitis, postictal states following febrile convulsions in children, and the obtundation and delirium commonly found with high fever. These conditions are relatively easy to exclude in a nonimmune adult. However, because asymptomatic malarial infections are common in endemic areas, the finding of *P. falciparum* in the blood smear of an immune, comatose patient does not definitively establish the diagnosis of cerebral malaria.

Unlike most of the life-threatening complications of falciparum malaria which typically are present on admission, *acute pulmonary insufficiency* may not develop until the third or fourth day of therapy. Nevertheless, it is highly lethal, killing approximately 80 percent of those involved. Pulmonary distress frequently accompanies cerebral malaria; pregnant women and patients with intense parasitemia are also at increased risk. Although overhydration is responsible for this syndrome in some patients, the pulmonary capillary wedge pressure is normal in most. This suggests that the major pathogenic mechanism is a malaria-induced change in the pulmonary capillary bed, not unlike that found in the adult respiratory distress syndrome (ARDS). Pathologic studies performed in patients dying with respiratory distress have demonstrated marked swelling of the pulmonary endothelial cells with narrowing of the capillary lumen, septal edema, and the presence of interstitial macrophages harboring phagocytized malaria pigment.

The splanchnic capillaries can become obstructed with consequent vomiting, abdominal pain, diarrhea, or melena. Such patients are sometimes thought to have bacillary dysentery or cholera. Hepatic dysfunction leads to a reduction in clotting factor synthesis, reduced clearance of antimalarial drugs, and impaired gluconeogenesis, and contributes to the jaundice seen in severe falciparum malaria. Marked dysfunction resulting in ''liver failure'' seldom occurs. Fever in patients with predominantly gastrointestinal manifestations may be low or absent.

The blood urea nitrogen (BUN) is commonly elevated in severe falciparum malaria. Dehydration, increased protein catabolism, and transient renal impairment all contribute. The BUN and serum creatinine fall to normal levels in most patients following appropriate rehydration and antimalarial treatment. A serum creatinine level of more than 3 μg/mL on admission, urine output of less than 400 mL in the first 24 h of hospital stay, and the presence of another *pernicious syndrome* strongly suggest the patient has developed acute tubular necrosis. Recovery of renal function is usual provided the patient survives the acute phase of the disease and there are facilities for intensive care management and dialysis.

Blackwater fever This is a disorder that occurs in association with malaria, particularly and perhaps only with *P. falciparum* infections. The usual attack begins with a rigor and fever followed by massive intravascular hemolysis, icterus, hemoglobinuria, collapse, and often acute renal failure and uremia. The pathologic findings in the kidney are necrosis of tubules and occasionally hemoglobin casts. The mortality is 20 to 30 percent, and survivors are very likely to experience hemolytic episodes with subsequent malarial infections.

Although blackwater fever is often classified as one of the ''pernicious'' complications of falciparum malaria, its cause is obscure. In many patients, parasitemia is absent at the time hemolysis occurs. In the past blackwater fever has usually occurred in nonimmune or partially immune patients with falciparum infections who received quinine intermittently, suggesting that the hemolysis results from an autoimmune reaction to the red blood cells that have been altered by the drug, parasite, or both. However, blackwater fever can occur in patients with glucose 6-phosphate dehydrogenase (G6PD) deficiency who have received oxidant antimalarial therapy and in those with severe malaria prior to the initiation of treatment. The institution of an appropriate regimen for acute renal failure will reduce the fatality rate considerably.

Miscellaneous complications Rupture of the spleen is relatively rare, but malaria is by far the commonest cause of spontaneous rupture and predisposes to traumatic rupture of this organ. It is most commonly seen in vivax infections.

Chronic malaria or repeated infection in an endemic area leads to anemia, debility, cachexia, and macrophage and T cell–mediated immunosuppression. These manifestations are particularly severe in children under the age of 3. Falciparum malaria during pregnancy is extremely dangerous to both mother and fetus. The immunosuppression of pregnancy enhances parasite multiplication. Intense parasitemia with its associated complications, particularly hypoglycemia and acute pulmonary insufficiency, is common. Sequestration of parasitized erythrocytes in the placental circulation may lead to fetal distress and death. Surviving children have low birth weights and a high neonatal mortality. Congenital malaria, although rare, does occur; it is probably most common in the offspring of nonimmune individuals. Secondary bacterial infection is frequent and is often the immediate cause of death. Bacillary dysentery, cholera, and pyogenic pneumonia are common. Tuberculous foci often extend in malarial patients, and miliary tuberculosis is occasionally observed.

Patients living in endemic malarious areas commonly present with chronic hepatosplenomegaly of unknown cause. In some of these, there is infiltration of hepatic sinusoids by lymphocytes, very high levels of serum IgM, and high malaria antibody titers. This condition, which is known as the *tropical splenomegaly syndrome,* is seldom seen before the age of 8. It differs from the ordinary hepatosplenomegaly of malaria in that parasitemia is rare. It has been suggested that the condition results from defective T-cell control of immunoglobulin production, leading to excessive macroglobulin production and immune-complex formation. Long-term antimalarial therapy leads to a decrease in spleen size and a disappearance of hepatic sinusoidal lymphocytosis. The epidemiologic evidence implicating malaria as a contributory factor in the etiology of Burkitt's lymphoma has increased. It has been suggested that continuous stimulation of the lymphoid system in chronic malaria makes it more susceptible to neoplastic transformation in the presence of Epstein-Barr virus.

LABORATORY FINDINGS The blood leukocyte count is low or normal. The platelet count is often reduced, especially in falciparum malaria. The erythrocyte sedimentation rate is very high. Plasmodia are demonstrable in smears of peripheral blood from the vast majority of patients with symptomatic malaria. When the disease is suspected, appropriately stained blood films should be examined diligently. For the inexperienced examiner, a thin smear of fingertip blood on a clean glass slide should be stained with Wright's or Giemsa's stain. Parasitized erythrocytes are most frequent at the edges of a smear; extracellular parasites are not found. Thick smears should be thoroughly dried and stained with diluted Giemsa's or Field's stain. This method has the advantage of concentrating the parasites, but artifacts are numerous, and correct interpretations of these preparations require much experience.

The morphology of the four species of plasmodia that infect humans is specific enough to allow identification in blood smears. The parasitized red blood cells in *P. vivax* infections are enlarged and pale and may contain diffuse bright-red dots (Schüffner's dots), and the parasite presents in a wide variety of shapes and sizes; in *P. ovale* infections, the red blood cells containing parasites are oval but otherwise resemble those in *P. vivax;* in *P. malariae* the red blood cells are of normal size and do not contain dots. The parasites often present in "band" forms, and the merozoites are arranged in a rosette around central pigment; in *P. falciparum* infections the rings are very small, may contain two rather than one chromatin dot, and often are found lying flat against the margin of the cell. Only the ring stages of the asexual forms are found in the peripheral smear, and there may be more than one ring in a single red blood cell. The gametocytes are distinctively large and banana-shaped. A parasitemia of more than 2 percent is strongly suggestive of *P. falciparum* infection.

There is no advantage of blood over material obtained by splenic or sternal puncture. Serologic tests are used primarily for epidemiologic rather than diagnostic purposes but are also helpful in screening potential blood donors. The indirect immunofluorescent test seems to be the most sensitive and specific. Monoclonal antibodies and DNA probes have been shown to be capable of detecting extremely low levels of parasitemia. Their ultimate role in clinical diagnosis, epidemiologic studies, and blood screening remains to be determined.

DIAGNOSIS The most important diagnostic test is a careful medical history. The diagnosis must be considered in any febrile patient who has resided in or traveled to Haiti, Latin America, Asia, or Africa within the previous 12 months. History of previous attacks of malaria, typical malarial paroxysms, or some artificial exposure (blood transfusion, narcotic injections in an addict) should also suggest the disease. Splenomegaly is a very common finding during the second week of illness. Leukocytosis is *not* a feature of malaria. The diagnosis is confirmed by demonstrating the parasites in the peripheral blood. Because the intensity of parasitemia varies greatly from hour to hour, particularly in *P. falciparum* infections, blood smears should be examined repeatedly over 2 or 3 days before the diagnosis is abandoned.

While final cure of malaria may be difficult, particularly in *P. vivax* infections, almost all cases will respond symptomatically to quinine or one of the newer antimalarial drugs, and failure of response to a therapeutic trial argues strongly against the diagnosis.

TREATMENT The use of appropriate chemotherapy can suppress symptoms in individuals exposed in endemic areas or cure malarial infection completely. However, the emergence of drug-resistant falciparum malaria in southeast Asia, including Burma, Indonesia, and the Philippines, in the Indian subcontinent, South America, and east and central Africa necessitates the use of drug combinations in the treatment of this infection.

Treatment of acute attack Treatment of an acute attack can be accomplished with chloroquine for all types of malaria except drug-resistant falciparum infection (Table 154-1). The drug usually produces complete subsidence of symptoms and destruction of the erythrocytic forms of the parasite. If vomiting is present, chloroquine hydrochloride should be given intramuscularly or, in the case of shock, by slow intravenous infusion. Oral therapy should be resumed as soon as possible. Although side effects are uncommon, this agent may produce nausea, epigastric distress, agranulocytosis, and neurotoxicity, including involuntary movements and convulsion. Pruritus occurs in up to 50 percent of dark-skinned patients.

If patients have transfusion-induced malaria or have contracted the disease in an area known to harbor drug-resistant *P. falciparum,* they should be treated with quinine administered in combination with one or more additional antimalarial agents. In uncomplicated infections, quinine sulfate, an extremely bitter, unpleasant oral medication is given in a dose of 650 mg three times daily for 3 days. If nausea and vomiting, shock, or one of the pernicious syndromes preclude oral therapy, quinine dihydrochloride diluted in saline or glucose should be administered by slow intravenous therapy. This intravenous drug is no longer commercially available in the United States and must be obtained from the Centers for Disease Control. However, another cinchona alkaloid, the readily available antiarrhythmic agent quinidine gluconate, has proved to be a highly satisfactory substitute. Although roughly four times more cardiotoxic than quinine, quinidine

TABLE 154-1 Malaria treatment

Purpose	Drug	Dosage
Cure chloroquine-resistant *P. falciparum* infection	Quinine sulfate*	650 mg PO tid for 10–14 days
	or quinine dihydrochloride†	600 mg in 300 mL normal saline IV over 1 h; repeat in 6–8 h; maximum 1800 mg per day‡
	plus pyrimethamine	25 mg PO bid for 3 days
	plus sulfadiazine	500 mg PO bid for 5 days
	or quinine as above	
	plus tetracycline	250 mg qid for 7 days
	or quinine as above	
	plus clindamycin	900 mg tid for 3 days
Cure *P. malariae* and chloroquine-sensitive *P. falciparum* infection	Chloroquine phosphate	1 g (600-mg base) PO, then 500 mg in 6 h, then 500 mg per day for 2 days
	or chloroquine hydrochloride†	250 mg (200-mg base) IM or IV every 6 h; administer IV dose as for quinine dihydrochloride above; maximum 900 mg per day
Cure *P. vivax* and *P. ovale* infection	Same as for *P. malariae*	
	plus primaquine phosphate	26.3 mg (15-mg base) PO qd for 14 days

* *If quinine is not immediately available, begin with chloroquine and switch when quinine arrives.*
† *For use when patient cannot take oral drug. Switch to oral therapy as soon as possible. If quinine dihydrochloride is unavailable, quinidine gluconate can be used in the dose of 800 mg, administered as described for quinine. See text.*
‡ *In southeast Asia, loading dose should be 20 mg/kg.*

can be used safely in the treatment of malaria if careful electrocardiographic monitoring is employed. It should be started if quinine dihydrochloride is not immediately available. In critical situations, the initial dose of either drug should be doubled to achieve parasiticidal blood levels as rapidly as possible. Oral therapy should be instituted as soon as possible. Because only 20 percent of the drugs are cleared by the kidney, acute renal failure does not require immediate dose reduction. After the third day of therapy, however, the maintenance dose should be reduced by one-third if renal failure is established or the patient has failed to demonstrate clinical improvement. Even in the absence of overt kidney failure, concentrations of both quinine and quinidine may be high in severe malaria due to a decrease in the total apparent volume of distribution. When plasma concentrations exceed 5 μg/mL, tinnitus and then nausea, dysphonia, and occasionally deafness result. However, this symptom complex, known as "cinchonism," is seldom dose-limiting. Quinine-induced hyperinsulinemia with hypoglycemia may develop in pregnant women. Thrombocytopenic purpura, neuromuscular blockade, and fever are rare adverse effects. The appearance of a Coombs-positive hemolytic anemia requires the immediate withdrawal of the drug. Mefloquine, a quinoline methanol structurally related to quinine, has proved to be effective in chloroquine-resistant falciparum malaria, but is not licensed for use in the United States

Pyrimethamine plus one of the sulfonamides is the most commonly used supplemental agent. It is given orally in dosage of 25 mg two times daily for 3 days. Because pyrimethamine is an antifolate agent, it may cause megaloblastic anemia; folate supplementation should be provided for pregnant and poorly nourished patients. Sulfisoxazole or sulfadiazine, 2.0 g initially and then 0.5 g every 6 h for 5 days, should be given concurrently with the pyrimethamine and quinine. A variety of other combinations of antifolate agents and sulfonamides have also been used with quinine to good effect. Fansidar, a fixed drug combination containing 25 mg pyrimethamine and 500 mg sulfadoxine has been particularly effective. Tetracycline 250 mg qid for 7 days or clindamycin 900 mg tid for 3 days plus quinine are also acceptable combinations.

Patients with uncomplicated disease who are capable of taking oral medications do not require hospital admission unless pregnant, poorly nourished, or very young. All should be followed for 1 month to detect recrudescence of the infection. If there are circulating asexual erythrocytic forms, retreatment with pyrimethamine and a sulfonamide should be instituted. The presence of gametocytes is not, however, an indication for retreatment.

Radical cure *Plasmodium vivax* and *P. ovale* persist in the liver in the exoerythrocytic stage and in this form are not affected by drugs used in the treatment of the acute attack. Unless destroyed, they will eventually reinvade the bloodstream. Primaquine base, 15 mg by mouth daily for 14 days, will effect a radical cure in most cases. If relapse occurs after primaquine therapy, a second course of the drug at twice the dosage should be given. Alternatively, 45 mg primaquine base can be given in combination with 300 mg chloroquine once weekly for 8 weeks. Primaquine may cause oxidant hemolysis in patients with G6PD deficiency; this is less likely to occur if the drug is administered once weekly.

Treatment of severe falciparum malaria Patients with severe malaria require intensive monitoring and nursing care. Immediately after the diagnosis has been confirmed and the parasitemia quantitated, the patient should be weighed and an intravenous infusion of quinine, quinidine, or chloroquine begun. Blood should be drawn for culture, type and cross match, hematocrit, blood glucose, BUN, and creatinine. Arterial blood gases are also obtained if the patient shows evidence of hyperventilation, cyanosis, or postictal aspiration pneumonia. Unconscious patients should have a lumbar puncture to exclude bacterial meningitis.

Comatose patients should be nursed on their side, because vomiting and convulsion are common. Although their value has not been determined in severe malaria, prophylactic anticonvulsants are employed by some experts. Rectal temperature is kept below 38.5°C with tepid sponging, fanning, and nonaspirin antipyretics. Urine output should be monitored hourly. If there is any doubt as to the state of hydration or fluid balance, a central venous catheter is inserted and the patient cautiously rehydrated to maintain urine output. Because overly enthusiastic fluid administration can precipitate pulmonary edema, central venous pressure should be maintained below 5 cmH_2O. Patients whose oliguria advances to acute renal failure can be managed with either peritoneal or hemodialysis. Hemodialysis is preferred because there is some evidence that peritoneal solute clearance is decreased in falciparum infections; dialysis-induced peritonitis is also common in the rural tropics. Indications for dialysis are the same as those in any other hypercatabolic infection complicated by renal failure. If acute pulmonary insufficiency develops, it should be managed as ARDS, although if there is any possibility of volume overload, intravenous diuretics should be given. Blood transfusion is indicated when the hematocrit falls below 20 percent; whole fresh blood is preferable. There have been several case reports documenting the dramatic clinical recovery of patients with severe falciparum malaria and hyperparasitemia following exchange transfusion. This form of therapy should be considered if the parasite count exceeds 10 percent. Gastrointestinal bleeding may occur in severe disease, but the incidence appears to have decreased since use of heparin and corticosteroids has been discontinued. Although thrombocytopenia is usual, clinically significant disseminated intravascular coagulation is uncommon, occurring in less than 5 percent of cases of cerebral malaria. Dexamethasone, mannitol, urea, and heparin have been shown to be either deleterious or unhelpful in the treatment of cerebral malaria and should be avoided.

The response to treatment is assessed by resolution of abnormal physical signs (such as recovery of consciousness in cerebral malaria), defervescence, and clearance of parasitemia. Parasite counts should be checked at least twice daily until negative, and rechecked if fever recurs. Hypoglycemia or bacteremia should be suspected in any severely ill patient who fails to improve or suddenly deteriorates on treatment. The management of hypoglycemia is often difficult, as it tends to recur, particularly in the presence of quinine-induced hyperinsulinemia.

PREVENTION General In areas of the world such as Africa where eradication is presently impractical, limited residual insecticides plus chemoprophylaxis for pregnant women and children are recommended. The long-term hope for eradication depends on the introduction of new technologies. Until recently, the development of a practical and effective vaccine has been hampered by the lack of a suitable in vitro culture system for plasmodia, difficulty in identifying the parasitic antigens responsible for the induction of protective immunity, and the wide antigenic differences found between malaria species, strains, and even life cycle stages. The achievement of continuous culture of *P. falciparum* in red blood cells and the application of monoclonal antibody and recombinant DNA procedures to the characterization of plasmodial antigens has permitted identification of short repeated amino acid sequences in the polypeptide surface coat of all falciparum sporozoites that are capable of stimulating the production of protective antibodies. These peptides have now been artificially synthesized and coupled with a carrier molecule to produce a "sporozoite" vaccine; it is anticipated that field trials will be conducted in the near future. Work on merozoite and gametocyte-based vaccines continues.

Personal protection The traveler to malarious areas should attempt to reduce the frequency of mosquito bites by avoiding exposure at peak feeding times (usually early morning or evening), use of house screens, bed netting, insect repellents, pyrethrum-containing insect spray, and appropriate clothing. In addition, chemoprophylaxis should be utilized as described below.

Chemoprophylaxis (Table 154-2) Although it is not possible to prevent infection with chemotherapeutic agents, it is possible to

TABLE 154-2 Malaria chemoprophylaxis

Purpose	Drug	Dosage
To suppress clinical malaria in areas *without* chloroquine-resistant strains	Chloroquine phosphate	500 mg (300 mg base) PO once weekly, continued 6 weeks after leaving malarious area
	or amodiaquine dehydrochloride	520 mg (400 mg base) PO once weekly, continued 6 weeks after leaving malarious area
To suppress clinical malaria in areas *with* chloroquine-resistant strains	Same as above	
	plus pyrimethamine-sulfadoxine* (Fansidar, Hoffmann-LaRoche)	25 mg pyrimethamine and 500 mg sulfadoxine PO once weekly, continued 6 weeks after leaving malarious area
	or mefloquine	250 mg PO once weekly, continued 6 weeks after leaving malarious area
To prevent relapses of *P. vivax* and *P. ovale* infection	Primaquine phosphate†	26.3 mg (15-mg base) PO daily for 14 days or 79 mg (45-mg base) for 8 weeks; start during last 2 weeks of suppressive therapy or immediately upon its completion

* *Given only in areas of intense exposure as described in the text.*
† *Recommended only for travelers without G6PD deficiency who have had heavy exposure.*

suppress symptoms while the patient is residing in an endemic area with the use of appropriate drugs. Because of its safety and efficacy, chloroquine remains the drug of choice for travelers to all malarious areas. Cases of retinopathy have been reported in patients who have taken this agent in prophylactic dosage over periods of 5 to 20 years. This, however, is rare, and the danger to individuals planning shorter stays in malarious areas is probably nonexistent. It is recommended that chloroquine be initiated 1 or preferably 2 weeks prior to departure for an endemic area. This allows time for the early adverse effects to develop and for therapeutic blood concentrations to be achieved. If this is not possible, the prophylactic dose should be doubled for the first few weeks in the malarious zone. Travelers must be warned that protection is not complete, and that malaria should be considered in the differential diagnosis of any febrile illness developing during the stay in an endemic area. Following departure from an endemic area, chloroquine should be continued for an additional 6 weeks. This will eradicate *P. malariae* and sensitive strains of *P. falciparum*. The hepatic forms of *P. ovale* and *P. vivax* will not be affected, however, and may produce relapse with clinical manifestations some weeks or months after chloroquine is discontinued. This can be circumvented by administration of primaquine during the final 2 weeks of chloroquine administration.

Chloroquine is not effective in suppressing chloroquine-resistant *P. falciparum* (CRPF) infections. Nevertheless, it should be used by travelers to malarious areas with CRPF because malaria caused by other plasmodium species that remain sensitive to chloroquine are also present in such areas. Fansidar, a fixed-combination tablet containing 25 mg of pyrimethamine and 500 mg of sulfadoxine, may be combined with the chloroquine for the suppression of CRPF. This is contraindicated in pregnant women, persons allergic to sulfonamides, and children under 2 months. Leukopenia and megaloblastic anemia is a hazard of long-term pyrimethamine therapy. Several cases of severe cutaneous reactions (erythema multiforme, Stevens-Johnson syndrome, and toxic epidermal necrolysis) have been documented among American travelers using pyrimethamine-sulfadoxine prophylaxis. Because of the potential untoward effects related to the prophylactic administration of this agent, it should be reserved for individuals planning prolonged visits to areas of intense CRPF transmission. These include the CRPF areas of Africa, Oceania (Papua, New Guinea, Irian Jaya, the Solomon Islands, and Vanuatu) and certain rural areas of China, southeast Asia, and South America. For visits of 3 weeks or less to these areas, a therapeutic dose of Fansidar can be carried with the traveler for presumptive treatment of any febrile illness occurring during travel when professional medical care is not readily available. The serious cutaneous side effects reported during Fansidar prophylaxis have not been seen with single-dose therapy.

Of the several alternatives to Fansidar for CRPF prophylaxis, mefloquine, the methanol quinoline mentioned in the treatment section above, holds the most promise. Both safe and effective, it has been used extensively in southeast Asia where Fansidar-resistant falciparum malaria is common. It has not yet been approved for use in the United States and its availability in other areas of the world is still limited. Amodiaquine, a 4-aminoquinoline related to chloroquine, may provide somewhat more protection than chloroquine against African strains of CRPF. Although not marketed in the United States, it is widely available in Africa.

Transfusions Transfusion malaria continues to occur in the United States; *P. malariae* and *P. falciparum* have been the most common causes. Adherence to recommendations of the American Association of Blood Banking will prevent most of these cases.

REFERENCES

BRUCE-CHWATT LJ: Man against malaria; conquest or defeat. Trans R Soc Trop Med Hyg 73:517, 1979

Drugs for parasitic infections. Med Lett 26:27, 1984

GALBRAITH RM et al: The human materno-faetal relationship in malaria. Trans R Soc Trop Med Hyg 74:52 and 61, 1980

GUERRERO IC et al: Transfusion malaria in the United States, 1972–1981. Ann Intern Med 99:221, 1983

HARINASUTA T et al: Trials of mefloquine in vivax and of mefloquine plus "Fansidar" in falciparum malaria. Lancet 1:885, 1985

LOBEL HO et al: Recent trends in the importation of malaria caused by *Plasmodium falciparum* into the United States from Africa. J Infect Dis 152:613, 1985

LOOAREESUWAN S et al: Quinine and severe falciparum malaria in late pregnancy. Lancet 2:4, 1985

LUZZATTO L: Genetics of red cells and susceptibility to malaria. Blood 54:961, 1979

MACPHERSON GG et al: Human cerebral malaria: A quantitative ultrastructural analysis of parasitized erythrocyte sequestration. Am J Pathol 119:385, 1985

MCLAUGHLIN GL et al: Detection of *Plasmodium falciparum* using a synthetic DNA probe. Am J Trop Med Hyg 34:837, 1985

MILLER LH: Hypothesis on the mechanism of erythrocyte invasion by malaria merozoites. Bull WHO 55:157, 1977

MOLINEAUX L, GRAMICCIA G: *The Garki Project. Research on the Epidemiology and Control of Malaria in the Sudan Savanna of West Africa.* Geneva, WHO, 1980

NIELSON RL et al: The use of exchange transfusions: A potentially useful adjunct in the treatment of fulminant falciparum malaria. Am J Med Sci 277:325, 1979

PHILLIPS RE et al: Intravenous quinidine for the treatment of severe falciparum malaria: Clinical and pharmacokinetic studies. N Engl J Med 312:1273, 1985

Revised recommendations for preventing malaria in travelers to areas with chloroquine-resistant *Plasmodium falciparum*. Morb Mort Week Rep 34(14):185, 1985

STILMA JS: Chloroquine retinopathy in a rural hospital in Ghana. Trop Geogr Med 32:221, 1980

WARRELL DA et al: Dexamethasone proves deleterious in cerebral malaria: A double blind trial in 100 comatose patients. N Engl J Med 306:313, 1982

WATKINS WM et al: Effectiveness of amodiaquine as treatment for chloroquine-resistant *Plasmodium falciparum* infections in Kenya. Lancet 1:357, 1984

WYLER DJ: Malaria—resurgence, resistance and research. N Engl J Med 308:875 and 934, 1983

ZAVALA F et al: Rationale for development of a synthetic vaccine against *Plasmodium falciparum* malaria. Science 228:1463, 1985

155 LEISHMANIASIS

RICHARD M. LOCKSLEY / JAMES J. PLORDE

DEFINITION Four major clinical syndromes are caused by protozoa of the genus *Leishmania*—visceral leishmaniasis (kala azar), cutaneous leishmaniasis of the old and new world, mucocutaneous leishmaniasis (espundia), and diffuse cutaneous leishmaniasis. These parasites of canines and rodents are transmitted from animal to human and occasionally from person to person by the bite of phlebotomine sandflies.

ETIOLOGY A large number of *Leishmania* species may infect humans. Morphologically these different organisms appear identical and are generally distinguished by clinical and geographic characteristics. Definitive speciation may require determination of isoenzyme patterns, kinetoplast DNA buoyant densities, or specific phlebotomine vectors. Newer methods using monoclonal antibodies, DNA hybridization, and DNA restriction endonuclease fragment analysis are being evaluated.

In the sandfly and in culture media, *Leishmania* exist as motile, spindle-shaped promastigotes (1.5 to 4 μm by 14 to 20 μm) with a single anterior flagellum. On inoculation into a mammalian host the organisms enter mononuclear phagocytes, lose their flagella, and multiply as small (2 by 5 μm), oval, intracellular amastigotes (Leishman-Donovan bodies). In stained preparations a dark, slightly flattened nucleus and rod-shaped kinetoplast may be discerned.

EPIDEMIOLOGY Leishmaniasis is a zoonotic infection which involves the rodents and canines of every inhabited continent except Australia. The prevalence varies; 4 to 10 percent of dogs in the Mediterranean littoral and 80 to 95 percent of the gerbils in the southern U.S.S.R. are infected, many subclinically. The disease is spread when female sandflies of the genus *Phlebotomus* (old world) or *Lutzomyia* (new world) ingest amastigotes while taking a blood meal from an infected mammal. These transform into promastigotes within the insect's gut, migrate to the proboscis, and are deposited on the skin of the new host when the insect next engorges. Phlebotomines breed in warm, humid microclimates and are typically found in rodent burrows, termite hills, and rotting vegetation. Humans may acquire the disease when they encroach upon this sylvatic cycle. Establishment of infection in the domestic dog provides an important urban reservoir of leishmaniasis. Person-to-person transmission is infrequent except in the Indian form of kala azar. Rarely, transmission can occur by blood transfusion, contact inoculation, and coitus. It is estimated that worldwide over 12 million people are infected with these parasites.

PATHOGENESIS Promastigotes are deposited on the skin into a small pool of blood drawn by the probing sandfly. The organisms fix complement onto their surface by the alternative pathway, and rapidly enter macrophages via the type 3 complement receptor (CR3) and the mannosyl/fucosyl receptor. The promastigotes transform into amastigotes within phagolysosomes and replicate by binary fission. They eventually rupture the cell and invade adjacent macrophages.

The course of the subsequent disease is determined by the host's cellular immunity as well as the species of the parasite. In cutaneous leishmaniasis, there is a marked lymphocytic infiltration associated with a reduction in the number of parasites, the development of a delayed skin (leishmanin) reaction, and, frequently, spontaneous cure. In mucocutaneous disease, the complete or partial resolution of the primary lesion may be followed by metastatic mucocutaneous lesions at some later date. The destructiveness of the metastatic lesions is attributed to the development of hypersensitivity to parasite antigens. An exception to the general pattern in cutaneous disease is diffuse cutaneous leishmaniasis in which there is no infiltration of lymphocytes and plasma cells or reduction in the number of parasites, the leishmanin reaction remains negative, and the skin lesions become chronic, progressive, and disseminated. The patients appear to have a selective anergy to leishmania antigens which is mediated at least in part by adherent suppressor cells. In visceral leishmaniasis, the cellular changes are similar, but the parasites spread to macrophages throughout the body, perhaps due to the greater resistance of *L. donovani* to the spontaneous cidal activity present in normal serum. Although antibodies are present, they are nonprotective. The ability of the organism to cause progressive disease may be related to the development in the host of suppressor T lymphocytes. Cure of leishmaniasis confers immunity to the infecting strain.

DIAGNOSIS Establishing a diagnosis of leishmaniasis requires demonstrating the organism by smear or culture of aspirates or tissue. Although Novy-MacNeal-Nicolle (NNN) medium traditionally has been used to culture *Leishmania,* several commercially available liquid media offer improved storage capability and enhanced recovery of organisms. Cultures are maintained at 22 to 28°C for 21 days and examined microscopically for the presence of the motile promastigotes. Inoculation of hamsters with infected clinical material results in infections after a period of months.

Species-specific diagnosis of human cutaneous new world isolates has been achieved by hybridization of tissue touch blots with radiolabeled kinetoplast DNA probes, but the method is not readily available.

Antibodies are detectable in all forms of leishmaniasis. The direct agglutination test[1] detects IgM antibody and is a sensitive indicator of acute disease. The test is group-specific, but the titer is generally greatest to the homologous strain. A positive test (>1:32) varies from 97 percent in visceral leishmaniasis to 81 percent in new world cutaneous leishmaniasis. Other serologic tests, including complement fixation, hemagglutination, microenzyme-linked immunoabsorbent assays, and indirect immunofluorescence, are less commonly available. Direct agglutination antibodies decline and may disappear with cure.

VISCERAL LEISHMANIASIS (KALA AZAR) *Leishmania donovani* causes kala azar, a disease that may be endemic, epidemic, or sporadic. Although the characteristics of the disease are similar throughout the world, certain local peculiarities in its behavior justify the classification of visceral leishmaniasis into three main types. These differences are attributed principally to the length of time that the disease has been endemic in a population.

African kala azar is found in the eastern half of Africa from the Sahara in the north to the equator in the south. Sporadic cases have been reported from west Africa. It is a disease of older children and young adults (10 to 25 years); males are involved more commonly than females. It is endemic in dogs and several wild carnivores in many areas and is more resistant to therapy with antimony compounds than the forms of kala azar found in the rest of the world.

Mediterranean, or infantile, kala azar, is seen primarily in the Mediterranean area, China, U.S.S.R, and Latin America. It is a disease of children under the age of 4, but adults, particularly travelers to endemic areas, are not spared. Dogs, jackals, and foxes serve as reservoirs. Rats have been identified as a potential reservoir in Italy. The strains responsible for the Eurasian and American disease are sometimes referred to as *L. infantum* and *L. chagasi,* respectively.

Indian kala azar has an age and sex distribution similar to African kala azar. Humans are the only known reservoir, and transmission is carried out by anthropophilic sandflies.

Manifestations The incubation period is generally about 3 months (3 weeks to 18 months). A primary cutaneous lesion (leishmanioma) is not uncommon in Africa. The onset of disease may be insidious or abrupt; the latter occurs more frequently in individuals from nonendemic areas. Fever, typically nocturnal and occasionally double-quotidian, is almost universal and is accompanied by tachycardia without signs of toxemia. Daily fever progresses to recurrent febrile

[1] *The leishmanin skin test (Montenegro test), performed by the intradermal injection of promastigote antigens, is nonstandardized and generally unavailable.*

waves. Diarrhea and cough are frequent. Nontender splenomegaly becomes dramatic by the third month. The liver enlarges less conspicuously. Cirrhosis and portal hypertension occur in about 10 percent of patients. Lymphadenopathy accompanies some cases of African kala azar. Atypical forms, including isolated tonsillar infections and cervical adenopathy, have been reported. Asymptomatic or subclinical disease has been suspected.

Pancytopenia is characteristic. Anemia is multifactorial: autoimmune hemolysis, splenomegaly, and gastrointestinal blood loss all contribute. The latter is exacerbated by thrombocytopenia. Agranulocytosis, cancrum oris, and superinfections complicate untreated cases. Extensive leishmanial infiltration of the gastrointestinal tract may lead to malabsorption. Hypoalbuminemia and polyclonal hypergammaglobulinemia (IgG and IgM) are constant features. Circulating immune complexes are frequently present. Immune-complex glomerulonephritis and interstitial nephritis have been described. Amyloidosis may occur in patients with chronic infections. Edema, cachexia, and hyperpigmentation (kala azar means "black fever") are late manifestations. Without treatment death occurs within 3 to 20 months in 90 to 95 percent of adults and 75 to 85 percent of children, usually due to superinfections or gastrointestinal hemorrhage.

After successful treatment, 3 percent of African cases and up to 10 percent of Indian cases develop post-kala azar dermal leishmaniasis (PKDL), characterized by a spectrum of lesions ranging from depigmented macules to wartlike nodules over the face and extensor surfaces of the limbs. PKDL appears shortly after symptoms subside in African cases and typically disappears after several weeks. In the Indian disease, PKDL appears after a latent period of 1 to 2 years and may last for years, creating a persistent human reservoir.

Diagnosis Buffy coat preparations may demonstrate the parasite, particularly in Indian kala azar (90 percent). Bone marrow aspirate and biopsy are positive in over 85 percent of cases. In Kenya, splenic aspiration (95 percent) has proved quite safe and has been used serially to assess the response to therapy. In general, however, aspiration of the spleen or liver (75 percent) is not recommended because of the risk of fatal hemorrhage. Aspirates or biopsy of enlarged lymph nodes will show parasites in 60 percent of cases. Suspicious skin lesions should be biopsied as well. The direct agglutination test is positive early in the disease. The leishmanin skin test becomes positive 6 to 8 weeks after recovery. Other causes of fever in the tropics, including malaria, brucellosis, tuberculosis, typhoid, and hepatic abscess, can be distinguished by appropriate testing. PKDL must be differentiated from leprosy, syphilis, and yaws.

Treatment Transfusions and treatment of complicating superinfections must supplement specific therapy. Pentavalent antimonials are highly effective against leishmania and are relatively nontoxic. Sodium antimony gluconate (Pentostam;[2] 100 mg Sb^{5+} per milliliter) is given intravenously or intramuscularly in a single daily dose of 10 mg/kg for adults and 20 mg/kg for patients under 18 years of age. Treatment should be given for at least 20 days in Indian kala azar and 30 days in other forms. Meglumine antimoniate (Glucantime; 85 mg Sb^{5+} per milliliter) can also be used. Therapy should be repeated using 20 mg/kg for 40 to 60 days in patients with relapses or incomplete responses. The addition of oral allopurinol (20 to 30 mg/kg per day in three divided doses) has been effective. Resistant cases must be treated with intravenous amphotericin B (0.5 to 1 mg/kg on alternate days) or pentamidine (3 to 4 mg/kg three times per week for 5 to 25 weeks, depending on the response). Adjunctive splenectomy has been successful in some cases of drug-resistant kala azar. Mortality remains 15 to 25 percent in advanced cases, although the cure rate is over 90 percent when therapy is given early. Follow-up at 3 and 12 months is recommended to detect relapses. PKDL should be treated in the same fashion as the initial illness.

[2] *Available from the Centers for Disease Control, Atlanta, Georgia.*

Prevention Preventive measures include early treatment of human cases, elimination of diseased dogs, and the use of DDT against sandflies. Application of insect repellents and the use of fine netting are important for travelers. There are no useful prophylactic agents.

CUTANEOUS AND MUCOCUTANEOUS LEISHMANIASIS This form of leishmaniasis is caused by a number of species in both the old world and the new world. Disease is characterized by the development of single or multiple localized lesions on exposed areas of skin that typically ulcerate. Although spontaneous healing is the rule for old world cutaneous leishmaniasis, this is less common in new world disease.

Old world cutaneous leishmaniasis *L. tropica* causes anthroponotic (urban, chronic, dry) cutaneous leishmaniasis, an endemic disease of children and young adults in areas bordering the Mediterranean, the Middle East, the southern U.S.S.R., and India. The principal reservoirs are humans, although domestic dogs are synanthropic hosts. The incubation period ranges from 2 to 24 months. Usually the lesion begins as a single, red pruritic papule on the face (oriental sore). The central area ulcerates and slowly enlarges centrifugally, reaching a size of approximately 2 cm. Lymphadenopathy is unusual. Healing occurs over 1 to 2 years and leaves a small depigmented scar. The disease can be complicated by the development of leishmaniasis recidiva, a condition marked by persistent facial lesions containing a scant number of parasites, and by an exaggerated delayed hypersensitivity response to parasite antigens. Rarely, the organism may spread to the viscera.

L. major causes zoonotic (rural, acute, moist) cutaneous leishmaniasis, which is endemic to the desert areas of the Middle East, the southern U.S.S.R., and Africa. The reservoir is maintained in burrowing rodents. The incubation period ranges from 2 to 6 weeks. The initial lesions are often multiple and located on the lower extremities. Regional lymphadenopathy and satellite lesions are common. Healing with scarring occurs within 3 to 6 months. *L. major* has been implicated in cases of mucocutaneous leishmaniasis in Saudi Arabia. Although *L. major* confers immunity to *L. tropica*, the converse is not true.

L. aethiopica, maintained in rock hyraxes of the Ethiopian and Kenyan highlands, causes cutaneous leishmaniasis which may pursue a relatively prolonged course and can be complicated by the development of diffuse cutaneous leishmaniasis (see below).

DIAGNOSIS Lesions should first be cleansed with alcohol to reduce bacterial contamination, which hinders recovery of the organisms. Aspirates should be obtained from the outer edge of the ulcer. If the aspirated smears are negative, full-thickness skin biopsies from the ulcer margin should be taken for touch smears, histology, and culture. The direct agglutination test and the leishmanin skin test become positive within 4 to 6 weeks.

TREATMENT Specific therapy should be withheld in endemic areas until ulceration takes place, thereby conferring immunity. Exceptions include disfiguring or disabling lesions and lesions persisting for longer than 6 months. Treatment is with antimonials as described for kala azar, although shorter courses (10 days) are effective. Higher doses of antimony may be required for *L. aethiopica* infections (20 mg/kg twice a day for 30 days). Ulcers should be covered to prevent infection of vectors and other canine and human hosts.

New world cutaneous and mucocutaneous leishmaniasis Leishmania causing new world cutaneous disease is divided into subspecies within the *L. mexicana* and *L. braziliensis* groups. The natural reservoirs for these organisms include a wide variety of mammals inhabiting the forests of South and Central America. Organisms are transmitted to humans entering the jungle to gather chicle or to clear land for new settlements. Disease is most prevalent in the Amazon basin but occurs in most countries of the area. *L. mexicana* species are endemic in south-central Texas.

L.m. mexicana causes chiclero's ulcer, or bay sore. Chicle gatherers who work in forests during the rainy season when sandflies are abundant develop isolated cutaneous lesions on the hand or head. These show little tendency to ulcerate and generally heal spontaneously within 6 months. Ear lesions, however, persist for years and may cause extensive destruction of the pinna.

L.m. venezuelensis causes indolent nodular lesions, *L.m. garnhami* causes ulcerating lesions that usually heal spontaneously, and *L.m. amazonensis* causes persistent lesions that may be multiple and seldom heal spontaneously. About 30 percent of patients infected with the last organism have diffuse cutaneous leishmaniasis (see below).

L.b. peruviana causes uta, a disease consisting of single or multiple ulcers typically on the face. Spontaneous healing within 3 months to a year is the rule. The reservoir is the domestic dog. The disease occurs on the western slopes of the Peruvian Andes at altitudes above 2000 ft. With widespread use of insecticides, the disease has become uncommon.

Mucocutaneous leishmaniasis, or espundia, is caused primarily by *L.b. braziliensis*, which typically produces one or several lesions on the lower extremities that undergo extensive ulceration; complete healing seldom occurs spontaneously. After months to years, metastatic lesions may appear in the nasopharynx and, less frequently, in the perineum. Nasal obstruction and epistaxis are frequent presenting symptoms. Extensive destruction of soft tissue structures ensues, with painful mutilating erosions (espundia). Fever, anemia, and weight loss are common. Death is caused by bacterial infection, inanition, aspiration, and respiratory obstruction.

L.b. panamensis causes nonhealing ulcerative lesions and *L.b. guyanensis* causes nodular lesions that persist and metastasize along lymphatics (pian bois). These strains may cause mucocutaneous leishmaniasis in Colombia.

DIAGNOSIS Speciation of the infecting organism should be attempted because of the marked differences in outcome. Skin biopsies are the preferred means of obtaining tissue for stains and culture. Parasites may be scant, particularly in mucocutaneous lesions. In espundia, organisms have been cultured from the blood when the cutaneous sites have been negative. The direct agglutination test and the leishmanin skin test become positive within 4 to 6 weeks. Syphilis, yaws, blastomycosis, paracoccidioidomycosis, sporotrichosis, leprosy, and carcinoma must be considered in the differential diagnosis.

TREATMENT Inconspicuous lesions due to *L.b. peruviana* or *L. mexicana* subspecies other than *L.m. amazonensis* may heal spontaneously or be treated with intralesional injections of antimonials. Local heat (40 to 41°C) may accelerate healing. Disfiguring or disabling lesions, cartilaginous involvement or lymphatic spread, and lesions due to *L.m. amazonensis* or other *L. braziliensis* subspecies should be treated with systemic antimonials as described for kala azar.

Espundia should be treated with antimonials (20 mg/kg per day) for at least 30 days. Cases that fail to respond should be treated with amphotericin. Reconstructive facial prostheses should not be used until the disease has been in remission for at least 1 year without therapy. A rising antibody titer may predict relapse and indicate that further therapy is required.

PREVENTION Vaccination of forest workers with *L.m. mexicana* has been successful in establishing immunity and preventing disfiguring ear lesions.

Diffuse cutaneous leishmaniasis Diffuse cutaneous leishmaniasis is found in Venezuela, Brazil, and the Dominican Republic in the new world and in Ethiopia in the old world. Patients display a specific deficiency of cell-mediated immunity to leishmanial antigens. *L.m. pifanoi* (Venezuela), *L.m. amazonensis* (Brazil), members of the *L. mexicana* complex (Dominican Republic), and *L. aethiopica* (Africa) are responsible. Disease is characterized by massive dissemination of skin lesions without visceral involvement. The clinical picture often bears a striking resemblance to lepromatous leprosy. The diagnosis is not difficult, because the lesions contain large numbers of organisms. In contrast to all other types of cutaneous leishmaniasis, the leishmanin skin test remains negative. The disease is progressive and very refractory to treatment. High doses of antimony (20 mg/kg twice a day for 30 days) and multiple courses of amphotericin or pentamidine are often required to produce remission, but cures are rare.

REFERENCES

CARVALHO EM et al: Absence of gamma interferon and interleukin 2 production during active visceral leishmaniasis. J Clin Invest 76:2066, 1986

CHULAY JD et al: High-dose sodium stibogluconate treatment of cutaneous leishmaniasis in Kenya. Trans Roy Soc Trop Med Hyg 77:717, 1983

GUSTAFSON TL et al: Human cutaneous leishmaniasis acquired in Texas. Am Soc Trop Med Hyg 34:58, 1985

KAGER PA et al: Clinical, hematological and parasitological response to treatment of visceral leishmaniasis in Kenya: A study of 64 patients. Trop Geog Med 36:21, 1984

LAINSON R: The American leishmaniases: Some observations on their ecology and epidemiology. Trans Roy Soc Trop Med Hyg 77:569, 1983

MARSDEN PD: Selective primary health care: Strategies for control of disease in the developing world. XIV. Leishmaniasis. Rev Infect Dis 6:736, 1984

PEARSON RD et al: The immunobiology of leishmaniasis. Rev Infect Dis 5:907, 1983

SAMPAIO RNR et al: Pentavalent antimonial treatment in mucosal leishmaniasis. Lancet 1:1097, 1985

WHO EXPERT COMMITTEE: *The Leishmaniases*. Geneva, WHO Tech Rep Ser 701, 1984, pp 1–140

WIRTH DF, PRATT DM: Rapid identification of *Leishmania* species by specific hybridization of kinetoplast DNA in cutaneous lesions. Proc Natl Acad Sci USA 79:6999, 1982

156 TRYPANOSOMIASIS

JAMES J. PLORDE

SLEEPING SICKNESS

DEFINITION African trypanosomiasis, or sleeping sickness, is a disease caused by the hemoflagellate *Trypanosoma brucei*, which is transmitted to human beings by several species of tsetse fly belonging to the genus *Glossina*. Clinically, the untreated disease is characterized by an acute febrile lymphadenopathy followed, after a variable period, by a chronic lethal meningoencephalomyelitis. It occurs in two principal epidemiologic patterns: Gambian, or mid- and west African, sleeping sickness, and Rhodesian, or east African, sleeping sickness.

ETIOLOGY Trypanosomes are polymorphic flagellates which undergo developmental change as they pass from vertebrate to invertebrate host. *T. brucei* trypanosomes, which circulate in the blood of infected mammals, are ingested by feeding tsetse flies, multiply in their midgut, migrate to the salivary glands, and assume the *epimastigote* form. Here, after a period of weeks, they are transformed into infectious (metacyclic) *trypomastigotes* and injected into another mammalian host when the insect again takes a blood meal. Within the mammal, the fusiform trypomastigotes are distinguished by an undulating membrane which extends along the length of the cell and terminates in an anterior flagellum. Multiplication occurs extracellularly by longitudinal fission. Initial generations are long (20 to 30 μm), slender, and delicately curved. In later generations, the flagellum becomes rudimentary and the parasite stumpy and graceless in appearance. Both forms are surrounded by a thick, antigenic glycoprotein coat. The morphologic characteristics of many varieties are so nearly identical that they are distinguishable only by biologic behavior, isoenzyme pattern, and mitochondrial structure.

The Gambian and Rhodesian forms of sleeping sickness were previously thought to be caused by two distinct species of trypanosomes, *T. gambiense* and *T. rhodesiense*. However, they, along with the animal trypanosome responsible for *nagana* in cattle, are all variants of a single species. The individual varieties are referred to as *T. brucei gambiense, T. brucei rhodesiense,* and *T. brucei brucei.*

EPIDEMIOLOGY Sleeping sickness occurs only in Africa. It is estimated that 50 million people live in the endemic areas and 10 to 20 thousand acquire the infection annually. Over the past decade severe outbreaks have occurred in the Cameroons, Central African Republic, Ivory Coast, the Sudan, Uganda, and Zaire. Gambian sleeping sickness is found in tropical, west, and central Africa extending from the Sahara to the Kalahari deserts and east to the Rift Valley. It is transmitted by the riverine tsetses, *G. palpalis, G. fuscipes,* and *G. tachinoides,* which live in shaded areas near water. Less than 5 percent of the flies are infected even in the most notorious endemic foci. Although pigs and other domestic animals have been shown to harbor *T. brucei gambiense,* human beings are thought to be the major reservoir. A few asymptomatic carriers have been reported, and it is possible that they play a role in the survival of the parasite during interepidemic periods.

Rhodesian trypanosomiasis is found in tropical east Africa from Ethiopia in the north to Botswana in the south. It is primarily a zoonosis transmitted to humans from the bushbuck, a small antelope, by the bite of *G. morsitans* and related savanna *Glossina.* It is seen typically in individuals who travel away from their villages to hunt or fish. Domestic cattle and sheep may also serve as reservoirs, and transmission from human to fly to human can occur.

In some situations trypanosomes can be mechanically transmitted from host to host by other hematophagous arthropods or by blood transfusion.

PATHOLOGY AND PATHOGENESIS The tsetse fly inoculates the organism into the subcutaneous pool of blood that forms during its feeding. Some of the parasites may reach the bloodstream directly, but most remain at the site of inoculation, where they multiply to produce a local chancre. Following the appearance of this lesion, the trypanosomes spread through tissue spaces and lymphatics, eventually spilling over into the general circulation where they continue to multiply. The parasitemia is of low intensity and typically occurs in waves; each wave disappears with the production of antibody to the parasite's glycoprotein surface antigen and reappears in 3 to 8 days as a new antigenic variant arises. A single trypanosomal strain can produce hundreds of antigenic variants, each encoded by a distinct gene and selected by the host's antibody response. The waves of parasitemia, which are accompanied by fever and mononuclear leukocytosis, tend to become more infrequent and irregular in the later stages of the disease. At some time during this stage of dissemination, trypanosomes localize in the small vessels of the heart and the central nervous system. In the central nervous system, it presents first as a diffuse leptomeningitis and later by a perivascular cerebritis. If untreated, this parenchymal inflammation gives rise to a demyelinating panencephalitis. Amastigote (leishmanial) forms have been demonstrated in experimental *T. brucei* infections, suggesting that this organism has an intracellular tissue phase in its developmental cycle. This could be of significance in occult infections.

The mechanism by which the trypanosome elicits tissue damage is unknown. The parasitemia stimulates the production of large quantities of IgM immunoglobulin, perhaps in response to the rapid antigenic variation of the parasite. A small part represents specific protective antibody; the remainder is nonspecific heterophil antibody and rheumatoid factor. High levels correlate well with the presence of circulating immune complexes which may, in turn, activate the kallikrein system and produce the vasculitis seen in this disease.

CLINICAL MANIFESTATIONS The Gambian and Rhodesian forms of sleeping sickness are both characterized by the presence of an entry lesion or chancre, a febrile period of parasite dissemination, and a stage of central nervous system involvement. They differ somewhat in symptoms, severity, and duration; Rhodesian trypanosomiasis is the more acute and severe of the two forms, usually terminating fatally within a year.

The *trypanosomal chancre* appears as an erythematous, tender nodule at the site of inoculation 2 to 7 days after the bite of an infected fly. It may occur anywhere on the body but is most commonly seen on the head or limbs and is accompanied by regional lymphadenopathy. The lesion may ulcerate, but it eventually heals spontaneously. It is noted more frequently in Rhodesian sleeping sickness, perhaps because of the acute nature of the illness.

The onset of systemic manifestations secondary to the dissemination of the parasite generally becomes apparent within 1 to 2 weeks, but in *T. brucei gambiense* may be delayed for several years. In the usual case the patient develops a high remittent fever, severe headache, insomnia, and inability to concentrate. Tachycardia out of proportion to the fever is common. In whites a characteristic circinate erythema resembling erythema marginatum is frequent. Transient firm areas of painful subcutaneous edema localized to the hands, feet, and periorbital tissues may appear. Discrete, nontender lymphadenopathy with gradual induration of the nodes and splenomegaly are almost invariably present. The nodes of the posterior cervical triangle are often prominent; this is referred to as *Winterbottom's sign.*

In the Gambian form of the disease there may be successive bouts of clinical activity with intervening latent periods that persist for a number of years. The early stages may be mild, and the disease may go unrecognized until the central nervous system is involved. In the Rhodesian form, fever is usually higher, emaciation more rapid, and lymphatic involvement less evident. Arrhythmia and other evidence or myocardial involvement are common; death from intercurrent infections or myocarditis usually occurs before the typical sleeping sickness syndrome appears.

Eventually the parasites enter the central nervous system. This may occur early in the course of the disease or may be delayed for as long as 8 years. Cerebral trypanosomiasis can be explosive, causing repeated convulsions or deep coma and death within a few days. Most patients show gradual progression to the classic picture of *sleeping sickness.* A vacant expression develops, the eyelids droop, the lower lip hangs loosely, and it becomes more and more difficult to gain the patient's attention or prod him or her to any activity. Patients will eat when offered food, but they never ask for it or engage in spontaneous conversation, and speech gradually becomes slurred and indistinct. Tremors of the hands and tongue, choreiform movements, seizures with transient paralysis, loss of sphincter control, ophthalmoplegia, extensor plantar responses, and finally death in coma, in status epilepticus, or from hyperpyrexia follows inexorably. Death may also occur from intercurrent infection, of which bacillary and amebic dysentery, malaria, and bacterial (often pneumococcal) pneumonia are the most important.

DIAGNOSIS AND LABORATORY FINDINGS *Anemia* and *hypermacroglobulinemia* are invariably present, and spontaneous clumping of erythrocytes in blood specimens is grossly evident in many cases. The sedimentation rate is rapid, and peripheral monocytosis is frequent. When there has been invasion of the central nervous system, the *cerebrospinal fluid* shows mononuclear pleocytosis and increased protein concentration. The protein concentration is a better index of severity of disease and therapeutic response than the number of cells. The presence of IgM in the spinal fluid is almost pathognomonic of cerebral trypanosomiasis.

The definitive diagnosis depends upon finding the trypanosomes in the blood, aspirate of lymph node, or cerebrospinal fluid. These should be examined first in wet mounts; actively motile organisms are seen easily under high power. For final identification thin and thick blood films should be stained with Wright's or Giemsa's stain. Parasitemia fluctuates daily and, particularly in the Gambian form of disease, may be difficult to detect by direct smears. If these procedures prove negative, concentrated specimens are examined. A variety of techniques, including differential centrifugation, microhematocrit buffy coat centrifugation, anion-exchange centrifugation, and membrane filtration, have been developed for field use. If these methods are negative, inoculation of rats or mice can be helpful in the diagnosis of Rhodesian disease. A severalfold increase in IgM globulins in the serum is of confirmatory value. Complement fixation, indirect fluorescent antibody, indirect hemagglutination, and enzyme-linked immunosorbent assay (ELISA) tests utilizing stable antigens are useful for screening patients in endemic areas. A card agglutination test for trypanosomiasis (CATT) can be performed on finger-stick blood within a few minutes. Positive serologic results must be confirmed by the direct demonstration of the parasite.

TREATMENT *Suramin* (Bayer 205, Antrypol) is the most effective agent before central nervous system involvement has occurred. The initial dose should be limited to 0.2 g intravenously because of possible idiosyncrasy. If there is no evidence of sensitivity, a full course of therapy can be instituted the following day. One gram (10 mL fresh 10% solution) is given intravenously on the first, third, seventh, fourteenth, and twenty-first days for a total of 5 g. If red blood cells, casts, or significant amounts of protein occur in the urine, therapy should be discontinued. Pentamidine given in water intramuscularly each day for 10 injections is also effective in early disease. The dose is 3 to 4 mg pentamidine base per kilogram for each injection. When the agent is given too rapidly by the intravenous route, it may cause hypotension.

Lumbar puncture should always be performed in patients who are about to undergo therapy for trypanosomiasis. If the central nervous system is involved, agents that will penetrate the blood-brain barrier must be used; for this purpose the most effective is *melarsoprol* (Mel B). This drug, an arsenic derivative of British antilewisite (BAL), is effective at all stages of the disease but is more toxic than suramin. It is given intravenously in the dose of 1.8 to 3.6 mg/kg on 3 consecutive days. This 3-day course is repeated in 7 days and again after 10 to 21 days. In frail patients the initial dose should be limited to 18 mg; subsequent doses are progressively increased to the daily maximum described above. If signs of arsenic toxicity occur, the drug should be discontinued. A reactive encephalopathy, probably due to the release of trypanosomal antigen, occurs early in the course of treatment in 5 to 10 percent of patients; it is fatal in 1 to 5 percent. Pretreatment with suramin may help avert this complication. A hemorrhagic encephalopathy, a direct arsenic toxic reaction, may also occur and is usually fatal. BAL may be of some use in this situation. An experimental ornithine decarboxylase inhibitor, DL-α-difluoromethylornithine (DFMO), is undergoing clinical trial in Africa. It appears effective in acute trypanosomiasis and, when used in combination with suramin, curative in CNS infection. It appears free of serious side effects.

PROGNOSIS The disease is probably always fatal if untreated. If the infection is treated with suramin prior to central nervous system involvement, the cure rate is high and recovery is rapid and complete. When the nervous system becomes involved, the prognosis is less bright, and in far-advanced disease the survivors may suffer neurological damage. Relapses may occur, particularly following treatment with suramin, if the central nervous system was already involved at the time therapy was instituted. Less commonly they may be the result of drug resistance. Examination of the spinal fluid 6 and 12 months after therapy, or earlier if symptoms recur, is helpful in detecting relapse. Such patients must be re-treated with a second therapeutic agent.

PREVENTION Personal protection is achieved by the use of repellents and protective clothing. A single intramuscular injection of pentamidine in a dosage of 3 to 4 mg base per kilogram (maximum 300 mg) will protect against the Gambian form of disease for 6 months or more. Because of the danger of cryptic infections occurring during chemoprophylaxis, it has been generally restricted to populations or work groups at particularly high risk. Wide-scale disease control projects employ active surveillance and treatment of infected individuals to decrease the size of the human reservoir. Use of insecticide-impregnated traps after an initial application of a residual insecticide to resting sites of flies has proved effective in controlling tsetse fly densities. During acute outbreaks of disease, aerosol application of insecticides from aircraft can temporarily interrupt transmission.

CHAGAS' DISEASE

DEFINITION American trypanosomiasis is an infection caused by *T. cruzi* that is characterized by an acute, often asymptomatic illness followed, after a latent period that may span decades, by chronic cardiac and gastrointestinal sequelae.

ETIOLOGY *Trypanosoma cruzi* circulates in the blood as a slender, fusiform trypomastigote measuring 20 μm in length. In stained preparations, its narrow undulating membrane, large kinetoplast, and characteristic C shape are easily recognized. Unlike the trypanosomes of sleeping sickness, it does not multiply within the bloodstream. After invading tissue cells, it loses its undulating membrane and flagellum, assumes its amastigote form, and divides by binary fission. Eventually, new flagellated forms are produced which reenter the general circulation to initiate another cycle.

Strains of *T. cruzi* vary widely in their host preference, geographic distribution, virulence, and tissue tropism. They may be distinguished by specific antiserum, zymotype, and DNA restriction pattern.

EPIDEMIOLOGY This infection is found in scattered foci from Chile and Argentina to Mexico. Within these endemic areas it affects 15 to 20 million people and is the leading cause of heart disease, responsible for one-quarter of all deaths in the 25- to 44-year age group. *Trypanosoma cruzi* has been found in insect vectors and wild animals in several areas of the southern United States, and serologic studies have documented that acquisition of human infection occurs within this country. There are to date, however, only a handful of clinically apparent autochthonous cases reported from Texas and California.

The disease is transmitted to humans by reduviid (''assassin'' or ''kissing'') bugs, primarily those of the genera *Triatoma, Panstrongylus,* and *Rhodnius.* These winged, hematophagous insects can be found in the burrows of animals and in the cracks and thatch of poorly constructed rural dwellings. The insect attacks human beings at night, usually biting the face at the mucocutaneous junction (most frequently the lip or outer canthus of the eye). The flagellated trypanosomes are ingested by the bug while feeding, and after multiplying and developing in the midgut of the insect for 8 to 10 days, are discharged in the feces following a subsequent feeding; human infection occurs through contamination of the bite wound. This is referred to as transmission by the ''posterior station.'' The reduviid may remain infected as long as 2 years.

Human beings, domestic animals (cats and dogs), and wild animals, especially the opossum and armadillo, may serve as reservoirs for the infection. The close association of human beings, domestic animals, and the vector within human dwellings is of prime epidemiologic importance, but the disease is also transmitted by a blood transfusion and via the placenta to newborn infants. Occasional laboratory infections have also been reported.

PATHOGENESIS AND CLINICAL MANIFESTATIONS Only one-third of newly infected patients have clinical manifestations. In them a local inflammatory reaction, manifested clinically as an erythematous nodule or *chagoma,* appears within 1 to 3 weeks at the site of inoculation of the protozoan. If the portal of entry has been the conjunctiva, the presenting manifestations are a unilateral, painless conjunctivitis, palpebral edema, and preauricular lymphadenopathy (Romaña's sign). This primary complex may persist for 1 to 2 months during which parasites can be demonstrated in the lesion.

Following an incubation period of 2 weeks, trypanosomal forms reach the general circulation, producing a parasitemia and initiating the acute phase of the illness. After circulating in the blood for some time, the trypanosomes invade tissue cells of mesenchymal origin, assume the amastigote form, and multiply, producing intracellular pseudocysts. In 4 to 6 days these pseudocysts rupture, releasing both amastigotes and newly formed trypomastigotes. The amastigotes disintegrate, eliciting an intense inflammatory reaction, while the flagellated forms regain the bloodstream to maintain the infection and invade new tissues, particularly the heart, skeletal muscle, smooth muscle, and nervous system. *Trypanosoma cruzi* antigens can absorb to the surface of both normal and infected cells, possibly rendering them susceptible to destruction by the host's hormonal and cellular immune response.

Clinically, the patient experiences a continuous or recurrent fever, generalized lymphadenopathy, hepatosplenomegaly, and in some cases extensive gelatinous edema of the face and trunk. A transient morbilliform or urticarial skin eruption may occur early in the acute phase. Although trypanosomes frequently can be demonstrated in the cerebrospinal fluid at this time, acute meningoencephalitis is relatively rare; newborn infants and young children are affected most commonly. Myocarditis characterized by tachycardia and nonspecific electrocardiographic changes is very common. In severe cases, there may be conduction disturbances, cardiac dilatation, and heart failure. The duration of the acute illness is variable. In 5 to 10 percent of cases, meningoencephalitis or severe heart disease results in a fatal outcome within a few days or weeks. Most often, the disease, in response to the development of humoral antibody, resolves slowly over a period of several weeks. Parasites become extremely scanty in both the tissues and blood, the patient appears well, and the persistent infection is detectable only by serological means. Rarely, in the face of leukemia or immunosuppression, parasitemia and acute manifestations reappear. In the overwhelming majority of patients, however, the infection remains latent for the remainder of life. In approximately 10 percent, progressive immunologic destruction of mesenchymal tissue eventually leads to the development of chronic organ damage. Most patients presenting with late manifestations deny a history of acute illness, suggesting that subclinical infections often result in chronic disease. It has been suggested that host cell antigens released during the acute phase of the illness initiate an autoimmune inflammatory reaction, and antibodies reactive with endocardium, striated muscle, and vascular tissues have been described. Self-reactive cytotoxic lymphocytes have also been demonstrated in experimental animals, and lymphocytic infiltrates are commonly seen in patients dying of chagasic cardiopathy. Some authors have suggested that the late manifestations of disease are primarily due to neuropathies caused by the destruction of ganglionic nerve cells during this phase of the disease, resulting in the dilatation and malfunction of the affected organs.

The most important late manifestation is heart disease. Symptoms and signs range from precordial pain, arrhythmias, and heart block to chronic congestive heart failure (predominantly right-sided). Thromboembolic phenomena and sudden cardiac arrest are relatively common. Right bundle branch block and left anterior hemiblock, premature ventricular contractions, and inverted T waves are frequently seen on ECG. Echocardiography has been shown to be of value both in screening patients with infection for evidence of cardiac involvement and in following the progress of those with established cardiomyopathy. At autopsy the hearts of patients with Chagas' disease may show a peculiar herniation of the endocardium through the apical muscle bundles. Megacolon and megaesophagus are sequelae seen in southern South America. In patients with megaesophagus, regurgitation and aspiration pneumonia are common; the incidence of esophageal cancer is increased. Neurologic manifestations including mental deficiency and cerebellar symptoms also have been reported in chronic Chagas' disease.

DIAGNOSIS The diagnosis depends on the demonstration of *T. cruzi* in the patient or upon serologic tests. In the acute phase of the disease the parasite may be seen in the peripheral blood by means of the same direct methods described for African trypanosomiasis. A microhematocrit concentration procedure has proved useful. If these are negative, blood may be cultured in a variety of artificial media, or inoculated into rats, mice, or guinea pigs.

Trypanosoma cruzi is easily grown in blood broth and incubated at 28°C. The technique of *xenodiagnosis* is often used in endemic areas; a laboratory-reared vector, known to be parasite-free, is allowed to feed on subjects with suspected cases, and 2 weeks later, the insect's intestinal contents are examined for parasites. Confusion sometimes arises from the finding of trypanosomes in blood. Many children in Venezuela and other South American countries are infected with a harmless species, *T. rangeli,* which produces no symptoms but may be present in the blood for many months. By utilization of both culture and xenodiagnosis repeatedly, organisms can be recovered from most acute cases and from up to 40 percent of chronic ones. Biopsy of an involved lymph node or calf muscle may reveal the organism during the initial illness when the parasites cannot be recovered from the blood. The Machado-Guerreiro test (a complement fixation reaction) is most helpful in the diagnosis of chronic cases and in survey work. Fluorescent antibody and hemagglutination inhibition tests appear more sensitive, but less specific. Rapid slide agglutination tests have been developed for use in blood banks. Most of these serologic tests employ crude epimastigote antigens which cross-react with serums from patients with leishmaniasis or *T. rangeli* infection. A new enzyme-linked immunosorbent assay utilizing a purified glycoprotein antigen eliminates these false-positive results.

TREATMENT AND PREVENTION There is no satisfactory treatment for Chagas' disease. Several drugs shorten the period of parasitemia, prevent seroconversion, and decrease both the duration of symptoms and the mortality in acute Chagas' disease; there is some doubt whether any have the capacity to destroy intracellular parasites at tolerable doses. Nifurtimox, a nitrofurazone derivative given in the dose of 10 mg/kg per day in four divided doses for 3 or 4 months, shows the greatest promise, but is frequently associated with serious side effects. Benznidazole, a nitroimidazole not presently available in the United States, is similar in efficacy. Ketoconazole has shown significant effectiveness against intracellular amastigotes in experimental infections but has not been tested in humans. Chronic organ damage is generally thought irreversible.

Prevention consists of using residual insecticides on the walls and roofs of houses, the main habitat of the vectors. The addition of latex to the insecticide creates a colorless paint which significantly prolongs the activity of the insecticide. The use of fumigant canisters can prevent reinfestation. Patching wall cracks, cementing over dirt floors, and moving firewood piles away from human habitations will also dramatically decrease the concentration of reduviid vectors within the home. Transfusion infections can be prevented by adding gentian violet or one of its analogues to the blood. Leukemia patients from endemic areas should be serologically screened before immunosuppressive therapy is initiated.

REFERENCES

Sleeping sickness

CLARKSON AB et al: New drug combination for experimental late-stage African trypanosomiasis: DL-α-difluoromethylornithine (DFMO) with suramin. Am J Trop Med Hyg 33:1073, 1984

DONELSON JE, TURNER MJ: How the trypanosome changes its coat. Sci Am 252:44, 1985

MOLYNEUX DH: Selective primary health care: Strategies for control of disease in the developing world. VIII. African trypanosomiasis. Rev Infect Dis 5:945, 1983

SEED JR et al: A physiologic mechanism to explain pathogenesis in African trypanosomiasis. Contrib Microbiol Immunol 7:83, 1983

WERY M et al: Hematologic manifestations, diagnosis, and immunopathology of African trypanosomiasis. Semin Hematol 19:83, 1982

Chagas' disease

APT W et al: Natural history of chagasic cardiopathy in Chile. Follow-up of 71 cases after 4 years. J Trop Med Hyg 86:217, 1983

HAMMERMEISTER KE et al: Left ventricular wall motion in patients with Chagas' disease. Br Heart J 51:70, 1984

LORCA M et al: *Trypanosoma cruzi* in blood banks of 12 Chilean hospitals. Bull Pan Health Organ 17:269, 1983
MARSDEN PD: Selective primary health care: Strategies for control of disease in the developing world. XVI. Chagas' disease. Rev Infect Dis 6:855, 1984
MARTINI-CAMPOS JV, TAFURI WL: Chagas' enteropathy. Gut 14:910, 1973
MILES MA: The epidemiology of South American trypanosomiasis—biochemical and immunological approaches and their relevance to control. Trans R Soc Trop Med Hyg 55:5, 1983
Status of Chagas' disease in the region of the Americas. Epidemiol Bull 5:5, 1984

157 TOXOPLASMOSIS

RIMA McLEOD / JACK S. REMINGTON

DEFINITION The term *toxoplasmosis* refers to disease caused by the obligate intracellular protozoan *Toxoplasma gondii* and must be differentiated from the more common asymptomatic infection caused by this organism. The infection and disease in older children and adults are discussed below. The reader is referred to the reference by Remington and Desmonts for information on congenital toxoplasmosis.

ETIOLOGY *Toxoplasma gondii* is classified among the coccidia and exists in three forms: tachyzoite, cyst, and oocyst.

Tachyzoites *Tachyzoites* are crescent or oval, approximately 3 by 7 μm in size, and stain well with either Wright's stain or Giemsa's stain. Tachyzoites invade all mammalian cells except nonnucleated erythrocytes and are found in tissues during the acute stage of infection.

Cysts Tissue cysts are formed within host cells and may contain thousands of organisms. They are 10 to 100 μm in size and stain well with periodic acid Schiff stain; the cyst wall stains with silver stain. Cysts are important in transmission, as they may be present in animal tissues ingested by carnivores. They may persist in virtually every organ, but skeletal and heart muscle and the central nervous system appear to be the most common sites of chronic (latent) infection.

Oocysts Oocysts are oval and 10 to 12 μm in diameter. They are formed only in the mucosal cells of the intestines of members of the cat family and are subsequently excreted in the feces. The cat is the only animal in which the organism has a sexual cycle in the intestine, and cats have systemic infection with *T. gondii* as well. The time of appearance of oocysts in the feces depends on the form of the organism with which the cat becomes infected and varies from 3 to 24 days. Excretion continues for 7 to 20 days, and as many as 10 million oocysts are shed in the feces in a single day. Except under unusual conditions, once a cat has been infected and has excreted oocysts, it will not shed oocysts again. When a cat becomes infected with *Isospora felis,* renewed oocyst excretion has been reported to occur. Sporulation, which occurs from 2 to 3 days (at 24°C) after the oocysts are excreted, is required for the oocysts to become infectious and does not occur below 4°C or above 37°C. Oocysts may remain infectious for more than 1 year under favorable conditions (e.g., in warm, moist soil). They presumably play a major role in transmission by the oral route since their ingestion has been shown to transmit infection.

EPIDEMIOLOGY *Toxoplasma gondii* is ubiquitous and infects herbivorous, omnivorous, and carnivorous animals, including mammals, birds, and reptiles. Prevalence of infection varies with locale; prevalence of positive serologic reaction increases with age. In the United States, approximately 5 to 30 percent of individuals 10 to 19 years old and 10 to 67 percent of individuals over 50 years old have serologic evidence of infection. Generally, less infection occurs in cold regions, in hot and arid areas, and at high elevations. No particular genetic susceptibility has been documented for humans. Epidemics of toxoplasmosis have occurred in humans and in domestic animals. Simultaneous occurrence of infection in multiple members of the same household has been reported to occur commonly.

The natural mechanism of infection is by ingestion of cysts or oocysts or by transplacental transmission. Infection may also be acquired through blood transfusion, leukocyte transfusion, organ transplantation, and laboratory accident. Clinical illness due to reinfection from an exogenous source has not been reported.

Oral transmission Cysts are present in approximately 10 percent of lamb and 25 percent of pork used for human consumption; cysts have been isolated from beef, but their prevalence in beef has not been defined. Direct contact with any material contaminated by infected cat feces may result in ingestion of oocysts, and this form can be transmitted to food by insects. When humans or other animals (including cats) eat infected tissues (from any animal) or mature oocysts (excreted only by cats), the life cycle is completed. Approximately 1 percent of cats have been found to be excreting oocysts in their feces.

Transplacental transmission Accumulated data support the concept that *Toxoplasma* is transmitted to the fetus in utero when the pregnant woman acquires infection during the current pregnancy. Most often, when a mother is infected during pregnancy, the outcome is a normal uninfected infant, but spontaneous abortion, stillbirth, or delivery of a premature or full-term infected infant may result. Congenital infection will occur in approximately one-third of infants born to mothers who acquire their infection during the current pregnancy. In infants born to mothers infected during the first trimester, congenital infection is least common (approximately 17 percent) but disease is most severe; in infants born to mothers infected during the third trimester, congenital infection is most common (approximately 65 percent) but is usually asymptomatic. The fetus is at risk whether or not the infection is symptomatic in the mother.

The following are general guidelines for ascertaining the risk of transmission of the organism to the fetus of a woman who is known to have been infected *prior to the pregnancy in question.* If a woman acquires *Toxoplasma* infection more than 6 months before gestation, she will not deliver an infected infant. When conception occurs less than 6 months after acquisition of *Toxoplasma,* the risk to the fetus is exceedingly low, but transplacental transmission has been documented in this setting. *Toxoplasma* has been isolated on rare occasions from abortuses of women with chronic (latent) infection. The frequency of chronic *Toxoplasma* infection as a cause of abortion has not been defined and is the subject of considerable controversy.

Transmission by blood or leukocyte transfusion or organ transplantation *Toxoplasma* may be transmitted by blood or leukocyte transfusion. The organism has been isolated from leukocytes of individuals without recognized clinical evidence of *Toxoplasma* infection, and parasitemia has been reported to persist in otherwise normal individuals for as long as 1 year after acquisition of infection. The high incidence of isolation of the organism from the blood of patients who have chronic myelogenous leukemia and high antibody titers to *Toxoplasma* is particularly noteworthy. The organism has survived for 50 days in whole citrated blood stored at 4°C. Immunodeficient patients who require multiple blood transfusions may be particularly at risk for transmission of infection by this route. *Toxoplasma* has also been transmitted by transplantation of hearts from acutely infected donors to recipients who were not previously infected with *Toxoplasma.*

PATHOGENESIS Organisms released from cysts or oocysts enter cells of the gastrointestinal tract, multiply, cause cell disruption, and then infect neighboring cells. Extracellular organisms or organisms within leukocytes are transported throughout the body via the lymphatic system and bloodstream and are capable of invading every organ and tissue. Proliferation of tachyzoites usually leads to death of invaded cells, resulting in foci of necrosis, surrounded by an intense cellular reaction. The immune response of the host primarily governs the outcome of the acute process. Both humoral and cell-mediated immunity are important. In some apparently normal individuals and in immunodeficient patients, the acute infection may progress with acute necrotizing encephalitis, pneumonitis, or myocarditis which may be fatal. Tachyzoites disappear from the tissues with development of the normal immune response. Organisms may continue to proliferate and to cause destruction in the central nervous system and eye while they are disappearing from extraneural tissues because of the barrier to transfer of antibody in the eye and central nervous system.

A unique aspect of the infection is that organisms persist in cysts in many organs during the life span of the host. Either persistence of viable tachyzoites within cells of the reticuloendothelial system or disruption of cysts may be the source of the recurrent parasitemias that occur in some asymptomatic individuals with chronic infection. Cysts are the probable origin of the organisms that cause recrudescent disease in immunocompromised patients or chorioretinitis in older children and adults with congenital toxoplasmosis.

PATHOLOGY The histopathologic changes in toxoplasmic lymphadenitis are characteristic and consist of reactive follicular hyperplasia with irregular clusters of epithelioid histiocytes that have vesicular nuclei and abundant eosinophilic cytoplasm and that encroach upon and blur the margins of germinal centers; numerous mitoses in the germinal centers; many necrotic cells and an associated focal distention of subcapsular and trabecular sinuses with monocytoid cells. Tachyzoites or cysts are only rarely observed in conventionally stained sections.

Single or multiple foci of necrosis occur as the earliest manifestations of involvement of the eye. Infiltrates are composed largely of lymphocytes, plasma cells, and mononuclear phagocytic cells. There are intra- and extracellular tachyzoites and cysts in the retinal lesions. Granulomatous inflammation of the choroid occurs secondary to necrotizing retinitis. Iridocyclitis, glaucoma, and cataracts may be complications of the chorioretinitis.

In cases of acute central nervous system infection, there is a focal or diffuse meningoencephalitis with necrosis and microglial nodules. In immunodeficient adults other than those with acquired immunodeficiency syndrome (AIDS), the major finding is necrotizing encephalitis. Often these lesions are multiple, small, and diffusely distributed, although large single lesions also occur. Margins of areas of necrosis may be infiltrated with monocytes, lymphocytes, and plasma cells. Perivascular mononuclear inflammation frequently is present contiguous to areas of necrosis, and occasionally there is necrosis of vessel walls. Intra- and extracellular tachyzoites are usually found at the periphery of areas of necrosis, and these areas of necrosis may mimic mass lesions. Cysts may be present after the first week of infection. In patients with AIDS, cysts are often found in normal brain adjacent to areas of necrosis in autopsy specimens. Cysts are seen less frequently in biopsy specimens. Polymorphonuclear leukocytes are present in addition to lymphocytes, plasma cells, and histiocytes in the toxoplasmic central nervous system lesions of patients with AIDS and mononuclear leukocytes in the toxoplasmic central nervous system lesions of other immunocompromised adults. The size of lesions and extent and location of central nervous system involvement vary considerably.

In cases of disseminated infection, pathologic changes occur in the heart, lungs, kidney, and multiple other organs. They consist of necrosis and the presence of tachyzoites, cysts, and inflammatory cells alone or in combination. Glomerulonephritis with deposits of gamma-M globulin (IgM), fibrinogen, and *Toxoplasma* antigen and antibody has been reported. Involvement of the pancreas has been a prominent finding in infection in immunocompromised patients. Findings in skeletal muscle vary from parasitized fibers without pathologic changes to focal areas of infiltration to widespread myositis with necrosis.

There are prolonged and marked changes in T-lymphocyte subpopulations associated with *T. gondii* infection. These changes can be correlated with particular disease syndromes but not with disease outcome: Some patients with prolonged fever and malaise have lymphocytosis, elevation in number of suppressor T cells, and depression of the ratio of helper to suppressor cells. Significant depression in the number of helper cells may persist when the patient is clinically asymptomatic. The number of helper cells may be significantly decreased in some patients with lymphadenopathy. Depression in the number of helper cells has persisted for more than 6 months after the onset of infection. T-cell subpopulations are normal in patients with asymptomatic infection. There is a marked reduction in the number of T cells and a marked depression of the ratio of helper to suppressor lymphocytes in some patients with disseminated disease.

CLINICAL MANIFESTATIONS **Lymphadenopathy and other manifestations in the immunocompetent individual** Lymphadenopathy is the most commonly recognized clinical manifestation of acute acquired toxoplasmosis. Cervical nodes are involved most frequently. Nodes may be single or multiple, and involvement may be symptomatic or asymptomatic. Asymptomatic lymphadenopathy may mimic lymphoma, and involvement of a pectoral node has been suspected to be carcinoma of the breast. Suboccipital, supraclavicular, axillary, inguinal, and mediastinal nodes may be involved. When mesenteric or retroperitoneal nodes are involved, abdominal pain and significant temperature elevation (e.g., up to 40°C) may occur. Involved lymph nodes vary in firmness, may be tender, do not suppurate, and are usually discrete. Confusion, malaise, fever, stiff neck, myalgias, arthralgias, headache, sore throat, maculopapular rash (which spares the palms and soles), urticaria, hepatosplenomegaly, hepatitis, or reactive lymphocytes may occur. In one epidemic, 35 of 37 individuals with serologic evidence of acute acquired *Toxoplasma* infection had signs or symptoms of infection. Although 25 individuals sought medical advice from physicians, only 3 were correctly diagnosed as having toxoplasmosis. Lymphadenopathic toxoplasmosis is self-limited, but malaise and/or lymphadenopathy may persist or recur for months. Recrudescent lymphadenopathy has also been described.

Individuals who appear to be normal immunologically rarely may present with any of the following, alone or in combination: pneumonitis, myocarditis, pericarditis, pericardial effusion, hepatitis, polymyositis, encephalitis, or meningoencephalitis. Signs or symptoms of involvement of these organs are nonspecific. Significant morbidity has occurred, and some of these patients have died of the infection.

Ocular involvement *Toxoplasma* has been estimated to be the cause of approximately 35 percent of cases of chorioretinitis in children and adults. Although chorioretinitis has been estimated to occur in approximately 1 percent of patients with the acute acquired infection, ocular disease is most often a consequence of congenital *Toxoplasma* infection. Chorioretinitis is usually unilateral with the acute acquired infection and as a sequel of congenital infection which occurs in adolescents or adults. Blurred vision, scotomas, pain, photophobia, or epiphora may be due to active chorioretinitis. If the macula is involved, impairment or loss of central vision may occur. In children, strabismus may be an early sign of chorioretinitis. Associated signs of systemic infection occur only rarely. Vision improves, but frequently visual acuity recovers only partially as inflammation subsides. Commonly, episodic flares of chorioretinitis cause destruction of irreplaceable retinal tissue. The peak incidence of symptomatic disease is in the second and third decades, and it is uncommon for clinically apparent reactivation to occur after the age of 40. These multiple recurrences may result in glaucoma or loss of vision and ultimately may necessitate enucleation. The acute lesions appear as yellowish-white, cotton-like patches that have elevated, indistinct margins surrounded by a zone of hyperemia. Papillitis is usually associated with overt central nervous system disease. Inflammatory exudate in the vitreous may obscure the fundus. Older lesions characteristically appear as atrophic, whitish-gray plaques with distinct borders and black spots of choroidal pigment. Lesions usually are located near the posterior pole of the retina, although they may be peripheral. They may be single but are more commonly multiple, and lesions of varying age may be seen simultaneously. Panuveitis and papillitis with optic atrophy occur less commonly. Isolated anterior uveitis due to *Toxoplasma* infection has never been proved. The typical ocular lesion of congenital toxoplasmosis in the newborn consists of bilateral congenital chorioretinitis.

Toxoplasmosis in the immunocompromised patient (non-AIDS) All forms of toxoplasmosis that occur in normal individuals may also occur in immunocompromised individuals. Patients receiving immunosuppressive therapy for lymphoproliferative disorders (especially Hodgkin's disease), for hematologic malignancy, or for prevention of organ graft rejection have the greatest predilection for life-threatening toxoplasmosis. Individuals who have not been infected previously with *T. gondii* and who receive a cardiac transplant from an infected individual have developed signs and symptoms of toxoplasmosis. The untreated infection in these patients is frequently fulminant and rapidly fatal. Central nervous system involvement, present in greater than 50 percent of documented cases, is the most characteristic clinical feature of toxoplasmosis in immunocompromised patients. Therefore, the diagnosis of toxoplasmosis must be excluded in any immunosuppressed patient with symptoms or signs referable to the central nervous system. Symptoms and signs are manifestations of diffuse encephalopathy, meningoencephalitis, or cerebral mass lesions and include changes in mental status, headache, focal neurologic deficits, and seizures. Brain involvement has been established by demonstration of tachyzoites in material from brain biopsy or in material aspirated from mass lesions that may have the characteristic appearance of a brain abscess on computerized tomography (CT) scan. CT scan may detect multiple, diffusely distributed or single lesions. Delayed (30 min or 1 h after infusion of contrast material) films may be important for detection of such lesions. Typically, the cerebrospinal fluid shows a mononuclear pleocytosis, a moderate elevation in protein, and a normal glucose. Some patients have had hypoglycorrhachia. Immunocompromised patients also may have other nonspecific manifestations of the infection which are reflections of inflammation and necrosis of the organs involved, particularly the heart and lungs. Toxoplasmosis may simulate rejection of a transplanted heart. Tachyzoites have been seen in endomyocardial biopsy, which established the diagnosis of toxoplasmosis.

Toxoplasmic encephalitis and AIDS Toxoplasmic encephalitis is a major cause of morbidity and mortality in patients with AIDS. The incidence of toxoplasmic encephalitis in patients with AIDS who have antibody to *T. gondii* has been reported to be between 6 and 12 percent. Based on this observation, an estimate is that there have been approximately 170 cases of toxoplasmic encephalitis among the 7000 patients with AIDS reported by 1984 and another 170 cases would be expected to develop in the 7000 patients projected to develop AIDS in 1985. The incidence of *T. gondii* as a cause of encephalitis in patients with AIDS and encephalitis has been reported to be between 25 and 80 percent. The diagnosis of toxoplasmic encephalitis should be considered in individuals who have central nervous system disease but who do not have the usual risk factors for AIDS, since heterosexual transmission of human T-cell leukemia virus (HTLV III) has resulted in AIDS in individuals who are not the usual high-risk groups.

Prominent signs and symptoms of toxoplasmic encephalitis in patients with AIDS include chills, fever, headache, seizures, depressed mental status, and neurologic findings; these may occur in conjunction with chorioretinitis. The majority of patients with AIDS and toxoplasmic encephalitis fail to produce a serum antibody response indicative of acute infection with *T. gondii*. Demonstration of a rising titer of antibody to *T. gondii* present in cerebrospinal fluid but not present in serum has been associated with toxoplasmic encephalitis in a patient with AIDS.

Cerebrospinal fluid abnormalities have included pleocytosis, elevated protein content, and hypoglycorrhachia; tachyzoites have been seen in cytocentrifuge preparations of cerebrospinal fluid. When cerebrospinal fluid (or brain) is cultured for viruses, tissue cultures should also be examined for *T. gondii*, which may form plaques or widespread cytopathic effects. The cultures can be stained with Giemsa stain.

On CT scans of the brain, findings include diffuse encephalitis and/or one or more mass lesions. Contrast infusion may produce ring, nodular, target, or no enhancement of the lesions. Lesions may be in the cortex or white matter, and there is some proclivity for these lesions to be deep within the basal ganglia. Initially, no abnormalities may be observed on CT scan of the brain of symptomatic individuals: abnormalities may first appear several weeks later. One-hour delayed, double-dose contrast studies have detected lesions which were isodense on plain scans.

Brain biopsy of lesions seen in CT scan of brain should be performed when feasible because the differential diagnosis of these lesions includes encephalitis due to *Candida* species, *Aspergillus* species, *Mycobacterium*, and *Cryptococcus neoformans*, as well as multifocal leukoencephalopathy and lymphoma. When conventional stains are used, *T. gondii* is seen in only 50 percent of brain biopsies from such patients with toxoplasmic encephalitis. When specific immunohistologic stains are used, however, the presence of *T. gondii* tachyzoites, cysts, and/or antigens are found in brain biopsies obtained from most infected patients (see under "Pathology").

If the CT scan of brain is normal or without focal lesions in a patient with AIDS who has neurologic signs or symptoms, and the patient has either a positive Sabin-Feldman dye test, or an IgG indirect fluorescent antibody (IFA) level that is high, empiric therapy for toxoplasmic encephalitis seems warranted. If there is a focal abnormality on CT scan, serology positive for antibodies to *Toxoplasma,* and the lesion is inaccessible for biopsy or the patient's clinical condition contraindicates biopsy, presumptive therapy for *T. gondii* should be instituted. In patients who are started on presumptive therapy, a therapeutic response within 7 to 10 days supports the diagnosis of toxoplasmic encephalitis. If the patient is being treated with corticosteroids, radiographic improvement does not provide reliable evidence of a therapeutic response.

If the standard therapy with 25 mg per day of pyrimethamine and 6 to 8 g per day of trisulfapyrimidines or sulfadiazine is not effective, the daily dose of pyrimethamine should be increased to 50 mg. If therapy is limited by adverse reactions to the sulfonamide, pyrimethamine (50 mg per day) alone may be used. Folinic acid dosage may need to be as high as 15 mg per day, especially when there is marrow depression caused by pyrimethamine. However, the mechanism for the marrow suppression in patients with AIDS may be immunologic, and prophylactic folinic acid may not reverse the leukopenia. Optimal duration of therapy is not known (see "Therapy"), but relapse of toxoplasmic encephalitis is frequent in patients with AIDS when therapy is discontinued, and treatment for the duration of the patient's life may be warranted.

Toxoplasmosis and *Toxoplasma* infection in the pregnant woman *Toxoplasma* infection acquired by the mother during pregnancy is symptomatic in only about 10 to 20 percent of cases. See also "Transplacental Transmission" above.

DIAGNOSIS Acute infection with *Toxoplasma* may be diagnosed by isolation of *T. gondii* from body fluids or blood (see qualification under "Isolation Procedures" below), demonstration of tachyzoites in histologic sections or in impression smears of tissue or body fluids, demonstration of characteristic lymph node histology, and serologic tests.

Isolation of the organism The organism can be isolated by inoculation of leukocytes, body fluids, or tissue specimens into tissue culture or by subcutaneous or intraperitoneal inoculation into mice. Body fluids should be processed and inoculated immediately, but blood and tissues may be stored at 4°C overnight. Freezing or treatment of specimens with formalin kills the organism. Mice should be examined for organisms in the peritoneal fluid 6 to 10 days after inoculation, or earlier if they die. Mice that survive 6 weeks should be tested for *Toxoplasma* antibody in serum. When antibody is present, visualization of *Toxoplasma* cysts in the mouse brain establishes the diagnosis. If cysts are not demonstrable in brains of mice with *Toxoplasma* antibody, portions of brain, liver, and spleen should be inoculated into other mice.

Isolation of *T. gondii* from body fluids reflects the acute stage of infection, as does isolation from blood in most patients. Although persistent parasitemia has been described in asymptomatic individuals with latent infection, this appears to be a rare occurrence, except, perhaps, in patients with chronic myelogenous leukemia. Isolation from tissues (e.g., skeletal muscle, lung, brain, or eye) obtained by biopsy or at autopsy may reflect the presence of tissue cysts and does not prove that infection is acute.

Histologic diagnosis Demonstration of tachyzoites in tissue sections (e.g., endomyocardial biopsy in cardiac transplant recipients) or smears (e.g., brain biopsy, bone marrow aspirate) or in body fluids (e.g., cerebrospinal fluid, amniotic fluid) establishes the diagnosis of the acute infection. It is difficult to identify tachyzoites by ordinary staining methods; direct and indirect immunofluorescent antibody techniques and a peroxidase-antiperoxidase (PAP) immunohistochemical staining technique have been used successfully for this purpose. Demonstration of tissue cysts does not differentiate between acute or chronic infection. When there are numerous cysts in any organ, infection is usually of recent onset. Characteristic histologic criteria establish toxoplasmic lymphadenitis (see "Pathology" above).

Serologic tests Methods most widely used to establish the diagnosis of acute *Toxoplasma* infection are the Sabin-Feldman dye test, indirect fluorescent antibody (IFA) test, and indirect hemagglutination (IHA) test. Measurement of antibodies by enzyme-linked immunosorbent assay (ELISA) or radioimmunoassay is potentially valuable because these techniques may be automated.

The dye test, which measures primarily IgG antibodies, is sensitive and specific. The World Health Organization has recommended that dye test titers be expressed in international units (IU/mL) and will supply a standard reference serum.

The IFA test appears to measure the same antibodies as the dye test and is the most widely available procedure. In both tests, titers tend to be parallel. Dye test IgG-neutralizing antibody and IFA test antibodies usually appear 1 to 2 weeks after infection, reach high titers (≥1:1000) in 6 to 8 weeks, and gradually decline over months to years; low titers (e.g., 1:4 to 1:64) commonly persist for life. The magnitude of the antibody titer does not correlate with severity of illness.

The agglutination test is available commercially in Europe (Bio-Merieux, Lyons, France). It detects IgG antibody. Formalin-preserved whole parasites are used. Because the test is very sensitive to IgM antibodies, "natural" IgM antibodies frequently cause nonspecific agglutination in serum of individuals who are negative when tested in the dye and IFA tests. Including 2-mercaptoethanol in the test obviates this problem. This method should not be used for measurement of IgM antibodies. The method is simple, accurate, inexpensive, excellent for screening sera of pregnant women, and useful in detection of antibodies to *T. gondii* in patients with AIDS.

The IgM–fluorescent antibody (IgM-IFA) test is useful in establishing the diagnosis of acute infection with *T. gondii* because IgM antibodies appear early (as early as 5 days after infection) and disappear early as contrasted with gamma-G globulin (IgG) antibodies. In most cases, IgM-IFA test antibodies rise rapidly (to levels of 1:80 to ≥1:1000) and fall to low titers (1:10 or 1:20) or disappear within a few weeks or months. However, in some patients they are present at low titer for several years. Some immunodeficient patients with acute toxoplasmosis and most patients with only active ocular toxoplasmosis may not have IgM *Toxoplasma* antibodies. Rheumatoid factor may cause false-positive reactions in the IgM-IFA test. Removal of rheumatoid factor (e.g., by absorption) will eliminate false-positive test results in the IgM-IFA test. Antinuclear antibodies may cause false-positive reactions in both the IFA and IgM-IFA tests.

The double-sandwich enzyme-linked immunosorbent assay (DS-IgM-ELISA) is more sensitive and specific than the IgM-IFA test for detection of IgM antibodies. Antinuclear antibodies and rheumatoid factor do not cause false-positive test results. As a guideline in adults, a serum level of IgM antibodies against *T. gondii* of 6 to 10 in this test indicates that *T. gondii* infection has most likely been acquired recently (i.e., within the prior 5 months); levels of 2 or 3 indicate infection has been acquired several months or more in the past; levels of 4 or 5 are intermediate; and levels of 0 or 1 are negative.

The DS-IgM-ELISA is a more specific and sensitive test that the IgM-IFA test to establish the diagnoses of congenital and acute acquired toxoplasmosis: The DS-IgM-ELISA detects approximately 75 percent of babies with congenital *Toxoplasma* infection whereas the IgM-IFA test detects only 25 percent of infants with proven congenital infection. The DS-IgM-ELISA avoids false-positive results due to the presence of rheumatoid factor (which the infant can produce in utero) and false-negative results due to competition from high levels of maternal IgM antibody (which occur in the IgM-IFA test).

The IgM-immunosorbent assay (IgM-ISA) combines trapping of the patient's IgM to a solid surface and formalin-fixed organisms or antigen-coated latex particles to detect the IgM antibodies. It is specific, sensitive, does not require use of an enzyme conjugate, and is simple to perform.

The antibodies measured in the IHA test may persist for years and are different than those measured in the IFA and dye tests. The IHA test may be helpful when titers in the IFA or dye test have stabilized since IHA test titers rise later. However, the rise in titer may occur so late that it is not helpful in diagnosis of the acute infection. Because of the frequency of false-negative results, the IHA test should not be used in infants with suspect congenital infection or in screening to determine if the infection has been acquired during pregnancy, since the test may be negative for too long a period early in the infection.

Titers in the complement fixation (CF) test also may appear several weeks later than those measured in the IFA and dye tests and also may persist for years. A negative CF test titer does not exclude acute or chronic infection, and a single positive CF test titer does not prove acute infection. A significant rise in CF test titer (i.e., of two serial dilutions performed at the same time on serums obtained several weeks apart) establishes recent infection.

Acute acquired *Toxoplasma* infection in the immunocompetent individual In settings in which acute acquired infection is suspected in an immunocompetent individual, a negative dye test or IFA test virtually excludes the diagnosis. The diagnosis of recent acute acquired infection is confirmed if there is a serial two-tube rise in titer when serums drawn at 3-week intervals are run at the same time or if there is seroconversion from a negative to a positive titer (in the absence of transfer of antibody by transfusion). A single high titer in any test does not prove the presence of active infection.

Guidelines for interpretation of test results are presented below and in Table 157-1. Exceptions to these generalizations may occur.

A dye test or IFA test titer of ≥1:1000, a high IgM-IFA test titer (≥1:80), or high DS-IgM-ELISA or IgM-ISA titer (≥6, as a guideline) are probably diagnostic of recent acute infection whether or not symptoms are present. In an individual with a positive titer in the dye test or IFA test, absence of IgM-IFA test or DS-IgM-ELISA or IgM-ISA antibodies almost always excludes very recent infection.

Ocular toxoplasmosis The diagnosis of ocular toxoplasmosis in older children and adults may be difficult because the level of antibody titer in serum does not necessarily correlate with presence of active lesions in the fundus. A patient with active *Toxoplasma* chorioretinitis usually has low serologic test titers (1:4 to 1:64). If a serologic test is negative when performed on undiluted serum, toxoplasmic chorioretinitis is excluded. If retinal lesions are characteristic and serologic tests are positive (see also "Serologic Tests" above), the diagnosis can be made with a high degree of confidence. If retinal lesions are atypical and serologic tests are positive, the diagnosis of toxoplasmosis is only presumptive; the high prevalence of *Toxoplasma* antibodies in the normal population precludes assumption of a causal relationship.

Active infection in the immunocompromised patient Because antibody formation may be deficient in immunocompromised patients, available serologic methods, including the IgM-IFA, DS-IgM-ELISA, and IgM-ISA tests, are at times insufficient for detection of active infection. For example, in patients with AIDS, dye test antibody titers are <1:1000 in many cases, and IgM antibody is rarely demonstrable. These patients do make IgG antibody when measured by other methods, such as in the IFA and agglutination tests. Serologic tests to screen for *Toxoplasma* infection are useful in asymptomatic immunocompromised individuals in order to identify those patients who are at risk for primary infection or reactivation of latent infection (see also "Prevention" below). Detection of *Toxoplasma* antigen in serum and possibly in cerebrospinal fluid by an ELISA appears to be promising as an adjunct method for establishing the diagnosis of disseminated *Toxoplasma* infection in immunocompromised individuals.

Toxoplasmosis and *Toxoplasma* infection in the pregnant woman It seems advisable to perform serology in any woman considering becoming pregnant to determine whether she has *Toxoplasma* infection prior to pregnancy and to provide essential information when tests are performed during pregnancy (see "Transplacental Transmission" above).

In the absence of a routine screening program in which *Toxoplasma* serology is performed frequently during pregnancy, an IgM-IFA, DS-IgM-ELISA, or IgM-ISA test should be performed if any other serologic test is found to be positive in any titer at any time during gestation. If the IgM-IFA test, DS-IgM-ELISA, or IgM-ISA is not available, a repeat serologic test should be obtained in 3 weeks to determine if the titer is stable or rising. No further evaluation is necessary if the IgM-IFA, DS-IgM-ELISA, or IgM-ISA test is negative and an IFA or dye test titer is stable and <1:1000 (<300 IU). If the dye test or IFA test is ≥1:1000 (≥300 IU) and stable (regardless of titer in the IgM-IFA test), the infection should be considered to have been acquired *at least* 4 weeks earlier and probably more than 8 weeks before the serum was obtained. For practical purposes, risk to the fetus is very low if the dye test or IFA test titer is ≥ 1:1000 and stable in the first 2 months of pregnancy.

Whereas titers in the dye test or IFA test may have peaked and stabilized by 8 weeks after onset of infection, titers in the CF or IHA test may continue to rise for 4 to 6 months or longer after acquisition of infection. Therefore, rises in these latter two tests may not be helpful in defining when infection occurred relative to the time of conception and should not be used as the sole test for this purpose.

A common problem arises when an asymptomatic woman is tested for *Toxoplasma* antibody late in the first trimester or in the second trimester of pregnancy and her IFA or dye test titer is found to be in the vicinity of 1:2000, her IgM-IFA, DS-IgM-ELISA or IgM-ISA test titer is found to be negative, and no significant rise in titer in any test is demonstrable. It is not possible to establish whether infection occurred before, at, or after conception in this situation. Detection of *Toxoplasma* antigen in amniotic fluid may become a useful adjunct in determining whether the fetus of a woman who acquired *Toxoplasma* during the current pregnancy is infected. Its use in this setting is experimental at this time, however.

THERAPY **Therapy in specific clinical settings** The need for and duration of therapy are determined by the clinical severity of illness and by the underlying medical problem.

Most immunologically normal patients with lymphadenopathic toxoplasmosis do not require specific treatment. Indication for treatment in these cases is severe and persistent symptoms. Evidence of serious damage to vital organs is also an indication for therapy. Infections acquired via transfusions or in laboratory accidents may be more severe than naturally acquired infections and probably should be treated.

TABLE 157-1 Guidelines for interpretation of commonly employed serologic tests in the diagnosis of toxoplasmosis*

	IgG Sabin-Feldman dye test	Indirect fluorescent antibody (IFA) test	Indirect fluorescent antibody test for IgM *Toxoplasma* antibodies (IgM-IFA)	DS-IgM-ELISA or IgM-ISA	Indirect hemagglutination (IHA) test	Complement fixation (CF) test	Direct agglutination
Positive titer	1:4, undiluted†	1:10‡	1:2 infants‡ 1:10 adults‡	≥2	1:16‡	1:4‡	≥1:20
Titer in acute infection	≥1:1000	≥1:1000	≥1:80	≥6	≥1:1000	Varies among laboratories	Relatively low, usually <1:1000
Titer in chronic (latent) infection	1:4–1:2000	1:8–1:2000	Negative to 1:20	0–1	1:16–1:256	Negative to 1:8	Later may be ≥1:6000
Duration of elevation of titer	Years	Years	Weeks to months; occasionally years	Unknown, often >1 year	Years	Years	
Special considerations	*1* No known cross-reactions or false-positive results in humans.	*1* Antibody measured is same as that measured in dye test. *2* Antinuclear antibodies may cause false-positive results.	*1* Either antinuclear antibodies or rheumatoid factor (IgM) may cause false-positive results. Rheumatoid factor may be absorbed from serum.	*1* Limited experience with this new test. *2* No cross-reaction with rheumatoid factor or antinuclear antibody if Fab_2 conjugate used.	*1* Not useful for diagnosis of congenital toxoplasmosis. *2* IHA antibodies rise later than in dye test and IFA. May be especially useful if rising IHA titer can be demonstrated.	*1* Antigen preparations have not been standardized. *2* CF antibodies also rise later than dye test and IFA; see special consideration *2* under IHA.	*1* Measures IgG. *2* Titer more often less than dye test in early weeks of acute infection. *3* Titer more often higher than dye test in older infection and much greater in chronic infection.

* *These guidelines are useful in the interpretation of test results, but exceptions to these generalizations may occur.*
† *In some cases of eye disease, the dye test may be positive only in undiluted serum.*
‡ *These values are representative, but normal values for each laboratory may differ significantly.*

Patients with active chorioretinitis should be treated with specific therapy. When there is potential for serious visual impairment secondary to macular or optic nerve involvement, corticosteroids are added to the regimen. For treatment of active ocular toxoplasmosis, pyrimethamine and sulfadiazine should be administered for 1 month. Within 10 days, the borders of retinal lesions should become sharper and the vitreous haze should disappear. In 60 to 70 percent of cases, there is a favorable clinical response. If the response is not favorable, repeated courses of pyrimethamine and sulfadiazine are needed. If vision is endangered by lesions involving the macula, optic nerve head, or papillomacular bundle, systemic corticosteroids should be added. Since the majority of new lesions appear contiguous to old ones, photocoagulation has been used to treat active lesions and to prevent spread of lesions. Occasionally, vitrectomy and removal of the lens may be needed to restore visual acuity.

Because of the high mortality rate associated with toxoplasmosis in patients whose resistance to infection is compromised by underlying disease or by therapy (e.g., corticosteroids or cytotoxic drugs), toxoplasmosis should be treated in all immunocompromised individuals. In immunocompromised patients, serologic evidence of acute infection (with or without signs and symptoms of infection) or demonstration of tachyzoites in tissue (with or without serologic test titers or signs and symptoms) is an indication for therapy. Improvement has been reported to occur in the majority of patients to whom specific therapy was administered. Considering the diagnosis early enough to institute treatment is the major problem.

When a pregnant woman who acquired infection at any time during pregnancy is treated, the chance of congenital infection in her infant is decreased but not eliminated. Pyrimethamine is a potential teratogen; therefore, sulfadiazine (which is highly effective in animal models when used alone) should be used alone if a decision is made to treat during the first trimester of pregnancy. When infection occurs during the first trimester, some authorities have recommended therapeutic abortion because of the high probability of severe damage when infection occurs early in fetal life. Other authorities recommend treatment rather than abortion because the risk of transmission of the infection to the fetus is low (approximately 15 percent) in the first trimester and because the incidence of congenital toxoplasmosis can be reduced significantly by intrapartum therapy.

Pyrimethamine plus sulfadiazine or trisulfapyrimidines In vivo, pyrimethamine and sulfadiazine act synergistically against *Toxoplasma.* Clinical experience confirms the efficacy of this combination. Comparative tests have shown that sulfapyrazine, sulfamethazine, and sulfamerazine are about as effective as sulfadiazine. In general, other sulfonamides are much less effective.

Pyrimethamine In adults, a loading dose of 100 to 200 mg pyrimethamine is given orally in two divided doses on the first 2 days of treatment. In young children, a loading dose of 2 mg per kilogram of body weight (not to exceed adult loading dose) is given for the first 2 to 3 days of treatment. The maintenance dose is 1 mg per kilogram of body weight (with a usual maximum of 25 mg) in a single dose. The dosage may be raised to 50 mg per day to treat severe disease in immunodeficient patients. In view of the drug's half-life of 4 to 5 days, administration of the maintenance dose at 3- to 4-day intervals has been suggested. Daily administration is recommended for the patient who is very ill, since there are no data concerning absorption of the drug in this situation. Daily therapy is also recommended for active ocular infection. Pyrimethamine is available only in tablet form.

Pyrimethamine is a folic acid antagonist and produces a dose-related, usually gradual, and reversible depression of the bone marrow. Anemia, leukopenia, and thrombocytopenia may occur. Platelet and peripheral blood cell counts should be evaluated twice weekly in any patient receiving pyrimethamine.

Folinic acid To prevent suppression of the bone marrow, folinic acid (calcium leucovorin) is administered in conjunction with pyrimethamine therapy. Optimal frequency for administration of folinic acid has not been established. A single oral dose of 5 to 20 mg daily is recommended. If folinic acid is not available, bakers' yeast (three to four cakes daily) may be used to prevent toxicity due to pyrimethamine. Neither folinic acid nor bakers' yeast inhibits the action of pyrimethamine on *T. gondii,* whereas folic acid does.

Sulfadiazine and trisulfapyrimidines The loading dose is 50 to 75 mg per kilogram of body weight; thereafter, a total daily dose of 75 to 100 mg per kilogram of body weight is administered in four divided doses at intervals of approximately 6 h. Tablet and liquid oral forms as well as an intravenous form of sulfadiazine are available. The potential toxicities of sulfonamides (e.g., crystalluria, hematuria, and rash) must be carefully monitored. Hypersensitivity reactions to sulfonamides are a particular problem in patients with AIDS. In this case, 50 mg per day of pyrimethamine has been administered alone. If standard therapy with 25 mg per day of pyrimethamine and 6 to 8 g per day of trisulfapyrimidines or sulfadiazine is not effective, the daily dose of pyrimethamine should be increased to 50 mg. If therapy is limited by adverse reaction to the sulfonamide, pyrimethamine (50 mg per day) may be used alone.

Other drugs Trimethoprim alone or in combination with a sulfonamide has not been proved to be effective in treatment of toxoplasmosis in humans, but the activity of this combination in vitro and in vivo in animal models warrants carefully designed and controlled clinical trials. This combination is significantly less active than the combination of pyrimethamine with sulfadiazine.

Spiramycin is less active and less toxic than the combination of pyrimethamine and sulfadiazine. This antibiotic can be obtained through the Food and Drug Administration in the United States and is available in most other countries in North America and Europe. The usual dose of 2 to 4 g per day for adults is administered orally in two to four divided dosages. Spiramycin can reduce the incidence of congenital transmission. Clindamycin is concentrated in the choroid and has been used to treat ocular toxoplasmosis, but efficacy has not been demonstrated in controlled clinical trials.

Duration of therapy Optimal duration of specific therapy has not been defined for any form of toxoplasmosis. Specific therapy should be continued for 4 to 6 weeks in a patient who appears to be immunologically normal but who requires treatment for severe and persistent symptoms or evidence of damage to vital organs (e.g., chorioretinitis, myocarditis). Longer treatment may be necessary.

It seems advisable to treat an immunocompromised patient for at least 4 to 6 weeks *beyond* complete resolution of all signs and symptoms of active disease. Careful follow-up of these patients is imperative because relapse may occur and requires prompt reinstitution of therapy. Relapse of central nervous system disease is frequent in patients with AIDS. There are no data as to whether prolonged therapy or prophylaxis should be used. Pyrimethamine plus sulfadoxine administered once or twice a week has been used in attempts to prevent relapse after therapy, but no controlled data are available to determine whether this is useful. Although therapy may be effective against *T. gondii* tachyzoites and may induce a beneficial clinical response, it does not eradicate cysts from the central nervous system.

Desmonts and Couvreur suggest that an acutely infected pregnant woman should be treated with spiramycin and use a total dose of 2 to 3 g daily, administered orally in four divided doses. A 3-week course of treatment is alternated with 2 weeks without treatment from the time of diagnosis until term.

PREVENTION Measures for prevention of infection involve intervention in the cycle of transmission and are most important for immunodeficient patients and seronegative pregnant women. It is important that patients at high risk be educated concerning the avoidance of cysts (in undercooked meat) and contact with sporulated oocysts (from cats). To kill cysts, meat should be heated to 60°C or frozen at −20°C. (Commercial freezers do not reach or maintain this temperature reliably.) Hands should be washed after touching uncooked meat, and fruits and vegetables that may be contaminated with oocysts should be washed. Dry heat (66°C) or boiling water renders oocysts noninfectious. Contact with cat feces should be avoided.

There are no definitive data to allow for a firm recommendation regarding the use of whole blood, leukocyte transfusions, or organ transplants when a donor is seropositive for *Toxoplasma* antibodies. It seems reasonable, however, not to use blood or blood products donated by an individual with *Toxoplasma* antibody in an immunosuppressed individual, and an organ transplanted to a seronegative recipient should be from an individual without serologic evidence of *Toxoplasma* infection.

No effective vaccine to prevent infection with *Toxoplasma* has been developed.

REFERENCES

Araujo FG, Remington JS: Antigenemia in recently acquired acute toxoplasmosis. J Infect Dis 141:144, 1980

Conley FK, Remington JS: *Toxoplasma gondii* infection of the central nervous system. Use of the PAP method to demonstrate *Toxoplasma* in formalin-fixed paraffin-embedded tissue sections. Hum Pathol 12:690, 1981

Desmonts G, Couvreur J: Congenital toxoplasmosis: A prospective study of 378 pregnancies. N Engl J Med 290:1110, 1974

Dorfman RF, Remington JS: Value of lymph node biopsy in the diagnosis of acute acquired toxoplasmosis. N Engl J Med 289:878, 1973

Dubey JP et al: Characterization of the new fecal form of *Toxoplasma gondii*. J Parasitol 56:447, 1970

Kimball AC et al: Congenital toxoplasmosis: A prospective study of 4048 obstetric patients. Am J Obstet Gynecol 111:211, 1971

Luft BJ et al: Primary and reactivated *Toxoplasma* infection in patients with cardiac transplants. Ann Intern Med 99:27, 1983

——— et al: Toxoplasmic encephalitis in patients with acquired immune deficiency syndrome. JAMA 252:913, 1984

———, Remington JS: Acute *Toxoplasma* infection among family members of patients with acute lymphadenopathic toxoplasmosis. Arch Intern Med 144:53, 1984

———, ———: Toxoplasmosis of the central nervous system, in *Current Clinical Topics in Infectious Diseases 6*, JS Remington, MN Swartz (eds). New York, McGraw-Hill, 1985, pp 315–358

Naot Y, Remington JS: An enzyme-linked immunosorbent assay for detection of IgM antibodies to *Toxoplasma gondii:* Use for diagnosis of acute acquired toxoplasmosis. J Infect Dis 142:757, 1980

O'Connor GR: Manifestations and management of ocular toxoplasmosis. Bull NY Acad Med 50:192, 1974

Remington JS, Desmonts G: Toxoplasmosis, in *Infectious Diseases of the Fetus and Newborn Infant*, 2d ed. JS Remington, JO Klein (eds). Philadelphia, Saunders, 1983

Ruskin J, Remington JS: Toxoplasmosis in the compromised host. Ann Intern Med 84:193, 1976

Townsend JJ et al: Acquired toxoplasmosis. Arch Neurol 32:335, 1975

158 PNEUMOCYSTIS CARINII PNEUMONIA

PETER D. WALZER

DEFINITION *Pneumocystis carinii* is an opportunistic pathogen whose natural habitat is the lung. The organism is an important cause of pneumonia in the compromised host.

ETIOLOGY The taxonomy of *P. carinii* is unsettled, but the generally accepted view is that it is a protozoan. The organism exists in two basic forms: the small (1 to 4 μm), pleomorphic, more numerous trophozoites; the 5- to 7-μm cyst, which has a thick wall and contains up to eight daughter forms, termed *sporozoites*. The sporozoites excyst and appear to develop into trophozoites. The life cycle of *P. carinii* is poorly understood, but may involve different forms of reproduction for the trophozoite and cyst stages; an intracellular phase in the life cycle of *P. carinii* has not been identified. *P. carinii* of animal origin has been grown in tissue culture. Ultrastructurally, *P. carinii* has a primitive organelle system, but little is known about its metabolism.

EPIDEMIOLOGY *P. carinii* has a worldwide distribution among humans and has been found in a variety of animals. Organisms for these hosts are morphologically identical, but species or strain differences probably exist. Data about environmental sources of *P. carinii* are lacking. Serologic surveys indicate that most normal children have been exposed to the organism by 3 to 4 years of age. Animal model experiments have demonstrated that *P. carinii* is transmitted by the airborne route. Human-to-human transmission has been suggested by the occurrence of outbreaks of pneumocystis pneumonia among institutionalized debilitated infants and in hospitals caring for immunosuppressed patients. Based on animal studies, the incubation period is thought to be 4 to 8 weeks.

PATHOGENESIS *P. carinii* pneumonia occurs in the following hosts: premature, malnourished infants; children with primary immunodeficiency diseases; patients receiving immunosuppressive therapy (particularly corticosteroids) for cancer, organ transplantation, and other disorders; and patients with the acquired immunodeficiency syndrome (AIDS). AIDS is currently the most common underlying disease for *P. carinii;* conversely, *P. carinii* is the most common opportunistic infection in AIDS and the leading cause of death (see Chap. 257).

Available data suggest that impaired cellular immunity is the major host predisposing factor in the development of pneumocystis pneumonia. Antibodies are produced locally and systemically in response to exposure to *P. carinii,* but do not appear to have a protective role. Pneumocystis pneumonia which develops with the use of immunosuppressive drugs probably represents reactivation of latent infection. At some institutions the incidence of the disease has been related to the intensity of the immunosuppression. *P. carinii* pneumonia which develops in patients with primary immunodeficiency diseases and AIDS could arise from latent infection with the progressive breakdown of host defenses, or could be acquired by contagion.

PATHOLOGY The histopathologic features of *P. carinii* pneumonia in humans and experimental animals are identical. Early in the infection the organisms line up along walls of alveoli in close apposition to the type I pneumocyte. The interaction of *P. carinii* with this alveolar cell plays a major role in the host-parasite relationship in the infection. The organisms slowly propagate and, as seen on methenamine silver–stained lung sections, gradually fill the alveolar spaces. With hematoxylin and eosin staining there is the typical foamy, vacuolated alveolar exudate which consists of organisms, host serum proteins, debris, and surfactant. On electron microscopy in the animal model there is a series of changes in alveolar microenvironment which culminate in damage to the type I cell. Very rarely, *P. carinii* has been found in tissue beyond the lungs.

The host inflammatory changes are mild and nonspecific, even with extensive infection. Hypertrophy of alveolar type II cells can frequently be found and has been interpreted as a reparative response. Alveolar macrophages are present but usually not prominent in phagocytosis of the organism. In most compromised hosts there is a mild mononuclear cell interstitial cell infiltrate. However, malnourished infants display an intense interstitial plasma cell infiltrate which was responsible for the disease's early name of "interstitial plasma cell pneumonia."

CLINICAL FEATURES Patients with *P. carinii* pneumonia complain of dyspnea, fever, and nonproductive cough. When corticosteroids have been administered, symptoms frequently begin after the dose has been tapered. The duration of illness until diagnosis is typically 1 to 2 weeks, although considerable variation exists, particularly among patients with AIDS in whom this time span may be much longer (see Chap. 257). Physical findings include tachypnea, tachycardia, and cyanosis but lung auscultation reveals few abnormalities. The white blood count is variable and usually governed by the patient's underlying disease. Arterial blood gases demonstrate hypoxemia, increased alveolar-arterial oxygen gradient, and respiratory alkalosis. Alterations in pulmonary function tests (e.g., vital capacity, diffusing capacity) are also present. The classic findings on chest radiograph consist of bilateral diffuse infiltrates beginning in the perihilar regions; with time, air bronchograms develop. Variants (e.g., nodular densities, unilateral infiltrates) to this picture have also been reported. Some patients may have a normal chest radiograph early in the course of the disease but demonstrate increased uptake on gallium scan.

P. carinii pneumonia in AIDS follows a more chronic and indolent course. The average duration of pulmonary symptoms is about 4 weeks, but some patients may be ill for several months. The cough and shortness of breath may be overlooked unless a careful history is taken, and fever may be present with other infectious complications of AIDS. Objective measurements (e.g., respiratory rate and arterial oxygenation) are also less severely impaired in AIDS patients.

DIAGNOSIS Since the clinical picture of *P. carinii* can be produced by many different infectious and noninfectious agents, diagnosis must be made by specific identification of the organism. Culture of human *P. carinii* is not yet feasible, and serology, whether based on antibody or antigen detection, is not reliable. Definitive diagnosis is made by histopathologic staining. Stains which selectively stain the cell wall of *P. carinii* cysts are the most popular. Methenamine silver is the prototype; toluidine blue and cresyl echt violet are simpler, more rapid alternatives. Stains such as Giemsa's or Diff Quik stain both the trophozoite and cyst forms of *P. carinii;* these stains also stain host tissues, and hence require a greater degree of experience for proper interpretation. Recently, *P. carinii* has been observed in Wright's and Gram's stains.

P. carinii is present rarely in sputum, and infrequently in transtracheal aspiration, so a more invasive procedure is usually necessary to obtain adequate specimens. This is best performed early in the patient's hospitalization according to an organized protocol with close cooperation between clinicians and laboratories. In recent years, fiberoptic bronchoscopy with bronchoalveolar lavage and/or transbronchial biopsy has become the most widely used procedure in adults with a diagnostic yield of ≥90 percent in patients with AIDS and about 40 percent in other immunocompromised hosts. The reasons for higher diagnostic efficacy in AIDS patients are unclear but may possibly reflect a higher organism burden. Open lung biopsy is generally performed when bronchoscopy is nondiagnostic or when infection with an additional organism is suspected.

COURSE AND PROGNOSIS According to current concepts, *P. carinii* causes an asymptomatic infection in the normal host but an almost invariably fatal pneumonia in the compromised host unless treatment is given. In premature infants the mortality of *P. carinii* pneumonia is 50 percent, and in the animal model the disease is reversible with removal of corticosteroids. The prognosis of *P. carinii* pneumonia in response to therapy is influenced by such factors as the status of the underlying disease, host nutrition, degree of abnormalities in respiratory function, prior lung damage (e.g, radiation), and total leukocyte and lymphocyte counts. Concomitant infection with other opportunistic pathogens frequently occurs and may adversely affect treatment of *P. carinii*.

TREATMENT The two major drugs used in the treatment of *P. carinii* pneumonia have been trimethoprim-sulfamethoxazole (TMP-SMX) and pentamidine isethionate. These drugs are equally effective, with success rates of 50 to 80 percent in different series. TMP-SMX inhibits folic acid synthesis, and pentamidine affects several different systems in cell replication; however, their mode of action against *P. carinii* is unknown. TMP-SMX is administered orally or intravenously in a dose of 20 mg/kg per day TMP and 100 mg/kg per day SMX in four divided doses for 14 days. Optimal serum levels in adults are ≥5 μg/mL TMP and 100 to 150 μg/mL SMX; these guidelines can be used to adjust the dose of TMP-SMX in renal insufficiency. TMP-SMX is preferred over pentamidine in non-AIDS patients because it is much better tolerated.

Pentamide is given intramuscularly or by slow intravenous infusion in a dose of 4 mg/kg per day for 14 days. Side effects occur in about 50 percent of patients and include painful induration at injection sites and systemic reactions, such as hypoglycemia, hyperglycemia, hypocalcemia, azotemia, and hepatic dysfunction.

Response to TMP-SMX or pentamidine begins on the average after 4 days of treatment and is characterized by improvement in fever, respiratory symptoms, and blood gases; chest radiograph findings usually lag behind. If a response fails to occur with one drug within 5 to 7 days, it is best to substitute the other agent. The combination of TMP-SMX and pentamidine does not appear to improve efficacy and may increase the risk of toxicity. General supportive measures including maintenance of adequate oxygenation, fluid and electrolyte balance, and nutrition are also important. Corticosteroids and other immunosuppressive drugs should be tapered to as low a dose as permitted by the patient's underlying disease. Except for patients with AIDS, recurrence of *P. carinii* pneumonia is generally uncommon, but has occurred in about 10 percent of pediatric patients at selected institutions.

Success rates for the treatment of the initial episode of *P. carinii* pneumonia in AIDS are similar to those for other immunocompromised hosts. However, AIDS patients respond more slowly and appear to require longer duration of therapy. Organisms can be found in the lungs even after 4 to 6 weeks of treatment. *P. carinii* pneumonia recurs in 20 to 30 percent of AIDS patients and is usually refractory to any form of therapy. AIDS patients have a high frequency (60 to 80 percent) of adverse reactions (rash, leukopenia, fever) to TMP-SMX which often requires discontinuation of the drug. The mechanism of these effects is unclear, and treatment with folinic acid has not been helpful. AIDS patients may also be somewhat more prone to developing leukopenia with pentamidine.

The experience in the treatment of *P. carinii* infection in AIDS has stimulated a search for alternative drugs. Pyrimethamine and sulfadiazine appear to be effective but have the same potential problems as TMP-SMX. Dapsone and difluoromethylornithine (DFMO), an inhibitor of polyamine biosynthesis, are undergoing clinical evaluation.

PREVENTION Controlled studies have shown that TMP-SMX in a dose of 5 mg/kg per day TMP and 25 mg/kg per day SMX can prevent *P. carinii* pneumonia in selected high-risk populations. Although chronic administration of TMP-SMX is well-tolerated in non-AIDS patients, a high incidence of side effects has limited its use in patients with AIDS. TMP-SMX is not lethal to *P. carinii,* and hence is only effective as long as it is being taken. Since *P. carinii* may be communicable, patients with the disease should be separated from direct contact with other susceptible hosts.

REFERENCES

Cushion MT et al: *Pneumocystis carinii:* Growth variables and estimates in the A549 and WI-38 VA 13 cell lines. Exper Parasitol 60:43, 1985

Gordin FM et al: Adverse reactions to trimethoprim-sulfamethoxazole in patients with the acquired immunodeficiency syndrome. Ann Intern Med 100:495, 1984

Haverkos HW: Assessment of therapy for *Pneumocystis carinii* pneumonia. Am J Med 76:501, 1984

Helmick CG, Green JK: Pentamidine-associated hypotension and route of administration. Ann Intern Med 103:480, 1985

Hughes WT: Natural mode of acquisition for de novo infection with *Pneumocystis carinii*. J Infect Dis 145:842, 1982

———: Trimethoprim-sulfamethoxazole therapy for *Pneumocystis carinii* pneumonitis in children. Rev Infect Dis 4:602, 1982

Kovacs JA et al: *Pneumocystis carinii* pneumonia: A comparison between patients with the acquired immunodeficiency syndrome and patients with other immunodeficiencies. Ann Intern Med 100:663, 1984

Murray JF et al: Pulmonary complications of the acquired immunodeficiency syndrome: Report of a National Heart, Lung and Blood Institute workshop. N Engl J Med 310:1682, 1984

Shelhamer JH et al: Persistence of *Pneumocystis carinii* in lung tissue of acquired immunodeficiency syndrome patients treated for *Pneumocystis* pneumonia. Am Rev Resp Dis 130:1161, 1984

Walzer PD et al: Lymphocyte changes during chronic administration and withdrawal of corticosteroids: Relevance to *Pneumocystis carinii* pneumonia. J Immunol 133:2502, 1984

——— et al: *Pneumocystis carinii* pneumonia in the United States: Epidemiologic, clinical and diagnostic features. Ann Intern Med 80:83, 1974

———, YOUNG LS: The clinical relevance of animal models of *Pneumocystis carinii* pneumonia. Diag Microbiol Infect Dis 2:1, 1984

YOUNG LS (ed): *Pneumocystis carinii Pneumonia: Pathogenesis, Diagnosis, Treatment*. New York, Dekker, 1984

159 BABESIOSIS

JAMES J. PLORDE

DEFINITION AND HISTORY Known since biblical times, this cosmopolitan infection of domestic and wild animals is caused by protozoa of the genus *Babesia*. These organisms are transmitted by ticks, multiply in red blood cells, and produce an acute febrile hemolytic anemia, the most prominent manifestation of which is hemoglobinuria.

EPIDEMIOLOGY AND CLINICAL MANIFESTATIONS The first human infection was described in Yugoslavia by Skrabalo in 1957. This and six other European cases were particularly severe with high fever, hemoglobinuria, jaundice, and renal failure. Both in their clinical presentation and in the presence of small intraerythrocytic parasites they closely resembled falciparum malaria with which they were originally confused. All seven occurred in splenectomized patients and five ended fatally. The causative agents were bovine parasites (*B. bovis, B. divergens*). Some 100 cases have now been documented in the United States. Two California cases resembled the European infections and were thought to be caused by equine babesia. The remaining cases have been acquired during the summer months on Cape Cod and the offshore islands lying between New York and Massachusetts, including Long Island, Fire Island, Shelter Island, Nantucket, and Martha's Vineyard. All were caused by a rodent parasite, *B. microti,* and approximately 80 percent occurred in patients with intact spleens. The patients experienced a prolonged illness characterized by the insidious onset of fever, chills, sweating, myalgia, and mild to moderate hemolytic anemia presumably caused by direct, parasite-induced damage to the erythrocytic membrane. The physical examination was usually negative except for occasional splenomegaly. In general, clinical manifestations have been more severe in asplenic subjects. Most patients were over 50 years of age and all but one recovered. The carrier state persisted for weeks to months in some patients and in three resulted in subsequent transfusion-induced infections. Two of the three recipients were asplenic; the third was an elderly individual who represents the only fatality in the series. Serologic studies suggest that most patients infected with *B. microti* are asymptomatic; seroconversion rates of nearly 6 percent and point prevalence rates of 2 to 4.4 percent have been noted in endemic areas. All age groups seem equally susceptible. Like their symptomatic counterparts, patients with subclinical infections may remain parasitemic for several months.

B. microti has been found in field moles and deer mice in New York State, Utah, and California. On the offshore islands of New England, however, the principal reservoir is the white-footed mouse. The northern deer tick, *Ixodes dammini,* which also serves as the vector in Lyme disease, is responsible for the transmission of *B. microti.* This hard-bodied tick takes a blood meal during each of its three developmental stages: larva, nymph, and adult. Rodents are the principal hosts of the first two stages while deer host the adult ticks. Only the nymphs, which feed from May through September, are capable of transmitting *B. microti* to humans. Since the engorged nymph measures 2 mm in diameter, infested patients may be oblivious to its presence. Transovarial transmission does not occur.

DIAGNOSIS The diagnosis depends on the demonstration of the intraerythrocytic parasite in Giemsa-stained peripheral blood smears. Like malaria parasites, these organisms measure 2 to 3 μm in diameter and demonstrate red-staining nuclear material with blue cytoplasm. In contrast to malaria parasites, however, neither gametocytes nor pigment are seen. As the parasites multiply by a nonsynchronous budding process, the organism displays marked pleomorphism; a single red cell may contain multiple parasites in different developmental stages. Unique basket shapes, tetrads, and trophozoites with multiple chromatin dots are helpful distinguishing features. In heavy infections, organisms can be seen outside red blood cells. Serologic diagnosis can be made with the indirect fluorescent antibody test or enzyme-linked immunosorbent assay. Because the disease is insidious in onset, most infected patients have titers ≥1024 at the time they present for medical care. There is no correlation between disease severity and the titer level; cross reactions with other *Babesia* species and malaria may be seen, but titers with homologous antigens are generally higher. Active infections have been demonstrated in smear-negative, serology-positive infections by inducing infection in experimental animals.

TREATMENT Mild disease should be managed symptomatically with antipyretics. If significant hemolysis ensues, transfusion may be warranted. In more severe infections specific therapy should be attempted. Although chloroquine provides symptomatic improvement, it appears to have little activity against this parasite. Quinine and clindamycin therapy has been successful in several patients. Antitrypanosomal agents also appear effective, and, in life-threatening infections, pentamidine should be considered. This agent appears to be effective in controlling the clinical manifestations of babesiosis and decreasing parasitemia; it may not eradicate the organism. Exchange transfusions are helpful in fulminant infections.

PREVENTION The prevention of *B. microti* infections in humans is difficult. Individuals summering on the offshore islands of New England should consider the use of insect repellents containing diethyltoluamide and examine themselves daily for the presence of the 2- to 3-mm nymphs. A pilot tick control program has been initiated on one of the islands. Asplenic patients should be advised to avoid endemic areas. To avoid transfusion-transmitted babesiosis, blood donors should be screened serologically for evidence of *B. microti* infection.

REFERENCES

CHISHOLM ES et al: *Babesia microti* infection in man: Evaluation of an indirect immunofluorescent antibody test. Am J Med Hyg 27:14, 1978

DAMMIN GJ et al: Babesiosis, in *Seminars in Infectious Diseases,* L Weinstein, J Fields (eds). New York, Stratton, 1978, pp 169–199

———: The rising incidence of clinical *Babesia microti* infections. Hum Pathol 12:398, 1981

FRANCIOLI PB et al: Response of babesiosis to pentamidine therapy. Ann Intern Med 94:326, 1981

JACOBY GA et al: Treatment of transfusion-transmitted babesiosis by exchange transfusion. N Engl J Med 303:1098, 1980

ROSNER F et al: Babesiosis in splenectomized adults: Review of 22 reported cases. Am J Med 76:696, 1984

RUEBUSH TK II et al: Development and persistence of antibody in persons with *Babesia microti*. Am J Trop Med Hyg 30:291, 1981

——— et al: Epidemiology of human babesiosis on Nantucket Island. Am J Trop Med Hyg 30:937, 1981

STEKETEE RW et al: Babesiosis in Wisconsin: A new focus of disease transmission. JAMA 253:2675, 1985

SUN T et al: Morphologic and clinical observations in human infection with *Babesia microti*. J Infect Dis 148:239, 1983

WITTER M et al: Successful chemotherapy of transfusion babesiosis. Ann Intern Med 96:601, 1982

160 GIARDIASIS

JAMES J. PLORDE

ETIOLOGY AND EPIDEMIOLOGY *Giardia lamblia* is a pear-shaped multiflagellar protozoan that parasitizes the human duodenum and jejunum of humans and other animals where it multiplies by longitudinal fission. Under a microscope, its pyriform shape, two nuclei, and central parabasal body give the organism the appearance of a face with two large eyes. It may actively browse the unstirred mucous layer at the bases of the microvilli or attach to the intestinal mucosa by means of a large ventral sucking disk. Unattached trophozoites may be carried in the fecal stream to the large bowel. If their passage through the gut is hurried, they will exit unchanged in the liquid stool and perish rapidly. With normal colonic transit times, however, the organisms retract their flagella, envelop themselves in a protective membrane, and undergo nuclear division. The resulting quadrinucleate cysts are infectious and may be transmitted to new hosts by a number of fecal-oral routes. Cysts deposited in cold water can survive for more than 2 months and have been shown to be resistant to chlorine concentrations (0.4 mg per liter) routinely used in community purification systems. The ingestion of water contaminated with as few as 10 cysts is sufficient to establish human infection. Not surprisingly, waterborne outbreaks in humans have been documented repeatedly during the past two decades. In fact, *G. lamblia* is now the single most frequently defined cause of waterborne outbreaks of diarrhea in the United States. They have involved campers who have drunk from remote surface waters, skiers who have used well water, and ordinary citizens served by chlorinated municipal systems. Contamination of the water supply with raw sewage has been found in several outbreaks. In others, *G. lamblia*–infected beavers were located within the watershed, suggesting that these mammals may serve as alternate reservoirs. Waterborne cysts are also thought to be responsible for the high incidence of giardiasis in travelers returning from third-world countries. Food may also serve as a transmission vehicle in these areas as well.

Direct person-to-person spread occurs with some frequency. This is most dramatically evident among male homosexuals practicing anilingus and groups of ambulatory, non-toilet-trained children. It also appears to be responsible for the secondary cases seen in families of infected children.

Giardiasis is a cosmopolitan infection that is particularly common in areas with poor sanitation and among populations unable to maintain adequate levels of hygiene. In developing countries, the prevalence of giardiasis often exceeds 10 percent. In the United States, *G. lamblia* is the most frequently identified intestinal parasite, being found in over 4 percent of stools submitted for parasitologic examination. Young children are three times more likely to be involved than adults; the prevalence may be particularly high among toddlers attending day-care centers and the institutionalized retarded, in whom rates exceeding 50 percent have been reported. Giardiasis is also frequent in individuals with immunoglobulin deficiencies and may be a major cause of intestinal abnormalities in this population. It has been suggested that the parasite is able to persist in such patients because of a relative deficiency of secretory IgA. Similarly, the immune deficiencies accompanying protein-calorie malnutrition are thought to enhance the susceptibility of involved individuals to parasitization with *G. lamblia*.

Among adults, parasitism is common in parents of infected children, travelers, and campers, but the precise prevalence in these populations is unknown. Achlorhydric individuals may be more susceptible to infection. Several studies have emphasized the association between male homosexuality and intestinal parasitosis; infection rates for *G. lamblia* and/or *Entamoeba histolytica* have ranged from 11 to 40 percent. In a New York study, all nontraveled immunocompetent males with giardiasis were homosexual.

PATHOLOGY AND PATHOGENESIS Clinical manifestations appear to be caused by an impairment of the absorptive capacity of the gut, particularly for fat and carbohydrates. The mechanism responsible for these changes is unknown. Mechanical blockage of the intestinal mucosa by large numbers of trophozoites, competition for essential nutrients, altered jejunal mobility with or without overgrowth of enteric bacteria or yeasts, pancreatic or biliary dysfunction, and organism-induced deconjugation of bile salts have been implicated. None, however, correlates well with disease severity, and eradication of associated microorganisms does not uniformly result in clinical improvement. Disaccharidase deficiency with lactose intolerance, altered levels of peptide hydrolyase and enteropeptidase, and decreased vitamin B_{12} absorption indicate that *G. lamblia* produces direct or indirect damage to the microvillar structure of the small bowel. Mechanical irritation to the fuzzy coat by the trophozoite's sucking disk might induce an accelerated turnover of the mucosal epithelium, resulting in functional immaturity of the transport systems. Excretion of a soluble toxin that interacts with the epithelial cell has been hypothesized, but never documented. Mucosal invasion may provoke a T cell–mediated insult to the jejunal mucosa. In experimentally infected nude mice immunologic reconstitution with lymphoid cells from previously infected animals results in marked mucosal changes including cellular infiltration and a decreased villus/crypt ratio. Similar pathologic findings have been reported in humans with giardial malabsorption. Both the structural changes and the malabsorption are reversible with specific therapy.

Although reinfection is common, the frequent occurrence of giardiasis in patients with immunologic defects, and the rarity with which it is seen in older adults, suggest that protective immunity, albeit incomplete, does develop with time. Animal experiments suggest humoral, secretory, and cellular mechanisms are all involved. The diversity of surface antigens, secretory products, and DNA banding patterns in *Giardia* isolates could influence the effectiveness of the host immune response in preventing reinfection.

CLINICAL MANIFESTATIONS In endemic situations, over two-thirds of infected patients may be asymptomatic. This ratio is usually reversed in point-source outbreaks. From 1 to 3 weeks after exposure, the patient notes the explosive onset of watery diarrhea. The stool is foul smelling, greasy in appearance, and floats. There is neither blood nor mucus. Abdominal cramping is present and is epigastric in location. The formation of large quantities of intestinal gas produces distention, sulfuric eructation, and flatulence. Anorexia, nausea, vomiting, and low-grade fever may be present. Typically, acute symptoms continue for at least 5 to 7 days. In an occasional patient, they may persist for months, leading to significant malabsorption and weight loss. More commonly, the illness resolves spontaneously in 1 to 4 weeks or lapses into a chronic phase characterized by intermittent bouts of flatulence, epigastric pain, and the passage of mushy stools. It is not unusual for patients to present in this fashion without having experienced the more acute manifestations described above. Chronic giardiasis is associated with reduced growth in preschool children. Eventually, both parasites and symptoms disappear. Lactose intolerance, however, may persist, producing a clinical picture easily confused with the parasitologic disease and subjecting the patient to unnecessary therapy.

DIAGNOSIS The diagnosis is made by identifying the cyst in formed feces or the trophozoite in diarrheal stools, duodenal secretions, or jejunal biopsies. In the majority of acute cases, the parasite can be demonstrated easily in a series of stool specimens collected and examined in the manner described for amebiasis (see Chap. 153). In acute illness, the onset of clinical manifestations may antedate the excretion of organisms by 5 to 7 days while in chronic infections the discharge of parasites is often scanty or intermittent, making laboratory confirmation more difficult. Purgation does not improve the yield. Many of these patients, however, can be diagnosed by examining specimens collected at weekly intervals for a period of 4 to 5 weeks. Alternatively, the duodenal contents can be sampled with a nylon string (Enterotest) or gastric tube and cultured by direct wet-mount preparation. Occasionally, jejunal biopsy is required to establish the diagnosis in patients with typical clinical manifestations. Immunodiagnostic methods for the rapid detection of *Giardia* antigen in feces appear both highly sensitive and specific, but are not commercially available. Enzyme-linked immunosorbent and indirect fluorescent serologic tests using axenically cultured *G. lamblia* have been developed. Their diagnostic usefulness remains to be established.

TREATMENT Treatment is usually carried out with quinacrine hydrochloride or metronidazole. Tinidazole, a more effective agent, is presently not available in the United States. Quinacrine, 0.1 g given three times daily for 5 days, eliminates the organisms in 70 to 95 percent of cases. Although the drug is usually well tolerated, it may produce gastrointestinal disturbances, exacerbate psoriasis, and, rarely, produce toxic psychosis. Metronidazole appears to be better tolerated and equally effective. A single oral dose of 2.0 g given on 3 consecutive days, 750 mg tid for 5 days, and 250 mg tid for 5 days give cure rates of 95, 95, and 70 percent, respectively. However, this drug is not currently licensed for giardiasis, and there is concern over its mutagenicity. Household contacts and sexual partners of infected patients should be examined; individuals harboring the parasite should be treated even if asymptomatic to prevent the spread to others. Pregnant women, however, should receive therapy only if severely symptomatic and never in the first trimester. Because parasitologic and clinical relapse can occur up to 7 weeks after the completion of therapy, long-term follow-up is essential.

PREVENTION Chemoprophylactic drugs are not effective in preventing the acquisition of giardiasis. Individuals visiting endemic areas should avoid the ingestion of potentially contaminated food and water. The latter may be made potable by boiling or by treating with a suitable halogen disinfectant. Most of the commercially available tablets appear effective when appropriate concentrations and contact times are utilized; they are temperature-dependent, and their dose should be increased when dealing with cold water. Custodial institutions for children should screen new admissions for the presence of *G. lamblia* and treat those found to be positive. Handwashing by children and staff must be emphasized. Community water purification systems should provide for adequate filtration as well as disinfection. Breast feeding appears to protect infants from giardiasis; this may be related to the known presence of antigiardial substances, including specific IgA antibodies, in breast milk.

REFERENCES

Black RE et al: Giardiasis in day-care centers—Evidence of person to person transmission. Pediatrics 60:486, 1977

Dykes AC et al: Municipal waterborne giardiasis: An epidemiologic investigation. Ann Intern Med 93:165, 1980

Gupta MC, Urrutia JJ: Effect of periodic antiascaris and antigiardia treatment on nutritional status of preschool children. Am J Clin Nutr 36:79, 1982

Jarroll EL Jr et al: *Giardia* cyst destruction: Effectiveness of six small-quantity water disinfection methods. Am J Trop Med Hyg 29:8, 1980

Osterholm MT et al: An outbreak of foodborne giardiasis. N Engl J Med 304:24, 1981

Solomons NW: Giardiasis: Nutritional implications. Rev Infect Dis 4:859, 1982

Speelman P: Single-dose tinidazole for the treatment of giardiasis. Antimicrob Ag Chemother 27:227, 1985

Stevens DP: Giardiasis: Host-pathogen biology. Rev Infect Dis 4:851, 1982

———: Selective primary health care: Strategies for control of disease in the developing world. XIX. Giardiasis. Rev Infect Dis 7:530, 1985

Unger LP et al: Enzyme-linked immunosorbent assay for the detection of *Giardia lamblia* in fecal specimens. J Infect Dis 149:90, 1985

161 CRYPTOSPORIDIOSIS AND OTHER PROTOZOAN INFECTIONS

JAMES J. PLORDE

CRYPTOSPORIDIOSIS

DEFINITION Cryptosporidiosis is a diarrheal disease of vertebrates produced by protozoa of the genus *Cryptosporidium.* These parasites inhabit the microvillous border of the intestinal epithelium, where they produce clinical illness ranging from an acute, self-limited, watery diarrhea in normal individuals to chronic, severe, life-threatening gastroenteritis in the immunocompromised. Unknown as human pathogens prior to 1976, cryptosporidia now rank with *Salmonella, Shigella, Campylobacter,* enterotoxigenic *Escherichia coli,* rotavirus, and *Giardia lamblia* as major enteric pathogens of humans.

ETIOLOGY Regardless of animal host, all strains of this tiny (2- to 6-μm) parasite appear morphologically identical. In the absence of firm evidence for host specificity, they can reasonably be regarded as a single species. Cryptosporidia exhibit alternating cycles of sexual and asexual reproduction and are thereby classified as sporozoan protozoa. As is true for *Toxoplasma, Isospora,* and other members of the sporozoan subgroup known as Coccidia, both cycles are completed within the gastrointestinal tract of a single host. The infective forms or oocysts are shed into the intestinal lumen of the parasitized animal. Unlike those of *Toxoplasma* and *Isospora,* cryptosporidia oocysts are fully mature and immediately infective upon passage in the feces. Following ingestion by another animal, *sporozoites* are released from the oocyst, attach themselves to the epithelial surface, and begin a series of developmental changes. Although excluded from the cytoplasm of the epithelial cell, *trophozoites* and all subsequent developmental stages are surrounded by a double membrane of host origin and are, by definition, intracellular parasites. The trophozoites divide asexually by a process of multiple fission (*schizogony*) to form *schizonts* containing eight daughter cells known as type I *merozoites.* Upon release from the schizont, each merozoite attaches itself to another epithelial cell, where it repeats the schizogony cycle, producing another generation of type I merozoites. Eventually, schizonts containing only four daughter cells are seen. Incapable of continued asexual reproduction, these type II merozoites are transformed into male (*microgamete*) and female (*macrogamete*) sexual forms. Following fertilization, the resulting *zygote* develops into an oocyst. The majority possess a thick protective cell wall which ensures their intact passage in the feces and survival in the external environment. Approximately 20 percent of the oocysts, however, fail to develop such a wall. Their thin cell membrane ruptures, releasing infective sporozoites directly into the intestinal lumen and initiating a new "autoinfective" cycle within the original host. In the normal host, the presence of innate or acquired immunity dampens both the cyclic production of type I merozoites and the formation of thin-walled oocysts, halting further parasite multiplication and terminating the acute infection. In the immunocompromised both presumably continue, explaining why such individuals develop severe, persistent infections in the absence of repeated reinfections.

EPIDEMIOLOGY Cryptosporidiosis appears to involve most vertebrate groups; the available prevalence studies demonstrate that although rare in adult animals, infection rates can be high in immature pets and farm stock. Experimental transmission of human *Cryptosporidium* strains to rodents, kittens, and puppies, and an outbreak of infection in human handlers of infected calves clearly suggest that domestic animals constitute an important reservoir of disease for humans. Disease outbreaks in day-care centers, hospitals, and urban family groups, however, indicate that most human infections result from person-to-person transmission rather than zoonotic spread. As in animals, human disease is more common in the young. In western countries, 1.4 to 4.1 percent of small children presenting to medical centers with gastroenteritis have been shown to harbor cryptosporidia oocysts; in third world countries the rates have varied from 4 to 11 percent. Up to 63 percent of children attending day-care centers during outbreaks of diarrhea have had oocysts detected in their stool. Infection rates in adults suffering from gastroenteritis are approximately one-third those reported for children and have been highest in family members of infected children, medical personnel caring for patients with cryptosporidiosis, male homosexuals, and travelers to foreign countries. Asymptomatic carriage is uncommon; other enteric pathogens, particularly *Giardia lamblia,* are recovered from a significant minority of infected patients. Since oocysts are found almost exclusively in stool, the principal transmission route is undoubtedly fecal-oral. In day-care centers and among male homosexual groups the spread is probably direct. The hardy nature of the oocysts makes it likely that there is also indirect transmission via contaminated food, water, and fomites. The increase in infection rates seen during the summer months is compatible with this hypothesis. On rare occasions oocysts have been recovered from the pharynx or found in expectorated sputum, raising the possibility that cryptosporidiosis may be acquired through contact with the respiratory secretions of infected patients.

PATHOGENESIS AND PATHOLOGY Although the jejunum is most heavily involved, cryptosporidia have been found in the pharynx, esophagus, stomach, duodenum, gallbladder, ileum, appendix, colon, and rectum of immunocompromised subjects. They appear as small, basophilic, spherical structures arranged in rows or clusters along the brush border of the epithelial cells. They color readily with Giemsa and hematoxylin-eosin, but not with acid-fast stains; they may be mistaken for epithelial blebs. Electron microscopy reveals the entire gamut of developmental forms including trophozoites, schizonts, merozoites, and macrogametes. All are covered by a double membrane derived from the reflection, fusion, and attenuation of the microvilli over the parasite. The attachment site is electron dense. Multiple, dense, membrane-bound bodies located within the apexes of the epithelial cells can be seen in the immediate vicinity. Some resemble degenerating parasites, raising the possibility that cryptosporidia can, in fact, invade the epithelial cytoplasm. By light microscopy, bowel changes appear minimal, consisting of mild-to-moderate villous atrophy, crypt enlargement, and a mononuclear infiltrate of the lamina propria.

The pathophysiology of the diarrhea that accompanies cryptosporidiosis is unknown, but its nature and intensity suggest a cholera-like enterotoxin. The vital role played by the host's immune status in the pathogenesis of the disease is indicated by both the enhanced susceptibility of the young to infection and the prolonged, severe clinical disease seen in inmmunocompromised patients. Animal studies with related coccidian parasites suggest that resistance to reinfection is mediated by T lymphocytes while the severity and duration of the primary infection are influenced by both cellular and humoral mechanisms.

CLINICAL MANIFESTATIONS Immunocompetent hosts Following an incubation period of 4 to 14 days, the patient notes the onset of an explosive, profuse, watery diarrhea accompanied by abdominal cramping. Typically, these manifestations persist for 5 to 11 days before rapidly abating; rarely, purging may continue for up to 4 weeks. When this happens, mild malabsorption with weight loss may be seen. Its shorter duration, more prominent abdominal pain and relative lack of flatulence help to distinguish cryptosporidiosis from the clinically similar *Giardia lamblia* infection. A small percentage of patients describe nausea, anorexia, low-grade fever, or vomiting. Routine laboratory work is unremarkable. Radiographic and endoscopic examinations of the gut either are normal or demonstrate mild, nonspecific abnormalities. Recovery is complete, and neither relapse nor reinfection has been reported.

Immunocompromised hosts Cryptosporidiosis has been described in patients with a broad range of immunodeficiencies. In third world countries, marasmus and other forms of childhood malnutrition have been most common. In the United States, the acquired immunodeficiency syndrome (AIDS), congenital hypogammaglobulinemia, cancer chemotherapy, and immunosuppressive management of organ transplantation patients have been the abnormalities noted most frequently. In patients with these conditions, cryptosporidiosis is usually indolent in onset and prolonged in duration. The abdominal cramping and systemic manifestations are similar to those seen in normal hosts. The diarrhea, however, is characteristically more severe; fluid losses of 1 to 17 liters a day have been described. Unless the patient's immunologic defect is reversed, the disease usually continues in a persistent or remittent fashion for the duration of life. In two-thirds, the diarrhea has lasted for more than 4 months; in a few it has persisted unabated for a number of years. Weight loss is often prominent. The prognosis depends upon the nature of the underlying immunologic abnormality; the 6-month survival rate in patients with AIDS is 50 percent. Although other intercurrent infections are usually the direct cause of death, malnutrition and complications of parenteral nutrition are often thought to play a contributory role.

DIAGNOSIS The diagnosis of cryptosporidiosis must be pursued in any immunocompromised patient who develops diarrhea. Before 1978, the diagnosis required small-bowel biopsy. The development of effective concentration and staining techniques, as well as the growing experience of clinical laboratories with this parasite, have made the recovery and identification of cryptosporidia oocysts from the stool the procedure of choice. Oocyst excretion is most intense during the first 4 or 5 days of illness, tapers during the second week, and generally stops within 2 or 3 days of the cessation of diarrhea; oocysts are rarely recovered from solid stool. Specimens should be examined immediately after passage or preserved in 2.5% potassium dichromate or 10% buffered formalin. Fresh and dichromate-preserved specimens are infectious and must be handled with care. The specimen may contain small amounts of mucus, but fecal erythrocytes or white cells are uncommon. Initially, an iodine wet mount can be made from the unconcentrated specimen and examined microscopically; the spherical 5-μm oocysts are differentiated from yeasts, which they resemble in size and morphology, by their failure to take up the iodine. As cryptosporidia oocysts are one of the few acid-fast particles found in feces, identification can be confirmed with any one of the many acid-fast staining procedures developed for mycobacteria. If the direct examinations are negative, the stool should be concentrated using either Sheather's sugar flotation or Ritchie's formalin-diethyl-acetate sedimentation procedure. The two are equally sensitive; use of both will improve yield in specimens with few oocysts. Supernatant from the former is examined by light or phase microscopy for the typical pink-tinged, refractile oocysts. Sediment from the formalin-diethylacetate procedure is acid-fast–stained before examination.

A highly sensitive and specific indirect immunofluorescent test has been described. Seroconversion occurs within 60 days of acute infection in both immunocompetent patients and those with AIDS; antibodies persist for at least 1 year. The usefulness of such tests for the diagnosis of acute infection remains undetermined.

TREATMENT AND PREVENTION In the immunocompetent patient, the disease is self-limited, and attempts at specific antiparasitic therapy are not warranted. Oral, and occasionally parenteral, rehydration may be required in small children. In the immunocompromised host, the severity and chronicity of the diarrhea warrants therapeutic intervention. The only uniformly successful approach has been the reversal of underlying immunologic abnormalities. Withdrawal of cancer chemotherapy agents, discontinuation of immunosuppressive drugs, and successful bone marrow transplantation have all resulted in cure. Specific anticryptosporidial therapy has been attempted with a large number of drugs; most have been ineffective. Some patients have experienced an amelioration or complete resolution of symptoms following treatment with spiramycin, furazolidone, or alpha-difluoromethylornithine (DFMO); however, clinical failures have been common, and parasitologic cures have been reported in few. In patients who responded clinically but continued to excrete oocysts, relapses have followed discontinuation of the therapeutic agent. Because spontaneous remissions can occur, the value of these drugs in the treatment of cryptosporidiosis remains uncertain.

The stools of patients with cryptosporidiosis are infectious. Stool precautions should be instituted at the time the diagnosis is first suspected; for the immunosuppressed patient this should be whenever diarrhea, regardless of presumed etiology, is first noted. This is particularly important in cancer chemotherapy and transplantation units, where spread of the disease, directly or indirectly, from a symptomatic patient to other immunosuppressed patients can have life-threatening consequences.

TRICHOMONIASIS

Trichomoniasis is a venereal infection caused by the protozoan *Trichomonas vaginalis*. Of the many members of the genus *Trichomonas,* three are parasites of human beings: *T. hominis* in the intestine, *T. tenax* in the oral cavity, and *T. vaginalis,* the only established pathogen, in the vagina, urethra, and prostate. All three exist only in the trophozoite stage and resemble one another morphologically. *Trichomonas vaginalis* is the largest, however, and confusion in diagnosis is rare because of the anatomic specificity of their habits. Strains varying in size, growth rates, virulence, and antigenic characteristics have been described.

Trichomonas vaginalis is transmitted by sexual intercourse. Although the organism is viable for up to 24 h in urine, semen, and water and may survive on moist washcloths for a few hours, transmission by fomites is probably uncommon. Approximately 5 percent of children born to infected mothers acquire the infection. The parasite is cosmopolitan in its distribution. It is estimated that 3 million women in the United States and 180 million worldwide are infected annually; 30 to 70 percent of their male sexual partners are parasitized, at least transiently. Prevalence correlates directly with the number of sexual contacts. The incidence in adult virgins is zero; rates as high as 70 percent have been seen in prostitutes, individuals with other venereal disease, and sexual partners of infected patients. Women with trichomoniasis are, on the average, a decade older than those with gonorrhea. Although the peak incidence is between 16 and 35 years, there is a relatively high prevalence among the 30- to 40- and 40- to 50-year-old age groups.

In the female, trichomoniasis usually presents as a persistent vaginitis. It is estimated that half of women with *Trichomonas* are asymptomatic when first diagnosed. A significant proportion, however, go on to develop clinical manifestations within 6 months. In approximately two-thirds a discharge is present and is frequently accompanied by vulvar itching (50 percent), dyspareunia (50 percent), odor (10 percent), and dysuria. This acute stage may persist for a week or months, often fluctuating in intensity; it may worsen following menstruation. Eventually the discharge and other symptoms subside and may actually disappear completely, even though the patient still harbors trichomonads. Examination shows inflammation ranging from mild hyperemia of the vaginal vault and endocervix to extensive erosion, petechial hemorrhages, and perianal intertrigo. The finding of a granular, friable, reddened endocervix (strawberry cervix) is a highly characteristic, although uncommon, finding. A discharge, typically thin, gray to yellow, and frothy in nature, is found pooled in the posterior vaginal fornix.

The prostate and urethra are the usual sites of infection in the male. Most commonly the infection is completely asymptomatic, but may present as persistent or recurring nonspecific urethritis. Approximately 5 percent of all episodes of nongonococcal urethritis in males is caused by *T. vaginalis*. The prevalence is higher among those failing tetracycline therapy. Acute purulent urethritis occurs rarely.

The diagnosis is made by examining vaginal, prostatic, or urethral secretions for the presence of *Trichomonas*. The organism may also be found in the sedimented urine. A wet mount reveals squamous epithelial cells, polymorphonuclear nucleocytes, and *T. vaginalis* with its characteristic twitching motility; although highly specific when positive, it is often negative in asymptomatic women and in patients who have douched in the previous 24 h. Stained smears provide little additional help. Culture is more sensitive but is not generally available.

Trichomonas is sometimes responsible for confusing changes in the cytologic pattern of exfoliated vaginal cells. Moreover, ordinary Papanicolaou preparations are not well suited to the diagnosis, and when trichomoniasis is suspected, fresh material should be looked at immediately.

Oral metronidazole (Flagyl), given either in dosage of 250 mg three times daily for 7 days or in a single 2-g dose, is an extremely effective therapeutic agent. Concurrent treatment of sexual partners is very important, particularly when single-dose therapy is given, if recurrent infection is to be avoided. A small number of *T. vaginalis* strains with high levels of resistance to metronidazole have been isolated from patients failing multiple courses of therapy.

The evidence that metronidazole is carcinogenic in rodents and mutagenic in bacteria mandates that the drug should not be used in the first trimester of pregnancy until further information on its teratogenicity is available. Because of the agent's antabuse-like action, alcohol consumption is contraindicated during therapy and for 24 h following its completion. Topical therapy with clotrimazole, an imidazole antifungal agent, can be employed in situations where systemic metronidazole therapy is contraindicated. The drug is applied intravaginally, in a dose of 100 mg daily for 6 days.

ISOSPORIASIS

This is an infrequently recognized disease characterized by fever, diarrhea, abdominal pain, and weight loss which results from ingestion of the oocysts of coccidia belonging to the genus *Isospora.* These sporozoan protozoa are widespread in the animal kingdom. *I. hominis* and *I. belli* have been shown to infect humans. Parasitization is much more common in children and is worldwide in distribution, particularly in tropical areas. In this country, a disproportionately large percentage of reported cases have occurred in male homosexuals.

Like the related plasmodia, there is both an asexual and sexual stage of multiplication in *I. belli* infections. However, both occur within a single host. Following the ingestion of an oocyst, *sporozoites* are released which invade the epithelial cells of the intestine to become trophozoites. These multiply asexually producing a large number of *merozoites,* which in turn invade other epithelial cells to continue the cycle. In some cells sexual gametocytes are produced. With the fertilization of the female gametocyte, an oocyst is formed which is then passed in the stool. Transmission is by the fecal-oral route. Volunteers develop symptoms about 1 week after the ingestion of viable oocysts. The illness usually has an acute onset with fever, headache, abdominal cramps, and diarrhea. Stools are often fatty and weight loss is common. Isosporiasis may be associated with a malabsorption syndrome and abnormalities of the mucosa in the small bowel. Symptoms, which presumably continue as long as the asexual cycle of multiplication continues, usually subside spontaneously within a few weeks. In the immunocompromised host, however, they are often severe, and may persist for months or even years, eventually resulting in death.

A peripheral eosinophilia occurs in approximately half of the infected patients. The diagnosis can be made by examination of stool for oocysts. These are often scanty, and concentration techniques such as zinc sulfate flotation or the formol-ether method must usually be employed. Incubation of the stool for 2 days at room temperature improves the recovery rate. Duodenal aspiration and jejunal biopsy are less cumbersome and more reliable. The oocysts stain well with the acid-fast techniques described for the closely related *Cryptosporidium* species (see above). *Isospora belli* infections have been successfully treated with combinations of pyrimethamine-sulfonamide and trimethoprim-sulfamethoxazole. The dose for the latter combination is 160/800 mg qid for 10 days, then bid for 3 weeks.

Isospora hominis is probably identical with *Sarcocystis fusiformis*. Its oocysts are believed to be infectious only for pigs and cattle in which it produces tissue sarcocysts. Humans become infected by eating undercooked pork or beef containing the cysts. These liberate trophozoites which invade intestinal epithelial cells to undergo gametogony with the formation of new oocysts. The disease in humans is usually asymptomatic, but mild self-limited gastrointestinal manifestations have been described. Therapy is not required.

BALANTIDIASIS

Balantidium coli, the largest protozoan of human beings, inhabits the large intestine. In addition to producing an asymptomatic carrier state, it elicits disease ranging from mild recurrent diarrhea to fulminant ulceration with perforation and death. In many respects the disease is similar to amebiasis in its range of manifestations, exclusive of spread to the liver.

The illness has been reproduced by feeding the organism to volunteers. The diagnosis is made by finding the trophozoite or cyst in the stool, but repeated examinations may be required because shedding of *Balantidium* is intermittent. The disease is more likely to occur in tropical areas, but at least 60 cases have been reported in the United States. Swine and rats are frequent carriers of *B. coli* and may play an important role in the spread of the disease to humans. Outbreaks have been noted in mental institutions where coprophagy implicated direct person-to-person transmission.

The tetracyclines in ordinary doses are highly effective in treatment, as is iodoquinol given in the dosage of 650 mg three times daily for 20 days. Metronidazole in the dosage used for amebiasis has also been effective (see Chap. 153).

DIENTAMEBIASIS

Dientamebiasis is an intestinal infection produced by a flagellated ameba, *Dientamoeba fragilis*. The genus and species names derive, respectively, from the binucleate nature of the trophozoite and the fragmented appearance of its nuclear chromatin. Like the related *Trichomonas* genus, the protozoan lacks a cyst stage. By virtue of its location in the large bowel, it has been thought to be spread from person to person by the fecal-oral route. However, the prevalence of the organism does not parallel that of other intestinal protozoa, its incidence in homosexual men does not correlate with the frequency of oral-anal sex, and the trophozoite is rapidly destroyed in both water and gastric juice. A mechanism of transmission compatible with these facts was suggested when *D. fragilis*–like structures were noted inside the eggs of pinworms. Several studies have now demonstrated that coinfection with these two intestinal parasites is 9 to 20 times higher than that expected by random occurrence, reinforcing the possibility that the helminth eggs may serve as a vector for the protozoan trophozoite. *D. fragilis* is a cosmopolitan parasite. Studies in this country report prevalence rates ranging from 1.4 to 18.6 percent. Rates are highest among children between 0 and 10 years of age, institutionalized individuals, communal groups, and missionaries serving in tropical areas. While *D. fragilis* was thought to be a harmless commensal of the colonic mucosal crypts, and probably is not capable of tissue invasion, it may act as a chronic irritant producing excess mucous secretion and hypermotility. Pathologic studies of surgically removed appendices shown to harbor *D. fragilis* demonstrated fibrosis that encroached upon the mucosal lymphoid tissue. Patients free of intestinal pathogens other than *D. fragilis* have reported a variety of clinical manifestations including diarrhea (58 percent) with blood or mucus (11 percent), abdominal pain (54 percent), and anal pruritus (11 percent).

The diagnosis is established by the identification of the parasite in stool. As the number of organisms varies greatly from day to day, at least three stool samples should be collected over a period of 3 to 6 days. Because the trophozoites are rapidly destroyed in the external environment, the stool should be examined immediately or preserved in polyvinyl alcohol. The use of permanent stains increases both the yield and identification accuracy of the examination. Tetracycline, iodoquinol, or metronidazole in the doses recommended for *E. histolytica* infections have all been used. There is little data available on their relative efficacy.

BLASTOCYSTIS HOMINIS INFECTION

Previously considered a commensal yeast, it now appears that *Blastocystis hominis* is a protozoan that, at least on occasion, may act as an agent of human disease. Evidence of its protozoan nature includes the lack of a cell wall, the capacity for pseudopod formation and particulate matter ingestion, multiplication by binary fission or sporulation, and possession of a well-demarcated smooth and rough endoplasmic reticulum, membrane-bound central body, and protozoan-like mitochondria and Golgi apparatus. Physiologically the organism is a strict anaerobe that requires the presence of bacteria for growth; it grows best at a neutral pH and a temperature of 37°C. The organism is resistant to high concentrations of amphotericin B.

Evidence of pathogenicity rests on the experimental induction of diarrhea in guinea pigs, its assocation with diarrhea in nonhuman primates, and a small number of reports describing human diarrheal disease, one fatal, for which no other cause could be established. A retrospective study designed to evaluate the pathogenicity and clinical relevance of *B. hominis* found the organism in 12 percent of all stools submitted for parasitologic examination; in 90 percent the numbers of *Blastocystis* were judged to be few or moderate. In approximately two-thirds of the positive stools, *B. hominis* was the only parasite present. An evaluation of case histories of a subset of patients whose stools were also known to be free of bacterial pathogens revealed that 67 percent had gastrointestinal complaints including nausea, vomiting, abdominal pain, and diarrhea, most for a period of 3 to 10 days. Only a single patient had received therapy; in none had the stools been screened for viral agents. Over half of the patients had an underlying, immunosuppressive disease.

Routine stool examinations utilizing concentration and permanent staining procedures are adequate for the identification of *B. hominis*. Some authorities recommend treating symptomatic patients shown to have more than five organisms per oil immersion field if other causes of disease cannot be identified. Metronidazole, used in the dose described for *E. histolytica* appears to be a suitable agent.

REFERENCES

Balantidiasis

KNIGHT R: Giardiasis, isosporiasis and balantidiasis. Clin Gastroenterol 7:31, 1978

NICHOLSON NW: Case report of *Balantidium coli* infection. East Afr Med J 55:133, 1978

WALZER PD et al: Balantidiasis outbreak in Truk Islands. Am J Trop Med Hyg 22:33, 1973

Blastocystis hominis infection

CALLAGHER PG et al: *Blastocystis hominis* enteritis. Pediatr Infect Dis 4:556, 1985

GARCIA LS et al: Clinical relevance of *Blastocystis hominis*. Lancet 1:1233, 1984

ZIERDT CH: *Blastocystis hominis*, A protozoan parasite and intestinal pathogen of human beings. Clin Microbiol Newsletter 5:57, 1983

Cryptosporidiosis

D'ANTONIO RG et al: A waterborne outbreak of cryptosporidiosis in normal hosts. Ann Intern Med 103:886, 1985

KOCH KL et al: Cryptosporidiosis in hospital personnel. Evidence for person-to-person transmission. Ann Intern Med 102:593, 1985
LEFKOWITCH JH et al: Cryptosporidiosis of the human small intestine: A light and electron microscopic study. Hum Pathol 15:746, 1984
NAVIN TR, JURANEK DD: Cryptosporidiosis: Clinical, epidemiologic, and parasitologic review. Rev Infect Dis 6:313, 1984
PORTNOY D et al: Treatment of intestinal cryptosporidiosis with spiramycin. Ann Intern Med 101:202, 1984
SOAVE R et al: Cryptosporidiosis in homosexual men. Ann Intern Med 100:504, 1984
WOLFSON JS et al: Cryptosporidiosis in immunocompetent patients. N Engl J Med 312:1278, 1985

Dientamebiasis

SHEIN R, GELB A: Colitis due to *Dientamoeba fragilis*. Am J Gastroenterol 78:634, 1983
SPENCER MJ et al: *Dientamoeba fragilis*. Gastrointestinal protozoan infection in adults. Am J Gastroenterol 77:565, 1982
YANG J et al: *Dientamoeba fragilis:* A review with notes on its epidemiology, pathogenicity, mode of transmission and diagnosis. Am J Trop Med Hyg 26:16, 1977

Isosporiasis

FORTHAL DN, GUEST SS: *Isospora belli* enteritis in three homosexual men. Am J Trop Med Hyg 33:1060, 1984
NG E et al: Demonstration of *Isospora belli* by acid-fast stain in a patient with acquired immune deficiency syndrome. J Clin Microbiol 20:384, 1984
TRIER JS: Chronic intestinal coccidiosis in man: Intestinal morphology and response to treatment. Gastroenterology 66:923, 1974
WESTERMAN EL, CHRISTENSEN RP: Chronic *Isospora belli* infection treated with co-trimoxazole. Ann Intern Med 91:413, 1980

Trichomoniasis

FOUTS AC, KRAUS SF: *Trichomonas vaginalis:* Reevaluation of its clinical presentation and laboratory diagnosis. J Infect Dis 141:137, 1980
KRIEGER JN et al: Geographic variation among isolates of *Trichomonas vaginalis:* Demonstration of antigenic heterogeneity by using monclonal antibodies and the indirect immunofluorescence technique. J Infect Dis 152:979, 1985
REIN MF, MÜLLER M: *Trichomonas vaginalis*, in *Sexually Transmitted Diseases*, KK Holmes et al (eds). New York, McGraw-Hill, 1984, pp 525–536
WAITKINS SA, THOMAS DJ: Isolation of *Trichomonas vaginalis* resistant to metronidazole. Lancet 2:590, 1981

162 TRICHINOSIS

JAMES J. PLORDE

DEFINITION Trichinosis is an intestinal and tissue infection of humans and other mammals caused by the nematode *Trichinella spiralis*. The disease is characterized by diarrhea during the development of the adults in the intestine and by myositis, fever, prostration, periorbital edema, eosinophilic leukocytosis, and, occasionally, evidence of myocarditis, pneumonitis, or encephalitis during the stage of larval migration in tissue.

ETIOLOGY Trichinosis in humans is contracted by ingestion of meat containing the encysted larvae of *T. spiralis*. The meat has almost always been pork, but for the past several years about 10 percent of cases reported in this country have been attributed to feral meat, usually bear or walrus. This has been particularly frequent in the northern and western states including Alaska, California, and Idaho. There are no intermediate hosts, and both the adult and larval stages develop in the same animal. Infection has been produced or observed in the bear, wild boar, wolf, coyote, fox, muskrat, horse, cow, dog, cat, rabbit, guinea pig, mouse, and marine mammals, in addition to the rat and the pig. Humans are particularly susceptible; most fowl are resistant. Among pigs, infection is contracted following feeding of the uncooked scraps, less often by eating infected rats. The incidence of infection in pigs has been reduced by laws requiring that garbage be cooked thoroughly before being fed. Rats also feed on uncooked pork scraps and, in addition, maintain a high incidence of infection by their cannibalism.

Soon after ingestion, the larvae are liberated from their cysts by gastric digestion and migrate into the intestinal mucosa, where copulation takes place. The male dies, and within a week, the viviparous female is discharging larvae (100 by 6 μm), which enter vascular channels and are distributed throughout the body. Larviposition continues for about 4 to 16 weeks, each female producing approximately 1500 offspring. The larvae enter skeletal muscle, grow, and begin encysting within 3 weeks; calcification of cysts begins in 6 to 18 months. The life span of the encysted organism has been estimated at 5 to 10 years. The muscles of the diaphragm, tongue, and eye, and the deltoid, pectoral, gastrocnemius, and intercostal muscles are most often affected. Larvae carried to sites other than skeletal muscles do not encyst but disintegrate, often stimulating a granulomatous inflammatory reaction. The life cycle can be carried further only if a new host ingests the encysted larvae.

The description of a fatal case of trichinosis in an immunosuppressed patient emphasizes the importance of the immune response in limiting the intensity of infection. Apparently, it does so by acting directly on circulating larvae, inhibiting the reproduction of the female worms, and accelerating the expulsion of the adult parasites from the intestine. Eosinophils as well as B- and T-cell lymphocytes are involved in the response. The T cells appear to have a "helper" function in promoting the production of IgG and IgM antibodies which, in collaboration with eosinophils, induce fracture of the larval cuticle and disintegration of its internal structures. Once safely encysted in striated muscle, the larvae appear resistant to immunologic attack.

EPIDEMIOLOGY Trichinosis is particularly common in Europe and North America, but with the exception of Australia it is found worldwide. In the United States its prevalence as measured by finding cysts in human diaphragms at autopsy has declined from 16.1 to 4.2 percent over the past 30 years. This decline has been accompanied by a similar reduction of trichinosis in pigs. The prevalence appears highest in the New England states, New Jersey, Louisiana, Hawaii, and Alaska. It is estimated that 1.5 million Americans carry live trichinae in their musculature and that somewhere between 150,000 and 300,000 acquire new infections annually. The overwhelming majority of these infections are asymptomatic, and many of those that become clinically manifest are never correctly diagnosed. In 1982 only 95 cases were officially reported in the United States; over the last 5 years the case fatality rate has been 0.6 per 1000. Large outbreaks are usually caused by consumption of ready-to-eat pork sausage prepared in noninspected facilities or at home. The incidence appears highest among Americans of Italian, German, Polish, or Portuguese descent, presumably because of their inclination to make and eat pork sausage over the holiday season. Although pork products are not currently inspected for trichinosis, U.S. Department of Agriculture–inspected "ready-to-eat" products are processed in a manner designed to destroy trichina larvae. Outbreaks have been reported among southeast Asian refugees living in the United States following the ingestion of undercooked pork obtained from private farms. Notable epidemics have also followed the ingestion of trichinae-infected wild pig in Hawaii and California and walrus in Alaska. The latter is the first reported outbreak caused by this host in North America. Each year, a few cases are acquired from ground beef, attesting to the frequency with which this meat is adulterated with pork.

PATHOLOGY The most striking lesions are in the skeletal muscles, where there is a severe myositis with basophilic granular degeneration of the invaded muscle fiber. Adjacent fibers exhibit hyalin or hydropic degeneration, and the focus becomes infiltrated with neutrophilic and eosinophilic leukocytes, some lymphocytes, and mononuclear macrophages. Hyperemia, edema, and hemorrhages are constant features.

Larvae do not encyst in cardiac muscle, but an intense myocarditis has been observed in fatal cases.

In cases of central nervous system involvement, there may be granulomatous nodules, and vasculitis involving small arterioles and capillaries of the brain and meninges. Encystment of larvae in the brain is unusual.

CLINICAL MANIFESTATIONS The severity of the clinical manifestations generally relates to the number of larvae disseminated to the tissues of the host; patients with severe disease usually harbor 50 to 100 larvae per gram of muscle, while those with 10 or less are often asymptomatic. The first symptoms usually appear within 1 to 2 days after ingestion of the uncooked or undercooked meat containing encysted larvae. At that time diarrhea, abdominal pain, nausea, and sometimes prostration and fever develop. Although generally brief, the intestinal phase may be prolonged in infections produced by arctic strains of trichina (*T. spiralis* var. *nativa*). The next stage, that of muscular invasion, typically begins about the end of the first week and may last as long as 6 weeks. During this period, patients have fever, periorbital edema, conjunctivitis and subconjunctival hemorrhages, muscle pain and tenderness, and often severe weakness. There may be a maculopapular rash which lasts for several days and subungual "splinter hemorrhages." More serious manifestations accompany lung, heart, or central nervous system invasion. Lung involvement is manifested by hemoptysis and consolidation on chest x-rays. Central nervous system involvement may be evident as polyneuritis, poliomyelitis, myasthenia, meningitis, encephalitis, focal or diffuse pareses, delirium, psychosis, and coma. Despite the severity of central nervous system involvement in some patients, the cerebrospinal fluid remains normal.

Myocarditis is characterized by persistent tachycardia or development of congestive heart failure. There are marked electrocardiographic alterations, including ST-T wave changes and conduction abnormalities in 20 percent of patients. High levels of circulating eosinophils may produce damage to the ventricular endothelium with superimposed thrombosis.

A causal relationship between trichinosis and polyarteritis nodosa has been reported, presumably related to the presence of circulating immune complexes.

LABORATORY FINDINGS The most constant finding, and one of significance early in the course of the disease, is the eosinophilic leukocytosis (over 500 eosinophilic leukocytes per cubic millimeter) which generally appears before the end of the second week. In cases of moderate severity, the proportion of eosinophilic leukocytes ranges between 15 and 50 percent. In severe cases, particularly terminally, the eosinophilic leukocytosis may disappear entirely.

The skin test to larval antigen becomes positive early in the third week of infection and may remain so for up to 20 years. The usual positive response is a wheal of 5 mm or more appearing within 30 min. Unfortunately, the commercially available skin test preparations are not reliable and should not be used.

There are a variety of serologic tests for trichinosis, including the countercurrent electrophoresis test, the complement fixation test, the indirect fluorescent antibody test, and the bentonite flocculation test, which is probably the most widely used. A commercially available latex agglutination test appears as sensitive but is somewhat less specific. These serologic tests all become positive during the third week of the disease and may remain positive for a few years. A newly introduced, highly sensitive enzyme-linked immunosorbent test is able to detect specific antibody in the first week of infection. Since each may occasionally be falsely negative, two or more tests should be used. The serologic tests are most valuable if they are negative initially and then in turn positive or if there is a change in titer.

Muscle biopsy when carried out during the third week of infection remains the most useful test for demonstration of larvae or cysts. The deltoid or gastrocnemius muscles are the most useful sites for biopsy. A 1-g portion of the excised muscle should be compressed between glass slides and examined under a low-power microscope for the presence of larvae. Calcified cysts or larvae represent an old infection. The remainder of the biopsy should be submitted for routine processing because myositis is a significant finding even in the absence of larvae or cysts.

In severe trichinosis there may be marked hypoalbuminemia, probably because of protein leakage from damaged capillaries. During the fourth, fifth, and sixth weeks of the disease, concomitant with a rise in antibody, diffuse hypergammaglobulinemia occurs. Elevated levels of circulating IgE have been reported. There may be moderate rises in serum glutamic oxaloacetic transaminase, serum aldolase, and creatine phosphokinase, probably related to myositis; electromyography may show evidence of altered motor function. Typically the sedimentation rate is slow.

DIFFERENTIAL DIAGNOSIS Trichinosis must be differentiated from diseases which are characterized by eosinophilia (such as Hodgkin's disease, eosinophilic leukemia, and periarteritis nodosa) and from entities which are characterized by myopathy, such as dermatomyositis. When the central nervous system is involved, the diagnosis may be very difficult.

TREATMENT Thiabendazole, in dosage of 25 mg/kg bid for 5 to 7 days, has resulted in apparent improvement in a number of patients, with relief of muscle pain and tenderness and with lysis of fever. The results have not been uniform, however, and the use of this drug in trichinosis has been associated with nausea, vomiting, abdominal discomfort, dermatitis, and drug fever. Mebendazole, given in the dosage of 400 mg tid for 2 weeks, has also been employed; its role in human disease has not been established.

Patients with "allergic" manifestations of trichinosis, including angioedema and urticaria as well as myocardial or central nervous system involvement, should be treated with prednisone in dosage of 20 to 60 mg per day. Response to steroids usually has been prompt, particularly in central nervous system trichinosis. Not all focal lesions have resolved, however.

Other measures should be directed at relief of pain and maintenance of adequate caloric and fluid intake.

PROGNOSIS The prognosis in trichinosis has improved markedly, and even when the central nervous system is involved, the mortality rate has fallen to under 10 percent. The overall mortality rate is now less than 1 percent.

PREVENTION The responsibility for control rests with the consumer. Adequate cooking of pork involves heating all portions of the meat to 170°F (77°C). Freezing procedures to kill porcine larvae require a temperature of −15°C for 20 days or −18°C for 24 h. Larvae isolated from arctic animals appear much more resistant to freezing. Proper smoking and pickling will also destroy the larvae. Important in control is the cooking of garbage fed to hogs. The enzyme-linked immunosorbent procedure described above is sufficiently sensitive, specific, and simple to be used for the routine inspection of pork. To date, however, such screening tests have not been made mandatory.

REFERENCES

BARRETT-CONNOR E et al: An epidemic of trichinosis after ingestion of wild pig in Hawaii. J Infect Dis 133:473, 1976

CAMPBELL WC (ed): *Trichinella and Trichinosis*. New York, Plenum, 1983

FRAYHA RA: Trichinosis-related polyarteritis nodosa. Am J Med 71:307, 1981

KAZURA JW, AIKAWA M: Host defense mechanisms against *Trichinella spiralis* infection in the mouse: Eosinophil mediated destruction of newborn larvae *in vitro*. J Immunol 124:355, 1980

KOLATA G: Testing for trichinosis: A new serological test should make it quick and easy to detect trichinosis in meat—a feat of no small economic importance. Science 227:621, 1985

LEVIN ML: Treatment of trichinosis with mebendazole. Am J Trop Med Hyg 32:980, 1983

MARGOLIS HS et al: Trichinosis: Two Alaskan outbreaks from walrus meat. J Infect Dis 139:102, 1979

METZLER MH et al: Second-degree atrioventricular block in acute trichinosis. Am J Dis Child 124:598, 1972

MOST H: Current concepts in parasitology. Trichinosis—preventable yet still with us. N Engl J Med 298:1178, 1978

PUN KK et al: The first documented outbreak of trichinellosis in Hong Kong Chinese. Am J Trop Med Hyg 32:772, 1983

163 FILARIASIS

JAMES J. PLORDE

DEFINITION Filariasis is a group of disorders produced by infection with the threadlike nematodes of the superfamily Filarioidea. These worms invade the lymphatics and subcutaneous and deep tissues of humans producing reactions ranging from acute inflammation to chronic scarring. The viviparous female discharges microfilariae into the blood or subcutaneous tissues where they live for weeks or months until taken up by hematophagous arthropods. Within these vectors they are transformed into filariform larvae which then infect a new host when the arthropod takes another blood meal. The clinical pictures produced by various species in this group are more or less specific. The term *lymphatic filariasis* is commonly used to designate the disease produced by *Wuchereria bancrofti, Brugia malayi,* and *Brugia timori,* the organisms responsible for lymphatic blockade and elephantiasis. *Loa loa* causes loiasis, a disease characterized by transient subcutaneous (Calabar) swellings, and *Onchocerca volvulus* produces the blindness and pruritic skin rash typical of onchocerciasis. *Mansonella ozzardi, M. perstans,* and *M. streptocerca* cause infections of questionable clinical significance to humans.

These parasites are identified by the location, periodicity, and morphologic characteristics of their microfilariae. Those of *W. bancrofti, B. malayi, B. timori, L. loa, M. perstans,* and *M. ozzardi* are all found in the blood, and, with the exception of the last, all display nocturnal or diurnal periodicity. *Onchocerca volvulus* and *M. streptocerca* are found in the subcutaneous tissues and are nonperiodic. Morphologically, the microfilariae are distinguished by the presence or absence of a sheath and by the distribution of their deeply staining column of nuclei. The sheath, which is an elongation of the original eggshell, can be seen extending beyond the head and tail only in the microfilariae of *W. bancrofti, B. malayi, B. timori,* and *L. loa.* The nuclear column extends to the very tip of the microfilariae of *B. malayi, B. timori, L. loa, M. perstans,* and *M. streptocerca.*

Skin and serologic tests are group-specific, lack sensitivity, and may be falsely positive in other nematode infections. In the absence of microfilariae and other helminthic infections, however, they may be helpful in establishing a diagnosis in clinically suspect cases.

LYMPHATIC FILARIASIS (BANCROFTIAN AND MALAYAN) Etiology and epidemiology The threadlike adult worms live coiled together in human lymphatics. The male *W. bancrofti* measures 35 mm and the female 80 to 100 mm. The *Brugia* adults are about one-half as long. Gravid females release microfilariae in large numbers into the lymphatics. These embryos, which are sheathed, measure approximately 200 to 300 μm. They eventually reach the peripheral blood, where further development depends on their ingestion by a proper mosquito vector. Species of *Culex, Aëdes,* and *Anopheles* transmit Bancroftian filariasis; *Mansonia, Anopheles,* and *Coquillettidia* serve as vectors in Brugian disease. After further development in the vector, larvae migrate to the mouthparts. If the mosquito feeds on a human host, they penetrate the puncture site and reach maturity in about a year. In the absence of reinfection, humans harbor microfilariae for 5 to 10 years, the reproductive life of the adult worms. In most *W. bancrofti* and *Brugia* infections, the microfilariae are found in the blood in greatest numbers between 9 P.M. and 2 A.M. During the day, apparently in response to changes in oxygen tension, they accumulate in the pulmonary vessels and disappear from the peripheral blood. However, in Polynesia and New Caledonia there is an *Aëdes*-transmitted variety of *W. bancrofti* (*W. pacifica*) in which microfilaria circulate for 24 h with a peak concentration at midday (diurnal subperiodicity). A nocturnally subperiodic form of *B. malayi* is present in Malaysia, Thailand, and Indonesia. Periodicity is of epidemiologic significance because it determines which species of mosquito serves as the vector. The human is the only known vertebrate host for *W. bancrofti* and the periodic strains of *B. malayi;* subperiodic *B. malayi* is found in monkeys and cats as well as humans.

It has been estimated that 100 million persons throughout the world are infected, and both the prevalence and distribution of the disease seem to be increasing in many parts of Africa and Asia.

Wuchereria bancrofti infection is endemic between latitudes 41°N and 30°S involving primarily Africa, the Pacific Islands, and southeastern Asia from Korea on the north to India in the west. The West Indies, Central America, and the eastern coastal plains of South America are also involved. Distribution is irregular, and there are many peculiar ''skip areas'' in this geographic pattern, presumably because the endemic disease can be maintained only where human infection and mosquitoes are prevalent. *B. malayi* infection is much more restricted in its distribution and occurs in India, Burma, Thailand, Vietnam, China, South Korea, Japan, Malaysia, Indonesia, Borneo, New Guinea, and the Philippines. The parasite has disappeared from Sri Lanka. *B. timori* is limited to the eastern Indonesian archipelago.

Pathogenesis Pathologic changes are caused primarily by the presence of the adult worm in the lymphatics and may be divided into inflammatory and obstructive. The inflammatory response, thought to be due to an immediate-type hypersensitivity reaction to molting larvae, consists of infiltration with lymphocytes, plasma cells, and eosinophils. There are hyperplasia of lymphatic endothelium, acute lymphangitis, and thrombosis. Obstructive phenomena are thought to be caused by a granulomatous reaction to dead or dying adults which may lead to reversible lymphatic obstruction. Repetition of this process over a period of years leads to permanent lymphatic blockade. The tissues become edematous, thickened, and fibrotic. Secondary streptococcal infections are common and may contribute to lymphatic blockade. Dilated lymphatics may rupture into surrounding tissue. Elephantiasis is actually a relatively unusual complication of filarial infections and is actually more common in immigrants to endemic areas. Apparently, exposure to filarial antigens early in life provides some protection against elephantiasis. If repeated reinfections do not occur, the disease is self-limited.

Manifestations The clinical manifestations vary with the geographic area, species of parasite, immune response of the infected patient, and intensity of infection. Light infections may be completely asymptomatic. Symptoms may occur within 3 months of infection, but ordinarily the incubation period is 8 to 12 months. The clinical findings closely reflect the pathological changes, with inflammation early in the disease followed by obstruction later. Inflammatory filariasis consists of a series of brief febrile attacks occurring over a period of weeks. Fever is usually low grade but may reach 40.6°C (105°F) and be accompanied by chills and sweats. Other symptoms include headache, nausea and vomiting, photophobia, and muscle pain. If the involved lymphatics lie close to the surface, the local symptoms dominate the clinical picture. Lymphangitis is very common, involving the legs more frequently than the arms. It often begins as a tender spot in the region of the malleoli or femoral area and spreads centrifugally. The involved vessels are palpably tender and painful. The overlying skin is red and swollen. When abdominal lymphatics are involved, the picture may simulate that of an acute abdomen. In Bancroftian filariasis the vessels of the spermatic cord and testes may be involved, resulting in painful orchitis, epididymitis, or funiculitis. Lymphadenitis almost always accompanies and may sometimes precede lymphangitis. The inguinal, femoral, and epitrochlear nodes are involved. Abscesses which may form about involved lymphatics and lymph nodes may discharge to the surface, resulting in persistently draining sinus tracts. The acute manifestations last only a few days and then subside spontaneously, only to recur at irregular intervals over a period of weeks or months. Recovery finally ensues. With repeated infections, slowly progressive lymphatic obstruction may develop in areas where the inflammatory reactions have occurred previously. Edema, ascites, lymph scrotum, hydrocele, pleural effusion, or joint effusion may appear as a result of interference with lymphatic drainage. Lymphadenopathy persists. The lymphatic vessels become palpably enlarged as tense elastic masses beneath the skin, especially in the femoral, inguinal, and scrotal areas. They may rupture and form draining sinuses. Internal rupture of lymphatics may give rise to chylous ascites or chyluria. In a small percentage of cases elephantiasis develops. This complication is rare below the age of 20 even in natives of heavily infested areas. The chronic obstructive phase of the disease often is punctuated by acute inflammatory episodes.

TROPICAL EOSINOPHILIA Attention has been focused on an aberrant type of filariasis which is characterized by the presence of hypereosinophilia, circulating filarial antibodies, microfilariae in tissue but *not in the blood,* and a chronic, clinical course that can be terminated with specific antifilarial treatment. These amicrofilaremic forms were originally thought to be caused by zoonotic parasites, but it is more likely that they represent an atypical host response to various filariae including *W. bancrofti* and *B. malayi.* The syndrome is most commonly seen in India, Indonesia, Sri Lanka, Pakistan, and southeast Asia, all areas of intense transmission for these organisms. Involved patients lack the IgG-blocking antibodies present in the patients with circulating microfilariae. Animal models suggest that microfilariae are removed from the peripheral circulation and trapped in various tissue sites by an IgG-dependent cell-mediated effector mechanism. Antigens released when the parasites are destroyed initiate an immediate IgE-mediated reaction. The eosinophilic inflammatory reaction, in time, progresses to granuloma formation and fibrosis. Clinically there may be marked enlargement of the lymph nodes and spleen (Meyers-Kouwenaar syndrome) and/or chronic cough, nocturnal bronchospasm, and miliary pulmonary infiltrates (Weingarten syndrome). The former syndrome is most frequently seen in children, and the latter in young male adults. Only one-quarter of the patients with pulmonary manifestations demonstrate obstructive defects on pulmonary function testing. All show restrictive disease, and irreversible pulmonary hypertension has been described in a few. A number of diseases characterized by pulmonary infiltration and eosinophilia (PIE) must be considered in the differential diagnosis of this disease. They include other helminthic infections, Loeffler's syndrome, chronic eosinophilic pneumonia, allergic aspergillosis, vasculitis, idiopathic hypereosinophilia, and drug allergies.

Diagnosis A history of exposure, the long incubation period, the occurrence of typical inflammatory episodes, and the finding of regional lymphadenopathy, thickening of the spermatic cord, or swelling of an extremity should suggest the diagnosis. There is usually eosinophilia during acute episodes. Lymphangiography may reveal dilated afferent and small efferent lymphatics. The definitive diagnosis depends on demonstration of the parasite. Although adult worms can be demonstrated in biopsied lymph nodes, biopsy is not recommended because it may interfere further with lymphatic drainage. Microfilariae are found in the blood during intermediate stages but not early or late in the disease. As they are motile, they can often be seen in a wet mount. Definite identification, however, requires staining with Giemsa. As in malaria, both thin and thick smears should be prepared. Either the Knott concentration, counting chamber, or membrane filtration technique should be employed if the parasite is not found in thick smears. Because the appearance of microfilariae in peripheral blood is periodic, it is essential to obtain blood at appropriate times. When this proves difficult, the oral administration of 100 mg diethylcarbamazine usually produces positive blood specimens within 30 to 60 min. Microfilariae may also be found in lymphatic fluid, hydrocele fluid, ascites, and pleural fluid. Indirect hemagglutination, bentonite flocculation, and soluble antigen fluorescent antibody tests are available and, although not completely reliable, are helpful when microfilariae cannot be demonstrated. An indirect immunofluorescent test utilizing adult *B. malayi* as the source of antigen is both more sensitive and specific than previously developed procedures. Filarial antigens are present in the blood and urine of most microfilaremic and in some seropositive–microfilaremic-negative patients, suggesting antigen detection may provide a more definitive indicator of active diseases than do standard serologic procedures. At present, such techniques are available only in research laboratories.

The diagnosis of *tropical eosinophilia* is confirmed by (1) a history of prolonged residence in an endemic area, (2) lack of microfilariae in the peripheral blood despite examination of both day and night specimens by concentration techniques, (3) peripheral eosinophilia in excess of 3000 cells per milliliter, (4) high titers of filarial antibodies, (5) IgE levels of at least 1000 units per milliliter, and (6) response to diethylcarbamazine within 7 to 10 days of initiating therapy. Recovery of microfilariae from the tissues is uncommon, and biopsy is not warranted.

Treatment Diethylcarbamazine rapidly eliminates microfilariae from the blood. It probably also kills or injures adult worms, impairing their ability to reproduce, and clears microfilariae permanently from the bloodstream of many patients. The drug is given in doses of 2 mg/kg three times a day for 3 or 4 weeks. Treatment with this agent is often followed by allergic reactions to the dying parasite. These reactions may be quite severe, especially in Malayan filariasis. They can be controlled with aspirin, antihistamines, or corticosteroids. In heavy infections, it may be desirable to begin treatment with antihistamines before administration of diethylcarbamazine.

Reassurance of the patient is very important in this disease. Effective and safe vaccines are presently not available. Pressure bandages and surgery sometimes benefit elephantiasis. The prognosis for life is excellent, particularly if infected individuals leave endemic areas or otherwise avoid reinfections. Disease control is accomplished by combining mass treatment with mosquito control measures.

ONCHOCERCIASIS ("RIVER BLINDNESS")

Definition Onchocerciasis is a cutaneous filariasis caused by *Onchocerca volvulus.* It is characterized by subcutaneous nodules, a pruritic skin rash, sclerosing lymphadenitis, and ocular lesions.

Etiology and epidemiology The disease is found in focal areas within Mexico, Guatemala, Colombia, Venezuela, Ecuador, Surinam, Brazil, Saudi Arabia, and Yemen, and throughout tropical Africa. It is estimated that at least 40 million individuals in Africa and 200,000 in the new world are infected and that about 5 percent of these are blind as a result of the disease.

The infection is transmitted by black flies of the genus *Simulium,* which breed along turbulent, fast-moving streams. An inoculated larva matures into a single male or female in approximately 1 year. Since larvae do not multiply within the human host, heavy parasite loads are the result of repeated infections. The adult worms are found coiled together in fibrous subcutaneous nodules. The gravid females, which may live as long as 15 years, release thousands of unsheathed microfilariae daily. These migrate in the skin, subcutaneous tissue, and eye for up to 30 months until they either degenerate or are ingested by a feeding *Simulium.*

Pathogenesis and clinical manifestations The subcutaneous nodules which enclose the adult worms are usually 2 to 3 cm in diameter when fully developed. Generally found over the bony prominences, they are firm, nontender, and freely movable, although occasionally they may be adherent to underlying tissue. Their location on the body is related to the biting habits of the vector. In Central America, where the fly bites on the upper part of the body, the nodules are frequently over the head; in Africa they are primarily on the trunk and thighs. They usually number less than 10, but more than 100 have been reported in a single patient.

The important pathologic changes occur as a result of an immediate hypersensitivity reaction to the dead or dying microfilariae. Specific antibody, complement, and eosinophils are all thought to be involved. Pruritus is often severe and constant. The skin lesion may appear as an erysipelas-like reaction over the face or a papular rash over one extremity. In chronic cases thickening, lichenification, and depigmentation may be present. In Africa microfilariae produce a fibrosing obstructive lymphadenitis, possibly by stimulating the deposition of immune complexes. This lesion is frequently associated with large folds of skin called *hanging groins* and with elephantiasis. Children living in endemic areas may not demonstrate these changes for decades even though microfilariae are present. The most serious complications of onchocerciasis are eye lesions which are usually found in patients repeatedly infected on the upper part of the body. A punctate and later sclerosing keratitis, iridocyclitis, optic atrophy, or chorioretinitis may eventually lead to blindness.

Diagnosis The diagnosis is made by demonstrating microfilariae in a skin snip taken from an involved area. A thin sliver of superficial skin is removed with a razor or punch. Care must be taken to prevent bleeding and possible contamination with blood microfilariae. The skin is weighed and is then placed in saline, teased with a pair of sharp dissecting needles, and observed for emerging microfilariae over the next hour. The results should be expressed in microfilariae per milligram of tissue. Multiple skin snips may be necessary. In patients with eye lesions, microfilariae can sometimes be seen in the anterior chamber with a slit lamp. If organisms cannot be detected by the above methods, the patient may be given 50 mg diethylcarbamazine orally. The occurrence of a pruritic rash within 24 h strongly suggests the presence of cutaneous microfilariae (Mazzotti's test). Several filarial serologic tests are available. Most use crude antigen preparations and lack specificity. The anticipated availability of more specific antigens in the near future may ameliorate this problem. Techniques for the detection of onchocercal antigens in blood and urine require further development.

Treatment and prevention Diethylcarbamazine is effective in destroying microfilariae but has little effect on the adult worm. The drug must be used with great care as rapid destruction of the parasites may cause a severe allergic reaction. If the eye is involved, this can result in further ocular damage. The initial adult dose is 50 mg orally. It is increased to 50 mg three times daily on the second day, 100 mg three times daily on the third day, and finally 200 mg three times a day for an additional 7 days. Antihistamines, or in rare cases corticosteroids, can be used to control allergic reactions. In ocular reactions, the pupil should be dilated and topical steroids applied.

The adult worms may be eliminated by excision of nodules on the head and neck, a procedure which is useful in preventing ocular complications, or by chemotherapy with suramin. Details of the administration and toxicity of this drug are given in Chap. 156. The dosage is 0.1 g given intravenously to detect drug idiosyncrasy, followed by 1.0 g intravenously once weekly for five to six doses.

Ivermectin, a macrocyclic antibiotic, is a slightly more effective microfilaricidal agent, and its administration does not appear to induce the severe allergic reactions seen with diethylcarbamazine. Although further studies are required to establish optimum dosage, it appears that this agent may be suitable for use in mass treatment programs.

Chemoprophylaxis is not practical, and personal protection depends upon the use of protective clothing. Insecticides, mass therapy, and nodulectomies have been used but have not been very satisfactory. A massive control project in west Africa utilizing insecticides dropped by airplane and helicopter has been more successful.

LOIASIS This form of filariasis is produced by *Loa loa* and is prevalent in west and central Africa. The infection is transmitted by deerflies of the genus *Chrysops*. The adult worms, which like the other filariae may live for 10 to 15 years, migrate continuously through the subcutaneous tissue. The resulting localized areas of allergic inflammation, *Calabar swellings*, are the hallmark of the disease. Occasionally the adult worms may be seen crossing the eye subconjunctivally. This usually results in intense lacrimation, pain, and anxiety. Infestation may, however, be completely asymptomatic. An association between loiasis, the nephrotic syndrome, and endomyocardial fibrosis has been reported; these conditions are considered autoimmune disorders. The diagnosis can be made by finding the adult worm or by demonstrating the distinctive sheathed microfilariae in contents of the Calabar swellings or in the bloodstream during the daytime. Microfilariae are often not found. In these cases, there are usually marked eosinophilia and a positive filarial complement fixation test. Diethylcarbamazine, administered for 2 to 3 weeks in the manner described for onchocerciasis, will kill both adult worms and microfilariae. This drug must be used with great care as it may induce a severe meningoencephalitis in patients with intense microfilaremia; this presumably reflects an allergic reaction to dead or dying parasites. It is taken in a dose of 200 mg twice daily for 3 days each month and is also effective as a chemoprophylactic agent.

MANSONELLIASIS PERSTANS *Mansonella perstans* (*Dipetalonema perstans, Acanthocheilonema perstans*) is a filarial parasite of humans and other primates inhabiting the tropical areas of Africa and Latin America. The adult worm lives encysted in the subserosal tissues of the pericardium, pleura, and peritoneum, particularly the mesentery. The unsheathed microfilariae, which can be found in the peripheral blood throughout the day, measure 200 μm in length and have four to six nuclei in their tail. They are transmitted from host to host by blood-sucking gnats of the genus *Culicoides*. Most infections are asymptomatic, and their principal significance lies in the fact that they may be confused with other, more serious, forms of filariasis. Nevertheless, some patients complain of fever, pruritus, Calabar swellings, erysipelas-like rashes, and abdominal pain. Although microfilariae are frequently seen in the cerebrospinal fluid, neurologic manifestations are rare. Peripheral eosinophilia is common, but filarial complement fixation tests are generally negative. The diagnosis is made by finding the characteristic microfilariae in the peripheral blood. Treatment with diethylcarbamazine is of doubtful benefit.

MANSONELLIASIS STREPTOCERCA *Mansonella streptocerca* (*Dipetalonema streptocerca*) is found in equatorial Africa where it inhabits the dermis and subcutaneous tissues of chimpanzees and humans. Like *M. perstans,* it is transmitted by *Culicoides*. The microfilariae inhabit the dermal collagen where they elicit a lymphocytic and eosinophilic inflammatory response, fibrosis, lymphatic dilatation, pruritus, hypopigmented macules, and a papular rash. The diagnosis is made by recovering the nonperiodic microfilariae from skin snips as described for onchocerciasis above. They are unsheathed and possess a sharply crooked tail with nuclei. Diethylcarbamazine, as described for Bancroftian filariasis above, is effective. Treatment often provokes a reaction similar to the Mazzotti reaction described for onchocerciasis.

MANSONELLIASIS OZZARDI *Mansonella ozzardi* are found as adult worms in the mesentery and visceral fat of people living in the tropical areas of Latin America and the Caribbean. This species is thought to be transmitted by flies of the genus *Simulium* and gnats of the genus *Culicoides*. The nonperiodic microfilariae are released into the peripheral blood where they can be identified by their lack of a sheath or caudal nuclei. Occasionally, they may also be found in skin snips, producing confusion with onchocerciasis. This common infection is thought to be asymptomatic, but reports of patients presenting with fever, pruritus, lymphadenopathy, hydroceles, and chronic arthritis have been published. There are conflicting reports on the efficacy of diethylcarbamazine therapy.

DIROFILARIASIS *Dirofilaria immitis* (canine heartworm) is a large, cosmopolitan filaria of dogs which lives in their right ventricle and pulmonary arteries and releases its microfilariae into the peripheral blood. It is transmitted by several types of mosquitoes. Human infections are increasingly reported, particularly from the eastern and southern United States, the Mississippi Valley, and California. The worm does not mature in humans, and hence microfilaremia is not present. Although cardiac infections have been noted at autopsy, most human infections present as well-defined pulmonary nodules, the result of an embolic infarct produced by an immature worm. The patients are most frequently asymptomatic and are discovered to have a "coin lesion," 2 cm or less in diameter, on pulmonary roentgenography. Less commonly they complain of cough and chest pain or, rarely, of hemoptysis, fever, chills, and myalgia. The diagnosis is usually made by the microscopic examination of excised pulmonary nodules. Eosinophilia is mild or absent and serologic tests are not helpful.

Other *Dirofilariae* may rarely invade humans producing subcutaneous eosinophilic granulomas of the eyelid, trunk, or extremities. The nodules, which measure 1 to 2 cm in diameter, may be painful or completely asymptomatic. In the southern United States, the filaria most frequently involved is *D. tenuis,* a parasite of raccoons. The nodules are removed by surgical excision.

REFERENCES

CHERNIN E: Sir Patrick Manson's studies on the transmission and biology of filariasis. Rev Infect Dis 5:148, 1983

CIFERRI F: Human pulmonary dirofilariasis in the United States: A critical review. Am J Trop Med Hyg 31:302, 1982

CONNOR DH et al: Pathologic changes of human onchocerciasis: Implications for future research. Rev Infect Dis 7:809, 1985

GREENE BM et al: Comparison of ivermectin and diethylcarbamazine in the treatment of onchocerciasis. N Engl J Med 313:133, 1985

GROVE DI: Selective primary health care: Strategies for the control of disease in the developing world. VII. Filariasis. Rev Infect Dis 5:933, 1983

HAWKING F: The 24-hour periodicity of microfilariae: Biological mechanisms responsible for its production and control. Proc R Soc Lond [Biol] 169:59, 1967

KOCHAR AS: Human pulmonary dirofilariasis. Report of three cases and brief review of the literature. Am J Clin Pathol 84:19, 1985

MEYERS WM et al: Human streptocerciasis. A clinico-pathological study of 40 Africans (Zaireans) including identification of the adult filaria. Am J Trop Med Hyg 21:528, 1972

NEGESSE Y et al: Loiasis: "Calabar" swellings and involvement of deep organs. Am J Trop Med Hyg 34:537, 1985

NEVA FA, OTTESON EA: Current concepts in parasitology. Tropical (filarial) eosinophilia. N Engl J Med 298:1129, 1978

ONKEL TC: Infections with *Dipetalonema perstans* and *Mansonella ozzardi* in the aboriginal Indians of Guyana. Am J Trop Med Hyg 16:628, 1967

OTTESEN EA: Immunologic aspects of lymphatic filariasis and onchocerciasis in man. Trans R Soc Trop Med Hyg 78(suppl):9, 1984

RAO CK, KUMAR S: Role of filariasis in endomyocardial fibrosis. J Commun Dis 14:91, 1982

THYLEFORS B: Ocular onchocerciasis. Bull WHO 56:63, 1978

WELLER PF et al: Tourism-acquired *Mansonella ozzardi* microfilaria in a regular blood donor. JAMA 240:858, 1978

WORLD HEALTH ORGANIZATION: Lymphatic filariasis. Fourth report of the WHO Expert Committee on Filariasis. Technical Report Series 702, Geneva:WHO, 1984

YANGCO BG et al: A survey of filariasis among refugees in south Florida. Am J Trop Med Hyg 33:246, 1984

164 SCHISTOSOMIASIS

THEODORE E. NASH

INTRODUCTION Three major schistosome species, *Schistosoma mansoni, Schistosoma haematobium,* and *Schistosoma japonicum,* and a number of less prevalent species of the genus *Schistosoma* infect humans. Both *Schistosoma mansoni* and *Schistosoma japonicum* adults reside in the venules of the intestine, and the major disease manifestations of these parasites are hepatic. *S. mansoni* is found in parts of South America (Brazil, Venezuela, and Surinam), some Caribbean islands, Africa, and the Middle East while infections with *S. japonicum* occur in the Far East, mostly in China and the Philippines. *S. haematobium* adults are found mostly in the venules of the urinary tract and cause disease primarily of the ureters and bladder. Infections with this species occur in Africa and the Middle East. Of lesser importance are *Schistosoma mekongi,* a newly recognized parasite related to *S. japonicum* which is found along the Mekong River in Indochina, and *Schistosoma intercalatum,* found in certain areas of central West Africa. Worldwide, as many as 200 million persons may be infected, and infection of entire communities is common. However, most infected persons experience few, if any, signs and symptoms, and only a small minority develop significant disease.

LIFE CYCLE The schistosome species infecting humans all share the same basic life cycle but are unique in a number of important ways which account for some of the different clinical and pathologic findings. Important differences include the length of time before egg laying begins (prepatent period), location of the adult worms, number of eggs produced by each pair of worms, response by the host to the ova, and eventual fate of retained eggs. The morphology of the various stages of the parasites and the types of intermediate host snail are also distinct. Humans become infected after contact with water containing the infective stage of the parasite, called a cercaria, which is a microscopic form of the schistosome possessing a forked tail used for swimming and a head which is the anlage of the future worm. Cercariae penetrate the unbroken skin, with the help of secreted enzymes, and in the skin transform into schistosomules or developing schistosomes. After 2 to 3 days the schistosomules migrate to the lungs and then to the portal vein, probably by an intravascular route. In the portal vein the maturing male and female schistosomes pair and migrate to the venules of the mesentery, bladder, or ureters, depending on the species of schistosome, and begin to deposit eggs. The time spent in migration and maturation differs. *S. mansoni* and *S. japonicum* begin depositing eggs around 4 to 5 weeks after infection, while egg deposition begins after 2 to 3 months for *S. haematobium.* Adult worms are about 1 to 2 cm in length and migrate in the blood vessels without eliciting a local inflammatory reaction. Adult worms do not multiply in humans, and immunosuppressive therapy does not result in increased numbers of worms. Once released, eggs are either retained in the tissues at the site of deposition or swept back, mostly to the liver, by way of the venous portal system in the case of the intestinal schistosomes. Eggs are deposited mainly in the bladder and ureters by *S. haematobium.* A portion of the mature schistosome ova are extruded into the lumen of the intestines, bladder, or ureters and after contact with water hatch, releasing a miracidium. This free-swimming ciliated stage seeks out the proper intermediate snail vector and burrows into the soft tissues of the snail. After 1 to 2 months, depending on the species of parasite, the miracidium develops into a primary and then secondary sporocyst which, after further development, begins releasing cercariae into the surrounding water. Thousands of cercariae can be released daily from each infected snail. Therefore one miracidium produces many cercariae, and this amplifies the number of infective parasites and the risk of infection. Cercariae are most infectious immediately after shedding and are not viable 48 h after release so storing water for 48 h before contact prevents exposure and infection. Unlike most other trematodes the sexes are separate in schistosomes, but this is only evident in the adult stage. Ova are laid only when males and females infect the same individual.

PATHOPHYSIOLOGY There are a number of factors which determine the disease manifestations of the host. These include the duration and intensity of infection, location of egg deposition, host genetics, concurrent infections, and other still undefined factors.

In individuals from endemic areas initial infection goes unnoticed. There are a number of possible reasons for this, including age of initial exposure, manner of exposure, and transfer of maternal immunity. However, in visitors to endemic areas initial infection with schistosomes commonly results in an acute febrile illness (Katayama fever or acute schistosomiasis) which is a manifestation of the immune response to the developing schistosomes and eggs. There is a good immune response which becomes suppressed. These individuals have elevated levels of eosinophils and immune complexes and react markedly to schistosome antigens as measured by lymphocyte blastogenesis. Despite ongoing infection, symptoms subside, as do blastogenic responses to antigens but not to unrelated antigens such as purified protein derivative of tuberculin (PPD). The exudative acute granulomatous response to schistosome eggs is also suppressed.

A major factor in determining the development of disease in humans is the worm burden of the host, which determines the number of eggs produced. It is the inflammatory and fibrotic response to these eggs which is responsible for most of the morbidity and mortality associated with schistosomiasis. Those factors which limit parasite survival will limit the development of disease. In human schistosome infections it is not known if protective immunity develops, but immunity clearly exists in experimental animals. In the first few days after infection the schistosomule is relatively susceptible to immune attack. A number of systems employing antibody and/or eosinophils, neutrophils, macrophages, and complement have been used to kill schistosomules in vitro. However, as the schistosomules mature, they become refractory to these immune responses. In addition, schistosomes coat their tegument with host proteins and evade recognition by the host. A number of pertinent schistosomule and adult antigens have been defined with the hope of developing vaccines; the administration of murine monoclonal antibodies to some of these antigens has reduced worm burdens in challenge infections by about 50 percent, and immunization with one antigen has produced similar levels of protection. Successful vaccination with anti-idiotypes has also been reported.

All schistosome eggs elicit a granulomatous response which is best understood in *S. mansoni* infections. The host becomes sensitized to the egg proteins by a T-cell-mediated mechanism which induces a larger granuloma. However, with continued infection the granuloma decreases in size due to the recruitment of suppressor T cells, while antibody has no effect on granuloma size. The regulation of granulomas due to *S. japonicum* eggs differs from that of granulomas from *S. mansoni* eggs. Immune modulation is mediated by serum factors, at least in the chronic stage of infection. Both eggs and granulomas release factors which induce fibroblast proliferation in vitro. The early cellular response induced by granulomas is followed by fibrosis in vivo; however, liver fibrosis in humans probably involves more than simple fusion of fibrotic granulomas. After years of continued infection, a minority of heavily infected individuals develop end-stage fibrotic lesions; mainly portal fibrosis (Symmers's fibrosis), esophageal varices, and splenomegaly in *S. mansoni, S. japonicum,* and *S. mekongi* infections and fibrosis of the ureters and bladder in *S. haematobium* infections. After the development of portal fibrosis eggs are shunted to the lungs via portal-systemic collateral veins resulting in cor pulmonale. Immune complexes shunted to the systemic circulation cause glomerulonephritis.

Host genetic factors have been found to influence the development of Symmers's fibrosis although there is no general agreement as to which factors are important. Schistosomes even of the same species are also genetically diverse, as shown by endonuclease restriction analysis, but the effect of this on disease in humans is unknown.

CLINICAL SYNDROMES **Acute schistosomiasis** Acute schistosomiasis, or Katayama fever, occurs following initial exposure and infection with *S. mansoni* and *S. japonicum*. It rarely follows infection with *S. haematobium*. Acute schistosomiasis is seldom recognized in endemic populations and therefore is noted primarily in visitors to endemic areas. Immediately following exposure patients frequently complain of intense transient itching. From 2 to 6 weeks or longer after exposure the patient may complain of a variety of symptoms including fever, chills, headache, hives or angioedema, weakness, weight loss, nonproductive cough, abdominal pain, and diarrhea. Sometimes symptoms abate but return with increased intensity about the time egg laying commences. These symptoms gradually diminish but may last as long as 2 to 3 months. Other newly infected individuals may be asymptomatic or have only minimal symptoms. In these individuals the diagnosis is established only after further evaluation prompted by suggestive laboratory test results or exposure history. More severe symptoms occur with heavier infections, but light infections may cause severe illness. Central nervous system lesions may occur during acute schistosome infection. The diagnosis of acute schistosomiasis is suggested by the clinical findings and the presence of eosinophilia, which is sometimes greater than 50 percent. Leukocytosis, increased immune complexes, and elevated IgM, IgG, and IgE immunoglobulins are found commonly. Although immune complexes have been suggested to play a role in the pathophysiology of acute schistosomiasis, glomerulonephritis and vasculitis are not present. The specific diagnosis can be established even before the shedding of ova by the detection of antibodies to adult schistosome gut antigens, or after egg excretion (5 to 6 weeks following exposure) by appropriate serologic testing and the finding of eggs in the stool or rectal biopsy. Clinically, acute schistosomiasis is frequently misdiagnosed as typhoid fever but can be confused with any prolonged febrile illness. Although these patients seem to tolerate chemotherapy well, it is unclear if therapy shortens the course of disease or decreases symptoms. Corticosteroids may be useful, but this has not been demonstrated in controlled studies.

Liver fibrosis The most important complication of intestinal schistosome infection is the development of periportal or Symmers's fibrosis and portal hypertension (hepatosplenic schistosomiasis). This pathognomonic finding occurs in *S. mansoni, S. japonicum,* and *S. mekongi* infections but has been best studied in *S. mansoni* infections, where it normally develops after 10 to 15 years of prolonged exposure and infection. The liver is usually but not always enlarged, firm, and nodular, and the left lobe is characteristically prominent. Macroscopically, finger-sized bands of fibrosis (''pipe-stem'' fibrosis) encompass the portal tracts. The portal venous tracts are replaced with fibrous tissue leading to presinusoidal blockage, portal hypertension, splenomegaly, and esophageal and gastric varices. The intrahepatic pressure is normal. Hepatic function is generally well preserved, and patients commonly present with hematemesis and/or signs and symptoms of splenomegaly. Ascites, hepatic coma, edema, spider angiomas, gynecomastia, and other signs of liver failure occur less frequently than in alcoholic and postnecrotic cirrhosis. Despite repeated episodes of hematemesis, patients may do reasonably well.

The diagnosis of periportal fibrosis is established by wedge biopsy of the liver; needle biopsy specimens are inadequate. Ultrasonograms of the liver show characteristic findings. The fibrotic bands appear as dense echogenic areas surrounding the portal vein and its tributaries. Further studies of the correlation between the pathologic and ultrasound findings are necessary to establish the sensitivity and specificity of this technique.

Patients with periportal fibrosis may not have schistosome eggs in their feces because of previous treatment and/or attrition of adult worms without subsequent reinfection. Since schistosome infections are practically universal in many populations, the mere presence of schistosome eggs in the feces of a patient does not establish the diagnosis of schistosomal periportal fibrosis; other liver diseases may be present. It is not clear whether there is any benefit from shunting procedures or splenectomy although these procedures are used commonly. The mortality of patients with portal fibrosis has not been well studied but in one group was 8.2 percent after 3.6 years.

Glomerulonephritis and pulmonary hypertension These two complications occur almost exclusively in patients with periportal fibrosis and portal hypertension, probably as a result of eggs and circulating antigens or immune complexes bypassing the liver. Pulmonary hypertension appears to be due to obliteration of pulmonary arterioles by granulomatous inflammation induced by shunted and embolized schistosome eggs. This is most frequently recognized with *S. mansoni* and *S. japonicum* infections but also occurs with *S. haematobium*. The association of glomerulonephritis and schistosomiasis has been noted in humans and in experimentally infected animals. This complication is manifested clinically as proteinuria and/or renal failure. Schistosome-specific antibodies and antigens have been detected in the glomeruli of infected patients.

Other complications Focal dense deposits of eggs of *S. mansoni* in the large intestine (and less commonly of *S. haematobium* and probably of *S. japonicum*) incite an exudative granulomatous response resulting in the formation of inflammatory polyps. Histologically, these consist of masses of eggs, inflammatory cells, and fibrosis. The major clinical presentation is bloody diarrhea, sometimes associated with protein-losing enteropathy and anemia. This type of involvement of the bowel is recognized primarily in Egypt and the Sudan. However, gastrointestinal symptoms are not increased in most chronically infected patients compared to control populations. In addition, granulomatous masses involving the bowel wall may mimic carcinoma of the bowel. Central nervous system (CNS) involvement with *S. mansoni* and *S. haematobium* has a predilection for the spinal cord while the brain is involved more commonly in *S. japonicum* infections.

Patients infected with the three major species of schistosomes and subsequently infected with salmonella may develop a prolonged intermittent febrile illness. In *S. haematobium* infections prolonged excretion of salmonella in the urine is common. Many times treatment of the salmonella infection alone is not effective, and specific antischistosomal chemotherapy is also required. Salmonella may be protected from host immune responses by residing in schistosome gut or by adhering to the surface tegument of the schistosome.

***SCHISTOSOMA MANSONI* Epidemiology and manifestations** *S. mansoni* is found in South America and certain islands of the Caribbean Sea, Africa, and the Middle East. The prepatent period is about 4 to 5 weeks. The intermediate hosts are various species in the genus *Biomphalaria*.

S. mansoni is the most common schistosome species infecting humans, and more is known about this parasite and human infection and disease than about the other schistosome species. Although infection is frequent and sometimes universal in endemic areas, the development of disease is relatively uncommon and depends on a number of factors which include the duration and intensity of infection. In endemic populations chronic infections are usual, many times lasting decades, and disease manifestations develop in a predictable manner. For the most part, the initial infection of persons living in endemic areas goes unnoticed. In endemic populations, throughout the first decade of life the intensity of infection as measured by the number of eggs excreted in the feces increases, and prevalence rates often approach 100 percent in highly endemic communities. Few if any symptoms are attributable to schistosomiasis during this time. The liver, particularly the left lobe, gradually enlarges and becomes firm in consistency. Between 10 and 15 years of age, some heavily infected persons develop splenomegaly which partly reflects the presence of portal fibrosis and portal hypertension. At about the same time, the number of eggs in the feces decreases, and there is some evidence to suggest that immune factors as well as decreased water contact are responsible for this. During the next three decades, persons with portal fibrosis and hypertension may experience repeated bouts of hematemesis secondary to esophageal varices or symptoms secondary to a massively enlarged spleen. Not infrequently, either because of prior chemotherapy, decreased exposure, or increased host immunity, patients with end-stage portal fibrosis no longer excrete viable eggs. Adult schistosomes can survive 20 years or more in the human host but usually live 5 to 8 years. The prognosis and the potential for reversing complications of infection after appropriate chemotherapy depend on the stage of disease. End-stage fibrotic lesions are not reversible after chemotherapy. Glomerulonephritis and cor pulmonale secondary to schistosomiasis occur exclusively in patients with portal fibrosis. Central nervous system (CNS) involvement can occur in any stage of the infection and is not related to the intensity of infection. Other complications are noted in Table 164-1 and in the pathophysiology section.

TABLE 164-1 Clinical manifestations of schistosomiasis from various *Schistosoma* species*

Manifestation	*S. mansoni*	*S. japonicum*	*S. haematobium*
Acute toxemic schistosomiasis	+	+	+
Chronic asymptomatic schistosomiasis	+	+	+
Hepatosplenic schistosomiasis	+	+	0
Cor pulmonale	+	+	±
Glomerulonephritis (clinically significant)	+	+	0†
Colonic polyposis	+	+	±
Ectopic lesions			
Brain	±	+	±
Spinal cord	+	±	+
Skin	+	+	+
Chronic cystitis and ureteritis	0	0	+
Mass lesions, bladder and ureters	0	0	+
Bladder cancer	0	0	+
Association with salmonella	+	+	+
Prolonged fever	+	+	+
Urinary carrier stage	?	?	+
Swimmer's itch‡	+	+	+

* *+ = recognized complications of infections by this species; ± = findings much less prominent in individuals infected by this species; 0 = complications not present in infections by this species.*

† *Except with associated salmonella infections.*

‡ *Usually from schistosomes that do not infect humans.*

Diagnosis The diagnosis of schistomiasis mansoni is established by identification of *S. mansoni* ova in the feces or tissues. The ova are 114 to 175 μm in length and 45 to 68 μm in width and have a prominent lateral spine. In light infections with less than 50 eggs per gram of feces, ova may not be detectable in the stool without the use of techniques which sample large quantities of stool. Even in light infections, ova can usually be detected in rectal biopsies and are best identified by squashing a small amount of tissue between two glass slides and searching for ova microscopically.

Many serologic tests have been employed in the diagnosis of schistosomiasis. These tests are not standardized and differ in sensitivity and specificity. In general, most currently employed tests have greater than 90 percent sensitivity, and a positive serology is indicative of a present or past infection. An immunofluorescent antibody test employing sections of adult schistosomes to determine the presence of antibodies to schistosome gut antigens has been extremely useful in identifying recently infected expatriates and persons with acute schistosomiasis.

Treatment In previous years, chemotherapy was offered to more heavily infected individuals who were more likely to develop disease. Although the risks of continued infection have not been clearly defined, with the availability of easily administered and safe drugs, most infected persons are likely to benefit from treatment. Patients with active infections have live eggs which can be identified microscopically by experienced parasitologists or by the presence of flame cells, or by their ability to hatch after contact with water. Although a number of drugs are available for the treatment of schistosomiasis mansoni, praziquantel and oxamniquine are the drugs of choice (Table 164-2). Both drugs are equally safe and effective in schistosomiasis mansoni found in the Caribbean and South America. Because some strains of *S. mansoni* in Africa are relatively resistant to oxamniquine, praziquantel is the better drug in treating these individuals. Both drugs can be used in patients with portal fibrosis. The side effects of praziquantel and oxamniquine are frequent but transient and mild. For praziquantel they include abdominal pain, lethargy, diarrhea, and fever and for oxamniquine, dizziness, tiredness, nausea and vomiting, neuropsychiatric manifestations, and rarely convulsions.

***SCHISTOSOMA JAPONICUM* Epidemiology and clinical manifestations** *Schistosoma japonicum* is found in southeast Asia and is an important health concern in areas of China and the Philippines. The intermediate hosts are amphibious snails of the genus *Oncomelania*. Besides humans, numerous mammals such as cattle and water buffalo are naturally infected and serve as reservoirs of infection. The prepatent period is about 4 weeks.

The course of infection and clinical manifestations of *S. japonicum* are similar to those of *S. mansoni*, but the epidemiology and disease manifestations are less well studied. Experimental infections are more virulent, probably because each worm pair produces 10 times as many eggs as *S. mansoni*. The granulomas contain clusters of eggs and are larger and frequently show central necrosis. As in *S. mansoni* infections, periportal fibrosis is the major clinical manifestation. The other clinical syndromes described in *S. mansoni* also occur as complications of this infection (see above). However, there are some notable differences in disease manifestations, particularly CNS involvement. In acute schistosomiasis associated with *S. japonicum* infections, about 2 to 3 percent of patients experience CNS symptoms and signs that mimic acute encephalitis or a focal neurologic process. Computerized axial tomography shows multiple enhancing lesions. In chronic infections, patients may present with focal lesions of the brain which mimic brain tumors. These lesions contain masses of eggs and granulomas. Uncontrolled studies suggest that treatment with antischistosomal drugs and corticosteroids is effective.

Diagnosis The principles of diagnosis are similar to those of *S. mansoni* and require the demonstration of the typical ova in the tissues or feces of infected individuals. The eggs are oval in shape, 70 to 100 μm by 50 to 65 μm, and have a vestigial spine. Old, calcified, dead eggs are commonly retained in the tissues for long periods of time and do not indicate active infection (see *S. mansoni*).

Treatment Most infected persons should be treated. The only safe and effective therapy for *S. japonicum* infections is praziquantel (Table 164-2).

SCHISTOSOMA MEKONGI *Schistosoma mekongi* occurs in the Mekong River in Indochina (Laos, Cambodia, and Thailand). The intermediate host is an aquatic snail, *T. aperta*. The eggs are similar to *S. japonicum's* but are slightly smaller and round, about 56 μm by 64 μm. Dogs and human beings are frequently naturally infected. The prepatent period is about 5 weeks. The disease manifestations appear to be similar to those of *S. japonicum* but are not fully documented. Praziquantel is effective therapy for this infection (Table 164-2).

SCHISTOSOMA HAEMATOBIUM **Epidemiology and clinical manifestations** *S. haematobium* infections occur in extensive areas of Africa and in the Middle East. The intermediate hosts are of the genus *Bulinus*. The prepatent period is 2 to 3 months. Natural infection is primarily limited to human beings.

As in *S. mansoni* infections, the prevalence and intensity of infection in endemic areas increases until 10 to 15 years of age. Thereafter, the intensity decreases markedly while the prevalence rate falls moderately. The signs and symptoms due to *S. haematobium*, owing to its predilection for the veins of the urinary tract, result from involvement of the ureters and bladder. In contrast to the asymptomatic period following initial infection with the intestinal schistosomes, dysuria and hematuria are frequently noted 2 to 3 months after infection. These findings may continue throughout the course of active infection. Initially, the eggs invoke an intense inflammatory and granulomatous response which may cause anatomic and/or functional obstruction, hydroureter and hydronephrosis, and masses in the bladder or ureters. Cystoscopic examination may reveal friable masses extending into the bladder, ulceration, petechiae, and granulomas. These early lesions are reversible after antischistosomal chemotherapy. Eggs shed into the urine are usually easily demonstrable. As the infection progresses, the inflammatory component lessens, possibly due to a modulating effect of the host's immune response, and fibrosis increases, most likely due to the accumulation of many old and some new lesions. Still later, a majority of the lesions consist of masses of dead and calcified eggs in fibrous tissue. When the concentration of calcified eggs in the tissues is large enough, radiographic opacification of the affected areas of the urinary tract becomes evident. Old fibrotic lesions which cause hydroureter and hydronephrosis are not reversible by antischistosomal chemotherapy. Renal failure occurs in a surprisingly small proportion of infected individuals.

Portal fibrosis and clinically significant glomerulonephritis are not complications of this infection, but passage of eggs into the lungs may result in pulmonary hypertension. Prolonged excretion of salmonella in the urine and intermittent bacteremias are well documented. Urinary tract infections with other bacteria do not appear to be increased in frequency unless there is instrumentation of the urinary tract; however, they may be difficult to eradicate once established. Central nervous system infection most commonly involves the spinal cord, as in *S. mansoni* infections. Although eggs of *S. haematobium* are frequently detected in the feces in low numbers and are often found in rectal biopsies, intestinal polyposis is uncommon. In certain geographic areas squamous cell cancer of the bladder is felt to be associated with *S. haematobium* infection and is a significant cause of morbidity and mortality.

Diagnosis The diagnosis of *S. haematobium* is established by demonstrating the characteristic eggs in the tissues or urine. These are 112 to 170 μm by 40 to 70 μm, have a prominent terminal spine, and are easily seen in the urine. An increased number of eggs is excreted around midday, and microscopic examination of a centrifuged urine specimen collected at this time usually reveals ova. In light infections, examination of increased quantities of urine is sometimes required. Gross or microscopic hematuria is common in endemic populations, and its presence should always suggest the diagnosis in exposed individuals. Antibodies to *S. haematobium* can be detected using *S. mansoni* antigen preparations.

Treatment Infected persons should be treated. Dead and calcified eggs are common in tissue, are often seen in urine specimens, and

TABLE 164-2 Treatment of schistosomiasis

Species	Drug	Total dose* (mg per kilogram body weight)	Regimen
S. haematobium	Praziquantel	40	Single dose or two 20 mg/kg doses
	Metrifonate†	22.5–30	Single dose of 7.5 to 10 mg per kilogram body weight administered every other week × 3
S. mansoni			
Americas and Caribbean	Oxamniquine	15	Single oral dose with food
	Praziquantel	40	Single or two 20 mg/kg doses 4 h apart with food
Africa and Middle East	Oxamniquine	60	15 mg per kilogram body weight twice a day for 2 days with food
	Praziquantel	40	Single dose or two 20 mg/kg doses 4 h apart with food
S. japonicum or *S. mekongi*	Praziquantel	60	20 mg per kilogram body weight every 4 h with food

* *All recommended drugs are given orally.*
† *Available from the Parasitic Diseases Division, Centers for Infectious Diseases, Centers for Disease Control, Atlanta, GA 30333.*

should be differentiated from viable eggs. Although a number of drugs have been used to treat *S. haematobium* in the past, praziquantel is the treatment of choice (Table 164-2). Metrifonate, a safe, orally administered agent, is also effective. Its major advantage is low cost, and the major disadvantage is that it is optimally given in three doses 2 weeks apart.

SCHISTOSOMA INTERCALATUM *Schistosoma intercalatum* infection is limited to areas of West Africa. Eggs, 140 to 240 μm by 50 to 85 μm, are found in the stool and have a terminal spine. Few symptoms can be attributable to this infection, and no cases of portal fibrosis have been reported. Praziquantel is effective treatment (Table 164-2).

SCHISTOSOME DERMATITIS (SWIMMER'S ITCH) When cercariae penetrate the skin, they may provoke a reaction known as schistosome dermatitis. Symptoms occur most commonly after penetration of nonhuman schistosomes of birds and mammals. In previously unexposed persons, the initial invasion causes transient itching and uncommonly urticaria followed by the development of macules within 24 h and papules after 24 h. Following repeated exposures, the signs and symptoms increase dramatically and occur earlier. Large pruritic, erythematous papules and uncommonly vesicles develop within 24 h. The lesions are most intense 2 to 3 days following exposure and subside after a few days. These lesions represent a delayed hypersensitivity reaction to the invading schistosome. Nonhuman schistosomes do not fully develop in humans, and the signs and symptoms are limited to the skin. A similar dermatitis also occurs after infection with human schistosomes.

Schistosome dermatitis occurs in many freshwater areas of the world but is particularly common in the north central and western United States. A dermatitis following seawater exposure (clam digger's itch) has also been described.

Treatment is symptomatic. Since cercariae need some time to invade the skin (15 min or less), rapid removal of cercariae-containing droplets after water contact will decrease exposure. Limiting the numbers of the intermediate host snail in frequented areas can effectively control exposure.

CONTROL OF SCHISTOSOMIASIS Theoretically, schistosome infections can be controlled by a variety of methods, but their application has generally been only partially successful. Simple and effective health education measures such as the elimination of indiscriminate urination and defecation are difficult to implement in endemic areas. Elimination of the intermediate molluscan host can be accomplished with the use of molluscicides or by destroying the habitat of the snail. Both methods require dedication of resources and personnel often not readily available. Mass chemotherapy of populations has been tried, and repeated treatments will be needed depending on the degree of reinfection. Some advocate the treatment of those likely to develop serious disease (e.g., those heavily infected). The methods employed will depend on the nature of the endemic area and the resources available.

REFERENCES

Cheever AW, Andrade ZA: Pathological lesions associated with *Schistosoma mansoni* infection in man. Trans R Soc Trop Med Hyg 61:626, 1968

Davis A, Wegner DHG: Multicenter trials of praziquantel in human schistosomiasis: Design and techniques. Bull WHO 57:767, 1979

Forsyth DM: A longitudinal study of endemic urinary schistosomiasis in a small East African community. Bull WHO 40:771, 1969

Hiat RA et al: Factors in the pathogenesis of acute schistosomiasis mansoni. J Infect Dis 139:659, 1979

Kolata G: Avoiding the schistosome's tricks. Science 227:285, 1985

Lehman JS et al: Urinary schistosomiasis in Egypt: Clinical, radiological, bacteriological, and parasitological correlations. Trans R Soc Trop Med Hyg 67:384, 1973

McCutchan TF et al: Differentiation of schistosome by species, strain, and sex by using cloned DNA markers. Proc Natl Acad Sci 81:889, 1984

Nash TE et al: Schistosome infections in humans: Perspective and recent findings. Ann Intern Med 97:740, 1982

——— et al: Treatment of *Schistosoma mekongi* with praziquantel: A double-blinded study. Am J Trop Med Hyg 3:977, 1982

Schistosomiasis, Epidemiology, Treatment and Control, P Jordan, G Webbe (eds). London, Heinemann Medical, 1982

165 TISSUE NEMATODES

JAMES J. PLORDE

ANGIOSTRONGYLIASIS CANTONENSIS Definition *Angiostrongylus cantonensis,* the rat lungworm, is the etiologic agent of the common form of *eosinophilic meningitis* found in southeast Asia and the tropical areas of the Pacific.

Etiology The delicate filariform adults (20 mm in length) reside and lay their eggs in the pulmonary arterioles of rats and certain other rodents. After hatching, the larvae break into the alveoli, migrate up the respiratory tract, are swallowed, and pass in the feces. They develop into infective third-stage larvae within snails and slugs, their natural intermediate host. Viable third-stage organisms may also be found in land planarians, crabs, and freshwater prawns. These carriers appear to acquire the larvae by feeding on the tissues of infected mollusks. Humans, like rodents, become parasitized when they ingest raw intermediate or carrier hosts containing the infective stage. In rodents the larvae migrate to the brain where they grow into young adults. After a period of further maturation, the worms travel to the lungs and begin to deposit eggs. The nematode does not complete its life cycle in humans and dies after reaching the central nervous system.

Epidemiology The majority of human infections with *A. cantonensis* have been found in Thailand, Vietnam, Cambodia, Indonesia, the Philippines, Taiwan, Hawaii, and several smaller Pacific islands from Okinawa in the north to New Caledonia, American Samoa, and Tahiti in the south. Cases have been described in Cuba, Egypt, and the Ivory Coast. In addition, rodent infections have been found in the islands of East Africa, Sri Lanka, India, and China. The rat lungworm may have been spread from Madagascar to Asia and to the Pacific by the recent dispersal of the giant African land snail, *Achatina fulica.*

Pathology and pathogenesis The nematode can produce extensive tissue damage by moving through the brain when alive and provokes a marked inflammatory reaction when dead. The pathologic lesions are characterized by (1) marked lymphocyte and eosinophilic infiltration of the meninges, (2) hemorrhagic and nonhemorrhagic worm tracts through the brainstem and spinal cord, (3) granuloma formation around dead parasites and necrotic debris which sheathes the worm, and (4) engorgement of almost all blood vessels, particularly the veins. Necrosis of vessel walls, aneurysmal dilatation of arteries, and perivascular hemorrhages have been noted. Living worms have been removed from the eyes of patients without central nervous system involvement.

Clinical manifestations The eosinophilic meningitis usually presents as an acute severe headache. Fever is usually mild or absent, and only 15 percent of patients show signs of meningeal irritation. Patients frequently complain of visual impairment and, in a majority of these, visual defects or blurring of the optic disk can be demonstrated. Paresthesias and exquisite pains of the trunk and lower extremities are a common complaint, and paralysis of the sixth and seventh nerves is seen in 3 to 7 percent of cases. Paralysis of the limbs, convulsions, and loss of consciousness are rare. Although some patients have experienced significant neurologic residua, the disease usually ends in complete spontaneous recovery. Death is rare. The cerebrospinal fluid contains several hundred cells per cubic millimeter and many eosinophils, and the cerebrospinal fluid protein is elevated. There may or may not be an eosinophilia in the peripheral blood.

A second clinically distinct form of eosinophilic meningitis has been reported. This presents as a radiculomyeloencephalitis with limb pain, paresis, and bowel and bladder dysfunction. This syndrome may be more common in heavy infections. In Thailand, this syndrome is thought to be caused by the nematode *Gnathostoma spinigerum.* The cerebrospinal fluid eosinophilic leukocytosis is less marked than in the meningitic form of the disease. The fluid is often xanthochromic. Death may occur from cerebral hemorrhage or destruction of vital centers.

Diagnosis The diagnosis is made on the basis of the clinical manifestations in an endemic area. Rarely, the adult worm is found in the cerebrospinal fluid. Angiostrongyliasis must be differentiated from other ectopic worm infections of the central nervous system including strongyloidiasis, filariasis, paragonimiasis, hydatid disease, schistosomiasis japonicum, trichinosis, cysticercosis, toxocariasis, and gnathostomiasis. A case of visceral larva migrans with eosinophilic meningitis has been described, in which the raccoon ascarid, *Baylisascaris procyonis,* was implicated.

Treatment and prevention There is no known effective treatment. Anthelmintic therapy has been thought by some authors to be dangerous since the simultaneous death of many worms might produce a severe inflammatory reaction. Steroids may be beneficial in severe cases. Prevention depends upon avoidance or proper cooking of such foods as snails, prawns, and crabs. Raw vegetables should be carefully inspected for the presence of planarians and mollusks before they are eaten. Freezing of crustaceans and mollusks at −15°C for 12 h will destroy infective larvae of *A. cantonensis.*

ANGIOSTRONGYLIASIS COSTARICENSIS *Angiostrongylus costaricensis* is a nematode that dwells in the mesenteric arteries of Central American rats. Larvae pass in the stool and develop in slugs, the intermediate hosts. Rats, and incidentally humans, are infected when they ingest slugs or vegetables contaminated with third-stage larvae deposited in the mucous trail of these mollusks. The larvae mature in the lymphatics and move to the mesenteric radicals of the cecum. Here they may cause arterial thrombosis, ischemic necrosis, ulceration, and eosinophilic granuloma formation. Infected patients present with fever, eosinophilic leukocytosis, abdominal pain, and a right lower quadrant mass. Occasionally perforation of the bowel and generalized peritonitis occur. The fever may persist for up to 2 months. Children are more frequently involved than adults. Neither larvae nor eggs are seen in the stool of the human host. No specific therapy is available.

GNATHOSTOMIASIS Definition Gnathostomiasis is a tissue infection of humans caused by *Gnathostoma spinigerum,* an intestinal nematode of carnivores. Clinically it is manifest as migratory subcutaneous swellings, creeping eruption, or a lethal eosinophilic meningitis.

Etiology and epidemiology The parasite, which is found throughout the Far East, lives encysted in the gastric mucosa of dogs, cats, and wild felines. The ova are passed to the external environment via the feces, hatch in water, and are ingested by *Cyclops,* the first intermediate hosts. These in turn are eaten by freshwater fish, frogs, snakes, and eels in whose flesh the infective third-stage larvae develop. Ducks and chickens fed on these second intermediate hosts may also come to harbor infective larvae. Human infections, which are most commonly seen in Thailand and Japan, occur when humans ingest infected uncooked fish (somfak, sashimi), duck, or chicken.

Pathogenesis and manifestations The parasite cannot complete its cycle in humans, and the immature worms migrate through the abdominal and thoracic organs producing localized areas of inflammation and hemorrhage. Clinically, this is manifest as fever, eosinophilic leukocytosis, urticaria, and pain. Typically, the systemic manifestations subside within a month as the worms make their way to the subcutaneous tissues. Here, their continued migration results in the production of transient serpiginous pruritic swellings, subcutaneous tunnels, and abscesses. If the worm invades the epidermis, the resulting lesions closely resemble those of cutanea larva migrans. Rarely the eye may be involved with orbital cellulitis, iritis, or uveitis. Migration into the central nervous system results in a lethal eosinophilic meningitis (see "Angiostrongyliasis Cantonensis" above). This presents as a radiculomyeloencephalitis with limb pain and paresis. The cerebrospinal fluid eosinophilic leukocytosis is present but less marked than in *Angiostrongylus* infections. The fluid is often xanthochromic. Death may occur from cerebral hemorrhage or destruction of vital centers.

Diagnosis and treatment Painless, recurrent migratory subcutaneous swellings and eosinophilic leukocytosis occurring in an endemic area make the diagnosis likely. It must be differentiated from cutanea larva migrans, however, and from angiostrongyliasis cantonensis when the central nervous system is involved. Definitive diagnosis depends upon the removal and identification of the worm. Other than excision, there is no specific therapy. The disease can be prevented by the adequate cooking of fish, chicken, and duck in endemic areas.

DRACUNCULIASIS Definition Dracunculiasis is an infection of human connective and subcutaneous tissues by the guinea worm, *Dracunculus medinensis.* The gravid female produces symptoms when she ruptures the skin to discharge her eggs.

Etiology and epidemiology Dracunculiasis affects about 50 million people in west, central, and northeast Africa, the Middle East, Iran, Pakistan, India, northeastern South America, and the Caribbean islands. Humans acquire the parasite when they ingest raw drinking water containing infected copepods (*Cyclops* spp.) which serve as the intermediate host. Shallow ponds, cisterns, and wells are the usual habitat of these crustaceans. In the stomach the copepod is digested and the larvae are released. The larva penetrates the intestinal wall and matures in the connective tissue of the retroperitoneal space. The adult male is small, seldom seen, and presumably dies after mating. In contrast, the female *Dracunculus* is one of the largest nematodes known—1 to 2 mm in diameter and 300 to 800 mm in length. The female reaches gravidity in approximately one year and then migrates to the subcutaneous tissue of the lower extremities. When the anterior end of the worm approaches the skin, a blister forms. This breaks down in a few days, forming a superficial ulcer. When the protruding portion of the worm comes in contact with water, the uterus prolapses through the body and discharges large numbers of motile rhabditiform larvae. Following ingestion by one of several species of *Cyclops,* the larvae undergo further development, becoming infective in 10 to 12 days. Mammals other than humans may be infected, but their importance as a disease reservoir is uncertain.

Pathogenesis and manifestations The infection is asymptomatic until the gravid female appears in the subcutaneous tissues, where it may, on occasion, be palpable. A few days before the formation of the blister, the patient frequently has fever, generalized urticaria, periorbital edema, and wheezing. Blister formation is accompanied by intense local pain and pruritus; like the systemic manifestations, this is thought to represent an allergic reaction to prematurely liberated larvae. The local lesion is usually found over the feet and ankles but may occur on the trunk or the upper extremities. Multiple infections are common. With the rupture of the blister and the release of embryos, the systemic manifestations abate, and the worm is slowly extruded over a period of 4 to 5 weeks. Secondary infection and cellulitis are common, particularly if the worm is ruptured during the process of extraction. In Nigeria, guinea worm ulcers are a common portal of entry for the spores of *Clostridium tetani.* The female worm often fails to reach the surface and discharge her larvae. In most of these cases, it dies without producing symptoms. The calcified appearance on roentgenograms is characteristic. Occasionally the worm may invade the deep tissues, causing serious symptoms, and sterile abscesses may follow the release of embryos. Invasion of joint spaces by the adult worm or larvae results in arthritis.

Diagnosis The clinical picture is characteristic. Placing a small amount of water on the worm results in discharge of larvae which can then be examined microscopically. A fluorescent antibody test may permit the diagnosis to be made prior to emergence of the gravid female.

Treatment and prevention If the outline of the worm can be clearly seen or palpated, it may sometimes be completely removed with a single incision. The gradual extraction of the worm can be accomplished by winding a few centimeters onto a stick each day. Administration of niridazole (Ambilhar) results in prompt remission of symptoms. The dose is 25 mg per kilogram of body weight given in three divided doses for 7 days. Thiabendazole in dosage of 25 mg/kg twice daily for 2 days or metronidazole 250 mg three times a day for 7 days is also effective in the relief of symptoms. At present, there is serious question whether any of the above agents hasten worm extrusion or death. Some authorities suggest the rapid symptomatic improvement induced by these agents is secondary to their anti-inflammatory rather than anthelmintic properties. Dracunculiasis can be prevented by the chemical treatment of drinking water or the provision of piped water.

REFERENCES

Editorial: After smallpox, guineaworm? Lancet 1:61, 1983

Fox AS et al: Fatal eosinophilic meningoencephalitis and visceral larva migrans caused by the raccoon ascarid *Baylisascaris procyonis*. N Engl J Med 312:1619, 1985

Kliks MM et al: Eosinophilic radiculomyeloencephalitis: An angiostrongyliasis outbreak in American Samoa related to ingestion of *Achatina fulica* snails. Am J Trop Med Hyg 31:1114, 1982

Loria-Cortes R, Lobo-Sanahuja JF: Clinical abdominal angiostrongylosis. A study of 116 children with intestinal eosinophilic granuloma caused by *Angiostrongylus costaricensis*. Am J Trop Med Hyg 29:538, 1980

Pascual JE et al: Eosinophilic meningoencephalitis in Cuba caused by *Angiostrongylus cantonensis*. Am J Trop Med Hyg 30:960, 1981

Punyagupta S et al: Eosinophilic meningitis in Thailand. Am J Trop Med 24:921, 1975

166 INTESTINAL NEMATODES

JAMES J. PLORDE

ENTEROBIASIS Definition Enterobiasis (pinworm, seatworm, or threadworm infection, oxyuriasis) is an intestinal infection of humans caused by *Enterobius vermicularis* and characterized by perianal pruritus. Eggs of this parasite have been found in a 10,000-year-old coprolith, making it the oldest demonstrated infection of humans. It has been estimated that the worm infects 200 million people, 30 to 40 million of them in the United States and Canada.

Etiology The female averages 10 mm in length, the male 3 mm. They live with their heads attached to the mucosa of the cecum, appendix, and adjacent parts of the bowel. The gravid female migrates through the anal canal at night, deposits her 10,000 eggs on the perianal skin, and dies. In female patients the worm may enter the vagina and occasionally gain access to the peritoneal cavity through the fallopian tubes. Each egg contains an embryo which, within a few hours, develops into an infective larva. After the egg has been ingested, the larva is released in the small intestine and migrates down the bowel lumen to the cecum. In less than 1 month from the time of ingestion, newly developed gravid females are again discharging eggs. They are planoconvex and measure approximately 20 by 50 μm. The shell is clear and doubly contoured.

Epidemiology Humans are usually infected by the direct transfer of eggs from the anus to the mouth by way of contaminated fingers. Retroinfection, which is seen primarily in adults, may occasionally take place when eggs hatch in the perianal area and the larvae migrate back into the bowel to mature. The eggs, which are relatively resistant to desiccation, also contaminate nightclothes and bed linen, where they remain viable and infective for 2 to 3 weeks. Airborne transmission is possible, and spread within family and children's groups occurs readily. Enterobiasis is found in all climates and is probably the most common helminthic infection of humans. Its low incidence in some tropical areas, however, is not fully explained.

Clinical manifestations The most common symptom is pruritus ani, which is most troublesome at night, being related to the migration of the gravid female worms. Irritability, insomnia, enuresis, and other minor complaints are probably secondary to the pruritus. Scratching may lead to perianal eczema or pyogenic infection. Vaginal discharge has been reported, and rarely a chronic granulomatous salpingitis or endometritis results from the presence of ectopic adults. An association between enterobiasis and cystitis in young females has been reported. This, it is suggested, results from the transport of enteric bacteria into the bladder by the migrating worm. Other rare ectopic locations include the lung, liver, and peritoneum. Probably the worms can penetrate the bowel wall only if its continuity has been compromised by some other disease.

Laboratory findings Examination for ova of material obtained from the perianal skin by means of a Scotch brand cellophane tape swab is the preferable method for the detection of enterobiasis. The tape is folded sticky-side out over the end of a tongue blade, pressed firmly against the perianal area, and then spread on a glass slide and examined under the lower power of a microscope. The swab should be taken at home by the patient on three to five consecutive mornings prior to bathing and brought to the laboratory for examination. Searching for ova in the feces is rarely helpful, but scrapings from under the nails may reveal ova. The diagnosis is sometimes made by finding adult worms in the perianal area or in the feces following a laxative or an enema. Eosinophilic leukocytosis may occur but is not a typical finding.

Treatment All infected individuals in a family or communal group should be treated simultaneously. The frequently recommended sanitary measures aside from daily bathing and hand washing before meals and after stools are of dubious benefit. It is relatively easy to eradicate the worms, but reinfection is frequent. Retreatment does not appear necessary unless symptoms recur.

Two highly satisfactory drugs are available. Pyrantel pamoate given in a single oral dose of 11 mg/kg (maximum 1.0 g) is probably the drug of choice. Alternatively, a single 100-mg oral dose of mebendazole can be used. This drug is not recommended for infants or pregnant women. Pyrvinium pamoate is equally effective but less convenient. It is given orally as a single dose of 5 mg/kg in tablet or liquid form. This compound turns the stool red and may stain bedclothes or undergarments. In heavily contaminated environments, treatment with the above drugs may be repeated after an interval of 2 weeks to eliminate any new infections.

Prevention Methods of preventing autoinfection and dissemination within a group involving children are extremely difficult to enforce. Personal environmental hygiene should be stressed, and anthelmintic and symptomatic treatment of pruritus ani should be instituted. To control infection within a group, simultaneous treatment of all cases is mandatory.

TRICHURIASIS Definition Trichuriasis (whipworm infection, trichocephaliasis) is an intestinal infection of humans caused by *Trichuris trichiura* and is characterized by invasion of the colonic mucosa by the adult trichuris. Five hundred million persons are thought to be infected with this parasite including 2 million in the United States. It may be the most commonly encountered helminthic infection in Americans returning from tropical areas.

Etiology The adult whipworms are found in the large intestine with their anterior ends deeply embedded in the mucosa. They are 30 to 50 mm in length and possess a threadlike anterior two-thirds with a stouter posterior third, giving them a whiplike structure. The female produces about 5000 eggs each day. They are characteristically barrel-shaped (20 to 50 μm), brown, thick-walled, and translucent with knoblike ends. The eggs, like those of *Ascaris*, must incubate at least 3 weeks in soil before they become infective. After ingestion, the eggs hatch in the small intestine and the larvae become embedded in the intestinal villi. After several days they migrate to the large intestine where they mature in about 3 months. The adult worms may live for 4 to 8 years. Occasionally, *T. vulpis*, the whipworm of dogs, may infect humans. The eggs are larger (35 by 75 μm) but otherwise identical to those of the human parasite.

Epidemiology Whipworm is a cosmopolitan parasite but is most commonly found in the tropics where the level of sanitation is low and environmental conditions necessary for the incubation of the eggs are optimal. In the United States, it is found throughout the rural areas of the southeast. Its distribution is similar to that of *Ascaris* and hookworm, but the eggs are less resistant than those of *Ascaris* to sunlight and drying. Because of their general lack of sanitary habits, children and the mentally retarded have the highest incidence of infection. For example, 13 percent of patients confined to hospitals for the mentally subnormal were found to harbor *Trichuris*.

Pathogenesis and clinical manifestations Symptomatic infection generally requires the presence of large numbers of adult whipworms and may be correlated in part with the degree of mucosal involvement. Heavy infections usually occur only in children and may be accompanied by finger clubbing, nausea, abdominal pain, diarrhea, and dysentery. It has been estimated that infected patients lose 0.005 mL blood per worm per day. Infections with more than 800 worms often result in anemia. In heavier infections, the distribution of worms throughout the colon and rectum may result in rectal prolapse while straining at stool. Some investigators also feel that *Trichuris* infections predispose to amebic dysentery and bacterial gastroenteritis.

Laboratory findings In symptomatic infection, large numbers of eggs are present in the feces, and there may be eosinophilic leukocytosis and anemia. In light infections, concentration techniques may be necessary to recover the eggs. Quantitation of egg output is helpful since only counts above 3000 eggs per gram of feces are likely to be associated with symptoms. Stools should be cultured for bacterial pathogens and examined for the presence of *Entamoeba histolytica*.

Treatment Treatment is unsatisfactory. Mebendazole in the oral dose of 100 mg twice daily for 3 days is the drug of choice. Its cure rate is 60 to 70 percent, and it achieves a 90 percent reduction in egg burden. The dose may have to be repeated in patients with heavy infections. It is not recommended for children under the age of 2 or pregnant women.

Prognosis Whipworm infection, unless characterized by severe diarrhea, blood loss, and systemic reaction, usually responds well to treatment. Serious infections may require supportive treatment as well as chemotherapy.

Prevention Measures recommended for ascariasis apply also to trichuriasis.

ASCARIASIS Definition Ascariasis is an infection of humans caused by *Ascaris lumbricoides* and characterized by an early pulmonary phase related to larval migration and a later, prolonged intestinal phase. It is estimated that 25 percent of the world's population, including 4 million Americans, are infected with this nematode.

Etiology The adult ascarids are large (15 to 40 cm in length), cylindric worms with blunt ends which maintain themselves in the lumen of the jejunum by virtue of their muscular activity. Despite a life span of only 6 to 18 months, the female releases millions of eggs, both fertile and infertile, into the fecal stream; the daily output is estimated to be 200,000 per worm. Fertilized eggs are elliptic (30 to 40 μm by 50 to 60 μm) with an irregular, dense outer shell and a regular, translucent inner shell. They require a period of soil incubation before they become infective. Under optimum conditions of warmth and moisture this occurs in 2 to 3 weeks. The eggs may then remain viable for up to 6 years in temperate climates and may survive freezing. When an infective egg is ingested, the larva is liberated in the small intestine. It migrates through the wall and is carried by the bloodstream or lymphatics to the lung. After about 10 days in the pulmonary capillaries and alveoli, the larvae pass in turn up the bronchioles, bronchi, trachea, and epiglottis, are swallowed, and return to the jejunum. There they develop into mature adult worms within 2 to 3 months of ingestion. *Ascaris suum*, a roundworm of pigs, may occasionally complete a similar life cycle in humans.

Epidemiology Infection follows the ingestion of the embryonated eggs contained in contaminated food, or, more commonly, the introduction of the eggs into the mouth by the hands after contact with contaminated soil. Geophagia may produce massive infections. In endemic areas, the infection is maintained primarily by small children who defecate indiscriminately in the area of the home. In dry, windy climates, eggs may become airborne, get into the mouth, and be swallowed. Since the eggs are relatively resistant to desiccation and wide variations in temperature, the disease is worldwide. In the developing areas of the world where the lack of sanitary facilities exposes populations to the greatest risk, the prevalence of infection may be as high as 80 to 90 percent. Children are almost universally infected in these areas, with peak infection rates achieved by age 5. In temperate areas, the infection occurs in family clusters.

Pathogenesis and clinical manifestations Because of the extensive migration of which both the larvae and adults are capable, the manifestations may be diverse. Bronchopneumonia characterized by fever, cough, dyspnea, wheeze, eosinophilic leukocytosis, and migratory pulmonary infiltrates may occur during the passage of the larvae through the lung. This is most commonly seen in communities where *Ascaris* transmission is seasonal. The severity of symptoms is apparently related to both intensity of infection and the degree of sensitization resulting from previous exposures. Significant arterial oxygen desaturation and, rarely, death may occur. Adult worms may produce no symptoms if the infection is light and may be detected accidentally when the adult worm is vomited or passed in the stool. Heavier infections may cause abdominal pain and malabsorption of fat, protein, carbohydrate, and vitamins. In marginally nourished children this may produce growth retardation. Occasionally a bolus of worms may result in volvulus, intussusception, or intestinal obstruction in the iliocecal area. Children are most likely to have these complications because of their anatomically smaller intestine and larger worm loads. Up to 2000 worms have been found in children, although the usual load is less than 20. In the United States where worm loads are usually modest, the incidence of obstruction is 2 per 1000 infected children per year. It often follows a febrile illness or drug therapy which stimulates the worms to increase motility. Rarely, an adult worm will migrate into the appendix, bile ducts, or pancreatic ducts, causing obstruction and inflammation of these organs. Biliary tract obstruction may be associated with bacterial cholangitis and liver abscess. Worms may also penetrate the intestinal wall, particularly at a site of surgical anastomosis, and patients should be dewormed prior to elective surgery. Migration of the worms into the oral pharynx and mouth may lead to acute respiratory distress.

Laboratory findings The diagnosis is usually made by finding the ova in the feces. The fertilized eggs are usually numerous, characteristic, and not easily confused with those of other helminths. The occasional unisexual infection may pose diagnostic problems. The male produces no eggs, and the unfertilized ova produced by a single female may be atypical and difficult to recognize. Occasionally the worms may be seen after a barium meal, either as negative images or after ingesting barium themselves. In biliary ascariasis an intravenous cholangiogram will often demonstrate dilatation of the common duct and/or the negative image of the parasite. Ascaris pneumonia may be diagnosed by finding larvae and eosinophils in the sputum or gastric aspirate. Eggs will usually not be found until after the larvae have matured in the intestine. Eosinophilic leukocytosis is usually noted during larval migration, but diminishes and often disappears during the chronic intestinal phase of infection.

Treatment Only symptomatic treatment can be used during the period of pulmonary involvement by the migrating larvae. For removal of the adult worms from the intestines, either pyrantel pamoate or mebendazole should be used. Pyrantel is given as a single oral dose of 11 mg/kg (maximum 1.0 g). Mebendazole is given as described for trichuriasis and is the preferred agent if both *Ascaris* and *Trichuris* are present. An older agent, piperazine citrate, is highly effective, less expensive, but slightly more toxic than the above two agents. It is given as a flavored syrup administered in a single dose after breakfast on two successive days and will cure the majority of cases. The drug acts by paralyzing the ascarids, which are then passed in the stool. The dose of piperazine is 75 mg/kg with a maximum of 3.5 g. No particular dietary regulation is necessary. The drug must be administered with caution to patients with renal insufficiency, because impaired elimination may produce neurotoxic signs. In intestinal obstruction, nasogastric suction should be initiated. After vomiting is controlled, piperazine should be given through the nasogastric tube every 12 to 24 h in dosage of 65 mg/kg (maximum 1.0 g) for six doses. Surgery usually is not required.

Prognosis The prognosis in intestinal infection is generally good. When acute or chronic obstruction of ducts or hollow viscera has occurred, the immediate prognosis is determined by the promptness of diagnosis and treatment. The case fatality rate of intestinal obstruction in the United States is 3 percent.

Prevention Ascariasis is primarily a household infection of rural areas. All infections should be treated, personal hygiene stressed, and adequate toilet facilities provided. Mass therapy administered at 6-month intervals may be effective in controlling ascariasis in small communities.

TOXOCARIASIS (VISCERAL LARVA MIGRANS) **Definition** This is a human infection with *Toxocara canis*. The animal ascarid is usually unable to complete its life cycle in humans, but they may be widely disseminated in the body, producing a variety of clinical manifestations, collectively referred to as *visceral larva migrans*.

Etiology and epidemiology The large adult toxocaral worms live in the intestine of dogs. Their eggs must be passed in the stool and incubate in soil for 2 to 3 weeks before they become infective. When ingested by a mammal, larvae are liberated in the intestine, penetrate the wall, and are carried in the blood to the liver, where most remain, and lung. If the host is a young puppy, the larvae burst into the alveoli and complete their life cycle in a manner analogous to *A. lumbricoides* in humans. In humans and fully grown dogs, *Toxocara* larvae, which are approximately one-half the size of those of *A. lumbricoides*, pass through the pulmonary capillaries to reach the systemic circulation. Larvae leave the circulatory system when their gradually increasing size approaches the diameter of the vessel through which they are traveling. They migrate extensively in the surrounding tissue; some may become dormant for years, only to resume migration at a later time. *Toxocara* infections of dogs are common and widespread. Transplacental and transmammary migration of larvae account for infection rates of 80 percent or more in young puppies; they can shed a large number of ova within 4 weeks of birth. Viable ova were found in 25 percent of soil samples taken from public parks in the United States and Great Britain. Although most of the 2000 documented human infections have occurred in the United States and Europe, cases have been reported from 48 countries around the world. Children from the age of 2 to 5 years, because of their sanitary habits, predilection to geophagia, and intimate association with domestic pets, are most frequently involved. The seroprevalence of human *Toxocara* infection in the United States is approximately 3 percent; the rates are highest in the south and northeast.

Pathogenesis and clinical manifestations The larvae migrate freely in tissues, causing hemorrhage, necrosis, eosinophilic inflammatory reaction, and eventually granuloma formation. The most frequently involved organs are the liver, lungs, brain, eye, heart, and skeletal muscles. Symptoms and signs are related to the number and location of the granulomas as well as sensitization to the parasite antigen. Commonly, only asymptomatic eosinophilia marks the presence of infection. Symptomatic patients most frequently present with fever and tender hepatomegaly. Splenomegaly, skin rash, and recurrent pneumonitis with wheezing respirations may occur in more severe infections. Respiratory failure with death has been reported. Most fatalities, however, result from involvement of the myocardium or central nervous system; the latter may result in convulsions, behavior disorders, or focal neurological defects. There is often a history of dirt eating and contact with puppies. Leukocytosis with eosinophilia to high levels (over 60 percent) and hypergammaglobulinemia with raised levels of IgG, IgM, and IgE are common. These manifestations may persist for months or years. At surgery or autopsy the liver may be studded with small granulomas. A granulomatous endophthalmitis, which may be mistaken for retinoblastoma, may be observed in older children and adults. Typically, this is unilateral and occurs in the absence of other clinical manifestations of visceral larva migrans. Decreased visual acuity or strabismus brings the patient to the attention of the physician.

Diagnosis The diagnosis can usually be made on the basis of clinical findings. Infections with *A. lumbricoides,* hookworm, and *Strongyloides stercoralis,* as well as other nonhuman nematodes, may also on occasion present as visceral larva migrans, making the etiologic diagnosis difficult. Eosinophilic leukemia, trichinosis, trematode infections, and periarteritis nodosa must be ruled out. Isoagglutinin, particularly anti-A, titers of 1:1024 or greater are present in 85 percent of patients with visceral but in very few with ocular disease. The adaption of larval antigens to the enzyme-linked immunosorbent assay has, for the first time, provided clinicians with a serologic test of diagnostic value. In one study, the sensitivity and specificity were 78 and 92 percent, respectively. A definitive diagnosis depends on the identification of the larvae in sputum or tissue granuloma. Biopsy of the liver with serial sections of the specimen may reveal eosinophilic granulomas or a *Toxocara* larva.

Treatment No uniformly effective therapy is available. Diethylcarbamazine as used in Bancroftian filariasis (see Chap. 163) is probably the drug of choice. Thiabendazole in dosage of 25 to 50 mg/kg for 7 to 10 days may be helpful. Adrenocortical steroids may be beneficial when respiratory difficulty is pronounced. Control measures are directed toward preventing ingestion of eggs. Removal and repeated worming of infected dogs must be considered. Animals less than 6 months of age should be wormed monthly; older ones every 2 or 3 months.

ANISAKIASIS Ascarids belonging to family Anisakidae infect seals, dolphins, porpoises, whales, and other large sea mammals. Their larval stages are found in the flesh of squid and several marine fish including cod, mackerel, salmon, herring, and various rock fishes, including "Pacific red snapper." Humans are infected by eating raw, pickled, or slightly salted fish delicacies such as "green herring," sushi, sashimi, sunomono, ceviche, and gravlax which contain the third-stage larvae. The infection may be asymptomatic and noted only when the worm is coughed or vomited up. More characteristically, the larvae burrow into the mucosa of the stomach, small intestine, or more rarely the colon. Here they produce eosinophilic granulomatous tumors with edema, thickening, and induration of the bowel wall which may be mistaken for gastric carcinoma or regional enteritis. Occasionally, larvae may penetrate the intestinal wall to involve other abdominal organs. Perforations of the bowel with peritonitis have also been described. The pathologic changes are thought to be the result of a hypersensitivity reaction. In the acute gastric syndrome common in Japan, the patient may develop epigastric pain, nausea, and vomiting within a few hours of ingesting infected fish. With a gastroscope 2- to 4-cm larvae can be seen penetrating the mucosa and can sometimes be removed. In Europeans, the small intestine has been the site most frequently involved. The clinical picture may be severe enough to simulate an acute surgical abdomen. More commonly, colicky pain, diffuse abdominal tenderness, fever, and leukocytosis develop a week or more after the ingestion of fish. Peripheral eosinophilia is not always present, and a definitive diagnosis can be made only by the identification of larvae in tissue. Serologic tests are being developed, but are neither highly reliable nor generally available. The disease usually subsides spontaneously with conservative therapy. Occasionally, a chronic illness develops which requires surgical resection of the lesion.

Over 1000 cases have been recognized in the Netherlands and Japan, and several cases have been reported from North America. The disease can be prevented by storing marine fish at $-20°C$ for a single day or by cooking it at normal cooking temperatures.

HOOKWORM DISEASE **Definition** Hookworm disease is a symptomatic infection caused by *Necator americanus, Ancylostoma duodenale,* or, less commonly, *A. ceylanicum.* Asymptomatic infection may be termed simply *hookworm infection,* and the individual with such infection is called a *carrier.*

Etiology *Ancylostoma duodenale,* also known as the "old world" hookworm, possesses four prominent hooklike teeth in its adult stage. The adults are about 1 cm long and inhabit the upper part of the human small intestine, where they attach to the mucosa by means of the mouth parts and suck blood. Each adult extracts approximately 0.20 mL blood daily. The adults migrate within the small intestine, and each site of attachment persists temporarily as a bleeding point. Following fertilization, the female liberates approximately 20,000 eggs per day. They measure about 40 by 60 μm and are usually in the two- to four-celled stage when discharged in the feces.

Necator americanus, the "new world" hookworm, has a buccal capsule containing dorsal and ventral plates rather than teeth. It is slightly smaller, deposits fewer eggs, and causes much less blood loss than *A. duodenale* (0.03 mL per worm daily). *Ancylostoma ceylanicum,* a hookworm of cats found in the Far East, may occasionally reach maturity in humans.

The life cycles of the hookworms are similar. Under appropriate conditions, the eggs hatch in 24 to 48 h, releasing free-living or rhabditiform larvae. Within a few days, these develop into infective or filariform larvae which may remain viable in the soil for several weeks. These, in turn, penetrate the skin to enter vessels which carry them to the lungs. The larvae leave the alveolar capillaries, enter the alveoli, ascend the respiratory tree, enter the pharynx, and are swallowed. They reach the intestine about 1 week after penetration of the skin and mature within 5 weeks. Larval development of *Ancylostoma* may be arrested or retarded in the human host. This may result in a prolonged latent period between the onset of infection and the appearance of gravid females in the intestine. Adults have been known to survive in the human intestine for as long as 14 years, but *A. duodenale* seldom persists beyond 6 to 8 years, and most *N. americanus* infections are eliminated within 2 to 4 years.

Epidemiology It has been estimated that hookworms infect 700 million people and cause the loss of 7 million liters of blood daily throughout the world from 45°N to 30°S latitude. *Necator americanus* is found predominantly in the tropical areas of Africa, Asia, and the Americas, while *A. duodenale* occurs in the Mediterranean Basin, the Middle East, northern India, China, and Japan. In many areas both species are found. In general, *Ancylostoma* presents a greater public health hazard than *N. americanus,* the species which is most prevalent in the southern United States, because it is more persistent in the environment, more harmful to the host, and less amenable to treatment. Conditions conducive to the development of the hookworm egg into infective filariform larvae are a mean temperature between 23 and 33°C, abundant rainfall, shade, and well-drained sandy soil. Hookworm infection occurs where there is opportunity for direct contact of the skin with soil contaminated by promiscuous defecation. The disease may also be acquired by oral ingestion of infective larvae, particularly those of *A. duodenale.* Lactogenic transmission may also occur with this species; presumably this results from the activation of larvae whose development within the tissues of the host has been arrested or retarded. Probably because of greater exposure, males show a higher incidence of infection than females. Infections are particularly common in closed, heavily populated communities such as coffee or tea plantations.

Repeated infections of hookworm in dogs result in immunity and elimination of the parasite. It seems probable that a similar phenomenon occurs in human infections. When the possibility of reinfection is eliminated, the majority of worms is eliminated spontaneously within 1 or 2 years.

Pathogenesis and clinical manifestations During the invasion of the exposed skin by the larvae, there may be an erythematous maculopapular skin rash and edema with severe pruritus. These manifestations, which may persist for several days, are more marked in *N. americanus* infection. The lesions are most common about the feet, particularly between the toes, and have been termed "ground itch."

During migration through the lungs, cough, pneumonia, and, in severe infections, fever may occur. Usually, however, pulmonary involvement does not give rise to clinical symptoms.

Various gastrointestinal symptoms, ranging from vague epigastric distress and pica to typical ulcer pain, have been reported in association with hookworm infection. Roentgenographic studies may reveal nonspecific changes such as excessive peristalsis and "puddling," particularly in the proximal jejunum. However, gross and microscopic examination of the bowel itself reveals conspicuously little damage. Previous reports of absorptive abnormalities in hookworm infection have not been supported.

The major clinical manifestations of hookworm disease clearly are those of iron-deficiency anemia and hypoalbuminemia consequent to chronic intestinal blood loss. Whether anemia develops and how severe it becomes depends on the balance between iron lost in the gut and iron absorbed from the diet. In many endemic areas, dietary iron is largely of vegetable origin and is absorbed poorly. General dietary deficiency also may lower resistance to parasitic infections. The severity of the disease and the prognosis depend on such factors as the age of the patient, the magnitude of the worm burden, the duration of the disease, and diet. Young children often have extreme anemia, with cardiac insufficiency and anasarca. These conditions may precipitate kwashiorkor. Those who survive to puberty show retarded physical, mental, and sexual development. Milder degrees of the disease, as seen in older children and adults, are characterized by lassitude, dyspnea, palpitation, tachycardia, constipation, and pallor of the skin and mucous membranes.

Asymptomatic infections outnumber symptomatic infections, considering all age groups, 20 to 40 times in endemic areas. The worm burden is small in asymptomatic infections, and the carrier state may be indicative of some degree of acquired host resistance.

Laboratory findings In symptomatic infection, hookworm eggs are usually numerous enough to be detected by microscopic examination of a direct or concentrated fecal smear. A quantitative egg count, using the Stoll or Beaver technique, allows an estimation of the intensity of infection. If a stool specimen is allowed to stand for several hours before examination, the eggs may hatch, releasing larvae which are easily confused with those of *Strongyloides.* The eggs must be differentiated from those of *Trichostrongylus* and *Ternidens diminutus,* which are larger and in a later stage of maturation when observed in a fresh fecal specimen than are those of *Necator* or *Ancylostoma.* Abdominal and pulmonary symptoms appear before the eggs are discharged, although a presumptive diagnosis may be made on the basis of the clinical history and the eosinophilic leukocytosis. The feces seldom contain gross blood in hookworm disease, although tests for occult blood are usually positive.

Generally, the leukocyte count is normal. However, in some early cases, leukocytosis may be marked, with an eosinophilia as high as 70 or 80 percent. The anemia is characteristically hypochromic and microcytic.

The species of hookworm may be determined by the identification of the adult worm passed in the stool following treatment or by culturing the feces and identifying the third-stage larvae. This is seldom important in clinical practice.

Differential diagnosis Since hookworm disease occurs in areas in which beriberi and malaria are also common, these diseases must be differentiated from hookworm disease, or their coexistence must be established.

Treatment Therapy specific for the infection and directed toward the improvement of nutrition and the anemia should be considered simultaneously. In areas where reinfection is likely, administration of anthelmintics to patients with light infections (less than 2000 eggs per milliliter of feces) is probably not beneficial. In most cases requiring specific therapy, anthelmintics may be administered immediately, followed by iron and a high-protein diet. A number of satisfactory anthelmintic agents are available, but two, pyrantel pamoate (see "Ascariasis" above) and mebendazole (see "Trichuriasis" above) are currently favored. Where expense remains a major consideration, the drug of choice is tetrachloroethylene (TCE). It is highly effective, nontoxic, inexpensive, and ideal for mass treatment. (The USP tetrachloroethylene available to veterinarians may be used.) In most instances a single dose of this agent will decrease the worm load substantially. Complete cure may require several courses of treatment but is not necessary in endemic areas; the aim of therapy is reduction of the worm load to an asymptomatic level. Tetrachloroethylene is administered as a single 5-mL oral dose. Children should receive 0.12 ml/kg (to a maximum of 5 mL) by the same route. The night before treatment, the patient is permitted a light fat-free meal. The following morning, breakfast is omitted and the drug is administered. No food is permitted for 4 h and no alcohol for 24 h. Treatment can be repeated in a week if complete cure is desired and has not been accomplished.

The anemia requires iron replacement. When anemia is severe and there is malnutrition with anasarca, blood transfusions and a high-protein diet should be given before drug treatment is begun. Blood should be given in an amount sufficient to raise the hemoglobin level to 10 g/dL. In advanced cases it may be necessary to delay drug treatment for 2 to 3 weeks.

Prognosis The immediate prognosis is good. When opportunity for reinfection persists and nutrition cannot be maintained, a state of chronic debility develops. Maturation of children is impaired, and intercurrent disease is a serious problem in adults.

Prevention Many of the measures required are obvious but difficult to apply on a large scale. Even if facilities for proper disposal of feces are provided, it is no simple matter to educate the population in their use. Soil pollution must be eliminated. Avoidance of direct skin contact with the soil (by wearing shoes) is often not practical in endemic areas. Periodic mass treatment of the population has been used in some hookworm control programs.

CUTANEOUS LARVA MIGRANS (CREEPING ERUPTION)

Definition Creeping eruption is an infection of human skin caused by the larvae of the dog and cat hookworm, *A. brasiliense*. The other dog hookworms, *A. caninum* and *Uncinaria stenocephala,* as well as the human parasites, *Strongyloides stercoralis* and *Necator americanus,* may also produce the disease. The larvae of *Gnathostoma spinigerum,* a nematode found in the Orient, and *Gasterophilus,* the horse botfly, may produce a similar cutaneous infection.

Etiology *Ancylostoma brasiliense* reaches adulthood regularly only in the dog and cat. The larvae emerging from eggs discharged in the feces develop to the filariform stage and then are capable of penetrating the skin. In humans, the larvae usually remain in the skin and migrate, producing an irregular erythematous tunnel visible on the skin surface.

Epidemiology and distribution Transmission to humans requires environmental temperature and humidity appropriate for development of the egg to the infective filariform larva stage. Beaches and other moist, sandy areas are hazardous, because animals choose such areas for defecation, and the *A. brasiliense* eggs develop well in such soil. In the United States infection is found in the southern Atlantic and Gulf states.

Pathogenesis and clinical manifestations The site of penetration of the skin by the larvae becomes apparent in a few hours. The migration of the larvae in the skin is accompanied by severe itching. Scratching may lead to bacterial infection. In the course of 1 week, the initial red papule develops into an irregular, erythematous, linear lesion which may attain a length of 15 to 20 cm. The larvae may persist for weeks to months without treatment.

Loeffler's syndrome has been observed in 26 of 52 cases of creeping eruption. Transient, migratory pulmonary infiltrations associated with an increased number of eosinophils in the blood and sputum were interpreted as an allergic reaction to the helminthic infection but may have reflected pulmonary migration of the larvae.

Laboratory findings Eosinophils occur in the lesion, but eosinophilic leukocytosis is slight, except when Loeffler's syndrome appears. The percentage of eosinophils in the blood may then rise to 50 percent and in the sputum to 90 percent. Only rarely are larvae found on skin biopsy.

Treatment Thiabendazole is the drug of choice; it should be given orally in the dosage suggested for strongyloidiasis (see below). It may be repeated if necessary. Alternatively, it may be applied topically as a 10% aqueous suspension. Topical administration avoids systemic toxicity. Superficial bacterial infections are improved by the application of wet dressing and elevation of the extremity. For intense itching, oral antihistaminics may be of aid.

Prognosis Untreated infections last several months. Treatment, which is usually sought because of severe pruritus, is usually successful.

Prevention Dogs and cats should be prevented from contaminating recreation areas and children's sandboxes.

TRICHOSTRONGYLIASIS

Definition Trichostrongyliasis is an intestinal infection of herbivorous animals throughout the world. Humans are incidental hosts.

Etiology Almost a dozen species of *Trichostrongylus* are known to have infected humans. The disease is common in Asia, the Middle East, and South America, but few human infections have been reported in the United States. In view of the high frequency of animal infections here, the low incidence of human infections is difficult to understand. The possibility exists that some such infections are mistaken for hookworm infections.

The ova resemble those of the hookworm but are larger, have more pointed ends, and, when observed in a fresh fecal specimen, show a more advanced stage of segmentation (16- to 32-cell stage).

Pathogenesis Infection is acquired by ingestion of green leafy plants contaminated with third-stage larvae. On reaching the small intestine, they attach themselves to the mucosa and develop into adult worms within 4 weeks. The adult at that time sucks blood and maintains residence in the intestine for long periods. Sandground, who infected himself, observed infection to last more than 8 years.

Manifestations Most infections are asymptomatic, but massive infections may result in epigastric distress and anemia. The parasite owes its importance primarily to the resemblance of its ova to those of the hookworms. Moreover, because the trichostrongylidae do not respond to some of the anthelmintics effective in hookworm infection, it may be assumed incorrectly that refractory hookworm infection is present.

Laboratory diagnosis The diagnosis depends on the finding of the ova in the feces. Since they are few, they are usually found only when a concentration method is used. In symptomatic infections, there may be leukocytosis with marked eosinophilia (for example, 80 percent).

Treatment These infections do not respond to tetrachloroethylene. Thiabendazole 25 mg/kg twice daily for 2 or 3 days, or pyrantel pamoate as used in hookworm infections, is effective in symptomatic infections. Both are considered investigational drugs for this condition by the U.S. Food and Drug Administration.

Prevention Leafy vegetables should be cooked before ingestion in endemic areas.

STRONGYLOIDIASIS Definition Strongyloidiasis is an intestinal infection of humans caused by *Strongyloides stercoralis* or, on occasion, the primate species, *S. fuelleborni*. Extraintestinal involvement may occur in severe cases.

Etiology The tiny (2 mm in length) adult female resides and lays her eggs in the mucosa of the upper part of the jejunum. In heavy infections, the biliary and pancreatic ducts, the entire small bowel, and the colon may be parasitized. The eggs quickly hatch, releasing rhabditiform larvae which enter the lumen of the bowel and are passed in the feces. On reaching the soil, the larvae develop into the infective filariform stage. There, as in the case of the filariform larvae of hookworm, they penetrate the skin and small blood vessels of humans. They are then carried to the lungs where they leave the alveolar capillaries, ascend the respiratory tree, enter the pharynx, and are swallowed. On reaching the small intestine, they mature and copulate. The fertilized female burrows into the jejunal mucosa, while the male is excreted in the stool. Oviposition (up to 40 eggs per day) begins 17 to 28 days after the initial infection. It is likely that the females also reproduce parthenogenetically. In addition to the *direct* host-soil-host cycle, *Strongyloides* has two alternative cycles. In the first, or *indirect*, cycle, the rhabditiform larvae, after passing from the host, develop into free-living adults which reside and reproduce in the soil, thus creating a reservoir of infection independent of the human host. Under certain environmental conditions, the free-living larvae are capable of transforming back into filariform larvae which initiate a new cycle in humans. In the second, or *autoinfection*, cycle, the rhabditiform larvae develop into filariform larvae before they are passed in the stool. They may then invade the intestinal mucosa or perianal skin of the same host without first going through a soil phase. This may explain the long persistence (20 to 30 years) of strongyloidiasis in patients who have left endemic areas and may also account for the extremely heavy worm loads in some individuals. The early transformation of the filariform larvae is probably also responsible for the frequency with which strongyloidiasis is seen in crowded, unsanitary institutions for the mentally retarded. It appears to occur frequently in patients with achlorhydria, delayed intestinal transit time, and blind loops or diverticula.

Epidemiology The usual mode of infection is the penetration of the skin by larvae. Some infections may result from ingestion of contaminated food and drink, and some are believed to be transmitted by contact. Transmission between sexual partners, however, appears to be uncommon. Transmammary passage in humans has been demonstrated for *S. fuelleborni*. This disease is endemic in the tropics, where the warmth, moisture, and lack of sanitation favor its spread. Sporadic cases appear among Puerto Ricans and throughout the rural south of the continental United States. Former British and American soldiers imprisoned in southeast Asia during World War II were examined for the presence of this parasite. Over one-quarter were found infected nearly four decades after exposure; the majority were symptomatic. Chronic strongyloidiasis has been reported in Vietnam veterans.

Pathogenesis and clinical manifestations The initial cutaneous penetration of the filariform larvae usually produces no symptoms. However, *larva currens*, transitory skin eruptions characterized by blotchy erythema, serpiginous lesions, and urticaria, may be seen. These may recur at irregular intervals thereafter and are particularly common following recovery from an acute febrile illness. In these situations the lesions are generally found over the lower back and buttocks and are related to episodes of autoinfection. Cough, dyspnea, gross hemoptysis, and bronchospasm may accompany migration through the lungs. Chest x-rays may show pulmonary infiltration at this time. The intestinal infestation is usually asymptomatic or productive only of vague abdominal complaints. In heavier infections, epigastric pain and tenderness, nausea, flatulence, vomiting, and diarrhea alternating with constipation may be observed. Peptic ulcer may be simulated, but food often aggravates the pain. The mucosal inflammation may be severe enough to produce subacute obstruction, segmental ileus, and impaired absorption. Chronic, relapsing intestinal and pulmonary manifestations have been noted in a few patients. A severe form of ulcerative colitis, accompanied by intestinal perforation and peritonitis, has also been encountered. In debilitated, immunodepressed, steroid-treated, alcoholic, and hemodialyzed patients, massive autoinfection with widespread dissemination of larvae to the extraintestinal organs including the central nervous system may occur. This hyperinfection is often associated with pulmonary manifestations, severe enterocolitis, persistent gram-negative bacteremia, and occasionally gram-negative meningitis. Unrecognized, it usually leads to death. Disseminated strongyloidiasis should be considered in any compromised host with unexplained gram-negative bacteremia, abdominal complaints, and pulmonary infiltrates with or without eosinophilia.

Laboratory findings Although clinical findings may be suggestive, the definitive diagnosis can be made only in the laboratory. Fresh fecal specimens should be examined to avoid confusion with hookworm infection; generally, fresh specimens contain *larvae* in strongyloidiasis infections, while in hookworm infection they contain *eggs*. Since the number of larvae in the stool is small and varies from day to day, several samples should be checked, using concentration and culture techniques. If pulmonary involvement is present, the sputum should be examined for larvae. Microscopic examination of the duodenal aspirates and jejunal biopsies may also establish the diagnosis. Alternatively, a weighted string can be passed into the duodenum, allowed to remain for a short time, and then withdrawn. The bile-stained section of the string is stripped of fluid which is then examined for the presence of larvae. An enzyme-linked immunosorbent assay utilizing *S. stercoralis* larval antigens was shown to be positive in approximately 80 percent of patients and may have some diagnostic utility.

Eosinophilic leukocytosis is common, except in very severe cases. When eosinophilia occurs in association with peptic ulcer symptoms, strongyloidiasis should be suspected.

Treatment All infected patients should be treated to prevent the occurrence of severe invasive disease. The drug of choice is thiabendazole, which should be given orally in dosage of 25 mg/kg twice a day for 2 or 3 days. In disseminated strongyloidiasis, treatment should be continued for 7 days or more. Lightheadedness, nausea, and vomiting are common accompaniments of therapy with this agent. Delayed aminophylline excretion may result in toxicity. Hypersensitivity reactions may occur but usually respond to treatment with antihistamines. The stools should be rechecked at intervals of 3 months because the parasite is not easily eradicated and retreatment may be necessary.

Prognosis In the usual case, the prognosis is good. Since the occurrence of hyperinfection is unpredictable, every effort should be made to eradicate the infection in each case. In severe cases with hyperinfection, the prognosis is poor.

Prevention In general, the measures are those for the control of hookworm infection. In addition, it is well to remember that infection may be contracted by ingestion of contaminated food (especially uncooked vegetables) or of contaminated drinking water and by contact. Patients who have a history of residence in an endemic area should be carefully checked for the presence of the parasite prior to the initiation of steroid or immunosuppressive therapy. Because the larvae may not appear in the stool for several weeks after the initiation of such therapy, repeated examinations of stool and upper intestinal aspirates are indicated. Since sputum, vomitus, stool, and body fluids of patients with disseminated disease may contain infective filariform larvae, gloves and gowns should be worn by hospital personnel caring for such patients.

INTESTINAL CAPILLARIASIS Definition Intestinal capillariasis is an infection of humans caused by the roundworm *Capillaria philippinensis*. This species of *Capillaria* was first discovered in 1963 from a fatal human infection occurring in the Philippines. The infection results in intractable diarrhea with a high mortality rate. Clinical studies have shown a severe protein-losing enteropathy and malabsorption of fats and sugars.

Etiology *Capillaria* are nematodes of the family Trichuroidea and are closely related to comembers *Trichuris* and *Trichinella*. Adult *C. philippinensis* are small, measuring 2 to 4 mm in length. The peanut-shaped eggs have flattened bipolar plugs and an average size of 42 by 20 μm. The adults inhabit the mucosa of the small intestine, especially the jejunum. Adults, larval forms, and eggs are found in the stool.

Epidemiology The infection has been found almost exclusively in persons residing along the north and west coastal areas of Luzon, Philippines. Several cases from Thailand have also been reported. Since 1966 the disease has occurred in epidemic form, and more than 2000 cases and 100 deaths have been reported. Males are infected more frequently than females, perhaps because of occupational exposure. Prior to the discovery of an effective chemotherapeutic agent, the mortality rate in untreated cases was about 30 percent. With chemotherapy, the case fatality rate has been reduced to 6 percent.

The mode of transmission and life cycle of the parasite are incompletely understood. First-stage larvae have been found in several species of freshwater fish. When these fish or the larvae are fed to gerbils, they develop to adulthood within their intestinal lumina. These adults rapidly produce new larvae which mature to a second generation of adults. Most of the females from this generation are oviparous, the resulting eggs passing in the gerbil's stool. Some, however, remain larviparous, leading to another generation of intestinal adults. Eggs must presumably embryonate in fresh water before being ingested by the fish host. No naturally infected mammal other than humans has been found, but both birds and rats can be experimentally infected. The presence of many adult worms, larviparous females, embryonated eggs, and all larval stages in human intestinal contents suggests that the parasitic cycles in gerbils and humans are the same. The mechanism by which humans originally became infected remains unproven. However, it is known that many of the naturally infected lagoon fish, particularly "bagsit" or *Hypselotris bipartita*, are eaten raw by the people of Luzon.

Pathogenesis and manifestations Adult worms in large numbers invade the small-intestinal mucosa and cause a severe protein-losing enteropathy and malabsorption. Hypokalemia, hypocalcemia, and hypoproteinemia are the rule. Autopsy studies have failed to show extraintestinal spread of the parasite. Initial symptoms of intestinal "gurgling" (borborygmi) and recurrent vague abdominal pain are followed, usually within 2 to 3 weeks, by a voluminous watery diarrhea. Other findings, consistent with the basic pathophysiologic process, are anorexia, vomiting, weight loss, muscle wasting and weakness, hyporeflexia, and edema. Abdominal tenderness and distention may occur. The period between onset of symptoms and death is usually 2 to 3 months. Subclinical infection has not been noted.

Diagnosis The diagnosis is made by finding ova in the stool. The ova of *C. philippinensis* must be differentiated from those of *T. trichiura,* which are similar. Care must be taken that capillaria are not overlooked in patients with *Trichuris* infections because in the endemic area most patients with capillariasis have coexistent *Trichuris* infection.

Treatment Administration of mebendazole combined with fluid and electrolyte replacement leads to dramatic improvement; 400 mg per day in divided dosage should be given for 20 days to prevent relapse.

REFERENCES

BANWELL JG, SCHAD GA: Hookworm. Clin Gastroenterol 7:129, 1978

CROSS JH, BASACA-SEVILLA V: Experimental transmission of *Capillaria philippinensis* to birds. Trans R Soc Trop Med Hyg 77:511, 1983

EMBIL JA et al: Prevalence of *Ascaris lumbricoides* infection in a small Nova Scotian community. Am J Trop Med Hyg 33:595, 1984

FISHMAN JA, PERRONE TL: Colonic obstruction and perforation due to *Trichuris trichiura*. Am J Med 77:154, 1984

GILLES HM: Selective primary health care: Strategies for control of disease in the developing world. XVII. Hookworm infection and anemia. Rev Infect Dis 7:111, 1985

GLICKMAN LT, SCHANTZ PM: Epidemiology and pathogenesis of zoonotic toxocariasis. Epidemiol Rev 3:230, 1981

IRGA-SIEGMAN Y et al: Syndrome of hyperinfection with *Stronglyoides sterocoralis*. Rev Infect Dis 3:397, 1981

KLIKS MM: Anisakiasis in the western United States: Four new case reports from California. Am J Trop Med Hyg 32:526, 1983

LITTLE MD et al: *Ancylostoma* larva in a muscle fiber of man following cutaneous larva migrans. Am J Trop Med Hyg 32:1285, 1983

MILDER JE et al: Clinical features of *Strongyloides stercoralis* infection in an endemic area of the United States. Gastroenterology 80:1481, 1981

NEVA FA et al: Comparison of larval antigens in an enzyme-linked immunosorbent assay for strongyloidiasis in humans. J Infect Dis 144:427, 1981

PAWLOWSKI Z: Ascariasis. Clin Gastroenterol 7:157, 1978

PELLETIER LL JR: Chronic strongyloidiasis in World War II Far East ex-prisoners of war. Am J Trop Med Hyg 33:55, 1984

SMITH B et al: Pulmonary strongyloidiasis. Diagnosis by sputum Gram stain. Am J Med 79:663, 1985

STEPHENSON LS: The contribution of *Ascaris lumbricoides* to malnutrition in children. Parasitology 81:221, 1980

WAGNER ED, EBY WC: Pinworm prevalence in California elementary school children, and diagnostic methods. Am J Trop Med Hyg 32:998, 1983

WOLFE MS: *Oxyuris, Trichostrongylus* and *Trichuris*. Clin Gastroenterol 7:201, 1978

WORLD HEALTH ORGANIZATION: Intestinal protozoan and helminthic infections. WHO Tech Rep Ser 1981, no 666

WORLEY G et al: *Toxocara canis* infection: Clinical and epidemiological association with seropositivity in kindergarten children. J Infect Dis 149:591, 1984

167 OTHER TREMATODES OR FLUKES

JAMES J. PLORDE

The trematodes of humans are long-lived parasites which produce progressive damage to the tissues of their hosts. With the exception of schistosomes, they are similar in morphology and life cycle. The adult flukes are flat, leaflike hermaphrodites that vary in length from a few millimeters to several centimeters. Their digestive tract, unlike that of the nematodes, ends blindly. As their name indicates, they have two "holes" in the form of oral and ventral suckers which are used as organs of attachment and locomotion. The operculated eggs, which are passed in the feces or sputum, hatch in the water to produce a ciliated, free-swimming *miracidium*. The miracidium reaches and penetrates the tissue of an intermediate snail host to undergo a period of development, eventuating in the release of thousands of swarms of free-living *cercariae* from the snail. These thousands of tail-bearing larvae must, in turn, reach a second intermediate host, usually an aquatic animal or vegetation, where they encyst forming *metacercariae*. The definitive host is infected when he or she ingests the parasitized second intermediate host. The distribution of flukes is usually limited by the location of their molluscan intermediate host. With the exception of *Opisthorchis* and *Fasciola*, most hermaphroditic flukes are found only in tropical or subtropical areas.

PARAGONIMIASIS Definition Paragonimiasis (endemic hemoptysis) is a chronic infection of the lung caused by trematodes of the genus *Paragonimus*. Clinically, the disease is characterized by cough and hemoptysis. Ectopic worms may cause a variety of other manifestations. Geographically, it is probably the most widely distributed disease caused by hermaphroditic flukes.

Etiology and epidemiology Although *P. westermani*, which is widely distributed in the far east, is the most common cause of human paragonimiasis, a number of other species, including *P. skrjabini, P. heterotremus* (China), *P. africanus, P. uterobilateralis* (central and west Africa), *P. kellicotti* (North America), *P. mexicanus, P. ecuadoriensis*, and *P. caliensis* (Central and South America), may cause the disease. Approximately 1 percent of Indochinese immigrants to the United States harbor *P. westermani*. The short, plump adults (7 to 12 mm in length, 4 to 6 mm in width) have a life span of 4 to 5 years which they typically spend encysted in the lung parenchyma of the host. Their golden-brown operculated eggs (50 by 90 μm) reach the bronchioles from where they are coughed up and excreted in the sputum or swallowed and passed in the feces. They must embryonate several weeks in fresh water before hatching to release the miracidia.

The infection is acquired by ingestion of cysts in the second intermediate host, a freshwater shrimp, crab, or crayfish. The metacercariae excyst in the duodenum, burrow through the intestinal wall into the peritoneal cavity, and then usually migrate through the diaphragm and into the lung. The worms also may be found in the intestinal wall, liver, pancreas, kidney, epididymis, mesentery, skeletal muscle, subcutaneous tissues, and central nervous system, particularly the brain. The dog, cat, pig, rat, and wild carnivores are definitive hosts for the parasite in addition to humans. In some of these, very young adults can be found in their striated muscles. Human infection has been reported following the ingestion of this undercooked flesh.

The incidence of paragonimiasis is often affected by food shortages or local customs. The metacercariae survive in vinegar, and lightly pickled or inadequately cooked food usually serves as the source of infection in the far east. Fresh crab juice used for the treatment of measles in Korea and for infertility in the Cameroons may also transmit the parasite. Children may acquire the disease in endemic areas while handling or eating raw crabs during play.

Pathogenesis and clinical manifestations An eosinophilic granuloma forms about the adult worm, eventually leading to the formation of a fibrous cyst. The pulmonary lesions which measure up to 1 cm in diameter frequently communicate with a bronchiole, resulting in secondary bacterial infection. Small, fibrous nodules representing reaction around deposited eggs also occur. Clinically the picture is one of chronic bronchitis and bronchiectasis with production of brownish sputum and hemoptysis. A poorly resolving pulmonary infiltrate, lung abscess, or pleural effusion may be present in heavy infections. Effusions are often large, may occur in the absence of parenchymal disease, and are typically exudative with eosinophils and cholesterol crystals. The roentgenographic findings vary with the stage of infection. Initially diffuse or segmental infiltrates, with or without pleural effusions, may be seen in lower or midlung fields. These are then gradually replaced by round 2- to 4-cm nodules which not infrequently cavitate. Eventually, cystic rings, fibrosis, and calcification occur, presenting a picture closely resembling tuberculosis, a disease which often coexists with paragonimiasis.

An abdominal mass, pain, and dysentery characterize intestinal or peritoneal infections. Various types of paralysis and epilepsy occur in cerebral involvement. Homonymous hemianopsia, optic atrophy, and papilledema are common. The cerebrospinal fluid usually shows an eosinophilic leukocytosis and elevated protein. Cerebral calcifications are seen on x-ray in 50 percent of cases. *Paragonimus skrjabini* and, perhaps, *P. ecuadoriensis* infections are characterized by migratory subcutaneous nodules that contain adult flukes.

Laboratory findings Eosinophilia is a constant finding. Definitive diagnosis depends upon finding the characteristic operculated ova in the sputum, stool, pleural fluid, or tissue. Eggs may be rare or totally absent from the sputum during the first 3 months of infection but are eventually found in 75 to 85 percent of infected patients. Their presence correlates well with the roentgenographic appearance of cavities. Even later, however, repeated examinations using concentration techniques may be required for their recovery. Ziehl-Neelsen staining, often carried out for suspected tuberculosis, usually will not demonstrate the eggs. In fact, the sputum concentration techniques for tuberculosis may destroy the eggs that are present. Since many patients have concomitant tuberculosis, the diagnosis may be overlooked. Stool examination is frequently helpful in children. A complement fixation test is available, and the results correlate well with active infection. It usually becomes negative within 6 months of successful therapy. The skin test does not distinguish present and past infections and is used primarily for epidemiologic purposes.

Treatment and prevention Praziquantel is the drug of choice. A total of 75 mg/kg is given in three divided doses for 1 or 2 days. Alternatively, bithionol may be administered. From 30 to 40 mg/kg in divided doses should be given every other day for a total of 10 to 15 treatment days. The symptoms disappear rapidly, and most infiltrates resolve within 3 months. Side effects are minor and consist of nausea, vomiting, and urticaria. Concomitant bacterial infection must be treated. Prevention of superinfection by the same parasite is important, because the disease is self-limiting.

The most practical control measure is the adequate cooking of all shellfish before they are eaten.

CLONORCHIASIS Definition Clonorchiasis is an infection of the biliary passages caused by *Clonorchis sinensis*, the most important liver fluke of humans. Although the infection is usually asymptomatic, heavy worm loads may produce manifestations of biliary obstruction.

Etiology and epidemiology *Clonorchis sinensis* is a small fluke (5 by 15 mm) that lives as long as 50 years in the biliary tree of its host. Here the flukes feed on mucosal secretions and pass operculated eggs into the feces. On reaching fresh water, the eggs are ingested by the intermediate snail host. After multiplication and development within the snail, the cercariae are released and penetrate freshwater fish. Infections result from ingestion of the raw, dried, salted, or pickled flesh of freshwater fish containing encysted metacercariae. The larva is released in the duodenum. It enters the common bile duct and migrates to the second-order bile ducts, where it develops into the adult form in about 1 month. In addition to humans, dogs, cats, pigs, and rats serve as disease reservoirs. The main endemic areas are Korea, Japan, Taiwan, Hong Kong, southern China, and Vietnam where, in previous years, clonorchiasis was perpetuated by the practice of fertilizing fish ponds with manure and human feces. Improvements in the disposal of human feces have dramatically decreased transmission in most areas, but the infection rate has remained high due to the prolonged life span of the adult worm. Twenty-five percent of the population of Hong Kong and a small proportion of Chinese immigrants to this country have been shown to be infected. The disease may also be acquired in the United States by the ingestion of infected, dried, frozen, or pickled fish imported from the far east. Clinically apparent cases are restricted to the adult population in whom the accumulated worm load eventually produces pathologic effects.

Pathogenesis and clinical manifestations Light infections are usually asymptomatic, but worm loads of 500 to 1000 flukes often result in clinical manifestations. During the migration of the larvae, the patient may have fever, chills, tender hepatomegaly, mild jaundice, and eosinophilia. The mature worm causes proliferation of the biliary epithelium, increased mucin production, adenoma formation, chronic pericholangitis, and periductal fibrosis. Hepatic parenchymal damage and portal hypertension are not seen in uncomplicated infections. Recurrent attacks of suppurative cholangitis with or without intrahepatic choledocholithiasis may follow biliary obstruction with dead flukes. These occasionally present as hypoglycemic coma. The occurrence of biliary stones in clonorchiasis is associated with an increased incidence of chronic *Salmonella typhi* carriage. Cholangiocarcinoma may occur in patients with severe, long-standing infections. The adult worms may infest the pancreatic ducts, where they can cause squamous metaplasia, periductal fibrosis, and acute pancreatitis.

Laboratory diagnosis Clinical and epidemiologic findings often suggest the diagnosis. There may be elevation of the alkaline phosphatase and hyperbilirubinemia. Eosinophilia is variable. Occasionally, a plain film of the abdomen will demonstrate intrahepatic calcification. Liver scan is usually negative in asymptomatic infections but may show multiple areas of diminished uptake in acute symptomatic disease. Percutaneous transhepatic cholangiography in such patients often reveals dilatation of the peripheral intrahepatic bile ducts. The adult worms appear as round filling defects several millimeters in diameter. Definitive diagnosis depends on the demonstration of the eggs in the feces or the duodenal contents. They measure 29 by 16 μm, possess a conspicuous opercular rim as well as a posterior knob, and can be distinguished from the eggs of *Metagonimus, Heterophyes,* and *Opisthorchis* only with difficulty. An antigen extracted from adult worms can be used in a complement fixation or enzyme-linked immunosorbent test for the detection of the host's antibody response.

Treatment and prevention The introduction of praziquantel has provided an effective chemotherapeutic agent for clonorchiasis. It is administered in a dosage of 25 mg/kg tid for a single day. Thorough cooking of freshwater fish will prevent infection.

OPISTHORCHIASIS Opisthorchiasis is caused by *Opisthorchis felineus* or *O. viverrini* and is characterized by hepatic lesions produced by adult worms in the larger bile ducts. The life cycle resembles that of *C. sinensis*. The geographic distribution differs in that *O. felineus* is endemic in eastern and central Europe and in Siberia and occurs in some parts of Asia, while *O. viverrini* is found in Thailand and Laos. Cats and wild carnivores act as the principal reservoir hosts, and the infection is found most commonly along rivers and lakes which harbor an abundant fish life. Up to 90 percent of inhabitants of some villages in northeastern Thailand are purported to carry the parasite. The clinical lesions are similar to those seen in clonorchiasis except that gallstones are rare. Cholangiocarcinoma occurs in approximately 50 percent of infected patients who come to autopsy. The diagnosis usually is based on the finding of the eggs in the feces or duodenal contents. Treatment as recommended for clonorchiasis may be used. Infection can be prevented by eating only well-cooked fish.

FASCIOLIASIS Fascioliasis is caused by *Fasciola hepatica,* which, like *Clonorchis,* inhabits the bile ducts of the definitive host. When fully matured, the adult measures about 3 by 1 cm and discharges large operculate eggs 140 by 70 μm which must embryonate in fresh water before hatching.

Fascioliasis produces so-called liver rot in sheep, the principal definitive host. The disease is most common in sheep- and cattle-raising countries but has been reported from many parts of the world. In North America it occurs in the southern and western United States, Central America, and in the Caribbean Islands, including Puerto Rico.

Infection is contracted by ingestion of the encysted forms of the fluke attached to edible aquatic plants such as watercress. The larvae excyst in the duodenum, migrate through the intestinal wall, pass into the peritoneal cavity, penetrate the liver capsule, and finally reach the bile ducts, where they mature. Occasionally larvae may migrate to and mature in ectopic locations including the pancreas, subcutaneous tissue, chest cavity, or brain.

Early clinical manifestations are related to the migration of the larval form to and within the liver. Epigastric pain, fever, diarrhea, jaundice, urticaria, pruritus, arthralgia, and eosinophilia may be observed during this stage. Fibrosis of the liver similar to that found in clonorchiasis appears only after prolonged residence of many adult worms in the bile ducts. Obstruction of the bile duct occurs frequently and may be the presenting manifestation of disease. A pharyngeal form of the disease, called *halzoun,* can result from eating infected raw liver, the young adults attaching themselves to the pharyngeal mucosa, occasionally interfering with respiration.

The diagnosis usually is based on the finding of the eggs in the feces or in the duodenal contents. It is difficult to distinguish the eggs from those of *Fasciolopsis buski*. Complement fixation, hemagglutination, and precipitin tests have been reported to be helpful. A skin test is also available.

Treatment is as described above for clonorchiasis.

To prevent infection, aquatic plants such as watercress should not be eaten, vegetables grown in fields irrigated with polluted water should be boiled, and safe drinking water should be provided.

FASCIOLOPSIASIS Fasciolopsiasis is caused by the large intestinal fluke *F. buski,* which inhabits the upper part of the intestine of its definitive host. The principal definitive host is the pig. China, Thailand, India, and other areas in the far east are the major endemic loci. Infection of humans occurs following ingestion, or peeling with the teeth, of water chestnuts, water lotus, and other edible aquatic plants. The large adults attach themselves to the intestinal mucosa, and these sites may later ulcerate. The infection is usually asymptomatic. In heavy infections, diarrhea, abdominal pain, gastrointestinal hemorrhage, and intestinal obstruction may appear early. Later, asthenia with ascites and anasarca occurs. Diagnosis is based upon the history and the finding of eggs in the feces. The eggs resemble those of *Fasciola hepatica*. The prognosis in untreated heavy infections, especially in children, is poor. Praziquantel as given for clonorchiasis is the treatment of choice. Tetrachloroethylene as given for hookworm infections may also be used.

HETEROPHYIASIS AND METAGONIMIASIS *Heterophyes heterophyes* and *Metagonimus yakagawa* are small intestinal flukes of humans and other fish-eating mammals. They are found in the far east and, in the case of *Heterophyes,* in India, Egypt, and Tunisia. Both are acquired by ingesting the raw or undercooked flesh of metacercarial-infected freshwater fish. The 2- to 3-mm adults attach themselves to the mucosa of the small intestine. If present in sufficient numbers, they may cause abdominal pain and/or diarrhea. Rarely the eggs have been found in sites such as the brain, spinal cord, or heart where they produce granulomatous lesions. Most commonly, they are passed in the stool where they very closely resemble those of *Clonorchis*. Both species can be treated with praziquantel as described for clonorchiasis or tetrachloroethylene as outlined in Chap. 166 for hookworm. As the life span of these trematodes is limited to a year or less, treatment is not indicated unless the patient is symptomatic.

REFERENCES

FLAVELL DJ: Liver-fluke infection as an aetiologic factor in bile-duct carcinoma of man. Trans R Soc Trop Med Hyg 75:814, 1981

HOOVER R et al: Seasonal transmission of *Fasciola hepatica* to cattle in northwestern United States. J Am Vet Med Assoc 184:695, 1984

JOHNSON RJ, JOHNSON JR: Paragonimiasis in Indochinese refugees: Roentgenographic findings with clinical correlations. Am Rev Resp Dis 128:534, 1983

——— et al: Paragonimiasis: Diagnosis and the use of praziquantel in treatment. Rev Infect Dis 7:200, 1985

JONES EA et al: Massive infection with *Fasciola hepatica* in man. Am J Med 63:842, 1977

JONG EC et al: Praziquantel for the treatment of *Clonorchis/Opisthorchis* infections. Report of a double-blind, placebo-controlled trial. J Infect Dis 152:637, 1985

KOENIGSTEIN RP: Observations on the epidemiology of infections with *Clonorchis sinensis*. Trans R Soc Trop Med Hyg 42:503, 1949
KOOMPIROCHANA C et al: Opisthorchiasis: A clinicopathologic study of 154 autopsy cases. Southeastern Asian J Trop Med 9:60, 1978
MCFADZEAN AJS, YEUNG RTT: Hypoglycemia in suppurative pancholangitis due to *Clonorchis sinensis*. Trans R Soc Trop Med Hyg 59:179, 1965
PACHUCKI CT et al: American paragonimiasis treated wtih praziquantel. N Engl J Med 311:582, 1984
PLANT AG et al: A clinical study of *Fasciolopsis buski* in Thailand. Trans R Soc Trop Med Hyg 63:470, 1969
UPATHAM ES et al: Morbidity in relation to intensity of infection in *Opisthorchiasis viverrini:* Study of a community in Khon Kaen, Thailand. Am J Trop Med Hyg 31:1156, 1982
YOKOGAWA M: *Paragonimus* and paragonimiasis, in *Advances in Parasitology*, B Dawes (ed). London, Academic, 1969, vol 7, p 375

168 CESTODE (TAPEWORM) INFECTIONS

PAUL G. RAMSEY / JAMES J. PLORDE

The tapeworms, or cestodes, are ribbon-shaped segmented hermaphroditic worms which inhabit the intestinal tract of many vertebrates. Unlike other helminths, they lack a digestive tract but absorb food through their entire surface. Tapeworms have a primitive nervous system, a muscular system, and excretory canals. Attachment to the host's intestinal mucosa is accomplished by sucking cups or grooves located on the head, or *scolex*. In some species, attachment is aided by hooklets located on the scolex. Behind the globular scolex lies a short, narrow neck from which segments or *proglottides* develop to form the chainlike *strobila* of the worm. The proglottides progressively mature as they are displaced further from the neck by new segments. As each section becomes gravid, eggs are released either through a uterine pore, by splitting open, or by disintegrating. Because the eggs of many tapeworms appear identical, species identification depends on the morphological characteristics of the scolex or gravid proglottides.

Except for *Hymenolepis nana* the human tapeworms require one or more intermediate hosts for larval development. After ingestion by a susceptible intermediate host, the eggs develop into larvae or *oncospheres* which are capable of penetrating the intestinal mucosa, migrating in tissues, and developing into encysted forms. If the cyst contains a single scolex, it is called a *cysticercus*, or *cysticercoid* in the case of *H. nana*. A *coenurus* is a cyst which contains several scolices, and a *hydatid* is a structure with daughter cysts each containing several scolices. Ingestion of tissues containing cysts with viable scolices by a definitive host allows development of the larval stage into an adult tapeworm. Cestodes in the *Diphyllobothrium* genus have a more complex life cycle involving two intermediate hosts (see below).

Human tapeworm infections may be divided into two major clinical groups. In the first, humans act as the definitive host and harbor the adult tapeworm in their intestines. The important species in this group include *Taenia saginata, Diphyllobothrium latum, Hymenolepis* species, and *Dipylidium caninum*. In the second group, humans are intermediate hosts and harbor the larval forms in their tissues. This is exemplified by echinococcosis, sparganosis, and coenurosis. *Taenia solium* is unique because humans may act as both the definitive and intermediate hosts.

TAENIASIS SAGINATA Definition Taeniasis saginata is an intestinal infection of humans caused by the beef tapeworm.

Epidemiology Infection with *Taenia saginata* occurs in all countries where raw or undercooked beef is eaten. It is particularly prevalent in Ethiopia, Kenya, Yugoslavia, the Middle East, Mexico and parts of South America, and the U.S.S.R. Indigenously acquired infection is uncommon in the United States except in areas where cattle and humans are concentrated such as around feedlots in the southwest.

Etiology and pathogenesis Humans are the only definitive host for the adult stage of *T. saginata* which inhabits the upper jejunum for as long as 25 years. The cestode is 5 to 10 m long and has a small, unarmed scolex with four prominent suckers and 1000 to 2000 proglottides. The gravid segments are longer than they are wide (5 by 20 mm) and have 15 to 30 lateral uterine branches (*T. solium* has 8 to 12). The eggs, which are indistinguishable from *T. solium* eggs, measure 30 by 40 μm, have a thick brown radially striated shell, and contain a fully developed embryo with three pairs of hooklets. After the egg-containing proglottides are deposited on soil or vegetation, they are ingested by cattle or other herbivores. The embryo is released in the intestine, invades the intestinal wall, and is carried by vascular channels to striated muscle in the hind limbs, diaphragm, and tongue where it is transformed over a period of 3 to 4 months into an ovoid bladder worm, or cysticercus. This form, which may be viable for 1 to 3 years, measures about 5 by 10 mm and consists of one scolex suspended in a fluid-filled sac. After ingestion of the cyst in raw or undercooked beef by humans, the adult worm develops in the intestine in about 2 months.

Clinical manifestations Most patients have minimal or no symptoms. Mild epigastric discomfort, nausea, and hunger sensations may occur. Weight loss, diarrhea, irritability, and an increase in appetite are more unusual. Movements of the worm are sometimes apparent, and occasionally proglottides may crawl through the anus, appearing in the bed linen or underclothing of the distraught host. Rarely segments become impacted in the appendix or cystic or pancreatic duct producing obstruction and inflammation of these organs.

Diagnosis After the adult tapeworm has been established for 2 to 3 months, several proglottides are shed daily in the stool and can be detected readily. Eggs may be distributed in the stool or on the perianal area if a proglottid ruptures during defecation and should be looked for in the absence of segments. The perianal region may be examined as for pinworm infection, using a Scotch brand cellophane tape swab. By this method 85 to 95 percent of infections may be detected, whereas by stool examination only 50 to 75 percent are recognized. Since egg morphology is not diagnostic, examination of mature proglottides or the scolex is necessary to identify the tapeworm species correctly. Reliable serologic tests are not available.

Treatment Niclosamide (Yomesan) is a highly effective taenicide which kills the scolex and immature segments of the worm on contact. Four 0.5-g tablets are thoroughly chewed at one time and swallowed with a small amount of water. No preparation or purge is necessary, and few side effects have been reported. As the worm is digested before it is passed in the stool, no attempt should be made to recover the scolex. Stool should be examined at 3 and 6 months for test of cure. Paromomycin (Humatin), 1.0 g orally every 15 min for four doses, is an alternative drug. Mebendazole in a dose of 300 mg twice daily for 3 days or a single dose of praziquantel (10 mg/kg) is effective, but these agents have not been approved for treating taeniasis in the United States.

Prevention Thorough cooking of beef is the major means of preventing taeniasis saginata. Temperatures as low as 56°C for as little as 5 min will destroy cysticerci. Refrigeration and salting for prolonged periods or freezing at −10°C for 9 days also destroys the cysticercus. General preventive measures include adequate meat inspection and proper disposal of human feces.

TAENIASIS SOLIUM AND CYSTICERCOSIS Definition *Taenia solium,* the pork tapeworm, inhabits the intestinal lumen of humans, its only definitive host. The hog is the usual intermediate host, although humans, dogs, cats, and sheep may harbor the larval form. When human tissue is invaded by the larval form, the condition is referred to as *cysticercosis*.

Epidemiology Taeniasis solium is worldwide but is most common in Mexico, Africa, southeast Asia, eastern Europe, and South America. *T. solium* has been found in swine in Colorado and New

Mexico, but autochthonously acquired human disease is rare in the United States. Cysticercosis has been recognized more frequently in industrialized nations due to migration of infected persons from endemic areas.

Etiology and pathogenesis The adult worm is about 3 m in length, resides in the upper jejunum, and may live for decades. The globular scolex contains a rostellum with two rows of hooklets. There are usually fewer than 1000 proglottides. The gravid proglottid is about 6 by 12 mm and contains a uterus with 8 to 12 lateral branchings. The eggs are infective for both human and hog. Infection usually occurs by the fecal-oral route, but humans may be autoinfected when gravid segments are returned to the stomach by reverse peristalsis. In the intermediate host, the embryo is released from the egg, penetrates the intestinal wall, and is carried by vascular channels to all parts of the body. Localization with development over 60 to 70 days to the encysted larval stage ("bladder worm") occurs primarily in striated muscle of the tongue, neck, and trunk. The cysticerci are ovoid, gray-white opalescent structures about 1 cm in diameter. They can survive for 5 years. Humans become infected with the adult stage following ingestion of undercooked pork containing cysticerci.

Clinical manifestations Clinical manifestations of adult worm infestation resemble those with *T. saginata.* When humans serve as the intermediate host (cysticercosis), the clinical picture is entirely different. Cysticerci develop in the subcutaneous tissues, in muscles, in viscera, and, most importantly, in the eye and brain. Only a moderate tissue reaction occurs while the scolex is viable, but the dead larvae invoke a marked tissue response with muscular pains, weakness, fever, and eosinophilia. Brain cysts are usually located in the cerebrum, ventricles, or subarachnoid space. The cerebral cysts are often less than 2 cm in diameter but may rarely be as large as 5 cm. If the cysticerci are widely distributed, the patient has signs and symptoms of meningoencephalitis. Epilepsy, brain tumors, and other types of neurologic or psychiatric disorders may also be simulated. Clinical findings may change during the course of infection due to changes in the inflammatory response.

Diagnosis Infection with the adult worm can be detected by finding eggs in perianal scrapings or in the feces. However, to differentiate *T. solium* from *T. saginata,* proglottides or the scolex must be examined. Cysticercosis should be suspected in an individual who has lived in a hyperendemic area and who develops neurologic findings. Subcutaneous cysts may be found in approximately 50 percent of patients, and roentgenograms of soft tissue may show typical calcifications later in the course of cysticercosis. Contrast-enhanced computerized tomography (CT) scans are valuable for identifying brain lesions, which may appear as solid nodules or cystic or calcified lesions. In some patients, only hydrocephalus may be seen. Cerebrospinal fluid is often abnormal but not diagnostic. Enzyme-linked immunosorbent assay (ELISA) provides a sensitive serologic test for diagnosis of cysticercosis, but cross-reactive antibodies occur in some patients with other infections. Brain, subcutaneous nodule, or skin biopsy specimens are needed to establish a specific diagnosis.

Treatment The stage and location of the parasite determine the prognosis and treatment. For removal of the adult worm in the human intestine, niclosamide, paromomycin, mebendazole, or praziquantel may be given as for *Taeniasis saginata.* However, because these drugs cause maceration of the proglottides with release of ova, cysticercosis could theoretically occur. To prevent this, some authorities recommend that a saline purge be administered 1 h after the medication. Treatment of ocular cysticercosis should be surgical.

Praziquantel has been used to treat cerebral cysticercosis with promising results. A dose of 50 mg of praziquantel per kilogram given daily in three divided doses for 15 days has been recommended. Corticosteroids have been used with praziquantel to treat fever, headache, and meningismus which presumably occur secondary to an inflammatory response to dying cysticerci. The optimal dose and duration of praziquantel, the long-term side effects, and the need for concomitant corticosteroid treatment have not been studied adequately.

HYMENOLEPIASIS NANA Definition Hymenolepiasis nana is an intestinal infection of humans, rats, and mice by *Hymenolepis nana,* the dwarf tapeworm. The life cycle is unique in that both the larval and adult phases occur in the same host.

Epidemiology Dwarf tapeworm infection has been reported in temperate and tropical regions around the globe. It is the most common autochthonously acquired tapeworm in the United States, most of the infections occurring in the southern states. The infection is spread by the direct fecal-oral route and is particularly common in children and institutional populations.

Etiology and pathogenesis The adult worm is small, about 2 cm, and lives for only a few weeks in the proximal ileum. Its proglottides are very small and are rarely seen in the stool. The gravid segments break apart in the fecal stream releasing spherical eggs. These measure 30 to 44 μm in diameter and have a double membrane enclosing the embryo which has six hooklets. The inner vitelline membrane has four to eight slender filaments arising from each pole. The eggs are immediately infective, and when ingested by a new host, the freed oncospheres penetrate the intestinal villi, becoming cysticercoids. Larvae migrate back into the intestinal lumen, attach to the mucosa, and mature into adult worms. The eggs may also hatch before passing in the stool, causing internal autoinfection with gradually increasing numbers of worms in the host.

Clinical manifestations Dwarf tapeworm infection may be asymptomatic even with many adult worms in the intestine. When infection is massive, abdominal cramps and diarrhea occur. Rarely, dizziness or seizures have been seen in children and have been attributed to a neurotoxic product of the worms.

Treatment Niclosamide, 2 g per day, must be given for 5 to 7 consecutive days. The dosage for children must be adjusted for body weight. The longer treatment course is necessary because niclosamide is not effective against the cysticercoid stage, and the encysted larvae continue to release organisms for 4 days. A repeat treatment course may be required in 2 weeks for patients with heavy infections. Paromomycin, 45 mg/kg daily for 5 to 7 days, may also be effective.

Prevention With a single host involved and the eggs being immediately infective, eradication of the disease presents problems similar to those encountered with enterobiasis. Personal hygiene is imperative. In an institution, epidemics can be avoided by proper screening programs.

HYMENOLEPIASIS DIMINUTA *Hymenolepis diminuta* is a cestode of rats and mice that occasionally infects small children. Larval development occurs in a wide variety of insects including fleas and mealworms. Humans become infected with the adult worm when they ingest uncooked cereal foods contaminated by these insects. Infection is usually asymptomatic, and the diagnosis is made only when characteristic eggs are found in the stool. The eggs resemble those of *H. nana* but are longer and lack polar filaments. Niclosamide, as prescribed for *H. nana,* results in approximately a 90 percent cure rate.

DIPYLIDIASIS *Dipylidium caninum* is the common tapeworm of cats and dogs. The orange-brown proglottid, which resembles a pumpkin seed, is often passed intact in the stool or migrates through the anal canal. This may cause animals harboring the parasite to drag their buttocks across the floor. The characteristic egg packets are then expelled by the proglottides and ingested by fleas to develop into infective larval forms. The definitive host becomes infected by swallowing involved fleas. Human infections occur primarily in small children who ingest fleas while playing with their pets. The diagnosis is made by recovering the characteristic proglottid or egg packet. Treatment is the same as for *T. saginata* described above. Periodic deworming of pets provides the best prevention.

DIPHYLLOBOTHRIASIS Definition *Diphyllobothrium latum* and other *Diphyllobothrium* species, the fish or broad tapeworms, produce an intestinal infection in the definitive host (including humans).

Epidemiology Diphyllobothriasis is common in the Baltic and Scandinavian countries, Japan, U.S.S.R., Switzerland, Italy, Chile, and central Africa. It occurs in the north central United States, Florida, and with increased frequency along the Pacific coast. The prevalence of infection is enhanced by the disposal of raw sewage into freshwater lakes. Anadromous Alaskan salmon have been implicated in an outbreak along the west coast. The popularity of raw fish dishes such as Japanese sushi and sashimi may lead to increased prevalence of the disease in the United States.

Etiology and pathogenesis The adult worm lies attached to the mucosa of the ileum and occasionally the jejunum by a pair of sucking grooves located on the scolex. It can live 20 years and achieve a length of more than 10 m. The 3000 to 4000 proglottides are wider than they are long. Unlike *Taenia,* the gravid segments are retained by the worm, and each day a million operculated ova are passed directly in the stool. On reaching water, the egg hatches, releasing a free-swimming embryo. This is eaten by small freshwater crustaceans belonging to the species *Cyclops* or *Diaptomus,* in which it develops into a *procercoid.* When the infected crustacean is swallowed by a fish, the larva migrates into the flesh and grows into a *plerocercoid,* or *sparganum,* larva. Humans acquire disease by ingesting raw infected fish. In 3 to 5 weeks the tapeworm matures in the intestine into an adult capable of discharging eggs. Several *Diphyllobothrium* species can infect humans, and *D. latum* cannot be distinguished from other species by its eggs or proglottides. Species determination requires examination of the scolex.

Clinical manifestations Most infections are asymptomatic or produce slight, transient abdominal discomfort. Rarely, there may be severe cramping abdominal pain, diarrhea or constipation, vomiting, weakness, and loss of weight. Intestinal obstruction has been reported in multiple infections. In 0.1 to 2 percent of infected patients, an anemia develops, and about 40 percent of fish tapeworm carriers will have low serum vitamin B_{12} levels. The anemia appears to result from the ability of the tapeworm to compete successfully with its host for vitamin B_{12} and resembles pernicious anemia including central nervous system involvement. A worm located high in the jejunum may take up 80 to 100 percent of labeled vitamin B_{12} ingested by a patient with anemia. These patients tend to be elderly, have diminished production of intrinsic factor, and have worms located in the proximal small bowel. Folate absorption may also be decreased and contribute to the anemia. Lysolecithin, a product of the tapeworm, may contribute to the severity of the disease. Neurologic manifestations are more common than in pernicious anemia and may occur in the absence of hematologic findings. Typically, they include paresthesias, impaired vibration sense, numbness, weakness, and, less commonly, central scotomas secondary to optic atrophy. These findings are reversible with proper treatment.

Diagnosis The characteristic eggs are present in the stool in large numbers, making the diagnosis easy. They measure 55 to 76 by 41 to 56 μm and possess a single shell with an operculum at one end and a knob on the other. Mild eosinophilia may be present.

Treatment Niclosamide or paromomycin as prescribed for taeniasis saginata will cure most infections. In the presence of macrocytic anemia, parenteral vitamin B_{12} should be given.

Prevention Fish tapeworm infection can be prevented by cooking to a temperature of at least 56°C for 5 min. Freezing at −10°C for 72 h or placing the fish in a brine solution with appropriate salt concentration and exposure time can also prevent disease. Commercially prepared lox is usually brined appropriately before smoking.

SPARGANOSIS The *sparganum,* or plerocercoid larva, of *Diphyllobothrium*-related tapeworms belonging to the genus *Spirometra* will develop in humans following ingestion (usually in drinking water) of a *Cyclops* bearing the procercoid larva. Sparganosis also follows ingestion of infected frogs or application of infected fresh frog flesh as a poultice. The frog tissues contain the sparganum, which is capable of invading human tissues. The dog and cat are definitive hosts for *Spirometra.* The infection often presents as a painful subcutaneous swelling. The periorbital tissues may be involved with marked palpebral edema and destruction of the globe. A marked eosinophilia is usually present. The location of the larvae determines the prognosis of the infection in humans. Surgery and injection of ethyl alcohol with epinephrine-free procaine to kill worms is the preferred method of treatment.

COENUROSIS This is a rare infection of humans by the larval stage, or coenurus, of the dog tapeworm *Taenia multiceps.* As in cysticercosis, the subcutaneous tissue, eye, and central nervous system may be involved. In tropical areas the brain has often been invaded, and the cases have been fatal. The clinical presentation is that of a slowly growing space-occupying lesion. Diagnosis and treatment both rely on surgical excision of the lesion. Treatment with drugs including mebendazole has not been effective.

ECHINOCOCCIASIS Definition Echinococciasis is a tissue infection of humans caused by the larval stage of *Echinococcus granulosus* or *E. multilocularis.* These species of echinococcus are distinct morphologically and biologically. In humans, *E. granulosus* produces cystic lesions primarily involving the liver and lungs, whereas *E. multilocularis* causes multilocular (alveolar) lesions that are locally invasive. A "sylvatic" form of *E. granulosus* differs significantly in clinical findings from a "pastoral" form.

Epidemiology Canines are the definitive hosts for *E. granulosus.* Sheep, cattle, and, in the Middle East, camels are the common intermediates for the pastoral form. This form of the disease has its highest incidence in countries where sheep and cattle raising is carried out with the help of dogs, particularly in the Middle East, Australia, New Zealand, east and south Africa, South America, and central Europe. Approximately 200 cases per year of echinococciasis are diagnosed in the United States, but most are imported. Autochthonously acquired cases have been reported from a few well-defined populations, including Basque sheep farmers in California, southwestern Indians, and sheep raisers in Utah.

The sylvatic focus of *E. granulosus* exists primarily in Alaska and western Canada, where wolves act as the definitive host and caribou and moose as the intermediate. A second sylvatic cycle involving deer and coyotes has been reported from California. A domestic cycle can be established when humans kill the herbivores and feed their viscera to dogs.

In *E. multilocularis* infections, rodents such as deer mice are the natural intermediate hosts, while wolves, foxes, coyotes, and domestic dogs and cats may serve as definitive hosts. An urban cycle involving the cat and common house mouse has been described. Human infection in the United States is most common in Alaska but has also been described in Minnesota. Large series of patients with *E. multilocularis* have been reported from Siberia and Switzerland.

Etiology The adult *E. granulosus* is a small worm measuring 5 mm in length which resides in the jejunum of canines for 5 to 20 months. In addition to the scolex and neck, it has three proglottides, one immature, one mature, and one gravid. The gravid segment splits, either before or after passage in the stool, to release eggs which appear identical with those of *T. saginata.* When ingested by an appropriate intermediate host, the embryos escape from the eggs, penetrate the intestinal mucosa, and enter the portal circulation. Most are filtered out by the liver or lung, but some escape into the general circulation to involve brain, kidney, bones, and other tissues. The larvae that are not phagocytosed and destroyed develop into hydatid cysts which are unilocular and consist of an external laminated cuticula and an inner germinal layer. The laminated membrane in the sylvatic form may be semitranslucent in appearance and more fragile than in the pastoral type. Fluid fills and distends the cyst. Brood capsules and second- or third-generation daughter cysts develop from the germinal layer. "Hydatid sand" found in the cyst consists of scolices liberated from ruptured brood capsules. The cysts grow slowly over a period of years. In the pastoral type cysts often reach a diameter of over 10 cm, while cysts in the sylvatic form are usually only 3 to 5 cm. When the hydatid cyst is ingested by a canine, the cycle is complete.

The life cycle of *E. multilocularis* is similar except that small rodents serve as the natural intermediate host. However, the cyst is quite different. The larval stage of *E. granulosus* develops normally in humans, and the unilocular cyst remains unattached to host tissue. In contrast, humans do not provide optimal conditions for development of *E. multilocularis,* and the larval form remains in the proliferative phase. The hydatid cyst is always multilocular or alveolar in type. Its vesicles progressively invade the host tissue, usually the liver, by extension of processes from the germinal layer. In general, the growth pattern is like a neoplasm, and the lesions may metastasize when growth extends into blood vessels.

Clinical manifestations Echinococciasis is usually acquired in childhood, but a latent period of 5 to 20 years occurs before diagnosis. In one patient the latent period of a hepatic cyst was 75 years. Enlarging cysts usually produce tissue damage by mechanical means. The resulting symptoms depend upon the site, type, and rate of growth of the cystic lesions.

Patients with the sylvatic form of *E. granulosus* are usually asymptomatic at the time of diagnosis. Approximately 60 percent of the cysts are found in the lung and 40 percent in the liver. The cysts are diagnosed as an incidental finding on routine x-ray. Rarely, a patient may present with hemoptysis or a palpable mass in the liver. Morbidity and mortality are almost never seen.

With the pastoral type the ratio of pulmonary to liver cysts is reversed, and the hydatids may reach enormous size. In as many as 20 percent of patients, the pulmonary hydatid may rupture producing cough, chest pain, or hemoptysis. Hepatic lesions often present as abdominal pain or a palpable mass. Rupture through the diaphragm or into the peritoneal cavity can occur. Intrabiliary extrusion of calcified hepatic cysts has been reported in 5 to 15 percent of affected patients and mimics recurrent cholecystitis. Obstruction of the bile duct may result in jaundice. Rupture of a hydatid into the bile duct, peritoneal cavity, lung, pleura, or bronchus may produce fever, pruritus, urticarial rash, or an anaphylactoid reaction which may be fatal. Release of the numerous scolices leads to disseminated infection. Most patients initially have one or more hydatids in a single site, but in about 10 percent other tissues are involved. In bone, the cysts are semisolid, invade the medullary cavity, and slowly erode bone, producing pathologic fractures. Central nervous system involvement may produce epilepsy or blindness. Cardiac cysts can lead to conduction blocks, pericarditis, and ventricular rupture. Hydatid antigen has been shown by fluorescent antibody in the glomerulus and has been related to membranous glomerulonephritis. Many other sites can be involved including spleen, ovary, prostate, and thyroid.

The alveolar cyst of *E. multilocularis* usually presents as a slowly growing hepatic tumor, with a minority of patients having metastatic disease to lung, brain, or other tissues. The natural course is one of malignant growth with massive destruction of the liver and extension into vital structures. If untreated, the disease is fatal in 70 percent of cases, but there is considerable individual variation in the course of the disease.

Diagnosis If a hydatid cyst ruptures or leaks fluid, an anaphylactoid reaction associated with eosinophilia and increased IgE levels may suggest the diagnosis. However, the clinical picture is usually not characteristic, and eosinophilia is seen in fewer than 25 percent of cases. Echinococciasis is most commonly discovered by routine x-ray. Pulmonary lesions usually are round, somewhat irregular masses of uniform density. They do not calcify. In contrast, hepatic cysts of *E. granulosus* show a smooth rim of calcification in about 50 percent of cases. Diffuse radiolucencies (2 to 4 mm) outlined by calcific densities may be seen in the liver with *E. multilocularis.* CT can be useful in demonstrating more details of the hydatid. In some cases of *E. granulosus,* simple, fluid-filled cysts indistinguishable from benign hepatic cysts are seen. In others, the findings of daughter cysts and hydatid sand strongly suggest echinococciasis. Thin eggshell calcification may indicate active disease. With alveolar hydatids, CT reveals indistinct solid masses, often with central necrosis, and plaque-like calcification. Ultrasound can also be helpful in distinguishing hydatid structure, and angiography may be necessary prior to surgical therapy.

Specific diagnosis is best accomplished by histologic examination. However, diagnostic aspiration should not be attempted because of potential anaphylactoid reactions to leakage of cyst fluid. Occasionally scolices may be found in sputum, stool, or urine and are best shown by Ziehl-Neelsen stain. The skin test (Casoni's test) is sensitive but gives 40 percent false-positive results. Serologic tests including indirect hemagglutination and latex agglutination are more useful if positive, but many cyst carriers will not develop an immune response. Indirect hemagglutination should be positive in 90 percent of patients with hepatic cysts but in only 50 to 60 percent of those with pulmonary hydatids. The presence of "arc 5" in the immunoelectrophoresis test provides the most specific serologic diagnosis of hydatid disease, and the adaptation of this technique to an enzyme-linked immunoelectrodiffusion assay may provide a more sensitive, rapid test. Following surgical removal of cysts, serologic tests may be helpful in screening for residual or recurrent disease. The Clq assay has also been employed for this purpose.

Treatment Surgical treatment remains the standard therapy. Patients with small calcified hepatic cysts and pulmonary hydatids of the sylvatic type need to be operated on only if the cysts are symptomatic or enlarge dramatically over time. All others should have their cysts excised if possible, or sterilized and drained. With a large cyst, the contents should be sterilized with hypertonic saline before an attempt is made to open it. The entire endocyst should then be removed if possible, and all biliary or bronchial fistulas carefully closed. The residual space must be obliterated to prevent postoperative infection or prolonged drainage. Aspergillomas have been seen in residual cavities of pulmonary cysts.

Medical therapy with "high-dose" mebendazole (40 mg/kg per day) may be considered in patients with other medical problems that preclude surgery or in patients with extensive disease that makes surgical cure impossible. In selected patients, it may also be considered in conjunction with definitive surgery to reduce the risk of metastatic spread of viable organisms. In animal models, mebendazole is larvacidal for *E. granulosus* but not for *E. multilocularis.* In human trials, all forms of echinococciasis appear to respond to the agent, although the experience with *E. multilocularis* is limited. Significant side effects including neutropenia have been reported. At present, the agent should be used only with the patient's informed consent. The absorption is erratic and drug levels should be followed. The drug is contraindicated in pregnancy.

Prevention The incidence of echinococciasis can be reduced by appropriate control measures as demonstrated in Iceland. Contact with infected dogs must be avoided, infected carcasses and offal should be burned or buried, and infected dogs should be treated.

REFERENCES

BEAVER PC et al: *Clinical Parasitology,* 9th ed. Philadelphia, Lea and Febiger, 1984

BENGER A et al: A human coenurus infection in Canada. Am J Trop Med Hyg 30:638, 1981

DE GHETALDI et al: Cerebral cysticercosis treated biphasically with dexamethasone and praziquantel. Ann Intern Med 99:179, 1983

GAMBLE WG et al: Alveolar hydatid disease in Minnesota: First human case acquired in the contiguous United States. JAMA 241:904, 1979

GHARBI HA et al: Ultrasound examination of the hydatidic liver. Radiology 139:459, 1981

GROLL E: Praziquantel for cestode infections in man. Acta Trop 37:293, 1980
JONES TC: Cestodes. Clin Gastroenterol 7:105, 1978
JONES WE: Niclosamide as a treatment for *Hymenolepis diminuta* and *Dipylidium caninum* infection in man. Am J Trop Med Hyg 28:300, 1979
KATZ R et al: Pulmonary echinococcosis: A pediatric disease of the southwestern United States. Pediatrics 65:1003, 1980
LOO L, BRAUDE A: Cerebral cysticercosis in San Diego. A report of 23 cases and a review of the literature. Medicine 61:341, 1982
MOHAMMED IN et al: Enzyme-linked immunosorbent assay for the diagnosis of cerebral cysticercosis. J Clin Microbiol 20:775, 1984
NASH TE, NEVA FA: Recent advances in the diagnosis and treatment of cerebral cysticercosis. N Engl J Med 311:1492, 1984
PINON JM et al: Immunological study of hydatidosis. Am J Trop Med Hyg 28:318, 1979
PORAT S, JOSEPH KN: Hydatid disease of bone. Israel J Med Sci 14:223, 1978
TAYLOR RL: Sparganosis in the United States. Report of a case. Am J Clin Pathol 66:560, 1976
WERCZBERGER A et al: Disseminated echinococcosis with repeated anaphylactic shock treated with mebendazole. Chest 76:482, 1979
WILSON JF et al: Cystic hydatid disease in Alaska. Am Rev Resp Dis 98:1, 1968
———, RAUSCH RL: Alveolar hydatid disease. A review of clinical features of 33 indigenous cases of *E. multilocularis* infection in Alaskan Eskimos. Am J Trop Med Hyg 29:1340, 1980
XANTHAKIS D et al: Hydatid disease of the chest. Report of 91 cases surgically treated. Thorax 27:517, 1972

section 10 Disorders caused by environmental agents

169 SCABIES, CHIGGERS, AND OTHER ECTOPARASITES

JAMES J. PLORDE

SCABIES Scabies is a cosmopolitan skin infection commonly referred to as the "seven-year itch." It is caused by a burrowing mite, *Sarcoptes scabiei* var. *hominis,* and is transmitted from person to person by close bodily contact, particularly among family members and bed partners. Although the disease is more common in the poor and unclean, sporadic cases involve individuals of all socioeconomic groups. Children under 15 years of age have the highest prevalence of scabies and are usually the first members of families to contract the disease. Those who spend nights with friends or exchange clothing with others are at increased risk. Institutional outbreaks in hospitals, nursing homes, mental institutions, and aboard naval vessels have been reported. There has been a worldwide resurgence of this infection over the past 20 years, and in the United States it currently involves 2 to 4 percent of patients seen in dermatologists' offices.

The turtle-shaped female measures 0.4 mm in length and possesses four pairs of legs. With the help of the two anterior pairs and her mouth, she burrows into the superficial layer of the epidermis. Here she deposits two or three enormous eggs daily until she dies 30 to 60 days later. The newly hatched larvae mature to adulthood on the skin surface within 2 weeks to continue the cycle of infection. Although an involved person may harbor thousands or occasionally millions of adult mites, the average number of adult females per infection is 11.

Two-thirds of the burrows are found in the upper extremities, particularly on the interdigital spaces of the hands and the flexor surface of the wrists. In heavy infections, other sites are typically involved. These include the dorsal surfaces of the elbows, anterior axillary folds, female breasts, periumbilical area, penis, scrotum, and buttocks. In bedridden patients, lesions are often concentrated over pressure points. The face, head, palms, and soles are seldom involved in adults; in infants, any area of the skin can be involved. Characteristically, a burrow appears as a short dark wavy line which may end in a small vesicle, the site of the adult female.

Sensitization (type IV) to the mites and their products begins approximately 1 month after infection and results in a papular or eczematous reaction at the sites of involvement. Itching is often severe and tends to be more marked at night or after a hot bath. Scratching frequently leads to secondary infection with pustulation; acute glomerulonephritis has followed infection with nephritogenic strains of streptococci. Occasionally, reddish pruritic nodules are seen in the groin and axillary regions. Infected individuals with good personal hygiene usually have few lesions, and burrows may be difficult to identify. In mentally retarded, debilitated, or immunosuppressed patients, a particularly virulent infection known as *Norwegian scabies* is sometimes seen. Millions of mites may be present, producing a highly infectious exfoliative dermatitis; itching is often mild or absent. Scabies usually terminates spontaneously in a few months, but chronic cases do occur.

The diagnosis should be considered in any patient presenting with a pruritic eruption, particularly if it involves several members of a living group. The occurrence of symmetric lesions at the sites of predilection should initiate a search for the characteristic burrows. These should be vigorously scraped with a sterile needle or scalpel blade, and the scrapings transferred to a drop of 10% potassium hydroxide on a glass slide. A coverslip is placed over the top, and the preparation examined for adults, larvae, and eggs. The diagnosis can also be made on histologic sections prepared from a punch biopsy. Considering the mode of disease transmission, adults shown to have scabies should also be checked for venereal disease.

All sexual contacts and household members should be treated simultaneously with the patient to prevent the occurrence of "ping-pong infections." The therapeutic agents are applied topically, covering the skin thinly but completely from the neck down. Although the patient is rendered noninfectious within 24 h, up to 2 months may be required for the clinical manifestations of the disease to disappear completely. Needless retreatment during this period can lead to contact dermatitis. Bed linen and clothes used by the patient the day prior to therapy should be washed in hot water.

A number of effective agents are available for use. Gamma benzene hexachloride (Gamene, Kwell) is left on for 12 h and then thoroughly washed off. Care must be taken to keep it away from eyes and mucous membranes. It should not be used in infants or pregnant adults. Benzyl benzoate (25%) is administered in a similar fashion. Crotamiton (Eurax) is massaged into the skin, and a second dose applied 24 h later. Antihistamines or salicylates are helpful in counteracting pruritus. Topical steroids may potentiate the infection and should not be used. Antibiotics are required occasionally when there is a significant bacterial superinfection.

CHIGGER MITES The term *chigger* is used to refer to larvae of harvest mites belonging to the family Trombiculidae. The cosmopolitan adults feed on vegetable matter and deposit their eggs upon the ground. The tiny (0.4 mm) emergent larvae crawl along the ground and upward onto vegetation. Here, they await the passage of a vertebrate host, upon which they must feed before again dropping to the ground and molting. In humans, the chigger usually attaches about the ankles, but some advance along the skin until they are stopped by tight-fitting clothing. It then pierces the skin, releases a digestant to liquefy tissue cells, and feeds for 3 or 4 days. Within a few hours, the chigger's secretions have produced an intensely pruritic papule 0.5 to 2 cm in diameter. This usually vesiculates, resulting in a chickenpox-like lesion. Occasionally, subcutaneous bleeding results in a surrounding area of ecchymosis. The lesion and itching may persist for several weeks. In the United States, most clinical cases are seen during the summer months; in warm climates, the seasonal pattern is missing. Treatment is directed at the relief of itching and the prevention of secondary infections. Insect repellants are highly effective prophylactic agents.

FLEAS Fleas are small wingless laterally compressed ectoparasites of humans and other warm-blooded animals. They tend to be found on the hairy portions of the host where they feed and deposit their eggs. The active larvae which hatch in 3 days can be found on the host, in its nest, or in dust. They eventually pupate and may remain dormant for weeks or months before completing their development to adults.

Medically, fleas serve as both vectors and agents of disease. Rodent fleas of the genus *Xenopsylla* are the most important. They are responsible for the transmission of both plague (*Yersinia pestis*) and murine typhus (*Rickettsia mooseri*) from animal reservoirs to humans. Humans may also acquire the rat tapeworm *Hymenolepis diminuta* by swallowing fleas containing the cysticeroid. The dog tapeworm *Dipylidium caninum* may be transmitted in a similar fashion. The bites of these and other species of fleas belonging to the family Pulicidae can induce an irritating dermatitis. In addition, the tungidae (*Tunga penetrans*) may burrow into the subcutaneous tissues, producing a painful and debilitating disease.

Flea dermatitis The fleas of humans (*Pulex irritans*), cats and dogs (*Cetenocephalides*), and rodents (*Xenopsylla*) may all induce dermatitis. In many individuals, the bites seem completely innocuous, but in sensitive persons, the saliva induces an erythematous raised pruritic papule. Repeated scratching may result in secondary infection with pustulation or ulceration. The intense pruritus, the ability of the flea to escape capture by virtue of its prodigious jumping ability, and the difficulty involved in crushing their hard chitinous bodies has led to many a frustrating nocturnal safari dedicated to the destruction of this unwanted bed partner. Control is effected by the use of frequent vacuuming to remove eggs, larvae, pupae, and adults from the environment. Insecticide sprays are also of help, but fleas have developed resistance to many of these. Dogs and cats should be washed, flea collars should be applied, and kennels should be dusted or sprayed with DDT or malathion. If rat runs can be located, they should also be dusted.

Tunga penetrans, sometimes referred to as a *jigger* or *chigoe flea,* is a burrowing flea found in the tropical areas of South America and Africa. These small (1 mm) free-living insects reside in sandy soil. The fertilized female burrows into the skin of the first warm-blooded animal encountered. In humans, they usually embed on the sole of the foot or under a toenail with only their anal pore exposed to the outside. Multiple infections are common. As the female becomes engorged with blood and eggs, a painful and pruritic pea-sized swelling is produced. Eventually, the overlying skin ulcerates, the flea dies, and the eggs are extruded. Secondary bacterial infections including tetanus and gas gangrene occur commonly. Autoamputation of the toes has been reported from Africa. The intact flea can usually be extracted by gently enlarging the entrance hole with a sterile needle and then applying pressure from the side. Alternatively, the lesion can be soaked in Lysol, the flea penetrated with a needle, and the lesion resoaked to kill the eggs and sterilize the wound. Antibiotics may be required to treat secondary bacterial infections.

PEDICULOSIS Lice are obligate human ectoparasites that complete their entire 30- to 40-day life cycle on the body of the host. *Pediculus humanus* var. *capitis* infests the head, *P. humanus* var. *corporis* the body and clothing, and *Phthirius pubis* (crab lice) the genital and occasionally other hairy areas of the body. All three are flattened dorsoventrally and measure 2 to 3 mm in length. The crab louse is broader and flatter than *Pediculus* and possesses powerful claws on its second and third legs with which it clings to the pubic hair. The females lay five or six eggs daily which they firmly attach to the hairs or, in the case of the body louse, the clothing of the host. These clearly visible tiny white nits hatch in 8 to 10 days. The resulting nymph matures to adulthood in an additional 2 weeks. Both the larvae and adults take two blood meals daily, leaving behind a small purpuric puncture site. With repeated exposure, the host develops an inflammatory hypersensitivity reaction manifested as a small red papule at each new feeding site. Pruritus results in scratching, a weeping dermatitis, and secondary infection. Chronic infections of the scalp may result in a fetid mass of matted hair and exudate. On the body and genital areas, the lesions may become pigmented—so-called vagabond disease. Heavy infections with *P. pubis* may involve the eyebrows and eyelids leading to blepharitis.

Lice can be transferred from person to person by direct contact or via discarded clothing in which the body louse can survive for up to a week. Migration is stimulated by fever, making *P. humanus* var. *corporis* an efficient vector of relapsing fever (*Borrelia recurrentis*), typhus (*R. prowazekii*), and trench fever (*R. quintana*). *Phthirius pubis* is not known to be a vector of human disease.

Pediculosis corporis is typically seen in the poor and transient who are unable to maintain even minimal levels of personal hygiene. In contrast, head and pubic lice are found on patients of all socioeconomic classes and are currently enjoying a resurgence in the United States. *P. capitis* most frequently infests white schoolchildren; blacks are seldom involved. Pubic lice are more common among the sexually active; their presence should stimulate a search for venereal disease.

The diagnosis is suggested by the typical dermatitis and confirmed by finding the adults or nits on the hair or clothing of the patient. Treatment may be carried out with pyrethrins with piperonyl butoxide (RID) or 1% gamma benzene hexachloride (lindane, Kwell). The latter agent may be absorbed through the skin, resulting in central nervous system toxicity if inappropriately applied. It should not be used in infants and pregnant women. In head infections, the hair should first be shampooed with ordinary soap. RID is then rubbed in for at least 10 min (Kwell shampoo, 4 min), the hair is rinsed, dried, and combed with a fine-tooth comb to remove the nits. The process should be repeated in 7 days. Combs and brushes should be heated in water to 65°C for 5 min or soaked in 2% Lysol. The clothing and bedding of the patient with body lice are heat-sterilized. The patient's body should be lathered for 10 min with RID or 4 min with Kwell and then rinsed thoroughly. The therapy may be repeated in 7 days. In crab louse infestations, RID or Kwell cream or lotion should be used on the involved areas and left for 24 h. In hirsute individuals, the treatment can be repeated in 1 week. If the eyelashes are involved, 0.25% physostigmine ophthalmic ointment is applied twice daily for 10 days. Lice and nits are carefully removed with a cotton-tipped applicator. Narrow-angle glaucoma should be ruled out before the physostigmine is used.

MYIASIS Infections with maggots or fly larvae are seen worldwide in a variety of animals. Human involvement occurs most frequently where people live in close contact with domestic animals. Many different species of flies are involved. In some, an animal host is required for larval development; in these, the larvae are capable of invading normal tissue or enter the body through the nose, mouth, or ears. Others are opportunists, depositing their eggs or larvae in the open wounds of debilitated patients. The clinical manifestations vary with the species of fly and site of involvement. Four of the more common clinical syndromes are described below.

Localized cutaneous myiasis In tropical America the lesions are produced by *Dermatobia hominis,* the human botfly. This remarkable forest-dwelling Diptera captures a mosquito or other blood-feeding insect on which to deposit its packet of eggs. When this unwilling vector then lands on a warm-blooded animal to feed, the eggs hatch and penetrate the feeding site. Within the skin of the host, the larva develops for 2 or 3 months. Finally, it emerges, drops to the ground, and pupates. The lesions are most frequently seen on unprotected areas of the body including the hands, feet, head, and neck. During the first week of infection, the pruritic lesion closely resembles a mosquito bite. As the larva grows and begins to move, it produces severe pain and itching. Tissue destruction and inflammation results in the development of a furuncle-like lesion. Generally, a central opening is present through which the posterior end of the larva protrudes. A dark serosanguinous discharge containing the feces of the insect may be noted.

In Africa, a similar lesion is produced by *Cordylobia anthropophaga* (tumbu fly). These flies deposit their eggs on sandy soil or laundry laid out to dry. The larvae hatch and invade the unbroken skin of humans or wild rodents, where they mature in 8 or 9 days. In either case, the larvae can be surgically extracted without difficulty. In tumbu fly infections, letting the larvae mature and drop off spontaneously may be appropriate. This process can occasionally be hastened by applying mineral oil to the central opening. This results in the suffocation of the larva and stimulates its early exodus.

Cutanea larva migrans This is usually caused by the large (1 to 2 cm) horse botflies belonging to the genus *Gasterophilus*. When the larvae hatch on the skin, they penetrate to the lower epidermis. Because they do not mature in humans, they may migrate in the skin for several months. Clinically, the infection presents as a pruritic serpiginous band of erythema closely resembling cutanea larva migrans produced by *Ancylostoma braziliense*. The diagnosis can be made by placing a small drop of mineral oil on the skin just in advance of the worm tract. This allows visualization of black backward-directed spines on its body segments. The parasite can be easily removed with a sharp needle. Occasionally, the larvae may penetrate the eye. A similar clinical picture is sometimes produced by the larvae of *Hypoderma* spp. (cattle botfly). These, however, often penetrate deeply into the subcutaneous tissue and produce more pain and less pruritus than *Gasterophilus* larvae.

Deep-tissue myiasis Screwflies of several genera can deposit large batches of eggs on unbroken skin or in wounds, ears, or the nose. After hatching, the larvae burrow into the tissues and develop for 2 or 3 weeks. The mature 1- to 2-cm larvae then drop to the ground and pupate. At times, they penetrate deep tissues, including the eye, nasal sinuses, and cranium, where they produce destructive foul-smelling lesions. Bacterial superinfection is common. In India and Africa, the flies are usually of genus *Chrysomyia*. In the western hemisphere, *Callitroga* spp. are involved. The occurrence of human cases in the United States often accompanies epizootics of screwworm activity. Flesh flies of the family Sarcophagidae have also been implicated in deep-tissue myiasis both in the United States and elsewhere. In all the above infections, the lesions should be surgically incised and debrided, the larvae removed, and secondary infections treated.

Intestinal myiasis When humans ingest food contaminated with the eggs or larvae of several genera of flies, some survive passage through the stomach and later mature in the intestine before they are extruded in the stool. In the United States, *Tubifera tenax* is the most frequently implicated species. Invasion of the intestinal mucosa may occur with *Sarcophaga* infections.

REFERENCES

BARKIN JS: Intestinal myiasis. Am J Gastroenterol 78:560, 1983

BURKHART CG: Scabies: An epidemiologic reassessment. Ann Intern Med 98:498, 1983

Drugs for parasitic infections. Med Lett 26:27, 1984

LEIBOWITZ M et al: Keratotic scabies (Norwegian scabies): Case reports and literature review. S Afr Med J 57:363, 1980

MAGNARELLI LA, ANDREADIS TG: Human cases of furuncular, traumatic and nasal myiasis in Connecticut. Am J Trop Med Hyg 30:894, 1981

STRICKLAND GT: *Hunter's Tropical Medicine*, 6th ed. Philadelphia, Saunders, 1984

170 DISORDERS CAUSED BY VENOMS, BITES, AND STINGS

JAMES F. WALLACE

Humans have the propensity to come into contact with a great variety of venomous animals. These contacts occur with many zoologic classes including snakes, lizards, sea animals, spiders, scorpions, and numerous species of insects. In general two types of injuries result: those due to the direct effect of venom on the victim, as exemplified in snakebite, and those due to indirect effects of the poison, of which hypersensitivity reaction to bee stings is an example. Each year in the United States at least 50 persons die as the result of venomous injuries. Three groups of animals—hymenopterous insects, snakes, and spiders—account for over 90 percent of the fatalities. Of even greater public health significance is the loss in economic productivity and human potential resulting from the many serious, nonfatal envenomations which occur annually in otherwise healthy children or working adults.

SNAKE BITE Epidemiology Fewer than one-tenth of the nearly 3500 known species of snakes are venomous. These poisonous varieties belong to five families or subfamilies: Elapidae (cobras, kraits, mambas, and coral snakes) found in all parts of the world except Europe; Viperidae (true vipers) found in all parts of the world except the Americas; Hydrophidae (sea snakes); Crotalidae (pit vipers) found in Asia and the Americas; and Colubridae (boomslangs, bird snakes) of the African continent. The poisonous varieties of the United States, with the single exception of the coral snake, are pit vipers and include rattlesnakes, the water moccasin, and the copperhead. Although this discussion centers around these species, most of the therapeutic measures outlined are applicable to snakes in all parts of the world.

The number of individuals bitten by poisonous snakes in the United States is estimated to be about 8000 per year, with a relatively large number occurring in the southeastern and Gulf states, particularly Texas. Deaths are not reported separately but are undoubtedly rare, numbering fewer than 20 per year, and most are due to bites of various species of rattlesnake. In many European countries deaths from snakebite have averaged only one every 3 to 5 years for the last half-century. In contrast, the estimate of annual deaths from snakebite throughout the world is between 30,000 and 40,000 with the largest number occurring in the countries of Burma and Brazil, where 2000 deaths are estimated to occur each year.

Etiology The *coral snake* is found in the southern states from Florida to Arizona. It is usually marked by alternating red and black bands separated by yellow rings; however, black and albino forms exist. Coral snakes are generally nocturnal in their activities, shy and elusive, and rarely bite humans. Their fangs are short and permanently erect; the highly toxic venom is injected into multiple puncture wounds produced by a series of chewing movements.

The *pit vipers* are so named because of a small pit between the eye and the nostril. Large venom glands in the temporal regions give the head a triangular appearance. They are generally aggressive and likely to strike if disturbed. The fangs are long and hinged, folding posteriorly when the mouth is closed. Pit vipers strike suddenly with a forward thrust of the head. The instant that the erect fangs make contact, venom is expressed by sudden muscular contraction.

The *rattlesnakes*, recognized by the horny rattle on the tail, which buzzes when the snake is disturbed, are widely distributed. The diamondbacks (*Crotalus adamanteus* in the southeast and *C. atrox* in the southwest) are the largest and most dangerous snakes in this country. Others include the prairie rattler (*C. confluentus*), the timber rattler (*C. horridus*), and the pigmy rattlers.

The *water moccasin*, or cottonmouth (*Agkistrodon piscivorus*), is found in swampy areas or along the banks of streams. It is a strong swimmer and can bite under water. This snake is notorious for inflicting severe facial bites when disturbed in the branches of small trees. The copperhead, or highland moccasin (*A. mokasen*), is a closely related species. Its bite is painful but rarely fatal.

Pathogenesis SNAKE VENOMS The venoms of most species which have been analyzed have been found to be mixtures of several toxic proteins and enzymes with diversified and complicated pharmacologic effects. As an example, the venom of the Indian cobra (*Naja naja*) contains these distinct and separate substances: a neurotoxin, a hemolysin, a cardiotoxin, a cholinesterase, at least three phosphatases, a nucleotidase, and a potent inhibitor of cytochrome oxidase. Several venoms, including those of the pit vipers, contain hyaluronidase and numerous proteolytic enzymes. Although the exact roles of these components in toxicity are incompletely understood, the venom of a given species is usually predominantly neurotoxic or necrotizing and is frequently associated with hemolysis, abnormalities of blood coagulation, changes in cardiac dynamics, and alterations in vascular resistance. Venoms of elapids, including the coral snake, are neurotoxic, with death resulting from respiratory paralysis probably caused by damage to brain centers and a curariform interference with transmission at the neuromuscular junction. Venoms of crotalid snakes produce local tissue injury, hemorrhage, and hemolysis. Death is often preceded by circulatory collapse associated with a marked fall in circulating blood volume resulting from pooling of blood in the microcirculation, and loss of plasma due to increased capillary permeability. Systemic absorption of venom occurs through the lymphatics, and therapeutic measures designed to reduce lymphatic function are helpful in controlling symptoms.

FACTORS AFFECTING SEVERITY OF SNAKE BITE Several factors affect the outcome of snake bite:

1 The age, size, and health of the patient. Envenomation in children is usually serious, and a fatal outcome is more likely, since a relatively large dose of poison is injected into a small victim.
2 Location of bite. Bites on extremities or into adipose tissue are less dangerous than those on the trunk, face, or directly into a blood vessel. A direct strike of the fangs is more dangerous than a scratch, a glancing blow, or one hitting a bone. The discharge orifice of a fang is well above its tip so that the point of the fang can penetrate the skin without envenomation; even a thin layer of clothing may afford great protection. Because of the superficial nature of the wound as many as one-fifth of patients bitten by venomous snakes will have no evidence of envenomation, even though the fangs have penetrated the skin.
3 The size of the snake (a large pit viper can inject over 1000 mg venom, six times a lethal dose for an adult), the extent of its anger or fear (if hurt it may inject a larger amount of venom), the condition of the fangs (broken or recently renewed), and the condition of the venom glands (recently discharged or full). All these factors are important. Contrary to popular belief, the bite of a snake which has recently killed and fed is not necessarily less venomous for humans; the snake usually does not exhaust its venom in a single bite.
4 The presence of various bacteria, particularly clostridia and other anaerobic organisms, in the mouth of the snake or on the skin of the victim. This may lead to serious infection in the necrotic tissues at the local site.
5 Exercise or exertion, such as running, immediately after the bite. This speeds systemic absorption of toxin.

Manifestations Following the bite of a pit viper, severe burning pain develops within a few minutes at the site of the wound. Local swelling rapidly develops and spreads in all directions, accompanied by the appearance of ecchymoses and bullae over the involved area. As the edema spreads, serosanguinous fluid oozes from the puncture wounds. Later gangrene of the skin and subcutaneous tissues may develop. Systemic effects resulting from the absorption of venom and local tissue destruction may include fever, nausea and vomiting, circulatory collapse, bleeding into the skin and from all body orifices, low-grade jaundice, neuropathic muscle cramping, pupillary constriction, disorientation, delirium, and convulsions. Death may occur after 6 to 48 h. Survival may be attended by massive local tissue loss from gangrene or secondary infection, or may be complicated by acute renal failure, secondary to disseminated intravascular clotting and cortical necrosis, or by tubular necrosis following circulatory collapse.

The bite of the coral snake causes little pain and local swelling. There are usually multiple fang marks. Within 10 to 15 min numbness and weakness begin in the region of the bite, followed by ataxia, ptosis, pupillary dilatation, palatal and pharyngeal paralysis, slurring of speech, salivation, and occasionally nausea and vomiting. The patient becomes comatose, develops respiratory paralysis and seizures, and dies within 8 to 72 h.

Cobra bites are painful and are often accompanied by severe hemolysis, local necrosis, and sloughing in addition to their neurotoxic effects. There is little pain and no edema at the site of a sea snake bite. Symptoms of systemic envenomation follow a latent period which may vary from 15 min to 8 h. Although the venom is both myotoxic and neurotoxic, the injury to skeletal muscle is most prominent and is characterized by generalized muscle pain, weakness, and myoglobinuria. Hemorrhagic manifestations predominate following envenomation by colubrids (boomslangs and bird snakes) and many pit vipers including certain species of rattlesnake.

Laboratory abnormalities In severe cases, laboratory abnormalities may include progressive anemia, polymorphonuclear leukocytosis of 20,000 to 30,000 cells per cubic millimeter, thrombocytopenia, hypofibrinogenemia, disordered tests of coagulation, proteinuria, and azotemia.

Treatment An attempt should be made to determine with certainty that the patient has been bitten by a poisonous snake. Absence of distinct fang punctures and failure of local pain, edema, numbness, or weakness to appear within 20 min are strong evidence against snake venom poisoning. If the species of snake is not known, the offending reptile should be killed for the purpose of identification.

FIRST AID This consists of reassuring and calming the victim, instituting measures to retard the absorption of venom and to remove it from the tissues as quickly as possible after the bite, and arranging for transportation to the nearest hospital. The patient should be promptly placed at rest and the bitten extremity immobilized to reduce the rate of spread of the venom. If anatomically feasible, a wide constriction band should be placed a few centimeters above the bite and made tight enough to allow one finger to pass beneath with difficulty. The purpose is to impede lymph flow; it is not necessary to obstruct venous return. The band should be loosened and moved proximally when local swelling causes it to tighten. If the victim is more than 30 min from the hospital and is seen within 5 min following the bite, incision and suction of the wound should be started prior to evacuation. By use of whatever antisepsis is available, 1.0-cm *linear* (not cruciate) incisions about 0.3-cm deep should be carefully made through each fang mark and suction applied. A rubber bulb, breast pump, or heated jar are all preferable to mouth suction, but if other means are not available and no oral lesions are present, this method may be employed. Suction should be continued for up to 1 h following the bite, or until antivenin has been administered. The practice of making multiple incisions along the advancing edge of edema as swelling progresses has not been found to be beneficial and is no longer advised. *Incision and suction are extremely important and should be diligently carried out.* When begun promptly, they may result in the removal of up to 50 percent of subcutaneously injected venom.

While the patient is being transported to a hospital, immobilization of the affected part is important in controlling lymph flow. This is best achieved by splinting. Although ice packs relieve pain and slow lymphatic drainage, they do not neutralize venom, and even a small amount of cooling may result in irreparable damage to already injured tissues by causing ischemia. For this reason, it is recommended that no form of cryotherapy be used.

IMMEDIATE HOSPITAL CARE This should include appropriate treatment for shock and respiratory difficulty, antivenin, measures to combat infection, and general supportive care. Initial laboratory studies in a patient with obvious crotalid envenomation should include blood typing and cross-matching, a complete blood count, urinalysis, coagulation screening tests, blood urea nitrogen (BUN), blood glucose, and serum electrolytes. In severe envenomations it is also advisable to obtain an electrocardiogram. None of these tests are particularly helpful in the initial evaluation of a patient with a coral snake bite.

Antivenin is the only specific treatment of snake venom poisoning, and its use in severe bites is vital. In the United States polyvalent crotaline antivenin effective against all American pit vipers and antivenin for North American coral snake poisoning are commercially available. Both products are a lyophilized powder of refined horse serum. Kits are available containing antivenin powder (reconstituted by diluting with water to 10 mL per vial), syringe, normal horse serum for prior sensitivity testing of the patient, and detailed instructions. Intravenously administered antivenin leads to the most rapid and effective response. It is not advisable to infiltrate antivenin at the local site. The initial dose should depend upon an estimate of the amount of envenomation. For pit viper bites accompanied by progressive local swelling but no systemic symptoms (minimal envenomation), 5 vials (50 mL) are usually sufficient. When swelling has progressed beyond the site of the bite, and mild systemic symptoms and/or hematologic and coagulation abnormalities are present, moderate envenomation has occurred, and initial treatment should be 5 to 10 vials (50 to 100 mL). For severe poisonings, associated with rapidly progressive and extensive local effects as well as systemic symptoms and evidence of hemolysis or coagulopathy, 10 to 20 vials (100 to 200 mL) or more should be administered. Up to 50 percent greater doses of antivenin should be given to children or small adults to neutralize the relatively higher venom concentrations. Reconstituted antivenin is diluted in 500 mL of intravenous fluid and administered as rapidly as tolerated over 1 to 2 h. Additional infusions containing 5 to 10 vials (50 to 100 mL) should be repeated hourly until progressive swelling in the bitten part ceases and systemic signs and symptoms have disappeared. When an adequate dose has been achieved, improvement in the victim's clinical signs is often extremely rapid.

If *any* evidence of envenomation appears during the first several hours following a coral snake bite, antivenin should be given without waiting for systemic manifestations to develop. Three vials of antivenin should be given intravenously for bites associated only with minimal swelling and/or local paresthesias. If evidence of a bite is more definitive, particularly if there was initial pain, 5 vials of antivenin should be given as soon as possible.

In the patient with severe envenomation who is allergic to horse serum, the relative risks of death from anaphylaxis rather than from venom poisoning should be carefully weighed before undertaking desensitization with small doses of diluted horse serum.

No antivenin for other snakes is manufactured in the United States, but antiserum for various types is usually kept on hand at large zoos all over the world. A national antivenin index is maintained by the Oklahoma Poison Information Center in cooperation with the Oklahoma City Zoo [(405) 271–5454], and provides 24-h telephone consultation service for physicians needing advice in handling snakebite accidents.

Maintaining *respiration* by mechanical or other means is important. In patients bitten by elapid snakes, respiratory failure is usually reversible. *Tetanus toxoid* or *tetanus immune globulin* of human origin should be given. If wound infections appear, antibiotics should be used with the knowledge that the predominant microorganisms in the mouths of snakes are gram-negative pathogens. Treatment should be preceded by appropriate aerobic and anaerobic cultures. *Fasciotomy* occasionally may be necessary to prevent further ischemic injury to a massively swollen limb. Whenever possible, intracompartmental tissue pressures should be monitored, with surgical decompression undertaken only if pressure exceeds 30 to 40 mmHg. *Surgical debridement* of vesicles and superficial necrotic tissue should be instituted near the end of the first week following the bite. *Relief of pain* with salicylates or meperidine, moderate sedation, maintenance of fluid balance, measures to combat shock and hemorrhagic diathesis, and appropriate management of coma or convulsions are all important.

The usefulness of corticosteroids to prevent tissue damage or systemic intoxication has not been convincingly demonstrated. However, these drugs may be of value in the management of severe shock associated with envenomation and for allergic reactions, particularly serum sickness, following the administration of antivenin.

Prevention In snake-infested regions long trousers, high shoes, boots, or leggings, and gloves should be worn. Most important of all is to look where one steps or reaches. A sharp knife or lancet, constriction band, suction bulb, and antiseptic suffice for an emergency kit, and in inaccessible areas, antivenin should also be carried.

POISONOUS LIZARD BITE Of the nearly 3000 species of lizard in the world, only two are venomous: the Gila monster (*Heloderma suspectum*) of the arid southwestern United States and the closely related Mexican beaded lizard (*H. horridum*) which inhabits the lowland forests of western Mexico. These reptiles are not aggressive, and virtually every instance of their attacking a human has involved teasing or handling the animals in captivity. The venom is elaborated in eight glands in the floor of the mouth and secreted directly into the oral cavity, where it bathes the teeth, which are grooved posteriorly. The lizard clings tenaciously and is often dislodged only after considerable effort; envenomation occurs by contamination of the wound. The venom contains a potent neurotoxin which is undoubtedly responsible for its lethal effect on experimental animals. Death in humans following a bite is extremely rare. Most often, human envenomation results in tissue injury, excruciating pain, massive edema, and patchy erythema. Acute systemic symptoms may last for 3 to 4 days and include nausea, vomiting, hematemesis, blurred vision, dyspnea, dysphonia, and profound weakness. Intense hyperesthesia of the bitten extremity may persist for several weeks. There is no antivenin available. Treatment should consist of constriction band, incision, suction, cooling of the bitten area, measures to prevent or combat infection, including tetanus, and supportive measures. Parenteral meperidine (Demerol) or infiltration of local anesthetic around the bite may be necessary to relieve pain.

SPIDER BITES The bite of many spiders is locally irritating, and several species can cause severe, even fatal systemic poisoning in humans. In North America, only two types of spiders are of medical importance: the widow spiders (*Latrodectus* species) and the recluse spiders (*Loxosceles* species).

Widow spider bite The most numerous and important of the venomous spiders are members of the genus *Latrodectus,* widely distributed throughout the world. In the United States and Canada, *L. mactans,* the black widow or show-button spider, causes a majority of clinically significant arachnidism. In Florida, *L. bishopi,* the red-legged widow spider, has been reported to produce human poisoning resembling mild black widow bite.

It is the female *L. mactans,* the black widow, that bites humans. She is glossy black with a body 1 cm in diameter, a leg span of 5 cm, and a characteristic red hourglass mark on her abdomen. She spins her web in woodpiles, sheds, basements, or outdoor privies, is very aggressive, and will bite on slight provocation. The venom produces diffuse central and peripheral nervous excitement, autonomic activity, muscle spasm, hypertension, and vasoconstriction.

In the United States, most black widow bites occur between April and October, and many patients are males bitten on the genitalia or buttocks while using a privy. After a momentary sharp pain at the site, there is cramping pain that begins locally within 15 to 60 min and gradually spreads. It may involve all extremities and the trunk. The abdomen is boardlike, and the waves of pain become excruciating, causing the patient to turn, toss, and cry out. Respirations are often labored and grunting. There are also nausea, vomiting, headache, sweating, salivation, hyperactive reflexes, twitching, tremor, paresthesias of the hands and feet, and occasionally, systolic hypertension. A mild polymorphonuclear leukocytosis is usual, and many patients have slight fever. After several hours, the pains subside, although mild recurrences for 2 or 3 days are common. It may be a week before well-being is restored. Deaths due to cardiac or respiratory failure have occurred, mostly in children and the aged.

Because the bite itself is not prominent, patients are often thought to have some abdominal catastrophe such as perforated ulcer, pancreatitis, or appendicitis. Renal colic, myocardial infarction, tetanus, strychnine poisoning, tabetic crisis, lead colic, and porphyria are other conditions to be ruled out. The abdomen is not tender to palpation in arachnidism, and pains in the extremities are not typical of most of these other disorders.

Treatment For *Latrodectus* poisoning, treatment consists of measures to relieve pain and administration of antivenin. Initial treatment should include a hot tub bath which affords prompt, although temporary, relief. A vial (10 mL) of 10% calcium gluconate slowly injected intravenously over 10 to 20 min usually produces dramatic, but transient, cessation of cramps. A solution of 10% methocarbamol administered intravenously also may be effective in treatment of muscle spasms. Opiates are sometimes necessary. When symptoms are severe or when the patient is a small child or is at special risk due to other associated medical problems, treatment with *Latrodectus* antivenin is indicated. An intravenous injection of 1 vial (2.5 mL) diluted in 50 mL of saline and administered over a 15-min period is usually quite effective within a few hours and can be repeated if symptoms recur. Since the antivenin is prepared from horse serum, appropriate testing for hypersensitivity should be undertaken prior to its administration.

***Loxosceles* spider bite** During the past 30 years in the United States, there have been increasing numbers of reports of severe necrotizing bites due to *Loxosceles* spiders. Originally thought to be a problem only in the midwestern states and associated only with the brown recluse spider, necrotic arachnidism has now been seen in many of the southern and southwestern states as well as in California and has been attributed to at least six species of *Loxosceles* spider. The bite of these spiders may initially produce only a mild stinging discomfort. In severe bites, intense local pain appears within 2 to 8 h, accompanied by bullae formation and erythema at the site of the wound. Subsequently, ischemic necrosis occurs leaving a deep ulcer with a necrotic base. The pathogenetic mechanism for the local reaction is not completely understood but is thought to involve complement-activated tissue damage. Some patients also experience a systemic reaction characterized by fever, myalgias, and a morbilliform rash 24 to 48 h after the bite. Intravascular hemolysis is seen occasionally, and in severe cases hemoglobinuria and acute renal failure may occur. Fatalities have been reported, mostly in children.

Treatment depends upon the severity of the bite. If bullae formation, intense pain, and signs of rapidly progressing ischemic necrosis do not appear within the first 6 to 8 h, the bite is probably not severe and treatment is unnecessary. When symptoms of more serious local reaction are present, the parenteral use of corticosteroids within the first 24 h following a bite has been advocated to prevent progression of the lesion, but convincing evidence that this is effective is lacking. Dapsone has been reported to prevent extensive ulceration in rapidly progressing *Loxosceles* spider bites. However, use of the drug in this setting should be considered experimental. Other therapeutic measures consist mainly of local wound care, timely surgical debridement, and treatment of secondary infection, if it occurs. The ulcer usually heals spontaneously, although skin grafting may be required on occasion. Patients with systemic loxoscelism should be hospitalized and monitored closely for signs of hemolysis, disseminated intravascular coagulation and acute renal failure. Although of unproven efficacy, systemic corticosteroids are usually given for the duration of the acute phase of the illness, which lasts 2 to 4 days. Renal failure should be treated as advised in Chap. 219.

SCORPION STING Scorpions are eight-legged arthropods. Glands in the terminal segment produce venom, which is injected into the victim by a stinger located on the tip of the tail. Scorpions often enter dwellings. During the day they retreat into crevices; emerging at night, they often get into shoes and clothing and even into bedding. They do not deliberately attack humans, but accidental contact results in a sting.

Of about 650 species, roughly 40 occur in the United States, distributed over three-fourths of the nation. They are most numerous in the south from Florida to California, but the only dangerous species, *Centruroides exilicauda,* is limited to Arizona, New Mexico, southern California, parts of Texas, and northern Mexico. This species reaches a maximal length of about 7 cm. Their sting may be fatal to young children or old people, but seldom to a healthy adult.

Most of the nonlethal species of scorpions in the United States cause only minor reactions, like a bee sting. Some in the southwest, however, produce local edema and ecchymosis, with burning pain. In contrast, many species whose venom has potentially lethal systemic effects, including the Arizona *Centruroides,* evoke little or no visible reaction at the site of the sting. There is an immediate burning sensation followed by local paresthesia (''pins and needles''), hyperesthesia, or numbness. These sensations spread to involve the whole extremity, and within an hour or two, malaise, restlessness, neurologic hyperexcitability, lacrimation, rhinorrhea, salivation, perspiration, nausea, and vomiting may appear.

The patient passes from an agitated state with hyperactive reflexes into coma; convulsions follow. Release of catecholamines may result in tachycardia, various arrhythmias, and hypertension. Myocarditis and pancreatitis have also been reported. Death usually occurs within 12 h, but sometimes as late as 2 days after the sting.

Treatment Despite the reputation for lethality associated with envenomation by *C. exilicauda,* most often the symptoms consist only of pain and paresthesias lasting less than 4 h. These patients can be treated at home with cold compresses and mild analgesics. There is no clear consensus on the management of more severe envenomations. Although constriction bands, incision, and suction as in the treatment of snake bite have been recommended, the amount of venom is minute; it produces no local necrotizing effect and is absorbed very rapidly.

Specific antivenin, reconstituted from lyophilized goat serum, is available in some areas and should be considered if the victim develops signs of central nervous system or cardiac involvement. Supportive therapy is directed at combating shock and dehydration. Diazepam or phenobarbital are useful in reducing restlessness, and adrenergic blockers in managing symptoms secondary to catecholamine release.

Prevention This depends upon alertness in avoiding contact with scorpions in infested areas. Clothing and shoes should be well shaken before being put on in the morning. Towels and bedclothes should be inspected. A house infested with scorpions can in time be rid of them by closing all obvious ways of ingress; picking up debris in the environment, such as piles of brush, logs, stones; introducing a mixture of fuel oil or kerosene, containing a small amount of creosote, between the earth and the house foundation; and spraying with a mixture of 2% chlordane, and 0.2% pyrethrins in an oil base.

HYMENOPTERA STINGS Each year in the United States, nearly twice as many people die as a result of bites by hymenopterous insects (including bees, wasps, hornets, yellow jackets, and fire ants) as from poisonous snake bites. Occasionally, multiple stings in enormous numbers (500 to 1000) are the cause of death. However, the majority of systemic reactions and deaths are due to allergic reactions to the venoms of these insects.

Hymenoptera venoms contain many nonallergenic amines and peptides such as histamine and various kinins which contribute to the local sting reaction through their inflammatory and vasoactive properties. The allergenic venom proteins, which elicit an IgE antibody response in those who are stung, include phospholipases, hyaluronidases, acid phosphatases, and melittin. Venoms are distinctly different for each of the three genera of hymenoptera capable of causing allergic sting reactions: Apidae (various species of bees), Vespidae (hornets, yellowjackets, and wasps), and *Solenopsis* (fire ants).

The usual reaction to a single bee or wasp sting is sharp pain, which lasts for several minutes, local wheal and erythema, followed by intense itching. All signs of the sting normally subside within a few hours. Only in the rare case when a bee is swallowed or inhaled and edema of the laryngopharynx or glottis develops is there danger. A sting directly into a peripheral nerve can destroy its function for a time, much as does an injection of alcohol. Bell's palsy has followed a sting into the trunk of the facial nerve. Unusual reactions such as optic neuritis, generalized polyneuropathy, and myasthenia gravis may follow a sting. The etiology of these reactions is unknown.

In hypersensitive individuals, the response to a single sting may vary from an exaggerated local reaction, unassociated with systemic symptoms, to serious anaphylaxis with urticaria, nausea, abdominal or uterine cramps, bronchospasm, massive edema of the face and glottis, dyspnea, cyanosis, hypotension, coma, and death. These symptoms usually appear within a few minutes of the sting. Other patients may experience delayed reactions of the serum-sickness type occurring 10 to 14 days after envenomation. Sensitization is usually the result of previous stings although may fatalities have occurred in individuals who experienced no apparent allergic reaction to earlier envenomation. It has been estimated that 10 to 15 percent of the general population in this country has hymenoptera venom allergy. Those who have experienced a previous systemic allergic reaction to a sting, such as respiratory difficulty, hypotension, or generalized urticaria, are at greatest risk for serious reactions if stung again by the same type of insect.

Many species of ant can produce stinging bites with local redness and swelling. The most notorious of these are the fire ants (*Solenopsis*), particularly two "imported" South American species (*S. invicta* and *S. richteri*). The *invicta* species is now found in thirteen southern states and has largely supplanted all others, including several domestic species. In addition to being a major agricultural pest, fire ants, whose bites may result in extensive vesiculation and skin necrosis or cause serious hypersensitivity reactions, have become a significant health hazard to humans. Unlike other hymenoptera venoms, fire ant venom is mostly a simple insoluble alkaloid rather than a complex mixture of proteins. Although associated with life-threatening allergic reactions of the type seen with IgE-mediated immediate hypersensitivity, there is limited cross-sensitivity between fire ant venom and the venoms of bees, wasps, hornets, and yellowjackets.

Treatment The wound site should be examined for a stinger which, if present, should be carefully removed in order to prevent further envenomation from the attached gland. The local reaction to the usual sting is treated by local cool application and antipruritic lotions or oral antihistamines. Fire ant stings, which are frequently multiple, should be thoroughly cleaned with soap and water. Secondary bacterial infection is common and should be anticipated and treated promptly. Epinephrine, 0.3 to 0.5 mL of a 1:1000 aqueous solution subcutaneously repeated every 20 to 30 min, may be lifesaving in patients with an anaphylactic reaction to a sting. A tourniquet to slow the absorption of venom and ice packs to relieve pain may be used. Oxygen, endotracheal intubation, vasopressors, and other supportive measures should be used as needed. In addition, corticosteroids should be employed in severe cases, although their maximum effect is not achieved until several hours after administration.

Prevention Allergic persons should make every effort to avoid contact with these insects, including wearing shoes when outside and not wearing perfumes or bright colors which may attract them. In addition, they should keep epinephrine readily available for immediate use in case of a sting, without waiting for symptoms to develop. Sting kits containing premeasured doses of 1:1000 epinephrine in disposable syringes, tourniquets, and antihistamine tablets are commercially available. Careful instruction in their use should be provided by the person's physician.

Immunotherapy Desensitization by injection of preparations containing venom of the specific insect has long been recommended for any patient who has had a systemic or generalized reaction to hymenopterous insect sting. For many years, the only products available for this purpose were extracts of the crushed whole bodies of the stinging insect. However, skin testing with whole-body extracts was frequently unreliable in identifying persons at risk for systemic reactions, and immunization with these materials did not increase IgG-blocking antibodies to venom proteins, a response felt to be essential for protection against insect allergy. In contrast, purified hymenopterous venoms, which were approved for clinical use in the United States in 1979, have proved to be highly accurate in the diagnosis of sting allergy by skin testing. In addition, venom immunotherapy has been shown consistently to stimulate production of circulating venom-specific IgG antibodies, and to provide much better protection than whole-body extracts. The purified venoms have not been associated with a greater number of adverse reactions than treatment with whole-body extracts or with desensitization for pollinosis. These venom antigens are the materials of choice for diagnosis and immunotherapy of high-risk patients, those who have had previous systemic sting reactions and who have positive venom skin tests.

TICK BITE Although ticks may be vectors for such serious diseases as Rocky Mountain spotted fever, Q fever, tularemia, borreliosis, human babesiosis, and Lyme disease, the local reaction to the bite of a tick may be nothing more than an itching papule which subsides within a few days unless there is secondary bacterial infection. However, incomplete removal of a tick, with retention of the mouthparts, may result in the local formation of a nodule which continues to grow and is sometimes annoyingly pruritic. The definitive treatment is surgical excision of the nodule. Histologically, the nodule is a granuloma, but the inflammatory response is sometimes so bizarre and changes in the overlying epithelium are so striking that, in the absence of a history of tick bite, a mistaken diagnosis of malignant tumor may be made.

Ticks should always be removed intact, using gentle, steady traction. Application of a drop of oil, petrolatum, nail polish, or other organic solvent may facilitate removal without leaving embedded remnants. However, touching with a hot object such as a glowing cigarette should be discouraged because of the likelihood of injuring the host.

Tick paralysis A progressive, ascending, flaccid paralysis, acute ataxia, or a combination of both sometimes develops in humans and certain other mammals while a tick is engorging upon them. Human cases have most frequently been reported from the northwestern United States and western Canada, where the wood tick, *Dermacentor andersoni* Stiles, is responsible. The dog tick, *D. variabilis* Say, has been identified in a number of cases occurring in the southeastern states. *Amblyomma americanum*, the Lone Star tick, *A. maculatum*, the Gulf Coast tick, and *Ixodes scapularis*, the black-legged deer tick, have also been incriminated.

This disorder is caused by a neurotoxin secreted in the saliva of the engorging tick which acts upon spinal and bulbar nuclei, slowing motor nerve conduction without affecting neuromuscular transmission. The tick must feed for several days before symptoms develop.

Most human cases occur in children, generally in young girls. The tick is usually attached to the scalp and hidden by the hair, but may be found on any part of the body, especially the ear, axilla, groin, vulva, or popliteal region.

The patient may be irritable or restless for up to 24 h before frank motor involvement appears. Weakness usually is noted first in the distal muscles of the lower extremities, progressing over the next 24 to 48 h to flaccid paralysis, which may extend to involve the trunk, arms, neck, tongue, pharynx, and bulbar centers. Sensory changes are typically absent, and there is little or no fever unless a secondary infection is present. Results of routine laboratory tests including cerebrospinal fluid examination are normal. Nerve conduction studies may reveal decreased velocities and compound action potentials of nerves and their corresponding muscles.

Tick paralysis is apt to be confused with poliomyelitis, the more so because ticks are active in warm weather when poliomyelitis is most prevalent. Among other diseases which might be considered in differential diagnosis are diphtheritic polyneuropathy, transverse myelitis, the Guillain-Barré syndrome, myasthenia gravis, the Eaton-Lambert syndrome, and botulism.

Definitive treatment is removal of the tick, including any mouthparts retained in the skin. After this is done, there is striking improvement of motor function within a few hours and complete recovery within 48 h.

The patient should be observed until the recovery trend is established, because if other ticks or retained mouthparts have been overlooked, the paralysis may progress. When bulbar or respiratory paralysis is present, death may occur if the tick is not removed in time. The mortality rate is 10 percent; nearly all who die are children.

OTHER ARTHROPOD BITES AND ENVENOMATIONS **Flea bite** There are many fleas that attack humans, including *Pulex irritans* and chicken fleas. In sensitive individuals, the salivary secretion of these bloodsuckers produces large, itching papules. It is thought that much of the papular urticaria of children is probably due to flea bites. Treatment is symptomatic only. Elimination of fleas from the environment may be very difficult, but persistent treatment of animals and of premises with appropriate insecticides is usually successful.

Centipede bite The giant desert centipede, which reaches 15 cm in length, is responsible for most centipede bites in the United States. It is capable of inflicting an intensely painful bite, associated with erythema, edema, and sometimes with regional lymphangitis. Rhabdomyolysis and acute renal failure have occurred following the bite of this arthropod. Pain usually disappears within a few hours, but may require oral or parenteral analgesics. The wound should be washed well with soap and water to help prevent secondary infection.

Caterpillar rash Contact with the early larval or caterpillar stage of several species of moth produces irritation of skin and mucous membranes resulting in a pruritic, erythematous rash, occasionally accompanied by urticaria and bullae. Symptoms come on rapidly after direct contact with caterpillars, after handling cocoons, or on being exposed to windblown fuzz. The pathogenesis is thought to be due to the direct irritant effects of insect hairs or appendages, although other mechanisms, including intracutaneous injection of toxins or hypersensitivity to insect antigens, have been suggested. The symptoms usually subside within a few days. Local soaks and oral antihistamines are often indicated.

Bedbug bite Members of the genus *Cimex* inflict bites that leave reactions varying from a simple puncture to large urticarial lesions, apparently depending on the sensitivity of the bitten individual. There is no specific treatment.

Kissing bug bite Of the many species of true bugs, those in the family Reduviidae are relatively commonly associated with severe bite reactions. The most important reduviid bug in this country is the kissing bug (genus *Triatoma*), which is found throughout the southern crescent of the United States. The bites of this bug, which is a nocturnal feeder, are characteristically inflicted in multiple groups. Reactions which follow are thought to be allergic in nature and may include intensely pruritic and painful papules with a central punctum, grouped vesicles with moderate swelling and redness but no central lesions, giant urticaria, generalized allergic reactions, including systemic anaphylaxis, and hemorrhagic nodular-to-bullous lesions on a hand or foot, appearing several days after the bite. These may be confused with necrotizing spider bites or with erythema multiforme. However, the former are usually single lesions and the latter rarely has a unilateral distribution. The possibility of kissing bug bites should be considered in patients who awaken in the middle of the night with intense itching, hives, and other signs of a systemic allergic reaction.

Treatment of the local reaction is symptomatic. More severe reactions should be managed similarly to other allergic sting reactions. Patients who have had accelerated reactions to reduviid bites should be provided with sting kits and instructions in their use.

Chiggers or redbugs These are tiny mites which are commonly found in foliage or grass in many parts of the world. In the United States, the larval form of *Eutrobicula alfreddugesi* attacks the skin by secreting a substance which digests tissue, creating a red papule that itches intensely. The tiny reddish larva can be seen in the center of the lesion. Treatment is palliative and consists of antipruritic applications. The use of insect repellents, appropriate protective clothing, and prompt bathing after exposure reduce the risk of infestation considerably.

Bloodsucking-fly bite Many species of flies, particularly the horsefly and the deerfly, viciously attack and feed upon warm-blooded animals, including humans. Occasionally, transmission of diseases such as anthrax, tularemia, loiasis, and trypanosomiasis has been attributed to horseflies and deerflies. More commonly in North America, however, their bites are responsible for painful, intensely pruritic cutaneous lesions which may be followed by delayed localized allergic reactions characterized by erythema, edema, and urticaria. Treatment should include thorough cleaning of the bite sites, topical corticosteroids, and oral antihistaminics for severe itching. Antibiotics may be necessary if the wounds become secondarily infected.

MARINE ANIMAL VENOM DISEASES The venoms of certain marine animals are known to cause illness in humans after injection or inoculation under naturally occurring conditions. Information concerning these toxins is limited; most appear to be composed of proteins and peptides as well as other substances that are pharmacologically active. Although probably less complex than the venoms of reptiles, many marine animal venoms are capable of causing several pathologic effects including neurotoxicity as well as local necrosis.

Portuguese man-of-war and jellyfish stings The burning discomfort induced by contact with sea nettles or jellyfish is familiar to most surf bathers. Contact with the tentacles of the colorful Portuguese man-of-war (*Physalia* species), which is found mainly in or near the Gulf of Mexico, or the more toxic jellyfish (*Chiropsalmus* of the Indian Ocean and *Rhizostoma* of the Atlantic) is followed by burning pain, swelling, and erythema. Severe, generalized muscular cramps, nausea, vomiting, and pulmonary edema may occur. Victims have died as a result of jellyfish stings, sometimes within minutes after contact. In nonfatal cases, systemic symptoms usually subside within several hours. Treatment consists of bathing the wound in salt water, taking care not to rub the area of the sting. Next, any tentacles still clinging to the skin should be scraped off after first inactivating any remaining nematocysts to prevent discharge of additional venom into the victim. This can be done by sprinkling baking soda over the wound to form a slurry for sea nettle stings or by bathing with vinegar or isopropyl alcohol for man-of-war stings. Rinsing with fresh water or household ammonia, or rubbing with sand are not recommended since these measures may actually cause nematocysts to discharge. Analgesics should be used for pain control, and antihistaminics if there is an accompanying pruritic rash. Severe envenomations may require advanced life support measures. Corticosteroids may be helpful in these cases. An antivenin is now available for treatment of stings by the highly lethal Australian sea wasp, *Chironex fleckeri*.

Coral wounds and stings The colorful structures known as coral are composed of thousands of small marine animals of the coelenterate phylum, surrounded by a stony exoskeleton of calcium carbonate. Several species, including the fire coral, found in many parts of the world, contain microscopic nematocysts capable of producing painful stings similar to those caused by jellyfish. Often more serious are wounds resulting from abrasions and cuts by the sharp edges of the outer skeleton. These frequently contain small pieces of animal protein and skeletal material which act as foreign bodies, and may lead to chronic, suppurative wound infections if not promptly and adequately debrided.

Sea anemone sting ("sponge diver's disease") Contact with certain sea anemones (especially *Sargatia elegans*) in Mediterranean and African waters produces extensive dermatitis with chronic ulceration. Occasionally, especially during August and September, systemic symptoms of headache, sneezing, nausea, chills, fever, and collapse are noted. Rare fatalities have occurred. No specific therapy is known; symptomatic treatment with topical steroids or oral antihistaminics may provide temporary relief.

Cone shell poisoning The colorful cone shells are highly prized by collectors. However, many species in the Pacific are venomous, a great danger to unwary hobbyists who pick them up. The poison, a neurotoxin, is delivered into a wound inflicted by pointed hollow teeth resembling darts in the long proboscis of the animal. Local manifestations include sudden intense pain, followed by swelling and numbness which may persist for several days. Symptoms of serious poisoning include muscular incoordination and weakness progressing to respiratory paralysis. Death may occur within 3 to 6 h, but recovery within 24 h is the rule. There is no specific therapy; recommended treatment is the use of tourniquet, incision, and suction (as for snake bite), and supportive measures which may include artificial respiration and administration of oxygen.

Sponge dermatitis Direct contact with several species of sponge results in a painful dermatitis, which may persist for several weeks. The lesions appear to be caused by mechanical irritation from the exoskeleton of the sponge as well as by toxins within its tissues. Delayed hypersensitivity reactions may also occur. Antihistaminics provide relief from the pruritus; dilute acetic acid ameliorates local pain, while alkali will intensify it. The lesions are self-limited.

Sea urchin wounds and stings Contact with the spines of some species of sea urchin results in painful erythema and ulceration, occasionally accompanied by neurotoxic symptoms of weakness and frank paralysis of lips, tongue, and face lasting for several hours. Treatment is purely symptomatic and supportive. The toxins isolated from sea urchins have produced paralysis in animals and are notably resistant to heat. Deaths from paralysis and drowning have been reported. Occasionally, fragments of sea urchin spines may remain in the skin, leading to granulomatous reactions, or they may migrate into a joint or lodge against a nerve, causing intractable pain. Treatment of these complications is surgical.

Paralytic and neurotoxic shellfish poisoning Certain dinoflagellates, which make up part of the marine phytoplankton, elaborate a potent neurotoxin. Occasionally, conditions in coastal waters become favorable for the growth of excessive numbers of these organisms, causing the water to develop an amber appearance termed the "red tide" and killing massive numbers of fish by exhausting their oxygen supply. When humans ingest shellfish which have themselves ingested toxic dinoflagellates, an illness occurs that is characterized by paresthesias of the face and extremities, dysphonia, and generalized muscular weakness, often accompanied by nausea, vomiting, and diarrhea and occasionally by paralysis and respiratory arrest. The more severe syndrome, known as paralytic shellfish poisoning, is encountered along the Pacific northwest and New England coasts. A milder form, not associated with paralysis in humans, is seen along the Gulf and Atlantic coasts of Florida. Treatment should include induced emesis and purgation to remove unabsorbed toxin from the gastrointestinal tract and whatever additional supportive measures are necessary. Spontaneous recovery usually takes place within 24 h. There is a standardized mouse bioassay procedure for demonstrating and quantitating toxin in shellfish but no diagnostic test for detecting toxin in clinical specimens.

Venomous fish injuries The dorsal fins or spines of bullhead sharks, dogfish, and ratfish and the dorsal and other fins of the lionfish, weeverfish, toadfish, and catfish are grooved, and at their bases are found venom glands. Little is known of the venoms involved except that they contain highly unstable proteins of variable molecular weights and are capable of causing toxic as well as allergic reactions.

Envenomation results in immediate, severe local pain and edema which, if untreated, reaches greatest intensity in 60 to 90 min and resolves within 8 to 12 h. Local necrosis with extensive tissue loss may occur, particularly following lionfish and catfish stings. Systemic reactions, including cardiac arrhythmias, hypotension, muscular weakness, seizures, and paralysis, have been reported and attributed to the effects of the venom.

Treatment should be immediate immersion of the wound in water as hot as the patient can stand for at least 1 h or until symptoms subside. The venoms are extremely heat labile, accounting for the usefulness of this procedure. Although rarely needed, an antivenin is available for patients with severe systemic reactions from stonefish envenomation. It can be obtained from the Health Services Department, Sea World of San Diego [(619) 222–0411]. Tetanus prophylaxis should be given as needed. Narcotics may be required to control pain. Secondary pyogenic infection is a frequent complication.

Probably the most frequent type of fish envenomation in the United States is that produced by the lashing tail of the stingray of the California coast (*Urobatis halleri*). The bony spine is encased in a sheath of epithelial cells containing venom which is expressed into the puncture wound. The wound may be several centimeters deep; portions of the bony spine may break off in it, or, more often, the integumentary sheath remains in the wound. The venom is a circulatory depressant in animals, but local injury predominates in humans. Severe pain and blanching followed by erythema and edema occur immediately. Symptoms due to systemic absorption of venom are infrequent but may include salivation, muscle cramps and weakness, cardiac arrhythmias, seizures, and death. Treatment consists of application of a constriction band (the vast majority of these injuries occur on the legs) and copious syringing of the wound with salt water to remove fragments of sheath. Additional therapeutic measures are the same as for other fish envenomations, including immersion of the injured area in hot water for up to 1 h.

REFERENCES

Hymenoptera stings

GOLDEN DBK, VALENTINE M: Insect sting allergy. Ann Allergy 53:444, 1984

LIGHT WC et al: Unusual reactions following insect stings. J Allergy Clin Immunol 59:391, 1977

PATTERSON R, VALENTINE M: Anaphylaxis and related allergic emergencies including reactions due to insect stings. JAMA 248:2632, 1982

PAULL BR: Imported fire ant allergy: Perspectives on diagnosis and treatment. Postgrad Med 76:155, 1984

Marine animal venoms

AUERBACH PS, HALSTEAD BW: Hazardous marine life, in *Management of Wilderness and Environmental Emergencies,* PS Auerbach, HR Gee (eds). New York, Macmillan, 1983

BURNETT JW et al: First aid for jellyfish envenomation. South Med J 76:870, 1983

GUESS HA et al: Hemolysis following a Portuguese man-of-war sting. Pediatrics 70:979, 1982

HUGHES JM, MERSON MH: Fish and shellfish poisoning. N Engl J Med 295:1117, 1976

KIZER KW et al: Scorpaenidae envenomation: A 5-year poison center experience. JAMA 253:807, 1985

SCOGGIN CH: Catfish stings. JAMA 231:176, 1975

Other arthropod bites and stings

FRAZIER CA: *Insect Allergy: Allergic and Toxic Reactions to Insects and Other Arthropods.* St Louis, Grace, 1969

HILLIER FF, WARM RP: Caterpillar dermatitis. Br Med J 1:346, 1967

HUNT GR: Bites and stings of uncommon arthropods: 2. Reduviids, fire ants, puss caterpillars, and scorpions. Postgrad Med 70:107, 1981

LOGAN JL, OGDEN DA: Rhabdomyolysis and acute renal failure following the bite of the giant desert centipede *Scolopendra heros.* West J Med 142:549, 1985

SHELLEY ED et al: The diagnostic challenge of non-burrowing mite bites. JAMA 251:2690, 1984

WIRTZ RA: Allergic and toxic reactions to non-stinging arthropods. Ann Rev Entomol 29:47, 1984

Scorpion stings

LIKES K et al: *Centruroides exilicauda* envenomation in Arizona. West J Med 141:634, 1984

RIMSZA ME et al: Scorpion envenomation. Pediatrics 66:298, 1980

Snake and lizard bites

GARFIN SR et al: Rattlesnake bites and surgical decompression: Results using a laboratory model. Toxicon 22:177, 1984

KITCHENS CS, VANMIEROP LHS: Mechanisms of defibrination in humans after envenomation by the eastern diamondback rattlesnake. Am J Hematol 14:345, 1983

LOPRINZI CL et al: Snake antivenin administration in a patient allergic to horse serum. South Med J 76:501, 1983

MINTON SA JR: *Venom Diseases.* Springfield, Ill, Charles C Thomas, 1974

MITRAKUL C, DHAMKRONG A: Clinical features of neurotoxic snake bite and response to antivenom in 47 children. Am J Trop Med Hyg 33:1258, 1984

RUSSELL FE: *Snake Venom Poisoning.* New York, Scholium International, 1983

STAHNKE HL et al: Bite of the Gila monster. Rocky Mt Med J 67:25, 1970

Spider bites

HUNT GR: Bites and stings of uncommon arthropods: 1. Spiders. Postgrad Med 70:91, 1981

KING LE JR, REES RS: Dapsone treatment of a brown recluse bite. JAMA 250:648, 1983

KOBERNICK M: Black widow spider bite. Am Fam Physician 29:241, 1984

REES RS et al: Management of the brown recluse spider bite. Plast Reconstr Surg 68:768, 1981

Tick bite and tick paralysis

GOTHE R et al: The mechanism of pathogenicity in the tick paralysis. J Med Entomol 16:357, 1979

SPIELMAN A: How to diagnose and treat tick and mite infestations. Drug Therapy 11:77, 1981

171 POISONING AND ITS MANAGEMENT

PAUL A. FRIEDMAN

GENERAL PRINCIPLES

In the United States accidental poisoning by chemical agents causes about 5000 deaths each year while suicides by chemical agents annually number more than 6000. In addition to the victims of fatal poisoning there is a much greater number of persons who are made seriously ill by chemical agents but recover after appropriate therapy. Unfortunately, some such patients are left with permanent sequelae of their intoxication.

Accidental poisonings occur far more frequently in the home than through industrial exposure and are usually acute; industrial intoxication is more often the result of chronic exposure. Accidental poisoning results most commonly from ingestion of toxic substances and involves children in the majority of cases. Each year 1 to 2 million American children accidentally swallow toxic materials, and approximately 1 ingestion in 1000 is fatal. Medicines are involved in 50 percent of all ingestions. Cleaning and polishing agents are ingested by 15 percent, while cosmetics, pesticides, petroleum products, and turpentine paints account for 20 percent.

Despite all precautions, accidental, suicidal, and criminal poisonings will remain an important problem which every physician must be prepared to treat promptly and effectively. Besides their immediate therapeutic responsibilities, physicians have legal obligations in cases of attempted suicide, homicide, criminal abortion, and industrial exposure. The physician should also obtain psychiatric care for any patient who has attempted suicide by poison.

DIAGNOSIS OF CHEMICAL POISONING

Optimal management of the poisoned patient requires a correct diagnosis. Although the toxic effects of some chemical substances are quite characteristic, most poisoning syndromes can simulate other diseases.

Poisoning usually is included in the differential diagnosis of coma, convulsions, acute psychosis, acute hepatic or renal insufficiency, and bone marrow depression. Although it should be, poisoning may not be considered when the major manifestation is a mild psychiatric disturbance or neurologic disorder, abdominal pain, bleeding, fever, hypotension, pulmonary congestion, or skin eruption. Furthermore, the patient may be unaware of exposure to poison, as in chronic, insidious intoxications, or, as after attempted suicide or abortion, may be unwilling to admit it. Physicians always should remember the variegated manifestations of poisoning and maintain a high index of suspicion.

In every case of poisoning, identification of the toxic agent should be attempted. Specific antidotal therapy is obviously impossible without such identification. In cases of homicide, suicide, or criminal abortion the identity of the poison may be of legal importance. When poisoning results from industrial exposure or therapeutic mishap, accurate knowledge of the responsible agents is essential for future prevention.

In acute accidental poisoning the offending substance may be known to the patient. In many other cases information can be obtained from relatives or acquaintances, by a search for containers at the scene of the poisoning, or by questioning the patient's physician or pharmacist. Frequently such efforts yield only the trade name of a product, which gives no clue to its component chemicals. A number of books which identify the active ingredients of household products, agricultural compounds, proprietary medicines, and poisonous plants are listed in the references to this chapter. A small handbook of this type should be carried in every physician's bag. Poison control centers and manufacturers' representatives are other useful sources of such information. When poisoning is chronic, rapid identification of the toxic agent from the history is often impossible. The lesser therapeutic urgency of such cases usually permits the required painstaking exploration of the patient's habits and environment.

Some poisons can produce clinical features characteristic enough to strongly suggest the diagnosis. Careful examination of the patient may reveal the unmistakable odor of cyanide; the cherry-colored flush of carboxyhemoglobin in skin and mucous membranes; the pupillary constriction, salivation, and gastrointestinal hyperactivity produced by cholinesterase-inhibitor insecticides; or the lead line and extensor paralyses of chronic lead poisoning. Unfortunately, these features are not always present, and in any case telltales are the exception in chemical poisonings.

Chemical analysis of body fluids provides the most definite identification of the intoxicating agent. Some common poisons, such as aspirin and barbiturates, can be identified and even quantitated by relatively simple laboratory procedures. Others require more complex toxicologic techniques, such as gas or high-performance chromatography, which are carried out only in specialized laboratories. Furthermore, the results of toxicologic determinations are rarely available in time to guide the initial treatment of acute poisoning. Nevertheless, specimens of vomitus, gastric aspirate, blood, urine, and feces should be saved for toxicologic study if diagnostic or legal questions are likely to arise. Chemical analyses of body fluids or tissues are of particular value in the diagnosis and evaluation of chronic intoxications. Finally, they are useful in following the success of some forms of therapy.

TREATMENT OF CHEMICAL POISONING

Correct treatment of the poisoned patient requires knowledge of both the general principles of management and the details of therapy for specific poisons. Treatment involves four steps: (1) prevention of further absorption of the poison, (2) removal of absorbed poison from the body, (3) symptomatic supportive therapy or symptomatic treatment of circulatory, respiratory, neurologic, and renal function, and (4) administration of systemic antidotes (Table 171-1). The first three are applicable to most types of poisoning. The fourth is most often used only when the toxic agent is known and a specific antidote is available. However, naloxone is given sometimes if the index of suspicion is high that the patient has had an overdose of an opiate. It should be recognized both that most poisons do not have a specific antidote and that essential supportive care does not require knowledge of the toxic agent. Thus, although the physician should always try to identify the poison, such attempts must never delay vital therapeutic measures.

PREVENTION OF ABSORPTION OF INGESTED POISONS If appreciable amounts of a poison have been ingested, one should attempt to minimize its absorption from the gastrointestinal tract. The success of such endeavors depends upon the time elapsed since ingestion and upon the site and speed of absorption of the poison.

Evacuation of the stomach Attempts to empty the stomach are always worthwhile unless specifically contraindicated. They can be highly successful if made soon after ingestion. Significant amounts of poison still may be recovered from the stomach hours after ingestion because gastric emptying may be delayed by gastric atony or pylorospasm. Such is the case with phenothiazines, antihistamines, and tricyclic antidepressants.

Emesis occurs spontaneously after the ingestion of many poisons. In a minority of instances it may be induced in the home by mechanical stimulation of the posterior pharynx. The emetic action of syrup of ipecac (not the 14 times more concentrated fluid extract) in 15- to 30-mL dosage is more effective and is safe enough for home use. Its action has an average latent period of 20 min and depends in part on gastrointestinal absorption, so that concurrent administration of charcoal, to which it adsorbs, is to be avoided. A second dose of ipecac should be given if the patient fails to vomit after 20 min (90 to 95 percent of patients will vomit after two doses). If ipecac is not available at home, every effort should be made to locate some, even if this requires taking the patient to the hospital. Apomorphine, 0.06 mg/kg intramuscularly, acts within 5 min but may cause prolonged vomiting. When given intravenously in doses of 0.01 mg/kg, apomorphine tends to produce almost immediate vomiting which is not followed by any other central nervous system effects. On occasion it is impossible to induce vomiting, and valuable time should not be lost with hopeful waiting. Induction of vomiting should not be attempted in convulsing patients, in patients with severe central nervous system depression, or (because of the danger of gastroesophageal perforation or tracheal aspiration of vomitus) in patients who have ingested strong caustics or small amounts (<100 mL) of liquid hydrocarbons which are potent lung irritants (e.g., kerosene, furniture polish).

In comparison with emesis, *gastric lavage* is more predictably and immediately active but usually no more effective in removing poison from the stomach. It can be employed in unconscious patients, and removal of gastric contents reduces the risk of aspiration of vomitus in such patients. It is, however, contraindicated after the ingestion of strong corrosives because of danger of perforating injured tissues. When properly performed, gastric lavage carries little risk of aspiration of gastric contents into the lungs. The patient should be prone, with head and shoulders lowered. A mouth gag is placed, and a gastric tube of sufficient diameter to permit withdrawal of particulate matter (size 30) is passed into the stomach. If central nervous system function is depressed, if introduction of the tube produces retching, or if pulmonary irritants have been ingested, it is wise to place a *cuffed endotracheal tube* before performing lavage. Gastric contents are withdrawn with a large syringe and usually contain most of the poison that will be removed. Thereafter 200 mL (less in children) of warm water or dilute solution alternately is instilled and withdrawn until the aspirate becomes clear.

Interference with gastrointestinal absorption Since neither emesis nor gastric lavage empties the stomach completely, one should attempt to minimize absorption by administering substances which trap ingested poisons. Many poisons are adsorbed by powdered, activated charcoal. A good grade of activated charcoal can adsorb as much as half its weight of many common poisons. A slurry of activated charcoal (20 to 50 g in 100 to 200 mL) should be administered after evacuation of the stomach.

Adsorption by charcoal is reversible, and the effectiveness of adsorption of many poisons varies with the pH. Acidic substances are adsorbed better in acid solutions and therefore may be released in the small intestine. It is desirable to speed the charcoal with its adsorbed poison through the intestine as quickly as possible. This will also decrease intestinal absorption of any unadsorbed poison which has passed beyond the pylorus. In patients with good renal and cardiac function this is best accomplished by oral or gastric administration of an osmotic cathartic such as magnesium or sodium sulfate (10 to 30 g given in solution at a concentration of 10% or less).

PREVENTION OF ABSORPTION OF POISON FROM OTHER SITES Most topically applied poisons can be removed by copious flushing with water. In certain instances weak acids or bases or alcohol plus soap or detergent are more effective, but rapid and voluminous washing with water should always proceed while they are being obtained. Chemical antidotes can be hazardous because tissue injury may result from the heat of the chemical reaction.

The systemic distribution of injected poisons can be slowed by the application of cold to the injection site or by the proximal application of a tourniquet.

Following inhalation of toxic gases, vapors, or dusts, the victim should be moved to clean air and adequate ventilation should be maintained. If the patient cannot be moved, a protective mask should be applied.

REMOVAL OF ABSORBED POISON FROM THE BODY Unlike prevention or retardation of absorption, measures to speed removal of the toxic agent from the body rarely have much influence on the peak poison concentration. However, they can significantly abbreviate the time during which the concentration of many poisons remains above any given level and may thereby reduce morbidity, avoid

TABLE 171-1 Treatment of acute chemical poisoning

- *I* Prevention of further absorption of poison
  - *A* Poisoning by ingestion
    - *1* Emptying the stomach
      - *a* Induction of vomiting
      - *b* Gastric lavage
    - *2* Minimizing gastrointestinal absorption
      - *a* Adsorption
      - *b* Catharsis
  - *B* Poisoning by other routes
- *II* Removal of absorbed poisons from body
  - *A* Detoxification—enzyme induction?
  - *B* Biliary excretion—interruption of enterohepatic circulation
  - *C* Urinary excretion
    - *1* Forced diuresis
    - *2* Alteration of urinary pH
  - *D* Dialysis
    - *1* Peritoneal dialysis
    - *2* Hemodialysis
  - *E* Charcoal or resin hemoperfusion
  - *F* Exchange transfusion
  - *G* Chelation and chemical binding
- *III* Supportive therapy
- *IV* Administration of systemic antidotes
  - *A* Chemical agents
  - *B* Pharmacologic antagonists

complications, and save lives. In judging the need for such measures, one must consider the patient's clinical state, the properties and metabolic fate of the poison, and the amount absorbed as judged by the history and the blood level. Removal of some poisons can be accelerated by several methods; selection depends on the clinical urgency, the amount in the body, and the skills and equipment available.

Biliary excretion Certain organic acids and active drugs are secreted into the bile against large concentration gradients. This process takes time and cannot be accelerated. However, the intestinal resorption of substances already secreted into the bile, such as glutethimide, can be decreased by the administration of charcoal every 6 h. The organochlorine pesticide chlordecone is eliminated slowly from the body (blood half-life 165 days). Cholestyramine (16 g per day) significantly accelerates elimination (blood half-life 80 days).

Urinary excretion Acceleration of renal excretion is applicable to a much larger number of poisons. Renal excretion of toxic substances depends on glomerular filtration, active tubular secretion, and passive tubular resorption. The first two processes should be protected by maintenance of adequate circulation and renal function, but for practical purposes they cannot be accelerated. On the other hand, passive tubular resorption of many poisons plays an important role in the prolongation of their action and can frequently be decreased by readily available methods. The effectiveness of forced diuresis by administration of large volumes of electrolyte solutions together with intravenous furosemide in increasing renal excretion has been demonstrated for drugs such as salicylates and long-acting barbiturates.

Alteration of the urinary pH can also inhibit passive back-diffusion of some poisons and increase their renal clearance. The renal tubular epithelium is more permeable to uncharged molecules than to ionized solutes. Weak organic acids and bases readily diffuse out of the tubular fluid in their un-ionized form but are trapped in it when ionized. Acidic poisons are ionized only at pHs above their pK_a. Alkalinization of the urine greatly increases the ionization in the tubular fluid of such organic acids as phenobarbital and salicylate. In contrast, the pK_a of pentobarbital (8.1) and secobarbital (8.0) are so high that renal clearance is not increased greatly by raising the urinary pH into the physiologic alkaline range. Alkalinization of the urine is achieved by the infusion of sodium bicarbonate at a rate determined by the urinary and blood pH. Excessive systemic alkalosis or electrolyte disturbances must be prevented. A combination of forced diuresis and alkalinization of the urine can raise the renal clearance of some acidic poisons tenfold or more and has been found highly effective in poisoning by salicylate, phenobarbital, barbital, and 2,4-dichlorophenoxyacetic acid. Conversely, depression of the urinary pH below its usual range has been shown to augment the clearance of amphetamines, phencyclidines, fenfluramine, and quinine.

Finally, the renal excretion of certain poisons can be increased in a highly specific fashion. An example is the removal of bromide by administration of chloride and chloriuretics. Such methods are discussed with the individual poisons.

Dialysis and hemoperfusion Dialysis has been found effective in the removal of many compounds, including barbiturates, borate, chlorate, ethanol, glycols, methanol, salicylate, sulfonamides, theophylline, and thiocyanate. Theoretically, it should accelerate the removal from the body of any dialyzable toxin which is not bound irreversibly to tissues. Its effectiveness does not extend to large-molecule, nondialyzable poisons and is decreased by a high degree of protein binding or lipid solubility of the toxic substance.

Peritoneal dialysis can be performed easily in any hospital and may be continued for long periods. It is valuable for the removal of poisons only if renal function is impaired, hemodialysis or hemoperfusion is not possible, or forced diuresis cannot be carried out.

Hemodialysis is unquestionably a more effective procedure for removing large amounts of dialyzable poisons. For barbiturates dialysance rates of 50 to 100 mL/min have been achieved, a removal rate 2 to 10 times faster than during peritoneal dialysis or forced diuresis. Perfusion of blood through activated charcoal or exchange resin achieves even higher clearance rates than hemodialysis for most poisons. Extracorporeal dialysis and hemoperfusion are clearly the procedures of choice for the rapid removal of poisons from patients who have absorbed amounts which make survival unlikely even with the best supportive care. Since the required equipment and skilled personnel are not available in every hospital, the possibility of transfer of such patients to an institution with these capabilities should be considered.

Chelation and chemical binding The removal of some poisons is accelerated by chemical interaction with other substances followed by renal excretion. These substances are considered systemic antidotes and are discussed with the individual poisons.

SUPPORTIVE THERAPY Most chemical poisonings are reversible, self-limited disease states. Skillful supportive therapy can keep many seriously poisoned patients alive and their detoxifying and excretory mechanisms functioning until the concentration of poison in the body has fallen to safe levels. Symptomatic measures are especially important when the poison is one of the many compounds for which no specific antidote is known. Even when an antidote is available, disturbances of vital functions must be prevented or controlled by appropriate supportive care.

The poisoned patient may suffer a variety of physiologic disturbances. Most of these are not peculiar to chemical intoxications, and their therapeutic management is described elsewhere in this text. Only those aspects of supportive therapy specially relevant to poisonings are discussed briefly here.

Central nervous system depression Specific therapy directed against the depressant effects of poisons on the central nervous system is usually both unnecessary and difficult. Most poisoned patients will emerge from coma as from a prolonged anesthesia. During the period of unconsciousness, meticulous nursing care and close observation are essential. If depression of medullary centers results in circulatory or respiratory failure, these vital functions must be immediately and vigorously supported by chemical or mechanical means. The use of analeptics in the treatment of poison-induced central nervous system depression has been largely abandoned. Certainly these agents should never be employed to restore consciousness, and it is doubtful whether their use to hasten the restoration of spontaneous breathing and active reflexes is ever justified. By contrast, the narcotic antagonist naloxone administered intravenously in adequate doses generally will reverse central nervous system depression secondary to narcotic overdosage.

Convulsions Many poisons (e.g., chlorinated hydrocarbons, insecticides, strychnine) cause convulsions by their specific excitatory effects. Poisoned patients also may have convulsions because of hypoxia, hypoglycemia, cerebral edema, or metabolic disturbances. In such cases these abnormalities should be corrected as far as possible. Regardless of the cause of the convulsions, anticonvulsant drugs often are required. Intravenously administered diazepam, phenobarbital, or phenytoin is usually effective.

Cerebral edema Intracranial hypertension due to cerebral edema is also a characteristic effect of some poisons and a nonspecific result of other chemical intoxications. For example, cerebral edema is seen in poisoning by lead, carbon monoxide, and methanol. Symptomatic treatment consists of use of adrenocortical steroids and, when necessary, the intravenous administration of hypertonic solutions of mannitol or urea.

Hypotension The causes of hypotension and shock in the poisoned patient are legion, and often several of them coexist. Poisons can depress the medullary vasomotor centers, block autonomic ganglia or adrenergic receptors, directly depress the tone of arterial or venous smooth muscle, reduce myocardial contractility, or induce cardiac arrhythmias. Less specifically, the poisoned patient may be in shock because of tissue hypoxia, extensive tissue destruction from corrosives, loss of blood or fluids, or metabolic disturbances. When possible, these abnormalities should be corrected. If the central venous pressure is low, fluid replacement should be the first therapeutic approach. Vasoactive drugs are often helpful and sometimes essential in the hypotensive poisoned patient, particularly in shock resulting from central depression. As in shock from other causes, choice of the most appropriate agent requires an analysis of the hemodynamic disturbance which goes beyond determination of the arterial pressure.

Cardiac arrhythmias Disturbances of cardiac impulse generation or conduction in the poisoned patient arise from the effects of certain poisons on the electrical properties of cardiac fibers or from myocardial hypoxia or metabolic disturbances. The latter should be corrected, and antiarrhythmic agents administered as indicated by the nature of the arrhythmia (see Chap. 184).

Pulmonary edema The poisoned patient may develop pulmonary edema because of depressed myocardial contractility or because of alveolar injury from irritant gases or aspirated fluids. The latter type of edema is less responsive to treatment and may be associated with laryngeal edema. Therapeutic measures include suctioning, administration of high concentrations of oxygen under positive pressure, aerosols of surface-active agents, bronchodilators, and adrenocortical steroids (see Chap. 26).

Hypoxia Poisoning may cause tissue hypoxia by various mechanisms, and several of these may operate in one patient. Inadequate ventilation can result from central respiratory depression, from muscular paralysis, or from airway obstruction by retained secretions, laryngeal edema, or bronchospasm. Alveolar-capillary diffusion may be impaired by pulmonary edema. Anemia, methemoglobinemia, carboxyhemoglobinemia, or shock can interfere with oxygen transport. Cellular oxidation may be inhibited (e.g., cyanide, fluoroacetate). Maintenance of an adequate airway is essential to treatment. The clinical situation and the site of obstruction may indicate frequent suctioning, insertion of an oropharyngeal airway or of an endotracheal tube, or a tracheotomy. If, despite a clear airway, ventilation remains inadequate, as judged by clinical appearance or by measurement of minute volume or blood gases, artificial ventilation by appropriate mechanical means is imperative. Administration of high concentrations of oxygen is indicated whenever tissue hypoxia occurs. When the central nervous system is severely depressed, oxygen administration often results in apnea and must be combined with artificial ventilation.

Acute renal insufficiency Renal failure with oliguria or anuria may occur in the poisoned patient because of shock, dehydration, or electrolyte disturbances. More specifically, it may be due to the nephrotoxic potential of some poisons (e.g., mercury, phosphorus, carbon tetrachloride, bromate), many of which are concentrated and excreted by the kidney. Renal damage due to poisons is usually reversible. The management of acute renal insufficiency is outlined in Chap. 219.

Electrolyte and water disturbances Imbalances of fluid and electrolytes are common features of chemical poisoning. They may result from vomiting, diarrhea, renal insufficiency, or therapeutic maneuvers such as catharsis, forced diuresis, or dialysis. These disturbances are corrected or, ideally, prevented by appropriate therapy. Certain poisons produce more specific defects, such as metabolic acidosis (e.g., methanol, phenol, salicylate) or hypocalcemia (e.g., fluoride, oxalate). These abnormalities and any specific treatment are described under the individual poisons.

Acute hepatic insufficiency The primary manifestation of some poisonings (e.g., chlorinated hydrocarbons, phosphorus, cinchophen, certain mushrooms) is acute hepatic failure. Its management is described in Chap. 247.

ADMINISTRATION OF SYSTEMIC ANTIDOTES Specific antidotal therapy is available for only a few poisons. Some systemic antidotes are chemicals which exert their therapeutic effect by reducing the concentration of the toxic substance. They may do this by combining with the poison (e.g., ethylene diaminetetraacetate with lead, dimercaprol with mercury, sulfhydryl-containing reagents with a toxic metabolite of acetaminophen) or by increasing its excretion (e.g., chloride or mercurial diuretics in bromide poisoning). Other systemic antidotes compete with the poison for its receptor site (e.g., atropine with muscarine, naloxone with morphine; physostigmine reverses some of the anticholinergic effects of the tricyclic antidepressants, as well as those of the antihistamines, belladonna, and other atropinic substances). Specific antidotes are discussed with the individual poisons.

COMMON POISONS

The poisons discussed in this section are some of those encountered by the general population such as commonly used nonprescription drugs, household products, solvents, pesticides, and poisonous plants. It has been necessary to disregard many uncommon toxic materials and products to which exposure occurs only in specialized industrial environments. Details concerning poisoning by such compounds may be found in some of the references to this chapter. In addition, toxic effects of many drugs are considered throughout this text in conjunction with their therapeutic and illicit uses as well as with overdose (see especially Chaps. 364 to 367). Manifestations of hypersensitivity to chemicals are described in Chap. 65. The following discussions of specific poisons stress those details of their action which are pertinent to the recognition or treatment of clinical poisoning.

ACETAMINOPHEN Termed *paracetamol* in the United Kingdom, acetaminophen, a popular alternative to salicylates as an analgesic and antipyretic, is a frequent cause of poisoning. While the toxic and lethal doses of acetaminophen may vary from patient to patient, hepatic damage may be expected if an adult has taken more than 8 g as a single dose. A plasma concentration of greater than 200 μg/mL at 4 h after ingestion is also cause for concern. Clinical manifestations of acetaminophen poisoning are nonspecific. In the first few hours after ingestion lethargy, pallor, nausea, vomiting, and diaphoresis may occur; there are no acid-base derangements like those which may accompany aspirin overdose. Hepatic damage, the most important manifestation of acetaminophen toxicity, becomes evident 1 to 2 days after ingestion. While some patients show only elevation of serum transaminase and others show tender hepatomegaly and jaundice, more severe damage can lead to hyperammonemia, asterixis, mental confusion, coma, bleeding, and death from acute liver failure. Acute tubular necrosis, pancreatitis, hypoglycemia, cardiac damage, and hypersensitivity reactions sometimes are seen. Damage to tissue (especially liver) is caused by metabolites of acetaminophen and not the drug itself. At therapeutic doses acetaminophen is eliminated mainly conjugated to sulfate or glucuronic acid. After an overdose, the pathways of conjugation to the sulfate and glucuronic acid become saturated, an increasing fraction of the drug is activated by the P_{450} system, glutathione stores are depleted, and the reactive intermediates then become free to bind covalently to liver macromolecules and cause necrosis.

Treatment should begin with induction of emesis or gastric lavage followed by administration of activated charcoal. Since endogenous glutathione appears to have a protective effect, the administration of one of several other sulfhydryl compounds has been studied for protection against acetaminophen hepatotoxicity. When administered orally within 10 h of ingestion, either *N*-acetylcysteine or cysteamine is effective in decreasing hepatotoxicity. A potentially toxic dose (>7.5 g) ingested within the previous 24 h is an indication for *N*-acetylcysteine therapy. Since early treatment is paramount, a patient suspected of having ingested a potentially hepatotoxic dose should be started on sulfhydryl therapy while awaiting the plasma acetaminophen level. A 5% solution of *N*-acetylcysteine in a cola beverage or fruit juice is given with a loading dose of 140 mg/kg and a maintenance dose of 70 mg/kg every 4 h for 3 days. If sulfhydryl therapy is to be instituted, charcoal and osmotic cathartic administration are contraindicated since both may reduce absorption of the antidote. In a mixed poisoning, charcoal may be removed by lavage prior to administration of the antidote.

ACIDS Corrosive acids are used widely in industry and laboratories. Ingestion is almost always with suicidal intent. Toxic effects are due to their direct chemical action. Ingestion of acids may produce irritation, bleeding, and sloughing in the mouth and esophagus with more severe burns occurring in the stomach, particularly in the pylorus. Perforations with peritonitis, though uncommon, may occur. Mouth and pharynx may be brownish black and may have a charred appearance. Yellow staining is seen after ingestion of nitric and picric acids. Severe pain in mouth, pharynx, chest, and abdomen is the rule and soon is followed by hematemesis and bloody diarrhea. Frequently profound shock develops and may be fatal. Survivors can develop mediastinitis or peritonitis from early or delayed esophageal or gastric perforation. Recovery from acid ingestion can be associated with stricture formation which most commonly involves the pylorus.

Ingested acid should be diluted immediately with large amounts of water or milk (when possible, in a hundredfold excess). The danger of perforation contraindicates the use of emesis or gastric lavage. Diagnostic esophagoscopy, if performed, should be done in the first 24 h after ingestion. Following the emergency measures, appropriate supportive therapy is administered for the relief of pain and the treatment of shock, perforation, and infection.

ALKALIES Strong alkalies such as ammonium hydroxide, potassium hydroxide (potash), potassium carbonate, sodium hydroxide (lye, Clinitest tablets), and sodium carbonate (washing soda) are used widely in industry and in cleansers and drain cleaners. Sodium and potassium phosphates find use as water softeners. Strong alkalies form soaps with fats and proteinates with proteins, resulting in penetrating necrosis of tissues. Fatalities have occurred from the ingestion of 5 to 30 g of such compounds.

The toxic effects of alkalies are due to irritation and destruction of local tissues. Ingestion is followed by severe pain in mouth, pharynx, chest, and abdomen. Vomiting of blood and sloughed mucosa and diarrhea are common. Reflex loss of vascular tone frequently leads to profound shock. Perforation of the esophagus or stomach may be immediate or delayed for several days. Mouth and pharynx show erythema and gelatinous necrotic areas. After ingestion of water softeners profound reduction in serum calcium may be seen and lead to tetany and hypotension. Survivors usually suffer from esophageal strictures.

Treatment consists of immediate administration of large amounts of water or milk. Because of the danger of perforation, both induction of emesis and gastric lavage are contraindicated. Esophagoscopy should be done within the first 24 h in patients with significant esophageal or gastric burns. Steroids usually are administered for about 3 weeks to decrease the incidence of stricture formation, although definitive evidence of efficacy is lacking. After the ingestion of water softeners (phosphates), calcium gluconate should be administered intravenously as needed. Treatment is otherwise symptomatic and directed at the relief of pain, respiratory obstruction due to edema of the hypopharynx, fluid loss, and shock.

Inhalation of ammonia, which is used as a refrigerant, results in irritation of the upper and lower parts of the respiratory tract. Laryngeal and pulmonary edema may occur and must be treated symptomatically.

ANILINE This substance is used in printing and clothmarking inks, paints, and paint removers. Both aniline and its derivatives, such as toluidine, nitroaniline, and nitrobenzene, are widely used in industrial synthesis. Aniline is absorbed from the gastrointestinal tract and through the lungs or skin. Ingestion of 1 g has been fatal. Methemoglobinemia is the most important manifestation. Headache, dizziness, hypotension, convulsions, and coma may occur. If the acute period is survived, jaundice and anemia may appear. Treatment consists of correction of methemoglobinemia (see Chap. 288) and supportive measures.

Antihistamines The common and unprescribed use of antihistamines makes them readily available for accidental overdosage and suicide attempts. There is wide variation among patients in tolerance to these drugs and in the manifestations of poisoning. Manifestations of poisoning are central nervous system excitement or depression. In adults drowsiness, stupor, and coma predominate, but convulsions followed by further depression may occur.

Treatment is supportive and directed toward removal of the unabsorbed drug and maintenance of vital functions. Convulsions may be controlled with phenobarbital or diazepam. Some antihistamines have prominent atropine-like properties. Patients poisoned with these drugs may show manifestations of atropine poisoning and are treated accordingly (see below).

ANTIMUSCARINIC COMPOUNDS Atropine, related belladonna alkaloids (hyoscyamine and scopolamine), and synthetic substitutes (e.g., benztropine, cyclopentolate, homatropine, methantheline, propantheline) are widely prescribed drugs and occur in many proprietary mixtures.

Individual sensitivity to the toxic effects of belladonna alkaloids varies widely; fatalities have occurred from as little as 10 mg atropine, but doses of 500 mg have been nonfatal. Young children are particularly susceptible to poisoning with belladonna alkaloids. Older persons appear to be more sensitive to the central nervous system effects of these drugs. Since atropine is both hydrolyzed in the liver and excreted unchanged in the urine, hepatic or renal insufficiency may lead to poisoning with otherwise therapeutic doses.

The most characteristic manifestations of atropine poisoning are those of parasympathetic blockade: dryness of mucous membranes, thirst, dysphagia, hoarseness, xerophthalmia, dilated pupils, blurring of vision, rise in intraocular tension, flushing, dryness and increased temperature of the skin, fever, tachycardia, hypertension, urinary retention, and abdominal distention. This widespread parasympatholysis is almost diagnostic of belladonna poisoning, but the diagnosis can be strengthened further by the reversal of blockade by physostigmine (2 mg administered intravenously over several minutes).

Central nervous system symptoms are also very common; atropine and scopolamine produce similar toxic psychoses. Restlessness, excitation, confusion, and incoordination precede mania, hallucinations, and delirium. Patients intoxicated by scopolamine not infrequently show lethargy and somnolence rather than excitement. In severe intoxication, central nervous system depression and coma are the rule. When death results, it is because of circulatory collapse and respiratory failure.

In the *treatment* of belladonna poisoning, emesis or gastric lavage should be followed by the administration of activated charcoal. Symptomatic treatment is directed at the reduction of body temperature, the moistening of mucous membranes, and urethral catheterization in the presence of urinary retention. Excitement or convulsions may require appropriate pharmacotherapy. Patients with deep coma, life-threatening cardiac arrhythmias, severe hallucinations, or severe hypertension have been treated with physostigmine with some reversal of these effects. It has not been established whether physostigmine reduces mortality.

Death occurs in fewer than 1 percent of cases of atropine or scopolamine poisoning. No permanent sequelae have been observed, but manifestations may persist for several days.

BENZENE, TOLUENE These solvents are used in paint removers, dry-cleaning solutions, and rubber or plastic cements. Benzene is also present, to some extent, in most gasolines. Poisoning may result from ingestion or from the breathing of concentrated vapors. Toluene is an ingredient in some cement used by glue sniffers.

Acute poisoning by these compounds causes central nervous system manifestations. With sufficient exposure, symptoms progress from an initial period of restlessness, excitement, euphoria, and dizziness to coma, convulsions, and respiratory failure. Ventricular arrhythmias may occur. Renal tubular acidosis can occur following repeated inhalation of toluene. Chronic poisoning by benzene or toluene results from repeated exposure to their vapors in low concentration. Central nervous system symptoms include irritability, insomnia, headache, tremors, and paresthesias. Anorexia and nausea are also common. Fatty degeneration of the heart, liver, and kidneys may occur. By far the most important manifestation of chronic exposure to benzene is bone marrow depression, which may progress to aplastic anemia and complete aplasia of the bone marrow. Individual susceptibility to this effect varies greatly and may not become apparent for months after the initial exposure to the poison.

Treatment of both acute and chronic poisoning is symptomatic. Neurologic, pulmonary, or cardiovascular problems are treated as in poisoning by petroleum distillates.

BLEACHES Industrial strength bleaching solutions contain 10% or more sodium hypochlorite, while household products (e.g., Clorox, Purex, Sanichlor) contain 3 to 6%. The solution used for chlorinating swimming pools is 20%. Their corrosive action in mouth, pharynx, and esophagus is similar to that of sodium hydroxide. Acid gastric juice releases hypochlorous acid from such solutions. This compound is very irritating to mucous membranes, and inhalation of its fumes causes severe pulmonary irritation and pulmonary edema. However, the systemic toxicity of hypochlorous acid is low. Perforation and stricture formation are rare after the ingestion of household bleaching solutions.

Treatment consists of dilution of the ingested bleach with water or milk. The usual household bleaching solutions do not cause enough corrosive injury to the esophagus to preclude the induction of emesis or gastric lavage, but one should be wary of this possibility if one of the more concentrated solutions has been ingested. Although sodium thiosulfate (100 mL of a 1 to 2.5% solution by lavage), which will reduce hypochlorite to nontoxic products, has been administered routinely to these patients, there is great doubt that it is of any use except very early after ingestion of very large quantities of bleach.

CARBON MONOXIDE (CO) Carbon monoxide is a colorless, odorless, tasteless, and nonirritating gas produced by the incomplete combustion of carbonaceous materials. Almost any flame or combustion device emits carbon monoxide. The gas is present in the exhaust of internal combustion engines in a concentration of 3 to 7 percent. Much higher concentrations are generated during the burning of most illuminating and heating gases, but normally not in the burning of natural gas. However, if gas appliances are defective, incomplete combustion of natural gas and the generation of toxic amounts of carbon monoxide can occur. CO annually is responsible for about 3500 accidental and suicidal deaths in the United States.

The toxic effects of CO are the result of tissue hypoxia. CO combines with hemoglobin to form carboxyhemoglobin. Since CO and O_2 react with the same group in the hemoglobin molecule, and since the affinity of hemoglobin for CO is 200 times greater than for O_2, carboxyhemoglobin is incapable of carrying O_2. (At equilibrium 1 part of CO in 1500 parts of air will result in 50 percent conversion of hemoglobin to carboxyhemoglobin.) Carboxyhemoglobin also interferes with the release of O_2 from oxyhemoglobin. This further reduces the amount of O_2 available to the tissues and explains why tissue anoxia appears in the CO-poisoned person at levels of arterial oxyhemoglobin concentration well tolerated by the anemic patient.

The extent of saturation of hemoglobin with CO depends on the concentration of the gas in inspired air and on the time of exposure. The severity of hypoxic symptoms depends further on an individual's state of activity, tissue O_2 needs, and hemoglobin concentration. As a general rule, no symptoms will develop at a concentration of 0.01% CO in inspired air, since this will not raise blood saturation above 10%. Exposure to 0.05% for 1 h during light activity will produce a blood concentration of 20% carboxyhemoglobin and result in a mild or throbbing headache. Greater activity or longer exposure to the same concentration causes a blood saturation of 30 to 50%. At this point headache, irritability, confusion, dizziness, visual disturbances, nausea, vomiting, and fainting on exertion may be observed. After exposure for 1 h to concentrations of 0.1% in inspired air, the blood will contain 50 to 80% carboxyhemoglobin, which results in coma, convulsions, respiratory failure, and death. On inhalation of high concentrations of CO, saturation of the blood proceeds so rapidly that unconsciousness may occur suddenly and without warning. When poisoning is more gradual, the individual may notice decreased exercise tolerance and dyspnea on exertion or even at rest. Patients with such subacute or chronic exposure can present with vague "flu-like" symptoms. Excessive sweating, fever, hepatomegaly, skin lesions, leukocytosis, bleeding diathesis, albuminuria, and glycosuria also have been described. Cerebral edema and intracranial hypertension may result from the increased permeability of hypoxic capillaries. Myocardial hypoxia is reflected by electrocardiographic abnormalities.

The most characteristic sign of severe CO poisoning is the cherry color of skin and mucous membranes, which results from the bright red carboxyhemoglobin. If the characteristic flush is not present and CO poisoning is suspected, 1 mL of the patient's blood can be diluted with 10 mL water; when 1 mL of 5% sodium hydroxide is added to this dilution, an oxyhemoglobin solution will turn brown. If significant amounts of carboxyhemoglobin are present, the solution will turn straw yellow (<20% carboxyhemoglobin) or will remain pink (>20% carboxyhemoglobin).

Treatment of CO poisoning requires effective ventilation in the presence of high O_2 tensions and in the absence of CO. If necessary, ventilation should be supported artificially. Pure O_2 should be administered. This will result not only in the replacement of CO by O_2 in the hemoglobin molecule but also in the partial relief of tissue hypoxia by O_2 dissolved in the plasma. For the same reasons hyperbaric O_2 is helpful in seriously poisoned patients. Transfusion of blood or packed cells is also of value. In order to reduce tissue needs for O_2, the patient must be kept absolutely quiet. Induction of hypothermia is not indicated. Cerebral edema should be treated with diuretics and steroids.

If severe tissue hypoxia has obtained too long, neurologic symptoms such as tremors, mental deterioration, and psychotic behavior may persist. Histologic changes characteristic of hypoxia may be observed in cerebral cortex, medulla, myocardium, and other organs.

CHLORINATED INSECTICIDES These compounds are ingredients of dusts, sprays, and solutions used as insecticides. The great majority of these compounds are chlorinated diphenyls (e.g., DDT, TDE, DFDT, DMC, Neotran) or chlorinated polycyclic compounds (e.g., aldrin, chlordane, dieldrin, endrin, hepatochlor). Lindane is a hexachlorobenzene. Their toxicity has led to their greatly diminished use in recent years, and many are banned in certain locales, including the United States. The chlorinated insecticides are soluble in lipid and organic solvents but not in water. They are poorly absorbed unless dissolved in a vehicle such as kerosene, petroleum distillates, or other organic solvents and can readily enter the body through the skin, lungs, or gastrointestinal tract. These compounds vary considerably in toxicity, and the toxicity of the dissolving vehicle must also be considered. The effects of the solvent may overshadow or modify those of the insecticide.

The initial symptoms of acute poisoning are nausea, vomiting, headache, dizziness, apprehension, excitement, and muscular tremors and weakness. These symptoms progress to generalized central nervous system hyperexcitability and delirium and clonic or tonic convulsions. This stage is in turn followed by progressive depression with paralysis, coma, and death. Except for endrin, which is strongly hepatotoxic, liver toxicity occurs only at extreme dosage levels. *Treatment* consists of induction of emesis or gastric lavage, activated charcoal administration, catharsis, anticonvulsive therapy, artificial ventilation, and other supportive measures. Sympathomimetic compounds should be avoided, since chlorinated insecticides apparently increase susceptibility to ventricular fibrillation. Cholestyramine accelerates the excretion of the chlorinated hydrocarbon chlordecone by preventing reabsorption following biliary excretion, and it may well have a similar effect on the excretion of pesticides such as DTT, dieldrin, chlordane, and heptachlor which remain in the body for prolonged periods.

CHOLINESTERASE INHIBITOR INSECTICIDES Many substances used in agriculture for control of soft-bodied insects are potent inhibitors of cholinesterase. Most of these compounds are organic phosphates (e.g., Parathion, Malathion, Guthion), others are carbamates (e.g., Carbaryl, Mactacil). The toxicity of these compounds varies widely. Usually they are prepared for use by dilution with powders, organic solvents, or water. Formulations containing 1 to 95 percent of the active ingredient are available. The cholinesterase inhibitor insecticides are absorbed rapidly through the intact skin and after inhalation or ingestion.

The toxicity of these agents results from inactivation of acetylcholinesterase which allows accumulation of excessive amounts of acetylcholine at a number of sites: central nervous system, autonomic ganglia, parasympathetic nerve endings, and motor nerve endings. In the central nervous system coma and respiratory depression and, less commonly, seizures can occur. Toxic muscarinic effects include nausea, vomiting, diarrhea, involuntary defecation and urination, blurring of vision due to miosis, sweating, lacrimation, and salivation. Nicotinic effects include muscle twitching, fasciculations, weakness, and flaccid paralysis. Cardiac arrhythmias and pulmonary edema, as well as EEG abnormalities, also occur.

Treatment consists of emesis or lavage, charcoal instillation, catharsis, and washing of contaminated skin with soap and water. Atropine should be given immediately to block the parasympathetic and central nervous system effects. A dose of 2 mg is injected intramuscularly and repeated every 10 min until parasympathetic manifestations are controlled and signs of atropinization appear. The same dosage must be repeated frequently to maintain xerostomia and mild tachycardia. Fatal respiratory failure or pulmonary edema may occur quickly upon cessation of atropine therapy, and the drug should be withdrawn judiciously. Atropine is virtually ineffective against the autonomic ganglionic actions of acetylcholine and against the peripheral neuromuscular paralysis. Relief of muscle weakness, in particular respiratory paralysis, can be achieved with certain oximes which can reactivate cholinesterase by reversing the phosphate ester bond formed by the organic phosphate at the enzyme active site. Pralidoxime is useful in the treatment of organic phosphate cholinesterase inhibition but should not be used if the inhibition is due to a carbamate. A dose of 1 g pralidoxime in aqueous solution is administered intravenously over a 5-min period, and this dose is repeated up to four times every 8 to 12 h. Supportive therapy includes administration of oxygen with artifical ventilation if necessary, removal of pulmonary secretions by suction, and treatment of convulsions with diazepam and phenobarbital. Energetic therapy with artificial ventilation, atropine, and pralidoxime allows survival after doses of organic phosphate esters vastly exceeding the usual fatal dose.

CYANIDE The cyanide ion is an exceedingly potent and rapid-acting poison, but one for which specific and effective antidotal therapy is available. Cyanide poisoning may result from the inhalation of hydrocyanic acid or from the ingestion of soluble inorganic cyanide salts or cyanide-releasing substances such as cyanamide, cyanogen chloride, and nitroprusside. Parts of many plants also contain substances such as amygdalin which release cyanide on digestion. Among these are the seeds of certain stone fruits (chokecherry, pin cherry, wild black cherry, peach, apricot, bitter almond), cassava roots, the berries of the jet berry bush, the leaves and shoots of elderberry, and all parts of hydrangea. The controversial drug Laetrile, composed in part of an extract of apricot kernels, has been responsible for fatal cyanide poisoning. Cyanides are widely used in industry and for fumigation and may reach the home in photographic chemicals or silver polishes. As little as 300 mg potassium cyanide may cause death.

The extreme toxicity of cyanide is due to its ready reaction with the trivalent iron of cytochrome oxidase. Formation of the cytochrome oxidase—cyanide complex blocks electron transport, thus inhibiting oxygen utilization. This results in cellular dysfunction and death. Inhalation of hydrogen cyanide may cause death within a minute. Oral doses act more slowly, requiring several minutes for the appearance of symptoms and up to several hours for death. The first effect is an increase in ventilation because of the blockade of oxidative metabolism in the chemoreceptor cells. As more cyanide is absorbed, there are headache, dizziness, nausea, drowsiness, hypotension, profound dyspnea, characteristic electrocardiographic changes, coma, and convulsions.

Cyanide poisoning is a true medical emergency. However, *treatment* is highly effective if given rapidly. The chemical antidotes should be immediately available wherever emergency medical care is dispensed. The diagnosis may be made by the characteristic "bitter almond" odor on the breath of the victim, and physicians should familiarize themselves with this smell. Since the saturation of hemoglobin is not disturbed by cyanide, cyanosis is not seen until respiratory depression supervenes. The objective of treatment is the production of methemoglobin by the administration of nitrite. The trivalent iron of methemoglobin competes with cytochrome oxidase for the cyanide ion. The cytochrome oxidase—cyanide complex dissociates, and enzymatic function and cell respiration are restored. Further detoxification then is achieved by the administration of thiosulfate. The enzyme rhodanese catalyzes the reaction of thiosulfate with cyanide liberated by the dissociation of cyanmethemoglobin; thiocyanate, which is relatively nontoxic, is formed and readily excreted in the urine.

Since speed is of the essence, nitrite should be immediately administered by inhalation of amyl nitrite perles, one every 2 min unless blood pressure is below 80 mmHg. This is followed as soon as possible by the intravenous injection of 10 mL of 3% sodium nitrite over a 3-min period. An intravenous infusion of norepinephrine may be necessary to maintain blood pressure during this injection period. After the administration of sodium nitrite, 50 mL of 25% sodium thiosulfate should be administered intravenously over a 10-min period. Supportive measures, especially artificial respiration with 100% O_2, should be instituted as soon as possible, but unless methemoglobinemia is produced promptly, other forms of treatment are of no value. Administration of sodium nitrite and sodium thiosulfate may have to be repeated. Ideally, dosage should be based on methemoglobin determinations, and the methemoglobin should not exceed 40%. If the patient survives 4 h, recovery is likely but residual cerebral symptoms may persist.

DETERGENTS AND SOAPS These substances fall into the three groups of anionic, nonionic, and cationic detergents. The first group contains common soaps and household detergents. They may cause vomiting and diarrhea but have no serious effects, and no treatment is required. However, some laundry compounds contain phosphate water softeners whose ingestion may cause hypocalcemia. The ingestion of nonionic detergents also requires no treatment.

Cationic detergents, such as benzalkonium chloride and many others, are commonly used for bactericidal purposes in hospitals and homes. These compounds are well absorbed from the gastrointestinal tract and interfere with cellular functions. The fatal oral dose is approximately 3 g. Concentrated preparations (>20% detergent) are corrosive to mouth and esophagus. Ingestion produces nausea and vomiting, and shock, coma, convulsions, and death may occur in a few hours. Treatment after ingestion of dilute preparations consists of minimizing gastrointestinal absorption by emesis and gastric lavage with ordinary soap solution, which rapidly inactivates cationic detergents. Emesis and lavage are contraindicated in the presence of esophageal injury which is unlikely to occur except after ingestion of concentrated preparations. Activated charcoal and an osmotic cathartic should be administered. If significant absorption has occurred, intensive supportive therapy may be required.

FLUORIDES Fluoride salts are used in insecticides. The gases fluorine and hydrogen fluoride are used in industry; the latter is a strong corrosive. Fluorine and fluorides are cellular poisons which inhibit a number of enzymatic reactions, probably the most important of which is the glycolytic degradation of glucose. Fluorides also form an insoluble precipitate with calcium and cause hypocalcemia. Finally, in an acid medium fluorides form the corrosive hydrofluoric acid. Ingestion of 1 to 2 g sodium fluoride may be fatal.

Inhalation of fluorine or hydrogen fluoride produces coughing and choking. After an asymptomatic period of a day or two, fever, cough, cyanosis, and pulmonary edema may develop. Ingestion of fluoride salts is followed by nausea, vomiting productive of corroded tissues, diarrhea, and abdominal pain. Consequent to the decrease in serum calcium the victim develops muscular hyperirritability, fasciculations, tremors, spasms, and convulsions. Death results from respiratory paralysis or circulatory collapse. If the patient survives the acute period, jaundice and oliguria may appear. Chronic fluoride poisoning (fluorosis) is characterized by weight loss, weakness, anemia, brittle bones, and stiff joints. Mottling of teeth is seen when exposure occurs during enamel formation.

Treatment of acute fluoride poisoning consists of immediate administration of milk, lime water, calcium gluconate, or calcium lactate solution to precipitate calcium fluoride. After lavage or emesis and charcoal instillation, calcium (e.g., calcium gluconate, 10 g) can be given again followed by an osmotic cathartic. Then 10% calcium gluconate or 1% calcium chloride should be slowly injected intravenously and repeated as needed to prevent a positive Chvostek's sign. Symptomatic and supportive therapy is administered as indicated.

FORMALDEHYDE This gas is available as 40% solution (formalin) which is used as a disinfectant, fumigant, or deodorant. Poisoning by formalin may be diagnosed by the characteristic odor of formaldehyde. Formaldehyde reacts chemically with cellular constituents, depresses cellular functions, and causes cell death. The fatal dose of formalin is about 60 mL. Ingestion of formalin immediately causes severe abdominal pain, nausea, vomiting, and diarrhea. This may be followed by collapse, coma, severe metabolic acidosis, and anuria. Death is usually the result of circulatory failure.

Since any organic material can inactivate formaldehyde, milk, bread, soup, etc., should be administered immediately unless activated charcoal is available. Formaldehyde is a corrosive, and emesis and lavage are not recommended. Parenteral administration of sodium bicarbonate is indicated to combat acidosis. The treatment is otherwise supportive.

GLYCOLS Ethylene glycol and diethylene glycol are used in antifreeze solutions. The more than 50 annual deaths from these compounds usually result from intentional drinking of antifreeze by alcoholics. The fatal dose of ethylene glycol is about 100 g while that of diethylene glycol is somewhat lower. Glycols are metabolized by alcohol dehydrogenase to the aldehyde, which is ultimately converted to oxalate. It is the metabolites of the glycols (particularly the aldehyde and oxalate) which are most responsible for toxicity after glycol ingestion.

The initial symptoms of acute poisoning by these glycols resemble those of alcoholic intoxication. They may progress to vomiting, stupor, coma with absent reflexes and anisocoria, and convulsions. Tachypnea, bradycardia, and hypothermia are seen commonly, as are metabolic acidosis and hyocalcemia. After massive ingestion death may occur from respiratory failure within a few hours or from pulmonary edema within a day or two. If the patient survives this stage, acute tubular necrosis often develops.

Intravenous infusion of ethanol to maintain a blood level of 100 mg/dL is effective in competing for alcohol dehydrogenase, thus slowing the conversion of glycol to the more toxic aldehyde. Pyridoxine (100 mg daily administered intravenously) and thiamine (100 mg daily administered intravenously) are given to stimulate conversion of glyoxalate, the immediate metabolic precursor of oxalate, to the nontoxic metabolites, glycine and α-hydroxy-β-ketoadipate, respectively. However, the effectiveness of these latter procedures has not been established. Dialysis is highly effective in the removal of ethylene and diethylene glycol from the body. Acidosis and hypocalcemia must be treated vigorously.

HALOGENATED HYDROCARBONS Halogenated hydrocarbons (carbon tetrachloride, ethylene chlorohydrin, ethylene dichloride, methyl halides, trichloroethane, trichloroethylene) find wide industrial use as solvents, refrigerants, and fumigants, and in chemical synthesis. They enter the home in household cleaners, floor waxes, fire extinguishers, and rubber or plastic cements. These compounds are highly fat-soluble and produce cell damage either directly or after conversion in the body to other compounds. Individual halogenated hydrocarbons differ considerably in the degree and the exact manifestations of their toxicity, but in sufficient concentration all these compounds are capable of inducing central nervous system depression and varying amounts of hepatic and renal toxicity. Myocardial depression, vascular damage, and pulmonary edema also may occur.

The most important halogenated hydrocarbon is carbon tetrachloride, which still is employed widely as a nonflammable solvent and fire extinguisher fluid but which largely has been replaced in products intended for household use by the less toxic trichloroethane. Poisoning may occur from inhalation of the vapor, ingestion, or, rarely, percutaneous absorption. An oral dose of as little as 4 mL may be fatal. Absorption from the gastrointestinal tract is slow and unpredictable but is increased by the presence of fats and alcohol. Abdominal pain, hematemesis, and hepatic damage are more common and severe after ingestion than when the poison is inhaled. Inhalation may lead to irritation of the upper part of the respiratory tract.

Acute systemic absorption of carbon tetrachloride results in nausea, dizziness, confusion, and headache within a few minutes. Depending upon the quantity absorbed, the symptoms may quickly progress to stupor, coma, convulsions, respiratory failure, hypotension, or ventricular fibrillation. The patient may recover from these immediate manifestations until evidence of hepatic or renal toxicity appears several hours to several days after the exposure. Liver and kidney damage also may occur in the absence of any severe early central nervous system effects. Initially tender hepatomegaly may be present, jaundice may be rapidly progressive, and death due to severe centrilobular necrosis may occur within days. The renal lesion has the characteristics of acute tubular necrosis, and manifests itself by proteinuria, hematuria, oliguria, or anuria. Uremia, acidosis, hypertension, and pulmonary edema may develop as complications of renal failure. Optic neuritis, pancreatitis, and adrenal cortical necrosis are less common manifestations of carbon tetrachloride intoxication.

Chronic poisoning may occur after repeated exposures to low concentrations of carbon tetrachloride and may also lead to liver or kidney damage. Usually it manifests itself by vague symptoms of fatigue, weakness, mental confusion, abdominal pain, anorexia, nausea, blurring of vision, and paresthesias.

Treatment of acute poisoning by halogenated hydrocarbons includes vigorous efforts at minimizing gastrointestinal absorption by lavage or emesis and catharsis. Treatment is otherwise symptomatic. Sympathomimetic drugs should be avoided because of the danger of inducing ventricular arrhythmias in the sensitized myocardium. Acute renal and hepatic failure must be managed carefully. Often, hemodialysis is required and may be lifesaving until kidney function returns 3 or more weeks after poisoning. Both hemodialysis and hemoperfusion will effectively remove carbon tetrachloride and trichloroethane from the body but are potentially useful in preventing severe toxicity and death only when begun early in the postingestion period.

IODINE The traditional antiseptic iodine tincture is an alcoholic solution of 2% iodine and 2% sodium iodide. Strong iodine solution (Lugol's solution) is an aqueous solution of 5% iodine and 10% potassium iodide. The fatal dose of tincture of iodine is approximately

2 g. Iodides are very much less toxic, and no fatalities have been reported.

The diagnosis of iodine poisoning is suggested by the brown staining of the oral mucous membranes. The effects largely result from the corrosive effects of the compound on the gastrointestinal tract. Burning abdominal pain, nausea, vomiting, and bloody diarrhea may occur soon after ingestion. If the stomach contained starch, the vomitus is blue or black. Tissue trauma from corrosive gastroenteritis and fluid loss by vomiting and diarrhea may result in shock. Severe edema of the glottis, fever, delirium, stupor, and anuria also have been observed.

Treatment consists of the immediate administration of milk, starch, bread, etc., or activated charcoal to provide a source other than human tissue with which the iodine can react. Catharsis should be induced. Sodium thiosulfate will reduce iodine to less toxic iodide; 100 mL of a 5% solution should be given orally followed by an osmotic cathartic. A 10-mL dose of a 10% thiosulfate solution also should be given intravenously every 4 h. Induction of emesis and lavage should not be attempted if esophageal injury is suspected. With appropriate treatment most patients poisoned by iodine survive, but esophageal strictures may complicate their recovery.

IRON SALTS (See Chap. 172)

ISOPROPYL ALCOHOL This compound is used as a sterilizing agent or as rubbing alcohol. Ingestion produces gastric irritation and raises the danger of vomiting with aspiration. The systemic effects of isopropyl alcohol are similar to those of ethyl alcohol, but it is approximately twice as potent as the latter. Coma is produced readily but rarely lasts longer than 12 h. About 15 percent of an ingested dose of isopropanol is metabolized to acetone; transient acetonuria is common, but significant acidosis does not occur. Emesis should be induced, or gastric lavage should be performed. Supportive therapy is required only after ingestion of massive amounts, and there are no sequelae other than transient gastritis.

MAGNESIUM Magnesium sulfate is used intravenously as a hypotensive agent and orally as a cathartic. The magnesium ion is a profound depressant of the central nervous system and of neuromuscular transmission. Poisoning after oral or rectal administration is unlikely in the presence of normal renal function, because the kidney removes magnesium more rapidly than it is absorbed by the gastrointestinal tract. In the presence of impaired renal function an oral dose of 30 g may be fatal. Symptoms begin at a serum magnesium level of 4 meq per liter, and concentrations of over 12 meq per liter may be fatal. Oral ingestion of concentrated solutions may cause gastrointestinal irritation. Manifestations of systemic poisoning are depression of reflexes, flaccid paralysis, hypotension, hypothermia, coma, and respiratory failure. Respiratory death usually precedes significant myocardial depression. The actions of magnesium on neurologic and neuromuscular function are antagonized by calcium. *Treatment* of magnesium poisoning therefore includes the intravenous administration of 10 mL of a 10% solution of calcium gluconate, which may be repeated as necessary.

METHYL ALCOHOL This simplest of alcohols, also called wood alcohol or methanol, is used as a solvent, antifreeze, paint remover, and as a denaturant in ethyl alcohol. Denatured ethyl alcohol preparations, such as Sterno or Solox, contain 5 to 15% methyl alcohol as well as other denaturants. Methyl alcohol poisoning results almost entirely from its ingestion as a substitute for ethanol or to the drinking of denatured ethyl alcohol. The toxic dose is quite variable: death has occurred after a dose of 20 mL, but 250 mL has been ingested with survival. As little as 15 mL methanol has caused permanent blindness.

Methanol is less inebriating than ethyl alcohol, and inebriation is not a prominent symptom of methyl alcohol intoxication. Methanol is oxidized in the body by alcohol dehydrogenase first to formaldehyde and then to formic acid; these metabolites cause the toxic mainfestations of methanol poisoning. At equivalent concentrations the rate of its metabolism is only 15 percent that of ethanol for which alcohol dehydrogenase has a greater affinity and which can inhibit competitively the rate of metabolism of methanol. Formic acid and especially formaldehyde have toxic actions on many cells; the retina and optic nerve are damaged specifically. The toxic metabolites of methyl alcohol are also responsible for the severe acidosis which is the most prominent feature of methyl alcohol poisoning. This acidosis results partly from the accumulation of formic acid, but formate also appears to exert an inhibitory effect upon enzymes involved in the oxidation of carbohydrate with consequent accumulation of acid intermediates.

Symptoms of methanol poisoning usually do not appear until 12 to 24 h after ingestion, when sufficient toxic metabolites have accumulated. Manifestations include headache, dizziness, nausea, vomiting, vasomotor disturbances, central nervous system depression, and respiratory failure. Visual disturbance is almost universal and ranges from mild blurring of vision to total blindness. Impairment of vision may be transient, but permanent blindness may follow survival of the acute intoxication. The pupils are dilated and nonreactive, and there is hyperemia of the optic disc and retinal edema. Acidosis is commonly severe.

In the *treatment* of methyl alcohol intoxication emesis and gastric lavage are of use only within the first 2 h after ingestion. Intravenous administration of large amounts of sodium bicarbonate combats acidosis. Return of acidosis is frequent after initial correction, and additional alkali must be administered as indicated by close observation of the patient and laboratory determinations. It is most useful to obtain a blood methanol level as soon as possible. At any time after ingestion, levels between 20 and 50 mg/dL are associated with acidosis and significant symptomatology and are an indication for intravenous ethanol therapy (1 g ethanol per kilogram of body weight in 5% dextrose in water over 30 min to load, then 7 to 10 g/h in adults to maintain the blood ethanol level at about 100 mg/dL). Severely symptomatic patients should be treated even if a methanol level cannot be obtained. A methanol level exceeding 50 mg/dL is an indication for hemodialysis as well as ethanol therapy; dialysis also is indicated in the presence of severe acidosis with lower blood levels.

MUSHROOMS There are many species of poisonous mushrooms, but in the United States most poisoning is due to the *Amanita*. More than 100 deaths result each year from consumption of wild poisonous mushrooms, 90 percent being due to *A. phalloides* (death cap) or closely related species. Fatalities have occurred after ingestion of only part of one mushroom.

A usually less severe poisoning follows ingestion of *A. muscaria* (fly agaric) which contains the parasympathomimetic alkaloid muscarine, as well as variable amounts of a substance active on the central nervous system and a parasympatholytic alkaloid. Symptoms are largely those of parasympathetic stimulation: lacrimation, pupillary constriction, perspiration, salivation, nausea, vomiting, diarrhea, abdominal pain, bronchorrhea, wheezing, dyspnea, bradycardia, and hypotension. Muscular tremors, confusion, excitement, and delirium are common in severe poisoning. Very rarely symptoms of atropine poisoning have predominated. After ingestion of *A. muscaria*, symptoms appear within minutes to 2 h. The patient may die within a few hours, but with appropriate therapy complete recovery in 24 h is the rule.

A. phalloides, A. virosa (destroying angel), some other *Amanita* species, and *Galerina venenata* contain heat-stable cyclopeptide cytotoxins which are rapidly bound to tissues. The principal toxin is α-amanitin, which binds to and inhibits specifically the mammalian RNA polymerase responsible for messenger RNA synthesis. Severe cell damage and fatty degeneration may occur in liver, kidneys, striated muscle, and brain. Ingestion of these dangerous mushrooms is followed by a latent period of 6 to 20 h. Manifestations of cytotoxicity then may appear suddenly and consist of severe nausea, violent abdominal pain, bloody vomiting and diarrhea, and cardiovascular collapse. Headache, mental confusion, coma, or convulsions are common. Painful and tender hepatomegaly, jaundice, hypoglycemia, dehydration, and oliguria or anuria frequently appear on the first or second day after ingestion. The victim may die from acute hepatic necrosis (yellow atrophy) within 4 days. About one-half of all poisonings with *A. phalloides* have a fatal outcome in 5 to 8 days. Recovery tends to be slow.

Ingestion of other poisonous mushrooms may cause gastrointestinal symptoms, visual disturbances, ataxia, disorientation, convulsions, coma, fever, hemolysis, and methemoglobinemia.

Treatment of mushroom poisoning depends upon the species ingested. If parasympathomimetic manifestations are prominent, atropine in doses of 1 to 2 mg is given intramuscularly and repeated every 30 min until symptoms are controlled. Poisoning by cytotoxic mushrooms is treated mainly symptomatically. Fluid and electrolyte balance must be carefully maintained. Hypoglycemia should be avoided; large quantities of carbohydrate may exert some protective effect on the liver. Excitement, convulsions, pain, hypotension, and fever may need symptomatic therapy. Early intensive hemoperfusion can remove α-amanitin from the body and probably is indicated in *A. phalloides* poisoning. Both thioctic acid (α-lipoic acid) and cytochrome c have been advocated as antidotes for α-amanitin poisoning, but convincing data as to their efficacy are lacking.

NAPHTHALENE Poisoning by this substance almost always results from ingestion of moth repellents. An oral dose of 2 g has been fatal. Nausea, vomiting, and diarrhea are the initial symptoms. Larger doses may produce hepatic damage with jaundice and renal toxicity which may progress to hematuria, oliguria, or anuria. Depending upon the amount ingested, central nervous system manifestations may range from headache, mental confusion, and excitement to coma and convulsions. In persons with glucose 6-phosphate dehydrogenase-deficient red blood cells the ingestion of naphthalene will produce hemolysis. *Treatment* consists of emesis or gastric lavage, catharsis, and supportive measures.

NICOTINE This alkaloid is an exceedingly potent and rapidly acting poison. It is a component of many insecticides. Nicotine is absorbed readily from the oral and gastrointestinal mucosa, from the respiratory tract, and through the skin. The lethal dose for an adult is approximately 50 mg, the quantity contained in two cigarettes. However, tobacco is much less toxic than would be anticipated on the basis of its nicotine content. Nicotine is poorly absorbed from ingested tobacco, and on smoking, most of the nicotine is burned. Nicotine acts on chemoreceptors, on synapses in the central nervous system and in autonomic ganglia, on the adrenal medulla, and on neuroeffector junctions. Furthermore, its transient initial stimulant effects are followed by a more persistent depressant phase of action. It is not surprising that the manifestations of nicotine poisoning are highly complex and somewhat unpredictable.

Small doses of nicotine produce nausea, vomiting, diarrhea, headache, dizziness, and neurologic stimulation manifested by tachycardia, hypertension, hyperpnea, tachypnea, sweating, and salivation. Larger doses also cause cortical irritability, progressing to convulsions, and myocardial arrhythmias. Finally coma, respiratory depression and arrest, and cardiac arrest or fibrillation may supervene. Severe poisoning may cause death from respiratory failure within a few minutes.

Treatment consists of induction of emesis or gastric lavage, followed by the instillation of activated charcoal and the administration of an osmotic cathartic. Potassium permanganate will oxidize nicotine, and a 1:10,000 solution can be used for lavage. Atropine, 2 mg, and phentolamine, 5 mg, may be given intramuscularly or intravenously and repeated as often as required to control signs and symptoms of parasympathetic or sympathetic hyperactivity. These compounds are ineffective in preventing paralysis of the respiratory muscles and disturbances in cardiac rhythm. Careful attention must be given to artificial ventilation with oxygen and to therapy of catecholamine-induced cardiac tachyarrhythmias. Propranolol is the drug of choice for the latter purpose. Nicotine is rapidly detoxified in the liver, and recovery will be prompt if the patient can be tided over the initial period.

NITRITES Poisoning by the nitrite ion may result from the ingestion of large amounts of drugs such as amyl, butyl, isobutyl, or sodium nitrite. Ingested nitrates may be reduced to nitrite by intestinal bacteria, especially *Escherichia coli*. Except after the ingestion of very large amounts, adults usually absorb all nitrate before this reduction takes place. However, in children nitrite poisoning may result from the ingestion of nitrates or nitrate-containing well water. Fatalities have occurred from the oral ingestion of 2 to 4 g nitrites.

Acute nitrite poisoning may lead to severe headache, flushing, dizziness, hypotension, and syncope. Usually the patient only need be positioned to facilitate venous return to the heart. Pressor agents seldom are required. The most important toxic effect of the nitrite ion is its ability to oxidize hemoglobin to methemoglobin (Chaps. 53 and 288).

PARAQUAT Paraquat is a dipyridilium compound which is used in 5 to 20% aqueous solutions as a herbicide. An oral dose of 5 mg/kg may be fatal. Some victims die within 24 h in respiratory failure, often with refractive pulmonary edema. In others a serious toxic effect is the delayed (3 days to 2 weeks postingestion) development of progressive pulmonary fibrosis. The lungs selectively accumulate paraquat from the blood over several days until a critical concentration is reached, after which pulmonary edema and fibrosis ensue. Progressive respiratory failure is the usual cause of death. The metabolism of paraquat by lung tissue leads to the production of radical intermediates as well as the superoxide radical; the latter appears to be at least partly responsible for the toxicity of the compound.

Prolonged absorption (up to several days) of paraquat from the gastrointestinal tract is common. After gastric emptying, diluted bentonite (Fuller's earth) or activated charcoal should be administered followed by an osmotic cathartic twice daily for 48 h. Forced diuresis, hemodialysis, and hemoperfusion significantly augment clearance of paraquat. Oxygen administration to animals experimentally poisoned with paraquat is associated with increased mortality; it would seem prudent to avoid, if possible, oxygen-enriched breathing mixtures in patients poisoned with paraquat. Intravenous administration of superoxide dismutase has been reported to decrease lung toxicity from paraquat in animals, but no beneficial effect has been demonstrated yet in humans.

PETROLEUM DISTILLATES Petroleum distillates (diesel oil, gasoline, kerosene, paint thinner, solvent distillate) are liquids with a boiling point between 50 and 325°C. They contain variable amounts of branched or straight-chain aliphatic and aromatic hydrocarbons. Kerosene is used widely as a fuel and as a vehicle for cleaning agents, furniture polishes, insecticides, and paint thinners. Not surprisingly, each year petroleum distillates cause about 100 accidental deaths in the United States, 90 percent of these in young children. Furthermore, these products are annually responsible for almost 20,000 hospitalizations. Ingestion of 10 mL kerosene has been fatal, but adults have recovered from as much as 250 mL. Petroleum distillates are central nervous system depressants; they damage cells by dissolving cellular lipids. Pulmonary damage manifested by pulmonary edema or pneumonitis is a common and serious complication.

Inhalation of gasoline or kerosene vapors induces a state resembling alcoholic intoxication. Headache, nausea, tinnitus, and a burning sensation in the chest may also be present. When aliphatic hydrocarbons are inhaled, these symptoms may progress to profound drowsiness or coma with absence of deep reflexes. If the distillate contains a high proportion of aromatic hydrocarbons, the coma is characterized by tremors, muscle jactitations, hyperactive reflexes, and convulsions. Death usually results from respiratory depression, rarely from ventricular fibrillation.

The oral ingestion of petroleum distillates causes irritation of the mucous membranes of the upper part of the intestinal tract. When large amounts have been ingested, the same manifestations as after inhalation may appear. Frequently eructation or vomiting results in aspiration of petroleum distillates into the trachea. Because of their low surface tension, minute amounts of these substances then may spread widely throughout the lungs and produce pulmonary edema and pneumonitis. Pulmonary damage also may arise because of absorption of ingested petroleum distillates from the gastrointestinal tract. However, kerosene is at least 100 times more toxic by the intratracheal route than when ingested.

In the *treatment* of poisoning by petroleum distillates extreme care must be used to prevent aspiration. If the patient is coughing when seen, aspiration is likely already to have occurred. When large amounts (>100 mL) have been ingested, gastric emptying is indicated. In the alert patient emesis may be induced; when vomiting occurs, the head of the patient should be lower than the hips. Otherwise, gastric lavage should be performed but only after insertion of an endotracheal tube with an inflatable cuff. A saline cathartic may be administered. All victims of kerosene poisoning should be hospitalized for at least 24 h for observation. If signs or symptoms of pulmonary irritation appear, oxygen should be given. Steroids do not appear useful in treatment of this pulmonary lesion and may be detrimental. Prophylactic antibiotics are not indicated. Symptomatic therapy for central nervous system depression or treatment of convulsions may be necessary. Sympathomimetic amines should be avoided because of the danger of inducing ventricular fibrillation in the hydrocarbon-sensitized heart.

PHENOL Phenol and related compounds (creosote, cresols, hexachlorophene, hydroquinone, Lysol, resorcinol, tannic acid) are used as antiseptics, caustics, and preservatives. These substances poison all cells by denaturing and precipitating cellular proteins. The approximate fatal oral dose ranges from 2 mL for phenol and cresols to 20 mL for tannic acid.

Ingestion of phenolic compounds produces erosion of mucosa from mouth to stomach. The corroded areas may have a characteristic dead-white appearance. Hematemesis and bloody diarrhea may occur. After an initial phase of hyperpnea due to stimulation of the respiratory center, stupor, coma, convulsions, pulmonary edema, and shock are seen. The initial respiratory alkalosis is soon followed by a profound acidosis which results from the renal excretion of base during the alkalotic stage, from the acidic nature of phenol, and from disturbances in carbohydrate metabolism, presumably the result of defects in enzymatic function. If the patient survives the acute stage, acute tubular necrosis may lead to oliguria or anuria and hepatic toxicity to jaundice. Poisoning by phenolic compounds often may be diagnosed by their characteristic odor. Development of a violet or blue color of the urine after addition of a few drops of ferric chloride indicates the presence of a phenolic compound.

Emesis and lavage are indicated for *treatment* in the absence of significant corrosive injury to the esophagus. Activated charcoal should be administered. Although definitive proof of efficacy is lacking, olive oil or castor oil, which dissolve phenol and are reputed to retard its absorption, may be given, followed by an osmotic cathartic. Supportive therapy consists of correction of the acidosis, the control of shock and convulsions, and the maintenance of a patent airway in the face of glottal edema by intubation or tracheotomy.

PHOSPHORUS Phosphorus occurs in two forms: a red, nonpoisonous form and a yellow, fat-soluble, highly toxic form. The latter is used in rodent and insect poisons and in fireworks. Yellow phosphorus and phosphides cause fatty degeneration and necrosis of tissues, particularly of the liver. The lethal ingested dose of yellow phosphorus is approximately 50 mg.

Ingestion of yellow phosphorus is followed within 1 h by burning pain in the upper part of the gastrointestinal tract, vomiting, diarrhea, and a garlic odor of the breath and excreta. The patient may die in coma during the first day or two, or symptoms may subside after a few hours. Then, 1 to 2 days later, the victim may develop tender hepatomegaly, jaundice, hypocalcemia, hypotension, and oliguria and may die following convulsions and coma. Death from acute hepatic necrosis may occur in a few days.

Treatment consists of induction of emesis or gastric lavage, instillation of activated charcoal, and administration of an osmotic cathartic. Calcium gluconate is given intravenously to maintain the serum calcium level. Treatment is otherwise supportive.

SALICYLATES Each year 30 million pounds of aspirin is consumed in the United States, and salicylates can probably be found in most American households. Aspirin is found in many compound analgesic tablets. Methyl salicylate (oil of wintergreen) is present in most skin liniments, and salicylic acid is used in ointments and corn plasters. The ingestion of 10 to 30 g aspirin or sodium salicylate may be fatal to adults, but survival has been reported after an oral dose of 130 g aspirin.

Salicylate intoxication may result from the cumulative effect of therapeutic administration of high doses. There is considerable individual variation: toxic symptoms may begin at dosages of 3 g per day or may not appear when 10 g per day is given. Toxic symptoms are also poorly correlated with the serum salicylate concentration, but few patients become intoxicated at levels less than 15 mg/dL and most at levels over 35 mg/dL. Therapeutic salicylate intoxication is usually mild and is called *salicylism.* The earliest symptoms are vertigo, tinnitus, and impairment of hearing. Further overdosage causes nausea, vomiting, sweating, diarrhea, fever, drowsiness, headache, dimness of vision, and mental aberrations. The latter may be characterized by confusion, excitement, restlessness, and talkativeness; this ''salicylate jag'' resembles alcoholic intoxication without the euphoria. The central nervous system effects may progress to hallucinations, convulsions, and coma. Toxic doses of salicylates also have a direct stimulant effect on the respiratory center, resulting in hyperventilation, loss of carbon dioxide, and respiratory alkalosis. Renal excretion of bicarbonate may compensate partially for this.

In acute salicylate poisoning due to accidental or suicidal ingestion of massive amounts, the same manifestations may be seen in more rapid succession. However, they usually are overshadowed by severe disturbances in the acid-base balance which follow a definite sequence. Early in the course of intoxication there may be only hyperpnea, and the seriousness of the poisoning may not be appreciated at that time. The hyperventilation causes a fall in blood P_{CO_2} and an increase in pH. Renal excretion of bicarbonate, sodium, and potassium will bring the pH back toward normal and produce a compensated respiratory alkalosis. At that point the buffering capacity of the extracellular fluid will have been decreased significantly. In young children and after large doses in adults further developments may then produce a combination of respiratory acidosis and metabolic acidosis which stems from a number of factors. High concentrations of salicylate depress the respiratory center and cause CO_2 retention. Renal function becomes impaired because of dehydration and hypotension, and inorganic metabolic acids accumulate. Furthermore, salicylic acid derivatives may displace several milliequivalents of blood bicarbonate. Finally, salicylates impair carbohydrate metabolism and cause accumulation of acetoacetic, lactic, and pyruvic acids. Severe acidosis and disturbances in electrolyte balance are seen most commonly in febrile young children.

Blood salicylate levels are of value in the estimation of the severity of poisoning. Serious poisoning is rare at levels less than 50 mg/dL but usual at levels between 50 and 100 mg/dL. Levels above 100 mg/dL during the first 6 h after poisoning signify severe intoxication and may be fatal. Excretion of salicylates is renal, and in the presence of normal renal function about 50 percent will be excreted in 24 h. Addition of a few drops of ferric chloride solution to 5 mL boiled acidified urine containing salicylate yields a violet color and may aid in diagnosis.

Treatment of salicylate poisoning consists initially of inducing emesis or of gastric lavage after which activated charcoal and then an osmotic cathartic are administered. Disturbances of acid-base or electrolyte balance and hypoglycemia are corrected by the intravenous administration of appropriate solutions. Respiratory depression may require artificial ventilation with oxygen. Convulsions may be treated with diazepam or phenobarbital. The renal clearance of salicylate is enhanced ten- to twentyfold if the pH of the urine can be kept between 7 and 8. In addition to intravenous bicarbonate and a diuretic to raise the pH above 7, it may be necessary to give potassium to prevent paradoxical aciduria. Peritoneal dialysis and hemodialysis are also highly effective in removing salicylate from seriously poisoned patients, but forced alkaline diuresis is so effective in clearing salicylate that these maneuvers most often are not required.

SMOKE Poisoning by smoke is usually due to carbon monoxide inhalation. However, burning material may also release irritant fumes. Many irritant gases combine with water to form corrosive acids or alkalies and cause chemical burns of exposed skin and of the upper part of the respiratory tract. Such gases (and the corrosives formed) are ammonia (ammonium hydroxide), nitrogen oxide (nitric acid), sulfur dioxide (sulfurous acid), and sulfur trioxide (sulfuric acid). These irritating gases as well as hydrogen sulfide also may be present in smog. Another highly toxic gas which may be inhaled by firefighters or victims is phosgene. This compound is formed by the high-temperature decomposition of chlorinated hydrocarbons and is released when carbon tetrachloride from fire extinguishers comes into contact with hot surfaces.

After inhalation of irritant gases the victim may notice burning pain in the throat and chest and severe coughing. These symptoms may subside completely, but from several hours to a day after exposure dyspnea and cyanosis may appear and progress rapidly to severe pulmonary edema and death from respiratory and circulatory failure. Treatment consists of administration of oxygen and adrenal steroids and appropriate therapy of pulmonary edema, should that develop.

REFERENCES

General

ARENA JM: *Poisoning: Toxicology, Symptoms, Treatments,* 4th ed. Springfield, Ill, Charles C Thomas, 1979

ARLEFF AL et al: Coma following nonnarcotic drug overdosage—management of 208 adult patients. Am J Med Sci 266:405, 1973

BOURNE PG: *Acute Drug Abuse Emergencies.* New York, Academic, 1976

Casarett and Doull's Toxicology: The Basic Science of Poisons, 2d ed, J Doull, CD Klaasen, MO Amdur (eds). New York, Macmillan, 1980

DREISBACH RH: *Handbook of Poisoning: Prevention, Diagnosis and Treatment,* 11th ed. Los Altos, CA, Lange, 1983

HADDAD LM, WINCHESTER JF: *Clinical Management of Poisoning and Drug Overdose.* Philadelphia, Saunders, 1983

LOOMIS TA: *Essentials of Toxicology,* 3d ed. Philadelphia, Lea & Febiger, 1978

LOVEJOY FH JR: Acute poisoning, in *Current Pediatric Therapy,* 9th ed, SS Gellis, BM Kegan (eds). Philadelphia, Saunders, 1980, p 654

TURK MH: *Occupational Medicine: Surveillance, Diagnosis and Treatment.* Cambridge, MA, Ballinger, 1982

WINCHESTER JF et al: Dialysis and hemoperfusion of poisons and drugs—update. Trans Am Soc Artif Intern Organs 23:762, 1977

Toxic product information

BILINGS NF, BILLINGS SM: *American Drug Index,* Philadelphia, Lippincott, 1984

GOODMAN and GILMAN: *The Pharmacological Basis of Therapeutics,* 7th ed, AG Gilman et al (eds). New York, Macmillan, 1985

GOSSELIN RE: *Clinical Toxicology of Commercial Products: Acute Poisoning,* 5th ed. Baltimore, Williams & Wilkins, 1984

HAYES WJ: *Pesticides Studies in Man.* Baltimore, Williams & Wilkins, 1982

The Merck Index, 9th ed. Rahway, NJ, Merck & Co, 1976

Poisonous Plants and Fungi. Philadelphia, Rittenhouse, 1976

SCHERZ RG: The history of poison control centers in the United States. Clin Toxicol 12:291, 1978

COMMON POISONS

Acetaminophen

PRESCOTT LF et al: Treatment of paracetamol poisoning with *N*-acetylcysteine. Lancet 2:432, 1977

RUMACK LF et al: Acetaminophen overdose: 662 cases with evaluation of oral acetylcysteine therapy. Arch Intern Med 141:380, 1981

ZIEVE L et al: Acetaminophen liver injury: Sequential changes in two biochemical indices of regeneration and their relationship to histologic alterations. J Lab Clin Med 105:619, 1985

Antimuscarinic compounds

RUMACK BH: Anticholinergic poisoning: Treatment with physostigmine. Pediatrics 52:449, 1973

Benzene, toluene

HAYDEN JW: The clinical toxicology of solvent abuse. Clin Toxicol 9:169, 1976

STREICHER HZ et al: Syndromes of toluene sniffing in adults. Ann Intern Med 94:758, 1981

Carbon monoxide

DOLAN MC: Carbon monoxide poisoning. Can Med Assoc J 133:392, 1985

REMICK RA, MILES JE: Carbon monoxide poisoning: Neurologic and psychiatric sequelae. Can Med Assoc J 117:654, 1977

TURINO GM: Effect of carbon monoxide on the cardiorespiratory system. Circulation 63:253A, 1981

Caustics

CAMPBELL GS et al: Treatment of corrosive burns of the esophagus. Arch Surg 112:495, 1977

RUMACK BH, BURLINGTON JD: Caustic ingestions: A rational look at diluents. Clin Toxicol 11(1):27, 1977

Chlorinated insecticides

BOYLAN JJ et al: Cholestyramine: Use of a new therapeutic approach for chlordecone (Kepone) poisoning. Science 199:893, 1978

STARR GH, CLIFFORD NJ: Acute lindane intoxication. Arch Environ Health 25:374, 1972

TAYLOR JR, CALABRESE VP: Organochlorine and other insecticides. Handbook Clin Neurol 36:391, 1979

Cholinesterase inhibitor insecticides

LUZHNIKOR EA et al: Plasma perfusion through charcoal in methylparathion poisoning. Lancet 1:38, 1977

MILBY TH: Prevention and management of organophosphate poisoning. JAMA 216:2131, 1971

WYCKOFF W et al: Diagnostic and therapeutic problems of parathion poisonings. Ann Intern Med 68:875, 1968

Cyanide

BRAICO KT et al: Laetrile intoxication: Report of a fatal case. N Engl J Med 300:238, 1979

UITTI RJ et al: Cyanide-induced parkinsonism: A clinicopathologic report. Neurology 35:921, 1985

VICK JA, FROEHLICH HL: Studies of cyanide poisoning. Arch Int Pharmcodyn Ther 273:314, 1985

WESSON DE et al: Treatment of acute cyanide intoxication with hemodialysis. Am J Nephrol 5:121, 1985

Detergents

TEMPLE AR, VELTRI JC: Outcome of accidental ingestions of soaps, detergents, and related household products. Vet Hum Toxicol 21:9, 1979

WILSON, JT, BURR, IM: Benzalkonium chloride poisoning in infant twins. Am J Dis Child 129:1208, 1975

Fluorides

BAYLESS JM, TINANOFF N: Diagnosis and treatment of acute fluoride toxicity. J Am Dent Assoc 110:209, 1985

SMITH GE: Toxicity of fluoride-containing dental preparations: A review. Sci Total Environ 43:41, 1985

Glycols

CATCHINGS TT et al: Adult respiratory distress syndrome secondary to ethylene glycol ingestion. Ann Emerg Med 14:594, 1985

DAROZA R et al: Acute ethylene glycol poisoning. Crit Care Med 12:1003, 1984

Halogenated hydrocarbons

BAERG RD, KIMBERG DV: Centrilobular hepatic necrosis and acute renal failure in "solvent sniffers." Ann Intern Med 73:713, 1970

RECHNAGEL RO: Carbon tetrachloride hepatotoxicity. Pharmacol Rev 19:145, 1967

SCHWARZBECK A, KOSTERS W: Extracorporeal hemoperfusion in acute carbon tetrachloride intoxication. Arch Toxicol 35:207, 1976

Isopropyl alcohol

LACOUTURE PG et al: Acute isopropyl alcohol intoxication. Diagnosis and management. Am J Med 75:680, 1983

Methyl alcohol

BENNET H JR et al: Acute methyl alcohol poisoning: A review based on experiences in an outbreak of 323 cases. Medicine 32:431, 1953

KAPLAN K: Methyl alcohol poisoning. Am J Med Sci 244:170, 1982

RAVICHANDRAN R et al: Methyl alcohol poisoning. J Postgrad Med 30:69, 1984

Mushrooms

CURRY SC, ROSE MC: Intravenous mushroom poisoning. Ann Emerg Med 14:900, 1985
HANRAHAN JP, GORDON MA: Mushroom poisoning. Case reports and a review of therapy. JAMA 251:1057, 1984
VESCONI S et al: Therapy of cytotoxic mushroom intoxication. Crit Care Med 13:402, 1985

Naphthalene

HAGGERTY RJ: Naphthalene poisoning. N Engl J Med 255:919, 1956

Nicotine

GEHLBACH SH et al: Nicotine absorption by workers harvesting green tobacco. Lancet 1:478, 1975

Nitrites

KEATING JP et al: Infantile methemoglobinemia caused by carrot juice. N Engl J Med 288:824, 1973

Paraquat

GAUDREAULT P et al: Efficacy of activated charcoal and magnesium citrate in the treatment of oral paraquat intoxication. Ann Emerg Med 14:123, 1985
VANDENBOGAERDE J et al: Paraquat poisoning. Forensic Sci Int 26:103, 1984

Petroleum distillates

BROWN J et al: Experimental kerosene pneumonia: Evaluation of some therapeutic regimens. J Pediatr 84:396, 1974
PEARLSON GD: Psychiatric and medical syndromes associated with phencyclidine (PCP) abuse. Johns Hopkins Med J 1:25, 1981
SHIRKEY H: Treatment of petroleum distillate ingestion. Mod Treat 8:580, 1971
TAUSSIG LN et al: Pulmonary function 8 to 10 years after hydrocarbon pneumonitis. Clin Pediatr 16:57, 1977

Phosphorus

SIMON FA, PICKERING LK: Acute yellow phosphorus poisoning. JAMA 235:1343, 1976
TALLEY RC et al: Acute elemental phosphorus poisoning in man: Cardiovascular toxicity. Am Heart J 84:139, 1972
WINEK CL et al: Yellow phosphorus ingestions: Three fatal poisonings. Clin Toxicol 6:541, 1973

Salicylates

ANDERSON RJ et al: Unrecognized adult salicylate intoxication. Ann Intern Med 85:745, 1976
BUSCHANUN N, RABINOWITZ L: Infantile salicylism: A reappraisal. J Pediatr 84:391, 1974
DONE AK, TEMPLE AR: Treatment of salicylate poisoning. Mod Treat 8:528, 1971
HILL JB: Salicylate intoxication. N Engl J Med 288:1110, 1973
PROUDFOOT AT, BROWN SS: Acidaemia and salicylate poisoning in adults. Br Med J 2:537, 1969
SEGAR WE, HOLLIDAY MA: Physiologic abnormalities of salicylate intoxication. N Engl J Med 259:1191, 1958

172 HEAVY METAL POISONING

JOHN W. GRAEF / FREDERICK H. LOVEJOY, JR.

ARSENIC

SOURCE Inorganic arsenic compounds such as arsenic trioxide and arsenic pentoxide as well as sodium and potassium arsenite and arsenate are found in insecticides, rodenticides, fungicides, wood preservatives, and herbicides, and in glass manufacturing. Organic arsenic compounds are present in the environment. Arsine gas poisonings have occurred in industry in the smelting and refining of metals, in galvanizing and etching, in lead plating, and in the silicon microchip industry. Historically, organic arsenical compounds have been used in the treatment of syphilis, epilepsy, psoriasis, and amebiasis. Currently, acute toxicity is encountered following accidental ingestion, industrial accidents, or suicidal or homicidal intoxications. Chronic exposures occur most commonly following low-dose exposure in industry or chronic consumption of contaminated food, water, or medications.

METABOLISM Arsenic is absorbed through the skin, lungs, and gastrointestinal tract. Inorganic compounds are absorbed more readily than organic. Arsine is efficiently absorbed through the lungs. Arsenic is distributed from blood to liver, kidney, lung, and spleen within 24 h of ingestion and within 2 weeks to skin, hair, and bone. Inorganic arsenic compounds are found in high levels in leukocytes. Inorganic arsenic does not cross the blood-brain barrier but does cross the placenta. Five to ten percent is excreted in feces and 90 to 95 percent in the urine. Arsenic may be detected in urine for 7 to 10 days following a single dose.

CLINICAL TOXICOLOGY Arsine gas combines with hemoglobin in red blood cells to produce severe hemolysis with anemia, hemoglobinuria, and subsequent gross hematuria occurring within 3 to 4 h of ingestion. Subsequent jaundice may be severe. Signs and symptoms of toxicity include nausea, vomiting and diarrhea, apprehension and malaise, tachycardia, and dyspnea. Acute renal failure is common and often fatal.

Manifestations of acute toxicity following arsenic ingestion include in the gastrointestinal tract—burning in the throat, difficulty swallowing, nausea, vomiting, diarrhea, abdominal pain, and a garlic odor on the breath; in the cardiovascular system—cyanosis, difficulty breathing, hypotension; in the central nervous system—delirium, coma, seizures; in the kidney—acute tubular necrosis; in the hematologic system—hemolysis, eosinophilia, and rarely bone marrow depression. Manifestations of chronic arsenic poisoning occurring 2 to 8 weeks following ingestion include in the skin and nails—erythroderma, hyperkeratosis, hyperpigmentation, exfoliative dermatitis, Aldrich-Mees lines in the nails; in the mucous membranes—laryngitis, tracheitis, bronchitis; in the central nervous system—polyneuritis (sensory and motor) occurring 1 to 3 weeks following ingestion. Skin basal cell carcinomas, squamous cell carcinomas, and Bowen's disease as well as lung carcinomas have been associated with chronic arsenic exposure.

Arsenic produces its toxicity by binding with tissue sulfhydryl groups. Other effects include capillary injury and direct toxic effects on large organs. Of lesser importance is uncoupling of oxidative phosphorylation. Pathologic findings include necrosis of the stomach and small bowel and vasculature and degenerative changes in the liver and kidneys.

LABORATORY FINDINGS Arsenic is radiopaque and is demonstrable on x-ray of the abdomen. It may also be detected in hair and nails for months following exposure. With specific organ system involvement the following may be seen: abnormal liver function tests; in the blood—anemia, leukocytosis, leukopenia, hemoglobinemia; in the urine—proteinuria, hematuria, hemoglobinuria, and urinary casts. Normal blood arsenic levels should not exceed 3 μg/dL or 100 μg per liter in urine.

TREATMENT Acute ingestion should be treated by inducing vomiting with ipecac syrup if the patient is alert. Gastric lavage is indicated if the patient is obtunded. Activated charcoal is ineffective, and cathartics are contraindicated. Cardiovascular stabilization is critical. Dimercaprol chelates arsenic by producing insoluble complexes that are excreted by the kidneys. For mild symptoms and elevated serum or urinary levels, 2 to 3 mg/kg per dose is given every 6 h for 24 h and then every 12 to 24 h for 10 days. Adequacy of urinary mobilization is confirmed by measurement of serum levels. Toxic manifestations of dimercaprol (increased blood pressure, tachycardia, nausea, vomiting, headache, burning sensation in the lips, mucous membrane irritation, coma, and convulsions) occur with increasing doses. For patients with severe symptoms and significantly elevated arsenic levels 3 to 5 mg/kg per dose of dimercaprol is administered in a similar regime.

D-Penicillamine has been successfully used in chronic poisoning, administered orally, up to 1 g per day in four divided doses for 5 days. Side effects of penicillamine include rashes, leukopenia, eosinophilia, thrombocytopenia, and nephrotoxicity. Hemodialysis removes arsenic with a clearance of 80 to 90 mL/min and is indicated if renal failure occurs.

Exchange transfusion and, if renal failure develops, hemodialysis are the preferred treatments for arsine poisoning. Dimercaprol does not appear to be useful.

CADMIUM

SOURCE Exposure to cadmium is usually occupational or via pollution from mining or smelting operations. Commercially produced as a by-product of copper and lead or zinc smelting, cadmium is used in the manufacture of batteries, in ceramics, in electroplating, and as a pigment in paints and plastics. In contaminated areas, high concentrations may be found in shellfish.

METABOLISM Absorption occurs via ingestion or inhalation. The normal range of daily oral intake is 2 to 200 μg with an estimated mean of 20 to 40 μg per day. Only 5 to 10 percent of this is absorbed, although like lead, absorption may be increased in the presence of calcium and iron deficiency. Similarly, about 5 percent of inhaled cadmium is absorbed depending on particle size. Small, highly soluble particles are absorbed at a rate of 25 to 50 percent.

About 50 percent of absorbed cadmium is concentrated in the liver and kidneys. In erythrocytes and soft tissues cadmium is bound to metallothionein, a low-molecular-weight protein containing a large number of available sulfhydryl groups which thereby exert a protective effect. With large single cadmium exposures saturation of the protein may be exceeded with loss of protective effect. Cadmium does not pass the placenta and gradually accumulates in the body with age. Biologic half-life has been estimated at more than 20 years except in the presence of kidney damage when urinary excretion is increased. In the kidney, metallothionein-bound cadmium is filtered at the glomerulus and is then reabsorbed by the proximal tubules into the renal cortex. The daily urinary excretion rarely exceeds 0.5 μg.

CLINICAL TOXICOLOGY Acute cadmium intoxication may occur after either ingestion or inhalation. Ingestion of water containing concentrations of 15 mg per liter or foods containing as little as 30 mg of cadmium can induce vomiting, abdominal pain, and severe diarrhea. Shock may ensue. Acute inhalation produces dyspnea, weakness, chest pain, shortness of breath, and cough. A chemical pneumonitis produces pulmonary edema and respiratory failure. Clinical symptoms may occur with air exposure as low as 1 mg/m^2 over 8 h. During the same time period inhalation of 5 mg/m^2 may be fatal. A latent period of 4 to 24 h from exposure to onset of symptoms may complicate accurate diagnosis. Death usually occurs in 5 to 10 days. Chemical pneumonitis may continue for several months, and pulmonary function can be abnormal for longer than 1 year after exposure.

Chronic intoxication usually occurs by industrial inhalation and produces emphysema and characteristic renal tubular damage with proteinuria and increased excretion of beta$_2$ microglobulin. Cadmium's inhibitory effect on alpha$_1$ antitrypsin may be the explanation for cadmium-induced emphysema. Relatively minor changes in liver function, a microcytic hypochromic anemia unresponsive to iron therapy, and hypertension are associated findings. Chronic oral intake of contaminated food and drinking water has produced a syndrome in Japan called *itai-itai* (ouch-ouch) disease wtih renal tubular damage and osteomalacia.

LABORATORY FINDINGS Measurement of blood cadmium levels are not useful because of preferential deposition of cadmium in the kidney. Urinary cadmium excretion exceeding 10 μg per liter is associated with renal tubular damage especially when accompanied by elevated urinary beta$_2$ microglobulin and metallothionein levels. Kidney cadmium content obtained by renal biopsy can be assessed by neutron activation analysis. A renal cadmium concentration exceeding 200 μg per gram of net weight is associated with renal disease.

TREATMENT Treatment is controversial. Although chelating agents bind cadmium, they may effectively shift cadmium to the kidney, where further damage can occur. In acute exposure, ethylenediaminetetraacetic acid (EDTA) in a dose of 1 g/m^2 daily can be beneficial. Dimercaprol has not been effective. A new investigational oral chelating agent, dimercaptosuccinic acid, appears promising. Acute inhalation pneumonitis should be treated with steroids and diuretics. Itai-itai disease appears to respond to large doses of vitamin D in the presence of adequate dietary calcium and phosphate. Long-term sequelae of chronic cadmium exposure include emphysema and chronic renal insufficiency.

IRON

SOURCE Iron preparations are used in the treatment of iron-deficiency anemia, as a dietary supplement during pregnancy, and in conjunction with multivitamin preparations. They are accidentally ingested with high frequency by children and occasionally purposefully by adults. They are available by prescription or over the counter.

PATHOPHYSIOLOGY Iron is essential for the synthesis of hemoglobin and myoglobin and is contained in cytochrome systems throughout the body. Of the total content of iron in the body, 70 percent is present in hemoglobin, 20 percent as ferritin or hemosiderin, 5 percent as myoglobin, and 5 percent coupled with enzymes in multiple tissues. Iron in its ferrous state is absorbed through the gastrointestinal mucosa and is carried in the blood in its ferric state bound to transferrin, a specific beta$_1$ globulin. Ferric iron is either transferred to specific sites in the bone marrow for use in erythropoiesis or is stored in ferritin or hemosiderin pools. Each day 1 mg is lost from the body through the intestine, skin, and urine. In overdose, binding sites in the blood are exceeded and free iron is available to cause toxicity. Iron injures cells through peroxidation leading to mitochondrial injury and alteration in oxidative enzymes of the Krebs cycle.

Pathologic findings in fatal cases include necrosis and inflammation of stomach and small bowel, fatty degeneration of hepatocytes, myocardial cells, and renal tubules, and pulmonary atelectasis and emphysema. Iron deposition is demonstrable histologically in intestines, liver, and spleen.

CLINICAL TOXICOLOGY Ingested doses of greater than 30 mg/kg are toxic; greater than 250 mg/kg may be fatal. Signs of poisoning occur within 6 h of ingestion, and the subsequent course of illness follows four stages. Stage I includes injury to the gastrointestinal mucosa with resultant vomiting and diarrhea. A consequent decrease in plasma volume leads to hemoconcentration and decreased cardiac output. Vasodilation from high iron levels and ferritin release augment hypovolemia with resultant clinical evidence of shock. Decreased cerebral perfusion and a possible direct effect of excess iron on the central nervous system cause lethargy and coma. Stage II may involve a quiescent period in milder cases of variable duration, but generally 6 to 24 h. Stage III includes shock, evidence of liver injury with jaundice and elevated liver enzymes, renal failure, and evidence of pulmonary injury. Stage IV occurs several months following the initial insult and involves pyloric scarring with subsequent intestinal obstruction.

LABORATORY FINDINGS Iron is radiopaque and is demonstrable on a flat plate of the abdomen. Efficacy of gastrointestinal decontamination may be confirmed by a follow-up x-ray. A white blood cell count greater than 150,000 per cubic millimeter or a blood sugar of greater than 120 mg/dL are correlated with a serum iron level in excess of 300 μg/dL, a figure associated with clinical evidence of serious systemic toxicity. A provocative chelation challenge test using deferoxamine may be used to determine when the serum iron level has exceeded the iron-binding capacity. Deferoxamine in a dose of 25 mg/kg (not to exceed 1 g) is given intramuscularly. If the serum iron has exceeded the iron-binding capacity, free circulating unbound iron is chelated to deferoxamine. The complex ferrioxamine is excreted as a *"vin rosé"* color in the urine. The most accurate index of severity of iron overdose is the serum iron level. Serum iron levels peak 2 to 4 h after ingestion in most patients. Levels less than 500 μg/dL are associated with a 6 percent risk of shock and coma; levels of 500 to 1000 μg/dL with a 20 percent risk of shock and coma, levels of greater than 1000 μg/dL with a 60 percent risk of shock and coma. Levels exceeding 5000 μg/dL are usually fatal.

TREATMENT Ingested doses of elemental iron greater than 30 mg/kg are best removed with syrup of ipecac (if the patient is alert) or gastric lavage with a large orogastric tube (if the patient is unconscious). Lavage should be carried out with half-normal saline followed by instillation of 50 to 100 mL of 1% bicarbonate to form the ferrous carbonate salt which is less irritating than iron and is poorly absorbed. If an x-ray of the stomach shows presence of iron tablets following gastrointestinal decontamination, repetition of this procedure is recommended. Activated charcoal is ineffective. Calcium phosphate salts, which precipitate iron in the gastrointestinal tract, are associated with significant systemic toxicity, and thus should not be used. Oral deferoxamine forms a ferrioxamine complex which is poorly absorbed and is a useful adjunct to therapy in cases of a large overdose.

Colloid or blood products should be used to correct hypotension. Intravenous sodium bicarbonate may be needed to correct metabolic acidosis. Correction of coagulation defects secondary to hepatic injury may require administration of vitamin K or fresh frozen plasma.

Deferoxamine, the chelating agent of choice, binds free iron in the plasma resulting in excretion of the ferrioxamine complex through the urine. Deferoxamine does not bind iron in ferritin or hemosiderin pools or iron bound to hemoglobin or cytochrome oxidase systems. If the patient is normotensive, deferoxamine 50 mg/kg per dose, up to a total of 1 to 2 g per dose, may be given intramuscularly every 4 to 6 h. If the patient is hypotensive, deferoxamine should be given intravenously at an infusion rate not to exceed 15 mg/kg per hour. A lessening in the *vin rosé* color of the urine and a decline in serum iron levels are used to document the efficacy of therapy. Adverse reactions to deferoxamine include flushing, blotchy erythema, or urticaria; hypotension may occur if the infusion rate is excessively rapid. Therapy should be continued until serum iron levels are less than the iron-binding capacity.

The intensity of therapy with deferoxamine is determined by the serum iron level. A patient with a level of less than 300 μg/dL will require only general supportive care. A level between 300 to 500 μg/dL will require brief chelation therapy, while a level greater than 500 μg/dL will require vigorous chelation therapy. Levels in excess of 1000 μg/dL may require continuous intravenous deferoxamine treatment coupled with close monitoring of serum iron and deferoxamine concentrations. Neither exchange transfusion nor hemodialysis is effective since they remove only a small portion of the total ingested dose (total-body burden) of iron.

LEAD

SOURCE Lead constitutes about 2 percent of the earth's crust and is ubiquitous throughout the world. The increased use of lead during the Industrial Revolution caused extensive disease among lead workers; the addition in the 1870s of lead salts to paints as coloring agents and stabilizers set the stage for what is now the largest epidemic of lead poisoning in history, that of childhood plumbism. This syndrome, caused by ingestion by small children of lead from paint, soil, or household dust, affects an estimated 2,000,000 preschool children annually in the United States alone. Evidence of permanent neurologic sequelae from levels of lead previously thought to be safe has raised fears of possible damage to the fetus and newborn as well. The nature of this epidemic has forced prohibition against the addition of organic lead salts to gasoline as well as extensive prohibitions against the use of lead in consumer products.

METABOLISM Inorganic lead salts are absorbed through ingestion or inhalation. Organic lead salts may also be absorbed through the skin. Gastrointestinal absorption is enhanced by deficiency of iron, calcium, and zinc. Generally, gastrointestinal absorption is about 10 percent of an ingested dose. Absorption through the lung varies with tidal volume and particle size. Particles smaller than 1 μm may be absorbed if they reach the alveoli. Adults may ingest up to 150 μg per day of lead from normal exposure to food and drinking water. Positive lead balance may occur at these levels since renal excretion normally does not exceed 80 to 100 μg per day. In children, no more than 5 μg per kilogram of body weight is tolerated without increasing the body lead burden.

Under steady state conditions, 5 to 10 percent of ingested lead may be found in blood; 95 percent of that fraction is associated with the erythrocyte. Up to 80 to 90 percent is taken up by bone and incorporated into hydroxyapatite crystals where it is relatively inactive. The remainder is found in soft tissues, principally the kidneys and brain. The principal route of excretion is stool (80 to 90 percent), and the remainder is found in the urine (10 percent). The half-life of lead in blood and soft tissues is 24 to 40 days, while that in bone is 104 days.

Lead is a poison of enzymes, binding to the disulfide groups of protein. In high concentration, lead alters the tertiary structure of intracellular proteins, denaturing them and causing cell death with resultant tissue inflammation.

CLINICAL TOXICOLOGY The toxic effects of lead differ between children and adults. The adult form is generally characterized by abdominal pain, anemia, renal disease, headache, peripheral neuropathy with demyelination of long neurons, ataxia, and memory loss. Symptoms are usually associated with prolonged elevation of lead levels above 80 to 100 μg per deciliter of whole blood. A subclinical form is recognized in adults, and affects primarily the peripheral nervous system and the kidneys. A linear association between hypertension and elevated lead levels (i.e., greater than 30 μg/dL) has been reported. Encephalopathy is rare in adults.

Childhood lead poisoning is manifested by anemia and abdominal pain, but the central nervous system effects are most important. As an enzymatic poison, lead affects susceptible developing tissues more than tissues with stable metabolism. Hence, a subclinical form of lead poisoning is most dangerous to children because its effects emerge without associated symptoms that bring the victim to medical attention. In the acute clinical form, signs and symptoms are thought to reflect both the direct effect of high concentrations of lead (i.e., blood lead greater than 80 to 100 μg/dL) and consequent severe alterations in porphyrin synthesis. Signs and symptoms include pallor (anemia), abdominal pain, irritability followed by lethargy, anorexia, ataxia, and slurred speech. In severe cases, convulsions, coma, and death are usually due to severe generalized cerebral edema and renal failure. Almost always associated with this syndrome is a ''high-dose'' exposure to lead (usually paint chips), pica (the ingestion of nonfood substances) and malnutrition (iron, calcium, and zinc deficiency).

The subclinical form of childhood plumbism is associated with elevated blood lead and increased erythrocyte protoporphyrin. However, no symptoms are usually detected. The syndrome is widespread, and its effects on the developing central nervous system are irreversible. These include mental retardation and selective deficits in language, cognitive functions, and behavior, depending on the age and duration of exposure.

LABORATORY FINDINGS Laboratory abnormalities include blood lead levels greater than 25 μg/dL associated with free erthrocyte protoporphyrin (FEP) greater than 35 μg/dL when determined by ethylacetate extraction. Although a hemolytic anemia is associated with acute plumbism, chronic plumbism produces a microcytic hypochromic anemia with associated or secondary iron deficiency. Other heme prescursors are increased in plasma and urine (e.g., coproporphyrin, delta aminolevulinic acid).

Renal abnormalities include pyuria, the Fanconi syndrome, and azotemia. In plumbism, 24-h urinary excretion of lead exceeds 80 to

100 μg. In adults, demyelination of long nerves produces prolonged nerve conduction time and subsequent paralysis of extensor muscles with atrophy (wrist drop or foot drop). While slight prolongation of nerve conduction can be seen in children, it is clinically evident only in those with sickle cell disease. This observation is not completely understood but may be due to an associated zinc deficiency. Abnormalities of cardiac, thyroid, and hepatic function have been observed in adults. In children, a characteristic laboratory finding is increased density at the metaphyseal plate of growing long bones, so-called lead lines. These are generally seen in association with prolonged blood lead levels greater than 50 μg per deciliter of whole blood. They are not seen in adults.

TREATMENT The *sine qua non* of treatment is removal of the source of exposure. Cases of industrial lead poisoning should be reported to the Occupational Safety Hazards Administration (OSHA). Cases of childhood plumbism should be reported to the local board of health to initiate examination of housing for sources of lead.

Reduction of the body burden of lead is accomplished by use of chelating agents, principally the calcium salt of EDTA, dimercaprol, and D-penicillamine (Cuprimine). A new oral chelating agent, dimercaptosuccinic acid (DMSA), is undergoing clinical trials. The lead mobilization test is used to determine the size of the "chelatable" pool of lead. In this test, administration of a calculated dose of chelating agent, usually EDTA, induces a lead diuresis which is then compared to the dose of chelating agent. The test is positive when greater than 1 μg lead is excreted per milligram of chelating agent administered per 24 h. The mobilization test can be useful in determining the utility of chelation therapy in patients with borderline lead levels or in those patients who have been previously treated.

In acute encephalopathy, double therapy (dimercaprol and EDTA) is used until blood lead levels are less than 40 μg/dL. Urine flow must be established, and even in the presence of cerebral edema, fluids must be sufficient to produce a lead diuresis. Mannitol and dexamethasone can reduce cerebral edema, but removal of the metal is essential. In symptomatic adults and children, double therapy should be used for 5 days at EDTA doses of 0.5 to 1 g/m² up to 1.5 g/m² daily. If further chelation is required, a minimum interval of 48 to 72 h should intervene between courses of therapy. The D-penicillamine dose is 20 to 40 mg/kg per day, not to exceed 1 g. Adverse effects, particularly allergy, may be reduced by beginning therapy with one-quarter of the total dose for 1 week, then doubling and redoubling the dose until full dose is reached. D-Penicillamine can be administered for 3 to 6 months until the body lead burden is depleted. Only D-penicillamine and, to a lesser extent, EDTA remove lead directly from bone. If EDTA is indicated, as many separate 5-day courses as are needed may be given provided that the total safe dose is not exceeded and proper intervals between courses are observed.

MERCURY

SOURCE Human beings may encounter mercury in an inorganic (elemental or mercuric salt) or an organic (usually methyl) form. All three are toxic, but organic mercury is most widespread and potentially dangerous. Elemental mercury is used in thermometers, sphygmomanometer, and dental amalgams. It is volatile at room temperature and rapidly oxidized to mercuric mercury when exposed to oxygen. Toxicity usually occurs from inhalation of mercury vapor during industrial exposure. Mercuric salts are found in topical medicines, as catalytic agents in the manufacture of plastics, as cathartics (e.g., Calomel), and in foodstuffs. Toxicity is usually through gastrointestinal exposure. Organic mercury is found in paints, fungicides, seeds, foods, medicines, and cosmetic agents. Because mercuric salts are methylated by bacteria in the environment, large amounts of methyl mercury are formed from inorganic mercury waste as occurred in the methyl mercury epidemic in Minamata Bay, Japan, following ingestion of mercury-laden fish.

METABOLISM Elemental mercury is absorbed primarily as vapor through the lungs, where 80 to 100 percent of inhaled mercury enters the bloodstream through the alveoli. Gastrointestinal absorption of elemental mercury is low. Volatilization of ingested elemental mercury is reduced by oxidation of surface mercury to mercuric sulphide, preventing vapor formation from the residual metallic mass. Absorbed mercury vapor is lipid-soluble and readily crosses the blood-brain barrier and the placenta. However, it is rapidly oxidized to the mercuric form, which combines readily with sulfhydryl groups of proteins and has limited mobility. Thus, an acute single exposure contributes to brain mercury levels more than similar doses ingested chronically. Excretion is similar to that of mercuric salts. Small amounts of mercury vapor may be excreted via the lungs. In humans, the half-life of elemental mercury is approximately 60 days.

Inorganic mercury is absorbed through the gastrointestinal tract and percutaneously. High intake produces corrosive effects on the gastrointestinal tract with consequent increased absorption. Normal uptake is less than 10 percent of an intravenous dose. Mercuric salts accumulate primarily in the kidney, but are distributed to the liver, erythrocytes, bone marrow, spleen, lung, intestine, and skin. Excretion is via the urine and feces. The half-life of inorganic mercury is approximately 40 days.

Organic (methyl) mercury is readily absorbed through the intestines and the skin. Short-chain alkyl and methyl mercury penetrate the erythrocyte membrane and bind to hemoglobin. The ratio of red blood cell to plasma methyl mercury may be as high as 9:1. Because of its high lipid solubility, methyl mercury freely passes the placenta and blood-brain barrier and enters breast milk. Organic mercury also concentrates in the kidneys and the central nervous system. Metallothionein synthesis is induced by mercury exposure, the augmented protein concentrations exerting a protective effect against tissue damage. Excretion is complex. A portion is excreted through renal tubules into urine, but this represents only 1 percent of the body burden. Methyl mercury is also acetylated in the liver or may be conjugated with cysteine or glutathione. The *N*-acetyl-homocysteine–methyl mercury complex then enters the enterohepatic circulation and is ultimately excreted in the urine. The half-life of organic mercury in humans is about 70 days.

CLINICAL TOXICOLOGY Mercury is a poison of enzymes with an affinity for thiol groups. Acute metallic mercury (vapor) poisoning causes inflammation of large and small airways with interstitial pneumonitis leading to respiratory failure. The rapid uptake of mercury vapor into the central nervous system produces associated symptoms including tremor and increased excitability. Chronic mercury vapor poisoning primarily affects the central nervous system. Initial symptoms include lassitude, anorexia, weight loss, and gastrointestinal disturbances. Increasing exposure produces the characteristic intention tremor of mercury poisoning. Initially peripheral, the tremor may become generalized and is accompanied by mercurial *erethism* (timidity, memory loss, insomnia, excitability, and, in severe cases, delirium). This neurologic picture in felt-hat workers exposed to mercury vapor and mercuric salts led to the phrase "mad as a hatter."

While chronic inorganic mercury poisoning also produces the above neurologic constellation, excessive salivation, loosening of the teeth, gingivitis, and stomatitis are also seen. When applied to the skin, mercuric salts may cause hypersensitivity reactions ranging from mild erythema to full-blown exfoliative dermatitis. Acrodynia, or pink disease, occurs in young children and may be mistaken for Kawasaki's disease. Symptoms include generalized rash, irritability, photophobia, hypertrichosis, and profuse perspiration associated with desquamation of the feet and hands. There may be hyperkeratosis of the skin and swelling of the hands and feet.

Acute inorganic mercury poisoning is characterized by the corrosive effect of mercuric salts on the gastrointestinal tract. Mild or, more often, severe gastrointestinal inflammation produces nausea, vomiting, hematemesis, and abdominal pain followed by tenesmus, bloody diarrhea, and necrosis of intestinal mucosa. Acute fluid loss in massive overdose can produce shock and death. Acute inorganic mercury poisoning causes acute tubular necrosis, while chronic inorganic mercury poisoning produces a nephrotic syndrome.

Acute organic mercury poisoning cannot be distinguished from the chronic form. Rather, the long half-life coupled with a latent period before onset of symptoms due to acute exposure produce a syndrome which varies more with species and gestational age than with duration of exposure. Prenatal poisoning produces cerebral palsy due to cortical and cerebellar atrophy. Postnatal poisoning causes paresthesias, headache, pain, visual, hearing, and speech disorders, neurasthenia, loss of memory and coordination, erethism, spasticity, paralysis, stupor, coma, and death. These neurologic abnormalities are often permanent.

The daily intake of methyl mercury should not exceed 100 parts per billion. In several studies of normal blood and urinary mercury levels, more than 90 percent of samples showed urinary mercury below 10 μg per liter. Blood mercury levels were below 20 ng/mL in 89 percent of samples. Thus, blood mercury levels above 35 ng/mL and urine mercury levels above 150 μg per liter are abnormal. Abnormalities may, of course, be associated with somewhat lower concentrations depending on when exposure occurred. Symptoms may be seen with blood mercury levels above 500 ng/mL and urine mercury levels above 600 μg per liter.

TREATMENT Treatment is aimed at reducing the absorption of mercury, protecting susceptible tissues from distribution of absorbed mercury, and eliminating absorbed mercury. In the case of ingestion of mercuric salts, initial treatment consists of removing mercury from the stomach by inducing emesis or by gastric lavage. Polythiol resins have been shown effective in binding mercury in the gastrointestinal tract. Activated charcoal, however, does not bind metals.

Generally, chelation therapy is indicated in mercury poisoning when high urine or blood mercury levels are present. Chelating agents with active mono- or dithiol groups are most effective. These include dimercaprol and D-penicillamine. The experimental oral chelating agent dimercaptosuccinic acid shows promise. Because D-penicillamine and dimercaprol form a toxic complex, they should not be used together. In acute inorganic mercury poisoning, dimercaprol should be used at a dose not exceeding 24 mg/kg per 24 h intramuscularly, in divided doses. Generally, therapy should not exceed 5 days at a time but can be reinstituted after a suitable rest period. D-Penicillamine can be used in the treatment of inorganic mercury poisoning but *N*-acetyl-DL-penicillamine is recommended as equally effective, stable, and less toxic. The dose is 30 mg/kg per day in two to three divided doses. Peritoneal dialysis and hemodialysis have also been used with some success. Neither is as effective as chelation therapy but may be useful in the presence of renal failure.

In chronic inorganic mercury poisoning, the use of dimercaprol does not appear to be beneficial in reducing the mercury burden and either *N*-acetyl-DL-penicillamine or D-penicillamine are the drugs of choice. *N*-acetyl-DL-penicillamine also appears to have an advantage in organic mercury poisoning and is more effective than either dimercaprol or EDTA. The goal of therapy is the reduction of symptoms and enhanced urinary excretion of mercury.

THALLIUM

SOURCE Thallium has been used as an insecticide and rodenticide, as a catalyst in fireworks, in optical lenses, in industry as an alloy, and in cardiac perfusion imaging. Accidental as well as purposeful ingestions of thallium occur. Epidemic poisoning has followed the ingestion of grain impregnated with thallium. Thallium is available as iodide, sulfate, and nitrate salts.

METABOLISM Thallium is absorbed percutaneously, by inhalation, and by oral ingestion. It has a large volume of distribution of 10 liters per kilogram with distribution to body organs including kidney, pancreas, spleen, liver, lung, muscles, and brain. Thallium is bound to sulfhydryl groups on mitochondrial membranes at intracellular sites. The elimination half-life is variable ranging from 3 to 15 days. The major pathway of elimination in human beings is through the urine, conforming to first-order pharmacokinetics; 3 percent of a dose is eliminated per day.

Thallium interferes with oxidative phosphorylation by inhibition of ATPase. Pathologic findings at postmortem include cerebral edema, loss of myelin in peripheral nerves, fatty infiltration of the liver, and degenerative changes in the myocardium.

CLINICAL TOXICOLOGY Severe poisoning occurs following a single ingested dose greater than 1 g or 8 mg/kg. Death has occurred following an ingested dose of 15 mg/kg.

Immediate signs and symptoms (occurring within 3 to 4 h of ingestion) include nausea and vomiting, abdominal pain, diarrhea, and hematochezia. Intermediate manifestations (within 1 week of ingestion) include involvement of the central nervous system with confusion, psychosis, choreoathetosis, organic brain syndrome, convulsions, and coma. Peripheral neurologic involvement is both motor and sensory and includes paresthesias, myalgias, weakness, tremor, and ataxia. Autonomic manifestations are less common and include tachycardia, hypertension, and salivation. Ophthalmologic abnormalities include neuritis, ophthalmoplegia, ptosis, strabismus, and cranial nerve palsies. Late manifestations (occurring 2 to 4 weeks after ingestion) include diffuse hair loss (with sparing of pubic and body hair and the lateral one-third of the eyebrows) with regrowth occurring as body burden decreases over time. Residual effects include memory loss, ataxia, tremor, and foot drop.

LABORATORY FINDINGS Thallium is radiopaque and is evident on an x-ray of the abdomen. Thallium levels with severe ingestion range from 30 to 200 μg/dL, and thallium excretion in excess of 10 to 20 μg per 24 h. The electroencephalogram (EEG) is diffusely abnormal, and peripheral nerve conduction may be delayed.

TREATMENT Therapeutic modalities include gastrointestinal decontamination, enhanced renal excretion by potassium chloride, hemodialysis, and the antidote diethyldithiocarbamate (Dithiocarb). Gastric lavage or ipecac syrup is indicated within 4 to 6 h of acute ingestion. Adequacy of removal of thallium can be documented by follow-up abdominal x-ray. Prussian blue absorbs thallium in the gastrointestinal tract by exchanging potassium for thallium on its crystal lattice network thereby preventing absorption. The oral dose is 250 mg/kg, administered once. Mannitol or magnesium citrate are used as a laxative to enhance gastrointestinal removal. The efficacy of this treatment has been demonstrated by a 50 percent shortening in serum half-life.

Potassium chloride–induced renal excretion of thallium occurs through the exchange of potassium for thallium thereby releasing thallium from tissue sites into blood and augmenting urinary excretion. Two- to threefold increases in urinary excretion of thallium have been demonstrated with quantitative thallium excretion rates of 20 to 30 mg per day. Efficacy of this method has been documented by shortening half-life in human studies, but this therapy has risks, and the amount of thallium removed as compared to the total ingested dose is small. Peritoneal dialysis removes 15 to 20 mg of thallium per day and hemodialysis 8 mg for each 8 h of dialysis. Prolonged hemodialysis can remove up to 25 mg of thallium per day, and while an increase over endogenous clearance, the total amount removed is relatively small. Hemoperfusion with activated charcoal may be useful.

Diethyldithiocarbamate has been advocated for early use in overdose because it leads to increased thallium blood levels and a two- to threefold increase in thallium excretion. However, Dithiocarb-thallium complexes diffuse into the brain with subsequent clinical and EEG worsening; therefore diethyldithiocarbamate is contraindicated in thallium intoxication.

CHELATING AGENTS

Chelating agents are used to bind toxic metals in stable, cyclic compounds with relatively low toxicity and enhanced renal excretion.

DIMERCAPROL (BAL) Dimercaprol was first developed during World War II as an antidote for the arsenical war gas lewisite; its chelating capacity is due to its four sulfhydryl groups which bind in a complex to polyvalent metal ions. Affinity of dimercaprol for metals is strong enough to reverse a significant portion of toxic metal enzyme binding. Dimercaprol diffuses well into erthrocytes and enhances fecal as well as urinary metal excretion. It is given intramuscularly in oil every 4 to 8 h in a dose of 12 to 24 mg/kg per 24 h. Toxicity includes mild febrile reactions, nausea, headache, lacrimation, conjunctivitis, salivation, and rhinorrhea. The drug emits a strong sulfide odor, and patients may complain of metallic taste. Contraindications to dimercaprol include glucose 6-phosphate dehydrogenase deficiency, allergy to peanut oil, and concurrent use of medicinal iron, which forms a toxic complex with dimercaprol.

ETHYLENEDIAMINETETRAACETATE (EDTA) Because the sodium salt of EDTA can produce profound hypocalcemia, only the calcium disodium salt should be used in therapy of metal poisoning. EDTA forms a sexadentate complex with divalent cations exchanging one atom of calcium for each metal ion. It enhances urinary excretion of lead twenty- to fiftyfold but also increases excretion of zinc and, to a lesser extent, iron. It does not enter the erythrocytes but removes metals from the extracellular compartment. Oral administration is contraindicated because it enhances absorption of metals from the gastrointestinal tract. The drug is given parenterally either by constant intravenous infusion or intramuscular injection in a dose of 500 to 1000 mg/m^2 per day. The drug can be used safely in conjunction with other chelating agents. Toxicity increases after 4 to 5 days of administration with concomitant reduction in metal excretion; as a consequence, the drug is given for several "courses" of from 3 to 5 days each.

Toxicity is principally renal, dose-related, and usually reversible. It can be reduced by maintaining adequate urine flow. During treatment renal function should be carefully monitored.

D-PENICILLAMINE D-Penicillamine (Cuprimine) is the only commercially available oral chelating agent. Not presently licensed by the Federal Drug Administration for treatment of lead poisoning, it is licensed for use in the treatment of rheumatoid arthritis, Wilson's disease, and cystinuria. Nevertheless, there is extensive experience in its use in chelation of other metals. The *N*-acetyl form is particularly helpful in the treatment of inorganic mercury poisoning.

Penicillamine enhances excretion of heavy metals in the urine by an unclear mechanism. The drug is given orally in a dose of 20 to 40 μg/kg per day. By initiating therapy at low doses (usually 25 percent of the anticipated maximum dose) and gradually increasing the dose, the frequency of side effects can be reduced substantially.

Side effects may be seen in up to 20 percent of patients receiving D-penicillamine. The most common resemble penicillin hypersensitivity and include rash, fevers, thrombocytopenia, and leukopenia. Rare side effects include autoimmune hemolytic anemia and Stevens-Johnson syndrome. Anorexia, nausea, sleep disturbances, and urinary frequency may be seen occasionally. Nephrotoxicity is reported in adults receiving large doses and in one case has been reported in a child. Patients receiving D-penicillamine should, therefore, be carefully monitored for signs of renal, hematologic, or allergic side effects.

DEFEROXAMINE Deferoxamine (Desferal) binds iron in a 9:1 molar ratio. It exerts its effect primarily on free iron in the plasma. It does not chelate iron bound to hemoglobin in red blood cells, iron present in hemosiderin or ferritin, or, finally, iron in myoglobin or the cytochrome oxidase systems of the body. The complex ferrioxamine, stable and resistant to dissociation in water, is soluble and readily excreted in the urine. The dose may be given intramuscularly or intravenously at a dose of 50 mg/kg (up to 2 g per dose) or 1 to 2 g per dose in an adult not to exceed 6 to 8 g total dose per day. Intravenous deferoxamine should be administered slowly not exceeding 15 mg/kg per hour, thereby preventing hypotension.

REFERENCES

Arsenic

FOWLER BA, WEISSBERG JB: Arsine poisoning. N Engl J Med 291:1171, 1974
HEYMAN A et al: Peripheral neuropathy caused by arsenical intoxication. N Engl J Med 254:402, 1956
MASSEY EW et al: Arsenic: Homicidal intoxication. South Med J 77:848, 1984
PETERSON RG, RUMACK BH: D-Penicillamine therapy of acute arsine poisoning. J Pediatr 91:661, 1977

Cadmium

FRIBERG L et al: *Cadmium in the environment*, 2d ed. Cleveland, CRC Press, 1974
——— et al: *Handbook on the Toxicology of Metals*. Amsterdam, Elsevier, 1979
MORGAN WD: New ways of measuring cadmium in man. Nature 282:673, 1979

Iron

LACOUTURE PG et al: Emergency assessment of severity in iron overdose by clinical and laboratory methods. J Pediatr 99:89, 1981
PROPPER R, NATHAN D: Clinical removal of iron. Ann Rev Med 35:509, 1982
ROBOTHAM JL, LIETMAN PS: Acute iron poisoning. Am J Dis Child 134:874, 1980
WHITTEN CF et al: Studies in iron poisoning: Parts I and II. Pediatrics 36:322, 1965, 38:102, 1966

Lead

BYERS RK: Lead poisoning: Review of the literature and report on 45 cases. Pediatrics 23:585, 1959
CANTAROW A, TRUMPER M: *Lead Poisoning*. Baltimore, Williams & Wilkins, 1944
CARNOW B (ed): *Health Effects of Occupational Lead and Arsenic Exposure, A Symposium*. Chicago, US Department of Health, Education, and Welfare, 1976
CDC: *Preventing Lead Poisoning in Young Children*, US Department of Health and Human Services, 1985
CHISOLM JJ JR: The use of chelating agents in the treatment of acute and chronic lead intoxication in childhood. J Pediatr 73:1, 1968
NATIONAL ACADEMY OF SCIENCES: *Lead in the Human Environment*, A Report Prepared by the Committee on Lead in the Human Environment, Environmental Studies Board, Commission on Natural Resources, National Research Council, Washington, DC, 1980
KEHOE RA: The metabolism of lead in man in health and disease. The Harben Lectures, 1960. J R Inst Pub Health 24:1, 101; 129; 177, 1961
WALDRON HA, STOFEN D: *Sub-Clinical Lead Poisoning*. New York, Academic, 1974

Mercury

FRIBERG L, VOSTAL J (eds): *Mercury in the Environment*. Cleveland, CRC Press, 1972
NATIONAL ACADEMY OF SCIENCES: *An Assessment of Mercury in the Environment*, Washington, DC, 1978
WHO Environmental Health Criteria, Mercury, Geneva, World Health Organization, 1976

Thallium

BANK WJ et al: Thallium poisoning. Arch Neurol 26:456, 1972
SADDIQUE A, PETERSON CD: Thallium poisoning. Vet Hum Toxicol 25:1, 1983
VAN KESTEREN RG et al: Thallium intoxication: An evaluation of therapy. Intensivmed 17:293, 1980

173 TOBACCO

JOHN H. HOLBROOK

Tobacco smoke is a ubiquitous personal and environmental pollutant. Although tobacco has been used in western culture for more than 400 years, human inhalation of cigarette smoke is a twentieth century phenomenon with major medical and economic consequences. In industrialized nations cigarette smoking is the principal cause of preventable disease, disability, and premature death. In the United States the estimated costs for smoking-related medical care and loss of productivity exceed $55 billion per year.

Important changes in smoking trends are occurring in the United States. In general, there is less smoking. For example, annual per capita cigarette consumption in adults declined from its 1963 peak of 4345 cigarettes to a 1984 estimate of 3454 cigarettes. Between 1965 and 1983, the proportion of adult cigarette smokers in the United States declined from 52 to 36 percent of men and 34 to 29 percent of women (Table 173-1). There are 51 million current adult smokers and 36.1 million former smokers in the United States; the distribution of smokers between the sexes is approximately equal with 26.4 million men and 24.5 million women. Among teenagers, smoking is slightly more prevalent in females than in males. While consumption of cigar and pipe tobacco has decreased, use of smokeless tobacco has increased.

CIGARETTE SMOKE Large prospective epidemiologic studies have shown a strong association between cigarette smoking and several diseases. More than 4000 substances have been identified in cigarette smoke, including some that are pharmacologically active, antigenic, cytotoxic, mutagenic, and carcinogenic; these diverse biologic effects provide a framework for understanding the adverse consequences of smoking.

Cigarette smoke is a heterogeneous aerosol produced by incomplete combustion of the tobacco leaf. It is composed of gases and uncondensed vapors in which droplets are dispersed. Mainstream smoke emerges from the mouthpiece during puffing. Sidestream smoke is emitted between puffs at the burning cone and from the mouthpiece. The composition of the smoke is influenced by several factors including type of tobacco, temperature of combustion, length of the cigarette, porosity of the paper, additives, and filters. The major tobacco leaf constituents are carbohydrates, nonfatty organic acids, nitrogen-containing compounds, and resins. Cigarette temperatures vary greatly from 30°C at the mouthpiece to 900°C at the burning cone. In the presence of intense heat some tobacco constituents undergo thermic decomposition (pyrolysis). Volatile substances are distilled directly into the smoke. Unstable molecules recombine to generate new compounds (pyrosynthesis). Concentration of smoke constituents occurs as the smoke is filtered by unburnt tobacco and is redistilled by the burning cone. Some substances found in tobacco pass unchanged into cigarette smoke.

Approximately 92 to 95 percent of the total weight of mainstream smoke is present in a gas phase. Nitrogen, oxygen, and carbon dioxide account for 85 percent of the smoke's weight. The remaining gases, uncondensed vapors, and particulate matter are the substances of medical importance (Table 173-2). Mainstream smoke contains 0.3 to 3.3 billion particles per milliliter; the mean particle size is 0.2 to 0.5 μm, which is within the respirable range.

Because a pack-a-day cigarette smoker puffs more than 70,000 times a year, the membranes of the mouth, nose, pharynx, and tracheobronchial tree are exposed repetitively to tobacco smoke. Some constituents act directly on the membranes, while others are absorbed into the blood or are dissolved in saliva and swallowed.

PHARMACOLOGY Tissue and organ system responses to cigarette smoke inhalation are multiple and complex. Most studies in humans have dealt with exposure to whole smoke or to selected constituents thought to pose the greatest risk to health, such as nicotine and carbon monoxide. Relatively little is known about the individual effects and interactions of other potentially toxic smoke constituents that are present in low concentrations.

TABLE 173-1 Estimated percentage of current cigarette smokers in the United States

Year	Percent current smokers 20 years of age and over		
	Females	Males	Both sexes
1965	34.1	52.4	42.7
1976	32.0	41.9	36.4
1980	29.4	38.3	33.6
1983	29.1	35.7	32.0

Nicotine, the component most characteristic of tobacco, is a highly toxic alkaloid that is both a ganglionic stimulant and depressant. Many of its complex effects are mediated by catecholamine release. Acute cardiovascular responses to nicotine observed in normal smokers include increases in systolic and diastolic blood pressure, heart rate, force of myocardial contraction, myocardial oxygen consumption, coronary artery blood flow, myocardial excitability, and peripheral vasoconstriction. Nicotine has also been shown to increase serum concentrations of glucose, cortisol, free fatty acids, and antidiuretic hormone and to increase platelet aggregation. Nicotine plays an important but not exclusive role in maintaining the smoking habit.

Carbon monoxide is a toxic gas that interferes with oxygen transport and utilization. Because cigarette smoke contains 2 to 6 percent carbon monoxide, smokers inhale concentrations as high as 400 parts per million (ppm) and develop elevated carboxyhemoglobin (COHb) levels. While the range of COHb found in smokers is 2 to 15 percent, levels for nonsmokers are near 1 percent. The average COHb level of moderate cigarette smokers is 5 percent. Carbon monoxide produces its adverse effects by reducing the amount of available oxyhemoglobin and myoglobin, and displacing the oxygen-hemoglobin dissociation curve to the left. Chronic, mild elevations of COHb due to smoking are a common cause of mild polycythemia and may produce subtle impairment of central nervous system function.

Cigarette smoke and its condensate are carcinogenic in several species of animals. The major identified carcinogens in cigarette smoke are polynuclear aromatic hydrocarbons, aromatic amines, and nitrosamines (Table 173-2). Cocarcinogens present in cigarette smoke, such as catechol, greatly enhance its carcinogenicity. The sister chromatid exchange rate, a sensitive indicator of mutagenic effects, is higher in the lymphocytes of smokers than in nonsmokers. Cigarette smoke condensate is also mutagenic in a microbial test system.

Potent pulmonary irritants and ciliotoxins are found in cigarette smoke (Table 173-2). These substances increase bronchial mucus secretion and mediate acute and chronic decreases in pulmonary and mucociliary function. Cigarette smoke also increases lung epithelial permeability.

EPIDEMIOLOGY Data from large prospective studies of populations in several countries show that cigarette-smoking men have 70 percent higher death rates than nonsmokers. This excess male mortality is present in all groups over the age of 35, but it is proportionately greatest in the age group 45 to 54. In a study of British physicians it was shown that 40 percent of 35-year-old men who smoked more than 25 cigarettes per day died before the age of 65, compared with 15 percent of nonsmokers in the same category. The excess mortality of female smokers has been somewhat less than that of male smokers, but recent trends suggest it is increasing. Smoking is responsible for an estimated 350,000 premature deaths each year in the United States. Coronary heart disease (CHD) is the chief contributor to smoking-related excess mortality. In the United States cigarette smokers experience more disability due to chronic illness and report 45 percent more days absent from work than do nonsmokers.

A strong dose-response relationship exists between tobacco exposure and excess mortality, as measured by age at onset of smoking, cigarette consumption, and smoke inhalation. Cessation of smoking is associated with a decrease in the excess mortality. These observations together with clinical, experimental, and pathologic studies indicate that smoking, per se, causes the excess mortality.

CHARACTERISTICS OF SMOKERS Demographic, anthropometric, physiologic, and laboratory features which distinguish cigarette smokers from nonsmokers are due both to baseline differences between these groups and to the effects of smoking. Smokers drink more alcohol, coffee, and tea than do nonsmokers. Their weight and blood pressure are slightly less and their heart rate is slightly faster than those of nonsmokers. In women the menopause comes earlier in smokers than in nonsmokers. Smokers have impaired maximum exercise performance and impaired immune systems. A markedly increased number of pulmonary alveolar macrophages is present in smokers, and the function and metabolism of these cells are abnormal. Serum thiocyanate concentrations are much higher in smokers. When compared with nonsmokers, smokers show small increases in the total white blood cell count and serum IgE levels as well as small decreases in leukocyte vitamin C levels, serum uric acid, and albumin. In smokers, the ratio of high-density lipoprotein cholesterol to low-density lipoprotein cholesterol is reduced. Smokers also show reduced levels of prostacyclin (PGI_2).

CLINICAL CORRELATIONS Individual patient risks due to cigarette smoking vary widely. Factors which influence these risks include the duration, intensity, and type of smoke exposure; genetically mediated susceptibility; occupational and environmental exposures; use of medication; and coexisting risk factors and diseases.

Cardiovascular disease Premature CHD is the most important medical consequence of cigarette smoking (see Chap. 189). Approximately 25 percent of the more than 500,000 CHD deaths occurring each year in the United States is attributable to smoking. Cigarette smoking is the most important modifiable CHD risk factor, acting both independently of and synergistically with other CHD risk factors. There is a dose-response relationship between CHD risk and cigarette smoking. The risk of CHD is 60 to 70 percent greater in male smokers than nonsmokers. Sudden death may be the first manifestation of CHD, and it is two to three times more likely to occur in 35- to 54-year-old male cigarette smokers than in nonsmokers. Women cigarette smokers are also at greater risk of developing CHD than nonsmokers, and the use of both cigarettes and oral contraceptives increases this risk approximately tenfold. Cessation of smoking is associated with decreased CHD mortality, an effect which is measurable within 1 year. Those who continue to smoke after an acute myocardial infarction are more likely to die from CHD than are those who quit smoking. Smokers who undergo coronary artery bypass surgery have increased perioperative mortality compared to nonsmokers. Cigarette smoking produces an imbalance between myocardial oxygen supply and demand, a decrease in the threshold for ventricular fibrillation, and an increase in platelet aggregation; avoidance of these effects may explain the prompt cardiac benefits of quitting smoking. Coronary atherosclerosis and intimal thickening of intramyocardial arteries and arterioles are more frequent in smokers than in nonsmokers.

Cigarette smoking is the most powerful risk factor for arteriosclerosis obliterans (see Chap. 195) and thromboangiitis obliterans (see Chap. 198). It also aggravates peripheral ischemia and may adversely affect peripheral bypass grafts. The mortality rate for atherosclerotic aortic aneurysm is greater in male smokers than nonsmokers. Cigarette smoking is not a risk factor for the development of hypertension; however, hypertensives who smoke appear to be at greater risk to develop malignant hypertension and renal artery stenosis. Cigarette smoking decreases cerebral blood flow and appears to increase the risk for cerebrovascular disease. Among women, subarachnoid hemorrhage is more likely to occur in smokers than nonsmokers, and the use of both cigarettes and oral contraceptives greatly increases this risk. Because of the association with chronic obstructive lung disease, cigarette smoking is an important factor leading to chronic pulmonary heart disease.

Cancer Cigarette smoking is the single most important cause of cancer mortality in the United States, accounting for 30 percent of all cancer deaths. In spite of the well-documented cause-and-effect relationship between cigarette smoking and lung cancer, more Americans continue to die from this cancer than from any other tumor (see Chap. 213). In 1985 an estimated 107,000 lung cancer deaths occurred in the United States; approximately 85 percent of these deaths were attributable to cigarette smoking. The risk of developing lung cancer is quantitatively related to cigarette smoke exposure. Men who smoke one pack a day increase their risk tenfold compared with nonsmokers; men who smoke two packs a day may increase their risk more than 25 times compared with nonsmokers. Asbestos workers who smoke cigarettes are at especially high risk for developing lung cancer. Cigarette consumption by women increased rapidly in the United States during the past 50 years, and lung cancer mortality is currently increasing at a faster rate in women than in men. Lung cancer has become the leading cause of cancer death among American women. Because 5-year survival rates for lung cancer are less than 10 percent, emphasis must be placed on prevention. Giving up cigarettes is associated with a gradual decline in the risk of developing lung cancer.

Cigarette smoking is causally associated in men and women with cancer of the larynx, oral cavity, and esophagus; alcohol consumption acts synergistically with cigarette smoking to increase the risk for these neoplasms. Carcinoma of the bladder, kidney, pancreas, stomach, and uterine cervix is also associated with cigarette smoking.

Respiratory disease Cigarette smoking is the major cause of chronic obstructive lung disease (COLD), that is, chronic bronchitis and emphysema (see Chap. 208). Of the estimated 60,000 deaths from COLD that occurred in the United States in 1983, approximately 85 percent were attributable to smoking, and many of these deaths were preceded by prolonged respiratory disability. There is a dose-response relationship between COLD death rates and cigarette smoking. Depending upon the extent of smoke exposure, male cigarette smokers experience from 4 to 25 times higher mortality secondary to COLD than do nonsmokers. Although the death rate from COLD among female smokers is somewhat lower than among male smokers, it is increasing much more rapidly in female than in male smokers. Chronic cough, sputum production, and breathlessness are much more common in smokers. Smokers are more likely than nonsmokers to show abnormalities in a number of pulmonary function tests including measurements of elastic recoil, airflow in large and small airways, and diffusing capacity. Mild airflow obstruction in small airways may be present even in teenage smokers. When compared with continuing smokers, ex-smokers experience a decrease in mortality from COLD, a decrease in prevalence of pulmonary symptoms, and a slowing of the rate of decline of lung function to approximately that seen in age-matched nonsmokers. Chronic inhalation of pulmonary irritants and ciliotoxins (Table 173-2) may contribute to the development of COLD. Studies of the pathogenesis of emphysema suggest that smoking results in an excess of pulmonary

TABLE 173-2 Selected cigarette smoke constituents

Substance	Effect
PARTICULATE PHASE	
"Tar"*	Carcinogen
Polynuclear aromatic hydrocarbons	Carcinogens
Nicotine	Ganglionic stimulator and depressor, cocarcinogen
Phenol	Cocarcinogen and irritant
Cresol	Cocarcinogen and irritant
β-Naphthylamine	Carcinogen
N-Nitrosonornicotine	Carcinogen
Benzo[a]pyrene	Carcinogen
Trace metals (e.g., nickel, arsenic, polonium 210)	Carcinogens
Indole	Tumor accelerator
Carbazole	Tumor accelerator
Catechol	Cocarcinogen
GAS PHASE	
Carbon monoxide	Impairs oxygen transport and utilization
Hydrocyanic acid	Ciliotoxin and irritant
Acetaldehyde	Ciliotoxin and irritant
Acrolein	Ciliotoxin and irritant
Ammonia	Ciliotoxin and irritant
Formaldehyde	Ciliotoxin and irritant
Oxides of nitrogen	Ciliotoxin and irritant
Nitrosamines	Carcinogen
Hydrazine	Carcinogen
Vinyl chloride	Carcinogen

* *The aggregate of particulate matter in cigarette smoke after subtracting nicotine and moisture.*

proteases, which may produce pulmonary damage. The damage is apparently mediated via release of elastase from increased numbers of lung leukocytes and partial inactivation of pulmonary antiproteases by oxidants present in smoke. For most people in the United States cigarette smoking is a more important cause of COLD than are occupational or environmental factors; however, factors such as cotton dust exposure may act independently or conjointly with smoking to produce COLD. In a rare disorder, homozygous α_1-antitrypsin deficiency, smoking greatly accelerates the tendency to panacinar emphysema; furthermore, smoking may play an additive role in individuals heterozygous for this state.

Cigarette smoking has been associated with an increased incidence of respiratory infections and deaths from pneumonia and influenza. Postoperative respiratory complications and spontaneous pneumothorax are also more common in smokers. Because tobacco smoke may increase airway obstruction, asthmatics should be urged not to smoke. Chronic stomatitis and chronic laryngitis occur more frequently in smokers than in nonsmokers.

Pregnancy Smoking may delay conception, and smoking during pregnancy may affect the fetus adversely. Infants whose mothers smoked during pregnancy weigh, on an average, 170 g less than infants whose mothers did not smoke. This effect probably results from impaired uteroplacental circulation. Maternal smoking during pregnancy increases the risk of spontaneous abortion, fetal death, neonatal death, and the sudden infant death syndrome. This increased risk may be much greater in pregnancies already at high risk due to other factors. Smoking by a woman during pregnancy may also adversely affect the long-term physical growth and intellectual development of the child.

Gastrointestinal disorders Gastric and duodenal ulcer disease is more prevalent in male than female cigarette smokers and causes more deaths in male smokers than in nonsmokers. Smoking impairs spontaneous and drug-induced healing of peptic ulcers, increases the likelihood of duodenal ulcer recurrence, inhibits pancreatic bicarbonate secretion, and decreases the pressure of esophageal and pyloric sphincters. Histamine-2-receptor antagonist inhibition of nocturnal gastric secretion is also prevented by smoking.

Involuntary smoke inhalation Indoor atmospheres and other confined spaces are often contaminated by tobacco smoke which is inhaled involuntarily by both smokers and nonsmokers. Most of the atmospheric pollutants arise from sidestream smoke. It contains greater concentrations of many smoke constituents than does mainstream smoke, but since sidestream smoke is diluted in a large volume of air, the smoke exposure from involuntary inhalation is less than that associated with smoking.

Initially, involuntary or passive smoking was thought to cause primarily an irritant effect such as ocular burning. It is now recognized as an important cause of air pollution. Approximately two-thirds of the adults in one survey reported some involuntary smoke exposure. The levels of smoke constituents or their metabolites measured in nonsmokers may be comparable to those found in ''light'' smokers. Parental smoking in the home is associated with an increased risk of respiratory illness in infants and impaired development of lung function in children. Asymptomatic nonsmokers who are chronically exposed to smoke-contaminated air may develop small-airways dysfunction. Several studies suggest that passive smoking increases the risk for lung cancer. In addition, patients with symptomatic CHD or COLD may experience exacerbation of symptoms when exposed to smoke-contaminated air.

Drug interactions Tobacco smoke constituents induce hepatic microsomal enzyme systems that are important in the metabolism of many drugs. For example, cigarette smoking increases the metabolism of propranolol, propoxyphene, and theophylline. Smokers may also demonstrate decreased insulin absorption compared to nonsmokers. With smoking cessation, adjustment of drug dose may be necessary.

TYPES OF SMOKING During the past 20 years the amount of tar and nicotine delivered by cigarettes made in the United States decreased by more than 50 percent. In 1980 the average American cigarette delivered 1 mg nicotine and 14 mg tar. The paucity of scientific data concerning the relative risks of lower-tar and -nicotine cigarettes compared with higher-tar and -nicotine cigarettes is of concern, because filter-tipped cigarettes and lower-tar and -nicotine cigarettes now account for more than 90 and 50 percent of sales, respectively. Lung cancer and laryngeal cancer are the only tobacco-related diseases for which the use of lower-tar and -nicotine cigarettes has been shown to result in risk reduction, compared with the use of higher-tar and -nicotine cigarettes; however, compared with not smoking or quitting, the benefits are minimal. Consumers who choose lower-tar and -nicotine cigarettes and then smoke a larger number of cigarettes or inhale more frequently or deeply may actually increase their exposure to harmful substances. There is also concern because unidentified flavoring agents are added to these cigarettes to enhance consumer acceptance. Their presence represents an undefined risk for both active and passive smokers.

Cigar and pipe smokers usually inhale less smoke than cigarette smokers, presumably because the alkaline pH of cigar and pipe tobacco makes it more irritating to the respiratory tract. The smoke exposure and overall mortality rates of pipe and cigar smokers in the United States are substantially less than those of cigarette smokers. Death rates of cigarette, cigar, and pipe smokers are approximately equal for carcinoma of the oral cavity, larynx, and esophagus, sites where exposures to cigarette, cigar, and pipe smoke are similar. The mortality rates of most cigar and pipe smokers for cancer at other sites, CHD, and COLD are not greatly elevated above the rates of nonsmokers, but cigar and pipe smokers who inhale consistently may experience adverse health effects comparable with those of cigarette smokers. The use of smokeless tobacco increases the risk for oral and pharyngeal cancer and may produce plasma nicotine levels comparable to those of smokers.

CESSATION OF SMOKING Psychosocial forces lead to initiation of smoking, especially among teenagers. Later, drug addiction and psychological factors help maintain dependence on tobacco. It is estimated that more than 36 million people in the United States have stopped smoking; 95 percent of these succeeded without formal assistance. Many long-term smokers quit because of smoking-related health problems. This seems to explain the observation that the death rate of men smoking more than 20 cigarettes a day was somewhat higher in the months immediately after quitting than that of continuing smokers. Thereafter, a gradual decline in death rates was observed in ex-smokers. Ten or more years after quitting, the death rate of those who had smoked more than 20 cigarettes a day decreased about two-thirds, and the death rate of individuals who had smoked 20 cigarettes a day or less was about the same as that of nonsmokers. Ex-smokers usually experience prompt symptomatic improvement. On the average they also gain approximately 5 lb.

In the United States more than 80 percent of cigarette smokers would like to stop smoking. Many self-care and organized programs are available to assist these individuals. Organized programs employ several techniques including instruction, counseling, withdrawal clinics, behavioral modification, hypnosis, aversive conditioning, self-monitoring, and drug therapy. In these programs 1-year abstinence rates of 20 to 30 percent are common. Relapse usually occurs during the 3-month interval after quitting. Successful programs emphasize maintenance of the nonsmoking state during this critical period.

Although only 10 percent of physicians smoke, a minority of patients report receiving advice from their physician to quit. Controlled trials have shown that physician counseling increases long-term smoking cessation rates. Polls also show that patients are inadequately informed about the hazards of smoking. All smokers should be encouraged to quit, especially those in high-risk groups with chronic pulmonary disease, coronary artery disease, and pregnancy. Physicians can help their smoking patients in the following manner:

1 Obtain a quantitative smoking history.
2 Explain the health risks in a personally relevant fashion.
3 Emphasize the benefits associated with cessation.
4 Advise and assist the patient to quit smoking.
5 Provide self-help reading materials.
6 Consider referring the patient to a formal treatment program.
7 Support the patient in a maintenance program.

A nicotine-containing chewing gum, which helps alleviate withdrawal symptoms, may be a useful adjunct in medically supervised programs. Patients who are unable or unwilling to stop cigarette smoking should be assisted to reduce their smoke exposure by smoking fewer cigarettes, inhaling less, taking fewer puffs, and leaving a longer stub.

Political, social, and cultural forces play a critical role in the individual decision to start or stop smoking. For this reason, physicians should lead and support efforts to increase tobacco excise taxes, to eliminate all tobacco advertisements and promotional activities, and to ban smoking in public places.

Ultimately, primary smoking prevention in the pediatric and adolescent age groups may be the most effective program. Young people who have been trained to resist social pressures, who understand the consequences of smoking to their health, and who appreciate the difficulty of quitting are less likely to start smoking.

REFERENCES

HOLBROOK JH et al: Cigarette smoking and cardiovascular disease. A statement for health professionals by a Task Force appointed by the Steering Committee of the American Heart Association. Circulation 70:1114A, 1984

LOEB LA et al: Smoking and lung cancer: An overview. Cancer Res 44:5940, 1984

REPACE JL, LOWREY AH: A quantitative estimate of nonsmoker's lung cancer risk from passive smoking. Environ Int 11:3, 1985

US DEPARTMENT OF HEALTH, EDUCATION, AND WELFARE: *Smoking and Health: A Report of the Surgeon General.* DHEW(PHS) Publication no 79-50066, 1979

US DEPARTMENT OF HEALTH AND HUMAN SERVICES: *The Health Consequences of Smoking: Cancer. A Report of the Surgeon General.* DHHS(PHS) Publication no 82-50179, 1982

———: *The Health Consequences of Smoking: Cardiovascular Disease. A Report of the Surgeon General.* DHHS(PHS) Publication no 84-50204, 1983

———: *The Health Consequences of Smoking: Chronic Obstructive Lung Disease. A Report of the Surgeon General.* DHHS(PHS) Publication no 84-50205, 1984

174 ELECTRICAL INJURIES

JAMES F. WALLACE

EPIDEMIOLOGY Since the first human fatality from accidental electrocution was reported in 1879, electrical injury has become progressively more common. In recent years, nearly 4000 electricity-related injuries have occurred annually in the United States, and major electrical burns have constituted nearly 5 percent of all admissions to burn centers. There are approximately 1000 deaths each year from electric current accidents, while another 200 persons die as a result of being struck by lightning. Electrical injuries occur most commonly among agricultural workers, utility pole linemen, crane and heavy equipment operators, and construction workers who come into contact with high-tension current, but nearly a third result from accidents in the home or other settings including the hospital with its many electrically powered instruments and appliances.

PATHOGENESIS For an electric current to flow, there must be a closed pathway or circuit, and a difference in potential or voltage must exist between two points in this completed circuit. The flow of current is directly related to the voltage difference and inversely proportional to the electrical resistance between two points in the circuit (Ohm's law). High-resistance paths allow relatively small currents to flow, while low resistances permit large currents to flow. When the voltage is very high, the flow of current will likewise be relatively great, unless the resistance is increased proportionally to the voltage; however, if the potential difference between the two points can be minimized, the current flow can also be minimized regardless of resistance.

Although the end result of passage of an electric current through the human body is unpredictable in the individual case, many factors are known to influence the nature and severity of electrical injuries. Body tissues vary considerably in their resistance to the flow of current, with conductivity being roughly proportional to water content. Bone and skin offer relatively high resistance, while blood, muscle, and nerve are good conductors. The resistance of normal skin can be lowered by moisture, and this factor alone can convert what might ordinarily be a mild injury to a fatal shock. Of importance at the time of contact is grounding which, if effective, can minimize the voltage difference between two points in the electric circuit and lower the intensity of current passing through the body. The pathway of the current through the body is also crucial. An accident involving passage of a current between a point of contact on the leg and the ground is less likely to be injurious than one between the head and the foot, in which the heart lies between the two poles of the circuit. Similarly, a small current leak which would be innocuous when applied to the surface of the intact body may result in a fatal arrhythmia when conducted directly to the heart via a low-resistance intracardiac catheter. Duration of contact also influences the outcome of electrical injury. Alternating current is much more dangerous than direct current, partly because of its ability to produce tetanic muscular contractions which prevent the victim from being able to release contact with the circuit. This is usually accompanied by sweating, which lowers skin resistance, allowing current of still greater intensity to pass into the body until fatal cardiac arrhythmia results.

In general, when sudden death occurs following low-voltage shock, it is due to the direct effect of relatively small amounts of current upon the myocardium resulting in ventricular fibrillation. With high-tension injury (greater than 1000 V), cardiac asystole and respiratory arrest occur probably as a result of injury to the medullary centers of the brain.

In addition, contact with high-intensity current may cause three types of thermal injuries. Current coursing externally to the body from the contact point to the ground may generate temperatures as high as 10,000°C and cause extensive carbonification of skin and immediately underlying tissues termed *arc* or *flash burns*. Such burns often ignite surrounding clothing or nearby objects which result in *flame burns*. Finally, there is injury due to the *direct heating* of tissues by electric current. As it traverses the skin, energy from current is converted into heat which produces coagulation necrosis at the points where it enters and exits from the skin as well as in striated muscle and blood vessels through which it passes. The associated vascular injury results in thromboses, often at sites distant from the body surface, and accounts for the observation that a greater amount of tissue destruction characteristically occurs in an electrical injury than is apparent on first inspection.

PATHOLOGY In patients who die immediately, autopsy findings are limited to burns and generalized petechial hemorrhages. If patients survive for a period of days or longer, postmortem examination reveals focal necrosis of bone, large blood vessels, muscle, peripheral nerves, spinal cord, or brain. Renal tubular necrosis may also be seen when acute renal failure follows extensive tissue destruction.

CLINICAL MANIFESTATIONS Immediately after a severe electrical shock, patients are usually comatose, apneic, and in circulatory collapse from ventricular fibrillation or cardiac standstill. If they survive this stage, they often are disoriented, combative, and frequently have seizures. Often they will be found to have fractures of bone caused either by convulsive muscular contractions accompanying the shock or from falls at the time of the accident. Hypovolemic shock often appears soon after high-tension electrical injury and is due to the rapid loss of fluid into areas of tissue damage, and from body surface burns. Hypotension, direct injury to the kidneys by the electric current, and renal tubular damage from myoglobin and hemoglobin pigments liberated during massive muscle necrosis and hemolysis may lead to acute renal failure.

Besides the extensive destruction of tissue occurring instantly in electrical burns, additional injury from ischemia produced by swelling of damaged tissues may appear later and is often accompanied by severe metabolic acidosis. Other serious complications are gastrointestinal hemorrhage from preexisting or acute Curling-type ulcers, neurogenic pulmonary edema, disseminated intravascular coagulation, and both anaerobic and aerobic infections originating in inadequately debrided necrotic muscle masses. Lightning injury may result in cerebral edema with coma lasting from several minutes to several days. Rupture of one or both tympanic membranes is seen in over half of lightning victims.

Late effects include various neurologic disabilities, visual disturbances, and the residual damage left by burns. Nervous system injuries are frequent and include peripheral neuropathies, incomplete transection of the spinal cord, and reflex sympathetic dystrophies, as well as late convulsive disorders and intractable headache. Psychological effects, particularly disturbances in memory and mood, are common in survivors of lightning strikes and may last for several months. The development of cataracts of one or both eyes has been reported to occur up to 3 years following electrical injury.

LABORATORY FINDINGS Immediately following major electrical injury the hematocrit is elevated and the plasma volume reduced, reflecting sequestration of fluid in the wound. Unless extensive flame burns are also present, serial determinations of either of these parameters provide a good means of monitoring the adequacy of fluid replacement therapy. Myoglobinuria is seen frequently in association with severe shocks, and when it persists following establishment of urine flow, usually indicates massive muscle injury. In many patients arterial blood pH determinations will indicate the presence of metabolic acidosis. Lumbar puncture may show elevated pressure associated with cerebral edema or bloody spinal fluid as a result of intracerebral hemorrhage. The electrocardiogram not infrequently shows tachycardia and minor ST-segment alterations which can persist for several weeks following injury. Unexplained acute hypokalemia leading to respiratory arrest and cardiac arrhythmias has developed in some patients between the second and fourth weeks following injury.

TREATMENT Removal of victims from contact with the current should be accomplished immediately without touching them directly. Rescuers should use a rubber sheet, a leather belt applied as a sling, a wooden pole, or other nonconductive material to detach them, and this should be preceded by cutting off the source of current when possible. If the victim is not breathing, mouth-to-mouth ventilation should be instituted at once. Although most cases who survive develop spontaneous respiration within half an hour, complete recovery after longer periods occurs often enough that respiratory support should be continued for at least 4 h. If there is no evidence of heartbeat, external cardiac massage should accompany ventilatory resuscitation. Persons struck by lightning frequently have cardiac asystole which responds to a manual blow to the chest, or which spontaneously resolves after several minutes of closed-chest cardiac massage and mouth-to-mouth resuscitation, while victims of low-voltage shocks will usually require defibrillation to restore heart action. During cardiopulmonary resuscitation and evacuation to the hospital, attention should be paid to possible broken bones and spinal cord injuries incurred at the time of the accident.

Subsequent hospital management of patients with electrothermal injuries requires considerable specialized care; whenever feasible, they should be referred to an appropriate burn or trauma unit.

Rapid institution of fluid and electrolyte therapy for hypovolemic shock and acidosis is essential, with guidelines being the patient's urine output, hematocrit, osmolality, central venous pressure, and arterial blood gases. Standard burn formulas should not be used to estimate fluid therapy since these are based only upon extent of body surface area injury and do not take into account the extensive damage to muscle which is usually present. Instead, fluid replacement principles used in the treatment of crush injury, which electrical injury closely resembles, should be followed. Large volumes of fluid, preferably lactated Ringer's solution, should be administered in order to maintain urine output greater than 50 mL/h. If myoglobinuria persists after adequate urine flow has been established, the use of furosemide or an osmotic diuretic such as mannitol along with alkalinization of the urine is indicated. Management of the electrical wound should include adequate debridement of necrotic tissue and often will require fasciotomy to prevent further ischemic injury. Anticlostridial prophylaxis, including tetanus toxoid and high doses of penicillin, should be administered to all severely injured patients, while topical antimicrobial chemotherapy with mafenide acetate or silver sulfadiazine may be useful in preventing or delaying infections in extensive surface burns. Survivors of the acute episode often require extensive treatment for infection, visceral injury, and delayed hemorrhage as devitalized tissues slough. If acute renal failure occurs, it should be managed as described in Chap. 219. Patients who remain comatose after being struck by lightning should undergo monitoring of intracranial pressure and cerebral perfusion and be treated for cerebral edema if it should develop.

PREVENTION Proper installation of appliances, grounding of telephone lines and radio and television aerials, and the use of rubber gloves and dry shoes when working with electric circuits should be routine. Unused wall sockets should be kept plugged and live extension cords not left unattended, particularly in households where there are young children. Electrical appliances used in bathrooms should be disconnected when not in use and never used in wet bathtubs. During a severe thunderstorm, refuge near hilltops, riverbanks, hedges, telephone poles, and trees should be avoided. The safest shelter is the closed house, while a closed automobile, cave, ditch, or even lying on the ground curled up with hands close together is relatively secure. In hospitalized patients, the hazard of ventricular fibrillation precipitated by minute current leaks conducted directly to the myocardium from monitoring equipment via pacemakers or intravascular manometric catheters should be more widely appreciated. Hospital personnel should be aware that, in addition to medical instruments, patient contact with two or more other power line–operated devices such as television sets, radios, electric razors, lamps, and especially electric beds can also result in electrocution if the heart lies within the current path through the patient. These hazards can be minimized by proper grounding of equipment *before* a patient is connected to the instrument, periodic measurement for leakage of current supplied by each device, and by instruction in the principles of electrical safety for hospital personnel who use the complex and dangerous equipment that is so much a part of modern medical practice.

REFERENCES

AMY BW et al: Lightning injury with survival in 5 patients. JAMA 253:243, 1985

APFELBERG DB et al: Pathophysiology and treatment of lightning injuries. J Trauma 14:453, 1974

BUDNICK LD: Bathtub-related electrocutions in the US, 1979–1982. JAMA 252:918, 1984

HUNT J et al: Acute electric burns: Current diagnostic and therapeutic approaches to management. Arch Surg 115:434, 1980

SAFFLE JR et al: Cataracts: Long-term complication of electrical injury. J Trauma 25:17, 1985

SOLEM L et al: The natural history of electrical injury. J Trauma 17:487, 1977

175 DROWNING AND NEAR-DROWNING

JAMES F. WALLACE

EPIDEMIOLOGY In the United States, drowning accounts for approximately 7000 fatalities per year and is the third leading cause of accidental death among all age groups, and the second among individuals aged 5 to 44 years. Although no national statistics are available, it has been estimated that as many as 48,000 persons annually are near-drowning victims: those who live at least temporarily following an immersion incident. Children and young adults are most often the victims, and nearly 80 percent are males. Other risk factors are epilepsy, mental retardation, and alcohol abuse. With the increasing popularity of boating and water sports in this country nearly half the population is at risk of drowning each year, especially during the summer months.

PATHOPHYSIOLOGY Ten to twenty percent of drowning victims have no evidence of water aspiration in their lungs at autopsy (''dry drowning''). Death is due to asphyxia secondary to reflex laryngospasm and glottic closure. It is probable that a similar number of near-drowning victims also do not aspirate. If ventilation is reestablished before they sustain irreversible anoxic brain damage, prompt and complete recovery can be anticipated.

When aspiration accompanies drowning (''wet drowning''), the clinical situation is further complicated by the amount of surrounding water that is introduced into the respiratory tract as well as by the solutes and solids contained in it. A severe pulmonary injury often occurs, resulting in persistent arterial hypoxia and metabolic acidosis even after ventilation has been restored.

In the past, an important distinction was made between the pathophysiology of saltwater and freshwater drowning with respect to changes in blood volume, serum electrolyte concentrations, and cardiovascular function. However, it has been established that the most important problem in human near-drowning is hypoxia and that the other disturbances are of considerably less significance in determining survival.

The mechanisms by which hypoxia develops in near-drowning with aspiration are often multiple: laryngospasm, bronchospasm, airway obstruction secondary to aspirated particulate matter, and pulmonary edema following prolonged hypoxia can take place regardless of the composition of the water aspirated, while other types of lung injury causing hypoxia depend upon the osmolar and chemical characteristics of the immersion fluid. Aspiration of seawater, which is hypertonic compared with blood and chemically irritating to the pulmonary alveolocapillary membrane, causes a rapid shift of plasma proteins and water from the circulation into the alveolar lumen. Continued perfusion of these nonventilated, edema-filled alveoli results in an intrapulmonary right-to-left shunt and arterial hypoxia. When hypotonic fresh water is aspirated, fluid is rapidly absorbed from the lung into the circulation. Injury to alveolar lining cells takes place, altering or destroying the properties of pulmonary surfactant that maintains surface tension, and leading to alveolar collapse. Ventilation-perfusion ratios change in these atelectatic areas of lung, and hypoxia is the result. Metabolic acidosis, which is present in as many as 70 percent of near-drowning victims, is a consequence of tissue hypoxia and may be severe.

Although changes in electrolyte concentrations occur, depending upon the type and volume of fluid aspirated, these disturbances are rarely life-threatening. Most persons who aspirate sufficient quantities to produce marked electrolyte abnormalities do not survive the immersion incident. Similarly, profound changes in circulating blood volume are unusual. However, hypovolemia requiring treatment may be seen in massive saltwater aspiration accompanied by shifts of fluid from the vascular space into the lung.

Although rarely of clinical significance, some hemolysis of red blood cells often takes place, especially with freshwater aspiration. Free hemoglobin may be found in the urine and blood, but the abnormality requires no specific therapy. Disseminated intravascular coagulation has been reported as a complication of freshwater near-drowning. It is thought that with extensive pulmonary injury, ''tissue factor'' in lung parenchyma and plasminogen activator from pulmonary endothelium are released, triggering the extrinsic clotting and fibrinolytic systems. Other pathophysiologic events in near-drowning include the development of renal failure secondary to acute tubular necrosis, probably due to the combined effects of hypoxia and hypotension, and neurologic deficits secondary to cerebral anoxia. Although the extent of the central nervous system injury tends to correlate with the duration of hypoxia, hypothermia accompanying the incident may be a moderating factor by reducing cerebral oxygen requirements. Complete neurologic recovery has been reported in victims submerged as long as 40 min in water temperatures less than 20°C.

CLINICAL MANIFESTATIONS The clinical features in near-drowning are variable and depend upon many factors including the amount and type of water aspirated and the promptness and effectiveness of treatment. Pulmonary and neurologic abnormalities usually predominate. Patients may present with mild cough and tachypnea, or with fulminant pulmonary edema. At least a third will require endotracheal intubation and some type of ventilatory therapy for the management of pulmonary injury. Instead of gradual recovery during the first 48 to 72 h of treatment, some patients will develop the adult respiratory distress syndrome, associated with progressive respiratory failure and reduction in lung compliance (see Chap. 216). Other pulmonary complications often include regional atelectasis due to aspirated particulate matter; secondary bacterial pneumonia; lung abscess; empyema; and injuries such as pneumothorax or pneumomediastinum sustained during resuscitation or related to ventilator therapy.

Early neurologic manifestations include seizures, especially during resuscitative efforts, and altered mental status, ranging from normal alertness to agitation, combativeness, or coma. Patients may present with speech, motor, or visual abnormalities or with more diffuse organic brain syndromes. Some of these neurologic deficits will improve gradually and resolve over several months. However, 5 to 20 percent of patients will have permanent sequelae, many of which prove ultimately fatal. Neurologic status usually does not continue to worsen after a near-drowning victim is admitted to the hospital unless there has been a preceding deterioration in pulmonary status. The possibility of unrecognized head trauma coincident with the drowning episode or a subdural hematoma should be considered as well.

Near-drowning victims often require treatment for cardiac as well as respiratory arrest during resuscitation. If this is successfully accomplished, most patients experience few additional cardiovascular problems. Supraventricular arrhythmias are common but usually resolve promptly when acidosis and hypoxia are treated. Heart failure secondary to myocardial ischemia or acutely expanded blood volume is unusual. Instead, pulmonary edema and low cardiac output states are usually due to the pulmonary injury from water aspiration with extravasation of fluid into the lung, resulting in hypovolemia.

Fever, frequently greater than 38°C, is seen in most patients within the first 24 h following significant aspiration. Its appearance later in the hospital course usually indicates a complicating infection. Vomiting is common during and after resuscitation. This often is associated with gastric distention by large quantities of fluid and air swallowed during the near-drowning episode and may result in additional aspiration. Other rare, but clinically important, features which may be encountered include acute renal failure and a severe hemorrhagic diathesis.

LABORATORY FINDINGS Arterial blood gas and pH determinations on admission reveal varying degrees of hypoxia and acidosis; follow-up values are the most reliable indicators of the effectiveness of ventilatory therapy. In 25 percent of near-drowning victims the initial chest x-ray film may be normal; however, this finding does not exclude the possibility that the patient has significant hypoxia. In the remainder of cases, radiologic findings range from fine, symmetric, perihilar infiltrates with relative sparing of apexes, bases, and lateral lung fields to massive bilateral pulmonary edema with little or no areas of sparing. Marked clearing of these abnormalities usually takes place within 72 to 96 h.

Alterations in serum sodium and potassium are generally mild and require no corrective treatment. Although leukocytosis up to 40,000 white blood cells per cubic millimeter is common during the first 24 to 48 h following near-drowning, significant changes in hematocrit and hemoglobin are rare, irrespective of the type of fluid aspirated. A *falling* hematocrit should raise the possibility of bleeding, not hemolysis, which, if it has occurred, should be apparent at the time of initial evaluation. Thrombocytopenia, prolonged prothrombin and partial thromboplastin times, hypofibrinogenemia, and elevated fibrin degradation products may be seen if disseminated intravascular coagulation takes place (see Chap. 281).

THERAPY The primary objective of therapy is to correct hypoxia and acidosis as rapidly as possible. On-the-scene efforts should include immediate institution of mouth-to-mouth breathing and, if necessary, closed-chest cardiac massage. Time should not be wasted with attempts to drain water from the victim's lungs. However, it is important to establish and maintain a clear airway at the onset of resuscitation in order to avoid accidental overdistention of the stomach which might result in regurgitation and aspiration. One hundred percent oxygen should be administered by inhalation as soon as possible, and other necessary resuscitative efforts continued during evacuation to the hospital. Even if spontaneous ventilation returns and the patient seems coherent, high concentrations of oxygen should be continued, since severe hypoxia and acidosis may be present even in persons who are alert and without cyanosis.

All near-drowning victims should be taken to a hospital for further evaluation. Initial diagnostic studies should include arterial blood gas and pH determinations, hemogram, serum electrolytes, and chest x-ray. Patients who are alert, have normal chest x-rays, and show no evidence of hypoxia or acidosis usually require no further therapy. Nevertheless they should be observed for several hours for evidence of deterioration in blood gas and acid-base status prior to discharge. Metabolic acidosis should be treated by intravenous administration of sodium bicarbonate ($NaHCO_3$), and hypoxia with supplemental oxygen. If bronchospasm is present, aerosol inhalation of a bronchodilator may be given. Patients with pulmonary edema or hypoxia which fails to respond to increasing inspired oxygen tensions up to 40 percent should be intubated endotracheally and have positive end-expiratory pressure (PEEP) applied to the airways. When respiratory failure is present, lung compliance is markedly reduced, or the patient is unable to breathe spontaneously, mechanical ventilatory support should be used in addition to PEEP. Arterial blood gas tensions and pH should be determined frequently to assess the adequacy of respiratory therapy. Treatment with PEEP should be continued long enough for the lung injury to stabilize before it is withdrawn. This may take 48 to 72 h or even longer. Monitoring the magnitude of the intrapulmonary shunt, the pulmonary wedge pressure, and cardiac output by means of a Swan-Ganz intraarterial catheter is often very helpful in weaning patients from PEEP as well as in managing cases complicated by low cardiac output and hypotension.

Comatose near-drowning victims frequently are found to have elevated intracranial pressure, which is caused by cerebral edema and loss of cerebrovascular autoregulation. Prolonged elevations over 15 to 20 mmHg lead to reductions of cerebral blood flow, adding ischemic injury to already damaged brain tissue. In order to preserve cerebral function in such patients, aggressive therapy termed *cerebral resuscitation,* and including controlled hyperventilation, deliberate hypothermia, and the use of barbiturates, corticosteroids, and osmotic and loop diuretics, has been advocated while the intracranial pressure is closely monitored via subarachnoid bolts and intraventricular catheters. Although several investigators have reported that there are fewer major neurologic sequelae, particularly in children treated in this manner, the need for such aggressive and potentially hazardous therapy requires further study before it can be recommended for all patients in deep coma following near-drowning.

Other therapeutic measures are largely supportive. Patients should be observed closely for evidence of pulmonary infection and treated with appropriate antibiotics on the basis of results of cultures of respiratory secretions. Prophylactic use of antibiotics and corticosteroids has been of no benefit in near-drowning victims. Fluid and electrolyte balance should be carefully maintained. If hypovolemia is associated with low urinary output or hypotension, plasma expanders may be required. Transfusion with packed red blood cells or whole blood, depending upon circulating blood volume status, may be used for significant anemia. Acute renal failure should be managed as described in Chap. 219.

PROGNOSIS The prognosis depends largely upon the extent and duration of the hypoxic episode. In addition, such factors as the temperature of the submersion medium, the availability and appropriate application of specific treatment, and coexisting medical illness or trauma are often important in determining the outcome. In general, patients who are alert and have normal chest x-rays upon arrival at the hospital can be expected to recover fully. Those who are obtunded but arousable and have normal respirations have nearly as good a prognosis, while approximately two-thirds of those who present in coma or cardiopulmonary arrest die or are left with significant neurologic deficits. Prediction of outcome on the basis of other presenting neurologic features or laboratory abnormalities is unreliable. The fact that nearly 90 percent of victims who live long enough to receive definitive hospital care will survive should serve to emphasize that extensive resuscitative efforts are advisable in all cases of near-drowning.

REFERENCES

Centers for Disease Control: Drownings—Georgia, 1981–1983. Morb Mort Week Rep 34:281, 1985

Conn AW et al: Cerebral salvage in near-drowning following neurologic classification by triage. Can Anaesth Soc J 27:201. 1980

Davis S et al: Drownings of children and youth in a desert state. West J Med 143:196, 1985

Frates RC Jr: Analysis of predictive factors in the assessment of warm-water near-drowning in children. Am J Dis Child 135:1006, 1981

Martin TG: Near-drowning and cold water immersion. Ann Emerg Med 13:263, 1984

Modell JH: Biology of drowning. Ann Rev Med 29:1, 1978

Oakes DD et al: Prognosis and management of victims of near-drowning. J Trauma 22:544, 1982

Pfenninger J, Sutter M: Intensive care after freshwater immersion accidents in children. Anesthesia 37:1157, 1982

Young RSK et al: Neurological outcome in cold water drowning. JAMA 244:1233, 1980

PART FOUR DISORDERS OF THE CARDIOVASCULAR SYSTEM

section 1 Disorders of the heart

176 APPROACH TO THE PATIENT WITH HEART DISEASE

EUGENE BRAUNWALD

The symptoms caused by heart disease result most commonly from myocardial ischemia, from disturbance of the contractile activity of the myocardium, or from an abnormal cardiac rhythm or rate. Ischemia is manifest most frequently as chest discomfort, while reduction of the pumping ability of the heart commonly leads to weakness and fatigability or, when severe, produces cyanosis, hypotension, syncope, and elevated intravascular pressure behind a failing ventricle; the latter results in abnormal fluid accumulation, which in turn leads to dyspnea, orthopnea, and edema. Cardiac arrhythmias often develop suddenly, and the resulting signs and symptoms—palpitation, dyspnea, angina, hypotension, and syncope—generally occur abruptly and may disappear as rapidly as they develop.

A cardinal principle useful in the evaluation of the patient with suspected heart disease is that myocardial or coronary function which may be adequate at rest may be inadequate during exertion. Thus, a history of chest discomfort and/or dyspnea which appears only during activity is characteristic of heart disease, while the opposite pattern, i.e., the appearance of these symptoms at rest and their remission during exertion, is rarely observed in patients with organic heart disease.

Patients with cardiocirculatory disease may also be entirely asymptomatic, both at rest and during exertion, but may present an abnormal physical finding, such as a heart murmur, elevated systemic arterial pressure, or an abnormality of the electrocardiogram or of the cardiac silhouette on the chest roentgenogram.

Diseases of the heart and circulation are so common and the laity is so well acquainted with the major symptoms resulting from these disorders that patients, and occasionally physicians, erroneously attribute many complaints to organic cardiovascular disease. Furthermore, the combination of the widespread fear of heart disease in the western world with the deep-seated emotional connotations concerning this organ's function results in the frequent development in persons with normal cardiovascular systems of symptoms which mimic those of organic disease. Sometimes it is difficult to interpret correctly the symptoms of patients with recognized organic cardiovascular disturbances. Such patients, in addition to having symptoms resulting from their disease, may also develop functional complaints referable to the cardiovascular system. The unraveling of symptoms and signs due to organic heart disease from those which are not directly related is an important and challenging task in these patients.

It must be recognized that dyspnea, one of the cardinal manifestations of diminished cardiac reserve, is not limited to disease of the heart, but is also characteristic of conditions as diverse as pulmonary disease, marked obesity, and anxiety (Chap. 26). Similarly, chest discomfort (Chap. 4) may result from a variety of causes other than myocardial ischemia. Whether heart disease is responsible for these symptoms can frequently be determined by carrying out a detailed clinical examination. Noninvasive testing using electrocardiography at rest and during exercise (Chap. 178), roentgenography, and echocardiography (Chap. 179) usually provide important additional information to permit the correct interpretation of symptoms; more specialized invasive examinations (catheterization and angiography) are occasionally necessary.

DIAGNOSIS In every branch of medicine the establishment of the prognosis and development of a rational plan of management are based on a correct diagnostic appraisal. In patients with disorders of the cardiocirculatory system, particular care must be taken to establish not only a correct but also a *complete* diagnosis. As outlined by the New York Heart Association, the elements of a complete cardiac diagnosis include consideration of:

1 *The underlying etiology.* Is the disease congenital, rheumatic, hypertensive, or arteriosclerotic in origin?
2 *The anatomic abnormalities.* Which chambers are enlarged? Which valves are affected? Is there pericardial involvement? Has there been a myocardial infarction?
3 *The physiologic disturbances.* Is an arrhythmia present? Is there evidence of congestive heart failure or of myocardial ischemia?
4 *The extent of functional disability.* How strenuous is the physical activity required to elicit symptoms?

Two simple examples may serve to illustrate the importance of establishing a complete diagnosis. The identification of myocardial ischemia as the cause of exertional chest discomfort is of great clinical importance. However, this diagnosis is insufficient to develop either a strategy of specific treatment or prognosis until the underlying disease process, e.g., coronary atherosclerosis or aortic stenosis, which is responsible for the myocardial ischemia, is identified and a judgment made as to whether severe anemia, thyrotoxicosis, or supraventricular tachycardia plays a contributory role. Similarly, determining that heart disease is congenital provides an important starting point, but the decision about whether surgical treatment is advisable depends upon the specific anatomic defect present and often upon the nature of the physiologic disturbance and the functional impairment as well.

The establishment of a correct and complete cardiac diagnosis often requires the use of six different methods of examination: (1) history, (2) physical examination (Chap. 177), (3) electrocardiogram (Chap. 178), (4) chest roentgenogram (Chap. 179), (5) noninvasive graphic examinations (echocardiogram, radionuclide scanning techniques, and other "noninvasive" tests, Chap. 179), and occasionally (6) specialized "invasive" examinations, such as cardiac catheterization or angiocardiography (Chap. 180). In order to be most effective, the results obtained from each of these six modalities should be analyzed independently of one another as well as with the information derived from the other methods clearly in mind. Only in this way can one avoid overlooking a subtle, though extremely significant, finding. For example, an electrocardiogram should be obtained in every patient suspected of having heart disease. It may provide the critical clue in establishing the correct diagnosis, e.g., the finding of an atrioventricular conduction disturbance in a patient with unexplained syncope, even when all other methods of examination reveal no abnormal findings. On the other hand, when combined intelligently with the results of other methods of examination, the electrocardiogram may provide essential confirmatory data. Thus, the knowledge that a patient has an apical diastolic rumbling murmur may direct particular attention to the P waves, and the recognition of left atrial enlargement electrocardiographically supports the suggestion that the murmur is caused by mitral stenosis. Under these circumstances the additional finding on the electrocardiogram of right ventricular hypertrophy suggests that pulmonary hypertension is present and that the mitral stenosis is severe.

Although the electrocardiogram is an invaluable aspect of every cardiovascular examination, with the exception of the identification of arrhythmias it rarely permits establishment of a specific diagnosis. In the absence of any other abnormal findings, electrocardiographic changes must not be overinterpreted. The range of normal electrocardiographic findings is wide, and the tracing can be affected significantly by many noncardiac factors, such as age, body habitus, and serum electrolyte concentrations.

In obtaining the history of the patient with known or suspected cardiovascular disease, particular attention should be directed to the family history. Familial clustering is common in many forms of heart disease. Genetic transmission may occur, as in hypertrophic cardiomyopathy (Chap. 192) or Marfan's syndrome (Chap. 319). In patients with essential hypertension or coronary atherosclerosis the genetic component may be less obvious but also of considerable importance. Familial clustering of cardiovascular diseases may not only occur on a genetic basis but may also be related to familial, dietary, or behavior patterns.

When an attempt is made to ascertain the severity of functional impairment in a patient with heart disease, it is essential to determine the precise extent of activity and the rate at which it is performed before symptoms develop. Thus, breathlessness which occurs after running up two long flights of stairs denotes far less functional impairment than similar symptoms occurring after taking a few steps on the level. Also, the degree of customary physical activity at work and during recreation should be considered. The development of two-flight dyspnea in a marathon runner may be more significant than the development of dyspnea on far less exertion in a previously sedentary person. Similarly, the history must include a detailed consideration of the patient's therapeutic regimen. For example, the persistence or development of edema in a patient whose diet is rigidly restricted in sodium content and who is receiving optimum doses of diuretics must be interpreted quite differently from the finding of edema in the absence of these measures. In an effort to ascertain the rate of progression of symptoms, and thereby of the severity of the underlying illness, it may be useful to ascertain what, if any, specific tasks the patient could carry out 1 year earlier which he or she cannot carry out now.

PITFALLS IN CARDIOVASCULAR MEDICINE Increasing subspecialization in internal medicine and the perfection of advanced diagnostic techniques in cardiology may sometimes be accompanied by several undesirable consequences, which can be summarized as follows:

1 Failure by the *noncardiologist* to recognize cardiac manifestations of systemic illnesses. The latter include but are by no means limited to (*a*) the Down syndrome (associated with endocardial cushion defect); (*b*) gonadal dysgenesis, i.e., Turner's syndrome (associated with a variety of congenital defects, particularly coarctation of the aorta); (*c*) bony abnormalities of the upper extremities (associated with atrial septal defect); (*d*) muscular dystrophies (associated with cardiomyopathy); (*e*) hemochromatosis and glycogen storage disease (associated with myocardial infiltration); (*f*) congenital deafness (associated with serious cardiac arrhythmias); (*g*) Raynaud's disease (associated with primary pulmonary hypertension and coronary vasospasm); (*h*) connective tissue disorders, i.e., Marfan's syndrome, Ehlers-Danlos syndrome, Hurler's syndrome, and related disorders of mucopolysaccharide metabolism (aortic dilatation, prolapsed mitral valve, a variety of arterial abnormalities); (*i*) chronic hemolytic anemia (cardiac dilatation); (*j*) Refsum's disease (myocardial failure and conduction defects); (*k*) acromegaly (accelerated coronary atherosclerosis, conduction defects, cardiomyopathy); (*l*) hyperthyroidism (heart failure, atrial fibrillation); (*m*) rheumatoid arthritis (pericarditis, aortic valve disease); (*n*) Whipple's disease (pericarditis and endocarditis); (*o*) scleroderma (cor pulmonale, myocardial fibrosis, pericarditis); (*p*) systemic lupus erythematosus (valvulitis, myocarditis); (*q*) polymyositis (pericarditis, myocarditis); (*r*) sarcoidosis (arrhythmias, cardiomyopathy); (*s*) Fabry's disease (myocardial ischemia, heart failure); (*t*) exfoliative dermatitis (high-output heart failure). In patients in whom these and other systemic disorders in which cardiovascular involvement may occur, a detailed cardiovascular examination should be carried out.

2 Failure by the cardiac specialist to recognize an underlying systemic illness, such as those listed above, among patients with a cardiac disorder. Patients known or suspected of having heart disease require a detailed general assessment and a search for the frequent noncardiac manifestations of systemic disorders with cardiovascular manifestations. Indeed, the cardiovascular abnormality may provide the clue critical to the recognition of these systemic disorders. Closely related is the failure to appreciate the profound effects of stress, such as that resulting from an intercurrent infection, of pregnancy, or from emotional disturbances, on cardiovascular performance and symptoms.

3 Overreliance on and overutilization of laboratory tests, particularly specialized invasive techniques for the examination of the cardiovascular system. Catheterization of the right and left sides of the heart, selective angiography, and coronary arteriography (Chap. 180), provide precise diagnostic information under many circumstances. For example, they aid in establishing a specific anatomic diagnosis and in determining the physiologic consequences of the abnormalities in patients with congenital heart disease, in patients with chest pain of uncertain etiology in whom coronary artery disease is suspected, and in determining the functional significance of valvular abnormalities in patients with rheumatic heart disease being considered for surgical treatment. Although a great deal of attention has been lavished on the newer specialized laboratory examinations, it should be recognized that they serve to *supplement*, not *supplant*, a careful examination carried out by clinical and noninvasive examination. There is an unfortunate tendency to carry out procedures such as coronary arteriography, in patients with chest pain suspected of having coronary artery disease, instead of taking a detailed and thoughtful history; although it may be established whether the coronary arteries are obstructed, the results often do not provide a definite answer to the question of whether a patient's complaint of chest pain is clearly attributable to coronary arteriosclerosis. Coronary arteriography is often carried out unnecessarily in patients with mild symptoms and signs of myocardial ischemia during exertion with normal left ventricular function who are not likely to be candidates for coronary bypass surgery. Similarly, catheterization of the left side of the heart is all too frequently employed to determine whether operative treatment of valvular disease is indicated, even before the patient has had a trial of medical therapy. Despite their enormous value, it must not be overlooked that these specialized examinations entail some small risk to the patient, involve discomfort and substantial cost, and place a strain on existing medical facilities. Therefore, *they should be carried out not as part of a "fishing expedition" or as evidence to the patient and the family that "everything is being done," but only if, after detailed clinical examination and assessment by noninvasive tests, the results of the invasive examination can be expected to modify or aid in the patient's management.*

Treatment After a complete diagnosis has been established, a number of therapeutic options are usually available. Several examples may be used to demonstrate some of the principles of modern cardiovascular therapeutics:

1 In the absence of evidence for the existence of heart disease a clear, definitive statement to that effect should be made and the patient should *not* be asked to return at intervals for repeated examinations. If there is no evidence for disease, such attention may lead to the patient developing an abnormal fixation on the heart.

2 If there is no evidence of cardiovascular disease but the patient has one or more risk factors for the development of ischemic heart disease (Chap. 195), a plan for their reduction should be developed and the patient should be retested at intervals to assess that he or she is complying and that these risk factors are in fact being reduced.

3 Asymptomatic or mildly symptomatic patients with established organic heart disease, e.g., valvular heart disease, should be evaluated periodically, e.g., every 6 to 12 months, by clinical and noninvasive examinations (Chap. 179). Early warning signs of deterioration of ventricular function can be detected in this manner and in appropriate patients may signify the need for surgical treatment despite the absence of disabling symptoms (Chap. 187).

4 It is critical for the physician to establish clear criteria for deciding on the form of treatment (medical, angioplasty, or surgical revascularization) in patients with ischemic heart disease (Chap. 189). Surgical treatment represents a major therapeutic advance in the treatment of this most common form of heart disease, but operation has probably been employed too widely in the United States; the mere presence of angina pectoris and/or the demonstration of coronary arterial narrowing at angiography should not reflexly evoke a decision to treat the patient surgically. Instead, this form of treatment should be limited to those patients with ischemic heart disease in whom it has been demonstrated that surgical treatment is superior to medical treatment.

REFERENCES

BRAUNWALD E (ed): *Heart Disease*, 2d ed. Philadelphia, Saunders, 1984

FOWLER NO: *Cardiac Diagnosis and Treatment*, 3d ed. Hagerstown, Harper & Row, 1980

HORWITZ LD, GROVES BM (eds): *Signs and Symptoms in Cardiology*. Philadelphia, Lippincott, 1985

HURST JW et al (ed): *The Heart*, 6th ed. New York, McGraw-Hill, 1986

NEW YORK HEART ASSOCIATION, INC, CRITERIA COMMITTEE: *Nomenclature and Criteria for Diagnosis of Diseases of the Heart and Great Vessels*, 8th ed. Boston, Little, Brown, 1981

PERLOFF JK (ed): *Physical Examination of the Heart and Circulation*. Philadelphia, Saunders, 1982

177 PHYSICAL EXAMINATION OF THE HEART

ROBERT A. O'ROURKE / EUGENE BRAUNWALD

The general examination of a patient with cardiac disease often provides important information concerning the status of the cardiovascular system. The general physical appearance should first be assessed. The patient may appear tired because of a persistently low cardiac output; the respiratory rate may be increased, indicating pulmonary venous congestion. Central cyanosis, often associated with clubbing of the fingers and toes, indicates right-to-left shunting of blood in the heart or great vessels or inadequate oxygenation of blood by the lungs. Cyanosis in the distal extremities, cool skin, and increased sweating result from vasoconstriction in patients with severe heart failure (Chap 27). Noncardiovascular details can be equally important. For example, the diagnosis of infective endocarditis is highly likely in patients with petechiae, Osler's nodes, and Janeway lesions (Chap. 188).

The blood pressure should be taken in both arms and with the patient supine and upright; the heart rate should be timed for 1 min. Orthostatic hypotension and tachycardia may indicate a reduced blood volume, while resting tachycardia may be a clue to the presence of severe heart failure.

Careful examination of the optic fundi is essential (Chap. 196), and the retinal vessels may show evidence of systemic hypertension, arteriosclerosis, or embolism. The latter may result from atherosclerosis in larger arteries (e.g., carotid) or may represent a complication of valvular heart disease (e.g., endocarditis).

Palpation of the peripheral arterial pulses in the upper and lower extremities is necessary to define the adequacy of systemic blood flow and to detect the presence of occlusive arterial lesions. It is also important to examine both legs for evidence of edema, varicose veins, or thrombophlebitis (Chap. 198). The cardiovascular examination includes careful evaluation of both the carotid arterial and the jugular venous pulses, as well as deliberate precordial palpation and attentive cardiac auscultation. An understanding of the events of the cardiac cycle (Fig. 179-1, page 882) is vital to performing an accurate cardiovascular examination.

ARTERIAL PRESSURE PULSE The normal central aortic pulse wave is characterized by a fairly rapid rise to a somewhat rounded peak (Fig. 177-1). The anacrotic shoulder, present on the ascending limb, occurs at the time of peak rate of aortic flow just before maximum pressure is reached. The less steep descending limb is interrupted by a sharp downward deflection, synchronous with aortic valve closure, called the *incisura*. As the pulse wave is transmitted peripherally, the initial upstroke becomes steeper, the anacrotic shoulder becomes less apparent, and the incisura is replaced by the smoother dicrotic notch. Accordingly, palpation of a peripheral pulse (e.g., the radial arterial) frequently gives less information than examination of a more central pulse (e.g., the carotid arterial) regarding alterations in left ventricular ejection or aortic valve function. However, certain findings such as the bounding pulses of aortic regurgitation or pulsus alternans are more readily evident in peripheral than in central arteries (Fig. 177-2). The carotid pulse usually is best examined with the sternocleidomastoid muscle relaxed

FIGURE 177-1 *A. Schematic representation of electrocardiogram, aortic pressure pulse (AOP), phonocardiogram recorded at the apex, and apexcardiogram (ACG). On the phonocardiogram, S_1, S_2, S_3, and S_4 represent the first through fourth heart sounds; OS represents the opening snap of the mitral valve, which occurs coincident with the O point of the apexcardiogram. S_3 occurs coincident with the termination of the rapid-filling wave (RFW) of the ACG, while S_4 occurs coincident with the a wave of the ACG. B. Simultaneous recording of electrocardiogram, indirect carotid pulse (CP), phonocardiogram along the left sternal border (LSB), and indirect jugular venous pulse (JVP). ES, ejection sound; SC, systolic click.*

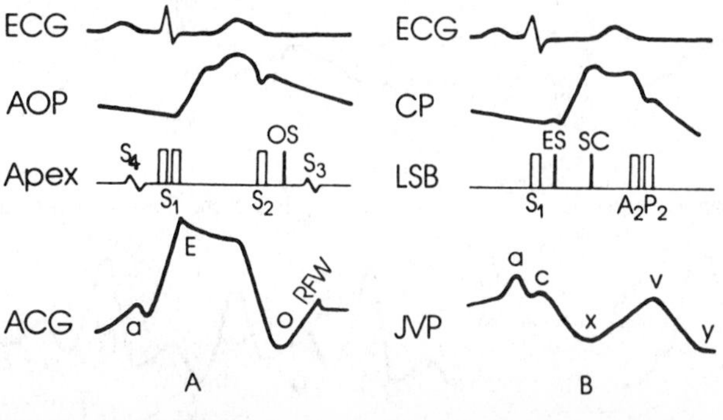

and with the head rotated slightly toward the examiner. In examining the brachial arterial pulse, the examiner can support the subject's relaxed elbow with his or her right arm while compressing the brachial pulse with the thumb. The usual technique for palpating the pulse is to compress the artery with the thumb or forefinger until the maximum pulse is sensed. The examiner should apply varying degrees of pressure while concentrating on the separate phases of the pulse wave. This method, referred to as *trisection,* is useful for assessing the sharpness of the upstroke, systolic peak, and diastolic slope of the arterial pulse. In most normal persons a dicrotic wave is not palpable.

A small weak pulse, *pulsus parvus,* is frequently present in conditions with a diminished left ventricular stroke volume, a narrow pulse pressure, and increased peripheral vascular resistance (Fig. 177-2). A hypokinetic pulse may be due to hypovolemia, to left ventricular failure secondary to myocardial disease or myocardial infarction, to restrictive pericardial disease, or to mitral valve stenosis. In aortic valve stenosis the delayed systolic peak, *pulsus tardus,* is the result of mechanical obstruction to left ventricular ejection and is often accompanied by the transmission of a coarse systolic thrill. In contrast, a large bounding pulse is usually associated with an increased left ventricular stroke volume, a wide pulse pressure, and a decrease in peripheral vascular resistance. This occurs characteristically in patients with abnormally elevated stroke volumes as in complete heart block, hyperkinetic circulation due to anxiety, anemia, exercise, or fever, or in patients with an abnormally rapid runoff of blood from the arterial system (patent ductus arteriosus, peripheral arteriovenous fistula). Patients with mitral regurgitation or a ventricular septal defect may also have a bounding pulse, since vigorous left ventricular ejection produces a rapid upstroke in the arterial pulse even though the duration of systole and the forward stroke volume may be diminished. In aortic regurgitation the rapidly rising, bounding arterial pulse results from increased left ventricular stroke volume and the associated increased rate of ventricular ejection.

The *bisferiens pulse,* which consists of two systolic peaks, is characteristic of aortic regurgitation (with or without accompanying stenosis) and of hypertrophic cardiomyopathy (Chap. 192). In the latter the pulse wave upstroke rises rapidly and forcefully, producing the first systolic peak ("percussion wave"). A brief decline in pressure follows because of the sudden decrease in the rate of left ventricular ejection during midsystole, when severe obstruction often develops. This pressure trough is followed by a smaller and more slowly rising positive pulse wave ("tidal wave") produced by continued ventricular ejection and by reflected waves from the periphery. The *dicrotic pulse* has two palpable waves, one in systole and one in diastole. It occurs most frequently in patients with a very low stroke volume, particularly in those with dilated (congestive) cardiomyopathy.

Pulsus alternans refers to a pattern in which there is regular alteration of the pressure pulse amplitude, despite a regular rhythm (Fig. 177-2). It is due to alternating left ventricular contractile force, usually denotes severe left ventricular decompensation, and commonly occurs in patients who also have a loud third heart sound. Pulsus alternans may also occur during or following paroxysmal tachycardia or for several beats following a premature beat in patients without heart disease. In *pulsus bigeminus* there is also regular alteration of pressure pulse amplitude, but it is caused by a premature ventricular contraction that follows each regular beat. *Pulsus paradoxus* is an accentuation of the decrease in systolic arterial pressure accompanying the reduced amplitude of the arterial pulse which normally occurs during inspiration. In patients with pericardial tamponade, airway obstruction, or superior vena cava obstruction, the decrease in systolic arterial pressure frequently exceeds the normal of 10 mmHg and the peripheral pulse may disappear completely during inspiration.

Simultaneous palpation of the radial and femoral arterial pulses, which normally are virtually coincident, is important to rule out aortic coarctation, in which the latter is weaker and delayed (Chap. 185).

JUGULAR VENOUS PULSE (JVP) The two main objectives of the bedside examination of the neck veins are inspection of their waveform and estimation of the central venous pressure (CVP). In most patients, the right internal jugular vein is superior for both purposes, but occasionally examination of the left internal jugular vein, the external jugular veins, or the venous pulsations in the supraclavicular fossae may yield more information. In most normal subjects, maximum pulsation of the internal jugular vein is observed when the trunk is inclined by less than 30°. In patients with elevated venous pressure it may be necessary to elevate the trunk further, sometimes to as much as 90°. When the neck muscles are relaxed, shining a beam of light tangentially across the skin overlying the vein exposes the pulsations of the internal jugular vein. Simultaneous palpation of the left carotid artery aids the examiner in deciding which pulsations are venous and in relating the venous pulsations to their timing in the cardiac cycle.

The normal JVP reflects phasic pressure changes in the right atrium and consists of two or sometimes three positive waves and two negative troughs (Fig. 177-1). The positive presystolic *a* wave is produced by venous distention consequent to right atrial contraction and is the dominant wave in the JVP, particularly during inspiration. Large *a* waves indicate that the right atrium is contracting against an increased resistance (Fig. 177-3), such as occurs with obstruction at the tricuspid valve (tricuspid stenosis) or more commonly with increased resistance to right ventricular filling (pulmonary hypertension or pulmonic stenosis). Large *a* waves also occur during dysrhythmias whenever the right atrium contracts while the tricuspid valve is closed by right ventricular systole. Such "cannon" *a* waves may occur regularly (as during junctional rhythm) or irregularly (as in atrioventricular dissociation with ventricular tachycardia or complete heart block). The *a* wave is absent in patients with atrial fibrillation, and there is an increased temporal delay between the *a* wave and the carotid arterial pulse in patients with first-degree atrioventricular block.

The *c* wave, often but not invariably observed in the JVP, is a positive wave produced by the bulging of the tricuspid valve into the right atrium during right ventricular isovolumetric systole and by the impact of the carotid artery adjacent to the jugular vein. The *x* descent is due to a combination of atrial relaxation and the downward displacement of the tricuspid valve during ventricular systole. In

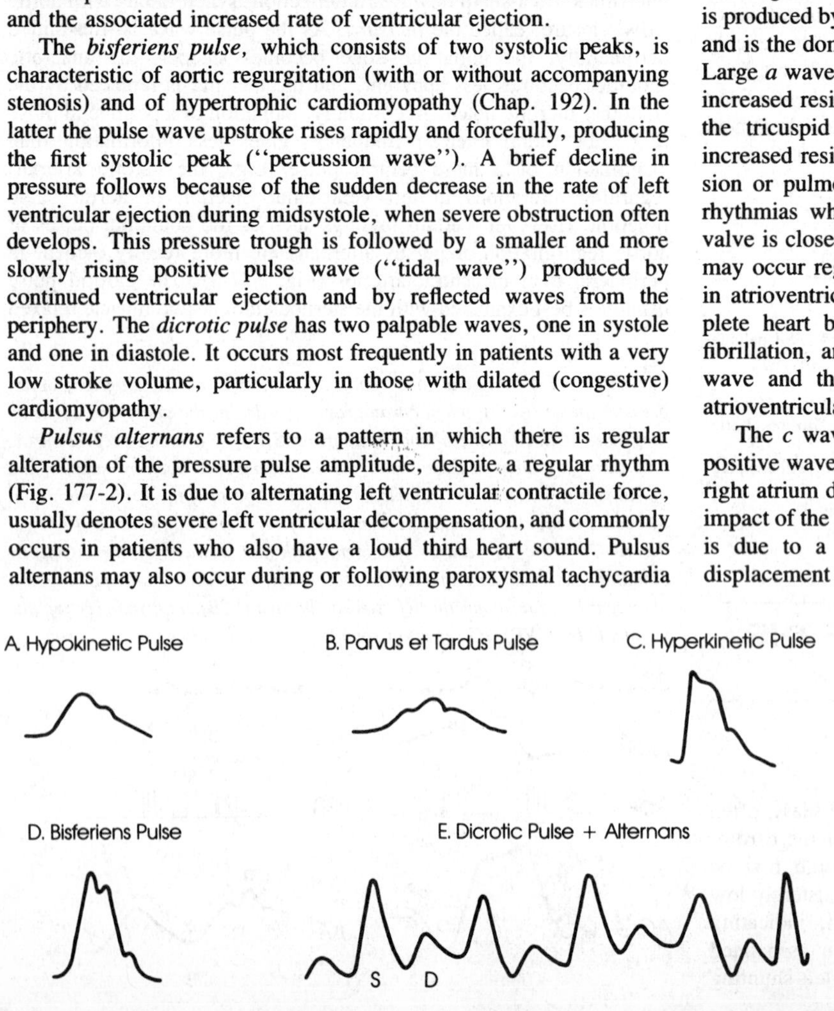

FIGURE 177-2 *Schematic representation of arterial pulse waveforms that occur with alterations in cardiac hemodynamics which may result from normal physiologic responses or may be due to cardiac disease S, systole; D, diastole.*

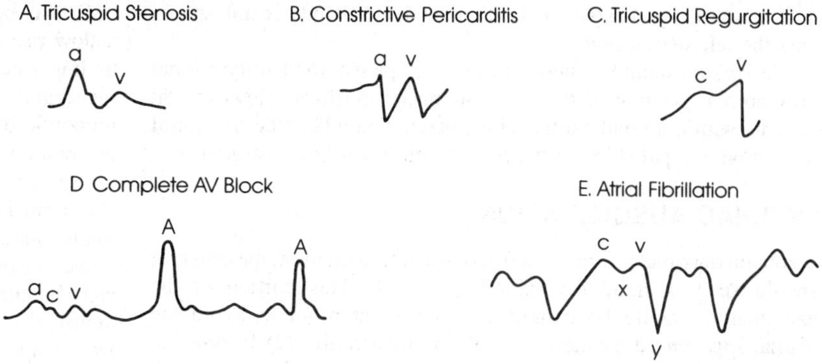

FIGURE 177-3 *Abnormal jugular venous pulse waveforms commonly present in patients with cardiac disease and/or arrhythmias. See text.*

patients with constrictive pericarditis (Fig. 177-3), there is often increased prominence of the *x* descent wave during systole, but this wave is reduced with right ventricular dilatation and may even be reversed in tricuspid regurgitation. The positive, late systolic *v* wave results from the increasing volume of blood in the venae cavae and right atrium during ventricular systole when the tricuspid valve is closed. With mild tricuspid regurgitation the *v* wave becomes more prominent, and when tricuspid regurgitation becomes severe, the prominent *v* wave and the obliteration of the *x* descent result in a single large positive systolic wave (''ventricularization''). After the peak of the *v* wave is reached, the right atrial pressure diminishes because of the decreased bulging of the tricuspid valve into the right atrium as right ventricular pressure declines and the tricuspid valve opens (Fig. 177-3).

Following the summit of the *v* wave there is a negative descending limb, referred to as the *y* descent or ''diastolic collapse,'' which is produced mainly by the tricuspid valve opening and the rapid inflow of blood into the right ventricle. A rapid, deep *y* descent in early diastole occurs with severe tricuspid regurgitation. A venous pulse characterized by a sharp *y* descent, a deep *y* trough, and a rapid ascent to the baseline is seen in patients with constrictive pericarditis or with severe failure of the right side of the heart and a high venous pressure. A slow *y* descent in the JVP suggests an obstruction to right ventricular filling, as occurs with tricuspid stenosis or right atrial myxoma.

For accurate estimation of the CVP, the right internal jugular vein is best utilized, with the sternal angle as the reference point, since in the average patient the center of the right atrium lies approximately 5 cm below the sternal angle, regardless of body position. The patient is examined at the optimum degree of trunk elevation for visualization of venous pulsations. The vertical distance between the top of the oscillating venous column and the level of the sternal angle is determined and generally found to be less than 3 cm (3 cm + 5 cm = 8 cm blood). The most common cause of an elevated venous pressure is an elevated right ventricular diastolic pressure. In patients suspected of having right ventricular failure who have a normal CVP at rest, the abdominojugular reflux test may be helpful. The palm of the hand is placed over the abdomen and firm pressure is applied for 30 to 60 s. Normally, the jugular venous pressure is not significantly altered, but with impaired function of the right side of the heart the upper level of venous pulsation usually increases. Also, abdominal compression may elicit the typical JVP of tricuspid regurgitation when the resting pulse wave is normal. Kussmaul's sign, an increase rather than the normal decrease in the CVP during inspiration, is most commonly caused by severe right-sided heart failure; it is a frequent finding in patients with constrictive pericarditis or right ventricular infarction.

PRECORDIAL PALPATION The location, amplitude, duration, and direction of the cardiac impulse can usually be best appreciated by using the fingertips. The normal left ventricular apex impulse is located at or medial to the left midclavicular line in the fourth or fifth intercostal space and is a tapping, early systolic outward thrust localized to a point not more than 3 cm in diameter. It is due primarily to recoil of the heart as blood is ejected and should be evaluated with the patient supine and in the left lateral decubitus position. Left ventricular hypertrophy results in an exaggerated amplitude and duration of the normal left ventricular thrust. The impulse may be displaced laterally and downward into the sixth or seventh interspace, particularly in patients with a left ventricular volume load such as occurs in aortic regurgitation.

Additional abnormal features of the left ventricular apex include marked presystolic distention of the left ventricle, often accompanying a fourth heart sound in patients with an excessive left ventricular pressure load or myocardial ischemia/infarction, and a prominent early diastolic rapid-filling wave, often accompanying a third heart sound in patients with left ventricular failure or mitral valve regurgitation (Fig. 177-1). A double systolic impulse is frequently palpable in patients with hypertrophic cardiomyopathy.

Right ventricular hypertrophy results in a sustained systolic lift at the lower left parasternal area which starts in early systole and is synchronous with the left ventricular apical impulse. In patients with chronic obstructive pulmonary disease a right ventricular impulse may often be detected by sliding the fingers up under the rib cage just beneath the sternum. The enlarged right ventricle strikes the ends of the fingertips as an inferiorly directed movement.

Abnormal precordial pulsations occur during systole in patients with abnormal left ventricular wall motion due to ischemic heart disease or to diffuse myocardial disease from some other cause. These pulsations often occur in patients with a recent transmural myocardial infarction and may be present in some patients only during episodes of anginal pain. They are most commonly felt in the left midprecordium one or two interspaces above and/or 1 to 2 cm medial to the left ventricular apex. When a systolic bulge occurs in the region of the apex, it is difficult to distinguish it from the impulse of left ventricular hypertrophy.

A left parasternal lift is present frequently in patients with severe mitral regurgitation. This pulsation occurs distinctly later than the left ventricular apical impulse, is synchronous with the *v* wave in the left atrial pressure curve, and is due to anterior displacement of the right ventricle by an enlarged, expanding left atrium. A similar impulse occurring to the right of the sternum has been noted in some patients with severe tricuspid regurgitation and a giant right atrium. Pulsation of the right sternoclavicular joint may indicate a right-sided aortic arch or aneurysmal dilatation of the ascending aorta. Pulmonary artery pulsation is often visible and palpable in the second left intercostal space and may be normal in children or thin young adults. However, this pulsation usually denotes pulmonary hypertension, increased pulmonary blood flow, or poststenotic pulmonary artery dilatation.

Thrills are palpable, low-frequency vibrations associated with heart murmurs. The diastolic rumble of mitral stenosis and the systolic murmur of mitral regurgitation may be palpated at the cardiac apex. When the palm of the hand is placed over the precordium, the thrill of aortic stenosis crosses the palm of the hand toward the right side of the neck, while the thrill of pulmonic stenosis radiates more often to the left side of the neck. The thrill due to a ventricular septal defect is usually located in the third and fourth intercostal spaces near the left sternal border.

Percussion should be performed in each patient to identify normal or abnormal position of the heart, stomach, and liver. However, in patients with a normal cardiac situs, percussion adds little to careful inspection and palpation in the recognition of cardiac enlargement.

CARDIAC AUSCULTATION

To obtain maximal information from cardiac auscultation, the observer should keep in mind several principles: (1) This portion of the examination should be carried out in a quiet room to avoid the distractions caused by the noises of normal activity. (2) In order to hear a faint heart sound or murmur, it is necessary to focus attention on that phase of the cardiac cycle during which the auscultatory event may be expected to occur. (3) The accurate timing of a heart sound or murmur necessarily involves ascertaining its relation to other observable events in the cardiac cycle—the carotid arterial pulse, the JVP, or the apical impulse. (4) To determine the significance of a cardiac sound or murmur, it is often necessary to observe alterations in its timing or intensity during various physiologic and/or pharmacologic interventions (Table 177-1).

HEART SOUNDS The major components of heart sounds are vibrations associated with the abrupt acceleration or deceleration of blood within the cardiovascular system, but there is continuing controversy regarding the relative significance of the vibrations of valves, muscles, vessels, and supporting structures in the production of the heart sounds. Recent studies using simultaneous echocardiographic-phonocardiographic recordings indicate that the first and second heart sounds are produced primarily by the closure of the AV and semilunar valves and the events that accompany these closures. The intensity of the *first heart sound* (S_1) is influenced by (1) the position of the mitral leaflets at the onset of ventricular systole, (2) the rate of rise of the left ventricular pressure pulse, (3) the presence or absence of structural disease of the mitral valve, and (4) the amount of tissue, air, or fluid between the heart and the stethoscope. S_1 is increased in intensity if diastole is shortened because of tachycardia, if atrioventricular flow is increased because of high cardiac output or prolonged because of mitral stenosis, or if atrial contraction precedes ventricular contractions by a short PR interval. The loud S_1 in mitral stenosis usually signifies that the valve is pliable and that it remains open at the onset of isovolumetric contraction because of the elevated left atrial pressure. A reduction in the intensity of S_1 may be due to poor conduction of sound through the chest wall, a slow rise of the left ventricular pressure pulse, a long PR interval, or imperfect closure due to reduced valve substance, as in mitral regurgitation. S_1 is also soft when the anterior mitral leaflet is immobile because of rigidity and calcification even in the presence of predominant mitral stenosis.

Splitting of the two high-pitched components of S_1 by 10 to 30 ms is a normal phenomenon (Fig. 177-1). The first component of S_1 normally is attributed to mitral valve closure and the second to tricuspid valve closure. A widened split of S_1 is most often due to complete right bundle branch block and the resulting delay in onset of the right ventricular pressure pulse. Reversed splitting of the S_1 with the mitral component following the tricuspid component has occasionally been noted in complete left bundle branch block and frequently is present in patients with severe mitral stenosis or a left atrial myxoma.

Splitting of S_2 into audibly distinct aortic (A_2) and pulmonic (P_2) components occurs normally during inspiration when augmented inflow into the right ventricle increases its stroke volume and ejection period and delays closure of the pulmonic valve. P_2 is coincident with the incisura of the pulmonary artery pressure curve, which is separated from the right ventricular pressure tracing by an interval termed the "hangout time." The absolute value of this interval reflects the resistance to pulmonary blood flow and the impedance characteristics of the pulmonary vascular bed. This interval is prolonged, and physiologic splitting of S_2 is accentuated in conditions associated with right ventricular volume overload and a distensible pulmonary vascular bed. However, in patients with an increase in pulmonary vascular resistance, the "hangout time" is markedly reduced and narrow splitting of S_2 is present. Splitting that persists with expiration, heard best at the pulmonic area or left sternal border, is usually abnormal when the patient is in the upright position. Such splitting may be due to delayed activation of the right ventricle (right bundle branch block), to prolongation of right ventricular contraction with an increased right ventricular pressure load (pulmonary embolism or pulmonic stenosis), or to delayed pulmonic valve closure because of right ventricular volume overload associated with diminished impedance of the pulmonary vascular bed and a prolonged "hangout time" (atrial septal defect). In pulmonary hypertension, P_2 is increased in intensity and splitting of the second heart sound may be diminished, normal, or accentuated, depending on the cause of the pulmonary hypertension, the pulmonary vascular resistance, and the presence or absence of right ventricular decompensation. Early aortic valve closure, occurring with mitral regurgitation or a ventricular septal

TABLE 177-1 Effects of physiologic and pharmacologic interventions on the intensity of heart murmurs and sounds*

Intervention	Changes in heart murmurs and sounds
Respiration	Systolic murmurs due to TR or pulmonic blood flow through a normal or stenotic valve and diastolic murmurs of TS or PR generally increase with inspiration or the Mueller maneuver as do right-sided S_3 and S_4. Left-sided murmurs and sounds usually are louder during expiration.
Valsalva maneuver	Most murmurs decrease in length and intensity. Two exceptions are the systolic murmur of HCM, which usually becomes much louder, and that of MVP, which becomes longer and often louder. Following release of the Valsalva, right-sided murmurs tend to return to control intensity earlier than left-sided murmurs.
Post VPB or AF	Murmurs originating at normal or stenotic semilunar valves increase in the cardiac cycle following a VPB or in the cycle after a long cycle length in AF. By contrast, systolic murmurs due to AV valve regurgitation do not change, diminish (papillary muscle dysfunction), or become shorter (MVP).
Positional changes	With *standing* most murmurs diminish, two exceptions being the murmur of HCM, which becomes louder, and that of MVP, which lengthens and often is intensified. With *squatting* most murmurs become louder but those of HCM and MVP usually soften and may disappear.
Exercise	Murmurs due to blood flow across normal or obstructed valves (e.g., PS, MS) become louder with both isotonic and submaximal isometric (handgrip) exercise. Murmurs of MR, VSD, and AR also increase with handgrip exercise. However, the murmur of HCM often decreases with near maximum handgrip exercise. Left-sided S_4 and S_3 are often accentuated by exercise, particularly when due to ischemic heart disease.
Pharmacologic interventions	During the initial relative hypotension following amyl nitrite inhalation, murmurs of MR, VSD, and AR decrease while murmurs of aortic stenosis or sclerosis increase. During the later tachycardia phase, murmurs of MS and right-sided lesions also increase. The response in MVP often is biphasic (softer then louder than control). The arterial constrictor phenylephrine tends to produce the opposite effects.
Transient arterial occlusion	Transient external compression of both arms by bilateral cuff inflation to 20 mmHg > peak systolic pressure augments the murmurs of MR, VSD, and AR but not murmurs due to other causes.

* *TR, tricuspid regurgitation; TS, tricuspid stenosis; PR, pulmonic regurgitation; HCM, hypertrophic cardiomyopathy; MVP, mitral valve prolapse; PS, pulmonic stenosis; MS, mitral stenosis; MR, mitral regurgitation; VSD, ventricular septal defect; AR, aortic regurgitation; VPB, ventricular premature beat; and AF, atrial fibrillation.*

defect, may also produce splitting that persists during expiration. It may also occur with constrictive pericarditis. In patients with large atrial septal defects the proportion of right atrial filling contributed by the left atrium and the venae cavae varies reciprocally during the respiratory cycle so that right atrial inflow remains relatively constant. Therefore, the volume and duration of right ventricular ejection are not significantly increased by inspiration, and there is little inspiratory exaggeration of the splitting of S_2. This phenomenon, termed "fixed splitting" of the second heart sound, is of considerable diagnostic value.

A delay in aortic valve closure causing P_2 to precede A_2 results in so-called reversed (paradoxic) splitting of S_2. Splitting is then maximal in expiration, and decreases during inspiration with the normal delay of pulmonic valve closure. The commonest causes of reversed splitting of S_2 are left bundle branch block and delayed excitation of the left ventricle from a right ventricular ectopic beat. Mechanical prolongation of left ventricular systole, resulting in reversed splitting of S_2, may be caused by severe aortic outflow obstruction, a large aorta-to-pulmonary artery shunt, systolic hypertension, and ischemic heart disease or cardiomyopathy with left ventricular failure. P_2 is normally softer than A_2 in the second left intercostal space; when P_2 is greater than A_2 in this area, it suggests pulmonary hypertension, except in patients with atrial septal defect.

The *third heart sound* is a low-pitched sound produced in the ventricle 0.14 to 0.16 s after A_2, at the termination of rapid filling. This sound is frequent in normal children and in patients with high cardiac output. However, in patients over 40 years of age, an S_3 usually indicates ventricular decompensation, AV valve regurgitation, or other conditions which increase the rate or volume of ventricular filling. The left-sided S_3 is best heard with the bell piece of the stethoscope at the left ventricular apex during expiration and with the patient in the left lateral position. The right-sided S_3 is best heard at the left sternal border or just beneath the xiphoid and is increased with inspiration. Often it is accompanied by the systolic murmur of functional tricuspid regurgitation. Third heart sounds often disappear with treatment of heart failure.

An earlier (0.10 to 0.12 s after A_2), higher-pitched third heart sound (pericardial knock) often occurs in patients with constrictive pericarditis; its presence is dependent upon the restrictive effect of the adherent pericardium, which halts diastolic filling abruptly.

The opening snap (OS) is a brief, high-pitched, early diastolic sound which is usually due to stenosis of an AV valve, more commonly the mitral valve. It is usually heard best at the lower left sternal border and radiates well to the base of the heart. The A_2-OS interval during exercise is inversely related to the height of the mean left atrial pressure, and ranges from 0.04 to 0.12 s. At the base an OS is often confused with P_2. However, careful auscultation at the upper left sternal border will reveal both components of the second heart sound, followed by the opening snap. The OS of tricuspid stenosis occurs later in diastole than the mitral OS. Since most patients with tricuspid stenosis also have severe mitral valve disease, the tricuspid OS is often overshadowed by the diastolic rumble and OS originating in the stenotic mitral valve. An OS also may occur when there is increased flow across an AV valve, such as exists with left-to-right intracardiac shunts and mitral or tricuspid regurgitation.

The *fourth heart sound* is a low-pitched, presystolic sound produced in the ventricle during the ventricular filling associated with an effective atrial contraction, and is heard best with the bell piece of the stethoscope. The sound is absent in patients with atrial fibrillation. The S_4 occurs when diminished ventricular compliance increases the resistance to ventricular filling, and it is present frequently in patients with systemic hypertension, aortic stenosis, hypertrophic cardiomyopathy, coronary artery disease, and acute mitral regurgitation. Most patients with an acute myocardial infarction and sinus rhythm have an audible S_4. The fourth heart sound is frequently accompanied by visible and palpable presystolic distention of the left ventricle. It is maximal in intensity at the left ventricular apex with the patient in the left lateral position, and is accentuated by mild supine exercise. The right-sided S_4 is present in patients with right ventricular hypertrophy, secondary to either pulmonic stenosis or pulmonary hypertension, and frequently accompanies a prominent presystolic *a* wave in the JVP.

Audible fourth heart sounds also may be present during increased ventricular filling and normal ventricular compliance such as occurs in patients with severe anemia, thyrotoxicosis, or a peripheral arteriovenous fistula. An S_4 frequently accompanies delayed AV conduction even in the absence of clinically detectable heart disease. The incidence of an audible S_4 increases with increasing age. Whether an audible S_4 in adults without other evidence of cardiac disease is abnormal remains controversial.

The *ejection sound* is a sharp, high-pitched event occurring in early systole closely following the first heart sound. Ejection sounds occur in the presence of semilunar valve stenosis, i.e., opening snaps of the aortic or pulmonic valves, and in conditions associated with dilatation of the aorta or pulmonary artery. The aortic ejection sound is usually heard best at the left ventricular apex and the second right interspace; the pulmonary ejection sound is of maximal intensity at the upper left sternal border. The latter, unlike most other right-sided acoustical events, is heard better during expiration.

Nonejection systolic clicks, occurring with or without a late systolic murmur, often denote prolapse of one or both leaflets of the mitral valve. They may also be caused by tricuspid valve prolapse (Chap. 187). They probably result from functionally unequal length of the chordae tendineae of either or both AV valves and are heard best along the lower left sternal border and at the left ventricular apex. Systolic clicks may be single or multiple, and they may occur at any time in systole but usually later than the systolic ejection sound. Frequently the midsystolic click is misinterpreted as S_2, and the actual second heart sound is called an OS or S_3.

HEART MURMURS Cardiac murmurs result from vibrations set up in the bloodstream and the surrounding heart and great vessels as a result of turbulent blood flow, the formation of eddies, and cavitation (bubble formation as a result of sudden decrease in pressure).

The intensity or loudness of murmurs may be graded from I to VI. A grade I murmur is so faint that it can be heard only with special effort, and a grade VI murmur is audible with the stethoscope removed from contact with the chest. The configuration of a murmur may be crescendo, decrescendo, crescendo-decrescendo (diamond-shaped), or plateau. The precise time of onset and time of cessation of a murmur depend on the instant in the cardiac cycle at which an adequate pressure difference between two chambers appears and disappears (Fig. 177-4).

FIGURE 177-4 *Schematic representation of ECG, aortic pressure (AOP), left ventricular pressure (LVP), and left atrial pressure (LAP). HSM is a holosystolic murmur; PSM, a presystolic murmur; MDM, a middiastolic murmur; MSM, a midsystolic murmur; EDM, an early diastolic murmur; LSM, a late systolic murmur; and CM, a continuous murmur.*

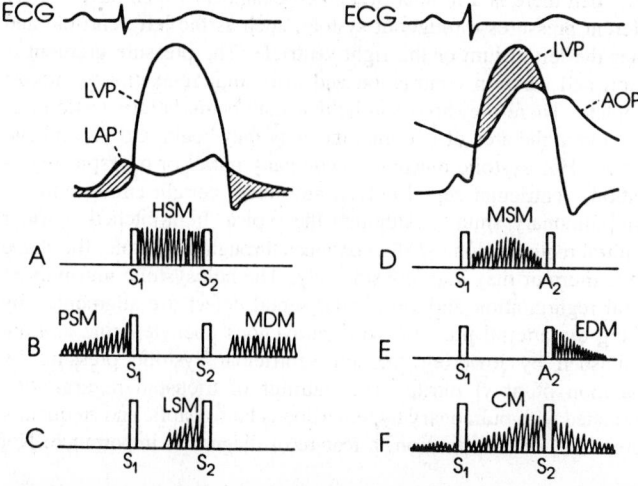

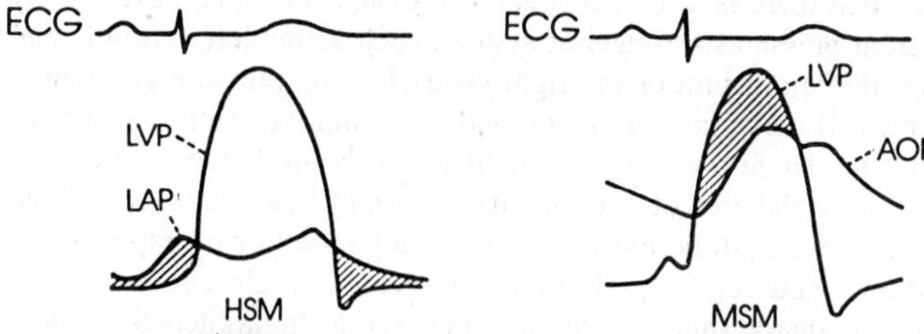

The location on the chest wall where the murmur is best heard and the areas to which it radiates can be helpful in identifying the cardiac structure from which the murmur originates. For example, the murmur of aortic valve stenosis is loudest usually in the second right intercostal space and radiates to the carotid arteries. By contrast, the murmur of mitral regurgitation is most often loudest at the cardiac apex and may radiate to the left sternal border and base of the heart when the posterior mitral leaflet is predominantly involved or to the axilla and back when the anterior leaflet is more severely affected. In the former case, the regurgitant blood is directed toward the posterior left atrial wall.

Many times it is difficult to classify with certainty a cardiac murmur based on its timing, configuration, location, radiation, pitch, or intensity. However, by noting changes in the characteristics of the murmur during maneuvers which alter cardiac hemodynamics, the auscultator often can identify its correct origin and significance (Table 177-1).

Accentuation of a murmur during inspiration with the augmentation of systemic venous return implies that it originates on the right side of the circulation; expiratory exaggeration has less significance. Prolonged expiratory pressure against a closed glottis, the Valsalva maneuver, reduces intensity of most murmurs by diminishing both right and left ventricular filling. The systolic murmur associated with *hypertrophic cardiomyopathy* and the late systolic murmur due to a *mitral valve prolapse* are exceptions and may be accentuated during the Valsalva maneuver. Murmurs due to flow across a normal or obstructed semilunar valve increase in intensity in the beat following a premature ventricular beat or a long RR interval in atrial fibrillation. In contrast, murmurs due to AV valve regurgitation or a ventricular septal defect do not change appreciably during the beat following a prolonged diastole. Standing, which decreases heart size, accentuates the murmur of hypertrophic cardiomyopathy and occasionally the murmur due to a prolapse of the mitral valve. Squatting, which increases both venous return and systemic arterial resistance, increases most murmurs, except those due to hypertrophic cardiomyopathy and mitral regurgitation due to a prolapsed mitral valve, which often decrease. Sustained handgrip exercise, which increases the systemic arterial pressure and heart rate, often accentuates the murmurs of mitral regurgitation, aortic regurgitation, and mitral stenosis but usually diminishes those due to aortic stenosis or hypertrophic cardiomyopathy. Pharmacologic interventions include inhalation of amyl nitrite, which reduces systemic arterial pressure and increases blood flow, thereby increasing the intensity of murmurs due to valvular stenosis while diminishing those due to aortic or mitral regurgitation (Table 177-1). Transient external arterial occlusion by the inflation of bilateral arm cuffs to 20 mmHg above systolic blood pressure for 5 s has been shown to intensify murmurs due to left-sided regurgitant lesions; this method is applicable to almost all patients and does not require administration of any drug.

Systolic murmurs *Holosystolic (pansystolic) murmurs* are generated when there is a flow between two chambers which have widely different pressures throughout systole, such as the left ventricle and either the left atrium or the right ventricle. The pressure gradient is established early in contraction and lasts until relaxation is almost complete. Therefore, holosystolic murmurs begin before aortic ejection, and at the area of maximal intensity they begin with S_1 and end after S_2. Holosystolic murmurs accompany mitral or tricuspid regurgitation, ventricular septal defect, and under certain circumstances, aortopulmonary shunts. Although the typical high-pitched murmur of mitral regurgitation usually continues throughout systole, the shape of the murmur may vary considerably. The holosystolic murmurs of mitral regurgitation and ventricular septal defect are augmented by raising the arterial pressure with intravenous phenylephrine and are diminished by lowering the left ventricular systolic pressure by inhalation of amyl nitrite. The murmur of tricuspid regurgitation associated with pulmonary hypertension is holosystolic and frequently increases during inspiration, a feature of diagnostic importance. Not all patients with mitral or tricuspid regurgitation or ventricular septal defect have holosystolic murmurs (Chap. 187).

Midsystolic murmurs, often crescendo-decrescendo in shape, occur when blood is ejected across the aortic or pulmonic outflow tracts. The murmur starts shortly after S_1 when the ventricular pressure rises sufficiently to open the semilunar valve. Ejection then begins and with it the onset of the murmur; as ejection increases, the murmur is augmented, and as ejection declines, it diminishes. The murmur ends before the ventricular pressure falls enough to permit closure of the aortic or pulmonic leaflets. In the presence of normal semilunar valves and increased flow rate, as may occur in states of elevated cardiac output, ejection into a dilated vessel beyond the valve, or increased transmission of sound through a thin chest wall may be responsible for the production of this murmur. Most benign, functional murmurs are midsystolic and originate from the pulmonary outflow tract. Valvular or subvalvular obstruction to either ventricle may also cause such a midsystolic murmur, the intensity being related to the flow.

The murmur of aortic stenosis is the prototype of the left-sided midsystolic murmur. The location and radiation of this murmur appear to be influenced by the direction of the high-velocity jet within the aortic root. In *valvular aortic stenosis* the murmur is usually maximal in the second right intercostal space, with radiation into the neck. In *supravalvular aortic stenosis* the murmur is occasionally loudest even higher, with disproportionate radiation into the right carotid artery. In hypertrophic cardiomyopathy, the murmur originates within the left ventricular cavity, and is usually maximal at the lower left sternal edge and apex, with relatively little radiation to the carotids. When the aortic valve is immobile (calcified), the aortic closure sound (A_2) may be soft and inaudible so that the length and configuration of the murmur are difficult to determine. Midsystolic murmurs also occur in patients with mitral regurgitation or, less frequently, tricuspid regurgitation resulting from papillary muscle dysfunction. Murmurs due to mitral regurgitation are often confused with those originating in the aorta, particularly in elderly patients.

The patient's age and the area of maximal intensity aid in determining the significance of midsystolic murmurs. Thus, in a young adult with a thin chest and high velocity of blood flow, a faint or moderate midsystolic murmur heard only in the pulmonic area is usually without clinical significance, while a somewhat louder murmur in the aortic area may indicate congenital aortic stenosis. In elderly patients pulmonic flow murmurs are rare, while aortic systolic murmurs are frequent and may be due to aortic dilatation, to a significant degree of valvular aortic stenosis, or to nonstenotic deformity of the aortic valve. Midsystolic aortic and pulmonic murmurs are intensified by amyl nitrite inhalation and during the cardiac cycle following a premature ventricular contraction, while those due to mitral regurgitation are unchanged or softer. Aortic systolic murmurs are diminished by interventions which increase systemic arterial resistance, such as intravenous phenylephrine. Echocardiography or cardiac catheterization may be necessary to separate a prominent and exaggerated functional murmur from one due to congenital semilunar valve stenosis.

Early systolic murmurs begin with the first heart sound and end in midsystole. They may be due to a very small *ventricular septal defect, a large defect with pulmonary hypertension,* or *severe acute mitral* or *tricuspid regurgitation.* In large ventricular septal defects with pulmonary hypertension, the shunting at the end of systole may be small or absent, resulting in an early systolic murmur. A similar murmur may occur with very small muscular ventricular septal defects, the shunt being interrupted in late systole. An early systolic murmur is a feature of tricuspid regurgitation occurring in the absence of pulmonary hypertension. This lesion is common in drug addicts with infective endocarditis, in whom a tall regurgitant right atrial *v* wave reaches the level of the normal right ventricular pressure in late systole, confining the murmur to early systole. In patients with acute mitral regurgitation and a large *v* wave in a noncompliant left atrium, a loud early systolic murmur is frequently heard which diminishes as the pressure gradient between left ventricle and left atrium decreases in late systole (Chap. 187).

Late systolic murmurs are faint or moderately loud high-pitched apical murmurs, which start well after ejection and do not mask either heart sound. They are probably related to papillary muscle dysfunction caused by infarction or ischemia of these muscles or to their distortion by left ventricular dilatation. They may appear only during angina but are common in patients with myocardial infarction or diffuse myocardial disease. Late systolic murmurs following mid-systolic clicks are associated with late systolic mitral regurgitation caused by prolapse of the mitral valve into the left atrium (Chap. 187).

Diastolic murmurs *Early diastolic murmurs* begin with or shortly after the second heart sound as soon as the corresponding ventricular pressure falls sufficiently below that in the aorta or pulmonary artery. The high-pitched murmurs of aortic regurgitation or pulmonic regurgitation due to pulmonary hypertension are generally decrescendo, since there is a progressive decline in the volume or rate of regurgitation during diastole. Faint, high-pitched murmurs of aortic regurgitation are difficult to hear unless they are specifically sought by applying firm pressure with the diaphragm over the left midsternal border while the patient sits, leans forward, and holds a breath in full expiration. The diastolic murmur of aortic regurgitation is enhanced by an acute elevation of the arterial pressure such as occurs with handgrip exercise; it diminishes with a decrease in arterial pressure which may be induced during amyl nitrite inhalation. The diastolic murmur of congenital pulmonic regurgitation in the absence of pulmonary hypertension is low- to medium-pitched. The onset of this murmur is delayed because at the onset of pulmonic valve closure the regurgitant flow is minimal, since the reverse pressure gradient responsible for the regurgitation is negligible at this time.

Middiastolic murmurs usually arise from the AV valves, occur during early ventricular filling, and like most midsystolic murmurs, are due to disproportion between valve orifice size and flow rate. Such murmurs may be loud despite only slight AV valve stenosis when there is normal or increased blood flow. Conversely, the murmur may be soft or even absent despite severe obstruction if the cardiac output is markedly reduced. When stenosis is marked, the diastolic murmur is prolonged and the duration of the murmur is more reliable than its intensity as an index of the degree of valve obstruction.

The low-pitched, middiastolic murmur of mitral stenosis characteristically follows the opening snap. It should be specifically sought by placing the bell of the stethoscope at the site of the left ventricular impulse, which is best localized with the patient on the left side. Frequently the murmur of mitral stenosis is present only at the left ventricular apex, and it may be increased in intensity by mild supine exercise or by inhalation of amyl nitrite. In tricuspid stenosis the middiastolic murmur is localized to a relatively limited area along the left sternal edge and may increase in intensity during inspiration.

Middiastolic murmurs may be generated across the mitral valve in ventricular septal defect, patent ductus arteriosus, or mitral regurgitation, and across the tricuspid valve in atrial septal defect or tricuspid regurgitation. These murmurs are related to the torrential flow across an AV valve, usually follow a third heart sound, and tend to occur with large left-to-right shunts or severe AV valve regurgitation. A soft middiastolic murmur may sometimes be heard in patients with acute rheumatic fever (Carey-Coombs murmur). It has been attributed to inflammation of the mitral valve cusps or excessive left atrial blood flow as a consequence of mitral regurgitation.

In acute aortic regurgitation, the left ventricular diastolic pressure may exceed the left atrial pressure, resulting in a middiastolic murmur due to "diastolic mitral regurgitation." In severe chronic aortic regurgitation a murmur is frequently present which may be either middiastolic or presystolic (Austin Flint murmur). This murmur appears to originate at the anterior mitral valve leaflet when blood simultaneously enters the left ventricle from both the aortic root and the left atrium.

Presystolic murmurs begin during the period of ventricular filling that follows atrial contraction and therefore occur in sinus rhythm. They are usually due to AV valve stenosis and have the same quality as the middiastolic filling rumble but are usually crescendo, reaching peak intensity at the time of a loud S_1. The presystolic murmur corresponds to the AV valve gradient, which may be minimal until the moment of right or left atrial contraction. It is the presystolic rather than the middiastolic murmur which is most characteristic of tricuspid stenosis and sinus rhythm. A right or left *atrial myxoma* may occasionally cause either middiastolic or presystolic murmurs that resemble the murmurs of mitral or tricuspid stenosis.

Continuous murmurs begin in systole, peak near S_2, and continue into all or part of diastole. These murmurs signify continuous flow due to communication between high- and low-pressure areas which persists through the end of systole and the beginning of diastole. A *patent ductus arteriosus* causes a continuous murmur as long as the pressure in the pulmonary artery is much below that in the aorta. The murmur is intensified by elevation of the systemic arterial pressure and is reduced by amyl nitrite inhalation. When pulmonary hypertension is present, the diastolic portion may disappear, leaving the murmur confined to systole. A continuous murmur is uncommon in aortopulmonary septal defects, since this malformation is generally associated with severe pulmonary hypertension. Surgically produced aortopulmonary connections and the subclavian–pulmonary artery anastomosis result in murmurs similar to that of a patent ductus.

Continuous murmurs may result from congenital or acquired *systemic arteriovenous fistula, coronary arteriovenous fistula,* anomalous origin of the left coronary artery from the pulmonary artery, and communications between the *sinus of Valsalva and the right side of the heart.* Continuous murmurs may also occur when high left atrial pressure results in continuous flow across a small defect in the atrial septum. Murmurs associated with *pulmonary arteriovenous fistulas* may be continuous but are usually only systolic. Continuous murmurs may also be due to disturbances of flow pattern in constricted systemic (e.g., renal) or pulmonary arteries when marked pressure differences between the two sides of the narrow segment persist; a continuous murmur in the back may be present in *coarctation of the aorta; pulmonary embolism* may cause continuous murmurs in partially occluded vessels.

In nonconstricted arteries continuous murmurs may be due to rapid flow through a tortuous bed. Such murmurs typically occur within the bronchial arterial collateral circulation in cyanotic patients with severe pulmonary outflow obstruction. The "mammary souffle," an innocent murmur heard during late pregnancy and early postpartum, may be systolic or continuous. The innocent cervical venous hum is a continuous murmur usually heard over the medial aspect of the right supraclavicular fossa with the patient upright. The hum is usually louder during diastole and can be instantaneously abolished by digital compression of the ipsilateral internal jugular vein. Transmission of a loud venous hum to the area below the clavicles may result in a mistaken diagnosis of patent ductus arteriosus.

The *pericardial friction rub,* which may have presystolic, systolic, and early diastolic scratchy components, may be confused with a murmur or extracardiac sound when heard only in systole. It is best appreciated with the patient upright and leaning forward and may be accentuated during inspiration.

REFERENCES

Baragan J et al (eds): *Dynamic Auscultation and Phonocardiography*. Maryland, Charles Press Publishers, 1979

Braunwald E: Physical examination, in *Heart Disease,* 2d ed, E Braunwald (ed). Philadelphia, Saunders, 1984, p 14

Craige E: Echophonocardiography and other noninvasive techniques to elucidate heart murmurs, in *Heart Disease,* 2d ed, E Braunwald (ed). Philadelphia, Saunders, 1984, p 68

———: Heart Sounds: Phonocardiography pulse tracings; and systolic time intervals, in *Heart Disease*, 2d ed, E Braunwald (ed). Philadelphia, Saunders, 1984, p 40

Dell Italia LJ et al: Physical examination for exclusion of hemodynamically important right ventricular infarction. Ann Intern Med 99:608, 1983

Eilen SD, Crawford MH, O'Rourke RA: Accuracy of precordial palpation for detecting increased left ventricular volume. Ann Intern Med 99:628, 1983

Fowler NO: Cardiac auscultation, in *Cardiac Diagnosis and Treatment*, 3d ed, NO Fowler (ed). Hagerstown, Harper & Row, 1980, p 62

Leatham A: *Auscultation of the Heart and Phonocardiography*, 2d ed. New York, Churchill Livingstone, 1976

Perloff JK (ed): *Physical Examination of the Heart and Circulation*. Philadelphia, Saunders, 1982

Reddy PS, Salerni R, Shaver JA: Normal and abnormal heart sounds in cardiac diagnosis, Part II: Diastolic sounds. Curr Probl Cardiol 10(4):1, 1985

Rothman A, Goldberger AL: Aids to cardiac auscultation. Ann Intern Med 99:346, 1983

Shaver JA, Salerni R, Reddy PS: Normal and abnormal heart sounds in cardiac diagnosis, Part I: Systolic sounds. Curr Probl Cardiol 10(3):1, 1985

Tavel ME: *Clinical Phonocardiography and External Pulse Recordings*, 4th ed. Chicago, Year Book, 1985

178 ELECTROCARDIOGRAPHY

ROBERT J. MYERBURG

INTRODUCTION The electrocardiogram (ECG) is a graphic description of the electrical activity of the heart, recorded from the body surface by electrodes positioned to reflect activity from a variety of spatial perspectives. The source of cardiac electrical activity resides within the working (contracting) myocardial cells as well as within the automatic and specialized cells as described in Chap. 183.

The magnitude and direction of the electrical activity recorded on the body surface are an average of the numerous cell depolarizations or repolarizations occurring at a given instant. Although much of the electrical activity from individual cells is canceled out before reaching the body surface by opposing forces from other cells, the resultant recording is a reasonably reproducible and accurate approximation of net cardiac electrical activity. However, the signals recorded at the body surface do not identify sites of origin because a given vector at the body surface can be accounted for by innumerable combinations of cellular signals at their source in the heart.

Early in the development of the ECG, Einthoven popularized the concept that the human body represents a large volume conductor having the source of cardiac electrical activity at its center. While this theory is not strictly accurate, it provides the clinician with a practical point from which to work. As an extension of this concept, the *net* electrical activity at any instant in the cardiac cycle may be viewed as originating from a polarized point source at a theoretical "electrical center" of the heart. Since this "equivalent dipole" would have direction and magnitude, one might then extend the pattern into a sequence of instantaneous vectors recordable from the body surface. The application of this concept to ECG analysis is discussed below.

LEAD SYSTEMS The ECG lead system is composed of five electrodes, one on each of the four limbs and one placed at various sites on the precordium. Each lead is a continuous recording of the change in electrical potential during the cardiac cycle between two of the electrodes, or between one electrode and a combination of the others. The right-leg electrode is an inactive ground electrode in all leads.

The original lead system developed by Einthoven is based on assumptions of (1) the homogeneity of the body volume conductor, (2) the symmetry of the leads, and (3) a single equivalent dipole at the center of the volume conductor. The *standard limb leads* (I, II, and III) are composed of three permutations of the right arm (RA), left arm (LA), and left leg (LL) electrodes [Fig. 178-1*A* (1)]. Lead I records the potential difference between the LA and the RA, the positive electrode on the LA, and the negative electrode on the RA [Fig. 178-1*A* (2)]. Lead II records the potential difference between the electrodes on the RA and the LL, the positive electrode on the LL. Lead III records the potential difference between the LA and the LL, with the positive electrode on the LL. It is likely that Einthoven arbitrarily selected the relationships between positive and negative electrodes in the three leads in order to have the major deflection of the QRS complex (see below) moving in an upward (positive) direction in most normal individuals.

The central terminal of Wilson (CTW) is constructed by connecting the RA, LA, and LL electrodes through 5000-Ω resistances, in order to cancel out the potentials from these three points. With the forces canceled out, the CTW theoretically remains inactive during the entire cardiac cycle, and an exploring electrode will function as a unipolar lead [Fig. 178-1*B* (1)]. The selection of the positions for the six *unipolar chest leads* [Figs. 178-1*B* (2) and 178-2] was based on the concept that the proximity of the heart to the anterior chest wall resulted in the unipolar chest leads functioning as "semidirect" leads, being influenced primarily by the tissue immediately beneath the electrode. While this concept does not have the quantitative signifi-

FIGURE 178-1 *Lead systems. A. Standard limb leads, showing (1) electrode positions, (2) the equilateral triangle of Einthoven, and (3) the conversion of the triangle to a triaxial reference system with positive (+) and negative (−) polarity. B. The unipolar chest leads, showing (1) the central terminal of Wilson (CTW) (or the indifferent electrode −i) and the chest electrode (C) (or the exploring electrode −E). The 5000 Ω between CTW and each limb electrode is not shown. The relationship between CTW and V_1 to V_6 in the horizontal plane is shown in B (2). C. The augmented unipolar limb leads, using the modified CTW. D. The hexaxial frontal plane reference system. Normal ranges are described in the text, and applications are derived in Figs. 178-5 and 178-6. RA, right arm; LA, left arm; LL, left leg; RL, right leg.*

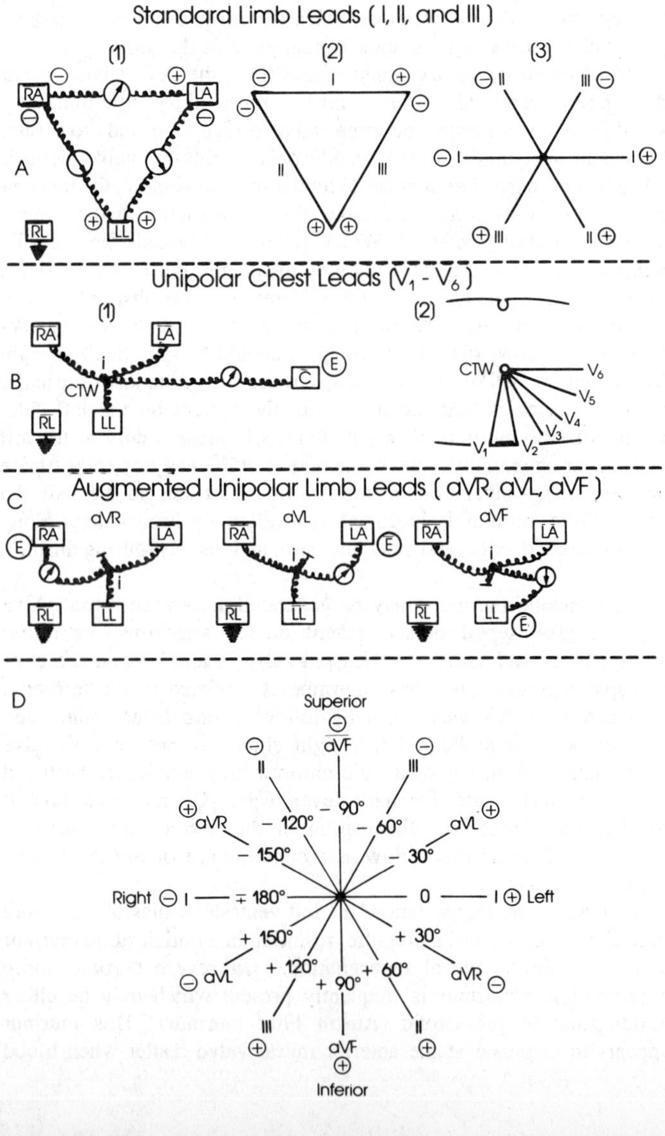

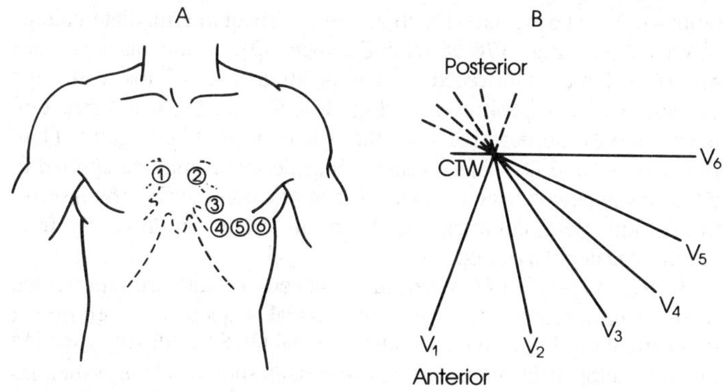

FIGURE 178-2 *The unipolar chest leads. A. The position of the chest electrode for V_1 to V_6. B. The relationship between the CTW and the chest electrode (C) in the horizontal plane.*

cance originally assumed, and the recordings do reflect the activity of the total heart, there is weighting of the voltages recorded by the tissue closest to the exploring electrode. The six standard chest leads (V_1 to V_6) are recorded by positioning the exploring chest electrode as follows: V_1 in the fourth intercostal space (4ICS) at the right sternal border; V_2 in the 4ICS at the left sternal border; V_4 in the 5ICS at the midclavicular line; V_3 midway between V_2 and V_4; V_5 at the left anterior axillary line at the level of V_4 horizontally; and V_6 at the left midaxillary line at the level of V_4 horizontally (Fig. 178-2). The CTW is the indifferent electrode, and the exploring chest electrode is the active electrode.

Unipolar limb leads may be recorded by a system in which the CTW constitutes the indifferent electrode and the exploring electrode is one of the three active limb electrodes. These leads are referred to as VR, VL, and VF. By disconnecting the input to the CTW from the extremity being explored, the voltage of the unipolar limb leads is augmented by as much as 50 percent. This modification is universally used for clinical ECGs, and the leads are labeled aVR, aVL, and aVF (Fig. 178-1*C*).

In recent years, the clinical value of chest wall mapping has been studied by a number of investigators. Multiple electrodes (32 to 192) are used for simultaneous recording, and computer processing for data reduction and display. This procedure yields information not available from the standard 12-lead ECG. New insights into normal and abnormal depolarization and repolarization patterns are evolving, and the value of sequential changes in ST segments during acute myocardial infarction is being studied.

ELECTROCARDIOGRAPHIC WAVEFORMS, DURATIONS, AND INTERVALS Clinical ECGs are recorded on paper having a graphic background (Fig. 178-3) to permit rapid measurement of standardized time intervals and voltages. Time lines are 1 mm apart, with every fifth line intensified. Standard paper speed is 25 mm/s. Thus, 1 mm = 0.04 s (lighter lines), and 5 mm = 0.20 s (heavier lines). The horizontal lines, 1 mm apart, permit calibration of the voltage deflections of the ECG. Usual standardization is ↑ 10 mm = +1 mV (Fig. 178-3).

The P wave reflecting atrial depolarization is normally the initial wave of activity during the cardiac cycle (Fig. 178-4). Ventricular muscle depolarization is represented by the *QRS complex*. A Q wave is an initial negative wave; an R wave is an initial positive wave or a positive wave following a Q wave; and an S wave is a negative deflection following an R wave (Fig. 178-4). A QRS complex having a Q wave which returns to the baseline but does not produce a positive wave is labeled a QS complex, and the second R wave in a QRS complex having more than one R wave is labeled R′. The T wave represents ventricular muscle repolarization and is sometimes followed by a small wave, the U wave, the mechanism of which remains uncertain. Repolarization of atrial muscle is represented by the T_a (or T_p) wave, which occurs during the PR interval and QRS complex, and is usually difficult to identify. The interval between

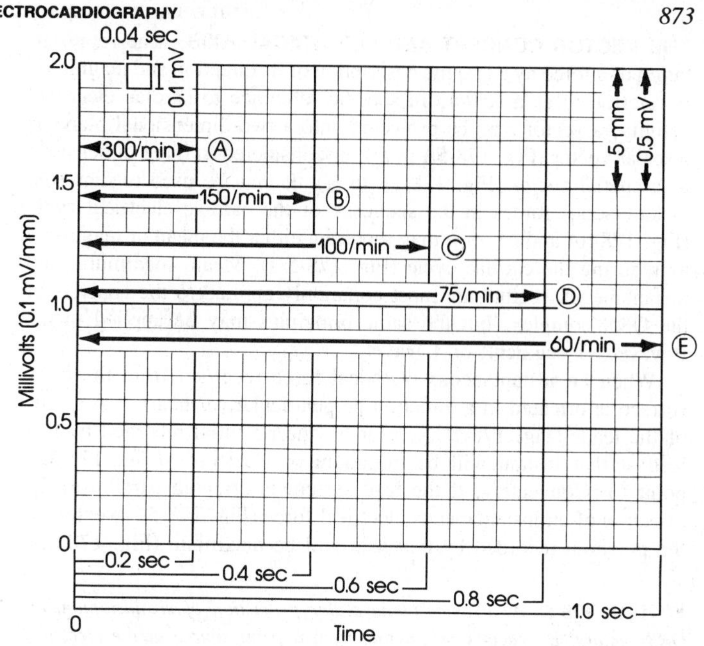

FIGURE 178-3 *Standardization of the ECG. Standard time calibration is 1 mm = 0.04 s or 5 mm = 0.20 s. Standard voltage is 0.1 mV/mm. A repetitive event occurring every 5 mm (A) on time axis (0.20 s) is occurring at 300 per minute. A repetitive event occurring every 10 mm (B) (0.40 s) is occurring at 150 per minute. C, D, and E indicate that repetitive events at 0.60, 0.80, and 1.00 s are occurring at rates of 100, 75, and 60 per minute, respectively.*

the end of the QRS complex and the onset of the T wave is the ST segment, representing the period of time between depolarization of the ventricles and the period of rapid repolarization of ventricular muscle.

The interval between the P wave and the QRS complex is the PR (or PQ) interval, measured from the *onset* of atrial depolarization (P) to the *onset* of ventricular depolarization (Q or R) (Fig. 178-4). The duration is 0.12 to 0.20 s in the adult. Since AV nodal activation begins before the end of depolarization of atrial muscle, the PR interval may be used as a rough approximation of AV conduction time.

The duration of the QRS complex (0.04 to 0.10 s) reflects the time required for depolarization of ventricular muscle. It may be slightly prolonged by regional block in a portion of the intraventricular SCT or by delayed conduction in a region of ventricular muscle. Block in a bundle branch prolongs the QRS to a greater extent. An approximation of the refractory period of the ventricles may be obtained by measuring the QT interval (from the onset of the QRS to the end of the T wave) (Fig. 178-4). The QT interval is rate-dependent, and may be altered by numerous pathophysiologic or pharmacologic influences.

FIGURE 178-4 *The waves of the electrocardiogram—P, QRS, T, and U—are indicated. The measurements of the PR interval, QRS complex, ST segment, and QT interval are identified on the right.*

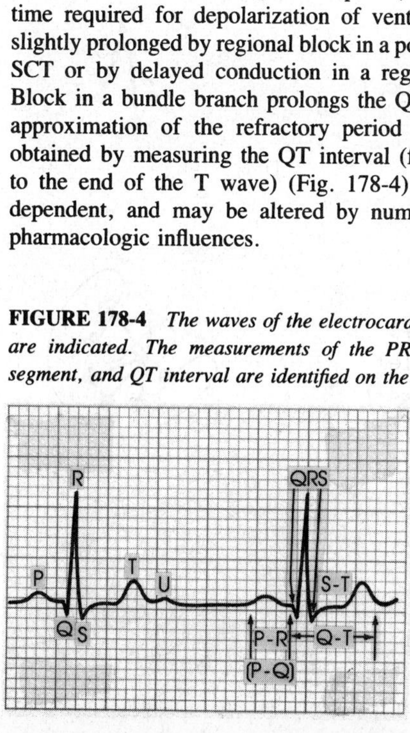

THE VECTOR CONCEPT AND ELECTRICAL AXIS The representation of a force by a graphic description of its direction and magnitude is referred to as a *vector*. In specific reference to cardiac electrical activity, a vector may be projected onto a two-dimensional plane as a scalar vector (Fig. 178-5*A* to *D*), or considered in three dimensions as a spatial vector (Fig. 178-5*E* to *H*). It may be used to represent instantaneous forces in the sequence of the cardiac electrical cycle (Fig. 178-5*A* and *E*), or it may represent either the mean or maximum axis during the cardiac cycle (Fig. 178-5*H*). Mean, maximum, and instantaneous vectors are most commonly applied to the analysis of the QRS complex, but the same principles may be applied to the P wave, ST segment, or T wave.

When an instantaneous electrical force recorded from the body surface is oriented in a direction perpendicular (or nearly so) to one of the leads (Fig. 178-5*C*, vector 6), the potential recorded by that lead at that instant will be minimum or isoelectric (Fig. 178-5*D*, point 6). Conversely, if the lead system is oriented parallel to the direction of an instantaneous electrical force (Fig. 178-5*C*, vector 4), the potential recorded by that lead will be maximum (Fig. 178-5*D*, point 4). An intermediate direction will record an intermediate voltage (for example, Fig. 178-5*C* and *D*, vector 2). If the instantaneous electrical force is oriented to the positive side of the lead, the deflection will be positive (4 in Fig. 178-5*C* and *D*); if the direction is oriented to the negative side, the deflection will be negative (1 in Fig. 178-5*C* and *D*). These general considerations may be applied to either instantaneous vectors occurring at any point during the inscription of the QRS complex, or the mean vector produced by total ventricular depolarization.

FIGURE 178-5 *A. Frontal plane scalar projection of six instantaneous QRS vectors. B. Vectors originating from a point source at the electrical center of the heart. C. Projection of the vectors on the lead I axis. D. Lead I QRS produced by the instantaneous vectors in panel C (see text). E. Spatial representation of ventricular depolarization. Seven instantaneous vectors in the sequence of depolarization indicated in spatial orientations. F. Spatial vectors originating from the electrical center of the heart. G. A line drawn through the terminations of the spatial vectors produces a spatial QRS loop (vector loop). H. The mean spatial QRS vector, average of all the instantaneous vectors—to the left, slightly inferiorly, and posteriorly. (See text.) (From JW Hurst, RJ Myerburg, Introduction to Electrocardiography, 2d ed, New York, McGraw-Hill, 1973; modified and reproduced by permission of the publisher.)*

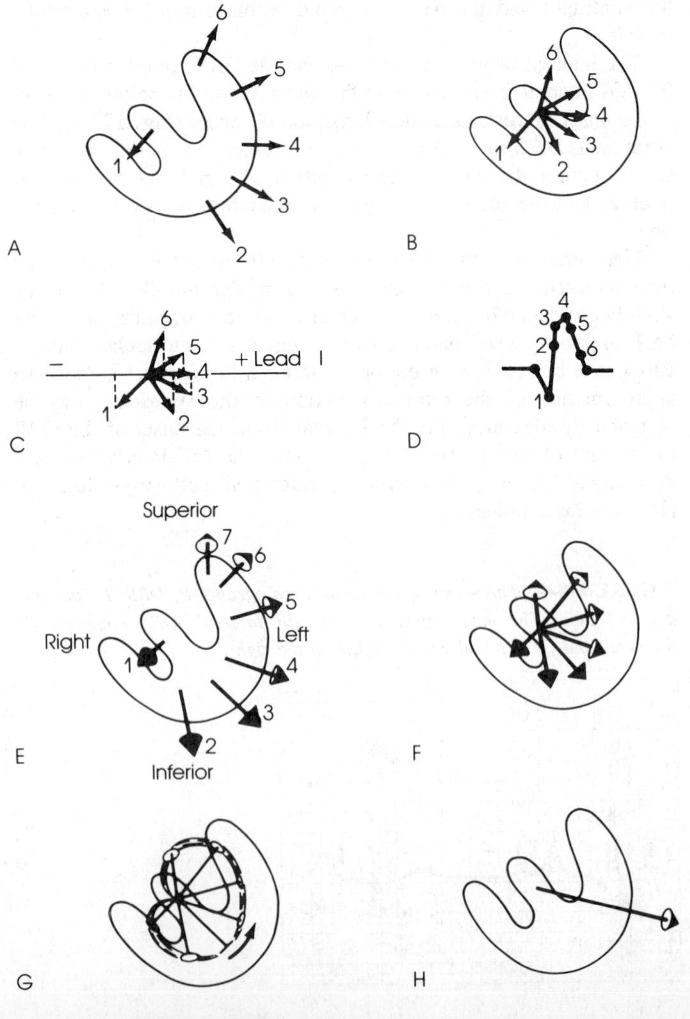

In Fig. 178-5*E* to *H*, seven instantaneous vectors are represented in three dimensions, indicating the spatial sequence of ventricular depolarization. In panel *H*, the mean spatial QRS vector, representing the net vector of all instantaneous forces, is shown. If the principles described above were applied, the QRS voltage would be large in lead I and small in aVF in the frontal plane (limb leads), and oriented posteriorly in the horizontal plane (chest leads).

When a triaxial system representing the augmented unipolar limb leads is superimposed on the triaxial system of Einthoven, a hexaxial system is obtained which is convenient for estimating the mean QRS axis, or any of the instantaneous vectors, in the frontal plane (Fig. 178-1*D*). When the appropriate positive and negative voltage orientations are assigned to each of the leads, the hexaxial reference system becomes a simple means of scalar vector analysis, requiring a minimum of two leads for estimation of the mean axis. An ECG which reveals a maximum positive QRS deflection in lead I and an isoelectric deflection in aVF would be oriented at 0°. Conversely, if the QRS voltage is positive and maximum in lead II and isoelectric in aVL, it would be oriented at +60°. The mean QRS axis in the frontal plane in normal adults ranges from −30 to +110°. Overlap between normal and abnormal occurs in the range of +90 to +110°. Generally, an axis $>$ +90° is referred to as *right axis deviation,* and more negative than −30° as *abnormal left axis deviation.* The determination of the mean QRS axis in the horizontal plane (Fig. 178-2*B*) is similarly derived, normal orientation being to the left and posteriorly.

Three normal ECGs are shown in Fig. 178-6. Analysis of the mean QRS axis in the *frontal plane* (I, II, III, aVR, aVL, aVF) reveals the axis of *A* to be oriented horizontally, of *C* to be oriented vertically, and of *B* to be oriented in an intermediate range. In *A* the net voltage of the QRS complex is largest in lead I, almost isoelectric in lead III, and low in aVF, placing the mean axis in a direction almost perpendicular to lead III. In *B*, the voltages in lead I and aVF are almost identical, and maximum in lead II and aVR. The mean QRS axis is between lead II (+) and aVR (−). In *C*, net voltage is largest in leads II and aVF and almost isoelectric in lead I, placing the mean QRS axis almost perpendicular to lead I. A similar approach is applied to QRS axis determination in the *horizontal plane*. In *C*, the lead in which the net forces are isoelectric is V_3. Therefore, as shown in the axial representation of the horizontal plane of tracing *C*, the QRS is oriented to the left and posteriorly. If this information is added to that obtained from the frontal plane axis, it is apparent that the mean QRS vector of electrocardiogram *C* is oriented inferiorly, to the left, and posteriorly. Similar principles may be applied to the analysis of the mean T-wave axis, which is normally oriented in the same general direction as the QRS axis. An angle between the QRS and T axes $>$45° in the frontal plane, or $>$60° in the horizontal plane, is abnormal.

ELECTRICAL ACTIVITY OF THE ATRIA The mean P-wave vector is normally directed to the left, inferiorly, and slightly anteriorly; the frontal plane P axis is usually oriented between +30 and +60°. Right atrial enlargement causes tall, peaked P waves ($\geq$0.25 mV), most prominent in standard leads II and V_1 (Fig. 178-7). Left atrial enlargement causes broad, notched P waves in lead II, and inverted or biphasic P waves (with the inverted portion of the biphasic P wave broader and deeper than the upright portion) in lead V_1. The upper limit of normal for P-wave duration is 0.11 s, and the broad P wave of left atrial enlargement usually is $\geq$0.12 s. However, criteria for left atrial enlargement are nonspecific, similar changes occurring in

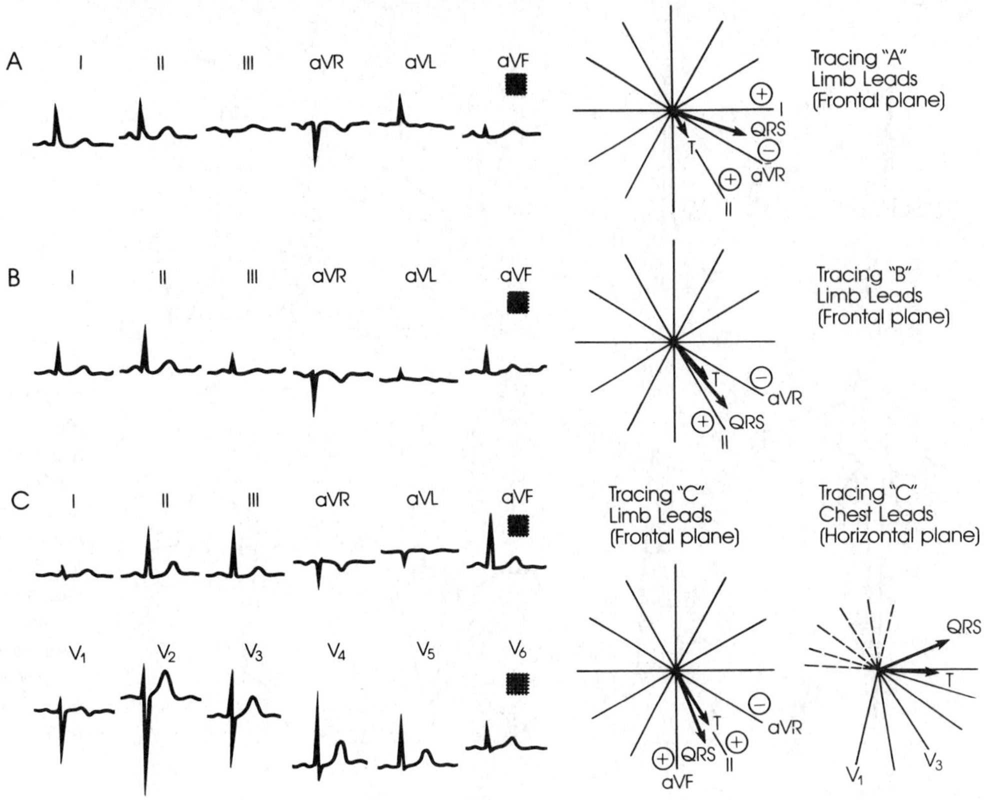

FIGURE 178-6 *Three normal ECGs demonstrating: (A) horizontal, (B) intermediate, and (C) vertical mean frontal plane QRS axes constructed on the hexaxial system. In addition, the horizontal plane vector in C is constructed on an axial system and is posteriorly oriented. T-wave vectors are similarly constructed.*

intraatrial conduction disturbances (Fig. 178-7), and the two must be distinguished on clinical grounds.

ABNORMALITIES OF VENTRICULAR DEPOLARIZATION: QRS COMPLEX Since the QRS complex is the ECG representation of the sequence, time, and synchronization of total ventricular muscle depolarization, focal or diffuse abnormalities in ventricular muscle or in the SCT may cause changes in QRS form. Abnormalities may be confined to initial depolarization (Fig. 178-8*B*), terminal depolarization (Fig. 178-8*C*), or mid and late depolarization (Fig. 178-8*D*), or they may be diffuse (Fig. 178-8*E* to *G*).

The normal earliest site of activation is in the midportion of the left side of the interventricular septum, followed closely by a site on the lower portion of the right side of the interventricular septum and the adjacent free wall endocardium. The dominant wavefront is that one arising on the left septum, which results in a small initial R wave in V_1 (anterior movement), and a small initial Q wave in I, aVL, and/or V_6 (rightward movement). Small initial Q waves in II, III, and aVF may be observed as an indication of a small superior movement of the initial wavefront. Normal septal Q waves are $\leq$0.02 s and of low amplitude. A normal R in V_1 is $\leq$0.4 mV.

After septal depolarization has been initiated, rapid endocardial propagation occurs through both ventricles. In the normal heart, the greater mass of the left ventricle predominates, and the magnitude and direction of the electrical vectors reflect this fact (Fig. 178-6). During normal depolarization, the sequence of instantaneous vectors rotates from rightward and anterior to leftward, posterior, and superior, as illustrated in Fig. 178-5*E* to *G*. Most individuals will have maximum QRS duration (i.e., the lead having the longest measurable QRS) of 0.05 to 0.08 s (normal range is 0.04 to 0.10 s). A QRS duration of 0.09 or 0.10 s may be a normal variant or may represent a conduction delay to limited regions of either ventricle. QRS durations $\geq$0.12 s represent left or right bundle branch block or severe degrees of diffuse intraventricular conduction delay (see Fig. 178-13).

Abnormal initial Q waves or an abnormal initial R in V_1 usually represents (1) a loss of muscle mass; (2) abnormal sequence of depolarization; or (3) a change in the relative muscle mass in the two ventricles.

The *intrinsicoid deflection* of the QRS complex is the major deflection *returning* to the baseline in a left (for example, 2→3 in Fig. 178-8*D*) or a right (S wave→2, Fig. 178-8*E*) precordial lead. Its *onset* should not exceed 0.035 s from the *onset* of the QRS complex in V_1, or 0.055 s from the *onset* of the QRS in V_5 or V_6. Delayed onset of the intrinsicoid deflection may indicate hypertrophy or conduction abnormalities (see Fig. 178-8).

The AV node and His bundle constitute the one normal pathway for impulse conduction from atria to ventricles. However, *accessory pathways* are present in some hearts. These are bands of muscle parallel to the AV junction, named Kent bundles, which form the

FIGURE 178-7 *P waves of right atrial enlargement (RAE) and left atrial enlargement (LAE).*

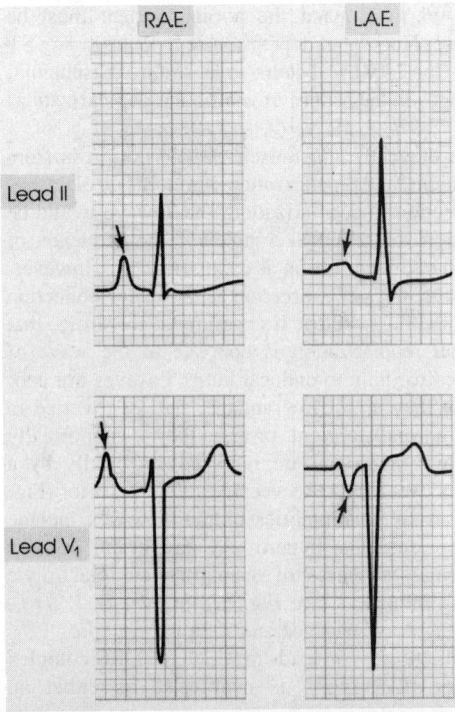

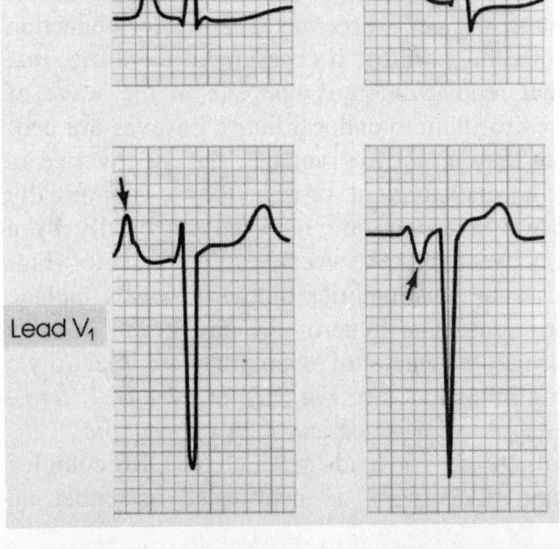

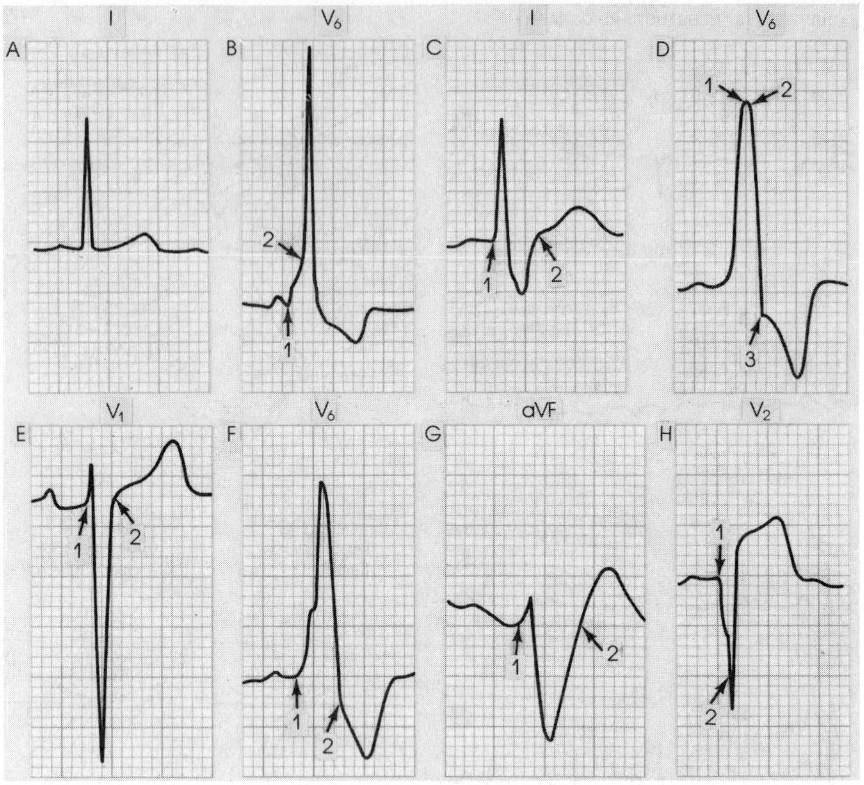

FIGURE 178-8 *QRS complexes. The lead is indicated above each example. A. Normal. B. Prolongation due to initial QRS delay between arrows (1→2) in Wolff-Parkinson-White syndrome (see Chap. 183). C. Prolongation due to terminal delay (1→2) in right bundle branch block. D. Prolongation due to mid (1→2) and late (2→3) delay in left bundle branch block. E. Minor uniform prolongation (1→2) in left ventricular hypertrophy. F. Distortion of total QRS pattern (1→2) in a cardiomyopathy. G. Uniform prolongation (1→2) in an electrolyte abnormality. H. Pathologic Q wave (1→2) in myocardial infarction. Intrinsicoid deflection = 2→3 in D and S→2 in E.*

anatomic substrate for the Wolff-Parkinson-White syndrome (see Chap. 184). The ECG manifestation is the *delta wave* (Fig. 178-8*B*).

ABNORMALITIES OF VENTRICULAR REPOLARIZATION: ST SEGMENT, T WAVE, AND U WAVE In the normal ECG, the ST segment is "isoelectric," resting at the same potential as the interval between the T wave and the next P wave. Deviations of the ST segment from the baseline may occur as a result of injury to cardiac muscle, changes in the synchronization of ventricular muscle depolarization, or drug or electrolyte influences. Elevations of the ST segment, in association with an elevation of the takeoff point of the ST segment from the QRS complex (the J point), may occur as a normal variant, especially in young individuals (Fig. 178-9*A*). The most common pathologic causes of ST-segment elevation are acute myocardial infarction and pericarditis (Fig. 178-9*B* to *F*), and the normal variant must be differentiated from these. Horizontal depression or a downsloping ST segment merging into the T wave occurs as a result of ischemia, ventricular strain, changes in the pattern of ventricular depolarization, or drug effects (Fig. 178-9*H*, *I*, *M*, *N*, *Q*, and *R*).

Since the sequence of ventricular muscle *de*polarization is from endocardium to epicardium, and *re*polarization represents an electrical current opposite in direction to depolarization, the T wave would be in the opposite direction to the QRS complex if the sequence of repolarization were in the same direction as depolarization. However, T waves generally assume the same direction as the major deflection of the QRS complex (see Fig. 178-6). It is assumed, therefore, that the direction of normal repolarization is opposite to the wave of depolarization—from epicardium to endocardium. T waves are considered abnormal when they are of low voltage, flat, or inverted in leads in which they are normally upright, or when they are abnormally tall and peaked. T-wave inversions are reflected vectorially by a widening of the angle between the QRS vector and the T vector (Fig. 178-6). Common causes of abnormalities of the T waves include ischemic heart disease, ventricular hypertrophy and strain, primary muscle disease, abnormal sequences of depolarization, electrolyte abnormalities, and drug influences (see Fig. 178-9*C*, *D*, *F*, *I*, *K*, *L*, and *N* to *R*). However, T-wave changes are often not specific.

The U wave is usually positive in leads in which the QRS complex is positive. The abnormal U wave is manifested as either an exaggeration of normal U-wave voltage, the appearance of a U wave in leads in which it is not normally seen, or inversion of a U wave. U-wave abnormalities occur in ischemic heart disease, left ventricular strain, and electrolyte disturbances. Unfortunately, the information they provide is usually nonspecific.

ECG MANIFESTATIONS OF VENTRICULAR HYPERTROPHY The normal dominance of the left ventricle on the features of the QRS complex is decreased or reversed in right ventricular hypertrophy (RVH) and exaggerated in left ventricular hypertrophy (LVH) (Fig. 178-10). RVH causes a shift of the net forces of depolarization from the left and posterior toward the right and anteriorly. On the ECG, this produces tall R waves in V_1 (≥0.5 mV), with an abnormal S wave in V_5 or V_6 (≥0.7 mV). In the frontal plane, the mean QRS axis shifts to the right of vertical (usually >110°). Less extreme degrees of RVH may result in preservation of a moderately deep S wave in V_1, with an R-wave voltage exceeding the S-wave voltage, or a normal R wave with a shallow S wave and prominent terminal S waves in V_5 and V_6. The primary QRS manifestation of LVH is an increase in voltage in those leads which reflect the electrical activity of the left ventricle. R waves in the standard limb leads may increase beyond the normal limit of 2.0 mV. Concomitantly, there is a tendency for a shift of the frontal plane QRS axis to the left. It is not likely that LVH alone will cause a shift in the QRS axis beyond −30°, but it commonly causes a shift in the range of 0 to −30° (Fig. 178-10). LVH causes a deep S wave in lead V_1 or V_2 (>2.5 mV) or an abnormal R wave in lead V_5 or V_6 (>2.5 mV). When T waves are normal, the presence of voltage criteria for LVH must be interpreted in terms of body habitus of an individual. Young, healthy, thin-chested individuals will frequently exceed the QRS voltage criteria for LVH in its absence. However, when the ST-segment and T-wave changes associated with "strain" are present (Figs. 178-9*Q* and 178-10), the diagnosis of LVH is clarified. Similarly, borderline voltage criteria are more specific for LVH when associated with the ST-segment and T-wave changes of left ventricular strain.

ACUTE MYOCARDIAL INFARCTION Three pathophysiologic events occur, either in sequence or simultaneously, in an acute myocardial infarction—ischemia, injury, and infarction. The ECG manifestations

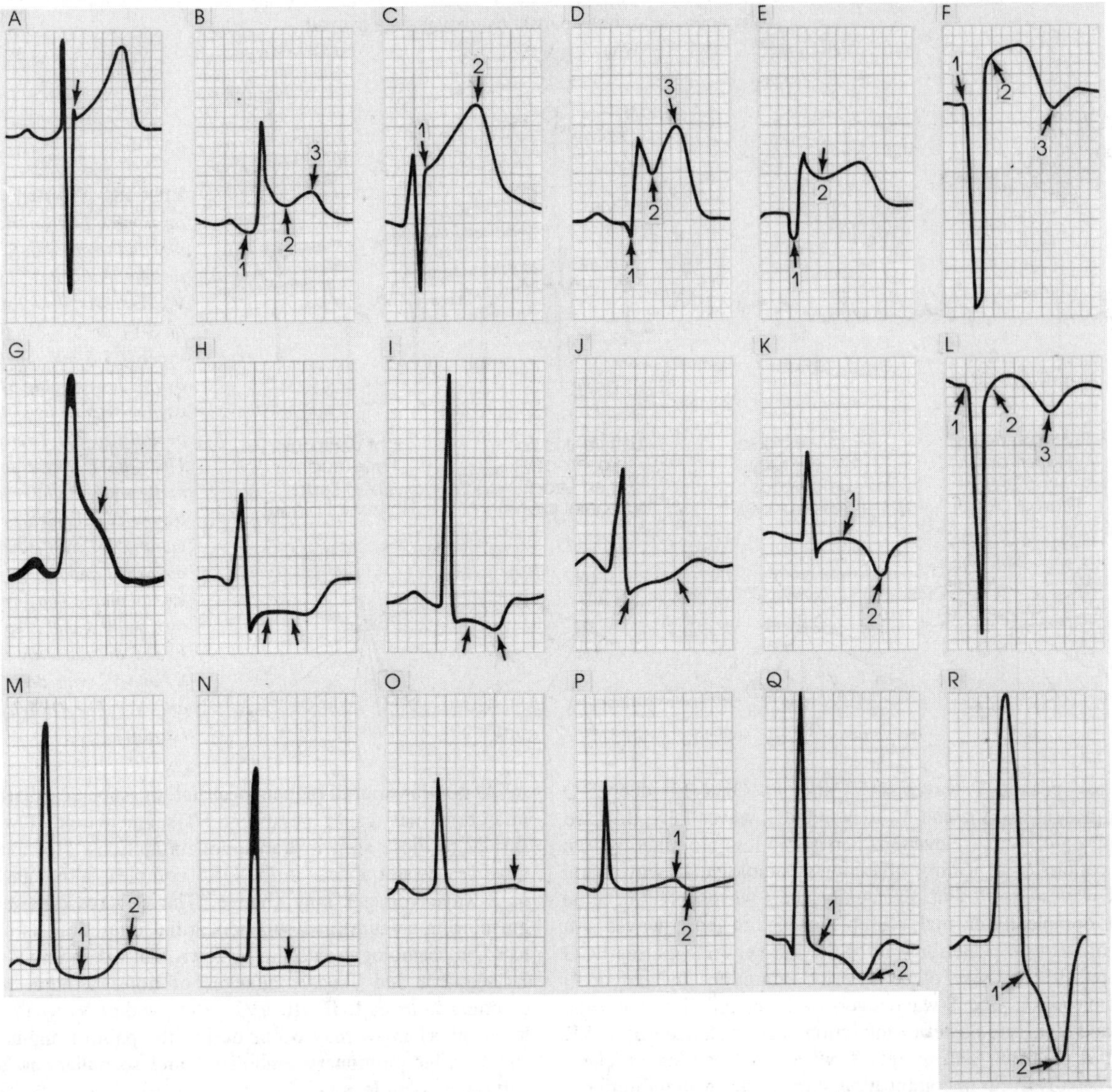

FIGURE 178-9 *ST-segment and T-wave changes. Arrows in each panel indicate the major features of each complex. A. Early repolarization (J-point elevation), normal variant. B. Acute pericarditis: (1) depressed* T_a*; (2) elevated ST; (3) normal T. C. Early acute myocardial infarction (AMI): (1) elevated ST; (2) tall, peaked T wave; steep angle between 1 and 2. D. AMI: (1) small Q wave; (2) elevated ST segment; (3) tall, peaked T wave with steep 2→3 angle. E. AMI: (1) pathologic Q wave; (2) elevated ST segment. F. AMI: (1) Q wave; (2) elevated ST segment; (3) terminal T-wave inversion. G. Angina pectoris (Prinzmetal variant) with ST elevation during pain. H and I. Angina pectoris (usual form) with horizontal or downward sloping ST segment during pain or exercise. J. J-point depression with upsloping ST segment during exercise, normal response. K. Primary T-wave inversion (2) in ischemia or primary muscle disease. L. Myocardial infarction (healed): (1) pathologic Q; (2) ST returning to baseline; (3) symmetrically inverted T wave. M. Digitalis effect: (1) downward coving of ST segment, merging into (2) an upright T wave. N to P. Nonspecific ST-segment and T-wave changes often seen in chronic ischemic heart disease. Q. Left ventricular strain pattern with (1) downsloping ST segment and (2) asymmetrically inverted (secondary) T wave. R. Downsloping ST segment merging into a deeply inverted T wave in ventricular conduction abnormality.*

of these processes include changes in the T waves (ischemia), ST segments (injury), and QRS complexes (infarction). The earliest T-wave changes of acute myocardial ischemia are tall, peaked T waves (''hyperacute'') (Fig. 178-9*C* and *D*), followed later by symmetrically inverted T waves (Fig. 178-9*F* and *K*). When the electrical integrity of the cell membranes is affected, currents of injury develop. The injury pattern on ECG during evolution of a transmural infarction is an elevation of the ST segments in the leads facing the infarcting area (Fig. 178-9*C* and *F*). The combination of ischemia and injury causes elevated ST segments, followed by either tall, peaked T waves (in the very early stages) or inverted T waves (Fig. 178-11). In leads opposite the region of the acute infarction, reciprocal changes occur: depressed ST segments and upright or isoelectric T waves (Figs. 178-11 and 178-12). There is some controversy about the distinction between ''reciprocal changes'' and nearly identical changes reflecting coexistent ischemia in a vascular bed remote from the infarction, i.e., ''ischemia at a distance.'' It is likely that remote ST depressions could be due to either. As the period of active injury resolves, the ST segments return to the baseline, but the inverted T waves may persist for months or years (Fig. 178-9*L*). Pathologic Q waves are the QRS manifestation of a transmural myocardial infarction. Q waves are pathologic when they appear in a lead in which Q waves were previously not present, or when the Q waves of normal septal depolarization become exaggerated (>20 ms; >0.2 mV).

The ECG in an acute inferior wall myocardial infarction is shown in Fig. 178-11. Leads II, III, and aVF, which face the inferior surface of the left ventricle (see Fig. 178-1*D*), demonstrate the direct patterns of infarction (pathologic Q waves), injury (elevated ST segments), and ischemia (inversion of the T waves). Reciprocal changes (depressed ST, tall T) are demonstrated in aVL. The evolution of an acute anterior myocardial infarction is demonstrated in Fig. 178-12. The most obvious direct changes occur in aVL, V_2, and V_3, and reciprocal changes in II, III, and aVF. In the tracing of 4/11, ST elevations (most prominent in aVL, V_2, and V_3) are accompanied by

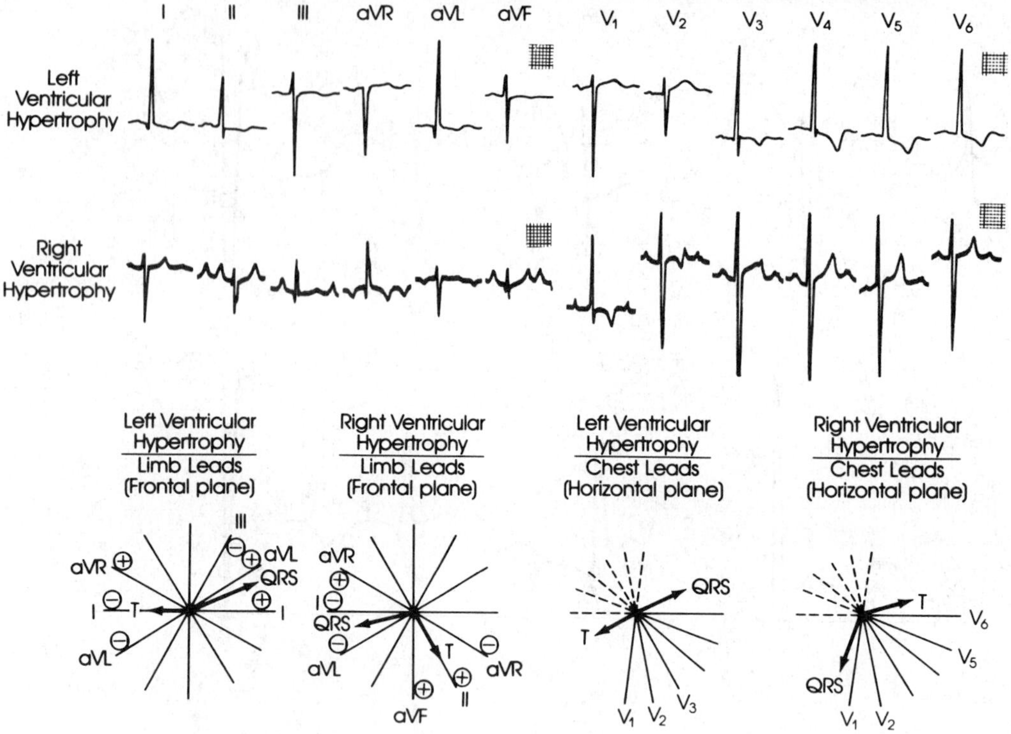

FIGURE 178-10 *Ventricular hypertrophy. Left ventricular hypertrophy and strain with R wave >2.0 mV in limb leads; R >2.5 mV in V_5 and V_6, and S in V_1 >2.5 mV. The sum of S-V_1 or S-V_2 and R-V_5 or R-V_6 exceeds 3.5 mV. Strain is indicated by the downsloping ST segments and asymmetrically inverted T waves, especially in the lateral chest leads. The QRS-T vector angle is abnormally wide. Right ventricular hypertrophy is indicated by right axis deviation in the frontal plane and abnormal anterior forces in the horizontal plane. The former is indicated by a small R and deep S wave in lead I, and the latter by tall R waves in V_1 and V_2 with deep S waves in V_5 and V_6. The QRS-T angle is wide (strain).*

''hyperacute'' peaked T waves in V_2 and V_3. On 4/12, deeper Q waves are present in aVL and V_1 to V_3, and T waves have inverted in aVL and V_2 to V_5. ST elevations persist but less prominently. On 4/25, the pattern of a healing infarction—pathologic Q waves and ischemic T waves—is present. Eventually, the T waves might become partially or completely normal, with persistence of the Q waves. An infarction of the true posterior wall of the left ventricle causes ECG changes opposite to those of an anterior infarction. Instead of Q waves, ST elevation, and T-wave inversion in the anterior precordial leads (V_1 and V_2), true posterior infarction is characterized by tall R waves, ST depression, and upright T waves in these leads. These infarctions usually occur in combination with inferior wall infarctions. Right ventricular myocardial infarction occurs infrequently and is almost always associated with inferior and/or posterior infarction of the left ventricle. Right ventricular infarction has no specific pattern on the standard 12-lead ECG; however, ST elevations on special right-sided precordial leads (V_4R to V_6R) may identify acute RV infarcts.

FIGURE 178-11 *Acute inferior wall myocardial infarction. The ECG of 11/29 shows minor nonspecific ST-segment and T-wave changes. On 12/5 an acute myocardial infarction occurred. There are pathologic Q waves (1), ST-segment elevation (2), and terminal T-wave inversion (3) in leads II, III, and aVF indicating the location of the infarct on the inferior wall (see text). Reciprocal changes in aVL (small arrow). Increasing R-wave voltage with ST depression and increased voltage of the T wave in V_2 is characteristic of true posterior wall extension of the inferior infarction.*

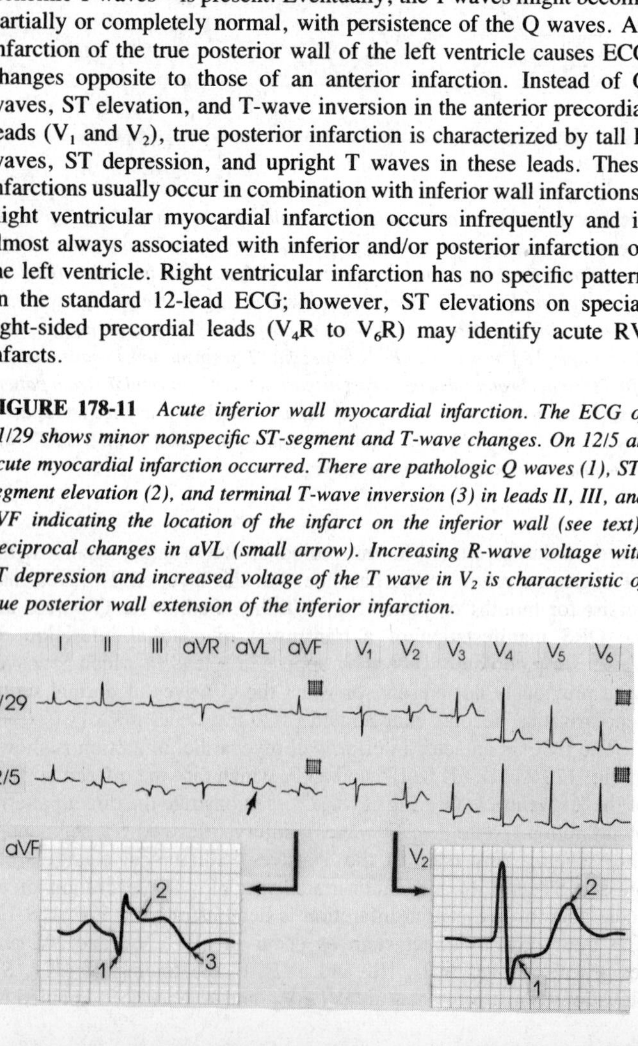

A nontransmural (subendocardial or subepicardial) myocardial infarction may cause persistent ST-segment and T-wave changes similar to those seen in transmural infarctions. However, abnormal Q waves do not appear in the QRS complex, although R-wave and/or S-wave voltages may change. The Q-wave criterion for distinguishing transmural and subendocardial infarctions is a useful ECG tool, but pathologic data have shown that exceptions do occur. The ST-segment and T-wave changes of nontransmural infarction are common in leads I, II, III, aVL, aVF, and/or V_4 to V_6. Similar, but transient, changes may occur during the pain of angina pectoris, in shock, after pulmonary embolism, and secondary to acute central nervous system lesions.

CHRONIC ISCHEMIC HEART DISEASE The ECG in chronic ischemic heart disease is often nonspecific. The patterns of chronic myocardial ischemia are intrinsically variable, and this is compounded by the problem of coexistent ECG changes related to pharmacologic interventions and/or LVH. Chronic ischemic heart disease causes a broad range of ST-segment and T-wave changes (Fig. 178-9*G* to *I*, *K*, *L*, and *N* to *P*). There may be moderate degrees of horizontal ST-segment depression or a downward sloping ST segment, flattening of inversion of T waves, and prominent U waves. It is difficult to define an abnormal ST-segment depression in precise quantitative terms. However, if the J point is more than 0.5 mm below the isoelectric line, the ST segment is horizontal or downsloping, and

FIGURE 178-12 *Acute anterior wall myocardial infarction. On 4/11, changes of a very early acute myocardial infarction in leads I, aVL, V_2, and V_3, with reciprocal changes in II, III, and aVF. On 4/12, ST segments remain elevated in the anterior leads, but T waves are inverted. On 4/25, a completed large anterior myocardial infarction is recorded—Q in I, aVL, V_1 to V_4.*

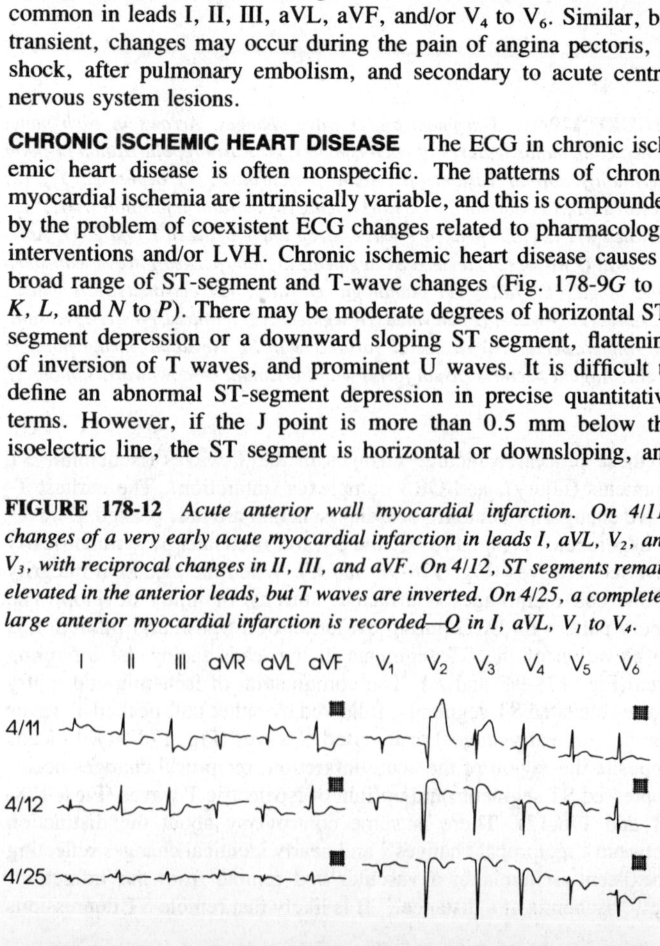

there is an associated T-wave abnormality, myocardial ischemia should be considered. The common clinical expression of chronic ischemic heart disease, angina pectoris, may be accompanied by a normal resting ECG or nonspecific ST-segment and T-wave changes. However, during spontaneous or exercise-induced pain, the ECG may demonstrate the horizontal or downward sloping ST-segment depressions shown in Fig. 178-9*H* and *I*, or rarely the variant pattern of spontaneous transient ST elevations (Prinzmetal variant) (Fig. 178-9*G*).

INTRAVENTRICULAR CONDUCTION DISTURBANCES The complex anatomy of the specialized conducting system of the ventricles, in conjunction with the focal nature of most cardiac diseases, is reflected in the multiplicity of ECG patterns which result from disorders of the sequence of activation of the ventricles. Disease of both the SCT and ventricular myocardium plays a role in the various patterns. The universal feature of ventricular conduction disturbances is a prolongation of the time required for depolarization of a portion of a ventricle, an entire ventricle, or both ventricles. Delayed or slow conduction may be diffuse or may be confined to a portion of the QRS complex (Fig. 178-8). Prolongation of the QRS may be modest, as in left ventricular hypertrophy, or extreme, as in cardiomyopathies or metabolic abnormalities (Fig. 178-8).

The classic bundle branch block patterns are associated with specific lesions in the left or right bundle branch in the majority of cases. Complete right bundle branch block (RBBB) (Fig. 178-13) is characterized by prolongation of the QRS complex (≥0.12 s) with the delayed activation of the right ventricle accounting for a terminal delay on the ECG. Since septal activation from the left bundle branch system normally precedes right ventricular activation, *the initial forces of ventricular depolarization are not disturbed in RBBB*, and the ability to identify coexistent pathologic Q waves is not hindered. The delayed activation of the right ventricle is reflected by the presence of terminal forces directed anteriorly and to the right.

The rightward direction of the slow terminal forces is indicated by the broad terminal S wave in leads I, aVL, and V_6 (Fig. 178-13). The anterior orientation of these forces is indicated by a large terminal R wave (R′) in V_1. Since initial forces are not disturbed, the normal initial R wave in V_1 persists, followed by an S wave. Incomplete RBBB is present when the waveform criteria for RBBB (rSR′) are present, but the QRS duration is <0.12 s.

Left bundle branch block (LBBB) is also characterized by a QRS duration ≥0.12 s. However, since normal initial ventricular depolarization is dependent upon the LBB to deliver the impulses of initial depolarization to the left septum, the patterns produced by LBBB are more complex. Normal septal depolarization is disturbed, and delay of the normally dominant left ventricular forces produces a more generalized disturbance of QRS morphology. The septal Q wave in standard leads I, aVL, and V_6 is typically lost. In addition, the initial anterior force reflected by the small R wave in lead V_1 may be lost because of a less anterior orientation of the initial forces. The delay in left ventricular activation produces the greatest degree of slowing in the mid and late portion of the QRS complex. This often results in notching at the peak of the upstroke in leads I and V_6 (see Figs. 178-8*D* and 178-14), with a late intrinsicoid deflection (>0.055 s) in V_5 and V_6. Most cases of LBBB produce secondary T-wave abnormalities as demonstrated in Fig. 178-14. Because of the changes in the initial forces, and the secondary ST-segment and T-wave changes, it is usually difficult to evaluate the QRS-complex, ST-segment, and T-wave changes of coexistent ischemic heart disease. When the intrinsicoid deflection is delayed in leads V_5 or V_6, but the QRS duration is <0.12 s, incomplete LBBB may be present. LBBB may be associated with either a normal QRS axis (Fig. 178-13) or left axis deviation.

In recent years a great deal of attention has been given to the ECG patterns referred to as the *left hemiblocks*. As the name implies, *left anterior hemiblock* (LAH) has been proposed to result from disease in the anterior radiation of fibers referred to as the anterior division of the LBB. *Left posterior hemiblock* (LPH) has been assumed to result from disease in the left posterior radiation. The complex nature of the LBB system has thus far defied a determination of whether focal proximal disease or diffuse distal disease in the distribution of these portions of the LBB is the mechanism responsible for the hemiblock patterns, although it is known that the pathologic process tends to be diffuse in those cases studied at autopsy.

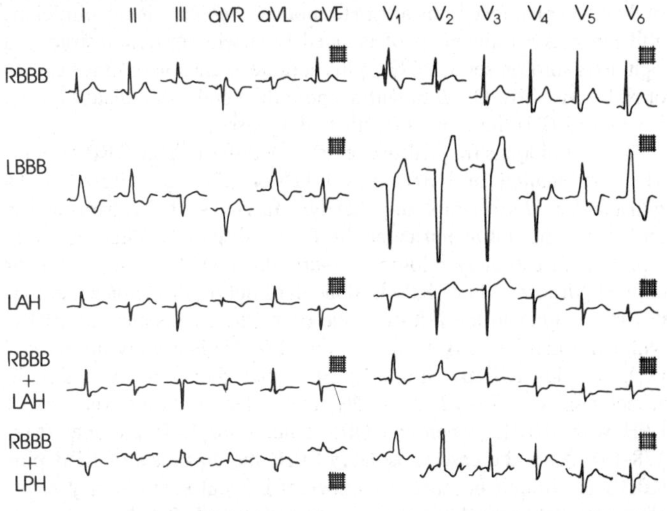

FIGURE 178-13 *Intraventricular conduction abnormalities. Illustrated are right bundle branch block (RBBB); left bundle branch block (LBBB); left anterior hemiblock (LAH); right bundle branch block with left anterior hemiblock (RBBB + LAH); and right bundle branch block with left posterior hemiblock (RBBB + LPH) (see text).*

LAH results in a moderate delay of activation of the superior portion of the left ventricular free wall, causing a modest prolongation of the QRS complex and shift of the front plane axis to the left. Initial septal depolarization is undisturbed (Fig. 178-13), and the QRS complex rarely exceeds 0.09 to 0.10 s. The differentiation between LAH and left ventricular hypertrophy (LVH) may occasionally be difficult. In general, LVH alone will not produce a left axis shift beyond −30°, and LAH will often produce left axis deviation ≥−60°. The key QRS features in left anterior hemiblock include small Q waves in leads I and aVL, with small initial R waves and deep S waves in leads II, III, and aVF.

LPH results in a moderate delay of activation of the posterior-inferior portion of the left ventricular free wall. Again, there is a modest prolongation of the QRS complex, but a shift of the frontal plane QRS axis to the *right*. Thus, the initial septal forces, though generally undisturbed, may be oriented more superiorly, producing small initial Q waves in leads II, III, and aVF. Since the specificity

FIGURE 178-14 *A. Acute pericarditis with ST-segment elevations in all leads except III, aVR, and V_1. B. Myocarditis: diffuse ST-segment and T-wave changes, with low-voltage T waves in the limb leads and primary T-wave changes in the chest leads. C. Cardiomyopathy: gross distortion of the QRS complex.*

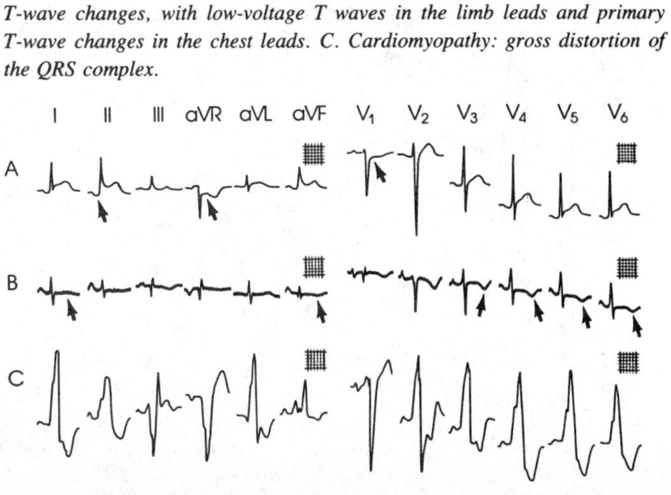

of the ECG manifestations of LPH is not very reliable, many clinicians will not make a diagnosis of isolated LPH without demonstrating a right axis shift on serial ECGs, plus definite exclusion of other causes of right axis shift. Of all the intraventricular conduction disturbances, isolated LPH is the most difficult to diagnose.

The hemiblocks frequently coexist with disease in the RBB system. The combination of RBB, plus LAH or LPH, is referred to as *bifascicular block*—implying that two fascicles of the trifascicular model of the intraventricular SCT are diseased. This probably represents a pathophysiologic oversimplification, but it is useful for clinical purposes. Since RBBB alone does not produce abnormal axis deviation either to the left or to the right, the coexistence of RBBB with abnormal left axis deviation (Fig. 178-13) is usually interpreted as LAH plus RBBB. Similarly, abnormal right axis deviation in association with RBBB is usually interpreted as the coexistence of LPH with RBBB, when the QRS criteria for LPH are met (Fig. 178-13). As is the case in isolated LPH, the diagnosis of LPH plus RBBB is difficult because a number of clinical settings may cause abnormal right axis deviation in conjunction with RBBB.

Trifascicular block describes abnormal conduction in all three divisions of the intraventricular SCT. The ECG diagnosis can be made only by inference when a patient has bifascicular block and a prolonged PR interval. Confirmation can be achieved only with His bundle electrocardiography (Chap. 183).

PERICARDITIS, MYOCARDITIS, AND THE CARDIOMYOPATHIES Acute pericarditis causes elevation of the ST segments in many leads without the reciprocal changes seen in acute myocardial infarction (Fig. 178-14*A*). ST-segment elevation may occur in all leads except aVR and rarely involves V_1. After a period of days, the diffuse ST elevations return to the baseline, and T-wave inversions may occur. Coexistent ST elevations and T-wave inversions do not occur as often as they do in myocardial infarction (compare Figs. 178-11 and 178-14*A*). T-wave abnormalities may persist for weeks or months after the acute episode of pericarditis. If the pericarditis is accompanied by significant degrees of pericardial effusion, electrical alternans may occur. On alternate beats, ECG voltage shifts in magnitude. There also may be low voltage of the QRS complexes and T waves in all leads. Finally, the T_a waves may be transiently depressed because of atrial involvement by the inflammatory process [see Fig. 178-9*B* (1)].

The ECG changes of myocarditis (Chap. 192 and Fig. 178-14*B*) are often difficult to differentiate from the late phase of pericarditis, in which symmetric T-wave inversions are present. However, myocarditis may occur in many other settings, and an appreciation of the range of the ECG changes is important. Almost all systemic infections may produce minor myocardial involvement. Measles, mumps, influenza, hepatitis, infectious mononucleosis, and scarlet fever, just to name a few diseases, may be associated with ECG abnormalities and with histopathologic evidence of myocardial inflammation. When the myocardial involvement is subclinical, the ECG changes are usually subtle and nonspecific. There are minor T-wave changes, manifested as flattening or perhaps shallow inversion of the T waves in multiple leads (Fig. 178-9*O* and *P*). The conducting system may be involved, and prolongation of the PR interval may be noted.

In clinically evident myocarditis, the ECG demonstrates symmetrically inverted T waves in most of the standard limb leads and in the lateral precordial leads (Fig. 178-14*B*). When the specialized conducting system is involved, bundle branch block or patterns of nonspecific intraventricular conduction defects may occur.

The ECG may be helpful in distinguishing types of cardiomyopathies (Chap. 192). In the hypertrophic cardiomyopathies, the most common ECG pattern is LVH and strain (Fig. 178-10). When asymmetric septal hypertrophy is present, abnormal septal depolarization may be indicated by the presence of deep abnormal Q waves in leads I, aVL, V_5, and/or V_6, and a tall initial R wave in V_1. In the congestive cardiomyopathies, nonspecific intraventricular conduction abnormalities, indicated by broad, notched QRS complexes without a specific bundle branch block pattern, are common (Fig. 178-14*C*). Nonspecific ST-segment and T-wave abnormalities are almost universal in congestive cardiomyopathies. In the restrictive cardiomyopathies, intraventricular conduction defects, low-voltage QRS complexes, or loss of R-wave progression across the precordium may occur.

ECG ABNORMALITIES IN METABOLIC AND ELECTROLYTE DISTURBANCES The electrically active tissues of the heart are particularly sensitive to changes in the extracellular concentration of K^+, and dramatic ECG changes may accompany abrupt changes in K^+. The initial effect of acute *hyper*kalemia is the appearance of tall, peaked T waves (Figs. 178-15 and 41-1). As the severity of hyperkalemia increases, the QRS complex widens and blends into the tall, peaked T waves, P-wave voltage decreases and may disappear entirely, and the PR interval is prolonged. As these changes evolve, there is marked prolongation of the QRS complex (Fig. 178-15) with the evolution of continuity between the S wave and T wave, ultimately producing a sine wave configuration. This pattern is a very late and ominous manifestation of hyperkalemia. Equally dangerous is the occurrence of severe *hypo*kalemia, which also produces characteristic ECG changes. Instead of the tall, peaked T waves of hyperkalemia, hypokalemia produces a flattening or inversion of the T wave with concomitant prominence of the U wave. In its fully developed state, the ECG gives the appearance of a very long QT interval. Careful analysis reveals that the QT interval is not so prolonged, and the U wave has assumed the appearance of the T wave (Fig. 178-15). Thus, the major prolongation is a "QU" prolongation. This ECG manifestation of hypokalemia may forewarn of the occurrence of serious ventricular arrhythmias, especially in the presence of digitalis. One must be careful to differentiate the ECG effects of hypo*calcemia* from hypo*kalemia*. Whereas hypokalemia may produce the appearance of a long ST segment and late T wave because of flattening of the T

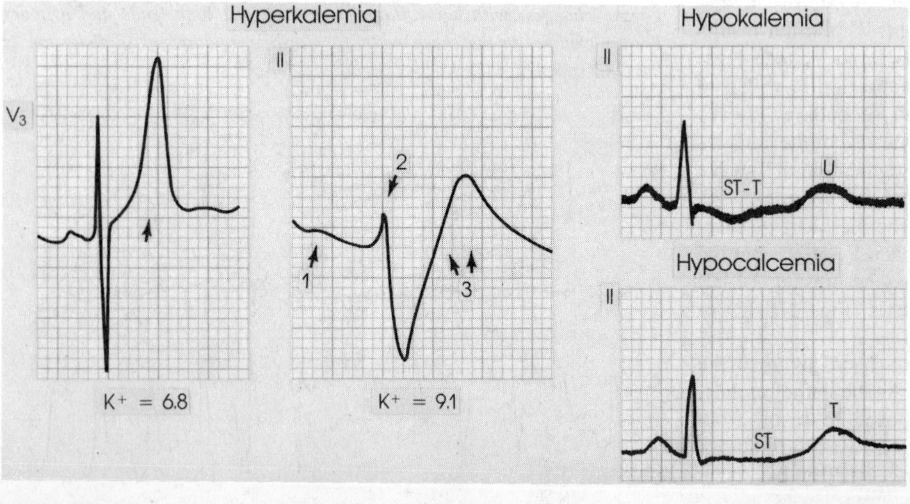

FIGURE 178-15 *Electrolyte disturbances.* Hyperkalemia *(K^+ = 6.8) with tall, peaked T waves. Severe hyperkalemia (K^+ = 9.1) with (1) flattening of the P wave, and ↑ PR interval (1→2), (2) marked widening of the QRS complex (2→3), and (3) merging of the S wave into the T wave.* Hypokalemia *produces flat or inverted T waves with prominent U waves, causing prolonged "QU" interval, while hypocalcemia produces true prolongation of the ST segment with marked QT prolongation.*

wave and prominence of the U wave, hypocalcemia does, in fact, produce prolongation of the ST segment with a late T wave (Fig. 178-15). Hypocalcemia is not as immediately ominous as hypokalemia in regard to potentially serious ventricular arrhythmias. Most of the other electrolyte imbalances produce ECG changes too nonspecific to be clinically useful.

Abnormalities of metabolism, such as hyper- or hypothyroidism, Addison's disease, diabetic ketoacidosis, and infiltrative diseases, such as amyloidosis and hemochromatosis, all may produce ECG abnormalities which may be helpful in the recognition of the disease process but are often nonspecific.

Many drugs, especially the antiarrhythmics and psychotropics, can influence the ECG. The most common effects are on the AV node (prolonged PR interval) and on repolarization (ST-T wave changes and prolonged QT intervals).

VECTORCARDIOGRAPHY

A vectorcardiogram (VCG) is a continuous loop representing the sequence of instantaneous electrical vectors in a two-dimensional plane (shown diagrammatically in Fig. 178-5*G*). This form of recording, requiring simultaneous voltage information from two leads, is achieved by recording one ECG lead on the vertical axis and replacing time by a second lead on the horizontal axis. The resulting loop is photographed on an oscilloscope screen. Most VCG systems today employ an XYZ lead system in which X is analogous to lead I (left-right), Y is analogous to lead aVF (superoinferior), and Z represents a lead in the anteroposterior orientation, most closely analogous to lead V_2. The XY plane records a vectorial loop in the frontal plane, projected on the hexaxial reference in Fig. 178-1*D*. The XZ plane records the horizontal loop in which the left-right orientation is plotted against the anteroposterior orientation on a reference system similar to that in Fig. 178-2*B*. In the YZ plane, the loop is in the sagittal orientation—the anteroposterior orientation (Z) plotted against the superoinferior orientation (Y). Recording in three planes provides information about spatial vectors, as in Fig. 178-5*F*. Loops consist of comma-shaped dots, the orientation of the comma indicating the direction of rotation, and the frequency of interruption providing a measurement of time. Closely grouped dots indicate a slow change in the magnitude and direction of the vector, while widely spread dots indicate rapid changes. Vectorial information of P waves, QRS complexes, ST segments, and T waves may be obtained.

The greatest value of the VCG today lies in the analysis of Q waves of uncertain significance and of certain intraventricular conduction abnormalities. When normal septal Q waves are absent in lead I or V_6, and no other evidence of septal infarction is present, the VCG may demonstrate either that the normal Q loop in the horizontal plane is absent, indicating a septal infarction or scarring, or conversely that the Q loop in the horizontal plane is morphologically normal but oriented directly anteriorly, accounting for the absence of the initial rightward forces. Similarly, the VCG can be helpful in assessing confusing initial forces or poor R-wave progression in the anterior precordial leads.

The VCG is particularly useful in identifying inferior wall myocardial infarctions. When the ECG is equivocal, the VCG may show the superior displacement of initial forces in the frontal plane and the clockwise rotation that is characteristic of inferior wall myocardial infarction. Furthermore, the difficulty in differentiating inferior wall infarctions from left anterior hemiblock on ECG, or recognizing their coexistence, may be aided by a VCG. In left anterior hemiblock, the initial forces are often normal, but there is superior displacement of the major portion of the frontal plane loop. However, the rotation is counterclockwise, in contrast to the clockwise rotation of inferior wall myocardial infarction. When the combination of inferior wall myocardial infarction and left anterior hemiblock is present, the infarction may be masked on the ECG; but the VCG may show the distinctly abnormal superiorly displaced initial forces of inferior wall myocardial infarction plus the counterclockwise rotation in the frontal plane characteristic of left anterior hemiblock.

REFERENCES

BERNE RM (ed): Electrophysiology of the heart, in *Handbook of Physiology*, sec 2: *The Cardiovascular System*, vol 1: *The Heart*. Washington, DC, American Physiological Society, 1979, pp 187–428

CASTELLANOS A, MYERBURG RJ: The resting electrocardiogram, in *The Heart*, 6th ed, JW Hurst et al (eds). New York, McGraw-Hill, 1986, p 206

COOKSEY JD et al: *Clinical Vectorcardiography and Electrocardiography*, 2d ed. Chicago, Year Book, 1977

FISCH C (ed): *Cardiovascular Clinics*, vol 5, no 3: *Complex Electrocardiography I*. Philadelphia, Davis, 1973

———: Electrocardiography and vectorcardiography, in *Heart Disease*, 2d ed, E Braunwald (ed). Philadelphia, Saunders, 1984, p 195

GOLDMAN MJ: *Principles of Clinical Electrocardiography*, 12th ed. Los Altos, California, Lange Medical Publishers, 1986

HOFFMAN BF, CRANEFIELD PF: *Electrophysiology of the Heart*. New York, McGraw-Hill, 1960

SILVERMAN ME et al: *Electrocardiography: Basic Concepts and Clinical Application*. New York, McGraw-Hill, 1983

179 NONINVASIVE METHODS OF CARDIAC EXAMINATION

Roentgenography, phonocardiography, echocardiography, radionuclide techniques, and magnetic resonance imaging

PATRICIA C. COME / JOSHUA WYNNE / EUGENE BRAUNWALD

ROENTGENOGRAPHY

The chest roentgenogram provides pathoanatomic information about the size and configuration of the heart and great vessels and pathophysiologic information about pulmonary arterial and venous pressures and flow. Chamber dilatation usually produces changes in cardiac size and contour. Myocardial hypertrophy, in contrast, often results in wall thickening at the expense of cavity size, producing only a slight alteration of the cardiac silhouette. Although standard 6-ft posteroanterior (PA) and lateral chest roentgenograms are routinely obtained, a cardiac series (Fig. 179-1) permits better assessment of chamber sizes and shapes. Image-intensification fluoroscopy may be used to detect calcification, recognize pericardial effusion or thickening if epicardial fat can be identified, assess movement of radiopaque valvular prostheses, or define further the size and motion of cardiac chambers and great vessels.

CARDIAC SILHOUETTE The *right atrium* is the most difficult chamber to evaluate. Enlargement, however, may cause bulging of the heart to the right and an increased curvature of the right heart border on PA and left anterior oblique views. The *right ventricle* is best seen on the lateral view, where its anterior wall lies behind the lower third of the sternum. As it enlarges, it displaces lung tissue, filling in the upper retrosternal space. Further dilatation may passively displace other chambers, particularly the left ventricle.

Enlargement of the *left atrial appendage* may be suspected by a bulge beneath the pulmonary artery on the PA film. Dilatation of the body of the *left atrium* is best demonstrated by posterior displacement of the barium-filled esophagus in the lateral or right anterior oblique view. As the left atrium dilates further, its right border contacts right lung posteriorly, forming a second border or "double density" adjacent to the right atrial wall. The left bronchus may be displaced posteriorly and superiorly. The *left ventricle* enlarges inferiorly, posteriorly, and to the left, often increasing the cardiothoracic ratio

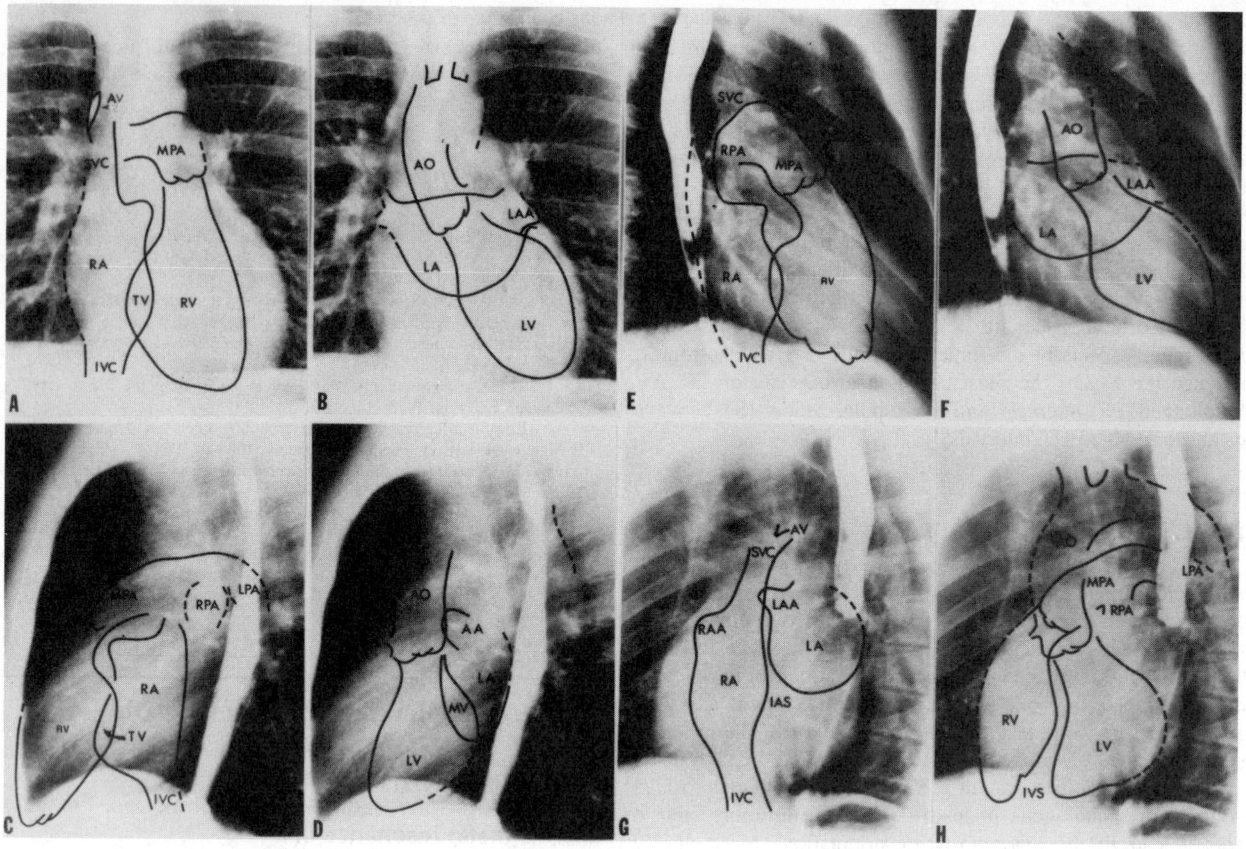

FIGURE 179-1 *Posteroanterior (A,B), lateral (C,D), right anterior oblique (E,F), and left anterior oblique (G,H) views of the heart, demonstrating the positions of the cardiac chambers, valves, and interatrial and interventricular septa. AV = azygos vein; SVC = superior vena cava; RA = right atrium; IVC = inferior vena cava; TV = tricuspid valve; RV = right ventricle; MPA = main pulmonary artery; RPA = right pulmonary artery; LPA = left pulmonary artery; AO = aorta; LA = left atrium; LAA = left atrial appendage; LV = left ventricle; MV = mitral valve; IVS = interventricular septum; IAS = interatrial septum; RAA = right atrial appendage. [From PC Come (ed): Diagnostic Cardiology. Reprinted with permission of Robert E. Dinsmore, M.D., and J.B. Lippincott Company.]*

(maximal cardiac diameter divided by maximal internal thoracic diameter, normally less than 0.50). The chest roentgenogram is a useful screening or initial test, but other imaging techniques, such as echocardiography, provide more definitive assessment of individual cardiac chambers.

PULMONARY VASCULATURE Since pulmonary vessel size is proportional to flow, vessels normally taper from central to peripheral and from dependent to nondependent portions of the lungs. Increased flow, as with left-to-right shunts, results in enlargement and tortuosity of all vessels. Regional or global reduction of flow, due to pulmonary emboli, emphysematous blebs, or a right-to-left shunt, results in decreased vessel caliber.

Increases in pulmonary venous pressure produce perivascular edema in the dependent portions of the lungs, causing loss of vessel wall definition and redistribution of flow to nondependent areas. Further increases cause interstitial edema, with peribronchial cuffing, perihilar and peripheral lung haziness, and linear densities (Kerley B lines) perpendicular to the pleura. They represent fluid collection in the dependent interlobular septa. Alveolar pulmonary edema, with air bronchograms, may ultimately develop. There may be considerable temporal delay between hemodynamic changes and roentgenographic findings.

Pulmonary artery hypertension produces dilatation of the main pulmonary artery and its central branches. When associated with conditions increasing pulmonary arteriolar resistance, such as primary pulmonary hypertension, the distal pulmonary arteries often appear small (''pruned'').

SPECIALIZED RADIOGRAPHIC METHODS *Digital subtraction angiography* (DSA) uses computer processing to digitize high-resolution fluoroscopic images. An image of the region of interest is subtracted from images obtained following intravenous, intracardiac, or intraarterial injection of contrast medium. Elimination of radiographic densities resulting from soft tissues and bone permits excellent definition of vascular structures using a concentration of contrast medium lower than that necessary for routine angiography. Vascular applications include recognition of vascular tumors, pulmonary emboli, and abnormalities of the aorta or of peripheral, cerebral, and renal arteries. Study of the heart permits assessment of ventricular function, intracardiac shunts, other congenital abnormalities, and bypass graft patency.

Computed tomography provides thin, cross-sectional images of the body by measuring attenuation of x-rays passing through the bodily planes of interest. The x-rays, generated by a rotating source, are detected by an array of detectors surrounding the patient. Digitized data accrued from contiguous, horizontal planes can subsequently be used to construct multiple two-dimensional projections. Contrast enhancement and electronic gating permit high-resolution images of the beating heart. Regions of infarction and ischemia, ventricular aneurysms, intracardiac thrombi, diseases of the aorta and pericardium, and patency of bypass grafts have been recognized.

PHONOCARDIOGRAPHY, SYSTOLIC TIME INTERVALS, AND PULSE TRACINGS

Although imaging techniques have largely replaced phonocardiography and pulse tracings as diagnostic tests, the latter may be useful, especially in combination with M-mode echocardiography, in clarifying the origin and timing of abnormalities noted on auscultation and palpation. The indirect recordings of the jugular, carotid, and apex pulses resemble the right atrial, central aortic, and left ventricular

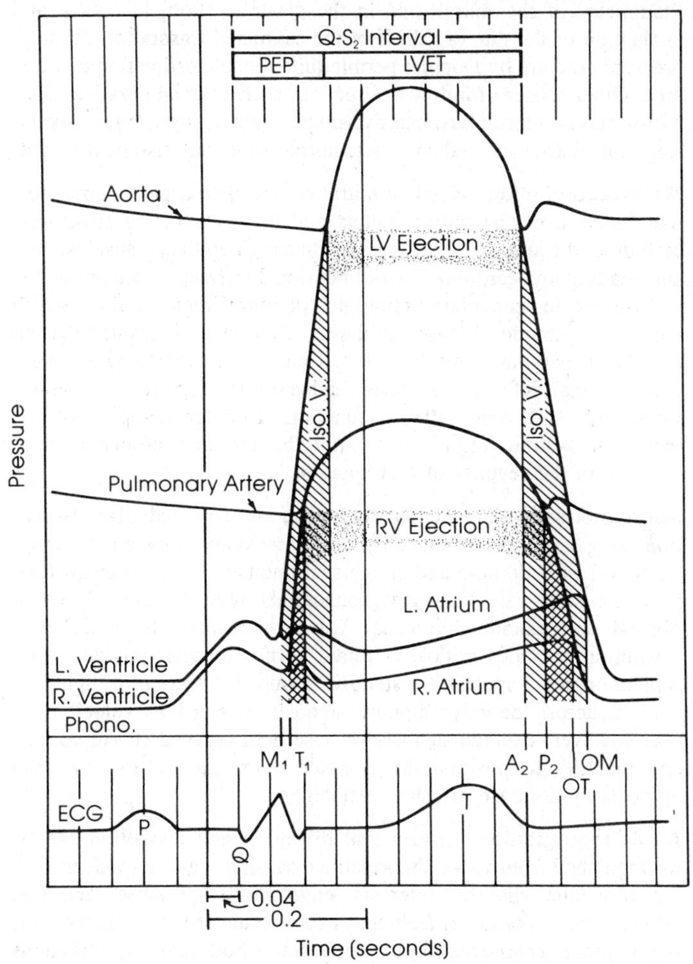

FIGURE 179-2 *Diagrammatic representation of intracardiac and aortic pressure tracings correlated with the ECG and phonocardiogram (Phono). The striped and cross-hatched areas labeled IsoV represent the isovolumetric phases of contraction and relaxation of the left and right ventricles, respectively; M_1, T_1, A_2, and P_2, sounds produced by closure of the mitral, tricuspid, aortic, and pulmonary valves, respectively; OT and OM, sounds produced by tricuspid and mitral opening. The QS_2 interval includes the preejection period (PEP) and the left ventricular ejection time (LVET), all of which can be measured noninvasively (see text).*

pressure tracings, respectively. The phonocardiogram provides a graphic display of heart sounds and murmurs.

The *carotid pulse morphology* and derived *systolic time intervals* may provide information about left ventricular function and outflow obstruction. The systolic time intervals consist of electromechanical systole (QS_2), measured from the onset of the QRS complex to the aortic component of S_2; the left ventricular ejection time (LVET), which begins with the upstroke of the carotid pulse and ends with the dicrotic notch; and the preejection period (PEP = QS_2 − LVET) (Fig. 179-2). In left ventricular failure, the PEP lengthens (reflecting primarily a decrease in rate of ventricular pressure generation) and the LVET shortens (reflecting a reduced stroke volume), increasing the PEP/LVET ratio. In fixed left ventricular outflow obstruction (e.g., valvular aortic stenosis) the carotid upstroke may be slow, while in dynamic obstruction (hypertrophic obstructive cardiomyopathy) it is brisk due to unimpeded early systolic flow. In the absence of concomitant heart failure, the LVET is generally prolonged in both forms of outflow obstruction.

ECHOCARDIOGRAPHY

Echocardiography uses ultrasound to image the heart and great vessels. A transducer containing a piezoelectric crystal, which interconverts electrical and mechanical (i.e., sound) energy, functions both as the transmitter of sound and as the receiver of reflected waves. Three types of studies are performed: M-mode, two-dimensional, and Doppler. In *M-mode echocardiography,* a single transducer, emitting 1000 to 2000 pulses per second along a single line, provides an "ice-pick" view of the heart, with excellent *temporal* resolution. When beam direction is changed, the heart can be scanned from the ventricles to the aorta and left atrium (Fig. 179-3). *Two-dimensional*

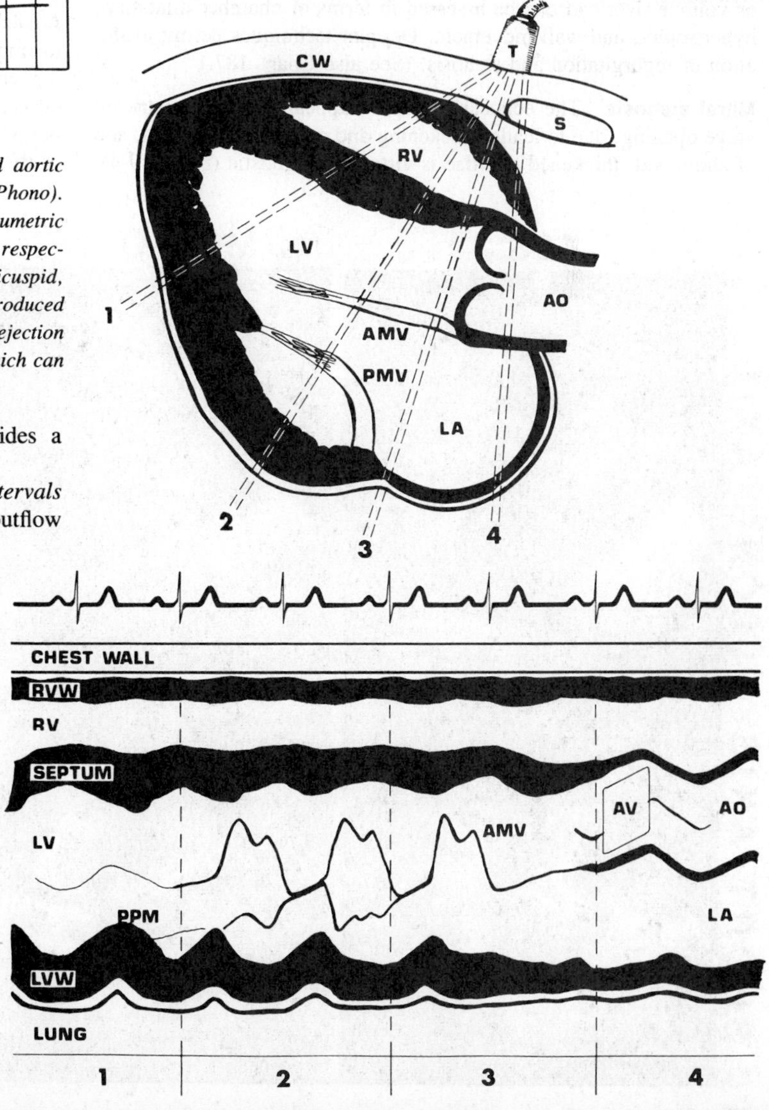

FIGURE 179-3 *Schematic diagrams of an M-mode echocardiographic scan through a normal heart. A long-axis section of the heart is depicted in the upper diagram. The echocardiographic movement patterns that arise from the corresponding anatomic structures are illustrated in the bottom diagram. CW = chest wall; T = echocardiographic transducer; S = sternum; RV = right ventricle; LV = left ventricle; AO = aortic root; AMV = anterior mitral leaflet; PMV = posterior mitral leaflet; LA = left atrium; RVW = right ventricular wall; AV = aortic valve; PPM = posterior papillary muscle; LVW = left ventricular wall. [From Come PC: Echocardiography in diagnosis and management of cardiovascular disease. Compr Ther 6(5):58, 1980. Courtesy The Laux Company, Inc., Ayer, MA.]*

echocardiography (Figs. 179-4 and 179-5) produces an image in two distance dimensions by steering the sound beam through an arc of up to 90° some 30 times per second. It provides excellent *spatial* resolution, permitting analysis of structural movement in real time, from multiple transducer positions.

Doppler echocardiography detects blood flow velocity and turbulence. When sound encounters moving red blood cells, the frequency of its reflected signal is altered. The magnitude of the change *(Doppler shift)* indicates the velocity V of blood flow with respect to the sound beam:

$$V = \frac{C \times \text{(Doppler shift)}}{(2 \times \text{emitted frequency}) \cos \theta}$$

where C is the speed of sound in tissue, and θ is the angle between the Doppler beam and the mean axis of blood flow. An upward shift (increased frequency of the reflected sound) indicates blood motion toward the transducer and a downward shift, motion away. High-flow velocities, such as across stenotic semilunar valves, can be measured, enabling calculation of transvalvular pressure gradients (P) using the modified Bernoulli equation, $P = 4V^2$. Recording of flow signals from small, preselected areas permits spatial localization of turbulence resulting from valvular stenosis and regurgitation and from shunts. Combined Doppler and imaging techniques permit calculation of cardiac output. Unfortunately, not all patients can be successfully studied by echocardiography. Sound penetration may be suboptimal in many elderly, obese, and emphysematous patients.

VALVULAR HEART DISEASE Imaging echocardiography can detect abnormalities of valve thickness and movement responsible for stenosis and regurgitation. In addition, the heart's response to pressure or volume overload can be assessed in terms of chamber dilatation, hypertrophy, and wall movement. Doppler techniques permit evaluation of regurgitation and stenosis. (See also Chap. 187.)

Mitral stenosis The echocardiographic appearance of a restricted valve opening, due to leaflet thickening and commissural fusion, and of shortened, thickened chordae is virtually diagnostic (Fig. 179-4). Planimetry of the mitral area in the diastolic short axis view and evaluation of the rate of falloff of the estimated transmitral diastolic pressure gradient by Doppler permit quite reliable estimation of valve area. Other causes of inflow obstruction, such as atrial myxoma (Fig. 179-4, right) or thrombus, massive annular calcification, supravalvular ring, cor triatriatum, and parachute mitral valve may also be detected.

Mitral regurgitation Systolic mitral competence depends upon normal function of the mitral leaflets and their supporting structures, including the annulus, chordae tendineae, papillary muscles, and surrounding myocardium. Two-dimensional techniques are preferable to M-mode in recognizing etiologies of mitral regurgitation, which include rheumatic disease, prolapse, flail leaflets resulting from chordal or papillary muscle rupture, annular calcification, atrioventricular canal defects, myxomas, endocarditis, hypertrophic cardiomyopathy, and ventricular dysfunction. Doppler mapping of the extent of systolic turbulence within the atrium provides a gross estimate of the severity of regurgitation.

Aortic stenosis Subvalvular, valvular, and supravalvular obstruction can generally be detected by two-dimensional echocardiography. Systolic leaflet doming and an unusual number or size of cusps (two in a bicuspid valve) suggest congenital valve disease. Acquired fibrosis and calcification cause valve thickening. Normal leaflet separation excludes critical acquired aortic stenosis, but decreased separation is not specific for stenosis. Doppler detection of high-flow velocity across the valve supports stenosis. Lesser flow velocities do not, however, exclude stenosis because both reduced stroke volume and inability to position the Doppler beam parallel to flow may appreciably decrease measured velocities.

Aortic regurgitation Aortic root dilatation and dissection can be distinguished from valve abnormalities causing regurgitation, including congenital disease, sclerosis, endocarditis, prolapse, and flail cusps. Two-dimensional techniques best define structural pathology, but M-mode techniques more readily detect both diastolic vibrations of the anterior mitral leaflet, a very sensitive sign of aortic regurgi-

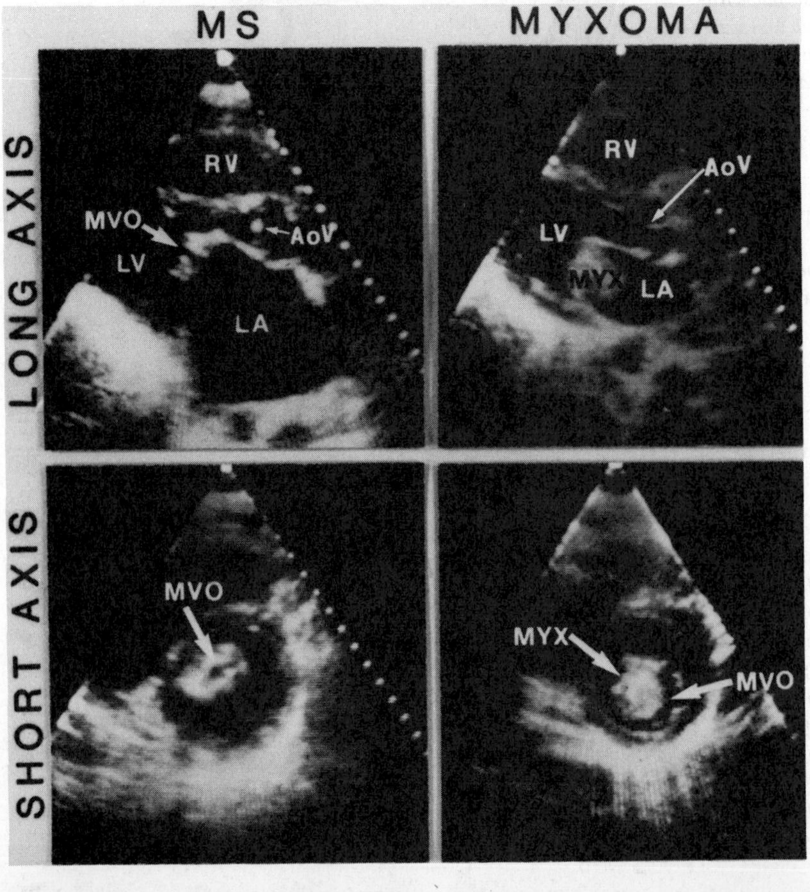

FIGURE 179-4 *Two-dimensional long- and short-axis views in diastole from patients with marked reduction of effective mitral valve orifice area (MVO) due to mitral stenosis (MS) and left atrial (LA) myxoma (MYX). In the MS patient, the valve leaflets are thickened, particularly at their tips, and there is markedly reduced diastolic separation of the anterior and posterior leaflets. The LA is enlarged. The LA MYX is seen to prolapse into the MVO during diastole, causing obstruction. RV = right ventricle; LV = left ventricle; AoV = aortic valve.*

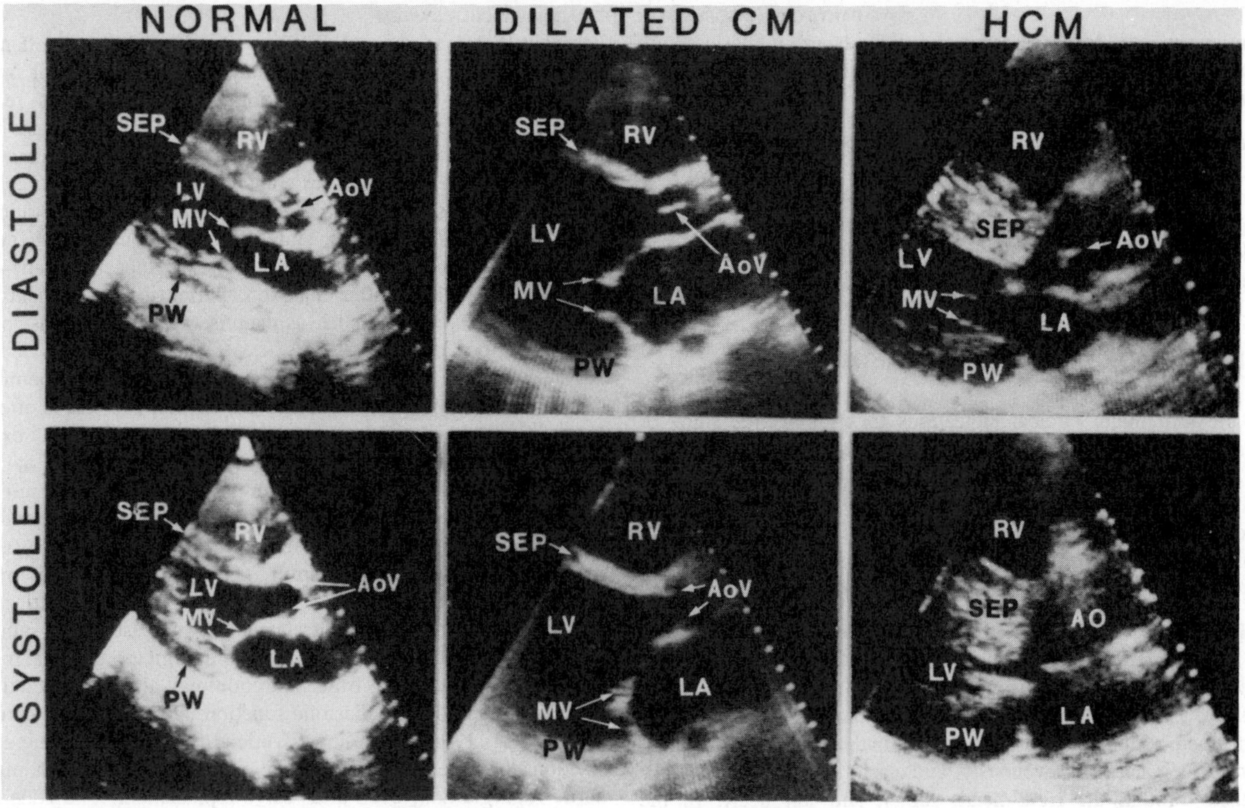

FIGURE 179-5 *Long-axis parasternal views of the left ventricle in diastole and systole in a normal individual and in patients with dilated cardiomyopathy (CM) and hypertrophic cardiomyopathy (HCM). Normal diastolic wall thicknesses and normal systolic wall thickening and excursion are illustrated in the left panels. In the patient with dilated CM, left ventricular (LV) and left atrial (LA) diameters are increased, and there is markedly reduced systolic thickening and excursion of the septum (SEP) and posterior wall (PW). In the patient with HCM, the SEP is abnormally thick and highly echogenic. The LV cavity is small in diastole and almost disappears during systolic contraction. RV = right ventricle; MV = mitral valve; AoV = aortic valve.*

tation, and premature mitral closure, produced by the marked elevation of left ventricular diastolic pressure which may accompany severe, acute regurgitation.

Tricuspid and pulmonary valve disease Two-dimensional scanning has improved visualization of right-sided valves. Changes in structure and movement may permit detection of rheumatic deformity, Ebstein's malformation, prolapse, flail cusps, endocarditis, congenital dysplasia, and thickening due to carcinoid, amyloid, Loeffler's endocarditis, or endocardial fibrosis. Systolic doming of the pulmonic valve is characteristic of pulmonic stenosis.

Prosthetic valves Mechanical prostheses are difficult to evaluate, because their intrinsically high echogenicity interferes with the recognition of vegetations and thrombi. Abnormal timing of valve opening and closure, best assessed using combined phonocardiography and M-mode techniques, and abnormalities on Doppler study may suggest dysfunction, but angiography and hemodynamic assessment are often necessary for full evaluation. Abnormalities of bioprostheses, including fibrosis, calcification, vegetations, and tears, are more easily recognized.

Endocarditis Valvular vegetations, characterized by masses of shaggy-appearing echoes, are evident in over half of patients with endocarditis. While their detection is associated with an increased risk of complications, many patients recover uneventfully with antibiotic therapy alone. (See also Chap. 188.)

Left ventricle M-mode echocardiography is widely used to measure left ventricular size, wall thickness, and function. The rate of wall thinning in diastole may permit assessment of diastolic function, and the percentage of shortening of the minor axis, normally greater than 28 percent, and the mean velocity of circumferential fiber shortening are useful measurements of systolic performance. These indexes of systolic performance are influenced, however, by preload and afterload as well as by myocardial contractility. Analyses of end-systolic pressure-dimension relations, which are independent of preload and incorporate afterload, provide better information regarding contractile function. Estimates of global ventricular performance, based on ice-pick M-mode views, are useful, however, only when ventricular shape is normal and systolic movement relatively symmetric in extent and timing. Two-dimensional echocardiography, which images the ventricle in a number of different planes, improves assessment of volumes and function, particularly in patients with asymmetric contraction resulting from ischemic heart disease. The left ventricular apex, the most common site of wall movement abnormalities and thrombi, can be adequately visualized only by two-dimensional techniques.

Echocardiography permits recognition of *cardiomyopathy* and classification into dilated, hypertrophic, and restrictive-obliterative types (Fig. 179-5). In dilated cardiomyopathy, both ventricles are generally enlarged and poorly contracting, and wall thicknesses are normal or only slightly increased. In contrast, appreciable ventricular hypertrophy, usually involving the septum asymmetrically, small ventricular size, enhanced systolic performance and impaired diastolic relaxation, characterize hypertrophic cardiomyopathy. Systolic anterior movement of the mitral valve to abut the septum and partial midsystolic closure of the aortic valve correlate with dynamic obstruction. Increased wall thickness also characterizes infiltrative disorders. In amyloidosis, the thick walls are often "speckled" in appearance and are associated with diminished voltage on electrocardiogram (ECG).

Pericardial effusion Echocardiography can detect effusions as small as 15 to 20 mL. While certain findings, such as diastolic compression of the right atrium and ventricle, may suggest tamponade, decisions regarding therapy are best based on clinical and hemodynamic observations.

Cardiac masses Most masses involving the heart and pericardium are easily recognized. They include myxomas (Fig. 179-4), other primary and secondary tumors, and thrombi.

Congenital heart disease Since valvular abnormalities and relationships of atria, valves, ventricles, and great vessels can easily be recognized by two-dimensional echocardiography, this technique has revolutionized the diagnosis of congenital heart disease. Contrast and Doppler echocardiography facilitate detection of shunts and of valvular stenosis and regurgitation.

RADIONUCLIDE IMAGING OF THE HEART

There are four major clinical indications for radionuclide study of the heart: (1) assessment of systolic and diastolic ventricular function using radionuclide ventriculography; (2) identification and quantification of intracardiac shunts using radioangiocardiography; (3) assessment of myocardial perfusion using ionic tracers, principally thallium 201; and (4) detection of acute myocardial infarction with infarct-avid radionuclides.

VENTRICULAR PERFORMANCE Radionuclide ventriculography (RVG) uses a radioactive intravascular indicator to delineate heart chambers and great vessels (Fig. 179-6). The radionuclide, usually technetium 99m, is generally attached to red blood cells. RVGs may be performed using two different methods. In the *first-pass* technique, radiotracer is injected intravenously, and a scintillation camera tracks its transit through the right heart, lungs, and left heart. In the *equilibrium,* or *gated, method,* counts are recorded from several hundred cardiac cycles following uniform distribution of radiotracer throughout the blood pool. The scintigraphic information in each cycle is divided into multiple frames (often 30 or more), using the ECG as a timing reference. Counts from corresponding frames of each cycle are then summed by computer to provide images of the spatial distribution and density of counts over time. Images are generally obtained in at least two views [anterior and left anterior oblique (LAO)]. Gated scans are frequently obtained after first-pass scans, since no additional injection of radionuclide is required. Because detected counts, after background subtraction, are proportional to blood volume, equilibrium studies permit estimation of chamber volumes, enabling calculation of left and right ventricular ejection fractions, left-to-right ventricular stroke volume ratios, and rates of ventricular ejection and filling. Agreement with standard catheterization methods has been excellent. Repeated scans can be obtained up to 20 h after injection, permitting assessment of the effects of interventions, such as exercise and medications, on ventricular performance.

RVG may be used to detect patients with chronic ischemic heart disease. Since resting function may be normal, exercise is often used to provoke ischemia. Scans are obtained at rest and at peak exercise. Failure to increase left ventricular ejection fraction by at least 5 percent and development of one or more regional wall movement abnormalities have a sensitivity and specificity of approximately 90 and 60 percent, respectively, for detection of significant coronary disease. The test is most helpful in patients with an intermediate pretest probability of disease. Low resting ejection fractions after acute infarction have been correlated with increased short- and long-term morbidity and mortality. Mitral regurgitation, septal rupture, and aneurysms resulting from infarction may also be detected. RVG can assess systolic and diastolic function in patients with cardiomyopathy (Fig. 179-6) or volume overload. A reduced resting ejection fraction correlates with a poor prognosis in patients with mitral or aortic regurgitation, even after valve replacement. The added value of exercise RVG in detecting reduced myocardial reserve due to volume overload remains controversial. Thrombi and other tumors may be recognized, but RVG is less sensitive than echocardiography.

SHUNT SCINTIGRAPHY Assessment of left-to-right shunts utilizes a modification of the first-pass RVG in which the "region of interest" is focused over an area of lung. Following rapid injection of radiotracer

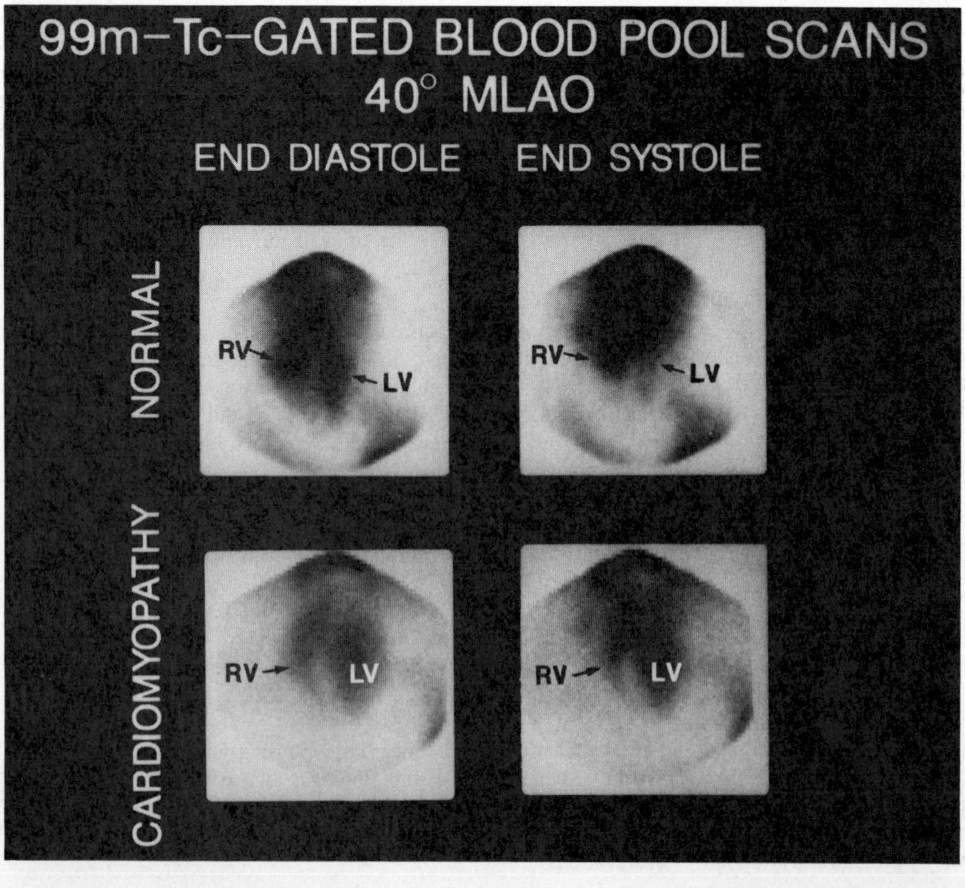

FIGURE 179-6 *End-diastolic and end-systolic gated blood pool images from a normal individual (with estimated left and right ventricular ejection fractions of 69 and 45 percent, respectively) and from a patient with idiopathic dilated cardiomyopathy and marked, global reduction of left ventricular systolic function (left ventricular ejection fraction of 23 percent). In the patient with cardiomyopathy, there is very little change in left ventricular cavity size or count density from diastole to systole. The right ventricle, however, shows normal function, with an ejection fraction of 57 percent. RV = right ventricle; LV = left ventricle.*

into a large vein, usually the external jugular, the pulmonary time-activity curve is recorded by a gamma camera-computer system. Normally, counts increase sharply as the bolus reaches the lung underlying the detector. Following peak activity, there is a smooth descent and a later, smaller increase in counts representing normal recirculation of the radiotracer following systemic circulation. Left-to-right shunts cause premature interruption of the descent, due to early reappearance of radioactivity within the lung. Computer analysis of the areas under the curve permits reliable determination of the ratio of pulmonic-to-systemic blood flow. Right-to-left shunts may also be recognized and quantified.

MYOCARDIAL PERFUSION IMAGING Certain radiolabeled monovalent cations, especially the potassium analogue thallium 201 (half-life of 72 h), are widely used to assess myocardial perfusion since their active uptake by normal myocardial cells is proportional to regional blood flow. Areas of myocardial necrosis, fibrosis, and ischemia show reduced thallium accumulation (''cold spots'') on images obtained soon after injection. Following its initial accumulation within cells, however, thallium 201 continues to exchange with the systemic pool. After several hours, all viable myocardial cells with intact membrane function will contain nearly equal concentrations.

Thallium 201 scintigraphy is most commonly used to detect exercise-induced ischemia (Fig. 179-7). Thallium is injected intravenously at peak exercise, and images are obtained in several projections 5 to 10 min later. Normal scans show relatively homogeneous distribution of activity, while those of patients with infarction or ischemia typically demonstrate one or more ''cold spots.'' Due to continued exchange of thallium between viable cells and the systemic pool, however, initial defects due to ischemia ''fill in'' on repeat imaging several hours later. Areas of infarction demonstrate persistent reduction of uptake. Compared to routine exercise electrocardiography, exercise thallium scintigraphy increases the sensitivity for detection of coronary disease from approximately 60 to 80 percent and increases specificity slightly from about 80 to 90 percent. It is most useful in patients with atypical chest pain in whom the exercise ECG is nondiagnostic or uninterpretable due to left bundle branch block, ventricular hypertrophy, or drug and electrolyte effects; in patients who fail to achieve 85 percent of predicted maximal heart rate; and in patients with a high likelihood of a false-positive exercise ECG study. Thallium scanning improves localization of ischemia and provides prognostic information, since the presence and number of redistributing defects correlate with the incidence of future cardiac events. Thallium scintigraphy has also been used to detect ischemia during pacing, dipyridamole-induced coronary vasodilatation, or spontaneous pain.

Thallium scanning does not distinguish new from old infarcts and is less accurate than serum enzyme analysis in detecting acute necrosis. It does, however, offer prognostic information. Patients with smaller defects have better survival rates. On submaximal exercise thallium tests following infarction, the presence of multiple or redistributing defects or increased lung uptake of thallium (probably representing transudation into the lung during periods of high pulmonary capillary pressure) identifies patients at higher risk for postinfarction morbidity and mortality.

Computed tomography using positron-emitting isotopes of potassium analogues permits quantitative assessment of radiotracer uptake. The short half-lives of such isotopes permit multiple studies over short periods of time, allowing assessment of changes in myocardial perfusion induced by therapeutic interventions.

ACUTE INFARCT SCINTIGRAPHY Pyrophosphate appears to bind to calcium and organic macromolecules in irreversibly damaged myocardial cells. If coronary flow is sufficient for its delivery to necrotic myocardium (10 to 40 percent of normal flow is required), technetium 99m stannous pyrophosphate will bind there, producing an image with increased uptake (''hot spot''). Scans are most likely to be positive when injections are performed 48 to 72 h after suspected infarction, when the elevated creatine kinase activity has often returned to normal. The major clinical indication is the detection of acute infarction in patients in whom traditional diagnostic methods cannot be interpreted or have provided equivocal results. Sensitivity and specificity for transmural infarcts are both about 90 percent. Uptake is often fainter and more poorly localized in subendocardial infarcts, and myocardial damage from causes other than coronary disease may result in a positive scan.

MAGNETIC RESONANCE IMAGING (MRI)

Certain atomic nuclei, which possess an odd number of either protons or neutrons (or both), absorb and reemit electromagnetic energy when they are placed in a strong magnetic field and have their net magnetization vector deflected by application of a radiofrequency pulse. Signals emitted during return of the magnetization vector to its equilibrium position can be analyzed to provide spectral and imaging information. Since blood flowing at normal velocities produces virtually no MR signal, there is a high natural contrast between the walls of the heart and great vessels and the moving blood. ECG gating of signals from ^{1}H has permitted excellent structural definition of myocardial, pericardial, great vessel, and congenital cardiac abnormalities. Advantages of MR imaging relative to computed

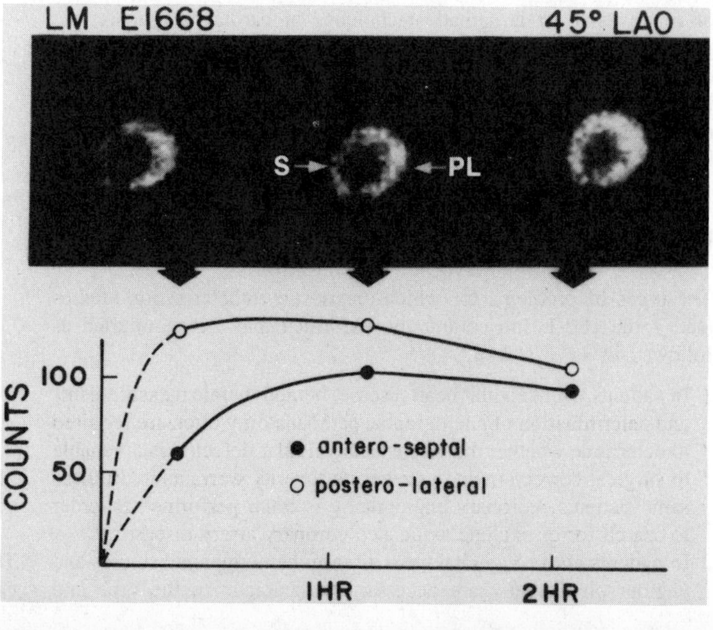

FIGURE 179-7 *Serial thallium 201 scintigrams obtained in the 45° LAO projection in a patient undergoing exercise testing for evaluation of chest pain. The immediate post-exercise image* (left) *demonstrates decreased perfusion of the septum. The 1- and 2-h delayed images* (middle and right) *demonstrate ''filling in'' of the defect, reflecting redistribution. The computer-derived time-activity curves* (bottom) *confirm the significant reduction in initial counts in the septum, relative to the posterolateral wall, and demonstrate near equalization of activity by 2 h. S = septum; PL = posterolateral wall. [From PC Come (ed): Diagnostic Cardiology. Reprinted with permission of George A. Beller, M.D., and J.B. Lippincott Company.]*

tomography include the lack of both ionizing radiation and the need for contrast administration. Advantages relative to echocardiography include the ability to image in any desired plane, the capability for transmission of signals through bone and air, a wider field of view, and improved spatial resolution. Disadvantages include the relatively long duration of the imaging procedure, the greater sensitivity of MR imaging to body movement, and the high cost and lack of portabililty of the required equipment. ^{1}H imaging also provides potential for tissue characterization. Areas of acute myocardial ischemia and infarction in experimental animals and in humans have been identified as locations of high signal intensity relative to normal myocardium, probably reflecting the greater number of hydrogen nuclei in areas of myocardial edema. Conversely, areas of fibrosis produce signals of lesser intensity. ^{31}P MR spectroscopy permits quantification of high-energy phosphate compounds and of intracellular pH. It is therefore a powerful research tool for evaluation of intracellular metabolism.

REFERENCES

Berger HJ, Zaret BL: Nuclear cardiology. N Engl J Med 305:799; 305:855, 1981
Come PC (ed): *Diagnostic Cardiology: Noninvasive Imaging Techniques*. Philadelphia, Lippincott, 1985
Feigenbaum H: *Echocardiography*, 4th ed. Philadelphia, Lea & Febiger, 1986
Higgins CB et al: Magnetic resonance imaging of the cardiovascular system. Am Heart J 109:136, 1985
Kisslo J et al (eds): *Basic Doppler Echocardiography*, vol 17. New York, Churchill Livingstone, 1986
McNamara MT, Higgins CB: Magnetic resonance imaging of chronic myocardial infarcts in man. AJR 146:315, 1986
Nanda NC (ed): *Doppler Echocardiography*. New York, Igaku-Shoin, 1985

180 CARDIAC CATHETERIZATION AND ANGIOGRAPHY

KIRK L. PETERSON / JOHN ROSS, JR.

Catheterization of the right and left sides of the heart and selective injection of contrast media into the coronary arteries and cardiac chambers during exposure of high-speed x-ray motion pictures (cineangiography) remain the most reliable methods for defining the dynamic physiology and anatomy of the heart in the normal state and a variety of cardiac disorders. When performed after the application of noninvasive or atraumatic techniques of cardiac diagnosis, the great majority of disorders of the heart can be accurately and fully defined and a rational decision made for medical or surgical therapy. In addition, in the past half-decade, cardiac catheterization techniques have been developed which provide therapeutic benefit and are now being applied on a broad scale.

DIAGNOSTIC INDICATIONS

The types of problems for which diagnostic catheterization studies (see Table 180-1) are commonly performed may be summaried as follows:

1 In patients with valvular heart disease, hemodynamic measurements and determination of angiographic pathoanatomy often are required to determine whether the mechanical valvular defect(s) is amenable to surgical correction and whether its severity warrants it. In these same patients, coronary angiography is often performed in order to search for or exclude associated coronary artery disease.

2 In patients with congenital heart disease, hemodynamic studies and angiography usually are necessary to characterize the type and severity of the primary defect and to determine whether associated lesions are present.

TABLE 180-1 Diagnostic information that can be obtained by cardiac catheterization and angiography

1	Intracardiac and intravascular pressure measurements and determination of pressure gradients across the cardiac valves
2	Cardiac output, pulmonary vascular resistance, and systemic vascular resistance
3	Radiographic anatomy of the cardiac chambers and great vessels (aorta, pulmonary artery)
4	Radiographic anatomy of the coronary arteries and detection of coronary artery spasm
5	Detection and quantification of intracardiac shunts
6	Intracardiac electrograms, His bundle electrograms, electrical pacing studies, and intracardiac phonocardiograms
7	Acute effects (hemodynamic and electrophysiologic) of cardioactive drugs
8	Quantification of coronary blood flow
9	Histology of myocardium from endomyocardial catheter biopsies

3 In patients with known coronary artery disease, angiographic visualization of the coronary arteries may be indicated to obtain useful prognostic information and help determine whether operative treatment is feasible. In other patients with a chest pain syndrome of undetermined cause, coronary angiography may be indicated to define the presence or absence of atherosclerotic coronary disease or coronary artery spasm.

4 In patients who have undergone cardiac operations, cardiac catheterization and angiography may be indicated to evaluate the success of the operation, particularly when residual symptoms are present. Such studies may reveal malfunction of a prosthetic valve, residual obstruction or regurgitation of a surgically reconstructed native valve, loss of patency of a coronary artery bypass graft, inadequate correction of a congenital defect, or residual disease of the ventricular myocardium.

5 In patients with suspected myocardial or pericardial disease, hemodynamic and angiographic information may be needed to detect or exclude lesions potentially amenable to surgical treatment, such as mitral regurgitation, coronary heart disease, constrictive pericarditis, or obstructive hypertrophic cardiomyopathy.

6 In patients with evidence of pulmonary hypertension, cardiac catheterization is needed to search for possible mitral stenosis, pulmonary venous obstruction, left-to-right shunts, multiple pulmonary emboli, or peripheral pulmonary artery stenosis, or to establish, by exclusion, the diagnosis of primary pulmonary hypertension.

7 In some patients in an intensive care setting (e.g., for hypotension or heart failure following acute myocardial infarction), catheterization of the right side of the heart by means of a balloon-tipped flotation catheter (Swan-Ganz catheter) often is employed to measure the pulmonary artery pressure, the pulmonary artery wedge pressure (as a measure of the left ventricular filling pressure), and the cardiac output. Such studies permit proper diagnosis, and repeated measurements allow accurate assessment of the effects of treatment.

8 In patients with known myocardial failure, or in the transplanted human heart, an endomyocardial biopsy specimen(s) is used to detect histologic evidence of inflammation, an infiltrative process (e.g., amyloidosis, hemochromatosis, granuloma, neoplasm), or immune rejection.

9 In patients with rhythm disturbances, recordings of intracardiac electrograms via electrode catheters provide insight into the anatomic locus of a conduction abnormality (e.g., accessory pathway), or stimulation of the right atrium or ventricle to produce extrasystoles over a spectrum of coupling intervals is used to test the efficacy of antiarrhythmic therapy for controlling repetitive tachycardias (Chap. 184).

THERAPEUTIC INDICATIONS

These are the major categories of cardiac problems for which catheterization techniques are applied for therapeutic benefit:

1 In patients with obstructive single- or multi-vessel coronary heart disease, passage of a balloon-dilation catheter (transluminal coronary angioplasty) is performed when judged feasible (Chap. 189).

2 In patients with recent (generally less than 6 h) myocardial infarction due to coronary thrombosis, selective coronary artery infusion of a thrombolytic agent (streptokinase or tissue plasminogen activator) serves to lyse the offending clot and reperfuse the jeopardized area of myocardium (Chap. 190). In some instances, successful clot lysis is followed by balloon angioplasty in order to relieve the atherosclerotic obstruction responsible for the thrombosis.

3 In some patients, particularly children with coarctation of the aorta or congenital aortic or pulmonic stenosis, a large balloon-dilation catheter can be utilized to relieve an anatomic obstruction to blood flow (Chap. 185).

4 In patients with congenital heart disease and inadequate pulmonary blood flow, balloon atrial septostomy (enlargement of an existing interatrial communication) serves to improve delivery of desaturated blood to the lungs (Chap. 185).

5 In patients with pulmonary arteriovenous fistulas, selective embolization of the artery with beads can serve to close off a right-to-left shunt.

6 In patients with knotted or fragmented intracardiac or intravascular catheters (due to iatrogenic manipulation), "snare" or "basket" devices can be used to uncurl and extract the offending segments of catheter.

TECHNIQUES

CATHETERIZATION OF THE RIGHT SIDE OF THE HEART Catheterization of the right side of the heart is now a safe and well-standardized procedure. With the patient under local anesthesia an antecubital or saphenous vein is isolated and a long, flexible radiopaque catheter is introduced. Alternatively, the percutaneous approach is employed, in which a needle is positioned in the vessel, a small, flexible wire is passed through the needle, and with a vein dilator, a sheath is then passed over the dilator into the femoral, internal jugular, or other vein. The guidewire is removed, leaving the sheath in place, and through it a catheter is guided sequentially into the right atrium, right ventricle, the pulmonary artery, and pulmonary arterial wedge positions. When fluoroscopy is not available (e.g., at the bedside, operating room, intensive care unit) a balloon-flotation catheter may be passed through the sheath, or directly into an exposed vein, and advanced by tactile sense until it is considered to be near the right atrium. Then while intracardiac pressure is being monitored, the balloon is inflated and the catheter advanced further, whereupon it is usually carried by the bloodstream directly into the right ventricle, the pulmonary artery, and into a second- or third-order pulmonary artery branch, from which a pulmonary arterial wedge tracing is obtained. Also, with a thermistor-tipped balloon catheter, cardiac output can be measured serially by using the indicator-dilution principle discussed subsequently in this chapter.

The course of the catheter in the right side of the heart on fluoroscopy or cineangiography may provide a clue to the diagnosis of certain congenital malformations. The catheter may enter an anomalous pulmonary vein or left superior vena cava; it may directly traverse a patent ductus arteriosus or an atrial septal defect; inability to cross the tricuspid valve may indicate tricuspid atresia; and passage of the catheter from the right ventricle to the aorta may indicate a ventricular septal defect or a form of transposition of the great vessels.

CATHETERIZATION OF THE LEFT SIDE OF THE HEART Various methods for catheterization of the left side of the heart have been devised, and each has found application under certain circumstances. Currently, the *retrograde arterial* approach is used most widely for entrance into the ascending aorta, left ventricle, and, less frequently, the left atrium; the catheter usually is inserted via the femoral artery by the percutaneous method, or through a small incision directly into the exposed brachial artery. The *transseptal* approach may be employed to gain access to the left atrium and left ventricle, particularly when severe obstruction of the aortic valve, obstructive hypertrophic cardiomyopathy, or a mechanical aortic prosthesis are present or suspected. With this method, a catheter is inserted via the right saphenous or femoral vein, and its tip positioned in the right atrium. A long needle, curved at its tip, is introduced through the catheter and employed to puncture the intact interatrial septum in the region of the fossa ovalis. The catheter then is advanced over the needle into the left atrium; preshaping of the catheter also allows ready entrance across the mitral valve into the left ventricle.

Other methods of catheterization of the left side of the heart are used less commonly; e.g., with the *anterior percutaneous* approach a needle is introduced directly into the left ventricle in the region of the cardiac apex. This procedure is occasionally useful for measuring the left ventricular pressure in patients with valvular aortic stenosis, or in postoperative patients with prosthetic valves in both the aortic and mitral positions.

CARDIAC ANGIOGRAPHY Right side of heart Selective injection of radiopaque contrast media at various sites within the right side of the heart also may be performed during cardiac catheterization. Injections into the superior or inferior vena cava are useful for detecting the thickened right atrial wall of constrictive pericarditis and for defining certain congenital lesions such as Ebstein's malformation of the tricuspid valve and tricuspid atresia (Chap. 185). Selective right ventriculography is used to detect tricuspid regurgitation and to delineate congenital cardiac lesions such as pulmonic stenosis and tetralogy of Fallot. Injection into the main pulmonary artery permits visualization of pulmonary thromboemboli, congenital pulmonary arterial branch stenoses, and anomalous pulmonary venous connections, and during the levophase of contrast passage may be useful in the detection of tumor or thrombus within the left atrium.

Left side of heart Selective left ventriculography is employed to define congenital and acquired lesions affecting the mitral valve and the left ventricular outflow tract and to assess the adequacy of left ventricular function. Mitral stenosis may be detected by left ventriculography as thickening and/or calcification of the valve leaflets, shortening of the chordal subvalvular apparatus, and reduced excursion and delayed closure of the leaflets. Mitral regurgitation may be detected and its degree estimated by noting the amount and density of contrast agent which enters the left atrium after left ventricular injection (Fig. 180-1). In addition systolic prolapse into the left atrium of one or both of the mitral valve leaflets, secondary to either chordal malfunction or primary myxomatous degeneration, and redundancy of the leaflets themselves may be identified. The site of discrete subvalvular, valvular, or supravalvular aortic stenosis may be visualized, and the abnormal apposition of the ventricular septum and the anterior mitral valve leaflet in hypertrophic cardiomyopathy can be defined.

Both regional and global left ventricular function can be determined from analysis of the silhouette of the left ventricular cavity on the left ventriculogram. Regions of absent contraction (akinesis), reduced contraction (hypokinesis), or paradoxical systolic expansion (dyskinesis), as well as frank aneurysm formation, can thereby be detected and assessed as to severity (Fig. 180-2). Mural thrombi also may be visualized within such areas where wall motion is disordered. In addition, by determination of a magnification factor, the area of the left ventricular cavity can be measured accurately, and by assumption of a geometric model of an ellipse, the volume of the chamber at end diastole and end systole can be determined (Fig. 180-1), and the total stroke volume can be calculated. The total stroke volume minus the forward stroke volume (calculated by an independent method for determining cardiac output, as discussed below) can then be used to derive the amount of aortic or mitral regurgitation per beat.

Values for end-diastolic volume greater than 90 mL per square meter of body surface area (average normal, plus 1 SD) generally indicate left ventricular dilatation due to heart failure, or to a volume overload such as occurs in aortic or mitral regurgitation. The ejection

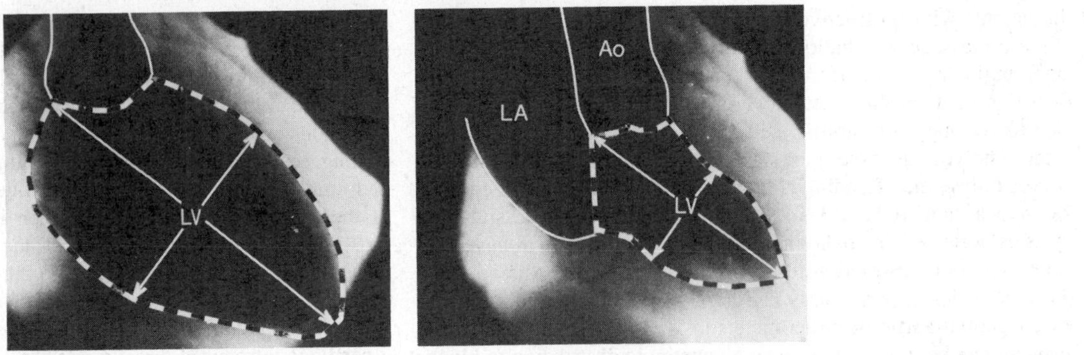

FIGURE 180-1 *Cineangiogram with injection of contrast medium into the left ventricle (LV). End diastole is on the left and end systole on the right. Study is performed in the right anterior oblique projection in a patient with severe mitral regurgitation in whom the left atrium (LA) is densely opacified simultaneously with the aorta (Ao) during ventricular systole.*

Volume (V) and LV is determined by planimetry of chamber area (enclosed by dashed line) and measurement of longest length (solid line between base and apex), using a geometric model of an ellipsoid. Thus, $D = 4A/\pi L$ *and* $V = \pi(D^2L/6)$*, where D = calculated diameter, L = longest measured length, A = area, and V = LV volume. Mean velocity of circumferential fiber shortening (mean* V_{cf}*, normalized to per unit circumference) can also be calculated by direct measurement of the minor axis (indicated by line with arrows) perpendicular to the midpoint of the long axis, and determination of the ejection time from cine frame rate and number of frames exposed from the beginning to the end of ejection.*

$$\textit{Ejection fraction} = \frac{\textit{end-diastolic } V - \textit{end-systolic } V}{\textit{end-systolic } V}$$

$$\textit{Mean } V_{cf} = \frac{\textit{end-diastolic } D - \textit{end-systolic } D}{\textit{end-diastolic } D \times \textit{ejection time}}$$

where V = ventricular volume, D = minor axis diameter

fraction, the ratio of stroke volume to end-diastolic volume, reflects the percent shortening of the left ventricular myocardium (normal range of ejection fraction = 0.56 to 0.78). When the ejection fraction is reduced, the presence of depressed left ventricular contractile function is suggested. A further useful index of myocardial function is the mean velocity of circumferential fiber shortening (mean V_{cf}), the fractional shortening per unit time of the minor axis of the left ventricular chamber (Fig. 180-1). Mean V_{cf} values below 1.2 end-diastolic circumferences per second in the basal state are considered indicative of depressed myocardial contractility. (Other measures of depressed contractility are discussed below in ''Measurement of Intravascular and Intracardiac Pressures.'')

Selective ascending aortography is used for assessing the severity of aortic regurgitation, for determining the size and location of aortic aneurysms, and for visualizing less common congenital or acquired malformations such as sinus of Valsalva aneurysm, paraaortic sinus tract or aortic valvular vegetation (infective endocarditis), or dissection of the aorta due to cystic medial necrosis. Direct injection of contrast medium into the left atrium has been used to study left atrial function or the movement of the mitral valve, and to detect thrombi or tumor (myxoma, rhabdomyoma, rhabdomyosarcoma) within that chamber.

FIGURE 180-2 *Diagrammatic representation of end-diastolic (solid line) and end-systolic (dashed line) silhouettes of left ventricular cineangiograms in various forms of localized wall motion disorder in patients with coronary heart disease, Normal patient exhibits relatively symmetrical contraction; patient with hypokinesis exhibits reduced contraction over anterior and apical surfaces; patient with dyskinesis exhibits paradoxic, outward movement over anterior surface during systole.*

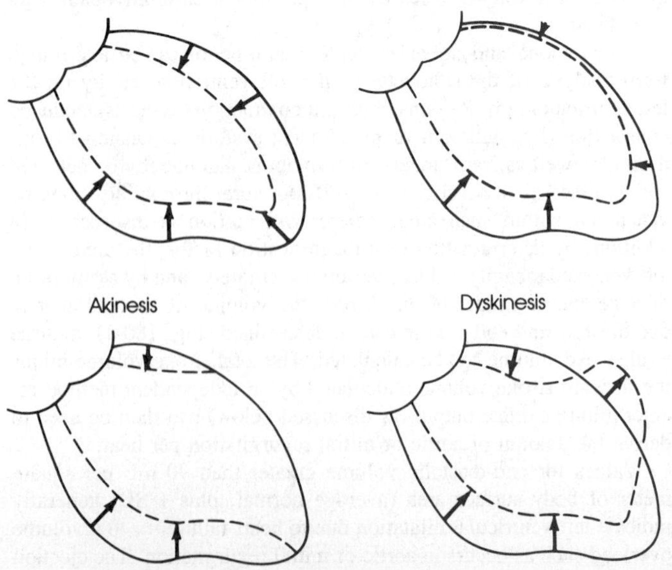

CORONARY ARTERIOGRAPHY Selective angiographic visualization of the coronary arterial tree is one of the most commonly applied diagnostic procedures in the cardiac catheterization laboratory. Accurate visualization of coronary artery atherosclerotic lesions has significantly increased understanding of the pathogenesis and natural history of ischemic heart disease. Moreover, this procedure has contributed in large measure to the advent of surgical procedures for bypassing obstructive lesions within the coronary arteries. Visualization of coronary artery anatomy is useful, likewise, for defining congenital abnormalities such as anomalous origin of the coronary arteries, or coronary arteriovenous fistula. Administration of ergonovine maleate during coronary arteriography is useful for inducing focal coronary artery spasm, particularly in patients with chest pain at rest in whom Prinzmetal's variant angina is suspected.

Coronary arteriography is performed by selective injection of 5 to 10 mL of contrast medium directly into each coronary artery orifice with cinefilming in multiple oblique and angulated projections at 30 to 60 frames per second and/or large film or photospot exposures at 4 to 6 frames per second, thereby obtaining dynamic as well as high-resolution images of the coronary arterial tree (Fig. 180-3). Specially designed catheters are used: one type, which has an open, tapered tip and multiple side holes, is inserted via a brachial arteriotomy (Sones technique); another type is advanced over a guidewire inserted percutaneously via the femoral artery and is preshaped to allow ready access to the right or left coronary artery orifices (Judkins technique). Both techniques provide diagnostic visualization of obstructive lesions within the main branches of the coronary vessels (Fig. 180-4*A* and *B*). In addition, collateral vessels, or new vascular pathways which serve to carry blood around a significant obstruction, can often be seen, and the vessel beyond a complete obstruction thereby visualized (Fig. 180-4*A*). The latter finding has obvious importance in determining the site for implantation of the distal end of a bypass graft.

DIGITAL ANGIOGRAPHY Digital computer processing of fluoroscopic or cineangiographic images is now being used to provide

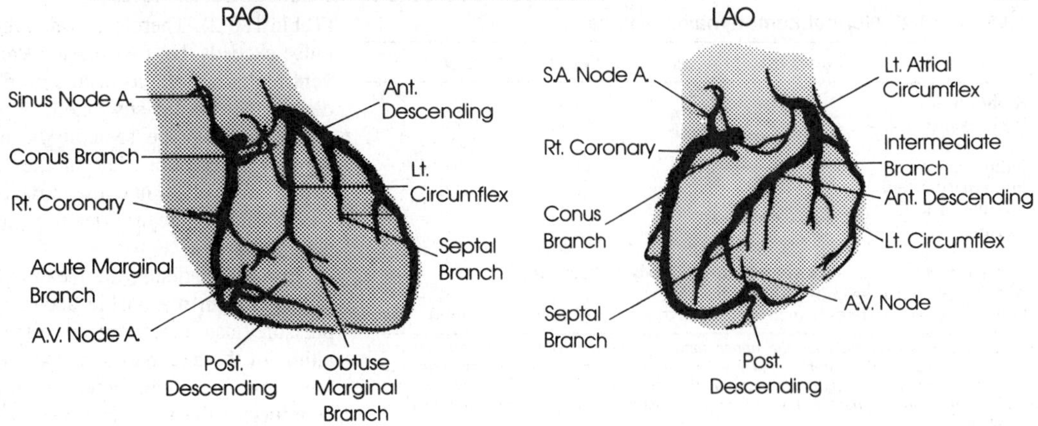

FIGURE 180-3 *Diagram of the coronary arterial tree as viewed in two projections commonly used in coronary arteriography, the right anterior oblique (RAO) and left anterior oblique (LAO) projections. A., artery; Ant., anterior, A.V., atrioventricular; Lt., left; Post., posterior; Rt., right; S.A., sinoatrial.*

visual enhancement of structures on both the right and left sides of the heart. In many of these studies the radiopaque contrast material is injected into a peripheral or central vein, obviating the need for a direct left-sided injection. This new approach to cardiac angiography has to date revealed the following advantages: (1) it allows definition of cardiac chamber size and geometry while using less contrast agent; (2) it facilitates computer generation of quantitative indexes of left ventricular function; (3) premature systoles generally are not induced during the recording of the angiographic images; (4) so-called functional or parametric images can be readily constructed which portray visually in one frame a physiologic or pathophysiologic parameter, e.g., regional wall motion (Fig. 180-2), global shortening of the left ventricle, rapidity of contrast wash-in and wash-out through the coronary arteries or into the myocardium.

COMPLICATIONS Catheterization of the right side of the heart is rarely associated with morbidity or mortality when performed under proper laboratory or bedside conditions. However, catheterization and angiography of the left side of the heart are procedures which unavoidably, although uncommonly, can lead to serious complications. Diagnostic cardiac catheterization procedures nevertheless have been increasingly applied in recent years, primarily in response to the need for precise functional and anatomic information prior to carrying out cardiac operations. In the pediatric age group great attention has been paid to preventing metabolic disorders (hypoxia and acidemia) and pulmonary difficulties, utilization of small amounts of contrast agents, and use of flexible catheters; such precautions have significantly reduced the incidence of major complications and markedly decreased the overall mortality rate in infants. In adults, the advent of coronary artery bypass graft surgery has brought about a predominance in the application of coronary arteriography and left ventriculography by retrograde aortic catheterization compared with other catheterization procedures. A prospective survey in 7553 patients of complications due to coronary arteriography reported in 1979 by the Collaborative Study of Coronary Artery Surgery (CASS) reported an overall mortality rate of 0.2 percent, an incidence of myocardial infarction of 0.025 percent, and an incidence of systemic embolization and vascular injury of 0.09 and 0.74 percent, respectively (all figures apply to 0 to 48 h after completion of the procedure). The brachial artery (Sones) technique increased the risk of death 3.6 times compared with the femoral approach, but this excess risk did not apply if a given laboratory performed greater than 80 percent of its procedures via the arm approach.

It seems clear that specialized invasive cardiac procedures in any age group should be performed only in well-equipped laboratories by highly experienced personnel, and the risks of cardiac catheterization and angiography should be weighed carefully in relation to the potential therapeutic benefits to be derived from an accurate anatomic and functional diagnosis.

MEASUREMENT OF INTRAVASCULAR AND INTRACARDIAC PRESSURES

The upper limits of normal for intracardiac pressures and certain other hemodynamic variables are shown in Table 180-2. In under-

FIGURE 180-4 *Selective coronary arteriograms obtained in the right anterior oblique projection. A and B show a normal subject, and C, a patient with severe stenosis of the right coronary artery. LMCA, left main coronary artery; CCA, circumflex coronary artery; LADCA, left anterior descending coronary artery; RCA, right coronary artery. In C, arrow 1 indicates the area of narrowing in the right coronary artery, and arrow 2 shows retrograde filling of the anterior descending coronary artery via collateral vessels, indicating that a severe obstruction is present in that vessel as well. (Courtesy of MP Judkins.)*

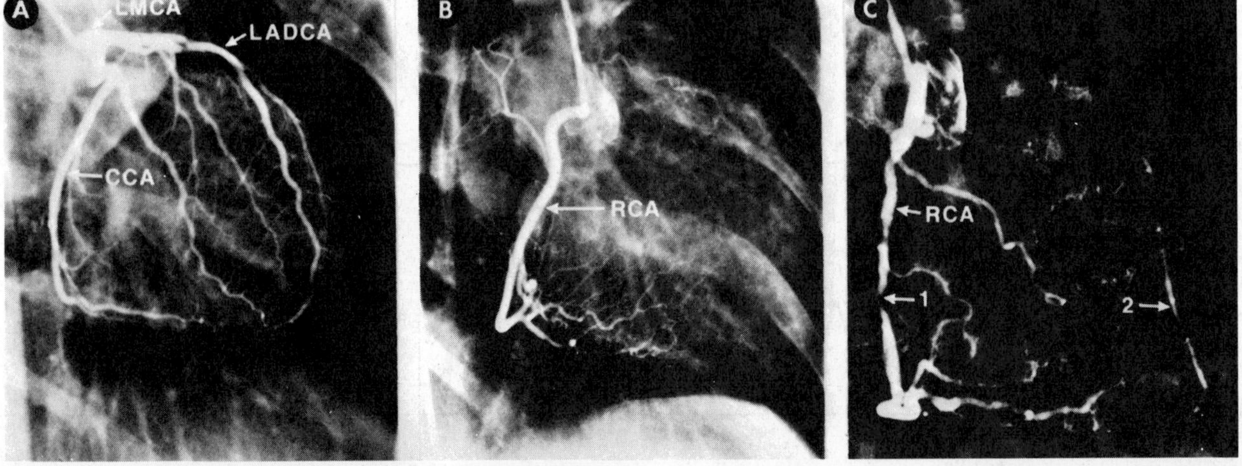

TABLE 180-2 Normal hemodynamic values*

	a wave	*v* wave	Mean	S/D
Right atrium	8	7	6	
Right ventricle				30/7
Left ventricle				145/12
Pulmonary artery			17	30/14
Pulmonary artery wedge or left atrium	10	15	12	

Cardiac index = 2.4–3.8 (liters/min)/m² body surface area
AV O_2 difference = 3.5–5.0 mL/dL
Pulmonary vascular resistance = 250 (dyn·s)/cm⁵ (3 resistance units)

* *The figures shown indicate the upper limits of pressure (mmHg) in normal adult subjects. The values for the pressure waves, the mean pressures, and the systolic and diastolic pressures (S/D) are shown; in the ventricles, D = end-diastolic pressure. The ranges for cardiac index and arterial–mixed venous (AV) O_2 differences are shown.*

standing the contours of the intracardiac pressure pulses, thorough knowledge of the temporal relations between the electrical and mechanical events of the cardiac cycle is important (Fig. 179-2).

The amplitude of the *a* wave in the right atrium normally is larger than the *v* wave, whereas in the left atrium the *v* wave is dominant (Table 180-2). Therefore, when the *v* wave in the right atrial pressure pulse exceeds the *a* wave, abnormal filling of the right atrium during ventricular systole, as occurs in tricuspid regurgitation or atrial septal defect, should be suspected. A characteristic right atrial pressure pulse also may be seen in the presence of tricuspid stenosis, the contour resembling that in the left atrium in mitral stenosis (see below), as well as in constrictive pericarditis, when an early diastolic ''dip'' and ''plateau'' elevation of pressure in mid and late diastole occur.

In many patients, the mean level of pressure in the left atrium is reflected with reasonable accuracy by the pulmonary artery wedge pressure (also sometimes termed the pulmonary ''capillary'' pressure), although the excursions of the wedge tracing often do not coincide with those measured directly within the left atrium. The characteristic contours of the left atrial pressure pulse in a normal subject and in patients with several forms of mitral valve disease are shown in Fig. 180-5. In the normal pressure pulse, or in the presence of mitral regurgitation without stenosis, there is a rapid fall in pressure during early diastole (the *y* descent), and a slow rise in pressure occurs during late diastole (diastasis), reflecting equilibration between the atrial and ventricular pressures during this slow phase of ventricular filling (Fig. 180-5*A*). In contrast, in patients with mitral stenosis

FIGURE 180-5 *Simultaneously recorded left ventricular (LV) and left atrial (LA) pressure tracings in a normal subject (A) and in patients with various forms of mitral valve disease (B to D). The tracings are recorded at high sensitivity (0 to 40 mmHg), and therefore the top portion of the left ventricular pressure tracing is cut off. The electrocardiogram is recorded in the upper portion of each panel.*

A. In the normal heart, diastole is initiated by a rapid-filling wave, which is followed by a period of slow ventricular filling, or diastasis (bracket D), in which atrial and ventricular pressure rise together slowly. This period of diastasis is followed by the atrial contraction (a), which precedes the onset of isometric contraction in the ventricle, the end-diastolic pressure. The c wave occurs during the phase of isometric ventricular contraction and is followed by the x descent. The v wave occurs during late systole, and the downslope of the v wave, constituting the y descent, occurs immediately after opening of the mitral valve.

B. Tracings obtained in a patient with mitral stenosis and atrial fibrillation. The pressure gradient from left atrium to left ventricle during diastole is indicated by the diagonally shaded area. The a wave is absent, and the c-v wave is prominent, and the y descent is slowed.

C. Tracings from a patient with mitral stenosis and normal sinus rhythm. The pressure gradient is indicated by the diagonally shaded area. A large pressure gradient occurs at the time of atrial contraction. No pressure rise during the period of diastasis is evident in the left atrial pressure tracings of panels B and C.

D. Tracings from a patient with isolated, severe mitral regurgitation and atrial fibrillation. The c wave is not evident, and the giant v wave in the left atrial pressure is nearly 70 mmHg. There is a small pressure gradient during the phase of rapid ventricular filling, because of the large volume of antegrade flow across the mitral valve.

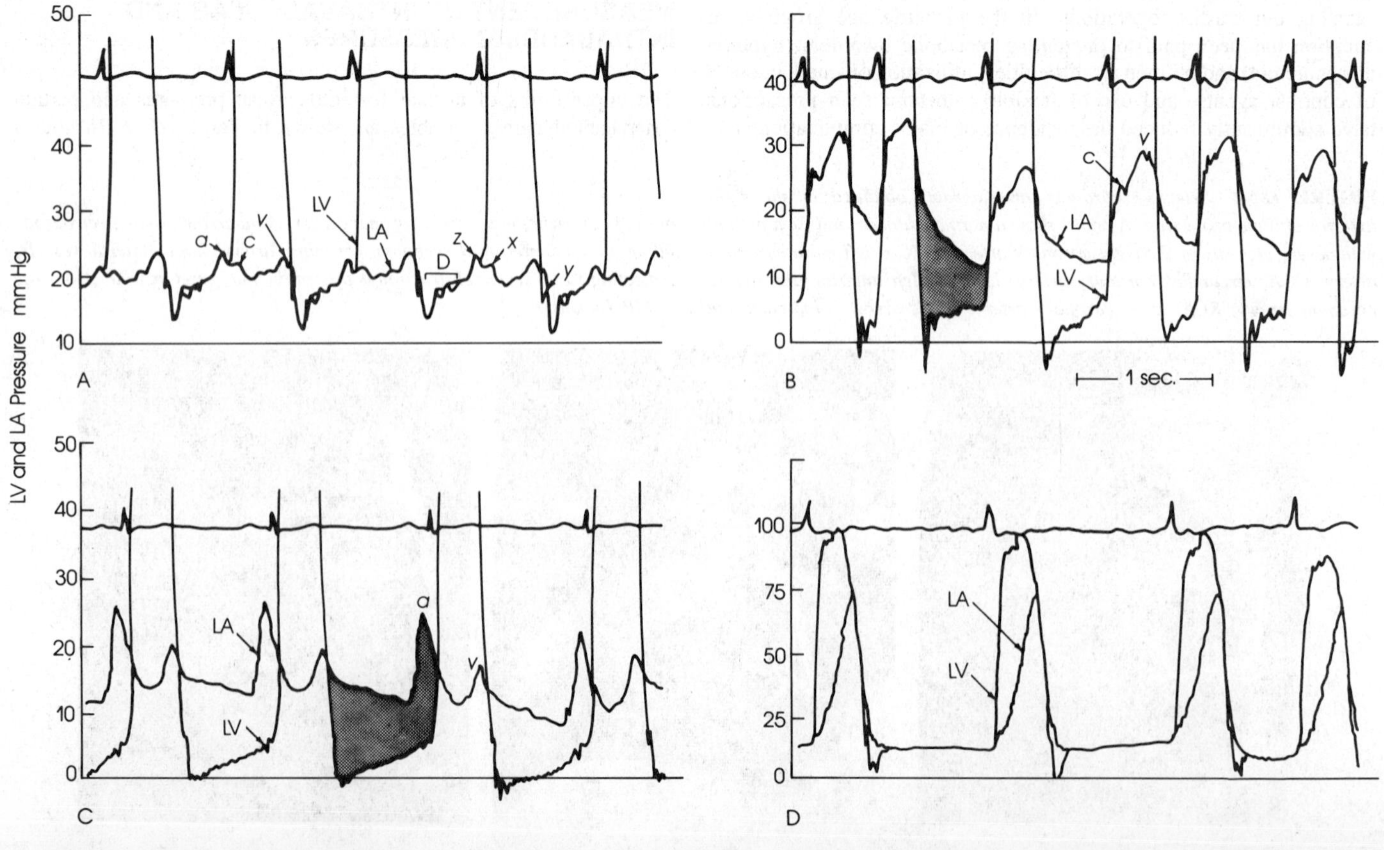

(Chap. 187) the y descent is slow and prolonged; pressure in the left atrium continues to fall throughout diastole, and evidence of diastasis on the left atrial pressure pulse is absent because of the persistent atrioventricular pressure gradient (Fig. 180-5*B*). When mitral stenosis is present with normal sinus rhythm (Fig. 180-5*C*), the *a* wave is present, and a large pressure gradient accompanies atrial contraction. In patients with pure mitral regurgitation, the *v* wave is prominent, and the descending limb of this wave (the y descent) is rapid (Fig. 180-5*D*).

The left ventricular end-diastolic pressure immediately precedes the onset of isometric contraction in the left ventricular pressure pulse. This pressure point therefore follows the *a* wave and precedes the *c* wave, and the coincident pressure point in time in the left atrial tracing is termed the *z* point (Fig. 180-5*A*). The left ventricular end-diastolic pressure may be elevated in several situations: (1) in the presence of myocardial failure, (2) when the ventricle bears a high flow load (as in aortic or mitral regurgitation), (3) when the ventricle is hypertrophied and/or relatively noncompliant (restrictive myocardial disease), (4) in the presence of constrictive pericarditis, and (5) with cardiac tamponade secondary to a pericardial effusion.

The systolic pressure in the left ventricle exceeds that in the aorta in any of the forms of aortic stenosis which produce significant obstruction to ventricular outflow (Chap. 187). In patients with severe valvular aortic stenosis, the left ventricular pressure pulse resembles that of an isometric contraction, the contour being more symmetric and the pressure peak more delayed than normal (a similar phenomenon is observed in the right ventricle in patients with pulmonic stenosis). The characteristics of the peripheral arterial pressure tracing also may be distinctive in patients with different types of aortic stenosis. Thus, when valvular stenosis is present, a slow and delayed rise of the peripheral arterial pulse wave is seen, while in hypertrophic obstructive cardiomyopathy an initially sharp upstroke is followed first by a rapid decline in pressure and then by a secondary positive wave, which reflects the development of the obstruction during systole (Chap. 192).

Derivatives of pressure pulses The rate of change, or slope, of the isovolumetric phase of the right or left ventricular pressure pulse, called the first derivative, or dp/dt, frequently is used in addition to ejection phase measures mentioned above (ejection fraction, mean V_{cf}) to characterize the contractile behavior of the ventricular myocardium. The dp/dt may be measured manually by determining the slope of the pressure rise, but it is recorded more accurately by means of an electronic circuit or by digital computer processing. The peak of this derivative tracing (maximum dp/dt) as well as the maximum value of the ratio of dp/dt to the corresponding instantaneous ventricular pressure [peak $(dp/dt)/p$] provide indexes of the speed of contraction of the ventricle and therefore can help to define the level of the inotropic or contractile state of the heart. These measures tend to be below 1200 mmHg/s and 32 per second, respectively, in the left ventricles of patients with disease of the myocardium, and they may be augmented strikingly by agents which improve the contractility of the heart, such as digitalis or catecholamines.

MEASUREMENT OF CARDIAC OUTPUT

The direct Fick and indicator-dilution methods presently are widely used in patients for the determination of volume blood flow, or the cardiac output. In general, the equations used with these techniques are derived from the principle proposed by Adolf Fick, which states that the rate at which a substance distributed in a fluid is delivered to an area by the moving fluid stream is equal to the product of the flow rate and the difference between the concentration of the substance at sites proximal and distal to the area. Thus,

$$Q = F(C_a - C_v)$$

where Q = quantity of substance delivered per unit time
F = flow rate
$C_a - C_v$ = concentrations of the substance at proximal and distal sampling sites, respectively

(The same equation is applicable to the measurement of the removal rate, or clearance, of a substance.) When flow is the quantity to be derived, the equation is rearranged to

$$F = \frac{Q}{C_a - C_v}$$

DIRECT FICK METHOD In this method for measuring the cardiac output it is assumed that at rest the oxygen uptake in the lungs is equal to that used by the tissues, and systemic flow, i.e., left ventricular output, is equated with blood flow through the lungs. It is essential to this method that a sample of mixed venous blood be obtained, because blood samples in the venae cavae and the coronary sinus have widely different oxygen concentrations, and therefore the venous blood sample generally is withdrawn from the right ventricular outflow tract or preferably the pulmonary artery. In practice, arterial and venous blood samples ($C_a - C_v$) are obtained during the measurement of oxygen consumption Q over a 3-min period by spirometry and subsequent chemical analysis of the expired gas. Flow F, or cardiac output, is then calculated. The subject must be in a steady state throughout the period of measurement to avoid transient changes in systemic blood flow or in the rate of ventilation that can negate the assumption that oxygen uptake in the lungs equals that taken up in the tissues.

INDICATOR-DILUTION METHOD This is a special application of Fick's principle. A variety of relatively nondiffusible indicators have been employed, the indicator substance being injected into the circulation and its concentration measured at a downstream sampling site by a suitable detector. For example, the dye indocyanine green is injected intravenously and blood is withdrawn from an artery at a constant rate through a calibrated densitometer, which provides direct measurement of the dye concentration. Generally, a single bolus of the indicator is injected rapidly and is thoroughly mixed in one of the vascular spaces, such as a ventricular chamber; the concentration versus time curve then provides a measure of the rate at which indicator is washed out of the mixing site. Prior to recirculation of the indicator, the downslope of this curve is exponential, and therefore extrapolation of the curve using semilog paper permits the elimination of recirculated indicator. The mean concentration c of the dye is determined from the area of this corrected curve and its duration. The rate of blood flow F then is directly related to the quantity of indicator injected i and is inversely related to the mean concentration of the indicator c and the duration of the curve t (in seconds) by the formula $F = 60\ i/ct$. A simple example will serve to illustrate this principle: if 8 mg dye is injected and a mean concentration of 2 mg per liter is recorded, and if the indicator takes 60 s to pass the sampling site, then the flow is 4 liters per minute.

Cold saline is another indicator which is used commonly when a thermodilution catheter is situated in the pulmonary artery. A standard amount of saline is injected at the junction of the superior or inferior vena cava with the right atrium, and the resultant change in temperature (analogous to concentration) is measured in the pulmonary artery by a small thermistor located 2 to 5 cm from the tip of the catheter. The thermodilution technique has demonstrated empirically an excellent correlation with other methods of measuring cardiac output. Cardiac output can also be computed by continuous infusion. Single thermodilution curves provide certain advantages: (1) no arterial entry is required, (2) the indicator is inexpensive, (3) recirculation is minimal, and (4) the analogue signal is well suited to rapid calculation of the cardiac output by computer analysis.

MEASUREMENT OF PULMONARY AND SYSTEMIC VASCULAR RESISTANCE The formula for calculation of pulmonary vascular resistance in simplified form (omitting consideration of vessel length and blood viscosity) states that resistance is directly proportional to the pressure drop across the bed and inversely proportional to the rate of blood flow. This ratio of mean pressure difference (expressed in dynes per square centimeter) to volume flow (expressed in cubic centimeters per second) is expressed in units of dyne-seconds per centimeter to the fifth power [(dyn·s)/cm^5]; e.g., the mean pressure difference across the pulmonary bed is obtained by subtracting the mean left atrial or pulmonary artery wedge pressure from the mean pulmonary artery pressure:

$$\text{Resistance} = \frac{[P_{pa}(\text{mmHg}) - P_{la}(\text{mmHg})] \times 1332 \text{ dyn/cm}^2}{\text{cardiac output (mL/s)}}$$

$$\text{where } P_{pa} \text{ and } P_{la} = \text{mean pulmonary artery and left atrial pressures, respectively}$$
$$1 \text{ mmHg} = 1.36 \text{ cmH}_2\text{O}$$
$$1 \text{ cmH}_2\text{O} = 980 \text{ dyn/cm}^2 \text{ force}$$

The resistance unit (i.e., the pressure difference in millimeters of mercury divided by the cardiac output in liters per minute and expressed in arbitrary units) also has been employed as an index of arteriolar resistance (Table 180-2). Estimation of the pulmonary vascular resistance, which normally is about 15 percent of that in the systemic vascular bed, is of particular importance in patients with congenital heart disease and circulatory shunts, as well as in certain forms of acquired cardiac and pulmonary diseases. Its calculation provides a useful means of interpreting the level of pulmonary arterial pressure relative to pulmonary blood flow, high pressure and high flow obviously bearing a different connotation than high pressure and low flow.

VALVE ORIFICE SIZE AND VALVULAR REGURGITATION When the cardiac output is normal, the severity of a stenotic valve lesion may be estimated from the magnitude of the pressure gradient across the valve. When the cardiac output is elevated or reduced, however, reliance on the pressure gradient alone may lead to an erroneous estimate of the degree of mechanical obstruction. In addition, it is of importance to consider the heart rate in assessing the significance of a pressure gradient. When the heart rate is rapid, systole occupies a disproportionate amount of time in each cardiac cycle, diastolic filling time is limited, and a large pressure gradient across an atrioventricular valve may exist in the face of relatively mild stenosis. The application of the hydraulic formulas devised by Gorlin and Gorlin to the calculation of valve orifice size has proved helpful in analyzing the degree of valve stenosis in these situations. These formulas state that

$$\text{Aortic valve area (cm}^2) = \frac{F/\text{systolic s}}{44.5\sqrt{\Delta P}}$$

$$\text{Mitral valve area(cm}^2) = \frac{F/\text{diastolic s}}{38.0\sqrt{\Delta P}}$$

$$\text{where } F = \text{flow across the orifice}$$
$$\Delta P = \text{the mean pressure gradient across the orifice}$$

These formulas state that the area of a short-bore orifice is directly proportional to the rate of blood flow across the orifice and inversely proportional to the square root of the pressure gradient. For example, if the flow rate across a narrowed valve orifice of fixed size doubles, as occurs frequently when the cardiac output increases during exertion, the pressure gradient will quadruple, often leading to a striking elevation of pressure in the chamber upstream to the stenotic valve. Conversely, when the flow rate is reduced, as in patients with heart failure, a small pressure gradient may exist in the presence of a severe degree of valve stenosis. This relationship differs from the general resistance equation discussed above and reflects the fact that the kinetic energy losses across a stenotic valve are high, a large pressure head being expended in developing the rapid flow velocity across the narrowed orifice.

The use of the above orifice formulas is not valid when significant valvular regurgitation is present and forward (systemic) cardiac output alone is measured, since an unknown volume of blood is regurgitated and recrosses the valve during the subsequent cardiac cycle. Application of the formulas under these circumstances leads to an underestimation of the valve orifice area, since forward flow across the valve is underestimated. However, when regurgitant flow is determined, generally by angiographic techniques, and total flow across the stenotic orifice is calculated, these orifice formulas may be applied.

DETECTION AND QUANTIFICATION OF CIRCULATORY SHUNTS When a communication exists between the left and the right sides of the heart, and when pulmonary vascular resistance and right ventricular stiffness are lower than systemic vascular resistance and left ventricular stiffness, respectively, a left-to-right shunt of oxygenated blood will occur. Conversely, when the resistance in the pulmonary bed is higher than that in the systemic circuit, or an obstruction such as pulmonic stenosis exists distal to an intracardiac communication, and right ventricular diastolic stiffness has increased, a right-to-left shunt of venous blood may occur.

Many types of indicators have been employed for the detection of circulatory shunts. The indicator may be the oxygen in room air, blood samples being withdrawn from various sites in the systemic venous bed, right heart, and pulmonary arteries, and analyzed for oxygen concentration manometrically or by an oximeter. A foreign, inert gas such as hydrogen may also be employed; this, like oxygen, is "injected" into the pulmonary circulation by inhalation and sampled from the right side of the heart by a catheter-tip sensor placed sequentially in the pulmonary artery, right ventricle, right atrium, and venae cavae. An inappropriate increase in concentration or early appearance of these indicators indicates the site of entry of a left-to-right shunt. Sometimes indicator-dilution curves are obtained by injecting indocyanine green into the right side of the circulation sampling through a densitometer from a peripheral artery; an early appearance of the indicator indicates a right-to-left shunt beyond (downstream to) the site of dye injection. Thereafter, sequential repeat injections into right atrium, right ventricle, and pulmonary artery until early appearance of contrast at the sampling site is no longer detected allow localization of the site of shunting. In most patients, however, the sites of shunting can be readily visualized and localized by exposure of cineangiograms during selective injections of contrast medium.

For quantification of left-to-right and right-to-left shunts, the oxygen content or saturation of the blood samples taken from the inferior and superior vena cava, the chambers of the right heart, pulmonary veins, left heart chambers, ascending aorta, and peripheral artery are used within the Fick equation to calculate the relative magnitude of pulmonary and systemic flow rates and the absolute amounts of right-to-left and left-to-right shunting. Generally, a pulmonary to systemic flow ratio of 1.5 to 1.0 or greater is considered to indicate a left-to-right shunt of clinical importance.

TRANSLUMINAL CORONARY ANGIOPLASTY

Following his development of a balloon catheter system for transluminal dilatation of peripheral arterial stenoses, Gruentzig designed a similar system for the coronary arterial tree and first applied it to a lesion of the anterior descending artery in 1977. This technique is now being used instead of surgery to treat coronary arterial obstruction in approximately 10 to 30 percent of those patients who, following diagnostic coronary angiography, are considered potential candidates for coronary artery bypass graft surgery (Chap. 189). The relief of obstruction is brought about by several mechanisms including (1) splitting of the plaque with development of a localized, partial circumferential dissection, (2) compression of the surrounding media and adventitia, and (3) remodeling of the "injured" artery over time as the small area of dissection heals (Fig. 180-6). The procedure is performed by passing a small, inflatable balloon-dilation catheter through a larger guiding catheter into the coronary artery ostium (Fig. 180-7*B*). A flexible guidewire passed through the balloon-dilation

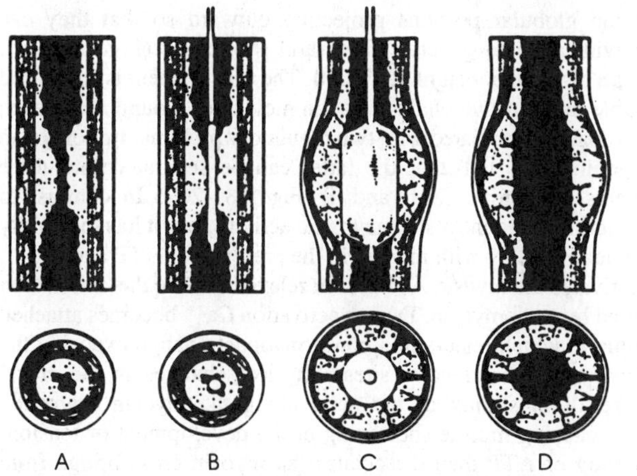

FIGURE 180-6 *Diagrammatic representation of the currently proposed mechanism by which angioplasty increases the luminal diameter of an atherosclerotic vessel is shown in two planes. A corresponds to the original stenosis, B to the introduction of the deflated balloon catheter, C to inflation of the balloon, and D to the final vessel appearance. Note extensive cracking of the intimal plaque, stretching of the media and adventitia, and expansion of the outer diameter of the vessel. (From W Castaneda-Zuniga, The mechanism of balloon angioplasty, Radiology 135:565–571, 1980.)*

catheter is then advanced down the appropriate coronary artery branch and across the stenosis until it reaches close to the cardiac apex. Thereafter, the deflated dilation catheter is advanced over the guidewire until it is situated within the stenotic segment of coronary artery, and the balloon is inflated with several atmospheres of pressure and for as long as 30 to 40 s. After two or more sequential inflations, the result is assessed by measuring the transstenotic gradient and by repeat coronary angiography (Fig. 180-7*C*).

The most comprehensive analysis of the results of transluminal coronary angioplasty has come from the Registry of the National Heart, Lung, and Blood Institute, which encompassed data from 105 centers in 3079 patients. The procedure was considered successful in approximately 66 percent of the total procedures attempted with a decrease in the degree of stenosis from approximately 80 to 30 percent by angiographic measurement. Emergency coronary artery bypass graft surgery was necessary in 6.6 percent of the patients analyzed, and the incidences of acute myocardial infarction and mortality were found to be 5.0 percent and 0.9 percent, respectively. Approximately 20 percent of patients later developed symptoms or signs of restenosis; many of this subgroup later underwent a successful redilation of the obstructed segment. With improvement in equipment design, patient selection, and operator experience, the primary (initial) success rate has now reached approximately 90 percent in many centers, and the need for emergency coronary bypass surgery and the incidence of infarction have each fallen to the neighborhood of 3 percent. Successful coronary angioplasty has been shown to result in enhanced myocardial perfusion, improvement in global left ventricular function, loss of electrocardiographic signs of ischemia during exercise, and an overall improvement in exercise capacity.

OTHER SPECIAL CARDIAC CATHETERIZATION TECHNIQUES

Miniaturization of electronics has permitted the construction and application of cardiac catheters with special measuring devices mounted on, or close to, the tip. For example, a catheter-tip micromanometer permits the measurement of intracardiac pressure free of the artifacts produced by fluid-filled manometer systems and catheter motion. Accurate high-fidelity pressure measurements are of particular utility in the assessment of the contractile and distensibility properties of the left ventricle. Micromanometer-tipped catheters also can be used for highly sensitive recordings of intracardiac sounds and murmurs. Electromagnetic or ultrasonic catheter-tip velocity probes also are available and have proved useful for study of phasic blood flow patterns in the venae cavae and pulmonary artery in patients with constrictive pericarditis and cardiac tamponade, and for analysis of the pattern and velocity of left ventricular ejection into the ascending aorta in patients with disorders of left ventricular function.

Other special catheters have been designed to record the intracardiac electrocardiogram and have made it possible to record selective potentials from the right atrium, right ventricle, and along the bundle of His. Recordings from the latter area are useful, for example, in determining whether a conduction delay or block on the surface electrocardiogram is located at or below the atrioventricular junction. His bundle recordings also have improved understanding of the mechanisms underlying paroxysmal atrial tachycardia and the preexcitation syndromes. Electrophysiologic studies with cardiac pacing are now being used in the diagnosis and selection of therapy for refractory cardiac tachyarrhythmias (Chap. 184). Electrode catheters have also been utilized to deliver a localized, high-intensity electrical discharge in order to ablate the atrioventricular node or an accessory pathway.

Transvenous intracardiac biopsy The subendocardium of the right and left ventricles may be biopsied safely by specially designed catheters. The specimens have proved to have some value from a diagnostic standpoint in uncommon varieties of infiltrative cardiomyopathy, e.g., those due to amyloid, iron, glycogen, granuloma, and neoplasm, and for identifying histologically differing patterns of inflammation. Endomyocardial biopsy is particularly useful in the detection of early cardiac rejection following cardiac transplantation.

REFERENCES

BAIM DS: Percutaneous transluminal angioplasty, in *Treatment Modalities. Harrison's Principles of Internal Medicine*, RG Petersdorf et al (eds), New York, McGraw-Hill, 1985, p 133

FIGURE 180-7 *Cine coronary arteriographic frames in right anterior oblique projection in patient undergoing percutaneous transluminal coronary angioplasty of the proximal left anterior descending branch of the left coronary artery. A. Before balloon dilation. B. During inflation of the contrast-filled balloon on the dilation catheter which has been passed over a tiny guidewire. C. After balloon catheter is withdrawn, demonstration of significant relief of stenosis.*

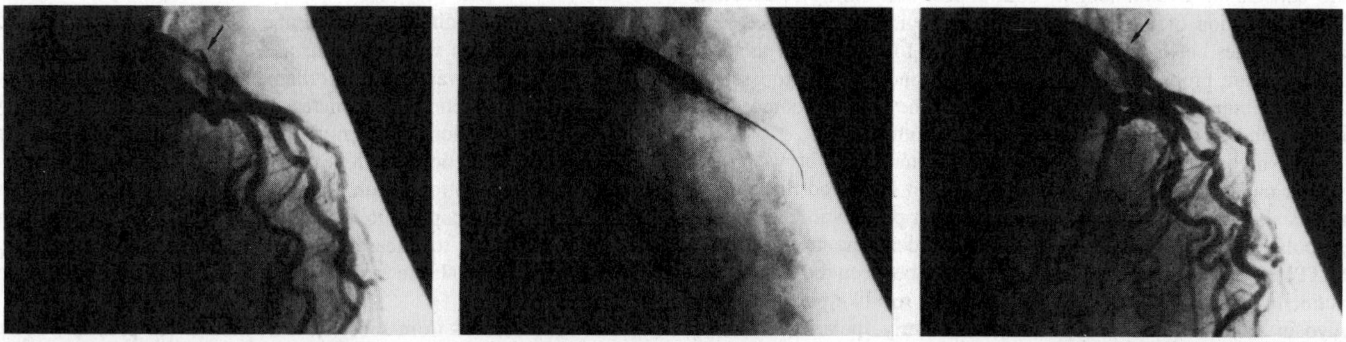

BARRY W, GROSSMAN W: Cardiac catheterization, in *Heart Disease*, 2d ed, E Braunwald (ed). Philadelphia, Saunders, 1984, p 279
BREDLAU CE et al: In-hospital morbidity and mortality in patients undergoing elective coronary angioplasty. Circulation 72:1044, 1985
DAVIS K et al: Complications of coronary arteriography from the Collaborative Study of Coronary Artery Surgery (CASS). Circulation 59:1105, 1979
FOWLES RE, MASON JW: Role of cardiac biopsy in the diagnosis and management of cardiac disease. Prog Cardiovasc Dis 27:153, 1984
GROSSMAN W (ed): *Cardiac Catheterization and Angiography*, 3d ed. Philadelphia, Lea & Febiger, 1986
KENT KM, MULLIN SM, PASSAMANI ER: Proceedings of the National Heart, Lung, and Blood Institute Workshop on the Outcome of Percutaneous Transluminal Coronary Angioplasty. Am J Cardiol 53(12):1C–146C, 1984
RACKLEY CE: Quantitative evaluation of left ventricular function by radiographic techniques. Circulation 54:862, 1976

181 NORMAL AND ABNORMAL MYOCARDIAL FUNCTION

EUGENE BRAUNWALD

CELLULAR BASIS OF CARDIAC CONTRACTION

The *myocardium* is composed of individual striated muscle cells (fibers), normally 10 to 15 μm in diameter and 30 to 60 μm in length (Fig. 181-1*A*). Each fiber contains multiple cross-banded strands (myofibrils), which run the length of the fiber and are composed of a serially repeating structure, the sarcomere. The remainder of the cytoplasm, lying between the myofibrils, contains other cell constituents, such as the single centrally located nucleus, numerous mitochondria, and intracellular membrane systems.

The *sarcomere*, the structural and functional unit of contraction, is delimited by two adjacent dark lines, the Z lines (Fig. 181-1). The distance between Z lines varies with the degree of contraction or stretch of the muscle and ranges between 1.6 and 2.2 μm. Within the confines of the sarcomere, alternating light and dark bands are seen, giving the myocardial fibers their striated appearance under the light microscope. At the center of the sarcomere is a broad dark band of constant width (1.5 μm), the A band, which is flanked by two lighter bands, the I bands, which are of variable width. The sarcomere of heart muscle, like that of skeletal muscle, is made up of two sets of myofilaments. Thicker filaments, composed principally of the protein myosin, traverse and are limited to the A band. They are about 100 Å in diameter, with tapered ends, and measure 1.5 to 1.6 μm in length. Thinner filaments, composed primarily of actin, course from the Z line through the I band into the A band. They are approximately 50 Å in diameter and 1.0 μm in length. Thus, there is overlapping of thick and thin filaments only within the A band, while the I band contains only thin filaments (Fig. 181-1). On electron-microscopic examination, bridges may be seen to extend between the thick and thin filaments within the A band.

The contractile process The "sliding" model for muscle rests on the fundamental observation that both the thick and thin filaments are constant in overall length, both at rest and during contraction. With activation of the sarcomere, repetitive interactions take place at the bridges between the actin and myosin filaments, and the actin filaments are propelled further into the A band. In the process, the A band remains constant in width, whereas the I band becomes more narrow and the Z lines move toward one another.

The myosin molecule is a complex, asymmetric fibrous protein with a molecular weight of about 500,000; it has a rod-like portion that is about 1500 Å in length with a globular portion at its end. This globular portion of the myosin contains adenosine triphosphatase (ATPase) activity and also forms the bridges between the myosin and actin. In forming the thick myofilament, the rod-like portions of the myosin molecules are laid down in an orderly, polarized manner, leaving the globular portions projecting outward so that they can interact with actin to generate force and shortening (Fig. 181-2*A*). Actin has a molecular weight of 47,000. The thin filament is composed of a double helix of two chains of actin molecules wound about each other, intimately associated with two regulatory proteins, tropomyosin and troponin (Fig. 181-2*B*); the latter can be separated into three components, troponins C, I, and T (Fig. 181-2*C*). In contrast to myosin, actin has no intrinsic enzymatic activity, but it has the ability to combine reversibly with myosin in the presence of ATP and Mg^{2+}, which activates the myosin ATPase. In relaxed muscle this interaction is inhibited by tropomyosin. During activation Ca^{2+} becomes attached to troponin C which results in a conformational change exposing the actin cross-bridge interaction sites. Physical changes in the cross-bridges result in sliding of the actin along the myosin filaments, ultimately causing muscle shortening or the development of tension. The splitting of ATP then dissociates the myosin cross-bridge from the actin. Linkages between actin and myosin filaments are made and broken cyclically as long as sufficient Ca^{2+} is present; these linkages are broken when Ca^{2+} concentration falls below a critical lead, and the troponin-tropomysin complex once more prevents interactions between the myosin cross-bridges and the actin filaments. Ionic calcium is a principal mediator of the inotropic state of the heart; most positive inotropic drugs, including the digitalis glycosides and catecholamines, act by increasing delivery of Ca^{2+} to the myofilament.

The *sarcoplasmic reticulum*, (Fig. 181-1*B*), a complex network of anastomosing, membrane-lined intracellular channels, which invests the myofibrils and which is less profuse in cardiac than in skeletal muscle, consists of a series of interconnecting longitudinally disposed membrane tubules closely applied to the surfaces of the individual sarcomeres; it has no direct continuity with the outside of the cell. Closely related, both functionally and structurally, are the transverse tubules or T system, formed by tubelike invaginations of the sarcolemma, which extend into the myocardial fiber, along the Z lines, i.e., the ends of the sarcomeres.

Cardiac activation At rest, the cardiac cell is polarized; i.e., the interior has a negative charge relative to the outside of the cell, with a transmembrane potential of −80 to −100 mV (Chap. 183). The sarcolemma, which in the resting state is largely impermeable to Na^+ and has a Na^+- and K^+-stimulated pump requiring adenosine triphosphate (ATP) which extrudes Na^+ from the cell, plays a critical role in establishing this resting potential. Thus, the inside of the cell has relatively large quantities of K^+ with far less Na^+, while the extracellular milieu is high in $[Na^+]$ and low in $[K^+]$. At the same time, in the resting state, the extracellular $[Ca^{2+}]$ greatly exceeds the free intracellular $[Ca^{2+}]$.

During the plateau of the action potential (phase 2) there is a slow inward current which reflects primarily a movement of Ca^{2+} into the cell (Fig. 181-3), although the absolute quantity of Ca^{2+} that crosses the surface membrane is relatively small and in and of itself appears to be incapable of bringing about full activation of the contractile apparatus. However, the depolarizing current not only extends across the surface of the cell but penetrates deeply into the cell by way of the ramifying T system. As a consequence of the transsarcolemmal movement of Ca^{2+}, much larger quantities of Ca^{2+} are released from the sarcoplasmic reticulum, a process termed "regenerative release" of Ca^{2+}.

The Ca^{2+} then diffuses toward the sarcomere, and as already described, combines with troponin, and, by repressing the inhibitor of contraction, activates the myofilaments to produce contraction. The sarcoplasmic reticulum then reaccumulates Ca^{2+}, thereby lowering its concentration in the myofibril to a level that inhibits the actin-myosin interaction which is responsible for contraction, and in this manner leads to relaxation. Thus, the cell membrane, transverse tubules, and the sarcoplasmic reticulum, with their ability to transmit an action potential, to release and then reaccumulate Ca^{2+}, appear to play a fundamental role in the rhythmic contraction and relaxation of heart muscle.

The ATP formed from substrate oxidation is the principal source

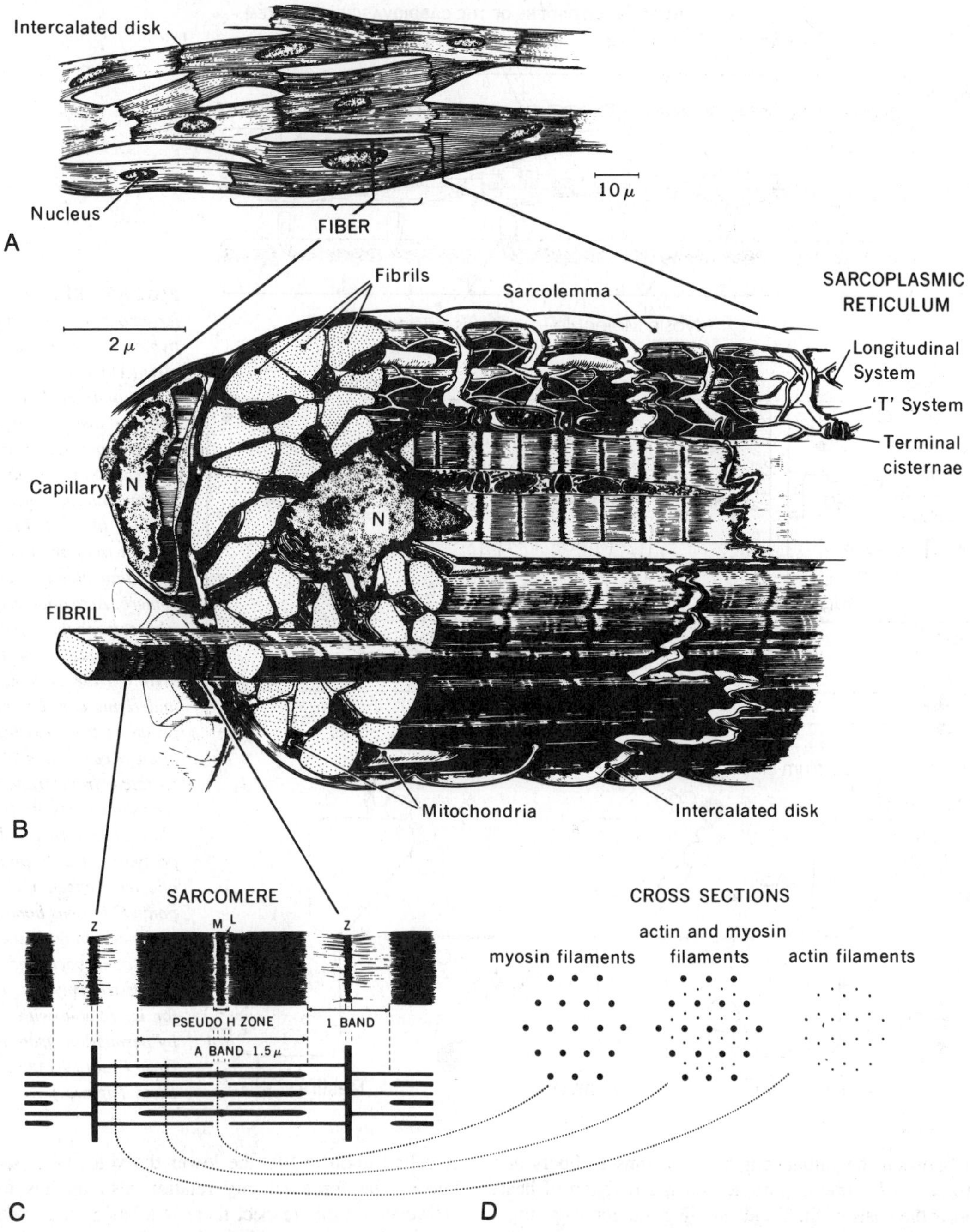

FIGURE 181-1 *Microscopic structure of heart muscle. A. Myocardium as seen under the light microscope. Branching of fibers is evident. Each fiber, or cell, contains a centrally located nucleus. B. Myocardial cell, reconstructed from electron micrographs. Each cell is composed of multiple parallel fibrils. Each fibril is composed of serially connected sarcomeres (N, nucleus). C. Sarcomere from a myofibril, with diagrammatic representation of myofilaments. Thick filaments (1.5 μm long, composed of myosin) form the A band, and thin filaments (1 μm long, composed primarily of actin) extend from the Z line through the I band into the A band. The overlapping of thick and thin filaments is seen only in the A band. D. Cross sections of the sarcomere indicate the specific lattice arrangements of the myofilaments. In the center of the sarcomere only the thick, or myosin, filaments arranged in a hexagonal array are seen. In the distal portions of the A band, both thick and thin, or actin, filaments are found, with each thick filament surrounded by six thin filaments. In the I band only thin filaments are present. (From Braunwald et al, 1976.)*

of energy for almost all of the mechanical work of contraction performed by the myocardial cell. The high-energy phosphate stores in ATP are in equilibrium with those in the form of creatine phosphate. The activity of the myosin ATPase determines the rate of forming and breaking the actin-myosin cross-bridges and ultimately the velocity of muscle contraction.

The role of muscle length In all forms of striated muscle, including cardiac muscle, the force of contraction depends on initial muscle length. The sarcomere length associated with the most forceful contraction is 2.2 μm. It is at this length that the two sets of myofilaments of the sarcomere are most ideally situated to provide the greatest area for their interaction. In support of the sliding-filament hypothesis, force development diminishes in direct proportion to the decrease in the overlap between thick and thin filaments, and the resultant reduction in the number of reactive sites. The length of the sarcomere also appears to regulate the extent of activation of the contractile system, i.e., its sensitivity to Ca^{2+}, which is greatest at 2.2 μm. When sarcomere length is increased to 3.65 μm, developed tension falls to zero, and it is at this point that the thin filaments are entirely withdrawn from the A band. Similarly, when the sarcomeres are shorter than 2.0 μm, the thin filaments bypass one another, producing a double overlap of the thin filaments, a reduction of sensitivity of the contractile sites to Ca^{2+}, and force also falls.

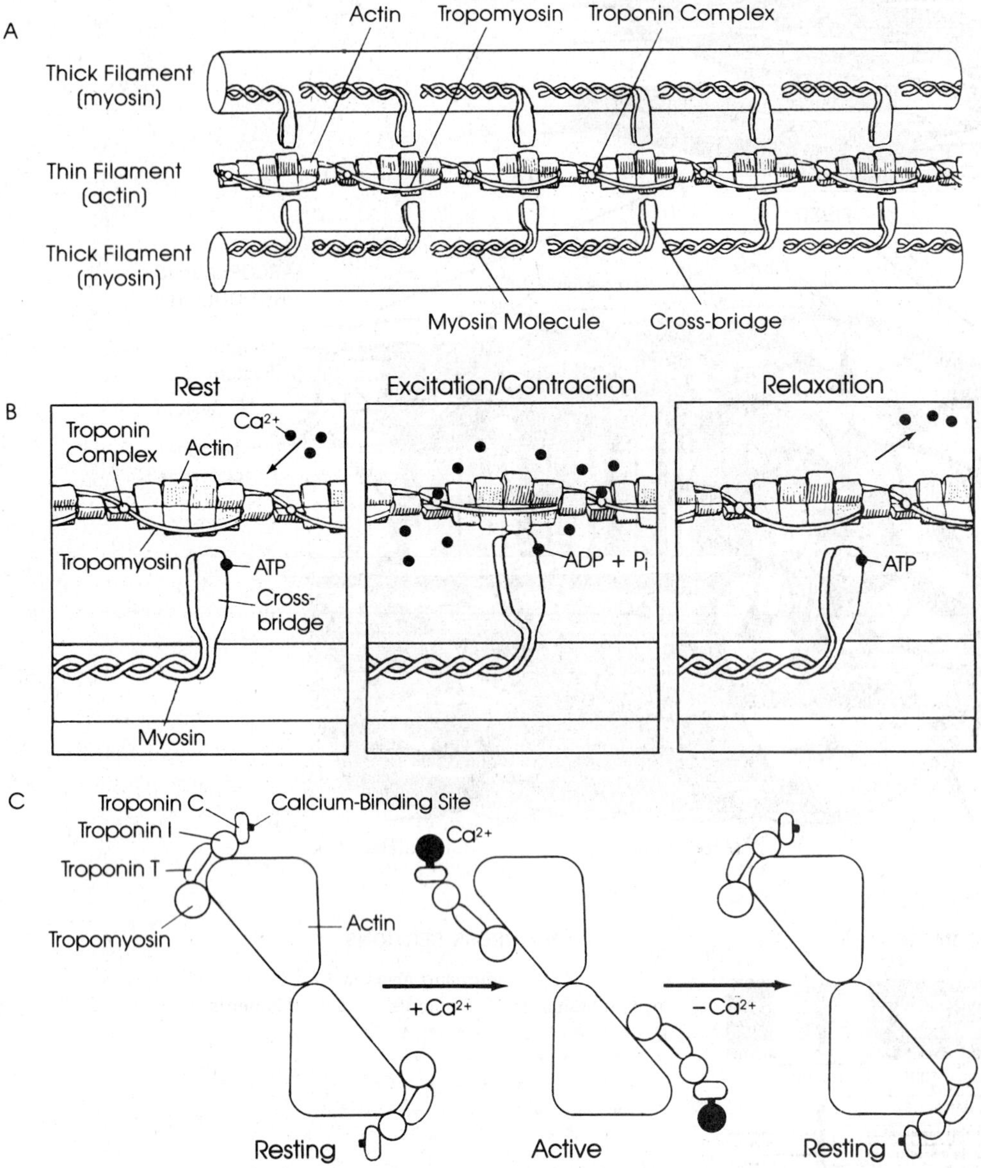

FIGURE 181-2 *Contractile protein interactions and the role of calcium as activator messenger are shown schematically: (A) Contractile proteins (myosin and actin) and regulatory proteins (troponin complex and tropomyosin) are shown in relative positions on myofilaments. (B) Contraction takes place when the heads of myosin molecules, which form cross-bridges of thick filament, bind to actin, followed by shift in orientation of cross-bridge that pulls thin filament toward center of sarcomere. Activation requires calcium binding to troponin complex, reversing inhibition of interaction between myosin and actin. In the cycle of chemical reactions underlying contraction, hydrolysis of ATP produces the cross-bridge motion. Relaxation occurs when calcium becomes dissociated from troponin. (C) Molecular rearrangements at the level of the thin filament involve regulatory proteins (tropomyosin and troponins C, I, T) in an allosteric effect. Calcium binding to troponin C loosens bond linking troponin I to actin; resulting dissociation of troponin T from actin backbone of thin filament displaces tropomyosin, exposing active sites for interaction with myosin. (Reproduced by permission, from AM Katz, VE Smith, Hosp Prac, 19(1):69, 1984. Illustration by Bunji Tagawa.)*

The relation between the initial length of the muscle fibers and the developed force is of prime importance for the function of heart muscle. This forms the basis of the Frank-Starling relation (Starling's law of the heart), which states that, within limits, an augmentation of initial volume of the ventricle, which is a function of the initial length of the muscle, results in an increase in the force of ventricular contraction. It has been shown for heart muscle that sarcomere length is directly proportional to muscle length along the ascending limb of the length–active tension curve. As muscle length decreases to the point at which developed tension approaches zero and at which sarcomere length approaches 1.5 μm, the I bands at first narrow, then disappear while the A band remains constant in length. At this latter point, the Z lines abut on the edges of the A bands. Thus, the sarcomere length–active tension curve forms the ultrastructural basis of Starling's law of the heart.

MYOCARDIAL MECHANICS

The mechanical activity of all muscle may be expressed externally in two ways: shortening and the development of tension. Hill showed in skeletal muscle that the velocity of shortening is inversely related to the magnitude of tension development, an expression of the so-called force-velocity relation, now acknowledged to be a fundamental property of muscle. Expressed simply, the greater the load the muscle is called upon to lift, the lower the velocity of shortening and vice versa. The force-velocity relation also applies to cardiac muscle. However, in this respect there is a basic difference between skeletal and cardiac muscle. Skeletal muscle has a single, essentially fixed, force-velocity curve; i.e., at any given muscle length, force and velocity are always related to each other in the same manner. The contractile activity of skeletal muscle is increased by the recruitment of additional muscle fibers, i.e., motor units, and by increasing the frequency of nerve impulses, while the contractile properties of each individual fiber remain constant. Although resting length also influences the characteristics of contraction, this variable remains essentially fixed in vivo because of the skeletal muscles' attachment to bone. In contrast, the number of cardiac cells and within them the myofibrils and sarcomeres which become activated during each contraction is constant. However, the contractile activity of the myocardium may be readily altered under physiologic conditions by changes in resting fiber length and by changes in the inotropic state, i.e., the contractility, both of which shift the myocardial force-velocity curve.

Variations in myocardial contractile activity may be expressed as displacements of the force-velocity curve in two fundamental ways. Figure 181-4*A* shows a family of force-velocity curves obtained from an isolated cardiac muscle; each curve was obtained at a different preload, i.e., with a different degree of stretch on the muscle. Note that changing the preload alters the intercept of the force-velocity curve on the horizontal axis; i.e., it increases the isometric force developed by the muscle. However, within limits, these alterations in preload do not appear to alter the velocity of shortening, since all the curves extrapolate to the same intercept on the vertical axis. Thus, a change in initial length of heart muscle shifts the force-velocity curve primarily by altering the total force which can be developed by the muscle, as illustrated by the isometric length-tension curve, shown in the insert of Fig. 181-4*A*.

This type of shift in the force-velocity curve may be contrasted with that obtained when a positive inotropic agent, such as Ca^{2+}, digitalis, or norepinephrine (which act ultimately, by increasing either the concentration of Ca^{2+} in the vicinity of the myofilaments and/or their sensitivity to Ca^{2+}) is added to the muscle while the initial length is held constant (Fig. 181-4*B*). These agents not only increase the force which the muscle is capable of developing, i.e., the intercept of the force-velocity curve on the horizontal axis, therefore shifting the isometric length-tension curve upward, but they also increase the velocity of shortening of the unloaded muscle, i.e., the extrapolated intercept on the vertical axis.

It has been postulated that an increase in initial muscle length up to an optimal length brings about an increase in the number of effective force-generating sites as a consequence of a more advantageous overlap of interdigitating contractile filaments within the sarcomere and in the extent of activation of the contractile sites, i.e., their sensitivity to Ca^{2+}. A change in the inotropic state, characterized by an increase in the velocity of shortening of the unloaded muscle, can also result from an increase in the rate of cyclic force-generating processes at the contractile sites, without a change in the number of these sites, i.e., at a constant muscle length. Increased contractility appears to be related primarily to an increased availability of Ca^{2+} within the cell.

CONTRACTION OF THE INTACT VENTRICLE

Analysis of the heart as a pump has classically centered upon the relation between the filling pressure, or diastolic volume, of the ventricle (length of the muscle fibers) and its stroke volume (the Frank-Starling relation). In the heart-lung preparation the stroke volume is a function of diastolic fiber length, and the failing heart delivers a smaller-than-normal stroke volume from a normal or elevated end-diastolic volume. The relation between the mean atrial or the ventricular end-diastolic pressure and the stroke work of the corresponding ventricle (the ventricular function curve) provides a useful definition of the level of the contractile, or inotropic, state of the ventricle. Significant increases in the level of ventricular contractility are accompanied by shifts of the ventricular function curve upward and to the left, while depression of contractility is identified by downward and rightward displacement of this relation.

It has been observed that during the adrenergic stimulation of the

FIGURE 181-3 *Calcium fluxes that activate contraction are downhill, and those that cause relaxation are uphill. As depicted in heart muscle at rest, calcium channels in the sarcolemmal membrane are closed, and intracellular calcium is stored in the sarcoplasmic reticulum. With excitation and membrane depolarization, voltage-sensitive sodium channels (not shown) and calcium channels in the sarcolemma open to allow rapid entry of extracellular sodium and calcium. Entry of calcium is now believed to cause release of calcium from the sarcoplasmic reticulum that initiates contraction. Reuptake of calcium by the sarcoplasmic reticulum by an ATP-dependent calcium pump is essential for the heart to relax. Importantly, contraction is activated mainly by passive calcium fluxes from the sarcoplasmic reticulum. By contrast, during diastole calcium must be pumped actively out of the cytosol to accomplish relaxation. Energy also must be expended during diastole to restore sodium and calcium gradients across the sarcolemma, which provide for the depolarizing ionic currents that generate the action potential. Sodium transport is accomplished by the sarcolemmal sodium pump (Na^+-K^+-ATPase), which utilizes ATP to pump sodium out of the cell in exchange for potassium. The resultant sodium gradient is largely responsible for active transport of calcium out of the cell during relaxation, via sodium-calcium exchange. (Reproduced by permission from AM Katz, VE Smith, Hosp Prac, 19(1):69, 1984. Illustration by Bunji Tagawa.)*

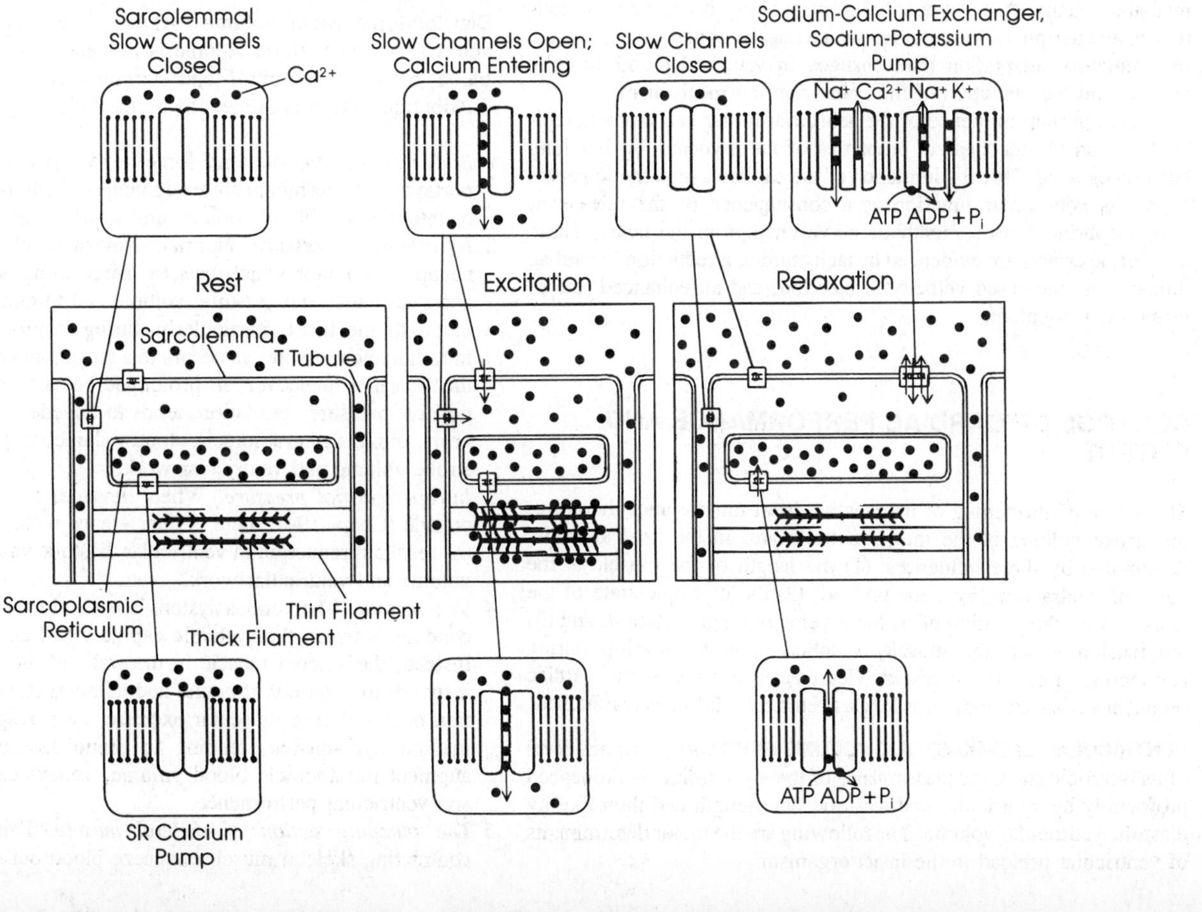

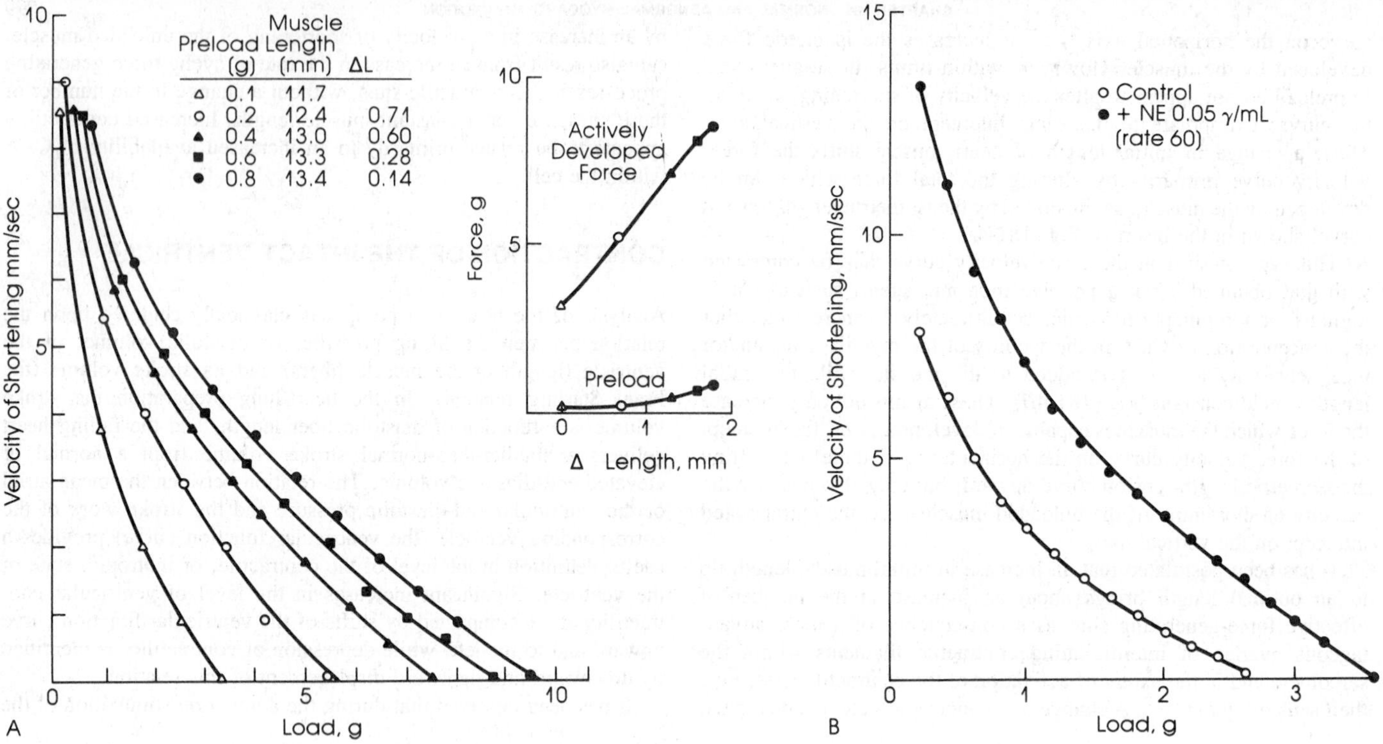

FIGURE 181-4 *A. Effects of increasing initial muscle length on the force-velocity relation of cat papillary muscle. Initial velocity of shortening has been plotted as a function of load for five different muscle lengths. The maximum velocity of shortening is essentially unchanged, whereas the maximum force of contraction is augmented. The insert shows the places along the length-tension curves at which these force-velocity curves were determined. B. Effects of norepinephrine on the force-velocity relation of the cat papillary muscle. Both the maximum velocity of shortening and the force of contraction are increased. (From Braunwald et al, 1976.)*

myocardium accompanying a stress such as exercise, relatively little change in ventricular end-diastolic size occurs, while cardiac output, aortic flow velocity, stroke work, and the rate of ventricular pressure development are all greatly augmented. Thus, neural and humorally mediated changes in myocardial contractility, heart rate, venous return, and peripheral vascular resistance may be of greater importance in circulatory adaptation than changes in ventricular end-diastolic volume and the operation of the Frank-Starling mechanism.

The important influence of the neurotransmitter substance norepinephrine on the mechanical properties of the myocardium has long been recognized. Direct stimulation of the cardiac sympathetic nerves augments ventricular function as a consequence of the release of norepinephrine from sympathetic nerve endings in the heart. These adrenergic effects are evidenced by tachycardia, a reduction in cardiac dimensions, increased velocity of ejection, and an enhanced rate of tension development.

CONTROL OF CARDIAC PERFORMANCE AND OUTPUT

The extent of shortening of mammalian heart muscle and, therefore, the stroke volume of the intact ventricle are, in the final analysis, determined by three influences: (1) the length of the muscle at the onset of contraction, i.e., the preload; (2) the inotropic state of the muscle, i.e., the position of its force-velocity-length relation; and (3) the tension which the muscle is called upon to develop during contraction, i.e., the afterload. Heart rate determines the cardiac output at any stroke volume as long as ventricular filling is maintained.

VENTRICULAR END-DIASTOLIC VOLUME (PRELOAD) At any level of its inotropic state, the performance of the myocardium is influenced profoundly by ventricular end-diastolic fiber length and therefore by diastolic ventricular volume. The following are the major determinants of ventricular preload in the intact organism:

Total blood volume When depleted, as in hemorrhage or prolonged vomiting, venous return to the heart declines (Chap. 29) and ventricular end-diastolic volume falls, as does ventricular performance, as reflected in ventricular work.

Distribution of blood volume At any given total blood volume, the ventricular end-diastolic volume is influenced by the distribution of blood between the intra- and extrathoracic compartments. This distribution in turn is influenced by the following:

1 *Body position*. Gravitational forces tend to pool blood in dependent portions. The upright posture augments extrathoracic at the expense of intrathoracic blood volume, and reduces ventricular work.
2 *Intrathoracic pressure*. Normally, mean intrathoracic pressure is negative, a factor which acts to increase thoracic blood volume and ventricular end-diastolic volume and to enhance the return of blood to the heart, particularly during inspiration. Elevation of intrathoracic pressure, as occurs in a tension pneumothorax, during the Valsalva maneuver, in prolonged bouts of coughing, or with positive-pressure ventilation, tends to impede venous return to the heart, diminish intrathoracic blood volume, and ultimately reduce stroke volume and ventricular work.
3 *Intrapericardial pressure*. When elevated, as in pericardial tamponade (Chap. 194), there is interference with cardiac filling, and the resultant reduction in ventricular diastolic volume lowers stroke volume and ventricular work.
4 *Venous tone*. The venous system is not a simple system of passive conduits between the systemic capillary bed and the right atrium. Instead, the smooth muscle in the walls of the venules and veins responds to a variety of neural and humoral stimuli. Venoconstriction occurs during muscular exercise, deep respiration, fright, or marked hypotension, tending to diminish extrathoracic and to augment intrathoracic blood volume, venous return to the heart, and ventricular performance.
5 *The pumping action of skeletal muscle*. During exercise the contracting skeletal muscles squeeze blood out of the venous bed

and, with the aid of the venous valves, displace it centrally, thereby increasing intrathoracic blood volume, ventricular end-diastolic volume, and ventricular work.

Atrial contraction Vigorous, appropriately timed atrial contraction augments ventricular filling and end-diastolic volume. The atrial contribution to ventricular filling is of particular importance in patients with ventricular hypertrophy, in whom the loss of atrial systole (as in atrial fibrillation) tends to reduce ventricular end-diastolic pressure and volume, ultimately lowering myocardial performance.

INOTROPIC STATE (MYOCARDIAL CONTRACTILITY) A number of factors determine the level of ventricular performance at any given ventricular end-diastolic volume, i.e., the position of the ventricular function curve. These influences may be considered to operate by modifying myocardial force-velocity-length relations.

Sympathetic nerve activity The quantity of norepinephrine released by sympathetic nerve endings in the heart is, under ordinary circumstances, dependent on the sympathetic nerve impulse traffic, and alterations in the frequency of nerve impulses modify the quantity of norepinephrine released and acting upon the beta-adrenergic receptors in the myocardium. This mechanism is the most important one which acutely modifies the position of the force-velocity and ventricular function curves under physiologic conditions.

Circulating catecholamines The adrenal medulla and other sympathetic ganglia outside the heart, when stimulated by sympathetic nerve impulses, release catecholamines, which, when they reach the heart, augment the inotropic state.

The force-frequency relation The position of the myocardial force-velocity curve is influenced by the rate and rhythm of cardiac contraction; e.g., ventricular extrasystoles result in post-extrasystolic potentiation, presumably by increasing the Ca^{2+} which enters the cardiac cell.

Exogenously administered inotropic agents The cardiac glycosides, isoproterenol and other sympathomimetic agents, calcium, caffeine, theophylline, and their derivatives, all improve the myocardial force-velocity relation and therefore may be used therapeutically to augment ventricular performance at any given ventricular end-diastolic volume.

Physiologic depressants Included among these are severe myocardial hypoxia, hypercapnea, ischemia, and acidosis. Acting either singly or in combination, these influences exert a depressant effect on the myocardial force-velocity curve and lower the level of the left ventricular work at any given ventricular end-diastolic volume.

Pharmacologic depressants These include quinidine, procainamide, barbiturates, and other local and general anesthetics, as well as many other drugs.

Loss of ventricular substance When a portion of ventricular myocardium becomes nonfunctional or necrotic, as occurs temporarily during ischemia (Chap. 189), and permanently in myocardial infarction (Chap. 190), total ventricular performance at any given level of end-diastolic volume is depressed, even if the remaining myocardium functions normally.

Intrinsic myocardial depression Although the fundamental mechanisms responsible for depression of myocardial contractility in chronic congestive heart failure still remain to be elucidated, it is now apparent that in this condition the inotropic state of each unit of myocardium is depressed and that the level of ventricular performance at any ventricular end-diastolic volume is thereby lowered.

VENTRICULAR AFTERLOAD The stroke volume is ultimately a function of the extent of ventricular fiber shortening. As in isolated cardiac muscle, the velocity and extent of shortening of ventricular muscle fibers at any given level of diastolic fiber length and myocardial inotropic state are inversely related to the afterload imposed on the muscle. The afterload on the intact heart is dependent on the level of aortic pressure, but it may be defined as the tension or stress developed in the wall of the ventricle during ejection. Therefore, the afterload on the ventricular muscle fibers also is dependent on the size of the heart, according to Laplace's law, which indicates that the tension of the myocardial fiber is a function of the product of the intracavitary ventricular pressure and ventricular radius divided by the wall thickness. Thus, at the same level of aortic pressure, the afterload faced by a dilated left ventricle is higher than that encountered by a ventricle of normal size. Furthermore, at any level of aortic pressure and left ventricular volume the afterload placed on any wall fiber varies inversely with wall thickness. The aortic pressure, in turn, is influenced largely by the peripheral vascular resistance, the physical characteristics of the arterial tree, and the volume of blood it contains at the onset of ejection. At any given ventricular end-diastolic volume and level of the inotropic state, the left ventricular stroke volume is a function of the afterload.

The critical role played by the ventricular afterload in cardiovascular regulation is summarized in Fig. 181-5. As already noted, increases in both preload and contractility increase myocardial fiber shortening, while increases in afterload reduce it. The extent of myocardial fiber shortening and left ventricular size are the determinants of stroke volume. Arterial pressure, in turn, is related to the product of cardiac output and systemic vascular resistance, while afterload is a function of left ventricular size and arterial pressure. An increase in arterial pressure induced by vasoconstriction, for example, augments afterload, which through a negative feedback depresses myocardial fiber shortening, stroke volume, and cardiac output; this in turn tends to restore arterial pressure to its previous level.

When left ventricular function becomes impaired, and the chamber dilates, i.e., when there is no preload reserve, left ventricular afterload

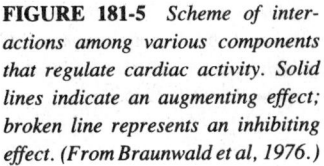

FIGURE 181-5 *Scheme of interactions among various components that regulate cardiac activity. Solid lines indicate an augmenting effect; broken line represents an inhibiting effect. (From Braunwald et al, 1976.)*

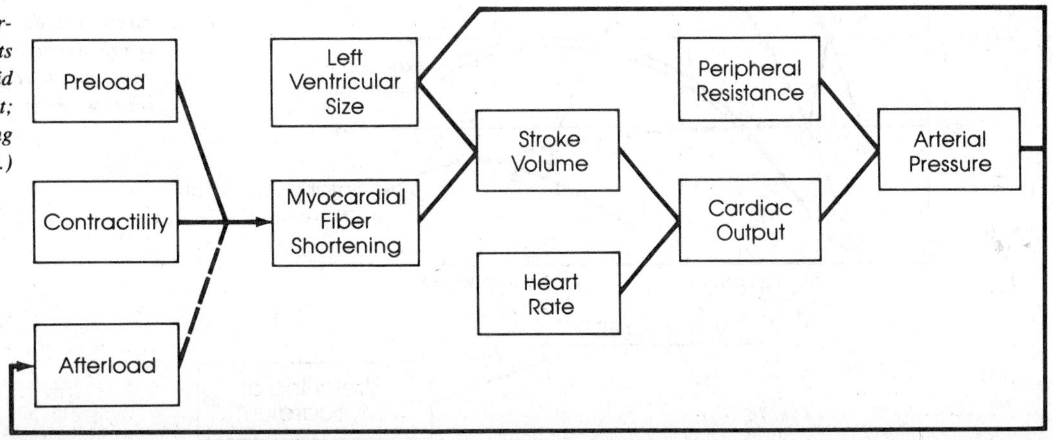

becomes increasingly important in determining cardiac performance. Increases in afterload may result from the influence on the arterial bed of neural, humoral, or structural changes which can occur in response to a fall in cardiac output. This increased afterload may further reduce cardiac output while myocardial oxygen requirements are increased. Treatment with vasodilators (Chap. 182) has the opposite effect. In this way, alterations in the peripheral vascular bed probably play an important role in the hemodynamic and metabolic events which usually are attributed to progressive impairment of the myocardium.

All of the influences acting on cardiac performance enumerated above interact in a complex fashion to maintain cardiac output at a level appropriate to the requirements of the metabolizing tissues, and in a normal person interference with one of these mechanisms may not influence the cardiac output. For example, a moderate reduction of blood volume or the loss of the atrial contribution to ventricular contraction can ordinarily be sustained without a reduction in the resting cardiac output. Presumably other factors, such as an increase in the frequency of sympathetic nerve impulses to the heart and an increase in heart rate, will, in the normal person, augment contractility and sustain cardiac output. Mechanisms are also available which prevent elevation of the cardiac output when there is no physiologic demand for augmented flow. For example, augmentation of myocardial contractility by means of cardiac glycosides does not increase the cardiac output in normal humans. Thus, in analyzing the effect of an intervention on cardiac output, it is important to recognize that it is the preload, which in turn is related to the volume of blood available for filling the heart, rather than the inotropic state of the myocardium or the afterload which limits cardiac output in the normal individual and that an improvement of myocardial contractility by a drug such as digitalis or the reduction of afterload with nitroprusside would not be expected to elevate the output in a normal subject. On the other hand, in the presence of congestive heart failure, the cardiac output usually is limited by the depressed contractile state of the myocardium, and a positive inotropic drug or reduction of afterload would be expected to raise cardiac output, and, indeed, does so.

EXERCISE The hemodynamic changes which normally occur during exercise in the upright position are complex (Fig. 181-6). The hyperventilation, the pumping action of the exercising muscles, and the venoconstriction which occur all tend to augment venous return and hence ventricular filling and preload. Simultaneously, the increase in the sympathetic nerve impulses to the myocardium, the increased concentration of circulating catecholamines, and the tachycardia which occur during exercise all combine to augment the contractile state of the myocardium (Fig. 181-6, curves 1 and 2) and lead to an elevation of stroke volume, with no change or even a decrease of end-diastolic pressure and volume (Fig. 181-6, points A and B). Vasodilatation occurs in the exercising muscles, thus tending to offset the marked increase in arterial pressure which would otherwise occur as cardiac output rises. This ultimately allows the achievement of a greatly elevated cardiac output during exercise, at an arterial pressure usually only slightly higher than in the resting state.

THE FAILING HEART

Though heart failure may be readily described as a clinical syndrome, characterized by well-known symptoms and physical signs, a precise physiologic or biochemical definition is far more difficult. However, from the clinical point of view, heart failure may be considered to be the condition in which *an abnormality of cardiac function is responsible for the inability of the heart to pump blood at a rate commensurate with the requirements of the metabolizing tissues or can do so only from an abnormally elevated filling pressure.* Abnormalities during systole and/or diastole may be present in heart failure (Fig. 181-7). In so-called *systolic heart failure,* i.e., classical heart failure, an impaired inotropic state leads to weakened systolic contraction, which leads, ultimately, to a reduction in stroke volume and cardiac dilatation. Idiopathic dilated cardiomyopathy is the prototype of systolic heart failure. In *diastolic heart failure* the principal abnormality involves impaired relaxation of the ventricle and leads to an elevation of ventricular diastolic pressure at a normal diastolic volume. Failure of relaxation can be functional, i.e., as during transient ischemia, or it can be caused by a stiffened, thickened ventricle. Typical conditions in which diastolic failure occurs are restrictive cardiomyopathy secondary to infiltrative conditions, such as amyloidosis or hemochromatosis (Chap. 192). In many patients with cardiac hypertrophy and dilatation, systolic and diastolic failure coexist; the ventricle both empties and fills abnormally. There may be cardiac dilatation, but the ventricle's pressure-volume relation is shifted, raising the ventricular diastolic pressure at any given volume.

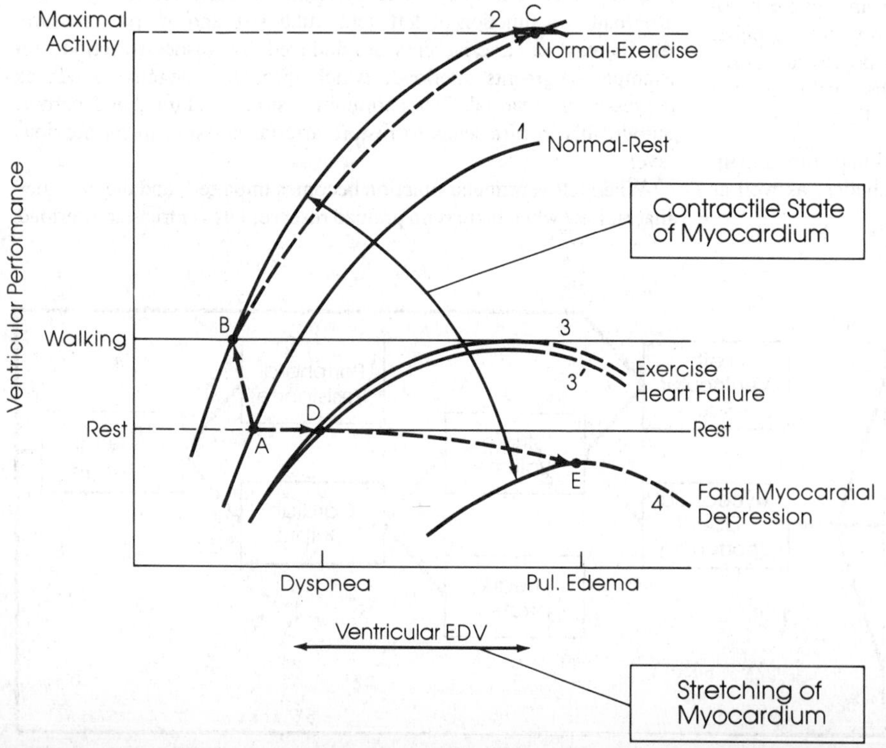

FIGURE 181-6 *Diagram showing the interrelations among influences on ventricular end-diastolic volume (EDV) through stretching of the myocardium and the contractile state of the myocardium. Levels of ventricular EDV associated with filling pressures that result in dyspnea and pulmonary edema are shown on the abscissa. Levels of ventricular performance required when the subject is at rest, while walking, and during maximal activity are designated on the ordinate. The dotted lines are the descending limbs of the ventricular-performance curves, which are rarely seen during life but which show the level of ventricular performance if end-diastolic volume could be elevated to very high levels. For further explanation see text. (From Braunwald et al, 1976.)*

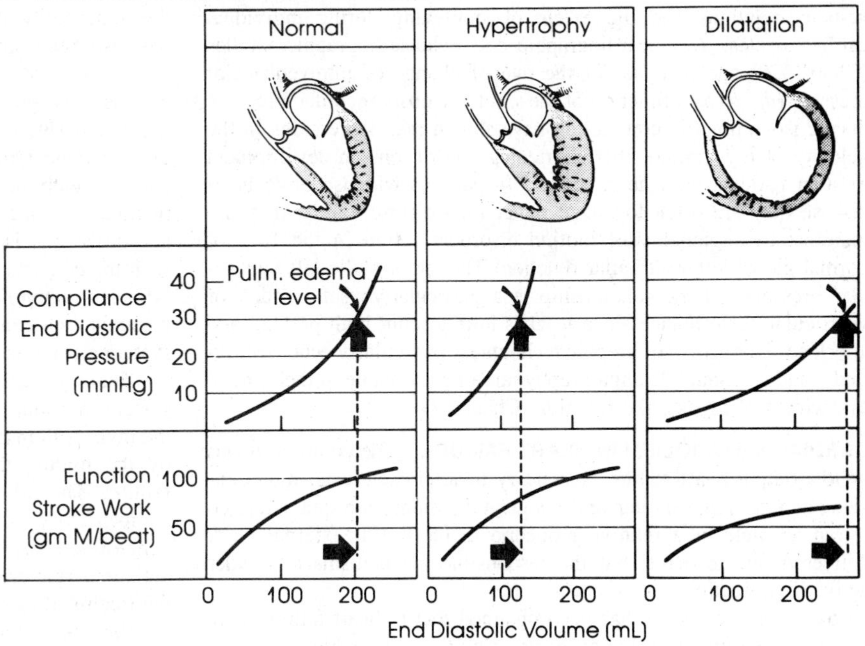

FIGURE 181-7 *Relationship between left ventricular end-diastolic volume and (1) end-diastolic pressure (top), describing the* compliance *of the left ventricle, i.e., its* diastolic *properties; and (2) left ventricular stroke work (bottom), describing the ventricle's* systolic *function curve. The normal left ventricle (left) reaches an end-diastolic pressure of 30 mmHg (pulmonary edema level) when its end-diastolic volume is elevated to 200 mL. The concentrically hypertrophied left ventricle (center), exhibits normal systolic function since the relation between left ventricular end-diastolic volume and stroke work is unchanged, but there is "diastolic failure" in that end-diastolic pressure reaches pulmonary edema level (i.e., 30 mmHg) at a lower level than normal (i.e., 130 mL). The dilated ventricle (right) exhibits "systolic failure" in that the maximal stroke work and the stroke volume at any level of end-diastolic volume are depressed. The left ventricle displays increased diastolic compliance, i.e., distensibility, with a higher than normal end-diastolic volume (280 mL) required to reach the pulmonary edema level. (Reprinted with permission from Gorlin R, Prim Cardiol 6:84, 1980.)*

Though a defect in myocardial contraction is characteristic of systolic heart failure, this defect may result from a primary abnormality in the heart muscle, as in cardiomyopathy, or it may be secondary to a chronic excessive work load as in hypertension and valvular heart disease, as well as in many forms of congenital heart disease. In ischemic heart disease systolic heart failure results from a loss in the quantity of normally contracting cells. It is important to distinguish heart failure from (1) states of circulatory insufficiency in which myocardial function is not primarily impaired, such as cardiac tamponade or hemorrhagic shock, (2) conditions in which there is circulatory congestion because of abnormal salt and water retention but in which there is no serious disturbance of the heart's function, and (3) conditions in which a normally contracting myocardium is suddenly presented with a load which exceeds its capacity, e.g., accelerated hypertension or rupture of a valve cusp secondary to infective endocarditis.

The intrinsic contractile state of myocardium removed from normal, hypertrophied, and failing animal hearts has been evaluated, and both ventricular hypertrophy and heart failure were shown to reduce the maximum isometric tension and velocity of shortening to subnormal levels; the changes are more marked in the myocardium of animals in which heart failure had been present than in those with hypertrophy alone. However, ventricular hypertrophy, in the absence of heart failure, also appears to be associated with a depression of the inotropic state per unit of myocardium, although the absolute increase of total muscle mass maintains overall cardiac compensation. Papillary muscles removed from the left ventricles of patients with heart failure have also shown a depression of the maximum degree of active tension which they can develop. Electron-microscopic analysis of failing cat papillary muscles fixed at the apexes of the length–active tension curves revealed sarcomere lengths averaging 2.2 μm. Thus, the abnormalities of contractility do *not* appear to be produced by an alteration in the overlap of filaments within the sarcomere.

The failing ventricle may still eject a normal or nearly normal stroke volume despite considerable depression of function, when its end-diastolic volume increases, i.e., through the operation of the Frank-Starling mechanism. As outlined above, an increase in the initial volume of the ventricle is associated with stretching of the sarcomere, a process which augments the number of sites at which the actin and myosin filaments can interact and/or which increases their sensitivity to Ca^{2+}. Furthermore, the development of ventricular hypertrophy may be considered to provide additional contractile units, and thereby constitutes an important compensatory mechanism when the myocardium's intrinsic inotropic state is depressed.

ASSESSMENT OF CARDIAC PERFORMANCE Several techniques are available for defining impaired cardiac performance in intact humans. With the patient at rest, the cardiac output and stroke volume may be depressed, but not uncommonly these variables are within normal limits. A more sensitive index is the ejection fraction, i.e., the ratio of stroke volume to end-diastolic volume, which may be estimated by standard radiologic or radionuclide angiography (Chaps. 179 and 180), and which is frequently depressed in heart failure even when the stroke volume itself is normal. A limitation of the ejection fraction (and of cardiac output) in the assessment of cardiac function is that these variables are influenced by ventricular loading conditions. Thus, a depressed ejection fraction and lowered cardiac output may be observed in patients with normal ventricular function but reduced preload, as occurs in hypovolemia, or with acutely elevated arterial pressure. An even more sensitive method for detecting impaired ventricular performance is based on the measurement of the circulatory changes occurring during stresses such as exercise or increased afterload. Thus, left ventricular performance may be estimated accurately by measuring the left ventricular end-diastolic pressure, cardiac output, and total body O_2 consumption at rest and during exercise. In normal persons, the cardiac output rises by more than 500 mL/min for each 100-mL increase in minute O_2 consumption. The left ventricular end-diastolic pressure at rest is less than 12 mmHg and rises slightly, remains unchanged, or decreases slightly during exercise, while stroke volume usually rises. The failing left ventricle, on the other hand, is characterized by an elevation of end-diastolic pressure during exercise, which reaches a value exceeding 12 mmHg, accompanied by either no change or a fall in stroke volume and a subnormal increase in cardiac output related to the increase in minute O_2 consumption. Various degrees of impairment intermediate between the normal response and that of the failing left ventricle during the stress of exercise also have been described.

The potential value of stressing the left ventricle is emphasized by the fact that the basal values for left ventricular end-diastolic pressure, cardiac index, and ventricular stroke work may be in the same range in patients with depressed ventricular function as in normal persons. The response to stress may prove useful not only in the detection of the impairment of myocardial function, but also in expressing the severity of this impairment quantitatively.

The performance of the left ventricle in humans may also be characterized by examining the instantaneous myocardial force-velocity relations and the extent of shortening during individual cardiac cycles. Angiocardiographic and echocardiographic studies (Chap. 179) and analyses of the rate of change of intraventricular pressure (*dp/dt*) as a function of the simultaneously recorded pressure during isovolumetric contraction have shown that depressions in the velocity of myocardial fiber shortening and of tension development exist in patients with heart failure. In patients with ischemic heart disease they are often localized rather than diffuse. Thus, they are manifest by regional wall motion disorders, often in the face of normal global left ventricular function. The end-systolic left ventricular pressure-volume relationship is a particularly useful index of ventricular performance since it takes into account both preload and afterload. Noninvasive, graphic techniques, particularly echocardiography and radionuclide angiography, are of great value in the clinical assessment of myocardial function (Chap. 179).

CARDIAC METABOLISM IN HEART FAILURE The common forms of low-output heart failure, secondary to arteriosclerosis, hypertension, and certain valvular and congenital lesions, are characterized by an absolute or a relative reduction in the useful external work delivered by the heart, but the responsible mechanisms are under active investigation.

Substantial evidence has been obtained that in heart failure there is an *abnormality of excitation-contraction coupling,* which alters the delivery of Ca^{2+} to the contractile sites, thereby impairing cardiac performance. The molecular basis of this abnormality, indeed its site, i.e., the sarcolemma, T tubules, and/or sarcoplasmic reticulum, has yet to be defined.

Considerable attention has also been directed to the question of whether cardiac failure is due to a defect in the production of energy, its conservation, or its utilization. Only in isolated instances of heart failure, such as those associated with beriberi, are there clear-cut disturbances of myocardial energy production. The major pathway by which pyruvate enters the citric acid cycle and some reactions within the cycle itself are dependent on the presence of adequate concentrations of thiamine (Chap. 76). Thiamine deficiency results in diminished pyruvic acid utilization by heart slices, and in abnormally low pyruvate extraction coefficients in intact dogs and in humans.

In the second phase of cardiac metabolism, energy conservation, the energy of substrate oxidation is converted into the terminal-bond energy of creatine phosphate (CP) and of ATP, the immediate source of chemical energy utilized by heart muscle. This process, known as oxidative phosphorylation, occurs in the mitochondria. The effectiveness of the combined energy production-conservation mechanisms may be studied by measuring the stores of ATP and CP existing in the myocardium, while energy conservation may be evaluated by determining (1) the P/O ratio, i.e., the ratio of high-energy phosphate produced to oxygen consumed in the mitochondria, and (2) the degree of coupling between electron transport and the generation of high-energy phosphate compounds. Although lively controversy exists concerning the status of this phase of metabolism in heart failure, it now appears that severe impairment of myocardial performance may occur *without* disturbances of mitochondrial function or reduction of high-energy phosphate stores, although abnormalities in these processes do occur in some forms of experimental heart failure.

In the absence of a definitive abnormality of energy liberation or conservation in the failing myocardium, attention has naturally been directed to the possibility that energy *utilization* is abnormal. An abnormality of energy liberation could certainly occur if the contractile proteins themselves were altered. A cardiac myosin isoenzyme characterized by immunologic and electrophoretic properties exhibiting a lower Ca^{2+}-dependent ATPase activity has been shown in some forms of experimentally produced heart failure, particularly those produced by mechanical overloading. It is possible that this depression may be responsible for a defect in the breakdown of ATP, the process which leads to contraction.

THE ADRENERGIC NERVOUS SYSTEM IN HEART FAILURE In view of the importance of the adrenergic nervous system in stimulating the contractility of the normal myocardium, the activity of this system has also been studied intensively in patients with congestive heart failure. An index of the activity of this system, at rest and during exercise, is provided by measurements of the concentration of norepinephrine (NE) in arterial blood. Relatively small increases in the NE concentration occur during exercise in normal subjects. In patients with heart failure the levels of circulating NE may be markedly elevated at rest, indicating that the activity of the adrenergic nervous system is augmented at rest, and the prognosis varies inversely with the concentration. Also, much greater increments in circulating NE occur when patients with congestive heart failure exercise, again presumably because of an increased activity of the adrenergic nervous system during exercise in these patients.

The importance of the increased activity of the adrenergic nervous system in maintaining ventricular contractility when the function of the myocardium is depressed in congestive heart failure also is shown by the finding that beta-adrenergic blockade may intensify heart failure. The adrenergic nervous system thus plays an important compensatory role in the circulatory adjustments of patients to congestive heart failure, and caution must be exercised in the use of antiadrenergic drugs, particularly beta-adrenergic blocking agents, in the treatment of patients with limited cardiac reserve (Chap. 182).

The concentration and content of the NE in cardiac tissue of patients with heart failure are reduced, sometimes to only 10 percent of normal. The mechanism responsible is not entirely clear, but a prolonged increase in cardiac sympathetic tone appears to play a critical role and to interfere in some manner with the biosynthesis of NE. Also, there is evidence that the beta-adrenergic receptor density and myocardial cyclic AMP concentration are reduced in chronic, severe heart failure.

In view of the strongly positive inotropic effect exerted by the NE released from these nerves, the adrenergic nervous system may be considered to provide an important potential source of support to the failing myocardium. However, the increments of heart rate and contractile force which occur in animals with experimental heart failure and cardiac NE depletion are abolished or markedly reduced with stimulation of the cardiac sympathetic nerves. Thus, it is likely that when congestive heart failure is accompanied by depletion of cardiac NE stores, the quantity of NE released by the sympathetic nerve endings in the heart is deficient relative to the impulse traffic along these nerves. Furthermore, whatever NE is released may not elicit a normal effect due to reduction of myocardial adrenergic receptor-effector mechanisms.

Cardiac stores of NE are not fundamentally necessary for maintaining the intrinsic contractile state of the myocardium. However, since the reduction of NE stores in heart failure is associated with a diminished release of neurotransmitter, this depletion of NE may be responsible for loss of the much-needed adrenergic support in the failing heart. In the later stages of heart failure, when the levels of circulating catecholamines are elevated and the cardiac NE stores depleted, the myocardium is largely dependent on a more generalized adrenergic stimulation derived from extracardiac sources, presumably the adrenal medulla; this would explain the deterioration of cardiac performance which may occur in patients with heart failure who are treated with beta-adrenergic blocking drugs. This generalized adrenergic stimulation resulting from circulating catecholamines may, however, also exert undesirable side effects, because it elevates vascular resistance and may present the heart with an afterload which is higher than optimal.

In the final analysis, in heart failure, the fundamental abnormality resides in depressions of the myocardial force-velocity relationship and of the length-active tension curve, reflecting reductions in the contractile state of the myocardium (Fig. 181-6, curves 1 to 3). In many instances, cardiac output and external ventricular performance at rest are within normal limits but are maintained at these levels only by an increased end-diastolic fiber length and an elevated ventricular end-diastolic volume, i.e., through the operation of the Frank-Starling mechanism (Fig. 181-6, points A to D). The elevation of left ventricular preload is associated with similar changes in the pulmonary capillary pressure, contributing to the dyspnea experienced by patients with heart failure. The normal improvement of contractility due to augmented sympathetic activity during exercise is attenuated or even prevented by norepinephrine depletion which occurs in severe heart failure (Fig. 181-6, curves 3 and 3′). The factors which tend to augment ventricular filling during exercise in the normal subject push the failing myocardium even farther along its flattened length-active tension curve, and although the left ventricle may perform somewhat better, this occurs only as a consequence of an inordinate elevation of ventricular end-diastolic volume and pressure and, therefore, of the pulmonary capillary pressure. The elevation of the latter intensifies dyspnea and therefore plays an important role in limiting the intensity of exercise which the patient can perform. Left ventricular failure becomes fatal when the myocardial length-active tension curve is depressed (Fig. 181-6, curve 4) to the point at which cardiac performance fails to satisfy the requirements of the peripheral tissues even at rest, and/or the left ventricular end-diastolic and pulmonary capillary pressures are elevated to levels which result in pulmonary edema (Fig. 181-6, point E).

REFERENCES

BRAUNWALD E et al (eds): *Congestive Heart Failure: Current Research and Clinical Applications.* New York, Grune & Stratton, 1982

———, et al: *Mechanisms of Contraction of the Normal and Failing Heart,* 2d ed. Boston, Little, Brown, 1976

———, SONNENBLICK EH, ROSS J: Contraction of the normal heart, in *Heart Disease,* 2d ed, E Braunwald (ed). Philadelphia, Saunders, 1984, p 409

BRISTOW MR et al: Decreased catecholamine sensitivity and beta-adrenergic-receptor density in failing human hearts. N Engl J Med 307:205, 1982

COHN, JN et al: Plasma norepinephrine as a guide to prognosis in patients with chronic congestive heart failure. N Eng J Med 311:819, 1984

GROSSMAN W: Evaluation of systolic and diastolic function of the myocardium, in W Grossman (ed): *Cardiac Catheterization and Angiography,* 3d ed. Philadelphia, Lea & Febiger, 1986, p 301

KASS DA et al: Determination of left ventricular end-systolic pressure-volume relationships by the conductance (volume) catheter technique. Circulation 73:586, 1986

LOMPRE AM et al: Myosin isoenzyme redistribution in chronic heart overload. Nature 282:105, 1979

MORGAN JP et al: Intracellular calcium transients in human working myocardium as detected with aequorin. J Am Coll Cardiol 3:410, 1984

SPIRITO P et al: Noninvasive assessment of left ventricular diastolic function: Comparative analysis of Doppler echocardiographic and radionuclide angiographic techniques. J Am Col Cardiol 7:518, 1986

182 HEART FAILURE

EUGENE BRAUNWALD

Heart failure may be defined as the pathophysiologic state in which an abnormality of *cardiac* function is responsible for the failure of the heart to pump blood at a rate commensurate with the requirements of the metabolizing tissues or can do so only from an abnormally elevated filling pressure. Heart failure is frequently, but not always, caused by a defect in myocardial contraction, and then the term *myocardial failure* is appropriate. The latter may result from a primary abnormality in the heart muscle, as occurs in the cardiomyopathies (Chap. 192). Myocardial failure may also result from extramyocardial abnormalities, such as coronary atherosclerosis which leads to myocardial ischemia, as well as from abnormalities of the heart valves in which the heart muscle is damaged by the long-standing excessive hemodynamic burden imposed by the valvular abnormality, and/or by the rheumatic process (Chap. 187). In patients with chronic constrictive pericarditis, myocardial damage resulting from infiltration of the heart muscle by pericardial inflammation and calcification is common (Chap. 194).

In other patients with heart failure, however, a similar clinical syndrome is present, but without any detectable abnormality of *myocardial* function. In these patients the normal heart is suddenly presented with a load that exceeds its capacity, such as an acute hypertensive crisis, rupture of an aortic valve cusp, or massive pulmonary embolism. Heart failure, in the presence of normal myocardial function, also occurs in chronic conditions in which there is impairment of filling of the ventricles due to tricuspid and/or mitral stenosis, constrictive pericarditis without myocardial involvement, and endocardial fibrosis.

Heart failure should be distinguished from (1) conditions in which there is circulatory congestion consequent to abnormal salt and water retention but in which there is no disturbance of cardiac function per se (the latter syndrome, termed the *congested state,* may result from the abnormal salt and water retention of renal failure, or from excess parenteral administration of fluids and electrolytes), and (2) from noncardiac causes of inadequate cardiac output, including shock due to hypovolemia and redistribution of blood volume (Chap. 29).

The ventricles respond to a chronically increased hemodynamic burden with the development of hypertrophy. With volume overload when the ventricle is called upon to deliver an elevated cardiac output, as in valvular regurgitation, it develops *eccentric* hypertrophy, i.e., cavity dilatation, with an increase in muscle mass so that the ratio between wall thickness and ventricular cavity size remains constant. With pressure overload when the ventricle is called upon to develop increased pressure, as in valvular aortic stenosis, it develops *concentric* hypertrophy, in which the ratio between wall thickness and ventricular cavity size increases. In both conditions, a stable hyperfunctioning state may exist for many years but myocardial function may ultimately deteriorate, leading to heart failure.

CAUSES OF HEART FAILURE

In evaluating patients with heart failure, it is important to identify not only the *underlying cause* of the heart disease but the *precipitating cause* of heart failure as well. The cardiac abnormality produced by a congenital or acquired lesion such as valvular aortic stenosis may exist for many years and produce no or only trivial disability. Frequently, however, the manifestations of clinical heart failure appear for the first time in the course of some acute disturbance which places an additional load on a myocardium that chronically is excessively burdened and while compensated has no additional reserves, resulting in further deterioration of cardiac function. Identification of such precipitating causes is of critical importance because their prompt alleviation may be lifesaving. However, in the absence of underlying heart disease these acute disturbances do not usually, by themselves, lead to heart failure.

PRECIPITATING CAUSES

1 *Pulmonary embolism.* Patients with low cardiac output and physical inactivity are at increased risk of developing thrombi in the veins of the lower extremities or the pelvis. Pulmonary embolization may result in further elevation of pulmonary arterial pressure, which in turn may produce or intensify failure of the right ventricle. In the presence of pulmonary vascular congestion, such emboli may also cause infarction of the lung (Chap. 211).

2 *Infection.* Patients with pulmonary vascular congestion are also more susceptible to pulmonary infections, but any infection may precipitate heart failure. The resulting fever, tachycardia, hypoxemia, and the increased metabolic demands may place a further burden on the overloaded, but compensated, myocardium of a patient with chronic heart disease.

3 *Anemia.* In the presence of anemia the oxygen needs of the metabolizing tissues can be satisfied only by an increase in the cardiac output (Chap. 53); though such an increase in the cardiac output might be sustained by a normal heart, a diseased, overloaded, but otherwise compensated heart may be unable to augment sufficiently the volume of blood which it delivers to the periphery. In this manner the combination of anemia and heart disease can lead to inadequate oxygen delivery and precipitate heart failure.

4 *Thyrotoxicosis and pregnancy.* As in anemia and fever, in these

conditions adequate tissue perfusion requires an increased cardiac output. The development or intensification of heart failure may actually be one of the first clinical manifestations of hyperthyroidism in a patient with underlying heart disease (Chap. 324). Similarly, heart failure not infrequently occurs for the first time during pregnancy in women with rheumatic valvular disease in whom cardiac compensation may return following delivery.

5 *Arrhythmias*. These are among the most frequent precipitating causes of heart failure in patients with underlying but compensated heart disease for a variety of reasons: (*a*) tachyarrhythmias reduce the time period available for ventricular filling; (*b*) the dissociation between atrial and ventricular contractions characteristic of many arrhythmias result in the loss of the atrial booster pump mechanism, thereby tending to raise atrial pressures; (*c*) in any arrhythmia associated with abnormal intraventricular conduction, myocardial performance may become further impaired because of the loss of normal synchronicity of ventricular contraction; (*d*) the marked bradycardia associated with complete atrioventricular block requires a greatly elevated stroke volume if a marked reduction in cardiac output is to be prevented.

6 *Rheumatic and other forms of myocarditis*. Acute rheumatic fever and a variety of infectious or inflammatory processes affecting the myocardium may further impair myocardial function in patients with preexisting heart disease (Chaps. 186 and 192).

7 *Infective endocarditis*. The additional valvular damage, anemia, fever, and myocarditis which often occur as a consequence of infective endocarditis may, singly or in concert, precipitate heart failure (Chap. 188).

8 *Physical, dietary, environmental, and emotional excesses*. The augmentation of sodium intake, the discontinuation of medications to treat heart failure, physical overexertion, excessive environmental heat or humidity, and emotional crises may all precipitate cardiac decompensation.

9 *Systemic hypertension*. Rapid elevation of arterial pressure, as may occur in some instances of hypertension of renal origin or upon discontinuation of antihypertensive medication, may result in cardiac decompensation (Chap. 196).

10 *Myocardial infarction*. In patients with chronic but compensated ischemic heart disease, a fresh infarct, sometimes otherwise silent clinically, may further impair ventricular function and precipitate heart failure (Chap. 190).

A systematic search for these precipitating causes should be made in every patient with heart failure, particularly if it is refractory to the usual methods of therapy. If properly recognized, the precipitating cause of heart failure can usually be treated more effectively than the underlying cause. Therefore, the prognosis in patients with heart failure in whom a precipitating cause can be identified, treated, and eliminated is more favorable than in patients in whom the underlying disease process has advanced to the point of producing heart failure.

FORMS OF HEART FAILURE

Heart failure may be described as *high-output* or *low-output, acute* or *chronic, right-sided* or *left-sided, forward* or *backward,* and *systolic* or *diastolic*. These descriptors are often useful in a clinical setting, particularly early in the patient's course, but they do not signify fundamentally different disease states, and late in the course the differences between some of these forms become blurred.

HIGH-OUTPUT VERSUS LOW-OUTPUT HEART FAILURE It is useful to classify patients with heart failure into those with a low cardiac output, i.e., *low-output heart failure,* and those with an elevated cardiac output, i.e., *high-output heart failure*. The cardiac output is often depressed in patients with heart failure secondary to ischemic heart disease, hypertension, cardiomyopathy, valvular and pericardial disease, but tends to be elevated in patients with heart failure and hyperthyroidism, anemia, arteriovenous fistulas, beriberi, and Paget's disease. In clinical practice, however, it is not always easy to distinguish between low-output and high-output heart failure. The normal range of cardiac output is wide [2.5 to 3.8 (liters/min)/m^2], and in many patients with so-called low-output heart failure the cardiac output may actually be just within the normal range at rest, although it is lower than it had been previously and fails to rise normally during exertion. On the other hand, in patients with so-called high-output heart failure the output may not be excessive, although it would have been found to be so had it been measured before heart failure supervened, but rather may be close to the upper limit of normal, particularly when heart failure is severe. Regardless of the absolute level of the cardiac output, however, cardiac failure may be said to be present when the characteristic clinical manifestations described below are accompanied by a depression of the curve relating ventricular end-diastolic volume to cardiac performance (Fig. 181-6, p. 902).

An integral part of systolic heart failure (p. 903) is evidence that the heart does not deliver the quantity of oxygen required by the metabolizing tissues. In the absence of peripheral shunting of blood, such inadequate delivery of oxygen to the metabolizing tissues is reflected in an abnormal widening of the normal arterial–mixed venous oxygen difference (3.5 to 5.0 mL/dL in the basal state), relative to the total-body oxygen consumption. In mild cases, such an abnormality may not be present at rest but becomes evident only during exertion or other hypermetabolic states. In patients with the high-output cardiac states associated with arteriovenous fistula, beriberi, thyrotoxicosis, Paget's disease, etc., the arterial–mixed venous oxygen difference is normal or low. The mixed venous oxygen saturation is raised by the admixture of blood which has been diverted from the metabolizing tissues, and it may be presumed that even in these patients the delivery of oxygen to the latter is reduced despite the normal or even elevated mixed venous oxygen saturation. When heart failure occurs in such patients, the arterial–mixed venous oxygen difference, regardless of the absolute value, still exceeds the level which existed prior to the development of heart failure, and therefore the cardiac output, though normal or elevated, is lower than before heart failure occurred.

The mechanisms responsible for the development of heart failure in patients whose cardiac outputs are initially high are complex and depend on the underlying disease process. In most of these conditions the heart is called upon to pump abnormally large quantities of blood in order to deliver the normal quota of oxygen to the metabolizing tissues. The burden placed on the myocardium by the increased flow load resembles that produced by regurgitant valvular lesions. In addition, thyrotoxicosis and beriberi may impair myocardial metabolism directly, while severe anemia may interfere with myocardial function by producing myocardial anoxia.

ACUTE VERSUS CHRONIC HEART FAILURE The prototype of acute heart failure develops in patients with large myocardial infarctions or valve rupture, while chronic heart failure is typically observed in patients with slowly progressive dilated cardiomyopathy or multivalvular heart disease. In acute failure, the sudden reduction in cardiac output often results in systemic hypotension without peripheral edema, while in chronic heart failure, arterial pressure tends to be well maintained, but there is accumulation of edema. Despite these differences in clinical presentation, there is no fundamental distinction between acute and chronic failure. For example, intensive efforts to prevent expansion of blood volume by means of dietary sodium restriction and the administration of diuretics will frequently delay the development of exertional dyspnea and edema in patients with chronic valvular heart disease, i.e., it will mask the clinical manifestations of chronic heart failure, until an acute episode, such as an arrhythmia or infection precipitates acute heart failure. Without intensive efforts to restrict blood volume the same patients would have been considered to have been suffering from chronic heart failure, even though their underlying myocardial disease was no further advanced.

RIGHT-SIDED VERSUS LEFT-SIDED HEART FAILURE Many of the clinical manifestations of heart failure result from the accumulation of excess fluid behind one or both ventricles (Chaps. 26 and 28). This fluid usually localizes upstream to the specific cardiac chamber which is initially affected. For example, patients in whom the left ventricle is mechanically overloaded (e.g., aortic stenosis) or weakened (e.g., postmyocardial infarction) develop dyspnea and orthopnea as a result of pulmonary congestion, a condition referred to as *left-sided heart failure*. In contrast, when the underlying abnormality affects the right ventricle primarily, e.g., valvular pulmonic stenosis or pulmonary hypertension secondary to pulmonary thromboembolism, symptoms resulting from pulmonary congestion such as orthopnea or paroxysmal nocturnal dyspnea are less common, and edema, congestive hepatomegaly, and systemic venous distention, i.e., clinical manifestations of *right-sided heart failure*, are more prominent. However, when heart failure has existed for months or years, such localization of excess fluid behind the failing ventricle may no longer exist. For example, patients with long-standing aortic valve disease or systemic hypertension may have ankle edema, congestive hepatomegaly, and systemic venous distention late in the course of their disease, even though the abnormal hemodynamic burden initially was placed on the left ventricle, in part because of the secondary pulmonary hypertension and resultant right-sided heart failure, but also because of the persistent retention of salt and water. It is also useful to recall that the muscle bundles composing both ventricles are continuous and both ventricles share a common wall, the interventricular septum. Also, biochemical changes which occur in heart failure and which may be involved in the impairment of myocardial function, such as norepinephrine depletion and alterations in the activity of myosin ATPase, occur in the myocardium of both ventricles, regardless of the specific chamber on which the abnormal hemodynamic burden is placed.

BACKWARD VERSUS FORWARD HEART FAILURE For many years a controversy has revolved around the question of the mechanism of the clinical manifestations resulting from heart failure. The concept of *backward heart failure*, propounded by James Hope in 1832, contends that when heart failure occurs, one or the other ventricle fails to discharge its contents normally, the end-diastolic volume of the ventricle rises, the pressures and volumes in the atrium and venous system behind the failing ventricle become elevated, and retention of sodium and water occurs as a consequence of the elevation of systemic venous and capillary pressures and the resultant transudation of fluid into the interstitial space (Chap. 28). In contrast, the proponents of the *forward heart failure* hypothesis, expounded by MacKenzie in 1913, maintain that the clinical manifestations of heart failure result directly from an inadequate discharge of blood into the arterial system. Salt and water retention, then, is a consequence of diminished renal perfusion and excessive proximal tubular sodium reabsorption and of excessive distal tubular reabsorption, through activation of the renin-angiotensin-aldosterone system.

A rigid distinction between *backward* and *forward heart failure* is artificial, since both mechanisms appear to operate to varying extents in most patients with heart failure. However, the rate of onset of heart failure often influences the clinical manifestations. For example, when a large portion of the left ventricle is suddenly destroyed, as in myocardial infarction, acute pulmonary edema may develop rapidly, and although stroke volume is reduced, the patient may die of acute pulmonary edema, a manifestation of backward failure, before the reduced cardiac output can be responsible for the renal retention of salt and water. However, if the patient survives the acute insult, clinical manifestations resulting from the abnormal retention of fluid within the systemic vascular bed might develop. Similarly, the right ventricle may dilate and the systemic venous pressure may rise to high levels immediately following acute massive pulmonary embolism, but this state may have to be maintained for some days before sodium and water retention sufficient to produce peripheral edema occurs.

SYSTOLIC VERSUS DIASTOLIC FAILURE The distinction between these two forms of heart failure, described on page 903 and in Fig. 181–7, relates to whether the principal abnormality is the inability to expel sufficient blood (systolic failure) or to relax and fill normally (diastolic failure). The major clinical manifestations of systolic failure relate to an inadequate cardiac output with weakness, fatigue, and other symptoms of hypoperfusion, while in diastolic failure they relate principally to an elevation of filling pressures. In many patients, particularly those who have both ventricular hypertrophy *and* dilatation, abnormalities both of contraction and relaxation coexist.

REDISTRIBUTION OF CARDIAC OUTPUT The redistribution of cardiac output also serves as an important compensatory mechanism when flow is reduced. This redistribution is most marked when a patient with heart failure exercises, but as heart failure advances, redistribution occurs even in the basal state. Blood flow is redistributed so that the delivery of oxygen to vital organs, such as the brain and myocardium, is maintained at normal or near-normal levels, while flow to less critical areas, such as the cutaneous and muscular beds and splanchnic viscera, is reduced. Vasoconstriction mediated by the sympathetic nervous system is largely responsible for this redistribution, which in turn may be responsible for many of the clinical manifestations of heart failure, such as fluid accumulation (reduction of renal flow), low-grade fever (reduction of cutaneous flow), and fatigue (reduction of muscle flow).

SALT AND WATER RETENTION (See also Chap. 28)

When the volume of blood pumped by the left ventricle into the systemic vascular bed is chronically reduced, and when one or both ventricles fail to expel the normal fraction of their end-diastolic volumes, a complex sequence of adjustments occurs which ultimately results in the abnormal accumulation of fluid. Though, on the one hand, many of the clinical manifestations of heart failure are secondary to this excessive retention of fluid, on the other hand, this abnormal fluid accumulation and the expansion of blood volume which accompanies it also constitute an important compensatory mechanism which tends to maintain cardiac output and therefore perfusion of the vital organs. Except in the terminal stages of heart failure, the ventricle operates on an ascending, albeit depressed and flattened function curve (Fig. 181-6), and the augmented ventricular end-diastolic volume and pressure characteristic of heart failure must be regarded as aiding the maintenance of cardiac output, despite causing pulmonary and systemic venous congestion.

In the presence of heart failure, effective filling of the systemic arterial tree is reduced, a condition which initiates the complex hemodynamic, renal, and hormonal adjustments that interact to promote reduced renal sodium and water excretion. Patients with severe heart failure may exhibit a reduced capacity to excrete a water load, which may result in dilutional hyponatremia. These abnormalities may be caused, in part, by excess antidiuretic hormone activity and/or factors that prevent sodium reabsorption in the distal tubule, such as avid proximal tubular reabsorption of sodium or the action of a diuretic acting on the distal tubule.

The importance of elevated systemic venous pressure and of the alterations of renal and adrenal function characteristic of heart failure vary in their relative importance in the production of edema in different patients with heart failure. The renin-angiotensin-aldosterone axis is activated most intensely by acute heart failure, and its activity tends to decline as heart failure becomes chronic. In patients with tricuspid valve disease or constrictive pericarditis the elevated venous pressure and the transudation of fluid from systemic capillaries appear to play the dominant role in edema formation. On the other hand, severe edema may be present in patients with ischemic or hypertensive heart disease, in whom systemic venous pressure is within normal limits or is only minimally elevated. In such patients, the retention of salt and water is probably due primarily to a redistribution of cardiac output and a concomitant reduction in renal perfusion, as well as activation of the renin-angiotensin-aldosterone axis. Regardless of the mechanisms involved in fluid retention, untreated patients with chronic congestive heart failure have elevations of total blood volume, interstitial fluid volume, and body sodium. These abnormalities diminish after clinical compensation has been achieved by treatment.

CLINICAL MANIFESTATIONS OF HEART FAILURE

Dyspnea Respiratory distress which occurs as the result of increased effort in breathing is the most common symptom of heart failure (Chap. 26). In early heart failure, dyspnea is observed only during activity, when it may simply represent an aggravation of the breathlessness which normally occurs under these circumstances. As heart failure advances, however, it appears with progressively less strenuous activity. Ultimately, breathlessness is present even when the patient is at rest. The principal difference between exertional dyspnea in normal persons and in cardiac patients is the degree of activity necessary to induce the symptom. Cardiac dyspnea is observed most frequently in patients with elevations of pulmonary venous and capillary pressures. Such patients have engorged pulmonary vessels and interstitial pulmonary edema, which reduces the compliance of the lungs and thereby increases the work of the respiratory muscles required to inflate the lungs. The activation of receptors in the lungs results in the rapid, shallow breathing of cardiac dyspnea. The oxygen cost of breathing is increased by the excessive work of the respiratory muscles. This is coupled with the diminished delivery of oxygen to these muscles, which occurs as a consequence of the reduced cardiac output, and which may contribute to fatigue of the respiratory muscles and the sensation of shortness of breath.

Orthopnea Dyspnea in the recumbent position occurs in part because of the redistribution of fluid from the abdomen and lower extremities into the chest causing an increase in the pulmonary capillary hydrostatic pressure. Patients with orthopnea generally elevate their heads on several pillows at night and frequently awaken short of breath if their heads slip off the pillows. The sensation of breathlessness usually is relieved by sitting bolt upright, since this position reduces venous return and pulmonary capillary pressure, and many patients report that they find relief from sitting in front of an open window. As heart failure advances, orthopnea may be so severe that patients cannot lie down at all and must spend the entire night in a sitting position. On the other hand, in other patients with long-standing, severe left ventricular failure, symptoms of pulmonary congestion may actually diminish with time as the function of the right ventricle becomes impaired.

Paroxysmal (nocturnal) dyspnea This term refers to attacks of severe shortness of breath which generally occur at night and usually awaken the patient from sleep. Though simple orthopnea may be relieved by sitting upright at the side of the bed with legs dependent, in the patient with paroxysmal nocturnal dyspnea coughing and wheezing often persist even in this position. The depression of the respiratory center during sleep may reduce ventilation sufficiently to lower arterial oxygen tension, particularly in patients with interstitial lung edema and reduced pulmonary compliance. Also, ventricular function may be further impaired at night because of reduced adrenergic stimulation of myocardial function. Acute pulmonary edema (Chap. 26) is a severe form of cardiac asthma due to further elevation of pulmonary capillary pressure leading to alveolar edema, associated with extreme shortness of breath, rales over the lung fields, and the transudation and expectoration of blood-tinged fluid. If not treated promptly acute pulmonary edema may be fatal.

Cheyne-Stokes respiration Also known as *periodic* or *cyclic respiration,* Cheyne-Stokes respiration is characterized by diminished sensitivity of the respiratory center. There is an apneic phase, during which the arterial P_{O_2} falls and the arterial P_{CO_2} rises. These changes in the arterial blood stimulate the depressed respiratory center, resulting in hyperventilation and hypocapnia, followed in turn by apnea. Cheyne-Stokes respiration occurs most often in patients with cerebral atherosclerosis and other cerebral lesions, but the prolongation of the circulation time from the lung to the brain which occurs in heart failure, particularly in patients with hypertension and coronary artery disease and associated cerebral vascular disease, also appears to precipitate this form of breathing.

Fatigue and weakness These nonspecific but common symptoms of heart failure are related to the reduction of perfusion of skeletal muscle. Anorexia and nausea associated with abdominal pain and fullness are frequent complaints which may be related to the congested liver and portal venous system.

Cerebral symptoms In severe heart failure, particularly in elderly patients with accompanying cerebral arteriosclerosis, arterial hypoxemia, and reduced cerebral perfusion, there may be alterations in the mental state characterized by confusion, difficulty in concentration, impairment of memory, headache, insomnia, and anxiety.

PHYSICAL FINDINGS In moderate heart failure the patient appears to be in no distress at rest except that it may be uncomfortable to lie flat for more than a few minutes. In more severe heart failure the pulse pressure may be diminished, reflecting a reduction in stroke volume, and occasionally the diastolic arterial pressure may be elevated as a consequence of generalized vasoconstriction. There may be cyanosis of the lips and nail bed and sinus tachycardia. *Systemic venous pressure* is often abnormally elevated in heart failure and may be recognized most readily by observing the extent of distention of the jugular veins. In the early stages of heart failure the venous pressure may be normal at rest but may become abnormally elevated during and immediately after exertion as well as with sustained pressure on the abdomen (positive abdominojugular reflux).

Third and fourth heart sounds (Chap. 177) are often audible but are not specific for heart failure, and *pulsus alternans,* i.e., a regular rhythm in which there is alternation of strong and weak cardiac contractions and therefore alternation in the strength of the peripheral pulses, may be present. Pulsus alternans may be detected by sphygmomanometry and in more severe instances by palpation; it frequently follows an extrasystole and is observed most commonly in patients with cardiomyopathy or with hypertensive or ischemic heart disease. It is caused by a reduction in the number of contractile units during weak contractions and/or by alternation in the ventricular end-diastolic volume.

Basal pulmonary rales Moist, inspiratory, crepitant rales and dullness to percussion over the posterior lung bases are common in patients with heart failure and elevated pulmonary venous and capillary pressures. In patients with pulmonary edema, rales may be heard widely over both lung fields; they are frequently coarse and sibilant and may be accompanied by expiratory wheezing. Rales may, however, be caused by many conditions other than left ventricular failure.

Cardiac edema Cardiac edema is usually dependent, occurring in the legs symmetrically, particularly in the pretibial region and ankles in ambulatory patients, and in the sacral region of individuals at bed rest. Pitting edema of the arms and face occurs rarely and only late in the course of heart failure.

Hydrothorax and ascites Pleural effusion in congestive heart failure results from the elevation of pleural capillary pressure and transudation of fluid into the pleural cavities. Since the pleural veins drain into both the systemic and pulmonary veins, hydrothorax occurs most commonly with marked elevation of pressure in both venous systems, but may also be seen with marked elevation of pressure in either venous bed. It is more frequent in the right pleural cavity than the left. *Ascites* also occurs as a consequence of transudation and results from increased pressure in the hepatic veins and the veins draining the peritoneum (Chap. 39). Marked ascites occurs most frequently in patients with tricuspid valve disease and with constrictive pericarditis.

Congestive hepatomegaly An enlarged, tender, pulsating liver also accompanies systemic venous hypertension and is observed not only in the same conditions in which ascites occurs, but also in milder forms of heart failure from any cause. With prolonged, severe hepatomegaly, as in patients with tricuspid valve disease or chronic constrictive pericarditis, enlargement of the spleen may also occur.

Jaundice This is a late finding in congestive heart failure and is associated with elevations of both the direct- and indirect-reacting bilirubin levels; it results from impairment of hepatic function secondary to hepatic congestion and the hepatocellular hypoxia associated with central lobular atrophy. Serum enzyme concentrations, particularly SGOT and SGPT, are frequently elevated. If hepatic congestion occurs acutely, the jaundice may be severe and the enzymes strikingly raised.

Cardiac cachexia With severe chronic heart failure there may be serious weight loss and cachexia because of (1) elevation of the metabolic rate, which results in part from the extra work performed by the respiratory muscles, the increased oxygen needs of the hypertrophied heart, and the discomfort associated with severe heart failure; (2) anorexia, nausea, and vomiting due to central causes, to digitalis intoxication, or to congestive hepatomegaly and abdominal fullness; (3) some impairment of intestinal absorption due to congestion of the intestinal veins; and (4) rarely, in patients with particularly severe failure of the right side of the heart, a protein-losing enteropathy.

Other manifestations With reduction of blood flow the extremities may be cold, pale, and diaphoretic. Urine flow is depressed, and the urine contains protein and has a high specific gravity and a low concentration of sodium. In addition, prerenal azotemia may be present. In patients with long-standing severe heart failure impotence and depression are common.

ROENTGENOGRAPHIC FINDINGS In addition to the enlargement of the particular chambers characteristic of the lesion responsible for heart failure, vascular changes in the lung fields are common in patients with heart failure and elevated pulmonary vascular pressures (Chap. 179). Also, pleural effusions may be present and associated with interlobar effusions.

DIFFERENTIAL DIAGNOSIS The diagnosis of congestive heart failure may be established by observing some combination of the clinical manifestations of heart failure, enumerated above, together with the findings characteristic of one of the etiologic forms of heart disease. Since chronic heart failure is often associated with cardiac enlargement, the diagnosis should be questioned, but is by no means excluded, when all chambers are normal in size. Heart failure may be difficult to distinguish from pulmonary disease, and the differential diagnosis is discussed in Chap. 26. Pulmonary embolism also presents many of the manifestations of heart failure, but hemoptysis, pleuritic chest pain, a right ventricular lift, and the characteristic mismatch between ventilation and perfusion on lung scan should point to this diagnosis (Chap. 211).

Ankle edema may be due to varicose veins, cyclic edema, or gravitational effects (Chap. 28), but in these patients there is no jugular venous hypertension at rest or with pressure over the abdomen. Edema secondary to renal disease can usually be recognized by appropriate renal function tests and urinalysis and is rarely associated with elevation of the venous pressure. Enlargement of the liver and ascites occur in patients with hepatic cirrhosis, but may also be distinguished from heart failure by normal jugular venous pressure and absence of a positive abdominojugular reflux.

TREATMENT OF HEART FAILURE

The treatment of heart failure may be divided into three components: (1) removal of the precipitating cause, (2) correction of the underlying cause, and (3) control of the congestive heart failure state. The first two are discussed together in subsequent chapters with each specific disease entity or complication. In many instances surgical treatment will correct or at least improve the underlying cause. The third component of the treatment of heart failure may, in turn, also be divided into three categories: (1) reduction of cardiac work load, including afterload; (2) control of excessive salt and water retention; and (3) enhancement of myocardial contractility. The vigor with which each of these measures is pursued in any individual patient should depend upon the severity of the heart failure state. Following effective treatment, recurrence of the clinical manifestations of heart failure can often be prevented by continuing those measures that were originally effective. While a simple rule for the treatment of all patients with heart failure cannot be formulated because of the varied etiologies, hemodynamic features, and clinical manifestations of heart failure, insofar as the treatment of chronic congestive failure is concerned, simple measures such as moderate restriction of activity and sodium intake should be tried first. If these are insufficient, therapy with a thiazide and/or a glycoside is then begun. The next step is more rigorous restriction of salt intake and a loop diuretic in place of the thiazide. If heart failure persists, then a vasodilator is added. Hospitalization with rigid salt restriction, bed rest, intravenous vasodilators, and positive inotropic agents comes next. In some patients the order in which these measures are applied may be altered.

REDUCTION OF CARDIAC WORK LOAD This consists of reducing physical activity, instituting emotional rest, and reducing afterload. The latter is generally instituted *after* the use of diuretics and cardiac glycosides. Modest restriction of physical activity in mild cases and rest in bed or in a chair in severe failure remain cornerstones in the treatment of heart failure. Meals should be small in quantity, and every effort should be made to diminish the patient's anxiety. Physical and emotional rest tend to lower arterial pressure, and reduce the load on the myocardium by diminishing the requirements for cardiac output. These influences act in concert to diminish the need for redistribution of the cardiac output, and in many patients, particularly those with mild heart failure, simple bed rest and mild sedation often result in an effective diuresis.

Rest at home or in the hospital should be maintained for 1 to 2 weeks in patients with overt congestive failure and should be continued for several days after the patient's condition has stabilized. The hazards of phlebothrombosis and pulmonary embolism which occur with bed rest may be reduced with anticoagulants, leg exercises, and elastic stockings. In any event, absolute bed rest rarely is required, and the patient should be encouraged to sit in a chair and be given toilet privileges unless heart failure is extreme. Heavy sedation should be avoided, but small doses of tranquilizers may be helpful in calming the emotionally disturbed patient through the first few days of therapy and in permitting much-needed sleep. In patients with chronic, mild heart failure, bed rest on weekends will frequently allow continuation of gainful employment. Following recovery from heart failure, the patient's activities must be carefully assessed, and often his or her professional, family, and/or community responsibilities must be reduced. Intermittent rest during the day and the avoidance of strenuous exertion are often helpful once compensation has been restored. Weight reduction by restriction of caloric intake in the obese patient with heart failure also diminishes cardiac work load and is an essential component of the therapeutic program.

ENHANCEMENT OF MYOCARDIAL CONTRACTILITY—DIGITALIS The improvement of myocardial contractility by means of cardiac glycosides is the second of the cornerstones in the control of heart failure. The basic molecular structure of the digitalis glycosides is a steroid nucleus to which an unsaturated lactone ring is attached at C-17. These two elements together are called *aglycone* or *genin,* and it is this portion of the molecule which is responsible for the cardiotonic activity. The addition of sugar residues to this basic structure determines water solubility and pharmacokinetic properties for individual glycosides.

Pharmacokinetics In the absence of severe malabsorption, most digitalis glycosides are adequately absorbed from the intestinal tract even in the presence of vascular congestion secondary to heart failure. Oral absorption is close to complete within 2 h. The bioavailability (i.e., percent of intravenous dose) of orally administered glycoside varies. Considerable variability of bioavailability has been found in different commercial preparations of digoxin. The bioavailability of Lanoxin elixir is 70 to 85 percent, Lanoxin tablets 60 to 80 percent, and Lanoxicaps 90 to 100 percent. Digitoxin tablets have a bioavailability of virtually 100 percent. Cholesterol-lowering resins, antidiarrheal agents containing pectin and kaolin, nonabsorbable antacids, and neomycin can reduce the absorption of digoxin and digitoxin. Varying degrees of protein-binding of glycosides occur in the bloodstream (for example, 97 percent for digitoxin and 25 percent for digoxin), and though these differences may account in part for the varying durations of the effect of different glycosides, they are not related to the speed of action of these drugs. The plasma contains only approximately 1 percent of the body stores of digoxin; therefore, digoxin is not effectively removed from the body by dialysis, exchange transfusions, or during cardiopulmonary bypass, presumably because of tissue binding. The major fraction of the glycosides is directly bound by various tissues including the heart, in which the concentration is approximately 30 times that in the plasma for digoxin and 7 times for digitoxin; the latter is less polar and more lipid-soluble than digoxin.

Digoxin, which has a half-life of 1.6 days, is filtered in the glomeruli and secreted by the renal tubules; 85 percent is excreted in the urine, most in unchanged form; only 10 to 15 percent of digoxin is eliminated in the stool through biliary excretion in the presence of normal renal function. The ratio of digoxin clearance to endogenous creatinine clearance is 0.8, and the percentage of the body's total stores of digoxin lost per day can be calculated as $(14 \pm 0.2) \times$ creatinine clearance in milliliters per minute. In patients with normal renal function a plateau concentration in the blood and tissue is reached after 5 days of daily maintenance treatment without a loading dose (Fig. 64-2). Therefore, significant reductions of the glomerular filtration rate reduce the elimination of digoxin (but not of digitoxin) and, therefore, may prolong digoxin's effect, allowing it to accumulate to toxic levels if it is administered as in patients with normal renal function. The administration of most diuretics does not alter the excretion of digoxin significantly, but spironolactone can inhibit tubular secretion of digoxin, resulting in significant accumulation of the drug. Serum levels and pharmacokinetics are essentially unchanged by massive weight loss. In about 10 percent of patients receiving digoxin, large amounts of digoxin reduction products are formed by bacterial flora in the gastrointestinal tract. Antibiotic therapy that alters gut flora reverses this tendency to metabolize digoxin to cardioinactive products and can result in striking alterations in the state of digitalization. *Digitoxin,* with a half-life of approximately 5 days, is metabolized chiefly in the liver; only 15 percent is excreted in the urine unchanged and an equal fraction in the stool. Drugs such as phenobarbital and phenylbutazone that increase the activity of hepatic microsomal enzymes accelerate the metabolism of digitoxin. To reach a steady state, digitoxin requires maintenance doses for 3 to 4 weeks. *Ouabain* is very rapidly acting, exhibiting an onset of action in 5 to 10 min and a peak effect within 60 min following intravenous injection. It is poorly absorbed from the gastrointestinal tract and, therefore, is not suitable for oral use; it is excreted by the kidneys, has a half-life of 21 h, and is useful in emergencies.

Mechanism of action The cardiac actions of all digitalis glycosides are alike. The clinical effects result from augmenting contractility and from slowing heart rate and atrioventricular conduction.

The most important effect of digitalis on cardiac muscle is to shift its force-velocity relation upward (Chap. 181). This positive inotropic effect is exhibited in normal, nonfailing hypertrophied as well as in failing hearts. In the absence of heart failure, however, when cardiac output is not limited by cardiac contractility, the drug does not elevate the output. The finding that digitalis increases the contractility of the nonfailing heart has led to its use (1) in patients with heart disease but without heart failure prior to operation or other stressful situations such as serious infections, and (2) in the presence of a chronically increased load, such as hypertension without heart failure. However, definitive evidence of its efficacy in these circumstances is not available.

Excitation-contraction coupling is the membrane and intracellular process most likely involved in producing the positive inotropic effect of digitalis glycosides. These drugs inhibit transmembrane sodium and potassium movement by inhibition of the monovalent cation transport enzyme–coupled Na^+,K^+-ATPase. The latter, localized to the sarcolemma, appears to be the receptor for cardioactive glycosides whose action results in an increase in intracellular sodium content, and this in turn increases intracellular calcium concentration through a Na^+-Ca^{2+} exchange carrier mechanism. The increased myocardial uptake of calcium augments calcium released to the myofilaments during excitation and, therefore, invokes a positive inotropic response. There is a correlation between the degree of enzyme inhibition and the inotropic potency of the glycoside.

Cardiac glycosides also produce alterations in the electrical properties of both the contractile cells and the specialized automatic cells. While low concentrations of glycosides produce little effect on the action potential, high concentrations result in a reduction in the resting potential (phase 4, see Fig. 183-1, p. 916) and an augmented rate of diastolic depolarization. The reduction in the resting potential brings the cell closer to the threshold for depolarization. These two effects lead to increased automaticity and ectopic impulse activity. With the lowering of the resting potential, the rate of rise of the action potential is reduced, resulting in a slowing of conduction velocity, which is conducive to the development of reentry. Thus, the known electrophysiologic effects of digitalis glycosides are capable of explaining the development of both reentry and ectopic foci and the resultant arrhythmias associated with digitalis intoxication.

The glycosides also prolong the effective *refractory period* of the atrioventricular node, largely as a result of an enhanced vagal effect. Digitalis also shortens the refractory period of the atrial and ventricular muscle. Small action potentials are propagated in a decremental fashion in the atrioventricular junction. Most do not reach the ventricles but leave some of the atrioventricular junctional cells in a refractory state. This helps to explain the slowing of ventricular rate produced by digitalis in supraventricular tachycardias. In atrial fibrillation, the slowing of ventricular rate is explained by prolongation of the effective refractory period of the atrioventricular node and increased concealed conduction with fewer impulses penetrating the atrioventricular junction owing to both vagal and possibly direct effects of glycosides on junctional tissue.

Digitalis exerts a clinically significant negative chronotropic action, usually only in the setting of ventricular failure. In heart failure, slowing of the sinus rate following the administration of digitalis results also from withdrawal of sympathetic activity secondary to general improvement in circulatory status due to the positive inotropic effect of the glycoside. In the nonfailing heart the slowing effect is negligible, and digitalis should not be used for the treatment of sinus tachycardia unless heart failure is present. The apparent suppression of pacemaker activity which may take place following large doses of digitalis is probably due not to arrest of the pacemaker but rather to a sinoatrial block related to a depression of conduction of impulses out of the sinus node.

In addition, the digitalis glycosides also exert an action on the peripheral vasculature, causing venous and arterial constriction in normal individuals and reflex dilatation resulting from withdrawal of sympathetic constrictor activity in patients with congestive heart failure.

Use in heart failure By stimulating the contractile function of the heart, digitalis improves ventricular emptying; i.e., it augments the ejection fraction, increases cardiac output, promotes diuresis, and reduces the elevated diastolic pressure and volume and end-systolic volume of the failing ventricle with consequent reduction of symptoms resulting from pulmonary vascular congestion and elevated systemic venous pressure. It is most beneficial in patients in whom ventricular contractility is impaired secondary to chronic ischemic heart disease, or when hypertensive, valvular, or congenital heart disease imposes an excessive volume or pressure load. It is helpful in slowing the rapid ventricular rate of patients with atrial flutter and fibrillation. It is of relatively little value in most forms of cardiomyopathy, myocarditis, beriberi with heart failure, mitral stenosis, thyrotoxicosis and sinus rhythm, cor pulmonale when the lung disease is not being treated concurrently (Chap. 191), and chronic constrictive pericarditis (Chap. 194). Nonetheless, when used in proper doses, it is not contraindicated in these disorders and is frequently used since it may exert a beneficial effect, albeit not a striking one.

Digitalis intoxication Although digitalis is one of the cornerstones of the treatment for heart failure, it is a two-edged sword, because intoxication due to digitalis excess is a common, serious, and potentially fatal complication of its use. The therapeutic-to-toxic ratios are identical for all cardiac glycosides. In most patients with heart failure the lethal dose of most glycosides is probably 5 to 10 times the minimal effective dose and only about twice the dose which leads to minor toxic manifestations. In addition, old age, acute myocardial infarction or ischemia, hypoxemia, magnesium depletion, renal insufficiency, hypercalcemia, electrical cardioversion, and hypothyroidism all may reduce the tolerance of the patient to the digitalis glycosides or provoke latent digitalis intoxication. The most common precipitating cause of digitalis intoxication, however, is depletion of potassium stores, which often occurs as a result of diuretic therapy and secondary hyperaldosteronism. Since it is not necessary for a patient to receive a maximally tolerated dose of digitalis to derive a beneficial effect, even small doses provide some therapeutic action; this point should be considered if these drugs are to be used in patients prone to toxicity.

Anorexia, nausea, and vomiting, which are among the earliest signs of digitalis intoxication, are caused by direct stimulation of centers in the medulla and are not of gastrointestinal origin. The most frequent disturbance of cardiac rhythm caused by digitalis is premature ventricular beats, which may take the form of bigeminy because of increased myocardial irritability or facilitation of reentry. Atrioventricular block of varying degrees of severity may occur. Nonparoxysmal atrial tachycardia with variable atrioventricular block is quite characteristic of digitalis intoxication. Sinus arrhythmia, sinoatrial block, sinus arrest, and atrioventricular junctional and multifocal ventricular tachycardia may also occur. These arrhythmias are due to action of the glycoside both on cardiac tissues and on the central nervous system. Chronic digitalis intoxication may be insidious in onset and characterized by exacerbations of heart failure, weight loss, cachexia, neuralgias, gynecomastia, yellow vision, and delirium. Digitalis-toxic cardiac arrhythmias precede extracardiac (gastrointestinal or central nervous system) toxicity in about one-half of cases.

Digitalis intoxication has been reported to occur in as many as 20 percent of hospitalized patients receiving a cardiac glycoside, which emphasizes the importance of the ability to diagnose this condition. The administration of quinidine to patients receiving digoxin raises the serum concentration of the latter by reducing both the renal and nonrenal elimination of digoxin and by reducing its volume of distribution and thereby increasing the propensity to digitalis intoxication. The calcium channel antagonist verapamil and the experimental antiarrhythmic agent amiodarone also appear to raise serum digoxin levels. Therefore, serum digoxin concentrations and electrocardiograms should be followed carefully when these drugs are administered to digitalized patients. The radioimmunoassays for digoxin and digitoxin make possible the correlation of serum glycoside levels with the presence of toxicity. In patients receiving standard maintenance doses of digoxin and digitoxin and in whom no sign of intoxication is present, serum concentrations approximate 1 to 1.5 and 20 to 25 ng/mL, respectively. When signs of intoxication are present, serum levels of more than 2 and 30 ng/mL, respectively, of these glycosides are often found. Since many factors other than the serum concentration determine digitalis intoxication, and since there is overlap in serum glycoside concentrations in patients with and without toxicity, it is clear that these levels cannot be used as a sole guide to digitalis dosage. However, when taken together with findings on the clinical examination and electrocardiogram, they add useful information to the clinical evaluations of digitalis intoxication. In addition they will indicate whether a patient for whom the history of digitalis intake is in doubt has, in fact, been receiving the drug.

Treatment of digitalis intoxication When tachyarrhythmias result from digitalis intoxication, withdrawal of the drug and treatment with potassium, phenytoin, propranolol, or lidocaine are indicated. Potassium should be administered cautiously and by the oral route whenever possible if hypokalemia is present, but small doses may also be helpful when serum potassium levels are normal; *potassium must not be employed in the presence of atrioventricular block or hyperkalemia.* Propranolol should not be used to treat digitalis toxicity in the presence of severe heart failure or atrioventricular block but may be useful otherwise; lidocaine is effective in the treatment of digitalis-induced ventricular tachyarrhythmias in the absence of preceding atrioventricular block. A cardiac pacemaker may be required in digitalis-induced atrioventricular block. Electrical conversion may not only be ineffective in treating these arrhythmias but may induce more serious arrhythmias. However, it may be lifesaving in digitalis-induced ventricular fibrillation. Quinidine and procainamide are of only limited value in the treatment of digitalis intoxication. Fab fragments of purified, intact digitalis antibodies represent a potentially lifesaving approach to the treatment of severe intoxication.

SYMPATHOMIMETIC AMINES (See also Chap. 66) Four sympathomimetic amines which act largely on beta-adrenergic receptors—epinephrine, isoproterenol, dopamine, and dobutamine—improve myocardial contractility in various forms of heart failure. The latter two agents appear to be most effective; they must be administered by constant intravenous infusion and are useful in patients with intractable heart failure, particularly in those with a reversible component, such as exists in patients who have undergone cardiac surgery, and in some instances of myocardial infarction and shock or pulmonary edema. While they improve the hemodynamics in that condition, it is not clear that they improve survival. Their administration must be accompanied by careful and continuous monitoring of the electrocardiogram, intraarterial pressure, and if possible pulmonary artery wedge pressure, in an intensive care unit.

Dopamine, the naturally occurring immediate precursor of norepinephrine, has a combination of actions which make it particularly useful in the treatment of a variety of hypotensive states and congestive heart failure. At very low doses, that is, 1 to 2 (μg/kg)/min, it dilates renal and mesenteric blood vessels through stimulation of specific dopaminergic receptors, thereby augmenting renal and mesenteric blood flow and sodium excretion. In the range of 2 to 10 (μg/kg)/min, dopamine stimulates myocardial beta receptors but induces relatively little tachycardia, while at higher doses it also stimulates alpha-adrenergic receptors and elevates arterial pressure.

Dobutamine is a synthetic catecholamine which acts on $beta_1$, $beta_2$, and alpha receptors. It exerts a potent inotropic action, has only a modest cardioaccelerating effect, and lowers peripheral vascular resistance, but since it raises cardiac output, it has little effect on systemic arterial pressure. Dobutamine, given in continuous infusions of 2.5 to 10 (μg/kg)/min, is useful in the treatment of acute heart failure without hypotension. Like the other sympathomimetic amines it may be particularly valuable in the management of patients requiring relatively short-term inotropic support—up to 1 week—in conditions which are reversible, such as the cardiac depression which sometimes follows open-heart surgery, or in patients with acute heart failure who are being prepared for operation. Adverse effects include sinus tachycardia, tachyarrhythmias, and hypertension.

A major problem with all sympathomimetics is the loss of responsiveness, apparently due to "downregulation" of adrenergic receptors, which becomes evident within 8 h of continuous administration.

Amrinone This bipyridine, a noncatecholamine, nonglycoside exerts both positive inotropic and vasodilator actions by inhibiting a specific phosphodiesterase. It is suitable for intravenous use only, and by simultaneously stimulating cardiac contractility and dilating the systemic vascular bed it reverses the major hemodynamic abnormalities associated with heart failure. Milrinone, a derivative of amrinone, and several other active phosphodiesterases are under active investigation for chronic oral administration.

CONTROL OF EXCESSIVE FLUID RETENTION Many of the clinical manifestations of heart failure result from hypervolemia and expansion of the interstitial fluid volume. By the time fluid retention due to heart failure first becomes clinically evident, considerable expansion of the extracellular space has already occurred, and heart failure usually is already advanced. Treatment aimed at reducing extracellular fluid volume is dependent primarily on lowering total body sodium stores, while fluid restriction is of less importance. A negative sodium balance can be achieved by reducing the dietary intake and increasing the urinary excretion of this ion with the aid of diuretics. In severe heart failure mechanical removal of extracellular fluid by means of thoracentesis, paracentesis, and rarely hemodialysis or peritoneal dialysis may also be employed.

Diet In patients with mild heart failure, considerable improvement in symptoms may result from simply reducing the sodium intake, particularly if accompanied by periods of rest. In patients with more severe heart failure the sodium intake must be controlled more rigidly, and other measures, such as diuretics and glycosides, are used. Even following recovery from a bout of heart failure, at least moderate sodium restriction should be maintained. The normal diet contains approximately 6 to 10 g sodium chloride; this intake can be reduced by half simply by excluding salt-rich foods and salt which is added at the table. Reduction of the ordinary dietary intake to approximately one-fourth of normal may be achieved if, in addition, all salt is omitted from cooking. In patients with severe heart failure, in whom the daily sodium chloride intake should be reduced to between 500 and 1000 mg, milk, cheese, bread, cereals, canned vegetables and soups, some salted cuts of meat, and some fresh vegetables, including spinach, celery, and beets, must be eliminated. A variety of fresh fruit, green vegetables, specially processed breads and milk, and salt substitutes are permissible, but such diets are difficult to keep palatable. Water intake may be ad libitum in all but the most severe forms of congestive heart failure. However, late in the course of heart failure, dilutional hyponatremia may develop in patients who are unable to excrete a water load, sometimes because of excessive secretion of antidiuretic hormone. In such cases water intake as well as sodium intake must be restricted.

Attention must also be directed to the caloric content of the diet. Substantial improvement can result from caloric restriction in obese patients with heart failure, in whom weight loss will reduce the load placed on the myocardium. On the other hand, in individuals with severe heart failure and cardiac cachexia, an attempt must be made to maintain nutritional intake and to avoid caloric and vitamin deficiencies.

Diuretics A variety of diuretic agents is available, and in patients with mild heart failure almost all are effective. However, in the more severe forms of heart failure, the selection of diuretics is more difficult, and any existing abnormalities in serum electrolytes must be taken into account. Overtreatment must be avoided, since the resultant hypovolemia may reduce cardiac output, interfere with renal function, and produce profound weakness and lethargy.

THIAZIDE DIURETICS These agents are widely used in clinical practice because of their effectiveness when administered orally. In patients with chronic heart failure of mild or moderate severity the continued administration of chlorothiazide or one of its many analogues abolishes or diminishes the need for very rigid dietary sodium restriction, although salty foods and table salt should still be avoided. Thiazides are well absorbed following oral administration; chlorothiazide and hydrochlorothiazide reach their peak action in 4 h, and diuresis persists for approximately 12 h. Thiazide diuretics reduce the reabsorption of sodium and chloride in the first half of the distal convoluted tubule and a portion of the cortical ascending limb of the loop of Henle, and water follows the unreabsorbed salt. Thiazides fail to increase free water clearance, and in some instances reduce it, supporting the hypothesis that these drugs inhibit selective sodium chloride reabsorption in the distal cortical diluting segment, at a site where the urine is normally diluted (Chap. 218). This may result in the excretion of a hypertonic urine and may contribute to dilutional hyponatremia. As a consequence of increased delivery of sodium to the distal nephron, sodium-potassium ion exchange is enhanced and kaliuresis results. The weak carbonic anhydrase–inhibiting properties of the thiazides are of limited importance and need not be invoked to account for most of the diuretic action. In contrast to the loop diuretics which enhance calcium excretion, the thiazides have the opposite effect. These drugs are effective and useful in the treatment of heart failure as long as the glomerular filtration rate exceeds 50 percent of normal.

Chlorothiazide is administered in doses of up to 500 mg every 6 h. Many derivatives of this compound are available but differ principally in dosage and duration of action and therefore offer few, if any, significant advances over the parent compound, except for chlorthalidone which may be administered once daily. Potassium depletion and metabolic alkalosis (the latter due to increased H^+ secretion as a substitute for the depleted intracellular stores of potassium and increased proximal tubular reabsorption of filtered HCO_3^- when there is relative depletion of the extracellular fluid volume) are the chief adverse metabolic effects following prolonged administration of the thiazides (as well as of metolazone and of the loop diuretics), and may seriously enhance the dangers of digitalis intoxication and induce fatigue and lethargy. Hypokalemia may be prevented by the oral supplementation of potassium chloride. However, the solution is not palatable and may be hazardous in patients with renal failure. Therefore, to control potassium depletion, intermittent dosage schedules, e.g., omitting the diuretic every third day, and the addition of a potassium-retaining diuretic, such as a spironolactone or triamterene, may be preferable. Other side effects of thiazides include reduction of the excretion of uric acid, which may lead to hyperuricemia, and a hyperglycemic effect, which rarely may precipitate hyperosmolar coma in the poorly regulated diabetic. Skin rashes, thrombocytopenia, and granulocytopenia have also been reported.

METOLAZONE This quinethazone derivative has a site of action and potency similar to that of the thiazides, but has been reported to be effective in the presence of moderate renal failure. The usual dose is 5 to 10 mg/day.

FUROSEMIDE, BUMETANIDE, AND ETHACRYNIC ACID These "loop" diuretics are similar physiologically but differ chemically. These extremely powerful diuretics reversibly inhibit the reabsorption of sodium, potassium, and chloride in the thick ascending limb of Henle's loop, apparently by blocking a cotransport system in the luminal membrane. These agents may induce renal cortical vasodilatation and can produce rates of urine formation which may be as high as one-fourth of the glomerular filtration rate. While other diuretics lose their effectiveness as blood volume is restored to normal levels, the loop diuretics remain effective despite the elimination of excessive extracellular fluid volume. The major side effects of these agents are due to this marked diuretic potency, which on rare occasions may result in contraction of the plasma volume, circulatory collapse, reductions in the renal blood flow and glomerular filtration rate, and the development of prerenal azotemia. Metabolic alkalosis is produced by a large increase in the urinary excretion of chloride, hydrogen, and potassium ions. Hypokalemia (see discussion of thiazides, above) and hyponatremia may occur, and hyperuricemia and hyperglycemia are observed occasionally, as with thiazide diuretics. The reabsorption of free water is decreased.

All three drugs are readily absorbed orally and are excreted in the bile and urine. They are usually effective by mouth and intravenously. Weakness, nausea, and dizziness may complicate the administration of all three loop diuretics; ethacrynic acid has been associated with skin rash and granulocytopenia, as well as with transient or permanent deafness.

These extremely effective diuretics are useful in all forms of heart failure, particularly in otherwise refractory heart failure and pulmonary edema. They have been shown to be effective in patients with hypoalbuminemia, hyponatremia, hypochloremia, hypokalemia, and reductions in the glomerular filtration rate, and to produce a diuresis in patients in whom thiazide diuretics and aldosterone antagonists, alone and in combination, are ineffective.

In patients with refractory heart failure the action of furosemide, bumetanide, and ethacrynic acid may be potentiated by intravenous administration and the addition of thiazide diuretics, carbonic anhydrase inhibitors, osmotic diuretics, and the potassium-sparing diuretics—spironolactone, triamterene, and amiloride. These latter agents act on the cortical collecting ducts, are relatively weak, and therefore are rarely indicated as sole agents. However, their potassium-sparing properties make them particularly useful in conjunction with the more potent kaliuretic agents, the loop diuretics and thiazides. These agents fall into two classes, as noted below.

ALDOSTERONE ANTAGONISTS The 17-spironolactones resemble aldosterone structurally and act on the distal half of the convoluted tubule and the cortical portion of the collecting duct by competitive inhibition of aldosterone, thereby blocking the exchange between sodium and both potassium and hydrogen in the distal tubules and collecting ducts. These agents produce a sodium diuresis, and, in contrast to the thiazides, ethacrynic acid, and furosemide, they result in potassium retention. Although secondary hyperaldosteronism exists in some patients with congestive heart failure, the spironolactones are effective even in patients in whom the serum aldosterone concentration is within normal limits. Aldactone A may be administered in doses of 25 to 100 mg three to four times daily by mouth. The maximal effect of this regimen is not observed for approximately 4 days. Spironolactones are most effective when administered in combination with thiazide and loop diuretics. The opposing action of these drugs on urine and serum potassium makes possible a sodium diuresis without either hyper- or hypokalemia when spironolactone and one of these other agents are administered in combination. Also, since spironolactone (as well as triamterene and amiloride) acts on the distal tubule, it is particularly effective when used in combination with one of these other diuretics which acts more proximally.

Spironolactone should not be administered alone to patients with hyperkalemia, renal failure, or hyponatremia. Reported complications include nausea, epigastric distress, mental confusion, drowsiness, gynecomastia, and erythematous eruptions.

TRIAMTERENE AND AMILORIDE These two drugs exert renal effects similar to those of the spironolactones; i.e., they block sodium reabsorption and secondarily inhibit potassium secretion in the distal tubules. However, their fundamental mechanism of action differs from those of the spironolactones, since they are active in adrenalectomized animals and their action does not depend on the presence of aldosterone. The effective dose of triamterene is 100 mg once or twice daily and that of amiloride is 5 mg daily. Side effects include nausea, vomiting, diarrhea, headache, granulocytopenia, eosinophilia, and skin rash. Both triamterene and the chemically unrelated diuretic amiloride resemble Aldactone A in that their diuretic potency is not great, and they are effective in preventing the hypokalemia characteristic of the administration of thiazides, furosemide, and ethacrynic acid. A number of diuretic preparations contain a combination of a thiazide and either triamterene or amiloride in a single capsule. They may be useful in patients who develop hypokalemia with a thiazide but should not be used in patients with impaired renal function and/or hyperkalemia.

CHOICE OF DIURETICS Orally administered thiazides or metolazone are the agents of choice in the treatment of chronic cardiac edema of mild to moderate degree in patients without hyperglycemia, hyperuricemia, or hypokalemia. Spironolactones, triamterene, and amiloride are not potent diuretics when used alone, but they potentiate other diuretics, particularly the thiazides and loop diuretics. However, in patients with heart failure and severe secondary hyperaldosteronism, spironolactone may be quite effective. Ethacrynic acid, bumetanide, or furosemide, given alone or with spironolactone or triamterene, are the agents of choice in patients with severe heart failure refractory to other diuretics. In very severe heart failure the combination of a thiazide, a loop diuretic (ethacrynic acid or furosemide), and a potassium-sparing diuretic (spironolactone, triamterene, or amiloride) is required.

VASODILATOR THERAPY In many patients with heart failure, left ventricular afterload is increased as a consequence of the several neural and humoral influences which act to constrict the peripheral vascular bed. These include increased activity of the adrenergic nervous system, elevation of circulating catecholamines, and activation of the renin-angiotensin system, and perhaps of increased circulating antidiuretic hormone as well. In addition to the vasoconstriction, the ventricular end-diastolic volume rises and as a consequence of the operation of Laplace's law, which relates myocardial wall tension to the product of intraventricular pressure and radius, the aortic impedance, i.e., the force which opposes left ventricular ejection, or the ventricular afterload, rises. The maintenance or even the elevation of arterial pressure is generally considered to be a useful compensatory mechanism that allows blood flow to vital organs to persist in the presence of hypovolemia, despite inadequacy of the total cardiac output. While this is the case in many forms of shock (Chap. 29), when there is no preload reserve in the presence of severely impaired cardiac function, the increase in afterload may reduce cardiac output and elevate myocardial oxygen consumption further.

As shown in Fig. 181-5, afterload is a major determinant of cardiac function. When cardiac function is normal, a moderate elevation in afterload does not alter stroke volume, because the resultant increase in left ventricular end-diastolic volume, i.e., preload, can be tolerated easily. However, when myocardial function is impaired, such an increase in preload evoked by an elevation of afterload may raise ventricular end-diastolic and pulmonary capillary pressures to levels that may produce severe pulmonary congestion or pulmonary edema. In many patients with heart failure, the ventricle is already operating at the peak, flat portion of its Frank-Starling curve (Fig. 181-6), and any additional increase in aortic impedance (afterload) will reduce stroke volume (page 902). Conversely, a reduction of afterload will tend to restore hemodynamics to normal by elevating the stroke volume of the failing ventricle, and may reduce the elevated ventricular filling pressure.

The pharmacologic reduction of impedance to left ventricular ejection with vasodilator drugs represents an important adjunct in the management of heart failure. This approach may be particularly helpful in patients with acute heart failure due to myocardial infarction (Chap. 190), valvular regurgitation, elevated systemic vascular resistance and/or arterial pressure, and marked cardiac dilatation. The reduction of afterload by means of a variety of vasodilators reduces left ventricular end-diastolic pressure, volume, and oxygen consumption, while raising stroke volume and cardiac output and causing only modest reduction in aortic pressure. Vasodilators should not be used in patients with hypotension.

In patients with both acute and chronic heart failure secondary to coronary artery disease, cardiomyopathy, or valvular regurgitation who are treated with vasodilators, cardiac output increases, the pulmonary wedge pressure falls, the signs and symptoms of heart failure are relieved, and a new steady state is achieved in which cardiac output is higher and afterload lower with no or only mild

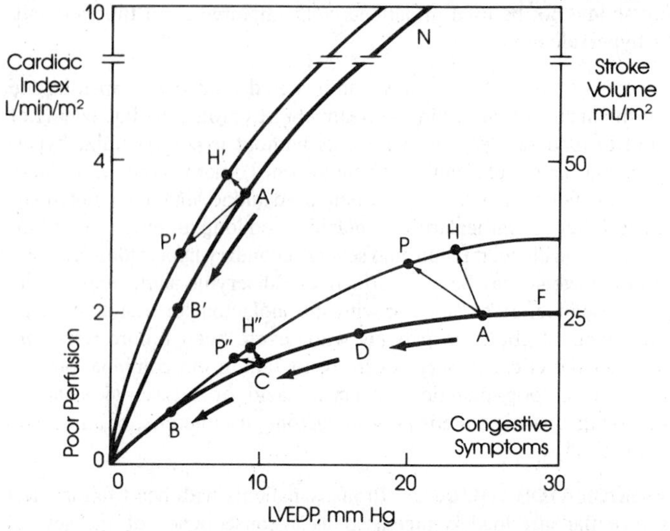

FIGURE 182-1 *Effects of various vasodilators on the relationship between left ventricular end-diastolic pressure (LVEDP) and cardiac index or stroke volume in normal (N) and failing (F) hearts. H represents hydralazine or any other pure arterial dilator. It produces only a minimal increase in cardiac index in the normal subject (A' → H') or in the patient with heart failure with normal LVEDP (C → H"). In contrast, it elevates output in the patient with heart failure and elevated LVEDP (A → H). P represents a balanced vasodilator, such as sodium nitroprusside or prazosin. It reduces filling pressure in all patients, elevates cardiac output in patients with heart failure and elevated LVEDP (A → P), lowers cardiac output in normal subjects (A' → P'), and has little effect on cardiac output in heart failure patients with normal filling pressures (C → P"). (Reprinted with permission from TW Smith, E Braunwald, in Heart Disease: A Textbook of Cardiovascular Medicine, 2d ed. Philadelphia, Saunders, 1984.)*

reduction of arterial pressure (Fig. 182-1). Furthermore, the reduction of elevated left end-diastolic pressure may improve subendocardial perfusion.

Vasodilator therapy is particularly useful in the treatment of acute pulmonary edema, which, if not precipitated by myocardial infarction, is often associated with hypertension. Also, vasodilator therapy is often helpful in refractory congestive heart failure; when heart failure is acute, the addition of an inotropic agent such as dobutamine may be required.

The several available vasodilators vary in their hemodynamic effects, locus and duration of action, and mode of administration (Table 182-1). Some vasodilators, such as hydralazine, minoxidil,

TABLE 182-1 Spectrum of vasodilators used for the treatment of heart failure*

	Principal site of action	Mode of administration	Duration of action
Phentolamine	Arterial	Continuous intravenous	Minutes
Hydralazine	Arterial	Oral	Hours
Minoxidil	Arterial	Oral	Hours
Captopril, enalapril	Arterial and venous	Oral	Hours
Nitroprusside	Arterial and venous	Continuous intravenous	Minutes
Prazosin	Arterial and venous	Oral	Hours
Nitroglycerin	Venous	Intravenous or sublingual	Minutes
		Ointment, patch	Hours
Isosorbide dinitrate	Venous	Sublingual	Minutes to hours

* *Although all these drugs have been demonstrated to be effective vasodilators in the treatment of heart failure, only captopril has been approved for this use in the United States at the time of this writing.*

and the alpha-adrenergic blocking agents, act predominantly on the arterial bed and primarily increase stroke volume while others, such as nitroglycerin and isosorbide dinitrate, act almost entirely on the venous side of the circulation; the latter agents cause pooling of blood in the venous bed and act primarily to reduce ventricular filling pressures. Captopril, prazosin, and sodium nitroprusside are "balanced vasodilators" which act on both the arterial and venous beds. Some agents, such as sodium nitroprusside, must be administered by continuous intravenous infusion, nitroglycerin requires administration in ointment or patch form when a prolonged effect is desired, while isosorbide dinitrate is most effective when it is administered by the sublingual route.

The ideal vasodilator for the treatment of *acute* heart failure should have a rapid onset and brief duration of action when administered by intravenous infusion; sodium nitroprusside qualifies as such a drug, but its use requires careful monitoring of the intraarterial pressure and electrocardiogram, and if possible of the pulmonary artery wedge pressure, in an intensive care unit. For the treatment of chronic congestive heart failure, the agent should be effective on oral administration, and its action should persist for at least 6 h. Captopril (an angiotensin-converting enzyme inhibitor), hydralazine (a smooth muscle dilator), prazosin (an alpha-adrenergic blocking agent), and hydralazine (a direct relaxant of vascular smooth muscle) satisfy these requirements. It is advisable to commence therapy with very low doses in order to avoid hypotension and gradually increase them as needed and tolerated.

In view of the spectrum of actions of available vasodilators, the selection of the specific agent or combinations of agents for any given patient should depend on the pathophysiologic state. For example, when the primary defect is a reduction of cardiac output and/or mitral regurgitation, an arterial vasodilator such as hydralazine or minoxidil is the drug of choice; when pulmonary congestion is the principal problem, a venodilator would be preferable. When it is desired both to elevate cardiac output and to reduce pulmonary vascular pressures, an agent which acts both on the arterial and venous beds, such as captopril or prazosin, or the combination of hydralazine and a nitrate is indicated. Vasodilators are potent and effective in acutely improving the deranged hemodynamics of heart failure and there is some evidence in favor of a beneficial chronic effect as well. Some studies with captopril have demonstrated a favorable long-term reduction of symptoms and enhancement of exercise tolerance. It has been reported that the combination of hydralazine and isosorbide dinitrate prolong survival of patients with heart failure.

Vasodilators are ineffective, indeed they may even exert a deleterious action, in patients without heart failure (Fig. 182-1). Arterial dilators may produce postural hypotension with little effect on cardiac output. Venodilators lower arterial pressure and cardiac output in patients with normal cardiac function, and in patients with heart failure whose ventricular filling pressures have previously been restored to normal by diuretic therapy.

REFRACTORY HEART FAILURE When the response to ordinary treatment is inadequate, heart failure is considered to be refractory. Before assuming that this state simply reflects advanced, perhaps preterminal, myocardial depression, careful consideration must be given to several possibilities: (1) an underlying and overlooked cause of the heart disease that may be amenable to specific surgical or medical therapy, such as silent aortic or mitral stenosis, constrictive pericarditis, infective endocarditis, hypertension, or thyrotoxicosis; (2) one or a combination of the precipitating causes of heart failure, such as pulmonary or urinary tract infection, recurrent pulmonary emboli, arterial hypoxemia, anemia, or arrhythmia; and (3) complications of overly vigorous therapy, such as digitalis intoxication, hypovolemia, or electrolyte imbalance.

Recognition and proper treatment of the aforementioned complications are likely to make the patient responsive to therapy again. Perhaps the most common complication results from overzealous treatment with diuretics. When administered too rapidly, these drugs can produce sudden hypovolemia before edema fluid can be mobilized to replace the loss of blood volume, the result being a shocklike state with evidence of systemic hypoperfusion in the presence of edema. The chronically excessively diuresed patient has exchanged the hazards of pulmonary edema and the inconvenience of systemic edema for a persistently depressed cardiac output with its associated weakness, lethargy, prerenal azotemia, and sometimes cardiac cachexia. Temporarily easing up on salt restriction and diuretic administration may overcome this difficulty, but as heart failure worsens, this course of action may lead to increased pulmonary congestion which is equally unacceptable.

Hyponatremia is a late manifestation of refractory heart failure. It, too, may be a complication of overaggressive diuresis leading to reduced glomerular filtration rate and decreased delivery of NaCl to the diluting sites in the distal tubule. Hyponatremia may also result from nonosmotic stimuli for the continued secretion of antidiuretic hormone. Therapy involves improvement of the cardiovascular status, if possible, as well as temporary cessation of diuretic therapy particularly of thiazides, and restriction of oral water intake. Hypertonic saline is very rarely indicated because total body sodium is usually elevated, not depressed.

The combination of an intravenously administered vasodilator, such as sodium nitroprusside, along with a potent sympathomimetic amine, such as dopamine or dobutamine, often results in an additive effect, raising cardiac output and lowering filling pressure. Intravenous amrinone, sometimes accompanied by oral captopril, may also be useful in patients with refractory heart failure. Once compensation is established, therapy can be continued with the combination of oral hydralazine or captopril to reduce afterload and one of the orally active nonglycoside inotropic agents, such as milrinone, a derivative of amrinone, which is available only for clinical investigation at the time of this writing.

Cardiac transplantation When patients with heart failure become unresponsive to a combination of all of the aforementioned therapeutic measures, are in New York Heart Association class IV, and are deemed unlikely to survive 1 year, they should be considered for cardiac transplantation. To qualify for this procedure, patients should be under 55 years of age, be stable psychologically, and possess a strong family support system. Contraindications include severe pulmonary hypertension, parenchymal lung disease, recent pulmonary emboli, active infection, insulin-requiring diabetes mellitus, and other diseases which may limit survival. As in renal transplantation (Chap. 221) the principal problem is graft rejection and the combination of cyclosporin A and corticosteroids has been helpful in reducing the severity of this complication; a second serious problem is infection as a consequence of the immunosuppression. In the hands of a skilled, experienced team, the 1-year survival rate is approximately 80 percent with a subsequent attrition of approximately 3 percent per year. The shortage of donor hearts and the enormous expense associated with this procedure have limited its application.

TREATMENT OF ACUTE PULMONARY EDEMA Pulmonary edema secondary to left ventricular failure or mitral stenosis is described in Chap. 26. It is life-threatening and must be considered a medical emergency. As is the case for the more chronic forms of heart failure, in the treatment of pulmonary edema, attention must be directed to identifying and removing any precipitating causes of decompensation, such as an arrhythmia or infection. However, because of the acute nature of the problem, a number of additional nonspecific measures are necessary. When possible, and if it does not delay treatment unduly, recording pulmonary vascular pressures through a Swan-Ganz catheter and intraarterial pressure directly is advisable. The first six measures listed below are ordinarily applied simultaneously.

1. Morphine is administered intravenously repetitively, as needed in doses from 2 to 5 mg. This drug reduces anxiety, reduces adrenergic vasoconstrictor stimuli to the arteriolar and venous beds, and thereby helps to break a vicious cycle. Naloxone should be available in case respiratory depression occurs.
2. Because the alveolar fluid interferes with oxygen diffusion, resulting in arterial hypoxemia, 100% oxygen should be administered, preferably under positive pressure. The latter increases intraalveolar pressure and therefore reduces transudation of fluid from the alveolar capillaries and impedes venous return to the thorax, reducing pulmonary capillary pressure.
3. The patient should be maintained in the sitting position, with the legs dangling along the side of the bed, if possible, which also tends to reduce venous return.
4. Intravenous loop diuretics, such as furosemide or ethacrynic acid (40 to 100 mg), or bumetanide (1 mg) will, by rapidly establishing a diuresis, reduce circulating blood volume and thereby hasten the relief of pulmonary edema. In addition when given intravenously, furosemide also exerts a venodilator action, reduces venous return, and reduces pulmonary edema even before the diuresis commences.
5. Afterload reduction is achieved with intravenous sodium nitroprusside at 20 to 30 μg/min in patients whose systolic arterial pressures exceed 100 mmHg.
6. If digitalis has not been administered previously, three-fourths of a full dose of a rapidly acting glycoside, such as ouabain, digoxin, or lanatoside C, should be administered intravenously.
7. Sometimes, aminophylline (theophylline ethylenediamine), 240 to 480 mg intravenously, is effective in diminishing bronchoconstriction, increasing renal blood flow and sodium excretion, and augmenting myocardial contractility.
8. If the above mentioned measures are not sufficient, rotating tourniquets should be applied to the extremities.

After these emergency therapeutic measures have been instituted, and the precipitating factors treated, the diagnosis of the underlying cardiac disorder responsible for the pulmonary edema must be established if it is not already known. After stabilization of the patient's condition a long-range strategy for prevention of future episodes of pulmonary edema must be established, and this may require surgical treatment.

PROGNOSIS

The prognosis in heart failure depends primarily on the nature of the underlying heart disease and on the presence or absence of a precipitating factor which can be treated. Also, the long-term prognosis for heart failure is most favorable when the underlying forms of heart disease can be treated. When one of the latter can be identified and removed, the outlook for immediate survival is far better than if heart failure occurs without any obvious precipitating cause. In the latter situation, median survival ranges between 6 months and 5 years depending on the severity of the heart failure. The prognosis can also be estimated by observing the response to treatment. When clinical improvement occurs with only modest dietary sodium restriction and small doses of diuretics or digitalis, then the outlook is far better than if, in addition to these measures, intensive diuretic therapy and vasodilators are necessary.

REFERENCES

ARNOLD SB et al: Long-term digitalis therapy improves left ventricular function in heart failure. N Engl J Med 303:1443, 1980

BERGER BE, WARNOCK DG: Mechanisms of action and clinical use of diuretics, in *The Kidney*, 3d ed, BM Brenner, FC Rector (eds). Philadelphia, Saunders, 1986, p 433

BRAUNWALD E (ed): Newer positive inotropic agents. Circulation 73(Suppl III):1, 1986

——— et al (eds): *Congestive Heart Failure: Current Research and Clinical Applications*. New York, Grune & Stratton, 1982

BRISTOW MR: The adrenergic nervous system in heart failure. N Engl J Med 311:850, 1984

CHERNIACK NS, LONGOBARDO GS: Cheyne-Stokes breathing: An instability in physiologic control. N Engl J Med 288:952, 1973

CREAGER MA et al: The acute and long-term effects of enalapril on the cardiovascular response to exercise tolerance in patients with congestive heart failure. J Am Coll Cardio 6:163, 1985

DZAU VJ et al: Angiotensin converting enzyme inhibition in the treatment of congestive heart failure and hypertension, in *Update IV: Harrison's Principles of Internal Medicine*, KJ Isselbacher et al (eds). New York, McGraw-Hill, 1982, p 137

FISCH C (guest ed): An account of the foxglove and some of its medical uses: 1785–1985. J Am Coll Cardiol 5 (Suppl A):1A, 1985

GOODMAN LS, GILMAN A (eds): Cardiovascular drugs, in *The Pharmacological Basis of Therapeutics*, 7th ed. New York, Macmillan, 1985, pp 716, 887

HUMPHREYS MH, RECTOR FC JR: Pathophysiology of edema formation, in *The Kidney: Physiology and Pathophysiology*, 2d ed, DW Seldin, G Giebisch (eds). New York, Raven Press, 1985, p 1163

ISKANDRIAN AS, HAKKI A-H, MATTLEMAN SJ: Predicting left ventricular function: Bedside examination. Prim Cardiol (Suppl) 10:3A, 1984

LEE WH, PACKER M: Prognostic importance of serum sodium concentration and its modification by converting-enzyme inhibition in patients with severe chronic heart failure. Circulation 73:257, 1986

MAKABALI C et al: Dobutamine and other sympathomimetic drugs for the treatment of low cardiac output failure. Semin Anesth 1:63, 1982

SMITH TW (ed): *Digitalis Glycosides*. New York, Grune & Stratton, 1986

———, BRAUNWALD E: Management of heart failure, in *Heart Disease*, 2d ed, E Braunwald (ed). Philadelphia, Saunders, 1984, p 503

SUKI WN et al: Physiology of diuretic action, in *The Kidney: Physiology and Pathophysiology*, 2d ed, DW Seldin, G Giebisch (eds). New York, Raven Press, 1985, p 2127

183 THE BRADYARRHYTHMIAS

MARK E. JOSEPHSON / ALFRED E. BUXTON / FRANCIS E. MARCHLINSKI

ANATOMY OF THE CONDUCTING SYSTEM Under normal conditions the pacemaker function of the heart resides in the sinoatrial node which lies at the junction of the right atrium and superior vena cava. The node is approximately 1½ cm long and 2 to 3 mm wide and is supplied by the sinus node artery, which arises from either the right coronary artery (60 percent of cases) or the left circumflex coronary artery (40 percent). Once the impulse exits the sinus node and perinodal tissue, it traverses the atrium until it reaches the atrioventricular (AV) node, whose blood supply is derived from the posterior descending coronary artery in 90 percent of cases and which lies at the base of the interatrial septum just above the tricuspid annulus and anterior to the coronary sinus. The electrophysiologic properties of the AV node result in slow conduction, which is responsible for the normal delay in AV conduction, i.e., the PR interval.

The bundle of His emerges from the AV node, enters the fibrous skeleton of the heart, and courses anteriorly across the membranous interventricular septum. It has a dual blood supply from the AV nodal artery and a branch of the anterior descending coronary artery. The branching (distal) portion of the bundle of His gives rise to a broad sheet of fibers which course over the left side of the interventricular septum to form the left bundle branch and a narrow, cablelike structure on the right side to form the right bundle branch. The arborization of both the right and left bundle branches gives rise to the distal His-Purkinje system, which ultimately extends throughout the endocardium of the right and left ventricles.

The sinus node, atrium, and AV node are significantly influenced by autonomic tone. Vagal influences depress automaticity of the sinus node, depress conduction, and prolong refractoriness in the perinodal tissue surrounding the sinus node and prolong AV nodal conduction and refractoriness. Sympathetic influences exert the opposite effect.

ELECTROPHYSIOLOGIC PRINCIPLES

In the resting state, the interior of most cardiac cells, with the exception of the sinus and AV nodes, is approximately 80- to 90-mV negative with respect to a reference extracellular electrode. The resting membrane potential is primarily determined by the concentration gradient of potassium across the cell membrane. Activation of cardiac cells results from movement of ions across the cell membrane, causing a transient depolarization known as the *action potential*. The ionic species responsible for the action potential vary among the cardiac tissues, and the configuration of the action potential is therefore unique to each tissue (Fig. 183-1).

The action potential of the bundle of His–Purkinje system and ventricular myocardium has five phases (Fig. 183-2). The rapid depolarizing current (phase 0) is mainly determined by an influx of sodium into myocardial cells with a secondary, slower, influx of calcium. The repolarization phases of the action potential (phases 1 to 3) are primarily related to outward potassium flux. The resting membrane potential is phase 4.

The bradyarrhythmias result from abnormalities either of impulse formation, i.e., automaticity, or of conduction. *Automaticity*, which is normally observed in the sinus node, the specialized fibers of the His-Purkinje system, and some specialized atrial fibers, is the property of a cardiac cell to depolarize spontaneously during phase 4 of the action potential, leading to the generation of an impulse. To exhibit automaticity the resting membrane potential must decrease spontaneously until threshold potential is reached and an all-or-none regenerative response occurs. The ionic components producing spontaneous diastolic depolarization appear to involve the inward current of either sodium or calcium. The velocity of conduction, i.e., impulse propagation through cardiac tissues, is influenced by the rate of rise and amplitude of phase 0 of the action potential. The more positive the threshold potential and the slower the rate of depolarization

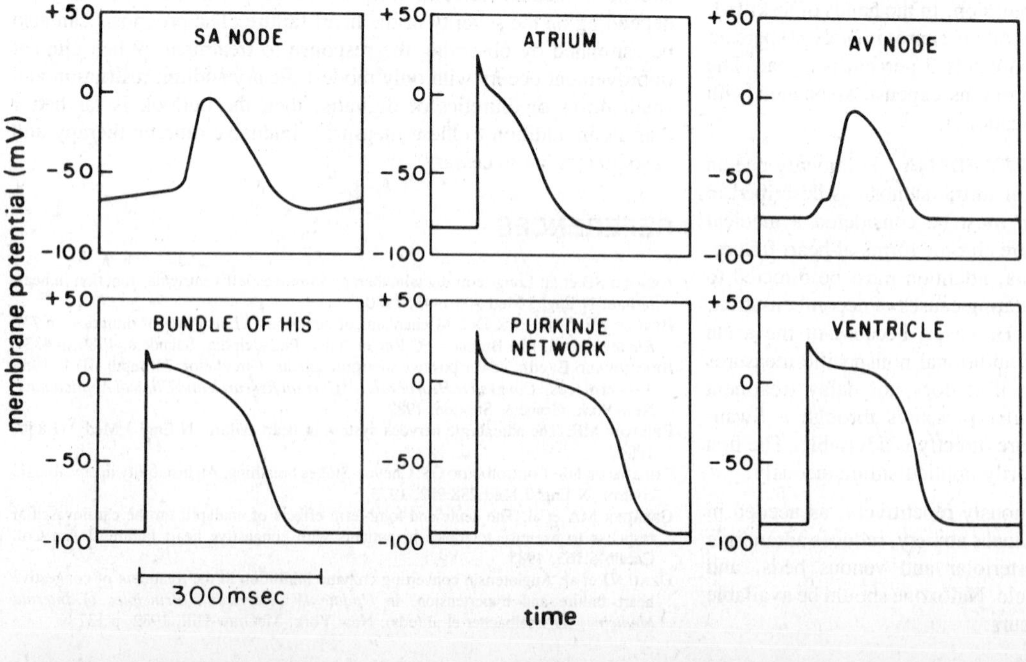

FIGURE 183-1 *Action potential configurations in different regions of the mammalian heart. (From AM Katz:* Physiology of the Heart, *New York, Raven Press, 1977.)*

FIGURE 183-2 *Schematic representation of the action potential in normal ventricle depicting the direction, strength, and period of flow of the ionic currents underlying the action potential. The arrows' direction and size indicate whether current is inward- or outward-directed and the approximate current strength, respectively, of the ion identified at the arrow's base. The horizontal position of the arrow corresponds to the same moment in the time course of action potential* (see text). *The five phases of the action potential are indicated by the numerals placed next to the corresponding portion of the waveform. (Originally published in Ten Eick et al: Ventricular dysrhythmia: Membrane basis or currents, channels, gates, and cables, in Progress in Cardiovascular Diseases, vol XXIV, no 2, pp 157–188. New York, Grune & Stratton, 1981, by permission.)*

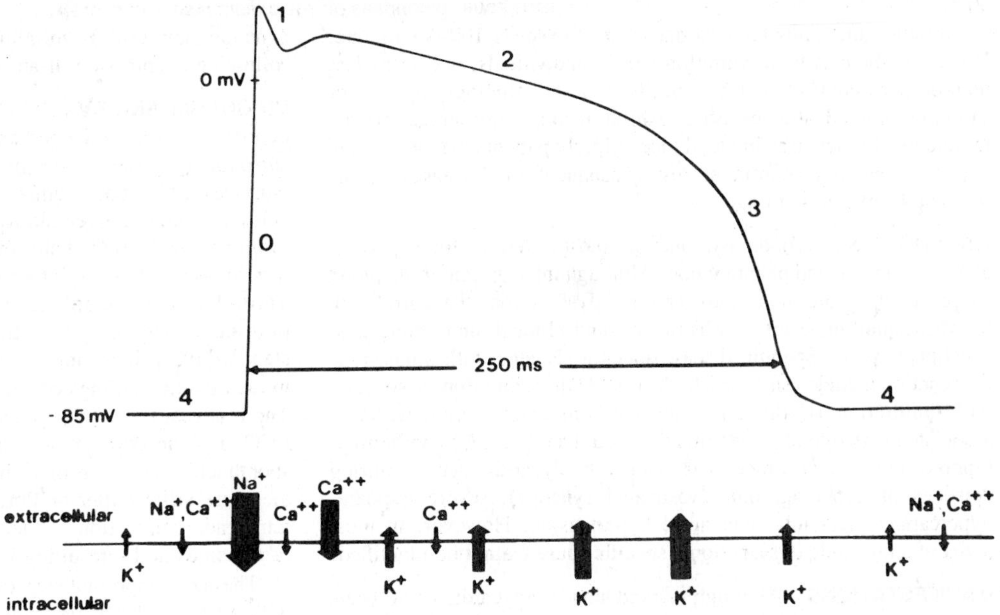

toward threshold, the slower the rate of rise of phase 0 of the action potential and the slower the conduction velocity. Disease states or drugs may result in lower rates of rise of phase 0 at any given membrane potential.

Refractoriness is a property of cardiac cells which defines the period of recovery that cells require before they can be reexcited by a stimulus after being discharged. The *absolute refractory period* is defined by that portion of the action potential during which no stimulus, regardless of its strength, can evoke another response. The *effective refractory period* is that part of the action potential at which time a stimulus can only evoke a local nonpropagated response. The *relative refractory period* extends from the end of the effective refractory period to the time that the tissue is fully recovered. During this time a stimulus of greater than threshold strength is required to evoke a response which is propagated more slowly than normal. After completion of the action potential, excitability recovers and evoked responses have characteristics similar to the spontaneous normal response.

INTRACARDIAC RECORDINGS OF THE SPECIALIZED CONDUCTING SYSTEM Electrode catheters allow the recording of activation of portions of the specialized conducting system including the bundle of His. To obtain a recording from the bundle of His the electrode catheter is positioned across the tricuspid valve (Fig. 183-3). The interval from local atrial depolarization in the His bundle recording to the onset of depolarization of the His bundle deflection is called the AH interval (normal = 60 to 125 ms) and represents an indirect method of assessing AV nodal conduction time. The interval from the beginning of the His bundle deflection to the earliest onset of ventricular activation, as measured from any of the multiple-surface electrocardiogram (ECG) leads or the intracardiac ventricular electrogram (the HV interval, normal = 35 to 55 ms), represents conduction time through the His-Purkinje system. Electrode catheters can be positioned in the area of the sinus node to record high right atrial activity. Left atrial activity may be recorded directly via a catheter placed across a patent foramen ovale, or indirectly using a catheter inserted into the coronary sinus. The atrial activation sequence may be "mapped," and sites of intra- and interatrial conduction abnormalities may be ascertained.

SINUS NODE DYSFUNCTION

The sinus node is normally the dominant cardiac pacemaker because its intrinsic discharge rate is the fastest of all potential cardiac pacemakers. Its responsiveness to alterations in autonomic nervous system tone is responsible for the normal acceleration of heart rate during exercise and the slowing which occurs during rest and sleep. Increases in sinus rate normally result from an increase in sympathetic tone acting via beta-adrenergic receptors and/or a decrease in parasympathetic tone acting via muscarinic receptors; slowing of the heart rate is normally due to opposite alterations. In adults, the normal sinus rate under basal conditions is 60 to 100 beats per minute. Sinus bradycardia is said to exist when the sinus rate is less than 60 beats

FIGURE 183-3 *Normal intracardiac recording. Surface ECG leads I, II, and V_1 are displayed with intracardiac ECGs from the high right atrium (HRA), left atrium from the coronary sinus (CS), and AV junction to obtain a His bundle electrogram (HBE). T = time lines. Atrial activation begins in the high right atrium and spreads inferiorly to the low atrial septum as recorded in the HBE and left atrium as recorded in the CS. The AH and HV intervals represent AV nodal and His-Purkinje conduction time, respectively. Vertical lines = 0.10 s. (From Josephson and Seides.)*

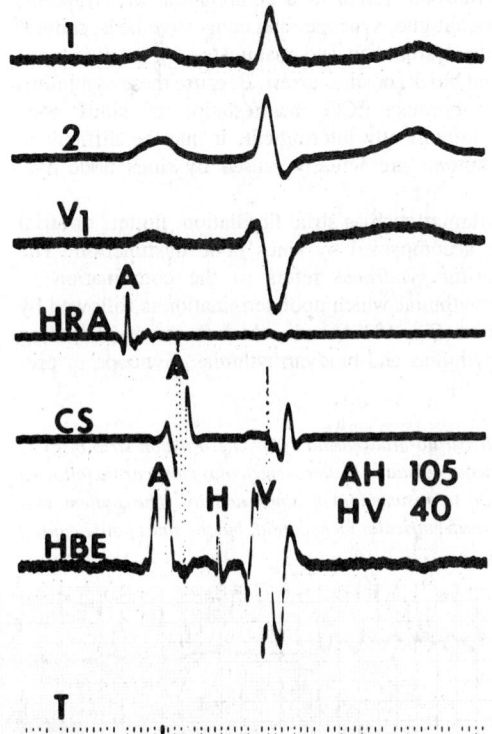

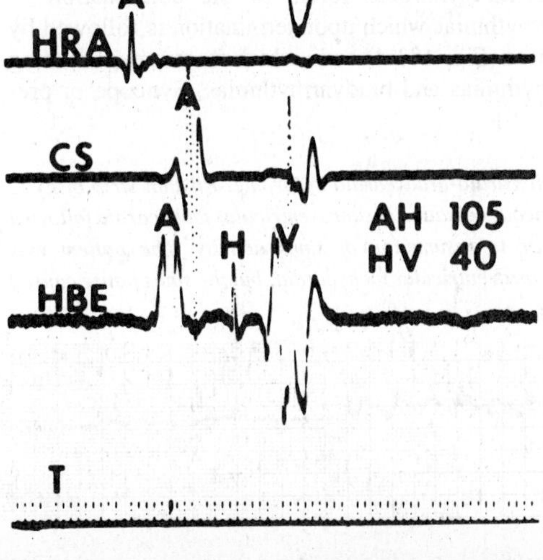

per minute, and sinus tachycardia when it exceeds 100 per minute. However, there is wide variation among individuals, and rates less than 60 per minute do not necessarily indicate pathologic states. For example, trained athletes often exhibit resting rates under 50 per minute due to increases in vagal tone. Elderly patients may also show marked sinus bradycardia at rest consequent to decreases in the intrinsic heart rate with age.

ETIOLOGY Sinus node dysfunction most often is found in the elderly as an isolated phenomenon. Although interruption of the blood supply to the sinus node may produce dysfunction, the correlation between sinus node artery obstruction and clinical sinus node dysfunction is poor. Specific disease states associated with sinus node dysfunction include senile amyloidosis and other conditions associated with infiltration of the atrial myocardium. Sinus bradycardia is associated with hypothyroidism, advanced liver disease, hypothermia, typhoid fever, and brucellosis. Sinus bradycardia occurs during episodes of hypervagotonia (vasovagal syncope), severe hypoxia, hypercapnia, acidemia, and acute hypertension. However, in most cases of sinus node dysfunction a specific cause cannot be identified.

MANIFESTATIONS Although marked sinus bradycardia (<50 beats per minute) may cause fatigue and other symptoms due to inadequate cardiac output, more commonly sinus node dysfunction is manifested as paroxysmal dizziness, presyncope, or syncope. These symptoms usually result from abrupt, prolonged sinus pauses caused by failure of sinus impulse formation (sinus arrest) or block of conduction of sinus impulses to the surrounding atrial tissue (sinus exit block). In either case, the ECG manifestation is a prolonged period (>3 s) of atrial asystole. In some patients sinus node dysfunction is accompanied by abnormalities in AV conduction. In addition to the absence of atrial activity, lower pacemakers fail to emerge during the sinus pauses, resulting in periods of ventricular asystole and syncope. Occasionally, sinus node dysfunction is manifested initially by the failure of the sinus rate to accelerate in response to conditions such as exercise or fever, which normally cause increases in the sinus rate. In some people sinus node dysfunction may become manifest only in the presence of certain cardioactive drugs: cardiac glycosides, beta-adrenergic blocking drugs, quinidine and other antiarrhythmic agents, and verapamil or diltiazem. These agents, which do not cause sinus node dysfunction in otherwise normal people, may unmask evidence of sinus node dysfunction in susceptible individuals.

The *sick-sinus syndrome* refers to a combination of symptoms (dizziness, confusion, fatigue, syncope, and congestive heart failure) caused by sinus node dysfunction and manifested by marked sinus bradycardia, sinoatrial block, or sinus arrest. Because these symptoms are nonspecific and because ECG manifestation of sinus node dysfunction are not infrequently intermittent, it may be difficult to prove that such symptoms are actually caused by sinus node dysfunction.

Atrial tachyarrhythmias such as atrial fibrillation, flutter, or atrial tachycardia may be accompanied by sinus node dysfunction. The *bradycardia-tachycardia syndrome* refers to the combination of paroxysmal atrial arrhythmias which upon termination is followed by prolonged sinus pauses (Fig. 183-4) or in which there are alternating periods of tachyarrhythmias and bradyarrhythmias. Syncope or presyncope may result from failure of the sinus node to recover function following suppression of automaticity by atrial tachyarrhythmias.

DIAGNOSIS AND EVALUATION First-degree *sinoatrial exit block* denotes a prolonged conduction time from the sinus node to the surrounding atrial tissue. It cannot be recognized on a standard (surface) ECG but requires invasive intracardiac recordings (see below). Second-degree sinoatrial exit block denotes the intermittent failure of conduction of sinus impulses to the surrounding atrial tissue; it is manifested as the intermittent absence of P waves (Fig. 183-5). Third-degree, or complete, sinoatrial block is characterized by a lack of atrial activity or by an ectopic subsidiary atrial pacemaker. On the standard ECG, it cannot be distinguished from sinus arrest, but direct intracardiac recordings of sinus node activity permit this distinction. The bradycardia-tachycardia syndrome is manifested on the standard ECG as inappropriate (>3 s) pauses in sinus activity following spontaneous cessation of tachyarrhythmias (Fig. 183-4). Most often these are atrial flutter or fibrillation, although any tachycardia with retrograde conduction to the atria may cause overdrive suppression of the sinus node, resulting in clinical appearance of this syndrome.

The most important step in the diagnosis is to correlate symptoms with ECG evidence of sinus node dysfunction. While ambulatory ECG (Holter) monitoring remains a mainstay in evaluating sinus node function, most episodes of syncope are paroxysmal and unpredictable. Single and even multiple 24-h Holter monitor recordings may fail to include a symptomatic episode. Therefore, noting the response to carotid sinus pressure and pharmacologic autonomic "denervation" of the heart is frequently helpful. Carotid sinus pressure is particularly useful in patients in whom paroxysmal dizziness or syncope is compatible with the hypersensitive carotid sinus syndrome (see Chap. 12). In such patients, the response can be dramatic, and sinus pauses in excess of 5 s may occur. Normally a sinus pause of ≤3 s results from 5 s of unilateral carotid sinus massage. If atropine can prevent the effects of carotid sinus pressure, autonomic dysfunction, not primary sinus node dysfunction, is responsible. The other noninvasive test of sinus node function involves the use of pharmacologic agents to manipulate the autonomic nervous system and assess the balance of parasympathetic and sympathetic activity on the sinus node. Vagomimetic (Valsalva maneuver or phenylephrine-induced hypertension) and vagolytic (atropine) agents as well as sympathomimetic (isoproterenol or hypotension by nitroprusside) and beta-adrenergic blocking agents can be utilized, singly and in combination. These studies are designed to test the response of the sinus node to autonomic stimulation and inhibition and thereby characterize the status of autonomic regulation of the sinus node. Abnormalities of the autonomic control of sinus function are particularly common in patients in whom the only presenting arrhythmias are sinus bradycardia.

Intrinsic heart rate This is a manifestation of the primary activity of the sinus node, and its determination requires chemical denervation of the heart. Complete autonomic blockade is achieved with 0.2 mg/kg propranolol intravenously, followed after 10 min by 0.04 mg/kg of atropine sulfate intravenously. Normal values of intrinsic heart rate = 118.1 − (0.57 × age) beats per min. The use of autonomic blockade can separate patients with asymptomatic sinus bradycardia into a group with primary sinus node dysfunction (slow intrinsic heart rate) and a group with autonomic imbalance (normal intrinsic heart rate). Autonomic blockade is particularly useful when combined with invasive assessment of sinus node function (see below). Autonomic blockade may depress conduction in patients with intrinsic disease of the conduction system and should be carried out only in a setting where arrhythmias can be monitored and rapidly treated.

FIGURE 183-4 *Tachycardia-bradycardia syndrome. Rhythm strip of ECG lead II showing spontaneous cessation of supraventricular tachycardia followed by a 5.6-s pause prior to resumption of sinus activity. The patient was asymptomatic during supraventricular tachycardia, but the sinus pause caused severe lightheadedness.*

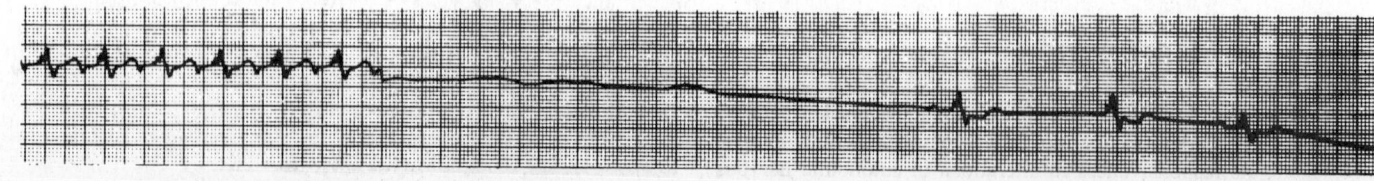

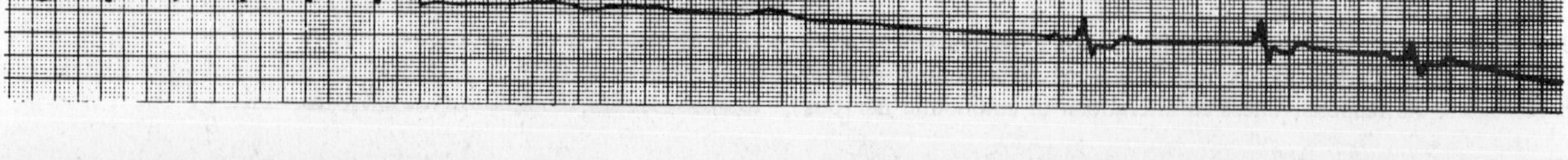

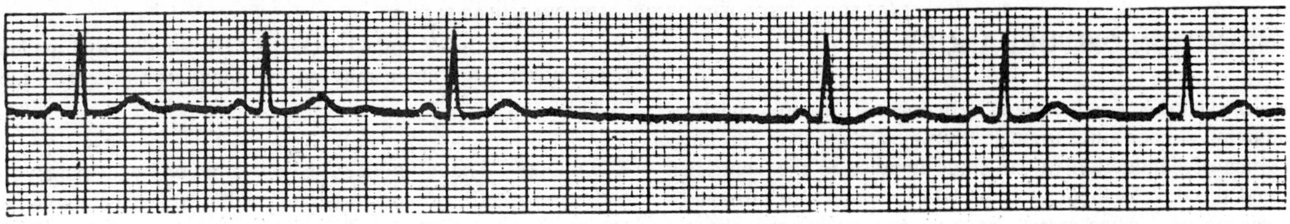

FIGURE 183-5 *Second-degree sinoatrial exit block. Surface ECG denoting abrupt absence of P wave during sinus rhythm. Prior to the pause the sinus rate is regular. The interval of the pause is exactly twice the basal sinus cycle length.*

Sinus node recovery time Sinus node recovery time is evaluated by assessing the response of the sinus node to rapid atrial pacing (Fig. 183-6). When atrial pacing is discontinued, a pause, the *sinus node recovery time,* occurs prior to resumption of spontaneous sinus rhythm. When the sinus recovery time is prolonged, the results of this test mimic the prolonged sinus pauses seen following termination of atrial tachyarrhythmias in the bradycardia-tachycardia syndrome (see Fig. 183-4). The corrected sinus node recovery time (sinus recovery time − sinus cycle length) normally is less than 550 ms, and the uncorrected sinus node recovery time less than 150 percent of the spontaneous cycle length. In patients with sinus node dysfunction, prolongation of the sinus node recovery time is often observed. Marked prolongation of the sinus node recovery time is rare in the absence of symptoms. Patients with abnormally slow intrinsic heart rates usually have abnormal sinus node recovery times, while those with normal intrinsic heart rates have normal recovery times.

Sinoatrial conduction time Determination of the conduction time from the sinus node to the atrium allows for the differentiation of abnormalities of sinoatrial conduction from abnormalities of sinus impulse formation. The conduction time equals one-half of the pause following termination of brief periods of pacing, minus the sinus cycle length. Alternatively, the sinus node electrogram can be recorded directly by a catheter electrode placed near the sinoatrial node.

EVALUATION Electrophysiologic investigation of sinus node dysfunction should be undertaken in patients who have had symptoms compatible with sinus node dysfunction and in whom no documentation of the arrhythmia responsible for these symptoms has been obtained by prolonged Holter monitoring. Asymptomatic patients with sinus bradycardia need not be tested since no therapy is indicated. Similarly, symptomatic patients with ECG documentation of asystole, sinoatrial block or arrest, or the bradycardia-tachycardia syndrome do not require electrophysiologic tests for diagnosis. However, in symptomatic patients *without* documentation of an arrhythmia, electrophysiologic assessment of sinus node function can yield information which may be used to guide appropriate therapy. Electrophysiologic studies may also be useful in assessing the effects of pharmacologic therapy. If a pacemaker is indicated, the site of pacemaker implantation for maximum hemodynamic effects can be guided by the results of electrophysiologic investigation. However, the results of tests of sinus node function must be interpreted with caution. Sinus node dysfunction coexists frequently with other disorders such as AV conduction disturbances or ventricular tachycardia which may cause symptoms such as syncope. Thus, electrophysiologic evaluation of patients with symptoms such as undiagnosed syncope must not stop with the demonstration of abnormalities of sinus node dysfunction or carotid sinus hypersensitivity. Instead, complete evaluation, including programmed atrial and ventricular stimulation (see Chap. 184) is necessary to search for additional electrophysiologic abnormalities which could be responsible for symptoms.

TREATMENT Permanent pacemakers (page 922) are the mainstay of therapy for patients with symptomatic sinus node dysfunction. Patients with intermittent paroxysms of bradycardia or sinus arrest and with the cardioinhibitory form of the hypersensitive carotid sinus syndrome are usually adequately treated by demand ventricular pacemakers. These devices are reliable, relatively inexpensive, and suffice to prevent episodic symptoms due to abrupt bradycardia. Patients with symptomatic chronic sinus bradycardia or frequent prolonged episodes of sinus node dysfunction may do better with dual-chamber pacemakers that preserve the normal AV activation sequence. Although theoretically an atrial demand pacemaker should be adequate for patients with sinus node dysfunction, the frequent accompaniment of dysfunction in other portions of the cardiac conduction system and its progressive nature usually mandates placement of a pacemaker capable of ventricular pacing.

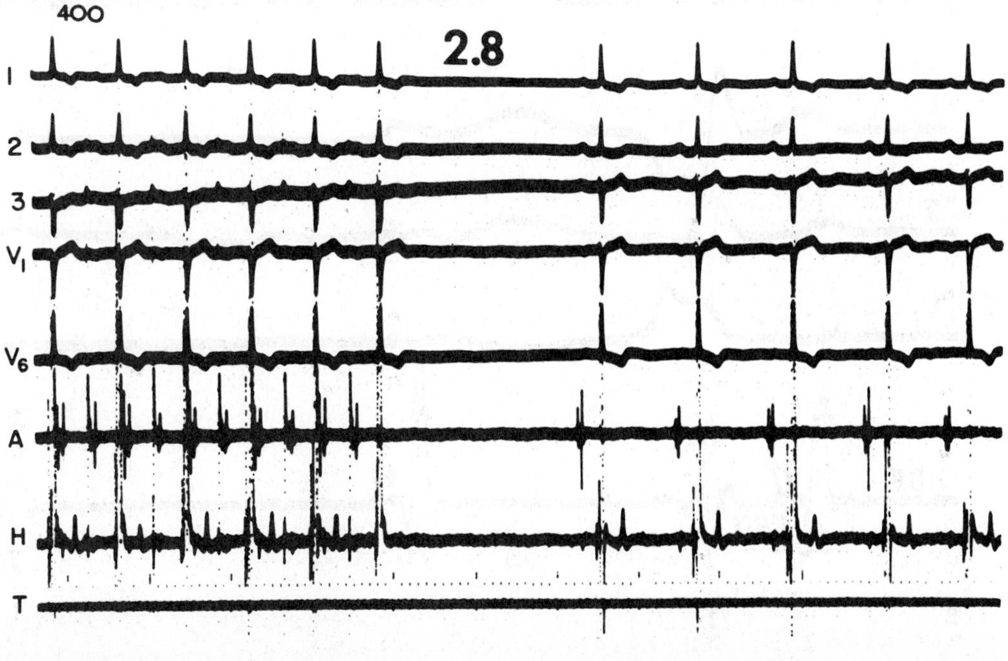

FIGURE 183-6 *Example of sinus node recovery time in a patient with symptomatic sinus node dysfunction. Cessation of atrial pacing at 150 beats per minutes (cycle length, 400 ms) results in a prolonged sinus pause. Surface ECG leads I, II, III, V_1, and V_6, are shown in addition to intracardiac recordings at the high right atrium (A) and His bundle (H). T = time lines.*

AV CONDUCTION DISTURBANCES

The specialized cardiac conducting system normally assures synchronous conduction of each sinus impulse from the atria to the ventricles. Abnormalities of conduction of the sinus impulse to the ventricles may portend the development of heart block, which can ultimately lead to syncope or cardiac arrest. In order to evaluate the clinical significance of conduction abnormalities the physician must determine (1) the site of conduction disturbance, (2) the risk of progression to complete block, and (3) the probability that a subsidiary escape rhythm arising distal to the site of block will be electrophysiologically and hemodynamically stable. This latter point is perhaps the most important since the rate and stability of the escape pacemaker determine what symptoms result from heart block. The escape pacemaker following AV nodal block is in the His bundle, which generally has a stable rate of 40 to 60 beats per minute and is associated with a QRS complex of normal duration (in the absence of a preexisting intraventricular conduction defect). This contrasts with escape rhythms arising in the distal His-Purkinje system, which have lower intrinsic rates (25 to 40 beats per minute), manifest QRS complexes with prolonged duration, and are unstable. Although prolonged QRS complexes are invariable when the distal His-Purkinje pacemakers form the escape mechanism, wide QRS complexes can also coexist with AV nodal block and a His bundle rhythm. Therefore, QRS morphology alone may not be adequate to identify the site of block.

ETIOLOGY The AV node is heavily supplied by the parasympathetic and sympathetic nervous systems and is sensitive to variations in autonomic tone. Chronic AV nodal dysfunction may be seen in highly trained athletes with hypervagotonia. A variety of diseases can also influence AV nodal conduction. These include acute processes, such as myocardial infarction (particularly inferior); coronary spasm (usually of the right coronary artery); digitalis intoxication; excesses of beta and/or calcium blockers; acute infections such as viral myocarditis; acute rheumatic fever; infectious mononucleosis; and miscellaneous disorders such as Lyme disease, sarcoidosis, amyloidosis, and neoplasms, particularly cardiac mesotheliomas. AV nodal block may also be congenital.

Two degenerative diseases are commonly responsible for damage to the specialized conducting system and produce AV block usually associated with bundle branch block (see Chap. 178). In *Lev's disease,* there is calcification and sclerosis of the fibrous cardiac skeleton, which frequently involves the aortic and mitral valves, the central fibrous body, and the summit of the ventricular septum. *Lenegre's disease* appears to be a primary sclerodegenerative disease

FIGURE 183-7 *A. Mobitz type I second-degree AV block. Intracardiac recordings of AV Wenckebach demonstrate that the PR prolongation (320, 615 ms) is localized to the AV node (AH 240, 535 ms, respectively). HBE = His bundle electrogram; A = atrium; H = His; V = ventricle. (Adapted from Josephson and Seides.) B. Mobitz type II second-degree AV block. Intracardiac recordings document block below the His bundle. HBE = His bundle electrogram; A = atrium; H = His; V = ventricle.*

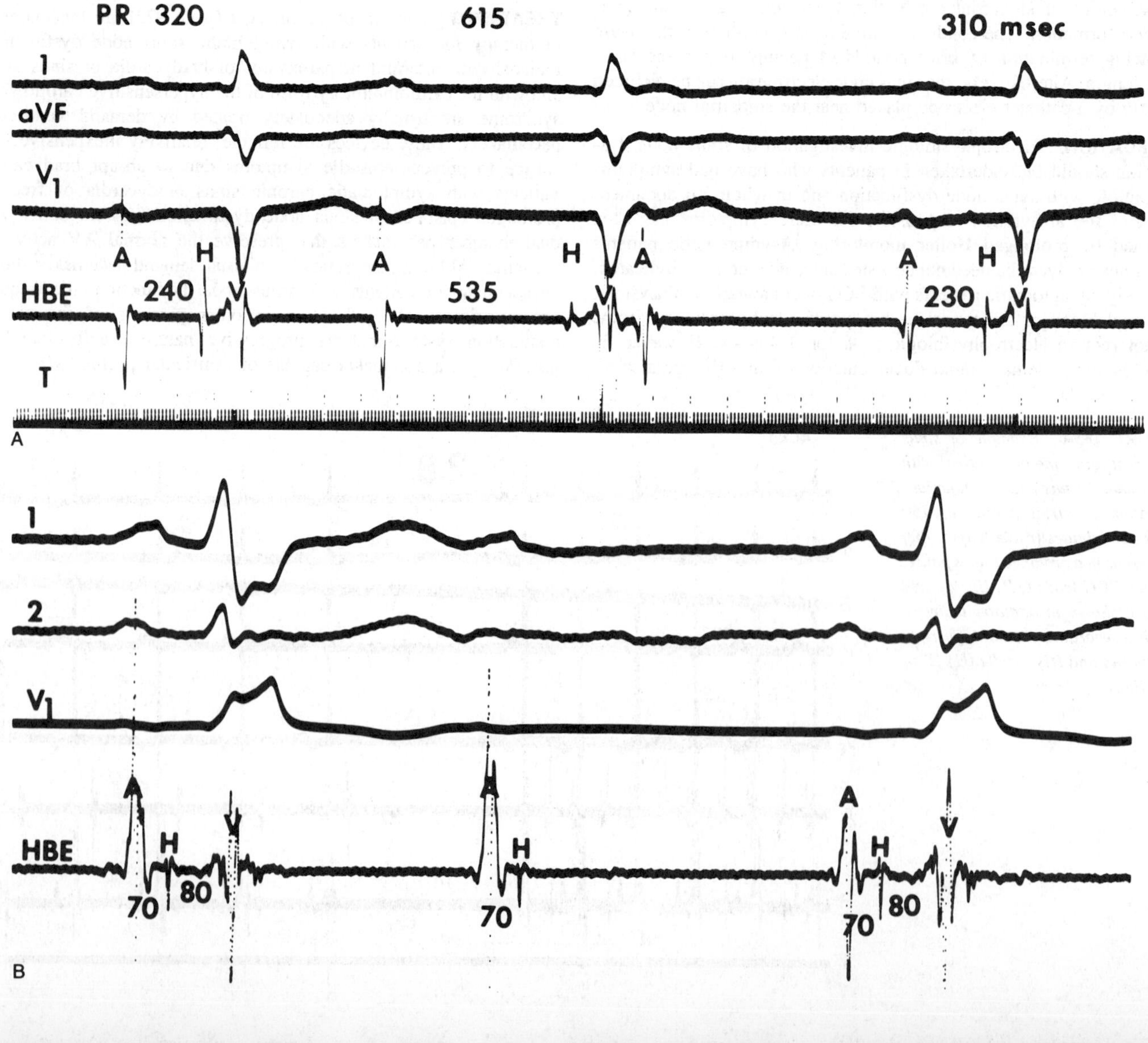

within the conducting system itself without involving the myocardium or fibrous skeleton of the heart. These latter two diseases are probably the most common causes of isolated chronic heart block in adults. Hypertension and aortic and/or mitral stenosis are specific disorders which either accelerate the degeneration of the conducting system or have a direct effect by calcification and fibrosis of the conducting system.

First-degree AV block, more properly termed prolonged AV conduction, is characterized by a PR interval >0.20 s. Since the PR interval is determined by atrial, AV nodal, and His-Purkinje activation, delay in any one or more of these structures can contribute to a prolonged PR interval. In the presence of a QRS complex of normal duration, a PR interval >0.24 s almost invariably is due to a delay within the AV node. If the QRS is prolonged, delays may be present at any of the levels mentioned above. Delay within the His-Purkinje system is always accompanied by prolonged QRS duration in addition to a prolonged PR interval. However, as indicated below, it is only with intracardiac recordings that the exact site of delay can be determined.

Second-degree heart block (intermittent AV block) is present when some trial impulses fail to conduct to the ventricles. Mobitz type I second-degree AV block (AV Wenckebach block) is characterized by progressive PR-interval prolongation prior to block of an atrial impulse (Fig. 183-7*A*). The pause that follows is less than fully compensatory (i.e., is less than two normal sinus intervals), and the PR of the first conducted impulse is shorter than the last conducted atrial impulse prior to the blocked P wave. This type of block is almost always localized to the AV node and associated with a normal QRS duration. It is most often seen as a transient abnormality with inferior wall infarction or with drug intoxication, particularly digitalis, beta blockers, and occasionally calcium channel antagonists. This type of block can also be observed in normal individuals with heightened vagal tone. Although Mobitz type I block can progress to complete heart block, this is uncommon. Even when it does, however, the heart block is usually well tolerated because the escape pacemaker usually arises in the proximal His bundle and provides a stable rhythm. As a result, the presence of Mobitz type I second-degree AV block usually does not mandate aggressive therapy. Therapeutic decisions depend upon the ventricular response and the symptoms of the patient. If the ventricular rate is adequate and the patient is asymptomatic, observation is sufficient.

In Mobitz type II second-degree AV block, conduction fails suddenly and unexpectedly without a preceding change in PR intervals (Fig. 183-7*B*). It is usually due to disease of the His-Purkinje system and is most often associated with a prolonged QRS complex. It is important to recognize this type of block since it has a high incidence of progression to complete heart block with an unstable, slow, lower escape pacemaker. Therefore, pacemaker implantation is necessary in this condition. Mobitz type II block may occur in the setting of anteroseptal infarction or in the primary or secondary sclerodegenerative or calcific disorders of the fibrous skeleton of the heart.

In 2:1 block, intracardiac recordings are necessary in order to ascertain the site of the conduction disturbance because the typical ECG features of Mobitz type 1 or Mobitz type 2 block cannot be discerned during a 2:1 pattern of AV conduction on the surface ECG. In so-called high-degree AV block there are periods of two or more consecutively blocked P waves. Regardless of the site of origin of the escape rhythm, if it is slow and the patient is symptomatic, a cardiac pacemaker is mandatory.

Third-degree AV block is present when no atrial impulse propagates to the ventricles. If the QRS complex of the escape rhythm is of normal duration and occurs at a rate of 40 to 55 beats per minute and increases with atropine or exercise, AV nodal block is probable. Congenital complete AV block is usually localized to the AV node (Fig. 183-8). If the block is within the His bundle, the escape pacemaker usually is less responsive to these perturbations. If the escape rhythm of the QRS is wide and associated with rates ≤40, block is usually localized in, or distal to, the His bundle and mandates a pacemaker since the escape rhythm in this setting is unreliable.

AV DISSOCIATION AV dissociation exists whenever the atria and ventricles are under the control of two separate pacemakers and, while present in complete AV block, can occur in the absence of a primary conduction disturbance. AV dissociation *unrelated* to heart block may occur under two circumstances: (1) an AV junctional rhythm in response to severe sinus bradycardia. When the sinus rate and the escape rate are similar and the P waves occur just before, in, or following the QRS, *isorhythmic AV dissociation* is said to be present. Treatment usually consists of removal of the offending cause of sinus bradycardia (i.e., discontinuation of digitalis, beta blockers, or calcium antagonists), accelerating the sinus node by vagolytic agents, or insertion of a pacemaker if the escape rhythm is slow and results in symptoms. (2) AV dissociation can be caused by an enhanced lower (junctional or ventricular) pacemaker which competes with normal sinus rhythm and frequently exceeds it. This has been called *interference AV dissociation* because the rapid lower pacemaker results in bombardment of the AV node in a retrograde fashion, rendering it refractory to the normal sinus impulses. Thus failure of antegrade conduction is a physiologic response in this circumstance, which commonly occurs during ventricular tachycardia, digitalis intoxication, myocardial ischemia and/or infarction, or local irritation

FIGURE 183-8 *Third-degree AV block. Complete heart block with a slow, wide complex escape rhythm is present. Block in this instance is usually intra-His. See text.*

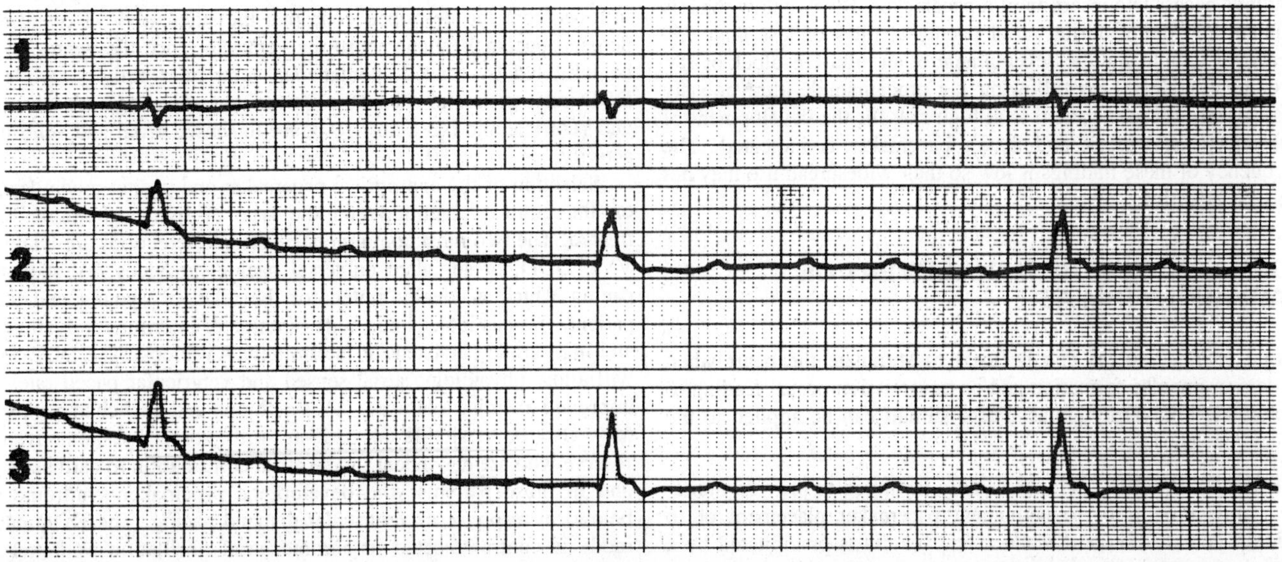

following cardiac surgery. The accelerated rhythm should be treated with either antiarrhythmic drugs (see Chap. 184), removal of the offending drug, or correction of the metabolic abnormality.

INTRACARDIAC ELECTROCARDIOGRAPHIC RECORDINGS IN DIAGNOSIS AND MANAGEMENT The main therapeutic decision in patients with AV conduction disturbance is whether or not a permanent pacemaker is required, and a number of circumstances exist in which His bundle electrocardiography can provide a useful diagnostic tool upon which to base this decision. It is unquestionable that patients with symptomatic second- or third-degree AV block should be paced, and therefore these patients do not require electrophysiologic study. However, intracardiac ECG recordings can be useful in at least the following four groups of patients:

1 Patients with syncope and bundle branch block without documentation of AV block. In such patients the demonstration of marked infra-His conduction disturbances, i.e., a prolonged HV interval (>80 ms) may usually be taken as an indication of the need for the insertion of a permanent pacemaker. With intervals ranging from 55 to 80 ms, the indications for pacing are equivocal. In this group observation appears most reasonable for those patients with normal HV intervals (<55 ms).
2 Patients with bundle branch block and second-degree AV block. When such patients are symptomatic, intracardiac recordings may demonstrate that AV nodal block, intra-His block, infra-His block, or combinations of block may be responsible. A finding that suggests an infra-His lesion is the presence of alternating bundle branch block associated with changing PR intervals. Intracardiac recordings in such patients show that when block is present in these patients, it is almost always in the His-Purkinje system. The finding of infra-His block in patients with asymptomatic second-degree AV block mandates pacemaker therapy because of the high likelihood of their developing symptomatic high-grade AV block and syncope.
3 Asymptomatic patients with third-degree AV block. In such patients electrophysiologic studies may be useful in assessing the stability of the junctional pacemaker. Pacing is indicated when the His bundle escape pacemaker is shown to be unstable by an inadequate response to excercise, atropine, or isoproterenol or by a prolonged junctional recovery time following ventricular pacing.
4 Patients with bundle branch block, particularly bifascicular block (see Chap. 178). Intracardiac recordings may be helpful in predicting whether these patients are at increased risk of developing AV block. HV intervals, even in excess of 80 ms, are not predictive of subsequent intra-His block. However, patients who have *extremely prolonged* HV intervals, i.e., >100 ms, and those in whom alternating bundle branch block is associated with changing HV intervals frequently develop complete AV block; therefore, these findings necessitate insertion of a pacemaker. Block below the His bundle developing during atrial pacing at rates of less than 150 beats per minute and the development of an infra-His block or HV prolongation >100 ms following 1 g procainamide intravenously also signify that the patient is at high risk for the development of subsequent AV block and that a pacemaker is indicated. The frequency of these findings is low so their widespread use may not be cost effective.

PACEMAKERS IN THE MANAGEMENT OF BRADYARRHYTHMIAS

External energy sources can be used to stimulate the heart when disorders in impulse formation and/or transmission occur, leading to symptomatic bradyarrhythmias. Pacer stimuli can be applied to the atria and/or ventricles.

TEMPORARY PACING This is usually instituted to provide immediate stabilization prior to permanent pacemaker placement or to provide pacemaker support when a bradycardia is precipitated by a transient event such as ischemia or drug toxicity. Temporary pacing is usually achieved by the transvenous insertion of an electrode catheter with the catheter positioned in the right ventricular apex and attached to an external generator. This procedure is associated with a small risk of cardiac perforation, infection at the insertion site, and thromboembolism; the risk of the latter two complications increases markedly after 48 h. The development of an entirely external transthoracic cardiac pacing system may preclude the need for transvenous pacing in selected patients. However, occasional failure of venticular capture and significant discomfort related to the large current required for effective transthoracic ventricular stimulation precludes the uniform use of this approach.

PERMANENT PACING This mode of pacing is instituted for persistent or intermittent symptomatic bradycardia not related to a self-limiting precipitating factor or for documented infranodal second- or third-degree AV block. Permanent pacing leads are usually inserted transvenously through the subclavian vein with the leads positioned in the right atrial appendage for atrial pacing and the right ventricular apex for ventricular pacing. The leads are then attached to the pulse generator, which is inserted into a subcutaneous pocket below the clavicle. Epicardial lead placement is used when: (1) transvenous access cannot be obtained; (2) the chest is already open, i.e., in the course of a cardiac operation; and (3) if adequate endocardial lead placement cannot be achieved. Two separate leads must be placed if both atrial and ventricular chambers are to be sensed and/or paced.

Most pacemaker generators are powered by lithium batteries. The life expectancy of the generator is related to (1) current output required for capture; (2) requirements for incessant or intermittent pacing; and (3) the number of cardiac chambers paced. Life expectancy of the simple ventricular demand pacemaker can exceed 10 years.

PACING CODE A code consisting of three to five letters has been developed for describing pacemaker type and function. The first letter indicates the chamber(s) paced and is designated *V* for ventricular pacing, *A* for atrial pacing, or *D* for dual chamber (both atrial and ventricular) pacing. The second letter indicates the chamber in which electrical activity is sensed and is also indicated by *A, V,* or *D*. An additional designation, *O*, has been used when pacemaker discharge is not dependent on a sensed electrical activity. The third letter refers to the response to a sensed electrical signal: *O* represents no response to an underlying electrical signal, usually related to the absence of associated sensing function; *I* represents inhibition of pacing function; *T* represents triggering of pacing function; and *D* indicates a dual response, i.e., spontaneous atrial and ventricular activity inhibiting atrial and ventricular pacing and atrial activity triggering a ventricular response. Additional fourth and fifth letters of the pacing code have been recommended to indicate whether the pacemaker is programmable and whether special antitachycardia functions are available. It follows from the described code that the standard VVI (ventricular demand pacemaker) can sense the ventricle, pace the ventricle, and be inhibited by sensed spontaneous ventricular activity, while the DDD pulse generator is capable of sensing and pacing both the atrium and ventricle and has a dual response to sensed atrial and ventricular activity.

Selection of the appropriate pacemaker and pacing mode depends on the clinical condition and the type of bradyarrhythmia being treated. The two most common pacing mode selections are DDD and VVI. DDD, or so-called universal pacing, provides AV sequential pacing which is ideally suited for the relatively young and active patient who has intact sinus node function or intermittent dysfunction and high-grade persistent or intermittent AV block. The DDD mode will allow physiologic atrial sensed and ventricular paced rates and improved exercise tolerance. AV synchrony and dual chamber pacing may also be desirable in patients with borderline hemodynamic reserve who are dependent on the atrial contribution to cardiac output and in those patients who develop the pacemaker syndrome (see below) in response to ventricular demand pacing. The DDD pacing mode is contraindicated in chronic atrial fibrillation or flutter and

TABLE 183-1 Programmable pacemaker functions

Rate*
Energy output
Sensitivity
Lead polarity
Hysteresis
Refractory period
Mode of function
AV Delay

* *Lower-end upper rate limits apply to dual-chamber pacing.*

atrial asystole. In these situations, ventricular demand (VVI) pacing is indicated. The DDD pacing mode may also be contraindicated in patients with intermittent or persistent ventriculoatrial (VA) conduction, who may develop pacemaker-mediated tachycardia (see below).

PROGRAMMABILITY OF PACEMAKERS This allows for modification of pacing function after implantation and thereby for adaptation to changes in clinical needs. Pacemaker programming is accomplished by activation of the programming head positioned over the implanted pulse generator after making the desired changes in programmable parameters (Table 183-1). A radiofrequency system is routinely used to communicate the program to the pacemaker.

COMPLICATIONS Adverse effects of permanent pacing are usually associated with failure or malfunction of the pacing system. These problems are usually secondary to over- or undersensing, output failure, and/or lead fracture or displacement. Two other problems may occur. The *pacemaker syndrome* consists of fatigue, dizziness, syncope, and distressing pulsations in the neck and chest and can be related to adverse hemodynamic effects of ventricular pacing. The pathophysiologic contributors to the pacemaker syndrome include (1) loss of atrial contribution to ventricular systole; (2) vasodepressor reflex initiated by cannon *a* waves; (3) systemic and pulmonary venous regurgitation due to atrial contraction against a closed AV valve. The symptoms associated with the pacemaker syndrome can be obviated by maintaining AV synchrony by dual chamber pacing or, in the case of a ventricular demand pacemaker, by programming an escape rate 15 to 20 beats per minute below that of the paced rate. The second major problem peculiar to dual chamber pacemakers is the development of *pacemaker-mediated tachycardia,* which is caused by ventriculoatrial conduction. In this instance, retrograde depolarization of the atria, resulting from a premature ventricular depolarization or a paced ventricular complex, is sensed and leads to subsequent triggering of ventricular pacing. This, in turn, can result in repetition of the phenomenon of ventriculoatrial conduction with the development of an endless-loop, pacemaker-mediated tachycardia. It may be corrected by programming the atrial refractory period.

REFERENCES

AUSTIN JL et al: Analysis of pacemaker malfunction and complications of temporary pacing in the coronary care unit. Am J Cardiol 49:301, 1982

BECKER AE et al: Functional anatomy of the cardiac conducting system, in *Cardiac Arrhythmias, A Decade of Progress*, DC Harrison (ed). Boston, G.K. Hall, 1981

CHUNG EK: Sick sinus syndrome: Current views. Mod Concepts Cardiovasc Dis 49:61, 1980

FURMAN S: Newer modes of cardiac pacing: Description of pacing modes. Mod Concepts Cardiovasc Dis 52:1, 1983

JOSEPHSON ME, SEIDES SF: *Clinical Cardiac Electrophysiology: Techniques and Interpretations*. Philadelphia, Lea & Febiger, 1979

LUDMER PL, GOLDSCHLAGER N: Cardiac pacing in the 1980's. N Engl J Med 311:1671, 1984

NARULA OS, SHANTHA N: Atrioventricular block: Clinical concepts and His bundle electrocardiography, in *Cardiac Arrthythmias*, WJ Mandel (ed). Philadelphia, Lippincott, 1980

PARSONETT V et al: Indications for dual chamber pacing. PACE 7:318, 1984

TONKIN AM, HEDDLE WF: Electrophysiological testing of sinus node function. PACE 7:735, 1984

ZOLL PM et al: External noninvasive temporary cardiac pacing: Clinical trials. Circulation 71:937, 1985

184 THE TACHYARRHYTHMIAS

MARK E. JOSEPHSON / ALFRED E. BUXTON / FRANCIS E. MARCHLINSKI

MECHANISMS OF TACHYARRHYTHMIAS

Tachyarrhythmias may be divided into disorders of impulse propagation and disorders of impulse formation. Disorders of impulse propagation (reentry) are generally considered to be the most common mechanism of sustained paroxysmal tachyarrhythmias. The requirements to initiate reentry include: (1) electrophysiologic inhomogeneity (i.e., differences in conduction and/or refractoriness) in two or more regions of the heart connected with each other to form a potentially closed loop; (2) unidirectional block in one pathway; (3) slow conduction over an alternative pathway, allowing time for the initially blocked pathway to recover excitability; and (4) reexcitation of the initially blocked pathway to complete a loop of activation. Repetitive circulation of the impulse over this loop can produce a sustained tachyarrhythmia. While anatomic obstacles may underlie reentry and provide an inexcitable center around which the impulse can circulate, they are not essential. Reentrant arrhythmias can be initiated as well as terminated by premature complexes and can be interrupted by rapid stimulation (overdrive suppression), which can help distinguish them from arrhythmias caused by triggered activity.

Disorders of impulse formation can be subdivided into tachyarrhythmias caused by enhanced automaticity and those caused by triggered activity. In addition to the sinus node, automatic pacemaker activity can be observed in specialized atrial fibers, fibers of the atrioventricular (AV) junction, and Purkinje fibers (see Chap. 183). Myocardial cells do not normally possess pacemaker activity. *Enhancement of normal automaticity* in latent pacemaker fibers or the development of abnormal automaticity due to partial depolarization of the resting membrane occurs as a consequence of a variety of pathophysiologic states, which include (1) increased endogenous or exogenous catecholamines; (2) electrolyte disturbances (e.g., hypokalemia, hypercalcemia); (3) hypoxia or ischemia; (4) mechanical effects (e.g., stretch); and (5) drugs (e.g., digitalis). Tachycardia caused by abnormal automaticity cannot be started or stopped by pacing.

Triggered activity has been observed in atrial, ventricular, and His-Purkinje tissue under conditions such as increased local catecholamine concentration, hyperkalemia, hypercalcemia, and digitalis intoxication. All of these conditions produce an accumulation of intracellular calcium which causes depolarizations following the action potential, termed *afterdepolarizations*. With increasing amplitude of the afterdepolarizations, threshold can be reached and repetitive activity produced. In contrast to automatic rhythms, triggered activity requires preceding activity for initiation and therefore can be initiated by pacing. In contrast to tachyarrhythmias caused by automaticity and reentry, the response of triggered activity to overdrive pacing is acceleration.

The use of electrophysiologic (EP) studies, i.e., intracardiac recordings and programmed stimulation, has greatly expanded our understanding of the mechanisms of tachyarrhythmias. In addition to helping in the diagnosis of arrhythmias, these techniques may be of value in determining the most appropriate types of therapy. EP studies of tachycardias require the positioning of multiple electrode catheters at critical areas within the heart; these electrodes must be capable of both stimulating and recording from multiple sites in the atria and/or ventricles.

PREMATURE COMPLEXES

ATRIAL PREMATURE COMPLEXES (APCs) APCs can be found on 24-h Holter monitoring in over 60 percent of normal adults. APCs are usually asymptomatic and benign, although at times they may be associated with palpitations. In susceptible patients, they can initiate paroxysmal supraventricular tachycardias. APCs may originate from any location in either atrium, and they are recognized on the ECG as early P waves with a morphology which differs from the sinus P wave. While APCs conduct to the ventricles normally when they occur late in the cardiac cycle, those appearing relatively early may reach the AV conduction system while it is still in its relative refractory period, resulting in a conduction delay manifested by a prolonged PR interval following the premature P wave (Fig. 184-1*A*). Very early APCs may even block in the AV node if this structure is encountered during its effective refractory period. APCs, whether conducted or not, are usually followed by a pause before a return to sinus activity. Most commonly, an APC enters and resets the sinus node, so that the sum of the pre- and postextrasystolic PP intervals is less than the sum of two sinus PP intervals (Fig. 184-1*A*). In this

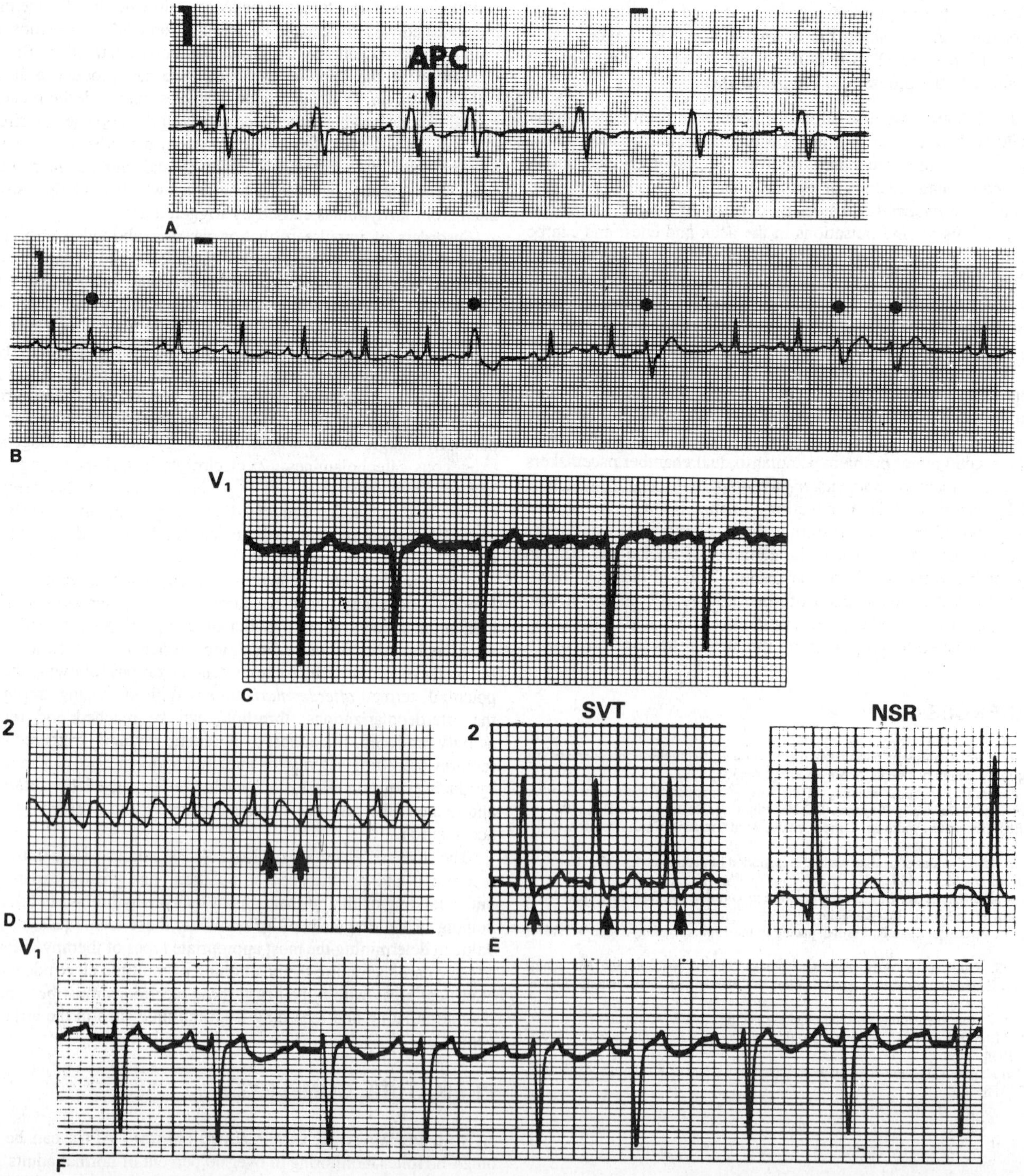

FIGURE 184-1 *A. Atrial premature complex. Lead I. Following a third sinus beat an atrial premature complex (APC) occurs which conducts slowly (prolonged PR interval) to the ventricles. The pause that follows the APC is less than compensatory. B. Complex ventricular ectopy. Lead II. Multiformed ventricular premature complexes (VPCs) and a couplet are shown (see dots). C. Atrial fibrillation. AF is characterized by an undulating baseline with an irregular ventricular response. D. Atrial flutter. Lead II. Note the sawtooth configuration of the flutter waves (arrows). E. AV nodal reentrant supraventricular tachycardia. Lead II is shown during supraventricular tachycardia (SVT) and normal sinus rhythm (NSR). The characteristic findings during SVT are pseudo S waves in lead II, which represent retrograde atrial activation. F. Proxysmal atrial tachycardia with block due to digitalis intoxication. A V_1 rhythm strip is shown at a paper speed of 50 mm/s. Atrial tachycardia is present at a rate of approximately 170 beats per minute. Every other P wave conducts to the ventricles, producing a ventricular response of 85 beats per minute.*

case the pause is said to be less than fully compensatory. The QRS complex following most APCs is normal, although early APCs may be followed by aberrantly conducted QRS complexes.

Since most APCs are asymptomatic, treatment is not required. When they cause palpitations or trigger paroxysmal supraventricular tachycardias (see below), treatment may be useful. Factors which precipitate APCs such as alcohol, tobacco, or adrenergic stimulants should be identified and eliminated, and in their absence mild sedation or the use of a beta blocker may be tried. If this fails, quinidine, procainamide, or a similar agent (Table 184-2) may be used.

AV JUNCTIONAL COMPLEXES The site of origin of these complexes is thought to be in the bundle of His, since the AV node itself possesses no automaticity (page 916). AV junctional complexes are less common than either atrial or ventricular premature complexes and are more often associated with cardiac disease or digitalis intoxication. Junctional premature impulses can conduct both antegradely to the ventricles and retrogradely to the atrium and, on rare occasions, may fail to conduct in either direction. Premature AV junctional complexes can be recognized by normal-appearing QRS complexes that are not preceded by a P wave. Retrograde P waves (inverted in leads II, III, and aV_F) may be observed after the QRS complex.

While often asymptomatic, junctional premature complexes may be associated with palpitations and cause cannon *a* waves which may result in distressing pulsations in the neck. When symptomatic, they should be treated like APCs.

VENTRICULAR PREMATURE COMPLEXES (VPCs) These are among the most common arrhythmia's and occur in patients with or without heart disease. Of adult males ≥60 percent will exhibit VPCs during a 24-h Holter monitoring. In patients without heart disease, VPCs have not been shown to be associated with any increased incidence in mortality or morbidity. VPCs may occur in up to 80 percent of patients with previous myocardial infarction, and in this setting, if frequent (>10 per hour) and/or complex (occurring in couplets or triplets), they have been associated with increased mortality. However, cardiac mortality in such patients usually occurs in association with significantly impaired ventricular function. While frequent and complex ventricular ectopy is an independent risk factor, it is not as strong a risk factor as is impaired ventricular function. Morever, even though ventricular tachycardia and/or fibrillation may be the basis for the sudden death in these patients, this does not a priori establish a cause-and-effect relation between spontaneous ectopy and life-threatening ventricular fibrillation. Very early VPCs have been stated by some to increase the risk of sudden death. Although this has been observed during acute ischemia and in the setting of QT prolongation, frequently ventricular tachycardia or fibrillation is precipitated by VPCs which occur after the T wave of the prior beat.

VPCs are recognized by wide (usually >0.14 s), bizarre QRS complexes that are not preceded by P waves (Fig. 184-1*B*). Often they bear a relatively fixed relationship to the preceding sinus complex and are thus considered *fixed coupled* VPCs. When fixed coupling is not present and the interval between VPCs has a common denominator, *ventricular parasystole* is said to be present. Under these circumstances the VPCs are a manifestation of abnormal automaticity of a ventricular focus which is protected so that it is not penetrated by sinus impulses which therefore do not reset this parasystolic focus, thereby allowing the interectopic intervals to remain fixed.

VPCs may occur singly in patterns of bigeminy, in which every sinus beat is followed by a VPC; trigeminy, in which two sinus beats are followed by a VPC; quadrigeminy, etc. Two successive VPCs are termed *pairs* or *couplets,* while three or more consecutive VPCs are termed *ventricular tachycardia*. Morphologically, VPCs may have a similar morphology (monomorphic) or may have different morphologies (multiformed or polymorphic) (Fig. 184-1*B*).

Most commonly VPCs are not conducted retrogradely to the atrium and the sinoatrial node and produce a fully compensatory pause, so that the interval between conducted beats which bracket the VPC equals two basic RR intervals. Ventricular impulses may also manifest retrograde conduction to the atrium and cause inverted P waves in leads II, III, and aV_F. The pause that results may therefore be less than compensatory. In many instances, the QRS complex will not be associated with retrograde ventriculoatrial (VA) conduction but may block in the AV node. This renders the AV node refractory to the subsequent sinus beat and causes a block of the sinus P wave or conduction with a markedly prolonged PR interval. This prolonged PR interval is said to be a manifestation of *concealed retrograde conduction* of the ventricular impulse into the AV node. A VPC which does not produce any manifestation of retrograde concealed conduction and fails to influence the oncoming sinus impulse is termed an *interpolated VPC*.

VPCs can cause palpitations or neck pulsations secondary to either the occurrence of cannon *a* waves or the increased force of contraction due to post extrasystolic potentiation of ventricular contractility. Patients with frequent VPCs or bigeminy may develop syncope because the VPCs do not result in an adequate stroke volume and the cardiac output is reduced.

Management In the absence of cardiac disease, isolated asymptomatic VPCs, regardless of configuration and frequency, need no treatment. When arrhythmias are symptomatic, the symptoms should first be addressed by either allaying the patient's anxiety with reassurance, or if this is not successful, reducing the frequency of the VPCs with antiarrhythmic agents. Beta-adrenergic blockers (page 366) may be successful in managing VPCs which occur primarily in the daytime or under stressful situations and in specific settings such as mitral valve prolapse and thyrotoxicosis. Quinidine or quinidine-like agents may be tried should this be unsuccessful. In patients with cardiac disease, frequent VPCs are often associated with an increased risk of sudden and nonsudden cardiac death, and many physicians attempt to eliminate or reduce the frequency of these VPCs in an attempt to reduce this risk. However, the cause-and-effect relationship of the VPCs to fatal events has not been established, and it has not been shown definitively that the suppression of VPCs with antiarrhythmic drugs prevents sudden death. In addition, it is important to recognize that the antiarrhythmic agents can also produce the lethal arrhythmias which they are given to prevent. Thus, therapy directed toward VPCs in the setting of chronic cardiac disease may result in an inappropriate and costly use of agents without proven efficacy and with potential side effects in many patients. The high incidence of side effects and the frequent exacerbation of arrhythmias caused by all antiarrhythmic drugs by them makes it mandatory for one to monitor patients being treated with such agents.

In the presence of acute myocardial infarction the greatest incidence of primary ventricular fibrillation occurs within the first 24 h. Temporary prophylactic antiarrhythmic therapy has therefore been recommended for all patients with this condition, regardless of the presence and/or degree of spontaneous ectopy (see Chap. 190).

TACHYCARDIAS

Tachycardias refer to arrhythmias with three or more complexes at rates exceeding 100 beats per minute and occur more often in structurally diseased than in normal hearts. Those paroxysmal tachycardias that are initiated by APCs or VPCs are considered to be due to reentry. Some of the digitalis-induced tachyarrhythmias are due to triggered activity (see below).

If the patient is hemodynamically stable, an attempt should be made to determine the mechanism and origin of the tachycardia since this will usually lead to an appropriate therapeutic decision. It is useful first to compare the ECG during the tachycardia with one recorded during sinus rhythm, and it is often desirable to record long rhythm strips using surface leads with the largest P waves, usually lead II or V_1. One can also utilize electrodes situated at the end of a flexible pacing catheter inserted into the esophagus behind the left atrium to record atrial activity. Information to be obtained from the ECG includes (1) the presence, frequency, morphology, and regularity of P waves and QRS complexes; (2) the relationship between atrial and ventricular activity; (3) a comparison of the QRS morphology during sinus rhythm and during the tachycardia; and (4) the response to carotid sinus massage or other vagal maneuvers.

Carotid sinus pressure should only be performed while the patient is electrocardiographically monitored with resuscitative equipment available to manage the rare episode of asystole and/or ventricular fibrillation. Carotid sinus massage should not be performed in patients with carotid arterial bruits. The patient should be positioned flat with the neck extended. Massage of one carotid bulb at a time should be performed by applying firm pressure just underneath the angle of the jaw for up to 5 s. Alternative vagomimetic maneuvers include the Valsalva maneuver, immersion of the face in cold water, and the administration of 5 to 10 mg edrophonium.

Observation of the jugular venous pulse can provide clues to the presence of atrial activity and its relationship to ventricular ectopy. Intermittent cannon *a* waves suggest AV dissociation, while persistent cannon *a* waves suggest 1:1 VA conduction. Flutter waves may be seen or no atrial activity may be apparent, as in the presence of atrial flutter and fibrillation, respectively. The arterial pulse may also manifest AV dissociation by demonstrating variations in amplitude. A first heart sound of variable intensity during a regular rhythm also suggests AV dissociation.

SINUS TACHYCARDIA In the adult sinus tachycardia is said to be present when the heart rate exceeds 100 beats per minute; sinus tachycardia does not usually exceed 200 beats per minute and is not a primary arrhythmia; instead, it represents a physiologic response to a variety of stresses, such as fever, volume depletion, anxiety, exercise, thyrotoxicosis, hypoxemia, hypotension, or congestive heart failure. Sinus tachycardia has a gradual onset and offset. The ECG demonstrates P waves with sinus contour preceding each QRS complex. Carotid sinus pressure usually produces modest slowing with a gradual return to the previous rate upon cessation. This contrasts with the paroxysmal supraventricular tachycardias which may slow slightly and terminate abruptly.

Sinus tachycardia should not be treated as a primary arrhythmia, since it is always a physiologic response to a demand placed on the heart. As such, the therapy should be directed to the primary disorder. This may involve institution of digitalis and/or diuretics for heart failure, oxygen for hypoxemia, treatment of thyrotoxicosis, volume repletion, aspirin for fever, or tranquilizers for emotional upset.

ATRIAL FIBRILLATION (AF) This common arrhythmia may occur in paroxysmal and persistent forms. It may be seen in normal subjects, particularly during emotional stress or following surgery, exercise, or acute alcoholic intoxication. It may also occur in patients with heart or lung disease who develop acute hypoxia, hypercapnia, or metabolic or hemodynamic derangements. Persistent AF usually occurs in patients with cardiovascular disease, most commonly rheumatic heart disease, nonrheumatic mitral valve disease, hypertensive cardiovascular disease, chronic lung disease, atrial septal defect, and a variety of miscellaneous cardiac abnormalities. AF may be the presenting finding in thyrotoxicosis. So-called lone AF, which occurs in elderly patients without underlying heart disease, is considered to represent the tachycardiac phase of the bradycardia-syndrome (page 918).

The morbidity associated with AF is related to (1) excessive rate of the ventricular response, which in turn may lead to hypotension or angina pectoris in susceptible individuals; (2) the pause following cessation of AF (page 918), which can cause syncope; (3) systemic embolization, which occurs most commonly in patients with rheumatic heart disease; (4) loss of the contribution of atrial contraction to cardiac output, which may cause fatigue; and (5) anxiety secondary to palpitations. In patients with severe cardiac dysfunction, particularly those with hypertrophied, noncompliant ventricles, the combination of the loss of the atrial contribution to ventricular filling and the abbreviated filling period due to the rapid ventricular rate in AF can produce marked hemodynamic embarrassment, syncope, or heart failure. In patients with mitral stenosis in whom filling time is critical, development of AF with a rapid ventricular rate may precipitate pulmonary edema (see Chap. 187).

AF is characterized by disorganized atrial activity without discrete P waves on the surface ECG (Fig. 184-1*C*). Atrial activation is manifested by an undulating baseline or by more sharply inscribed atrial deflections of varying amplitude and frequency ranging from 350 to 600 per minute. The ventricular response is irregularly irregular. This results from the large number of atrial impulses which penetrate the AV node, making it partially refractory to subsequent impulses. This effect of nonconducted atrial impulses to influence the response to subsequent atrial impulses is termed *concealed conduction*. As a result, the ventricular response is relatively slow, considering the actual atrial rate. If AF converts to atrial flutter, which has a slower atrial rate, the effect of concealed conduction may be diminished and a paradoxic increase in the ventricular response may occur. The main factor determining the rate of the ventricular response is the functional refractory period of the AV node or the most rapid paced rate at which 1:1 conduction through the AV node can be observed.

If, in the presence of AF, the ventricular rhythm becomes regular and slow (e.g., 30 to 60 beats per minute), complete heart block is suggested, and if the rhythm is regular and rapid ($\geq$100 beats per minute), a tachycardia arising in the AV junction or ventricle should be suspected. Digitalis intoxication is a common cause of both of these phenomena.

Patients with AF exhibit a loss of *a* waves in the jugular venous pulse and variable pulse pressures in the carotid arterial pulse. The first heart sound usually varies in intensity. On echocardiography, the left atrium is frequently enlarged, and in patients in whom the left atrial diameter exceeds 4.5 cm, it may not be possible to convert AF to sinus rhythm or to maintain the latter despite therapy.

Management In acute AF, a precipitating factor such as fever, pneumonia, alcoholic intoxication, thyrotoxicosis, pulmonary emboli, or pericarditis should be sought. When such a factor is present, therapy should be directed toward the primary abnormality. If the patient's clinical status is severely compromised, electrical cardioversion is the treatment of choice. In the absence of severe cardiovascular compromise, slowing of ventricular rate becomes the initial therapeutic goal. This may be accomplished with digitalis, calcium channel antagonists, or beta-adrenergic blockers, all of which prolong the refractory period of and slow conduction in the AV node. Conversion to sinus rhythm may then be attempted, using quinidine or quinidine-like (type IA) agents (Table 184-1). It is important to slow AV node conduction *prior* to administering such drugs because their vagolytic effect and ability to convert AF to atrial flutter may reduce the concealed conduction and lead to an excessively rapid

TABLE 184-1 Classification of antiarrhythmic drugs

Type I	Drugs that reduce maximal velocity of phase 0 depolarization ($\dot{V}_{max}$) due to block of inward Na^+ current in tissue with fast response action potentials A $\downarrow$ $\dot{V}_{max}$ at all heart rates and $\uparrow$ action potential duration e.g., quinidine, procainamide, disopyramide B Little effect at slow rates on $\dot{V}_{max}$ in normal tissue; $\dot{V}_{max}$ in partially depolarized cells with fast response action potentials Effects increased at faster rates No change or $\downarrow$ in action potential duration, e.g., lidocaine, phenytoin, tocainide, mexiletine C $\downarrow$ $\dot{V}_{max}$ at normal rates in normal tissue Minimal effect on action potential duration, e.g., encainide, lorcainide, flecainide
Type II	Antisympathetic agents, e.g., propranolol and other beta-adenergic blockers; automaticity, AV nodal refractoriness, and conduction velocity
Type III	Agents that prolong action potential duration in tissue with fast response action potentials, e.g., bretylium, amiodarone
Type IV	Calcium (slow) channel blocking agents—decrease conduction velocity and increase refractoriness in tissue with slow response action potentials, e.g., verapamil, diltiazem

ventricular response. Beta-adrenergic blockers are especially useful in this regard. If medical therapy fails to convert AF, electrical cardioversion is useful; it generally requires 100 to 200 W·s of energy. Anticoagulation should be started at least 2 weeks prior to and continued for 2 weeks following any attempt at electrical cardioversion, either pharmacologic or electrical, in patients with long-standing AF. Anticoagulation appears to decrease the incidence of systemic embolization associated with cardioversion. It is less likely for chronic AF to convert to or remain in sinus rhythm in the presence of long-standing rheumatic heart disease and/or when the atria are markedly enlarged. It is also unlikely for patients with lone AF to be converted to and maintained in sinus rhythm.

If sinus rhythm is restored electrically or pharmacologically, quinidine or related agents may be used to prevent recurrence. In patients in whom cardioversion is unsuccessful or in whom AF is likely to recur, it is probably wisest to allow the patient to remain in AF and to control the ventricular response with calcium antagonists, beta-adrenergic blockers, or digitalis. Since they are always at risk of systemic embolization, chronic anticoagulation must be considered for such patients.

ATRIAL FLUTTER This arrhythmia occurs almost invariably in patients with organic heart disease. Flutter may be paroxysmal, in which case there is usually a precipitating factor, such as pericarditis or acute respiratory failure, or it may be persistent. Atrial flutter (as well as AF) is very common during the first week following open heart surgery. Atrial flutter is usually less long-lived than is AF, although on occasion it may persist for months to years. Most commonly, if it lasts for more than a week, atrial flutter will convert to AF. Systemic embolization is less common in atrial flutter than AF.

Atrial flutter is characterized by an atrial rate between 250 and 350 beats per minute. Typically, the ventricular rate is half the atrial rate, i.e., approximately 150 beats per minute. If the atrial rate is slowed to <220 per minute by antiarrhythmic agents such as quinidine, which also possess vagolytic properties, the ventricular rate may rise suddenly because of the development of 1:1 AV conduction. Classically, flutter waves are seen as regular sawtooth-like atrial activity, most prominent in the inferior leads (Fig. 184-1*D*). When the ventricular response is regular and not a simple fraction of the atrial rate, AV block is present. Activation mapping suggests that atrial flutter is a form of atrial reentry localized to the low right atrium.

Management The most effective treatment of atrial flutter is dc cardioversion, which can be accomplished with low energy (10 to 50 W·s) under mild sedation. In patients who develop atrial flutter following open heart surgery or recurrent flutter in the setting of acute myocardial infarction, particularly when they are being treated with digitalis, atrial pacing (using temporary pacing wires implanted at the time of operation or using a pacing lead inserted into the atrium pervenously) at rates of 115 to 130 percent of the atrial flutter rate can usually convert the atrial flutter to sinus rhythm. Atrial pacing may also result in the conversion of atrial flutter into AF, which allows for easier control of the ventricular response. If immediate conversion of atrial flutter is not mandated by the patient's clinical status, the ventricular response should first be slowed by blocking the AV node with a beta blocker, calcium antagonist, or digitalis; the latter drug occasionally converts atrial flutter into AF. Once AV nodal conduction is delayed with any of these drugs, an attempt to convert flutter to sinus rhythm using quinidine or quinidine-like agents should be made. Increasing doses of the drug selected are administered until the rhythm converts or side effects occur.

Quinidine, quinidine-like drugs, and amiodarone, an experimental drug, (Table 184-2) are useful in preventing recurrences of both atrial flutter and fibrillation.

PAROXYSMAL SUPRAVENTRICULAR TACHYCARDIAS (PSVT) In most cases functional differences in conduction and refractoriness in the AV node or the presence of an AV bypass tract provide the substrate for the development of PSVT (previously termed paroxysmal atrial tachycardia). Electrophysiologic studies have demonstrated that *reentry* is the mechanism responsible for the vast majority of PSVT. Reentry has been localized to the sinus node, atrium, AV node, or to a macroreentrant circuit involving normal conduction in the antegrade direction through the AV node and retrograde conduction through an AV bypass tract. Such a bypass tract may also conduct antegradely, in which case the Wolff-Parkinson-White (WPW) syndrome is said to be present. More frequently, however, the bypass tract manifests only retrograde conduction, and therefore it is termed a *concealed* bypass tract. In the absence of the WPW syndrome, reentry through the AV node or through a *concealed* bypass tract makes up more than 90 percent of all PSVTs.

AV nodal reentrant tachycardia There is no age, sex, or disease predisposition for the development of AV nodal reentrant tachycardia, the most common cause of supraventricular tachycardia. This usually presents as a narrow QRS complex with regular rates ranging from 120 to 250 per minute. APCs which initiate the arrhythmia are almost always associated with a prolonged PR interval. Retrograde P waves may be absent, buried in the QRS complex, or appear as distortions at the terminal parts of the QRS complex.

AV nodal reentrant PSVT (Fig. 184-1*E*) can be reproducibly initiated and terminated by appropriately timed atrial premature extra stimuli. The onset of the tachycardia is almost always associated with prolongation of the PR interval due to marked AV nodal conduction delay (prolonged AH interval) that is critical for the genesis of the arrhythmia. The sudden prolongation of the AH interval is consistent with the concept of dual AV nodal pathways as the substrate for AV nodal reentry. This concept (Fig. 184-2) assumes that the AV node is longitudinally dissociated into two functionally different pathways: (1) a beta pathway which exhibits rapid conduction and a long refractory period (fast pathway), and (2) an alpha pathway which has a short refractory period but conducts slowly (slow pathway). During sinus rhythm the atrial impulse travels over the beta pathway to produce a single QRS complex with a normal PR interval. The impulse which simultaneously conducts down the slow pathway reaches the His bundle after it has been depolarized and is therefore refractory. Atrial extra stimuli are blocked in the beta pathway because of its longer refractory period and are conducted slowly through the alpha pathway. If conduction down the alpha pathway is slow enough to allow the previously refractory beta pathway time to recover excitability, a single atrial echo or sustained tachycardia ensues. A critical balance between conduction velocity and refractoriness within the node is required to sustain AV nodal reentry. Atrial and ventricular activation occur simultaneously, explaining why no P waves may be apparent on the surface ECG.

CLINICAL FEATURES AV nodal reentry may produce palpitations, syncope, and heart failure, depending on the rate and duration of the arrhythmia and the presence and severity of any underlying heart disease. Hypotension and syncope may occur because of the sudden loss of the atrial contribution to ventricular filling; this can also lead to a marked increase in atrial pressure, acute pulmonary edema, and a reduction in ventricular filling. Simultaneous atrial and ventricular contraction produces cannon *a* waves with each heart beat.

TREATMENT In patients without hypotension, vagal maneuvers, particularly carotid sinus massage, can terminate the arrhythmia in 80 percent of cases. If hypotension is present, raising the blood pressure by the cautious use of phenylephrine may terminate the arrhythmia alone or may aid termination with carotid sinus pressure. If these maneuvers are unsuccessful, verapamil (2.5 to 10 mg intravenously) is the agent of first choice. Propranolol (0.05 to 0.2 mg/kg, intravenously) or other beta blockers may be used. Digitalis glycosides have a slower onset of action. When these drugs fail to terminate the tachycardia or when the tachycardia is recurrent, pacing via a temporary pacemaker inserted pervenously may be used to terminate the arrhythmia.

AV nodal reentry can usually be prevented by the use of drugs

TABLE 184-2 Electrophysiologic effects

Drug	Sinus node	Atrium and ventricle	AV node	His-Purkinje system	Atrioventricular bypass tracts
Digoxin and other cardiac glycosides (also see p. 910)	No change; patients with sinus node disease may develop sinus exit block or arrest	Controversial	Increase in ERP; decreased conduction velocity	No change	No change or decrease in ERP
Propranolol and other beta-adrenoreceptor blockers (also see p. 980)	Decreased sinus rate; increased sinus node recovery time	No change	Increase in ERP; decreased conduction velocity	No change	No change
Verapamil	Decreased sinus rate; sinus exit block in patients with sinus node disease	No change	Increase in ERP; decreased conduction velocity	No change	Indirect effects may decrease ERP when given IV
Quinidine	No change; may suppress sinus node in patients with underlying sinus node disease	Increase in ERP; decreased conduction velocity	Decrease or no change in ERP, no change in conduction velocity	Decreased automaticity; decreased conduction velocity; increased ERP	Increase in ERP
Procainamide	No change	Increase in ERP; decreased conduction velocity	Decrease or no change in ERP; decrease or no change in conduction velocity	Decreased automaticity; decreased conduction velocity; Increased ERP	Increase in ERP
Disopyramide	No change	Increase in ERP; decreased conduction velocity	Decrease or no change in ERP; no change in conduction velocity	Decreased automaticity; increased ERP; decreased conduction velocity	Increase in ERP
Lidocaine	No change	No change in ERP	No change or decrease in ERP	No change or decrease in ERP	No change, decrease, or increase in ERP
Phenytoin	No change	No change in ERP	No change or decrease in ERP; no change or increased conduction velocity	Decrease in ERP; decreased automaticity	
Tocainide	No change	No change	No change	No change; decreased automaticity	Increase in ERP
Bretylium	Initial increase in sinus rate followed by decrease	Increase in ERP	No change	No change	
Amiodarone*	Decreased sinus rate	Increase in ERP	Increase in ERP; decreased conduction velocity	Increase in ERP; decreased conduction velocity	Increase in ERP
Mexiletine*	No change; patients with sinus node disease may develop sinus arrest	No change	Variable and inconsistent effects on conduction and refractoriness	Increase in ERP; no change or decreased conduction velocity	

* *Investigation.*

NOTE: *AV = atrioventricular, ERP = effective refractory period, IV = intravenous, SVT = supraventricular tachycardia, VT = ventricular tachycardia, AF = atrial fibrillation, VF = ventricular fibrillation.*

which act primarily on the antegrade slow pathway (such as digitalis, beta blockers, or calcium antagonists) or on the fast pathway (such as quinidine). Drugs most likely to prevent recurrences prevent induction of the arrhythmias by programmed stimulation. This technique utilizes temporary pacemaker catheters connected to a physiologic stimulator capable of variable rate pacing and stimulation with one or more precisely timed premature impulses. If episodes of PSVT are frequent and produce disabling symptoms, therapy based on electrophysiologic studies is preferable to empiric drug trials. Antitachycardia pacemakers can be used to terminate PSVT due to AV nodal reentry when these arrhythmias occur infrequently. Ablation of the AV junction (page 937) has been developed as a method of controlling AV nodal reentry, but this approach should only be considered as a last resort since it usually mandates insertion of a permanent pacemaker.

AV reentrant tachycardia PSVT due to AV reentry incorporates an AV bypass tract which conducts only retrogradely as part of the tachycardia circuit. Thus, the impulse passes antegradely from the atria through the AV node and His-Purkinje system to the ventricles, then retrogradely through the (concealed) bypass tract back to the atrium. Patients with this disorder manifest the same type of PSVT as do patients with the WPW syndrome (see below), but the bypass tract does not conduct in an antegrade direction in AV reentry tachycardia.

AV reentrant tachycardia can be initiated and terminated by either APCs or VPCs. Alternation of the QRS complexes and/or T wave occurs in approximately one-third of such tachycardias. Since atrial activation must follow ventricular activation during AV reentry, the P wave usually occurs after the QRS complex.

Atrial activation mapping is of major value in evaluating the origin

Indications	Side effects and toxicity
Slowing of ventricular rate during AF, atrial flutter, and other atrial tachycardias in the absence of preexcitation; SVT due to AV nodal reentry and AV reentry utilizing bypass tracts	Atrial tachycardia, VT, AV nodal block, accelerated junctional rhythms, atrial and ventricular premature depolarizations, VT, ventricular fibrillation, anorexia, nausea, vomiting; acceleration of ventricular rate during atrial fibrillation/flutter in the presence of preexcitation causing ventricular fibrillation
Slowing of ventricular rate during AF, atrial flutter, and other atrial tachycardias in the absence of preexcitation; SVT due to AV nodal reentry, reentry utilizing bypass tracts; arrhythmias induced by exercise, arrhythmias occurring in the presence of hyperthyroidism; polymorphic VT associated with congenital long QT syndrome	Sinus bradycardia, AV nodal block, congestive heart failure, bronchospasm, masking symptoms of hypoglycemia
Same as digoxin	Sinus arrest in patients with sinus node dysfunction; AV nodal block in patients with AV nodal dysfunction; exacerbation of congestive heart failure (may be potentiated in presence of beta-adrenergic blocking agents); elevation of digoxin levels; hypotension following IV administration; IV administration during AF/flutter in the presence of preexcitation may cause acceleration of ventricular response rate and VF or hemodynamic collapse; IV administration to patients with VT may cause hemodynamic collapse
Atrial and ventricular extrasystoles; atrial and ventricular tachyarrhythmias; all types of SVT; control of ventricular rate in patients with preexcitation and AF and flutter	Anorexia, nausea, vomiting, diarrhea; cinchonism: tinnitus, confusion, hearing and visual changes; thrombocytopenia, hemolytic anemia, rash; drug interactions: elevation of digoxin levels; phenytoin and phenobarbital will decrease quinidine levels; QT prolongation associated with polymorphic VT (torsade de pointes); conversion of nonsustained to sustained VT; acceleration of ventricular response to atrial flutter and fibrillation
Same as quinidine	Anorexia, nausea, confusion, hallucinations; agranulocytosis; lupus erythematosus-like syndrome; QT prolongation associated with polymorphic VT (torsade de pointes); marked elevations in the primary metabolite (NAPA) may be more likely to cause polymorphic VT; conversion of nonsustained into sustained VT; acceleration of ventricular response to atrial flutter and fibrillation
Same as quinidine	Anticholinergic actions including dry mouth, blurred vision, urinary retention or hesitancy, constipation, narrow angle glaucoma; congestive heart failure, especially in patients with abnormal ventricular function; QT prolongation associated with polymorphic VT (torsade de pointes)
VT and VF especially during acute ischemia and myocardial infarction	Dizziness, paresthesias, confusion, delirium, seizures, coma; may depress sinus node in patients with underlying sinus node disease; may suppress escape foci in patients with complete heart block; congestive heart failure or liver disease increase risk of side effects
Tachyarrhythmias induced by digitalis; occasionally effective for ventricular tachyarrhythmias not induced by digitalis alone or in combination with other antiarrhythmic agents; polymorphic VT associated with increased QT	Gingival hypertrophy, rash, blood dyscrasias, nystagmus, ataxia, stupor coma, lupus erythematosis syndrome; lymph node hyperplasia, peripheral neuropathy, hypocalcemia, hyperglycemia; phlebitis and hypotension during IV administration
VT, VF, frequent VPCs	Ataxia, tremor, paresthesias, lightheadedness, nausea, rash, lupus erythematosus syndrome, pulmonary fibrosis, bone marrow suppression; may exacerbate heart failure in patients with ventricular dysfunction
Refractory ventricular VT and VF, especially due to acute ischemia	Initially, transient hypertension; subsequently, hypotension increased in the upright position; the hypotensive effect can be prevented by tricyclic drugs; nausea, vomiting
Refractory atrial and ventricular tachyarrhythmias; refractory SVT due to AV nodal reentry and AV reentry utilizing bypass tracts	Marked sinus bradycardia, complete heart block; IV administration may cause hypotension; increased QT associated with polymorphic VT; increased T_4, hypo- and hyperthyroidism; peripheral neuropathy, proximal myopathy; pulmonary fibrosis; increased liver enzymes, hepatitis; photodermatitis, blue-gray skin discoloration; corneal microdeposits; elevation of digoxin levels; potentiation of oral anticoagulants
Ventricular tachyarrhythmias	Nausea, vomiting, ataxia, tremor, gait disturbances, rash

of these tachycardias. Most concealed bypass tracts are left-sided. Thus, during supraventricular tachycardia or during ventricular pacing, the earliest activation sequence is recorded in the left atrium, usually via a catheter in the coronary sinus (Fig. 184-3). This eccentric atrial activation is quite distinct from the normal retrograde activation sequence in which the earliest activation of the atria is in the area of the AV junction. The ability of a ventricular stimulus to conduct to the atrium at a time when the bundle of His is refractory and termination of the tachycardia by a ventricular stimulus which does not reach the atrium are diagnostic of retrograde conduction over a concealed bypass tract.

Treatment is similar to that for AV nodal reentry tachycardia.

Sinus node reentry and other atrial tachycardias Reentry in the region of the sinus node or within the atria is invariably initiated by APCs. These arrhythmias are less common than AV nodal or AV reentry and are more often associated with underlying cardiac disease. During sinus node reentry the P-wave morphology is identical to that occurring in sinus rhythm, and the PR interval is prolonged. This is in contrast to sinus tachycardia, in which the PR interval tends to shorten. With intraatrial reentry the P-wave configuration differs from that during sinus rhythm, but the PR interval is prolonged.

TREATMENT Sinus node and atrial reentrant arrhythmias are managed like other reentrant PSVTs.

NONREENTRANT ATRIAL TACHYCARDIAS These may be a manifestation of digitalis intoxication or may be associated with severe pulmonary or cardiac disease, with hypokalemia, or with the administration of theophylline or adrenergic drugs. The digitalis-induced arrhythmias may be caused by triggered activity and/or enhanced automaticity. In such atrial tachycardias with AV block secondary to

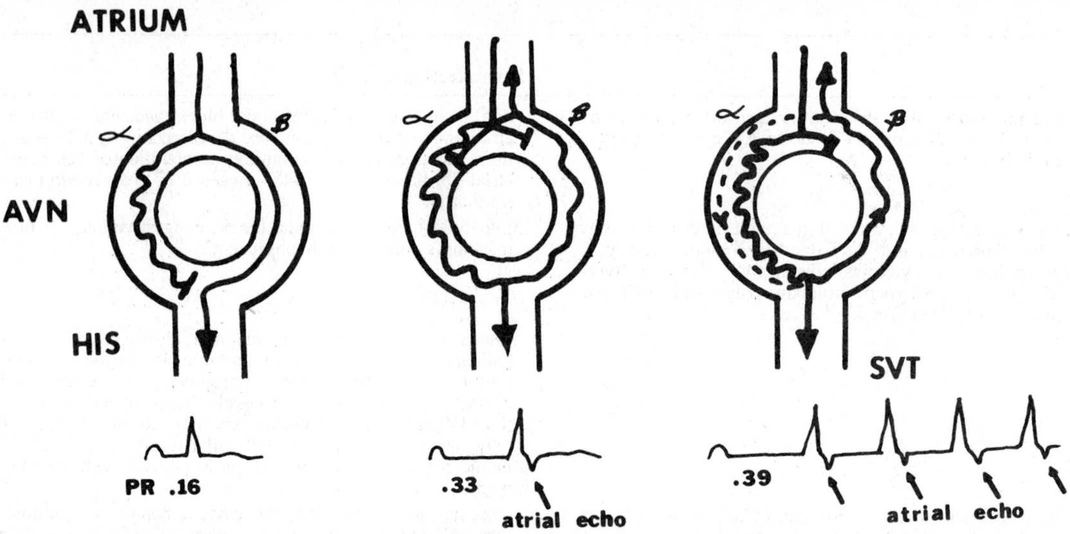

FIGURE 184-2 *Mechanism of AV nodal reentry. The atrium, AV node (AVN), and His bundle are schematically shown. The AV node is longitudinally dissociated into two functionally different pathways, alpha and beta (see text). During sinus rhythm the impulse conducts down the beta pathway to produce a normal PR interval. Conduction down the alpha pathway cannot be completed because the His bundle is refractory. With a premature atrial impulse, block occurs in the fast beta pathway and slow conduction occurs to the ventricle over the slow alpha pathway. The impulse can then return to the chamber of origin (atrium) to produce an atrial echo. This is schematically shown on the bottom, which is dissociation of a long PR interval with an atrial echo. In the tracing on the far right a more premature atrial impulse will again block in the fast pathway, but this time conduction will be so slow down the slow pathway that it will be able to recover to maintain a sustained circus movement within the AV node. This is schematically shown on the bottom where a premature atrial impulse associated with a PR interval of 0.39 s is followed by the initiation of supraventricular tachycardia (SVT).*

digitalis intoxication (Fig. 184-1*F*), the atrial rate rarely exceeds 180 per minute, and typically 2:1 block is present. Atrial arrhythmias precipitated by digitalis can usually be treated by withdrawal of the drug.

Automatic trial tachycardias not caused by digitalis are difficult to terminate, and in such cases the main goal of therapy should be to control the ventricular response, either by drugs which affect the AV node, such as digitalis, beta blockers, or calcium channel antagonists, or by ablation techniques. Surgery has been employed in resistant cases.

PREEXCITATION (WPW) SYNDROME The most frequently encountered type of ventricular preexcitation is that associated with AV bypass tracts. These connections are composed of strands of atrial-

FIGURE 184-3 *Intracardiac recordings during supraventricular tachycardia using a left-sided AV bypass tract. Intracardiac recordings during sinus rhythm (NSR) in supraventricular tachycardia (SVT) are shown. ECG leads I, aVF, and* V_1 *are displayed with electrograms from the high right atrium (HRA), coronary sinus (CS), His bundle (HBE), and right ventricle (RV). During NSR, the QRS complex and the AH and HV intervals are normal. During SVT the retrograde atrial activation sequence is abnormal. The earliest site of atrial activation is in the CS, which is followed by activation in the HBE and HRA. This activation sequence is diagnostic of a left-sided AV bypass tract conducting retrogradely from ventricle to atrium. [From ME Josephson, in* Update IV, Harrison's Principles of Internal Medicine, *KJ Isselbacher et al (eds). New York, McGraw-Hill Book Company, 1983, by permission.]*

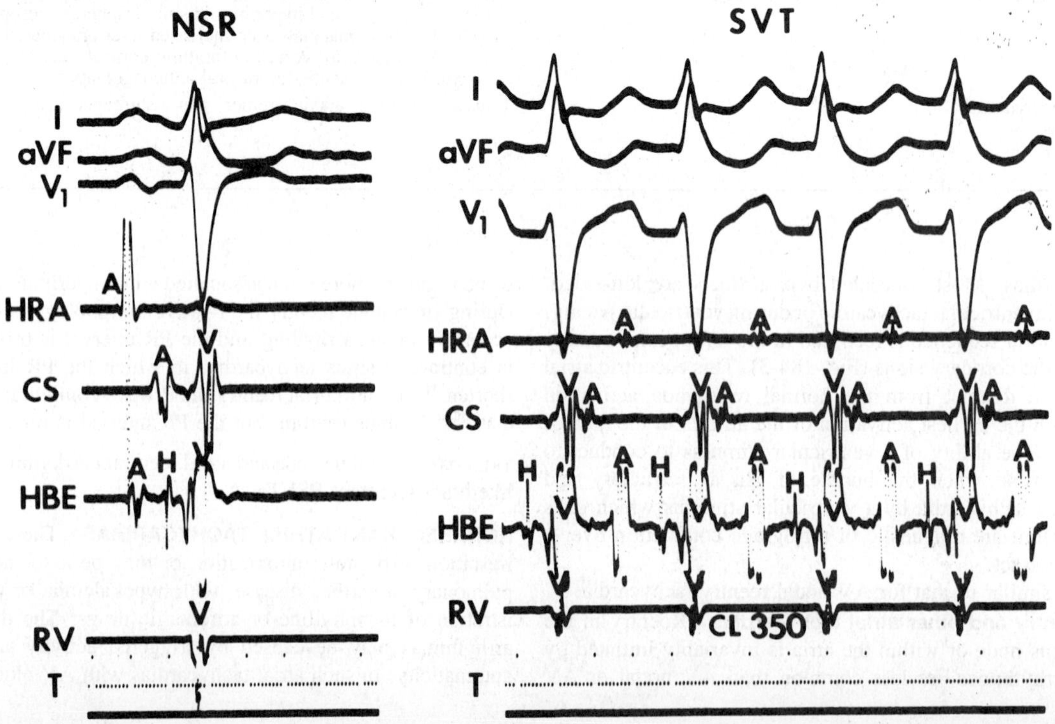

like muscle which may occur almost anywhere around the AV rings. The term WPW syndrome is applied to patients with both preexcitation on the ECG and paroxysmal tachycardias. AV bypass tracts can be associated with certain congenital abnormalities, the most important of which is Ebstein's anomaly (see Chap. 185).

AV bypass tracts which conduct in an antegrade direction produce a typical ECG pattern of a short PR interval (<0.12 s), a slurred upstroke of the QRS complex (delta wave), and a wide QRS complex. This pattern results from a fusion of activation of the ventricles over both the bypass tract and the AV nodal His-Purkinje system (Fig. 184-4). The relative contribution of activation over each system determines the amount of preexcitation.

During PSVT in WPW the impulse is usually conducted antegrade along the normal AV system and retrograde through the bypass tract. The characteristics are identical to those described on page 928 under "AV Reentrant Tachycardia." Rarely (approximately 5 percent) tachycardias occurring in patients with WPW will exhibit a reverse pattern with antegrade conduction through the bypass tract and retrograde conduction through the normal AV system. This produces a tachycardia with a wide QRS complex in which the ventricles are totally activated by the bypass tract. Atrial flutter and AF also occur commonly in patients with the WPW syndrome. Since the bypass tract does not have the same decremental conducting properties as the AV node, the ventricular responses during atrial flutter or fibrillation may be unusually rapid and may cause ventricular fibrillation.

The goals of electrophysiologic evaluation in patients suspected of having the WPW syndrome are to (1) confirm the diagnosis; (2) localize the bypass tract; (3) demonstrate the role of the bypass tract in the genesis of the arrhythmias; (4) determine the refractory period of the bypass tract and its role in the development of potential life-threatening rates during atrial flutter or fibrillation; and (5) evaluate therapeutic options, such as specific pharmacologic agents, pacing therapy, and surgery.

Management This should be aimed at (1) decreasing the occurrence of the APCs and VPCs responsible for the initiation of the tachycardia; (2) increasing the refractory period of the bypass tract (refractory periods <220 ms are associated with rapid ventricular responses during AF); and (3) blocking conduction down the normal AV conduction system. Specific antiarrhythmic therapy can be assessed by electrophysiologic studies, as described on page 935.

In patients with the WPW syndrome and AF, dc cardioversion should be carried out if there is a life-threatening, rapid ventricular response. Alternatively, lidocaine (2 to 4 mg/kg) or procainamide (15 mg/kg) administered intravenously over 15 to 20 min will usually slow the ventricular response. Caution should be employed when using digitalis, verapamil, or beta blockers in patients with the WPW syndrome and AF, since these drugs can shorten the refractory period of the accessory pathway and can increase the ventricular rate, thereby placing the patient at increased risk for ventricular fibrillation. Although atrial or ventricular pacing can almost always terminate PSVT in patients with the WPW syndrome, they can induce AF. Successful surgical ablations of bypass tracts is possible in more than 90 percent of cases (page 938) and offers a permanent cure.

ACCELERATED AV CONDUCTION IN THE ABSENCE OF MANIFEST PREEXCITATION The ECG pattern of a short PR interval (≤0.12 s) and a normal QRS complex is due to a partial or complete bypass of the AV node. Such patients may develop PSVT due to reentry in the AV node or through a concealed AV bypass tract (the *Lown-Ganong-Levine syndrome*). Treatment should be the same as for patients with normal PR intervals and these arrhythmias. Serial drug testing using the response to programmed stimulation can be utilized to tailor treatment specifically for those patients in whom initial empiric therapy fails.

NONPAROXYSMAL JUNCTIONAL TACHYCARDIA This rhythm usually results from conditions which produce enhanced automaticity or triggered activity in the AV junction and is most common due to digitalis intoxication, inferior wall myocardial infarction, myocarditis, endogenous or exogenous catecholamine excess, acute rheumatic fever, or following valve surgery.

The onset of nonparoxysmal junctional tachycardia is usually

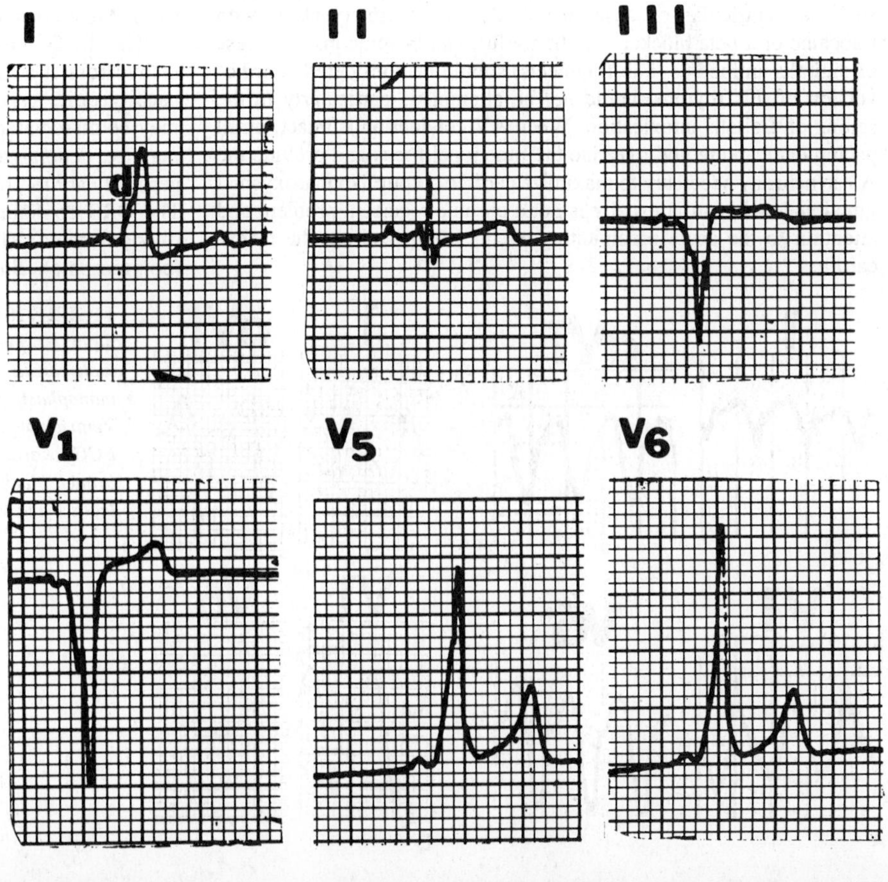

FIGURE 184-4 *ECG in WPW syndrome. There is a short PR interval (0.11 s), a wide QRS complex (0.12 s), and slurring on the upstroke of the QRS produced by early ventricular activation over the bypass tract (delta wave, d in lead I). The negative delta waves in V_1 are diagnostic of a right-sided bypass tract.*

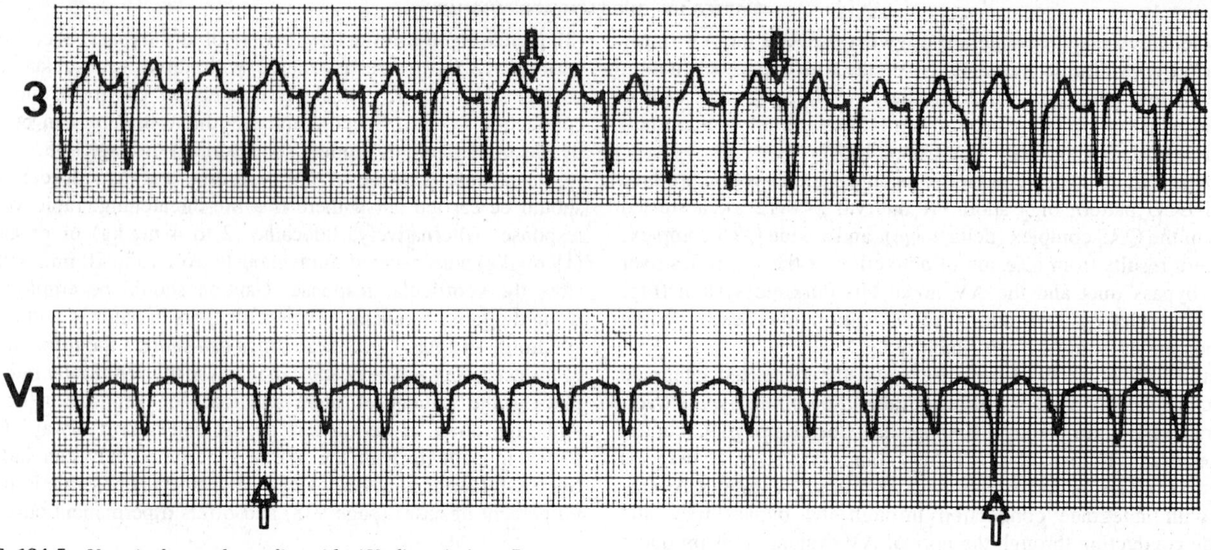

FIGURE 184-5 *Ventricular tachycardia with AV dissociation. P waves which are totally dissociated from the underlying ventricular rhythm can be noted (arrows). AV dissociation is highly suggestive of ventricular tachycardia.*

gradual with a ''warm-up'' period prior to stabilization of the rate, which can range from 70 to 150 per minute with faster rates usually being associated with digitalis intoxication. Nonparoxysmal junctional tachycardia is recognized by a QRS complex identical to that in sinus rhythm. The rate can be influenced by autonomic tone and can be increased by catecholamines, vagolytic agents, or exercise and can be slowed somewhat by carotid sinus pressure. When this rhythm is due to digitalis intoxication, it usually is associated with AV block and/or disassociation. Early after cardiac surgery, retrograde conduction is more likely to be present due to heightened sympathetic state.

Management This is directed toward elimination of the underlying etiologic factors. Since digitalis is the most common cause of this rhythm, discontinuation of this drug is indicated. If the rhythm is associated with other serious manifestations of digitalis intoxication, such as ventricular or atrial irritability, active intervention with lidocaine or a beta blocker may be useful, and in some instances use of digitalis antibodies (Fab fragments) should be considered. Cardioversion of this rhythm should *not* be attempted, particularly in the setting of digitalis intoxication. When AV conduction is intact, atrial pacing can capture and override the junctional focus and provide the AV synchrony necessary to maximize cardiac output. Nonparoxysmal junctional tachycardia usually is not a chronic recurrent problem and attention to the acute precipitating events often resolves the tachycardia.

VENTRICULAR TACHYCARDIA (VT) *Sustained* VT is defined as one which persists for more than 30 s or requires termination because of hemodynamic collapse. VT generally accompanies some form of structural heart disease, most commonly chronic ischemic heart disease associated with a prior myocardial infarction. Sustained VT may also be associated with nonischemic cardiomyopathies, metabolic disorders, drug toxicity, or prolonged QT syndrome, and it occurs occasionally in the absence of heart disease or other predisposing factors. Nonsustained VT (3 beats to 30 s) is also associated with cardiac disease but occurs in its absence more often than the sustained arrhythmia. While nonsustained VT usually does not produce symptoms, sustained VT is almost always symptomatic and is often associated with marked hemodynamic embarrassment and/or the development of myocardial ischemia. A fixed anatomic substrate, not acute ischemia, is responsible for most recurrent episodes of sustained VT. Acute ischemia appears to have little role in the genesis of sustained uniform VT associated with chronic infarction but may play a role in the degeneration of stable VT into ventricular fibrillation (VF). Most episodes of VF in fact begin with VT.

The ECG diagnosis of VT is suggested by a wide complex tachycardia at a rate exceeding 100 per minute. While the rhythm is usually quite regular, slight irregularity may exist. Atrial activity may be dissociated from ventricular activity (Fig. 184-5) or the atria may be depolarized retrogradely. The onset of the tachycardia is generally abrupt, but in nonparoxysmal tachycardias it can be gradual. The QRS configuration during any episode of VT may be uniform (monomorphic) (Fig. 184-6), or it may vary from beat to beat (polymorphic). *Bidirectional tachycardia* refers to VT which shows

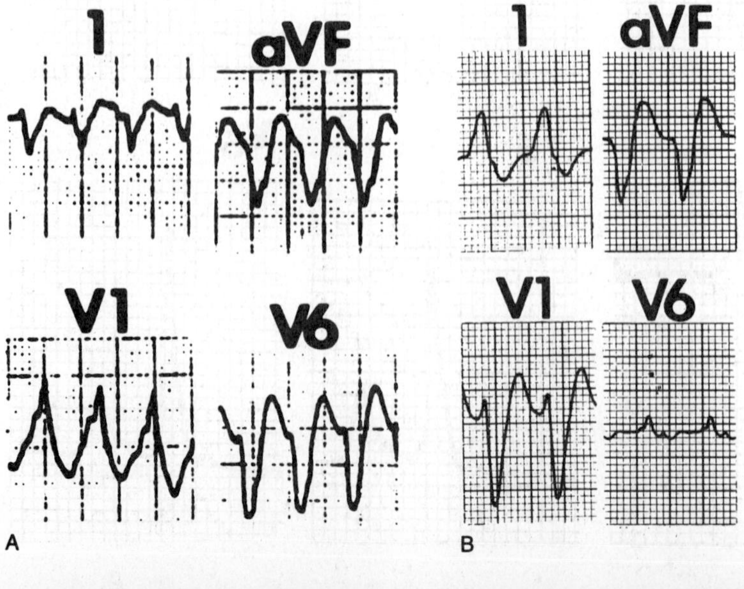

FIGURE 184-6 *A. Ventricular tachycardia with right bundle branch block morphology. ECG characteristics compatible with ventricular tachycardia are wide QRS complexes (≥0.14 s), superior axis, monophasic R waves in lead V_1, and R:S ratio <1 in lead V_6. B. Ventricular tachycardia with left bundle branch block morphology. ECG characteristics of ventricular tachycardia with a left bundle branch block morphology are the broad, slowly inscribed R waves in leads I and V_6.*

an alternation in QRS amplitude and direction. *Paroxysmal* VT is usually initiated by a VPC.

It is important to distinguish supraventricular tachycardia with aberration of intraventricular conduction from VT since the clinical implications and management of these two arrhythmias are totally different. It is always useful to have a 12-lead ECG recorded during sinus rhythm for comparison with that during the tachycardia. When the tracing obtained during sinus rhythm demonstrates a bundle branch block pattern with the same morphologic features as those during the tachycardia, the diagnosis of supraventricular tachycardia is favored. In addition, an infarction pattern on the sinus rhythm tracing suggests the presence of the anatomic substrate necessary for VT. Characteristics of the 12-lead ECG during the tachycardia which support a ventricular origin for the arrthymia are (1) a QRS complex >0.14 s in the absence of antiarrhythmic therapy; (2) AV dissociation or variable retrograde conduction; (3) a superior QRS axis; (4) concordance of the QRS pattern in all precordial leads (i.e., all positive or all negative deflections); and (5) other QRS patterns with prolonged duration but inconsistent with typical right or left bundle branch block patterns. A wide, complex, bizarre tachycardia that is very irregular suggests AF with conduction over an AV bypass tract (page 930). Similarly, a QRS complex in excess of 0.20 s is uncommon during VT in the absence of drug therapy and is more common with preexcitation.

The diagnosis of VT can be made by analyzing the relationship between the electrogram recording His bundle and ventricular activity. In three-fourths of the cases of VT, no consistent His deflection is observed (Fig. 184-7). Occasionally one may identify His bundle activity either just preceding or following the QRS, due to retrograde activation over the His-Purkinje system. In patients with a wide, complex tachycardia the diagnosis of VT is confirmed when atrial pacing produces normalization of the QRS complex with a normal HV interval. Regardless of QRS morphology [left or right bundle branch block patterns (Fig. 184-6)] VT due to ischemic heart disease arises from the *left* ventricular endocardium.

It has been possible to replicate sustained VT in more than 95 percent of patients with this arrhythmia using programmed stimulation. In most patients the tachycardia is initiated with ventricular premature stimuli. A sustained monomorphic VT with a morphology identical to that of the spontaneous arrhythmia is the rule. The clinical significance of polymorphic VT initiated by programmed stimulation is not clear. It has been shown that when more aggressive stimulation is performed (i.e., the use of three or four extra stimuli), polymorphic VT and even VF can be induced in some normal subjects and in patients who have never had a clinical arrhythmia.

Sustained uniform VT can be terminated by programmed stimulation or rapid pacing in at least 75 percent of patients; the remainder require cardioversion. The ability to initiate and terminate a sustained, uniform VT reproducibly permits assessment of pharmacologic and electric therapy of these arrhythmias. Serial testing of antiarrhythmic agents over a period of several days can be accomplished and predicts the likelihood of success of the agents or devices tested (page 936).

The reproducible termination of VT by programmed stimulation permits evaluation of the effectiveness of antitachycardia pacemakers for long-term therapy of paroxysmal episodes of arrthythmia. Unfortunately, rapid pacing, which is the most effective form of therapy, can cause acceleration of the tachycardia and/or produce ventricular fibrillation.

Clinical features Symptoms resulting from VT depend on the ventricular rate, duration of the tachycardia, and presence and extent of underlying cardiac disease. When the tachycardia is rapid and associated with severe myocardial dysfunction and cerebrovascular disease, hypotension and syncope are common. The loss of the atrial contribution to ventricular filling and an abnormal sequence of ventricular activation are important factors producing a decreased cardiac output during VT.

The *prognosis* of VT depends on the underlying disease state. If sustained VT develops within the first 6 weeks following acute myocardial infarction, the prognosis is poor, with an 85 percent mortality rate at 1 year. Nonsustained VT following myocardial infarction is associated with a threefold risk of death over a comparable group of patients without this arrhythmia. However, a cause-and-effect relationship between the nonsustained tachycardia and subsequent sudden death has not been established.

Management The risk/benefit ratio of treating each specific type of VT should be considered before beginning therapy. This is important because antiarrhythmic agents can produce or exacerbate the very arrhythmias which they are given to prevent. In general, patients with VT but without organic heart disease have a benign course; such patients with asymptomatic, nonsustained VT need not be treated since their prognosis will not be affected. Patients with sustained VT in the absence of heart disease usually require therapy because the arrhythmia causes symptoms. These tachycardias may respond to beta blockers, verapamil, or quinidine-like agents. Among patients with VT and organic heart disease, if marked hemodynamic embar-

FIGURE 184-7 *Intracardiac recordings distinguishing supraventricular tachycardia from ventricular tachycardia. ECG leads I, aVF, and V_1 are shown with a His bundle electrogram (HBE) and time line (TL). Wide QRS complex tachycardias with a right bundle branch block morphology are shown on the left and right panels. On the left, supraventricular tachycardia is diagnosed by the presence of His deflection (H) preceding each QRS complex with a normal HV interval. During ventricular tachycardia no His bundle deflections can be seen (arrow) and AV dissociation is observed [note single atrial deflection (A)]. (From JA Kastor et al. Reprinted by permission of The New England Journal of Medicine 304:1004, 1981.)*

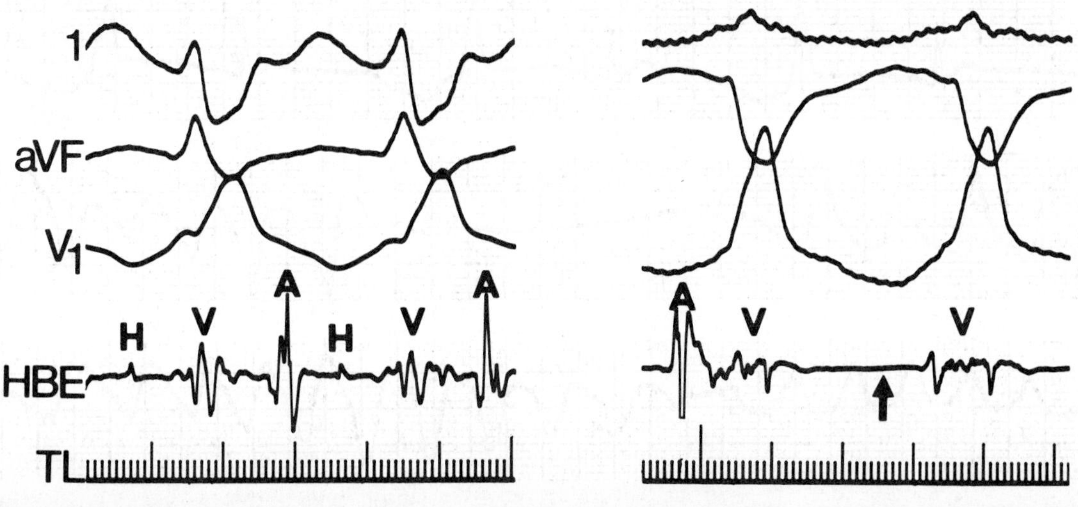

rassment is present or if there is evidence of ischemia, congestive heart failure, or central nervous system hypoperfusion, the rhythm should be promptly terminated by dc cardioversion (see below). If the patient with organic heart disease tolerates the VT well, pharmacologic therapy may be tried. Procainamide is probably the most effective agent. It may or may not terminate the tachycardia, but almost always slows the rate. In stable patients in whom these drugs do not terminate the arrhythmia, a pacing catheter can be inserted pervenously into the right ventricular apex, and the tachycardia can be terminated by rapid pacing.

Therapy guided by programmed stimulation is probably the most efficacious method for selecting the appropriate antiarrhythmic agent to prevent recurrent, sustained VT. In this controlled situation, drugs can be serially studied, and the drug which prevents initiation of the tachycardia can be selected and long-term successful prevention of the arrhythmia can be expected (see Pharmacologic Antiarrhythmic Therapy, page 936).

Antitachycardia pacing has been used as a means to terminate drug-resistant tachycardia. This usually requires that the tachycardia be stable and slow and the patient be aware of it. No automatic antitachycardia device has been approved for the therapy of VT at the time of this writing. Radiofrequency pacemakers which are best activated by a physician have been used in occasional patients.

The advent of endocardial catheter and intraoperative mapping has led to the development of new surgical techniques in the management of VT. In centers in which expertise in mapping is available, operation has been successfully employed to cure tachycardias in the majority of patients in whom it has been undertaken. Even though most patients with VT and ischemic heart disease have markedly impaired left ventricular function and multivessel coronary artery disease, the operative mortality rate has ranged between 8 and 15 percent. Following operation 85 to 90 percent of survivors are controlled either off (two-third of patients) or on (one-third) antiarrhythmic agents which were previously ineffective in controlling these rhythms.

Specific types of VT TORSADE DE POINTES (''twisting of the points'') (Fig. 184-8) This refers to VT characterized by polymorphic QRS complexes which change in amplitude and cycle length, giving the appearance of oscillating around the baseline. This rhythm is by definition associated with QT prolongation. The latter may result from electrolyte disturbances (particularly hypokalemia and hypomagnesemia), use of a variety of antiarrhythmic drugs (especially quinidine), phenothiazines and tricyclic antidepressants, liquid protein diets, intracranial events, and bradyarrhythmias, particularly third-degree AV block.

The electrocardiographic hallmark is polymorphic VT preceded by marked QT prolongation, often in excess of 0.60 s. These patients often have multiple episodes of nonsustained polymorphic VT associated with recurrent syncope, but they may also develop VF and sudden cardiac death.

Therapy should be directed at removing the precipitating factors, i.e., correcting metabolic abnormalities and removing drugs which have induced the prolonged QT interval. In the setting of drug-induced torsade de pointes, atrial or ventricular pacing and the administration of magnesium have also been useful in terminating and preventing the arrhythmia. For patients with the congenital prolonged QT interval syndrome, beta-adrenergic blocking agents have been the mainstay of therapy; agents which shorten the QT interval may also be useful. Cervicothoracic sympathectomy has been proposed as a form of therapy for congenital prolonged QT syndrome, but it is not often effective as the sole therapy.

Polymorphic tachycardias associated with *normal QT intervals* in patients with ischemic heart disease which are initiated by ''R on T'' VPCs are probably caused by reentry, and their treatment is totally different. These are not true ''torsade de pointes.'' In such cases, quinidine-like agents are the most effective form of therapy and should be administered in full antiarrhythmic doses.

ACCELERATED IDIOVENTRICULAR RHYTHM (Fig. 184-9) This arrhythmia, also termed *slow VT,* with a rate which ranges from 60 to 120 per minute, usually occurs in acute myocardial infarction. It may also be seen following cardiac operations, in patients with cardiomyopathy or rheumatic fever or with digitalis intoxication as well as in patients with no evidence of heart disease. The rhythm is usually transient and in and of itself rarely causes significant hemodynamic compromise.

Regardless of whether accelerated idioventricular rhythm occurs in the setting of acute myocardial infarction, in which case the rates are generally slow, or during exercise when it may be more rapid, the arrhythmia is usually transient, rarely causes symptoms and the prognosis is generally excellent.

Treatment is rarely necessary and should usually be considered only if symptoms arise due to impaired hemodynamics, most commonly due to AV dissociation. In most cases, atropine can accelerate the sinus rate to overdrive the ventricular rhythm.

VENTRICULAR FLUTTER AND VENTRICULAR FIBRILLATION (VF) (Fig. 184-9, also see Chap. 30), Ventricular flutter and VF occur

FIGURE 184-8 *Torsade de pointes. During sinus rhythm a markedly prolonged QT interval (0.74 s) was present. The arrhythmia commences with ventricular bigeminy (aVL) followed by progressively longer runs of polymorphic ventricular tachycardia (V_1, lead I).*

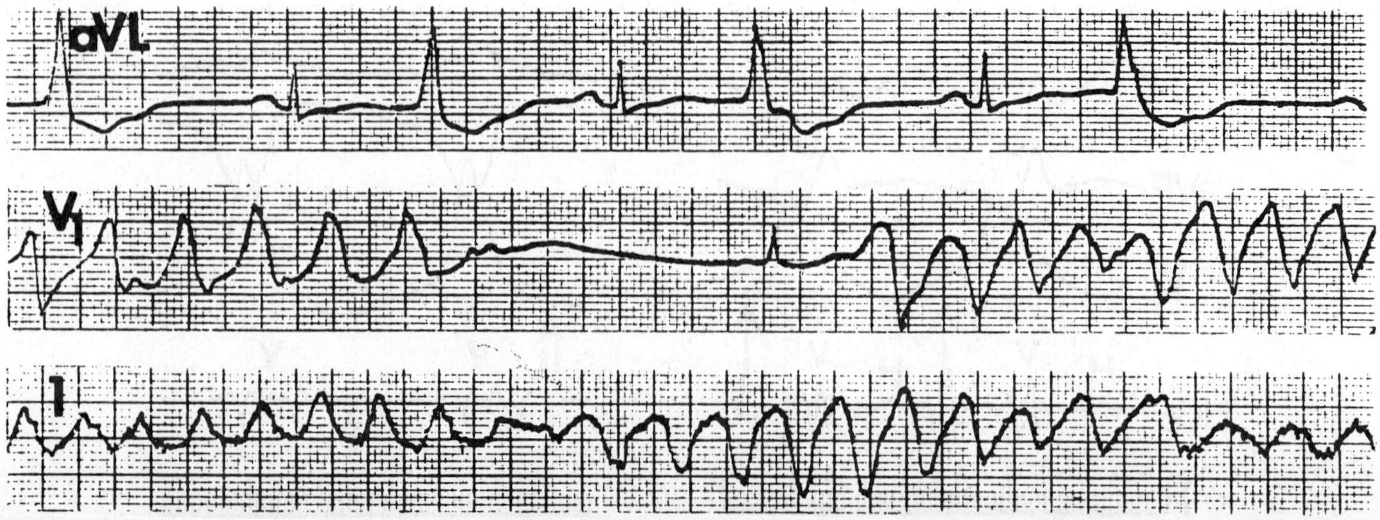

most often in patients with ischemic heart disease. They also occur following administration of antiarrhythmic drugs, particularly those which induce prolonged QT intervals and torsade de pointes (see above), with severe hypoxia or ischemia, and in patients with WPW who develop AF with an extremely rapid ventricular response (page 931). Electrical accidents frequently cause cardiac arrest due to the development of VF. The onset of these arrhythmias is rapidly followed by loss of consciousness and, if untreated, death. Episodes of cardiac arrest recorded during Holter monitoring reveal that approximately three-fourths of the patients have VT or VF producing the sudden cardiac death.

In patients with VF, the onset almost always begins with a short run of rapid VT, which is initiated by a relatively late coupled VPC. In patients with acute myocardial infarction or ischemia, however, VF is usually precipitated by a single early ventricular complex beat falling on the T wave (the vulnerable period), which produces a rapid VT which degenerates into VF (Fig. 184-9).

The clinical setting in which VF occurs is important, since most patients who have primary VF associated with an acute infarction have a good prognosis with a very low recurrence rate of sudden cardiac death. In contrast, most patients who experience VF unassociated with the development of acute myocardial infarction have a recurrence rate of 20 to 30 percent in the year following the event (see Chap. 30).

Ventricular flutter usually appears as a sine wave with rates between 150 and 300 beats per minute. These oscillations make it impossible to assign a specific morphology to the arrhythmia and in some cases to distinguish it from rapid VT. VF is recognized by grossly irregular undulations of varying amplitudes, contours, and rates (Fig. 184-9). Electrophysiologic studies have demonstrated that regardless of the apparent gross irregularity on the surface ECG, VF usually starts out with the rapid repetitive sequence of VT which ultimately breaks down into multiple wavelets of reentry.

Electrophysiologic studies have been useful in patients who have been resuscitated from cardiac arrest. Programmed stimulation has demonstrated that in approximately 70 percent of such patients one can reproducibly initiate a sustained VT. Treatment is discussed in Chap. 30.

PHARMACOLOGIC ANTIARRHYTHMIC THERAPY

Prior to initiation of pharmacologic antiarrhythmic therapy, potential aggravating factors such as transient metabolic abnormalities, congestive heart failure, or acute ischemia must be corrected and in some cases may suffice to control arrhythmias. In addition, the potential role of drugs as a cause or exacerbating factor in the development of the arrhythmia must be considered.

Antiarrhythmic drugs are used in three principal situations: (1) to terminate an acute arrhythmia, (2) to prevent recurrence of an arrhythmia, and (3) to prevent a life-threatening arrhythmia for which the patient is perceived to be at risk, but which has never occurred.

Most currently available antiarrhythmic agents have a relatively low toxic/therapeutic ratio; all can exert proarrhythmic effects, and therefore they may exacerbate underlying arrhythmias. Serum levels can be determined for most currently available antiarrhythmic agents. Standards for therapeutic and toxic levels can serve only as a rough guide for selecting the appropriate dose in any individual patient. In the final analysis, the therapeutic level in a given patient is that concentration which achieves the desired antiarrhythmic effect, and the toxic level for each patient is that at which undesirable side effects occur. Since many adverse effects are directly related to drug concentrations, the minimal serum level which achieves an effective antiarrhythmic response should be chosen.

In order to determine the therapeutic level for a patient, one must have a standard to judge drug efficacy. For a patient with an incessant arrhythmia, antiarrhythmic drugs may be administered empirically until the arrhythmia is suppressed. If a reproducible precipitating factor such as exercise can be identified, serial drug testing during such a provocative maneuver may be performed. Unfortunately, most arrhythmias are sporadic and occur unpredictably without identifiable precipitating factors. In these cases, assessment of drug efficacy may require months, if one waits to observe spontaneous recurrences on each antiarrhythmic drug. This type of assessment of efficacy may be adequate for arrhythmias which are not life-threatening. However, this mode of assessment is inadequate for arrhythmias which compromise hemodynamic stability, result in syncope, or are potentially life-threatening. In such cases two methods for determination of antiarrhythmic drug efficacy have been utilized. The first, which consists of continuous ECG monitoring in the control state and then in the presence of antiarrhythmic drugs, has been used in order to determine the effect which each drug has on spontaneous atrial or ventricular ectopy. This method presupposes that the mechanism responsible for sustained arrhythmias is the same as that causing isolated premature depolarizations (which may or may not be true) and that therefore eradication of isolated ectopy will correlate with prevention of sustained arrhythmias. This method has a number of limitations. First, patients frequently show marked degrees of spontaneous variation in frequency of ectopy, which may mimic antiarrhythmic drug effects. Second, 25 to 30 percent of patients with

FIGURE 184-9 *Top: Accelerated idioventricular rhythm. The lead II strip demonstrates the gradual onset and offset of a wide complex rhythm that is slightly faster than the sinus rhythm. Middle and bottom: Ventricular fibrillation. In a patient with coronary disease ventricular fibrillation is initiated by a VPC which produces a rapid polymorphic ventricular tachycardia which rapidly degenerates to ventricular fibrillation (note the undulating baseline with the inability to distinguish systole and diastole).*

2

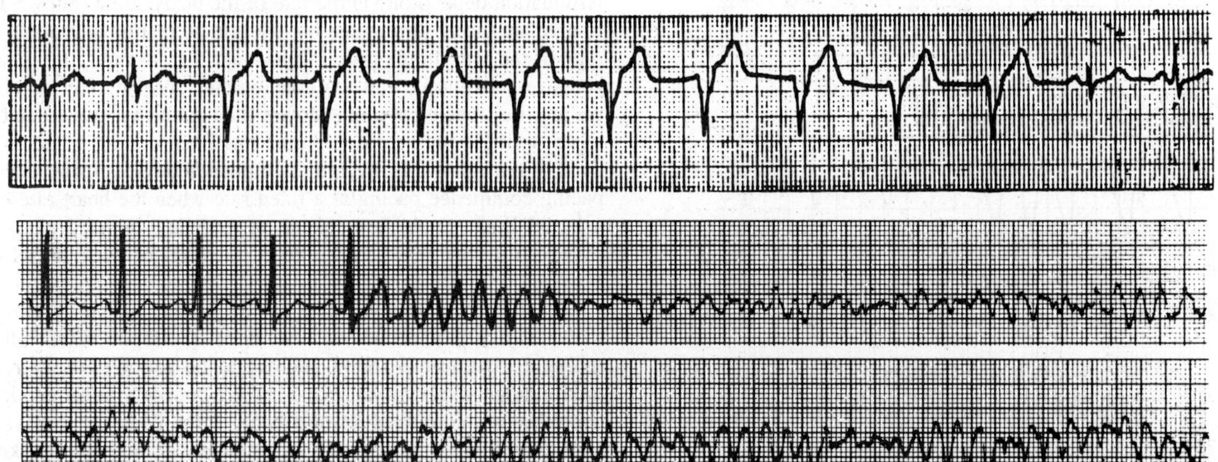

sustained ventricular arrhythmias such as VT or VF demonstrate only rare spontaneous ectopy. Finally, many patients demonstrate a dissociation between the effects of antiarrhythmic agents on spontaneous ectopy and the effects of the same agent on sustained arrhythmias.

An alternative method to assess drug efficacy is programmed stimulation. Numerous studies have demonstrated that most clinically occurring supraventricular and ventricular tachyarrhythmias may be reproducibly initiated and terminated safely using this technique. Studies are performed initially in a control state in the absence of antiarrhythmic drugs (Fig. 184-10). If the patient's clinical arrhythmia can be reproducibly initiated, then the ability of individual antiarrhythmic drugs to prevent reinduction of the arrhythmia can be assessed after the drug is administered either intravenously or after several days of oral loading in order to achieve a steady-state serum concentration, and induction of the arrhythmia is attempted once again. Use of this method assumes that (1) the induced and spontaneous arrhythmias are identical, and (2) prevention of induction of arrhythmias will correlate with prevention of recurrent spontaneous tachycardias on the same drug regimen. This technique has been validated in patients with a variety of PSVTs secondary to reentry, as well as VT and VF. The technique is safe when carefully performed, the potential complications being those of any intravascular catheterization. Appropriate interpretation of the results of programmed stimulation is critically dependent on correlating the patient's spontaneous arrhythmias with those induced in the laboratory, with regard to rate and morphology.

FIGURE 184-10 *Selection of an effective antiarrhythmic drug for ventricular tachycardia by programmed stimulation. From top to bottom, the effects of programmed stimulation during the control state and following administration of several antiarrhythmic agents. During the control state two ventricular extrastimuli initiate the ventricular tachycardia at a rate of 230 per minute. Lidocaine, phenytoin, and disopyramide at the plasma levels shown failed to prevent induction of the tachycardia. Both procainamide and quinidine at the plasma levels shown prevented initiation of sustained tachycardia. Chronic oral quinidine therapy effectively prevented recurrences of the arrhythmia. (From JA Kastor et al. Reprinted by permission of The New England Journal of Medicine 304:1004, 1981.)*

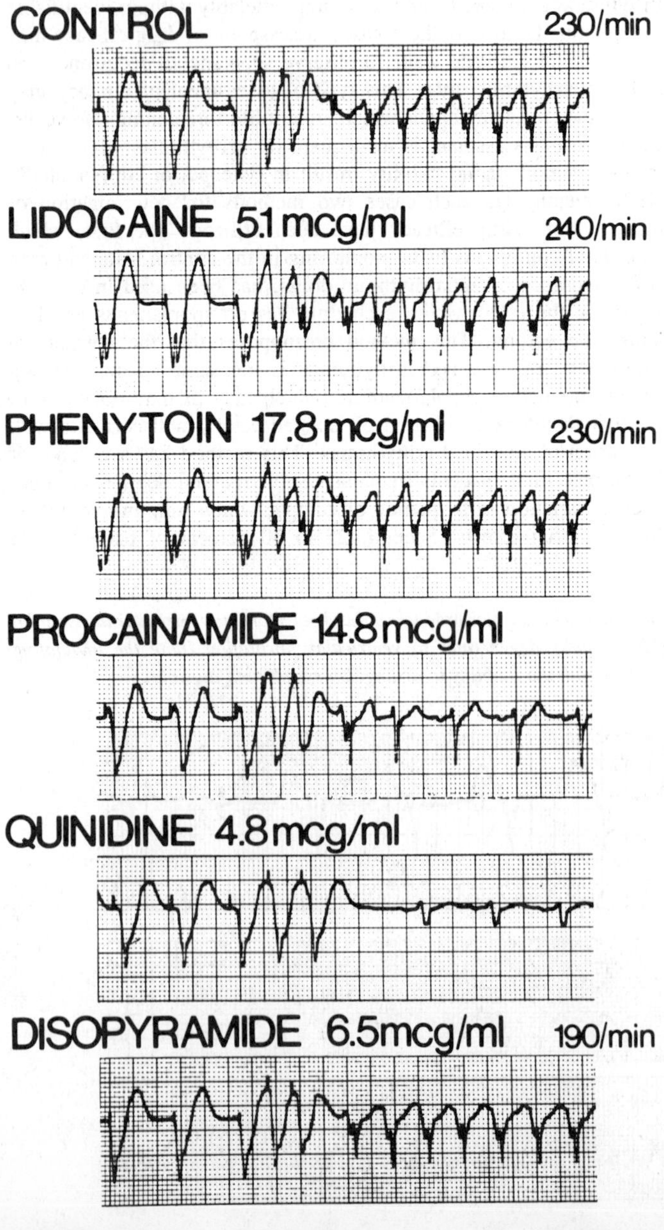

A number of classifications of antiarrhythmic drugs have been proposed, the most frequently used of which is a modification of that proposed by Vaughn-Williams (Table 184-1). This classification is based in part on the ability of antiarrhythmic drugs to modify the cardiac cellular (1) excitatory currents (Na^+ or Ca^{2+}), (2) action potential duration, and (3) automaticity (phase 4 depolarization). These effects of the drugs on isolated cardiac cells are thought to account for some of the antiarrhythmic effects of the drugs. Thus, depression of excitatory currents in so-called type I and type IV antiarrhythmics results in slowing of conduction velocity and may interrupt arrhythmias by blocking conduction in areas of marginal excitability, where conduction velocity is already slow. Type III antiarrhythmics exert their action by increasing refractoriness through prolongation of the action potential duration. However, such classifications are limited in that the electrophysiologic effects of these drugs in vivo may differ from their effects on isolated cells. The uses and actions of currently available antiarrhythmic drugs are summarized in Tables 184-2 and 184-3.

ELECTRICAL THERAPY OF TACHYARRHYTHMIAS

PACEMAKERS Cardiac pacing can be used to terminate and in selected cases prevent recurrent supraventricular and ventricular arrhythmias. Because many tachyarrhythmias appear to be due to a reentrant mechanism with the impulse traveling in a circuit, a properly timed paced impulse can penetrate and prematurely depolarize part of the circuit, rendering it refractory to the next circulating wavefront, thereby interrupting the circus movement. Pacing therapy for arrhythmias is generally reserved for patients whose arrhythmias are refractory to drug therapy. All forms of pacing therapy require repeated demonstration of their effectiveness and reliability in terminating the arrhythmias during electrophysiologic testing prior to implantation of the pacing device.

The type of pacing device and modality selected for arrhythmia termination depend on (1) the rate of the tachycardia (rates >160 per minute are rarely terminated by a single premature stimulus); (2) the type of the arrhythmia (atrial flutter and VT are rarely terminated by single extrastimuli); and (3) concomitant drug therapy. Underdrive pacing, i.e., pacing at a rate slower than the tachycardia, can be used when a single premature stimulus has been demonstrated to reproducibly terminate a tachycardia. Implanted devices using underdrive pacing commence pacing at a fixed rate when the heart rate exceeds a preset limit. Such pacemakers, termed dual-demand pacemakers, may also discharge when the heart rate falls below a preset critical level.

Because many tachycardias cannot be terminated by single premature stimuli, pacemakers have been developed which allow for multiple extrastimuli (burst pacing) to be introduced. In reentrant tachycardias involving an accessory AV connection, sequential, near simultaneous activation of the heart from both the atria and the ventricle using a dual-chamber pacemaker will increase the likelihood of bidirectional block and termination of the tachycardia.

TABLE 184-3 Dose, serum half-life ($t_{½}$) following oral administration, and route of metabolism of drugs used in the treatment of arrhythmias

Drug	Mode of administration	$t_{½}$ (oral), h	Route of metabolism
Digoxin	IV 0.75–1.5 mg Oral, 0.75–1.5 mg loading dose over 12–24 h Maintenance, 0.25–0.50 mg/day	36	Renal
Propranolol	IV, 0.5–1 mg/min to total dose of 0.15–0.2 mg/kg Oral, 10–200 mg every 6 h	3–6	Hepatic
Verapamil	IV, 2.5–10 mg over 1–2 min to total 0.15 mg/kg Oral, 80–120 mg every 6–8 h	3–8	Hepatic
Quinidine	IV, 20 mg/min to total 10–15 mg/kg Oral, 200–400 mg every 6 h	5–9	Hepatic
Procainamide	IV, 40–50 mg/min to total 10–20 mg/kg Oral, 500–1000 mg every 4 h	3–5	Hepatic-renal
Disopyramide	Oral, 100–300 mg every 6–8 h	8–9	Renal
Lidocaine	IV, 20–50 mg/min to total dose of 5 mg/kg loading followed by 1–4 mg/min	1–2	Hepatic
Phenytoin	IV, 20 mg/min total dose to 1000 mg Oral, 1000-mg loading over 24 h Maintenance, 100–400 mg/day	18–36	Hepatic
Tocainide	Oral, 400 to 600 mg every 8–12 h	10–17	Hepatic-renal
Bretylium	IV, 1–2 (mg/kg)/min to total load, 5–10 mg/kg Maintenance, 0.5–2 mg/min	8–14	Renal
Amiodarone*	IV, 5–10 mg/kg Oral, load 800–1400 mg/day for 1–2 weeks Maintenance, 100–600 mg/day	Unknown	Hepatic
Mexiletine*	Oral, 100–300 mg every 6–8 h	9–12	Hepatic

* *Investigational.*

Cardiac pacing has also been used to prevent ventricular tachyarrhythmias. Polymorphic VT associated with a long QT interval and bradycardias (torsade de pointes, page 934) is most likely to respond. Pacing the atrium and/or ventricle at rates between 90 and 120 per minute appears to increase the homogeneity of electrical recovery and markedly reduces the propensity for a recurrence of arrhythmias. Regardless of the arrhythmia being treated and the pacing mode selected, the potential for alterations in pacing requirements for termination of tachycardia and therefore programmability of pacing modes (e.g., underdrive, dual-demand, dual-chamber, burst) as well as rate and coupling interval of introduced extrastimuli are probably essential features for pacemakers used to terminate tachycardias.

Pacemakers may be self-contained or energized by an external radiofrequency source. The self-contained pacemaker may function automatically [i.e., it incorporates an arrhythmia recognition program (circuit) or it is activated by an external magnet]. The major advantage of a fully automatic system is that there is no need for the patient to recognize the arrhythmia in order for termination to occur. The advantages of the externally activated system include (1) the decreased risk of unnecessary treatment because of faulty sensing; and (2) the opportunity to initiate monitoring at the time of attempted arrhythmia termination. This type of monitoring is frequently helpful if pacing techniques are employed to terminate VT, given the risk of acceleration of the arrhythmia by pacing.

The limitations of pacing therapy are primarily related to (1) the changes in the characteristics of the arrhythmia over time such that programmed pacing parameters no longer terminate the tachycardia; and (2) the risk of acceleration of the tachycardia with the development of AF when stimulating the atrium and the development of rapid VT and VF when stimulating the ventricles. In the future, pacing generators which can also deliver a larger amount of energy and perform cardioversion and defibrillation of accelerated arrhythmias are likely to increase the applicability of pacing therapy for the treatment of arrhythmias.

CARDIOVERSION AND DEFIBRILLATION Electrical cardioversion and defibrillation remain the most reliable method for terminating arrhythmias. By depolarizing all or at least a large portion of excitable myocardium in a near homogeneous fashion, the electric shock can interrupt reentrant arrhythmias. External cardioversion is routinely performed by placing two paddles 12 cm in diameter in firm contact with the chest wall, with one paddle usually located to the right of the sternum at the level of the second rib and the other in the left midclavicular line in the fifth intercostal space. If the patient is conscious, a short-acting barbiturate to act as an anesthetic or an amnesic drug such as diazepam should be administered to prevent patient discomfort. A person skilled in maintaining an airway should be present. Energy is delivered synchronously with the QRS complex for all arrhythmias except ventricular flutter and VF; sinoasynchronous shocks can produce VF. The amount of energy used will vary with the type of tachycardia being treated. With the exception of AF, supraventricular tachycardias can frequently be terminated with energy levels in the range of 25 to 50 W·s, while AF usually requires ≥100 W·s for termination. For terminating VT, energy levels ≥100 W·s should probably be employed. While energies as low as 25 W·s may be successfully used, they also have a higher incidence of producing VF. At least 200 W.s of energy should be used for initial attempts at terminating VF. All repeated attempts at defibrillation should be with the maximum energy that the defibrillator is capable of delivering (320 to 400 W·s).

Indications for cardioversion depend upon the clinical setting and the patient's general condition. Any tachycardia (except sinus tachycardia) that produces hypotension, myocardial ischemia, or heart failure warrants consideration of prompt termination using external cardioversion. Arrhythmias that fail to terminate with pharmacologic therapy may also be terminated by electrical cardioversion. Transient bradycardias and supraventricular and ventricular irritability following cardioversion are common and usually do not warrant antiarrhythmic intervention.

AUTOMATIC INTERNAL DEFIBRILLATION An automatic implanted cardioverting-defibrillating device has been developed to allow for prompt recognition and termination of life-threatening ventricular arrhythmias. The device delivers 25 to 33 W·s of energy. Clinical trials testing the function of the device in patients with drug refractory ventricular arrhythmias have demonstrated survival from sudden death at 1 year ranging between 92 and 100 percent. Based on the results of the initial trials, it appears that an automatic sensing, implanted cardioverter-defibrillator will play an important role in arrhythmia management. At the time of this writing, use of this device should be reserved for patients with VT which is not hemodynamically tolerated or for patients with VF whose arrhythmias are refractory to drug therapy and who are not candidates for surgical intervention (see below). The most frequent problem with the device has been its inappropriate discharge in the absence of sustained ventricular arrhythmias.

CATHETER ABLATION FOR ARRHYTHMIAS Catheter ablation of tachyarrhythmias, a technique which involves the delivery of large amounts of energy (25 to 400 W·s) through a catheter to effect closed-chest electroablation of the bundle of His has been primarily used to interrupt AV conduction and prevent a rapid ventricular response to supraventricular arrhythmias. Although not yet approved by the Food and Drug Administration, catheter ablation of the AV junction has become the procedure of choice for creating AV block to control supraventricular arrhythmias. However, the introduction of complete heart block necessitating a pacemaker following His bundle ablation and the small risk of sudden death associated with the procedure make catheter ablation a procedure of "last resort" at this time.

SURGICAL TREATMENT OF ARRHYTHMIAS

Programmed stimulation and endocardial activation mapping have provided a better understanding of the mechanisms and sites of origin of many supraventricular and ventricular tachyarrhythmias, so that in selected patients surgical treatment may be considered.

WPW SYNDROME Surgery may be preferable to other forms of therapy in some patients, particularly those with the WPW syndrome and recurrent arrhythmias. Advances made in the localization and surgical ablation of bypass tracts now allow for an extremely high success rate with minimal morbidity. As a result, surgery can now be considered not only in patients with drug-refractory arrhythmias but also as a reasonable alternative in (1) patients with symptomatic arrhythmias who require long-term drug therapy; (2) patients with AF and a life-threatening rapid ventricular response; and (3) patients undergoing cardiac surgery for other reasons in whom a bypass tract is present.

SUPRAVENTRICULAR TACHYCARDIA AND OTHER ATRIAL ARRHYTHMIAS Although atrial flutter, AF, and PSVT are usually not life-threatening, they may be refractory to pharmacologic or pacing interventions. In such cases surgery may be considered as a method of removing the abnormal focus, interrupting the reentry circuits, and curing the tachycardia or controlling the ventricular response by creating AV block. In atrial flutter and AF the pathophysiologic substrate cannot be identified; thus, the only surgical option is to destroy the AV node–His bundle region by cryosurgery or transvenous catheter electroablation (page 936). Similarly, surgery, cryoablation, or electrode catheter ablation for the treatment of AV nodal reentrant tachycardia usually results in the production of AV block and requires concomitant implantation of a permanent pacemaker. Focal atrial tachycardias have been treated surgically by discrete resection or ablation by cryothermal injury. Mapping the tachycardia is mandatory if a primary direct approach on the arrhythmia is to be performed.

Surgery should only be performed for patients with arrhythmias refractory to other treatment modalities and should only be performed for tachycardias in whom the tachycardia has been localized.

VENTRICULAR TACHYCARDIA The demonstration that VT due to ischemic heart disease can often be reliably induced by programmed stimulation and that the arrhythmia is localized to a small region of endocardium in the area of prior infarction has permitted the development of specific surgical techniques for the cure of the arrhythmia.

Preoperatively all morphologically distinct tachycardias which occur spontaneously are induced by programmed stimulation and their respective sites of origin are determined by catheter activation mapping. Catheter mapping may be supplemented by intraoperative mapping, involving similar techniques. These studies have shown that tachycardias arise in the scar tissue near the endocardium.

Subendocardial resection and endocardial encircling ventriculotomy, the surgical techniques that have been applied to the management of ventricular tachycardia, are aimed at removing or isolating the pathophysiologic substrate of the arrhythmia, as identified by mapping. The major factor responsible for surgical success is the ability to localize the site from which the arrhythmias arise. These procedures are associated with a 10 percent operative mortality rate but have prevented recurrences of VT and VF in 85 to 90 percent of survivors without drugs or with drugs that had been previously ineffective.

REFERENCES

BHANDARI AK, SCHEINMAN M: The long QT syndrome. Mod Concepts Cardiovasc Dis 54:45, 1985

BOINEAU JP: Atrial flutter: A synthesis of concepts. Circulation 72:249, 1985

———, COX JL: Rationale for a direct surgical approach to control ventricular arrhythmias. Relation of specific intraoperative techniques for mechanism and location of arrhythmia circuit. Am J Cardiol 49:381, 1982

CHAROS GS et al: A theoretically and practically more effective method for interruption of ventricular tachycardia: Self-adapting autodecremental overdrive pacing. Circulation 73:309, 1986

ECHT DS et al: Clinical experience, complications and survival in 70 patients with the automatic implantable cardioverter defribrillator. Circulation 71:289, 1985

FRAME LN, HOFFMAN BF: Mechanisms of tachycardia. In *Tachycardias*, B Surawicz (ed). Boston, Martinus Nijhoff, 1984

GALLAGHER JJ et al: The preexcitation syndromes. Prog Cardiovasc Dis 20:285, 1978

JOSEPHSON ME: Paroxysmal supraventricular tachycardia: An electrophysiologic approach. Am J Cardiol 41:1123, 1978

———, SEIDES SF: *Clinical Cardiac Electrophysiology: Techniques and Interpretations*. Philadelphia, Lea & Febiger, 1979

———, WELLENS HJJ (eds): *Tachycardias: Mechanisms, Diagnosis, Treatment*. Philadelphia, Lea & Febiger, 1984

ROSEN MR, HOFFMAN BF (eds): *Cardiac Therapy*. Boston, Martinus Nijhoff, 1983

SCHEINMAN MM, EVENS-BELL T: Catheter ablation of the atrioventricular junction: A report of the percutaneous mapping and ablation registry. Circulation 70:1024, 1984

TORRES V et al: QT prolongation and the antiarrhythmic efficacy of amiodarone. J Am Coll Cardiol 7:142, 1986

WALDECKER B et al: Dysrhythmias after direct-current cardioversion. Am J Cardiol 57:120, 1986

WIT AL, ROSEN MR: Cellular electrophysiology of cardiac arrhythmias. Mod Concepts Cardiovasc Dis 50:1, 1981

185 CONGENITAL HEART DISEASE

WILLIAM F. FRIEDMAN

GENERAL CONSIDERATIONS

INCIDENCE Approximately 1 percent of all live births have a cardiovascular malformation. If recognized early, the anomalies can now be diagnosed accurately, and most patients can be salvaged by medical and surgical management.

Congenital heart disease shows an overall male preponderance, but specific defects may exhibit a specific sex preponderance; patent ductus arteriosus and atrial septal defect are common in females, whereas valvular aortic stenosis, congenital aneurysms of the sinus of Valsalva, coarctation of the aorta, tetralogy of Fallot, and transposition of the great arteries are more common in males.

ETIOLOGY Congenital cardiovascular malformations are generally the result of aberrant embryonic development of the heart or a failure of such a structure to progress beyond an early stage. Malformations are due to complex multifactorial genetic and environmental causes; only rarely may a single causal factor be identified (Table 185-1).

A single gene mutation (Chap. 57) may be causal in the familial forms of atrial septal defect, mitral valve prolapse, ventricular septal defect, congenital heart block, situs inversus, the combination of supravalvular aortic stenosis and peripheral pulmonary arterial stenosis, idiopathic hypertrophic subaortic stenosis, and the syndromes of Noonan, Holt-Oram, Ellis–van Creveld, and Kartagener. Table 185-1 provides a partial list of syndromes in which cardiovascular anomalies are due to the pleiotropic effects of single genes or examples of gross chromosomal defects. Recognized chromosomal aberrations and mutations of single genes account for less than 10 percent of all cardiac malformations.

The fact that only one of a pair of monozygotic twins may be affected by congenital heart disease indicates that the majority of cardiovascular malformations are not inherited in a simple manner. Family studies indicate a two- to fivefold increase in the incidence of congenital heart disease in the siblings of affected patients. The malformations are concordant or partially concordant in at least half of such cases. Nonetheless, the incidence of congenital heart disease in the siblings of an index patient is only 2 to 5 percent. Most patients with isolated heart defects have a negative family history for malformations and a normal chromosome pattern, and it is rarely wise to discourage the parents of one affected child from having additional children. The low recurrence rate and the increasing possibilities for effective therapy for most cardiac lesions usually justify a positive approach to family counseling. If, however, two or more members of a family are affected, the recurrence risk may be quite high, and a detailed family history should be obtained prior to further counseling. If a dominant or recessive mendelian pattern is present, the risk of recurrence in each pregnancy can be predicted (Chap. 57).

PREVENTION The feasibility of preventive programs will depend upon what is learned in the future about the cause of the majority of cardiovascular anomalies for which no cause is known. An effective rubella vaccine is available, and immunization of children with this vaccine may lessen maternal rubella and its cardiac consequences. Strict testing in animals of new drugs that can be teratogenic when taken early in pregnancy may reduce the chances of another thalidomide tragedy. In this regard, no medications should be taken during pregnancy without prior consultation with a physician. Physicians should be aware of known teratogens, as well as of drugs for which inadequate information exists as to teratogenic potential. Similarly, appropriate use of radiologic equipment and techniques for reducing gonadal and fetal radiation exposure may reduce the hazards of this likely cause of birth defects.

The presence of a cardiac malformation as one component of a multiple system involvement in Down's, Turner's, and the trisomy 13-15 (D_1) and 17-18 (E) syndromes (see Chap. 60) may be anticipated in occasional pregnancies at risk by fetal cells obtained from amniotic fluid or chorionic villus biopsy. Similarly, identification in such cells of the enzyme disorders characteristic of Hurler's syndrome, homocystinuria, or type II glycogen storage disease may allow one to predict cardiac disease.

THE FETAL AND TRANSITIONAL CIRCULATIONS

The fetus has a single circulation in which the pulmonary vasculature exists in parallel, not in series, with the systemic circulation. Prenatal survival is not endangered by severe cardiac anomalies as long as one side of the heart can drive blood from the great veins to the aorta. Inferior vena caval blood is deflected across the foramen ovale into the left atrium. Most of the blood that reaches the right ventricle bypasses the high-resistance, unexpanded lungs and passes through the ductus arteriosus into the descending aorta. In fetal life, pulmonary arteries and arterioles are surrounded by a fluid medium, have relatively thick walls and small lumens, and resemble comparable arteries in the systemic circulation.

Normally, at birth this single circulation is divided into two separate circulations in series. Inflation of the lungs at the first inspiration produces a reduction in pulmonary vascular resistance. Fetal pulmonary vessels, heretofore supported by fluid media, are suddenly suspended in air, reducing extravascular pressure. New vessels are opened, and already patent vessels enlarge. Pulmonary arterial pressure falls, and pulmonary blood flow increases, primarily because pulmonary arteriolar vasodilatation results from the increase in oxygen tension to which these vessels are exposed. The systemic vascular resistance rises because clamping the umbilical cord removes the low-resistance placental circulation. Increased pulmonary blood flow increases the return of blood to the left atrium and raises left atrial pressure, which in turn closes the foramen ovale. The shift in oxygen dependence from the placenta to the lungs produces a sudden increase in arterial blood oxygen tension, which, in concert with alterations in the local prostaglandin milieu, initiates constriction of the ductus arteriosus, and total anatomic closure follows within a few days.

PULMONARY HYPERTENSION Pulmonary hypertension is a common accompaniment of many congenital cardiac lesions, and the status of the pulmonary vascular bed is often the principal determinant of the clinical manifestations, the course, and the feasibility of surgical repair. Increases in pulmonary arterial pressure result from elevation of pulmonary blood flow and/or resistance, the latter due sometimes to an increase in vascular tone but usually the result of obstructive, obliterative structural changes within the pulmonary vascular bed. Fortunately, most patients with congenital heart disease are suitable for surgical repair because only a few isolated or combined malformations remain physiologically or anatomically uncorrectable by cardiovascular surgery. Moreover, there has been a remarkable advance in surgical techniques for infants and very young children and an enhanced awareness of the need to operate early on patients at risk for pulmonary vascular obstructive disease. These developments will reduce the number of older children and adults whose pulmonary vascular obstructive disease is the consequence of delayed operation or progression of pulmonary vascular obstruction after complete closure of the defect in childhood.

As in the other vascular beds, the pressure in the pulmonary artery is determined by the product of the volume of blood flow per unit of time and of the resistance to that flow. Equalization of pressures in the systemic and pulmonary circulations occurs if a large communication exists between the two great arteries or between the two ventricles in the absence of semilunar valve obstruction. Pulmonary vascular resistance is calculated as the transpulmonary pressure difference per unit of pulmonary blood flow (Chap. 180). When blood flow increases, existing patent vessels are distended, and additional vessels are opened, so that calculated vascular resistance diminishes. Therefore, in a normal pulmonary vascular bed, pressure rises substantially only if flow is greatly increased. In most patients with congenital heart disease and elevated pulmonary vascular resistance, the pulmonary arterioles are the principal locus of this abnormal resistance.

The causes of pulmonary vascular obstructive disease are unknown, although increased pulmonary blood flow, increased pulmonary arterial blood pressure, elevated pulmonary venous pressure, polycythemia, systemic hypoxia, acidosis, and the bronchial circulation have been implicated. In many patients with pulmonary vascular obstruction the cardiac anomaly places them at risk early in life, precluding survival to adulthood. Patients at particular risk for significant pulmonary vascular obstruction are those with cyanotic congenital heart disease, such as complete transposition of the great arteries, single ventricle, and double-outlet right ventricle without pulmonary stenosis and truncus arteriosus. Other conditions in which pulmonary vascular obstruction progresses rapidly include a large ventricular septal defect and the less common conditions of complete atrioventricular canal defects and congenital left-to-right shunts in an environment of high altitude or in association with Down's syndrome.

Variability among patients whose cardiac lesions have the same or similar time of appearance exists in the rate of progression of the pulmonary vascular obstructive process. Although genetic influences may be operative (witness the apparent acceleration of pulmonary vascular disease in patients with congenital heart disease and trisomy 21), important pre- and postnatal modifiers of the pulmonary vascular bed appear, at least in part, to be lesion-dependent. Thus, a quantitative variability exists in the pulmonary vascular bed as to the number, not just the size and wall structure, of arterial vessels within the pulmonary circulation. Modeling of the blood vessels proximal to and within terminal bronchioles (preacinar and intraacinar vessels, respectively) occurs continuously from before birth. The intraacinar vessels, in particular, increase in size and number from late fetal life throughout childhood with minimal muscularization of the walls. The

TABLE 185-1 Syndromes with associated cardiovascular involvement

Syndrome	Major cardiovascular manifestations	Major noncardiac abnormalities
HERITABLE AND POSSIBLY HERITABLE		
Ellis–van Creveld	Single atrium or atrial septal defect	Chondrodystrophic dwarfism, nail dysplasia, polydactyly
TAR (thrombocytopenia-absent radius)	Atrial septal defect, tetralogy of Fallot	Radial aplasia or hypoplasia, thromocytopenia
Holt-Oram	Atrial septal defect (other defects common)	Skeletal upper limb defect, hypoplasia of clavicles
Kartagener	Dextrocardia	Situs inversus, sinusitis, brochiectasis
Laurence-Moon-Biedl-Bardot	Variable defects	Retinal pigmentation, obesity, polydactyly
Noonan	Pulmonary valve dysplasia, cardiomyopathy (usually hypertrophic)	Webbed neck, pectus excavatum, cryptorchidism
Tuberous sclerosis	Rhabdomyoma, cardiomyopathy	Phacomatosis, bone lesions, hamartomatous skin lesions
Multiple lentigines (leopard) syndrome	Pulmonic stenosis	Basal-cell nevi, broad facies, rib anomalies
Rubenstein-Taybi	Patent ductus arteriosus (others)	Broad thumbs and toes, hypoplastic maxilla, slanted palpebral fissures
Familial deafness	Arrhythmias, sudden death	Sensorineural deafness
Osler-Rendu-Weber	Arteriovenous fistuals (lung, liver, mucous membranes)	Multiple telangiectasia
Apert	Ventricular septal defect	Craniosynostosis, midfacial hypoplasia, syndactyly
Incontinentia pigmenti	Patent ductus arteriosus	Irregular pigmented skin lesions, patchy alopecia, hypodontia
Alagille (arteriohepatic dysplasia)	Peripheral pulmonic stenosis, pulmonic stenosis	Biliary hypoplasia, vertebral anomalies, prominent forehead, deep-set eyes
DiGeorge	Interrupted aortic arch, tetralogy of Fallot, truncus arteriosus	Thymic hypoplasia or aplasia, parathyroid aplasia or hypoplasia, ear anomalies
Friedreich's ataxia	Cardiomyopathy and conduction defects	Ataxia, speech defect, degeneration of spinal cord dorsal columns
Muscular dystrophy	Cardiomyopathy	Pseudohypertrophy of calf muscles, weakness of trunk and proximal limb muscles
Cystic fibrosis	Cor pulmonale	Pancreatic insufficiency, malabsorption, chronic lung disease
Sickle cell anemia	Cardiomyopathy, mitral regurgitation	Hemoglobin SS
Conradi-Hünermann	Ventricular septal defect, patent ductus arteriosus	Asymmetric limb shortness, early punctate mineralization, large skin pores
Cockayne	Accelerated atherosclerosis	Cachectic dwarfism, retinal pigment abnormalities, photosensitivity dermatitis
Progeria	Accelerated atherosclerosis	Premature aging, alopecia, atrophy of subcutaneous fat, skeletal hypoplasia
CONNECTIVE TISSUE DISORDERS		
Cutis laxa	Peripheral pulmonic stenosis	Generalized disruption of elastic fibers, diminished skin resilience, hernias
Ehlers-Danlos	Arterial dilatation and rupture, mitral regurgitation	Hyperextensible joints, hyperelastic and friable skin
Marfan	Aortic dilatation, aortic and mitral incompetence	Gracile habitus, arachnodactyly with hyperextensibility, lens subluxation
Osteogenesis imperfecta	Aortic incompetence	Fragile bones, blue sclera
Pseudoxanthoma elasticum	Peripheral and coronary arterial disease	Degeneration of elastic fibers in skin, retinal angioid streaks
INBORN ERRORS OF METABOLISM		
Pompe's disease	Glycogen storage disease of heart	Acid maltase deficiency, muscular weakness
Homocystinuria	Aortic and pulmonary arterial dilatation, intravascular thrombosis	Cystathionine synthetase deficiency, lens subluxation, osteoporosis
Mucopolysaccharidosis:		
Hurler, Hunter	Multivalvular and coronary and great artery disease, cardiomyopathy	Hurler: Deficiency of α-L-iduronidase, corneal clouding, coarse features, growth and mental retardation Hunter: Deficiency of L-iduranosulfate sulfatase, coarse facies, clear cornea, growth and mental retardation
Morquio, Scheie, Morateaux-Lamy	Aortic incompetence	Morquio: Deficiency of *N*-acetylhexosamine sulfate sulfatase, cloudy cornea, normal intelligence, severe bony changes involving vertebrae and epiphyses Scheie: Deficiency of α-L-iduronidase, cloudy cornea, normal intelligence, peculiar facies Morateaux-Lamy: Deficiency of arylsulfatase B, cloudy cornea, osseous changes, normal intelligence
CHROMOSOMAL ABNORMALITIES		
Trisomy 21 (Down's syndrome)	Endocardial cushion defect, atrial or ventricular septal defect, tetralogy of Fallot	Hypotonia, hyperextensible joints, mongoloid facies, mental retardation
Trisomy 13 (D)	Ventricular septal defect, patent ductus arteriosus, double-outlet right ventricle	Single midline intracerebral ventricle with midfacial defects, polydactyly, nail changes, mental retardation
Trisomy 18 (E)	Congenital polyvalvular dysplasia, ventricular septal defect, patent ductus arteriosus	Clenched hand, short sternum, low-arch dermal-ridge pattern on fingertips, mental retardation
Cri-du-chat (short-arm delection-5)	Ventricular septal defect	Cat cry, microcephaly, antimongoloid slant of palpebral fissures, mental retardation

TABLE 185-1 Syndromes with associated cardiovascular involvement *(continued)*

Syndrome	Major cardiovascular manifestations	Major noncardiac abnormalities
XO (Turner)	Coarctation of aorta, bicuspid aortic valve	Short female, broad chest, lymphedema, webbed neck
XXXY and XXXXX	Patent ductus arteriosus	XXXY: hypogenitalism, mental retardation, radial-ulnar synostosis XXXXX: small hands, incurving of fifth fingers, mental retardation
SPORADIC DISORDERS		
VATER association	Ventricular septal defect	Vertebral anomalies, anal atresia, tracheoesophageal fistula, radial and renal anomalies
CHARGE association	Tetralogy of Fallot (other defects common)	Colobomas, choanal atresia, mental and growth deficiency, genital and ear anomalies
Williams	Supravalvular aortic stenosis, peripheral pulmonic stenosis	Mental deficiency, "elfin" facies, loquacious personality, hoarse voice
Cornelia de Lange	Ventricular septal defect	Micromelia, synophrys, mental and growth deficiency
Shprintzen (velocardiofacial)	Ventricular septal defect, tetralogy of Fallot, right aortic arch	Cleft palate, prominent nose, slender hands, learning disability
TERATOGENIC DISORDERS		
Rubella	Patent ductus arteriosus, pulmonic valvular and/or arterial stenosis, atrial septal defect	Cataracts, deafness, microcephaly
Alcohol-induced	Ventricular septal defect (other defects)	Microcephaly, growth and mental deficiency, short palpebral fissures, smooth philtrum, thin upper lip
Phenytoin-induced	Pulmonic stenosis, aortic stenosis, coarctation, patent ductus arteriosus	Hypertelorism, growth and mental deficiency, short phalanges, bowed upper lip
Thalidomide-induced	Variable	Phocomelia

ensuing increase in the cross-sectional area of the pulmonary arterial circulation allows the cardiac output to rise substantially without an increase in pulmonary arterial pressure or resistance. If, however, the presence of a cardiac lesion does not permit these most peripheral arteries to grow and multiply normally, the resulting elevation of pulmonary vascular resistance may first be related to failure of the intraacinar pulmonary circulation to develop fully and then secondarily to the morphologic changes of obliterative vascular disease. The latter are described by the grading system of Heath and Edwards and encompass anatomic changes that include medial thickening, intimal proliferation, hyalinization and fibrosis, angiomatoid and plexiform lesions, and, ultimately, arterial necrosis.

Because pulmonary vascular obstructive disease can be the factor limiting a decision concerning the advisability of operation, it is important to quantify and compare pulmonary to systemic flows and resistances in patients with severe pulmonary hypertension. Furthermore, the lability of the pulmonary vascular resistance should be evaluated; a marked reduction with the infusion of tolazoline or the inhalation of oxygen suggests that resistance is not fixed and may fall after successful operation. Some defects between the left and right sides of the heart should be closed to eliminate a sizable left-to-right shunt, which, in turn, may cause a drop in pulmonary arterial pressure because of reduction of pulmonary blood flow. Conversely, little or no benefit and high mortality rates may be expected from the closure of defects associated with bidirectional or predominant right-to-left shunts in patients with high-resistance and obstructive pulmonary hypertension. The designation *Eisenmenger's reaction* is applied to this condition in patients who may have a large communication between the two circulations at the aortopulmonary, ventricular, or atrial levels.

Pregnant women with pulmonary vascular obstruction, whether pre- or postoperative, are at risk of dying during delivery or in the immediate postpartum period. The cause of the increased mortality rate is poorly understood. A particularly high mortality rate has been reported for those undergoing cesarean section, although such surgery should cause less cardiovascular stress than that of labor and vaginal delivery. Irrespective of approach to delivery, some simple guidelines include both continuous administration of oxygen and avoidance of inhalant anesthetic agents. Arterial blood gases and, if possible, pulmonary arterial and systemic blood pressure should be monitored periodically throughout delivery and the early postpartum period.

Some physicians advise early abortion in patients with pulmonary vascular obstruction because of the risks of pregnancy, and all such women should receive counseling on birth control. Intrauterine devices should be avoided because of the risks of bleeding and infection. Oral contraceptive agents are contraindicated because they are associated with the tendency to develop pulmonary vascular thrombosis. Use of a barrier method of birth control is preferable. Prevention of pregnancy is safer than any form of management during pregnancy, labor, delivery, and the postpartum period.

The clinical manifestations of the hyperkinetic form of pulmonary hypertension, i.e., that associated with a large left-to-right shunt, reflect the specific malformation responsible. When a significant right-to-left shunt exists, cyanosis, polycythemia, and clubbing of the digits may be present (Chap. 27). A dominant *a* wave in the jugular venous pulse may be seen, reflecting vigorous right atrial contraction due to diminished compliance of the right ventricle; in some instances large systolic *c-v* waves suggest tricuspid regurgitation. A prominent right ventricular parasternal lift and palpable systolic expansion of the pulmonary artery are present. On auscultation, one often hears a soft pulmonary systolic ejection murmur following a loud ejection sound, marked accentuation of the pulmonic component of the second heart sound, and a fourth heart sound. The decrescendo diastolic murmur of pulmonary valvular regurgitation may be heard. The electrocardiogram shows right ventricular hypertrophy. Roentgenologic examination reveals enlargement of the right ventricle, a conspicuously enlarged pulmonary artery, prominent hilar pulmonary vascular markings, and attenuated peripheral vessels. The site of the underlying defect may be localized by means of two-dimensional and Doppler echocardiography and/or cardiac catheterization and angiocardiography (Chap. 180). Pressures in the right side of the heart are essentially identical to systemic pressures in cyanotic patients if the shunt is at the ventricular or aortopulmonary levels, but they are usually lower than systemic pressure in patients with an interatrial shunt. No specific treatment has proved beneficial for obstructive pulmonary vascular disease.

CIRCULATORY SHUNTS

Although equal quantities of blood flow through the pulmonary and systemic circulations in normal subjects postnatally, the systemic circulation has a flow resistance approximately six times that of the pulmonary circuit, which is reflected in the higher arterial and ventricular systolic pressures in the systemic circulation; the lower compliance of the thicker left ventricle is reflected in higher ventricular end-diastolic and mean atrial pressures on the left side of the heart. Therefore, if an abnormal communication is present, blood flows from the left to the right side of the heart. The size of the opening and the pressures on either side determine the direction and magnitude of the shunt flow. A right-to-left shunt usually requires either an obstructive lesion at some point in the right-sided circulation (i.e., tricuspid stenosis or atresia, pulmonary valvular or infundibular stenosis, elevated pulmonary vascular resistance), a mixing of systemic venous and arterialized blood (i.e., total anomalous pulmonary venous drainage, a single atrium or ventricle, or a persistent truncus arteriosus), or some form of obligatory recirculation of systemic venous blood (e.g., transposition of the great arteries). The location, direction, and magnitude of the right-to-left shunt may be determined during hemodynamic study by measuring the admixture of venous and arterial blood at various sites in the central circulation, by indicator-dilution curves, and by angiocardiography, as outlined in Chap. 180.

CLINICAL MANIFESTATIONS OF RIGHT-TO-LEFT SHUNTS Cyanosis and polycythemia These signs are discussed in Chap. 27.

Clubbing A prominent accompaniment of arterial hypoxemia is widening and thickening of the terminal phalanges of the fingers and toes, accompanied by convex nails. These digits have an increased number of capillaries, an increased blood flow through extensive arteriovenous aneurysms, and an increase of connective tissue.

Hypoxic spells and squatting A sudden increase in cyanosis due to an abrupt reduction in pulmonary blood flow can occur in children with certain types of cyanotic heart disease, particularly tetralogy of Fallot. The spells may lead to convulsions and may even be fatal and can be precipitated by fluctuations in intravascular volume or in arterial P_{CO_2} and pH, a sudden fall in systemic or increase in pulmonary vascular resistance, or an acute increase in the severity of right ventricular outflow tract obstruction, either by augmented contraction of the hypertrophied muscle in the right ventricular outflow tract or by a decrease in right ventricular cavity volume due to tachycardia. Treatment consists of placing the child in the knee-chest position, oxygen administration, and intravenous administration of fluids and of sodium bicarbonate to correct the accompanying acidosis. Additional medications that may prove of value include morphine, alpha-adrenergic receptor stimulants such as phenylephrine to raise peripheral resistance and diminish right-to-left shunting, and beta-adrenergic blocking agents, which may increase ventricular volume by reducing heart rate and lessen infundibular obstruction by reducing contractility.

Patients with cyanotic heart disease, especially tetralogy of Fallot, typically assume a squatting posture after exertion to obtain relief from breathlessness. Squatting appears to hasten an increase in the arterial oxygen saturation by increasing systemic vascular resistance and thereby diminishing the right-to-left shunt and by trapping markedly unsaturated blood in the legs. Also, systemic venous return and therefore pulmonary blood flow may rise.

"Paradoxic" embolus and brain abscess In patients with cyanotic congenital heart disease, venous blood bypasses the normal filtering action of the lungs, and emboli arising in systemic veins may pass directly to the systemic circulation. Patients with severe cyanosis or polycythemia often have occlusive microcirculatory damage to the central nervous system and are predisposed (2 to 4 percent) to brain abscess.

Impaired growth Physical underdevelopment and a delayed onset of adolescence are common features of cyanotic and, to a lesser extent, acyanotic forms of congenital heart disease. Mental development is rarely affected. Possible explanations for the growth interference include malnutrition, tissue anoxia, diminished peripheral blood flow, hypermetabolic state, chronic cardiac decompensation, genetic and endocrine factors, and frequent upper and lower respiratory infections.

SPECIFIC CARDIAC DEFECTS

Various classifications of congenital cardiovascular lesions have been proposed, depending on hemodynamic, anatomic, and radiographic factors. Table 185-2 provides a classification of cardiac anomalies that recognizes the general categories of clinical presentation, functional consequences, and site of origin of congenital defects.

The text of this chapter focuses on common cardiac malformations, whereas Table 185-2 presents a more comprehensive list of lesions. Cardiac lesions are organized into those which do or do not result in cyanosis. The acyanotic group is subdivided into malformations with and without a left-to-right shunt. The shunt lesions are further classified with respect to the principal site of communication between the systemic and pulmonary circulations. The acyanotic lesions without a shunt are categorized with respect to the location of the lesion in the left or right heart and from inflow to outflow regions on either side of the circulation. Cyanotic lesions are classified with respect to pulmonary blood flow, since the radiographic determination of the magnitude of the latter provides an insight into whether the cyanosis is the result of an obligatory admixture of systemic and pulmonary venous return (increased pulmonary blood flow) or of reduced pulmonary blood flow.

GENERAL Congenitally corrected transposition The two fundamental anatomic derangements composing this malformation are transposition of the ascending aorta and pulmonary trunk and inversion of the ventricles. This arrangement permits functional correction, so that systemic venous blood passes into the pulmonary trunk while arterialized pulmonary venous blood flows into the aorta. The systemic veins drain into the right atrium; hence venous blood flows across an atrioventricular valve, which has the structure of a normal *mitral* valve, into the right-sided "venous ventricle." This chamber ejects blood into the pulmonary trunk, which arises *posterior* to the ascending aorta. Oxygenated blood returns from the lungs to the left atrium, from which it flows into the left-sided "arterial ventricle" across an atrioventricular valve, which has the structure of a normal *tricuspid* valve. The arterial ventricle ejects blood into the aorta, which arises anterior to the pulmonary trunk.

Patients in whom corrected transposition is an isolated anomaly present no functional alterations and have no symptoms. Ebstein-type anomalies of the left-sided, tricuspid atrioventricular valve, ventricular septal defect, obstruction to outflow from the venous ventricle, and congenital heart block are often associated with corrected transposition. An accentuated, single second heart sound in the second left intercostal space, representing closure of the aortic valve, which lies lateral and anterior to the pulmonic valve is often present. The His bundle is elongated, often leading to atrioventricular conduction disturbances. Roentgenographic examination characteristically reveals absence of the normal pulmonary artery segment and a smooth convexity of the left supracardiac border produced by the displaced ascending aorta. The displaced aorta may be visualized by cross-sectional echocardiography and by radionuclide scintillation scans of the central circulation. The diagnosis of corrected transposition can usually be established by selective angiocardiography.

Malpositions of the heart Positional anomalies of the heart refer to conditions in which the cardiac apex is in the right side of the chest (dextrocardia) or at the midline (mesocardia) or in which there is a normal location of the heart in the left side of the chest but abnormal position of the viscera (isolated levocardia). Knowledge of the position of the abdominal organs is important in diagnosing these malpositions. For example, a mirror-image dextrocardia is usually observed in a patient with complete situs inversus; this condition occurs more frequently in people whose hearts are otherwise normal. In contrast, when dextrocardia occurs without situs inversus, associated cardiac malformations are the rule. When the heart occupies its normal position but situs inversus of the viscera is present, the heart is usually seriously malformed. Moreover, when the visceral situs is indeterminate, there is a striking association of asplenia or polysplenia

TABLE 185-2 Classification of congenital heart disease

GENERAL

Congenitally corrected transposition of the great arteries
The cardiac malpositions
Congenital complete heart block

ACYANOTIC WITH LEFT-TO-RIGHT SHUNT

Atrial level shunt:
- *1* Atrial septal defect
  - *a* Ostium secundum
  - *b* Ostium primum
  - *c* Sinus venosus
- *2* Atrial septal defect with mitral stenosis (Lutembacher's syndrome)
- *3* Partial anomalous pulmonary venous connection

Ventricular level shunt:
- *1* Ventricular septal defect
  - *a* Inlet septum
  - *b* Muscular septum
  - *c* Perimembranous septum
  - *d* Infundibular septum
- *2* Ventricular septal defect with aortic regurgitation
- *3* Ventricular septal defect with left ventricular to right atrial shunt

Aortic root to right heart shunt:
- *1* Ruptured sinus of Valsalva aneurysm
- *2* Coronary arteriovenous fistula
- *3* Anomalous origin of the left coronary artery from the pulmonary trunk

Aortopulmonary level shunt:
- *1* Aortopulmonary window
- *2* Patent ductus arteriosus

Multiple level shunts:
- *1* Complete common atrioventricular canal
- *2* Ventricular septal defect with atrial septal defect
- *3* Ventricular septal defect with patent ductus arteriosus

ACYANOTIC WITHOUT A SHUNT

Left heart malformations:
- *1* Congenital obstruction to left atrial inflow
  - *a* Pulmonary vein stenosis
  - *b* Mitral stenosis
  - *c* Cor triatriatum
- *2* Mitral regurgitation
  - *a* Endocardial cushion defect
  - *b* Congenitally corrected transposition of the great arteries
  - *c* Anomalous origin of the left coronary artery from the pulmonary trunk
  - *d* Miscellaneous (double-orifice mitral valve, congenital performations, accessory commissures with anomalous chordal insertion, congenitally short or absent chordae, cleft posterior leaflet, parachute mitral valve, etc.)
- *3* Primary dilated endocardial fibroelastosis
- *4* Aortic stenosis
  - *a* Discrete subvalvular
  - *b* Valvular
  - *c* Supravalvular
- *5* Aortic valve regurgitation
- *6* Coarctation of the aorta

Right heart malformations:
- *1* Acyanotic Ebstein's anomaly of the tricuspid valve
- *2* Pulmonic stenosis
  - *a* Subinfundibular
  - *b* Infundibular
  - *c* Valvular
  - *d* Supravalvular (stenosis of pulmonary artery and its branches)
- *3* Congenital pulmonary valve regurgitation
- *4* Idiopathic dilatation of the pulmonary trunk

CYANOTIC

Increased pulmonary blood flow:
- *1* Complete transposition of the great arteries
- *2* Double-outlet right ventricle of the Taussig-Bing type
- *3* Truncus arteriosus
- *4* Total anomalous pulmonary venous connection
- *5* Single ventricle without pulmonic stenosis
- *6* Common atrium
- *7* Tetralogy of Fallot with pulmonary atresia and increased collateral arterial flow
- *8* Tricuspid atresia with large ventricular septal defect and no pulmonic stenosis
- *9* Hypoplastic left heart (aortic atresia, mitral atresia)

Normal or decreased pulmonary blood flow:
- *1* Tricuspid atresia
- *2* Ebstein's anomaly with right-to-left atrial shunt
- *3* Pulmonary atresia with intact ventricular septum
- *4* Pulmonic stenosis or atresia with ventricular septal defect (tetralogy of Fallot)
- *5* Pulmonic stenosis with right-to-left atrial shunt
- *6* Complete transposition of the great arteries with pulmonic stenosis
- *7* Double-outlet right ventricle with pulmonic stenosis
- *8* Single ventricle with pulmonic stenosis
- *9* Pulmonary arteriovenous fistula
- *10* Vena caval to left atrial communication

SOURCE: *Modified from JK Perloff, in The Clinical Recognition of Congenital Heart Disease, 2d ed. Philadelphia, Saunders, 1978.*

with complex, multiple cardiac anomalies, which usually include a combination of systemic and pulmonary venous abnormalities, defects in the atrial and ventricular septa, and endocardial cushion defects. Transposition of the great arteries occurs frequently in cardiac malposition, and double-outlet right ventricle is common in asplenia. It is important to recognize these complex syndromes in order to distinguish them from forms of cyanotic heart disease that are more amenable to corrective surgical therapy. The diagnosis is suggested by a symmetric liver shadow roentgenographically, and by the presence of Howell-Jolly and Heinz bodies in red blood cells demonstrated by blood smear, and confirmed by a negative or abnormal radioactive spleen scan.

Congenital complete heart block The atrioventricular node and the His bundle originate during fetal development as separate structures and later join together. The basic lesion in congenital complete heart block consists of discontinuity between the atrial musculature and the atrioventricular node or the His bundle if the atrioventricular node is absent. Occasionally, the anatomic interruption may be between the atrioventricular node and the main His bundle or within the bundle itself. No known etiology exists for the majority of cases of congenital heart block in infants who usually have otherwise anatomically normal hearts. However, fetal myocarditis, idiopathic hemorrhage and necrosis involving conduction tissue, and degeneration and fibrosis related in some instances to the transplacental passage of immune complexes from mothers with systemic lupus erythematosus are all capable of causing congenital heart block. Less often, congenital heart block may be associated with congenital heart disease, the most common malformation being corrected transposition of the great arteries.

Detection of consistent fetal bradycardia (heart rate 40 to 80 beats per minute) by auscultation, ultrasound, or electronic monitoring allows anticipation of the correct diagnosis. The newborn, especially with a ventricular rate less than 50 beats per minute and an atrial rate in excess of 150 beats per minute, is at highest risk; the presence of an associated cardiovascular anomaly greatly lessens the chances of survival. Treatment is not required for the asymptomatic infant. Digitalization is recommended for the baby in congestive heart failure, irrespective of the presence of complete heart block.

Isoproterenol and other sympathomimetic drugs and atropine do not have permanent or beneficial effects. Congestive heart failure and Stokes-Adams attacks require pacemaker treatment at any age. Initial management of the child in whom permanent epicardial pacemaker insertion is indicated usually involves preoperative insertion of a transvenous intracardiac electrode into the right ventricle in order to protect the patient from serious arrhythmias during the induction of anesthesia. After pacemaker implantation, one may anticipate a variety of problems related to growth of the patient, which stresses the lead system; the fragility of the lead system in a physically active young patient; and the limited life span of the pulse generator. Patients with congenital complete heart block who survive infancy usually remain asymptomatic until late in childhood or adolescence.

ACYANOTIC WITH A LEFT-TO-RIGHT SHUNT **Atrial septal defect** Atrial septal defect is a commonly recognized congenital cardiac anomaly in adults and occurs more frequently in females than in males. Defects of the *sinus venosus* type occur high in the atrial septum near the entry of the superior vena cava and are associated frequently with anomalous connection of pulmonary veins from the right lung to the junction of the superior vena cava and right atrium. Most often, an atrial defect involves the fossa ovalis, is midseptal in location, and is of the *ostium secundum* type. This type of defect should not be confused with a patent foramen ovale. Anatomic obliteration of the foramen ovale ordinarily follows its functional closure soon after birth, but residual "probe patency" is a normal variant; atrial septal defect denotes a true deficiency of the atrial septum and implies functional and anatomic patency. *Ostium primum* anomalies are a form of endocardial cushion defect that lie immediately adjacent to the atrioventricular valves, either of which may be deformed and incompetent or which may form together a common atrioventricular valve; this defect may also involve the basal portion of the interventricular septum. *Ostium primum defects* occur commonly in patients with *Down's syndrome,* although the more complex endocardial cushion anomalies are more characteristic. *Lutembacher's syndrome* is the term applied to the rare combination of atrial septal defect and mitral stenosis; this component of the malformation is usually the result of acquired rheumatic valvulitis.

The magnitude of the left-to-right shunt through an atrial septal defect depends on the size of the defect, the relative compliance of the ventricles, and the relative resistances in the pulmonary and systemic circulations. The left-to-right shunt causes diastolic overloading of the right ventricle and increased pulmonary blood flow. The pulmonary vascular resistance is usually normal or low in the child and young adult with atrial septal defect, and the volume load is usually well tolerated even though pulmonary blood flow may be three to six times greater than systemic.

Patients with atrial septal defect are usually asymptomatic in early life, although there may be some physical underdevelopment and an increased tendency for respiratory infections; cardiorespiratory symptoms occur in many older patients. Beyond the fourth decade, a significant number of patients develop atrial arrhythmias, pulmonary arterial hypertension, bidirectional and then right-to-left shunting of blood, and cardiac failure. Patients exposed to the chronic environmental hypoxia of high altitude tend to develop pulmonary hypertension at younger ages. Historical features suggesting that the defect is of the endocardial cushion variety include the onset of disability, pulmonary hypertension, and heart failure in infancy or childhood.

Physical examination usually reveals a prominent right ventricular cardiac impulse and palpable pulmonary artery pulsation. The first heart sound is normal or split, with accentuation of the tricuspid valve closure sound. Increased flow across the pulmonic valve is responsible for a midsystolic pulmonary ejection murmur. The second sound is widely split and is relatively fixed in relation to respiration, because of reciprocal changes in the magnitude of the left-to-right shunt and of the systemic venous inflow into the right ventricle during respiration, so that filling of the right ventricle remains constant and the stroke volume of the right ventricle exceeds that of the left throughout the respiratory cycle. With pulmonary hypertension the splitting is still fixed throughout respiration, although the width may be reduced. A middiastolic rumbling murmur at the fourth intercostal space and along the left sternal border reflects increased flow across the tricuspid valve. In patients with ostium primum defects, an apical thrill and holosystolic murmur indicate associated mitral or tricuspid incompetence or a ventricular septal defect.

The *physical findings* are altered when an increase in the pulmonary vascular resistance results in diminution of the left-to-right shunt. Both the pulmonary and tricuspid murmurs decrease in intensity, the pulmonic component of the second heart sound and a systolic ejection sound are accentuated, the two components of the second heart sound may fuse, and a diastolic murmur of pulmonic incompetence appears. Cyanosis and clubbing accompany the development of a right-to-left shunt.

The *electrocardiogram* in patients with an ostium secundum defect usually shows right axis deviation and an rSr′ pattern in the right precordial leads, representing delayed posterobasal activation of the ventricular septum. Right ventricular hypertrophy is common in children but not adults. An ectopic atrial pacemaker or first-degree heart block occurs occasionally in patients with defects of the sinus venosus type. In patients with an ostium primum defect, the right ventricular conduction defect is characteristically accompanied by left axis deviation and by superior orientation and counterclockwise rotation of the QRS loop in the frontal plane. Varying degrees of right ventricular and right atrial hypertrophy may occur with each type of defect, depending on the height of the pulmonary artery pressure; prolongation of the PR interval is most common with ostium primum defects. Chest roentgenograms reveal enlargement of the right atrium and ventricle, dilatation of the pulmonary artery and its branches, and increased pulmonary vascular markings. Left atrial enlargement is uncommon. Echocardiographic assessment should include an attempt at direct visualization of the defect from subcostal right parasternal or apical windows. Indirect features include pulmonary arterial and right ventricular dilatation and anterior systolic (paradoxic) or "flat" interventricular septal motion if significant right ventricular volume overload is present. Mitral valve prolapse may occur in 10 to 20 percent of patients with secundum defects. A cleft (trileaflet) mitral valve and abnormal septal-atrioventricular valve relationships are common in endocardial cushion anomalies; Doppler assessment of the severity of any mitral regurgitation is valuable.

The diagnosis can be confirmed at cardiac catheterization by passage of the catheter across the atrial defect. The site at which the catheter crosses, if high in the cardiac silhouette, may suggest a sinus venosus defect, or, if low, a primum defect. Serial determinations of the oxygen saturation or indicator-dilution curve techniques can be used to estimate the magnitude of the shunt. In young patients, pressures in the right side of the heart are often normal despite a large shunt; pulmonary arterial hypertension is more common in the older patients. If an endocardial cushion defect is present, a left ventricular angiogram frequently demonstrates a "gooseneck" deformity of the left ventricular outflow tract caused by an abnormal anterior mitral valve leaflet; it may also show mitral regurgitation. When oxygen saturation is high in the superior vena cava or when the catheter enters pulmonary veins directly from the right atrium, a sinus venosus defect is likely, and indicator-dilution curves and selective angiography will aid in identifying the number and location of the anomalous veins. *Partial anomalous pulmonary venous connection,* although generally associated with a sinus venosus defect, may accompany primum and secundum defects or be unassociated with any defect of the interatrial septum.

Endocardial cushion anomalies more complex than the ostium primum defect are associated with marked pulmonary hypertension and high morbidity and mortality rates in infancy and childhood. Patients with atrial septal defect of the sinus venosus or secundum types rarely die before the fifth decade. During the fifth and sixth decades, the incidence of progressive symptoms, often leading to severe disability, increases substantially. Medical management should include prompt treatment of respiratory tract infections, antiarrhythmic medications for atrial fibrillation or supraventricular tachycardia, and the usual measures for heart failure (Chap. 182) if these complications occur. Although the risk of subacute bacterial endocarditis is low, antibiotics should be administered prophylactically prior to dental procedures (see Chap. 188).

Operative repair, ideally in patients between 3 and 6 years of age, should be advised for all patients with uncomplicated atrial septal defects in whom there is significant left-to-right shunting, i.e., with pulmonary-to-systemic flow ratios exceeding approximately 1.5:1.0. Excellent results may be anticipated, at low risk, even in patients beyond 40 years of age in the absence of pulmonary hypertension. The defect is closed by suture or with a patch of prosthetic material with the patient on cardiopulmonary bypass. Symptomatic infants with complex endocardial cushion defects require corrective operation. Special attention must be given to the atrioventricular valves in patients with endocardial cushion defects; cleft, deformed, and incompetent valves may require repair or replacement to prevent significant regurgitation and failure in the postoperative period. The operative risk and the incidence of such complications as complete heart block and persistent mitral regurgitation are higher in patients with endocardial cushion defects. Electrophysiologic mapping of the course of the conduction system during operation may reduce the risk of postsurgical heart block. Operation should not be carried out in patients with small defects and trivial left-to-right shunts, or in those with severe pulmonary vascular disease without a significant left-to-right shunt.

Partial anomalous pulmonary venous connection In this condition, one of the pulmonary veins (or more than one) is connected to the right atrium or to one or more of its tributaries. An atrial septal defect, particularly one of the sinus venosus type, usually accompanies partial transposition of the pulmonary veins, and the usual connection involves the veins of the right upper and middle lobes and the superior vena cava. The hemodynamic state and physical findings are usually similar to those in atrial septal defect.

Ventricular septal defect Defects of the ventricular septum are common as isolated defects and as one component of a combination of anomalies. The opening is usually single and situated in the membranous portion of the septum. The functional disturbance is dependent primarily on its size and on the status of the pulmonary vascular bed, rather than on the location of the defect. A substantial left-to-right ventricular pressure gradient occurs in the presence of a small defect (*maladie de Roger*), and a small shunt, limited by the size of the defect, occurs throughout systole. Larger defects offer less resistance to flow, while in the presence of very large defects both ventricles function hemodynamically as a single pumping chamber with two outlets, equalizing the pressures in the systemic and pulmonary circulations. In such patients, the magnitude of the left-to-right shunt varies inversely with the ratio of pulmonary-to-systemic vascular resistance. In patients with large defects and large left-to-right shunts, the left ventricle is overloaded and may fail. Survival through infancy depends on delayed regression of the fetal pulmonary vascular pattern, the development of an elevated pulmonary vascular resistance, or the secondary development of infundibular hypertrophy and obstruction to right ventricular outflow. Irreversible obliterative changes in the pulmonary vessels with dominant right-to-left shunts and cyanosis become manifest in many patients with large defects after the second decade of life. Spontaneous closure of small and even large ventricular defects may occur, especially before the age of 3 years. In others the relative size of the interventricular communication may diminish as normal growth of the heart occurs with advancing age. Rarely, incompetence of the aortic valve resulting from insufficient cusp tissue or prolapse of a cusp through the interventricular defect complicates and dominates the clinical course of patients with ventricular septal defect.

The clinical picture varies, depending on the age, the size of the defect, and the level of the pulmonary vascular resistance. Patients with small defects are generally asymptomatic; moderate left-to-right shunts may be associated with effort intolerance and fatigue. Large defects are commonly accompanied by frequent pulmonary infections, growth retardation, and cardiac failure in infancy, but survival past this period is often associated with an amelioration of symptoms until adulthood. In patients with severe pulmonary vascular obstruction, symptoms in adult life consist of exertional dyspnea, chest pain, syncope, and hemoptysis. The right-to-left shunt leads to cyanosis, clubbing, and polycythemia.

Patients with moderate-sized defects exhibit cardiomegaly with a forceful left ventricular impulse and a prominent systolic thrill along the lower left sternal border. The second heart sound is normally or closely split, with moderate accentuation of the pulmonic component; a third heart sound and diastolic rumbling murmur, reflecting increased flow across the mitral valve during rapid ventricular filling, are often audible at the cardiac apex. The characteristic holosystolic murmur results from flow across the defect; it is best heard along the third and fourth interspaces to the left of the sternum and is widely transmitted over the precordium. A basal midsystolic ejection murmur may also be heard, because of increased flow across the pulmonic valve. In patients with pulmonary vascular obstruction and small left-to-right shunts, both the systolic thrill and murmur decrease in intensity and duration and may disappear entirely, to be replaced by a marked right ventricular precordial lift, pulmonary ejection sound and soft systolic ejection murmur, a closely split second heart sound with accentuation of the pulmonic component, and the diastolic murmur of pulmonic incompetence.

The electrocardiographic pattern, the relative size and contour of the two ventricles roentgenographically, and the appearance of the lung fields serve as indicators of the underlying pathophysiologic condition. The electrocardiogram is generally normal in patients with small defects. Left or combined ventricular hypertrophy is seen with large left-to-right shunts; right ventricular hypertrophy occurs with pulmonary vascular obstruction. The roentgenograms may be normal with small defects; large defects are characterized by an enlarged left atrium, biventricular hypertrophy, a prominent pulmonary artery segment, and increased pulmonary vascular markings. Relative diminution and attenuation of the peripheral pulmonary vasculature occur in patients with obstructive pulmonary vascular disease. The features of a ventricular septal defect on M-mode echocardiography are those of left atrial and left ventricular enlargement from the shunt. Two-dimensional imaging allows a scan of the ventricular septum from multiple acoustic windows.

In approximately 90 percent of patients, the defect occurs in the membranous septum. A shunt from the left ventricle to the right atrium may occur with a defect in the most superior portion of the ventricular septum, since the tricuspid valve is lower than the mitral valve. The clinical, electrocardiographic, and radiologic findings in these patients often do not differ from those with a simple ventricular septal defect, although right atrial enlargement and evidence of right ventricular volume overload may be present; the diagnosis can be established by left ventriculography. Prolapse of an aortic valve leaflet through a subpulmonary ventricular defect or the combination of subcristal ventricular septal defect and underdevelopment of an aortic valve commissure may produce aortic regurgitation that is frequently progressive and is the most significant hemodynamic lesion. In these patients complete operative repair may necessitate insertion of a prosthetic aortic valve.

The pathophysiology of a single or common ventricle may resemble that of a large ventricular septal defect, although the two lesions are dissimilar embryologically. There is an obligatory admixture of systemic and pulmonary venous return in patients with a single ventricle, but little or no cyanosis may result if selective streaming and increased pulmonary blood flow occur. Severe pulmonary hypertension occurs unless pulmonic stenosis coexists. A large ventricular septal defect should be differentiated from a single ventricle by echocardiography and angiography, because operative correction of the latter is more difficult.

The risk of bacterial endocarditis is higher in patients with small or moderate-sized defects than in those with large ones, but appropriate prophylaxis is essential in all. In the small infant with a large left-to-right shunt, congestive failure may be severe and intractable despite intensive medical management; this problem is managed best by primary closure of the defect. Operation is indicated in children and adults when there is a moderate or large left-to-right shunt with a pulmonary to systemic flow ratio that exceeds 1.5:1.0 or 2.0:1.0 regardless of the level of pulmonary artery pressure. Operation is contraindicated in patients with small defects and left-to-right shunts and in patients in whom the pulmonary vascular resistance is elevated to a level which eliminates the net left-to-right shunt. Indeed, operation carries an increased risk whenever pulmonary resistance is significantly elevated.

Aortic sinus aneurysm and fistula Congenital aneurysm of an aortic sinus of Valsalva, particularly the right coronary sinus, is uncommon; it consists of a separation, or lack of fusion, between the media of the aorta and the annulus fibrosus of the aortic valve. Progressive aneurysmal dilatation of the weakened area may not be recognized until the third or fourth decade of life, when rupture into a cardiac chamber occurs. The receiving chamber of the aorticocardiac fistula is usually the right ventricle, but occasionally the fistula drains into the right atrium.

The unruptured aneurysm generally does not produce symptoms or a hemodynamic abnormality. Rupture is often abrupt, causes chest pain, and creates continuous arteriovenous shunting and volume overloading of both right and left heart chambers, with resultant heart failure. This anomaly should be suspected in a patient with a history of recent onset of chest pain, symptoms of diminished cardiac reserve, bounding pulses, a loud, superficial, continuous murmur accentuated in diastole when the fistula opens into the right ventricle, and a thrill along the right or left lower parasternal area. The diagnosis may be established by two-dimensional and Doppler echocardiography, and by retrograde thoracic aortography. Operation is indicated in patients with large left-to-right shunts.

Coronary arteriovenous fistula Coronary arteriovenous fistula is an unusual anomaly that most often consists of a communication between the right coronary artery and the right atrium or ventricle. The shunt is usually of small magnitude, and myocardial blood flow is not usually compromised. Potential complications include bacterial endocarditis, thrombus formation with occlusion or distal embolization, rupture of an aneurysmal fistula, and rarely, pulmonary hypertension and congestive failure. The finding of a loud, superficial, continuous murmur at the lower or midsternal border usually prompts a further evaluation of asymptomatic patients. Doppler echocardiography demonstrates the site of drainage; if the site of origin is proximal, it may be detectable by two-dimensional echocardiography. Retrograde thoracic aortography or coronary arteriography permits identification of the size and anatomic features of the fistulous tract, which may be closed by suture obliteration.

Anomalous pulmonary origin of coronary artery The left coronary artery rarely originates from the pulmonary artery. As the elevated pulmonary vascular resistance declines immediately after birth, perfusion of the left coronary artery from the pulmonary artery ceases and the direction of flow in the anomalous vessel reverses. Total myocardial perfusion must pass through the right coronary artery and may be sufficient for normal activity if adequate collateral channels develop between the two coronary circulations. Myocardial infarction and fibrosis commonly develop during the first 6 months of life, leading to death within the first year. From 10 to 20 percent of patients survive to childhood or adolescence without surgical correction. Occasionally, in older children or adults mitral regurgitation may result from dysfunction of ischemic or infarcted papillary muscles.

The diagnosis of anomalous origin of the coronary artery is supported by the electrocardiographic findings of an anterolateral myocardial infarction. Aortic root or coronary angiography demonstrates the retrograde drainage of the coronary vessel into the pulmonary artery and the presence of a single right coronary artery arising from the aorta.

Ideal operative management of adult patients employs a saphenous vein–coronary artery graft. The outcome of operation and ultimate prognosis are influenced by the degree of preoperative myocardial damage.

Patent ductus arteriosus The ductus arteriosus is a vessel leading from the bifurcation of the pulmonary artery to the aorta just distal to the left subclavian artery. Normal closure of the ductus immediately after birth may be due to the sudden increase in arterial oxygen tension that accompanies ventilation and abrupt alterations in the disposition of vasoactive substances, particularly prostaglandins. Intimal proliferation and fibrosis proceed more gradually, so that anatomic obliteration may not be completed until several months after birth. Persistent patency of the ductus after birth is relatively common, occurring more frequently in females, in the offspring of women whose pregnancies were complicated by first-trimester rubella, in premature infants, and in children born at high altitudes. A distinction should be made between patency of the ductus arteriosus in the preterm infant who lacks the normal mechanisms for postnatal ductal closure because of immaturity and the full-term newborn in whom patency of the ductus is a true congenital malformation related, most likely, to a primary anatomic defect of the elastic tissue within the wall of the vessel. Although the latter anomaly occurs most frequently in the isolated form, it may coexist with other malformations, particularly coarctation of the aorta, ventricular septal defect, pulmonic stenosis, and aortic stenosis. Patency of the ductus may provide the only route for maintaining pulmonary or systemic blood flow in the presence of such lesions as pulmonary atresia or aortic arch interruption.

The flow across the ductus is determined by the pressure and resistance relationships between the systemic and the pulmonary circulations, and by the cross-sectional area and length of the ductus. Most commonly, pulmonary pressures are normal, and a gradient and shunt from aorta to pulmonary artery persists throughout the cardiac cycle. Physical examination reveals a characteristic thrill and a continuous "machinery" murmur with a late systolic accentuation at the upper left sternal border. The left atrium and ventricle enlarge to accommodate the increased pulmonary venous return, and flow murmurs across the mitral and aortic valves may be present. With large or moderate-sized left-to-right shunts, the runoff of blood through the ductus causes a widened systemic pulse pressure and bounding peripheral pulses. The hemodynamic abnormality is reflected by left ventricular and, occasionally, left atrial hypertrophy on the electrocardiogram and by left atrial and ventricular enlargement, a prominent ascending aorta and pulmonary artery, and pulmonary vascular engorgement on the chest roentgenogram. Determination of left atrial and ventricular size by echocardiography provides an estimate of the magnitude of left-to-right shunting.

The recognition of patent ductus arteriosus may be difficult in infancy and in patients with pulmonary hypertension or heart failure. In these circumstances, the pressure gradient between the aorta and pulmonary artery is reduced or absent, as is the typical continuous murmur, and there may be only a systolic ejection murmur at the base, a diastolic blowing murmur of pulmonary regurgitation (Graham Steell), or no murmur. When severe, pulmonary vascular disease results in reversal of flow through the ductus, unoxygenated blood is shunted to the descending aorta, and the toes, but not the fingers, become cyanotic and clubbed, a finding termed *differential cyanosis*.

A large ductus can cause cardiac failure and pulmonary edema in the premature infant, but in the full-term baby it is often compatible with survival until adult life. The symptomatic *preterm* infant may be managed either by pharmacologic inhibition of prostaglandin synthesis with indomethacin to constrict and close the ductus or by surgical ligation. Pharmacologic approaches are ineffective in full-term infants or children in whom patency is a true malformation. The leading causes of death in adults with patent ductus are cardiac failure and bacterial endarteritis and less frequently, severe pulmonary vascular obstruction may cause aneurysmal dilatation, calcification, and rupture of the ductus.

In the absence of severe pulmonary vascular disease and predominant right-to-left shunting of blood, the patent ductus should be surgically repaired, at least in patients over 2 years of age. Ligation or division of the ductus is associated with a low risk (under 2 percent) when it is performed electively in a healthy person. The operative risk is also reduced if cardiac failure, when present, can be treated successfully before operation. Operation should be deferred for several months in patients treated successfully for bacterial endarteritis, because the ductus may remain somewhat edematous and friable.

ACYANOTIC WITHOUT A SHUNT Congenital aortic stenosis Malformations that cause obstruction to the ejection of blood from the left ventricle include congenital valvular aortic stenosis, the discrete form of congenital subaortic stenosis, congenital narrowing of the supravalvular ascending aorta, and hypertrophic cardiomyopathy with outflow tract obstruction (Chap. 192).

Valvular aortic stenosis Valvular aortic stenosis is a relatively rare congenital cardiovascular defect that occurs three to four times more often in males than in females. However, the congenital bicuspid aortic valve, which is not necessarily stenotic, may actually be the most common congenital malformation of the heart, although it may go undetected in early life. Because bicuspid valves may become stenotic with time or be the site of infective endocarditis, the lesion may be difficult to distinguish in adults from acquired rheumatic aortic stenosis. Commonly associated anomalies include patent ductus arteriosus and coarctation of the aorta.

The dynamics of blood flow associated with a congenitally deformed, rigid aortic valve commonly lead to thickening of the cusps and, in later life, to calcification. Hemodynamically significant obstruction causes concentric hypertrophy of the left ventricular wall and dilatation of the ascending aorta.

The hemodynamic abnormalities are discussed in Chap. 187. A peak systolic pressure gradient exceeding 70 mmHg, in association with a normal cardiac output, or an effective aortic orifice less than 0.6 cm^2 per square meter of body surface, is considered to represent critical obstruction to left ventricular outflow. In children and young adults, the resting cardiac output is generally normal but often fails to rise normally during muscular exercise.

Most children with congenital aortic stenosis are asymptomatic. Usually, a murmur is detected on a routine examination. Moderately severe obstruction should be suspected if there is a history of fatigability and exertional dyspnea. With severe obstruction, the inability of the left ventricle to increase its output and maintain cerebral flow during exercise may result in exertional syncope, and the disparity between the oxygen supply and myocardial oxygen requirements may cause angina. The symptomatic patient with valvular aortic stenosis generally has critical stenosis, although a lack of symptoms does not preclude the presence of moderately severe obstruction. Sudden death occurs in patients with critical stenosis, and ventricular arrhythmias, perhaps initiated by acute myocardial ischemia, may be responsible.

Hemodynamically significant obstruction is associated with a left ventricular lift and a precordial systolic thrill over the base of the heart, with transmission to the jugular notch and along the carotid arteries. Presystolic expansion is often palpable. A systolic aortic ejection sound, signifying opening of the aortic valve, is typical at the cardiac apex when the valve is mobile, particularly with mild to moderate stenosis. Delayed closure of the stenotic aortic valve leads to a single or a closely split second heart sound, and paradoxic splitting may be present. A fourth heart sound is generally associated with severe obstruction. The systolic murmur starts after the completion of left ventricular isometric contraction, is rhomboid-shaped, loud, harsh, and best heard at the base of the heart. The murmur, like the thrill, radiates to the jugular notch and carotid vessels and to the apex. An early diastolic blowing murmur of aortic regurgitation may be present, but unless the valve has been eroded by infective endocarditis, the regurgitation is usually not hemodynamically significant; occasionally, in patients with a congenital bicuspid valve, severe aortic regurgitation may be the dominant hemodynamic lesion.

The electrocardiographic evidence of left ventricular hypertrophy tends to reflect the severity of obstruction, although a *normal or near-normal electrocardiogram does not exclude severe aortic stenosis*. The left ventricular "strain pattern" generally indicates that severe aortic stenosis is present.

The overall heart size is most often normal or only slightly enlarged. Left atrial enlargement and concentric left ventricular hypertrophy accompany moderate or severe obstruction. Poststenotic dilatation of the ascending aorta is common. Echocardiographic findings include multiple eccentric diastolic closure lines in the aortic lumen, thickening of the left ventricular posterior wall and septum, reduced separation of thickened aortic valve leaflets, and aortic dilatation. Two-dimensional echocardiography demonstrates the aortic value morphology; Doppler echocardiography is the most accurate means of noninvasively estimating the magnitude of obstruction. Cardiac catheterization is indicated when the clinical diagnosis of aortic stenosis has been established and when the history, clinical examination, roentgenogram, electrocardiogram, or echocardiogram suggests severe obstruction. The site and severity of obstruction are established, and any associated malformations are identified. With mild or moderate obstruction repeat left-sided heart catheterization should be carried out every 5 to 10 years because stenosis may progress.

The medical management of congenital valvular aortic stenosis includes prophylaxis against infective endocarditis and, in patients with diminished cardiac reserve, the administration of digitalis and diuretics and sodium restriction while awaiting operation. If severe aortic stenosis is present, strenuous physical activity should be avoided even when the patient is asymptomatic, and participation in competitive sports should probably be restricted in patients with milder degrees of obstruction. The decision concerning the advisability of operation depends on the severity of obstruction rather than on the symptoms. Operation is carried out under direct vision with the aid of cardiopulmonary bypass, and in children without valvular calcification the fused commissures are opened. Commissurotomy may result in aortic regurgitation that can progress to require prosthetic valve replacement. Moreover, since the valves remain deformed after valvulotomy, further degenerative changes, including calcification, may lead to significant stenosis later. The treatment of congenital aortic stenosis in the adult is described in Chap. 187.

Subaortic stenosis The most common form of subaortic stenosis is the *idiopathic hypertrophic* variety, also termed *hypertrophic cardiomyopathy,* which occurs in a congenital form in about one-third of the patients and is discussed in Chap. 192. Both clinically and physiologically, the *discrete* form of subaortic stenosis resembles valvular aortic stenosis. The lesion usually consists of a membranous diaphragm or fibrous ring encircling the left ventricular outflow tract just beneath the base of the aortic valve. It is less common than isolated valvular obstruction and occurs more frequently in males than in females. There are no reliable clinical criteria to distinguish the two forms of obstruction, although a systolic ejection sound is rare and the diastolic murmur of aortic regurgitation is more common in patients with discrete subvalvular aortic stenosis than with valvular aortic stenosis. Valvular calcification does not occur with subaortic stenosis. Echocardiography often demonstrates the subaortic obstruction; Doppler echocardiography demonstrates turbulence proximal to the aortic valve and may also detect aortic regurgitation. Definitive differentiation between valvular and subvalvular obstruction is accomplished at cardiac catheterization by recording pressure tracings as a cardiac catheter is withdrawn across the outflow tract and by left ventricular angiocardiography.

Because of the likelihood of progressive obstruction and aortic regurgitation, the presence of even mild or moderate subaortic stenosis warrants consideration of elective surgery to excise the membrane or fibrous ridge.

Occasionally, valvular and subvalvular aortic stenosis coexist in the same patient, producing a tunnel-like narrowing of the left ventricular outflow tract. Common associated findings are a small ascending aorta, hypoplasia of the aortic valve ring, and thickened valve leaflets. It may be recognized by angiography. Operative treatment frequently involves prosthetic replacement of the aortic valve, as well as enlarging the aortic annulus, proximal aorta, and left ventricular outflow tract, or the interposition of a valved conduit between the left ventricular apex and the aorta.

Supravalvular aortic stenosis Supravalvular aortic stenosis is a localized or diffuse narrowing of the ascending aorta, originating just above the level of the coronary arteries at the superior margin of the sinuses of Valsalva. In contrast to other forms of aortic stenosis, the coronary arteries are subjected to the elevated pressures that exist within the left ventricle and are often dilated and tortuous. Adherence of the free edges of the aortic cusps to the sites of supravalvular stenosis may interfere with coronary arterial inflow.

William's or the *supravalvular aortic stenosis syndrome* is the coexistence of the cardiovascular lesion and idiopathic infantile hypercalcemia, which is probably due to deranged cholecalciferol metabolism. Other manifestations include mental retardation, a peculiar "elfin facies," craniosynostosis, strabismus, narrowing of peripheral systemic and pulmonary arteries, inguinal hernias, cryptorchidism (in males), premature development of secondary sexual characteristics in females, auditory hyperacusis, and abnormalities of dental development. Supravalvular aortic stenosis and peripheral pulmonary arterial stenosis are also seen in familial and sporadic forms unassociated with the other features of the syndrome. The familial disorder is transmitted as an autosomal dominant trait with variable expressivity.

The physical findings resemble those in valvular aortic stenosis, except that the sound of aortic valve closure is accentuated, ejection sounds are infrequent, and transmission of the thrill and murmurs into the jugular notch and along the carotid vessels is more prominent; the systolic pressure in the right arm is characteristically higher than in the left. Poststenotic dilatation of the ascending aorta is rare.

The electrocardiogram reveals left ventricular hypertrophy. The diagnosis is confirmed by the demonstration at retrograde aortic catheterization of a pressure gradient just above the aortic valve, and a constriction at this level as revealed by aortography.

Surgical treatment consists of widening the lumen of the aorta by the insertion of a fabric prosthesis, and operative treatment is indicated if the obstruction is severe and discrete without generalized hypoplasia of the ascending aorta and arch.

Coarctation of the aorta Narrowing or constriction of the lumen of the aorta may occur anywhere along its length but is most common distal to the origin of the left subclavian artery near the insertion of the ligamentum arteriosum. Coarctation occurs in about 7 percent of patients with congenital heart disease and is twice as common in males as in females, although the lesion occurs frequently in patients with gonadal dysgenesis (Chap. 331). Clinical manifestations depend on the site and extent of obstruction and the presence in the majority of associated cardiac anomalies. These include bicuspid aortic valve, congenital aortic stenosis, patent ductus arteriosus, ventricular septal defect, and mitral regurgitation. When diffuse narrowing of the aorta is proximal to the ductus arteriosus, right ventricular hypertrophy develops in utero, and pulmonary hypertension and congestive heart failure are common in early life. *Differential cyanosis* may result from preferential shunting of unsaturated pulmonary arterial blood through a patent ductus to the lower part of the body.

More commonly, the coarctation is at or just distal to the attachment of the ductus or ligamentum arteriosus. The majority of children and young adults with isolated juxta- or postductal coarctation are asymptomatic. Headache, epistaxis, cold extremities, and claudication with exercise may occur, and attention is usually directed to the cardiovascular system when a heart murmur or hypertension in the upper extremities is detected on physical examination. In childhood, mechanical rather than renal factors play the primary role in hypertension.

Absence, marked diminution, or delayed pulsations in the femoral arteries and a low or unobtainable arterial pressure in the lower extremities with hypertension in the arms are clues to diagnosis. In adults, enlarged and pulsatile collateral vessels may be palpated in the intercostal spaces anteriorly, in the axillae, or posteriorly in the interscapular area. The upper extremities and thorax may be more developed than the lower extremities. A midsystolic murmur over the anterior part of the chest, back, and spinous processes may become continuous if the lumen is narrowed sufficiently to result in a high-velocity jet across the lesion throughout the cardiac cycle. Additional systolic and continuous murmurs over the lateral thoracic wall may reflect increased flow through dilated and tortuous collateral vessels. The *electrocardiogram* reveals left ventricular hypertrophy of varying degree, depending on the height of the arterial pressure proximal to the obstruction and the patient's age; predominant right or combined ventricular hypertrophy in infants and children usually implies a complicated lesion. *Roentgenograms* may show a dilated left subclavian artery high on the left mediastinal border and a dilated ascending aorta. Indentation of the aorta at the site of coarctation and pre- and poststenotic dilatation (the "3" sign) along the left paramediastinal shadow are almost pathognomonic. Notching of the ribs, an important radiographic sign, is due to erosion by dilated collateral vessels, increases with age, and usually becomes apparent between the sixth and twelfth years of life. Two-dimensional echocardiography from para- or suprasternal windows usually identifies the site and length of coarctation. Cardiac catheterization and aortography may be indicated to localize the site of obstruction, determine the length of the coarctation, and identify associated malformations.

The *treatment* of uncomplicated coarctation of the aorta is surgical; resection and end-to-end anastomosis or subclavian flap angioplasty can usually be accomplished with excellent results, although it may be necessary to use a tubular graft or patch if the narrowed segment is long. Paradoxic hypertension of short duration is common in the immediate postoperative period, and necrotizing panarteritis of the small vessels of the gastrointestinal tract of uncertain cause may complicate the recovery. In those who survive the first 2 years of life complications are uncommon before the second or third decade; operation on asymptomatic patients is recommended between the ages of 3 and 6. The chief hazards result from severe hypertension and include the development of cerebral aneurysms and hemorrhage, rupture of the aorta, left ventricular failure, and infective endocarditis. Systemic hypertension in the absence of residual coarctation postoperatively appears to be related to the duration of preoperative hypertension; lifelong observation is desirable because of the late onset of hypertension in some postoperative patients.

Pulmonary stenosis with intact ventricular septum Obstruction to right ventricular outflow is relatively common; it may be localized to the supravalvular, valvular, or subvalvular levels or occur at a combination of these sites. Multiple sites of narrowing of the peripheral pulmonary arteries are a feature of rubella embryopathy and may occur with both the familial and sporadic forms of supravalvular aortic stenosis. Valvular pulmonic stenosis is the most common form of isolated right ventricular obstruction.

The severity of the obstructing lesion, rather than the site of narrowing, is the most important determinant of the course. In the presence of a normal cardiac output, a peak systolic transvalvular pressure gradient between 50 and 80 mmHg is considered to be moderate stenosis; levels below and above that range are classified as mild and severe, respectively. Patients with mild pulmonic stenosis are generally asymptomatic and demonstrate little or no progression in the severity of obstruction with age. In patients with more significant stenosis, the severity may increase with time. Atresia of the pulmonary valve is commonly associated with a hypoplastic right ventricle and interatrial communications. Symptoms vary with the degree of obstruction. Infants with pulmonary atresia often die from hypoxia. Fatigue, dyspnea, right ventricular failure, and syncope may limit the activity of older patients, in whom moderate or severe obstruction may prevent an augmentation of pulmonary blood flow with exercise.

In patients with severe obstruction, the systolic pressure in the right ventricle may exceed that in the left ventricle, since the ventricular septum is intact. Right ventricular ejection is prolonged with moderate or severe stenosis, and the sound of pulmonary valve closure is delayed and soft. Right ventricular hypertrophy reduces the compliance of that chamber, and a forceful right atrial contraction is necessary to augment right ventricular filling. A fourth heart sound, prominent *a* waves in the jugular venous pulse, and occasionally, presystolic pulsations of the liver reflect the vigorous atrial contraction. The clinical diagnosis is supported by a right parasternal lift and harsh systolic ejection murmur and thrill at the upper left sternal border, typically preceded by a systolic ejection sound if the obstruction is valvular. The systolic murmur becomes louder, and its crescendo occurs later in systole, and more severe degrees of valvular obstruction result in a greater prolongation of right ventricular systole. The holosystolic decrescendo murmur of tricuspid regurgitation may accompany severe pulmonic stenosis, especially in the presence of congestive heart failure. Cyanosis usually reflects venoarterial shunting through a patent foramen ovale or atrial septal defect. In patients with supravalvular or peripheral pulmonary arterial stenosis, the murmur is systolic or continuous and is best heard over the area of narrowing, with radiation to the peripheral lung fields.

The electrocardiogram may be helpful in assessing the degree of obstruction to right ventricular output. In mild cases, the electrocardiogram is often normal, whereas moderate and severe stenoses are associated with right axis deviation and right ventricular hypertrophy. A ventricular strain pattern, as well as high-amplitude P waves in leads II and V_1, indicating right atrial enlargement, is associated with severe stenosis. The chest roentgenogram with mild or moderate pulmonic stenosis often shows a heart of normal size and normal vascularity of the lungs. In the presence of valvular stenosis, poststenotic dilatation of the main and left pulmonary arteries may be evident. With severe obstruction and resultant right ventricular failure, right atrial and right ventricular enlargement are generally evident. The pulmonary vascularity may be reduced with severe stenosis, right ventricular failure, and/or a venoarterial shunt at the atrial level.

Two-dimensional echocardiographic visualization of pulmonary value morphology from a parasternal window is usually possible. The outflow tract pressure gradient can usually be estimated by Doppler ultrasonography. Cardiac catheterization and angiocardiography with right ventricular injection localize the site of obstruction, establish its severity, and document the coexistence of additional cardiac malformations. Catheter techniques are also available for therapeutic balloon valvuloplasty. Treatment of moderate and severe degrees of pulmonary valvular and subvalvular stenosis is usually surgical. Direct surgical relief of the obstruction is accomplished at a low risk. Multiple stenoses of the peripheral pulmonary arteries are usually inoperable, but narrowing of a single branch or at the bifurcation of the main pulmonary trunk may be corrected.

CYANOTIC—INCREASED PULMONARY BLOOD FLOW Complete transposition of the great arteries The aorta arises from the right ventricle to the right of and anterior to the pulmonary artery, which emerges from the left ventricle. This results in two separate and parallel circulations, and some communication between the two circulations must exist after birth to sustain life. Most patients have an interatrial communication, two-thirds have a patent ductus arteriosus, and about one-third have an associated ventricular septal defect. Transposition is more common in males and occurs more frequently in the offspring of diabetic mothers. It is a leading cause of death due to congenital heart disease in the first 2 months of life and accounts for approximately 10 percent of cyanotic heart disease.

The course is determined by the degree of tissue hypoxia, the ability of each ventricle to sustain an increased work load in the presence of reduced coronary arterial oxygenation, the nature of the associated cardiovascular anomalies, and the status of the pulmonary vascular bed. Severe morphologic alterations develop in the pulmonary vascular bed by 1 to 2 years of age in most patients who also have an associated large ventricular septal defect or large patent ductus arteriosus in the absence of obstruction to left ventricular outflow.

The usual manifestations are dyspnea and cyanosis from birth, retardation of growth, and congestive heart failure. The roentgenographic findings are often highly suggestive and consist of (1) progressive cardiac enlargement in early infancy, (2) characteristic oval or egg-shaped cardiac configuration in the anteroposterior view and a narrow vascular pedicle, and (3) increased pulmonary vascular markings. In the absence of dextrocardia, two-dimensional echocardiography provides the diagnosis by demonstrating that the anterior great artery (aorta) is to the right of the posterior greater artery (pulmonary). Angiocardiography is also diagnostic and demonstrates that the anteriorly placed aorta arises from the right ventricle and that the posteriorly placed pulmonary artery in continuity with the mitral valve arises from the left ventricle.

The creation or enlargement of an interatrial communication is the simplest procedure for providing increased intracardiac mixing of systemic and pulmonary venous blood; it may be achieved surgically or, preferably, by rupturing the valve of the foramen ovale with a balloon catheter during cardiac catheterization (Rashkind's procedure). Systemic-pulmonary artery anastomosis may be indicated in the patient with severe obstruction to left ventricular outflow and diminished pulmonary blood flow. Intracardiac repair may be accomplished by rearranging the venous return so that the systemic venous blood is directed to the mitral valve and thence to the left ventricle and pulmonary artery, while the pulmonary venous blood is diverted through the tricuspid valve and right ventricle to the aorta (Mustard or Senning operation). For those patients with a ventricular septal defect in whom it is necessary to bypass a severely obstructed left ventricular outflow tract, corrective operation employs an intracardiac ventricular baffle and extracardiac prosthetic conduit to replace the pulmonary artery (Rastelli's procedure). The management of patients with a large ventricular septal defect is a subject of debate. In some centers pulmonary artery banding is advocated early in life, followed by definitive intracardiac repair at 1 to 2 years of age. In others, a one-stage operation is utilized to close the ventricular septal defect, transpose both coronary arteries to the posterior artery, and transect, contrapose, and anastomose the aorta and pulmonary arteries (Jatene or arterial switch operation).

Total anomalous pulmonary venous connection When all the pulmonary veins connect either to the right atrium directly or to the systemic veins or their tributaries, the condition is called total anomalous pulmonary venous connection (TAPVC). Because all venous blood returns to the right atrium, an interatrial communication is an integral part of this malformation. Most infants with TAPVC fail to thrive, are subject to repeated respiratory infections, and have congestive heart failure by the age of 6 months. Cyanosis is not prominent in the absence of congestive failure unless the patient survives long enough to acquire secondary pulmonary vascular changes and a reduction in pulmonary blood flow.

A characteristic finding is the presence of multiple heart sounds, consisting of a first sound followed by an ejection click, a fixed, widely split second heart sound with an accentuated pulmonic component, and a third, and often a fourth, heart sound. The electrocardiogram shows right axis deviation, as well as right atrial and ventricular hypertrophy. Roentgenograms of the chest reveal increased pulmonary blood flow; the right atrium and ventricle are dilated and hypertrophied, and the pulmonary artery segment is enlarged. Echocardiography demonstrates marked enlargement of the right ventricle and may reveal the course and level of entry of the anomalous pulmonary venous channels. Selective pulmonary arteriography is helpful in determining the drainage pathways of the pulmonary veins.

Balloon atrial septostomy may provide dramatic palliation for the infant in whom the small size of the interatrial communication limits the amount of blood reaching the left side of the heart and systemic circulation. Unless serious pulmonary vascular disease is present, results of operation for TAPVC in patients more than 1 year of age are good. The procedure consists of creating an anastomosis between the common pulmonary venous channel and the left atrium and of closing the atrial defect and the anomalous venous pathway.

CYANOTIC—DECREASED PULMONARY BLOOD FLOW Tetralogy of Fallot Tetralogy is responsible for about 10 percent of all forms of congenital heart disease and is the most common cause of cyanosis after 1 year of age. The four components of the tetralogy of Fallot are ventricular septal defect, obstruction to right ventricular outflow, aortic override (straddle) of the ventricular septal defect, and right ventricular hypertrophy. The basic anomaly results from an anterior deviation of the infundibular ventricular septum away from its usual location in the heart between the limbs of the trabecular septum. The ventricular defect is typically large and located just below the right cusp of the aortic valve, separated from the pulmonic valve by the crista supraventricularis. The aortic root may be displaced anteriorly, overriding the septal defect but, as in a normal heart, to the right of the pulmonary artery. In most cases, the overriding of the aorta is due to the subaortic location of the ventricular septal defect.

The severity of obstruction to right ventricular outflow determines the clinical presentation. The degree of hypoplasia of the outflow tract of the right ventricle varies from mild to complete (pulmonary atresia). Pulmonary valve stenosis and supravalvular and peripheral pulmonary arterial obstruction may coexist, and unilateral absence of the pulmonary artery (usually the left) occurs rarely. Circulation to the abnormal lung is by systemic arterial collaterals. Atresia of the pulmonic valve, infundibulum, or main pulmonary artery is occasionally referred to as *pseudotruncus arteriosus*. True truncus arteriosus with absent pulmonary arteries (truncus type 4) differs from tetralogy of Fallot in which pulmonary artery branches are present and are perfused by systemic arterial collaterals or a patent ductus arteriosus. A right-sided aortic arch and descending aorta occur in about 25 percent of patients with tetralogy. The coronary arteries may have variations that are surgically important. The anterior descending artery sometimes originates from the right coronary artery, which may also give rise to a left branch coursing anterior to the infundibulum; a single left coronary artery may give rise to a branch that crosses the outflow tract of the right ventricle. Associated cardiac anomalies occur in about 40 percent, and noncardiac anomalies are present in 20 to 30 percent of patients.

When right ventricular outflow obstruction is severe, the pulmonary blood flow is markedly reduced, and a large volume of unsaturated systemic venous blood is shunted from right to left across the ventricular septal defect, severe cyanosis and polycythemia occur, and symptoms of systemic anoxia are prominent. The term *pink,* or *acyanotic, tetralogy of Fallot* is used often to describe an interventricular communication and a milder degree of obstruction to right ventricular outflow with no appreciable venoarterial shunting. In many patients the obstruction to right ventricular outflow is mild but progressive, so that early in life pulmonary exceeds systemic blood flow, and the symptoms resemble those produced by a simple ventricular septal defect.

Most children with tetralogy of Fallot are cyanotic from birth or develop cyanosis before 1 year of age. Dyspnea with exertion, retarded growth and development, clubbing, and polycythemia are common. When resting after exertion, infants with tetralogy characteristically assume a squatting posture. Spells of severe anoxia and cyanosis (see ''Hypoxic Spells'' above) constitute a major threat to survival.

Physical examination reveals variable degrees of underdevelopment and cyanosis. Clubbing of the digits may be prominent after the first year of life. A right ventricular impulse and systolic thrill may be palpable along the left sternal border; there is no generalized cardiomegaly. The second heart sound is single, and the pulmonic component is rarely audible. A systolic ejection murmur is produced by flow across the narrowed right ventricular outflow tract or pulmonic valve. The intensity and duration of the murmur vary inversely with the severity of obstruction, the opposite of the relation existing in patients with an intact ventricular septum and pulmonary stenosis. Polycythemia, decreased systemic vascular resistance, and increased obstruction to right ventricular outflow may all be responsible for a decrease in the intensity of the murmur. A continuous murmur over the paravertebral area may indicate collateral circulation to the lungs through bronchial arteries.

The electrocardiogram ordinarily shows right ventricular and, less often, right atrial hypertrophy. Radiologic examination characteristically reveals a normal-sized, boot-shaped heart (*coeur en sabot*) with prominence of the right ventricle and a concavity in the region of the pulmonary conus. The pulmonary vascular markings are typically diminished, and the aortic arch and knob may be on the right side. Two-dimensional echocardiography from the parasternal or subcostal windows demonstrates the malalignment of the ventricular septal defect and the subpulmonary stenosis. The presence or absence of stenoses at the origins of the branch pulmonary arteries can also be assessed. Selective angiocardiography with right ventricular injection is necessary to confirm the diagnosis and to evaluate the architecture of the right ventricular outflow tract, pulmonary valve and annulus, and caliber of the main branches of the pulmonary artery.

Factors that may complicate the management of patients with tetralogy include infective endocarditis, paradoxic embolism, polycythemia, coagulation defects, and cerebral infarction or abscess. The paroxysmal cyanotic spells may respond to oxygen, placing the child in the knee-chest position, and morphine. If the spell persists, metabolic acidosis will develop from prolonged anaerobic metabolism, and infusion of sodium bicarbonate may be necessary to interrupt the attack. Vasopressors, beta-adrenergic blockade, or general anesthesia may occasionally be necessary.

In infants with pulmonary atresia cardiac catheterization is often done as an emergency. Because survival in this setting usually depends on patency of the ductus arteriosus, intravenous infusion of prostaglandin E_1 (0.1 mg per kilogram of body weight per minute) may dramatically reverse clinical deterioration and improve arterial blood gases and pH.

Primary correction is advisable at some point for almost all patients who have tetralogy of Fallot. Early intracardiac repair, even in infancy, is advocated in most centers properly equipped for infant cardiac operations. Successful early correction avoids progressive infundibular obstruction, acquired pulmonary atresia, delayed growth, and complications due to hypoxemia and polycythemia. The size of the pulmonary arteries rather than the age or size of the infant or child is the most important determinant in establishing candidacy for primary repair. Pronounced hypoplasia of the pulmonary arteries is a relative contraindication for an early corrective surgical procedure. When this problem is present, a palliative operation, such as creation of a systemic arterial–pulmonary arterial shunt, is carried out and is usually followed by complete correction, which can be carried out at a lower risk later in childhood.

Ebstein's anomaly In this anomaly there is abnormal morphogenesis of the tricuspid valve, with redundancy of tricuspid valve tissue, and the attachment of portions of the septal and posterior leaflets of the tricuspid valve is lower than normal; the leaflets originate from the right ventricular wall rather than from the atrioventricular ring. Hence, the portion of the right ventricle that lies between the atrioventricular ring and the origin of the valve is continuous with the right atrial chamber. The tricuspid valve is usually incompetent, the foramen ovale is patent, and the right ventricle exhibits varying degrees of hypoplasia. The clinical manifestations of Ebstein's anomaly are variable, depending on the severity of the anatomic changes in the tricuspid valve. Ultimately, however, progressive cyanosis resulting from the right-to-left shunt across the interatrial communication, symptoms resulting from right ventricular dysfunction, and/or paroxysmal arrhythmias develop.

A prominent systolic pulsation of the liver and a large *v* wave in the jugular venous pulse accompany the systolic thrill and murmur of tricuspid regurgitation. Wide splitting of the first and second heart sounds and prominent third and fourth heart sounds may produce a characteristically rhythmic auscultatory cadence. The electrocardiogram shows giant P waves, a prolonged PR interval, and complete or incomplete right bundle branch block. Roentgenography usually demonstrates an enlarged right atrium and a small right ventricle and pulmonary artery and reduced pulsations; the pulmonary vascularity may be reduced if a large right-to-left shunt is present. The principal echocardiographic findings include a large anterior tricuspid leaflet with delayed tricuspid valve closure with respect to mitral closure. Two-dimensional echocardiography best demonstrates the morphologic features. At cardiac catheterization the intracavitary electrocardiogram recorded just proximal to the tricuspid valve shows a right ventricular type of complex, while the pressure recorded is that of the right atrium.

Most patients survive to the third decade at least. In some disabled patients moderate improvement has resulted from anastomosis of the superior vena cava to the right pulmonary artery to divert systemic venous return from the right atrium and to increase pulmonary blood flow. Patients beyond early childhood have occasionally benefited from prosthetic replacement of the tricuspid valve; at all ages, however, patients with Ebstein's anomaly are poor surgical risks.

Tricuspid atresia Atresia of the tricuspid valve, an interatrial communication, and, frequently, hypoplasia of the right ventricle and pulmonary artery exist in this malformation. The clinical picture is usually dominated by severe cyanosis as a result of greatly diminished pulmonary blood flow.

Blood atrial septostomy and palliative operations consisting of increasing pulmonary blood flow, often by systemic arterial or venous–pulmonary artery anastomosis, may allow survival to the age of 10 to 20 years; functional correction of the anomaly can then be accomplished in those with normal or low pulmonary arterial pressure by anastomosis of the right atrial appendage to the right ventricle with the aid of a pericardial patch or by insertion of a prosthetic conduit or direct anastomosis between the right atrium and pulmonary artery and closure of the interatrial communication.

REFERENCES

General

ADAMS FH, EMMANOUILIDES GC: *Moss' Heart Disease in Infants, Children and Adolescents*, 3d ed. Baltimore, Williams and Wilkins, 1983

BOROW KM et al: Congenital heart disease in the adult, in *Heart Disease*, 2d ed, E Braunwald (ed). Philadelphia, Saunders, 1984, p 1024

ENGLE MA, PERLOFF JK (eds): *Congenital Heart Disease After Surgery*. New York, Yorke, 1983

FREEDOM RM: *Angiocardiography of Congenital Heart Disease*. New York, Macmillan, 1984

FRIEDMAN WF: Congenital heart disease in infancy and childhood, in *Heart Disease*, 2d ed, E Braunwald (ed). Philadelphia, Saunders, 1984, p 941

———, HIGGINS CB: *Pediatric Cardiac Imaging*. Philadelphia, Saunders, 1984

STARK J, DELEVAL M: *Surgery for Congenital Heart Defects*. New York, Grune and Stratton, 1983

Specific malformations

BARBER G et al: Pulmonary atresia with ventricular septal defect. J Am Coll Cardiol 7:630, 1986

BEHL P: Ebstein's anomaly: 16 years experience with valve replacement without plication of the right ventricle. Thorax 39:8, 1984

BISSET GS: Aortic valve replacement in childhood: Evaluation of left ventricular function by electrocardiography, echocardiography and graded exercise testing. Am J Cardiol 52:568, 1983

DISESSA TG et al: Systemic venous and pulmonary arterial flow patterns after Fontan's procedure for tricuspid atresia or single ventricle. Circulation 70:898, 1984

DOTY DB et al: Aortic pulmonary septal defect: Hemodynamics, angiography and operation. Ann Thorac Surg 32:244, 1981

FOSTER ED: Reoperation for aortic coarctation. Ann Thorac Surg 38:81, 1984

FREED MD et al: Repair of secundum and sinus venosus atrial septal defects. J Am Coll Cardiol 4:333, 1984

FRIEDMAN WF: Patent ductus arteriosus in respiratory distress syndrome: A historical review. Pediatr Cardiol 4:3, 1983

———, GEORGE BL: Medical progress—Treatment of congestive heart failure by altering loading conditions of the heart. J Pediatr 106:697, 1985

HAWKINS JA: Total anomalous pulmonary venous connection. Ann Thorac Surg 36:548, 1983

HENZE A et al: Ruptured sinus of Valsalva aneurysms. Scand J Thorac Cardiovasc Surg 17:249, 1983

KIRKLIN JW: Surgical results and protocols in the spectrum of tetralogy of Fallot. Ann Surg 198:251, 1983

MACRI R et al: Congenital coronary artery fistula. Thorac Cardiovasc Surg 30:167, 1982

MARX GR et al: Transposition of the great arteries with intact ventricular septum. J Am Coll Cardiol 1:476, 1983

MOODIE DS et al: Anomalous origin of the left coronary artery from the pulmonary artery in adult patients; long term follow-up after surgery. Am Heart J 106:381, 1983

POLANSKI DB: Pulmonary stenosis in infants and young children. Ann Thorac Surg 39:159, 1985

ROSENTHAL A: Long-term prognosis (15 to 26 years) after repair of tetralogy of Fallot. Ann Thorac Surg 38:151, 1984

STARK J: Transposition of the great arteries: Which operation? Ann Thorac Surg 38:429, 1984

TENORIO A et al: The spectrum of atrioventricular discordance: A clinical study. Br Heart J 51:498, 1984

VAN PRAAGH R: Diagnosis of complex congenital heart disease: A morphologic-anatomic method and terminology. Cardiovasc Intervent Radiol 7:115, 1984

WRIGHT GB et al: Subaortic stenosis in the young: Medical and surgical course in 83 patients. Am J Cardiol 52:830, 1983

186 RHEUMATIC FEVER

GENE H. STOLLERMAN

DEFINITION Rheumatic fever is an inflammatory disease which occurs as a delayed sequel to pharyngeal infection with group A streptococci. It involves principally the heart, joints, central nervous system, skin, and subcutaneous tissues. The usual manifestations in the acute form are migratory polyarthritis, fever, and carditis. Sydenham's chorea, subcutaneous nodules, and erythema marginatum may occur as other typical manifestations. No single symptom, sign, or laboratory test is pathognomonic of rheumatic fever, although several combinations of them are diagnostic. Although the name *acute rheumatic fever* emphasizes involvement of the joints, rheumatic fever owes its importance to the involvement of the heart, which can be fatal during the acute stage of the disease or can lead to rheumatic heart disease, a chronic condition due to scarring and deformity of the heart valves.

ETIOLOGY AND PATHOGENESIS The etiologic relationship of group A streptococci to rheumatic fever can be summarized briefly, as follows. (1) Numerous clinical and epidemiologic studies have shown a close association of group A streptococcal infections and rheumatic fever. (2) Antecedent streptococcal infection can almost always be demonstrated immunologically in the acute stage of rheumatic fever by increased titers of antibodies to streptococcal antigens. Moreover, in long-term prospective follow-up studies, rheumatic fever recurs only as a result of intercurrent streptococcal infections. (3) Both primary and secondary attacks of the disease can be prevented by prompt treatment or prevention of streptococcal infections with antimicrobial therapy. The pharyngeal route of infection is necessary to initiate the rheumatic process. Streptococcal skin infections do not do so. Furthermore, throat infections with some group A strains appear to produce rheumatic fever rarely or not at all.

The mechanism by which the group A streptococcus initiates the disease process remains unknown. A relatively small percentage of persons who suffer from streptococcal sore throats subsequently develop rheumatic fever. The organism is not demonstrable in the lesions when rheumatic fever appears several days or weeks after the acute streptococcal infection. No one product of the streptococcus has been incriminated as a cause of the lesions, either as a direct tissue toxin or as an antigen inducing hypersensitivity. Several streptococcal antigens have demonstrated cross-reactivity with cardiac and other tissues. Their direct relationship to pathogenesis is, however, unproven, and streptococcus-induced autoimmunity as a mechanism to explain the rheumatic process remains a popular but unestablished pathogenetic concept.

INCIDENCE AND EPIDEMIOLOGY Although rheumatic fever may occur at any age, it is extremely rare in infancy; it appears most commonly between the ages of 5 and 15 years, when streptococcal infection is most frequent and intense. Similarly, the geographic distribution, incidence, and severity of rheumatic fever are, in general, a reflection of the frequency and severity of streptococcal pharyngitis. The attack rate of rheumatic fever following exudative streptococcal pharyngitis in epidemics averages approximately 3 percent. When streptococcal pharyngitis is sporadic and mild or due to strains of lesser rheumatic potential, the attack rate of rheumatic fever may be very much lower. Strains of group A streptococci that cause epidemics of streptococcal pharyngitis are most likely to be rheumatogenic. Following such infections, the attack rate of rheumatic fever is directly correlated with the magnitude of the streptococcal immune response. Analysis of reported epidemics of acute rheumatic fever caused by a variety of serotypes shows some, such as type 5, to be overrepresented, and others to be conspicuously absent. In some populations, such as in Trinidad, strains responsible for rheumatic fever and acute glomerulonephritis are serotypically distinct.

Environmental, bacterial, and host factors which appear to play a role in the development of rheumatic fever are important primarily as they are related to the incidence and severity of preceding streptococcal infection. Such factors as latitude, altitude, dampness, economic factors, and age all affect the incidence of rheumatic fever because they are related to the incidence of streptococcal infection in general. Crowding is, however, the major environmental factor relating to the occurrence of this disease because, regardless of other variables, it promotes interpersonal spread of the most virulent group A streptococcal strains. Such crowding as occurs in military barracks, closed institutions, large families in small quarters, and those massed in the densely populated core of major urban centers is most likely to be associated with an increase in incidence of rheumatic fever.

The attack rate of rheumatic fever following streptococcal infections in patients who have had previous attacks of rheumatic fever is increased to as high as 5 to 50 percent and is also related to the virulence of the reactivating infection. Furthermore, the frequency of rheumatic recurrences following streptococcal infection is consistently greater in those with rheumatic heart disease than in those who escaped cardiac injury during prior attacks. The tendency to suffer recurrences of rheumatic fever following streptococcal infections declines with the passage of years since the preceding attack. It appears, therefore, that certain host variables, as well as probable qualitative and quantitative differences in the nature of the antecedent streptococcal infection, also influence the development of rheumatic fever. To what extent such variables are genetic or acquired has not been settled. It is common to obtain a family history of rheumatic fever as well as to encounter multiple cases among siblings of a single family. However, the concordance of rheumatic fever in identical twins is approximately 20 percent, suggesting only a limited penetrance of genetic predisposition to rheumatic fever. Although investigations of the distribution of haplotypes in rheumatic hosts have been limited in scope and number, there has been so far no consistent association of rheumatic fever, or any of its major manifestations, with any predominant histocompatibility locus antigens.

The mortality of acute rheumatic fever has been declining steadily for the past 30 years. It is still, however, a major cause of death and disability in children and adolescents in socioeconomically depressed areas of the world. The incidence of rheumatic fever has been decreasing for several years in countries where housing and economic conditions have been improving steadily. The rate of decrease may have been accelerated by the wide use of antimicrobial therapy. The decrease also may be due to a change in the prevalence of rheumatogenic streptococcal strains. Rheumatic fever remains, however, a worldwide disease having its greatest incidence wherever poor economic conditions, overcrowding, and substandard housing are most common.

PATHOLOGY The lesions of rheumatic fever are disseminated widely throughout the body, with special predilection for connective tissues. Focal inflammatory lesions occur particularly around small blood vessels.

Cardiovascular lesions The heart is the site of the most characteristic and consequential involvement, and all its layers—endocardium, myocardium, and pericardium—may be involved. This generalized involvement gives rise to the term *rheumatic pancarditis.* The most characteristic and specific pattern of rheumatic inflammation is found in the *myocardial Aschoff body,* a submiliary granuloma. This lesion, when present in its classic form, is generally considered to be pathognomonic of rheumatic fever. In many areas the inflammatory lesion is accompanied by swelling and fragmentation of the collagen fibers and alteration in the staining properties of the ground substances of the connective tissues. This change is described as *fibrinoid degeneration of collagen,* but its chemical basis has not been established. Aschoff bodies with less exudative and more productive changes may persist for many years as the lingering traces of chronic rheumatic inflammation in patients with rheumatic heart disease, long after rheumatic fever has become clinically quiescent. The persistence of such lesions is most common in patients who develop severe mitral stenosis. Eventually the Aschoff body is converted into a spindle-shaped or triangular scar lying between the muscle bundles and surrounding blood vessels.

Rheumatic endocarditis produces the verrucous valvulitis of acute rheumatic fever which leads to the most serious permanent cardiac damage. It may heal with fibrous thickening and adhesion of the valve commissures and chordae tendineae, leading to variable degrees of valvular regurgitation and stenosis. Deformity resulting in functional impairment of the heart occurs most commonly in the mitral and aortic valves, less frequently in the tricuspid, and almost never in the pulmonic valves. *Rheumatic pericarditis* (Chap. 194) produces a serofibrinous effusion, with the deposit of shaggy elements of fibrin on the surface of the heart. The pericardium may become calcified, but pericardial constriction does not occur.

Extracardiac lesions Involvement of the *joints* is characterized by exudative rather than proliferative changes, and healing of these structures occurs without significant scarring or deformity. *Subcutaneous nodules,* seen during the acute phase of the disease, are composed of granulomas with localized areas of "fibrinoid" swelling of subcutaneous collagen bundles, and perivascular collections of large cells with pale nuclei and prominent nucleoli. Synovitis is usually mild and nonspecific. *Pulmonary* and *pleural* lesions are less definite and less characteristic. Fibrinous pleurisy and rheumatic pneumonitis may occur with exudative and proliferative lesions but without definite Aschoff bodies. Patients with active *chorea* rarely die. The pathologic findings which have been reported in the central nervous system are not consistent, and no characteristic lesion has been reported to explain this clinical manifestation. During active chorea the spinal fluid remains normal, being free of cells, with no increase in total protein and no change in the relative concentration of various proteins.

CLINICAL FEATURES The major clinical manifestations by which rheumatic fever can be recognized are polyarthritis, carditis, chorea, erythema marginatum, and subcutaneous nodules.

Arthritis The classic attack of rheumatic fever appears as an acute migratory polyarthritis accompanied by signs and symptoms of an acute febrile illness. The large joints of the extremities are most frequently affected, but no joint is impervious to the inflammatory process; one may find arthritis of the hands and feet but only rarely of the spine or of the sternoclavicular or temporomandibular joints. Joint effusions occur but are not persistent. As pain and swelling subside in one joint, others tend to become involved. Although such "migratory" involvement is characteristic, it is not invariable, and several large joints may be inflamed at one time. To be acceptable as a criterion for the diagnosis of rheumatic fever, the polyarthritis should involve two or more joints, should be associated with at least two minor manifestations such as fever and elevation of sedimentation rate, and should be associated with high titer of antistreptolysin O or some other streptococcal antibody (Table 186-1). There is nothing

TABLE 186-1 Jones criteria (revised)

Major manifestations	Minor manifestations
Carditis	Fever
Polyarthritis	Arthralgia
Chorea	Previous rheumatic fever or rheumatic heart disease
Erythema marginatum	Elevated ESR or positive CRP
Subcutaneous nodules	Prolonged PR interval

Two major criteria or one major and two minor criteria indicate a high probability of the presence of rheumatic fever with supporting evidence of preceding streptococcal infection: history of recent scarlet fever; positive throat culture for group A streptococcus; increased ASO titer or other streptococcal antibodies.

SOURCE: *American Heart Association, 1965.*

distinctive about the arthritis of rheumatic fever, and other causes of migratory polyarthritis that may be associated only fortuitously with high streptococcal antibody levels must, of course, be excluded.

Acute rheumatic carditis Acute rheumatic carditis first manifests itself by the appearance of the heart murmurs of either mitral or aortic regurgitation, the former most frequently. Signs and symptoms of pericarditis and of congestive heart failure may supervene in more severe cases. Death may result from heart failure during the acute stage of the disease, or permanent valvular damage may be sustained which results ultimately in serious disability. Carditis may vary from a fulminating, fatal course to a low-grade, inapparent inflammation. *It is well to bear in mind that the vast majority of patients with carditis do not have symptoms referable to the heart.* The latter occur only in more severe cases when heart failure or pericardial effusions produce characteristic symptoms. For this reason, unless extracardiac manifestations, such as polyarthritis and chorea, are present, patients whose rheumatic fever is manifested only by carditis are frequently not diagnosed and in later life may be discovered to have rheumatic heart disease without a definite history of rheumatic fever.

When carditis is manifest, there is usually tachycardia disproportionate to the degree of fever, gallop rhythms are often heard, and the heart sounds may become fetal or "tic-tac" in quality. Occasionally, arrhythmias and/or a pericardial friction rub may be present. Prolongation of the conduction time may lead to dropped beats with varying degrees of heart block. Prolongation of the PR interval and other changes in the electrocardiogram are very common, but these findings, in the absence of clinical manifestations of carditis, have a benign prognosis. Therefore, changes in the electrocardiogram alone, unassociated with significant murmurs or cardiac enlargement, do not by themselves constitute an acceptable criterion for the diagnosis of rheumatic carditis. Pericarditis may cause precordial pain, and a friction rub may be audible.

A definite clinical diagnosis of carditis can be made if one or more of the following can be demonstrated: (1) the appearance of, or change in the character of, organic heart murmurs; (2) definite increase in heart size demonstrated by radiogram or fluoroscopy; (3) pericardial friction rub or effusion best demonstrated by echocardiography; or (4) signs of congestive heart failure. Rheumatic carditis is almost always associated with a significant murmur.

Subcutaneous nodules These are usually small, pea-sized, painless swellings over bony prominences and therefore frequently go unnoticed by the patient. The skin moves freely over them. Characteristic locations are the extensor tendons of the hands and feet, the elbows, margins of the patellae, the scalp, over the scapulae, and over the spinous processes of the vertebrae.

Chorea (Sydenham's chorea, chorea minor, Saint Vitus' dance) This is a disorder of the central nervous system characterized by sudden, aimless, irregular movements, often accompanied by muscle weakness and emotional instability. Chorea is a delayed manifestation of rheumatic fever, and other manifestations may or may not still be present at the time it appears. Polyarthritis, when part of the same attack, always subsides before chorea appears. Carditis is often discovered for the first time when the presenting feature of rheumatic fever is chorea. Chorea usually appears after a long latent period (up to several months) from the antecedent streptococcal infection and at a time when all other manifestations of rheumatic fever have abated. When no previous rheumatic manifestations are noted, such cases are called *pure chorea.*

The clinical onset of chorea is often gradual. Patients may be unusually nervous and fidgety and may have difficulty in writing, drawing, and handiwork. They may stumble or fall, drop things, and grimace. As symptoms become more severe, spasmodic movements extend to all parts of the body, and muscular weakness may become so marked that patients cannot walk, talk, or sit up. Often the weakness is severe enough to simulate paralysis. The irregular, jerky, spasmodic movements may become so violent that cribs and beds must be padded to prevent injury. Symptoms are exaggerated by excitement, effort, or fatigue but subside during sleep. Emotional instability is almost invariable in patients with chorea. All degrees of speech disturbance are seen. Central nervous stimulants exacerbate and sedatives suppress choreiform activity.

Erythema marginatum This evanescent pink rash is characteristic of rheumatic fever. The erythematous areas often have clear centers and round or serpiginous margins. They vary greatly in size and occur mainly on the trunk and proximal part of the extremities, never on the face. The erythema is transient, migratory, and may be brought out by the application of heat; it is nonpruritic, not indurated, and blanches on pressure.

Minor clinical criteria These are clinical features which occur frequently in rheumatic fever but are also common to many other diseases and are therefore of minor diagnostic value. They include fever, arthralgia, abdominal pain, tachycardia, and epistaxis.

LABORATORY FINDINGS There is no specific laboratory test to indicate the presence of rheumatic fever. The appraisal of rheumatic activity by laboratory findings is, however, of value, since various tests may indicate *continued* rheumatic inflammation when clinical features are not apparent.

Streptococcal antibody tests to disclose preceding streptococcal infection Streptococcal antibody titers differentiate preceding streptococcal from other acute respiratory infections and are increased following asymptomatic as well as symptomatic streptococcal infections. These antibody levels are increased in the early stages of acute rheumatic fever. They may be declining, or low, if the interval between the acute streptococcal infection and the detection of rheumatic fever has been longer than 2 months, a situation which occurs most often in patients whose presenting rheumatic manifestation is chorea. However, patients whose only major manifestation is rheumatic carditis also may have low antibody titers when first seen. Their rheumatic attack may have been in progress several months before becoming symptomatic and recognized. Except in these two instances, *one should be reluctant to make the diagnosis of acute rheumatic fever in the absence of serologic evidence of a recent streptococcal infection.* The antistreptolysin O test (ASO) is the most widely used and best-standardized streptococcal antibody test. In general, single titers of at least 250 Todd units in adults and at least 333 units in children over 5 years of age are considered to be increased. Depending on the general prevalence of streptococcal infections, a varying percentage of the normal population may show titers of this magnitude.

About 20 percent of patients in the early stages of acute rheumatic fever, and most patients who present with chorea, have a low or borderline ASO titer. In these instances, it is advisable to obtain a different streptococcal antibody test such as anti-DNase B, or antihyaluronidase (AH). The antistreptozyme test (ASTZ) is a hemagglutination reaction to a concentrate of extracellular streptococcal antigens absorbed to red blood cells. It is a very sensitive indicator of recent streptococcal infection; virtually all patients with acute rheumatic fever have titers greater than 200 units per milliliter. The real value of the ASTZ test is in *ruling out* rheumatic fever when the titer is low in patients with isolated polyarthritis. To date, the specific antigens involved in the ASTZ test remain unidentified and therefore the test has not yet been adequately standardized. A rise in titer of two dilution tubes or more can be demonstrated for at least one of the streptococcal antibodies in almost all recurrent as well as primary attacks of rheumatic fever (Table 186-2). Increased streptococcal antibodies, however, do not reflect rheumatic activity per se, and their rate of decline is independent of the course of the rheumatic attack.

Isolation of group A streptococci Some patients continue to harbor group A streptococci at the onset of acute rheumatic fever, but these organisms are usually present in small numbers and may be difficult to isolate by a single throat culture. The administration of penicillin or other antibodies may also result in failure to isolate the infecting organism. In addition, a significant number of *normal* individuals, particularly children, may harbor group A streptococci in the upper respiratory tract. For these reasons, throat cultures are less satisfactory than antibody tests as supporting evidence of recent streptococcal infection.

Acute phase reactants These tests offer objective but nonspecific confirmation of the presence of an inflammatory process. *The erythrocyte sedimentation rate* (ESR) and the test for *C-reactive protein* (CRP) in serum are used most commonly. Unless the patient has received corticosteroids or salicylates, these reactions are almost always abnormal in patients presenting with polyarthritis or acute carditis, whereas they are often normal in patients with chorea. Other laboratory findings which reflect inflammation include reactions such as leukocytosis, and increases in serum complement, mucoproteins, and $alpha_2$ and gamma globulins. Prolongation of the PR interval of the electrocardiogram, although neither specific for rheumatic fever nor diagnostic of serious cardiac involvement, is frequent in acute rheumatic fever (about 25 percent of all cases), and other nonspecific electrocardiographic changes are also common. Anemia, due to the suppression of erythropoiesis characteristic of chronic inflammatory diseases, is another feature of rheumatic activity.

COURSE AND PROGNOSIS The course of rheumatic fever varies greatly and is impossible to predict at the onset of the disease. In general, however, approximately 75 percent of acute rheumatic attacks subside within 6 weeks, 90 percent within 12 weeks, and less than 5 percent persist more than 6 months. These last usually consist of severe, intractable forms of rheumatic carditis or stubborn, prolonged attacks of Sydenham's chorea, both of which may persist for as long as several years. Once acute rheumatic fever has subsided and more than 2 months has elapsed after withdrawal of treatment with salicylates or adrenal corticosteroids, rheumatic fever does not recur in the absence of new streptococcal infections. Recurrences are most common within the first 5 years of the initial attack and tend to decline with increasing duration of freedom from rheumatic activity. The frequency of recurrences is dependent upon the frequency and severity of streptococcal infection, the presence or absence of rheumatic heart disease following an attack, and the duration of freedom from the last attack.

TABLE 186-2 Serologic results in patients with streptococcal disease

	Percent of patients whose serums were "positive"				
Patient group (no.)	ASO	AH	Anti-DNase B	At least 1 of 3	ASTZ
Acute rheumatic fever (20)	90	65	85	95	100
Acute glomerulonephritis (22)	50	63	72	91	95
Convalescent pharyngitis (11)	81	54	54	91	91
Convalescent pyoderma (23)	35	35	91	96	91
Total (76)	61	54	79	93	95

SOURCE: *AL Bisno, I Ofek, Am J Dis Child 127:676, 1974.*

Approximately 70 percent of patients who develop carditis do so within the first week of the disease, 85 percent within the first 12 weeks of the disease, and almost all within 6 months from the onset of the acute attack. Thereafter, if significant murmurs have not appeared, the prognosis for a patient in whom recurrences are prevented is excellent.

Chronic rheumatic carditis and the course of rheumatic heart disease The remarkable variability in the course of rheumatic carditis and rheumatic valvular disease stems from several factors: (1) the variability in the duration and severity of the rheumatic inflammation; (2) the amount of scarring of the valves and myocardium following the abatement of the acute inflammation; (3) the location and severity of the hemodynamic lesion due to valvular insufficiency or stenosis; (4) the frequency of recurrent bouts of carditis; and (5) the progression of valvular calcification and sclerosis, which occurs as a secondary phenomenon in a deformed or injured valve without recurrent or persistent rheumatic inflammation (as seen in congenital valvular disease or following healed acute bacterial endocarditis). These factors, and possibly others not yet appreciated, produce striking variations in the clinical syndromes of rheumatic heart disease.

Chronic rheumatic myocarditis In this syndrome, the presenting picture is one of chronic heart failure in a patient with a markedly dilated heart and with physical, roentgenographic, and electrocardiographic findings of mitral regurgitation. The differentiation of this syndrome from other forms of chronic myocarditis may be very difficult, if not impossible, when the associated extracardiac features of rheumatic fever (chorea, polyarthritis, and so forth) are not present (Chap. 192). Although rheumatic fever does not produce *isolated* myocarditis, and is almost invariably a pancarditis, the pericardial inflammation may not be clearly evident, and the mitral valvulitis may not be distinguishable from mitral regurgitation due to dilation of the mitral ring. In such cases one must search diligently for an evanescent friction rub, evidence of pericardial effusion, appearance of a soft aortic regurgitation murmur, and extracardiac clues such as fever responding promptly to salicylates, arthralgias, transient subcutaneous nodules, evanescent erythema marginatum, and subtle signs of chorea.

The course of chronic rheumatic carditis may be intractable and end fatally after months or even several years. Often, however, the patient improves rather suddenly and even recovers cardiac reserve dramatically in association with the disappearance of systemic manifestations of the inflammatory process. The heart may remain large, may decrease somewhat in size, or in occasional instances may return to normal size with varying degrees of residual valvular deformity. Such a course signals the termination of the "toxic" phase of the rheumatic process, and thereafter the course of rheumatic heart disease depends on the variables in healing cited above.

DIFFERENTIAL DIAGNOSIS Early cases of rheumatic fever may be confused with other diseases which begin with acute polyarthritis. It is wise to exclude *bacteremia* by blood cultures, particularly because such infections may be masked by penicillin given for presumed acute rheumatic fever. Polyarthritis due to *infective endocarditis* in a patient with preexisting rheumatic heart disease may be mistaken for a recurrence of acute rheumatic fever. If streptococcal antibodies are not increased, polyarthritis should be attributed to some cause other than rheumatic fever. Gonococcal polyarthritis may be distinguished from rheumatic fever by the dramatic response of the former to a therapeutic trial of penicillin. In rheumatoid arthritis, joint involvement will persist and characteristic joint deformities may appear. The latter are not seen in rheumatic fever. The rheumatoid factor so characteristic of rheumatoid arthritis is not present in rheumatic fever. Antibodies against nuclear components and other autoantibodies are absent in rheumatic fever. Rheumatic pericarditis and myocarditis, associated with cardiac enlargement and heart failure, are both almost invariably associated with valvular lesions which produce significant murmurs.

Overdiagnosis of rheumatic fever should be avoided. Unless ill-defined febrile syndromes are clearly associated with a major manifestation of rheumatic fever, the diagnosis of rheumatic fever should not be made. A common error is the premature, vigorous administration of corticosteroids or salicylates before the signs and symptoms of rheumatic fever are unmistakable. In the absence of a curative agent, one should not suppress the signs and symptoms of rheumatic fever until they are clearly expressed.

Particularly confusing in the differential diagnosis of rheumatic fever is the drug sensitivity with fever and polyarthritis which may occur after administration of penicillin for a previous pharyngitis. Urticaria or angioneurotic edema, if present, helps identify penicillin sensitivity in such cases. The abdominal pain of rheumatic fever may be mistaken for appendicitis, and the crisis of sickle cell anemia may also be associated with joint pain, enlargement of the heart, and cardiac murmurs. The rapidity with which the arthritis symptoms of rheumatic fever are controlled with salicylates is characteristic of this disease. Dramatic response to salicylates does not in itself, however, establish a diagnosis of rheumatic fever.

In order to help clarify the diagnosis of rheumatic fever, the American Heart Association has accepted and modified criteria usually referred to as the *Jones criteria* (Table 186-1). They are not to be used as a substitute for good medical judgment but are recommended as a guide for careful study of questionable cases. The finding of two major criteria, or of one major and two minor criteria, indicates a high probability of the presence of rheumatic fever if supported by evidence of a preceding streptococcal infection. The absence of the latter should always make the diagnosis questionable, except in the situation in which rheumatic fever is first discovered after a long latent period from the antecedent infection (Sydenham's chorea or low-grade carditis). Because the prognosis may differ according to the major manifestations, for recording purposes the diagnosis of rheumatic fever should be followed by a list of the major manifestations present, e.g., rheumatic fever manifested by polyarthritis and carditis. An indication of the severity of carditis in terms of presence or absence of congestive heart failure and cardiomegaly is also advisable.

TREATMENT There is no specific cure for rheumatic fever, and no known measures change the course of the attack. Good supportive therapy, however, can reduce the mortality and morbidity of the disease.

Chemotherapy After rheumatic fever is first diagnosed, a course of penicillin should be given to eliminate group A streptococci. This course is advisable even if bacteriologic examination yields throat cultures negative for streptococci, since the organisms may be present in areas inaccessible to swabs. It is preferable to administer penicillin parenterally. An effective course is a single injection of 1.2 million units of benzathine penicillin intramuscularly or 600,000 units of procaine penicillin intramuscularly daily for 10 days. Attempts to reduce ultimate heart damage by administering penicillin early in the acute rheumatic attack in larger doses have not been successful. After completion of the therapeutic course of penicillin, continuous protection from reinfection with streptococci should be provided by instituting one of the prophylactic regimens described below.

Suppressive therapy For patients without carditis treatment with adrenal corticosteroids is unnecessary. Acute arthritis can be relieved with codeine or with salicylate, the latter being preferable to reduce fever and joint inflammation. When salicylate is used in the therapy of rheumatic fever, the dosage should be increased until the drug produces either a clinical effect or systemic toxicity characterized by tinnitus, headache, or hyperpnea. A starting dose of 100 to 125 mg/kg per day in children and 6 to 8 g in adults given in four or five divided doses is recommended. Of the various salicylate preparations ordinary aspirin is cheapest and most effective.

Many physicians prefer corticosteroids to salicylates for the treatment of carditis, despite the lack of a demonstrated advantage of these adrenal hormones in controlled clinical trials. Corticosteroids are more potent anti-inflammatory agents but are more likely to be followed by posttherapeutic "rebounds," and they have the additional disadvantage of more frequent side effects, particularly acne, hirsutism, and cushingoid changes in facies and habitus. For this reason it is preferable to begin treatment of patients who have carditis with salicylates; if these drugs fail to reduce fever and to ameliorate heart failure, therapy with corticosteroids may be initiated promptly. Prednisone is administered in doses of 60 to 120 mg or higher when necessary in four divided doses daily. After the inflammation has been brought under control by either salicylates or corticosteroids, treatment should be continued until the sedimentation rate approaches near-normal values and should be maintained for several weeks thereafter. To prevent poststeroid rebounds, an "overlap" course of salicylate therapy may be added when steroids are tapered off over a 2-week period. A useful method for tapering steroids is outlined in Chap. 325. Salicylates may then be continued for an additional 2 to 3 weeks. Rebounds of rheumatic activity are usually of short duration and, when mild, are best managed without resuming anti-inflammatory treatment, because a second or even a third rebound may occur when suppressive therapy is discontinued. About 5 percent of rheumatic attacks persist for 6 months or longer, either in the form of spontaneous acute recrudescences or as posttherapeutic rebounds. These "chronic" attacks are most likely to occur in patients with cardiac damage and with previous rheumatic episodes. Weekly tests for C-reactive protein in blood and for erythrocyte sedimentation rate are useful in following the healing process, particularly while treatment with corticosteroids or salicylates is gradually withdrawn.

Treatment of chorea The signs and symptoms of chorea usually do not respond well to treatment with antirheumatic agents. Because the patient with chorea is frequently emotionally unstable and because the manifestations of chorea may be exaggerated by emotional trauma, complete mental and physical rest is essential. Patients with chorea should be kept in a quiet room and cared for by sympathetic attendants. Corticosteroids or salicylates have little or no effect on chorea. Sedatives and tranquilizers, particularly diazepam and chlorpromazine, are useful. Chorea, no matter how severe, disappears during sleep, which should therefore be ensured by adequate sedation. Padded sideboards for the bed may be necessary to avoid injury to the patient. In the absence of other evidence of acute rheumatic disease, it is advisable to allow gradual resumption of physical activity when improvement is apparent rather than waiting for all choreiform movements to disappear, which may require many months.

Because of the great variability in the course of chorea, evaluating the effectiveness of various therapeutic measures is difficult. It is well to remember that chorea is a self-limited disease which is usually not followed by significant neurologic sequelae and that good results are almost invariably obtained by patient, attentive nursing care and by conservative medical management.

PREVENTION OF RECURRENCE The most efficient regimen for continuous prophylaxis against group A streptococci is a monthly intramuscular injection of 1.2 million units of benzathine penicillin. The disadvantages and discomfort of this regimen have to be weighed against the individual patient's susceptibility to recurrences. Those with rheumatic heart disease, recent rheumatic fever, and exposure to an environment in which the incidence of streptococcal infection is frequent deserve the most effective protection. As a second choice, prophylaxis may be administered orally with either 1 g sulfadiazine daily in a single dose or 200,000 units of penicillin given twice daily on an empty stomach. The duration of continuous prophylaxis cannot be fixed arbitrarily. Certainly, those under the age of 18 years should receive a continuous prophylactic regimen. A minimum period of 5 years is recommended for patients who develop rheumatic fever without carditis over the age of 18 years. The decision to continue prophylaxis beyond this period should take into account a number of variables. Patients with rheumatic heart disease are more susceptible to reactivation of rheumatic fever if they contract a streptococcal infection. Moreover, patients who have had carditis in a previous attack are much more likely to suffer carditis again in a subsequent attack. Climate, age, occupation, household situation, cardiac status, and length of time since the previous attack are all significant variables which influence the risk of recurrence. The decline in recurrence rates with increasing age is due to (1) decreased rate of streptococcal infection and (2) decrease in the rate of rheumatic reactivation following streptococcal infection in older rheumatic subjects. Despite this decreased rate, however, the risk of rheumatic recurrence in adults remains relatively high when the streptococcal disease encountered is severe or epidemic.

PREVENTION OF INITIAL RHEUMATIC ATTACKS Early and adequate treatment of pharyngeal infection due to group A streptococci will prevent initial attacks of rheumatic fever. If clinical streptococcal disease were properly detected by throat cultures and adequately treated, the spread of infection in a given population would be prevented, the epidemiology of streptococcal disease would be modified markedly, and the incidence of rheumatic fever in the community would be diminished. In communities where group A streptococcal disease has been diagnosed early and treated well and where socioeconomic standards are high, the group A organisms cultured frequently from schoolchildren's throats may be of relatively low virulence and may cause rheumatic fever less frequently than do more virulent strains prevalent in many epidemics.

Streptococcal pharyngitis is adequately treated by a single intramuscular injection of 600,000 units of benzathine penicillin in children less than 10 years of age or 1.2 million units in older children and adults. Any alternate plan of parenteral therapy or combined parenteral and oral therapy should provide for treatment over a period of 10 days. If oral penicillin is employed, at least 800,000 units per day in four divided doses must be given for no less than 10 days to achieve results comparable with a single injection of benzathine penicillin. Erythromycin in daily doses of 1 g for 10 days may be substituted in penicillin-sensitive individuals. Tetracycline is not recommended because some strains of group A streptococci have acquired resistance to it. All group A streptococci have so far remained extremely sensitive to penicillin.

REFERENCES

American Heart Association: Jones criteria (revised) for guidance in the diagnosis of rheumatic fever. Circulation 69:204A, 1984

Ayoub EM: The search for host determinants of susceptibility to rheumatic fever: The missing link. Circulation 69:197, 1984

Bisno AL: Acute rheumatic fever: Current concepts and controversies, in *Current Clinical Topics in Infectious Diseases*, JS Remington, MN Swartz (eds). New York, McGraw-Hill, 1984

Joint Report of UK-US Cooperative Study: The natural history of rheumatic fever and rheumatic heart disease. 10 year report of a cooperative clinical trial of ACTH, cortisone and aspirin. Circulation 32:457, 1965

Land MA, Bisno AL: Acute rheumatic fever: A vanishing disease in suburbia. JAMA 249:895, 1983

McDanald EC, Weisman MH: Ventricular manifestations of rheumatic fever in adults. Ann Intern Med 89:917, 1978

Persellin RH: Acute rheumatic fever: Changing manifestations. Ann Intern Med 89:1002, 1978

Read S, Zabriskie JB (eds): *Streptococcal Diseases and the Immune Response.* New York, Academic, 1980

Stollerman GH: *Rheumatic Fever and Streptococcal Infection.* New York, Grune & Stratton, 1975

———: Global changes in group A streptococcal diseases and strategies for their prevention, in *Advances in Internal Medicine* 27:373. Chicago, Year Book Medical Publishers, 1982

187 VALVULAR HEART DISEASE

EUGENE BRAUNWALD

The role of physical examination in the evaluation of patients with valvular disease is considered in Chap. 177; of roentgenography, echocardiography, phonocardiography and other indirect graphic techniques in Chap. 179; of electrocardiography in Chap. 178; and of cardiac catheterization and angiography in Chap. 180.

MITRAL STENOSIS

PATHOPHYSIOLOGY In normal adults the mitral valve orifice is 4 to 6 cm^2. In the presence of significant obstruction, i.e., when the orifice is less than one-half of normal, blood can flow from the left atrium to the left ventricle only if propelled by an abnormally elevated left atrioventricular pressure gradient, the hemodynamic hallmark of mitral stenosis. When the mitral valve opening is reduced to 1 cm^2, a left atrial pressure of approximately 25 mmHg is required to maintain a normal cardiac output. The elevated left atrial pressure in turn raises pulmonary venous and capillary pressures, reducing pulmonary compliance and causing exertional dyspnea. The first bouts of dyspnea are usually precipitated by clinical events which increase the rate of blood flow across the mitral orifice, which results in further elevation of the left atrial pressure (see below). In order to assess the severity of obstruction, it is essential to measure both the transvalvular pressure gradient and the flow rate. The latter is dependent not only on the cardiac output but on the heart rate as well. An increase in heart rate shortens diastole proportionately more than systole, and diminishes the time available for flow across the mitral valve. Therefore, at any given level of cardiac output tachycardia augments the transvalvular gradient and elevates further the left atrial pressure.

The left ventricular diastolic pressure is normal in isolated mitral stenosis; coexisting mitral regurgitation, aortic valve disease, the residua of damage produced by rheumatic myocarditis, systemic hypertension, or ischemic heart disease may be responsible for elevations which reflect impaired left ventricular function and/or reduced left ventricular compliance. Left ventricular dysfunction, as reflected in reduced ejection fraction and circumferential fiber shortening rate, occurs in about one-fourth of patients with mitral stenosis, as a consequence of chronic reduction of preload and extension of the scarring from the valve into the adjacent myocardium. In pure mitral stenosis and sinus rhythm, the mean left atrial and pulmonary artery wedge pressures are usually elevated and the pressure pulse shows a prominent atrial contraction (*a* wave), and a gradual pressure decline after mitral valve opening (*y* descent). In patients with mild to moderate mitral stenosis without elevation of the pulmonary vascular resistance, the pulmonary arterial pressure may be normal at rest and may rise only with exercise. In severe mitral stenosis and whenever the pulmonary vascular resistance is significantly increased, the pulmonary arterial pressure is elevated even when the patient is at rest, and in extreme cases it may exceed the systemic arterial pressure. Further elevations of left atrial, pulmonary capillary, and pulmonary arterial pressures occur during exercise. When the pulmonary arterial systolic pressure exceeds approximately 50 mmHg in patients with mitral stenosis, or for that matter with any valvular lesion, the increased right ventricular afterload impedes the emptying of this chamber, and right ventricular end-diastolic pressure and volume usually rise as a compensatory mechanism.

The cardiac output at rest varies considerably in patients with mitral stenosis. Thus, the hemodynamic response to a given degree of mitral obstruction may be characterized by a normal cardiac output and a high left atrioventricular pressure gradient or, at the opposite end of the hemodynamic spectrum, by a reduced cardiac output and low transvalvular pressure gradient. In a small fraction of patients with moderately severe mitral stenosis, the cardiac output is normal at rest and rises normally during exertion; under these circumstances, the high atrioventricular pressure gradient elevates the left atrial and pulmonary capillary pressures markedly, and this elevation is responsible for symptoms of relatively severe pulmonary congestion. In the majority of patients, however, the cardiac output is normal at rest but rises subnormally during exertion. In patients with severe stenosis, particularly those in whom the pulmonary vascular resistance is strikingly elevated, the cardiac output is subnormal at rest and may fail to rise or may even decline during activity. The depressed cardiac output in patients with mitral stenosis is related primarily to the obstruction of the mitral orifice but may also be due to the impairment of the function of either ventricle.

The clinical and hemodynamic features of mitral stenosis are dictated largely by the level of the pulmonary artery pressure. Pulmonary hypertension results from (1) the passive backward transmission of the elevated left atrial pressure, (2) pulmonary arteriolar constriction, which presumably is triggered by left atrial and pulmonary venous hypertension (reactive pulmonary hypertension), and (3) organic obliterative changes in the pulmonary vascular bed. The elevation of pulmonary vascular resistance may be considered to be a complication of long-standing and severe mitral stenosis; in time, the resultant severe pulmonary hypertension results in tricuspid and pulmonary incompetence as well as right-sided heart failure. However, the changes in the pulmonary vascular bed may also be considered to exert a protective effect; the elevated precapillary resistance reduces the likelihood of symptoms of pulmonary congestion by reducing the surge of blood into the pulmonary capillary bed which then dams up behind the stenotic mitral valve during activity. However, this protection occurs at the expense of a decreased cardiac output.

ETIOLOGY AND PATHOLOGY Mitral stenosis is generally rheumatic in origin. Pure or predominant mitral stenosis occurs in approximately 40 percent of all patients with rheumatic heart disease; two-thirds of all patients with mitral stenosis are females. The valve leaflets are diffusely thickened by fibrous tissue and/or calcific deposits. The mitral commissures fuse, the chordae tendineae fuse and shorten, the valvular cusps become rigid, and these changes in turn lead to narrowing at the apex of the funnel-shaped valve. While the initial insult to the mitral valve is rheumatic, the later changes may be a nonspecific process resulting from trauma to the valve caused by altered flow patterns due to the initial deformity. Calcification of the stenotic mitral valve immobilizes the leaflets and narrows the orifice. Thrombus formation and arterial embolization may arise from the calcific valve itself. Rarely, mitral stenosis is congenital in origin.

SYMPTOMS In temperate climates the latent period between the initial attack of rheumatic carditis, in the rare circumstances in which a history of one can be elicited, and the development of symptoms due to mitral stenosis is generally on the order of two decades; most patients begin to experience disability in the fourth decade. Once a patient with mitral stenosis becomes seriously symptomatic, continuous progression of the disease to death usually occurs in 2 to 5 years unless the stenosis is relieved by operation. In economically deprived areas, particularly on the Indian subcontinent, in Central America, and the Middle East, mitral stenosis tends to progress more rapidly and frequently causes serious symptoms before the age of 20 years. On the other hand, slowly progressive mitral stenosis in the elderly is also being recognized with increasing frequency in the United States and western Europe.

When valvular obstruction is mild, many of the physical signs of mitral stenosis may be present in the absence of any symptoms. However, even in those patients whose mitral orifices are large enough to accommodate a normal blood flow with only mild elevations of left atrial pressure, extreme exertion, excitement, fever, severe anemia, paroxysmal tachycardia, sexual intercourse, pregnancy, and thyrotoxicosis all may precipitate elevations of pulmonary capillary pressure and lead to dyspnea and cough. As stenosis progresses, the stresses that precipitate dyspnea become less severe, and the patient becomes limited in his or her daily activities. Redistribution of blood from the dependent portions of the body to the lungs, which occurs when the recumbent position is assumed, leads to orthopnea and paroxysmal nocturnal dyspnea. *Pulmonary edema* develops when there is a sudden increase in flow rate across a markedly narrowed mitral orifice (Chap. 26). When moderately severe mitral stenosis has existed for several years, *atrial arrhythmias*—premature contractions, paroxysmal tachycardia, flutter, and fibrillation—occur with increasing frequency. The rapid ventricular rate associated with untreated or inadequately treated atrial fibrillation is frequently responsible for acute exacerbations of dyspnea. The development of permanent atrial fibrillation often marks a turning point in the patient's course and is generally associated with acceleration of the rate at which symptoms progress.

Hemoptysis (Chap. 25) results from rupture of pulmonary-bronchial venous connections secondary to pulmonary venous hypertension. It occurs most frequently in patients who have elevated left atrial pressures without markedly elevated pulmonary vascular resistances and is almost never fatal. True hemoptysis must be distinguished from the bloody sputum that occurs with pulmonary edema, pulmonary infarction, and bronchitis, three conditions that occur with increased frequency in the presence of mitral stenosis.

When the pulmonary vascular resistance rises or when tricuspid stenosis or regurgitation develops, symptoms secondary to pulmonary congestion may diminish, and the episodes of acute pulmonary edema and hemoptysis become reduced in frequency and severity. Elevation of pulmonary vascular resistance further increases right ventricular systolic pressure, leading to right ventricular failure, fatigue, weakness, abdominal discomfort due to hepatic congestion, and edema.

Recurrent pulmonary emboli with infarction (Chap. 211) are an important cause of morbidity and mortality late in the course of mitral stenosis, occurring most frequently in patients with right ventricular failure. *Pulmonary infections,* i.e., bronchitis, bronchopneumonia, and lobar pneumonia, commonly complicate untreated mitral stenosis. *Infective endocarditis* (Chap. 188) is rare in pure mitral stenosis but is not uncommon in patients with combined stenosis and regurgitation. *Chest pain* occurs in about 10 percent of patients with severe mitral stenosis; it may be due to pulmonary hypertension, or myocardial ischemia secondary to coronary atherosclerosis; often the cause cannot be discovered.

In addition to the aforementioned changes in the pulmonary vascular bed, fibrous thickening of the walls of the alveoli and pulmonary capillaries occurs commonly in mitral stenosis. The vital capacity, total lung capacity, maximal breathing capacity, and oxygen uptake per unit of ventilation are reduced, and in patients with severe stenosis the latter fails to rise normally during exertion. The reduction of pulmonary compliance that occurs generally correlates directly with the severity of the dyspnea and with the heightened pulmonary capillary pressure, and these changes are intensified during exercise. In some patients airway resistance is abnormally increased. These alterations in pulmonary mechanics contribute to an increase in the work of breathing and play an important role in the genesis of dyspnea. The changes in the lungs are due, in part, to increased transudation of fluid from the pulmonary capillaries into the interstitial and alveolar spaces as a consequence of the elevated pulmonary capillary pressure. The distribution of blood flow and ventilation may be uneven; as in other conditions in which left atrial pressure is elevated, pulmonary blood flow in the erect position is displaced from the basal to the superior segments of the lung (Chap. 200). The diffusing capacity may be reduced, particularly during exertion, as a result of structural changes in the diffusing surface and reduction of the pulmonary capillary blood volume. The thickening of the alveolar and capillary walls impedes the transudation of fluid into the alveoli and the development of pulmonary edema at times when the pulmonary capillary pressure exceeds the plasma oncotic pressure. The increased capacity of the pulmonary lymphatic system to drain excess fluid also retards the development of pulmonary edema.

Thrombi may form in the left atria, particularly in the enlarged atrial appendages of patients with mitral stenosis. When they embolize, they do so most commonly to the brain, kidneys, spleen, and extremities. This complication occurs much more frequently in patients with atrial fibrillation or unstable rhythms, in older patients, and in those with a reduced cardiac output, but it is also seen in patients with relatively mild as well as severe obstruction. Thus, systemic embolization may be the presenting complaint in otherwise asymptomatic patients with mild mitral stenosis. At operation, thrombi are not found more frequently in the left atria of patients with past history of embolization than in those without this complication, indicating that it is usually the freshly formed clots that dislodge. Patients who have had one or more systemic emboli have the predilection to have further embolic episodes more often than patients with stenosis of comparable severity without previous embolization. Rarely, a large pedunculated thrombus or a free-floating clot may suddenly obstruct the stenotic mitral orifice. Such ''ball valve'' thrombi produce syncope, angina, and changing auscultatory signs with alterations in position, findings that resemble those produced by a left atrial myxoma (Chap. 193).

PHYSICAL FINDINGS (See also Chap. 177) Peripheral and facial *cyanosis* may occur in patients with extremely severe mitral stenosis. In advanced cases there is a malar flush and the facies appear pinched and blue. The jugular venous pulse reveals prominent *a* waves due to vigorous right atrial systole in patients with sinus rhythm who have severe pulmonary hypertension or associated tricuspid stenosis. When atrial fibrillation is present, the jugular pulse reveals only a single expansion during systole (*c-v* wave). The systemic arterial pressure is usually normal or slightly low. A right ventricular tap is present along the left sternal border, signifying an enlarged right ventricle. The first heart sound may be palpable in patients with pliable valve leaflets. In patients with pulmonary hypertension, the impact of pulmonary valve closure can usually be felt in the second and third left intercostal spaces just left of the sternum; the left ventricle is not palpable in severe, pure mitral stenosis. A diastolic thrill is frequently present at the cardiac apex, particularly if the patient is turned into the left lateral recumbent position.

The first heart sound is generally accentuated and snapping, and since the mitral valve does not close until the left ventricular pressure reaches the level of the elevated left atrial pressure, this sound is often slightly delayed on phonocardiography, particularly in patients with severe stenosis. In patients with pulmonary hypertension, the pulmonary component of the second heart sound is often accentuated, and the two components of the second heart sound are closely split. A pulmonary systolic ejection click may be heard in patients with severe pulmonary hypertension and marked dilatation of the pulmonary artery. The opening snap of the mitral valve is most readily audible in expiration at, or just medial to, the cardiac apex but may also be easily heard along the left sternal edge or at the base of the heart. This sound generally follows the sound of aortic valve closure by 0.06 to 0.12 s, that is, it follows the pulmonic valve closure sound. Since the opening snap of the mitral valve occurs at the instant at which the left ventricular pressure falls below the left atrial pressure, the time interval between aortic closure and the opening snap varies inversely with the severity of the mitral stenosis. It tends to be short, that is, 0.06 to 0.07 s, in patients with severe obstruction and long, that is, 0.10 to 0.12 s, in patients with mild mitral stenosis. The intensities of the opening snap and the first heart sound correlate with the mobility of the anterior mitral leaflet.

The opening snap usually ushers in a low-pitched, rumbling, diastolic murmur, heard best at the apex with the patient in the left lateral recumbent position, and often accentuated by exercise carried out just before auscultation. In general, the duration of this murmur correlates with the severity of the stenosis. In patients with sinus rhythm the murmur often reappears or becomes reaccentuated during atrial systole, as atrial contraction reelevates the rate of blood flow across the narrowed orifice. Soft (grade I or II/VI) systolic murmurs are commonly heard at the apex or along the left sternal border in patients with pure mitral stenosis and do not necessarily signify the presence of mitral regurgitation. Hepatomegaly, ankle edema, ascites, and pleural effusion, particularly in the right pleural cavity, may occur in patients with mitral stenosis and right ventricular failure.

Associated lesions With severe pulmonary hypertension a loud pansystolic murmur produced by functional tricuspid regurgitation may be audible along the left sternal border. This murmur may be accentuated by inspiration, diminishes during forced expiration or during performance of the Valsalva maneuver, diminishes or disappears as compensation is restored, and must not be confused with the apical pansystolic murmur of mitral regurgitation, since management is quite different if mitral regurgitation is present.

The recognition of associated mitral regurgitation is of considerable clinical importance in patients with mitral stenosis. A presystolic murmur and an accentuated first heart sound speak against the presence of serious associated mitral regurgitation, but when the first heart sound and/or the opening snap are soft or absent in a patient with mitral valve disease, it is likely that significant mitral regurgitation and/or serious calcification of the deformed mitral valve leaflets are present. A third heart sound at the apex often signifies that the mitral regurgitation is serious; this sound is generally duller and lower pitched and follows the opening snap. Occasionally, in patients with pure mitral stenosis, physical signs may falsely suggest mitral regurgitation. Thus, in the presence of severe pulmonary hypertension and right ventricular failure, a third heart sound may originate from the right ventricle. The enlarged right ventricle may rotate the heart in a clockwise direction and form the cardiac apex, giving the examiner the erroneous impression of left ventricular enlargement. Under these circumstances the rumbling diastolic murmur and the other auscultatory features of mitral stenosis become less prominent or may even disappear and be replaced by the systolic murmur of functional tricuspid regurgitation. When cardiac output is markedly reduced in a patient with mitral stenosis, none of the typical auscultatory findings may be detectable, but they may reappear as compensation is restored. Associated tricuspid stenosis also tends to obscure many of the physical signs of mitral stenosis.

The Graham Steell murmur of pulmonary regurgitation, a high-pitched, diastolic, decrescendo blowing murmur along the left sternal border, results from dilatation of the pulmonary valve ring and occurs in patients with mitral valve disease and severe pulmonary hypertension. This murmur may be indistinguishable from the more common murmur produced by mild aortic regurgitation except that it is rarely audible at the second right intercostal space, and may disappear following successful surgical treatment of the mitral stenosis.

Electrocardiogram In mitral stenosis and sinus rhythm the P wave usually suggests left atrial enlargement (Chap. 178). It may become tall and peaked in lead II and upright in lead V_1 when severe pulmonary hypertension or tricuspid stenosis complicates mitral stenosis and right atrial enlargement occurs. The QRS complex may be normal, even in patients with critical mitral stenosis. However, with severe pulmonary hypertension, right axis deviation and right ventricular hypertrophy are usually found. When left ventricular hypertrophy is present in patients with mitral stenosis, it generally indicates that an additional lesion which places a burden on the left ventricle, such as mitral regurgitation, aortic valve disease, or hypertension, is present.

Echocardiogram (see also Chap. 179) The echocardiogram is the most sensitive and specific noninvasive method for diagnosing mitral stenosis. The M-mode tracing reveals that the anterior and posterior mitral leaflets do not separate widely in early diastole (i.e., less than 15 mm) and they maintain a fixed relation to each other throughout diastole. A reduction in the EF slope reflects failure of the anterior leaflet of the mitral valve to float back to midposition in middiastole.

Calcification and thickening of the mitral valve are detected as multilayered echoes or a thickening of the echo pattern. Mitral orifice area may be estimated with cross-sectional (two-dimensional) echocardiography. The left atrium is usually enlarged. Doppler studies reveal increased turbulence and transvalvular flow velocity and may be used both in the diagnosis of mitral stenosis and in estimating the transvalvular gradient.

Roentgenographic features (Chap. 179) The earliest changes are straightening of the left border of the cardiac silhouette, prominence of the main pulmonary arteries, dilatation of the upper lobe pulmonary veins, and backward displacement of the esophagus by an enlarged left atrium. In patients with mild or moderate stenosis, the heart is not grossly enlarged. In severe mitral stenosis, however, all chambers and vessels upstream to the narrowed valve are prominent, including the two atria, the pulmonary arteries and veins, right ventricle, and superior vena cava. Kerley B lines are fine, dense, opaque, horizontal lines which are most prominent in the lower and midlung fields and which result from distention of interlobular septa and lymphatics with edema when the resting mean left atrial pressure exceeds approximately 20 mmHg. As the pulmonary arterial pressure rises, the smaller pulmonary arteries become attenuated, at first in the lower, then in the mid-, and finally in the upper lung fields. Deposits of hemosiderin occur in the lungs of patients who have had multiple hemoptyses; the hemosiderin-containing macrophages fill the air spaces, and if they become confluent result in a fine, diffuse nodulation most prominent in the lower lung fields.

DIFFERENTIAL DIAGNOSIS Significant mitral regurgitation may be associated with a prominent diastolic murmur at the apex, but this murmur commences slightly later than in patients with stenosis, and there is often clear-cut evidence of left ventricular enlargement on physical examination, roentgenography, and electrocardiography. In addition, an apical pansystolic murmur of at least grade III/VI intensity as well as a third heart sound should arouse the suspicion of significant associated regurgitation. Similarly, the apical middiastolic murmur associated with aortic regurgitation (Austin Flint murmur) may be mistaken for mitral stenosis. However, in a patient with aortic regurgitation the absence of an opening snap or of presystolic accentuation if sinus rhythm is present points to the absence of mitral stenosis. Tricuspid stenosis, a valvular lesion that occurs very rarely in the absence of mitral stenosis, may mask many of the clinical features of mitral stenosis. Echocardiography is particularly useful in detecting mitral stenosis in patients who have or are suspected of having other valve lesions.

Exertional dyspnea and recurrent pulmonary infections may be falsely ascribed to pulmonary emphysema in patients with both *chronic lung disease* and mitral stenosis. Careful auscultation, however, will generally reveal the characteristic opening snap and rumbling diastolic murmur. Similarly, the hemoptysis that occurs in many otherwise asymptomatic patients with mitral stenosis may be improperly attributed to bronchiectasis or tuberculosis. Actually, the latter condition is uncommon in patients with significant mitral obstruction.

Primary pulmonary hypertension (Chap. 210) results in a number of the clinical and laboratory features observed in mitral stenosis. It occurs most frequently in young women; however, the opening snap and diastolic rumbling murmur are absent, there is no left atrial enlargement, and the pulmonary artery wedge and left atrial pressures are *normal. Atrial septal defect* (Chap. 185) may also be mistaken for mitral stenosis; in both conditions there is often clinical, electrocardiographic, and roentgenographic evidence of right ventricular enlargement and accentuation of the pulmonary vascularity. The widely split second heart sound of atrial septal defect may be confused with the mitral opening snap, and the diastolic flow murmur across the tricuspid valve mistaken for the mitral diastolic murmur. However, the absence of left atrial enlargement and of Kerley B lines and the demonstration of fixed splitting of the second heart sound all favor atrial septal defect over mitral stenosis. *Cor triatriatum* is an unusual congenital malformation that consists of a fibrous ring within the left atrium (Chap. 185). It results in elevation of the pulmonary venous, capillary, and arterial pressures. This lesion can be recognized most readily by means of left atrial angiography.

Left atrial myxoma (Chap. 193) may obstruct left atrial emptying, resulting in dyspnea, a diastolic murmur, and hemodynamic changes resembling those of mitral stenosis. However, patients with left atrial myxoma often demonstrate findings suggestive of a systemic disease, with weight loss, fever, anemia, systemic emboli, and elevated erythrocyte sedimentation rate and serum gamma-globulin concentration. Usually an opening snap is not audible, there is no clinical evidence of associated aortic valve disease, and the auscultatory findings frequently change with body position. The diagnosis can be established by demonstrating a characteristic echo-producing mass in the left atrium by echocardiography and a lobulated filling defect by angiocardiography.

Specialized techniques Catheterization of the left side of the heart (Chap. 180) is extremely helpful in deciding whether valvulotomy is necessary in patients in whom it is difficult to estimate the severity of obstruction by clinical means and noninvasive tests. When combined with aortography and left ventricular angiocardiography, this procedure serves as the ultimate method for detecting and estimating associated mitral regurgitation and coexisting lesions such as aortic stenosis and regurgitation as well as left ventricular dysfunction. Left atrial thrombi and tumors may be detected or excluded by angiocardiography, particularly when the contrast medium is injected directly into the left atrium. These "invasive" methods are also helpful in the detection of accompanying conditions, such as coronary artery disease, that impair left ventricular function and would thereby contraindicate or reduce the effectiveness of mitral valvulotomy. Catheterization and left ventricular angiography are indicated in most patients who have undergone previous mitral valve operations and who have redeveloped serious symptoms; in such patients clinical assessment may be particularly difficult, and the hemodynamic studies allow determination of the severity of the lesion, intelligent planning of the operative procedure when it is indicated, and a more accurate estimate of the risk.

MANAGEMENT In the asymptomatic adolescent with mitral valve disease, penicillin prophylaxis of beta-hemolytic streptococcal infections (Chap. 186), prophylaxis for infective endocarditis (Chap. 188), and vocational counseling are particularly important; physically strenuous occupations should be avoided so that premature retirement will not be necessary should symptoms develop later. In symptomatic patients some improvement usually occurs with restriction of sodium intake and maintenance doses of oral diuretics. Digitalis glycosides do not alter the hemodynamics and usually do not benefit patients with pure stenosis and sinus rhythm, but they are necessary for slowing the ventricular rate of patients with atrial fibrillation and for reducing the manifestations of right-sided heart failure in the advanced stages of the disease. Small doses of beta blockers (e.g., atenolol 25 to 50 mg qd) may be added when cardiac glycosides fail to control ventricular rate in patients with atrial fibrillation or flutter. Particular attention should be directed to detecting and treating any accompanying anemia and infections. Hemoptysis is treated by measures designed to diminish pulmonary venous pressure, including bed rest, the sitting position, salt restriction, and diuresis. Anticoagulants should be administered for at least 1 year in patients with mitral stenosis who have suffered systemic and/or pulmonary embolization and those with intermittent atrial fibrillation.

If atrial fibrillation is of relatively recent origin in a patient whose mitral stenosis is not severe enough to warrant surgical treatment, reversion to sinus rhythm, pharmacologically or by means of electrical countershock is indicated. Usually this should be undertaken following 4 weeks of anticoagulant treatment. Conversion to sinus rhythm is rarely helpful in patients with severe mitral stenosis, particularly those in whom the left atrium is especially enlarged or in whom atrial fibrillation has been present for more than 1 year, since reversion to atrial fibrillation is common.

Surgical treatment Unless there is a specific contraindication, operative treatment is indicated in the symptomatic patient with pure mitral stenosis whose effective orifice is less than approximately 1.2 cm^2. Operation not only usually results in striking symptomatic and hemodynamic improvement but also prolongs survival. In uncomplicated cases, the surgical mortality rate should be 0 to 2 percent. However, there is no evidence that surgical treatment improves the prognosis of patients with slight or no functional impairment. Therefore, unless recurrent systemic embolization has occurred, valvulotomy is *not* recommended for patients who are entirely asymptomatic, regardless of hemodynamic findings. When there is little symptomatic improvement following valvulotomy, it is likely that the procedure was ineffective, that it induced mitral regurgitation, or that associated valvular or myocardial disease was present. The recurrence of symptoms several years after what appeared to be a satisfactory initial result is usually due to an inadequate valvulotomy, but progression of other valvular lesions, the development of myocardial disease, restenosis of the mitral valve, or some combination of these conditions may also be responsible. In the *pregnant patient* with mitral stenosis operative treatment should be carried out if pulmonary congestion occurs despite intensive medical treatment.

An "open" operation using cardiopulmonary bypass is usually preferable for patients with pure mitral stenosis who have not been operated upon previously. In addition to opening the valve commissures, it is important to loosen any subvalvular fusion of papillary muscles and chordae tendineae and to remove large deposits of calcium, thereby improving valvular function, and to remove atrial thrombi. In patients with significant associated mitral regurgitation, those in whom the valve has been severely distorted by previous operative manipulation, or those in whom the surgeon does not find it possible to improve valve function significantly, the valve may have to be replaced with a prosthesis or a heterograft. Since the operative mortality of replacement of the mitral valve is still approximately 5 to 10 percent and since there are long-term complications of valve replacement, patients in whom preoperative evaluation suggests the possibility that replacement may be required should be operated on only if they have *critical* mitral stenosis, i.e., an orifice $<1.0\ cm^2$, and are in the New York Heart Association class III, i.e., symptomatic with ordinary activity, despite optimal medical therapy.

VALVE REPLACEMENT The results of replacement of any valve are dependent primarily on (1) the patient's myocardial function at the time of operation, (2) the technical abilities of the operative team and the quality of the postoperative care, and (3) the durability, hemodynamic characteristics, and thrombogenicity of the prosthesis. Increased operative mortality is associated with the degree of preoperative functional disability and pulmonary hypertension. Late complications of replacement of any valve, which fortunately are declining in incidence, include paravalvular leakage, thromboemboli, bleeding due to anticoagulants, mechanical dysfunction of the prosthesis, and infective endocarditis.

The considerations regarding the choice between a bioprosthetic and artificial mechanical valve are similar in the mitral and aortic positions and in the treatment of stenotic, regurgitant, or mixed lesions. All patients who have undergone replacement of any valve with a mechanical prosthesis must be maintained permanently on anticoagulants. The primary advantage of bioprostheses (tissue valves) over mechanical prostheses is the reduction of thromboembolic complications and, except for patients with chronic atrial fibrillation, few such instances have been associated with their use. Bioprosthetic valves are contraindicated in younger patients (<35 years) because of accelerated deterioration and are particularly useful in the elderly (>65 years) in whom there is more concern about chronic anticoagulation than about long-term (>15 years) valve durability. These valves are also indicated in women who expect to become pregnant as well as others in whom anticoagulation may be contraindicated. In patients without such contraindications, particularly those under 60 years, a mechanical prosthesis may be preferable. Many surgeons now select the St. Jude prosthesis, a double-disk tilting prosthesis, for replacement of both aortic and mitral valves because of somewhat more favorable hemodynamic characteristics and a suggestion of lower thrombogenicity.

The overall 9-year survival of operative survivors following mitral valve replacement is approximately 60 percent. Long-term prognosis is worse in subgroups of older patients and those with marked disability and striking depression of the cardiac index preoperatively.

MITRAL REGURGITATION

PATHOPHYSIOLOGY The regurgitant mitral orifice may be considered to be in parallel with the aortic orifice, and therefore the resistance to left ventricular emptying is reduced in patients with mitral regurgitation. As a consequence, the left ventricle decompresses itself into the left atrium during ejection, and with the reduction in left ventricular size there is a rapid decline in left ventricular tension, allowing a greater proportion of the contractile activity of the left ventricle to be expended in shortening. Thus, the initial compensation to mitral regurgitation consists of more complete systolic emptying of the left ventricle. However, a progressive increase in left ventricular end-diastolic volume occurs as the severity of the regurgitation increases and the function of the left ventricle deteriorates. The atrial contraction wave in the left atrial pressure pulse (*a* wave) is usually not as prominent as it is in mitral stenosis, but the *v* wave is often much taller, since it is inscribed during ventricular systole, when the left atrium fills from the pulmonary veins as well as from the left ventricle. During early diastole, as the distended left atrium suddenly empties, there is a particularly rapid *y* descent as long as there is no associated mitral stenosis. Left ventricular end-diastolic pressure may be slightly elevated. However, in chronic mitral regurgitation, there is often an increase in left ventricular compliance, so that ventricular volume may be greatly increased with little elevation in end-diastolic pressure. The effective cardiac output usually declines in seriously symptomatic patients. Although a left atrioventricular pressure gradient persisting throughout diastole signifies the presence of significant associated mitral stenosis, a brief, early diastolic gradient may occur in patients with pure regurgitation as a result of the torrential flow of blood across a normal-sized mitral orifice.

The prompt appearance of contrast material in the left atrium following its injection into the left ventricle signifies the presence and can be useful in the diagnosis of mitral regurgitation. The regurgitant volume can be measured by determining the difference between the total left ventricular stroke estimated angiocardiographically and the effective forward stroke volume determined by the Fick method. The results of such studies suggest that the regurgitant volume may be of the same magnitude as the effective forward stroke volume or may even exceed it in patients with severe regurgitation. Qualitative, but clinically useful, estimates of the severity of regurgitation may be made by Doppler echocardiography and by observation on cineangiograms of the degree of left atrial opacification following the injection of contrast material into the left ventricle.

Patients with severe mitral regurgitation may be divided into several subgroups, depending on the compliance, i.e., the pressure-volume relationship, of the left atrium and pulmonary venous bed. Among patients with severe mitral regurgitation, three major groups have been identified:

1 *Normal or reduced compliance*. These patients usually have *acute* mitral regurgitation. There is little enlargement of the left atrium, but marked elevation of the mean left atrial pressure, particularly of the *v* wave. In these patients severe mitral regurgitation has usually developed suddenly, as when it follows rupture of chordae tendineae, infarction of one of the heads of a papillary muscle, or tear of a mitral leaflet. Pulmonary edema is common. After several months the pulmonary vascular resistance may become markedly

elevated, presumably as a consequence of the left atrial hypertension, and right-sided heart failure may also occur; sinus rhythm is usually present.

2 *Marked increase in compliance.* At the opposite end of the spectrum from group 1 are those patients with severe long-standing mitral regurgitation, massive enlargement of the left atrium, and normal or only slightly elevated left atrial pressure. The pulmonary artery pressure and pulmonary vascular resistance are also normal or only slightly elevated at rest. Clinically, these patients usually complain of severe fatigue and exhaustion secondary to a low cardiac output, while symptoms resulting from pulmonary congestion are less prominent; atrial fibrillation is almost invariably present. The association of a near-normal left atrial pressure with a markedly enlarged, thin-walled left atrium indicates that this chamber is far more compliant than normal. Thus, long-standing mitral regurgitation may, in some instances, alter the physical properties of the left atrial wall and thereby displace the atrial pressure-volume curve, allowing a normal pressure to exist in a greatly enlarged left atrium.

3 *Moderate increase in compliance.* By far the most common group are patients whose clinical and hemodynamic features are between those in the other two groups with variable degrees of enlargement of the left atrium and with significant elevation of the left atrial pressure. Symptoms are secondary to both reduced cardiac output and pulmonary congestion.

ETIOLOGY In about half the patients mitral regurgitation is caused by chronic *rheumatic heart disease,* but in contrast to mitral stenosis, pure or predominantly rheumatic mitral regurgitation occurs more frequently in males. The rheumatic process produces rigidity, deformity, and retraction of the valve cusps, and commissural fusion, as well as shortening, contraction, and fusion of the chordae tendineae. Mitral regurgitation may also occur as a congenital anomaly (Chap. 185), most commonly as (1) a defect of the endocardial cushions or in association with (2) corrected transposition, (3) endocardial fibroelastosis, and (4) the ''parachute'' mitral valve deformity. Mitral regurgitation may occur with fibrosis of a papillary muscle in patients with healed myocardial infarction as well as in patients with a ventricular aneurysm involving the base of a papillary muscle. Transient regurgitation may also occur during periods of ischemia involving a papillary muscle or the adjacent myocardium and may accompany bouts of angina pectoris. Mitral regurgitation may occur with marked left ventricular enlargement of any cause in which dilatation of the mitral annulus and lateral displacement of the papillary muscles interfere with coaptation of the valve leaflets. In hypertrophic cardiomyopathy the anterior leaflet of the mitral valve is displaced anteriorly during systole, leading to regurgitation (Chap. 192). Massive calcification of the mitral annulus of unknown cause, which occurs most commonly in elderly women, can also be responsible for significant mitral regurgitation. Systemic lupus erythematosus, rheumatoid arthritis, and ankylosing spondylitis are less common causes. *Acute* mitral regurgitation may occur secondary to infective endocarditis involving the valve or chordae tendineae, in acute myocardial infarction with rupture of a papillary muscle or one of its heads as a consequence of trauma, or as a complication of cardiac surgery.

Abnormal elongation of chordae tendineae and/or redundant posterior cusps of the mitral valve with prolapse of the cusps into the left atrium, the so-called floppy valve, leading to the syndrome of midsystolic click and midsystolic murmur, also referred to as the *prolapsing mitral valve leaflet syndrome* (see below), is another important cause of mitral regurgitation.

Regardless of etiology, serious mitral regurgitation tends to be progressive since enlargement of the left atrium places tension on the posterior mitral leaflet, pulling it away from the mitral orifice, thereby aggravating the valvular dysfunction. Similarly, the dilatation of the left ventricle increases the regurgitation, which in turn further enlarges the left atrium and ventricle, resulting in a vicious cycle; hence the aphorism, ''mitral regurgitation begets mitral regurgitation.''

SYMPTOMS Only a fraction of patients with chronic mitral regurgitation ever experience any reduction of cardiac reserve, but in those who do become symptomatic, fatigue, exertional dyspnea, and orthopnea may be prominent complaints. Symptoms resulting from pulmonary congestion tend to be less episodic in nature in patients with chronic severe mitral regurgitation than mitral stenosis, since fluctuations of the mean pulmonary capillary pressure are less marked. Indeed, acute paroxysmal pulmonary edema is quite rare in patients with chronic mitral regurgitation. Hemoptysis and systemic embolism also occur far less frequently in mitral regurgitation than in stenosis. On the other hand, fatigability, weakness, exhaustion, weight loss, and even cachexia are more prominent and occur most frequently in patients with marked reduction of cardiac output. Right-sided heart failure, with painful hepatic congestion, ankle edema, distended neck veins, ascites, and tricuspid regurgitation, may be observed in patients with mitral regurgitation who have associated pulmonary vascular disease. In patients with *acute* severe mitral regurgitation, left ventricular failure with acute pulmonary edema and/or cardiovascular collapse is common.

PHYSICAL FINDINGS The arterial pressure is usually normal, and the arterial pulse is often characterized by a sharp upstroke. The jugular venous pulse shows abnormally prominent *a* waves in patients with sinus rhythm and marked pulmonary hypertension. A systolic thrill is often palpable at the cardiac apex, the left ventricle is hyperdynamic with a brisk systolic impulse and a palpable rapid-filling wave, and the apex beat is often displaced laterally. When the left atrium is markedly enlarged, it may extend anteriorly, and its expansion may be palpable along the sternal border late during ventricular systole, resembling a right ventricular lift. The combination of the retraction of the left ventricle and expansion of the left atrium during systole may produce a characteristic rocking motion of the chest with each cardiac cycle. A right ventricular tap and the shock of pulmonary valve closure may be palpable in patients with marked pulmonary hypertension.

The first heart sound is generally absent, soft, or buried in the systolic murmur, and an accentuated mitral closure sound is useful in excluding severe regurgitation. A pulmonary ejection sound is often audible in patients with associated pulmonary hypertension. Splitting of the second heart sound is usually normal, but in patients with severe regurgitation, the aortic valve may close prematurely, resulting in wide splitting of the second heart sound. An opening snap indicates associated mitral stenosis but does not exclude predominant regurgitation. A low-pitched third heart sound, occurring 0.12 to 0.17 s after the aortic valve closure sound, at the completion of the rapid-filling phase of the left ventricle, is believed to be caused by the sudden tensing of the papillary muscles, chordae tendineae, and valve leaflets and is an important auscultatory feature of severe mitral regurgitation. The absence of a third heart sound indicates that if mitral regurgitation exists, it may not be severe. The third heart sound may be followed, often after a brief interval, by a short, rumbling, diastolic murmur, even in the absence of mitral stenosis. A fourth heart sound is often audible in patients with acute severe regurgitation of recent onset who are in sinus rhythm. A presystolic murmur is not ordinarily heard in patients with pure regurgitation and sinus rhythm but is present when there is significant associated mitral stenosis.

A systolic murmur, grade III/VI in intensity or louder, is the most characteristic auscultatory finding in severe mitral regurgitation. It is usually holosystolic (Chap. 177), but it may be decrescendo because the tall *v* wave in the left atrial pressure pulse results in a reduced late systolic left ventricular–atrial pressure gradient in patients with acute severe mitral regurgitation. Although the systolic murmur usually radiates into the axilla, in a minority of patients, particularly those with ruptured chordae tendineae or primary involvement of the posterior mitral leaflet, the regurgitant jet strikes the left atrial wall adjacent to the aortic root, and the systolic murmur is referred to the base of the heart and therefore may be confused with the murmur of aortic stenosis. In patients with ruptured chordae tendineae the systolic murmur may have a cooing or "sea gull" quality; in patients with a flail leaflet the murmur may have a musical quality.

Electrocardiogram In patients with sinus rhythm there is evidence of left atrial enlargement, but right atrial enlargement may also be present when pulmonary hypertension is extreme. Chronic, severe mitral regurgitation with left atrial enlargement is generally associated with atrial fibrillation. In many patients there is no clear-cut electrocardiographic evidence of enlargement of either ventricle. In severe regurgitation the signs of left ventricular hypertrophy are often present, although in patients with pulmonary hypertension combined ventricular hypertrophy or rarely pure right ventricular hypertrophy may be present.

Echocardiogram The left atrium is usually enlarged and/or exhibits increased pulsations; the left ventricle may be hyperdynamic. With ruptured chordae tendineae or a flail leaflet coarse, erratic motion of the involved leaflets may be noted. Two-dimensional echocardiography usually shows incomplete coaptation of the anterior and posterior mitral leaflets. Annular calcification can be readily identified, as can left ventricular dilatation, aneurysm, or dyskinesis, which may be causally associated. Doppler echocardiography is the most accurate noninvasive technique for the detection and estimation of mitral regurgitation. The echocardiogram in patients with mitral valve prolapse is described below.

Roentgenographic features The left atrium and left ventricle are the dominant chambers; in chronic cases the latter may be enlarged to aneurysmal proportions and forms the right border of the cardiac silhouette. On fluoroscopy the left ventricle is hyperdynamic and the left atrium exhibits vigorous systolic expansions. Marked calcification of the mitral leaflets occurs commonly in patients with long-standing combined regurgitation and stenosis but is uncommon in patients with pure regurgitation. Contrast left ventriculography is useful in the detection and quantification of mitral regurgitation.

TREATMENT The nonsurgical management of mitral regurgitation is directed toward restricting those physical activities which regularly produce extreme fatigue and dyspnea, reducing sodium intake, and enhancing sodium excretion with the appropriate use of diuretics (Chap. 182). Digitalis glycosides and vasodilators increase the output of the failing left ventricle. The same considerations as in patients with mitral stenosis apply to the reversion of atrial fibrillation to sinus rhythm. In the late stages anticoagulants and leg binders are used to diminish the likelihood of venous thrombi and pulmonary emboli. Effective surgical treatment of rheumatic mitral regurgitation generally requires valvular replacement with a suitable prosthesis or tissue valve. Though most patients who survive operation appear to be greatly improved, some degree of myocardial dysfunction may persist.

When surgical treatment is contemplated, right- and left-sided heart catheterization and selective left ventricular angiocardiography are generally indicated. These studies are helpful in confirming the presence of severe regurgitation and aid in the identification of patients with primary myocardial disease and relatively mild, functional mitral regurgitation, who usually do not benefit from operation. Hemodynamic studies are also helpful in detecting and assessing the severity of any associated valve lesions, which may have to be dealt with at the time of operation or which might limit the patient's ultimate improvement if they are left untreated.

Surgical treatment of mitral regurgitation usually requires replacement of the valve with a prosthesis, although in selected patients, particularly those with severe annular dilatation, flail leaflets, or ruptured chordae, mitral annuloplasty or reconstruction of the mitral valve apparatus may be possible.

In the selection of patients for surgical treatment, the chronic, often slowly progressive nature of the disease must be balanced against the immediate risks and long-term uncertainties attendant upon valve replacement. Patients with mitral regurgitation who are asymptomatic or who are limited only during strenuous exertion are not considered to be candidates for surgical treatment, since they may live for many years with little deterioration. On the other hand, unless there are contraindications, surgical treatment should be offered to patients with severe mitral regurgitation whose limitations do not allow them to work full time or carry out normal household activities despite optimal medical management. The risks of valve replacement rise sharply, the recovery of impaired left ventricular function is incomplete, and the long-term survival is reduced in patients with congestive heart failure. However, conservative management has little to offer these patients, so that operative treatment may be indicated even at these advanced stages of the disease, and occasionally the clinical and hemodynamic improvement following surgical treatment is dramatic. It is likely that the immediate results of surgical treatment will continue to improve considerably and will lead to recommendations of operative treatment for selected patients with mitral regurgitation before they become severely disabled.

MITRAL VALVE PROLAPSE This is also variously termed the *systolic click-murmur syndrome, Barlow's syndrome, floppy-valve syndrome,* and *billowing mitral leaflet syndrome,* a common, but highly variable, clinical syndrome resulting from diverse pathogenic mechanisms of the mitral valve apparatus. Among these are excessive or redundant mitral leaflet tissue, which is commonly involved with myxomatous degeneration and greatly increased concentration of acid mucopolysaccharide. This is a frequent finding in patients who have the typical features of Marfan's syndrome or cystic medial necrosis (Chap. 197), although in most patients myxomatous degeneration is confined to the mitral valve leaflets without other clinical or pathologic manifestations of disease; the posterior leaflet is usually more affected than the anterior, and the mitral valve annulus is often greatly enlarged. In many patients, elongated redundant chordae tendineae have been identified. There are probably several subsets of these patients, who differ in regard to the etiology and hemodynamic and clinical sequelae of abnormal mitral valve function. In the majority of patients, the etiology is unknown, but mitral valve prolapse may be a genetically determined collagen tissue disorder. It may be associated with thoracic skeletal deformities similar to but not as severe as those in Marfan's syndrome, including a high arched palate, and alterations of the chest and thoracic spine. Mitral valve prolapse may also occur in acute rheumatic fever, chronic rheumatic heart disease, and following mitral valvulotomy, in ischemic heart disease, and cardiomyopathies as well as in 20 percent of patients with ostium secundum atrial septal defect.

Mitral valve prolapse is usually a benign abnormality that may progress to a stage involving significant regurgitation and ventricular dilatation in some individuals. In these, prolapse of the valve leads to excessive stress on the papillary muscles, which in turn leads to dysfunction and ischemia of the papillary muscles and subjacent ventricular myocardium; rupture of chordae tendineae and progressive annular dilatation also contribute to valvular regurgitation. The electrocardiographic changes (see below) and ventricular arrhythmias appear to result from regional ventricular dysfunction related to increased stress placed on the papillary muscles.

Mitral valve prolapse is more common in females and occurs in a wide age range but most commonly between the ages of 14 and 30. Echocardiographic surveys have suggested that it may occur in as many as 7 percent of this group. There is an increased familial incidence suggesting an autosomal dominant form of inheritance. In many patients the echocardiographic abnormality is not accompanied by any other clinical manifestation of cardiac disease, and the significance of this finding is uncertain.

Most of the patients are asymptomatic and remain so for their entire lives. Although severe mitral regurgitation is an uncommon complication of mitral valve prolapse, the latter has become the most common cause of isolated severe mitral regurgitation. Arrythmias, most commonly ventricular premature contractions and paroxysmal supraventricular and ventricular tachycardia, have been reported. Patients with arrhythmias complain of palpitations, light-headedness, and syncope. Sudden death is a very rare complication. Many patients have chest pain which is difficult to evaluate. It is often substernal, prolonged, poorly related to exertion, and rarely resembles typical angina pectoris. Transient cerebral ischemic attacks secondary to emboli from the roughened surface of the valve have been reported. Infective endocarditis may occur in patients with mitral regurgitation associated with mitral valve prolapse.

Physical examination The most common finding is the mid- or late (nonejection) systolic click, which occurs 0.14 s or more after the first heart sound, and is thought to be generated by the sudden tensing of slack, elongated chordae tendineae or by the prolapsing mitral leaflet when it reaches its maximum excursion; systolic clicks may be multiple and are often followed by a high-pitched late systolic crescendo-decrescendo murmur, occasionally "whooping" or "honking," which is heard best at the apex. The click and murmur occur earlier with standing, the Valsalva maneuver, or inhalation of amyl nitrate, interventions which decrease left ventricular volume, exaggerating the propensity of mitral leaflet prolapse. Conversely, squatting or isometric exercise, which increases left ventricular end-diastolic volume, diminish the propensity for the mitral valve leaflets to prolapse, and the click-murmur complex is delayed and may even disappear. Some patients have a midsystolic click without the murmur; others have the murmur without a click.

Laboratory examination The *electrocardiogram* most commonly shows biphasic or inverted T waves in leads II, III, and aVF. The *echocardiogram* characteristically shows an abrupt posterior displacement of the posterior or sometimes of both mitral valve leaflets in mid- to late systole, immediately after the click, and during the systolic murmur. Two-dimensional echocardiography is particularly useful in identifying the abnormal position of the mitral valve leaflets, and Doppler studies are helpful in revealing and evaluating accompanying mitral regurgitation. *Angiocardiography* generally shows prolapse of the posterior and sometimes of both mitral valve leaflets and, rarely, severe mitral regurgitation. Many patients have bulging of the posteroinferior wall of the left ventricle into the left ventricular cavity during systole and/or hypokinesis of the anterolateral left ventricular wall. Others display prolapse of other valves, particularly the tricuspid, as well.

Treatment The management of patients with mitral valve prolapse is directed toward reassurance of the asymptomatic patient, the prevention of infective endocarditis with antibiotic prophylaxis, and the relief of the atypical chest pain; beta blockers have been found to be helpful in this regard, although their use is empiric. Antiarrhythmic agents are administered if frequent ventricular premature contractions are present or if tachyarrhythmias have occurred. If mitral regurgitation is severe, mitral valve replacement is indicated. Antiplatelet aggregation agents (aspirin and dipyridamole) should be given to patients with transient ischemic attacks, and if these are not effective, anticoagulants should be employed.

AORTIC STENOSIS

This lesion occurs in about one-fourth of all patients with chronic valvular heart disease; approximately 80 percent of adult patients with symptomatic valvular aortic stenosis are male.

PATHOPHYSIOLOGY The primary hemodynamic abnormality is obstruction to left ventricular outflow which leads to a systolic pressure gradient between the left ventricle and aorta. When severe obstruction is suddenly produced experimentally, the left ventricle responds by dilatation and reduction of stroke volume. However, in patients the obstruction may be present at birth or it increases gradually over the course of many years, and left ventricular output is maintained by the presence of left ventricular hypertrophy, which serves as a useful compensatory mechanism since it reduces toward normal the systolic stress developed by each segment of myocardium. A large transaortic valvular pressure gradient may exist for many years without a reduction of cardiac output, left ventricular dilatation, or the development of any symptoms. As aortic stenosis progresses in severity, the left ventricular systolic pressure continues to rise, but rarely exceeds 300 mmHg.

A peak systolic pressure gradient exceeding 50 mmHg in the face of a normal cardiac output or an effective aortic orifice less than 0.5 cm^2 per square meter of body surface area, i.e., less than approximately one-third of the normal orifice, is generally considered to represent critical obstruction to left ventricular outflow. The left ventricular pressure pulse exhibits a rounded summit as the contraction of this chamber becomes progressively more isometric. The elevated left ventricular end-diastolic pressure observed in many patients with severe aortic stenosis does not necessarily signify the presence of left ventricular dilatation or failure, but may instead reflect diminished compliance of the hypertrophied left ventricular wall.

A large *a* wave in the left atrial pressure pulse is usually present with severe stenosis, because of enhanced atrial contraction and diminished ventricular compliance. Atrial contraction tends to raise left ventricular end-diastolic pressure without producing a similar elevation of mean left atrial pressure. This "booster pump" function of the left atrium prevents the pulmonary venous and capillary pressures from rising to levels which would produce pulmonary congestion, while at the same time maintaining left ventricular end-diastolic pressure at the elevated level necessary for effective left ventricular contraction. Loss of an appropriately timed, vigorous atrial contraction, as occurs in atrial fibrillation or atrioventricular dissociation, may result in a rapid aggravation of symptoms.

Although the cardiac output at rest is within normal limits in the majority of patients with severe aortic stenosis, it may fail to rise normally during exercise. Late in the disease the cardiac output and left ventricular–aortic pressure gradient decline, and the mean left atrial, pulmonary artery wedge, pulmonary arterial, and right ventricular pressures become elevated.

The hypertrophied left ventricular muscle mass elevates myocardial oxygen requirements. In addition, even in the absence of obstructive coronary artery disease, there may be interference with coronary blood flow, because the pressure compressing the coronary arteries exceeds the coronary perfusion pressure. Metabolic evidence of myocardial ischemia, i.e., lactate production, can be demonstrated in patients with aortic stenosis both in the presence and in the absence of coronary arterial narrowing, when myocardial oxygen needs are stimulated by isoproterenol.

A significant fraction of patients with rheumatic aortic stenosis has associated mitral valve disease. Aortic stenosis intensifies the severity of mitral regurgitation by increasing the pressure driving blood from the left ventricle to the left atrium.

Etiology Aortic stenosis may be congenital in origin, secondary to rheumatic inflammation of the aortic valve, or due to degenerative calcification of the aortic cusps of unknown cause. The *congenitally affected valve* may already be stenotic at birth and may gradually become calcified during the first three decades of life, becoming progressively more stenotic. In others, the valve may also be congenitally bicuspid without serious narrowing of the aortic orifice during childhood; its abnormal architecture makes its leaflets susceptible to otherwise ordinary hemodynamic stresses, which ultimately lead to valvular calcification, increased rigidity, and narrowing of the aortic orifice.

Rheumatic endocarditis of the aortic leaflets produces commissural fusion, resulting, sometimes, in a bicuspid valve. This, in turn, also makes the leaflets more susceptible to trauma, and ultimately leads to calcification and further narrowing. By the time the obstruction to left ventricular outflow causes serious clinical disability, the valve is usually a rigid calcified mass, and careful examination may make it difficult or even impossible to determine whether the underlying process was rheumatic or congenital. Rheumatic aortic stenosis is almost always associated with rheumatic involvement of the mitral valve. A rheumatic etiology is also favored by a history of active rheumatic fever and by associated severe aortic regurgitation. *Idiopathic calcific aortic stenosis* occurs most often in the elderly and is occasionally associated with fibrosis and fusion of the valve cusps; the pathologic process is considered to be a degenerative one—a "wear-and-tear" phenomenon. It may produce many of the characteristic physical signs of aortic stenosis. The valvular obstruction is usually relatively mild and of little if any hemodynamic significance; it may, however, on occasion, produce critical obstruction.

OTHER FORMS OF OBSTRUCTION TO LEFT VENTRICULAR OUTFLOW Besides valvular aortic stenosis, three other lesions may be responsible for obstruction to left ventricular outflow.

1 *Hypertrophic cardiomyopathy*. This is the most important of these conditions numerically. It is characterized by marked hypertrophy of the left ventricle, involving in particular the interventricular septum of the left ventricular outflow tract, and may cause subaortic obstruction, as described in Chap. 192.
2 *Discrete congenital subvalvular aortic stenosis*. This condition is produced by either a membranous diaphragm or a fibrous ridge just below the aortic valve (Chap. 185).
3 *Supravalvular aortic stenosis*. This uncommon congenital anomaly is produced by narrowing of the ascending aorta or by a fibrous diaphragm with a small opening just above the aortic valve (Chap. 185).

SYMPTOMS Aortic stenosis is rarely of hemodynamic or clinical importance until the valve orifice has narrowed to approximately one-third of normal. In contrast to mitral stenosis, which results in symptoms as soon as the obstruction becomes severe because the chamber just proximal to the narrowed valve, i.e., the left atrium, provides little compensation, severe aortic stenosis may exist for many years without producing any clinical disability because of the ability of the hypertrophied left ventricle to generate the elevated intraventricular pressures and the presence of a competent mitral valve behind the left ventricle.

Most patients with pure or predominant aortic stenosis have gradually increasing obstruction for years but do not become symptomatic until the fifth to seventh decades. Exertional dyspnea, angina pectoris, and syncope are the three cardinal symptoms. Often there is a history of insidious progression of fatigue and dyspnea associated with gradual curtailment of activities. Dyspnea results primarily from elevation of the pulmonary capillary pressures, which in turn is caused by elevations of left atrial and left ventricular end-diastolic pressures. Angina pectoris usually develops somewhat later and reflects an imbalance between the augmented myocardial oxygen requirements and reduced oxygen availability; the former results from the increased myocardial mass and intraventricular pressure, while the latter may result from accompanying coronary artery disease which is not uncommon in patients with aortic stenosis, as well as from compression of the coronary vessels by the hypertrophied myocardium. Therefore, angina may occur in severe aortic stenosis without organic coronary obstruction, but the *absence* of angina usually signifies that severe coronary obstructive disease is unlikely. Exertional syncope may result from a decline in arterial pressure caused by vasodilatation in the exercising muscles and inadequate vasoconstriction in nonexercising muscles in the face of a fixed cardiac output, or from a sudden fall in cardiac output produced by an arrhythmia.

Since the cardiac output is usually well maintained at rest until late, marked fatigability, weakness, peripheral cyanosis, and other clinical manifestations of a low cardiac output are usually not prominent until this stage is reached. Orthopnea, paroxysmal nocturnal dyspnea, and pulmonary edema, i.e., symptoms of left ventricular failure, also occur only in the advanced stages of the disease. Severe pulmonary hypertension leading to right ventricular failure and systemic venous hypertension, hepatomegaly, atrial fibrillation, and tricuspid regurgitation are usually preterminal findings.

When aortic stenosis and mitral stenosis coexist, the latter lesion masks many of the clinical findings of the former. The reduction of cardiac output induced by mitral stenosis lowers the pressure gradient across the aortic valve, diminishes the frequency of anginal episodes, and retards the development of severe left ventricular hypertrophy. On the other hand, symptoms considered more characteristic of mitral stenosis, such as pulmonary congestion and hemoptysis, may be present. Physical, electrocardiographic, radiologic, and echocardiographic examinations in patients with aortic and mitral stenosis generally reveal more evidence of left ventricular enlargement than in patients with pure mitral stenosis, and catheterization of the left side of the heart is helpful in defining the relative importance of each valvular abnormality.

PHYSICAL FINDINGS AND GRAPHIC TRACINGS The systemic arterial pressure is usually within normal limits. In the late stages, however, when stroke volume declines, the systolic pressure may fall and the pulse pressure narrow. Systemic hypertension is unusual in patients with marked aortic stenosis, and a basal systolic arterial pressure exceeding 200 mmHg practically excludes severe narrowing of this valve. The peripheral arterial pulse, as palpated in the carotid or brachial arteries, rises slowly to a delayed sustained peak. Indirect recordings of the carotid pulse exhibit a gradually ascending limb, often with a prominent anacrotic notch or shoulder on the upstroke, as well as a delayed peak, with coarse systolic vibrations. The left ventricular ejection period is prolonged, the preejection period is abbreviated, and the ratio of these two, i.e., the preejection period/systolic ejection period, is characteristically reduced (Chap. 179). Late in the course of the disease, in the presence of heart failure, the ratio may be normal. A palpable double systolic arterial pulse, the so-called bisferiens pulse, excludes pure or predominant aortic stenosis and signifies dominant or pure aortic regurgitation or obstructive hypertrophic cardiomyopathy (Chap. 192). In the late stages of valvular aortic stenosis, when the pulse pressure is reduced, the pulse amplitude may be so small that the anacrotic nature of the pulse and the delay in its upstroke may become more difficult to appreciate. The jugular venous pulse may be normal, although in many patients the *a* wave is accentuated. This results from the diminished distensibility of the right ventricular cavity caused by the bulging, hypertrophied interventricular septum and/or the presence of pulmonary hypertension.

The apex beat is usually active and displaced inferiorly and laterally, reflecting the presence of left ventricular hypertrophy. A double apical impulse may be appreciated, particularly with the patient in the left lateral recumbent position; the first outward expansion occurs during atrial systole and reflects the important contribution made by atrial contraction to ventricular systole, while the second occurs during ventricular systole, usually is forceful and sustained during ejection. The right ventricle is usually palpable only when pulmonary hypertension develops in the late stages of the disease. A systolic thrill is generally present at the base of the heart, in the jugular notch, and along the carotid arteries, but occasionally it is palpable only during expiration and with the patient leaning forward. In patients who do not have marked pulmonary emphysema, a thick chest wall, thoracic deformity, or heart failure, the absence of a systolic thrill suggests that the aortic stenosis is relatively mild.

The rhythm is generally regular until very late in the course; at other times, atrial fibrillation should suggest the possibility of associated mitral valve disease. An early systolic ejection sound, actually the opening snap of the aortic valve, is frequently audible in children and adolescents with congenital noncalcific valvular aortic stenosis. This sound usually disappears when the valve becomes calcified and rigid. The sound of aortic valve closure can also be identified most frequently in patients with aortic stenosis who have pliable valves, and calcification diminishes the intensity of this sound as well. As aortic stenosis increases in severity, left ventricular systole may become prolonged so that the aortic valve closure sound no longer precedes the pulmonic valve closure sound, and the two components may become synchronous, or aortic valve closure may even follow pulmonic valve closure, causing paradoxic splitting of the second heart sound (Chap. 177). In patients with aortic stenosis without a left intraventricular conduction defect, this finding usually signifies severe obstruction to left ventricular outflow. A fourth heart sound is audible at the apex in many patients with severe aortic stenosis, and reflects the presence of left ventricular hypertrophy and an elevated left ventricular end-diastolic pressure; a third heart sound generally occurs when the left ventricle dilates and fails.

The murmur of aortic stenosis is characteristically an ejection systolic murmur which commences shortly after the first heart sound, increases in intensity to reach a peak toward the middle of the ejection period, and diminishes progressively thereafter to end just before aortic valve closure (Chaps. 177 and 179). The murmur is usually low-pitched, rough, and rasping in character and is loudest at the base of the heart, most commonly in the second right intercostal space. It is transmitted to the jugular notch and upward along the carotid arteries. In patients with mild degrees of obstruction or in those with severe stenosis with heart failure in whom the stroke volume and therefore the transvalvular flow rate is reduced, the murmur may be relatively soft and brief. However, in almost all patients with severe obstruction, the murmur is at least grade III/VI. Occasionally, the murmur is transmitted downward and to the apex and may be confused with the systolic murmur of mitral regurgitation. However, the latter is usually holosystolic (Chap. 177).

Electrocardiogram This reveals left ventricular hypertrophy in the majority of patients with severe aortic stenosis (Chap. 178). In advanced cases, ST-segment depression and T-wave inversion in standard leads I and aVL and in the left precordial leads are evident. However, there is no close correlation between the electrocardiogram and the hemodynamic severity of obstruction, and the absence of electrocardiographic signs of left ventricular hypertrophy does not exclude severe obstruction. Left bundle branch block or the presence of intraventricular conduction defects suggests diffuse fibrotic involvement of the myocardium. The presence of left atrial enlargement should suggest the possibility of associated mitral valve disease.

Echocardiogram This reveals left ventricular hypertrophy, and in patients with valvular calcification, multiple, bright, thick, echoes from within the aortic root. While cusp calcification does not necessarily indicate significant valve stenosis, its absence can usually be used to exclude such a diagnosis after the age of 25. Eccentricity of the aortic valve cusps is characteristic of congenitally bicuspid valves (Chap. 179). Left ventricular dilatation and reduced systolic shortening reflecting impairment of left ventricular function can be recognized. The severity of aortic stenosis can be estimated from the ratio of end-systolic wall thickness to ventricular diameter on an M-mode study, from the degree of aortic leaflet separation on a two-dimensional echocardiogram, and most accurately by estimating the transvalvular pressure gradient using Doppler techniques. Echocardiography is particularly useful for identifying valvular abnormalities such as mitral stenosis and aortic regurgitation which sometimes accompany aortic stenosis, and for differentiating valvular from obstructive hypertrophic cardiomyopathy.

Roentgenographic features The chest roentgenogram may show no or little overall cardiac enlargement for many years, since the development of concentric left ventricular hypertrophy is the initial response to obstruction to left ventricular outflow. Hypertrophy without dilatation may produce some rounding of the cardiac apex in the frontal projection and slight backward displacement in the lateral view; critical aortic stenosis is often associated with poststenotic dilatation of the ascending aorta. Aortic calcification is usually readily apparent on fluoroscopic examination with an image intensifier or by echocardiography; *the absence of valvular calcification in an adult suggests that severe valvular aortic stenosis is not present.* In later stages of the disease as the left ventricle dilates, there is progressively more evidence of left ventricular enlargement, and there may also be roentgenologic signs of pulmonary congestion, as well as enlargement of the left atrium, pulmonary artery, right ventricle, and right atrium.

Catheterization and angiocardiography Catheterization of the left side of the heart should generally be carried out in patients suspected of having severe aortic stenosis, particularly before a final decision concerning operative treatment is made. The goals are to assess (1) the severity of the aortic obstruction, (2) the status of left ventricular function, and (3) the location of left ventricular outflow obstruction. These investigations are especially indicated in the following:

1 Young, asymptomatic patients with noncalcific congenital aortic stenosis (Chap. 185), in order to define the severity of obstruction to left ventricular outflow, since operation may be indicated in them even in the absence of symptoms if severe aortic stenosis is present.
2 Patients in whom it is suspected that the obstruction to left ventricular outflow may not be at the aortic valve, but rather in the sub- or supravalvular regions.
3 Patients with clinical signs of aortic stenosis and symptoms of myocardial ischemia, in whom associated coronary artery disease is suspected. An effort should be made to determine whether aortic stenosis or coronary atherosclerosis is primarily responsible for the symptoms, and coronary arteriography should be carried out in addition to catheterization of the left side of the heart.
4 Patients with multivalvular disease, in whom the role played by each valvular deformity must be defined before operative treatment is planned.

Angiographic studies are helpful in defining the size of the left ventricular cavity, the thickness of the wall, the site of obstruction, the degree of deformity and mobility of the aortic valve cusps, the diameter of the ascending aorta, and the presence and degree of accompanying mitral and aortic regurgitation and of obstructive coronary disease. In patients with severe narrowing, a jet of contrast substance passing through the aortic orifice is readily visualized.

NATURAL HISTORY Death in patients with severe aortic stenosis occurs most commonly in the seventh decade. Based on analysis of data obtained at postmortem examination, the average duration of various symptoms was as follows: angina pectoris, 3 years; syncope, 3 years; dyspnea, 2 years; and congestive heart failure, 1.5 to 2 years. Moreover, in more than 80 percent of patients who died with aortic stenosis, symptoms had existed for less than 4 years. Congestive heart failure was considered to be the cause of death in one-half to two-thirds of patients. Among adults dying with valvular aortic stenosis, sudden death, which presumably results from an arrhythmia, occurred in 10 to 20 percent, and at an average age of 60 years (Chap. 30).

TREATMENT Strenuous physical activity should be avoided even in the asymptomatic stage in patients with *severe* aortic stenosis. Digitalis glycosides, sodium restriction, and diuretics are indicated in the treatment of congestive heart failure. While nitroglycerin is helpful in relieving angina pectoris, vasodilator therapy for heart failure is usually of little value. The most critical decision in the management of aortic stenosis, indeed of any valvular lesion, concerns the advisability of surgical treatment. The indications and results of operation, as well as the techniques, differ considerably, depending on the patient's age and the nature of the valvular deformity.

In children and adolescents with noncalcific congenital aortic stenosis, considerable hemodynamic improvement can be anticipated from simple commissural incision under direct vision (Chap. 185). When carried out by an experienced surgical team, this procedure may be expected to be hemodynamically effective and to be associated with a mortality rate of less than 2 percent. This operation is recommended not only for symptomatic patients but also for asymptomatic children and adolescents with hemodynamic evidence of severe obstruction to left ventricular outflow, with a peak systolic pressure gradient exceeding 50 mmHg when the cardiac output is normal, or a calculated effective orifice less than 0.6 cm^2 per square meter of body surface area. Though this procedure can be expected to result in complete or almost complete relief of obstruction in the majority of patients, the valve cannot be rendered entirely normal anatomically, and it may become deformed, calcified, and stenotic again, and may require valve replacement at some later date.

In the majority of adults with calcific aortic stenosis, satisfactory valve function cannot be restored, even by deliberate sculpturing procedures carried out under direct vision, and replacement of the valve is necessary. In most instances, it is prudent to postpone operation in patients with severe calcific aortic stenosis who are asymptomatic, since their future course is difficult to predict and they may continue to do well for many years. However, they should be followed carefully by clinical examination for the development of symptoms and by the various noninvasive tests, such as echocardiograms and/or radionuclide angiograms (Chap. 179), for evidence of deteriorating left ventricular function. It is likely that as the results of surgical replacement of the aortic valve continue to improve, many of these patients will become candidates for operation before their disease reaches the symptomatic stage. At the present, replacement of the aortic valve should be undertaken in patients with symptoms, even when relatively mild, that are believed to result primarily from aortic stenosis and who have hemodynamic evidence of severe obstruction. In such patients the operative risk is relatively low (<5 percent) in centers with experience.

When angina pectoris, syncope, or left ventricular decompensation develops in adults with valvular aortic stenosis, the outlook, despite medical treatment, is very poor and can be improved significantly by replacement of the aortic valve with a mechanical or bioprosthetic valve. Therefore, the risk entailed by operation in this group of patients is considerably lower than the risk involved by nonoperative treatment; moreover, the symptomatic improvement in many survivors of operation has been remarkable.

Operation should, if possible, be carried out before frank left ventricular failure supervenes; at this late stage, the operative risk is high (approx. 15 percent), and evidence of myocardial disease may persist even when the operation is technically successful. Furthermore, long-term postoperative survival also correlates inversely with preoperative functional disability. Nonetheless, in view of the very poor prognosis of such patients when they are treated medically, there is usually little choice but to advise immediate surgical treatment. In patients in whom severe aortic stenosis and coronary artery disease coexist, relief of the aortic stenosis and revascularization of the myocardium by means of aortocoronary bypass grafting may result in striking clinical and hemodynamic improvement. Since many patients with calcific aortic stenosis are elderly, particular attention must be directed to the adequacy of hepatic, renal, and pulmonary function before valve replacement is recommended. The mortality rate depends to a substantial extent on the patient's preoperative clinical and hemodynamic state. The 9-year survival rate of operative survivors following aortic valve replacement is approximately 67 percent. Approximately 15 percent of bioprosthetic valves evidence primary valve failure in 10 years, requiring re-replacement, and an approximately equal percentage of patients with mechanical prostheses develop significant hemorrhagic complications as a consequence of treatment with anticoagulants. Fortunately, there is evidence that regression of left ventricular hypertrophy may occur following relief of obstruction.

AORTIC REGURGITATION

PATHOPHYSIOLOGY The total stroke volume expelled by the left ventricle (i.e., the sum of the effective forward stroke volume and the volume of blood which regurgitates back into the left ventricle) is increased in aortic regurgitation. In patients with free aortic regurgitation the volume of regurgitant flow may be of the same order of magnitude as the effective forward stroke volume. In contrast to mitral regurgitation, in which a fraction of the left ventricular stroke volume is delivered into the low-pressure left atrium, in aortic regurgitation the entire left ventricular stroke volume must be ejected into a high-pressure zone, the aorta. Although the low aortic diastolic pressure facilitates ventricular emptying during early systole, an increase of the left ventricular end-diastolic volume constitutes the major hemodynamic compensation to aortic regurgitation. The dilatation of the left ventricle allows this chamber to expel a larger stroke volume without requiring any increase in the relative shortening of each myofibril. Therefore, severe aortic regurgitation may occur with a normal effective forward stroke volume and a normal ejection fraction [total (forward plus regurgitant) stroke volume/end-diastolic volume], together with an elevated left ventricular end-diastolic pressure and volume. On the other hand, through the operation of Laplace's law (which indicates that myocardial wall tension is the product of intracavitary pressure and left ventricular radius), left ventricular dilatation increases the left ventricular systolic tension required to develop any given level of systolic pressure. As left ventricular function deteriorates, the end-diastolic volume increases without further elevation of the aortic regurgitant volume; the ejection fraction and forward stroke volume decline. Deterioration of left ventricular function often precedes the development of symptoms. Considerable thickening of the left ventricular wall also occurs with chronic aortic regurgitation, and at autopsy the hearts of these patients may be among the largest encountered, occasionally exceeding 1000 g in weight.

The reduction of the aortic diastolic pressure in aortic regurgitation shortens the left ventricular isometric contraction period, which is advantageous since it prolongs the left ventricular ejection period. The reverse pressure gradient from aorta to left ventricle, which is responsible for the aortic regurgitant flow, falls progressively during diastole, accounting for the decrescendo nature of the diastolic murmur. Equilibration between aortic and left ventricular pressures may occur toward the end of diastole, particularly when the heart rate is slow, and the left ventricular end-diastolic pressure may be elevated, occasionally to extremely high levels (>40 mmHg). Rarely, the left ventricular pressure exceeds the left atrial pressure toward the end of diastole, and this reversed pressure gradient closes the mitral valve prematurely, or may cause diastolic mitral regurgitation.

In patients with free aortic regurgitation the effective forward cardiac output usually is normal or only slightly reduced at rest, but often it fails to rise normally during exertion. Early signs of left ventricular dysfunction include reductions of the fraction of systolic shortening and of the ejection fraction determined by echocardiography or radionuclide or contrast angiography. In advanced stages there may be considerable elevation of the left atrial, pulmonary artery wedge, pulmonary arterial, and right ventricular pressures, and lowering of the forward cardiac output at rest.

Myocardial ischemia occurs in patients with aortic regurgitation because both left ventricular dilatation and the elevated left ventricular systolic pressure tend to augment myocardial oxygen requirements. However, the major portion of coronary blood flow occurs during diastole, when arterial pressure is subnormal, thereby reducing coronary perfusion pressure. The result is a combination of increased oxygen demand and reduced supply.

ETIOLOGY Approximately three-fourths of all patients with pure or predominant regurgitation are males; however, females predominate among patients with aortic regurgitation who have associated mitral valve disease. In approximately two-thirds of patients with aortic regurgitation the disease is rheumatic in origin, resulting in a chronic form of the disorder with thickening, deformation, and shortening of the individual aortic valve cusps, changes which prevent their proper closure during diastole. A rheumatic etiology is less common in patients with isolated aortic regurgitation. Acute aortic regurgitation may also result from infective endocarditis, which may attack a valve previously affected by rheumatic disease, a congenitally deformed valve, or rarely a normal aortic valve, and may result in the perforation or erosion of one or more of the leaflets. Patients with discrete membranous subaortic stenosis may develop thickening of the aortic valve leaflets, which in turn leads to mild or moderate degrees of aortic regurgitation and makes these valves particularly susceptible to endocarditis. Aortic regurgitation may also occur in patients with congenital bicuspid aortic valves. Prolapse of an aortic cusp, resulting in progressive chronic aortic regurgitation, occurs in approximately 15 percent of patients with ventricular septal defect (Chap. 185). Congenital fenestrations of the aortic valve occasionally produce mild aortic regurgitation. Although traumatic rupture of the aortic valve is an uncommon cause of acute aortic regurgitation, it does represent the most frequent serious lesion observed in patients surviving nonpenetrating cardiac injuries. In patients with aortic regurgitation due to primary valvular disease, dilatation of the aortic annulus may occur secondarily and intensify the regurgitation.

Aortic regurgitation, both acute and chronic, may also be due entirely to marked aortic dilatation, without primary involvement of the valve leaflets; widening of the aortic annulus and separation of the aortic leaflets are responsible for the aortic regurgitation. Syphilis and ankylosing rheumatoid spondylitis may be associated with cellular infiltration and scarring of the media of the thoracic aorta, leading to aortic dilatation, aneurysm formation, and severe regurgitation. In syphilis of the aorta (Chap. 197), the involvement of the intima may narrow the coronary ostia, which in turn may be responsible for myocardial ischemia. Cystic medial necrosis of the ascending aorta, which may or may not be associated with other manifestations of the Marfan syndrome (Chap. 197), idiopathic dilatation of the aorta, and severe hypertension all may also widen the aortic annulus and lead to progressive aortic regurgitation. Occasionally, retrograde dissection of the aorta involving the aortic annulus produces aortic regurgitation.

The coexistence of hemodynamically significant aortic stenosis with aortic regurgitation usually excludes all of the rarer forms of aortic regurgitation because it occurs almost exclusively in patients whose aortic regurgitation is on a rheumatic or congenital basis.

HISTORY A family history may frequently be elicited from patients with the Marfan syndrome, and a history of a heart murmur heard early in life may be obtained from patients with congenital aortic regurgitation. Patients with aortic regurgitation of obscure cause should also be questioned about a positive serologic test for syphilis, and about prior chest trauma; a history compatible with infective endocarditis may sometimes be elicited from patients with rheumatic or congenital involvement of the aortic valve, and the infection often precipitates or seriously aggravates preexisting symptoms. Ankylosing spondylitis is usually self-evident.

The interval between the first episode of acute rheumatic fever and the development of hemodynamically significant aortic regurgitation averages approximately 7 years, and this period is followed by an asymptomatic interval of approximately 10 to 20 years, during which the severity of the aortic regurgitation usually increases. Thus, asymptomatic severe aortic regurgitation may exist for many years.

In chronic severe aortic regurgitation, uncomfortable awareness of the heartbeat, especially on lying down, is often an early complaint. Sinus tachycardia during exertion or with emotion, or premature ventricular contractions, may produce particularly uncomfortable palpitations, as well as head pounding. These complaints may persist for many years before the development of exertional dyspnea, usually the first symptom of diminished cardiac reserve. This is followed by orthopnea, paroxysmal nocturnal dyspnea, and excessive diaphoresis. Chest pain occurs frequently, even in younger patients, and it is not necessary to invoke the presence of coronary artery disease to explain this symptom in patients with aortic regurgitation. It may be due to myocardial ischemia, or it may originate from excessive cardiac pounding on the chest wall. Anginal pain may develop at rest as well as during exertion. Nocturnal angina may be a particularly troublesome symptom and is frequently accompanied by marked diaphoresis. The anginal episodes may be prolonged and often do not respond satisfactorily to sublingual nitroglycerin. Late in the course of the disease, evidence of systemic fluid accumulation, including congestive hepatomegaly, ankle edema, and ascites, may develop. Patients with severe aortic regurgitation tolerate high fevers, infections, or cardiac arrhythmias poorly, and may die in pulmonary edema as a result of one of these complications.

In patients with acute severe aortic regurgitation, as may occur in trauma or infective endocarditis, the left ventricle rapidly exhausts its ability to dilate, and left ventricular diastolic pressure rises rapidly with associated elevations of left atrial and pulmonary capillary pressures.

PHYSICAL FINDINGS The examination should be directed toward the detection of causes predisposing to aortic regurgitation, such as the Marfan syndrome, rheumatoid spondylitis, syphilis, essential hypertension, and ventricular septal defect. Even prior to the examination of the heart of the patient with free aortic regurgitation, the jarring of the entire body and the bobbing motion of the head with each systole can be appreciated, and the abrupt distention and collapse of the larger arteries are easily visible. A rapidly rising "water-hammer" pulse, which collapses suddenly as arterial pressure falls rapidly during late systole and diastole (Corrigan's pulse), and capillary pulsations (Quincke's pulse), an alternate flushing and paling of the skin at the root of the nail while pressure is applied to the tip of the nail, are characteristic of free aortic regurgitation. A booming, "pistol-shot" sound can be heard over the femoral arteries, and a to-and-fro murmur (Duroziez's sign) is audible if the femoral artery is lightly compressed with a stethoscope.

The arterial pulse pressure is widened, with an elevation of the systolic pressure, sometimes to as high as 300 mmHg, and a depression of the diastolic arterial pressure. The measurement of arterial diastolic pressure with a sphygmomanometer may be complicated by the fact that systolic sounds are frequently heard with the cuff completely deflated. However, the level of cuff pressure at the time of muffling of the Korotkoff sounds generally corresponds fairly closely to the true intraarterial diastolic pressure. The severity of aortic regurgitation does not always correlate directly with the arterial pulse pressure, and severe regurgitation may exist in patients with arterial pressures in the range of 140/60. As the disease progresses, and the left ventricular end-diastolic pressure becomes markedly elevated, the arterial diastolic pressure may actually rise since the aortic diastolic pressure cannot fall below the left ventricular end-diastolic pressure.

The apex beat is displaced laterally and inferiorly. The left ventricle is hyperdynamic in patients with free regurgitation, and the systolic expansion and subsequent retraction of the apex are prominent and contrast sharply with the sustained systolic thrust characteristic of severe aortic stenosis. A diastolic thrill is often palpable along the left sternal border, and a prominent systolic thrill may be palpable in the jugular notch and transmitted upward along the carotid arteries. This thrill and the accompanying systolic murmur are due to the markedly increased blood flow across the aortic orifice, and do not necessarily signify the coexistence of aortic stenosis. In many patients with pure aortic regurgitation, or with combined stenosis and regurgitation, palpation, or indirect recording of the carotid arterial pulse, reveals it to be bisferiens, i.e., with two systolic waves separated by a trough.

In patients with severe regurgitation the aortic valve closure sound is usually diminished or absent, and the indirectly recorded carotid arterial pulse does not usually show a clear-cut incisura. A third heart sound is common, and occasionally a fourth heart sound may also be heard. A loud systolic ejection sound is frequently audible; presumably it results from the sudden dilatation of the aorta by a greatly increased stroke volume.

The murmur of aortic regurgitation is typically a high-pitched, blowing, decrescendo diastolic murmur which is usually heard best in the third left intercostal space. In patients with mild regurgitation this murmur is brief, but as the severity increases, the murmur generally becomes louder and longer, and in patients with free aortic regurgitation it is usually holodiastolic. When the murmur is soft, it can be heard best with the diaphragm of the stethoscope and with the patient sitting up, leaning forward, and with the breath held in forced expiration. As it increases in intensity it tends to radiate widely, particularly down the lower sternal edge. In patients in whom the regurgitation is caused by primary valvular disease, the diastolic murmur is usually louder along the left than the right sternal border. However, when the decrescendo diastolic murmur is heard best along the right sternal border, it suggests that the aortic regurgitation is caused by dilatation or an aneurysm of the aortic root. "Cooing" or musical diastolic murmurs suggest eversion of an aortic cusp vibrating in the regurgitant stream. A diastolic blowing murmur along the left sternal border is much more commonly caused by aortic than by pulmonic regurgitation. Unless it is trivial in magnitude, the aortic regurgitation is usually accompanied by peripheral signs such as a widened pulse pressure or a collapsing pulse. On the other hand, with the Graham Steell murmur of pulmonary regurgitation there usually is clinical evidence of severe pulmonary hypertension, including a loud and palpable pulmonary component of the second heart sound. In addition, the phonocardiogram reveals that the murmur of aortic regurgitation begins with the aortic second sound and therefore commences somewhat before the murmur of pulmonary regurgitation.

A midsystolic ejection murmur is generally heard best at the base of the heart and is transmitted to the jugular notch and along the carotid vessels. This murmur may be as loud as grade V/VI without indicating the presence of organic obstruction; it is often higher pitched, shorter, and less rasping in quality than the ejection systolic murmur heard in patients with predominant aortic stenosis. A third murmur which is frequently heard in patients with aortic regurgitation is the Austin Flint murmur, a soft, low-pitched, rumbling middiastolic or presystolic bruit. It is probably produced by the displacement of the anterior leaflet of the mitral valve by the aortic regurgitant stream but does not appear to be associated with hemodynamically significant obstruction to left ventricular filling; earlier onset of and longer Austin Flint murmurs correlate with more severe aortic regurgitation. Both the Austin Flint murmur and the rumbling diastolic murmur of mitral stenosis are loudest at the apex, but the murmur of mitral stenosis is usually accompanied by a loud first heart sound and immediately follows the opening snap of the mitral valve, while the Austin Flint murmur is often shorter in duration than the murmur of mitral stenosis, and in patients with sinus rhythm the latter more frequently is characterized by presystolic accentuation. The auscultatory features of aortic regurgitation are intensified by isometric exercise such as strenuous handgrip, which augments systemic resistance, and reduced by inhalation of amyl nitrite, which evokes the opposite effect. A blowing holosystolic murmur at the apex, which is transmitted to the axilla, may also be heard in patients with aortic regurgitation who have marked left ventricular dilatation and functional mitral regurgitation.

In *acute* severe aortic regurgitation, the elevation of left ventricular end-diastolic pressure may lead to early closure of the mitral valve, an associated middiastolic sound, a soft or absent S_1, a pulse pressure that is not particularly wide, and a soft, short diastolic murmur.

Electrocardiogram In patients with mild aortic regurgitation there may be no electrocardiographic abnormalities, but as the severity of chronic aortic regurgitation increases, so do the electrocardiographic signs of left ventricular hypertrophy (Chap. 178). In addition to the abnormally tall R waves over the left precordium and deep S waves over the right precordium, patients with severe aortic regurgitation frequently exhibit ST-segment depressions and T-wave inversions in leads I, aVL, V_5, and V_6. Left axis deviation and/or QRS prolongation denote diffuse myocardial disease, generally associated with patchy fibrosis, and usually denote a poor prognosis.

Echocardiogram This reveals increased systolic excursion of the posterior left ventricular wall; the extent and velocity of wall motion is supernormal or normal, until myocardial contractility declines. A rapid, high-frequency fluttering of the anterior mitral leaflet produced by the impact of the aortic regurgitant jet is a characteristic finding. The echocardiogram is also useful in detecting dilatation of the aortic annulus, and of the left atrium. Thickening of the aortic valve and failure of coaptation of the leaflets may be noted in patients with primary valve disease. Doppler studies are most sensitive, both in detecting aortic regurgitation and in quantifying it.

Roentgenogram Moderate or severe degrees of chronic aortic regurgitation are associated with varying degrees of left ventricular enlargement. The apex is displaced downward and to the left in the frontal projection, and frequently the cardiac shadow extends below the left diaphragm. Left ventricular enlargement may also be apparent in the left anterior oblique and lateral projections, in which the left ventricle is displaced posteriorly and encroaches on the spine. On fluoroscopic examination the aorta and left ventricle pulsate vigorously and in opposite directions. In patients in whom primary valvular disease is responsible for the aortic regurgitation, the ascending aorta and aortic knob may be moderately dilated. When aortic regurgitation is caused by primary disease of the aortic wall, aneurysmal dilatation of the aorta may be noted roentgenographically, and the aorta may fill the retrosternal space in the lateral view.

TREATMENT In deciding upon the advisability and proper timing of surgical treatment, two points should be kept in mind: (1) patients with chronic aortic regurgitation usually do not become symptomatic until *after* the development of myocardial dysfunction; and (2) surgical treatment often does not restore normal left ventricular function. Therefore, careful clinical follow-up and noninvasive testing, preferably with echocardiography, at approximately 6-month intervals, are necessary if operation is to be undertaken at the optimal time, i.e., with the onset of left ventricular dysfunction but prior to the development of severe symptoms. Operation can be deferred as long as the patient remains asymptomatic *and* retains normal left ventricular function.

Replacement of the aortic valve with a suitable mechanical or tissue prosthesis is generally necessary in patients with rheumatic aortic regurgitation and in many patients with other forms of regurgitation. Rarely, when a leaflet has been perforated during an episode of infective endocarditis, or torn from its attachments to the aortic annulus, surgical repair may be possible. When aortic regurgitation is due to aneurysmal dilatation of the annulus and ascending aorta, rather than to primary valvular involvement, it may be possible to reduce the regurgitation by narrowing the annulus or by excising a portion of the aortic root without replacing the valve. More frequently, however, regurgitation can be eliminated only by replacing the aortic valve, excising the aneurysm responsible for the regurgitation, and replacing the latter with a graft. This formidable procedure entails a higher risk than aortic valve replacement alone.

As in patients with aortic stenosis, both the operative risk of aortic valve replacement and late mortality are largely dependent on the stage of the disease and on myocardial function at the time of operation; patients with marked cardiac enlargement and prolonged left ventricular dysfunction have a late mortality of approximately 5 percent per year despite a technically satisfactory operation.

Although operation constitutes the principal treatment of aortic regurgitation, and should be carried out before the development of heart failure, the latter usually does respond initially to treatment with digitalis glycosides, salt restriction, and diuretics. Digitalis may also be indicated in patients with severe regurgitation and dilated left ventricles without symptoms of frank left ventricular failure. Cardiac arrhythmias and infections are poorly tolerated in patients with free aortic regurgitation, and must be treated promptly and vigorously. Although nitroglycerin and long-acting nitrates are not as helpful in relieving anginal pain as in patients with coronary artery disease or aortic stenosis, they are worth a trial. Patients with syphilitic aortitis should receive a full course of penicillin therapy (Chap. 122).

ACUTE AORTIC REGURGITATION Infective endocarditis, aortic dissection, and trauma are the most common causes of severe, acute aortic regurgitation. Since the left ventricle has not had time to dilate, stroke volume declines and ventricular diastolic pressure rises markedly; the arterial pulse pressure is often not markedly widened and the physical signs characteristic of severe chronic regurgitation may be absent. Premature closure of the mitral valve is common and can be recognized by echocardiography. The first heart sound is soft or absent; the aortic diastolic murmur is characteristically brief. Patients present with pulmonary congestion and edema, and cardiovascular collapse secondary to a low cardiac output. Acute, severe regurgitation requires prompt surgical treatment, which may be lifesaving.

TRICUSPID STENOSIS

Tricuspid stenosis, a relatively uncommon valvular lesion, is generally rheumatic in origin and is much more common in women than in men. It does not usually occur as an isolated lesion or in patients with pure mitral regurgitation, but most commonly is observed in association with mitral stenosis, and sometimes with combined mitral and aortic stenosis. Hemodynamically significant tricuspid stenosis occurs in 5 to 10 percent of patients with severe mitral stenosis; rheumatic tricuspid stenosis is commonly associated with some degree of regurgitation.

PATHOPHYSIOLOGY A diastolic pressure gradient between the right atrium and ventricle is present. This gradient can be recorded most accurately and conveniently with a double-lumen cardiac catheter. It is augmented when the transvalvular blood flow increases during inspiration, and reduced during expiration. A mean diastolic pressure gradient exceeding 5 mmHg is usually sufficient to elevate the mean right atrial pressure to levels which result in systemic venous congestion and, unless sodium intake has been restricted or diuretics have been given, is associated with ascites and edema. In patients with sinus rhythm, the right atrial *a* wave may be extremely tall and may even approach the level of the right ventricular systolic pressure. The resting cardiac output is usually quite low and fails to rise during exercise. The low cardiac output is responsible for the normal or only slightly elevated left atrial, pulmonary arterial, and right ventricular systolic pressures despite the presence of even moderately severe mitral stenosis.

SYMPTOMS Since mitral stenosis generally precedes the development of tricuspid stenosis, many patients initially have symptoms of pulmonary congestion. Amelioration of the latter should raise the possibility that tricuspid stenosis may be developing. Characteristically, patients complain of relatively little dyspnea for the degree of hepatomegaly, ascites, and edema which they present. Weakness secondary to a low cardiac output and discomfort due to refractory edema, ascites, and marked hepatomegaly are common in patients with tricuspid stenosis and/or regurgitation. In some patients tricuspid stenosis may be suspected for the first time when symptoms of right ventricular failure persist after an adequate mitral valvulotomy.

PHYSICAL FINDINGS The diagnosis is often missed unless it is specifically considered and searched for. Severe tricuspid stenosis is associated with marked hepatic congestion, often resulting in cirrhosis, jaundice, serious malnutrition, severe edema, and ascites. Congestive hepatomegaly and, in cases of severe tricuspid valve disease, splenomegaly are present. The jugular veins are distended, and in patients with sinus rhythm there may be giant *a* waves. The *v* waves are less conspicuous, and since tricuspid obstruction impedes right atrial emptying during diastole, there is a slow *y* descent. In patients with sinus rhythm there may be prominent presystolic pulsations of the enlarged liver as well.

The right ventricle and the shock of pulmonary valve closure are usually not easily palpable. Indeed, a giant *a* wave in the jugular venous pulse without palpatory evidence of pulmonary hypertension or right ventricular enlargement suggests the possibility of tricuspid stenosis. The pulmonic closure sound is not accentuated on auscultation, and occasionally an opening snap of the tricuspid valve may be heard or recorded phonocardiographically approximately 0.06 s after pulmonary valve closure. The diastolic murmur of tricuspid stenosis has many of the qualities of the mitral diastolic murmur, and since tricuspid stenosis almost always occurs in the presence of mitral stenosis, the less-common valvular lesion may be missed. However, the tricuspid murmur is generally heard best along the left lower sternal margin and over the xiphoid process and is most prominent during presystole in sinus rhythm. In patients with sinus rhythm the presystolic component is often loudest. It is augmented during inspiration, and it is reduced during expiration and particularly during the Valsalva maneuver, when tricuspid blood flow is reduced. This finding (Carvallo's sign) is often most easily elicited when the patient is in the erect position. The diastolic murmur is reduced in amplitude as the stethoscope is inched laterally, only to intensify or reappear as the mitral murmur at the apex.

Noninvasive examinations The features of right atrial enlargement (Chap. 178) include tall, peaked P waves in lead II, as well as prominent, upright P waves in lead V_1. The *absence* of electrocardiographic evidence of right ventricular hypertrophy in a patient with right-sided heart failure who is believed to have mitral stenosis should suggest associated tricuspid valve disease. The chest roentgenograms in patients with combined tricuspid and mitral stenosis show particular prominence of the right atrium and superior vena cava without much enlargement of the pulmonary artery and with less evidence of pulmonary vascular congestion than occurs in patients with pure mitral valve disease. On echocardiographic examination the tricuspid valve is usually thickened with reduction of the EF slope.

TREATMENT Patients with tricuspid stenosis generally exhibit marked systemic venous congestion; intensive salt restriction and diuretic therapy are required during the preoperative period. Such a prolonged preparatory period may diminish hepatic congestion and thereby improve hepatic function sufficiently so that the risks of operation are diminished. Surgical treatment of the tricuspid valve is not ordinarily indicated at the time of mitral valve surgery in patients with mild tricuspid stenosis. On the other hand, definitive surgical relief of the tricuspid stenosis should be carried out, preferably at the time of mitral valvulotomy, in patients with moderate or severe tricuspid stenosis who have mean diastolic pressure gradients exceeding 5 mmHg and tricuspid orifices less than 1.5 to 2.0 cm^2. Tricuspid stenosis is almost always accompanied by significant tricuspid regurgitation. Open-heart operations utilizing cardiopulmonary bypass may permit substantial improvement of tricuspid valve function. If this cannot be accomplished, the tricuspid valve may have to be replaced with a prosthesis, preferably a tissue valve.

TRICUSPID REGURGITATION

Most commonly, tricuspid regurgitation is functional and secondary to marked dilatation of the right ventricle and the tricuspid valve ring. Functional tricuspid regurgitation may complicate right ventricular failure of any cause, including inferior wall infarcts that involve the right ventricle, and is commonly seen in the late stages of heart failure due to rheumatic or congenital heart disease with severe pulmonary hypertension, as well as in ischemic heart disease, cardiomyopathy, and cor pulmonale. It is in part reversible if pulmonary hypertension is relieved. Rheumatic fever may produce organic tricuspid regurgitation, often associated with tricuspid stenosis. Less commonly, regurgitation results from congenitally deformed tricuspid valves, and it occurs with defects of the atrioventricular canal, as well as with Ebstein's malformation of the tricuspid valve (Chap. 185). Infarction of right ventricular papillary muscles, tricuspid valve prolapse, carcinoid heart disease, endomyocardial fibrosis, infective endocarditis, and trauma may also produce tricuspid regurgitation.

As is the case for tricuspid stenosis, the clinical features of tricuspid regurgitation result primarily from systemic venous congestion and reduction of cardiac output. With the onset of tricuspid regurgitation in patients with pulmonary hypertension, as cardiac output declines, symptoms of pulmonary congestion diminish, but the clinical manifestations of right-sided heart failure become intensified. The neck veins are distended, with prominent *v* waves, and marked hepatomegaly, ascites, pleural effusions, edema, systolic pulsations of the liver, and positive hepatojugular reflux are common. A prominent right ventricular pulsation along the left parasternal region and a blowing holosystolic murmur along the lower left sternal margin which is generally intensified during inspiration and reduced during expiration or the Valsalva maneuver are characteristic findings; atrial fibrillation is usually present.

The electrocardiogram may show changes characteristic of the lesion responsible for the enlargement of the right ventricle which leads to this form of valvular dysfunction. In the rare instances of isolated tricuspid regurgitation the electrocardiogram often shows incomplete right bundle branch block. Roentgenographic examination usually reveals enlargement of both the right ventricle and right atrium, and the latter chamber expands during systole. Echocardiography may be helpful by demonstrating right ventricular dilatation and prolapsing or flail tricuspid leaflets; the diagnosis of tricuspid regurgitation can be made by contrast echocardiography.

The cardiac output is usually markedly reduced, and the right atrial pressure pulse may exhibit no *x* descent during early systole, but a prominent *c-v* wave, with a rapid *y* descent. The mean right atrial and the right ventricular end-diastolic pressures are often elevated.

Isolated tricuspid regurgitation, without pulmonary hypertension, such as that occurring as a consequence of infective endocarditis or trauma, is usually well tolerated and does not require operation. Indeed, even total excision of an infected tricuspid valve is often well tolerated. Treatment of the underlying cause of heart failure usually reduces the severity of functional tricuspid regurgitation. In patients with mitral valve disease and tricuspid regurgitation due to pulmonary hypertension and massive right ventricular enlargement, effective surgical correction of the mitral valvular abnormality results in lowering of the pulmonary vascular pressures and gradual reduction or disappearance of the tricuspid regurgitation without direct treatment of the tricuspid valve. However, recovery may be much more rapid in patients with severe secondary tricuspid regurgitation if, at the time of mitral replacement, tricuspid annuloplasty or, if necessary, tricuspid valve replacement is performed. Surgical treatment of the tricuspid regurgitation, consisting of either valve replacement or narrowing of the annulus, should be carried out in patients with severe regurgitation secondary to deformity of the tricuspid valve due to rheumatic fever, particularly those without severe pulmonary hypertension.

PULMONIC VALVE DISEASE

The pulmonic valve is affected by rheumatic fever far less frequently than the other valves and is uncommonly the seat of infective endocarditis. The most common acquired abnormality affecting the pulmonic valve is regurgitation secondary to dilatation of the pulmonary valve ring as a consequence of severe pulmonary hypertension of any cause. This produces the Graham Steell murmur, a high-pitched, decrescendo, diastolic blowing murmur along the left sternal border, which is difficult to differentiate from the far more common murmur produced by aortic regurgitation. It is of little hemodynamic significance; indeed surgical removal or destruction of the pulmonic valve by infective endocarditis does not produce heart failure unless serious pulmonary hypertension is also present.

Congenital pulmonic stenosis is discussed in Chap. 185.

REFERENCES

Braunwald E: Valvular heart disease, in *Heart Disease*, 2d ed, E Braunwald (ed). Philadelphia, Saunders, 1984, p 1063

Cohn LH et al: Early and late risk of aortic valve replacement: A 12-year concomitant comparison of the porcine bioprosthetic and tilting disc prosthetic aortic valves. J Thorac Cardiovasc Surg 88:695, 1984

Come PC: Echocardiographic evaluation of valvular heart disease, in *Diagnostic Cardiology: Noninvasive Imaging Techniques*, PC Come (ed). Philadelphia, Lippincott, 1985, p 407

Frankl WS, Brest AN (eds): *Valvular Heart Disease: Comprehensive Evaluation and Management*. Philadelphia, FA Davis, 1986

Greenberg BH et al: Arterial dilators in mitral regurgitation: Effects on rest and exercise, hemodynamics and long-term clinical follow-up. Circulation 65:181, 1982

Grossman W: Aortic and mitral regurgitation: How to evaluate the condition and when to consider surgical intervention. JAMA 252:2447, 1984

Ionescu MI, Cohn LH (eds): *Mitral Valve Disease: Diagnosis and Treatment*. London, Butterworths, 1985

Jeresaty RM: Mitral valve prolapse: An update. JAMA 254:793, 1985

Kirklin JW, Barratt-Boyes BG: Part III. Acquired valvular heart disease, in *Cardiac Surgery*, JW Kirklin, BG Barratt-Boyes (eds). New York, Wiley, 1986, p 323

Lingameni R et al: Tricuspid regurgitation: Clinical and angiographic assessment. Cath Cardiovasc Diag 5:7, 1979

Mahapatra RK et al: Rheumatic tricuspid stenosis. Indian Heart J 30:1381, 1978

Masuyama T et al: Noninvasive evaluation of aortic regurgitation by continuous-wave Doppler echocardiography. Circulation 73:460, 1986

Morganroth J et al: Acute severe aortic regurgitation. Ann Intern Med 87:223, 1977

Ohlsson J, Wranne B: Noninvasive assessment of valve area in patients with aortic stenosis. J Am Coll Cardiol 7:501, 1986

Richards KL: Doppler echocardiographic diagnosis and quantification of valvular heart disease. Curr Probl Cardiol 10:7, 1985

Ross J Jr: Left ventricular function and the timing of surgical treatments in valvular heart disease. Ann Intern Med 94:498, 1981

Sagar KB et al: Doppler echocardiographic evaluation of Hancock and Bjork-Shiley prosthetic valves. J Am Coll Cardiol 7:681, 1986

188 INFECTIVE ENDOCARDITIS

LAWRENCE L. PELLETIER, JR. / ROBERT G. PETERSDORF

DEFINITION Infective endocarditis is a microbial infection of the heart valves or of the endocardium in proximity to congenital or acquired cardiac defects. A similar clinical illness develops when there is infection of arteriovenous fistulas or aneurysms. The infection may develop abruptly or insidiously, may pursue a fulminant or prolonged course, and is fatal unless treated. Infection caused by indigenous microorganisms with low pathogenicity is ordinarily subacute, whereas infection by microorganisms with high pathogenicity is often acute. Fever, cardiac murmurs, splenomegaly, anemia, hematuria, mucocutaneous petechiae, and embolic manifestations are characteristic of the disease. Valve destruction may result in acute mitral or aortic regurgitation requiring urgent surgical intervention. Mycotic aneurysms may develop in the aortic root, cerebral artery bifurcations, or other remote sites.

ETIOLOGY AND EPIDEMIOLOGY In the preantimicrobial era 90 percent of infections were due to *Streptococcus viridans* acquired as a consequence of transient bacteremias originating from the upper respiratory tract, most often in young patients with rheumatic valvular heart disease. These individuals were usually seen after prolonged infection and possessed most of the classic physical manifestations of infective endocarditis. In contrast, patients with infective endocarditis today are more likely to be older, male, have other forms of congenital or valvular heart disease, have acquired the infection in hospital or from drug abuse, and have infections with organisms other than the *S. viridans*. Patients often present early in the course of infection without clubbing of the digits, splenomegaly, Osler's nodes, or Roth's spots.

Certain clinical settings are associated with specific etiologic agents as outlined in Table 188-1. Parenteral drug addicts may have sepsis without any evident portal of entry, but often will have signs of phlebitis, septic pulmonary emboli, and tricuspid regurgitation. The use of intravascular devices for prolonged periods has increased the incidence of nosocomial endocarditis. Patients with prosthetic heart valves are at risk of acquiring infection from organisms implanted at the time of surgery, or from transient bacteremias that colonize the heart valves months or years after operation.

PATHOGENESIS Hemodynamic events are important in the development of infective endocarditis. Bacteria in the circulation are often deposited on the endothelium at sites at high flow rates distal to an obstruction where lateral pressure is decreased, such as the pulmonary side of a ventricular septal defect (in the absence of pulmonary hypertension and reversal of the shunt) or patent ductus arteriosus. Alterations in blood flow at such sites or other areas of structural change or abnormality may cause changes in the endothelial surface resulting in the formation of a sterile vegetation consisting of platelets and fibrin. This vegetation becomes the nidus on which microorganisms are implanted.

Most often, endocardial infections are initiated by transient bacteremias that seed abnormal endothelial surfaces. Transient *S. viridans* bacteremias are common following dental manipulation or extraction, tonsillectomy, use of a water jet, or chewing of food. Bacteremia is increased in the presence of gingival disease or dental infection. Enterococcal bacteremia may result from manipulation of an infected genitourinary tract, such as urinary catheterization or cystoscopy. Bacteremia may occur spontaneously or as a result of manipulation of localized infections at other sites. Although gram-negative rod bacteremia occurs frequently, gram-negative rod endocarditis is relatively rare. The low incidence of gram-negative rod endocarditis may be due to protection offered by nonspecific complement-fixing antibodies, or the relative lack of adherence of gram-negative bacteria to fibrin-platelet aggregates and fibronectin-coated endothelial surfaces.

Infective endocarditis occurs most often in persons with preexisting heart disease, but virulent organisms can seed normal cardiac valves. Infection most commonly involves the left side of the heart with the mitral, aortic, tricuspid, and pulmonary valves involved in decreasing order of frequency. Congenital bicuspid aortic valves, mitral and aortic valves damaged by rheumatic fever, calcific mitral and aortic valves in the elderly with arteriosclerosis, mitral valve prolapse, mechanical and bioprosthetic heart valves, Marfan's syndrome, idiopathic hypertrophic subaortic stenosis, coarctation of the aorta, arteriovenous shunt, ventricular septal defect, and a patent ductus arteriosus all predispose to the development of endocarditis. Infective endocarditis rarely involves interatrial septal defects.

Prolonged intravascular infection results in high titers of antibodies against the infecting microorganisms. Circulating antigen-antibody complexes are commonly found, and are sometimes associated with immune-complex glomerulonephritis and cutaneous vasculitis.

Intravascular organisms adherent to endothelium are rapidly covered with a coat of fibrin and platelets, forming a vegetation. Large numbers of organisms within a vegetation exhaust available nutrients producing a static growth phase less susceptible to antimicrobial agents that inhibit cell wall development and require rapidly proliferating organisms for maximal killing. Highly pathogenic microorganisms often cause rapid valvular destruction and ulceration associated with valvular regurgitation. Less pathogenic microorganisms usually cause less valvular destruction or ulceration but can lead to the development of large polypoid vegetations that may obstruct the valve or become dislodged, producing emboli. The infection may extend from the valve to the surrounding mural endocardium or penetrate the valve ring to produce a mycotic aneurysm, myocardial abscess, or cardiac conduction defect. Involvement of the chordae tendineae may lead to rupture and acute valvular insufficiency. Infected vegetations are poorly vascularized and heal by granulation tissue forming on the surface of the vegetation, sometimes trapping within the vegetation viable organisms that may be grown months after successful treatment if the valves are cultured after removal at surgery.

The microbemia of intravascular infections is usually continuous unless interrupted by antimicrobial therapy. For this reason, few blood cultures are required to demonstrate the microorganisms. The microorganisms are primarily cleared from the blood by the reticuloendothelial cells of the liver and spleen, often producing splenomegaly. There is no reduction in the number of bacteria in the blood during circulation through the extremities, so that arterial blood cultures are no more likely to show bacteremia than venous blood cultures.

Embolization is a characteristic feature of infective endocarditis. The friable fibrin vegetations may separate from the site of infection and be propelled into the systemic or pulmonary circulation, depending on whether the endocarditis involves the left or right side of the heart. Emboli vary in size and most often involve the brain, spleen, kidney, gastrointestinal tract, heart, or extremities. Emboli in fungal endocarditis tend to be large and occlude major vessels. Pulmonary infarction or abscess is common in right-sided endocarditis. Septic infarction is uncommon in endocarditis caused by organisms of low pathogenicity, such as *S. viridans,* although osteomyelitis has been described as a complication of viridans streptococcal and enterococcal endocarditis. *Staphylococcus aureus* and other virulent microorganisms often produce septic infarction with metastatic abscesses and may result in meningitis. Involvement of major arteries by emboli produces mycotic aneurysms, which may rupture. Focal myocarditis may be due to emboli. Myocardial infarction may develop after coronary embolization. Three types of renal lesions may be produced: segmental infarction due to large emboli, focal glomerulitis from small emboli, and a diffuse glomerulonephritis indistinguishable from other types of immune-complex disease most commonly seen with group A streptococcal endocarditis. Petechial skin lesions characterized histologically by acute vasculitis are probably immunologic in origin. Other skin lesions associated with pain, tenderness, and cellulitis may be embolic.

MANIFESTATIONS Subacute infective endocarditis Infections are commonly caused by organisms with lesser virulence, *S. viridans* in patients with native valves, and diphtheroid organisms or *Staphylococcus epidermidis* in individuals with prosthetic valves. Enterococci and numerous other microorganisms also can produce the syndrome. Even *S. aureus* may on occasion follow a subacute course. Symptoms usually begin insidiously, and patients find it difficult to date the onset of infection. In some individuals the onset of infection can be related to a recent dental extraction, urethral instrumentation, tonsillectomy, acute respiratory infection, or abortion.

Weakness, fatigability, weight loss, feverishness, night sweats, anorexia, and arthralgia are the usual symptoms of subacute bacterial endocarditis. Emboli may produce paralysis, chest pain due to myocardial or pulmonary infarction, acute vascular insufficiency with pain in the extremities, hematuria, acute abdominal pain, or sudden blindness. Painful fingers or toes and painful skin lesions may also be important symptoms. Chills are not common. Transient cerebral ischemic attacks, toxic encephalopathy, headache, brain abscess, subarachnoid hemorrhage from rupture of a mycotic aneurysm, or purulent meningitis may develop.

Physical examination may reveal a variety of findings, none of which alone is pathognomonic of subacute infective endocarditis. Physical examination may be normal early in the course of infection. The association of the different manifestations, however, usually provides a characteristic picture of the disease. The patient usually appears chronically ill and pale and has an elevated temperature. The fever is most often remittent, with afternoon or evening peaks. The pulse is usually rapid, and if cardiac failure complicates the infection, it may be greater than expected with the degree of fever.

Mucocutaneous lesions are common and vary in type. Petechiae are most frequent and may be found in the mucosa of the mouth, pharynx, or conjunctivas. These small, red, hemorrhagic-appearing lesions do not blanch on pressure and are not tender or painful. On the mucous membranes or conjunctivas these petechiae may have a pale center. Petechiae may be found anywhere on the skin but are most common over the upper part of the trunk anteriorly. They are frequently difficult to distinguish from angiomas, but they gradually become brownish and disappear. Frequently, petechiae continue to appear, even during convalescence. Linear hemorrhages (splinter hemorrhages) may be found under the nails, but these are difficult to differentiate from traumatic lesions, particularly in manual laborers. These mucocutaneous lesions are not specific for bacterial endocarditis but may be found in patients with other conditions such as profound anemia, leukemia, trichinosis, and sepsis without endocarditis. Erythematous or purple, painful, tender nodules (Osler's nodes) may develop on the palms of the hands, soles of the feet, pulp of the fingers, or other sites. These are probably embolic lesions. Emboli to larger peripheral arteries may result in gangrene of the fingers, toes, or larger portions of the extremities. Clubbing of the fingers is observed in long-standing or prolonged infective endocarditis. Mild jaundice is found occasionally.

Findings in the heart are usually those of underlying heart disease. Major changes in cardiac murmurs, primarily development of a new diastolic murmur, may be attributable to ulceration of a valve, dilatation of the heart or valve ring, rupture of chordae tendineae, or development of a very large vegetation. Minor changes in systolic bruits are usually of little significance. In rare instances, no cardiac murmurs are detected. In this situation, right-sided endocarditis or an infected mural thrombus, or pulmonary, or peripheral arteriovenous fistula should be suspected.

Splenomegaly is common in subacute infective endocarditis. Rarely is the spleen tender, but a friction rub may be heard over it when there is infarction. Hepatomegaly is not characteristic unless heart failure develops.

Arthralgia is relatively common, and arthritis resembling acute rheumatic fever may occur.

Embolic phenomena may precipitate awareness of the infection. Sudden development of hemiplegia, flank pain with hematuria, abdominal pain with melena, pleuritic pain and hemoptysis, left upper abdominal pain with splenic friction rub, blindness, or monoplegia in a patient with fever and cardiac murmurs makes infective endocarditis suspect. Pulmonary emboli in right-sided endocarditis may be confused with pneumonia.

Acute bacterial infective endocarditis Suppurative infection commonly antedates the onset of endocarditis. For example, infection of the heart may develop as a complication of pneumococcal meningitis, septic thrombophlebitis, group A streptococcal cellulitis, or staphylococcal abscesses. The source of cardiovascular infection, therefore, is often evident.

Acute endocarditis often involves the normal heart, in contrast to the subacute infection, which almost invariably involves the abnormal heart. It is particularly common in intravenous drug users and individuals with previously undetected abnormalities of the aortic valve. The acute infection is fulminant and pursues a rapid course. Fever is often greater, may be intermittent, and in certain instances (as in gonococcal endocarditis) may be characterized by a twice daily temperature elevation. Chills are common. Petechiae may be numerous, and embolic phenomena are prominent. Small, occasionally flame-shaped hemorrhages that may have pale centers (Roth's spots) are found in the retina. Osler's nodes are uncommon, but the pulp of the fingers may show nontender subcutaneous erythematous maculopapular lesions (Janeway's spots) that may ulcerate. Hematuria is seen with embolic lesions of the kidney, and diffuse glomerulonephritis may occur. Destruction of the cardiac valves can be complicated by rupture of chordae tendineae or perforation of cusps, leading to rapidly progressing cardiac failure. Metastatic abscesses following septic emboli are frequent.

TABLE 188-1 Organisms causing infective endocarditis

Predisposing condition	Organism	Comment
Dental manipulations	Viridans streptococci	
Parenteral drug addicts	*S. aureus* Group A streptococcus Gram-negative rods *Candida* spp.	Septic phlebitis and right-sided endocarditis are common.
Prosthetic valve recipients		
< 2 months after surgery	*S. epidermidis* Diphtheroids Gram-negative rods *Candida* spp. Enterococcus *S. aureus*	Early-onset infections tend to be resistant to prophylactic antimicrobials administered at surgery.
> 2 months after surgery	*Streptococcus* spp. *S. epidermidis* Diphtheroids Enterococcus *S. aureus*	Some low-virulence infections implanted at surgery are slow to develop.
Urinary tract infections	Enterococcus Gram-negative rods	Associated in older males with prostatism and in women with genitourinary tract infections.
Catheter-related phlebitis	*S. aureus* *S. epidermidis* *Candida* spp. Gram-negative rods	An increasingly common source of endocarditis in hospitalized patients.
Alcoholism	Pneumococcus	May be associated with simultaneous pneumonia and meningitis.
Colon cancer	*Streptococcus bovis*	

Right-sided endocarditis Tricuspid valve and rarely pulmonary valve endocarditis or pulmonary artery mycotic aneurysm are seen in parenteral drug addicts with skin cellulitis or septic phlebitis. Infected peripheral or central venous catheters or transvenous pacing wires may also result in right-sided infective endocarditis. The infecting organisms originate from the skin (*S. aureus, Candida albicans*) or presumably from injected materials (*Pseudomonas aeruginosa, Serratia marcescens*). *S. aureus* is the most frequently isolated organism, and the tricuspid valve the most common site of involvement in parenteral drug addicts. The clinical presentation is that of acute endocarditis with pulmonary infarction and abscess formation. The most frequent symptoms are high fever of several weeks' duration, pleuritic chest pain, hemoptysis and sputum production, dyspnea on exertion, malaise, anorexia, and fatigability. A tricuspid valve regurgitant murmur accentuated by inspiration with pulsatile neck veins and liver may be present, but more often there is no audible murmur at all or the murmur is difficult to detect. Two-dimensional echocardiogram may be required to confirm the presence of endocardial vegetations. Blood cultures are as likely to be positive in right-sided endocarditis as in left-sided lesions. The chest roentgenograph usually shows peripheral wedge-shaped pulmonary infiltrates with cavitation. Due to the absence of emboli to vital organs, acute hemodynamic decompensation secondary to valve destruction, and a generally younger, healthier patient population, and perhaps because of a better response to antimicrobial agents, patients with right-sided endocarditis have a better prognosis. Large (greater than 1-cm diameter) vegetations or infection caused by resistant microorganisms may require valve debridement or excision in conjunction with antimicrobial therapy to eradicate the infection.

Prosthetic valve endocarditis Prosthetic valve infections develop in 2 to 3 percent of patients the first year following prosthetic valve placement, and 0.5 percent per year subsequently. About one-third of infections in the first year develop *within 2 months of surgery* and are probably due to colonization of the prosthesis or suture sites during surgery. Organisms that cause early infections (Table 188-1) are often resistant to antimicrobial agents; such infections are associated with a high mortality due to septic shock, valve dehiscence, and myocardial invasion. Gram-negative bacteremia in the immediate postoperative period may originate from the urinary tract, wound, pulmonary infections, or septic phlebitis and is often not associated with prosthetic valve infection.

Prosthetic valve infections that occur *more than 2 months after surgery* (Table 188-1) may result from implantation at surgery or colonization of the prosthesis or its site of attachment during transient bacteremias. Patients with prosthetic valves should receive prophylactic antimicrobial agents when undergoing procedures known to produce bacteremia, and minor infections that might produce bacteremia should be treated promptly. Late onset infections caused by streptococci have a better prognosis than early infections and may be controlled with antibiotics alone.

Prosthetic valve infections often produce symptoms and signs indistinguishable from infections on natural valves, but there is a greater frequency of valve ring infection that may involve part or all of the circumference producing valve dehiscence or penetration into the myocardium or surrounding tissues. Myocardial abscess, conduction disturbances, sinus of Valsalva aneurysm, or fistulas into the right side of the heart or pericardium may result. Prolongation of the PR interval, a new left bundle branch block, or right bundle branch block with left anterior hemiblock should suggest involvement of the ventricular septum in aortic valve infections. Extension of infection from the mitral valve annulus may be associated with nonparoxysmal junctional tachycardia, or second- or third-degree heart block with a narrow QRS complex. Prosthetic valve stenosis due to vegetations narrowing the orifice or interfering with valve excursion may be detected by auscultation or echocardiography. A postoperative regurgitant murmur or abnormal position or movement of the valve on fluoroscopic examination or echocardiogram may indicate partial dehiscence of the prosthesis. Prosthetic valve infections complicated by valve stenosis, valve dehiscence with congestive heart failure, recurrent emboli, resistance to antimicrobial therapy, or evidence of myocardial invasion require early surgical intervention. Patients receiving anticoagulants to prevent embolism who develop endocarditis should continue to take the medication if the risk of embolization without anticoagulation is high and accept a 36 percent risk of intracranial hemorrhage with 80 percent consequent mortality. Relapse following appropriate antimicrobial treatment or fungous infections also requires early surgical removal of the infected prosthesis.

LABORATORY FINDINGS Leukocytosis with neutrophilia is the rule but is by no means invariable. Macrophages (histiocytes) may be found in the blood, particularly in the first drop obtained from the earlobe. Normocytic, normochromic anemia is almost always found in subacute infective endocarditis but may not be present early in acute bacterial endocarditis. The erythrocyte sedimentation rate is rapid. Serum immunoglobulins are increased but return to normal during convalescence. The anti-gamma globulin latex fixation test is commonly positive due to IgM and IgA factors. Circulating immune complexes are usually present and titers often decline with successful antimicrobial therapy, but may remain elevated in bacteriologic cures when associated with arthritis, glomerulitis, or drug reactions. Mild bilirubinemia is detected occasionally. Proteinuria is common, and microscopic hematuria is frequently present. Serum total hemolytic complement and the third component of complement may be decreased. Antiteichoic acid antibody titers in *S. aureus* endocarditis are usually 1:4 or greater after 2 weeks of antimicrobial therapy.

An echocardiogram may identify high-risk patients with large vegetations or unsuspected preexisting valvular lesions, or it may provide an indication for early operation in patients with acute aortic insufficiency and severe volume overload of the left ventricle. The echocardiogram does not detect vegetations smaller than 2 mm, nor does it differentiate active from healed lesions. Two-dimensional scanners are more sensitive than M-mode echocardiography but demonstrate vegetations in only 43 to 80 percent of patients with endocarditis. Degenerative bioprosthetic valve changes may mimic echocardiographic changes of infective endocarditis.

Blood cultures are positive in the majority of cases. Three to five cultures of 20 to 30 mL of blood, taken at intervals determined by the patient's clinical status, are usually adequate to demonstrate the bacteremia, if it is demonstrable at all. Blood cultures may not become positive for several days, if at all, in patients who have received antibiotics prior to the time when cultures are obtained. Failure to demonstrate bacteremia or delayed growth in blood cultures also may be due to infection by unusual microorganisms such as *Hemophilus parainfluenzae, Cardiobacterium hominis, Corynebacterium* spp., *Histoplasma capsulatum, Brucella, Pasteurella,* or anaerobic streptococci that require special nutrient media or extended (up to 4 weeks) incubation. Thiol-requiring streptococcal variants may require pyridoxine- or cysteine-supplemented broth. Castañeda-type culture bottles assist in the recovery of fungi and *Brucella. Aspergillus* endocarditis is seldom associated with positive blood cultures. *Coxiella burnetii* endocarditis and *Chlamydia psittaci* endocarditis are diagnosed by serologic tests, since blood cultures are always negative. Bone marrow cultures and serologic testing for *Candida, Histoplasma,* and *Brucella* may be helpful in culture-negative endocarditis.

DIFFERENTIAL DIAGNOSIS When several of the manifestations of infective endocarditis occur together, the diagnosis is not difficult. In particular, the presence of fever, petechiae, splenomegaly, microscopic hematuria, and anemia in a patient with cardiac murmurs is most suggestive of infection. When only a few manifestations are present, however, the diagnosis is not simple. Prolonged fever in a patient with rheumatic heart disease is particularly troublesome, but the diagnosis of bacterial endocarditis should be considered in every patient with fever and a heart murmur. The diagnosis becomes even more difficult when blood cultures show no growth.

Acute rheumatic fever with carditis is often difficult to distinguish from infective endocarditis, and in a few instances, active rheumatic fever has been found to coexist with the valvular infection. The diagnosis of rheumatic carditis hinges on a combination of clinical and laboratory criteria (see Chap. 186).

Subacute infective endocarditis is no longer a common cause of "fever of undetermined origin" (see Chap. 9). However, occasionally it may be mistaken for a hidden neoplasm, systemic lupus erythematosus, periarteritis nodosa, poststreptococcal glomerulonephritis, and intracardiac tumors such as myxoma of the atrium. Aortic dissection with acute aortic regurgitation also may mimic bacterial endocarditis. Postoperative endocarditis should be suspected in patients who develop fever, anemia, and leukocytosis after cardiovascular surgery. In these postoperative patients, the various postthoracotomy and postcardiotomy syndromes must also be considered.

PROGNOSIS Recovery from untreated infective endocarditis is rare. With appropriate antibiotic therapy, however, over 70 percent of the patients with infection on endogenous valves and 50 percent with infection on prosthetic valves survive the infection. Intravenous drug users with right-sided staphylococcal endocarditis generally have a good prognosis. Factors that suggest a less favorable outcome are the presence of congestive heart failure, extreme age of the patient, involvement of the aortic valve or multiple heart valves, polymicrobial bacteremia, failure to identify the etiologic agent owing to negative blood cultures, antimicrobial resistance to nontoxic bactericidal drugs, and delay in initiating therapy. Prosthetic valve, gram-negative bacillus, and fungal endocarditis are associated with the poorest prognosis.

The commonest cause of death in treated endocarditis is congestive heart failure, attributable either to valve destruction or to myocardial damage. Additionally, death may be precipitated by embolization to vital organs, by renal insufficiency, by rupture of a mycotic aneurysm, or by complications following cardiac surgery. Many patients recover completely without apparent worsening of the underlying cardiovascular disease. When recurrent endocarditis develops, it usually involves the same valve and is due to failure to kill microorganisms in an environment of suboptimal host resistance.

Further reduction in the mortality rate of infective endocarditis will depend primarily on the increased use of cardiac surgery in combination with antimicrobial therapy to eliminate refractory infections, and the early replacement of damaged valves in patients with congestive heart failure.

PROPHYLAXIS Patients with suspected congenital or acquired valvular heart disease, prosthetic heart valves, ventriculoseptal patches, or prior history of infective endocarditis should receive antimicrobial prophylaxis for viridans streptococci immediately before any dental manipulation that causes bleeding, oral surgery, and tonsillectomy or adenoidectomy. Likewise, patients with similar cardiac risks undergoing urinary catheterization, cystoscopy, prostatectomy, obstetrical or gynecologic manipulation of infected tissues, or rectal or colon surgery should receive prophylaxis directed against the enterococcus. Patients with mitral valve prolapse, asymmetric septal hypertrophy, and tricuspid or pulmonary valve lesions are at lower risk of developing endocarditis but should also receive antimicrobial prophylaxis. Prophylaxis is not required for atherosclerotic arterial plaques, coronary artery bypass grafts, systolic clicks, isolated atrial septal defects, or transvenous pacemakers. The high-risk patients mentioned above undergoing surgical manipulation of infected tissues at other sites should receive an antimicrobial active against the most likely infecting organism.

The rationale for antimicrobial prophylaxis is that when these patients develop bacteremia, they are more likely to develop endocarditis. The best experimental evidence available holds that for prevention of endocarditis caused by viridans streptococci with penicillin, both a high concentration and relatively prolonged duration of action are necessary. It has been shown that penicillin and streptomycin act synergistically in killing viridans streptococci. These data suggest a regimen consisting of a single dose of 1.2 million units of aqueous procaine penicillin G plus 1.0 g streptomycin administered intramuscularly within 30 min of dental surgery, followed by penicillin V 0.5 g orally at 6-h intervals for four doses, is effective. A single oral preoperative dose of 3 g amoxicillin is probably equally effective. Patients who are allergic to penicillin should receive vancomycin, 1.0 g intravenously over 30 min, 1 h before the procedure or erythromycin, 1.0 g orally 1 h before the procedure. Either antibiotic should be followed with erythromycin, 0.5 g orally every 6 h for four doses. The best regimen for preventing enterococcal endocarditis is ampicillin plus gentamicin. Ampicillin, 1 g, plus gentamicin, 1.0 mg/kg (not over 80 mg), should be given intramuscularly or intravenously 30 to 60 min before the procedure, and both agents should be repeated every 8 h for two doses. Penicillin-allergic patients should receive vancomycin, 1.0 g intravenously, and gentamicin 1.0 mg/kg intramuscularly, 30 to 60 min before the procedure; administration of both agents is repeated 12 h later. Antistaphylococcal prophylaxis is indicated during surgery associated with implantation of prosthetic heart valves, intracardiac materials, or vascular prostheses. Cefazolin, 1.0 g intravenously, every 6 h should be given 30 min prior to surgery and continued no longer than 24 h.

The prophylactic doses of penicillin used to prevent group A streptococcal infection and recurrent rheumatic fever will not prevent bacterial endocarditis. The dose of benzathine penicillin given for rheumatic fever prophylaxis does not predispose to bacterial endocarditis caused by penicillin-resistant microorganisms, whereas oral penicillin V does promote the emergence of penicillin-resistant oral flora. All high-risk patients should be cautioned to maintain a high level of oral hygiene, avoid the use of a water jet in the mouth, and seek prompt treatment of infections that occur at any site.

TABLE 188-2 Recommended treatment for infective endocarditis

S. viridans and nonenterococcal group D streptococci (penicillin G MIC < 0.1 μg/mL)	Penicillin G 10–20 million units per day IV in divided doses every 4–6 h × 4 weeks
	Penicillin G 10–20 million units per day IV with streptomycin 7.5 mg/kg IV or IM every 12 h or gentamicin 1 mg/kg IV every 8 h × 2 weeks
	Penicillin G 10–20 million units per day IV × 2 weeks, followed by amoxacillin 1 g PO every 6 h × 2 weeks
	Cefazolin 2 g IV every 6–8 h × 4 weeks if allergic to penicillin
	Vancomycin 15 mg/kg IV every 12 h × 4 weeks if allergic to penicillin
Enterococcus or relatively penicillin-resistant viridans streptococci (penicillin G MIC > 0.1 μg/mL)	Penicillin G 15–24 million units per day IV in divided doses every 4–6 h with gentamicin 1 mg/kg IV every 8 h × 4–6 weeks
	Ampicillin 2 g IV every 6 h possible substitute for penicillin G
	Streptomycin 7.5 mg/kg IV or IM possible substitute for gentamicin if the MIC for streptomycin is < 2000 μg/mL
	Vancomycin 15 mg/kg IV every 12 h with gentamicin 1 mg/kg IV every 8 h × 4–6 weeks, if allergic to penicillin
Pneumococcus or group A streptococcus	Penicillin G 6–12 million units per day IV in divided doses every 4–6 h × 4 weeks
	Cefazolin 2 g IV every 6–8 h × 4 weeks if allergic to penicillin
Methicillin-susceptible *S. aureus* or *S. epidermidis*	Nafcillin 2 g IV every 4 h × 4–6 weeks or longer
	Cefazolin 2 g IV every 6 h × 4–6 weeks or longer, if allergic to penicillin
	Vancomycin 15 mg/kg IV every 12 h × 4–6 weeks or longer, if allergic to penicillin
Methicillin-resistant *S. aureus, S. epidermidis,* or *Corynebacterium* spp.	Vancomycin 15 mg/kg IV every 12 h × 4–6 weeks or longer
	Vancomycin in combination with rifampin 900–1200 mg PO once daily for 4–6 weeks or longer with gentamicin 1 mg/kg IV every 8 h × 2 weeks

TREATMENT Intravascular infections must be treated with antimicrobial agents that kill microorganisms at concentrations attainable in serum because organisms within endocardial vegetations are protected by surrounding fibrin and platelet aggregates against the bactericidal action of host neutrophils, complement, and antibodies. Infective endocarditis is the prototype infection for which bacteriostatic agents that inhibit but do not kill organisms are ineffective, and bactericidal drugs are necessary for cure. The best results occur when a microbicidal agent active against the infecting organism is administered early in the course of the infection in high dosage, and treatment is continued for a relatively long period of time. When a prosthetic valve is infected, the microorganism is relatively resistant to available agents; or when a mycotic aneurysm or myocardial abscess develops, surgery in addition to antimicrobial therapy is often required to eliminate the infection.

The initial step in selecting the correct antimicrobial agent begins with obtaining blood cultures before empiric antimicrobial therapy is begun so that the organism can be isolated and identified, and antimicrobial susceptibilities determined. It is generally advisable to obtain macrotube or microtube dilution minimum inhibitory concentration measurements for therapeutic agents, although this is not always necessary for microorganisms with large zones of inhibition on disc diffusion susceptibility tests. Penicillin-susceptible *Streptococcus bovis* group D organisms should be differentiated from enterococci; and methicillin-resistant *S. aureus* and *S. epidermidis* separated from methicillin-susceptible strains. Determination of the bactericidal activity of antimicrobial agents against the infecting organism would be desirable, but since there is no standardized reproducible laboratory measurement of bacterial killing, routine use of minimum bactericidal concentration (MBC) tests to select antimicrobial agents or serum bactericidal activity (SBA) tests to adjust dosage is usually not recommended.

Table 188-2 outlines recommended treatment programs for the most common causes of endocarditis. Two weeks of penicillin and streptomycin are as effective as 4 weeks of penicillin alone in the treatment of penicillin-susceptible *S. viridans* infections. When streptomycin is administered, the minimum inhibitory concentration (MIC) of streptomycin should be determined, and gentamicin used instead of streptomycin if the streptomycin MIC is greater than 2000 μg/mL. Elderly patients and individuals with deafness or renal insufficiency are likely to have increased aminoglycoside renal and ototoxicity and should be treated with penicillin alone for 4 weeks. If 2 weeks of parenteral penicillin are followed by 2 weeks of oral therapy, then serum levels of the oral agent should be measured to demonstrate adequate absorption. Amoxicillin provides better oral absorption than penicillin V. In patients allergic to penicillin, cefazolin may be administered with caution if the reaction was a mild drug rash or fever. If there is a history of a life-threatening anaphylaxis to penicillin, then vancomycin should be given. Skin testing with major and minor penicillin antigens may be used to guide antimicrobial selection in patients with an unclear history of penicillin allergy. In view of the availability of effective alternative drugs, penicillin desensitization by frequent sequential administrations of increasing concentrations of penicillin under close supervision with readiness to treat anaphylactic reactions is seldom required.

Penicillin alone is not bactericidal against enterococcal organisms (*Streptococcus fecalis, S. faecium, S. durans*), and requires combination with an aminoglycoside to cure endocarditis. The combination of penicillin and gentamicin is synergistic against almost all enterococci, whereas 30 to 40 percent of enterococci are resistant to penicillin and streptomycin. Resistance to penicillin and streptomycin synergy is predicted by a streptomycin MIC greater than 2000 μg/mL. Ampicillin may be substituted for penicillin G. Lower doses of gentamicin (3 mg/kg per day) are as effective as higher doses and are less toxic. Cephalosporin antimicrobials are not active against the enterococcus and should not be used to treat enterococcal endocarditis. Vancomycin and gentamicin or streptomycin should be used to treat patients allergic to penicillin. Many patients can be treated for 4 weeks, but those with prosthetic valves, mitral valve involvement, or symptoms for longer than 3 months should be treated for 6 weeks.

Nafcillin should be used to treat *S. aureus* bacteremia while waiting for antimicrobial susceptibility results unless methicillin-resistant *S. aureus* is epidemic, in which case vancomycin should be administered instead. The addition of gentamicin to a penicillinase-resistant penicillin or cephalosporin results in enhanced killing of methicillin-susceptible staphylococci in the test tube and in animal models, but does not seem to improve the clinical outcome for most patients. Combination therapy for staphylococcal endocarditis is controversial and should not be used routinely except in the treatment of methicillin-resistant *S. epidermidis* prosthetic valve endocarditis. In staphylococcal endocarditis in particular, attention must be given to possible metastatic abscesses requiring surgical drainage and especially prolonged antimicrobial therapy to prevent relapse.

Prosthetic valve infections should be treated for 6 to 8 weeks, and patients should be monitored closely for signs of valve dysfunction and embolism. Mechanical valves are more likely to require placement than bioprostheses.

Patients with suspected endocarditis but negative blood cultures present a difficult clinical decision since treatment must be based on a guess about the likely organism. Patients with a native valve and no obvious portal of entry should be treated for enterococcal endocarditis with penicillin G and gentamicin. Parenteral drug addicts should be treated for staphylococcal and gram-negative bacilli endocarditis with nafcillin, ticarcillin, and gentamicin. The extended-spectrum penicillin should be adapted to gram-negative organisms usually encountered locally in drug addicts. Culture-negative prosthetic valve infections should be treated for methicillin-resistant *S. epidermidis* and enterococcal endocarditis with vancomycin and gentamicin.

Usually, fever begins to disappear within 3 to 7 days after the start of treatment of infective endocarditis. Embolic complications of the disease, heart failure, phlebitis, and infection with resistant microorganisms, however, may delay defervescence. If a drug fever or rash to penicillin develops during the course of therapy, antihistamines or corticosteroids may be used to alleviate the manifestations of the reaction; or more commonly, penicillin is discontinued and an alternative agent initiated. When attempting to discern the cause of a fever, cessation of all therapy for 72 h is not hazardous and may identify such a drug reaction readily. Sterile emboli or late valve rupture occurs occasionally up to 12 months after cessation of therapy.

Many patients with arteriovenous fistulas, valve ring abscess, recurrent embolization, endocarditis produced by resistant organisms, or infected cardiac prostheses require surgical intervention before the infection can be controlled. In addition, early valve replacement should be considered in patients who develop congestive heart failure associated with marked valve damage (particularly aortic or mitral regurgitation) as a consequence of infective endocarditis. Valve replacement may be lifesaving and must be undertaken before intractable heart failure ensues. Whether operation can be based entirely on cardiac ultrasound results or whether cardiac catheterization always needs to be performed remains controversial.

Fungal endocarditis is usually fatal. However, a few survivors have been reported after surgical debridement and replacement of infected valves combined with amphotericin B therapy.

When infective endocarditis recurs, it usually develops within 4 weeks after treatment is terminated. Reinstitution of antimicrobial therapy is required, and the sensitivity of the microorganisms should be reevaluated. Relapse may indicate inadequate or inappropriate treatment, or the need for surgical intervention. Recrudescence of infective endocarditis more than 6 weeks after cessation of treatment usually connotes a new infection.

REFERENCES

DiNubile MJ: Surgery in active endocarditis. Ann Intern Med 96:650, 1982

Freedman LR: *Infective Endocarditis and other Intravascular Infections.* New York, Plenum, 1982

Karchmer AW et al: *Staphylococcus epidermidis* causing prosthetic valve endocarditis: Microbiologic and clinical observations as guides to therapy. Ann Intern Med 98:447, 1983

Kaye D (ed): *Infective Endocarditis.* Baltimore, University Park Press, 1976

———: Prophylaxis for infective endocarditis: An update. Ann Intern Med 104:419, 1986

Korzeniowski O et al: Combination antimicrobial therapy for *Staphylococcus aureus* endocarditis in patients addicted to parenteral drugs and in non-addicts. Ann Intern Med 97:496, 1982

Petersdorf RG, Pelletier LL: Prevention of infective endocarditis, in *Cardiology 2: Preventive Cardiology,* DG Julian, JO Humphries (eds). London, Butterworth, 1983, pp 86–122

Shulman ST et al: Prevention of bacterial endocarditis. Circulation 70:1123A, 1984

Von Reyne CF et al: Infective endocarditis: An analysis based on strict case definitions. Ann Intern Med 94:505, 1981

Weinstein L: Infective endocarditis, in *Heart Disease: A Textbook of Cardiovascular Medicine,* E Braunwald (ed). Philadelphia, Saunders, 1984, pp 1136–82

Weinstein MP et al: Multicenter collaborative evaluation of a standardized serum bactericidal test as a prognostic indicator in infective endocarditis. Am J Med 78:262, 1985

Wilson WR et al: Short-term therapy for streptococcal infective endocarditis. JAMA 245:360, 1981

——— et al: Treatment of streptomycin-susceptible and streptomycin-resistant enterococcal endocarditis. Ann Intern Med 100:816, 1984

Wolfson JS, Swartz MN: Serum bactericidal activity as a monitor of antibiotic therapy. N Engl J Med 312:968, 1985

189 ISCHEMIC HEART DISEASE

ANDREW P. SELWYN / EUGENE BRAUNWALD

Ischemia refers to a lack of oxygen due to inadequate perfusion. *Ischemic heart disease* is a condition of diverse etiologies all having in common a disturbance of cardiac function due to an imbalance between oxygen supply and demand.

ETIOLOGY AND PATHOPHYSIOLOGY

The most common cause of ischemia is atherosclerotic disease of epicardial coronary arteries, which by reducing the lumen of these vessels causes an absolute decrease in myocardial perfusion in the basal state or limits appropriate increases in perfusion when demand for flow is augmented. Coronary blood flow can also be limited by arterial thrombi, spasm, and rarely coronary emboli, arteritis, and ostial narrowing due to luetic aortitis. Congenital abnormalities, such as anomalous origin of the left anterior descending coronary artery from the pulmonary artery (Chap. 185), may cause myocardial ischemia and infarction in infancy but this is a very rare cause in adults. Myocardial ischemia can also occur if myocardial oxygen demands are abnormally increased, as in severe ventricular hypertrophy due to hypertension or aortic stenosis. The latter can present with angina that is indistinguishable from that caused by coronary atherosclerosis. Myocardial ischemia occurs rarely if the oxygen-carrying capacity of the blood is reduced, as in extremely severe anemia or in the presence of carboxyhemoglobin. Not infrequently, two or more causes of ischemia will coexist, such as an increase in oxygen demand due to left ventricular hypertrophy and a reduction in oxygen supply secondary to coronary atherosclerosis.

The normal coronary circulation is dominated and controlled by the myocardial requirements for oxygen. This need is met by the ability to vary considerably the coronary vascular resistance (and therefore blood flow) while the myocardium extracts a high and relatively fixed percentage of oxygen (Chap. 4). Normally, intramyocardial resistance arterioles demonstrate an immense capacity for dilation. With exercise and emotional stress, the changing oxygen needs affect coronary vascular resistance and in this manner regulate the supply of blood and oxygen (metabolic regulation). These same vessels adapt to physiologic alterations in blood pressure in order to maintain coronary blood flow at levels appropriate to myocardial needs (autoregulation). Although the large epicardial coronary arteries are capable of constriction and relaxation, in healthy persons they serve as conduits, and are referred to as *conductance vessels,* while the intramyocardial arterioles normally exhibit striking changes in tone and are therefore referred to as *resistance vessels.*

CORONARY ATHEROSCLEROSIS (See also Chap. 195) Epicardial coronary arteries are a major site of atherosclerotic disease. Subintimal collections of abnormal fat, cells, and debris, i.e., atherosclerotic plaques, develop at irregular rates in different segments of the epicardial coronary tree and lead eventually to segmental reductions in cross-sectional area. The relationship between pulsatile flow and luminal stenosis is complex, but experiments have shown that when a stenosis reduces the cross-sectional area by approximately 75 percent, a maximal increase in flow to meet increased myocardial demand is not possible. When the luminal area is reduced by more than approximately 80 percent, blood flow at rest may be reduced and minor further reductions of the stenotic orifice can cause dramatic limitations of coronary flow and myocardial ischemia.

Segmental atherosclerotic narrowing of epicardial coronary arteries is caused most commonly by the formation of a plaque, which is subject to fissuring, hemorrhage, and thrombosis. Any of these events can temporarily worsen the obstruction, reduce coronary blood flow, and cause clinical manifestations of myocardial ischemia, as described below. In addition, the location of the stenosis will influence the quantity of myocardium rendered ischemic and this will determine the severity of the clinical manifestations. Severe coronary narrowing and myocardial ischemia are frequently accompanied by the development of collateral vessels, especially when the narrowing develops gradually. When well developed, such vessels can provide sufficient blood flow to sustain the viability of the myocardium at rest, but not during circumstances of increased demand.

Once severe stenosis of a proximal epicardial artery has reduced the cross-sectional area by more than ~70 percent the distal resistance, vessels will dilate to reduce vascular resistance to maintain coronary blood flow. A pressure gradient develops across the proximal stenosis, poststenotic pressure falls, and when the resistance vessels are maximally dilated, myocardial blood flow becomes dependent on the pressure in the coronary artery distal to the obstruction. Once the resistance vessels are maximally dilated, alterations in myocardial oxygenation can be caused by changes in myocardial oxygen demand, by alterations in the caliber of the stenosed coronary artery caused by physiologic vasomotion, by pathologic spasm, or by small platelet plugs. All of these transient events can upset the critical balance between oxygen supply and demand and thus precipitate myocardial ischemia.

EFFECTS OF ISCHEMIA The inadequate oxygenation induced by coronary atherosclerosis may cause transient disturbances of the mechanical, biochemical, and electrical function of the myocardium. The abrupt development of ischemia usually affects a segment of left ventricular myocardium with almost instantaneous failure of normal muscle relaxation and contraction. The relatively poor perfusion of the subendocardium causes more intense ischemia of this portion of the wall. Ischemia of large segments of the ventricle will cause transient left ventricular failure and if the papillary muscles are involved, mitral regurgitation can complicate this event. When ischemic events are transient, they may be associated with angina pectoris, but if prolonged they can lead to myocardial necrosis and scarring with or without the clinical picture of acute myocardial infarction. Coronary atherosclerosis is a focal process that causes nonuniform ischemia. The resulting focal disturbances of ventricular contractility cause segmental bulging or dyskinesia and can greatly reduce the efficiency of myocardial pump function.

Underlying these mechanical disturbances are a wide range of abnormalities in cell metabolism, function, and structure. When oxygenated, the normal myocardium metabolizes fatty acids and glucose to carbon dioxide and water. With severe oxygen deprivation, fatty acids cannot be oxidized and glucose is broken down to lactate; intracellular pH becomes reduced as do the myocardial stores of high-energy phosphates, adenosine triphosphate (ATP), and creatine phosphate. Impairment of cell membrane function leads to leakage of potassium and uptake of sodium by myocytes. The severity and duration of the imbalance between myocardial oxygen supply and demand will determine whether the damage is reversible or whether it is permanent with the development of myocardial necrosis.

Ischemia also alters the electrical properties of the heart. The most characteristic early electrocardiographic changes represent repolarization abnormalities, as evidenced by inversion of the T wave and later by displacement of the ST segment (Chap. 178). Transient ST-segment depression often reflects subendocardial ischemia, while transient ST-segment elevation is thought to be caused by more severe transmural ischemia. Another important consequence of myocardial ischemia is electrical instability, since this may lead to ventricular tachycardia or ventricular fibrillation (Chap. 184). Most patients who die suddenly from ischemic heart disease do so because of the occurrence of ischemia-induced malignant ventricular arrhythmias (Chap. 30).

CLINICAL MANIFESTATIONS

ASYMPTOMATIC VERSUS SYMPTOMATIC CORONARY ARTERY DISEASE Postmortem studies on accident victims and military casualties in western countries have shown that coronary atherosclerosis often starts prior to age 20 and is widespread among adults who were asymptomatic during life. In addition, exercise stress tests in asymptomatic persons may show evidence of silent myocardial ischemia, i.e., exercise-induced electrocardiographic changes not accompanied by angina, and coronary angiography in such persons frequently reveal obstructive coronary artery disease. Postmortem studies in patients with obstructive coronary artery disease who had no history of myocardial ischemia frequently show macroscopic scars of myocardial infarction in regions supplied by diseased coronary arteries. In addition, population studies have shown that approximately 25 percent of patients with acute myocardial infarctions may not reach medical attention and that these carry the same adverse prognosis as those in whom the classic clinical syndrome (Chap. 190) develops. *Sudden death* may be unheralded and is a common presenting manifestation of coronary disease (Chap. 30). Patients can also present with cardiomegaly and heart failure secondary to ischemic damage to left ventricular myocardium that caused no symptoms prior to the development of heart failure, a condition referred to as *ischemic cardiomyopathy*. In contrast to the asymptomatic phase of ischemic heart disease, the *symptomatic* phase presents with chest pain due either to angina pectoris or acute myocardial infarction (Chap. 190). Once having entered the symptomatic phase, the patient may exhibit a stable or progressive course, revert to the asymptomatic stage, or die suddenly.

Angina pectoris This is an episodic clinical syndrome resulting from transient myocardial ischemia. Various diseases that result in myocardial ischemia as well as the numerous pain syndromes with which it may be confused are discussed in Chap. 4. Approximately 80 percent of patients with angina pectoris, and an even greater fraction of those younger than 50 years of age, are male. The typical patient with angina is a 50- to 60-year-old man who seeks medical help for troublesome or frightening chest discomfort, usually described as heaviness, pressure, squeezing, smothering, or choking, and only rarely as frank pain. When the patient is asked to localize the sensation, he or she will typically press on the sternum, sometimes with a clenched fist, to indicate a squeezing central, substernal site of the discomfort. This symptom is usually crescendo-decrescendo, lasting 1 to 5 min. Angina can radiate to the left shoulder and to both arms, and especially to the ulnar surfaces of the forearm and hand. It can also arise in or radiate to the back, neck, jaw, teeth, and epigastrium.

Although angina is typically caused by exertion (e.g., exercise, hurrying, or sexual activity) or emotion (e.g., stress, anger, fright, or frustration) and is relieved by rest, it may also occur at rest and at night while the patient is recumbent (angina decubitus). The patient may be awakened at night distressed by typical chest discomfort and dyspnea. The pathophysiology of nocturnal angina may be similar to that of paroxysmal nocturnal dyspnea (Chap. 182) with the development of transient left ventricular failure due to expansion of the intrathoracic blood volume that occurs with recumbency and a resultant increase in cardiac size and myocardial oxygen demand.

The threshold for the development of angina pectoris may vary with the time of day and the patient's emotional state. The typical patient may have to stop because of symptoms at exactly the same spot on the way to work each morning, yet by midday may be able to cover many times that distance without symptoms. After experiencing chest discomfort while shaving in the morning, a man might be able to perform moderately heavy manual labor later in the day after he has "warmed up." Angina is frequently precipitated by unfamiliar tasks, by a heavy meal, or by exposure to cold.

Sharp fleeting chest pain or prolonged dull aches localized to the left submammary area are rarely due to myocardial ischemia. However, angina pectoris may be atypical in location and may not be strictly related to provoking factors. This symptom can also exacerbate and remit over days, weeks, or months, and its occurrence can be seasonal.

Systematic questioning of the patient with suspected ischemic heart disease is important to uncover a positive family history of ischemic heart disease, diabetes, hyperlipidemia, hypertension, cigarette smoking, and other risk factors for coronary atherosclerosis.

In *variant (Prinzmetal's) angina,* the chest discomfort characteristically occurs at rest or awakens the patient from sleep. It can be accompanied by palpitations or severe shortness of breath, may be explosive in onset, severe, and frightening. It may also be brought on by effort, although the workload at which it is precipitated usually varies considerably. Variant angina is caused by focal spasm of proximal epicardial coronary arteries; in approximately three-fourths of the patients atherosclerotic coronary artery obstruction is present, and in them the vasospasm occurs near the stenotic lesion.

PHYSICAL EXAMINATION The physical examination is usually normal. The patient's general appearance may reveal signs and risk factors associated with coronary atherosclerosis such as xanthelasma, xanthomas (Chap. 195), or diabetic skin lesions. There may also be signs of anemia, thyroid disease, and nicotine stains on the fingertips from cigarette smoking. Palpation can reveal thickened or absent peripheral arteries, signs of cardiac enlargement, and abnormal contraction (akinesia or dyskinesia) of the cardiac impulse. Examination of the fundi may reveal increased light reflexes and arteriovenous nicking as evidence of hypertension, while auscultation can uncover arterial bruits, a third and/or fourth heart sound, and when acute ischemia or previous infarction impairs papillary muscle function, a late apical systolic murmur due to mitral regurgitation. These ausculatory signs are best appreciated with the patient in the left decubitus position. Aortic stenosis, aortic regurgitation (Chap. 187), and hypertrophic cardiomyopathy (Chap. 192) must be excluded, since these disorders may cause angina even in the absence of coronary artery disease. Examination during an anginal attack is useful, since ischemia can cause transient left ventricular failure with the appearance of a third and/or fourth heart sound, a dyskinetic cardiac apex, mitral regurgitation, and even pulmonary edema.

LABORATORY EXAMINATION Although the diagnosis of ischemic heart disease can be made with confidence from a typical history, a number of simple laboratory tests can be most helpful. The urine should be examined for evidence of diabetes mellitus and renal disease, since both of these conditions may accelerate atherosclerosis. Similarly, examination of the blood should include measurements of lipids (cholesterol and high-density lipoproteins), glucose, creatinine, hematocrit, and, if indicated from the physical examination, thyroid function. The chest x-ray is an important test, since the consequences of ischemic heart disease, i.e., cardiac enlargement, ventricular aneurysm, or signs of heart failure, may be evident. Calcification of the coronary arteries can sometimes be identified by chest fluoroscopy. These signs can provide confirmation of the diagnosis of coronary artery disease and are important in assessing the degree of cardiac damage and the effects of treatment.

ELECTROCARDIOGRAM A normal ECG does not exclude the diagnosis of ischemic heart disease; however, certain characteristic abnormalities in tracings obtained at rest can confirm it. A 12-lead ECG recorded at rest is normal in about half of the patients with typical angina pectoris, but there may be signs of old myocardial infarction (Chap. 178). Serial tracings are particularly useful to look for evolving signs of infarction. Repolarization abnormalities, i.e., T-wave and ST-segment changes and intraventricular conduction disturbances at rest, are suggestive of ischemic heart disease but they are nonspecific, since they can also occur in pericardial, myocardial, and valvular heart disease or with anxiety, changes in posture, drugs, or esophageal disease. Typical ST-segment and T-wave changes which accompany episodes of angina pectoris and which disappear thereafter are more specific. The most characteristic changes include displacement of the ST segment that is similar in every way to that induced during a stress test (see below). The ST segment is usually depressed during angina but may be elevated, sometimes strikingly so, as in the early stages of myocardial infarction and in Prinzmetal's angina.

STRESS TESTING The most widely used test in the diagnosis of ischemic heart disease involves recording the 12-lead ECG before, during, and after exercise on a treadmill or using a bicycle ergometer. The patient undergoes a standardized incremental increase in external workload while the ECG, symptoms, and arm blood pressure are continuously monitored. The test is usually symptom-limited, and is discontinued with the onset of chest discomfort, severe shortness of breath, dizziness, fatigue, ST-segment depression of greater than 2 mm, a fall in systolic blood pressure exceeding 15 mmHg or the development of ventricular tachyarrhythmias. This test seeks to establish the relationship between chest discomfort and the typical electrocardiographic signs of myocardial ischemia. The ischemic ST-segment response is generally defined as flat depression of the ST segment of *more* than 0.1 mV below the baseline (i.e., the PR segment) and lasting *longer* than 0.08 s. This type of depression is designated a square wave or ''plateau'' type and is flat or downsloping. Upsloping or junctional ST-segment changes are not considered characteristic of ischemia and do not constitute a positive test. T-wave abnormalities, conduction disturbances, and ventricular arrhythmias developing during exercise should be noted but are also not diagnostic.

Based on the above criteria, the rate of false-positive diagnoses, using the coronary arteriogram as the ''gold standard,'' is approximately 15 percent, and an approximately equal percentage of patients with severe, multivessel coronary artery will not have a positive test (false-negative). The incidence of false-negative tests is higher in young women without angina and much lower in men over 45 years with typical angina pectoris. There is an increased incidence of false-positive tests in women, in patients taking cardioactive drugs such as digitalis and quinidine, or in those with conduction disturbances, resting abnormalities of the ST segment and the T wave, myocardial hypertrophy, or abnormal serum potassium levels. It should be noted that the posterior surface of the heart is less accessible to the electrocardiogram and therefore more silent clinically. Negative exercise tests in which the target heart rate (85 percent of maximal heart rate for age and sex) is not achieved are considered to be nondiagnostic. It is important to emphasize that according to Bayes' theorem the probability that ischemic heart disease exists in the population under study (pretest probability) must be considered in accord with the diagnostic features of the test in order to interpret a positive or negative test result (Fig. 2-2). For example, a positive exercise result indicates that the likelihood of coronary artery disease is 98 percent in patients with typical angina pectoris, 88 percent in those with atypical chest pain, 44 percent in those patients with nonanginal chest pain, and 33 percent in asymptomatic persons.

The physician should be present throughout the exercise test, and it is important to measure total duration of exercise, the external work performed, and the internal cardiac work performed, as represented by the heart rate–blood pressure product with the time to the onset of ischemic ST-segment change and chest discomfort. It is also important to note the depth of the ST-segment depression and the time for recovery of these electrocardiographic changes. Because the risks of exercise testing are small but real, equipment for resuscitation should be available. The risks are estimated at one fatality and two nonfatal complications per 10,000 tests. Modified (heart rate–limited rather than symptom-limited) exercise tests can be performed safely in patients as early as 10 days after myocardial infarction.

The normal response to exercise includes a progressive increase in heart rate and blood pressure. Failure of the blood pressure to increase or an actual decrease in blood pressure during the test is an important adverse prognostic sign, since it may reflect ischemia-induced global left ventricular dysfunction. The presence of pain or severe ST-segment depression at a low workload and ST-segment depression persisting for more than 5 min after the termination of exercise all increase the specificity of the test and point to the presence of severe ischemic heart disease.

The exercise test can be enhanced by the intravenous administration of a radioisotope such as thallium 201 to assess regional myocardial perfusion by means of a gamma camera, with images recorded immediately after exercise (to identify acute ischemia) and 2 to 4 h later to discriminate between reversible ischemia and infarction (Fig. 179-7). Another radioisotope, most often technetium 99m, can be used to label the blood pool for gated radioisotope angiography. This technique (Fig. 179-6) can provide a measure of ventricular volume, ejection fraction, and regional ventricular wall motion at rest and during exercise, and can identify transient global and regional left ventricular dysfunction due to myocardial ischemia. A reduction in ejection fraction during exercise with the appearance of regional wall motion abnormalities represent important signs of myocardial ischemia and suggests the presence of severe ischemia and/or multivessel coronary disease.

The two-dimensional echocardiogram records cross-sectional images of the left ventricle and can identify regional wall motion abnormalities resulting from myocardial infarction (Chap. 179). In this way this test too can be used as an aid in the diagnosis of ischemic heart disease.

CORONARY ARTERIOGRAPHY (Chap. 180) This invasive diagnostic method outlines the coronary anatomy and can provide important evidence of coronary atherosclerosis or can exclude this condition. The severity of obstructive lesions and the global and regional function of the left ventricle can be assessed. Coronary arteriography is indicated in (1) patients with chronic stable or unstable angina pectoris who are refractory to medical therapy and who are being considered for revascularization, i.e., percutaneous transluminal coronary angioplasty or coronary artery bypass graft surgery; (2) patients with troublesome symptoms that present diagnostic difficulties and in whom there is need to establish or rule out coronary artery disease; and (3) patients suspected of having left main stem or three-vessel coronary artery disease, regardless of the presence or severity of symptoms.

Examples of other particular clinical situations include:

1 Patients with chest discomfort suggestive of angina pectoris but a negative exercise test who require a definitive diagnosis for guiding medical management, alleviating psychological stress, career or family planning, or for insurance purposes.

2 Patients who have been admitted to the hospital several times for suspected acute myocardial infarction but in whom this diagnosis has not been established and in whom the presence or absence of coronary artery disease should be determined.

3 Patients with responsible careers that involve the safety of others (e.g., airline pilots) who have questionable symptoms and suspicious or positive noninvasive tests and in whom there are reasonable doubts about the state of the coronary arteries.

4 Patients with aortic stenosis or hypertrophic cardiomyopthy and angina in whom the pain could be due to coronary artery disease.

5 Patients after myocardial infarction who are at high risk because of an unstable state characterized by angina, heart failure, or frequent ventricular premature contractions.

6 Patients with angina pectoris, regardless of severity, in whom noninvasive testing reveals signs of severe ischemia [e.g., marked (>2 mm) ST-segment depression], development of one large or multiple perfusion defects in thallium-201 scintigrams during exercise, and/or global left ventricular dysfunction at rest or precipitated by exercise.

PROGNOSIS The three principal prognostic indicators in patients with ischemic heart disease are the functional state of the left ventricle, the location and severity of coronary arterial narrowing, and the severity or activity of myocardial ischemia. Compromise of left ventricular function may be indicated by symptoms and signs of heart failure, roentgenographic evidence of cardiac enlargement, and by angiographic evidence of elevated left ventricular end-diastolic pressure and ventricular volume, and reduced ejection fraction. Patients with chest discomfort but normal left ventricular function and normal coronary arteries have an excellent prognosis. In patients with normal left ventricular function, mild angina, and critical (>70 percent luminal diameter) stenoses of one, two, or three epicardial coronary arteries, the 5-year mortality rates are approximately 2, 8, and 11 percent, respectively. Critical stenosis of the left main coronary artery is accompanied by a mortality of about 15 percent per year. With any degree of obstructive coronary artery disease, mortality is greatly increased when left ventricular function is impaired; conversely at any level of left ventricular function, prognosis is influenced importantly by the quantity of myocardium perfused by critically obstructed vessels. In addition, at any level of left ventricular function and degree of obstructive coronary artery disease the mortality is related to the rate of progression of the underlying atherosclerotic process. The development of unstable angina and severe ischemia in an exercise stress test reflects rapid progression.

It is useful to consider coronary atherosclerosis to be a process that destroys myocardial tissue, thereby reducing cardiac reserve at an unpredictable rate. The larger the amount of myocardial necrosis, the less the ability to tolerate additional damage and the poorer the prognosis. In this light, the various indexes of ischemic damage, such as an ECG showing evidence of old infarction or symptoms or signs of heart failure or cardiac enlargement, should be taken as indications of myocardial damage. Obstructive lesions of the proximal left anterior descending coronary artery are associated with a greater risk than are lesions of the right or left circumflex coronary artery since they usually perfuse a greater quantity of myocardium.

Frequent angina pectoris that is difficult to control with medical therapy, angina following myocardial infarction, a fall in ejection fraction associated with the development of regional wall motion abnormalities during exercise, and a strongly positive exercise test for myocardial ischemia at low workloads (>2 mm ST segment depression) all indicate that myocardial ischemia is severe and reflect a poor prognosis.

The segmental atherosclerotic plaques in epicardial arteries show phases of cellular activity, degeneration, endothelial instability, vasomotion, platelet aggregation, and fissuring or hemorrhage. These factors could also temporarily cause worsening of the stenosis and abnormal reactivity of the vessel and thus exacerbate the manifestations of ischemia.

MANAGEMENT

Each patient must be evaluated individually with respect to life patterns, risk factors, control of symptoms, and prevention of damage to left ventricular myocardium. The degree of the patient's disability and the specific physical and emotional stresses that precipitate pain must all be carefully recorded in order to set the proper goals for treatment. The management plan should consist of (1) explanation and reassurance, (2) reduction of risk factors in an attempt to slow the progression of coronary atherosclerosis, (3) treatment of coexisting conditions capable of aggravating angina, (4) sensible adaptations of activities to minimize anginal attacks, (5) a program of drug therapy, and (6) definition of end points that will indicate the need to consider mechanical revascularization.

EVALUATION AND REASSURANCE Patients with ischemic heart disease need to understand their condition as best they can and to realize that a long and useful life is possible even though they suffer from angina pectoris or have experienced and recovered from an acute myocardial infarction. Offering case histories of persons in public life who have lived with coronary disease can be of great value when encouraging patients to resume or maintain activity and return to their occupation.

REDUCTION OF RISK FACTORS (See also Chap. 195) Although there is no definitive proof that the lesions of coronary atherosclerosis in human beings can be made to regress, extrapolation from animal experiments makes this appear possible. Even more likely, the rate of progression of coronary atherosclerosis may be retarded by reduction of risk factors, which is important in the management of patients with coronary atherosclerosis. Ideal weight should be attained and maintained, hypertension treated if present, and cigarette smoking forbidden. Diabetes and hyperlipidemia, when present, should be treated. Unless angina is provoked, the patient should be encouraged to engage in steady dynamic exercise such as walking; isometric exercise may be hazardous. By maintaining good physical condition, the patient will be able to perform physical work more efficiently and at a lower pulse rate, thus reducing the frequency of anginal episodes. Patients in good physical condition may also have a better chance of surviving a myocardial infarction.

ELIMINATION OF COEXISTING ILLNESS A number of illnesses that are not primarily cardiac in nature may either increase oxygen demand or decrease oxygen supply to the myocardium and may precipitate or exacerbate angina. In the former category, hypertension and hyperthyroidism may be treated successfully in order to reduce anginal frequency. Decreased myocardial oxygen supply may be due to reduced oxygenation of the blood (e.g., with intrinsic pulmonary disease or carboxyhemoglobin due to cigarette or cigar smoking) or decreased oxygen-carrying capacity (e.g., in anemia). Correction of these abnormalities, if present, may reduce or even eliminate angina pectoris.

ADAPTATION OF ACTIVITIES Therapy of ischemic heart disease consists of eliminating the discrepancy between the demand of the heart muscle for oxygen and the ability of the coronary circulation to meet this demand. Most patients will understand this fundamental concept and utilize it in the rational programming of activity. Many tasks that ordinarily evoke angina may be accomplished without symptoms simply by reducing the speed at which they are performed. Patients must appreciate the diurnal variation in their tolerance of certain activities and should reduce their energy requirements in the morning and immediately after meals. It is sometimes helpful to alter the eating pattern and take small and more frequent meals.

It may be necessary to recommend a change in employment or residence to avoid physical stress; however, with the exception of manual laborers, most patients with ischemic heart disease can usually continue to function merely by allowing more time to complete each task. In some patients, anger and frustration may be the most important factors precipitating myocardial ischemia. If these cannot be avoided, tranquilizing and sedative drugs should be used, although caution is necessary when prescribing any of these agents for a prolonged time. A treadmill exercise test to determine the approximate heart rate at which ischemic electrocardiographic changes or symptoms develop may be helpful in the development of a specific exercise program. Ambulatory electrocardiography during daily activities may also be helpful in this regard.

DRUG THERAPY **Nitrates** This is the most valuable class of drugs in the management of angina pectoris. These drugs act by causing systemic venodilatation, thereby reducing myocardial wall tension and oxygen requirements, as well as by dilating the epicardial coronary vessels and increasing blood flow in collateral vessels. The activity of these agents depends on their absorption, which is most rapid and complete through the mucous membranes. For this reason, nitroglycerin is administered sublingually in tablets of 0.4 or 0.6 mg. Patients with angina should be instructed to take the medication both to relieve an attack and also in anticipation of stress that is likely to induce an attack. When the patient experiences discomfort on exertion, he or she should cease activity and place a tablet under the tongue. The discomfort generally disappears more rapidly with nitroglycerin than would be expected if the drug were not administered. Walking up a flight of stairs or up a hill or sexual intercourse may produce angina consistently, and this can often be prevented by the anticipatory use of nitroglycerin. The value of this *prophylactic* use of the drug cannot be overemphasized.

The dose of nitroglycerin should be sufficient to relieve discomfort but not so large as to produce hypotension, headache, or a feeling of pulsating fullness in the head. The latter is the most common side effect of nitroglycerin and fortunately only rarely becomes disturbing at a dose required to relieve or prevent angina. Nitroglycerin deteriorates with exposure to air, moisture, and sunlight, so that if it produces neither relief of discomfort nor headache, nor a slight sensation of burning at the sublingual site of absorption, the preparation may be inactive and a fresh supply should be obtained. If relief is not attained with the first dose of nitroglycerin, a second or third dose may be given, but the patient should be instructed not to continue to take the medication if the first few doses prove unsuccessful. If discomfort continues for more than 7 to 10 min despite nitroglycerin, the patient should consult the physician or report promptly to a hospital emergency room for evaluation of possible acute myocardial infarction (Chap. 190).

Asking the patient with recently diagnosed angina pectoris to keep a diary of the time of occurrence of pain relative to activity and other precipitating factors with nitroglycerin consumption is often helpful to the physician attempting to tailor a management program. A diary may also be valuable for detecting changes in the frequency or severity of discomfort that may signify the development of unstable angina pectoris (p. 981) and/or herald an impending myocardial infarction.

Unfortunately, none of the long-acting nitrates is as effective as sublingual nitroglycerin for the relief of angina. These preparations can be swallowed, chewed, or administered as a patch or paste by the transdermal route. They can provide effective plasma levels for up to 24 h, but the therapeutic response is highly variable, and tolerance often develops. Different preparations and increased dosage should be used in an attempt to relieve discomfort in the individual patient while avoiding side effects. Useful preparations include isosorbide dinitrate (5 to 20 mg sublingual every 3 h or 5 to 40 mg PO tid), nitroglycerin ointment (0.5 to 2.0 in qid), or sustained-release transdermal patches (5 to 25 mg per day). Individual dose titration is important in order to avoid headache and dizziness. Long-acting nitrates are relatively safe and can be used together with intermittent sublingual nitroglycerin to relieve discomfort and prevent attacks of angina.

Beta-adrenoceptor blockade (see also Chap. 66) Beta-adrenoceptor blockade represents an important component of the pharmacologic treatment of angina pectoris. These drugs reduce myocardial oxygen demand by inhibiting the increases in heart rate and myocardial contractility caused by adrenergic activity. Beta blockade reduces these variables most strikingly during exercise while causing only small reductions in heart rate, cardiac output, and arterial pressure at rest. Propranolol is usually administered in an initial dose of 20 to 40 mg four times a day and is increased as tolerated to 320 mg per day in divided doses; sometimes higher doses are required. Long-acting beta-blocking drugs (atenolol 50 to 100 mg per day and nadolol, 40 to 80 mg per day) offer the advantage of once-a-day dosage (see Table 66-1). The therapeutic aims include relief of angina and effective inhibition of exercise-induced increases in heart rate. These drugs can produce fatigue, impotence, cold extremities, intermittent claudication, and bradycardia, and can worsen disturbed cardiac conduction, left ventricular failure, bronchial asthma, or intensify the hypoglycemia produced by oral hypoglycemic agents and insulin. Reducing the dose or even discontinuation of the drug may be necessary if these side effects develop and persist.

Calcium channel antagonists Nifedipine (10 to 40 mg qid), verapamil (80 to 120 mg tid), and diltiazem (30 to 90 mg qid) are all coronary vasodilators that produce a variable and dose-dependent reduction in myocardial oxygen demand, contractility, and arterial pressure. These combined pharmacologic effects are of advantage and make these agents quite effective in the treatment of angina pectoris. Verapamil and diltiazem can produce symptomatic disturbances in cardiac conduction and bradyarrhythmias and all three of these agents can cause left ventricular failure, particularly when used in combination with beta-adrenergic blockers in patients with underlying left ventricular dysfunction. Although useful effects are usually achieved when calcium channel antagonists are combined with beta-adrenoreceptor blockers and nitrates, individual titration of doses is essential with these potent combinations. Variant (Prinzmetal's) angina responds particularly well to calcium channel antagonists, supplemented when necessary by nitrates.

Treatment of angina and heart failure Patients with angina pectoris may also have evidence of cardiac enlargement and elevated ventricular diastolic pressures and volume. This increases left ventricular wall tension and thereby raises myocardial oxygen demand. Agents that are useful in the treatment of congestive heart failure, such as digitalis and diuretics (Chap. 182), may also be useful in the management of patients with angina and heart failure since they decrease heart size, wall tension, and myocardial oxygen demands. Nocturnal angina can often be favorably affected by these agents; however, there is no benefit and possibly aggravation of angina when these drugs are used in patients with a normal heart size and no evidence of heart failure. The nitrates can also have beneficial effects on angina and heart failure.

MECHANICAL REVASCULARIZATION It is important to appreciate that the basic management of patients with a lifelong condition such as ischemic heart disease is medical. The years of medical management may be punctuated by mechanical revascularization, as described below, but these important interventions do not replace the continuing need to ease symptoms and modify risk factors.

Percutaneous transluminal coronary angioplasty (PTCA) PTCA is a widely used method to achieve revascularization of the myocardium in patients with symptomatic ischemic heart disease and suitable proximal stenoses of epicardial coronary arteries. Whereas patients with stenosis of the left main coronary artery and those with distal three-vessel coronary artery disease who require revascularization are best treated by coronary artery bypass surgery (CAS), the use of PTCA in patients with symptomatic proximal stenoses of one or two vessels, and even selected cases with three-vessel disease, is widely employed and may have many advantages over CAS.

The method is described in Chap. 180 and illustrated in Figs. 180-6 and 180-7. After a flexible guidewire is advanced into a coronary artery and across the stenosis to be dilated, a miniature balloon catheter is advanced over the guidewire and into the stenosis followed by repeated inflations until the stenosis is decreased or relieved. The development of a range of guiding catheters, steerable guidewires, and low-profile balloon catheters and the use of high inflation pressures have all helped to decrease complications, reach more distal lesions, and dilate more complex stenoses.

INDICATIONS AND PATIENT SELECTION The most common clinical indication is angina pectoris, stable or unstable, which should be accompanied by evidence of ischemia in an exercise test. This symptom should be sufficiently severe to warrant the consideration of bypass graft surgery. Some physicians will perform angioplasty on asymptomatic or mildly symptomatic patients with suitable stenosis of the left anterior descending coronary artery and severe ischemia on an exercise stress test. PTCA can also be used to dilate stenoses in native coronary arteries and in bypass grafts in patients who have recurrent angina following CAS. This is an important indication when considering the technical difficulties and the increased mortality that accompanies reoperation. Angioplasty has also been carried out in patients with recent total occlusion (within 3 months) of a coronary artery and severe angina; in this group the primary success rate is decreased to approximately 50 percent.

RISKS Two and three vessels can be dilated in sequence with a modest increase in risk. Female gender, the presence of left ventricular damage, a stenosis of an artery which perfuses a large segment of myocardium without collaterals, long eccentric or irregular stenoses, and calcified plaques all increase the likelihood of complications. The major complications are usually due to dissection or thrombosis with vessel occlusion, uncontrolled ischemia, and ventricular failure. In the most experienced hands, the overall mortality rate should be less than 1 percent, the need for emergency coronary surgery is 3 to 5 percent, and myocardial infarction occurs in approximately 3 percent of cases. Minor complications occur in 5 to 10 percent of patients and include occlusion of a branch of a coronary artery, and complications of arterial catheterization.

EFFICACY Primary success, i.e., adequate dilation with relief of angina, occurs in 85 to 90 percent of cases. Recurrent stenosis of the dilated vessels occurs in 15 to 40 percent of cases within 6 months of the procedure, and angina will recur within 6 to 12 months in 25 percent of cases. This recurrence of symptoms and restenosis is more common in patients with unstable angina and with incomplete dilatation of the stenosis. It is usual clinical practice to administer aspirin, persantine, and a calcium blocker for months after the procedure; however, there are no controlled clinical trials that prove that these medications reduce the incidence of restenosis.

If patients do not develop restenosis or angina during the first year following angioplasty, the prognosis for maintenance of improvement for the subsequent 4 years is excellent. If restenosis occurs, the success rate of repeat PTCA is marginally better than the first procedure.

Between 15 and 30 percent of patients with symptomatic coronary artery disease who require revascularization can be treated by PTCA and need not undergo CAS. Successful angioplasty is less invasive and expensive than CAS, requires only 2 to 3 days in the hospital, and permits considerable savings in the cost of care. Successful PTCA also allows earlier return to work and the resumption of an active life.

Coronary artery surgery (CAS) A section of a vein (usually the saphenous) is used to form a connection between the aorta and the coronary artery distal to the obstructive lesion. Alternatively, anastomosis of the left internal mammary artery to the coronary artery distal to the obstructive lesion may be employed.

Some indications for CAS are controversial, but certain areas of agreement exist:

1 The operation is relatively safe, with mortality rates less than 1 percent when it is performed by an experienced surgical team in selected patients with normal left ventricular function.

2 Intraoperative and postoperative mortality increase with ventricular dysfunction and surgical inexperience. The effectiveness and risk of CAS vary widely depending on the skill and experience of the surgical team. Therefore the selection of patients must take into account the results of the team which will perform the procedure.

3 Occlusion is observed in 10 to 20 percent of vein grafts during the first year, the incidence is ~2 percent per year during 5 to 7 year follow-up and ~5 percent per year thereafter. Long-term patency rates are higher for internal mammary artery implantations, and in patients with left anterior descending coronary artery obstruction coronary bypass with an internal mammary artery results in better survival than venous bypass grafting.

4 Angina is abolished or unequivocally reduced in 85 percent of patients following complete revascularization. Although this is usually associated with graft patency and restoration of blood flow, the pain may also be improved as a result of infarction of the ischemic segment or a placebo effect.

5 CAS does not appear to reduce the incidence of myocardial infarction in patients with chronic ischemic heart disease; perioperative myocardial infarction occurs in 5 to 10 percent of cases but in most instances these infarcts are small.

6 Mortality is reduced by operation in patients with stenosis of the left main coronary artery. Some reduction in mortality also occurs in patients with three-vessel coronary artery disease and impaired left ventricular function. There is no evidence that CAS reduces mortality in patients with one- or two-vessel disease who have chronic stable angina and normal left ventricular function or in patients with one-vessel disease and impaired left ventricular function. There is conflicting evidence concerning the effects of operation on survival in patients with impaired left ventricular function and obstructive disease of two coronary arteries, one of which is the proximal left anterior descending artery.

7 Other important considerations which affect the outcome include the age of the patient as well as accompanying medical problems such as diabetes mellitus, obesity, and renal disease.

Indications for CAS are usually based on the severity of symptoms, coronary anatomy, and ventricular function. The ideal candidate is less than 70 years of age, has no other complicating disease, has troublesome or disabling symptoms which are not adequately controlled by medical therapy, wants to lead a more active life, and has severe stenoses of several epicardial coronary arteries with objective evidence of myocardial ischemia as a cause of the chest discomfort. Great symptomatic benefit can be anticipated in such patients. When disturbance of left ventricular function coexists, CAS may, in addition, prolong life.

UNSTABLE ANGINA PECTORIS

This condition includes four groups of patients: (1) patients with angina pectoris of recent onset (within 6 weeks) that is troublesome and frequent; (2) patients with angina of any duration that occurs at rest; (3) patients with chronic stable angina with a recent increase in intensity, frequency, or duration of pain; and (4) patients with angina pectoris developing or becoming more severe within days or weeks of acute myocardial infarction. Unstable angina, particularly groups 2 and 4 defined above, carries an adverse prognosis, with a high risk of acute myocardial infarction, sudden death, and the development of intractable chronic stable angina. In short, the course tends to be unstable in these patients—hence its name. When unstable angina is accompanied by objective electrocardiographic evidence of transient myocardial ischemia, it is almost always associated with critical stenoses in one or more major epicardial coronary arteries. Less than 10 percent of such patients have normal coronary arteries at arteriography. The atherosclerotic lesions may have a complicated morphology with evidence of superimposed thrombosis in approximately one-fourth of cases. Segmental spasm in the vicinity of atherosclerotic plaques may also play a role in the development of unstable angina. The diagnosis of unstable angina is made on the basis of the history and transient ST-segment changes, most commonly depressions, and/or T-wave inversions occurring during episodes of chest pain.

Management The patient should be admitted promptly to the hospital for observation, further diagnosis, and treatment. It is important immediately to identify and treat concomitant conditions which can intensify ischemia such as uncontrolled hypertension and diabetes, cardiomegaly, heart failure, arrhythmias, and any acute febrile illness. Acute myocardial infarction should be ruled out using serial electrocardiograms and measurements of plasma cardiac enzyme activity.

Continuous elecrocardiographic monitoring should be carried out and the patients should receive reassurance and sedation. Beta-adrenergic blocking drugs and calcium channel antagonists should be administered, but with caution, noting all of the side effects discussed above. Dosages must be titrated to avoid bradycarida, heart failure, and hypotension. Nitroglycerin should be given by the sublingual route. In addition, intravenous nitroglycerin is quite effective, but requires continuous monitoring of intraarterial pressure. It is begun at a dosage of 5 μg/min and raised in 5-μg/min increments to a level at which chest pain is abolished, but systolic arterial pressure is maintained or reduced only slightly and other side effects are avoided. Thrombus formation frequently complicates the atheromatous narrowing of coronary arteries in this condition. Therefore, intravenous heparin should be given for 3 to 5 days to maintain the partial thromboplastin time at 2 to 2.5 times control, followed by oral coumadin and aspirin at a dose of 325 mg per day.

The majority of patients will improve on this treatment. However, the clinical outcome is highly variable. If angina and objective evidence of ischemia do not diminish within 24 to 48 h of treatment in patients in whom there are no obvious contraindications for revascularization, then cardiac catheterization and coronary arteriography should be performed. If the anatomy is suitable, PTCA can be performed with surgical standby. If this cannot be done, CAS should be considered to relieve symptoms and myocardial ischemia and as a means of preventing myocardial damage. If the patient's symptoms and signs are controlled on medical therapy, a diagnostic exercise electrocardiogram should be obtained at the time of discharge from hospital, and the patient can be managed as outlined above for chronic stable angina pectoris. However, it should be recognized that among those patients with unstable angina who respond to medical therapy, severe coronary artery disease is usually present, and although angina may become stable, it often remains severe and ultimately mechanical revascularization is necessary.

ASYMPTOMATIC ISCHEMIA

Both obstructive coronary artery disease and myocardial ischemia are frequently asymptomatic. During continuous ambulatory electrocardiographic (Holter) monitoring, the majority of patients with typical chronic stable angina are found to have objective evidence of myocardial ischemia (ST-segment deviation) during episodes of chest discomfort while they are active outside of the hospital, but most of these patients also appear to have more frequent episodes of asymptomatic ischemia. In addition, there is a large, but as yet unknown, number of totally asymptomatic people with severe coronary atherosclerosis who exhibit ST-segment changes during activity.

The widespread use of exercise electrocardiography during routine examinations has defined some of these heretofore unrecognized patients with asymptomatic coronary artery disease. Longitudinal studies of young military personnel have demonstrated an increased incidence of coronary events (sudden death, myocardial infarction, and angina) in asymptomatic patients with positive exercise tests. In addition, patients who are asymptomatic after suffering a myocardial infarction are nonetheless at far greater risk for a second coronary event than is the general population. Patients with asymptomatic ischemia should be subjected to a detailed noninvasive examination, utilizing stress electrocardiography and radionuclide scintigraphy.

Management of patients with asymptomatic ischemia must be individualized. Thus, the physician should consider the following: (1) the degree of positivity of the exercise test, the stage of exercise at which electrocardiographic signs of ischemia appear, and/or the magnitude of the perfusion defect on thallium scintigraphy; (2) the electrocardiographic leads showing a positive response, with changes in the anterior precordial leads indicating a less favorable prognosis than changes in the inferior leads; (3) the patient's age and occupation. Most would agree that an asymptomatic 45-year-old commercial airline pilot with 4-mm ST-segment depression in leads V_1 to V_4 during mild exercise should undergo coronary arteriography, while the asymptomatic, sedentary 75-year-old retiree with 1-mm ST-segment depression in leads II and III during maximal activity need not. However, there is no consensus about the appropriate procedure in the majority of patients for whom the situation is less extreme. Patients with evidence of severe ischemia on noninvasive testing should be subjected to coronary arteriography and depending on the findings should be considered for revascularization. Thus, asymptomatic patients with three-vessel coronary disease and impaired left ventricular function and asymptomatic patients with left main coronary artery disease may be considered appropriate candidates for CAS.

While the incidence of asymptomatic ischemia can be reduced by treatment with beta blockers and calcium antagonists, it is not clear whether this is necessary or desirable in patients who have not suffered a myocardial infarction. However, there is evidence that beta-adrenoceptor blockade begun 7 to 35 days after acute myocardial infarction improves survival. This therapy is recommended in asymptomatic patients as long as there are no contraindications such as heart failure, bradycardia, heart block, and asthma.

REFERENCES

AMBROSE JA et al: Angiographic evolution of coronary artery morphology in unstable angina. J Am Coll Cardiol 7:472, 1986

BRAUNWALD E (ed): Symposium on experimental and clinical aspects of coronary vasoconstriction. Am J Cardiol 56(Suppl):1E, 1985

——— et al (eds): Surgery in the treatment of coronary artery disease. Circulation 72(Suppl):V1, 1985

BREDLAU CE et al: In-hospital morbidity and mortality in patients undergoing elective coronary angioplasty. Circulation 72:1044, 1985

CHRISTIE LG et al: Systematic approach to evaluation of angina-like chest pain: Pathophysiology and clinical testing with emphasis on objective documentation of myocardial ischemia. Am Heart J 102:897, 1981

COHN PF, BRAUNWALD E: Chronic ischemic heart disease, in *Heart Disease*, 2d ed, E Braunwald (ed): Philadelphia, Saunders, 1984, p 1334

——— (ed): *Diagnosis and Therapy of Coronary Artery Disease*, 2d ed. Boston, Little, Brown, 1985

GOTTLIEB SO et al: Effect of the addition of propranolol to therapy with nifedipine for unstable angina pectoris: A randomized, double-blind, placebo-controlled trial. Circulation 73:331, 1986

HOMMA A et al: Usefulness of oral dipyridamole suspension for stress thallium imaging without exercise in the detection of coronary artery disease. Am J Cardiol 57:503, 1986

HULTGREN HN et al: Treatment of unstable angina. JAMA 253:2555, 1985

MADDAHI J et al: Noninvasive identification of left main and triple vessel coronary artery disease: Improved accuracy using quantitative analysis of regional myocardial stress distribution and washout of thallium-201. J Am Coll Cardiol 7:53, 1986

190 ACUTE MYOCARDIAL INFARCTION

RICHARD C. PASTERNAK / EUGENE BRAUNWALD / JOSEPH S. ALPERT

Myocardial infarction is one of the commonest diagnoses occurring in hospitalized patients in western countries. In the United States, approximately 1.5 million myocardial infarctions occur each year. Mortality with acute infarction is approximately 35 percent, with slightly more than half of the deaths occurring before the stricken individual reaches the hospital. An additional 15 to 20 percent of survivors die in the first year following myocardial infarction. Risk of excess mortality persists in patients who recover; indeed, the age-corrected risk of death is increased 3.5 times as long as 10 years after infarction.

CLINICAL PRESENTATION *Pain* is the most common presenting complaint in patients with myocardial infarction. In some instances, the discomfort may be severe enough to be described as the worst pain the patient has ever experienced (Chap. 4). The pain of myocardial infarction is deep and visceral; adjectives commonly used to describe it are *heavy, squeezing,* and *crushing*. It is similar in character to the discomfort of angina pectoris but is usually more severe and lasts much longer. Typically the pain involves the central portion of the chest and/or epigastrium, and in about 30 percent of cases it radiates to the arms. Less common sites of radiation include the abdomen, back, lower jaw, and neck. The location of the pain beneath the xiphoid and patients' denial that they may be suffering a heart attack are chiefly responsible for the mistaken diagnosis of indigestion. The pain of myocardial infarction may radiate as high as the occipital area but not below the umbilicus. The pain is often accompanied by weakness, sweating, nausea, vomiting, giddiness, and anxiety. The discomfort usually commences with the patient at rest and more commonly in the morning than at any other time of day. However, when it begins during a period of exertion, in contrast to angina pectoris, it does not usually subside with cessation of activity.

Although pain is the most common presenting complaint, it is by no means always present; a minimum of 15 to 20 percent of myocardial infarcts are *painless*. The frequency of such silent infarcts is probably even higher than this estimate because patients without pain may not seek medical attention. The incidence of painless infarcts is greater in patients with diabetes mellitus, and it increases with age. In the elderly, myocardial infarction may present as sudden-onset breathlessness, which may progress to pulmonary edema. Other less common presentations, with or without pain, include sudden loss of consciousness, a confusional state, a sensation of profound weakness, the appearance of an arrhythmia, or merely an unexplained drop in arterial blood pressure.

PHYSICAL FINDINGS In many instances the dominant feature of the patient's presentation is the reaction to the chest pain. Patients are typically anxious and restless, attempting to relieve the pain by moving about in bed, squirming, stretching, belching, or even inducing vomiting. This is in contrast to the discomfort of angina pectoris, which causes the patient to remain relatively immobile for fear of making the discomfort reappear. Pallor is common and is often associated with perspiration and coolness of the extremities. The combination of substernal chest pain persistent for more than 30 min and diaphoresis strongly suggests acute myocardial infarction. Although many patients have a normal pulse rate and blood pressure, within the first hour of infarction about one-fourth of patients with anterior infarction have manifestations of sympathetic nervous system hyperactivity (tachycardia and/or hypertension), and up to one-half with inferior infarction show evidence of parasympathetic hyperactivity (bradycardia and/or hypotension).

The precordium is usually quiet, and the apical impulse may be difficult to palpate. In about one-fourth of patients with anterior wall infarction, an abnormal systolic pulsation develops in the periapical area within the first days of the illness and then may resolve. Other physical signs of ventricular dysfunction that may be present include, in decreasing incidence, fourth (S_4) and third (S_3) heart sounds, decreased intensity of heart sounds, and, rarely, paradoxical splitting of the second sound (Chap. 177). A transient apical systolic murmur, presumably due to mitral regurgitation secondary to papillary muscle dysfunction during acute infarction, may be midsystolic or late systolic in timing. A pericardial friction rub is heard in many patients with transmural myocardial infarction at some time in their course if they are examined frequently. Jugular venous distention occurs commonly in patients with right ventricular infarction. The carotid pulse is often decreased in volume despite a normal upstroke. Temperature elevations in the range of 37 to 38°C may be observed during the first week following acute myocardial infarction; however, a temperature exceeding 38°C should prompt a search for other causes. The arterial pressure is variable; in most patients with transmural infarction systolic pressure declines approximately 10 to 15 mmHg from the preinfarction state.

LABORATORY DIAGNOSIS The laboratory tests of value in confirming the diagnosis of myocardial infarction may be divided into three groups: (1) nonspecific indexes of tissue necrosis and inflammation, (2) the electrocardiogram, and (3) serum enzyme changes.

The *nonspecific reaction* to myocardial injury is associated with polymorphonuclear leukocytosis, which appears within a few hours after the onset of pain, persists for 3 to 7 days, and often reaches levels of 12,000 to 15,000 leukocytes per cubic millimeter. The erythrocyte sedimentation rate rises more slowly than the white blood cell count, peaking during the first week, and sometimes remaining elevated for 1 or 2 weeks.

The *electrocardiographic manifestations* of acute myocardial infarction are described in Chap. 178. Although electrocardiographic/pathologic correlations are not excellent, transmural infarction is diagnosed if the electrocardiogram demonstrates Q waves or loss of R waves; nontransmural infarction is said to be present if the electrocardiogram shows only transient ST-segment and sustained T-wave changes. However, these changes are variable and nonspecific and should not form the sole basis for the diagnosis of infarction. Therefore, a more rational nomenclature for designating electrocardiographic infarction would be *Q-wave* or *ST-T-wave infarction* in place of the terms *transmural* or *nontransmural infarction*, respectively.

SERUM ENZYMES Enzymes are released in large quantities into the blood from necrotic heart muscle following myocardial infarction. The rate of liberation of specific enzymes differs following infarction, and the temporal pattern of enzyme release is of diagnostic importance. The time course of the serum concentration of the most commonly used enzymes is shown in Fig. 190-1. Levels of two of the enzymes, serum glutamic oxaloacetic transaminase (SGOT) and creatine phosphokinase (CK), rise and fall rapidly, while that of lactic dehydrogenase (LDH) rises later and remains elevated longer. SGOT has the disadvantage that it is also present in skeletal muscle, liver, and red blood cells and may be liberated from these extracardiac stores. SGOT is less widely used than heretofore because of its lack of specificity and because of its time course, which is intermediate between CK and LDH, making the information redundant in most cases. The MB isoenzyme of CK has an advantage over SGOT in that it is not present in significant concentrations in extracardiac tissue, and therefore it is more specific than SGOT. Since rises in serum concentration of CK and SGOT are short-lived, they may be missed if initial blood samples are obtained more than 48 h after the infarct develops. MB-CK isoenzymes are particularly useful when skeletal muscle and/or brain damage are suspected since both tissues contain large quantities of the enzyme but none of the MB isoenzyme. The myocardial specificity of the MB isoenzyme determination depends on the technique used for measurement. Radioimmunoassay techniques are most specific, but the more commonly employed gel electrophoresis technique is significantly less specific and therefore prone to more frequent false positives. In myocardial infarction, the level of LDH rises during the first day, peaks at 3 to 4 days, and returns to normal in 14 days. Five common LDH isoenzymes may be separated by starch-gel electrophoresis. Tissues differ with respect to the specific isoenzyme patterns; the rapidly migrating isoenzyme which predominates in the heart is referred to as LDH_1, while the slowly migrating components predominate in liver and skeletal muscle. LDH_1 rises before total LDH in patients with myocardial infarction and may rise when there is no change in total LDH. Therefore, increased LDH_1 is a more sensitive indicator of myocardial infarction than total LDH; sensitivity exceeds 95 percent.

Of particular clinical importance is the fact that a two- to threefold elevation of total CK (not MB-CK) may follow an intramuscular injection. This may lead to the erroneous diagnosis of myocardial infarction in a patient who has been given an intramuscular injection of a narcotic for chest pain of noncardiac origin. Other potential sources of total CK elevation worthy of note are (1) muscular diseases including muscular dystrophy, myopathies, and polymyositis, (2) electrical cardioversion, (3) cardiac catheterization, (4) hypothyroidism, (5) stroke, (6) surgery, and (7) skeletal muscle damage secondary to trauma, convulsions, and prolonged immobilization. Cardiac surgery and electrical cardioversion often result in elevation of serum levels of MB isoenzyme.

It has long been recognized that the amount of enzyme released correlates with the size of the infarct. It has been demonstrated that the mass of heart muscle infarcted can be estimated from analysis of

FIGURE 190-1 *The time course of serum enzyme concentration changes following a typical myocardial infarction. CK, creatinine phosphokinase; LDH, lactic dehydrogenase; GOT, glutamic oxaloacetic transaminase.*

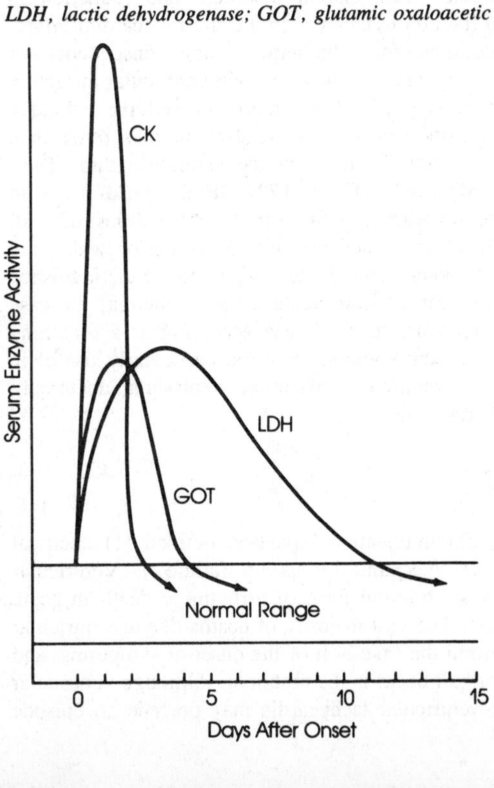

the concentration-time curve of the enzyme if the kinetics of the release, degradation, disposal, etc., of the enzyme are known. The size of an infarct in terms of grams of infarcted tissue can be estimated from an analysis of the MB-CK–time curve. While the *area* under the MB-CK–time curve is related to infarct size, the *absolute* value of the peak MB-CK and its time to peak are related to the kinetics of MB-CK washout from myocardium. The opening of a coronary artery occlusion (either spontaneously, or by mechanical or pharmacologic means) in the early hours of myocardial infarction will cause early peaking (at about 1 to 3 h following reperfusion) of the MB-CK–time curve. However, the total area under the curve may be smaller than without reperfusion, reflecting smaller overall infarction size.

Characteristic rises occur in serum enzyme concentration in more than 95 percent of patients with clinically proven myocardial infarction. CK, LDH, and SGOT levels generally do not rise in unstable angina. Many patients with suspected infarction have baseline enzyme levels which are normal and increase threefold in a pattern consistent with infarction, although the absolute level of enzyme in the blood never exceeds the upper limits of normal. This situation is most commonly observed in patients with small infarctions and, although not diagnostic, is highly suggestive of acute infarction. Isoenzyme studies are particularly helpful in this situation.

Several radionuclide imaging techniques are of value in the diagnosis or assessment of the patient with acute myocardial infarction (Chap. 179). Acute infarct scintigraphy (''hot-spot'' imaging) is carried out with an infarct-avid imaging agent such as ^{99m}Tc stannous pyrophosphate. Scans are usually positive 2 to 5 days after infarction, particularly in patients with transmural infarcts; although they aid in *localizing* infarcts and provide a measure of infarct size (page 887), these scans are less accurate than CK determination for making the *diagnosis* of myocardial infarction. Myocardial perfusion imaging with thallium 201, which is taken up and concentrated by viable myocardium, reveals a defect (''cold spot'') in most patients during the first few hours after development of a transmural infarct. This localized area of decreased radioactivity may fill in during the following hours (page 887). However, it is not possible to distinguish acute infarcts from chronic scars. Therefore, while thallium scanning is extremely sensitive for the detection of myocardial infarction, it is not specific for *acute* myocardial infarction. Radionuclide ventriculography, carried out with ^{99m}Tc-labeled red blood cells (page 886), frequently demonstrates wall motion disorders and reduction in ventricular ejection fraction in patients with acute myocardial infarction. While of value in assessing the hemodynamic consequences of infarction, and in aiding in the diagnosis of right ventricular infarction when the right ventricular ejection fraction is depressed, the technique is quite nonspecific, since many cardiac abnormalities other than myocardial infarction alter the radionuclide ventriculogram. Two-dimensional echocardiography (Chap. 179) can also be of value in patients with acute myocardial infarction. Abnormalities of wall motion, particularly of the septal and inferior-posterior walls, are readily detectable. Although acute infarction cannot be distinguished from old myocardial scar or from acute severe ischemia, the ease and safety of the procedure make its use appealing as a screening tool. Additionally, echocardiography may be particularly useful in the diagnosis of right ventricular infarction, ventricular aneurysm, and left ventricular thrombus.

MANAGEMENT

Two general classes of complications have been defined: (1) electrical (arrhythmias) and (2) mechanical (''pump failure''). Ventricular fibrillation is the most common form of arrhythmic death in acute myocardial infarction. The vast majority of deaths due to ventricular fibrillation occur within the first 24 h of the onset of symptoms, and of these deaths, over half occur in the first hour. Although ventricular premature beats or ventricular tachycardia may precede an episode of ventricular fibrillation, the latter often occurs without warning arrhythmias. This observation has led to the use of lidocaine in the prophylactic treatment of ventricular ectopic activity in acute myocardial infarction. The focus of coronary care has shifted from resuscitation to prevention, and the incidence of primary ventricular fibrillation has diminished markedly in the last two decades. Reduction of in-hospital mortality for acute myocardial infarction from about 30 to less than 10 percent is in large measure the result of institution of measures such as rapid transfer of patients with acute myocardial infarction to facilities with ECG monitoring capability staffed by personnel (not necessarily physicians) knowledgeable in the recognition and immediate treatment of ventricular arrhythmias.

With sudden and unexpected in-hospital arrhythmic deaths essentially eliminated by the preventive approach to ventricular arrhythmias, attention has turned to the other major complication of acute myocardial infarction, i.e., pump failure. Although advances have been made in the treatment of pump failure, it remains the primary cause of in-hospital death from acute myocardial infarction. The extent of ischemic necrosis correlates well with the degree of pump failure and with mortality, both early, i.e., within 10 days of infarction, and later as well. A clinical classification dependent on the status of cardiac pump function originally proposed by Killip divides patients into four groups as follows: class I, no signs of pulmonary or venous congestion; class II, moderate heart failure as evidenced by rales at the lung bases, S_3 gallop, tachypnea, or signs of failure of the right side of the heart including venous and hepatic congestion; class III, severe heart failure, pulmonary edema; class IV, shock with systolic pressure less than 90 mmHg and evidence of peripheral constriction, diaphoresis, peripheral cyanosis, mental confusion, and oliguria. The expected hospital mortality rate of patients in these clinical classes has been established by a number of investigators as follows: class I, 0 to 5 percent; class II, 10 to 20 percent; class III, 35 to 45 percent; and class IV, 85 to 95 percent.

GENERAL CONSIDERATIONS Given the information summarized above, the principal objectives of management of the patient with myocardial infarction are to prevent death from arrhythmia and to minimize the mass of infarcted tissue.

Arrhythmias can usually be managed successfully if trained personnel and appropriate equipment are available when this complication develops. Since mortality from arrhythmia is greatest during the first few hours after infarction, it is obvious that the effectiveness of coronary care units relates directly to the speed with which patients come under medical observation. The biggest delay usually is not in transportation to the hospital but rather between the onset of pain and the patient's decision to call for help. This delay can best be reduced by education of the public concerning the significance of chest pain and the importance of seeking early medical attention.

A number of ''common sense'' rules in the management of acute myocardial infarction deserve particular emphasis. First and foremost, it is mandatory to maintain an optimal balance between myocardial oxygen supply and demand in order to salvage as much as possible of the jeopardized zone of myocardium surrounding the center of the infarct. Therapeutic strategies that help to attain this goal include rest, analgesia, mild sedation, and a quiet atmosphere in order to reduce anxiety and thereby lower heart rate, a major determinant of myocardial oxygen consumption.

Marked sinus bradycardia (heart rate less than approximately 45 beats per minute) should be treated by leg elevation and atropine or by electrical pacing, particularly if the bradycardia is associated with a fall in blood pressure or with worsening ventricular arrhythmias. However, routine administration of atropine, with resultant increase in heart rate, to patients without serious bradycardia is not recommended. Patients with acute myocardial infarction who have a hyperdynamic state, i.e., tachycardia and elevation of arterial pressure, should be treated with a beta-adrenergic blocking agent. Initially, 0.1 mg/kg propranolol or 15 mg metoprolol given intravenously in three divided doses is safe, if there are no contraindications, such as heart failure, AV block, or asthma. All forms of tachyarrhythmias require prompt and direct treatment. Drugs that exert a positive inotropic effect, such as digitalis glycosides and cardioactive sympathomimetics, should be administered only if there is evidence of pronounced heart failure; they should not be given prophylactically. Of the various sympathomimetic amines available, isoproterenol with its chronotropic and vasodilator effects is the least desirable. Dobutamine (page 911), which has less effect on heart rate and systemic vascular resistance, is more desirable when it is necessary to augment cardiac contractility. Dopamine (page 911) is useful in patients with left ventricular failure and systemic hypotension (systolic pressure <90 mmHg. Diuretics are indicated in the presence of heart failure and should, in fact, be used prior to cardiac stimulants unless the patient is hypovolemic or hypotensive.

All patients should inhale oxygen-enriched air (see below). Particular attention must be paid to preserving arterial oxygenation in patients with hypoxemia, as occurs in patients with chronic pulmonary disease, pneumonia, or left ventricular failure. Severe anemia, which can also extend the area of ischemic injury, should be corrected by cautious administration of packed red blood cells, sometimes accompanied by a diuretic. Associated conditions, particularly infections with accompanying tachycardia and elevated myocardial oxygen demand, require immediate attention. Systolic arterial pressure should not be allowed to deviate by more than 25 to 30 mmHg from the patient's usual level.

Coronary care units Coronary care units have resulted in improved care of patients with myocardial infarction, reduction in mortality rates, and major increases in knowledge about myocardial infarction. The coronary care unit is a specially designed *nursing unit,* the most important feature of which is a staff of highly trained nursing personnel with authority to take immediate action in emergency situations. The unit should be equipped with a system which permits continuous monitoring of the electrocardiogram of each patient and hemodynamic monitoring in selected patients. Defibrillators, respirators, and facilities for introducing pacing catheters and flow-directed balloon-tipped catheters should be available. However, equipment alone does not ensure an effective coronary care unit. Of prime importance is the organization of a highly trained team of nurses who can recognize arrhythmias, adjust the dosage of antiarrhythmic drugs, and perform cardiac resuscitation, including the application of electroshock, when necessary. A physician should be available at all times, but many lives have been saved because nurses have treated ventricular tachycardia or fibrillation before the physician's arrival.

The policies and procedures for admission to a coronary care unit should ensure that patients are admitted early in their illness when they may expect to derive maximum benefit from the care provided. In order to accomplish this, the threshold for admission of patients with suspected infarction should be low, and this is best monitored in terms of the fraction of total admissions in whom myocardial infarction is eventually proven. In the past, all patients with suspected myocardial infarction were admitted to the coronary care unit. Currently, however, several factors have led to a change in this rule. The availability of electrocardiographic monitoring and trained personnel in "intermediate care units" has allowed admission of lower-risk patients (e.g., those not hemodynamically compromised or without active arrhythmias) to such units. For economic reasons, and to utilize limited facilities optimally, many institutions have developed guidelines to aid in triaging patients with suspected myocardial infarction. While most such patients in the United States are admitted to the hospital, in other countries, such as the United Kingdom, the patients at lowest risk may be cared for at home. Once admitted to the hospital the fraction of patients actually admitted to the coronary care unit may depend on a balance between the clinical status of the patient and bed availability. In some units beds are utilized primarily for patients with a complicated course, particularly those who require hemodynamic monitoring. Mortality rates for myocardial infarction treated in coronary care units vary from 5 to 20 percent; this variation can be explained, in part, by variations in admission policies as regard age limitations, the type of population being served, the nature of the hospital (tertiary care referral center versus community hospital), and other as yet unidentified factors.

REPERFUSION An occlusive or near-occlusive thrombus overlying or adjacent to an atherosclerotic plaque in a coronary artery appears to be the cause of most transmural infarcts. Therefore, reperfusion of the ischemic zone by the prompt dissolution of the thrombus with a thrombolytic agent is a logical approach to the reduction of infarct size. There is considerable evidence that if reperfusion is to be effective in salvaging jeopardized myocardium, it must be carried out immediately after the onset of the clinical event; certainly within 4 h, and preferably within 2 h.

Streptokinase (SK), administered via a coronary catheter, has been approved by the Food and Drug Administration (FDA) in the treatment of acute myocardial infarction. While the administration of this agent is effective in lysing the offending thrombus in about 75 percent of cases, many questions, such as whether or not this therapy reduces mortality or morbidity, remain unanswered, and its role in therapy remains to be established. Intravenous administration of SK appears to be less effective than intracoronary administration, but has the advantage of not requiring cardiac catheterization. Tissue plasminogen activator (tPA), when administered intravenously, lyses approximately two-thirds of recent coronary thrombi; it has the theoretical advantage of causing fibrinolytic activity predominantly at the site of a fresh thrombus, and thus may be safer than SK by virtue of causing a less intensive systemic lytic state than that produced by intravenous SK. However, even while the ideal thrombolytic agent is sought, it remains unclear whether such therapy will be effective in routinely salvaging myocardium, whether mechanical revascularization by means of coronary angioplasty or coronary bypass surgery will be required following successful thrombolysis in the majority of patients, and whether the mortality and morbidity of acute myocardial infarction can actually be reduced by this intervention. Studies are underway to address these issues. At the time of writing, as tPA is not available for widespread clinical use or approved by the Bureau of Biologics, the very early (<4 h from the onset of chest pain) administration of intravenous or, if possible within this time interval, intracoronary SK, followed by percutaneous transluminal coronary angioplasty (PTCA) if a severe (>80 percent luminal diameter) obstruction persists appears to be a reasonable approach to therapy. The necessity of having a well-trained angiography team "stand by" at all times, will limit this approach to a small fraction of patients with acute myocardial infarction. However, if studies which are presently underway indicate that the intravenous infusion of tPA, followed by coronary arteriography within 1 or 2 days, and if necessary by PTCA, salvages substantial myocardium in the majority of patients, a practical approach for the treatment of acute myocardial infarction will have been found. The tPA would be given intravenously as soon as the diagnosis was established; it could be administered in an emergency room, ambulance, physician's office, even in the patient's home or work site. The patient would then be taken to a center where coronary arteriography or PTCA could be carried out within 2 days. This would not require standby of trained personnel and specialized facilities.

Acute primary PTCA, i.e., without preceding thrombolysis, has also been reported to be effective in restoring effective reperfusion in acute myocardial infarction, but this technique is very expensive in terms of personnel and facilities.

The amount of myocardial tissue which becomes necrotic secondary to a vascular occlusion is determined by factors other than just the site of occlusion. One such important factor is the status of collateral blood supply to ischemic tissue. Myocardium well supplied by collaterals clearly has the capacity to survive hours longer than poorly collateralized areas. Infarct size is now known to vary with time and be affected by a number of therapeutic agents currently in use. The balance between myocardial oxygen supply and demand in areas rendered ischemic determines the ultimate fate of these areas of jeopardized myocardium. While no routine therapeutic approach to reduce infarct size in all patients is currently recommended, the realization that infarct size may be increased by interventions which adversely alter the supply-demand balance has prompted the reevaluation of previously accepted therapeutic maneuvers in the management of patients with acute infarction.

TREATMENT OF THE PATIENT WITH AN UNCOMPLICATED INFARCT **Analgesia** Since myocardial infarction usually presents with severe pain, one of the important initial therapeutic objectives is the relief of pain. Morphine, the agent traditionally used for this purpose, is an extremely effective analgesic for the pain associated with myocardial infarction. However, it may lower arterial pressure by reducing sympathetically mediated arteriolar and venous constriction. The resultant venous pooling may produce a reduction in cardiac output. This must be recognized but does not necessarily contraindicate its use. Hypotension associated with venous pooling usually responds promptly to elevation of the legs, but in some patients volume expansion with intravenous saline is required. The patient may experience diaphoresis and nausea, but these events usually pass and are replaced by a feeling of well-being associated with the relief of pain. It is important to recognize this syndrome as one attributable to morphine, rather than as a manifestation of the shock syndrome, so that inappropriate vasoconstrictor therapy is not initiated. Morphine also has a vagotonic effect and may cause bradycardia or advanced degrees of heart block, particularly in patients with posteroinferior infarction. These side effects of morphine usually respond to atropine (0.4 mg intravenously). Morphine is routinely administered by repetitive (every 5 min) intravenous injection of small doses of drug (2 to 4 mg) rather than by administration of a larger quantity by the subcutaneous route, by which absorption may be unpredictable. Meperidine hydrochloride or hydromorphone hydrochloride may be effectively employed in place of morphine.

Prior to administering morphine, sublingual nitroglycerin can be given safely to most patients with myocardial infarction. As long as hypotension does not occur, up to three 0.3-mg doses should be administered at about 5-min intervals. In addition to diminishing or abolishing chest discomfort, this form of therapy, once considered contraindicated in the setting of acute myocardial infarction, may be capable of both decreasing myocardial oxygen demand (by lowering preload) and increasing myocardial oxygen supply (by dilating infarct-related coronary vessels or collateral vessels). However, therapy with nitrates should be avoided in patients who present with a low systolic arterial pressure ($<$100 mmHg). The potential for an idiosyncratic reaction to nitrates, consisting of sudden marked hypotension and bradycardia, should be recognized. This problem, occurring more frequently in patients with inferior wall infarction, can usually be promptly reversed by the rapid administration of intravenous atropine.

Intravenous beta blockers are also useful in the control of the pain of acute myocardial infarction. These drugs have been shown to control pain effectively in some patients, presumably by diminishing ischemia consequent to lowering myocardial oxygen demand. More importantly, there is some evidence that intravenous beta blockers reduce in-hospital mortality, particularly in high-risk patients. Dosing similar to that used to treat the hyperdynamic state (see above) may be utilized.

Oxygen The routine use of oxygen is supported by the observation that the arterial P_{O_2} is reduced in many patients with myocardial infarction and that oxygen inhalation reduces the area of ischemic injury in experimental animals. Inhalation of oxygen increases arterial P_{O_2} and hence increases the concentration gradient responsible for the diffusion of oxygen into the ischemic myocardium from adjacent, better-perfused areas. Although oxygen therapy has been associated with theoretically deleterious effects such as elevation of systemic vascular resistance and slight reduction of cardiac output, the weight of evidence favors its administration. It should be administered by face mask or nasal prongs for the first day or two after infarction.

Activity Factors which increase the work of the heart may increase the size of the infarct. Circumstances in which heart size, cardiac output, or myocardial contractility are increased should be avoided. It has been demonstrated that 6 to 8 weeks are required for complete healing, i.e., replacement of the infarcted myocardium by scar tissue. The purpose of reduced physical activity is to provide the most favorable possible circumstances for this healing.

Most patients with myocardial infarction should be admitted to a coronary care unit or suitable monitoring facility and remain there for 2 to 4 days under constant observation by trained personnel utilizing continuous electrocardiographic monitoring. A catheter should be introduced into a peripheral vein, firmly fixed so that it is not easily dislodged, and be kept open either by the slow infusion of isotonic glucose solution or by a closed heparin lock. This provides a route of administration for antiarrhythmic or other drugs which may be necessary. In the absence of heart failure or other complications during the first 2 to 3 days, the patient should be in bed most of the day, with one or two periods of 15 to 30 min in a bedside chair. The patient may use a bedside commode and should be bathed but may eat unassisted. Bedside commode privileges are given to all hemodynamically stable patients with a stable rhythm from the first day. The bed should be equipped with a footboard, and the patient should push both feet against the footboard firmly 10 times during each waking hour to prevent venous stasis and thromboembolism and to maintain muscle tone in the legs.

By the third or fourth day the patient with an uncomplicated course should be spending at least 30 to 60 min in a chair twice a day. At this time the patient's blood pressure should be measured when standing in order to be aware of postural hypotension, which may be a problem when ambulation is begun. Standing and gradual ambulation are usually begun between the third and fifth days post infarction in patients with uncomplicated myocardial infarction. Initial walking is to the bathroom if it is in the patient's room or nearby. Ambulation is progressively increased, eventually including walks about the hospital floor. In many hospitals a cardiac rehabilitation program with progressive exercise is initiated in the hospital and continued after discharge. The total duration of hospitalization in uncomplicated cases is usually 7 to 12 days, but some physicians still hospitalize patients with Q-wave infarction for 3 weeks. Patients in clinical class II or higher may require 3 or more weeks of hospitalization, depending upon the rapidity with which heart failure resolves and the home situation to which the patient is returning. Many physicians perform a limited (heart rate–limited) exercise tolerance test just prior to discharge in selected patients with myocardial infarction. Such testing identifies high-risk patients as those who develop angina, ST-segment change, hypotension, or serious ventricular ectopic activity during or immediately following exercise. These patients require special attention, including measures such as antiarrhythmic drugs for ectopic activity, and beta-adrenergic blockers, long-acting nitrates, and/or calcium channel blocking agents for evidence of ischemia. If ischemia occurs at rest, or if during limited exercise ischemia and/or hypotension occur, coronary arteriography should be carried out. If a large quantity of viable myocardium, perfused by critically narrowed vessel(s), is found at angiography, then revascularization (either by operation or by angioplasty) may be required. Exercise tests also aid in formulating an individualized exercise prescription, which can be much more vigorous in patients who tolerate exercise without any of the above-mentioned adverse signs. Additionally, predischarge stress testing may provide an important psychological benefit related to building the patient's confidence through the demonstration of reasonable exercise tolerance. Furthermore, particularly when no arrhythmias or signs of ischemia are identified, the patient benefits by the physician's reassurance that objective evidence suggests no immediate jeopardy.

The remainder of the convalescent phase of myocardial infarction may be accomplished at home. From 3 to 8 weeks, the patient should be encouraged to increase activity by walking about the house and outdoors in good weather. Patients should still spend 8 to 10 h in bed each night. Additional rest periods in the morning and afternoon may be advisable for selected patients.

From 8 weeks onward, the physician must regulate the patient's activity on the basis of his or her exercise tolerance. It is during this period of increasing activity that the patient may become aware of profound fatigue. Postural hypotension may still be a problem. Most patients will be able to return to work after 12 weeks, and many patients much earlier. A maximal exercise test is frequently performed after 6 to 8 weeks or prior to returning to work. A trend toward earlier ambulation, hospital discharge, and resumption of full activity for patients recuperating from acute myocardial infarction has developed in recent years.

Diet During the first 4 or 5 days, a low-calorie diet divided into multiple small feedings is preferred. Cardiac output increases following ingestion of food, and therefore the quantity of individual feedings should be kept low. If heart failure is present, sodium intake should be restricted. Since constipation is common, it is reasonable to give average or even increased amounts of bulk in the diet. In addition, the ingestion of potassium-rich foods should be encouraged in patients receiving diuretics. During the second week, increasing amounts of food may be introduced into the diet. At this time, the importance of restriction of calories, cholesterol, and saturated fat may be explained to the patient, and he or she can be started on an appropriate diet. Willingness to accept dietary restriction and to discontinue cigarette smoking is usually never greater than it is during this early period of convalescence.

Bowels Bed rest of 3 to 5 days and the effect of the narcotics utilized for the relief of pain often lead to constipation. Most patients are not comfortable using a bedpan, which frequently results in excessive straining. A bedside commode, a diet rich in bulk, and the routine use of a stool softener such as dioctyl sodium sulfosuccinate, 200 mg daily, are recommended. If the patient remains constipated despite these measures, a laxative can be safely used. It is safe to perform a gentle rectal examination on patients with acute myocardial infarction.

Sedation Most patients require sedation during hospitalization in order to withstand the period of enforced inactivity with tranquillity. Diazepam 5 mg or oxazepam 15 to 30 mg given four times daily is usually effective. Appropriate sleeping medication may be given at night to ensure adequate sleep. Triazolam 0.25 to 0.5 mg is a rapid-onset, short-acting benzodiazepine ideal for inducing sleep. If maintenance of sleep is required, then temazepam 15 to 30 mg or flurazepam 15 to 30 mg can be used. Attention to this problem is especially important during the first few days in the coronary care unit, where the atmosphere of 24-h vigilance may interfere with the patient's sleep. Sedation is no substitute for reassuring, quiet surroundings.

Anticoagulants Few topics are more controversial than the use of anticoagulants in the routine treatment of acute myocardial infarction. The lack of a confirmed, statistically clear-cut demonstration of a lower mortality rate in the first few weeks following myocardial infarction suggests that the benefit of anticoagulant therapy, if any, is small. The use of anticoagulant therapy to retard the process of coronary occlusion during the initial phases of the illness, while not clearly justified, is undergoing renewed interest as a result of the recognition that thrombosis plays an important role in the pathogenesis of acute myocardial infarction. However, there is agreement that anticoagulant therapy does reduce the incidence of both arterial and venous thromboembolic complications. Since the incidence of venous thromboembolic disease is known to be increased in patients with heart failure, shock, and previous venous or thromboembolic disease, the routine, prophylactic use of anticoagulant drugs to prevent pulmonary embolism in the coronary care unit is recommended for those patients at high risk for this complication. Routine anticoagulation as prophylaxis against venous thromboembolism is not recommended in class I patients. Patients in classes III and IV are at greater risk for pulmonary embolism, and therefore systemic anticoagulation should be considered during the initial 10 to 14 days of hospitalization, or until they are ambulatory. This is best accomplished initially by the continuous intravenous administration of heparin with a constant infusion pump with measurement of the clotting time or partial thromboplastin time to define the need for increasing or decreasing the infusion rate. Once the patient is out of the intensive care area, oral anticoagulants may be substituted for heparin. Alternatively, small subcutaneous doses of heparin (5000 units every 8 to 12 h) can be employed. Controversy as to the need for anticoagulant therapy in class II patients persists. It seems appropriate to anticoagulate these patients if the signs of congestive heart failure persist for more than 3 or 4 days or if they have large anterior infarctions.

The incidence of arterial embolism from clot originating in the ventricle at the site of infarct is small but definite. Two-dimensional echocardiography allows for the early detection of left ventricular thrombi in about one-third of patients with anterior wall infarction but rarely in patients with inferior or posterior infarction. Arterial embolism often presents as a major complication, such as hemiparesis when the cerebral circulation is involved, or hypertension if the renal circulation is compromised. The low incidence of these complications, contrasted with their severity, renders it impractical to establish firm guidelines for the use of anticoagulant drugs as prophylaxis against arterial embolism in acute myocardial infarction. The likelihood of arterial embolism appears to increase with the extent of infarction and the resultant inflammation and endocardial stasis due to akinesis. Therefore, as is the case with venous thromboembolism, the indication for anticoagulation as prophylaxis against arterial embolism increases with the extent of infarction. When a thrombus has been clearly demonstrated by echocardiographic or other techniques, systemic anticoagulation should be undertaken (in the absence of contraindications), for the incidence of embolic complications appears to be markedly lowered by such therapy. The appropriate duration of therapy is unknown, but probably should be carried out for 3 to 6 months.

Beta-adrenergic blockers Use of intravenous beta-adrenergic blockers is discussed on page 986. The chronic routine use of oral beta-adrenergic blockers for at least 2 years following acute myocardial infarction is supported by several well-conducted placebo-controlled trials which have demonstrated reductions in total mortality, sudden death, and in some instances, the reinfarction rate. Patients are ordinarily begun on oral beta blockers 5 to 28 days following the acute event. Propranolol in a dose of 60 to 80 mg tid, or an equivalent dose of a more slowly acting beta blocker, is usually prescribed. Contraindications include congestive heart failure, bradyarrythmias, heart block, hypotension, asthma, and "brittle" insulin-dependent diabetes mellitis.

TREATMENT Arrhythmias (see also Chaps. 183 and 184) The improved management of arrhythmias constitutes a most significant advance in the treatment of myocardial infarction.

VENTRICULAR PREMATURE SYSTOLES Infrequent, sporadic ventricular premature depolarizations occur in almost all patients with infarction and do not require therapy. Suggested indications for suppression of ventricular ectopic beats are generally considered to be the following: (1) the presence of more than five isolated ectopic beats per minute, (2) the occurrence of consecutive or multifocal ventricular extrasystoles, and (3) the occurrence of ectopic ventricular beats early in diastole and hence superimposed on the T wave of the preceding beat (the so-called R-on-T phenomenon). Intravenous lidocaine has become the treatment of choice for ventricular premature beats and ventricular arrhythmias, because it acts rapidly and side effects disappear soon (15 to 20 min) after its administration is discontinued. Lidocaine is given as an intravenous bolus of 1 mg/kg to establish adequate blood levels quickly. This initial dose usually eliminates the ectopic activity, if present, and is followed by an infusion of 2 to 4 mg/min. An additional bolus of 0.5 mg/kg is given 10 min after the initial bolus if ectopy is still present. The dose should be reduced by half in patients with congestive heart failure, shock, or hepatic disease. Usually, ventricular premature beats spontaneously disappear after 72 to 96 h. If significant ventricular ectopic activity persists past this time, chronic antiarrhythmic therapy is often initiated.

Procainamide, tocainide, and quinidine are commonly used for the treatment of persistent ventricular ectopic activity; beta-adrenergic blocking agents and disopyramide are also effective in abolishing ventricular ectopic activity in infarction patients. The latter agent should be used with great care in patients with left ventricular failure since it has a significant negative inotropic action. If the usual doses of these drugs (Chap. 184), singly or in combination, are not effective, blood levels should be measured to ensure that adequate blood concentrations are being obtained. Frequent clinical and electrocardiographic assessment of the patient for signs of drug toxicity is mandatory when higher doses of these agents are employed.

VENTRICULAR TACHYCARDIA AND VENTRICULAR FIBRILLATION Within the first 24 h of myocardial infarction, ventricular tachycardia and fibrillation often occur without prior warning arrhythmias. The occurrence of such primary arrhythmias can be materially reduced by prophylactic administration of intravenous lidocaine. The use of prophylactic antiarrhythmic drug therapy is particularly well suited to patients who cannot reach a hospital or those treated in hospitals that lack constant physician presence in the coronary care unit. Sustained ventricular tachycardia is treated first with lidocaine, and if it cannot be terminated by one or two 50- to 100-mg doses, electroconversion should be employed (Chap. 184). Electroshock is used immediately in patients with ventricular fibrillation, or when ventricular tachycardia causes hemodynamic deterioration. If fibrillation has persisted for more than a few seconds, the first shock may be unsuccessful, and in this situation it is advisable to administer closed-chest massage, mouth-to-mouth respiration, and intravenous sodium bicarbonate solution (40 to 90 meq) before attempting electroconversion again. Improvement of oxygenation and perfusion and correction of acidosis increase the likelihood of successful defibrillation (see also Chap. 30). Bretylium is useful in the treatment of both refractory ventricular fibrillation and ventricular tachycardia. For ventricular fibrillation, bretylium is given as a 5-mg/kg bolus and defibrillation is again attempted. If the latter fails, a second bolus of 10 mg/kg is given to facilitate electroconversion of ventricular fibrillation. Ventricular tachycardia can be treated with bretylium 5 to 10 mg/kg injected slowly over 10 min. In either situation, the initial dose of bretylium may be followed by a continuous infusion of 2 mg/min if the arrhythmia is recurrent. Severe postural hypotension occurs after intravenous bretylium administration; therefore, patients should always be supine when and immediately after the drug is given, and intravenous fluids should be available for rapid administration if needed.

Long-term survival is good in patients with *primary* ventricular fibrillation, i.e., ventricular fibrillation resulting as a primary response to acute ischemia and not associated with predisposing factors such as congestive heart failure, shock, bundle branch block, or ventricular aneurysm. In one series, 87 percent of patients with primary ventricular fibrillation left the hospital alive. This prognosis is in sharp contrast to that for patients who develop ventricular fibrillation *secondary* to severe pump failure. Only 29 percent of patients in this group survived.

In patients who develop ventricular tachycardia late in their hospital course, the mortality in 1 year may be as high as 85 percent. Such patients warrant electrophysiologic study (Chap. 184).

ACCELERATED IDIOVENTRICULAR RHYTHM Accelerated idioventricular rhythm (AIVR, "slow ventricular tachycardia"), a ventricular rhythm with a rate of 60 to 100 beats per minute, occurs in 25 percent of patients with myocardial infarction. It is especially frequent in inferoposterior infarction, where it is usually associated with sinus bradycardia. The rate of AIVR is usually similar to that of the sinus rhythm which precedes and follows it, and this similarity of rate and the relatively minor hemodynamic effects make this rhythm difficult to detect other than by electrocardiographic monitoring. The rhythm comes and goes spontaneously as fluctuation in sinus rate causes the atrial rate to fall below the accelerated escape level. For the most part, this rhythm is benign and does not presage the development of classic ventricular tachycardia. However, a number of cases have been documented wherein AIVR was associated with more dangerous forms of ventricular ectopic activity or where AIVR degenerated into a potentially fatal ventricular arrhythmia. Most AIVR does not require treatment if the patient is monitored carefully since degeneration into a more serious arrhythmias is rare, and if it occurs, the AIVR can generally be readily treated with a drug which decreases the ventricular escape rate, such as tocainide, and/or one that increases the sinus rate (atropine).

SUPRAVENTRICULAR ARRHYTHMIAS The common arrhythmias in this group are junctional rhythm and tachycardia, atrial tachycardia, atrial flutter, and atrial fibrillation. These rhythm disturbances are often secondary to left ventricular failure. The administration of digoxin is usually the treatment of choice. If the abnormal rhythm persists for more than 2 h with a ventricular rate in excess of 120 beats per minute, or at any time when tachycardia induces heart failure, shock, or ischemia (as manifested by recurrent pain or ECG changes), electroshock should be utilized.

Junctional arrhythmias are of diverse etiology, are not indicative of any specific abnormality, and from a therapeutic viewpoint must be considered on an individual basis. Digitalis excess must be ruled out as a cause of junctional tachycardia. In some patients with severely compromised left ventricular function, the loss of appropriately timed atrial systole results in a marked decrease in cardiac output. Right atrial or coronary sinus pacing is indicated in such instances. The hemodynamic effects of these two modes of pacing are identical, but coronary sinus pacing offers the advantage of better catheter stability.

SINUS BRADYCARDIA The significance of bradycardia as a factor predisposing to ventricular fibrillation in acute myocardial infarction is controversial. While the incidence of ventricular tachycardia in patients with sustained bradycardia is twice that observed in patients with normal heart rates, sinus bradycardia has also been identified in hospitalized patients as an index of a favorable prognosis. Experience with mobile coronary care units indicates that sinus bradycardia occurring within the first hour after infarction is more consistently associated with ventricular ectopic rhythms than that occurring later in the course of the illness. Treatment of sinus bradycardia is indicated if significant ventricular ectopic activity is present or if hemodynamic compromise results from the slow heart rate. Elevation of the legs and/or the foot of the bed is frequently helpful in the treatment of sinus bradycardia. Atropine is the most useful drug for increasing heart rate and should be given intravenously in doses of 0.4 to 0.6 mg. If the rate remains below 60 beats per minute, additional doses of 0.2 mg, up to a total of 2.0 mg, may be given in divided doses. Persistent bradycardia ($<$ 40 beats per minute) despite atropine may be treated with electrical pacing. Isoproterenol should be avoided.

CONDUCTION DISTURBANCES Failure of conduction may develop at three different levels in the conduction system: the atrioventricular (AV) node, the bundle of His, or the more peripheral portions of the conduction system (Chap. 183). If the block occurs in the AV node, the escape rhythm usually originates in the AV junction, and the QRS complexes are usually of normal duration; but when the block occurs distal to the AV node, the escape site is ventricular, and the QRS configuration is abnormal and its duration is prolonged. Disturbances of conduction may occur in the three peripheral branches (fascicles) of the conduction system, and their recognition is of value in identifying patients at risk of developing complete heart block. When block occurs in any two of the three fascicles, bifascicular block is said to exist; complete AV block often develops in such patients. Thus, patients who develop the combination of right bundle branch block and either left anterior or left posterior hemiblock or patients with new left bundle branch block have a particularly high risk of progression to complete heart block.

The mortality rate of patients with complete AV block in association with anterior infarction (80 to 90 percent) is almost three times that of patients who develop AV block with inferior infarction (30 percent), and the risk of subsequent death in those who survive to leave the hospital is also increased in the former group. This difference is related to the fact that heart block in inferior infarction is usually caused by AV nodal ischemia. The AV node is a small discrete structure, and thus a small amount of ischemia or necrosis can result in AV nodal dysfunction. In anterior wall infarction, heart block is related to ischemic malfunction of all three fascicles of the conduction system and thus results only from extensive myocardial necrosis.

Electrical pacing provides an effective means of increasing the heart rate of patients with bradycardia due to AV block, but it is not possible to be sure that such acceleration is always beneficial. For example, in patients with anterior wall infarction and complete heart block, the large size of the infarct is the major factor determining the outcome, and correction of the conduction deficit does not clearly improve the poor prognosis in this group. Pacing does appear to be beneficial, however, in patients with inferoposterior infarction who have complete heart block associated with heart failure, hypotension, marked bradycardia, or significant ventricular ectopic activity. A subgroup of these patients, those with right ventricular infarction, often respond poorly to ventricular pacing because of the loss of the atrial "kick." In such patients, dual chamber, atrioventricular sequential pacing may be required.

Some cardiologists advocate the placement of a pacing catheter prophylactically in patients with conduction disturbances known to be precursors of complete heart block. Unanimity of opinion does not exist on this point. Permanent pacing has been advocated for patients who develop the combination of persistent bifascicular and transient third-degree heart block during the acute phase of myocardial infarction. Retrospective studies in small numbers of such patients suggest that the incidence of sudden death is decreased in those in whom permanent pacing was instituted.

Heart failure Some degree of transient impairment of left ventricular function occurs in over half of patients with myocardial infarction. The most common clinical signs are pulmonary rales and S_3 and S_4 gallop rhythms. Pulmonary congestion is also frequently seen on chest roentgenogram. However, roentgenographic signs of pulmonary congestion often fail to parallel, temporally, clinical evidence of pulmonary congestion, i.e., the presence of rales and dyspnea. Elevation of left ventricular filling pressure and pulmonary artery pressure are the characteristic hemodynamic findings, but it should be appreciated that these findings may result from a reduction of diastolic ventricular compliance (diastolic failure) and/or a reduction of stroke volume with secondary cardiac dilatation (systolic failure) (Chap. 181). The therapy of heart failure in association with myocardial infarction is similar to that of heart failure secondary to other forms of heart disease, with a few exceptions (Chap. 182). The major difference concerns the use of cardiac glycosides. The benefit following the administration of digitalis in acute myocardial infarction is unimpressive. This is not surprising since the function of the noninfarcted tissue may be normal and digitalis would not be expected to improve the systolic or diastolic dysfunction of infarcted or ischemic tissue. On the other hand, diuretic agents are extremely effective in the treatment of heart failure following myocardial infarction, since they diminish pulmonary congestion in the presence of systolic and/or diastolic heart failure. A fall in left ventricular filling pressure and an improvement in orthopnea and dyspnea follow the intravenous administration of furosemide. This drug should be used with caution, however, as it can result in a massive diuresis with associated decrease in plasma volume, cardiac output, systemic blood pressure, and hence coronary perfusion. Nitrates in various forms may be used to decrease preload and congestive symptoms. Oral isosorbide dinitrate or topical nitroglycerin ointment have the advantage over a diuretic of lowering preload through venodilatation without decreasing the total plasma volume. Additionally, nitrates may improve ventricular compliance if concurrent ischemia is present, since ischemia causes an elevation of left ventricular filling pressure. The patient with pulmonary edema is treated in the manner described in Chap. 182. Studies with vasodilators to reduce cardiac afterload indicate that the reduction in cardiac work, which results from the lowered afterload, may significantly improve left ventricular performance with a reduction of ventricular filling pressure and pulmonary congestion concomitant with an elevation of cardiac output.

Hemodynamic monitoring Hemodynamic evidence of abnormal left ventricular function becomes apparent when contraction is seriously impaired in 20 to 25 percent of the left ventricle. Infarction of 40 percent or more of the left ventricle usually results in the syndrome of cardiogenic shock (see below). Pulmonary capillary wedge pressure and pulmonary artery diastolic pressure correlate well with left ventricular diastolic pressure and are therefore often referred to as left ventricular filling pressures. Positioning of a balloon flotation catheter in the pulmonary artery enables the physician to monitor left ventricular filling pressure constantly, a technique which is useful in patients who exhibit clinical evidence of hemodynamic abnormalities or instability. Cardiac output can also be determined with a pulmonary artery catheter. With the addition of intraarterial pressure monitoring, systemic vascular resistance can be calculated as a guide to adjusting vasopressor and vasodilator therapy. Some patients with acute myocardial infarction have markedly elevated left ventricular filling pressures (>22 mmHg) and normal cardiac outputs [>2.6 and <3.6 (liters/min)/m²], while others have relatively low filling pressures (<15 mmHg) and reduced cardiac outputs. The former usually benefit from diuresis, while the latter respond to volume expansion by means of intravenous administration of colloid-containing solutions.

Cardiogenic shock—power failure With the development of effective methods for treating arrhythmias, cardiogenic shock has become the most important fatal complication of acute myocardial infarction for patients who reach the hospital. It occurs in approximately 10 percent of such patients and now accounts for about two-thirds of in-hospital deaths. Unfortunately, improvements in care have not affected the mortality rate in patients with acute myocardial infarction and cardiogenic shock (Killip class IV), which continues to be in the 85 to 95 percent range.

It is useful to consider cardiogenic shock as a form of severe left ventricular failure. This syndrome is characterized by marked hypotension with systolic arterial pressure <80 mmHg and a marked reduction of cardiac index [<1.8 (liters/min)/m²] in the face of elevated left ventricular filling (pulmonary capillary wedge) pressure >18 mmHg. Hypotension alone is not a basis for the diagnosis of cardiogenic shock, because many patients who make an uneventful recovery will have serious hypotension (systolic pressure <80 mmHg) for several days. Such patients often have low left ventricular filling pressures, and their hypotension usually resolves with intravenous administration of colloid-containing solutions. In cardiogenic shock hypotension is accompanied by other clinical signs of circulatory inadequacy. The following *clinical* criteria for cardiogenic shock define a population of patients with a mortality rate of >85 percent: (1) systolic arterial blood pressure <90 mmHg which has declined by at least 30 mmHg below the previous level; (2) clinical signs of peripheral circulatory insufficiency, e.g., cold, moist skin and cyanosis; (3) dulled sensorium; (4) oliguria with urine flow of less than 20 mL/h; and (5) failure of improvement following relief of pain and administration of oxygen. Specifically *excluded* are patients with hypotension secondary to vasovagal reaction, hypovolemia, arrhythmia, drug reaction, or sepsis.

PATHOPHYSIOLOGY OF PUMP FAILURE Marked reduction in the quantity of contracting myocardium is the cause of cardiogenic shock in myocardial infarction, although all organ systems are ultimately involved. The function of the heart is impaired by the initial insult; this results in a decrease in arterial pressure and hence in coronary blood flow because of its dependence on aortic perfusion pressure (Fig. 190-2). The reduction in coronary perfusion pressure and myocardial blood flow further impairs myocardial function and may increase the size of the myocardial infarction. Arrhythmias and metabolic acidosis also contribute to this deterioration because they are the result of inadequate perfusion, and both tend to perpetuate the precipitating conditions. It is this positive feedback loop which accounts for the high mortality rate associated with the shock syndrome.

Arterial blood pressure is a function of two factors—cardiac output and systemic vascular resistance—and a decrease in either without a compensatory rise in the other will result in a fall in arterial blood pressure. Cardiac output is lower in a population of patients with myocardial infarction and shock. However many patients with myocardial infarction without shock have cardiac outputs in the same range as those in patients with shock, and therefore it is not possible to characterize these patients on the basis of reductions of cardiac output alone. Systemic vascular resistance, the other factor important in determining blood pressure, may be either normal or increased in myocardial infarction. Normally, a fall in cardiac output is accompanied by a compensatory rise in systemic vascular resistance, but in patients with shock due to myocardial infarction, the appropriate elevation in resistance may fail to occur. However, it is necessary to return to the heart itself as the site of the fundamental physiologic alteration in cardiogenic shock.

A simple schematic diagram depicting the relationship between left ventricular work and filling pressure is seen in Fig 190-3. The upper curve represents the familiar Frank-Starling relationship in the normal heart; the lower curve shows the relation which might be expected in the patient with shock secondary to myocardial infarction. It is obvious that, at all levels of end-diastolic pressure, the left ventricular work of the patient with myocardial infarction is depressed. At point C, the end-diastolic pressure is elevated, but at point B, it may be normal despite the fact that myocardial work is well below that expected of the normal heart at this diastolic pressure, as indicated by point A.

FIGURE 190-2 *Diagram depicting the sequence of events in the vicious cycle in which coronary artery obstruction leads to cardiogenic shock and progressive circulatory deterioration.*

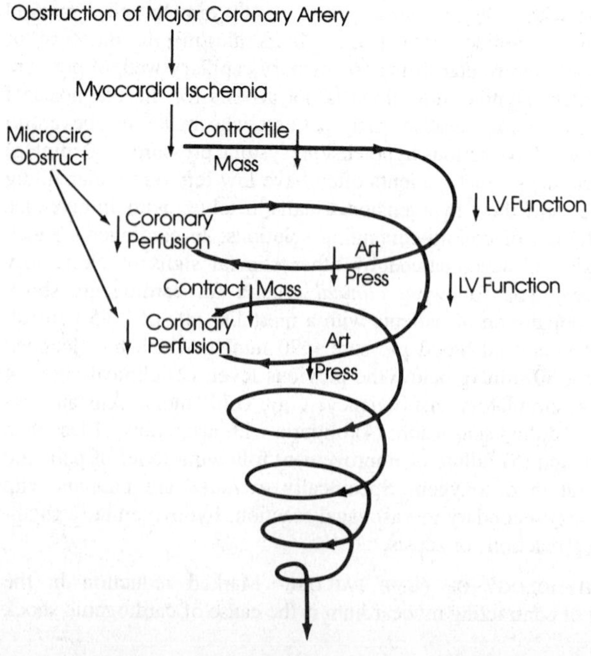

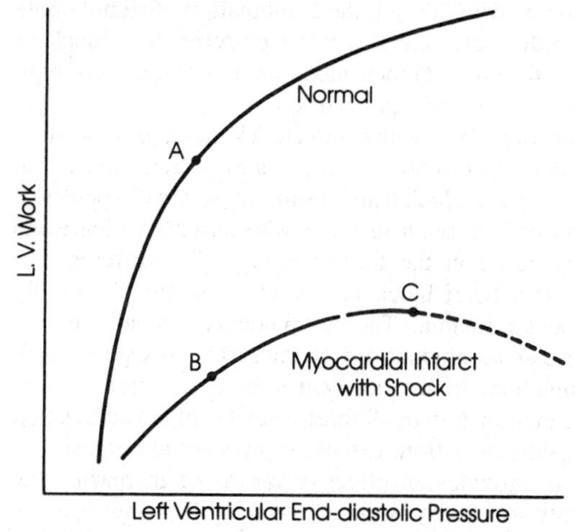

FIGURE 190-3 *Schematic representation of the Frank-Starling relationship as applied to patients with the shock syndrome in myocardial infarction.*

TREATMENT OF PUMP FAILURE The physiology and ominous prognosis associated with this condition dictate that all patients with shock should, if possible, have continuous monitoring of arterial pressure and of left ventricular filling pressure (as reflected in the pulmonary capillary wedge pressure measured with a pulmonary artery balloon catheter) as well as frequent determinations of cardiac output. All patients with the shock syndrome should receive 100% oxygen continuously to help combat the hypoxemia which is universally present. When pulmonary edema coexists, endotracheal intubation may be necessary to ensure oxygenation. The relief of pain is important, as some vasodepressor reflex activity may be a response to severe pain. However, narcotics should be used cautiously in view of their propensity to lower arterial pressure.

Treatment is directed at the interruption of the feedback loop (Fig. 190-2), whereby impaired myocardial function leads to a reduction in arterial pressure, decreased coronary blood flow, and further depression of left ventricular function. This objective is approached by attempting to maintain coronary perfusion by raising the arterial blood pressure with vasopressors (see below), intraaortic balloon counterpulsation, and manipulation of blood volume to a level that ensures an optimum left ventricular filling pressure (approximately 20 mmHg). The latter may require either infusion of crystalloid or diuresis. In patients seen within the first 4 h of the onset of infarction, reperfusion by thrombolytic therapy and/or PTCA (page 985) may improve left ventricular function dramatically.

Hypovolemia This is an easily corrected condition which may contribute to the hypotension and vascular collapse associated with myocardial infarction in some patients. Fluid loss may be secondary to previous diuretic use, to reduced fluid intake during the early stages of the illness, and/or to vomiting associated with pain or medications. In addition, a state of relative hypovolemia may exist; i.e., with the acute reduction in contractile function and ventricular compliance resulting from infarction an increase in vascular volume is needed to maintain cardiac output. Owing to the acute nature of the process, there is insufficient time for compensatory fluid retention to accommodate this need, and relative hypovolemia in a normally hydrated patient results. Consequently, hypovolemia should be identified and corrected in patients with acute myocardial infarction and hypotension before embarking upon more vigorous forms of therapy. If left ventricular filling pressure is in the normal range, fluid should be administered until the cardiac output is maximized. This usually occurs at a left ventricular filling pressure of approximately 20 mmHg. However, the optimal left ventricular filling or pulmonary artery wedge pressure may vary considerably among different patients. Each patient's ideal level is reached by cautious fluid administration during careful monitoring of oxygenation and cardiac output. When the cardiac output plateaus (Fig. 190-3, point C), further increases in left ventricular filling pressure will only increase congestive symptoms and decrease systemic oxygenation. Central venous pressure measurements reflect right rather than left ventricular filling pressure and are inadequate in this situation, since left ventricular function is almost always affected much more adversely than is right ventricular function in acute myocardial infarction.

VASOPRESSORS A variety of intravenous drugs may be used to augment arterial pressure and cardiac output in patients with cardiogenic shock. Unfortunately, all have important disadvantages or problems associated with their use, and none have been shown to change the outcome in patients with established shock. *Isoproterenol* is a synthetic sympathomimetic amine which is now rarely used in the treatment of shock due to myocardial infarction. Although this agent increases contractility, it also produces peripheral vasodilatation and increases heart rate. The resultant increase in myocardial oxygen consumption and reduction of coronary perfusion pressure may extend the area of ischemic injury. *Norepinephrine* is a potent alpha-adrenergic agent with powerful vasoconstrictive properties. It also possesses beta-adrenergic activity and therefore enhances contractility. Norepinephrine can be effective in raising arterial pressure, but usually the increase in afterload and contractility associated with its use cause a marked increase in myocardial oxygen consumption as well. It should be reserved for relatively desperate situations or for patients with cardiogenic shock and lowered systemic vascular resistance. It should be used at the lowest dose possible (begin infusion at 2 to 4 μg/min) to maintain systolic blood pressure near 90 mmHg. If pressure cannot be maintained with a dosage of 15μg/min, it is unlikely that a further increase will be beneficial.

Dopamine (Chap. 66) is useful in many patients with power failure. At low doses [2 to 10 (μg/kg)/min] the drug has positive chronotropic and inotropic effects as a consequence of stimulation of beta receptors. At higher doses, a vasoconstrictive effect as a result of the stimulation of alpha receptors is also noted. Dopamine at lower doses [≤2 (μg/kg)/min] also has the unique effect of dilating the renal and splanchnic vascular beds and apparently has little effect on myocardial oxygen consumption. Intravenous dopamine is started at an infusion rate of 2 to 5 (μg/kg)/min with increments in dosage every 2 to 5 min up to a maximum of 20 to 50 (μg/kg)/min. Systolic arterial blood pressure should be maintained at approximately 90 mmHg. *Dobutamine* is a synthetic sympathomimetic amine with positive inotropic action and minimal positive chronotropic or peripheral vasoconstrictive activity in the usual dosage range [2.5 to 10 (μg/kg)/min]. It should not be employed when a vasoconstrictor effect is deemed desirable. However, in patients with less profound degrees of hypotension, dobutamine may be an extremely useful agent, particularly if positive chronotropy is to be avoided.

Amrinone (see page 912) is a positive inotropic agent without catecholamine structure or activity. It resembles dobutamine in its pharmacologic activity, although its vasodilating effect appears to be more potent. Initially a loading dose of 0.75 mg/kg is given. If effective, this is followed by an infusion of 10 (μg/kg)/min, followed if necessary 30 min later by an additional bolus of 0.75 mg/kg.

Patients with global left ventricular ischemia as the cause of power failure and profound hypotension, such as those with critical left main coronary artery obstructive disease, may benefit from brief treatment with a pure vasoconstrictor in preference to a positive inotropic agent. In such cases coronary perfusion may be improved by the vasoconstrictor-induced increase in arterial pressure, whereas a positive inotropic agent may only increase ischemic injury in muscle that is incapable of performing more work. In this situation a vasoconstrictor such as *neosynephrine*, 10 to 100 μg/min, should be used, as briefly as possible, usually only as interim therapy while preparations are made for counterpulsation with an interaortic balloon pump and/or emergency coronary artery surgery.

CARDIAC GLYCOSIDES (Chap. 182) Consideration of the central role of impaired myocardial function in the shock syndrome leads to the conclusion that cardiac glycosides should be administered to patients with this condition. Controlled studies, however, have failed to demonstrate significant beneficial effects of glycoside therapy in the early phases (0 to 48 h) of acute myocardial infarction. Hemodynamic improvement has been documented at later times, but this effect, too, is marginal. Since cardiac glycosides cannot improve the function of necrotic myocardium and since pump failure is thought to be related to the total mass of infarcted tissue, digitalis therapy does not result in dramatic improvement in patients with acute myocardial infarction. Nonetheless, it may be useful to treat patients with signs and symptoms of left ventricular failure with digitalis. It has been demonstrated that when scrupulous attention is paid to the dosage, the incidence of arrhythmias and cardiac rupture is no higher in patients with myocardial infarction treated with digitalis than in a control group, and therefore digitalis can be administered with relative safety.

AORTIC COUNTERPULSATION The basic defect in the shock syndrome is impaired myocardial function; therefore, mechanical assist devices have been developed to supplement the pumping action of the heart. The largest body of clinical experience has been obtained with the intraaortic balloon system of diastolic pressure augmentation. A sausage-shaped balloon at the end of a catheter is introduced into the aorta via the femoral artery, and the balloon is inflated during early diastole, thereby enhancing both coronary blood flow and peripheral perfusion. The balloon collapses in early systole, thereby reducing the afterload against which left ventricular ejection takes place. Improvement in hemodynamic status has been observed with balloon pumping in a large number of patients, but long-term survival following this mode of therapy in patients with cardiogenic shock is still disappointing. The balloon counterpulsation system may best be reserved for patients whose condition merits surgical intervention (e.g., continuing ischemia, ventricular septal rupture, or mitral regurgitation) and in whom a successful surgical result is likely to result in the reversal of cardiogenic shock.

There is reason to believe that results of therapy of the shock syndrome secondary to myocardial infarction, while improving gradually as a result of meticulous attention to the details of therapy outlined above, will continue to be disappointing overall because a large fraction of patients with the syndrome have large areas of infarcted myocardium with severe, diffuse coronary atherosclerosis. Although occasional dramatic results have been reported with emergency revascularization surgery alone, or in combination with infarctectomy, the overall results with this approach, too, have been disappointing. It is hoped that early thrombolytic therapy will reduce the amount of myocardium which becomes necrotic and thereby reduce the incidence of this syndrome.

Other complications MITRAL REGURGITATION Apical systolic murmurs of mitral regurgitation appear in more than one-fourth of patients during the first 5 days after the onset of a myocardial infarction, but mitral regurgitation is of hemodynamic importance in only a minority of these patients. In most patients the murmur is present during the acute phase of infarction, disappearing with recovery. The most common cause of mitral regurgitation following myocardial infarction is dysfunction of the papillary muscles of the left ventricle due to ischemia or infarction.

Mitral regurgitation may also be the result of alteration in the size or shape of the ventricle due to impaired contractility or to aneurysm formation. Either papillary muscle may rupture, the posterior one twice as frequently as the anterior. Left ventricular function may deteriorate dramatically with superimposition of mitral regurgitation. The differential diagnosis includes perforation of the ventricular septum (see below), and the differentiation from mitral regurgitation is conveniently made at the bedside with a flow-directed balloon catheter. Large *v* waves may be recorded in the pulmonary capillary wedge position in patients with hemodynamically significant mitral regurgitation, and there is no oxygen "step up" as the catheter is advanced from the right atrium to the right ventricle. Surgical replacement of the mitral valve may be followed by dramatic improvement in patients in whom acute heart failure results primarily from severe mitral regurgitation due to papillary muscle rupture or dysfunction and in whom myocardial function is relatively well maintained.

If aortic systolic pressure is lowered in patients with mitral regurgitation, a greater fraction of the left ventricular output will be ejected antegrade, thus lessening the regurgitant fraction. To this end, both intraaortic balloon counterpulsation, which lowers the aortic systolic pressure mechanically, and the infusion of sodium nitroprusside, 0.5 to 8.0 (μg/kg)/min, which reduces systemic vascular resistance, have been used with success for the interim management of patients with severe mitral regurgitation in the setting of acute myocardial infarction. Ideally, definitive operative treatment should be postponed for 4 to 6 weeks after the infarct. However, if the patient's hemodynamic and/or clinical condition does not improve and stabilize, surgical treatment should be undertaken, even in the acute stage.

CARDIAC RUPTURE Myocardial rupture is a dramatic complication of myocardial infarction most likely to occur during the first week after the onset of symptoms; its frequency increases with the age of the patient. First infarction, female sex, and hypertension are associated with a higher incidence of cardiac rupture. The clinical presentation may often be that of a sudden disappearance of the pulse, blood pressure, and consciousness while the electrocardiogram continues to show sinus rhythm (*apparent* electromechanical dissociation). The myocardium continues to contract, but forward flow is not maintained as blood escapes into the pericardium. Cardiac tamponade (Chap. 194) ensues, and closed-chest massage is ineffective. Although almost universally fatal, there have been a few instances in which cardiac rupture has been recognized and successfully treated by pericardiocentesis and emergency cardiac surgery.

SEPTAL PERFORATION The pathogenesis of perforation of the ventricular septum is similar to that of external rupture of the myocardium, but the therapeutic potential is greater. Patients with ventricular septal rupture present with severe heart failure in association with the sudden appearance of a pansystolic murmur, often accompanied by a parasternal thrill. It is often impossible to differentiate this condition from rupture of a papillary muscle with resultant mitral regurgitation, and a tall *v* wave in the pulmonary capillary wedge pressure in both conditions further complicates the differentiation. The diagnosis can be established by the demonstration of a left-to-right shunt (i.e., an oxygen step-up at the level of the right ventricle) by limited cardiac catheterization performed at the bedside using a flow-directed balloon catheter. Rupture of the ventricular septum is amenable to immediate surgical treatment, albeit at a relatively high mortality rate, but this form of therapy is ordinarily indicated on an urgent basis in patients whose condition cannot be stabilized rapidly. A prolonged period of hemodynamic compromise may produce end-organ damage and other complications that can be avoided by early intervention including nitroprusside infusion and intraaortic balloon counterpulsation. If stabilization occurs, surgical intervention can be postponed for 4 to 8 weeks, to allow for formation of scar tissue at the margins of the defect, rendering surgical closure easier. However, mortality is primarily a function of the overall extent of myocardial damage rather than the timing of surgical treatment.

The physiology of acute mitral regurgitation and acute ventricular septal perforation are similar in that the level of aortic systolic pressure determines in part the regurgitant volume, the principal difference being the chamber into which the regurgitant fraction is ejected. In septal perforation, a fraction of left ventricular output is ejected into the right ventricle. In a manner analogous to mitral regurgitation, lowering of aortic systolic pressure by mechanical (intraaortic balloon counterpulsation) and/or pharmacologic (nitroglycerin or nitroprusside) means can decrease the hemodynamic compromise caused by perforation.

VENTRICULAR ANEURYSM The term *ventricular aneurysm* is usually used to describe *dyskinesis* or local expansile paradoxical wall motion. Normally functioning myocardial fibers must shorten more if stroke volume and cardiac output are to be maintained in patients with ventricular aneurysm, and if they are unable to do so, overall ventricular function is impaired. Aneurysms are composed of scar tissue and neither predispose to nor are associated with cardiac rupture.

The complications of left ventricular aneurysm do not usually occur for weeks to months following myocardial infarction; they include congestive heart failure, arterial embolism, and ventricular arrhythmias. Apical aneurysms are the most common and the most easily detected by clinical examination. The physical finding of greatest value is a double, diffuse, or displaced apical impulse. The standard roentgenogram frequently reveals an abnormal bulge distorting the contour of the left heart border, but the roentgenogram may be entirely normal, especially with posterior aneurysms. The electrocardiographic finding of ST-segment elevation at rest is present in precordial leads in 25 percent of patients with either apical or anterior aneurysms. Ventricular aneurysms are readily detectable by two-dimensional echocardiography, which may also reveal a mural thrombus in aneurysms involving the anterior wall and/or apex. Ventricular aneurysms may cause sustained ventricular tachycardia which requires treatment with antiarrhythmic drugs or endocardial resection (Chap. 184).

RIGHT VENTRICULAR INFARCTION Approximately one-third of patients with inferoposterior infarction demonstrate at least a minor degree of right ventricular necrosis. An occasional patient with inferoposterior left ventricular infarction also has extensive right ventricular myocardial infarction. These patients often present with signs of severe right ventricular failure (jugular venous distention, hepatomegaly) with or without hypotension. ST-segment elevations of the right-sided precordial electrocardiographic leads, particularly lead V_4R, are present in the majority of patients with right ventricular infarction. Radionuclide ventriculography and two-dimensional echocardiography are also sensitive in the detection of right ventricular damage associated with acute myocardial infarction. Catheterization of the right side of the heart often reveals a distinctive hemodynamic pattern resembling cardiac tamponade or constrictive pericarditis (Chap. 194). Volume expansion is often successful in treating low cardiac output and hypotension associated with extensive right ventricular infarction.

THROMBOEMBOLISM Clinically apparent thromboembolism complicates myocardial infarction in approximately 10 percent of cases, but embolic lesions are found in 45 percent of patients in necropsy series, suggesting that thromboembolism is often clinically silent. Thromboembolism is considered to be at least an important contributing cause of death in 25 percent of infarct patients who die following admission to the hospital. Arterial emboli originate from left ventricular mural thrombi, but most pulmonary emboli arise in the leg veins. Thromboembolism most commonly occurs in association with large infarcts in the presence of heart failure. Thromboembolism occurs extremely commonly in patients with echocardiographic evidence of a left ventricular thrombus, but only rarely if a thrombus is not present on the echocardiogram. Although well-controlled trials do not exist, the incidence of embolization appears to be decreased by anticoagulation.

PERICARDITIS (see also Chap. 194) Pericardial friction rubs and/or pericardial pain are frequently encountered in patients with acute transmural myocardial infarction. This complication can usually be managed with aspirin (650 mg qid). It is important to diagnose the chest pain of pericarditis accurately, since failure to appreciate it may lead to the erroneous diagnosis of recurrent ischemic pain and/or infarct extension with resultant inappropriate use of anticoagulants, nitrates, beta blockers, or narcotics. No definite cause and effect relationship between administration of anticoagulants and pericarditis or tamponade has been proved. Nonetheless, the possibility that anticoagulants can cause tamponade in the presence of acute pericarditis is sufficiently high to contraindicate their use in patients with pericarditis, as manifested by either pain or persistent rub, unless there is a compelling indication.

POSTMYOCARDIAL INFARCTION SYNDROME—DRESSLER'S SYNDROME (see also Chap. 194) This syndrome, characterized by fever and pleuropericardial chest pain, is thought to be due to an autoimmune pericarditis, pleuritis, and/or pneumonitis. It may begin from a few days to 6 weeks after myocardial infarction. The occurrence of Dressler's syndrome may be etiologically related to the early use of anticoagulants and appears to have decreased markedly in the last decade as anticoagulants are used less frequently in acute myocardial infarction. The syndrome usually responds promptly to therapy with salicylates. On occasion, corticosteroids may be required to relieve discomfort of an unusual, refractory nature. Effusions associated with Dressler's syndrome may become hemorrhagic if anticoagulants are administered.

REFERENCES

ALPERT JS, FRANCIS GS: *Manuel of Coronary Care*, 3d ed. Boston, Little, Brown, 1984

———, BRAUNWALD E: Acute myocardial infarction: Pathological and clinical manifestations, in *Heart Disease*, 2d ed, E Braunwald (ed). Philadelphia, Saunders, 1984, p 1262

CALIFF RM, WAGNER GS (eds): *Acute Coronary Care: Principles and Practice*. Boston, Martinus Nijhoff, 1985

CHADDA K et al: Effect of propranolol after acute myocardial infarction in patients with congestive heart failure. Circulation 73:503, 1986

COHN PF: The role of noninvasive cardiac testing after an uncomplicated myocardial infarction. N Engl J Med 390:90, 1983

DAVIES MJ, THOMAS AC: Plaque fissuring—The cause of acute myocardial infarction, sudden ischaemic death, and cresendo angina. Br Heart J 53:363, 1985

DEBUSK RF et al: Stepwise risk stratification soon after acute myocardial infarction. Am J Cardiol 52:1161, 1983

FRIEDMAN LM et al: Effect of propranolol in patients with myocardial infarction and ventricular arrhythmia. J Am Coll Cardiol 7:1, 1986

FRISHMAN WH et al: Beta-adrenergic blockade for survivors of acute myocardial infarction. N Engl J Med 310:830, 1984

GOLD HK et al: Acute coronary reocclusion after thrombolysis with recombinant human tissue-type plasminogen activator: Prevention by a maintenance infusion. Circulation 73:347, 1986

HJALMARSON A (ed): Miami: Metoprolol in acute myocardial infarction. Am J Cardiol 56:1G, 1985

KEEFE DL et al: Prophylactic tocainide or lidocaine in acute myocardial infarction. Am J Cardiol 57:527, 1986

KRONE RJ et al and the Multicenter Postinfarction Research Group: Low-level exercise testing after myocardial infarction: Usefulness in enhancing clinical risk stratification. Circulation 71:80, 1985

LAFFEL GL, BRAUNWALD E: Thrombolytic therapy: A new strategy for the treatment of acute myocardial infarction. N Engl J Med 311:710, 770, 1984

PAPAPRETRO SE et al: Percutaneous transluminal coronary angioplasty after intracoronary streptokinase in evolving myocardial infarction. Am J Cardiol 55:48, 1985

SOBEL BE, BRAUNWALD E: Management of acute myocardial infarction, in *Heart Disease*, 2d ed, E Braunwald (ed). Philadelphia, Saunders, 1984, p 1301

The TIMI Study Group: The thrombolysis in myocardial infarction (TIMI) trial: Phase I findings. N Engl J Med 312:932, 1985

191 COR PULMONALE

ALFRED P. FISHMAN

Cor pulmonale denotes enlargement of the right ventricle secondary to malfunctioning lungs. However, the abnormal performance of the lungs is not always due to intrinsic lung disease: in some instances, an abnormal chest bellows or a depressed ventilatory drive from the respiratory centers (Table 191-1) is the cause. If the cause is intrinsic to the lungs, the disease will be diffuse, bilateral, and extensive, in most cases affecting airways as well as parenchyma. As a rule, hypertrophy and dilatation contribute to the right ventricular enlargement; in chronic cor pulmonale hypertrophy is more apt to predominate than in acute cor pulmonale.

Pulmonary arterial hypertension invariably precedes cor pulmonale. In practice, cor pulmonale is synonymous with pulmonary hypertensive heart disease, even though hypoxemia and polycythemia, as well as pulmonary hypertension, often contribute to overloading the right ventricle. But before making the diagnosis of cor pulmonale, *primary disease of the left side of the heart* and *congenital heart disease* must be excluded. It is worth emphasizing that the term *cor pulmonale* does not automatically imply heart failure. However, it is understood that if the pulmonary hypertension that led to enlargement of the right ventricle is not relieved, cor pulmonale will become associated with right ventricular failure.

Hypertrophy and/or dilatation of the right ventricle are usually much more difficult to detect and to quantify, both clinically and at autopsy, than are left ventricular hypertrophy and dilatation. Moreover, in dealing with right ventricular enlargement it is essential to understand the mechanisms that operated during life to impose an abnormal hemodynamic load upon it.

The definitions and reservations above have several practical implications. By underscoring the critical role that is played by some abnormality of the respiratory system in the pathogenesis of cor pulmonale, they underscore that prognosis and treatment of cor pulmonale *depend more on relieving the respiratory disorder than on improving the performance of the right ventricle*. Moreover, by stressing *enlargement* of the right ventricle as the hallmark of cor pulmonale—without distinguishing between dilatation and hypertrophy—they stress that pulmonary hypertension is an antecedent of cor pulmonale and that right ventricular failure is a consequence of both.

TYPES OF COR PULMONALE By tradition, the designation *acute* is generally reserved for the dilatation of the right side of the heart which follows acute embolization of the lungs. The designation *chronic* is less specific. Usually chronicity is judged by the type and duration of the respiratory disorder that led to the cardiac enlargement (Table 191-1). Just how long, and to what degree, the heart remains enlarged will depend on fluctuations in its workload, i.e., primarily pulmonary arterial pressure, but also cardiac output, polycythemia, heart rate, and the level of arterial hypoxemia.

FREQUENCY Reliable estimates of the prevalence of chronic cor pulmonale are sparse. After the age of 50, cor pulmonale is the most common cardiac disorder except for coronary and hypertensive heart disease. Most instances are secondary to obstructive disease of the airways and the pulmonary hypertension that it elicits. Indeed, in parts of the world where cigarette smoking and air pollution have resulted in a high incidence of chronic bronchitis and emphysema (described in detail in Chap. 208), cor pulmonale may comprise up to one-quarter of all types of heart failure. Men are more often affected than women presumably because of greater exposure to air pollutants, including cigarette smoke. Chronic cor pulmonale is a

TABLE 191-1 Respiratory disorders predisposing to chronic cor pulmonale*

1 Intrinsic disease of the lungs and intrapulmonary airways
- *a* Chronic obstructive lung disease (COLD)
- *b* Diffuse pulmonary interstitial disease
- *c* Pulmonary vascular disease

2 Upper airways obstruction
- *a* Tracheal stenosis
- *b* Obstructive sleep apnea syndromes
- *c* Congenital anatomic abnormalities of oropharynx

3 Malfunctioning chest bellows
- *a* Kyphoscoliosis
- *b* Neuromuscular incompetence
- *c* Marked obesity (''Pickwickian syndrome'')

4 Inadequate ventilatory drive from respiratory centers
- *a* Primary or idiopathic alveolar hypoventilation (''Ondine's curse'')
- *b* Chronic mountain sickness
- *c* Central sleep apnea syndromes

* *The term* respiratory disorders *includes not only the diseases and disorders of the lungs, airways, and chest bellows, but also malfunctioning of the centers that control breathing and the support structures of the oropharynx. In essence,* respiratory disorders *refers to malfunctioning of any part or parts of the entire respiratory system and of the structures that impinge upon it.*

common sequel to cystic fibrosis (Chap. 207) but an unusual complication of allergic asthma.

Most diffuse pulmonary diseases are either too limited in extent or too circumscribed in their effects on alveolar-capillary gas exchange to set in motion the train of events leading to cor pulmonale. Even patients with extensive silicosis, emphysema, or diffuse fibrosis usually fail to develop appreciable pulmonary hypertension or cardiomegaly even though the disease may suffice to evoke breathlessness for years.

PATHOGENESIS

Pulmonary hypertension is a prerequisite for cor pulmonale. Although a high cardiac output, tachycardia, and an expanded blood volume may contribute to the pulmonary hypertension, the crux in the pathogenetic sequence is right ventricular overload due to an increase in pulmonary vascular resistance to blood flow through small muscular arteries and arterioles. The increase in vascular resistance may be anatomic or vasomotor in origin; often both mechanisms are involved (Table 191-2). In contrast to the situation in left ventricular failure, cardiac output is often normal or high, the peripheral pulses strong, and the extremities warm in the face of overt signs of systemic venous congestion. Peripheral edema complicating cor pulmonale is generally attributed to the heart failure, but the explanation is not entirely satisfying because pulmonary arterial pressures rarely exceed 65 to 80 kPa except during the acute exacerbation when hypoxia and acidosis are severe.

It has been noted above that the increase in the work of the right ventricle imposed by the pulmonary hypertension may cause it to fail. However, even in patients in whom the right ventricular stroke volume is decreased due to pulmonary hypertensive overloading, the myocardium of the right ventricle seems capable of responding normally when the overload is relieved.

ANATOMIC INCREASE IN PULMONARY VASCULAR RESISTANCE In the normal resting individual, the pulmonary circulation is a highly distensible, low-resistance circuit, accommodating the same blood flow as the systemic circulation at approximately one-fifth the mean blood pressure; during moderate exercise, tripling the blood flow elicits only slight increments in pulmonary arterial pressure. Even after pneumonectomy, the residual pulmonary vascular bed accepts considerable increments in pulmonary blood flow with only a slight increase in pulmonary artery pressure as long as the lung is free of fibrosis, emphysema, or pulmonary vascular change. Similarly, amputation of large portions of the pulmonary capillary bed in emphysema generally fails to elicit pulmonary hypertension.

However, when pulmonary vascular reserve has been exhausted by progressive reduction in the extent and distensibility of the pulmonary vascular tree, even the modest increments in pulmonary blood flow associated with daily living may suffice to elicit marked pulmonary hypertension. For this to occur the cross-sectional area of the pulmonary resistance vessels must be considerably reduced. Restriction of the pulmonary vascular bed stems from widespread narrowing and obstruction of small pulmonary arteries and arterioles, usually accompanied by a decrease in the distensibility not only of the vessels but also of the adjacent lung.

VASOMOTOR INCREASE IN PULMONARY VASCULAR RESISTANCE (HYPOXIA AND ACIDOSIS) The most potent stimulus for pulmonary vasoconstriction is alveolar hypoxia, which acts directly on adjacent small pulmonary arteries and arterioles; systemic arterial hypoxemia supplements the local effects of alveolar hypoxia indirectly by way of the sympathetic nerves to the pulmonary circulation. Experiments in dogs indicate that severe acidosis ($pH < 7.2$) also elicits pulmonary vasoconstriction. In humans, acidosis acts synergistically with hypoxia, whereas alkalosis diminishes the pressor response to hypoxia. The biologic basis for this interplay remains unclear. In chronic hypoxia, the effects of these pulmonary hypertensive stimuli are often intensified by increased viscosity of the blood arising from secondary polycythemia.

HYPERCAPNIA In contrast to the effects of hypoxia and acidosis, the effects of CO_2 on the pulmonary circulation appear to be by way of the acidosis that it generates rather than by a direct action on pulmonary vessels. However, because heart failure in cor pulmonale is often associated with respiratory insufficiency, and because management of the respiratory insufficiency generally determines the outcome of the heart failure, the extracardiac effects of hypercapnia merit consideration.

Hypercapnia affects mainly the central nervous system, producing cerebral vasodilatation, increased cerebrospinal fluid pressure, and neurologic derangements ranging from weakness, irritability, lassitude, and cloudy sensorium to somnolence, confusion, and coma. These derangements are most apt to occur if hypercapnia is acute in onset and severe, or if chronic hypercapnia is acutely aggravated. In contrast, during chronic hypercapnia, the patient may be virtually free of central nervous system disturbances if respiratory acidosis is fully compensated. When severe hypoxemia and hypercapnia coexist, it may be impossible to distinguish between their neurologic effects because severe hypoxia causes anatomic damage to nervous tissues.

Carbon dioxide retention, with elevated CO_2 tensions in the blood and tissues, is self-perpetuating. On the one hand, hypercapnia from any cause blunts the responsiveness of the respiratory center to the

TABLE 191-2 Pathogenetic mechanisms in chronic pulmonary hypertension and cor pulmonale

Pathogenetic mechanism	Intermediaries	Examples
PRIMARY MECHANISMS		
Anatomic increase in pulmonary vascular resistance	Obliteration, obstruction, reduction, and stiffening of pulmonary vascular tree	*Vascular disease:* Primary pulmonary hypertension; recurrent pulmonary emboli *Extravascular disease:* Diffuse interstitial disease; fibrosing alveolitis; pneumoconiosis
Vasomotor increase in pulmonary vascular resistance	Pulmonary vasoconstriction by hypoxia and acidosis	*General alveolar hypoventilation with normal lungs:* *1* Disorders of chest bellows: neuromuscular; extreme obesity; kyphoscoliosis *2* Diminished ventilatory drive: primary alveolar hypoventilation; sleep; hypercapnia
Combined anatomic restriction and vasomotor	Combination of above	*Net alveolar hypoventilation with abnormal lungs:* Chronic obstructive lung disease: ''blue bloater''; cystic fibrosis of pancreas
SECONDARY MECHANISMS		
Increase in cardiac output	Increase in metabolic rate; acute hypoxia	Daily activities; acute respiratory infection
Increase in blood viscosity	Secondary polycythemia	Chronic hypoxia
Tachycardia	Aggravation of hypoxia	Heart failure

CO_2 stimulus; on the other, hypercapnia promotes retention of bicarbonate by the kidney. Not only the hypercapnia originating in disorders of the lungs or ventilation, but also the hypercapnia of metabolic alkalosis, such as that produced by powerful diuretics, causes ventilatory depression. This is why patients with chronic hypercapnia are particularly vulnerable to the effects of sedatives or oxygen breathing, both of which may cause calamitous increments in the degree of hypercapnia: sedatives by depressing further the respiratory centers in the brain, and oxygen by abolishing the hypoxic peripheral drive to ventilation. A large diuresis in which the loss of chloride is inordinate for the output of bicarbonate may be equally effective in depressing the ventilation. It is usually in the severely hypoxic, hypercapnic patient that right-sided heart failure occurs.

ALVEOLAR HYPOVENTILATION A large disparity commonly exists between the degree of pulmonary hypertension recorded during life and the anatomic changes in the lungs and pulmonary vessels at autopsy. This discrepancy is particularly marked in patients with obstructive disease of the airways, in whom the anatomic changes in the gas-exchanging parts of the lungs consistently appear to be inadequate to explain either the blood-gas abnormalities or the pulmonary arterial pressor response. Similarly, the most extensive emphysema may be associated with normal levels of blood gases and normal pulmonary arterial pressures. Much of this discrepancy disappears when account is taken of alveolar hypoventilation, an important functional disorder which cannot be quantified at autopsy. Recognizing that alveolar hypoventilation is an essential component in the pathogenesis of cor pulmonale is critical for two reasons: (1) elimination of the initiating mechanism (e.g., acute respiratory infection) usually reverses the alveolar hypoventilation, and (2) unless alveolar ventilation is improved, other therapeutic measures are apt to be ineffective.

The importance of alveolar hypoventilation in the pathogenesis of cor pulmonale has been underscored in recent years by observations of its occurrence in patients with sleep apnea syndromes in whom hypoxia is a consequence of inadequate ventilatory drive (central apnea) or of upper airways obstruction (peripheral apnea) whereas the lungs and chest bellows are normal. Dramatic improvements have often followed relief of the initiating mechanism, e.g., hypertrophied tonsils and adenoids, or bypass of an area of obstruction, e.g., tracheostomy for tracheal stenosis.

PULMONARY HYPERTENSION

Two distinct patterns characterize the natural history of cor pulmonale at sea level: (1) The pattern of *episodic* pulmonary hypertension, due to exacerbations of the underlying pulmonary disorder, is more common. Generally, each bout leaves its imprint and predisposes to continuing hypertension even though recovery from the *early* bouts frequently is associated with the return of pulmonary arterial pressures to normal. (2) The pattern of *progressive,* unremitting pulmonary hypertension and cor pulmonale leading inexorably to right-sided heart failure is generally a consequence either of progressive pulmonary vascular or interstitial disease or of unremitting hypoxia (as in continuing alveolar hypoventilation). Distinction between the two sequences tends to become blurred if intercurrent respiratory infections decrease the intervals between bouts of hypoxia and pulmonary hypertension. Also, each bout of pulmonary hypertension seems to predispose to a subsequent bout of cor pulmonale because of residual hypertrophy of the muscular pulmonary arteries or further curtailment of the extent and distensibility of the pulmonary vascular tree. Consequently, although relief of hypoxia may restore the pulmonary arterial pressure to normal or near-normal levels, with each attack the pulmonary vascular tree seems to lose some of its adaptability and the patient moves a little closer to the verge of persistent pulmonary hypertension and cor pulmonale.

As a general rule, pulmonary hypertension appears in a predisposed individual either when blood flow is increased (exercise, fever) or during a bout of acute hypoxia (bronchopulmonary infection). In time, pulmonary hypertension is present even at rest. The highest pulmonary artery pressures occur in pulmonary vascular and interstitial disease; the levels of pulmonary hypertension are neither as high nor as fixed in chronic obstructive diseases of the airways, even during an acute exacerbation.

The pulmonary hypertension that comes on only during exercise or hypoxia is associated with normal end-diastolic pressure in the right ventricle. However, as pulmonary hypertension becomes persistent and severe, abnormally high filling (end-diastolic) pressure develops in the right ventricle as a result either of incomplete emptying of the ventricle as it dilates or of the decrease in ventricular compliance associated with hypertrophy; cardiac output is still normal at rest and increases normally during exercise (cor pulmonale without heart failure). Finally, the onset of right-sided heart failure is identified by abnormally high end-diastolic pressures in the right ventricle. At this stage, the cardiac output, which may still be normal at rest, fails to increase normally during exercise; the systemic veins are engorged, reflecting the inability of the right ventricle to empty normally.

Interest is high in developing techniques to permit the diagnosis of pulmonary hypertension, using noninvasive techniques, especially echocardiography. Approaches to the problem have differed in that some aim to predict pulmonary arterial pressure whereas others attempt inferences based on right ventricular dimensions and hypertrophy and on the motions of the pulmonic valve. The diverse patient populations complicate extrapolation and generalization. But it does seem that some noninvasive procedures can detect pulmonary hypertension that is moderate or severe even though none are reliable or of sufficient accuracy to substitute for direct determinations by cardiac catheterization. Attention is currently shifting to a combination of approaches in the hope that indirect determinations of multiple aspects of right ventricular performance and of the pulmonary circulation will provide more accurate and reproducible measurements of the level of pulmonary hypertension than any single measure alone. It is perhaps worth reiterating that evaluations of accuracy require simultaneous determinations of cardiac output since in pulmonary hypertensive states the level of pulmonary blood flow strongly influences the level of pulmonary arterial pressure.

THE LEFT VENTRICLE IN COR PULMONALE Recent observations on the interplay between the two ventricles (''interdependence'') have served as a reminder that not only are both ventricles encased in common muscle bundles and pericardium, but they also have one wall in common, i.e., the ventricular septum. Increasing pressures in the right ventricle displace the septum into the left ventricle, thereby encroaching upon its lumen and modifying left ventricular pressures as well as volumes. However, the clinical significance of these changes is uncertain.

Except in the case of the few severely hypoxemic high-altitude dwellers who develop mountain sickness, the left ventricle does not seem to share in the cardiomegaly of high altitude. Consequently, *tolerable* levels of hypoxia do not exert serious noxious effects on the myocardium; nor are they associated with an inordinate hemodynamic load on the left ventricle. Conversely, severe, intolerable levels of hypoxia and arterial hypoxemia at altitude may impair myocardial function of both ventricles as well as produce right ventricular overload. The left ventricle then enlarges and fails, primarily because of inadequate oxygen delivery to the myocardium. These observations at high altitude suggest that right ventricular overload, per se, does not interfere with left ventricular function unless pulmonary hypertension is severe and accompanied by severe hypoxemia.

At sea level, cor pulmonale is not associated with left ventricular enlargement as long as the respiratory disorder is not long-standing and arterial hypoxemia is modest in degree. But in pulmonary disorders associated with chronic severe hypoxemia, left ventricular enlargement and malfunction may become evident, presumably due to independent disease of the left ventricle—particularly arteriosclerotic heart disease—aggravated by the direct effects of inadequate oxygen delivery to the myocardium plus the noxious effect of severe hypoxemia and acidosis on the myocardium. In turn, the consequences of respiratory insufficiency, which contributed to impaired myocardial performance by way of arterial hypoxemia and acidosis, are intensified by interstitial and alveolar pulmonary edema if the left ventricle should fail.

CLINICAL MANIFESTATIONS

The likelihood that a physician will recognize that a patient has cor pulmonale depends on his or her awareness that the underlying respiratory disorder can culminate in pulmonary hypertension. The diagnosis is generally straightforward in obliterative diseases of the pulmonary circulation, e.g., multiple pulmonary emboli. It is much more elusive in obstructive disease of the airways because chronic bronchitis and bronchiolitis may be more subtle in their clinical manifestations, and clinical indexes of pulmonary hypertension are not always reliable. Indeed, the first bout of pulmonary hypertension and cor pulmonale secondary to chronic bronchitis may be appreciated only retrospectively, i.e., after an episode of frank right ventricular failure. Detection may be particularly difficult if the systemic venous congestion and peripheral edema develop insidiously, over days to weeks, rather than suddenly in the course of an acute bronchopulmonary infection. Attention has recently been focused on the gradual onset of cor pulmonale and right ventricular failure by patients who develop alveolar hypoventilation as part of a sleep apnea syndrome rather than as a consequence of intrinsic pulmonary disease.

DIFFERENTIAL DIAGNOSIS Cor pulmonale is particularly important to recognize in the elderly patient who is old enough to have arteriosclerotic heart disease, has had cough and sputum for many years ("chronic bronchitis"), and clearly manifests right ventricular failure. Analyses of arterial blood gases are then most helpful in deciding whether the primary cardiac disorder is in the right or left ventricle, since appreciable arterial hypoxemia, hypercapnia, and acidosis are unusual in left-sided heart failure unless frank pulmonary edema is also present.

Support for the diagnosis of cor pulmonale may be adduced from roentgenographic and electrocardiographic evidence of right ventricular enlargement. Rarely is catheterization of the right side of the heart needed to settle the question, once suspicion of cor pulmonale is aroused. But, if necessary, cardiac catheterization will typically show pulmonary arterial hypertension, normal left atrial ("pulmonary wedge") pressures, and the classic hemodynamics of right ventricular failure.

The conventional signs of right ventricular enlargement include a cardiac thrust along the left sternal border, or immediately below the sternum, and a fourth heart sound arising in the hypertrophied ventricle. Concomitant pulmonary hypertension is suggested by a thrust in the second left interspace adjacent to the sternum, an unusually loud second component of the second heart sound in the same area, and occasionally the murmur of pulmonary valvular insufficiency. If the right ventricle fails, tricuspid insufficiency and a right ventricular gallop sound are often added. Hydrothorax is uncommon, even after the advent of overt right ventricular failure. Permanent arrhythmias, such as atrial flutter or fibrillation, are unusual, but transitory arrhythmias are common during severe hypoxia or when respiratory alkalosis has been induced by mechanical hyperventilation.

TABLE 191-3 ECG patterns in chronic cor pulmonale

1 Chronic obstructive lung disease (suggestive, but not diagnostic, of right ventricular enlargement)*
  a "P pulmonale" (in leads II, III, aVF)
  b Right axis deviation $\geq 110°$
  c R/S ratio in $V_6 \leq 1$
  d rSR′ in right chest leads
  e Right bundle branch block (partial or complete)
2 Pulmonary vascular or interstitial disease; general alveolar hypoventilation (diagnostic of right ventricular enlargement)
  a Classic pattern in V_1 or V_3R (dominant R or R′ with inverted T waves in right chest leads)
  b Often associated with "suggestive" criteria above

* *Among the "suggestive" criteria, it is difficult to distinguish right ventricular enlargement (hypertrophy and dilatation) from changes in the anatomic and electrical positions of the heart produced by the hyperinflated lungs. Consequently, the "suggestive" criteria are more useful as confirmatory, than as diagnostic, evidence.*

The diagnostic value of the *electrocardiogram* in cor pulmonale depends on the underlying pulmonary or ventilatory disorder (Table 191-3). It is most valuable in pulmonary vascular or interstitial disease, particularly if unassociated with obstructive disease of the airways, or in alveolar hypoventilation with normal lungs. Conversely, because of the hyperinflated lungs and the episodic nature of the pulmonary hypertension and right ventricular overload, patterns diagnostic of right ventricular hypertrophy are uncommon in cor pulmonale secondary to chronic bronchitis and emphysema. Consequently, even if right ventricular enlargement in the course of chronic bronchitis and emphysema is marked, as during a bout of acute upper respiratory infection, electrocardiographic evidence may be inconclusive because of rotation and displacement of the heart, widened distances between electrodes and the cardiac surface, and the predominance of dilatation over hypertrophy in the cardiac enlargement. Thus a reliable diagnosis of right ventricular enlargement can be expected in one-third of patients with chronic bronchitis and emphysema whose hearts show right ventricular hypertrophy at autopsy, whereas the diagnosis is easily and reliably made in the great majority of patients with cor pulmonale originating in pulmonary disorders other than chronic bronchitis and emphysema. With these qualifications in mind, the more reliable criteria for right ventricular hypertrophy in a patient who has chronic bronchitis and emphysema have proved to be an S_1Q_3 pattern; right axis deviation $\geq 110°$; an $S_1S_2S_3$ pattern; and an R/S ratio in $V_6 \leq 1.0$. Combinations of these criteria enhance their diagnostic sensitivities.

Roentgenography has more diagnostic value in arousing suspicion of, or in confirming, enlargement of the right ventricle than in detecting it. Suspicion is aroused by evidences of an antecedent predisposing pulmonary disorder coupled with large central pulmonary arteries and a pruned peripheral arterial tree, i.e., evidence of pulmonary hypertension. Serial x-rays are generally more useful than a single examination for heart size, particularly in obstructive disease of the airways, where dramatic changes in heart size may occur between a bout of acute respiratory insufficiency and recovery.

Echocardiography has recently come into play as a tool for detecting pulmonary hypertension on the basis of movements of the pulmonic valve. The technique is not easy but is gaining in popularity.

CLINICAL FORMS OF COR PULMONALE AND THEIR TREATMENT

Regardless of the mechanism of initiation—anatomic, vasomotor, or both—chronic pulmonary hypertension tends to be self-perpetuating because of anatomic changes that cause continuing narrowing of small arteries and arterioles and obliteration of the pulmonary vascular bed by muscular hypertrophy, arteriosclerosis, and thrombosis. Often the impact of these anatomic changes is heightened by increased pulmonary vasomotor tone.

ANATOMIC INCREASE IN PULMONARY VASCULAR RESISTANCE These abnormalities may be sorted into two general categories (Table 191-2): vascular disease and extravascular disease, as described below.

Vascular disease; occlusive disease of the small pulmonary arteries In these disorders, widespread occlusion of the small pulmonary vessels takes place over months to years. Most often, the cause is multiple pulmonary emboli (Chap. 211); less common are multiple thromboses such as those which complicate sickle cell anemia. A rare cause is primary (unexplained) pulmonary hypertension (Chap. 210).

Tachypnea, persisting during sleep, is an outstanding feature of multiple pulmonary emboli. This increase in respiratory frequency is associated with alveolar hyperventilation as indicated by characteristically low values for alveolar and arterial P_{CO_2} and for serum bicarbonate. Incapacitating breathlessness occurs on mild exertion. Precordial or thoracic pain is not uncommon: occasionally the pain mimics angina; at other times it is clearly pleuritic, intensifying during inspiration. The clinical roentgenographic and electrocardiographic signs of right ventricular enlargement are present. Cyanosis, which is rarely impressive before heart failure, usually becomes striking after the right ventricle fails. Objective evidence for pulmonary emboli is conventionally sought by photoscanning and pulmonary angiography (Chaps. 201 and 211).

Of all patients who develop cor pulmonale, those with multiple pulmonary emboli or primary pulmonary hypertension have the highest pulmonary arterial pressures; these may equal or even exceed systemic arterial pressures. The cardiac output tends to be low. Mild arterial hypoxemia is the rule and seems to arise from shunting within the lungs. Whether the shunts represent blood flow through recanalized vessels that divert mixed venous blood from contact with alveoli, or too-rapid passage of the entire cardiac output through unoccluded and dilated portions of the pulmonary vascular tree, or blood flow through anatomic pulmonary arteriovenous channels that are ordinarily inoperative is conjectural. During right-sided heart failure, these shunts cause profound arterial hypoxemia because the shunted (mixed venous) blood has an extremely low O_2 content.

Once pulmonary hypertension is fixed, treatment directed at the process in the lungs is rarely effective, since organization of emboli has led to irreversible occlusions of innumerable small arteries. Continuous administration of O_2-enriched mixtures is standard. Caution must be exercised to avoid oxygen toxicity by administering as little additional oxygen as possible. Unfortunately, compromises are often required, since arterial blood is not easily restored toward normal levels of oxygenation because of the magnitude of the venous shunts.

The grim outlook for treating the cor pulmonale of multiple pulmonary emboli, as well as the ever-present prospect of catastrophic pulmonary embolization, has emphasized the need for prophylactic measures in patients judged to be candidates for pulmonary emboli (Chap. 211). Heart failure is treated by the usual cardiotonic measures in conjunction with measures directed at improving arterial oxygenation. Rarely does it respond dramatically as long as the hemodynamic overload persists.

Diffuse interstitial fibrosis and granuloma Among the diverse entities included in this category are (1) sarcoidosis, berylliosis, and the "nonspecific" granulomatoses (Chap. 209); (2) scleroderma of the lung (Chap. 209); (3) the various interstitial or alveolar-septal fibroses such as "fibrosing alveolitis," radiation fibrosis, or pulmonary asbestosis, and the special progressive form of interstitial disease known as the Hamman-Rich syndrome (Chap. 209); (4) immunopathologic disease of the lungs, exemplified by "farmer's lung" (Chap. 203); and (5) diffuse carcinomatous infiltration of the lung, such as "alveolar cell" or lymphangitic carcinoma (Chap. 213).

Clinically, the respiratory difficulty is often manifested by an acute respiratory illness that fails to resolve. Tachypnea persists. The roentgenogram shows fine nodular or fibrotic lesions widely disseminated throughout both lung fields. In the resting subject, the arterial P_{O_2} is sustained at near-normal levels by chronic hyperventilation; during exercise, it drops precipitously. The arterial P_{CO_2} is normal or slightly low, reflecting the balance between the augmented ventilation, the oxygen consumption, which is often increased, and the partition of the augmented ventilation between the alveoli and the dead space.

As long as hypoxemia is mild, pulmonary hypertension is modest. But as the disease progresses and as hypoxemia increases—in part because of ventilation-perfusion abnormalities—the level of pulmonary hypertension also increases, and cor pulmonale begins to evolve. Right ventricular failure generally occurs late in the course of the disease. At first, it responds well to oxygen mixtures and the usual forms of treatment of heart failure (Chap. 182). Oxygen therapy is quite useful since it affords relief of dyspnea and improves oxygenation without threat of carbon dioxide retention. However, oxygen dependence may become marked, and the hazards of oxygen toxicity increase pari passu with the increasing concentrations of inspired oxygen and the duration of exposure.

Relief of heart failure is usually transient unless the initiating mechanism is controlled. Rarely is the underlying lesion in the lung reversible, even though steroids occasionally have been associated with dramatic benefit, especially in some of the granulomatoses and "fibrosing alveolitis." More apt to be rewarding is the successful treatment of superimposed respiratory infection which has toppled a stable patient into heart failure.

VASOMOTOR INCREASE IN PULMONARY VASCULAR RESISTANCE For convenience, alveolar hypoventilation, a prime cause of elevated pulmonary vascular resistance, can be identified by a value for arterial P_{CO_2} greater than 60 kPa; the disorder may be regarded as either "general" or "net."

Alveolar hypoventilation: general The critical importance of abnormal values for blood gases in the pathogenesis of cor pulmonale is illustrated by the syndrome of alveolar hypoventilation coexistent with normal lungs ("general alveolar hypoventilation"). In these patients, some abnormality, either in the regulation of ventilation or in the neuromuscular apparatus, rather than intrinsic pulmonary disease, is responsible for the hypoxia and hypercapnia. The syndrome may have diverse etiologies. Sleep apnea syndromes associated with alveolar hypoventilation are currently receiving considerable attention. These disorders and the pathways by which they lead to alveolar hypoventilation and cor pulmonale are considered in Chap. 215.

Alveolar hypoventilation: net The common denominator in this group of disorders is the imbalance between alveolar ventilation, blood flow, and diffusion, resulting in hypercapnia and hypoxemia. In contrast to *general* alveolar hypoventilation, in which the same abnormalities of arterial blood-gas levels occur despite normal lungs, intrinsic lung disease is the basis for the abnormal values for blood gases in *net* alveolar hypoventilation.

The assortment of obstructive airways diseases predisposing to cor pulmonale has been pictured as a spectrum of bronchopulmonary disorders, ranging from pure obstruction of the airways at one end to pure emphysema at the other; between the two ends are the mixtures which are most prevalent (Chap. 208). Most likely to develop cor pulmonale is the patient with bronchitis and bronchiolitis, usually with some emphysema, in whom obstructive disease of the airways has so deranged the balance between alveolar ventilation, blood flow, and diffusion as to cause the characteristic syndrome of cyanosis (hypoxemia), somnolence (hypercapnia), and right ventricular failure; these are the "blue bloaters." In contrast, the "pink puffers," with comparable degrees of airways obstruction by conventional tests, do not develop hypoxia in the course of their breathless existence; only during an intercurrent respiratory infection, as hypoxia is superimposed, do they become candidates for cor pulmonale. Emphysema without bronchitis is rarely associated with cor pulmonale since alveolar ventilation and capillary blood flow seem to be commensurately curtailed, as after pulmonary resection, so that neither hypoxia nor pulmonary hypertension becomes appreciable.

Treatment of the "blue bloater" with cor pulmonale is directed at relieving the bronchitis and bronchiolitis (Chap. 216); the mainstays are antibiotics for respiratory infection and bronchodilators for bronchoconstriction. Prolonged oxygen therapy (on the order of 15 h per day by nasal catheter) relieves pulmonary hypertension due to alveolar and arterial hypoxia. Cardiac glycosides are useless unless oxygenation is improved. If the patient succeeds in maintaining good oxygenation, digitalis and diuretics can usually be discontinued.

Relief of airways obstruction is more readily accomplished in some disorders than in others. For example, it is generally easier in chronic bronchitis than in cystic fibrosis, in which most of the airways remain plugged with abnormal thick, tenacious sputum despite heroic therapeutic efforts.

Cor pulmonale is uncommon in uncomplicated silicosis or tuberculosis. On the other hand, it is not uncommon when silicosis, anthrosilicosis, or long-standing fibrotic tuberculosis is complicated by extensive, conglomerate, massive fibrosis, distorted adjacent parenchyma, shrunken lobes, and bronchitis. The likelihood of cor pulmonale is increased further by chronic pleurisy, fibrothorax, or excisional surgery. In such cases, a combination of anatomic restriction of the vascular bed and disturbances in gas exchange is involved in the pathogenesis of the pulmonary hypertension. Indeed, the disturbances in gas exchange, often brought to clinical levels by an acute respiratory infection, are the most reversible element of this disorder.

Although it is convenient to separate "net" from "general" alveolar hypoventilation on pathogenetic grounds, the therapeutic principles are basically the same for both and are described in Chap. 216. The present section will deal only with the circulatory abnormalities.

Since the pulmonary hypertension in the most prevalent pulmonary disorders is rarely anatomically fixed but arises mainly from hypoxia and acidosis, relief of alveolar hypoventilation is usually remarkably successful in restoring the circulation to normal. Measures to improve alveolar ventilation vary considerably. In mild cases, simple measures, such as hydration, antibiotics, and bronchodilators, often suffice; in more severe degrees of hypoxemia and hypercapnia, in which heart failure is associated with respiratory insufficiency, mechanical aids to respiration are usually needed.

It has been noted above that treatment of right-sided heart failure is less important than restoring the blood gas values to tolerable levels. The usual therapeutic measures for heart failure (Chap. 182) apply: low-salt regimen, digitalis, diuretics. However, measures to decrease the circulating blood volume (and hematocrit) are of greater importance. Several phlebotomies, each draining 300 to 400 mL, may be needed within a period of 2 to 3 weeks to bring hematocrit and blood volume back to normal; repeated phlebotomies at monthly or bimonthly intervals may have to be instituted to prevent return of the hypervolemia. Diuretics have to be given with more care than usual because the metabolic alkalosis, which may complicate the use of potent diuretics such as ethacrynic acid, aggravates ventilatory insufficiency by depressing the effectiveness of the CO_2 stimulus on the respiratory centers.

The effects of vigorous therapy, directed mainly to the pulmonary disorder, are often dramatic in improving the blood gas abnormalities and heart failure. Other manifestations usually clear more slowly. Indeed, several weeks to a month may elapse before the arterial blood gases, hematocrit, cardiac output, and pulmonary arterial pressures return to optimal levels. But therapy throughout is guided by the fact that the final outcome in cor pulmonale usually depends on the ability to cope with the underlying respiratory disorder rather than with the changes in the heart and circulation.

Vasodilators in pulmonary hypertension and cor pulmonale In recent years, vasodilator agents, such as hydralazine, nitroprusside, prostaglandins, and nifedipine, have been given to patients with pulmonary hypertension of diverse etiologies. These trials have been undertaken with some trepidation, particularly in patients with intrinsic lung disease, in whom relaxation of vascular tone in diseased areas might exaggerate ventilation–blood flow abnormalities and, thereby, increase arterial hypoxemia. As a rule, in acute experiments pulmonary vasodilators do decrease pulmonary arterial pressures toward normal, and the fear of increasing arterial hypoxemia has not been realized. Instead, cardiac output and oxygen delivery to the tissues do increase at the same time that pulmonary arterial pressure decreases. Symptomatic improvement, at rest and during exercise, accompanies the increase in cardiac output and oxygen delivery to the tissues. However, periods of observation have been brief, and long-term consequences of this therapy are still unknown. Moreover, as far as the work of the heart is concerned, the increase in cardiac output often nullifies the direct vasodilator effect of the agent, leaving pulmonary arterial pressure unchanged and occasionally increased; often, the heart rate increases concomitantly. The end result of increase in cardiac output, unchanged pulmonary arterial pressure, and tachycardia is an increase in the work of the heart, raising questions about the extent to which the evolution of cor pulmonale can be favorably influenced by the use of pulmonary vasodilators that also exert direct and reflex stimulatory effects on the heart. Finally, the proper place of pulmonary vasodilator agents in therapy remains to be defined since antibiotics, bronchodilators, and oxygen still remain the essential ingredients.

REFERENCES

FISHMAN AP: Chronic cor pulmonale: State of the art. Am Rev Resp Dis 114:775, 1976

——— (ed): *Pulmonary Diseases and Disorders,* 2nd ed. New York, McGraw-Hill, 1987

———, PIETRA GG: Vasodilator treatment of primary pulmonary hypertension, in *Update: Pulmonary Diseases and Disorders,* AP Fishman (ed). New York, McGraw-Hill, 1982, p 396

HEATH D, WILLIAMS DR: *Man at High Altitude.* Edinburgh, Churchill Livingstone, 1977

LUPI-HERRERA E et al: Hemodynamic effect of hydralazine in interstitial lung disease patients with cor pulmonale. Immediate and short-term evaluation at rest and during exercise. Chest 87:564, 1985

MATTHAY RA, BERGER HJ: Cardiovascular function in cor pulmonale. Clin Chest Med 4:269, 1983

MCFADDEN ER, BRAUNWALD E: Cor pulmonale and pulmonary thromboembolism, in *Heart Disease,* 2d ed, E Braunwald (ed). Philadelphia, Saunders, 1984, p 1572

MIDGREN B et al: Nocturnal hypoxaemia and cor pulmonale in severe chronic lung disease. Bull Eur Physiopathol Respir 21:527, 1985

RUBIN LJ, PETER RH (eds): *Pulmonary Heart Disease.* Hingham, Mass, Martinus Nijhoff-MTP Press, 1984

STERN RC et al: Heart failure in cystic fibrosis. Am J Dis Child 134:267, 1980

WAGENVOORT CA, WAGENVOORT N: *Pathology of Pulmonary Hypertension.* New York, Wiley, 1977

WEIR EK, REEVES JT (eds): *Pulmonary Hypertension.* Mt Kisco, NY, Futura, 1984

WEITZENBLUM E et al: Long-term course of pulmonary arterial pressure in chronic obstructive lung disease. Am Rev Resp Dis 130:993, 1984

192 THE CARDIOMYOPATHIES AND MYOCARDITIDES

JOSHUA WYNNE / EUGENE BRAUNWALD

CARDIOMYOPATHY

The cardiomyopathies are diseases involving the myocardium primarily, not as the result of hypertension or of congenital, valvular, coronary, arterial, or pericardial abnormalities.[1] Although not a leading cause of heart disease in western countries, cardiomyopathy in some of the underdeveloped parts of the world may account for 30 percent or more of all deaths due to heart disease. When the cardiomyopathies are classified on an etiologic basis, two fundamental forms are recognized: (1) a primary type, consisting of heart muscle disease of unknown cause; (2) a secondary type, consisting of myocardial disease of known cause, or associated with a disease involving other organ systems (Table 192-1). In many cases it is not possible to arrive at an etiologic diagnosis on clinical grounds, and thus it is often more desirable to classify the cardiomyopathies on the basis of differences in their pathophysiology and clinical presentation (Tables 192-2 and 192-3). The distinction between the

[1] *Diffuse myocardial fibrosis secondary to multiple myocardial scars produced by extensive coronary arterial narrowing and occlusion can impair left ventricular function and is frequently referred to as ischemic cardiomyopathy. According to the definition given above, however, the term* cardiomyopathy *should be restricted to a condition* primarily *involving heart muscle. In ischemic cardiomyopathy the* primary involvement *is in the coronary vessels.*

TABLE 192-1 Etiologic classification of cardiomyopathies

I Primary myocardial involvement
- *A* Idiopathic (D,R,H)
- *B* Familial (D,H)
- *C* Eosinophilic endomyocardial disease (R)
- *D* Endomyocardial fibrosis (R)

II Secondary myocardial involvement
- *A* Infective (D)
  - *1* Viral myocarditis
  - *2* Bacterial myocarditis
  - *3* Fungal myocarditis
  - *4* Protozoal myocarditis
  - *5* Metazoal myocarditis
- *B* Metabolic (D)
- *C* Familial storage disease (D,R)
  - *1* Glycogen storage disease
  - *2* Mucopolysaccharidoses
- *D* Deficiency (D)
  - *1* Electrolytes
  - *2* Nutritional
- *E* Connective tissue disorders (D)
  - *1* Systemic lupus erythematosus
  - *2* Polyarteritis nodosa
  - *3* Rheumatoid arthritis
  - *4* Scleroderma
  - *5* Dermatomyositis
- *F* Infiltrations and granulomas (R,D)
  - *1* Amyloidosis
  - *2* Sarcoidosis
  - *3* Malignancy
  - *4* Hemochromatosis
- *G* Neuromuscular (D)
  - *1* Muscular dystrophy
  - *2* Myotonic dystrophy
  - *3* Friedreich's ataxia (H,D)
  - *4* Refsum's disease
- *H* Sensitivity and toxic reactions (D)
  - *1* Alcohol
  - *2* Radiation
  - *3* Drugs
- *I* Peripartum heart disease (D)
- *J* Endocardial fibroelastosis (R)

NOTE: *The principal clinical manifestation(s) of each etiologic grouping is denoted by D (dilated), R (restrictive), or H (hypertrophic) cardiomyopathy.*
SOURCE: *Adapted from the WHO/ISFC task force report on the definition and classification of cardiomyopathies, 1980.*

functional categories is not absolute, however, and there is often some overlap.

DILATED (CONGESTIVE) CARDIOMYOPATHY Systolic pump function is impaired, leading to cardiac enlargement and often producing symptoms of congestive heart failure. Mural thrombi are often present, particularly in the left ventricular apex. Histologic examination reveals extensive areas of interstitial and perivascular fibrosis, with minimal necrosis and cellular infiltration. Although no

TABLE 192-2 Clinical classification of cardiomyopathies

1 Dilated (congestive): Left and/or right ventricular enlargement, impaired systolic function, congestive heart failure, arrhythmias, emboli
2 Restrictive: Endomyocardial scarring or myocardial infiltration resulting in restriction to left and/or right ventricular filling
3 Hypertrophic: Disproportionate left ventricular hypertrophy, typically involving septum more than free wall, with or without obstruction to ventricular outflow; usually of a nondilated left ventricular cavity

etiology is apparent in many cases, dilated cardiomyopathy (formerly called congestive cardiomyopathy) is probably the end result of myocardial damage produced by a variety of toxic, metabolic, or infectious agents. There is increasing evidence to suggest that in at least some patients dilated cardiomyopathy may be the late sequel of acute viral myocarditis, possibly mediated through an immunologic mechanism. Although most commonly a disease of middle-aged men, it may occur in any patient population. A reversible form of dilated cardiomyopathy may be found with selenium deficiency.

CLINICAL MANIFESTATIONS Symptoms of left- and right-sided congestive failure, manifested by dyspnea on exertion, fatigue, orthopnea, paroxysmal nocturnal dyspnea, peripheral edema, and palpitations, develop gradually in most patients. Some patients have left ventricular dilatation for months or even years before becoming symptomatic. Although vague chest pain may be present, typical angina pectoris is unusual and suggests the presence of concomitant coronary artery disease.

PHYSICAL EXAMINATION Variable degrees of cardiac enlargement and findings of congestive heart failure are noted. In patients with advanced disease, the pulse pressure is small, and the jugular venous pressure is elevated. Third and fourth heart sounds are common, and mitral or tricuspid regurgitation may occur. Diastolic murmurs, valvular calcification, hypertension, and changes of vascular disease in the optic fundi militate *against* the diagnosis of cardiomyopathy.

LABORATORY EXAMINATIONS The chest roentgenogram demonstrates left ventricular enlargement, although generalized cardiomegaly is often seen, sometimes due to a concomitant pericardial effusion. The lung fields may demonstrate evidence of pulmonary venous hypertension and interstitial or alveolar edema. The electrocardiogram often shows sinus tachycardia or atrial fibrillation, ventricular arrhythmias, left atrial enlargement, diffuse nonspecific ST-T-wave changes, and sometimes intraventricular conduction defects. Echocardiography and radionuclide ventriculography show left ventricular enlargement, with normal or minimally thickened or thinned walls, and systolic dysfunction (reduced ejection fraction); a pericardial

TABLE 192-3 Laboratory evaluation of the cardiomyopathies

	Dilated (congestive)	Restrictive	Hypertrophic
Chest roentgenogram	Moderate to marked cardiac enlargement Pulmonary venous hypertension	Mild cardiac enlargement	Mild to moderate cardiac enlargement
Electrocardiogram	ST-segment and T-wave abnormalities	Low-voltage Conduction defects	ST-segment and T-wave abnormalities Left ventricular hypertrophy Abnormal Q waves
Echocardiogram	Left ventricular dilatation and dysfunction	Increased left ventricular wall thickness Normal systolic function	Asymmetric septal hypertrophy (ASH) Systolic anterior motion (SAM) of the mitral valve
Radionuclide studies	Left ventricular dilatation and dysfunction (RVG)	Normal systolic function (RVG)	Vigorous systolic function (RVG) Asymmetric septal hypertrophy (RVG or ^{201}Tl)
Cardiac catheterization	Left ventricular dilatation and dysfunction Elevated left- and often right-sided filling pressures Diminished cardiac output	Normal systolic function Elevated left- and right-sided filling pressures	Vigorous systolic function Dynamic left ventricular outflow obstruction Elevated left- and right-sided filling pressures

NOTE: *RVG = radionuclide ventriculogram; ^{201}Tl = thallium 201.*

effusion is often noted. Radioisotopic imaging with gallium 67 may identify patients with dilated cardiomyopathy and myocarditis.

Hemodynamic studies reveal a cardiac output that is moderately or severely reduced at rest, and that does not increase normally with exercise. The left ventricular end-diastolic, left atrial, and pulmonary capillary wedge pressures usually are elevated; when failure of the right side of the heart supervenes, the right ventricular end-diastolic, right atrial, and central venous pressures are also elevated. Angiography reveals a dilated, diffusely hypokinetic left ventricle, often with some degree of mitral regurgitation; the coronary arteries are normal, thereby excluding so-called ischemic cardiomyopathy. Transvenous endomyocardial biopsy (Chap. 180) may be helpful in excluding certain conditions such as myocardial infiltration by amyloid; in some patients there is biopsy evidence of myocardial round cell inflammation, suggesting an inflammatory etiology and compatible with previous viral myocarditis.

TREATMENT Most patients pursue an inexorably downhill course, and the majority, particularly those over 55 years of age, die within 2 years of the onset of symptoms. Death is due to either congestive heart failure or ventricular arrhythmia; sudden death, presumably arrhythmic in etiology, is a constant threat. Systemic embolization is common, and all patients without contraindications should receive anticoagulants. Since the cause of primary dilated cardiomyopathy is, by definition, unknown, specific therapy is not possible. Prolonged strict bed rest for up to 1 year or more has been advocated, but the effectiveness of this form of therapy remains controversial and such therapy is not feasible in most patients; strenuous exertion should, however, be interdicted. Treatment of heart failure in dilated cardiomyopathy should be considered palliative and directed toward improvement in symptoms; there is no convincing evidence that therapy alters prognosis. Standard therapy of heart failure with salt restriction, diuretics, digitalis, and vasodilators may produce symptomatic improvement, at least in the initial phases of the illness; however, these patients appear to be at increased risk of digitalis toxicity. Newer cardiotonic agents, such as amrinone and the related experimental agent milrinone, may provide additional clinical improvement (Chap. 182). Some patients with dilated cardiomyopathy who have evidence of myocardial inflammation have been treated with corticosteroids, often in association with azathioprine; others have been treated cautiously with gradually increasing doses of beta-adrenergic blockers. However, the indications and value of such experimental therapy remain controversial. Antiarrhythmic agents may be used to treat symptomatic or serious arrhythmias, although they may be extremely resistant to the usual as well as investigational agents. Because of this, alternative experimental therapies, such as surgical interruption of the arrhythmic circuit or implantation of an automatic internal defibrillator, have gained favor. In patients with advanced disease who are refractory to medical therapy and who have no contraindications to the procedure (Chap. 182), cardiac transplantation should be considered.

The preceding discussion emphasized clinical features of the dilated cardiomyopathies, regardless of whether they are primary or secondary in etiology. Many cases of dilated cardiomyopathy are primary (without a definable cause), but a number of specific conditions may also cause dilated cardiomyopathy secondarily. Since some of these conditions are reversible, features peculiar to these disorders will be considered in turn.

Alcoholic cardiomyopathy Individuals who consume large quantities of alcohol over many years may develop a clinical picture identical to idiopathic dilated cardiomyopathy; indeed, alcoholic cardiomyopathy is the major form of secondary dilated cardiomyopathy in the western world. Ceasing alcohol consumption before severe heart failure has developed may halt the progression, or even reverse the course of this disease, unlike the idiopathic variety which is marked by progressive deterioration. Alcoholics with advanced heart failure have a poor prognosis, particularly if they continue to drink; less than one-quarter survive 3 years. The key to the treatment of alcoholic cardiomyopathy is total and permanent abstinence. Although thiamine deficiency may be present in some of these patients, alcoholic cardiomyopathy is associated with a low cardiac output and systemic vasoconstriction. In contrast, beriberi heart disease (Chaps. 76 and 193) is characterized by elevated cardiac output and diminished peripheral vascular resistance, so that thiamine deficiency per se does not appear to cause alcoholic cardiomyopathy. A second presentation of alcoholic cardiotoxicity may be found in individuals without overt heart failure, and consists of recurrent supraventricular or ventricular tachyarrhythmias. Termed the "holiday heart syndrome," it typically appears after a drinking binge; atrial fibrillation is seen most frequently, followed by atrial flutter and ventricular premature depolarizations.

Peripartum cardiomyopathy Cardiac dilatation and congestive heart failure of unexplained cause may develop during the last month of pregnancy or within the first few months after delivery. The etiology of this disorder is unknown but may relate to a preexisting cardiomyopathy that was not apparent prior to pregnancy. Necropsy shows cardiac enlargement, often with mural thrombi, along with histologic evidence of myocardial degeneration and fibrosis. The patient who develops peripartum cardiomyopathy is typically multiparous, black, and over the age of 30. While some patients are malnourished, there is no conclusive evidence that dietary deficiencies are etiologically involved. The symptoms, signs, and treatment are similar to those in patients with idiopathic dilated cardiomyopathy. The prognosis in these patients appears to be closely related to whether the heart size returns to normal after the first episode of congestive heart failure. If it does, subsequent pregnancies may sometimes be well tolerated; if the heart remains enlarged, however, further pregnancies frequently produce increasing myocardial damage, ultimately leading to refractory congestive heart failure and death. Those who recover should be encouraged to avoid further pregnancies, particularly if cardiomegaly persists.

Neuromuscular disease (see also Chap. 357) Cardiac involvement is common in many of the muscular dystrophies. In *Duchenne's progressive muscular dystrophy,* myocardial involvement is most frequently indicated by a distinctive and unique electrocardiographic pattern consisting of tall R waves in right precordial leads with an R/S ratio greater than 1.0, often associated with deep Q waves in the limb and lateral precordial leads, and is not found in other forms of muscular dystrophy. These electrocardiographic abnormalities appear to result from selective transmural necrosis of the posterobasal left ventricle and associated papillary muscle. A variety of supraventricular and ventricular arrhythmias is frequently found. Rapidly progressive congestive heart failure may supervene after years of apparent circulatory stability during which the only detectable abnormalities are in the electrocardiogram. *Myotonic dystrophy* is characterized by a variety of electrocardiographic abnormalities, especially disorders of impulse formation and conduction, but other overt clinical evidence of heart disease is uncommon. Because of the abnormalities of impulse generation and conduction, syncope and sudden death are major hazards; in appropriate patients, insertion of a permanent pacemaker may be efficacious. In *limb-girdle* and *fascioscapulohumeral dystrophy,* cardiac involvement is uncommon and seldom severe. Involvement of the heart is very common in *Friedreich's ataxia,* with as many as half of the patients developing cardiac symptoms. It is now generally accepted that the heart disease in Friedreich's ataxia is similar to hypertrophic cardiomyopathy (page 1002), although typically of the concentric form (with symmetric hypertrophy of left ventricular septum and free wall) and without the cellular disarray found in the usual case of hypertrophic cardiomyopathy. The electrocardiogram may demonstrate inappropriate sinus tachycardia and a variety of arrhythmias, as well as ventricular hypertrophy and ST-segment and T-wave abnormalities. The echocardiogram usually demonstrates left ventricular hypertrophy, and dynamic left ventricular outflow tract obstruction is seen on occasion.

Drugs A variety of pharmacologic agents may damage the myocardium acutely, producing a pattern of inflammation (myocarditis), or they may lead to chronic damage of the type seen with idiopathic dilated cardiomyopathy. Certain drugs produce only electrocardiographic abnormalities, while others may precipitate fulminant congestive heart failure and death. The anthracycline derivatives, particularly *doxorubicin* (Adriamycin), are powerful antineoplastic agents, which, when given in high doses (more than 550 mg/m^2 for doxorubicin), may produce fatal heart failure. The incidence of heart failure is related not only to the dose of the drug but to the presence or absence of several risk factors (cardiac irradiation, age greater than 70 years, underlying heart disease, hypertension, treatment with cyclophosphamide); at any dose patients with these risk factors have an eight- to tenfold greater frequency of developing heart failure than do patients lacking them. Radionuclide ventriculography (Chap. 179) may document preclinical deterioration of left ventricular function and allow appropriate dose adjustments; half of asymptomatic patients treated with standard doses may demonstrate left ventricular dysfunction for years after treatment. Recent efforts to modify the dose schedule by giving the drug more slowly have reduced the risk of cardiotoxicity further. High-dose *cyclophosphamide* may produce congestive heart failure acutely or within 2 weeks of administration; a characteristic histopathologic feature is myocardial edema and hemorrhagic necrosis. Rarely, patients treated with *5-fluorouracil* will develop chest pain and electrocardiographic changes of myocardial ischemia or infarction. Electrocardiographic changes and arrhythmias may result from treatment with tricyclic antidepressants, the phenothiazines, emetine, lithium, and various aerosol propellants.

RESTRICTIVE CARDIOMYOPATHY The hallmark of the restrictive cardiomyopathies is abnormal diastolic function; the ventricular walls are excessively rigid and impede ventricular filling. Myocardial fibrosis, hypertrophy, or infiltration secondary to a variety of etiologies is usually responsible. The infiltrative diseases, which represent important etiologies for secondary restrictive cardiomyopathy, may also show some impairment of systolic function. Myocardial involvement with *amyloid* is a common cause of secondary restrictive cardiomyopathy, although restriction is also seen in hemochromatosis, glycogen deposition, endomyocardial fibrosis, fibroelastosis, the eosinophilias, neoplastic infiltration, and myocardial fibrosis of diverse causes. In many of these conditions, particularly those with substantial concomitant endocardial involvement, partial obliteration of the ventricular cavity by fibrous tissue and thrombus contributes to the abnormally increased resistance to ventricular filling. As a result of persistently elevated venous pressure these patients commonly have dependent edema, ascites, and an enlarged, tender liver. The jugular venous pressure is elevated and does not fall normally, or it may rise with inspiration (Kussmaul's sign). The heart sounds may be distant, and third and fourth heart sounds are common. In contrast to constrictive pericarditis, which these diseases resemble, the apex impulse is usually easily palpable. The electrocardiogram shows low-voltage, nonspecific ST-T-wave changes and various arrhythmias. Pericardial calcification on x-ray, which would suggest constrictive pericarditis, is absent. Echocardiography typically reveals symmetrically thickened left ventricular walls and normal or slightly reduced systolic function. Cardiac catheterization shows a decreased cardiac output, elevation of the right and left ventricular end-diastolic pressures, and a dip-and-plateau configuration of the diastolic portion of the ventricular pressure pulse resembling that seen in constrictive pericarditis.

Differentiation from constrictive pericarditis, at the bedside and even after cardiac catheterization, may be difficult or impossible (Chaps. 180 and 194). This distinction is of importance because the latter condition is potentially curable by operation. Right ventricular transvenous endomyocardial biopsy may be helpful in the differentiation of these two diseases by revealing interstitial infiltration or fibrosis in restrictive cardiomyopathy, but exploratory thoracotomy is occasionally necessary to distinguish restrictive cardiomyopathy from chronic constrictive pericarditis.

Endomyocardial fibrosis This is a progressive disease of unknown etiology which occurs most commonly in children and young adults residing in tropical and subtropical Africa, particularly Uganda and Nigeria. The disease is characterized by fibrous endocardial lesions of the inflow portion of the right or left ventricle (or both) and often involves the atrioventricular valves, producing valvular regurgitation. The apex of the ventricles may be obliterated by a mass of thrombus and fibrous tissue. In many ways this disease resembles eosinophilic endomyocardial disease, although they occur in quite different geographic areas and age groups. Endomyocardial fibrosis is a frequent cause of heart failure in Africa, accounting for up to one-quarter of deaths due to heart disease.

The clinical picture depends upon which ventricle and atrioventricular valve show predominant involvement; left-sided involvement results in symptoms of pulmonary congestion, while predominant right-sided disease presents features of a restrictive cardiomyopathy. Medical treatment is often disappointing, and surgical excision of the fibrotic endocardium and replacement of the involved atrioventricular valve has led to substantial symptomatic improvement in a small number of patients.

Eosinophilic endomyocardial disease Also called *Loeffler's endocarditis* and *fibroplastic endocarditis,* this disease appears to be a subcategory of the hypereosinophilic syndrome in which the heart is predominantly involved. Typically, the endocardium of either or both ventricles thickens markedly, with involvement of the underlying myocardium. Large mural thrombi may develop in either ventricle, thereby compromising the size of the ventricular cavity and serving as a source of pulmonary and systemic emboli. Hepatosplenomegaly and localized eosinophilic infiltration of other organs are usually present. Once the disease becomes clinically evident, survival is usually brief, although recent reports have suggested a more benign course, with average survival exceeding 5 years. The reason for this improvement in prognosis is unclear but may be related to therapy with corticosteroids and immunosuppressive drugs.

Differential diagnosis Involvement of the heart is the most frequent cause of death in *primary amyloidosis* (Chap. 259), while clinically significant cardiac involvement is uncommon in the secondary form. Biopsy of the rectal mucosa, gingiva, liver, kidney, and myocardium permits the diagnosis to be made before death in over three-quarters of cases. The heart is firm, rubbery, and noncompliant, and four clinical presentations (alone or in combination) are seen: (1) diastolic dysfunction (restrictive cardiomyopathy); (2) systolic dysfunction; (3) arrhythmias; and (4) orthostatic hypotension. The two-dimensional echocardiogram may be helpful in making the diagnosis of amyloidosis and may show a thickened myocardial wall with a distinctive "speckled" appearance. *Hemochromatosis* (Chap. 310) should be suspected if cardiomyopathy occurs in the setting of diabetes mellitus, hepatic cirrhosis, and increased skin pigmentation. Phlebotomy may be of some benefit if employed early in the course of the disease. Continuous subcutaneous administration of desferrioxamine may reduce body iron stores in advanced cases, but whether this produces clinical improvement is unclear. Myocardial *sarcoidosis* (Chap. 270) is generally associated with other manifestations of systemic disease and may have restrictive as well as congestive features, since cardiac infiltration by sarcoid granulomata results not only in increased stiffness of the myocardium but also in diminished systolic contractile function. A variety of arrhythmias, including atrioventricular block, have been noted. *Endocardial fibroelastosis* is a disease seen in infants, characterized by a thickened endocardium that shows proliferation of elastic tissue. It is most unusual in adult patients, although small patches of it may be found in patients with endomyocardial fibrosis.

Transvenous biopsy of the endocardium (Chap. 180), usually right ventricular, has been used increasingly to obtain tissue specimens for histologic and electron-microscopic study. This relatively simple and safe technique is important in the diagnosis of myocardial disease, particularly in the recognition of infiltrative diseases such as amyloidosis, hemochromatosis, and sarcoidosis.

HYPERTROPHIC CARDIOMYOPATHY This disease is characterized by left ventricular hypertrophy, typically of a nondilated chamber, without obvious antecedent cause. The hypertrophy is thus not secondary to a cardiovascular or systemic disease, such as hypertension or aortic stenosis, that places a hemodynamic burden on the left ventricle. Two features of the disease which are common, but by no means universal, have attracted the greatest attention: (1) asymmetric septal hypertrophy (ASH), wherein the upper portion of the interventricular septum is preferentially hypertrophied in comparison to the thickness of the posterobasal left ventricular free wall; and (2) dynamic left ventricular outflow tract obstruction, due to narrowing of the subaortic area usually resulting from the midsystolic apposition of the anterior mitral valve leaflet against the hypertrophied septum, i.e., systolic anterior motion of the mitral valve (SAM). Initial studies of this disease emphasized the dynamic obstructive features, and it has been termed idiopathic hypertrophic subaortic stenosis (IHSS), hypertrophic obstructive cardiomyopathy (HOCM), and muscular subaortic stenosis. It has become clear, however, that many and perhaps most patients with hypertrophic cardiomyopathy do not, in fact, demonstrate outflow tract obstruction. The ubiquitous pathophysiologic abnormality is not systolic but rather *diastolic* dysfunction, characterized by increased stiffness of the hypertrophied muscle. This results in elevated diastolic filling pressures and is present despite a hypercontractile left ventricle.

The pattern of hypertrophy is distinctive in hypertrophic cardiomyopathy and differs from that seen in secondary hypertrophy (as in hypertension). Most patients demonstrate a ventricular septum whose thickness is disproportionately increased when compared with the free wall. Other patients may demonstrate disproportionate involvement of the apex or left ventricular free wall; 10 percent or more of patients have concentric involvement of the ventricle. All, however, show a bizarre and disorganized arrangement of cardiac muscle cells in the septum, whether or not obstruction is present. Patients without obstruction may demonstrate similar derangements of the left ventricular free wall.

At least half of all cases of hypertrophic cardiomyopathy appear to be transmitted as autosomal dominants with a high degree of penetrance; the remainder occur sporadically. Echocardiographic studies have confirmed that up to one-half the first-degree relatives (i.e., parents, siblings, and children) of patients with familial hypertrophic cardiomyopathy have evidence of septal hypertrophy, although many of these are without evidence of obstruction and are asymptomatic.

In contrast to the obstruction produced by a fixed narrowed orifice, such as valvular aortic stenosis, the obstruction in hypertrophic cardiomyopathy, when present, is dynamic and may change between examinations and even from beat to beat. Obstruction appears to result from further narrowing of an already small left ventricular outflow tract by systolic anterior motion of the mitral valve against the hypertrophied septum. While SAM may be found in a variety of other conditions besides hypertrophic cardiomyopathy, it is *always* found when obstruction is present in hypertrophic cardiomyopathy. Three basic mechanisms are involved in the production of dynamic obstruction: (1) increased left ventricular contractility, which reduces ventricular systolic volume and increases the ejection velocity of the blood moving through the outflow tract, thus drawing the anterior mitral valve leaflet against the septum as a result of reduced distending pressure; (2) decreased ventricular volume (preload), which reduces further the size of the outflow tract; and (3) decreased aortic impedance and pressure (afterload), which increases the velocity of flow through the subaortic area and also reduces ventricular systolic volume. Interventions that increase myocardial contractility, such as exercise, isoproterenol, and digitalis glycosides, and those that reduce ventricular volume, such as the Valsalva maneuver, sudden standing, nitroglycerin, amyl nitrite, or tachycardia, all may cause an increase in obstruction. Conversely, elevation of arterial pressure by phenylephrine, squatting, sustained handgrip, augmentation of venous return by raising the legs, and expansion of the blood volume all increase ventricular volume and ameliorate the obstruction. Sometimes the hypertrophied septum bulges into the outflow tract of the right ventricle, thereby impeding the ejection of blood from this chamber as well. Hypertrophic cardiomyopathy has been found in association with *lentiginosis* and other disorders of neural crest tissue. Similar gross anatomic and hemodynamic patterns may be found in the infants of diabetic mothers and in patients with *Friedreich's ataxia*.

CLINICAL FEATURES Many patients with hypertrophic cardiomyopathy are asymptomatic and may be relatives of patients with known disease. Unfortunately, the first clinical manifestation of the disease may be sudden death, frequently occurring in children and young adults, often during or after physical exertion. In symptomatic patients the most common complaint is dyspnea, largely due to increased stiffness of the left ventricular walls, which impairs ventricular filling and leads to elevated left ventricular diastolic and left atrial pressures. Other symptoms include angina pectoris, fatigue, syncope, and near syncope (''graying-out spells''). Symptoms are not related to the presence or severity of outflow obstruction. Most patients with obstruction demonstrate a double or triple apical impulse, a rapidly rising carotid arterial pulse, and a fourth heart sound. The hallmark of obstructive hypertrophic cardiomyopathy is a systolic murmur, which is typically harsh, diamond-shaped, and usually begins well after the first heart sound, since ejection is unimpeded early in systole. The murmur is best heard at the lower left sternal border as well as at the apex, where it is often more holosystolic and blowing in quality, no doubt due to the mitral regurgitation that usually accompanies obstructive hypertrophic cardiomyopathy.

LABORATORY EVALUATION The *electrocardiogram* commonly shows left ventricular hypertrophy and widespread, deep, broad Q waves that suggest an old myocardial infarction but apparently result from the abnormal electrophysiologic properties of the hypertrophied septum. Many patients demonstrate arrhythmias, both atrial (supraventricular tachycardia or atrial fibrillation) as well as ventricular (ventricular tachycardia) during ambulatory (Holter) monitoring. *Chest roentgenography* may be normal, although a mild to moderate increase in the cardiac silhouette is common. Aortic root enlargement and valvular calcification are not seen, helping to differentiate this condition from valvular aortic stenosis. The mainstay of the diagnosis of hypertrophic cardiomyopathy is the *echocardiogram,* which demonstrates left ventricular hypertrophy, typically with the septum 1.3 or more times the thickness of the high posterior left ventricular free wall. The septum may demonstrate an unusual ground-glass appearance, probably related to its abnormal cellular architecture and myocardial fibrosis. Systolic anterior motion of the mitral valve is found in patients with obstruction. The left ventricular cavity is typically small in hypertrophic cardiomyopathy, with vigorous posterior wall motion, but reduced septal excursion. A rare form of hypertrophic cardiomyopathy is characterized by massive apical hypertrophy, often associated with giant negative T waves on the electrocardiogram and a ''spade-shaped'' left ventricular cavity on angiography. The two-dimensional *echocardiogram* is particularly useful in identifying all of the characteristic changes, including the size and shape of the left ventricular cavity. The indirectly recorded *carotid arterial pulse* tracing rises unusually rapidly and often displays a ''spike-and-dome'' configuration when an outflow pressure gradient is present. *Radionuclide scintigraphy* with thallium 201 and blood pool scans permits visualization of the size and orientation of the interventricular septum.

The two typical *hemodynamic* features are an elevated left ventricular diastolic pressure due to diminished left ventricular compliance and, when obstruction is present, a systolic pressure gradient between the body of the left ventricle and the subaortic region. When a gradient is not present, it often can be induced by provocative maneuvers such as infusion of isoproterenol, inhalation of amyl nitrite, or the Valsalva maneuver.

TREATMENT Beta-adrenergic blockers are often used and may ameliorate to some degree the symptoms of angina pectoris and syncope. Resting intraventricular pressure gradients are usually unchanged, although these drugs may limit the increase in the gradient that occurs during exercise. However, there is no evidence that beta blockers protect against sudden death, which is presumably arrhythmic in origin. It is unestablished whether any antiarrhythmic agent is efficacious in this setting. However, the experimental agent amiodarone appears to be effective in reducing the frequency of supraventricular as well as life-threatening ventricular arrhythmias. The calcium channel blocking drugs, particularly verapamil and nifedipine, are promising agents that may reduce the stiffness of the ventricle, reduce the elevated diastolic pressures, increase exercise tolerance, and in some instances reduce the severity of outflow tract obstruction. Disopyramide has been used in some patients to reduce left ventricular contractility and the outflow gradient. Surgical myotomy/myectomy of the hypertrophied septum may result in lasting symptomatic improvement, but the mortality of approximately 10 percent limits the operation to severely symptomatic patients with high-grade obstruction unresponsive to medical management. Digitalis, diuretics, nitrates, and beta-adrenergic agonists are best avoided if possible, particularly in patients with known left ventricular outflow tract pressure gradients.

PROGNOSIS The natural history of hypertrophic cardiomyopathy is variable, although many patients demonstrate an improvement or stabilization of symptoms with time. Atrial fibrillation is common late in the course of the disease; its onset usually leads to a striking increase in symptoms, presumably due to loss of the atrial contribution to filling of the thickened ventricle. This rhythm, when sustained, is associated with a poor prognosis. Infective endocarditis occurs in less than 10 percent of patients, and endocarditis prophylaxis is indicated, particularly in patients with resting obstruction and mitral regurgitation. Progression of obstructive hypertrophic cardiomyopathy to left ventricular dilatation and dysfunction without an outflow gradient has been reported but is unusual. The major cause of mortality in hypertrophic cardiomyopathy is sudden death, which may occur in asymptomatic patients or interrupt an otherwise stable course in symptomatic ones. Paradoxically, younger patients and those with mild or no obstruction appear to be at particular risk of sudden death. Since sudden death often occurs during or just after physical exertion, strenuous exercise should be avoided in all patients, regardless of symptoms. Although hemodynamic factors may play a role, it is likely that most deaths, particularly those that are sudden, are due to ventricular arrhythmias. Beta-adrenergic blockade appears to be ineffective in preventing sudden death. The protective effect of calcium channel blockers or antiarrhythmic agents has not been established, but of the agents available, amiodarone appears to be the most promising in this regard.

MYOCARDITIS

Myocarditis is said to be present when the heart is involved in an inflammatory process. Most commonly the result of an infectious process, myocarditis may also be present in hypersensitivity states such as acute rheumatic fever (Chap. 186) or may be caused by radiation, chemicals, physical agents, and drugs. Myocarditis may be acute or chronic. In an unknown number of cases, acute myocarditis progresses to chronic dilated cardiomyopathy. While almost every infectious agent is capable of producing myocarditis, clinically significant acute myocarditis in the United States is caused most commonly by viruses. Coxsackie B is the most frequent etiologic agent of viral myocarditis, but Coxsackie A, poliomyelitis, influenza, adeno, echo, rubeola, and rubella viruses also cause the disease. In most cases, the presence of myocarditis is inferred only by the finding of transient electrocardiographic ST-T-wave abnormalities, but arrhythmias, heart failure, and death may occur in fulminant cases, particularly in infants and pregnant women. Myocarditis is frequently associated with acute pericarditis, particularly when it is caused by Coxsackie B strains or echoviruses (Chap. 140).

Physical examination may be normal in patients who have only electrocardiographic abnormalities, although more severe cases may show a muffled first heart sound, along with a third heart sound and a murmur of mitral regurgitation. A pericardial friction rub may be audible in patients with associated pericarditis.

Experimental studies suggest that exercise may be deleterious in patients with myocarditis, and strenuous activity should be proscribed until the electrocardiogram has returned to normal. Prolonged bed rest has been advocated for more severe cases, although its efficacy remains to be established. Patients who develop congestive heart failure respond to the usual measures (digitalis, diuretics, salt restriction), but they appear to be unusually sensitive to digitalis. Arrhythmias are common and are occasionally difficult to manage. Deaths attributed to heart failure, tachyarrhythmias, and heart block have been reported, and it seems prudent to monitor the electrocardiogram of patients with arrhythmias, especially during the acute illness.

Though viral myocarditis is most often self-limited and without sequelae, active disease may recur, and it is likely that acute viral myocarditis occasionally progresses to a chronic form. Patients with viral myocarditis often give a history of a preceding upper respiratory febrile illness, and viral nasopharyngitis or tonsillitis may be evident clinically. The isolation of virus from the stool, pharyngeal washings, or other body fluids, and changes in specific antibody titers are helpful clinically. Many instances of apparent *idiopathic* dilated cardiomyopathy (page 999) appear to arise from mild or subclinical episodes of myocarditis. While corticosteroids may exacerbate heart damage in animals with acute viral myocarditis, a small number of humans with congestive heart failure and inflammatory myocarditis appear to respond to an experimental protocol utilizing immunosuppression with prednisone and azathioprine. Serial right ventricular endomyocardial biopsies have shown regression of inflammatory infiltrates in some patients so treated. However, the effects of this treatment program have not been rigorously compared to a comparable control group.

Bacterial myocarditis Bacterial involvement of the heart is uncommon, but when it does occur, it is usually as a complication of bacterial endocarditis (typically due to *Staphylococcus aureus* and enterococci). Myocardial abscess formation may involve the valve rings and interventricular septum. *Diphtheritic myocarditis* develops in over one-quarter of the patients with diphtheria, is one of the most serious complications, and is the most common cause of death due to diphtheria (Chap. 96). Cardiac damage is due to the liberation of a toxin that inhibits protein synthesis, and leads to a dilated, flabby, hypocontractile heart; the conducting system is frequently involved as well. Cardiomegaly and severe congestive heart failure typically appear after the first week of illness. ST-segment and T-wave abnormalities on the electrocardiogram are the rule, but atrial and ventricular arrhythmias, bundle branch block, and abnormalities of atrioventricular conduction are also common. Prompt therapy with antitoxin is crucial; antibiotic therapy is also indicated but is of less urgency.

Chagas' disease Chagas' disease, caused by the protozoan *Trypanosoma cruzi* (Chap. 156), produces an extensive myocarditis that typically becomes evident years after the initial infection. It is one of the most common causes of heart disease encountered in Central and South America; in rural areas up to 20 percent of the population may be affected. Although only a minority of infected individuals have an acute illness, upwards of one-third develop chronic myocardial damage, typically appearing 20 years after the initial infection. The chronic form is characterized by dilatation of several cardiac chambers, fibrosis and thinning of the ventricular wall, aneurysm formation in the areas of thinning (especially at the apex), and mural thrombi. Chronic progressive heart failure, often predominantly right-sided, is the rule. The electrocardiogram typically shows right bundle branch block and left anterior hemiblock, which may progress to complete atrioventricular block. The echocardiogram may reveal a unique pattern of hypokinesis of the posterior left ventricular wall and relatively preserved septal motion. Ventricular arrhythmias are common and are seen particularly during and after exertion; oral amiodarone appears to be particularly effective in treating ventricular tachyarrhythmias. The cause of death is either intractable congestive heart failure or an arrhythmia. Therapy is directed toward amelioration of the congestive heart failure and arrhythmias; the latter may require implantation of a pacemaker.

Toxoplasmic myocarditis (see also Chap. 157) This uncommon form of protozoal myocardial involvement occurs most frequently in immunosuppressed adults; congenital toxoplasmal infections are much more common, but myocarditis is not a prominent feature. Myocardial involvement may lead to cardiac dilatation, pericarditis, and percardial effusion. Heart failure, arrhythmias, and conduction abnormalities may be seen. Because of the difficulty in diagnosing this condition, it may be a more common problem than is usually appreciated. Treatment is with pyrimethamine and sulfonamides, but the response to treatment is variable.

Giant cell myocarditis This rare myocarditis of unknown etiology is characterized by the presence of multinucleated giant cells in the myocardium. It usually causes rapidly fatal congestive heart failure and arrhythmia in young to middle-aged adults. At necropsy, the distinctive features include grossly visible serpiginous areas of myocardial necrosis in both ventricles and microscopic evidence of giant cells within an extensive inflammatory infiltrate. The cause of giant cell myocarditis remains obscure, although it occurs in association with thymoma, systemic lupus erythematosus, and thyrotoxicosis.

Lyme carditis (see also Chap. 127) Lyme disease is a newly described condition, caused by a tick-borne spirochete. Conduction abnormalities are the most common manifestations of cardiac involvement and may progress to complete atrioventricular block with syncope. Concomitant myopericarditis is not uncommon, and mild left ventricular dysfunction may occur. Prednisone may be efficacious in ameliorating the heart block; penicillin is used to treat the accompanying skin rash, arthritis, and neurologic abnormalities.

Radiation myocarditis A variety of acute and chronic cardiac complications may result from the use of ionizing radiation in the treatment of carcinoma of the lung or breast, lymphoma, or Hodgkin's disease. Only an occasional patient manifests acute cardiac abnormalities; typically such an abnormality consists of acute pericarditis. The most common presentation is that of chronic pericardial effusion or constriction occurring months or years after exposure (in rare cases up to 10 years) (Chap. 194). Myocardial fibrosis, resulting from damage to the microvasculature, often with formation of atherosclerotic plaques of the epicardial coronary arteries, is also common.

REFERENCES

ABELMANN WH: Classification and natural history of primary myocardial disease. Prog Cardiovasc Dis 27:73, 1984

BROSIUS FC III et al: Radiation heart disease. Am J Med 70:519, 1981

CUETO-GARCIA L et al: Echocardiographic findings in systemic amyloidosis: Spectrum of cardiac involvement and relation to survival. J Am Coll Cardiol 6:737, 1985

DALY K et al: Acute myocarditis: Role of histological and virological examination in the diagnosis and assessment of immunosuppressive treatment. Br Heart J 51:30, 1984

DEC GW JR et al: Active myocarditis in the spectrum of acute dilated cardiomyopathies: Clinical features, histologic correlates, and clinical outcome. N Engl J Med 312:885, 1985

FENOGLIO JJ JR et al: Diagnosis and classification of myocarditis by endomyocardial biopsy. N Engl J Med 308:12, 1983

FIGUILA HR et al: Spontaneous hemodynamic improvement or stabilization and associated biopsy findings in patients with congestive cardiomyopathy. Circulation 71:1095, 1985

GOTTDIENER JS et al: Doxorubicin cardiotoxicity: Assessment of late left ventricular dysfunction by radionuclide cineangiography. Ann Intern Med 94:430, 1981

GREENSPON AJ, SCHAAL SF: The "holiday heart": Electrophysiologic studies of alcohol effects in alcoholics. Ann Intern Med 98:135, 1983

HARTZ AJ et al: The association of smoking with cardiomyopathy. N Engl J Med 311:1201–1206, 1984

KNOCHEL JP: Cardiovascular effects of alcohol. Ann Intern Med 98:849, 1983

KOWEY PR et al: Sustained arrhythmias in hypertrophic obstructive cardiomyopathy. N Engl J Med 310:1566, 1984

LANGE RM et al: Adverse effects of acute alcohol ingestion in young adults. Ann Intern Med 102:742, 1985

MASON JW: Endomyocardial biopsy: The balance of success and failure. Circulation 71:185, 1985

MCKENNA WJ: Arrhythmia and prognosis in hypertrophic cardiomyopathy. Eur Heart J 4:225, 1983

OLSEN EG, SPRY CJ: Relation between eosinophilia and endomyocardial disease. Prog Cardiovasc Dis 27:241, 1985

PARRILLO JE et al: The results of transvenous endomyocardial biopsy can frequently be used to diagnose myocardial diseases in patients with idiopathic heart failure: Endomyocardial biopsies in 100 consecutive patients revealed a substantial incidence of myocarditis. Circulation 69:93, 1984

POLL DS et al: Sustained ventricular tachycardia in patients with idiopathic dilated cardiomyopathy: Electrophysiologic testing and lack of response to antiarrhythmic drug therapy. Circulation 70:451, 1984

REGAN TJ: Alcoholic cardiomyopathy. Prog Cardiovasc Dis 27:141–152, 1984

REYES MP, LERNER AM: Coxsackie-virus myocarditis: With special reference to acute and chronic effects. Prog Cardiovasc Dis 27:373–394, 1985

SIEGEL RJ et al: Idiopathic restrictive cardiomyopathy. Circulation 70:451, 1984

STEERE AC et al: Lyme carditis: Cardiac abnormalities of Lyme disease. Ann Intern Med 93:8, 1980

TEN CATE FJ (ed): *Hypertrophic Cardiomyopathy: Clinical Recognition and Management*. Vol. 4, Basic and Clinical Cardiology. New York, Marcel Dekker, 1985

TORTI FM et al: Reduced cardiotoxicity of doxorubicin delivered on a weekly schedule: Assessment by endomyocardial biopsy. Ann Intern Med 99:745, 1983

VEILLE J-C: Peripartum cardiomyopathies: A review. Am J Obstet Gynecol 148:805, 1984

WYNNE J: Hypertrophic cardiomyopathy: A broadened concept of the disease and its management, in *Update III: Harrison's Principles of Internal Medicine*, KJ Isselbacher, et al (eds). New York, McGraw-Hill, 1982, p 129

———, BRAUNWALD E: The cardiomyopathies and myocarditides, in *Heart Disease*, 2d ed, E Braunwald (ed). Philadelphia, Saunders, 1984, p 1399

193 CARDIAC TUMORS, CARDIAC MANIFESTATIONS OF SYSTEMIC DISEASES, AND TRAUMATIC CARDIAC INJURY

WILSON S. COLUCCI / EUGENE BRAUNWALD

TUMORS OF THE HEART

PRIMARY TUMORS Primary tumors of the heart are rare and are often classified as "benign" histologically (Table 193-1). However, since all cardiac tumors have the potential for causing life-threatening complications, and many are now curable by surgery, it is important that this diagnosis be made whenever possible. Approximately three-quarters are *histologically* benign, and the remainder are malignant, in almost all cases sarcomas.

Clinical presentation Cardiac tumors may present with a wide array of cardiac and noncardiac manifestations. There may be signs and symptoms of all the more common forms of heart disease, including chest pain, syncope, heart failure, murmurs, arrhythmias, conduction disturbances, and pericardial effusion or tamponade. The specific signs and symptoms produced are most closely related to the location of the tumor.

Myxoma Myxomas are the most common type of primary cardiac tumor, accounting for one-third to one-half of all cases. They occur at all ages, show no sex preference, and may be familial. Most authorities consider the myxoma a true neoplasm, while others have suggested that it is formed by organization of an intracardiac thrombus attached to the endocardium. The large majority of myxomas are located in the atria, particularly the left, and arise from the interatrial septum in the vicinity of the fossa ovalis. Myxomas may also occur in the ventricles or be multiple in location. Most are pedunculated on a fibrovascular stalk and average 4 to 8 cm in diameter. The most common clinical presentation resembles that of mitral valve disease,

TABLE 193-1 Relative incidence of primary tumors of the heart

Type	Percent
BENIGN	
Myxoma	30.5
Lipoma	10.5
Papillary fibroelastoma	9.9
Rhabdomyoma	8.5
Fibroma	4.0
Hemangioma	3.5
Teratoma	3.3
Mesothelioma of the AV node	2.8
Other benign tumors	2.1
Total	75.1
MALIGNANT	
Sarcomas	18.6
Lymphoma	1.6
Other malignant tumors	4.7
Total	24.9

SOURCE: *Modified from HA McAllister, JJ Fenoglio, in Atlas of Tumor Pathology, Washington, Armed Forces Institute of Pathology, 1978, fasc 15, 2d series.*

either stenosis as a result of tumor prolapse into the mitral orifice during diastole or regurgitation as a consequence of injury to the valve by tumor-induced trauma. Ventricular myxomas may cause outflow obstruction and may therefore mimic subaortic or subpulmonic stenosis. Characteristically, the symptoms and signs are highly dependent on position, intermittent, and sudden in onset as a result of changes in tumor position with gravity. On auscultation, a characteristic low-pitched sound, termed a "tumor plop," is audible during early or middiastole and is thought to result from the tumor abruptly stopping as it strikes the ventricular wall. Myxomas may also present with peripheral or pulmonary emboli, or any of several noncardiac signs and symptoms including fever, weight loss, cachexia, malaise, arthralgia, rash, clubbing, Raynaud's phenomenon, hypergammaglobulinemia, anemia, polycythemia, leukocytosis, elevated erythrocyte sedimentation rate, thrombocytopenia, or thrombocytosis. Not surprisingly, myxomas are frequently misdiagnosed as endocarditis, collagen vascular disease, or noncardiac tumor.

Both M-mode and two-dimensional echocardiography are useful in the diagnosis of cardiac myxoma, the latter having the advantage of allowing determination of the site of tumor attachment and tumor size, important considerations in the planning of surgical excision. While cardiac catheterization and angiography are often performed prior to surgery, catheterization of the chamber from which the tumor originates is attended by the risk of dislodgment of tumor emboli. In many centers catheterization is no longer considered mandatory when adequate noninvasive information is available.

Surgical excision utilizing cardiopulmonary bypass is indicated in all patients and is generally curative. Occasional reports of tumor recurrence are most likely due to inadequate excision of multiple tumor sites.

Other benign tumors Cardiac *lipomas,* although relatively common, are usually incidental findings at postmortem examination and seldom result in symptoms. However, they may grow as large as 15 cm and present with symptoms due to mechanical interference with cardiac function, arrhythmias, or conduction disturbances, or as an abnormality of the cardiac silhouette on chest x-ray. *Papillary fibroelastomas,* similarly, are relatively common findings on cardiac valves or the adjacent endothelium but seldom result in clinical symptoms. Occasionally, these growths may cause mechanical interference with valvular function. *Rhabdomyomas* and *fibromas,* the most frequent tumors in infants and children, most commonly occur in the ventricles, and therefore produce signs and symptoms by mechanical obstruction which may mimic valvular stenosis, congestive heart failure, restrictive or hypertrophic cardiomyopathy, and pericardial constriction. Rhabdomyomas are probably hamartomatous growths, are multiple in about 90 percent of cases, and may be associated with tuberous sclerosis, adenoma sebaceum, and benign kidney tumors. *Hemangiomas* and *mesotheliomas* are generally small tumors, most often intramyocardial in location, and may cause atrioventricular (AV) conduction disturbances and even sudden death as a result of their propensity for location in the region of the AV node.

Sarcomas Cardiac sarcomas may be of several histologic types, but in general are characterized by a rapidly downhill course leading to the patient's death in weeks to months from the time of presentation as a result of hemodynamic compromise, local invasion, or distant metastases. Sarcomas commonly involve the right side of the heart, and because of their rapid growth, invasion of the pericardial space and obstruction of the cardiac chambers or venae cavae are common. At the time of presentation these tumors have often spread too extensively for surgical excision. While there are scattered reports of palliation with surgery, radiotherapy, and chemotherapy, the overall experience with cardiac sarcomas is poor. The one exception to this appears to be cardiac lymphosarcomas, which may respond to a combination of chemo- and radiotherapy.

TUMORS METASTATIC TO THE HEART Tumors metastatic to the heart are several times more common than primary tumors, and as the life expectancy of patients with various forms of malignant neoplasms is extended by more effective therapy, it is likely that the frequency of cardiac metastases will also increase. Although cardiac metastases occur in all tumor types with an incidence ranging from 1 to 20 percent, the incidence is especially high in malignant melanoma, and to a somewhat lesser extent in leukemia and lymphoma. In absolute numbers, cardiac metastases are most common in carcinoma of the breast and lung, reflecting the high incidence of these cancers. Cardiac metastases almost always occur in the setting of widespread primary disease, and most often there is either primary or metastatic disease elsewhere in the thoracic cavity. Nevertheless, occasionally a cardiac metastasis may be the initial presentation of a tumor elsewhere in the body.

Cardiac metastases reach the heart via the bloodstream, lymphatics, or direct invasion and generally are small, firm nodules; although diffuse infiltrations may also occur, especially with sarcomas or hematologic neoplasms. The pericardium is most often involved, followed by myocardial involvement of any chamber, and, rarely, by involvement of the endocardium or cardiac valves.

Cardiac metastases result in clinical manifestations only about 10 percent of the time, and rarely are they the cause of death. In most patients they are *not* the cause of the presenting clinical features but occur in the setting of a previously recognized malignant neoplasm. While cardiac metastases may present a large number of nonspecific signs and symptoms, the most common are dyspnea, a new systolic murmur, signs of acute pericarditis, cardiac tamponade, a rapid increase in the cardiac silhouette on chest x-ray, the new onset of an ectopic tachyarrhythmia, AV block, and congestive heart failure. As with primary cardiac tumors, the clinical presentation is more closely related to the location and size of the tumor than to its histologic type. Many of these signs and symptoms may also occur with myocarditis, pericarditis, or cardiomyopathy resulting from radiotherapy or chemotherapy.

The electrocardiographic findings are entirely nonspecific and may include ST-T–wave changes, decreased QRS voltage, arrhythmias, and conduction disturbances. On chest roentgenography the cardiac silhouette is most often normal but may reveal a pericardial effusion or bizarre contour. Echocardiography is useful for the diagnosis of pericardial effusion and the visualization of larger metastases. Angiography may delineate discrete lesions, and pericardiocentesis can allow a specific cytologic diagnosis. Since most patients with cardiac metastases have widespread disease, therapy generally consists of pericardiocentesis when there is hemodynamic compromise, and treatment directed at the primary tumor. The removal of a malignant effusion by pericardiocentesis with or without concomitant instillation of a sclerosing agent (e.g., tetracycline) may palliate symptoms and delay or prevent reaccumulation of the effusion.

CARDIAC EFFECTS OF CANCER THERAPY See Chap. 192.

CARDIOVASCULAR MANIFESTATIONS OF SYSTEMIC DISEASES

DIABETES MELLITUS (see Chap. 327) In patients with insulin-dependent diabetes mellitus there is an increased incidence of large-vessel atherosclerosis and myocardial infarction, and diabetics are more likely to have an abnormal or absent pain response to myocardial ischemia, probably as a result of generalized autonomic nervous system dysfunction. Diabetic patients may also have myocardial dysfunction characteristic of a restrictive cardiomyopathy in the absence of large-vessel coronary artery disease, as evidenced by elevated left ventricular filling pressures. Histologically, these patients have increased amounts of collagen, glycoprotein, triglycerides, and cholesterol in the myocardial interstitium, and in some cases intimal thickening, hyaline deposition, and inflammatory changes have been observed in small intramural arteries. While these changes alone seldom result in clinical heart failure, it is likely that they contribute to the excessive cardiovascular morbidity and mortality of diabetics. There is some evidence that insulin therapy results in an amelioration of the myocardial dysfunction.

MALNUTRITION AND THIAMINE DEFICIENCY (BERIBERI)
Malnutrition (see Chap. 72) In patients whose intake of protein, calories, or both is severely deficient, the heart may become thin, pale, and flabby with myofibrillar atrophy and interstitial edema. The systolic pressure and cardiac output are low, and the pulse pressure narrow. Generalized edema is common and is due to a combination of factors, including reduced serum oncotic pressure and myocardial dysfunction. Such profound states of malnutrition, termed *marasmus* in the case of caloric deficiency, or *kwashiorkor* in the case of relative protein deficiency, are most common in underdeveloped countries. However, significant nutritional heart disease may also occur in developed nations, particularly in patients with severe cardiac failure in whom gastrointestinal hypoperfusion and venous congestion may cause anorexia and malabsorption. Open-heart surgery poses an increased risk in such patients, who may benefit from preoperative intensive hyperalimentation. Deficient nutrients and minerals should be replaced gradually since rapid expansion of the intravascular space may stress the weakened heart and result in overt congestive heart failure.

Thiamine deficiency (see Chap. 76) In many cases, malnutrition is accompanied by thiamine deficiency, although this hypovitaminosis may also occur in the presence of an adequate protein and caloric intake, particularly in the far east, where polished rice deficient in thiamine is a major dietary component. The widespread use of thiamine-enriched flour in western nations confines this disease primarily to alcoholics and food faddists. Clinically, there is usually evidence of generalized malnutrition, peripheral neuropathy, glossitis, and anemia. The characteristic cardiovascular syndrome is that of high-output heart failure with tachycardia, increased cardiac output, and often elevated filling pressures in the left and right side of the heart. It appears that the major cause of the high-output state is vasomotor depression, the precise mechanism of which is not understood, but which leads to a reduced systemic vascular resistance. The cardiac examination reveals a wide pulse pressure, tachycardia, a third heart sound, and, frequently, a systolic murmur at the apex. The electrocardiogram may show decreased voltage, a prolonged QT interval, and T-wave abnormalities; the chest x-ray generally shows a large heart with signs of congestive heart failure. The response to thiamine is often dramatic, with diuresis and a reduction in heart size. Although the response to digitalis and diuretics may be poor prior to thiamine therapy, these agents may be important *after* thiamine is given since the left ventricle may not be capable of dealing with the increased workload presented by the return of vascular tone.

OBESITY (see Chap. 317) Although not defined as a disease per se, severe obesity is associated with an increase in cardiovascular morbidity and mortality, due in part to hypertension, glucose intolerance, and atherosclerotic coronary artery disease, all of which are more prevalent in obese patients. In addition, these patients have a distinct abnormality of the cardiovascular system characterized by increases in total and central blood volumes, cardiac output, and left ventricular filling pressure. It appears that cardiac output is elevated in order to help supply the metabolic needs of the excessive adipose tissue. Left ventricular filling pressure is often at the upper limits of normal and rises excessively with exercise. As a result of chronic volume and pressure overload, abnormal ventricular function may develop. Pathologically, there is left and, in some cases, right ventricular hypertrophy and generalized cardiac enlargement, which is not due simply to fatty infiltration of the myocardium. Clinically, these patients may develop pulmonary congestion, peripheral edema, and exercise intolerance, findings which may be difficult to recognize in massively obese patients. Weight reduction is the most effective therapy and results in reduction in blood volume and in return of cardiac output toward normal. Digitalis, sodium restriction, and diuretics may also be useful. This form of heart disease should be distinguished from the Pickwickian syndrome (Chap. 215), which may share several of the cardiovascular features but, in addition, frequently has components of central apnea, hypoxemia, pulmonary hypertension, and cor pulmonale.

THYROID DISEASE (see Chap. 324) Thyroid hormone exerts a major influence on the cardiovascular system by a number of direct and indirect mechanisms, and not surprisingly, cardiovascular effects are prominent in both hypo- and hyperthyroidism. Thyroid hormone causes increases in total-body metabolism and oxygen consumption which indirectly place an increased workload on the heart. In addition, although the exact mechanism has not been defined, thyroid hormone exerts direct inotropic and chronotropic effects which are similar to those seen with adrenergic stimulation (e.g., tachycardia, increased cardiac output). It has been shown that thyroid hormone increases the synthesis of myosin and of Na^+, K^+-ATPase, as well as the density of myocardial beta-adrenergic receptors.

Hyperthyroidism Excess thyroid hormone results in increases in heart rate, cardiac output, and pulse pressure. Patients may present with palpitations, systolic hypertension, fatigue, or, in patients with underlying heart disease, angina, or heart failure. Sinus tachycardia is found in about 40 percent of patients, and atrial fibrillation in about 15 percent. Other findings include a hyperactive precordium, an increase in the intensity of the first heart sound and the pulmonic component of the second heart sound, a third heart sound, and, in some cases, a midsystolic murmur heard best at the left sternal border with or without a systolic ejection click. A systolic scratchy sound, the *Means-Lerman scratch,* may occasionally be heard at the left second intercostal space during expiration and is thought to result from the rubbing of the hyperdynamic pericardium against the pleura. Elderly patients with hyperthyroidism may present with only the cardiovascular manifestations of thyrotoxicosis, which may be resistant to therapy until the hyperthyroidism is controlled. Both angina pectoris and congestive heart failure are unusual, unless there is coexistent underlying heart disease, and in many cases will resolve with therapy of the hyperthyroidism.

Hypothyroidism There is a reduction in cardiac output, stroke volume, heart rate, blood pressure, and pulse pressure. In about one-third of patients there is a pericardial effusion which only rarely results in tamponade. Clinically, there is cardiomegaly, bradycardia, weak arterial pulses, and distant heart sounds. Biochemical abnormalities, including elevations of creatine kinase (CK), serum glutamic oxaloacetic transaminase (SGOT), and lactic dehydrogenase (LDH), may lead to a mistaken diagnosis of myocardial infarction. The electrocardiogram generally shows sinus bradycardia and low voltage and may show prolongation of the QT interval, decreased P-wave voltage, prolonged AV conduction time, intraventricular conduction disturbances, and nonspecific ST-T–wave abnormalities. Chest x-ray shows cardiomegaly, often with a "water bottle" configuration, pleural effusions, and, in some cases, evidence of congestive heart failure. Pathologically, the heart is pale, dilated, and flabby, often with myofibrillar swelling, loss of striations, and interstitial fibrosis.

Patients with hypothyroidism frequently have elevations of cholesterol and triglycerides and severe atherosclerotic coronary artery disease. Prior to treatment with thyroid hormone, patients with hypothyroidism frequently do not have angina pectoris, presumably because of the low metabolic demands made by their condition. However, such patients, especially when elderly, are prone to angina and myocardial infarction during replacement of thyroid hormone, and this should always be done with extreme care, starting with very low doses which are increased gradually.

MALIGNANT CARCINOID (see Chap. 299) These tumors elaborate a variety of vasoactive amines, kinins, indoles, and other substances which are believed to be responsible for the diarrhea, flushing, and labile blood pressure seen in these patients. The cardiac lesions due to gastrointestinal carcinoids are almost exclusively in the right side of the heart and occur only when there are hepatic metastases, suggesting that the substance responsible for the cardiac lesions is inactivated by passage through the liver and lungs. Similar lesions occur in the left side of the heart when there is a right-to-left shunt or the tumor is located in the lungs. Fibrous plaques are found on the endothelium of the cardiac chambers, valves, and great vessels. These plaques, which result in distortion of the cardiac valves, consist of smooth muscle cells imbedded in a stroma of acid mucopolysaccharide and collagen, and presumably result from healing of endothelial injury. The clinical syndrome is most often that of tricuspid regurgitation, pulmonic stenosis, or both. In some cases a high-output state may occur, presumably as a result of a decrease in systemic vascular resistance due to a vasoactive substance released by the tumor. Progression of the cardiac lesions does not appear to be affected by treatment with serotonin antagonists, and in some cases valve replacement is indicated. Coronary artery spasm, presumably due to a circulating vasoactive substance, may occur in patients with carcinoid syndrome.

PHEOCHROMOCYTOMA (see Chap. 326) In addition to causing hypertension, which may be labile or sustained, the high circulating levels of catecholamines may also cause direct myocardial injury. Focal myocardial necrosis and inflammatory cell infiltration are seen in about 50 percent of patients who die with pheochromocytoma and may contribute to clinically significant left ventricular failure and pulmonary edema. In addition, hypertension results in left ventricular hypertrophy.

RHEUMATOID ARTHRITIS AND THE COLLAGEN VASCULAR DISEASES **Rheumatoid arthritis** (see Chap. 263) There may be inflammation of any or all parts of the heart in patients with rheumatoid arthritis. *Pericarditis* is the most common cause of clinically apparent disease and may be found in 30 to 50 percent of all patients with rheumatoid arthritis, particularly those with subcutaneous nodules, if carefully searched for by echocardiography or at postmortem examination. However, only a small fraction of these patients will have clinical evidence of pericarditis, which usually follows a benign course, but occasionally may progress to cardiac tamponade or constrictive pericarditis. The pericardial fluid is generally an exudate, with decreased concentrations of complement and glucose and elevated cholesterol. Treatment is directed at the underlying rheumatoid arthritis and may include corticosteroids. Pericardiectomy is usually required in cases of tamponade or persistent effusion. *Coronary arteritis* with intimal inflammation and edema is present in about 20 percent of cases but only rarely results in angina pectoris or myocardial infarction. The cardiac valves, most often the mitral and aortic, may be involved by inflammation and granuloma formation which in some cases may cause clinically significant regurgitation due to valve deformity. Myocarditis rarely results in cardiac dysfunction.

Seronegative arthropathies The seronegative arthropathies (Chaps. 267 and 276), ankylosing spondylitis, Reiter's syndrome, psoriatic arthritis, and the arthritides associated with ulcerative colitis and regional enteritis may be accompanied by a pancarditis with tachycardia, cardiomegaly, and prolongation of the AV conduction time. These patients are particularly likely to develop aortic regurgitation due to an aortitis and consequent dilatation of the aortic root and AV block, both of which are more common in patients with peripheral joint involvement and long-standing disease. Up to one-fifth of patients with peripheral joint involvement and disease for more than 30 years have significant aortic regurgitation. Occasionally, aortic regurgitation precedes the onset of arthritis, and, therefore, the diagnosis of a seronegative arthritis should be considered in young males with isolated aortic regurgitation.

Systemic lupus erythematosus (SLE) (see Chap. 262) Pericarditis is common, occurring in about two-thirds of patients, and generally pursues a benign course, although rarely tamponade or constriction may result. The characteristic *endocardial lesions* of SLE, described by Libman and Sacks, consist of wartlike lesions most often located at the angles of the AV valves or on the ventricular surface of the mitral valve. Although arteritis of large coronary arteries may rarely result in myocardial ischemia, there is also an increased frequency of coronary atherosclerosis which may be related to hypertension or corticosteroid therapy.

TRAUMATIC HEART DISEASE

Cardiac damage may be due to both penetrating and nonpenetrating injuries. The most frequent cause of a *nonpenetrating injury* is impact of the chest against the steering wheel of an automobile. Serious injury of the heart may ensue even though no external sign of thoracic trauma is evident. Although the commonest injury is myocardial contusion, any structure of the heart may be affected by the trauma. If the valvular apparatus is ruptured, a loud heart murmur produced by valvular regurgitation may appear, followed by the development of rapidly progressive heart failure. The most serious consequence of nonpenetrating injury is rupture, either of the atria or of the ventricles, which is generally fatal. Hemopericardium may also follow tearing of a pericardial vessel or coronary artery.

Myocardial contusion may cause arrhythmias, bundle branch block, or electrocardiographic abnormalities resembling those of infarction, and so it is important to bear trauma in mind as a cause of otherwise unexplained electrocardiographic changes. Similarly, myocardial contusion may produce positive radionuclide scans and regional impairment of ventricular function, as occurs in patients with acute myocardial infarction (Chap. 179). Pericardial effusion may occur weeks or even months after the accident. In these cases, the pericardial effusion is a manifestation of the postcardiac injury syndrome, which resembles the postpericardiotomy syndrome (Chap. 194).

Acute myocardial failure resulting from rupture of a valve usually requires operative correction. Myocardial infarction due to trauma is treated similarly to that due to ischemic heart disease (Chap. 190). Pericardial hemorrhage often leads to constriction which must be treated by decortication.

Penetrating injuries of the heart, produced by bullets or stab wounds, usually result in immediate or very rapid death because of hemopericardium or massive hemorrhage. However, sometimes the patient survives the acute incident and presents with a cardiac murmur and congestive heart failure. A left-to-right shunt due to traumatic ventricular septal defect, aortopulmonary artery fistula, or coronary arteriovenous fistula may be suspected and confirmed by cardiac catheterization and angiocardiography. Operation is indicated if hemodynamically significant abnormalities are present or if a foreign body, e.g., a bullet, is lodged in the heart. Immediate thoracotomy should be carried out if there is cardiac tamponade and/or shock, whether the trauma was penetrating or nonpenetrating. Pericardiocentesis may be helpful in patients with tamponade, but usually only as a holding maneuver. Patients who suffer penetrating injuries of the heart should be carefully examined several weeks after the event to rule out a ventricular septal defect or mitral regurgitation which may have gone undetected at the time of emergency surgery.

Rupture of the aorta is a common consequence of chest trauma. Indeed, rupture of the aorta at the isthmus or just above the aortic valve is the most common vascular deceleration injury. The clinical presentation is similar to that in aortic dissection (Chap. 197). The arterial pressure and pulse amplitude may be increased in the upper extremities and decreased in the lower extremities, and on chest roentgenogram there may be widening of the mediastinum. Occasionally, the rupture is limited by the aortic adventitia and results in a silent false aneurysm which may be discovered months or years after the injury. When great vessel rupture is due to a penetrating injury, there is usually a hemothorax and, less often, a hemopericardium. Hematoma formation may compress major vessels, and arteriovenous fistulae may be formed, sometimes resulting in high-output congestive heart failure.

REFERENCES

AYZENBERG O et al: Beriberi heart disease. S Afr Med J 68:263, 1985

BRANCH CL JR, et al: Left atrial myxoma with cerebral emboli. Neurosurgery 16:675, 1985

BULKLEY BH, ROBERTS WC: The heart in systemic lupus erythematosus and the changes induced in it by corticosteroid therapy. A study of 36 necropsy patients. Am J Med 58:243, 1975

COHN PF, BRAUNWALD E: Traumatic heart disease, in *Heart Disease*, 2d ed, E Braunwald (ed). Philadelphia, Saunders, 1984, p 1528

COLUCCI WS, BRAUNWALD E: Primary tumors of the heart, in *Heart Disease*, 2d ed,E Braunwald (ed). Philadelphia, Saunders, 1984, p 1457

FEIN FS, SONNENBLICK EH: Diabetic cardiomyopathy. Progr Cardiovasc Dis 27:255, 1985

FYKE FE et al: Primary cardiac tumors: Experience with 30 consecutive patients since the introduction of two-dimensional echocardiography. J Am Coll Cardiol 5:1465, 1985

KLEIN I, LEVEY GS: New perspectives on thyroid hormone, catecholamines, and the heart. Am J Med 76:167, 1984

LOCKWOOD WB, BROGHAMER WL JR: The changing prevalence of secondary cardiac neoplasms as related to cancer therapy. Cancer 15:2659, 1980

PERLOFF JK: Cardiac rhythm and conduction in Duchenne's muscular dystrophy: A prospective study of 20 patients. J Am Col Cardiol 3:1263, 1984

ROBERTS WC, SJOERDSMA A: The cardiac disease associated with the carcinoid syndrome. Am J Med 36:5, 1969

SEMB RK et al: Angiographic and echocardiographic observations in surgical patients with atrial myxoma. Cardiovasc Intervent Radiol 8:119, 1985

STOLLERMAN E: Rheumatic fever, connective tissue disorders and heart disease, in *Heart Disease*, 2d ed, E Braunwald (ed). Philadelphia, Saunders, 1984, p 1641

SUTHERLAND GR et al: Hemodynamic adaptation to acute myocardial contusion complicating blunt chest injury. Am J Cardiol 57:291, 1986

194 PERICARDIAL DISEASE

EUGENE BRAUNWALD

NORMAL FUNCTIONS OF THE PERICARDIUM The visceral pericardium is a serous membrane, separated by a small amount of fluid, an ultrafiltrate of plasma, from a fibrous sac, the parietal pericardium. The pericardium prevents sudden dilatation of the cardiac chambers during exercise and hypervolemia, and as the result of the development of a negative intrapericardial pressure during ejection it facilitates atrial filling during ventricular systole. The pericardium also restricts the anatomic position of the heart, minimizes friction between the heart and surrounding structures, prevents displacement of the heart and kinking of the great vessels, and probably retards the spread of infections from the lungs and pleural cavities to the heart. Notwithstanding the foregoing, total absence of the pericardium does not produce obvious clinical disease. In partial left pericardial defects the main pulmonary artery and left atrium may bulge through the defect; rarely herniation and subsequent strangulation of the left atrium may cause sudden death.

ACUTE PERICARDITIS

It is useful to classify the types of pericarditis both clinically and etiologically (Table 194-1), as this disorder is by far the most common pathologic process involving the pericardium.

Pain, a pericardial friction rub, electrocardiographic changes, and pericardial effusion with cardiac tamponade and paradoxic pulse are cardinal manifestations of many forms of acute pericarditis and will be considered prior to a discussion of the most common forms of the disorder.

Pain is an important but not invariable symptom in various forms of acute pericarditis; it is usually present in the acute infectious types and in many of the forms presumed to be related to hypersensitivity or autoimmunity. Pain is often absent in a slowly developing tuberculous, postirradiation, neoplastic or uremic pericarditis. The pain of pericarditis is often severe; its character and location have been described in Chap. 4. It is characteristically in the center of the chest, referred to the back and the trapezius ridge. Often the pain is pleuritic, i.e., sharp and aggravated by inspiration, coughing, and changes in body position, but occasionally it is a steady, constrictive pain, which radiates into either arm or both arms and resembles that

TABLE 194-1 Classification of pericarditis

I Clinical classification
- *A* Acute pericarditis (<6 weeks)
  - *1* Fibrinous
  - *2* Effusive (or bloody)
- *B* Subacute pericarditis (6 weeks to 6 months)
  - *1* Constrictive
  - *2* Effusive-constrictive
- *C* Chronic pericarditis (>6 months)
  - *1* Constrictive
  - *2* Effusive
  - *3* Adhesive (nonconstrictive)

II Etiologic classification
- *A* Infectious pericarditis
  - *1* Viral
  - *2* Pyogenic
  - *3* Tuberculous
  - *4* Mycotic
  - *5* Other infections (syphilitic, parasitic)
- *B* Noninfectious pericarditis
  - *1* Acute myocardial infarction
  - *2* Uremia
  - *3* Neoplasia
    - *a* Primary tumors (benign or malignant)
    - *b* Tumors metastatic to pericardium
  - *4* Myxedema
  - *5* Cholesterol
  - *6* Chylopericardium
  - *7* Trauma
    - *a* Penetrating chest wall
    - *b* Nonpenetrating
  - *8* Aortic aneurysm (with leakage into pericardial sac)
  - *9* Postirradiation
  - *10* Associated with atrial septal defect
  - *11* Associated with severe chronic anemia
  - *12* Infectious mononucleosis
  - *13* Familial Mediterranean fever
  - *14* Familial pericarditis
    - *a* Mulibrey nanism*
  - *15* Sarcoidosis
  - *16* Acute idiopathic
- *C* Pericarditis presumably related to hypersensitivity or autoimmunity
  - *1* Rheumatic fever
  - *2* Collagen vascular disease
    - *a* Systemic lupus erythematosus
    - *b* Rheumatoid arthritis
    - *c* Scleroderma
  - *3* Drug-induced
    - *a* Procainamide
    - *b* Hydralazine
    - *c* Other
  - *4* Postcardiac injury
    - *a* Postmyocardial infarction (Dressler's syndrome)
    - *b* Postpericardiotomy

* *An autosomal recessive syndrome, characterized by growth failure, muscle hypotonia, hepatomegaly, ocular changes, enlarged cerebral ventricles, mental retardation, and chronic constrictive pericarditis.*

of myocardial ischemia; confusion with myocardial infarction is common. Characteristically, however, the pericardial pain is relieved by sitting up and leaning forward. This problem becomes even more perplexing when, with acute pericarditis, the serum transaminase level rises to about 80 units. However, the MB isoenzyme of creatine kinase does not rise in acute pericarditis.

The *pericardial friction rub* is the most important physical sign; it may have up to three components per cardiac cycle, as described in Chap. 177, and can sometimes be elicited only when firm pressure with the diaphragm of the stethoscope is applied to the chest wall. It is heard most frequently during expiration, but an independent pleural friction rub may be audible during inspiration, with the patient leaning forward or in the left lateral decubitus position. The rub is likely to be inconstant and transitory, and a loud to-and-fro leathery sound may disappear within a few hours, possibly to reappear the following day.

The *electrocardiogram* in acute pericarditis without massive effusion (see also Chap. 178) usually displays widespread elevation of the ST segments, involving two or three standard limb leads and V_2 to V_6, with reciprocal depressions only in aVR and V_1 and without significant changes in QRS complexes, except occasionally for some diminution in voltage. Several days later, the ST segments return to normal and the T waves *then* become inverted. In contrast, in acute myocardial infarction, reciprocal depression of ST segments is usually more prominent; QRS changes occur, particularly the development of Q waves, and notching and loss of the amplitude of R waves; and T-wave inversions usually occur *before* the ST segments have become isoelectric. Sequential electrocardiograms are useful in distinguishing acute pericarditis from acute myocardial infarction. Early repolarization is a normal variant and may also cause widespread ST-segment elevation, most prominent in left precordial leads. However, in this condition the T waves are usually tall and the ST/T ratio is under 0.25, but exceeds this number in acute pericarditis. Depression of the PR segment (below the TP segment) also is common in acute pericarditis. With large pericardial effusions, the QRS voltage is reduced. Atrial premature beats and atrial fibrillation are sometimes noted.

PERICARDIAL EFFUSION Usually associated with one or more of the above-mentioned manifestations of pericarditis and an enlargement of the cardiac silhouette, pericardial effusion is especially important clinically when it develops within a relatively short time. Differentiation from cardiac enlargement may be difficult, but heart sounds tend to become faint; the friction rub may disappear or remain clearly audible, and the apex impulse may vanish, but sometimes it is palpable well medial to the left border of cardiac dullness. The chest roentgenogram may show a "water bottle" configuration of the cardiac silhouette, but it may also be normal or almost so. Lucent pericardial fat lines may be seen deep within the cardiopericardial silhouette. Fluoroscopic examination may show the ventricular pulsations to be diminished. When the effusion is large, an area of dullness and tubular breath sounds is often encountered at the angle of the left scapula, probably caused by compression of the lung (Ewart's sign).

Diagnosis of pericardial effusion Echocardiography (Chap. 179) is the most effective laboratory technique available, since it is sensitive, specific, simple, innocuous, and noninvasive, and may be performed at the bedside. The presence of pericardial fluid is recorded as a relatively echo-free space between the posterior pericardium and the posterior left ventricular epicardium in patients with small effusions and such a space between the anterior right ventricle and the parietal pericardium just beneath the anterior chest wall with larger effusions (Fig. 194-1). In patients with large effusions the heart may swing freely within the pericardial sac; when severe, this motion may be associated with electrical alternans. While M-mode echocardiography is usually adequate for the diagnosis of pericardial effusion, two-dimensional echocardiography is often superior since it allows more precise localization and estimation of the quantity of pericardial fluid. In tamponade, during inspiration, right ventricular diameter increases while left ventricular diameter and mitral valve opening decrease. Often there is late diastolic inward motion (collapse) of the right ventricular free wall, and of the right atrium. The diagnosis of pericardial fluid or thickening may be confirmed by one of the following:

1 *Cardiac catheterization*. A catheter is introduced into the right atrium and rotated so that its tip makes contact with the lateral right atrial wall. In the presence of an effusion, or pericardial thickening, the tip of the catheter is seen to be separated from the radiolucent lungs by an opaque band.
2 *Angiocardiography*. Contrast medium is injected rapidly into the right atrium; again the lateral wall is separated from the edge of the cardiac silhouette.

When it is deemed desirable to remove pericardial fluid for diagnostic and/or therapeutic purposes, a needle attached to a properly grounded electrocardiographic lead is inserted into the pericardial

FIGURE 194-1 *Two-dimensional (upper panel) and short-axis (lower panel) parasternal scans in systole in a patient with a large pericardial effusion surrounding the entire heart. Fluid is seen to extend behind the left atrium (white arrowhead) and anterior to the descending thoracic aorta (DA). AoV = aortic valve; LA = left atrium; LV = left ventricle; PE = pericardial effusion; RV = right ventricle. (Modified from PC Come (ed), Diagnostic Cardiology: Noninvasive imaging techniques, Philadelphia, Lippincott, 1985.)*

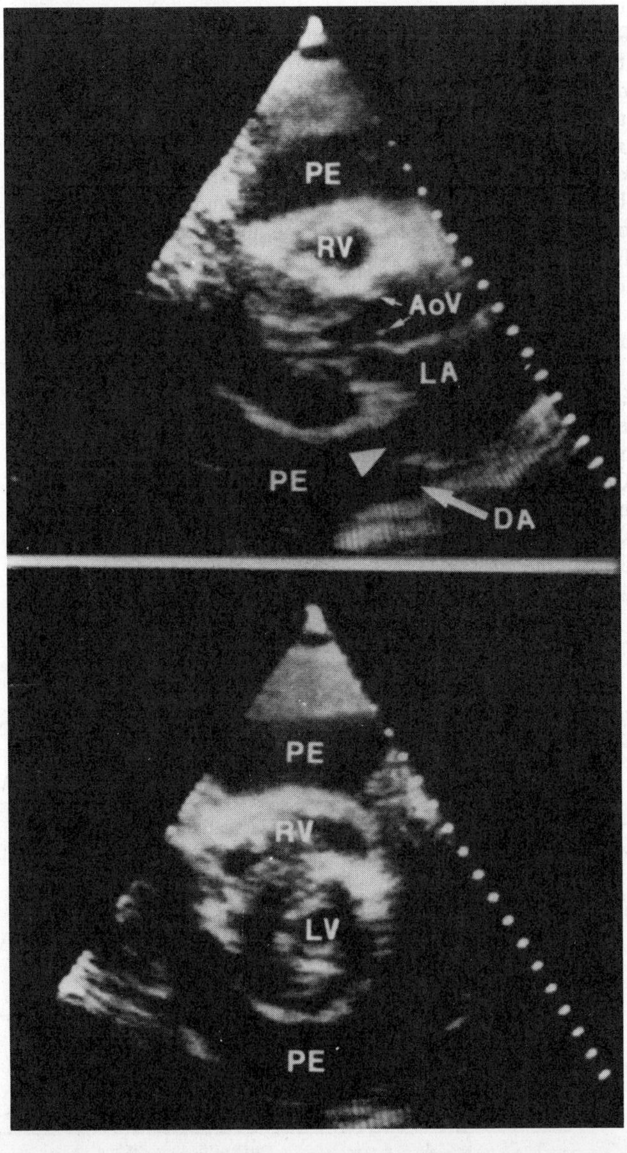

space, usually through a subxiphoid approach, and if possible using echocardiographic control. Intrapericardial pressure should be measured before fluid is withdrawn. When an effusion develops, the fluid nearly always has the physical characteristics of an exudate. Bloody fluid is commonly due to tuberculosis or tumor, but it may also be found in the effusion of rheumatic fever or in the post-cardiac injury syndrome (see below). Occasionally, bloody fluid may be found in the effusion of uremic pericarditis and in the hemopericardium following myocardial infarction, especially following the administration of anticoagulants.

CARDIAC TAMPONADE The accumulation of fluid in the pericardium in an amount sufficient to cause serious obstruction to the inflow of blood to the ventricles results in cardiac tamponade. The amount of fluid necessary to produce this critical state may be as small as 250 mL, when the fluid develops rapidly; or it may be over 1000 mL in slowly developing effusions when the pericardium has had the opportunity to stretch and adapt to the increasing volume of fluid. The volume of fluid required to produce tamponade varies directly with the thickness of the ventricular myocardium and inversely with the thickness of the parietal pericardium. Tamponade results most often from bleeding into the pericardial space following cardiac operations, trauma (including cardiac perforation during diagnostic procedures), tuberculosis, and tumor (most commonly carcinoma of the lung and breast and lymphoma), but it may occur in acute viral or idiopathic pericarditis, postirradiation pericarditis, renal failure during dialysis, and hemopericardium which may result when a patient with any form of acute pericarditis is treated with anticoagulants.

The clinical manifestations are due to the fall in cardiac output and to systemic venous congestion. However, the classic findings of falling arterial pressure, rising venous pressure, and a small quiet heart with faint heart sounds usually are seen only with severe tamponade occurring within minutes, as happens with cardiac trauma. More frequently, tamponade develops more slowly and the clinical manifestations, resembling those of heart failure, include dyspnea, orthopnea, hepatic engorgement, and jugular venous hypertension. A high index of suspicion is required, since, in many instances, no obvious cause for pericardial disease is apparent, and tamponade should be considered in any patient with hypotension and elevation of jugular venous pressure with a prominent x descent; often the y descent is diminutive or absent. A widening of the area of flatness to percussion across the anterior aspect of the chest wall, a paradoxical pulse (see below), relatively clear lung fields, diminished pulsations of the cardiac silhouette on fluoroscopy, reduction in amplitude of the QRS complexes, and *electrical alternans* of the P, QRS, and T waves should raise the suspicion of cardiac tamponade. A positive Kussmaul's sign (see below) is rare in cardiac tamponade, as is a pericardial knock. Their presence suggests that the beginning of an organizing process and epicardial constriction are present in addition to effusion. Since immediate treatment may be lifesaving, prompt measures to establish the diagnosis definitely, i.e., echocardiography followed by cardiac catheterization, should be undertaken. The latter reveals elevation of the right atrial pressure with prominence of the x but not of the y descent. When measured, the pericardial pressure is also elevated and equal to the right atrial pressure. There is "equalization" of pressures, i.e., the pulmonary artery wedge is equal, or close, to right atrial, right ventricular, and pulmonary artery diastolic pressures. The "square root" sign in the ventricular pressure pulses and the prominent y descent in atrial and jugular venous pressure characteristic of constrictive pericarditis (see below) are usually absent.

Paradoxical pulse This important clue to the presence of cardiac tamponade consists of *a greater than normal (10 mmHg) inspiratory decrease in systolic arterial pressure*. When severe, it may be detected by palpating weakness or disappearance of the arterial pulse during inspiration, but usually sphygmomanometric measurement of systolic pressure during slow respiration is required (Fig. 194-2).

The mechanism of paradoxical pulse in cardiac tamponade is complex. Normally, the inspiratory decline in intrathoracic pressure enhances right ventricular filling by virtue of the increased pressure gradient between the extrathoracic veins and the chambers of the right side of the heart. As a consequence right ventricular diastolic volume and stroke output increase, and this increase is transmitted to the left side of the heart several cardiac cycles later, leading to an increase in systemic arterial pressure during the following expiration. Therefore, normally a small pressure fall occurs during inspiration. Also, left ventricular afterload rises during inspiration as intrapericardial pressure falls, and left ventricular stroke volume and therefore arterial pressure decline slightly during inspiration. In cardiac tamponade, since both ventricles share a tight incompressible covering, the pericardial sac, the inspiratory increase in right ventricular volume compresses and reduces left ventricular volume; leftward bulging of the interventricular septum may further reduce the left ventricular cavity as the right ventricle enlarges during inspiration. Thus, in cardiac tamponade the inspiratory augmentation of right ventricular volume causes an exaggerated reciprocal reduction in left ventricular volume. Also, respiratory distress increases the fluctuations in intrathoracic pressure, which exaggerates the mechanism just described.

Low-pressure tamponade refers to mild tamponade in which the intrapericardial pressure is increased from its slightly subatmospheric levels to +5 to +10 mmHg; in some instances hypovolemia coexists. As a consequence the central venous pressure is slightly elevated while arterial pressure is unaffected. The patients are asymptomatic or complain of mild weakness and dyspnea. The diagnosis is aided by echocardiography, and both hemodynamic and clinical manifestations improve following mild pericardiocentesis.

Paradoxical pulse occurs in only approximately one-third of patients with *constrictive pericarditis*. It is important to bear in mind

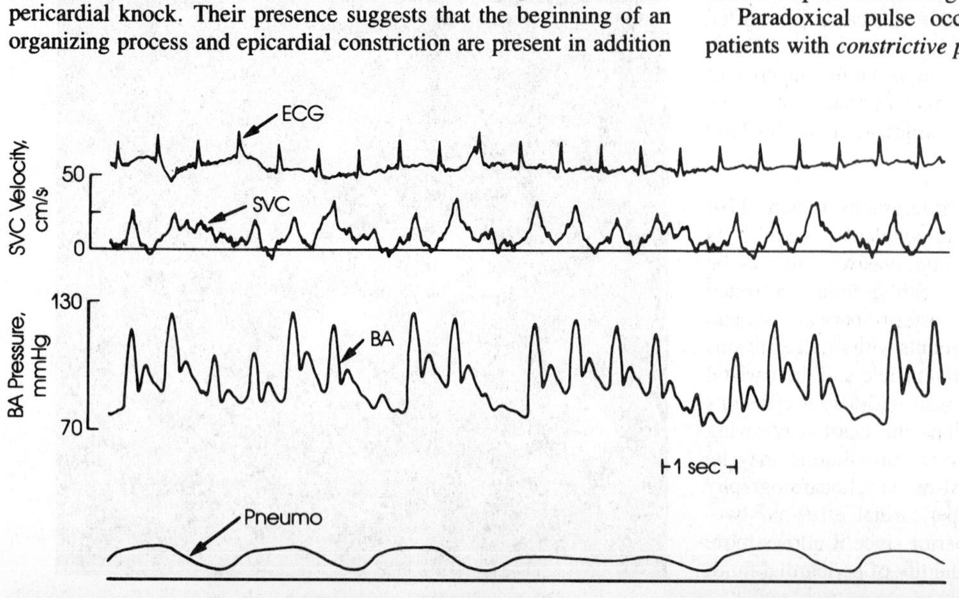

FIGURE 194-2 *Simultaneous recording of electrocardiogram (ECG), blood flow velocity in the superior vena cava (SVC), brachial arterial pressure (BA), and the pneumogram (Pneumo) in a patient with cardiac compression and paradoxical pulse. A downward deflection of the pneumogram denotes inspiration, when SVC blood velocity rises and arterial pressure falls (paradoxical pulse). Arterial pressure is maintained during prolonged expiratory pause.*

that paradoxical pulse is not pathognomonic of pericardial disease because it may be observed in various forms of restrictive cardiomyopathies (Chap. 192) and, in some cases of hypovolemic shock, chronic obstructive airways disease, and severe bronchial asthma.

TREATMENT All patients with acute pericarditis should be observed frequently and carefully for the possibility of a developing effusion or, if effusion is already present, for signs of tamponade. In the presence of an effusion, arterial and venous pressures and heart rate should be monitored continuously or carefully followed and serial echocardiograms obtained. If manifestations of tamponade appear, pericardiocentesis must be carried out at once, since relief of the intrapericardial pressure may be lifesaving. A small catheter advanced over the needle inserted into the pericardial cavity may be left in place if fluid accumulation persists and allows draining of the pericardial space.

VIRAL OR IDIOPATHIC FORM OF ACUTE PERICARDITIS This disorder is an important clinical entity because of its frequency and because it may be confused with other more serious illnesses. In some cases an A or B coxsackievirus or the virus of influenza, echovirus type 8, mumps, herpes simplex, chickenpox, or adenovirus has been isolated from pericardial fluid and/or appropriate elevations in viral antibody titers have been noted; in other instances, acute pericarditis has occurred in association with illnesses of known viral origin and, presumably, was caused by the same agent. More commonly there is an antecedent infection of the respiratory tract, but in many patients such an association is not evident and viral isolation and serologic studies are negative. Most frequently, a viral causation cannot be established nor can it be excluded; the term *acute idiopathic pericarditis* is then appropriate. However, regardless of the specific causative factor, the clinical manifestations are similar. This form of acute pericarditis occurs at all ages but is more frequent in young adults; it is often associated with pleural effusions and pneumonitis. The appearance of fever and precordial pain at about the same time, often 10 to 12 days after a presumed viral illness, constitutes an important feature in the differentiation of acute pericarditis from myocardial infarction, in which pain precedes fever. The constitutional symptoms are usually mild to moderate, but occasionally the initial symptoms are stormy, the temperature rising to 40°C. The disease ordinarily runs its course in a few days to 2 weeks, but occasionally after the patient has apparently recovered he or she may have one or several recurrences, weeks or even months later. Tamponade is unusual, although accumulation of some pericardial fluid is common, and constrictive pericarditis develops rarely. A pericardial friction rub is often audible. The ST-T–wave alterations in the electrocardiogram are usually transitory, but the abnormal T waves may persist for several years or indefinitely and be a source of confusion in persons without a clear history of pericarditis. Pleuritis and pneumonitis frequently accompany pericarditis. The erythrocyte sedimentation rate is elevated. Granulocytosis followed by lymphocytosis is common.

There is no specific therapy, but anti-inflammatory treatment with aspirin, if necessary up to 900 mg qid, may be given. If this is ineffective, one of the nonsteroidal anti-inflammatory agents, such as indomethacin (25 to 75 mg qid) or a corticosteroid (e.g., prednisone, 20 to 80 mg daily) effectively suppresses the clinical manifestations of the acute illness and may be useful in patients in whom the purulent and tuberculous forms of pericarditis have been excluded. After the patient has been asymptomatic for 1 week, the dose of the anti-inflammatory agent is gradually tapered. Recurrences occur in about one-fourth of patients, but the tendency to relapse decreases within 2 years after the initial episode. When recurrences continue to occur beyond this period and are frequent and disabling, pericardiectomy may be effective in terminating the illness.

POST-CARDIAC INJURY SYNDROME During the past few years, it has been recognized that an acute form of pericarditis may appear under a variety of circumstances which have one common feature: previous injury to the myocardium, with blood in the pericardial cavity. The syndrome has been observed when the injury has been induced in the course of a cardiac operation (postpericardiotomy syndrome or, as it was originally designated, postcommissurotomy syndrome). It may also follow myocardial infarction (Dressler's syndrome) or develop after trauma of the heart (e.g., stab wound, contusions following a nonpenetrating blow to the chest, and following perforation of the heart with a pacemaker catheter).

The principal symptom is the pain of acute pericarditis, which usually develops after an interval of 1 to 4 weeks following the cardiac injury but sometimes appears only after a lapse of months. Recurrences are common and may occur up to 2 years or more after the injury. Fever up to 40°C, pericarditis, pleuritis, and pneumonitis are the outstanding features, the bout of illness usually subsiding in 1 or 2 weeks. The pericarditis, which appears to be the most constant lesion, may be of the fibrinous variety, or it may be a pericardial effusion, which is often serosanguineous and sometimes causes tamponade. Rarely, the pericarditis may be accompanied by arthralgias. Leukocytosis, an increased sedimentation rate, and electrocardiographic changes typical of acute pericarditis may also occur.

The mechanism whereby the clinical manifestations are induced is not certain, but there is a likelihood that they are the result of a hypersensitivity reaction in which the antigen originates from injured myocardial tissue and/or pericardium; the suggested designation of post-cardiac injury syndrome for this group of disorders implies that they may have a common pathogenetic mechanism. Circulating autoantibodies to myocardium occur frequently, but their precise role in this syndrome has not been defined. Viral infection may also play an etiologic role, since antiviral antibodies are often elevated in patients who develop this syndrome following cardiac surgery.

The clinical picture mimics acute viral or acute idiopathic pericarditis. Moreover, it is possible that the recurrences that occur so frequently in the latter condition are not always caused by an exacerbation of the original (presumably viral) infection, but that the original injury may have initiated the sequence of events that culminates in the post-cardiac injury syndrome.

Often no treatment is necessary aside from aspirin, nonsteroidal anti-inflammatory drugs, or analgesics. The management of pericardial effusion and tamponade has already been discussed. When the illness is severe and is followed by a series of disabling recurrences, therapy with a nonsteroidal anti-inflammatory agent or a corticosteroid is usually effective.

Differential diagnosis Differential diagnosis of *acute idiopathic pericarditis* is primarily one of exclusion, as there is no specific test for this disorder. Consequently all other disorders that may be associated with acute fibrinous pericarditis must be considered. When associated with *acute myocardial infarction,* acute fibrinous pericarditis may be confused with acute viral or idiopathic pericarditis; this complication of infarction, described on page 992, must be differentiated by the occurrence of fever, pain, and a friction rub in the first 4 days following the development of the infarct. Electrocardiographic abnormalities (such as the appearance of Q waves and earlier T-wave changes in myocardial infarction), the extent of the elevations of myocardial enzymes, and the total clinical picture are helpful in the identification of the pericarditis of acute myocardial infarction. A common error is assuming that acute viral or idiopathic pericarditis represents acute myocardial infarction.

Acute pericarditis occurring as a component of the *post-cardiac injury* syndrome is most likely to be confused with acute idiopathic pericarditis when it follows myocardial infarction or a nonpenetrating bruise to the chest. Such pericarditis is differentiated from acute idiopathic pericarditis chiefly by timing. If it occurs within a few weeks of an infarction or a chest blow, it may be justified to conclude that the two are probably related. If the infarct has been silent or the chest blow forgotten, the relationship to the pericarditis may not be recognized.

It is important to distinguish *pericarditis due to collagen disease* from acute idiopathic pericarditis. Most important in the differential diagnosis is the pericarditis due to systemic lupus erythematosus (Chap. 262). Sometimes the latter appears as an asymptomatic effusion; more often pain is present, and rarely tamponade develops. Very rarely, when pericarditis occurs in the absence of other evidence of any underlying disorder, differentiation from acute viral and idiopathic pericarditis or tuberculous pericarditis may be made on discovery of lupus erythematosus (LE) cells, a rise in antinuclear antibodies, or by the specific methods for diagnosing tuberculosis. Acute pericarditis is also an occasional complication of *rheumatoid arthritis, scleroderma,* and *periarteritis nodosa,* but again, other evidence of these diseases is usually obvious. Asymptomatic pericardial effusion is also frequent in these disorders. It is important to question every patient with acute pericarditis about the ingestion of procainamide, hydralazine, isoniazid, cromolyn, and minoxidil, since these drugs can cause this syndrome.

The pericarditis of *acute rheumatic fever* is generally associated with evidence of severe pancarditis and with cardiac murmurs (Chap. 186). *Pyogenic (purulent) pericarditis* is usually secondary to cardiothoracic operations, immunosuppressive therapy, rupture of the esophagus into the pericardial sac, and rupture of a ring abscess in a patient with infective endocarditis and with septicemia complicating aseptic pericarditis. It is now uncommonly due to pneumococcal pneumonia and pleuritis, previously the most common cause. *Tuberculous pericarditis* (see Chap. 119) may present as an acute pericarditis, associated with fever, weight loss, and other clinical manifestations of active systemic tuberculosis; the diagnosis may be aided by a positive tuberculin test and evidence of pulmonary or mediastinal tuberculosis. Tubercle bacilli can be cultured from the pericardial space only infrequently, and a biopsy of the pericardium with bacteriologic and histologic examination may be required. Alternatively, tuberculous pericarditis may present as a chronic asymptomatic effusion, as subacute effusive-constrictive pericarditis, or frank chronic constrictive pericarditis (see below). *Uremic pericarditis* (Chap. 220) occurs in up to one-third of patients with chronic uremia, and is seen most frequently in patients undergoing chronic hemodialysis. It may be fibrinous or associated with a bloody effusion. A friction rub is common, but pain is usually absent. Treatment with an anti-inflammatory agent and intensification of hemodialysis is usually adequate therapy. Occasionally, when tamponade occurs, pericardiocentesis is required. When pericarditis is recurrent or persistent, pericardiectomy is necessary. Pericarditis due to *neoplastic diseases* results from irradiation or extension of primary or metastatic tumors (most commonly carcinoma of the lung and breast, malignant melanoma, and lymphoma) to the pericardium or from invasion by a lymphomatous or leukemic process; pain, atrial arrhythmias, and tamponade are complications which occur occasionally. *Mediastinal irradiation* for neoplasm may cause pericarditis after eradication of the tumor. Unusual causes of acute pericarditis include syphilis, fungous infection (histoplasmosis, blastomycosis, aspergillosis, and candidiasis), and parasitic infestation (amebiasis, toxoplasmosis, echinococcosis, trichinosis).

CHRONIC PERICARDIAL EFFUSIONS Chronic pericardial effusions are often encountered in patients without an antecedent history of acute pericarditis. They may cause few symptoms per se, and may be suspected by finding an enlarged cardiac silhouette on chest roentgenogram which may be obtained in the course of the workup of a patient with symptoms related to the underlying illness.

Tuberculosis This is the most common cause of chronic pericardial effusion (Chap. 119). The symptoms are often those of a chronic, systemic illness in an individual with effusion. It is important to bear this condition in mind when a middle-aged or elderly person with fever has apparent enlargement of the heart of undetermined origin, with or without elevation of venous pressure. Weight loss, fever, and fatigability are sometimes observed. Inasmuch as effective specific methods of therapy have now reduced strikingly the mortality rate from the previous figures of about 70 percent, overlooking a tuberculous pericardial effusion is a serious error. Consequently, no method of examination should be omitted to establish this diagnosis. Included are chest roentgenograms for pulmonary tuberculosis and a search for tuberculosis in other organs; tuberculin skin tests, repeated after several weeks; cultures and smears of gastric washings and of pleural and pericardial fluid. Finally, if the diagnosis is still obscure, a pericardial biopsy, preferably by a limited thoracotomy, should be performed after 1 or 2 weeks of preliminary antituberculous chemotherapy. If definitive evidence is then still lacking, but the specimen shows caseation necrosis, antituberculous chemotherapy for at least 24 months is justified (Chap. 119). Pericardiectomy should be carried out in order to prevent the development of constriction if the biopsy specimen shows a thickened pericardium.

Other causes of chronic pericardial effusion *Myxedema* may be responsible for a pericardial effusion that is sometimes massive but rarely, if ever, causes cardiac tamponade. The other manifestations of myxedema should clarify the diagnosis, but unfortunately, even when they are present, the diagnosis is frequently overlooked. It is important, therefore, to carry out appropriate tests for thyroid function (Chap. 324) in patients with an enlarged cardiac outline of undetermined origin. The cardiac silhouette is markedly enlarged and an echocardiogram is necessary to distinguish cardiomegaly from pericardial effusion. *Cholesterol pericardial disease* produces large pericardial effusions with a high cholesterol content, which may induce an inflammatory response and constrictive pericarditis.

Neoplasms, systemic lupus erythematosus, rheumatoid arthritis, mycotic infection, radiation therapy, pyogenic infections, severe chronic anemia, and chylopericardium may also cause chronic pericardial effusion and should be considered and specifically looked for in such patients.

Aspiration and analysis of the pericardial fluid are often helpful in diagnosis. In infections the organism can often be identified by smear or culture. Grossly sanguineous pericardial fluid results most commonly from a neoplasm, tuberculosis, uremia, or slow leakage from an aortic aneurysm.

CHRONIC CONSTRICTIVE PERICARDITIS

This disorder results when the healing of an acute fibrinous or serofibrinous pericarditis is followed by obliteration of the pericardial cavity, with the formation of granulation tissue which gradually contracts and forms a firm scar, encasing the heart and interfering with filling of the ventricles. In some reports, a high percentage of all cases has been of tuberculous origin. In other series, particularly those reported in the United States in the last decade, tuberculosis has been an infrequent cause. The condition also may follow purulent infection, trauma, cardiac operation of any type, mediastinal irradiation, histoplasmosis, neoplastic disease, and acute viral or idiopathic pericarditis, rheumatoid arthritis, lupus erythematosus, and chronic renal failure with uremia treated by chronic dialysis. In many patients the cause of the pericardial disease is undetermined, and in them it is presumed that an asymptomatic or forgotten bout of acute pericarditis, acute or idiopathic, was the inciting event. Rarely, routine radiographic examination may reveal calcification of the pericardium in a person who is free of all symptoms referable to the heart.

The basic physiologic abnormality in symptomatic patients with chronic constrictive pericarditis, as in those with cardiac tamponade, is the inability of the ventricles to fill adequately during diastole because of the limitations imposed by the rigid, thickened pericardium or the tense pericardial fluid. Stroke volume is reduced, and the end-diastolic pressures in both ventricles, as well as the mean pressures in the atria, pulmonic veins, and systemic veins, are all elevated to about the same levels. Despite these hemodynamic changes myocardial function may be normal; instead, the ventricles may be considered to be underloaded. In constrictive pericarditis the central venous and right and left atrial pressure pulses display an M-shaped contour, with prominent x and y descents; the y descent is the most prominent deflection and is interrupted by a rapid rise in pressure during early diastole, when ventricular filling is impeded by the constricting pericardium. In cardiac tamponade the pressure contour differs in that the most prominent deflection is the x trough, while the y descent is usually absent. These characteristic changes are transmitted to the jugular veins, where they may be recognized by inspection or recorded. In constrictive pericarditis, both ventricular pressure pulses exhibit characteristic "square root" signs during diastole. These hemodynamic changes, although characteristic, are not pathognomonic of constrictive pericarditis but are also observed in cardiomyopathies characterized by restriction of ventricular filling, as discussed on page 1001.

CLINICAL FINDINGS Weakness, fatigue, weight loss, and anorexia are common. The patients often appear to be chronically ill with decreased muscle mass, a protuberant abdomen, and peripheral edema. Contrary to a widely held impression, dyspnea, though absent or slight at rest, is often present on exertion, and orthopnea is common in chronic constrictive pericarditis, although it is not severe. Attacks of acute left ventricular failure (acute pulmonary edema) practically never occur. The cervical veins are distended and may remain so even after intensive diuretic treatment, and venous pressure may fail to decline during inspiration (Kussmaul's sign). In about one-third of the cases a paradoxical pulse may be observed. Congestive hepatomegaly is pronounced and may impair hepatic function; ascites is common and is usually more prominent than dependent edema. In about half of the patients, the heart is normal in size; if it is enlarged, the enlargement is rarely extreme. The apical pulse is reduced in intensity. The heart sounds may be distant, an early third heart sound, i.e., a pericardial knock, occurring 0.06 to 0.12 s after aortic valve closure which coincides with a sudden deceleration in ventricular filling, is often conspicuous, and murmurs are usually absent. The apex beat is poorly defined, and cardiac pulsations under fluoroscopic examination are diminished. Because of the high sustained venous pressure, congestive splenomegaly may be sufficiently pronounced to make the spleen palpable. In the absence of infective endocarditis or tricuspid valve disease, splenomegaly in a patient with congestive heart failure should arouse suspicion of constrictive pericarditis. Protein-losing gastroenteropathy due to impaired lymphatic drainage from the small intestine, and the nephrotic syndrome, or sometimes only marked proteinuria or hypoalbuminemia, may complicate chronic constrictive pericarditis. The electrocardiogram frequently displays low voltage of the QRS complex and diffuse flattening or inversion of the T waves. P mitrale may be present in patients with sinus rhythm; atrial fibrillation is present in about one-third of these patients.

Systemic and/or pulmonary venous congestion is initially the result of impaired filling of the ventricles caused by the restrictive action of the inelastic pericardium. However, the fibrotic process may extend into the myocardium, and venous congestion may then be due to the combined effects of the myocardial and pericardial lesions. The interference with filling reduces the work of the heart and perhaps this leads to myocardial atrophy. The latter probably accounts for the delayed beneficial effects of operative treatment observed in some patients with advanced disease.

Inasmuch as the usual physical signs of cardiac disease (murmurs, cardiac enlargement) may be inconspicuous or absent, hepatic enlargement and dysfunction associated with intractable ascites may lead to a mistaken diagnosis of cirrhosis of the liver. This error should be avoided if the neck veins are inspected carefully in all patients with ascites and hepatomegaly. *Given a clinical picture resembling that of cirrhosis, but with the added feature of distended neck veins, careful search for calcification of the pericardium by chest roentgenograms, fluoroscopy, and echocardiography should be carried out and may disclose a curable or remediable form of heart disease.* Calcification occurs in only about one-half of these patients and usually in those with long-standing pericardial constriction. Most patients with chronic constrictive pericarditis show pericardial thickening on echocardiographic examination. Surgical exploration of the pericardium is justifiable if the clinical picture and echocardiographic and cardiac catheterization findings are suggestive even in the absence of pericardial calcification.

DIFFERENTIAL DIAGNOSIS Like cor pulmonale (Chap. 191), chronic constrictive pericarditis may be associated with severe systemic venous hypertension but with little or no pulmonary congestion; the heart may not appear to be enlarged, and a striking inspiratory fall in arterial pressure may be present. However, in cor pulmonale advanced parenchymal pulmonary disease is usually evident and venous pressure *falls* during inspiration. *Tricuspid stenosis* may also simulate the picture of chronic constrictive pericarditis; congestive hepatomegaly and ascites may be equally prominent, and the manifestations of left-sided heart failure may be inconspicuous. However, in tricuspid stenosis, the characteristic murmur, the frequent coexistence of mitral stenosis, the absence of a paradoxic pulse, as well as the absence, in the jugular venous pulse, of the steep, deep y descent followed by a rapid ascent (manifested by the diastolic shock on palpation and its audible equivalent, the pericardial knock), should make the clinical differentiation possible.

It is of the greatest importance, though often difficult, to distinguish chronic constrictive pericarditis from various forms of heart disease which are characterized by a similar physiologic abnormality, i.e., restriction of ventricular filling, leading to a similar clinical picture. Described in Chap. 192, these include endomyocardial fibrosis, infiltrative cardiomyopathies such as amyloidosis, hemochromatosis, sarcoidosis, scleroderma and idiopathic myocardial hypertrophy, in which the marked thickening of the ventricular wall is responsible for the diminished compliance.

The features favoring the diagnosis of one of the above forms of cardiomyopathy are a well-defined apex beat, conspicuous enlargement of the heart, and pronounced orthopnea with attacks of acute left ventricular failure, left ventricular hypertrophy, gallop sounds, bundle branch block, and significant Q waves in the electrocardiogram. The echocardiogram shows ventricular thickening, sometimes with a granular sparkling appearance. At catheterization, patients with chronic constrictive pericarditis usually have left atrial or pulmonary arterial wedge pressure equaling right atrial pressure, the latter often exceeding 15 mmHg despite intensive medical treatment for heart failure; the pulmonary artery systolic pressure is often less than 50 mmHg, and the right ventricular end-diastolic pressure often reaches one-third of the systolic pressure; the cardiac output is slightly depressed. In contrast, in patients with cardiomyopathy, the left atrial usually exceeds the right atrial pressure by more than 5 mmHg, the mean right atrial pressure often falls to below 15 mmHg following intensive treatment, the pulmonary artery systolic pressure often exceeds 50 mmHg, and the right ventricular end-diastolic pressure is usually less than one-third of the systolic pressure, while the cardiac output is markedly depressed. The volumes of both ventricles, as determined by angiography or echocardiography, are characteristically reduced or normal in constrictive pericarditis, and the ejection fractions are normal; the left ventricular end-diastolic volume may be normal in some cardiomyopathies but is frequently elevated in others, in whom the ejection fraction is reduced; the latter finding militates strongly against the diagnosis of constrictive pericarditis. The echocardiogram in chronic constrictive pericarditis characteristically shows pericardial thickening, i.e., a distinct echo posterior to the left ventricular wall, and paradoxical septal motion. The left ventricular wall moves sharply outward in early diastole and then remains flat. The definitive diagnosis of restrictive cardiomyopathy, when it is due to an infiltrative disease such as amyloidosis, can often be established by endomyocardial biopsy.

It is important to emphasize that when a patient has progressive, disabling, and unresponsive congestive failure, and if he or she displays any of the phenomena of constrictive heart disease, the most careful and detailed clinical and laboratory studies must be carried out in order to detect or exclude constrictive pericarditis, which is potentially a curable condition. In many instances cardiac catheterization, selective angiocardiography, coronary arteriography, and endomyocardial biopsy may be required. However, when even these examinations do not yield a definitive diagnosis, surgical exploration of the pericardium is the only decisive method of determining whether constrictive pericarditis is responsible for the clinical manifestations of heart failure.

Occult constrictive disease Patients with this condition may have unexplained fatigue, dyspnea, and chest pain. No overt manifestations of pericardial disease are present, but following the rapid intravenous infusion of 1 liter of saline solution, atrial and ventricular pressure pulses and diastolic equilibration of intracardiac pressures, as in overt constrictive pericarditis, occur. Although symptomatic improvement may follow pericardiectomy, this procedure should not be carried out in asymptomatic persons.

TREATMENT Pericardial resection is the only definitive treatment of constrictive pericarditis, but diuretics and sodium restriction are useful during preoperative preparation. Digitalis may be beneficial in the prevention of heart failure when resection of the thickened pericardium permits an increased inflow into the ventricles and hence places an enhanced burden on an atrophic myocardium. The benefits derived from a complete cardiac decortication are often striking, and frequently the improvement, though slight at first, is progressive over a period of many months.

Many instances of constrictive pericarditis are of tuberculous origin. Antituberculous therapy during the phase of effusion may prevent the development of constriction, and such therapy should be carried out before and after operation, if a tuberculous origin is suspected or cannot be excluded in a patient with chronic constrictive pericarditis (Chap. 119).

SUBACUTE EFFUSIVE-CONSTRICTIVE PERICARDITIS This form of pericardial disease is characterized by a combination of a tense effusion in the pericardial space, as well as constriction of the heart by thickened pericardium, and thus it shares a number of features both with pericardial effusion producing cardiac compression and with pericardial constriction. It may be caused by tuberculosis, multiple attacks of acute idiopathic pericarditis, radiation, traumatic pericarditis, uremia, and scleroderma. The heart is generally enlarged, and there are a paradoxical pulse and a prominent x descent in the atrial pressure pulse. Following pericardiocentesis, the physiologic findings may change from those of cardiac tamponade to those of pericardial constriction, with a ''square root sign'' in the ventricular pressure pulse and a prominent y descent in the atrial and jugular venous pressures. In many patients the condition progresses to the chronic constrictive form of the disease. Wide excision of both the visceral and parietal pericardium is usually effective.

OTHER DISORDERS OF THE PERICARDIUM

Pericardial cysts appear as rounded or lobulated deformities of the cardiac silhouette, most commonly at the right cardiophrenic angle. They do not cause symptoms, and their major clinical significance lies in the possibility of confusion with a tumor, ventricular aneurysm, or massive cardiomegaly. *Tumors* involving the pericardium are most commonly secondary to malignant neoplasms originating in or invading the mediastinum, including carcinoma of the bronchus and breast, lymphoma, and melanoma. The most common *primary* malignant tumor is the mesothelioma. The usual clinical picture of malignant pericardial tumor is an insidiously developing, often bloody, pericardial effusion. Surgical exploration is required to establish a definitive diagnosis and to carry out definitive or, more commonly, palliative treatment.

REFERENCES

BOLTWOOD CM, SHAH PM: The pericardium in health and disease. Cur Probl Cardiol 9:1, 1984

BUSH CA et al: Occult pericardial disease. Circulation 56:924, 1977

HANCOCK EW: Subacute effusive-constrictive pericarditis. Circulation 43:183, 1971

LORELL B, BRAUNWALD E: Pericardial disease, in *Heart Disease,* 2d ed. Philadelphia, Saunders, 1984, p 1470

MCCAUGHAN BC et al: Early and late results of pericardiectomy for constrictive pericarditis. J Thorac Cardiovasc Surg 89:340, 1985

NISHIMURA RA et al: Constrictive pericarditis: Assessment of current diagnostic procedures. Mayo Clin Proc 60:397, 1985

REDDY et al (eds): *Pericardial Disease.* New York, Raven, 1982

RIBEIRO P et al: Constrictive pericarditis as a complication of coronary artery bypass surgery. Br Heart J 51:205, 1984

section 2 Disorders of the vascular system

195 ATHEROSCLEROSIS AND OTHER FORMS OF ARTERIOSCLEROSIS

EDWIN L. BIERMAN

Arteriosclerosis, a generic term for thickening and hardening of the arterial wall, is responsible for the majority of deaths in the United States and most westernized societies. One type of arteriosclerosis is *atherosclerosis,* the disorder of the larger arteries that underlies most *coronary artery disease, aortic aneurysm,* and *arterial disease of the lower extremities* and also plays a major role in *cerebrovascular disease.* Atherosclerosis is by far the leading cause of death in the United States, both above and below age 65 (Table 195-1).

Other types of arteriosclerosis include focal calcific arteriosclerosis (*Mönckeberg's sclerosis*) and *arteriolosclerosis.* The major arterial diseases other than arteriosclerosis include *congenital structural defects, inflammatory* or granulomatous diseases (e.g., syphilitic aortitis), and disorders affecting mainly the smaller vessels, such as *hypersensitivity* or autoimmune diseases.

THE NORMAL ARTERY

STRUCTURE The normal artery wall consists of three reasonably well-defined layers: the intima, the media, and the adventitia.

Intima A single continuous layer of *endothelial cells* lines the lumen of all arteries. The intima is delimited on its outer aspect by a perforated tube of elastic tissue, the *internal elastic lamina.* This tube of elastic tissue is particularly prominent in the large elastic arteries and the medium-caliber muscular arteries, and it disappears in capillaries. The endothelial cells are attached to one another by a series of junctional complexes and are also attached, apparently somewhat tenuously, to an underlying meshwork of loose connective tissue, the *basal lamina*. These lining endothelial cells normally form a barrier that controls the entry of substances from the blood into the artery wall. Such substances usually enter the cells by specific transport systems. Normally, no other cell type is present in the intima of most arteries.

Media The media consists of only one cell type, the *smooth-muscle cell,* arranged in either a single layer (as in small muscular arteries) or multiple lamellae (as in elastic arteries). These cells are surrounded by small amounts of collagen and elastic fibers, which they elaborate, and usually take the pattern of diagonal concentric spirals through the vessel wall. They are closely apposed to one another and may be attached by junctional complexes. The smooth-muscle cell appears to be the major connective tissue–forming cell of the artery wall, producing collagen, elastic fibers, and proteoglycans. In that sense it is analogous to the fibroblast in skin, the osteoblast in bone, and the chondroblast in cartilage. The media is bounded on the luminal side by the internal elastic lamina and on the abluminal side by a less continuous sheet of elastic tissue, the *external elastic lamina.* In *elastic arteries,* like the aorta and the major pulmonary arteries, elastic lamellae are prominent. Such arteries expand and increase their elastic tension with the pulse of systole. In diastole, the elastic fibers recoil, helping to propel the blood distally and progressively damping the pulsatile character of flow toward more terminal vessels. In *muscular arteries,* in which smooth-muscle cells predominate, peripheral flow is regulated, particularly in arterioles, by contraction (vasoconstriction) and relaxation (vasodilatation). Located about midway through the media of most arteries is a "nutritional watershed." The outer portion is nourished from the small blood vessels (vasa vasorum) in the adventitia; the inner layers receive their nutrients from the lumen.

Adventitia The outermost layer of the artery is the adventitia, which is delimited on the luminal aspect by the external elastic lamina. This external coat consists of a loose interwoven admixture of collagen bundles, elastic fibers, smooth-muscle cells, and fibroblasts. This layer also contains the vasa vasorum and nerves.

METABOLISM AND FUNCTION The artery wall is a metabolically active organ that must meet a steady demand for energy to maintain smooth-muscle tension and endothelial cell function and to repair and replenish tissue constituents. The mechanical forces on the arterial wall are complex, and considerable tensile stresses are imposed on it, mainly by hydraulic force. Shear or frictional stresses are especially prominent near the entrance regions of branches. The form and manner in which these forces are dissipated depend upon flow, the amount of elastic tension developed, and the tethering or external support provided by surrounding structures. Arteries are also permeable pipes, which constantly exchange fluid and solutes with the blood they carry.

Maintenance of the endothelial cell lining is critical. Endothelial cell turnover occurs at a slow rate but may be accelerated in focal areas by changing patterns of flow along the vessel wall. When intact, these cells selectively control the passage of circulating substances by active transport (endocytosis and exocytosis) through their cytoplasm, and they elaborate connecting tissue components to form their own substratum. In addition, intact endothelial cells function to prevent clotting partly by elaboration of a particular prostaglandin (prostacyclin or PGI_2) that inhibits platelet function, thereby enhancing unimpeded flow of blood. When the lining is damaged, platelets adhere to it, in part as the result of production of a different class of prostaglandins, the thromboxanes, and form a clot; endothelial cells function in the clotting process by elaboration of key substances, including factor VIII.

The metabolism of arteries reflects the biochemistry of smooth-muscle cells. Arterial smooth-muscle cells form abundant collagen, elastic fibers, soluble and insoluble elastin, and glucosaminoglycans (mainly dermatan sulfate). Multiple anabolic and catabolic pathways are present. These cells metabolize glucose by both anaerobic and aerobic glycolysis. A variety of catabolic enzymes are present including fibrinolysins, mixed-function oxidases, and lysosomal hydrolases. Because of the prominence of lipids in atherosclerotic lesions, much attention has been directed to lipid metabolism in arteries. Arterial wall cells can synthesize fatty acids, cholesterol, phospholipids, and triglycerides from endogenous substrates to satisfy their structural needs (membrane replenishment), but smooth-muscle cells appear preferentially to utilize lipids from plasma lipoproteins transported into the wall. Circulating lipoproteins traverse endothelial cells in pinocytotic vesicles. Smooth-muscle cells possess specific high-affinity surface receptors for certain apoproteins on the surface of lipid-rich lipoproteins, thus facilitating the entry of lipoproteins into the cell by adsorptive endocytosis. As has been shown for cultured skin fibroblasts, in arterial smooth-muscle cells these vesicles fuse with lysosomes, resulting in catabolism of lipoprotein components (Chap. 315). Free cholesterol entering the cell in this manner inhibits endogenous cholesterol synthesis, facilitates its own esterification, and partially limits further entry of cholesterol by regulating the number of lipoprotein receptors. However, lipoprotein cholesterol can gain entry into arterial smooth muscle cells by non-receptor-mediated pathways, potentially causing cholesterol ester accumulation.

Thus, many complex and interrelated metabolic processes are present in arterial wall cells. Although some of these may play a role in the production of arteriosclerosis, no one biochemical reaction can be singled out as culpable. Physiologic factors, such as transfer processes across the endothelial lining, the flux of oxygen and substrates from both the luminal and adventitial sides of the wall, and the reverse flow of catabolic products, need to be considered as well. The ability of the arterial wall to maintain the integrity of its endothelium, prevent platelet aggregation, prevent adherence of blood mononuclear cells, and ensure the nutrition of its middle portion may be the critical determinants of the arteriosclerotic process.

CHANGES WITH AGING The major change that occurs with normal aging in the arterial wall in humans is a slow, apparently continuous, symmetric increase in the thickness of the intima. This intimal thickening results from a gradual accumulation of smooth-muscle cells (presumably resulting from migration of these cells from the media and their subsequent proliferation), surrounded by additional connective tissue. In the nondiseased artery wall, lipid content, mainly cholesterol ester and phospholipid (particularly sphingomyelin), also progressively increases with age. Phospholipid synthesis rises with aging (perhaps in response to the need for more membrane formation for plasma membranes, vesicles, lysosomes, and other intracellular organelles) followed by a compensatory increase in activity of all phospholipases except sphingomyelinase. While most of the phospholipid in the normal artery wall appears to be derived from in situ synthesis, the cholesterol ester that accumulates with aging appears to be derived from plasma, since it contains principally linoleic acid, the major plasma cholesterol ester fatty acid. Furthermore, low-density lipoproteins (LDL) are immunologically detectable in the intima of normal arteries in direct relation to their concentration in

TABLE 195-1 Deaths, by cause, in the United States, 1982

	No. of deaths, thousands			
	Below age 65		Age 65 and above	
Causes of death	Male	Female	Male	Female
All causes	396	224	660	695
All cardiovascular diseases	130	57	359	421
Ischemic heart disease	86	29	216	223
Cerebrovascular disease	11	11	52	84
Hypertensive disease*	1	1	3	4
All infectious disease	6	9	6	7
All cancer	85	75	149	125
Accidents	54	17	12	11

* *A substantial proportion of deaths of hypertensive persons occurs with ischemic heart disease or cerebrovascular disease; such deaths are classified in those categories.*
SOURCE: *National Center for Health Statistics, Vital Statistics Report, Final Mortality Statistics, 1982.*

plasma. It has been estimated that between the second and sixth decade, the normal intima accumulates approximately 10 mg cholesterol per gram of tissue. Thus, as the normal artery ages, smooth-muscle cells and connective tissue accumulate diffusely in the intima, leading to progressive thickening of this layer, coupled with progressive accumulation of sphingomyelin and cholesterol linoleate. This diffuse age-related intimal thickening is to be distinguished from focal discrete raised fibromuscular plaques, a characteristic feature of atherosclerosis.

Functionally, these changes with aging result in gradually increasing rigidity of vessels. The larger arteries may become dilated, elongated, and tortuous, and aneurysms may form in areas of an encroaching degenerating arteriosclerotic plaque. Such "wear-and-tear" changes are frequently proportional to the vessel diameter and correlated with branching, curvature, and anatomic points of attachment. The amount of external support also determines the ability of vessels, weakened by loss of elasticity, to withstand hydrostatic pressure. The unsupported cerebral arteries may be particularly vulnerable in this regard. Although senescence is accompanied by the intimal thickening that is a feature of localized atheromatosis, the changes of aging and arteriosclerosis appear to be separate and distinct processes.

NONATHEROMATOUS FORMS OF ARTERIOSCLEROSIS

Atherosclerosis involves primarily the intimal layer and occurs most commonly in the abdominal aorta and its large renal and lower extremity branches, the coronary arteries, and the cerebral vasculature. It may accompany or accelerate the other major forms of arteriosclerosis, *focal calcification* and *arteriolosclerosis* (Table 195-2).

FOCAL CALCIFICATION Not to be confused with atherosclerosis is focal calcification of the media, particularly in the medium-sized muscular arteries. This type of arteriosclerosis is called *Mönckeberg's sclerosis* and is common in the lower extremities, upper extremities, and the arterial supply of the genital tract in both sexes. This disorder is rare in individuals below age 50 and affects both sexes indiscriminately. The process involves degeneration of smooth-muscle cells, followed by calcium deposition. The vessels become hard and tortuous, so that palpable vessels such as the radial artery can be felt as rigid tubes. Its characteristic radiologic appearance consists of regular concentric calcifications, commonly seen in pelvic and femoral vessels. The medial changes alone do not narrow the lumen, have little effect on the circulation, and have relatively little clinical significance. However, in the lower extremities, medial sclerosis is often associated with atherosclerosis, leading to arterial occlusion.

TABLE 195-2 Disorders associated with early arteriosclerosis

ATHEROSCLEROSIS
Diabetes mellitus
Hypertension
Familial hypercholesterolemia
Familial combined hyperlipidemia
Familial dysbetalipoproteinemia
Hypothyroidism
Werner's syndrome
Cholesterol ester storage disease
Systemic lupus erythematosus
NONATHEROMATOUS ARTERIOSCLEROSIS
Diabetes mellitus
Chronic renal insufficiency
Chronic vitamin D intoxication
Pseudoxanthoma elasticum
Idiopathic arterial calcification in infancy
Aortic valvular calcification in the elderly
Werner's syndrome
Homocystinuria

These changes are common in the elderly, and in patients on long-term corticosteroid therapy, but in individuals with diabetes mellitus, focal calcification may be accelerated and severe. It is much more common in diabetics with neuropathy, and sympathetic denervation of medial smooth muscle has been implicated in its etiology.

Focal calcification also can produce the arteriosclerotic aortic valve in the elderly. Progressive calcium deposition occurs on the aortic surface of normal trileaflet aortic valves with age, resulting in a spectrum of clinical findings ranging from an innocent systolic murmur to severe calcific aortic stenosis (Chap. 187).

ARTERIOLOSCLEROSIS This disorder involves hyaline and degenerative changes affecting both the intima and media of small arteries and arterioles, particularly in the spleen, pancreas, adrenal, and kidney. In the kidney, but not necessarily elsewhere, arteriolosclerosis is almost invariably associated with hypertension. Lesser degrees of sustained hypertension characteristically cause *hyalinization* of renal arterioles; more severe or malignant hypertension produces a typical *fibrous and elastic hyperplasia,* and even necrosis, of the media and intima.

ATHEROSCLEROSIS

LESIONS Morbid anatomy Atherosclerosis is a patchy nodular type of arteriosclerosis. The lesions are commonly classified as *fatty streaks, fibrous plaques,* and *complicated lesions. Fatty streaks* may be the earliest lesions of atherosclerosis, but the evidence is very uncertain. They are characterized by an accumulation of lipid-filled smooth-muscle cells and macrophages (foam cells) and fibrous tissue in focal areas of the intima. They are stained distinctly by fat-soluble dyes but may be visible without staining as yellowish or whitish patches on the intimal surface. The lipid is mainly cholesterol oleate, partly derived from synthesis in situ. The fatty streak is usually sessile and causes little obstruction and no symptoms. The lesion is universal, appearing in various segments of the arterial tree at different ages beginning in the aorta in infancy. In all children, regardless of race, sex, or environment, fatty streaks are present in the aorta by age 10 and increase to occupy as much as 30 to 50 percent of the aortic surface by age 25, but they do not appear to extend further with aging. Despite a presumed relation between fatty streaks and fibrous atherosclerotic plaques, aortic fatty streaks are not correlated with the location and extent of fibrous lesions. In the coronary arteries, the extent of fatty streaks may be a better indicator of the development of clinically significant raised lesions later in life. They are usually observed by age 15 and continue to involve more surface area with increasing age. Fatty streaks in the cerebral arteries are also present in all populations, develop during the third and fourth decade, and are more extensive in those populations having a higher incidence of cerebrovascular disease. It is generally believed that fatty streaks may be reversible, but the evidence is inconclusive.

Fibrous plaques, also called raised lesions or pearly plaques, are palpably elevated areas of intimal thickening and represent the most characteristic lesion of advancing atherosclerosis. They do not share with fatty streaks the ubiquitous distribution among populations. These plaques first appear in the abdominal aorta, coronary arteries, and carotid arteries in the third decade and increase progressively with age. They appear in men before women, in the aorta before the coronary arteries, and much later in the vertebral and intracranial cerebral arteries. Reasons for the difference in susceptibility of various segments of the arterial tree and the nonuniform distribution of lesions are not known. Typically, the fibrous plaque is firm, elevated, and dome-shaped, with an opaque glistening surface that bulges into the lumen. It consists of a central core of extracellular lipid and necrotic cell debris ("gruel") covered by a fibromuscular layer or cap containing large numbers of smooth-muscle cells, macrophages, and collagen. Thus the plaque is much thicker than is normal intima. Although the lipid, like that of fatty streaks, is mainly cholesterol ester, the principal esterified fatty acid is linoleic rather than oleic. Thus plaque cholesterol ester composition differs from fatty streaks but resembles plasma lipoproteins.

The *complicated lesion* is a calcified fibrous plaque containing various degrees of necrosis, thrombosis, and ulceration. These are the lesions frequently associated with symptoms. With increasing necrosis and accumulation of gruel, the arterial wall progressively weakens, and rupture of the intima can occur, causing aneurysm and hemorrhage. Arterial emboli can form when fragments of plaque dislodge into the lumen. Stenosis and impaired organ function result from gradual occlusion as plaques thicken and thrombi form.

Localization Although the term *generalized atherosclerosis* is commonly used clinically, lesions are actually irregularly distributed; different vessels are involved at different ages and to varying degrees. The aorta, especially its abdominal portion, is involved earliest and most severely by atherosclerotic lesions, and it is the bellwether of lesions elsewhere. The *aorta* is usually most heavily involved in its abdominal portion, about the orifices of its branches (particularly at the level of the coronary and intercostal arteries), in the aortic arch, and frequently at its bifurcation into the iliac arteries. There is more atherosclerosis in the lower than in the upper limbs. In the legs, the incidence decreases peripherally, as the musculoelastic vessels give way to large muscular arteries and these become smaller vessels, such as the plantar or digital arteries. Plaques and thromboses are particularly common in the *femoral* artery, in Hunter's canal, and in the *popliteal* artery just above the knee joint. The *anterior* and *posterior tibial* arteries are often occluded together, but in different sites—the posterior where it rounds the internal malleolus and the anterior where it is superficial and becomes the dorsalis pedis artery. The peroneal artery, which is well embedded in muscle, often escapes when other major vessels are occluded, and it may be the main blood supply to the extremity (*peroneal leg*). Atherosclerosis in abdominal branches, except for the renal and mesenteric arteries, causes less difficulty than in coronary and cerebral vessels.

In the *coronary arteries,* raised lesions are most prominent in the main stems, the highest incidence being a short distance beyond the ostia. Atherosclerosis is nearly always found in the epicardial (extramural) portions of the vessels, while the intramural coronary arteries are spared. Coronary atherosclerosis is often diffuse. The degree to which the lumen is narrowed varies, but once the process is present, all the intima of the extramural portions of the vessel is usually involved. A single tiny plaque occluding an otherwise normal coronary artery is rare. Selective involvement of the coronary arteries may relate to the unique hemodynamic forces, unlike those of other major arteries, resulting from greater flow in diastole than systole. The implications of these flow patterns for atherogenesis are as yet unknown. Typical atheromatous fibrous plaques also develop in saphenous vein aortocoronary bypass grafts.

In the cervical and cerebral arteries the distribution of atherosclerosis is patchy, as it may be in other arteries. It first appears in the base of the brain in the carotid, basilar, and vertebral arteries. The proximal portion of the internal carotid artery in the neck is a site of special predilection. There is a concentration of lesions near bifurcations. Atherosclerosis in the *pulmonary artery* bears no relation to the severity of the disease in the aorta or other systemic arteries. There is some involvement in about half of adults over 50 years of age who have no reason to have pulmonary hypertension. Pulmonary hypertension per se, however, is associated with medial hypertrophy, intimal thickening, and great acceleration of atheroma formation.

THEORIES OF ATHEROGENESIS One generally accepted theory for the pathogenesis of atherosclerosis consistent with a variety of experimental evidence is the *reaction to injury* hypothesis. According to this idea the endothelial cells lining the intima are exposed to repeated or continuing insults to their integrity. The injury to the endothelium may be subtle or gross, resulting in a loss of the ability of the cells to function normally or to attach to one another and to the underlying connective tissue. In the extreme, the cells may desquamate. Examples of types of "injury" to the endothelium include chemical injury, as in chronic hypercholesterolemia or homocystinemia, mechanical stress associated with hypertension, and immunologic injury, as may be seen after cardiac or renal transplantation. Loss of functional endothelial cells at susceptible sites in the arterial tree would lead to exposure of the subendothelial tissue to increased concentrations of plasma constituents and a sequence of events including platelet adherence, platelet aggregation and formation of microthrombi, and release of platelet granular components, including a potent mitogenic factor. This platelet factor, in conjunction with other plasma constituents, including lipoproteins and hormones such as insulin, could stimulate both the migration of medial smooth-muscle cells into the intima and their proliferation at these sites of injury. These proliferating smooth-muscle cells would deposit a connective tissue matrix and accumulate lipid, a process that would be particularly enhanced with hyperlipidemia. Macrophages derived from circulating blood monocytes can also accumulate lipid.

Adherence of monocytes and their migration into the arterial wall to become resident macrophages may be the earliest cellular abnormality in atherogenesis. Thus repeated or chronic injury could lead to a slowly progressing lesion involving a gradual increase in smooth-muscle cells, macrophages, connective tissue, and lipid. Areas where the shearing stress on endothelial cells is increased, such as branch points or bifurcation of vessels, would be at greater risk. As the lesions progress and the intima becomes thicker, blood flow over the sites will be altered and will potentially place the lining endothelial cells at even greater risk for further injury, leading to an inexorable cycle of events culminating in the complicated lesion. However, a single or a few injurious episodes may lead to a proliferative response that could regress, in contrast to continued or chronic injury. This hypothesis of reaction to injury thus is consistent with the known intimal thickening observed during normal aging, would explain how many of the etiologic factors implicated in atherogenesis might enhance lesion formation, might explain how inhibitors of platelet aggregation could interfere with lesion formation, and fosters some optimism regarding the possibility of interrupting progression or even producing regression of these lesions.

Other theories of atherogenesis are not mutually exclusive. The *monoclonal hypothesis* suggests, on the basis of single isoenzyme types found in lesions, that the intimal proliferative lesions result from the multiplication of single, individual smooth-muscle cells, as do benign tumors. In this manner, mitogenic, and possibly mutagenic, factors that might stimulate smooth-muscle cell proliferation would act on single cells. Focal *clonal senescence* may explain how intrinsic aging processes contribute to atherosclerosis. According to this theory, the intimal smooth-muscle cells that proliferate to form an atheroma are normally under feedback control by diffusible agents (mitosis inhibitors) formed by the smooth-muscle cells in the contiguous media, and this feedback control system tends to fail with age as these controlling cells die and are not adequately replaced. This is consistent with the recent observation that cultured human arterial smooth-muscle cells, like fibroblasts, show a decline in their ability to replicate as a function of donor age. If this loss of replicative potential applies to a controlling population of smooth-muscle cells, then cells that are usually suppressed would be able to proliferate.

The *lysosomal theory* suggests that altered lysosomal function might contribute to atherogenesis. Since lysosomal enzymes can accomplish the generalized degradation of cellular components required for continuing renewal, this system has been implicated in cellular aging and the accumulation of lipofuscin or "age pigment." It has been suggested that increased deposition of lipids in arterial smooth-muscle cells may be related in part to a relative deficiency in the activity of lysosomal cholesterol ester hydrolase. This would result in increased accumulation of cholesterol esters within the cells, perhaps accentuated by lipid overloading of lysosomes, eventually leading to cell death and extracellular lipid deposition. Consonant with this idea, patients with the rare cholesterol ester storage disease, caused by a defect in lysosomal cholesterol ester hydrolase, may have accelerated atherosclerosis. However, lipid droplets in foam cells are often cytoplasmic rather than lysosomal.

RECOGNITION OF ATHEROSCLEROSIS Angiographic visualization of deformity in the lumen of a vessel remains the best presumptive test of silent atherosclerosis. Coronary angiography now permits visualization and assessment of arteries as small as 0.5 mm in diameter. Several sophisticated noninvasive techniques have been developed for demonstrating its presence. Doppler probes for measuring velocity and amount of blood flow have been used noninvasively and adapted to determine vessel outlines. Ultrasonic techniques are not yet clinically useful for detection of plaques in the coronary arteries.

Functional tests based on pathophysiologic or metabolic effects of a narrowed arterial lumen often give indirect clues. Assessment of electrocardiographic changes induced after standardized exercise is a relatively simple noninvasive aid to the diagnosis of coronary atherosclerosis with significant narrowing. Similarly, myocardial perfusion defects demonstrable with imaging techniques using radionuclides are usually attributable to atherosclerosis (Chap. 179). Digit plethysmography with exercise often unmasks significant atherosclerotic involvement of lower extremity arteries.

Radiographic demonstration of calcification in the location of arteries does not always indicate the presence of atherosclerosis. Although calcified coronary vessels usually indicate atherosclerosis, complete luminal obstruction may occur in the absence of any calcification. Calcification or beading of peripheral arteries is not correlated directly with atherosclerosis. Abnormalities in retinal arterioles evident upon funduscopic examination are not well correlated with atherosclerosis in arteries. Thus despite the availability of a variety of tests, detection of atherosclerosis usually awaits one of the clinical complications attending a critical decrease of blood flow in an involved vessel. As yet there is no blood test for atherosclerosis. Knowledge of the prevalence and incidence of arteriosclerosis and most of the inferences concerning its causes are derived from tabulations of the appearance of its complications.

Ischemic heart disease (IHD), synonymous with *coronary heart disease* or *arteriosclerotic heart disease* (Chap. 189), is the most reliable indicator of atherosclerosis available today. Practically all patients with myocardial infarction, as defined by electrocardiographic and enzyme changes, have coronary atherosclerosis. Rare exceptions are due to congenital anomalies of the coronary vessels, emboli, or ostial occlusion due to other types of cardiac or vascular disease. Nontraumatic *sudden death* (Chap. 30) makes up a sizable portion of all deaths eventually certified as due to IHD. At autopsy, evidence of fresh myocardial infarction or of *coronary thrombosis* is usually absent. While ventricular fibrillation may have been due to sudden closure of a partially compromised vessel by a small thrombus or embolus, or to *spasm,* none of these need have preceded a fatal arrhythmia. The majority of victims of sudden death have had a previous diagnosis of IHD; the number who had diabetes or hypertension is also significant. In epidemiologic studies of IHD, *angina pectoris* and electrocardiographic changes attributable to ischemia without infarction are considered "softer end points" and treated separately.

Cerebrovascular disease (stroke) is a less reliable criterion for the presence of atherosclerosis. It includes *cerebral hemorrhage* and *cerebral thrombosis* (Chap. 343). Cerebral thrombosis, including infarction or softening without evidence of embolus, is usually due to atherosclerosis. On the other hand, cerebral hemorrhage is most often the result of congenital aneurysms or of vascular defects peculiar to hypertension and diabetes. Dissections of the aorta (Chap. 197), *peripheral vascular disease* (Chap. 198), thrombosis of other major vessels, and ischemic renal disease (Chap. 227) likewise are not used to determine the prevalence of atherosclerosis in a population or as an index of atherosclerosis elsewhere. Therefore, from an epidemiologic standpoint, consideration of atherosclerosis focuses on IHD.

TABLE 195-3 Age-adjusted death rates by cause in the United States, 1968 and 1982

	Rate per 100,000 population		
Cause of death	1968	1982	Percent change
All deaths	744	554	−26
All cardiovascular diseases	362	238	−34
Ischemic heart disease	242	139	−42
Cerebrovascular disease	71	36	−50
Rheumatic heart disease	7	2	−69
Cancer	129	133	+3
Accidents and violence	77	58	−24

SOURCE: *The National Center for Health Statistics, Vital Statistics Report, Final Mortality Statistics, 1982.*

INCIDENCE AND PREVALENCE According to the National Health Examination Survey, about 5 million Americans have IHD. It is the leading cause of death in males after age 35 and in all persons after age 45. Premature deaths from IHD, arbitrarily defined as those appearing before age 65, occur preponderantly in men, and a third of all deaths from IHD in males occur before age 65. In fact nearly all the excess premature mortality in American males is due to IHD. Between the ages of 35 and 55 the death rate is five times higher in white men than in white women in the United States. The exceptions are women with hypertension, diabetes, hyperlipidemia, or premature (usually iatrogenic) menopause, who are at increased risk and often share the risk of the male. For both sexes, there is more than a fivefold increase in the average annual incidence of myocardial infarction between ages 40 and 60. A distressing higher mortality rate in younger nonwhite women is probably due mainly to a greater incidence of hypertension in blacks. There is less difference between men and women in the prevalence of angina pectoris than in that of myocardial infarction; after age 65 more women than men have angina without a history of infarction.

Changing death rates Death rates in the United States from IHD rose appreciably between 1940 and 1960. Mortality peaked in 1963 and started to decline, with the rate of decline accelerating in recent years for all ages, for both sexes, and for whites and nonwhites. This recent decline in mortality from coronary atherosclerosis (Table 195-3) is the first recorded in American history and is almost unique among industrialized countries. In other parts of the world, including the Soviet Union and many countries in Europe, IHD death rates are still climbing. In 1980 the reduction in IHD death rate averaged more than 20 percent for persons age 35 to 74. The trend remains unexplained, but there has been a concurrent change in living habits including reduced smoking among middle-aged males, decreased consumption of animal fats and cholesterol, better control of hypertension, and improved treatment of IHD.

International comparisons In most industrialized countries, IHD is the major single cause of premature cardiovascular deaths. There are, however, marked differences in premature death rates among them. The seven having the highest rates in males between 35 and 74 years of age are Finland, Scotland, Northern Ireland, Australia, New Zealand, England, and the United States. Much lower age-adjusted death rates from IHD are found in Latin America and Japan. The rates in Japan are about one-sixth of those in the United States. Subsamples obtained in many countries convey the strong impression that upper socioeconomic classes that have adopted the culture of western industrialized countries have far more IHD than do lower socioeconomic classes. Among the most obvious cultural differences between these groups are total calories, fat content of the diet, and amount of physical work. Extensive epidemiologic studies have not revealed the reasons for differences between cultures that are superficially similar. Migrants to the United States tend to have a higher risk of death from premature IHD than do age-matched relatives who remain at home. Although there are many instances in which different ethnic groups in the same locality have widely differing prevalences of IHD, the available data suggest that cultural factors are more important than genetic determination of IHD. Nevertheless, genetic heterogeneity undoubtedly underlies many of the striking differences in susceptibility seen among individuals sharing the same ethnic and cultural setting.

ETIOLOGIC FACTORS A number of conditions and habits present more frequently in individuals who develop atherosclerosis than in the general population; these factors have been termed *risk factors*. The majority of people below age 65 afflicted with atherosclerosis have one or more identifiable risk factors other than aging per se (Table 195-4). The risk factor concept implies that a person with at least one risk factor is more likely to develop a clinical atherosclerotic event and is likely to do so earlier than a person with no risk factors. The presence of multiple risk factors further accelerates atherosclerosis. They vary in terms of importance in the population of the United States. There is general agreement from an epidemiologic perspective that hypercholesterolemia, hypertension, and cigarette smoking may be the most potent factors involved in causation of atherosclerosis. Risk factors also vary in terms of their potential reversibility with current techniques of preventive management.

Thus age, gender, and genetic factors are currently considered to be irreversible risk factors, whereas continually emerging evidence suggests that elimination of cigarette smoking and treatment of hypertension reverses the high risk for atherosclerosis attributable to those factors. A major multicenter trial has shown that reduction of hypercholesterolemia reduces the risk of IHD. Life insurance policyholder data suggest that reduction of marked obesity reduces total mortality, presumably by diminishing the sequelae of atherosclerosis. Other potentially reversible factors are currently under study.

These factors are not mutually exclusive since they clearly interact. For example, obesity, particularly of the abdominal type (assessed by the waist/hip circumference ratio), appears to be causally associated with hypertension, hyperglycemia, hypercholesterolemia, and hypertriglyceridemia. Genetic factors may play a role by exerting direct effects on arterial wall cell structure and metabolism, or they may act indirectly via such factors as hypertension, hyperlipidemia, diabetes, and obesity. Aging appears to be one of the more complex factors associated with the development of atherosclerosis, since many of the risk factors in themselves are related to aging, e.g., elevated blood pressure, hyperglycemia, and hyperlipidemia. Thus in addition to the possible involvement of intrinsic aging in atherogenesis (perhaps through effects on arterial wall metabolism), a variety of associated metabolic factors are also age-dependent.

TABLE 195-4 Risk factors for atherosclerosis

1 Not reversible
- *a* Aging
- *b* Male sex
- *c* Genetic traits—positive family history of premature atherosclerosis

2 Reversible
- *a* Cigarette smoking
- *b* Hypertension
- *c* Obesity

3 Potentially or partially reversible
- *a* Hyperlipidemia—hypercholesterolemia and/or hypertriglyceridemia
- *b* Hyperglycemia and diabetes mellitus
- *c* Low levels of high-density lipoproteins (HDL)

4 Other possible factors
- *a* Physical inactivity
- *b* Emotional stress and/or personality type

Hyperlipidemia Both *hypercholesterolemia* and *hypertriglyceridemia* appear to be important risk factors for atherosclerosis. While there is no absolute quantitative definition of hyperlipidemia, statistical definitions, based on the upper 5 or 10 percent of the distribution of plasma lipid levels within a population, are often used. Such definitions are likely to detect affected individuals from families with one of the familial hyperlipidemias or having hyperlipidemia associated with other diseases or drugs; they also are useful for prediction of emergence of premature atherosclerosis and institution of preventive measures. However, these upper limits of "normality" are too high for defining those cholesterol and triglyceride levels that are correlated with increasing risk of IHD in whole populations. Thus, correlations between the cholesterol concentrations in young men in North America and the incidence of premature IHD indicate that an increasing risk can be detected when the cholesterol level is higher than 220 mg/dL, a value close to the mean for men from 40 to 49 years of age in this population. Extrapolation of similar data from other populations suggests that a cholesterol level at birth averages 60 mg/dL. Within a month the average has risen to about 120 and by the first year to 175. A second rise begins in the third decade and continues to about age 50 in men and somewhat later in women.

A similar age-related increase in plasma triglyceride levels is also observed. The increases in cholesterol are associated mainly with a rise in *low-density lipoprotein* (LDL) concentrations, the increases in triglyceride with a rise in *very low density lipoproteins* (VLDL). Adiposity may play a key role in this age-associated rise in triglyceride and cholesterol levels since the increases in triglyceride, cholesterol, and body weight with age in whole populations occur concurrently. In primitive people who remain thin throughout adulthood, plasma lipids do not increase with age. Metabolic mechanisms have been postulated whereby obesity, which is associated with insulin resistance of peripheral tissues and compensatory hyperinsulinemia, promotes enhanced production of triglyceride- and cholesterol-rich lipoproteins by the liver. Current concepts of plasma lipoprotein transport suggest that accumulation of cholesterol in the circulation may in part be secondary to excessive production of triglyceride-rich lipoproteins.

Hypercholesterolemia is associated unequivocally with increased incidence of premature IHD; however, its importance varies in relation to age. In the Framingham Study, cholesterol levels in males below age 40 were closely related to the future development of IHD; this relation was much less pronounced in older individuals. For both sexes combined, the relative incidence of myocardial infarction in individuals between the ages of 30 and 49 with cholesterol levels greater than 260 mg/dL was three to five times that for individuals with cholesterol levels less than 220. There appears to be a continuous gradient of risk as the cholesterol level ascends. These data are supported by comparisons of the prevalence of IHD and cholesterol (or LDL) in many other populations. The relationship of triglycerides and VLDL to IHD is confounded by a rise in cholesterol as VLDL increases. Nevertheless, in several, but not all, population studies, increased triglycerides (or VLDL) are independently correlated with premature IHD.

Hypertriglyceridemia may be associated with premature atherosclerosis in some specific disorders; this association may not be apparent in studies of whole populations. Patients with high VLDL who come from families with familial combined hyperlipidemia appear to be at the same increased risk as those affected members of these families with elevated LDL levels. In contrast, patients with comparably elevated VLDL levels who come from families with pure monogenic familial hypertriglyceridemia do not appear to have an increased risk. In addition, high VLDL may increase the risk for premature atherosclerosis when associated with other risk factors for coronary artery disease, such as in diabetes, and in patients on chronic hemodialysis who smoke and are hypertensive. Individuals in whom remnant lipoproteins accumulate, with resulting elevations in both cholesterol and triglycerides (Chap. 315), also seem to be at risk for early development of atherosclerosis.

Some of these relationships were clarified in a comprehensive study in Seattle of the role of the genetics of hyperlipidemia in clinical atherosclerosis in which 500 consecutive survivors of myocardial infarction were tested. Hyperlipidemia was present in about one-third of the group. Approximately one-half of the males and two-thirds of the females below age 50 had either hypertriglyceridemia, hypercholesterolemia, or both. On the other hand, in individuals over age 70 the prevalence of atherosclerotic coronary disease was very high, yet virtually no males (and only about one-fourth of the females) had hyperlipidemia. Thus, in both sexes there appeared to be a progressive decline with age in the association of hyperlipidemia with myocardial infarction. More than half of the hyperlipidemic atherosclerotic survivors appeared to have simple monogenic familial disorders inherited as an autosomal dominant trait (*familial combined hyperlipidemia, familial hypertriglyceridemia,* and *familial hypercholesterolemia,* in descending order of frequency, Table 195-5). These simply inherited hyperlipidemias (particularly hypercholesterolemia) were more frequent in myocardial infarction survivors below age 60 than in those who were older. In contrast, nonmonogenic forms of hyperlipidemia occurred with equal frequency above and below age 60. Thus it appears that genes associated with the simply inherited hyperlipidemias accelerate changes seen with age, leading to atherosclerosis at an earlier age than usual. All studies indicate that hyperlipidemia is a more meaningful risk factor below age 50 and that it operates independently of, and in addition to, hypertension, diabetes, obesity, and other factors. For men and women over age 65, there is no evidence of a correlation between hyperlipidemia and atherosclerosis or its complications.

When the screening of individuals for hyperlipidemia occurs after a myocardial infarction, it is several decades too late. Screening at birth or in childhood for genetic hyperlipidemia is not practical or useful except in the instance of familial hypercholesterolemia, which may affect about 1 in 1000 children. This is detectable by LDL elevations in cord blood when one already knows that a parent is affected. Other genetic or nongenetic primary hyperlipidemia is often not apparent until the third decade. *Today, good health maintenance practice includes a test for detection of hyperlipidemia in all persons between 20 and 30 years of age. It is especially important in all young persons who have a family history of premature IHD.*

Hyperlipidemia is best detected by measurement of the concentration of cholesterol and triglycerides in serum or plasma in a sample obtained after an overnight fast. The measurements should be made by a reliable laboratory that follows a program of standardization. Routine use of lipoprotein electrophoresis provides little additional information, is nonspecific, and is not recommended for screening or for management. In adults less than 55 years of age, a cholesterol concentration (C) greater than 240 mg/dL or a triglyceride concentration (TG) greater than 250 mg/dL clearly indicates hyperlipidemia sufficient to require some attention by the physician to the items listed in Table 195-6. If hyperlipidemia is absent, the tests need not be repeated for several years in an adult who maintains body weight and does not otherwise change in health or life-style. Vigor in pursuing the "causative factors" in Table 195-6 should increase in proportion to the degree of hyperlipidemia. If causes of *secondary hyperlipidemia* or offending drugs are absent, attention to the origin of *primary hyperlipidemia* turns mainly to diet and genetic causes. Severe hyperlipidemia ($C > 300$ mg/dL or $TG > 500$ mg/dL) usually reflects a genetic disorder; when xanthomas are present, it practically always does. Diagnosis always includes examination of first-degree relatives and proceeds according to information contained in Chap. 315.

Reduction of hypercholesterolemia results in a decrease in progression of atherosclerosis in humans and other primates. Several controlled trials of different diets which have been accompanied by fall in mean cholesterol levels in small test populations have shown a favorable effect on incidence of the overall complications of IHD. The drug clofibrate given to a normal population reduced the incidence of nonfatal myocardial infarctions associated with a reduction of cholesterol levels; however, total mortality was not lowered. In the recent Lipid Research Clinics trial, the drug cholestyramine given to hypercholesterolemic asymptomatic men reduced morbidity and mortality from myocardial infarction in direct relation to the degree of cholesterol lowering; again, however, total mortality was not reduced. The weight of evidence strongly favors conservative measures to reduce cholesterol levels in patients through middle age and aggressive measures in patients who are frankly hypercholesterolemic.

The first step in treatment of primary hyperlipidemia is attention to diet. All patients with mild to moderate hyperlipidemia should first be brought to normal weight if they exceed it and then be maintained on a diet emphasizing decreases in intake of saturated fat and cholesterol. If hypertriglyceridemia is present, alcohol intake should be limited or eliminated. A single dietary approach to all forms of hyperlipidemia, including reduced intake of calories, cholesterol, and saturated fat, is appropriate for most patients. The degree of dietary restriction would be proportional to the degree and nature of the hyperlipidemia. The maximum effect of such a regimen will be observed within 2 months after body weight has stabilized. If at that time C is greater than 260 mg/dL, a 2-month trial of a bile acid–binding resin (cholestyramine or colestipol) should be considered. If TG remains greater than 300 mg/dL, a fibric acid derivative (clofibrate or bezafibrate) may be tried. These two types of drugs may be used simultaneously if both C and TG are high; their use remains empirical. In patients with familial hypercholesterolemia (Chap. 315) combined therapy with a resin and nicotinic acid has achieved dramatic normalization of LDL cholesterol levels. New cholesterol synthesis inhibitors (e.g., mevinolin), which are more specific and more effective than nicotinic acid, are currently being studied. Continued therapy with any hypolipidemic drug is dependent upon the demonstration that, when added to diet at stable weight, it is associated with at least a 15 percent further decrease in hyperlipidemia. However, further studies are needed to define the long-term efficiency of various hypolipidemic agents in the prevention of atherosclerosis and its sequelae in specific disorders. The long-term effects of these drugs used before puberty are unknown, and their use during pregnancy is not advocated.

High-density lipoproteins (HDL) HDL, a complex family of particles that carry about 20 percent of the total plasma cholesterol, is inversely associated with the development of premature atherosclerosis and therefore can be considered an "antirisk factor." HDL levels can be assessed simply by measurement of cholesterol in the supernatant fluid after the other lipoproteins in plasma have been

TABLE 195-5 Frequency of hyperlipidemia in survivors of myocardial infarction

Disorder	% of total myocardial infarction survivors: Under age 60	Over age 60	Ratio
1 Monogenic hyperlipidemias	20.6	7.5	—
a Familial hypercholesterolemia	4.1	0.7	6:1
b Familial hypertriglyceridemia	5.2	2.7	2:1
c Familial combined hyperlipidemia	11.3	4.1	3:1
2 Polygenic hypercholesterolemia	5.5	5.5	1:1
3 Sporadic hypertriglyceridemia	5.8	6.9	1:1

SOURCE: *Goldstein et al. 1973.*

TABLE 195-6 Factors to consider in patients with hyperlipidemia

1 Disorders to which hyperlipidemia is secondary
- *a* Uncontrolled diabetes mellitus (insulin deficiency)
- *b* Hypothyroidism
- *c* Uremia
- *d* Nephrotic syndrome (hypoproteinemia)
- *e* Obstructive liver disease
- *f* Dysproteinemia (multiple myeloma, lupus erythematosus)

2 Drugs producing or aggravating hyperlipidemia
- *a* Oral contraceptives
- *b* Estrogens
- *c* Glucocorticoids
- *d* Antihypertensives

3 Dietary factors
- *a* Caloric intake (recent weight gain)
- *b* Content of saturated fats and cholesterol
- *c* Alcohol intake

4 Genetic disorders (primary hyperlipidemias)
- *a* Family history of hyperlipidemia or xanthomas
- *b* History of pancreatitis or recurrent abdominal pain

precipitated. Thus individuals whose HDL cholesterol is elevated may be less likely to develop IHD; conversely, low HDL cholesterol is associated with increased risk of IHD. In the Framingham Study, low HDL cholesterol was a more potent lipid risk factor than was high cholesterol or LDL. At least five diverse population studies have confirmed a close correlation between IHD and low HDL, independent of other factors.

Consistent with differences in risk between the sexes, HDL cholesterol averages about 25 percent higher in women than in men. Estrogens tend to raise and androgens tend to lower HDL levels. In women, low HDL, particularly when associated with diabetes and obesity, markedly raises the risk of IHD. Octogenarians tend to have high HDL, which may be partly familial. Of interest for preventive measures, cigarette smoking decreases and regular strenuous exercise increases HDL cholesterol. Regular exercise increases HDL even in individuals after myocardial infarction. A small daily intake of alcohol has been associated with both reduced risk of IHD and high HDL levels. Mechanisms for these effects remain unknown.

HDL cholesterol measurements are usually not very helpful since the analytical error in most laboratories exceeds the differences in HDL levels associated with risk. HDL measurements are most helpful in individuals, especially women, with only a mild increase in plasma cholesterol and normal triglyceride levels to determine whether the increase is in HDL rather than in LDL. Because of the close inverse relationship between plasma triglycerides (or VLDL) and HDL, HDL in hypertriglyceridemic persons, with or without hypercholesterolemia, will be predictably low and gives little additional useful information.

Hypertension (see Chap. 196) High blood pressure is an important risk factor for atherosclerosis, mainly IHD and cerebrovascular disease. The risk increases progressively with increasing blood pressure; in the Framingham Study, IHD incidence in middle-aged men with blood pressures exceeding 160/95 was more than five times that in normotensive men (blood pressure 140/90 or less). Hypertensive men and women are both affected, with the diastolic pressure perhaps being more important. In industrialized populations, blood pressure appears to increase inexorably with age; however, the nature of this age relation varies among populations, since there are remote primitive populations that age without any changes in blood pressure levels. The age-associated blood pressure increase might be related to physical activity or dietary factors, particularly sodium and total caloric content. In contrast to the other age-related risk factors, hypertension appears to increase atherosclerosis throughout the age span. Thus, after the age of about 50, hypertension may be more potent than hypercholesterolemia as a risk factor.

Conversely, the risk for atherosclerosis appears diminished by therapeutic reduction of blood pressure. Recent intervention studies have shown convincingly that reduction of diastolic levels that had been greater than 105 mmHg significantly reduces the incidence of strokes, IHD, and congestive heart failure in men. Even when patients with diastolic pressures between 90 and 105 mmHg are similarly maintained on adequate treatment, the incidence of some of these complications may be reduced. Special urgency for relief of hypertension obtains when hyperlipidemia or other risk factors are present.

Cigarette smoking Not only is cigarette smoking one of the more potent risk factors for atherosclerosis, it is also one of the factors that when reduced or eliminated clearly decreases the risk of developing atherosclerosis. Ample statistical evidence supports a mean increase of about 70 percent in the death rate, and a three- to fivefold increase in risk of IHD, in men who smoke one pack of cigarettes per day compared with nonsmokers. In general, the increase in death rate is proportional to the amount smoked and decreases with age. Excess morbidity from myocardial infarction is also present in women smokers, but the relationship is somewhat less firm than in men. However, there is an impressive accentuation of IHD mortality in women over age 35 taking oral contraceptives who in addition smoke cigarettes. In some atherosclerosis-prone populations, such as patients maintained on long-term hemodialysis, cigarette smoking interacts with other risk factors, resulting in a marked enhancement of atherosclerosis mortality. Such interaction is also likely for diabetic and hypertensive populations.

The association of smoking and increased IHD remains unexplained. Pipe and cigar smokers have a lesser increase in risk of IHD, presumably because less smoke is inhaled. Smokers dying of causes other than IHD have been found at autopsy to have more coronary atherosclerosis than nonsmokers. The major influence of smoking is upon the incidence of sudden death, however. Those who stop smoking show a prompt decline in risk and may reach the risk level of nonsmokers as early as after 1 year of abstention.

Hyperglycemia and diabetes mellitus (see Chap. 327) Studies in a variety of populations have shown an association of hyperglycemia with clinically evident atherosclerotic disease, suggesting a role of hyperglycemia in atherogenesis. In known diabetics, both insulin-dependent and non-insulin-dependent types, there is at least a twofold increase in incidence of myocardial infarction compared with nondiabetics. This risk is markedly increased in younger diabetics, and diabetic women are even more prone to IHD than are diabetic men. There is an increased tendency toward cerebral thrombosis and infarction but not toward cerebral hemorrhage in diabetes. Gangrene of the lower extremities has been variously estimated to be from 8 to 150 times as frequent in diabetics as in nondiabetics and is most often found in diabetics who smoke. Diabetes is associated with an increase in atherosclerosis observed at autopsy in a variety of populations worldwide, whether the prevalence of atherosclerosis in a particular population is high or low. The approximately twofold increase in the frequency of hypertension among diabetics, particularly adult females, may accentuate the risk. This relationship is presumably associated with obesity.

The risk for atherosclerotic disease, however, does not appear to be grossly related to the degree of hyperglycemia among diabetics. Results in the University Group Diabetes Program Study have suggested that reduction of blood glucose by insulin does not appear to influence mortality from established atherosclerosis during a 5-year period. Thus, hyperglycemia and atherosclerosis are associated, since there is an increased prevalence of large-vessel disease in known diabetics and, conversely, an increased prevalence of hyperglycemia in association with atherosclerotic disease. These associations remain unexplained and reversibility undocumented. Clinical and experimental studies also support a role for high circulating insulin levels in IHD. The capillary microangiopathy, pathognomonic of diabetes and causing important dysfunction of the kidneys and retina, has unknown clinical significance in relation to atherosclerotic disease in larger arteries.

Obesity In general, morbidity and mortality from IHD are higher in direct relation to the degree of overweight beyond about 30 percent. Furthermore, from data obtained in the Framingham Study, it appears that obesity may accelerate atherosclerosis since its effect is more apparent before age 50. Nevertheless, some of the major epidemiologic studies of coronary heart disease have not demonstrated an independent relationship between this condition and anything less than very severe obesity. Recent studies have shown a close relation between type of obesity (i.e., abdominal) and IHD. Furthermore, obesity is a disorder closely associated with four other potent risk factors, i.e., hypertriglyceridemia, hypercholesterolemia, hyperglycemia, and hypertension. The relationship between obesity and atherosclerosis is thus multifaceted; since in practice obesity does not occur "independently," it is of considerable importance as a risk factor.

Physical inactivity Study of the relationship of the prevalence of IHD to daily (occupational) physical activity is made difficult because so many variables are involved. Among prospective studies the Framingham data do indicate that the less sedentary an individual is, the less susceptible that individual is to sudden death. Physical work may be the major determinant of greatly differing incidences of IHD in southern black and white males in the United States and in populations that move from rural areas to urbanized environments. How physical activity may operate to decrease death from IHD, or possibly to decrease atherogenesis, is not known. Beyond the amelioration of hyperlipidemia by increasing caloric expenditure, no mechanism has been demonstrated. The meaning of the physical activity–induced increase in HDL, the antirisk factor for IHD, remains mysterious. Physical training has been shown to improve exercise performance in patients with IHD and angina pectoris. Regular physical activity is supported as a desirable element in a program of preventive health maintenance.

Stress and personality There is a valid clinical impression that psychic or emotional stress and anxiety are associated with precipitation of overt IHD and sudden death. Debate continues as to whether there may be distinct personality types prone to or relatively immune to premature IHD (the so-called personality types A and B), and whether the presumably more deleterious type is amenable to correction beyond elimination of cigarette smoking, adverse dietary patterns, and avoidance of stressful life situations. Many social and demographic analyses have so far failed to reach any agreement about the etiologic relationships of occupation and similar situational factors and the incidence of IHD.

Genetic factors Premature atherosclerosis often appears to be familial. In many instances this can be attributed to the inheritance of risk factors such as hypertension, diabetes mellitus, and hyperlipidemia. Occasionally, families with excessive premature vascular disease can be found in which none of the known risk factors appears to be operating. Genetic determinants of protective factors, such as HDL, need to be understood; undoubtedly other important determinants remain to be discovered. Nevertheless, family history is one of the more important factors to be weighed in assessment of risk in helping the physician to avoid missing treatable risk factors and in institution of appropriate preventive measures.

ROLE OF DIET IN RISK FOR ATHEROSCLEROSIS The relationship of diet to IHD remains an area of intense interest and persistent controversy. In epidemiologic studies, no population habitually subsisting on a diet low in saturated fat and cholesterol has an appreciable amount of IHD. These populations also tend to have lower plasma lipid concentrations. There is a general upward shift of average cholesterol and triglyceride levels in highly developed countries, which is an effect of change in total culture and life-style as well as in diet. Dietary changes in migrant populations who move from more primitive to more industrialized societies commonly include increased intake of total calories, animal fats, cholesterol, and salt, leading to a diet-accentuated emergence of risk factors such as obesity, hyperlipidemia, diabetes, and hypertension. There is no question that the plasma cholesterol (and LDL) level is sensitive to the amount of saturated fat and cholesterol in the diet. The ''average'' adult male in the United States eats about 140 g fat per day and about 500 mg cholesterol. The mixture of fats ingested usually contains about three times as much saturated fatty acids (mainly palmitic and stearic) as polyunsaturated fatty acids (mainly linoleic and linolenic). If a healthy young adult switches from this diet to one containing the same amount of total fat in which the ratio of polyunsaturates to saturates is closer to unity and the cholesterol content is less than 300 mg per day, the cholesterol concentration will usually drop by 10 to 15 percent within 2 weeks and remain depressed on continuation of the diet.

The average cholesterol level in most populations is most closely related to the amount of animal fats (meat, eggs, and milk products, major sources of long-chain saturated fatty acids and cholesterol) in the diet. Increased animal fat consumption also tends to be correlated with a greater proportion of dietary fats being saturated and with lesser intake of complex carbohydrates and vegetable fibers; these are dietary changes that may lead to a rise in plasma cholesterol levels. The average triglyceride level is more sensitive to total caloric balance and to alcohol intake. It is important to note that physical activity, emotional stress, smoking, and intake of coffee or tea have only weak or indirect influences on total cholesterol and triglyceride concentrations.

In experimental animals added dietary cholesterol and fat are essential for the production of atherosclerosis. Typical American diets fed to nonhuman primates produce aortic and coronary atherosclerosis which is reversible when a cholesterol-free diet is fed. Controlled metabolic studies in humans show a direct relation between dietary and plasma cholesterol below intakes of about 600 mg per day; no relation is observed at higher intakes when plasma cholesterol is already high. There appear to be marked genetic variations in the ability of dietary cholesterol to influence plasma cholesterol among individuals and among populations. The relation between dietary polyunsaturated/saturated fat ratio (P/S) and both cholesterol and triglyceride levels also has been amply established. The unique lipid-lowering effects of the particular long-chain polyunsaturated fatty acids in large ocean fish are currently under study.

A definitive prospective study of the effect of diet on IHD in the general population has never been undertaken. Nevertheless, preliminary reports of newer studies of alterations of diet in high-risk populations, coupled with published findings of studies in selected populations, provide strong evidence of a reversible relation among diet, plasma lipids, and IHD. On this basis, although without definite proof of effectiveness, numerous authoritative nutrition councils have recommended prudent dietary modifications for the general population of western countries to be instituted early in life and to include a caloric intake adjusted to achieve and maintain ideal body weight, a reduction in total fat calories to 30 to 35 percent of total calories achieved by a substantial reduction in dietary saturated fat to less than 10 percent of total calories, and a reduction in cholesterol intake to less than 300 mg per day. Although a causal relationship in humans between sodium intake and hypertension has not been firmly established, avoidance of excessive dietary sodium has also been recommended.

RISK FACTORS AND MECHANISMS OF ATHEROGENESIS *Adiposity* produces insulin resistance in peripheral tissues (mainly muscle and adipose), which leads to compensatory hyperinsulinemia. The liver is not resistant to some effects of insulin, and enhanced production of triglyceride-rich lipoproteins results, leading to elevated plasma triglyceride and cholesterol levels. Thus it has been demonstrated that body weight is related not only to triglyceride levels but also to cholesterol levels. Concomitantly, obesity is associated with increased total body cholesterol synthesis. Obesity produces higher circulating levels of insulin, both in the basal state and after stimulation with glucose or other secretagogues. Since obesity is related to atherosclerosis—both directly and via hypertension, hypertriglyceridemia, hypercholesterolemia, and hyperglycemia—it is not surprising that many studies show a relationship between serum insulin levels, particularly after oral glucose intake, and atherosclerotic disease of the coronary and peripheral arteries. A few studies, however, suggest that this association between insulin and atherosclerosis occurs independently of obesity. It has been postulated that insulin may directly affect arterial wall metabolism, leading to increased endogenous lipid synthesis and thus predisposing to atherosclerosis. Insulin has been shown in physiologic concentrations to stimulate proliferation of arterial smooth-muscle cells and enhance binding of LDL and VLDL to fibroblasts; it therefore may be one of the plasma factors involved in atheroma formation.

Hypertension may enhance atherogenesis by directly producing injury via mechanical stress on endothelial cells at specific high-pressure sites in the arterial tree. This would allow the sequence of events in the chronic injury hypothesis of atherogenesis to take place. In addition, hypertension might allow more lipoproteins to be transported through intact endothelial lining cells by altering permeability. Hypertension markedly increases lysosomal enzyme activity, presumably owing to stimulation of the cellular disposal system by the internalization of increased amounts of plasma substances. This might lead to increased cell degeneration and release of the highly destructive enzymes (within the lysosomes) into the arterial wall. Experimental hypertension also increases the thickness of the intimal smooth-muscle layer in the arterial wall and increases connective tissue elements. It is still not known if continued high pressure within the artery produces changes in the ability of smooth-muscle cells or stem cells to proliferate.

Diabetes could provide a unique contribution to atherogenesis. Although the fundamental genetic abnormality in human diabetes mellitus remains unknown, it has been suggested that genetic diabetes in humans represents a primary cellular abnormality intrinsic to all cells, resulting in a decreased life span of individual cells, which in turn results in increased cell turnover in tissues. If arterial endothelial and smooth-muscle cells are intrinsically defective in diabetes, accelerated atherogenesis can be readily postulated on the basis of any one of the current theories of pathogenesis. Platelet dysfunction in diabetes might also play a role.

The role of glucose in atheroma formation, if any, is poorly understood. Hyperglycemia is known to affect aortic wall metabolism. Sorbitol, a product of the insulin-independent aldose reductase pathway of glucose metabolism (the polyol pathway) accumulates in the arterial wall in the presence of high glucose concentrations, resulting in osmotic effects including increased cell water content and decreased oxygenation. Increased glucose also appears to stimulate proliferation of cultured arterial smooth-muscle cells.

The development of atherosclerosis accelerates in approximate quantitative relation to the degree of *hyperlipidemia*. A long-established theory suggests that the higher the circulating levels of lipoprotein the more likely they are to gain entrance to the arterial wall. By an acceleration of the usual transendothelial transport, large concentrations of lipoproteins within the arterial wall could overwhelm the ability of smooth-muscle cells to metabolize them. Lipoproteins have been immunologically identified in atheroma, and in humans there is a close relationship between plasma cholesterol and arterial lipoprotein cholesterol concentration. Chemically modified lipoproteins, possibly produced in hyperlipidemic disorders, could gain access to the scavenger arterial wall macrophages, leading to formation of foam cells as in xanthomas. It is possible that the lipid that accumulates in the arterial wall with increasing age results from infiltration of plasma lipoproteins. However, atheromatous lesions are associated with a more marked increase in arterial wall lipids, which may result in part from injury to the endothelium possibly produced by chronic hyperlipidemia, as demonstrated in cholesterol-fed monkeys. A further mechanism for accelerated atherogenesis in hyperlipidemia is related to the ability of LDL to stimulate proliferation of arterial smooth-muscle cells.

The effect of *chronic smoke inhalation* from cigarettes could result in repetitive injury to endothelial cells, thereby accelerating atherogenesis. Hypoxia stimulates proliferation of cultured human arterial smooth-muscle cells; thus, since cigarette smoking is associated with high levels of carboxyhemoglobin and low oxygen delivery to tissues, another mechanism for atherogenesis is suggested. Hypoxia could produce diminished lysosomal enzyme degradative ability, as evidenced by impaired degradation of LDL by smooth-muscle cells, causing LDL to accumulate in the cells. Consistent with this suggestion is the fact that aortic lesions that resemble atheroma have been produced in experimental animals by systemic hypoxia, and lipid accumulation in the arterial wall of cholesterol-fed rabbits and monkeys appears to be increased by hypoxia.

RISK FACTOR REVERSAL AND REGRESSION OF ATHEROSCLEROSIS Although the emergence of clinical consequences of atherosclerosis can be lessened, no convincing instance of regression or interruption of progression of atherosclerosis, determined by direct or indirect examination of lesions, by removal or reversal of any single risk factor or group of risk factors has yet been proved in humans. Nevertheless, feasibility of such demonstrations is becoming established, and preliminary results are encouraging. Through mass-media educational efforts, whole communities can be influenced to reduce smoking, change diet, and lower blood pressure levels. Adult males in the United States have lowered cigarette consumption, although increases among teenage girls have kept total usage high. There has been a trend toward lower cholesterol and saturated fat consumption in the United States, coupled with increasing attention to reducing overweight and the use of exercise programs. Concomitantly, and perhaps causally, there has been the noted decline in IHD mortality. Treatment of hyperlipidemia in some instances has been shown to reduce atherosclerotic involvement of peripheral vessels by both invasive and noninvasive measurement. There is also some encouraging evidence in animals, most notably in primates, that relatively complicated plaques induced by hyperlipidemia will regress, and that further progression of atherosclerosis will cease when hyperlipidemia is removed. Therefore efforts to prevent atherogenesis, to interrupt progression, and perhaps to promote regression of existing lesions by risk factor reduction seem warranted.

PREVENTION Although premature IHD is overall the most costly and common of the untimely complications of atherosclerosis, preoccupation with IHD should not obscure the fact that angina pectoris and myocardial infarction are expressions of late-stage atherosclerotic lesions. Factors precipitating these clinical events may be independent of those leading to initiation of plaque formation or its progression to a complicated lesion. Steps taken to prevent recurrence of myocardial infarction or fatal arrhythmia, termed *secondary prevention,* will not necessarily be the same as those taken to delay or prevent formation of atherosclerosis (*primary prevention*). Since atherosclerotic plaques have been detected in the coronary arteries of American males as early as the second decade in autopsy studies of Korean and Vietnam war deaths, primary prevention of atherosclerosis must begin early in life, long before there is any suspicion of IHD.

Thus, *prevention of atherosclerosis, rather than treatment, is the goal.* Although an effective program has not been established with certainty, enough is known to act as a guide both in identification of those with a higher risk and in development of conservative measures that probably will reduce that risk. Thus prevention currently is equated with risk factor reduction.

The decline of American death rates from premature IHD today coincides with two trends in health practices. One is the increasing acceptance of the importance of detecting and attempting to correct some of the risk factors correlated with atherosclerosis. The other is a greater awareness of the dietary sources of cholesterol and saturated fats and a tendency of the public to restrict their intake somewhat. Whether these trends are causally related to the decline in death rate is not known. While a rigorous approach to changes in life-style for the general population may be debatable, it is desirable to continue finding and helping those most susceptible to early atherosclerosis. The physician's role in risk factor reduction involves treatment of hypertension and advice regarding diet, body weight, smoking, and exercise. Drug treatment of hyperlipidemia should be limited to those individuals at risk who do not respond adequately to dietary management. Although preliminary trials are encouraging, the long-term value of antiplatelet drugs in reducing either the mortality rate or incidence of myocardial infarction in individuals with IHD remains unproved, and trials are continuing.

TREATMENT There is no agent proven to have any value in "treatment" of atherosclerosis unless it clearly reduces severe hyperlipidemia or obvious hypertension. In fact, there is no treatment of atherosclerosis, only of its complications. While end-stage treatment technology has reduced morbidity (Chap. 189), prevention remains the long-term goal of both research and health care practice.

REFERENCES

Bierman EL: Aging and atherosclerosis, in *Principles of Geriatric Medicine,* R. Andres et al (eds). New York, McGraw-Hill, 1985, p 42

Brunzell JD et al: Pathophysiology of lipoprotein transport. Metabolism 27:1109, 1978

GOLDSTEIN JL et al: Hyperlipidemia in coronary heart disease. J Clin Invest 52:1533, 1544, 1973

——— et al: Defective lipoprotein receptors and atherosclerosis. N Engl J Med 309:288, 1983

GORDON T et al: Diabetes, blood lipids, and the role of obesity in coronary heart disease risk for women. The Framingham Study. Ann Intern Med 87:393, 1977

——— et al: High density lipoprotein as a protective factor against coronary heart disease. The Framingham Study. Am J Med 62:707, 1977

KANNEL WB et al: Optimal resources for primary prevention of atherosclerotic diseases. Circulation 70:155A, 1984

LEVY RI: Declining mortality in coronary heart disease. Arteriosclerosis 1:312, 1981

MCGILL HC: Persistent problems in the pathogenesis of atherosclerosis. Arteriosclerosis 4:443, 1984

PELL S, FAYERWEATHER WE: Trends in the incidence of myocardial infarction and in associated mortality and morbidity in a large employed population, 1957–1983. N Engl J Med 312:1005, 1985.

ROSS R: The pathogenesis of atherosclerosis—an update. N Engl J Med 314:488, 1986

STEINBERG D: Lipoproteins and atherosclerosis: A look back and a look ahead. Arteriosclerosis 3:283, 1983

196 HYPERTENSIVE VASCULAR DISEASE

GORDON H. WILLIAMS / EUGENE BRAUNWALD

An elevated arterial pressure is probably the more important public health problem in developed countries—being common, asymptomatic, readily detectable, usually easily treatable, and often leading to lethal complications if left untreated. As a result of extensive educational programs in the late 1960s and 1970s by both private and governmental agencies, the number of undiagnosed and/or untreated patients has been significantly reduced. This factor may be the most important one responsible for the decline in cardiovascular mortality which has taken place during the past 15 years (Chap. 195). Although our understanding of the pathophysiology of an elevated arterial pressure has increased, in 90 to 95 percent of cases the etiology (and thus potentially the prevention or cure) is still largely unknown.

DEFINITION

Since there is no dividing line between normal and high blood pressure, arbitrary levels have been established to define those who have an increased risk of developing a morbid cardiovascular event and/or will clearly benefit from medical therapy. These definitions should consider not only the level of diastolic pressure but also systolic pressure, age, sex, and race. For example, patients with a diastolic pressure greater than 90 mmHg will have a significant reduction in morbidity and mortality with adequate therapy. These, then, are patients who have hypertension and who should be considered for treatment.

The level of *systolic* pressure is also important in assessing arterial pressure's influence on cardiovascular morbidity. Males with normal diastolic pressures (<82 mmHg) but elevated systolic pressures (>158 mmHg) have a $2\frac{1}{2}$-fold increase in their cardiovascular mortality rates when compared with individuals with similar diastolic pressures but whose systolic pressures are normal (<130 mmHg). Other significant factors which modify blood pressure's influence on the frequency of morbid cardiovascular events are age, race, and sex with young black males being most adversely affected by hypertension.

When hypertension is suspected, blood pressure should be measured at least twice on two separate examinations. In adults, a *diastolic* pressure below 85 mmHg is considered to be normal; between 85 and 89 is high normal; 90 to 104 is mild hypertension; 105 to 114 moderate hypertension; 115 or greater is severe hypertension. When the diastolic pressure is below 90 mmHg, a *systolic* pressure below 140 mmHg indicates normal blood pressure; between 140 and 159 is borderline isolated systolic hypertension; 160 or higher is isolated systolic hypertension.

Arterial pressure fluctuates in most persons, whether they are normotensive or hypertensive. Those who are classified as having *labile* hypertension are patients who sometimes, but not always, have arterial pressures within the hypertensive range. These patients are often considered to have borderline hypertension.

Sustained hypertension can become accelerated or enter a malignant phase. Though a patient with *malignant hypertension* often has a blood pressure above 200/140, it is papilledema, usually accompanied by retinal hemorrhages and exudates, and not the absolute pressure level, that defines this condition. *Accelerated hypertension* signifies a significant recent increase over previous hypertensive levels associated with evidence of vascular damage on funduscopic examination but without papilledema.

FREQUENCY The prevalence of hypertension depends on both the racial composition of the studied population and the criteria used to define the condition. In a white suburban population as used in the Framingham Study, nearly one-fifth have blood pressures greater than 160/95, while almost one-half have pressures greater than 140/90. An even higher prevalance has been documented in the nonwhite population.

ETIOLOGY

The cause of elevated arterial pressure is unknown in most cases. The prevalence of various forms of secondary hypertension depends on the nature of the population studied and how extensive the evaluation is. There are no available data to define the frequency of secondary hypertension in the general population, although in middle-aged males it has been reported to be 6 percent. On the other hand, in referral centers where patients undergo an extensive evaluation, it has been reported to be as high as 35 percent. The various forms of hypertension are outlined in Table 196-1, and their relative frequencies are given in Table 196-2.

ESSENTIAL HYPERTENSION Patients with arterial hypertension and no definable cause are said to have *primary, essential,* or *idiopathic hypertension.* Undoubtedly, the primary difficulty in uncovering the mechanism(s) responsible for the hypertension in these patients is attributable to the variety of systems that are involved in the regulation of arterial pressure—peripheral and/or central adrenergic, renal, hormonal, and vascular—and to the complexity of the relationships of these systems to one another. Several abnormalities have been described in patients with essential hypertension, often with a claim that one or more of these are primarily responsible for the hypertension. While it is still uncertain whether these individual abnormalities are primary or secondary, varying expressions of a single disease process or reflective of separate disease entities, the accumulating data increasingly support the latter hypothesis. Thus, just as pneumonia is caused by a variety of infectious agents, even though the clinical picture observed may be similar, so essential hypertension likely has a number of distinct causes. Therefore, the distinction between primary and secondary hypertension has become blurred, and the approach to both the diagnosis and therapy of hypertensive patients have been modified. For example, as a group of patients with essential hypertension are separated into a distinct subset (e.g., low-renin essential hypertension), they have not been reclassified as a form of secondary hypertension but rather remain in the essential hypertensive group. In this chapter, we define those individuals with a specific organ defect responsible for hypertension as having a *secondary* form of hypertension. In contrast, individuals who may have generalized or functional abnormalities causing their hypertension are defined as having *essential* hypertension.

Heredity Genetic factors have long been assumed to be important in the genesis of hypertension. Data supporting this view can be found in animal studies as well as population studies in humans. One approach has been to assess the correlation of blood pressures within families (familial aggregation). From these studies the minimum size of the genetic factor can be expressed by a correlation coefficient of approximately 0.2. However, the variation in the size of the genetic factor in different studies reemphasizes the likely heterogeneous nature of the essential hypertensive population. Additionally, most studies support the concept that the inheritance is probably multifactoral.

Environment A number of environmental factors have been specifically implicated in the development of hypertension including salt intake, obesity, occupation, family size, and crowding. These factors have all been assumed to be important in the increase in blood pressure with age in more affluent societies, in contrast to the decline in blood pressure with age in more primitive cultures.

SALT-SENSITIVITY The environmental factor which has received the greatest attention is salt intake. Even this factor illustrates the heterogeneous nature of the essential hypertensive population in that the blood pressure in only approximately 60 percent of hypertensives is particularly responsive to the level of sodium intake. The etiologic basis for this special sensitivity to salt varies, with primary aldosteronism, bilateral renal artery stenosis, renal parenchymal disease, or low-renin essential hypertension accounting for about half of the patients. In the remainder, the pathophysiology is still uncertain, but recent postulated contributing factors include chloride, calcium, a generalized cellular membrane defect, and "nonmodulation" (vide infra).

Most studies assessing the role of salt in the hypertensive process have assumed that it is the sodium ion which is important. However, some investigators have suggested that the chloride ion may be equally important. This suggestion is based on the observation that feeding chloride-free sodium salts to salt-sensitive hypertensive animals fails to increase arterial pressure. Calcium has also been implicated in the pathogenesis of some forms of essential hypertension. A low calcium intake has been associated with an increase in blood pressure in epidemiologic studies; an increase in leukocyte cytosolic calcium levels has been reported in some hypertensives; and finally calcium entry blockers are effective antihypertensive agents. Several studies have reported a potential link between the salt-sensitive forms of hypertension and calcium. It has been postulated that with salt loading and a defect in the kidney's ability to excrete it, a secondary increase in circulating natriuretic factors may occur. One of these, the so-called digitalis-like natriuretic factor, inhibits ouabain-sensitive sodium-potassium ATPase and thereby leads to intracellular calcium accumulation and a hyperreactive vascular smooth muscle.

A third postulated explanation for salt-sensitive hypertension is a generalized membrane defect. This hypothesis derives most of its data from studies on circulating blood elements, particularly red blood cells, in which abnormalities in the transport of sodium across the cell membrane have been documented. Since both increases and decreases in the activity of different transport systems have been reported, it is likely that some abnormalities are primary and some secondary processes. It has been assumed that this abnormality reflects a defect in the cellular membrane and that this defect occurs in many, perhaps all cells of the body, particularly the vascular smooth muscle. Because of this defect, there is then an abnormal accumulation of calcium within vascular smooth muscle, resulting in a heightened vascular responsivity to vasoconstrictor agents. This defect has been proposed to be present in 35 to 50 percent of the essential hypertensive population based on studies using red cells. Other studies suggest that the abnormality in the red cell sodium transport is not a fixed abnormality but can be modified by environmental factors. Finally, the mechanisms underlying salt sensitivity in some patients may be a defect in the kidney's ability to excrete sodium appropriately, secondary to an abnormality in the control of the renal circulation and aldosterone secretion with changes in sodium intake. Sodium intake normally modulates adrenal and renal vascular responses to angiotensin II. With dietary sodium restriction, the adrenal response is enhanced and the renal vascular response reduced. Sodium loading has the opposite effect. In this subset of hypertensives this adjustment is absent, thus leading to the term "nonmodulators" to describe those patients in whom the excretion of a sodium load is impaired.

Each of these hypotheses has as a common final pathway an increase in cytosolic calcium resulting in increased vascular reactivity. However, as described above, several mechanisms might produce the increase in calcium accumulation.

Factors modifying the course of essential hypertension Age, race, sex, smoking, serum cholesterol, glucose intolerance, weight, and perhaps renin activity may all alter the prognosis of this disease. The younger the patient when hypertension is first noted, the greater the reduction in life expectancy if left untreated. In the United States,

TABLE 196-1 Classification of arterial hypertension

I Systolic hypertension with wide pulse pressure
- *A* Decreased compliance of aorta (arteriosclerosis)
- *B* Increased stroke volume
  - *1* Aortic regurgitation
  - *2* Thyrotoxicosis
  - *3* Hyperkinetic heart syndrome
  - *4* Fever
  - *5* Arteriovenous fistula
  - *6* Patent ductus arteriosus

II Systolic and diastolic hypertension (increased peripheral vascular resistance)
- *A* Renal
  - *1* Chronic pyelonephritis
  - *2* Acute and chronic glomerulonephritis
  - *3* Polycystic renal disease
  - *4* Renovascular stenosis or renal infarction
  - *5* Most other severe renal disease (arteriolar nephrosclerosis, diabetic nephropathy, etc.)
  - *6* Renin-producing tumors
- *B* Endocrine
  - *1* Oral contraceptives
  - *2* Adrenocortical hyperfunction
    - *a* Cushing's disease and syndrome
    - *b* Primary hyperaldosteronism
    - *c* Congenital or hereditary adrenogenital syndromes (17α-hydroxylase and 11β-hydroxylase defects)
  - *3* Pheochromocytoma
  - *4* Myxedema
  - *5* Acromegaly
- *C* Neurogenic
  - *1* Psychogenic
  - *2* "Diencephalic syndrome"
  - *3* Familial dysautonomia (Riley-Day)
  - *4* Poliomyelitis (bulbar)
  - *5* Polyneuritis (acute porphyria, lead poisoning)
  - *6* Increased intracranial pressure (acute)
  - *7* Spinal cord section (acute)
- *D* Miscellaneous
  - *1* Coarctation of aorta
  - *2* Increased intravascular volume (excessive transfusion, polycythemia vera)
  - *3* Polyarteritis nodosa
  - *4* Hypercalcemia
- *E* Unknown etiology
  - *1* Essential hypertension (>90% of all cases of hypertension)
  - *2* Toxemia of pregnancy
  - *3* Acute intermittent porphyria

TABLE 196-2 Prevalence of various forms of hypertension in the general population and in specialized referral clinics*

Diagnosis	General population, %	Specialty clinic, %
Essential hypertension	92–94	65–85
Renal hypertension:		
Parenchymal	2–3	4–5
Renovascular	1–2	4–16
Endocrine hypertension:		
Primary aldosteronism	0.3	0.5–12
Cushing's syndrome	<0.1	0.2
Pheochromocytoma	<0.1	0.2
Oral contraceptive–induced	2–4	1–2
Miscellaneous	0.2	1

* *Estimates based on a number of reports in the literature.*

urban blacks have about twice the prevalence rate for hypertension as whites and more than four times the hypertension-induced morbidity rate. At all ages and in both white and nonwhite populations, females with hypertension fare better than males. Yet, females with hypertension run the same relative risk of a morbid cardiovascular event compared with their normotensive counterparts as males do. Accelerated atherosclerosis is an invariable companion of hypertension. Thus, it is not surprising that independent risk factors associated with the development of atherosclerosis, e.g., an elevated serum cholesterol, glucose intolerance, and/or cigarette smoking, significantly enhance the effect of hypertension on mortality rates regardless of age, sex, or race (Chap. 195). There also is no question that there is a positive correlation between obesity and arterial pressure. A gain in weight is associated with an increased frequency of hypertension in subjects with normal pressures, and weight loss in obese subjects with hypertension lowers their arterial pressure and, if they are being treated, the intensity of therapy required to maintain them normotensive. However, there are no convincing data that obesity adversely affects the hypertension-associated mortality rate. Plasma renin activity has also been reported by some to influence and correlate with the development of morbid cardiovascular events in patients with hypertension.

Natural history Because essential hypertension is a heterogeneous disorder, variables in addition to the level of arterial pressure modify its course. Thus, the probability of developing a morbid cardiovascular event with a given arterial pressure may vary by as much as twentyfold depending on whether associated risk factors are present (Table 196-3). Although exceptions have been reported, most untreated adults with hypertension will develop further increases in their arterial pressure with time. Furthermore, both from actuarial data and from experience in the era prior to effective therapy, it has been documented that untreated hypertension is associated with a shortening of life by 10 to 20 years, usually related to an acceleration of the atherosclerotic process, with the rate of acceleration in part related to the severity of the hypertension. Even individuals with relatively mild disease, i.e., without evidence of end organ damage, left untreated for 7 to 10 years have a high risk of developing significant complications. Nearly 30 percent will exhibit atherosclerotic complications, and more than 50 percent will have end organ damage related to the hypertension itself, e.g., cardiomegaly, congestive heart failure, retinopathy, a cerebrovascular accident, and/or renal insufficiency. Thus, even in its mild forms, hypertension is a progressively lethal disease, if left untreated.

SECONDARY HYPERTENSION

As noted earlier, in only a small minority of patients with an elevated arterial pressure can a specific cause be identified. Yet, they should not be ignored for at least two reasons: (1) with correction of the cause their hypertension may be cured, and (2) the secondary forms may provide insight into the etiology of essential hypertension. Nearly all the secondary forms are related to an alteration in hormone secretion and/or renal function and are discussed in detail in other chapters.

TABLE 196-3 Factors indicating an adverse prognosis in hypertension

I Black race
II Youth
III Male
IV Persistent diastolic pressure >115 mmHg
V Smoking
VI Diabetes mellitus
VII Hypercholesterolemia
VIII Obesity
IX Evidence of end organ damage
- *A* Cardiac
  - *1* Cardiac enlargement
  - *2* ECG changes of ischemic or left ventricular strain
  - *3* Myocardial infarction
  - *4* Congestive heart failure
- *B* Eyes
  - *1* Retinal exudates and hemorrhages
  - *2* Papilledema
- *C* Renal: impaired renal function
- *D* Nervous system: cerebrovascular accident

X High-renin hypertension?

RENAL HYPERTENSION (see also Chap. 227) Hypertension produced by renal disease is the result of either (1) a derangement in the renal handling of sodium and fluids leading to volume expansion or (2) an alteration in renal secretion of vasoactive materials resulting in a systemic or local change in arteriolar tone. The main subdivisions of renal hypertension are renovascular hypertension, including preeclampsia and eclampsia, and renal parenchymal hypertension. A simple explanation for *renal vascular hypertension* is that decreased perfusion of renal tissue due to stenosis of a main or branch renal artery activates the renin-angiotensin system, described in Chap. 325. Circulating angiotensin II elevates arterial pressure by direct vasoconstriction, by stimulation of aldosterone secretion with resultant sodium retention (Chap. 29), and/or by stimulating the adrenergic nervous system. In actual practice only about one-half of patients with renovascular hypertension have elevated absolute levels of renin activity in peripheral plasma, although when renin measurements are referenced against an index of sodium balance, a much higher fraction have inappropriately high values. The use of the competitive angiotensin antagonist, saralasin (1-sar, 8-ala angiotensin II), has further clarified the role of angiotensin in the genesis of the hypertension in this disease. Nearly all patients with surgically correctable disease have exhibited a reduction of arterial pressure when given this agent in the sodium- or volume-depleted state.

Activation of the renin-angiotensin system also has been offered as an explanation for the hypertension in both acute and chronic *renal parenchymal disease*. In this formulation the only difference between renovascular and renal parenchymal hypertension is that the decreased perfusion of renal tissue in the latter case results from inflammatory and fibrotic changes involving multiple small intrarenal vessels. There are enough differences between the two conditions, however, to suggest that there are other mechanisms active in renal parenchymal disease: (1) peripheral plasma renin activity is elevated far less frequently in renal parenchymal than in renovascular hypertension; (2) cardiac output is said to be normal in the renal parenchymal type (unless uremia and anemia are present), but slightly elevated in renovascular hypertension; (3) circulatory responses to tilting and to the Valsalva maneuver are exaggerated in the latter condition; and (4) blood volume tends to be high in patients with severe renal parenchymal disease and low in patients with severe renovascular hypertension. Alternate explanations for the hypertension in renal parenchymal disease include the possibilities that the damaged kidneys (1) produce an unidentified vasopressor substance other than renin, (2) fail to produce a necessary humoral vasodilator substance (perhaps prostaglandin or bradykinin), (3) fail to inactivate circulating vasopressor substances, and/or (4) are ineffective in disposing of sodium, and the retained sodium is responsible for the hypertension as outlined earlier. Though all these explanations, including participation of the renin-angiotensin system, probably have some validity in individual patients, the hypothesis involving sodium retention is particularly attractive. It is supported by the observation that those patients with chronic pyelonephritis or polycystic renal disease who are salt wasters do not develop hypertension, and by the observation that removal of salt and water by dialysis or diuretics is effective in controlling arterial pressure in the majority of patients with renal parenchymal disease.

A rare form of renal hypertension results from the excess secretion of renin by juxtaglomerular cell tumors or nephroblastomas. The initial presentation is similar to that of hyperaldosteronism with hypertension, hypokalemia, and overproduction of aldosterone. However, in contrast to primary aldosteronism, peripheral renin activity is *elevated instead of subnormal*. This disease can be distinguished from other forms of secondary aldosteronism by the presence of normal renal function and with unilateral increases in renal vein renin concentration without a renal artery lesion.

ENDOCRINE HYPERTENSION Adrenal hypertension Hypertension is a feature of a variety of adrenal cortical abnormalities. In *primary aldosteronism* (Chap. 325) there is a clear relationship between the aldosterone-induced sodium retention and the hypertension. Normal individuals given aldosterone develop hypertension only if they also ingest sodium. Since aldosterone causes sodium retention by stimulating renal tubular exchange of sodium for potassium, hypokalemia is a prominent feature in most patients with primary aldosteronism, and therefore the measurement of serum potassium provides a simple screening test. The effect of sodium retention and volume expansion in chronically suppressing plasma renin activity is critically important for the definitive diagnosis. In most clinical situations plasma renin activity and plasma or urinary aldosterone levels parallel each other, but in patients with primary aldosteronism, aldosterone levels are high and relatively fixed because of autonomous aldosterone secretion, while plasma renin activity levels are suppressed and respond sluggishly to sodium depletion. Primary aldosteronism may be secondary either to a tumor or bilateral adrenal hyperplasia. It is important to distinguish between these two conditions preoperatively, as usually the hypertension in the latter is not modified by operation.

The sodium-retaining effect of large amounts of glucocorticoids also offers an explanation for the hypertension in severe cases of Cushing's syndrome (Chap. 325). Moreover, increased production of mineralocorticoids also has been documented in some patients with Cushing's syndrome. However, the hypertension in many cases of Cushing's syndrome does not seem volume-dependent, leading investigators to speculate that it may be secondary to glucocorticoid-induced production of renin substrate (angiotensin-mediated hypertension) or a steroid-induced change in vascular reactivity. In the forms of the adrenogenital syndrome due to C-11 or C-17 hydroxylase deficiency (Chap. 325) deoxycorticosterone accounts for the sodium retention and the resultant hypertension, which is accompanied by suppression of plasma renin activity.

In patients with pheochromocytoma (Chap. 326) increased secretion of epinephrine and norepinephrine by a tumor most often located in the adrenal medulla causes excessive stimulation of adrenergic receptors, which results in peripheral vasoconstriction and cardiac stimulation. This diagnosis is confirmed by demonstrating increased urinary excretion of epinephrine and norepinephrine or their metabolites.

Acromegaly (see also Chap. 321) Hypertension, coronary atherosclerosis, and cardiac hypertrophy are frequent complications of this condition.

Hypercalcemia (see also Chap. 335) The hypertension which occurs in up to one-third of patients with hyperparathyroidism ordinarily can be attributed to renal parenchymal damage due to nephrolithiasis and nephrocalcinosis. However, increased calcium levels can also have a direct vasoconstrictive effect. In some cases, the hypertension disappears when the hypercalcemia is corrected. Thus, paradoxically the increased serum calcium level in hyperparathyroidism raises blood pressure, while epidemiologic studies suggest that a high calcium intake lowers blood pressure. To further confuse the issue, calcium entry blocking agents are effective antihypertensive agents. Additional studies are needed to resolve these seemingly conflicting observations.

Oral contraceptives The most common cause of endocrine hypertension is that resulting from the use of estrogen-containing oral contraceptives. Indeed, this may be the most common form of secondary hypertension. The mechanisms producing the hypertension is likely to be secondary to activation of the renin-angiotensin-aldosterone system. Thus, both volume (aldosterone) and vasoconstrictor (angiotensin II) factors are important. The estrogen component of oral contraceptive agents stimulates the hepatic synthesis of the renin substrate angiotensinogen, which in turn favors the increased production of angiotensin II and secondary aldosteronism. Women taking oral contraceptives have increased plasma concentrations of angiotensin II and aldosterone with some increase in arterial pressure. However, only about 5 percent actually have an increase in arterial pressure greater than 140/90, and in about half of these the hypertension will remit within 6 months of stopping the drug.

Why some women taking oral contraceptives develop hypertension and others do not is unclear but may be related to (1) increased vascular sensitivity to angiotensin II, (2) the presence of mild renal disease, (3) familial factors (over one-half have a positive family history for hypertension), (4) age (hypertension is significantly more prevalent in women over age 35), and/or (5) obesity. Indeed some investigators have suggested that the oral contraceptives are simply unmasking patients with essential hypertension.

COARCTATION OF THE AORTA (See also Chap. 185) The hypertension associated with coarctation may be caused by the constriction itself, or perhaps by the changes in the renal circulation which result in an unusual form of renal arterial hypertension. The diagnosis of coarctation is usually evident from physical examination and routine x-ray findings.

LOW-RENIN ESSENTIAL HYPERTENSION Approximately 20 percent of patients who by all other criteria have essential hypertension have suppressed plasma renin activity. This occurs more frequently in black than in white patients. Though these patients are not hypokalemic, they have been reported to have expanded extracellular fluid volumes, and it is tempting to implicate sodium retention and renin suppression due to excessive production of an unidentified mineralocorticoid. Involvement of the adrenal cortex is suggested by the observation that large doses of spironolactone, the mineralocorticoid antagonist, and the inhibition of steroidogenesis by aminoglutethimide can result in sodium loss and lowering of blood pressure in these patients. A search for other mineralocorticoids occasionally reveals increased secretion of 18-hydroxy-11-deoxycorticosterone or 16-hydroxydehydroepiandrosterone in some patients. However, the frequency of these abnormalities is no greater than in patients with normal renin hypertension. Some studies have suggested that many of these patients have an increased sensitivity of their adrenal cortex to angiotensin II which may be the underlying mechanism. Since this altered sensitivity has been reported even in patients with normal renin hypertension, it is likely that patients with low-renin hypertension are not a distinct subset but rather form part of a continuum of patients with essential hypertension.

HIGH-RENIN ESSENTIAL HYPERTENSION Approximately 15 percent of patients with essential hypertension have plasma renin levels elevated above the normal range. It has been suggested that plasma renin plays an important role in the pathogenesis of the elevated blood pressure in these patients. However, most studies have documented that saralasin significantly reduces blood pressure in less than half of these patients. This has led some investigators to postulate that the elevated renin levels and blood pressure may both be secondary to an increased activity of the adrenergic system. It has been proposed that, in those patients with angiotensin-dependent high-renin hypertension whose arterial pressures are lowered by saralasin, the mechanism responsible for the increased renin and, therefore, the hypertension is a compensatory hyperreninemia secondary to a decreased adrenal responsiveness to angiotensin II. Additional studies have documented that patients with high-renin hypertension are the same as the nonmodulators described on page 1025.

EFFECTS OF HYPERTENSION

Patients with hypertension die prematurely; the most common cause of death is heart disease, with stroke and renal failure also frequent, particularly in those with significant retinopathy.

EFFECTS ON HEART Cardiac compensation for the excessive work load imposed by increased systemic pressure is at first sustained by concentric left ventricular hypertrophy, characterized by an increase in wall thickness. Ultimately, the function of this chamber deteriorates, the cavity dilates, and the symptoms and signs of heart failure appear (Chap. 182). Angina pectoris may also occur because of the combination of accelerated coronary arterial disease and increased myocardial oxygen requirements as a consequence of the increased myocardial mass (Chap. 189). On physical examination the heart is enlarged and has a prominent left ventricular impulse. The sound of aortic closure is accentuated, and there may be a faint murmur of aortic regurgitation. Presystolic (atrial, fourth) heart sounds appear frequently in hypertensive heart disease, and a protodiastolic (ventricular, third heart) sound or summation gallop rhythm may be present. Electrocardiographic changes of left ventricular hypertrophy (Chap. 178) are common; evidence of ischemia or infarction may be observed late in the disease. The majority of deaths due to hypertension result from myocardial infarction or congestive heart failure.

NEUROLOGIC EFFECTS The neurologic effects of long-standing hypertension may be divided into retinal and central nervous system changes. Because the retina is the only tissue in which the arteries and arterioles can be examined directly, repeated ophthalmoscopic examination provides the opportunity to observe the progress of the vascular effects of hypertension (Table 196-4). The Keith-Wagener-Barker classification of the *retinal changes* in hypertension has provided a simple and excellent means for serial evaluation of hypertensive patients. Increasing severity of hypertension is associated with focal spasm and progressive general narrowing of the arterioles, as well as the appearance of hemorrhages, exudates, and papilledema. These retinal lesions often produce scotomata, blurred vision, and even blindness, especially in the presence of papilledema or hemorrhages of the macular area. Hypertensive lesions may develop acutely and, if therapy results in significant reduction of blood pressure, may show rapid resolution. Rarely, these lesions resolve without therapy. In contrast, retinal arteriolosclerosis results from endothelial and muscular proliferation, and it accurately reflects similar changes in other organs. Sclerotic changes do not develop as rapidly as hypertensive lesions, nor do they regress appreciably with therapy. As a consequence of increased wall thickness and rigidity, sclerotic arterioles distort and compress the veins as they cross within their common fibrous sheath, and the reflected light streak from the arterioles is changed by the increased opacity of the vessel wall.

Central nervous system dysfunction also occurs frequently in patients with hypertension. Occipital headaches, most often in the morning, are among the most prominent early symptoms of hypertension. Dizziness, lightheadedness, vertigo, tinnitus, and dimmed vision or syncope may also be observed, but the more serious manifestations are due to vascular occlusion, hemorrhage, or encephalopathy (Chap. 343). The pathogeneses of the former two disorders are quite different. *Cerebral infarction* is secondary to the increased atherosclerosis observed in hypertensive patients, while *cerebral hemorrhage* is the result of both the elevated arterial pressure and the development of cerebral vascular microaneurysms (Charcot-Bouchard aneurysms). Only age and arterial pressure are known to influence the development of the microaneurysms. Thus, it is not surprising that the association of arterial pressure with cerebral hemorrhage is much better than with either cerebral or myocardial infarction.

Hypertensive encephalopathy consists of the following symptom complex: severe hypertension, disordered consciousness, increased intracranial pressure, retinopathy with papilledema, and seizures. The pathogenesis is uncertain but probably not related to arteriolar spasm or cerebral edema. Focal neurologic signs are infrequent, and if present, suggest that infarction, hemorrhage, or transient ischemic attacks are more likely diagnoses. Although some investigators have suggested that prompt lowering of arterial pressure in these patients may adversely affect cerebral blood flow, most studies indicate that this is not the case.

RENAL EFFECTS (See also Chap. 227) Arteriolosclerotic lesions of the afferent and efferent arterioles and the glomerular capillary tufts are the most common renal vascular lesions in hypertension and result in decreased glomerular filtration rate and tubular dysfunction. Proteinuria and microscopic hematuria occur because of glomerular lesions, and approximately 10 percent of the deaths secondary to hypertension result from renal failure. Blood loss in hypertension occurs not only from renal lesions; epistaxis, hemoptysis, and metrorrhagia also occur frequently in these patients.

APPROACH TO THE PATIENT WITH HYPERTENSION

In evaluating patients with hypertension, the initial history, physical examination, and laboratory tests should be directed at (1) uncovering correctable secondary forms of hypertension (Table 196-1), (2) establishing a pretreatment baseline, (3) assessing factors which may influence the type of therapy or which may be adversely modified by therapy, and (4) determining whether other risk factors for the development of arteriosclerotic cardiovascular disease are present (Chap. 195). Ideally, this evaluation would also determine the

TABLE 196-4 Classification of hypertensive and arteriolosclerotic retinopathy

	Hypertension					Arteriolosclerosis	
	Arterioles						
Degree	General narrowing AV ratio*	Focal spasm†	Hemorrhages	Exudates	Papilledema	Arteriolar light reflex	AV crossing‡ defects
Normal	3:4	1:1	0	0	0	Fine yellow line, red blood column	0
Grade I	1:2	1:1	0	0	0	Broadened yellow line, red blood column	Mild depression of vein
Grade II	1:3	2:3	0	0	0	Broad yellow line, "copper wire," blood column not visible	Depression or humping of vein
Grade III	1:4	1:3	+	+	0	Broad white line, "silver wire," blood column not visible	Right-angle deviation, tapering, and disappearance of vein under arteriole; Distal dilatation of vein
Grade IV	Fine, fibrous cords	Obliteration of distal flow	+	+	+	Fibrous cords, blood column not visible	Same as grade III

* *This is the ratio of arteriolar to venous diameters.*
† *This is the ratio of diameters of region of spasm to proximal arteriole.*
‡ *Arteriolar length and tortuosity increase with severity.*

underlying mechanism(s) in essential hypertension, particularly if such information leads to a more specific therapeutic program. Unfortunately, at the present time this aspect of the evaluation is limited either by lack of knowledge of the underlying mechanisms, uncertainty as to the specificity of therapy for a distinct subset even if the underlying mechanisms are known, or the prohibitive expense in defining a subset of hypertensive patients even if specific therapy were available. However, with the accumulation of additional information a fifth component in the evaluation of patients with hypertension may become increasingly more important.

SYMPTOMS AND SIGNS The majority of patients with hypertension have no symptoms referable to their blood pressure elevation and will be identified only in the course of a physical examination. When symptoms do bring the patient to the physician, they fall into three categories. They are related to (1) the elevated pressure itself, (2) the hypertensive vascular disease, and (3) the underlying disease in the case of secondary hypertension. Though popularly considered a symptom of elevated arterial pressure, headache is characteristic only of severe hypertension; most commonly it is localized to the occipital region, is present when the patient awakens in the morning, and subsides spontaneously after several hours. Other possibly related complaints include dizziness, palpitations, and easy fatigability. Complaints referable to vascular disease include epistaxis, hematuria, blurring of vision owing to retinal changes, episodes of weakness or dizziness due to transient cerebral ischemia, angina pectoris, and dyspnea due to cardiac failure. Pain due to dissection of the aorta or to a leaking aneurysm is an occasional presenting symptom.

Examples of symptoms related to the underlying disease in secondary hypertension are polyuria, polydipsia, and muscle weakness secondary to hypokalemia in patients with primary aldosteronism, or weight gain and emotional lability in patients with Cushing's syndrome. The patient with a pheochromocytoma may present with episodic headaches, palpitations, diaphoresis, and postural dizziness.

CLINICAL EVALUATION **History** A strong family history of hypertension, along with the reported finding of intermittent pressure elevation in the past, favors the diagnosis of essential hypertension. Secondary hypertension often develops before the age of 35 or after the age of 55 years. The history of use of adrenal steroids or estrogens is of obvious significance. A history of repeated urinary tract infections suggests chronic pyelonephritis, although this condition may occur in the absence of symptoms; nocturia and polydipsia suggest renal or endocrine disease, while trauma to either flank or an episode of acute flank pain may be a clue to the presence of renal injury. A history of weight gain is compatible with Cushing's syndrome, and weight loss with pheochromocytoma. A number of aspects of the history aid in determining whether vascular disease has progressed to dangerous stages. These include angina pectoris and symptoms of cerebrovascular insufficiency, of congestive heart failure, and/or of peripheral vascular insufficiency. Other risk factors that should be elicited include cigarette smoking, diabetes mellitus, lipid disorders, and a family history of early deaths due to cardiovascular disease.

Physical examination The physical examination starts with the patient's general appearance. For instance, are the round face and trunkal obesity of Cushing's syndrome present? Is muscular development in the upper extremities out of proportion to that in the lower extremities, suggesting coarctation of the aorta? The next step is to compare the blood pressures and pulses in both upper extremities. Also, measurements in the supine position should be compared with measurements taken during standing. A rise in diastolic pressure when the patient goes from the supine to the standing position is most compatible with essential hypertension; a fall, in the absence of antihypertensive medications, suggests secondary forms of hypertension. Detailed examination of the ocular fundi is mandatory, since funduscopic findings provide one of the best indications of the duration of hypertension and of prognosis. The Keith-Wagener-Barker classification of funduscopic changes (Table 196-4) is useful; the specific changes in each fundus should be recorded and a grade assigned. Palpation and auscultation of the carotid arteries for evidence of stenosis or occlusion are important; narrowing of a carotid artery may be a manifestation of hypertensive vascular disease, and it may also be a clue to the presence of a renal arterial lesion, since these two lesions may occur together. In examination of the heart and lungs, one should search for evidence of left ventricular hypertrophy and cardiac decompensation. Is there a left ventricular lift? Are third and fourth heart sounds present? Are there pulmonary rales? Chest examination also includes a search for extracardiac murmurs and palpable collateral vessels that may result from coarctation of the aorta.

The most important part of the abdominal examination is auscultation for bruits originating in stenotic renal arteries. Bruits due to renal arterial narrowing nearly always have a diastolic component or may be continuous and are best heard just to the right or left of the midline above the umbilicus, or in the flanks; they are present in many patients with renal artery stenosis due to fibrous dysplasia and in 40 to 50 percent of those with functionally significant stenosis due to arteriosclerosis. The abdomen also should be palpated for abdominal aneurysm and for the enlarged kidneys of polycystic renal disease. The femoral pulses must be carefully felt, and, if they are decreased and/or delayed in comparison to the radial pulse, the blood pressure in the lower extremities must be measured. Even if the femoral pulse is normal to palpation, arterial pressure in the lower extremities should be recorded at least once in patients in whom hypertension is discovered before the age of 30 years. Finally, examination of the extremities for edema and a search for evidence of a previous cerebrovascular accident and/or other intracranial pathology should be performed.

Laboratory investigation Controversy exists as to what laboratory studies should be performed in patients presenting with hypertension. In general, the disagreement resides in how extensively to evaluate the patient for secondary forms of hypertension or subsets of essential hypertension. In the following discussion laboratory studies are divided into those which should be performed in all patients with sustained hypertension (basic studies) and those which should be added if (1) from the initial evaluation a secondary form of hypertension is suggested and/or (2) arterial pressure is not controlled after initial therapy (secondary studies).

BASIC STUDIES Renal status is evaluated by assessing the presence of protein, blood, and glucose in the urine and measuring serum creatinine and/or blood urea nitrogen (BUN). Microscopic examination of the urine is also helpful. A serum potassium level is needed both as a screen for mineralocorticoid-induced hypertension and as a baseline prior to initiating diuretic therapy.

Other blood chemistries may also be useful, particularly since they can often be ordered as a battery of automated tests at minimal cost to the patient. For example, a blood glucose is helpful both because diabetes mellitus may be associated with accelerated arteriosclerosis, renal vascular disease, and diabetic nephropathy in patients with hypertension, and because primary aldosteronism, Cushing's syndrome, and pheochromocytoma all may be associated with hyperglycemia. Furthermore, since antihypertensive therapy with diuretics, for example, can raise the blood glucose level, it is important to establish a baseline. The possibility of hypercalcemia may also be investigated. Serum uric acid is useful because of the increased incidence of hyperuricemia in patients with renal and essential hypertension and because, as with blood glucose, the level subsequently may be raised by treatment with diuretics. Serum cholesterol and triglycerides may be measured to identify other factors which predispose to the development of arteriosclerosis. An electrocardiogram should be obtained in all cases as an assessment of cardiac status, particularly if left ventricular hypertrophy is present, and as a baseline. The chest roentgenogram may also be helpful by providing the opportunity to identify aortic dilatation or elongation and the rib notching that occurs in coarctation of the aorta.

SECONDARY STUDIES (Table 196-5) Certain clues from the history, physical examination, and basic laboratory studies suggest an unusual cause for the hypertension and dictate the need for special studies. For example, the abrupt onset of severe hypertension and/or the onset of hypertension of any severity under the age of 25 or after the age of 50 years should lead to laboratory tests to exclude renovascular hypertension and pheochromocytoma. A history of headaches, palpitations, anxiety attacks, unusual sweating, hyperglycemia, and weight loss should also lead to tests to exclude pheochromocytoma. The presence of an abdominal bruit should lead to workup for renovascular hypertension, and the finding of bilateral upper abdominal masses on physical examination, consistent with polycystic renal disease, to the performance of an intravenous pyelogram. An elevated creatinine or blood urea nitrogen, associated with proteinuria and hematuria, should initiate a detailed workup for renal insufficiency (Chap. 218). Special studies for secondary hypertension are also indicated if there is therapeutic failure with the initial drug program. The specific diagnostic measures depend on the most likely causes of secondary hypertension.

Pheochromocytoma (see also Chap. 326). The easiest and best screening procedure for pheochromocytoma is the measurement of catecholamines or their metabolites in a 24-h urine collected during the time the patient is hypertensive. Measurement of plasma catecholamine levels may also be useful. These tests may be indicated even in patients who do not have episodic hypertension, since over half the patients with pheochromocytoma have fixed hypertension. Provocative tests are seldom if ever indicated, although occasionally a suppressive test may be useful.

Cushing's syndrome (see also Chap. 325). A 24-h urine test for cortisol or the administration of 1 mg dexamethasone at bedtime, followed by measurement of plasma cortisol at 7 to 10 A.M. is the best test for the presence of this condition. A urine cortisol less than 100 μg or suppression of the plasma cortisol level to below 5 μg/dL effectively rules out Cushing's syndrome.

Renovascular hypertension (see also Chap. 227). The standard screening test for renal vascular hypertension has been the rapid-sequence intravenous pyleogram (IVP). Features suggestive of renal ischemia include (1) unilateral delayed appearance and excretion of contrast material, (2) a difference in kidney size greater than 1.5 cm, (3) irregular contour of the renal silhouette, suggesting partial infarction or atrophy, (4) indentations on the ureter or renal pelvis, possibly due to dilated ureteral arteries (collateral notching), and (5) hyperconcentration of contrast medium in the collecting system of the smaller kidney. When these criteria are used, the false-positive rate is 11 percent and the false-negative rate 12 percent. The digital subtraction angiogram has been received with considerable enthusiasm as a more precise screening test for renal vascular disease. Its ultimate place as a screening test is unclear, however, because of its relatively high cost and as yet unproven greater sensitivity and specificity relative to an IVP. The isotope renogram and saralasin infusion test, both enthusiastically endorsed in the past as screening procedures, are now used infrequently either because of lower sensitivity and specificity or limited availability.

TABLE 196-5 Laboratory tests and special studies for evaluation of hypertension

I Basic studies
- *A* Always included
  - *1* Urine for protein, blood, and glucose
  - *2* Hematocrit
  - *3* Serum potassium
  - *4* Serum creatinine and/or blood urea nitrogen
  - *5* Electrocardiogram
- *B* Usually included, depending on cost and other factors
  - *1* Microscopic urinalysis
  - *2* White blood cell count
  - *3* Plasma/blood glucose, cholesterol, and triglycerides
  - *4* Serum calcium, phosphate, and uric acid
  - *5* Chest x-ray

II Special studies to screen for secondary hypertension
- *A* Renovascular: rapid sequence IVP or digital subtraction angiogram
- *B* Pheochromocytoma: 24-h urine for creatinine, metanephrines, and catecholamines or plasma catecholamines
- *C* Cushing's syndrome: overnight dexamethasone suppression test or 24-h urine cortisol

The definitive test of surgically correctable renal disease is the combination of a renal angiogram and renal vein renin determinations. The renal arteriogram both establishes the presence of a renal arterial lesion and aids in determining whether the lesion is due to atherosclerosis or to one of the fibrous or fibromuscular dysplasias. It does not, however, prove that the lesion is responsible for the hypertension, nor does it permit prediction of the chances of surgical cure; it must be noted that (1) renal artery stenosis is a frequent finding by angiography and at postmortem in normotensive individuals, and (2) essential hypertension is a common condition and may occur in combination with renal arterial stenosis which actually may not be responsible for the hypertension. Bilateral renal vein catheterization for measurement of plasma renin activity is, therefore, used to assess the functional significance of any lesion noted on arteriography. When one kidney is ischemic and the other is normal, all the renin released comes from the involved kidney. In the most straightforward situation, the ischemic kidney has a significantly higher venous plasma renin activity than the normal kidney by a factor of 1.5 or more. Moreover, the renal venous blood draining the uninvolved kidney exhibits levels similar to those in the inferior vena cava below the entrance of the renal veins. Significant benefit from operative correction may be anticipated in at least 80 percent of patients with the findings described above if care is taken to prepare the patient properly prior to renal vein blood sampling, i.e., discontinuing renin-suppressing drugs, such as beta blockers, for at least 10 days, placing the patient on a low sodium intake for 4 days, and/or giving a converting enzyme inhibitor for 24 h. When obstructing lesions in the *branches* of the renal arteries are demonstrated by arteriography, an attempt to obtain blood samples from the main *branches* of the renal vein should be made in an effort to identify a localized intrarenal arterial lesion responsible for the hypertension.

Primary aldosteronism (see also Chap. 325). These patients almost always exhibit hypokalemia. Diuretic therapy often complicates the picture when the hypokalemia is first observed and needs to be assessed. Given hypokalemia, the relation between plasma renin activity and the aldosterone level becomes the key to the diagnosis of primary aldosteronism. The aldosterone concentration or excretion is high and plasma renin activity is low in primary aldosteronism, and these levels are relatively unaffected by changes in sodium balance. A critical part of the evaluation after primary aldosteronism has been established is to determine whether unilateral or bilateral disease is present since surgical removal of the lesion usually reduces arterial pressure only in those with unilateral disease.

Plasma renin activity measurements. Some studies have suggested that most hypertensive patients should have a plasma renin level measured and related to a 24-h urine sodium excretion rate to assess whether high, low, or normal levels are present. It has been proposed that this information may be important for both therapeutic and prognostic reasons. However, it is unclear, on the basis of presently available data and treatment programs, that these random measurements are really useful except in patients with findings suggestive of renal vascular disease or mineralocorticoid excess in whom lateralizing renal vein renin levels or suppressed peripheral renin levels may be of diagnostic and/or therapeutic significance.

TREATMENT

Virtually every patient with a diastolic arterial pressure which persistently exceeds 90 mmHg is a candidate for diagnostic studies and for subsequent treatment. Furthermore, at any given level of blood pressure elevation, the ultimate risk of developing hypertensive vascular complications is greater in men than in women, and in younger than in older persons. It may be argued, then, that it is hard to justify producing the uncomfortable side effects of therapy in, for example, an asymptomatic woman over 70 years of age with a diastolic pressure of 90 mmHg. On the other hand, it is easy to justify side effects in a man of 30 with a diastolic pressure exceeding 110 mmHg, because such a person may be expected to receive the greatest benefit from therapy. Fortunately, the choice of treatment is such that a satisfactory program to control arterial pressure with minimal side effects can be developed for most patients. A reasonable guideline would be that all patients with diastolic pressure repeatedly above 90 mmHg should be treated unless specific contraindications exist. There is controversy regarding the advisability of treating isolated *systolic* hypertension. Until the results of a well-controlled prospective study provide evidence to the contrary, treatment of isolated systolic hypertension is not recommended. Patients with labile hypertension or isolated systolic hypertension who are not treated should have regular follow-up examinations at 6-month intervals, because of the frequent development of progressive and/or sustained hypertension.

The identification of an operable form of secondary hypertension does not automatically mean that surgical treatment is indicated. The decision depends upon the age and general health of the patient, the natural history of the lesion, and the response of the pressure to drug therapy. In patients with renovascular hypertension the feasibility of renal angioplasty, surgical repair versus nephrectomy, and the degree of overall renal function impairment must be considered. Age and general health are important in patients with renovascular hypertension due to arteriosclerosis, because there is no evidence that repair of the stenosis increases life expectancy in the elderly patient with other evidence of vascular disease. Knowledge of the natural history of the disease is especially important when approaching the decision in the young patient with renal-artery stenosis due to fibrous dysplasia. If the arteriographic appearance suggests that the stenosis is due to intimal or subadventitial fibroplasia, the lesion may be expected to progress and operation or angioplasty is required. Medial fibroplasia, on the other hand, often remains stable, and operation or angioplasty may not be necessary if pressure can be controlled by drug therapy. The decision regarding operation should also be considered carefully in patients with primary aldosteronism when bilateral adrenal venography does not demonstrate a tumor, because such patients may prove to have multinodular hyperplasia. This means that bilateral adrenalectomy would be required to eliminate the aldosterone excess, and, even then, hypertension usually persists. If hypokalemia can be controlled by spironolactone or other drug therapy, and arterial pressure lowered with antihypertensive agents, then it is reasonable to withhold operative treatment.

GENERAL MEASURES Nondrug therapeutic intervention is probably indicated in all patients with sustained hypertension and probably most with labile hypertension. The general measures employed include (1) relief of stress, (2) diet, (3) regular exercise, and (4) control of other risk factors contributing to the development of arteriosclerosis. Relief of emotional and environmental stress is one of the reasons for the improvement in hypertension that occurs when the patient is hospitalized. Though it is usually impossible to extricate the hypertensive patient from all internal and external stresses, he or she should be advised to avoid any unnecessary tensions. In rare instances, it may be appropriate to recommend a change of job or of life-style. Recently it has been suggested that relaxation techniques may also lower arterial pressure. However, it is uncertain that these techniques alone have much long-term effect.

Dietary management has three aspects:

1 Because of the documented efficacy of sodium restriction and volume contraction in lowering blood pressure, patients previously were instructed to curtail sodium intake drastically. Some investigators have suggested this is no longer necessary. They base their conclusion on two observations: (1) In many patients the blood pressure is not sensitive to the level of sodium intake, and (2) diuretics provide another method of decreasing body sodium stores in those individuals whose blood pressure may be sodium-sensitive. However, a number of reports have documented that while mild sodium restriction has little, if any, direct action on blood pressure, it significantly potentiates the efficacy of nearly all antihypertensive agents and thereby by allowing blood pressure control with lower doses of drugs, side effects are reduced. In addition, it is quite clear that in some hypertensive patients, as noted above, the level of sodium intake does influence the blood pressure. Thus, since there is no apparent risk to mild sodium restriction, the most practical approach now is to advise mild dietary sodium restriction (up to 5 g NaCl per day), which can be achieved by eliminating all additions of salt to food which is prepared normally. Some studies have also reported lowering of arterial pressure by *increasing* calcium intake. While the advisability of this form of dietary alteration is still controversial, since a high calcium intake probably also reduces the extent of age-related osteoporosis, it is probably a useful adjunct.
2 Caloric restriction should be urged for the patient who is overweight. Some obese patients will show a significant reduction in pressure simply as a consequence of weight loss.
3 A restriction in intake of cholesterol and saturated fats is recommended on the suggestive evidence that such a diet may diminish the incidence of arteriosclerotic complications. Regular exercise is indicated within the limits of the patient's cardiovascular status. Not only is exercise helpful in controlling weight, but in addition there is evidence that physical conditioning itself may lower arterial pressure. Isotonic exercises (jogging, swimming) are better than isometric exercises (weight lifting) since, if anything, the latter raises arterial pressure. The dietary management outlined above is aimed at the control of other risk factors. Probably the most significant additional step that could be taken in this area would be to convince the smoker to give up cigarettes.

DRUG THERAPY (Table 196-6) To make rational use of antihypertensive drugs, the sites and mechanisms of their action must be understood. In general, there are four classes of drugs: diuretics, antiadrenergic agents, vasodilators, and angiotensin-converting enzyme (ACE) inhibitors.

Diuretics (see also Chap. 182) The thiazides are the most frequently used and most extensively investigated members of this group, and their early effect certainly is related to sodium diuresis and volume depletion. A reduction in peripheral vascular resistance also has been reported by some workers to be important in the long term. Traditionally, thiazide diuretics have formed the cornerstone of most therapeutic programs designed to lower arterial pressure and are usually effective within 3 to 4 days. However, in recent years increasing resistance to their routine use has occurred primarily because of their adverse metabolic effects, which include hypokalemia due to renal potassium loss, hyperuricemia due to uric acid retention, carbohydrate intolerance, and hyperlipidemia. The more potent diuretics, furosemide and ethacrynic acid, also have been shown to be antihypertensive but have been less extensively used for this purpose primarily because of their shorter duration of action. Spironolactone causes renal sodium loss by blocking the effect of endogenous mineralocorticoids, and therefore it may be more effective in patients whose mineralocorticoids are present in excess, e.g., primary or secondary aldosteronism. Although they do not compete directly with aldosterone, triamterene and amiloride act at the same site as spironolactone to impede sodium reabsorption and are effective in the same situations as spironolactone, except triamterene has little intrinsic antihypertensive effect. Their major disadvantage is that they can produce hyperkalemia, particularly in patients with impaired renal function. Any of these three potassium-sparing diuretics can also be given along with thiazide diuretics to minimize renal potassium loss.

Antiadrenergic agents (see also Chap. 66) These drugs act at one or more sites either centrally on the vasomotor center, in peripheral neurons modifying catecholamine release, or by blocking adrenergic

TABLE 196-6 Drugs used in treatment of hypertension—listed according to site of action

Site of action	Drug	Dosage	Indications	Contraindications	Frequent or peculiar side effects
DIURETICS					
Renal tubule	Thiazides: e.g., hydrochlorothiazide	Depends on specific drug Oral: 25 mg daily or twice daily	Mild hypertension as adjunct in treatment of moderate to severe hypertension	Diabetes mellitus, hyperuricemia, primary aldosteronism	Potassium depletion, hyperglycemia, hyperuricemia, dermatitis, purpura
	Loop acting: e.g., furosemide	Oral: 40–80 mg 2 or 3 times a day	Mild hypertension as adjunct in severe or malignant hypertension	Hyperuricemia, primary aldosteronism	Potassium depletion, hyperuricemia, nausea, vomiting, diarrhea
	Potassium-sparing: Spironolactone	Oral: 25 mg 2 to 4 times daily	Hypertension due to hypermineralocorticoidism, adjunct to thiazide therapy	Renal failure	Hyperkalemia, diarrhea, gynecomastia, menstrual irregularities
	Triamterene Amiloride	Oral 50–100 mg 1 or 2 times daily Oral 5–10 mg daily	Hypertension due to hypermineralocorticoidism, adjunct to thiazide therapy	Renal failure	Hyperkalemia, nausea, vomiting, leg cramps, nephrolithiasis, hyperkalemia, GI disturbances
ANTIADRENERGIC AGENTS					
Central	Clonidine Guanabenz	Oral: 0.1–0.6 mg twice daily Oral: 4–16 mg twice daily	Mild to moderate hypertension, renal disease with hypertension		Postural hypotension, drowsiness, dry mouth, rebound hypertension after abrupt withdrawal, insomnia, lupuslike syndrome
	Methyldopa (also acts by blocking sympathetic nerves)	Oral: 250–1000 mg twice daily IV: 250–1000 mg every 4–6 h (tolerance may develop)	Mild to moderate hypertension (oral), malignant hypertension (IV)	Pheochromocytoma, active hepatic disease (IV), during MAO inhibitor administration	Postural hypotension, sedation, fatigue, diarrhea, impaired ejaculation, fever, gynecomastia, lactation, positive Coombs tests (occasionally associated with hemolysis), chronic hepatitis, acute ulcerative colitis
Autonomic ganglia	Trimethaphan	IV: 1–6 mg/min	Severe or malignant hypertension	Severe coronary artery disease, cerebrovascular insufficiency, diabetes mellitus (on hypoglycemic therapy), glaucoma, prostatism	Postural hypotension, visual symptoms, dry mouth, constipation, urinary retention, impotence
Nerve endings	Rauwolfia alkaloids: Reserpine	Oral: 0.05–0.25 mg daily	Mild to moderate hypertension in young patient	Pheochromocytoma, peptic ulcer, depression, during MAO inhibitor administration	Depression, nightmares, nasal congestion, dyspepsia, diarrhea, impotence
	Guanethidine Guanadrel	Oral: 10–300 mg daily Oral 5–75 mg twice daily	Moderate to severe hypertension	Pheochromocytoma, severe coronary artery disease, cerebrovascular insufficiency, during MAO inhibitor administration	Postural hypotension, bradycardia, dry mouth, diarrhea, impaired ejaculation, fluid retention, asthma
Alpha receptors	Phentolamine	IV: 1–5 mg	Suspected or proved pheochromocytoma	Severe coronary artery disease	Tachycardia weakness, dizziness, flushing
	Phenoxybenzamine	Oral: 10–50 mg once or twice daily (tolerance may develop)	Proven pheochromocytoma		Postural hypotension, tachycardia, miosis, nasal congestion, dry mouth
	Prazosin	Oral: 1–10 mg twice daily	Mild to moderate hypertension		Sudden syncope, headache, sedation dizziness, tachycardia anticholinergic effect
Beta receptors	Propranolol Metoprolol Nadolol Atenolol Timolol	Oral: 10–120 mg 2 to 4 times daily Oral: 25–150 mg twice daily Oral: 20–120 mg daily Oral 25–100 mg daily Oral: 10–30 mg twice daily	Mild to moderate hypertension (especially with evidence for hyperdynamic circulation), adjunct to hydralazine therapy	Congestive heart failure, asthma, diabetes mellitus (on hypoglycemic therapy), during MAO inhibitor administration	Dizziness, depression, bronchospasm, nausea, vomiting, diarrhea, constipation, heart failure
	Pindolol Labetalol	Oral: 5–30 mg twice daily Oral: 100–600 mg twice daily			Less resting bradycardia than other beta blockers

TABLE 196-6 Drugs used in treatment of hypertension—listed according to site of action *(continued)*

Site of action	Drug	Dosage	Indications	Contraindications	Frequent or peculiar side effects
VASODILATORS					
Vascular smooth muscle	Hydralazine	Oral: 10–75 mg 4 times daily IV or IM: 10–50 mg every 6 h (tolerance may develop)	As adjunct in treatment of moderate to severe hypertension (oral), malignant hypertension (IV or IM), renal disease with hypertension	Lupus erythematosus, severe coronary artery disease	Headache, tachycardia, angina pectoris, anorexia, nausea, vomiting, diarrhea, lupus-like syndrome
	Minoxidil	Oral 2.5–50 mg twice daily	Severe hypertension	Severe coronary artery disease	Tachycardia, aggravates angina, marked fluid retention, hair growth on face and body, coarsening of facial features, possible pericardial effusions
	Diazoxide	IV: 1–3 mg/kg up to 150 mg rapidly	Severe or malignant hypertension	Diabetes mellitus, hyperuricemia, congestive heart failure	Hyperglycemia, hyperuricemia, sodium retention
	Nitroprusside	IV:0.5–8 (μg/kg)/min	Malignant hypertension		Apprehension, weakness, diaphoresis, nausea, vomiting, muscle twitching
ANGIOTENSIN-CONVERTING ENZYME INHIBITORS					
	Captopril	Oral: 12.5–75 mg twice daily	Mild to moderate and treatment-resistant hypertension, renal artery stenosis	Renal failure (reduction of dose)	Leukopenia, pancytopenia, proteinuria, nephrotic syndrome, membranous glomerulopathy, urticarial rash, fever, loss of taste, acute renal failure in bilateral renal artery stenosis
	Enalapril	Oral: 5–40 mg daily			Same as captopril, but no evidence for leukopenia, nephrotic syndrome, or taste loss

receptor sites on target tissue. Drugs that appear to have predominant *central actions* are *clonidine, methyldopa*, and *guanabenz*. These drugs and their metabolites are predominantly alpha-receptor agonists. Stimulation of $alpha_2$ receptors in the vasomotor centers of the brain *reduces* sympathetic outflow, thereby reducing arterial pressure. Usually a fall in cardiac output and heart rate also occurs, more commonly with clonidine and guanabenz, but the baroreceptor reflex is intact. Thus, postural symptoms are absent. However, rebound hypertension may rarely occur when these drugs, particularly clonidine and guanabenz, are stopped. This is probably secondary to the increase in norepinephrine release which had been inhibited by these agents secondary to their agonist effect on presynaptic alpha receptors.

Another class of antiadrenergic agents is the *ganglionic blocking* drugs, which have little effect when the patient is supine but prevent reflex vasoconstriction in the upright position. Ganglionic blocking agents interfere with parasympathetic as well as sympathetic function, and this results in such side effects as impairment of visual accommodation, paralytic ileus, retention of urine, and failure of erection and ejaculation. Because of these problems, ganglionic blocking agents are now usually reserved for the rapid lowering of arterial pressure by parenteral administration of the short-acting agent *trimethaphan* in patients with severe hypertension.

Various drugs act at *postganglionic adrenergic nerve endings*. The *rauwolfia alkaloids* such as reserpine are the oldest members of the group; their long-term effect results from their ability to inhibit the storage of norepinephrine within the vesicles in adrenergic nerve endings, thus leading to depletion of catecholamine stores. The frequent side effects including depression, nasal congestion, diarrhea, impairment of sexual function, and increased gastric secretion have limited the use of these drugs. *Guanethidine* and its shorter-acting analogue guanadrel block the release of norepinephrine from adrenergic nerve endings. They have a greater postural effect than the other drugs that act at the nerve endings, and orthostatic hypotension is a frequent side effect. However, centrally mediated side effects (sedation, depression) are infrequently observed since they are poorly soluble in lipids and, therefore, do not readily enter the central nervous system.

The last group of drugs affecting the adrenergic system are those which block the *peripheral adrenergic receptors*, alpha, beta, or both (see also Chap. 66). *Phentolamine* and *phenoxybenzamine* block the action of norepinephrine at *alpha*-adrenergic receptor sites. While the above two compounds block both presynaptic ($alpha_2$) and postsynaptic ($alpha_1$) alpha receptors, the former action accounts for the tolerance which develops, while *prazosin* is more effective because it selectively blocks only *postsynaptic alpha* receptors, i.e., $alpha_1$ receptors. Thus, presynaptic alpha activity remains, suppressing norepinephrine release. Accordingly, prazosin produces less tachycardia but more postural hypotension than direct-acting vasodilators, e.g., hydralazine.

A variety of effective *beta-adrenergic receptor blocking agents* are available which block sympathetic effects on the heart and should be most effective in reducing cardiac output and in lowering arterial pressure when there is increased cardiac sympathetic nerve activity. In addition, they block the adrenergic nerve-mediated release of renin from the renal juxtaglomerular cells, and this action may be an important component of their blood pressure–lowering action. Beta-adrenergic blockers are particularly useful when employed in conjunction with vascular smooth-muscle relaxants, which tend to evoke a reflex increase in myocardial contractility, and with diuretics, the administration of which often results in an elevation of circulating renin activity. In practice, beta blockers appear to be effective even when there is no evidence of increased sympathetic tone with about one-half or more of all hypertensive patients showing a fall in pressure. However, these agents can precipitate congestive heart failure and asthma in susceptible individuals and must be used with caution in diabetics receiving hypoglycemic therapy because they inhibit the usual sympathetic responses to hypoglycemia. Cardioselective beta-blocking agents (so-called $beta_1$ blockers) have been developed (metoprolol, atenolol) which may be superior to nonselective beta blockers such as propranolol and timolol in patients with bronchospasm. Nadolol, a nonselective beta blocker, unlike other drugs of this class is excreted unchanged in the urine and has a half-life of 14 to 20 h. Therefore, only one dose a day is required. Atenolol also usually only needs to be given once a day. Pindolol is a nonselective beta blocker with partial agonist activity and, therefore, produces less bradycardia. Labetalol exerts both alpha- and beta-adrenergic blocking actions. Thus, it lowers arterial pressure by the same complex actions as do beta blockers, but also directly by reducing systemic vascular resistance.

Vasodilators *Hydralazine* is the most versatile of the drugs that cause direct relaxation of vascular smooth muscle; it is effective both orally and parenterally, acting mainly on arterial resistance, rather than on venous capacitance vessels, as evidenced by lack of postural changes. Unfortunately, the effect of hydralazine on peripheral resistance is partly negated by reflex increases in sympathetic discharges that raise heart rate and cardiac output. These limit the usefulness of hydralazine, especially in patients with severe coronary artery disease. However, the efficacy of hydralazine can be increased if it is given in conjunction with beta blockers or drugs such as methyldopa or clonidine, all of which block reflex sympathetic stimulation of the heart. A serious side effect of doses of hydralazine exceeding 300 mg per day has been the production of a lupus erythematosus-like syndrome.

Minoxidil is even more potent but unfortunately produces significant hirsutism and, therefore, is mainly limited to patients with severe hypertension and renal insufficiency.

Diazoxide, a thiazide derivative, is restricted in its application to acute situations. It is not a diuretic; in fact, it causes sodium retention. However, like other thiazides, it reduces carbohydrate tolerance. It must be given rapidly intravenously to guarantee effect. It begins to act immediately to lower blood pressure, and its effects may last for several hours. *Nitroprusside* given intravenously also acts as a direct vasodilator, with onset and offset of actions that are almost immediate. These latter two drugs are useful only for the treatment of hypertensive emergencies (Table 196-7).

Angiotensin-converting enzyme inhibitors Drugs from several of the categories discussed above have been shown to possess an additional action resulting in inhibition of renin secretion. These include clonidine, reserpine, methyldopa, and beta blockers. A second group of drugs in this class are those which inhibit the enzyme converting angiotensin I into angiotensin II, e.g., captopril and enalapril. These agents are useful because they not only inhibit the generation of a potent vasoconstrictor (angiotensin II) but also may retard the degradation of a potent vasodilator (bradykinin), alter prostaglandin production, and can modify the activity of the adrenergic nervous system. They are especially useful in renal or renovascular hypertension, as well as in accelerated and malignant hypertension. They are also effective in milder, uncomplicated hypertension with minimal side effects, although caution still needs to be exercised until their long-term safety is determined.

APPROACH TO DRUG THERAPY (Fig. 196-1) The aim of drug therapy is to use the agents just described, alone or in combination, to return arterial pressure to normal levels with minimal side effects. Ideally, one would choose a therapeutic program which specifically corrects the underlying defect resulting in the elevated blood pressure, e.g., spironolactone for patients with primary aldosteronism. As our knowledge of the mechanisms underlying the hypertension in individual patients increases, more specific drug programs will become available. This presumably will result in normalization of blood pressure with fewer side effects. In the absence of that information an empiric approach is used. When used in combination, drugs are chosen for their different sites of action. However, except for those individuals with severe hypertension (average diastolic blood pressure greater than 130 mmHg) in whom intensive therapy with several agents simultaneously usually is required, most patients should initially be treated with a single agent. Since many effective antihypertensive agents are available, a number of useful therapeutic regimens have been developed, with the ideal program still unclear. Previously, the step-care program suggested by the Joint National Committee on Detection, Evaluation and Treatment of High Blood Pressure was the primary approach. This program assumed that nearly all hypertensives should be treated similarly, beginning with a thiazide diuretic and adding other agents in a fixed pattern until the blood pressure was normalized. Recently, deviations from this standard approach have been advocated because of concern regarding the potential long-term adverse effects of thiazide diuretics and increasing evidence that other classes of drugs, e.g., beta blockers and angiotensin-converting enzyme inhibitors, may also be effective monotherapeutic agents. We believe that the first choice is between a beta blocker and a thiazide diuretic. The reason for choosing one over the other is empiric, although in general older individuals and blacks may be particularly responsive to diuretics while younger individuals and whites respond well to beta blockers.

The schema outlined in Fig. 196-1 takes into account the presently available data on effectiveness, adverse reactions, and cost in deciding when to use a given agent. This approach is applicable to all patients in whom an indication for a specific form of therapy is lacking. Because of its lower cost, low-dose thiazide therapy, e.g., 25 mg of hydrochlorothiazide or its equivalent, daily often is the first choice rather than a beta blocker. If a beta blocker is chosen, it also should be started at a low dose, e.g., equivalent to 25 mg of atenolol daily. If with either agent, seated blood pressure is lowered to less than 140/90, no further therapy is indicated. If not controlled, the next step is to combine these two agents in a low-dose program, e.g., 25

TABLE 196-7 Therapeutic agents used to treat malignant hypertension

		Time course of action			
Drug	Route	Onset	Peak	Duration	Oral preparation available
IMMEDIATE ONSET					
Diazoxide	IV bolus	1–3 min	2–4 min	4–12 h	No
Nitroprusside	Continuous IV	<1 min	1–2 min	2–5 min	No
Trimethaphan	Continuous IV	<1 min	1–2 min	2–5 min	No
DELAYED ONSET					
Hydralazine	IV, IM	10–20 min	20–40 min	2–6 h	Yes
Methyldopa	IV	1–3 h	3–5 h	2–12 h	Yes
Reserpine	IM	2–3 h	3–4 h	6–24 h	Yes

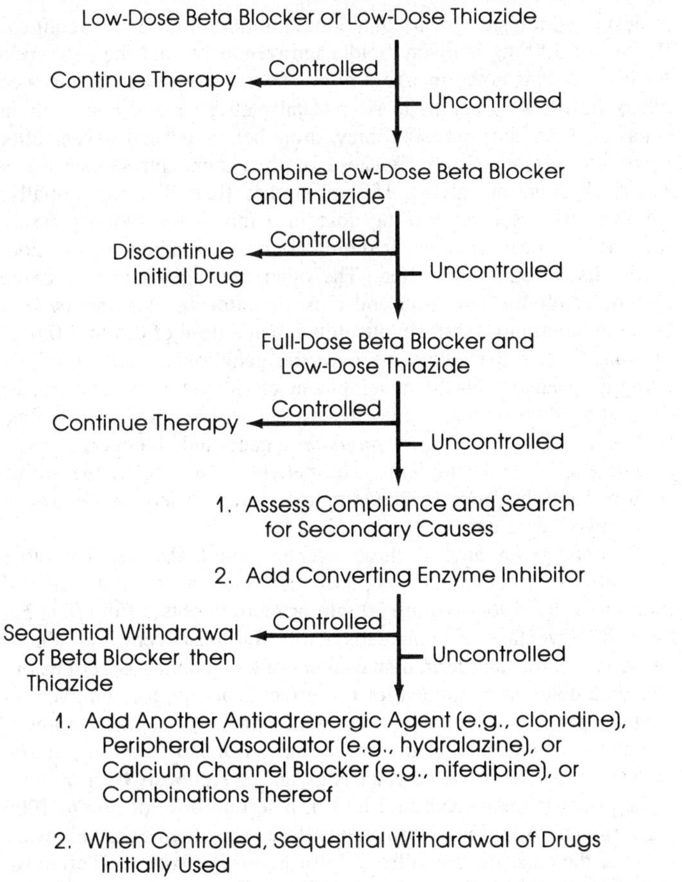

FIGURE 196-1 *Schematic approach to the treatment of the patient with hypertension in whom a specific form of therapy is unavailable or unknown.*

or 50 mg of atenolol (or its equivalent) and 25 mg of hydrochlorothiazide (or its equivalent) daily. Alternatively, the beta blocker could be increased to full dose, e.g., 100 mg of atenolol daily. Since the blood pressure response is often delayed, at least 8 weeks should elapse before changing the therapeutic program.

If combining low doses of a thiazide with a beta blocker does not achieve blood pressure control, the beta blocker is increased to a full dose. Rarely, increasing the thiazide to the equivalent of 50 mg of hydrochlorothiazide daily also may bring about control of the hypertension. However, thiazide doses higher than this are seldom, if ever, warranted since they almost invariably produce significant side effects, including reduction of serum potassium levels, hyperuricemia, and abnormalities in glucose metabolism with little increase in efficacy. If the hypertension is still uncontrolled despite treatment with a thiazide and full-dose beta blockers, then a detailed search for secondary causes of hypertension as outlined above is indicated. If none is found, then a converting enzyme inhibitor should be added. If control of blood pressure is achieved, then the beta blocker and/or thiazide is withdrawn or reduced in order to determine the minimum therapeutic program that will maintain the blood pressure at 140/90 mmHg or less.

Fewer than 5 percent of patients will still be hypertensive at this point. In them, one first should consider the reasons for therapeutic failure as shown in Table 196-8. If none can be identified, then one of the other agents such as a vasodilator listed in Table 196-6 (e.g., hydralazine) or an antiadrenergic agent (e.g., prazosin or clonidine) should be added. If blood pressure is controlled, previous drugs are sequentially withdrawn in order to determine the minimal therapeutic program that maintains a normal blood pressure.

While the recommendations outlined above are satisfactory for a large majority of patients, it is important to use a flexible approach since individual patients may respond differently to individual drugs and drug combinations. For those patients requiring multiple drugs, once the appropriate combination has been found, the use of a single formulation with the appropriate combination of drugs may simplify the regimen and thereby increase compliance. Every effort should be made to reduce the number of times each day the patients must interrupt his or her schedule for the medication. Pharmacologic treatment of essential hypertension is usually lifelong, and since most patients are asymptomatic, compliance with a complex regimen may be a serious problem.

Special considerations Four groups of patients with hypertension require special consideration because of associated conditions.

RENAL DISEASE Reduction of arterial pressure in hypertensive patients with impaired renal function is often accompanied initially by an increase in serum creatinine. This change does not represent further structural renal damage and should not deter continuation of therapy, since achievement of blood pressure control may eventually reduce the value toward normal. However, if serum creatinine increases in patients treated with a converting enzyme inhibitor, care needs to be exercised since these patients may have bilateral renal artery disease. Their renal function will continue to deteriorate as long as the converting enzyme inhibitor is given. Thus, converting enzyme inhibitors should be used cautiously in patients with impaired renal function and renal function should be assessed frequently (every 4 to 5 days) for the first 3 weeks. While converting enzyme inhibitors are contraindicated in patients with bilateral renal artery stenosis, these are the drugs of choice in patients with unilateral renal artery stenosis and a normally functioning contralateral kidney.

CORONARY ARTERY DISEASE In these patients who may also be taking cardiac glycosides, thiazides should be used judiciously and a reduction in serum potassium levels should be looked for and if found, should be corrected rapidly. Beta blockers should be withdrawn carefully, if at all, in these patients. Finally, calcium channel antagonists and converting enzyme inhibitors may be particularly useful in these patients since they minimize a number of potential adverse reactions accompanying other therapeutic agents, particularly nonspecific vasodilators.

DIABETES MELLITUS The diabetic patient with hypertension is particularly challenging since many of the agents used to lower blood pressure can affect glucose metabolism adversely. Converting enzyme inhibitors may be particularly useful in these individuals. They have no known adverse effects on glucose or lipid metabolism and may actually minimize the development of diabetic nephropathy by reducing renal vascular resistance and renal perfusion pressure—the primary factor underlying renal deterioration in these patients.

PREGNANCY The patient who is pregnant and hypertensive or who develops hypertension during pregnancy (pregnancy-induced hypertension, preeclampsia, eclampsia) is particularly difficult to treat. Because it is uncertain that autoregulation of uterine blood flow occurs, lowering blood pressure in the pregnant hypertensive may result in reduced placental and fetal perfusion. Thus, a conservative approach to lowering blood pressure is usually indicated. In the second and third trimesters, antihypertensives often are not indicated unless the diastolic pressure exceeds 95 mmHg. In general, severe

TABLE 196-8 Reasons for poor therapeutic response in patients with hypertension

1 Inadequate patient compliance
2 Volume expansion
  a Excessive sodium intake
  b Secondary to nondiuretic antihypertensive agent
3 Excessive weight gain
4 Inadequate doses
5 Drug antagonism
  a Cold remedies
  b Sympathomimetics
  c Oral contraceptives (estrogens)
  d Adrenal steroids
6 Secondary forms of hypertension

salt restriction and/or diuretics are not given because of the associated increase in fetal wastage. Beta blockers need to be used cautiously, if at all, for similar reasons. Methyldopa and hydralazine are the most frequent antihypertensives used since they have no known adverse effects on the fetus. Little is known about the safety of other antihypertensives in pregnancy except that nitroprusside and converting enzyme inhibitors may cause adverse effects on the fetus and should be avoided.

Probably fewer than one-third of hypertensive patients in the United States are being treated effectively. Only a small number of these failures is related to drug unresponsiveness. The majority is related to (1) failure to detect hypertension, (2) failure to institute effective treatment of the asymptomatic hypertensive subject, and (3) failure of the asymptomatic hypertensive subject to adhere to therapy. In order to improve this deficiency, patients must be educated to continue treatment once an effective regimen has been identified. Side effects and inconveniences of treatment must be minimized or counteracted in order to obtain the patient's continued cooperation.

MALIGNANT HYPERTENSION

In addition to marked blood pressure elevation in association with papilledema and retinal hemorrhages and exudates, the full-blown picture of malignant hypertension may include manifestations of hypertensive encephalopathy, such as severe headache, vomiting, visual disturbances (including transient blindness), transient paralyses, convulsions, stupor, and coma. These have been attributed to spasm of cerebral vessels and to cerebral edema. In some patients who have died, multiple small thrombi have been found in the cerebral vessels. Cardiac decompensation and rapidly declining renal function are other critical features of malignant hypertension. Oliguria may, in fact, be the presenting feature. The vascular lesion characteristic of malignant hypertension is fibrinoid necrosis of the walls of small arteries and arterioles, and this can be reversed by effective antihypertensive therapy.

The pathogenesis of malignant hypertension is unknown. However, at least two independent processes, dilatation of cerebral arteries and generalized arteriolar fibrinoid necrosis, contribute to the associated signs and symptoms. The cerebral arteries dilate because the normal autoregulation of cerebral blood flow decompensates secondary to the markedly elevated arterial pressure. As a result, cerebral blood flow is excessive, producing the encephalopathy associated with malignant hypertension. Many patients also show evidence of a microangiopathic hemolytic anemia; this secondary phenomenon could contribute to the deterioration of renal function. Most patients also have elevated levels of peripheral plasma renin activity and increased aldosterone production, and these may be involved in causing vascular damage.

About 1 percent of hypertensive patients develop the malignant phase, which occurs in the course of both essential and secondary hypertension. Rarely it is the first recognized manifestation of the blood pressure problem. The average age at diagnosis is 40, and men are more often affected than women. Prior to the availability of effective therapy, life expectancy after diagnosis of malignant hypertension was less than 2 years, with most deaths being due to renal failure, cerebral hemorrhage, or congestive heart failure. With the advent of effective antihypertensive therapy, at least half of the patients survive for more than 5 years.

Malignant hypertension is a medical emergency and requires immediate therapy. The initial aim of therapy should be to reduce diastolic pressure toward, but not below, 90 mmHg. The drugs available for treatment of malignant hypertension can be divided into two groups on the basis of time of onset of action (Table 196-7). Those in the first group act within a few minutes but are not satisfactory for long-term management. If the patient is having convulsions, if arterial pressure must be reduced rapidly, then one from the immediate-acting group should be used. *Diazoxide* is the easiest to administer, for no individual titration of dosage is required. A dose of 300 mg is given rapidly intravenously, and the antihypertensive effect is noted in 1 to 3 min. The same dose can be repeated when the pressure begins to rise, usually after several hours. In an occasional patient, pressure may drop below normal levels after diazoxide administration. Because of this, some physicians use a modified program, giving 150 mg rather than 300 mg initially, followed by a second 150-mg dose in 5 min if the blood pressure response has been minimal. It should not be used in patients in whom aortic dissection is suspected. The other two agents in this group require continuous infusion and close monitoring. *Nitroprusside* is given by continuous intravenous infusion at a dose of 0.5 to 8.0 (μg/kg)/min. It has the advantage over the ganglionic blockers of not being associated with the development of tachyphylaxis and can be utilized for days with few side effects. The dosage must be controlled with an infusion pump. *Trimethaphan,* a ganglionic blocker, is given at a rate of 1 to 15 mg/min. The patient should be in the sitting position, and the pressure should be monitored closely, preferably in an intensive care unit.

Patients given any of these agents should also receive other medications effective for long-term control. Those in the second group in Table 196-7 require 30 min or more to obtain full effect but have the advantage of being satisfactory for subsequent oral administration and for long-term management of the patient's hypertension. If such a delay in attainment of full effect is acceptable, intravenous *methyldopa* is an effective drug with which to begin therapy if symptoms of encephalopathy are absent. A dose of 500 mg in 100 to 200 mL 5% dextrose in water is given intravenously over 30 min; if the effect is inadequate in 2 to 4 h, a second dose of 500 to 1000 mg is given. Additional intravenous doses may then be given every 6 h until the pressure is stabilized. Intravenous *hydralazine* is effective in many patients within 10 min; an effective protocol involves giving 10-mg doses intravenously every 10 to 15 min until the desired effect has been obtained or until a total of 50 mg has been administered. The total required for response may then be repeated intramuscularly or intravenously every 6 h. Hydralazine should be used with caution in patients with significant coronary artery disease and should be avoided in patients evidencing myocardial ischemia or aortic dissection.

Furosemide is an important adjunct to the therapy just discussed. Given either orally or intravenously, it serves to maintain sodium diuresis in the face of a falling arterial pressure and thus will speed recovery from encephalopathy and congestive heart failure as well as maintain sensitivity to the primary antihypertensive drug. Digitalis (Chap. 182) also is indicated if there is evidence of cardiac decompensation.

In patients with malignant hypertension in whom the existence of pheochromocytoma is suspected, urine should be collected for measurement of the products of catecholamine metabolism, and drugs which might release additional catecholamines, such as methyldopa, reserpine, and guanethidine, must be avoided. The parenteral drug of choice in these patients is phentolamine, administered with care to avoid a precipitous reduction in arterial pressure.

There is hope even for patients who fail to respond sufficiently to any of the forms of therapy and who show progressive deterioration in renal function. In some, a period of peritoneal dialysis or hemodialysis to deplete extracellular fluid has resulted in better blood pressure control and eventual improvement in renal function. In other patients with refractory hypertension and renal failure who do not respond to volume depletion or hypotensive therapy, including minoxidil, particularly those with marked elevation of plasma renin activity, bilateral nephrectomy has resulted in amelioration of hypertension; subsequently these patients have been maintained on chronic dialysis or have received renal homografts. However, bilateral nephrectomy should be avoided where possible since (1) the loss of renal erythropoietin will contribute to the associated anemia, (2) vitamin D metabolism may be adversely affected, and (3) all residual renal function will be lost.

REFERENCES

AMERY A et al: Mortality and morbidity results from the European working party on high blood pressure in the elderly trial. Lancet 1:1349, 1985

BERGLUND G et al: Prevalence of primary and secondary hypertension: Studies in a random population sample. Br Med J 2:554, 1976

BLAUSTEIN MP: Role of a natriuretic factor in essential hypertension: An hypothesis. Ann Intern Med 98:785, 1983

BOUDOULAS H et al: Left ventricular mass and systolic performance in chronic systemic hypertension. Am J Cardiol 57:232, 1986

CAMPESE VM et al: Role of sympathetic nerve inhibition and body sodium-volume state in antihypertensive action of clonidine in essential hypertension. Kidney Int 18:351, 1980

CHALMERS MJ: The nervous system and the pathogenesis of essential hypertension, in *Handbook of Hypertension: Clinical Aspect of Essential Hypertension,* JIS Robertson (ed). Amsterdam, Elsevier, 1983, p 64

FUJITA I et al: Factors influencing blood pressure in salt-sensitive patients with hypertension. Am J Med 69:334, 1980

GENEST J: Personal views of the mechanisms of essential hypertension, in *Hypertension,* 2d ed, J Genest et al (eds). New York, McGraw-Hill, 1983

HOLME I et al: Treatment of mild hypertension with diuretics. The importance of ECG abnormalities in the Oslo study and in MRFIT. JAMA 251:1298, 1984

KAPLAN NM: Systemic hypertension: Therapy, in *Heart Disease,* E Braunwald (ed). Philadelphia, Saunders, 1984, p 902

KOTCHEN TA et al: Effect of chloride on renin and blood pressure responses to sodium chloride. Ann Intern Med 98:817, 1983

LINAS SL et al: Minoxidil. Ann Intern Med 94:61, 1981

MCCARRON DA: Calcium in the pathogenesis and therapy of human hypertension. Am J Med 78:27, 1985

RAM CVS et al: Moderate sodium restriction and various diuretics in the treatment of hypertension. Arch Intern Med 141:1015, 1981

STRANDGAARD S: Autoregulation of cerebral blood flow in hypertensive patients. Circulation 53:720, 1976

THE 1984 REPORT OF THE JOINT NATIONAL COMMITTEE ON DETECTION, EVALUATION, AND TREATMENT OF HIGH BLOOD PRESSURE. Arch Intern Med 144:1045, 1984

VETERANS ADMINISTRATION COOPERATIVE STUDY ON ANTI-HYPERTENSIVE AGENTS: Racial differences in response to low-dose captopril are abolished by the addition of hydrochlorothiazide. Br J Clin Pharmacol 14:97S, 1982

VIDT DG, GIFFORD RW JR: A compendium for the treatment of hypertensive emergencies. Cleve Clin Q 51:421, 1984

VLASSES PH et al: Double-blind comparison of captopril and enalapril in mild to moderate hypertension. J Am Coll Cardiol 7:651, 1986

WILLIAMS GH, HOLLENBERG NK: Abnormal adrenal and renal responsiveness to angiotensin II, in *Essential Hypertension as an Endocrine Disease,* CRW Edwards, RMC Carey (eds). London, Butterworths, 1985

197 DISEASES OF THE AORTA

JAMES E. DALEN

The walls of the aorta must withstand the shearing effect of each systolic thrust of blood. With its large diameter, the aorta is under greater tension than the rest of the arterial system because wall tension is a direct function of both diameter and pressure. For this reason, the effects of hypertension are particularly deleterious. In addition, the aorta is subject to infection, trauma, necrosis of the media, and, most notably, arteriosclerosis, which has replaced syphilis as the disease most frequently affecting the aorta. Arising from these stresses are four major diseases of the aorta: aneurysm, dissection, arteriosclerotic occlusive disease, and aortitis. The number of deaths due to disease of the aorta is uncertain because other cardiovascular diseases, such as ischemic heart disease, hypertensive disease, and cerebrovascular disease, often coexist and take priority in the coding of death certificates.

ANEURYSMS A "true" aortic aneurysm is an abnormal widening that involves all three layers of its wall. The basic defect is destruction of elastic fibers in the media, which permits the remaining fibrous tissue to stretch and leads to an increase in diameter, which in turn raises wall tension. As this process leads to further enlargement, rupture becomes increasingly possible. "False" aneurysms, which are usually caused by trauma, are those disruptions of the inner and medial segments of the wall which permit expansion of the aorta so that the wall of the aneurysm consists of only adventitia and/or perivascular clot.

The commonest aneurysms are *fusiform,* in which a segment of the aorta becomes diffusely dilated, its total circumference being affected. In contrast, *saccular* aneurysms involve a portion of the circumference and consist of an outpouching with a mouth.

The commonest underlying cause of aneurysm is arteriosclerosis, but cystic medial necrosis, trauma, and syphilis and other infections must also be noted as causes.

Aneurysms of the abdominal aorta Three-fourths of all aortic aneurysms occur in the abdominal aorta, just below the renal arteries. Nearly all aneurysms in the abdominal aorta are caused by arteriosclerosis. Multiple aortic aneurysms occur in more than 10 percent of these patients. A familial occurrence of abdominal aortic aneurysms in males has recently been reported. The majority of victims are men older than age 60; more than one-half have associated hypertension. The incidence is increased in cigarette smokers.

The *diagnosis* is often made by physical examination, which reveals a pulsating mass in the midepigastrium. The diagnosis may first be suspected by x-ray of the abdomen, which demonstrates curvilinear calcification in the wall of the aneurysm. The diagnosis is confirmed by *ultrasound.* Continuous ultrasonic B scanning can visualize the abdominal aorta in longitudinal and transverse sections. This permits delineation of the size of the abdominal aorta and the thickness of its walls. It also allows detection of intraluminal clot (Fig. 197–1). Its noninvasive nature permits serial estimation of the size of the aneurysm. Abdominal aortic aneurysms increase their

FIGURE 197-1 *Aortic aneurysm. A. Longitudinal midline scan. B. Transverse scan just caudal to umbilicus. 1. Aortic aneurysm, 2. mural thrombus, 3. urinary bladder. [Reprinted with permission from HH Holm et al (eds): Abdominal Ultrasound: Static and Dynamic Scanning, 2d ed. Baltimore, University Park Press, 1980.]*

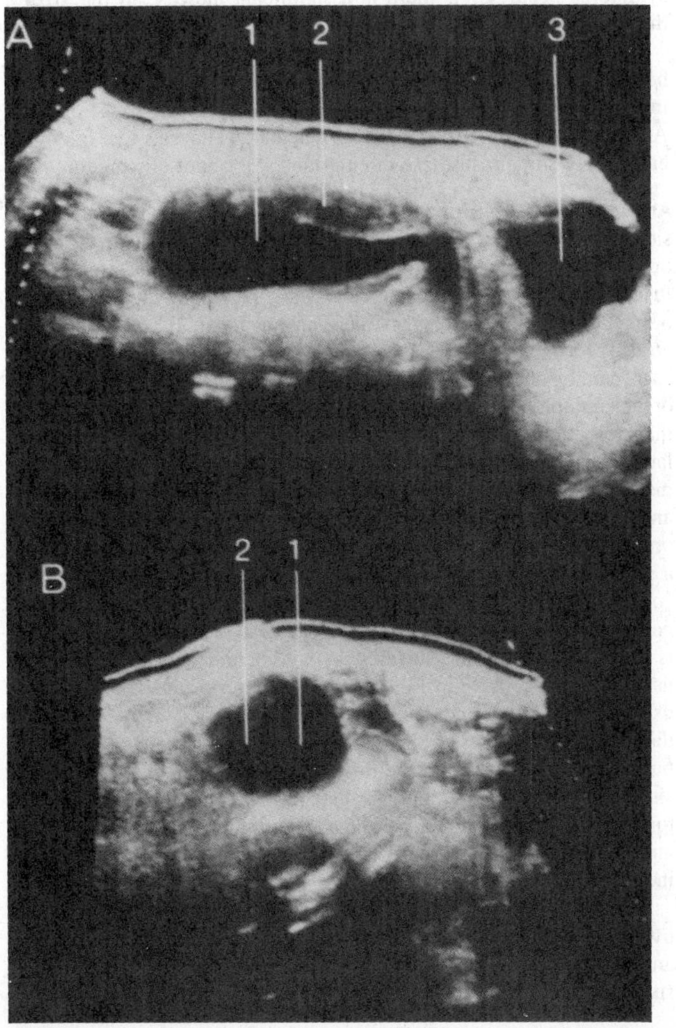

diameter at a rate of approximately 0.5 cm per year. Computed tomography can also accurately delineate abdominal aneurysms and may identify those that are at risk of rupture. Most patients are asymptomatic when the diagnosis is first made. When symptoms do occur, they consist of abdominal or low back pain.

The *prognosis* depends upon the size of the aneurysm and, very importantly, the presence of other arteriosclerotic cardiovascular diseases. The diameter of the normal abdominal aorta is 2.5 cm. When the diameter of the aneurysm is greater than 6 cm, the probability of rupture in a 10-year period is 45 to 50 percent, whereas it is only 15 to 20 percent when the diameter is less than 6 cm.

Ischemic arteriosclerotic heart disease, which is present in more than one-half of patients with abdominal aneurysm, has a profound impact on the prognosis. In one series of patients who did not have surgery, 5-year survival without clinically evident associated coronary disease was 50 percent. With ischemic heart disease, 5-year survival was only 20 percent. Follow-up of patients without surgery for abdominal aneurysms has shown that about one-third die of rupture of the aneurysm and one-third die of associated cardiovascular disease.

In properly selected patients operation prolongs life by preventing rupture. Symptomatic or expanding aneurysms and aneurysms more than 6 cm in diameter should have prompt surgical correction. The therapeutic decision for patients with asymptomatic aneurysms of moderate size (4 to 6 cm) is more difficult. Operative mortality with elective surgery, that is, before rupture, is about 5 to 10 percent. It is influenced by the size of the aneurysm but far more by the presence of associated cardiovascular disease. If there is no significant associated cardiovascular disease, small (4 to 6 cm) asymptomatic aneurysms should usually have surgical correction. With significant associated disease, it may be appropriate to follow the patient with serial ultrasound examinations. Surgery should be performed if symptoms occur, or if there is a significant increase in the size of the aneurysm.

Some patients with ruptured aneurysms survive long enough to become candidates for emergency surgical repair. They usually present in shock with severe pain in the abdomen, the lower back, or both. A tender pulsatile mass may be palpated. The salvage rate with emergency surgery in these circumstances is about 50 percent.

Aneurysms of the descending aorta The second most frequent site of aortic aneurysms is in the descending aorta just distal to the origin of the left subclavian artery. These aneurysms are usually fusiform and due to arteriosclerosis. Many patients with an aneurysm of the descending aorta also have an aneurysm of the abdominal aorta. Most patients are asymptomatic when the diagnosis is first suspected by chest x-ray and then confirmed by computed tomography or aortography. Resection of thoracic aneurysms is more difficult than resection of abdominal aneurysms. The risk of operation is in large part determined by associated cardiovascular or pulmonary disease. Operative therapy to prevent rupture is indicated if the aneurysm is symptomatic, larger than 10 cm in transverse diameter, or enlarging rapidly, unless associated cardiovascular disease presents a prohibitive risk.

Traumatic, false aneurysms of the descending aorta may occur in patients who survive rupture of the aorta. The most frequent cause is deceleration injuries suffered in automobile accidents. Rupture usually occurs at the site of the ligamentum arteriosum. These patients usually note chest and back pain similar to that associated with dissection. Blood pressure may be increased in the upper extremities but absent or decreased in the lower extremities. Chest x-ray usually shows mediastinal widening. The diagnosis is confirmed by computed tomography or angiography. These patients are likely to be young and without associated cardiovascular disease. Surgical repair is indicated.

Less frequently, aneurysms of the descending aorta are saccular owing to *syphilis* or other *infection* (mycotic aneurysms). Saccular aneurysms are particularly likely to rupture and should be treated surgically.

Aneurysms of the ascending aorta In a prior era, nearly all aneurysms of the ascending aorta were due to *syphilis*. They were readily recognized by x-ray by the presence of calcification in the wall of the ascending aorta. Luetic aneurysms can become huge, causing signs and symptoms by compression of adjacent structures. At the present time, the commonest cause of aneurysms of the ascending aorta is *cystic medial necrosis*, which may occur in association with Marfan's syndrome or as a response to hypertension and/or aging of the aorta, or may be of unknown etiology.

Aneurysms of the ascending aorta, particularly when they are due to cystic medial necrosis, may cause aortic regurgitation and lead to left ventricular failure. In this circumstance, resection of the aneurysm and replacement of the ascending aorta and aortic valve and coronary artery reimplantation are indicated.

The most common symptom of large aneurysms of the ascending aorta is chest pain, usually described as a deep, diffuse, aching sensation. The decision to resect an asymptomatic aneurysm to prevent rupture depends upon its size, the presence and severity of aortic regurgitation, and the presence of associated cardiovascular disease. More than half of these patients have additional aortic aneurysms.

Aneurysms of the aortic arch These aneurysms—the least frequent of all—are the most likely to cause symptoms because they compress adjacent structures, thus causing dysphagia, dry cough, hoarseness, dyspnea, or pain. Arch aneurysms may be fusiform due to arteriosclerosis, or saccular due to syphilis or other infection. Surgical correction of aneurysms of the aortic arch carries an operative risk as high as 40 to 50 percent.

Management of concurrent hypertension Hypertension, which is present in more than half of patients with aortic aneurysms, needs optimal management. Persistent systolic hypertension abets further enlargement of aneurysms and may predispose to their rupture. In addition to standard antihypertension medications, beta blockers are appropriate to help control hypertension and, in addition, decrease stress to the aortic wall by blunting myocardial contractility.

DISSECTION OF THE AORTA This occurs when the intima is interrupted so that blood enters the wall of the aorta and separates its layers. Dissection is the most frequent and the most important acute disease involving the aorta and without treatment is almost always fatal. With prompt diagnosis and appropriate therapy, the majority of patients survive.

As with aneurysm of the aorta, the basic defect that permits dissection is disease of the media. The commonest risk factor for dissection is hypertension. In patients with dissection of the ascending aorta severe arteriosclerosis is uncommon, but severe medial degeneration (cystic medial necrosis) is present in about one-fifth of cases. Cystic medial necrosis may be associated with Marfan's syndrome, which is present in about 10 percent of dissections. This inheritable connective tissue disorder (Chap. 319) is characterized by ocular and skeletal abnormalities in addition to the cardiovascular complications of dissection, aortic aneurysm, and mitral or aortic valve regurgitation. The majority of patients with Marfan's syndrome die of these cardiovascular complications, often before age 40. Coarctation of the aorta and bicuspid aortic valves also increase the risk of dissection of the ascending aorta.

Dissection of the descending aorta is often associated with severe arteriosclerosis as well as hypertension. Cystic medial necrosis is less common in the descending aorta.

Nearly all aortic dissections begin as a tear in the intima at one of two sites: the ascending aorta (2 to 5 cm above the aortic valve) or the descending aorta, just distal to the origin of the left subclavian artery. The aorta is relatively fixed in each of these two positions, but is mobile on each side. Thus, at these two points, the hemodynamic stress of each systolic pressure wave is maximal, and the intima overlying diseased media may tear there, permitting blood to enter and separate the layers of the aorta.

The signs and symptoms and, importantly, the therapeutic implications are quite different when dissection involves the ascending aorta as opposed to the descending aorta only.

Dissection of the ascending aorta Dissection usually begins as an intimal tear in the proximal ascending aorta. The so-called DeBakey type I dissection extends antegrade around the arch into the descending and abdominal aorta, while type II is confined to the ascending aorta. Dissection of the ascending aorta is the most common and the most lethal. In other cases, the intimal tear may occur in the aortic arch or descending aorta, and the dissection may progress retrograde to involve the ascending aorta. The majority of these patients are men under age 60. About one-half have hypertension.

Dissection of the ascending aorta is heralded by the abrupt onset of very severe chest pain. Unlike the pain of myocardial infarction, the pain is maximal at the onset. The pain is most frequent in the anterior chest, but may radiate to, or even be limited to, the midscapular area of the back. The pain is nearly always initially attributed to acute myocardial infarction. There are several ways that the appropriate diagnosis may be made. Since dissection of the ascending aorta involves the great vessels in the majority of cases, a discrepancy between the carotid pulses, or a difference in the blood pressure in the two arms, should lead to a search for other evidence of aortic dissection. Dissection involving the carotids can cause a sudden neurologic deficit that may be intermittent. If the dissection compromises the right coronary artery, arrhythmias may occur, and occasionally there may be electrocardiographic signs of acute inferior myocardial infarction. In approximately one-half of patients, the dissection causes acute aortic regurgitation. The presence of a new murmur of aortic regurgitation in the setting of apparent myocardial infarction should suggest the possibility of dissection of the ascending aorta. In the most severe cases, dissection causes hemopericardium. The appearance of a pericardial friction rub may be rapidly followed by pericardial tamponade.

Chest x-rays provide the most important clue to the presence of dissection of the ascending aorta. The most consistent finding is widening of the superior mediastinum. The ascending aorta may be enlarged out of proportion to the descending aorta. Once dissection is suspected by physical examination or chest x-ray, preparations for aortography to confirm the diagnosis should be made at once. Dissection of the ascending aorta can also be recognized by computed tomography or echocardiography. Unless hypotension is present, medical treatment, aimed at lowering blood pressure and depressing myocardial contractility, should be begun. This is most appropriately effected by beginning an infusion of nitroprusside, 20 to 400 ng/min, or trimethaphan, 1 to 2 mg/min, with intraarterial pressure monitoring in place.

Cineangiography of the aorta performed by the retrograde arterial technique will usually demonstrate a false lumen, and possibly an intimal flap separating the true and false lumina in the ascending aorta. If the blood in the false lumen has clotted, the principal finding will be an abnormal narrowing of the true lumen.

Once the diagnosis of dissection involving the ascending aorta has been established by aortography, the majority of patients should have surgical correction, which consists of resection of the portion of the aorta containing the intimal tear and replacement with a prosthetic graft. Concomitant aortic valve replacement may be required if severe aortic regurgitation is present. Surgical correction can be performed at a risk of about 20 percent. Although medical treatment is vital to stabilize the patient prior to operation, it rarely is definitive in patients with dissection involving the ascending aorta because the majority develop life-threatening complications, such as hemopericardium, hypotension, compromise of the carotid or coronary arteries, or aortic regurgitation. Without treatment, death is usually due to rupture into the pericardium.

Dissection of the descending aorta (DeBakey type III dissection) Dissection limited to the descending aorta is most likely to occur in elderly hypertensive patients with arteriosclerosis of the aorta. Dissection ordinarily begins with an intimal tear just beyond the origin of the left subclavian artery, and the hematoma proceeds distally to the diaphragm or into the abdominal aorta. Dissection of the descending aorta usually does not proceed in retrograde fashion. Therefore, aortic regurgitation and hemopericardium do not occur. The carotid pulses and blood pressure in the arms are usually not altered. The primary symptom is the sudden onset of chest pain, often interscapular, often radiating to the anterior chest. The prime supporting evidence of dissection is to be found in the chest roentgenogram, which usually shows a widening of the superior mediastinum and may show the descending to be larger than the ascending aorta. If there is intimal calcification in the aortic knob, its distance from the outer border of the aortic shadow may be increased.

The diagnosis of dissection of the descending aorta should be confirmed by aortography. As with dissection involving the ascending aorta, hypotensive treatment should begin when the diagnosis is first suspected. Nitroprusside or trimethaphan, in a continuous intravenous drip at an infusion rate sufficient to keep systolic pressure at 100 to 120 mmHg are the ideal first drugs. A beta blocker or reserpine should also be begun.

Patients with dissection of the descending aorta usually do not have urgent indications for surgical correction. Medical treatment to lower systolic pressure, and to depress myocardial contractility so as to blunt the force of systole, may control the dissection. If medical treatment does not relieve the pain, or if there is evidence of progression of the dissection by x-ray or the appearance of a left pleural effusion (due to hemothorax), surgical resection should be performed. Surgical correction of dissection of the descending aorta poses a higher risk than dissection of the ascending aorta because the patients are older and are more likely to have associated cardiovascular disease. Elective surgical correction may be indicated after the dissection is controlled with medical therapy.

Prolonged, optimal control of hypertension is essential in patients with dissection of the ascending or descending aorta. In the absence of overt or latent congestive heart failure, it is advisable to include beta blockers in the regimen to help prevent recurrent dissection. An important complication of aortic dissection is formation of aneurysms. Rupture of these aneurysms is the commonest cause of late death. Follow-up of patients treated for dissection should include periodic computerized tomography of the chest to detect the formation or enlargement of a thoracic aortic aneurysm.

ARTERIOSCLEROTIC OCCLUSIVE DISEASE The majority of adults in the United States have some degree of arteriosclerosis of the aorta. However, the disease remains silent unless it causes aneurysm, or unless it is sufficiently advanced to cause occlusive disease. The mildest form of arteriosclerosis of the aorta, longitudinal fatty streaks of the intima, may be seen in children (Chap. 195). Elevated intimal plaques begin to appear in adult life. Occlusive disease of the aorta may occur if these plaques are complicated by hemorrhage, ulceration, calcification, or overlying thrombus formation.

Arteriosclerotic occlusive disease is most frequent in the abdominal aorta, where it involves the terminal part of the aorta and extends for a variable distance into the iliac and femoral arteries. Diabetes and cigarette smoking increase the severity of arteriosclerotic occlusive disease. Arteriosclerosis of the aorta may be complicated by superimposed thrombosis. Depending upon the adequacy of collateral circulation, arteriosclerotic occlusive disease may cause ischemia of the lower extremities.

The classic symptom is claudication, which is present in the buttocks and thighs or in the calves. If the occlusive disease is severe, or the collateral circulation is poor, severe ischemia may lead to pain at rest or tissue necrosis and gangrene. Impotence may also occur. The femoral pulses are absent or diminished in the majority of cases. The diagnosis of arteriosclerotic occlusive disease is confirmed by measuring segmental systolic pressure in the lower extremities with

Doppler ultrasound before and after exercise. Arteriography is needed to delineate the extent of the disease if surgical correction is indicated.

Surgical treatment consists of aortic-femoral bypass grafting. The results of operation are usually excellent; symptoms are relieved or decreased in more than 90 percent of the patients in some series. Patency rates of 80 to 90 percent at 10 years have been reported. Endarterectomy may be indicated when the disease is limited to the terminal aorta and proximal iliac arteries. Transluminal angioplasty performed by the percutaneous technique may also be effective in patients with iliac disease. As with aneurysms, operative and late death is usually due to associated ischemic heart disease, which is present in up to one-half of the patients. The status of the coronary and cerebrovascular circulations should be assessed prior to operation.

Symptomatic arteriosclerotic occlusive disease is rare in the ascending or descending thoracic aorta but may occur in the arch, where it becomes symptomatic by compromising the origin of one or more of the arch vessels. The carotid pulses, and/or pulses of the upper extremities, may be obliterated; thus, arteriosclerotic occlusive disease is one of the causes of the aortic arch syndrome. Other causes of this syndrome (also called "pulseless disease") include Takayasu's arteritis, syphilis, trauma, and neoplasm. Symptoms may include ischemia of the upper extremities or, more commonly, cerebrovascular ischemia, dependent upon the location of the disease. Surgical correction is usually feasible, utilizing a bypass graft; however, its appropriateness depends upon the extent of the disease, and the status of the coronary and cerebral circulations.

AORTITIS Several different diseases may cause aortitis, i.e., an inflammatory process involving the wall of the aorta. The pathophysiology of aortitis depends on the severity of the process and upon its location. Aortitis becomes most evident when it involves the origins of the vessels of the aortic arch. Under these circumstances, it can, as noted above, cause the aortic arch syndrome.

The best understood cause of aortitis is *syphilis*. Only 10 percent of patients with luetic aortitis develop complications that permit its detection during life: saccular thoracic aneurysms, aortic valvulitis causing aortic regurgitation, and stenosis of the coronary ostia. Uncomplicated luetic aortitis is recognized at postmortem as a chronic panarteritis that causes patchy destruction of smooth muscle and elastic tissue of the media, endarteritis obliterans of the vasa vasorum, and intimal atherosclerosis. The process is most marked in the ascending aorta because of the predilection of treponemas for its rich lymphatic supply. The only clinical correlates of uncomplicated luetic aortitis are dilatation of the ascending aorta with or without calcification and a tambour-like aortic second sound.

TAKAYASU'S DISEASE Takayasu's disease is a nonspecific obstructive arteritis that has a particular predilection for young females. It is more common in the orient than in the west. Although it is suspected to be an autoimmune disease, its exact etiology is unknown. In the majority of cases, the disease begins in the second or third decade of life. In its initial stage, constitutional symptoms may occur. These may include fever, malaise, anorexia, weight loss, night sweats, and at times arthralgias. The erythrocyte sedimentation rate is elevated.

These constitutional symptoms are then replaced by signs and symptoms secondary to involvement of the large arteries, particularly the aortic arch and its main branches. The pathologic lesion is a panarteritis that seems to begin with inflammation of the adventitia, with subsequent disruption and fibrotic changes in the media, and marked proliferation of the intima. Involvement of the arch vessels may be heralded by local pain and the presence of bruits. The activity of the disease is variable over time. Increased activity is usually associated with an increase in the erythrocyte sedimentation rate. Progression of the aortitis causes stenosis at, or obliteration of, the origins of the arch vessels, thereby causing the aortic arch syndrome. Obstruction of the carotid arteries causes ischemic retinopathy, blurred vision, syncope, and dizziness secondary to cerebral ischemia. Involvement of the subclavian arteries causes paresthesias, intermittent claudication, and loss of pulses of the upper extremities. In addition to segmental obstructions, aneurysms and aortic regurgitation may occur. The pulmonary arteries may be involved in some cases. Hypertension occurs in the majority of cases owing to involvement of the renal arteries or to suprarenal obstruction of the aorta. The presence of hypertension, with absent pulses in the upper extremities, has caused this syndrome to be called *reversed coarctation*. The diagnosis is confirmed by angiographic study of the aorta.

Although some studies have shown that corticosteroid therapy may alleviate some of the constitutional symptoms of this disease, there is no evidence that treatment improves life expectancy. Reconstructive vascular surgery may relieve symptoms; however, the disease follows a relentless course so that death from congestive failure or stroke usually occurs within 5 years of diagnosis.

REFERENCES

Crawford ES, Cohen ES: Aortic aneurysm: A multifocal disease. Arch Surg 117:1393, 1982

Dalen JE et al: Dissection of the aorta: Pathogenesis, diagnosis, and treatment. Prog Cardiovasc Dis 23:237, 1980

DeBakey ME et al: Aneurysms of the thoracic aorta. Mod Concepts Cardiovasc Dis 10:53, 1975

——— et al: Dissection and dissecting aneurysms of the aorta: Twenty-year follow-up of five hundred twenty-seven patients treated surgically. Surgery 92:1118, 1982

Dinsmore RE et al: Magnetic resonance imaging of thoracic aortic aneurysms: Comparison with other imaging methods. AJR 146:309, 1986

Grossman E et al: Clinical use of captopril in Takayasu's disease. Arch Intern Med 144: 95, 1984

Hall S et al: Takayasu arteritis. A study of 32 North American patients. Medicine 64:89, 1985

Larson EW, Edwards WD: Risk factors for aortic dissection: A necropsy study of 161 cases. Am J Cardiol 53:849, 1984

Lupi-Herrera E et al: Takayasu's arteritis: Clinical study of 107 cases. Am Heart J 93:94, 1977

Malone JM et al: The natural history of bilateral aortofemoral bypass grafts for ischemia of the lower extremities. Arch Surg 110:1300, 1975

Miller DC et al: Operative treatment of aortic dissections: Experience with 125 patients over a sixteen-year period. J Thorac Cardiovasc Surg 78:365, 1979

Norrgard O et al: Familial occurrence of abdominal aortic aneurysms. Surgery 95:650, 1984

Slater EE, DeSanctis RW: Disease of the aorta, in *Heart Disease*, 2d ed, E Braunwald (ed). Philadelphia, Saunders, 1984, p 1540

Smuckler AL et al: Echocardiographic diagnosis of aortic root dissection by M-mode and two-dimensional techniques. Am Heart J 103:897, 1982

White RD et al: Noninvasive evaluation of suspected thoracic aortic disease by contrast-enhanced computed tomography. Am J Cardiol 57:282, 1986

198 VASCULAR DISEASES OF THE EXTREMITIES

D. EUGENE STRANDNESS, JR.

The correct approach to patients with suspected peripheral vascular disease is to identify the system involved (arterial, venous, or lymphatic), estimate the degree of disability, and determine if special tests are required to clarify further the extent of the involvement. The therapy employed depends upon a knowledge of the natural history of the disorder as related to known risk factors, the potential for further complications, and the likelihood that available therapy will be successful.

ARTERIAL DISORDERS

ACUTE ARTERIAL OCCLUSION Sudden interruption of the blood supply results in a spectrum of symptoms and signs which are dependent upon the location and extent of the occlusion and existing collateral circulation. The major causes are embolism, thrombosis, and injury. In the arm, the heart is the source of emboli in 95 percent of the patients. Less common causes include emboli from ulcerated plaques in the subclavian artery, aneurysms of the arch vessels, and paradoxical emboli via a patent foramen ovale.

In the leg, the heart is again the most common source of emboli, but they may also arise from ulcerated plaques and aneurysms of the thoracic, abdominal, femoral, and popliteal arteries. Over half of the large emboli from the heart lodge in the femoral or popliteal arteries. The iliac arteries are involved in approximately one-fifth, the abdominal aorta in one-sixth. The remainder will occlude the tibial or peroneal vessels.

When the heart is the source, the causes include mural thrombi from the left atrium or ventricle and the aortic or mitral valve. Mural thrombi arise secondary to atrial fibrillation or on the endocardial surface of the ventricle secondary to myocardial infarction. A prosthetic valve in either the aortic or mitral position may also be the source. While uncommon, the possibility of an atrial myxoma must always be kept in mind. When emboli arise from ulcerated plaques or aneurysms, they are often small and lodge in the small arteries of the distal limb. When they arise from the abdominal or thoracic aorta, bilateral involvement is the rule.

Arterial thrombosis occurs secondary to injury, arteriosclerosis obliterans, femoral or popliteal aneurysms, collagen vascular diseases, myeloproliferative disorders, disseminated intravascular coagulation, and the dysproteinemias.

Symptoms and signs Acute arterial occlusion results in symptoms and signs related to the site of involvement and the immediately available collateral circulation. If the pressure distal to the obstruction falls to below 40 mmHg, the clinical picture will be dramatic. The initial complaint is pain in the most distal part of the limb, followed by pallor, coldness, and a sensation of numbness. Cutaneous sensation is lost within the first hour. Within 6 h, ischemic muscular contracture develops associated with subcutaneous hemorrhage and focal areas of gangrene. Fixed staining of the skin is the most certain sign of irreversible tissue death.

If limb viability is not in question, pallor, a decrease in temperature, and numbness may be the only complaints. The appearance of rest pain in the digits and forefoot indicates that arterial inflow is marginal. Pulses are absent distal to the site of occlusion.

Though the diagnosis is rarely difficult when the extent of the ischemia is as outlined above, there are important variations in the clinical picture. If the immediately available collateral circulation is sufficient to maintain viability, the patient may complain only of a sensation of numbness, usually accompanied by a decrease in the temperature of the part. Under these circumstances, the circulation will nearly always improve, with these minor symptoms disappearing over the course of several hours.

Diagnosis The most important elements include a history of the sudden onset of pain, coldness, and numbness. If a combination of pain, pallor, and paralysis is noted, limb viability will be lost unless the responsible lesion can be corrected within a time frame of 6 h or less. If the limb remains viable, the only complaints may be coldness and numbness. Detection of a bruit is common when an arterial plaque or aneurysm is the source of the embolus.

When the leg is affected, it is important to determine if there is a history of intermittent claudication since under these circumstances, the acute ischemia may be due to thrombosis on an ulcerated plaque. When cholesterol emboli occur, the symptoms may be confusing depending upon the source. The most common situation is the "blue-toe" syndrome, which may be bilateral if the origin is the abdominal or thoracic aorta. Ischemic rest pain is often present and accompanied by prominent livedo reticularis of the feet. Peripheral pulses are nearly always present, since emboli rarely pass through collateral arteries in sufficient quantity to produce serious foot ischemia. When these tiny emboli originate from the thoracic aorta, abdominal pain and hematuria may also occur. Aneurysms of the femoral and popliteal arteries must always be kept in mind. The initial manifestation is often thrombosis or embolization. The diagnosis may be suspected by physical examination and verified by B-mode ultrasound.

Arteriography is rarely necessary to make the diagnosis of major artery occlusion and results in needless, dangerous delay when severe ischemia is present.

Treatment When limb viability is threatened, immediate operation is required for occlusion of the major arteries. Heparin should be given immediately. The occlusion may usually be removed under local anesthesia, but in some instances it may be necessary to bypass the obstructed area. If limb viability is not in doubt, streptokinase to urokinase should be considered, since lysis may be achieved by infusion of low doses directly into the thrombosis via an arterial catheter. When the acute occlusion is secondary to thrombosis in proximity to a stenosis, the underlying defect may be corrected by either transluminal angioplasty or bypass grafting after lysis of the thrombus. If the cause of the problem is embolic, long-term anticoagulation with coumadin should be employed. Chronic subcutaneous heparin, while also effective, should be used with caution since it may lead to the development of osteoporosis. Patients with microemboli should be treated expectantly with aspirin. On occasion it may be necessary to remove or bypass an ulcerated plaque responsible for the emboli, but usually surgery is reserved for those patients with aneurysms (particularly femoral and popliteal) that might be the source of emboli. Vasodilator drugs are not useful.

ARTERIOSCLEROSIS OBLITERANS The primary lesion of arteriosclerosis is the intimal plaque, which progressively narrows and, in many instances, leads to complete occlusion of large and medium-sized arteries (Chap. 195). In the abdomen the disease has its highest incidence in the aorta and common iliac arteries. The external iliac arteries are often spared. Distal to the inguinal ligament, occlusions are most common in the adductor canal, with the popliteal artery itself down to the level of its three major branches having a much lower incidence of involvement. In the lower leg, the posterior tibial artery at the ankle and the anterior tibial at its origin are most commonly diseased. Arteriosclerosis obliterans is usually a segmental disease, with marked variation from patient to patient in its extent.

Clinical features Unless complicated by thrombosis, the symptoms and signs that develop secondary to arteriosclerosis obliterans rarely have an abrupt onset, since the process is a gradual, progressive one. The most common symptom occurs with exercise and is termed *intermittent claudication,* i.e., the pain that occurs in a muscle(s) with an inadequate blood supply that is stressed by exercise. The patient often describes the discomfort as a cramp which disappears within 1 or 2 min after stopping the exercise. Occasionally, profound weakness will be noted as exercise progresses. The walk-pain-rest cycle is constant from day to day, which is the hallmark of this particularly troublesome complaint. The pain never occurs with standing or sitting. The pain is more severe and the walking distance is always shortened when the patient walks upstairs and up a hill.

A point not often appreciated is that, with arteriosclerosis obliterans, claudication does not occur with occlusions in the anterior tibial, posterior tibial, or peroneal arteries. The location of the involved muscle group(s) is useful in predicting the most proximal level of occlusion. For example, calf and thigh claudication suggests that the primary involvement is proximal to the origin of the thigh muscles, i.e., the profunda femoris artery. The combination of hip, thigh, and buttock claudication with impotence in a middle-aged male indicates terminal aortic occlusion, the *Leriche syndrome.*

The second important group of symptoms consists of those which occur at rest and are the result of either multiple levels of occlusion or involvement of a critical arterial segment where the major collaterals are also obstructed. Paresthesias and indeed numbness may occur but are less common than continuous pain in the toes or foot, which may be partially or completely relieved by dependency. Ulceration and gangrene of the toes and distal foot are a common occurrence when the disease reaches this advanced stage.

The patient with diabetes mellitus often presents variations in the clinical picture. Approximately 30 percent of patients with diabetes have a peripheral neuropathy which results in loss of deep pain sensation and sympathetic tone. When diabetics with a neuropathy develop ulcers with or without arterial occlusion, the lesions are typically painless. The combination of chronic arterial occlusion, peripheral neuropathy, and a nonhealing ulcer is a difficult therapeutic problem.

The physical examination is useful in substantiating the diagnosis and localizing the levels of disease. Patients with single occlusions in the aortoiliac or superficial femoral artery often have limbs which are normal in appearance. Patients with far-advanced disease secondary to multiple levels of disease often have ulcers, gangrene, loss of hair, trophic nail changes, and dependent rubor. Chronic arterial narrowing and occlusion lead to loss of pulses distal to the most proximal level of disease. The pulses should be examined in the groin, in the popliteal fossa, and at the level of the ankle. If the involvement results in narrowing only, bruits are commonly heard which are transmitted for varying distances downstream from the stenosis. Auscultation should be performed from the level of the midabdomen to the popliteal artery; one should listen for the characteristic sound which is diagnostic of arterial narrowing.

Special diagnostic tests The magnitude of the physiologic derangement can be assessed simply by measuring the ankle systolic blood pressure at rest and following exercise to the point of claudication. Since arterial occlusion forces the blood to follow alternate pathways (collaterals) whose resistance to flow exceeds that of the normal vessel, an abnormal pressure gradient develops which lowers the pressure recorded at the ankle. The pressure may be measured by a variety of plethysmographs or the ultrasonic velocity detector. In general, if the systolic pressure at the ankle is greater than one-half that recorded from the arm, occlusion of one segment is most likely. Ankle pressures less than one-half of the arm systolic pressure are most often observed with multiple levels of disease.

When the patient with intermittent claudication exercises to the point of pain, the postexercise ankle blood pressure falls, often to unrecordable levels, requiring several minutes to return to the prewalking level. With exercise there is a marked fall in arterial resistance in the muscle. The amount of inflow available through the collateral arteries is inadequate because of their high resistance to flow. As a consequence, distal arterial pressure falls and blood is shunted away from the foot. These changes explain the pallor in the foot which is so commonly observed during and immediately following exercise to the point of claudication. This test is most useful in following the progress of disease with and without therapy and is the most sensitive index of change available. Its great utility lies in the fact that each patient can serve as his or her own control.

Arteriography is essential prior to operation to localize precisely the disease and the extent of the involvement. With the introduction of ultrasonic duplex scanning, it is now feasible to scan the arterial system from the level of the celiac artery to the popliteal artery. Segments which are narrowed or occluded are readily identified. This method is useful in selecting patients for transluminal angioplasty and surgery and documenting the results of therapy.

Differential diagnosis It is rarely difficult to make the diagnosis of chronic arterial narrowing or occlusion when the clinical impression is combined with measurements of ankle blood pressure. However, there is a recognized subset of conditions, lumped under the title of "pseudoclaudication," that are not uncommon and may be a source of some confusion.

The features of the symptom complex which are useful in distinguishing it from true intermittent claudication include the following: (1) the exercise-pain-rest cycle is not constant; (2) the symptoms may include numbness, tingling, weakness, incoordination, and clumsiness; (3) patients with pseudoclaudication may have to sit down or even lie down for relief; and (4) the time required for the pain to disappear often exceeds the few minutes observed in claudication due to arterial occlusion. When it becomes clear that chronic arterial disease is not the basis for the leg pain, it is necessary to investigate the back and hip areas since diseases such as spinal stenosis, herniated nucleus pulposus, spinal cord tumors, and degenerative joint disease may be responsible for the patient's complaints.

Therapy Patients with mild or moderate intermittent claudication may benefit from a rigorous, daily exercise training program. The essential features of this program include (1) repetitive daily walks to 75 percent of the claudication distance with interspersed periods of rest (1 to 2 min); (2) weekly retesting of maximum walking time with readjustment of walking distance; and (3) continuation of the exercise program—this is essential, since evidence suggests that cessation of the daily walking periods will result in loss of improvement. A new drug, pentoxifylline, has become available which may improve muscle perfusion by decreasing blood viscosity. A multicenter trial in this country showed use of this drug resulted in a modest (59 percent) increase in the initial claudication distance over placebo in a group of patients with claudication. Vasodilator drugs are of no value.

Weight reduction can be useful in patients with intermittent claudication by simply reducing the workload involved. It is also important that *smoking be stopped* entirely. All patients with arteriosclerosis should have their serum lipid levels determined, since they may be found to have a treatable disorder (Chap. 195). Direct arterial surgery may be effective in bypassing or removing areas of occlusion but should be reserved for those patients with disabling claudication.

Transluminal angioplasty provides an excellent method of dealing with stenoses involving the aortoiliac segments, giving results comparable to those obtained by direct arterial surgery. The long-term patency below the groin is not as good as with the iliac arteries, but the procedure can be used when a short-term flow increase may be of benefit in providing the necessary increased blood flow to heal open, painful ulcers.

Most patients with ischemic rest pain, ulcers, or gangrene present serious problems which can be helped only by direct arterial surgery. Lumbar sympathectomy may be useful but should be used *only* in patients with mild rest pain. If the rest pain is controlled by nonnarcotic analgesics and transient dependency, about 50 percent of these patients can obtain permanent pain relief by lumbar sympathectomy.

The majority of patients with arteriosclerosis obliterans will never require surgical therapy even though they do suffer some disability. The nondiabetic will have a limb loss rate of about 2 percent per year; this rate increases to 7 percent per year if the patient has diabetes mellitus. Meticulous foot care, which includes properly fitting shoes, and immediate attention to cuts and blisters are critical in proper management. This is particularly true in patients with diabetes and a peripheral neuropathy who are unable to appreciate deep pain.

Selected patients with isolated stenoses of the iliac arteries or superficial femoral artery may be candidates for transluminal dilatation with a balloon catheter. The early results are promising, but performance of the procedure must be a joint decision between the radiologist and vascular surgeon.

THROMBOANGIITIS OBLITERANS (BUERGER'S DISEASE) In 1908 Buerger described a nonatheromatous lesion involving arteries, veins, and nerves occurring in young males and frequently leading to nonhealing ulcers and gangrene. The exact pathogenesis is obscure, but there appears to be a definite relationship with tobacco smoking or chewing. Recent studies have shown that patients with Buerger's disease may have abnormal cellular and humoral immune responses to type I and type III collagen. This provides further support for its existence as a distinct vascular disease and its diagnosis by means of immunologic testing.

The disease typically occurs in young males and has a characteristic location and set of clinical manifestations. Whereas arteriosclerosis obliterans is a segmental disease of large and medium-sized arteries, Buerger's disease starts in the smaller arteries of the hands and feet. There is usually an intense inflammatory component, which in later stages results in arterial and venous occlusion as well as fibrous encasement of the entire neurovascular bundle.

Clinical features The diagnosis of Buerger's disease should be suspected when male patients in the 20- to 40-year age range give the following history: A superficial, migratory nodular phlebitis may occur early in the disease. These nodules are well localized, associated with cutaneous erythema, and tender to touch. Cold sensitivity of the Raynaud's type occurs in about one-half the patients and is frequently confined to the hands. The fingers turn white when exposed to cold, then blue, and finally red—the so-called triphasic color response.

One of the most characteristic and typical symptoms of Buerger's disease is *instep claudication*. Exercise results in pain in the instep, promptly relieved by rest. Calf claudication may occur but is unusual, since the disease does not commonly progress proximally to involve and occlude either the popliteal or superficial femoral artery. When there is hand involvement, the occlusions may be bilateral, are often symmetric, and may lead to the development of hand claudication and fingertip ulcers which are exquisitely painful and difficult to heal.

The following findings during *physical examination* should lead one to suspect Buerger's disease: (1) intense rubor of the feet; (2) absent foot pulses in the presence of a normal femoral and popliteal pulse; and (3) reduction or absence of the radial and/or ulnar pulses.

Therapy There is only one effective treatment, and that is permanent, complete abstinence from tobacco. However, for some unknown reason, patients with Buerger's disease rarely discontinue smoking even though amputation is usually the inevitable consequence and the only method available of controlling the severe rest pain and ulceration which ultimately develop.

ARTERIOVENOUS FISTULAS **Acquired** Most acquired arteriovenous fistulas occur secondary to penetrating injuries; however, they may in certain circumstances occur secondary to blunt trauma. Malignancy, infection, and arterial aneurysms have also been responsible for the development of arteriovenous communications.

CLINICAL PICTURE Patients with penetrating injuries of an extremity should all be suspected of having an arteriovenous fistula. Initially there are no distinguishing symptoms which alert the physician to the presence of the fistula. The diagnosis is made by noting a continuous murmur and palpable thrill over the abnormal communication. Compression of the feeding artery will obliterate the murmur and thrill. With large fistulas compression of the feeding artery results in an abrupt slowing of the heart rate (Branham's sign). In rare instances distal arterial perfusion may be so severely impaired that gangrene develops.

With chronic fistulas the clinical manifestations may mimic those of venous disease, with varicose veins, stasis pigmentation, and cutaneous ulcers. Cardiac enlargement with or without failure may be seen in long-standing fistulas. Infection (bacterial endarteritis) may complicate large fistulas.

THERAPY The proper treatment of arteriovenous fistulas is division of the communication with maintenance of arterial continuity. Immediate operation may be indicated with large fistulas between such vessels as the abdominal aorta and inferior vena cava where cardiac failure may develop very quickly.

Congenital The development of anomalous communications between arteries and veins can pose both diagnostic and therapeutic difficulties. When there is an arrest in the development of the circulation during the stage of an undifferentiated capillary network, a *cavernous hemangioma* results. There is at this period an interlacing system of blood spaces which contain mixed blood, and it is impossible to distinguish the arterial and venous components.

When the development is arrested at the stage of differentiation, intercommunicating arteriovenous channels may persist. If the fistulas are large enough to be visualized arteriographically, the term used is congenital *macrofistulous arteriovenous aneurysm*. When the fistulas are too small to be visualized by arteriography, the term *microfistulous communication* should be used. This classification, based upon the size of the communications, is useful from a therapeutic standpoint.

CLINICAL MANIFESTATIONS The clinical manifestations are extremely variable and largely depend upon the location and extent of the abnormal communications. The most common symptoms are (1) cosmetic changes due to the presence of the fistulas in the subcutaneous tissue and skin, (2) limb swelling and hypertrophy, (3) visible pulsations in some cases with macrofistulous communications, and (4) varicose veins in atypical locations. In long-standing cases stasis pigmentation and cutaneous ulcers may develop in response to the continued venous hypertension.

DIAGNOSIS The presence of arteriovenous fistulas should be suspected when the following findings are presented: (1) unilateral leg or arm swelling, (2) cutaneous hemangioma of the "port-wine" variety, (3) varicose veins in atypical locations, and (4) an increase in temperature of the part. An important syndrome which may be confused with congenital arteriovenous fistulas is the *Klippel-Trénaunay* syndrome. The triad of this syndrome consists of varicose veins, "port-wine" hemangioma of the skin, and bone and soft-tissue hypertrophy. The arteriovenous communications are rarely demonstrable by arteriography.

THERAPY The management of congenital arteriovenous fistulas depends entirely upon location, extent, and clinical manifestations. Treatment is largely conservative, with support stockings used to control the venous hypertension and valvular incompetence which often produce symptoms identical with those of the postthrombotic syndrome. If the fistulas are limited in extent, it may be possible to excise the lesions in their entirety, but this is usually not feasible.

THORACIC OUTLET SYNDROMES The neurovascular bundle, by virtue of its course from the neck and thorax, is subject to compression by both muscular and skeletal structures. The symptoms which may develop include numbness and paresthesias (usually in the ulnar distribution) and pain which is brought on by a position of the arm that results in compression of the brachial plexus. From a diagnostic standpoint, obliteration of the radial pulse in a variety of arm positions has been considered the distinguishing feature of the underlying problem. This should no longer be considered the key diagnostic test since it frequently occurs in normal subjects. Further, the symptoms are generally due to compression of the brachial plexus and not the subclavian artery.

Those patients with the most prominent symptoms and signs will have cervical ribs with an associated fibrous band which attaches to the first rib producing compression of the neurovascular bundle. The key diagnostic features in these patients are (1) prompt appearance of paresthesias and numbness with the arm abducted to 90° and externally rotated, (2) appearance of a prominent bruit in the supraclavicular fossa, and (3) immediate disappearance of the symptoms when the arm is returned to the neutral position. There is little doubt that chronic arterial compression can lead to aneurysmal dilatation of the subclavian artery with occlusion and/or emboli, but this is rare.

In the absence of a *clear-cut* relationship between arm position and the symptoms, it is essential to rule out other causes for the clinical picture, which includes a cervical disc, degenerative joint disease, and the carpal tunnel syndrome. If cold sensitivity is also present, the vasospastic syndromes discussed in the next section must be ruled out. Removal of the first rib is performed too frequently and must be reserved for only those patients in whom the diagnosis is clear and other causes have been ruled out. The best results will be obtained in patients with cervical ribs in whom the relationship between arm position and neurovascular compression is easily demonstrated.

VASOSPASTIC DISORDERS The diseases in this category include primary and secondary cold sensitivity of the Raynaud's type, livedo reticularis, and acrocyanosis. The challenge in dealing with these entities is not in making the correct diagnosis but rather in determining if there is an associated disease responsible for the symptoms and signs. Those that are primary, e.g., without underlying disease, are generally benign, rarely lead to digit ulcers, and never terminate fatally.

Cold sensitivity of the Raynaud's type To establish this diagnosis, it is necessary to determine if a "triphasic" color response occurs, i.e., pallor, cyanosis, and rubor in that sequence. The most important element is the pallor, during which the digits turn absolutely white.

Livedo reticularis Livedo reticularis presents with a persistent cyanotic mottling of the skin which has a typical "fishnet" appearance. In contrast to Raynaud's disease, a phenomenon which is confined to the digits, livedo reticularis may involve all parts of the extremities and trunk. This cutaneous pattern is often accentuated by exposure to cold.

Acrocyanosis The most uncommon of the vasospastic disorders is acrocyanosis, which is characterized by a persistent diffuse cyanosis of the fingers, hands, toes, and feet. This disease is benign and not associated with an underlying disorder. The involved parts are nearly always cold, with excessive perspiration being a common accompanying feature.

Diagnosis Primary cold sensitivity of the Raynaud's type is more common in women, often starting in the late teens, is bilateral and symmetric, and rarely leads to fingertip ulcers or gangrene. The hands are more commonly affected than the feet. Those factors which should lead the clinician to suspect an underlying disorder include (1) abrupt onset with rapid progression to tissue necrosis; (2) late onset in life (age greater than 50 years), particularly in men; (3) unilateral or asymmetric involvement; and (4) associated symptoms compatible with a systemic disease.

Sorting out the underlying causes is often difficult because of the wide variety of diseases which may have cold sensitivity as a part of their clinical picture. The following diseases must be kept in mind: (1) chronic arterial disease, most particularly thromboangiitis obliterans; (2) the collagen vascular disorders, with scleroderma being the most common; (3) occupational and industrial exposure to vibrating instruments; (4) poisoning with lead and arsenic; (5) ingestion of drugs, namely, the ergotamine preparations, methysergide, and propranolol; (6) hematologic disorders, namely, cryoglobulins, cold agglutinins, and dysproteinemias; (7) bilateral thoracic outlet syndromes; (8) late sequelae of bilateral cold injury; (9) primary pulmonary hypertension; and (10) occult carcinoma.

The secondary causes of livedo reticularis include (1) collagen diseases, in particular periarteritis nodosa and disseminated lupus erythematosus; (2) hematologic disorders, i.e., hyperviscosity syndrome, macroglobulinemia, and cryoglobulinemia; (3) cholesterol emboli arising from ulcerated plaques in the thoracic and abdominal aorta; (4) Cushing's syndrome; (5) drug ingestion, i.e., adrenal corticosteroids; (6) prolonged dependency or immobilization; (7) late result of cold injury; and (8) prolonged exposure to or the local application of heat.

Therapy The primary forms of cold sensitivity, i.e., livedo reticularis and acrocyanosis, rarely require treatment other than assurance and instruction relative to the dangers of prolonged exposure to cold. Sympathectomy has been widely applied, with inconsistent results, in the treatment of Raynaud's disease. Lumbar sympathectomy, probably because of the higher incidence of permanent denervation, is more likely to give good results than cervicodorsal sympathectomy. Sympathectomy, particularly in the upper extremity, should be performed only when conservative measures fail to control the symptoms. Vasodilator drugs have been used but with limited success. Nifedipine has been reported to be of benefit, but carefully controlled, randomized trials are not available. Biofeedback techniques may be used to lessen the severity of the attacks. When an underlying disease has been found, treatment is directed at the cause of the problem.

ERYTHROMELALGIA This rare disorder of unknown etiology expresses itself as burning, tingling, and often itching of the foot and lower leg which appears as the ambient temperature increases. There is usually a critical temperature for each patient above which the symptoms appear [usually in the range of 31.7 to 36.1°C (89 to 97°F)]. During the attack the patient's feet and lower legs become bright red. The patient quickly finds that the symptoms are related to temperature and will assiduously avoid those circumstances which bring out the symptoms. Characteristically, patients wear sandals, avoid stockings, sleep with their feet outside the bedcovers, and use fans to reduce skin temperature.

The *diagnosis* is established by the history and the examination of the extremities during an attack. The pedal pulses are intact, and the skin is warm and bright red. The disease is usually primary but has, in rare instances, been associated with myeloproliferative disorders.

Therapy is usually unsuccessful, but some patients have reported relief with aspirin or methysergide maleate.

VENOUS DISORDERS

VARICOSE VEINS Varicose veins are dilated, tortuous superficial veins with incompetent valves. The greater and lesser saphenous systems are most commonly involved, but it is not unusual for secondary branches of the superficial system of veins also to become dilated. They most often appear after the age of 20, but in women often develop in relation to puberty, during pregnancy, and with commencement of the menopause. In men there is a fairly even distribution in the onset of symptoms by decades up to age 70.

The etiology remains largely obscure, but varicose veins are known to be aggravated by hormonal factors in the female, increased intraabdominal pressure, and in rare instances, arteriovenous fistulas. Hereditary factors are important but have been poorly studied.

Classification It is important to classify varicose veins as either primary or secondary. Primary varicose veins occur in the absence of deep venous disease and generally have a benign course. Varicosities which occur secondary to obstruction and valvular incompetence of the deep venous system are much more serious.

Clinical features Primary varicose veins are brought to the attention of the patient first by the cosmetic deformity and second by the symptoms which develop with prolonged standing. The patient complains of a feeling of heaviness in the leg, combined with fatigue, that gets progressively worse toward the end of the day. Elevation of the legs will result in rapid and impressive relief from the symptoms. When the varicose veins are secondary to deep venous obstruction, loss of valves, and incompetent perforating veins, the symptoms are more severe and accompanied by swelling (see "Postthrombotic Syndrome" below).

Diagnosis The diagnosis of primary varicose veins is made largely by inspection of the legs in the upright position. The varicosities appear as dilated, often tortuous channels which are most commonly observed in the greater and lesser saphenous systems. When isolated clusters are observed in atypical locations, the possibility of an underlying incompetent perforating vein or arteriovenous fistula should be considered. To assess whether or not incompetent valves in the deep venous system and perforating veins are contributing factors, the Doppler velocity detector may be used. Valvular incompetence is detected by reflux (reversal of flow) in the vein when a Valsalva maneuver is performed.

Therapy The majority of patients with symptomatic primary varicose veins should be treated initially with compression stockings. It is rare for primary varicose veins to lead to stasis pigmentation and ulceration. In those rare instances in which treatment with compression stockings is inadequate, high ligation and stripping of the long and/or short saphenous veins may be required.

ACUTE VENOUS OCCLUSION Obstruction of superficial or deep veins occurs in two settings. The first is associated with an intense inflammatory component as usually observed with involvement of superficial veins. More common and potentially lethal is thrombosis of the deep veins where inflammation as either the inciting event or a clinical manifestation is uncommon. Thus, it is appropriate to separate these two entities since the clinical course and treatment are different.

Superficial thrombophlebitis Except for so-called chemical phlebitis secondary to direct intimal injury, the etiology remains obscure, but the clinical presentation is dramatic. The involved vein is exquisitely tender with surrounding erythema and edema. A fever is often present. While concern has been expressed regarding propagation of the thrombus into the deep venous system with subsequent pulmonary embolization, this rarely occurs. Treatment is directed at local measures to reduce the inflammation—application of heat, elevation of legs, and administration of anti-inflammatory agents such as indomethacin. It is important to be certain that the presenting symptoms are not signs due to a bacterial cellulitis or lymphangitis. The Doppler velocity detector is useful in making the distinction, since thrombophlebitis is always associated with thrombosis of the involved segment.

Acute venous thrombosis The most common in-hospital vascular disorder is thrombosis of the minor and major deep veins of the leg. In the initial stages, the soleus plexus of veins and sinus of the venous valve are the sites most commonly involved. When the thrombi remain confined to these areas, they are not detectable unless prospective screening with ^{125}I-labeled fibrinogen has been carried out (Chap. 211).

Upper extremity thrombosis is uncommon but may be associated with strenuous effort. The site of involvement is most commonly at the level of the axillary-subclavian vein as it enters the thorax.

ETIOLOGY There are definite known precipitating factors, which include trauma and bacterial infection, but these are not the most common causes. The much larger group of these patients develop this problem as a result of one or more of the following conditions or circumstances: (1) prolonged bed rest associated with a medical or surgical illness; (2) malignancy, particularly of the pancreas, lung, or gastrointestinal system; (3) administration of estrogens including oral contraceptives; (4) disseminated intravascular coagulation; (5) the postpartum period; and (6) paralysis.

CLINICAL FEATURES The most important factor concerning the symptoms and signs that develop is that they are not specific and may result from a variety of other diseases. Although edema and local tenderness with associated pain have been considered the most important findings, they are not sufficient to warrant either making the diagnosis of venous thrombosis or instituting therapy. Pulmonary embolization (Chap. 211) may, in fact, be the first clue that deep venous thrombosis is present.

DIAGNOSIS The bedside diagnosis of deep venous thrombosis is so inaccurate that it *must* be established by some independent means. The ^{125}I-labeled fibrinogen test is used for prospective studies but has limited application since it must be given prior to the initiation of the thrombosis. The most useful available noninvasive tests include Doppler ultrasound and plethysmography. Properly used, these tests have a rate of false-positive and false-negative results in the range of 5 to 10 percent. These methods are insensitive to thrombi confined to the muscular veins but can be used for sequential study to detect propagation into the major deep veins. If a vascular laboratory is present which has experience with these noninvasive tests, therapy can be based upon the results. However, if the tests are unavailable or the findings equivocal, contrast venography should be performed. A simpler test is radionuclide venography with simultaneous lung scanning. With this technique excellent visualization of the major deep veins from the popliteal to the vena cava can be obtained. The procedure is of no value for evaluating the venous segments below the knee.

THERAPY The treatment is directed at control of the thrombotic process already initiated. There is agreement that intravenous heparin is the most effective therapy. The preferred method is continuous administration, starting with a loading dose of 5000 to 10,000 units and varying the dosage depending upon the partial thromboplastin time, which should be kept between two and three times the control time. The two major advantages of this approach are a more uniform level of anticoagulation and a lower incidence of hemorrhagic complications.

The duration of heparin therapy depends upon the degree of involvement and whether pulmonary embolization has occurred. With the latter, treatment must be continued for 10 to 14 days and even longer if the patient remains at risk. Oral therapy with one of the coumarin preparations should be started while the patient is still on heparin, which is discontinued only when a satisfactory level of anticoagulation has been achieved. The maintenance level varies considerably between 2 and 15 mg daily. It appears that adequate protection against recurrent episodes can be obtained by keeping the one-stage prothrombin time at 1.5 to 2.0 times the control level.

Fibrinolytic therapy may be of value in that small group of patients with spontaneous venous thrombosis not associated with surgery or trauma. Streptokinase may be effective in lysing thrombi that have been present for less than 10 days, but its efficacy in preserving valve function remains an open question.

The duration of oral anticoagulation is dependent upon the severity of the problem. For isolated calf vein thrombosis, therapy of 4 to 6 weeks is sufficient. However, for femoropopliteal or iliofemoral thrombosis, with or without pulmonary embolism, anticoagulation should be continued for 3 to 6 months.

PROPHYLACTIC MEASURES There is conflicting evidence that low-dose heparin (5000 units subcutaneously 2 h prior to operation, then three times daily) is effective in reducing the incidence of deep venous thrombosis as well as the occurrence of fatal and nonfatal pulmonary embolism.

Patients with pulmonary embolism that has occurred with adequate doses of heparin, or who have developed bleeding complications, should be considered for transvenous placement of an ''umbrella'' in the vena cava below the renal veins. This is effective and obviates the need for ligation of the inferior vena cava or for partial occlusion by the direct placement of a plastic clip.

POSTTHROMBOTIC SYNDROME Patients who have single or multiple episodes of deep venous thrombosis will frequently have irreversible changes in the veins which lead to further morbidity. The acute venous thrombosis often leads to residual chronic occlusion and destruction of the venous valves.

The loss of the valvular mechanism in the deep venous system forces the blood to follow abnormal pathways, particularly during exercise. In the standing position or during walking the muscle pump pushes the blood proximally, distally, and out through the perforating veins into the superficial system. By increasing venous and capillary pressures, this sequence of events, over a period of many years, leads to edema, and to rupture of small superficial veins in the vicinity of the perforating veins. The subcutaneous hemorrhage leads to deposition of hemosiderin pigment (stasis pigmentation), subcutaneous fibrosis, cutaneous atrophy, and lymphatic obstruction. These chronic changes lead to the development of stasis ulcers, which are difficult to manage.

Clinical features and diagnosis The important features of this disorder consist of swelling which is always worse at the end of the day, pain, cutaneous pigmentation (usually in the region of the medial malleolus), and nonhealing ulcers which develop secondary to minor trauma. Repeated trauma, subcutaneous hemorrhage, and cellulitis can produce changes in the skin and subcutaneous tissues that are indistinguishable from those of the postthrombotic state. In questionable cases venography is useful in establishing the cause of the problem.

Therapy The most important factor in the treatment of the postphlebitic syndrome is to reduce the hydrostatic pressure and to prevent "high-pressure leaks" through the perforating veins when the patient is erect. This can best be accomplished by a tailored pressure-gradient stocking, which must be worn at all times that the patient is ambulatory, and by elevating legs when possible.

When an ulcer is present, healing may be accomplished by applying an impregnated gauze dressing from the base of the toes to below the knee. This is changed weekly and permits healing in 90 percent of patients. The remaining patients require excision of the ulcer with skin grafting. Support stockings must be worn regardless of the therapy directed at the ulcer, because the deep venous system remains incompetent and edema will continue to develop without adequate external support.

LYMPHATIC DISORDERS

LYMPHEDEMA Lymphedema, an abnormal accumulation of lymph in the extremities, occurs from multiple causes which include (1) lymphedema from organisms such as *Wuchereria bancrofti*; (2) infectious lymphedema resulting in thrombosis of lymphatics; (3) congenital lymphedema with arrest in lymph growth, which is apparent at birth or shortly thereafter; (4) traumatic lymphedema secondary to direct injury, burns, operations, and radiation; (5) essential lymphedema—so-called Milroy's disease, which appears at puberty and is most commonly observed in women; (6) allergic lymphedema occurring secondary to exposure to drugs and pollens; (7) postthrombotic lymphedema, which represents combined venous and lymphatic obstruction; and (8) malignant lymphedema, which occurs secondary to either direct invasion or obstruction of the lymphatics by tumor cells.

Clinical features Painless swelling of the involved extremity is the earliest and most common symptom and sign with most types of lymphedema. The swelling usually starts in the foot and ankle and then progresses proximally. Initially the swelling tends to subside somewhat at night, but as the process progresses, the swelling becomes permanent secondary to fibrosis of both the skin and subcutaneous tissues. Skin color and texture are normal until the late stages, when the skin becomes thickened and brown and has multiple papillary projections—so-called lymphostatic verrucosis.

Diagnosis The location and nature of the edema readily separate lymphedema from edema due to other causes. In the legs, the dorsa of the toes and foot are nearly always involved; this is uncommon in other causes of swelling. The edema is often brawny in character and pits only with difficulty. Though the other forms of edema often improve with bed rest, elevation, and diuretics, lymphedema, even in early stages, responds poorly to these measures. In later stages when fibrosis develops in the skin and subcutaneous tissues, these conservative measures are of little, if any, value. Lymphangiography in selected cases may be of value in localizing and elucidating the cause of the lymphedema.

Therapy Therapy is directed at minimizing the amount of edema and preventing recurrent attacks of cellulitis when this is a problem. Pressure-gradient stockings and the use of intermittent-pressure devices at night are helpful in controlling the edema. Since recurrent attacks of cellulitis due to the beta-hemolytic streptococcus are not uncommon and always result in further lymphatic destruction, prophylactic penicillin should be used indefinitely. Excision of the edematous tissue is reserved for only the most advanced stage of the disease when there is marked, irreversible swelling and disfigurement.

ANTERIOR TIBIAL COMPARTMENT SYNDROMES

Acute swelling of the anterior tibial compartment may occur secondary to intensive exercise, increased capillary permeability (with ischemia), or hematoma in the enclosed space. When arterial revascularization has been successful for prolonged ischemia, muscular swelling resulting in an increase in compartment pressure may lead to nerve damage and muscle necrosis. This is recognized by the severe pain in the compartment, swelling, and local tenderness. If the anterior compartment is involved, there is anesthesia of a triangular area on the dorsum of the foot at the base of the first and second toes. *Immediate* fasciotomy is indicated, since a delay of even a few hours may result in irreversible changes.

REFERENCES

ADAR R et al: Cellular sensitivity to collagen in thromboangiitis obliterans. N Engl J Med 308:1113, 1983

BERNI GA et al: Streptokinase treatment of acute arterial occlusion. Ann Surg 198:185, 1983

BERNSTEIN EF (ed): *Noninvasive Diagnostic Techniques in Vascular Disease,* 3d ed. St Louis, Mosby, 1985

BROWSE NL: The diagnosis and management of primary lymphedema. J Vasc Surg 3:181, 1986

DAVL G et al: Inhibition of platelet function by ticlopidine in arteriosclerosis obliterans of the lower limbs. Throm Res 40:275, 1985

GERBRACHT DD et al: Evolution of primary Raynaud's phenomenon (Raynaud's disease) to connective tissue disease. Arthritis Rheum 28:87, 1985

HULL R et al: Adjusted subcutaneous heparin versus warfarin sodium on the long-term treatment of venous thrombosis. N Engl J Med 306:189, 1982

PORTER JM et al: Pentoxifylline efficacy in the treatment of intermittent claudication: Multicenter controlled double-blind trial with objective assessment of chronic occlusive arterial disease patients. Am Heart J 104:66, 1982

RICHMOND DM et al: Sequential pneumatic compression for lymphedema. A controlled trial. Arch Surg 120:1116, 1985

RUTHERFORD RF (ed): *Vascular Surgery,* 2d ed. Philadelphia, Saunders, 1984

STEININGER H: Thromboangiitis obliterans (Buerger's disease). Pathologe 6:204, 1985

STRANDNESS DE JR: The case against low-dose heparin, in *Current Controversies in Cardiovascular Disease,* E Rapaport (ed). Philadelphia, Saunders, 1980

———, THIELE BL: *Selected Topics in Venous Disorders.* New York, Futura, 1981

——— et al: Long-term sequelae of acute venous thrombosis. JAMA 250:1289, 1983

WESSLER SW: The case for low-dose heparin, in *Current Controversies in Cardiovascular Disease,* E Rapaport (ed). Philadelphia, Saunders, 1980

Harrison's

PRINCIPLES OF INTERNAL MEDICINE

Eleventh Edition

VOLUME 2

PART FIVE
THROUGH
PART THIRTEEN

PART FIVE DISORDERS OF THE RESPIRATORY SYSTEM

199 APPROACH TO THE PATIENT WITH DISEASE OF THE RESPIRATORY SYSTEM

EUGENE BRAUNWALD

As in other branches of medicine, a careful and detailed history and physical examination are the cornerstones for establishing an accurate diagnosis in patients with disorders of the respiratory system. In addition, the roentgenographic examination occupies a particularly important role in the evaluation of patients with lung disease. Since abnormalities of the respiratory system are frequently a manifestation of a systemic process, attention must be focused not only on the chest but also a comprehensive evaluation of the patient's entire health status is essential. For example, the presence of a pulmonary lesion on x-ray may be due to metastatic disease with the primary disease elsewhere, and hemoptysis may be due to a disorder of hemostasis. Diffuse scleroderma may result in diffuse pulmonary infiltrative disease (Chaps. 209 and 264), and multiple pulmonary cavities may be a manifestation of Wegener's granulomatosis (Chap. 269). All of the so-called collagen vascular diseases may have prominent pulmonary manifestations. Carcinoma of the lung (Chap. 213) may be accompanied by prominent extrathoracic manifestations, which may overshadow the pulmonary lesion. These include myopathy, peripheral neuropathy, hypertrophic pulmonary osteoarthropathy, and a variety of endocrine and metabolic manifestations, including Cushing's syndrome, the carcinoid syndrome, a hyperparathyroid-like picture, inappropriate secretion of antidiuretic hormone, gonadotropin (Chap. 303), and increased frequency of pulmonary infections.

HISTORY In eliciting the history of patients with pulmonary disease, it must be appreciated that an increasing fraction of the population is exposed to materials which are potentially toxic to the lung (Chap. 204). The history must therefore contain a detailed *occupational and personal history* with a description of exposure to hazards such as asbestos, coal, silica, beryllium, bagasse, iron oxide, tin oxide, cotton dust, titanium oxide, silver, nitrogen dioxide, animals, moldy hay, air conditioners, and furnace humidifiers. It is useful to construct a work history, which includes the patient's duties, duration of exposure, use of protective devices, and illness in fellow workers. The occupational history should include information on a job-by-job basis as well as the military service. Contact with both wild and domestic animals may result in pulmonary symptoms, such as bronchospasm in subjects allergic to pets, or, less commonly, acute pneumonitis in patients with psittacosis (Chap. 150), tularemia (Chap. 113), or Q fever. Because it is such an important risk factor for many forms of lung disease, history of tobacco consumption must be sought and should be quantified. The habits of the patient with pulmonary disease must be gone into. Aspiration pneumonia and pneumococcal and *Klebsiella* pneumonia are often seen in alcoholics, lung abscess occurs in intravenous drug abusers, and *Pneumocystis carinii* pneumonia is a frequent complication of the acquired immunodeficiency syndrome. (Chap. 257). A record of the patient's *previous residence* is of considerable importance in the diagnosis of histoplasmosis (the south and midwestern United States), coccidioidomycosis (the southwestern United States), tropical eosinophilia, and South American blastomycosis. For example, pulmonary mass lesions in patients in the Mediterranean Basin may be due to hydatid cysts, hemoptysis in patients from central China may be caused by paragonimiasis (Chap. 167), and cor pulmonale in Egypt frequently results from schistosomiasis (Chap. 164).

It is vitally important to elicit a history of *drug exposure* since essentially every class of drugs can produce pulmonary toxicity (Chap. 203), and all parts of the respiratory apparatus can be affected, including the alveoli, tracheobronchial tree, mediastinum, pleural cavities, pulmonary vessels, respiratory muscles, and the medullary respiratory center. Examples include the interstitial infiltrative diseases caused by bleomycin, cyclophosphamide, methotrexate, and nitrofurantoin; noncardiogenic pulmonary edema caused by aspirin; bronchospasm caused by beta-adrenergic blockers and nonsteroidal anti-inflammatory drugs; pulmonary vasculitis from intravenous drug abuse; pulmonary thromboembolism in women receiving oral contraceptives; (drug-induced) systemic lupus erythematosus with pleural involvement caused by hydralazine and procainamide; and weakness of the respiratory muscles caused by the aminoglycoside antibiotics.

The *family history* should consider pulmonary diseases which may be genetic, such as cystic disease of the lung, pulmonary emphysema due to alpha$_1$ antitrypsin deficiency (Chap. 208), cystic fibrosis (Chap. 207), asthma (Chap. 202), hereditary telangiectasia, Kartagener's syndrome, and alveolar microlithiasis, as well as infections due to the tubercle bacilli, fungi, and schistosoma where exposure to involved family members is important.

Dyspnea is a cardinal manifestation of diseases involving the respiratory and cardiovascular systems (Chap. 26). A detailed physical examination of both organ systems is therefore mandatory in every patient with this symptom. Dyspnea secondary to cardiac disease is often recognized by the presence of other evidence of heart failure, such as cardiac enlargement, gallop rhythms, and cardiac murmurs. It may be difficult to differentiate paroxysmal nocturnal dyspnea due to pulmonary edema of cardiac origin from nocturnal attacks of bronchial asthma, but a detailed description of the circumstances in which this symptom occurs is most useful. Dyspnea also is a common functional complaint, and an important clue in the identification of this form is the observation that shortness of breath often occurs at rest and is relieved during exertion; the opposite is the case in patients in whom this symptom is secondary to disease of the lungs or heart. Equally important in the differential diagnosis is a careful elucidation of the relationship of dyspnea to other symptoms such as cough or angina pectoris.

Patients with diseases involving the respiratory system may also present with *chest pain* which is frequently caused by inflammation of the pleura, occurring in pneumonia, pulmonary thromboembolism, tuberculosis, and malignancy (Chap. 4). Pleuritic pain is usually localized to one side of the chest and is related to respiration and to movements of the thorax. Lesions confined to the pulmonary parenchyma do not produce pain, while diseases involving the organs in the mediastinum (Chap. 214) may cause local discomfort with radiation characteristic of the specific organ. Pain may also originate in or be referred to the chest wall; it may be due to intercostal neuritis, as in herpes zoster, or to compression of the intercostal nerves as they leave the spinal cord. Such pain is often superficial in character and may be related to coughing and straining. Thoracic pain may also be due to myositis, costochondral disturbances, myocardial ischemia, pericarditis, esophageal disease, and aortic dissection and aneurysm (Chap. 4).

Cough and *expectoration* are also cardinal features of pulmonary disease (Chap. 25). Few patients can describe the severity of cough or quantity of expectoration reliably, and it is therefore desirable for the physician to inspect a 24-h collection of sputum. Cough is often precipitated by foreign materials irritating nerve endings in airways and is frequently caused by inflammation of the bronchi; the latter may be persistent (as in patients with a cigarette cough and chronic bronchitis) or acute (as in a variety of viral and bacterial infections). The time of occurrence of the cough and the character and quantity of expectorated material may point to the diagnosis. For example, bronchiectasis and lung abscess produce purulent sputum which may have an offensive odor or be streaked with blood (Chaps. 205 and 206). In pulmonary edema, the sputum is pink, frothy, and watery (Chap. 26). Mucoid (translucent, viscid, shiny, white or gray) or mucopurulent (mucoid with flecks of yellow or green pus) sputum is characteristic of acute and chronic bronchitis. Sputum is bloody or rusty in pneumonia; it is thick, gelatinous, brick red, and laced with pus in *Klebsiella* pneumonia. Paroxysmal cough may also be the presenting feature in patients with bronchial asthma, in whom physical examination reveals wheezing respirations and squeaking musical sounds (Chap. 202), as well as in patients with left ventricular failure, in whom it generally occurs at night and in the recumbent position (Chap. 182). Pulmonary tuberculosis (Chap. 119), though less common than previously, remains a common cause of chronic cough, as does primary neoplasm of the lung (Chap. 213). A change in the character of a chronic cough, unaccompanied by an acute infection, should alert the physician to the need of carrying out a detailed examination.

Hemoptysis is often a frightening symptom (Chap. 25). Faint streaking of the sputum with blood may be observed in acute infections of the respiratory tract. However, many patients with bloody sputum have serious disease, such as pulmonary thromboembolism, tuberculosis, critical mitral stenosis, neoplasm of the lung, or bronchiectasis. In all instances it is necessary to exclude sources of blood in the nasopharynx and bleeding of gastric or esophageal origin. The character of the bloody expectorate should be defined, since it may be helpful in identifying the underlying disease process. Sputum which is frankly bloody without mucus or pus may be due to pulmonary thromboembolism (Chap. 211). When pus is present, pneumonia, bronchiectasis, or lung abscess should be considered. Dilute, pink, frothy sputum is observed in acute pulmonary edema (Chap. 26).

PHYSICAL EXAMINATION In addition to a careful examination of the thorax, a meticulous *general physical examination* is mandatory in patients with disorders of the respiratory system. Disturbances of mentation or even coma occur in patients with acute carbon dioxide retention and hypoxemia. Telltale stains on the fingers point to heavy cigarette smoking; infected teeth and gums may occur in patients with aspiration pneumonitis and lung abscess; characteristic cutaneous lesions may point to sarcoidosis (Chap. 270), collagen vascular disease, Wegener's granulomatosis, and berylliosis, all of which may have prominent pulmonary manifestations. Clubbing of the fingers or, when advanced, osteoarthropathy (Chap. 278) may suggest carcinoma (Chap. 213) or suppurative disease (Chap. 205) of the lung; chronic hypoxemia, as occurs in patients with chronic bronchitis (Chap. 208); pulmonary arteriovenous fistula; or congenital heart disease with right-to-left shunt (Chap. 185). However, clubbing is also seen in some patients with biliary cirrhosis, regional enteritis, and ulcerative colitis. A careful search for infection in the teeth, gums, tonsils, or sinuses is recommended in patients known to have or to be suspected of having bronchiectasis or lung abscess. Neurologic findings including headache, drowsiness, papilledema, and other evidence of increased intracranial pressure may occur in patients with pulmonary disease who have hypoxemia and hypercapnia. Vascular collapse is a late complication of carbon dioxide intoxication and is characterized by hypotension, flushed skin, sweating, and tachycardia.

DIAGNOSTIC TESTS The *roentgenographic examination* of the chest represents the cornerstone of the diagnostic workup of the patient with suspected pulmonary disease, and it is the integration of the information obtained from the clinical examination and the roentgenogram which often provides the key to diagnosis. Unfortunately, physical examination of the chest has been deemphasized, largely because of the recognition of the enormous value of radiographic techniques. However, abnormalities such as small or moderate amounts of fluid in the alveoli or in the mediastinum, bronchospasm, and pleural effusions can often be detected more accurately by physical examination than by chest roentgenography. Tracheal deviation can be readily recognized on physical examination and may be observed in obstruction of a major bronchus and in atelectasis.

Chest roentgenograms obtained in the lateral decubitus position frequently reveal small pleural effusions not evident in the upright posture. A number of other abnormalities may be associated with normal roentgenograms. These include solitary lesions less than 6 mm in diameter, acute pulmonary thromboembolism without infarction, early interstitial pneumonia, diffuse granulomatous disease such as miliary tuberculosis, interstitial disease such as scleroderma and systemic lupus erythematosus, bronchiectasis, acute chronic bronchitis, mild to moderate emphysema, endobronchial masses only partially obstructing the airways, and the majority of instances of hypoventilation due to disorders of the central nervous system or neuromuscular disease. On the other hand, gross abnormalities of thoracic structure; pulmonary, mediastinal, and pleural masses; parenchymal consolidation, cysts, cavities, and abnormalities of the pulmonary vascular bed are all detected more reliably by roentgenographic than by physical examination.

An abnormal chest roentgenogram may be the presenting feature in an asymptomatic patient. In such circumstances the physician must make every effort to obtain earlier films in order to determine whether the lesion is new or old. Laminography, computerized tomography, angiocardiography, and pulmonary scintigraphy are additional procedures which may be helpful in establishing a diagnosis in a patient with an abnormality on the plain chest roentgenogram.

A variety of other diagnostic procedures are helpful in the workup of the patient with known or suspected pulmonary disease. These are presented in Chap. 201 and include skin tests for tuberculosis; scratch or intradermal tests to detect atopic reactions; appropriate serum complement fixation tests; and examination and culture of the sputum, pleural fluid, and bronchial washings. Bronchoscopy, bronchial brushings, and bronchoscopic biopsy have been greatly facilitated by the development of the fiberoptic bronchoscope. Mediastinoscopy, scalene node and mediastinal node biopsy, and pleural and lung biopsy may also be instrumental in establishing a diagnosis in an otherwise asymptomatic patient. Particularly important points which must be investigated in the history of the asymptomatic patient with an abnormality discovered on a routine chest roentgenogram include exposure to individuals with tuberculosis; previous tuberculin and fungous skin tests; residence in or visits to areas where fungal disease is endemic; a history of smoking and of exposure to dusts; and symptoms of systemic disease such as fever, sweat, fatigue, and weight loss. Physiologic (lung function) studies (Chap. 200) are of limited value in establishing an etiologic diagnosis in the patient with pulmonary diseases. They are, however, very helpful in assessing the physiologic consequences of disorders of the respiratory system and chest wall, as well as in following the effects of their progression or remission. Simple functional tests, such as observing the patient climbing one or two flights of stairs, are often valuable in determining whether or not the patient is grossly disabled.

In the approach to a patient with pulmonary disease, consideration must be given to the observation that substantial changes in the relative incidence of disease affecting the respiratory system have taken place in the United States during the past three decades. The prevalence of chronic infectious disorders such as tuberculosis, lung abscess, and bronchiectasis have decreased. On the other hand, patients with chronic bronchitis and with emphysema now survive longer and form an increasing fraction of patients with chronic respiratory disease, as do patients with environmental lung disease and with drug-induced disease. Modern intercontinental travel has increased the appearance in the western world of parasitic infestations of the lung. Also, the reduction of immunologic competence which occurs in patients with the acquired immunodeficiency syndrome (Chap. 257) and in diabetics as well as in the treatment of patients with a variety of malignancies and following organ transplantation has led to an increasing incidence of opportunistic infections of the lungs with a variety of microorganisms rarely pathogenic in the past.

REFERENCES

FISHMAN AP (ed): *Pulmonary Diseases and Disorders*, 2d ed. New York, McGraw-Hill, 1987

SNIDER GL (ed): *Clinical Pulmonary Medicine*. Boston, Little, Brown, 1981

200 DISTURBANCES OF RESPIRATORY FUNCTION

JOHN B. WEST

The prime function of the lung is to exchange gas between the inspired air and the venous blood. A convenient starting point, therefore, for a discussion of disturbances of respiratory function is the alveolar membrane across which gas exchange occurs (Fig. 200-1). This blood-gas barrier is less than 1 μm thick and has a surface area of some 100 m². It is therefore ideally suited to its gas exchange function.

Air is pumped to one side of this membrane and blood to the other. The air flows through conducting tubes, the bronchi; these are not lined with blood capillaries, with the result that no gas exchange can occur within them. These conducting airways, therefore, comprise the *anatomic dead space*. Beyond these airways is the *alveolar gas*, which makes up most of the volume of the lung. This gas is in a constant state of agitation because of molecular diffusion, and thus all the alveolar gas has access to the capillary blood via the alveolar membrane.

On the other side of the membrane, blood is pumped from the right side of the heart to the pulmonary capillaries. These delicate vessels have diameters of only about 10 μm, so that the blood is spread out in a thin film, one or two red blood cells thick, around the air sacs.

It is worth emphasizing two features of the basic lung unit shown in Fig. 200-1: (1) its symmetry, i.e., air and blood are equally important in the central process of gas exchange (this simple fact is sometimes forgotten in clinical medicine, where the patient's difficulties in moving air in and out of the lung often dominate the picture); (2) the simplicity of the lung unit compared with, say, the nephron. The structure of the lung is simple because its main role is simple; i.e., it brings together air and blood so that gas exchange can occur by passive diffusion. By contrast, the kidney carries out many functions involving active transport, and its structure is correspondingly complicated (compare Fig. 218-2).

VENTILATION

This is the process of moving inspired air into the alveolar gas compartment, where the gas exchange with the blood occurs. Some typical values for ventilation are shown in Fig. 200-1. A normal breath is about 500 mL, so that with a breathing frequency of 15 per minute some 7 to 8 liters of air enters the lung each minute. This is the *total ventilation*. However, because the volume of the conducting airways (anatomic dead space) is about 150 mL, only 350 of the 500 mL of air inhaled with each breath reaches the alveolar gas compartment. The rest remains behind in the airways and is subsequently exhaled. Thus, the volume of fresh gas entering the alveoli each minute is about 350 mL × 15, or some 5 liters. This is known as the *alveolar ventilation* and is of key importance to gas exchange. Of the 5 liters of fresh air entering the alveoli, some 300 mL of oxygen moves across into the blood each minute to be replaced by about 250 mL of carbon dioxide. Thus less than 5 percent of the gas volume inhaled is exchanged with the blood.

The above figures apply to resting conditions. On exercise, the oxygen uptake may rise as high as 4 to 6 liters per minute and the total ventilation inspired may increase twentyfold. This is accomplished by an increase in both tidal volume and frequency of breathing.

It should be noted that inspired air passes only a limited distance down the airways by ordinary bulk flow. Before it gets to the alveoli, its forward velocity is reduced to something like a millimeter per second, because of the enormous combined cross-sectional area of the small airways. In addition, the volume of gas in the bronchioles is so large that the alveoli and their ducts have completed their expansion before the fresh inspired air reaches them. The last few millimeters of its travel are therefore accomplished by molecular diffusion within the small airways. This process is very rapid for gas molecules but exceedingly slow for dust particles if they are over 0.5 μm in diameter. For this reason most inhaled dusts and aerosols never reach the alveoli, and many are deposited in the region of the terminal bronchioles.

MEASUREMENT OF VENTILATION The total volume of air passing the lips is easily measured by connecting a large bag or spirometer to the patient via a mouthpiece and one-way valve. The resting and exercise ventilations are increased when disease impairs the efficiency of pulmonary gas exchange, but the measurement of ventilation by itself is often unreliable because it is partly under voluntary control and is often changed by the stress of the measurement.

CONTROL OF VENTILATION The rhythmic act of breathing is initiated in the respiratory centers of the pons and medulla. The level of ventilation is controlled by the arterial P_{CO_2}, P_{O_2}, and pH and by reflexes originating in the lung and elsewhere. The chief regulation is carried out by the medullary chemoreceptors which respond to changes in the partial pressure of carbon dioxide, P_{CO_2}, in arterial blood. There is evidence that these chemoreceptors are exquisitely sensitive to a fall in pH of the extracellular fluid around them, which occurs when carbon dioxide diffuses across the blood-brain barrier. This dissolved gas moves easily across the blood-brain barrier,

FIGURE 200-1 *Simplified diagram of the lung showing typical volumes and flows. There is considerable variation around these values. (From West, 1985.)*

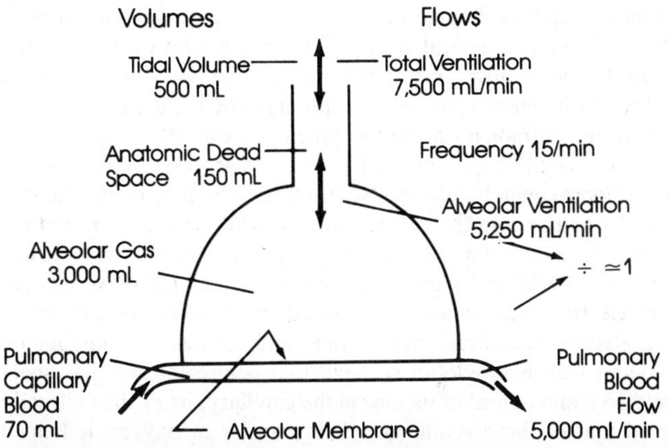

whereas H^+ and HCO_3^- do not. The composition of extracellular fluid is similar to that of cerebrospinal fluid.

Arterial hypoxemia also increases the ventilation through its action on the peripheral chemoreceptors in the carotid bodies. This hypoxic stimulus is normally relatively weak and variable but may dominate during chronic hypoxemia—for example, following ascent to high altitude. This is also often the situation in patients with chronic respiratory failure, with the result that the administration of oxygen may cause hypoventilation and severe carbon dioxide retention.

The pH of the arterial blood has an effect on ventilation which is independent of the P_{CO_2}. This is why ventilation may be increased during metabolic acidosis, thus reducing the arterial P_{CO_2}.

Reflexes from the lung from stretch receptors, irritant receptors, and receptors situated in the alveolar walls (juxtacapillary or J) also influence ventilation under some conditions.

HYPOVENTILATION When inspired air reaches the alveoli, oxygen is removed from it and carbon dioxide is added. The concentrations, or partial pressures, of these two gases in the alveoli depend on a balance between two processes. On the one hand, the removal of oxygen from (or addition of carbon dioxide to) the alveolar gas is determined by the metabolic demands of the body. On the other hand, the addition of oxygen to (or removal of carbon dioxide from) the alveolar gas depends on the amount of alveolar ventilation. Thus, if the alveolar ventilation is low in relation to oxygen uptake and carbon dioxide output, the partial pressure of oxygen in alveolar gas and arterial blood falls, and the level of carbon dioxide rises. This is hypoventilation.

Hypoventilation is commonly caused by disease outside the respiratory system and often exists in the presence of normal lungs. Causes include depression of the respiratory center by drugs or anesthesia, damage to the medulla by disease, diseases affecting the nerve supply to the muscles of the thorax or the muscles themselves, injury to the chest wall, and obstruction to the airways. Because the lungs themselves are often (though not always) normal, the prognosis may be excellent if the precipitating cause is removed. Note that hypoventilation always causes both hypoxemia and hypercapnia, although the first can be abolished by adding oxygen to the inspired air. The carbon dioxide retention can be relieved only by increasing the ventilation, e.g., by using a ventilator. Disorders leading to hypoventilation are discussed in more detail in Chap. 215.

HYPERVENTILATION If the alveolar ventilation is abnormally high for the carbon dioxide production of the body, the arterial P_{CO_2} falls. This may occur in metabolic acidosis, e.g., uremia, where the chemoreceptors respond to the low blood pH. Hysterical hyperventilation also occurs. For more information on hyperventilation see Chap. 215. The sensation of respiratory distress, or *dyspnea,* which should be clearly distinguished from *hyperpnea,* is considered in detail in Chap. 26.

DIFFUSION ACROSS THE BLOOD-GAS BARRIER

Oxygen and carbon dioxide move across the blood-gas barrier by a process of simple physical diffusion from a region of high partial pressure to one of low, just as water runs downhill. Consider a red blood cell as it enters a pulmonary capillary. The P_{O_2} in mixed venous blood (in the pulmonary artery) is typically about 40 mmHg, and as the cell enters the capillary the P_{O_2} in alveolar gas less than 1 μm away is approximately 100 mmHg. Oxygen therefore moves rapidly across the barrier into the cell to combine with hemoglobin, and the P_{O_2} rises. As a consequence, the oxygen pressure difference between the cell and the alveolar gas falls, and the rate of inflow of oxygen is reduced. However, under normal conditions, the diffusion properties of the alveolar membrane are so good and the rate of combination of oxygen with hemoglobin so rapid that before the cell has spent more than about a third of its time in the capillary, its P_{O_2} has virtually reached that of the alveolar gas. This transfer of oxygen is helped by the shape of the oxygen dissociation curve; the nearly flat upper part of the curve (see Fig. 283-4) ensures that the driving pressure difference is maintained until almost all the oxygen has moved across. Thus, under ordinary circumstances, there is no measurable difference between the P_{O_2} of alveolar gas and that of the blood at the end of the pulmonary capillary. Indeed, the normal lung has plenty of reserve diffusion.

Two factors which stress the diffusion ability of the lung are exercise and alveolar hypoxia. During strenuous exercise, the time spent by the red blood cells in the capillaries is greatly reduced, perhaps to a half or a third of that at rest, so that the time available for the diffusion process is curtailed. Even so, the P_{O_2} in the capillary blood almost reaches that of the alveolar gas, except possibly during the most exhausting work. Additional stress occurs if the lung inspires a low oxygen mixture, thus reducing the alveolar P_{O_2}. Because the pressure difference between the oxygen in the gas and that in the red blood cells as they enter the capillary is lowered, the rate of movement of oxygen across the membrane is slowed. There is evidence that heavy work when the inspired P_{O_2} is very low (e.g., at high altitude) causes lowering of the arterial P_{O_2} because of inadequate diffusion into the pulmonary capillary. It is generally argued that carbon dioxide transfer is never limited by diffusion across the alveolar membrane because of the much higher diffusion rate of this gas in tissue, but recent work suggests that this may not always be the case.

MEASUREMENT OF DIFFUSING CAPACITY This can be done using carbon monoxide. The subject inspires a low concentration (approximately 0.1 percent), and the rate of uptake of the gas by the blood is calculated from the difference between the inspired and expired concentrations. The measurement can be made during the course of a single 10-s breath-holding period or during a minute or so of steady breathing. In both cases, the diffusing capacity is expressed as the milliliters per minute of carbon monoxide taken up by the lung per millimeter of mercury of partial pressure of carbon monoxide in the alveolar gas. Normal values are in the region of 20 (mL/min)/mmHg at rest, rising to 60 (mL/min)/mmHg or more on exercise.

The reason why the uptake of carbon monoxide measures the diffusing capacity is the remarkable avidity of blood for this gas. This means that appreciable amounts of carbon monoxide can be combined with hemoglobin in the blood at an exceedingly low partial pressure. As a result, the rise in partial pressure of carbon monoxide in the red blood cells as they pass along the pulmonary capillaries is negligible, and the amount of the gas which is transferred into the blood is determined only by the diffusion properties of the alveolar membrane and the rate of combination of carbon monoxide with hemoglobin. This rate depends on the P_{O_2} in the alveoli; by measuring the carbon monoxide uptake at various inspired oxygen partial pressures, it is possible to determine separately the diffusing capacity of the alveolar membrane itself and the volume of blood in pulmonary capillaries. In patients who smoke, the level of carboxyhemoglobin in the blood may not be negligible and should be allowed for.

The measurement of carbon monoxide uptake is a relatively simple procedure, and there is no problem in following changes of diffusing capacity in the normal lung under a variety of conditions. Unfortunately, however, it is very difficult to say how far the carbon monoxide uptake reflects the true diffusion characteristics of the alveolar membrane and the capillary blood in the presence of appreciable lung disease. The reason for this is that inequalities of ventilation, diffusion properties of the alveolar membrane, and blood volume within the lung reduce the carbon monoxide in an unpredictable way. For this reason, the term *transfer factor* is sometimes used (especially in Europe), and the test should be looked upon as a general index of the efficiency of gas exchange in the lung rather than as a specific test of diffusion.

IMPAIRMENT OF DIFFUSION The diffusion properties of the alveolar membrane depend on its thickness and area. Thus, the diffusing capacity is reduced by diseases in which the thickness is increased, including diffuse interstitial fibrosis (Chap. 209), sarcoidosis (Chap.

270), asbestosis (Chap. 204), and alveolar cell carcinomatosis (Chap. 213). The diffusing capacity also falls when the area of the membrane is reduced. This occurs following pneumonectomy and in emphysema. In addition, as we saw above, the diffusing capacity falls when the capillary blood volume or the number of red blood cells in the capillaries is reduced. This is the case in anemia and in diseases such as pulmonary embolism.

The importance of diffusion impairment as a cause of hypoxemia has long been disputed. In those lung diseases such as diffuse interstitial fibrosis in which microscopically the alveolar wall is thickened, it is tempting to attribute all the hypoxemia to defective diffusion. The term *alveolar-capillary block* was coined for this situation, and it is certainly an easy one to remember. However, more recent work indicates that impaired diffusion is not the principal cause of the hypoxemia in these patients. It is probably impossible for normal ventilation and blood flow to occur in an alveolus which has a thickened wall. Studies in which it is possible to assess the extent of ventilation-perfusion inequality in patients with interstitial lung disease using the multiple inert gas technique indicate that, at rest, all the hypoxemia can be attributed to uneven ventilation and blood flow. However, on exercise, a small component of the hypoxemia is apparently caused by diffusion impairment. Thus, most of the hypoxemia in patients with so-called alveolar-capillary block must be attributed to ventilation-perfusion inequality.

BLOOD FLOW

Mixed venous blood is pumped to the pulmonary capillaries directly from the right side of the heart so that the total *pulmonary blood flow* is equal to the cardiac output, say 5 or 6 liters per minute in a normal adult. Figure 200-1 shows that the volume of fresh inspired air entering the alveoli each minute, the *alveolar ventilation,* is some 5 liters. Thus, the overall ratio of ventilation to blood flow, or *ventilation/perfusion ratio,* is about 1.

Even though the volumes of fresh gas and blood reaching the alveoli each minute are about the same, the volumes involved in exchanging gas at any instant are very different. Thus, while the alveolar gas volume is 2 to 3 liters at the end of a normal expiration, the capillary blood volume is only some 70 mL.

The pressures in the pulmonary circulation have long been considered the domain of the cardiologist, but they have an important bearing on gas exchange in the lung. The normal pulmonary arterial pressure is only just sufficient to raise blood to the top of the upright lung; if the pressure is reduced, as in hemorrhagic shock, the upper part of the lung is unperfused and gas exchange is impaired. Alterations in the pulmonary venous pressure, too, affect the distribution of blood flow in the lung.

VENTILATION-PERFUSION RELATIONSHIPS

Life would be much simpler if all lung units behaved identically. In practice, however, the lung is not homogeneous, and the differences in behavior between the millions of units are responsible for the greater part of the hypoxemia and carbon dioxide retention seen in clinical practice. We shall see that even in the normal lung, there are marked regional differences in blood flow and ventilation which affect gas exchange, while in diseased states, the inhomogeneity becomes so severe that respiratory failure may ultimately develop.

NORMAL DISTRIBUTION OF BLOOD FLOW It is possible to measure the regional distribution of blood flow and ventilation in the lung by using radioactive gases. In one technique, the inert gas xenon 133 is employed. To measure blood flow, the xenon is dissolved in saline and injected into a peripheral vein. On reaching the lung, it is evolved into alveolar gas because of its poor solubility; there it remains during breath holding, and its radiation can be detected by external counters. To measure ventilation, the patient inhales a single breath of the radioactive gas and again its regional distribution is measured. In both instances, a further measurement after a period of rebreathing of xenon allows a correction for lung volume to be made.

In the normal upright lung, blood flow per unit volume decreases rapidly from bottom to top, reaching very low values at the apex. This pattern is affected by change of posture and exercise. When the subject lies supine, the apical and basal blood flows become the same, but the posterior (dependent) part of the lung has a higher blood flow than the anterior region. In the lateral position, the dependent regions are best perfused. On exercise in the upright position, both apical and basal blood flows increase, so that the proportion of the total flow going to the apex rises.

The cause of this uneven distribution of blood flow lies in the hydrostatic pressure differences within the lung. The pulmonary circulation is unique in that air and blood are separated by a very delicate membrane over a vertical distance of some 30 cm in the upright position, and consequently, the hydrostatic effect of this large column of blood determines the caliber of the small vessels. The distribution of blood flow depends on the relative magnitudes of the pulmonary arterial, venous, and alveolar pressures. In particular, if pulmonary arterial pressure falls (as in hemorrhage, shock, and anesthesia) or alveolar pressure is raised (as in positive-pressure ventilation), the distribution of blood flow becomes more uneven. The normal pattern is also commonly affected by both heart and lung disease.

NORMAL DISTRIBUTION OF VENTILATION Ventilation also increases down the upright lung, though the changes are less marked than for blood flow. This distribution of ventilation which is seen under normal resting conditions is altered at low lung volumes. It has been shown that when a normal subject exhales as far as possible (to *residual volume*) and then gradually inhales in small steps, initially very little air goes into the lower zones, but the upper zones are well ventilated. However, before the subject reaches a normal resting lung volume (*functional residual capacity*), this distribution is reversed and the lower zones are better ventilated than the upper. This pattern is then maintained right up to maximal volumes. The poor ventilation of the dependent regions of the lung at low lung volumes is seen in the erect, supine, and lateral situations, and it has important implications in clinical situations in which the lung volume is low, e.g., in obesity or following abdominal surgery. Since the dependent regions are the best perfused, the impairment of gas exchange may then be severe.

The cause of the normal uneven distribution of ventilation has to do with the weight of the lung and the way it is supported inside the chest. It is known that the expanding pressure on the lung is less in the dependent zones, because these regions help to support the lung above them. Thus, the intrapleural pressure is less negative at the bottom of the lung than at the top. The reason for the greater ventilation of the dependent regions at normal volumes is twofold: (1) these alveoli have a smaller resting volume, and (2) their increase in volume is relatively large because, having a smaller volume, they are more distensible. By contrast, these dependent regions are poorly ventilated at low lung volumes because the expanding forces on them are then too weak to inflate them. Indeed, under these conditions, the airways to these alveoli may close and the alveoli become unventilated.

The volume at which the lower zone airways close (the *closing volume*) is considerably less than the functional residual capacity in normal young subjects. However, as the lung ages, and especially in the presence of chronic obstructive lung disease, the closing volume increases until it encroaches on the normal breathing range. Thus elderly normal subjects and patients with chronic bronchitis and emphysema frequently close their lower zone airways during resting breathing; this results in a poorly ventilated region which impairs gas exchange.

The closing volume can be measured from the single-breath nitrogen test (see "Measurement of Ventilation Inequality" below). There is some evidence that the measurement of closing volume is a sensitive test of early disease affecting the small airways, though this is disputed.

VENTILATION/PERFUSION RATIO We have seen that while blood flow increases greatly down the upright lung, the change in ventilation is less. As a result, the ventilation/perfusion ratio varies from a high value at the top of the lung to a low value at the bottom. The ventilation/perfusion ratio is of key importance because it determines the gas exchange which occurs in any part of the lung.

We saw earlier that the partial pressure of oxygen in the alveolar gas (and therefore in the end-capillary blood) is set by a balance between the rate of its removal by the blood flow, on the one hand, and the rate of its replenishment by the ventilation on the other. Thus, if the ventilation is gradually reduced but the blood flow is maintained, the oxygen partial pressure will gradually fall. The limit is reached when the unit is not ventilated, and the P_{O_2} becomes that of venous blood. This is a ventilation/perfusion ratio of zero. By contrast, if perfusion is gradually reduced, the P_{O_2} will rise. The limit now occurs when the unit is unperfused and the P_{O_2} in the alveolus is the same as that of inspired air. This is a ventilation/perfusion ratio of infinity.

Thus, the crucial factor determining the oxygen partial pressure is the ventilation/perfusion ratio; this is also true for the partial pressure of carbon dioxide, and indeed of any other gas that might be present. It can be shown that marked regional differences of gas exchange occur in the normal upright lung as a consequence of the uneven ventilation/perfusion ratios.

OVERALL GAS EXCHANGE Though such regional differences in gas exchange are of interest, more important is the effect of uneven ventilation/perfusion ratios on overall gas exchange, i.e., the ability of the lung to take up oxygen and put out carbon dioxide. The reason why gas transfer is impaired by uneven ventilation and blood flow is that those lung units which are overperfused in relation to their ventilation, and which therefore have a low P_{O_2}, contribute a disproportionate amount of the blood flow to the systemic arterial system. The net result is that the arterial P_{O_2} is depressed because it is loaded with less well oxygenated blood. In the same way, because these lung units have a relatively high P_{CO_2}, they tend to elevate the arterial P_{CO_2}. It is as if uneven ventilation/perfusion ratios set up a barrier between the gas and the blood, with the result that the arterial P_{O_2} is depressed and the P_{CO_2} is raised. The effects of ventilation/perfusion ratio inequality on arterial P_{O_2} are exaggerated by the nonlinearity of the oxygen dissociation curve.

In the normal lung, the effects of uneven ventilation/perfusion ratios on overall gas exchange are trivial; the arterial P_{O_2} is reduced by only a few millimeters of mercury and the P_{CO_2} is raised by less than 1 mmHg, if all else remains the same. Both these liabilities can be met if the total ventilation of the lung and thus its overall ventilation/perfusion ratio are increased. Indeed, the level of overall ventilation is normally set by the medullary respiratory center via the arterial P_{CO_2}. Thus, if uneven ventilation/perfusion ratios elevate the arterial P_{CO_2}, this is brought back by the increased respiratory drive and the consequently higher overall ventilation.

In the diseased lung, the effects of ventilation/perfusion ratio inequality on gas transfer may be very severe because the degree of uneven ventilation and blood flow is far greater than in the normal lung. The arterial P_{O_2} may be depressed by 50 mmHg or more, and in practice no amount of increased ventilation can return it to its normal level. The P_{CO_2}, however, is often maintained at the normal level by an increase in total ventilation. The reason why an increase in ventilation to diseased lungs can reduce the arterial P_{CO_2} but cannot increase the P_{O_2} to normal levels lies in the different shapes of the two dissociation curves. If the ventilation is not increased, the P_{CO_2} remains elevated. Ventilation/perfusion ratio inequality is much the commonest cause of hypoxia and hypercapnia in generalized lung disease.

MEASUREMENT OF VENTILATION/PERFUSION INEQUALITY Unfortunately, it is difficult to derive much information about the pattern of uneven ventilation and blood flow in the diseased lung. Because much of the inequality is at the microscopic level, radioactive gas detectors which ''see'' relatively large regions of lung give little indication of the extent of the unevenness. The simplest way to obtain information about the amount of ventilation/perfusion inequality is by the analysis of expired gas and arterial blood.

One valuable measurement is the *alveolar-arterial P_{O2} difference*. This is obtained by subtracting the arterial P_{O_2} from the so-called ideal alveolar P_{O_2}. The latter is the P_{O_2} which the lung would have if there were no ventilation/perfusion inequality. It is calculated from the arterial P_{CO_2} and the respiratory exchange ratio; specialized texts should be consulted for details.

An increased alveolar-arterial P_{O_2} difference is caused both by abnormally low and abnormally high ventilation/perfusion ratios within the lung. It is possible to assess separately the approximate contribution of these two groups to the impairment of gas exchange. For the units with low ventilation/perfusion ratios, we can calculate the *physiologic shunt*. To do this we assume that all the hypoxemia is caused by blood passing through unventilated alveoli (although we know this is an oversimplification). The calculation is made using a modified shunt equation.

The effect of lung units with abnormally high ventilation/perfusion ratios is assessed by calculating the *physiologic dead space*. Here we assume that all the reduction of P_{CO_2} in expired gas is caused by unperfused alveoli together with the anatomic dead space. A modified dead space equation is used for the calculation. Again, a specialized text should be consulted for details.

Another method of measuring ventilation/perfusion inequality uses a continuous infusion of six foreign inert gases into the venous blood. After a steady state of gas exchange has been established, the consequent partial pressures in arterial blood and expired gas are then measured. From this information, it is possible to derive an almost continuous distribution of ventilation/perfusion ratios. Young normal subjects have very narrow distributions centered on the normal value of about 1. Patients with chronic obstructive lung disease and asthma, for example, often have bimodal distributions with substantial amounts of blood flow going to lung units with very low ventilation/perfusion ratios.

MEASUREMENT OF VENTILATION INEQUALITY Because the measurement of ventilation/perfusion ratio inequality is a relatively difficult procedure, the simpler measurement of uneven ventilation is often made. Although it would be theoretically possible for a patient to have ventilatory inequality but no mismatch of ventilation and blood flow, this is not seen in practice.

The simplest method of measuring uneven ventilation is the single-breath nitrogen wash-out test. For this, the patient takes a vital capacity inspiration of pure oxygen and then exhales fully. A rapid nitrogen meter at the lips measures expired nitrogen concentration, and expired volume is recorded simultaneously. After 750 mL has been expired (sufficient to clear the dead space), the rise in nitrogen concentration over the next 500 mL is measured. This is less than 1.5 percent in normal subjects. However, in patients with uneven ventilation, the nitrogen concentration rises more rapidly because the degree of dilution of the nitrogen by the inhaled oxygen varies throughout the lung, and also because the poorly ventilated regions (which receive little oxygen and therefore have the most nitrogen) always empty last. This is a simple, quick, and useful test, and it may also be used to give the closing volume (see earlier under ''Normal Distribution of Ventilation'').

Uneven ventilation can also be detected by a multibreath nitrogen wash-out test, but this is now usually confined to the research laboratory.

VENTILATION/PERFUSION RATIO INEQUALITY IN DISEASE Virtually all generalized diseases of the lung, such as emphysema, chronic bronchitis, diffuse interstitial fibrosis, and the pneumoconioses, result in mismatch of ventilation and blood flow. As yet little is known about the pattern of unevenness in these conditions, though it is not difficult to imagine that an area of fibrosis or a bulla, for example, must interfere with both ventilation and blood flow.

There is evidence that, in general, areas of the lung which are poorly ventilated are also poorly perfused. One reason for this is that local pathologic change tends to disturb both processes by its mechanical effects. However, there are other physiologic mechanisms which reduce the mismatch of ventilation and perfusion. One is the reduction in blood flow to a poorly ventilated, hypoxic region of the lung, which has now been demonstrated on many occasions. The precise mechanism is unknown, but the phenomenon appears to be a local response to alveolar hypoxia since it occurs in the isolated denervated lung. Another mechanism is the reduction of ventilation which has been shown to follow obstruction of a branch of the pulmonary artery. This is apparently due to an increase in resistance of the small airways caused by a fall in P_{CO_2} in the region. This mechanism is weak in human beings.

How far these two mechanisms operate in practice is unknown, but it has been shown that the administration of various bronchodilator and vasodilator drugs to patients with generalized lung disease can exaggerate their hypoxemia. For example, isoproterenol (by aerosol) and epinephrine and aminophylline (by injection) have been shown to reduce the arterial P_{O_2} of some patients with chronic obstructive lung disease and bronchial asthma. It is possible that one of the actions of these drugs is to interfere with these active mechanisms which reduce ventilation/perfusion ratio inequality.

MECHANICS OF BREATHING

The bellows function of the lung is one of the easiest to measure and also one of the most informative measurements in practice. Serious malfunction of the lung is almost always accompanied by a reduced ventilatory capacity.

LUNG AND CHEST WALL The lung is elastic and collapses if it is not held expanded. The pressure *inside* the lung (alveolar pressure) is the same as atmospheric pressure at the end of inspiration or expiration if the glottis is open. The pressure *outside* the lung (intrapleural pressure) is less than atmospheric pressure, or "negative." This pressure keeps the lung inflated and is developed because the chest wall, which is also elastic, tends to bow outward, whereas the lung tends to collapse inward. If air is introduced into this space and a pneumothorax is produced, the lung collapses and the chest wall moves outward.

MUSCLES OF RESPIRATION The most important muscle of inspiration is the diaphragm, a thin, dome-shaped sheet of muscle which is inserted into the lower ribs and spine. It is supplied by the phrenic nerves from cervical segments 3, 4, and 5. When the diaphragm contracts, the abdominal contents are forced downward and forward, and the vertical dimension of the chest cavity is increased. In addition, the rib margins are lifted and moved out, causing a widening of the transverse diameter of the thorax.

In normal tidal breathing, the dome of the diaphragm descends about 1 cm, but on forced inspiration and expiration, a total descent of up to 10 cm may occur. If the diaphragm is paralyzed, it moves up rather than down with inspiration because of the fall of intrathoracic pressure. This is known as *paradoxical movement* and can be demonstrated at fluoroscopy by asking the patient to sniff.

The external intercostal muscles connect adjacent ribs and slope downward and forward. When they contract, the ribs are pulled upward and forward, causing an increase in both the lateral and anteroposterior diameters of the thorax. The lateral dimension of the rib cage also increases because of the "bucket-handle" movement of the ribs. The intercostal muscles are supplied by intercostal nerves which come off the spinal cord at the same level. Paralysis of the intercostal muscles alone does not seriously affect breathing because the diaphragm is so effective.

The accessory muscles of inspiration include the scalene muscles, which elevate the first two ribs, and the sternocleidomastoid muscles, which raise the sternum. There is little if any activity in these muscles during quiet breathing, but during exercise they may contract vigorously. Other muscles which play a minor role include the alae nasi, which cause flaring of the nostrils, and the small muscles in the neck and head.

Expiration is passive during quiet breathing. The lung and chest wall tend to return to their equilibrium positions after being actively expanded during inspiration. During exercise and voluntary hyperventilation, expiration becomes active. The most important muscles of expiration are those of the abdominal wall, including the rectus abdominus, internal and external oblique muscles, and transversus abdominus. When these muscles contract, intraabdominal pressure is raised and the diaphragm is pushed upward. They also contract forcefully during coughing, vomiting, and defecation.

The internal intercostal muscles assist active expiration by pulling the ribs downward and inward (opposite to the action of the external intercostal muscles) thus decreasing the thoracic volume. In addition, they stiffen the intercostal spaces to prevent them from bulging outward during straining.

Disease affects the action of the respiratory muscles. In patients who have a greatly increased work of breathing, the diaphragm may become fatigued; this can result in inadequate ventilation and carbon dioxide retention. There is some evidence that diaphragmatic fatigue plays an important role in the respiratory failure of some patients.

In some newborns, the action of the various respiratory muscles may be poorly coordinated. This may be a factor in the sudden infant death syndrome (Chap. 215).

COMPLIANCE This is a term used to describe the elastic properties of the lung and chest wall. The normal lungs expand by about 200 mL when the expanding pressure (intrapleural pressure) falls by 1 cmH_2O. Thus the compliance (or distensibility) of the lungs is said to be 200 mL/cmH_2O. In fact, this figure only applies at normal resting lung volumes; at high lung volumes, the lungs are less easy to expand and their compliance falls. A more complete description of the elastic properties of the lungs, therefore, is the pressure-volume curve over the whole range of lung volumes; for this reason, this measurement is preferred in many pulmonary function laboratories. The compliance of the normal chest wall is about the same as that of the lungs, and the compliance of both lung and chest wall together is therefore about half this value, i.e., 100 mL/cmH_2O.

The compliance of the lung depends very much on how much tissue is present. A single lobe, for example, will clearly not change its volume as much as a whole lung for the same change in expanding pressure. Compliance is therefore sometimes corrected for lung volume and called *specific compliance*.

The normal elastic behavior of the lungs is partly caused by the elastic tissue within it. The two most important tissue components are elastin and collagen, and fibers of both kinds can be seen in the alveolar walls and around vessels and bronchi. Probably the elastic behavior of the lung has less to do with simple elongation of these fibers than with their geometric arrangement. An analogy is a nylon stocking which is very distensible because of its knitted makeup, although the individual nylon fibers are very difficult to stretch. The changes in elastic recoil that occur in the lung with age and in emphysema are presumably caused by changes in the configuration of these elastic tissue elements.

Another important component of the elastic behavior is the surface tension of the fluid lining the alveoli. The lungs may be regarded as composed of 300 million tiny bubbles which tend to collapse for the same reason that a soap bubble on the end of a bubble pipe does (although this is clearly an oversimplification). The surface forces which tend to reduce the area of the surface thus tend to reduce the volume of the bubble. These surface forces therefore contribute to the elastic force of the lung. Fortunately some of the cells lining the alveoli produce a phospholipid which lowers the surface tension of the lining fluid to extremely low values, especially at low lung volumes. The substance is known as a *surfactant*. This lowering of the surface tension is of great physiologic importance, because it helps to maintain the stability of the alveoli and discourage atelectasis. About half the normal elastic recoil force of the lung is due to these surface forces.

The exact composition of pulmonary surfactant is not known, but dipalmitoyl phosphatidyl choline (DPPC) is an important constituent. This is secreted by type 2 alveolar cells. Electron microscopy shows osmiophilic laminated bodies within the cells which are extruded into the alveoli and transform into surfactant. Some of the surfactant can be washed out of lungs by rinsing them with saline solution. Surfactant is formed relatively late in fetal life, and premature babies born without adequate amounts develop the infant respiratory distress syndrome (hyaline membrane disease).

The normal elastic behavior of the lung is disturbed by many diseases. Diffuse pulmonary fibrosis, pleural thickening, healed tuberculosis with scarring, and atelectasis all reduce the compliance of the lung. Heart disease such as mitral stenosis and left ventricular failure also commonly lowers compliance, although it is often difficult to be certain whether the volume of ventilating lung is reduced by edema in the airways, for example, or whether the elastic behavior of the lung tissue itself is altered. In emphysema and old age, the lungs become more compliant and have an abnormally large volume at normal expanding pressures.

Dynamic compliance refers to a measurement of compliance made at end inspiration and end expiration during breathing. In normal lungs, this is the same as the static compliance referred to above. However, when airway disease is present, dynamic compliance is smaller because some parts of the lung have not completely filled at the end of inspiration as a result of their increased airway resistance. Measurements of dynamic compliance can be used to infer increases in airway resistance.

AIRWAY RESISTANCE So far we have been looking at the static forces involved in maintaining the expansion of the lung. However, during ventilation, additional forces are required to move air along the airways, because of the resistance offered to flow. This is expressed as the pressure difference between the alveoli and the mouth per unit of airflow rate. The normal value is in the vicinity of 1 to 2 cmH_2O per liter per second of flow at normal flow rates. The resistance rises at higher flow rates.

Until recently it was thought that the chief site of resistance was the small airways. However, it is now known that most of the resistance lies in the medium-sized bronchi and that the bronchioles less than 2 mm in diameter contribute less than 20 percent of the total airway resistance. The reason for this is the prodigious number of small airways and their large collective cross-sectional area. As a consequence, substantial increases in resistance of these bronchioles will not be detected by the usual pulmonary function tests, and they are said to constitute a "silent zone." There are tests designed to detect changes in the small airways. These include the single-breath nitrogen test, the measurement of closing volume referred to above, and the measurement of "frequency-dependent compliance," i.e., the apparent fall in dynamic compliance which occurs at high breathing rates. Whether these tests are better at detecting early airway disease than is the time-honored forced expiratory volume (see below under "Measurements of Mechanics") has not yet been established.

Various factors alter airway resistance. For example, the resistance is higher during expiration than inspiration, and it is greater at small lung volumes because the airways are then not held open so much. A single deep inspiration often reduces the resistance, but the inhalation of cigarette smoke or other irritants increases it through reflex contraction of airway smooth muscle following stimulation of irritant receptors located in the airway wall.

A dramatic increase in airway resistance occurs during forced expiration. The cause of this is collapse of the airways, called *dynamic compression*. The explanation is that the high intrapleural pressure is applied not only to the alveoli in an effort to empty them but also to the outside walls of the airways which lie within the chest. Consequently the airways are compressed, and as a result, the expiratory flow rate is independent of respiratory effort over a large range, since the greater the effort, the more the collapse. In normal subjects, this phenomenon takes place only during forced expirations, but it occurs much more readily in patients with chronic bronchitis and emphysema. This is because the airway walls are diseased and weakened, or because the airways lose their support by radial traction from the surrounding lung. In addition, the pressure difference responsible for expiration during dynamic compression is alveolar pressure minus pleural pressure, and this difference is reduced when compliance is increased, as in emphysema.

Diseases which increase airway resistance during normal breathing include bronchial asthma and chronic bronchitis. The resistance may rise to many times its normal value and even during clinical remissions of the disease can be shown to be abnormally high. Lung volume increases in these conditions, and this has two helpful consequences: the airways are pulled open more, thus limiting the increase in resistance, and the higher passive recoil pressure of the lung assists expiration.

WORK OF BREATHING To move the lungs and chest wall and force air along the airways, work is required, and the respiratory muscles must consume oxygen. In normal subjects, the work of breathing is very small except during the large ventilation of heavy exercise. In patients with obstructive lung disease, however, the frictional resistance to airflow is high even at rest and the work of breathing is much increased, perhaps to 5 or 10 times its normal value. Under these conditions, the oxygen cost of breathing may become an appreciable fraction of the total oxygen consumption.

Patients with a reduced compliance of the lungs or chest wall have a higher work of breathing, because the stiffer structures are more difficult to move. These patients tend to use rapid shallow breaths, which reduce their oxygen cost of ventilation. However, if breathing becomes too shallow, the volume of air merely moved in and out of the anatomic dead space becomes disproportionately high, and gas exchange is consequently impaired. A compromise is therefore reached.

MEASUREMENTS OF MECHANICS One of the most useful tests in the armamentarium of the pulmonary function laboratory is the analysis of a single forced expiration. The patient makes a full inspiration and then exhales as hard and as fast as possible into a lightweight spirometer. Typical records are shown in Fig. 200-2. It can be seen that for a normal subject the total volume exhaled is large. This is called the vital capacity or, preferably, the *forced vital capacity* (FVC). (The word *forced* is added because the volume may be less than the vital capacity measured with a slow expiration.) Also, about 80 percent of this volume is exhaled in 1 s. This is called the *forced expiratory volume,* or FEV_1. In *obstructive lung disease,* e.g., chronic bronchitis and emphysema, the forced vital capacity is reduced because the airways close and limit expiration before the patient has breathed out fully. In addition, the FEV_1 is grossly reduced, as is the FEV/FVC percentage. This is because of the high airway resistance which slows the rate of expiration. In *restrictive lung disease,* e.g., sarcoidosis, the FVC is low because of the limited expansion of the lung or chest wall. However, the FEV_1 is often not reduced proportionately, because airway resistance is normal. Thus the FEV/FVC percentage is normal or high. Normal values for lung volumes and spirometric tests are found in the appendix.

Other indexes of ventilatory function can be derived from a forced expiration. One is the maximal midexpiratory flow ($FEF_{25-75\%}$), which is obtained by dividing the volume between 75 percent and 25 percent of the vital capacity by the corresponding elapsed time (Fig. 200-2). This correlates well with the FEV_1 but may be a more sensitive measure of airway obstruction in early chronic obstructive lung disease.

Impaired lung function is frequently associated with a reduced FEV_1, and the test is therefore a valuable screening procedure. It is also useful in assessing the efficacy of bronchodilator therapy and in following the progress of patients with asthma or chronic obstructive lung disease.

Other lung volumes can also be measured at the same time. The *total lung capacity* is the total volume of gas in the lung at full inspiration. The *inspiratory capacity* is the maximum volume that can be inspired from the resting volume of the lungs, which is called the *functional residual capacity*. The maximum volume that can be expired from the resting level is the *expiratory reserve volume*. This leaves the *residual volume* still in the lungs, and this and the functional residual capacity can only be measured indirectly. One technique is to connect the patient to a spirometer circuit containing helium and measure the degree of dilution of this gas which occurs after several minutes of rebreathing. Another is to use a body plethysmograph (see below).

These volumes are often altered by disease. The functional residual capacity and residual volume are typically increased in diseases in which there is an increased airway resistance, for example, in emphysema, chronic bronchitis, and asthma. Indeed, at one time an elevated residual volume was regarded as an essential feature of emphysema, but less emphasis is placed on this test now. A reduced functional residual capacity and residual volume are often seen in patients with a reduced lung compliance, for example, in diffuse interstitial fibrosis. Here the lung is stiff and tends to recoil to a much smaller resting volume.

The measurement of compliance and airway resistance is more difficult. In order to determine lung compliance, i.e., volume change per unit of pressure change, the pressure expanding the lungs must be known. In practice this can be found by passing a small latex balloon connected to a manometer down into the esophagus. Esophageal pressure is then taken as a measure of intrapleural pressure. To measure airway resistance, i.e., the pressure drop along the airways per unit of airflow, alveolar pressure must be known. This can be found by seating the patient in a large airtight box, or plethysmograph. First, the patient is asked to try to breathe against a complete obstruction, and from the change in box pressure, lung volume can be calculated. Next, the patient is asked to pant, and again box pressure is recorded. Alveolar pressure can then be derived and airway resistance calculated. This equipment is available only in specialized centers.

Aging has an important influence on lung function. With increasing age there is a fall in vital capacity and forced expiratory volume and an increase in functional residual capacity, residual volume, and closing volume. In addition, lung elastic recoil decreases. Some inequality of ventilation and ventilation/perfusion ratios develops and the arterial P_{O_2} falls almost linearly with age. It is therefore important to take account of the age of the patient when interpreting many pulmonary function tests.

ACID-BASE DISTURBANCES If pulmonary gas exchange is impaired, the P_{CO_2} in the arterial blood may rise, which tends to depress the pH and causes *respiratory acidosis*. A decrease in P_{CO_2} causes *respiratory alkalosis*. The compensatory mechanisms which are then brought into play are discussed in Chap. 42.

MEASUREMENT OF BLOOD GASES Blood gas measurements play a vital role in the management of respiratory failure. Arterial blood can be obtained by direct puncture, and the oxygen and carbon dioxide partial pressures and the pH can be measured by electrodes. Oxygen saturation can be derived by spectrophotometry.

HYPOXEMIA

The four main causes of a low arterial P_{O_2} are (1) ventilation/perfusion ratio inequality, (2) right-to-left shunt, (3) hypoventilation, and (4) impaired diffusion. In addition, living at high altitude or deliberately inspiring a low oxygen mixture causes hypoxia.

1 *Ventilation/perfusion ratio inequality* is the commonest cause and is responsible for almost all the hypoxemia seen in chronic lung disease. Specific tests of ventilation/perfusion inequality are not generally available, although the multiple inert gas infusion technique referred to earlier can be used in specialized centers. The demonstration of ventilatory inequality (see above) is a useful pointer. Mild degrees of ventilation/perfusion ratio inequality may be present without hypoxemia, and considerable inequality may exist without hypercapnia if overall ventilation is increased. However, carbon dioxide retention almost always develops eventually. The hypoxemia is eventually abolished by the administration of 100% oxygen. However, with severe inequality, the arterial P_{O_2} may take so many minutes to rise to normal values because of very poorly ventilated areas that, in practice, the levels seen in normal subjects may not be attained. Exercise may or may not aggravate the hypoxemia and hypercapnia (see Table 200-1). The response of the arterial P_{O_2} to exercise depends to a large extent on the changes in total ventilation and blood flow.

2 *Shunted blood,* i.e., blood which has bypassed ventilated areas of the lung, causes hypoxemia. Patients with right-to-left shunts through congenital heart defects or a pulmonary arteriovenous fistula belong to this group. Patients with ventilation/perfusion ratio inequality often have some parts of the lung completely unventilated, and the contribution of these regions is indistinguishable from that of a shunt. The hypoxemia due to shunt is not abolished (although it is reduced) by administering 100% oxygen, and this test will distinguish it from the other causes of hypoxemia. The level of the arterial P_{O_2} under these conditions allows the percentage of shunted blood to be measured. The arterial P_{O_2} rises

TABLE 200-1 Features helpful in distinguishing the various causes of hypoxemia and hypercapnia

	Hypoxemia	Hypercapnia	Hypoxemia on exercise	Hypercapnia on exercise	Hypoxemia on 100% O_2
Ventilation/perfusion ratio inequality	Yes	Yes or no	Yes	Yes or no	No
Shunt	Yes	No	Yes	Possible	Yes
Hypoventilation	Yes	Yes	Often severe	Often severe	No
Impaired diffusion	Yes (rarely)	No	Often severe	No	No

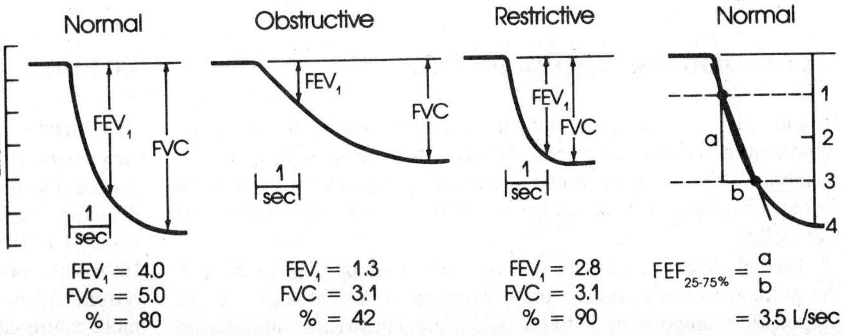

FIGURE 200-2 *Measurement of the forced expiratory volume, FEV_1; forced vital capacity, FVC; and maximum midexpiratory flow, $FEF_{25-75\%}$. The patient makes a full inspiration and then exhales as hard and as fast as possible. As the patient exhales the pen moves down. The FEV_1 is the volume exhaled in 1 s; the FVC is the total volume exhaled. The $FEF_{25-75\%}$ is the mean flow rate measured over the middle half of the FVC. Note the differences between the normal, obstructive, and restrictive patterns.*

to some extent because of the addition of dissolved oxygen to the pulmonary blood. The hypoxemia of shunt may be exaggerated by exercise. Hypercapnia does not occur unless the shunt is very gross, because the respiratory center increases the ventilation, thus holding the arterial P_{CO_2} down.

3 *Hypoventilation* always causes both hypoxemia and hypercapnia. Because of the shape of the oxygen dissociation curve, which means that a substantial fall in arterial P_{O_2} can occur with little reduction in oxygen saturation (see Fig. 283-4), considerable carbon dioxide retention may be present without recognizable cyanosis. If the patient is inhaling an enriched oxygen mixture, e.g., in the anesthetic recovery room, hypoxemia is not present but the hypercapnia may be severe.

4 *Impaired diffusion* rarely causes hypoxemia but does not cause hypercapnia. The hypoxemia is accentuated by exercise but abolished if an enriched oxygen mixture is administered. As we have seen, diffusion impairment may occur in normal subjects during work at very high altitude, but its importance as a cause of hypoxemia in disease is minimal.

HYPERCAPNIA

The two chief causes of carbon dioxide retention are ventilation/perfusion ratio inequality and hypoventilation. Ventilation/perfusion ratio inequality is the commonest cause, although many patients have some degree of uneven ventilation and blood flow without hypercapnia. A combination of the two causes can occur.

Why does a patient with chronic lung disease develop hypercapnia? Progressive lung disease (perhaps aggravated by an acute infection) causes increasing mismatch of blood flow and ventilation and greater impairment of carbon dioxide transfer. For a time, the respiratory center is able to hold the arterial P_{CO_2} down to the normal level by increasing the ventilation, but the work of breathing is usually high because of airway obstruction, so that eventually a compromise is reached and the arterial and alveolar partial pressures rise. This has the advantage that more carbon dioxide is put out for the same ventilation, so it may be looked upon as a compensatory mechanism, albeit a hazardous one. As the ventilation/perfusion ratio inequality becomes worse, the tendency is for the arterial P_{CO_2} to rise further.

A particularly dangerous situation may arise if such a patient is given oxygen to breathe. The chief stimulus to ventilation in these patients is often hypoxemia, and when this is suddenly relieved, the ventilation may drop precipitously and the arterial P_{CO_2} climb rapidly. The carbon dioxide retention and acidosis may then cause clouding of consciousness, muscular twitching, and a raised intracranial pressure. Drugs which depress the respiratory center may produce a similar effect. Thus while oxygen administration is indicated in these patients because of their severe hypoxemia, it should be given with caution and the blood gases should be frequently measured.

Another hazardous situation often arises when these patients are taken off oxygen because they are retaining too much carbon dioxide. Since the body stores of carbon dioxide are so large, many minutes elapse before the alveolar P_{CO_2} returns to reasonable levels. During this recovery period, this high alveolar carbon dioxide dilutes the alveolar oxygen and may cause profound hypoxia.

METABOLIC FUNCTIONS OF THE LUNG

In addition to its primary function of gas exchange, the lung has important metabolic functions. Several vasoactive substances are metabolized by the lung. Since it is the only organ that receives the whole circulation, it is uniquely suited to modify blood-borne substances.

The only known example of biologic activation by passage through the pulmonary circulation is the conversion of a relatively inactive polypeptide, angiotensin I, to the potent vasoconstrictor, angiotensin II. The latter, which is up to 50 times more active than its precursor, is unaffected by passage through the lung. The conversion of angiotensin I is catalyzed by angiotensin-converting enzyme (ACE), which is located in small pits in the surface of the capillary endothelial cells.

Many vasoactive substances are completely or partially inactivated during passage through the lung. Bradykinin is largely inactivated (up to 80 percent); the enzyme responsible is ACE. The lung is also the major site of inactivation of serotonin (5-hydroxytryptamine), but this is not by enzymatic degradation but by an uptake and storage process. Some of the serotonin may be transferred to platelets in the lung or stored in some other way and released during anaphylaxis. The prostaglandins E_1, E_2, and $F_{2\alpha}$ are also inactivated in the lung, which is a rich source of the responsible enzymes. Norepinephrine is also taken up by the lung to some extent. Histamine appears not to be affected by the intact lung but is readily inactivated by lung slices.

Some vasoactive materials pass through the lung without significant gain or loss of activity. These include epinephrine, prostaglandins A_1 and A_2, angiotensin II, and vasopressin (ADH).

Several vasoactive substances are normally synthesized or stored within the lung but may be released into the circulation in pathologic conditions. For example, in anaphylaxis or during an asthma attack, histamine, bradykinin, prostaglandins, and "slow-reacting substances" are discharged into the circulation (see Chap. 202). Other conditions in which the lung may release potent chemicals include pulmonary embolism and alveolar hypoxia.

In disease, the lung has a remarkable potential for hormone production and secretion. For example, neoplasms such as bronchial carcinomas can produce a variety of polypeptide hormones.

REFERENCES

COTES JF: *Lung Function,* 4th ed. St Louis, Mosby, 1979

WEST JB: *Pulmonary Pathophysiology—The Essentials,* 2d ed. Baltimore, Williams & Wilkins, 1982

———: *Respiratory Physiology—The Essentials,* 3d ed. Baltimore, Williams & Wilkins, 1985.

201 DIAGNOSTIC PROCEDURES IN RESPIRATORY DISEASES

KENNETH M. MOSER

In seeking a definitive diagnosis in the patient with respiratory disease, a wide choice of diagnostic procedures is available. These procedures vary considerably, not only in diagnostic reliability and specificity, but also in terms of the discomfort and hazard to the patient. Hence, an orderly sequence of test selection is mandatory. This sequence should begin with procedures involving little risk and, only if necessary, move on to those which entail higher morbidity and potential mortality.

NONINVASIVE PROCEDURES

RADIOGRAPHIC PROCEDURES The *chest roentgenogram* serves two major roles in the search for a diagnosis in the patient with respiratory disease: *detector* and *guide*. Occasionally, in its role as a detector, the routine chest roentgenogram initiates the diagnostic search by disclosing an abnormality in an asymptomatic individual. However, routine chest roentgenography (e.g., as an element of all hospital admissions) is neither necessary nor cost-effective. Therefore, more commonly, it detects pulmonary involvement in someone already ill. Rarely, detection may coincide with diagnosis; e.g., in spontaneous pneumothorax or when a radiopaque foreign body has been aspirated.

Far more frequently, however, the roentgenogram, having detected potential disease, provides a guide to the selection of subsequent diagnostic procedures. Many radiographic findings are quite characteristic of certain diseases. A number of radiographic patterns are sufficiently repetitive to warrant descriptive names, such as bilateral hilar adenopathy, solitary pulmonary nodule, diffuse interstitial infiltrate, alveolar filling pattern, multinodular lesion, and honeycomb lung. Thus, a particular radiographic finding, combined with other pertinent data, often permits establishment of a reasonable list of possible diagnoses. For example, the roentgenographic detection of bilateral hilar adenopathy in an asymptomatic, 26-year-old black male immediately places sarcoidosis at the top of the list. A chest roentgenogram disclosing upper lobe cavities in a febrile male whose brother recently was admitted to a tuberculosis sanitarium would make tuberculosis the most likely entity. Or a "diffuse interstitial" infiltrate—for which more than 100 causes exist—may yield a prompt diagnosis of varicella pneumonia when combined with the classical skin lesions. Multinodular lesions, with some cavitating, in a patient with sinusitis and red cell casts on urinalysis makes Wegener's granulomatosis a primary diagnostic possibility. However, no roentgenographic pattern is sufficiently specific to *establish* a diagnosis. Lung cancer (primary and metastatic) can present many roentgenographic patterns, as can both infectious and noninfectious lung disorders. For example, cardiogenic pulmonary edema may present as a perihilar or diffuse alveolar filling pattern, as an interstitial process and, rarely, as a lobar infiltrate or interlobar collection of fluid ("pseudotumor")—all with or without a pleural effusion.

In some instances, special radiographic techniques may provide valuable diagnostic insights.

Fluoroscopy allows visualization of the thoracic contents in a dynamic rather than static manner and also permits a wide range of special views. It also indicates whether a lesion is pulsatile, what its precise location in the thorax is, whether the hemidiaphragms move normally, i.e., whether they are fixed or move paradoxically, and how various zones of the lung behave during inspiration and expiration. Thus, fluoroscopy can define whether a roentgenographic density is actually in a rib or in the pleura rather than in the parenchyma; and may distinguish between a unilateral hyperlucent lung due to emphysema (mediastinum shifts toward the normal lung on expiration) or to unilateral pulmonary arterial obstruction (no shift).

Tomography (laminography, planigraphy) is a radiographic technique by which a sequence of roentgenograms, each representing a "slice of the lung" at a different depth, is obtained. Ordinarily, "cuts" are made at 0.5- to 1-cm distances through the area of interest. Tomograms can identify a number of features which were not appreciated on the "routine" roentgenogram, including calcium in a solitary nodule (which if diffuse or in concentric rings signifies a benign etiology); distinction between hilar adenopathy and dilated pulmonary arteries; a cavity in a mass lesion; and the contours of masses in the mediastinum.

Thoracic *computerized tomography* (*CT*) *scanning*, also may provide information not available through other techniques. It is particularly useful in the definition of pleural disease (e.g., differentiating fluid from tumor; identifying calcium in asbestos-exposed individuals); in evaluating hilar, paratracheal, and subcarinal node enlargement; with contrast injections, in differentiating tissue masses from vascular structures; and in identifying small parenchymal nodules. However, to some extent, the sensitivity of CT will be a mixed blessing until it is known how many "normal" individuals have pleural or parenchymal abnormalities by CT and how these small, benign, hitherto undetected lesions can be distinguished from neoplastic lesions.

Magnetic resonance imaging (MRI) remains, in terms of its potential value in pulmonary diseases, an investigational technique.

SKIN TESTS Having arrived at a tentative list of diagnostic possibilities based on the history, physical examination, and radiographic appearance, the physician should move to other procedures. One of the simplest and most commonly overlooked is the application of *skin tests* with specific antigens. Antigens are now available to assist in the diagnosis of tuberculosis, histoplasmosis, coccidioidomycosis, blastomycosis, trichinosis, toxoplasmosis, and aspergillosis. These tests vary with respect to sensitivity and cross-reactivity, and attention to scrupulous technique in performance and interpretation is vital. Also, some antigens (e.g., histoplasmosis) may confound serologic tests performed subsequently. A positive skin test indicates only that the antigen has been encountered previously by the host; it does not, regardless of reaction intensity, imply active disease. Furthermore, drugs or diseases which depress cell-mediated immunity (e.g., prednisone, cyclophosphamide, lymphomas, sarcoidosis, disseminated tuberculosis, or coccidioidomycosis) may cause skin anergy. Indeed, a negative battery of skin tests, if it incorporates antigens such as mumps, streptokinase-streptodornase, *Trichophyton,* and *Monilia,* suggests that a cause of skin anergy should be sought.

SEROLOGIC TESTS These tests also may be useful in the diagnosis of histoplasmosis, blastomycosis, coccidioidomycosis, toxoplasmosis, *Mycoplasma* pneumonia, Legionnaires' disease, a variety of other infectious diseases involving the lungs, and certain immunologically mediated lung diseases (e.g., lupus erythematosus). Often, more extensive diagnostic procedures can be avoided if appropriate serologic tests are obtained. However, there is substantial interinstitutional variability with respect to the sensitivity, specificity, and types of serologic tests available. Therefore, their appropriate use requires close interaction with the responsible laboratory.

SPUTUM EXAMINATION Another rapid, innocuous diagnostic procedure is *sputum examination.* It is important that the specimen contain sputum, not saliva, the latter being identified by the presence of squamous (mouth) rather than epithelial (bronchial) cells. The gross nature of the sputum—color, odor, and the presence of blood—may provide valuable clues; e.g., foul sputum suggesting anaerobic pulmonary infection and blood, in any amount, indicating an abnormality that mandates further investigation. Carefully stained smears of the sputum should be examined next, for these may disclose the causative organism in many bacterial pneumonias, in tuberculosis, and in some fungous infections. Sputum eosinophilia can suggest the presence of reversible airway disease responsive to corticosteroids; hemosiderin-laden macrophages suggest the possibility of Goodpasture's syndrome. Often valuable time is lost because the sputum smear is not examined and results of culture are awaited instead.

Culture of expectorated sputum (spontaneous or induced) has fallen into disrepute because of uncertain yield and, particularly, because of frequent and unavoidable contamination by the oropharyngeal bacterial flora. Although such cultures are invaluable for identification of organisms responsible for tuberculous and fungous infections, their utility in detection of other bacterial agents responsible for pulmonary infection is often uncertain and can be misleading, particularly in patients who are immunocompromised, intubated, or receiving antimicrobial therapy. Five procedures, described below, are now gaining wide acceptance because they limit oropharyngeal contamination and/or can be used to obtain representative samples of lung secretions from the area of lung involvement: (1) catheter-brush sampling, (2) bronchoalveolar lavage, (3) transtracheal aspiration, (4) transbronchial lung biopsy, and (5) percutaneous needle aspiration of the lung.

Exfoliative cytology of the sputum is helpful in the diagnosis of carcinoma of the lung (Chap. 213). Proper handling of such specimens is essential. Sputum samples often can be obtained in patients who are not coughing by having them inhale a heated mixture of a mildly irritative solution which induces cough.

PULMONARY FUNCTION TESTS (see also Chap. 200) Certain "patterns" of derangement in spirometric tests, arterial blood gases, diffusing capacity, and other functional parameters are particularly suggestive of certain pulmonary diseases. For example, diffuse interstitial fibrotic diseases of the lungs (Chap. 209) produce a "restrictive" spirometric defect, reduced pulmonary compliance, a reduced diffusing capacity, and an alveolar-arterial oxygen tension difference which is widened at rest and widens further with exercise. Emphysema (Chap. 208) characteristically causes expiratory obstruction, lung hyperinflation, decreased static elastic recoil (increased compliance), and a reduced diffusing capacity.

PULMONARY SCINTIPHOTOGRAPHY Scintiphotographs ("scans") of intrathoracic structures are obtained by a variety of "scanning" devices which record the pattern of intrathoracic radioactivity after intravenous injection or inhalation of gamma-emitting radionuclides. Direct photographic or computer-derived images, or digital data, reflecting radionuclide distribution are used for diagnostic purposes. The most commonly used images are those which reflect the distribution of pulmonary blood flow (perfusion) and ventilation. Such scans have multiple diagnostic applications. For example, a normal perfusion scan excludes the diagnosis of acute pulmonary embolism (Chap. 211). When perfusion scans showing defects are combined with ventilation scans, ventilation-perfusion patterns are provided which assist in the diagnosis of parenchymal lung diseases and vascular occlusive disorders, including pulmonary embolism.

Another type of scan involves intravenous injection of radionuclides which have an affinity for intrathoracic inflammatory and neoplastic tissues. Gallium 67 is the most useful of such radionuclides now available. Concentration of such agents, defined by scanning, may permit detection of neoplastic or inflammatory disease in the lungs or mediastinal lymph nodes. Uptake by the lungs may, in some patients, reflect the intensity of inflammatory activity associated with diffuse interstitial pneumonitis, sarcoidosis, and granulomatous infections. Inapparent extrapulmonary foci of granulomatous or neoplastic diseases also may be detected by body scanning.

New radionuclides continue to emerge which, when complexed with such materials as platelets, white blood cells (e.g. indium 111), fibrinogen, and albumin, may allow imaging of intrathoracic vessels, thrombi, inflammation, and neoplasms. Tomographic and other image-processing methods are emerging which may further extend the value of these techniques.

All the above procedures involve minimal risks and discomfort to the patient. Where applicable, these approaches should be considered before the more invasive techniques discussed below are considered, unless the condition of the patient demands immediate diagnosis.

INVASIVE PROCEDURES

BRONCHOSCOPY The primary objectives of bronchoscopy include direct visualization of the tracheobronchial tree, including abnormalities such as tumors or granulomatous lesions; biopsy of suggestive or obvious endobronchial lesions; and lavage, brushing, or biopsy of lung regions for cultural and cytologic examinations. Both the *diagnostic reach of* and *accessibility to* bronchoscopy have been expanded by the flexible fiberoptic bronchoscope (FOB). This can be understood best by comparing the FOB with the "standard" rigid bronchoscope.

The rigid bronchoscope is a wide-bore metal tube which incorporates a lighted mirror-lens system. The FOB is composed of fiberoptic bundles which provide both illumination and visualization pathways. A small channel with a diameter of 1 to 3 mm traverses the FOB, through which instruments can be passed, fluids delivered, and suction applied. The rigid bronchoscope comes in various external diameters limited only by the feasibility of introducing the rigid device orally and through the larynx. Biopsy and other procedures are carried out through the rather capacious interior of the rigid tube. The FOB also is available in various external diameters, but all are substantially smaller than rigid bronchoscopes (since no "wall" exists in the FOB). The distal tip of the FOB can be *flexed* easily to 90° and usually to 130° or more from the vertical.

Thus, the rigid bronchoscope permits visualization only of lobar bronchi and the orifices of some segmental bronchi. The flexible, smaller FOB extends the range of *view* to all segmental and subsegmental bronchi and the range for *biopsy and sampling* to the pulmonary parenchyma itself. A biopsy forceps, catheter, or brush passed through the FOB can be directed well beyond the tip of the bronchoscope itself, permitting *transbronchial lung biopsy, brushings,* or *aspiration of secretions* for culture and cytologic examination from the most distal regions of the lung. Indeed, both forceps and brush can reach and perforate the pleura, leading to pneumothorax. Therefore, when the lesion being approached is distal, fluoroscopic guidance is essential. Not only does this permit placement of the FOB, forceps, catheter, or brush directly into the area of interest, but also it ensures that the pleura will not be inadvertently reached and punctured. The FOB also allows *regional* lung lavage to obtain materials for cytologic examination and culture. The use of specially designed catheters (see below) placed through the FOB is quite useful in obtaining representative, noncontaminated secretions for culture, thus avoiding the problems mentioned previously with expectorated sputum.

Thus, the FOB has sharply increased the limited diagnostic reach previously available with rigid bronchoscopy. Equally important, the FOB has made bronchoscopy more available to the physician and more acceptable to the patient. The performance of rigid bronchoscopy requires the supine position for peroral insertion of the device; can be performed safely by a relatively few trained surgeons; and is often carried out under general anesthesia in an operating room. Therefore, it has been a procedure requiring significant preparation and hence delay. Fiberoptic bronchoscopy can be performed in the sitting or supine position, since the FOB is easily inserted transnasally; can be performed by a large number of trained pulmonary specialists as well as surgeons; usually requires only local anesthesia; and can be performed safely on the wards, in diagnostic rooms equipped with a "dentist-type" chair, and in intensive care units. The FOB can be used easily in intubated patients on ventilators with simple "side-arm" adapters attached to the endotracheal tube. Therefore, when bronchoscopy is indicated, it is not surprising that fiberoptic bronchoscopy is now commonly the first choice. The roomier rigid bronchoscope is now usually reserved for situations in which the small biopsy-suction channel in the FOB may be inadequate (e.g., for removal of large foreign bodies, for laser surgery). The FOB also has a widening range of therapeutic applications including aspiration or lavage of secretions in patients with airway obstruction or atelectasis due to retained secretions; obstruction of bleeding areas of the lung, with a wedged FOB itself or with a balloon catheter passed via the FOB, in patients who are poor surgical risks; removal of small foreign bodies; and placement of radionuclides in tumors. Transtracheal needle aspiration of paratracheal and subcarinal nodes also can be performed via the FOB, a procedure which is particularly useful in the staging of carcinoma of the lung.

The hazards of bronchoscopy are modest but should be recognized. In addition to the risk of general anesthesia which rigid bronchoscopy usually requires, they can include hypoxemia, laryngospasm, bronchospasm, pneumothorax, and, of course, bleeding following biopsy. Proper management before, during, and after bronchoscopy should prevent most of these complications. There is no absolute contraindication to FOB. Even in the presence of massive hemoptysis, FOB with appropriate precautions can yield useful information. Patients with bronchospasm (or a history of bronchospasm) are at particular risk of acute enhancement of spasm and should be approached after good preparation and with resources for intubation-ventilation at hand. The primary contraindication to both rigid and fiberoptic bronchoscopy is the same: performance by inexperienced personnel. Lack of experience sharply reduces diagnostic and therapeutic yield while increasing risks.

BRONCHOGRAPHY In this method, radiopaque material is instilled into the tracheobronchial tree via a catheter or bronchoscope. Positioning of the patient and catheter permits the material to coat all portions of the tracheobronchial tree for a sufficient period so that their outline can be recorded on chest roentgenograms. Bronchography is indicated for the diagnosis of bronchiectasis, for the identification of obstruction in distal bronchi, and for the detection of other types of congenital and acquired forms of tracheobronchial distortion or malformation. Like FOB, bronchography may induce bronchospasm; also, the irritative effects of the contrast medium may persist for some days.

TRANSTRACHEAL, CATHETER-BRUSH, AND PERCUTANEOUS NEEDLE ASPIRATION OF THE LUNG All three of these procedures are used to obtain material for culture and microscopic examination. In the case of culture, all three techniques bypass the oropharyngeal flora, though transtracheal aspiration is the least certain in this regard.

Transtracheal aspiration involves needle puncture of the cricothyroid membrane, insertion of a plastic cannula, and instillation of a saline solution, followed by suctioning of a sample. The procedure cannot be performed in intubated patients; contamination rates are high in previously intubated patients or those who have aspirated oropharyngeal contents. Because the procedure entails risks, although these are minimized by meticulous technique and experience, clear indications for its use should exist. These include patients with apparent pulmonary infection who are unable to cough, in whom cough is nonproductive, or in whom there has been a lack of response to therapy based on smears or cultures from expectorated sputum.

In these same contexts, *catheter-brush devices* specially designed with a distal plug to avoid oropharyngeal contamination can be used. These are manipulated (through an FOB or without it) under fluoroscopic guidance into the involved lung area. The distal absorbable plug is then ejected and the inner brush or catheter advanced for sampling. Finally, an alternative procedure is direct percutaneous aspiration, which can be performed using a small (23- or 25-gauge), thin-walled, *noncutting* needle. The needle, connected to a syringe, is introduced percutaneously into the area of the lung of interest; 2 to 3 mL saline is injected and then aspirated into the syringe and the needle withdrawn. Both the catheter-brush and needle approaches are high-yield, low-contamination procedures. In experienced hands, the risks are low, consisting chiefly of pneumothorax and bleeding. Patients should be carefully monitored for both.

The presence of a hemorrhagic diathesis is a relative contraindication to all three of the above procedures.

THORACENTESIS AND PLEURAL BIOPSY Thoracentesis should be performed to obtain pleural fluid in all pleural effusions of uncertain etiology and may be indicated for relief of symptoms in some patients with effusion of known cause. In effusions of uncertain cause, closed (needle) pleural biopsy should be performed as part of the same procedure.

When pleural fluid is small in amount or when its presence or location is uncertain from routine or lateral decubitus roentgenograms, performance of the thoracentesis and biopsy under fluoroscopic, ultrasound, or CT scan guidance enhances both yield and safety. Pleural fluid obtained should be examined for specific gravity, white blood cell count and differential, protein and glucose concentrations, lactic acid dehydrogenase (LDH), pH, P_{CO_2} (sample collected anaerobically), and amylase. Gram stain, cultures, and exfoliative cytologic specimens should be obtained; and in some instances, rheumatoid factor and complement levels are measured. The gross appearance of the fluid, the quantity obtained, and the precise location of the thoracentesis should be recorded. A combination of a pleural fluid LDH above 200 IU, a pleural fluid/serum protein ratio greater than 0.5, and a pleural fluid/serum LDH ratio greater than 0.6 all indicate that an "exudative" rather than "transudative" process is present. A low pH (<7.20) indicates that an empyema, probably requiring tube drainage, is present (Chap. 214). Specific diagnostic findings in pleural fluid may include the opalescent, pearly fluid characteristic of chylothorax; positive smears or cultures for tuberculosis or other infections; a marked elevation of amylase indicative of effusion secondary to pancreatitis or a ruptured esophagus; and the very low glucose values often seen in effusions associated with rheumatoid arthritis.

As already noted, closed (needle) pleural biopsy should follow thoracentesis whenever the diagnosis is uncertain. It is important to leave some fluid in the pleural space as this makes biopsy easier and safer. Bleeding, pneumothorax, and bronchopleural fistula induced by cutting through the visceral pleura are all more likely in the absence of fluid, and a satisfactory biopsy specimen is less likely to be obtained. Several special needles are available for biopsy of the parietal pleura. All have a cutting edge and some device for retaining the biopsy. The needle is inserted into the pleural effusion, then withdrawn until it is seated on the parietal pleura, from which a biopsy is obtained with the cutting edge. Usually, three biopsies are taken from different sites at the same session. Care should be exercised to place the needle in a position least likely to impinge on the intercostal vessels. All fluid to be used for diagnosis should be removed before biopsy since postbiopsy bleeding may obscure the true character of the fluid.

Pleuroscopy, using a modified FOB inserted through an intercostal trocar, also can be used for both direct inspection and biopsy of the pleura. In the absence of a pleural effusion, two other options exist for obtaining tissue from pleural-based lesions: aspiration needle biopsy and open biopsy. The technique for aspiration biopsy is the same as that described above, although some physicians use "cutting" needles (see "Lung Biopsy" below). Open pleural biopsy involves a limited thoracotomy, requiring anesthesia. A small intercostal incision is made, and the parietal pleura is biopsied under direct visualization. The incision is then closed, often without an intercostal tube. Open biopsy has several advantages because a larger specimen is obtained and the pleura and underlying lung can be seen and palpated. When pleural involvement is "spotty," open biopsy increases the possibility of establishing a diagnosis.

PULMONARY AND BRONCHIAL ANGIOGRAPHY Radiopaque materials are injected rapidly by vein or via a catheter into the systemic veins, right heart chambers, or the pulmonary artery. Magnification techniques allow visualization of smaller pulmonary vessels. *Digital* pulmonary angiography, providing computer-derived images of digital data, may allow imaging of the larger pulmonary arteries with contrast injected more proximally (into superior or inferior vena cava or peripheral vein) or at lower concentrations; however, motion artifacts limit its sensitivity and specificity. Angiography is frequently used to detect pulmonary emboli and a variety of congenital and acquired lesions of the pulmonary vessels. The procedure is not without risk, particularly in patients with pulmonary hypertension, and clear indication for it must exist as well as personnel experienced in its performance and interpretation.

Angioscopy, an experimental technique for direct visualization of the right cardiac chambers and pulmonary arterial system, can be accomplished by insertion of a fiberoptic device via a peripheral vein. The diagnostic role of this procedure in embolic and other disorders remains to be defined.

Bronchial arteriography is now used in some centers to identify otherwise obscure bleeding sites in the lungs. Transarterial placement of a catheter into the orifices or parent vessels of bronchial arteries can be accomplished by experienced operators. Radiopaque material is then injected so that these arteries can be visualized. If a bleeding site is identified, emboli can be injected via the catheter as a means for halting hemoptysis.

MEDIASTINOSCOPY AND MEDIASTINOTOMY Another favored site for biopsy is the lymph nodes in the mediastinum. Because they receive lymphatic drainage from the lungs, these nodes often disclose intrathoracic diseases such as carcinoma, granulomatous infections, and sarcoidosis. As noted above, transtracheal needle aspiration of mediastinal nodes via the FOB is one new approach to such nodes. Another is mediastinoscopy, which involves insertion of a lighted mirror-lens system, much like a bronchoscope, through an incision at the base of the neck anteriorly. The instrument is advanced under visual control into the mediastinum, where inspection and biopsy can be carried out. Because of its higher yield of diagnostic lymph nodes, mediastinoscopy has virtually replaced biopsy of the *scalene fat pad* for nodes of interest on the right side of the mediastinum. However, for anatomic reasons, mediastinoscopy on the left is less satisfactory and more hazardous. Nodes in this location are usually approached through a limited left anterior thoracotomy (mediastinotomy) or, occasionally, by scalene fat pad biopsy. Needle aspiration, mediastinoscopy, and mediastinotomy are low-risk, high-yield procedures. They are invaluable in the "staging" of patients with known or suspected pulmonary malignancy.

LUNG BIOPSY Finally, if the diagnosis still remains unclear, biopsy of the lung may be required. Again, "closed" and "open" approaches are available. Closed biopsies are of three types: transbronchial, aspiration, and "cutting needle." Transbronchial biopsy, carried out through the fiberoptic bronchoscope, is a highly useful procedure, particularly since larger forceps have been introduced and the taking of multiple biopsies during one procedure has become routine.

However, when lesions are small and/or anatomically located beyond the reach of the FOB, direct aspiration needle biopsy is often more rewarding. *Aspiration* biopsy, mentioned previously, provides cytologic material but does not actually obtain a specimen of lung whose architecture can be examined, a feature which may be necessary to establish a diagnosis. Various "cutting" needles are available which do provide a "core" of the involved lung. However, this approach has waned in popularity because of the high incidence of pneumothorax and bleeding, occasional deaths due to air embolism, and the small size of the biopsy specimen, which may limit diagnostic interpretation. Fluoroscopic guidance is essential in all these closed approaches, and they are contraindicated if pulmonary hypertension or a hemorrhagic diathesis is present.

Open lung biopsy, requiring thoracotomy, is the final diagnostic resort. It is, however, a relatively safe procedure even in patients with respiratory failure, hemorrhagic diathesis, or pulmonary hypertension if meticulous surgical and anesthetic techniques are observed. Direct visualization allows selection of an optimum biopsy site, and of course, a specimen of adequate size is obtained. In selecting among these closed and open options, consideration of local expertise in their performance is a key factor.

All specimens obtained by biopsy should be both cultured and processed for pathologic examination.

REFERENCES

BARON RL et al: Computed tomography in the pre-operative evaluation of bronchogenic carcinoma. Radiology 145:727, 1982

BARTLETT JG, FINEGOLD SM: Bacteriology of expectorated sputum with quantitative culture and wash technic compared to transtracheal aspirates. Am Rev Resp Dis 117:1019, 1979

BORDOW RA, MOSER KM: *Manual of Clinical Problems in Pulmonary Medicine*. Boston, Little, Brown, 1985

COLICE GL etal: Comparison of computerized tomography with fiberoptic bronchoscopy in identifying endobronchial abnormalities in patients with known or suspected lung cancer. Am Resp Dis 131:397, 1985

GODWIN D et al: Distinguishing benign from malignant pulmonary nodules by computed tomography. Radiology 144:349, 1982

HAYES DA et al: Evaluation of two bronchofiberoscopic methods of culturing the lower respiratory tract. Am Rev Resp Dis 122:319, 1980

POE RH: Sensitivity and specificity of the non-specific transbronchial lung biopsy. Am Rev Resp Dis 119:25, 1979

SACKNER MA (ed): *Diagnostic Technics in Pulmonary Disease*. New York, Dekker, 1981

SEGELMAN SS et al: *Pulmonary System: Practical Approaches to Pulmonary Diagnosis*. New York, Grune & Stratton, 1980

SHURE D, FEDULLO PF: The role of carinal biopsy via the fiberoptic bronchoscope in the routine staging of lung cancer. Am Rev Resp Dis 127:82, 1983

SNIDER GL (ed): *Clinical Pulmonary Medicine*. Boston, Little, Brown, 1981

WESSELIUS LJ et al: Computer-assisted versus usual lung gallium-67 index in normals and patients with interstitial lung disorders. Am Rev Resp Dis 128:1084, 1983

WILLIFORD ME et al: Computed tomography of pleural disease. Am J Roentgenol 140:909, 1983

202 ASTHMA

E. R. McFADDEN, JR.

DEFINITION Asthma is a disease of airways that is characterized by increased responsiveness of the tracheobronchial tree to a multiplicity of stimuli. Asthma is manifested physiologically by a widespread narrowing of the air passages which may be relieved spontaneously or as a result of therapy and clinically by paroxysms of dyspnea, cough, and wheezing. It is an episodic disease, acute exacerbations being interspersed with symptom-free periods. Typically, most attacks are short-lived, lasting minutes to hours, and after them the patient seems to recover completely clinically. However, there can be a phase in which the patient experiences some degree of airway obstruction daily. This phase can be mild, with or without superimposed severe episodes, or much more serious, with severe obstruction persisting for days or weeks, a condition known as *status asthmaticus*.

PREVALENCE AND ETIOLOGY The prevalence and incidence of asthma is difficult to assess with certainty because of the lack of reliable population-based figures which have used uniform diagnostic criteria. However, it has been suggested that approximately 5 percent of adults and 7 to 10 percent of children in the United States and Australia have the disorder. Bronchial asthma occurs at all ages but predominantly in early life. About one-half of the cases develop before age 10 and another third occur before age 40. In childhood, there is a 2:1 male/female preponderance which equalizes by age 30.

From an etiologic standpoint, asthma is a heterogeneous disease, and attempts to define it in etiologic or pathologic terms have proved difficult. It is useful for epidemiologic and clinical purposes to classify the forms of this disease by the principal stimuli that incite or are associated with acute episodes. However, it is important to emphasize that the distinction between various types of asthma may often be artificial, and the response of a given subclassification may be initiated by more than one type of stimulus. With this reservation in mind, one can describe two broad groups: allergic and idiosyncratic.

Allergic asthma is often associated with a personal and/or family history of allergic diseases such as rhinitis, urticaria, and eczema; positive wheal-and-flare skin reactions to intradermal injection of extracts of airborne antigens; increased levels of IgE in the serum; and/or positive response to provocation tests involving the inhalation of specific antigen.

A significant segment of the asthmatic population will present with negative family or personal histories of allergy, negative skin tests, and normal serum levels of IgE, and therefore cannot be classified on the basis of defined immunologic mechanisms. These we term *idiosyncratic*. Many of these will develop a typical symptom complex upon contracting an upper respiratory illness. The initial insult may be little more than a common cold, but after several days the patient begins to develop paroxysms of wheezing and dyspnea that can last for days to months. These individuals should not be confused with the so-called infective asthmatics or with persons in whom the symptoms of bronchospasm are superimposed upon chronic bronchitis (see Chap. 208).

Unfortunately, many patients will not clearly fit into either of the above categories but will fall into a mixed group with features of each. In general, those patients whose onset of disease is in early life will tend to have a strong allergic component to their illness, while those who develop their asthma late tend to be nonallergic or to have mixed etiologies.

PATHOGENESIS OF ASTHMA The common denominator underlying the asthmatic diathesis is a nonspecific hyperirritability of the tracheobronchial tree. This phenomenon is the cardinal feature of asthma and is thought to be the primary pathogenic event in the disease. The increased airway reactivity can be familial or acquired and is materially worsened by events that promote airway inflammation. Heightened airway responsiveness is also found in first-degree relatives of asthmatics who are free of the disease and in some individuals with allergic rhinitis, cystic fibrosis, and chronic bronchitis. In asthmatics it correlates well with the clinical features of the illness, and it rises with repeated exposures to inciting stimuli and falls with avoidance and therapy. As the disease process becomes more severe, as indicated by increasing symptoms and medication requirements, the airways become more irritable and so respond more to nonspecific stimuli. Pulmonary function then becomes more unstable with greater diurnal variation.

The stimuli that increase airway responsiveness and incite acute episodes of asthma can be grouped into seven major categories: allergenic, pharmacologic, environmental, occupational, infectious, exercise-related, and emotional.

Allergens Allergic asthma is dependent upon an IgE response controlled by T and B lymphocytes and activated by the interaction of antigen with mast cell–bound IgE molecules. Most of the allergens that provoke asthma are airborne, and in order to induce a state of sensitivity, they must be reasonably abundant for considerable periods of time. Once sensitization has occurred, however, the patient can then exhibit exquisite responsivity, so that minute amounts of the offending agent can produce significant exacerbations of the disease. Immunologic mechanisms appear to be causally related to the development of asthma in 25 to 35 percent of all cases, and contributory in perhaps another third. Allergic asthma is frequently seasonal, and it is most often observed in children and young adults. A nonseasonal form may result from allergy to feathers, animal danders, molds, and other antigens present continuously in the environment. Exposure to antigen typically produces an immediate response in which airway obstruction develops in minutes and then resolves. In 30 to 50 percent of patients a second wave of bronchoconstriction, the so-called late reaction, develops 6 to 10 h later. In a minority only a late reaction occurs. In some individuals following a single exposure marked cyclic changes in airway lability may recur daily for a variable period. This phenomenon is frequently associated with an increase in airway responsivity.

The mechanism by which an inhaled antigen can provoke an acute episode of asthma is unknown but seems to depend, in part, upon antigen-antibody interactions on the surface of pulmonary mast cells with the subsequent generation and release of the mediators of immediate hypersensitivity. Current postulates hold that very small antigenic particles penetrate the lung's defenses and come in contact with mast cells that are interdigitating with the epithelium at the luminal surface of the central airways. The subsequent elaboration of mediators produces an immediate direct effect on airway smooth muscle and bronchial capillary permeability, thereby allowing an intense local reaction that is then followed by a more chronic one. The mediators released—histamine; bradykinin; the leukotrienes C, D, and E; prostaglandins PGG_2, $PGF_{2\alpha}$, and PGD_2, and thromboxane A_2—produce an intense inflammatory reaction with bronchoconstriction, vascular congestion, and edema formation. In addition to their ability to produce prolonged contraction of airway smooth muscle and mucosal edema, the leukotrienes also produce some of the other pathophysiologic features of asthma such as increased mucus production and impaired mucociliary transport mechanisms. The chemotactic factors that are elaborated, such as eosinophil and neutrophil chemotactic factors of anaphylaxis and leukotriene B_4, bring eosinophils, platelets, and polymorphonuclear leukocytes to the site of the reaction, and they, plus plasma proteins, immunoglobulins, and complement, provide the essential ingredients for a severe humoral and cellular inflammatory reaction involving both components. Diffusion of mediators through the mucosal edema can disrupt more defenses and spread the reaction along the airways. Further amplification can also occur if the reaction takes place in the vicinity of neural receptors. In this fashion, reflex bronchoconstriction can develop, and so an event which began in a single airway can now extend to involve a large part of the tracheobronchial tree. Whether frequent, persistent, or chronic low-grade mediator release alone is sufficient to establish an acquired state of airway hyperreactivity has not yet been established.

Pharmacologic stimuli The drugs most commonly associated with the induction of acute episodes of asthma are aspirin, coloring agents such as tartrazine, beta-adrenergic antagonists, and sulfiting agents. The typical aspirin-sensitive respiratory syndrome primarily affects adults, although the condition may be seen in childhood. This problem usually begins with perennial vasomotor rhinitis that is followed by a hyperplastic rhinosinusitis with nasal polyps. Progressive asthma then appears. On exposure to even very small quantities of aspirin, affected individuals typically develop ocular and nasal congestion and acute, often severe, episodes of airway obstruction. The prevalence of aspirin sensitivity in asthmatic subjects varies from study to study, but many authorities feel that 10 percent is a reasonable figure. There is a great deal of cross-reactivity between aspirin and other nonsteroidal anti-inflammatory compounds. Indomethacin, fenoprofen, naproxen, zomepirac sodium, ibuprofen, mefenamic acid, and phenylbutazone are particularly important in this regard. On the other hand, acetaminophen, sodium salicylate, choline salicylate, salicylamide, and propoxyphene are well tolerated. The exact frequency of cross-reactivity to tartrazine and other dyes in aspirin-sensitive asthmatic subjects is also controversial, and again 10 percent is the commonly accepted figure. This peculiar complication of aspirin-sensitive asthma is particularly insidious, however, in that tartrazine and other potentially troublesome dyes can be present in many of the drugs used to treat airway and nasal diseases and may unknowingly be administered to sensitive patients.

Patients with aspirin sensitivity can be desensitized by daily administration of the drug. Following this form of therapy cross tolerance also develops to other nonsteroidal anti-inflammatory agents. The mechanism by which aspirin and other such drugs produce bronchospasm is unknown; however, immediate hypersensitivity does not seem to be involved.

Beta-adrenergic antagonists regularly produce airway obstruction in asthmatics as well as in others with heightened airway reactivity and should be avoided in such individuals. Even the selective $beta_1$ agents have this propensity, particularly at higher doses. In fact, even the local use of $beta_1$ blockers in the eye for the treatment of glaucoma has been associated with worsening asthma.

Sulfiting agents, such as potassium metabisulfite, potassium and sodium bisulfite, sodium sulfite, and sulfur dioxide, which are widely used in the food and pharmaceutical industry as sanitizing and preservative agents, can also produce wheezing in sensitive individuals. Exposure usually follows ingestion of food or beverages containing these compounds, e.g., salads, fresh fruit, potatoes, shellfish, and wine. Recently, however, exacerbation of asthma has been reported following the use of sulfite-containing topical ophthalmic solutions, intravenous glucocorticoids, and some inhalational bronchodilator solutions. The incidence and mechanism of action of this phenomenon are unknown. When suspected, the diagnosis can be confirmed by either oral or inhalational provocations.

Environment and air pollution (see Chap. 204) Environmental causes of asthma are usually related to climatic conditions that promote the concentration of atmospheric pollutants and antigens. These conditions tend to develop in heavy industrial or densely populated urban areas and are frequently associated with thermal inversions or other situations associated with stagnant air masses. In these circumstances, although the general population can develop respiratory symptoms, patients with asthma and other respiratory diseases tend to be more severely affected.

Occupational factors (see Chap. 204) Occupational-related asthma is a significant health problem, and acute and chronic airway obstruction has been reported to follow exposure to a large number of compounds used in many types of industrial processes: bronchoconstriction can result from working with, or exposure to, *metal salts* (platinum, chrome, and nickel); *wood and vegetable dusts* (oak, western red cedar, grain, flour, castor bean, green coffee bean, mako, gum acacia, karay gum, and tragacanth); *pharmaceutical agents* (antibiotics, piperazine, and cimetidine); *industrial chemicals and plastics* (tidoluene isocyanate, phthalic acid anhydride, trimellitic anhydride, persulfates, ethylenediamine, paraphenylenediamine, and various dyes); *biologic enzymes* (laundry detergents and pancreatic enzymes); and *animal and insect dusts, serums, and secretions*. It is important to recognize that exposure to sensitizing chemicals, particularly those used in paints, solvents, and plastics, can also occur during leisure or non-work-related activities.

The underlying mechanisms for this airway obstruction appear to be three in number: (1) in some cases the offending agent results in the formation of a specific IgE, and the cause seems immunologic (the immunologic reaction can be immediate, late, or dual); (2) materials being employed, in other cases, cause a direct liberation of bronchoconstrictor substances; and (3) work-related irritant substances, in still other cases, directly or reflexly stimulate the airways of either latent or frank asthmatics. With occupational exposures, other than those that give an immediate and dual immunologic reaction, the patients give a characteristic cyclic history. They are well when they arrive at work; symptoms develop toward the end of the shift, progress after leaving the work site, and then regress. Absence from work during weekends or vacation periods brings about a remission. Frequently, there are similar symptoms in fellow employees.

Infections Respiratory infections are the most common of the stimuli that evoke acute exacerbations of asthma. Well-controlled investigations have demonstrated that respiratory viruses and not bacteria are the major etiologic factors, and there is no evidence to support the concept that bacterial infections or allergy play any role in this phenomenon. In young children, the most important infectious agents are respiratory syncytial virus and parainfluenza virus. In older children and adults, rhinovirus and influenza virus predominate as pathogens. Simple colonization of the tracheobronchial tree is insufficient to evoke acute episodes of bronchospasm, and attacks of asthma occur only when symptoms of an ongoing respiratory tract infection are, or have been, present. The mechanism by which viruses induce asthma is unknown, but it is probable that the resulting inflammatory changes in the airway mucosa produce a reduction in the firing thresholds of the subepithelial vagal receptors. Supporting evidence for this concept is derived from the fact that the airway responsiveness of normal nonasthmatic subjects to nonspecific stimuli is transiently increased after a viral infection. Increased airway responsiveness can last from 2 to 8 weeks after the infection in both normals and asthmatics.

Exercise Asthma can also be induced or made worse by physical exertion. Provocation of bronchospasm by exercise is probably operative to some extent in every asthmatic patient, and in some it may be the only trigger mechanism that will produce symptoms. In the latter circumstance, when such patients are followed for sufficient periods of time, they often develop recurring episodes of airway obstruction independent of exercise: thus, the onset of this problem can frequently serve as the first manifestation of the full-blown asthmatic syndrome. Exercise-induced asthma is particularly troublesome in children and young adults because of their usual high level of physical activity. The mechanism by which exercise produces acute exacerbations of asthma is related to the thermal changes that develop in the intrathoracic airways as heat and water are transferred from the mucosa to the inspired air to bring the latter to body conditions before it reaches the alveoli. The higher the ventilation and the colder, hence drier, the inspired air, the more the airway temperature falls, and so there is a significant interaction between the stress of the exercise task, the climatic environment in which it is performed, and the magnitude of the postexertional obstruction. Thus, for the same inspired air conditions, running will produce a more severe attack of asthma than will walking. Conversely, for a given task, the inhalation of cold air during its performance will markedly enhance the response, while warm, humid air will blunt or abolish it. Consequently, activities such as ice hockey, cross-country skiing, or ice skating are more provocative than is swimming in an indoor heated pool. The mechanism by which airway thermal changes evoke obstruction is unknown.

Emotional stress Abundant objective data now exist which demonstrate that psychological factors can interact with the asthmatic diathesis to worsen or ameliorate the disease process. The pathways and nature of the interactions are complex but probably operational to some extent in almost half of the patients studied. Changes in airway caliber seem to be mediated through modification of vagal efferent activity. The most frequently studied variable has been that of suggestion, and the weight of current evidence is that it can be quite an important influence in selected asthmatics. When psychically responsive individuals are given the appropriate suggestion, they can actually decrease or increase the pharmacologic effects of adrenergic and cholinergic stimuli on their airways. The extent to which psychological factors participate in the induction and/or continuation of any given acute exacerbation is unknown but probably varies from patient to patient and in the same patient from episode to episode.

PATHOLOGY In a patient who has died of acute asthma, the most striking feature of the lungs at necropsy is their gross overdistention and failure to collapse when the pleural cavities are opened. When the lungs are cut, numerous gelatinous plugs of exudate are found in the majority of the bronchial branches down to the terminal bronchiole. Histologic examination shows hypertrophy of the bronchial smooth muscle, mucosal edema, denudation of the surface epithelium, pronounced thickening of the basement membrane, and eosinophilic infiltrates in the bronchial wall. In asthmatic patients who die from trauma and causes other than asthma itself, mucous casts, basement membrane thickening, and eosinophilic infiltrates are frequently observed. In both situations there is an absence of any of the well-recognized forms of destructive emphysema.

PATHOPHYSIOLOGY AND CLINICAL CORRELATES The pathophysiologic hallmark of asthma is a reduction in airway diameter brought about by contraction of smooth muscle, edema of the bronchial wall, and thick tenacious secretions. Although the relative contributions of each component to the patient's ventilatory impairment are unknown, the net result is an increase in airway resistance, decreased forced expiratory volumes and flow rates, hyperinflation of the lungs and thorax, increased work of breathing, alterations in respiratory muscle function, changes in elastic recoil, abnormal distribution of both ventilation and pulmonary blood flow, mismatched ratios, and altered arterial blood gases. Thus, although asthma is considered to be primarily a disease of airways, virtually all aspects of pulmonary function are compromised during an acute attack. In addition, in very symptomatic patients there frequently is electrocardiographic evidence of right ventricular hypertrophy, and pulmonary hypertension can be found. Quantification of the changes that develop during an acute episode of asthma demonstrate that when a patient presents for therapy, his or her forced vital capacity tends to be ≤ 50 percent of normal. The 1-s forced expiratory volume (FEV_1) averages 30 percent of predicted, while the maximum and minimum midexpiratory flow rates are reduced to 20 percent or less of expected. In keeping with the alterations in mechanics, the associated air-trapping is substantial. In acutely ill patients, residual volume (RV) frequently approaches 400 percent of normal, while functional residual capacity doubles. The patients tend to report that their attacks have ended clinically when their RV has fallen to 200 percent of its predicted value and when the FEV_1 rises to 50 percent.

Hypoxia is a universal finding during acute exacerbations, but frank ventilatory failure is relatively uncommon, being observed in 10 to 15 percent of patients presenting for therapy. Most asthmatics have hypocapnia and a respiratory alkalosis. Statistically, the finding of normal arterial carbon dioxide tension tends to be associated with quite severe levels of obstruction and consequently, when found in a symptomatic individual, should be viewed as impending respiratory failure and treated as such. Equally, the presence of metabolic acidosis in the setting of acute asthma heralds severe obstruction. Usually, there are no clinical counterparts to the derangements in blood gases. Cyanosis is a very late sign. Thus, a dangerous level of hypoxia can go undetected. Likewise the signs which are attributable to carbon dioxide retention such as sweating, tachycardia, and wide pulse pressure or to acidosis such as tachypnea do not tend to be of great value in predicting the presence of hypercapnia or hydrogen ion excess in individual patients, for they are too frequently seen in anxious patients with more moderate disease to be of much use. Consequently, trying to judge the state of an acutely ill patient's ventilatory status on clinical grounds alone can be extremely hazardous and should not be relied upon with any confidence. Arterial blood gas tensions, therefore, must be measured.

The symptoms of asthma consist of a triad of dyspnea, cough, and wheezing, the latter often being regarded as the sine qua non. In its most typical form asthma is an episodic disease, and all three symptoms coexist. Attacks often occur at night, for reasons which are not clear but may relate to fluctuations in airway receptor thresholds that may result from circadian variations in the circulating levels of endogenous catecholamines and histamine. Attacks may also abruptly follow exposure to a specific allergen, physical exertion, a viral respiratory infection, or emotional excitement. At the onset the patient experiences a sense of constriction in the chest, often with a nonproductive cough. Respiration becomes audibly harsh, and wheezing in both phases of respiration becomes prominent, expiration becomes prolonged, and patients frequently have tachypnea, tachycardia, and mild systolic hypertension. The lungs rapidly become overinflated, and the anterior-posterior diameter of the thorax increases. If the attack is severe or prolonged, the accessory muscles become visibly active and frequently a paradoxical pulse will develop. These two signs have been found to be extremely valuable in indicating the severity of the obstruction. In the presence of either, pulmonary function tends to be significantly more impaired than in its absence. It is important to note that the development of these signs depends upon the generation of large negative intrathoracic pressures. Thus, if the patient's breathing is shallow, these signs could be absent even though obstruction is quite severe. The other signs and symptoms of asthma imperfectly reflect the physiologic alterations that are present, so much so that if one relies upon the loss of subjective complaints, or even the sign of wheezing, as being the end point at which therapy for an acute attack should be terminated, an enormous reservoir of residual disease is missed.

Termination of the episode is frequently marked by a cough producing thick stringy mucus which often takes the form of casts of the distal airways (Curschmann's spirals), and when examined microscopically often shows eosinophils and Charcot-Leyden crystals. In extreme situations, wheezing may markedly lessen or even disappear completely, cough may become extremely ineffective, and the patient may begin a gasping type of respiratory pattern. These findings imply extensive mucous plugging and impending suffocation. Ventilatory assistance by mechanical means may be required. Atelectasis due to inspissated secretions may occasionally occur with asthmatic attacks. Other complications such as spontaneous pneumothorax and/or pneumomediastinum are rare.

Less typically, a patient with asthma may complain of intermittent episodes of nonproductive cough or dyspnea only on exertion. Unlike other asthmatics when examined during their symptomatic periods, these patients tend to have normal breath sounds but will wheeze after repeated forced exhalations and will show dynamic ventilatory impairments when tested in the laboratory.

The differentiation of asthma from other diseases associated with dyspnea and wheezing is usually not difficult, particularly if the patient is seen during an acute episode. The physical findings and symptoms listed above, and the history of periodic attacks, are quite characteristic. A personal or family history of allergic diseases such as eczema, rhinitis, or urticaria is valuable contributory evidence. *Upper airway obstruction by tumor* or *laryngeal edema* can occasionally be confused with asthma. Typically, such a patient will present with stridor, and the harsh respiratory sounds can be localized to the area of the trachea. Diffuse wheezing throughout both lung fields is usually absent. However, differentiation can sometimes be difficult, and indirect laryngoscopy or bronchoscopy may be required. Recently a group of patients with glottic dysfunction have been described. These individuals close their glottis during inspiration and produce episodic attacks of severe airway obstruction that mimic asthma, yet they do not respond to standard therapy. Frequently they produce enough obstruction to develop carbon dioxide retention. However, unlike asthma the arterial oxygen tension is well preserved, and the alveolar-arterial gradient for oxygen narrows during the episode and does not widen as is the case with lower airway obstruction.

Persistent wheezing localized to one area of the chest in association with paroxysms of cough indicates *endobronchial disease* such as foreign-body aspiration, neoplasms, or bronchial stenosis.

The signs and symptoms of *acute left ventricular failure* can occasionally mimic asthma, but the findings of moist basilar rales, gallop rhythms, blood-tinged sputum, and other signs of heart failure (Chap. 182) allow the appropriate diagnosis to be reached.

Recurrent episodes of bronchospasm can occur with *carcinoid tumors* (Chap. 299), *recurrent pulmonary emboli* (Chap. 211), and *chronic bronchitis* (Chap. 208). In the last there are no true symptom-free periods in that one can usually obtain a history of chronic cough and sputum production as a background upon which acute attacks of wheezing are superimposed. Recurrent emboli, particularly in young women on oral contraceptives, are occasionally very difficult to separate from asthma. Frequently, these patients will present with episodes of breathlessness, particularly on exertion, and they can sometimes wheeze. Pulmonary function studies may show evidence of peripheral airway obstruction (Chap. 200), and when these changes are present, lung scans may also be abnormal. The therapeutic response to bronchodilators, discontinuation of the contraceptives, and institution of anticoagulant therapy may be helpful, but pulmonary angiography may be necessary in order to establish the correct diagnosis.

Eosinophilic pneumonias (Chap. 203) are often associated with asthmatic symptoms as are various chemical pneumonias and exposures to insecticides and cholinergic drugs. Bronchospasm can occasionally be a manifestation of *systemic vasculitis* with pulmonary involvement.

LABORATORY FINDINGS It is difficult to establish the diagnosis of asthma in the laboratory, for no single test is conclusive. Positive wheal-and-flare reactions to skin tests can be demonstrated to various allergens, but that finding does not necessarily correlate with the intrapulmonary events. Sputum and blood eosinophilia and measurement of serum IgE levels are also helpful but are not specific for asthma. Chest roentgenograms showing hyperinflation are nondiagnostic, as are tests of pulmonary function. The latter, however, are quite useful in that one can measure the degree of obstruction present, document its reversible nature, and, when combined with provocational challenges, demonstrate the airway hyperirritability so characteristic of this disease. Furthermore, the performance of forced vital capacity maneuvers is very helpful in the evaluation of acute asthmatic attacks. A reduction in the FEV_1 to less than 25 percent of that predicted or to less than 750 mL with little or no response following the administration of a bronchodilator indicates that the patient should receive very careful surveillance in conjunction with intensive treatment.

THERAPY Elimination of the causative agent(s) from the environment of an allergic asthmatic is the most successful means available for treating this condition (for details on avoidance see Chap. 260). Desensitization or immunotherapy with extracts of the suspected allergens has enjoyed widespread favor, but controlled studies are limited and have not proved it to be highly effective.

Drug treatment The drugs used in the treatment of asthma may be conveniently grouped into five major categories: beta-adrenergic agonists, methylxanthines, glucocorticoids, chromones, and anticholinergics. No one group is effective against all of the pathologic processes producing the disease, and since the degree of relief of airway obstruction is frequently incomplete with the use of a single agent, multiple drug regimens are commonplace.

ADRENERGIC STIMULANTS The drugs in this category consist of the catecholamines, resorcinols, and saligenins. These agents are analogues and produce airway dilatation through stimulation of beta receptors with the resultant formation of cyclic AMP. The catecholamines in widespread clinical use are epinephrine, isoproterenol, isoetharine, rimiterol, and hexoprenaline. The latter two are not yet available in the United States. As a group these compounds are short-acting and effective only by inhalational or parenteral routes. Epinephrine and isoproterenol are not beta$_2$-selective and have considerable chronotrophic and inotrophic cardiac effects. Epinephrine also has substantial alpha-stimulating effects. The usual dose is 0.3 to 0.5 mL of a 1:1000 solution administered subcutaneously. Isoproterenol is devoid of alpha activity and is the most potent agent of this group. It is usually administered in a 1:200 solution by inhalation. Controlled studies have shown that repetitive doses of epinephrine or isoproterenol are considerably more efficacious than the use of methylxanthines in the therapy of acute exacerbations of asthma. Isoproterenol has been used by the intravenous route in the management of status asthmaticus. In these circumstances, extremely careful monitoring of heart rate, rhythm, and blood pressure is an absolute requirement; and this therapy is not recommended save for very dire emergencies. Isoetharine is the most beta$_2$-selective compound of this class, but is a relatively weak bronchodilator. It is employed as an aerosol and supplied as a 1% solution. The pharmacologies of hexoprenaline and rimiterol are similar to isoetharine.

The commonly used resorcinols are metaproterenol, terbutaline, and fenoterol, and the most widely known saligenin is albuterol, or salbutamol. With the exception of metaproterenol, these drugs are highly selective for the respiratory tract and virtually devoid of significant cardiac effects except in high doses. They are active by all routes of administration, and because their chemical structures allow them to bypass the metabolic processes used to degrade the catecholamines, their effects are long-lasting, exceeding 6 h in many studies.

The method by which beta agonists are administered is of great importance since it influences both the clinical response and the metabolic fate. Inhalation increases the bronchial selectivity of these drugs, allows maximal bronchodilation to occur with fewer side effects than other routes of administration, and is considered by many as the route of choice. Recent data indicate that this is true not just in maintenance therapy but also during the treatment of severe acute obstruction. A frequent side effect of these drugs is tremor.

METHYLXANTHINES Theophylline, and its various salts, are medium potency bronchodilators. Like the beta agonists, they improve the movement of airway mucus. Although efficacious, the drugs in this class are not as potent as the sympathomimetics, and they have a narrower therapeutic-toxic window. The mechanism responsible for the bronchodilator effect of the methylxanthines is unknown. It was formerly thought that these drugs increased cyclic AMP by the inhibition of phosphodiesterase. However, recent evidence no longer supports this concept. The therapeutic plasma concentrations of theophylline lie between 10 and 20 μg/mL. But the dose required to achieve this level varies widely from patient to patient due to differences in the metabolism of the drug. Theophylline clearance, and thus dosage requirements, is decreased substantially in neonates and the elderly and those with acute and chronic hepatic dysfunction, cardiac decompensation, and cor pulmonale. Clearance is also decreased during febrile illnesses. Clearance is increased in children. In addition a number of important drug interactions can alter theophylline metabolism. Clearance falls with the concurrent use of cigarettes, marijuana, erythromycin and troleandomycin, allopurinol, cimetidine, and propranolol. It rises with phenobarbital and phenytoin or any other drug that has the capability of inducing hepatic microsomal enzymes.

In contrast to the large number of oral compounds, aminophylline is the only compound available for intravenous use. The recommendations for intravenous therapy in children aged 9 to 16 and young adult smokers not currently receiving theophylline products are as follows: a loading dose of 6 mg/kg is given followed by an infusion of 1.0 (mg/kg)/h for the next 12 h and then 0.8 (mg/kg)/h thereafter. In nonsmoking adults, older patients, and those with cor pulmonale, congestive heart failure, and liver disease, the loading dose remains the same but the maintenance dose is reduced to between 0.1 and 0.5 (mg/kg)/h. In those patients already receiving theophylline, the loading dose is frequently withheld or in extreme situations given in a reduced amount at 0.5 mg/kg.

The most common side effects of theophylline are nervousness, nausea, vomiting, anorexia, and headache. At plasma levels greater than 30 μg/mL there is a risk of seizures and cardiac arrhythmias.

GLUCOCORTICOIDS Glucocorticoids have been used for many years in the treatment of asthma, but controversy still surrounds such basic issues as their specific indication and dose. Glucocorticoids are not bronchodilators, and their major use is in reducing airway inflammation. Although it is difficult to provide precise recommendations because objective data are lacking, there are several situations in the management of acute and chronic asthma in which all would agree that steroids should be employed. In acute illness, that is, when severe airway obstruction is not resolving, or is even worsening despite intense optimal bronchodilator therapy, and in chronic disease, steroids are most helpful when there has been failure of a previously optimal regimen with frequent recurrences of symptoms of progressive severity.

Although many dosage schedules have been proposed, few objective data on pulmonary function are available to support them. Those that are available indicate that plasma cortisol levels above 100 μg/dL may be required to produce an effect. In acute situations, this can be achieved by the intravenous administration of 4 mg per kilogram of body weight of hydrocortisone as a loading dose, followed several hours later by an infusion regulated to deliver 3 mg/kg every 6 h. It should be emphasized that the effects of steroids in acute asthma are not immediate and may not be seen for 6 h or more after their initial administration. Consequently, it is mandatory to continue vigorous bronchodilator therapy during this interval. After 24 to 72 h, depending upon response, the patient can be switched to oral agents. A usual starting point is 40 to 60 mg prednisone as a single daily morning dose. The amount can then be reduced by half every fourth to fifth day. In situations in which it appears that continued steroid therapy will be needed, an alternate-day schedule should be instituted to minimize side effects. This is particularly important in children, since continuous corticosteroid administration interrupts growth. Long-acting preparations such as dexamethasone should not be used in this approach for they defeat the purpose of alternate-day schedules by causing prolonged suppression of the pituitary-adrenal axis.

Several inhaled steroids of high topical potency are available and greatly facilitate the withdrawal of oral agents. They are also useful in reducing airway sensitivity and as an alternative to oral glucocorticoids in situations where asthma symptoms are escalating. Hyperadrenal corticism and adrenal suppression are not major issues, and the most frequent side effect is symptomatic oropharyngeal candidiasis. This can be controlled by the use of a spacing device on the metered-dose inhaler.

CHROMONES Cromolyn sodium is not a bronchodilator. Its major therapeutic effect is the inhibition of degranulation of mast cells, thereby preventing the release of the chemical mediators of anaphylaxis. The drug does not inhibit the combination of antigen with antibody, nor does it affect the fixation of IgE to mast cells. Cromolyn has been shown to be of use in atopic and nonatopic asthmatics, and it blunts exercise-induced asthma in both children and adults. Numerous trials have shown that about 75 percent of patients derive worthwhile benefits from the drug in terms of reduction of medications and improvement in symptoms. Therapy is best initiated between attacks or in periods of relative remission. If no response is noted by 4 to 6 weeks, the drug can be discontinued.

ANTICHOLINERGICS Anticholinergic drugs, such as atropine sulfate, are known to produce bronchodilatation in patients with asthma, but their use has been limited by systemic side effects. Recently, newer nonabsorbable quaternary ammonium (atropine methylnitrate and ipratropium bromide) aerosol agents have undergone extensive trials and have been found to be both effective and remarkably free of untoward effects. These new agents, when generally available, may be of particular benefit in patients with asthma and coexistent heart disease, in whom use of methylxanthines and beta stimulants may be dangerous. A chief disadvantage of the anticholinergics are their slow onset of action. Sixty to 90 min may be required before peak bronchodilatation is achieved.

MISCELLANEOUS Opiates, sedatives, and tranquilizers should be absolutely avoided in the acutely ill asthmatic because the risk of depressing alveolar ventilation is great and respiratory arrest has been reported to occur shortly after their use. Admittedly most individuals are anxious and frightened, but experience has shown that they can be calmed equally well by the physician's presence and reassurances. Beta-adrenergic blockers and parasympathetic agonists should be avoided, or used with great caution, for they can cause marked deterioration in lung function.

Expectorants and mucolytic agents have enjoyed great vogue in the past, but there is little evidence available to indicate that they add significantly to the treatment of the acute or chronic phases of this disease. Mucolytic agents such as acetylcysteine may actually produce bronchospasm when administered to susceptible asthmatics. This can be overcome by aerosolizing them in solution with a beta-adrenergic agent. The use of intravenous fluids in the treatment of acute asthma has also been advocated. There is little evidence to indicate that this adjunct hastens recovery, but it may prevent dehydration and through that forestall the inspissation of secretions, by replacing the larger insensible water losses that could occur with prolonged hyperventilation.

PROGNOSIS AND CLINICAL COURSE Death from asthma is uncommon. Available mortality statistics for the United States indicate a death rate of approximately 0.3 per 100,000 persons.

The available information on the clinical course of asthma suggests that somewhere between 50 to 80 percent of all patients can expect to have a reasonably good prognosis, particularly those whose disease is mild and develops in childhood. The number of children still having asthma 7 to 10 years after the initial diagnosis varies from 26 to 78 percent with an average of 46 percent; however, the percentage who continue to have severe disease is relatively low (6 to 19 percent). The natural course of asthma in adult life has been little investigated. Some studies suggest that spontaneous remissions occur in approximately 20 percent of those who develop the disease as adults and 40 percent or so can be expected to improve with less frequent and severe attacks as they grow older.

REFERENCES

FANTA CH, MCFADDEN ER JR: Status Asthmaticus, in *Current Therapy in Internal Medicine*, TM Bayless et al (eds). Philadelphia, Decker, 1984, pp 6–10

HENDELES L, WEINBERGER M: Theophylline. Pharmacotherapy 3:2–44, 1983

MCFADDEN ER JR: Beta$_2$ receptor agonists: metabolism and pharmacology. J Allergy Clin Immunol 68:91–97, 1981

———: Asthma. Airway dynamics, cardiac function, and clinical correlates, in *Allergies: Principles and Practice*, E Middleton et al (eds). St Louis, CV Mosby, 1983, pp 843–862

WASSERMAN SI: Mediators of immediate hypersensitivity. J Allergy Clin Immunol 72:191–115, 1983

203 HYPERSENSITIVITY PNEUMONITIS

GARY W. HUNNINGHAKE / HAL B. RICHERSON

DEFINITION Hypersensitivity pneumonitis (HP), or extrinsic allergic alveolitis, is an immunologically induced inflammation of the lung parenchyma, involving alveolar walls and terminal airways, secondary to repeated inhalation of a variety of organic dusts and other agents by a susceptible host. In contrast to many of the other interstitial lung diseases, the etiology of this interstitial and alveolar filling disease is known. Although a number of etiologic agents have been identified, most are rare, and a few well-documented syndromes are associated with the vast majority of cases. The diagnosis of HP requires a constellation of clinical, radiographic, physiologic, pathologic, and immunologic criteria, each of which by itself is rarely pathognomonic, and the preferred treatment is avoidance of the causative antigen.

ETIOLOGY Agents implicated as causes of HP include those listed in Table 203-1. Many cases of HP occurring in various occupations involve exposure to similar agents, particularly the thermophilic actinomycetes. Except for exotic occupational exposures, the usual sources of causative antigens are "moldy" hay, silage, or grain, pet birds, and heating, cooling, and humidification systems. Simple chemicals, such as isocyanates, may also cause hypersensitivity pneumonitis.

PATHOGENESIS The finding that precipitating antibodies against extracts of moldy hay were demonstrable in most patients with farmer's lung led to the early conclusion that HP was an immune-complex-mediated reaction. Subsequent investigations of HP in human beings and animal models also provided evidence for the importance of cell-mediated hypersensitivity. The early (acute) reaction is likely a result of the formation of immune complexes in the lung, and is characterized by an increase in polymorphonuclear leukocytes in the alveoli and small airways. This early lesion is followed by an influx of mononuclear cells into the lung and the formation of granulomas. The latter lesion appears to be a classic delayed hypersensitivity reaction to repeated inhalation of antigen and adjuvant-active materials.

Bronchoalveolar lavage in patients with HP has consistently demonstrated an increase in T lymphocytes in lavage fluid (a finding which is also observed in patients with other granulomatous lung disorders). Patients with recent or continual exposure to antigen may also have an increase in polymorphonuclear leukocytes in lavage fluid. In most patients examined during recovery from acute disease, the T lymphocytes in lavage fluid are predominantly the suppressor/cytotoxic T-cell subset, which expresses surface antigens detected by OKT8 or Leu 2a monoclonal antibodies. In patients with very recent exposure to antigen, however, the numbers of helper T cells (OKT4$^+$ or Leu 3a$^+$) may increase in lavage fluid. Similar findings may be present as well in similarly exposed, asymptomatic individuals. These observations suggest that there is an active modulation of granuloma formation in the lung by immunoregulatory T cells in this disorder.

CLINICAL PRESENTATION The *clinical picture* varies from patient to patient and is related to the frequency and intensity of exposure to the causative antigen and perhaps other host factors. The presentation can be *acute*, *subacute*, or *chronic*. In the *acute form*, symptoms such as cough, fever, chills, malaise, and dyspnea may occur 6 to 8 h after exposure to the antigen and usually clear within a few days if there is no further exposure to antigen. The *subacute form* often appears insidiously over a period of weeks marked by cough and dyspnea, and may progress to cyanosis and severe dyspnea requiring hospitalization. In some patients, a subacute form of the disease may persist after an acute presentation of the disorder, especially if there is continued exposure to antigen. In most patients with the acute or subacute form of HP, the symptoms, signs, and other manifestations

TABLE 203-1 Selected examples of hypersensitivity pneumonitis

Disease	Antigen	Source of antigen
Farmer's lung	Thermophilic actinomycetes*	Contaminated hay, grain, silage
Bird fancier's, breeders, or handler's lung	Parakeet, pigeon, dove, chicken, turkey proteins	Avian droppings
Humidifier or air-conditioner lung	Thermophilic actinomycetes, *Aureobasidium pullulans*, amoeba, other	Contaminated water in humidification aerosols, vaporizers, sprays
Woodworker's lung	Wood dust; *Alternaria*	Oak cedar, mahogany dusts; pine and spruce pulp
Sauna taker's lung	*A. pullulans*, other	Contaminated sauna steam
Bagassosis	Thermophilic actinomycetes	Contaminated bagasse (sugar cane)
Malt worker's lung	*Aspergillus fumigatus, A. clavatus*	Moldy barley
Mushroom worker's lung	Thermophilic actinomycetes, other	Mushroom compost
Sequoiosis	*Aureobasidium, Graphium* species	Redwood sawdust
Maple bark stripper's disease	*Cryptostroma corticale*	Maple bark
Coffee worker's lung	Coffee bean dust	Coffee beans
Miller's lung	Infested wheat flour	*Sitophilus granarius* (wheat weevil)
Bathtub refinisher's lung	Toluene diisocyanate (TDI)	Porcelain-surfacing catalyst
Chemical worker's lung	Toluene diisocyanate TDI, methylene diisocyanate (MDI), phthallic anhydride, vinyl chloride, other	Polyurethane foam and insulation, synthetic rubber manufacturing, meat wrapping and labeling, other

* *Thermophilic actinomycetes species include* Micropolyspora faeni, Thermoactinomyces vulgaris, T. saccharrii, T. viridis, *and* T. candidus.

of HP disappear within days, weeks, or months if the causative agent is no longer inhaled. Transformation to a chronic form of the disease may occur in patients with continued antigen exposure, but the frequency of such progression is uncertain. The *chronic form* of the disease may also present as a gradually progressive interstitial disease associated with cough and exertional dyspnea without a prior history consistent with acute or subacute disease. Such a gradual onset of the disease frequently occurs with low-dose exposure to the antigen.

DIAGNOSIS Following acute exposure to antigen, neutrophilia and lymphopenia are frequently present. All forms of the disease may be associated with elevations in erythrocyte sedimentation rate, C-reactive protein, rheumatoid factor, and serum immunoglobulins. Antinuclear antibodies are rarely present.

Examination for *serum precipitins* against suspected antigens, such as those listed in Table 203-1, is an important part of the diagnostic workup. If found, precipitins indicate sufficient exposure to the causative agent for generation of an immunologic response. The diagnosis of HP is not established solely by the presence of precipitins, however, since precipitins merely indicate a significant exposure to an antigen source. Precipitins are found in sera of many individuals exposed to appropriate antigens who demonstrate no other evidence of HP. False-negative results may occur because of poor quality antigens or an inappropriate choice of antigens. Extraction of antigens from the patient's environment may at times be helpful.

No specific or distinctive *chest roentgenogram* occurs in HP. It can be normal even in symptomatic patients. The acute or subacute phase may be associated with poorly defined, patchy or diffuse infiltrates or with discrete, nodular infiltrates. In the chronic phase, the chest x-ray usually shows a diffuse reticulonodular infiltrate. Honeycombing may eventually develop as the condition progresses. Abnormalities rarely seen in hypersensitivity pneumonitis include pleural effusion or thickening, and hilar adenopathy.

Pulmonary function studies in all forms of HP may show a restrictive pattern with loss of lung volumes, impaired diffusion capacity, decreased compliance, and an exercise-induced hypoxemia. Depending on the severity of the disease, a resting hypoxemia may be found. Functional abnormalities may gradually increase in severity or may occur rapidly following acute or subacute exposure to antigen. As the chronic stage progresses, changes consistent with airway obstruction may also become increasingly prominent.

Bronchoalveolar lavage is used in some centers to aid in diagnostic evaluation, and the characteristic features of the lavage fluid are described above.

Lung biopsy may be indicated in patients without sufficient other criteria to make a definitive diagnosis. The initial biopsy procedure is usually a transbronchial biopsy. In some patients, an open-lung biopsy may be necessary since this procedure will provide adequate material for pathologic studies, whereas transbronchial biopsy may not. Although the histopathology is distinctive, it may not be pathognomonic of HP. When the biopsy is taken during the active phase of disease, typical findings include an interstitial alveolar infiltrate consisting of plasma cells, lymphocytes, and occasional eosinophils and neutrophils, usually with accompanying granulomas. Interstitial fibrosis is common but most often mild in earlier stages of the disease. Some degree of bronchiolitis is found in about half the cases, whereas vasculitis is not a feature of the disorder.

The lack of standardized, nonirritating antigens and of proven controlled protocols makes *skin testing* and *inhalational challenge* useful only for experimental purposes. Similarly *in vitro tests of cell-mediated (delayed) hypersensitivity* have not been shown to consistently correlate with clinical HP and cannot be recommended in the routine diagnostic workup.

DIFFERENTIAL DIAGNOSIS The diagnosis of HP should be initially considered in any patient with a history of recurrent ''pneumonias'' or with interstitial lung disease, as well as in those with typical presentations of acute, subacute, or chronic HP. A condition termed *pulmonary mycotoxicosis* (or ''atypical'' farmer's lung) occurs in patients massively exposed to moldy silage and is manifested by fever, chills, and cough within a few hours. Precipitins are not present, suggesting this disease may occur in individuals not previously sensitized to the inhaled antigen.

Chronic HP may often be difficult to distinguish from a number of other interstitial lung disorders such as idiopathic pulmonary fibrosis, interstitial lung disease associated with a collagen vascular disorder, and drug-induced lung diseases. A negative history for use of appropriate drugs and no evidence of a systemic disorder usually exclude the presence of drug-induced lung disease or a collagen vascular disorder. In some patients, a lung biopsy may be required to differentiate chronic HP from idiopathic pulmonary fibrosis.

The lung disease associated with acute or subacute HP may resemble other disorders which present with systemic symptoms and recurrent pulmonary infiltrates. These disorders include the collagen vascular disorders, drug-induced lung disease, allergic bronchopulmonary aspergillosis and other eosinophilic pneumonias. Eosinophilic pneumonia is often associated with asthma and is typified by peripheral eosinophilia; neither of these are features of HP. Allergic bronchopulmonary aspergillosis is sometimes confused with HP because of the presence of precipitating antibodies to *Aspergillus fumigatus*.

TREATMENT Because effective treatment depends largely on avoiding the antigen, identification of the causative agent and its source is essential. This is usually possible if the physician takes a careful environmental and occupational history or, if necessary, visits the patient's environment.

The simplest way to avoid the incriminated agent is to remove the patient from the environment, or the source of the agent from the patient's environment. This recommendation cannot be taken lightly when it completely changes the life-style or livelihood of the patient. In many cases, however, the source of exposure (birds, humidifiers) can easily be removed. If occupational exposure is involved, an initial attempt can be made at antigen avoidance maneuvers least disruptive to the patient's livelihood, which usually means avoiding areas associated with heavy exposure, and wearing an appropriate mask. This will not suffice for small-molecular-weight agents such as isocyanates, which require elaborate filtration devices. Pollen masks, personal dust respirators, airstream helmets, and ventilated helmets with a supply of fresh air are increasingly efficient means of purifying inhaled air. If symptoms recur or physiologic abnormalities progress in spite of these measures, then more effective measures to avoid antigen exposure must be pursued.

Compromises with environmental control pertain only to the acute, recurrent, transient clinical form of HP and must be accompanied by careful follow-up. Subacute forms are ordinarily the result of a heavy, sustained exposure. The chronic form typically results from low-grade exposure over many months to years, and the lung disease may already be partially irreversible. These patients should be advised to avoid completely all possible contact with the offending agent.

Patients with the *acute*, recurrent form of HP usually recover without need for corticosteroids. *Subacute* HP may be associated with severe symptoms and marked physiologic impairment, and may continue to progress for several days despite hospitalization. Urgent establishment of the diagnosis and prompt institution of corticosteroid treatment are indicated in such patients. Corticosteroid therapy may also hasten recovery in patients with lesser involvement. Prednisone at a dosage of 1 mg/kg per day or its equivalent is continued for 7 to 14 days, and then tapered over the ensuing 2 to 6 weeks at a rate which depends on the patient's clinical status.

Patients with *chronic* extrinsic allergic alveolitis may gradually recover without therapy following environmental control. In many patients, however, a trial of prednisone may be useful to obtain maximal reversibility of the lung disease. Following initial prednisone therapy (1 mg/kg per day for 4 to 6 weeks), the drug is tapered to the lowest dosage that will maintain the functional status of the patient. Many patients will not require or benefit from long-term therapy if there is no further exposure to antigen.

THE EOSINOPHILIC PNEUMONIAS

The eosinophilic pneumonias are composed of distinct individual syndromes characterized by eosinophilic pulmonary infiltrates and, commonly, peripheral blood eosinophilia. Since Loeffler's initial description of a transient, benign syndrome of migratory pulmonary infiltrates and peripheral blood eosinophilia of unknown cause, this group of disorders has been enlarged to include diseases of known and unknown etiology (Table 203-2). These diseases may be considered as examples of hypersensitivity lung disease but are not to be confused with hypersensitivity pneumonitis (extrinsic allergic alveolitis) in which eosinophilia is not a feature.

When an eosinophilic pneumonia is associated with bronchial asthma, it is important to determine if the patient has extrinsic (allergic, atopic) asthma and has wheal-and-flare skin reactivity to *Aspergillus* allergens. If so, other criteria should be sought for diagnosis of *allergic bronchopulmonary aspergillosis* (ABPA) (Table 203-3). *Aspergillus fumigatus* is the most common etiologic agent although other *Aspergillus* species have also been implicated. The chest roentgenogram in ABPA may show transient, recurrent infiltrates or suggest the presence of central bronchiectasis. The bronchial asthma of ABPA likely involves an IgE-mediated hypersensitivity whereas the bronchiectasis associated with this disorder is thought to result from a deposition of immune complexes in proximal airways. Adequate treatment usually requires the long-term use of systemic corticosteroids.

Tropical eosinophilia is usually caused by filarial infection; however, eosinophilic pneumonias also occur with other parasites such as *Ascaris, Ancyclostoma* species, *Toxocara* species, and *Strongyloides stercoralis*. Tropical eosinophilia due to *Wuchereria bancrofti* or *W. malayi* occurs most commonly in southern Asia, Africa, and South America, and is treated successfully with diethylcarbamazine.

TABLE 203-2 The eosinophilic pneumonias

1 Etiology known
  a Allergic bronchopulmonary aspergillosis
  b Parasitic infestations
  c Drug reactions
2 Idiopathic
  a Loeffler's syndrome
  b Chronic eosinophilic pneumonia
  c Allergic granulomatosis of Churg and Strauss
  d Hypereosinophilic syndrome

Drug-induced eosinophilic pneumonias are typified by acute reactions to nitrofurantoin which may begin 2 h to 10 days after nitrofurantoin is started, with symptoms of dry cough, fever, chills, and dyspnea; an eosinophilic pleural effusion accompanying patchy or diffuse pulmonary infiltrates may also occur. Other drugs associated with eosinophilic pneumonias include sulfonamides, penicillin, chlorpropamide, thiazides, tricyclic antidepressants, hydralazine, mephenesin, mecamylamine, nickel carbonyl vapor, gold salts, isoniazid, para-aminosalicylic acid, and others. Treatment consists of withdrawal of the incriminated drugs and the use of corticosteroids, if necessary.

The idiopathic eosinophilic pneumonias consist of a group of diseases of varying severity. *Loeffler's syndrome* is a benign, acute eosinophilic pneumonia characterized by migrating pulmonary infiltrates and minimal clinical manifestations. *Chronic eosinophilic pneumonia* presents with significant systemic symptoms including fever, chills, night sweats, cough, anorexia, and weight loss lasting several weeks to months. The chest x-ray frequently shows peripheral infiltrates which have been described as a photographic negative of pulmonary edema. Some patients also have bronchial asthma which is of the intrinsic or nonallergic type. Dramatic clearing of symptoms and chest x-rays is often noted within 48 h after initiation of corticosteroid therapy.

Allergic angiitis and granulomatosis of Churg and Strauss is a multisystem vasculitic disorder which frequently involves the skin, kidney, and nervous system in addition to the lung (Chap. 269). The disorder may occur at any age and favors persons with a history of bronchial asthma. The asthma often is progressive until the onset of fever and exaggerated eosinophilia at which time the symptoms of asthma may ease. The illness may be fulminating and the prognosis grave unless treated aggressively with corticosteroids and immunosuppressive therapy.

The hypereosinophilic syndrome is characterized by a peripheral blood eosinophilia over 1500 eosinophils per cubic millimeter for 6 months or longer; lack of evidence for parasitic, allergic, or other known causes of eosinophilia; and signs or symptoms of multisystem organ dysfunction. Consistent features are blood and bone marrow eosinophilia with tissue infiltration by relatively mature eosinophils. The organs affected typically include the heart, lungs, liver, spleen, skin, and nervous system. Therapy of the disorder consists of corticosteroids and/or hydroxyurea plus therapy as needed for cardiac dysfunction, which is frequently responsible for much of the morbidity and mortality in this syndrome.

TABLE 203-3 Diagnostic features of allergic bronchopulmonary aspergillosis (ABPA)

MAIN DIAGNOSTIC CRITERIA

1 Bronchial asthma
2 Pulmonary infiltrates
3 Peripheral eosinophilia (>1000 per cubic millimeter)
4 Immediate wheal-and-flare response to *Aspergillus fumigatus*
5 Serum precipitins to *A. fumigatus*
6 Elevated serum IgE
7 Central bronchiectasis

OTHER DIAGNOSTIC FEATURES

1 History of brownish plugs in sputum
2 Culture of *A. fumigatus* from sputum
3 Elevated IgE (and IgG) class antibodies specific for *A. fumigatus*

REFERENCES

Hypersensitivity pneumonitis

HUNNINGHAKE GW, BEDELL GN: Interstitial lung disease: Concepts of pathogenesis. Sem Resp Med 6:31, 1984

——— et al: Inflammatory and immune processes in the human lung in health and disease: Evaluation by bronchopulmonary lavage. Am J Pathol 97:149, 1979

LEATHERMAN JW et al: Lung T cells in hypersensitivity pneumonitis. Ann Intern Med 100:390, 1984

RICHERSON HB: Hypersensitivity pneumonitis (extrinsic allergic alveolitis), in AP Fishman (ed), *Pulmonary Diseases and Disorders*. New York, McGraw-Hill, 1980, pp 691–698

———: Hypersensitivity pneumonitis—pathology and pathogenesis. Clin Rev Allergy 1:469, 1983

The eosinophilic pneumonias

MALO JL et al: Studies in chronic allergic bronchopulmonary aspergillosis. 1. Clinical and physiological findings. 2. Radiological findings. 3. Immunological findings. 4. Comparison with a group of asthmatics. Thorax 32:254, 262, 269, 275, 1977

MAYCOCK RL, SALDANA MJ: Eosinophilic pneumonia, in AP Fishman (ed), *Pulmonary Diseases and Disorders*, New York, McGraw-Hill, 1980, pp 926–939

SCHATZ M et al: The eosinophil and the lung. Arch Intern Med 142:1515, 1982

SCHOENBERGER CI, CRYSTAL RG: Drug-induced lung disease, in KJ Isselbacher et al (eds), *Update IV: Harrison's Principles of Internal Medicine*. New York, McGraw-Hill, 1983, pp 49–74

SLAVIN RG: Allergic bronchopulmonary aspergillosis. Clin Rev Allergy 3:167, 1985

204 ENVIRONMENTAL LUNG DISEASES

FRANK E. SPEIZER

This chapter is designed to provide a perspective on the approaches used to assess pulmonary diseases for which environmental causes are suspected. This assessment is important because removal of the patient from a harmful environment is often the only intervention that might prevent further significant deterioration or lead to improvement in a patient's condition. Furthermore, the identification of an environmentally associated disease in a single patient may lead to primary preventive strategies in other similarly exposed people who have not yet developed disease. Unless the physician specifically considers environmental exposures, these diseases and their causes will go undetected.

The exact magnitude of the problem is unknown, but there is no question that large numbers of people are at risk of developing serious respiratory disease as a result of occupational or environmental exposures. For example, even if only 5 percent (a conservative estimate) of workers currently exposed to asbestos, cotton dust, or silica are to suffer from respiratory disease as a result of their exposure, this represents more than 100,000 individuals in the United States. Although industries are required to spend substantial amounts of capital in efforts to protect their workers, occupationally related respiratory diseases continue to occur. These diseases are often attributed to exposures in the distant past at a time when we were not aware of or at least did not consider worker protection to the degree that we do today. We have, as a society, elected to pay compensation to affected individuals, and the physician is often called upon to judge not only the physical condition of such a patient but also the degree to which the illness can be related to, or aggravated by, a particular occupational exposure.

HISTORY AND PHYSICAL EXAMINATION The patient history is of paramount importance in assessing any potential occupational or environmental exposure. Often one is dealing with potential exposures in industries or environmental settings in which the physician has little personal experience. The physician must, therefore, ask the patient to describe a suspected environmental exposure in detail.

Inquiry into specific work practices should include questions about specific contaminants involved, the availability and use of personal respiratory protection devices, the size and ventilation of workspaces, the numbers of other workers potentially at risk of exposure, and whether other coworkers have similar complaints. In addition, the patient must be questioned about alternative sources for potentially toxic exposures, including hobbies or other environmental exposures at home. Short-term exposures to potential toxic agents in the distant past also must be considered. This information can be best elicited by a detailed occupational history which inquires about every job (beginning even with part-time jobs during schooling), about the nature of the work, the materials handled, and the duration and chronologic years of employment.

Many people are aware of the potential hazards in their workplaces, and recent legislation has made it a requirement in many states that employees be informed about potentially hazardous exposures. These requirements include the provision of specific educational materials, personal protective equipment, along with instruction in its use, and information on environmental control procedures. Reminders posted in the workplace may warn workers about hazardous substances. Protective clothing, lockers, and shower facilities may be considered necessary parts of the job. However, even in these ideal settings, the introduction of new processes, particularly when related to the use of new chemical compounds, may change exposure significantly, and often only the employee on the production line is aware of the change. For the physician who regularly sees patients from a particular industry, a visit to the work site can be very instructive.

The physical examination of patients with environmentally related lung diseases may help to determine the nature and severity of the pulmonary condition. Unfortunately, the pulmonary response to most injurious agents is the development of a limited number of nonspecific physical signs. These findings do not point to the specific causative agent, and other types of information must be used to arrive at an etiologic diagnosis.

PULMONARY FUNCTION TESTS AND CHEST RADIOGRAPH The use of pulmonary function tests and radiographic examinations of the chest can provide insight into the nature of the exposures which have led to the current condition of the patient and the level of impairment. Many mineral dusts produce characteristic alterations in the mechanics of breathing and lung volumes which clearly indicate a restrictive pattern (Chaps. 200 and 209). On the other hand, exposures to a number of organic dusts or chemical agents capable of producing occupational asthma result in pronounced obstructive patterns of pulmonary dysfunction that may be reversible (Chap. 202). Standardized approaches for measuring the mechanics of breathing and diffusion across the alveolar membrane (Chap. 200) have been proposed for screening large industrial groups. Measurement of change in forced expiratory volume (FEV_1) before and after a working shift can be used to detect an acute bronchoconstrictive response. An acute decrement of FEV_1 over the Monday work shift is a characteristic feature of cotton textile workers with byssinosis.

For many years the chest radiograph has been used to detect and monitor the pulmonary response to mineral dusts. To provide a standardized way of recording judgments about the kind and severity of radiographic abnormalities, the International Labour Organization (ILO)/International Classification of Radiographs of Pneumoconioses was developed. The ILO scheme involves classifying chest roentgenograms according to the nature and size of opacities seen and the extent of involvement of the parenchyma. Extensive description of the ILO system is beyond the scope of this chapter; however, judgments based only on chest radiographs may over- or underestimate the functional impact of pneumoconiosis. With dusts causing rounded, regular opacities, such as in coal worker's pneumoconiosis, the degree of involvement on the chest radiograph may be quite extensive, while pulmonary function may be only minimally impaired. In contrast, in pneumoconiosis causing linear, irregular opacities, as seen in asbestosis, the radiograph may lead to underestimation of the severity of the impairment. It is possible to have a history of exposure, moderately reduced forced vital capacity (FVC), and a reduced diffusion in asbestosis with a relatively normal chest radiograph. The radiographic findings of irregular or linear opacities are simply more difficult to separate from normal markings until relatively late in the disease. When shadows become large (radiographic lesions greater than 1 cm in diameter), the condition is termed *complicated pneumoconiosis*, sometimes called *progressive massive fibrosis* (PMF).

Other diagnostic procedures of use in identifying environmentally induced lung disease include evaluating heavy metal exposures (arsenic, cadmium in battery plant workers); bacteriologic studies (tuberculosis in medical care personnel, anthrax in wool sorters); fungal studies (coccidioidomycosis in southwestern farm workers, histoplasmosis in poultry or pigeon handlers); or serologic studies (psittacosis in pet shop workers or owners of sick birds, Q fever in tanners or slaughterhouse workers). Ultimately, a lung biopsy may be required both to make a morphologic diagnosis of the underlying pulmonary disease and to attempt to identify the specific etiologic agent.

MEASUREMENT OF EXPOSURE If reliable environmental sampling data are available, these sources of information should be used in assessing a patient's exposure. Since many of the chronic diseases result from exposure over many years, current environmental measurements should be combined with work histories to arrive at estimates of past exposure. However, the dose of any environmental agent is a complex interaction of chemical reaction, both at the emission source and in the ambient atmosphere, and physiologic factors, including ventilation rate and depth, which may affect transport and deposition of aerosols and gases in the lung. Even in acute conditions, when monitoring of exposure may be possible, little may be known about the actual dose received by the lung. Most of the research on health effects of air pollutants (discussed later in this chapter) has relied upon fixed-station monitoring of outdoor air, often at locations somewhat distant from the residences of the people being studied. In addition, most people spend less than 20 percent of their time outdoors. Efforts to determine the penetration rate of outdoor contaminants into the indoors suggest that these penetration rates are highly pollutant specific. Therefore, outdoor measurements can be used only in a relative sense, and they cannot be relied upon to estimate actual dose.

In situations where individual exposure to specific agents has been determined, either in a work setting or for ambient air pollutants, transport of these agents through the airways may be an important factor affecting dose. The upper airways are remarkably effective filters of both particles and gases. For example, virtually 100 percent of sulfur dioxide, a highly soluble gas, is absorbed in the upper airways in concentrations as high as 35 parts per million (ppm) during quiet breathing, and even during exercise sulfur dioxide is unlikely to penetrate beyond the large bronchi. On the other hand, nitrogen dioxide, which is less soluble, may reach the bronchioles and alveoli in sufficient quantities to result in an acute life-threatening disease in farmers exposed even briefly to the gas evolved from moldy hay in silos (silo filler's disease).

Particle size and chemistry of air contaminants also must be considered. Particles above 10 to 15 μm, because of their settling velocities in air, do not penetrate beyond the upper airways. These larger particles are often referred to as "fugitive dusts" and include pollens, other windblown dusts, and dusts resulting from mechanical industrial processes. They have little or no role in chronic respiratory disease except as possibly related to cancer (see below).

Particles below 10 μm in size are created by the burning of fossil fuel or high-temperature industrial processes resulting in condensation products from gases, fumes, or vapors. These particles are divided into two size fractions on the basis of their chemical characteristics. Particles approximately 2.5 to 10 μm (coarse-mode fraction) contain crustal elements, such as silica, aluminum, and iron. These particles mostly deposit relatively high in the tracheobronchial tree. Particles less than approximately 2.5 μm (fine-mode fraction or accumulation mode) contain sulfates, nitrates, and organic compounds. The deposition of the fine-mode particles is more often in the terminal bronchioles and alveoli. The smallest particles, those less than 0.1 μm in size, remain in the airstream and deposit in the lung only on a random basis as they come into contact with the alveolar walls through thermal forces and/or Brownian movement.

Besides the size characteristics of particles and the solubility of gases, the actual chemical composition, mechanical properties, and immunogenicity or infectivity of inhaled material determine in large part the nature of the diseases found among exposed persons.

OCCUPATIONAL EXPOSURES AND PULMONARY DISEASE

INORGANIC DUSTS **Asbestos exposure** Except in localized regions with single industrial exposures, such as coal-mining or granite-quarrying regions, the most frequent inorganic dust–related chronic pulmonary diseases are associated with industries using *asbestos fibers*. Asbestos is a generic term for several different mineral silicates, including chrysotile, amosite, anthophyllite, and crocidolite. Approximately 9.1 million workers in the United States who had exposure to the various forms of asbestos fibers were estimated to be alive in 1980 and therefore subsequently at risk of asbestos-related diseases. Besides mining, milling, and manufacturing of asbestos products, exposures occur in the construction trades (pipe fitters, boiler makers) because of the exceptional properties of asbestos fibers for use in thermal and electric insulation. In addition, asbestos is used in the manufacture of fire-smothering blankets and safety garments, as filler for plastic materials, in cement and floor tiles, and in friction materials, such as brake and clutch linings.

Exposure to asbestos is not limited to persons who directly handle the material. Cases of asbestos-related diseases have been encountered in individuals with only moderate exposure, such as the painter or electrician who works alongside the insulation worker in a shipyard, or the housewife who does no more than shake out and wash her husband's work clothes. Community exposure has probably resulted from the use of asbestos-containing material sprayed on steel girders in many large buildings as a safety feature to prevent buckling in case of fire. Clusters of cases of mesothelioma have been noted in the neighborhood of an asbestos plant in London and in the communities near asbestos mines in South Africa.

Asbestos was first used extensively in the 1940s. Starting in 1975 it has been replaced with alternatives, such as fiberglass or slag wool. The major health effects from exposure to asbestos are pulmonary fibrosis (asbestosis) and cancers of the respiratory tract and pleura and, rarely, peritoneum.

Asbestosis is a diffuse interstitial fibrosing disease of the lung which is directly related to the intensity and duration of exposure. Except for a history of exposure to asbestos (generally in a work setting), asbestosis resembles the other forms of diffuse interstitial fibrosis (Chap. 209). Usually at least 10 years of moderate to severe exposure has occurred before the disease becomes manifest.

Physiologic studies reveal a restrictive pattern with a decrease in lung volumes. Flow rates are commonly reduced less than would be predicted on the basis of the volume reduction. An early sign of severe disease may be a reduction in diffusing capacity.

Pulmonary fibrosis occurs following exposure to any of the four common types of asbestos fiber. The fibrotic lesions do not appear to relate to either shape or chemical composition of any of the four, although the prevalence of disease may be influenced by fiber type. Recent studies indicate that during phagocytosis of the asbestos fiber, the membrane of the macrophage is damaged, which results in the release of lysosomes containing enzymes which may act to damage the lung parenchyma. The clinical manifestations are typical of those physical findings in any patient with pulmonary fibrosis (Chap. 209).

The chest radiograph can be used to determine a number of manifestations of asbestos exposure, as well as to identify specific lesions. Past exposure is specifically indicated by pleural plaques, which are characterized by either thickening or calcification along the parietal pleura, particularly along the lower lung fields, the diaphragm, and the cardiac border. Without additional manifestations, pleural plaques imply only exposure, not pulmonary impairment. Benign pleural effusions may occur, particularly in patients with abestosis, but not necessarily restricted to those with overt disease. The fluid is sterile, but may be a serous or blood-stained exudate and may occur bilaterally. Often the effusion may be slowly progressive or may resolve spontaneously.

The radiographic diagnosis of asbestosis depends upon the presence of irregular or linear opacities, usually first noted in the lower lung fields and spreading into the middle and upper lung fields as the disease becomes progressively worse. An indistinct heart border or a "ground glass" appearance in the lung fields is seen in some cases. As the fibrotic changes in the parenchyma begin to coalesce, the patient develops obliteration of entire acinar units with eventual formation of the classical honeycombed lung, which appears on chest radiographs as coarse infiltrates with small (about 7- to 10-μm) air spaces. No specific therapy is available in the management of patients with asbestosis. The supportive care is that of any patient with diffuse interstitial fibrosis from any cause. In general, newly diagnosed cases will have resulted from exposure levels that were present many years before, and in spite of the patients' having left the industry, are attributable to that former exposure. Because of present-day occupational safety and health regulations protecting workers from exposure, in theory, at least, one need not advise currently exposed workers to leave their jobs. In contrast, because the association of smoking and asbestosis increases the risk of developing lung cancer (see below), it is extremely important to advise such patients to stop smoking.

Lung cancer (Chap. 213), either squamous cell or adenocarcinoma, is the most frequent cancer associated with asbestos exposure. The excess frequency of lung cancer in asbestos workers is associated with a minimum lapse of 15 to 19 years between first exposure and development of the disease. Persons with more exposure are at greater risk of disease. In addition, there appears to be a significant multiplicative effect which leads to a far greater risk of lung cancer in persons who are cigarette smokers and have asbestos exposure than would be expected by taking the sum of both risks. Efforts to consider these high-risk individuals for special surveillance studies, including sputum cytologic examinations and repeated chest x-rays as frequently as every 4 to 6 months, suggest that cancers can be detected at an earlier stage and that the survival of these patients is prolonged.

Mesotheliomas (Chap. 214), both pleural and peritoneal, are also associated with asbestos exposure. In contrast to lung cancer there does not appear to be any association with smoking. Relatively short-term exposures of 1 to 2 years or less occurring some 20 to 25 years in the past have been associated with the development of mesotheliomas (which stresses the point of obtaining a complete environmental exposure history). The risk for this type of tumor peaks 30 to 35 years after initial exposure. Although approximately 50 percent of mesotheliomas metastasize, the tumor generally is locally invasive, and death usually results from local extension. Most patients present with effusions that may obscure the underlying pleural tumor. In contrast to other causes of effusion, because of the restriction placed on the chest wall no shift of mediastinal structures toward the opposite chest will be seen. The major diagnostic problem is differentiation from peripherally spreading pulmonary adenocarcinoma or adenocarcinoma metastatic to pleura from an extrathoracic primary site. A needle or even open biopsy is helpful in diagnosis.

One concern in making a definitive diagnosis of a mesothelioma relates to potential compensation to the survivors of a patient with this usually fatal disease. Since epidemiologic studies have shown that up to 80 percent of mesotheliomas may be associated with asbestos exposure, documented mesothelioma in a worker with occupational exposure to asbestos may be compensable in many parts of the United States.

Silicosis In spite of the technical adequacy of existing protective equipment, *free silica* (SiO_2), or crystalline quartz, is still a major occupational hazard. In the United States estimates of potential numbers of exposed workers range between 1.2 to 3 million people. The major occupational exposures include mining, stone cutting, abrasive industries, blasting, road and building construction, farming, and quarrying, particularly of granite. Most often the progressive pulmonary fibrosis (silicosis) occurs in a dose-response fashion after many years of exposure.

Workers exposed to sandblasting in confined spaces, tunneling through rock with high quartz content (15 to 25 percent), and engaged in the manufacture of abrasive soaps may develop acute silicosis with as little as 10 months' exposure. The disease may be rapidly fatal in less than 2 years in spite of the worker being removed from exposure. A radiographic picture of profuse miliary infiltration or consolidation is characteristic of acute silicosis.

In long-term, relatively less intense exposure, radiographic changes of rounded, small opacities in the upper lobes with retraction and hilar adenopathy classically appear after 15 to 20 years of exposure. Calcification of hilar nodes may occur in as many as 20 percent of cases and produces the characteristic "eggshell" pattern. These changes may be preceded by or be associated with a reticular pattern of irregular densities which are uniformly present throughout the upper lung zones.

The nodular fibrosis may be progressive in the absence of further exposure, with coalescence and formation of nonsegmental conglomerates of irregular masses in excess of 1 cm in diameter. These masses become quite large and are characteristic of progressive massive fibrosis (PMF). Significant functional impairment with both restrictive and obstructive components may be associated with this form of silicosis. In the late stages of the disease ventilatory failure may develop. Patients with silicosis are at greater risk of acquiring *Mycobacterium tuberculosis* infections (silicotuberculosis), although tuberculosis is not always involved in the progression of the disease to PMF. Because the frequency with which tuberculosis has been found at autopsy in patients with PMF exceeds considerably the frequency of premorbid diagnosis, treatment for tuberculosis is indicated in any patient with silicosis and a positive tuberculin test.

Other less hazardous silicates include fuller's earth, kaolin, mica, diatomaceous earths, silica gel, soapstone, carbonate dusts, and cement dusts. The production of fibrosis in workers exposed to these agents is believed to be related to either the free silica content of these dusts or, for substances which contain no free silica, to the potentially large dust loads to which these workers may be exposed.

Other silicates, including *talc dusts,* may be contaminated with asbestos and/or free silica. Accidental exposure to significant quantities of talc may result in an acute syndrome with cough, cyanosis, and labored breathing (acute talcosis). Severe progressive fibrosis with respiratory failure may ensue within a few years. Far more common is the fibrosis and/or pleural or lung cancer associated with chronic exposure in rubber workers who use commercial talc as a lubricant in tire molds. Pure talc does not produce fibrosis; thus, it is difficult to sort out whether the effects are due to the contamination of commercial talc by asbestos or by free silica.

Coal worker's pneumoconiosis (CWP) *Coal dust* is associated with CWP, which has enormous social, economic, and medical significance in every nation in which coal mining is an important industry. Simple radiographically identified CWP is seen in 12 percent of all miners and in as many as 50 percent of anthracite miners with more than 20 years' work on the coal face. The prevalence of disease is lower in workers in bituminous coal mines. Since much of the western United States coal is bituminous, CWP is less prevalent in that region.

Much of the symptomatology associated with simple CWP appears to be similar and additive to the effects of cigarette smoking on the development of chronic bronchitis and obstructive ventilatory disease (Chap. 208). In the early stages of simple CWP, radiographic abnormalities consist of small, irregular opacities (reticular pattern). With prolonged exposure, one sees small, rounded, regular opacities, 1 to 5 mm in diameter (nodular pattern). Calcification is generally not seen, although approximately 10 percent of older anthracite miners have calcified nodules.

Complicated CWP is manifested by the appearance on the chest radiograph of nodules ranging from 1 cm in diameter to the size of an entire lobe, generally confined to the upper half of the lungs. This condition, considered a form of PMF, is associated with premature mortality and is accompanied by significant reduction in diffusing capacity. In contrast to patients with silicosis, only a relatively small percentage of underground miners with simple CWP (5 to 15 percent, depending on the type of coal) develop PMF.

The mechanism whereby PMF occurs in CWP is not fully understood. Several hypotheses have been proposed, including (1) sufficient free silica is present in the dust; (2) normal clearance mechanisms are unable to clear the excessive dust loads; (3) an interplay occurs between an intrinsic immunologic mechanism and the dust and/or damaged lung tissue; and (4) atypical reactions to *Mycobacterium tuberculosis* occur. As previously described, PMF in silicosis is associated with prolonged duration and high intensity of exposure to free silica. Heavy exposure to carbon particles free of silica occurs in carbon black, graphite, and charcoal workers. The prolonged exposure of these workers may result in sufficient accumulation of carbon in the lung to produce PMF. The mechanism appears to relate to a breakdown of the clearance capacity of the airways.

Caplan's syndrome, which includes seropositive rheumatoid arthritis with characteristic PMF, is consistent with an immunopathologic mechanism. The syndrome was first described in coal miners but subsequently has been found in a number of pneumoconioses. Similarly, the high prevalence of antinuclear antibodies in sandblasting workers with silicosis and the elevation of gamma globulin levels in silicotic individuals suggest an immunologic mechanism. Although mycobacterial infections are found more often in coal miners than PMF is found in silicotic patients, tuberculosis does not appear to be associated with most of the cases of PMF in coal miners.

Berylliosis Beryllium may produce an acute pneumonitis or, far more commonly, a chronic interstitial pneumonitis. Histologically, it may be difficult to differentiate the chronic form of the disease from sarcoidosis (Chap. 270). Nonspecific pulmonary function tests may be normal or may indicate evidence of restrictive disease. Between 2 and 15 years of exposure, depending on its intensity, is required for the disease to become manifest. Unless one inquires specifically about occupational exposures to beryllium in the manufacture of alloys, ceramics, high-technology electronics, and, before the 1950s, in the production of fluorescent lights, one may miss entirely the etiologic relationship to an occupational exposure.

Rarely, other hard metals, including aluminum powders, chromium, cobalt, titanium dioxide, and tungsten, may produce an interstitial pneumonitis.

Other inorganic dusts Other dusts are considered *nuisance dusts* because their major impact seems to be reduction in visibility and irritation of eyes, ears, nasal passages, and other mucous membranes. If they penetrate to the lower airways, they do not affect the architecture of the terminal bronchioles or acinar spaces or destroy collagen. Generally, clinical effects are reversible. Pulmonary function tests are usually normal unless another disease process coexists. If radiodense, macular collections of these dusts may produce striking radiographic pictures which are so characteristic that patients with a history of significant exposure are easily diagnosed as having the condition which bears the name reflecting the nature of the dust. Examples are iron and iron oxides from welding or silver finishing (*siderosis*); tin oxide used in metallurgy, color stabilization, printing, and the manufacture of porcelain, glass, and fabric (*stannosis*); and barium sulfate used as a catalyst for organic reactions, drilling mud components, and electroplating (*baritosis*). Other metal dusts producing similar radiodense pictures include *cerium dioxide* and *antimony salts*.

Most of the inorganic dusts discussed thus far are associated with the production of either dust macules or interstitial fibrotic changes in the lung. Another set of dusts (see Table 204-1), along with some of the dusts previously discussed, is associated with chronic mucous hypersecretion (chronic bronchitis), with or without reduction of expiratory flow rates. These conditions may be caused by cigarette smoking, and any effort to attribute some component of the disease to occupational and environmental exposures must take cigarette smoking into account. In some studies the evidence suggests an additive effect of dust exposure and smoking. Those exposures associated with obstructive syndromes are generally represented by one or two studies of specific occupational groups with a small number of affected nonsmokers. Cigarette smoke is usually the more noxious agent, and dust effects may be discernible only in nonsmokers.

ORGANIC DUSTS Some of the specific diseases associated with organic dusts are discussed in detail in the chapters on asthma (Chap. 202) and on hypersensitivity pneumonitis (Chap. 203). Many of these diseases are named for the specific setting in which the disease is found, e.g., farmer's lung, malt worker's disease, or mushroom worker's disease. Occupational and other environmental exposures must be sought when these conditions are suspected. Often the temporal relation of symptoms to exposure furnishes the best evidence for the diagnosis. Three occupational groups are singled out for discussion because they represent the largest proportion of people affected by the diseases resulting from organic dusts.

Cotton dust (byssinosis) Estimates of the number of exposed persons in the United States vary, but probably over 800,000 are exposed occupationally to cotton, flax, or hemp in the production of yarns for cotton, linen, and rope making. Although this discussion focuses on cotton, the same syndrome to a somewhat lesser degree has been reported in exposure to flax, hemp, and jute.

Although cotton dust–related disease was first described in the seventeenth century, it is only in the last 35 years that the disease has been recognized as a worldwide problem in the textile industry. Exposure occurs throughout the manufacturing process but is most pronounced in those portions of the factory involved with the treatment of the cotton prior to spinning—i.e., blowing, mixing, and carding (straightening of fibers). Cases reported from spinning rooms are believed to be due to secondary contamination from carding rooms. Recent attempts to control dust levels by use of exhaust hoods, general increase in ventilation, and wetting procedures in some settings have been highly successful. However, respiratory protective equipment appears to be required during certain operations to prevent workers from being exposed to levels of dust that exceed the current United States cotton dust standard.

Byssinosis is characterized clinically as occasional (early stage) and then regular (late stage) chest tightness toward the end of the first day of the workweek (Monday chest tightness). In epidemiologic studies, up to 80 percent of carding room employees may show a significant drop in their FEV_1 over the course of a Monday shift, depending on the level of exposure in the carding room air.

Initially the symptoms do not recur on subsequent days of the week. However, in 10 to 25 percent of workers, the disease may be progressive with chest tightness recurring or persisting throughout the workweek. After more than 10 years of exposure, workers with recurrent symptoms are more likely to have an obstructive ventilatory pattern on pulmonary function testing. These higher grades of impairment are seen in workers exposed both to high levels of dust and for greater durations. There is an additive effect of cotton dust exposure plus cigarette smoking. The highest grades of impairment are generally seen in smokers.

Treatment in the early stages of the disease is directed toward reversing the bronchospasm with bronchodilators; however, the chest tightness appears at least in part to relate to histamine release, and antihistamines have been shown to lessen anticipated fall in FEV_1 the first day of the week. Clearly, reduction of dust exposure is of primary importance. All workers with persistent symptoms or significantly reduced levels of pulmonary function should be moved to areas of lower risk of exposure. Regular surveillance of pulmonary function in the industry has made it easier to identify affected persons.

TABLE 204-1 Selected occupational dusts believed to be associated with mucous hypersecretion and/or obstructive airway disease and other respiratory diseases*

Agent	Exposure	Mucus hypersecretion	Obstruction	Other conditions†
INORGANIC DUST				
Antimony	Storage batteries, bearing, solder, ceramics, glass, plastics	X		P
Arsenic	Manufacture of pesticides, pigments, glass, alloys	X		C
Barium and compounds including BaO, $BaSO_4$, $BaCO_3$	Catalyst, drilling mud, electroplating	X		P
Cadmium dust	Electroplating, battery manufacture, welding, smelting, aluminum soldering	X	X	P
Cement dust	Construction trades, manufacture of cement blocks	X	X	
Chromium and CrO_3, CrF_2	Corrosion inhibitor pigment, metallurgy, electroplating	X		C
Coal dust	Mining	X		P
Coke oven emissions	Retort house, coke ovens	X	X	P, C
Graphite	Steelmaking, lubricants, pencils, paints, stove polish	X	X	P
Iron dust	Steel and nonferrous foundry workers, welding	X		P
Mica	Insulation, roofing shingles, oil refining, rubber manufacturing	X		P
Phosphorus, elemental chlorides, sulfides	Manufacture of fireworks, agricultural chemicals, insecticides, pesticides	X	X	
Rock dusts	Miners, tunnelers, quarry workers	X		P
Vanadium pentoxide	Welding electrodes, additive to steel, by-product in ash from oil burning	X	X	
ORGANIC DUST (see Chap. 203)				
Cotton dust, flax, hemp	Manufacture of yarns for linen, rope, cotton; ginning, cottonseed crushing; waste fiber processing	X	X	
Grain dusts	Farmers, workers in grain elevators, barge and grain ship crewmembers	X	X	
Moldy hay	Farmers, other animal attendants	X		HP

* *The table excludes agents associated with asthma as the primary disease (see Chap. 202).*
† *Other conditions include hypersensitivity pneumonitis (HP), pneumoconiosis (P), and cancers (C).*
NOTE: *X indicates that mucous hypersecretion or obstruction are associated with exposure.*

Persons with reduced pulmonary function, a personal history of respiratory allergy, and positive history of continued cigarette smoking should be considered at increased risk of developing byssinosis in association with working in the cotton industry.

Grain dust Although the exact number of workers at risk in the United States is not known, at least 500,000 people work in grain elevators, and over 2 million farmers are potentially at risk. The presentation of disease in grain elevator employees or workers in flour or feed mills is virtually identical to the characteristic finding in cigarette smokers, i.e., persistent cough, mucus hypersecretion, wheeze and dyspnea on exertion, and reduced FEV_1 and FEV_1/FVC ratio (Chap. 200).

Dust concentrations in grain elevators vary greatly but appear to be in excess of 10,000 $\mu g/m^3$ with approximately one-third of the particles by weight being in the respirable range. The effect of grain dust exposure is additive to that of cigarette smoking with approximately 50 percent of workers who smoke having symptoms. Among nonsmoking grain elevator operators, approximately one-quarter have mucous hypersecretion, about five times the number that would be expected in unexposed nonsmokers. However, evidence of obstruction is observed only in workers who smoke. It is not clear if this results from an enhancement of cigarette smoking effect in exposed workers or if smokers are more susceptible to the effects of grain dust.

Farmer's lung This condition results from exposure to moldy hay containing spores of thermophilic actinomycetes that produce a hypersensitivity pneumonitis (Chap. 203). There are few good population-based estimates of the frequency of occurrence of this condition in the United States. However, among farmers in Great Britain the rate of disease ranges from approximately 10 to 50 per 1000. The prevalence of disease varies in association with rainfall, which determines the amount of fungal growth, and with differences in agricultural practices related to turning and stacking hay.

The patient with acute farmer's lung presents 4 to 8 h after exposure with fever, chills, malaise, cough, and dyspnea without wheezing. The history of exposure is obviously essential to separate this disease from similar symptoms that might occur in influenza or pneumonia. In the chronic form of the disease, the history of repeated attacks after similar exposure is important to separate this syndrome from other causes of patchy fibrosis, e.g., sarcoidosis.

A wide variety of other organic dusts are associated with the occurrence of hypersensitivity pneumonitis (Chap. 203). For those patients who present with hypersensitivity pneumonitis, specific and careful inquiry about occupations, hobbies, or other home environmental exposures will, in most cases, reveal the source of the etiologic agent.

ASSESSMENT OF DISABILITY Significant reduction of dust levels in coal mines has resulted from federal legislation, enacted in the

United States in 1969, which requires that respirable dust levels in underground mines be reduced to less than 2000 μg/m³. This same legislation authorized payment to coal miners (or their survivors) totally disabled by CWP. The criteria for disability from CWP remain unclear and arbitrary. Much of the difficulty relates to the inability to determine in an individual with simple CWP what proportion of an observed respiratory impairment is related to coal dust and what proportion is due to cigarette smoking. The laws as currently interpreted suggest that to be eligible for payment of a claim, one need only show that an underlying condition (i.e., chronic bronchitis with obstruction, presumably due to cigarette smoking) is aggravated by CWP. Thus, it becomes critical that physicians involved in occupational lung disease claim cases be aware of detailed exposure histories of their patients, both in terms of occupational exposures and other environmental exposures (cigarette smoking). In addition, these physicians must understand that the extent to which the level of physiologic impairment incapacitates an individual may not be the sole criterion for determining disability. To assess disability properly may require input not only from physicians but also from experts in ergonomics and vocational rehabilitation, lawyers, and employer and employee representatives. Similar separate bills have been introduced into Congress to deal with other single occupational diseases, such as asbestosis and byssinosis.

TOXIC CHEMICALS Exposure to toxic chemicals affecting the lung generally occurs in the form of gases and vapors. A common accident is one in which the victim is trapped in a confined space where the chemicals have accumulated to toxic levels. In addition to the specific toxic effects of the chemical, the victim will often sustain considerable anoxia, which can play a dominant role in determining whether the individual recovers.

Table 204-2 lists a variety of toxic agents which can produce acute and sometimes life-threatening reactions in the lung. All of these agents in sufficient concentrations have been demonstrated, at least in animal studies, to affect the lower airways and disrupt alveolar architecture, either acutely or as a result of chronic exposure. Some of these agents may be generated acutely in the environment. For example, when plastics burn, a number of compounds, including hydrogen cyanide and hydrochloric acid, may be formed and released. The effects and treatment of exposure to these toxic gases are discussed elsewhere (Chap. 171).

Fire fighters and fire victims are at risk of *smoke inhalation,* a numerically important cause of acute cardiorespiratory failure. Smoke inhalation kills more fire victims than does thermal injury. Exposed victims may suffer some degree of lower respiratory tract inflammation, similar to that seen with exposure to irritant gases, e.g., chlorine. Severe cases may develop pulmonary edema. Carbon

TABLE 204-2 Selected common toxic chemical agents

Agents	Selected exposures	Acute effects from high or accidental exposure	Chronic effects from relatively low exposure
Acid fumes; H_2SO_4, HNO_3	Manufacture of fertilizers, chlorinated organic compounds, dyes, explosives, rubber products, metal etching, plastics	Mucous membrane irritation, followed by chemical pneumonitis 2–3 days	No data
Ammonia	Refrigeration, petroleum refining, manufacture of fertilizers, explosives, plastics, and other chemicals	Same as for acid fumes	Chronic bronchitis
Cyanides	Electroplating, extraction of gold or silver, manufacture of mirrors, fumigants, photo supplies	Increase in respiratory rate followed by respiratory arrest, lactic acidosis, pulmonary edema, death	No data
Diazomethane	Methylating agent for acid compounds; laboratory workers	Violent coughing, dyspnea, wheezing, pulmonary edema	No data
Formaldehyde	Manufacture of resins, leathers, rubber, metals, & woods; laboratory workers, embalmers; emission from urethane foam insulation	Same as for acid fumes	Cancers in one species of animals; no data on humans
Halides (Cl, Br, F)	Bleaching in pulp, paper, textile industry; manufacture of chemical compounds; synthetic rubber, plastics, disinfectant, rocket fuel, gasoline	Mucous membrane irritation, pulmonary edema; possible reduced FVC 1–2 yrs after exposure	Dryness of mucous membrane, epistaxis, dental fluorosis, tracheobronchitis
Hydrogen sulfide	By-product of many industrial processes, oil, other petroleum processes and storage	Low exposure: conjunctival irritation; higher: respiratory paralysis similar to cyanides	Chronic bronchitis, recurrent pneumonitis
Isocyanates (TDI, HDI, MDI)	Production of polyurethane foams, plastics, adhesives, surface coatings	Mucous membrane irritation, dyspnea, cough, wheeze, pulmonary edema	Upper respiratory tract irritation, cough, asthma, allergic alveolitis
Nitrogen dioxide	Silage, metal etching, explosives, rocket fuels, welding, by-product of burning fossil fuels	Cough, dyspnea, pulmonary edema may be delayed 4–12 h; possible result from acute exposure: bronchiolitis obliterans in 2–6 wks	Emphysema in animals, ? chronic bronchitis
Ozone	Arc welding, flour bleaching, deodorizing, emissions from copying equipment, photochemical air pollutant	Mucous membrane irritant, pulmonary hemorrhage and edema	Chronic eye irritation
Phosgene	Organic compound, metallurgy, volatization of chlorine-containing compounds	Delayed onset of bronchiolitis and pulmonary edema	Chronic bronchitis
Phthalic anhydride	Manufacture of resin esters, polyester resins, thermoactivated adhesives	Nasal irritation, cough	Asthma, chronic bronchitis
Sulfur dioxide	Manufacture of sulfuric acid, bleaches, coating of nonferrous metals, food processing, refrigerant, burning of fossil fuels, wood pulp industry	Mucous membrane irritant, epistaxis	? Chronic bronchitis

monoxide poisoning with resulting significant hypoxemia can be life-threatening (Chap. 171). Fire fighters may inappropriately use the "blackness" of the smoke to indicate the degree to which incomplete combustion and, thus, elevation of carbon monoxide levels are present. The increased use of synthetic materials (plastic, polyurethanes), which, when burned, may release a variety of other toxic agents, must be considered when evaluating smoke inhalation victims.

Fire fighters and victims also may be exposed to large quantities of particulate smoke. Significant long-term effects are not clearly associated with this particulate exposure except as related to the production of irritating effects on the upper airways. Studies attempting to demonstrate either an increased risk of cardiovascular events, presumably from recurrent exposure to carbon monoxide, or excess incidence of chronic respiratory disease from repeated smoke inhalation, are inconclusive, partly because of the difficulties in measuring exposure.

Some agents used in the manufacture of synthetic materials such as plastics, polyurethanes, and other polymers have resulted in some workers being sensitized to extremely low levels of *isocyanates, aromatic amines,* or *aldehydes.* Repeated exposure to these agents causes some workers to develop chronic cough and sputum production, asthma, or episodes of low-grade fever and malaise. Occasionally, as in byssinosis, these symptoms occur early in the workweek, but usually recur without workweek periodicity. In the case of exposure to diisocyanate in the production of polyurethane, chronic and persistent asthma in selected individuals appears to result from exposure to concentrations well below the recognized industrial standard. Methods to identify susceptible individuals are needed. At present, challenge testing is being used to determine if a given patient is sensitive. These challenges can be carried out in special environmental chambers where the physician can simulate the work exposure. Alternatively, nonspecific challenges with either pharmacologic agents, such as methacholine and histamine, or isocapneic cold air breathing are being used to identify patients with hyperreactive airways. The usefulness of this nonspecific approach as a method to screen potential workers has yet to be established.

An unusual route of exposure occurs in *polymer fume fever.* Polymers, notably fluorocarbons, which at normal temperatures produce no reaction, may be transmitted from a worker's hands to his or her cigarettes. Upon burning the cigarette, the polymer is volatilized, and the inhaled agent causes a characteristic syndrome of fever, chills, malaise, and occasionally mild wheezing. The same condition occurs in workers exposed to heated polymers without cigarette use. The syndrome is obviously controlled by proper attention to hygiene in the workplace. A similar self-limited, influenza-like syndrome—*metal fume fever*—results from acute exposure to fumes or smoke of zinc, copper, magnesium, and other volatilized metals. The syndrome may begin several hours after work and resolves within 24 h, only to return on repeated exposure. A proper occupational history should make the diagnosis evident.

ENVIRONMENTAL RESPIRATORY CARCINOGENS Historically, it has been the astute clinician who has recognized a higher incidence of malignant tumors associated with certain environmental exposures. When these observations are linked to an occupational setting, they must be pursued by epidemiologic studies of relatively large groups of both current and former workers. Often the concentration and/or exact nature of the substances contained in the putative exposures cannot be determined. Rarely, the possibility that a substance can play an etiologic role in cancer is supported by observing that a few cases of a very rare tumor in a particular group represent "an epidemic." Two best examples of this are nasal sinus and lung cancer in nickel workers and angiosarcomas in vinyl chloride workers.

Only in those few cases in which animal studies have been carried out can one confirm that a given suspected agent is really a carcinogen. For example, bis(chloromethyl) ether (BCME) has been shown to produce tumors in animals and oat cell cancer of the lung in humans. In this particular case, BCME, used as a chemical intermediary in the manufacture of a number of organic compounds, was known to produce tumors in animals almost before the substance was introduced into industry. (This case is one of the prime examples of why federal legislation was enacted in the United States in the 1970s to control the release of toxic substances, particularly new chemicals.)

In addition to the asbestos trades, other occupational exposures associated with either proven or suspected respiratory carcinogens include acrylonitrile, arsenic compounds, beryllium (animal studies only), BCME, chromium, coke ovens (exposure to polycyclic hydrocarbons), iron oxide, isopropyl oil (nasal sinuses), mustard gas, the various ores used to produce pure nickel, talc (possible asbestos contamination in both mining and milling), vinyl chloride, welding, wood used in woodworking (nasal cancer only), and uranium. The occurrence of excess cancers in uranium miners raises the possibility that there exists a large number of workers at risk by virtue of exposure to similar radiation hazards. This includes not only workers involved in processing uranium, up to and including its use in nuclear power plants and in military nuclear hardware, but also workers exposed in underground mining operations where radon daughters may be emitted from rock formations. In the latter case, the levels of exposure are generally considered to be relatively low; however, specific consideration must be given to the possibility of excess exposure for any hard rock miner.

GENERAL ENVIRONMENTAL EXPOSURES

AIR POLLUTION Dramatic and disastrous episodes of air pollution inversion have been documented in many industrialized centers in the world. Each of these episodes has been associated with excess acute mortality in the very old, the very young, and in those with chronic cardiopulmonary diseases. The most dramatic event was the London fog of 1952, in which approximately 4000 excess deaths occurred over a 2-week period following 5 days of severe cold and dense fog. Similar episodes in the United States, although less dramatic in terms of total deaths, occurred in Donora, Pennsylvania, in 1948, and in New York City in the 1960s. In these episodes, generally associated with cold temperature and air stagnation, patients with underlying cardiopulmonary disease were most severely affected.

In addition to significant excess mortality during these episodes, a large number of people required medical care for cardiorespiratory complaints. Subsequent follow-up studies failed to implicate these episodic disasters in the etiology of chronic respiratory disease in adults. On the other hand, many epidemiologic studies of both international and regional differences in the prevalences of chronic respiratory disease suggest that long-term exposures in polluted areas in the early to middle part of the twentieth century were associated with excess chronic respiratory disease.

In 1970, the U.S. federal government established air quality standards for several pollutants believed to be responsible for excess cardiorespiratory diseases. Primary standards regulated by the Environmental Protection Agency (EPA) designed to protect the public health with an adequate margin of safety exist for sulfur dioxide, total suspended particulates, nitrogen dioxide, ozone, lead, and carbon monoxide. These standards vary in their averaging times and levels, in part related to the differences in the known physiologic responses and epidemiologic evidence for each pollutant.

Pollutants are generated from both stationary sources (power plants and industrial complexes) and mobile sources (automobiles), and none of the pollutants occur in isolation. Thus, except for the change in carboxyhemoglobin from carbon monoxide exposure, it becomes extremely difficult to relate any specific health effect to any single pollutant. Furthermore, pollutants may be changed by chemical reactions after being emitted. For example, reducing agents, such as sulfur dioxide and particulate matter from a power plant stack, may react in air to produce acid sulfates and aerosol (acid rain), which can be transported long distances in the atmosphere. Oxidizing substances, such as oxides of nitrogen and oxidants from automobile exhaust, may react with sunlight to produce ozone. Although originally a problem confined to the southwestern part of the United States, in recent years, at least during the summertime, elevated ozone and sulfate levels can occur throughout the United States. Both acute and chronic effects of these exposures are currently under investigation.

The symptoms and diseases associated with air pollution are the same as the nononcogenic conditions commonly associated with cigarette smoking. In addition, respiratory illness in early childhood has been associated with chronic exposure to only modestly elevated levels of SO_2 and total suspended particulates. It is not known whether persistent chronic exposure to a relatively constant level of pollutant(s) and recurrent short-term peak exposures which average to the same mean level have different effects. For a patient with significant cardiopulmonary impairment, one can only advise the individual to stay indoors during periods when pollution exceeds current standards.

INDOOR EXPOSURE Because of increased concern about energy costs, efforts to become energy efficient have led to reduced air exchange rates in indoor environments. The effects of these efforts have been to increase exposures to a variety of air contaminants heretofore not considered important. Two examples of potential health effects from exposure to indoor pollutants are discussed to indicate the magnitude of possible problems.

For many years little attention, beyond its nuisance effect, has been given to the effects of *passive cigarette smoking*. The implication has been that passive smoking exposures were too low to be of any consequence. Recent studies have shown that the respirable particulate load in any household is directly proportional to the number of cigarette smokers living in the home. Increases in prevalence of respiratory illnesses and reduced levels of pulmonary function measured with simple spirometry have been found in children of smoking parents in a number of studies. The long-term consequences of these findings are unknown. Other potential health effects are discussed in Chap. 173.

A novel source of indoor exposure to *formaldehyde* results from the curing process involved in the placement of urea-formaldehyde insulating foam or in several wood products used in modern furniture and the construction of mobile homes. Natural "degassing" of formaldehyde occurs during the first few months after the foam has been blown into the walls, with concentrations of formaldehyde as high as 5 ppm rapidly dropping off to less than 0.1 ppm. Chronic exposure to low levels of urea-formaldehyde (generally less than 1 ppm) may result if the foam is improperly installed. Patients apparently sensitive to concentrations of formaldehyde generally well below 1 ppm will complain of upper airway irritation with occasional epistaxis and sore throats. Lower respiratory complaints, such as chest pain and wheeze, however, are uncommon, and often the most disturbing complaints are mild memory and mood disorders. Formaldehyde is a proven animal carcinogen. Whether it causes cancer in humans is not established.

PORTAL OF ENTRY The lung is a primary source of entry into the body for a number of toxic agents that affect other organ systems. For example, the lung is the route of entry for benzene (bone marrow), carbon disulfide (cardiovascular and nervous systems), cadmium (kidney), and mercury (kidney, central nervous system). Thus, in any disease state of obscure origin, it is important to consider possible inhaled environmental agents. Such consideration can sometimes furnish the clue needed to identify a specific external cause for a disorder that might otherwise be labeled "idiopathic."

REFERENCES

American Thoracic Society: *Update: Health Effects of Air Pollution.* New York, American Lung Association, (in press)

Attfield M et al: The incidence and progression of pneumoconiosis over nine years in U.S. coal miners. Am J Ind Med 6:407, 1984

Cochrane AL, Moore FA: A 20-year follow-up of men aged 55–64 including coal-miners and foundry workers in Stavley, Derbyshire. Br J Ind Med 37:226, 1980

Craighead JE, Mossman BT: The pathogenesis of asbestos-associated diseases. N Engl J Med 306:1446, 1982

Ferris BG Jr: Epidemiology Standardization Project. Am Rev Respir Dis 118(6)(2):1, 1978

Guidelines for the Use of International Labour Office Classification of Radiographs of Pneumoconiosis. Occupational Safety and Health Sciences 22 (Revised 1980). Geneva, ILO, 1980

Kilburn KH: Byssinosis: Causes and practical control. Ann Intern Med 101:252, 1984

Koskinen H: Symptoms and clinical findings in patients with silicosis. Scan J Work Environ Health 11:101, 1985

Mundie TG et al: Byssinosis: Serum immunoglobulin and complement concentrations in cotton mill workers. Arch Environ Health 40:326, 1985

Parkes WR: *Occupational Lung Disorders,* 2d ed. London, Butterworth, 1982

Peto R, Schneiderman M (eds): *Quantification of Occupational Cancer,* Banbury Report, 9. Cold Spring Harbor, 1981

Schmidt JA et al: Silica-stimulated monocytes release fibroblast proliferation factors identical to interleukin. A potential role for interleuken I in the pathogenesis of silicosis. J Clin Invest 73:1462, 1984

Weill J: Occupational pulmonary diseases and acute and accidental exposures to irritant gases, in *Pulmonary Diseases and Disorders,* 2d ed, A P Fishman (ed). New York, McGraw-Hill, 1987, chap. 54.

205 PNEUMONIA AND LUNG ABSCESS

JAN V. HIRSCHMANN / JOHN F. MURRAY

PNEUMONIA

DEFINITION Pneumonia is defined as inflammation in the lung parenchyma, the portion distal to the terminal bronchioles and comprising the respiratory bronchioles, alveolar ducts, alveolar sacs, and alveoli. Although the inflammation may have many different causes and varying durations, the term *pneumonia* most commonly refers to acute infections.

PATHOGENESIS Organisms reach the lung to cause pneumonia by one of four routes: (1) inhalation of microbes present in the air, (2) aspiration of organisms from the naso- or oropharynx, the most common cause of bacterial pneumonia, (3) hematogenous spread from a distant focus of infection, or rarely, (4) direct spread from a contiguous site of infection or penetrating injury.

Lung defense mechanisms Although inhalation of organisms and aspiration of oropharyngeal contents are probably common, even in healthy people, the airway distal to the larynx is normally sterile or possesses a sparse flora because of several protective mechanisms. The glottis reflexly closes when material is aspirated; whatever reaches the trachea and large bronchi usually evokes coughing, which expels the material from the tracheobronchial tree. The airways between the larynx and the terminal bronchioles are further protected by their lining of mucus-covered ciliated epithelium, which propels trapped inhaled matter from the smaller to the larger airways, where it can be eliminated by expectoration or swallowing.

The immunoglobulins constitute another defense mechanism. IgA, present in high concentrations in the upper respiratory tract, protects against viral infection. It is less abundant in the lower respiratory secretions, where it may help agglutinate bacteria, neutralize microbial toxins, and reduce bacterial attachment to mucosal surfaces. IgG in the serum and lower respiratory tract agglutinates and opsonizes bacteria; activates complement, promoting chemotaxis of granulocytes and macrophages; neutralizes bacterial toxins and viruses; and lyses gram-negative bacteria. Also present on the alveolar surface are alveolar macrophages, which ingest and kill organisms, and alveolar lining material, which may enhance phagocytic function. In addition, neutrophils, which ingest and kill organisms, and lymphocytes, providing humoral and cell-mediated immunity, migrate from the bloodstream into the parenchyma to help combat infection.

Predisposing conditions Pneumonia may occur in healthy people but is usually associated with conditions that impair one or more of the defense mechanisms listed above. Altered consciousness from alcoholism, cranial trauma, seizures, general anesthesia, drug overdose, cerebrovascular disease, or other causes, and old age depress the cough and glottic reflexes, allowing the aspiration of oropharyngeal contents. Pain from trauma or thoracic or upper abdominal surgery; weakness from malnutrition or neuromuscular disease; thoracic cage deformities such as serious kyphoscoliosis; or severe obstructive lung disease may prevent the full inspiration and brisk expiration necessary to generate an effective cough. An endotracheal tube or tracheostomy eliminates glottic closure and impedes effective coughing.

Mucociliary transport is impaired by alcohol, cigarette smoke, old age, and preceding viral respiratory infections, which may cause necrosis and desquamation of the tracheobronchial epithelium. Endobronchial obstruction from tumor, foreign body, or other causes compromises effective clearance mechanisms. Thick mucus from cystic fibrosis or chronic bronchitis makes the transport system less effective. Indeed, in chronic bronchitis, the tracheobronchial tree is typically colonized with an abundant flora, especially pneumococci and *Haemophilus influenzae*.

Lymphocyte disorders, including congenital and acquired immunodeficiencies, and granulocyte abnormalities may predispose to pneumonia (see Chaps. 56, 84, and 256). Pulmonary infection may also occur when alveolar macrophage function is impaired by cigarette smoke, hypoxia, starvation, anemia, pulmonary edema, and viral respiratory infections.

Oropharyngeal flora Most pneumonias arise from the aspiration of oropharyngeal flora, normally a complex assortment of aerobic and anaerobic bacteria. Which of these organisms causes the pneumonia seems to depend upon the identity of the microbes present and the quantity of material aspirated. *Streptococcus pneumoniae, H. influenzae, Staphylococcus aureus,* and even *Neisseria meningitidis,* all potential pathogens, are often found in the oropharynx of healthy adults. Each of these organisms, as single agents, may cause pneumonia when aspirated into alveoli. Anaerobes, however, which outnumber aerobes severalfold in the oral cavity, are weak pathogens individually and usually cause infection by an interaction among several species. These organisms, therefore, are likely to cause pneumonia, usually as a polymicrobial infection, only when aspirated in relatively large quantities.

Coliforms, such as *Escherichia coli, Klebsiella,* and *Proteus,* are uncommon in the oropharynx of healthy adults. Several conditions, especially hospitalization, however, favor their growth. Serious underlying illness, confinement in an intensive care unit, the use of an endotracheal tube or tracheostomy, contaminated respiratory equipment, and antimicrobial therapy, which frequently selects out organisms resistant to the agents used, especially encourage colonization with coliforms present in the hospital environment. Certain illnesses, such as acute granulocytic leukemia, alcoholism, and diabetes mellitus, are associated with an increased frequency of oropharyngeal colonization with aerobic gram-negative bacilli whether or not the patient is hospitalized.

Aspiration pneumonia Since most bacterial pneumonias originate from the aspiration of oropharyngeal flora into the lung parenchyma, they are, strictly speaking, examples of *aspiration pneumonia.* In common use, however, this term refers to the aspiration of *large* quantities of oropharyngeal contents, primarily in patients with impaired consciousness, altered swallowing, or feeble coughs. In aspirations occurring outside the hospital the organisms causing infections are likely to be pneumococci or a mixture of aerobes and anaerobes. These microbes are also common pathogens in hospitalized or institutionalized patients but because their oropharyngeal flora has often changed, infections with aerobic gram-negative rods are frequent.

The term *aspiration pneumonia,* however, has also been applied to the aspiration of *gastric* contents in patients with altered consciousness, gastric outlet obstruction, esophageal disorders, or vomiting. The initial pulmonary reaction is not an infection, but an inflammatory response to irritating chemicals, chiefly HCl, present in gastric fluid, which is usually sterile or contains only a sparse flora. Antimicrobial therapy is reserved for the uncommon and delayed complication of superinfection, suggested by fever and purulent sputum, with pathogens present on Gram's stain and culture. If the patient is seen to aspirate gastric contents, the major therapy is vigorous chest physiotherapy, nasotracheal suctioning, and maintenance of adequate oxygenation. Corticosteroids are not useful.

CLINICAL MANIFESTATIONS The major symptoms of pneumonia, occurring in varying combinations, are cough, fever, chest pain, dyspnea, and the production of sputum, which may be mucoid, purulent, or even bloody. In some patients, extrapulmonary features such as confusion or disorientation may predominate, and occasionally, especially in elderly, alcoholic, or neutropenic patients, respiratory symptoms and signs are absent altogether. Important in the history are inquiries about prodromal symptoms, the type of onset (abrupt or gradual), the presence of rigors and pleuritic chest pain, similar illness in family members or acquaintances, animal exposure, and recent travel.

Common physical findings are fever, tachycardia, and tachypnea. Severely hypoxic patients may be cyanotic. On chest examination there may be decreased respiratory excursion on the affected side because of pleuritic pain and dullness to percussion from pneumonic consolidation or an accompanying pleural effusion. Among the earliest auscultatory findings is the presence of high-pitched, end-inspiratory crackles, originating from fluid-filled alveoli, that are often increased by, or heard only after, coughing. Secretions in the airways may cause lower-pitched, early or midinspiratory crackles. Consolidated lung surrounding a patent bronchus often gives rise to bronchial breath sounds, an accentuation of both the inspiratory and expiratory phases of breathing. In some patients, despite impressive roentgenographic abnormalities, physical examination of the chest is entirely normal. In patients whose pneumonia is secondary to hematogenous spread, the primary site of infection may be apparent. Alternatively, bacteremia arising from pneumonia may cause infection in distant sites, such as meningitis, septic arthritis, or pustular skin lesions.

The arterial blood gases commonly reveal hypoxia and, in the absence of other pulmonary disease, hypocarbia and respiratory alkalosis. The hypoxia results from right-to-left shunting of blood, because of the continued perfusion of the nonventilated areas affected by the pneumonia.

ROENTGENOGRAPHIC FINDINGS The microbial etiology of a pneumonia cannot be accurately predicted by its roentgenographic characteristics. Nevertheless, certain appearances are more typical of some organisms than others. Pneumonias tend to conform to one of three pathologic and roentgenographic patterns (Fig. 205-1): (1) alveolar or air space pneumonia, (2) bronchopneumonia, or (3) interstitial pneumonia. In air space pneumonia the organism causes an inflammatory exudate that spreads from one alveolus to the next via the communicating channels, known as the pores of Kohn, and the canals of Lambert. Segmental boundaries are not preserved, and the bronchi, relatively uninvolved, remain patent. The roentgenographic result is nonsegmental consolidation with air bronchograms, the classic example being pneumococcal pneumonia. Some organisms produce bronchopneumonia, which consists of inflammation in the conducting airways, especially terminal and respiratory bronchioles, and the surrounding alveoli. Because interalveolar spread in the peripheral air spaces is minimal, the pneumonia tends to maintain a distribution corresponding to the involved pulmonary segment. Inflammation affects the bronchi themselves, sometimes causing atelectasis, and air bronchograms are absent. An example is staphylococcal pneumonia. *Mycoplasma pneumoniae* and viruses often cause an interstitial pneumonia, where inflammation is predominantly in the interalveolar septa, producing a reticular radiographic appearance.

DIAGNOSTIC TECHNIQUES Among the most useful procedures to define a pneumonia's etiology is the microscopic examination of a Gram-stained sputum specimen. Although precise speciation of bacteria is impossible by Gram's stain alone, the appearance of organisms allows reasonable inferences about their identity. An acceptable sputum sample, one genuinely arising from the lower respiratory tract rather than the oropharynx, has more than 25 leukocytes per low-power field (100×). Squamous epithelial cells from the oropharynx are sparse, and alveolar macrophages are often present. Specimens that fail to meet these standards represent mostly saliva and are useless for further examination or culture. Acceptable specimens should be cultured on appropriate media.

Adequate staining of acceptable specimens is crucial for accurate interpretation. If cells, including the nuclei of leukocytes, are not gram-negative (red), the sample is underdecolorized. If gram-positive (blue) organisms are present near the gram-negative leukocytes, the stain is suitable. If the cells and all the organisms are gram-negative, the slide may be overdecolorized and may require restaining. The slide should be examined carefully for the predominant organism; bacteria overlying squamous epithelial cells should be disregarded.

Usually, sputum expectorated after a deep cough is acceptable for stain and culture by the criteria outlined above. When the patient cannot produce a satisfactory specimen, inhalation of ultrasonically nebulized saline or suctioning with a catheter introduced through the nose into the posterior pharynx will often induce coughing and provide an adequate sample. Since sputum that is expectorated or obtained by nasotracheal suction is unavoidably contaminated by oropharyngeal flora, which normally contains anaerobic organisms, it is not appropriate for anaerobic cultures.

Another method of obtaining sputum is transtracheal aspiration with a polyethylene catheter inserted into the trachea through the cricothyroid membrane. This procedure is generally safe but should be accompanied by oxygen administration in those with hypoxia and avoided in uncooperative patients and those with serious clotting disorders or platelet defects. This method avoids contamination with the abundant, complex mouth flora and yields a specimen suitable for anaerobic culture. An alternate way of obtaining lower respiratory secretions is transthoracic aspiration of the lung with a spinal needle attached to a syringe. The major complications are pneumothorax or pulmonary hemorrhage. Lower respiratory secretions may also be obtained by bronchoscopy. Because contamination with oropharyngeal flora is generally unavoidable, even with preceding endotracheal intubation, these specimens are approximately equivalent to good expectorated sputum samples, unless specially designed catheters, which may provide uncontaminated specimens, are used.

Occasionally, lung biopsy may be necessary for accurate diagnosis and treatment, especially in immunocompromised patients. This procedure is discussed later in the chapter under "Treatment, Pneumonia in Compromised Hosts."

Since bacteremia sometimes accompanies pneumonia, blood cultures taken from two separate venipuncture sites may grow the responsible organism. Similarly, the presence of a pleural effusion requires a thoracentesis, which may yield infected fluid. Skin lesions, joint effusions, and cerebrospinal fluid should be cultured if these areas appear infected.

Although viruses, *M. pneumoniae, Coxiella burnetti, Legionella pneumophila,* and *Francisella tularensis,* may grow from sputum specimens cultured on appropriate media, pneumonias due to these agents are usually diagnosed by serology. Acute and convalescent serum samples should be obtained when these agents are suspected; seroconversion to *L. pneumophila* may take 6 weeks. Legionnaires' disease may also be diagnosed by direct immunofluorescence of respiratory tract secretions (see Chap. 117).

DIFFERENTIAL DIAGNOSIS Community-acquired pneumonias Pneumococcal pneumonia (see Chap. 93), the most common bacterial pneumonia, in its classic form frequently follows an upper respiratory infection and begins abruptly with a single shaking chill, fever, pleuritic chest pain, and a cough productive of purulent, often bloody sputum. In some patients, especially the elderly and those with serious underlying disorders such as alcoholism or chronic obstructive lung disease, the illness is often considerably less dramatic, with the insidious onset of fever, cough, and dyspnea or extrapulmonary features such as confusion or weakness. The white blood cell count is usually elevated, with increased immature forms, but may be normal or low. The typical sputum Gram's stain shows numerous neutrophils and abundant, gram-positive lancet-shaped diplococci as the predominant organism. The chest roentgenogram characteristically demonstrates a unilateral, homogeneous, nonsegmental air space consolidation, usually abutting against a visceral pleural surface. Unilateral or bilateral multilobar involvement may occur, and in patients with emphysema the consolidation may have an inhomogeneous appearance of multiple "holes" from the radiolucent, unconsolidated bullae. Cavitation rarely occurs, but parapneumonic pleural effusions, usually small but occasionally voluminous, are frequent.

Pneumonia from *S. pyogenes* (see Chap. 95) is very uncommon. It may follow pharyngitis or a viral illness, especially influenza, or occasionally occurs as outbreaks in closed populations, such as military recruits. The onset is typically abrupt, with multiple rigors, fever, a productive cough, and pleuritic chest pain. Pharyngitis is often present. The white blood cell count is commonly elevated, and immature forms increased. The sputum Gram's stain shows multiple neutrophils and gram-positive cocci in chains. The chest roentgenogram usually reveals a large pleural effusion, which develops rapidly after the onset of illness, and which tends to obscure any underlying pneumonia.

Pneumonia from *S. aureus* (see Chap. 94), also quite uncommon, tends to follow an influenza attack. The onset is generally abrupt and the course rapid, with fever, multiple rigors, purulent sputum production, and pleuritic chest pain. The white blood cell count is

FIGURE 205-1 *Roentgenographic appearances of pneumonia. A. Air space pneumonia. There is a dense, homogeneous, nonsegmental consolidation in the right lower lobe with a visible air bronchogram. B. Interstitial pneumonia. A linear or reticular pattern involves the lower lung fields bilaterally, more on the right. C. Bronchopneumonia. A segmental infiltrate without a visible air bronchogram appears in the left lower lung field.*

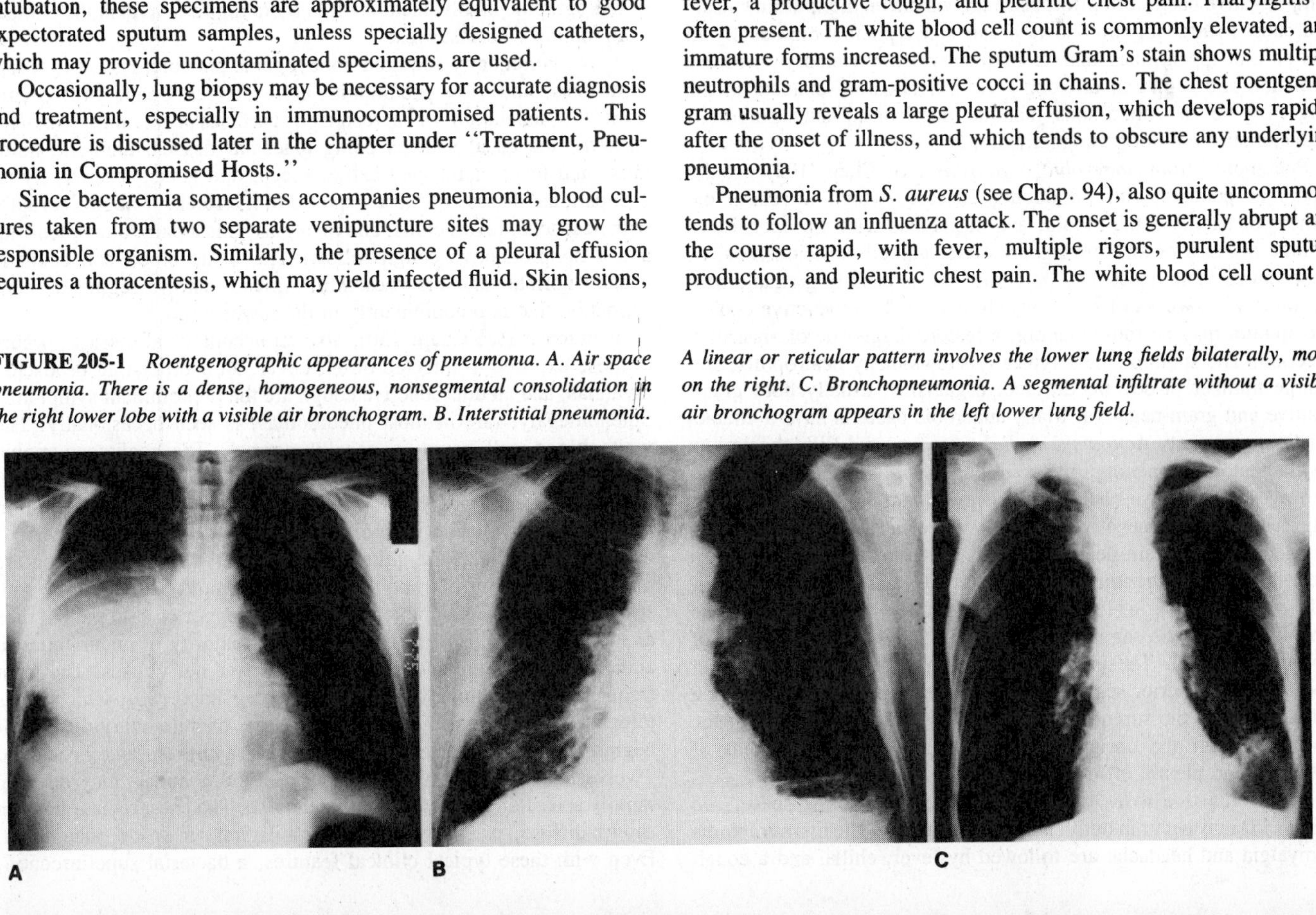

elevated, and immature forms are increased. The sputum smear shows numerous neutrophils and gram-positive cocci in clumps. The chest roentgenogram reveals bronchopneumonia, often bilateral, frequently with cavitation and pleural effusions. Pneumatoceles, thin-walled cystic spaces, may develop, primarily in children.

Pneumonia due to *N. meningitidis* (see Chap. 103) may occur in sporadic cases, following viral respiratory infections, or in closed populations, especially in military recruits. The onset may be abrupt, resembling pneumococcal pneumonia, or more gradual, with cough, fever, sore throat, and chest pain. Meningitis or cutaneous evidence of meningococcemia is uncommon, and blood cultures are typically sterile. Neutrophilic leukocytosis is usual. The sputum smear shows gram-negative diplococci that are often present within the cytoplasm of neutrophils. The chest film most commonly demonstrates patchy alveolar consolidation, predominantly in the lower lobes. Pleural effusions and pulmonary cavitation are rare.

Although *H. influenzae* (see Chap. 109) pneumonia may occur in healthy young adults, the typical patient is over 50 years old and has chronic obstructive lung disease or is an alcoholic. The onset may be abrupt but is more frequently gradual. The major complaints are fever, productive cough, chills, dyspnea, and pleuritic chest pain. Neutrophilic leukocytosis is usual. The sputum smear shows abundant neutrophils and many pleomorphic gram-negative organisms that range from cocci to bacilli of various sizes and are often especially predominant in the cytoplasm of the white blood cells. The bacilli are slender, unlike the typical plump appearance of enteric organisms. The chest film usually discloses diffuse bronchopneumonia, often bilateral, although air space consolidation sometimes occurs. Pleural effusions developing rapidly in the course of disease are common, but lung abscess is rare.

Klebsiella pneumoniae (see Chap. 105) pneumonia is very uncommon. It typically occurs in middle-aged or elderly patients with underlying chronic disease, especially alcoholism or diabetes mellitus. The illness begins abruptly with fever, rigors, productive cough, and dyspnea. Neutrophilic leukocytosis is usual, although neutropenia occasionally occurs. The sputum may be tenacious and bloody. Plump gram-negative bacilli of uniform size are visible on the sputum smear. The chest roentgenogram shows an air space pneumonia usually in one of the upper lobes that is frequently complicated by abscess formation and a pleural effusion. The inflammatory exudate in the lung may be so voluminous that the interlobar fissure bulges, a characteristic, but not pathognomonic, finding.

Pneumonia from *anaerobic organisms* (see Chap. 102) usually occurs in patients with periodontal disease, which increases the number of bacilli in the mouth, and in patients with a propensity to aspirate because of swallowing disorders, altered consciousness, or other causes. The onset may be abrupt but is usually gradual, with several days to weeks of fever, weight loss, and a productive cough. The sputum may be foul smelling, a feature diagnostic of anaerobic infection. The sputum smear typically shows many neutrophils, and a large number of several different organisms, usually both gram-positive and gram-negative. Many anaerobic bacteria have a characteristic appearance. *Actinomyces, Eubacterium,* and Bifidobacterium are filamentous, branching, thin gram-positive rods. Peptostreptococci are tiny gram-positive cocci in chains. *Fusobacterium* appears as a long, fusiform gram-negative rod with pointed ends, while *Bacteroides* are pleomorphic gram-negative bacilli that range from coccoid to long, filamentous structures. Understandably, aerobic cultures typically fail to grow a likely pathogen. Chest films demonstrate consolidation in the segments where gravitation favors the flow of aspirated material. These are the posterior segments of the upper lobes and the superior segments of the lower lobes, when aspiration has occurred in the supine position, and the basilar segments of the lower lobes for the upright position. Single or multiple areas of cavitation and pleural effusions are very common.

Pneumonia due to *L. pneumophila* (Legionnaires' disease, see Chap. 117) may occur in outbreaks or sporadically. The first symptoms of myalgia and headache are followed by fever, chills, and a cough that is nonproductive or yields small amounts of mucoid sputum. Diarrhea, chest pain that is often pleuritic, and confusion or delirium are common. Sputum smears show few leukocytes and rare bacteria. The organism itself is not visible on Gram's stain. The chest film reveals air space consolidation that may develop into unilateral or bilateral, poorly marginated, rounded opacities. Pleural effusions, if present, are usually small, and cavitation rarely occurs.

Pneumonia due to *Francisella tularensis* (see Chap. 113) follows tick bites or exposure to infected animals. A cutaneous ulcer and regional lymphadenopathy may be present but are absent in the typhoidal form. The illness typically begins abruptly with fever, chills, headache, and cough, which is usually nonproductive. The leukocyte count is usually normal but may be elevated. The sputum smear may show neutrophils, but the organism is rarely seen. The chest roentgenogram typically shows a bronchopneumonia, often with hilar adenopathy, a finding seldom seen in other bacterial pneumonias. Sometimes the pneumonia appears as a distinctive, oval, homogeneous consolidation. Pleural effusions are common, but cavitation is rare.

The most frequent cause of community-acquired, nonpyogenic pneumonia is *M. pneumoniae* (see Chap. 149). It occurs most commonly in children or young adults, but may develop in older persons, especially during outbreaks in a family group. It differs from the bacterial pneumonias described above in many respects. It has an insidious, rather than abrupt, onset and a cough that is nonproductive or yields only small amounts of mucoid sputum. Pleuritic chest pain, rigors, and hemoptysis are distinctly uncommon. The temperature is generally less than 38.9°C (102°F), and headache is a prominent symptom. As in other nonpyogenic pneumonias, the sputum smear typically demonstrates mononuclear leukocytes or neutrophils but few organisms, since the agent is not visible on Gram's staining. The white blood cell count is usually normal or only mildly elevated, with a normal differential. The chest roentgenogram demonstrates segmental bronchopneumonia, or sometimes a predominant interstitial pattern, mostly affecting the lower lung fields. Bilateral involvement is common, but, unlike many bacterial pneumonias, substantial pleural effusions or cavitation are rare. The extent of radiographic involvement is often more impressive than the clinical examination would suggest.

Other community-acquired nonpyogenic pneumonias are Q fever, psittacosis, and viral pneumonia. Q fever (see Chap. 148) occurs from the inhalation of aerosolized particles containing *Coxiella burnetti,* the usual sources being placental tissues, amniotic fluid, milk, and feces of infected cattle, sheep, and goats. It is largely an occupational disease of those exposed to livestock. It begins abruptly with headache, fever, chills, and myalgias. Chest pain, often pleuritic, and a nonproductive cough follow. The white blood cell count is usually normal, and the chest film typically shows segmental consolidation that is predominantly in the lower lobes.

Psittacosis (see Chap. 150), also an occupational disease, occurs in those exposed to infected birds. Fever, an excruciating headache, myalgias, and an unproductive cough are the predominant symptoms. Splenomegaly, rare in most pneumonias, is seen occasionally. The white blood cell count is usually normal. The roentgenographic appearance varies from homogeneous to patchy consolidation, which may be segmental or lobar in distribution. Sometimes the chest film shows nodular or miliary opacities.

Viral pneumonias are quite uncommon in civilian adults who are not immunosuppressed, and this diagnosis should be made only with strong clinical or epidemiologic evidence, supported by viral cultures and serologic studies. The overwhelming majority of pneumonias in adults are due to the agents discussed above, not viruses. The most frequent viral pneumonia is *influenza* (see Chap. 130), which tends to occur in patients with underlying cardiac or pulmonary disease. It begins as typical influenza, with fever, myalgias, and headache. Twelve to thirty-six hours later dyspnea and cyanosis may develop rapidly and often proceed to a fatal outcome. The chest roentgenogram shows diffuse, patchy, unilateral or bilateral air space pneumonia. Even with these typical clinical features, a bacterial superinfection, especially with pneumococci or *S. aureus,* may be responsible for the pneumonia, instead of the virus itself.

Varicella (see Chap. 135) can cause pneumonia in adults and typically begins 2 to 3 days after the vesicular eruption appears. Fever, cough, dyspnea, hemoptysis, and pleuritic chest pain are the major symptoms. The chest film demonstrates patchy, diffuse, generally discrete air space consolidations that are coarsely nodular.

Measles (see Chap. 132) pneumonia in adults generally occurs in military recruits and may begin just before, with, or after the skin rash. The chest film shows a diffuse bilateral reticular pattern.

Adenovirus (see Chap. 131) pneumonia also occurs predominantly in military recruits. Fever, cough, rhinitis, and pharyngitis are the major features. The chest film shows patchy consolidation, generally in the lower lung fields.

In endemic areas the fungi *Coccidioides immitis, Blastomyces dermatitidis,* and *Histoplasma capsulatum* (see Chap. 147) must be considered in the differential diagnosis of community-acquired pneumonia.

In chronic pneumonias—those lasting for weeks or months—the primary infectious causes are anaerobic bacteria, mycobacteria, *Nocardia asteroides*, and various fungi. Among the fungi, *Cryptococcus neoformans* and *Sporothrix schenckii* are found worldwide, while *Blastomyces dermatitidis*, *Coccidioides immitis*, *Histoplasma capsulatum*, and *Paracoccidioides brasiliensis* have limited geographic distributions. In southeast Asia one form of melioidosis, an infection caused by the bacterium *Pseudomonas pseudomallei*, presents as a chronic pneumonia. Previous travel history is very important in evaluating chronic pulmonary infections.

Hospital-acquired pneumonia Because of changes in oropharyngeal flora with hospitalization, hospital-acquired pneumonias, unlike community-acquired ones, are likely to be due to a wide variety of aerobic gram-negative bacilli with varying antimicrobial susceptibilities and, less frequently, *S. aureus,* pneumococci, or *H. influenzae*. Only rarely is it possible to distinguish among pneumonias caused by different species of gram-negative rods on the basis of the clinical or roentgenographic features. Adequate sputum Gram's stains and cultures, therefore, are especially important in defining the etiologic agent and suggesting the appropriate antibiotic therapy.

Hospitalized patients with endotracheal tubes or tracheostomies receiving mechanical ventilation are an important group in whom the diagnosis of pneumonia is particularly difficult to make. Shortly after intubation, the tracheobronchial tree becomes colonized with organisms, and a purulent tracheobronchitis commonly ensues. Even though there is purulent sputum with plentiful organisms, this tracheobronchitis requires no antimicrobial therapy, which only encourages the growth of drug-resistant organisms, unless pneumonia is present. The diagnosis of pneumonia requires evidence of parenchymal lung involvement and in this setting depends upon the presence of purulent tracheobronchial secretions *plus* fever, leukocytosis, and a new or progressive pulmonary infiltrate on chest films.

TREATMENT Community-acquired pneumonia Patients whose history or physical examination suggests the likelihood of pneumonia should have a chest roentgenogram to confirm the diagnosis and delineate the pattern and extent of pulmonary involvement. Most patients with mild to moderate disease on clinical and radiologic assessment can be treated as outpatients. In them, a white blood cell count may be useful in the differential diagnosis, but routine blood cultures and arterial blood gases are unnecessary. The clinical and radiographic features and the sputum Gram stain should dictate the choice of antimicrobial therapy. If sputum is unobtainable or unhelpful and the other information inconclusive, oral erythromycin, 500 mg qid, is a good choice. It is effective against pneumococci and *M. pneumoniae,* the two most frequent causes of community-acquired pneumonia, but also should be satisfactory to treat Legionnaires' disease and many cases of *H. influenzae* pneumonia and anaerobic pneumonias. Auxiliary measures should include adequate hydration, analgesics to relieve chest pain, if present, and cough suppressants for those with the harassing, unproductive cough characteristic of *M. pneumoniae*. In patients with good clinical improvement, a repeat chest film after 6 weeks is appropriate to document radiographic resolution. Failure to resolve by then indicates possible endobronchial obstruction and the necessity for bronchoscopy.

Reasons for hospitalization include severe dyspnea or hypoxia; evidence of empyema or extrapulmonary foci of infections, such as meningitis; shock; serious underlying disease, especially cardiac or pulmonary; severe systemic manifestations such as delirium, whose presence warrants a lumbar puncture to exclude concomitant meningitis; or social circumstances making treatment at home unfeasible. These patients should have two blood cultures obtained from separate venipuncture sites; a complete blood count, including white blood cell differential; and arterial blood gas measurements if there is marked tachypnea, severe dyspnea, altered mental status potentially attributable to hypoxia, cyanosis, or serious underlying cardiopulmonary disease. The clinical and radiographic features and, especially, the sputum Gram's stain should indicate the proper antibiotic choice. Since the most common community-acquired pneumonia requiring hospitalization is pneumococcal, the appropriate agent usually is penicillin, 2.4 million units daily, intramuscularly or intravenously. If the sputum smear is unsatisfactory or unobtainable by expectoration or nasotracheal suctioning, transtracheal aspiration may be indicated, particularly if the patient has an underlying illness like alcoholism that makes gram-negative pneumonia more likely.

In patients with unobtainable or uninformative sputum, penicillin remains the drug of choice in most circumstances, including suspected anaerobic infections following the aspiration of large quantities of oropharyngeal contents. Reasonable alternatives include clindamycin, 300 mg intravenously every 6 h, parenteral cefazolin, 500 mg every 8 h, or erythromycin, 1 g intravenously every 6 h, especially in suspected Legionnaires' disease, where it is the drug of choice. In drug addicts and in patients developing pneumonia after an influenza attack, pneumococcus or *S. aureus* are the likely pathogens, and a semisynthetic penicillinase-resistant penicillin like oxacillin or nafcillin, 8 to 12 g daily intravenously, is indicated. Alternatives include vancomycin, 2 g intravenously daily, or cephalothin, 8 to 12 g intravenously daily. In patients with chronic bronchitis complicated by acute pneumonia, pneumococcus and *H. influenzae* are the most common causes, and ampicillin, 2 to 6 g daily intravenously, is a good choice for therapy in the unusual patient whose sputum sample is inadequate for diagnosis. Alternatives include tetracycline, 2 g daily; chloramphenicol, 2 g daily; or cefamandole, 2 g daily, all given intravenously.

Auxiliary measures include adequate hydration, the administration of humidified oxygen, relief of chest pain by adequate analgesics or nonsteroidal anti-inflammatory drugs, and the encouragement of coughing to expectorate sputum. Intermittent positive pressure breathing (IPPB), however, is not helpful, and postural drainage should generally be reserved for those with bronchiectasis or lung abscess. Mechanical ventilation is required when the diffuseness of the pneumonia or the severity of underlying cardiopulmonary disease prevents adequate oxygenation with spontaneous respiration and supplemental oxygen by mask or nasal prongs.

Hospital-acquired pneumonia Since the range of organisms causing hospital-acquired pneumonias is so wide and their antimicrobial susceptibilities so variable, precise bacteriologic diagnosis is crucial. Patients with hospital-acquired pneumonias should have blood cultures, and vigorous attempts must be made to obtain sputum by expectoration, nasotracheal suctioning, or, if these are unsuccessful, transtracheal aspiration. When gram-negative rods are the predominant organism on Gram's stain, an aminoglycoside effective against *Pseudomonas aeruginosa,* like gentamicin, plus an antipseudomonal penicillin like ticarcillin or carbenicillin should be given. If gram-positive cocci resembling *S. aureus* are present, vancomycin or a penicillinase-resistant penicillin is appropriate. If a mixture of these organisms is present or no sputum is obtainable, a combination of an aminoglycoside plus a penicillinase-resistant penicillin or a cephalosporin is a good choice. Determination of the precise agents used should be guided by knowledge of the local hospital flora and its antimicrobial sensitivities. The regimen should be altered later according to the identity and susceptibility of the organisms isolated. If the sputum smear reveals organisms characteristic of pneumococci, anaerobes, or *H. influenzae,* which sometimes cause nosocomial pneumonias, the appropriate therapy for these organisms recommended in Chap. 88 should be given.

Pneumonia in compromised hosts (see also Chap. 84) Compromised hosts with pneumonia require special consideration. Patients who are severely neutropenic from acute leukemia or from cytotoxic agents generally develop pneumonia from aerobic gram-negative bacilli. Unless the Gram's stains strongly indicate otherwise, these patients should receive an aminoglycoside effective against *P. aeruginosa* and an antipseudomonal penicillin like ticarcillin or carbenicillin until the culture results return.

In severely immunosuppressed patients without neutropenia, the possible causes of fever and a new pulmonary infiltrate are legion. They fall into four categories: (1) the disease itself, such as Hodgkin's disease of the lung; (2) the effects of treatment, such as radiation pneumonitis or pulmonary toxicity from agents like methotrexate; (3) infections; and (4) miscellaneous disorders such as pulmonary emboli and intrapulmonary hemorrhage. Possible infectious causes include not only bacteria but also fungi, like *Candida* or *Aspergillus*; viruses, especially cytomegalovirus; and protozoa, particularly *Pneumocystis carinii* (see Chap. 158). In these patients unless the initial evaluation, including sputum smears, strongly indicates a specific diagnosis, further information obtained by bronchoscopic biopsy and lavage, transthoracic needle aspiration, or open-lung biopsy is necessary for definitive diagnosis.

For safe performance, all these procedures, except lavage, require correction of severe thrombocytopenia and clotting disorders. *Transthoracic needle aspiration* may be useful in peripheral, localized disease, but because it fails to provide tissue specimens, it is not recommended for diffuse infiltrates, where histologic examination rather than stains and cultures of aspirated material is so frequently necessary for specific diagnosis. Pneumothorax occurs in about 20 percent, requiring chest tube placement in about 10 percent; significant pulmonary hemorrhage develops in about 5 percent. Contraindications include uncorrectable hypoxia, lack of patient cooperation, bullous lung disease, and mechanical ventilation. *Fiberoptic bronchoscopy* with washings, sterile brushings, and transbronchial biopsy is appropriate for both localized and diffuse processes, but the quantity of tissue obtained is small and may be unrepresentative, especially in diffuse disease. The procedure yields a specific diagnosis in about 50 percent of cases. Pneumothorax or significant hemorrhage each occurs in about 5 to 10 percent, with about one-half of pneumothoraxes requiring chest tube drainage. Contraindications include uncorrectable hypoxia or an uncooperative patient. Bleeding complications are considerably greater in uremia, although it is not an absolute contraindication. In patients with acquired immunodeficiency syndrome (AIDS) (see Chap. 257), fiberoptic bronchoscopy demonstrates the cause of diffuse pulmonary infections in almost all cases. *Open-lung biopsy* yields accurately representative tissue in nearly all patients. A specific diagnosis is established in about 70 percent of immunodeficient patients without AIDS; in the remaining 30 percent nonspecific inflammation and fibrosis are found whose cause is unknown and for which there is no effective therapy. Such a finding allows antimicrobial agents to be withheld or discontinued. Open-lung biopsy is remarkably safe, with a mortality rate of less than 1 percent in these very ill patients. It can be performed even in patients requiring mechanical ventilation.

While many clinicians initiate these invasive diagnostic procedures in immunodeficient patients without AIDS as soon as the initial, rapid clinical evaluation and examination of sputum smears prove inconclusive, others reserve them for patients who fail to respond to "empiric" therapy within 48 to 72 h. Empiric treatment is initiated with an aminoglycoside combined with a cephalosporin, carbenicillin, or ticarcillin. With diffuse infiltrates sulfamethoxazole-trimethoprim is added to treat *P. carinii.* For those patients who fail to respond and are unable to undergo invasive diagnostic procedures, amphotericin B is added for focal infiltrates, especially if the patient has recently received prolonged broad-spectrum antibiotic therapy and is leukopenic. This empiric approach is usually less advisable than obtaining a specific diagnosis with invasive techniques. Patients with known or suspected AIDS and pulmonary complications should not be treated empirically but should undergo fiberoptic bronchoscopy.

TABLE 205-1 Classification of lung abscesses according to cause

1 Necrotizing infections
- *a* Pyogenic bacteria (*S. aureus, Klebsiella,* group A streptococcus, *Bacteroides, Fusobacterium,* anaerobic and microaerophilic cocci and streptococci, other anaerobes, *Nocardia)*
- *b* Mycobacteria (*Mycobacterium tuberculosis, M. kansasii, M. intracellularis)*
- *c* Fungi (*Histoplasma, Coccidioides, Aspergillus)*
- *d* Parasites (amoebas, lung flukes)

2 Cavitary infarction
- *a* Bland embolism
- *b* Septic embolism (various anaerobes, *Staphylococcus, Candida)*
- *c* Vasculitis (Wegener's granulomatosis, periarteritis)

3 Cavitary malignancy
- *a* Primary bronchogenic carcinoma
- *b* Metastatic malignancies (very uncommon)

4 Other
- *a* Infected cysts
- *b* Necrotic conglomerate lesions (silicosis, coal miner's pneumoconiosis)

LUNG ABSCESS

DEFINITION A lung abscess is a necrotic area of lung parenchyma containing purulent material. An etiologic classification appears in Table 205-1.

PATHOGENESIS The pathogenesis of infectious lung abscesses is nearly identical to that of pneumonia. Most arise from the aspiration of naso- or oropharyngeal contents. The development of a lung abscess, instead of just pneumonia, depends upon the infecting organism's ability to cause necrosis of lung tissue. Pneumococci, *H. influenzae, M. pneumoniae,* and viruses rarely cause necrosis, but it is common in pulmonary infections due to *K. pneumoniae* and other enteric gram-negative bacilli and *S. aureus.* Anaerobic organisms are the most frequent cause of pyogenic lung abscesses and tend to occur when large quantities of oropharyngeal material are aspirated because of disordered consciousness or impaired swallowing.

Processes that cause mechanical or functional obstruction of the bronchi may predispose to lung abscesses. Mechanical causes include tumor, foreign body, or bronchial stenosis. Lung cancer is particularly important because occult bronchogenic neoplasms may be complicated by a distal abscess, or a cavitating, uninfected carcinoma may mimic a lung abscess.

Less frequently, abscesses arise from hematogenous spread of organisms to the lung. This may occur during bacteremia originating from a distant site of infection or as a result of septic emboli either from right-sided endocarditis or from septic thrombophlebitis associated with infections in the extremities or the abdominal cavity.

Patients with tuberculosis (see Chap. 119), pulmonary fungal infections (see Chap. 147), and pleuropulmonary amebiasis (see Chap. 153) may develop one or more areas of lung necrosis. Although usually labeled "cavities," these lesions are really abscesses. While the clinical course typically distinguishes these conditions from pyogenic lung abscess, there may be many similarities that cause confusion in the differential diagnosis.

CLINICAL MANIFESTATIONS The clinical features of pulmonary infections due to staphylococci, streptococci, and aerobic gram-negative bacilli are discussed earlier in this chapter and in the chapters dealing with the specific organisms. These are usually rapidly progressive infections in which single or multiple cavities develop as complications of an acute pneumonia. Persistent fever, profuse sputum production, and hemoptysis are common. Occasionally, an abscess ruptures into the pleural cavity, causing an empyema or, rarely, a pneumothorax.

Anaerobic lung abscess Although the spectrum of illness in anaerobic lung abscess may vary from a mild productive cough to acute disease with severe systemic manifestations, the onset is usually insidious, with the symptoms gradually worsening over several weeks. The most common feature is a cough productive of moderate to large amounts of purulent sputum that is often fetid and bloody. Fever, pleuritic or dull chest pain, dyspnea, weakness, anorexia, and weight loss, which can be considerable, are common. A condition predisposing to aspiration, such as alcoholism or epilepsy, is usually present.

Most patients are febrile. Oral examination usually discloses poor dentition, with caries, gingivitis, and periodontal infection, conditions which increase the number of anaerobes in the oral cavity. The chest examination may be normal or may include signs of consolidation, rales, and, occasionally, amphoric or cavernous breath sounds over the involved area. An empyema, present in about one-third of cases, may cause dullness to percussion and decreased breath sounds. Clubbing, although uncommon, may occur. Neutrophilic leukocytosis with an increase in immature forms is usual, and, if the infection has persisted for several weeks, anemia and hypoalbuminemia may be present. The medical history, physical findings, and routine laboratory results are often nonspecific; foul-smelling sputum, which is present in about half the patients, however, clearly indicates an anaerobic pulmonary infection. Definitive diagnosis rests on the demonstration of an abscess cavity on chest films and the identification of the causative organisms on culture.

The chest roentgenogram reveals an area of consolidation containing a radiolucency. Not all radiolucent areas are abscesses, however, and either a wall or a border completely surrounding the lucent area or a fluid level within it should be present to diagnose an abscess cavity. Even these criteria are not definitive, since infected bullae or cysts or an empyema with a bronchopleural fistula may have an identical appearance. The abscess cavities are located in those segments that are most dependent at the time of aspiration: the posterior segment of the upper or superior segment of the lower lobes, especially on the right, when the patient is supine or the basilar segments of the lower lobes when upright.

Examination of the sputum by both microscopy and culture is essential to establish the correct diagnosis. In staphylococcal and aerobic gram-negative bacillary infections, the single causative organism clearly predominates on smear and culture. Gram's stain of sputum from an anaerobic abscess reveals abundant neutrophils and numerous organisms, including gram-positive cocci and rods and gram-negative rods of varying size and configuration. Since expectorated sputum is unavoidably contaminated by the normal anaerobic oral flora, anaerobic sputum cultures are appropriate only for specimens obtained by transtracheal or transthoracic aspiration. Secretions aspirated through the fiberoptic bronchoscope (unless a special catheter is used) are unsuitable because the instrument is contaminated as it passes through the naso- or oropharynx, even with preceding endotracheal intubation. Appropriately collected and cultured sputum specimens usually grow two or more anaerobic organisms, most commonly *Peptococcus, Peptostreptococcus, Fusobacterium nucleatum,* and *Bacteroides melaninogenicus*. In about 60 percent of cases the infecting flora is exclusively anaerobic; in 40 percent both aerobes and anaerobes are present. The most common aerobic isolates are *S. aureus* and enteric gram-negative bacilli.

Associated pleural effusions should be aspirated and cultured aerobically and anaerobically. Blood cultures are usually sterile.

Septic pulmonary emboli In patients with septic pulmonary emboli, the site of origin is usually tricuspid valve endocarditis, particularly in intravenous drug abusers, or septic thrombophlebitis, which may occur in the arm veins of patients with infected intravenous catheter sites, infected injection sites from intravenous drug abuse, or infected arteriovenous shunts used in hemodialysis. Other areas of septic thrombophlebitis include pelvic veins with postpartum or postoperative pelvic infections, peritonsillar and internal jugular veins with pharyngeal infections, and veins adjacent to undrained suppuration, such as soft tissue infections or osteomyelitis. Rigors, high fever, dyspnea, cough, tachycardia, and tachypnea are the major clinical manifestations in these acutely ill patients. Neutrophilic leukocytosis is usual. The chest film typically discloses multiple, bilateral, round, or wedge-shaped opacities. These frequently and rapidly excavate to form thin-walled cavities, often without fluid levels. Small pleural effusions on one or both sides are common. Blood cultures are usually positive. Patients may not produce sputum, but if they do, it usually reveals the responsible organism, most commonly *S. aureus,* on Gram's stain and culture.

TREATMENT The history, physical examination, chest roentgenograms, and most importantly, Gram's and acid-fast sputum stains usually indicate whether an abscess is caused by aerobic organisms, anaerobes, or tubercle bacilli. Abscesses caused by aerobic organisms usually require prolonged treatment with the antibiotics recommended in the chapters dealing with them.

Where septic pulmonary emboli from septic thrombophlebitis are suspected, it is important not only to institute appropriate antimicrobial therapy but also to identify the source. Removal of catheters, incision and drainage of systemic abscesses or infected veins, or ligation of the inferior vena cava may be necessary to prevent further embolization.

When the clinical findings and the sputum Gram's stain suggest an anaerobic abscess, clindamycin probably is the drug of choice. It is usually given in doses of 600 mg intravenously every 8 h until clinical improvement (return of appetite, defervescence) occurs. Oral clindamycin in doses of about 300 mg four times daily is then given for the duration of therapy. Some clinicians use oral medication from the start. Many physicians prefer penicillin as the initial treatment, reserving clindamycin for fulminant infections or those failing to respond to penicillin after 5 to 7 days. The dose is 10 to 12 million units intravenously daily, followed by oral penicillin V, 750 mg to 1 g four times a day. Because of relapses with shorter courses, antibiotics are usually given for 6 weeks.

Ancillary measures include postural drainage and chest physiotherapy to help drain the abscess cavity. The role of bronchoscopy is unsettled. Some physicians believe that every patient with a lung abscess deserves bronchoscopy; most others reserve its use for patients who fail to respond as anticipated to antibiotic therapy, who have evidence of an obstructing tumor or foreign body, or who have poorly communicating cavities that fail to drain adequately. Features that especially suggest the possibility of lung cancer and the necessity for bronchoscopy include a long history of smoking, lack of a predisposing cause to aspirate, good oral hygiene, evidence of volume loss or mediastinal or hilar lymph node enlargment on chest film, location of the cavity in a nondependent area, and failure to respond to appropriate antibiotic therapy.

Except for the tube thoracostomy drainage of an associated empyema, surgery for lung abscess is rarely necessary. Incomplete roentgenographic resolution is not a sufficient reason for resectional surgery since delayed closure is common. Resection is indicated for massive hemoptysis, malignancy, or associated symptomatic bronchiectasis. Rarely, tube thoracostomy or some other form of surgical drainage may be necessary to manage uncontrolled sepsis arising from a poorly draining abscess.

REFERENCES

Pneumonia

BARTLETT JG: Anaerobic bacterial pneumonitis. Am Rev Resp Dis 119:19, 1979

FRASER RG, PARE JAP: *Diagnosis of Diseases of the Chest.* Philadelphia, Saunders, 1978, vol II, chap 6
GEORGE WL, FINEGOLD SM: Bacterial infections of the lung. Chest 81:502, 1982
GREEN GM et al: Defense mechanisms of the respiratory membrane. Ann Rev Resp Dis 115:479, 1977
PIERCE AK, SANFORD JP: Aerobic gram-negative bacillary pneumonias. Am Rev Resp Dis 110:647, 1974
———: The gram-negative bacillary pneumonias, in *Update IV: Harrison's Principles of Internal Medicine,* KJ Isselbacher et al (eds). New York, McGraw-Hill, 1983, pp 75–86
REYNOLDS HY (ed): Respiratory infections. Clin Chest Med 2:1, 1981

Lung abscess

BARTLETT JG et al: Bacteriology and treatment of primary lung abscess. Am Rev Resp Dis 109:510, 1974
JOHANSON WG et al: Aspiration pneumonia, anaerobic infections, and lung abscess. Med Clin N Am 64:385, 1980
LEVISON ME et al: Clindamycin compared with penicillin for the treatment of anaerobic abscess. Ann Intern Med 98:466, 1983

206 BRONCHIECTASIS AND BRONCHOLITHIASIS

JOHN F. MURRAY

These disorders both involve branches of the tracheobronchial system, have numerous, rather than single, underlying causes, and occasionally coexist. However, the pathogenesis, clinical manifestations, treatment, and prognosis of the two conditions are remarkably different.

BRONCHIECTASIS

DEFINITION Bronchiectasis can be defined as a permanent abnormal dilatation of one or more bronchi, those airways that contain cartilage and bronchial glands, due to destruction of the elastic and muscular components of the bronchial wall. This definition is not completely satisfactory because bronchi are also abnormally dilated in chronic bronchitis. Thus chronic bronchitis merges into bronchiectasis, and the distinction between them depends upon the *degree* of dilatation. The semantic problem is complicated further by the fact that the two conditions frequently coexist.

Classification is therefore difficult and is not useful in indicating the clinical severity of the disease; however, certain descriptive terms are commonly used to describe the appearance of bronchi displayed by bronchography. *Saccular* (*cystic*) *bronchiectasis* occurs mainly in the proximal large bronchi; affected airways show marked dilatation ending in large sacs at about the fourth bronchial division. *Cylindrical* (*fusiform*) *bronchiectasis* involves airways from the sixth to the tenth generation; the bronchographic appearance shows mild to moderate uneven widening, without a great increase in diameter, of bronchi that often look beaded and end squarely and abruptly. *Varicose bronchiectasis* is intermediate between saccular and cylindrical changes and is used to describe bronchi that resemble varicose veins. Because all three types may be present in the same patient, these terms have little therapeutic or prognostic implication.

Although "true" bronchiectasis is not reversible, the concept of reversibility is important, because abnormalities displayed by bronchography in some patients with reversible lung diseases (atelectasis, tracheobronchitis) may simulate bronchiectasis. Atelectasis causes shortening and tortuosity of airways in the involved region, producing an accordion-like appearance on bronchography. Similarly, ulcerations of the bronchial mucosa, which are common in viral infections of the lower respiratory tract, appear as an irregular pattern on bronchography. Both conditions resemble cylindrical bronchiectasis. Reexpansion of the collapsed lung and/or regeneration of the epithelium results in reversibility of the "pseudobronchiectasis." Thus bronchography, if indicated, should be delayed for several months after an episode of tracheobronchitis, pneumonia, or atelectasis.

PATHOGENESIS Since bronchiectasis is defined by the presence of morphologic changes in the caliber of bronchi, its pathogenesis depends on antecedent factors that either cause or lead to necrosis of the bronchial wall and supporting tissues. Necrotizing inflammation, nearly always infectious in origin, seems clearly to be the most important cause of bronchiectasis. Local pressure on the bronchial wall from retained secretions may act as a contributing factor. Hereditary, congenital, or mechanical abnormalities that predispose to bronchopulmonary infection and sputum retention are often also present. The use of vaccines and antibiotic drugs has resulted in a marked decline in the incidence of severe necrotizing pneumonias and their bronchiectatic complications in developed countries, however, bronchiectasis as a complication of underlying systemic disorders appears to be increasing.

Hereditary and congenital factors Several hereditary and congenital disorders have been identified in which there is a high incidence of secondary bronchiectasis. *Congenital bronchiectasis* occurs at the site of a pre- or postnatal development defect of the bronchial system. The formation of cysts, cul-de-sacs, or bronchomalacia leads to pooling of secretions and bacterial infection. The generalized disorder of exocrine gland secretions in patients with *cystic fibrosis,* discussed in Chap. 207, affects the physical properties of tracheobronchial mucus and/or the adequacy of mucociliary clearance; this causes retention of secretions, with partial or complete plugging of airways, that provides a nidus for implantation and growth of bacteria. Most deaths (95 percent) of patients with cystic fibrosis who survive beyond 1 year of age are now caused by the consequences of bronchiectasis and accompanying chronic bronchopulmonary suppuration. The diffuse bronchiectasis rarely encountered with patients with *atopic bronchial asthma,* in whom there is often a strong familial association (Chap. 202), presumably is related to diffuse obstruction, as described below.

A variety of hereditary *immune-deficiency diseases,* secondary to either cellular or humoral defects, is associated with a high incidence of bacterial infections. Involvement of the sinuses and airways is particularly common, and the tendency for infections to recur in the lower airways often leads to bronchiectasis in patients with impaired immunologic mechanisms.

A group of genetically determined disorders called the *immotile cilia syndrome,* which includes *Kartagener's syndrome* (bronchiectasis, dextrocardia, and sinusitis) is characterized by ultrastructural changes causing immotility of cilia in the respiratory tract epithelium, sperm, and other cells. These abnormalities lead to recurrent sinopulmonary infections, infertility, and presumably disturbances during embryogenesis. This definition has recently been broadened to include patients with chronic sinobronchial disease from impaired mucociliary clearance who had "ciliary dyskinesia," not immotile cilia. The high incidence of unexplained bronchiectasis in Polynesians has been attributed to hereditary abnormalities of respiratory tract ciliary motility.

Obstruction Postobstructive bronchiectasis was much commoner in preantibiotic years than it is today. The availability of antimicrobial therapy and corrective surgical procedures accounts for the decreased incidence of this form of the disease. It is now recognized that obstruction per se does *not cause* bronchiectasis but *favors its development* by impairing clearance mechanisms, which enhances bacterial infection. Any process that leads to bronchial obstruction, therefore, may be associated with bronchiectasis distal to the site of involvement. Since the disorders causing obstruction are usually confined to one part of the bronchial system, postobstructive bronchiectasis is of the localized rather than the diffuse variety found in most forms of congenital-hereditary bronchiectasis. An exception is the bronchiectasis associated with diffuse obstruction of airways in patients with chronic bronchitis, atopic asthma, and cystic fibrosis. Patients with atopic asthma are liable to have secondary infections with *Aspergillus,* which produces the syndrome of bronchopulmonary aspergillosis characterized by proximal airway bronchiectasis, eosinophilia, and recurrent bouts of mucous plugging (Chap. 203).

Endobronchial tumors or foreign bodies, compression of airways from enlarged hilar lymph nodes or tumor masses, and bronchostenosis from endobronchial inflammatory disease (especially tuberculosis) all cause bronchial obstruction and may predispose to the development of postobstructive bronchiectasis.

Necrotizing inflammation Virtually all forms of bronchiectasis are associated with bacterial infections. If it were not for the presence of infection, the complications of bronchiectasis would be negligible. Although the development of the causative infection(s) is often precipitated by the presence of a hereditary disorder and/or bronchial obstruction that predisposes the patient to secondary bacterial involvement, bronchiectasis can occur as the result of necrotizing infections in a previously healthy individual. This presumably is the mechanism underlying the bronchiectasis that follows tuberculosis and staphylococcal or other suppurative pneumonias; furthermore, the tendency for necrotizing pneumonias occasionally to complicate measles, pertussis, adenovirus infections, and influenza accounts for the occurrence of bronchiectasis as a sequela of these disorders.

In rare instances, bronchiectasis may follow the introduction of corrosive chemical substances, commonly hydrocarbons, into the tracheobronchial tree. Similarly, the repeated aspiration of gastric fluid into the lungs may cause bronchiectasis. Since recurrent ulceration from chemical causes is invariably associated with secondary bacterial infection, it is difficult to dissociate the contributions of these two factors.

CLINICAL MANIFESTATIONS The signs and symptoms of bronchiectasis depend on the extent, severity, and location of the abnormal airways, and the presence of complications, but the hallmarks of the disease are chronic cough with sputum production, hemoptysis, and recurrent pneumonia. Even these vary greatly in frequency and severity and may be absent or intermittent if the disease is mild or involves only the upper lobes of the lung.

The most frequent symptom is a *chronic cough* that produces sputum. The amount of sputum varies considerably but may be voluminous and is apt to be purulent during bouts of intercurrent infections. Streaks of blood in the sputum are common, and frank hemoptysis of large amounts of blood may develop if necrosis of the mucosa is severe. Exacerbation of chronic bronchial infection is frequent and may progress to pneumonia, occasionally with lung abscess or empyema formation. Associated systemic features of bronchiectasis are fever, weight loss, anemia, and weakness; these usually indicate the presence of active sepsis from severe disease or untreated intercurrent bacterial infection.

In what was once the typical patient with bronchiectasis, symptoms developed during infancy or early childhood; the onset was usually acute and followed suppurative pneumonia or pulmonary infection complicating measles or pertussis. However, because of the success of antimicrobials and vaccines in treating or preventing these disorders, acute onset of bronchiectasis at an early age is becoming infrequent, except in those areas of the United States and other countries where, owing to isolation or poverty, good medical care is not available.

Although chronic childhood bronchiectasis is decreasing, another group of patients with a different form of the disease appears to be increasing: these patients have recurrent lower respiratory tract infections that initially respond to treatment, with symptom-free intervals between episodes. The infections usually begin during childhood or young adulthood. As the number of recurrent bouts increases, the time between them tends to shorten and the response to treatment becomes less complete. Finally, chronic symptoms of cough and sputum develop. Patients in this category are likely to have cystic fibrosis, immune-deficiency diseases, immotile cilia, or atopic asthma.

Sinusitis is a common accompaniment of diffuse bronchiectasis and may be an expression of the vulnerability of the entire respiratory tract in these patients. Development of digital clubbing, metastatic abscesses (often brain), and amyloidosis were common complications in the past but are less frequent now. If the disease is widespread, it may resemble other forms of chronic obstructive lung disease, with generalized wheezing and ultimate progression to cor pulmonale; this constellation is particularly apt to occur in patients with underlying systemic abnormalities that lead to diffuse pulmonary involvement.

DIAGNOSIS Bronchiectasis is defined as a morphologic disorder; hence its diagnosis depends on demonstrating the abnormal anatomy of the bronchial system. Ordinarily this is accomplished by roentgenographic techniques, either *bronchography* or *computed tomography*. The diagnosis should be *suspected* in any patient with chronic productive cough, especially if the sputum intermittently becomes more purulent and streaked with blood. The distinction between bronchiectasis and chronic bronchitis, which may cause identical symptoms and which may coexist, is unimportant except when surgery is contemplated. Physical examination seldom reveals the severity and extent of distribution of the disease. Inspiratory rales are often the only evidence of pulmonary involvement. Occasionally, advanced cases of saccular bronchiectasis can be diagnosed by routine (plain) chest roentgenography; in such cases multiple 1- to 2-cm cystic lesions or fluid levels in poorly delineated sacs can be seen. More often, however, plain chest roentgenograms show only streaky infiltrations and loss of volume in involved areas; at times the chest roentgenograms may appear completely normal.

Bronchography (Chap. 201) should not be performed routinely in all patients with suggestive symptoms but is indicated primarily in the evaluation of patients for possible operation, those with recurrent, localized pneumonias or severe hemoptysis. Since the information from bronchography contributes little to the management of patients in whom surgery is contraindicated, such as those with minimal disability, with generalized involvement, or with obstructive airways disease, the procedure should be avoided in these patients because of its hazards. When bronchography is indicated, it should not be performed in patients during exacerbations of their cough and sputum production, but only after the manifestations have been thoroughly treated (see next section) and the volume of secretions is minimal. It is safer and advisable to study one lung at a time, owing to alterations in pulmonary function and to occasional inflammatory reactions induced by the procedure. Filling must be adequate and all segments must be visualized if the study is to be considered satisfactory for diagnostic purposes.

Computed tomography is being increasingly used to diagnose bronchiectasis. At present, the procedure is not a substitute for bronchography in the evaluation of patients for surgery. Computed tomography appears to be a useful, noninvasive—but expensive—way of making the diagnosis in patients who are not candidates for bronchography.

Bronchoscopy does not establish the diagnosis of bronchiectasis but may be useful in identifying the source of secretions in patients with cough and sputum and in determining the site of bleeding in patients with hemoptysis.

All patients with multiple episodes of sinopulmonary infections should have an immunologic survey to detect immune-deficiency diseases. Similarly, patients with suspected cystic fibrosis should have measurements of the concentrations of sodium and chloride in two or more samples of sweat (Chap. 207). Electron photomicrographic studies of sperm or mucosal biopsies from the respiratory tract reveal characteristic abnormalities in patients with the immotile cilia syndrome in whom tracheobronchial clearance is delayed or absent. Patients with asthma and suspected bronchiectasis from bronchopulmonary aspergillosis should have sputum cultures for *Aspergillus,* serologic studies for aspergillin precipitins, and measurement of serum IgE values.

The sputum volume, color, cellular content, and bacterial inhabitants are useful guides to the presence of active infection. Sputum eosinophilia provides a clue to the presence of asthma and/or bronchopulmonary aspergillosis. During exacerbations of the disease, the sputum increases in volume, becomes more purulent, and contains large numbers of polymorphonuclear leukocytes and bacteria that can be identified by Gram's stain. Culture of the sputum often reveals normal nasopharyngeal flora and, less commonly, *Streptococcus pneumoniae* or *Haemophilus influenzae*. Fetid sputum signifies the presence of anaerobic microorganisms. Sputum from patients receiving prolonged or frequent treatment with broad-spectrum antibiotic drugs may grow *Staphylococcus* species or a mucoid strain of *Pseudomonas aeruginosa;* this finding is especially common in patients with cystic fibrosis, and indicates superinfection by an organism refractory to conventional treatment.

The blood count is usually within the normal range but may reveal anemia, reflecting chronic infection, or leukocytosis, signifying active suppuration. The urinalysis is normal except in the rare instances of *amyloidosis,* when proteinuria occurs. The electrocardiogram is normal until the late stages, when *cor pulmonale* may supervene and right ventricular hypertrophy develops. Owing to the wide variations in the extent and severity of the disease, only broad generalizations about pulmonary function abnormalities are possible, although a correlation exists between the overall impairment of lung function and the number of involved segments. Vital capacity and expiratory flow rates tend to be reduced but may be within normal limits if the disease is mild. In the late stages of diffuse bronchiectasis severe airflow obstruction can occur. A mild to moderate reduction in arterial oxygen tension (P_{O_2}) reflects regional abnormalities in the distribution of ventilation with respect to perfusion. Disturbances of ventilation in excess of those of perfusion, as expected in a disorder of the airways, are the physiologic hallmark of bronchiectasis and can now be examined in regions of the lung by the use of radioactive gases, e.g., ^{133}Xe (Chap. 200). Pulmonary function studies are helpful in defining the extent and severity of abnormalities, in assessing the need for and effects of bronchodilator therapy, and in evaluating patients for surgery.

TREATMENT Since bacterial infections are associated with most forms of bronchiectasis initially and are responsible for its exacerbation, antibiotics are the major weapons for its prevention and treatment. The choice of antimicrobial agents should be guided by the results of sputum culture; however, as indicated, these may reveal "normal flora" and no conspicuous pathogen. The drug of choice for patients with this finding is ampicillin or one of its derivatives; patients allergic to the penicillins usually respond to trimethoprim-sulfamethoxazole or one of the tetracyclines. When pneumococci are present, it is best to avoid the tetracycline drugs, as some pneumococcal strains are resistant to these agents. Antibiotics should be given until sputum production becomes minimal and purulence disappears; this desirable therapeutic result is usually achieved swiftly (5 to 7 days) if antibiotics are started early in the course of an exacerbation—as soon as the patient's cough increases and becomes productive of sputum in greater quantity and purulence than customary—but much longer periods are required if the infection is well established. Continuous treatment with antimicrobials or "prophylactic" schedules such as 1 week per month has not been shown to be beneficial and promotes the development of resistant organisms. Antibiotics should be administered either orally or by injection, *not* by nebulization (owing to failure of delivery, inactivation of the antibiotic, and risk of sensitization).

Adjuvant medical measures are useful in diminishing the consequences of bronchiectasis. Postural drainage and physical therapy are recommended for those with thick or tenacious sputum, especially if present in large amounts. Many patients with bronchiectasis have reversible bronchospasm as shown by the results of pulmonary function studies; these patients should be treated with bronchodilators. Expectorants and humidifiers are of questionable value. Adequate hydration is probably just as effective as the administration of expectorants. Fiberoptic bronchoscopy is useful in identifying sites of endobronchial disease (Chap. 201) and sources of secretions and hemoptysis, and permits removal of secretions by aspiration under direct vision. Repeated bronchoscopies are helpful in the management of the unusual patient with problems of sputum retention. Similarly, bronchial lavage has been tried as a "last resort" in patients with large volumes of inspissated secretions. Oxygen should be given to patients with hypoxia during acute exacerbations; it can be administered outside the hospital to patients who are severely and chronically hypoxic. Inflammation from any cause will aggravate the effects of chronic bronchiectasis; therefore, smoking should be prohibited, exposure to air which is excessively polluted should be avoided, and influenza and pneumococcal vaccines should be administered yearly.

Resectional surgery, once the mainstay of treatment, is used far less often now than previously for two reasons: (1) medical management is very effective in controlling bronchiectasis and preventing disability from it; (2) many patients with bronchiectasis have a generalized disorder that makes their entire tracheobronchial system vulnerable; although their bronchiectasis may appear well localized when evaluated initially, new sites of involvement may appear later. Operation should be considered in patients with localized (i.e., resectable) lesions who do not respond to medical management or who are so disabled by complications that either their livelihood or their emotional life is impaired. Bouts of hemoptysis, especially if massive, and recurrent localized pneumonias are the usual complications that require hospitalization, cause repeated disability, and require that the patient be evaluated for surgery.

PREVENTION The best approach to bronchiectasis is prevention. Patients with heritable diseases that predispose to bronchiectasis and their families should obtain genetic counseling to minimize the incidence of these disorders. Prompt diagnosis and effective antimicrobial treatment of bacterial infections of the lower respiratory tract constitute the best way of avoiding their potential chronic sequelae. The eradication of measles and pertussis by vaccines will eliminate these diseases as harbingers of bronchiectasis.

Prompt removal of foreign bodies, tumors, and other causes of bronchial obstruction should diminish postobstructive bronchiectasis.

BRONCHOLITHIASIS

The term *broncholith* has two meanings: in a general sense it indicates any calcification that impinges on and distorts the wall of a bronchus; in a restricted sense it refers to a calcified tissue fragment that is loose within the lumen of a bronchus. Intraluminal broncholiths can form in three ways: (1) calcification of aspirated food or tissue that was retained in the airway for a long time, (2) protrusion into the lumen and fragmentation of a calcified bronchial cartilage because of necrosis of the bronchial wall in bronchiectasis, and (3) erosion of a contiguous calcified granuloma through the wall. Numerous disorders leave calcified deposits that can be detected by chest roentgenography, but clinically significant broncholithiasis is rare. It is usually a late complication of one of the three common granulomatous infections: tuberculosis, histoplasmosis, and coccidioidomycosis. Of these, histoplasmosis has the greatest tendency to heal with multiple residual calcifications, and coccidioidomycosis has the least; hence broncholithiasis in the United States, especially in the central and eastern regions, is most likely to be related to previous infection with *Histoplasma capsulatum;* in Europe half the cases are caused by tuberculosis.

The clinical consequences of broncholithiasis are related to the movement of stones through the airway wall and their release into the lumen. The process of erosion is often accompanied by paroxysms of cough, intermittent hemoptysis, and bronchopulmonary infection. The overlying inflammatory reaction impairs bronchial clearance and narrows the lumen; these conditions may lead to distal bronchiectasis or, if the obstruction is complete, atelectasis. The hallmark of broncholithiasis is the coughing and expectoration of chalky sediment, sandy (gritty) particles, or stones. Such episodes are usually single but may be multiple.

Broncholithiasis should be suspected in any patient with recurrent cough and hemoptysis whose chest roentgenograms show multiple calcifications in the lung and/or mediastinal lymph nodes. The diagnosis can be established by recovering stones in the sputum, by visualizing broncholiths penetrating the bronchial wall at the time of bronchoscopy, or by establishing that calcified particles have disappeared on serial chest x-ray films. Computed tomography is helpful in determining with greater precision than routine roentgenograms the presence and location of calcifications in and around bronchi.

Treatment depends on the magnitude of the symptoms. The disorder is self-limiting once the stone has eroded into the lumen and is coughed up; however, ulceration by the particle may be slow and attended by significant symptoms. Antimicrobial agents are useful in the treatment of associated bacterial infection. Bronchoscopy should be performed and the stone removed if possible. At times, thoracotomy and lung resection are necessary, usually for obstructive complications or massive hemoptysis.

REFERENCES

Bronchiectasis

BREATNACH ES et al: Preoperative evaluation of bronchiectasis by tomography. J Comput Assist Tomogr 9:949, 1985

DAVIES PB et al: Bronchiectasis and oligospermia: Two families. Thorax 40:376, 1985

LEWISTON NJ: Bronchiectasis in childhood. Pediatr Clin North Am 31:865, 1984

MURPHY MB et al: Atopy, immunological changes, and respiratory function in bronchiectasis. Thorax 39:179, 1984

PROTO AV: Evaluation of the bronchi with CT. Semin Radiol 19:199, 1984

SWARTZ MN: Bronchiectasis, in *Pulmonary Diseases and Disorders*, 2d ed, AP Fishman (ed). New York, McGraw-Hill, 1987, chap 93

Broncholithiasis

DIXON GF et al: Advances in the diagnosis and treatment of broncholithiasis. Am Rev Respir Dis 129:1028, 1984

TRASTEK VF et al: Surgical management of broncholithiasis. J Thorac Cardiovasc Surg 90:842, 1985

207 CYSTIC FIBROSIS

HARVEY R. COLTEN

Cystic fibrosis (CF) is an inherited multisystem disorder which is characterized by an abnormality in exocrine gland function. Nearly all patients develop chronic progressive disease of the respiratory system. Pulmonary disease is the most common cause of death and morbidity in patients with cystic fibrosis. Pancreatic dysfunction (exocrine or endocrine) occurs in 85 percent of patients; hepatobiliary and genitourinary disease are also frequent. Prior to the 1930s the syndrome was confused with several other disorders with signs and symptoms of intestinal malabsorption.

CF is common in populations of European origin. Estimates of the incidence of the disorder range from about 1/500 in Amish (Ohio) to 1/90,000 in Hawaiian Orientals. For the white American population the disease occurs in 1/1600 to 1/2000 live births. The disease is recognized less frequently in black Americans (about 1/17,000) and rarely, if at all, among black Africans. Hence, although the "CF gene" is undetectable in the heterozygous state, from the apparent autosomal recessive mode of inheritance the gene frequency in white Americans is estimated at 1/20. The inability to detect heterozygous individuals has retarded more extensive genetic studies and limits the value of genetic counseling for relatives of patients with CF. On the other hand, several DNA probes localized to the long arm of chromosome 7 which detect restriction fragment length polymorphisms linked to the "CF gene" have been identified. These markers will be used for carrier detection, antenatal diagnosis, and ultimately determination of the molecular basis of this disorder. Most cases of CF appear to be due to defect(s) at a single locus, but the possibility of genetic heterogeneity has not been excluded.

Currently, the median survival for patients with CF is about 20 years, and many patients survive to the third and fourth decades. A few have survived to age 50 and beyond. Even though survival of CF patients has improved, the mutation is semilethal. More than 98 percent of males with CF are infertile (see below), and fertility is reduced in women with the disease. This, together with the high incidence of the disease suggests a selective advantage for the individual heterozygous for the CF gene, but there is a paucity of basic information about the genetic defect.

CLINICAL MANIFESTATIONS **General** The majority of CF patients are diagnosed in infancy or childhood, but some escape detection until adulthood. Table 207-1 summarizes the multiple clinical features of this disease. Substantial pancreatic disease is more common in patients diagnosed early in life, because acute intestinal obstruction (meconium ileus at birth) or malnutrition and poor growth or development alerts the pediatrician and family. Patients with minimal or absent gastrointestinal complaints and atypical respiratory symptoms may be diagnosed for the first time when adult. The finding of microorganisms typically isolated from sputum of CF patients (a mucoid form of *Pseudomonas aeruginosa*) or male infertility in association with evidence of obstructive pulmonary disease suggests CF in a previously undiagnosed adult.

Respiratory All levels of the respiratory tract may be affected in CF. Nasal polyposis, sinusitis, and lower respiratory tract disease are common. Abnormalities in water and electrolyte transport across the respiratory epithelium are said to be uniquely abnormal in patients with CF. Primary qualitative or quantitative alterations in mucous

TABLE 207-1 Principal clinical manifestations of cystic fibrosis

I Respiratory/cardiovascular
- *A* Bronchitis, bronchopneumonia, bronchiectasis, lung abscesses, aspergillosis (allergic)
- *B* Atelectasis
- *C* Sinusitis, nasal polyposis
- *D* Pulmonary hypertension
- *E* Cor pulmonale and congestive heart failure
- *F* Hemoptysis
- *G* Pneumothorax
- *H* Respiratory failure

II Gastrointestinal
- *A* Intestinal
  - *1* Meconium ileus
  - *2* Volvulus
  - *3* Ileal atresia
  - *4* Rectal prolapse
  - *5* Intussusception
  - *6* Fecal impaction
  - *7* Pneumatosis intestinalis
- *B* Pancreatic
  - *1* Nutritional deficit and growth failure due to pancreatic insufficiency
  - *2* Steatorrhea
  - *3* Diabetes mellitus
  - *4* Recurrent pancreatitis
- *C* Hepatobiliary
  - *1* Atrophic gallbladder, cholelithiasis
  - *2* Loss of bile salts
  - *3* Focal biliary cirrhosis
  - *4* Portal hypertension
    - *a* Esophageal varices
    - *b* Hypersplenism
    - *c* Hemorrhoids

III Reproductive system
- *A* Males: sterility; absent or defective vas deferens, epididymis, and seminal vesicles in about 99 percent of males
- *B* Females: decreased fertility; increased viscosity of vaginal secretions

IV Skeletal
- *A* Retardation of bone age
- *B* Demineralization
- *C* Hypertrophic osteoarthropathy

V Other
- *A* Salt depletion
- *B* Heat stroke
- *C* Salivary gland hypertrophy
- *D* Retinal hemorrhage
- *E* Hypertrophy of apocrine glands

secretion that are characteristic for CF have been suggested, but most if not all that have been experimentally determined appear similar to findings in patients with chronic bronchitis or bronchiectasis of diverse etiologies. Autopsy studies of infants dying of meconium ileus suggest that the lungs of newborns with CF are normal. The earliest pulmonary changes are hypertrophy of bronchial glands followed by mucous plugging and obstruction of small airways. Subsequent infection leads to a bronchiolitis, and centripetal progression of endobronchial disease results in chronic bronchitis, bronchiectasis, and peribronchial inflammation. The release of toxic oxygen species and proteolytic enzymes by bacterial and inflammatory cells probably contributes to the progression of airway disease. Specific and nonspecific systemic host defenses are normal or increased, though chronic inflammatory disease may lead to mechanical interference with local defense mechanisms.

Three major bacterial organisms chronically colonize or infect the airways of patients with CF. *Staphylococcus aureus* and *Haemophilus influenzae* are recovered from sputum in a minority, and *P. aeruginosa*, especially mucoid forms, are detected in more than 90 percent of CF patients. Once the *P. aeruginosa* is acquired, the organism is rarely if ever eliminated. Other bacteria (mucoid forms of *Escherichia coli, Legionella,* etc.) and other microorganisms, including viruses, mycoplasma, and fungi, may be present in the sputum of patients with CF. Colonization with *Pseudomonas cepacia* may herald a more unfavorable short-term prognosis. The mucoid *Pseudomonas* strains are detected almost exclusively in the CF population. Even family members of patients with CF are not colonized by this organism, so that recovery of a mucoid form of *P. aeruginosa* from patients with chronic pulmonary disease should prompt further diagnostic studies to rule out CF.

Acute and chronic pulmonary parenchymal involvement leads to loss of tissue, extensive fibrosis, and changes in lung and airway mechanics. The inflammatory and structural changes in airways and lung parenchyma lead to airway obstruction, hyperinflation, and ventilation-perfusion imbalance. The upper lobes are generally more involved than lower lobes. Pleural involvement is rare, and extrathoracic infection with respiratory pathogens is virtually absent. Secondary changes in pulmonary and bronchial vasculature in patients with advanced respiratory disease may lead to the substantial hemoptysis often observed in older patients. Pulmonary hypertension develops frequently in CF patients with severe airway obstruction and hypoxemia, resulting in progressive right ventricular failure (cor pulmonale). Clubbing is seen in nearly all patients.

TREATMENT Treatment of CF pulmonary disease is directed toward increasing mechanical drainage, as in patients with chronic bronchitis (Chap. 208), with the use of chest physiotherapy, exercise programs, etc. Control of bacterial infection or colonization is effected by antibiotic therapy specific for the common bacterial organisms isolated from CF sputum. Antibiotic-resistant strains of *P. aeruginosa* are frequently isolated from patients with advanced disease, but in general intravenously administered aminoglycosides in combination with modified penicillins or cephalosporins are employed for treatment of pulmonary exacerbations. Aerosolized antibiotics have been used as well. Management of the bronchospastic component of the disease involves the use of systemic and aerosolized bronchodilators. Occasionally surgery (e.g., lobectomy) is required when infection or tissue destruction is localized. Prompt attention to and specific therapy of complications of pulmonary disease have been important factors in the improved survival of patients with CF. Small pneumothoraxes can generally be managed expectantly, while many will respond to tube thoracostomy alone. However the best evidence suggests that this approach is associated with high recurrence rates. Therefore most episodes are treated with pleural sclerosis (with agents such as tetracycline or quinacrine), open pleurectomy, or pleurodesis. Massive hemoptysis is treated most safely and effectively by bronchial artery embolization via a percutaneous catheter. Congestive heart failure is managed as described elsewhere (Chaps. 182 and 191).

Gastrointestinal Pancreatic insufficiency leading to fat and protein malabsorption is a feature in the majority of cases (Chap. 255). Deficiencies of fat-soluble vitamins, caloric deprivation, failure to grow and develop, and other manifestations such as rectal prolapse occur in patients with untreated pancreatic insufficiency. About 5 percent of patients with CF are born with meconium ileus, i.e., intestinal obstruction secondary to inspissated meconium in the terminal ileum. Occasionally perforation and meconium peritonitis can occur. Treatment of pancreatic insufficiency with oral pancreatic enzymes corrects most of the deficits. For instance, it decreases the number and bulk of stools; the amount of flatulence, abdominal pain, and distention; and it largely corrects the malabsorption and hence corrects the nutritional deficiencies.

In patients with intact or partial pancreatic exocrine function, recurrent acute pancreatitis may occur. A minority of patients (2 to 5 percent) develop overt diabetes mellitus requiring exogenous insulin, but subclinical abnormalities in glucose metabolism can be detected in a much larger group of CF patients. The longer survival of patients with CF may allow the development of typical diabetic complications such as retinal and glomerular lesions. These should prompt more aggressive efforts to maintain optimal diabetic control.

Hepatobiliary disease is common in older patients. There is chronic cholestasis, inflammation, fibrosis, and even cirrhosis. All of the features of portal hypertension have been recognized. Extrahepatic disease of the biliary system is common.

Genitourinary Abnormalities of the genitourinary tract are present in 98 percent of males. These are due to an interruption in wolffian duct structures (atresia of the vas deferens) which results in azoospermia and decreased ejaculate volume (Chap. 330). Sexual development and potency are unaffected by the genitourinary abnormalities. Women have abnormal cervical mucus. Sexual development, the menstrual cycle, and fertility in women are less affected by direct effects of the mutation than by the effects of poor nutrition and/or chronic pulmonary disease. Women with CF can conceive and deliver healthy infants, but the maternal and fetal risks are functions of the extent of pulmonary disease and its complications. Close monitoring and prompt therapy in centers expert in high-risk obstetrical management are indicated.

Sweat glands The abnormality in the eccrine sweat gland function provides the most reliable diagnostic test for CF at present. Sodium, potassium, and chloride are elevated in sweat of patients with CF. The chloride concentration exceeds 70 meq per liter, and the sodium concentration is greater than 60 meq per liter in sweat of nearly all patients, though some individuals with "borderline values" may have many other manifestations of the disease. The corresponding values for chloride and sodium in normals rarely exceed 50 and 40 meq per liter, respectively. Sweat electrolytes are measured most reliably by the pilocarpine iontophoresis method. Even when qualitative screening methods are used, the diagnosis cannot be made without a quantitative sweat electrolyte measurement. The increased electrolyte content results from a failure of reabsorption in the sweat duct. Electrolyte losses may lead to significant salt depletion, especially in young children.

CONCLUSION Increasing survival of patients with typical findings of CF as well as patients undiagnosed until adult life requires an increased awareness of this disorder among physicians. The relatively high prevalence of this disorder and the enormous resources required to treat patients with CF has stimulated research activity to define the basic genetic defect responsible for the protean clinical manifestations of CF.

REFERENCES

Davis PB: Cystic fibrosis. Semin Resp Med 6:243, 1985

di Sant'Agnese PA, Davis PB: Cystic fibrosis in adults: 75 cases and a review of 232 cases in the literature. Am J Med 66:121, 1979

FELLOWS KE et al: Bronchial artery embolization in cystic fibrosis: Technique and long-term results. J Pediatr 95:959, 1979
KNOWLES M et al: Increased bioelectrical potential difference across respiratory epithelia in cystic fibrosis. N Engl J Med 305:1489, 1981
MATTHEWS WJ et al: Hypogammaglobulinemia in patients with cystic fibrosis. N Engl J Med 302:245, 1980
PARK RW, GRAND RJ: Gastrointestinal manifestations of cystic fibrosis: A review. Gastroenterol 81:1143, 1981
SCANLIN TF: Cystic fibrosis (including assessment of pulmonary performance), in *Pulmonary Diseases and Disorders,* 2d ed, AP Fishman (ed). New York, McGraw-Hill, 1987, chap 76
SHWACHMAN H et al: The sweat test: Sodium and chloride values. J Pediatr 98:576, 1981
TALAMO RC et al: Cystic fibrosis, in *Metabolic Basis of Inherited Disease,* 5th ed, JB Stanbury et al (eds). New York, McGraw-Hill, 1983

208 CHRONIC BRONCHITIS, EMPHYSEMA, AND AIRWAYS OBSTRUCTION

ROLAND H. INGRAM, JR.

Chronic bronchitis and emphysema are two distinct processes, often present in combination in patients with chronic airways obstruction. The diagnosis of chronic bronchitis is made by history, chronic airways obstruction is assessed physiologically, and emphysema can be diagnosed with certainty only by histologic examination of sections of whole lung fixed at inflation. Although the relationships between clinical characteristics, physiologic derangements, and morphologic changes have been diligently studied for many years, reasonably certain and uniform clinical criteria are still not available. Definitions and classifications have evolved, but these are not universally accepted. Nonetheless, the following definitions along with brief qualifications and descriptions are currently used by most persons involved in the diagnosis, treatment, and epidemiology of the chronic obstructive airways syndromes.

DEFINITIONS *Chronic bronchitis* is a condition associated with excessive tracheobronchial mucus production sufficient to cause cough with expectoration for at least 3 months of the year for more than 2 consecutive years. Several subclassifications have been proposed. *Simple chronic bronchitis* describes a condition characterized by mucoid sputum production. *Chronic mucopurulent bronchitis* is characterized by persistent or recurrent purulence of sputum in the absence of localized suppurative diseases such as bronchiectasis. Since there may or may not be obstruction as assessed by the use of the forced expiratory vital capacity maneuver, *chronic bronchitis with obstruction* deserves a separate classification. There is a further subset of patients with chronic bronchitis and obstruction who experience severe dyspnea and wheezing in association with inhaled irritants or during acute respiratory infections. Such patients are said to have *chronic infective asthma* or *chronic asthmatic bronchitis.* Confusion is possible between patients with this condition and those with asthma (Chap. 202) who may also have *chronic airways obstruction.* The patient with chronic asthmatic bronchitis has a long history of cough and sputum production with a later onset of wheezing, whereas the asthmatic with chronic obstruction gives a long history of wheezing with later onset of chronic productive cough.

Emphysema is defined as distention of the air spaces distal to the terminal bronchiole with destruction of alveolar septa. *Chronic obstructive lung disease* is defined as a condition in which there is chronic obstruction to airflow due to chronic bronchitis and/or emphysema (see below). Although the degree of obstruction may be less when the patient is free from respiratory infection and may improve somewhat with bronchodilator drugs, some obstruction is always present.

PREVALENCE Approximately 20 percent of adult males have chronic bronchitis, yet only a minority of these are clinically disabled. According to all surveys males are more often affected than females. With increased cigarette smoking in women, however, the prevalence of bronchitis in them is increasing. Although cigarette smoking is the single most important etiologic factor, occupational and environmental exposures are now receiving more attention.

Since no criteria have been agreed upon for making the diagnosis of emphysema during life, the incidence data are derived solely from postmortem surveys. It is rare to find adult lungs completely free of emphysema. There is a distinct increase in the extent of emphysema in the fifth decade with further increases through the seventh decade and little increase after that. Approximately two-thirds of adult males and one-fourth of females (most without recognized dysfunction) will have well-defined emphysema, which is often limited in extent. Therefore, the majority of those with emphysema will not have had disability or even symptoms associated with it. The situation is analogous to atherosclerosis in that the morphologic changes are far more frequent than the clinical manifestations attributable to the changes.

PATHOLOGY *Chronic bronchitis* is associated with hyperplasia and hypertrophy of the mucus-producing glands found in the submucosa of large cartilaginous airways. Quantitation of this anatomic change, known as the *Reid index,* is based upon the ratio of the thickness of the submucosal glands to that of the bronchial wall. In persons without a history of chronic bronchitis the mean ratio is 0.44 with a standard deviation ± 0.09, whereas in those with such a history the mean ratio is 0.52 ± 0.08. Although a low index is *rarely* associated with symptoms and a high index is commonly associated with symptoms during life, there is a great deal of overlap. Therefore many persons will have morphologic changes in large airways without having had chronic bronchitis.

Perhaps more important than the abnormalities in large airways are the changes often found in the small noncartilaginous airways. Goblet-cell hyperplasia, mucosal and submucosal inflammatory cells, and edema, peribronchial fibrosis, intraluminal mucus plugs, and increased smooth muscle are characteristic findings in small airways. The frequency of these latter findings in relation to premortem clinical and functional status has not been determined. However, in lungs from patients with chronic obstructive lung disease which have been studied at postmortem, the major site of airflow obstruction has been shown to be in the small airways.

Emphysema is classified according to the pattern of involvement of the gas-exchanging units (acini) of the lung distal to the terminal bronchiole. Although several morphologic patterns have been described, the two most important in the context of this discussion are those involving the respiratory bronchioles and alveolar ducts in the center of the acinus (centriacinar emphysema) and those involving the entire acinus (panacinar emphysema). Quite often both morphologic patterns are present in a single lung of a patient dying from chronic obstructive lung disease, although one type may predominate over the other.

With centriacinar emphysema the distention and destruction are mainly limited to the respiratory bronchiole and alveolar ducts, with relatively less change peripherally in the acinus. Because of the large functional reserve in the lung, many units must be involved in order for overall dysfunction to be detectable. The centrally destroyed regions of the acinus have a high ventilation/perfusion ratio because the capillaries are missing yet ventilation continues. This results in increased wasted ventilation (Vd/Vt), while the peripheral portions of the acinus have crowded and small alveoli with intact, perfused capillaries giving a low ventilation/perfusion ratio. This results in wasted blood flow to give a high alveolar-arterial P_{O_2} difference ($P_{A_{O_2}} - P_{a_{O_2}}$) (Chap. 200). Mild degrees of centriacinar emphysema, often limited to the lung apices, are extremely common in lungs from persons above age 50 and are practically considered a normal finding.

Panacinar emphysema involves both the central and peripheral portions of the acinus which results, if the process is extensive, in a reduction of the alveolar-capillary gas exchange surface and loss of elastic recoil properties. When emphysema is severe, it may be difficult to distinguish between the two types which most often coexist in the same lung.

CONTRIBUTORY FACTORS **Smoking** Cigarette smoking is the most commonly identified correlate with both chronic bronchitis during life and extent of emphysema at postmortem. Experimental studies have shown that prolonged cigarette smoking impairs ciliary movement, inhibits function of alveolar macrophages, and leads to hypertrophy and hyperplasia of mucus-secreting glands; massive exposure in dogs can produce emphysematous changes. In addition to these chronic effects it is probable that smoke causes polymorphonuclear leukocytes to release proteolytic enzymes acutely. Inhaled cigarette smoke can produce an acute increase in airways resistance due to vagally mediated smooth-muscle constriction, presumably by way of stimulating submucosal irritant receptors. The relationship of such recurrent episodes of acute bronchial constriction to the development and progression of chronic airways obstruction is uncertain. Recent studies, however, indicate that increased airways reactivity is associated with more rapid progression in those with chronic airways obstruction.

It is now well established that some young asymptomatic smokers have considerable obstruction in small airways without there being either an increase of airway resistance or a diminution in the forced expiratory volume in 1 s. Since small airways, because of their large total cross-sectional areas, contribute very little to overall airflow resistance, more sensitive tests must be used to detect mild degrees of small-airways obstruction. Some tests, such as a decrease in compliance and resistance at rapid breathing rates, are based upon nonuniform behavior of the lung which is apparent only at increased frequencies. Obstruction of small airways also results in airways closure at higher lung volumes than in persons of the same age with unobstructed airways (Chap. 200). The measurements of closing volume and frequency dependence of resistance and compliance require special equipment not often available to clinicians. However, the simple spirogram is useful since flow rates at or below the mid-vital capacity range are often diminished in persons with mild small-airways obstruction. It has been shown that obstruction of small airways is the earliest demonstrable mechanical defect in young cigarette smokers and that the obstruction may disappear after cessation of smoking. It is possible, but has not been established with certainty, that those with small-airways obstruction are at greater risk of developing disabling chronic airways obstruction at some future time.

Not only is cigarette smoking the most common single factor leading to chronic airways obstruction, it also interacts with virtually every other contributory factor to be discussed below.

Air pollution The incidence and mortality rates of both chronic bronchitis and emphysema may be higher in heavily industrialized urban areas. Exacerbations of bronchitis are clearly related to periods of heavy pollution with sulfur dioxide (SO_2) and particulate matter. While nitrogen dioxide (NO_2) can produce small-airways obstruction (bronchiolitis) in experimental animals exposed to high concentrations, there are no data convincingly implicating NO_2, at even the highest pollutant levels, in the pathogenesis or worsening of airways obstruction in humans (Chap. 204).

Occupation Chronic bronchitis is more prevalent in workers who engage in occupations exposing them to either inorganic or organic dusts or to noxious gases. Epidemiologic surveys have succeeded in demonstrating an accelerated decline in lung function in many such workers—e.g., workers in plastics plants exposed to toluene diisocyanate and carding room workers in cotton mills (Chap. 204)—suggesting that their occupational exposure contributes to their future disability.

Infection Morbidity, mortality, and frequency of acute respiratory illnesses are higher in patients with chronic bronchitis. Many attempts have been made to relate these illnesses to infection with viruses, mycoplasmas, and bacteria. However, only the rhinovirus is found more often during exacerbations; that is to say, pathogenic bacteria, mycoplasmas, and viruses other than rhinovirus are found just as often between as during exacerbations. It is intuitively appealing to assign some role to respiratory infections in the pathogenesis and progression of chronic obstructive lung disease, and although this question is under study, there has been no conclusion to date. Recent epidemiologic studies, however, implicate acute respiratory illness as one of the major factors associated with the etiology as well as the progression of chronic airways obstruction. It has been shown that cigarette smokers may either transitorily develop or worsen small-airways obstruction in association with even mild viral respiratory infections. There is also some evidence that severe viral pneumonia early in life may lead to chronic obstruction, predominantly in small airways.

Familial and genetic factors Familial aggregation of chronic bronchitis has been well demonstrated in the past. Recent surveys have shown that children of smoking parents may experience more frequent and severe respiratory illnesses and have a higher prevalence of chronic respiratory symptoms. In addition, nonsmokers who remain in the presence of cigarette smokers (passive smokers) have increased blood levels of carbon monoxide which indicate that they are significantly exposed to smoke. Another well-documented form of indoor air pollution relates to the use of natural gas for cooking. The role of such pollution, however, remains controversial. Thus a part of the familial aggregation may be related to home air pollution. However, some studies of monozygotic twins have suggested some genetic predisposition to the development of chronic bronchitis independent of personal or familial smoking habits and other indoor air pollution. The exact genetic mode of transmission, if it exists at all, is uncertain.

The protease inhibitor $alpha_1$ antitrypsin is an acute-phase reactant, and normally the serum levels rise in association with many inflammatory reactions and with estrogen administration. Either deficient or absent serum levels of $alpha_1$ antitrypsin are found in some patients with the early onset of emphysema. By use of the techniques of acid starch gel and immunoelectrophoresis, genetic typing of the protease inhibitor (Pi) types has been possible. Most of the normal population have two M genes, designated as Pi type MM, and have serum $alpha_1$ antitrypsin levels in excess of 250 mg/dL. Several genes are associated with alterations in levels of serum $alpha_1$ antitrypsin, but the commonest ones associated with emphysema are the Z and S genes. Individuals who are homozygous ZZ or SS have serum levels often near 0 but always less than 50 mg/dL and develop severe panacinar emphysema in the third and fourth decades of life. The panacinar process predominates at the lung bases. Progressive dyspnea with minimal cough characterizes the clinical presentation, although chronic bronchitis is prominent in smokers. Given that $alpha_1$ protease inhibitors can be chemically synthesized or biologically produced in significant quantities and can be shown with intravenous infusion to restore the protease-antiprotease balance in liquid lavaged from the lungs of ZZ patients, it has been suggested that replacement therapy should be of value in preventing the development of emphysema; limited clinical trials are underway. The MZ and MS heterozygotes have intermediate levels of serum $alpha_1$ antitrypsin (i.e., between 50 and 250 mg/dL); hence the genetic expression is that of an autosomal codominant allele. It is a matter of some controversy whether the heterozygous state is associated with lung function abnormalities. Published studies are in direct conflict on this point, and further data are needed to be certain. The matter is of some importance, since the heterozygous state is common, with incidence estimates varying between 5 and 14 percent of the general population.

The precise way in which antitrypsin deficiency produces emphysema is unclear. In addition to inhibition of trypsin, $alpha_1$ antitrypsin is an effective inhibitor of elastase and several other proteolytic enzymes. There is experimental evidence that the structural integrity of lung elastin depends upon this antienzyme, which protects the lung from proteases released from leukocytes. It is tempting to speculate that recurrent inflammatory reactions related to infection and pollutants play some role in pathogenesis by calling forth leukocytes whose released proteases are uninhibited and are free to cause the damage.

The role of proteolytic enzymes in the induction of emphysema is not restricted to patients with alpha$_1$ antitrypsin deficiency. Evidence is accumulating that proteolytic enzymes derived from neutrophilic leukocytes and alveolar macrophages can produce emphysema even in subjects with normal circulating levels of antiproteases. It is possible that local concentrations of proteolytic enzymes may exceed the inhibitory capacity of antiproteases, that some proteases present are not susceptible to the available antiproteases, or that some of the proteolytic enzymes may be physically inaccessible to the antiprotease activity. The ultimate clinical utility of exogenously produced protease inhibitors currently under development will undoubtedly depend upon which of the protease-antiprotease interactions predominates in the production of emphysema.

PATHOPHYSIOLOGY On the basis of the use of flow rates from forced expiratory vital capacity maneuvers and more sophisticated measures of airways resistance and elastic recoil properties of the lung, it has become clear that both chronic bronchitis and emphysema can exist without evidence of obstruction. However, by the time a patient begins to experience dyspnea as a result of these processes, obstruction is always demonstrable. Since chronic bronchitis and emphysema are usually combined, it might appear fruitless to determine the role of each in producing an individual patient's disability. However, one process may dominate over the other, and to the extent that inflammatory airways disease, secretions, and bronchospasm are present, there are therapeutic possibilities with some hope for improvement. Therefore it is of value to understand the mechanisms of airways obstruction in order to guide therapy and anticipate results.

Both chronic bronchitis and emphysema result in airways narrowing. In addition to the primary airways processes of chronic bronchitis, loss of elastic recoil of the lung in emphysema accounts for a decrease in airways caliber through loss of radial traction on airways. Narrowing of airways is often associated with both an increase in airways resistance and a diminution in maximal expiratory flow rates.

There are occasions in which a normal or only slightly elevated airways resistance is accompanied by low maximal expiratory flow rates. Under such circumstances an increase in the dynamic collapsibility of intrathoracic airways during forced exhalation is a possible explanation. Also in this context, the elastic recoil pressure of the lung must be considered in a slightly different way. In addition to providing radial support to airways during quiet breathing, the elastic recoil properties of the lung serve as a major determinant of maximal expiratory flow rates. The static recoil pressure of the lung is the difference between alveolar and intrapleural pressure. During forced exhalations, when alveolar and intrapleural pressures are high, there are points in the airway at which bronchial pressure equals pleural pressure. Flow does not increase with higher pleural pressure after these points become fixed so that the effective driving pressure between alveoli and such points is the elastic recoil pressure of the lung (Fig. 208-1). Hence maximal expiratory flow rates represent a complex and dynamic interplay between airways caliber, elastic recoil pressures, and collapsibility of airways. As a direct consequence of the altered pressure-airflow relationships, the work of breathing is increased in bronchitis and emphysema. Since flow-resistive work is flow rate–dependent, there is a disproportionate increase in the work of breathing with increased ventilation.

The designated subdivisions of the lung volume outlined in Chap. 200 are abnormal to varying degrees in both bronchitis and emphysema. The residual volume (RV) and functional residual capacity (FRC) are almost always higher than normal. Since the normal FRC is the volume at which the inward recoil of the lung is balanced by the outward recoil of the chest wall, loss of elastic recoil of the lung would clearly result in a higher static FRC. In addition, prolongation of expiration in association with obstruction would lead to a dynamic increase in FRC if inspiration is initiated before the respiratory system reaches its static balance point. Elevations of total lung capacity (TLC) are frequent. The exact cause is uncertain, but increases in TLC are often found in association with decreases in the elastic recoil of the lung. The vital capacity is frequently decreased, yet significant airways obstruction can be present with a normal to near-normal vital capacity.

The consequences of the airways and parenchymal processes are far more extensive than just the mechanical alterations discussed above. Maldistribution of inspired gas and blood flow is always present to some extent. When the mismatching is severe, impairment of gas exchange is reflected in abnormalities of arterial blood gases. There are regions of the lung with ventilation in excess of perfusion which increase the wasted ventilation ratio (that is, *Vd/Vt;* Chap. 200). At a normal resting CO_2 production, the net effective alveolar ventilation, as reflected by the arterial P_{CO_2}, may be excessive, normal, or insufficient depending upon the relationship of the overall minute volume to the wasted ventilation ratio. The net contribution of regions with perfusion in excess of ventilation can be assessed by either estimating or measuring the alveolar-arterial P_{O_2} difference (that is, $P_{A_{O_2}} - P_{a_{O_2}}$; Chap. 200). Whatever the clinical syndrome associated with chronic bronchitis and emphysema, there are to some degree increases in both wasted ventilation and wasted blood flow.

The clinical manifestations depend, in large part, upon the ventilatory response to the disordered lung function. Some patients, at the cost of extremely high effort of breathing and chronic dyspnea,

FIGURE 208-1 *A. A schematic diagram of the lung and intrathoracic airways with no airflow. The alveolar pressure (Palv) is greater than pleural pressure (Ppl) by an amount equal to the elastic recoil pressure of the lung (Pel)—i.e., Palv is the algebraic sum of Ppl + Pel. With no airflow Palv = P atmospheric, and for all of the intrathoracic airways, pressure outside is less than the pressure inside due to the Pel. B. The same schematic lung during forced exhalation when pleural pressure becomes quite positive. Palv is still greater than Ppl by an amount equal to Pel. However, there is a pressure drop along the airway associated with flow, and at some point Ppl equals local bronchial pressure (so-called equal pressure point, EPP). Mouthward from this point, Ppl exceeds local bronchial pressure and hence acts to compress the airways. C. Pressure within the airways from alveoli to the intrathoracic trachea is shown as a dashed line (---) and Ppl is shown as a constant (———). Therefore, the driving pressure from alveoli to EPP is equal to Pel, and a decrease in Pel (i.e., loss of elastic recoil) would mean a smaller driving pressure and smaller flow rates.*

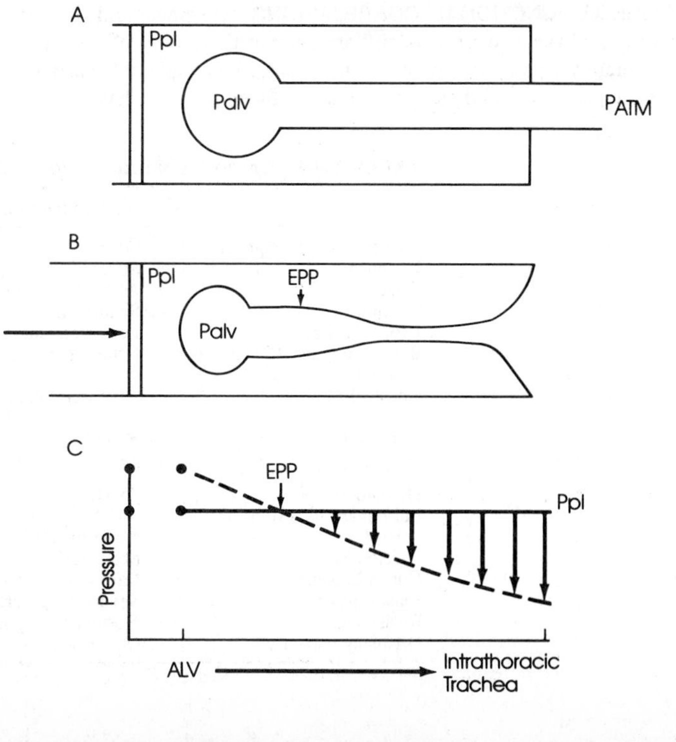

will maintain a strikingly increased minute volume, which results both in a normal to low arterial P_{CO_2}, despite the high *Vd/Vt*, and a relatively high arterial P_{O_2}, despite the high difference, $P_{A_{O_2}} - P_{a_{O_2}}$. Other patients with only modest increases in effort of breathing and less dyspnea will maintain a normal to only moderately elevated minute volume at the cost of accepting a high arterial P_{CO_2} and a severely depressed arterial P_{O_2}.

Factors which account for clear differences in ventilatory responses between patients have been studied and debated for years. The bulk of available evidence suggests that those patients who maintain relatively normal or low arterial P_{CO_2} levels are those with an increased ventilatory drive relative to their blood gas values and those who chronically maintain high arterial P_{CO_2} and lower P_{O_2} levels have a diminished ventilatory drive in relation to their more severely deranged blood gas values. It is not at all certain whether individual differences are accounted for by variations in peripheral or central chemoreceptor sensitivity or through other afferent pathways. Perhaps of more immediate value is the fact that patients with predominant emphysema are either normally or excessively responsive both to hypercapnia and to exercise, whereas those with predominant bronchitis are less responsive to both, despite similar degrees of airways obstruction by spirometry.

The pulmonary circulation malfunctions not only in terms of regional distribution of blood flow but in terms of abnormal overall pressure-flow relationships. There is often mild to severe pulmonary hypertension at rest with further increases disproportionate to cardiac output elevations during exercise. A reduction in the total cross-sectional area of the pulmonary vascular bed can be attributed to anatomic changes and constriction of vascular smooth muscle in pulmonary arteries and arterioles as well as destruction of alveolar septa with loss of capillaries. Rarely does loss of capillaries alone lead to severe pulmonary hypertension with cor pulmonale, except as a terminal event. Of more importance is the constriction of pulmonary vessels in response to alveolar hypoxia. The constriction is reversible upon increase in alveolar P_{O_2} with therapy. There is a synergism between hypoxia and acidosis which assumes importance during episodes of acute or chronic respiratory insufficiency. Chronic hypoxia leads not only to pulmonary vascular constriction but also to secondary erythrocytosis. The latter, although not proved to be a significant contributor to pulmonary hypertension, could add an unfavorable rheologic load. As discussed in Chap. 191, the chronic afterload on the right ventricle leads to hypertrophy and, in association with disordered blood gases, ultimately to failure.

CLINICAL-FUNCTIONAL CORRELATIONS Dyspnea and impairment of physical work capacity are characteristic only of severe to moderately severe airways obstruction. There is considerable variation among patients, and those with predominant emphysema have greater dyspnea and restriction of physical activity with lesser degrees of obstruction than those in whom chronic bronchitis predominates. The majority of patients have functionally mixed disease, will usually experience exertional dyspnea when the forced expiratory volume in 1 s (FEV_1) falls below 50 percent of that predicted, and will have dyspnea at rest when the FEV_1 is less than 25 percent of that predicted. In addition to dyspnea at rest, carbon dioxide retention and cor pulmonale frequently occur when the FEV_1 falls to 25 percent of that predicted. However, those with predominant bronchitis often have carbon dioxide retention and cor pulmonale with FEV_1 values above 25 percent of normal, in contrast to patients with predominant emphysema whose FEV_1 usually falls well below that level before the onset of carbon dioxide retention and cor pulmonale. With a respiratory infection, small changes in the degree of obstruction can make a large difference in symptoms and gas exchange. Thus small therapeutic gains have rewarding results.

In general, the more severe the obstruction, the poorer the prognosis. Despite the general relationship, 20 to 30 percent of patients with severe obstruction and carbon dioxide retention will survive beyond 5 years.

CLINICAL SYNDROMES It is clear that the clinical presentation can vary in severity from simple chronic bronchitis without disability to the severely disabled state with chronic respiratory failure. From a practical standpoint, it is well to consider that any symptom or any measurable abnormality may foreshadow the development of severe disabling disease; hence cessation of smoking and avoidance of environmental irritants and toxins are to be advised. However, the advice to modify behavior and life patterns is rarely taken, and most physicians are called upon to categorize and treat patients with fully developed, chronic airways obstruction. Thus the approach taken here is to describe two polar opposite types of fully developed, chronic obstructive pulmonary disease with the realization that the majority of patients will have some features of both types. The salient features of each type are outlined in Table 208-1.

Predominant emphysema These patients often give a long history of exertional dyspnea with minimal cough which is productive of only small amounts of mucoid sputum. Mucopurulent exacerbations in association with infections are not frequent. The body build is asthenic with evidence of weight loss. The patient appears distressed with obvious use of accessory muscles of respiration which serve to lift the sternum in an anterosuperior direction with each inspiration. There is tachypnea with a relatively prolonged expiration through pursed lips, or expiration is begun with a grunting sound. While sitting, these patients often lean forward, extending the arms to brace themselves. The neck veins may be distended during expiration, yet they collapse briskly with inspiration. The lower intercostal spaces

TABLE 208-1 Chronic obstructive lung disease: Salient features of the two types

	Predominant emphysema	Predominant bronchitis
Age at time of diagnosis, yrs	60±	50±
Dyspnea	Severe	Mild
Cough	After dyspnea starts	Before dyspnea starts
Sputum	Scanty, mucoid	Copious, purulent
Bronchial infections	Less frequent	More frequent
Respiratory insufficiency episodes	Often terminal	Repeated
Chest film	"Hyperinflation" ± bullous changes, small heart	Increased bronchovascular markings at bases, large heart
Chronic Pa_{CO_2}, mmHg	35–40	50–60
Chronic Pa_{O_2}, mmHg	65–75	45–60
Hematocrit, %	35–45	50–55
Pulmonary hypertension:		
Rest	None to mild	Moderate to severe
Exercise	Moderate	Worsens
Cor pulmonale	Rare, except terminally	Common
Elastic recoil	Severely decreased	Normal
Resistance	Normal to slight increase	High
Diffusing capacity	Decreased	Normal to slight decrease

retract with each inspiration, and by palpation the lower lateral chest wall can be felt to move inward. The percussion note is hyperresonant, and by auscultation the breath sounds are diminished, with faint, high-pitched rhonchi heard toward the end of expiration. The cardiac impulse, if at all visible, is seen only in the xiphoid and subxiphoid regions, and cardiac dullness is either absent or severely reduced. By palpation there is frequently a sustained forward and downward right ventricular impulse in the subxiphoid region, and a presystolic gallop accentuated during inspiration is commonly heard.

The arterial P_{O_2} is often in the mid-70s (mmHg), and the P_{CO_2} is low to normal. Because of the maintained increase in minute volume and the maintenance of arterial P_{O_2} sufficient to nearly saturate hemoglobin, these patients have been referred to as "pink puffers."

The TLC and RV are invariably increased, the vital capacity is low, and the maximal expiratory flow rates are diminished. The elastic recoil properties of the lung are severely impaired, and in direct proportion to this impairment, the capacity of the lung to transfer carbon monoxide is lowered.

On radiographic examination the diaphragms are low and flattened, the bronchovascular shadows do not extend to the periphery of the lung, and the cardiac silhouette is lengthened and narrowed. These findings in association with a large retrosternal translucency on lateral chest radiographs are interpreted as hyperinflation, which correlates well with increases in TLC and loss of elastic recoil. Peripheral attenuation of bronchovascular markings and increased retrosternal lucency correlate best with subsequent postmortem demonstration of extensive and severe emphysema which is predominantly of the panacinar type.

It is fortunate that the patient with predominant emphysema is less prone to mucopurulent relapses than is the patient with predominant bronchitis, since such relapses frequently lead to severe respiratory failure and death. That is to say, right-sided heart failure and hypercapnic respiratory failure are often terminal events in those patients with predominant emphysema. In the absence of such relapses, the clinical course is characterized by severe and progressive dyspnea for which little can be done. The physician's role is to seek out and treat any factor that is possibly reversible and strive to avoid pollutants and infections.

Predominant bronchitis The patient with predominant bronchitis usually has an impressive history of cough and sputum production for many years with an immodest history of cigarette smoking. Initially the cough is present only in the winter months, and the patient is apt to seek medical attention, if at all, only during the more severe of the frequent mucopurulent relapses. Over the years the cough progresses from hibernal to perennial, and mucopurulent relapses increase in frequency, duration, and severity. After beginning to experience exertional dyspnea, the patient often seeks medical help and will be found to have a severe degree of obstruction. Occasionally such a patient will seek out a physician only after the onset of peripheral edema secondary to overt right ventricular failure. More rarely the initial medical contact is made by family members who present the physician with a deeply cyanotic, edematous, and stuporous patient with acute respiratory insufficiency.

The patient with predominant bronchitis is often overweight and cyanotic. There is usually no apparent distress at rest, the respiratory rate is normal or only slightly increased, and there is no apparent usage of accessory muscles. The chest percussion note is normally resonant, and by auscultation, one can usually hear coarse rhonchi and wheezes which change in location and intensity after a deep and productive cough. There may be a sustained heave along the lower left sternal border which indicates right ventricular hypertrophy. In the presence of right ventricular failure there are often an early diastolic gallop and occasionally a holosystolic murmur, both of which are accentuated by inspiration. The latter finding is indicative of functional tricuspid regurgitation which is frequently accompanied by neck vein distention characterized by large *v* waves and brisk *y* descents. With right ventricular failure the cyanosis deepens and peripheral edema becomes prominent. Clubbing of the digits is unusual.

With or without right ventricular failure, the minute volume is only slightly increased. Failure to increase minute volume greatly in the face of significant proportions of wasted ventilation and blood flow results in severely deranged arterial blood gases, with arterial P_{CO_2} values which are chronically increased to the range of the high 40s to low 50s (mmHg). The lowered P_{O_2} produces desaturation of hemoglobin, serves to stimulate erythropoiesis, and results in hypoxic pulmonary vasoconstriction. Desaturation and erythrocytosis combine to produce the cyanosis, and hypoxic pulmonary vasoconstriction accentuates the right-sided heart failure. Because of cyanosis and edema secondary to heart failure, such patients have been referred to as "blue bloaters." It has been proposed, with some supporting data, that one of the pathophysiologic events in the blue bloaters is the occurrence of repeated episodes of severe nocturnal oxygen desaturation in association with sleep apnea.

The TLC is often normal, and there is a moderate elevation of RV. The vital capacity is mildly diminished, and maximal expiratory flow rates are invariably low. The elastic recoil properties of the lung are normal or only slightly impaired, and the capacity of the lung to transfer carbon monoxide is either normal or minimally decreased.

On radiographic examination the diaphragms are well rounded, the bronchovascular markings are increased in the lower lung fields, and the cardiac silhouette is somewhat enlarged. In association with right ventricular failure the cardiac silhouette enlarges further, pulmonary arteries become more prominent, and an antigravity distribution of perfusion is apparent.

Despite well-planned management (see below) the patient with predominant bronchitis may experience many episodes of respiratory failure from which recovery is frequent with proper therapy (see p. 1093). The ability to recover from such repeated episodes in those patients is in striking contrast to the frequently fatal outcome of such events in those with predominant emphysema. Ultimately, the lungs at postmortem will be found to have severe bronchitic changes in both large and small airways and only moderate emphysema, predominantly of the centriacinar variety.

PRINCIPLES OF MANAGEMENT Intelligent management must be based upon as complete knowledge as possible of the degree of obstruction, the extent of disability, and the relative reversibility of the patient's illness. To the extent that obstructive processes in the airways are contributory, there is a chance for treatment to be effective. Since emphysema is an irreversible process, prevention of progression and avoidance of acute insults constitute the only approach. History, physical examination, and chest radiographs should be supplemented by tests of lung function performed during a symptomatically stable period. Ideally, complete spirometry, plethysmographic lung volumes, airways resistance, transfer of carbon monoxide, arterial blood gases, and lung elastic recoil properties should be measured. Spirometry, lung volumes, and resistance should be remeasured after the administration of bronchodilators in order to assess the degree of acutely reversible airways obstruction. Failure to see an acute change with bronchodilator drugs does not rule out the possibility of improvement with more prolonged administration of these agents. In instances in which the degree of exertional dyspnea appears to be disproportionately greater than the degree of obstruction, measurements of blood gases, minute volume, CO_2 production, and O_2 consumption during exercise are indicated in order to determine whether impaired lung function is sufficient to account for the symptoms. After the initial assessment the physician has some idea of the relative emphasis to be placed upon patient education, preventive measures, and direct therapeutic interventions in management of the patient and the illness.

Cessation of smoking is the only certain means of influencing the progression of the chronic obstructive airways syndromes, and such behavior modification is most effective at early stages of the disease processes. In the instances in which occupational or environmental exposures are thought to play a significant role, change of occupation or relocation of dwelling is advisable. The validity of such advice should be carefully considered since the impact on both the patient and the family is likely to be great. A simpler environmental change is that of eliminating aerosol sprays such as deodorants, hair sprays, and insecticides from the household. Hair sprays have been shown to produce acute airways responses even in normal subjects. Other preventive measures include yearly vaccination against the common or expected influenza virus strains. The patient should be given pneumococcal polysaccharide vaccine only once. Recent evidence of severe Arthus-type immunologic reactions following repeat pneumococcal vaccination has led to this "once-in-a-lifetime" recommendation.

Infections cannot be totally avoided, and the patient should be made aware that increasing purulence, viscosity, or volume of secretions signals the onset of an infection which should be treated early. The commonest pathogenic bacteria found are *Haemophilus influenzae* and *Streptococcus pneumoniae*. As mentioned above, however, the role of such bacteria is in question since they are just as often isolated during periods of relative clinical quiescence. Nonetheless, tetracycline or ampicillin should be given for a 7- to 10-day course. It is practical to have the patient keep a 7- to 10-day supply of antibiotics at home and to begin treatment at the onset of symptoms. In Great Britain it is common practice to give continuous antibiotic therapy during winter months in order to prevent mucopurulent relapses. Although there is evidence that viruses are frequent causes of mucopurulent relapses, clinical studies have shown that the standard antibiotic regimens decrease the duration and severity of infective episodes unrelated to culturable bacterial pathogens. Microscopic examination and culture of sputum are indicated if there are chills, fever, or chest pain or if purulence fails to respond to usually administered antibiotics.

It has been shown repeatedly that exercise programs, although not accompanied by measurable improvement in lung function, result in increased exercise tolerance and an improved sense of well-being. The improvement is usually task-specific, so that most physicians advise walking in preference to the use of special apparatus, such as stationary bicycles or wall gyms.

Bronchodilator drugs are often quite helpful in alleviating symptoms, especially in those patients who respond to them acutely in the laboratory. These drugs form three categories: the methylxanthines, sympathomimetics with strong $beta_2$-adrenergic-stimulating properties, and anticholinergics. Theophylline, the most commonly used methylxanthine, can be given orally, rectally, or parenterally; in addition to bronchodilatation, it stimulates respiration and has cardiotonic and diuretic properties. Selective $beta_2$-stimulating drugs such as albuterol and metaproterenol can be given both orally and by aerosol with fewer cardiac side effects than are experienced with isoproterenol. Anticholinergic agents such as atropine have been avoided in the past because of their tendency to desiccate secretions, but such drugs are effective bronchodilators; new analogues that are given by inhalation with less effect on secretions are now being developed and tested and may be found useful in the future.

The use of glucocorticosteroids is, at our present state of knowledge, based upon very little scientific data from properly controlled clinical trials. Since these agents have time- and dose-related side effects that vary from deleterious to catastrophic, the almost invariable subjective benefit must be supported by objective measurements. There is little room for doubt in the minds of physicians that some patients respond well, even dramatically, to these agents in both objective and subjective terms. The real problem is how to select those most likely to benefit. Eosinophilia in the sputum, rather than in the blood, appears to help identify that subgroup in advance. However, the best guidelines are, first, to try these agents only after maximal bronchodilator and bronchopulmonary drainage measures have been tried without success; second, to begin prednisone 30 mg once per day; third, to confirm the objective change in terms of spirometry and gas exchange, stopping these agents if no objective benefit is seen; and fourth, to decrease to the smallest dose that will maintain the improved level of function.

Bronchopulmonary drainage should be maintained in patients with hypersecretion. If the coughing mechanism is ineffective or if paroxysms of coughing are exhausting, postural drainage is often a useful adjunct. Although liquefaction of secretions by means of orally administered expectorants or aerosol delivery of mucolytic agents is an appealing idea, it has never been shown by properly designed trials to be more effective than simple maintenance of total-body hydration.

Intermittent positive pressure breathing (IPPB) devices have long been advocated for home management. The various rationales include diminution in the work of breathing, promotion of bronchopulmonary drainage, and more efficient delivery of bronchodilator drugs. The first of the rationales has been shown to have no basis in fact, and the goals of the last two have been shown to be as well accomplished by postural drainage and use of less elaborate aerosol generators. Hence the use of IPPB for home management cannot be justified.

When arterial hypoxia is persistent and severe (Pa_{O_2} <55 mmHg) in association with cor pulmonale (see Chap. 191) and signs of right heart failure, continuous oxygen therapy is indicated. The available data indicate that supplemental oxygen improves both exercise tolerance and neuropsychological function and alleviates pulmonary hypertension and right heart failure. In patients with severe hypoxemia the need for hospitalization occurs less frequently and life span is lengthened by the use of supplemental oxygen. In view of the expense of such therapy and the dangers of uncontrolled oxygen delivery (see below), it should be given only when it can be carefully monitored and its beneficial effects objectively verified.

Since most patients with chronic airways obstruction, especially those with features of predominant bronchitis, can be shown to decrease their Pa_{O_2} values significantly during sleep, most prominently during the REM phase, nocturnal oxygen administration has been suggested. While the rationale is clear and the results quite good, a recent cooperative clinical trial that compared nocturnal with continuous O_2 supplementation in severely hypoxic patients found that continuous O_2 administration was associated with a significantly lower mortality rate. Patients in both treatment groups experienced neuropsychological and hemodynamic benefits. Thus, supplemental nocturnal oxygen is better than none, but continuous oxygen is better than nocturnal in such severely ill patients.

Secondary erythrocytosis with the hematocrit in excess of 50 percent is most easily viewed as a mechanism allowing greater oxygen delivery to compensate for the chronically lowered arterial Pa_{O_2}; hence improvement in oxygenation through improved lung function or by oxygen administration is the most physiologic means to reverse erythrocytosis. Since erythrocytosis results in elevation of blood viscosity at all shear rates, the proposal has been made that pulmonary vascular hypertension is aggravated by its presence. Although no study has demonstrated an objective improvement in hemodynamics, lung mechanics, or gas exchange at rest following phlebotomy, ventilatory and cardiovascular function during exercise improve. Some patients who complain of headaches and a sense of head fullness show a favorable subjective response to periodic phlebotomy when the hematocrit is in excess of 55 percent. In support of this subjective improvement is the demonstration that, following phlebotomy, cerebral blood flow, previously diminished, returns toward normal.

ACUTE RESPIRATORY FAILURE

DIAGNOSIS Although it may be strongly suspected on clinical grounds, the firm diagnosis of acute respiratory failure in chronic airways obstruction is based upon measurements of arterial blood gas (Pa_{O_2}, Pa_{CO_2}) and pH values that must be interpreted in relation to the patient's chronic status. Since many patients will have chronically lowered Pa_{O_2} levels and increased Pa_{CO_2} values, the diagnosis is based upon the degree of change from the usual state of the individual patient. With regard to oxygenation, an acute decrease in Pa_{O_2} from a usual mid-70-mmHg range to the low 60s (mmHg) is just as indicative of acute respiratory failure as is an acute drop from a chronic mid-50-mmHg range to the mid-40s (mmHg). Thus a drop in Pa_{O_2} equal to or greater than 10 to 15 mmHg indicates acute failure.

Since renal compensation for chronic hypercapnia results in adjustment of arterial pH to near-normal values, the acuteness of the increase in Pa_{CO_2} can often be judged by the pH, unless there is a concomitant metabolic acidemia. As a practical guide, any level of hypercapnia associated with an arterial pH value less than 7.30 should be considered as acute respiratory failure.

PRECIPITATING FACTORS Increases in volume, viscosity, and/or purulence of secretions, presumably due to infection of the tracheobronchial tree, are the most common antecedents of acute respiratory failure in chronic obstructive lung disease. Increasing airways obstruction with airways inflammation and secretion, especially in association with a relatively blunted ventilatory drive, leads to worsening hypoxia and increasing CO_2 retention. Agitation, insomnia, and increasing dyspnea with impending respiratory failure are occasionally treated, mistakenly, with either sedatives or narcotics, and these, too, may precipitate frank respiratory failure. In fact such depressant drugs which impair ventilatory drive should be avoided at all times in patients with severe chronic obstructive lung disease. Major episodes of air pollution can also lead to respiratory failure, and the physicians responsible for patients with severe bronchitis and emphysema should be alert to these environmental events.

Pneumonia, thromboembolism, left ventricular failure, and pneumothorax occasionally precipitate acute respiratory failure and are extremely difficult to detect unless considered and specifically sought. As a minimum, chest radiographs, electrocardiograms, and sputum examinations should be obtained in addition to arterial blood gas measurements in all patients with respiratory failure.

TREATMENT OF RESPIRATORY FAILURE The treatment of respiratory failure consists of two simultaneous processes: (1) maintaining acceptable levels of oxygenation and ventilation; and (2) treatment of infection, removal of secretions, and reversing any airway constriction present.

With regard to the first, these patients *need* oxygen when they are severely hypoxic, and while fears of respiratory depression due to the removal of the hypoxic respiratory stimulus are realistic, O_2 must be used, yet in the smallest concentration possible, to give a Pa_{O_2} in the mid-50-mmHg range while the patient's Pa_{CO_2}, pH, and clinical status are carefully monitored. It is best to begin with only modest increases in FI_{O_2} to approximately 0.24 (cf. air at 0.21), which can be accomplished using nasal prongs with O_2 flows at 1 to 2 liters per minute or, more precisely, with the use of a 0.24 Venturi mask. These latter masks, based upon Bernoulli's principle, deliver a fixed concentration of O_2 irrespective of the O_2 flow rate by entraining air in direct proportion to O_2 flow rate. They are high-flow masks (oxygen plus air entrained from the room), each designed for a specific FI_{O_2} (0.24, 0.28, 0.35, 0.40). Even small increases in Pa_{O_2} when starting from low levels result in significant increases in arterial oxygen content due to the shape of the oxygen-hemoglobin saturation curve over this range (Chap. 283). With improved oxygenation some patients will concomitantly increase their Pa_{CO_2} values. The standard explanation has been that this increase is due to the removal of the hypoxic drive to ventilation leading to further hypoventilation. While this is the most important mechanism, recent data indicate that worsening ventilation-perfusion relationships (Chap. 200) occur with O_2 treatment. This is attributed to reversal of hypoxic pulmonary arterial constriction in the more initially hypoxic, less well ventilated regions, which in turn leads to decreased perfusion of initially less hypoxic, better ventilated regions. The result is an increase in the wasted ventilation ratio (*Vd/Vt*, Chap. 200) leading to a smaller effective alveolar ventilation. In either case, the FI_{O_2} should be increased as little as possible to achieve a Pa_{O_2} in the mid-50-mmHg range. Some increase in Pa_{CO_2} can be expected and should not cause alarm if the patient is alert. The majority of patients can be managed in this conservative way with excellent results. However, occasionally large increases in Pa_{CO_2} occur and lead to stupor and coma. This can be explained by CO_2-induced cerebral vascular dilatation with increased intracranial pressure, including the development of papilledema, combined with the effect of hypercapnia and hypoxia on cerebral function. It must be emphasized that if stupor and coma supervene, stopping the administration of oxygen is the *worst possible* course of action. When CO_2 narcosis is present, respirations are sufficiently depressed from the CO_2 itself so that the patient will no longer respond to the rapidly worsening hypoxia, and fatal arrhythmias, generalized seizures, and death may ensue. The only alternative is to intubate the trachea and provide mechanical ventilatory support. Mechanical ventilators are described in Chap. 216.

Once mechanical ventilation has been instituted, the tidal volume and frequency should be set gradually to decrease the Pa_{CO_2} only down to the chronically elevated level rather than attempt to decrease it to or below a normal value. Since such patients have renal compensation for their chronic hypercapnia, Pa_{CO_2} values at or below the normal level result in significant alkalemia which in turn can lead to severe tachyarrhythmias and generalized seizures.

As mentioned above, maintaining oxygenation and ventilation serves to buy time while secretion removal, bronchial dilatation, and treatment of infection are instituted. Removal of secretions is accomplished by urging the patient to cough or by passing suction catheters into the trachea which, in addition to removing secretions that are present, stimulate cough that brings more secretions up to the region of the catheter tip. The advantage, if any, from the use of mucolytic agents in this process has yet to be demonstrated. However, $beta_2$-adrenergic bronchodilating agents have been shown to increase the rate of transport of particles by the mucociliary blanket, and, thus, in addition to bronchodilatation, such agents should improve the clearance of airway secretions. Postural drainage and chest percussion are other often-used adjuncts that have been shown, especially when secretions are voluminous, to improve tracheobronchial clearance, to increase sputum volume beyond that produced by cough, and to reduce airways obstruction.

Bronchodilatation with aminophylline given orally or by infusion and $beta_2$-adrenergic agonists by inhalation or subcutaneous injection has assumed a prominent role in treatment of acute respiratory failure in chronic airways obstruction. In addition to bronchodilatation these agents improve bronchopulmonary clearance and may help induce diuresis and hemodynamic improvement when there is cor pulmonale with failure (Chap. 191). Unless there is clearly an acute pneumonia, the use of antibiotics is more controversial in the setting of acute respiratory failure than in mucopurulent relapses without failure. Nonetheless, broad-spectrum antibiotics, if no single agent is suspected or isolated, or erythromycin, if legionellae or mycoplasmas are suspected, should be added to the regimen.

Complications arising in the course of treatment for acute respiratory failure are cardiac arrhythmias, most often multifocal supraventricular tachycardias, left ventricular failure, pulmonary emboli, and gastrointestinal hemorrhage from stress ulceration. Cardiac arrhythmias resulting from rapid decreases in oxygenation or increases in pH due to overventilation can be readily avoided. However, when giving multiple drugs having cardiotonic properties, the question always arises as to whether the arrhythmias are related to these. Keeping serum theophylline levels in the 10 to 20 mg per liter range and using relatively selective beta agonists, such as isoetharine by inhalation, can minimize these effects.

Left ventricular failure, usually attributable to coronary atherosclerosis with acute myocardial infarction, systemic hypertension, or aortic valvular disease, is difficult to detect in the presence of cor pulmonale. Fortunately, improving lung function and oxygenation most often reverse the pulmonary hypertension and right ventricular failure (Chap. 191) and induce a brisk diuresis. If signs of congestive failure persist or worsen after providing adequate oxygenation, consideration must be given to left ventricular failure; an assessment in such patients is best made through echocardiography or radioventriculography since the usual physical and radiographic findings are obscured in such patients. Only in the presence of adequate gas exchange and only with either the firm demonstration of, or strong clinical suspicion of, left ventricular failure should digitalis be used. Diuretic agents should also be reserved for left ventricular failure. They almost invariably produce hypokalemic, hypochloremic metabolic alkalemia that results in depression of ventilatory drive and interference with removal from mechanical ventilatory support.

Pulmonary emboli are suspected to be common in the setting of acute respiratory failure and are extremely difficult to detect since the lung scan is totally nonspecific and signs of cor pulmonale fluctuate in concert with the degree of lung dysfunction. Hence low-dose heparin prophylaxis should be used to prevent this complication. Gastrointestinal hemorrhage commonly complicates acute respiratory failure and is thought to be due to stress ulceration of the gastric mucosa. Awareness of this complication enhances the ability to detect it and act quickly. Antacids, nasogastric suction, and/or cimetidine have been used to diminish the frequency.

For those patients who have required mechanical ventilatory support, the process of removal from that support is largely empirical. In general, improving gas exchange and lung mechanics along with alertness and responsiveness of the patient signal that the support can be removed. Data such as maximal voluntary inspiratory mouth pressures greater than 20 cmH_2O, vital capacity greater than 10 mL per kilogram of body weight, and spontaneous tidal volume greater than 5 mL per kilogram of body weight are reassuring. However, many patients can be removed from such support with lesser values than these.

Failure to maintain gas exchange after removal of mechanical ventilatory support can usually be explained. *First* on the list is the continued administration or persistence of sedative and tranquilizing drugs that may have been prescribed earlier for agitation. These should be discontinued and time allowed for their metabolism. *Second* is the possibility that the endotracheal tube is of small bore and imposes a resistive load. If so, it should be replaced by a larger one. *Third* is worsening airways obstruction and accumulation of secretions; continued bronchial dilatation and airway suctioning avoid these. *Fourth* is a metabolic alkalemia, with or without diuretic therapy, that should be treated with potassium chloride. *Fifth* is having maintained a Pa_{O_2} and Pa_{CO_2} while being on mechanical ventilation that are too high and too low, respectively. This can be avoided by using an FI_{O_2} just sufficient to keep the Pa_{O_2} around 60 mmHg and using the assist mode with small enough tidal volumes to keep the Pa_{CO_2} at the expected chronic level (i.e., that associated with a normal or slightly low arterial pH) before discontinuing mechanical support. *Sixth* is poor nutrition, hypokalemia, or neuromuscular disease, making the patient too weak to maintain breathing or resulting in fatigue of the respiratory muscles. Nutrition, of course, is a longer range problem that should be anticipated, while hypokalemia is often handled along with the metabolic alkalemia. Muscle fatigue, especially diaphragmatic, has received a great deal of attention. From a practical standpoint, paradoxical (inward) movement of the upper abdomen with inspiration is the key clinical finding. Experimental evidence suggests that therapeutic levels of aminophylline reverse the manifestations of fatigue but the role of respiratory stimulants continues to be debated and the data to be inconclusive. In those patients with severely blunted ventilatory drive and improving lung function, stimulants may be tried cautiously. If there is severe metabolic alkalemia, acetazolamide can be tried as a stimulant while chloride replacement is being carried out. Medroxyprogesterone, a central stimulant, or almitrine, a peripheral chemoreceptor stimulant, appear to be safe and, in some instances, effective. Hypothyroidism is a metabolic condition with neuromuscular consequences and is difficult to detect in this clinical setting. Thus any prolonged and difficult weaning process should lead to the assessment of thyroid function.

PROGNOSIS On the average, data collected on large populations demonstrate a slow and relentless diminution in ventilatory function in patients with chronic airways obstruction. Although slow, the decrement in function with time far exceeds the rate of change seen with normal aging. In general, the likelihood of episodes of acute respiratory failure increases when the FEV_1 falls below 25 percent of predicted normal values. Although the in-hospital mortality rate averages 30 percent for a single episode and the 5-year survival rate after the initial episode of respiratory failure averages only 15 to 20 percent, the clinical syndrome is extremely important in determining both the short- and long-range prognosis. As noted above, those patients with predominant emphysema have a poorer prognosis after the onset of respiratory failure than do those with predominant bronchitis. In either case long-term oxygen treatment in those with severe hypoxemia results in prolongation of life and improvement in the quality of life.

BULLOUS EMPHYSEMA Confluent air spaces with diameters in excess of 1 cm are occasionally congenital but most often are found in association with generalized emphysema or progressive fibrotic processes. Gradual increases in size of such air spaces (or bullae) result from traction applied by regions with better elastic recoil properties, and such regions lose volume as the bullae become enlarged. If disability is severe, if the bulla is extremely large, and if either lobar gas sampling or ventilation and perfusion scans demonstrate that sufficient function remains in the nonbullous regions, surgical excision of the bulla may lead to functional improvement. Usually, however, improvement is relatively transitory because other emphysematous regions gradually enlarge into bullae after surgery.

VARIANTS OF EMPHYSEMA In addition to the centriacinar and panacinar forms of emphysema described above, other structural patterns have been described but are functionally less important. Often there is overdistention and alveolar septal destruction in lung regions surrounding scar tissue (paracicatricial or scar emphysema) or along the borders of the acinus (paraseptal emphysema). The latter form, when it occurs at the visceral pleural surface, may predispose to episodes of spontaneous pneumothorax (Chap. 214). Infants rarely develop a check valve mechanism in a lobar bronchus which leads to rapid and life-threatening overdistention (congenital lobar emphysema). Unilateral emphysema may be an incidental radiographic finding (Macleod's or Swyer-James's syndromes). Since, in this condition, the airways are normal in number and structure but the alveoli are reduced in number, this form of unilateral emphysema has been attributed to disease occurring before the age of 8 years when alveoli are normally increasing in number. Overdistention and alveolar septal destruction are not present, and so this condition does not fit the definition of true emphysema. Most often the pulmonary artery on the affected side is hypoplastic. Although usually an incidental finding, the affected lung may become repeatedly infected so that surgical excision may be indicated.

MISCELLANEOUS DIFFUSE OBSTRUCTIVE SYNDROMES *Bronchiolitis obliterans* is a term applied to widespread inflammatory and fibrotic obstruction of small airways. Initially this syndrome was thought to be restricted to those persons who had suffered severe viral infections in childhood, particularly those due to parainfluenza virus. However, recently this syndrome has also been described in adult patients with rheumatoid arthritis. The response to bronchodilator treatment is poor, as would be expected from the histopathologic findings, and fatal respiratory failure often ensues within 2 years. There have been reports suggesting a relationship between penicillamine therapy and the development of bronchiolitis obliterans in patients with rheumatoid arthritis; however, it is clear that this syndrome can develop in patients who have never received penicillamine.

A syndrome with similar histopathology has been described in recipients of autologous bone marrow transplants. Although most often interstitial pneumonitis and fibrosis are sequelae, it has been documented that some patients develop a bronchiolitis obliterans picture. It appears that the development of this process occurs most often in the setting of a chronic graft-versus-host syndrome; however, it is clear that diffuse airways obstruction has developed without evidence of this syndrome in bone marrow recipients.

Lymphangioleiomyomatosis is a rare disease affecting young women. It is characterized by proliferation of smooth muscle in the lymphatics of the abdomen and the thorax. The clinical syndrome is that of an obstructive ventilatory defect in association with disproportionately poor gas exchange and interstitial lung disease by radiography with recurring chylous pleural effusions and/or pneumothoraces. Recent evidence suggests that oophorectomy or progesterone administration halts the progression of this otherwise untreatable disease.

Cystic fibrosis in the adult with chronic airways obstruction is discussed elsewhere (Chap. 207).

REFERENCES

ANTHONISEN NR: Home oxygen therapy, in *Update VI: Principles of Internal Medicine*, RG Petersdorf et al (eds). New York, McGraw-Hill, 1985, p 203

BLOCK ER: Oxygen therapy, in *Update: Pulmonary Diseases and Disorders*, AP Fishman (ed). New York, McGraw-Hill, 1982, p 349

CAMPBELL AH et al: Factors affecting the decline of ventilatory function in chronic bronchitis. Throax 40:741, 1985

CATTERAL JR et al: Mechanism of transient nocturnal hypoxemia in hypoxic chronic bronchitis and emphysema. J Appl Physiol 59:1698, 1985

COHEN AB (ed): Proteases and antiproteases in the lung. Am Rev Resp Dis 127 (Suppl):S1, 1983

CHETTY KG et al: Improved exercise tolerance of the polycythemic lung patient following phlebotomy. Am J Med 74:415, 1983

FISHMAN AP: The spectrum of chronic obstructive disease of the airways, in *Pulmonary Diseases and Disorders*, 2d ed, AP Fishman (ed). New York, McGraw-Hill, 1987, Chap 68

HUGH-JONES P, WAIMSTER W: The etiology and management of disabling emphysema: State of the art. Am Rev Resp Dis 117:343, 1978

LAROS CD et al: Bullectomy for giant bullae in emphysema. J Thorac Cardiovasc Surg 91:63, 1986

PUSA T, TCHERZEWSKI H: Analysis of proteolytic enzymes and their natural inhibitors in serum and bronchial lavage fluid in atopic bronchial asthma, chronic bronchitis and pneumonia. Allerg Immunol 31:169, 1985

THURLBECK WM: A pathologist's approach to clinical bronchitis and emphysema, in *Update: Pulmonary Diseases and Disorders*, AP Fishman (ed). New York, McGraw-Hill, 1982, p 137

209 INTERSTITIAL LUNG DISORDERS

RONALD G. CRYSTAL

The interstitial lung disorders (ILD) are chronic, nonmalignant, noninfectious diseases of the lower respiratory tract characterized by inflammation and derangement of the alveolar walls. The major consequence of ILD is loss of functional alveolar-capillary units and thus a limitation in the transfer of O_2 from air to blood. Affected individuals have dyspnea, particularly with exercise, and are restricted in their activities. If the disease progresses, death usually results from O_2 deprivation of vital organs.

TABLE 209-1 Interstitial lung disorders of known etiology

Inhalation of environmental agents (see also Chaps. 203 and 204)
Inorganic dusts (the "pneumoconioses")
Organic dusts ("hypersensitivity pneumonitis" or "extrinsic allergic alveolitis")
Gases
Fumes
Vapors
Aerosols
Drugs (see also Chap. 65)
Secondary to the inflammation associated with lung infections
Radiation
Poisons (see also Chap. 171)
Recovery phase of adult respiratory distress syndrome (see also Chap. 216)

The ILD derive their name from the fact that all are characterized, to a variable extent, by derangements of the alveolar interstitium, the connective tissue matrix that forms the structural backbone of the alveolar walls. Because these derangements usually include the deposition of scar tissue, they are also called the "fibrotic lung diseases." Alternatively, because the widespread inflammation and fibrosis of the alveolar walls are reflected in the chest x-ray as "infiltration" of the lung parenchyma, the ILD are often grouped with the "diffuse infiltrative diseases" of the lung, a term that also includes infectious and neoplastic disorders. Since they are inflammatory disorders of the lower respiratory tract, the interstitial lung diseases are also called the "interstitial pneumonias" or "chronic pneumonitides."

Together, there are approximately 180 different ILD. Conveniently, they are categorized into those of known etiology (Table 209-1) and those of unknown etiology (Table 209-2). Despite this diversity, all are diffuse disorders associated with derangements of the lung parenchyma and loss of functioning alveoli and thus display certain common pathologic, physiologic, and clinical features. This chapter provides an overview of all of the ILD and discusses in detail the ILD of unknown etiology. Information on the specific disorders of known etiology are discussed in the chapters identified in Table 209-1.

NORMAL ANATOMY (See Fig. 209-1) The ILD of unknown etiology are diseases of the lower respiratory tract, structures that include alveoli, terminal bronchioles, alveolar ducts, and the small pulmonary arteries and veins that serve the pulmonary capillaries. Although all of these structures can be involved, it is the loss of functional alveoli that causes the respiratory dysfunction that characterizes these diseases.

The normal adult lung contains 300×10^6 alveoli. Together, they form a beehive-like structure, with each alveolus 200 to 300 μm in diameter, with walls 5- to 10-μm thick. The total surface area of the alveoli is approximately 150 m^2; it is through this surface that gas exchange takes place between alveolar air and the approximately 200

TABLE 209-2 Interstitial lung disorders of unknown etiology

Sarcoidosis (Chap. 270)	ILD associated with liver disease
Idiopathic pulmonary fibrosis	Chronic active hepatitis (Chap. 248)
ILD* associated with the collagen-vascular disorders	Primary biliary cirrhosis (Chap. 249)
Rheumatoid arthritis (Chap. 263)	ILD associated with bowel disease
Progressive systemic sclerosis (Chap. 264)	Whipple's disease (Chap. 237)
Systemic lupus erythematosus (Chap. 262)	Ulcerative colitis (Chap. 238)
Polymyositis-dermatomyositis (Chap. 356)	Crohn's disease (Chap. 238)
Sjögren's syndrome (Chap. 266)	Weber-Christian disease (Chap. 318)
Histiocytosis X	ILD associated with pulmonary vasculitis
Chronic eosinophilic pneumonia	Wegener's granulomatosis (Chap. 272)
Idiopathic pulmonary hemosiderosis	Lymphomatoid granulomatosis
Goodpasture's syndrome (Chap. 224)	Churg-Strauss syndrome (Chap. 269)
Hypereosinophilic syndrome	Systemic necrotizing vasculitis (overlap vasculitides) (Chap. 269)
Immunoblastic lymphadenopathy	Hypersensitivity vasculitis (Chap. 269)
Undefined lymphocytic infiltrative disorders	ILD associated with chronic cardiac disease
Lymphocytic interstitial pneumonitis	Left ventricular failure
Pseudolymphoma	Left-to-right shunt
Lymphangiomyomatosis	ILD associated with chronic renal disease with uremia
Amyloidosis (Chap. 259)	ILD associated with graft-versus-host reaction (Chap. 291)
Alveolar proteinosis	
Bronchocentric granulomatosis	
Inherited disorders	
Familial pulmonary fibrosis	
Tuberous sclerosis (Chap. 351)	
Neurofibromatosis (Chap. 351)	
Hermansky-Pudlak syndrome	
Niemann-Pick disease (Chap. 316)	
Gaucher's disease (Chap. 316)	

* *ILD = interstitial lung disease.*

mL of blood present at any one time in the pulmonary capillaries passing through the alveolar walls. In the normal lung, the capillaries are in close proximity to the alveolar air, so the path for gas exchange between air and blood is only 0.6 to 0.8 μm.

The alveolar walls are made up of four basic cell types: the type I and II epithelial cells, endothelial cells, and mesenchymal cells. The type I cells are flat, floppy, "fried-egg"–shaped cells that cover 95 percent of the alveolar epithelial surface. The type II cells are cuboidal cells responsible for producing surfactant, a lipid-protein aggregate stored in lamellar bodies in the cytoplasm; the surfactant is secreted onto the alveolar surface, where it reduces surface tension and stabilizes air space units. The junctions between the alveolar epithelial cells are tight, providing a barrier that protects the air surface from fluid that might leak from injured pulmonary capillaries. Together, the type I and II cells form a continuous epithelial layer, and both are attached to a continuous basement membrane sheet 0.1 μm thick. The endothelial cells that line the pulmonary capillaries are similar to capillary endothelial cells elsewhere. The endothelial cells also rest on a continuous 0.1-μm basement membrane; at sites where the capillaries and epithelial cells are in close apposition the respective basement membranes fuse. The mesenchymal cells are part of a family of cells that are dominated by fibroblasts, but include myofibroblasts, smooth muscle cells, and pericytes. These cells produce the bulk of the connective tissue matrix of the alveolar walls.

The connective tissue of the alveolar wall is called the "interstitium" and is composed of the epithelial and endothelial basement membranes surrounding a connective tissue matrix dominated by type I collagen but including type III collagen, fibronectin, elastic fibers, and proteoglycans. Together, these macromolecules provide the mechanical support that defines the architecture of the alveolar walls and dictate the mechanical properties of the lower respiratory tract.

DISEASE-RELATED CHANGES OF THE LUNG PARENCHYMA (See Fig. 209-2) To a variable degree, the morphologic changes of all ILD include an interstitial and/or intraalveolar inflammatory process superimposed upon derangements of the lower respiratory tract that include loss of pulmonary capillaries, alterations of the alveolar epithelial cells, and fibrosis of the alveolar walls. For most ILD, the extent and type of derangements are defined by the character of the injury and the ability, or inability, of the remaining parenchymal cells to reestablish the normal architecture. In some disorders, such as sarcoidosis, where the injury is usually mild, the normal architecture can be completely restored if the disease is suppressed. In contrast, in diseases like idiopathic pulmonary fibrosis, where the injury is more intense, the derangements to the affected alveoli are permanent. If the changes are extensive, the normal architecture is lost, leaving large masses of fibrotic tissue interspersed with cystic air spaces. Such regions of "end-stage lung" are not capable of mediating effective gas exchange.

The extent of the epithelial changes depends on the type and severity of the disease. Typically, there are losses in the numbers of type I epithelial cells and replacement with cuboidal epithelial cells, mostly type II cells but also bronchial cells migrating from the terminal brochioles. The loss of capillaries is not accompanied by new capillary growth, and there are changes in the pulmonary arteries secondry to pulmonary hypertension.

The alveolar walls can be thickened several-fold. Depending on the extent of these changes, the consequences include a widening of the distance between the air and blood, a reduction in the amount of air that can be contained in the alveolar air spaces, and an alteration of the mechanical properties of the lung parenchyma. In part, the thickening results from a mild edema of the alveolar walls. Most, however, results from the fibrosis, a process that includes an expansion in the numbers of mesenchymal cells and accumulation of their connective tissue products, particularly type I collagen. In some disorders, the fibrosis is entirely within the alveolar interstitium. In others, breaks in the epithelial basement membrane allow the fibrotic process to expand into the alveolar spaces. Sometimes the mass of this "intraalveolar fibrosis" is reincorporated into the alveolar walls, contributing to the thickening of the walls.

PATHOGENESIS The derangements to the alveoli that characterize most ILD are caused almost entirely by chronic inflammatory processes involving the lower respiratory tract, either exclusively or as part of a more generalized process. In the ILD of known etiology, the chronic inflammation is initiated by the causative agent. In some of these diseases, such as the drug-induced disorders or paraquat poisoning, the causative agent also directly injures the lung parenchyma, usually because it is cytotoxic to the parenchymal cells. For a few of the ILD of unknown etiology, the inflammation plays a minor role and

FIGURE 209-1 *Anatomy of the normal lower respiratory tract. A. Schematic low-power view showing a terminal bronchiole opening into the alveoli. B. Schematic high-power view of a cut surface of the alveolar wall. Shown are the flat type I epithelial cells, cuboidal type II epithelial cells, endothelial cells, mesenchymal cells, and interstitial connective tissue.*

A

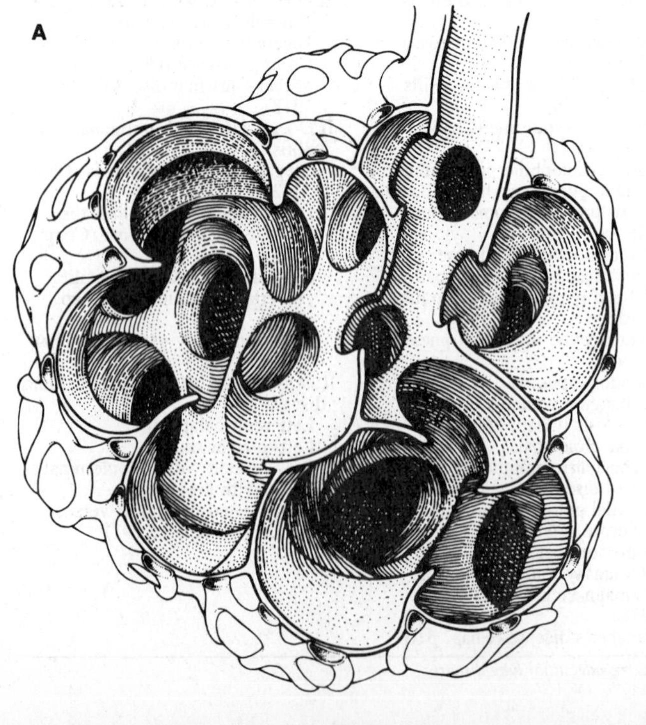

B

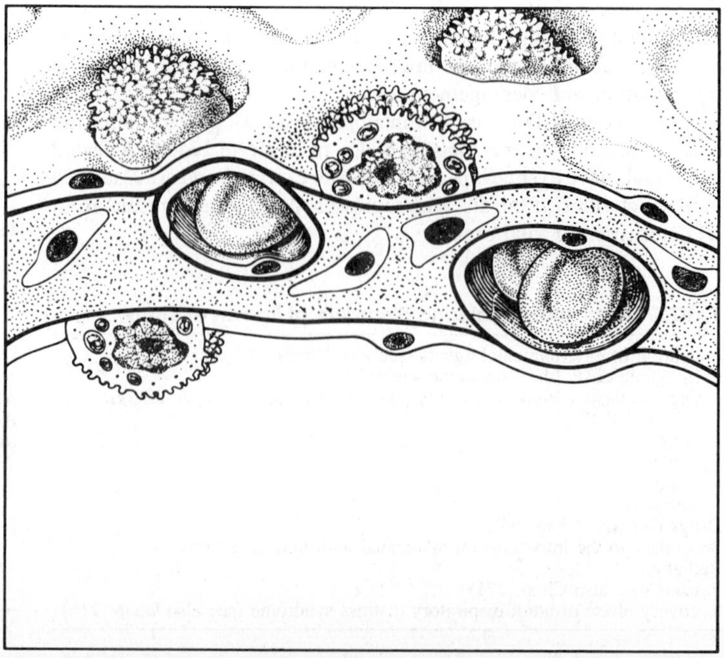

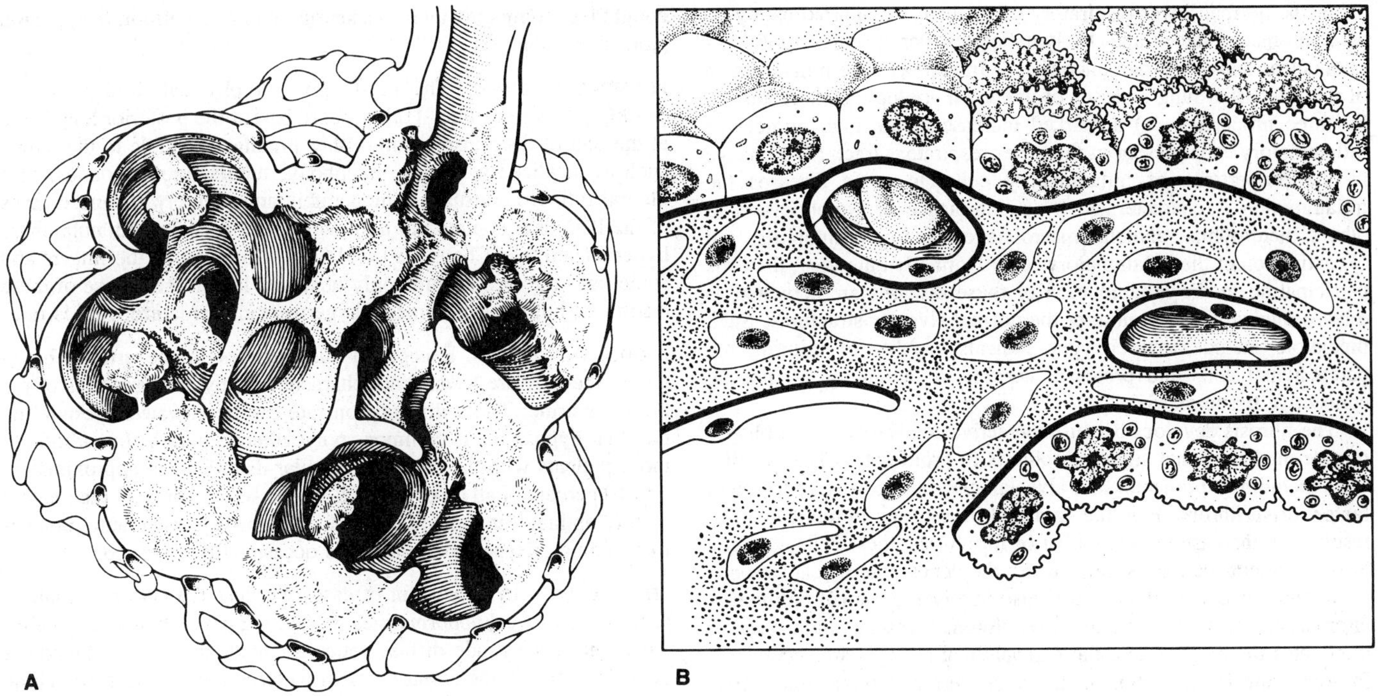

FIGURE 209-2 *Disease-related changes of the lung parenchyma in ILD. A. Schematic low-power view showing thickening of the alveolar walls, intraalveolar fibrosis, and areas where intraalveolar fibrosis has been incorporated into the alveolar walls. B. Schematic high-power view showing lost type I epithelial cells replaced by type II epithelial cells (cells with microvilli) and bronchiolar epithelial cells (smooth cuboidal cells). One capillary is compromised by the proliferation of fibroblasts and thickening of the alveolar walls with fibrosis. The basement membranes are thickened, but at one site the epithelial basement membrane is interrupted, allowing the interstitial components egress into the alveolar air space.*

the derangements of the lung parenchyma result from the abnormal proliferation of mesenchymal cells (e.g., lymphangioleiomyomatosis) or the deposition of an extracellular material not normally present in the lower respiratory tract (e.g., alveolar proteinosis).

The inflammatory cells derange the alveoli by two general mechanisms. First, the accumulation of the inflammatory cells in the confined regions of the alveolar walls distorts the normal architecture, thus altering the intimate relationship between air and blood. Second, the inflammatory cells release a battery of mediators that can injure the parenchymal cells and connective tissue matrix and stimulate fibroblasts to proliferate, thus promoting the development of fibrosis (Fig. 209-3).

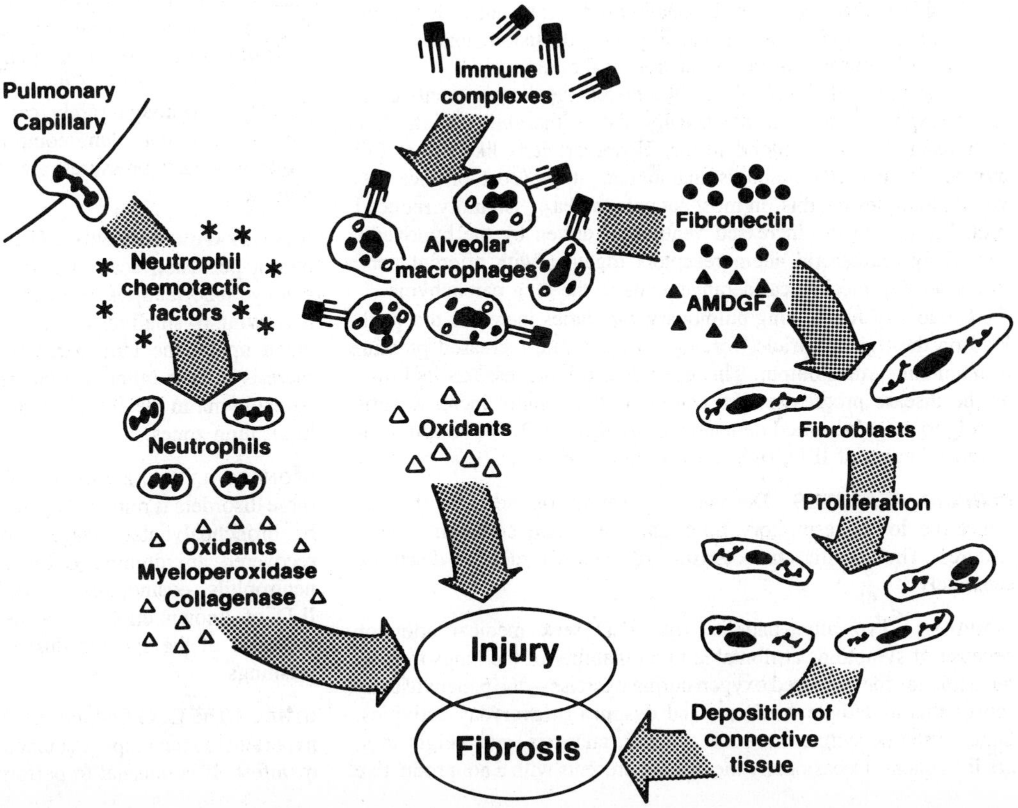

FIGURE 209-3 *Schematic concept of the pathogenesis of idiopathic pulmonary fibrosis, one of the major ILD of unknown etiology. Although the mechanisms shown are specific for IPF, and not applicable to all ILD, the concept of local inflammation causing the derangements and fibrosis serves as a paradigm for the pathogenesis of the ILD. AMDGF = alveolar macrophage–derived growth factor.*

In the normal lower respiratory tract, there are approximately 60 alveolar macrophages and 15 lymphocytes per alveolus; polymorphonuclear leukocytes are uncommon. In contrast, the inflammation of the interstitial lung diseases of unknown etiology is characterized by three properties: (1) a marked increase in the total number of inflammatory cells present in the lower respiratory tract; (2) a change in the proportions of inflammatory cells; in some diseases the inflammation is characterized by a dominance of lymphocytes, in others, neutrophils, alveolar macrophages, and/or eosinophils; and (3) activation of the inflammatory cells. Normally quiescent, the cells participating in the inflammation of these diseases are activated to release mediators that can alter the normal alveolar structures. Such mediators include toxic oxygen radicals capable of injuring the parenchymal cells and proteases capable of deranging the normal connective tissue matrix.

The fibrosis develops because the activated alveolar macrophages release mediators that signal fibroblasts to proliferate. These mediators, including fibronectin and alveolar macrophage–derived growth factor, drive fibroblasts in the damaged interstitium to replicate. The result is an increase in the number of fibroblasts; these cells continue to produce connective tissue, causing the deposition of scar tissue.

In some ILD the inflammation also involves the small pulmonary arteries and veins. Occasionally, the pulmonary vascular inflammation dominates the disease, and the parenchymal changes are secondary. In some, the inflammation includes the terminal bronchioles, thus limiting airflow to the associated alveoli, while in others it includes the visceral pleura, generating a pleuritis and pleural effusion.

PATHOPHYSIOLOGY The major consequence of the ILD is the inability of the lung to mediate the transfer of the normal amounts of O_2 from air to blood. The hypoxemia occurs by two mechanisms. First, some alveoli have insufficient ventilation to supply the capillary blood with the amount of O_2 necessary to saturate the red blood cells in the local capillaries. Second, there is an increased path for O_2 diffusion due to the thickening of alveolar walls. When this is combined with the fact that because of the loss of capillaries, the output of the right side of the heart can be maintained only by moving the blood through the remaining capillaries more quickly, the time the red blood cells remain in the proximity of the alveolar air is insufficient for the hemoglobin to be saturated with O_2. The hypoxemia resulting from these processes is usually mild at rest, but with exercise the ventilation-perfusion mismatching and diffusion abnormalities worsen and there is a further reduction in the Pa_{O_2}.

In contrast to their effects on O_2 transfer, the derangements in the lower respiratory tract do not usually disturb the ability of the lung to transfer CO_2 from blood to air. However, it is likely that CO_2 transfer is inefficient, and is maintained at the cost of increased ventilation. Despite this, in most patients the Pa_{CO_2} is mildly reduced, probably due to the increased ventilation driven by the hypoxemia sensed by the carotid chemoreceptors together with afferent nerve fibers sensing mechanical derangements in the lung parenchyma.

The loss of functioning pulmonary capillaries increases the workload on the right ventricle, forcing it to generate increased pressure to maintain cardiac output. This compensatory process has its limits; as the disease progresses, the cardiac output cannot increase sufficiently to meet increased demands for total-body O_2 consumption. In advanced cases of ILD, right heart failure may occur.

CLINICAL FEATURES Despite the diversity of the ILD, they all affect the lower respiratory tract and thus share common clinical features. The specific characteristics of each disorder are discussed separately.

SYMPTOMS Typically, patients with ILD seek medical attention because of symptoms attributable to an inability of the lungs to meet the demands for increased oxygen during exercise—the patient usually senses this as fatigue, malaise, and dyspnea in everyday activities. Other systemic symptoms, such as fever, anorexia, and weight loss, are infrequent. Occasionally the disease presents with a nonproductive cough; less commonly there is a sensation of chest discomfort, pleural pain, or hemoptysis.

PHYSICAL FINDINGS The most common physical finding is dry, crackling (''Velcro-like'') rales, heard best at the posterior lung bases at the end of deep inspiration. Other findings referable to the lungs, such as localized wheezing, egophony, tubular breath sounds, or a pleural rub, are unusual. In moderately and severely advanced cases of the ILD, it is common to find evidence consistent with pulmonary hypertension (see Chaps. 191 and 210). Clubbing of the fingers and sometimes the toes is commonly observed late in the course of these disorders, but the syndrome of hypertrophic osteoathropathy is rare.

BLOOD AND URINE Except for the changes in the arterial blood gases, the ILD are usually not characterized by abnormalities of the blood or urine. The sedimentation rate can be elevated. Despite the fact that hypoxemia is common, polycythemia is rare. In addition to those patients with the collagen-vascular disorders, in approximately 5 to 10 percent of all cases of the ILD, the serum contains rheumatoid factor, antinuclear antibodies, and occasionally other autoimmune-like findings. Hyperglobulinemia is occasionally observed.

CHEST X-RAY In 90 percent of cases the posteroanterior and lateral chest x-rays reveal abnormalities in the lung parenchyma. Typically, these changes include diffuse reticular, nodular, or reticulonodular patterns. Early in the disease, acinar patterns can be observed. These changes are diffuse but in most disorders are most apparent in the lower and midlung zones; occasionally they are localized. Small cystic spaces (''honeycombing'') are seen in some disorders and are common features of the late stages of most. Despite these ''classic'' x-ray features, a normal chest x-ray does not exclude the possibility of significant ILD. Alternatively, an abnormal chest x-ray does not necessarily mean that there is lung dysfunction resulting in abnormalities in gas exchange.

LUNG FUNCTION TESTS Typically, the ILD are characterized as ''restrictive'' disorders: there is a reduction in lung volumes (vital capacity, total lung capacity) together with a normal or supranormal ratio of expiratory volume in 1 s to forced vital capacity (FEV_1/FVC). There is usually a decrease in the diffusing capacity, reflecting a loss of functioning alveolar capillary units. Arterial blood-gas analysis reveals mild hypoxemia which worsens with exercise. The Pa_{CO_2} is mildly reduced and remains so with exercise. The pH is typically normal, but if O_2 delivery is insufficient to meet systemic demands with exercise, the arterial pH drops as metabolic acidosis develops. Although rarely carried out in routine clinical practice, evaluation of static lung compliance shows ''stiff'' lungs, i.e., high transpulmonary pressures are required to achieve maximum lung volumes.

SCINTIGRAPHIC FINDINGS The technetium-99m macroaggregated albumin perfusion scan and xenon-133 ventilation scan demonstrate patchy abnormalities reflecting dysfunction of capillary units and narrowing of small airways, respectively. Gallium-67 is not normally taken up by the lung parenchyma, but in circumstances in which there is diffuse inflammation, such as is typically found in the lung parenchyma in the ILD, the gallium-67 lung scan is usually positive in all lung zones.

BRONCHOALVEOLAR LAVAGE The inflammation that characterizes these disorders is reflected by the types of inflammatory cells recovered by bronchoalveolar lavage. Depending on the disorder, the cells recovered are dominated by alveolar macrophages, lymphocytes, neutrophils, eosinophils, or various mixtures of these cells. In the ILD of known etiology caused by inhalation of inorganic dusts, evidence of the specific dust may frequently be found in the lung washings.

OTHER The ECG findings are usually nonspecific, but as pulmonary hypertension develops, evidence of right heart abnormalities becomes manifest. It is unusual to perform right heart catheterization in these patients, but the findings typically include pulmonary hypertension, normal wedge pressure, and, late in the disease, a mild elevation of the right ventricular end-diastolic pressure. Despite the fact that there is progressive limitation of available pulmonary capillaries to handle the right ventricular output, frank right ventricular failure is rare.

DIAGNOSTIC EVALUATION The initial approach includes a history, physical examination, posteroanterior and lateral chest x-rays, and lung function tests, including vital capacity, total lung capacity, diffusing capacity, FEV_1/FVC, and arterial blood gases at rest. Together, the information derived should be sufficient to determine whether a diffuse parenchymal lung disorder is present. The age of the patient plays an important role in considering alternative diagnoses. For example, in the setting of a history of dyspnea and chest x-ray evidence of hilar adenopathy and a reticular nodular infiltrate, a 25-year-old would most likely have sarcoidosis while a 60-year-old is more likely to have a malignant neoplasm. A detailed exposure history with specific reference to inorganic or organic dusts, fumes, gases, aerosols, and drugs may help to identify or eliminate the known causes of ILD. Although routine blood screening occasionally helps to identify systemic disorders, with rare exceptions, blood studies do not help in making a specific diagnosis. The major noninterstitial lung disorders that may be confused with these diseases include congestive heart failure (Chap. 182) and the whole spectrum of malignant (Chap. 213) and infectious disorders of the lung parenchyma (Chaps. 205 and 206). Fiberoptic bronchoscopy is usually carried out to rule out infection and malignancy, and broncholveolar lavage helps to characterize the inflammation. Although helpful in judging disease activity, gallium-67 scans usually do not provide useful diagnostic information. For the ILD of known etiology, a lung biopsy is unnecessary if the relationship to the causative agent is "classic." In contrast, with few exceptions (see below), identification of the specific disorders of unknown etiology requires histologic evaluation of the lung parenchyma. If a lung biopsy is to be carried out, with the exception of sarcoidosis in which a transbronchial biopsy is adequate, an open lung biopsy is usually necessary.

Staging There are two aspects to staging these disorders: staging the extent of the derangements to the lung parenchyma and staging the activity of the disease. The extent of the parenchymal abnormalities is assessed with a combination of history, physical examination, chest x-ray, and routine lung function tests. Since it is the inflammation in the lower respiratory tract that causes these derangements to the lung parenchyma that, in turn, cause the loss of lung function, accurate assessment of disease activity must include an accurate assessment of the inflammation ongoing in the alveolar structures. Chest x-rays and lung function tests do not specifically evaluate the intensity of the inflammation in the lower respiratory tract and hence cannot be used to accurately judge the activity of the disease process. The best method is an open lung biopsy, but this is generally used only once in the course of the disease. Since the inflammation is compartmentalized in the lower respiratory tract, it is not reflected in abnormalities in blood tests. In major centers evaluating these disorders, gallium-67 scans and bronchoalveolar lavage are used to specifically document the extent and character of the inflammation.

THERAPY The most important therapy for the ILD of known etiology is to remove the individual from exposure to the causative agent. With the exception of the pneumoconioses, which generally are not treated, specific therapy for most of the ILD of known and unknown etiology is directed toward suppressing the inflammatory process in the lower respiratory tract. Typically, oral corticosteroids are used, starting with a high dose (usually 1 mg/kg of prednisone daily) for 4 to 6 weeks and then gradually taping to a low maintenance dose (0.25 mg/kg of prednisone) or, if the disease is suppressed, no therapy. Other anti-inflammatory and anti-immune agents such as cyclophosphamide are used for specific disorders (see below). Nonspecific therapeutic agents such as bronchodilators are used in those disorders accompanied by a component of reversible bronchospasm. Late in the course of the disease, once the Pa_{O_2} at rest is less than 50 to 55 mmHg, supplemental oxygen is used, first with exercise only and then continuously. Because the hypoxemia results from ventilation-perfusion inequalities and diffusion abnormalities, it is usually possible to reestablish a normal Pa_{O_2}. In most cases O_2 therapy can be given without concern for the complication of CO_2 retention.

Complications The ILD have a variable course depending on the specific disorder. While some are progressive and invariably fatal, others stabilize, while still others run a fluctuating course. Most complications are related to the inability of the lung to provide sufficient O_2 for systemic demands. As a result, these patients suffer the consequences of O_2 deprivation of vital organs; these consequences include stroke, cardiac arrhythmias, and myocardial infarction. Late in the course of the disease lung infections are common. Despite the fact that most patients are treated with corticosteroids, opportunistic infections are unusual.

INTERSTITIAL LUNG DISORDERS OF KNOWN ETIOLOGY Overall, the ILD of known etiology represent approximately one-third of all cases of ILD. The most common disorders in this group are those due to inhalation of inorganic dusts, inhalation or organic dusts, or to adverse reactions to pharmacologic agents. All of these disorders are discussed in separate chapters (see Table 209-1).

INTERSTITIAL LUNG DISEASE OF UNKNOWN ETIOLOGY

The ILD of unknown etiology represent two-thirds of all cases of ILD (Table 209-2). The most common disorder in this group, sarcoidosis, is discussed separately (Chap. 270). Among the other frequently encountered ailments are idiopathic pulmonary fibrosis and the ILD associated with the collagen-vascular disorders. Most others are relatively uncommon.

IDIOPATHIC PULMONARY FIBROSIS (IPF) This is a chronic, usually progressive disorder affecting only the lower respiratory tract. It is the "classic" interstitial lung disease of unknown etiology, with clinical features representative of this group of diseases. It was previously referred to as the "Hamman-Rich syndrome" and in the pathology literature as "desquamative interstitial pneumonitis" (early IPF) and "usual interstitial pneumonitis" (late IPF); in the British literature it is called "cryptogenic fibrosing alveolitis."

The derangements to the lung parenchyma in IPF result from a chronic inflammatory process initiated by immune complexes produced within the lower respiratory tract (Fig. 209-3). The immune complexes are directed against unknown antigens, likely components of the lung parenchyma. The inflammatory process is initiated by the immune complexes interacting with Fc receptors on alveolar macrophages; consequently the alveolar macrophages release mediators that amplify the inflammation, injure lung parenchymal cells, and stimulate fibroblasts to proliferate. Among these mediators are chemotactic factors, including leukotriene B4, that recruit neutrophils, and to a lesser extent, monocytes and eosinophils. Together with the recruited neutrophils and eosinophils, the activated macrophages release oxidants such as superoxide and hydrogen peroxide that injure the normal lung parenchymal cells. The neutrophils release type I collagenase, an enzyme that modifies the major connective tissue component of the alveolar walls, and myeloperoxidase, an enzyme that catalyzes the conversion of hydrogen peroxide to the hypohalide radical, an oxidant very toxic to the lung parenchymal cells. Among the alveolar macrophage mediators released in increased amounts in IPF are fibronectin and alveolar macrophage–derived growth factor, growth factors that together are sufficient to stimulate fibroblasts to proliferate, thus causing an expansion of numbers of fibroblasts in the alveolar walls, resulting in fibrosis. In some alveoli, the inflammation induces breaks in the epithelial basement membranes, allowing the interstitial components to protrude into the alveolar air spaces, causing intraalveolar fibrosis.

The *clinical findings* of IPF are those typical for ILD (see above). Males and females are affected equally. IPF most commonly develops in middle age but the disorder can occur in any age group. There is no history of exposure to the known causes of ILD. The chest x-ray, lung function tests, and blood findings are typical for diseases in this category. When the disease is active, the gallium-67 scan is moderately positive and bronchoalveolar lavage usually shows a dominance of alveolar macrophages and, to a lesser extent, neutrophils. Rarely, eosinophils and lymphocytes are major components of the inflammation.

The *diagnosis* of IPF requires an open lung biopsy. The morphology shows diffuse changes typical of ILD (Fig. 209-1) with a superimposed mononuclear phagocyte-neutrophil inflammatory process interspersed with lymphocytes and some eosinophils.

IPF is usually fatal 4 to 5 years after the onset of symptoms despite therapy. Approximately 10 percent die of bronchogenic carcinoma. Therapy for the ILD is directed toward suppressing the alveolitis. Corticosteroids are usually used, but a persistent neutrophil component of the inflammation can be suppressed by cyclophosphamide. Occasionally low-dose oral corticosteroids are supplemented with large doses of intravenous corticosteroids administered weekly.

ILD ASSOCIATED WITH DISORDERS OF IMMUNE-MEDIATED INJURY (COLLAGEN-VASCULAR DISORDERS) In most cases of ILD in association with the collagen-vascular disorders, the collagen-vascular disease is generally evident before the ILD becomes manifest. The ILD associated with the collagen-vascular disorders are usually mild and of little functional significance, but they can become the dominant feature of the disease and can be fatal. The pathogenesis of the ILD is assumed to be part of the systemic process, but the mechanisms causing the specific lung abnormalities are unknown.

The clinical features of these disorders are generally similar to a mild form of IPF in the presence of a systemic collagen-vascular disorder; occasionally other features dominate the clinical picture (see below). The diagnosis is made with the clinical, x-ray, and physiologic evidence of ILD in the presence of a diagnosis of a specific collagen-vascular disorder. Lung biopsy is usually not needed, but if the presentation is unusual, or if the ILD is clearly progressive, an open lung biopsy is often performed to confirm the diagnosis and help in making therapeutic decisions. Bronchoalveolar lavage analysis of inflammatory cells generally is dominated by macrophages, often with a mild neutrophil component, but occasionally lymphocytes are increased in numbers. The gallium-67 scan is usually mildly positive.

If the disease is mild, no therapy is used. If the ILD is progressive, corticosteroids are administered. There is no evidence that any other agents are effective, although there are anecdotal reports of cytotoxic drugs being used.

Rheumatoid arthritis (see Chap. 263) Lung function abnormalities are observed in about 50 percent of patients with rheumatoid arthritis, and 25 percent have x-ray evidence of ILD. The pulmonary abnormalities associated with rheumatoid arthritis are usually similar to IPF. Less commonly, the disease manifests as rheumatoid nodules in the lung parenchyma, pulmonary arterial arteritis with hypertension and secondary interstitial changes, or an acute, patchy inflammation associated with pleuritis and pericarditis. Coal workers with rheumatoid arthritis have an increased incidence of an interstitial lung disease referred to as "rheumatoid pneumoconiosis" or "Caplan's syndrome." In addition to the parenchymal disease, individuals with rheumatoid arthritis commonly develop pleural effusion, thickening, and adhesions. Rarely, rheumatoid arthritis is associated with a marked obstructive functional pattern along with inflammation, fibrosis, and obliteration of small airways, a condition termed *bronchiolitis obliterans*.

Progressive systemic sclerosis (see Chap. 264) Of individuals with progressive systemic sclerosis 30 to 50 percent have some form of ILD. Most commonly, the pulmonary disease is like IPF, but with less intense inflammation. Unique among the sufferers of ILD, these patients have an increased incidence of bronchoalveolar cell carcinoma. Alternatively, the ILD may be secondary to pulmonary arterial disease. If the diagnosis of ILD associated with progressive systemic sclerosis is considered, attention should be paid to the fact that these patients commonly have esophageal problems and therefore can have chronic aspiration. They also frequently develop cardiac disease, sometimes with left ventricular failure. Both of these entities may be mistaken for ILD. In rare cases, scleroderma of the chest wall restricts respiration, mimicking the functional abnormalities of ILD.

Systemic lupus erythematosus (see Chap. 262) ILD is less common in SLE than in the other collagen-vascular disorders. The pulmonary disease can be like IPF, but more commonly is an acute inflammatory process causing patchy infiltrates on the x-ray, sometimes with atelectasis. In the acute disease, concomitant parenchymal lung infections are common as are pleuritis and pleural effusion. Rarely, patients with lupus develop a lymphocytic infiltrative disease, small vessel pulmonary vasculitis, or a disorder similar to idiopathic pulmonary hemosiderosis.

Polymyositis-dermatomyositis (see Chap. 356) ILD is uncommon in this disorder, but when it occurs, it can precede the systemic disease. The ILD is usually like IPF. Since polymyositis can affect the muscles of respiration, the contribution of the ILD is sometimes difficult to separate from the functional abnormalities caused by the loss of intercostal muscle and diaphragm function.

Sjögren's syndrome (see Chap. 266) Patients with Sjögren's syndrome commonly develop a dry cough, usually due to the decreased secretions and resulting mucosal irritation in the airways. ILD is relatively uncommon; when it occurs, it is similar to IPF or characterized by a diffuse lymphocytic infiltrate.

Histiocytosis X This is a disorder of the mononuclear phagocyte system characterized by the accumulation of mononuclear phagocytes (described in the morphologic literature as "tissue histiocytes") in various organs. In the pediatric age group it usually manifests itself as Letterer-Siwe disease and Hand-Shüller-Christian disease. In adults it is usually an ILD referred to as histiocytosis X or eosinophilic granuloma.

The adult disease is characterized by a mixture of fibrotic and destructive changes in the lung parenchyma. The fibrotic changes are typical for ILD and the destruction is characterized by small cystic spaces. There is a focal but massive accumulation of mononuclear phagocytes in the lung parenchyma, often centered about terminal bronchioles. The mononuclear phagocytes are a mixture of alveolar macrophages and Langerhans cells (also called *HX cells*); the HX cell is normally present in skin but rarely in the lung parenchyma. It is characterized by a surface antigen identified by the OKT6 monoclonal antibody and 40- to 45-nm wide pentalamellar cytoplasmic inclusions called X bodies. Although they are known to be a derivative of the mononuclear phagocyte system, it is not known why HX cells accumulate in the lung in this disease or how they contribute to the derangements of the lung parenchyma.

Histiocytosis X usually develops in individuals 20 to 40 years of age. More than 90 percent are former current cigarrette smokers, but the relationship of smoking to the pathogenesis of the disease is unknown. The disease often presents insidiously with a nonproductive cough, dyspnea, and chest pain. Spontaneous pneumothorax occurs in 10 percent of cases and a small portion of individuals develop diabetes insipidus, bone involvement, and/or skin lesions.

The x-ray has a characteristic appearance with a reticulonodular infiltrate with superimposed small cystic spaces in the mid and upper lung zones. Lung function testing reveals a mixed restrictive-obstructive pattern with a decreased diffusing capacity and mild hypoxemia that worsens with exercise. Bronchoalveolar lavage reveals large numbers of mononuclear phagocytes including OKT6-positive HX cells. The gallium-67 scan is usually negative. There is no known treatment. Most individuals stabilize with some lung dysfunction, but the disease can be progressive and fatal.

Chronic eosinophilic pneumonia This disorder is characterized by fever, chills, weight loss, malaise, fatigue, dyspnea, and cough. Unlike most patients with ILD, many have chronic asthma. Females are affected more commonly than males. There is usually a blood eosinophilia and increased levels of immunoglobulins, particularly IgG. The x-ray shows patchy, nonsegmental infiltrates that are poorly defined and typically spare the central lung zones. A lung biopsy shows an eosinophilic inflammatory process in the lower respiratory tract, together with macrophages, lymphocytes, and neutrophils. There can be eosinophilic abscesses, a mild vasculitis, and occasional granulomas. The derangements to the lung parenchyma are usually mild but can be severe and progressive. Therapy with corticosteroids generally results in dramatic resolution, but the disorder often recurs spontaneously.

Hypereosinophilic syndrome This is a poorly understood disorder characterized by a persistent marrow and blood eosinophilia with eosinophilic infiltration of various organs, particularly the heart. A mild ILD occurs in about 20 to 40 percent of patients but is usually not a prominent feature of the disease. The disease has a variable course; therapy is usually with corticosteroids and/or hydroxyurea.

Idiopathic pulmonary hemosiderosis This ILD is characterized by recurrent pulmonary hemorrhage, dyspnea, and iron-deficiency anemia. It usually begins in childhood, but can occur in adults. The recurrent pulmonary hemorrhage may be life-threatening. The pathogenesis of the disease is unknown. There is usually a mild to moderate interstitial disease than can be progressive. The inflammation is dominated by alveolar macrophages containing deposits of hemosiderin, the normal epithelial cells are replaced by cuboidal cells, and a variable degree of fibrosis is seen. The lung function abnormalities are typical for an ILD, but the diffusing capacity can be falsely elevated secondary to the carbon monoxide test gas ''artifactually'' interacting with hemoglobin deposited in the lung parenchyma. The x-ray shows transient, patchy infiltrates that clear in a few weeks. Diagnosis of this disorder requires an open lung biopsy. Idiopathic pulmonary hemosiderosis is not associated with kidney disease or anti-basement membrane antibodies, thus differentiating it from Goodpasture's syndrome. Treatment includes iron for the anemia and corticosteroids for the lung disease, although there is no evidence that the latter alters the course of the disorder. The disease is often progressive and fatal but can stabilize.

Goodpasture's syndrome Patients with this disorder present with relapsing pulmonary hemorrhage, anemia, and renal disease (see Chap. 224). Adult males are most commonly affected. Renal failure is common and there are circulating antibodies that cross-react with glomerular and alveolar basement membranes. The kidneys show focal or diffuse proliferative or necrotizing glomerulonephritis. The lung disease is identical to idiopathic pulmonary hemosiderosis. While the lung hemorrhage can be life-threatening, the ILD is usually mild. Diagnosis is usually made by demonstrating circulating anti-basement membrane antibodies together with a renal biopsy showing the characteristic pattern of immunoglobulin staining; these findings differentiate this disorder from idiopathic pulmonary hemosiderosis, uremic pneumonitis, Wegener's granulomatosis, and systemic lupus erythematosus. Therapy is usually corticosteroids and cyclophosphamide, often combined with plasmapheresis to remove the circulating antibodies.

Immunoblastic lymphadenopathy Also called angioimmunoblastic lymphadenopathy, this is a disease of older individuals characterized by fever, malaise, generalized lymphadenopathy, hemolytic anemia, and, in some individuals, ILD. It is thought to be a disorder of the control of B lymphocytes. There is usually a polyclonal increase in immunoglobulins. Biopsy of lymph nodes shows a replacement of the normal architecture by pleomorphic lymphocytes in various stages of differentiation. Hilar and mediastinal lymph nodes are usually increased in size, and the lung parenchyma shows an accumulation of interstitial and intraalveolar lymphocytes, a deposition of intraalveolar eosinophilic material, and mild to moderate changes typical of ILD. Despite therapy with corticosteroids and cytotoxic drugs, most patients die within 1 year, often from lung infections or the development of a T-lymphocyte malignancy.

Lymphocytic infiltrative diseases These are poorly understood and inadequately classified ILD characterized by the accumulation of lymphocytes in the lung parenchyma, often in association with dysproteinemias and the eventual development of lymphoid malignancy. *Lymphocytic interstitial pneumonitis* is a term used to characterize patients with ILD showing a diffuse accumulation of mature lymphocytes in the alveolar walls and airspaces. There is often a coexisting systemic autoimmune disorder such as Sjögren's disease (Chap. 266). Occasionally there is a history of phenytoin usage. If the lymphocytes form germinal centers in the lung parenchyma, the disease is referred to as *pseudolymphoma*. The ILD may be mild but can progress and be fatal. Alternatively, the disease can develop into a lymphocytic malignancy. Therapy is usually with corticosteroids and/or cytotoxic agents.

Lymphangioleiomyomatosis This unusual disorder is found almost exclusively in women of childbearing age. It presents with progressive dyspnea, unilateral or bilateral chylous pleural effusions, pneumothoraxes, and occasional hemoptysis. The lung parenchyma shows an accumulation of smooth muscle cells in the alveolar walls and around bronchioles and venules. Thoracic and abdominal lymphatics and lymph nodes are frequently involved. In addition to the thickening of the alveolar walls, there is some lung destruction. There is a mild inflammation of the lung parenchyma dominated by macrophages. The chest x-ray shows a diffuse reticulonodular infiltrate intermixed with cystic spaces. Lung function testing usually reveals normal total lung capacity, reduced diffusing capacity, and limitation of airflow. Diagnosis requires an open-lung biopsy. There is no proven therapy, but, because the disease occurs in women 20 to 40 years of age, hormonal manipulation with progesterone or oophorectomy has been tried. Surgical intervention is occasionally used for the chylous effusions, but can result in a shifting of the effusion to other spaces. Death is invariable within 10 years of onset.

Amyloidosis (see Chap. 259) Although uncommon, amyloidosis can involve the lung parenchyma and/or airways diffusely or in a nodular fashion. When it occurs, it is usually associated with systemic primary amyloid or multiple myeloma and/or less frequently with secondary amyloid. Diagnosis is made by open-lung biopsy demonstrating deposits of amyloid in the alveolar walls, pulmonary vasculature, and/or airways. There is mild parenchymal inflammation dominated by macrophages. The clinical picture depends on the site of amyloid deposition; nodules are usually asymptomatic, airway deposition causes airflow obstruction, and parenchymal amyloid presents as typical ILD. There is no specific therapy available for the ILD.

Alveolar proteinosis This disorder is more properly conceptualized as an intraalveolar disorder rather than an ILD. It is rare, affects mostly males, and is characterized by diffuse filling of the air spaces with granular eosinophilic PAS-positive protein-lipid material. This intraalveolar material includes lamellated concentric structures similar to the cytoplasmic structures in type II epithelial cells. There is mild inflammation with changes in the alveolar epithelial cells typical of the ILD. There is dyspnea, cough, some sputum production, weight loss, and occasional fever. The chest x-ray shows diffuse, fine nodular infiltrates and can be confused with pulmonary edema. Lung function tests reveal decreased lung volumes associated with moderate to severe hypoxemia usually due to a large right-to-left shunt. Although lipid-laden macrophages recovered by bronchoalveolar lavage may suggest this disorder, diagnosis requires a lung biopsy. Although the disease is recurrent and can be life-threatening, the material can be removed from the lungs with whole-lung lavage under general anesthesia with temporary, and sometimes permanent, improvement in lung function. The pathogenesis of alveolar proteinosis is unknown, but since the intraalveolar material resembles the lipid componenet of surfactant, dysfunction of type II cells has been suggested. Rare cases are associated with massive silica exposure or with lung infections.

Bronchocentric granulomatosis This disorder is characterized by masses of granulomas centered in the walls of airways and the surrounding tissues, including pulmonary arteries. There is destruction of the bronchiolar walls, and, like the vasculitides involving the lung, there are varying degrees of parenchymal inflammation and derangement typical of the ILD. The disease was originally defined by morphologic criteria without regard for the associated specific clinical features, and it likely represents several different diseases, including a hypersensitivity-type disorder in response to fungi such as aspergilli. Treatment is usually with corticosteroids, but their efficacy and the natural history of this disorder have not been well defined.

Inherited disorders In addition to family clusters of sarcoidosis, there are some rare inherited disorders associated with ILD. Except for familial IPF, the pathogenesis of the lung derangements have not been defined, and there are no guidelines for their specific management.

FAMILIAL IPF This autosomal dominant disorder with incomplete penetrance is identical to IPF. The ILD with lung function abnormalities usually manifests itself in the fourth to fifth decades, but younger family members have been identified with evidence of alveolar inflammation but without derangements to the lower respiratory tract, supporting the concept that chronic inflammation plays a critical precursor role in the pathogenesis of the ILD.

TUBEROUS SCLEROSIS (see Chap. 351) This autosomal dominant disorder with incomplete penetrance is characterized by mental retardation, seizures, adenoma sebaceum, and proliferation of smooth muscle in various tissues including the lung parenchyma. The ILD is similar to lymphangioleiomyomatosis, but chylous effusions are rare.

NEUROFIBROMATOSIS (see Chap. 351) ILD, often in association with some lung destruction, occurs in 10 to 20 percent of patients with this autosomal dominant disorder characterized by skin and nervous system neurofibromas and cutaneous café au lait spots. There are no neurofibromas in the lung, and the pathogenesis of the ILD is unknown.

HERMANSKY-PUDLAK SYNDROME This is an autosomal recessive disorder manifesting as oculocutaneous albinism, platelet dysfunction, and the accumulation of a ceroid-like material in various organs including the lung parenchyma. The ILD is a prominent feature of the disease. It usually develops in the third to fourth decades.

NIEMANN-PICK DISEASE (see Chap. 316) This is an autosomal recessive storage disorder characterized by the accumulation of sphingomyelin in tissue. Although hepatosplenomegaly and central nervous system abnormalities dominate the clinical picture, ILD can be prominent, particularly in type B disease.

GAUCHER'S DISEASE (see Chap. 316) This is an autosomal recessive disorder associated with an accumulation of glucosylceramide in various tissues. The disease manifests primarily as hepatosplenomegaly and erosion of bones, but ILD can occur and cause respiratory failure.

ILD associated with liver disease Patients with chronic active hepatitis can have an IPF-like syndrome with systemic autoimmune features suggesting an overlap with the collagen-vascular disorders. Primary biliary cirrhosis also occurs in conjunction with ILD; the lung disease is usually like sarcidosis, but a disorder similar to IPF is occasionally seen.

ILD associated with bowel disease Whipple's disease (Chap. 237) is classically localized to the small intestine, but similar abnormalities can occur in other organs, including the lower respiratory tract, causing a mild form of ILD. Ulcerative colitis can be associated with a disorder like IPF, and Crohn's disease with a disorder like sarcoidosis. A systemic form of the relapsing panniculitis of Weber-Christian disease (Chap. 318) can involve the lung parenchyma; there are fat globules, necrosis, and changes typical of ILD.

ILD associated with pulmonary vasculitis Except for polyarteritis nodosa, most of the systemic vasculitides can involve the pulmonary arteries and/or veins. ILD usually plays an important role in the clinical picture of Wegener's granulomatosis, lymphomatoid granulomatosis, and the Churg-Strauss syndrome, but the inflammation and derangements in the alveolar structures are thought to be secondary to the primary vascular disease. The ILD associated with the pulmonary vasculitides are managed like the primary disorders.

ILD associated with chronic cardiac disease or chronic renal disease Prior to cardiac surgery for congenital cardiac lesions, mitral or aortic valvular disease and high-flow left-to-right shunts were occasionally associated with chronic ILD. Likewise, prior to widespread use of dialysis, chronic uremia was associated with a variety of derangements of the lower respiratory tract. Both categories of disease are rarely seen today.

ILD associated with graft-versus-host reaction One of the adverse reactions to bone marrow transplantation (Chap. 291) is a graft-versus-host syndrome with airway inflammation and injury, sometimes in association with ILD. Treatment is directed toward suppression of the immune reaction. Care must be taken to exclude infectious complications, which are frequently seen in immunosuppressed transplant recipients.

REFERENCES

CRYSTAL RG et al: Interstitial lung disease of unknown etiology: Disorders characterized by chronic inflammation of the lower respiratory tract. N Engl J Med 310:154, 235, 1984

——— et al: Interstitial lung disease: Current concepts of pathogenesis, staging, and therapy. Am J Med 70:542, 1981

DAVIS WB, CRYSTAL RG: Chronic interstitial lung disease, in *Current Pulmonology*, D Simmons, (ed). New York; Wiley, 1984, vol V, pp 347–473

FISHMAN AP: *Pulmonary Diseases and Disorders* 2d ed. New York, McGraw-Hill, 1987

FRASER RG, PARE JAP: *Diagnosis of Diseases of the Chest.* Philadelphia, Saunders, 1978

KATZENSTEIN A-L A, ASKIN FB: *Surgical Pathology of Non-neoplastic Lung Disease*, Philadelphia, Saunders, 1982

210 PRIMARY PULMONARY HYPERTENSION

JOHN ROSS, JR.

Primary (or idiopathic) pulmonary hypertension is an uncommon disease, the diagnosis of which can be established only after a thorough search for the usual causes of pulmonary hypertension. The patient with primary pulmonary hypertension typically is a young female between the ages of 20 and 40, although older and younger patients of either sex have been described. The clinical and laboratory features of severe pulmonary hypertension are present, but there is no evidence of parenchymal pulmonary disease or of primary heart disease, nor is there evidence for the occurrence of pulmonary emboli. Anatomic verification often has been necessary to distinguish clearly the primary form of pulmonary hypertension from that due to multiple pulmonary emboli, although angiography and radioisotope scanning methods have facilitated this differentiation considerably.

PATHOLOGY The findings on pathologic examination of patients with primary pulmonary hypertension usually are confined to the right side of the heart and lungs. The right atrium often is enlarged and the right ventricle is hypertrophied. Frequently, the large pulmonary arteries exhibit atherosclerotic plaques. The disease process involves the small pulmonary arteries (between 40 and 300 μm in diameter), which exhibit muscular hypertrophy and intimal hyperplasia, sometimes with fibrosis. On occasion, a necrotizing arteritis may be encountered. Other histologic studies have shown a reduced number of small arteries, as well as fewer capillaries in the alveolar wall. Electron-microscopic studies have documented an increase in thickness of the endothelial cells and basement membranes of alveolar capillaries, and some capillaries are blocked by the abnormal epithelial cells. Medial hypertrophy of muscular pulmonary arteries may be the first response to prolonged pulmonary vasoconstriction, but in later stages of the disease concentric laminar intimal fibrosis and plexiform lesions appearing as cellular, intraluminal tufts (so-called plexogenic pulmonary arteriopathy) may develop. Patients with recurrent pulmonary thromboembolism may clinically resemble patients with primary pulmonary hypertension, but histologic sections of the lung exhibit various degrees of organization of pulmonary thromboemboli; some may be recanalized, there may be fibrous septa and eccentric fibrosis in the vessels; secondary medial hypertrophy of muscular arteries may be marked, but plexiform lesions are not present. In infants and young children with pulmonary venoocclusive disease the clinical picture may suggest primary pulmonary hypertension, and the pulmonary wedge pressure may be normal. Organized thrombotic disease is found in the venules and small veins, together with proximal hypertrophy of the muscular venous wall and secondary medial hypertrophy in the pulmonary arterioles.

Rarely, disease of the systemic arterial vascular bed resembling that found in the pulmonary blood vessels has been described. The syncope and sudden death which may occur in this disease have been attributed in some patients to involvement of the coronary arterial branch supplying the sinoatrial node.

ETIOLOGY The cause of primary pulmonary hypertension is unknown, but a number of possible etiologic factors have been suggested. A few patients with primary pulmonary hypertension have been reported in whom minimal changes were found in the pulmonary vessels on pathologic examination, and this observation has raised the possibility that a neurohumoral vasoconstrictor mechanism is involved. Support for this view has been provided by the observation that the pulmonary vascular resistance can be acutely reduced in some patients with this disease by the infusion of vasodilators, or by administering oxygen. A febrile illness may precede the onset of the disease by a variable period and has been implicated in the etiology. In 15 to 20 percent of female patients with this disorder, symptoms begin soon after pregnancy, which has prompted the suggestion that unrecognized thromboemboli or amniotic fluid emboli during pregnancy may play a role. In other patients, it seems quite possible that the disease may represent an end stage of earlier, unrecognized emboli originating from the legs or pelvic veins. An apparent association between an increased occurrence of primary pulmonary hypertension and use of the anorectic agent aminorex fumarate, a drug having structural similarity to ephedrine, was observed in Europe between 1967 and 1970. The alkaloids in many species of crotalaria plants used in herbal brews may cause pulmonary hypertension in human beings, as demonstrated experimentally in rats. The use of oral contraceptives may bear a relation to the occurrence of pulmonary hypertension, particularly in patients with predisposing factors such as systemic lupus erythematosus or a family history of primary pulmonary hypertension.

Raynaud's phenomenon precedes the onset of primary pulmonary hypertensive disease by a number of years in an appreciable number of patients. This association and the occurrence of Raynaud's disease in scleroderma, disseminated lupus erythematosus, rheumatoid arthritis, and dermatomyositis have led to the speculation that primary pulmonary hypertension may represent a form of collagen vascular disease. Moreover, primary pulmonary hypertension and collagen vascular disease, including lupus erythematosus, have been reported to occur simultaneously in a number of patients. It also has been suggested that the disease may be congenital and present from birth; however, the closely packed, parallel elastic fibers in the main pulmonary arteries in patients having Eisenmenger's syndrome from birth, described by some investigators, usually have not been observed in patients with primary pulmonary hypertension. Finally, primary pulmonary hypertension has been reported in a number of families; sometimes more than two members and up to three generations have been affected. A fibrinolytic defect was reported in one family study.

PATHOPHYSIOLOGY Some studies have suggested that the response of the pulmonary vascular bed is labile early in the course of this disease, as evidenced by a response to vasodilating agents and oxygen. It also has been proposed that the disease tends to progress. Thus, serial cardiac catheterizations have shown a tendency for the pulmonary vascular resistance to increase and to become fixed. With the development of severe pulmonary vascular disease, abnormal elevation of the pulmonary arterial pressure occurs, often to a striking degree, and the pulmonary arterial pressure may be equal to that in the systemic arterial bed. The pulmonary arterial wedge pressure is normal in patients with primary pulmonary hypertension, the cardiac output is normal or reduced, and no intracardiac shunts are detected. In many patients the mean right atrial pressure is elevated, and the *a* wave in the right atrium may be markedly elevated, an indication of the forceful atrial contraction necessary to fill the hypertrophied right ventricle. With the long-standing overload on the right side of the heart, right ventricular failure finally develops. In some patients, peripheral cyanosis occurs secondary to reduced cardiac output, and occasionally central cyanosis becomes evident at the end stage of the disease because of right-to-left shunting through a patent foramen ovale. Mild systemic arterial desaturation is quite common, even in the absence of heart failure, and may be due to shunting within the lungs. Pulmonary function in patients with primary pulmonary hypertension generally is normal, although hyperventilation often is present, resulting in hypocapnia and a decreased serum bicarbonate concentration. A low carbon monoxide–diffusing capacity has been described in some patients.

CLINICAL PICTURE The patient, usually a young female, gives a history of relatively recent onset of symptoms. Ordinarily, the natural course of the disease encompasses less than 5 years, but occasionally survival for 25 years or more has been reported. In one large retrospective study, the median time from initial symptoms to diagnosis was about 2 years, and that from diagnosis to death was about 2 years, with over 75 percent of deaths occurring within 5 years after diagnosis. Not uncommonly, patients with primary pulmonary hypertension are classified as neurotic early in the course of their disease because of the hyperventilation, chest discomfort, and the relative paucity of objective findings. Precordial pain on exertion occurs in from 25 to 50 percent of patients, and occasionally severe chest pain has been associated with a dissection of the main pulmonary artery. Other common symptoms are weakness, fatigue, exertional dyspnea, and effort syncope, which usually results from peripheral vasodilatation in the presence of a fixed cardiac output. Hoarseness may be noted because of compression of the left recurrent laryngeal nerve by the enlarged pulmonary artery. Unexplained sudden death occurs relatively often. Sudden death also has occurred during cardiac catheterization or surgical procedures and after the administration of barbiturates or anesthetic agents. The terminal course usually is characterized by right-sided heart failure. Very rarely, spontaneous regression of the disease has been reported.

On physical examination, the jugular venous pulse usually shows a prominent *a* wave, there is a right ventricular heave, and an impulse may be felt over the region of the main pulmonary artery. An ejection click may be audible at the pulmonic area, the second heart sound is narrowly split, and the pulmonic closure sound is markedly accentuated and may be palpable. Often, an atrial gallop sound is heard at the lower left sternal border, and in some patients there is an ejection murmur at the pulmonic area or the early diastolic murmur of pulmonic regurgitation. The chest roentgenogram may show cardiac enlargement with right ventricular and right atrial prominence, and there is marked dilatation of the pulmonary artery segment. Peripherally, the pulmonary arteries taper sharply, and the lung fields may appear oligemic. The electrocardiogram almost always shows some evidence of right ventricular enlargement, with right axis deviation, right ventricular hypertrophy in the precordial leads, and sometimes inverted T waves over the right precordium. Right atrial enlargement also may be evident on the electrocardiogram. Echocardiography is useful for identifying right ventricular enlargement, and in pulmonary hypertension the pulmonic valve usually shows attenuation or absence of the *a* dip and midsystolic notching.

DIFFERENTIAL DIAGNOSIS It is imperative that the diagnosis of primary pulmonary hypertension not be made until potentially treatable causes of elevated pulmonary arterial pressure have been excluded. The presence of pulmonary hypertension and cor pulmonale caused by chronic pulmonary disease can be established readily by finding abnormalities in pulmonary function. In particular, interstitial lung diseases with fibrosis, such as sarcoidosis, and pneumoconioses, such as silicosis, as well as hypoxic pulmonary hypertension associated with impaired ventilation should be excluded. Cardiac catheterization and/or echocardiographic studies are necessary to search for a primary cardiac defect, and angiography or radioactive lung-scanning studies also may be indicated to detect emboli to relatively large pulmonary arteries (Chap. 211). In performing pulmonary arteriography, the use of small amounts of contrast medium, preferentially injected selectively into the branches of the main pulmonary artery, is advisable since sudden death during catheterization has occasionally occurred. Patients having chronic emboli to the lungs are difficult to distinguish from those with primary pulmonary hypertension, but the distinction is important because anticoagulants, inferior vena caval interruption, and pulmonary embolectomy sometimes have been effective in patients with embolic disease. The lung scan and pulmonary arteriogram are typically normal in primary pulmonary hypertension, but with thromboembolic pulmonary hypertension, perfusion defects on lung scan or pulmonary arterial occlusions and filling defects on angiography often are visible. With pulmonary embolism, serial chest x-rays may show evidence of pulmonary infarction. Open lung biopsy has been used occasionally to differentiate primary pulmonary hypertension from the thromboembolic variety. Sometimes a site of origin for emboli cannot be identified in the leg veins, and other possible sources should be considered, such as right atrial thrombus, or ovarian and pelvic vein thromboses. Occasionally, pulmonary hypertension is due to parasitic disease, such as schistosomiasis or filariasis, or to multiple pulmonary artery thromboses consequent to sickle cell disease. Although the importance of accurate diagnosis is emphasized, short of open lung biopsy clinical differentiation may be impossible between the three main pathologic types of pulmonary hypertension (pulmonary venoocclusive, thromboembolic or thrombotic, and plexogenic pulmonary arteriopathic types), and they are frequently categorized by the clinician as primary pulmonary hypertension.

Several congenital cardiac conditions must be considered and excluded by appropriate echocardiographic or cardiac catheterization studies. Valvular pulmonic stenosis usually can be distinguished from pulmonary hypertension by identification of the delayed, soft pulmonic closure sound, but peripheral stenoses of the pulmonary arteries may be associated with an increased second heart sound. A left-to-right shunt at the pulmonary arterial, ventricular, or atrial levels should be sought. The wide, fixed splitting of the second heart sound should be helpful in identifying patients with atrial septal defect. Eisenmenger's syndrome in a patient with ventricular septal defect or patent ductus arteriosus (Chap. 185) may be confused with primary pulmonary hypertension, but usually in Eisenmenger's syndrome cyanosis, polycythemia, and clubbing are present, and at cardiac catheterization a large right-to-left shunt at the ventricular, atrial, or pulmonary arterial level can be demonstrated.

The murmurs of tricuspid or pulmonic regurgitation and the atrial gallop sounds heard in patients with primary pulmonary hypertension may be mistaken for the murmurs of rheumatic mitral and aortic valve disease, or vice versa. Before making the diagnosis of primary pulmonary hypertension, the presence of left atrial hypertension due to undetected mitral stenosis, or to a more unusual lesion such as left atrial myxoma or cor triatriatum, should be specifically sought and excluded. This can be done by echocardiography, by obtaining pulmonary arterial wedge pressure tracings, or by catheterization of the left side of the heart, with angiography if necessary.

THERAPY In many patients with primary pulmonary hypertension the downhill course is progressive despite treatment, and therapy must be palliative. The use of anticoagulants has been considered of doubtful value, provided chronic pulmonary embolic phenomena can be excluded. However, in a retrospective natural history study of 120 patients, postmortem examinations in 56 patients showed organized thrombus in small arteries (embolic or in situ) to be present in over 50 percent of patients; the only apparent clinical difference between these patients and those with plexiform arteriopathy was a somewhat older average age. Anticoagulation within 12 months of diagnosis was an independent predictor of improved survival rate, and anticoagulant therapy was recommended for all patients. The diagnosis of chronic thrombotic obstruction of major pulmonary arteries is important because surgical thromboendarterectomy in such patients has been successful in a number of patients.

Right-sided heart failure should be treated with a cardiotonic and diuretic regimen (Chap. 182). Since there is no hypercapnia in these patients, the hypoxia which may accompany heart failure can be treated safely with oxygen therapy.

Recent reports have indicated that in some patients pharmacologic therapy can produce clinical and hemodynamic improvement. Although long-term observations concerning prolongation of life are not available, several categories of drugs have been found useful in small groups of patients: (1) direct vascular smooth-muscle relaxants (nitroprusside, diazoxide, nitroglycerine, and hydralazine); (2) beta agonists (sublingual isoproterenol, oral terbutaline); (3) alpha-adrenergic blocking agents (phentolamine and phenoxybenzamine); (4) calcium antagonists (nifedipine and verapamil); and (5) angiotensin converting enzyme inhibitors. Immunosuppressive agents and prostaglandin antagonists (indomethacin) have rarely been used. Prostacyclin (PGI_2) has been employed successfully intravenously as a test of vascular reactivity and for short-term therapy.

In some patients, favorable hemodynamic effects from orally administered drugs such as diazoxide or hydralazine have been sustained for many months, with clinical improvement manifested by relief of severe dyspnea and reduction in the number of syncopal episodes. Hydralazine and nifedipine are currently used most commonly. The calcium channel blocker nifedipine has been reported to lower pulmonary artery pressure and pulmonary vascular resistance and to increase cardiac output, as well as to improve exercise tolerance in some patients. Although few long-term studies are available, limited data suggest that the lowered pulmonary vascular resistance may be maintained over many months in some patients. Initial studies suggest that the angiotensin-converting enzyme inhibitor captopril may be effective in a few patients, but it appears to have its main effect on the systemic circulation to lower arterial pressure and increase cardiac output, with a less prominent action on the pulmonary circulation. Prior to instituting long-term therapy with such drugs, measurement of the acute responses of the pulmonary artery pressure, pulmonary vascular resistance, cardiac output, and arterial pressure is usually indicated in order to assess efficacy and to detect unfavorable effects. In some patients hemodynamic deterioration has been reported following the use of vasodilators.

Heart and lung transplantation has now been successful in a number of patients, with survival for several years. Although early mortality was relatively high (about 30 percent), the functional status of survivors has been good, and such treatment represents a possible approach in selected patients if suitable donors can be found.

REFERENCES

FUSTER V et al: Primary pulmonary hypertension: Natural history and the importance of thrombosis. Circulation 70:580, 1984

GROSSMAN W, BRAUNWALD E: Pulmonary hypertension, in *Heart Disease,* 2d ed, E Braunwald (ed). Philadelphia, Saunders, 1984, p 823

HAWORTH SG: Primary pulmonary hypertension. Br Heart J 49:517, 1983

HUGHES JD, RUBIN LJ: Primary pulmonary hypertension: An analysis of 28 cases and a review of the literature. Medicine 65:56, 1986

JAMIESON SW et al: Heart and lung transplantation for pulmonary hypertension. Am J Surg 147(6):740, 1984

MCGOON MD, VLIETSTRA RE: Vasodilator therapy for primary pulmonary hypertension. Mayo Clin Proc 59:872, 1984

MOSER KM et al: Chronic thrombotic obstruction of major pulmonary arteries. Results of thromboendarterectomy in 15 patients. Ann Intern Med 99:299, 1983

OLIVARI MT et al: Hemodynamic effects of nifedipine at rest and during exercise in primary pulmonary hypertension. Chest 86(1):14, 1984

PACKER M: Vasodilator therapy for primary pulmonary hypertension. Ann Intern Med 103:258, 1985

REITZ BA: Heart-lung transplantation, in *Pulmonary Diseases and Disorders,* 2d ed, AP Fishman (ed). New York, McGraw-Hill, 1987, Part 18

RICH S, BRUNDAGE BH: Primary pulmonary hypertension: Current update. JAMA 251:2252, 1984

VOELKEL N, REEVES JT: Primary pulmonary hypertension, in *Pulmonary Vascular Diseases,* KM Moser (ed). New York, Marcel Dekker, 1979

WAGENVOORT CA, WAGENVOORT N: *Pathology of Pulmonary Hypertension.* New York, Wiley 1977

211 PULMONARY THROMBOEMBOLISM

KENNETH M. MOSER

Pulmonary thromboembolism (PTE) is a leading cause of morbidity and mortality and can appear in many clinical contexts. Epidemiologic surveys indicate that PTE is responsible for more than 50,000 deaths in the United States annually. However, available data suggest that less than 10 percent of all pulmonary emboli result in death. Thus, the incidence of fatal plus nonfatal emboli in this nation probably exceeds 500,000 annually. This overall incidence seems verified by autopsy statistics. Evidence of recent or old embolism is detected in 25 to 30 percent of routine autopsies; with special techniques, this figure exceeds 60 percent. Even these data underestimate incidence, since many emboli resolve without trace and are not found at postmortem examination. The high incidence of PTE at autopsy contrasts sharply with the incidence of antemortem diagnosis. Available information suggests that an antemortem diagnosis has been made in only 10 to 30 percent of all cases in which old or recent embolism is demonstrated at autopsy.

VENOUS THROMBOSIS

PATHOGENESIS Available data indicate that more than 95 percent of pulmonary emboli arise from thrombi in the deep venous system of the lower extremities. Thrombi occurring in the right cardiac chambers or in other veins account for the remainder. In situ pulmonary arterial thrombosis is rare. Thus, embolism should be viewed as a *complication* of deep venous thrombosis (DVT). Furthermore, it appears that the larger leg veins (those above the knee) are the most common source of those pulmonary emboli which reach clinical attention. These facts have several important implications with respect to PTE: (1) prevention of DVT is the most effective approach to prevention of embolism; (2) prompt treatment of DVT may limit the frequency of embolism; (3) techniques which allow the diagnosis of DVT in the leg veins will allow identification of the vast majority of patients at high risk of embolism.

The three factors which promote DVT (and, therefore, embolic risk), as defined by Virchow in the nineteenth century, are stasis, abnormalities of the vessel wall, and alterations in the blood coagulation system. Coagulation alterations have been studied extensively, but as yet there is no reliable test for a state of "hypercoagulability," i.e., a test which will predict the risk of DVT (except for the infrequent patients with antithrombin III, protein C, or protein S deficiencies or cystinuria). In the absence of such a test, the risk of DVT is best assessed by recognizing the presence of known "clinical" risk factors. Conditions associated with a high risk of venous thromboembolism include the postpartum period, left and right ventricular failure, fractures or other injuries of the lower extremities, chronic deep venous insufficiency of the legs, prolonged bed rest, carcinoma, obesity, and the use of estrogens.

NATURAL HISTORY In the contexts noted above, deep venous thrombi usually develop in the region of a venous valve. Platelets aggregate, forming a nidus (white thrombus), followed by development of a large fibrin (red) thrombus. The process is apparently a rapid one; large, extensive thrombi can develop within minutes. Growth occurs by continued fibrin and platelet accretion. Beyond formation, two processes may contribute to resolution: fibrinolysis and organization. Fibrinolysis may result in complete resolution within hours to several days. Any remaining thrombus undergoes organization, leaving behind a fibrotic zone that becomes reendothelialized. Valves are often rendered incompetent by this process, and modest or extensive luminal narrowing may occur. Once thrombus growth has halted, fibrinolysis/organization reaches a stable state in 7 to 10 days. It is during the first few days after formation, therefore, that embolic risk is highest.

DETECTION The clinical diagnosis of DVT is difficult. DVT is frequently present in the absence of clinical signs (e.g., pain, heat, swelling), and it is absent in 50 percent of patients in whom clinical signs or symptoms suggest its presence. Therefore a number of diagnostic tests have been developed. There are three reliable noninvasive procedures available for the early detection and follow-up of DVT: (1) impedance plethysmography (IPG), which detects venous outflow obstruction, is highly sensitive to above-knee thrombosis, but fails to detect many below-knee thrombi; (2) the Doppler technique, which is highly operator-dependent; (3) the radiofibrinogen method, which is very sensitive to thrombus formation in calf veins and lower thigh veins, but not sensitive to thrombi which form in the upper thigh or above (also, 24 h is required for a definitive answer). The IPG and radiofibrinogen tests correlate well with the definitive (but invasive) standard for the diagnosis of DVT, i.e., *ascending contrast phlebography.* The combination of IPG and radiofibrinogen leg scanning is equal in accuracy to contrast venography. Radiovenography and the use of ^{111}indium-labeled platelets await validation.

PROPHYLAXIS Application of these noninvasive approaches to the early diagnosis and follow-up of patients at high risk of DVT has led to significant changes in the approach to the prevention of DVT (and therefore of PTE). One validated prophylactic method is the use of small doses of subcutaneous heparin. Multiple studies, utilizing chiefly radiolabeled fibrinogen, have shown the high incidence of DVT in certain groups: patients over the age of 40 years with fractures of the pelvis and/or lower extremities; patients with myocardial infarction and/or severe congestive heart failure; patients undergoing major abdominal, thoracic, or gynecologic surgery. Furthermore, in the last group of patients, investigations have demonstrated a significant reduction in the incidence of DVT, PTE, and lethal PTE when heparin is given subcutaneously, in a dose of 5000 units every 12 h, beginning *before* operation (or on admission to the hospital) and continued until the patient is ambulatory. There is general agreement that this prophylactic approach, which has limited effect on coagulation tests and is associated with little risk of hemorrhage, should also be applied to *medical* patients at high risk of DVT and PTE. In the case of acute myocardial infarction, high risk would be imposed by the development of congestive failure, the presence of severe obesity, chronic venous insufficiency, or a prior history of DVT or PTE. Devices which compress the calf intermittently (usually once a minute) appear an effective alternative for prophylaxis in patients at risk of hemorrhage with low-dose heparin (neurosurgery, spinal cord trauma) or in whom low-dose heparin has proved ineffective (hip surgery, prostate surgery).

NATURAL HISTORY OF EMBOLISM

THE ACUTE EVENTS The immediate result of thromboembolism is complete or partial obstruction of the pulmonary arterial blood flow to the distal lung. This obstruction leads to a series of pathophysiologic events which can be categorized as the "respiratory" and "hemodynamic" consequences of PTE.

Respiratory consequences Embolic obstruction produces a zone of the lung which is ventilated but not perfused—an intrapulmonary "dead space" (Chap. 200). Because it cannot participate in the process of gas exchange, ventilation of this nonperfused area is "wasted," in the functional sense. A potential consequence of embolic obstruction is constriction of the air spaces and airways in the affected lung zone. This pneumoconstriction, which might be viewed as a homeostatic mechanism to reduce wasted ventilation, appears to be due to the marked bronchoalveolar hypocapnia that results from cessation of pulmonary capillary blood flow, because it is abolished by inhalation of carbon dioxide–enriched air. While it occurs in animal experiments in which a double-lumen tube separates the ventilation from each lung, it probably occurs very rarely in patients who inhale dead space air (rich in carbon dioxide) into embolized lung zones.

Another disturbance caused by embolic obstruction—loss of alveolar surfactant—does not occur immediately. This surface-active lipoprotein is required to maintain alveolar stability. In its absence, alveolar collapse occurs. Cessation of pulmonary capillary blood flow leads to reduction in surfactant within 2 or 3 h, which becomes severe at 12 to 15 h. Frank atelectasis—the morphologic expression of alveolar instability—can be detected at 24 to 48 h after interruption of blood flow.

Arterial hypoxemia is a common, though by no means universal, consequence of embolism. Several mechanisms can contribute to hypoxemia: ventilation-perfusion disturbances; cardiac failure with a lowered mixed venous P_{O_2} (widened arteriovenous difference); and obligatory perfusion through hypoventilated lung zones. Such obligatory perfusion develops because elevation of pulmonary arterial pressure due to embolic obstruction can overcome the vasoconstriction normally present in hypoventilated lung zones.

Hemodynamic consequences The primary hemodynamic consequence of thromboembolic obstruction is a reduction in the cross-sectional area of the pulmonary arterial bed. This loss of vascular capacity increases the resistance to pulmonary blood flow, which, if marked, leads to pulmonary hypertension and acute failure of the right ventricle. Tachycardia and often a decline in cardiac output also occur.

The factors which determine the severity of these hemodynamic changes have been the subject of continued debate. There is agreement that the *extent of embolic obstruction* is a key factor. However, the reserve capacity of the pulmonary arteriocapillary bed is so extensive that more than 50 percent of the vascular area must be obstructed before significant elevation in pulmonary arterial pressure results. Because pulmonary hypertension occurs in some patients with occlusion of lesser extent, investigators have searched for reflex or humoral vasoconstrictor mechanisms associated with embolism. Despite long and careful search for such mechanisms, their extent and frequency in human PTE remains unknown. Hence, some workers maintain that the degree of embolic obstruction itself is the only determinant of hemodynamic impairment. They suggest that instances of apparent disparity between the extent of embolism and clinical response reflect only clinical underestimation of the magnitude of the embolism. Other investigators, however, have presented compelling evidence to support the occurrence of pulmonary vasoconstriction with embolism. Some have demonstrated that constriction is associated with obstruction of the smaller, but not the larger, pulmonary arterial vessels. Another thesis holds that serotonin or thromboxane, known pulmonary vasoconstrictive-bronchoconstrictive substances, are released from platelets, which coat fresh emboli as they lodge in the pulmonary tree. This thesis introduces the attractive concept that an embolus might be regarded, in part, as a packet with pharmacologic, as well as obstructive, potential. A consensus view is that, while the extent of embolism is a key factor, humoral and/or reflex influences probably operate in certain patients and compromise the pulmonary circulation to a greater extent than might be expected on an anatomic basis alone.

The cardiopulmonary status of the patient prior to embolism is also critical in determining the clinical severity of embolism. A small embolus may have limited impact upon an otherwise healthy individual but may have serious consequences in someone with advanced cardiac or pulmonary disease.

Both experimental and clinical studies have established that infarction—death of lung tissue—rarely accompanies embolic occlusion. It is likely that less than 10 percent of emboli in humans lead to infarction. That infarction rarely follows embolism should occasion little surprise. The lung has three avenues for obtaining oxygen: the pulmonary arterial circulation, the bronchial arterial circulation, and the airways. Thus, infarction occurs infrequently, and its appearance usually is associated with compromise of bronchial arterial flow and/or airways to the involved area. Such compromise is promoted by the existence of other cardiac or pulmonary diseases, such as left ventricular failure, mitral stenosis, and chronic obstructive lung disease. Thus, infarction may occur in 30 percent or more of such patients, while it is quite rare in individuals who are free of cardiopulmonary disease.

BEYOND THE ACUTE STATE The vast majority of pulmonary emboli resolve, and resolve rather quickly. Resolution of fresh emboli begins within the first few days and is well advanced in 10 to 14 days. As in DVT, two mechanisms promote restoration of vascular patency: the fibrinolytic system and the process of organization. However, the fibrinolytic system appears capable of more rapid dissolution of emboli than of venous thrombi.

The availability of these two efficient mechanisms raises the question as to why not all emboli resolve. There may be some impairment of the intrinsic fibrinolytic system. The emboli may have been well organized prior to their lodgment in the lung so that they are subject to neither fibrinolytic attack nor further organization. Alternatively, some emboli may be recurrent, so that their failure to resolve is more apparent than real.

Another important element of the natural history of thromboembolism is the development of bronchial arterial collateral circulation. If pulmonary arterial obstruction persists, bronchial arterial flow increases substantially over a period of several weeks, restoring flow to the capillary bed. With the return of flow, surfactant production is restored, so that alveolar stability is regained and atelectasis resolves.

DIAGNOSTIC FEATURES

While sequential studies of patients with venous thrombosis have demonstrated that embolism can occur without causing symptoms, *sudden onset of unexplained dyspnea* is the most common, and often the only symptom of pulmonary embolism. *Pleuritic chest pain and hemoptysis are present only when infarction has occurred* and, because bland embolism rarely leads to infarction, are usually absent.

With extensive embolism, severe substernal oppressive discomfort may be present, probably due to right ventricular ischemia. Patients also may present with syncope, suggesting a neurologic disorder. Other "occult" presentations in which embolism should be considered include repetitive bouts of otherwise unexplained supraventricular tachyarrhythmias; sudden onset or worsening of congestive heart failure (Chap. 182); sudden deterioration in the patient with chronic obstructive lung disease; and as an alternative to the diagnosis of "psychic" (anxiety-associated) hyperventilation. The most reliable symptom, however, is breathlessness. Severe, persistent dyspnea is an ominous sign, for it usually indicates extensive embolic occlusion.

PHYSICAL EXAMINATION Findings on physical examination, like the history, may be deceptively normal. Examination of the lungs may disclose a few atelectatic rales; localized wheezes rarely are heard. A pleural friction rub or evidence of pleural effusion will not be present unless infarction has occurred.

On cardiac examination, the single consistent finding is tachycardia. Only in the rare cases of massive embolism will signs such as a right ventricular gallop, a palpable "lift" over the right ventricle (along the left sternal border), a loud pulmonary closure sound, or prominent *a* waves in the jugular venous pulse be found. A scratchy systolic ejection-type murmur may be heard in the pulmonic area. Also, a systolic or continuous murmur accentuated by inspiration may be audible over the lung fields. These murmurs appear to be generated by turbulence of flow in vessels partially obstructed by emboli since they disappear after resection or resolution of emboli. They should be carefully sought in any patient suspected of having PTE. Wide splitting of the second heart sound may be present. This indicates extensive embolic obstruction and implies both severe pulmonary hypertension and right ventricular failure. As embolic resolution occurs, this finding disappears. Absence of an accentuated pulmonic closure sound is not a reliable guide to the severity of PTE, since when embolism is sufficiently massive to reduce cardiac output, pulmonary closure may be normal or diminished.

The detection of *deep venous thrombosis* qualifies as an excellent clue to the diagnosis of embolism, but its absence does not exclude embolism. Even when sought with diligence, *clinical* evidence of thrombophlebitis is found in less than half of patients with PTE. *Fever* in patients with pulmonary embolism is uncommon without complicating infection or infarction. With infarction, fever of 37.8 to 38.3°C (oral) is the rule; but temperature elevations to 39°C or above may occur, making the differentiation between pulmonary infarction and infection difficult.

On clinical grounds alone, then, a firm diagnosis of embolism cannot be made; the clinical *suspicion* of embolism requires confirmation by laboratory studies (Fig. 211-1).

LABORATORY STUDIES Routine laboratory studies contribute little toward the diagnosis. Leukocytosis and elevation of the sedimentation rate are rarely present in the absence of infarction. A variety of other blood tests, such as assay for specific fibrinopeptides, fibrin degradation products, or enzymes, have been proposed; none has been shown to be diagnostically sensitive or specific.

Aside from tachycardia, the *electrocardiogram* is normal in most patients. With extensive embolization, there may be evidence of acute pulmonary hypertension, rightward shift of the QRS axis, a tall, peaked P wave, and ST-T changes indicative of right ventricular strain (Chap. 178). These changes are often transient, lasting minutes to hours, but when persistent, suggest severe pulmonary vascular obstruction.

The *chest roentgenogram* may show a parenchymal infiltrate and evidence of a pleural effusion if *infarction* has occurred. Characteristically, the infiltrates caused by infarction abut against the pleura. However, their shape varies, and they do not usually appear until 12 to 36 h after the embolism has occurred. The effusion, which often

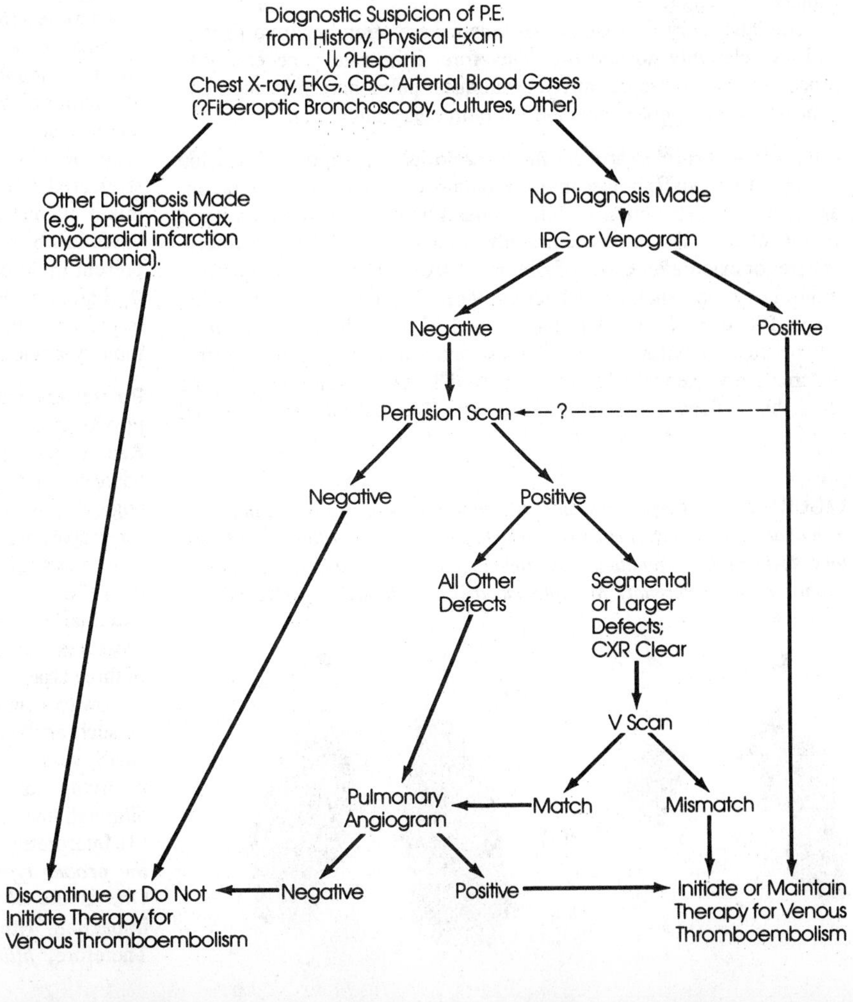

FIGURE 211-1 *Flow chart used in diagnosis of pulmonary embolism (PE). IPG, impedance plethysmogram; V scan, ventilation scan.*

precedes the infiltrate, is characteristically small. Thoracentesis usually, but by no means invariably, yields hemorrhagic fluid, with the characteristics of an exudate.

The radiographic findings with embolism alone are more subtle. *Differences in diameter between vessels which should be of equivalent size* should raise the suspicion of embolism. For example, embolic obstruction of the right main pulmonary artery can lead to dilation of the left main pulmonary artery because that vessel must accept the entire pulmonary flow. There may be *abrupt "cutoff"* of a vessel; i.e., as the vessel is traced distally, it suddenly disappears. Clot has the same radiodensity as blood, accounting for the proximal shadow; the absence of flow beyond the clot explains the sudden radiographic "disappearance" of the vessel.

Organization of a clot within a pulmonary artery may lead to retraction of the vessel's walls and a so-called rattail configuration, in which the vessel is relatively normal proximally and suddenly tapers to a sharp point. Finally, there may be *abnormal radiolucency* in some lung zones due to absent or decreased flow. Such abnormally lucent areas, indicative of proximal arterial obstruction, are best appreciated by examining comparable areas in the two lung fields.

Even in embolization without infarction, the roentgenogram may show small infiltrates, which appear in about 24 h and reflect atelectasis secondary to surfactant depletion. They are not associated with effusion, may fail to touch a pleural surface, and disappear without the linear scarring characteristic of infarction. It should be emphasized that a *normal chest roentgenogram does not exclude the diagnosis of PTE.* Indeed, a *normal* chest roentgenogram is the *most common* finding in embolic disease.

Analysis of arterial blood gases Massive embolism is commonly associated with arterial hypoxemia, hypocapnia, and respiratory alkalosis. In addition, the difference between alveolar P_{CO_2} and arterial P_{CO_2} ($PA_{CO_2} - Pa_{CO_2}$) may be widened owing to the increase in alveolar dead space (Chap. 200). However, a normal P_{O_2} does not exclude the diagnosis.

The laboratory tests discussed thus far are often negative in PTE and are relatively nonspecific. Therefore, it is usually necessary to proceed to two more definitive techniques: pulmonary perfusion and ventilation radiophotoscans and the pulmonary angiogram.

Pulmonary perfusion and ventilation scintiphotography Perfusion scintiphotographs (photoscans) are obtained by gamma camera imaging of the distribution of intravenously injected, gamma-emitting radionuclides. The most commonly used radionuclides are microspheres or macroaggregates of albumin (MAA), labeled with a gamma-emitting isotope such as technetium 99m. The radioactive particles, 50 to 100 μm in diameter, are trapped in the pulmonary capillary bed because the pulmonary capillaries approximate 10 μm in diameter. Alternatively, xenon 133 gas, dissolved in saline solution, may be used, but patients must hold their breath. The distribution of labeled particles entrapped in capillaries, or of xenon 133 evolved from them, accurately depicts the distribution of pulmonary blood flow.

The camera-generated perfusion image can be recorded on radiographic film, on special photographic film, on a television screen, or on videotape. Normal scans exhibit homogeneous distribution of radioactivity, smooth margins, and a configuration which corresponds to the normal anatomy of the lungs. Any deviation from these characteristics requires explanation because it represents an abnormality in blood flow distribution.

The perfusion lung photoscan is quite valuable in the diagnosis of embolism. A properly performed perfusion scan which is *normal* excludes the diagnosis of clinically significant pulmonary embolism. On the other hand, a scan demonstrating zones of absent or sharply decreased radioactivity in the patient whose other findings are compatible with PTE keeps the diagnosis of embolism among the possibilities. Scanning is simple, safe, and rapid. It can be repeated to define the resolution, or recurrence, of obstructive vascular phenomena. Like any laboratory test, however, the photoscan must be applied and interpreted with care. It is important, for example, to obtain multiple scan views because lesions not apparent in one view may be easily detected in others. Furthermore, the lung photoscan demonstrates only abnormalities of the *distribution of blood flow.* It does not provide anatomic information. Many disorders other than PTE are associated with abnormalities in the distribution of pulmonary blood flow. Any disease process, such as pneumonia, atelectasis, or pneumothorax, which reduces the ventilation of a lung zone will decrease its perfusion. Parenchymal diseases, such as emphysema, sarcoidosis, bronchogenic carcinoma, and tuberculosis, can all produce scan defects. Therefore a perfusion defect lacks specificity. One approach to enhancing specificity is the performance of a ventilation scan, best achieved by having patients breathe a radioactive gas such as xenon 127 or xenon 133. To assist in deciding whether a ventilation scan may be useful and when pulmonary angiography is required, two factors should be considered: the size of the perfusion defect(s) and the chest roentgenographic findings. If all defects are subsegmental in size *or* if all defects (of any size) are limited to areas of roentgenographic infiltration, ventilation scanning will not be useful, and pulmonary angiography is required. If defect(s) are segmental or larger in size, and one or more are in areas clear by x-ray, a ventilation scan should be done. If the radioactive gas enters ("washes in") and is cleared ("washes out") from the area(s) of perfusion defect(s), this "mismatch" of ventilation and perfusion is characteristic of vascular obstruction (Fig. 211-2). Pulmonary vascular obstruction is present in 90 percent or more of patients with this pattern. However, if ventilation is also abnormal (i.e., ventilation-perfusion "match" is present), no reliable diagnostic conclusion can be reached; pulmonary angiography is required.

Pulmonary angiography This is the only established means for providing anatomic information about the pulmonary vasculature. Radiopaque material is injected, preferably through a cardiac catheter advanced into the pulmonary artery. Cardiac catheterization and angiography require specialized personnel, and a reasonable period for preparation and performance, and they entail more risk than the procedures discussed above. However, angiography provides a visual image of the pulmonary vessels, and catheterization can provide potentially important hemodynamic data (pulmonary artery and wedge pressures, cardiac output). Interpretive limitations of angiography are of three types: (1) *Injection artifacts* may occur which suggest absence of flow to a vessel. Injection should be repeated whenever the question of such artifacts exists. (2) The inability to evaluate the patency of small vessels is another limitation. Emboli in vessels below the resolving capability of the method cannot be detected with certainty, although magnification techniques can extend resolving capability. (3) Interpretive errors may also be a consequence of *not looking for the proper type of defect.* There are only two diagnostic findings. One is the *abrupt "cutoff"* of a vessel at the point of embolic impaction. However, complete embolic obstruction is uncommon. Therefore, *filling defects* are the most frequent finding; i.e., the

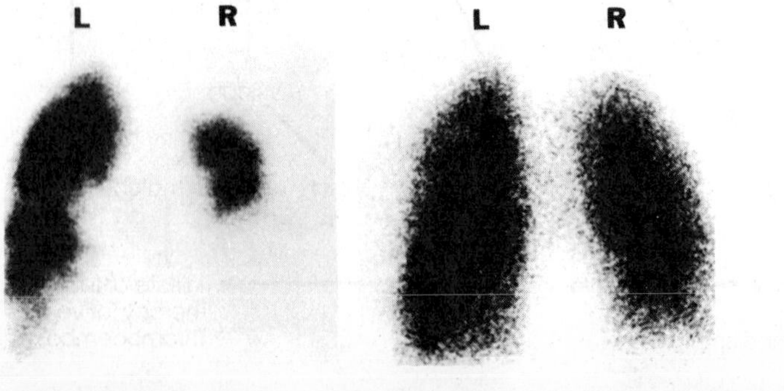

FIGURE 211-2 *Perfusion scan (left), posterior view, shows multiple segmental and larger perfusion defects in right upper and lower lobes, left lower lobe, and lingula. Ventilation scan (right) is normal at equilibrium. Xenon[133] washed in and out normally. Multiple emboli were confirmed angiographically. L, left; R, right.*

embolus creates a "negative" shadow as the radiopaque material flows around it. The major contraindication to angiography is the absence of personnel who are experienced in both performing the procedure and interpreting the results. Serious diagnostic errors are commonplace if optimal techniques are not used or the complexities of interpretation are not appreciated. However, the risks of angiography are low in experienced hands. Injection of large boluses of contrast medium into the main pulmonary artery should be avoided in favor of small injections into vessels supplying lung regions identified as abnormal on the perfusion scan.

How far one should proceed down the diagnostic pathway outlined above depends on many factors, the major ones being the presence or absence of documented venous thrombosis, the severity of the patient's symptoms, and the hazards of contemplated therapy. In each condition, there is a need for precise diagnosis. If IPG or venography already has documented deep venous thrombosis, one is committed to anticoagulant therapy; thus, proceeding beyond perfusion scanning is rarely necessary. This means that evaluation for venous thrombosis is an integral part of the evaluation of the embolic suspect. Unfortunately, the absence of venous thrombosis cannot be used to exclude the diagnosis of pulmonary embolism. More than 20 percent of patients with embolism have no evidence of venous thrombosis, apparently because the entire venous thrombus has embolized. Therefore, in such patients, if symptoms are severe and/or the hazards of therapy are substantial, diagnostic precision is mandatory, and there should be no hesitancy in proceeding to angiography. Substantial hazards of therapy which mandate angiography include a high risk of bleeding on, or absolute contraindication to, anticoagulant therapy and consideration of embolectomy, thrombolytic therapy, or vena caval interruption.

TREATMENT

Initial intravenous administration of heparin is the therapy of choice for PTE. With a strong *suspicion* of embolism based on clinical and routine laboratory tests, such therapy should be instituted immediately, without awaiting diagnostic confirmation, unless the initial dose of heparin places the patient at clear risk (i.e., in patients with recent or active bleeding or a known hemostatic defect). Except in such patients, heparin therapy should not await diagnostic confirmation; one can always stop therapy if such confirmation is not forthcoming.

There is consensus regarding the goals of therapy in both DVT and PTE: (1) immediate inhibition of the growth of thromboemboli, (2) promotion of thromboembolic resolution, and (3) prevention of recurrence. Heparin achieves the first goal; it encourages the second by allowing fibrinolytic dissolution to be achieved unopposed by thrombus growth; and it assists in, although it does not ensure, prevention of recurrence. In addition, heparin inhibits platelet aggregation (and therefore potential release of thromboxane and serotonin) at the embolic site, and its anticoagulant action is promptly reversible.

There is *not* consensus, however, regarding (1) heparin regimens which best combine safety and efficacy; (2) the need for, and type of, tests for monitoring coagulation behavior during heparin therapy; (3) how long, and with what agents, antithrombotic therapy should be maintained; or (4) in which patients thrombolytic therapy should antedate antithrombotic therapy.

REGIMENS In DVT, three methods of heparin administration have been advocated by various investigators: continuous intravenous, intermittent intravenous, intermittent subcutaneous. Continuous intravenous heparin is usually given in a dose of approximately 1000 units per hour. Intermittent intravenous heparin is commonly given in a dose of approximately 5000 units every 4 h or 7500 every 6 h. Subcutaneous heparin has been recommended as a dose of 5000 units every 4 h, 10,000 every 8 h, or 20,000 every 12 h. Studies exist which indicate that each of these regimens is more efficacious, safer, or both. Therefore, at this time, one can conclude only that *each* of these regimens (which approximate 30,000 units per 24 h) represents an acceptable treatment regimen. At present, the continuous intravenous regimen, delivered by an infusion pump, is the most popular. *Intramuscular* injection of heparin is to be avoided because hematomas will develop.

In PTE, the same options for heparin therapy exist. The only additional question is whether an initial large intravenous bolus (10,000 to 20,000 units) should be given to inhibit the aggregation (and release reaction) of platelets adherent to the embolus. Most workers advocate such a dose, with one of the "standard" regimens being started 2 to 4 h later.

MONITORING The value of clotting times (CT), partial thromboplastin times (PTT), or other coagulation tests to monitor heparin effect and guide alterations in dose is not clearly established. The risk of hemorrhage (the principal complication of heparin therapy) is not clearly related to coagulation test alterations; rather, it appears related to factors such as the coexistence of other diseases associated with bleeding risk (gastric or duodenal ulcer, coagulopathies, uremia) and advanced age. Likewise, achievement of the desired effect of heparin (cessation of thrombus growth in vivo) has not been related to coagulation tests. Therefore, it is questionable whether monitoring with such tests is superior to empiric use of one of the regimens described above. While animal investigations have disclosed that maintaining the PTT above 1.5 times control does prevent growth of venous thrombi, such data are not available for human patients. If done improperly or poorly timed, the CT or PTT tests are worthless and may be misleading. If used appropriately, the usual objective is to keep the CT or PTT, measured *just prior to the next* intermittent dose, at or above 1.5 times the baseline CT or PTT and at 1.5 to 2.0 times control with continuous infusion.

DURATION OF THERAPY In DVT, one of the "full-dose" regimens is usually maintained for 7 to 10 days, the rationale being that this is the period required for dissolution and/or organization of the thrombus. In PTE, for the same reasons, a similar duration of therapy is advised. Bed rest is indicated until cardiopulmonary or leg symptoms subside. Carefully applied elastic support hose should be used (to encourage venous flow) as soon as leg pain, if present, subsides.

Beyond the acute phase, there are three therapeutic options available: cessation of heparin, maintenance of low-dose heparin, or initiation of therapy with *prothrombinopenic drugs*. In deciding among these options, it should be recognized that the question being addressed is: Does the patient need continued protection against the risk of *recurrent* DVT (and, therefore, PTE)? If the risk factor(s) that precipitated the acute episode of DVT-PTE is no longer present, the patient is asymptomatic, and the IPG is normal, it is acceptable to reduce heparin to a lower dose starting on day 7, ambulate the patient, and, if no symptoms develop, discontinue heparin on day 9 or 10. If these criteria are not met, prolonged prophylactic therapy is warranted. There is no consensus regarding the optimal duration of such therapy because firm data on this point are lacking. If *reversible* risk factors are present (e.g., immobilization after a leg fracture), therapy should be continued until the risk factors present have resolved. If the risk factors present are nonreversible (e.g., severe left and/or right ventricular failure) or if the IPG remains positive, empiric decisions are made. At a minimum, 3 months of therapy seems wise because recurrence is relatively common during this period. Beyond 3 months, however, continuation depends upon the balance among specific risk factors exhibited by the patient, IPG results, and the risks of continued therapy. In some instances, this balance may warrant lifetime maintenance on anticoagulant drugs.

Prothrombinopenic drugs are not suitable for initial therapy in thromboembolism. Their only role is in maintaining anticoagulant protection for prolonged periods. If prothrombinopenic drugs are to be used, the patient should be "in range" as defined by a prothrombin time 1.5 to 2.0 times the control time for 3 to 5 days before heparin is discontinued. An alternative to the prothrombinopenic agents is the use of self-injected subcutaneous heparin. Current data suggest that a dose of 7500 to 10,000 units every 12 h is adequate for this type of prophylaxis, is well tolerated, and need not be monitored with coagulation tests.

Thrombolytic (fibrinolytic) agents such as streptokinase and urokinase can hasten the resolution of venous thrombi and pulmonary emboli. They do not replace antithrombotic therapy. When used, thrombolytic agents must be followed by a standard course of antithrombotic therapy. Despite extensive study and a clear demonstration that these agents can enhance the speed of resolution, it has not been established that their use alters the short- or long-term morbidity or mortality rates among patients with either DVT or PTE. Both drugs are associated with hemorrhagic risk, particularly in patients who recently have had, or require, any invasive procedure (e.g., venipuncture, arterial puncture, angiography, Swan-Ganz catheterization). If they do offer a therapeutic advantage, it would appear to be (1) in patients with extensive, large-vein DVT (e.g., iliofemoral); and (2) in patients with massive embolism and persistent systemic hypotension in whom embolectomy would otherwise be contemplated. The potential role of new thrombolytic agents (e.g., tissue plasminogen activator), which may pose less hemorrhagic risk and allow the concomitant use of heparin, remains to be determined.

Surgical therapy for DVT (thrombectomy) is now rarely considered because the results have not been encouraging. In PTE, surgical therapy should be reserved for those patients in whom heparin therapy is deemed inadequate or impractical. Anticoagulant therapy may be contraindicated by the presence of a bleeding diathesis, or the patient may be in such critical condition that it is felt unwise to await a response to medical therapy. In such instances *venous interruption* and *pulmonary embolectomy* must be considered.

The objective of venous interruption is to prevent immediate recurrence of embolism. Ligation of the superficial femoral vein offers no protection against embolization from the deep femoral venous system, and ligation of the common femoral vein is unacceptable because of severe obstruction to venous drainage. Furthermore, these procedures must be bilateral to grant protection from a suspected embolic focus in the legs. For these reasons, interruption of the inferior vena cava has replaced more distal ligation procedures. A number of surgical procedures have been applied to the inferior vena cava: simple ligation; plication, in which fine channels are preserved; and the application of totally or partially occlusive clips or filters. Nonsurgical interruption also can be accomplished by introducing "umbrella," balloon, or filter devices, attached to catheters, into the inferior vena cava via neck or upper extremity veins. Each procedure has advantages and disadvantages. For example, total interruption leads to a transient fall in cardiac output and variable degrees of edema of the legs; successful plication does not prevent small emboli from reaching the lungs; devices introduced into the inferior vena cava may migrate upward or be badly placed. Unfortunately, no form of inferior vena caval interruption precludes embolic recurrence. There are several reasons for this: sizable collateral channels develop weeks to months after complete occlusion of the cava, through which embolization may recur; thromboembolism may originate at the site of caval manipulation; caval blockade does not prevent embolization from foci within the right cardiac chambers; small emboli may traverse clips, filters, or plications, and such devices may themselves thrombose. Therefore, because most pulmonary emboli do resolve, caval interruption should be regarded as a *lifesaving procedure* to be restricted to patients who could not tolerate an *immediate* embolic recurrence or those with documented venous thrombosis in whom anticoagulant therapy is contraindicated.

There is one instance, however, in which prompt caval ligation is the therapy of choice: septic thrombophlebitis of pelvic origin with multiple septic pulmonary emboli. If these patients do not respond promptly to a heparin-antibiotic regimen, they may die unless caval (and left ovarian vein) ligation is carried out promptly.

Two criteria should be met before emergency pulmonary embolectomy is performed: (1) there must be evidence of severe hemodynamic compromise due to embolism, particularly sustained systemic hypotension, which is not responsive to supportive measures; and (2) the personnel and equipment required for embolectomy carried out with the aid of cardiopulmonary bypass must be available.

SPECIAL CONSIDERATIONS Total resolution of emboli does not always occur. If residual vascular obstruction is substantial, the patient may present, months or years after the actual embolic events, with dyspnea and pulmonary hypertension of uncertain cause, often with right ventricular failure. Such patients commonly are misdiagnosed, for months or years, as having "asthma," "chronic lung disease," "primary" pulmonary hypertension (Chap. 210), or cor pulmonale of unclear etiology (Chap. 191).

Such patients should be studied by appropriate techniques, since emboli in the main or lobar arteries can be surgically removed (thromboendarterectomy), allowing cure of this otherwise fatal form of pulmonary hypertensive disease.

PROGNOSIS IN PULMONARY EMBOLISM The prognosis of the patient with pulmonary embolism *in whom therapy is promptly instituted* is excellent. As stated at the outset of this chapter, less than 1 embolic event in 10 is lethal. The majority of these deaths occur suddenly and can be avoided only by prophylaxis (see above). The remainder appear to be due to embolic extension or recurrence, which therapy can moderate. Thus, for patients who survive long enough to reach medical attention and receive heparin, the outlook is quite good. Morbidity following embolism is uncommon since embolic resolution is the rule, and few patients develop the pulmonary hypertensive problem noted above.

Limited reliable data are available regarding recurrence rates in the months and years after a single embolic event (with or without prolonged postembolic anticoagulant therapy). In the absence of risk factors, or a positive IPG, recurrence appears to be uncommon, but more precise data are needed.

NONTHROMBOTIC EMBOLISM

Because the lung vasculature serves as a filter of the venous circulation, it is the recipient of diverse materials which can gain entry into venous blood, including bone marrow, foreign bodies, parasites, and tumor cells. The most frequently encountered form of nonthrombotic embolism is *fat embolism.* This dramatic and controversial entity follows the introduction of neutral fat into the venous circulation, most commonly after bone trauma or fracture (marrow fat), but occasionally after trauma to adipose tissue or liver infiltrated by fat. The clinical sequence is characteristic. After a latent period of 12 to 36 h or more, during which the patient is asymptomatic, sudden cardiopulmonary and neurologic deterioration appears. Mental aberrations, delirium, and coma develop. Dyspnea, tachypnea, and tachycardia occur, and the chest roentgenographic and physiologic components of the "adult respiratory distress syndrome" appear (see Chap. 216). Anemia and thrombocytopenia are common, as are petechiae on the upper thorax and arms. The pathogenesis of the syndrome is not clear, but it seems likely that two events occur: release of free fatty acids (by action of lipases on the neutral fat), which induces a toxic vasculitis, followed by platelet-fibrin thrombosis; and actual obstruction of small pulmonary arteries by macroaggregates of fat. Several forms of therapy have been proposed (corticosteroids, heparin, ethanol), but none has proved effective; treatment remains supportive and mortality rate high.

Another dramatic form of nonthrombotic embolism is *amniotic fluid embolism.* This occurs during both spontaneous delivery and cesarean section. Sudden and massive obstruction of the pulmonary microvasculature occurs, leading to shock and, often, death. With survival of the initial phase of the disease, the picture of disseminated intravascular coagulation appears. The syndrome is due to the entrance of a significant quantity of amniotic fluid into the venous circulation. This fluid is a potent thromboplastic agent which induces thrombosis in the pulmonary vasculature and elsewhere. The fluid also contains particulates which lodge in the lung. Treatment consists of supportive measures.

Nonembolic pulmonary arterial obstruction due to *vasculitis* has become a common problem among intravenous drug users. This vasculitis, caused by the drugs per se or materials (e.g., talc) mixed with the drugs, can induce thrombosis. This entity may be difficult to distinguish from PTE. Repetitive episodes may lead to irreversible and severe pulmonary hypertension.

REFERENCES

FEDULLO PF et al: [111]-Indium labelled platelets: Effect of heparin on uptake by venous thrombi and relationship to the activated partial thromboplastin time. Circulation 66:632, 1982

FISHMAN AP, KELLEY MA: Pulmonary thromboembolism (including prophylaxis, treatment, sickle cell disease and multiple pulmonary thrombi), in *Pulmonary Diseases and Disorders,* 2d ed, AP Fishman (ed). New York, McGraw-Hill, 1987, Chap 66.

GOLDHABER SZ (ed): *Pulmonary Embolism and Deep Venous Thrombosis*. Philadelphia, Saunders, 1985

HULL R et al: Pulmonary angiography, ventilation lung scanning and venography for clinically suspected pulmonary embolism in the abnormal perfusion scan. Ann Intern Med 98:891, 1983

——— et al: Adjusted subcutaneous heparin versus warfarin sodium in the long-term treatment of venous thrombosis. N Engl J Med 305:189, 1982

——— et al: Combined use of leg scanning and impedance plethysmography in suspected venous thrombosis. N Engl J Med 296:1497, 1977

KAKKAR VV et al: Prevention of post-operative embolism by low-dose heparin: An international multicenter trial. Lancet 2:45, 1975

KIPPER MS et al: Long-term follow-up of patients with suspected pulmonary embolism and a normal lung scan. Chest 82:411, 1982

MERCANDETTI A et al: Influence of perfusion and ventilation scans on therapeutic decision-making and outcome among embolic suspects. West J Med 142:208, 1985

MOSER KM: Pulmonary vascular obstruction due to embolism and thrombosis, in *Pulmonary Vascular Disease,* KM Moser (ed). New York, Dekker, 1979, p 341

——— et al: Chronic thrombotic obstruction of major pulmonary arteries: Results of thromboendarterectomy in 15 patients. Ann Intern Med 99:299, 1983

———, FEDULLO PF: Venous thromboembolism: Three simple decisions. Chest 83:117, 256, 1983

SALZMAN EW et al: Intraoperative external pneumatic calf compression to afford long-term prophylaxis against deep vein thrombosis in urologic patients. Surgery 87:239, 1980

SASAHARA AA, DALEN JE: Controversy: Should fibrinolytic drugs be used to treat acute pulmonary embolism? J Cardiovasc Med 5:793, 1980

212 DISEASES OF THE UPPER RESPIRATORY TRACT

LOUIS WEINSTEIN

Disorders of the upper respiratory tract (nose, nasopharynx, paranasal sinuses, and larynx) are among the commonest forms of human illness. In most instances, they result in discomfort which is more annoying and distracting than disabling, and while they may interfere with the individual's function sufficiently to prevent participation in normal activities, usually they are not life-threatening and do not lead to serious chronic disability.

NOSE

ANOSMIA Total loss of olfactory sense is most common as a transient manifestation of acute infections of the upper respiratory tract. It may be present with chronic nasal obstruction due to edema of the mucosa or marked swelling of the turbinates and with congenital defects, ozena, tumors (see below), trauma involving the olfactory nerves, and nasal polyps.

RHINITIS AND NASAL OBSTRUCTION Intermittent or persistent nasal discharge may be caused by a variety of disorders, including hay fever, vasomotor rhinitis and complicating nasal polyposis, acute coryza, and other forms of viral rhinitis, the upper respiratory manifestations of measles, syphilis (the "snuffles" of the congenital disease), tuberculosis, and nasal diphtheria, intranasal foreign bodies, and chronic use of vasoconstrictor drugs.

Acute and self-limited nasal obstruction is usually associated with acute upper respiratory tract infections, most commonly viral. Hypertrophy and inflammation of the turbinates leading to nasal obstruction, with or without persistent nasal discharge, may be caused by allergic reactions. A common reason for difficulty in breathing through the nose is a *deviated septum*. Menstruation is associated, in some instances, with bogginess of the turbinates to a degree sufficient to produce retardation of airflow through the nose; pregnancy may produce the same phenomenon.

RHINORRHEA Although unilateral nasal discharge may be caused by intranasal foreign bodies, when it is intermittent or persistent, the possibility that it is due to *cerebrospinal fluid (CSF) rhinorrhea* must be considered. This condition may be diagnosed by injecting a marker such as a dye (fluorescein) or a radioactive tracer into the CSF and following its appearance in nasal secretions.

EPISTAXIS Probably the commonest cause is nose picking, leading to tearing of the rich network of veins in the anterior nares (Kiesselbach's plexus). Minor epistaxis may also appear in the course of viral infections of the upper respiratory tract. Among the more serious infections in which acute nosebleed may develop are typhoid fever, unilateral nasal diphtheria, pertussis, and malaria. Other causes of intermittent epistaxis are uncontrolled hypertension, vicarious menstruation, bleeding diatheses, polycythemia vera, rhinoliths, acute sinusitis especially involving the ethmoid sinus with thrombosis of the ethmoidal vein, tumors of the nose and paranasal sinuses, and nasal angiomas. Episodes of bleeding or the severity of attacks are frequently increased in patients receiving aspirin. Vitamin C and prothrombin deficiency are *not* associated with isolated epistaxis, although this may occur with bleeding from other sites. In hereditary hemorrhagic telangiectasia (Osler-Rendu-Weber syndrome) the only site of bleeding may be the nose; a family history of repeated hemorrhages from this and other sites should suggest this diagnosis.

NASAL FURUNCULOSIS Furuncles involving the internal or external surfaces of the nose pose potential threats to life because of the possibility of spread to the cavernous sinus via the draining veins. When seen in their early stage, they respond rapidly to antimicrobial therapy which should be directed primarily against *Staphylococcus aureus* and given in large doses (Chap. 94). Oral treatment may be adequate in the early stages of the disease, but parenteral therapy is necessary when the constitutional reaction is severe and there is marked edema of the intra- or extranasal tissues. *Under no circumstances should these lesions be squeezed* because of the danger of spread of organisms to intracranial venous sinuses. Also, incision for drainage should not be carried out unless pain becomes severe or the lesion has become large.

PHARYNX

ACUTE PHARYNGITIS The outstanding symptom of acute pharyngitis, regardless of cause, is a sore throat. About two-thirds of all acute illnesses in families are viral infections of the upper respiratory tract, with varying degrees of pharyngeal discomfort present. The acute pharyngitides can be classified into three groups: (1) treatable infections, (2) untreatable infections, and (3) noninfectious disorders (Table 212-1).

Physical examination of the pharyngeal mucosa may reveal changes varying in intensity from mild redness and congestion of blood vessels (many viral infections) to intense red-purple color, patchy yellow exudate, hypertrophy of all the lymphoid tissue, and marked vascular injection (e.g., severe disease due to group A *Streptococcus pyogenes*). Symptoms may be variable and may range from a complaint of "scratchy throat" to pain so severe that swallowing of saliva is difficult. In some cases, the lingual tonsils, situated on the posterolateral surface of the tongue, may be infected in the course of streptococcal pharyngitis. This causes pain on movement of the tongue. The presence of exudate does not establish a specific etiology and may be noted in infections due to *S. pyogenes, Haemophilus influenzae, H. parainfluenzae* (children), *Corynebacterium diphtheriae, and Streptococcus pneumoniae* (rare) as well as in some viral diseases, such as those caused by adenovirus and Epstein-Barr (EB) virus. Ulcerations involving the posterior pharyngeal wall and/or tonsils are characteristically present in fusobacterial infections (Plaut-Vincent's angina), pharyngeal tularemia, syphilis (primary chancre), tuberculosis, following local trauma to the pharynx, and in immunosuppressed and agranulocytic patients in whom invasion by fusobacteria or other members of the indigenous pharyngeal microflora takes place. The presence of limited or extensive pseudomembrane does not always indicate a specific microbial cause. While most characteristic of faucial diphtheria, such lesions may be present in infectious mononucleosis (EB virus), agranulocytosis, staphylococcal pharyngitis, and diffuse injury to the pharyngeal mucosa following direct trauma or chemical or thermal burns.

The tonsils are often involved in the course of viral and bacterial pharyngitis; they may be markedly reddened and swollen and contain exudate in the crypts.

The etiologic diagnosis of acute pharyngitis is difficult to establish on the basis of visual examination of the throat. However, in some instances in which characteristic findings are present, such as the typical pseudomembrane and suggestive odor of diphtheria, severe group A streptococcal infection, the ulceration and anaerobic odor of fusobacterial disease, or the white irregular patches overlying shallow ulcers produced by *Candida,* a specific cause may be suspected.

TABLE 212-1 Etiology of pharyngitis

I Infectious
- *A* Treatable
  - *1* Group A *Streptococcus pyogenes*
  - *2* *Hemophilus influenzae*
  - *3* *H. parainfluenzae*
  - *4* *Neisseria gonorrhoeae*
  - *5* *N. meningitidis*
  - *6* *Corynebacterium diphtheriae*
  - *7* *Spirochaeta pallida*
  - *8* *Fusobacterium*
  - *9* *F. tularensis*
  - *10* *Candida*
  - *11* *Cryptococcus*
  - *12* *Histoplasma*
  - *13* *Mycoplasma pneumoniae*
  - *14* *Streptococcus pneumoniae* (?)
  - *15* *Staphylococcus aureus* or gram-negative bacilli (usually found in neutropenic patients or those treated with antibiotics)
  - *16* *Chlamydia trachomatis*
- *B* Untreatable
  - *1* Primary
    - *a* Influenza virus
    - *b* Rhinovirus
    - *c* Coxsackievirus A
    - *d* Epstein-Barr virus
    - *e* Echovirus
    - *f* Herpes simplex
    - *g* Reovirus
  - 2 Manifestation of systemic disease
    - *a* Poliomyelitis
    - *b* Measles
    - *c* Chickenpox
    - *d* Smallpox
    - *e* Viral hepatitis
    - *f* Rubella
    - *g* Pertussis

II Noninfectious
- *A* Trauma by heat, sharp objects, etc.
- *B* Inhalation of irritants
- *C* Dehydration—mouth breathing
- *D* Glossopharyngeal neuralgia
- *E* Subacute thyroiditis (tends to be prolonged or frequently recurrent, often associated with low-grade fever)
- *F* Psychogenic
- *G* Monomyelocytic leukemia
- *H* Immunosuppressed state

Cultures of the pharyngeal mucosa, tonsils, or exudate will usually reveal the bacteria responsible for the disease and determine the choice of antimicrobial agent. It should be stressed, however, that these are not always rewarding. For example, only 70 percent of single throat cultures yield *S. pyogenes,* even when pharyngitis due to this organism is severe. Patients suspected of having streptococcal pharyngitis but whose throat cultures fail to yield the organism should be treated if this kind of disease is known to be present in the community. The sore throat of subacute thyroiditis may be relieved occasionally by the administration of thyroid hormone or prednisone. None of the viral pharyngitides is treatable.

Gonococcal pharyngitis is almost always the result of orogenital contact. The incidence of the disease in heterosexual men varies from 0.2 to 1.4 percent. It ranges from 5 to 25 percent in homosexual males; 20 percent of those with genital infection have simultaneous involvement of the throat. From 5 to 18 percent of women with other manifestations of gonorrhea have pharyngitis; in 1 to 3 percent this is the only disease. While mild to severe sore throat is present in about 30 percent of patients, the majority are asymptomatic. Because the clinical features of gonococcal pharyngitis may mimic disease produced by other organisms, the diagnosis is based on isolation and identification of *Neisseria gonorrhoeae.* The isolated organism must be confirmed as the gonococcus by its biologic properties because of the presence of other *Neisseria* in the pharynges of most normal individuals.

PERITONSILLAR CELLULITIS AND ABSCESS (QUINSY) This condition is most often a complication of acute pharyngitis. The organisms commonly involved are *S. pyogenes* and *Staphylococcus aureus.* The first sign of this disease is marked enlargement of the tonsils, which are surrounded by red, edematous pillars. The tonsillar and peritonsillar hypertrophy may progress to a degree threatening occlusion of the upper airway. High-grade fever and leukocytosis are present, and severe rigors may occur. In its early stages, the process is a cellulitis, but, in the absence of therapy, abscess develops as infection progresses and involves one or both tonsils; at this time, soft grayish-white exudate may cover the tonsillar surfaces. The diagnosis is made on the basis of the physical findings. If detected early when only peritonsillar cellulitis is present, administration of a properly selected antimicrobial agent may clear the infection and abort the development of abscess. Antimicrobial therapy alone is inadequate after abscess has developed. The optimal treatment at this stage is incision and drainage of the involved tonsil(s).

PARAPHARYNGEAL SPACE ABSCESS This syndrome is always a complication of acute pharyngitis. Primary or secondary bacterial invasion of one of the tonsils results in the development of an intratonsillar abscess accompanied by considerable edema and inflammatory reaction in the parapharyngeal space. The lesion is usually unilateral and the involved tonsil protrudes toward the midline; there is frequently very little pharyngeal discomfort, but there is marked tenderness at the angle of the jaw on the same side as the tonsillar abscess. The remainder of the throat frequently has a benign appearance. There is usually considerable fever and leukocytosis. If unrecognized and not treated early in its course, the infection spreads through the tonsillar veins to the jugular vein, where it produces thrombophlebitis. Septic emboli from this source may be widely disseminated and cause widespread metastatic thrombosis and infection with single or multiple abscesses of the lungs, a highly fatal syndrome termed *postanginal sepsis.* Early recognition and institution of therapy before spread to the jugular vein results in rapid clearing of the infection.

RETROPHARYNGEAL ABSCESS Although retropharyngeal abscess is most common in children under the age of 4 years because of the presence of lymph nodes in the retropharynx that may become infected in the course of acute pharyngitis, the disease also occurs in adults. The factors that predispose to the development of a retropharyngeal abscess in adults include acute infections of the ears, nose, and throat, dental disease, regional trauma such as ingestion of a foreign body, oroendotracheal intubation, endoscopic procedures, external penetrating injuries, fracture of vertebral bodies, and blunt trauma to the neck. Diabetes mellitus, a poor nutritional state, or immunosuppression may predispose to development of this infection in adults. A very important lesion that may lead to development of a retropharyngeal abscess in adults is cervical or cervicodorsal vertebral osteomyelitis complicated by the development of paravertebral abscess. Among the organisms responsible for the infection of the bone and the related abscess are *Mycobacterium tuberculosis,* pyogenic bacteria, and *Coccidiodes immitis.*

TUMORS AND OTHER CAUSES OF CHRONIC SORE THROAT Although not always associated with pharyngeal pain, some patients with various neoplastic diseases are troubled by a persistent sore throat. The fever which may be present is not always caused by microbial invasion but rather by the pyrogenic activity of the tumor itself. Carcinoma of the tonsil is the second commonest tumor of the upper airway (osteoma is most common, see below). Other neoplasms that involve the pharynx and may cause pain are nasopharyngeal carcinoma, multiple myeloma, myelomonocytic leukemia, and Hodgkin's disease. The solid tumors often involve only one tonsil; leukemia tends to produce diffuse pharyngitis. Treatment of the neoplasms may induce a persistent sore throat not present earlier. Immunosuppression induced by the drugs used to treat the tumors, and may lead to the development of mucositis, or infection by uncommon organisms such as *Aspergillus, Mucor, Actinomyces,* and *Pseudomonas.*

Among a number of benign causes of chronic sore throat is ''mouth breathing.'' Many elderly persons breathe through an open mouth while asleep, and when they wake experience pharyngeal discomfort which usually disappears with intake of fluids. Another group of ''mouth breathers'' are patients with severe obstruction of the nasal passages due to marked deviation of the septum. In them, the pharyngeal discomfort is constant and not relieved without surgical correction of the septum. Exposure to irritants like tobacco smoke in those who are heavy smokers of cigars and pipes may induce persistent sore throat. Subacute thyroiditis is often associated with severe pain in the pharynx that may persist for weeks to months. Patients often seek medical attention because of the severe pharyngitis and are unaware that this is a manifestation of inflammation of the thyroid. A helpful diagnostic finding is the normal appearance of the pharyngeal mucosa at the time when the pain is severe. Emotional disorders may occasionally be associated with chronic low-grade discomfort in the pharynx. A rare cause of severe and persistent pain in the throat is glossopharyngeal neuralgia.

SINUSES

ACUTE SINUSITIS The organisms most often responsible for acute sinusitis are *S. pneumoniae, S. pyogenes,* and *H. influenzae.* Other bacteria may be involved in patients receiving immunosuppressive therapy, in those who have received antibiotics, or in whom penetrating trauma, local tumors, or vasculitis is a predisposing factor. The etiology of chronic sinusitis may be the same as that of the acute form, but more than one pathogen may be present. In many instances, however, cultures yield only members of the indigenous microflora of the upper respiratory tract.

The commonest predisposing factor of acute purulent sinusitis is viral infection of the upper respiratory tract, which may lead to obstruction of drainage of the paranasal sinuses and the development of localized pain, tenderness, and low-grade fever. These manifestations usually clear as the viral disease subsides. In a number of instances, however, invasion by pyogenic bacteria supervenes and is responsible for the development of purulent sinusitis. Obstruction of meatal drainage of any type or direct introduction of bacteria into the sinuses may lead to the development of acute infection of the paranasal sinuses. Abscesses of the roots of the upper bicuspid or molar teeth that rupture into the maxillary sinuses, swimming and diving, and direct local injury may be inciting mechanisms. Fractures of the bones encompassing the sinuses, especially the frontals and ethmoids, may be followed by infection. Wegener's granulomatosis and tumors of the meatuses of the turbinates may produce the clinical picture of acute or chronic sinusitis. In some of these patients, bacterial infection is superimposed, and when these patients are studied only after infection develops, the underlying lesion is often overlooked. This underscores the fact that recurrent or prolonged episodes of sinusitis that are refractory to antimicrobial therapy, or that relapse soon after treatment is discontinued, must be investigated thoroughly for the presence of a noninfectious obstructing lesion.

The diagnosis of acute purulent sinusitis is usually made when constitutional manifestations are present, such as fever, chills, pain and tenderness of the involved sinuses, nasal obstruction, and recurrent headaches that change in intensity with position and disappear shortly after getting out of bed. Isolation of a pathogenic organism from the nasal secretions or from material draining into the meatuses of the nasal turbinates may help to solidify the diagnosis. When there is marked swelling of the turbinates, they can be shrunk by the local application of cocaine or other potent vasoconstrictors. This exposes the meatuses and permits the collection of exudate draining directly from the involved sinus. Transillumination of the sinuses is also helpful, while radiologic study is of value in identifying the specific sinus involved.

Effective management of acute sinusitis rests on demonstration of a specific pathogenic organism in the secretion present in the nose or drained from the sinuses, testing of the organism for sensitivity to a variety of antimicrobial agents, and administration of the most active agent in adequate doses (Chap. 88). Vasoconstrictors are of help in producing transient relief of symptoms but must not be used excessively. Surgical drainage may be indicated when infection becomes prolonged or local or intracranial complications develop.

Frontal sinusitis is characterized by pain over the forehead approximately in the area of the underlying sinus. Although the overlying site is usually normal, it may be swollen and reddened over an area outlining the sinuses. Pressure applied over the sinuses and on the lateral edge of the orbital ridges produces pain. Examination of the nasal turbinates shows purulent exudate in the middle or superior meatus if drainage is not prevented by swelling of these structures. Pain, swelling, and tenderness in the anterior portions of the maxillae are the outstanding features of *maxillary sinusitis.* When the infection is severe, pain may be referred to the upper teeth which may become loosened, and hemorrhage may be present in the surrounding tissues. Pus is visible in the middle meatus of the turbinates. The symptoms and signs of *ethmoid sinusitis* are pain in the upper medial areas of the nose, frontal headache, and redness of the skin and tenderness to pressure over the superior areas of the nasal bones adjacent to the inner canthi of the eyes. Pus is visible in the middle meatus when the anterior cells of the sinus are involved, and in the superior meatus if the posterior cells are infected; in most instances, both areas of the sinus are involved and exudate is present in both meatuses. The manifestations of infection of the *sphenoid sinus* are tenderness and pain over the vertex of the skull, the mastoid bones (in the presence of normal tympanic membranes), and the occipital portion of the head. Rarely, streaks of redness may be detectable over both zygomas as a result of irritation of the maxillary branch of the trigeminal nerve that lies in close proximity to the sinus.

Osteomyelitis of the frontal bone is a rare complication of frontal sinusitis. This is characterized by fever, chills, leukocytosis, frontal headache, and the presence of cool, pale edema over the forehead (Pott's puffy tumor). Involvement of the bone in which the ethmoid sinus lies may be manifested by unilateral or bilateral exophthalmos when one or both sinuses are involved. This is usually due to a sterile or pyogenic orbital cellulitis secondary to a ''sympathetic'' inflammation or perforation of the lamina papyracea, the lateral wall of the sinus, and the medial wall of the orbit. Impairment of venous return from the orbits may lead to the development of retinal hemorrhages. Intracranial spread of infection from the sinuses through the diploic veins may lead to meningitis, infection, and thrombosis of the superficial cerebral veins or cavernous and sagittal venous sinuses, cranial nerve palsies, and extradural abscess.

Bacterial meningitis is also a rare complication of purulent sinusitis, usually involving the frontal sinuses, and associated with cranial osteomyelitis and subdural and brain abscess. Sudden onset of convulsions, hemiplegia, and aphasia in a patient with acute frontal sinusitis should suggest the possibility of subdural abscess with thrombophlebitis of the sagittal sinus or superficial cerebral veins. Infections of the ethmoid sinus may be complicated by paralysis of the third cranial nerve due to invasion of the dural sinuses, or profuse epistaxis as a result of thrombosis of the ethmoidal veins that drain into the cavernous sinus, which may become thrombosed. Chronic or recurrent purulent sinusitis may eventually be responsible for the development of bronchiectasis. An unusual form of chronic sinusitis in association with bronchiectasis and situs inversus is *Kartagener's syndrome*. Patients with this disorder have been noted to have delayed mucociliary transport in the lower airways—the immotile ciliary syndrome; this is accompanied in men by lack of motility of sperm, the numbers of which are normal.

TABLE 212-2 Differential diagnosis of hoarseness and other manifestations of laryngeal dysfunction

- *I* Intralaryngeal disease
  - *A* Infectious
    - *1* Common cold
    - *2* Viral laryngitis
    - *3* *Hemophilus influenzae*
    - *4* Membranous laryngitis (*Streptococcus pyogenes, Pseudomonas, Fusobacterium*)
    - *5* Diphtheria (laryngeal membrane)
    - *6* Herpes simplex
    - *7* Actinomycosis
    - *8* Candidiasis
    - *9* Blastomycosis
    - *10* Histoplasmosis
    - *11* Tuberculosis (ulcers)
    - *12* Leprosy
    - *13* Syphilis (secondary stage, chondritis, gumma)
    - *14* *Mycoplasma pneumoniae*
    - *15* *Syngamus laryngeus*
  - *B* Noninfectious
    - *1* Trauma (edema or hematoma)
    - *2* Vocal cord nodules (singer's nodes)
    - *3* Papillomas of vocal cords
    - *4* Pachyderma of vocal cords
    - *5* Inhalation of smoke, fire, irritating gases, tobacco smoke
    - *6* Leukoplakia of vocal cords
    - *7* Rheumatoid arthritis (involvement of cricoarytenoid joint)
    - *8* Chronic alcoholism
    - *9* Benign tumors
    - *10* Cancer
    - *11* Foreign bodies
- *II* Extralaryngeal disease
  - *A* Lesions in neck [produce hoarseness because of (1) pressure on larynx that interferes with movement of vocal cords, (2) edema secondary to decreased venous and lymphatic drainage, and (3) impingement on laryngeal nerves with paresis or paralysis of cords]
    - *1* Hemorrhages and/or edema due to trauma, severe traction of neck, thyroidectomy, tracheostomy, and biopsy of scalene node
    - *2* Tumors of hypopharynx
    - *3* Tumors of carotid body
    - *4* Thrombophlebitis of jugular bulb
  - *B* Local and systemic disorders outside neck (produce hoarseness by pressure on laryngeal nerves anywhere along the course outside the neck, or paresis or paralysis of the vocal cords as a manifestation of generalized neurologic dysfunction)
    - *1* Local lesions
      - *a* Bacterial meningitis
      - *b* Meningovascular syphilis
      - *c* Infectious mononucleosis (enlarged mediastinal nodes)
      - *d* Angioneurotic edema
      - *e* Mitral stenosis (enlarged pulmonary artery)
      - *f* Aneurysms of arch of aorta, carotid or innominate arteries
      - *g* Ligation of patent ductus arteriosus
      - *h* Tumors of mediastinal structures
      - *i* Tumors of parotid gland
      - *j* Relapsing polychondritis
      - *k* Neoplastic disease of meninges
      - *l* Fracture of base of skull
      - *m* Cancer or nodules of thyroid
      - *n* Goiter
    - *2* Systemic disorders
      - *a* Diphtheria (peripheral neuritis)
      - *b* Poliomyelitis (bulbar)
      - *c* Infectious mononucleosis (nervous system involvement)
      - *d* Herpes zoster
      - *e* Mucoviscidosis
      - *f* Myxedema
      - *g* Acromegaly
      - *h* Wegener's granulomatosis
      - *i* Lupus erythematosus
      - *j* Diabetic neuropathy
      - *k* Poisoning by lead, mercury, arsenic, botulinus toxin

CHRONIC SINUSITIS It is difficult to establish the diagnosis of chronic sinusitis in the absence of documented recurrences of acute purulent infection. Many patients complaining of headaches, often frontal in nature, and troubled by obstruction of the nasal airway, may have some degree of tenderness over any of the paranasal sinuses. X-ray examinations of the sinuses often reveal thickening of the mucous membranes. Cultures of the nose or nasal discharge frequently yield no pathogenic organisms. In many instances, an allergic background is present in individuals with this syndrome; in these cases, relief of symptoms is often produced by the judicious use of nasal vasoconstrictors, and treatment is directed to the specific allergy. The manifestations presented by many patients are not related to chronic infection, but are due to other factors such as irritating dusts or gases or excessive exposure to tobacco smoke.

TUMORS OF THE SINUSES The commonest benign tumor of the paranasal sinuses is osteoma. Fifty percent of cases involve the frontal, 40 percent the ethmoid, and 10 percent the maxillary and sphenoid sinuses. The malignant tumors include carcinoma of the maxilla, sarcoma, Burkitt's lymphoma, myeloma, and adenocarcinoma. Melanoma of the nasal cavity may extend into the paranasal sinuses. Other malignant diseases originating in the sinuses may invade the nasal cavity and, because they produce obstruction, lead to consideration of the nose as the primary site of the lesion. A neoplastic lesion should be ruled out in patients who experience repeated episodes of acute sinusitis or who have chronic symptoms, particularly repeated epistaxis in the absence of an identifiable pathogenic organism.

LARYNX

SYMPTOMS AND SIGNS OF LARYNGEAL DISEASE There are three main causes of laryngeal disease: (1) intralaryngeal lesions, (2) extralaryngeal processes that produce other manifestations by direct pressure on either the larynx or the nerves that supply the vocal cords, and (3) disorders in which either local or diffuse disease of the nervous system leads to dysfunction of the vocal cords. A differential diagnosis of the various disorders of the larynx is presented in Table 212-2.

Hoarseness is the commonest symptom of disorders of the larynx, regardless of etiology. The common denominator of the numerous causes of this symptom is interference with normal phonatory function of the larynx. Both inflammatory and noninflammatory diseases of this organ as well as functional disturbances (hysterical aphonia) may be causative factors. Although hoarseness is usually of short duration with acute self-limited processes such as infections, it may persist for long periods.

Cough is common with any type of laryngeal disease. *Pain* occurs occasionally, while *stridor* and *dyspnea* are uncommon manifestations of laryngeal involvement. However, when present, these are ominous because they indicate the development of airway obstruction which may rapidly become complete. Obstruction to breathing is not only associated with intralaryngeal lesions or those which exert pressure directly on this organ but may also occur as a result of neurologic disorders in which paralysis of both vocal cords develops.

The exact cause of laryngeal obstruction can be detected only by direct or indirect examination of the larynx. *This is usually necessary when manifestations have persisted for longer than 2 or 3 weeks.* However, if serious obstruction of the airway develops rapidly in acute disorders of the larynx, laryngoscopic examination should be carried out promptly and tracheostomy performed if necessary.

The disorders of the larynx described below require specific and early diagnosis because of their life-threatening potential.

EPIGLOTTITIS Although much less common than in children, epiglottitis may occur in adults. Some of the clinical and microbiologic features in the older age group are different from those in youngsters. Men are involved three times more often than women. Predisposing factors include multiple myeloma, Hodgkin's disease, myelomonocytic leukemia, laryngeal blastomycosis, and disorders that lead to immunosuppression. Among the organisms reported to be responsible for the disease are *H. influenzae, H. parainfluenzae, S. pneumoniae, S. pyogenes, Escherichia coli,* and ''normal flora''; primary blastomycosis of the larynx may extend to the laryngeal surface of the epiglottis. Bacteremia supervenes in about 50 percent of cases. The symptoms of epiglottitis in adults differ from those in children. Sore throat is present in all patients. Next, in order of decreasing frequency, are fever (80 percent), dyspnea, dysphagia, and hoarseness (about 15 percent). Objective evidence of pharyngitis and tenderness of the neck are relatively uncommon. Abscess of the epiglottis occurs in about 12 percent of cases. Examination discloses a red, swollen epiglottis that may be so large that it protrudes into the lower pharynx. The diagnosis is proved by ''cross-table'' radiographic study of the neck. Antimicrobial therapy is mandatory, and the choice is based on the nature of the responsible organism. Dyspnea that progresses to the point of threatening complete obstruction of the airway is an indication for tracheostomy.

FUNGAL LARYNGITIS Disease caused by *Candida* species is uncommon but occurs occasionally in patients with mucocutaneous candidiasis and those who have been receiving antibiotics or are immunosuppressed. Because it is almost always associated with candidal esophagitis, it has been suggested that all persons with involvement of the esophagus by *Candida* undergo laryngoscopy. Hoarseness is not common. Scarring of the larynx may develop if antifungal therapy is not administered.

Two true fungi, *Histoplasma capsulatum* and *Blastomyces dermatitidis,* may produce chronic laryngitis. Symptoms common to both include hoarseness, dyspnea, and dysphagia; obstruction of the airway and hemoptysis may occur in some cases. The lesions may appear as large masses. Ulcerations are common and are probably the reason for the bleeding.

TUBERCULOUS LARYNGITIS Although decreasing in incidence over many years, infection of the larynx by *Mycobacterium tuberculosis* is still a problem. Many of the clinical features of this disease have changed over the last 40 years. It is now most common in older patients (50 to 59 years), more frequent in men than in women (3:1), and may be present in the absence of radiographic evidence of pulmonary disease. Hoarseness is present in almost all cases. While multiple ulcers, present primarily on the posterior aspect of the vocal cords, were common in the past, they are now relatively infrequent. The vocal cords are involved in 50 percent of cases; disease of the false cords and ventricles is next most common. In some cases, only hyperemia and edema are present; this may lead to a misdiagnosis of nonspecific laryngitis.

SYNGAMOSIS OF THE LARYNX This disease, caused by the worm *Syngamus laryngeus,* is a problem in the Caribbean islands, Brazil, and the Philippines. The vectors of the parasite are domestic and wild birds and cattle. Infestation is initiated by inhalation of the worm, which attaches to the mucosa of the larynx, pharynx, or trachea. Symptoms include severe, paroxysmal, nonproductive cough, occasional hemoptysis, and a ''crawling'' sensation in the larynx. Diagnosis is established by washing out the trachea and demonstrating the characteristic eggs. There is no specific treatment. The disease usually clears when the eggs and worms are coughed out.

FOREIGN BODY Inhalation of a foreign body rapidly produces symptoms. *Pain* is ''sticking'' in quality and localized to the larynx. *Laryngeal spasm* is usually present. *Dyspnea* may develop as a result of edema and lead to a degree of obstruction sufficient to compromise the airway. There is often a *change in the quality of the voice;* complete *aphonia* may occur. If the inhaled object is sharp, as a chicken bone, there is rapid development of local swelling and progressive obstruction to breathing. Perforation of the larynx may occur and lead to infection that extends from the local site to other areas in the neck and mediastinum. Suspicion of a foreign body makes mirror or laryngoscopic examination an emergency procedure.

CANCER OF THE LARYNX This lesion develops at an average age of 60 years and is 10 times more common in men than in women. Cancers of the larynx are of two types: *intrinsic,* arising on the anterior segment of the vocal cords (70 percent of the cases), and *extrinsic,* extending beyond the vocal cords. Although hoarseness develops early in the course of intrinsic lesions, it is frequently late in onset with extrinsic ones. The treatment of choice for this disease is surgery.

Small lesions of the middle third of the cord often respond to radiation alone. Total or partial laryngectomy is required in the majority of cases. When the cancer involves the epiglottis and/or the false cords, partial supraglottic laryngectomy is the preferred operative procedure because it does not result in loss of normal speech and has a high chance of cure. In some instances, preoperative irradiation of the larynx and surrounding lymph nodes may help in the eradication of the tumor. About 90 percent of cancers of the larynx are cured if detected and treated early.

REFERENCES

Bailey CM, Windle-Taylor PC: Tuberculous laryngitis: A series of 37 patients. Laryngology 91:93, 1981

Donegan JO, Wood MD: Histoplasmosis of the larynx. Laryngoscope 94:206, 1984

Eliasson R et al: The immotile-cilia syndrome: A congenital ciliary abnormality as an etiologic factor in chronic airway infections and male sterility. N Engl J Med 297:1, 1977

Khilanani U, Khatib R: Acute epiglottitis in adults. Am J Med Sci 287:65, 1984

Koopmann CF Jr, Coulthard SW: Retropharyngeal abscess—a ten-year experience. Laryngoscope 94:455, 1984

Levenson MJ et al: Laryngeal tuberculosis: Review of twenty cases. Laryngoscope 94:1094, 1984

Morgan MA et al: Fungal sinusitis in healthy and immunocompromised individuals. Am J Clin Pathol 82:597, 1984

Paparella MM, Shumrick DA: *Otolaryngology.* Philadelphia, Saunders, 1980

Payne J, Koopmann CF Jr: Laryngeal carcinoma—Or is it laryngeal blastomycosis? Laryngoscope 94:608, 1984

Weinstein L, Molavi A: *Syngamus laryngeus* infection. Ann Intern Med 74:577, 1971

213 NEOPLASMS OF THE LUNG

JOHN D. MINNA

In 1984, primary carcinoma of the lung affected more than 96,000 males and 43,000 females in the United States, most of whom died within 1 year. The peak incidence occurs between ages 55 and 65 years, and lung cancer is the leading cause of cancer death. The incidence is increasing, causing the age-adjusted lung cancer death rate to double every 15 years. At the time of diagnosis, only 20 percent of all lung cancer patients will have local disease, while 25 percent will have disease spread to regional lymph nodes, and 55 percent will have distant metastatic sites. Even in those patients with supposedly localized disease, overall 5-year survival is only 30 percent for males and 50 percent for females, and this survival rate has not changed significantly over the past 20 years. Thus, primary carcinoma of the lung is a major health problem with a generally grim prognosis. However, an orderly approach to diagnosis, staging, and treatment based on knowledge of the clinical behavior of lung cancer, combined with a critical review of clinical treatment trials, allows selection of the best therapy for individual patients for either potential cure or optimal palliation. This approach should be multidisciplinary, involving the interaction of medical internists or chest physicians, medical, radiation, and surgical oncologists, pathologists, as well as diagnostic and supportive care personnel.

PATHOLOGY

The histologic classification of primary lung neoplasms recommended by the World Health Organization in 1977 should be used (see Table 213-1). Four major cell types make up 95 percent of all primary lung neoplasms. These are squamous or epidermoid carcinoma, small cell (also called "oat cell") carcinoma, adenocarcinoma (including bronchioloalveolar), and large cell (also called large cell anaplastic) carcinoma. The various cell types have different natural histories and responses to therapy, and thus a correct histologic diagnosis by an experienced pathologist is the first step to correct treatment.

Major treatment decisions are made on the basis of whether the tumor is histologically classified as a small cell carcinoma or one of the "non-small cell" varieties (which include epidermoid, adenocarcinoma, large cell carcinoma, bronchioloalveolar carcinoma, and mixed versions of these). Some of these distinctions are summarized in Tables 213-2 and 213-3.

In general, small cell carcinoma has spread beyond the bounds of resectional surgery at the time of presentation and is primarily managed with chemotherapy with or without radiotherapy, while if they are found to be localized at the time of presentation, the non-small cell varieties should be considered for a curative attempt with either surgery or radiotherapy.

Epidermoid cancer is the most common histologic type found in males, while adenocarcinoma is the most common type found in females. Ninety percent of patients with lung cancer of all histologic types are cigarette smokers, while the rare nonsmoking patient who develops lung cancer usually has adenocarcinoma. However, in nonsmokers with adenocarcinoma involving the lung, the possibility of other primary sites, particularly breast cancer, should be considered. Epidermoid and small cell cancers usually present as central masses with endobronchial growth, while adenocarcinomas and large cell cancers tend to present as peripheral nodules or masses with pleural involvement. Epidermoid and large cell cancers cavitate in 20 to 30 percent of cases. Bronchioloalveolar carcinoma can present as a single mass, a diffuse, multinodular lesion, or as a fluffy infiltrate.

TABLE 213-1 World Health Organization (WHO) classification of malignant pleuropulmonary neoplasms

I Epidermoid carcinoma
II Small cell carcinoma (including fusiform, polygonal, lymphocyte-like, and others)
III Adenocarcinoma (including acinar, papillary, and bronchioloalveolar)
IV Large cell carcinoma (including solid tumors with and without mucin and giant cell and clear cell tumors)
V Combined epidermoid and adenocarcinomas
VI Carcinoid tumors
VII Bronchial gland tumors (including cylindromas and mucoepidermoid tumors)
VIII Papillary tumors of the surface epithelium
IX "Mixed" tumors and carcinosarcomas
X Sarcomas
XI Unclassified
XII Mesotheliomas (including localized and diffuse)
XIII Melanomas

ETIOLOGY

The large majority of lung cancers are associated with and probably caused by cigarette smoking; benzo[*a*]pyrene is a major carcinogen in tobacco smoke. There is a dose-response relationship between the lung cancer death rate and the total amount (often expressed in "cigarette pack-years") of cigarettes smoked, such that the risk is increased sixty- to seventyfold for the man smoking two packs a day for 20 years compared to the nonsmoker. Conversely, the chance of developing lung cancer decreases with cessation of smoking but may never return to the nonsmoker level. The increase in lung cancer in women is also associated with a rise in female cigarette smoking. As a preventive measure, efforts to get persons to stop smoking should continue. Probably there is a cocarcinogenic effect of smoking and industrial or environmental pollutants. Also, peripheral adenocarcinomas occur more frequently in areas of chronic scarring caused by chronic inflammatory changes, chronic interstitial fibrosis, or scleroderma. Molecular genetic studies have revealed the presence of activated cellular oncogenes in lung cancer cells. These include point mutations in specific coding regions of *ras* oncogenes (*H, K,* and *N-ras* genes), occurring in 15 percent of all types of lung cancer; and amplified *myc* family oncogenes (*c, N,* and *L-myc*), occurring primarily in small cell lung cancer. Changes in the expression and function of the products of these genes are likely to account for the malignant behavior of lung cancer and represent targets for future efforts at prevention and treatment.

CLINICAL MANIFESTATIONS AND MODE OF PRESENTATION

The natural history of lung cancer begins with cytologic changes of atypia in bronchial epithelial cells progressing through carcinoma in situ to frank invasion. These changes usually occur before signs or symptoms have developed and are only seen in cytology (e.g., sputum and bronchial washings) or biopsies. Lung cancer gives rise to chest radiograph findings and other signs and symptoms from local tumor growth, invasion or obstruction of adjacent structures, growth in regional nodes via lymphatic spread, growth in distant metastatic sites after hematogenous dissemination, or as a remote effect of the tumor (paraneoplastic syndrome) usually resulting from peptide hormone secretion by the tumor. Appropriate identification of these signs and symptoms as tumor-related will guide further evaluation and therapy and be of prognostic importance.

If mass screening programs are excluded, 5 to 15 percent of patients are detected while asymptomatic, usually on a routine chest radiograph, while the vast majority of patients present with some sign or symptom. Signs and symptoms secondary to central or endobronchial growth of the primary tumor include cough, hemop-

TABLE 213-2 Incidence, frequency of metastases, and surgical resectability of the major lung cancer histologic types

Cell type	Incidence in autopsy series, %	Necropsy frequency of distant metastases when clinically localized, %*	Resectability rate (AJC study), %†	5-year survival after curative resection, %
Non-small cell carcinoma:				
Epidermoid	33	17	60	37
Adenocarcinoma	25	40	38	27
Large cell carcinoma	16	14	38	27
Small cell carcinoma	25	63	11	<1

* *Determined from autopsy studies of patients dying of causes other than cancer within 30 days following an apparent curative surgical resection.*
† *AJC = American Joint Committee Study for Cancer Staging and End Results Reporting, indicating percentage of cases thought to undergo a curative resection.*
SOURCE: *Adapted from Minna et al, 1985.*

tysis, wheeze and stridor, dyspnea, and pneumonitis (fever and productive cough) from obstruction. Signs and symptoms secondary to the peripheral growth of the primary tumor include pain from pleural or chest wall involvement, cough, dyspnea on a restrictive basis, and symptoms of lung abscess resulting from tumor cavitation. Signs and symptoms related to the regional spread of tumor in the thorax by contiguity or by metastasis to regional lymph nodes include tracheal obstruction, esophageal compression with dysphagia, recurrent laryngeal nerve paralysis with hoarseness, phrenic nerve paralysis with elevation of the hemidiaphragm and dyspnea, and sympathetic nerve invasion and paralysis with Horner's syndrome. *Pancoast's,* or *superior sulcus tumor, syndrome* results from local extension of a tumor (usually epidermoid) growing in the apex of the lung with involvement of the eighth cervical and first and second thoracic nerves, with shoulder pain which characteristically radiates in the ulnar distribution of the arm, and often with radiologic destruction of the first and second ribs. Often Horner's syndrome and Pancoast's syndrome will coexist. Other problems of regional spread include *superior vena cava syndrome* from vascular obstruction; pericardial and cardiac extension with resultant tamponade, arrhythmia, or cardiac failure; lymphatic obstruction with resultant pleural effusion; and lymphangitic spread through the lungs with hypoxemia and dyspnea. In addition, bronchioloalveolar carcinoma can spread transbronchially, producing tumor growing along multiple alveolar surfaces with resultant impairment of oxygen transfer, respiratory insufficiency, dyspnea, hypoxemia, and production of large amounts of sputum.

Extrathoracic metastatic disease is found at autopsy in over 50 percent of patients with epidermoid carcinoma, 80 percent of patients with adeno- and large cell carcinoma, and over 95 percent of patients with small cell cancer. These autopsy studies have found lung cancer metastases in virtually every organ system. Thus, the majority of lung cancer patients eventually need therapy to palliate symptoms. Common clinical problems related to metastatic disease of lung cancer include brain metastases with neurologic deficits; bone metastases with pain and pathologic fractures; bone marrow invasion with cytopenias or leukoerythroblastosis; liver metastases causing biochemical liver dysfunction, anorexia, biliary obstruction, and pain; lymph node metastases in the supraclavicular region and occasionally in the axilla and groin that can be painful and ulcerate; and spinal cord compression syndromes from epidural or bone metastases.

Remote effects of cancer or *paraneoplastic syndromes* are common in lung cancer patients and may be the presenting finding or first sign of recurrence. In addition, paraneoplastic syndromes may mimic metastatic disease and, unless detected, lead to inappropriate palliative rather than curative treatment. Often the paraneoplastic syndrome may be relieved with successful treatment of the tumor, and tumor treatment is the basis for correcting such syndromes. In some cases the pathophysiology of the paraneoplastic syndrome is known, particularly when a hormone with biologic activity is secreted by a tumor (Chap. 303). However, in many cases the pathophysiology is unknown. *Systemic symptoms* of anorexia, cachexia, and weight loss (seen in 30 percent of patients), fever (20 percent), and suppressed immunity are paraneoplastic syndromes of unknown etiology. *Endocrine syndromes* are seen in 12 percent of patients and have the best understood pathophysiology, including hypercalcemia and hypophosphatemia resulting from ectopic parathyroid hormone production by epidermoid cancer; hyponatremia with the syndrome of inappropriate secretion of antidiuretic hormone by small cell cancer; and Cushing's syndrome resulting from ectopic secretion of ACTH by small cell cancer. *Skeletal connective tissues syndromes* include clubbing in 30 percent (usually non-small cell), and hypertrophic pulmonary osteoarthropathy in 1 to 10 percent (usually adenocarcinomas) with periostitis and clubbing giving pain, tenderness, and swelling over the affected bones, and a positive bone scan. *Neurologic-myopathic syndromes* are seen in only 1 percent of patients but are dramatic and include the myasthenic *Eaton-Lambert syndrome* with small cell cancer, peripheral neuropathies, subacute cerebellar degeneration, cortical degeneration, and polymyositis seen with all lung cancer types. *Coagulation and thrombotic and hematologic manifestations* occur in 1 to 8 percent of patients and include migratory venous thrombophlebitis (*Trousseau's syndrome*); nonbacterial thrombotic (marantic) endocarditis with arterial emboli; disseminated intravascular coagulation with hemorrhage; and anemia, granulocytosis, and leukoerythroblastosis. *Cutaneous manifestations* such as dermatomyositis and acanthosis nigricans are uncommon (1 percent or less) as are the *renal manifestations* of nephrotic syndrome or glomerulonephritis (1 percent or less).

DIAGNOSIS AND STAGING

EARLY DIAGNOSIS Screening persons at high risk (males over 45 years of age smoking 40 or more cigarettes per day) for lung cancer with sputum cytologies and chest radiographs every 4 months has shown a prevalence rate of lung cancer in asymptomatic patients of 4 to 8 cases per 1000 persons. With follow-up screening, 4 new cases of lung cancer are found per 1000 persons followed per year. These lung cancers are detected 72 percent of the time by radiographs alone, 20 percent by cytology alone, while 6 percent are detected by both methods. In contrast to nonscreened patients, 90 percent of these screened patients who develop lung cancer are asymptomatic, 62 percent have resectable lung cancer, and 53 percent of all the new cases are American Joint Commission (AJC) postsurgical stage I (see below) with a 5-year survival probability of 45 percent. These results are being prospectively compared to a randomized control group not

TABLE 213-3 Comparison between small cell and "non-small cell" lung cancers

	Small cell	Non-small cell
HISTOLOGY		
	Scant cytoplasm, indistinct nucleoli, small hyperchromatic nuclei	Abundant cytoplasm, prominent nucleoli, enlarged, pleomorphic nuclei
BIOCHEMICAL		
	L-Dopa decarboxylase, neuron-specific enolase, creatinine kinase BB isoenzyme	Keratin (epidermoid) Mucin (adenocarcinoma)
CELL SURFACE ANTIGENS		
	Absent-low: HLA, B_2m Leu-7 expressed	HLA, B_2m expressed Leu-7 not expressed
CYTOGENETICS		
	Deletion 3p(14–23)	No known specific defect
HORMONE PRODUCTION		
	ACTH, AVP, calcitonin, bombesin, neurotensin	PTH (epidermoid)
RESPONSE TO RADIOTHERAPY		
	+ + + (often complete)	+ (uncommonly complete)
RESPONSE TO COMBINATION CHEMOTHERAPY		
Overall regression rate	90%	30%
Complete regression rate	50%	5%
OVERALL 5-YEAR SURVIVAL RATES		
	5%	8%

receiving this intensive screening. If the lung cancer death rate is reduced significantly in the screened group, screening should be generally practiced in high-risk patients.

ESTABLISHING A TISSUE DIAGNOSIS OF LUNG CANCER Once signs, symptoms, or screening studies suggest lung cancer, it is necessary to establish a tissue diagnosis of malignancy, determine the histologic cell type, and stage the patient for appropriate treatment. In the initial evaluation of each patient, tumor tissue should be obtained so that a histologic diagnosis of cancer and tumor cell type can be firmly made. Distinction of small cell from non-small cell lung cancer can sometimes be difficult in cytology preparations. Therefore, cytologic diagnoses from washings or needle aspirates should be reserved for very high risk patients or patients relapsing with cancer after initial treatment. Tumor tissue can be obtained at the time of definitive surgical resection, from a bronchial biopsy or transbronchial forceps biopsy at fiberoptic bronchoscopy, from node biopsy at mediastinoscopy, from percutaneous biopsy of an enlarged lymph node, soft tissue mass, lytic bone lesion, bone marrow, or pleural lesion; or from an adequate cell block from a malignant pleural effusion.

STAGING PATIENTS WITH LUNG CANCER Lung cancer staging consists of two parts: first, a determination of the location of tumor (anatomic staging) and second, an assessment of a patient's ability to withstand various antitumor treatments (physiologic staging). For example, in a patient with non-small cell lung cancer it is crucial to determine if the tumor can be resected by a standard surgical procedure such as a lobectomy or pneumonectomy (determination of "resectability") based on the anatomic stage of the tumor and whether the patient could tolerate such a surgical procedure (determination of "operability") based on the cardiopulmonary condition of the patient.

TABLE 213-4 TNM classification of lung cancer

PRIMARY TUMOR (T)	
TX	Occult cancer; only evidence in bronchial washings cytologically
T1	Less than 3 cm, surrounded by lung or visceral pleura, and without bronchoscopic invasion proximal to a lobar bronchus
T2	Tumor more than 3 cm; or tumor with atelectasis or pneumonitis extending to hilum but less than entire lung, within a lobar bronchus, and more than 2 cm distal to carina; no pleural effusion
T3	Tumor of any size with extension into parietal pleura, chest wall, diaphragm, mediastinum; less than 2 cm from carina; or atelectasis, pneumonitis of entire lung; pleural effusion with or without malignant cells
REGIONAL LYMPH NODES (N)(see Note)	
N0	Negative hilar and mediastinal nodes
N1	Positive ipsilateral hilar nodes
N2	Positive mediastinal nodes (also scored when vocal cord paralysis, SVC obstruction, and trachea or esophageal compression are present, all of which strongly indicate mediastinal node invasion)
DISTANT METASTASIS (M)	
M0	No known distant metastasis
M1	Distant metastasis present with site specified (e.g., brain)
STAGE GROUPING	
Occult carcinoma	TX, N0, M0
Stage I	T1, N0, M0; T1, N1, M0; T2, N0, M0
Stage II	T2, N1, M0
Stage III	T3 with any N or M; N2 with any T or M; M1 with any T or N

NOTE: *For planning surgical treatment and assigning postoperative prognosis, the ATS has recommended dropping the terms* hilar *(for N1) and* mediastinal *(for N2) nodal disease. They recommend that N1 include ipsilateral intrapulmonary, lobar, and segmental nodes; ipsilateral paratracheal and peribronchial (on the left) and tracheobronchial (on the right) nodes be assigned an uncertain prognosis (i.e., may be either N1 or N2); while all remaining nodes be scored as N2. In practical terms, the decision to resect N1 or N2 involved nodes will have to be made by the surgeon at the time of thoracotomy.*

Non-small cell lung cancer The TNM (tumor size, or T factor; regional nodal involvement, or N factor; and presence or absence of distant metastases, M factor) staging system developed by the AJC on End Results Reporting should be used in non-small cell lung cancer, particularly in preparing patients for curative attempts with surgery or radiotherapy (Table 213-4). The various T, N, and M factors are combined to form three different groups (stages I, II, and III) and a fourth group consisting of occult carcinoma detected on screening cytology exams but with no other evidence of tumor (Table 213-4). This stage grouping can be performed at different times.

Small cell lung cancer A simple two-stage system adapted from the Veterans Administration Lung Cancer Study Group is used. In this two-stage system, *limited stage disease* (about 40 percent of all small cell cancer patients) is defined as disease confined to one hemithorax and regional lymph nodes (including mediastinal, contralateral hilar, and usually ipsilateral supraclavicular nodes), while *extensive stage disease* (about 60 percent of all patients) is defined as disease beyond this. In part, the definition of *limited stage* relates to whether the known tumor can be encompassed within a tolerable radiation therapy port. Thus, contralateral supraclavicular nodes, recurrent laryngeal nerve involvement, and superior vena caval obstruction can all be limited stage disease. However, cardiac tamponade, malignant pleural effusion, and bilateral pulmonary parenchymal involvement are generally scored as extensive stage disease because of the size of the radiation therapy port required to cover all known disease.

GENERAL STAGING PROCEDURES All lung cancer patients should have a complete history and physical examination, with evaluation of all other medical problems and a determination of performance status and weight loss.

An ear, nose, and throat examination is necessary because of the frequent occurrence of second cancers in this area. Chest roentgenograms are needed to evaluate tumor size and nodal involvement, and it is very useful, if not mandatory, to obtain any old x-ray films for comparison. Tomograms are only used for specific diagnostic problems. Chest computerized tomography (CT) scans are now widely used in the staging and follow-up of lung cancer patients. CT scans are of use in non-small cell lung cancer in preoperative staging to detect mediastinal nodes and pleural extension, and in the planning of curative radiation therapy to allow design of fields to encompass all known tumor volume while avoiding as much normal tissue as possible. However, as recommended by the American Thoracic Society (ATS), definitive characterization of mediastinal nodal involvement should depend upon histologic proof when planning curative treatment. In small cell lung cancer, CT scans are used for chest radiation treatment planning and assessing the response to chemotherapy and radiation therapy. In following patients after surgery or radiotherapy, procedures which can make interpretation of conventional chest x-rays difficult, CT scans can provide good evidence of tumor recurrence.

A complete blood count with platelet determination, routine blood chemistries, skin test for tuberculosis, electrocardiogram, and pulmonary function studies are obtained. Arterial blood gas measurements are obtained if any signs or symptoms of respiratory insufficiency are present. If signs or symptoms suggest organ involvement by tumor, appropriate radionuclide scans (e.g., brain, liver, or bone) are performed, as well as radiographs of any suspicious bony lesions. Routine radionuclide scans are not obtained in the asymptomatic patient because of the high frequency of false-positive and false-negative studies. Any accessible lesions suspicious for cancer should be biopsied if a histologic diagnosis has not already been made, or if treatment or staging decisions would be based on whether or not the lesion contained cancer. In candidates for curative surgery or radiotherapy, a barium swallow is performed, if esophageal symptoms are present, followed by esophagoscopy if abnormalities are found.

In patients presenting with a mass lesion on chest x-ray and no obvious contraindications to a curative approach with surgery or radiotherapy after the initial evaluation and fiberoptic bronchoscopy (see below), the mediastinum must be investigated. This varies between different centers and includes (1) chest CT scan, and if this is positive, mediastinoscopy; (2) proceeding directly to mediastinoscopy (right-sided tumors) or lateral mediastinotomy (left-sided lesions) on all patients; (3) proceeding directly to thoracotomy with staging of the mediastinum at this time. In patients presenting with disease confined to the chest but not resectable, thus making them candidates for curative radiotherapy, other tests are only done as indicated to evaluate specific symptoms.

Pretreatment staging for patients with histologically documented small cell lung cancer includes the initial general lung cancer evaluation as well as fiberoptic bronchoscopy with washings and biopsies to determine the tumor extent before therapy; brain CT scan; bone marrow biopsy and aspiration since 20 to 30 percent of patients have tumor in the bone marrow; and radionuclide scans of liver and bone if symptoms or other findings are suggestive of disease involvement in these areas. Percutaneous or peritoneoscopy-directed liver biopsy may be performed if other findings are suggestive but not diagnostic of the presence of tumor in the liver, particularly if this would alter the planned therapy.

If signs or symptoms of spinal cord compression or leptomeningitis develop at any time in lung cancer patients of any histologic type, a myelogram and examination of the cerebrospinal fluid cytology are performed to determine the need for local therapy to the site of compression (usually with radiotherapy), and intrathecal chemotherapy (usually with methotrexate) if malignant cells are detected. In addition, a brain CT scan is performed to search for brain metastases that are often associated with compression or leptomeningitis.

STAGING OF NON-SMALL CELL CANCER WITH METASTATIC DISEASE In patients presenting with disease that is not curable by either surgery, radiotherapy, or their combination, all of the general procedures are done plus fiberoptic bronchoscopy as indicated to evaluate hemoptysis, obstruction, or pneumonitis; and pleurocentesis and cytologic examination if fluid is present.

A variety of other staging procedures including gallium 67 citrate scanning, computed tomography (outside the chest), tomograms, angiograms, venograms, scintiscans, sonography, and blind nodal biopsies at present should not be part of the routine staging evaluation of the lung cancer patient.

DETERMINATION OF RESECTABILITY AND OPERABILITY In patients with non-small cell lung cancer, the following are major contraindications to curative attempts by surgery or radiotherapy alone using standard treatment methods: extrathoracic distant metastases; superior vena cava syndrome; vocal cord and, in most cases, phrenic nerve paralysis; malignant pleural effusion; cardiac tamponade; tumor within 2 cm of the carina (not curable by surgery but potentially curable by radiotherapy); metastasis to the contralateral lung; bilateral endobronchial tumor (potentially curable by radiotherapy); metastasis to the supraclavicular lymph nodes; lymph node metastasis in the contralateral mediastinum (potentially curable by radiotherapy); involvement of the main stem pulmonary artery; and a histologic diagnosis of small cell lung cancer.

PHYSIOLOGIC STAGING Patients with lung cancer often have cardiopulmonary and other medical problems related to chronic obstructive pulmonary disease as well as other medical problems. Since it is not always possible to predict whether a lobectomy or pneumonectomy will be required until the time of operation, a conservative approach is to restrict resectional surgery to patients who could potentially tolerate a pneumonectomy. In addition to nonambulatory performance status, a myocardial infarction within the past 3 months is a contraindication to thoracic surgery because 20 percent of patients will die of reinfarction alone, while an infarction in the past 6 months is a relative contraindication. Other major contraindications include uncontrolled major arrhythmias; maximum breathing capacities of less than 40 percent predicted; an FEV_1 less than 1 liter, though an FEV_1 over 2.5 liters allows pneumonectomy (recommending surgery when the FEV_1 is 1.1. to 2.4 liters requires careful judgment); CO_2 retention (which is more serious than hypoxemia); and severe pulmonary hypertension. In patients with borderline pulmonary status or a question of pulmonary hypertension, split pulmonary function testing by ventilation-perfusion lung scans or bronchospirometry and right heart catheterization study with temporary unilateral pulmonary artery occlusion can define physiologic operability.

TREATMENT

After a histologic diagnosis is obtained and appropriate anatomic and physiologic staging studies are completed, the overall treatment approach to patients with lung cancer may be formulated (Table 213-5).

NON-SMALL CELL LUNG CANCER: LOCALIZED DISEASE In patients with non-small cell lung cancer of AJC clinical stages I and II (Table 213-4) who can tolerate operation, the treatment of choice is pulmonary resection. In some stage III cases with favorable age, cardiopulmonary function, and anatomy resection should also be considered. Currently, there is interest in carrying out resectional therapy followed by postoperative radiotherapy in some patients with positive ipsilateral N2 nodes that do not exhibit extracapsular tumor extension. If a complete resection is possible, the 5-year survival rate for N1 disease is about 50 percent, while it is about 30 percent for N2 disease. However, only 20 percent of all patients who have N2 disease are technically resectable, and in most cases these resectable patients are only discovered to have N2 disease at thoracotomy. Patients with contralateral or bilateral N2 nodes, extracapsular nodal involvement, or fixed nodes are not currently considered resectable. The extent of resection is a matter of surgical judgment based on findings at exploration. In general, conservative resection that encompasses all known tumor gives survival equal to that obtained with more extensive procedures. Thus, lobectomy is preferred to pneumonectomy, while wedge resections and segmentectomies are reserved for patients with poor pulmonary reserve and small peripheral lesions.

TABLE 213-5 Summary of treatment approach to lung cancer patients

NON-SMALL CELL LUNG CANCER
Resectable (AJC stage I, II, and selected T3, N2 lesions)
Surgery
Radiotherapy for "nonoperable" patients
Postoperative radiotherapy for N2 disease
Nonresectable (N2 and M1)
Confined to chest: high-dose chest radiotherapy (RT) if possible
Extrathoracic: RT to symptomatic local sites; chemotherapy (CT) (for good-performance-status patients, with evaluable lesions)
SMALL CELL LUNG CANCER
Limited stage (good performance status)
High-dose combination chemotherapy ± chest RT
Extensive stage (good performance status)
High-dose combination chemotherapy
Complete tumor responders all stages
Prophylactic cranial RT
Poor-performance-status patients (all stages)
Modified dose combination chemotherapy
Palliative RT
ALL PATIENTS
Radiotherapy for brain metastases, spinal cord compression, weight-bearing lytic bony lesions, symptomatic local lesions (nerve paralyses, obstructed airway, hemoptysis in non-small cell lung cancer and in small cell cancer not responding to chemotherapy)
Appropriate diagnosis and treatment of other medical problems and supportive care during chemotherapy
Encouragement to stop smoking

Approximately 43 percent of all lung cancer patients will undergo thoracotomy. Of these, 76 percent will have a definitive resection, 12 percent will only be explored for disease extent, and 12 percent will have a palliative procedure with known disease left behind. The fraction of long-term survivors following definitive surgical therapy is remarkably consistent throughout major centers performing lung cancer surgery in the United States. Approximately 30 percent of all patients resected for cure survive 5 years, and 15 percent survive 10 years. The 30-day hospital mortality following pulmonary resection at major centers is also very consistent, 3 percent for lobectomy and 6 percent for pneumonectomy. The 5-year survivals following resection for the different histologic types are epidermoid, 33 percent; adenocarcinoma, 26 percent; large cell carcinoma, 28 percent; bronchioloalveolar carcinoma, 51 percent; and small cell carcinoma, less than 1 percent. As a function of postsurgical treatment stage the AJC 5-year survival data are epidermoid: stage I, 54 percent, stage II, 35 percent, stage III N0–N1, 19 percent, stage III N2, 13 percent; adenocarcinoma and large cell carcinoma: stage I, 51 percent, stage II, 18 percent, stage III N0–N1, 10 percent, stage III N2, 2 percent. Thus, the majority of patients who were initially thought to have a "curative" resection ultimately died of metastatic disease (usually within 2 years of surgery), indicating the need for some form of adjuvant treatment.

MANAGEMENT OF OCCULT CARCINOMA When sputum cytology screening indicates malignant cells but a normal chest radiograph is found (TX tumor stage), the lesion must be localized. Over 90 percent can be localized by meticulous examination of the bronchial tree with a fiberoptic bronchoscope under general anesthesia and collection of a series of differential brushings and biopsies.

Often carcinoma in situ or multicentric lesions are found. Thus, current recommendations are for the most conservative surgical resection, allowing removal of the cancer and conservation of lung parenchyma even if the bronchial margins are positive for carcinoma in situ. The 5-year overall survival for these occult cancers is approximately 60 percent. Close follow-up of these patients is indicated because of the high incidence of second primary lung cancers (approximately 5 percent per patient per year).

SOLITARY PULMONARY NODULE When a patient presents with an asymptomatic, solitary pulmonary nodule (defined as an x-ray density completely surrounded by normal aerated lung, with circumscribed margins, of any shape, usually 1 to 6 cm in greatest diameter) a decision to resect or follow the nodule must be made. Approximately 35 percent of all such lesions in adults will be malignant, the majority being primary lung cancer, while less than 1 percent are malignant in nonsmoking patients under 35 years of age. A complete history, including a smoking history, physical examination, routine laboratory tests, fiberoptic bronchoscopy, and old chest x-rays are obtained. If no diagnosis is immediately apparent, the following risk factors would all argue strongly in favor of proceeding with resection to establish a histologic diagnosis: history of cigarette smoking; age 35 years or older; a relatively large-sized lesion; lack of calcification; chest symptoms; associated atelectasis, pneumonitis, or adenopathy; and growth of the lesion compared to old x-rays. At present, only two radiographic criteria are strongly reliable for benignity of a solitary pulmonary nodule: lack of growth over a period greater than 2 years and certain characteristic patterns of calcification. Calcification alone does not exclude malignancy. However, a dense central nidus, multiple punctate foci, "bull's eye" (granuloma), and "popcorn ball" (hamartoma) calcifications are all highly suggestive of a benign lesion.

When old x-rays are not available and the characteristic calcification patterns are absent, the following approach is reasonable: nonsmoking patients under 35 years can be followed with serial chest x-rays every 3 months for 1 year and then yearly. If any significant growth is found, a histologic diagnosis is needed. For patients over 35 and all patients with a smoking history, a histologic diagnosis must be made. This can either occur at the time of nodule resection or, if the patient is a poor operative risk, via transthoracic fine-needle biopsy. Some institutions would use preoperative fine-needle aspiration on all such lesions; however, all positive lesions will have to proceed to resection, and negative cytologic findings will in most cases have to be confirmed by histology on a resected specimen. While much has been made of sparing patients an operation, the high probability of finding a malignancy (particularly in smokers over 35) and the excellent chance for surgical cure when the tumor is small, all suggest an aggressive approach to these lesions.

RADIOTHERAPY Those patients who are AJC stage III M0, as well as those with AJC stages I and II disease who refuse surgery or appear not to be candidates for pulmonary resection for medical reasons, should be considered for radiation therapy with curative intent. The decision to administer high-dose and potentially curative radiotherapy is based upon the extent of disease and the volume of the chest that requires irradiation. Patients with distant metastases, positive supraclavicular nodes, pleural effusion, or cardiac involvement are generally not considered for such curative radiation treatment. The median survival for unresectable patients with non-small cell lung cancer localized to the chest undergoing primary radiotherapy with curative intent is less than 1 year. However, 5-year survival data show up to 6 percent of patients alive when treated with radiotherapy alone. In addition to potential cure, radiotherapy, by controlling the primary tumor, may increase the quality and length of life of noncured patients, although there are few data to support this latter consideration directly. Treatment usually involves midplane doses of 55,000 to 60,000 mGy (5500 to 6000 rad), and the major concern is the amount of lung parenchyma and other organs in the thorax included within the treatment plan, including the spinal cord, heart, and esophagus. Patients with a major degree of underlying pulmonary disease may have to have the treatment plan compromised because of the deleterious effect of radiation on pulmonary function. Either split course or continuous fraction radiotherapy can be given with similar survival results. The development of radiation pneumonitis is proportional to the dose of radiation and volume of lung incorporated within the radiation field. The full clinical syndrome (dyspnea, fever, and radiographic infiltrate corresponding to the treatment port) occurs in 5 percent of cases. Acute radiation esophagitis occurs during treatment but usually is self-limited, while spinal cord injury should be avoided by careful treatment planning.

COMBINED MODALITY THERAPY At present there appears to be no consensus for the routine use of pre- or postoperative radiation therapy, debulking surgery, or adjuvant chemotherapy. Currently, these forms of combined modality therapy should only be administered as part of approved clinical trials. However, many centers give high-dose, postoperative radiation if postsurgical staging documents N2 nodal disease. Another exception to this is the management of carcinomas of the superior pulmonary sulcus producing *Pancoast's syndrome*. These patients should have the usual preoperative staging procedures, including mediastinoscopy as well as CT scans to determine tumor extent and neurologic examination with electromyography to document neurologic findings. Often a histologic diagnosis is not made, and with the constellation of tumor location and pain distribution the diagnostic accuracy for cancer is better than 90 percent. If mediastinoscopy is negative, two curative approaches may be used in treating a Pancoast's syndrome tumor. The first preoperative irradiation [30,000 mGy (3000 rad) in 10 treatments] is given to the area followed by an en bloc resection of the tumor and involved chest wall 3 to 6 weeks later. At 3 years, survival figures of 42 percent for epidermoid and 21 percent for adeno- and large cell carcinomas have been reported. The second approach involves radiotherapy alone in curative doses and standard fractionation with similar survival to combined modality therapy reported. Data have now appeared suggesting a high frequency of brain metastases as isolated sites of relapse in patients with adenocarcinoma of the lung otherwise cured by surgery or radiotherapy. While there is no proven role for "prophylactic" cranial irradition, it is not unreasonable to follow potentially cured, asymptomatic adenocarcinoma patients with frequent brain CT scans to detect such recurrence at the earliest possible time.

DISSEMINATED NON-SMALL CELL LUNG CANCER The 70 percent of patients who turn out to have unresectable non-small cell cancer have a poor prognosis. For example, median survivals of 34, 25, 17, 8, and 4 weeks are seen for patients with performance status scores of 0 (asymptomatic), 1 (symptomatic, fully ambulatory), 2 (in bed $<$ 50 percent of the time), 3 (in bed $>$ 50 percent of the time), and 4 (bedridden), respectively. Standard medical management, the judicious use of pain medications, and the appropriate use of radiotherapy form the cornerstone of management. Patients whose primary tumors are causing symptoms such as bronchial obstruction with pneumonitis, hemoptysis, or upper airway or superior vena caval (SVC) obstruction should, in general, have radiotherapy to the primary tumor. The case for prophylactic treatment of the asymptomatic patient is to prevent major symptoms from occurring within the thorax, if follow-up is uncertain. However, if the patient can be followed closely, deferring treatment until the development of symptoms is appropriate. Usually a course of 30,000 to 40,000 mGy (3000 to 4000 rad) over 2 to 4 weeks is given to the tumor. The frequencies of relief by radiation therapy of intrathoracic symptoms are hemoptysis, 84 percent; SVC syndrome, 80 percent; dyspnea, 60 percent; cough, 60 percent; atelectasis, 23 percent; and vocal cord paralysis, 6 percent. Other symptoms of metastatic disease treated with radiotherapy include cardiac tamponade (treated with pericardiocentesis and radiation therapy to the entire cardiac silhouette); painful bony metastases (with relief in 66 percent of cases); and brain, spinal cord compression, or brachial plexus involvement. Usually, with brain and cord compression, dexamethasone (25 to 100 mg total per day in four divided doses) is also given and then rapidly tapered to the lowest dosage which relieves neurologic symptoms. In all cases, the key to effective palliation is to detect the complication and begin radiotherapy at the earliest possible time. Pleural effusions are common and are usually treated with thoracentesis as needed, but without radiotherapy. If they recur and are symptomatic, chest tube drainage with a sclerosing agent such as intrapleural tetracycline is used. The chest is first completely drained. Then 1000 mg of tetracycline is dissolved in 100 mL of normal saline, and 50 mL of 1% xylocaine added, and this is injected via the chest tube. The chest tube is clamped and the patient rotated onto different sides to distribute the sclerosing agent. Then 24 to 48 h later the chest tube is pulled when there is little drainage (usually less than 100 mL per 12 h).

Anticancer chemotherapy is not yet standard therapy for non-small cell lung cancer and, in general, should only be given as part of clinical trials approved by the local institutions. Approximately 10 to 20 percent of patients will have objective tumor shrinkage with the most active single agents, and 30 to 40 percent of patients will respond to combination chemotherapy. However, a complete clinical regression of tumor occurs (a "complete response") in less than 5 percent of cases. Those patients whose tumors respond to chemotherapy have significantly longer survivals (around 30 to 40 weeks median survival) compared to those patients who do not respond to therapy (10 to 20 weeks median). The problem is that the responding patients also have better prognostic features (such as good performance status), and it is difficult to separate the effect of these on survival from that of chemotherapy. However, in patients with good performance status, response to chemotherapy is also associated with prolonged survival, and in some cases, relief of symptoms. Nevertheless, such combination chemotherapy can have severe side effects including treatment-related mortality. Thus, in those patients with non-small cell lung cancer who desire nonprotocol chemotherapy, it is reasonable to give chemotherapy if the patient is fully ambulatory, has an evaluable tumor mass (to follow response to therapy), has not received prior chemotherapy, and is able to understand and accept the potential benefits and toxicities from such therapy. The chemotherapy should be delivered by an experienced physician or medical oncologist, and one of the published standard regimens such as "CAP" [cyclophosphamide, doxorubicin (Adriamycin), *cis*-platin] or vindesine (an experimental drug) or vinblastin plus *cis*-platin should be used.

SMALL CELL LUNG CANCER The goal of initial treatment is to obtain a complete clinical regression of tumor documented by repeating the initial positive staging procedures, particularly fiberoptic bronchoscopy with washings and biopsy. This initial response, determined 6 to 12 weeks after the start of therapy, predicts both median and long-term survival and potential cure. Patients obtaining a complete clinical regression of tumor survive longer than patients with an objective but only partial regression (tumor shrinkage of more than 50 percent of visible disease with no sign of tumor progression elsewhere), who in turn survive longer than patients with no response. In addition, all long-term (over 3 years) survivors come from the complete response group. Untreated patients with small cell lung cancer have median survivals of only 6 to 17 weeks, and randomized trials have shown that radiotherapy alone is superior to surgery alone, that chemotherapy is superior to radiotherapy, and that chemotherapy plus radiotherapy is superior to radiotherapy alone. Randomized trials comparing chemotherapy plus radiotherapy to chemotherapy alone are currently underway. Thus, the correct integration of chemotherapy with or without radiotherapy or surgery is the cornerstone of the treatment of small cell cancer.

Following initial staging, patients are grouped into the limited or extensive disease stages and classified as being physiologically able or not able to tolerate intensive combination chemotherapy or combined modality chemoradiotherapy. Such intensive therapy should be reserved for ambulatory patients, with no prior chemotherapy or radiotherapy, no other major medical problems, and adequate heart, liver, renal, and bone marrow function. The arterial P_{O_2} on room air should be above 50 mmHg, and there should be no CO_2 retention. All patients with some or more of these limitations must have their initial chemoradio- or chemotherapy modified to prevent undue toxicity. The overall mortality rate from initial high-dose combination chemotherapy even in these selected patients is about 5 percent at major centers. This figure is comparable to the operative mortality rate for pulmonary resection and indicates the need for physiologic staging of patients before chemotherapy.

In appropriate patients, high-dose combination chemotherapy with or without radiotherapy should be given ("induction therapy"). This must be coupled with supportive care for infectious, hemorrhagic, and other medical complications. Meticulous attention to the details of therapy and the day to day management of the patient through the initial 6 to 12 weeks of treatment is essential if therapy-related mortality is to be kept low. Because of this the induction period should be supervised by a medical oncologist.

Chemotherapy The current principles of primary chemotherapy may be summarized as follows: first, combination chemotherapy using three or four of the known active agents concurrently should be used. A variety of combination chemotherapies have been reported, including CMC (cyclophosphamide + methotrexate + CCNU), alternating with VAP (vincristine + doxorubicin + procarbazine); CAV (cyclophosphamide + doxorubicin + vincristine); CCMV (cyclophosphamide + CCNU + methotrexate + vincristine); CAVP-16 (cyclophosphamide + doxorubicin + VP-16); and VP-16 (etoposide) + *cis*-platin. At present there is no evidence that any one regimen is better than another if adequate drug dose and schedules are given. Second, the initial combination chemotherapy is given in high doses during the first 6 to 8 weeks such that severe granulocytopenia (e.g., granulocyte counts less than 500 per microliter) and moderate to severe thrombocytopenia (platelets less than 50,000 per microliter) are to be expected. Following the initial intense (or "induction") therapy, patients should be restaged to determine if they have entered a "complete clinical remission," including complete disappearance of all clinically evident lesions and paraneoplastic syndromes, or a "partial remission"; or have "no response" or tumor progression (seen in 10 percent of patients or less). Following this, "maintenance" chemotherapy is given to responding patients for periods of 6 to 12 months in 3-, 4-, or 6-week cycles, depending on the combination of chemotherapy used. Appropriate drug dose modifications are made to keep the white blood count above 2000 per microliter and the platelet count above 50,000 per microliter. The patients are restaged between 6 and 12 months, depending on the individual regimens; if they are still in a complete remission, chemotherapy is stopped. The value of more prolonged chemotherapy is not documented. Patients with a partial tumor regression are generally kept on chemotherapy until the time of objective tumor progression and then switched to new chemotherapy (either with known activity or on an experimental protocol). Patients not responding or with objective tumor progression should be switched to new chemotherapy, preferably with a non-cross-resistant combination in an attempt to get an objective tumor response. High-dose [40,000 mGy (4000 rad)] radiotherapy to the whole brain should be given to patients with documented brain metastases. Prophylactic cranial radiotherapy may be given to patients with complete responses, as this will significantly decrease the development of brain metastases (occurring in 60 to 80 percent of patients living 2 or more years who do not receive such prophylactic radiotherapy), but such prophylactic therapy has not been shown to prolong survival. In the case of symptomatic progressive lesions in the chest or at other critical sites, if radiotherapy has not yet been given to these areas, it may be administered in full doses (e.g., 40,000 mGy to the chest tumor mass). Occasionally, a "recall" phenomenon will be seen in the radiation field (manifested by esophagitis, or erythema) if the patient has received prior doxorubicin chemotherapy. The management of other metastatic disease is similar to that for non-small cell lung cancer.

There are definite toxicities of both an acute and chronic nature that should be expected with combined modality chemoradiotherapy, particularly if chemo- and radiotherapy are given concurrently. Thus, the role of radiotherapy in the primary treatment of small cell lung cancer is still undergoing clinical investigation. However, retrospective analysis of long-term survivors, and analysis of local failures in the chest following chemotherapy alone, are suggestive that chest radiotherapy is of benefit. If radiotherapy is to be given to the primary lesion, patients should be selected (limited stage disease with PS 0–1 and initial good pulmonary function) such that radiotherapy can be given in full doses, by conventional fractionation, and in a manner that will not compromise the needed combination chemotherapy or sacrifice too much lung. The radiation oncologist must be prepared to deliver tailored radiotherapy with shaping of fields during treatment, much the same as is done for Hodgkin's disease. In extensive stage disease, the routine use of chest radiotherapy is to be avoided. However, if chemotherapy is inadequate to relieve local tumor symptoms, a course of radiotherapy can be added.

Applying these principles, several centers around the world have reported potential cure rates of 15 to 25 percent for limited stage disease and 1 to 5 percent for extensive stage disease. Overall, approximately 50 percent of patients with limited stage and 30 percent with extensive stage disease will enter a complete remission, and 90 to 95 percent of all patients will have some objective tumor shrinkage (complete or partial response). These responses increase the median survival from 2 to 4 months for untreated patients to 10 to 12 months for extensive stage and 14 to 18 months for limited stage patients. In addition, most patients have relief of their tumor-related symptoms and improvement of performance status. However, the maintenance of good performance status by the patient while receiving outpatient chemotherapy requires judgment and skill on the part of the medical oncologist delivering the chemotherapy so as to avoid undue therapeutic toxicity. A variety of new drug treatments are being tried (such as new drug combinations, alternating combinations of drugs, very intensive initial or "reinduction" therapy with autologous bone marrow infusion), as well as novel forms of combining chemo- and radiotherapy and surgery, but these should all be reserved for approved clinical protocols.

While surgical resection is not routinely recommended for small cell lung cancer, occasional small cell cancer patients will either meet the usual AJC requirements for resectability (stage I or II with negative mediastinal nodes) or only have a histologic diagnosis made on review of the resected surgical specimen. Such patients have been reported to have high cure rates (above 25 percent) if adjuvant combination chemotherapy is used. Thus, such uncommon, resectable small cell lung cancer patients are candidates for combined modality surgery and chemotherapy.

CLINICAL TRIALS AND BIOLOGIC STUDIES

The current poor prognosis for most lung cancer patients requires the continued performance of well-designed clinical trials to test new forms of therapy. Such trials have shown that there is no survival benefit from currently available immunotherapies such as BCG or levamisole. In addition, the development of methods to culture tumor cells directly from patients will allow (1) the prospective testing of tumor sensitivity in vitro to drugs, radiation therapy, and biologic response modifiers such as monoclonal antibodies; (2) the analysis of tumor cell growth factors, hormone and other nutritional requirements including "autocrine" growth factors such as bombesin (gastrin-releasing peptide); and (3) the biochemical and genetic study of lung cancer cells, including the characterization of oncogenes and paraneoplastic syndromes. All of these should provide a more rational basis for treatment.

BENIGN LUNG NEOPLASMS

The benign neoplasms of the lung, representing less than 5 percent of all primary tumors, include bronchial adenomas and hamartomas (90 percent of such lesions) and a group of very uncommon neoplasms (chondromas, fibromas, lipomas, hemangiomas, leiomyomas, teratomas, pseudolymphomas, and endometriosis). The diagnostic and primary treatment approach is basically the same for all of these neoplasms. They can present as central masses causing airway obstruction, cough, hemoptysis, and pneumonitis with or without x-ray findings but be accessible to fiberoptic bronchoscopy. Alternatively, they can present without symptoms as solitary pulmonary nodules and thus will be evaluated as part of a solitary pulmonary nodule workup. In all cases, the extent of surgery must be determined at operation, and a conservative procedure with appropriate reconstructions is usually performed.

BRONCHIAL ADENOMAS Bronchial adenomas (80 percent of which are central) are slowly growing intrabronchial lesions which represent 50 percent of all benign pulmonary neoplasms. Eighty to ninety percent are carcinoids, 10 to 15 percent are adenocystic tumors (or cylindromas), and 2 to 3 percent are mucoepidermoid tumors. Adenomas present in patients 15 to 60 years old (average age 45) as intrabronchial lesions and are often symptomatic for several years. Patients may have chronic cough, recurrent hemoptysis, or obstruction with atelectasis, lobar collapse, or pneumonitis and abscess formation. Bronchial carcinoids, which usually follow a benign course, and small cell lung cancers, which are highly malignant, are both derived from the same normal bronchial epithelial component, the Kulchitsky cell. This cell is part of the amine precursor uptake and decarboxylation (APUD) system. Carcinoids, like small cell lung cancers, may secrete other hormones such as ACTH or arginine vasopressin and thus cause paraneoplastic syndromes which resolve with resection. In addition, bronchial carcinoids when metastatic (usually to the liver) may produce the carcinoid syndrome, with cutaneous flush, bronchoconstriction, diarrhea, and cardiac valvular lesions (see Chap. 299), which small cell lung cancer does not. Occasionally pathologists may have difficulty in distinguishing carcinoids from small cell lung cancers, and carcinoid tumors appearing more aggressive histologically (referred to as ''atypical carcinoids'') metastasize in 70 percent of cases to regional nodes, liver, or bone, compared to only a 5 percent metastasis rate of carcinoids with typical histology.

Bronchial adenomas of all types, because of their endobronchial and often central location, are usually visible via fiberoptic bronchoscopy, and tissue for histologic diagnosis is obtained in this manner. Because they are hypervascular, they can bleed profusely after bronchoscopic biopsy, and this should be anticipated. Bronchial adenomas must be dealt with as potentially malignant and thus require removal not only for symptom relief but also because they can be locally invasive or recurrent, potentially can metastasize, or because they produce paraneoplastic syndromes. Surgical excision is the primary treatment for all types of bronchial adenomas. The extent of surgery is determined at operation and should be as conservative as possible. Often bronchotomy with local excision, sleeve rejection, segmental resection, or lobectomy is sufficient. Five-year survival rates following surgical resection are 95 percent, decreasing to 70 percent if regional nodes are involved. The treatment of metastatic pulmonary carcinoids is currently unclear because they can either be indolent, growing slowly over several years, or behave more like small cell lung carcinoma. Assessment of the tempo and the histology of the disease in the individual patient is necessary to determine if and when chemotherapy or radiotherapy is indicated.

HAMARTOMAS Pulmonary hamartomas have a peak incidence at age 60 and are more frequent in men than women. Histologically, they contain normal pulmonary tissue components (smooth muscle and collagen) in a disorganized fashion. They are usually peripheral, clinically silent, and benign in their behavior. While it would be advantageous to avoid thoracotomy in these older patients, unless the radiographic findings are pathognomonic of hamartoma with ''popcorn'' calcification, the lesions will usually have to be resected for diagnosis, particularly if the patient is a smoker.

METASTATIC PULMONARY TUMORS

The lung is frequently the site of metastatic disease from primary cancers outside the lung. Usually such metastatic disease is considered incurable. However, two special situations may arise. First is the development of a solitary pulmonary shadow on chest x-ray in a patient known to have an extrathoracic neoplasm. This may represent a metastasis or a new primary lung cancer. Because the natural history of lung cancer is worse than for most other primary tumors, it is wise to approach the single pulmonary nodule in a patient with a known extrathoracic tumor as though the nodule were a primary lung cancer, particularly if the patient is over 35 years of age and a smoker. This means a vigorous evaluation looking for other sites of active cancer and, if none are found, surgical resection of the nodule. Second, multiple pulmonary nodules may be resected for cure as well. This is usually recommended if, after careful staging, (1) the patient can tolerate the contemplated pulmonary resection; (2) the primary tumor has been definitively and successfully treated; and (3) all known metastatic disease can be encompassed by the projected pulmonary resection. The key is selection and screening of patients to exclude patients with uncontrolled primary tumors and extrapulmonary metastases. Primary tumors whose pulmonary metastases have been successfully resected for cure include osteogenic and soft tissue sarcomas; colon, rectal, uterine, cervix, and corpus tumors; head and neck, breast, testis, and salivary gland cancer; melanoma; and bladder and kidney tumors. Five-year survival rates of 20 to 30 percent have been found in carefully selected patients, and the most dramatic results have been seen in osteogenic sarcomas, where resection of pulmonary metastases (sometimes requiring several thoracotomies) is becoming a standard curative treatment approach.

REFERENCES

ATTAR S et al: Bronchial adenoma: A review of 51 patients. Ann Thorac Surg 40:126, 1985

BUNN PA JR, MINNA JD: Paraneoplastic syndromes, in *The Principles and Practice of Oncology*, 2d ed, VT DeVita et al (eds). Philadelphia, Lippincott, 1985, p 1798

CARNEY et al: Cancer of the lungs, in *Pulmonary Diseases and Disorders*, 2d ed, AP Fishman (ed). New York, McGraw-Hill, 1987, Section 14

DEDRICK CG: The solitary pulmonary nodule and staging of lung cancer. Clin Chest Med 5:345, 1984

GAZDAR AF: The biology of endocrine tumors of the lung, in *The Endocrine Lung in Health and Disease*, KL Becker, AF Gazdar (eds). Philadelphia, Saunders, 1984

GOLUMB H: Non-small cell lung cancer. Semin Oncol 10:1, 1983

HAMPER UM et al: Pulmonary hamartoma: Diagnosis by transthoracic needle-aspiration biopsy. Radiology 155:15, 1985

LUKE WP et al: Prospective evaluation of mediastinoscopy for assessment of carcinoma of the lung. J Thorac Cardiovasc Surg 91:53, 1986

MARTINI N et al: Results of resection in non-oat cell carcinoma of the lung with mediastinal lymph node metastases. Ann Surg 198:386, 1983

MINNA JD et al: Lung cancer, in *The Principles and Practice of Oncology*, 2d ed. VT DeVita et al (eds). Philadelphia, Lippincott, 1985, p 507

RADFORD EP et al: Lung cancer in Swedish iron miners exposed to low doses of radon daughters. N Engl J Med 310:1485 1984

SAMET JM et al: Uranium mining and lung cancer in Navajo men. N Engl J Med 310:1481, 1984

TISI GM et al: Clinical staging of primary lung cancer. Am Rev Resp Dis 127:1, 1983

WEISS ST: Passive smoking and lung cancer. What is the risk? Am Rev Respir Dis 133:1, 1986

214 DISEASES OF THE PLEURA, MEDIASTINUM, AND DIAPHRAGM

ROLAND H. INGRAM, JR.

THE PLEURA

The visceral and parietal pleurae form a continuous membrane that encloses a potential space which normally contains only a small amount of liquid. This liquid is dynamic, and, as with all movements of liquid between the vascular and extravascular compartments, the principles of the Starling equation (Chap. 26) apply. Under normal circumstances, the liquid is filtered out of the parietal pleura, which is supplied by systemic capillaries at a mean pressure of 30 cmH_2O, and most is taken up at the visceral pleura, supplied by the pulmonary circulation that has a mean capillary pressure of 11 cmH_2O. For the removal of macromolecules plus some liquid there are, in addition, lymphatic stomata in the diaphragmatic and basilar portions of the parietal pleura. Abnormal accumulations of liquid, designated as pleural effusions, occur with changes in hydrostatic and oncotic forces (transudation) or with alterations in membrane permeability (exudation) such as occurs with inflammation or neoplastic involvement.

The parietal pleura is supplied by segmental nerves and when inflamed gives rise to pain which is referred to superficial regions supplied by the intercostal nerves and the thoracic segments. This pain is sharp and superficial, and is aggravated during inspiration (Chap. 4). Since the location of the pain is determined by the distribution of the somatic afferents, pain may be referred to the shoulder if the diaphragmatic pleura (C3 to C5) is involved or to the upper abdomen if the lower thoracic intercostals are affected. The visceral pleura is supplied by visceral afferents that do not produce sharp and localizable pain.

The patient with pleuritic chest pain frequently has shallow, rapid breathing, and there may be lesser excursion of the affected hemithorax than the unaffected side (splinting). Inflammation of the pleural surfaces may also cause a pleural friction rub which may be localized or may be best heard at the lower thorax posteriorly, the region where there is greatest respiratory excursion. A pleural friction rub has a harsh, scratchy quality and is heard throughout the respiratory cycle; it is maximal toward the end of inspiration and early in expiration.

PLEURITIS Inflammation of the pleura can occur with or without apparent underlying pulmonary disease and has many causes, including pneumonia, tuberculosis, pulmonary infarction, and neoplasm. Pleural pain in the *absence of physical and roentgenographic findings* suggests the diagnosis of epidemic pleurodynia (Bornholm's disease, Chap. 139), other viral infections of the pleura, or connective tissue disorders such as systemic lupus erythematosus. The *presence of parenchymal disease on the chest roentgenogram* in a patient with pleuritic chest pain and fever suggests an infectious process such as acute bacterial pneumonia (Chap. 205). Pulmonary infarction secondary to pulmonary embolism (Chap. 211) may also cause inflammation of the pleural surface. Under these circumstances, hemoptysis is a common presenting feature. The finding of a *pleural effusion in the absence of parenchymal disease* suggests postprimary tuberculosis, subdiaphragmatic abscess, mesothelioma, or primary bacterial infection of the pleural space.

Treatment of pleuritis is directed toward the underlying disease and relief of pain. Analgesics frequently suppress pain, but generally they do not completely eradicate the pain associated with deep breaths and coughing. If pain prevents the patient from coughing up secretions, regional anesthesia by blockade of the appropriate intercostal nerves with a medium-duration local anesthetic is helpful. Occasionally, acute pleuritis leads to chronic adhesive pleuritis as a sequela of tuberculosis, empyema, or hemothorax. Adhesive pleuritis is characterized by marked thickening of the pleura, which may interfere with pulmonary function. Under these circumstances, the thickened pleura encases the lung and "traps" it, so that the lung behaves as if it were small and stiff, despite having intrinsically normal mechanical properties. If symptoms such as dyspnea are severe, surgical removal of the thickened pleura (decortication) may be indicated.

PLEURAL EFFUSION Pleural effusions may or may not be associated with disease of the pleura. In general, effusions due to pleural disease more nearly resemble plasma (exudates), while those occurring with a normal pleura are ultrafiltrates of the plasma (transudates). Effusions in association with pleuritis are due to increased permeability of the parietal pleura secondary to inflammatory or neoplastic involvement. A good example of pleural effusion with a normal pleura is that associated with congestive heart failure. Both increased liquid formation from the parietal pleura due to systemic capillary hypertension and decreased reabsorption from the visceral pleura secondary to elevations in pulmonary capillary pressure account for the abnormal collection of pleural liquid in this condition. Hypoalbuminemia, as occurs in nephrosis or cirrhosis, also leads to increased formation and decreased resorption of pleural liquid on the basis of decreased intravascular oncotic pressures. An additional mechanism, lymphatic obstruction, also leads to effusions in the absence of pleural disease. In this case the sharp distinction between exudates and transudates may become fuzzy. Since the lymphatic channels provide the only route for reabsorption of protein from the pleural space, protein concentrations in the effusion are often high, even though the pleura is not abnormally permeable.

The extent to which a pleural effusion compromises lung volume will depend in part on the relative stiffness of the lung and chest wall. At lung volumes in the normal breathing range, the chest wall tends to recoil outward while the lung tends to recoil inward. Many pleural effusions are asymptomatic, but patients may complain of shortness of breath. Whatever the underlying cause, dyspnea that accompanies large pleural effusions is often relieved by the removal of 1 liter of liquid. The mechanism for this relief is not totally clear since the increase in gas volume of the lungs is usually less than half the amount of liquid removed; decrease in the volume of hemithorax by inward movement of the chest wall accounts for more than half the volume change. It is possible that the inward movement of the chest wall, which puts the muscles of inspiration at a better mechanical advantage, may account for the relief of dyspnea. Pleuritic chest pain or a dull sensation in the chest may also be present. The physical signs include deviation of the trachea away from the affected side, dullness to percussion, and diminished breath sounds over the affected side. Egophony may be heard at the upper border of the effusion.

The most common appearance of a pleural effusion on chest roentgenogram is obliteration of the sharp angle between the diaphragm and rib cage (costophrenic angle) with an upward concavity of the liquid level. Occasionally, effusions lie underneath the lung (*subpulmonic effusion*) and give the appearance of an elevated hemidiaphragm. A chest roentgenogram in the lateral decubitus position (affected side down) will show the pleural liquid layering out along the lateral chest wall, provided the liquid is not loculated. A clue to the presence of a subpulmonic effusion in the left hemithorax from the chest roentgenograph taken in the upright posture is a wide density between the gastric air bubble and the apparent upper border of the diaphragm. Another clue to the presence of a subpulmonic effusion in the upright position on either side is a lateral displacement and slight flattening of the apparent dome of the diaphragm as liquid moves laterally. Pleural effusions may be missed on anteroposterior roentgenograms taken in the supine posture since the liquid layers out posteriorly. In this case it produces a generally hazy shadow that is difficult to detect when unilateral and impossible to detect when bilateral. Occasionally, effusions may form between lobes of the lungs and produce a rounded opacity on the chest roentgenogram that resembles a solitary nodule. Since these often disappear with resolution of the effusion, they are referred to as *phantom tumors.*

Aspiration of the pleural effusion under local anesthesia should always be performed if the etiology of the effusion is in doubt, or if the effusion is causing dyspnea. If the diagnosis of neoplasm or tuberculosis is seriously considered, closed pleural biopsy with an Abrams or Cope needle should be performed at the time of the initial thoracentesis. Biopsy under direct visualization via a fiberoptic thorascope should be considered if liquid analysis and blind needle biopsy fail to provide a diagnosis and if someone experienced in the procedure is available.

Characteristics of pleural fluid Pleural fluid that is bloodstained is suggestive of neoplasm or pulmonary infarction; however, blood may also be present in effusions due to infection, congestive heart failure, and trauma. The differentiation of pleural effusions into *transudates* and *exudates* is of considerable diagnostic importance. Many different tests on the pleural liquid have been advocated (Table 214-1); however, no single test is diagnostic. Effusions which have a high protein content, high pleural liquid-to-serum lactic dehydrogenase (LDH) activity ratios, and many white blood cells are indicative of exudates. However, transudates secondary to congestive heart failure may have high protein contents after the volume of the effusion decreases with diuresis; any effusion that contains cellular debris may have a high pleural fluid-to-serum LDH ratio; and there is no absolute leukocyte count that clearly differentiates transudates from exudates. Clearly the diagnosis depends on interpretation of the test results in the context of the patient's illness. In addition to chemical tests, exudative pleural liquid should receive complete cytologic and microbiologic examinations. Figure 214-1 presents an approach to the evaluation of pleural effusions. Despite an orderly and complete approach, no cause will be found for the pleural effusion in up to 25 percent of patients.

Postprimary tuberculous effusions present as isolated pleural effusions in the absence of radiologically demonstrable parenchymal disease and occur within months of primary subclinical infection. The patient may be asymptomatic or, more commonly, presents with fever, malaise, and weight loss. Occasionally, high fever and pleuritic chest pain are present. More than 90 percent of patients have a positive tuberculin skin test. Thoracentesis reveals an *exudative* effusion, with predominant lymphocytosis. Acid-fast bacilli are rarely seen on direct smear, and cultures are positive in fewer than 20 percent of pleural effusions due to tuberculosis. The diagnostic yield is higher with closed pleural biopsy, which will reveal noncaseating granulomas and/or positive culture material in more than 50 percent of the cases.

TABLE 214-1 Constituents of pleural effusions

	Transudate	Exudate
ROUTINE TESTS		
Protein	<3.0 g/100 mL	>3.0 g/100 mL
Lactic dehydrogenase	Low	High
Pleural fluid/serum LDH ratio	<0.6	>0.6
SPECIAL TESTS		
RBC	<10,000/mm³	>100,000/mm³ suggests neoplasm, infarction, trauma; >10,000, <100,000/mm³ indeterminate
WBC	<1000/mm³	Usually >1000/mm³
Differential WBC	Usually >50% lymphocytes or mononuclear cells	>50% lymphocytes (tuberculosis, neoplasm) >50% polymorphonuclear (acute inflammation)
pH	>7.3	<7.3 (inflammatory)
Glucose	Same as blood (±)	Low (infection) Extremely low (rheumatoid arthritis, occasionally neoplasm)
Amylase		>500 units/mL (pancreatitis; occasionally neoplasm, infection)
Specific proteins		Low C3, C4 components of complement (SLE, rheumatoid arthritis) Rheumatoid factor Antinuclear factor

Neoplastic pleural effusions are common; they are usually exudative. *Bronchogenic carcinoma* is the commonest malignancy causing pleural effusions and may do so by direct extension to the pleural surface, obstruction to lymphatic drainage (secondary to mediastinal spread), or by pleural inflammation secondary to pneumonia behind an obstructed bronchus. Patients usually present with symptoms referable to the primary lesion (Chap. 213) but may present with dyspnea or pleuritic chest pain. The effusion is invariably an exudate with or without blood. Pleural liquid cytology and pleural biopsy will confirm the diagnosis in up to 60 percent of cases. *Metastatic carcinoma,* most commonly from the breast, may also cause pleural effusions and is a more frequent cause of bilateral pleural effusions than bronchogenic carcinoma. *Lymphoma* may directly involve the pleura or may obstruct lymphatic drainage leading to a pleural effusion. Malignant effusions reaccumulate rapidly after aspiration, and repeated aspirations are not warranted. Instillation of sclerosing compounds such as tetracycline or cytotoxic agents may succeed in producing adhesions between parietal and visceral pleural surfaces and decrease the rate of liquid accumulation.

Rheumatoid arthritis (Chap. 263) may cause exudative pleural effusions with or without nodular changes in the pulmonary parenchyma or on the pleural surface. Patients are most often males, and subcutaneous nodules are usually associated with the arthritis. The pleural liquid is characteristically turbid and greenish yellow and has a very low glucose concentration (less than 20 mg/dL) due to impaired glucose transport into the pleural liquid. These effusions are usually asymptomatic and do not require specific therapy. However, on occasion pleuritic chest pain and fever herald the onset of rheumatoid effusions, and, because of the acute presentation along with low glucose levels in the liquid, infectious empyema must be ruled out. Mononuclear pleocytosis and negative Gram stains and cultures aid in eliminating empyema.

Symptoms and signs referable to the chest very frequently accompany *subphrenic* (*subdiaphragmatic*) *abscess.* Fever, pleuritic chest pain, and an exudative pleural effusion are common. The chest roentgenogram usually reveals elevation of the hemidiaphragm, a small pleural effusion, and basal atelectasis, but is rarely diagnostic. Thoracentesis usually reveals sterile liquid, but an empyema due to direct extension of the infection may be present. It should be emphasized that pleural effusions following abdominal surgery are very common and should not be taken as a sign of a subdiaphragmatic abscess in the absence of other clinical features.

In *pancreatitis,* a left-sided pleural effusion may be present in up to 15 percent of patients with acute pancreatitis or pancreatic pseudocysts. Effusions are typically exudative and have a high amylase concentration. A high pleural fluid amylase concentration has occasionally been reported in neoplasm and infection, and may also be found in cases of esophageal rupture where the amylase is of salivary origin. No specific therapy of pleural effusion secondary to pancreatitis is indicated. An exception is the occurrence of a chronic effusion due to a fistula connecting a pancreatic pseudocyst to the pleural space. Surgical management of the primary pancreatic problem is indicated.

Pleural effusion and ascites in association with nonmetastatic pelvic tumors in women has been designated as *Meigs's syndrome.* The pleural effusion is most commonly right-sided, may be an exudate or transudate, and is thought to develop from movement of ascitic liquid across the diaphragm. Both the ascites and pleural liquid dramatically resolve following removal of the pelvic tumor.

Eosinophilic pleural effusion is defined as the finding of eosinophils in excess of 10 percent in the pleural liquid; this attention-getting yet nonspecific finding may be present in effusions due to acute bacterial pneumonia, viral pleuritis, pancreatitis, and trauma. Eosinophilic effusions, however, are uncommon with neoplasms and quite rare with tuberculosis.

Patients have been described with the triad of *yellow nails, lymphedema of the extremities, and pleural effusions.* The effusions have a high protein concentration and are thought to be due to impaired lymphatic drainage of the pleural space rather than to pleural disease.

CHYLOTHORAX Leakage of thoracic duct lymph into the pleural space may be due to trauma to the thoracic duct or obstruction of the duct by a malignant process (lymphoma, mediastinal spread of bronchogenic carcinoma) or mediastinal fibrosis. A rare disorder, *lymphangiomyomatosis,* is frequently accompanied by chylothorax. Thoracentesis reveals a milky white liquid which is characteristically an exudate. Fat globules may be seen microscopically on staining with Sudan III dye. Total fat content ranges from 1 to 4 g/dL. In cases of traumatic rupture of the thoracic duct, conservative man-

FIGURE 214-1 *Approach to the diagnosis of pleural effusions.*

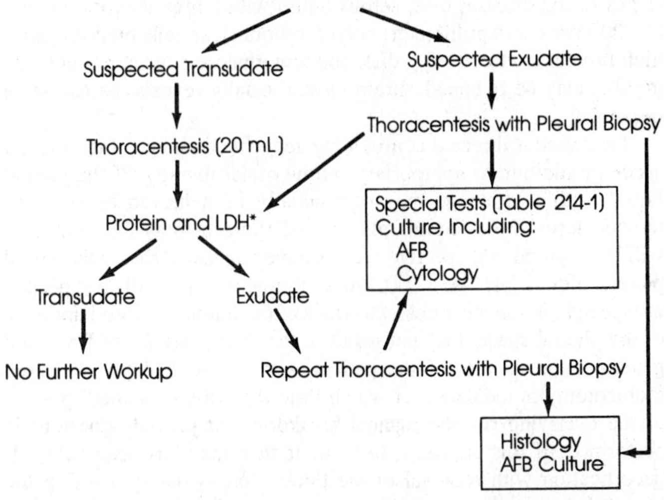

*Draw Blood Sample Simultaneously to Compare with Pleural Fluid Values agement by repeated aspiration or thoracostomy-tube drainage and by cessation of oral feedings is tried initially. If this fails, lymphangiography followed by surgical ligation of the thoracic duct may be indicated. A chylothorax secondary to malignancy should not be repeatedly aspirated, since it reaccumulates rapidly.

Pseudochylous effusions do not contain fat globules but have a cloudy, milky appearance due to high concentrations of cholesterol in the pleural liquid. Cholesterol crystals may give a metallic sheen to the pleural liquid. This condition most frequently occurs in long-standing pleural effusions, and the most frequent underlying diagnoses are tuberculosis and rheumatoid lung disease.

HEMOTHORAX Hemothorax due to frank bleeding into the pleural space most commonly follows blunt or penetrating trauma to the chest. A small amount of bleeding may complicate a spontaneous pneumothorax, producing a hemopneumothorax when preexisting adhesions are disrupted as air separates the parietal and visceral pleurae. Patients with hematologic disorders or who are taking anticoagulants may bleed into the pleural space following procedures such as closed pleural biopsy; therefore, a pleural biopsy should never be performed without first ensuring that the patient's coagulation status is adequate. Treatment of hemothorax is directed toward adequate drainage of the pleural space. Continued bleeding, inadequate drainage, or shock unresponsive to blood replacement require thoracotomy. Inadequate drainage of a hemothorax may lead to an intense, fibrous reaction (fibrothorax) where the thickened pleura encases the lung (trapped lung); early decortication is indicated.

EMPYEMA The presence of infected liquid or frank pus in the pleural space is termed an empyema. In the majority of cases it is the result of spread of infection from a contiguous structure and may complicate the course of bacterial pneumonia, subdiaphragmatic abscess, lung abscess, or esophageal perforation. Up to 20 percent of empyemas follow thoracic surgery or instrumentation of the pleural space (thoracentesis, inadvertent entry of the pleural space during puncture of the subclavian vein). Direct infection of the pleural space without involvement of the underlying lung by hematogenous spread of organisms from a distant site accounts for the remaining cases and is more common in children than adults. Bacteria implicated in the etiology of empyema include *Staphylococcus aureus* (most common in all ages), *Pseudomonas aeruginosa, Klebsiella pneumoniae, Escherichia coli, Pneumococcus* spp., and anaerobic bacteria.

Chest pain, fever and night sweats, cough, and weight loss are common complaints. These symptoms may be mild if an empyema develops during the course of antibiotic treatment for bacterial pneumonia; hence the empyema may go unrecognized. Signs of a pleural effusion will be present, and the chest roentgenogram will reveal pleural liquid and usually underlying parenchymal disease. Thoracentesis may reveal thick, purulent liquid, but in the early stages of the disease, thin, serous liquid with a high leukocyte count (>5000 per cubic millimeter; polymorphonuclear cells predominate), high protein content (>3 g/dL), and low glucose concentration (<20 mg/dL) may be obtained. Gram's stain usually reveals the causative organism.

Treatment is directed at providing adequate drainage of the pleural space in addition to appropriate antimicrobial therapy. If the pleural liquid is thin, drainage may occasionally be achieved by repeated thoracenteses. Most commonly, closed thoracostomy-tube drainage will be required. Prospective studies have suggested that if the initial pleural liquid pH is <7.0, tube thoracostomy will be needed irrespective of the other characteristics of the liquid. If closed drainage of the pleural space does not result in the disappearance of fever and general improvement of the patient within 4 to 5 days, a limited thoracotomy is indicated, at which time resection of a small portion of the overlying rib and manual breakdown of pleural adhesions is performed. If this approach fails, or if treatment has been delayed, decortication with removal of the thick, fibrous tissue covering the lung (pleural peel) may be necessary to obtain lung expansion and obliteration of the empyema cavity. Rarely, an unrecognized empyema may rupture through the chest wall and spontaneously drain onto the body surface (*empyema necessitans*).

Occasionally a loculated empyema and an edematous, inflamed pulmonary lobe or segment may resemble each other on routine radiographic examination. In such instances ultrasonography or computer-assisted tomography aid in making the differential diagnosis. In the case of a loculated empyema, drainage under guidance of such detection techniques is often successful.

The mortality rate of empyema is high among patients who are elderly, who have serious underlying disease, or in whom treatment is delayed.

PNEUMOTHORAX A pneumothorax is a collection of gas in the pleural space that results in complete or partial collapse of the lung. Normally, the pressure in the pleural space at the end of a quiet breath is subatmospheric due to a balance between the tendency of the lung to recoil inward and the tendency of the chest wall to recoil outward (Chap. 200). The lung may therefore be thought to be held in an expanded position by the surrounding negative pleural pressure much as a balloon would be held inflated when surrounded by a vacuum. When air enters the pleural space, pleural pressure in the affected hemithorax tends toward atmospheric pressure; the less negative the pleural pressure, the greater the degree of lung collapse. The mediastinum shifts toward the unaffected side as a result of the normal elastic recoil of the unaffected lung. If pressure inside the pneumothorax becomes above atmospheric, as may occur with a one-way leak into the pleural space ("ball-valve" leak) or when a pneumothorax occurs as a complication of positive pressure ventilation, a *tension pneumothorax* is present. Under these circumstances the affected lung is compressed, the mediastinum is further shifted toward the unaffected side, and cardiac output may be severely compromised due to the positive intrathoracic pressure decreasing venous return to the heart. Tension pneumothorax is a medical emergency.

A pneumothorax may occur spontaneously or may be secondary to underlying lung disease, chest trauma, mechanical ventilation, or perforated esophagus.

Spontaneous pneumothorax Spontaneous pneumothorax most commonly occurs in previously healthy adults between 20 and 40 years of age. In such patients there is a strong tendency toward recurrence of the pneumothorax. Air leaks into the pleural space due to rupture of small blebs on the surface of the visceral pleura; the etiology of these blebs is unclear. They tend to be at the apex of the lung, perhaps due to the more negative pleural pressure around the lung apex. Some patients have been found to have small pleural nodules consisting of histiocytes, giant cells, and other inflammatory cells (*reactive eosinophilic pleuritis*). These lesions should be differentiated from pulmonary eosinophilic granuloma.

Pleuritic chest pain and dyspnea are the commonest complaints in patients with pneumothorax. Physical examination reveals tachypnea, asymmetric expansion of the chest on the affected side (due to outward recoil of the chest wall as the lung collapses), mediastinal shift with deviation of the trachea and apex beat away from the pneumothorax, and hyperresonance to percussion and diminished breath sounds over the affected side. The chest roentgenogram reveals a visible visceral pleural edge with no lung markings between this edge and the chest wall. Chest roentgenograms should be taken in the upright position before a pneumothorax can be excluded, since in the supine posture upward movement of air with approximation of visceral and parietal pleurae laterally may obscure its presence. Small pneumothoraxes may be more easily seen if the chest roentgenogram is taken at the end of a maximal expiration. If pneumothorax is associated with tearing of adhesions in the pleural space, *hemopneumothorax* may develop, with a gas-liquid level visible in the pleural space.

Treatment depends on the size of the pneumothorax. A small pneumothorax needs only close observation, since the air leak has usually sealed by the time the patient presents. The air in the pleural space will be reabsorbed spontaneously, since the sum of the partial pressures of the gases in the pleural space (i.e., air = 760 mmHg at sea level) is greater than the sum of the partial pressures of gases in the end-capillary blood due to the low end-capillary P_{O_2}. Modestly sized pneumothoraxes can be easily evacuated using commercially available catheters prepackaged with insertion needles and one-way flutter valves that allow escape but not reentry of air. Larger pneumothoraxes should be aspirated or treated with closed thoracostomy-tube drainage. Failure of the lung to reexpand, despite application of suction to the chest tube, indicates that the lung is "trapped," that a major bronchus is occluded, or that there is a large continuing air leak through a major communication between the pleural space and lung (*bronchopleural fistula*). A bronchopleural fistula rarely occurs spontaneously unless there is underlying lung disease such as rupture of a lung abscess into the pleural space or necrotizing pneumonia, but may occur following lung resection or chest trauma or during mechanical ventilation (barotrauma). Spontaneous *tension* pneumothorax is unusual, but if present, it should be treated by immediate aspiration through a wide-bore needle placed in the pleural space at the level of the second intercostal space anteriorly at the midclavicular line. If there is circulatory collapse and severe dyspnea, tension pneumothorax should be suspected and treated without waiting for roentgenographic confirmation.

Approximately 50 percent of patients with spontaneous pneumothorax have a recurrence, and the incidence of further recurrence is even higher following the second episode. Repeated spontaneous pneumothorax should be treated surgically by application of irritants to the pleural surfaces so that they adhere to each other (*pleurodesis*) or by performing a *parietal pleurectomy*. Because of the tendency of pneumothorax to recur, if both sides are ever involved, even at different times, surgical intervention is indicated.

Patients with pneumothorax should not be moved in unpressurized aircraft because the decrease in atmospheric pressure may result in enlargement of the pneumothorax to an extent that it may seriously compromise ventilatory and cardiac function. Similarly, patients with a history of spontaneous pneumothorax should not pilot aircraft or undertake scuba diving. Should a pneumothorax occur underwater, enlargement of the pneumothorax on ascent may be catastrophic.

Pneumothorax may occur spontaneously in patients with a wide variety of lung diseases, such as asthma, emphysema, lung abscess, neoplasm, eosinophilic granuloma, and the adult respiratory distress syndrome. In the presence of underlying lung disease closed thoracotomy-tube drainage will almost always be needed. *Catamenial pneumothorax* is a rare disorder characterized by spontaneous pneumothorax at the time of the menstrual period. The right side is more frequently, but not invariably, affected. The pathogenesis of this disorder is not understood but may be related to intrathoracic endometriosis. Hormonal therapy with suppression of ovulation is usually successful.

PLEURAL TUMORS Two types of *mesothelioma,* a rare tumor of the visceral and parietal pleurae, are recognized. The *localized form* is a solitary growth on the pleural surface that only occasionally causes a pleural effusion and may be cured by surgical resection. Patients are often asymptomatic or may complain of chest pain and cough. The *diffuse mesothelioma* is a highly malignant tumor that is usually associated with a serous or blood-stained pleural effusion. There is no effective therapy for this tumor. Clubbing of the digits and hypertrophic pulmonary osteoarthropathy are associated with pleural-based tumors. The diagnosis of mesothelioma may be obtained from cytologic examination of the pleural liquid or closed pleural biopsy, but difficulty may be encountered distinguishing this tumor histologically from adenocarcinoma. There is an increased incidence of pleural and peritoneal mesotheliomas among persons exposed to asbestos; a higher incidence is found among those engaged in the processing and use of asbestos products than those in the mining industry. The interval between exposure and tumor development often exceeds 20 years; continuous exposure to asbestos is not necessary. In addition to primary tumors, the pleura is a common site for *metastases* from neoplasms of the bronchus, breast, ovary, and gastrointestinal tract.

MEDIASTINUM

The mediastinum occupies the central portion of the chest and is anatomically defined by the thoracic inlet above, the diaphragm below, the mediastinal pleura laterally, the paravertebral gutter and ribs posteriorly, and the sternum anteriorly. The mediastinum is divided into four compartments for descriptive purposes (Fig. 214-2). The *superior mediastinum* is bounded above by the plane of the first rib and below by an imaginary line drawn anteroposteriorly from the sternal angle to the lower edge of the fourth thoracic vertebra. It contains the trachea, upper esophagus, thymus gland, thoracic duct, great veins, arch of the aorta and its branches, and the phrenic, vagus, and left recurrent laryngeal nerves. Below the superior mediastinum lie three further compartments. The *anterior mediastinum* contains fibroareolar tissue and lymph nodes, but no major structures. The *middle mediastinum* contains the heart, ascending aorta, great veins, pulmonary artery, and phrenic nerves. The *posterior mediastinum* contains the esophagus, thoracic duct, descending aorta, sympathetic chain, and intercostal and vagal nerves.

TUMORS AND CYSTS The commonest mediastinal masses in adults are metastatic carcinomas (most commonly bronchogenic carcinoma) and lymphomas. These masses may represent enlargement of lymph nodes and the possibility of sarcoidosis, infectious mononucleosis, and the diffuse lymphadenopathy syndrome in association with the acquired immunodeficiency syndrome must be considered in addition to lymphoma and carcinoma. Neurogenic tumors, teratodermoids, thymomas, and bronchogenic cysts account for approximately two-thirds of the remaining mediastinal masses.

One-third of patients are asymptomatic, with the mediastinal mass detected on a routine chest roentgenogram. In the remainder, chest pain, cough, dyspnea, and symptoms due to compression or invasion of structures in the mediastinum may be present (e.g., dysphagia, hoarseness due to recurrent laryngeal nerve involvement, superior vena caval obstruction). Symptoms are more common with malignant tumors.

Investigation of a mediastinal mass begins with posteroanterior and lateral chest roentgenograms to which are added oblique views, a contrast study of the esophagus, and tomography, if needed, to define more clearly the anatomic location and borders of the mass. The anatomic site of the lesion is of diagnostic importance, and may determine the next step in the diagnostic workup (Fig. 214-2). Computerized tomography of the chest with injection of contrast material into a peripheral vein, or angiography of the pulmonary circulation or aorta may be needed to distinguish vascular from nonvascular lesions, a differentiation of particular importance if biopsy of the mass is considered. A further value of computerized tomography is the detection of the cystic nature of a lesion, a finding

FIGURE 214-2 *Common sites for mediastinal masses.*

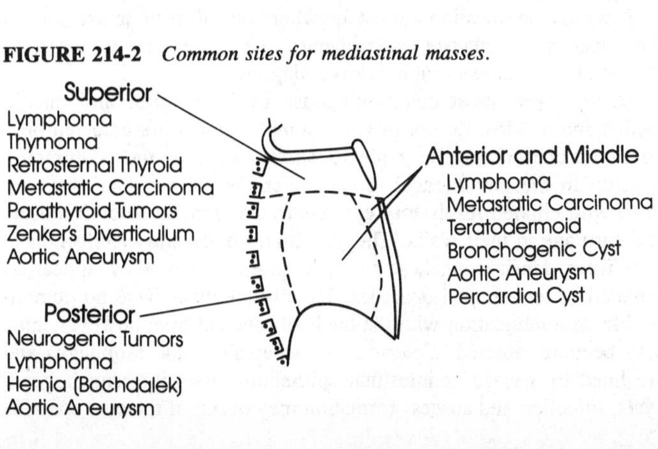

that strongly indicates that it is benign. Mediastinoscopy and biopsy are useful in the diagnosis of mediastinal masses if metastatic carcinoma, lymphoma, or sarcoidosis are considered likely. Lymph nodes behind the trachea and below the aortic arch on the left side are not accessible for biopsy using this approach. Scalene lymph node biopsy in the absence of palpable nodes may provide the diagnosis if lymphoma or metastatic carcinoma is suspected. Bronchoscopy is unlikely to be helpful in the diagnostic workup unless there are symptoms suggestive of an endobronchial lesion (e.g., hemoptysis) or unless there is evidence of lobar collapse, consolidation, or a mass lesion in the lung parenchyma on chest roentgenograph. Special tests such as radionuclide scanning with ^{131}I to detect an active retrosternal goiter may also be helpful.

Neurogenic tumors are the most common primary mediastinal neoplasms and are found almost exclusively in the posterior mediastinum near the paravertebral gutter. The majority of these neoplasms are benign; neurofibromas, schwannomas, and ganglioneuromas are the commonest tumors seen. Vague chest pain and cough may be present, but "root" pain is an infrequent complaint. *Paravertebral abscesses* also appear in the posterior mediastinum, and the clinical picture of infection often gives the major clue. Neurofibromas may occur singly or in association with von Recklinghausen's disease (Chap. 351). Occasionally these are accompanied by hypertrophic pulmonary osteoarthropathy. *Ganglioneuromas* arise from the sympathetic chain and, together with *neuroblastomas,* may secrete hormones which lead to diarrhea, flushing, and hypertension. Vanillylmandelic acid (VMA) may be found in the urine. Mediastinal *neuroblastoma* usually occurs in children, is particularly responsive to irradiation, and has a better prognosis than neuroblastomas of the abdomen or retroperitoneal space. *Pheochromocytoma* is a rare mediastinal tumor which may secrete catecholamines and present the same clinical picture as the more common (but still rare) abdominal form (Chap. 326). The treatment of all neurogenic tumors of the mediastinum is surgical, with postoperative irradiation for patients with neuroblastomas.

Teratodermoids most commonly arise in the anterior mediastinum. Most of these tumors are detected in early adult life and approximately 10 to 20 percent undergo malignant changes. Teratodermoids frequently contain linear calcification of the lining of a cyst, and bone and teeth may be evident on chest roentgenogram. They are treated by surgical excision.

Thymomas account for 10 percent of primary mediastinal neoplasms and are found in the superior and anterior mediastinum. Approximately one-fourth are malignant, but they rarely metastasize. Myasthenia gravis (Chap. 358) occurs in about 50 percent of patients with thymoma; however, the majority of patients with myasthenia gravis do not have a thymic tumor. Agammaglobulinemia, pure red blood cell aplasia, and Cushing's syndrome have been reported to be associated with thymoma. Because of compression of the trachea by the tumor, patients may complain of dyspnea in the supine posture. Symptoms may also arise from local invasion or compression of other surrounding structures. Treatment is by surgical excision; malignant thymomas are usually radiation-sensitive.

Lipomas can develop almost anywhere but most often are seen in the superior or anterior mediastinum. Computerized tomography almost always allows a noninvasive diagnosis.

Benign cysts most commonly arise in the anterior and middle mediastinum. Most do not produce symptoms and are detected only on routine chest roentgenography. *Bronchogenic cysts* most commonly develop in the paratracheal area or near the carina. The cysts are lined with ciliated respiratory epithelium and contain smooth muscle and cartilage in their walls. They are liquid-filled and therefore have a uniform density on chest roentgenogram, where they appear as rounded or tear-shaped opacities. Usually the cysts have no demonstrable communication with the tracheobronchial tree; however, they may become infected. *Enteric cysts* occur along the esophagus and are lined by gastric or intestinal epithelium. As with bronchogenic cysts, infection and abscess formation may occur. If the cyst contains acid-secreting cells, ulcer formation, perforation, and hemorrhage may occur. The *pericardial cyst* is a developmental anomaly and is attached to the pericardium but only rarely communicates with the pericardial cavity.

Hernias through the diaphragm produce mediastinal masses that may or may not contain intestinal gas. The commonest is through the esophageal hiatus as discussed below. More rarely a defect in the posterolateral portion (so-called foramen of Bochdalek) of the diaphragm allows herniation of intestine into the left side of the chest. More often presenting as a mediastinal mass is a retrosternal herniation through the foramen of Morgagni.

SUPERIOR VENA CAVAL SYNDROME Obstruction of the superior vena cava (SVC) secondary to compression or infiltration by superior mediastinal tumors results in a characteristic constellation of physical findings with dilatation of collateral veins of the upper thorax and neck, plethora and edema of the face and neck, conjunctival edema, and headache. Visual disturbances and alterations in the state of consciousness may occur. Compression of the adjacent esophagus and trachea may cause dysphagia, wheeze, and shortness of breath.

Obstruction of the SVC is most often due to malignant disease, approximately 75 percent of the cases being due to *bronchogenic carcinoma*. *Lymphoma* accounts for almost all the remaining cases. Right-sided tumors much more frequently produce the syndrome as would be expected on an anatomic basis. Rarely, this syndrome occurs with *fibrosing mediastinitis* that is either idiopathic or secondary to histoplasmosis or occurs in association with methylsergide ingestion. *Retrosternal thyroid* and *aortic aneurysms* are among the other benign causes of SVC obstruction. Using invasive diagnostic procedures such as bronchoscopy, esophagoscopy, and mediastinoscopy in an attempt to obtain a tissue diagnosis is contraindicated due to the risk of bleeding during the procedure. Unless clinical examination and noninvasive investigations suggest a benign cause for the obstruction, or unless there is tissue elsewhere to biopsy (e.g., lymphadenopathy, skin lesions), the patient should receive irradiation or chemotherapy before attempts are made to obtain a tissue diagnosis. Corticosteroids are sometimes given during the initial stages of management in an effort to decrease edema at the site of obstruction.

PNEUMOMEDIASTINUM (MEDIASTINAL EMPHYSEMA) Air within the planes of the mediastinum may appear spontaneously or may be secondary to chest trauma, perforation of the trachea, bronchus, or esophagus, spread of air from the fascial planes of the neck or pharynx, or from dissection of air from the retroperitoneal space. When pneumomediastinum occurs with no apparent cause, it is referred to as a *spontaneous pneumomediastinum*. In contrast to spontaneous pneumothorax, as discussed above, there is no tendency for recurrence. Air is thought to dissect from alveoli to the interstitial space and into the vascular adventitia to the hilum. From there it moves into the mediastinum, neck, or retroperitoneal space. Occasionally mediastinal air ruptures into the pleural space, giving a small pneumothorax, most often on the left side. Predisposing factors include raised intrathoracic pressure, as with coughing, vomiting, and Valsalva maneuvers. Rapid decompression such as occurs with sudden ascent during diving has also been implicated. Pneumomediastinum may also occur spontaneously during an attack of asthma. The patient with pneumomediastinum may be asymptomatic but usually complains of retrosternal pain and dyspnea; less commonly there is sore throat due to dissection of air into the retropharyngeal space. Examination may reveal subcutaneous crepitus in the upper body, and a crunching sound synchronous with the heart beat may be heard over the precordium (Hamman's sign). Fever and mild leukocytosis are common with uncomplicated pneumomediastinum. Occasionally, cardiac function is compromised with physical signs of cardiac tamponade (Chap. 194). A lateral chest roentgenogram should always be obtained if pneumomediastinum is suspected since abnormalities may be seen only on this view. Air is seen outlining the pulmonary artery trunk and root of aorta and may be seen tracking into the neck.

Pneumomediastinum secondary to *esophageal perforation* may follow endoscopy or may occur with vomiting (Boerhaave's syndrome). Esophageal perforation is a surgical emergency and should be suspected if there is increasing pain aggravated by swallowing or fever and when signs of increasing mediastinal width and left pleural effusion occur on chest roentgenogram. Acute and fulminant mediastinitis is a frequent sequela and should be treated with immediate surgical drainage, closure of the perforation site, and broad-spectrum antibiotic therapy.

THE DIAPHRAGM

The diaphragm is the major muscle of inspiration and is derived embryonically from the septum transversum and the pleuroperitoneal membranes. Its motor nerve supply is from the phrenic nerves (C3 to C5); the afferent supply is derived both from the phrenic and lower intercostal nerves. When the diaphragm contracts, intrathoracic pressure is lowered and intraabdominal pressure is increased. Thus, the diaphragm acts as if it were "pulling" on the lung (by lowering intrathoracic pressure) and "pushing" on the rib cage (by raising abdominal pressure), resulting in an increase in lung volume and outward movement of both rib cage and abdomen as it descends on inspiration.

DIAPHRAGMATIC PARALYSIS *Unilateral diaphragmatic paralysis* is often the result of injury to a phrenic nerve secondary to trauma or tumor in the mediastinum. However, slightly more than half the cases remain unexplained even after intensive investigation and several years of follow-up; some patients spontaneously recover function. The lesion is usually asymptomatic, but the patient may complain of dyspnea in the supine posture when the diaphragm, weakened by unilateral paralysis, must work against the added load of the abdominal contents. Unilateral paralysis results in only a small decrease in vital capacity. The diagnosis is suggested by the finding of an elevated hemidiaphragm on chest roentgenogram and can be confirmed by fluoroscopy. Paradoxical (i.e., upward) motion of the affected hemidiaphragm occurs when the patient is asked to sniff, a maneuver that suddenly lowers intrathoracic and raises intraabdominal pressure.

Bilateral diaphragmatic paralysis is less common than unilateral paralysis, but it has far greater consequences on respiration. Bilateral paralysis may be due to high cervical cord injury, motor neuron disease, poliomyelitis, polyneuropathies, or bilateral involvement of the phrenic nerve by mediastinal lesions. Recently the use of ice slush in the pericardium for cardioplegia during cardiac surgery has been associated with bilateral paralysis due to cold injury of the phrenic nerves. The patient with bilateral diaphragmatic paralysis usually has severe shortness of breath, particularly in the supine position, and often hypercapnic respiratory failure is present. In most of these patients there is paradoxical (i.e., inward) motion of the abdomen on inspiration, a finding easily observed at the bedside, particularly with the patient supine. This is due to passive ascent of the diaphragm as intrathoracic pressure is lowered by the intercostal and accessory muscles. In a few patients paradoxical abdominal motion may not be obvious with the patient erect due to use of the abdominal muscles during expiration. Here, abdominal motion will appear normal as contraction of the abdominal muscles causes inward abdominal motion on expiration and relaxation results in outward abdominal motion on inspiration. Under these circumstances the diaphragm may appear to move normally at fluoroscopy, and the diagnosis of diaphragmatic paralysis will be missed.

The vital capacity which is reduced in the upright posture is even more severely reduced when the patient is supine because the paralyzed diaphragm is sucked upward during a maximal inspiration with displacement of abdominal contents into the thorax. The diagnosis of bilateral diaphragmatic paralysis is established by assessment of transdiaphragmatic pressure obtained by comparison of simultaneous measurements of esophageal and gastric pressures. Treatment of this disorder may be conservative, using a rocking bed at night; in patients with intact phrenic nerves, electrical pacing of those nerves has been successful.

ELEVATION OF THE HEMIDIAPHRAGM ON CHEST ROENTGENOGRAPH Normally, the right side of the diaphragm is approximately 4 cm higher than the left due to displacement by the liver. *Apparent elevation* of one hemidiaphragm is due to a subpulmonic pleural effusion, and a lateral decubitus chest roentgenogram will establish this diagnosis. *True elevation* of one hemidiaphragm is most commonly due to upward displacement secondary to intraabdominal masses or ascites, or it may be due to loss of lung volume on the affected side secondary to pulmonary collapse or fibrosis. *Eventration of the diaphragm* is a rare congenital disorder more common on the left side. The anterior two-thirds of the diaphragm is replaced by a thin membrane, resulting in upward movement of abdominal contents into the thoracic cage. Patients are usually asymptomatic, and the diagnosis is made following a routine chest roentgenogram. No treatment is necessary. Rarely, eventration of the diaphragm may seriously compromise ventilatory function in the newborn. Plication of the hemidiaphragm is then performed. Eventration must be distinguished from *diaphragmatic hernias* through which abdominal contents are displaced into the chest. The most common location is at the esophageal hiatus with displacement of part of the stomach into the posterior mediastinum (Chap. 234).

MISCELLANEOUS DISEASES OF THE DIAPHRAGM Neoplasms of the diaphragm are rare; they include lipomas, fibromas, neurofibromas, and cysts. These benign tumors are approximately 1 to 1½ times more frequent than the malignant fibrosarcoma. The diaphragm may be involved by direct extension of primary lung or abdominal tumors and may be the site of metastases from distant tumors.

REFERENCES

AHMAN FR: A reassessment of the clinical implications of the superior vena caval syndrome. J Clin Oncol 2:961, 1984

CAMFFERMAN F et al: Idiopathic bilateral diaphragmatic paralysis. Eur J Respir Dis 67:65, 1985

HAUSHEER FH, YARBRO JW: Diagnosis and treatment of malignant pleural effusion. Semin Oncol 12:54, 1985

KOPECKY SL: Pneumomediastinum: Pitfalls in diagnosis and management. Minn Med 67:683, 1984

LIGHT RW et al: Parapneumonic effusions. Am J Med 69:507, 1980

MARVASTA MA et al: Misleading density of mediastinal cysts on computed tomography. Ann Thorac Surg 31:167, 1981

NEWSOM DJ et al: Diaphragm function and alveolar hypoventilation. Q J Med 177:87, 1976

SABISTON DC: Primary neoplasms and cysts of the mediastinum, in *Pulmonary Diseases and Disorders*, AP Fishman (ed). New York, McGraw-Hill, 1987, chap 130

SILVERMAN NA, SABISTON DC: Mediastinal masses. Surg Clin North Am 60:757, 1980

215 DISORDERS OF VENTILATION

JOHN B. WEST

The principles governing pulmonary ventilation and its regulation are discussed in Chap. 200. The fine control of ventilation is normally carried out by the central chemoreceptors near the central surface of the medulla which respond to changes in pH of the extracellular fluid around them. The composition of this fluid is mainly determined by the cerebrospinal fluid. For example, a fall in pH caused by diffusion of carbon dioxide across the blood-brain barrier increases respiratory drive, thus holding the arterial P_{CO_2}[1] within close limits (Fig. 215-1). The response of the central chemoreceptors is augmented by the effects of P_{CO_2} on the peripheral chemoreceptors. The extreme sensitivity of these feedback controls is seen when a normal subject

[1] *Unless otherwise stated, the partial pressures refer to arterial blood.*

inhales air containing carbon dioxide. Typically the ventilation may double for a rise in P_{CO_2} of only 2 to 3 mmHg.

Arterial hypoxemia constitutes a coarse control through its action on the peripheral chemoreceptors in the carotid bodies. Although this control is minor under normal conditions, it becomes very important during chronic hypoxia, as in people living at high altitude, or in patients with chronic lung disease. Under these conditions the increased ventilation lowers the P_{CO_2} of the arterial blood and cerebrospinal fluid, but the pH of the cerebrospinal fluid is reset to near its normal level of about 7.32 by outward movement of bicarbonate.

Additional control is afforded by changes in pH of the arterial blood irrespective of its P_{CO_2}. This relatively weak regulation apparently occurs through stimulation of the peripheral chemoreceptors, and although it is seldom seen under normal conditions, it may dominate in the control of ventilation in metabolic acidosis. Reflexes originating in the lung and elsewhere also affect ventilation under some circumstances.

Disorders of the regulation of respiration include hypoventilation, hyperventilation, and abnormal patterns of breathing. A cardinal feature of hypoventilation is carbon dioxide retention (Table 215-1), and indeed these terms are often used virtually interchangeably. This can be misleading, but following common usage, the various types of carbon dioxide retention are grouped here under the heading of hypoventilation.

FIGURE 215-1 *Scheme to illustrate the various causes of carbon dioxide retention. These include (1) disorders of the respiratory center, (2) disorders of the supplying nerves, (3) disorders of muscles of ventilation, or (4) some mechanical problem in lung or chest wall, including obstruction to the upper airways. All these conditions result in hypoventilation. However, chronic obstructive pulmonary disease (5) in effect diverts blood from the ventilated regions, so that carbon dioxide retention occurs in spite of a normal (or high) ventilation. In addition, the ventilatory response is inappropriate for the level of carbon dioxide in these patients because of the increased work of breathing and sometimes also because of a reduced sensitivity of the respiratory center.*

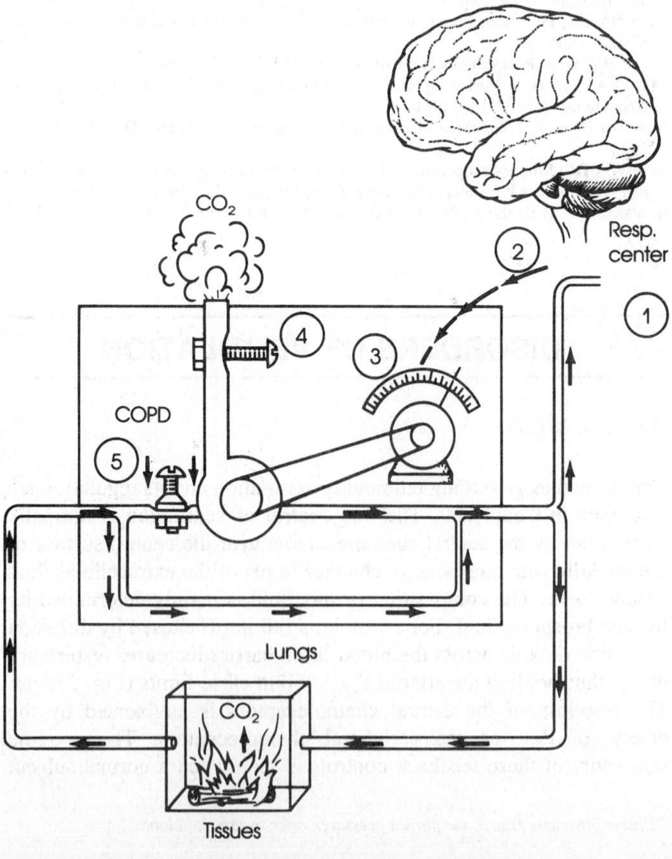

HYPOVENTILATION

CARBON DIOXIDE RETENTION CAUSED BY PURE HYPOVENTILATION (NORMAL LUNGS) In this group of diseases, the amount of air going into the lungs each minute is reduced. Strictly, it is the volume of air entering the alveoli, or *alveolar ventilation,* which is crucial (Chap. 200). However, in practice, the volume of the conducting airways remains fairly constant so that if the amount of air passing the lips is abnormally low, hypoventilation is said to be present.

The alveolar ventilation and alveolar P_{CO_2} are related by the following equation:

$$\text{Alveolar } P_{CO_2} = \frac{CO_2 \text{ output}}{\text{alveolar ventilation}}$$

In normal lungs, the P_{CO_2} of arterial blood is virtually the same as that in alveolar gas, and the carbon dioxide output at rest remains fairly constant. Thus the expression implies that if the alveolar ventilation is halved, the arterial P_{CO_2} is doubled.

The level of alveolar ventilation also influences the P_{O_2}. As the ventilation falls and the P_{CO_2} rises, the P_{O_2} falls. An important practical point is that if the P_{CO_2} is considerably increased by pure hypoventilation, say to 70 mmHg, the P_{O_2} may still be well above the level at which cyanosis can be detected clinically. Thus a patient may have serious carbon dioxide retention and yet appear a "healthy" pink color. Note also that if a patient is given an oxygen-enriched mixture to breathe, the hypoxia will be abolished, but the hypercapnia remains (Chap. 208).

Conditions affecting the respiratory center During normal *sleep,* the P_{CO_2} rises by 3 or 4 mmHg. Patients with idiopathic hypoventilation or with the Pickwickian syndrome (see below) are particularly likely to develop depressed breathing when they are asleep. One of the commonest causes of hypoventilation is depression of the respiratory center by *drugs.* These include many anesthetics, the barbiturates, and morphine and its derivatives. Respiratory center depression is often seen in the recovery room, before the effects of anesthesia and preoperative sedatives have worn off, and also in the emergency room in patients who have taken an overdose of barbiturate. In these circumstances, the arterial P_{CO_2} should be measured, and assisted ventilation following endotracheal intubation or tracheostomy may be lifesaving. Depression of the respiratory center is often accompanied by impairment of the cough reflex and difficulties with swallowing, so that aspiration of fluid into the lungs may occur and lead to pneumonia. An additional advantage of intubation is that it allows the airways to be sucked free of secretions and inhaled material (Chap. 216).

Brainstem abnormalities Conditions which may cause hypoventilation include inflammation, hemorrhage, trauma, and rarely neo-

TABLE 215-1 Causes of carbon dioxide retention

1 Pure hypoventilation (normal lungs)
- *a* Respiratory center depression—morphine derivatives, barbiturates, some general anesthetics
- *b* Diseases of the brainstem—encephalitis, hemorrhage, trauma, neoplasm (rare)
- *c* Abnormalities of spinal cord conducting pathways—high cervical dislocation
- *d* Anterior horn cell disease—poliomyelitis
- *e* Diseases of nerves to respiratory muscles—Guillain-Barré syndrome, diphtheria
- *f* Diseases of the myoneural junction—myasthenia gravis, anticholinesterase poisoning
- *g* Diseases of the respiratory muscles—progressive muscular dystrophy
- *h* Thoracic cage abnormalities—crushed chest, kyphoscoliosis (lungs may be abnormal)
- *i* Upper airway obstruction—thymoma, aortic aneurysm
- *j* Hypoventilation associated with extreme obesity (Pickwickian syndrome)
- *k* Idiopathic hypoventilation
- *l* Other causes—metabolic alkalosis

2 CO_2 retention associated with chronic lung disease

plasms. Encephalitis and acute bulbar poliomyelitis (even in the absence of involvement of the respiratory muscles) may cause slowing and shallowness of respiration. Irregularities of rhythm and periods of apnea may develop. The first signs of these abnormalities often appear during sleep. The ventilatory response to inhaled CO_2 mixtures is depressed. These patients can return their blood gases to normal by voluntarily increasing their ventilation, and indeed they can sometimes be managed by being reminded to breathe when periods of apnea develop. However, they may die because of apnea during sleep. Respiratory depression may be associated with loss of the cough and swallowing reflexes and consequent accumulation of secretions.

Neuromuscular disorders Neuromuscular disorders affecting the spinal conducting pathways, the anterior horn cells, the nerves to the respiratory muscles, and the respiratory muscles themselves are important causes of hypoventilation (Table 215-1). Examples include compression of the cervical cord, poliomyelitis, the Guillain-Barré syndrome, and myasthenia gravis. The most important muscle of respiration is the diaphragm, and patients with progressive disease often do not complain of dyspnea until the diaphragm is involved. By then their ventilatory reserve is severely compromised, and they must be carefully observed. The converse also occurs. Patients with neurologic disease such as amyotrophic lateral sclerosis may complain of dyspnea as their initial symptom at a time when their neurologic findings may be extremely subtle. The progress of the disease can be monitored by measuring the vital capacity and the arterial blood gases. Again, the treatment of hypoventilation in these conditions is assisted ventilation either by oropharyngeal intubation in acute states, or with a tracheostomy for long-term management (Chap. 208). Patients with chronic paresis of their respiratory muscles are likely to develop chest infections because of their difficulty in getting rid of secretions.

Thoracic cage abnormalities CRUSHED CHEST An increasingly common cause of hypoventilation is trauma to the thoracic cage resulting from automobile accidents. Frequently this is caused by impact of the steering wheel with the sternum, or the chest is crushed when a wheel of a car runs over it. Usually there are multiple injuries. There may be dissociation of movement of the chest wall, so that one region is sucked in while the remainder of the chest wall moves out during inspiration (''flail chest''). Prompt intubation and assisted ventilation is often required, and careful monitoring of the arterial blood gases is mandatory.

SCOLIOSIS Bony deformity of the chest can lead to respiratory failure with a raised arterial P_{CO_2}. *Scoliosis* refers to lateral curvature of the spine, and *kyphosis* to posterior curvature. The effects of scoliosis on cardiopulmonary function are the more serious, especially if the angulation is situated high in the vertebral column. Scoliosis is frequently associated with rotation of the spine and backward protuberance of the ribs, giving the appearance of an added kyphosis. In fact, the term *kyphoscoliosis* is often used for this condition, although true kyphoscoliosis is rare. Some 80 percent of cases of scoliosis are idiopathic in origin. The rest are caused by neuromuscular disorders such as poliomyelitis or are congenital in origin.

The initial complaint is dyspnea on exertion. Later hypoxemia develops; eventually carbon dioxide retention and signs of failure of the right side of the heart may supervene. Sometimes bronchitis may complicate the picture, especially in smokers. The chief cause of the CO_2 retention is the deformity of the chest wall which leads to an inefficient action of the respiratory muscles and a great increase in the work of breathing. The compliance of the chest wall is reduced (it is stiffer), especially in older patients, and this results in rapid, shallow breathing, so that an increasingly large fraction of the tidal volume is wasted in the dead space of the bronchi. The hypoventilation causes not only hypercapnia but also hypoxemia. Pulmonary vasoconstriction results, pulmonary artery pressure rises, and the work of the right side of the heart increases. This is exaggerated by the polycythemia which develops (Chap. 191).

It should be noted, however, that these patients also have abnormal lungs. These tend to be remarkably small, and the restricted pulmonary vascular bed probably also plays a role in the development of pulmonary hypertension. Areas of atelectasis are common, presumably because the volume of the thoracic cage is greatly reduced. Uneven ventilation of the lungs has been demonstrated in many cases, so that ventilation-perfusion inequality contributes to the hypoxemia.

Pulmonary function tests show a reduction in all lung volumes; indeed the total lung capacity may be reduced to half the predicted normal value. Some of the inequality of ventilation can be explained by airway closure in dependent regions of the lung as a result of the gross reduction of lung volume. Airway resistance in relation to lung volume is approximately normal, but the maximum breathing capacity is reduced because of the restricted vital capacity. The diffusing capacity of the lung for carbon monoxide is not markedly abnormal when related to lung volume. In advanced disease, a reduced ventilatory response to inhaled carbon dioxide can be demonstrated. This is probably related to the large increase in the work of breathing caused by the deformity of the chest wall. Not only is the chest wall stiff, but the respiratory muscles operate inefficiently.

Little specific therapy is available. Just as the cause of most cases of the disease is unknown, so are the factors determining its progression poorly understood. Some help can be obtained from orthopedic braces such as the Milwaukee brace, in the early stages of the disease. Corrective surgery such as the Harrington procedure during adolescence improves the appearance and may relieve back pain. However, the long-term effects on cardiopulmonary function are unknown. Any pulmonary infection should be promptly and vigorously treated with appropriate antibiotics. If hypoxemia is severe and O_2 therapy is required (Chap. 216), the patient should be carefully watched for evidence of increasing hypoventilation. Cor pulmonale and right-sided heart failure should be treated with diuretics, digitalis, and perhaps phlebotomy if the polycythemia is severe.

OTHER CONDITIONS Also associated with an abnormal chest wall are ankylosing spondylitis and pectus excavatum. In *ankylosing spondylitis* (Chap. 267) there is immobility of the vertebral joints and fixation of the ribs, so that movement of the chest wall may be grossly reduced. There is a reduction of vital capacity and total lung capacity, but good movement of the diaphragm is preserved so that the ventilatory capacity is unimpaired. Some fall in the compliance of the chest wall has been reported and also some uneven ventilation, the latter possibly caused by the reduced lung volume. In general, however, the lungs are virtually normal and do not show the pathologic changes seen in kyphoscoliosis. Hypoventilation is not a feature, and secondary heart failure does not occur.

Pectus excavatum is a congenital abnormality in which the lower part of the sternum is depressed toward the spine. In spite of the bizarre appearance of the chest, little interference with pulmonary function is the rule. There may be a slight reduction in vital capacity, total lung capacity, and maximum breathing capacity, but gas exchange is virtually normal, and hypoventilation does not occur. Surgical correction for cosmetic reasons may be considered.

Obstruction to the upper airways Tracheal stenosis can be caused by neoplasms such as thymoma in structures adjacent to the trachea, by scarring following injury, by aortic aneurysm, or by a congenital abnormality. Tumors originating in the upper airways and foreign bodies may also be responsible for airways obstruction. Hypoventilation with CO_2 retention may occur, and this may be of long standing. It is possible to distinguish tracheal obstruction from the airway obstruction of chronic obstructive lung disease by the stridor and by the reduced flow rates during both forced inspiration and expiration. In addition, pulmonary function tests show no inequality of ventilation. Intermittent upper airway obstruction may occur in obese and other people during sleep (see ''Sleep Apnea'' below).

Hypoventilation associated with extreme obesity (Pickwickian syndrome) Some extremely obese patients hypoventilate, and the association of obesity, somnolence, polycythemia, and excessive appetite has been dubbed the *Pickwickian syndrome,* after the fat boy, Joe, in Charles Dickens's *Pickwick Papers*. Apart from the obesity, the clinical features are similar to those in patients with idiopathic hypoventilation (see below). In the fully developed form they include marked obesity (body weight typically over 130 kg), somnolence, twitching, cyanosis, periodic respiration, secondary polycythemia, right ventricular hypertrophy, and right-sided heart failure.

The obesity may have been present for years, but in some cases a recent rapid gain in weight has been described. The somnolence may be a striking feature, the patient sometimes dozing off halfway through a sentence. The cyanosis and periodic breathing are particularly marked during sleep. Sleep apnea may occur (see below), and in some patients this is caused by upper airway obstruction as a result of collapse of the pharyngeal walls. Ankle edema is a common symptom, and an enlarged liver and engorged neck veins are seen.

Blood gas measurements show an elevated P_{CO_2} and depressed P_{O_2}; the former may be as high as 70 mmHg. Lung function tests show a reduction in lung volumes, particularly in the expiratory reserve volume (the volume which can be forcibly exhaled from normal end expiration). The vital capacity is also reduced, as is the compliance of the chest wall. The abdominal pressure is raised, especially when the patient is supine, thus forcing the diaphragm into the chest. There are no indications of airway obstruction and little inequality of ventilation, but the energy cost of moving the chest wall is abnormally high. The ventilatory response to inhaled CO_2 is therefore generally greatly decreased. In these respects the syndrome is similar to kyphoscoliosis. However, in addition, some patients have a diminished sensitivity of the respiratory center to CO_2. The reduction of lung volume causes airway closure in the dependent regions of the lung, and this contributes to the hypoxemia. There is an increase in the resting O_2 consumption of these patients which aggravates the effects of their impaired ventilation.

A striking feature of this syndrome is the dramatic improvement that takes place in all symptoms when the patient loses weight. Objective indices of improvement include a fall in arterial P_{CO_2}, a rise in P_{O_2}, increases in vital capacity, total lung capacity, and total ventilation, and an enhanced ventilatory response to inhaled CO_2. In addition, signs of heart failure often disappear. Even a loss of 15 to 20 kg is often sufficient to bring about a remarkable improvement in well-being. Treatment by caloric restriction is indicated. In addition, recent work shows that some patients respond well to progesterone, which stimulates ventilation. If upper airway obstruction causes sleep apnea, tracheostomy is often very beneficial.

It is important to note that not all extremely obese patients develop hypoventilation. Some investigators have suggested that the Pickwickian individual is simply a patient with idiopathic hypoventilation who happens to be obese. The term *Pickwickian syndrome* is often used rather loosely. It should be reserved for very obese patients who have an increased P_{CO_2} without evidence of lung disease. The cause of the hypoventilation is not clear but presumably is related to the high energy cost of moving the chest wall. In addition the reduction in lung volumes caused by elevation of the diaphragm causes shallow, inefficient breathing. However the association of marked somnolence and voracious appetite suggests that, in some patients at least, there is an abnormality in the central nervous system.

Idiopathic hypoventilation Idiopathic, or primary, hypoventilation is a rare disease of unknown cause occurring in patients whose lungs and chest wall are normal. A colorful name sometimes given to this condition is *Ondine's curse,* after the fairy whose human lover lost the ability to breathe automatically and had to will himself to do so. Most of the reported patients have been between 20 and 60 years of age, and there has been a preponderance of males. Typical symptoms include lack of energy, somnolence, headache, and some breathlessness on exertion. Cyanosis, especially when the patient is asleep, is a common observation, this being caused by a combination of the hypoxemia and polycythemia. Periodic breathing is often noted at night. Occasionally unusual sensitivity to sedatives or hypnotic drugs given preoperatively has been a feature. In some cases, an acute respiratory infection has prompted awareness of the condition. Several patients have had a past history of encephalitis, neurosyphilis, or schizophrenia. Signs of heart failure including engorged neck veins, enlarged heart, palpable liver, and peripheral edema have been described in severe cases.

The P_{CO_2} is elevated, generally in the range of 55 to 80 mmHg, and the P_{O_2} is depressed; these can rapidly be restored to near normal by asking the patient to increase ventilation voluntarily. Indeed some observers have found considerable variability in the P_{CO_2}, because when the patients are tested and become aware of their breathing, they tend to breathe more. For this reason the finding of a raised plasma bicarbonate indicating metabolic compensation of the chronic respiratory acidosis may be a useful diagnostic pointer. The hematocrit is typically between 50 and 70 percent. The ventilatory response to inhaled CO_2 is greatly impaired, though the work of breathing is not increased. Tests of pulmonary function are generally normal with no indication of airway obstruction. The pulmonary arterial pressure is typically increased because of the alveolar hypoxemia.

No specific pathologic changes have been found in the central nervous system of these patients. Congestive heart failure and respiratory infections should be treated vigorously.

Metabolic alkalosis A few patients with metabolic alkalosis hypoventilate, although this causes no symptoms and is difficult to detect clinically. The commonest causes include severe vomiting and potassium and chloride loss such as that caused by diuretics or steroid therapy. The arterial pH is always raised, indicating only partial respiratory compensation. Many patients with metabolic alkalosis do not hypoventilate at all.

Sleep apnea Over the last 15 years a number of patients have been described in whom breathing periodically stops during sleep. Sleep apnea is defined as cessation of airflow at the nostrils and mouth for at least 10 s. This can occur in normal subjects up to 10 times a night and then only during rapid eye movement (REM) sleep. But in the patients with sleep apnea syndrome there are usually over 10 apneic periods per hour of sleep.

Sleep apnea is of two types: obstructive and central. In *obstructive sleep apnea,* airflow (as measured by thermistors at the nose and mouth) ceases despite persistent respiratory efforts as shown by abdominal and thoracic inspiratory movements. These movements can be recorded by transducers around the abdomen and chest. Sometimes the patient seeks medical advice because of loud snoring and daytime somnolence. The airway obstruction can be caused by backward movement of the tongue, narrowing of upper airway by obesity, collapse of the pharyngeal walls due to failure of the genioglossus muscle, or greatly enlarged tonsils or adenoids. Arterial oxygen saturation (measured by ear oximeter) falls during the apneic periods, cardiac arrhythmias may develop, and acute elevations in systemic and pulmonary artery pressures can occur. There is often chronic sleep deprivation, and the patient may exhibit daytime somnolence, chronic fatigue, and morning headaches. Personality disturbances such as paranoia, hostility, and agitated depression may develop. Long-term tracheostomy has been shown to be beneficial in some of these patients. Weight loss is valuable if the patient is obese. Methoxyprogesterone has been used as a respiratory stimulant, but its value is uncertain.

Central sleep apnea is caused by a transient cessation of inspiratory muscle activity. It is recognized by the absence of both airflow and respiratory movements. Patients who tend to hypoventilate (see Table 215-1) may develop apneic episodes during sleep when respiratory drive is depressed. It is now known that during REM sleep breathing is often irregular and unresponsive to chemical and vagal drives. The exception is hypoxemia, which remains a powerful stimulus to breathe. Even during hypoxemia, irregular breathing and periods of apnea may develop if normal respiratory drive is altered by sleep. This is seen to a striking degree in the Cheyne-Stokes breathing of normal subjects at high altitude.

Sudden infant death syndrome This is sometimes known as ''crib death.'' Typically the infant is found dead in the crib with no apparent cause. The etiology of this is still obscure, but some investigators believe that this is a special case of the sleep apnea syndrome described above. In addition it is known that the rib cage collapses easily in some young infants and there may be paradoxical movement of the chest wall; that is, the rib cage moves in rather than out during inspiration. This may be accentuated by poor coordination of the respiratory muscles as a result of immaturity of the nervous system. It has also been shown that infants do not respond to transient airway obstruction by increasing their respiratory efforts, as occurs in the normal adult. This would make them abnormally vulnerable to upper respiratory tract infections. Finally, it is possible that some deaths are caused by cardiac arrhythmias during an apneic period.

CARBON DIOXIDE RETENTION ASSOCIATED WITH CHRONIC LUNG DISEASE The commonest clinical situation in which CO_2 retention is seen is chronic lung disease. Patients with this condition are often said to be ''hypoventilating,'' but the cause of their hypercapnia is clearly very different from that in patients with normal lungs whom we have considered so far. Historically it is easy to see how the term *hypoventilation* came to be applied so indiscriminately. When in the late 1950s it became possible to measure the P_{CO_2} of arterial blood in the clinical setting, CO_2 retention was found to be a common and serious complication of chronic lung disease which could always be abolished by artificially increasing the ventilation. Thus it was natural to say that these patients had a reduced ventilation, and this term had the advantage of keeping an important therapeutic option in the forefront.

It is important to understand the factors leading to CO_2 retention in these patients if their disease is to be managed most effectively. Figure 215-1 shows a scheme of the factors determining CO_2 elimination in patients with lung disease. CO_2 is produced in the tissues at a rate which depends on the level of metabolic activity; at rest there is little variation. It is transported to the lungs in the venous blood and pumped out by the ventilation. The speed of the pump is normally set by the level of the P_{CO_2} via the medullary chemoreceptors. In the presence of lung disease, the efficiency of the pump is impaired. Thus, for the same level of ventilation, less CO_2 is eliminated. This is principally because ventilation and blood flow are unevenly matched within the lung (see Chap. 200). In any event the result is that for a normal level of ventilation, inadequate amounts of CO_2 are excreted, and CO_2 retention occurs.

When the increased arterial P_{CO_2} causes a fall in the cerebrospinal fluid pH which is sensed by the medullary chemoreceptors, the ventilation is increased. The peripheral chemoreceptors also respond to the increased P_{CO_2}. The result is that the P_{CO_2} returns to normal, because fortunately even lungs with grossly mismatched ventilation and blood flow can greatly increase their elimination of CO_2 when their ventilation is raised. (Contrast this with the behavior of O_2 where uneven ventilation and blood flow invariably result in low P_{O_2}; this follows from the shape of the O_2 dissociation curve as discussed in Chap. 200.) Thus a common end result is a normal P_{CO_2}, but at the expense of increased ventilation. However, in the presence of severe disease, the ventilation may not be increased enough to restore the P_{CO_2} to normal, and CO_2 retention therefore occurs.

The ventilatory response to CO_2 in these patients can be reduced for two reasons. One is an increased work of breathing. It has been shown that if normal subjects breathe through a resistance, their ventilatory response to inhaled CO_2 is depressed. Indeed, the relationship between increase in ventilation and inspired CO_2 concentration may become indistinguishable from that observed in patients with chronic airway obstruction. In most cases of chronic obstructive lung disease, the resistance to airflow is high so that the increase in ventilation for a given rise in arterial P_{CO_2} is depressed. Such patients may have a normal neural output of the respiratory center in response to an increased P_{CO_2}, but nevertheless the ventilatory response is impaired.

However, some patients also have a reduced neural output of the respiratory center in response to an increased arterial P_{CO_2}. This can be established by specialized tests such as measurement of the mechanical work performed during inspiration or the inspiratory pressure developed during a brief period of airway occlusion. The reason for the diminished sensitivity of the respiratory center in these patients is not understood, though in some cases it may be congenital. There is evidence that the sensitivity of the respiratory center to CO_2 (and hypoxemia) varies considerably among normal subjects. It may be that those patients who have good respiratory center sensitivity are more distressed by dyspnea, while those who respond weakly may succumb to CO_2 retention and respiratory failure.

When CO_2 retention becomes established, the respiratory center becomes reset at a higher arterial P_{CO_2}. This can be explained by an increase in bicarbonate concentration in the cerebrospinal fluid because of transport of bicarbonate across the blood-gas barrier. As a result the pH of the cerebrospinal fluid is returned to near its normal value of 7.32 in spite of its increased P_{CO_2}. Since this pH apparently chiefly determines the response of the medullary chemoreceptors, respiratory drive may then not be much increased despite the raised P_{CO_2}.

Further CO_2 retention occurs in some patients with chronic lung disease following the administration of oxygen. These patients have chronic hypercapnia and hypoxemia but a near normal pH in their arterial blood (compensated respiratory acidosis) and in their cerebrospinal fluid. Their main stimulus to ventilation may be the arterial hypoxemia via the peripheral chemoreceptors, so that when this is relieved, ventilation almost ceases. The ensuing rise in P_{CO_2} may further depress ventilation because of the narcotic effect of high levels of CO_2. This extremely dangerous situation should be avoided by giving carefully controlled O_2 concentrations, for example, 24 to 28%, assiduously watching the patient, and measuring the arterial P_{O_2}, P_{CO_2}, and pH frequently. CO_2 retention in chronic obstructive lung disease is considered in Chap. 208, and the treatment of acute and chronic respiratory failure in Chap. 216.

MEASUREMENT OF CONTROL OF VENTILATION The cause of disorders of ventilation can sometimes be elucidated by studying the control of ventilation. The ventilatory response to CO_2 can be measured by means of a rebreathing technique. A bag is filled with a mixture of about 6% CO_2 in O_2, and the patient rebreathes from this over a period of several minutes. The P_{CO_2} in the bag increases at the rate of 4 to 6 mmHg per minute, and thus the change in ventilation per mmHg rise in P_{CO_2} can easily be determined. A similar technique can be employed to measure the ventilatory response to hypoxia. In this instance the bag is filled with 24% O_2, 7% CO_2, and the balance N_2. The P_{CO_2} in the bag is monitored and held constant. Rebreathing can be continued until the inspired P_{O_2} falls to about 40 mmHg.

Another method of assessing the output of the respiratory center is to measure the inspiratory pressure during a brief period of airway occlusion. The patient breathes through a valve box, the inspiratory port of which is provided with a shutter. This is closed during an expiration (the patient being unaware), so that the first part of the next inspiration is against an occluded airway. The shutter is opened after about 0.5 s. The pressure generated during the first 0.1 s of attempted inspiration ($P_{0.1}$) is taken as a measure of respiratory center output.

HYPERVENTILATION

Hyperventilation is most commonly caused by lesions of the central nervous system, metabolic acidosis, and anxiety states. In addition, hyperventilation may be seen in salicylate poisoning, acute or chronic hypoxemia (as at high altitude), severe hypoglycemia, and hepatic coma. A patient with severe cerebral hemorrhage causing coma may exhibit deep, regular respirations of a mechanical nature. This causes a reduced P_{CO_2} in the arterial blood, which initially shows a high pH and a normal base excess. Irregularities of breathing such as Cheyne-Stokes respiration may also occur. In metabolic acidosis caused, for example, by uncontrolled diabetes mellitus or by chronic renal insufficiency, deep regular respiration known as *Kussmaul breathing* is frequently seen. Active rather than passive expiratory movements are a feature of this pattern. Here the low P_{CO_2} is accompanied by reduction in base excess and a low pH (see Chap. 42).

In the hyperventilation of anxiety states, the patient may be very apprehensive and complain of shortness of breath, difficulty in taking a deep breath, a feeling of chest tightness, or a sense of suffocation. The patient is often a nervous, anxious woman who has other functional disturbances due to tension. There are often accompanying symptoms such as numbness in the limbs, palpitations, and epigastric discomfort. The fall in P_{CO_2} and the consequent alkalosis may be severe and may cause tetany with carpopedal spasm. The reduced plasma bicarbonate level and relatively normal arterial pH (compensated respiratory alkalosis) distinguish chronic hyperventilation from the acute hyperventilation with fall in P_{CO_2} which frequently accompanies an arterial puncture. The patient may complain of fainting spells and blurring of vision; these are probably related to the reduction in cerebral blood flow caused by low P_{CO_2}. The finding of slow waves of high voltage in the EEG suggests that these changes may be the result of hypoxemia. The changes can be reversed by hyperbaric oxygenation. The serum calcium level remains normal. It is likely that some of the cardiovascular symptoms are related to the release of epinephrine.

These patients are usually not aware of the overbreathing, although they may admit to periods of sighing. It is often possible to reproduce many of the symptoms of an attack by encouraging them to overbreathe spontaneously. It is also useful to demonstrate to these patients that they can hold a breath for a considerable period even during an attack. An attack can sometimes be terminated by having the patient breathe in and out of a plastic bag, or inhale a 5% CO_2 mixture. However, attention to the underlying anxiety state is indicated.

Hyperventilation also occurs in some types of lung disease, including interstitial lung disease and pulmonary edema. The hyperventilation of interstitial disease is particularly marked on exercise where the breathing is typically rapid and shallow, and the arterial P_{CO_2} may fall to the 20s. The cause of the hyperventilation is uncertain, but stimulation of the juxtacapillary (J) receptors in the alveolar wall by the process involving the lung has been suggested as a possible cause. Part of the hyperventilation may also be explained by the stimulation of the peripheral chemoreceptors by the severe arterial hypoxemia which may occur in these conditions.

ABNORMAL PATTERNS OF VENTILATION

CHEYNE-STOKES BREATHING This is a form of periodic breathing characterized by alternating periods of apnea and hyperpnea. The patient often lies motionless for 10 to 20 s and then begins to breathe shallowly at first, then with increasing amplitude, and finally shallowly again. The respirations during this period of breathing are regular in time.

The cause of this disturbance presumably lies in some abnormality in the control process which results in "hunting" for the equilibrium condition. Periodic breathing can be produced in experimental animals by lengthening the distance over which blood travels from the thorax to the brain. As a result, the response of the chemoreceptors lags behind the blood gas changes produced by the lungs, and a cyclic chain of events is created. Any increase in chemoreceptor gain also tends to make the system unstable. Conditions in which Cheyne-Stokes breathing is seen include congestive heart failure when the circulation time is prolonged (Chap. 182), brain damage caused by trauma or cerebral hemorrhage, and chronic hypoxia. It occurs in normal subjects living at high altitude, especially during sleep.

BIOT'S BREATHING This is another form of periodic breathing in which periods of apnea are punctuated by a few deep breaths which may be irregular and which do not have the waxing and waning pattern of Cheyne-Stokes respiration. It is most frequently associated with brain damage.

OTHER TYPES Brain injury can result in bizarre patterns of ventilation. These include apneustic breathing, which is characterized by a postinspiratory pause (rather than the usual postexpiratory), and ataxic breathing, which is irregular in timing and depth.

REFERENCES

CHOLLET S et al: Contribution of nocturnal polygraphy to the diagnosis of Pickwickian syndrome. Respiration 46:272, 1984

HORNBEIN TF: *Regulation of Breathing*, Part II. New York, Marcel Dekker, 1981

LISBOA C et al: Inspiratory muscle function in patients with severe kyphoscoliosis. Am Rev Respir Dis 132:48, 1985

MILLMAN RP, FISHMAN AP: Sleep apnea syndrome, in *Pulmonary Diseases and Disorders*, AP Fishman (ed). New York, McGraw-Hill, 1987, Section 17, Part III, chap 6

ROUSSOS C, MACKLEM PT: Disorders of the respiratory muscle function, in *Update III: Harrison's Principles of Internal Medicine*, KJ Isselbacher et al (eds). New York, McGraw-Hill, 1982, p 83

SAUNDERS NA, SULLIVAN CE: *Sleep and Breathing*. New York, Marcel Dekker, 1984

WEST JB: *Pulmonary Pathophysiology—The Essentials*, 2d ed. Baltimore, Williams & Wilkins, 1982

216 ADULT RESPIRATORY DISTRESS SYNDROME

ROLAND H. INGRAM, JR.

Adult respiratory distress syndrome is a descriptive term that has been applied to many acute, diffuse infiltrative lung lesions of diverse etiologies when they are accompanied by severe arterial hypoxemia. The term was chosen because of several clinical and pathologic similarities between such acute illnesses in adults and the neonatal respiratory distress syndrome. However, in the neonatal form, immaturity of alveolar surfactant production and a highly compliant chest wall are primarily involved in the pathophysiology, whereas in the adult, alveolar surfactant changes are secondary to the primary process, and the chest wall is not compliant. Despite the large number of causes (Table 216-1), the clinical characteristics, respiratory pathophysiologic derangement, and current techniques for management of these acute abnormalities are remarkably similar. It has been argued that the "lumping" of such processes of different etiologies obscures the unique features of each in terms of pathogenesis, prevention, and specificity of treatment. It is clear that the conditions listed do not always lead to respiratory failure and that specific treatment of the underlying processes will often be different. Therefore, the reader is urged to refer to the appropriate sections of this text for the unique characteristics of each condition and to recognize that only the common features at the onset of respiratory failure will be focused upon in this chapter. It should be further emphasized that many of the listed conditions are often present in combination and may come into play at different times in the clinical course of the adult respiratory distress syndrome.

PATHOPHYSIOLOGY Regardless of the initiating process, the adult respiratory distress syndrome is invariably associated with increased liquid in the lungs. Thus it is a form of pulmonary edema, yet it is distinct from cardiogenic pulmonary edema because pulmonary capillary hydrostatic pressures are not elevated (Chap. 26). Since hydrostatic pressures are not elevated, there is increased permeability of the alveolocapillary membranes that occurs via direct chemical injury in the case of inhaled toxic gases or aspirated acid or indirectly through activation and aggregation of formed elements of the blood within pulmonary capillaries in the case of septicemia and/or endotoxemia. Although platelet aggregation occurs, the major offenders appear to be the neutrophilic leukocytes that adhere to endothelial surfaces. These leukocytes undergo a respiratory burst to inflict oxidant injury and release mediators of inflammation such as leukotrienes, thromboxanes, and prostaglandins. Initially the injury to the alveolocapillary membrane results in leakage of liquid, macromolecules, and cellular components from the blood vessels into the

TABLE 216-1 Conditions which may lead to the adult respiratory distress syndrome

1 Diffuse pulmonary infections (e.g., viral, bacterial, fungal, *Pneumocystis*)
2 Aspiration (e.g., gastric contents with Mendelson's syndrome, water with near drowning)
3 Inhalation of toxins and irritants (e.g., chlorine gas, NO_2, smoke, ozone, high concentrations of oxygen)
4 Narcotic overdose pulmonary edema (e.g., heroin, methadone, morphine, dextropropoxyphene)
5 Nonnarcotic drug effects (e.g., nitrofurantoin)
6 Immunologic response to host antigens (e.g., Goodpasture's syndrome, systemic lupus erythematosus)
7 Effects of nonthoracic trauma with hypotension ("shock lung")
8 In association with systemic reactions to processes initiated outside the lung (e.g., gram-negative septicemia, hemorrhagic pancreatitis, amniotic fluid embolism, fat embolism)
9 Postcardiopulmonary bypass ("pump lung," "postperfusion lung")

interstitial space and, with increasing severity, into the alveoli. The increasing vascular permeability to proteins (decreased reflection coefficient, σ, discussed in Chap. 26) leaves the hydrostatic gradient unopposed so that even mild elevations in capillary pressures greatly increase interstitial and alveolar edema. Alveolar collapse occurs secondary to the effect of the alveolar liquid, especially its fibrinogen, that interferes with normal surfactant activity and because of possible impairment of further surfactant production by injury to the granular pneumocytes. Though radiographically diffuse, the regional dysfunction is nonhomogeneous; it leads to severe ventilation-perfusion imbalance and the shunting of blood through regions in which alveoli are collapsed or filled with liquid. The lungs become less compliant—i.e., stiffen because of interstitial edema, alveolar collapse, and increase in surface forces. Because of the decreased compliance, large inspiratory pressures must be generated by the respiratory muscles so that the work of breathing is elevated. The large mechanical loads lead to fatigue of the muscles of breathing with resulting diminution in tidal volumes and worsening gas exchange. Both hypoxemia and the stimulation of receptors in the stiff lung parenchyma cause an increase in respiratory frequency, decrease in tidal volume, and deterioration in gas exchange.

PATHOLOGY In the absence of specific demonstrable pathogens, the pathology is remarkably similar among the various conditions leading to the adult respiratory distress syndrome, since the lung has a limited number of ways in which it reacts to an almost limitless number of injuries. Grossly, the lungs are heavy, edematous, and almost airless with regions of hemorrhage, atelectasis, and consolidation. By light microscopy there is edema and cellular infiltration of interalveolar septa and interstitial spaces surrounding airways and blood vessels, atelectasis and hyaline membranes in many regions, engorgement of vessels with red blood cells, and aggregates of platelets and neutrophilic leukocytes along with interstitial and alveolar hemorrhage. In addition, both hyperplasia and dysplasia of the granular pneumocytes are often present.

If the illness has been prolonged beyond 10 days, there is often a surprising amount of fibrosis in addition to the acute changes. In instances of recovery and subsequent death from another cause, significant interstitial fibrosis and emphysematous changes may be found in the lung. A significant number of patients, however, will recover completely and have normal pulmonary function with no respiratory symptoms. Hence aggressive clinical management is both indicated and often rewarding.

CLINICAL CHARACTERISTICS At the time of initial injury and for several hours thereafter the patient may be free of respiratory symptoms or signs. The earliest sign often is an increase in respiratory frequency followed shortly by dyspnea. Arterial blood gas measurement in the earlier period will disclose a depressed P_{O_2} despite a decreased P_{CO_2} so that the alveolar-arterial difference for oxygen (Chap. 200) is increased. At this early stage, administration of oxygen by mask or nasal prongs results in a significant increase in the arterial P_{O_2}. The brisk rise in P_{O_2} indicates that ventilation-perfusion mismatching and, possibly, diffusion impairment account for the widened alveolar-arterial P_{O_2} difference ($P_{A_{O_2}} - P_{a_{O_2}}$) initially. Physical examination may be unremarkable, although a few fine inspiratory rales may be audible. Radiographically the lung fields may be clear or demonstrate only minimal and scattered interstitial infiltrates. With progression, the patient becomes cyanotic and increasingly dyspneic and tachypneic. Rales are more prominent and are easily heard throughout both lung fields along with regions of tubular breath sounds; the chest radiograph demonstrates diffuse, extensive bilateral interstitial and alveolar infiltrates (Fig. 216-1). At this point hypoxemia cannot be corrected by the simple expedient of increasing the oxygen concentration of the inspired gas, and mechanical ventilatory support must be started. Right-to-left shunting of blood through collapsed or filled alveoli becomes the major mechanism for arterial hypoxemia at this more advanced stage. In contrast to ventilation-perfusion mismatching and diffusion impairment, with right-to-left shunts, $P_{A_{O_2}} - P_{a_{O_2}}$ remains high with breathing of pure oxygen. Positive end-expiratory pressure (PEEP) serves to increase lung volume, which in turn opens collapsed alveoli and decreases shunting. With further progression, and if mechanical ventilator and PEEP therapy are delayed, the combination of increasing tachypnea and decreasing tidal volumes results in alveolar hypoventilation, a rising P_{CO_2}, and worsening hypoxemia; these represent a near-terminal constellation of findings.

MANAGEMENT OF HYPOXEMIC RESPIRATORY FAILURE The brief description given above contains the salient principles of management, integrated with the clinical events that lead to escalation of therapeutic interventions. Implicit in that description is that the simplest method and the lowest inspired fraction of oxygen ($F_{I_{O_2}}$) should be used to give the desired result. The oxyhemoglobin dissociation curve gives some guide as to the $P_{a_{O_2}}$ for which to aim. At a P_{O_2} of 60 mmHg, hemoglobin is approximately 90 percent saturated. Therefore, a reasonable objective is to achieve a $P_{a_{O_2}}$ of 60, since higher levels add little to oxygenation and introduce the risk of oxygen toxicity to the lung. In contrast to respiratory failure complicating chronic airways obstruction (Chap. 208), depression of ventilation is not an issue in hypoxemic respiratory failure.

There are multiple means to deliver O_2, in order of increasing

FIGURE 216-1 *A standard posteroanterior chest radiograph from a patient with the adult respiratory distress syndrome secondary to a severe viral pneumonitis. Such a diffuse radiographic change is typical of all conditions listed in Table 216-1 when they are severe enough to cause acute hypoxemic respiratory failure. A similar radiographic picture is also seen in pulmonary edema due to left ventricular failure (Chap. 26). Often in such acutely ill patients, the radiograph must be taken with a portable unit and the film exposed from the anterior direction. Both the anteroposterior exposure and the failure to take a deep inspiration result in an apparent enlargement of the cardiac silhouette which further obscures the reliable detection of left ventricular failure.*

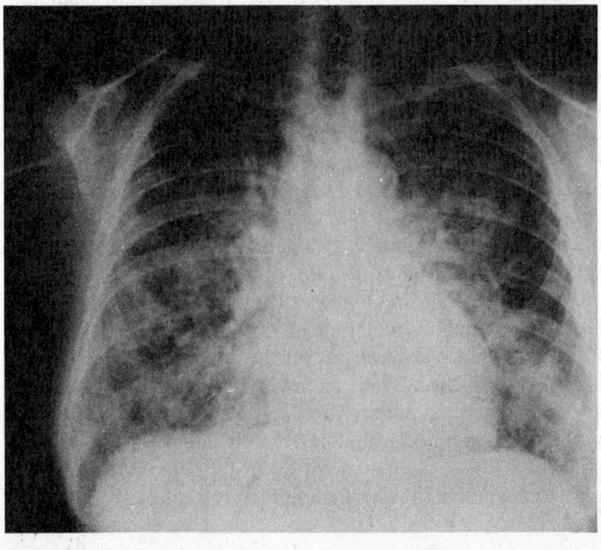

effectiveness: soft nasal prongs, simple face masks, and face masks with inspiratory reservoir bags. The effective $F_{I_{O_2}}$ (that is actually entering the trachea) will be determined by the concentration of O_2 delivered from the tank or wall device, its flow rate, and the minute ventilation of the patient. In the hypoxemic form of respiratory failure, it is reasonable to start with moderate flow rates (5 to 10 liters per minute of 100% O_2) and monitor arterial blood gases, adjusting flow rates and O_2 concentrations depending upon results.

If adequate oxygenation cannot be maintained with these less invasive measures, endotracheal intubation should be carried out and mechanical ventilatory support should be instituted. The rationale behind mechanical ventilatory support in a patient who is hyperventilating is *not* to increase ventilation but to increase mean lung volume, thereby opening previously closed airways and improving oxygenation. This is done by using large tidal volumes (approximately 15 mL per kilogram of lean body weight) at a slower breathing rate (12 to 15 breaths per minute) than the spontaneous one of the patient. Most often, at this juncture, the respiratory system is sufficiently stiff that high inflation pressures are required and a volume-cycled ventilator (in contrast to the pressure-cycled ones) is needed. If the patient makes expiratory efforts during the inflation cycle, peak inspiratory pressures will increase, possibly enough to activate the high-pressure pop-off valve, which results in delivery to the patient of a smaller tidal volume than selected. Under these circumstances consideration is often given to sedation and/or neuromuscular paralysis. However, a much more logical way to proceed is to institute synchronized intermittent mandatory ventilation (SIMV). In the SIMV mode, the patient is allowed to breathe spontaneously with periodic delivery of mandatory breaths that are synchronized with spontaneous inspiratory efforts. If the spontaneous breathing rate is so rapid that expiratory efforts occur before the mandatory breath is fully delivered, only then should sedation and/or paralysis be used.

Should the Pa_{O_2} be greater than 60 mmHg, the next step is to lower the $F_{I_{O_2}}$. If the $F_{I_{O_2}}$ can be lowered to 0.6 or less with a Pa_{O_2} equal to or greater than 60 mmHg, the mechanical ventilation should proceed at that $F_{I_{O_2}}$ as long as necessary. There are two basic indications for the addition of PEEP, the basic rationale for which is to increase lung volume further, thereby opening previously closed alveoli. First, if the $F_{I_{O_2}}$ cannot be lowered to or below 0.6, then PEEP should be added to allow a decrease of the $F_{I_{O_2}}$ below the toxic range. Second, if the Pa_{O_2} cannot be increased to or above 60 mmHg with an $F_{I_{O_2}}$ of 1.0, PEEP should be added. The optimal magnitude of the PEEP is determined by the response of the Pa_{O_2} and the extent of the cardiovascular alterations resulting from the higher pressure. The major alteration is a decrease in cardiac output due to two mechanisms. First, increased intrapleural pressures serve to impede venous return directly, an effect which is, to a variable extent, offset by peripheral venoconstriction. Second, increases in lung volume may increase pulmonary vascular resistance, leading to increased pressure and dilatation of the right ventricle, which in turn displaces the interventricular septum toward the left. This displacement, in effect, decreases left ventricular diastolic compliance; hence less filling leads to smaller stroke volumes. An additional mechanism for decreased diastolic filling of the ventricles is direct compression of the heart by the stiffened lung. In a physiologic sense optimal levels of PEEP are those associated with the greatest delivery of O_2 to the body; the latter is the product of cardiac output and arterial oxygen content.

In patients who are critically ill and/or unstable, insertion of a catheter into a radial artery and a balloon-tipped (Swan-Ganz) catheter into the pulmonary artery can provide valuable information in guiding supportive therapy such as requirements for intravenous fluids, the need for diuresis, and assessment of the effects of mechanical ventilation. From the Swan-Ganz catheter it is possible to measure pulmonary arterial and pulmonary capillary wedge pressures, cardiac output by the thermodilution technique, and to sample mixed venous blood as a means to assess the adequacy of O_2 delivery in relation to demand. Recognition of over-damping and accelerative artifacts in the pulmonary arterial pressure signal and learning the criteria for true wedging are essential if serious misinterpretations are to be avoided. Even with accurate pressure measurements, there is an additional precaution that must be taken with regard to interpretation of intrathoracic vascular pressures referenced to atmosphere when PEEP is being used. If pleural pressure is greater than atmospheric, as is most often the case with PEEP, the true effective (i.e., intravascular minus pleural) pressure will be overestimated and could lead to errors in both assessment and management. A reasonable estimate of the true value is gained by examining vascular pressures just before inflation and subtracting from these pressures an amount equal to one-half the value of PEEP. In view of the leaky alveolo-capillary membrane it is best to keep the pulmonary capillary wedge pressure as low as is compatible with a reasonable cardiac output, arterial pressure, and urinary output. Recently, inotropic and selective vasoactive agents (e.g., dopamine, page 911) have been used with some success to achieve this, but require careful monitoring to assess effects and adjust doses.

Mixed venous blood P_{O_2} values have long been considered to indicate the adequacy of oxygen delivery relative to demand. A low value (e.g., <20 mmHg) surely indicates that there is tissue hypoxemia irrespective of measured cardiac output and Pa_{O_2}. However, a high value does not exclude serious hypoxemia of the tissues, especially in gram-negative bacillary septicemia, in which systemic low-resistance shunts can develop and leave several capillary beds underperfused.

Body position may also affect the degree of arterial oxygenation. Although patients with the adult respiratory distress syndrome have diffuse lung disease, there may be some regional variation in the extent of disease such that one side is more severely involved than the other. In this instance the less involved lung should be the more dependent one when the patient is in a lateral position. Since the distribution of pulmonary blood flow is so heavily determined by gravity (Chap. 200), having the more involved lung, with its minimal ventilation, in the more dependent position results in a measurable increase in intrapulmonary shunt, manifested as a striking fall in Pa_{O_2}. The possible contribution of a positional effect on arterial oxygenation should always be considered before escalating therapeutic interventions.

Occasionally PEEP must be gradually increased to levels in excess of 20 cmH_2O in an attempt to maintain arterial oxygenation. At these high levels of PEEP there may be a paradoxic decrease in Pa_{O_2}. The explanation for this paradox is as follows: high levels of PEEP may not open some of the closed airways but will overdistend those units already open. Overdistention of units increases the vascular resistance in these regions and results in more blood perfusing regions with closed airways, thereby increasing the degree of shunt. The only alternative is to decrease PEEP back to that level associated with the greatest delivery of oxygen to the body (product of cardiac output and arterial oxygen content).

In the situations where maximal PEEP with $F_{I_{O_2}}$ of 1.0 does not supply sufficient oxygen, the possibility of utilizing extracorporeal membrane oxygenators (ECMO) has been both considered and tried. Despite the logical appeal of this form of supportive therapy, a randomized, large prospective study of ECMO therapy has demonstrated that, while it can support gas exchange, there is no effect on survival in acute hypoxemic respiratory failure.

Complications Increasing severity of the clinical illness and continued radiographic progressions in association with the primary process often obscure complications that arise during the course of acute hypoxemic respiratory failure. The development of *left ventricular failure* is a good example of a common, easily missed complication. This is because all patients are likely to have diffuse rales and rhonchi, even without left ventricular failure, and these sounds also serve to make it difficult to detect gallop rhythms. An additional difficulty is that portable chest films are taken in the anteroposterior direction, often at less than full lung inflation, so that the cardiac silhouette appears enlarged. Thus the ordinary physical and radiographic assessments are difficult to rely on. With deterioration, therefore, left ventricular failure should be suspected; it is helpful to insert a Swan-Ganz (see above) catheter which can be used to monitor pulmonary arterial pressure continuously and intermittently to assess pulmonary capillary wedge pressure and oxygen content of mixed venous blood.

With a diffuse radiographic pattern, a secondary bacterial infection is easily overlooked; therefore, frequent sputum smears and cultures should be obtained, especially when there is fever. With many conditions—e.g., gram-negative septicemia, acute hemorrhagic pancreatitis, and "shock lung"—there may be associated *disseminated intravascular coagulation,* which leads to gastrointestinal and intrapulmonary hemorrhage (Chap. 281). Frequent monitoring of platelet count, fibrinogen level, and partial thromboplastin and prothrombin times is helpful in the early detection of this complication and in guiding treatment.

Bronchial obstruction by endotracheal or tracheostomy tubes often occurs. These tubes, when too long or poorly anchored, slide into one main bronchus, usually the right one because of its less angulated origin from the trachea. The tube then blocks ventilation of the other main bronchus, and atelectasis may ensue. Such an event usually causes abrupt deterioration in the patient with respiratory failure. It is detected readily by physical examination, which reveals the absence of breath sounds over the occluded lung. The tube should immediately be pulled back slowly if this complication is suspected. Finally, in the course of treating the illness with mechanical ventilators and high inflation pressures, *pneumothorax* or *pneumomediastinum* may develop and may be impossible to detect except radiologically. Occasionally the presence of subcutaneous emphysema provides a clinical clue. Any deterioration should lead the physician to suspect this complication, repeat the chest radiograph, and institute immediate treatment should pneumothorax be present. If deterioration is sudden, *tension pneumothorax* should be suspected; if physical signs are present, a pleural catheter should be inserted immediately without radiographic confirmation. It is important to realize that high oxygen concentrations (>0.60) for prolonged periods can produce both the lesions and the clinical picture of the adult respiratory distress syndrome. Therefore, as discussed under clinical management above, the *minimal* oxygen concentration associated with acceptable arterial oxygenation should always be used.

Discontinuation of mechanical ventilatory support The ability of the patient to maintain adequate gas exchange without the support of a mechanical ventilator is most often heralded by a decreasing $F_{I_{O_2}}$ requirement, smaller inflation pressures for mandatory or assisted breaths, and a spontaneous respiratory rate below 30 per minute. Other useful guidelines are a spontaneous tidal volume $\geq$ 5 mL per kilogram of lean body weight, a vital capacity $\geq$ 15 mL/kg, and the ability to generate a static inspiratory pressure $\geq$ 20 cmH_2O. Despite these indicators and guidelines, some patients are unable to support themselves for long periods of time so that multiple weaning "trials" guided by mechanical and gas exchange data are carried out in a semiempirical way. Synchronized intermittent mandatory ventilation (SIMV) as described above has been advocated as a logical transitional mode whereby the frequency of the mandatory breaths is gradually decreased. There is a great deal of intuitive appeal to this approach, but it has not been appropriately tested and compared with more abrupt, intermittent withdrawal trials. As in patients with hypercapnic respiratory failure, the six mechanisms for failure to wean should be considered in these patients as well (p. 1094).

Prognosis Given the diversity of the etiologies and the frequency of associated diseases, it is difficult, if not impossible, to give meaningful prognostic figures for the adult respiratory distress syndrome. If all recently published series are taken together, the mortality rate runs between 50 and 60 percent. This represents an improved survival rate over the virtual 100 percent mortality rate of a few years ago and is a result of the application of modern treatment techniques described above. If the syndrome is due to drug overdose, the mortality rate is low; if associated with shock, the chances of a fatal outcome are much greater. Recently, it has become apparent that multiple organ system failure (e.g., renal, hepatic) supervenes when there is an extrapulmonic source of sepsis in need of surgical drainage and that almost all such patients succumb despite maximal support of the respiratory and cardiovascular systems. Other etiologies and associated diseases are between these two extremes. The following factors appear to be associated with a poor outcome: an increase in $P_{A_{O_2}} - P_{a_{O_2}}$, requiring increasing inspired O_2 concentrations and PEEP; decreasing compliance, requiring greater inflation pressures; either low or falling colloid osmotic pressures; and the onset of systemic arterial hypotension not responding to intravascular volume replacement.

In survivors with previously normal lung function, the long-term prognosis for recovery appears to be remarkably good. Lung volumes and arterial blood gases have been shown to return to normal levels within 4 to 6 months after respiratory failure. There are instances, however, when the fibrotic residua are sufficiently great that complete recovery is unlikely.

REFERENCES

BELL RC et al: Multiple organ system failure and infection in the adult respiratory distress syndrome. Ann Intern Med 99:293, 1983

FANTA CH: Pathophysiology and clinical recognition of the adult respiratory distress syndrome. Med Grand Rounds 2:284, 1983

HALL JB, WOOD LDH: Acute hypoxemic respiratory failure. Med Grand Rounds 3:183, 1984

HANLEY ME, BONE RC: Acute respiratory failure. Pathophysiology, causes, and clinical manifestations. Postgrad Med 79:166, 172, 1986

HYERS TM, FOWLER AA: Adult respiratory distress syndrome: Causes, morbidity and mortality. Fed Proc 45:25, 1986

MOLLOY WD et al: Effects of dopamine on cardiopulmonary function and left ventricular volumes in patients with acute respiratory failure. Am Rev Resp Dis 130:396, 1984

SCHUSTER DP et al: Prospective evaluation of the risk of upper gastrointestinal bleeding after admission to a medical intensive care unit. Am J Med 76:623, 1984

TATE RM, REPINE JE: Neutrophils and the respiratory distress syndrome. State of the art. Am Rev Resp Dis 128:552, 1983

VIIRES N et al: Effects of aminophylline on diaphragmatic fatigue during acute respiratory failure. Am Rev Resp Dis 129:396, 1984

PART SIX DISORDERS OF THE KIDNEY AND URINARY TRACT

217 APPROACH TO THE PATIENT WITH DISEASES OF THE KIDNEYS AND URINARY TRACT

FREDRIC L. COE / BARRY M. BRENNER

Specific diseases of the kidneys and urinary tract frequently give rise to consistent arrays, or clusters, of clinical signs, symptoms, and laboratory findings called *syndromes*. Syndromes are useful diagnostically because each has fewer causes than the individual clinical signs and symptoms it contains. For example, any injured capillary bed from glomerulus to the urethral meatus can cause hematuria, but only glomerular injury can also cause heavy albuminuria and erythrocyte casts (Chap. 40), and only a few of the diseases that injure the glomerular capillaries enough to cause hematuria and proteinuria also cause a rapid fall in glomerular filtration rate. Routine clinical evaluation is often sufficient to suggest that a particular syndrome may be present (Table 217-1), but additional laboratory measurements beyond the routine, as well as radiologic and/or urologic evaluation and sequential clinical observations, are usually required to establish the diagnosis. This chapter presents the general features of the syndromes, the clinical and laboratory data base required for their recognition, and outlines the diseases that cause them. Succeeding chapters in this section describe the diseases and their treatment in detail.

ACUTE (ARF) AND RAPIDLY PROGRESSIVE RENAL FAILURE (RPRF) Whether the glomerular filtration rate falls over a period of days (acute renal failure) or weeks (rapidly progressive renal failure) is a useful distinction, because the causes of these two syndromes are somewhat different (Tables to 217-1 and 217-2). For example, acute tubular necrosis, from sepsis, nephrotoxic materials, shock, or other cause (see Chap. 219), presents itself as, and is the usual cause of, acute renal failure, whereas extracapillary proliferative (crescentic) glomerulonephritis, due to immunologic injury or to vasculitis, is an important cause of rapidly progressive, but not acute, renal failure (Chap. 223).

Proof for the existence of either syndrome requires serial determination of the glomerular filtration rate (GFR), or blood urea nitrogen or serum creatinine level. Anuria or oliguria (Chap. 40) strongly suggest acute renal failure, as life cannot be sustained for very long with such inadequate renal function. Symptoms and signs of uremia of recent onset suggest rapidly progressive or acute renal failure, but could also result from chronic renal failure that has only recently become life-threatening. Although edema, hypertension, and abnormalities of electrolytes and the urine sediment (Table 217-1) are frequent in acute and rapidly progressive renal failure, they occur in other syndromes as well and are not specific.

The causes of these two important syndromes number about 36, but only 18 (indicated by T, Table 217-2) typically cause acute renal failure and 8, rapidly progressive renal failure. Urinary obstruction, acute tubular necrosis, some forms of vasculitis, major renal vascular accidents, and endogenous and exogenous nephrotoxins are the usual causes of acute renal failure. Vasculitis and crescentic forms of glomerulonephritis are the main causes of rapidly progressive renal failure. Hemolytic-uremic syndrome, malignant nephrosclerosis, and essential mixed cryoimmunoglobulinemia occasionally present as rapidly progressive renal failure. Idiopathic rapidly progressive glomerulonephritis—the prototype of a disease that produces rapidly progressive renal failure—sometimes causes acute renal failure. Chronic renal failure may occur in some patients with diseases that typically cause acute renal failure. Nevertheless, despite some variability of disease presentations, the finding of acute or rapidly progressive renal failure narrows the range of causes.

ACUTE NEPHRITIS (AN) A number of diseases involve the glomeruli and, to a generally lesser extent, the tubules in an acute but transient inflammatory process, manifested clinically by acute reduction in GFR, rapidly progressive renal failure, and salt and water retention. Expansion of the extracellular volume, if marked, causes hypertension, pulmonary vascular congestion, and facial and peripheral edema (Chap. 223). Since the causes of this syndrome all can damage the glomerular wall enough to permit red blood cells and plasma proteins to enter the urinary space and appear in the urine, gross or microscopic hematuria, red blood cell casts, and proteinuria are necessary for the diagnosis of acute nephritis, and their absence should suggest other diagnostic possibilities. Acute nephritis itself is a transient inflammatory process, so its clinical and laboratory manifestations wax and wane in synchrony over days to a few weeks. Many of the diseases that cause acute nephritis also cause acute or rapidly progressive renal failure (Table 217-2).

The fact that many diseases produce both acute nephritis and acute or rapidly progressive renal failure, some produce only acute nephritis, and some produce acute or chronic renal failure without acute nephritis is useful in diagnosis. Only two diseases, poststreptococcal glomerulonephritis and nonstreptococcal postinfectious glomerulonephritis, typically cause acute nephritis alone (Table 217-2), and only three of the diseases that typically cause acute renal failure, idiopathic rapidly progressive glomerulonephritis, Goodpasture's syndrome, and non-Goodpasture's antiglomerular basement membrane (anti-GBM) disease, also cause acute nephritis (Table 217-2). On the other hand, most of the diseases that cause acute nephritis also cause rapidly progressive renal failure.

Acute glomerulonephritis following infection with group A streptococci is the prototype of a disease that causes acute nephritis alone (Chap. 223). Immune complexes deposit in the subepithelial region of the glomerular capillary wall, between the basement membrane and the visceral epithelial cells that separate the membrane from the urinary space, and provoke an intense but transient inflammatory process. GFR falls, but returns to normal within weeks to months in the vast majority of affected patients. Deposition of immune complexes is also believed to be the cause of acute nephritis following other bacterial and viral infections, and of lupus nephritis, membranoproliferative glomerulonephritis, Henoch-Schönlein purpura, and Berger's disease, i.e., IgA nephropathy. That the typical presentations of the last four diseases are chronic renal failure, nephrotic syndrome, and asymptomatic urinary abnormalities (Table 217-2) illustrate the weakness of relationships between pathogenesis and final clinical manifestations.

TABLE 217-1 **Initial clinical and laboratory data base for defining major syndromes in nephrology**

Syndromes	Important clues to diagnosis	Findings which are common but not of diagnostic value	Location of discussion of diseases causing syndrome
Acute or rapidly progressive renal failure	Anuria Oliguria Documented recent decline in GFR	Hypertension, hematuria Proteinuria, pyuria Casts, edema	Chaps. 219, 223, 226, 227, 230
Acute nephritis	Hematuria, RBC casts Azotemia, oliguria Edema, hypertension	Proteinuria Pyuria Circulatory congestion	Chaps. 222 to 224
Chronic renal failure	Azotemia for > 3 months Prolonged symptoms or signs of uremia Symptoms or signs of renal osteodystrophy Kidneys reduced in size bilaterally Broad casts in urinary sediment	Hematuria, proteinuria Casts, oliguria Polyuria, nocturia Edema, hypertension Electrolyte disorders	Chaps. 218, 220
Nephrotic syndrome	Proteinuria > 3.5 g per 1.73 m^2 per 24 h Hypoalbuminemia Hyperlipidemia Lipiduria	Casts Edema	Chaps. 223, 224
Asymptomatic urinary abnormalities	Hematuria Proteinuria (below nephrotic range) Sterile pyuria, casts		Chap. 223
Urinary tract infection	Bacteriuria > 10^5 colonies per milliliter Other infectious agent documented in urine Pyuria, leukocyte casts Frequency, urgency Bladder tenderness, flank tenderness	Hematuria Mild azotemia Mild proteinuria Fever	Chap. 225
Renal tubule defects	Electrolyte disorders Polyuria, nocturia Symptoms or signs of renal osteodystrophy Large kidneys Renal transport defects	Hematuria "Tubular" proteinuria Enuresis	Chaps. 226, 228
Hypertension	Systolic/diastolic hypertension	Proteinuria Casts Azotemia	Chaps. 29, 196, 227
Nephrolithiasis	Previous history of stone passage or removal Previous history of stone seen by x-ray Renal colic	Hematuria Pyuria Frequency, urgency	Chap. 229
Urinary tract obstruction	Azotemia, oliguria, anuria Polyuria, nocturia, urinary retention Slowing of urinary stream Large prostate, large kidneys Flank tenderness, full bladder after voiding	Hematuria Pyuria Enuresis, dysuria	Chap. 230

Renal biopsy is usually required for the evaluation of patients with acute nephritis, whether or not acute or rapidly progressive renal failure is also present. The usual histologic picture is proliferative glomerulonephritis, often with extracapillary crescent formation, but prognosis and treatment are influenced strongly by the precise histologic and ultrastructural pattern, as well as the types of immune complexes and immunoglobulins deposited in the renal tissues.

CHRONIC RENAL FAILURE (CRF) Chronic renal failure is a syndrome which results from progressive and irreversible destruction of nephrons, regardless of cause (Chap. 220). This syndrome may be considered to exist when GFR is found to be reduced and is known to have been reduced for at least 3 to 6 months (Table 217-1). Often, in fact, a gradual decline in GFR can be documented over a period of years. Proof of chronicity is also provided by the demonstration by abdominal scout film, ultrasonography, intravenous pyelography, or tomography of bilateral reduction of kidney size. Other findings consistent with long-standing renal failure, such as renal osteodystrophy or signs and symptoms of uremia, also help to establish this syndrome (Table 217-1). Several laboratory abnormalities are often regarded as reliable indicators of chronicity of renal disease, such as anemia, hyperphosphatemia, or hypocalcemia, but these are not specific and may be misleading (Chap. 218). In contrast, the finding of broad casts in the urinary sediment (Chap. 40) is quite specific for chronic renal failure, the wide diameters of these casts reflecting the compensatory dilatation and hypertrophy of surviving nephrons. Proteinuria is a frequent but nonspecific finding, as is hematuria. Chronic obstructive uropathy, polycystic and medullary cystic diseases, analgesic nephropathy, and the inactive end stage of any chronic tubulointerstitial nephropathy are excellent examples of conditions in which the urine often contains little or no protein, cells, or casts even though nephron destruction has progressed to the stage of chronic renal failure.

When ARF occurs and there is also clear evidence of CRF, the acute component must be evaluated as if CRF were not present, largely because the acute component is potentially reversible. In most instances, depletion of extracellular fluid volume accounts for the acute deterioration of renal function, but other factors such as urinary tract obstruction, drug-induced nephrotoxicity, or exacerbation of the underlying renal disease may also be responsible (Chap. 220).

NEPHROTIC SYNDROME (NS) This syndrome is generally held to be present when a patient excretes more than 3.5 g protein per 1.73 m^2 per 24 h that consists mainly of albumin (massive proteinuria) and has reduced serum albumin concentration, edema, and hyperlipidemia (Table 217-1). Massive proteinuria alone has come to define the syndrome since this finding connotes serious renal disease whether or not the protein losses lead to hypoalbuminemia, lipid disturbances, or edema (Chap. 40). Provided the proteins appearing in the urine are not abnormal paraproteins readily excreted by the normal kidney (e.g., light chains in multiple myeloma), massive proteinuria is invariably a sign of injury to the glomeruli.

Common causes of the nephrotic syndrome include minimal change disease, idiopathic membranous glomerulopathy, focal glomerulosclerosis, and diabetic glomerulosclerosis (Chaps. 223 and 224). Because these diseases typically cause less inflammation than those that cause acute nephritis, the urine contains fewer cellular elements, and acute changes in GFR and urine volume are uncommon. Hematuria may be a frequent manifestation of some forms of nephrotic syndrome, however, especially chronic membranoproliferative glomerulonephritis (Chap. 223). The presence of many cellular or granular casts should suggest lupus nephritis (Chap. 224) or one of the other causes

TABLE 217-2 Syndromes produced by diseases of the kidneys and urinary tract

Diseases (Chap.)	Syndromes					
	ARF	RPRF	AN	CRF	NS	AUA
Bilateral arterial occlusion (227)	T					
Acute tubular necrosis (219)	T					
Bilateral acute renal vein thrombosis (227)	T					
Acute uric acid nephropathy (226)	T					
Hypovolemia (219)	T					
Cardiovascular collapse (219)	T					
Acute bilateral upper tract obstruction (230)	T					
Hypercalcemic nephropathy (226)	T			O		
Hemolytic uremic syndrome (227)	T	O	O			
Malignant nephrosclerosis (227)	T	O				
Essential mixed cyroimmunoglobulinemia (224)	T	O	O	O	O	
Nephrotoxic drugs and chemicals (226)	T			O		
Oxalate nephropathy (226)	T			O		
Cortical necrosis (219)	T			O		
Postpartum glomerulosclerosis (219)	T			O		
Hypersensitivity nephropathy (226)	T		O			P,H,L
Scleroderma (227)	T					P
Idiopathic rapidly progressive GN (223)	O	T	T		R	
Goodpasture's syndrome (223)	O	T	T	O		P,H
Non-Goodpasture's anti-GBM disease (223)	O	T	T	O		P,H
Acute bacterial endocarditis or visceral sepsis (223)		T	T	O	O	
Microscopic polyarteritis nodosa (224, 227)		T	T			
Wegener's granulomatosis (224, 227)		T	T			
Allergic granulomatosis (269)		T	T			
Acute radiation nephritis (226)		T	T			P
Poststreptococcal glomerulonephritis (223)		R	T	O	R	P,H
Nonstreptococcal postinfectious GN (223)		R	T	R	R	P,H
Macroscopic polyarteritis nodosa (269, 224, 227)				T		P,H
Diffuse proliferative lupus nephritis (224)	R	O	R	T	O	P,H,L
Chronic radiation nephritis (226)				T	O	
Balkan nephropathy (226)				T		P*,H
Analgesic nephropathy (226)				T		L,H
Heavy metals (lead, cadmium, mercury) (226)				T		P*
Cystinosis (226)				T		P*
Chronic obstructive uropathy (230)				T		H
Adult polycystic renal disease (228)				T		H,P
Medullary cystic renal disease (228)				T		
Gouty nephropathy (226)				T		
Minimal change disease (223)					T	
Idiopathic membranous nephropathy (223)				O	T	P,H
Membranoproliferative glomerulonephritis (223)		R	O	O	T	P,H
Renal amyloidosis (224)				O	T	P
Membranous lupus nephropathy (224)				O	T	P
Chronic renal vein thrombosis	O			O	T	
Rheumatoid arthritis (224)					T	
Congenital nephrotic syndrome (224)				O	T	
Dermatomyositis (223)					T	
Dermatitis herpetiformis (223)				O	T	P
Medullary sponge kidney (228)						T:H
Nephrolithiasis (229)						T:H
Neoplasms (226)						T:H
Arteriolar nephrosclerosis (227)				O		T:P
Waldenström's macroglobulinemia (224)	O					T:P
Multiple myeloma (224)	O	O		O	O	T:P
Reflux nephropathy (225, 227)				O	O	T:P
Diabetic nephropathy (224)				O	O	T:P
Toxemia of pregnancy (227)						T:P
Orthostatic proteinuria (223)						T:P
Sarcoid nephropathy (224)						T:P
Hypokalemic nephropathy (226)						T:P
Berger's (IgA) nephropathy (223)	R	R	O	O	O	T:H,P
Henoch-Schönlein purpura (224)		O	O	R	O	T:H,P
Fabry's disease (224)				O		T:H,P
Alport's syndrome (224)				O		T:H,P
Sickle cell nephropathy (224)				O	R	T:H,P
Subacute bacterial endocarditis (188)						T:H,P
Minimal and mesangial lupus nephritis (224)						T:P,H
Mesangial proliferative GN (223)				R	O	T:P,H
Mixed connective tissue disease (224)					R	T:P,H
Chronic glomerulonephritis (224)				O		T:P,H
Nail patella syndrome (224)				R		T:P,H
Focal glomerulosclerosis (223)		R	O	O	O	T:P,H,L
Focal and segmental lupus nephritis (224)				O	O	T:P,H,L
Sjögren's syndrome (224)						T:L,P
Urinary and renal infection (225)						T:L,H

NOTE: *T, typical presentation; O, occurs frequently, but not invariably; R, occurs rarely; P*, tubular proteinuria; P, proteinuria; H, hematuria; L, leukocyturia; ARF, acute renal failure; RPRF, rapidly progressive renal failure; AN, acute nephritis; CRF, chronic renal failure; NS, nephrotic syndrome; AUA, asymptomatic urinary abnormality.*

of acute nephritis associated with massive proteinuria such as essential mixed cryoimmunoglobulinemia, acute bacterial endocarditis, visceral sepsis, and Henoch-Schönlein purpura (Table 217-2).

ASYMPTOMATIC URINARY ABNORMALITIES (AUA) As indicated in Table 217-2, mild degrees of microscopic hematuria, pyuria, casts, or less than 3.5 g protein per 1.73 m² per 24 h may be present in the urine of a patient lacking concurrent evidence of other nephrologic syndromes. By exclusion, these patients are best considered to belong to the syndrome of asymptomatic urinary abnormalities. Isolated hematuria or proteinuria, or unexplained pyuria, are the most frequent abnormalities that occur in this syndrome.

Isolated hematuria, without proteinuria or casts, may be the sole clue to the presence of neoplasm, stone, or infection (e.g., tuberculosis) in any part of the urinary tract (Chaps. 40, 225, 229, and 231). Isolated hematuria may also arise from renal papillae in analgesic and sickle cell nephropathies (Chaps. 226 and 227). Persistent isolated hematuria often requires intravenous pyelography, cystoscopy, and, occasionally, renal arteriography to identify the source of bleeding. *Nephronal hematuria,* in which red blood cells or hemoglobin pigment is present in casts, indicates damage to the nephron (Chap. 40). It occurs without proteinuria, mainly in benign recurrent hematuria and Berger's disease (Chap. 223). *Nephronal hematuria and proteinuria* occur together in many specific renal diseases that may eventually lead to chronic renal failure (Chap. 220). In general, the combination of nephronal hematuria and proteinuria suggests a worse prognosis than either one alone.

Isolated proteinuria, without red blood cells or other formed elements in the urinary sediment, is characteristic of many renal diseases which manifest little or no inflammatory reaction within the glomeruli (e.g., diabetes mellitus, amyloidosis). Less than nephrotic-range proteinuria is common in mild forms of all the diseases that can cause overt nephrotic syndrome (Chaps. 223 and 224). "Tubular" proteinuria (Chap. 40) is the rule in cystinosis; in heavy metal intoxication from cadmium, lead, or mercury, and in the peculiar Balkan nephropathy localized to only a small region along the Danube River (Chap. 226).

Pyuria (leukocyturia) may also be a sole urinary abnormality and frequently reflects infection or inflammation of the lower urinary tract, rather than intrinsic parenchymal renal disease. Nevertheless, prominent pyuria can occur in any inflammatory disease of the kidneys, especially tubulointerstitial nephritis, lupus nephritis, pyelonephritis, and renal transplant rejection, but usually in association with mild proteinuria or hematuria. The finding of leukocyte casts (Chap. 40) establishes the kidney as the site of the inflammatory reaction.

Pyuria associated with urine that is sterile on routine bacteriologic culture presents a special problem. Certain causes of "sterile pyuria" that are clinically obvious include (1) recent bacterial urinary infection being treated with antibiotics, (2) adrenocortical steroid therapy, (3) acute febrile episodes, (4) cyclophosphamide administration, (5) pregnancy, (6) renal transplant rejection, (7) recent genitourinary trauma, and (8) prostatitis and cystourethritis. Leukocytes from vaginal secretions may contaminate the urine, so a midstream, clean-catch urine sample should be collected to substantiate a urinary origin. Pyuria associated with proteinuria, nephronal hematuria (Chap. 40), or casts probably signifies inflammatory disease of the renal glomeruli, tubules, interstitium, or microcirculation, and evaluation should focus not upon the pyuria but upon identifying the nature of the renal disease.

Persistent sterile pyuria that cannot be ascribed to any of the foregoing causes has a narrow differential diagnosis. Unusual infections, such as tuberculosis, fungi, atypical mycobacteria, *Haemophilus influenzae,* anaerobic bacteria, fastidious bacteria that grow only on enriched media, and L forms, all must be sought. Intravenous pyelography is needed to detect causes such as urinary tract calculi, papillary necrosis, and renal infiltration by lymphoma or myeloma cells. The latter is usually suspected because of other evidence of myeloma or lymphoma, for both rarely involve only the kidneys. If all tests are negative, cystoscopy may reveal cystitis or trigone inflammation.

URINARY TRACT INFECTION (UTI) This syndrome is defined by the demonstration in urine of pathogenic organisms, either bacteria, tubercle bacilli, or fungi (Chap. 225). When urine specimens are obtained for culture, the condition under which the urine is collected must minimize contamination from external genitourinary surfaces. Women should void into a wide-mouthed sterile container after preliminary cleansing of the vulva with a moist, sterile gauze pledget. In men, midstream collection is usually adequate. Bacterial colony counts of 10^5 organisms per milliliter or greater in urine generally indicate urinary tract colonization and infection. Levels above 10^2 colonies per milliliter are sufficient to indicate infection in symptomatic patients (Table 217-1) and in urine samples obtained by suprapubic aspiration or bladder catheter (Chap. 226). When the urinary tract is anatomically normal, *Escherichia coli* is the usual bacterial pathogen. After prolonged antibiotic treatment of persistent infections, particularly when urinary drainage is impaired or stones are present, *Klebsiella, Enterobacter,* and *Proteus* species predominate.

As discussed in Chap. 225, the presence of a positive urine culture need not imply that an organism is producing tissue inflammation or injury. In some patients, tissue effects may be trivial; in others, injury may be occurring even though symptoms or urinary abnormalities are not present at the time of evaluation. When bacteriuria is associated with tissue inflammation or injury, clinical manifestations usually depend upon the site(s) involved. Dysuria, frequency, urgency, and suprapubic tenderness are common symptoms of bladder and urethral inflammation (Chap. 40 and Table 217-1). Prostatitis also leads to frequency, dysuria, and urgency, and the prostate may be boggy and tender on rectal examination. Flank pain, chills, fever, nausea and vomiting, hypotension from sepsis, and leukocyte casts all suggest true renal parenchymal infection, i.e., pyelonephritis (Chap. 225); their absence, however, does not exclude pyelonephritis.

RENAL TUBULE DEFECTS (RTD) This syndrome encompasses a large number of acquired and hereditary disorders, all of which tend to affect tubules more than glomeruli. Hereditary anatomic defects, including such entities as polycystic renal disease, medullary cystic disease, and medullary sponge kidney, are readily detected by intravenous pyelography, which is usually performed because of hematuria, bacteriuria, flank pain, or unexplained azotemia (Chap. 228).

Defects in tubule transport functions, on the other hand, tend not to be associated with prominent renal anatomic defects and arise either as inherited traits (Chap. 228) or during the course of acquired renal disease (Chap. 226). In general, these functional defects impair secretion and/or reabsorption of electrolytes and organic solutes, or limit urinary concentrating and diluting ability (Table 217-1). Typical manifestations of such functional disturbances include polyuria and nocturia (Chap. 40), metabolic acidosis (Chap. 42), and various disorders of fluid and electrolyte balance (Chap. 41). Such defects are defined by direct physiologic measurements; their elucidation requires a sound understanding of normal renal physiology.

HYPERTENSION (H) The syndrome of hypertension is considered to exist when the average of a series of reliable blood pressure measurements exceeds 140 mmHg systolic or 90 mmHg diastolic (Table 217-1). The pathogenetic mechanisms, clinical and laboratory manifestations, and therapeutic approaches are discussed in detail elsewhere (Chaps. 29 and 196). In addition, a number of renal complications of hypertension are reviewed in Chap. 227, as is the entity of renal artery stenosis, an infrequent but potentially curable cause of hypertension.

NEPHROLITHIASIS (N) This syndrome is established with certainty when a stone is passed, visualized by x-ray, or removed at surgery or cystoscopy (Table 217-1 and Chap. 229). Less certain, but highly suggestive, evidence of nephrolithiasis exists in the patient with renal colic, painful hematuria, or unexplained pyuria, dysuria, and urinary frequency (Chap. 40). Colic varies in its symptomatology but usually begins suddenly in one flank, radiates downward toward the groin, and is excruciatingly painful.

Most renal stones are composed of calcium, uric acid, cystine, or struvite (magnesium ammonium phosphate). All are radiopaque except for those composed solely of uric acid and are, therefore, visible by routine abdominal radiography. Uric acid stones appear as radiolucent filling defects and can be mistaken for tumor or blood clot. The causes of stones are diverse; the approach to their detection, treatment, and prevention is discussed in Chap. 229.

URINARY TRACT OBSTRUCTION (UTO) Documentation of the various structural or functional causes of urinary tract obstruction usually requires radiologic or surgical visualization. The manifestations of obstruction, which initiate the search for its causes, are numerous (Table 217-1) and are reviewed in Chap. 230. Anuria in an adult is almost always due to obstruction of bladder outflow. Less commonly, blockage of upper urinary drainage from both kidneys, or from a solitary functioning kidney, accounts for total or near-total cessation of urine flow. A large bladder after voiding is a sign of outflow obstruction, usually due to urethral stricture, tumor, stone, neurogenic causes, or prostatic hypertrophy. Nocturia, frequency and overflow incontinence, and slowing or hesitancy of micturition are also suggestive of outflow obstruction (Chap. 40). Upper tract obstruction often produces few clinical manifestations. When it is incomplete or unilateral, urine volume may be normal, or even elevated because of a loss of renal concentrating ability (Chap. 40). Urinary stasis secondary to obstruction commonly predisposes to recurrent urinary tract infection, chronic obstruction to progressive loss of renal function (Table 217-2).

REFERENCES

BLACK DAK: Diagnosis and renal disease, in *Renal Disease*, 4th ed, DAK Black (ed). St. Louis, Blackwell, 1980

CAMERON JS: The natural history of glomerulonephritis, in *Renal Disease*, 4th ed, DAK Black (ed). St. Louis, Blackwell, 1980, p. 329

COE FL: The clinical and laboratory assessment of the patient with renal disease, in *The Kidney*, 3d ed, BM Brenner, FC Rector Jr (eds). Philadelphia, Saunders, 1986, p 703

218 DISTURBANCES OF RENAL FUNCTION

BARRY M. BRENNER / THOMAS H. HOSTETTER / STEVEN C. HEBERT

Near constancy of the composition of the internal environment, including the volume, tonicity, and compartmental distribution of the body fluids, is a state essential to human survival. With day-to-day variations in amount as well as composition of food and fluids, preservation of the internal environment requires the continuous excretion of these substances (and/or their by-products) in amounts that balance precisely the quantities acquired by ingestion and metabolic transformation. Although losses from skin, lungs, and intestine normally contribute to this excretory capacity, by far the greatest responsibility for solute and water excretion is borne by the kidneys.

The kidneys operate primarily to maintain the composition and volume of the *extracellular* fluid compartment. The continuous exchange of water and solutes that takes place across all cell membranes during life, however, permits the kidneys to contribute significantly to the regulation of the volume, composition, and tonicity of the *intracellular* fluids as well. To accomplish these tasks, the human kidney has evolved a number of physiologic mechanisms that enable the individual to excrete any excesses of water and nonmetabolized solute contained in the diet, as well as the nonvolatile end products of nitrogen metabolism, such as urea and creatinine. By contrast, when faced with deficits of water and/or any of the other major constituents of the body fluids, renal excretion of these substances can be curtailed, reducing the likelihood of severe volume or solute depletion. The purpose of this chapter is to review the major excretory functions of the normal kidney and to examine the way these functions are affected by disorders that impair the operations of this organ in humans.

MECHANISMS OF RENAL EXCRETORY FUNCTION WITH NORMAL AND REDUCED NEPHRON MASS

The volume of urine excreted per day (about 1.5 liters, or roughly 1 mL/min) is the small residuum of two very large, and in many ways opposing, processes—namely, *ultrafiltration* of 180 liters or more fluid per day (approximately 125 mL/min) across glomerular capillaries on the one hand and, on the other, *reclamation* (or *reabsorption*) of more than 99 percent of this ultrafiltrate by transport processes operating in the renal tubules. The enormity of the initial step in this process in humans is underscored by the fact that, under resting conditions, about 20 percent of the cardiac output passes through the kidneys, which together comprise less than 1 percent of body weight. Hence, per unit weight of tissue, the rate of blood flow to the kidneys is much greater than that to other solid organs generally considered to be well perfused, including the heart, brain, and liver.

GLOMERULAR ULTRAFILTRATION Urine formation begins with the elaboration of a protein-free ultrafiltrate of plasma across the walls of the glomerular capillaries. The rate of ultrafiltration (glomerular filtration rate, GFR) is determined by three factors: (1) the balance of pressures acting across the capillary wall (the glomerular capillary hydrostatic and Bowman's space oncotic pressures tend to favor filtration, while glomerular capillary oncotic and Bowman's space hydrostatic pressures tend to retard it), (2) the rate at which plasma flows through the glomeruli, and (3) the permeability and the total surface area of the filtering capillaries. A decrease in GFR can be expected when (1) glomerular hydrostatic pressure is reduced (as in hypotensive shock), (2) tubule (hence, Bowman's space) hydrostatic pressure is increased (ureteral or bladder neck obstruction), (3) plasma oncotic pressure rises to unusually high levels (hemoconcentration due to dehydration; multiple myeloma or other dysproteinemias), (4) renal (hence, glomerular) blood and plasma flow are decreased (circulatory collapse, profound heart failure), and (5) permeability and/or total filtering surface area is reduced (acute or chronic glomerulonephritis).

Despite the extraordinarily high rate of water movement across the glomerular capillary wall, all but the smallest of the circulating plasma proteins are normally excluded from passage through this barrier. Molecules the size of inulin (approximately 5200 mol wt), or smaller, normally appear in glomerular urine in the same concentrations as in plasma water, whereas the transport of substances of increasingly greater size diminishes progressively, normally approaching very low values as the size of serum albumin is approached. The *glomerular capillary basement membrane* and the *slitlike diaphragms* that connect adjacent epithelial cell foot processes on the urinary aspect of the glomerular capillary wall (Fig. 40-1, page 193) are believed to serve as major barriers to protein filtration. In addition to these mechanical gates, *electrostatic factors* also serve to retard the filtration of plasma proteins, especially albumin. The albumin molecule behaves as a polyanion in physiologic solution, and is therefore retarded by the highly anionic glycoproteins contained in the various component layers of the glomerular wall. With disruption of these mechanical and electrostatic barriers, as seen in many forms of glomerular injury (see Chaps. 222 to 224); abnormally large quantities of plasma proteins gain access to the urine.

BIOLOGIC CONSEQUENCES OF SUSTAINED REDUCTIONS IN GFR Measurement of total GFR of both kidneys provides a sensitive and commonly employed index of overall renal excretory function. When renal excretory function is impaired, either acutely or chronically, one or more of the determinants of GFR in affected nephrons is altered unfavorably so that total GFR declines. The magnitude of the decline is determined by the sum of the impairments of function of individual glomeruli. Initially, the effect of such impairments in single-nephron GFR (SNGFR), no matter how small, is to reduce the total rate of excretion of water and those solutes normally contained in the glomerular ultrafiltrate. In the steady state, these reduced rates of filtration, when accompanied by comparably reduced rates of excretion, lead to *retention* and *accumulation* of the unexcreted substances in the body fluids. Further reduction in GFR augments the degree to which these substances are retained.

Figure 218-1 depicts the major patterns of response to these impairments in filtration. The degree of reduction in total GFR is plotted on the abscissa, expressed as a percentage of normal (100 percent). For the various solutes normally contained in glomerular filtrate, three general types of response are common, depicted by curves A, B, and C. Curve A describes the pattern seen with substances, such as creatinine and urea, which normally depend largely on glomerular filtration for their excretion into the urine; i.e., secretion fails to influence urinary excretion appreciably. Therefore, as GFR falls, plasma levels of creatinine, urea, and other substances normally excreted largely by filtration rise progressively, albeit in the nonlinear manner illustrated.

The clinical course of chronic renal failure (CRF) usually also conforms to the pattern described by *curve A*. Patients with CRF usually pass from a long asymptomatic period of ''compensation'' to a more accelerated and clinically symptomatic terminal phase. In other words, chronic forms of renal injury which lead to slow but inexorable destruction of nephron mass usually lead to progressive but modest elevations in creatinine and urea levels in plasma, but not to levels beyond the range of normal, despite loss of as much as 50 percent of total GFR. With further loss of nephron mass, and further reduction in GFR, however (even though the rate of nephron destruction may not be accelerated), the limits of renal reserve are exceeded, and continued accumulation of *curve A–type solutes* leads to plasma concentrations clearly beyond the range of normal (Fig. 218-1). Because these retained solutes are believed to exert ''toxic'' effects on virtually all organ systems, manifestations of CRF now become overt. As a result, for patients with reduced renal mass, even small additional decrements in total GFR may spell the difference between ''compensation'' and overt uremia.

FIGURE 218-1 *Representative patterns of adaptation for different types of solutes in body fluids in chronic renal failure. (After NS Bricker et al, in Brenner and Rector, 2d ed.)*

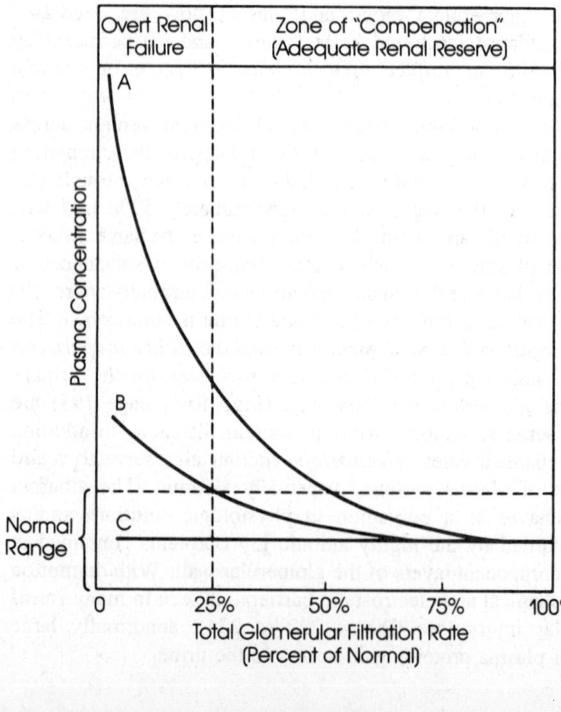

The accumulation of *curve A–type solutes* with progressive renal failure continues until external balance for these solutes is achieved, that is, until acquisition and/or production rates and excretion rates are exactly matched. In the case of creatinine, for example, assuming a constant rate of creatinine production, a 50 percent reduction in GFR results in an approximate doubling of the plasma creatinine concentration. The latter restores the filtered load of creatinine (that is, GFR × plasma creatinine concentration) to the preillness level, and urinary excretion rate again becomes equivalent to the rate of creatinine production. Unfortunately, since no mechanism exists in human beings for augmenting creatinine excretion beyond this level, elimination of retained creatinine is not possible, and plasma concentration remains twice normal. With progressive reduction in GFR, plasma creatinine levels continue to rise, due both to the most recent loss of nephron excretory function and to the retention associated with earlier nephron destruction (Fig. 218-1). *In practice, so long as the net rates of acquisition and production remain reasonably constant, the inverse relationship between plasma concentrations of solutes such as creatinine and urea and GFR is sufficiently reliable and predictable to allow plasma levels of such solutes to serve as useful clinical indexes of GFR.*

In contrast to solutes of the *curve A type*, plasma levels of substances such as phosphate, urate, and potassium (K^+) and hydrogen (H^+) ions usually fail to rise above the normal range until GFR falls to a small percentage of normal. With progressive renal failure this pattern of response, depicted by *curve B* in Fig. 218-1, reflects the participation of tubule transport mechanisms that contribute to the excretion of these substances. In other words, *as GFR declines, the tubules facilitate the excretion of progressively greater fractions of the filtered load of these solutes, either by enhancing their net secretion and/or by diminishing their net reabsorption.* Plasma levels of *curve B–type solutes,* therefore, rise much less than do those of *curve A* because, with progressive reduction in GFR, *excretion rate per nephron* and, therefore, *fractional excretion* both increase. Eventually, however, enhanced fractional excretion can no longer offset the reduction in the filtered load of these solutes caused by a markedly diminished GFR, and plasma levels rise above the normal range (Fig. 218-1). For urate, phosphate, and K^+ at least, increased fractional excretion usually serves to maintain normal plasma levels until GFR falls to less than one-fourth of normal.

Finally, for certain solutes, such as sodium chloride (NaCl), concentrations in plasma remain virtually constant, and at normal levels, throughout the entire course of CRF, despite continued ingestion of these substances in normal amounts. Such solutes conform to the pattern described by *curve C* in Fig. 218-1. The extent of compensation is nearly complete and represents a fundamental adaptation to renal injury. To illustrate the magnitude of the adaptation involved, it is useful to compare the excretion of Na^+ in an individual with normal renal excretory function (GFR of 125 mL/min) with that in an individual with advanced renal insufficiency (GFR of 2 mL/min). Both subjects are allowed to ingest a diet containing 7 g salt per day (120 meq Na^+). With a normal serum Na^+ concentration of 140 meq per liter, external Na^+ balance is achieved in the normal individual by excreting approximately 0.5 percent of the filtered load of Na^+. By contrast, for external balance to be maintained in the patient with CRF, fractional excretion of Na^+ must rise to 30 percent. *In other words, external balance for Na^+ demands that the same quantity of Na^+ (120 meq) be excreted into the urine each day in the subject with CRF as in the normal subject.* Given the drastic reduction in GFR faced by the patient with CRF, external balance can be achieved only by a progressive transformation of the Na^+ reabsorptive processes in surviving tubules, so that a progressively larger fraction of the filtered load of Na^+ escapes reabsorption and appears in final urine. In short, *the rate of excretion of Na^+ per surviving nephron increases in inverse proportion to the composite GFR of surviving nephrons.*

MECHANISMS OF TUBULE TRANSPORT WITH NORMAL AND REDUCED NEPHRON MASS Loss of renal function with nearly all forms of progressive renal disease is usually attended by a progressive distortion of renal morphology and architecture. Despite this structural disarray, glomerular and tubule functions often remain as closely integrated (i.e., *glomerulotubular balance*) in the diseased kidney as they do in the normal organ, at least until the final stages of CRF. A fundamental feature of this *intact nephron hypothesis* is that following loss of nephron mass, residual renal function derives primarily from the operation of surviving healthy nephrons, while the diseased nephrons are believed to cease functioning. Despite progressive nephron destruction, there is considerable evidence to suggest that many of the mechanisms that contribute to the maintenance of solute and water balance differ only quantitatively, and not qualitatively, from those believed to govern fluid and solute homeostasis under normal physiologic conditions. The most important of these are considered below.

Tubule transport of sodium chloride and water in health Most of the filtered water and Na^+ salts are reabsorbed by the tubules, leaving small and variable amounts, equivalent on a day-to-day basis to the quantities ingested, to reach the final urine. About two-thirds of the glomerular ultrafiltrate is reabsorbed in the *proximal tubule* with little change in the osmolality or Na^+ concentration of the unreabsorbed fraction (Fig. 218-2). In other words, fluid reabsorption in the proximal tubule is nearly *isosmotic* and is coupled to the active transport of Na^+. Since Cl^- and HCO_3^- are the primary anions in the extracellular fluid, most of the filtered Na^+ is reabsorbed with these anions. In the early convoluted portion of the proximal tubule, bicarbonate is the principal anion accompanying the reabsorption of sodium. This process occurs via a Na^+/H^+ exchange mechanism at the luminal brush border and is dependent upon both cystolic and brush border carbonic anhydrase. Glucose, amino acids, and other organic solutes (e.g., lactate) are also extensively reabsorbed in the proximal convoluted tubule by a cotransport process that links the cellular entry of these organic substrates with Na^+. Three processes appear to operate in parallel to couple water (i.e., volume) absorption with solute absorption in the proximal tubule. First, given the remarkably high water permeability of this nephron segment, very small transepithelial osmolality differences, that is, *luminal hypotonicity* on the order of 2 to 3 mosmol, produced by solute absorption, could drive volume absorption. Second, due to the *preferential* absorption of HCO_3^- and organic solutes in the early portions of the proximal tubule, the concentrations of these substances decrease while that of Cl^- increases along the length of the proximal tubule. Volume absorption would occur if the rate of Na^+ and Cl^- diffusion down their respective electrochemical gradients were more rapid than the back diffusion of sodium bicarbonate into the lumen. Finally, an *effective osmotic gradient* would be established (despite equal macroscopic osmolalities of luminal and peritubular fluids) if the effective osmolality produced by Cl^- in the lumen were greater than that for bicarbonate in the peritubular fluid.

The rate of reabsorption of fluid from proximal convoluted tubules and peritubular interstitium is sensitive to the effects of *physical factors,* i.e., the hydrostatic and colloid osmotic (or oncotic) pressures acting across the walls of the peritubular capillaries. Because the plasma proteins in glomerular capillaries are concentrated by ultrafiltration, there is a marked rise in the oncotic pressure as plasma flows along the glomerular capillary network. This step-up in plasma oncotic pressure is transmitted largely unchanged to the peritubular capillaries, via the efferent arterioles. These resistance vessels cause a substantial drop in hydrostatic pressure, however, so that when the plasma reaches the peritubular capillaries, oncotic pressure greatly exceeds hydrostatic pressure. These *Starling forces* are therefore oriented in an *uptake mode,* in contrast to the *filtration mode* at the glomerulus, where hydrostatic pressure exceeds oncotic. The extent to which oncotic pressure exceeds hydrostatic pressure in the peritubular capillary network is thought to modulate the overall rate of reabsorption of fluid by the proximal tubules. Therefore, when peritubular oncotic pressure falls, or hydrostatic pressure rises, uptake of fluid by these capillaries is reduced. As a result, fluid is retained in the interstitial space, altering the hydrostatic pressure in the space, and ultimately retarding the egress of fluid from the lateral intercellular channels. Without an adequate route of drainage, fluid in the channels leaks back into the tubule lumen and diminishes *net fluid reabsorption* by this tubule segment. The opposite occurs in states in which peritubular oncotic pressure increases (increased filtration fraction), or hydrostatic pressure decreases (enhanced efferent arteriolar tone). Under these circumstances, peritubular capillary uptake of reabsorbate is augmented, leading ultimately to *enhanced net fluid reabsorption* by the proximal tubule.

In contrast to the proximal tubule, active outward transport of NaCl from tubule lumen to peritubular blood has not been established for the *thin limbs of Henle's loop.* However, passive outward salt transport does occur, as indicated in Fig. 218-2. In the next segment of the nephron, the *medullary thick ascending limb of Henle,* the concentration of NaCl is reduced below the level that prevails at the beginning of this segment. Here Cl^- absorption occurs by an active process involving a furosemide-sensitive Na^+:K^+:$2Cl^-$ cotransport mechanism in the luminal membrane, with one-half of Na^+ absorption proceeding passively, driven by the lumen-positive transepithelial voltage. Since the ascending limb of Henle is always impermeable to water, net NaCl reabsorption not only generates hypotonic tubule fluid, but also gives rise to the high NaCl concentration of the outer medullary interstitium (Fig. 218-2). In certain animals the antidiuretic hormone (ADH) enhances NaCl absorption but not water permeability in the medullary portion of the thick ascending limb, but an effect of this hormone on this segment in human beings is uncertain.

The fluid leaving the thick ascending limb of Henle is normally low in NaCl concentration, a condition largely independent of the organism's diet or state of hydration. In the *distal convoluted tubule,* water reabsorption is variable, depending on the state of hydration or, more specifically, on the presence or absence of the ADH in plasma. In the absence of ADH, this and more distal nephron segments are impermeable to water, so that the hypotonic fluid entering this segment is excreted as *dilute urine.* Indeed, continued salt reabsorption along the distal convoluted tubule results in further dilution of the urine. In the presence of ADH, the permeability of the late portion of this segment to water increases, and as a result, the osmolality of the late distal tubule fluid rises to a value close to that of plasma. NaCl continues to be reabsorbed from the tubule lumen, against moderately steep chemical and electrical gradients. The reabsorptive process for NaCl at this site is enhanced by *aldosterone.*

The *cortical collecting tubule* possesses an extremely low permeability to water in the absence of ADH, whereas this permeability increases greatly in the presence of the hormone. The sensitivity of this segment to ADH appears to be more pronounced than that of the distal convoluted tubule. As with the distal convoluted tubule, the cortical collecting tubule is capable of further active reabsorption of NaCl.

The terminal segment of the distal nephron is the highly branched *papillary collecting duct.* Continued electrolyte transport in this segment results in the large ion concentration differences that normally exist between urine and plasma. As in the cortical collecting tubule, Na^+ transport appears to be active since reabsorption proceeds against sizable electrochemical gradients. The rate of Na^+ transport in this segment depends on the diet and on the load of Na^+ delivered from more proximal segments, and is affected by aldosterone. The permeability of this segment to water also increases markedly in the presence of ADH.

Effects of reduced nephron mass on sodium chloride transport in surviving nephrons With progressive destruction of nephrons, *maintenance of external balance for NaCl requires that fractional salt excretion increase as GFR decreases.* Very likely several mechanisms contribute to this adaptive increase in fractional salt excretion. With losses of functioning nephron units, peritubular capillary hydrostatic and oncotic pressures are probably altered in directions that serve to suppress proximal tubule reabsorption of NaCl and water. For example, a rise in peritubular capillary hydrostatic pressure, which tends to inhibit net proximal fluid reabsorption, might be anticipated with arterial hypertension, a common feature of renal insufficiency. Similarly, peritubular oncotic pressure might be expected to decline with renal injury, owing both to reductions in filtration fraction and to hypoalbuminemia. While such alterations in peritubular factors clearly account for diminution in proximal fluid reabsorption in response to falling levels of GFR in animals, such alterations have not been established with certainty in humans. Aldosterone, normally an important determinant of Na^+ reabsorption in distal portions of the nephron, is probably not a major factor responsible for reducing fractional Na^+ reabsorption, since aldosterone

FIGURE 218-2 *Transport functions of the various anatomic segments of the mammalian nephron. Fluid reabsorption across the proximal tubule is isosmotic and accounts for reabsorption of approximately two-thirds of the filtered Na^+ and H_2O. The major portions of the filtered HCO_3^-, amino acids, and glucose are reabsorbed in the early proximal convoluted tubule. Reabsorption of glucose and amino acids is coupled to Na^+ transport and thereby generates a negative potential difference within the tubule lumen. At the same time, HCO_3^- is reabsorbed by a nonelectrogenic mechanism, via H^+ secretion. The active transport of these solutes results in transepithelial concentration and effective osmotic pressure gradients promoting H_2O flow across the proximal tubule, into the peritubular capillaries. The rise in tubule fluid Cl^- concentration is a necessary reciprocal consequence of the decreased luminal HCO_3^- concentration. The resultant high concentration of Cl^- becomes an important force for the outward passive transport of Cl^- down its concentration gradient, resulting in a lumen positive potential difference in the late proximal convoluted tubule. The pars recta of the proximal tubule is capable of active electrogenic transport of Na^+ independent of organic solute transport. Under normal conditions, approximately one-third of the glomerular filtrate enters the descending limb of Henle's loop. Because the thin descending limb is incapable of active outward NaCl transport and is characterized by low permeability to Na^+ but high H_2O permeability, H_2O is abstracted passively as the fluid approaches the bend of Henle's loop. Hypertonic fluid with a greater NaCl concentration but lower urea concentration than the surrounding medullary interstitium thus enters the thin ascending limb of Henle. This segment differs from the descending limb in that it is largely impermeable to H_2O and urea but highly permeable to NaCl. These characteristics allow for passive diffusion of NaCl out of the ascending limb. Active electrogenic NaCl transport across the water-impermeable thick ascending limb of Henle allows for separation of solute and water. In consequence tubule fluid becomes dilute, and the medullary interstitium hypertonic. Irrespective of the final osmolality of the urine, the fluid that enters the distal convoluted tubule is always hypoosmotic. This segment exhibits active Na^+ reabsorption. All but the terminal portion of the distal convoluted tubule is water impermeable, even in the presence of ADH. Aldosterone exerts its effect in this segment by enhancing Na^+ reabsorption, which is variably coupled to K^+ and H^+ secretion. The cortical and papillary portions of the collecting duct are sites where ADH exerts its principal effect. The permeability of these segments to H_2O in the absence of ADH is very low but can be greatly enhanced in the presence of ADH. These segments are also characterized by active Na^+ reabsorption, which appears to depend on the presence of mineralocorticoid. In the absence of ADH, the collecting tubule is water impermeable so that hypotonic tubule fluid courses through it. However, in the presence of ADH, water is avidly reabsorbed here, resulting in hypertonic final urine.*

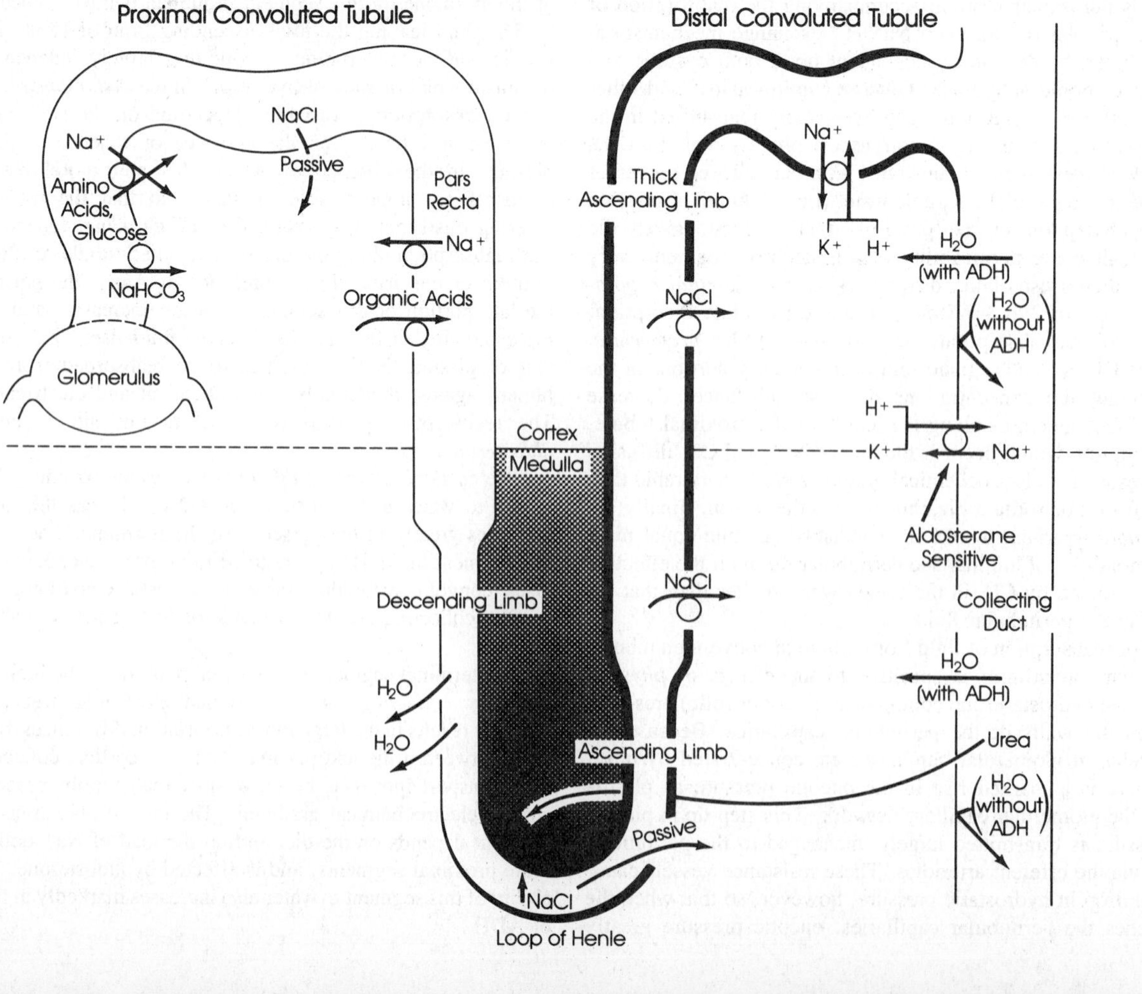

levels in plasma are rarely reduced in CRF. Furthermore, external Na^+ balance has been shown to be preserved in bilaterally adrenalectomized uremic dogs maintained on fixed doses of mineralocorticoid hormones. Yet another factor that has received attention in contributing to the suppression of fractional NaCl reabsorption in CRF relates to the retention of solutes as GFR declines. In addition to urea and creatinine, a host of *organic acids* (including *hippurates*) also accumulate. These substances are normally excreted by both filtration and tubule secretion; the latter process involves a carrier-mediated organic acid transport system in proximal tubule epithelia. When GFR is reduced and plasma levels of these organic acids increase, sufficient fluid may accompany the secretion of these organic anions into the proximal tubule lumen (by osmosis) to diminish net fluid reabsorption, and even favor net fluid secretion. Evidence in support of this intriguing mechanism derives from studies in which uremic serums were capable of inducing net fluid secretion in isolated proximal tubules of rabbits studied in vitro.

It has also been suggested that NaCl transport across the mammalian renal tubule may be governed, at least in part, by a *natriuretic hormone*. In support of this possibility, serums and urine from patients and dogs with uremia have been reported to contain factors capable of inhibiting NaCl transport across frog skin, toad bladder, and rat renal tubule. However, accumulation of natriuretic factors in uremia may not be without cost; the "trade-off" for maintenance of external Na^+ balance is the possibility of abnormalities occurring in Na^+ transport across cell membranes, which often occurs in advanced renal insufficiency. This possibility is discussed in greater detail in Chap. 220.

The obligatorily high rate of solute excretion per surviving nephron (so-called osmotic diuresis due to urea and other retained solutes) may also contribute to enhancing fractional NaCl excretion, much as occurs in normal subjects following administration of nonreabsorbable solutes such as mannitol. Finally, certain forms of CRF tend to be associated with unusually pronounced salt losses in urine. These *salt-wasting nephropathies* include chronic pyelonephritis and other tubulointerstitial diseases (see Chap. 226) as well as polycystic and medullary cystic diseases. These disorders have in common greater destruction of medullary and interstitial, than cortical and glomerular, portions of the renal parenchyma. Preferential impairment of tubule reabsorptive function, rather than a primary reduction in GFR, may, therefore, underlie the salt-losing tendency in these disorders. A number of clinical derangements associated with the altered renal handling of NaCl in CRF (including hypo- and hypervolemia, hypertension, etc.) are considered in Chap. 220.

Effects of reduced nephron mass on water reabsorption in surviving nephrons As with NaCl, there is a progressive increase in the fractional excretion of water with advancing renal insufficiency, so that even the patient with a total GFR of 5 mL/min or less can usually maintain external water balance. The adaptations in the handling of water by the tubules of the diseased kidney are of importance in the pathogenesis of the urinary concentrating defect and, hence, of the polyuria and nocturia seen commonly in CRF (see Chap. 40). To appreciate the mechanisms involved, the responses of a normal and a uremic subject in maintaining external water balance need to be compared. Assuming that both subjects ingest the same diet and also the same amount of fluid, total solute and volume excretion in each subject should be identical as well. If the *obligatory solute load* to be excreted in each is assumed to be 600 mosmol per day, and urine osmolality is 300 mosmol/kg, a urine volume of 2 liters per day will be required to excrete the total solute load in each subject. If GFR in normal and uremic subjects is 180 and 4 liters per day, respectively, urinary volume excretion of 2 liters per day represents excretion of slightly more than 1 percent of the filtered water in the normal individual, compared with a much larger value, 50 percent, in the uremic subject. Since the range of urine osmolalities that the diseased kidney can achieve (250 to 350 mosmol/kg) is much narrower than in the normal (40 to 1200 mosmol/kg), the individual with normal function is able to excrete the obligatory daily solute load of 600 mosmol in as little as 500 mL urine per day or as much as 15 liters per day, compared with the much narrower range in the patient with renal insufficiency, from about 1.7 to 2.4 liters per day.

In CRF, the limited ability to concentrate the urine usually correlates closely with other measures of impaired renal function. Isosthenuria is, therefore, a nearly universal finding when GFR falls below 25 mL/min. At this level of GFR and below, urine osmolality does not rise even with supramaximal parenteral doses of ADH, suggesting that the concentrating defect is related not only to loss of diseased nephrons but also to impaired concentrating ability in surviving nephrons. As has been discussed, with diminution in functioning nephron mass, there is a concurrent increase in fractional excretion of a number of solutes. As a consequence, solute diuresis per nephron obligates a nearly isosmotic amount of water and prevents the elaboration of either hypotonic or hypertonic urine. Disease-induced abnormalities of the architecture of the renal medulla (loops of Henle, vasa rectae), aberrations in renal medullary blood flow, and defective transport of NaCl in the ascending limb of Henle undoubtedly also contribute to this defect in urine concentration. Finally, there is suggestive evidence that uremia per se may impair the responsiveness of terminal nephron segments to ADH.

Since patients with renal insufficiency are usually unable to excrete concentrated urine, they must have access to adequate amounts of water in order to ensure the excretion of total daily solute loads. For this reason, restriction of fluid intake may prove extremely hazardous in patients with CRF. Likewise, impairment of diluting capacity may prevent many patients from excreting large amounts of ingested fluids. The consequences of the abnormal water excretion patterns in CRF, including the tendencies to development of hypo- and hypernatremia, are considered in Chaps. 41 and 220.

Tubule transport of phosphate with normal and reduced nephron mass Under normal physiologic conditions, about 80 to 90 percent of the filtered load of phosphate is reabsorbed, mainly in the proximal tubule. *Parathyroid hormone* (*PTH*), by augmenting phosphate excretion via inhibition of this proximal reabsorptive process (Chap. 335), plays a key role in phosphate homeostasis. In normal humans, when dietary phosphate intake increases, a *transient* rise in plasma phosphate concentration is usually observed. This results in a similarly transient reduction in the plasma ionized calcium concentration (due largely to calcium-phosphate deposition in bone), which, in turn, stimulates PTH secretion. By enhancing fractional phosphate excretion, PTH restores external phosphate balance and normophosphatemia. This then enables plasma ionized calcium levels to return to normal, thereby removing the stimulus to PTH release, and restoring all elements of the phosphate control system to the original steady state.

With advancing renal disease, and constant dietary intake of phosphate, external phosphate balance is achieved by progressive reduction in fractional phosphate reabsorption. Enhanced PTH secretion is an important determinant of this phosphaturic response to reduced nephron mass. With each succeeding decrement in GFR, the total amount of phosphate filtered by surviving glomeruli is reduced, leading to transient retention of phosphate and, therefore, a rise (albeit small) in the phosphate concentration in extracellular fluid, including plasma. This rise in plasma phosphate concentration leads to a reciprocal small decline in plasma ionized calcium concentration and a corresponding increase in PTH secretion. Although the phosphaturic response of surviving tubules to this elevation in circulating PTH is thought to restore plasma phosphate and, therefore, calcium levels to normal (at least in the "compensated" stage of CRF described by the relatively flat portion of curve B in Fig. 218-1), the biologic cost of this return to normophosphatemia and normocalcemia is a *persistent elevation in the plasma PTH level.* With successive decrements in GFR, each stage in this overall process is repeated, but at an ever-increasing cost, namely, *progressive elevation in the circulating level of PTH.* At least two additional processes are thought to contribute to elevated PTH levels in renal failure. One relates to the skeletal resistance to the calcemic effect of PTH seen in uremia. This resistance necessitates a greater than normal level of circulating PTH to effect an increment in serum calcium concentration. The other derives from the finding that reductions in renal mass impair the ability of the kidneys to degrade circulating PTH. The fact that phosphate conforms more to a curve B– than curve C–type solute in Fig. 218-1 indicates that these forms of adaptation are limited; ultimately phosphate retention occurs when GFR falls below about 25 mL/min.

Since PTH exerts major biologic effects on bone, as well as renal tubules, the external balance of phosphate in CRF is achieved at the expense of elevated PTH levels, which, in turn, account for many of the bone changes of renal osteodystrophy (i.e., *secondary hyperparathyroidism,* Fig. 220-1). In support of this ingenious *trade-off hypothesis,* studies in animals with CRF suggest that when dietary phosphate intake is reduced in proportion to the reduction in GFR, external balance of phosphate no longer requires augmentation of fractional phosphate excretion in surviving nephrons. Accordingly, circulating PTH levels no longer rise, and the typical bone changes of secondary hyperparathyroidism are diminished, if not prevented.

Destruction of renal mass also impairs phosphate, calcium, and skeletal metabolism by mechanisms largely independent of impaired excretory function. The kidneys are normally the major site of *metabolic conversion of vitamin D to its active metabolites.* Whereas the tendency to secondary hyperparathyroidism begins, at least theoretically, when a single nephron unit is destroyed, impaired vitamin D biotransformation is not usually apparent until GFR falls to below 25 percent of normal. As discussed in Chap. 336, precursors of the active form of vitamin D, synthesized in skin or acquired from foods, undergo initial hydroxylation in the liver to form 25-hydroxyvitamin D_3 [25(OH)D_3]. The kidney is the site of a second important hydroxylation step, to form 1,25-dihydroxyvitamin D_3 [1,25$(OH)_2D_3$]. This activated form of vitamin D operates to enhance intestinal calcium and phosphate absorption, as well as to promote resorption of these ions from bone. In addition, 1,25$(OH)_2D_3$ probably opposes the phosphaturic action of PTH at the level of the renal tubule by augmenting, rather than diminishing, phosphate reabsorption. With advancing renal disease, reduction in renal mass causes vitamin D hydroxylation to be impaired; phosphate retention has also been shown to suppress this important hydroxylation reaction. Reduction in circulating 1,25$(OH)_2D_3$ levels, by suppressing calcium absorption from gut, contributes further to the development of the hypocalcemia and PTH excess of CRF, the consequences of which are considered in Chap. 220.

Hydrogen and bicarbonate transport with normal and reduced nephron mass As discussed in Chap. 42, the pH of extracellular fluid in humans is normally maintained within a narrow range, 7.36 to 7.44, despite day-to-day variations in the quantity of acids entering the body fluids from dietary and metabolic sources (approximately 1 meq H^+ per kg per day). These acids consume both intracellular and extracellular buffers, of which bicarbonate (HCO_3^-) is the most important in the intracellular compartment. Such buffering minimizes the changes in pH that would otherwise occur. The HCO_3^- buffer system would be of little long-term benefit were it not for homeostatic mechanisms, however, since with unrelenting acquisition of nonvolatile acids from dietary and metabolic sources, buffering capacity would ultimately be exhausted, eventually culminating in fatal acidosis. The kidneys normally function to prevent this possibility by *regenerating* HCO_3^- and, thereby, maintaining the concentration of HCO_3^- in the plasma. In addition to generating HCO_3^-, the kidneys also *reclaim* essentially all the HCO_3^- present in the glomerular ultrafiltrate. This reabsorptive process takes place largely in the proximal tubule and is virtually complete below a critical serum HCO_3^- concentration—the threshold concentration—which in humans is normally about 26 meq per liter, identical to the concentration of HCO_3^- in plasma. As a consequence, urinary wastage of HCO_3^- is prevented. Alternatively, when plasma HCO_3^- concentration rises above this threshold level, reabsorption of HCO_3^- becomes less complete, and the excess HCO_3^- escapes into the final urine, returning the plasma HCO_3^- concentration to the threshold level. Despite reabsorption of all the filtered HCO_3^-, metabolic acidosis would still ensue if HCO_3^- consumed in buffering nonvolatile strong acids were not constantly regenerated.

The *reabsorption* of filtered HCO_3^- in the proximal tubule occurs by the following mechanism. In proximal tubule cells, H^+, formed by the splitting of water into H^+ and OH^-, is secreted into the tubule lumen, very likely in exchange for Na^+. The OH^- ion, under the influence of *carbonic anhydrase,* combines with CO_2 to form HCO_3^-, which diffuses across the peritubular cell membrane to enter the extracellular HCO_3^- pool. The H^+ secreted into the tubule lumen combines with a filtered HCO_3^-, forming H_2CO_3. Dehydration of the latter in the proximal tubule lumen leads to the formation of CO_2 which also diffuses from lumen to peritubular blood. As a result, *a filtered* HCO_3^- *ion is reclaimed.* Secreted H^+ ions are also free to combine with non-HCO_3^- buffers (e.g., phosphate or ammonia) in the tubule fluid and are excreted in these forms in the final urine. HCO_3^-, the other original product of the breakdown of H_2CO_3, formed within the tubule cell, enters the peritubular blood, and *a* HCO_3^- *ion is regenerated.*

Hydrogen ions in the urine are bound primarily to filtered buffers (e.g., phosphate) in an amount (the so-called titratable acid) equivalent to the amount of alkali required to titrate the pH of the urine to the pH of blood. It is usually not possible, however, to excrete all the daily acid load as titratable acid alone. To serve as an additional buffer, the cells of the renal tubules generate ammonia (NH_3), largely from the hydrolysis of glutamine. NH_3 diffuses from these cells into the tubule lumen, where it combines with H^+ to form NH_4^+. As noted above, each mole of NH_4^+ excreted into the urine is associated with the regeneration of 1 mol of HCO_3^-. *Ammoniagenesis,* a process which occurs within proximal tubule cells, is responsive to the acid-base needs of the individual. When faced with an acute acid burden and an increased need for HCO_3^- regeneration, the rate of renal ammonia synthesis increases sharply.

The quantity of hydrogen ions excreted as titratable acid and NH_4^+ is equal to the quantity of HCO_3^- regenerated in tubule cells and added to the plasma. Under steady-state conditions, the quantity of net acid excreted into the urine (the sum of titratable acid and NH_4^+ minus HCO_3^-) must equal the quantity of acid gained by the extracellular fluid from all sources. Metabolic acidosis and alkalosis result when this delicate balance is perturbed, the former the result of *insufficient* net acid excretion, the latter due to *excessive* acid excretion.

Progressive loss of renal function usually causes little or no change in arterial pH, plasma bicarbonate concentration, or arterial carbon dioxide tension (P_{CO_2}) until GFR falls below 50 percent of normal. Thereafter, all three quantities tend to decline as *metabolic acidosis* ensues. In general, the metabolic acidosis of CRF is not due to overproduction of endogenous acids, but is largely a reflection of the reduction in renal mass, which limits the amount of NH_3 (and therefore HCO_3^-) that can be generated. Although surviving nephrons are probably capable of generating supernormal quantities of NH_3 *per nephron,* the diminished nephron population causes overall NH_3 production to be reduced to an extent inadequate to permit sufficient buffering of H^+ in urine. Though patients with CRF may acidify the urine normally (i.e., urine pH as low as 4.5), the defect in NH_3 production limits total daily acid excretion to 30 to 40 meq, or half to two-thirds the quantity of nonvolatile acid formed in the same time period. Metabolic acidosis is the inevitable consequence of this positive balance for H^+, which in most patients with stable CRF is relatively mild and nonprogressive (arterial pH of approximately 7.33 to 7.37).

Given this substantial daily accumulation of H^+, and the typically stable and nonprogressive nature of the resulting acidosis, including the observed relative constancy of the plasma HCO_3^- concentration (albeit at reduced levels of 14 to 20 meq per liter), it follows that some large tissue source of buffering must account for the stability of the acidosis in CRF. Bone is the most likely candidate, particularly in view of its large reservoir of alkaline salts (calcium phosphate and calcium carbonate). Dissolution of this buffer source probably contributes to the osteodystrophy of CRF (see Fig. 220-1).

Although the acidosis of CRF is a consequence of the reduction in total renal mass and is therefore tubule in origin, it nevertheless depends to a large extent on the level of GFR. When GFR is reduced to only a moderate extent (i.e., to about 50 percent of normal), retention of anions, principally sulfates and phosphates, is not pronounced, so that as the plasma HCO_3^- level falls owing to tubule dysfunction, retention of Cl^- by the kidneys leads to the development of *hyperchloremic acidosis*. At this stage, therefore, *the anion gap is normal*. With further reduction in GFR and more pronounced azotemia, however, retention of phosphates, sulfates, and other *unmeasured* anions is the rule, and plasma Cl^- concentration falls to normal levels despite the reduction in plasma HCO_3^- concentration. *A moderate to large anion gap therefore develops*.

Tubule potassium transport with normal and reduced nephron mass As with H^+, the concentration of K^+ in extracellular fluid is normally maintained within a relatively narrow range, 4 to 5 meq per liter. Ninety-five percent or more of total body K^+ is in the intracellular fluid compartment, where the intracellular concentration is approximately 160 meq per liter. Normal individuals maintain external K^+ balance by excreting into the urine an amount of K^+ per day equivalent to the amount ingested, minus the relatively small amounts lost in stool and sweat. K^+ is freely filtered at the glomerulus, although the amount excreted usually represents no more than about 20 percent of the quantity filtered. The great bulk of the filtered K^+ is *reabsorbed* in the early portions of the nephron, about two-thirds in the proximal tubule, and an additional 20 to 25 percent in the loop of Henle. A K^+ *secretory process* operates in the distal tubule and terminal nephron segments. This process is largely dependent on exchange of K^+ for Na^+, the reabsorbed Na^+ creating an electrical gradient across the tubule wall, lumen negative. K^+ therefore diffuses from the cell interior into the lumens of distal tubules and collecting ducts, down this electrochemical gradient.

The ability to maintain external K^+ balance and normal plasma K^+ concentration as well, until relatively late in the course of CRF, is a consequence primarily of a progressive increase in fractional excretion of K^+. Greatly enhanced rates of K^+ secretion in distal portions of surviving tubules appear to underlie this adaptation. The augmented secretion rate of aldosterone is believed to contribute to enhanced tubule secretion of K^+, as do the increased distal tubule flow rates in residual functioning nephrons due to the osmotic diuresis and the enhanced luminal electronegativity created by the increased concentration of highly impermeable anions such as phosphate and sulfate. Aldosterone also stimulates net entry of K^+ into the lumen of the colon, a mechanism known to be enhanced in CRF. More detailed discussions of the abnormalities in K^+ homeostasis in acute and chronic forms of renal failure are given in Chaps. 219 and 220.

REFERENCES

BRENNER BM, RECTOR FC JR (eds): *The Kidney*, 3d ed. Philadelphia, Saunders, 1986

BRICKER NS: On the pathogenesis of the uremic state: An exposition of the "trade-off" hypothesis. N Engl J Med 286:1093, 1972

HAYSLETT JP: Functional adaptation to reduction in renal mass. Physiol Rev 59:137, 1979

HOSTETTER TH, BRENNER BM: Glomerular adaptations to renal injury, in *Contemporary Issues in Nephrology*, vol 8: *Chronic Renal Failure*. New York, Churchill Livingstone, 1981

MAXWELL MH et al: *Clinical Disorders of Fluid and Electrolyte Metabolism*, 4th ed. New York, McGraw-Hill, 1987

ROSE BD: *Clinical Physiology of Acid-Base and Electrolyte Disorders*, 2d ed. New York, McGraw-Hill, 1984

219 ACUTE RENAL FAILURE

ROBERT J. ANDERSON / ROBERT W. SCHRIER

Acute renal failure is broadly defined as a rapid deterioration in renal function sufficient to result in accumulation of nitrogenous wastes in the body. Approximately 5 percent of all hospitalized patients develop acute renal failure. The causes of such deterioration include renal hypoperfusion, obstructive uropathy, and intrinsic renal disease such as disease of renal vasculature, glomeruli, and interstitium. After exclusion of these entities, there remains a group of patients with acute renal failure commonly referred to as acute tubular necrosis. However, the histologic findings of tubular necrosis are not present in all of these patients. Many clinicians use the terms acute renal failure and acute tubular necrosis interchangeably to denote the clinical syndrome of reversible intrinsic acute renal failure in the absence of renal vascular, glomerular, and interstitial disease.

ETIOLOGY Sixty percent of all cases of acute renal failure are related to surgery or trauma. Forty percent occur in a medical setting, and 1 to 2 percent are related to pregnancy. The most common general cause of acute renal failure is *renal ischemia*. Clinical conditions associated with renal ischemia include severe hemorrhage, profound volume depletion, intraoperative hypotension, cardiogenic shock, and operative procedures associated with interruption of renal circulation. The duration of the renal ischemia is very important in the occurrence of acute renal failure. If ischemia is brief, then correction of the course of ischemia can restore renal function (i.e., prerenal azotemia). With longer duration of renal hypoperfusion, acute tubular necrosis may supervene. Recent studies suggest that removal of the vasodilating influence of renal prostaglandins with nonsteroidal anti-inflammatory agents can enhance renal ischemia. Thus, use of these agents in patients with diminished basal renal blood flow (cardiac failure, hepatic cirrhosis, nephrotic syndrome, glomerulonephritis, hypoalbuminemia, old age) may precipitate acute renal failure.

Nephrotoxic agents are a frequent cause of acute renal failure. In the past, heavy metals, organic solvents, and glycols were common inducers of acute renal failure. Although these toxins are less frequently encountered currently, their occasional occurrence serves to illustrate the importance of seeking a history of occupational and environmental toxin exposure in each patient with acute renal failure. More recent studies suggest that *aminoglycoside antibiotics* and radiographic contrast agents are now the leading nephrotoxic cause of acute renal failure. Acute renal failure occurs in 10 to 20 percent of patients receiving a course of an aminoglycoside. The acute renal failure associated with these drugs is enhanced by depletion of intravascular volume, advancing age, the presence of underlying renal disease, potassium depletion, and the concomitant use of other nephrotoxic agents or potent diuretics. Radiographic contrast agents have little nephrotoxicity in healthy individuals. However, in patients with underlying renal disease, particularly patients with diabetic nephropathy, contrast exposure is associated with a 10 to 40 percent frequency of acute renal failure. Some anesthetic agents (methoxyflurane and enflurane) also may induce acute renal failure.

Release of large amounts of *myoglobin* into the circulation is now recognized with increasing frequency as a cause of acute renal failure. Rhabdomyolysis and myoglobinuria are often due to extensive trauma with crush injuries. However, nontraumatic rhabdomyolysis associated with increased muscle oxygen consumption (heat stroke, severe exercise, and seizures), decreased muscle energy production (hypokalemia, hypophosphatemia, and genetic enzymatic deficiencies), muscle ischemia (arterial insufficiency, drug overdosage with resultant coma and muscle compression), infections (influenza, Legionnaires' disease), and direct toxins (alcohol) also can produce rhabdomyolysis resulting in acute renal failure. Careful questioning of patients with acute renal failure for muscular symptoms as well as examination for tender, swollen muscles is therefore important, although many of these patients may have muscle necrosis without muscle symptoms. The exact mechanism whereby myoglobinuria results in acute renal failure is uncertain. There is substantial evidence that myoglobin is not directly nephrotoxic. However, direct nephrotoxicity of other muscle breakdown products, as well as tubular obstruction due to myoglobin precipitation and cast formation, has been proposed. Most patients with rhabdomyolysis-associated acute renal failure also have concomitant depletion of intravascular volume and renal hypoperfusion.

Intravascular hemolysis may also cause acute renal failure. Although pure hemoglobin per se is not a potent nephrotoxin, toxic substances from red blood cell stroma and concomitant renal hypoperfusion may act synergistically to induce acute renal failure. Lastly, in spite of intensive investigation, experienced clinicians are often unable to establish a definite etiology for some cases of acute renal failure. In other cases, multiple etiologies are likely, as in patients with shock who are volume-depleted, have received blood transfusions, are septic, and have received nephrotoxic antibiotics.

PATHOPHYSIOLOGY (Fig. 219-1) Current pathogenic theories of acute renal failure have been developed largely in animal models. These theories can be divided into those suggesting either a tubular or a vascular basis for acute renal failure. One tubular theory suggests that casts and cellular debris obstruct tubular lumina with resultant increases in intratubular pressure sufficient to decrease net filtration pressure. Alternatively, some investigators feel that "back-leak" of glomerular filtrate across damaged renal tubular epithelium is responsible for azotemia in acute renal failure. Proponents of a vascular basis for acute renal failure suggest that marked decreases in renal perfusion pressure, severe afferent arteriolar constriction, or efferent arteriolar dilatation reduce glomerular plasma flow and hydrostatic pressure sufficiently to diminish glomerular filtration. This vascular theory has led some proponents to suggest that *vasomotor nephropathy* might be the preferred term for many cases of acute renal failure. Another theory of acute renal failure suggests that alterations in the permeability properties of the glomerular capillary wall are responsible for acute renal failure. While a precise pathogenic schema of acute renal failure is not available at present, it seems likely that both tubular and vascular events interact to cause acute renal failure. For example, ischemia may cause a lower glomerular capillary pressure, which then predisposes to slow tubular flow. Ischemic cellular necrosis with release of apical membrane into the tubular lumen results in sludging debris, and ultimately secondary tubular obstruction. Additional studies are required to define the relative importance of each factor and to differentiate between mechanisms that are involved in the initiation (early) and maintenance (late) phases of acute renal failure.

PATHOLOGY The histopathologic alterations observed in kidneys of patients with acute renal failure are variable. Frequently, no, or minimal, overt abnormalities are observed on light microscopy. However, varying degrees of tubular necrosis with disrupted, necrotic, or regenerating tubular epithelium, intratubular casts, interstitial edema, and interstitial cellular infiltration can be seen. Tubular collapse and dilated tubules both can be observed. Unless either disseminated intravascular coagulation or severe, prolonged ischemic insults are present, intrarenal blood vessels and glomeruli are normal by light and electron microscopy. Microdissection studies demonstrate two general types of renal lesions. Following direct nephrotoxic injury, a uniform, diffuse necrosis of proximal tubular cells, especially of proximal convoluted and straight tubules, is observed. The tubular basement membrane is unaltered. In contrast, following renal ischemia, mild, patchy necrosis occurs throughout the nephron, which tends to be most marked in tubular segments at the corticomedullary junction. The juxtamedullary proximal straight tubule and medullary thick ascending limb of Henle appear particularly vulnerable. Disruption of tubular basement membrane is also observed. Despite these histologic differences, the clinical courses of nephrotoxic and ischemic acute renal failure are similar. A striking lack of correlation between renal histopathologic changes and renal functional parameters is often noted in acute renal failure. Renal biopsies performed after recovery from acute renal failure either demonstrate minor abnormalities or are normal.

DIFFERENTIAL DIAGNOSIS (See Table 219-1) The diagnosis of acute renal failure is one of exclusion since prerenal (renal hypoperfusion), postrenal (obstruction of urine flow), and other intrarenal disorders (glomerulonephritis, renal interstitial and vascular diseases) may all lead to an identical clinical syndrome of deteriorating renal function. In contrast to acute renal failure, however, prerenal, postrenal, and other intrarenal glomerular or vascular disorders may be specifically treatable.

Impaired renal perfusion from extrarenal causes may result in sufficient reduction in glomerular filtration that the daily endogenous load of nitrogenous wastes cannot be excreted. The azotemia can be reversed if the cause of the renal ischemia is corrected. This may require expansion of extracellular fluid volume, improvement in cardiac output, or restoration of normal renal perfusion pressure. A careful history with regard to weight and volume loss or sequestration and symptoms of impaired cardiac output then is necessary in patients with declining renal function. In addition, physical examination with specific attention to orthostatic hypotension and tachycardia, jugular

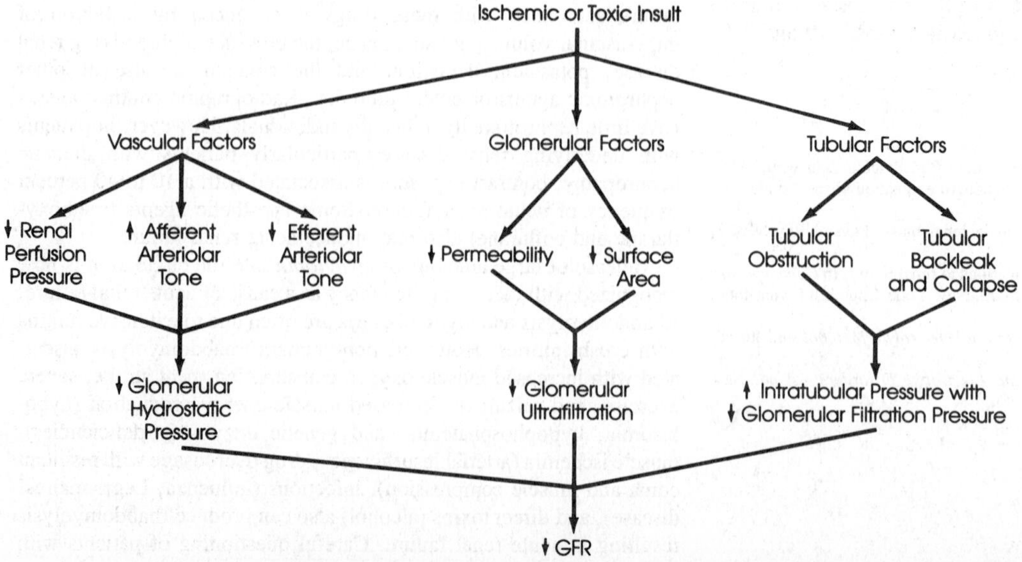

FIGURE 219-1 *Potential pathogenic schema in acute renal failure.*

venous pressure, cardiac function, skin turgor, and mucous membranes should be an initial undertaking in any patient with renal deterioration.

Obstruction to urine flow at any level of the urinary tract must be considered in every patient with renal failure. This form of acute deterioration in renal function is often reversible and will be encountered in 1 to 10 percent of patients with decreasing renal function. Urinary retention secondary to anatomic (prostatic disease) or functional (organic or drug-induced neuropathy) bladder neck obstruction is a relatively common cause of renal failure and can be evaluated by suprapubic palpation and percussion as well as by a single bladder catheterization to measure postvoiding residual volume. Obstruction of the upper urinary tract is a less common cause of renal failure since it requires simultaneous obstruction of both ureters or unilateral ureteric obstruction with absence of, or severe disease in, the contralateral kidney. Causes of bilateral urinary tract obstruction include retroperitoneal fibrosis and space-occupying processes such as tumor or abscess, surgical accident, and bilateral intraureteric occlusion (stones, papillary tissue, blood clots, or pus). A careful rectal and pelvic examination is essential in evaluation for postobstruction renal failure. A plain film of the abdomen may help detect retroperitoneal disease or radiopaque calculi. If obstruction of the upper urinary tract cannot be excluded by ultrasound, infusion pyelography, computerized tomography (CT scanning), or investigation of the patency of the ureter(s) by retrograde pyelography may be required. Obstruction to urine flow can also occur within the kidney. Such intrarenal obstruction is usually due to intratubular precipitation of poorly soluble material such as uric acid (tumor chemotherapy), oxalic acid (ethylene glycol overdose, methoxyflurane anesthesia, small bowel bypass), methotrexate (insoluble metabolites), sulfonamides (outdated, long-acting insoluble compounds), and perhaps myeloma proteins.

Once pre- and postrenal disorders have been excluded, it is appropriate to consider specific renal disorders such as renal vascular disorders, glomerulonephritis, and interstitial nephritis (Table 219-1). The frequency with which these specific renal disorders will be encountered as a cause of deteriorating renal function depends on the patient's age. In adults, only 5 to 10 percent of all cases of decreasing renal function can be attributed to these specific disorders, while this figure may be as high as 40 to 60 percent in the pediatric population. Although these disorders are less frequent than acute tubular necrosis, they are often amenable to specific therapy and should be considered in each case of deterioration in renal function.

The initial presentation of the patient with end-stage renal failure may be confused with acute renal failure when there is no information about renal function prior to presentation. Under these circumstances, the presence of uremic osteodystrophy, uremic neuropathy, small kidney size on abdominal films, and unexplained anemia suggests chronic renal failure. However, some end-stage renal diseases, such as amyloidosis, polycystic disease, diabetic glomerulosclerosis, scleroderma, and rapidly progressive glomerulonephritis, may present with normal-sized or enlarged kidneys, necessitating time for continued observation and rarely renal biopsy to distinguish between potentially reversible forms of acute renal failure and end-stage chronic renal failure.

Observation of the pattern of urine flow may provide a diagnostic clue as to the cause of declining renal function. Complete anuria (no urine by catheterization) is rare in acute tubular necrosis. Potential causes of total anuria include complete bilateral ureteric obstruction, diffuse cortical necrosis, rapidly progressive glomerulonephritis, and bilateral renal artery occlusion. Wide fluctuations in daily urine output suggest intermittent obstructive uropathy. Polyuria (>3 liters per day) can be a hallmark of partial urinary tract obstruction. This occurs secondary to the accompanying defect in renal concentrating ability. Although oliguria (<400 mL per day) has been considered to be a cardinal feature of acute renal failure, many patients have urine volumes of greater than 1 liter per day. This situation has been termed nonoliguric acute renal failure.

Examination of the urinary sediment is of great value in the differential diagnosis of acute impairment of renal function. Sediment containing few formed elements or only hyaline casts strongly suggests prerenal azotemia or obstructive uropathy. With acute tubular necrosis, brownish pigmented cellular casts and many renal tubular epithelial cells are observed in over 75 percent of patients. Red blood cell casts suggest the presence of glomerular or vascular inflammatory diseases of the kidney and rarely, if ever, occur with acute tubular necrosis. The presence of large numbers of polymorphonuclear leukocytes, singly or in clumps, suggests acute diffuse interstitial nephritis or papillary necrosis. Eosinophilic casts on Hansel's stain of urine sediment support a diagnosis of acute allergic interstitial nephritis. The combination of brownish pigmented granular casts and positive occult blood tests on urine in the absence of hematuria indicates either hemoglobinuria or myoglobinuria. In acute renal failure, the finding in fresh, warm urine of large numbers of uric acid crystals may suggest a diagnosis of acute uric acid nephropathy, while the finding of large numbers of oxalic acid or hippuric acid crystals suggests ethylene glycol toxicity. The presence of large numbers of broad casts (greater than two to three white blood cells in diameter) suggests chronic renal disease. Chemical analysis of urine composition is also helpful in differentiating acute tubular necrosis from prerenal azotemia in the oliguric patient and is depicted in Table 219-2. It is important to recall that other disorders associated with abrupt deterioration in renal function and intact renal tubular integrity, such as glomerulonephritis and early (few hours) obstructive uropathy, have urine chemical values similar to those encountered in prerenal azotemia. Prior administration of diuretic agents, osmotic diuresis due to glycosuria, bicarbonaturia, and ketonuria may interfere with avid renal tubular reabsorption of sodium and water and thus alter urinary chemical indexes. A urinary uric acid/creatinine concentration

TABLE 219-1 Major causes of acute renal failure

Disorder	Example
PRERENAL FAILURE	
Hypovolemia	Skin, gastrointestinal, or renal volume loss; hemorrhage; sequestration of extracellular fluid (burns, pancreatitis, peritonitis)
Cardiovascular failure	Impaired cardiac output (infarction, tamponade); vascular pooling (anaphylaxis, sepsis, drugs)
POSTRENAL FAILURE	
Extrarenal obstruction	Urethral occlusion; bladder, pelvic, prostatic, or retroperitoneal neoplasms; prostatism; surgical accident; medications; calculi; pus; blood clots
Intrarenal obstruction	Crystals (uric acid, oxalic acid, sulfonamides, methotrexate)
Bladder rupture	Trauma
SPECIFIC RENAL DISEASES	
Vascular diseases	Vasculitis; malignant hypertension; thrombotic thrombocytopenic purpura; scleroderma; arterial and/or venous occlusion
Glomerulonephritis	Immune-complex disease; antiglomerular basement membrane disease
Interstitial nephritis	Drugs; hypercalcemia; infections, idiopathic
ACUTE TUBULAR NECROSIS	
Postischemic	All conditions listed above for prerenal failure
Pigment-induced	Hemolysis (transfusion reaction, malaria); rhabdomyolysis (trauma, muscle disease, coma, heat stroke, severe exercise, potassium or phosphate depletion)
Toxin-induced	Antibiotics; contrast material; anesthetic agents; heavy metals; organic solvents
Pregnancy-related	Septic abortion; uterine hemorrhage; eclampsia

ratio of greater than 1 is compatible with acute uric acid nephropathy as a cause of the acute renal failure.

Rarely, the cause of declining renal function will not be readily apparent. In other cases, features considered atypical for acute tubular necrosis (gradual onset of renal failure; anuria in the absence of obstructive uropathy; the presence of marked hypertension, heavy proteinuria, significant hematuria, underlying systemic disease, and prolonged oliguria) will be present. Since such atypical features may indicate the presence of a potentially treatable form of renal parenchymal disease, e.g., secondary Wegener's disease, systemic lupus erythematosus, Goodpasture's syndrome, or rapidly progressive glomerulonephritis, a diagnostic renal biopsy may be indicated when the cause of renal failure is not apparent or such atypical features are present.

CLINICAL COURSE The clinical course in acute tubular necrosis can be divided into an initiating phase, a maintenance phase, and a recovery phase. The initiating phase is the period of time between the precipitating event and the appearance of acute renal failure which is no longer reversible by alteration in extrarenal factors. Recognition of the initiating phase of acute renal failure is extremely important since early correction of the underlying cause of renal failure may theoretically prevent the development of the maintenance phase. However, the initiating phase of acute renal failure may be evident to the clinician only in retrospect because it lacks characteristic signs and symptoms.

Oliguria has been considered the cardinal feature of the initiating and maintenance phases of acute renal failure. However, recent studies suggest that 40 to 50 percent of all patients with acute renal failure are nonoliguric (urine volume >400 mL per day). Although progressive acute renal failure without oliguria can result from any type of renal insult, including both ischemic and toxic insults, this form of renal failure appears to be particularly frequent following nephrotoxic (e.g., aminoglycoside) drug administration. Progressive azotemia occurs in nonoliguric patients owing to the marked impairment in glomerular filtration rate and renal concentrating capacity. For example, maximal urine osmolality of the nonoliguric patient averages only 350 mosmol per kilogram of water. Therefore, with a urine output of 1000 mL per day, a maximum of 350 mosmol solute can be excreted daily. In acute renal failure, daily solute loads may be increased from normal values of 600 mosmol to values as high as 1000 mosmol. Thus, a positive solute (predominately urea and creatinine) balance and azotemia would occur despite a daily urine output of 1 liter.

Oliguria characterizes the maintenance phase of acute renal failure in more than 50 percent of cases. When oliguria occurs, it starts shortly following the inciting event and lasts an average of 10 to 14 days. However, the oliguric phase may be as short as a few hours or as long as 6 to 8 weeks. Prolonged oliguria is common in the elderly patient with underlying vascular disease. If oliguria persists for longer than 4 weeks, the diagnosis of acute tubular necrosis should be reconsidered, and entities such as diffuse cortical necrosis, rapidly progressive glomerulonephritis, renal artery occlusion, renal vasculitis, and superimposed volume depletion are possible. Anuria is not characteristic of acute tubular necrosis. However, several days of severe oliguria with urine volume less than 100 mL per day may be encountered with acute tubular necrosis.

TABLE 219-2 Urine findings in prerenal azotemia and acute renal failure

Laboratory test	Prerenal azotemia	Acute renal failure
Urine osmolality (mosmol/kg)	>500	<400
Urine sodium (meq/liter)	<20	>40
Urine/plasma creatinine	>40	<20
Fractional excretion* of filtered sodium	<1	2
Urine sediment	Normal or occasional hyaline and granular casts	Brown granular casts, cellular debris

$$* \frac{\text{Urine Na/serum Na}}{\text{Urine creatinine/serum creatinine}} \times 100$$

Urinary elimination of nitrogenous wastes, water, electrolytes, and acid is impaired in the initiating and maintenance phases of acute renal failure. The magnitude of resultant abnormalities in blood chemistry depends on whether the patient is oliguric or nonoliguric and on the catabolic state of the patient. Nonoliguric patients have higher levels of glomerular filtration than do oliguric patients and thus excrete more nitrogenous waste, water, and electrolytes in their urine. Hence, abnormalities in blood chemistry are generally milder in nonoliguric than oliguric patients with acute renal failure.

In the afebrile, noncatabolic, oliguric patient with acute renal failure, the daily increments in blood urea nitrogen (BUN) and serum creatinine average 10 to 20 and 0.5 to 1.0 mg/dL, respectively. In catabolic patients with fever, sepsis, or extensive trauma, daily increments in BUN and serum creatinine may be as high as 40 to 100 and 2 to 5 mg/dL, respectively. In patients with acute renal failure due to rhabdomyolysis, the daily increment in serum creatinine may be disproportionately higher compared with the BUN. This is due to the release from muscle of creatine, which is converted by nonenzymatic hydrolysis to creatinine.

Salt and water overload with resultant hyponatremia, edema, and pulmonary congestion are ever-present dangers in patients with acute renal failure, particularly oliguric patients. Hyponatremia results from excessive water intake, and edema from excessive sodium and water intake. If urinary losses are not replaced, the nonoliguric patient with a relatively high rate of urine flow and high concentration of urine sodium will develop intravascular volume depletion which may retard recovery of renal function.

Hyperkalemia due to decreased renal elimination of potassium occurring with continued tissue potassium release is a frequent accompaniment of acute renal failure. The usual rate of increase in serum potassium in the noncatabolic, oliguric patient is 0.3 to 0.5 meq per day. Higher rates of rise in serum potassium concentration should suggest the possibility of an endogenous (tissue destruction, hemolysis) or exogenous (medication, diet, blood transfusion) potassium load or of cellular shift of potassium due to acidemia. Generally, hyperkalemia is asymptomatic until serum potassium increases to values greater than 6.0 to 6.5 meq per liter. Above that level, electrocardiographic abnormalities (bradycardia, recent appearance of left axis deviation, peaked T waves, prolonged QRS complexes, prolonged PR interval, and decreased amplitude of the P waves) and ultimately cardiac arrest can occur. Hyperkalemia can also result in muscle weakness and flaccid quadriparesis.

Hyperphosphatemia, hypocalcemia, and mild *hypermagnesemia* are usually present in acute renal failure. Hyperphosphatemia results from decreased renal phosphorus elimination in the presence of continued release of phosphorus from tissues. The serum phosphorus is usually in the range of 6 to 8 mg/dL, but much higher values may be encountered in the traumatized, catabolic patient as well as the patient with rhabdomyolysis. Hypocalcemia in the range of 6 to 9 mg/dL often develops during acute renal failure. The reason for this decrease in serum calcium concentration is not clear. Asymptomatic increases in serum magnesium to levels of 2 to 3 mg/dL are often observed in acute renal failure. The serum magnesium elevation is mild unless magnesium-containing compounds such as antacids are ingested.

Metabolic acidosis is a regular accompaniment of acute renal failure. The daily production of approximately 1 meq per kilogram of body weight of nonvolatile acid from endogenous metabolic sources can no longer be eliminated by the damaged kidney. A retention of organic acids results, which is sufficient to produce a daily decrease of 1 to 2 meq in plasma bicarbonate and metabolic acidosis with an anion gap.

Hyperuricemia in the range of 9 to 12 mg/dL due to decreased renal uric acid excretion is usually present in acute renal failure. In catabolic patients with extensive tissue damage, much higher values of serum uric acid may be observed. Elevation of serum amylase due to impaired renal amylase excretion may be observed in the absence of clinical evidence of pancreatitis. The elevations of amylase are mild and are usually less than twice the upper limit of normal.

Abnormalities in the hematologic examination are usually present in acute renal failure. A normocytic normochromic anemia occurs shortly following the onset of significant azotemia, and the hematocrit usually stabilizes between values of 20 to 30 volume percent. This anemia is due to impaired erythropoiesis as well as to a mild and variable degree of shortened red blood cell survival. Additional factors that often contribute to anemia include hemodilution, gastrointestinal blood loss, and suppressed erythropoiesis due to infections or drug administration. White blood cell production is not severely disturbed in acute renal failure. However, since acute renal failure usually occurs in the setting of stress and tissue damage, mild leukocytosis is usually present. Leukocytosis persisting after the initial week of acute renal failure should suggest the possibility of infection. Mild degress of thrombocytopenia due to reduction of bone marrow platelet production may be observed early in the course of acute renal failure. Qualitative defects in platelet function occur and, in association with additional poorly defined coagulation disturbances, contribute to the bleeding tendency of acute renal failure. Acute renal failure may follow intravascular hemolysis and may also be a complication of several primary hematologic or vascular disorders that have major hematologic manifestations such as disseminated intravascular coagulation, thrombotic thrombocytopenic purpura, hemolytic uremic syndrome, and systemic lupus erythematosus.

Infections complicate 30 to 70 percent of all cases of acute renal failure and are a leading cause of morbidity and mortality. The sites of infection include the respiratory tract, operative sites, and urinary tract. Resultant septicemia is frequent, and both gram-positive and gram-negative organisms are encountered. Operative site abscesses (especially intraabdominal) are associated with a poor prognosis if not recognized and treated promptly. Although the exact factors responsible for the high rate of infection remain to be determined, disruption of normal anatomic barriers with intravenous infusions and indwelling catheters may play a role. There is also evidence of impaired host defenses including leukocyte dysfunction in the setting of uremia. Minimization of use of catheters and intravenous lines, careful daily examination, and prompt thorough evaluation of fever is particularly important in patients with acute renal failure. It is also important to emphasize that uremia may obscure the fever associated with infections.

Cardiovascular complications of acute renal failure involve circulatory congestion, hypertension, arrhythmias, and pericarditis. Circulatory congestion is usually due to excessive sodium and water administration. Mild hypertension is seen in 15 to 25 percent of cases and usually appears in the second week of oliguria. This hypertension is usually a manifestation of extracellular fluid volume overload; however, the increased activity of the renin-angiotensin system may also be involved in some instances. Supraventricular arrhythmias may complicate 20 to 30 percent of cases of acute renal failure. Known causes for these arrhythmias include congestive heart failure, electrolyte abnormalities, digitalis intoxication, pericarditis, and anemia. Pericarditis currently occurs infrequently, probably because of the early institution of dialytic therapy.

Neurologic abnormalities are common in acute renal failure. In undialyzed patients, lethargy, somnolence, confusion, disorientation, asterixis, agitation, myoclonic muscle twitching, and generalized seizures may be observed. These neurologic abnormalities are most often encountered in the elderly patient and generally respond well to dialytic therapy. In addition to uremia per se, drug administration, metabolic and electrolyte abnormalities, and primary neurologic disease should be considered as potential causes of neurologic disturbances in the patient with acute renal failure.

Gastrointestinal complications of acute renal failure are common and include anorexia, nausea, vomiting, ileus, and poorly defined abdominal complaints. The combination of stress of acute illness and hemostatic abnormalities can lead to gastrointestinal hemorrhage in 10 to 30 percent of patients. Fortunately, the gastrointestinal hemorrhage is usually mild in nature and easily controlled with conservative therapy. Intravenous 1-deamino-8-arginine-vasopressin (DDAVP, 0.4 μg/kg intravenously) has been shown to lower the bleeding time and improve hemostasis in some patients with acute renal failure. Cryoprecipitate can also be used especially in cases refractory to DDAVP.

The recovery phase of acute renal failure commences when the glomerular filtration rate increases so that the BUN and serum creatinine concentrations no longer continue to increase. In oliguric acute renal failure, the recovery phase is heralded by a progressive increase in urine volume. Generally, in the first days the urine volume may double daily, and in some cases a daily urine volume of greater than 2 liters may be observed for a few days. In nonoliguric patients, a marked diuretic phase is usually not observed. The duration of the recovery phase in patients with BUN and serum creatinine concentrations greater than 50 and 5 mg/dL, respectively, averages 15 to 25 days in oliguric patients and 5 to 10 days in nonoliguric patients. The major complications of acute renal failure, such as infections, gastrointestinal hemorrhage, fluid and electrolyte disturbances, and cardiovascular dysfunction, may persist or first appear during the recovery phase of acute renal failure. In addition, during the recovery phase, persistent abnormalities in glomerular and tubular function can lead to over- or underhydration or electrolyte disturbances unless careful daily weight, intake and output, biochemical, and clinical monitoring are continued during the recovery phase of acute renal failure. Hypercalcemia may occur during the recovery phase, especially in patients with rhabdomyolysis. The cause of this complication remains obscure.

Although the major improvement in renal function occurs within the first 1 to 2 weeks of the recovery phase, renal function continues to improve for up to a year following acute renal failure. Sensitive tests of glomerular and tubular function also suggest that some mild defects in renal function may persist indefinitely following acute tubular necrosis. However, the vast majority of patients achieve clinically normal renal function, and there is no evidence of later progression of renal dysfunction or of complications such as hypertension.

The mortality rates in large series of patients with acute renal failure vary from 30 to 60 percent. The mortality rates are highest in postoperative or traumatized patients (50 to 70 percent), intermediate in patients with acute renal failure encountered in a medical setting (30 to 50 percent), and lowest in acute renal failure observed in an obstetrical setting (10 to 20 percent). Advanced age, the presence of serious underlying illness, and the development of multiple medical complications during the course of acute renal failure are associated with higher mortality rates. Nonoliguric acute renal failure is associated with a lower morbidity and mortality rate than oliguric acute renal failure. Infections, complications resulting from fluid and electrolyte disturbances, gastrointestinal hemorrhage, and progression of the primary underlying disease are the major causes of mortality in acute renal failure.

MANAGEMENT (Table 219-3) The first principle of therapy in acute renal failure is to exclude causes of deterioration in renal function which are potentially remedial. A search for prerenal factors, obstructive uropathy, glomerulonephritis, renal vascular and interstitial disease, and intrarenal crystal precipitation should be performed. Once the diagnosis of acute tubular necrosis is made by exclusion, little specific therapy is available. Dialysis for the removal of nephrotoxins, such as carbon tetrachloride, ethylene glycol, and heavy metals following chelation therapy, may be indicated. Even in the presence of acute tubular necrosis, any prerenal factors should be corrected both to improve the circulation and to avoid delay in the onset of the recovery phase. In the oliguric patient in whom prerenal factors have been corrected, it has become common clinical practice to administer either a potent loop diuretic or mannitol in an attempt to enhance urine flow. In patients who remain oliguric despite potent diuretics, low dose intravenous infusions of dopamine [1 to 3 (μg/kg)/min] may increase renal blood flow and allow a diuretic response to potent diuretics. The rationale for such therapy is based on the thought that there is an early phase of renal failure during which the correction of prerenal factors and establishment of urine flow can lead to a nonoliguric state. Prospective studies have demonstrated lower morbidity and mortality rates in nonoliguric as compared with oliguric acute renal failure. However, a prospective controlled study of the utility of potent diuretics and dopamine in early acute renal failure to convert oliguric to nonoliguric renal failure with attendant decrease in morbidity and mortality rates is needed.

Conservative therapy is capable of controlling many of the manifestations of acute renal failure. After any defects in intravascular volume have been corrected, fluid intake should equal measured output plus estimated insensible losses. Sodium and potassium administration should not exceed measured losses. Daily monitoring of fluid balance and body weight allow assessment of the patient's volume status. A daily weight loss of 0.2 to 0.3 kg occurs in the well-managed patient with acute renal failure. Greater weight loss suggests hypercatabolism or volume depletion, and lesser weight loss suggests excessive salt and water administration. Since most pharmacologic agents are eliminated at least in part by the kidney, careful attention to medication usage and dosage adjustment is needed. The serum sodium concentration provides a guideline for water administration. A decrease in serum sodium concentration indicates that an excess of total body water is present, while an abnormally high serum sodium concentration indicates a deficiency of body water.

In an effort to minimize catabolism, daily intake should include at least 100 g of carbohydrate. Recently some studies suggest that central intravenous administration of a mixture of amino acids and hypertonic glucose improves morbidity and mortality in patients with acute renal failure following surgical procedures or trauma. Since parenteral hyperalimentation may be associated with significant complications, this form of nutrition should be reserved for catabolic patients in whom the enteral routine of alimentation does not prove to be satisfactory. In the past, anabolic androgens have been utilized in an effort to decrease protein catabolism and diminish the rate of rise of BUN. Such therapy is not generally utilized at present. Additional means of minimizing catabolism include early removal or debridement of necrotic tissue, control of pyrexia, and early, specific antimicrobial therapy.

The mild metabolic acidosis associated with acute renal failure is generally not treated unless serum bicarbonate falls to below 10 meq per liter. Rapid correction of acidemia by acute alkali administration may decrease ionized calcium concentrations and precipitate tetany. Hypocalcemia is usually asymptomatic and rarely requires specific therapy. Hyperphosphatemia should be controlled with 30 to 60 mL aluminum hydroxide administered orally four to six times per day, since a high calcium-phosphorus product (>70) may cause soft tissue calcification. For the occasional patient with profound hyperphosphatemia, early dialysis therapy and alimentation may help control elevated serum phosphate concentration. Unless acute uric acid nephropathy is a diagnostic consideration, the secondary hyperuricemia of acute renal failure is usually not treated with allopurinol. Because of the decreased glomerular filtration rate, the filtered load of uric acid, and thus intratubular deposition, is low. Also, for unknown reasons, clinical gout rarely complicates acute renal failure, despite hyperuricemia. Careful observation of the hematocrit and stool for occult blood is important in the early detection of gastrointestinal blood loss. If a rapid decrease in hematocrit occurs which appears to be out of proportion to the degree of renal failure, alternative causes of anemia should be sought.

TABLE 219-3 General therapeutic approach to patient with acute renal failure

1 Exclude all specifically treatable causes of decreasing renal function including correction of prerenal and postrenal factors.
2 Attempt to establish a urine output.
3 Conservative therapy:
- *a* Decrease intake of nitrogen, water, and electrolytes to match output.
- *b* Provide adequate nutrition.
- *c* Alter medication therapy.
- *d* Maintain clinical monitoring (frequency of vital signs determined by patient status; intake and output, body weight, inspection of wound and intravenous sites, and physical examination required daily).
- *e* Maintain biochemical monitoring (frequency of BUN, creatinine, electrolytes, and blood counts will be dictated by patient status; in catabolic oliguric patients, daily determination will be needed; calcium, phosphorus, magnesium, and uric acid can often be determined less often).

4 Provide dialytic therapy.

Congestive heart failure and hypertension indicate the presence of volume overload and should be treated accordingly, recognizing, of course, that many drugs such as digoxin are largely excreted by the kidneys. As suggested earlier, hypertension occasionally may persist in the absence of volume overload; thus factors such as hyperreninemia may contribute to the hypertension. Selective histamine-2 receptor blockade (cimetidine, ranitidine) therapy has been of benefit in preventing gastrointestinal bleeding in some seriously ill patients but has not yet been studied in acute renal failure. Avoidance and early detection of infection require minimization of interruption of normal anatomic barriers, including avoidance of long-term catheterization of the urinary bladder, provision of mouth and skin care, promotion of early mobilization, utilization of aseptic techniques for intravenous and tracheostomy sites, and close clinical monitoring. Fever and suspected infection should be promptly evaluated with careful inspection of lung, wounds, urinary tract, and intravenous sites.

Hyperkalemia is an ever-present threat in acute renal failure. Mild elevations of serum potassium (<6.0 meq per liter) can best be treated by withdrawal of all sources of potassium and by continued close laboratory observation. If serum potassium increases to values greater than 6.5 meq per liter and particularly if any electrocardiographic changes appear, active therapy should be instituted. Therapy of such hyperkalemia can be divided into emergent and nonemergent forms. Emergent therapy includes intravenous administration of calcium (5 to 10 mL of 10% calcium chloride solution intravenously over 2 min with electrocardiographic monitoring), bicarbonate (44 meq intravenously over 5 min), and insulin and glucose (200 to 300 mL of 20% glucose with 20 to 30 units regular insulin given intravenously over 30 min). Nonemergent therapy includes administration of potassium-binding ion exchange resins such as sodium polystyrene sulfonate. This can be administered orally every 3 to 4 h in 25- to 50-g doses with 100 mL 20% sorbitol to avoid constipation. Alternatively, in the patient who cannot take oral medications, 50 g sodium polystyrene sulfonate and 50 g sorbitol in 200 mL water can be given as a retention enema at 1- to 2-h intervals. With refractory hyperkalemia, hemodialysis may be necessary.

Some patients with acute renal failure, particularly those who are nonoliguric and noncatabolic, can be successfully managed with minimal or no dialytic therapy. There has been an increasing tendency to use dialysis therapy early in acute renal failure in an attempt to minimize the development of complications. Early (prophylactic) use of dialysis frequently simplifies management, allowing more liberal fluid and potassium intake and improvement of the general well-being of the patient. Absolute indications for dialysis include symptomatic uremia (usually manifested by central nervous system and/or gastrointestinal symptomatology), development of resistant hyperkalemia, severe acidemia or fluid overload not responsive to medical therapy, and pericarditis. In addition, many centers attempt to keep predialysis levels of BUN and serum creatinine less than 100 and 8 mg/dL, respectively. Adequate prevention of uremic symptoms may require infrequent dialysis in the noncatabolic, nonoliguric patient or daily dialysis in the catabolic, traumatized patient. Often, peritoneal dialysis is an acceptable alternative to hemodialysis. Peritoneal dialysis may be especially useful in the patient with noncatabolic acute renal failure when the need for infrequent dialysis is anticipated. Slow, continuous arteriovenous filtration using highly permeable filters has been advocated as a means of controlling extracellular volume in patients with acute renal failure. Currently available filters connected to the patient via an arteriovenous shunt allow for removal of 5 to 12 liters of plasma ultrafiltrate per day without use of a pump. Thus, these devices appear particularly useful in the oliguric volume-overloaded patient with hemodynamic instability.

PREVENTION Because of the high mortality and morbidity of acute renal failure, prophylactic therapy deserves special mention. A fivefold reduction in deaths secondary to acute renal failure occurred from the Korean war to the Vietnamese conflict. This reduction in the acute renal failure mortality rate paralleled earlier evacuation from the field and early expansion of intravascular volume. Thus, identification of patients at high risk for the development of acute renal failure is important. Such high-risk patients include those with multiple trauma, burns, rhabdomyolysis, and intravascular hemolysis; those receiving potential nephrotoxins; and those undergoing operative procedures necessitating interruption of renal blood flow. In these patients, particular attention should be given to maintaining optimal intravascular volume, cardiac output, and urine flow rates. Care in the use of potential nephrotoxic drugs, early therapy of cardiogenic shock, sepsis, and eclampsia of pregnancy may also reduce the occurrence of acute renal failure.

ACUTE RENAL FAILURE IN PREGNANCY When acute renal failure occurs during pregnancy, it is usually in either the earlier or later stages of gestation. During the first trimester of pregnancy, acute renal failure usually occurs in the setting of nontherapeutic, nonsterile abortion. In these cases, volume depletion, sepsis, and nephrotoxins contribute to the acute renal failure. This form of acute renal failure has markedly declined with the current widespread availability of sterile abortion.

Acute renal failure can also occur because of either excessive postpartum hemorrhage or preeclampsia in the later stages of pregnancy. The majority of patients with this type of acute renal failure generally recover total renal function. A small number of pregnant patients with acute renal failure, however, have not recovered renal function, and in these cases histologic evidence of diffuse cortical necrosis is found. This entity usually complicates the severe hemorrhage of abruptio placentae and is associated with clinical and laboratory evidence of intravascular coagulation.

A rare form of acute renal failure occurring 1 to 12 weeks following uncomplicated pregnancy has been described and termed postpartum glomerulosclerosis. This form of renal failure is usually characterized by irreversible, rapidly progressive renal failure, although milder cases have been described. All of these patients have an associated microangiopathic hemolytic anemia. The renal histopathologic changes are indistinguishable from malignant hypertension or scleroderma. The pathophysiology of this disorder has not been defined. No therapeutic modality is consistently successful, although heparin therapy has been advocated.

HEPATORENAL SYNDROME The hepatorenal syndrome is a serious complication of advanced liver disease in which renal failure occurs in the absence of clinical, laboratory, or anatomic evidence of other causes of renal dysfunction. The renal failure is usually associated with oliguria, an unremarkable urinary sediment, and low urinary sodium concentrations (<10 meq per liter). Generally, the renal failure occurs in the setting of advanced hepatic cirrhosis complicated by jaundice, ascites, and hepatic encephalopathy. Occasionally, this syndrome may complicate fulminant hepatitis. The mechanism of the renal failure is not known. The lack of consistent histopathologic alterations in kidneys of patients with this syndrome and the restoration of normal renal function when kidneys from donors with hepatorenal syndrome are transplanted into recipients without liver disease suggest a functional defect.

Treatment of the hepatorenal syndrome is usually unsuccessful. Care should be taken in the cirrhotic patient not to induce major changes in intravascular volume by large paracentesis or aggressive diuresis, maneuvers which may precipitate hepatorenal syndrome. Since this syndrome mimics prerenal azotemia, a cautious trial of expansion of intravascular volume is warranted. In a few cases, recovery has followed portacaval shunting, insertion of an abdominal-venous (Leveen) shunt, or prolonged hemodialysis. These treatment modalities have not been subjected to controlled trials. The abdominal-venous shunt may be associated with peritonitis, intravascular coagulation, and pulmonary congestion. Improvement in hepatic function often results in parallel improvement in renal function. Every effort should be made to ensure that more specifically treatable causes of concomitant liver and renal dysfunction, such as infections (leptospirosis, hepatitis with immune-complex disease), toxins (aminoglycosides, carbon tetrachloride), and circulatory disorders (severe heart failure, shock), are not present. It should also be recalled that jaundiced patients with liver disease may be particularly susceptible to acute tubular necrosis.

REFERENCES

BENNETT WM et al: Drug prescribing in renal failure: Dose guidelines for adults. Am J Kid Dis 3:155, 1983

BRENNER BM, LAZARUS JM (eds): *Acute Renal Failure*. Philadelphia, Saunders, 1983

BREZIS M et al: Renal ischemia: A new perspective. Kid Int 26:375, 1984

CONGER JD, SCHRIER RW: Acute renal failure: Pathogenesis, diagnosis and management, in *Renal and Electrolyte Disorders*, RW Schrier (ed). Boston, Little, Brown, 1985

CRONIN RE: The patient with acute azotemia, in *Manual of Nephrology, Diagnosis and Therapy*, RW Schrier (ed). Boston, Little, Brown, 1985, p 135

GROSS PA, ANDERSON RJ: Acute renal failure and toxic nephropathy. Contemp Nephrol, 1986

HOU SH et al: Hospital-acquired renal insufficiency: A prospective study. Am J Med 74:243, 1983

220 CHRONIC RENAL FAILURE: PATHOPHYSIOLOGIC AND CLINICAL CONSIDERATIONS

BARRY M. BRENNER / J. MICHAEL LAZARUS

In contrast to the remarkable capacity of the kidney to regain function following the various forms of acute renal injury discussed in the preceding chapter, renal injury of a more sustained nature is often not reversible but leads instead to progressive destruction of nephron mass. Despite successful treatment of hypertension, urinary tract obstruction and infection, and systemic disease, many forms of renal injury associated with permanent nephron loss progress inexorably to chronic renal failure (CRF). Reduction of renal mass has been shown to cause structural and functional hypertrophy of remaining nephrons. Recent experimental evidence in animals suggests that this "compensatory" hypertrophy is due to adaptive hyperfiltration mediated by increases in glomerular capillary pressures and flows. Eventually these adaptations prove "maladaptive" in that they predispose to glomerular sclerosis, an enhanced functional burden on less affected glomeruli, leading in turn to their ultimate destruction.

Glomerulonephritis, in one of its several forms, is the most common initiating cause of CRF. The other major etiologies of chronic renal failure are listed in Table 220-1. These and other progressive forms of renal disease are considered in detail in the remaining chapters of this section. Irrespective of cause, the eventual impact of severe reduction in nephron mass is an alteration in function of virtually every organ system in the body. *Uremia* is the term generally applied to the clinical syndrome observed in patients suffering from profound loss of renal function. Although the cause(s) of the syndrome remain unknown, the term uremia was adopted originally because of

TABLE 220-1 Causes of chronic renal failure*

Diagnosis	Percent
Glomerulonephritis	24
Glomerulosclerosis	2
Diabetes mellitus	15
Polycystic kidney disease	9
Nephrosclerosis	8
Hypertension	9
Pyelonephritis	3
Other interstitial nephritis	5
Unknown etiology	6
Other	19

* *Patients presenting for treatment of end-stage renal disease in New England as of December 1982.*

the presumption that the abnormalities seen in patients with chronic renal failure (CRF) resulted from *retention* in the blood of urea and the other end products of metabolism normally excreted into the urine. It is clear that the uremic state represents more than failure of renal excretory function alone, because a host of metabolic and endocrine functions normally subserved by the intact kidney are also impaired in CRF. Furthermore, the inexorably progressive course to renal failure is often accompanied by severe malnutrition, impaired metabolism of carbohydrates, fats, and proteins, and defective utilization of energy. Because CRF involves more than just retention of normal urinary constituents in blood, the term *uremia* in current usage is devoid of any pathophysiologic connotation, but is employed instead to refer, in a general sense, to the constellation of signs and symptoms associated with CRF, regardless of etiology.

The presentation and severity of signs and symptoms of uremia often vary greatly from patient to patient, depending, at least in part, on the magnitude of the reduction in functioning renal mass as well as the rapidity with which renal function is lost. As discussed in Chap. 218, in the relatively early stage of CRF [i.e., when total glomerular filtration rate (GFR) is reduced but not to levels below about 35 to 50 percent of normal], overall renal function is sufficient to maintain the patient symptom-free, although renal reserve may be diminished. At this stage of renal impairment baseline excretory, biosynthetic, and other regulatory functions of the kidney are generally well maintained. At a somewhat later stage in the course of CRF (GFR about 20 to 35 percent of normal), *azotemia* occurs, and initial manifestations of renal insufficiency usually appear. Although patients are relatively asymptomatic at this stage, renal reserve is diminished sufficiently that any sudden stress, such as intercurrent infection, urinary tract obstruction, dehydration, or administration of a nephrotoxic drug, may compromise renal function still further, often leading to signs and symptoms of overt uremia. With further loss of nephron mass (GFR below 20 to 25 percent of normal), the patient develops *overt renal failure*. Uremia may be viewed as the final stage in this inexorable process, when many of or all the untoward manifestations of CRF become evident clinically. In this chapter the causes and clinical characteristics of the disturbances of the various organ systems seen in patients with CRF will be considered.

PATHOPHYSIOLOGY AND BIOCHEMISTRY OF UREMIA

ROLE OF RETAINED TOXIC METABOLITES The finding that serums from patients with uremia exert toxic effects in a variety of biologic test systems has motivated a diligent search to identify the responsible toxin(s). The most likely candidates thought to qualify as toxins in uremia are the *by-products of protein and amino acid metabolism*. Unlike fats and carbohydrates, which are eventually metabolized to carbon dioxide and water, substances which are easily excreted even in uremic subjects via lungs and skin, the products of protein and amino acid metabolism depend largely on the kidneys for excretion. A vast number of such products have been identified, with urea being quantitatively the most important. *Urea* represents some 80 percent or more of the total nitrogen excreted into the urine in patients with CRF maintained on diets containing 40 or more grams of protein per day. The *guanidino compounds* are the next most abundant of the nitrogenous end products of protein metabolism and include substances such as guanidine, methyl- and dimethylguanidine, creatinine, creatine, and guanidinosuccinic acid. As with urea, guanidines are derived, at least in part, from urea cycle amino acids. Other metabolic products of amino acid and protein catabolism that have been implicated as possible uremic toxins include *urates and other end products of nucleic acid metabolism, aliphatic amines,* a variety of *peptides,* and, finally, several *derivatives of the aromatic amino acids tryptophan, tyrosine, and phenylalanine.* The role of these substances in the pathogenesis of the clinical and biochemical abnormalities seen in CRF is unclear. It is generally believed that uremic symptoms correlate only in a rough and inconsistent way with concentrations of urea in blood. Nevertheless, although urea is probably not a major cause of overt uremic toxicity, it may account for some of the less serious clinical abnormalities, including anorexia, malaise, vomiting, and headache. On the other hand, elevated levels of plasma *guanidinosuccinic acid,* by interfering with activation of platelet factor III by adenosine diphosphate (ADP), have been shown to contribute to the impaired platelet function seen in CRF. *Creatinine,* generally regarded as a nontoxic substance, may cause adverse effects in uremic subjects following conversion to more toxic metabolites such as sarcosine and methylguanidine. Whether these substances, as well as *creatine,* a metabolic precursor of creatinine, and the other compounds cited above, are of clinical importance in the pathogenesis of uremic toxicity remains to be established.

Nitrogenous compounds of larger molecular weight are also retained in CRF. A toxic role for these substances has been suggested, on the impression that patients treated with intermittent peritoneal dialysis are less troubled with neuropathy than patients maintained on chronic hemodialysis, despite higher levels of urea and creatinine in blood in the former group. Since the clearance of small molecules depends mainly upon blood and dialysate flow rates, which are higher with hemodialysis, whereas clearance of larger molecules depends more on membrane surface area and time, which are greater with peritoneal dialysis, this latter form of therapy may be a more effective means of removing these substances of larger molecular weight. Using a variety of chemical separation procedures, several groups of workers have obtained evidence in support of this ''middle-molecule hypothesis'' by observing differences in composition between normal and uremic plasmas, with prominent abnormal ''uremic peaks'' in the molecular weight range of about 300 to 3500. Evidence from amino acid analysis suggests that these substances of larger molecular weight are polypeptides. Despite the foregoing, proof that efficient removal of middle molecules is associated with objective evidence of clinical well-being, and improvement in neuropathy in particular, remains to be provided. On the other hand, when there is insufficient removal of substances of smaller molecular weight (e.g., urea), symptoms of uremia are frequently aggravated.

Not all these middle-sized molecules accumulate in uremic plasma because of decreased renal excretion alone. The kidney normally *catabolizes* a number of circulating plasma proteins and polypeptides; with reduced renal mass, this capacity may be impaired greatly. Furthermore, plasma levels of many polypeptide hormones [including parathyroid hormone (PTH), insulin, glucagon, growth hormone, luteinizing hormone, and prolactin] rise with advancing renal failure, often markedly so, not only because of impaired renal catabolism but also because of enhanced endocrine secretion. The consequences of high circulating levels of many of these hormones in CRF are considered below and in Chap. 218.

EFFECTS OF UREMIA ON CELLULAR FUNCTIONS

Alterations in the composition of intracellular and extracellular fluids in CRF have long been recognized. Such abnormalities are believed to be a consequence, at least in part, of *defective ion transport* across cell membranes generally, with retained uremic toxins possibly mediating these alterations in transmembrane ion transport. Integrity of cellular volume and composition depends to a large extent on the active outward transport of Na^+ from cell interior to exterior, the resulting intracellular fluid being relatively low in Na^+ and high in K^+, whereas the reverse is true for extracellular fluid. Active Na^+ transport is a metabolically costly process, accounting for a major fraction of basal energy utilization and oxygen consumption. The consequences of this efflux of Na^+ from cells are many and include, most notably, (1) the generation of a resting electrical potential difference across the cell membrane (with this transcellular voltage oriented so that cell interior is electronegative to cell exterior), and (2) a mechanism for enhancing the influx of K^+ into cells.

In experimental animals, partial inhibition of this active efflux mechanism for Na^+ across cell membranes leads to alterations in body composition and cell functions similar to those demonstrable in erythrocytes, leukocytes, skeletal muscle, and other tissues obtained from uremic subjects. These include increased and decreased intracellular concentrations of Na^+ and K^+, respectively, and reduction in magnitude of the transcellular voltage. These alterations have been shown to be largely reversed by efficient hemodialysis and, for erythrocytes at least, to be recreated when cells from normal subjects are incubated in uremic serums. Other derangements in cellular function have also been implicated as causes for altered body composition in uremia. For example, *Na^+- and K^+-stimulated ATPase activity* has been shown to be decreased in erythrocytes and brain tissue derived from uremic patients and animals, respectively. Whether the "uremic toxins" which account for these derangements in cellular function represent abnormally retained products of metabolism which fail to be excreted, or normal substances present in increased quantities in response to reduced renal mass, remains unknown. *Parathyroid and natriuretic hormones,* examples of this category of substances, are discussed in this context in Chap. 218.

EFFECTS OF UREMIA ON WHOLE-BODY COMPOSITION

What is the impact of these disturbances in active transcellular Na^+ transport on the uremic organism as a whole? From the pathophysiologic considerations already discussed, CRF is likely to lead to abnormally high intracellular Na^+ concentrations, and hence to osmotically induced overhydration of cells generally, whereas these same cells are thought to be relatively deficient in K^+. With the inevitable onset of malaise, anorexia, nausea, vomiting, and diarrhea, patients with CRF may eventually develop classic protein-calorie malnutrition and negative nitrogen balance, often with profound losses of lean body mass and fat deposits. Owing to the concomitant tendency for salt and water retention, these losses often go unnoticed until the late stages of CRF. Whereas a large fraction of the increase in total body water in uremia is the result of expansion of intracellular volume, extracellular volume expansion also is observed commonly. With initiation of intermittent hemodialysis or renal transplantation, there is often an immediate and substantial loss of body weight, due primarily to correction of this overhydration. With successful transplantation, the initial diuresis is followed by a period of impressive weight gain, due to restoration of lean body mass and fat deposits to preillness levels. For patients on chronic dialysis, the anabolic response is less dramatic, even when therapy is regarded as optimal, involving mainly reaccumulation of fat deposits. The failure to restore lean body mass to normal with chronic dialysis may reflect insufficient intake of protein, which, in adequately dialyzed patients, should be maintained at levels of 0.8 to 1.4 g/kg per day.

The occurrence of deficits in intracellular K^+ concentration in CRF has already been mentioned and may result from inadequate intake (poor diet or overzealous K^+ restriction by the physician), excessive losses (vomiting, diarrhea, diuretics), reduction of Na^+- and K^+-stimulated ATPase, or a combination of these. In addition to promoting losses of K^+ into urine (which may be substantial if urine volume remains relatively normal in uremic subjects), the high levels of plasma aldosterone often seen in CRF may also augment net secretion of K^+ into the colon, thereby contributing to marked K^+ losses in stool or diarrheal fluids. Despite deficits in intracellular K^+ concentration, serum K^+ is usually normal or high in CRF, owing most often to metabolic acidosis, which induces an efflux of K^+ from cells. Additionally, uremic patients are relatively resistant to the action of insulin (see below), a hormone which normally enhances K^+ uptake by skeletal muscle.

EFFECTS OF UREMIA ON METABOLISM

HYPOTHERMIA In experimental animals injections of urine, urea, or other retained toxic metabolites can induce hypothermia, and basal heat production diminishes soon after nephrectomy. Since active Na^+ transport across cell membranes accounts for a major proportion of basal energy production, it is generally believed that the inverse relationship between body temperature and degree of azotemia is due, in part, to inhibition of the sodium pump by some retained toxin(s). Dialysis usually returns body temperature to normal.

CARBOHYDRATE METABOLISM The ability to metabolize an exogenous glucose load is impaired in most patients with CRF. The defect largely involves a slowing of the rate at which blood glucose concentration declines to the normal range after administration of a glucose load. Fasting blood sugar levels are usually normal or only slightly elevated; severe hyperglycemia and/or ketosis is uncommon. Consequently, the *glucose intolerance of CRF* usually does not require specific therapy (hence the term *azotemic pseudodiabetes*). Because insulin depends to a large extent on the kidney for its removal from plasma and eventual degradation, circulating insulin levels tend to be increased in uremia. Whereas insulin levels in plasma are only slightly to moderately increased in most fasting uremic subjects, levels considerably in excess of normal are usually found in response to a glucose load. The response to intravenous insulin in patients with CRF is also abnormal, and the rate of utilization of glucose by peripheral tissues often is diminished substantially. The glucose intolerance of uremia is thought to result largely from this peripheral resistance to the action of insulin. Other possible factors contributing to the glucose intolerance include intracellular deficits of potassium, metabolic acidosis, increased levels of glucagon and other hormones including catecholamines, growth hormone, and prolactin, as well as the myriad of potentially toxic metabolites retained in CRF. In true insulin-dependent diabetics, there is often a decrease in insulin requirement with progressive azotemia, a phenomenon not related solely to decreased caloric intake.

NITROGEN AND LIPID METABOLISM Given that the capacity to eliminate the nitrogenous end products of protein catabolism is reduced drastically, CRF may be regarded as a state of *protein intolerance*. As discussed above, retention of these end products of nitrogen metabolism is thought to represent a dominant cause of the signs and symptoms of uremic toxicity.

Hypertriglyceridemia and decreased high-density lipoprotein cholesterol are common in uremia, whereas cholesterol levels in plasma are usually normal. Whether uremia accelerates triglyceride production by the liver and intestine is unknown. The well-known lipogenic effect of hyperinsulinism may contribute to increased triglyceride synthesis. The rate of removal of triglycerides from the circulation, which depends in large part on the enzyme *lipoprotein lipase,* has been shown to be depressed in uremia, an effect not corrected appreciably by hemodialysis. The high incidence of premature atherosclerosis seen in patients on chronic dialysis (see "Cardiovascular and Pulmonary Abnormalities" below) may be related, at least in part, to these abnormalities in lipid metabolism.

CLINICAL SPECTRUM OF ABNORMALITIES IN UREMIA

The diagnosis of chronic renal failure is based on recognition of a constellation of signs and symptoms with or without reduced urine

TABLE 220-2 Clinical spectrum of abnormalities in uremia*

FLUID AND ELECTROLYTE DISTURBANCES
Volume expansion and contraction (I)
Hypernatremia and hyponatremia (I)
Hyperkalemia and hypokalemia (I)
Metabolic acidosis (I)
Hyperphosphatemia and hypophosphatemia (I)
Hypocalcemia (I)
ENDOCRINE-METABOLIC DISTURBANCES
Renal osteodystrophy (I or P)
Osteomalacia (D)
Secondary hyperparathyroidism (I or P)
Carbohydrate intolerance (I)
Hyperuricemia (I or P)
Hypothermia (I)
Hypertriglyceridemia (P)
Protein-calorie malnutrition (I or P)
Impaired growth and development (P)
Infertility and sexual dysfunction (P)
Amenorrhea (P)
NEUROMUSCULAR DISTURBANCES
Fatigue (I)
Sleep disorders (P)
Headache (I or P)
Impaired mentation (I)
Lethargy (I)
Asterixis (I)
Muscular irritability (I)
Peripheral neuropathy (I or P)
Restless legs syndrome (I or P)
Paralysis (I or P)
Myoclonus (I)
Seizures (I or P)
Coma (I)
Muscle cramps (D)
Dialysis disequilibrium syndrome (D)
Dialysis dementia (D)
Myopathy (P or D)
CARDIOVASCULAR AND PULMONARY DISTURBANCES
Arterial hypertension (I or P)
Congestive heart failure or pulmonary edema (I)
Pericarditis (I)
Cardiomyopathy (I or P)
Uremic lung (I)
Accelerated atherosclerosis (P or D)
Hypotension and arrhythmias (D)
DERMATOLOGIC DISTURBANCES
Pallor (I or P)
Hyperpigmentation (I, P, or D)
Pruritus (P)
Ecchymoses (I or P)
Uremic frost (I)
GASTROINTESTINAL DISTURBANCES
Anorexia (I)
Nausea and vomiting (I)
Uremic fetor (I)
Gastroenteritis (I)
Peptic ulcer (I or P)
Gastrointestinal bleeding (I, P, or D)
Hepatitis (D)
Refractory ascites on hemodialysis (D)
Peritonitis (D)
HEMATOLOGIC AND IMMUNOLOGIC DISTURBANCES
Normocytic, normochromic anemia (P)
Lymphocytopenia (P)
Bleeding diathesis (I or D)
Increased susceptibility to infection (I or P)
Splenomegaly and hypersplenism (P)
Leukopenia (D)
Hypocomplementemia (D)

* *Virtually all the abnormalities contained in this table are completely reversed in time by successful renal transplantation. The response of these abnormalities to hemo- or peritoneal dialysis therapy is more variable. (I) denotes an abnormality which usually improves with an optimal program of dialysis and related therapy. (P) denotes an abnormality which tends to persist or even progress, despite an optimal program. (D) denotes an abnormality which develops only after initiation of dialysis therapy.*

output but always with elevation in serum urea nitrogen and creatinine concentrations. Differentiation between acute and chronic renal failure can be difficult. The history is often most helpful, particularly if normal renal function existed prior to a sudden recent insult. The laboratory findings and physical examination may not be helpful in the differentiation. The hallmark of chronic renal failure is the presence of reduced kidney size on either ultrasound, abdominal scout film, or pyelogram. In the absence of small kidneys, renal biopsy may be necessary for diagnosis.

As noted earlier, CRF leads ultimately to disturbances in function of every organ system in the body. With the advent and increasingly greater application of chronic dialysis in the past two decades, the incidence and severity of these disturbances have been modified enormously, so that virtually everywhere that modern medicine is practiced, the overt and florid manifestations of uremia have largely disappeared. Unfortunately, however, even optimal dialysis therapy is not a panacea for the patient with CRF, because, as indicated in Table 220-2, some disturbances resulting from impaired renal function fail to respond fully, while others may even progress despite dialysis treatment. Furthermore, as with many modern and complex therapeutic modalities, intermittent dialysis may be responsible for the appearance of unique abnormalities not seen prior to initiation of therapy; these abnormalities should be viewed as complications of dialysis.

FLUID, ELECTROLYTE, AND ACID-BASE DISORDERS (See also Chaps. 41 and 42) **Sodium and volume homeostasis** In most patients with stable CRF, modest increases in total body Na^+ and water content can be documented, although objective signs of extracellular fluid (ECF) volume expansion may not be apparent clinically. With ingestion of excessive amounts of salt and water, however, control of excess volume becomes an important clinical and therapeutic consideration. In general, excessive *salt* ingestion contributes to, or aggravates, congestive heart failure, hypertension, ascites, and edema formation. On the other hand, hyponatremia and weight gain are the typical consequences of excessive ingestion of *water*, abnormalities which in most patients are relatively mild and asymptomatic. In the majority of patients, daily intake of fluid equal in volume to urine volume per day plus about 500 mL usually will maintain the serum Na^+ concentration at normal levels. Hypernatremia is encountered relatively infrequently in CRF. In the edematous patient with CRF not maintained on dialysis, diuretics and modest restriction of salt and water intake are the mainstays of therapy. In volume-expanded dialysis patients, management should include ultrafiltration and restriction of salt and water intake between dialyses.

Patients with CRF have grossly impaired renal mechanisms for conserving Na^+ and water (discussed in detail in Chap. 218). When confronted with an *extrarenal* cause for increased fluid loss (e.g., vomiting, diarrhea, fever), these patients are prone to develop ECF volume depletion, with signs and symptoms of dry mouth and other mucous membranes, dizziness, syncope, tachycardia, decreased filling of jugular veins, orthostatic hypotension, and even vascular collapse. Depletion of extracellular fluid volume typically results in deterioration of residual renal function and, in the previously stable and asymptomatic patient with mild CRF, signs and symptoms of overt uremia. Cautious fluid repletion usually restores extracellular and intravascular volumes to normal and often, but not always, returns renal function to previously stable levels.

Potassium homeostasis Derangements in K^+ balance (see also Chaps. 41 and 218) are occasionally documented by laboratory analysis in patients with CRF, but are rarely responsible for clinical symptoms unless GFR is below 5 mL/min or an endogenous (hemolysis, trauma, infection) or exogenous (stored blood, K^+-containing medications) K^+ load is administered. Despite progression of renal failure, most patients maintain normal serum K^+ concentrations until the final stages of uremia. As discussed in Chap. 218, this ability to sustain K^+ balance with advancing renal failure is due to adaptations in the renal distal tubules and colon, sites where aldosterone and other factors serve to enhance K^+ secretion. Not surprisingly, oliguria, or disruption of key adaptive mechanisms, can lead to *hyperkalemia* and its potentially ominous effects on cardiac function. Antikaliuretic drugs, such as spironolactone or triamterene, should be used with extreme caution in CRF. Hyperkalemia in CRF may also be induced by abrupt lowering of arterial blood pH, since acidosis is associated with efflux of K^+ from intracellular to extracellular fluids. A clinically useful index of the magnitude of this hydrogen-potassium exchange is that for every 0.1-unit change in blood pH, there will be a reciprocal change in serum K^+ concentration of approximately 0.6 meq per liter. Correction of acidosis-induced hyperkalemia with sodium bicarbonate is the treatment of choice. Intravenous insulin and dextrose are useful in lowering serum potassium acutely, while the ion exchange resin sodium polystyrene sulfonate (Kayexalate) is useful in longer-term control of hyperkalemia. Patients in whom hyperkalemia persists in the absence of excessive K^+ intake, oliguria, or acute acidosis should be evaluated for the possibility of *hyporeninemic hypoaldosteronism*. Patients with this syndrome have reduced circulating levels of renin and aldosterone in the plasma and often also have diabetes mellitus.

Hypokalemia due to diminished ability of the kidneys to conserve K^+ is uncommon in most forms of CRF. When hypokalemia occurs in these patients, poor dietary K^+ intake, usually in association with excessive diuretic therapy or gastrointestinal losses, is likely to be the underlying cause. When hypokalemia occurs as a result of primary K^+ wasting in urine, it may represent a solitary renal reabsorptive defect or, more commonly, be associated with other solute transport abnormalities, as in Fanconi's syndrome, renal tubular acidosis, or other forms of hereditary or acquired tubulointerstitial diseases (see Chaps. 226 and 228). A detailed discussion of the clinical consequences and management of hypokalemia and hyperkalemia is given in Chap. 41.

Metabolic acidosis With advancing renal failure, total daily acid excretion and buffer production fall below the level needed to maintain external balance of hydrogen ions. Metabolic acidosis is the inevitable result, and the mechanisms involved are considered in Chap. 218. In most patients with stable renal insufficiency, administration of 20 to 30 meq sodium bicarbonate or sodium citrate per day will usually correct the acidosis. In response to a sudden acid challenge (whether from an endogenous or exogenous source), however, patients with CRF are particularly susceptible to profound acidosis, which requires more substantial quantities of alkali for correction. Administration of sodium must be carried out with careful attention to the patient's volume status.

Phosphate, calcium, and bone As discussed in detail in Chap. 218, serum phosphate concentration begins to rise when GFR falls below about 25 percent of normal. Calcium deposition in bone is critically dependent upon the availability of phosphate; retention of phosphate in plasma, therefore, facilitates calcium entry into bone and thereby contributes to the *hypocalcemia* and *elevations in plasma PTH* levels seen in CRF. Hypocalcemia in CRF also results from the impaired ability of the diseased kidney to synthesize *1,25-dihydroxyvitamin* D_3 [$1,25(OH)_2D_3$], the active metabolite of vitamin D (Fig. 220-1). Reabsorption of calcium in the gut is impaired when circulating levels of this active metabolite are low. Finally, in patients with advanced CRF, the ability of PTH to mobilize calcium salts from bone may be altered. Despite these various causes of hypocalcemia, symptoms such as tetany are rare unless patients are treated with large amounts of alkali.

Overproduction of parathyroid hormone, disordered vitamin D metabolism, chronic metabolic acidosis, and excessive fecal losses of calcium all contribute to the occurrence of bone diseases in uremia (Fig. 220-1). *Renal* or *metabolic osteodystrophy* are broad and imprecise terms that encompass a number of distinct skeletal abnormalities, including osteomalacia, osteitis fibrosa cystica, osteosclerosis, and, in children especially, impaired bone growth. Although clinical symptoms of bone disease are uncommon, occurring in less than 10 percent of predialysis patients with advanced renal failure, radiologic and histologic abnormalities are observed in about 35 and 90 percent, respectively. In patients who have been treated by means of dialysis for several years, symptoms from bone disease are a major cause of morbidity. Renal osteodystrophy is seen more often in growing children than in adults, and especially in patients with congenital renal anomalies associated with very slowly progressive renal insufficiency. On radiologic examination, three types of lesions can be identified: (1) changes analogous to those described in children with nutritional rickets, namely, widened osteoid seams at the growth margin of bones (so-called renal rickets); (2) the bone changes of *secondary hyperparathyroidism* (*osteitis fibrosa cystica*), character-

FIGURE 220-1 *Pathogenesis of bone diseases in chronic renal failure.*

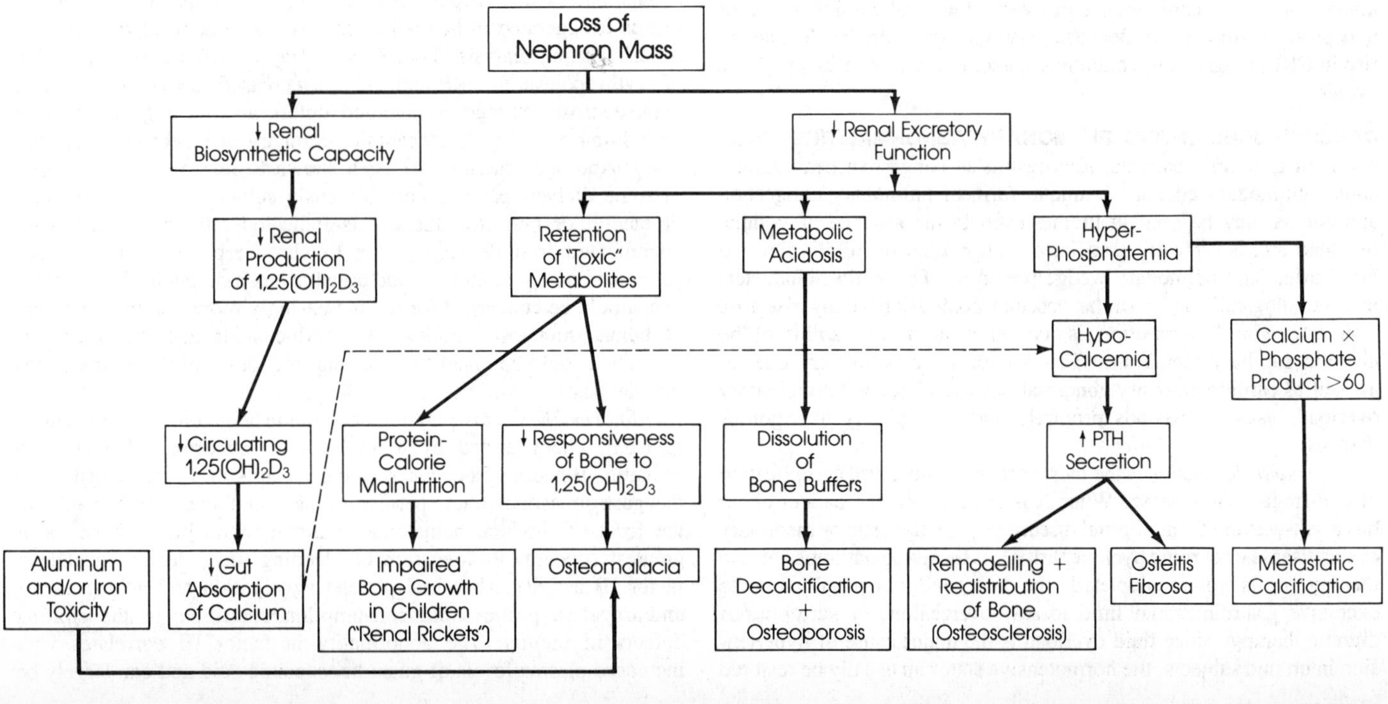

ized by osteoclastic bone resorption and manifested by subperiosteal erosions, especially of the phalanges, long bones, and distal ends of the clavicles; and (3) *osteosclerosis,* often best noted by enhanced bone density in the upper and lower margins of vertebrae, producing the so-called rugger jersey spine.

With renal osteodystrophy there is a tendency to *spontaneous fractures,* which are often slow to heal. The ribs are most commonly involved. Painful joints may occur in association with renal osteodystrophy due to calcium deposition in bursas and other periarticular structures. Bone pain is due to osteitis fibrosa cystica as well as to osteomalacia. Osteomalacia was initially thought to be secondary to decreased availability of 1,25-dihydroxycholecalciferol. There is now evidence that at least a component of osteomalacia is due to deposition of aluminum and/or iron at the calcification fronts. The aluminum is thought to be derived from increased aluminum in the dialysis fluid, as well as aluminum-containing phosphate-binding gels. Iron excess is usually secondary to frequent transfusions. When bone pain is severe, a proximal *myopathy* often coexists, giving rise to gait abnormalities and even leading to cessation of ambulation. The incidence of *aseptic necrosis of the hip* is increased in renal transplant recipients, probably related to such factors as chronic corticosteroid therapy, secondary hyperparathyroidism, and altered vitamin D metabolism. In CRF there is often a tendency to *extraosseous,* or *metastatic, calcification,* especially when the calcium-phosphate product exceeds 60. Medium-sized blood vessels; subcutaneous, articular, and periarticular tissues; myocardium; eyes; and lungs are common sites of metastatic calcification.

Management of patients with renal osteodystrophy includes reduction in dietary phosphate available for absorption through the use of restricted, 1 g phosphate, diet as well as phosphate-binding agents. Supplementation of calcium, primarily by judicious increase in the calcium ion concentration of the dialysate, but also by oral calcium intake (1 to 1.5 g per day) and efforts to enhance intestinal calcium absorption with 1,25-dihydroxycholecalciferol or dihydrotachysterol, may improve osteitis fibrosa cystica, osteomalacia, and myopathy. Treatment with phosphate binders, calcium, and vitamin D should be initiated early in chronic renal failure so that hyperparathyroidism and bone disease may be prevented. Serum phosphorus must be maintained below 4.5 mg/dL before administering calcium and/or vitamin D analogues, in order to avoid metastatic calcification.

Other solutes Other inorganic solute derangements in CRF include *hyperuricemia* and *hypermagnesemia.* Uric acid retention is a common feature of CRF but rarely leads to symptomatic gout. Hypophosphatemia is usually a consequence of overzealous oral administration of phosphate-binding gels. Because serum magnesium levels tend to rise in CRF, magnesium-containing antacids and cathartics should be avoided.

CARDIOVASCULAR AND PULMONARY ABNORMALITIES Fluid retention in uremic patients often results in congestive heart failure and/or pulmonary edema. A unique form of pulmonary congestion and edema may be seen in uremia even in the absence of volume overload and is typically associated with normal or mildly elevated intracardiac and pulmonary wedge pressures. This entity, characterized radiologically by perihilar vascular congestion giving rise to a "butterfly wing" distribution, is due to increased permeability of the alveolar capillary membrane. This low-pressure pulmonary edema, as well as cardiopulmonary abnormalities associated with circulatory overload, usually responds promptly and dramatically to vigorous dialysis.

Arterial hypertension is the most commonly observed complication of end-stage renal disease. When it is not present, the patient either has a salt-wasting form of renal disease (e.g., polycystic or medullary cystic disease or chronic pyelonephritis), is receiving antihypertensive therapy, or is volume-depleted, the last condition usually due to excessive gastrointestinal fluid losses, overzealous or surreptitious diuretic therapy. Since fluid overload is the major cause of hypertension in uremic subjects, the normotensive state can usually be restored by dialysis. Nevertheless, some patients remain hypertensive, despite rigorous salt and water restriction and ultrafiltration, because of hyperreninemia. In most cases, routine antihypertensive drug therapy is effective. A small minority of these patients develop *accelerated or malignant hypertension,* manifested by markedly elevated systolic and diastolic pressures, severe hyperreninemia, encephalopathy, seizures, retinal changes, and papilledema. Use of more potent drugs such as diazoxide, minoxidil, captopril, and nitroprusside, along with control of extracellular volume, will generally control such hypertension and has obviated the need for bilateral nephrectomy.

Pericarditis, once a common complication of CRF, is now seen infrequently because of early initiation of dialysis. Retained metabolic toxins are thought to be the cause of *pericarditis* in patients with CRF. The very unusual finding of pericarditis in the well-dialyzed patient is usually due to viral infection or systemic disease.

The clinical presentation of pericarditis in uremic subjects is generally similar to that of other etiologies (Chap. 194), except that pericardiocentesis for effusions usually yields hemorrhagic fluid. Treatment with intensive dialysis is recommended, and systemic anticoagulation should be avoided to minimize the possible occurrence of hemorrhagic tamponade. Oral indomethacin may be useful for relief of pain in pericarditis. In some patients, pericardiocentesis with intrapericardial instillation of air or steroids is effective for pericardial tamponade. Pericardiectomy should be considered only after more conservative treatment has failed.

Clinical experience with chronically dialyzed patients followed for the past decade or more has revealed the disturbingly high incidence of *accelerated atherosclerosis,* leading to development of significant coronary, cerebral, and peripheral vascular disease. There are seemingly ample causes for these complications, including long-term hypertension, hyperlipidemia, glucose intolerance, chronic high cardiac output, and metastatic vascular and myocardial calcification.

HEMATOLOGIC ABNORMALITIES *Normochromic, normocytic anemia* occurs regularly in CRF and contributes to fatigability and listlessness in these patients. Erythropoiesis is depressed in CRF, due both to the effects of retained toxins on bone marrow and to diminished biosynthesis of erythropoietin by the diseased kidney or to the presence of erythropoietin inhibitors. *Hemolysis* also occurs and involves an extracorpuscular defect since survival of erythrocytes from normal subjects is reduced when these cells are transfused into uremic patients, and erythrocytes from patients with CRF have relatively normal survival times when transfused into normal individuals. Gastrointestinal and chronic dialyzer *blood loss* contributes to anemia, as does *hypersplenism* in the occasional patient. Blood loss is exaggerated in hemodialysis patients because of the need for heparin during dialysis. Transfusions may contribute to suppression of erythropoiesis in CRF and, due to increased risk of hepatitis and hemosiderosis, should be avoided unless anemia aggravates other underlying disorders (for example, coronary or cerebrovascular disease). Androgen therapy has been shown to improve erythropoiesis in some dialysis patients not previously subjected to nephrectomy. Parenteral or oral iron therapy is indicated only in patients with documented iron deficiency due to chronic blood loss. In those patients in whom multiple blood transfusions have been administered, one should be concerned for the increasingly more common problem of hemachromatosis. Folic and ascorbic acids and the soluble B vitamins should be given to offset chronic losses of these substances via dialysis.

Abnormal hemostasis is another common hematologic derangement in CRF, characterized by a tendency to abnormal bleeding and bruising. Bleeding from the surgical wounds or spontaneously into the gastrointestinal tract, pericardial sac, and intracranial vault, in the form of subdural hematoma or intracerebral hemorrhage, is of greatest concern. Prolongation of bleeding time, decreased platelet factor III activity, abnormal platelet aggregation and adhesiveness, and impaired prothrombin consumption contribute to the clotting defects in uremia. The abnormality in factor III correlates with increased plasma levels of guanidinosuccinic acid and can largely be corrected by dialysis. Prolongation of the bleeding time continues to be a common finding even in the well-dialyzed patient.

A wide variety of changes in leukocyte formation and function also occur in uremia leading to *enhanced susceptibility to infection.* Lymphocytopenia and atrophy of lymphoid structures occur in CRF, whereas neutrophil production is relatively unimpaired. Nevertheless, there is evidence to suggest that all leukocyte cell types are affected adversely by uremic serum. Decreased chemotaxis is among the best documented of the defects occurring in uremic leukocytes, with resulting impairment of acute inflammatory response and decreased delayed hypersensitivity. There is a tendency for uremic patients to have less fever in response to infection. For these reasons, infections may be more difficult to recognize in uremia. Leukocyte function may also be impaired in patients with CRF because of such coexisting factors as acidosis, hyperglycemia, protein-calorie malnutrition, and serum and tissue hyperosmolarity (due to azotemia). Mucosal barriers to infection may also be defective, and, in dialysis patients, vascular access devices also serve as common portals of entry for pathogens, particularly staphylococci. Anti-inflammatory steroids and immunosuppressive drugs add further to the risk of serious infection in many of these patients. Leukopenia is a common transient finding in patients exposed to cellophane-derived membranes during dialysis (Chap. 221).

NEUROMUSCULAR ABNORMALITIES Subtle disturbances of central nervous system function, including inability to concentrate, drowsiness, and insomnia, are among the earliest symptoms of uremia. Mild behavioral changes, loss of memory, and errors in judgment soon follow and often are associated with signs of neuromuscular irritability, including hiccups, cramps, and fasciculations and twitching of large muscle groups. Asterixis, myoclonus, and chorea are common in terminal uremia, as are stupor, seizures, and coma. Many of these neuromuscular complications of severe uremia resolve with dialysis, although nonspecific EEG abnormalities may persist.

Peripheral neuropathy is a relatively common complication of advanced CRF. Initially, sensory nerve involvement exceeds motor, lower extremities are involved more than the upper, and the distal portions of the extremities more than proximal. The "restless legs syndrome," characterized by ill-defined sensations of discomfort in the feet and lower legs and frequent leg movement, is a disturbing complication in some uremic patients. If dialysis is not instituted soon after onset of sensory abnormalities, motor involvement follows, often leading to loss of deep tendon reflexes, weakness, peroneal nerve palsy (foot drop), and, eventually, flaccid quadriplegia. Accordingly, early evidence of peripheral neuropathy is generally taken as a firm indication to initiate dialysis or transplantation.

Two types of neurologic disturbances appear to be unique to patients on chronic dialysis. One is the syndrome of *dialysis dementia,* seen in patients who have been on dialysis for a number of years. This syndrome is characterized by speech dyspraxia, myoclonus, dementia, and eventually seizures and death. The possibility of aluminum intoxication has been suggested. Other factors are also likely to play a role in such patients since a very small percentage of the patients with increased aluminum exposure develop the syndrome. The other disturbance, dialysis disequilibrium, occurs during the first few dialyses, in association with rapid reduction of blood urea levels. Nausea, vomiting, drowsiness, headache, and even grand mal seizures have been attributed to the more rapid (dialysis-induced) pH change and reduction in osmolality of extracellular than intracellular fluids within the cranium, leading to cerebral edema and raised intracranial pressure.

GASTROINTESTINAL ABNORMALITIES Anorexia, hiccups, nausea, and vomiting are common and early manifestations of uremia. The use of carefully monitored protein restriction in the diet may be useful to slow progression of renal insufficiency if initiated early. Protein restriction is also useful in diminishing the frequent symptoms of nausea and vomiting late in the course. Protein restriction should not, of course, be implemented in those patients with severe protein-calorie malnutrition. *Uremic fetor,* a uriniferous odor to the breath, derives from the breakdown of urea in saliva to ammonia and is often associated with unpleasant taste sensation. Mucosal ulcerations leading to blood loss can occur at any level of the gastrointestinal tract in very late stages of CRF—so-called uremic gastroenteritis. Peptic ulcer disease is particularly common, occurring in as many as one-fourth of uremic subjects. Whether this high incidence is related to increased gastric acidity, hypersecretion of gastrin, or secondary hyperparathyroidism is unknown. Most of the gastrointestinal symptoms, except those related to peptic ulcer disease, usually improve with dialysis. A syndrome of idiopathic ascites is seen rarely in patients on chronic dialysis, presumably secondary to fluid overload and/or chronic passive hepatic congestion. Patients with chronic renal failure, particularly those with polycystic kidney disease, have an increased incidence of diverticulosis. Viral hepatitis is more commonly seen in patients on chronic dialysis and is discussed in detail in Chap. 221.

ENDOCRINE-METABOLIC DISTURBANCES The common disturbances in parathyroid function, glucose, and insulin metabolism, as well as the lipid, protein-calorie, and other nutritional abnormalities of uremia have already been considered. In general, pituitary, thyroid, and adrenal gland functions are relatively normal, often despite measurable abnormalities in circulating thyroxine, growth hormone, aldosterone, and cortisol levels. In women, estrogen levels are low and amenorrhea and inability to carry pregnancies to term are early manifestations of uremia. While menses frequently reappear after chronic dialysis is initiated, successful pregnancies remain rare. In men with CRF, including those on chronic dialysis, impotence, oligospermia, and germinal cell dysplasia are common, as are reduced plasma testosterone levels. As with growth, sexual maturation is often impaired in adolescent children, even among those on chronic dialysis.

DERMATOLOGIC ABNORMALITIES The skin shows many abnormalities. This is not surprising in view of anemia (pallor), defective hemostasis (ecchymoses and hematomas), calcium deposition and secondary hyperparathyroidism (pruritus, excoriations), dehydration (poor skin turgor, dry mucous membranes), and the general cutaneous consequences of protein-calorie malnutrition. A sallow, yellow cast may reflect the combined influences of anemia and retention of a variety of pigmented metabolites, or *urochromes.* In advanced uremia urea concentrations in sweat may reach sufficiently high levels that, after evaporation, a fine white powder can be found on the skin surface—so-called uremic (urea) frost. Although many of these cutaneous abnormalities improve with dialysis, *uremic pruritus* may persist and is usually resistant to most systemic and topical therapies. Hemochromatosis causes a slate-gray–bronze discoloration of the skin and is common in the dialysis patient who has received multiple transfusions.

REFERENCES

Acchiardo SR et al: Malnutrition as the main factor in morbidity and mortality of hemodialysis patients. Kidney Int 24:S199, 1983

Andrassy K, Ritz E: Uremia as a cause of bleeding. Am J Nephrol 5:313, 1985

Brenner BM et al: Dietary protein intake and the progressive nature of kidney disease: The role of hemodynamically mediated glomerular injury in the pathogenesis of progressive glomerular sclerosis in aging, renal ablation, and intrinsic renal disease. N Engl J Med 307:652, 1982

Deykin D: Uremic bleeding. Kidney Int 24:698, 1983

Dumbauld S et al: Carbohydrate metabolism during fasting in chronic hemodialysis patients. Kidney Int 24:222 1983

Gokal R et al: Iron metabolism in hemodialysis patients: A study of the management of iron therapy and overload. Q J Med 48:369, 1979

Goldblum SE, Reed WP: Host defenses and immunologic alterations associated with chronic hemodialysis. Ann Intern Med 93:597, 1980

Kopple JD, Massry SG: Uremic toxins: What are they? How are they identified? Semin Nephrol 3:263, 1983

Mahoney C et al: Central and peripheral nervous system effects of chronic renal failure. Kidney Int 24:170, 1983

Massry SG et al: Current status of the use of 1,25-$(OH)_2D3$ in the management of renal osteodystrophy. Kidney Int 18:409, 1980

MITCH WE et al: A simple method of estimating progression of chronic renal failure. Lancet 2:1326, 1976
PARKINSON IS et al: Dialysis encephalopathy, bone disease and anemia: The aluminum intoxication syndrome during regular hemodialysis. J Clin Pathol 34:1285, 1981
ROSTAND SG et al: Dialysis-associated ischemic heart disease: Insights from coronary angiography. Kidney Int 25:653, 1984

221 DIALYSIS AND TRANSPLANTATION IN THE TREATMENT OF RENAL FAILURE

CHARLES B. CARPENTER / J. MICHAEL LAZARUS

Over the past three and one-half decades, dialysis and transplantation have become effective treatment modalities in prolonging the life of patients with renal insufficiency. The approach to treatment in acute renal failure is different than in chronic renal failure because of the irreversible nature of the latter. Conservative medical management or dialysis are the mainstays of therapy for acute renal failure. Obviously, transplantation is not a treatment modality for this group of patients. Options for treatment of patients with *chronic* or *irreversible* renal failure are outlined in Fig. 221-1.

Initially patients are managed with conservative therapy, but eventually they require hemodialysis, peritoneal dialysis, or cadaver or related donor transplantation. Because of limited success with each of these treatment modalities, chronic renal failure should be approached with the concept of moving from one form of therapy to another as indicated by the degree of success and incidence of complications with each form of treatment.

Therapy for renal failure should be initiated at a time in the disease process when complications will be moderate, but not when the patient is completely asymptomatic. The advanced complications of uremia, as noted in Chap. 220, should be avoided by early treatment. Early dialysis is especially applicable to patients with acute renal failure in whom resumption of renal function can be expected and to patients with chronic renal failure who have a good immunologic match with a related donor in whom transplantation can be carried out promptly and will very likely lead to resumption of normal renal function. In the remainder of patients, the clinical judgment to move from conservative treatment to dialysis or transplantation is determined by the patient's quality of life and whether or not the benefits of treatment outweigh the risks. Treatment with protein restriction as described in Chap. 220 may prolong the time before dialysis and transplantation are required but should be carried out only if complications of such therapy do not negatively impact on long-term morbidity and mortality.

Selection of patients to receive dialysis and/or transplantation is a matter of some debate. Because of the reversible nature of acute renal failure, *all* patients with this diagnosis should be supported with dialysis, at least for some period of time, to allow return of renal function. In patients with irreversible or chronic renal failure, criteria for selection for transplantation are generally more stringent

FIGURE 221-1

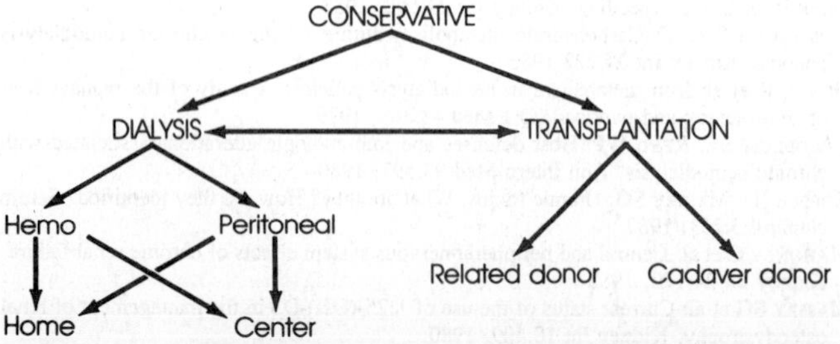

than those for dialysis and are guided by the possibility of complications related to immunosuppressive therapy. Table 221-1 lists practical considerations in the selection of a recipient for a human renal allograft. Such a procedure should be undertaken only when conservative treatment has failed, when there are no reversible elements in the patient's renal failure, and when the patient is too ill to be maintained comfortably with the usual methods of treatment. However, morbidity is less if transplantation is performed before the patient is critically ill. Transplantation should not be utilized in an attempt to salvage patients from failure to thrive on dialysis.

The recipient should be free of life-threatening extrarenal complications such as cancer, severe coronary artery disease, and cerebrovascular disease. Provided that diffuse vascular involvement is not present, diabetes itself is not a contraindication. Oxalosis may recur in relatively short order in a transplanted kidney and is generally a contraindication for this procedure. Although age may be a limiting factor, it is advanced ''physiologic'' rather than chronologic age which contraindicates transplantation. In general, patients reach a ''physiologic'' limit at approximately age 60 to 65 years when the incidence of complications due to prednisone become much higher than in younger patients. Although abnormalities of the bladder and urethra present additional hazards, successful renal allografts have been placed in individuals with these abnormalities by prior constitution of an artificial bladder (i.e., ileal conduit) into which the donor ureter is placed. Patients with any disease process which may be aggravated by prednisone, cyclosporine, azathioprine, or other immunosuppressive agents, or any patient with medical complications so severe that the risks of operation and drug therapy are high, should obviously not be offered transplantation. In evaluating potential exclusionary diseases, it should be kept in mind that quality of life and long-term results are superior in the *successful* renal transplantation.

Criteria for treatment with hemodialysis or peritoneal dialysis are more liberal since dialysis has less morbidity than transplantation in older patients and those with the aforementioned medical complications. Because of the cost of these programs, some have suggested restricted entry. These decisions, based on moral and social issues, continue to generate debate. In most areas of the world today, the cost of medical care for chronic renal failure is borne by government. With economic support from the government for dialysis and transplant programs, rules and regulations have been and will continue to be generated which will affect the selection and the type of treatment employed.

CONSERVATIVE TREATMENT As discussed in Chap. 220, conservative (nondialytic, nontransplant) therapy should be instituted early to control symptoms, minimize complications, prevent long-term sequelae of uremia, and slow the progression of renal insufficiency. Every effort should be made to correct any of the numerous reversible components which aggravate renal impairment. In patients with acute renal failure, prerenal factors, such as volume depletion, decreased cardiac output, or renal artery stenosis, or postrenal components, such as urethral or ureteral obstruction, must be sought and corrected. Such pre- and postrenal components may exacerbate

TABLE 221-1 Contraindications to kidney transplantation

1 Absolute contraindications
- *a* Reversible renal involvement
- *b* Ability of conservative measures to maintain useful life
- *c* Advanced forms of major extrarenal complications (cerebrovascular or coronary disease, neoplasia)
- *d* Active infection
- *e* Active glomerulonephritis
- *f* Previous sensitization to donor tissue

2 Relative contraindications (see text)
- *a* Age
- *b* Presence of vesical or urethral abnormalities
- *c* Iliofemoral occlusive disease
- *d* Diabetes mellitus
- *e* Psychiatric problems
- *f* oxalosis

underlying parenchymal disease in patients with chronic renal insufficiency and must be treated in this group as well. Most important is treatment of the underlying disease or complications of renal insufficiency which further hasten the loss of nephrons. Hypertension, urinary tract infections, nephrolithiasis, structural abnormalities of the urinary tract, or those forms of glomerulonephritis which may respond to therapy should be treated aggressively. Preventive aspects include avoidance of nephrotoxic drugs and large doses of radiopaque agents in the patient with already compromised renal insufficiency.

Modification of diet is an important aspect of conservative therapy. Early restriction of sodium and fluid may be important in the treatment of hypertension. As renal insufficiency progresses, restriction of foods high in phosphate and potassium is necessary. Reduction of protein content reduces anorexia, nausea, and vomiting and, if initiated early, may retard progression of the disease. Adult patients should receive no less than 0.6 g of protein per kilogram per day to avoid negative nitrogen balance. Supplementation of low-protein diets with essential ketoamino acid therapy may be useful in prolonging the period of conservative therapy by allowing utilization of urea as a source of nonessential nitrogen. Correction of electrolyte imbalance, e.g., use of sodium bicarbonate or calcium carbonate to correct mild acidosis, or bicarbonate, dextrose and insulin, and potassium exchange resins for treatment of hyperkalemia, will be necessary in more advanced states of uremia. Some chemical abnormalities occurring with renal failure do not require or are not amenable to treatment; hypermagnesemia, hyperamylasemia, hypertriglyceridemia, or mild carbohydrate intolerance generally do not require therapy. Treatment of hyperuricemia may be in order if the patient suffers from gout. However, hyperuricemia alone has not been shown to be detrimental. It has been suggested that secondary hyperparathyroidism may accentuate progression of renal failure. Whether this is due to hyperphosphatemia, an elevated calcium-phosphorus product, or parathyroid hormone itself is not clear. Nonetheless, vigorous efforts using phosphate-binding agents and calcium supplements and vitamin D products (dihydrotachysterol or 1,25-dihydroxycholecalciferol) to maintain the serum calcium are effective in suppressing parathyroid stimulation, perhaps in slowing renal insufficiency, and likely avoiding severe bone disease later (see Chap. 336). To avoid visceral and vascular calcification it is important to maintain the calcium-phosphorus product below 60. Fluid, sodium, potassium, phosphate, and protein restriction offer the patient a very restricted and often unacceptable diet. This, coupled with the administration of multiple medications, often occurs at a time when the complications of uremia appear and consideration for dialysis and/or transplantation is in order.

While conservative measures are being carried out, it is necessary to prepare the patient with an intensive educational program to explain the possibilities of eventual renal failure and the various forms of therapy available. The more knowledgeable patients are concerning hemodialysis, peritoneal dialysis, and transplantation, the easier and more appropriate will be their decisions at a later time. With hemodialysis, the major method of obtaining blood for treatment is from an arteriovenous fistula. Since these devices often take several months to develop, prophylactic placement of a fistula in a patient planning for hemodialysis is important in minimizing future complications of circulatory access. For those patients who select peritoneal dialysis (continuous ambulatory peritoneal dialysis—CAPD; or continuous cyclic peritoneal dialysis—CCPD), placement of the peritoneal catheter does not require preparation, and therapy can be instituted as soon as uremic signs and symptoms develop. In those patients who may perform home dialysis or undergo transplantation, early education of family members for selection and preparation as a home dialysis helper or a related donor for transplantation should occur well before the onset of symptomatic renal failure. In those patients who may have a good antigenic match with a willing donor, transplantation without intervening hemodialysis or peritoneal dialysis should be considered. In considering related donor transplantation, the risk of unilateral nephrectomy, including development of proteinuria and hypertension, should be considered. As discussed below, the success rate of cadaver donor transplantation has improved sufficiently that this form of therapy should be carefully considered both with the patient and with family members who are potential donors.

HEMODIALYSIS Hemodialysis employs the process of diffusion across a semipermeable membrane (cellophane, cellulose acetate, polyacrylnitrile, or polymethylmethacrylate) to remove unwanted substances from the blood while adding desirable components. A constant flow of blood on one side of the membrane and a cleansing solution–dialysate on the other allows removal of waste products in a fashion grossly similar to that of glomerular filtration. By altering the composition of the dialysate, the method of exposure of blood and dialysate (geometry of the dialyzer), the type and surface area of dialysis membrane, and the frequency and duration of exposure, patients without renal function can be maintained in a relatively healthy state. Hemodialysis equipment consists of three components—the blood delivery system, the composition and delivery system of the dialysate, and the dialyzer itself. Blood is pumped to the dialyzer by a roller pump through lines with appropriate equipment to measure flow and pressures within the system; blood flow should be approximately 250 to 300 mL/min. Hydrostatic pressure within the system can be manipulated to achieve desirable fluid removal, so-called ultrafiltration. The dialysate is delivered to the dialyzer from a storage tank or proportioning system which manufactures dialysate on line. In most systems dialysate passes once across the membrane, countercurrent to blood flow at a rate of 500 mL/min, or it may be recirculated multiple times at higher flow rates. The composition of the dialysate is similar to plasma water, but may be altered depending upon the patient's needs. There are two principal types of dialyzers—the flat plate dialyzer, in which flat sheets of membrane are layered one on another with intervening plastic templates; and the hollow fiber or capillary dialyzer, in which membrane material is spun into fine capillaries, thousands of which are packed into bundles with blood flowing through the capillaries while dialysate is circulated on the outside of the fiber bundle (Fig. 221-2).

Most patients require between 10 and 15 h of dialysis per week, equally divided into several sessions. The time depends upon body size, residual renal function, dietary intake, complicating illnesses, and the degree of anabolism or catabolism. The time, frequency of treatments, type and size of dialyzer, and dialysate composition, blood, or dialysate flow may all be altered to accomplish specific

FIGURE 221-2 *Hollow fiber or capillary dialyzer; the most commonly used artificial kidney.*

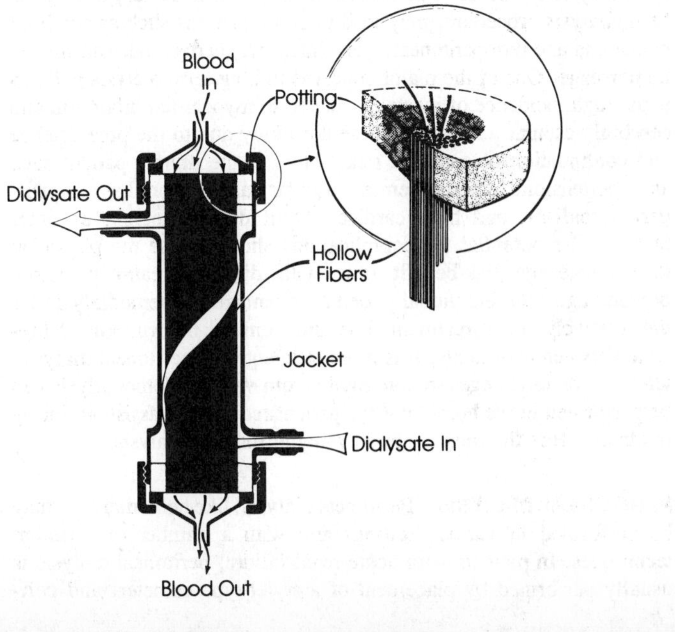

needs. In recent years, kinetic modeling, utilizing urea generation and protein catabolic rates, has lead to a more definite dialysis prescription.

Many complications in the chronic dialysis patient are related to underlying disease or those uremic conditions not reversed by dialytic therapy. These and other related problems of hemodialysis are discussed in Chap. 220. The Achilles' heel of hemodialysis is access to the circulation. In the early 1960s, development of the arteriovenous shunt made chronic dialysis possible. This device has had a high failure rate because of infection and thrombosis and led in 1966 to the development of the arteriovenous (AV) fistula. The fistula is preferably created from a native vein, but if not available, a prosthetic conduit (Dacron, extended polytetrafluoroethylene, bovine carotid arteries, human umbilical cord artery) subcutaneously placed between an artery and a nearby vein may be utilized. Cannulation of arteriovenous fistulas with 15- to 16-gauge needles allows blood flow sufficient to carry out hemodialysis. Unfortunately, infection, thrombosis, and aneurysm formation also occur in the arteriovenous fistula, particularly in prosthetic devices. There is a relatively high incidence of septicemia and septic embolization associated with shunt and fistula infection; the most common infecting agent is *Staphylococcus aureus*.

In addition, a significant psychological impact is related to the failure of the AV fistula. Depression and altered self-image are other common psychiatric problems. The rapid flux in osmolality may cause a disequilibrium syndrome, while rapid changes in electrolytes (particularly potassium) may lead to arrhythmia during dialysis. Hypotension is a common phenomenon during hemodialysis and is due to many factors—the size of the extracorporeal circulation, degree of ultrafiltration, change in serum osmolality, presence of autonomic neuropathy, concomitant use of antihypertensive agents, removal of catecholamines, or infusion of acetate (used as the dialysate buffer) which is a cardiac depressant and vasodilator. Syndromes of dialysis dementia and osteomalacia may be secondary to aluminum contamination of dialysate water or from oral intake of aluminum hydroxide. An increased incidence of HB-S (hepatitis B–surface) antigenemia is related to decreased immunologic integrity. Patients with chronic antigenemia are usually asymptomatic and have little derangement of liver function. There is a higher rate of non-A, non-B hepatitis and cytomegalovirus infection, but these, too, are usually of mild degree. Mechanical and/or iatrogenic complications such as hemolysis, air embolus, blood leaks, and contaminated dialysate have become less common with improved equipment. Device-induced adverse reactions may occur, as exemplified by complement-mediated leukopenia and hypoxemia due to exposure of blood to cellophane. More prominent symptoms such as back and chest pain, bronchospasm, and anaphylaxis may rarely occur in this reaction. Heparin, necessary during the hemodialysis procedure, may lead to complications such as subdural hematoma and retroperitoneal, gastrointestinal, pericardial, and pleural hemorrhage. One of the major concerns in long-term dialysis patients is the high incidence of mortality related to myocardial infarction and cerebral vascular accidents. These are likely due to the preexistence and continuation of common risk factors in the uremic patient such as hypertension, hyperlipidemia, vascular calcification due to hyperparathyroidism, and high cardiac output due to anemia or other factors. The potential for complications should cause the physician to evaluate the risk/benefit ratio with dialysis treatment before proceeding in the individual patient. Advantages of hemodialysis are the relatively short treatment time and minimal interruption of lifestyle between treatments. It is more efficient than peritoneal dialysis, allowing rapid changes in abnormal serum values. Hemodialysis can be performed in the home, but the patient requires an assistant during treatment. It is the most widely available form of dialysis.

PERITONEAL DIALYSIS Peritoneal dialysis, like hemodialysis, may be performed in various settings and with a number of different techniques. In patients with acute renal failure, peritoneal dialysis is usually performed by placement of a stylet-type catheter, and peritoneal lavage is constantly performed for 24 to 72 h. One- to two-liter exchanges every 20 to 60 min can be carried out until the desired clinical and/or chemical improvements are achieved. The catheter is then removed and the patient observed until symptoms or laboratory results dictate the need for a further 1 to 3 days of peritoneal dialysis. Chronic peritoneal dialysis has been attempted since the late 1940s but was relatively unsuccessful until development of a permanent peritoneal catheter in 1968—the Tenckhoff catheter. Use of this indwelling catheter and closed continuous-cycle dialysate delivery equipment led to treatment protocols with which patients were treated 2 to 3 times per week for a total of 30 to 40 h (intermittent peritoneal dialysis—IPD) to achieve clearances and fluid removal similar to those of hemodialysis. In 1978, the concept of constant peritoneal lavage with prolonged dwell times led to the development of CAPD, which differs from intermittent peritoneal dialysis in that patients instill fluid into the peritoneal cavity, seal the catheter, continue in an ambulatory mode, and every 4 to 6 h empty the peritoneal cavity and replace the dialysate. This technique utilizes 2-liter containers of dialysate and obviates the need for dialysis equipment. Modification of the technique using a cyclic dialysate delivery device to exchange dialysate during the night with chronic dwelling of fluid during the waking hours (CCPD) may be more acceptable to some patients.

Twenty-four– to seventy-two–hour acute peritoneal dialysis using a stylet-catheter is usually performed in a hospital setting. IPD or CCPD may be performed in a center or at home (usually overnight), while CAPD can be performed anywhere. As with hemodialysis, the composition of the dialysate can be modified to accommodate ultrafiltration and clearance needs. The major difference in peritoneal dialysate formulas is the larger quantity of dextrose used as an osmotic agent to achieve fluid removal. Advantages of peritoneal dialysis are avoidance of heparinization and vascular surgery and a slower clearance rate which may be advantageous in some patients with cardiovascular instability. It is more amenable to total self-treatment. Disadvantages include the longer treatment time—either longer periods intermittently or continuous involvement. It should not be used in patients with recent abdominal surgery or pulmonary compromise. Inadequate clearance may occur in some patients, e.g., those with scleroderma, vasculitis, malignant hypertension, or any disease involving the peritoneum. Complications include catheter tunnel infection, peritonitis, moderate protein loss, hypertriglyceridemia, hypercholesterolemia, obesity, and inguinal and abdominal hernias. CAPD requires a higher degree of patient compliance and has a higher rate of peritonitis than intermittent peritoneal dialysis because of multiple entries into the system, but is the predominant form of peritoneal dialysis.

RESULTS At the end of 1983, approximately 72,000 patients were on chronic dialysis, while over the past 15 years, nearly 55,000 patients have undergone renal transplantation in the United States. Approximately 85 to 90 percent of patients are on hemodialysis, while 15 percent perform some type of peritoneal dialysis. Of all new patients with end-stage renal disease, approximately 35 to 50 percent are physically and psychologically suitable for renal transplantation. Many of these patients are sensitized with high antibody titers and are on hemodialysis and peritoneal dialysis awaiting availability of a cadaver kidney. An acutely ill or medically complicated patient will likely undergo dialysis in a hospital dialysis unit or intensive care unit, while stable patients may be dialyzed as outpatients in the hospital dialysis unit, in an out-of-hospital dialysis center, or at home. Most centers attempt to have patients participate in their own care, so-called self-dialysis. Approximatley 14,000 patients were performing home dialysis at the end of 1983, this number representing 12 to 40 percent of all patients on dialysis, depending upon the area of the country and factors such as population density, economics, and social issues. Home dialysis (either hemodialysis or peritoneal) is preferable for many because of self-reliance and freedom from hospital or center dialysis schedules. Patient motivation is the primary factor in selection of home or in-center self-dialysis. Dialysis performed in the hospital setting is most expensive, while home dialysis with a nonpaid family assistant or alone (peritoneal dialysis only) is somewhat less expensive than in-center dialysis. Despite absence of equipment, peritoneal dialysis remains equally as expensive as home hemodialysis because of the cost of dialysate and hospitalization related to an increased incidence of peritonitis.

The mean age for patients on dialysis is the late fifties, partly because nephrosclerosis and eventual renal failure from other parenchymal diseases occur in older patients, but more likely because the selection process favors transplantation in younger patients.

Approximately 10 to 20 percent of patients with chronic renal failure are totally rehabilitated by dialysis, and another 30 to 40 percent of nondiabetic patients may be expected to be rehabilitated to a functional status even if not employed. Twenty percent of patients will be returned to a level of function not considered rehabilitated but able to care for themselves. The remainder (approximately 20 percent) are fully dependent on support from others. Diabetics, who have a rehabilitation rate and survival rate significantly lower than that of nondiabetic patients, make up much of the latter two groups. Determination of mortality rates is variable because of age and the disease process; however, most chronic dialysis programs have annual mortality rates of approximately 5 to 10 percent per year.

TRANSPLANTATION

Transplantation of the human kidney has become a justified procedure for the treatment of advanced chronic renal failure. Worldwide, tens of thousands of such procedures have been performed and occur at the rate of 50 to more than 100 per year in some medical centers. When azathioprine (Imuran) and prednisone are used as immunosuppresive drugs, the results with properly matched familial donors are superior to those obtained with organs from cadaveric donors, with 75 to 90 percent compared to 50 to 60 percent graft survival rates at 1 year, respectively. When antilymphocyte globulins (ALG) have been added to the treatment regimens in some centers, the results with cadaveric donors have approached those with living related donors, at least for the initial 1 to 2 years after transplantation. Most recently, the new fungal endecapeptide cyclosporine has significantly improved 1-year cadaveric survival rates to the 80 percent range, when used along with prednisone in place of azathioprine and ALG. With all therapies, the rate of graft loss from rejection is much slower after the first year, although occasionally an acute irreversible rejection episode may occur after many months of good function. This is especially likely if the patient neglects to take the immunosuppressive drugs. There has been a most striking improvement in clinical renal transplant results in recent years in patient morbidity and mortality rates, the latter declining to less than 5 percent in a number of centers. These findings represent an increasing tendency on the part of transplant teams to decrease immunosuppressive therapy so that in the case of severe rejection the kidney rather than the patient is lost. The beneficial effects of blood transfusions in the preconditioning of potential recipients are clearly established. Nontransfused recipients are at highest risk for rejecting their grafts, while multiple random transfusions or transfusions from specific donors can greatly improve chances for graft survival. An increasing number of second and even third transplants are being performed, and the overall results show only a 10 to 20 percent reduction in expected survival compared to first transplants; in other words, rejection of a graft does not necessarily prejudice the results of another transplant attempt.

DONOR SELECTION Donor sources are cadavers or volunteer blood-related living donors. Living volunteer donors should be normal on physical examination and of the same major ABO blood group, because there is good evidence that crossing major blood group barriers prejudices survival of the allograft. It is, however, possible to transplant a kidney of a type O donor into an A, B, or AB recipient. Selective renal arteriography should be performed on volunteer donors to rule out the presence of multiple or abnormal renal arteries, because the surgical procedure is inordinately difficult and the ischemic time of the transplanted kidney prohibitively long when vascular abnormalities exist. Cadaveric donors should be free of malignant neoplastic disease because of the possible transmission of cancer to the recipient.

A coordinated regional or national system of computerized information sharing and logistical support for the transportation of cadaver kidneys to suitable recipients is under development. It is now possible to remove cadaver kidneys and to maintain them for over 48 h on cold pulsatile perfusion or simple flushing and cooling. This permits adequate time for various typing, cross matching, transportation, and selection problems to be solved.

TISSUE TYPING AND CLINICAL IMMUNOGENETICS Matching for antigens of the HLA major histocompatibility gene complex (Chap. 63) has long been accepted as an ideal criterion for selection of donors for renal allografts. Each mammalian species studied has shown evidence for a single chromosomal region which encodes the strong, or major, transplantation antigens, and the analogous sixth chromosomal region is called *HLA* in human beings. Other antigens, called "minor," may nevertheless play crucial roles, especially the ABH(O) blood groups and an endothelial antigen which is shared with blood monocytes, but not lymphocytes. Evidence for designation of HLA as the genetic region encoding strong transplantation antigens comes from the success rate in living related donor renal and bone marrow transplantation, with superior results in HLA-identical sibling pairs. Nevertheless, 10 to 15 percent of HLA-identical renal allografts are rejected, often within the first weeks after transplantation. It is likely, though not proved, that these failures represent states of prior sensitization to non-HLA antigens. Non-HLA antigens are relatively weak and therefore suppressible by conventional immunosuppressive therapy. Once priming has occurred, however, secondary responses are much more refractory to treatment. In fact, ABH incompatibilities are hazardous because of the presence of natural anti-A and anti-B antibodies.

Living related donors For more than two decades, during which time azathioprine was the mainstay immunosuppressive drug, living related donors provided superior graft survivals. Among first-degree relatives, the general level of expected graft success was in direct proportion to matching for 2,1, or no HLA haplotypes, as defined by HLA serologic typing and the presence or absence of a proliferative response in the mixed lymphocyte response (MLR) (Chap. 63). HLA-incompatible siblings did barely better than the overall average with cadaveric donors (50 to 60 percent at 1 year), while HLA semi-identicals (haploidentical) were in the 70 to 75 percent range. Intrafamilial MLRs among haploidenticals were found to be a measure of responsiveness. Low responder donor-recipient pairs had a 1-year graft survival rate of 90 percent, while vigorous responders were at the level of 55 percent unless donor-specific blood transfusions were given to eliminate this disadvantage. The MLR is a relatively imprecise technique, but it has been repeatedly shown that for both living related and cadaveric donors, MLR reactivity with a specific donor is more predictive of graft outcome than serologic typing for HLA-A, -B, -C, or -DR antigens. Cyclosporine is having a major impact upon the assumption that living related donors are generally superior to cadaveric donors, because in most recent series the improvement in cadaveric results rivals the 80 percent 1-year result previously attained only with haploidentical relatives. One must now weigh the choices in light of the availability of organs and waiting times on dialysis, rather than on the initial rate of graft success. It must be pointed out that long-term survival rates, comparing the various donor types and treatment protocols, have yet to be discerned. With azathioprine, the half-life of graft function after the first year is 34 years with HLA-identical donors, 11½ years with haploidentical donors, and 7 years with cadaveric donors. Long-term use of cyclosporine, assuming that cumulative nephrotoxicity is not a problem, may or may not sustain a high rate of survival.

Cadaveric donors For first transplants receiving cyclosporine overall success rate for unrelated donors is 80 percent of grafts functioning at 1 year. It has been extremely difficult to assess the role of HLA matching in cadaveric donor grafting because of considerable variation in overall results from center to center, including, until recently, relatively high mortality rates. The so-called full-house match of two HLA-A and two HLA-B antigens between unrelated individuals does not ensure matching for other loci adjacent to HLA-A and -B, in contrast to first-degree relatives where the HLA-A and -B antigens are excellent markers for the other linked loci. The degree to which two-A and two-B antigen matching improves cadaveric renal graft survival is in the range of 10 percent and is most likely attributable to the fact that some of these matches will also include compatibility for HLA-D because of the nonrandomness of the association of linked alleles (linkage disequilibrium) in the population (Chap. 63). The more racially homogeneous the population, the greater the chances that any given marker will be in linkage disequilibrium with another.

Rapid assessment of MLR (e.g., within 24 h) is not possible; therefore, serologic techniques are used to approximate degrees of compatibility. Of the class II HLA molecules, DP, DQ, and DR, the last plays the major role in the MLR; indeed, matching for DR provides the most significant improvement in cadaveric renal transplantation. Pooled data from all over the world from over 5000 cadaveric transplants show a 20 percent improvement when the two DR antigens are matched compared to cases when both are mismatched. In addition, when HLA-B antigens are also matched, there is further improvement. The likelihood of obtaining a DR match depends upon the size of the waiting pool, and also on the willingness of transplant centers to share organs on this basis. A 20-percent DR match rate has been readily achieved in some transplant programs. Data on the impact of cyclosporine on the role of HLA matching show that it is additive to HLA-B and -DR matching. As results are improved by multiple approaches (therapy, matching, blood transfusions), it becomes more difficult to discern which factors may or may not be additive. A greater than 90 percent success rate for cadaveric grafts has not as yet been claimed, however.

Presensitization A positive cross match of recipient serum with donor T lymphocytes representing anti-HLA class I is usually predictive of an acute vasculitic event termed *hyperacute* rejection. A few years ago it was thought that patients making such antibodies against a surrogate panel of normal lymphocytes were at high risk for accelerated, if not hyperacute, rejection, even when the donor-specific cross match was negative. That this is no longer so can be attributed to the greater efforts being made in monitoring patients on dialysis, defining not only the presence or absence of antibodies but also the HLA antigens to which they are directed. Patients with anti-HLA antibodies can be safely transplanted if careful cross matching is performed. Patients sustained by hemodialysis often show fluctuating antibody titers and specificity patterns, sometimes, but not always, temporally related to receipt of blood transfusions. At the time of assignment of a cadaveric kidney, cross matches are performed with more than one highly reactive serum, and the previously analyzed antibody specificities are also taken into account. It has recently been found that anti-HLA antibody responses do not necessarily recur several months later when the incompatible antigen is given in a blood product transfusion. Indeed, it seems relatively safe to ignore positive cross matches with sera kept in storage for several months as long as recent sera are negative. The loss of anamnesis to HLA by chronic dialysis patients may result from development of specific unresponsiveness due to suppressor cell activation, or from anti-idiotypic immunity. Presensitization to antigens expressed on B lymphocytes, but not T lymphocytes, is not a contraindication to transplantation. Some of these antibodies are anti-DR, while others are non-HLA IgM antibodies active in the cold and at room temperature, but apparently not relevant to graft survival.

TABLE 221-2 Histocompatibility in renal transplantation

RELATIVE IMPORTANCE OF TYPING AND CROSS MATCHING FOR SEROLOGICALLY DEFINED ANTIGENS

Antigens	Typing (antigen matching)	Cross matching
Class I (HLA-A, -B, -C)	+	+ + +
Class II (HLA-DR)	+ + +	−
Endothelial-monocyte (non-HLA)	?−	+ + +

Endothelial-monocyte system In some cases of unexpected accelerated rejection, antibodies with reactivity to renal endothelium and blood monocytes have been found, both in the circulation and in eluates from rejected grafts. Practical aspects of typing and cross matching for this non-HLA system are difficult. Second transplants following rapid loss of the first graft seem to be particularly at risk.

Overview of transplantation immunogenetics In addition to the ABH(O) blood groups, the important histocompatibility antigens presently known are HLA-A, -B, -C, -DR, and the endothelial-monocyte system (Table 221-2). The best current data suggest that major immunogenicity lies in the DR antigens, while A, B, C, and endothelial-monocyte antigens provide the major targets for effector IgG, and in the case of A, B, and C, at least, for killer T lymphocytes. Hence the current emphasis is on A, B, and C cross matching and DR matching.

Blood transfusions At a time when it appeared that transfusion-induced sensitization against a random lymphocyte panel was predictive of a high graft failure rate, a number of transplantation units undertook a policy of withholding blood from as many dialysis patients as possible. The clinical need for blood was found to be less than originally thought, especially in nonnephrectomized patients, and avoidance of possible exposure to hepatitis was also a consideration. The overall experience with the nontransfused patients has been a dramatic one, confirmed many times over: such patients are at the *highest risk* for graft failure. Still at issue is the number of transfused units needed for optimal graft survival, with the bulk of the evidence showing that more than 5 units is optimal, although some studies claim an effect with 1 or 2 units, given in advance or at the time of transplantation. Data are presently lacking on the question of using fresh vs. frozen vs. washed cells, as well as the precise methods of storage employed. As in many areas of clinical transplantation, there are not a sufficient number of cases and/or carefully randomized trials. Nevertheless, the large number of cases included in prospective studies has already provided impressive overall evidence that avoidance of blood exposure reduces graft success rate by 20 to 30 percent.

The mechanisms of the transfusion effect are unknown but may involve a selection process of screening out responders to certain HLA antigens, or, alternatively, transfusions may induce states of specific suppression. Assessment of the combined effects of transfusions and DR matching shows that they are not additive. If there is a good match for HLA-DR antigens, prior priming to induce low responsiveness appears to be unnecessary. Alternatively, if the recipient is exposed to multiple units of blood, HLA-DR matching adds no further benefit. Living donor haploidentical grafts also benefit from blood transfusions. In particular, the use of blood from the intended donor on three occasions prior to transplantation results in superior graft survival in those 70 percent of recipients who do not become sensitized to HLA. Part of the effect is one of selection of antibody nonresponders; in addition, it is likely that specific suppression is induced. The preliminary data with donor-specific transfusions show a success rate of greater than 90 percent at 1 year, in the range attained by HLA identical grafts. Again, experience with cyclosporine may alter the impact of blood transfusion policies, but firm data are currently unavailable.

IMMUNOLOGY OF REJECTION Knowledge of the immunology of tissue transplantation stems largely from animal experimentation. However, enough evidence has accumulated in humans, particularly in kidney transplantation, to indicate that the evidence is similar though not identical for the different species. The immunologic mechanisms are not qualitatively different from those found in other areas of immunology (Chap. 62). The evidence is that early rejection is associated with T lymphocytes having direct specificity against donor antigens. These may be cytotoxic cells (T8+ or T4+) or cells which mediate DTH (T4+); however, significant numbers of B lymphocytes, null cells, natural killer (NK) cells, and macrophages appear in the early infiltrate, and cells capable of mediating antibody-dependent cell-mediated cytotoxicity (ADCC) are also present (Fig. 221-3). Many of the B lymphocytes produce immunoglobulins. The spectrum of cellular and humoral response and graft injury is quite varied, depending upon specific genetic differences between donor and recipient and states of presensitization. The greater the degree of presensitization, the more likely it is that one will find antibody-mediated vascular lesions. All of the processes shown in Fig. 221-3 are possible, but their relative contribution varies from case to case. Further dissection of the heterogeneity of the human allograft response, utilizing newer techniques for identification of lymphocyte subsets, is adding to the value of graft biopsy as a guide to therapy and prognosis. Monitoring of peripheral blood lymphocyte subsets, utilizing monoclonal antibodies (Chap. 62) to functionally related surface molecules, such as T4 (T-helper cells) and T8 (T-suppressor cells), has been related to the degree of rejection activity in some surveys, but the T4/T8 ratio has not always been clinically meaningful. Part of the problem may lie in the fact that these subsets are not as uniquely related to function as originally believed. Finally, the cytokine mediators of the cellular immune response (IL 1, IL 2, IL 3, IFNγ) (Chap. 62) have been shown to be importantly involved in the control and expression of the alloimmune rejection response. For example, T-cell production of IFNγ causes increased expression of HLA antigens upon endothelial cells. In normal immunobiology this effect may be to promote more efficient presentation of foreign antigen, while in the transplantation it enhances the immunogenicity of the vascularized transplant.

The failure of transplanted kidneys after 2 or even 3 years of adequate function is due to a form of "chronic rejection." In such kidneys the development of nephrosclerosis, with proliferation of the vascular intima of renal vessels, and intimal fibrosis, with marked decrease in the lumen of the vessels, takes place (Fig. 221-4). The result is renal ischemia, hypertension, widespread tubular atrophy, interstitial fibrosis, and glomerular atrophy with eventual renal failure.

IMMUNOSUPPRESSIVE TREATMENT When histocompatibility differences exist between donor and recipient, it is necessary to modify or suppress the immune response in order to enable the recipient to accept a graft. Immunosuppressive therapy, in general, suppresses all immune responses, including those to bacteria, fungi, and even malignant tumors. In the 1950s when clinical renal transplantation began, sublethal total-body irradiation was employed. Currently, immunosuppression is more safely induced pharmacologically. Agents used in humans to suppress the immune response are discussed in the following paragraphs.

Drugs *Azathioprine* (Imuran), an analogue of mercaptopurine, is the keystone to immunosuppressive therapy in humans. This agent can inhibit synthesis of deoxyribonucleic acid (DNA), ribonucleic acid (RNA), or both. Because cell division and proliferation are a necessary part of the immune response to antigenic stimulation, suppression by this agent may be mediated by the inhibition of mitosis of immunologically competent lymphoid cells, interfering with synthesis of DNA. Alternatively, immunosuppression may be brought about by blocking the synthesis of RNA (possibly messenger RNA), to inhibit processing of antigens prior to lymphocyte stimulation. Azathioprine metabolites block the formation of rosettes by T cells with sheep red blood cells. This latter phenomenon is produced by receptors on the T11 molecule, which is part of a system for activating T cells. This drug has little effect in suppressing a secondary immune response, however. Therapy with azathioprine is generally instituted 2 days prior to transplantation in the recipient of a living donor kidney and on the day of transplantation in the case of a cadaveric donor kidney recipient at a level of 4 mg/kg per day. The drug is later tapered to levels of 1.5 to 3 mg/kg per day, as long as the allograft functions. Because the drug is rapidly metabolized by the liver, its dosage need not be varied directly in relation to renal function, even though renal failure results in retention of the metabolites of azathioprine. Some patients are unusually sensitive to this drug, particularly when renal function is compromised, and reduction in dosage is required because of leukopenia and occasionally thrombocytopenia. Excessive amounts of azathioprine may also cause jaundice, anemia, and alopecia. If it is essential to administer allopurinol concurrently, the azathioprine dose must be drastically reduced, since inhibition of xanthine oxidase delays degradation. This combination is best avoided.

The *glucocorticosteroids* are important adjuncts to immunosuppressive therapy. Of all the agents employed, prednisone has effects that are easiest to assess, and in large doses it is unquestionably the most effective agent for the reversal of rejection. In general, 30 to 40 mg prednisone is given immediately prior to or at the time of

FIGURE 221-3 *Overall scheme of the development of effector mechanisms in graft rejection. Bone marrow stem cells differentiate under the influence of the thymus gland into mature thymus-derived (T) lymphocytes, or under the influence of an equivalent to the avian bursa of Fabricius into mature bone marrow–derived (B) lymphocytes. Exposure to antigen (Δ) results in an interaction between T cells and B cells, and often involves macrophages. The sensitized B cells, after mitoses, develop into immunoglobulin-secreting cells (e.g., plasma cells), illustrated here by IgG and IgM. Such immunoglobulins may form immune complexes with antigen in the circulation which activate the complement sequence, or they may react directly with antigens on the blood vessel surface. Elaboration of secondary mediators, including the products of complement activation, results in vascular damage as illustrated. Sensitized T lymphocytes are the primary effector cells in cell-mediated immunity (CMI) and may react directly with antigens in the graft to exert a cytotoxic effect. In addition, T cells release factors, such as macrophage migration inhibition factor (MIF), which may accelerate the rate of mononuclear cell infiltration. This process is similar to delayed-type hypersensitivity (DTH). It has also been shown that unsensitized non-T cells (K cells) can be activated to exert cytotoxic effects by the fixation of IgG to target cells, followed by interaction of the IgG (Fc portion) with a receptor on the K cell. Finally, platelet aggregation and thrombosis can occur following the endothelial damage induced by any of these mechanisms.*

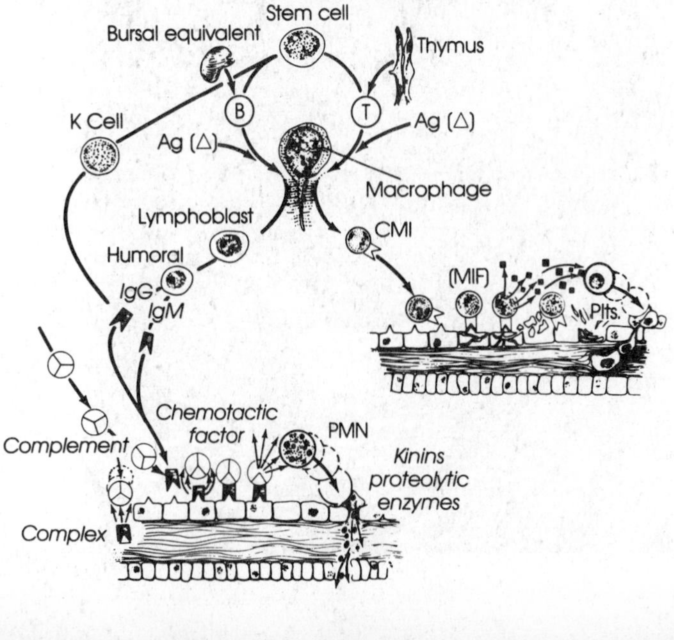

transplantation, and the dosage is gradually reduced. The well-known side effects of the glucocorticosteroids, particularly impairment of wound healing and predisposition to infection, make it desirable to taper the dose as rapidly as possible in the immediate postoperative period. Customarily methylprednisolone, 1 to 2 g intravenously, is administered immediately upon diagnosis of beginning rejection and continued once daily for 3 days. When the drug is effective, the results are usually apparent within 48 to 96 h. Such "pulse" doses are less effective in the slow rejection process, which may not become apparent until 2 to 3 years after transplantation. Most patients whose renal function is stable after 6 months or a year do not require large doses of prednisone; maintenance doses of 15 or 20 mg per day are the rule. Many patients tolerate an alternate-day course of steroids better than daily doses without an increased risk of rejection.

A major effect of steroids is upon the monocyte/macrophage system, preventing the release of IL 1. Although lymphopenia results from large doses of corticosteroids, this is primarily due to sequestration of recirculating blood lymphocytes to lymphoid tissue.

When jaundice or nephritis appears in patients maintained on azathioprine, *cyclophosphamide* may be substituted. It appears to be as effective in the maintenance of renal allografts as azathioprine and somewhat more effective in hepatic allografts. Leukopenia, alopecia, cystitis, ovarian fibrosis, and aspermia may result if the dosage is not carefully regulated. Prospective cadaveric *donors* have been treated with massive doses of cyclophosphamide and methylprednisolone in an attempt to decrease the antigenicity of the graft by eliminating "passenger leukocytes." The results of this technique are somewhat uncertain.

FIGURE 221-4 *Biopsy of the renal cadaveric allograft illustrating obliterative endarteritis. Loss of the media is associated with intimal thickening. The elastic tissue shows dissolution of the elastica. The evidence for arteritis with subsequent thrombosis is typically the gaps in the elastica and media. The intimal thickening probably represents organization of a thrombus formed in response to the arteritis. [From GJ Dammin, JP Merrill, in Structural Basis for Renal Disease, EL Becker (ed), New York, Hoeber-Harper, 1968.]*

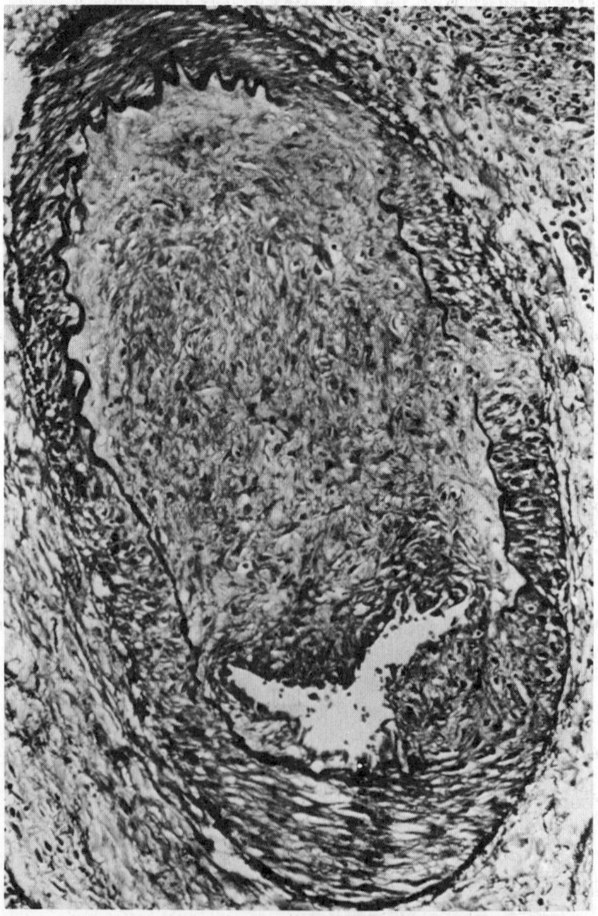

Cyclosporine A is a fungal peptide having potent immunosuppressive activity in animals and in in vitro systems. It appears to have a preferential effect upon early activation of helper-inducer T lymphocytes, thereby augmenting suppressor T-cell responses. Assessment of this agent in human renal transplantation has generally shown that it works well only in conjunction with corticosteroids. Since cyclosporine blocks production of IL 2 by helper-inducer (T4+) T cells, its combination with steroids is expected to produce a double block in the macrophage → IL 1 → T cell → IL 2 sequence. As noted, clinical results with several hundreds of renal transplants have been impressive. Of all its toxic effects (nephrotoxicity, hepatotoxicity, hirsutism, tremor, gingival hyperplasia), only nephrotoxicity presents a serious management problem, and is discussed further below.

Antilymphocyte globulin (ALG) When serum from animals made immune to host lymphocytes is injected into the recipient, a marked suppression of cellular immunity to the tissue graft results. The action upon cell-mediated immunity is considerably greater than upon humoral immunity. A globulin fraction of the serum is the agent generally employed. For use in humans, peripheral human lymphocytes, thymocytes, or lymphocytes from spleens or thoracic duct fistulas have been injected into horses, rabbits, or goats to produce antilymphocyte serum, from which the globulin fraction is then separated. Although ALG, or ATG (antithymocyte globulin), is unquestionably effective in prolonging grafts in experimental animals, its efficacy in the transplantation of human tissue is somewhat less clear, as it varies from source to source. Heterologous antibody against defined T-lymphocyte subsets, in the form of mouse antihuman monoclonal IgG, may offer a more precise approach to this form of therapy. Two such antibodies, OKT3 and anti-T12, directed against molecules expressed on virtually all mature T lymphocytes, have undergone initial trials in reversal of established rejection episodes. OKT3, while somewhat toxic initially, is generally effective, while anti-T12 does not work in all circumstances. These are considered prototypes of reagents having improved selectivity for immunologic manipulation in the future.

Other techniques Among other techniques of immunosuppression, thymectomy and splenectomy have not been widely accepted. Local irradiation of the transplanted kidney in two or three doses of 3500 mGy (350 rads) has also been utilized. This technique may result in fewer early rejection episodes in cadaveric transplants than in nonirradiated controls. Fractional total-lymph-node irradiation (TLI), as employed in the therapy of Hodgkin's disease, is an interesting new modality currently under investigation.

CLINICAL COURSE AND MANAGEMENT OF THE RECIPIENT Bilateral nephrectomy at some point prior to transplantation is performed for a specific cause but not as a routine. Hypertension which is difficult to control or infection involving the end-stage kidneys are the two most common indications. Nephrectomized patients maintain a much lower hematocrit level, but this is no longer considered a disadvantage per se, because blood transfusions need not be avoided in preparation for transplantation. Difficulties do arise when these multiply transfused patients become sensitized and must remain on dialysis. Nephrectomy per se does not appear to affect the survival of subsequent renal allografts.

Adequate hemodialysis should be performed within 48 h of surgery, and care should be taken that the serum potassium level is not markedly elevated so that intraoperative cardiac arrhythmias can be averted. The diuresis that commonly occurs postoperatively must be carefully monitored; in many instances it may be massive, reflecting the inability of ischemic tubules to regulate sodium and water excretion. Massive potassium losses may occur and occasionally result in cardiac arrhythmias. Most chronically uremic patients have some excess of extracellular fluid, and some degree of negative balance should be accomplished, provided circulatory hemodynamics remain stable. Acute tubular necrosis (ATN) may cause immediate oliguria or may follow an initial short period of graft function. ATN is most likely to occur when cadaveric donors have been hypotensive, or if the interval between cessation of blood flow and organ harvest (warm ischemic time) has been more than a few minutes. Recovery usually occurs within 3 weeks, although periods as long as 6 weeks have been reported. Superimposition of rejection upon ATN is common, and the differential diagnosis may be difficult. Cyclosporine therapy aggravates ATN, and some patients do not diurese until they are converted to azathioprine.

The rejection episode Early diagnosis of rejection allows prompt institution of therapy to preserve renal function and prevent irreversible damage due to fibrosis. Clinical evidence of rejection may be characterized by fever, swelling, and tenderness over the allograft, and by significant reduction in urine volume. In patients whose renal function is good initially, oliguria may be accompanied by decreased urinary sodium concentration and increased osmolarity. These changes may not be present in the more chronic stages of rejection or when renal function is impaired at the onset of rejection.

Arteriography and radioactive iodohippurate sodium (Hippuran) renograms of the transplanted kidney may be useful in ascertaining changes in the renal vasculature and in renal blood flow, even in the absence of urinary flow. Diagnostic ultrasound has become the procedure of choice to rule out urinary obstruction or to confirm the presence of perirenal collections of urine, blood, or lymph. When renal function has been good initially, a rise in the serum creatinine level and a decrease in the creatinine clearance is the most sensitive and reliable indicator of rejection.

Cyclosporine may cause deterioration in renal function in a manner similar to a rejection episode. In fact, rejection processes tend to be more indolent with cyclosporine, and the only way to make a diagnosis may be by renal biopsy. There is no universally accepted lesion(s) which makes a diagnosis of cyclosporine toxicity, although interstitial fibrosis and thickening of arteriolar walls have been noted by some pathologists. Basically, if the biopsy does not reveal moderate and active cellular rejection activity, the serum creatinine will most likely respond to a reduction in cyclosporine dose. Blood levels of drug can be useful if very high or very low, but precise correlation with renal function does not exist. If rejection activity is present in the biopsy, appropriate therapy is indicated.

Management problems Modification of the usual clinical manifestations of infection by immunosuppressive therapy is a major problem in the posttransplant period. The signs and symptoms of infection may be masked and distorted, and fever without obvious cause is common. Only after days or weeks will it become apparent that it has a viral or fungal origin. The importance of blood cultures in such patients cannot be overemphasized, because systemic infection without obvious foci is frequent, although wound infections with or without urinary fistulas are most common. Particularly important are rapidly occurring pulmonary lesions, which may result in death within 5 days of onset. When these become apparent, immunosuppressive agents should be discontinued except for maintenance doses of prednisone. The major toxic effect of azathioprine is bone marrow suppression, while cyclosporine has no marrow effects. They both may predispose to unusual opportunistic infections, however. In the case of *Pneumocystis carinii* (Chap. 158) trimethoprim-sulfamethoxazole is the treatment of choice; amphotericin B has been used effectively in systemic fungal infections. Involvement of the oropharynx with *Candida* (Chap. 147) may be treated with local nystatin. Small doses (a total of 300 mg) of amphotericin given over a period of 2 weeks may be effective in refractory oral candidiasis. *Aspergillus* (Chap. 147), *Nocardia* (Chap. 146), and cytomegalovirus (CMV) (Chap. 137) infections also occur. The latter are particularly common in transplant recipients, and active CMV infection is frequently associated with rejection episodes. The complications of corticosteroid therapy are well known and include gastrointestinal bleeding, impairment of wound healing, osteoporosis, diabetes, cataract formation, and hemorrhagic pancreatitis. The treatment of jaundice in transplant patients should include cessation of azathioprine or cyclosporine therapy. It is surprising that total cessation of azathioprine therapy often does not result in rejection of a graft. In some instances of jaundice, cyclophosphamide may be substituted for azathioprine. Antiplatelet agents and anticoagulants, although effective in theory, have not been successful in the prevention of the chronic vascular lesion. Persistent elevations of serum creatinine levels above 2.5 mg/dL in patients maintained on cyclosporine may be an indication for conversion to azathioprine, particularly if reduction in dose provokes either rejection activity or toxicity. Another indication for conversion would be in the patient recovering from a series of infections developing while cyclosporine is being administered. Our own experience with such conversions between 4 and 8 months after transplantation has been quite satisfactory; however, 30 percent of patients had temporally related rejection episodes requiring additional steroid therapy. Subsequent follow-up showed improved renal function in most cases. Hence, if the nephrotoxic potential of cyclosporine should indeed grow with each passing year, conversion to azathioprine remains an option.

In spite of the potential teratogenic effects of immunosuppressive agents, both women and men have become parents after transplantation. The incidence of congenital abnormalities in the offspring is not unusual.

Glomerular lesions Even identical twins who do not require immunosuppression may develop glomerular lesions after transplantation. These represent recurrence of a glomerulonephritic process. Glomerular lesions may occur in 10 to 15 percent of allografts, even when the original disease was accidental removal of a solitary kidney. The pathogenesis is related to a chronic rejection process. In other cases the lesions resemble those of the patient's own original disease. The recurrence of the nephrotic syndrome with "nil disease" in transplanted kidneys whose recipient's original nil disease had progressed to renal failure with focal sclerosis, and the recurrence in renal allografts of the classic lesions of IgA nephropathy and of membranoproliferative glomerulonephritis with electron-dense deposit disease are classic examples. In the last of these, the incidence of recurrence has been reported to be as high as 30 to 40 percent. In most instances, however, the recurrence of the original renal lesions represents no threat to the patient's immediate prognosis, and a primary diagnosis of glomerulonephritis is rarely taken as a contraindication to transplantation.

Malignancy The incidence of tumors arising in patients on immunosuppressive therapy is 5 to 6 percent, or approximately 100 times greater than that observed in the general population in the same age range. The most common lesions are cancer of the skin and lips and carcinoma in situ of the cervix, as well as lymphomas, particularly reticulum cell sarcoma in the central nervous system and gastrointestinal tract.

Other complications *Hypercalcemia* after transplantation may indicate failure of hyperplastic parathyroid glands to regress. Aseptic necrosis of the head of the femur is probably due to preexisting hyperparathyroidism. With improved management of calcium and phosphorus metabolism during chronic dialysis the incidence of parathyroid-related complications has fallen dramatically.

Both chronic dialysis and renal transplant patients have a higher incidence of death from myocardial infarction and stroke than in the population at large, and this is particularly true in diabetics. Contributing factors are hypertension and hypertriglyceridemia. Depressed high-density lipoprotein cholesterol (HDL) concentrations in dialysis patients may persist after transplantation.

REFERENCES

CARPENTER CB, MILFORD EL: Renal transplantation: Immunobiology, in *The Kidney*, 3d ed, B Brenner, F Rector (eds). Philadelphia, Saunders, 1986, p 1907

COHEN DJ, LOERTSCHER R et al: Cyclosporine: A new immunosuppressive agent for organ transplantation. Ann Intern Med 101:667, 1984

HAKIM RM, LAZARUS JM: Medical aspects of hemodialysis, in *The Kidney*, 3d ed, B Brenner, F Rector (eds). Philadelphia, Saunders, 1986, p 1791

———, ———: Hemodialysis in acute renal failure, in *Acute Renal Failure*, B Brenner, JM Lazarus (eds). Philadelphia, Saunders, 1983, p 643

LAZARUS JM: Complications in hemodialysis: An overview. Kidney Intern 18:783, 1980

———: Hemodialysis, in *Chronic Renal Failure, Contemporary Issues in Nephrology*, vol 7: B Brenner, J Stein (eds). New York, Churchill-Livingstone, 1981, p 153

MORRIS PJ (ed): *Kidney Transplantation. Principles and Practice*, 2d ed. New York, Grune & Stratton, 1983

NOLPH KD et al: Continuous ambulatory peritoneal dialysis: Three-year experience at one center. Ann Intern Med 92:609, 1980

OPELZ G: Correlation of HLA matching with kidney graft survival in patients with or without cyclosporine treatment. Transplantation 40:240, 1985

STROM TB, TILNEY NL: Renal transplantation: Clinical aspects, in *The Kidney*, 3d ed, B Brenner, FC Rector (eds). Philadelphia, Saunders, 1986, p 1941

222 IMMUNOPATHOGENIC MECHANISMS OF RENAL INJURY

RICHARD J. GLASSOCK / BARRY M. BRENNER

Recognition of the important role played by aberrant immunologic processes in many forms of renal injury, especially those involving the glomerular circulation, constitutes one of the most significant conceptual advances made in the understanding of renal diseases during the last quarter century. Although the fine details of these abnormal processes have been elucidated for many disease entities, large gaps in knowledge still exist concerning both the initiating events and the etiologic factors involved in renal disease.

In its broadest conceptual framework the immunopathogenesis of renal injury can be simplified to a few fundamental mechanisms, which are presented in Chap. 62. One involves the reaction of a circulating antibody with its respective renal antigen in situ. The antigen may be either an intrinsic constituent of the kidney or one which has been bound to the tissue by a particular biochemical or immunologic reaction. Antigens in basement membranes of glomerular capillaries or renal tubules and antibodies to these basement membranes are prime components of this mechanism. A variety of antigenic components of the glomerular capillary walls and renal tubules are now recognized. Binding of circulating antibody to these tissue antigens gives rise to several distinctive structural alterations and immunohistochemical appearances, as will be discussed below. This category of immune processes is often referred to as the *antitissue antibody–mediated diseases*.

Another pathogenic category, by far the most prevalent in human renal disease, involves the localization of circulating macromolecular aggregates composed of antigens and antibodies (i.e., circulating immune complexes) within renal structures, principally glomeruli. This mechanism is referred to as *immune-complex–mediated disease*. The immune complexes need not bear any special immunochemical relationships to renal structures; thus the kidney can be viewed as a passive participant or an innocent party, damaged by processes originating elsewhere. The source of the antigen may be either *endogenous* (*autologous*) or *exogenous* (*environmental*). Further, exogenous antigens may be biologically inert or derived from an organism capable of self-replication (e.g., bacteria, viruses, etc.). Under special circumstances environmental agents may also combine with autologous substances to result in new antigenic compounds (hapten-protein conjugates), which may act in concert with antibodies to form immune complexes. In contrast to the above mechanisms, *cell-mediated* immune processes are far less well established as possible mechanisms in glomerular and vascular diseases of the kidney. Finally, certain human glomerular diseases are prominently associated with abnormal activation of the *alternative pathway of the complement cascade*.

IMMUNOPATHOGENIC MECHANISMS Once initiated, immune injury is mediated by the interaction of a number of humoral and cellular factors. Activation of the complement (C) cascade may lead to the direct cytolysis of the cellular constituents of the glomerulus or may lead to the production of biologically active fragments capable of enhancing vascular permeability or attracting polymorphonuclear leukocytes and other cellular constituents. Coagulation may be directly initiated by alterations in the endothelial surface and exposure of collagen matrix, followed by localized platelet aggregation. Interactions between the complement cascade and the coagulation process are numerous and complex. Complement activation may trigger coagulation and vice versa. Activation of the Hageman factor may initiate the kallikrein-kinin system. Potent vasoactive peptides, prostaglandins, and leukotrienes may thus be released and may play a role in alterations in local and systemic hemodynamics observed in conjunction with immunologically induced renal diseases. Polymorphonuclear leukocytes, eosinophils, and monocytes (macrophages) and platelets all may be called forth to participate in immune-mediated injury to varying degrees. Polymorphonuclear leukocytes and monocytes appear to participate in glomerular injury by virtue of their ability to release factors locally which are capable of degrading basement membrane glycoproteins enzymatically and by facilitating the local production of toxic oxygen species (hydroxyl radical and superoxide anion). Activated monocytes may also express a membrane-bound procoagulant, thus fostering local fibrin deposition. Platelet deposition may be involved in the proliferation of glomerular cells via the release of a platelet-derived growth factor or may alter the anionic charge of the capillary wall by local release of cationic proteins, thus facilitating altered glomerular permselectivity. The composite result of these events is to alter the structural and functional integrity of the glomerular capillary and/or peritubular capillary wall, and lead to reduced filtration capacity, enhanced permeability to plasma proteins, and migration of cellular elements (i.e., erythrocytes and leukocytes) outside the intravascular compartment.

ANTITISSUE ANTIBODY–MEDIATED RENAL INJURY **Anti-basement membrane antibody disease** This form of renal injury is relatively rare in humans, accounting for less than 5 percent of all immunologically mediated glomerulonephritides. By mechanisms which remain obscure, autoantibodies (usually of the IgG isotype) which are directed to epitopes on noncollagenous domains of type IV (basement membrane) collagen arise in the circulation. These autoantibodies deposit in basement membranes of the kidney (glomerular basement membrane, GBM, and/or tubular basement membrane, TBM) and on occasion elsewhere (alveolar basement membrane, choroid plexus basement membrane). Since the epitope is a part of a repeating subunit uniformly expressed in basement membrane, the deposits of IgG will appear *linear* when studied by immunofluorescence microscopy (Fig. 222-1*A*). Electron-dense lattices of antigen and antibody complexes are not seen by electron microscopy. The local interaction of the autoantibody with the fixed and native basement membrane antigen leads to local activation of mediator systems as described above.

Although the activation of the complement cascade facilitates injury by virtue of chemotactic and cytolytic effects, glomerular injury may occur independent of complement activation. Proteinuria results from loss of glomerular anionic residues (see Chap. 40) and by structural defects in the capillary wall. Glomerular filtration rate may decline if the loss of filtering surface area is sufficient to overcome adaptive increases in capillary flows and pressures in remaining nephron units. Leakage of macromolecules and cells such as fibrinogen and monocytes into Bowman's space through gaps in the capillary wall may provoke extracapillary proliferation (crescents) as fibrinogen is polymerized to fibrin and monocytes divide, proliferate, and release monokines locally.

Renal disease due to anti-basement membrane autoantibody production is seen primarily in three circumstances: in connection with glomerulonephritis and pulmonary hemorrhage due to anti-GBM autoantibodies (Goodpasture's syndrome), in idiopathic crescentic glomerulonephritis due to anti-GBM antibodies (without pulmonary hemorrhage), and in idiopathic tubulointerstitial nephritis due to anti-TBM antibody production. In all instances, characteristic findings are present which serve to identify the pathogenic mechanism underlying the disease: (1) circulating autoantibodies reactive with basement membrane antigens in vitro are present; (2) linear deposits of IgG are found in the involved tissue; and (3) eluates of diseased tissue will contain Ig reactive with normal, native basement membrane antigens both in vivo and in vitro.

Other nonglomerular basement membrane–related antitissue antibody diseases It now seems clear that the glomerular capillary wall and mesangium are composed of a number of potentially immunogenic glycoproteins other than the classic GBM glycoprotein mentioned above. These antigens are distributed in various patterns along the glomerular capillary wall and/or within the mesangium and are probably biochemically distinct structural components of the glomerulus. Binding in situ of passively administered heterologous antibody or the actively induced autoantibody to these antigens will therefore produce differing patterns of immunoglobulin localization and functional and structural alterations of the capillary wall. If the antigen is localized in clusters in relation to the capillary wall the reaction with antibody in situ may give rise to discontinuous deposits of Ig detected by immunofluorescence and to electron-dense deposits noted on electron microscopy. While the number of possible antigen-antibody interactions in this category is quite large, very few have in fact been documented to be responsible for human glomerular or tubulointerstitial disease. Thus far, animal experimentation has proceeded at a greater pace than understanding of human analogues of this mechanism. The best-studied animal model is Heymann's nephritis, which is induced in rats by passive administration of a heterologous antibody to a particular glomerular capillary wall antigen or by active immunization with the antigen in complete Freund's adjuvant. The antigen-antibody interaction occurs in the subepithelial space of the glomerulus and at the brush border of the proximal tubule, where the antigen is synthesized as a component of endocytotic, clathrin-coated pits on the surface of the glomerular visceral and proximal tubular epithelial cells. A granular pattern of IgG deposits and subepithelial dense deposits are seen by immunofluorescence and electron microscopy, respectively. A similar mechanism might account for some instances of idiopathic membranous glomerulonephritis in man.

Finally, it is also now well recognized that circulating endogenous or environmental substances having special biologic or biochemical affinity for glomerular structures, including the glomerular capillary wall or mesangium, may deposit in these structures in a nonimmunologic fashion and thus act as a "planted" antigen. An antibody or cellular response to these planted nonglomerular antigens could result in disease upon the formation of antigen-antibody complexes in situ. The pattern of disease produced would depend upon the sites of deposition of the planted antigen and the nature of the immune response. Examples of such planted antigens thus far described include certain drugs, plant lectins, cationized plasma proteins, aggregated immunoglobulins, and deoxyribonucleic acid. Several experimental models of this pathogenic sequence have been described, but there is little definitive information concerning the prevalence of this mechanism in human renal disease.

IMMUNE-COMPLEX–MEDIATED RENAL INJURY (See Chap. 261) **Circulating immune-complex disease** The deposition in the kidney of immune complexes formed in the circulation accounts for the majority of diseases of the kidney for which there is clear evidence of participation of some immunologic process. In this category an immunogenic replicating or nonreplicating substance arises in the circulation either from an endogenous (autologous) or exogenous

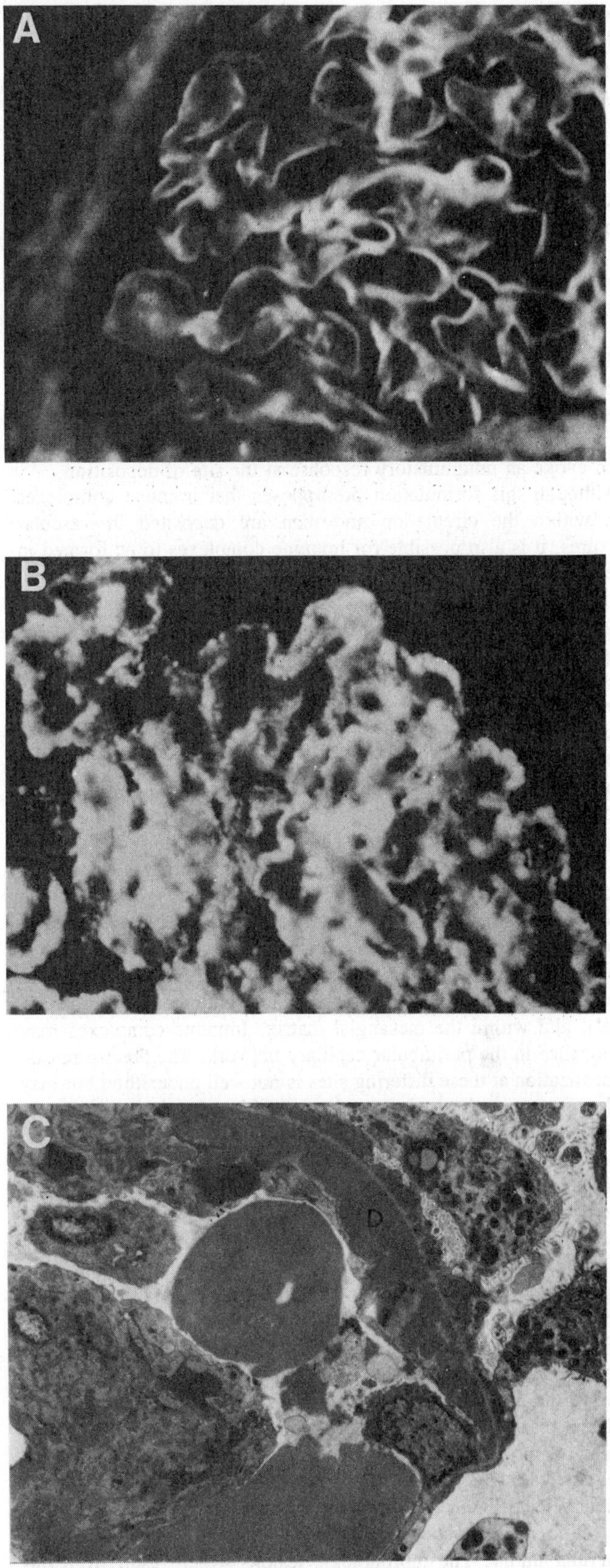

FIGURE 222-1 *A. Immunofluorescence photomicrograph of a portion of a glomerulus from a patient with antiglomerular basement membrane antibody–mediated glomerular injury. Note the linear deposits (fluorescein-labeled antihuman IgG). B. Immunofluorescence photomicrograph of a portion of a glomerulus from a patient with immune-complex–mediated glomerular injury. Note the irregular, granular deposits (fluorescein-labeled antihuman IgG). C. Electron micrograph of a portion of a glomerular capillary from a patient with immune-complex–mediated glomerular injury. Note the electron-dense deposits (D).*

(environmental) source. Antibody response to the antigen occurring while the antigen remains in the circulation leads to the formation of an aggregate of antigen and antibody known as a *circulating immune complex*. A small fraction of circulating immune complexes may escape removal by the mononuclear phagocyte system and instead be trapped by vascular structures including the glomeruli. Circulating immune complexes trapped in these sites have the capability of evoking inflammation utilizing many of the mediator systems described above. One of the best-studied examples of this circulating immune-complex disease involving a nonreplicating antigen is serum sickness, which results from the acute or chronic administration of an immunogenic, soluble, heterologous, foreign serum protein (see Fig. 261-1). A small portion of the immune complexes will then localize within the glomerular mesangium; in the walls of peripheral capillaries; and in joints, heart valves, choroid plexus, splenic sinusoids, and larger blood vessels, particularly at sites of turbulent flow. Once deposited, these complexes possess unique properties which evoke an inflammatory response at the site of deposition.

Although this formulation presupposes that immune complexes form within the circulation and then are deposited in vascular structures, it is also possible for immune complexes to be formed in the extravascular (interstitial) compartment by virtue of diffusion into this fluid compartment of cell-derived antigens and circulating antibody. Such a phenomenon may explain the deposition of immune complexes in the interstitial areas of the kidney, with relative sparing of the glomerular circulation. Regardless of the nature of the antibody or antigen or the particular circumstances surrounding the immunologic events, a valuable clue to the presence of immune-complex deposition is the morphologic pattern found when tissues are examined by immunofluorescence or electron microscopic techniques. Granular, discontinuous, and irregular deposits of Ig, often in conjunction with complement components, are found by immunofluorescence (Fig. 222-1*B*), whereas electron-dense deposits are seen by electron microscopy (Fig. 222-1*C*). Sometimes these deposits acquire a definite substructure, but for the most part they are rather homogeneous. The deposits may develop in several locations within the glomerulus: beneath the epithelial cells (subepithelial), within the basement membrane (intramembranous), beneath the endothelium (subendothelial), and within the mesangial matrix. Immune complexes may also localize in the peritubular capillary network. The precise reason for localization at these differing sites is not well understood but may involve factors such as size or charge of the complexes, receptors for the Fc or complement components within glomerular structures, or local hemodynamic events. The deposits appear to increase in size by aggregation, and there is some evidence that glomerular cells may participate in their removal. The persistence of deposits is related to the rate of formation balanced by the activity of removal systems. Ig itself in a circulating immune complex trapped in the glomerular circulation may behave as a planted antigen, either via the idiotypic determinants present in the antigen-binding sites of antibody or via the Fc portions evoking an anti-immunoglobulin (rheumatoid factor) response. The roles played by anti-idiotype antibody or rheumatoid factor in the evolution of glomerular lesions in immune-complex–mediated disease is not yet clear. Once deposited in glomeruli, circulating immune complexes evoke local inflammatory and functional changes, which at least for the glomerular circulation may be relatively independent of complement or polymorphonuclear leukocytes. Infiltrating monocytes may play a critical role in mediating glomerular injury. The morphologic lesions which result from immune-complex deposition may vary considerably, from diffuse proliferative to nonproliferative membranous or sclerosing lesions. Coagulation, platelet aggregation, activation of the complement cascade, and release of vasoactive amines may participate in determining the pattern of morphologic response.

The *exogenous* antigens involved in circulating immune-complex–mediated disease are derived chiefly from infectious agents such as bacteria, viruses, or parasites. Replication of the organism provides a continuing source of antigen. The best-studied examples of these in humans are *infective endocarditis, leprosy, syphilis, hepatitis B,* and *malaria*. The *endogenous* antigens involved in human disease vary considerably and include *DNA, thyroglobulin, autologous immunoglobulins, erythrocyte stroma, renal tubule antigens,* and *tumor-specific* or *tumor-associated* antigens.

COMPLEMENT-ASSOCIATED GLOMERULAR INJURY Although there is little evidence that complement activation, independent of antitissue antibody or circulating immune complexes, can bring about glomerular injury, there are certain associations between complement and renal disease in humans. The clinicopathologic entity known as *idiopathic mesangiocapillary glomerulonephritis* (see also Chap. 223) may be associated with patterns of serum complement component deposition within glomeruli suggestive of involvement of the alternative pathway of complement activation, perhaps independent of immune-complex deposition. These patterns are not, however, necessarily unique to this group of disorders since they may also be observed in a wide variety of postinfectious glomerulonephritides and in certain collagen-vascular diseases.

As discussed in greater detail in Chap. 62, the alternative pathway mechanism of complement activation depends upon the interaction of aggregated or immune-complex IgA, polysaccharides, or lipopolysaccharides with factors B, D of the alternative pathway system and C3 of the classical complement cascade. Subsequently, an enzyme capable of cleaving native C3 is assembled, composed of a fragment of C3 (C3b) and an altered form of factor B (Bb). This alternative pathway C3 convertase is analogous to the C3 convertase generated in the classic pathway of complement activation. The alternative pathway C3 convertase is stabilized by binding to properdin and degraded by several inactivators (C3b inactivator, β1H). Alternative pathway C3 convertase cleaves C3 into C3a (anaphylatoxin I) and C3b, which is further cleaved by C3 inactivator into C3c and C3d, biologically inactive fragments. The C3b formed in this manner can also autocatalytically form additional alternative pathway C3 convertase in the presence of factors B, D, and of Mg^{2+}. The hallmarks of activation of the alternative pathway are depressed serum levels of native C3, circulating fragments of C3 (C3c, C3d), low levels of factor B, and circulating fragments of B (Bb), all occurring in the absence of perturbations in the early classic components C1q, C4, and C2. The terminal complement components C5 through C9 may also be activated and even result in lysis of cells in the absence of antibody. Depression of the synthesis of C3 may also contribute to diminished serum levels, since circulating fragments of C3 may reduce cellular production.

In *idiopathic mesangiocapillary glomerulonephritis,* particularly the subset known as *dense deposit disease,* serum C3 levels are depressed; C4, C1, and C2 levels tend to be normal; and C3 may be deposited in glomeruli without Ig (see also Chap. 223). In addition, an oligoclonal autoantibody (an immunoconglutinin) to alternative pathway C3 convertase is frequently found in the circulation. This autoantibody reacts with a conformational neoantigen of the alternative pathway C3 convertase and acts to stabilize this enzyme from the influence of C3b inactivator and β1H in a fashion similar to properdin. As a result serums containing this autoantibody are capable of inducing C3 cleavage in vitro by permitting the assembly of a stable fluid phase C3 convertase. This antibody is also known as C3 nephritic factor (C3NeF) and was first described in the serums of patients with glomerulonephritis and persistent depression of C3 levels.

The relationship between these aberrations in the complement pathway and glomerular injury is uncertain. No experimental models of persistent activation of the alternative pathway have been associated with glomerulonephritis; thus, glomerular injury may be a closely associated but pathogenically unrelated phenomenon, perhaps genetically determined. The recognition that certain structural genes for complement components (C2, C4) are closely associated with the major histocompatibility complex provides a potential explanation for the association of disease susceptibility with defects in biosynthesis of complement proteins. On the other hand, some have suggested that persistent hypocomplementemia may interfere with the normal removal processes for environmental antigens such as viruses. Such a defect might favor the persistence of these antigens in the circulation and enhance the likelihood of formation of circulating immune complexes. The discovery that C3 and its degradation product (primarily C3b) are able to solubilize aggregates of antigen and antibody may provide an additional explanation for the occurrence of immune-complex disease in association with defects of complement synthesis or activation.

CELL-MEDIATED IMMUNITY IN GLOMERULAR AND TUBULOINTERSTITIAL DISEASES The roles of specifically sensitized cells acting independently of antibody (T cytotoxic cells), "armed" macrophages, and antibody-dependent cell-mediated cytotoxicity in the pathogenesis of glomerular and tubulointerstitial diseases have been difficult to establish firmly. The glomerulus and more than likely the cortical interstitium possess all of the necessary elements to support a cell-mediated response to an autologous or heterologous antigen. Mononuclear cells capable of processing antigen and activating T-helper inducer cells in a major histocompatibility complex–restricted fashion are present in the glomerular mesangium and interstitium. A number of experimental diseases of the kidney, most notably tubulointerstitial nephritis, have been developed which are uniquely the consequence of a cell-mediated immune response. However, at the present time, relatively few human diseases can be ascribed with certainty to cell-mediated immune processes exclusively. The rejection of renal allografts in nonsensitized recipients is clearly a cell-mediated process. This subject is dealt with in greater detail in Chap. 221.

It is true that by utilizing a variety of in vitro techniques cell-mediated hypersensitivity to both environmental and endogenous antigens may be demonstrable in several diseases of the kidney, including glomerulonephritis. The precise role such "sensitized" cells play in the actual tissue injury is unclear, especially in human glomerular disease. No doubt the burgeoning knowledge in the field of cell-cell interactions will eventually clarify these uncertainties. It is very likely that some diseases which do not fit into an antibody- or immune-complex–mediated category will find an explanation in reactions of the cell-mediated variety. One likely candidate for this category is so-called minimal change disease, one of the morphologic subsets of idiopathic nephrotic syndrome. Furthermore, because of the prominence of lymphoid cell infiltration, various forms of chronic tubulointerstitial nephritis have also been suggested as examples of cell-mediated reactions (see Chap. 226).

REFERENCES

BRENTJENS JR, et al: Immunologically mediated lesions of kidney tubules and interstitium of laboratory animals and man. Springer Semin Immunopathol 5:357, 1982

CUMMINGS NB et al: *Immune Mechanisms in Renal Disease.* New York, Plenum Medical Book Co., 1983

GLASSOCK RJ, COHEN AH: Immunologically mediated renal disease, in *Contemporary Nephrology,* S Klahr and S Massry (eds). New York, Plenum Medical Book Co., 1985, vol 3

NEALE TJ, WILSON CB: Glomerular antigens in glomerulonephritis. Springer Semin Immunopathol 5:221, 1982

WILLIAMS DG, PETERS DK: The immunology of nephritis, in *Clinical Aspects of Immunology,* 4th ed, PJ Lachmann and DK Peters (eds). Oxford, Blackwell, 1982, p 853

WILSON CB, DIXON FJ: Renal response to immunological injury, in *The Kidney,* 3d ed, BM Brenner and FC Rector Jr (eds). Philadelphia, Saunders, 1986, p 800

223 THE MAJOR GLOMERULOPATHIES

RICHARD J. GLASSOCK / BARRY M. BRENNER

Disease-induced alterations of the structural and functional integrity of the glomerular capillary circulation are often associated with the findings, either singly or in combination, of hematuria, proteinuria, reduced glomerular filtration rate (GFR), and hypertension. Five major glomerulopathic syndromes are recognized: *acute glomerulonephritis, rapidly progressive glomerulonephritis, chronic glomerulonephritis,* the *nephrotic syndrome,* and *asymptomatic urinary abnormalities.* This chapter deals with each of these syndromes in some detail, describing diseases in which the kidney is either the sole or predominant organ involved (i.e., the primary glomerulopathies) or is involved as a complication of infection or drug exposure. Glomerular injury associated with multisystem disorders or heredofamilial conditions is discussed in Chap. 224.

ACUTE GLOMERULONEPHRITIS (AGN)

The causes of AGN are given in Table 223-1. The "acute nephritic syndrome" consists of the abrupt onset of *hematuria* and *proteinuria,* accompanied by evidence of *azotemia* (i.e., reduced GFR) and renal *salt and water retention.* If GFR is reduced markedly, oligoanuria may be present (see also Chap. 219). Salt and water retention leads to circulatory congestion, hypertension, and edema. Hematuria is most likely the consequence of migration of erythrocytes across damaged glomerular and/or peritubular capillary walls leading to the addition of erythrocytes to tubule fluid in the early part of the nephron. Proteinuria is the consequence of either a loss of anionic charges of the capillary wall (charge-selective defect) or the appearance of a population of glomerular capillaries with larger-than-normal pore radius, permitting large plasma protein molecules to traverse the glomerular filter. Glomerular filtration rate is reduced presumably because of infiltration of the capillaries by inflammatory cells, which thereby reduce filtering surface area. Extensive crescentic disease may obliterate Bowman's space, further impeding filtration. Fluid retention is due in part to decreased glomerular filtration rate but also to persistence of avid distal nephron salt and water reabsorption. Extracellular and intravascular fluid volumes are expanded by primary renal salt and fluid retention.

The edema of acute glomerulonephritis tends to appear initially in areas of low tissue pressure, such as the *periorbital* areas, but may subsequently progress to involve dependent portions of the body and lead to *ascites* and/or *pleural effusions. Circulatory congestion* is manifested by an increase in systemic and pulmonary vascular pressures, normal or increased cardiac output, and a shortened circulation time. In the absence of underlying valvular, myocardial, or coronary artery disease or severe diastolic hypertension there is little likelihood that true left ventricular congestive heart failure will

TABLE 223-1 Causes of acute glomerulonephritis

I Infectious diseases
- *A* Poststreptococcal glomerulonephritis
- *B* Nonpoststreptococcal glomerulonephritis
  - *1* Bacterial: infective endocarditis, "shunt nephritis," sepsis, pneumococcal pneumonia, typhoid fever, secondary syphilis, meningococcemia
  - *2* Viral: hepatitis B, infectious mononucleosis, mumps, measles, varicella, vaccinia, echovirus, and coxsackievirus
  - *3* Parasitic: malaria, toxoplasmosis

II Multisystem diseases: systemic lupus erythematosus, vasculitis, Henoch-Schönlein purpura, Goodpasture's syndrome

III Primary glomerular diseases: mesangiocapillary glomerulonephritis, Berger's disease, "pure" mesangial proliferative glomerulonephritis

IV Miscellaneous: Guillain-Barré syndrome, irradiation of Wilms's tumor, self-administered diphtheria-pertussis-tetanus vaccine, serum sickness develop. If pulmonary capillary pressure rises above the opposing plasma oncotic pressure, however, pulmonary edema may ensue. *Arterial diastolic hypertension* is the consequence of several factors, including extracellular fluid volume expansion, enhanced cardiac output, and modest increases in peripheral vascular resistance. Plasma renin activity, aldosterone, and the sympathetic nervous system are relatively suppressed. Hypertension may at times be accompanied by encephalopathy, particularly in young children.

The extent and severity of urinary abnormalities in AGN vary considerably. Gross (macroscopic) *hematuria* is the most common, and is often described by the patient as smoky-, coffee-, or cola-colored urine. Lesser degrees of hematuria may go unrecognized by the patient or parent; for this reason, the features of fluid retention and hypertension may be ascribed erroneously to other illnesses if a careful examination of the urine sediment is omitted from the initial laboratory evaluation. Hematuria is often, but not invariably, accompanied by the excretion of *red cell casts.* The erythrocytes in the urinary sediment are characteristically distorted, fragmented, and hypochromic (dysmorphic hematuria). Leukocyturia and leukocyte casts may also occur, indicating the presence of inflammation in the glomerulus and interstitium. The degree of *proteinuria* varies according to the nature and severity of the underlying glomerular lesions. Rarely, protein excretion rates may fall within the normal range, but generally are between 0.2 and 3 g per day. If proteinuria is marked and sustained, features of the nephrotic syndrome may appear (see below).

The short-term evolution of acute nephritis generally depends upon the nature of the underlying glomerular lesion; however, within a week or so of onset most patients with postinfectious AGN will begin to experience spontaneous resolution of fluid retention and hypertension. Urinary abnormalities often take longer to resolve. A few patients with the acute nephritic syndrome will go on in the ensuing weeks or months to develop a rapidly progressive form of renal failure (i.e., rapidly progressive glomerulonephritis, discussed below). The long-term outlook for patients with AGN is considered below in the context of treatment of specific lesions. Renal biopsy is useful in characterizing the nature of the underlying lesion but need not be done in every case (see below).

ACUTE POSTSTREPTOCOCCAL GLOMERULONEPHRITIS (PSGN)

Clinical features and diagnosis This disorder can be viewed as the archetype of AGN. PSGN follows in the wake of *pharyngeal or cutaneous infection* with one of a limited number of strains of *group A β-hemolytic streptococci.* These potentially "nephritogenic" streptococci may be identified by serotyping of a cell wall antigen (M protein). Among outbreaks of infection with proved "nephritogenic" strains of streptococci the PSGN attack rate is relatively uniform, but because of variation in the nephritogenicity among group A streptococci, attack rates with outbreaks of infection may vary considerably. Among families, asymptomatic episodes of PSGN exceed symptomatic episodes by a factor of 3 or 4 to 1. Immunity to M protein is type-specific, long-lasting, and protective. Repeated episodes of PSGN are therefore unusual. Outbreaks of pharyngeal infection–associated PSGN are commonest in children aged 6 to 10. AGN following cutaneous streptococcal infection is more commonly associated with factors such as poor personal hygiene, overcrowding, and concomitant cutaneous disease, such as scabies infestation. Seasonal and geographic variations in prevalence of PSGN are more marked for pharyngeal- than for cutaneous-associated disease.

An important feature of PSGN is the existence of a *latent period* between the earliest manifestations of infection and the onset of recognizable signs and symptoms of nephritis. The latent period is more apparent following pharyngeal infections, where it usually is 6 to 10 days in duration. Cutaneous infections are associated with longer latent periods, averaging about 2 weeks. Definitive signs of glomerular inflammation occurring at the same time as, or shortly after, infection usually indicate an *exacerbation* of a preexisting chronic glomerular disease such as Berger's disease (IgA nephropathy) (see below).

The diagnosis of PSGN rests upon the demonstration of at least two of the following features: (1) The presence of a group A β-hemolytic streptococcus of a potentially nephritogenic M-protein type in a throat or skin lesion. (2) The demonstration of an immune response to one or more of the streptococcal *exoenzymes,* including anti-streptolysin O (ASO), antistreptokinase (ASK), anti-deoxyribonuclease B (ADNAase B), anti-nicotinyl adenine dinucleotidase (ANADase), or antihyaluronidase (AH). ASO responses are typically brisk in pharyngeal infections, but often absent in cutaneous infection; whereas AH, ADNAase, and ANADase responses occur after the latter. Testing for multiple antibody responses and serial determinations is necessary to achieve a diagnostic accuracy of 90 percent. Early antimicrobial therapy may prevent the antibody response to exoenzymes and render throat cultures negative, but may not interfere with the development of PSGN; this makes accurate serologic diagnosis difficult or impossible. (3) The demonstration of a transient decline in the serum concentration of the C3 component of complement, with a return to normal within 8 weeks after the first signs of renal disease. Other complement components (i.e., C1q and C4) are frequently less depressed. In addition to these laboratory features it is desirable to document a latent period appropriate to the nature of the infection. Furthermore, the patient should not have any known preexisting renal disease.

Other laboratory features commonly observed in PSGN include transient cryoimmunoglobulinemia, positive tests for circulating immune complexes, and circulating high-molecular-weight fibrinogen complexes. The erythrocyte sedimentation rate is usually elevated, while C-reactive protein and rheumatoid factor are generally normal or absent. Mild anemia and hypoalbuminemia, both largely dilutional in origin, may be present. Severe hypoalbuminemia may be encountered if heavy proteinuria is present and prolonged. Excretion rates of urinary protein in excess of 3.5 g per day occur in less than 20 percent of hospitalized patients. Proteinuria is usually of a nonselective character and frequently contains high concentrations of fibrin-degradation products (FDP) and C3 protein, particularly during the diuretic phase. Hyponatremia, hyperchloremia, hyperkalemia, and metabolic acidosis may be seen in azotemic or oliguric patients, especially those having free access to water or potassium. Urinary sodium concentration is usually low, reflecting avid salt reabsorption in the distal nephron. Abdominal films reveal normal or enlarged kidneys. The chest x-ray may be normal or reveal a slightly enlarged heart, often accompanied by signs of pulmonary congestion. The electrocardiogram may reveal nonspecific T-wave abnormalities. Rheumatic fever rarely coexists with acute PSGN.

The differential diagnosis of PSGN includes other infectious or primary renal diseases which may produce an identical acute nephritic syndrome (Table 223-1). Multisystem diseases such as SLE, Henoch-Schönlein purpura, and vasculitis may present initially as acute nephritis (Chap. 224). Predominantly nonglomerular diseases, including thrombotic thrombocytopenic purpura, hemolytic-uremic syndrome, atheroembolic renal disease, and acute hypersensitivity interstitial nephritis may also present the features of the acute nephritic syndrome (Chaps. 226 and 227).

Pathology and pathogenesis Renal biopsies performed early in the course of PSGN reveal *diffuse, endocapillary proliferative glomerulonephritis.* Infiltration of glomeruli with polymorphonuclear leukocytes and monocytes is also common. The glomerular capillary walls are usually thin and delicate and free of necrosis. Occasional discrete proteinaceous deposits projecting from the outer aspects of the capillary wall toward the urinary space (humps) may be recognized by light microscopy and coincide with the electron-dense deposits seen by electron microscopy. Segmental extracapillary proliferation (crescents) may involve a few glomeruli, but diffuse crescent formation is uncommon except among a subset of patients presenting with severe and rapidly progressive acute renal failure (see section below on rapidly progressive glomerulonephritis). Extraglomerular vessels and tubulointerstitial areas are usually normal. Red blood cells are frequently seen in the lumens of distal tubules, where they form red blood cell casts and dysmorphic erythrocytes.

By immunofluorescence microscopy, granular deposits of IgG are seen in peripheral capillary loops and mesangium, nearly always accompanied by C3 and properdin, but less commonly by C1q and C4 (Chap. 222). A variety of patterns of Ig and/or C3 deposition has been described. Extensive involvement of the peripheral capillary loops with deposits may be associated with a poorer prognosis, while deposits exclusively involving the mesangium usually indicate a more benign outcome. The precise nature of the antigen-antibody systems involved remains unknown. Most likely the antigen is derived from the streptococcal organism itself, but this has been difficult to verify. The profile of altered serum complement components described above, and the prominent C3 and properdin deposition in glomeruli, are suggestive of involvement of the alternative pathway of complement activation (Chap. 222).

Course and treatment The ultimate *prognosis* for PSGN appears to differ between sporadic and epidemic forms and between adults and children. *Epidemic* forms of the disease in *children* have a uniformly favorable short- and long-term prognosis. Few patients die of complications of renal failure (fewer than 1 percent), and nearly all experience a spontaneous resolution of abnormal clinical signs within a week after the onset of illness. Abnormalities in the urinary sediment and protein excretion subside slowly in the ensuing months; in a few cases, several years elapse before the urinary sediment becomes consistently normal. Among children with PSGN during epidemics of streptococcal infection, and in whom some form of preexisting chronic glomerular disease was absent, long-term follow-up has revealed little or no evidence of progression to chronic renal disease. A very small percentage may develop extensive crescentic glomerulonephritis with its relentlessly progressive course. The site of the streptococcal infection, the type of M protein, the severity in abnormalities of complement components or urinary sediment, or the extent of the rise in antibody response to exoenzymes have little or no bearing on the ultimate prognosis of PSGN. Prolonged and persistent heavy proteinuria and/or abnormal GFR imply a more unfavorable outcome. *Sporadic* cases of PSGN among *children* may have more serious long-term consequences, although this remains controversial. After the subsidence of the acute disease, some children subsequently develop slowly progressive glomerular capillary obliteration (glomerulosclerosis), reduced GFR, and hypertension; after several decades, end-stage renal failure from chronic glomerulonephritis may result. The persistence of abnormal proteinuria is the rule in such cases.

The prognosis for *adults* with PSGN seems to be less favorable than for children. The reason for this apparent age difference is poorly understood. Although the overall prognosis for PSGN in *epidemics* seems good, *sporadic* PSGN in adults appears to be associated with lasting and/or progressive deterioration in renal function in as many as one-third to one-half of all cases. This may take the form of persistent proteinuria and/or hematuria, or of slowly progressive glomerulosclerosis and renal failure, often accompanied by hypertension. This evolution seems more likely to occur when the initial disease has been unusually severe. Whether milder forms of sporadic PSGN can lead to chronic disease is an important but unresolved issue (see "Chronic Glomerulonephritis" below).

The *treatment* of acute PSGN is supportive. It seems reasonable to recommend bed rest until the signs of glomerular inflammation and circulatory congestion (primarily hypertension) subside, but prolonged forced periods of inactivity are of no demonstrable benefit in the healing process. Fluid retention, circulatory congestion, and edema may be treated with sodium and fluid restriction, or loop diuretics. Diuresis alone will often ameliorate mild to moderate hypertension. If severe hypertension is present, vasodilator drugs such as nitroprusside, nifedipine, hydralazine, or diazoxide may be useful. Encephalopathy and pulmonary congestion will generally improve with lowering of blood pressure and the relief of circulatory overload. Digitalis preparations should be avoided except in instances of well-documented organic heart disease with congestive failure. Treatment with ion exchange resins and/or dialysis may be required for cases of severe oliguria, fluid overload, and hyperkalemia. Mild protein restriction is desirable for azotemic patients. A 7- to 10-day course of antimicrobials (e.g., penicillin or erythromycin) should be given if streptococcal infection is documented. Long-term chemoprophylaxis is not indicated. Steroids and cytotoxic drugs have not been shown to be of value.

NONSTREPTOCOCCAL ACUTE GLOMERULONEPHRITIS Clinical features and diagnosis A variety of infectious illnesses other than those caused by group A β-hemolytic streptococci may also be associated with AGN (Table 223-1). These include *bacteremic states* and various *viral* and *parasitic* diseases. Ordinarily these diseases can be diagnosed by the presence of typical extrarenal clinical features or by bacteriologic or serologic findings. Infective endocarditis, visceral sepsis, typhoid fever, infectious mononucleosis, acute viral hepatitis (hepatitis B), falciparum malaria, and toxoplasmosis represent examples of infectious diseases capable of evoking AGN. A substantial body of evidence indicates that circulating immune complexes play an important role in the pathogenesis of AGN in these diseases. Bacteremic states are frequently associated with persistent depression of serum concentrations of complement components C1q, C4, and C3, elevated levels of rheumatoid factor, circulating cryoimmunoglobulins, and strongly positive tests for circulating immune complexes. Control of infection usually results in the resolution of the signs of glomerular inflammation, although, in occasional instances, rapidly progressive or chronic glomerulonephritis may ensue.

RAPIDLY PROGRESSIVE GLOMERULONEPHRITIS (RPGN)

Transient azotemia, often associated with a brief period of oliguria, is commonly observed in AGN. A diuresis usually follows within days or a few weeks and GFR returns to normal. On the other hand, some cases of AGN are characterized by a *rapidly progressive* form of renal failure, which often develops abruptly and displays little tendency for spontaneous or complete recovery. The clinical term *rapidly progressive glomerulonephritis* (*RPGN*) is often applied to this group to connote the development of renal failure in a period of weeks to months, rather than years or decades, as is typical of chronic glomerulonephritis (see below). Usually, but not invariably, extensive *extracapillary* (*crescentic*) *glomerulonephritis* is found as the pathologic lesion underlying the syndrome of RPGN, and the two terms are often used interchangeably.

RPGN can arise in three clinical settings (Table 223-2): (1) as a renal complication of an acute or subacute infectious disease, (2) as a renal complication of many multisystem diseases, and (3) as a

TABLE 223-2 Causes of rapidly progressive glomerulonephritis

I Infectious diseases
- *A* Poststreptococcal glomerulonephritis
- *B* Infective endocarditis
- *C* Occult visceral sepsis

II Multisystem diseases
- *A* Systemic lupus erythematosus
- *B* Henoch-Schönlein purpura
- *C* Vasculitis (including Wegener's granulomatosis)
- *D* Goodpasture's syndrome
- *E* Essential cryoimmunoglobulinemia
- *F* Malignancy (rare)

III Primary glomerular diseases
- *A* Idiopathic crescentic glomerulonephritis
- *B* Mesangiocapillary glomerulonephritis
- *C* Berger's disease (rare)
- *D* Membranous glomerulonephritis complicated by anti-glomerular basement membrane antibody formation (rare)

primary or idiopathic glomerular disease. The first category is discussed in Chap. 222, the second in Chap. 224, and the third will be considered here.

IDIOPATHIC RAPIDLY PROGRESSIVE GLOMERULONEPHRITIS

Clinical features and diagnosis This disorder affects individuals in a broad age distribution and has a predilection for males. Wide geographic differences in the prevalence of the disease have been noted, and outbreaks (''miniepidemics'') may occur. Some patients have had recent heavy exposure to volatile hydrocarbons, but there is little evidence to support a cause-and-effect relationship. While a flulike or viral prodrome may occur, frank arthritis, sinusitis, otitis, skin rash, neuritis, or encephalopathy are uncommon and are more in keeping with a multisystem disease. Symptoms of weakness, nausea, and vomiting (indicative of azotemia) usually dominate the clinical picture. Oliguria, abdominal or flank pain, and hemoptysis may also be present (see ''Goodpasture's Syndrome,'' Chap. 224). The blood pressure is usually normal or only modestly elevated. Urinalysis typically reveals dysmorphic hematuria and red cell casts, but exceptional cases with relatively benign urine sediments have been observed. Proteinuria is always present and may occasionally be massive. Other biochemical features of the nephrotic syndrome are uncommon, probably because of the concomitant reduction in GFR. Proteinuria is typically nonselective, and high concentrations of FDP are found in urine. Azotemia develops early and tends to progress at a rapid rate. Other clinical and laboratory features relate to the underlying pathology and pathogenesis.

Pathology and pathogenesis It is clear that idiopathic RPGN is far from a homogeneous disease. By light microscopy the characteristic abnormality found in the kidneys is *extensive extracapillary proliferation,* i.e., *crescents.* The extent and degree of glomerular involvement varies considerably; however, among patients with rapid deterioration of renal function it is usual for more than 70 percent of glomeruli to be involved with circumferential crescents. Endocapillary proliferation may also be seen but, if very prominent, suggests the presence of antigen-antibody complexes. Fibrin-related antigens are nearly always demonstrable within the crescents by special stains or by immunofluorescence. Gaps or focal discontinuities in the glomerular basement membrane (GBM) and/or Bowman's capsule are observed in association with crescents.

Variations in the underlying pathogenetic mechanisms responsible for RPGN are revealed by immunofluorescence studies of renal biopsies (Chap. 222). In approximately one-third of cases, *linear deposits* of IgG, often accompanied by C3, indicate involvement of *anti-GBM antibodies.* Circulating anti-GBM antibodies are found in this group by indirect immunofluorescence, hemagglutination, or radioimmunoassay techniques. Patients falling into this pathogenetic subgroup tend to have normal serum complement levels and a marked tendency to develop hemoptysis (see also ''Goodpasture's Syndrome,'' Chap. 224). About one-third of cases will have findings indicative of *immune-complex–mediated disease,* namely, *granular deposits* of immunoglobulin by immunofluorescence microscopy and electron-dense deposits by electron microscopy. This mechanism of RPGN tends to occur in older individuals, to produce more constitutional symptoms, and to result in more disturbances of the complement pathways than does anti-GBM antibody–mediated disease. Hemoptysis may also occur, but circulating anti-GBM antibodies are absent. The remainder of cases of RPGN reveal scanty or no immunoglobulins or complement by immunofluorescence; their pathogenesis is unknown. This group also tends to include older individuals, in whom serum complement concentrations are normal and anti-GBM antibodies are absent. Occasionally, mild hemoptysis may occur.

It is obvious from the foregoing discussion that lung hemorrhage may be observed in a variety of circumstances associated with RPGN. This subject is covered in greater detail in the section on Goodpasture's syndrome in Chap. 224. As noted in Table 223-2, other idiopathic (primary) renal diseases may, from time to time, be accompanied by a prominent tendency for crescent formation and a rapidly progressive course.

Course and treatment In general, the prognosis for preservation of renal function in RPGN is poor. Patients with crescent formation in 70 percent or more of glomeruli, oliguria or severe reduction in GFR (less than 5 mL/min) at the time of presentation, or an anti-GBM antibody–mediated process have the worst prognosis. Although advances in treatment are changing the outlook for patients with RPGN, at least one-half to two-thirds of patients currently require maintenance hemodialysis within 6 months of discovery of the illness. Exceptional patients with crescentic glomerulonephritis will have a more protracted illness. Spontaneous resolution is very uncommon, except among patients with infection as the basis for formation of antigen-antibody complexes, where removal of antigen can take place.

The treatment of RPGN is currently undergoing reevaluation. *Corticosteroids,* in the form of ''pulses'' of parenteral methylprednisolone in high doses, or continuous oral prednisone daily, often combined with *cytotoxic agents* (azathioprine or cyclophosphamide), have yielded varying degrees of success, particularly in the patients revealing granular or minimal Ig deposits in glomeruli. Since no controlled studies have yet been conducted, however, it is difficult to verify the exact value of these approaches. Nonetheless, more than two-thirds of patients treated with several ''pulses'' of intravenous methylprednisolone have experienced improvement in renal function often sufficient to avoid the necessity of dialysis for renal failure. The addition of *anticoagulants* (heparin or warfarin sodium) and antithrombotic agents (cyproheptadine, dipyridamole, sulfinpyrazone) seems rational on the basis of evidence suggesting involvement of the coagulation process in the genesis of crescent formation. However, objective evidence of benefit from such therapies in animals afflicted with experimentally induced crescentic glomerulonephritis has been inconsistent, in part because of variations in the severity of the disease models, the timing of treatment, and the nature of the anticoagulant or antithrombotic agent used. Anticoagulants may be hazardous in patients with advanced renal failure. *Ancrod,* a fibrinogenolytic agent not yet released in the United States, may also prove to be an effective agent. *Intensive plasma exchange* (plasmapheresis—2 to 4 liters of plasma daily or three times weekly), combined with steroids and cytotoxic agents, has been employed in patients with RPGN with very encouraging preliminary results, especially in patients revealing linear Ig deposits in glomeruli (anti-GBM antibody–mediated disease). Beneficial effects appear to be greatest when such combined therapy is instituted early in the course of disease, before glomerular abnormalities are advanced. Therefore, renal biopsy assessment of the nature, severity, and potential reversibility of disease is a vital aspect of evaluation of patients suspected of having rapidly progressive glomerulonephritis. Such renal biopsies should be performed early rather than late in the course of disease. Despite aggressive therapy, patients with oliguria continue to do poorly. Clearly, treatment must be individualized, and because regular dialysis therapy and/or transplantation are available to virtually all patients with RPGN, one should probably err on the side of a conservative approach, unless compelling evidence in support of potential reversibility is present.

RPGN may recur in the renal transplant. It is difficult to be certain of the precise risk in individual cases. At present it seems prudent to recommend that, after initiating dialysis, a period of 3 to 6 months be allowed to elapse before undertaking renal transplantation in patients who have circulating anti-GBM antibodies. There is no convincing evidence that bilateral nephrectomy in advance of transplantation reduces the risk of recurrent disease in the transplant.

THE NEPHROTIC SYNDROME (NS)

In its overt form, NS is characterized by *albuminuria, hypoalbuminemia, hyperlipidemia,* and *edema.* These abnormalities are direct or indirect consequences of excessive glomerular leakage of plasma proteins into the urine (see also Chaps. 28 and 40). The defects in the charge- or size-selective barriers of the glomerular capillary wall which underline the excessive filtration of plasma proteins can arise as a consequence of a wide variety of disease processes, including immunologic disorders, toxic injuries, metabolic abnormalities, biochemical defects, and vascular disorders. Thus, nephrotic syndrome should be viewed as a common end point of a variety of disease processes damaging the permeability properties of the glomerular capillary wall. *Heavy proteinuria* is the hallmark of the nephrotic state. Arbitrarily, protein excretion rates in excess of 3.5 g per 1.73 m^2 per day (or urinary protein concentration of greater than 3.5 mg/dL creatinine) are considered to be in the nephrotic range, primarily because proteinuria of this magnitude is seldom observed in tubulointerstitial and vascular diseases of the kidney. Sustained heavy proteinuria is often, but not invariably, accompanied by *hypoalbuminemia.* Excessive urinary losses, increased renal catabolism, and inadequate hepatic synthesis of albumin all contribute to this depression of plasma albumin. The resulting decrease in plasma oncotic pressure leads to a disturbance in the Starling forces acting across peripheral capillaries. Intravascular fluid migrates into the interstitial tissue (i.e., *edema*), particularly in areas of low tissue pressure. These disturbances initiate a series of homeostatic adjustments designed to correct the resulting deficit in effective plasma volume. These include activation of the renin-angiotensin-aldosterone system, enhanced antidiuretic hormone secretion, stimulation of the sympathetic nervous system, and perhaps a reduction in the secretion of a postulated "natriuretic hormone." These and other poorly understood adjustments lead to renal sodium and water retention, primarily because of avid reabsorption in distal nephron segments, resulting in unrelenting edema. The severity of edema correlates with the level of serum albumin and with the extent of urinary protein losses. The extent and severity of edema is significantly conditioned by the presence of other factors such as heart disease or peripheral vascular disease. Profound hypoalbuminemia may occasionally be associated with severe plasma volume reduction, postural hypotension, syncope, and shock. Very occasionally acute renal failure may occur. Although this formulation would indicate that nephrotic syndrome is invariably accompanied by a significant deficit in intravascular volume and homeostatically appropriate renal salt and water retention, this pattern is not always observed. In fact, measurements of plasma volume, renin, and aldosterone, and determination of the events underlying renal salt and water reabsorption have uncovered considerable heterogeneity in the pathophysiology of fluid volume homeostasis in the nephrotic syndrome. Some cases demonstrate expanded intravascular fluid volume and suppressed renin-aldosterone axis, presumably mediated by primary, non-aldosterone-dependent renal salt and fluid retention, resembling the pathophysiology of acute nephritis (see above). These patients often, but not invariably, have some decrease in GFR and structural glomerular lesions. At the other end of the spectrum are patients with overt hypovolemia, hyperreninemia, and avid, secondary renal salt retention. Serum albumin levels are low, extracellular fluid volume is expanded, and edema is usually present in both groups.

The diminished plasma oncotic pressure also appears to stimulate hepatic lipoprotein synthesis, and *hyperlipidemia* is a frequent accompaniment of the nephrotic state. Low-density lipoproteins and cholesterol are elevated most frequently, but as the plasma oncotic pressure falls to very low levels, very low density lipoproteins and triglycerides also increase. Excessive urinary losses of plasma protein factors regulating lipoprotein synthesis or disposal may also contribute to the hyperlipidemic state. Whether these lipid abnormalities contribute to accelerated atherosclerosis remains controversial. Lipid bodies (fatty casts, oval fat bodies) commonly appear in the urine.

Urine losses of plasma proteins other than albumin are also of importance in NS. Loss of thyroxine-binding globulin may produce abnormalities in thyroid function tests, including a low T4 and an enhanced resin T3 uptake. Loss of cholecalciferol-binding protein may lead to a vitamin D deficiency state, secondary hyperparathyroidism, and bone disease, and also may contribute to the hypocalcemia and hypocalciuria seen commonly in NS. Enhanced urinary excretion of transferrin may produce an iron-resistant microcytic, hypochromic anemia. Zinc and copper deficiency may result from urinary losses of metal-binding proteins. Loss of antithrombin III (heparin cofactor) in the urine may be associated with increased coagulability, which may or may not be balanced by losses of procoagulant factors in the urine. If it is not, it may produce a hypercoagulable state, and the increased tendency to thrombosis may lead to renal vein thrombosis.

Some patients with NS develop severe IgG deficiency, in part due to urinary losses and hypercatabolism. Low-molecular-weight complement components may also be lost in the urine and contribute to defects in the opsonization of bacteria. Various drug-binding proteins (chiefly albumin) may be decreased, altering the pharmacokinetic and toxicity properties of many drugs. Cellulose acetate electrophoresis of serum reveals, in addition to diminished albumin levels, increases of alpha and beta globulins.

COMPLICATIONS AND MANAGEMENT OF THE NEPHROTIC SYNDROME *Edema* should be managed cautiously and conservatively. Overly vigorous diuresis with potent loop diuretics (furosemide or ethacrynic acid) may result in an abrupt decline in effective plasma volume as the deficit in plasma oncotic pressure may preclude mobilization of the extracellular fluid into the intravascular compartment. This is more likely to occur if plasma volume is already diminished and may lead to further reduction in GFR, worsening azotemia, and postural hypotension. Severe extracellular volume depletion may predispose to the development of acute renal failure. The temptation to administer concentrated salt-poor albumin should be resisted, as nearly all the administered protein will be excreted in 24 to 48 h, so that any beneficial effect on plasma oncotic pressure will be transient. However, such treatment may be necessary in severely hypoalbuminemic patients suffering from profound postural symptoms or very refractory anasarca.

The treatment of *hyperlipidemia* is difficult at best and its influence on morbidity and mortality uncertain. Most agents effective in reducing cholesterol and/or triglyceride levels are either too toxic (e.g., clofibrate) or poorly tolerated (e.g., cholestyramine) for chronic use. The value of newer agents in the management of hyperlipidemia in NS is not well established.

The *thromboembolic complications* of NS are reasonably common and have a broad range of clinical manifestations, including spontaneous peripheral venous and/or arterial thromboses, as well as pulmonary arterial and renal venous occlusions. *Renal vein thrombosis* (RVT), either unilateral or bilateral, is a particularly distressing complication of NS. In the past, this was regarded as a cause rather than a consequence of NS, a conclusion no longer held to be true. Certain glomerular lesions are more likely than others to be associated with RVT. These include membranous glomerulonephritis, mesangiocapillary glomerulonephritis, and amyloidosis. Features which are suggestive of acute RVT include unilateral or bilateral flank or loin pain, gross hematuria, left-sided varicocele, widely fluctuating GFR and urinary protein excretion rates, and asymmetry of renal size and/or function. Scalloping of the ureters (due to collateral circulation) and evidence of pulmonary emboli and/or infarction (Chap. 227) may occur in chronic RVT.

Chronic forms of RVT are commonly asymptomatic. The approach to the patient with *chronic* RVT is widely debated. Some advocate an aggressive approach in patients with nephrotic syndrome due to lesions associated with inherently high prevalence of RVT (e.g., membranous glomerulonephritis), routinely employing selective renal venous angiography. If RVT is detected, long-term (optimal duration unknown) anticoagulants are prescribed. Such an approach might prevent later development of serious embolic complications, but since the true risk of pulmonary embolism in this group of patients is not known, but is probably low, the benefits/risk relationship of this approach cannot be determined. Long-term anticoagulation of nephrotic patients is not without risk, and the benefits for renal functional preservation are uncertain. A more conservative approach has also been advocated in which renal venous angiography is performed only in those patients who have a documented pulmonary embolism (e.g., symptoms, compatible laboratory findings, and a high-probability ventilation-perfusion scan or pulmonary angiogram) and who have negative noninvasive studies directed at detecting deep venous thrombosis in the lower extremities. Since such patients would receive anticoagulant therapy in any case, the value of localizing the site of thrombosis is not well established. Positive ventilation-perfusion scans in asymptomatic nephrotic patients are likely to have limited value, since subsegmental defects in perfusion may be observed even in the absence of renal vein or lower extremity deep venous thrombosis in nephrotic patients. These changes could conceivably be due to in situ pulmonary arterial thrombosis. The risk of renal vein thrombosis or deep venous thrombosis is increased primarily in patients with nephrotic syndrome and a very low serum albumin level (e.g., less than 2 g/dL). The presence of a documented thromboembolic complication of NS is usually regarded as a clear indication for long-term oral anticoagulation. The effectiveness of heparin may be impaired by concomitant antithrombin III deficiency, a plasma factor required for the full expression of the heparin-induced antithrombin effect.

High-protein diets are frequently prescribed; however, the beneficial effect of this approach can be challenged since the main effect of increasing dietary protein is to increase urinary protein excretion rate and the effect on serum albumin levels is very modest. Furthermore, such diets are difficult to manage with concomitant salt restriction, and at least theoretically, could aggravate the rate of progression of an underlying structural glomerular lesion. An alternative approach would be to prescribe modest protein restriction (e.g., 0.6 g/kg per day), particularly in azotemic patients; some also advocate adding a supplementary amount of dietary protein equal to urinary protein losses. Dietary protein should be of high biologic value and can be supplemented with amino acids. Plasma albumin and transferrin concentrations as well as urinary protein excretion rates should be monitored to evaluate the effect of dietary regimens on overall nutritional status. Correction of transport protein deficiencies is not feasible. Supplemental vitamin D might be desirable if overt deficiency is present, but this has not been fully evaluated clinically. In rare circumstances, profound protein malnutrition or other complications of massive proteinuria may justify ablation of renal function by medical or surgical means.

A classification of the causes of NS is provided in Table 223-3. The multisystemic, heredofamilial, neoplastic, and metabolic causes are discussed in Chap. 224. The primary (idiopathic) glomerular diseases associated with NS, as well as the diseases secondary to infectious or drug etiologies, are considered below.

TABLE 223-3 Causes of the nephrotic syndrome

I Primary glomerular diseases
- *A* Minimal change disease
- *B* Mesangial proliferative glomerulonephritis*
- *C* Focal and segmental glomerulosclerosis
- *D* Membranous glomerulonephritis
- *E* Mesangiocapillary glomerulonephritis
  - *1* Type I
  - *2* Type II
  - *3* Other variants
- *F* Other uncommon lesions
  - *1* Crescentic glomerulonephritis
  - *2* Focal and segmental proliferative glomerulonephritis*
  - *3* Unclassifiable lesions

II Secondary to other diseases
- *A* Infections: poststreptococcal glomerulonephritis, endocarditis, "shunt nephritis," secondary syphilis, leprosy, hepatitis B, HTLV-III, infectious mononucleosis, malaria, schistosomiasis, filariasis
- *B* Drugs: organic gold; inorganic, organic, and elemental mercury; penicillamine; "street" heroin; probenecid; captopril; Tridione; mesantoin; perchlorate; antivenom; antitoxins; contrast media
- *C* Neoplasia: Hodgkin's disease, lymphomas, leukemia, carcinomas, melanoma, Wilms's tumor
- *D* Multisystem: systemic lupus erythematosus, Henoch-Schönlein purpura, vasculitis, Goodpasture's syndrome, dermatomyositis, dermatitis herpetiformis, amyloidosis, sarcoidosis, Sjögren's syndrome, rheumatoid arthritis
- *E* Heredofamilial: diabetes mellitus, Alport's syndrome, sickle cell disease, Fabry's disease, nail-patella syndrome, lipodystrophy, congenital nephrotic syndrome
- *F* Miscellaneous: preeclamptic toxemia, thyroiditis, myxedema, malignant obesity, renovascular hypertension, chronic interstitial nephritis with vesicoureteric reflux, chronic allograft rejection, beestings

* *Includes Berger's disease (IgA nephropathy).*

IDIOPATHIC NEPHROTIC SYNDROME This diagnosis is arrived at by exclusion of known causes of NS, such as infections, drug exposure, malignancy, multisystem disease, or hereditary disorders. The idiopathic forms of NS are further classified according to the morphologic features found on renal biopsy (Table 223-4). Performance of a renal biopsy, at least among adults, is required for the accurate diagnosis of idiopathic NS and for the formulation of a rational plan of treatment. Children need not always be subjected to renal biopsy since careful clinical study can often lead to accurate diagnosis.

Minimal change disease This is often referred to as *lipoid nephrosis, nil lesion,* or *foot process disease.* In this form of idiopathic NS, although little or no alterations of the glomerular capillaries are demonstrable by light microscopy (hence the designation "minimal change"), *diffuse epithelial foot process effacement*[1] is evident by electron microscopy. Immunofluorescence microscopy reveals absent or irregular and nonspecific deposits of immunoglobulin and complement components. Minimal change disease is the most frequently encountered form of idiopathic NS in children, accounting for more than 70 to 80 percent of cases diagnosed before the age of 8. This lesion is not rare in adults, representing 15 to 20 percent of cases of idiopathic NS in patients over the age of 16. There is a slight predilection for males. Typically patients present with overt NS, normal blood pressure, normal or slightly reduced GFR, and a "benign" urinary sediment. Varying degrees of microscopic hematuria are found in up to 20 percent of cases. Urinary protein is typically highly selective in children (e.g., it contains principally albumin and minimal amounts of high-molecular-weight plasma proteins such as IgG, $alpha_2$ macroglobulin, or C3) but is variable in adults. The pattern of protein excretion indicates a major "charge-selective" defect in permselectivity. Fibrin split products and C3 are absent in the urine. Serum levels of complement components are normal, except for a slight reduction in C1q. IgG concentrations are often quite depressed during relapse, whereas IgM levels are modestly increased, both during remission and relapse. Some cases may have associated allergic diathesis (e.g., to milk, pollens, etc.), a history of recent immunization, or upper respiratory infection. Circulating immune complexes may be found in some patients using certain assays. The histocompatibility antigen HLA-B12 is more prevalent when minimal change disease is associated with atopy, indicating a possible genetically based predisposition to this disease. Thromboembolic manifestations occur, but renal vein thrombosis is uncommon.

Spontaneous remissions and relapses of heavy proteinuria may occur, usually for reasons which are unexplained. Interestingly, an identical lesion is encountered in patients with Hodgkin's disease in whom NS develops, suggesting a role for lymphocytes in its pathogenesis. Except for patients who develop focal and segmental sclerosing lesions (see below), a progressive decline in GFR does not occur. Acute renal failure is rare. In the preantibiotic era infection with encapsulated organisms (e.g., pneumococci) was a leading cause of death, but now the mortality rate is exceedingly low and most deaths are associated with complications of treatment rather than the disease itself. Rarely, acute renal failure may occur even in the absence of profound hypovolemia. The mechanism of this phenomenon is obscure but could relate to tubular obstruction from heavy proteinuria or severe glomerular epithelial cell effacement. The renal failure is responsive to steroids and diuretics.

[1] *The term "fusion" is often used to describe these changes in foot processes, although true fusion of cell membranes does not occur.*

Since the etiology and pathogenesis are unknown, treatment is empirical and symptomatic. A large body of evidence indicates that corticosteroids markedly enhance the natural tendency for this disease to undergo spontaneous remission. Daily or alternate-day oral steroid therapy seem to be equally effective, the latter associated with fewer steroid-related complications. Daily prednisone (60 mg/m² in children, 1 to 1.5 mg/kg in adults) for 4 weeks, followed by alternate-day prednisone (35 to 40 mg/m² in children, 1 mg/kg in adults) for 4 additional weeks is a regimen often recommended for initial treatment of this disorder. The vast majority of patients who respond do so within the first 4 weeks of treatment, but occasionally a favorable response requires more prolonged therapy. The absence of a response within 8 weeks is usually indicative of an error in diagnosis and should provoke a review of the renal biopsy. In many patients who respond, withdrawal of steroid treatment is often accompanied by relapse; this usually occurs within the first year after cessation of treatment. Such relapses may be re-treated with the initial regimen as described above, but with gradual withdrawal of prednisone and low-maintenance doses of 5 to 10 mg daily or on alternate days for 3 to 6 months. A steroid-dependent patient or one with multiple relapses may be benefited by a brief course of cyclophosphamide (2 to 3 mg/kg per day) or chlorambucil (0.1 to 0.2 mg/kg per day) for 8 to 10 weeks. When given with steroids to patients to induce remissions, either of these agents reduces the likelihood of a subsequent relapse. However, these agents have serious adverse effects on bone marrow and, in the case of cyclophosphamide, the gonads and urinary bladder. Careful monitoring of hematologic and urinary findings is mandatory. They may also be oncogenic. Azathioprine has been demonstrated to be ineffective in inducing prolonged remissions. The use of cytotoxic agents should be reserved for patients who develop serious or life-threatening complications of multiple courses of steroid therapy. The long-term prognosis of patients with the minimal change lesion is excellent; a 10-year survival in excess of 90 percent can be expected, but a few develop renal failure usually as a consequence of development of focal sclerosing glomerular lesions (see below).

Mesangial proliferative glomerulonephritis The lesion is characterized by a mild to moderate diffuse, but distinct, increase in the cellularity of the glomerular capillary bed. The peripheral glomerular capillary walls are thin and delicate, and extracapillary proliferation is not seen. The precise nature of the proliferating cells is not clearly understood but may represent combinations of proliferating mesangial cells, endothelial cells, and infiltrating mononuclear cells. Glomerular involvement is usually reasonably uniform, although there may be some segmental accentuation of hypercellularity. Necrosis of glomerular tufts is absent. Deposits of proteinaceous material, if seen, are confined to the mesangial areas. Interposition of mesangial cells and cytoplasm into the periphery of the glomerular capillary wall is not seen. By immunofluorescence, a variety of patterns are observed. If granular IgA deposits in the mesangium predominate, accompanied by C3 and fibrin-reactive antigens but not the early acting components of the complement cascade, then the lesion is categorized as IgA nephropathy, or Berger's disease (see below). Other patterns of immunofluorescence may be observed, including a predominance of IgM deposits in a granular pattern diffusely throughout the mesangium, isolated mesangial C3 deposits, scattered mesangial IgG deposits, and no immunoglobulin or complement deposits. Thus, the light-microscopic appearance of mesangial proliferative glomerulonephritis represents an extremely heterogeneous category of glomerular diseases with respect to underlying pathogenesis and undoubtedly to etiology. Some patients presenting with this morphologic lesion may in fact represent instances of resolving postinfectious glomerulonephritis, hereditary nephritis, or other multisystem diseases such as Henoch-

TABLE 223-4 Idiopathic nephrotic syndrome

SELECTED FEATURES OF UNDERLYING PRIMARY GLOMERULAR LESIONS

Lesion	Morphology* LM	Morphology* IFM	Morphology* EM	Approximate prevalence in children/adults, %	Common clinical/lab features	Response to therapy†	Likelihood of maintaining renal function‡
Minimal change	Normal or very mild proliferation	Negative–trace IgM	Foot process fusion, no deposits	70+/15–20	Highly selective proteinuria,§ *normal* C3, decreased IgG, increased IgM	Steroids ++ Cytotoxic drugs + (cyclophosphamide, chlorambucil) Frequent relapses	95+
Mesangial proliferative	Diffuse proliferation	Negative or variable mesangial IgM, IgG, C3	Mesangial deposits	15–20/5–10	Hematuria, *normal* C3	Steroids ± Cytotoxic drugs (?)	80 (?)
Focal sclerosis	Focal and segmental sclerosis	Focal and segmental IgM, C3	Foot process fusion, sclerosis, hyaline	10/10–20	Hematuria, leukocyturia, poorly selective proteinuria, *normal* C3	Steroids ± Cytotoxic drugs − Anticoagulants (?)	45–50
Membranous glomerulonephritis	Thick capillary wall, spikes of BM material	Diffuse granular capillary wall IgG	Subepithelial deposits	<5/30–40	Variable protein selectivity, *normal* C3, renal vein thrombosis	Steroids + Cytotoxic drugs (?)	50–70
Mesangial proliferative glomerulonephritis							
Type I	Mesangial interposition, lobular change	Diffuse C3; variable IgG, IgM	Subendothelial deposits	8/<5	Hematuria, *reduced* C3 (intermittent)	Steroids (?) Anticoagulants (?) Cytotoxic drugs (?) Antithrombotics +	60
Type II	Mesangial interposition	C3 capillary wall and mesangial nodules	Intramembranous deposits	3/<5	Hematuria, *reduced* C3 (persistent), +C3NF	Steroids − Cytotoxic drugs −	45

** LM = light microscopy, IFM = immunofluorescence microscopy, EM = electron microscopy, BM = basement membrane.*
† Response to therapy: ++ = highly responsive, + = variably responsive, ± = occasionally responsive, − = unresponsive.
‡ Percent of patients maintaining sufficient renal function to obviate need for chronic dialysis or transplantation within 5 years.

Schönlein purpura, vasculitis, or systemic lupus erythematosus. Electron-microscopic findings are nonspecific. Occasionally small electron-dense paramesangial deposits may be observed. The findings of large electron-dense deposits in the mesangium in association with the morphologic appearance of mesangial proliferative glomerulonephritis should heighten the suspicion of a multisystem disease or Berger's IgA nephropathy.

This lesion accounts for approximately 10 percent of instances of idiopathic nephrotic syndrome in adults and 15 percent in children. It tends to be more common in older children and young adults. Males tend to be affected slightly more often than females. Hematuria, either gross or microscopic, is commonly observed. Loin pain, bilateral or unilateral, may be seen in the idiopathic disorder but is more frequently observed in patients who have underlying IgA nephropathy. Laboratory features are not distinctive. Renal function may be modestly decreased at the time of diagnosis but is most often normal. Complement component levels are most often normal. IgG levels may be modestly reduced. IgA levels may be increased in IgA nephropathy. Circulating immune complexes may be found in some patients. Anti-streptolysin O titers are usually normal. Proteinuria is most often nonselective. No association with HLA antigens has yet been described for that category of patients who do not display predominant IgA mesangial deposits. The pathogenesis of this lesion is unknown and almost certainly the result of diverse pathogenetic processes. The presence of mesangial immunoglobulin deposits and circulating immune complexes in some, but not all, patients suggests an immune-complex pathogenesis, although the antigen(s) is unknown.

Among patients with well-developed nephrotic syndrome and moderate to severe diffuse mesangial proliferation, there is a tendency for persistence of proteinuria and progression to renal insufficiency. This is particularly true if areas of focal and segmental glomerular sclerosis are noted to be superimposed on the mesangial proliferative lesion at the time of the initial renal biopsy. Patients with milder forms of mesangial proliferative glomerulonephritis, particularly when unassociated with mesangial immunoglobulin deposition, may follow a more benign course. Some patients behave in a fashion quite similar to those with the minimal change lesion. Since renal biopsies from patients with the minimal change lesion may display mild degrees of glomerular hypercellularity, the apparently benign course followed by this subset of patients may indicate that they should be categorized as examples of minimal change lesion with more prominent mesangial proliferation rather than separately categorized under the heading of mesangial proliferative glomerulonephritis. Well-developed mesangial proliferative lesions, particularly in association with mesangial IgM deposits, tend to be unresponsive to corticosteroid therapy and to evolve with time into those of focal and segmental glomerular sclerosis. Indeed, the lesion of mesangial proliferative glomerulonephritis may be a predecessor of the lesion of focal and segmental glomerulosclerosis. Patients with mesangial proliferative glomerulonephritis who have complete remissions of proteinuria following treatment with corticosteroids in a fashion similar to that described for the minimal change lesion tend to do well with little inclination toward progressive renal insufficiency. Exacerbations and remissions of proteinuria may occur. Steroid-unresponsive patients with persistent nephrotic syndrome have a tendency to progress to renal insufficiency at variable rates. The role of adjunctive cytotoxic therapy (cyclophosphamide, chlorambucil, or azathioprine) has not yet been established in this category of lesions. Some studies have indicated that long-term therapy with indomethacin may be of benefit in this category of lesions, but no suitably controlled long-term studies have yet been performed.

Because of the highly variable pathogenesis in mesangial proliferative glomerulonephritis and its relative rarity, long-term prospective studies of natural history and therapy have not yet been conducted. Many patients, particularly those with mild degrees of proliferation and a remitting course following corticosteroid therapy, will have a very benign prognosis. Other patients, particularly those with steroid unresponsiveness and focal and segmental glomerulosclerosing lesions on the initial biopsy, will have a poor prognosis, often developing end-stage renal failure in 5 to 10 years following the initial diagnosis.

Focal and segmental glomerulosclerosis (focal sclerosis) This lesion is characterized by sclerosis and hyalinization of some, but not all, glomeruli (hence the term *focal*). Among affected glomeruli, only a portion of the glomerular tuft is abnormal (hence, *segmental*). There is a predilection for these lesions initially to affect the *juxtamedullary glomeruli* and to be associated with progressive tubulointerstitial damage. By immunofluorescence, granular and nodular deposits of IgM and C3 are found in the segmental sclerosing lesion. By electron microscopy, focal basement membrane collapse and denudation of epithelial surfaces are noted. All glomeruli reveal diffuse epithelial foot process effacement. This lesion accounts for 10 to 15 percent of cases of idiopathic NS seen among children and adults. Males tend to be affected slightly more often than females. Many investigators believe that focal sclerosis represents a stage in the evolution of a subgroup of patients with minimal change disease or "pure" mesangial proliferative glomerulonephritis (see above). In more than two-thirds of cases of focal sclerosis overt NS will be present at the time of diagnosis; in the remainder only isolated proteinuria in the nonnephrotic range is present. Hypertension, reduced GFR, abnormal tubule function, and abnormal urinary sediment occur commonly. It is important to emphasize that focal sclerosis may have clinical features indistinguishable from either minimal change disease, mesangial proliferative glomerulonephritis, or membranous glomerulopathy (see below). Proteinuria is nearly always nonselective or becomes so on follow-up. FDP and C3 may be present in the urine. Serum levels of C3 are normal and IgG levels are reduced, but not as severely as in minimal change disease. Similar lesions may be seen in association with "street" heroin abuse, vesicoureteral reflux, acquired immunodeficiency syndrome, solitary kidney, and renal allograft rejection and may complicate a variety of other primary glomerular diseases in the late stages. The occurrence of focal and segmental glomerulosclerosis in remnant glomeruli after extensive renal ablation has led to the suggestion that hyperfiltration (or some hemodynamic determinant thereof) may play a causative role in pathogenesis. Abnormalities in the prevalence of HLA antigens have not been consistently described. Renal vein thrombosis is uncommon.

There is little tendency for spontaneous remission, except among children. A progressive decline in GFR is the rule, albeit at variable rates. A subset of patients with focal sclerosis, who have extremely heavy proteinuria (i.e., greater than 15 to 20 g per day) and profound hypoalbuminemia, progress quite rapidly to end-stage renal failure, occasionally in a period of only a few months. Rarely, acute renal failure without recovery occurs.

The etiology and pathogenesis of focal sclerosis are unknown. Immune-complex–mediated disease has been postulated, primarily on the basis of immunofluorescence findings, and circulating immune complexes have been found in a small minority of cases.

Although very few prospective clinical trials have been conducted, a decline in the level of proteinuria concomitant with corticosteroid therapy and a lowered risk of progressive renal failure among patients experiencing a complete or partial remission of proteinuria suggest that corticosteroids may exert a beneficial effect on the natural history of the disorder. The effect of cytotoxic drugs and anticoagulants requires further study. At least 50 percent of patients with persistent heavy proteinuria develop end-stage renal failure or die of intercurrent illnesses within 10 years of diagnosis. The prognosis is much poorer for those patients with persistent NS in whom azotemia or hypertension is evident at time of diagnosis. This lesion has been found to recur in renal allografts, occasionally within a few hours of transplantation, suggesting the possibility of a circulating glomerular permeability "toxin" in its pathogenesis.

Membranous glomerulonephritis This lesion is characterized by the presence of irregular, discontinuous proteinaceous deposits along the outer (or subepithelial) aspect of the glomerular capillary wall.

These deposits contain IgG and appear dense by electron microscopy. Unlike focal sclerosis, *all glomeruli are involved uniformly*. At an early stage all glomeruli may appear normal by light microscopy, but as the disease progresses, immune deposits coalesce, causing the capillary wall to thicken. Eventually, increased amounts of basement membrane material project outward between deposits toward the urinary space, giving the appearance of "spikes." There is little proliferation of capillary endothelial or mesangial cells, although mesangial sclerosis may occur in advanced cases. Tubulointerstitial atrophy and vascular lesions are other late manifestations.

This disorder accounts for 30 to 40 percent of cases of idiopathic NS in adults but is quite rare in children. In over 80 percent of cases overt NS is present. In the remainder only isolated proteinuria is found. Males tend to be affected more often than females. Blood pressure, GFR, and urinary sediment tend to be normal early in the course, making it extremely difficult to distinguish membranous glomerulopathy from minimal change disease on clinical grounds alone. Urinary protein selectivity is quite variable. Serum complement components are normal, but IgG levels are usually modestly depressed. Membranous glomerulonephritis may develop in association with systemic lupus erythematosus (Chap. 224), certain chronic infections (e.g., malaria, hepatitis B), solid tumors (e.g., melanoma and cancer of the lung and colon), or after exposure to heavy metals (gold, mercury) or drugs (penicillamine, captopril). A careful search for these causes is warranted in every case of idiopathic NS due to membranous glomerulonephritis. There appears to be a high frequency of renal vein thrombosis in affected patients (see above).

Spontaneous complete remissions of NS are quite common in children but take place in only 20 to 25 percent of adults. Steroid treatment does not greatly influence the development of lasting complete remissions, but may induce a reduction of proteinuria to nonnephrotic levels. A beneficial effect of steroids is still a source of controversy, since spontaneous partial remissions also occur, although somewhat less frequently than in steroid-treated patients. There is presently no agreement about optimal dosage and duration of therapy; however, alternate-day steroid therapy seems to be the safest approach and may be associated with a lower risk of progressive renal failure. Regimens involving combinations of corticosteroids and alkylating agents have variable effects, but may be associated with a higher remission rate and a slower rate of progression of renal failure.

Slowly progressive renal functional impairment occurs almost exclusively among those patients with persistent proteinuria in the nephrotic range. Partial or complete spontaneous or treatment-associated remissions provide nearly complete protection from renal failure. Complete or partial remissions occur at variable times after the discovery of the disease, but renal failure is unlikely to develop in the first few years. Within 10 years of the time of the diagnosis, however, 35 to 50 percent of patients will die of intercurrent illness or develop end-stage renal failure. The vast majority of survivors will have had complete or partial remission of proteinuria. Rare cases have recurred in renal transplants. A few patients are known to have developed superimposed anti-GBM antibody–mediated disease and RPGN.

Mesangiocapillary glomerulonephritis This group of disorders is characterized by proliferation of mesangial cells, often with segmental or diffuse interposition of these cells or their cytoplasm into peripheral capillary loops. There is evidence of increased synthesis of mesangial matrix as well. The glomerular capillary wall is irregularly thickened, by virtue of the mesangial extensions and the attendant synthesis of basement membrane–like material. This group of disorders is also known as *membranoproliferative* or *lobular glomerulonephritis*. Several immunofluorescence and electron-microscopic patterns are present and are believed to reflect heterogeneous mechanisms of pathogenesis. In the ultrastructural *type I* lesion, subendothelial electron-dense deposits are present. C3 is deposited in a granular pattern indicative of immune-complex pathogenesis, but IgG and the early components of complement are present inconsistently. In the ultrastructural *type II* lesion the lamina densa of the GBM is transformed into an extremely electron-dense character, giving rise to the term *dense deposit disease*. Basement membranes in Bowman's capsules and in tubules are similarly affected. C3 is found irregularly in the GBM and in granules or rings in the mesangium. Small amounts of Ig (typically IgM) are present, but the early acting complement components are absent from the deposits. Properdin deposition is variable. Additional ultrastructural variants, based upon location of deposit and basement membrane changes, have also been described.

Mesangiocapillary glomerulonephritis, types I and II, is found in 5 to 10 percent of cases of idiopathic NS in children, particularly between the ages of 8 to 16 years, and somewhat less commonly in adults. Type I accounts for at least two-thirds of cases. Sexes are affected equally. In 50 to 75 percent of patients, a full-blown NS is present, often with features of AGN. In the remainder, proteinuria is in the nonnephrotic range and is nearly always accompanied by microscopic hematuria. Blood pressure and GFR are frequently abnormal, and the urinary sediment is typically active. Functional abnormalities of the renal tubules are common. Urinary protein selectivity is usually poor; FDP and C3 are found in the urine. Serum C3 levels are reduced in 70 to 80 percent of cases of type I and in over 90 percent of type II disease. The early acting complement components C1q, C4, and C2 are often normal, however, especially in type II disease. This pattern may be indicative of activation of the alternate complement pathway (see Chap. 222). C3 nephritic factor (C3NF) is often found in the serum of patients with type II, especially if the C3 level is quite low. Circulating immune complexes are found in type I. Lesions similar to type I membranoproliferative glomerulonephritis may also be found in SLE, hemolytic-uremic syndrome, transplant rejection, chronic hepatitis B antigenemia, and "shunt" nephritis. Renal vein thrombosis may occur. Type II nephritis may be associated with partial lipodystrophy.

Spontaneous remissions are uncommon. Long-term, alternate-day steroid therapy (0.3 to 0.5 mg/kg every other day) may delay the progression of the disease. Treatment regimens which combine steroids and cytotoxic agents are not of proven value. Recently, evidence suggesting a beneficial effect of anticoagulants and inhibitors of platelet aggregation (acetylsalicylic acid plus dipyridamole) has appeared. The course is usually relentlessly progressive, and approximately one-half of patients die or develop end-stage renal failure within 10 years of the diagnosis. The prognosis for type II lesions seems somewhat worse than for type I. Type II disease almost invariably recurs in the transplanted kidney but does not always result in the premature loss of the allograft.

Other forms of idiopathic nephrotic syndrome In a small percentage of adults and children with idiopathic NS (i.e., 5 to 10 percent) other lesions are encountered on renal biopsy. These include *crescentic glomerulonephritis* and *focal* and *segmental proliferative glomerulonephritis*. The pathogenetic mechanisms responsible for these lesions vary. For example, some of the cases of focal and segmental glomerulonephritis may have extensive mesangial IgA deposits and fit into the category of Berger's disease (see below). Serum C3 levels are usually normal. The clinical characteristics, natural history, and response to treatment of these lesions are not well defined. Hematuria is common and may be recurrent. Proteinuria tends to be nonselective. Spontaneous remissions of NS are uncommon. Since no controlled studies have been conducted, it is not possible to evaluate the effectiveness of treatment. Crescentic glomerulonephritis is likely to have a poor prognosis, whereas mesangial and focal and segmental proliferative glomerulonephritis have a more favorable long-term outlook.

NEPHROTIC SYNDROME CAUSED BY INFECTIOUS AGENTS, DRUGS, OR CHEMICALS Table 223-3 lists the common infectious and drug-related etiologies of NS. In many instances, NS will abate following cure of the infection or withdrawal of the offending medication. In patients receiving organic gold therapy for rheumatoid arthritis, or in those exposed to inorganic, organic, or elemental mercury or to penicillamine therapy, membranous glomerulonephritis is usually the lesion responsible for NS. NS is known to follow immunization and antiserum treatment of tetanus or snakebite and to occur in situations associated with atopy.

ASYMPTOMATIC URINARY ABNORMALITIES

This group of patients is identified principally by the findings of *proteinuria in the nonnephrotic range and/or hematuria,* unaccompanied by edema, reduced GFR, or hypertension. Abnormalities are often discovered incidentally and may be persistent or recurrent. This syndrome may, of course, be but a phase in the natural history of other glomerulopathic syndromes, especially nephrotic syndrome or chronic glomerulonephritis. Common glomerular disorders which present as asymptomatic proteinuria and/or hematuria at some point in their natural history are listed in Table 223-5. The heredofamilial and multisystem diseases are discussed in Chap. 224. The presence of dysmorphic erythrocytes and/or red cell casts is a very useful finding indicative of an underlying glomerular cause for the hematuria.

IDIOPATHIC RENAL HEMATURIA (See also Chap. 40) **Berger's disease (IgA nephropathy)** This disorder was first described by Berger and Hinglais in 1968 and is characterized by recurrent episodes of gross or microscopic hematuria. The diagnosis depends on the finding of prominent IgA deposits in the mesangium by immunofluorescence microscopy. Berger's disease is the most common cause of recurrent hematuria of glomerular origin. It most commonly affects young adults, mostly males. Typically, episodes of macroscopic hematuria are associated with minor flulike illnesses or vigorous exercise. Patients frequently complain of vague constitutional symptoms, but skin rash, arthritis, and abdominal pain are absent. Urine protein excretion rates are usually less than 3.5 g per day; not uncommonly protein excretion is normal or only mildly increased. The nephrotic syndrome develops occasionally. Blood pressure, GFR, and serum albumin are normal, at least early in the disease. Serum IgA levels are increased in about 50 percent of cases, while serum complement component levels remain normal. Biopsy of the skin of the volar surface of the forearm will often reveal dermal capillary deposits of IgA, C3, and fibrin, but not early acting complement components or IgA secretory fragments. Similar skin biopsy findings may be encountered in Henoch-Schönlein purpura (Chap. 224). Indeed, Berger's disease may be a monosymptomatic form of Henoch-Schönlein purpura.

Renal biopsy reveals a spectrum of changes by light microscopy, but diffuse mesangial proliferative or focal and segmental proliferative glomerulonephritis is found most often. In some cases glomerular morphology may be normal by light microscopy; rarely, crescents may be found. The distinguishing feature is the finding by immunofluorescence microscopy of *diffuse mesangial deposition of IgA,* often accompanied by lesser amounts of IgG and nearly always by C3 and properdin, but not by C1q or C4. Fibrin reactive antigens are also commonly demonstrable in the mesangium or in association with crescents if the latter are present. The pathogenesis of IgA nephropathy is unknown, but the systemic character of the IgA deposits (skin and glomerular capillaries), the presence of circulating IgG and IgA complexes in the majority of cases, and its similarity to Henoch-Schönlein purpura suggest that it is an immune-complex–mediated disease. The nature and source of the antigen are unknown.

The prognosis is variable, but, in general, the disease tends to progress slowly. It has been estimated that approximately 50 percent of patients can be expected to develop end-stage renal failure within 25 years of the time of diagnosis. Azotemia, hypertension, or proteinuria in the nephrotic range at the time of diagnosis are associated with a poor prognosis. At present, there is no evidence to suggest that any form of therapy greatly influences the natural history. Some have suggested that intermittent steroid therapy may reduce the frequency of episodes of gross hematuria. Corticosteroids may also result in remissions of proteinuria in those patients with nephrotic syndrome and mild glomerular abnormalities by light microscopy.

Other primary renal hematurias Some cases of recurrent hematuria do not reveal the typical immunofluorescence findings seen in Berger's disease. This group of patients is poorly defined, and in them the etiology and pathogenesis is varied. Some may represent resolving episodes of acute glomerulonephritis or early examples of mesangiocapillary or hereditary glomerulonephritis (Alport's syndrome, see Chap. 224). The morphologic lesions most commonly encountered are focal and segmental or diffuse mesangial proliferative glomerulonephritis, although mild and nonspecific glomerular changes may also be observed. Immunofluorescence studies reveal varying degrees of immunoglobulin and/or complement component deposition (principally IgM and/or C3) in the mesangium. Some cases show linear deposits of IgG, suggesting a possible anti-GBM antibody pathogenesis. Electron microscopy may reveal dense deposits in the mesangium or thin and attenuated glomerular basement membranes. Overall, this group of patients is believed to have an excellent prognosis, with spontaneous permanent remissions of recurrent hematuria. Progressive renal insufficiency is unusual. Because of the benign prognosis no treatment is indicated.

ISOLATED NONNEPHROTIC PROTEINURIA OF GLOMERULAR ORIGIN (See also Chap. 40) The discovery of mild to moderate degrees of proteinuria (i.e., greater than 150 mg but less than 2.0 g per day), unaccompanied by abnormalities in the urinary sediment or evidence of hypertension or reduced renal function, is a common problem in internal medicine. Such patients may display other features of heredofamilial or multisystem diseases, including diabetes mellitus, amyloidosis, rheumatoid arthritis, or cancer. Among cases of isolated proteinuria consequent to primary glomerular disease the abnormality may either be persistent or evanescent. Proteinuria may occur primarily in the upright posture (*orthostatic proteinuria*) or be present both in recumbent and erect positions (*constant proteinuria*). Fixed and reproducible orthostatic proteinuria is regarded as having a benign prognosis and frequently disappears on long-term follow-up. Renal biopsies will most often reveal normal glomeruli or trivial alterations of dubious significance. On the other hand, persistent and constant proteinuria may be indicative of a more serious disease, and renal biopsies will more often reveal definite evidence of a structural lesion. Some of the lesions which might be encountered have been discussed in the context of idiopathic nephrotic syndrome. Other patients may prove to have a clinically unsuspected disease such as amyloidosis or diabetes mellitus. In the remainder, the lesions are usually trivial and nonspecific and their long-term significance is quite uncertain. In the case of primary glomerular diseases, so long as urinary protein

TABLE 223-5 Glomerular causes of asymptomatic urinary abnormalities

I Hematuria with or without proteinuria
- *A* Primary glomerular diseases
  - *1* Berger's disease (IgA nephropathy)
  - *2* Mesangiocapillary glomerulonephritis
  - *3* Other primary glomerular hematurias accompanied by "pure" mesangial proliferation, focal and segmental proliferative glomerulonephritis, or other lesions
- *B* Associated with multisystem or heredofamilial diseases
  - *1* Alport's syndrome and other "benign" familial hematurias
  - *2* Fabry's disease
  - *3* Sickle cell disease
- *C* Associated with infections
  - *1* Resolving poststreptococcal glomerulonephritis
  - *2* Other postinfectious glomerulonephritides

II Isolated nonnephrotic proteinuria
- *A* Primary glomerular diseases
  - *1* "Orthostatic" proteinuria
  - *2* Focal and segmental glomerulosclerosis
  - *3* Membranous glomerulonephritis
- *B* Associated with multisystem or heredofamilial diseases
  - *1* Diabetes mellitus
  - *2* Amyloidosis
  - *3* Nail-patella syndrome

excretion remains modest, the prognosis is excellent and deterioration of renal function is uncommon. Renal biopsy is not commonly undertaken in patients with persistent and isolated nonnephrotic proteinuria, as determining underlying morphology seldom leads to specific therapy and adds information chiefly of a prognostic nature. Since patients having proteinuria over 2.0 g per day are more likely to have lesions which will later progress, many experienced nephrologists limit renal biopsies to this latter group of patients.

CHRONIC GLOMERULONEPHRITIS (CGN)

The syndrome of CGN is characterized chiefly by *persistent urinary abnormalities* (e.g., proteinuria and/or hematuria) and by *slowly progressive impairment of renal function,* eventuating in hypertension, contracted granular kidneys, and end-stage renal failure. With the possible exception of the minimal change lesion associated with idiopathic nephrotic syndrome (see above) all the disorders described in this chapter and in Chap. 224 can lead eventually to CGN. The pathophysiology of the syndrome of CGN as it appears in the context of renal failure is described in Chaps. 218 and 220.

The glomerular structural alterations that underlie this syndrome may be categorized as *proliferative* (including mesangial, endo- and/or extracapillary proliferative glomerulonephritis, and focal and segmental proliferative glomerulonephritis), *sclerosing* (including focal and diffuse glomerular sclerosis), and *membranous.* Such lesions are found in the vast majority of patients with CGN. In the small remainder, the underlying lesions are not readily categorized morphologically. These are often referred to as *chronic "nonspecific" glomerulonephritis.*

The clinical characteristics of the specific lesions are described in other sections of this chapter. The etiologic and pathogenetic origins of chronic nonspecific glomerulonephritis are unknown but are undoubtedly heterogeneous. Complicating vascular disease contributes to the glomerular obliteration seen in this group of disorders. It is quite reasonable to suspect that some of the patients categorized as having chronic nonspecific glomerulonephritis may have had an earlier unrecognized or undiagnosed episode of acute PSGN. However, such patients usually fail to recall a specific episode of acute nephritis.

The detection of CGN usually occurs in one of several ways: (1) by the incidental finding of abnormal urine, impaired renal function, or hypertension during multiphasic screening of asymptomatic individuals or during evaluation of such individuals for an unrelated illness; (2) as the result of the insidious onset of progressive symptoms or signs of advanced renal disease, especially anemia and hypertension; or (3) after an exacerbation of glomerulonephritis, usually during the course of a nonspecific viral or bacterial illness. In advanced stages of the syndrome, the clinical separation of CGN from other causes of renal failure may be difficult; however, the presence of symmetrically contracted kidneys, moderate to heavy proteinuria, abnormal urinary sediment (especially red blood cell casts), and x-ray evidence of normal pyelocalyceal systems are all suggestive of CGN.

The evolution of CGN varies considerably, depending upon the nature of the underlying disease and the presence or absence of complications, especially hypertension. Ten, fifteen, twenty, or more years may elapse from the first discovery of an abnormal urine sediment until the development of end-stage renal failure. Renal biopsy is necessary to define the precise nature of the underlying glomerular lesion. The principal advantage of a morphologic evaluation among patients presenting with the syndrome of CGN is to determine prognosis rather than therapy.

Treatment of patients with CGN is supportive and symptomatic. Despite many years of controlled and uncontrolled trials, unequivocal evidence of a favorable effect of treatment with steroids, cytotoxic agents, nonsteroidal anti-inflammatory agents, and anticoagulants has yet to be provided. The management of specific lesions is discussed in greater detail in the relevant sections of this chapter. Hypertension and symptomatic urinary tract infections should be treated vigorously, taking care to avoid nephrotoxic agents. Diuretics should generally be employed only as adjuncts to antihypertensive management or to deal with debilitating degrees of edema. Fluid and sodium should be provided according to the dictates of blood pressure control. Rigorous salt restriction is usually unnecessary and may be hazardous. In the absence of congestive heart failure or marked hypoalbuminemia, severe edema rarely occurs in CGN until the terminal phases of the illness. Potassium restriction is usually unnecessary. Protein and phosphate restriction may slow the rate of progression of renal failure.

REFERENCES

Brenner BM, Stein JH (eds): Nephrotic syndrome, in *Contemporary Issues in Nephrology,* vol 9. New York, Churchill Livingstone, 1982

Couser WG: Idiopathic rapidly progressive glomerulonephritis. Am J Nephrol 2:57, 1982

D'Amico G et al (eds): IgA mesangial nephropathy. Contrib Nephrol 40:1, 1984

Glassock RJ (ed): Primary glomerular diseases. Semin Nephrol 2:190, 1982

——— et al: Primary glomerular diseases, in *The Kidney,* 3d ed, BM Brenner, FC Rector Jr (eds). Philadelphia, Saunders, 1986, p 929

Madaio MP, Harrington JT: The diagnosis of acute glomerulonephritis. N Engl J Med 309:1299, 1983

Mallick NP et al: Clinical membranous nephropathy. Nephron 34:209, 1983

224 GLOMERULOPATHIES ASSOCIATED WITH MULTISYSTEM DISEASES

RICHARD J. GLASSOCK / BARRY M. BRENNER

Glomerular injury may be a prominent feature of diseases which affect multiple organs and systems. By and large the etiologies of these diseases are unknown, but aberrant immunologic processes, neoplasia, metabolic disturbances, and genetically based biochemical abnormalities are believed to be dominant factors in their pathogenesis. These processes lead to a variety of alterations in glomerular structure and function. Some of the glomerular lesions are specific for the underlying disease entity (e.g., amyloidosis, nodular diabetic glomerulosclerosis); however, the majority are nonspecific. Proteinuria results from defects in the charge- and/or size-selective glomerular permeability barriers. Reductions in glomerular filtration rate develop because of progressive loss of filtration surface area. Although the extrarenal manifestations of these diseases are useful in establishing a diagnosis, some may present with predominant or exclusive renal involvement and only covert extrarenal manifestations.

IMMUNOLOGICALLY MEDIATED MULTISYSTEM DISEASES

SYSTEMIC LUPUS ERYTHEMATOSUS (See also Chap. 262) Systemic lupus erythematosus (SLE) is the archetype of an immunologically mediated multisystem disease (see Chap. 222) and is representative of the multisystem diseases in which renal involvement is common. The etiology of SLE is unknown; however, viral infection, genetic factors, and abnormal immune responsiveness probably interact to produce the disease. The principal mechanism for tissue injury in SLE appears to be the deposition of circulating immune complexes, although other mechanisms may also play a role, including antitissue antibody and in situ immune-complex formation (see Chap. 222). The circulating immune complexes may be composed of a wide variety of endogenous antigens combined with autoantibodies. DNA (single-stranded and double-stranded) is a major antigenic component of immune complexes. The prevalence of clinically evident renal involvement in SLE ranges from as low as 35 percent to more than 90 percent in different series. Manifestations of renal disease range from mild abnormalities of the urinary sediment (predominantly hematuria) to massive proteinuria and from chronic indolent glomerulonephritis to a fulminant inflammatory process leading to rapidly progressive renal failure.

The diagnosis and extrarenal manifestations of SLE are described in Chap. 262. This section will deal with the renal involvement. Although extrarenal features often dominate the clinical picture, SLE may present initially solely with renal manifestations. Morphologic evidence of renal involvement may exist with or without clinical manifestations. If immunofluorescence and electron-microscopic studies of renal tissue are performed, abnormalities are present in virtually every patient with SLE. The abnormal glomerular morphologic lesions in SLE form a spectrum based upon such correlative light- and electron-microscopic and immunofluorescence studies of renal biopsies.

Minimal lupus glomerular lesion This pattern is characterized by few or no changes by light microscopy. Immunofluorescence studies reveal moderate immunoglobulin (Ig) and complement deposits exclusively in mesangium. Scattered electron-dense deposits are found in mesangium by electron microscopy. Clinical renal manifestations may include mild proteinuria and microscopic hematuria. Nephrotic syndrome is uncommon. Glomerular filtration rate (GFR) is almost always normal. Serologic manifestations vary depending upon the activity of extrarenal disease. Antibodies to DNA are usually present in low titer, and levels of C3 and C4 may be decreased, especially if dermatitis is severe. Circulating immune complexes may also be detected in patients with skin lesions.

Mesangial lupus glomerulonephritis This pattern is characterized by mild to moderate diffuse mesangial cell proliferation and/or mesangial sclerosis. Immunofluorescence studies reveal immunoglobulins (IgG, IgM, and IgA) and complement components (C1q, C4, and C3) deposited in a granular pattern principally in the mesangium. By electron microscopy, electron-dense deposits are also found to be confined to the mesangium. This morphologic appearance may be present in the absence of clinical renal disease or may be associated with minor abnormalities in the urinary sediment and modest proteinuria. Nephrotic syndrome and hypertension may occasionally be present. GFR is almost always normal. Mesangial lupus glomerulonephritis may be the initial renal involvement in SLE, from which other patterns evolve. Associated serologic abnormalities depend upon the degree of extrarenal activity. These include increased levels of antibody to denatured, single-stranded DNA (ssDNA) or native, double-stranded DNA (dsDNA); depressed serum levels of C3, C4, and C1q; and detectable levels of circulating immune complexes (CIC) (Table 224-1).

Focal and segmental lupus glomerulonephritis This pattern is characterized by focal and segmental cellular proliferation, often associated with necrosis, superimposed on diffuse mesangial hypercellularity. Granular deposits of immunoglobulins and complement components are more extensive than in the mesangial form and involve both the mesangium and occasional glomerular capillary loops. By electron microscopy, dense subendothelial deposits are found in the mesangium and in a few peripheral capillary loops. Clinical and laboratory evidence of renal injury is more common than in mesangial lupus glomerulonephritis. Nephrotic syndrome may occur in 10 to 20 percent of patients, but in general GFR is well preserved. This lesion may persist, resolve, or progress to diffuse proliferative lupus glomerulonephritis. Serologic features of active disease are often present in untreated patients.

Diffuse proliferative lupus glomerulonephritis This pattern is characterized by diffuse mesangial and endothelial cell proliferation which may include extensive peripheral capillary wall interposition of mesangial cells. In addition focal cellular necrosis, hematoxylinophilic bodies, fibrinoid necrosis, and "wire loops" (capillaries whose basement membranes are thickened markedly owing to subendothelial deposits) may be present. Extensive extracapillary proliferative (crescentic) glomerulonephritis, vasculitis, and interstitial nephritis may also be found. Granular deposits of immunoglobulins and complement components are extensive and involve the mesangium and nearly every capillary loop. Electron microscopy reveals extensive subendothelial and mesangial electron-dense deposits as well as occasional intramembranous or subepithelial deposits. Most patients have an active urinary sediment, heavy proteinuria, and progressive impairment of renal function; occasionally, clinical evidence of renal involvement is lacking. In the untreated patient evidence of serologic activity is usually present, including depressed serum C3 and C4 concentrations, high levels of precipitating and nonprecipitating complement-fixing antibody to dsDNA, cryoimmunoglobulinemia, and circulating immune complexes. This lesion is associated with an ominous prognosis, although vigorous treatment may modify the course (see below).

Membranous lupus glomerulonephritis This pattern is nearly identical with that described for idiopathic membranous glomerulonephritis (Chap. 223), except that mesangial deposits and mesangial proliferation are more frequent. There is thickening of the glomerular capillary wall due to the presence of immunoglobulin and complement-containing electron-dense deposits in the subepithelial space, often associated with a spike-like basement membrane reaction. Nearly all patients have heavy proteinuria and the nephrotic syndrome. Although GFR may be normal initially, most patients ultimately develop progressive renal failure. A proliferative lesion may occasionally evolve, and the prognosis then assumes that of diffuse proliferative glomerulonephritis. Serologic features of SLE may or may not be present at the time of diagnosis of this nephropathy. Antibody to dsDNA tends to be nonprecipitating. Some patients with membranous lupus glomerulonephritis may be erroneously categorized as having

TABLE 224-1 Serologic findings in selected multisystem diseases

Disease	C3	Ig	FANA	Anti-dsDNA	Anti-GBM	Cryo-Ig	CIC
Systemic lupus erythematosus	↓↓	↑ IgG	+ + +	+ +	–	+ +	+ + +
Goodpasture's syndrome	–	–	–	–	+ + +	–	±
Henoch-Schönlein purpura	–	↑ IgA	–	–	–	±	+ +
Polyarteritis	↓	↑ IgG	+	±	–	+ +	+ + +
Wegener's granulomatosis	↓↑	↑ IgA, IgE	–	–	–	±	+ +
Cryoimmunoglobulinemia	↓	±	–	–	–	+ + +	+ +
Multiple myeloma	–	↓↑ IgG, IgA, IgD, IgE	–	–	–	+	±
Waldenström's macroglobulinemia	–	↑ IgM	–	–	–	–	–
Amyloidosis	–	± Ig	–	–	–	–	–

NOTE: *C3 = C3 component of complement; Ig = immunoglobulin levels; FANA = fluorescent antinuclear antibody assay; anti-dsDNA = antibody to double-stranded (native) DNA; anti-GBM = antibody to glomerular basement membrane antigens; cryo-Ig = cryoimmunoglobulin; CIC = circulating immune complexes; – = normal; + = occasionally slightly abnormal; + + = often abnormal; + + + = severely abnormal.*

idiopathic membranous glomerulopathy (see Chap. 223). Measurements of the level of antibody to dsDNA or ssDNA and circulating immune complexes and biopsies of skin for dermal-epidermal deposits of Ig ("lupus band test") may be helpful for diagnosis in such cases.

Sclerosing or end-stage lupus glomerulonephritis This pattern is characterized by obliterative and sclerosing lesions of the glomeruli and probably represents a late stage of proliferative lesions. Immunofluorescence studies may be only weakly positive for immunoglobulins; subendothelial deposits are infrequent. Hypertension and impaired renal function are common. Serologic parameters of activity of SLE may or may not be present.

Prognosis and treatment The prognosis and treatment of SLE with renal involvement depends upon the nature of the underlying renal lesion especially with regard to the class and the activity of the morphologic disease and to the extent and severity of associated glomerulosclerosis and interstitial fibrosis. Patients with milder forms of renal disease (e.g., minimal, mesangial, or focal lupus glomerulonephritis) tend to do well if treatment is directed to control of the extrarenal manifestations of the disease. Corticosteroids in modest doses, salicylates, or antimalarials are usually sufficient. Potent nonsteroidal, anti-inflammatory agents may cause functional depression of GFR and should be used with caution in patients with known renal involvement. Serologic parameters, including anti-dsDNA and complement components (C3, C4), should be followed serially. Fluorescent antinuclear antibody tests have little value in prognosis or in following the effectiveness of treatment. A return to normal values for antibody to dsDNA and/or complement components is a favorable sign; however, persistently abnormal serologic features do not necessarily indicate worsening or progressive renal involvement, especially in patients with active extrarenal manifestations. For patients with mild lesions, 85 percent or more can be expected to survive at least 10 years. Patients with membranous lupus glomerulonephritis who receive treatment directed primarily at the extrarenal features also have favorable long-term prognosis. On the other hand, patients with diffuse proliferative lupus glomerulonephritis do less well and, therefore, warrant a more aggressive approach toward ameliorating the renal disease. High-dose, long-term oral glucocorticoid therapy, although capable of improving extrarenal signs of active disease and reducing the acute inflammatory component of the renal lesions, is not an altogether satisfactory regimen for lupus nephritis. Such treatment is associated with a high prevalence of side effects and may not prevent progression of chronic lesions. High-dose, short-term intravenous methylprednisolone is effective in reducing signs of systemic activity of the disease, especially in patients with recent deterioration. Adjunctive use of cytotoxic agents (azathioprine, cyclophosphamide, or chlorambucil) exerts a steroid-sparing effect and may prevent progression of chronic lesions, particularly among those with mild chronic lesions prior to therapy. The optimal regimen has not yet been established; however, intermittent intravenous cyclophosphamide plus low-dose oral prednisone (0.5 mg/kg per day) and combinations of azathioprine, cyclophosphamide, and low-dose oral prednisone appear to be more effective than azathioprine or cyclophosphamide combined with low-dose prednisone. Because prospective randomized trials have involved only small numbers of patients, it is premature to adopt any particular regimen as the treatment of choice. Even combinations of azathioprine and low-dose prednisone may exert a benefical effect in certain subsets of patients. Little is gained by using a combined steroid-cytotoxic approach in patients with advanced renal failure due to progressive glomerular capillary obliteration and sclerosis. These patients are best treated with dialysis and/or transplantation. Plasma exchange accompanied by immunosuppressive therapy for fulminating disease appears promising. Serologic studies, especially serial measurements of antibody to dsDNA, complement components, and circulating immune complexes, are useful parameters to follow in patients under therapy. Return of these parameters to normal usually indicates satisfactory control of disease and indicates that drug dosage can be safely diminished. These measurements also need to be monitored to guide more aggressive therapy when appropriate.

Overall, long-term prognosis for patients with SLE and renal involvement has improved. Whether improvements in methods of diagnosis, serologic monitoring, or treatment are responsible is unknown. Progression to end-stage renal disease is now relatively uncommon even for patients with diffuse proliferative glomerulonephritis. Cerebral involvement and infectious complications of therapy are now major causes of morbidity and mortality in SLE. Patients with SLE seem to do well on regular chronic dialysis; moreover, as uremia develops, some patients experience remissions of extrarenal activity. In transplanted patients, recurrence of SLE in the renal allograft is uncommon. Thus, patients with SLE and nephritis are satisfactory candidates for both dialysis and transplantation.

GOODPASTURE'S SYNDROME This disorder consists of *pulmonary hemorrhage, glomerulonephritis,* and *antibody to basement membrane antigens*. Its etiology is unknown. Goodpasture's syndrome may appear at any age and typically affects young men. However, an increasing number of affected women are being recognized.

Pulmonary hemorrhage may be mild and easily overlooked or severe and life-threatening. The initial manifestations of pulmonary involvement are cough, mild shortness of breath, and hemoptysis. Hilar pulmonary infiltrates may be seen by chest x-ray, and hypoxia is frequent. With marked intraalveolar hemorrhage pulmonary carbon monoxide uptake is increased, and the pulmonary clearance of radioactive carbon monoxide is depressed. Pulmonary iron sequestration may be documented by scanning of the lungs with ^{59}Fe. Hemosiderin-laden macrophages may be seen in the sputum, but this is a nonspecific finding. Iron-deficiency anemia may result if pulmonary bleeding is prolonged and severe. A history of recent inhalation of volatile hydrocarbons or of viral influenza may be obtained. Fever, arthralgias, and other systemic symptoms are mild or absent at the time of presentation. Pulmonary hemorrhage may also be associated with renal failure in SLE, polyarteritis, Wegener's granulomatosis, cryoimmunoglobulinemia, Henoch-Schönlein purpura, pulmonary embolism consequent to renal vein thrombosis, Legionnaires' disease, and congestive heart failure in patients with end-stage renal disease. These disorders can ordinarily be differentiated from Goodpasture's syndrome by their extrarenal features and by typical serologic findings (Table 224-1).

The glomeruli in Goodpasture's syndrome range from normal or nearly normal to focal proliferative and necrotizing glomerulonephritis; most often there is extensive extracapillary proliferation (crescents). Rapidly progressive renal failure is the common feature, although patients may initially have normal renal function and mild microscopic abnormalities in the urinary sediment. Immunofluorescence studies of renal biopsy material reveal the typical *linear deposits* of anti-basement membrane antibody, often but not necessarily always accompanied by C3 deposition. Electron-microscopic studies do not reveal electron-dense deposits.

Circulating antibody to glycopeptide antigens related to the noncollagenous domains on type IV (basement membrane) collagen are found in over 90 percent of cases if serums are examined early in the course by immunofluorescence or radioimmunoassay (Table 224-1). The level of circulating antibody does not correlate well with the severity of the renal or pulmonary manifestations. Measurements of circulating antibody are of diagnostic value and have no prognostic significance. Serum complement components are nearly always normal, and circulating immune complexes and cryoimmunoglobulins are absent.

The course is variable. Patients surviving an initial bout of severe hemoptysis may undergo long-term remissions or may have repeated bouts of pulmonary hemorrhage. Mild forms of glomerular injury may not progress, and the principal clinical problems may be related to recurrent hemoptysis. The diagnosis in such patients may be confused with idiopathic pulmonary hemosiderosis. More commonly the renal disease is progressive, sometimes fulminant, leading to oliguric renal failure in a matter of a few weeks or months (i.e., rapidly progressive glomerulonephritis).

Life-threatening degrees of pulmonary hemorrhage may respond temporarily to high doses of parenteral methylprednisolone (10 to 15 mg/kg) given over short periods. The effectiveness of such therapy in reversing extensive crescentic glomerular lesions is not established. Anticoagulants are contraindicated in the face of active pulmonary hemorrhage. Intensive plasma exchange (2 to 4 liters of plasma per day), in combination with cytotoxic drugs and modest doses of corticosteroids, has been associated with dramatic remissions of pulmonary hemorrhage and improvement of the glomerular lesions. This is particularly true if treatment is initiated early in patients with relatively acute disease in whom oliguria has not yet developed. The duration and frequency of plasma exchanges depend upon the response of the patient and the results of monitoring levels of circulating antibody to glomerular basement membrane antigens. Renal biopsy is helpful in guiding the management, but even in the presence of extensive crescent formation responses may be satisfactory. If irreversible glomerular obliteration, extensive interstitial fibrosis, and tubular atrophy are found, especially in the oliguric patient with long-standing disease, plasma exchange offers little hope for improving the renal lesion. Such patients are best managed by regular hemodialysis and/or transplantation. Although recurrences may occasionally develop, the diagnosis is not a contraindication to transplantation so long as the procedure is delayed until levels of circulating anti-basement membrane antibody decrease to undetectable levels.

HENOCH-SCHÖNLEIN PURPURA (See also Chap. 280) This disorder is characterized by nonthrombocytopenic purpura, arthralgias, abdominal pain, and glomerulonephritis. Renal involvement is common and is manifested chiefly by hematuria and proteinuria. In some instances renal involvement is severe, leading to rapidly progressive glomerulonephritis or nephrotic syndrome. The onset of the disease may resemble acute postinfectious glomerulonephritis. Serum complement component levels are usually normal. Serum IgA levels are increased in about half the patients (Table 224-1). Renal biopsy reveals a spectrum of abnormalities. Mild diffuse mesangial cell proliferation and/or focal and segmental proliferative glomerulonephritis is most common when bouts of macroscopic hematuria and proteinuria are present. More severe and diffuse proliferative glomerulonephritis, sometimes accompanied by extracapillary proliferation (crescents), arises in patients with heavy proteinuria and/or rapidly diminishing GFR. Characteristically, immunofluorescence studies reveal mesangial and peripheral capillary granular deposits of IgA, IgG, C3, and fibrinogen but not C1q, C4, or IgA secretory piece. Similar immunofluorescence findings are present in the dermal capillaries of biopsies of involved and uninvolved skin. Electron microscopy reveals electron-dense deposits principally in the mesangium. These findings suggest that Henoch-Schönlein purpura is due to circulating IgA-containing immune complexes. Circulating cryoimmunoglobulins and immune complexes may be present, but the nature of the antigen and the antibody reactivity of the IgA are unknown. Although food allergies and upper respiratory infections may be present, there is no clear-cut etiologic relationship. *Berger's disease* (IgA nephropathy, Chap. 223) may represent a form of Henoch-Schönlein purpura.

The diagnosis is ordinarily not difficult when the typical clinical features are present. The differential diagnosis includes SLE, polyarteritis, infective endocarditis, postinfectious glomerulonephritis, and essential cryoimmunoglobulinemia.

The course is usually benign; however, progressive renal failure may occur. Renal biopsy is a useful prognostic tool. Patients with persistent urinary abnormalities may experience deterioration of renal function several years after diagnosis. Treatment is symptomatic. There is no convincing evidence that corticosteroid or immunosuppressive therapy is beneficial for the renal lesion, although these treatments may ameliorate extrarenal features. Patients with rapidly progressive (crescentic) glomerulonephritis benefit from intensive plasma exchange or immunosuppressive drugs combined with anticoagulant and antithrombotic agents (see Chap. 223).

SYSTEMIC NECROTIZING VASCULITIS (See also Chap. 269) Glomerular involvement is common in the heterogeneous group of disorders which result from widespread inflammatory and necrotizing lesions of blood vessels. Several variations are recognized, including microscopic polyarteritis (hypersensitivity angiitis), macroscopic polyarteritis (periarteritis nodosa), Wegener's granulomatosis, allergic angiitis and granulomatosis, rheumatoid vasculitis, temporal arteritis, and Takayasu's arteritis. Henoch-Schönlein purpura and SLE can also be considered as examples of vasculitis.

MISCELLANEOUS IMMUNOLOGICALLY MEDIATED MULTISYSTEM DISEASES **Mixed connective tissue disease (MCTD)** In this disorder, which is described in Chap. 265, renal disease is uncommon and, if present, is usually mild. Clinical manifestations include hematuria and proteinuria and occasionally nephrotic syndrome. Pathologically, membranous glomerulonephritis or mesangiocapillary glomerulonephritis is seen. The prognosis is generally favorable, and treatment is directed at extrarenal manifestations. Corticosteroid therapy often results in improvement of the glomerular lesions.

Rheumatoid arthritis Several forms of glomerular injury may occur in rheumatoid arthritis (Chap. 263). Secondary amyloidosis is present in 5 to 10 percent of patients with long-standing arthritis. Nephrotic syndrome may arise as a complication of either gold or penicillamine therapy (see Chap. 223). In addition, the kidney may share in the vasculitis seen occasionally in severe rheumatoid arthritis. Finally, patients with rheumatoid arthritis (untreated with gold or penicillamine) may develop a mild proliferative glomerulitis or membranous glomerulonephritis which resembles lesions seen in SLE. Proteinuria, sometimes with nephrotic syndrome, is the principal clinical feature of such lesions. Prolonged and excessive use of analgesics may lead to renal papillary necrosis.

Other disorders *Sjögren's syndrome* (Chap. 266) may be associated with nephrotic syndrome due to membranous or mesangiocapillary glomerulonephritis (type I) or, more frequently, interstitial nephritis. *Sarcoidosis* is rarely complicated by membranous glomerulonephritis. *Partial or total lipodystrophy* may be associated with mesangiocapillary glomerulonephritis (type II, dense deposit disease) (see Chaps. 223 and 318). Complement abnormalities are found, consisting of depressed C3 levels, normal C1q and C4 levels, and circulating C3 nephritic factor.

Chronic liver disease may be complicated by glomerular disease. The nephrotic syndrome may appear in the course of *chronic active hepatitis* associated with persistent hepatitis B surface antigenemia. Glomerular lesions include membranous glomerulonephritis or mesangiocapillary (type I) glomerulonephritis. Immunofluorescence studies in such patients reveal granular deposits of immunoglobulins, complement components, and hepatitis B viral antigens, indicating an immune-complex disease. Serum C3 levels are often reduced, and tests for CIC and cryoimmunoglobulins are frequently positive. Occasionally patients with little clinical evidence of liver disease develop distinct glomerular lesions secondary to chronic hepatitis B infection. *Acute viral hepatitis* may be associated with transient hematuria or proteinuria and may resemble other postinfectious glomerulonephritides (see Chap. 223). Severe *chronic liver disease* (cirrhosis) may be associated with diffuse glomerulosclerosis. Few clinical manifestations of glomerular disease are found. Prominent mesangial IgA deposits, of unknown pathogenic significance, have been noted in patients with cirrhosis.

MULTISYSTEM DISEASES ASSOCIATED WITH PARAPROTEINEMIA AND NEOPLASIA

ESSENTIAL (MIXED) CRYOIMMUNOGLOBULINEMIA This disorder is associated with circulating cold precipitable immunoglobulins (cryoimmunoglobulins), usually consisting of IgG and IgM; the latter possesses rheumatoid factor activity. Purpura, necrotizing skin lesions in cold-exposed areas, arthralgias, fever, and hepatosplenomegaly are common. Hepatitis B infection and other occult fungal, bacterial, or viral infections may be the cause of this syndrome. Circulating cryoimmunoglobulins are also found in chronic infections and probably represent circulating immune complexes with unusual physical properties. Glomerular disease results from the precipitation of the cryoimmunoglobulin in the glomerular capillaries and may result in acute renal failure, rapidly progressive (crescentic) glomerulonephritis, or the nephrotic syndrome. Serum complement components are depressed, and circulating immune complexes are present (Table 224-1). Pathologically, a diffuse proliferative glomerulonephritis may be seen with findings consistent with the deposition of the circulating cryoimmunoglobulin. Eradication of the underlying infection, if possible, is of value in treatment. Intensive plasma exchange, accompanied by the administration of corticosteroids and cytotoxic agents, has been of some success in severe cases.

MONOCLONAL GAMMOPATHIES *Multiple myeloma* (Chap. 258) may be associated with at least three types of glomerular injury. Amyloidosis (Chap. 259) (see below) occurs in 10 to 15 percent of patients with multiple myeloma. Lesions may resemble nodular diabetic glomerular sclerosis, and monoclonal cryoimmunoglobulins may be deposited in glomeruli. Proteinuria and the nephrotic syndrome are common. In addition, a tubulointerstitial lesion (myeloma kidney) consisting of large, laminated intratubular casts, tubule cell atrophy, interstitial fibrosis, and inflammation is common in patients with multiple myeloma and acute or chronic renal failure. *Waldenström's macroglobulinemia* may cause acute renal failure when the IgM paraprotein precipitates in glomerular capillaries as "thrombi." Intensive plasma exchange and therapy with alkylating agents may be beneficial. Hyperviscosity may cause functional alterations in GFR. Renal amyloidosis is uncommon. *Benign monoclonal gammopathies* are seldom associated with glomerular complications, except for mild asymptomatic proteinuria and, rarely, nephrotic syndrome. Excessive production of *light chains of Ig* (especially kappa type) may evoke glomerular alterations (nodular glomerulosclerosis, focal sclerosis) due to deposition of the protein in mesangium or along the subendothelial aspect of the glomerular capillary wall.

AMYLOIDOSIS (See also Chap. 259) This disorder may occur in the absence of systemic disease (primary amyloidosis), may be secondary to chronic inflammatory processes (e.g., rheumatoid arthritis, osteomyelitis, paraplegia), multiple myeloma or other neoplastic diseases, or may occur in a heredofamilial form (e.g., familial Mediterranean fever). All forms may affect the glomeruli.

Primary amyloidosis commonly affects the kidneys and usually occurs in older age groups. Proteinuria, often of nephrotic proportions, is the most common manifestation of renal involvement. The urine sediment tends to be benign. The degree of proteinuria is not necessarily related to the extent of glomerular deposition of amyloid. Enlarged kidneys may be present in patients with well-preserved renal function, but this is a nonspecific finding. The blood pressure is normal unless advanced uremia is present. Typical pathologic features include hypocellular glomeruli infiltrated with amorphous deposits that stain with Congo red and exhibit green birefringence under polarized light. The fibrillar nature of the amyloid deposits can be demonstrated by electron microscopy. The fibrils in primary amyloidosis and in multiple myeloma are related immunologically to the immunoglobulin light chain. Immunofluorescence studies reveal amorphous deposits of immunoglobulin and complement in glomeruli. Renal vein thrombosis may complicate the course of amyloidosis.

Renal amyloidosis is a progressive disease for which there is no established treatment. Remissions may occur in secondary amyloidosis if the cause can be eliminated. Remissions in primary amyloidosis are exceedingly rare; a few reports describe remissions following the use of cytotoxic agents. Overall the 5-year survival for patients with primary amyloidosis is less than 20 percent. Azotemia, persistent nephrotic syndrome, and myocardial involvement confer an even more ominous prognosis.

NEOPLASTIC DISEASE Glomerular alterations may develop with a variety of neoplastic diseases. *Carcinomas,* especially adenocarcinoma of lung, colon, stomach, and breast, may be accompanied by glomerular lesions resembling idiopathic membranous glomerulonephritis, although, on occasion, crescentic or focal and segmental proliferative glomerulonephritis or amyloidosis may be present. Nephrotic syndrome is the most common clinical renal manifestation, and approximately 6 to 10 percent of patients with idiopathic nephrotic syndrome associated with membranous glomerulonephritis harbor an underlying malignancy. Successful treatment of the tumor, especially by surgical means, may lead to a remission of the renal manifestation. Presumably the glomerular lesions arise because of the deposition of circulating immune complexes that are composed of tumor antigen and antitumor antibody. Amyloidosis may occasionally occur.

Lymphomas and leukemias may also give rise to glomerular abnormalities. Hodgkin's disease is commonly associated with the findings of idiopathic nephrotic syndrome (minimal change disease). Other glomerular lesions may include membranous glomerulonephritis, focal proliferative and sclerosing glomerulonephritis, and amyloidosis. The mechanism of the association of Hodgkin's disease with minimal change disease may involve an underlying T-cell abnormality. Proteinuria may wax and wane with fluctuations in the clinical activity of the Hodgkin's disease. Remissions may be produced by local irradiation of involved lymph nodes or by systemic chemotherapy.

METABOLIC, BIOCHEMICAL, AND HEREDITARY DISORDERS

DIABETIC NEPHROPATHY (See also Chap. 327) Diabetes mellitus affects the structure and function of the kidney in many ways. The term *diabetic nephropathy* encompasses all the lesions occurring in the kidneys of patients with diabetes mellitus. These lesions include *glomerulosclerosis* (diffuse or nodular), *arterionephrosclerosis, chronic interstitial nephritis, papillary necrosis,* and various tubular lesions. Diabetic nephropathy is associated with a variety of clinical syndromes, including mild asymptomatic proteinuria, nephrotic syndrome, progressive renal failure (acute, rapidly progressive, or chronic), and hypertension. Glomerular lesions are particularly common and account for the majority of abnormal clinical findings referable to the kidney. *Diffuse diabetic glomerulosclerosis* (diffuse intercapillary glomerulosclerosis) is the most common lesion and can be identified in the vast majority of diabetic patients regardless of the presence of abnormal clinical findings referable to the kidney. This lesion consists of a mild diffuse increase in mesangial matrix accompanied by an increased width of the glomerular basement membrane. Various exudative lesions, such as capsular drops and fibrin caps, may also be present. Hyaline arteriosclerosis, particularly of the efferent arteriole, is also common. Taken together, these lesions suggest the diagnosis of diabetes mellitus, but individually they are not specific. *Nodular glomerulosclerosis* (Kimmelstiel-Wilson lesion), on the other hand, is reasonably specific for juvenile onset (type I) diabetes mellitus. This lesion consists of PAS-positive, laminated, intercapillary nodules on a background of an increase in mesangial matrix. At the periphery of the nodules open glomerular capillary loops are found. The nodules are relatively acellular, in contrast to the cellular lesions of membranoproliferative glomerulonephritis (often referred to as *lobular glomerulonephritis*). A variable percentage of glomeruli may be affected.

The pathogenesis of diffuse or nodular diabetic glomerulosclerosis is poorly understood. Evidence supporting a role for both the abnormal diabetic milieu (e.g., insulinopenia, hyperglycemia, glycosuria) and genetic factors is reviewed in Chap. 327.

The principal clinical manifestation of diabetic glomerular disease is proteinuria. Initially, only small amounts of albumin (20 to 40 μg/

min) are excreted, particularly following exercise (microalbuminuria). This amount of albumin excretion is undetectable by routine screening methods. Under ordinary circumstances, microalbuminuria develops within 10 to 15 years from the onset of hyperglycemia and usually progresses within 3 to 5 years to overt proteinuria and clinical diabetic nephropathy. With "tight" control of hyperglycemia, the development of microalbuminuria may be prevented or reversed. With time, the quantity of protein excreted usually increases and may progress to an overt nephrotic syndrome. Glomerular filtration rate is initially elevated and subsequently falls towards normal coincident with the onset of overt proteinuria. The urinary sediment is typically benign, although microhematuria and/or pyuria may also be present if a complicating urinary tract infection or papillary necrosis is present. Hypertension develops if GFR falls but is seldom of malignant proportions. When hypertension is severe or abrupt in onset, one should suspect a complicating atherosclerotic renal arterial stenosis. Typically, plasma renin activity is normal or decreased. Acquired hyporeninemic hypoaldosteronism with persistent hyperkalemia and mild hyperchloremic metabolic acidosis is common. Once azotemia develops, the disease progresses at variable rates. End-stage renal failure usually develops within 5 years of the onset of overt proteinuria and clinical nephropathy. Despite poor control of hyperglycemia, only about 50 to 60 percent of type I (insulin-dependent) diabetic patients develop clinical nephropathy. The factors that protect the remaining patients from renal failure are unknown. Patients with type II (non-insulin-dependent) diabetes mellitus may also develop clinical nephropathy.

Until the cause of diabetes mellitus is established, prevention of the glomerulopathy will not be feasible. If the abnormal diabetic milieu is responsible for the vascular complications (including glomerular disease), as some have suggested, then very precise regulation of blood sugar (e.g., meticulous attention to diet, exercise, and insulin dosage and servofeedback devices for insulin administration) may be effective in reducing the development of nephropathy. Once the nephropathy has reached a clinically recognizable stage, aggressive management of hypertension may slow the rate of loss of renal function, but strict control of blood sugar does not seem to retard the rate of progression. Patients with end-stage renal failure due to diabetic nephropathy are not ideal candidates for long-term dialysis because of concomitant multiple organ dysfunction secondary to widespread arteriovascular disease. Mortality rates among diabetics on chronic dialysis are about three times higher than among similarly treated nondiabetics of comparable age. Renal transplantation may be successful in the younger diabetic, especially if a living related donor is available. The success rate is somewhat less than in the nondiabetic population, but transplantation is a viable alternative to dialysis in selected patients. Recurrence of typical diabetic glomerular lesions has been documented in renal allografts, but thus far, progressive loss of GFR secondary to recurrent disease has not been noted.

ALPORT'S SYNDROME This disorder consists of sensorineural deafness associated with hereditary nephritis. Renal disease manifests itself at an early age, principally as recurrent hematuria. Men are more frequently and severely affected than women. Slowly progressive renal insufficiency in men commonly terminates in end-stage renal disease in the second to third decade. There is no clear-cut relationship between the onset or severity of the hearing abnormality and the extent of renal disease. Other associated abnormalities include two related ophthalmologic complications, spherophakia and lenticonus, as well as thrombocytopathia, hyperprolinemia, and cerebral dysfunction. Family studies have indicated autosomal dominant or X-linked modes of inheritance with variable expressivity. The pathogenesis may be due to defective synthesis of glycopeptide (noncollagenous) components of glomerular and tubular basement membranes.

The pathologic features detected by light microscopy are nonspecific, and a diagnosis cannot be established by optical microscopy alone. Both glomerular and interstitial lesions are present. Focal and diffuse glomerular proliferation, with segmental sclerosis, is common. Interstitial foam cells are nonspecific findings. Electron microscopy reveals thinning, splitting, and delamination of both glomerular and tubular basement membranes, thought by some to be specific for the syndrome. Immunofluorescence studies fail to reveal deposits of immunoglobulins or complement components. The autoantibody to basement membrane antigens found in patients with Goodpasture's syndrome does not react with the glomeruli of some patients with Alport's syndrome. Treatment is supportive; corticosteroids and cytotoxic agents are ineffective. The disease is not known to recur following transplantation.

FABRY'S DISEASE (See also Chap. 316) This disorder, angiokeratoma corporus diffusum, is an X-linked inborn error of glycosphingolipid metabolism that leads to the accumulation of neutral glycosphingolipids in many tissues including the kidney. A milder disease may develop in heterozygous females. Manifestations include angiokerotomas involving the lower trunk, scrotum, and buttocks; acroparesthesia; corneal opacities; tortuous retinal veins; and premature coronary and cerebral ischemic disease. Renal manifestations include hematuria and modest proteinuria, often associated with slowly progressive renal failure. Light-microscopic findings include foamy alterations of the epithelial cells of the glomerulus due to the accumulation of lipid. Electron microscopy reveals intracellular rounded laminated bodies ("myelin figures"). The disorder is untreatable unless replacement of the deficient enzyme can be ensured; successful renal transplantation may correct the enzyme deficiency. Perhaps transplantation of other tissues (e.g., bone marrow) may ultimately become the treatment of choice.

NAIL-PATELLA SYNDROME This autosomal dominant disease is characterized by dystrophic nails, absence of one or both patellae, iliac horns, and renal disease. The renal manifestations include isolated proteinuria and hematuria and occasionally the nephrotic syndrome. Progressive renal failure is uncommon. Glomerular lesions are nonspecific by light microscopy, but electron microscopy reveals a characteristic moth-eaten appearance of the glomerular basement membrane associated with intramembranous collagen fibrils. The prognosis is generally favorable. No treatment is known.

CONGENITAL NEPHROTIC SYNDROME This autosomal recessive trait is characterized by the development of nephrotic syndrome at the time of or shortly after birth. It occurs with highest frequency in families of Finnish origin. Affected individuals have very large placentas, low birth weight, anasarca, polycythemia, and initially normal GFRs. Levels of α-fetoprotein are increased in amniotic fluid and maternal serum. Proteinuria is marked and nonselective. Nephrotic syndrome appearing several months after birth is usually due to other causes, especially minimal change disease or focal glomerular sclerosis (Chap. 223). Congenital syphilis and congenital toxoplasmosis may produce similar syndromes and must be excluded. Pathologically, microcystic transformation of the cortical nephrons results in proximal tubular dilatation. Glomerular changes are nonspecific. Extensive effacement of the foot processes and sclerosis of the glomerular tufts are seen by electron microscopy. Immunofluorescence findings are nonspecific. The course is progressive, and few patients survive the first year of life. Treatment is ineffective. Death is usually due to inanition, infection, or renal failure. A few patients may survive long enough to be considered for renal transplantation.

SICKLE CELL DISEASE (See also Chap. 288) This disorder is an autosomal trait characterized by an abnormal hemoglobin (hemoglobin S). Glomerular lesions occur occasionally in homozygous disease. The medulla is affected, leading to impairment of concentrating ability and acid excretion and, occasionally, to papillary necrosis. Rarely, patients develop mainly glomerular lesions, either membranous or mesangiocapillary glomerulonephritis and are accompanied by proteinuria and a nephrotic syndrome. Immunofluorescence studies demonstrate renal deposition of immunoglobulin and complement in a granular pattern suggesting immune-complex–mediated disease. In a few instances, renal tubuloepithelial antigens are localized in these

TABLE 224-2 Drugs associated with glomerular lesions

Elemental, inorganic, or organic mercury compounds
Organic gold compounds
Penicillamine
Captopril
Heroin
Amphetamines
Probenecid
Oxazoladinedione derivatives (e.g., Trimethadione)
Antivenoms and antitoxins
Sulfonamides
Vaccinations

deposits, suggesting that ischemic damage of the kidney may release autologous antigens to provoke the immune-complex disease. The course in patients with the glomerulopathy of sickle cell disease is often relentless, leading to end-stage renal disease. No treatment is known to be effective. Transplantation has been successful occasionally.

LECITHIN: CHOLESTEROL ACYLTRANSFERASE DEFICIENCY (See also Chap. 315) This autosomal recessive trait leads to absence in plasma of the enzyme that catalyzes the conversion of lecithin and cholesterol to lysolecithin and cholesteryl ester. Multiple lipoprotein abnormalities develop, including absence of α and pre-β lipoproteins, hypertriglyceridemia, accumulation of abnormal lipoproteins, and increased plasma-esterified cholesterol. Corneal opacities, anemia, hyperuricemia, proteinuria and progressive renal failure are characteristic. Foam cells are present in bone marrow and glomeruli, and a picture resembling focal and segmental glomerulosclerosis may evolve. Treatment is generally ineffective, but plasma or blood transfusions may transiently correct the disorder. Renal failure has been corrected by renal transplantation, but recurrence of disease in allografts may occur.

DRUG-INDUCED GLOMERULAR DISEASE Many drugs have been associated with the development of glomerular disease; however, it is usually difficult to establish a direct cause and effect relationship. In a few situations the association is clear-cut, and reexposure has led to recurrence of disease. A partial listing of these drugs is provided in Table 224-2. Certain *heavy metals* (Hg, Au) and their inorganic salts or organic compounds may produce membranous glomerulonephritis and nephrotic syndrome. Removal of the drug is not invariably associated with resolution. *Sulfhydryl compounds* (penicillamine, captopril) may also cause membranous or proliferative glomerulonephritis. The risk of developing a renal complication following penicillamine or gold therapy for rheumatoid arthritis is influenced by genes in the major histocompatibility complex. *Nonsteroidal anti-inflammatory agents* may produce nephrotic syndrome (minimal change disease), interstitial nephritis, and acute renal failure. *Probenecid, trimethadione,* or *paramethadione* may be associated with nephrotic syndrome and a variety of glomerular lesions, including minimal change disease and membranous glomerulonephritis. *Heroin* abuse may be associated with focal and segmental glomerulosclerosis that may progress to nephrotic syndrome and progressive renal failure. *Intravenous amphetamine abuse* may be associated with systemic necrotizing vasculitis. Chronic hepatitis B infection may also participate in the development of glomerular lesions in association with intravenous drug abuse.

REFERENCES

CAMERON JS: Henoch-Schönlein purpura, in *Textbook of Nephrology,* SG Massry and RJ Glassock (eds). Baltimore, Williams & Wilkins, 1983, p. 6.104

FAUCI AS et al: Wegener's granulomatosis: Prospective clinical and therapeutic experience with 85 patients for 21 years. Ann Intern Med 98:76, 1983

GLASSOCK RJ et al: Secondary glomerular diseases, in *The Kidney,* 3d ed. BM Brenner and FC Rector Jr (eds). Philadelphia, Saunders, 1986, p 1014

HILL GS et al: Renal lesions in multiple myeloma: Their relationship to associated protein abnormalities. Am J Kidney Dis 2:423, 1983

HUGHES GRV (ed): Systemic lupus erythematosus. Clin Rheum Dis 8:1, 1982

SPEAR GS: Hereditary nephritis (Alport's syndrome), 1983. Clin Nephrol 21:3, 1983

WETZELS JF et al: The changing natural history of nephropathy in type I diabetes. Am J Med 80: A63, 1986

225 URINARY TRACT INFECTION, PYELONEPHRITIS, AND RELATED CONDITIONS

WALTER E. STAMM / MARVIN TURCK

DEFINITIONS Acute infections of the urinary tract can be subdivided into two general anatomic categories: lower tract infection (urethritis, cystitis, and prostatitis) and upper tract infection (acute pyelonephritis). Infections at these various sites may occur together or independently, and may be asymptomatic or present as the clinical syndromes outlined below.

Recurrent infections can be classified as relapses (a recurrence with the same strain, as judged by species identification, serotype, and antibiogram, that occurs within 1 to 2 weeks of stopping antibiotic therapy) or reinfections (a recurrence with a new strain). Most relapses are thought to result from unresolved renal or prostatic infection.

Symptoms of dysuria, urgency, and frequency unaccompanied by significant bacteriuria have been termed the acute urethral syndrome. Although widely used, this term lacks anatomic precision because many cases of urethral syndrome are in actuality bladder infections. Moreover, since the causative agent can usually be identified in these patients, the term *syndrome,* implying unknown causation, is inappropriate.

Chronic pyelonephritis refers to chronic interstitial nephritis believed to result from bacterial infection of the kidney (see Chap. 226). Many noninfectious diseases also cause an interstitial nephritis indistinguishable pathologically from chronic pyelonephritis.

Microbiologically, urinary tract infection exists when pathogenic microorganisms are detected in the urine, urethra, kidney, or prostate. In most instances, growth of more than 10^5 organisms per milliliter from a properly collected midstream "clean catch" urine sample indicates infection. However, significant bacteriuria may be absent in some circumstances when true urinary infection exists. Especially in symptomatic patients, a smaller number of bacteria (10^2 to 10^4 per milliliter of midstream urine) may accompany infection. In urine specimens obtained by suprapubic aspiration or "in and out" catheterization, or from a patient with an indwelling catheter, colony counts of 10^2 to 10^4 per milliliter generally indicate infection. Conversely, colony counts in excess of 10^5 per milliliter of midstream urine are occasionally due to specimen contamination.

ACUTE INFECTIONS OF THE URINARY TRACT: URETHRITIS, CYSTITIS, AND PYELONEPHRITIS

EPIDEMIOLOGY Epidemiologically, urinary tract infections should be subdivided into catheter-associated (or nosocomial) infections and noncatheter-associated (or community-acquired) infections. In either category, infections may be symptomatic or asymptomatic. Acute infections in noncatheterized patients occur very commonly, especially in women, and account for over 6 million office visits annually in the United States. These infections occur in 1 to 3 percent of schoolgirls, and then increase markedly in incidence with the onset of sexual activity in adolescence. The vast majority of acute symptomatic infections occur in young women. Acute symptomatic urinary infections are rare in men under the age of 50. The occurrence of asymptomatic bacteriuria parallels that of symptomatic infection and is rare in men under 50, but is common in women between the ages of 20 and 50.

ETIOLOGY Many different microorganisms can infect the urinary tract, but by far the most common agents are the gram-negative bacilli. *Escherichia coli* causes approximately 80 percent of acute infections in patients without urologic abnormalities or calculi. Other gram-negative rods, including *Proteus, Klebsiella, Enterobacter,*

Serratia, and *Pseudomonas,* account for a smaller proportion of uncomplicated infections. These organisms assume increasing importance in recurrent infections and infections associated with urologic manipulation, calculi, or obstruction. They play a major role in nosocomial, catheter-associated infections (see below). *Proteus* species, by virtue of urease production, and *Klebsiella* species, through production of extracellular slime and polysaccharides, predispose to stone formation and are isolated more frequently from patients with calculi.

Gram-positive cocci play a lesser role in urinary tract infections. However, *Staphylococcus saprophyticus,* a novobiocin-resistant, coagulase-negative staphylococcus, accounts for 10 to 15 percent of acute symptomatic urinary tract infections in young females. Enterococci and *Staphylococcus aureus* cause infections in patients with renal stones or previous instrumentation. Isolation of *S. aureus* should arouse suspicion of bacteremic infection of the kidney.

About one-third of women with dysuria and frequency have either a nonsignificant number of bacteria in midstream urine cultures or completely sterile cultures, and have been previously defined as having the urethral syndrome. About three-quarters of these women have significant pyuria, while one-quarter have no pyuria and little objective evidence of infection. In the women with pyuria, two groups of pathogens account for the majority of infections. Low quantities (10^2 to 10^4 bacteria per milliliter) of typical bacterial uropathogens such as *E. coli, S. saprophyticus, Klebsiella,* or *Proteus* in midstream urine specimens are found in the majority of these women, are probably the causative agents because they can usually be isolated from a suprapubic aspirate, are usually associated with pyuria, and respond to appropriate antimicrobial therapy. In other women with acute urinary symptoms, pyuria, and sterile urine (even on suprapubic aspiration), sexually transmitted urethritis-producing agents such as *Chlamydia trachomatis, Neisseria gonorrhoeae,* and herpes simplex virus are important etiologic agents. These sexually transmitted agents are more frequently found in young, sexually active women with new sexual partners.

Viruses can produce pyelonephritis in animals and may increase the kidney's susceptibility to infection with gram-negative bacteria. In humans, viruses (cytomegalovirus, for example) are most commonly recovered from the urine without evidence of acute urinary disease, although some adenoviruses cause acute hemorrhagic cystitis. Similarly, *Candida* and other fungi may colonize the urine of catheterized patients or diabetics, and rarely cause acute symptomatic infection.

PATHOGENESIS AND SOURCES OF INFECTION The urinary tract should be viewed as a single anatomic unit connected by a continuous column of urine that extends from the urethra to the kidney. In the vast majority of infections, bacteria gain access to the bladder via the urethra. Ascent of bacteria from the bladder may then follow and is probably the usual pathway for most renal parenchymal infections.

The distal urethra is normally colonized with diphtheroids, streptococcal species, and staphylococcal species but not with the enteric gram-negative bacilli that commonly cause urinary tract infections. In females prone to development of cystitis, however, enteric gram-negative organisms residing in the bowel colonize the introitus, the periurethral skin, and the distal urethra prior to and during episodes of bacteriuria. Factors predisposing to periurethral colonization with gram-negative bacilli remain poorly understood but may involve alteration of the normal perineal flora by antibiotics or by other genital infections, absence of local antibody, and/or enhanced attachment of organisms to the epithelial cells of infection-prone women. Small numbers of periurethral bacteria probably gain entry to the bladder frequently, facilitated in some women by urethral massage during intercourse. Whether bladder infection ensues then depends upon interaction between the pathogenicity of the strain, the inoculum size, and local and systemic host defense mechanisms.

Under normal circumstances, bacteria placed in the bladder are rapidly cleared in humans or experimental animals. This results partly from the flushing and dilutional effects of voiding, but also from direct antibacterial properties of urine and the bladder mucosa. Due mostly to high urea concentration and high osmolarity, the bladder urine of many normal persons inhibits or kills bacteria. Prostatic secretions possess antibacterial properties as well. Polymorphonuclear leukocytes in the bladder wall also appear to play a role in clearing bacteriuria. The role of locally produced antibody remains unclear. Hematogenous pyelonephritis occurs most often in debilitated patients who either have chronic illnesses or who are receiving immunosuppressive therapy. Staphylococcal pyelonephritis may follow bacteremia from distant foci of infection in the bone, skin, endothelium, or elsewhere.

CONDITIONS AFFECTING PATHOGENESIS **Gender and sexual activity** The female urethra appears particularly prone to colonization with colonic gram-negative bacilli, owing to its proximity to the anus, its short length (about 4 cm), and its termination beneath the labia. Urethral massage, as occurs during sexual intercourse, causes introduction of bacteria into the bladder, and appears to be very important in the pathogenesis of urinary infections in younger women. In addition, diaphragm use has been associated with a twofold increase in risk of urinary infection. In males, prostatitis or urethral obstruction due to prostatic hypertrophy are important factors predisposing to bacteriuria.

Pregnancy Depending on socioeconomic status, urinary infections are detected in 2 to 8 percent of pregnant women. In particular, symptomatic upper tract infections occur more commonly during pregnancy; fully 20 to 30 percent of pregnant women with asymptomatic bacteriuria subsequently develop pyelonephritis. This predisposition to upper tract infection during pregnancy results from the decreased ureteral tone, decreased ureteral peristalsis, and temporary incompetence of the vesicoureteral valves seen in pregnancy. Bladder catheterization during or after delivery causes additional infections. Cystitis and pyelonephritis are no more common in women with toxemia of pregnancy than in other pregnant women. An increased prevalence of prematurity and newborn mortality may result from urinary infections during pregnancy.

Obstruction Any impediment to the free flow of urine—tumor, stricture, stone, or prostatic hypertrophy—results in hydronephrosis and greatly increased frequency of urinary tract infection. Infection superimposed on urinary tract obstruction may lead to rapid destruction of renal tissue. It is of utmost importance, therefore, when infection is present, to repair obstructive lesions. On the other hand, with minor degrees of obstruction that are not progressive or associated with infection, great caution must be exercised in attempting surgical correction. The introduction of infection in such patients may be more damaging than uncorrected minor obstructions which do not significantly impair renal function.

Neurogenic bladder dysfunction Interference with the nerve supply to the bladder, as in spinal cord injury, tabes dorsalis, multiple sclerosis, diabetes, or other diseases, may be associated with urinary tract infection. The infection may be initiated by the use of catheters for bladder drainage and is favored by the prolonged standing of urine in the bladder. An additional factor often present in these patients is bone demineralization due to immobilization, which causes hypercalciuria, calculus formation, and obstructive uropathy.

Vesicoureteral reflux This condition is defined as reflux of urine from the bladder cavity up into the ureters and sometimes into the renal pelvis. It occurs during voiding or with elevation of pressure in the bladder. In practice, vesicoureteral reflux exists when retrograde movement of radiopaque or radioactive material can be demonstrated. However, since a fluid connection between the bladder and kidney always exists in the patent urinary system, during infections some retrograde movement of bacteria probably occurs normally but is not detected by radiologic techniques. An anatomically impaired ureterovesical junction facilitates reflux of bacteria.

Vesicoureteral reflux is common in children with anatomic abnormalities of the urinary tract and in children with anatomically normal but infected urinary tracts. In the latter group, reflux disappears with advancing age and probably results from rather than causes urinary infection. Follow-up of children with urinary tract infection who were found to have reflux establishes that renal damage correlates with massive reflux, not with infection.

The routine search for reflux would be aided by development of noninvasive tests applicable to young children, where the need is greatest. In the meantime, it appears reasonable to search for massive reflux in anyone with unexplained failure of renal growth or renal scarring, because urinary tract infection per se is an insufficient explanation for these abnormalities. On the other hand, it is doubtful that all children with recurrent urinary tract infections but normal urinary tracts on pyelography should be subjected to voiding cystoureterography merely to detect the rare patient with massive reflux that did not reveal itself on the intravenous pyelogram.

Bacterial virulence factors Bacterial virulence factors influence the likelihood that a given strain, once introduced into the bladder, will cause urinary tract infection. The majority of strains that cause symptomatic urinary tract infections in noncatheterized patients belong to a small number of serogroups, produce hemolysin, and share certain other properties. Adherence of bacteria to uroepithelial cells is a critical first step in the initiation of infection. For both *E. coli* and *Proteus,* fimbriae (hairlike surface appendages) mediate bacterial attachment to specific receptors on epithelial cells. Nearly all strains of *E. coli* that cause pyelonephritis in patients with anatomically normal urinary tracts possess a particular pilus (the P pilus or gal-gal pilus) that mediates attachment to a digalactoside portion of glycosphingolipids present on uroepithelium. Strains that produce pyelonephritis are also usually hemolysin producers and are resistant to the bactericidal action of human serum.

LOCALIZATION OF INFECTION Infections involving the upper urinary tract usually cause a significant rise in serum antibodies directed against the O antigen of the infecting strain. They also produce a temporary defect in renal concentrating ability in many patients, and may be associated with formation of leukocyte casts. Lower tract infections rarely result in increased antibody titers, concentrating defects, or white cell casts. Unfortunately, these methods of distinguishing renal parenchymal infection from cystitis are neither reliable nor convenient enough for routine clinical use. More sensitive tests for distinguishing pyelonephritis from cystitis (bilateral ureteral catheterization and the bladder wash-out technique originated by Fairley) are inherently invasive and too complex for clinical practice. The development of a simpler and clinically applicable test to separate upper and lower tract infections based upon antibody coating of bacteria in the urine has been studied. In this test, bacteria from patients with pyelonephritis demonstrate antibody coating on their surface when they have been exposed to a fluorescein-labeled antihuman globulin and are viewed under a fluorescence microscope. No surface antibodies can be seen on bacteria from patients with cystitis. This antibody response consists mainly of IgG and can be reproduced in an experimental pyelonephritis model in animals. However, false-negative results occur in 15 to 20 percent of patients who have upper tract infection as judged by direct localization procedures. These false-negatives probably occur because antibody production, particularly in first infections, requires 10 to 15 days, and most patients are treated before this length of time elapses. ~~False-positive results occur~~ in males with prostatitis and women with hemorrhagic cystitis, heavy proteinuria, and vaginal or fecal contamination of midstream urine. Infections with yeast or *Pseudomonas* cause false-positives due to autofluorescence, and staphylococci with protein A nonspecifically bind human immunoglobulin, also causing false-positives. The antibody-coated bacteria test does not have sufficient sensitivity and specificity to be of value in the routine clinical management of patients. An elevated C-reactive protein often accompanies acute pyelonephritis and rarely is seen in cystitis, but this acute phase reactant is nonspecific and occurs in infections other than pyelonephritis as well.

CLINICAL PRESENTATION Clinical signs and symptoms cannot be relied upon to diagnose urinary tract infection correctly or to localize the site of infection. Many patients with significant bacteriuria (including some with upper tract infection) have no symptoms at all. Of those with significant bacteriuria and symptoms of cystitis, about one-half have lower tract infection and about one-half have clinically silent upper tract infection that is evident only upon performing localization studies. Clinical symptoms and signs of pyelonephritis, though often suggestive, do not always indicate upper tract infection. Finally, among women presenting with acute dysuria and frequency, only 60 to 70 percent have significant bacteriuria, but the majority of those without significant bacteriuria also have urinary tract or urethral infections.

Enumeration of the number of bacteria in the urine is an extremely important diagnostic procedure. In symptomatic infections of the urinary tract, bacteria are usually demonstrable in the urine in large numbers. Quantitative estimation of the number of bacteria in voided urine specimens as a rule makes it possible to distinguish contaminants from true bacteriuria, and 10^5 or more bacteria per milliliter has been the criterion traditionally used for this purpose. However, in symptomatic women with pyuria, counts of 10^2 to 10^4 *E. coli, Klebsiella, Proteus,* or *S. saprophyticus* per milliliter of midstream urine usually indicate infection, not contamination, and should not be disregarded. In asymptomatic patients, two or three consecutive urine specimens should be examined bacteriologically before instituting therapy, and 10^5 or more per milliliter of a single species should be demonstrable in the repeated specimens. A quantitative estimate of the degree of bacteriuria can be made by direct microscopic examination of a Gram's stain of uncentrifuged, freshly voided urine. If bacteria can be found by this method, it may be assumed that the number present approximates 100,000 per milliliter. Since the large number of bacteria in the bladder urine is due in part to bacterial multiplication during residence in the bladder cavity, samples of urine from the ureters or renal pelvis might contain fewer than 10^5 bacteria per milliliter and yet indicate infection. Similarly, the presence of bacteriuria of any degree in suprapubic aspirates or of 10^2 or more bacteria per milliliter of urine obtained by catheterization usually indicates infection. In some circumstances (antibiotics, high urea concentration, high osmolarity, low pH), urine will inhibit bacterial multiplication, resulting in a lower number of bacteria in the presence of infection. For this reason, antiseptic solutions should not be used in washing the periurethral area prior to collection of the urine specimen. Water diuresis or recent voiding also reduces the bacterial counts in urine.

Cystitis Patients with dysuria, frequency, urgency, and suprapubic pain usually have cystitis. The urine often becomes grossly cloudy, malodorous, and, in about 30 percent of cases, bloody. Pyuria without leukocyte casts and bacteria should be present on examination of the unspun urine in most patients. However, some women with cystitis have only 10^2 to 10^4 bacteria per milliliter of urine, which cannot be seen on Gram's stain of unspun urine. Physical examination generally reveals only a tender urethra or suprapubic tenderness. If a genital lesion or a vaginal discharge is present, especially with fewer than 10^5 bacteria per milliliter on culture, causes of urethritis, vaginitis, or cervicitis such as *C. trachomatis,* gonorrhea, *Trichomonas, Candida,* and *Herpesvirus hominis* should be ruled out. Prominent systemic manifestations like fever over 101°F, nausea, vomiting, and costovertebral angle tenderness usually indicate concomitant renal infection. However, the absence of these findings does not ensure that infection is limited to the bladder and urethra.

Acute pyelonephritis Symptoms generally develop rapidly over a few hours or a day and include fever which is often 103°F or greater, shaking chills, nausea, vomiting, and diarrhea. Symptoms of cystitis may or may not be present. Besides fever, tachycardia, and generalized muscle tenderness, physical examination reveals marked tenderness on deep pressure in one or both costovertebral areas or on deep abdominal palpation. In some patients, signs and symptoms of gram-negative sepsis predominate. Most patients have significant leukocytosis, pyuria with leukocyte casts in the urine, and bacteria on a Gram's stain of unspun urine. Hematuria may be present during the acute phase of the disease, but if it persists after acute manifestations of infection have subsided, a stone, tumor, or tuberculosis should be considered.

Except in individuals with papillary necrosis or urinary obstruction, the manifestations of acute pyelonephritis usually subside within a few days, even without specific antibacterial therapy. However, despite the absence of symptoms, bacteriuria or pyuria may persist. With severe pyelonephritis, fever subsides more slowly and may not disappear for several days, even after appropriate antibiotic treatment has been instituted.

Urethritis Approximately 30 percent of women with acute dysuria, frequency, and pyuria have midstream urine cultures that show either no growth or nonsignificant bacterial growth. Clinically, these women cannot be readily distinguished from those with cystitis. In these women distinction should be made between those having sexually transmitted pathogens such as *C. trachomatis, Neisseria gonorrhoeae,* or herpes simplex virus, and those having low-count *E. coli* or staphylococcal infection. Women with a gradual onset of illness, no hematuria, no suprapubic pain, and a history of more than 7 days of symptoms should be suspected of having chlamydial infection. The additional history of a recent sex partner change, especially if the patient's partner has recently had chlamydial or gonococcal urethritis, should heighten the suspicion of a sexually transmitted infection, as would the finding of mucopurulent cervicitis. Gross hematuria, suprapubic pain, abrupt onset of illness, a duration of illness of less than 3 days, and a history of previous urinary tract infections favor *E. coli* or staphylococcal infection.

Catheter-associated urinary tract infections Bacteriuria occurs in at least 25 percent of hospitalized patients with indwelling urethral catheters. The risk of infection is about 5 percent per day of catheterization. *Proteus, Pseudomonas, Klebsiella,* and *Serratia,* in addition to *E. coli,* usually cause these infections. Many infecting strains show marked antimicrobial resistance compared with organisms that cause community-acquired urinary infections. Factors associated with an increased risk of infection include female sex, lengthy period of catheterization, severe underlying illness, faulty catheter care, and poorly trained nursing personnel.

Infection occurs when bacteria reach the bladder by one of two routes: by migrating through the column of urine in the catheter lumen (intraluminal route); or by moving up the mucous sheath outside the catheter (periurethral route). Hospital-acquired pathogens reach the patient's catheter or urine-collecting system on the hands of hospital personnel, in contaminated solutions or irrigants, and via contaminated instruments or disinfectants. Entry of bacteria into the catheter system usually occurs at the catheter–collecting tube junction or at the drainage bag portal. Bacteria then ascend intraluminally into the bladder. More often, the patient's own bowel flora migrate to the perineal skin and periurethral area and reach the bladder via the external surface of the catheter. This route is particularly common in women.

Most catheter-associated infections appear to be benign. They cause minimal symptoms, no fever, and often resolve after withdrawal of the catheter. The frequency of upper tract infection associated with catheter-induced bacteriuria is unknown. Gram-negative bacteremia, which follows 1 to 2 percent of cases of catheter-associated bacteriuria, is the most significantly recognized complication of catheter-induced urinary infections. The catheterized urinary tract has repeatedly been demonstrated to be the most common source of gram-negative bacteremia in hospitalized patients. It has also been suggested that bacteriuria in catheterized patients is associated with an adjusted increased relative risk of death of approximately threefold compared with similar patients without bacteriuria.

Catheter-associated urinary tract infections can be partially prevented in patients catheterized less than 2 weeks by use of a sterile closed collecting system, attention to aseptic technique during insertion and care of the catheter, use of meatal antiseptic ointments, and by measures to minimize cross infection. Despite these precautions, the majority of patients catheterized longer than 2 weeks develop bacteriuria. The optimal treatment for such patients has not been established. Removal of the catheter and a short course of antibiotics to which the organism is susceptible is probably the best course of action and nearly always eradicates the bacteriuria. If the catheter cannot be removed, antibiotic therapy usually proves to be unsuccessful and may result in infection with a more resistant strain. In this situation, the bacteriuria should be ignored unless the patient develops symptoms or is at high risk of developing bacteremia. In these cases, systemic antibiotics or urinary bladder antiseptics may reduce the degree of bacteriuria and the likelihood of bacteremia. In patients who require long-term catheterization, sterile intermittent in-and-out catheterization performed by a nurse or by the patient results in fewer infections than does continuous indwelling catheterization.

TREATMENT Several therapeutic principles should underlie treatment of urinary tract infections:

1. A quantitative urine culture, a positive Gram stain, or an alternative rapid diagnostic test should be obtained to confirm infection before starting treatment, and antimicrobial sensitivity testing should be used to direct therapy in these patients.
2. Factors predisposing to infection, such as obstruction, neurogenic bladder, calculi, etc., should be identified and corrected if possible.
3. Relief of clinical symptoms does not always indicate bacteriologic cure.
4. After completion of therapy, each treatment episode should be classified as a failure (bacteriuria not eradicated during therapy or upon the immediate posttreatment culture) or a cure (resolution of symptoms and elimination of bacteriuria). Recurrent infections should be classified as relapses or reinfections.
5. In general, uncomplicated infections confined to the lower urinary tract respond to low doses and short courses of therapy, while upper tract infections require longer periods of treatment. Relapses usually indicate an upper tract focus of infection while reinfection more often indicates lower tract infection.
6. Community-acquired infections, especially initial infections, are nearly always due to antibiotic-sensitive strains.
7. Patients with repeated infections, instrumentation, or recent hospitalization should be suspected of harboring resistant strains.

The anatomic location of a urinary tract infection greatly influences success or failure of a therapeutic agent. Bladder bacteriuria (cystitis) can usually be eliminated with nearly any antimicrobial to which the infecting strain is sensitive; as little as a single dose of 500-mg intramuscular kanamycin eliminates bladder bacteriuria in most patients. A 7-day course of therapy with oral drugs appears more than adequate. With upper tract infections, however, single-dose therapy fails in the majority of cases and even a 7-day course will be unsuccessful in many patients. Longer periods of treatment (2 to 6 weeks) aimed at eradicating a persistent focus of infection may be necessary in cases of relapse.

In *acute uncomplicated cystitis,* more than 90 percent of infections are due to *E. coli,* and although resistance patterns vary geographically, most strains are sensitive to many antibiotics. Single-dose amoxicillin (3.0 g), trimethoprim-sulfamethoxazole (4 to 6 single-strength tablets), trimethoprim (400 mg), and sulfa alone (2.0 g) have been successfully used to treat acute uncomplicated episodes of cystitis. Amoxicillin appears to result in a lower cure rate than the other three agents. The advantages of single-dose therapy include less expense, ensured compliance, fewer side effects, and perhaps less intense selective pressure for emergence of resistant organisms in the gut, vaginal, or perineal flora. Although some studies suggest more relapses occur after single-dose therapy than after longer treatment, it does appear safe and efficacious for women presenting with acute uncomplicated cystitis. Single-dose therapy should be used only in reliable patients in whom posttreatment follow-up can be ensured, and in patients in whom symptoms have been present for less than 10 days. It should not be used in women with symptoms or signs of pyelonephritis or in women with urologic abnormalities or stones. In women with previous infections due to antibiotic-resistant organisms, single-dose therapy may be less appropriate. Further evaluation of single-dose therapy in children and pregnant women with bacteriuria is needed before it can be recommended in these populations. In these populations, 7 days of therapy with the antimicrobials listed above should be given. Males with urinary tract infection often have urologic abnormalities or prostatic involvement and positive antibody-coated-bacterial bacteriuria, and hence are not candidates for single-dose therapy.

Treatment of the acute urethritis in women depends upon the etiologic agent involved. In chlamydial infection, tetracycline (500 mg orally qid for 7 days) should be used. Women with acute dysuria and frequency, negative urine cultures, and no pyuria do not usually respond to antimicrobial agents.

Acute pyelonephritis without accompanying clinical evidence of calculi or urologic disease is due to *E. coli* in most cases. Although the optimal route and duration of therapy have not been established, a 10- to 14-day course of trimethoprim-sulfamethoxazole, trimethoprim alone, an aminoglycoside, or a cephalosporin usually provides adequate therapy. Ampicillin should not be used as initial therapy since 20 to 30 percent of *E. coli* are now resistant in vitro. Intravenous antibiotics, at least for the first several days of treatment, should probably be given to all but minimally symptomatic patients. Some patients relapse following therapy and should be investigated to determine whether unrecognized calculi or urologic disease is present. If not, treatment should be extended to 2 to 6 weeks to eliminate a presumed upper tract focus causing recurrent bacteriuria.

When suspected *gram-negative sepsis* complicates acute pyelonephritis, hospitalization, prompt parenteral therapy with an aminoglycoside, and ancillary measures to treat sepsis should be provided (see Chap. 86). When the antibiotic sensitivities of the infecting strain are available, therapy can be changed to a less toxic agent. Similar therapy should be used for infected patients with calculi or urologic abnormalities who have suspected sepsis.

In *pregnancy,* acute cystitis can be managed with 7 days of amoxicillin, nitrofurantoin, or a cephalosporin. After treatment, a culture should be obtained to ensure cure and repeated monthly thereafter. Acute pyelonephritis in pregnancy should be managed by hospitalization and parenteral antibiotics, generally a cephalosporin or an extended-spectrum penicillin. Continuous low-dose prophylaxis with nitrofurantoin should be given to women who have recurrent infections during pregnancy.

Asymptomatic bacteriuria should be documented with at least two positive cultures before treatment is given. Seven days of an oral agent to which the organism is sensitive should be given initially. If bacteriuria persists, it can be followed without further treatment in most patients. In patients who may be at high risk because of neutropenia, compromised host defenses, renal transplant, or previous development of pyelonephritis or bacteremia, further treatment with either 6 weeks of oral therapy or 4 to 6 weeks of combined parenteral and oral therapy should be given.

Optimal treatment regimens for patients with *catheter-associated urinary tract infections* have not been well established. These infections often remit spontaneously or with short-term antibiotic therapy if the catheter can be removed. If the catheter cannot be removed, systemic antibiotics or urinary antiseptics may reduce bacteriuria, but do not usually eliminate it. Asymptomatic bacteriuria in catheterized patients can probably be left untreated in most patients who are not immunosuppressed or who are not at high risk for sepsis because of old age, severe underlying disease, diabetes, or pregnancy.

UROLOGIC EVALUATION Very few women with recurrent urinary tract infections have correctable lesions discovered at cystoscopy or upon intravenous pyelography, and these procedures should not be routinely performed in such patients. In selected women, namely those with relapsing infection, those with a history of childhood infections, those with stones or painless hematuria, and those with recurrent pyelonephritis, urologic evaluation should be performed. All males with urinary infection should be evaluated urologically. Men or women presenting with acute infection and signs or symptoms suggestive of an obstruction or stones should undergo urologic evaluation, generally ultrasound.

PROGNOSIS In patients with uncomplicated cystitis or pyelonephritis, treatment ordinarily results in complete resolution of symptoms. In fact, symptoms usually remit even without specific therapy. Lower tract infections in adult women are of concern mainly because they cause discomfort, minor morbidity, and time lost from work. Cystitis may also result in upper tract infection or in bacteremia (especially during instrumentation), but there is little evidence to suggest that renal impairment follows. When repeated episodes of cystitis occur, they are nearly always reinfections, not relapses. Why a significant subpopulation of adult women develops a predisposition to multiple recurrent infections remains poorly understood. In some cases, residual urine, urethral stenosis, or other anatomic explanations exist, but most women with recurrent infections have no such demonstrable abnormality. Their uroepithelial cells appear highly prone to persistent colonization with *E. coli;* the explanation for this phenomenon is not clear.

Uncomplicated acute pyelonephritis in adults rarely progresses to functional impairment and chronic renal disease. Repeated upper tract infections often indicate relapse rather than reinfection, and a vigorous search for renal calculi or an underlying urologic abnormality should be undertaken. If neither is found, 6 weeks of chemotherapy may be useful in eradicating an unresolved focus of infection.

Repeated symptomatic urinary tract infections in children, and in adults with obstructive uropathy, neurogenic bladder, structural renal disease, or diabetes more often progress to chronic renal disease. Asymptomatic bacteriuria in these groups, as well as in adults without urologic disease or obstruction, predisposes to increased episodes of symptomatic infection but does not result in renal impairment in most instances.

PREVENTION Patients with frequent symptomatic infections may benefit from long-term low-dose antibiotics directed at preventing recurrences. A single dose of trimethoprim-sulfamethoxazole (80 mg trimethoprim and 400 mg sulfamethoxazole daily), trimethoprim alone (100 mg daily), or nitrofurantoin (50 mg daily) have been particularly effective. Suppressive therapy should be initiated only after bacteriuria has been eradicated with a full-dose treatment regimen. Women having more than two infections every 6 months should be considered for preventive antibiotics. Low-dose antibiotics (nitrofurantoin 50 to 100 mg) after sexual intercourse may also be of benefit in preventing episodes of symptomatic infections. Other situations in which prophylaxis appears to have some merit include men with chronic prostatitis; patients undergoing prostatectomy, both during the operation and postoperative periods; and pregnant women with asymptomatic bacteriuria. All pregnant women should be screened for bacteriuria in the first trimester, and should be treated if bacteriuria is found.

CHRONIC PYELONEPHRITIS

Chronic interstitial nephritis thought to result from bacterial infection of the kidney has been termed *chronic pyelonephritis*. It may occur in patients with predisposing urologic abnormalities (obstruction, vesicoureteral reflux, or neurogenic bladder) or in patients with apparently normal urinary tracts. Unlike acute urinary tract infections, for which simple diagnostic criteria and characteristic clinical syndromes exist, no pathognomonic clinical, laboratory, or pathologic criteria can be used to identify cases of chronic pyelonephritis, and few reliable data on the incidence or prevalence of this condition have been collected. Many patients with renal lesions that fulfill the pathologic criteria for chronic pyelonephritis at autopsy have sterile urine cultures and were not known to have had clinical episodes of bacterial urinary tract infection or urinary obstruction during life. Such cases suggest that other forms of renal injury result in morphologic changes indistinguishable from those produced by bacterial infection. Conversely, relatively few individuals with acute urinary infection develop chronic infection or progressive renal impairment. Most often, this occurs in patients with anatomic obstruction, neurogenic bladder, or vesicoureteral reflux.

Patients with many episodes of urinary tract infection; impaired renal function; pyuria with white cell casts; bacteriuria; an intravenous pyelogram showing an irregularly outlined renal pelvis with caliectasis and cortical scars; and typical pathologic changes can be diagnosed as having chronic pyelonephritis. In less typical patients, the relationship of infection to renal damage is uncertain and the diagnosis often remains unclear.

PATHOLOGY Characteristically, the kidneys are asymmetric in size, scarred, and irregularly pitted on the surface. Pathologic changes usually begin in the interstitial tissue of the medulla and papillae, with connective tissue, lymphocytes, and plasma cells completely replacing interstitium and tubules. Foci of active interstitial inflammation may be seen throughout the medulla, and leukocyte casts are found in some tubules. Other tubules contain large amounts of eosinophilic material and colloid casts, and may be dilated. Early in the disease, most glomeruli appear relatively normal. A proliferative endarteritis may be present. With progression, involvement of glomeruli and vessels becomes more pronounced and uniform, eventually resulting in an "end-stage" kidney.

None of the foregoing changes is pathognomonic for chronic pyelonephritis. Similar morphologic features may result from the nephropathy of chronic hypokalemia, nephrocalcinosis, chronic analgesic abuse, primary vascular disease of the kidneys, obstruction, diabetes mellitus, and Balkan nephropathy (see Chap. 226).

CLINICAL FEATURES Early signs and symptoms are minimal and nonspecific and often include hypertension. Later, as glomerular filtration and renal blood flow decline, the characteristic clinical and laboratory features of uremia appear (see Chap. 220).

The appearance of white blood cell casts in the urine suggests the diagnosis of chronic pyelonephritis. However, bacteria, leukocytes, and leukocyte casts may appear only intermittently and often are not present during the chronic stage of the disease. Intravenous pyelography is often normal early in the course of the disease but subsequently shows bilateral small kidneys with irregular outlines, calyceal blunting or dilatation, and cortical scarring. Renal biopsy may be normal owing to the focal nature of the disease early in its course.

PROGNOSIS The course of chronic pyelonephritis may be prolonged and compatible with a comfortable life even after considerable impairment of renal function. Associated hypertension generally worsens the prognosis. In perhaps no other renal disease can fluctuations in renal function be so marked or frequent. During acute infections or episodes of dehydration, renal decompensation may progress to the stage of advanced uremia; yet the patient may recover and regain adequate renal function for years. Correction of obstructing lesions may prevent progression of the disease.

TREATMENT Surgically approachable obstructive lesions should be promptly corrected. Antibiotic therapy for proven infections should be given and should be based on antimicrobial sensitivity tests. Hypertension should be controlled to reduce renal vascular complications. The treatment of chronic renal failure is discussed in Chap. 220.

PAPILLARY NECROSIS

The renal papilla is of major importance in the pathogenesis of chronic interstitial nephritis and, when complicated by bacterial infection, pyelonephritis. It has become evident that a variety of underlying conditions cause primary renal papillary damage, resulting eventually in the renal lesions of chronic interstitial nephritis. When urinary infection does not supervene, the resulting renal disease may progress slowly and silently to the point of renal insufficiency. The pathology of this renal injury may be indistinguishable from that of pyelonephritis. In addition to common diseases such as gout and diabetes mellitus, which cause renal papillary damage, many medications, which achieve enormous concentrations in the urine traversing the renal papilla, may be toxic for that zone of the kidney. The best known of these are phenacetin-containing analgesic mixtures. This problem is much more common than generally recognized, and diagnosis requires a careful history.

It is not known how many other substances may be important in the pathogenesis of primary renal papillary disease. However, in view of the benignity of urinary infection in persons without underlying renal papillary damage, it is reasonable to assume the presence of primary underlying renal papillary damage in any patient with urinary infection who shows the development or progression of renal damage.

When severe infection of the renal pyramids is present in association with vascular diseases of the kidney or with urinary tract obstruction, renal papillary necrosis is likely to result. Patients with diabetes, sickle cell disease, chronic alcoholism, and vascular disease seem peculiarly susceptible to this complication. Hematuria, pain in the flank or abdomen, and chills and fever are the most common presenting symptoms. Acute renal failure with oliguria or anuria sometimes occurs. Rarely, sloughing of a pyramid may take place without symptoms in a patient with chronic urinary infection, and the diagnosis is made when the necrotic tissue is passed in the urine or identified as a "ring shadow" on pyelography. If renal function deteriorates suddenly in a diabetic or a patient with chronic obstruction, the diagnosis of renal papillary necrosis should be entertained, even in the absence of fever or pain. Although renal papillary necrosis is often bilateral, when it is unilateral, nephrectomy may be lifesaving in the management of overwhelming infection.

RENAL AND PERINEPHRIC ABSCESS

See Chap. 87.

PROSTATITIS

The term *prostatitis* has been used for various inflammatory conditions affecting the prostate, including acute and chronic infections with specific bacteria and, more commonly, instances in which signs and symptoms of prostatic inflammation are present but no specific organisms can be detected. To classify patients with suspected prostatitis correctly, each patient should be evaluated using first-void and midstream urine specimens, a prostatic expressate, and a post-massage urine specimen. All specimens should be quantitatively cultured and evaluated for numbers of leukocytes. Based on the results of these studies, patients can be classified as having acute bacterial prostatitis, nonbacterial prostatitis, or prostatodynia. Patients with suspected prostatitis usually have low back pain, perineal or testicular discomfort, mild dysuria, and lower urinary obstructive symptoms. Microscopic pyuria may be the only objective manifestation of prostatic disease.

ACUTE BACTERIAL PROSTATITIS This disease generally affects young male adults when it occurs spontaneously, but it may also be associated with an indwelling urethral catheter. It is characterized by fever, chills, dysuria, and a tense or boggy, extremely tender, prostate on examination. Although prostatic massage usually produces purulent secretions with a large number of bacteria on culture, bacteremia may result from manipulation of the inflamed gland. For this reason, and because the etiologic agent can usually be identified on urine

Gram stain and culture, vigorous prostatic massage should be avoided. In noncatheter-associated cases, the infection is generally due to one of the common gram-negative urinary tract pathogens or *Staphylococcus aureus*. Initially, intravenous trimethoprim-sulfamethoxazole, a cephalosporin or an aminoglycoside can be utilized if gram-negative rods are seen in the urine Gram stain, and a cephalosporin or nafcillin if gram-positive cocci are seen. Although these drugs do not readily diffuse into the noninflamed prostate gland, the response to antibiotics is usually prompt, perhaps because drugs penetrate more readily into the acutely inflamed prostate. In catheter-associated cases, a broader spectrum of etiologic agents is seen, including hospital-acquired gram-negative rods and enterococci. In such cases, an aminoglygoside or a third-generation cephalosporin should be used for initial therapy until the organism has been isolated and susceptibilities determined. The long-term prognosis is good, although in some instances acute infection may result in abscess formation, epididymoorchitis, seminal vesiculitis, septicemia, and residual chronic bacterial prostatitis. Since the advent of antibiotics, the frequency of acute bacterial prostatitis has diminished markedly. Many so-called cases of acute prostatitis are probably posterior urethritis.

CHRONIC BACTERIAL PROSTATITIS This entity is a major cause of recurrent bacteriuria in males but may be difficult to diagnose. Symptoms are usually absent, the prostate feels normal on palpation, and although many white blood cells may be seen in the urinary sediment, results of conventional bacteriologic studies are often negative. Bacteria may be cultured from the expressed prostatic secretion or postmassage urine. The presence of these bacteria can be determined only by careful quantitative bacteriologic techniques when the bladder urine is sterile, employing the method used by Stamey and colleagues. Intermittently, symptoms of frequency, urgency, and dysuria occur when infection spreads to the bladder urine. The pattern of recurrent bladder infection in the male with chronic bacterial prostatitis is clinically not very different from that seen in the recurrent cystourethritis of the female. Antibiotics are of limited value in eradicating the focus of chronic infection in the prostate, but they do relieve the symptoms of the acute exacerbations promptly. The relative ineffectiveness of antimicrobials in part results from the poor penetration of most antibiotics into the prostate because the low pH which prevails in this organ precludes solubility of most drugs. The macrolide group of drugs (erythromycin) do enter the prostatic secretions, but these agents are generally ineffective against gram-negative organisms. Sulfonamide-trimethoprim has been employed successfully in some of these infections. Patients with frequent episodes of acute cystitis should be treated with prolonged courses of antimicrobials (usually sulfonamide, trimethoprim, or nitrofurantoin), with a view toward suppressing symptoms and keeping the bladder urine sterile. Total prostatectomy produces cure of chronic prostatitis but is associated with considerable morbidity. Transurethral prostatectomy is safer but cures only one-third of patients.

NONBACTERIAL PROSTATITIS Patients who present with symptoms and signs of prostatitis, increased leukocytes in their expressed prostatic secretions and postmassage urine, and no bacterial growth in cultures are classified as having nonbacterial prostatitis. Prostatic inflammation can be considered present when the expressed prostatic secretion and postmassage urine contain at least tenfold more leukocytes than the first-void and midstream specimens, or when the expressed prostatic secretion contains ≥ 1000 leukocytes per cubic millimeter. The presumed infectious etiology of this condition remains unidentified. Evidence for the causative role of both *Ureaplasma urealyticum* and *Chlamydia trachomatis* has been presented, but is not conclusive. Since most cases of nonbacterial prostatitis occur in young, sexually active men, and since many cases arise following an episode of nonspecific urethritis, the causative agent may well be sexually transmitted. The effectiveness of antimicrobial agents in this condition remains uncertain. Some patients benefit from a 4- to 6-week course of erythromycin, doxycycline, or trimethoprim-sulfamethoxazole.

PROSTATODYNIA Patients who have symptoms and signs of prostatitis but no evidence of prostatic inflammation (normal leukocyte counts) and negative urine cultures should be classified as having prostatodynia. Despite their symptoms, these patients most likely do not have prostatic infection and should not be given antimicrobial agents.

REFERENCES

BAILEY RR: Single-dose therapy for uncomplicated urinary tract infections. NZ Med J 98:327, 1985

BRUMFITT W, ASSCHER AW: *Urinary Tract Infection.* New York, Oxford University Press, 1973

FRANCOIS B, PERRIN P: *Urinary Infection: Insights and Prospects.* London, Butterworth, 1983

JONES SR et al: Localization of urinary tract infection by detection of antibody-coated bacteria in urine sediment. N Engl J Med 290:591, 1975

KOMAROFF AL: Acute dysuria in women. N Engl J Med 310:368, 1984

KRIEGER JN: Prostatitis syndromes: Pathophysiology, differential diagnosis, and treatment. Sex Transm Dis 11:100, 1984

KUNIN CM: *Detection, Prevention and Management of Urinary Tract Infections,* 3d ed. Philadelphia, Lea & Febiger, 1979

MEARES EM: Prostatitis syndromes: New perspectives about old woes. J Urol 123:141, 1980

PLATT R et al: Mortality associated with nosocomial urinary tract infection. N Engl J Med 307:637, 1982

RONALD AR: Current concepts in the management of urinary tract infections in adults. Med Clin N Am 68:335, 1984

———, HARDING GKM: Urinary prophylaxis in women. Ann Intern Med 94:268, 1981

———: Current concepts in the management of urinary tract infections in adults. Med Clin North Am 68:335, 1984

STAMEY TA: *Urinary Infections.* Baltimore, Williams & Wilkins, 1972

STAMM WE et al: Causes of the acute urethral syndrome in women. N Engl J Med 303:409, 1980

——— et al: Diagnosis of coliform infection in acutely dysuric women. N Engl J Med 307:463, 1982

WONG ES, HOOTON TM: Guidelines for prevention of catheter-associated urinary tract infections. Infect Control 2:125, 1980

226 TUBULOINTERSTITIAL DISEASES OF THE KIDNEY

BARRY M. BRENNER / THOMAS H. HOSTETTER

A large and etiologically diverse group of bilateral renal diseases can be distinguished from those considered in Chaps. 223 and 224 because the histologic and functional abnormalities involve the tubules and interstitium to a greater degree than the glomeruli and renal vasculature (see Table 226-1). Morphologically, acute forms of these tubulointerstitial disorders are characterized predominantly by interstitial edema, often associated with cortical and medullary infiltration by polymorphonuclear leukocytes and patchy areas of tubule cell necrosis. In more chronic forms, interstitial fibrosis predominates, inflammatory cells are typically mononuclear, and abnormalities of the tubules tend to be more widespread, as evidenced by atrophy, luminal dilatation, and thickening of tubule basement membranes. In the past, the diagnosis of chronic pyelonephritis was almost universally applied when these chronic tubulointerstitial abnormalities were found. It is now apparent that only a small proportion of these lesions results from infection. Nonbacterial factors, including exogenous toxins and metabolic and immunologic derangements, constitute the major pathogenic mechanisms thought to be involved. Because of the nonspecific nature of the histology, particularly in chronic tubulointerstitial diseases, biopsy specimens rarely provide a specific diagnosis. The urine sediment is also unlikely to be diagnostic, except in allergic forms of acute tubulointerstitial disease in which eosinophils may predominate in the urinary sediment (see below).

Defects in tubule function often accompany these alterations of tubule and interstitial structure. Proximal tubule dysfunction may be manifested as selective reabsorptive defects leading to hypokalemia, aminoaciduria, glycosuria, phosphaturia, uricosuria, or bicarbonaturia (proximal or type II renal tubular acidosis, see Chap. 228). In combination these defects constitute the *Fanconi syndrome*. Protein excretion is usually modest, rarely exceeding 2 g per 24 h. The excreted proteins are typically of low molecular weight and include $beta_2$ microglobulin, lysozyme, and immunoglobulin light chains. Defective proximal tubule reabsorption of these readily filtered small-molecular-weight proteins accounts for their augmented excretion in these disorders. Tubule sodium reabsorption may also be deranged in patients with advanced tubulointerstitial diseases, predisposing them to the tendency to salt wasting and the threat of overt hypovolemia. One or more of these reabsorptive defects are commonly encountered with heavy metal poisoning, multiple myeloma, and other tubulointerstitial processes affecting the renal cortex diffusely.

Defects in urinary acidification and concentrating ability often represent the most troublesome of the tubule dysfunctions encountered in patients with tubulointerstitial disease. Metabolic acidosis of the hyperchloremic type often develops at a relatively early stage in the course of the renal insufficiency. Patients with this finding generally elaborate urine of maximal acidity (pH of 5.3 or less). In such patients the defect in acid excretion usually proves to be caused by a reduced capacity to generate and excrete ammonia due to the reduction in renal mass. Preferential damage to the collecting ducts, as in amyloidosis or chronic obstructive uropathy, may also predispose to distal or type I renal tubular acidosis, characterized by abnormally high urine pH (>5.5) during spontaneous or NH_4Cl-induced metabolic acidosis. Patients with tubulointerstitial diseases affecting medullary and papillary structures predominantly may also evidence substantial concentrating defects, with resultant nocturia and polyuria. The impairment in maximal concentration is typically unresponsive to the administration of antidiuretic hormone, hence a form of nephrogenic diabetes insipidus. Analgesic nephropathy and sickle cell disease are prototypes of this form of injury.

Although the major structural defects originate in the tubules and interstitium, progressive reduction in glomerular filtration rate (GFR) is a common functional accompaniment of most, if not all, forms of tubulointerstitial damage, reflecting secondary injury to glomeruli and other elements of the renal microcirculation. Indeed oliguric, acute renal failure may be caused by acute forms of tubulointerstitial disease, and as many as one-third of patients with chronic renal insufficiency suffer from a primary chronic tubulointerstitial disease.

TABLE 226-1 Principal causes of tubulointerstitial disease of the kidney

I Toxins
- *A* Exogenous toxins
  - *1* Analgesic nephropathy
  - *2* Lead nephropathy (see Chap. 172)
  - *3* Miscellaneous nephrotoxins (e.g., antibiotics, radiographic contrast media, heavy metals)
- *B* Metabolic toxins
  - *1* Acute uric acid nephropathy (see Chap. 309)
  - *2* Gouty nephropathy (see Chap. 309)
  - *3* Hypercalcemic nephropathy (see Chap. 336)
  - *4* Hypokalemic nephropathy (see Chap. 41)
  - *5* Miscellaneous metabolic toxins (e.g., hyperoxaluria, cystinosis, Fabry's disease)

II Neoplasia
- *A* Lymphoma (see Chap. 294)
- *B* Leukemia (see Chap. 292)
- *C* Multiple myeloma (see Chap. 258)

III Immune disorders
- *A* Hypersensitivity nephropathy
- *B* Sjögren's syndrome (see Chap. 266)
- *C* Amyloidosis (see Chap. 259)
- *D* Transplant rejection (see Chap. 221)
- *E* Tubulointerstitial abnormalities associated with glomerulonephritis (see Chaps. 223 and 224)

IV Vascular disorders (see Chaps. 219 and 227)
- *A* Arteriolar nephrosclerosis
- *B* Atheroembolic disease
- *C* Sickle cell nephropathy
- *D* Acute tubular necrosis

V Hereditary renal diseases
- *A* Hereditary nephritis (Alport's syndrome) (see Chap. 224)
- *B* Medullary cystic disease (see Chap. 228)
- *C* Medullary sponge kidney (see Chap. 228)

VI Infectious injury (see Chap. 225)
- *A* Acute pyelonephritis
- *B* Chronic pyelonephritis

VII Miscellaneous disorders
- *A* Chronic urinary tract obstruction (see Chap. 230)
- *B* Vesicoureteral reflux
- *C* Radiation nephritis
- *D* Balkan nephropathy

TOXINS

A number of factors make the renal tubules and interstitium particularly prone to toxic injury. Although the kidneys constitute less than 1 percent of total body mass, they receive approximately 20 percent of the cardiac output, and 90 percent or more of this very large renal blood flow is distributed to the renal cortex. Exposure of tubules and interstitium of the renal cortex to circulating toxins is, therefore, quantitatively greater than is that of most other tissues. Transport processes operating in renal tubules contribute further to the intrarenal accumulation of toxins, thereby enhancing local concentrations of noxious agents. Furthermore, the urinary concentrating mechanism can establish high levels of toxins within medullary and papillary portions of the kidney, predisposing these regions to chemical injury. Finally, the relatively acid pH of the fluid within most nephron segments may affect the ionization characteristics of potentially toxic compounds and thereby influence local concentration and solubility. Although these normal physiologic processes render the kidney particularly vulnerable to toxic injury, the role of nephrotoxins in the causation of renal damage often goes unrecognized, largely because the manifestations of such injury are usually nonspecific in nature and insidious in onset. Diagnosis largely depends upon obtaining a history of exposure to a certain toxin, a difficult matter since exposure may be occult. Particular attention should, therefore, be paid to the patient's occupational history, as well as to an assessment of exposure, current as well as remote, to pharmaceutical agents, especially antibiotics and analgesics. The clinical recognition of a potential association between a patient's renal disease and exposure to a nephrotoxin is of crucial importance because, unlike many other forms of renal disease, progression of the functional and morphologic abnormalities associated with toxin-induced nephropathies may be prevented, and even reversed, simply by eliminating additional exposure.

EXOGENOUS TOXINS Analgesic nephropathy Over the past three decades, numerous studies have established that individuals who ingest large quantities of analgesic drugs are particularly prone to develop tubulointerstitial damage and papillary necrosis. Indeed, in Australia, Switzerland, and Sweden, analgesic abuse ranks as one of the most common causes of chronic renal failure, and it is now recognized as an important cause of renal insufficiency in the United States as well. Studies in animals have demonstrated that *phenacetin* and *aspirin* can induce papillary necrosis when either of these drugs is given in quantities far in excess of usual therapeutic doses. However, these chemicals are most likely to cause renal damage, and clinically apparent renal disease, when ingested in combination. Epidemiologic studies leave no doubt that the chronic ingestion of mixtures of these analgesics produces permanent and irreversible renal injury in humans.

Morphologically, analgesic nephropathy is characterized by papillary necrosis and tubulointerstitial inflammation. At an early stage prior to overt papillary necrosis, damage to the vascular supply of the inner medulla (vasa recta) leads to a local interstitial inflammatory reaction and, eventually, to papillary ischemia, necrosis, fibrosis, and calcification. Destruction of papillae usually precedes extension of the tubulointerstitial abnormalities to the renal cortex and, therefore, occurs before renal size and GFR are reduced significantly. It is important to recognize that although papillary necrosis is a common finding in patients with the nephropathy of analgesic abuse, necrosis of papillae may also be seen in patients with chronic pyelonephritis, diabetes mellitus, sickle cell disease, and obstructive uropathy. The susceptibility of the renal papillae to damage by analgesic compounds which contain phenacetin is believed to be related to the establishment of a renal corticomedullary gradient for the phenacetin metabolite *acetaminophen,* resulting in papillary tip concentrations which are more than tenfold higher than those present in renal cortex. Hydration serves to dissipate this gradient and may explain the protective effect of this maneuver in preventing phenacetin-induced papillary necrosis in animals. The aspirin in these analgesic compounds is also believed to contribute to renal injury, by uncoupling oxidative phosphorylation in renal mitochondria and by inhibiting the synthesis of renal prostaglandins, which are potent endogenous renal vasodilator hormones. Both effects of aspirin favor hypoxia in renal tissues and, therefore, enhance the susceptibility of the inner medulla to nephrotoxic injury.

Clinically, analgesic nephropathy occurs some three to five times more commonly in women than men. A direct relationship exists between the total amount of analgesic compounds ingested and the degree of renal impairment. An intake of 1.0 g phenacetin per day for 1 to 3 years, or total ingestion of 2 kg phenacetin in combination with other analgesics, appears to represent minimum requirements for the development of analgesic nephropathy. In such patients, renal function usually declines gradually, in association with chronic necrosis of papillae and diffuse tubulointerstitial damage to the renal cortex. Occasionally, papillary necrosis may be associated with gross hematuria, and even renal colic, due to obstruction of a ureter by a fragment of necrotic tissue. More than half of patients with analgesic nephropathy have pyuria, which, if persistently associated with sterile urine, provides an important clue to the diagnosis. Nonetheless, active pyelonephritis may coexist in patients with analgesic nephropathy. Proteinuria, if present, is typically mild (less than 1 g per 24 h). Patients with analgesic nephropathy are usually unable to generate maximally concentrated urine, reflecting the underlying medullary and papillary damage. An acquired form of distal renal tubular acidosis has been described and may contribute to the development of *nephrocalcinosis.* The occurrence of anemia out of proportion to the degree of azotemia may also provide a useful clue to the diagnosis of analgesic nephropathy. Occult gastrointestinal bleeding (usually secondary to analgesic-induced gastritis) and, in an occasional patient, hemolysis (particularly in those with glucose 6-phosphate dehydrogenase deficiency) are believed to contribute to the severity of the anemia. Vague abdominal complaints, as well as nonspecific headaches and arthralgias, are common in these patients. Moderate hypertension is also a common finding, which progresses to a malignant phase in only a small minority of patients. When analgesic nephropathy has progressed to the stage of moderate to severe renal insufficiency, the kidneys usually appear bilaterally shrunken on intravenous pyelography, and the calyces are deformed. A "ring sign" on the pyelogram is pathognomonic of papillary necrosis and represents the radiolucent sloughed papilla surrounded by the radiodense contrast material which fills the calyx. Also, transitional cell carcinoma may develop in the urinary pelvis or ureters as a late complication of analgesic abuse.

Every effort must be made to convince the patient who ingests excessive quantities of analgesics to discontinue this hazardous practice. When renal damage is at an early stage, cessation of drug abuse will usually arrest the progression of the nephrotoxic process; not infrequently, overall renal function will improve with time. With continued abuse of these drugs, however, progressive renal damage leads invariably to chronic renal failure.

Lead nephropathy (see also Chap. 172) Children and adults suffering from lead intoxication often develop a chronic form of tubulointerstitial renal disease. In children, lead poisoning usually results from ingestion of lead-based paints (pica). The oxide of lead liberated from paint, or present in the vapor arising from the welding of metals covered with lead-based paint, may be inhaled in substantial quantities, thereby constituting an industrial form of exposure in adults. Alcohol, illegally distilled in an apparatus constructed from automobile radiators (so-called moonshine), is yet another source of lead poisoning. Tubule transport processes enhance the accumulation of lead within renal cells, particularly of the proximal convoluted tubule, leading to cell degeneration, mitochondrial swelling, and eosinophilic intranuclear inclusion bodies rich in lead. In addition to tubule degeneration and atrophy, lead nephropathy is associated with ischemic changes in the glomeruli, fibrosis of the adventitia of small renal arterioles, and focal areas of cortical scarring. Eventually, the kidneys become grossly atrophic. In addition to progressive azotemia, abnormalities of tubule function may occur, particularly *renal glycosuria* and *aminoaciduria.* Urinary excretion of lead, bile pigments, and porphyrin precursors, particularly δ-aminolevulinic acid, coproporphyrin, and urobilinogen, may be increased. Patients with chronic lead nephropathy are characteristically *hyperuricemic,* a consequence of enhanced reabsorption of filtered urate. Acute gouty arthritis (so-called saturnine gout) occurs in about 50 percent of patients with lead nephropathy, in striking contrast to other forms of chronic renal failure in which gout is rare. Hypertension is also a frequent complication of this disorder. Therefore, in any patient with slowly progressive renal failure, atrophic kidneys, gout, and hypertension, the diagnosis of lead intoxication should be seriously considered. In addition to these manifestations, patients with chronic lead poisoning often complain of frequent episodes of abdominal colic and have evidence of anemia, peripheral neuropathy, and encephalopathy. The diagnosis may be suspected by finding elevated serum levels of lead. However, because blood levels may not be elevated even in the presence of a toxic total-body burden of lead, the quantitation of lead excretion following a standardized infusion of the chelating agent calcium disodium ethylenediaminetetraacetic acid (EDTA) is a more reliable indicator of serious lead exposure. Urinary excretion of more than 0.6 mg of lead per day is indicative of overt or potential toxicity. Treatment includes removing the patient from the source of exposure and augmenting lead excretion with a chelating agent such as calcium disodium EDTA.

Miscellaneous nephrotoxins Therapeutic use of lithium salts for manic-depressive illness has been associated with evidence of tubulointerstitial disease. The most frequent clinical finding is a mild to moderate form of nephrogenic diabetes insipidus resulting in polyuria and polydipsia. It is more controversial whether long-term lithium therapy produces irreversible chronic tubulointerstitial lesions and impairment of glomerular filtration rate. Though present evidence suggests that some patients develop histologic evidence of such injury, there are only rare reports of chronic renal insufficiency attributable to this agent. In any case, renal function should be followed in patients taking this drug, and extreme caution should be exercised if lithium is employed in patients with underlying renal disease.

Many agents which commonly lead to acute renal failure are also capable of producing tubulointerstitial injury (see Chap. 219). These include antibiotics (e.g., aminoglycosides, amphotericin B), radiographic contrast agents, various hydrocarbons (e.g., carbon tetrachloride), and heavy metals (e.g., mercury, cadmium, and bismuth).

METABOLIC TOXINS Acute uric acid nephropathy (see also Chap. 309) Disorders characterized by acute overproduction of uric acid and extreme hyperuricemia often lead to a rapidly progressive form of renal insufficiency, so-called acute uric acid nephropathy. This tubulointerstitial disease is usually seen in patients given cytotoxic drugs for the treatment of lymphoproliferative or myeloproliferative disorders, but may also occur in these patients even before such treatment is begun. The pathologic changes associated with acute uric acid nephropathy are largely the result of deposition of uric acid crystals in the kidneys and their collecting systems leading to partial or complete obstruction of collecting ducts, renal pelvis, or ureter. Since obstruction is often bilateral, patients typically show the clinical course of acute renal failure, characterized by oliguria and rapidly rising serum creatinine concentration. In the early phase of this disorder, uric acid crystals can often be found in urine, usually in association with microscopic or gross hematuria. Peak serum uric acid levels vary but are almost always above 20 mg/dL and may even exceed 60 mg/dL.

Prevention of hyperuricemia in patients at risk, by treatment with allopurinol in doses of 200 to 800 mg per day prior to cytotoxic therapy, greatly reduces the danger of acute uric acid nephropathy. Once hyperuricemia develops, however, efforts should be directed to preventing deposition of uric acid within the urinary tract. Increasing urine volume with potent diuretics (furosemide or mannitol) effectively lowers intratubular uric acid concentrations, and alkalinization of the urine to pH 7 or greater with sodium bicarbonate and/or a carbonic anhydrase inhibitor (acetazolamide) enhances uric acid solubility. If these efforts, together with allopurinol therapy, are ineffective in preventing acute renal failure, dialysis should be instituted to lower the serum uric acid concentration as well as to treat the acute manifestations of uremia. The combination of conservative therapy and hemodialysis allows most patients with acute uric acid nephropathy to survive this form of acute renal failure and ultimately recover renal function essentially completely.

Gouty nephropathy (see also Chap. 309) Patients with less severe but more prolonged forms of hyperuricemia are predisposed to a more chronic tubulointerstitial disorder, often referred to as *gouty nephropathy*. Since other conditions associated with hyperuricemia, such as hypertension, nephrolithiasis, pyelonephritis, and even lead poisoning, may contribute to renal damage, the effect of chronic hyperuricemia per se on renal function is unclear. Nevertheless, the severity of renal involvement in this disorder correlates well with the duration and magnitude of the elevation of the serum uric acid concentration. Histologically, the distinctive feature of gouty nephropathy is the presence of crystalline deposits of uric acid and monosodium urate salts in kidney parenchyma. These deposits are believed to represent the primary pathogenic process in gouty nephropathy, with intraluminal crystallization of uric acid taking place in distal tubules and collecting ducts where urine pH is generally quite low and where uric acid concentrations are considerably in excess of levels in plasma. These deposits not only cause intrarenal obstruction, but also incite an inflammatory response, leading to lymphocytic infiltration, foreign-body giant cell reaction, and eventual fibrosis, especially of medullary and papillary regions of the kidney. Bacteriuria and pyelonephritis occur in about one-fourth of cases, presumably as complications of intrarenal urinary stasis. Since patients with gout frequently suffer from hypertension and hyperlipidemia, degenerative changes of the renal arterioles may constitute a striking feature of the histologic abnormality, often out of proportion to other morphologic defects. Clinically, gouty nephropathy is an insidious cause of renal insufficiency. Early in its course, GFR may be near normal, often despite focal morphologic changes in medullary and cortical interstitium, proteinuria, and diminished urinary concentrating ability. Whether reducing serum uric acid levels with allopurinol exerts a beneficial effect on the kidney remains to be demonstrated. Although such undesirable consequences of hyperuricemia as gout and uric acid stones respond well to allopurinol, use of this drug in asymptomatic hyperuricemia has not been shown to improve renal function consistently. On the other hand, uricosuric agents such as probenecid, which may increase uric acid stone production, clearly have no role in the treatment of renal disease associated with hyperuricemia.

Hypercalcemic nephropathy (see also Chap. 336) Chronic hypercalcemia, as occurs in primary hyperparathyroidism, sarcoidosis, multiple myeloma, vitamin D intoxication, or metastatic bone disease, is a well known cause of tubulointerstitial damage and progressive renal insufficiency. Pathologically, the earliest renal lesion induced by hypercalcemia is a focal degenerative change in renal epithelia, primarily in collecting ducts, distal convoluted tubules, and loops of Henle. Tubule cell necrosis leads to nephron obstruction and stasis of intrarenal urine, favoring local precipitation of calcium salts and infection. Dilatation and atrophy of tubules eventually occur, as do interstitial fibrosis, mononuclear leukocyte infiltration, and interstitial calcium deposition (nephrocalcinosis). Calcium deposition may also occur in glomeruli and the walls of renal arterioles. Clinically, the most striking defect is an inability to concentrate the urine maximally, resulting in polyuria and nocturia. Defective transport of chloride in the ascending limb of Henle's loop is believed to be responsible, at least in part, for this concentrating defect. Additionally, reduced collecting duct responsiveness to ADH may contribute to this abnormality. Reductions in GFR and renal blood flow also occur, both in states of acute severe hypercalcemia as well as with prolonged hypercalcemia of lesser severity. Distal renal tubular acidosis and sodium and potassium wasting have also been described in these chronic states. Eventually, uncontrolled hypercalcemia leads to severe tubulointerstitial damage and overt renal failure. Urinalysis is rarely a clue to the presence of hypercalcemic renal failure, but abdominal x-rays may demonstrate nephrocalcinosis as well as nephrolithiasis, the latter due to the hypercalciuria which often accompanies hypercalcemia. Treatment for hypercalcemic nephropathy consists of reducing the serum calcium concentration toward normal and correcting the primary abnormality of calcium metabolism. The management of hypercalcemia is discussed in Chap. 336. Prognosis for recovery of renal function depends upon the severity of the renal lesion at the time hypercalcemia is corrected. Renal dysfunction of recent onset secondary to acute hypercalcemia may be completely reversible. Gradual, progressive renal insufficiency related to chronic hypercalcemia, however, may not improve with correction of the calcium disorder. Nonetheless, every effort should be made to return serum calcium concentration to normal in order to minimize further loss of renal function.

Hypokalemic nephropathy (see also Chap. 41) Disturbances of renal structure and function are observed commonly in patients with moderate to severe potassium depletion of at least several weeks' duration. Histologically, renal epithelial cells are often seen to contain numerous vacuoles, most marked in proximal, and to a lesser extent, distal convoluted tubules. These findings usually disappear with potassium repletion. Glomeruli are reduced in size and may become sclerotic while larger blood vessels are usually uninvolved. Whether prolonged or recurrent potassium deficiency results in irreversible tubulointerstitial fibrosis, scarring, and atrophy is still a controversial issue. Loss of urinary concentrating ability is the most commonly encountered functional defect. Experimental studies in animals have shown that this urinary concentrating abnormality is preceded by a period of primary polydipsia. The reduced concentrating capacity which eventually develops is due, at least in part, to defective operation of the countercurrent multiplier system. Elevated rates of intrarenal prostaglandin synthesis may also contribute to this concentrating defect, since prostaglandins are known to antagonize the hydroosmotic action of antidiuretic hormone on collecting-duct epithelium. Symptoms of nocturia, polyuria, and polydipsia are frequently encountered in patients with chronic potassium depletion, although, occasionally, patients with severe hypokalemia have no complaints referable to the urinary tract. It has been suggested that patients with hypokalemic nephropathy have an enhanced susceptibility to pyelonephritis, but this issue remains unresolved. The polydipsia is probably due to both the impaired renal concentrating ability and a primary disorder of the thirst mechanism, which is believed to be a common feature of most chronic potassium depletion states. Urinalysis often reveals no abnormalities except for mild proteinuria. Serum creatinine and urea nitrogen concentrations usually remain within normal limits. Treatment should be directed at repleting body potassium stores and correcting the primary process responsible for potassium loss. With correction of body potassium stores, functional and histologic abnormalities of the kidneys usually disappear, although maximal urinary concentrating ability may not return to normal for several months.

Miscellaneous metabolic toxins Urinary oxalate, derived from the metabolism of glycine and, to a variable extent, from ingested oxalate, may deposit as insoluble intratubular calcium oxalate crystals and result in chronic tubulointerstitial damage in patients with hereditary or acquired forms of *hyperoxaluria*. *Cystinosis* and *Fabry's disease* are other hereditary depositional disorders affecting the renal tubules and interstitium. The reader is referred to Chaps. 224, 228, and 229 for more detailed discussions of these and other uncommon metabolic causes of tubulointerstitial injury.

RENAL PARENCHYMAL DISEASE ASSOCIATED WITH EXTRARENAL NEOPLASM

In addition to being the site of origin of several benign and malignant neoplasms (see Chap. 231), the kidneys are frequently affected by neoplasms arising outside the urinary tract. Except for the glomerulopathies associated with lymphomas and several solid tumors (see Chap. 224), the renal manifestations of primary extrarenal neoplastic processes are confined mainly to the interstitium and tubules. Although metastatic renal involvement by solid tumors is unusual, the kidneys are often invaded by neoplastic cells in various lymphomas and leukemias and in multiple myeloma. In postmortem studies of patients with *lymphoma,* renal involvement is found in approximately one-half of cases. The involvement may be focal, in the form of multiple discrete nodules, or diffuse, with lymphomatous infiltration throughout the renal parenchyma. Diffuse infiltration is seen most commonly in lymphomas other than Hodgkin's disease. There may be flank pain related to massive renal infiltration, and x-rays may show enlargement of one or both kidneys. Renal insufficiency occurs in a distinct minority of cases, and overt uremia is rare. Treatment of the primary disease may improve renal function in these cases.

The kidneys are also commonly involved in various forms of *leukemia.* At postmortem examination, bilateral renal involvement can be demonstrated in approximately 50 percent of cases. As with lymphoma, uremia is rarely, if ever, a consequence of leukemic infiltration of the kidneys. The kidneys can also be involved in leukemias because of the associated high incidence of hyperuricemia, hypercalcemia, and lysozymuria. The myelogenous leukemias, particularly of the monocytic type, may be complicated by tubule defects involving potassium and magnesium wasting.

In contrast, infiltration of the kidneys with *myeloma* cells is infrequent (see also Chap. 258). When it occurs, the process is usually focal, so that renal insufficiency from this cause is also uncommon. The more usual lesion is *myeloma kidney,* which is characterized histologically by atrophic tubules, many with eosinophilic intraluminal casts, and numerous multinucleated giant cells within tubule walls as well as in the interstitium. The frequent occurrence of myeloma kidney in patients with Bence-Jones proteinuria has suggested a causal relation. Bence-Jones proteins are thought to cause myeloma kidney through direct toxicity to renal tubule cells. In addition, Bence-Jones proteins may precipitate within the distal nephron where the high concentrations of these proteins and the acid composition of the tubule fluid favor intraluminal cast formation and intrarenal obstruction. Indeed, positive immunofluorescence staining for light chains can often be demonstrated in casts found in myeloma kidneys. Occasionally, acute renal failure occurs after intravenous pyelography in patients with multiple myeloma and is believed to result from the further precipitation of Bence-Jones proteins induced by dehydration prior to radiographic study. Routine dehydration of the patient with myeloma in preparation for intravenous pyelography should, therefore, be avoided. Multiple myeloma may also affect the kidneys indirectly. Hypercalcemia or hyperuricemia may occur and lead to the nephropathies described above. Proximal tubule disorders are also seen occasionally in patients with myeloma, including type II proximal renal tubular acidosis and the Fanconi syndrome. Additionally, intrarenal deposits of *amyloid* (see below) may contribute to impaired excretory function in patients with multiple myeloma.

IMMUNE DISORDERS

HYPERSENSITIVITY NEPHROPATHY An acute diffuse tubulointerstitial reaction may result from hypersensitivity to a number of drugs. First reported after the use of sulfonamides, acute tubulointerstitial damage is now seen most often with the antibiotic *methicillin,* although other drugs, including *ampicillin, penicillin, cephalothin, phenindione, thiazides, furosemide,* and nonsteroidal anti-inflammatory drugs have also been implicated. Of note, the tubulointerstitial nephropathy which develops in some patients taking nonsteroidal anti-inflammatory drugs may be associated with nephrotic-range proteinuria and histologic evidence of minimal change glomerulopathy. Grossly, the kidneys are usually enlarged. Histologically, the glomeruli appear normal. The principal pathologic abnormalities are in the interstitium of the kidney, which reveals pronounced edema and infiltration with polymorphonuclear leukocytes, lymphocytes, plasma cells, and, in some cases, large numbers of eosinophils. If the process is severe, tubule cell necrosis and regeneration may also be apparent. Immunofluorescence studies in a number of cases either have been unrevealing or have demonstrated a linear pattern of immunoglobin and complement deposition along tubule basement membranes. In a few cases of methicillin-induced acute tubulointerstitial disease, circulating antitubule basement membrane antibodies have also been found, suggesting that autoantibody formation may have been induced by the penicilloyl hapten of methicillin (by conjugation of hapten with tubule basement membrane proteins, thereby altering the native antigenicity of the basement membrane). In cases associated with nonsteroidal, anti-inflammatory drugs a role for cell-mediated immunity has been proposed, since renal infiltration by both T and B lymphocytes has been observed with a relative predominance of cytotoxic T cells. Evidence for an immunologic basis for these various drug-related nephropathies also derives from the facts that the onset of nephropathy does not appear to be dose-related, often follows a second exposure to the drug presumed to be responsible for the renal injury, and often is associated with increased levels of serum IgE. In the case of methicillin, the patients usually develop evidence of renal injury after about 2 weeks of drug administration. Hematuria, fever, skin rash, and eosinophilia are prominent. Many patients develop azotemia which typically resolves after withdrawal of the offending drug. Proteinuria and pyuria often accompany the hematuria, and occasionally eosinophils are found in the urine sediment. The clinical picture may be confused with acute glomerulonephritis, but when acute azotemia and hematuria are accompanied by eosinophilia, skin rash, and a history of drug exposure, a hypersensitivity reaction leading to acute tubulointerstitial nephritis should be regarded as the leading diagnostic possibility. Discontinuation of the drug usually results in complete reversal of the renal injury; rarely, renal damage may be irreversible. Corticosteroids have been used, but their value in this disorder has not been established with certainty.

SJÖGREN'S SYNDROME (See also Chap. 266) Keratoconjunctivitis sicca, or Sjögren's syndrome, is an immunologic disorder characterized by dryness of mucous membranes and mononuclear cell infiltration of salivary and lacrimal glands; it is often seen in patients with rheumatoid arthritis. When the kidneys are involved in Sjögren's syndrome, the predominant histologic findings are those of chronic tubulointerstitial disease. Interstitial infiltrates are composed primarily of lymphocytes, causing the histology of the renal parenchyma in these patients to resemble that of the salivary and lacrimal glands. Renal functional defects associated with this disorder include diminished urinary concentrating ability and distal (type I) renal tubular acidosis. Urinalysis may show pyuria (predominantly lymphocyturia) and mild proteinuria.

AMYLOIDOSIS (See also Chaps. 224 and 259) Glomerular pathology usually predominates and leads to heavy proteinuria and azotemia. However, tubule function may also be deranged, giving rise to a nephrogenic form of diabetes insipidus and to distal (type I) renal tubular acidosis. In several cases these functional abnormalities have been correlated with peritubular deposition of amyloid, particularly in areas surrounding vasa rectae, loops of Henle, and collecting ducts. Bilateral enlargement of the kidneys, especially in a patient with massive proteinuria and evidence for tubule dysfunction, should raise the possibility of amyloid renal disease.

TUBULOINTERSTITIAL ABNORMALITIES ASSOCIATED WITH GLOMERULONEPHRITIS A number of primary glomerulopathies may also be associated with damage to tubules and interstitium. Pathogenetically, the extraglomerular component in these renal disorders often involves the same mechanisms that are responsible for the more pronounced glomerular injury. For example, in more than half of patients with the nephropathy associated with systemic lupus erythematosus, deposits of immune complexes can be identified in tubule basement membranes, usually accompanied by an interstitial mononuclear inflammatory reaction. Similarly, in many patients with glomerulonephritis associated with antiglomerular basement membrane antibody, the same antibody can be shown to be reactive against tubule basement membranes as well.

MISCELLANEOUS DISORDERS

VESICOURETERAL REFLUX (See also Chaps. 225 and 230) Normally, the junction of the terminal ureter with the urinary bladder provides a competent sphincter so that during micturition urine leaves the bladder only via the urethra. However, when the function of the ureterovesical junction is impaired, urine may reflux into the ureters due to the high intravesical pressure that develops during voiding. Clinically, reflux is often detected on the voiding and postvoiding films obtained during intravenous pyelography, although voiding cystourethrography may be required for definitive diagnosis. Bladder infection may ascend the urinary tract to the kidneys through incompetent ureterovesical sphincters. Not surprisingly, therefore, reflux is often discovered in patients with acute and/or chronic urinary tract infections. In children particularly, reflux of minor degree may disappear with time and standard therapy of intercurrent urinary infection. With more severe degrees of reflux, characterized by marked dilatation of ureters and renal pelves, progressive renal damage often appears, and although active infection may also be present, uncertainty exists as to the necessity of infection in producing the scarred kidney of reflux nephropathy. In contrast to those with other forms of chronic tubulointerstitial disease, patients with renal insufficiency and scarring due to reflux often demonstrate substantial proteinuria. Indeed, in such cases glomerular lesions similar to those of idiopathic focal glomerulosclerosis (Chap. 223) are often present in addition to the more usual changes of chronic tubulointerstitial disease. Surgical correction of reflux is usually necessary only with the more severe degrees of reflux since renal damage appears to best correlate with the extent of reflux. Obviously, if extensive glomerulosclerosis already exists, urologic repair may no longer be warranted.

RADIATION NEPHRITIS Clinical renal dysfunction can be expected to occur if 2300 R or more of x-ray irradiation is administered to both kidneys during a period of 5 weeks or less. Histologic examination of the affected kidneys reveals hyalinized glomeruli, atrophic tubules, extensive interstitial fibrosis, and hyalinization of the media of renal arterioles. Radiation-induced renal ischemia is believed to be the main pathogenic factor responsible for the widespread tubulointerstitial damage, which may not become evident clinically for weeks to months after completion of irradiation. The clinical presentation of acute radiation nephritis includes rapidly progressive azotemia, moderate to malignant hypertension, anemia, and proteinuria which may reach the nephrotic range. More than 50 percent of these cases progress to chronic renal failure. A more insidious form of radiation nephritis may also occur; it is characterized by slower development of azotemia, anemia, and nephrotic syndrome. Malignant hypertension has also been known to follow unilateral renal irradiation and to resolve with ipsilateral nephrectomy. Radiation nephritis in recent years has all but vanished because of heightened awareness of its pathogenesis by radiotherapists.

BALKAN NEPHROPATHY Balkan nephropathy is an acquired, endemic disorder restricted to the small geographic region where Yugoslavia, Romania, and Bulgaria meet to form the Danubian basin. The renal lesions seen in affected patients from this region progress from focal tubular atrophy, interstitial edema, and mononuclear cell infiltration to diffuse interstitial fibrosis, leading eventually to bilaterally shrunken, atrophic kidneys. Epidemiologic studies point to an environmental toxin as the cause, but the offending agent has not yet been identified. Defects in urinary concentrating ability, low-molecular-weight ("tubular") proteinuria, and renal tubular acidosis are common. In most cases, the disease is progressive, leading eventually to chronic renal failure. A high incidence of papillary transitional carcinoma of the renal pelvis and upper ureter appears to be a late complication in patients with this endemic nephropathy.

REFERENCES

BATUMEN V et al: The role of lead in gout nephropathy. N Engl J Med 304:520, 1981

BUCKALEW VM JR, SCHEY HM: Analgesic nephropathy: A significant cause of morbidity in the United States. Am J Kidney Dis 7:164, 1986

COTRAN RS: Glomerulosclerosis in reflux nephropathy. Kidney Int 21:528, 1982

——— et al: Tubulointerstitial diseases, in *The Kidney,* 3d ed, BM Brenner, FC Rector Jr (eds). Philadelphia, Saunders, 1986, p 1143

CUSHNER HM et al: Acute interstitial nephritis associated with mezlocillin, nafcillin, and gentamicin treatment for *Pseudomonas* infection. Arch Intern Med 145:1204, 1985

DITLOVE J et al: Methicillin nephritis. Medicine 56:483, 1977

HALL PW, DAMMIN GJ: Balkan nephropathy. Nephron 22:281, 1978

HUMES HD, WEINBERG J: Toxic nephropathies, in *The Kidney,* 3d ed, BM Brenner, FC Rector Jr (eds). Philadelphia, Saunders, 1986, p 1491

KINCAID-SMITH P: Analgesic abuse and the kidney. Kidney Int 17:250, 1980

MURRAY T, GOLDBERG M: Chronic interstitial nephritis: Etiologic factors. Ann Intern Med 82:453, 1975

RUBIN RH et al: Urinary tract infection, pyelonephritis, and reflux nephropathy, in *The Kidney,* 3d ed, BM Brenner, FC Rector Jr (eds). Philadelphia, Saunders, 1986, p 1085

SINGER I: Lithium and the kidney. Kidney Int 19:374, 1981

TORRES VE et al: The progression of vesicoureteral reflux nephropathy. Ann Intern Med 92:776, 1980

WILSON CB, DIXON FJ: Renal response to immunological injury, in *The Kidney,* 3d ed, BM Brenner, FC Rector Jr (eds). Philadelphia, Saunders, 1986, p 800

227 VASCULAR INJURY TO THE KIDNEY

NORMAN K. HOLLENBERG

Processes ranging from renal artery stenosis and occlusion to arteriolar nephrosclerosis, polyarteritis nodosa, the hemolytic uremic syndromes, scleroderma, and preeclampsia share a sufficient number of clinical features, morphologic characteristics, and pathogenetic consequences to justify their consideration together. The clinical, functional, and morphologic expressions of interrupting the renal blood supply depend on the degree of obstruction to flow, the rate at which the occlusion occurs, the level of vessel involved, and the total mass of ischemic parenchyma. Because the intrarenal arterial tree is made up of end arteries, sudden occlusion results in infarction with clinical manifestations that vary with the level at which the occlusion occurs. More gradual partial occlusion, on the other hand, results in ischemic atrophy and a different functional and clinical picture.

Renal blood flow, averaging 4.0 (mL/g)/min, exceeds by three- to fivefold the flow in such metabolically active organs as the heart, liver, and brain. Renal blood flow is not adjusted to satisfy metabolic need, but rather to provide the plasma flow and pressure to the glomerular capillary bed required to sustain glomerular filtration. Renal perfusion is also an important determinant of sodium handling by the kidney. For these reasons, a reduction in renal blood flow too small to result in cell death has important consequences including a reduction in filtration rate, increased sodium reabsorption, increased renin release, and hypertension. To a varying extent all are features common to the syndromes resulting from abnormalities in the renal circulation.

ACUTE ARTERIAL OCCLUSION Acute, complete occlusion of the main renal artery or a major intrarenal arterial branch may follow blunt trauma to the abdomen or back or embolism in patients with mitral stenosis and atrial fibrillation, infective endocarditis, mural thrombi overlying myocardial infarcts, or ulcerating atherosclerotic disease of the aorta. The kidneys receive about one-fifth of the cardiac output, making embolic occlusion of the small intrarenal arteries relatively common. Acute occlusion results in coagulation necrosis in the region supplied by the obstructed artery, the size of the wedge-shaped infarct varying with the level of the occlusion.

The clinical features also depend on the size of the infarct. Small infarcts, involving a portion of the renal cortex, are often clinically silent. Larger infarcts may induce a sudden, sharp unremitting pain in the flank or upper abdomen associated with fever, leukocytosis, and gross or microscopic hematuria. The impact on renal function also varies. Even total occlusion of one main renal artery may leave the blood urea nitrogen (BUN) and serum creatinine in the normal range in the presence of a healthy contralateral kidney which can undergo hypertrophy. When the patient has only a solitary functioning kidney, arterial occlusion enters the differential diagnosis of acute oliguric renal failure. Although total destruction of the kidney will generally occur within hours of occlusion, at least a dozen case reports of restoration of renal function after days to weeks of total occlusion have appeared, generally in a setting in which prior partial occlusion has led to a rich collateral arterial blood supply sufficient for nutrition although inadequate to maintain renal function. Angiography is necessary to establish the diagnosis. Evidence of collateral filling of the intrarenal arterial tree suggests that operation may restore renal function.

RENAL ARTERY STENOSIS (See also Chap. 196) Partial occlusion of the renal artery or its major branches by atherosclerotic narrowing or by fibromuscular dysplasia is responsible for about 1 to 2 percent of cases of hypertension; its importance lies in the fact that it represents the most common curable form of hypertension. *Renal arterial atherosclerosis,* as with atherosclerosis elsewhere, is more frequent in males, and its incidence increases with advancing age, previous hypertension, or diabetes mellitus. The *fibromuscular dysplasias* of the renal artery are a heterogeneous group of lesions in which fibrous or fibromuscular thickening may involve the intima, the media, or the subadventitial region. The process is frequently bilateral and may extend into the intrarenal tree. The fibrous dysplasias are 10 times more common in females, appear most often in the third and fourth decades, and, presumably because the individuals are younger, are associated with a lower surgical morbidity and a higher cure rate than are atherosclerotic renal arterial lesions.

The clinical features which may be helpful in detecting renal artery stenosis include a history of the onset of hypertension at an age which is unusual for essential hypertension, i.e., under 30 or over 50 years of age, a poor response to medical therapy, and a bruit in the flank or upper abdominal region. Routine laboratory evaluation often reveals evidence of secondary hyperaldosteronism including hypokalemia and metabolic alkalosis. As in primary aldosteronism, hypokalemia may be masked by a restricted sodium intake.

The intravenous pyelogram (IVP) and the radionuclide Hippuran renogram are still the most widely used screening tests for renovascular hypertension. Characteristics in the pyelogram suggesting renal artery stenosis include a reduction in renal size of at least 1.5 cm compared with the opposite kidney, a delay in the appearance of contrast in the involved kidney when films are obtained at 1, 2, and 3 min after injection of the contrast agent, hyperconcentration of contrast on the involved side in the late films, and filling defects in the renal pelvis and ureter reflecting the local effects of dilated collateral arteries. In the Cooperative Study on Renovascular Hypertension, the characteristic features of the late appearance of contrast medium in a small kidney which showed late hyperconcentration of contrast in the renal pelvis was never seen in patients with essential hypertension. Unfortunately, only 22 percent of patients with renovascular hypertension had this triad, and so it was relatively insensitive. The presence of any single abnormality was found in 78 percent of patients with renovascular hypertension, but with a sharp reduction in specificity since 11 percent of patients with essential hypertension had at least one of these manifestations, most commonly a significant difference in renal size. The characteristics of a radiohippuran renogram which suggest renal artery stenosis include a delay in the rate of rise of the tracer in the kidney, a delay in the time to reach the peak, and a reduced rate of disappearance from the kidney. The renogram identified 75 percent of patients with renovascular hypertension, with a false-positive rate of 24 percent. Because both the IVP and the renogram compare the two kidneys, they are less often positive when stenosis is bilateral. Digital subtraction angiography is finding increased use, but it is still more invasive and expensive than the IVP, and its specificity and sensitivity have not yet been defined clearly.

Because of the prevalence of hypertension and the low yield of renovascular hypertension when a detailed evaluation is undertaken, the clinical indications for laboratory investigations in search of renovascular hypertension are gradually undergoing modification. No more than 1 to 2 percent of patients with hypertension have a curable renal arterial lesion. The evaluation is costly. Finally, operation, especially in patients with atherosclerosis, carries considerable risk. For these reasons a detailed evaluation for renal artery stenosis is currently recommended only when the yield is likely to be high, including patients in whom the onset of hypertension has occurred before the age of 30 years, in the presence of a bruit, or when hypertension is severe and responds poorly to medical therapy.

If the screening test is positive, identification of renal artery stenosis is accomplished only by arteriography. Because all arterial lesions are not hemodynamically significant, ancillary tests are used to assess the hemodynamic significance of the stenosis. The most widely used test involves the measurement of renin activity in blood samples obtained from both renal veins and either the lower inferior vena cava or the aorta. A positive test, strongly suggestive of curable renovascular hypertension, reveals a plasma renin activity from the involved renal veins which exceeds the contralateral renal vein concentration by at least 50 percent, and evidence of suppression of renin-release from the intact contralateral kidney, i.e., identical renin activity in the arterial and contralateral renal venous plasma. With these criteria the false-positive rate is only 7 percent, but there is a quantitatively important false-negative rate. At present we employ renal arteriography and renal vein renin determinations in patients in whom the history, physical examination, and screening tests make renovascular hypertension likely.

The Cooperative Study on Renovascular Disease has provided a clear picture of the current results of operation. When renal artery stenosis was due to fibromuscular disease, the cure rate exceeded 90 percent with a mortality of no more than 3 percent—probably reflecting the youth of the population, which was largely free of additional systemic disease. In patients with atherosclerotic disease, on the other hand, the mortality was 9 percent and the failure rate exceeded 25 percent. For these reasons evaluation for renal artery surgery in older patients who are likely to have atherosclerotic disease is restricted in many centers to patients in whom medical management fails.

If medical therapy is selected because of surgical risk, the converting enzyme inhibitor captopril is particularly effective in renovascular hypertension and is recommended for the patient with hypertension which is resistant to a standard regimen. Medical therapy, while it may control the hypertension, will not prevent the progress of the renal arterial lesion. The agent should be used cautiously or avoided in the patient with advanced bilateral renal artery disease or with stenosis of the artery to a single kidney as it may precipitate functional renal failure. Percutaneous transluminal angioplasty, in which a balloon-tipped catheter is employed to dilate the stenotic area during renal arteriography, has been most successful in renal vascular hypertension due to fibromuscular dysplasia. When atherosclerosis has been at the origin of the renal artery, i.e., is ostial, the results of angioplasty have been much poorer.

ARTERIOLAR NEPHROSCLEROSIS Small-vessel changes in the kidney are so intimately associated with both long-standing hypertension and the normal aging process that it is difficult to define the boundary between normal and disease and to discuss the vascular lesion without discussing hypertension. At least some degree of small-vessel lesion is found in about 70 percent of normotensive individuals who die after the age of 60 years. The frequency and severity is increased in younger age groups with predisposing factors, hypertension and diabetes. Large and medium-sized arteries at the interlobar and arcuate levels show intimal thickening of variable degree. Typically, more widespread and more severe abnormalities are seen in the small arteries and arterioles where, in addition, there is an eosinophilic hyalin thickening which results in a variable degree of vascular narrowing. As a consequence there is patchy ischemic atrophy which parallels that of the vascular change.

The vascular changes presumably account for most of the loss of renal function which accompanies normal aging and which is accentuated in the patient with hypertension. The reductions in renal plasma flow and glomerular filtration rate account for the loss of an element of functional reserve, making older individuals more prone to develop azotemia when faced with volume depletion or surgical stress. The increased incidence of drug-induced complications in the elderly presumably reflects the important role played by glomerular filtration in the excretion of drugs and metabolites. Some examples are the propensity of the elderly to suffer toxicity with streptomycin and digoxin. Other features of arteriolar nephrosclerosis include a moderate loss of concentrating power and often mild proteinuria. Occasionally more profound renal functional abnormalities occur, but marked renal insufficiency is uncommon.

On the other hand, "accelerated nephrosclerosis" associated with malignant hypertension is a dramatic complication of all forms of hypertension in which an abrupt change in course, renal insufficiency, and a uremic death were common before effective therapy became available (Chap. 196). The onset of the malignant phase is characterized by a sharp increase in blood pressure, with diastolic pressures typically exceeding 130 mmHg. In essential hypertension, the malignant phase is usually preceded by a benign period of variable duration, but occasionally occurs de novo. This process also occurs as a complication of all forms of secondary hypertension. Until recently it was suggested that accelerated nephrosclerosis does not complicate the course of primary aldosteronism, but several well-documented cases now exist. In pheochromocytoma accelerated hypertension is typically associated with preserved renal function.

The renal lesions of malignant hypertension include petechial hemorrhages of the cortical surface, responsible for the characteristic "flea-bitten" appearance; fibrinoid necrosis of afferent arterioles; a hyperplastic endarteritis of the interlobular and arcuate arteries; and severe ischemic atrophy or infarction distal to the abnormal vessels. Immunofluorescent and electron-microscopic studies have shown that the amorphous material in the arteriolar wall consists of fibrin. Severe hypertension, per se, is probably responsible for the vascular necrosis resulting from endothelial injury and leakage of fibrin and other plasma constituents into the arteriolar wall.

The clinical features include severe hypertension, neuroretinopathy with blurring of vision, retinal hemorrhages, exudates, and papilledema. Hypertensive encephalopathy is evidenced by severe headache, changes in the sensorium, and seizures. Congestive heart failure and rapidly progressive uremia are common. The renal manifestations include gross or microscopic hematuria, marked proteinuria, and a rapid rise in BUN and creatinine. As in renal artery stenosis, evidence of secondary aldosteronism is common with hypokalemia and a metabolic alkalosis, until the metabolic acidosis of renal failure supervenes.

Prior to the availability of effective therapy for the hypertension, the mortality in patients with this syndrome approximated 50 percent in 3 months and 90 percent within 1 year. In the past two decades, the availability of effective antihypertensive therapy (Chap. 196) has greatly improved the prognosis of accelerated nephrosclerosis. In the early 1950s a BUN which exceeded 30 mg/dL at the time the diagnosis was made guaranteed a rapid demise. Today a patient with a BUN which exceeds this level by three- or fourfold may have a stable course with effective therapy.

SCLERODERMA RENAL CRISIS (PROGRESSIVE SYSTEMIC SCLEROSIS) (See also Chap. 264) The renal aspects of scleroderma are considered in some detail here because renal involvement is second only to that of heart and lungs as a cause of death, and the characteristic morphologic lesions and clinical course closely resemble those associated with accelerated nephrosclerosis.

As in accelerated nephrosclerosis, the morphologic features include kidneys which are only slightly reduced in size even in patients who have died with renal failure. Petechial hemorrhages and wedge-shaped cortical infarcts are common. The most striking and distinctive abnormality is seen in the intralobular arteries, which are markedly narrowed or occluded as a result of fibrinoid change and deposition of fibrin and acid mucopolysaccarides. The afferent arterioles in some patients also show fibrinoid necrosis and occasional occlusion by fibrin thrombi. Distal to the occlusion, ischemic atrophy and infarction are evident. Although the renal vascular lesions may be secondary to the hypertension, they have been documented at necropsy in patients with scleroderma who have never been hypertensive.

Renal involvement is rarely the presenting feature. In one study renal involvement was found at presentation in only 3 percent of patients with scleroderma. However, in a 20-year longitudinal survey, 47 percent of patients ultimately developed a clinically important renal lesion. Renal failure contributes to or is primarily responsible for 40 to 50 percent of all deaths. Most patients with clinically evident renal disease die in less than 1 year and often within 3 months. Indeed, in the aforementioned longitudinal study only 10 percent of patients without renal involvement died, whereas 60 percent of patients with proteinuria, azotemia, or hypertension succumbed.

Renal involvement in scleroderma is usually characterized clinically by an abrupt onset and an explosive course; accelerated hypertension is followed by oliguria and a uremic death within months. Clinical evidence of major renal involvement is typically noted 3 to 5 years after the onset of manifestations in the skin and other systems. Occasionally, however, renal disease antedates obvious skin involvement.

A second, less distinct clinical expression of renal involvement is also being recognized. Isolated proteinuria unaccompanied by either hypertension or azotemia adversely affects prognosis but less strikingly than does the syndrome of malignant hypertension. Mild hypertension, without proteinuria or azotemia, occurs with greater frequency in scleroderma than would be anticipated from known prevalence of essential hypertension. Mild hypertension without proteinuria or azotemia occurs later than the malignant form and has a much less grave prognosis.

No specific therapy exists for scleroderma. A series of reports have indicated that very aggressive antihypertensive therapy sometimes makes renal failure avoidable. Presumably because the hypertension is renin-mediated, the converting enzyme inhibitor, captopril, has been especially effective. Furthermore, renal transplantation has been successful in a limited number of patients with scleroderma.

SICKLE CELL NEPHROPATHY (See also Chaps. 224 and 288) Patients with sickle cell disease, sickle cell trait, sickle thalassemia, and other combinations of hemoglobin S with abnormal hemoglobins often have clinically important disorders of renal structure and function. The most dramatic of the renal manifestations is gross painless hematuria. The bleeding arises from miliary gross and microscopic infarcts in the papillae, renal pelvis, and renal cortex. For unknown reasons the bleeding occurs from the left side in 80 percent of cases and, despite the systemic nature of the primary process, is bilateral in only 11 percent. Abnormalities in the IVP, most commonly a pelvic filling defect reflecting blood clot, are frequent and have led to unnecessary surgical intervention. Most cases remit spontaneously. Because causes other than sickle cell anemia may be responsible for hematuria in these patients, a complete urologic assessment is generally performed (Chap. 40). When filling defects are found, serial studies are recommended; surgical exploration should be considered only if they persist. Operation may also be required in rare instances of life-threatening hemorrhage.

Failure of urinary concentration is the most consistent feature of sickle cell nephropathy. In very young children with sickle cell anemia the concentrating defect can be reversed by multiple transfusions, but the capacity for improvement is lost with age, becoming negligible in patients after 15 years of age. In older adults the maximal concentration of the urine rarely exceeds 400 mosmol per liter. The failure of urinary concentration is typically attributed to a disorder of perfusion of the renal medulla, perhaps due to the sickling process per se. Both hypoxia and an increased osmolality precipitate the sickling phenomenon and sickle cells increase blood viscosity significantly, so this condition may impede the normal circulation through the vasa recta, which normally have a very high resistance to flow. Microangiographic studies have revealed obliteration and distortion of the remaining vasa recta.

Appreciable proteinuria is common in sickle cell disease and occurred in 31 percent of patients in one series. On occasion proteinuria is sufficiently severe that the nephrotic syndrome develops. Distal renal tubular acidosis has also been reported as an uncommon complication.

With increasing age, the growing number and size of cortical infarcts result in a progressive reduction in glomerular filtration rate and renal plasma flow, which are typically higher than normal in the young patients with sickle cell disease. Deterioration of renal function caused by sickle cell anemia to the point at which dialysis becomes necessary has not been described. However, it has been shown that patients with sickle cell disease can be maintained on chronic hemodialysis without encountering undue complications.

HEMOLYTIC-UREMIC SYNDROMES (See also Chap. 287) The coincidence of acute renal failure, hemolytic anemia, and thrombocytopenia has emerged as a clearly defined, relatively common entity in which infants or children develop acute anemia, signs of renal and central nervous system injury, and gastrointestinal bleeding after a prodrome of digestive, respiratory, and systemic symptoms. The hallmarks of the syndrome are hemolysis due to red blood cell fragmentation, a reduction in platelet count, and biochemical and pathologic evidence of intravascular coagulation. The differential diagnosis includes thrombotic thrombocytopenic purpura (TTP), renal cortical necrosis as part of the Shwartzman reaction in gram-negative sepsis, and severe vasculitis. Differentiation among these entities may be extremely difficult, even at necropsy. TTP, which has a worse prognosis, is more likely if the patient is a young adult, if there is a continuing fever, and if the central nervous system involvement is more severe than the renal failure.

Initially only severe, generally fatal cases were recognized, but with increasing familiarity patients with mild or moderate lesions have been identified. The immediate prognosis is related to the degree of renal failure and the severity of involvement of the central nervous system. If the patient survives, the hematologic abnormality is short-lived and does not recur. In some patients the extent of renal destruction precludes prolonged survival without dialysis. In a few others severe neurologic sequelae have been permanently disabling. In many patients the renal lesions heal completely, but on occasion slowly progressive renal failure occurs after the initial insult.

Although primarily a disease of children, there has been increasing recognition of this syndrome in adults. In adults the prodrome, which resembles a nondescript viral illness, is less striking, but associations have been found with pregnancy and the postpartum period, use of oral contraceptive agents, and infection, including typhoid fever, gram-negative bacteremia, mumps, and infectious mononucleosis. The clinical manifestations are similar to those in children, and the prognosis appears to be poorer, although that may reflect confusion with TTP.

Because evidence of coagulation disturbances and fibrin deposition in small arteries and arterioles is common and because the syndrome is accompanied by a microangiopathic hemolytic anemia, there is widespread belief that intravascular coagulation plays a major role. The commonly observed coagulation disturbances include thrombocytopenia, a prolonged prothrombin time, and accumulation of fibrin degradation products in the serum. For unknown reasons the kidney is the most extensively involved organ in the hemolytic-uremic syndrome. Because in adults pregnancy and oral contraceptive agents appear to predispose to cortical necrosis and pregnancy also predisposes to the Shwartzman reaction induced by endotoxin in animals, it has been suggested that the Shwartzman reaction and the hemolytic-uremic syndrome share a common mechanism. The morphologic lesions are also strikingly similar; immunofluorescent studies have revealed intense staining with antibody to fibrin in both conditions.

The treatment is largely supportive. There is controversy as to whether heparin therapy modifies the natural history. Controlled studies have been disappointing, but in individual patients heparin therapy has been temporally associated with improvement in renal function. Other forms of therapy including corticosteroids, immunosuppressive agents, antiplatelet agents, exchange transfusions, and dextran have met with equivocal results.

RENAL VEIN THROMBOSIS Thrombosis of one or both of the renal veins is an uncommon cause of the nephrotic syndrome. Occlusion of both renal veins usually, but not necessarily, implies thrombosis of the inferior vena cava as well. Renal vein thrombosis is most commonly associated with membranous glomerulonephritis. It is not clear whether the glomerulonephritis predisposes to renal vein thrombosis or vice versa, but the weight of evidence favors the former (Chap. 223). Other causes of renal vein thrombosis include local trauma, invasion of the renal vein by hypernephroma, and severe dehydration, especially in children.

Clinical and morphologic features depend on the availability of an adequate collateral venous drainage. Sudden complete thrombosis of a renal vein, without adequate collateral drainage, causes severe lumbar pain, hematuria, and loss of function of the involved kidney. The kidney is enlarged and suffers hemorrhagic infarction. When the process is bilateral or involves a solitary kidney, this sequence leads to oliguria and renal failure. If the occlusion is more gradual, especially if adequate collateral venous channels develop, renal function is preserved, and massive proteinuria results in the nephrotic syndrome. Hypertension is uncommon, and the urinary sediment may be entirely normal or contain only a few red blood cells.

The diagnosis is suggested by a history of trauma, pain, or a predisposing factor such as prolonged travel in a cramped position. A history of pulmonary embolism should also lead to suspicion of this diagnosis. Physical examination may reveal a venous collateral map on the anterior abdominal wall if the inferior vena cava is involved. The intravenous pyelogram may show filling defects in the renal pelvis and ureter reflecting collateral draining veins. The diagnosis is established by inferior vena caval and selective renal venography. Diagnostic ultrasound is playing an increasing role in diagnosis.

Surgical removal of a clot from the renal venous system has been successful in a small number of patients, especially in children in whom the onset is often in association with dehydration and occurs acutely. In most circumstances, however, medical management with anticoagulants has been used. Recanalization of the renal veins has led to amelioration of the nephrotic syndrome in occasional patients. Typically, however, anticoagulants are employed to prevent pulmonary embolism and extension of the thrombus into the open collateral veins.

PREECLAMPSIA AND ECLAMPSIA: TOXEMIAS OF PREGNANCY Toxemia of pregnancy is characterized by the appearance, during gestation or within 7 days of delivery, of a constellation of abnormalities which includes hypertension, edema, and proteinuria (preeclampsia). When hypertension is more severe, convulsions and coma may occur (eclampsia). Preeclampsia usually begins after the thirty-second week of pregnancy but may begin earlier, particularly in women with preexisting renal disease or hypertension. Preeclampsia in the first trimester occurs in hydatidiform mole. Toxemia has a bimodal frequency with peak incidence in the young primipara and in multiparous women over 35 years of age. In the United States toxemia occurs in approximately 7 percent of pregnancies. There is an increased prevalence in the economically underprivileged. Most series include many patients in whom preexisting renal disease or hypertension either begins during or is exacerbated by pregnancy. In addition, there is a specific process affecting the kidney and the vascular system which in most patients improves dramatically when, or soon after, pregnancy is terminated.

The morphologic features in the kidney include reversible generalized swelling of the glomerular tufts and apparent thickening of the glomerular basement membrane due to an increase of the cytoplasm of the endothelial cells with narrowing of the capillary lumina, a finding termed *glomerular endotheliosis,* and sub- or interendothelial fibrinoid deposition. In patients who die of acute toxemia of pregnancy, necrosis of renal tubules and of liver cells is frequent, along with evidence of disseminated intravascular coagulation and petechial hemorrhage in the brain.

The pathogenesis is not clearly understood. Sodium retention and an increase in blood volume are normal concomitants of pregnancy. Considerable evidence suggests that plasma volume is *lower* in the toxemic than in the normal pregnancy, and from this observation debate about the role of too little or too much sodium intake has emerged. Whether the reduced plasma volume is a cause or consequence of the process is unclear. Uteroplacental ischemia occurs with toxemia. The uterus, like the kidney, synthesizes both vasoconstrictors (renin) and vasodilators (prostaglandins of the E series). One current hypothesis is that an imbalance in their action is responsible for the severe hypertension. Recent studies have also demonstrated production of a sodium-potassium ATPase inhibitor in such patients that could lead to hypertension by enhancing vascular responsiveness to constrictor stimuli.

The onset is typically insidious but may be abrupt. Because arterial blood pressure normally falls during pregnancy, pressures which exceed 125/75 mmHg should be considered abnormal, especially if they are rising. Headache, visual disturbances, epigastric distress, and apprehension are frequently associated with toxemias. Edema usually appears coincident with hypertension; it is typically generalized, being particularly evident in the face and hands. Proteinuria generally follows the onset of the syndrome within several days but occasionally precedes the hypertension and edema. Examination of the optic fundi reveals segmental arteriolar narrowing and a glistening retinal sheen indicative of edema. Hemorrhages and exudates occur late and only in severe cases.

The urine contains trace to 10 g protein per 24 h, as well as granular and hyalin casts, but red blood cells and cellular casts are infrequent. Because of the physiologic increase of glomerular filtration rate and reduction in serum urea and creatinine concentration which occurs in a normal pregnancy, a blood urea nitrogen of 20 mg/dL is usually indicative of a sharp diminution in filtration rate. A more striking increase in blood uric acid is common, reflecting a reduction in urate clearance.

Treatment varies with the severity of the process. In patients with mild hypertension and minimal proteinuria, bed rest and mild sedation are routinely used: whether restriction of sodium intake, which may be required to control edema, is a precipitating factor in preeclampsia is debated. Diuretics are generally avoided. If the process is more severe, patients are admitted to the hospital for sustained bed rest and closer control of sodium intake and blood pressure. Antihypertensive agents employed include hydralazine, methyldopa, and beta blockers. Marked hypertension and involvement of the central nervous system with convulsions are unequivocal indications for termination of pregnancy, which is usually followed by prompt improvement of the mother. At this stage parenteral magnesium sulfate is widely used for its central nervous system and antihypertensive effects. Emptying of the uterus is the most effective treatment. Proteinuria and hypertension usually disappear within weeks but on occasion may persist for as long as 6 months. A substantial fraction of multiparous patients over the age of 35 years with preeclampsia are left with a process that is undistinguishable from essential hypertension. Whether such patients were candidates for development of essential hypertension which became apparent during, or was precipitated by, pregnancy is not yet clear.

VASCULITIS (See also Chaps. 224 and 269) Because renal involvement occurs in at least 80 percent of patients with vasculitis and contributes to death in a substantial number, they are considered here, although some vasculitides such as rheumatic arteritis and temporal arteritis rarely involve the kidney. An expanded classification for the vasculitides with a discussion of the distinctions and overlaps among various syndromes is contained in Chap. 269. They are generally thought to be a form of immune complex disease, and the rate, site, and size of the vessel involved may reflect the physiochemical properties of the complex and events in the vessel such as flow turbulence.

Polyarteritis nodosa (PAN) is a recurrent or progressive, necrotizing inflammatory disease of the medium and small-sized muscular arteries. The kidney is the most common organ involved, with estimates ranging upward of 70 percent, and renal failure is one of the major causes of death. Hypertension occurs in at least 50 percent of patients and often terminates in a malignant phase with hypertensive encephalopathy or heart failure. Renal involvement may be manifested by proteinuria, microscopic or gross hematuria, urinary casts, azotemia, and edema.

In classic PAN (see Chap. 269), the lesions involve only the medium and small muscular arteries, especially at sites of branching. Classically there are subendothelial and medial edema and fibrinoid necrosis; infiltration of all vessel coats with an inflammatory exudate including polymorphonuclear leukocytes, eosinophils, lymphocytes, and plasma cells; destruction of the media and internal elastica; proliferation of fibroblasts, which generally starts in the adventitia and progresses during a stage of granulation through the vessel wall with healing, and a reduction in the acute inflammatory process; and healed lesions in which the vessel wall is replaced by fibrous tissue and the lumen is generally narrowed or occluded. Glomerular lesions are common. Any or all of these stages may be present at any time in the kidney. Renal insufficiency and hypertension characteristically develop during the healing stages. Because larger vessels are involved, a renal biopsy of the cortex may miss the characteristic lesion.

The pathogenetic factors responsible for polyarteritis are becoming clearer. Multiple lines of evidence have implicated an immunologic mechanism involving immune complexes and hepatitis B as the responsible antigen in as many as 30 percent of patients with necrotizing vasculitis and the PAN syndrome. A vasculitis indistinguishable from PAN is also recognized in intravenous drug abusers. Because of the multiplicity of the chemical agents injected, and the high probability of contamination, the exact etiologic agent has not been unequivocally defined, but methamphetamine appears to be a common denominator.

Hypersensitivity angiitis includes many identifiable groups such as drug-related, Henoch-Schönlein purpura, that associated with serum sickness, or that underlying primary disease such as systemic lupus erythematosus. It is often an acute illness characterized by an acute necrotizing inflammatory process involving small vessels, particularly postcapillary venules; however, small arteries, arterioles, and capillaries may also be involved. Proteinuria and hematuria are present in many patients, but hypertension is generally absent and azotemia substantially less common than in the polyarteritis group.

Therapy of the vasculitides is discussed in Chap. 269. General supportive measures include control of hypertension, which is required in most patients with renal involvement. The pathogenesis of the hypertension is similar to that in scleroderma renal crisis, as is the therapy. Corticosteroids are widely employed and with immunosuppressive agents are the only presently available therapy of any potential value. In patients with renal involvement, steroids may have an initial adverse effect on the clinical course because vascular healing is frequently associated with obliteration of arteries, resulting in focal renal infarction, increasing hypertension, and azotemia. The addition of cyclophosphamide has been shown to be useful in the patient in whom steroids are ineffective, especially when there is renal involvement.

REFERENCES

ALLEYNE GAQ et al: The kidney in sickle cell anemia. Kidney Int 7:371, 1975

BECKETT VL et al: Use of captopril as early therapy for renal scleroderma: A prospective study. Mayo Clin Proc 60:763, 1985

FAUCI AJ: Systemic vasculitis, in *Current Therapy in Allergy and Immunology*, LM Lichtenstein, AS Fauci (eds). Decker, Philadelphia, 1983, p 130

FERRIS TF: Toxemia and hypertension, in *Medical Complications During Pregnancy*, GN Burrow, TF Ferris (eds). Philadelphia, Saunders, 1975

GIANANTONIO CA et al: The hemolytic-uremic syndrome. Nephron 11:174, 1973

HUMPHREYS MH, ALFREY AC: Vascular diseases of the kidney, in *The Kidney*, 3d ed, BM Brenner, FC Rector Jr (eds). Philadelphia, Saunders, 1986, p 1175

KEATING MA, ALTHAUSEN AF: The clinical spectrum of renal vein thrombosis. J Urol 133:938, 1985

MAXWELL MH: Cooperative study of renovascular hypertension: Current status. Kidney Int 8:S153, 1975

MILLAN VG et al: Percutaneous transluminal renal angioplasty in nonatherosclerotic renovascular hypertension. Long-term results. Hypertension 7:668, 1985

OLIVER JA, CANNON PJ: The kidney in scleroderma. Nephron 18:141, 1977

RATLIFF NB: Renal vascular disease: Pathology of large blood vessel disease. Am J Kidney Dis 5:A93, 1985

STIMPEL M et al: The spectrum of renovascular hypertension. Am J Med 79:14, 1985

THIND GS: Role of renal venous renins in the diagnosis and management of renovascular hypertension. J Urol 134:2, 1985

228 HEREDITARY TUBULAR DISORDERS

FREDRIC L. COE / SATISH KATHPALIA

POLYCYSTIC RENAL DISEASE IN ADULTS

ETIOLOGY AND PATHOLOGY This disease is found in 1 in 500 autopsies and 1 in 3000 hospital admissions and accounts for approximately 5 percent of end-stage renal failure. Inheritance is autosomal dominant. The cortex and medulla of both kidneys are usually filled with thin-walled, spherical cysts, ranging from millimeters to centimeters in diameter, that enlarge the organs and interfere with their functioning, presumably by compressing the nephrons and causing localized obstruction. The cysts, which are lined by a low cuboidal epithelium, contain straw-colored fluid that becomes hemorrhagic with trauma or infection. The intervening renal parenchyma may be normal or show changes of nephrosclerosis or interstitial nephritis.

CLINICAL FEATURES Symptoms usually begin in the third or fourth decades. Flank pain is frequent. Other common symptoms include gross and microscopic hematuria, especially after trauma, and nocturia due to impaired concentrating ability. Ten percent of patients pass renal calculi whose composition and pathogenesis have not been well studied. Stones and blood clots both cause renal colic. Usually the kidneys are palpable and asymmetric and have a knobby surface. Hypertension develops in 75 percent of patients, and progression to chronic renal failure usually occurs (Table 228-1).

Proteinuria is common, but rarely exceeds 2 g per day. Urinary infection ultimately occurs in most patients, especially as a consequence of instrumentation and renal calculi. Erythrocytosis may occur because of high erythropoietin levels; in other patients blood loss anemia may result from the hematuria.

Acute renal failure can result from infection, ureteral obstruction due to clots or stone, or sudden angulation of a ureter by a nearby cyst. Azotemia progresses slowly in the absence of these complications. Patients with end-stage chronic renal failure tend to have higher hematocrits than their counterparts with other renal diseases. Fluid overload is infrequent because of a tendency for renal salt wasting.

Hepatic cysts are present in about 30 percent of patients. Hepatic function is usually normal, and the liver cysts can be asymptomatic or cause epigastric discomfort or biliary colic or become infected. Cysts also may occur in the spleen, pancreas, lungs, ovaries, testes, epididymis, thyroid, uterus, broad ligament, and bladder. Subarachnoid hemorrhage from intracranial aneurysm is the cause of death in about one-tenth of patients.

DIAGNOSIS Palpable kidneys, hypertension, or asymptomatic abnormalities of urine are often the only manifestations. Excretory or retrograde urography typically shows large kidneys with elongated pelvises and flat calyces indented by cysts. Ultrasonography and radioisotopic renal scanning can both demonstrate the cysts quite well. Gray scale sonography may be an alternative to intravenous pyelography for screening individuals at risk, especially when genetic counseling is desired. Computerized tomography may be useful.

TREATMENT Superimposed renal damage such as is produced by analgesics, obstruction, urinary infection, nephrotoxic antibiotics, and hypertension must be guarded against. Dehydration and inadequate intake of sodium chloride (less than 100 mmol per day) should be avoided. The management of chronic renal failure is simplified because fluid overload is not a usual problem and the hypertension is usually amenable to treatment, but the cysts can cause special problems, such as pain, bleeding, infection, or ureteral obstruction. Puncture of cysts, and in some instances even nephrectomy, may be necessary.

POLYCYSTIC RENAL DISEASE IN INFANTS AND CHILDREN

CLINICAL FEATURES The *infantile form* manifests itself at birth by diffusely enlarged kidneys, renal failure, and maldevelopment of intrahepatic bile ducts. The *childhood form* consists of medullary ductal ectasia which is usually asymptomatic, in association with congenital hepatic fibrosis and portal hypertension. Inheritance of both the infantile and childhood forms is autosomal recessive. Renal failure develops frequently in both forms, but death in the childhood form usually results as a consequence of hepatic disease.

MORPHOLOGY In the infantile form, the distal tubules and collecting ducts are dilated into elongated cysts that are arranged in a radial fashion, particularly in the cortex, and make the kidneys large and spongy. In the childhood form, cysts are fewer in number, cortical collecting ducts are less involved, and the kidneys are not as large. Small intrahepatic bile ducts are irregularly dilated, and large interconnecting spaces, lined by hyperplastic epithelium, fill the portal areas. There is portal fibrosis rather than dilatation and proliferation of small bile ducts, and portal hypertension is the rule by late childhood.

DIAGNOSIS AND TREATMENT Infantile polycystic kidneys may be large enough to cause dystocia. At birth they do not function and cause oliguric renal failure, respiratory distress, hypertension, and congestive heart failure. Intravenous pyelography may reveal a mottled nephrogram with variable retention of contrast material in cysts that correspond to dilated cortical and medullary collecting ducts. On retrograde urography the calyces are blunted, and pyelotubular reflux may be seen. In the childhood type the intravenous pyelogram may suggest medullary sponge kidney, because medullary tubular ectasia is prominent. Renal failure and chronic infection are common.

TABLE 228-1 Renal tubule defects

Disease	Renal morphologic abnormalities	Functional abnormalities	Mode*	Associated abnormalities and system consequences
Adult polycystic disease	Cortical and medullary cysts	Chronic renal failure	AD	Hepatic cysts, intracranial aneurysms
Infantile polycystic disease	Distal tubule and collecting duct cysts	Renal failure in the newborn	AR	Intrahepatic bile duct abnormalities
Childhood polycystic disease	Medullary ductal ectasia	Variable chronic renal failure	AR	Hepatic fibrosis and portal hypertension
Medullary sponge kidneys	Ectatic ducts of Bellini	Nephrocalcinosis	AD + S	None
Medullary cystic disease, recessive	Distal tubule and collecting duct cysts	Chronic renal failure, <20 yr salt wasting polyuria	AR	Variable retinal degeneration (renal retinal dysplasia)
Medullary cystic disease, dominant	Same	Chronic renal failure, >20 yr salt wasting, polyuria	AD	None
Bartter's syndrome	Hyperplasia of juxtaglomerular and medullary interstitial cells	Hypokalemia, high renin and aldosterone levels, polyuria	AR	None
Liddle's syndrome	None	Hypokalemia, low aldosterone levels	AR	None
Familial nephrogenic diabetes insipidus	None	Vasopressin-resistant renal concentrating defect	XLR	None
Renal tubular acidosis, type 1	Papillary nephrocalcinosis	Inability to lower urine pH normally, reduced acid excretion	AD	Periodic paralysis, hypokalemia, non-anion-gap metabolic acidosis, growth retardation, rickets
Renal tubular acidosis, type 2	None	Reduced bicarbonate reabsorption	AR AD XLR	Non-anion-gap metabolic acidosis, growth retardation rickets, Fanconi syndrome
Renal tubular acidosis, type 4	Underlying renal disease (HTN, DM, OBST)	Reduced proton and potassium secretion	ACQ	Azotemia
X-linked vitamin D–resistant rickets	None	Reduced phosphate reabsorption, hypophosphatemia	XLR	Rickets, osteomalacia, normal serum 1,25-D
Vitamin D–dependent rickets, type 1	None	Defective renal 1,25-D production	AR	Rickets, osteomalacia, low serum 1,25-D
Vitamin D–dependent rickets, type 2	None	Defective cell, 1,25-D receptors	AR	Rickets, osteomalacia, high serum 1,25-D, variable alopecia
Oncogenic osteomalacia	None	Reduced phosphate reabsorptions, hypophosphatemia	ACQ	Osteomalacia; mesenchymal tumors; cancer of the prostate or lung
Renal glucosuria	None	Reduced glucose reabsorption	AD	None
Isolated hypouricemia	None	Reduced urate reabsorption	AR	Variable hypercalciuria, bone demineralization
Cystinuria	Cystine stones	Reduced reabsorption of dibasic amino acids	AR	Short stature
Hartnup's disease	None	Reduced reabsorption of monoamino and carboxylic amino acids	AR	Pellagra-like rash, ataxia, delirium
Iminoglycinuria	None	Reduced reabsorption of proline, hydroxyproline, and glycine	AR	None
Adult Fanconi syndrome	Swan neck deformity of the proximal tubule	Reduced proximal tubule reabsorption of bicarbonate, glucose, uric acid, phosphate, and amino acids	AR	Rickets, osteomalacia, acidosis, dwarfism, low serum potassium
Lowe's syndrome (oculocerebrorenal syndrome)	Same	Same	XLR	Ocular and cerebral malformations

* *AR, autosomal recessive; AD, autosomal dominant; XLR, X-linked recessive; ACQ, acquired; HTN, hypertension; DM, diabetes mellitus; OBST urinary tract obstruction; S, sporadic.*

MEDULLARY SPONGE KIDNEY

PATHOLOGY In this condition the ducts of Bellini, i.e., the terminal collecting ducts that reach to the ends of the papillae and drain the urine into the renal pelvis, are dilated to cystic proportions and frequently contain calcium oxalate calculi. The kidneys are asymmetric, and the more abnormal kidney is usually the larger. One or more medullary cysts are found near the tip of each involved papilla, and calculi form in the terminal collecting ducts in, or proximal to, the cysts (Fig. 228-1). Parenchymal alterations are secondary to intrarenal obstruction. The cysts are lined by cuboidal and, sometimes, pseudostratified and stratified squamous epithelium.

CLINICAL DIAGNOSIS AND TREATMENT Medullary sponge kidney is present in 1 of 200 unselected intravenous pyelograms. Although most cases are sporadic, autosomal dominant inheritance has been described. The disease has a bimodal pattern of appearance, the first in adolescence and the second during the third and fourth decades. Calculi, infection, and hematuria occur in 60, 35, and 30 percent of patients, respectively. Papillary nephrocalcinosis due to clusters of stones in cysts is common. Hypercalciuria occurs in nearly half of stone-forming patients but is equally common in other forms of calcium stone disease (Chap. 229). Hypertension is no more common than in the general population. Renal failure is rare, unless nephrolithiasis and/or renal infections are severe.

The diagnosis of medullary sponge kidney is made by intravenous urography. The magnitude of pyelotubular backflow may vary from a simple papillary blush to frank tubular ectasia at the tips of the papillae. Small pyramidal cysts and nephrocalcinosis are frequent, and papillary concretions are obscured by the urographic contrast medium. Ectatic collecting ducts are difficult to fill during retrograde pyelography, and so the contrast material remains separate from papillary concretions in the cysts.

Asymptomatic patients require no treatment except advice to avoid dehydration and thereby reduce the risk of stone formation. The metabolic etiology of stones should be sought and treated conventionally, while infection and urologic consequences of stones should be treated as described in Chap. 229. Medullary sponge kidneys are vulnerable to infection, and urologic instrumentation should, therefore, be minimized.

MEDULLARY CYSTIC DISEASE (NEPHRONOPHTHISIS COMPLEX)

ETIOLOGY Several hereditary medullary cystic diseases have similar morphology but differing patterns of inheritance. The recessive form is associated with renal failure before 20 years of age (early-onset type), whereas the dominant form causes renal failure only after the second decade (adult-onset type). When renal disease is associated with retinal degenerative changes (renal retinal dysplasia), inheritance is always recessive, but renal failure occurs during adult life.

PATHOLOGY In both forms, most of the cysts are in the medulla and the corticomedullary region and have been localized to collecting ducts and distal convoluted tubules. Cysts have a low, frequently atrophic, epithelium and range in size from microscopic dimensions to millimeters. The kidneys usually are asymmetrically scarred and shrunken. Both tubular atrophy and periglomerular fibrosis are present, but the former is more severe. In advanced cases, glomeruli become sclerotic and hyalinized, cortical fibrosis and cellular interstitial infiltration appear, and the histology is difficult to differentiate from that of chronic interstitial nephritis.

DIAGNOSIS AND TREATMENT Concentrating ability, acid excretion, and sodium conservation are defective as might be expected from a lesion that damages distal segments of the nephron. The disease is marked by polyuria, progressive renal failure, stunted growth, severe anemia, hyperchloremic metabolic acidosis, and poor sodium conservation. In adults, the inability to conserve sodium may cause a salt-wasting syndrome that resembles adrenal insufficiency but is unresponsive to mineralocorticoids. Hypertension usually is a terminal event. The urinalysis is normal at first, but proteinuria may develop. On intravenous pyelography, the kidneys are small, scarred, and without calcification. The calyces are distorted by numerous cysts in the corticomedullary area.

High sodium and water intake, and alkali replacement for acidosis, are needed. Treatment of infections, anemia, hypertension, and other aspects of end-stage renal failure are as discussed in Chap. 220. Genetic counseling may be helpful in family planning and in selection of an unaffected related donor for renal transplantation.

FIGURE 228-1 *A. Radiographic appearance of medullary sponge kidney. Abdominal flat plate reveals multiple bilateral calcifications. B. Radiographic contrast material accumulates in the dilated and cystic terminal collecting ducts and obscures the calcifications.*

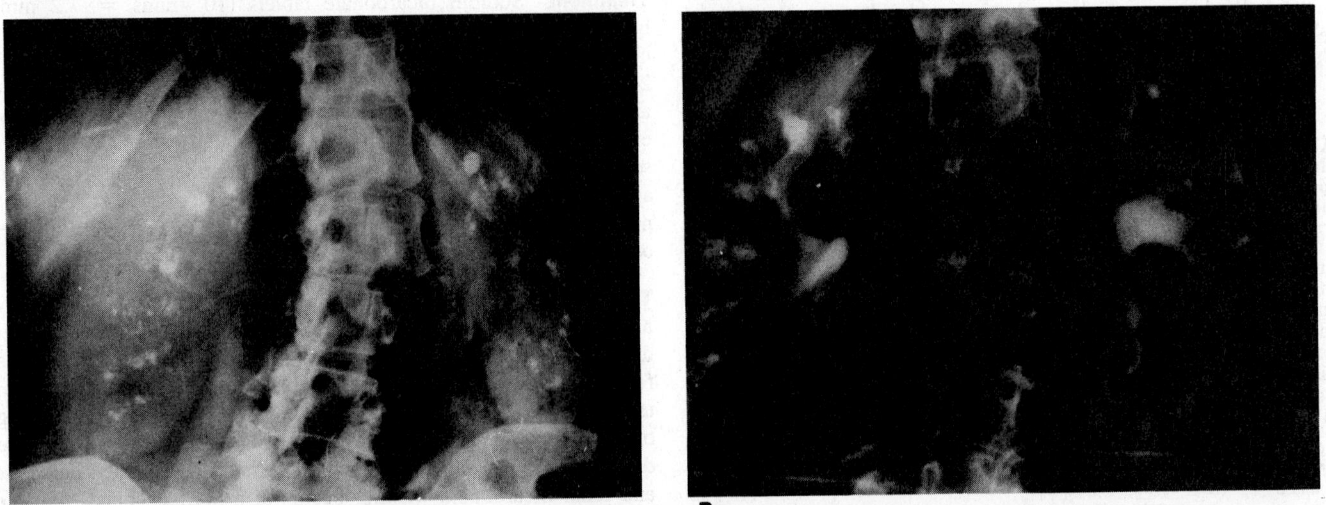

A B

BARTTER'S SYNDROME

Bartter's syndrome consists of hypokalemia due to renal potassium wasting, elevated plasma renin activity and aldosterone secretion, normal blood pressure, hyporesponsiveness of blood pressure to infused angiotensin II, and hyperplasia of the granular cells of the juxtaglomerular apparatus of the kidney. Weakness or periodic paralysis and polyuria occur because of chronic potassium depletion. Hyperplasia of renal medullary interstitial cells, which produce prostaglandins PGE and PGF, has been described, along with elevated PGE_2 production. Inheritance is autosomal recessive, and manifestations commonly begin in childhood.

PATHOGENESIS While the pathogenetic sequence is not understood with certainty, there is some evidence for a defect of tubular chloride or potassium transport. Either may produce hypokalemia, which stimulates release of prostaglandins E_2 and I_2, which in turn results in increased secretion of renin, leading to enhanced concentration of circulating angiotensin II and thus aldosterone. Both angiotensin II and aldosterone increase renal kallikrein, which increases plasma bradykinin, while aldosterone further enhances renal potassium loss. The normality of blood pressure results from the vasodepressor actions of PGE_2 and bradykinin, despite increased production of renin, angiotensin, and aldosterone.

Excessive production of PGE_2 resulting from hypokalemia, a known stimulator of PGE_2 synthesis, may therefore be a secondary consequence of the syndrome. In some cases blockade of PGE_2 production with indomethacin lowers renin levels and restores vascular response to angiotensin II infusion, but does not reduce potassium wasting.

TREATMENT The dietary intake of sodium chloride and potassium should be liberal; potassium supplements may be required. Pharmacologic blockade of aldosterone effects on distal tubules with spironolactone can prevent potassium wasting, though sodium intake must be increased. Inhibition of prostaglandin synthesis with indomethacin, ibuprofen, or aspirin has met with varying success, as indicated above. Beta-adrenergic blockade may lower renin production.

LIDDLE'S SYNDROME (PSEUDOHYPERALDOSTERONISM)

This rare inherited disorder is characterized by hypertension, hypokalemic alkalosis, and negligible aldosterone secretion. It appears to be due to an unusual tendency of distal tubules or collecting ducts to conserve sodium and excrete potassium despite the virtual absence of aldosterone. No other biochemical abnormalities have been described. However, transport rates of sodium in red blood cells are altered. These patients respond to 100 mg per day of triamterene (Chap. 182), a diuretic agent that blocks sodium and potassium exchange in the distal tubule.

FAMILIAL NEPHROGENIC DIABETES (DI)

In this disease the distal tubules and collecting ducts are unresponsive to vasopressin because of an X-linked recessive disease, with variable expressivity in heterozygous females. Affected individuals excrete large volumes of hypotonic urine even when plasma osmolality and vasopressin concentration are both high. Polyuria, polydipsia, and hypertonic dehydration following restriction of fluid intake all result from renal tubular insensitivity to antidiuretic hormone (ADH) (also see Chap. 323). Unresponsiveness to vasopressin may be secondary to reduced production of cyclic adenosine 5′-monophosphate (cyclic AMP) in the epithelium of the collecting ducts, to the inability of cyclic AMP to increase the permeability of collecting duct luminal cell membranes to water, or to a combination of the two. Other hereditary tubular defects such as juvenile nephronophthisis, medullary cystic and polycystic diseases, cystinosis, and congenital or acquired chronic urinary tract obstruction can also cause vasopressin-resistant (nephrogenic) DI, but in these syndromes the characteristic features of the underlying disorder are present.

Affected infants easily become dehydrated, hypernatremic, and hyperthermic, and damage of the central nervous system, including mental retardation, may result. In the absence of dehydration, overall renal function is normal. On intravenous pyelography the renal pelvis, ureters, and bladder are dilated, as in any form of DI, because of massive diuresis.

Oral hydration usually is adequate treatment except during early infancy, when hypotonic parenteral fluids may be required. Vasopressin and its synthetic analogues are ineffective, but diuretic agents such as chlorothiazide reduce polyuria. This drug inhibits NaCl reabsorption in the cortical portions of the thick ascending limb of the loop of Henle, thereby reducing production of free water. In addition, chlorothiazide produces a diuresis that causes contraction of extracellular fluid volume which, in turn, stimulates reabsorption of NaCl and water in the proximal tubule and limits their delivery to the thick ascending limb. Sodium restriction enhances its effect.

RENAL TUBULAR ACIDOSIS (RTA)

In this group of disorders renal excretion of acid is reduced out of proportion to any reduction of glomerular filtration rate. Metabolic acidosis results, but in contrast to renal failure the anions that accompany surplus hydrogen ions in the blood, such as sulfate and phosphate, are excreted normally and are unavailable to balance the fall in serum bicarbonate. Therefore, the kidneys reabsorb chloride in unusually large amounts, and serum chloride rises to preserve electroneutrality in the extracellular fluid. The result is *hyperchloremic acidosis,* and the unmeasured anion gap is normal. There is general agreement that four types of RTA exist (Table 228-2). Types 1 and 2 are often hereditary. Type 3 is a rare mixture of types 1 and 2. Type 4 is acquired and is associated with either hyporeninemic hypoaldosteronism or tubular hyporesponsiveness to circulating mineralocorticoids.

TABLE 228-2 Comparison of three types of renal tubular acidosis*

Finding	Type 1	Type 2	Type 4
Non-anion-gap acidosis	Yes	Yes	Yes
Minimum urine pH	>5.5	<5.5	<5.5
% filtered HCO_3 excreted	<10	>15	<10
Serum potassium	Low	Low	High
Fanconi syndrome	No	Yes	No
Stones/nephrocalcinosis	Yes	No	No
Daily acid excretion	Low	Normal	Low
Ammonium excretion	High for pH	Normal	Low for pH
Daily HCO_3 replacement needs	<4 mmol/kg	>4 mmol/kg	<4 mmol/kg

* *HCO_3, bicarbonate. Type 3 renal tubular acidosis is a rare form of a mixture of types 1 and 2.*

TYPE 1 (DISTAL) RTA Sporadic cases occur, but autosomal dominant inheritance is usual. The kidney does not lower urine pH normally, either because the collecting ducts permit excessive back-diffusion of hydrogen ions from lumen to blood or fail to transport hydrogen ions against a steep pH gradient. Since titration of urine buffers and diffusion trapping of NH_4^+ in the tubules both depend upon a low intraluminal pH, excretion of acid is deficient. However, urine ammonium excretion is as high or higher than in normal people whose urine is equally alkaline. Urinary osmotic concentration and potassium conservation also tend to be impaired.

Chronic acidosis lowers tubule reabsorption of calcium, causing renal hypercalciuria and mild secondary hyperparathyroidism. The hypercalciuria, alkaline urine, and low levels of urine citrate—which normally serves to complex about 40 percent of urine calcium—cause calcium phosphate stones and papillary nephrocalcinosis. Growth is stunted in children because of rickets; this growth defect responds to amelioration of the acidosis with sodium bicarbonate or other alkali. In the adult, bone disease takes the form of osteomalacia. In both children and adults, bone disease may result, in part, from acidosis-induced loss of bone mineral and from inadequate production of 1,25-dihydroxyvitamin D_3 [$1,25(OH)_2D_3$]. Since the kidney does not conserve potassium or concentrate the urine normally, polyuria and hypokalemia occur. Given the stress of an intercurrent illness, acidosis and hypokalemia can become life-threatening.

The diagnosis is suggested by osteomalacia or rickets, hyperchloremic acidosis associated with alkaline urine, and calcium phosphate stones or nephrocalcinosis. To prove that the urine pH cannot be lowered normally, the oral ammonium chloride (NH_4Cl) loading test should be carried out: 0.1 g (1.9 mmol) NH_4Cl per kilogram is administered, and the blood and urine pH are followed with time. Although systemic acidosis worsens, urine pH does not fall below 5.5. Urinary infection must not be present during this test because bacteria may possess urease, which hydrolyzes urea to ammonia and produces a very alkaline urine. When hyperchloremic acidosis is severe and the urine is grossly alkaline, the test is unnecessary.

A confusing situation may occur when type 1 RTA results from nephrocalcinosis due to hereditary idiopathic hypercalciuria. In this circumstance, stones usually are composed of calcium oxalate, and hypokalemia is absent. Other hereditary diseases that cause RTA, such as medullary sponge kidney, galactosemia, Ehler-Danlos syndrome, Fabry's disease, and hereditary elliptocytosis, can be excluded by clinical findings. The relatives of patients with type 1 RTA should be screened for this treatable cause of renal damage.

Treatment Sodium bicarbonate tablets (10 grains = 7.2 mmol base) and Shohl's solution (1 mmol base per milliliter, as Na and K citrate) are both convenient for treatment; the dose should be 0.5 to 2.0 mmol/kg in four or five divided doses daily. The total dose of alkali should be raised until acidosis and hypercalciuria are both eliminated, and the patients should be followed by measurements of serum chloride and CO_2 content and of urine calcium excretion approximately twice yearly. Potassium supplementation usually is not required. Requirements for alkali usually increase during intercurrent illnesses but are usually below 4 mmol/kg per day.

TYPE 2 (PROXIMAL) RTA Proximal RTA usually occurs as part of a generalized disorder of proximal tubule function. It can be a transient disorder of infancy which usually disappears in childhood. An isolated form, i.e., without accompanying phosphaturia, aminoaciduria, and uricosuria, has been described in one family. The pathophysiology of proximal RTA is the same whether isolated or part of a generalized disorder. Bicarbonate reabsorption in the proximal tubule is defective, and renal bicarbonate wasting occurs at a normal concentration of plasma bicarbonate. As plasma bicarbonate falls, the filtered load drops to a level that the defective tubule can reabsorb. Then the urine is free of bicarbonate and has a low pH. Potassium wasting and hypokalemia occur, especially when supplementary alkali is given, because bicarbonate is excreted in the urine partly as the potassium salt. Hypercalciuria is moderate, and stone formation is rare. During the NH_4Cl loading test, urine pH falls below 5.5.

Treatment is often not required. When acidosis is severe, bicarbonate must be given in large amounts daily, often above 4 mmol/kg, and even up to 10 mmol/kg per day, because bicarbonate is rapidly excreted in the urine. Another approach is to use a thiazide diuretic and a low-salt diet, which induce mild volume depletion and enhance proximal bicarbonate reabsorption, thereby reducing the required dose. Potassium supplements are needed during treatment because excessive sodium bicarbonate reaches the distal nephron, where much of the sodium is exchanged for potassium, which is then lost in the urine.

TYPE 4 RTA Some patients have a form of renal tubular acidosis that differs from types 1 and 2 and has been called type 4. They have metabolic acidosis without an elevation of the anion gap but differ from type 1 patients in having an acid urine during periods of severe acidosis (Table 228-2), and from type 2 patients in having low urine excretion of bicarbonate and a daily replacement alkali requirement of <4 mmol per kilogram of body weight. They differ from both types 1 and 2 in having a high serum potassium level and a low urine ammonia excretion rate. They have neither Fanconi syndrome nor stone disease. Because potassium and hydrogen excretion are abnormal, they are considered to have generalized distal nephron dysfunction that is due either to intrinsic renal disease or to abnormal aldosterone levels. Hyperkalemia worsens acidosis by suppressing renal production of ammonia, which is the most important urinary buffer, and thereby limiting acid excretion.

The most common patients with type 4 renal tubular acidosis have hyporeninemic hypoaldosteronism; plasma levels of renin and aldosterone are subnormal, even during extracellular volume depletion. Diabetic nephropathy, nephrosclerosis from hypertension, and chronic tubulointerstitial nephropathies are the usual causes. Hyperkalemia and acidosis can be treated with replacement doses of a mineralocorticoid hormone such as fludrocortisone, 0.1 to 0.2 mg per day; some patients may require 0.3 to 0.5 mg per day, suggesting tubule unresponsiveness to the hormone. Furosemide can also improve the hyperkalemia and acidosis, provided salt intake is sufficient to prevent extracellular volume contraction.

A less common condition is *mineralocorticoid-resistant hyperkalemia;* hyperkalemia and acidosis do not improve despite mineralocorticoid hormone treatment. This occurs in occasional patients with underlying renal disease who also have severe salt wasting, as a consequence of distal nephron damage. Plasma renin and aldosterone levels are elevated, and patients are prone to extracellular fluid volume depletion. Treatment requires salt supplements and alkali, but mineralocorticoid hormones are not necessary. Other patients with mild acidosis have no evidence of renal disease and do not waste salt in their urine. Plasma renin and aldosterone levels are low, but hyperkalemia and acidosis do not respond to mineralocorticoid hormone treatment. The cause is thought to be abnormally high distal tubule permeability to chloride ion; sodium chloride reabsorption is elevated, the potential across the distal tubule epithelium is presumed to be below normal, potassium secretion is reduced because it is driven by the transepithelial voltage, hyperkalemia causes acidosis by suppressing ammonia production, and extracellular volume expansion from sodium chloride absorption suppresses renin and aldosterone levels and causes hypertension. The main evidence for this formulation is that infusion of sodium with anions such as bicarbonate or sulfate raises potassium excretion to normal or supranormal levels. Treatment of this rare condition is with thiazide diuretic agents or low-sodium diet.

Primary mineralocorticoid deficiency from diseases of the adrenals also causes hyperkalemia and acidosis. Evaluation and treatment of adrenal disorders is discussed in Chap. 325.

VITAMIN D DISORDERS

FAMILIAL X-LINKED HYPOPHOSPHATEMIC VITAMIN D–REFRACTORY RICKETS (See also Chap. 337) Reduced tubular reabsorption of phosphate by the proximal tubule and hypophosphatemia occur in this X-linked dominant disease, which can also be termed *renal phosphate leak.* Patients may be asymptomatic but are usually short and have rachitic bones; their legs are particularly short and deformed, and they develop osteomalacia in adult life. Bone age and dentition are retarded, and the teeth are poorly developed. The skull becomes deformed, and the maxillofacial region may be abnormal. Overgrowth of bone at sites of muscular attachment can limit movement or compress nerves. Bony abnormalities are less common in women. Serum alkaline phosphatase levels are elevated, serum parathyroid levels are normal or high, serum calcium concentration is usually normal, and urinary calcium excretion rate is normal or low.

The hypophosphatemia arises in part from decreased tubular reabsorption of phosphate and increased fractional excretion of phosphate. Intestinal absorption of calcium and phosphate may be decreased in untreated patients but increased during treatment with vitamin D. Although glycinuria and mild glucosuria may occur, most patients exhibit only a defect in excretion of phosphate. Absence of hyperchloremic acidosis and a normal serum calcium concentration help to exclude RTA, malabsorption syndrome, and nutritional rickets.

Treatment requires oral neutral phosphate, 1 to 4 g daily, in divided doses, and 10,000 to 50,000 units of vitamin D; one must watch for hypercalcemia. Combination of oral phosphate with calcitriol [$1,25(OH)_2D_3$] may be more beneficial. Bony deformities require orthopedic management, but corrective surgery, except for genu valgum, should be postponed until active growth is completed.

VITAMIN D–DEPENDENT RICKETS TYPE 1 (See also Chap. 337) Also known as hereditary pseudovitamin D–deficiency rickets, this disease is inherited as an autosomal recessive trait. Defective production of $1,25(OH)_2D_3$ by the kidneys, perhaps because of a genetic defect in 25-hydroxycholecalciferol 1α-hydroxylase, has been proposed as the basis for the disease. But the dose of calcitriol required to heal rickets is higher than that for vitamin D–deficiency rickets, suggesting an attenuated response to, or excessive degradation of, $1,25(OH)_2D_3$.

Rickets usually appears before 2 years of age. Serum calcium is low, parathyroid hormone concentration and alkaline phosphatase are high, and plasma phosphorus is variable. Urinary calcium is decreased, fecal calcium is increased, and tubular phosphate reabsorption is reduced. Serum levels of $1,25(OH)_2D_3$ are undetectable. Aminoaciduria and hyperchloremic acidosis can occur, but urinary cyclic AMP increases normally in response to PTH infusion.

The 1α-hydroxylated metabolites of vitamin D bypass the enzyme defect and produce a dramatic healing of rickets. Vitamin D_2, 10,000 to 40,000 units per day, is also effective, but oral calcium, 0.5 to 2.0 g per day, is needed as well. The need for vitamin D persists throughout life. Calcitriol, an ideal replacement therapy, is the drug of choice, but one must watch for hypercalcemia.

VITAMIN D–DEPENDENT RICKETS TYPE 2 Like type 1, this disease causes rickets, hypocalcemia, hypophosphatemia, and secondary hyperparathyroidism, but serum levels of $1,25(OH)_2D_3$ are elevated, and treatment with additional $1,25(OH)_2D_3$ does not increase the serum calcium level or heal the bone disease even though it can reduce serum levels of parathyroid hormone. Generalized alopecia is often present and may be either a linked defect or the result of the mineral disorder. The cause appears to be an autosomal recessive defect of the $1,25(OH)_2D_3$ receptor. Treatment with a high dose of calcitriol and mineral supplements may achieve healing of bone, but relapse may occur despite continued treatment.

ONCOGENIC OSTEOMALACIA Mesenchymal tumors, usually benign, can cause renal phosphate wasting similiar to that of X-linked hypophosphatemic rickets, with resulting osteomalacia. Carcinoma of the prostate and oat cell carcinoma of the lung also have caused this syndrome. The disease almost always occurs in adults and develops gradually, over years. The tumors occur mainly in the extremities, scalp, nose, and mandible, in close association with bone. Their removal cures the phosphate wasting and leads to healing of the osteomalacia.

RENAL GLUCOSURIA

See Chap. 308.

ISOLATED HYPOURICEMIA (See also Chap. 308)

This disorder, in which there is a defect in proximal tubular reabsorption of sodium urate, appears to be inherited as an autosomal recessive trait. Hypouricemia can occur in the Fanconi syndrome, Hartnup's disease, and Wilson's disease. Uric acid clearance is high, and urine oxypurine levels are normal, excluding hereditary xanthinuria. Patients are asymptomatic except for occasional uric acid nephrolithiasis. No specific treatment is needed except the avoidance of dehydration. Coexistent hypercalciuria and decreased bone density have been described in a few patients, who may have a related disease.

SELECTIVE DISORDERS OF AMINO ACID TRANSPORT

HARTNUP'S DISEASE (See also Chap. 308) In this rare autosomal recessive disorder, renal and intestinal transport of monoamino–monocarboxylic amino acids is defective. An erythematous, scaly, pellagra-like rash appears after exposure to sunlight, and episodic cerebellar ataxia, emotional instability, delirium, and aminoaciduria all occur. The prevalence is 1 in 15,000 newborns and is higher in the offspring of consanguineous marriages.

Dietary monoamino–monocarboxylic amino acids remain in the intestinal lumen where they undergo bacterial degradation. At the same time, they are lost in the urine. Inadequate tryptophan availability limits nicotinamide synthesis and leads to pellagra. Decreased absorption and urine loss of the other monoamino–monocarboxylic amino acids can cause generalized malnutrition.

The diagnosis is based upon demonstration of massive urine losses of alanine, serine, threonine, asparagine, glutamine, valine, leucine, isoleucine, phenylalanine, tyrosine, tryptophan, histidine, glycine, and citrulline. Hypouricemia may occur. Renal function is otherwise normal. Most patients respond to treatment with oral nicotinamide, 40 to 200 mg per day, and a high-protein diet to compensate for amino acid malabsorption and loss. The ultimate prognosis is good, and the disease often improves with age.

FAMILIAL IMINOGLYCINURIA (See also Chap. 308) This autosomal recessive trait is characterized by excessive urinary excretion of proline, hydroxyproline, and glycine despite normal plasma levels of these amino acids, probably because of deletion or alteration of a membrane transport protein of the renal tubule cells. The patients are well. Iminoglycinuria can occur in normal newborn infants for up to 3 months.

FANCONI SYNDROME

Fanconi syndrome is a constellation of transport defects in the proximal tubule involving amino acids, monosaccharides, sodium, potassium, calcium, phosphate, bicarbonate, uric acid, and proteins. Generalized aminoaciduria, glucosuria, salt wasting, hypercalciuria, hypophosphatemia, proximal renal tubular acidosis, hypouricemia, and tubular proteinuria (Chap. 40) may result. Fanconi syndrome can be acquired secondary to diseases such as cystinosis, tyrosinemia, galactosemia, fructose intolerance, glycogen storage disease (type 1), Wilson's disease, familial nephrosis, and hereditary amyloidosis. Lowe's (or oculocerebrorenal) syndrome is an X-linked recessive form of the Fanconi syndrome associated with ocular and cerebral abnormalities.

An autosomal recessive disease, *adult Fanconi syndrome,* occurs in the absence of any systemic disorder. The term *adult* is misleading since cases are recognized in childhood, but no abnormalities are apparent at birth. Dwarfism and hypophosphatemic rickets occur along with the laboratory abnormalities of Fanconi syndrome. Renal failure is rare, and the prognosis is good when the systemic manifestations are treated. Typically, there is a "swan neck" deformity of the initial portion of the proximal tubule which is probably the anatomic basis of this tubular disorder. There is cellular atrophy in the deformed tubular segment. The consequences of the defects in the transport of water, sodium, potassium, acid, and phosphate excretion often require treatment. Water, sodium, and potassium intake must be liberal, and phosphate supplements may be needed. Metabolic acidosis can be corrected by the administration of alkali. Vitamin D helps promote bone healing. Glucosuria, uricosuria, and tubular proteinuria do not require treatment.

CYSTINURIA

See Chap. 308.

REFERENCES

AVIOLI LV: Vitamin D–resistant rickets, in *Diseases of the Kidney,* 3d ed, LE Earley, CW Gottschalk (eds). Boston, Little, Brown, 1979, p 1055

BATLLE DC, ARRUDA JAL: Renal tubular acidosis syndromes. Miner Electrolyte Metab 5:83, 1981

BERNSTEIN J, KISSANE JM: Hereditary disorders of the kidney. Part 1: Parenchymal defects and malformations. Perspect Pediatr Pathol 1:117, 1973

BRENES LG et al: Familial proximal renal tubular acidosis. Am J Med 52:244, 1977

CANTANI A et al: Familial juvenile nephronophthisis: A review and differential diagnosis. Clin Pediatr 25:90, 1986

CULPEPPER RM et al: Nephrogenic diabetes insipidus, in *The Metabolic Basis of Inherited Disease,* 5th ed, JB Stanbury et al (eds). New York, McGraw-Hill, 1983, p 1867

DANOVITCH GM: Clinical features and pathophysiology of polycystic disease in man, in *Cystic Diseases of the Kidney,* KD Gardner (ed). New York, Wiley, 1976, p 123

DEFRONZO FA, THIER SO: Inherited disorders of renal tubule function, in *The Kidney,* 3d ed, BM Brenner, FC Rector Jr (eds). Philadelphia, Saunders, 1986, p 1297

GAMBLIN GT et al: Vitamin D–dependent rickets type 2. J Clin Invest 75:954, 1985

GARRICK R et al: Bartter's syndrome: A unifying hypothesis. Am J Nephrol 5:379, 1985

HALPERIN EC, THIER SO: Cystinuria, in *Contemporary Issues in Nephrology,* BM Brenner, JH Stein (eds), FL Coe (guest ed). New York, Churchill Livingstone, 1980, vol 5, p 208

——— et al: Distal renal tubular acidosis syndromes: A pathophysiological approach. Am J Nephrol 5:1, 1985

JEPSON JB: Hartnup disease, in *The Metabolic Basis of Inherited Disease,* 5th ed, JB Stanbury et al (eds). New York, McGraw-Hill, 1983, p 1804

KUPIER JJ: Medullary sponge kidney, in *Cystic Diseases of the Kidney,* KD Gardner Jr (ed). New York, Wiley, 1976, p 151

LIBBER S et al: Treatment of nephrogenic diabetes insipidus with prostaglandin synthesis inhibitors. J Pediatr 108:35, 1986

LIDDLE GW et al: A familial renal disorder simulating primary aldosteronism but with negligible aldosterone secretion. Trans Assoc Am Phys 76:199, 1963

RASMUSSEN H, ANAST C: Familial hypophosphatemic rickets and vitamin D–dependent rickets, in *The Metabolic Basis of Inherited Disease,* 5th ed, JB Stanbury et al (eds). New York, McGraw-Hill, 1983, p 1743

RYAN EA, REISS E et al: Oncogenous osteomalacia. Am J Med 77:501, 1984

SCRIVER CR: Familial iminoglycinuria, in *The Metabolic Basis of Inherited Disease,* 5th ed, JB Stanbury et al (eds). New York, McGraw-Hill, 1983, p 1792

——— et al: Genetic aspects of renal tubular transport: Diversity and topology of carriers. Kidney Int 9:149, 1976

SEGAL S: Disorders of renal amino acid transport. N Engl J Med 294:1044, 1976

TOFUKU Y et al: Hypouricemia due to renal urate wasting: Two types of tubular transport defects. Nephron 30:39, 1982

229 NEPHROLITHIASIS

FREDRIC L. COE / MURRAY J. FAVUS

TYPES OF STONES

Calcium salts, uric acid, cystine, and struvite ($MgNH_4PO_4$) are the basis of virtually all kidney stones formed by patients residing in the western hemisphere. Calcium oxalate and calcium phosphate stones make up 75 to 85 percent of the total (Table 229-1) and may be admixed in the same stone. Calcium phosphates in stones are usually hydroxyapatite [$Ca_5(PO_4)_3OH$] or, less commonly, brushite ($CaHPO_4 \cdot H_2O$).

Calcium stones are formed mainly by men; the average age of onset is the third decade. Most persons who form a single calcium stone will eventually form another, and the intervals between successive stones shorten or remain constant, suggesting that stone-forming activity usually does not wane with time. The average rate of new stone formation in patients who have previously formed a stone is about one stone every 2 or 3 years. Calcium stone disease is strongly familial.

In the urine, calcium oxalate monohydrate crystals (whewellite) usually grow as biconcave ovals that resemble red blood cells in shape and size, but also occur in a larger, ''dumbbell'' form. In polarized light the crystals appear bright against a dark background with an intensity dependent upon orientation, a property known as *birefringence*. Calcium oxalate dihydrate crystals (weddellite) are bipyramidal and only weakly birefringent. Apatite crystals do not exhibit birefringence and appear amorphous, because the actual crystals are too small to be resolved by light microscopy. Brushite produces elongated lathlike (narrow, long, rectangular) crystals.

Uric acid stones are radiolucent, account for 5 to 8 percent of all stones (Table 229-1), and are also formed mainly by men. Half of the patients who form uric acid stones have gout; whether or not gout is present, uric acid lithiasis is usually familial. In urine, uric acid crystals become red-orange in color because they adsorb the pigment uricine. Anhydrous uric acid produces very small crystals that appear amorphous by light microscopy. They are indistinguishable from apatite crystals, except for their birefringence. Uric acid dihydrate tends to form teardrop-shaped crystals as well as flat, square plates; both are strongly birefringent. Uric acid gravel appears like red dust, and the stones are also orange or red on some occasions. *Cystine stones* are very uncommon (less than 1 percent of all stones), are lemon yellow, and sparkle; they are radiopaque because they contain sulfur. Cystine crystals appear in the urine as flat, hexagonal plates.

Struvite ($MgNH_4PO_4$) *stones* are common (Table 229-1) and potentially dangerous. These stones, formed mainly by women, result from urinary tract infection with bacteria that produce urease, usually *Proteus* species. The stones can grow to a large size and fill the renal pelvis and calyces to produce a ''staghorn'' appearance. They are radiopaque and have a variable internal density. In urine, struvite crystals are rectangular prisms that have been likened to coffin lids.

MANIFESTATIONS OF STONES

As stones grow upon the surfaces of the renal papillae or within the urinary collecting system, they need not produce symptoms. Accordingly, asymptomatic stones are often discovered during the course of abdominal radiographic studies undertaken for unrelated reasons. Sometimes stones cause only gross or microscopic hematuria. In fact, stones rank, along with benign and malignant neoplasms, renal cysts, and genitourinary tuberculosis, as among the most common causes of isolated hematuria. Much of the time, however, stones break loose

TABLE 229-1 Major causes of renal stones

Stone type and causes	Percent of all stones*	Percent occurrence of specific causes*	Ratio of men to women	Etiology	Diagnosis	Treatment
Calcium stones	75–85		2:1 to 3:1			
Idiopathic hypercalciuria		50–55	2:1	Hereditary (?)	Normocalcemia, unexplained hypercalciuria†	Thiazide diuretic agents
Hyperuricosuria		20	4:1	Diet	Urine uric acid >750 mg per 24 h (women), >800 mg per 24 h (men)	Allopurinol or diet
Primary hyperparathyroidism		5	3:10	Neoplasia	Unexplained hypercalcemia	Surgery
Distal renal tubular acidosis		Rare	1:1	Hereditary	Hyperchloremic acidosis, minimum urine pH >5.5	Alkali replacement
Intestinal hyperoxaluria		~1–2	1:1	Bowel surgery	Urine oxalate >50 mg per 24 h	Cholestyramine or oral calcium loading
Hereditary hyperoxaluria		Rare	1:1	Hereditary	Urine oxalate and glycolic or L-glyceric acid increased	Fluids and pyridoxine
Idiopathic stone disease		20	2:1	Unknown	None of the above present	Oral phosphate, fluids
Uric acid stones	5–8					Alkali to raise urine pH
Gout		~50	3:1 to 4:1	Hereditary	Clinical diagnosis	Allopurinol if daily urine uric acid above 1000 mg
Idiopathic		~50	1:1	Hereditary (?)	Uric acid stones, no gout	
Dehydration		?	1:1	Intestinal, habit	History, intestinal fluid loss	Alkali, fluids, reversal of cause
Lesch-Nyhan syndrome		Rare	Men	Hereditary	Reduced hypoxanthine-guanine phosphoribosyltransferase level	Allopurinol
Malignant tumors		Rare	1:1	Neoplasia	Clinical diagnosis	Allopurinol
Cystine stones	1		1:1	Hereditary	Stone type; elevated cystine excretion	Massive fluids, alkali, D-penicillamine if needed
Struvite stones	10–15		2:10	Infection	Stone type	Antimicrobial agents and judicious surgery

* *Values are percent of patients who form a particular type of stone and who display each specific cause of stones.*
† *Urine calcium above 300 mg per 24 h (men), 250 mg per 24 h (women), or 4 mg/kg per 24 h either sex. Hyperthyroidism, Cushing syndrome, sarcoidosis, malignant tumors, immobilization, vitamin D intoxication, rapidly progressive bone disease, and Paget's disease all cause hypercalciuria and must be excluded in diagnosis of idiopathic hypercalciuria.*

and enter the ureter, or occlude the ureteropelvic junction, causing pain and obstruction.

STONE PASSAGE A stone can traverse the ureter without symptoms, but most of the time passage produces pain and bleeding. The pain begins gradually, usually in the flank, but increases over the next 20 to 60 min to become so severe that narcotic drugs are often needed for its control. The pain may remain in the flank or spread downward and anteriorly toward the ipsilateral loin, testicle, or vulva. Pain that migrates downward always indicates that the stone has passed to the lower third of the ureter, but if the pain does not migrate, the position of the stone cannot be predicted. A stone in the portion of the ureter within the bladder wall causes frequency, urgency, and dysuria that may be confused with urinary tract infection. Hematuria is the rule with passage of a stone.

OTHER SYNDROMES **Staghorn calculi** Struvite, cystine, and uric acid stones often grow too large to enter the ureter. They gradually fill the renal pelvis and may extend outward through the infundibula to the calyces themselves.

Nephrocalcinosis Calcium stones grow on the renal papillae. Most break loose and cause colic, but sometimes they remain in place so that multiple papillary calcifications are found by x-ray, a condition termed *nephrocalcinosis*. Papillary nephrocalcinosis is very common in hereditary distal renal tubular acidosis and in other states characterized by severe hypercalciuria. In medullary sponge kidney disease (Chap. 228) calcification may occur in dilated distal collecting ducts.

Sludge There can be enough uric acid or cystine in the urine to plug both ureters with precipitate. Calcium oxalate crystals do not do this because usually less than 100 mg oxalate is excreted daily in the urine in even severe hyperoxaluric states, compared with 1000 mg uric acid in patients with ordinary hyperuricosuria and 400 to 800 mg cystine in patients with homozygous cystinuria. Calcium phosphate crystals can render the urine milky but do not plug the urinary tract.

INFECTION Although urinary tract infection is not a direct consequence of stone disease, it is a frequent complication that arises from instrumentation and surgery of the urinary tract, which are frequently required in the treatment of stone disease. Stone disease and urinary infection can enhance the seriousness of one another and interfere with treatment. Obstruction of an infected kidney by a stone may lead to sepsis and extensive damage of renal tissue, since it converts the urinary tract proximal to the obstruction into a closed, or partially closed, space that can become an abscess. On the other hand, some forms of infection, those due to bacteria that possess the enzyme urease, can produce stones composed of struvite.

ACTIVITY OF STONE DISEASE *Active disease* means that new stones are forming or that preformed stones are growing. Sequential radiographs of the renal areas are needed to document the growth or appearance of new stones and to ensure that stones which pass are actually newly formed, not preexistent ones.

PATHOGENESIS OF STONES

Urinary stones usually arise because of the breakdown of a delicate balance. On the one hand the kidneys must conserve water, but they must also excrete materials that have a low solubility. These two opposing requirements must be balanced against one another during adaptation to a particular combination of diet, climate, and activity. The problem is mitigated to some extent by the fact that urine contains some substances that inhibit crystallization of calcium salts and others that bind calcium in soluble complexes. But these protective mechanisms are less than perfect. When the urine becomes supersaturated with insoluble materials, because their excretion rates are excessive, and/or because water conservation is extreme, crystals form and may grow and aggregate with one another to form a stone.

SUPERSATURATION Consider a solution that is in equilibrium with crystals of calcium oxalate. The product of the chemical activities of the calcium and oxalate ions in the solution is termed the *equilibrium solubility product,* because it is the activity product that is unique to the equilibrium condition. If the crystals are removed, and if either calcium or oxalate is added to the solution, the activity product will rise, but the solution will remain clear; no new crystals form. Such a solution is considered to be *metastably supersaturated.* If new calcium oxalate seed crystals are now added, they will grow in size. Ultimately, the activity product will reach a critical value at which a solid phase begins to develop spontaneously. This value is called the *upper limit of metastability,* or the *formation product.* Stone growth in the urinary tract requires a urine that, on the average, is above the equilibrium solubility product. Persistence of a stone requires an average activity product at least equal to the solubility product. In general there is agreement that excessive supersaturation is a factor common to the formation of most stones.

Calcium, oxalate, and phosphate form many stable soluble complexes among themselves and with other substances in urine, such as citrate. As a result, their free ion activities are considerably below their chemical concentrations and can be measured only by indirect techniques. Reduction in ligand such as citrate can increase ion activity without changing measurably total urinary calcium. Urine supersaturation can be increased by dehydration or by overexcretion of calcium, oxalate, or phosphate. Supersaturation of the urine with cystine or uric acid also occurs when overexcretion or low urine volume is present. Urine pH can also be an important factor; phosphate and uric acid are weak acids that dissociate readily over the physiologic range of urine pH. Alkaline urine contains more urate and dissociated phosphate, favoring deposits of sodium hydrogen urate, octocalcium phosphate, and apatite. Below a urine pH of 5.5, uric acid crystals (pK 5.47) predominate, whereas phosphate crystals are rare. The solubility of calcium oxalate, on the other hand, is not influenced by changes in urine pH. Measurements of supersaturation in a 24-h urine sample are averages that probably underestimate the risk of precipitation. Transient dehydration or postprandial bursts of overexcretion may cause values that are considerably above the average.

NUCLEATION **Homogeneous nucleation** In urine that is supersaturated with respect to calcium oxalate, these two ions come together and form clusters. The higher the supersaturation, the larger and more numerous the clusters become. Most small clusters eventually disperse because the internal forces between ions that hold them together are too weak to overcome the random tendency of ions to move away. Clusters of over 100 ions can remain stable because attractive forces balance surface losses. Once they are stable, nuclei can grow at a supersaturation far below that needed for their creation. The formation product marks the point at which stable nuclei become frequent enough to create a permanent solid phase.

Heterogeneous nucleation If a supersaturated urine is seeded with preformed nuclei of a crystal that is similar in structure to calcium oxalate, calcium and oxalate ions in solution will bind to the crystal's surface as they would upon a seed crystal of calcium oxalate itself. The organized growth of one crystal on the surface of another is called *epitaxial growth,* and the seeding of a supersaturated solution by foreign nuclei is called *heterogeneous nucleation.* Sodium hydrogen urate, uric acid, and hydroxyapatite crystals can serve as heterogeneous nuclei that permit calcium oxalate stones to form even though urine calcium oxalate supersaturation never exceeds the metastable limit.

INHIBITORS OF CRYSTAL GROWTH AND AGGREGATION Stable nuclei must grow and aggregate to produce a stone of clinical significance. Urine contains potent inhibitors of both of these processes for calcium oxalate and calcium phosphate, but not for uric acid, cystine, or struvite crystals. Inorganic pyrophosphate is a potent inhibitor which appears to affect calcium phosphate more than calcium oxalate crystals. Other urine inhibitors that appear to be glycoproteins strongly inhibit the growth of calcium oxalate crystals. Slowing of crystal growth must raise the apparent upper limit of metastability, because the critical growth of ion clusters into stable nuclei is hindered. As a consequence of the presence of these inhibitors, crystal growth in urine is very slow compared with simple salt solutions, and the upper limit of metastability is higher. Urine citrate may also inhibit crystal growth or nucleation.

EVALUATION AND TREATMENT OF PATIENTS WITH NEPHROLITHIASIS

A majority of patients with nephrolithiasis harbor remediable metabolic disorders that cause stones and can be detected by chemical analysis of the serum and urine. A practical outpatient evaluation consists of three 24-h urine collections, each with a corresponding blood sample. Serum and urine calcium, uric acid and creatinine, urine oxalate and citrate, and serum electrolyte measurements should be made. Whenever possible, the composition of kidney stones should be determined because treatment depends on stone type (Table 229-1). No matter what disorders are found, every patient should be counseled to avoid dehydration and to drink six to eight glasses of water daily. Since treatment is prolonged, the use of medications must be justified by the activity and severity of stone disease and the desire the patient may have for protection against new stones.

The management of stones that are already present in the kidneys or urinary tract requires a combined medical and surgical approach. The specific treatment for any individual patient depends upon the details of the location of the stone, the extent of obstruction, the function of the affected and unaffected kidneys, the presence or absence of urinary tract infection, the progress of stone passage, and the risk of operation or anesthesia, given the overall clinical state of the patient. In general, severe obstruction, infection, intractable pain, or serious bleeding are indications for removal of a stone.

In the past, stones could be removed only by operation upon the kidney, renal pelvis, or ureter or by passing a flexible basket retrograde up the ureter from the bladder during cystoscopy. However, there now are three new alternatives. Stones can be fragmented in situ by exposing them to extracorporeal shock waves. The patient is submerged in a water tank, the kidney with the stone is centered at the focal point of parabolic reflectors, and high-intensity shock waves are created by high-voltage discharge. The waves are focused by the reflectors so that they pass through the patient. The rigid stone fractures as the shock wave passes by. After many discharges, most stones are reduced to powder that passes through the ureter into the bladder. Larger fragments are removed by cystoscopy. Extracorporeal lithotripsy is used for stones in the kidney, renal pelvis, or proximal ureter. A second method is percutaneous ultrasonic lithotripsy, in which a rigid cystoscope-like instrument is passed into the renal pelvis through a small incision in the flank. Stones can be disrupted by a small ultrasound transducer, and fragments removed directly. The last method is endoscopic passage of an ultrasonic transducer into the ureter via a cystoscope; ureteral stones that are inaccessible to extracorporeal or percutaneous lithotripsy can be fragmented and removed. Extracorporeal, percutaneous, and endoscopic lithotripsy seem to be replacing pyelolithotomy and ureterolithotomy.

CALCIUM STONES **Idiopathic hypercalciuria** (see also Chap. 336) This condition appears to be hereditary, and its diagnosis is straightforward (Table 229-1). In some patients, primary intestinal hyperabsorption of calcium causes transient postprandial hypercalcemia that suppresses secretion of parathyroid hormone. The renal tubules are deprived of their most potent normal stimulus to reabsorb calcium at the same time that the filtered load of calcium is increased. In other patients, reabsorption of calcium by the renal tubules appears to be defective, and secondary hyperparathyroidism is evoked by urinary losses of calcium. Renal activation of 1,25-dihydroxyvitamin D is increased, producing intestinal hyperabsorption of calcium. In the past, the separation of "absorptive" and "renal" forms of hypercalciuria has been used to guide treatment. However, these may not be separate entities but the extremes of a continuum of behavior. Hypercalciuria contributes to stone formation by raising urine saturation with respect to calcium oxalate and calcium phosphate.

Thiazide diuretics lower urine calcium in both types of hypercalciuria and are very effective in preventing the formation of stones. The drug effect requires slight contraction of the extracellular fluid volume, and massive use of NaCl will reduce its therapeutic effect. Potassium citrate is useful to prevent hypokalemia and raise urine citrate; the latter lowers urine calcium ion levels.

Hyperuricosuria About 20 percent of calcium oxalate stone formers are hyperuricosuric, primarily because of an excessive intake of purine from meat, fish, and poultry. The mechanism of stone formation probably is heterogeneous nucleation of calcium oxalate by crystals of sodium hydrogen urate or uric acid that lodge in the terminal ends of the collecting ducts and produce an anchored site on which calcium oxalate can deposit. A change in diet is ideal treatment but difficult for many patients to achieve. The alternative is allopurinol, usually 100 mg bid. Some patients eventually alter their diets so that allopurinol can be withdrawn.

Primary hyperparathyroidism (see also Chap. 336) The diagnosis of this condition, which is more common in women than men, is established by documenting hypercalcemia that cannot be otherwise explained accompanied by inappropriately elevated serum concentrations of parathyroid hormone. Hypercalciuria, which is usually present, raises the urine supersaturation of calcium phosphate and/or calcium oxalate (Table 229-1). It is important to establish the diagnosis since parathyroidectomy is effective treatment and should be carried out before renal damage has occurred.

Distal renal tubular acidosis (see also Chap. 228) The defect in this condition seems to reside in the distal nephron, which cannot establish a normal pH gradient between urine and blood, leading to hyperchloremic acidosis. The minimum urine pH in response to an oral challenge with NH_4Cl, 1.9 mmol/kg, is above 5.5. Hypercalciuria, an alkaline urine, and a low urine citrate excretion cause supersaturation with respect to calcium phosphate. Calcium phosphate stones are formed, nephrocalcinosis is common, and osteomalacia or rickets may occur. Renal damage is frequent, and a gradual fall in glomerular filtration rate usually occurs. Treatment with supplemental alkali reverses hypercalciuria and limits the production of new stones. The usual dose of sodium bicarbonate is 0.5 to 2.0 meq/kg, in four to six divided doses. An alternative is Shohl's solution, which contains citrate and citric acid. Incomplete renal tubular acidosis (RTA) refers to a disease in which systemic acidosis is absent, but the kidneys cannot lower urine pH below 5.5 when patients are given an exogenous acid load such as ammonium chloride. Incomplete RTA may be acquired by some patients who form calcium oxalate stones because of idiopathic hypercalciuria; the importance of the RTA in producing stones is uncertain, and thiazide treatment is a reasonable alternative. Some patients with incomplete RTA form calcium phosphate stones because of low urine citrate and an abnormally alkaline urine, and are best treated as if RTA were complete: with alkali.

Hyperoxaluria Overabsorption of dietary oxalate and consequent oxaluria, i.e., so-called intestinal oxaluria, has been ascribed to fat malabsorption (Chap. 237). The latter can be caused by a variety of conditions, including bacterial overgrowth syndromes, chronic disease of the pancreas and biliary tract, jejunoileal bypass in treatment of obesity, or ileal resection greater than 22 cm for inflammatory bowel disease. With fat malabsorption, calcium in the bowel lumen is bound by fatty acids instead of precipitating with oxalate, which is left free for excessive absorption in the colon. Delivery of unabsorbed fatty acids and bile salts to the colon may injure the colonic mucosa and permit excessive oxalate absorption. Dietary excess of oxalate, ascorbic acid loading, and hereditary hyperoxaluric states due to overproduction of oxalate are much less common causes of hyperoxaluria. Ethylene glycol intoxication and methoxyflurane, an anesthetic agent, can also cause oxalate overproduction and hyperoxaluria. Hyperoxaluria from any cause can produce tubulointerstitial nephropathy (Chap. 226) and lead to stone formation.

Cholestyramine, a resin that can bind oxalate, at a dose of 8 to 16 g per day, correction of fat malabsorption, and a low-fat diet are effective treatments for oxaluria secondary to intestinal absorption. Calcium lactate, 8 to 14 g per day, which acts by precipitating oxalate in the gut lumen is an alternative form of therapy. Both treatments require additional study to assess their effectiveness. There is no effective treatment for hereditary hyperoxaluria, a disorder characterized by an enzymatic defect involving the metabolism of the precursor of oxalate and transmitted as an autosomal recessive. A high fluid intake, phosphate, and pyridoxine (200 mg per day) are recommended, but irreversible renal failure secondary to recurrent stone formation usually occurs before the age of 20 years.

Idiopathic calcium lithiasis At least 20 percent of patients have no obvious cause for stones (Table 229-1). The best treatment for them appears to be a high fluid intake, so that the urine specific gravity remains below approximately 1.005 throughout the day and night. Oral phosphate at a dose of 2 g phosphorus daily may lower urine calcium and increases urine pyrophosphate excretion, and thereby may bring about a reduction in the rate of recurrence of stones. Orthophosphate causes mild nausea and diarrhea initially, but tolerance may improve with continued intake. Thiazide treatment to reduce calcium excretion and allopurinol to diminish uric acid output may also be helpful. There are no adequate studies to support the use of supplemental magnesium, pyridoxine, or methylene blue, commonly mentioned remedies.

URIC ACID STONES These stones form because the urine becomes supersaturated with undissociated uric acid, uric acid that is protonated at its N-9 position. This proton has a p*K* of 5.35 in urine. In gout, idiopathic uric acid lithiasis, and dehydration, the average pH is abnormally low, usually below 5.4, and often below 5.0. Undissociated uric acid therefore predominates, and can dissolve in urine in concentrations of only 100 mg per liter. Concentrations above this level represent supersaturation that causes crystals and stones to form. Hyperuricosuria, when present, increases supersaturation; but urine of low pH can be excessively supersaturated with undissociated uric acid even though the daily excretion rate is normal. Myeloproliferative syndromes, chemotherapeutic treatment of malignant tumors, and the Lesch-Nyhan syndrome cause such massive production of uric acid and consequent hyperuricosuria that stones and uric acid sludge occur even at a normal urine pH. The renal collecting tubules can be plugged by uric acid crystals with consequent acute renal failure.

The two goals of treatment are to raise urine pH and to lower urine uric acid excretion when it is very high, i.e., above 1000 mg per day. Supplemental alkali, 1 to 3 meq/kg per day, should be given in three or four evenly spaced divided doses, one of which should be reserved for bedtime. The form of the alkali may be important. Potassium citrate may reduce the risk of calcium salts crystallizing when urine pH is increased, whereas sodium citrate or sodium bicarbonate may increase the risk. If the overnight urine pH is below 5.5, the evening dose of bicarbonate may be raised, or 250 mg acetazolamide added at bedtime. With massive overexcretion of uric acid, high doses of allopurinol, exceeding 300 mg daily, may be needed. Treatment with allopurinol should be instituted before chemotherapy of highly cellular tumors, since massive hyperuricosuria can be expected. Alkali treatment must be avoided if hypercalciuria is also present.

TABLE 229-2 Classification of cystinuria

	Type I	Type II	Type III
Intestinal transport:			
Cystine	0	↓↓	N—↓
Lysine	0	0	↓
Arginine	0	–	–
Urine excretion in heterozygotes:			
Cystine	N	↑	↑
Lysine	N	↑	↑

NOTE: ↑ = *increased;* ↓ = *reduced;* ↓↓ = *very reduced; 0 = absent transport; N = normal urinary excretion rates;* – = *not known.*

CYSTINURIA AND CYSTINE STONES (See also Chap. 308) Proximal tubular and jejunal transport of cystine and the other dibasic amino acids, lysine, arginine, and ornithine, are defective, and excessive amounts are lost in the urine. Clinical disease is due solely to the insolubility of cystine, which forms stones. Patients are short, probably because of a linked inherited tendency rather than amino acid losses. Cystinuria is transmitted as an autosomal recessive trait whose prevalence in newborns is 1 in 7000.

Pathogenesis The weight of available evidence indicates that cystinuria occurs because of defective transport of amino acids by the brush borders of renal tubule and intestinal epithelial cells. Cystine, lysine, arginine, and ornithine appear to share a common renal transport pathway, because infusion of lysine decreases tubular reabsorption of the other three. But cystine also seems to be transported by a separate transport mechanism, because cystinuria and dibasic aminoaciduria can each occur independently. The inheritance of the brush border transport defects is complex. The intestinal defects are not similar in all patients who are homozygous for cystinuria, and the extent of aminoaciduria in those relatives of cystinuric patients who are heterozygous carriers of the defect, for example, their siblings, varies from family to family. Thus far three types of inheritance have been described (Table 229-2).

Diagnosis and treatment Cystine stones are formed only by patients with cystinuria, but 10 percent of stones formed by cystinuric patients do not contain cystine; therefore, every stone former should be screened for the disease. The sediment from a first morning urine specimen in many patients with homozygous cystinuria reveals typical flat hexagonal platelike cystine crystals. Cystinuria can also be detected using the sodium nitroprusside test on a urine sample. The test gives a positive response to 75 to 125 mg cystine per gram of creatinine, a concentration lower than that found in the urine of patients with homozygous cystinuria but well above the levels encountered in normal urine. Because the test is sensitive, it will be positive in many individuals who are heterozygous for cystinuria, most of whom do not form cystine stones (Table 229-2). A positive nitroprusside test or the finding of cystine crystals in the urine sediment should be evaluated by measurement of daily cystine excretion. Normal adults excrete 40 to 60 mg per gram of creatinine; heterozygotes usually excrete less than 300 mg/g; and patients with homozygous cystinuria almost always excrete above 250 mg/g.

Treatment consists of a high fluid intake, even at night. Daily urine volume should exceed 3 liters. Raising urine pH with alkali is helpful, provided the resulting daily urine pH exceeds 7.5. Because drug side effects are frequent, D-penicillamine, which forms the soluble mixed disulfide cysteine-penicillamine, should be used only when fluid loading and alkali therapy have been ineffective. *N*-Acetyl-D-penicillamine has a similar mode of action and may have fewer side effects, but is not available for routine use. Mercaptopropinylglycine has been used to dissolve renal calculi by perfusion of the renal pelvis and has been given by mouth to prevent stones, but also is experimental. Low-methionine diets have not proved to be practical for clinical use.

STRUVITE STONES These stones are always a result of urinary infection with bacteria, usually *Proteus* species, which possess urease, an enzyme that degrades urea to NH_3 and CO_2. The NH_3 hydrolyzes to NH_4^+ and raises pH, usually to 8 or 9. The CO_2 hydrates to H_2CO_3 and then dissociates to CO_3^{2-} which precipitates with calcium as $CaCO_3$. The NH_4^+ precipitates PO_4^{3-} and Mg^{2+} to form the triple salt $MgNH_4PO_4$. The result is a stone of calcium carbonate admixed with struvite. It is impossible to form struvite in urine without infection, because NH_4^+ concentration is very low in urine that is alkaline in response to physiologic stimuli. Chronic *Proteus* infection can occur because of impaired urinary drainage, infection of retained stones of any type, urologic instrumentation or surgery, and especially chronic antibiotic treatment, which can favor the emergence of *Proteus* as the predominant urinary tract flora.

Treatment Mandelamine, which lowers urine pH and liberates formaldehyde, is used for chronic suppression of infection when a stone is present. More extreme lowering of urine pH with chronic administration of NH_4Cl may retard stone growth but may also raise urine calcium level and promote the formation of calcium oxalate stones. Antimicrobial treatment is best reserved for dealing with acute exacerbation of infection and for maintenance of a sterile urine after surgery, in the hope of preventing recurrence or minimizing stone growth. Surgery should be reserved for severe obstruction, intractable pain, bleeding, or serious manifestations of urinary infection. Since stones can regrow from any infected fragment which is left behind, recurrences following operation are quite common. In some centers, it is possible to irrigate the renal pelvis and calyces with Renacidin, a solution that dissolves struvite, using a catheter passed through a cutaneous flank incision into the kidney.

REFERENCES

COE FL: Nephrolithiasis: Pathogenesis and treatment. Chicago, Year Book, 1978

——— et al: Effect of low calcium diet on urine calcium excretion, parathyroid function, and serum 1,25(OH)$_2$D$_3$ levels in patients with idiopathic hypercalciuria and in normal subjects. Am J Med 72:25, 1982

FLEISCH H et al (eds): *Urolithiasis Research.* New York, Plenum, 1976

———, FAVUS MJ: Disorders of stone formation, in *The Kidney,* 3d ed, BM Brenner, FC Rector Jr (eds). Philadelphia, Saunders, 1986, p 1403

GRANTHAM JR et al: Renal stone disease treated with extracorporeal shock wave lithotripsy: Short-term observations in 100 patients. Radiology 158:203, 1986

NAKAGAWA Y et al: Purification and characterization of the principal inhibitors of calcium oxalate monohydrate crystal growth in human urine. J Biol Chem 258:12594, 1983

PAK CYC (ed): Urolithiasis. Kidney Int 13:341, 1978

———: Kidney stones, in *Williams' Textbook of Endocrinology,* 7th ed, JD Wilson, DW Foster (eds). Philadelphia, Saunders, 1985, p 1256

STRAUSS AL et al: Factors that predict relapse of calcium nephrolithiasis during treatment. Am J Med 72:25, 1982

WEBB DR et al: Extracorporeal shockwave lithotripsy, endourology and open surgery: The management and follow-up of 200 patients with urinary calculi. Ann R Coll Surg Engl 67:337, 1985

230 URINARY TRACT OBSTRUCTION

BARRY M. BRENNER / EDGAR L. MILFORD / JULIAN L. SEIFTER

Obstruction to the flow of urine, with attendant stasis and elevation in urinary tract pressure, impairs renal and urinary conduit functions and represents a common cause of acute and chronic renal failure. With early relief of obstruction, these defects in function usually disappear completely. However, chronic obstruction may produce profound and permanent loss of renal mass (renal atrophy) and excretory capability, as well as enhanced susceptibility to local infection and stone formation. Early and accurate diagnosis and prompt and appropriate therapy are, therefore, essential to minimize the otherwise devastating effects of obstruction on urinary tract structure and function.

ETIOLOGY Obstruction to urine flow can result from *intrinsic* or *extrinsic mechanical blockade* as well as from *functional defects* not associated with fixed occlusion of the urinary drainage system. Lesions causing mechanical obstruction can occur at any level of the urinary tract, from the renal calyces to the external urethral meatus. Normal points of narrowing, such as the ureteropelvic and ureterovesical junctions, bladder neck, and urethral meatus, are common sites of obstruction. When blockage is above the level of the bladder, unilateral dilatation of the ureter (*hydroureter*) and renal pyelocalyceal system (*hydronephrosis*) occur; when the lesion is at or below the level of the bladder, bilateral involvement is the rule.

Common forms of obstruction are listed in Table 230-1. In childhood, *congenital malformations,* including marked narrowing of the ureteropelvic junction, anomalous (retrocaval) location of the ureter, and posterior urethral valves predominate. The latter defect is the most common cause of bilateral hydronephrosis in the male child. Children may also have bladder dysfunction secondary to congenital urethral stricture, urethral meatal stenosis, or bladder neck obstruction. In adults, urinary tract obstruction is due mainly to *acquired defects.* Pelvic tumors, calculi, and urethral stricture predominate. Ligation of, or injury to, the ureter during pelvic or colonic surgery can lead to hydronephrosis which, if unilateral, may remain relatively silent and undetected. Obstructive uropathy may also result from extrinsic neoplastic (carcinoma of cervix or colon, retroperitoneal lymphoma) or inflammatory disorders. One such inflammatory disorder is retroperitoneal fibrosis, a process of unknown cause seen most commonly in middle-aged males, which occasionally leads to bilateral ureteral obstruction. Occurring in some patients taking methysergide for relief of migraine, retroperitoneal fibrosis must be distinguished from other retroperitoneal causes of ureteral obstruction, particularly lymphomas and pelvic neoplasms.

Functional impairment of urine flow usually results from disorders which involve both the ureter and bladder. Common functional lesions include neurogenic bladder, often with adynamic ureter, and vesicoureteral reflux. Reflux of urine from bladder to ureter(s) is more common in children than adults and may result in severe unilateral or bilateral hydroureter and hydronephrosis. Abnormal insertion of the ureter into the bladder is the most common cause of vesicoureteral reflux in children. Reflux occurring in the absence of urinary tract infection or bladder neck obstruction usually does not lead to renal parenchymal damage and often resolves spontaneously as the child matures. Surgical reinsertion of the ureter into the bladder is indicated if reflux is severe and unlikely to improve spontaneously, if renal function deteriorates, or if urinary tract infections recur despite chronic antimicrobial therapy.

TABLE 230-1 Common mechanical causes of urinary tract obstruction

Ureter	Bladder outlet	Urethra
CONGENITAL		
Ureteropelvic junction narrowing or obstruction Ureterovesical junction narrowing or obstruction Ureterocele Retrocaval ureter	Bladder neck obstruction Ureterocele	Posterior urethral valves Anterior urethral valves Stricture Meatal stenosis Phimosis
ACQUIRED INTRINSIC DEFECTS		
Calculi Inflammation Trauma Sloughed papillae Tumor Blood clots Uric acid crystals	Benign prostatic hypertrophy Cancer of prostate Cancer of bladder Calculi Diabetic neuropathy Spinal cord disease	Stricture Tumor Calculi Trauma Phimosis
ACQUIRED EXTRINSIC DEFECTS		
Pregnant uterus Retroperitoneal fibrosis Aortic aneurysm Uterine leiomyomata Carcinoma of uterus, prostate, bladder, colon, rectum Retroperitoneal lymphoma Accidental surgical ligation	Carcinoma of cervix, colon Trauma	Trauma

CLINICAL FEATURES The pathophysiology and clinical features of urinary tract obstruction are summarized in Table 230-2. Pain is the symptom which most commonly provokes the need for medical attention. The pain of urinary tract obstruction is due to distention of the collecting system or renal capsule. The severity of the pain is influenced more by the rate at which distention develops than the degree of distention. Acute supravesical obstruction, as from a stone lodged in a ureter (Chap. 229), is associated with excruciatingly severe pain, usually called *renal colic*. This pain is relatively steady and continuous, with little fluctuation in intensity, and often radiates to the lower abdomen, testes, or labia. By contrast, more insidious causes of obstruction, such as chronic narrowing of the ureteropelvic junction, may produce little or no pain, yet result in total destruction of the affected kidney. Flank pain which comes on only with micturition is pathognomonic of vesicoureteral reflux.

Azotemia develops in urinary tract obstruction when overall excretory function is impaired. This may occur in the setting of bladder outlet obstruction, bilateral renal pelvic or ureteric obstruction, or unilateral disease in a patient with a solitary functioning kidney. Complete bilateral obstruction should be suspected when acute renal failure is accompanied by anuria. Any patient with renal failure otherwise unexplained or with a history of nephrolithiasis, hematuria, prostatic enlargement, pelvic surgery, trauma, or tumor should be evaluated for urinary tract obstruction.

Symptoms of *polyuria* and *nocturia* commonly accompany chronic partial urinary tract obstruction and result from impaired renal concentrating ability. This defect usually does not improve with administration of exogenous vasopressin and is therefore a form of acquired nephrogenic diabetes insipidus. Disturbances in sodium chloride transport in the ascending limb of Henle and, in azotemic patients, the osmotic (urea) diuresis per nephron lead to decreased medullary hypertonicity and, hence, a concentrating defect. Partial obstruction, therefore, may be associated with increased rather than decreased urine output. Indeed, wide fluctuations in urinary output in a patient with azotemia should always raise the possibility of intermittent or partial urinary tract obstruction. If fluid intake becomes inadequate in these patients, severe dehydration and hypernatremia may develop. Hesitancy and straining to initiate the urinary stream, postvoid dribbling, urinary frequency, and (overflow) incontinence are complaints common to patients with obstruction at or below the level of the bladder (see Chap. 40).

TABLE 230-2 Pathophysiology of bilateral ureteral obstruction

Hemodynamic effects	Tubule effects	Clinical features
ACUTE		
↑ Renal blood flow ↓ GFR ↓ Medullary blood flow ↑ Vasodilator prostaglandins	↑ Ureteral and tubule pressures ↑ Reabsorption of Na^+, urea, water	Pain (capsule distention) Azotemia Oliguria
CHRONIC		
↓ Renal blood flow ↓ ↓ GFR ↑ Vasoconstrictor prostaglandins ↑ Renin-angiotensin production	↓ Medullary osmolarity ↓ Concentrating ability Structural damage ↓ Transport functions for Na^+, K^+, H^+	Azotemia Hypertension ADH-insensitive polyuria Natriuresis Hyperkalemic, hyperchloremic acidosis
RELEASE OF OBSTRUCTION		
Slow ↑ in GFR (variable)	↓ Tubule pressure ↑ Solute load per nephron (urea, NaCl) Natriuretic factors present	Postobstructive diuresis Potential for volume depletion and electrolyte imbalance (Na^+, K^+, PO_4^{2-}, Mg^{2+})

In addition to loss of urinary concentrating ability and azotemia, partial bilateral urinary tract obstruction often results in other derangements of renal function, including *acquired distal renal tubular acidosis, hyperkalemia,* and *renal salt wasting*. These defects in tubule function are often accompanied by histologic evidence of widespread renal tubulointerstitial damage. Morphologic abnormalities appear early in the course of obstruction; initially the interstitium becomes edematous and infiltrated with mononuclear inflammatory cells. With continued obstruction, the interstitium becomes fibrotic; scarring and atrophy of the papillae and medulla occur and precede these processes in the cortex.

The possibility of urinary tract obstruction must always be considered in patients with urinary tract infections or urolithiasis. Urinary stasis encourages the growth of organisms as well as the formation of crystals, especially magnesium ammonium phosphate (struvite). *Hypertension* is seen frequently in acute and subacute forms of unilateral obstruction and is usually a consequence of increased release of renin by the involved kidney. Chronic unilateral or bilateral hydronephrosis, in the presence of extracellular volume expansion or other forms of renal disease, may result in significant hypertension. *Polycythemia,* an infrequent complication of obstructive uropathy, is probably secondary to increased erythropoietin production by the obstructed kidney.

DIAGNOSIS A history of difficulty in voiding, pain, infection, or changes in urinary volume is common. Evidence for distention of the kidney or urinary bladder often can be obtained by palpation and percussion of the abdomen. A careful rectal examination may reveal enlargement or nodularity of the prostate, abnormal rectal sphincter tone, or a rectal or pelvic mass. The penis should be inspected for evidence of meatal stenosis or phimosis. In the female, vaginal, uterine, and rectal lesions responsible for urinary tract obstruction are usually revealed by inspection and palpation.

Urinalysis and examination of the urine sediment may reveal hematuria, pyuria, and bacteriuria. Often, however, the urine sediment is devoid of abnormal elements, even when obstruction leads to marked azotemia and extensive structural damage. An abdominal scout film should be obtained to evaluate the possibility of nephrocalcinosis or a radiopaque stone at any level of the urinary collecting system. As indicated in Fig. 230-1 if urinary tract obstruction is suspected, abdominal ultrasonography should be performed to evaluate renal and bladder size, as well as pyelocalyceal and ureteral contours. If distention of these structures is absent, functionally significant urinary tract obstruction can safely be excluded in differential diagnosis. Abdominal ultrasound may also detect an obstructing pelvic mass.

Intravenous pyelography is frequently employed if an obstructive abnormality is revealed by ultrasound. If the patient is not azotemic, a standard dose of contrast medium usually provides adequate information. With renal insufficiency, however, high-dose (drip-infusion) pyelography with nephrotomography is usually required for adequate visualization. In the presence of obstruction, the appearance time of the nephrogram is often delayed but eventually becomes more dense than normal because of slow tubular fluid flow rate which results in enhanced water reabsorption by the nephrons and greater concentration of contrast medium within tubules. The kidney involved by an acute obstructive process is usually slightly enlarged, and there is dilatation of the calyces, renal pelvis, and ureter above the obstruction. The ureter, however, is not tortuous, as is the case when the obstruction is chronic. In comparison with the nephrogram, the pyelogram may be extremely faint, especially if the dilated renal pelvis is voluminous, causing dilution of the contrast medium. The radiographic study should be continued until the site of obstruction is determined or the contrast medium is excreted. Delayed films taken as long as 48 h after contrast administration may be necessary to determine the exact site of obstruction.

Patients suspected of having intermittent ureteropelvic obstruction (whether functional or mechanical) should have radiologic evaluation while they are in pain, since a normal pyelogram is commonly seen during asymptomatic periods. Hydration or mannitol infusion often helps to provoke a symptomatic attack. Voiding cystourethrography is of great value in the diagnosis of vesicoureteral reflux and bladder neck and urethral obstructions. Patients with obstruction at or below the level of the bladder exhibit thickening, trabeculation, and diverticula of the bladder wall. Postvoiding films reveal residual urine. If these radiographic studies fail to provide adequate information for diagnosis, endoscopic visualization by the urologist often permits precise identification of lesions involving the urethra, prostate, bladder, and ureteral orifices. To facilitate visualization of a suspected lesion in a ureter or renal pelvis, *retrograde* or *antegrade pyelography* should be attempted. These diagnostic studies may be preferable to the intravenous pyelogram in the azotemic patient in whom poor excretory function precludes adequate visualization of the collecting system. Furthermore, intravenous pyelography carries the risk of contrast-induced renal failure in some patients with renal insufficiency, diabetes mellitus, and multiple myeloma, particularly when performed under conditions of dehydration. For these reasons retrograde and antegrade pyelography may offer advantages over the intravenous approach in the diagnostic evaluation of the azotemic patient. The retrograde approach involves catheterization of the involved ureter under cystoscopic control, while the antegrade technique necessitates placement of a catheter into the renal pelvis via a needle inserted percutaneously under ultrasonic or fluoroscopic guidance. While the antegrade approach carries the added advantage of providing immediate and certain decompression of a unilateral obstructing lesion, many urologists initially attempt the retrograde approach and resort to the antegrade method only when attempts at retrograde catheterization have been unsuccessful or when cystoscopy or general anesthesia is contraindicated.

TREATMENT AND PROGNOSIS An individual with any form of urinary tract obstruction complicated by infection requires relief of obstruction as soon as possible to prevent development of generalized sepsis and progressive renal damage. On a temporary basis, depending on the site of obstruction, drainage is often satisfactorily achieved by nephrostomy, ureterostomy, or ureteral, urethral, or suprapubic catheterization. When infection is not present, immediate surgery often is not required, even in the presence of complete obstruction and anuria (because of the availability of dialysis), at least until acid-base, fluid and electrolyte, and cardiovascular status have been restored to normal. Nevertheless, the site of obstruction should be ascertained as soon as feasible, in part because of the possibility that sepsis may occur and necessitate prompt urologic intervention. Elective relief of obstruction is usually recommended in patients with urinary retention, recurrent urinary tract infections, persistent pain, or progressive loss of renal function. Infrequently, mechanical obstruction can be alleviated by nonsurgical means, as with radiation therapy for retroperitoneal lymphoma. Likewise, functional obstruction secondary to neurogenic bladder may be decreased with the combination of frequent voiding and cholinergic drugs. The approach to obstruction secondary to renal stones is discussed in Chap. 229.

FIGURE 230-1 *Diagnostic approach for urinary tract obstruction in unexplained renal failure. Circles represent diagnostic procedures and squares indicate clinical decisions based on available data (CT, computerized tomography; IVP, intravenous pyelogram).*

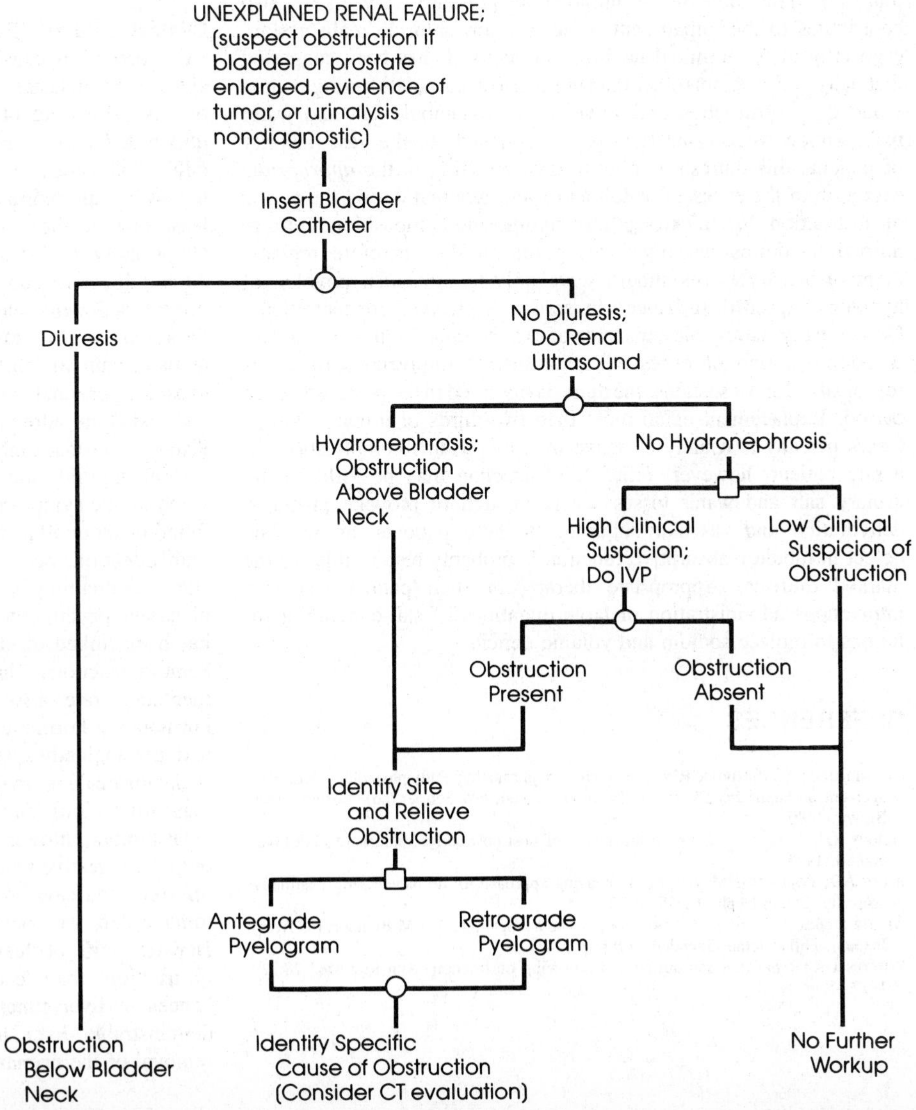

With relief of obstruction, the *prognosis* regarding return of renal function depends largely upon whether irreversible renal damage has occurred. When obstruction is not relieved, the patient's course will depend mainly on whether the obstruction is complete or incomplete, bilateral or unilateral, and whether urinary tract infection is also present. Complete obstruction with infection can lead to total destruction of the kidney within days. Experimental studies in dogs suggest that relief of complete obstruction of 1 and 2 weeks' duration restores glomerular filtration rate to 60 and 30 percent of normal, respectively; after 8 weeks, recovery does not occur. Nevertheless, in the absence of definitive evidence of irreversibility, every effort should be made to facilitate decompression in the hope of restoring renal function at least partially.

In patients undergoing cystectomy for bladder cancer, the ileal conduit is the currently preferred urinary diversionary procedure. In benign disease a sigmoid conduit may result in less ureteral reflux and secondary chronic renal insufficiency. These approaches are preferable to ureterosigmoidostomy, a procedure complicated by a high incidence of ureteral obstruction, reflux, hypokalemic metabolic acidosis, pyelonephritis, and neoplasms developing at the ureteral anastomotic site.

POSTOBSTRUCTIVE DIURESIS Relief of bilateral, but not unilateral, complete urinary tract obstruction commonly leads to a postobstructive diuresis, characterized by polyuria, which may be massive. The urine is usually hypotonic and may contain a large amount of sodium chloride. The natriuresis is due, at least in part, to the excretion of retained urea, which acts as a poorly reabsorbable solute and diminishes salt and water reabsorption in the tubules (osmotic diuresis). The increase in intratubular pressure very likely also contributes to the impairment in net sodium chloride reabsorption, especially in the terminal nephron segments. It has been suggested that natriuretic factors (other than urea) also accumulate during uremia induced by obstruction and serve to depress tubule salt and water reabsorption when urine flow is reestablished. In the vast majority of patients this diuresis is physiologic, resulting in the *appropriate* excretion of the excesses of salt and water retained during the period of obstruction. When extracellular volume and composition return to normal, the diuresis usually abates spontaneously. Therefore, replacement of urinary losses should serve only to prevent hypovolemia, hypotension, or disturbances in serum electrolyte concentrations. Occasionally, iatrogenic expansion of extracellular volume, secondary to administration of excessive quantities of intravenous fluids, is responsible for, or sustains, the diuresis observed in the postobstructive period. Replacement of no more than two-thirds of urinary volume losses per day is usually effective in avoiding this complication. In a rare patient, however, relief of obstruction may be followed by urinary salt and water losses severe enough to provoke profound dehydration and vascular collapse. In these patients, an intrinsic defect in tubule reabsorptive function is probably responsible for the marked diuresis. Appropriate therapy in such patients includes intravenous administration of large quantities of salt-containing solutions to replace sodium and volume deficits.

REFERENCES

GUGGENHEIM SJ, SCHRIER RW: Obstructive nephropathy: Pathophysiology and management, in *Renal and Electrolyte Disorders,* 2d ed, RW Schrier (ed). Boston, Little, Brown, 1980

HARRIS RH, YARGER WE: The pathogenesis of post-obstructive diuresis. J Clin Invest 56:880, 1975

KAYE AD, POLLACK HM: Diagnostic imaging approach to the patient with obstructive uropathy. Semin Nephrol 2:55, 1982

KLAHR S et al: Urinary tract obstruction, in *The Kidney,* 3d ed, BM Brenner, FC Rector Jr (eds). Philadelphia, Saunders, 1986, p 1443

WILSON DR: Renal function during and following obstruction. Ann Rev Med 28:329, 1977

231 TUMORS OF THE URINARY TRACT

MARC B. GARNICK / BARRY M. BRENNER

TUMORS OF THE KIDNEY

RENAL CELL CARCINOMA Renal cell carcinoma (renal adenocarcinoma—formerly "hypernephroma") accounts for 85 percent of all primary renal neoplasms. Approximately 18,000 new cases are diagnosed annually with 8000 deaths in the United States. The peak age incidence is between 55 and 60 years; the male-to-female ratio is 2:1. Environmental risk factors include exposure to cigarette smoke and cadmium. Genetically transmitted forms of renal cell carcinoma, which are commonly multifocal and bilateral, occur in a high proportion of patients with von Hippel–Lindau disease (retinal and central nervous system hemangiomas, autosomal dominant transmission). Marker chromosomal translocations between chromosomes 3 and 8 and 3 and 11 have been found in several kindreds with familial renal cancer. Patients with end-stage renal disease on chronic dialysis may develop renal cystic disease and associated renal carcinomas. Using electron-microscopic and immunologic techniques, renal cell carcinoma has been shown to arise from the proximal convoluted tubular epithelium. The term "hypernephroma" for renal cell carcinoma (reflecting the previously held notion of cellular origin from adrenal "rests") should be abandoned.

Clinical features Renal cell carcinoma has been called the "internist's tumor" because the lesion is often diagnosed, even in the absence of metastases, by its *systemic* rather than urologic manifestations. The triad of *gross hematuria, flank pain,* and a *palpable abdominal mass,* although considered as classic evidence for the clinical diagnosis, is encountered in less than 10 percent of cases; however, approximately one-third of patients will demonstrate at least one of these manifestations. The most common presenting abnormality is *hematuria,* which occurs in 60 percent of cases. Although microscopic hematuria is a consistent abnormality of the urinary sediment, bleeding is not usually evident grossly, allowing the tumor to grow to a large size before clinical manifestations such as flank pain and fullness appear. Contiguous extension to the renal capsule, perirenal fat, lymph nodes, renal vein, inferior vena cava, and ipsilateral adrenal gland is common. The most common sites of distant metastases include lung, mediastinum, bone, central nervous system, thyroid, and liver.

Systemic symptoms of fatigability, weight loss, and cachexia are found in about 50 percent of patients. Intermittent fever, unassociated with infection, occurs occasionally and may be the only presenting sign. Anemia may be present at the onset in approximately 50 percent of cases. Erythrocytosis is seen in about 5 percent of patients and has been linked to elaboration of erythropoietin. Eosinophilia, leukemoid reactions, thrombocytosis, and increased erythrocyte sedimentation rate also occur. Renal cell carcinomas may produce hormones or hormone-like substances, including parathyroid hormone and prostaglandins (which may lead to hypercalcemia), prolactin (galactorrhea), renin (hypertension), gonadotropins (feminization and masculinization), and glucocorticoids (Cushing's syndrome). In vascular tumors, intrarenal arteriovenous fistulas may predispose to high-output congestive heart failure. Tumor invasion of the renal vein and inferior vena cava may result in the development of abrupt, symptomatic left varicocele and lower extremity edema, respectively. Hepatic vein occlusion by tumor, with or without vena caval obstruction, may lead to hepatosplenomegaly and ascites. Disturbances in liver function are sometimes found in patients without demonstrable liver metastases and are often reversed following removal of the primary tumor.

Diagnosis (see Fig. 231-1) Although intrarenal calcifications and/or alterations in renal contours seen on the abdominal scout film may suggest the presence of a renal cell carcinoma, *intravenous pyelography* (IVP) with *nephrotomography* is the primary examination by which most renal masses are detected and evaluated. The major task is to differentiate cystic lesions from renal neoplasms. Splaying, distortion or nonvisualization of the collecting system, and distorted renal outlines suggest cancer. Nephrotomography provides clear delineation of renal borders and further aids in distinguishing cystic from solid lesions. *Ultrasonography* has greatly improved the ability to distinguish simple sonographic cysts from renal neoplasms. When combined with nephrotomography, the accuracy of ultrasonography in diagnosing a benign cyst approaches 97 percent. If a cystic lesion on IVP, combined with a benign-appearing sonolucent cystic lesion on ultrasound, is found in an asymptomatic patient without hematuria, cyst puncture is probably unnecessary. Repeat IVP or ultrasound should then be performed periodically.

If diagnostic accuracy beyond 97 percent is required or if there are changes on repeat IVP or ultrasound, needle aspiration with evaluation of the aspirated fluid for cytology can be performed. A renal cystogram following aspiration can provide additional valuable information. Although renal cell carcinoma may coexist within a simple cyst, this is a rare occurrence.

If the IVP or ultrasound examination demonstrates a lesion which does not satisfy the criteria for a benign, simple cyst, *computerized tomography* (CT) is the next modality employed. CT is comparable and possibly superior to selective renal arteriography in both diagnosing and staging renal cell carcinoma. In addition, CT is equivalent to selective renal arteriography in the determination of renal vein involvement and superior to arteriography in determining whether regional nodes are enlarged (representing either tumor or hyperplasia) and/or the liver is involved. CT is the preferred modality for the diagnosis and staging of renal cell carcinoma. If, however, the findings on CT are equivocal or additional definition of vascular anatomy is required, renal arteriography should complement CT studies.

OTHER STUDIES Evaluation of urinary cytology is not useful in the diagnosis of renal adenocarcinomas. Retrograde pyelography may be a useful adjunct for opacifying the collecting systems that are not filled by standard IVP and may suggest the diagnosis of transitional cell carcinoma of the renal pelvis. In patients who present with hematuria and a renal mass, cystoscopy is an important adjunct to exclude the coexistence of an unsuspected urothelial tumor, such as carcinoma of the bladder.

If the diagnosis of renal cell carcinoma is considered likely, the patient should then undergo routine chest x-ray, bone scan, and liver function studies, in addition to the abdominal CT, to evaluate other potential sites of tumor spread.

Staging, primary treatment, and prognosis If there is no evidence of metastatic disease following the preoperative evaluation, the treatment of choice for renal cell carcinoma is radical nephrectomy. In addition to en bloc removal of the kidney with the surrounding Gerota's fascia, many urologic surgeons advocate regional lymphadenectomy to help determine prognosis. Preoperative arterial embolization of the main renal artery with a variety of agents may help to simplify the operative approach for large lesions. There is no role for localized pre- or postoperative radiation therapy.

Following surgical and pathologic evaluation, renal cell cancers are staged as follows: stage I, tumor confined within the kidney

FIGURE 231-1 *Diagnostic evaluation for renal mass.*

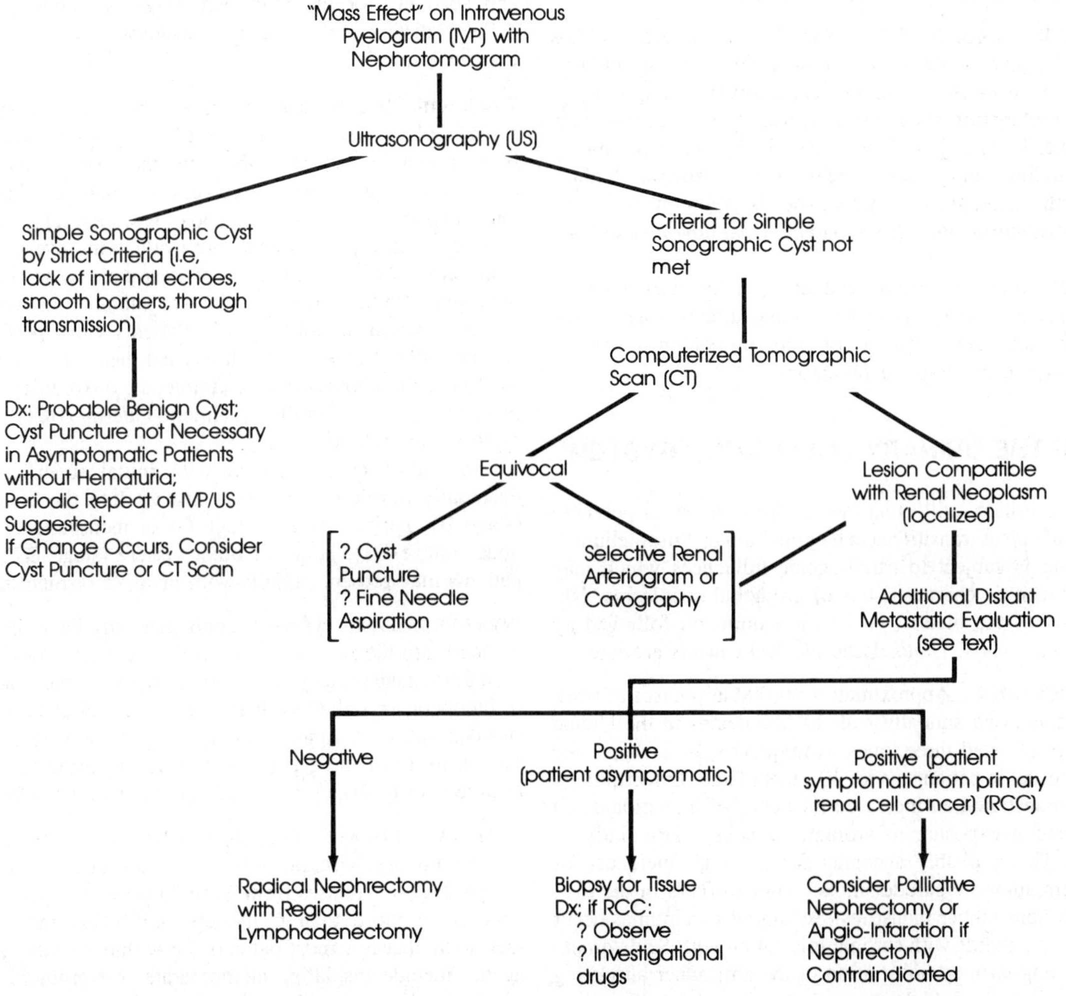

capsule; stage II, invasion through the renal capsule but confined within Gerota's fascia; stage III, involvement of regional lymph nodes, ipsilateral renal vein, or vena cava; stage IV, distant metastases. Five-year survival rates for stage I range from 60 to 75 percent; for stage II, 47 to 65 percent; for stage III without regional lymph node involvement, 25 to 50 percent; with regional lymph node involvement, 5 to 15 percent; for stage IV, less than 5 percent.

Systemic therapy for metastatic disease There is no standard chemotherapeutic, hormonal, or immunologic program for patients with metastatic renal cancer. Although early reports demonstrated a favorable effect using progestational or androgenic agents, there seems to be very little role for hormonal therapy of renal cell carcinoma. Commonly employed chemotherapy programs include the use of vinblastine sulfate, with or without the use of nitrosoureas. Interferons have been used with limited success. The systemic management of patients with renal adenocarcinoma remains investigational, and entry of patients into phase II clinical trials is encouraged.

Selected surgical management of patients with metastatic disease There is little wisdom in hoping for spontaneous regression of metastases by removing the kidney of a patient who presents with stage IV renal cell carcinoma who is otherwise asymptomatic. If, however, the primary lesion is associated with pain, bleeding, or other paraneoplastic phenomena, it is sometimes useful to remove the primary tumor or consider angioinfarction for local therapy despite the presence of metastatic disease. In patients who have had renal cell cancer in the past who then present with an isolated pulmonary or central nervous system metastasis, it is often useful to surgically resect these metastases. Generally, patients selected for surgical nodulectomy have been disease-free for at least 1 year from the original diagnosis to the time of metastatic development and have tumors which demonstrate a slow doubling time.

MISCELLANEOUS TUMORS OF THE KIDNEY In children, Wilms tumor (nephroblastoma) is the most common cancer of the kidney. These tumors respond well to multimodality therapy including surgery, radiation, and combination chemotherapy, usually with actinomycin D and vincristine. Metastatic lesions to the kidney occur commonly in patients with lung and breast cancer, and melanoma. Kidney involvement with malignant lymphoma, too, is common; however, functional renal abnormalities from parenchymal involvement are unusual.

Benign renal tumors do occur and are usually recognized as incidental findings at autopsy. In newborns and infants, mesoblastic nephroma (fetal hamartoma) is the most common benign tumor and is successfully treated by simple nephrectomy.

TUMORS OF THE URINARY COLLECTING SYSTEM

The lining of the urinary collecting system from the renal pelvis to the urethra is made up of transitional cell epithelium or "urothelium." This entire lining is subject to carcinogenic influences which may explain the multicentric characteristics of urothelial neoplasms. Numerically, cancer of the bladder is the most common followed by tumors of the renal pelvis. Ureteral and urethral cancers are rare.

BLADDER CARCINOMA Approximately 40,000 new cases of bladder cancer are diagnosed annually with 11,000 deaths in the United States. Males are affected three times as frequently as females, and the disease is unusual in patients under 40 years of age. Epidemiology studies have demonstrated an increased incidence of transitional cell carcinoma following exposure to aromatic amines, particularly 2-naphthylamine. This probably accounts for the high incidence of urothelial cancers among cigarette smokers and workers in the dye, chemical, and certain rubber industries. Squamous carcinomas occur more frequently in patients with chronic infestation with *Schistosoma haematobium*. Long-term administration of the anticancer alkylating agent cyclophosphamide, which is metabolized to the active compounds acrolein and phosphoramide mustard, has been associated with the development of urothelial neoplasms.

Clinical features While gross and microscopic hematuria are the most common presenting complaints, other features include dysuria, urinary frequency, or urgency, which may be the only manifestations of bladder carcinoma, and the persistence of these symptoms in a previously asymptomatic patient deserves careful attention. Other manifestations, such as ureteral obstruction, pelvic pain, or symptoms from visceral or osseous metastases, occur in a minority of patients at presentation.

Diagnosis and staging Urinary cytology, obtained by bladder washing, catheterized or voided urine, IVP, and cystoscopic evaluation with tumor biopsies and selected mucosal biopsies, as well as bimanual examination under anesthesia, have been the mainstays for diagnosis of bladder cancer. Findings on IVP which suggest a bladder carcinoma include unilateral or bilateral ureteral obstruction with hydronephrosis, filling defect, or lack of distensibility of the bladder. Additional staging information may be obtained with abdominal or pelvic CT scanning. Following endoscopic resection of a bladder neoplasm, the depth of penetration into the bladder wall is assessed. If additional staging workup, including physical examination, chest x-ray, and routine serum chemistries, are within normal limits, the patient is clinically staged, based upon the cystoscopic biopsy, as having either *superficial* or *invasive* disease. Additional information about perivesical extension or nodal metastases can be obtained at the time of cystectomy and indicates the true pathologic stage of disease. A substantial number of patients who are clinically staged endoscopically as having muscle-invasive disease will have occult lymphatic or distant metastases if pathologically staged at the time of cystectomy. Such occult micrometastatic disease indicates systemic involvement and accounts for the high percentage of patients who eventually develop distant metastatic disease despite treatment of the primary bladder lesion.

Treatment Bladder cancer can be subdivided conceptually as being *superficial, invasive,* or *metastatic. Superficial carcinoma* of the bladder includes patients with carcinoma in situ, mucosal involvement (stage O), or submucosal involvement (stage A). These patients are generally treated with endoscopic resection and selected bladder biopsies with repeat cystoscopic evaluations every 3 to 6 months. Approximately 50 to 70 percent of these patients will have a superficial recurrence (limited to the mucosa or submucosa) within a period of 3 years following initial diagnosis. Patients with superficial recurrences are then often treated with intravesical therapies, including *N,N′,N″*-triethylenethiophosphoramide (thiotepa), doxorubicin hydrochloride, mitomycin C, or bacillus Calmette-Guérin (BCG) in addition to cystoscopic resection.

An additional 12 percent with initial superficial disease will eventually develop progressive disease into the bladder muscularis (stage B), perivesical fat (stage C) or metastatic disease to lymph nodes (stage D1), bone, or other viscera (stage D2). Alternatively, patients may present initially with invasive or metastatic disease.

INVASIVE DISEASE These patients generally have disease which has invaded into the muscle and/or perivesical fat. Traditional treatment modalities have been cystectomy (radical or simple), radiation therapy, or preoperative radiation therapy followed by cystectomy. Five-year survival rates are approximately 45 percent with such treatments. The majority of these patients will die of distant metastatic disease despite radical surgery or radiation rather than from local recurrences.

METASTATIC DISEASE For patients who have distant metastatic disease in lymph nodes, viscera, or bone, the use of systemic chemotherapy has produced responses from 30 to 70 percent of patients, but usually not lasting more than 6 months. Following the development of metastatic disease, most patients die within 2 years. The most active agents include cisplatin, methotrexate, doxorubicin hydrochloride, cyclophosphamide, and vinblastine, and combinations of these agents have recently produced meaningful and durable remissions. One current therapeutic strategy for patients with invasive disease consists of initiating chemotherapy followed by definitive local treatment to the bladder (surgery or radiation). The goal of such programs is to eradicate micrometastases which are commonly present in patients with invasive disease.

TRANSITIONAL CELL CANCER OF THE RENAL PELVIS Renal pelvic tumors account for approximately 10 percent of all primary renal cancer. Nearly 90 percent are transitional cell carcinomas. In addition to the etiologic associations implicated for bladder carcinoma, renal pelvic tumors occur with analgesic abuse nephropathy. These patients are usually middle-aged women with a psychiatric history or chronic headaches who ingest >3 kg of analgesics over years. The exact amount and type of analgesic which induces transitional cell cancer of the renal pelvis is unknown, although aspirin and/or phenacetin can induce the disease experimentally. Balkan nephropathy (see also Chap. 226) is associated with a high incidence of renal pelvic and ureteral tumors, especially in women.

Most patients present with painless, gross hematuria. Ureteral obstruction and pain secondary to clots are unusual. The diagnosis is suggested by IVP, which may demonstrate an obstructed, poorly functioning, or nonvisualized kidney or filling defects in a visualized kidney, and a positive urinary cytology. Cystoscopy and retrograde pyelography with brush biopsy generally will establish the nature and location of the renal pelvic or ureteral tumor. For low-grade, low-stage tumors, conservative treatment with local excision and preservation of the kidney parenchyma has been associated with very favorable 5-year survival rates. For high-stage, high-grade lesions, the treatment of choice is radical nephroureterectomy and removal of the cuff of the bladder containing the ipsilateral ureteral orifice. This latter operative approach has been dictated by the high likelihood of recurrence in the ureteral stump and orifice if the ureter or orifice are not removed. In addition, routine follow-up with cystoscopies and urinary cytologies are mandatory to help detect the subsequent development of metachronous bladder carcinomas and/or contralateral ureteral and renal pelvic tumors. Five-year survival rates range from 10 to 50 percent. Although chemotherapy programs employed for bladder cancer have been used for patients with metastatic transitional cell carcinoma of the renal pelvis, the overall results are not as successful.

REFERENCES

Chisholm GD, Roy RR: The systemic effects of malignant renal tumors. Br J Urol 43:687, 1971

Cronin RE et al: Renal cell carcinoma: Unusual systemic manifestations. Medicine 55:291, 1976

Garnick MB (ed): *Genitourinary Cancer. Contemporary Issues in Clinical Oncology*, vol 5. New York, Churchill Livingstone, 1985

———, Richie JP: Renal neoplasia, in *The Kidney*, 3d ed, BM Brenner, FC Rector Jr (eds). Philadelphia, Saunders, 1986, p 1533

Heney NM et al: Superficial bladder cancer: Progression and recurrence. J Urol 130:1083, 1983

Pathak S et al: Familial renal cell carcinoma with a 3;11 chromosome translocation limited to tumor cells. Science 217:939, 1982

Richie JP et al: Computed tomography scan for diagnosis and staging of renal cell carcinoma. J Urol 129:1114, 1983

Rieselbach RE, Garnick MB (eds): *Cancer and the Kidney*. Philadelphia, Lea & Febiger, 1982

Skinner DG et al: Diagnosis and management of renal cell carcinoma. A clinical and pathologic study of 309 cases. Cancer 28:1165, 1971

Whitmore WF Jr (ed): Urothelial tumors. Semin Oncol 1:1, 1983

PART SEVEN DISORDERS OF THE GASTROINTESTINAL SYSTEM

section 1 Disorders of the alimentary tract

232 APPROACH TO THE PATIENT WITH GASTROINTESTINAL DISEASE

KURT J. ISSELBACHER / ROGER J. MAY

GENERAL CONSIDERATIONS Gastrointestinal symptoms occur not only with primary gastrointestinal tract disease but frequently as manifestations of other organic and functional disorders. Thus anorexia, nausea, and vomiting may be seen in patients with anxiety or depression, congestive failure, and uremia; diarrhea or constipation may be seen as a consequence of metabolic derangements such as electrolyte changes or alterations in thyroid function. With advances in medical technology, all too often physicians are willing to diagnose (or misdiagnose) gastrointestinal disease simply by relying on routine procedures such as x-ray studies of the upper and lower parts of the gastrointestinal tract. Such an overwhelming dependence on technical procedures often leads to great pitfalls. It cannot be overemphasized that the proper initial approach still demands a carefully obtained history and thorough physical examination before proceeding with any diagnostic tests.

IMPORTANCE OF THE HISTORY To evaluate gastrointestinal symptoms, a careful history is crucial. Pain or indigestion is the most common intestinal complaint. Correlation between pain and gastrointestinal function must of necessity be chronologic. There should be a meticulous inquiry as to the frequency and specificity of the complaint. The questioning should include the location of the pain and whether it is circumscribed or diffuse. It is important to determine what factors aggravate or relieve the discomfort. *Does eating produce the symptom?* If so, determine whether the discomfort occurs *while eating* (as in esophageal disorders and abdominal angina), shortly *after the meal* (as often occurs in biliary tract disease), or *30 to 90 min later* (as typically seen with peptic ulcer). *Does eating relieve the symptom,* and if so, for how long? Temporary relief of epigastric pain is characteristic of gastritis and peptic ulceration. Many patients have tried or taken antacids by the time they come to the physician, and a history indicating relief of epigastric pain by antacids is suggestive of peptic disease of the upper part of the intestine. *What is the relation of pain to bowel movements?* The patient with ulcerative colitis often obtains temporary relief from lower abdominal cramps by defecation.

Attention should be paid to *anorexia* and *weight loss;* their combined occurrence should make one suspicious of an underlying depression as well as of an occult malignancy. If *weight* loss is accompanied by an increased appetite, one must consider the diagnosis of malabsorption or maldigestion as well as of a hypermetabolic state, such as thyrotoxicosis. If *diarrhea* is present, one should determine the average number of the stools, their consistency, and their timing. To some patients, diarrhea means an increased number of stools, even though they are relatively normal in consistency; to others, diarrhea means watery stools. The occurrence of nocturnal diarrhea is suggestive of organic rather than functional bowel disease. In a patient with diarrhea one should ask about stool *odor* (malodorous stools being typical of pancreatic insufficiency and sprue), change in stool *color* (light-colored stools are seen with steatorrhea or cholestasis), and whether blood or mucus has been noted (blood is characteristic of inflammatory bowel disease or infectious dysentery but is hardly ever noted in functional bowel disease).

In the evaluation of male patients, especially those with diarrhea, a tactful inquiry into sexual activity is essential. Homosexual males are at increased risk for a large variety of gastrointestinal infections as well as the acquired immunodeficiency syndrome, which may present with gastrointestinal symptoms. Finally, careful attention must be given to a ''drug history.'' Unless asked, patients may forget to mention that they take aspirin almost daily for headache, and this may indeed account for occult blood in the stool. Many patients take daily laxatives, which may explain chronic diarrhea and colonic changes on x-ray. Still others may be taking illicit drugs, and this history may be difficult to obtain.

PHYSICAL EXAMINATION, ENDOSCOPY, AND RADIOLOGY A vague history of abdominal distress may be brought into focus by a thorough physical examination. Upper abdominal distress together with tenderness in the right upper quadrant suggests that cholecystitis or hepatitis may be present. In a young patient, a history of intermittent abdominal pain together with a palpable mass or tender loop of bowel in the right lower quadrant should make one suspicious of regional enteritis. All too often, however, in gastrointestinal diseases the routine physical examination is negative, and other techniques for examining the intestine are needed. Among the techniques which should almost be routine as an extension of the physical examination is *sigmoidoscopy*. This procedure may be performed with the customary rigid instrument or with the flexible fiberoptic sigmoidoscope. Sigmoidoscopy is important in the diagnosis of colonic cancer because (1) 50 percent or more of large-intestine malignancies are within the reach of the sigmoidoscope; and (2) small rectosigmoid tumors may be missed on barium enema examination because of the tortuosity and redundancy of the intestine in this area. Sigmoidoscopy also permits inspection of the mucosa for edema, erythema, friability, or ulceration. In a patient with diarrhea due to nonspecific causes, the mucosa may be normal; with dysentery due to agents such as *Shigella,* the mucosa may become friable, edematous, and hyperemic; if the latter findings are combined with extensive ulcerations, ulcerative or amebic colitis may be present. In almost all patients with diarrhea, sigmoidoscopy should be done before barium studies.

As discussed in Chap. 233, the use of fiberoptic instruments has assumed increasing importance in the assessment of patients with gastrointestinal disorders. Routine upper gastrointestinal endoscopy permits evaluation of the esophagus, stomach, and duodenum, while the colonoscope permits direct inspection of the entire large bowel and frequently the terminal ileum. The appropriate use of these techniques with respect to the more limited examination obtained via a rigid or flexible sigmoidoscope remains to be fully clarified. Specialized fiberoptic instruments may be used to identify the ampulla of Vater, permitting peroral opacification of pancreatic and/or biliary ducts (ERCP). These techniques and their related merits are discussed in detail in Chap. 233. Increasingly, fiberoptic examination is supplementing conventional radiologic studies, permitting direct visual inspection and the opportunity to obtain samples for microbiologic and histologic studies.

The roles of endoscopic versus radiologic examination remains an area of debate. While routine barium studies remain the most effective way to assess mucosal and other structural lesions in the small intestine, increasingly, proximal and distal portions of the GI tract are more efficiently studied for the presence of anatomic disease using fiberoptic instruments. However, these tools are not useful in assessing GI tract motility, which can be more effectively appreciated fluoroscopically or by using manometric techniques. With the decreasing use of conventional x-ray studies, other modalities have become increasingly important. These newer techniques include most notably ultrasound (US), computed tomography (CT), and radionuclide scanning. Both US and CT are useful in the delineation of abdominal mass lesions. While the latter is more expensive, it may be more effective in evaluation of the lower abdomen. Both are useful in the assessment of the structure and function of the gallbladder and bile ducts, but lower cost and lack of ionizing radiation tends to make US preferable.

While the use of barium studies has diminished, these x-rays continue to play a role in GI tract evaluation. In preparing a patient for *barium enema*, preparation or prior cleansing is important for a proper examination, but the physician must keep in mind that with obstructing lesions of the colon or small intestine or in the presence of active ulcerative colitis, the use of strong cathartics may be hazardous and even life-threatening. *No x-ray preparation should be considered routine*. In fact, the barium examination itself may aggravate an acute ulcerative colitis or precipitate colonic perforation or the onset of toxic megacolon. Similarly, if partial obstruction of the intestine is detected by plain x-ray of the abdomen, the physician must be wary of introducing barium from above for fear of producing further or complete intestinal obstruction. In patients with active GI bleeding, barium studies should be avoided lest they preclude subsequent angiographic evaluation.

Consultation with the radiologist Finally, one cannot overemphasize the importance of providing the radiologist with as much information as possible about the nature of the disease process under investigation. This will focus the attention of the radiologist on the appropriate region of the GI tract and optimize the information gained from the study.

All too often the busy physician allows a negative x-ray report to be the decisive factor in the diagnosis. It is essential to recognize the limitations of any diagnostic modality. With regard to routine radiologic studies, a negative barium enema may simply reflect that too much fecal material has been retained in the colon or that the area of concern was never well visualized. Similarly, if the patient has typical symptoms of biliary colic, the physician should not discard the diagnosis merely because of a negative x-ray report.

On the other hand the physician must be able to determine whether the abnormal finding is causally related to the symptoms. This is especially true in older patients where the presence of a hiatus hernia, gallstones, or diverticulosis is not unusual and hence may be coincidental.

DIAGNOSTIC APPROACHES **Problems of swallowing** The approach should be as follows:

1 *Careful visual and neurologic examination* of the pharynx, with tests for myasthenia gravis if indicated.
2 *Routine esophageal x-rays* in the upright and lateral or Trendelenburg position. The horizontal views are essential for demonstration of the swallowing mechanism, unaided by gravity, and of the esophagogastric junction. For details of the pharyngoesophageal area cineradiography is necessary because of the rapidity with which the contrast media passes through. Hiatus hernia is extremely common (in 15 to 35 percent of persons over 50) and often asymptomatic unless spontaneous reflux of gastric contents can be demonstrated to occur repeatedly.
3 *Esophagoscopy*. This procedure is desirable to describe lesions suggested by x-ray or, if the lesion is unsuspected, to obtain biopsies from masses or abnormal mucosa and to obtain washings for exfoliative cytologic study. The diagnosis of peptic esophagitis is best made endoscopically. Esophageal varices can be identified by this approach when they are too small to be seen radiologically, although the latter technique will pick up 70 percent of large varices.
4 *Manometric studies* of the upper esophagus, particularly in conjunction with cineradiography. At present, this procedure offers the best differential between disorders primary in the central nervous system, primary pharyngeal muscular disease, and cricopharyngeal dystonia. Manometry of the lower esophagus is useful in the diagnosis of diffuse esophageal spasm, achalasia, and infiltrative diseases which can alter esophageal motility.

Peptic or digestive disorders The approaches to these disorders include:

1 *Insertion of a nasogastric tube*. This is used to establish whether significant gastric retention (more than 75 mL of gastric contents in the fasting state) exists, and whether there is acid, bile, blood, or other material in these contents. If pyloric obstruction or gastric atony is present, the tube is used to maintain suction while the patient's electrolyte and fluid balance is restored to normal; the stomach is kept as clean as possible so that reliable diagnostic investigation may be carried out.
2 *Upper intestinal endoscopy*. This procedure is most helpful in identifying the diffuseness of the mucosal response in gastritis or, together with biopsy and brushings for cytology, in differentiating between peptic and neoplastic ulcerating lesions. Gastroscopy may permit the diagnosis of superficial erosive gastritis and the Mallory-Weiss syndrome as a cause of bleeding when the x-ray examination is negative. It may identify a specific bleeding site in clinical situations where several potential bleeding sites could exist, such as in the patient with portal hypertension. Gastroscopy is also particularly helpful in inspecting the postoperative stomach, especially in detecting stomal ulceration or alkaline reflux gastritis. The first and second portions of the duodenum can also be examined with the fiberoptic gastroscope, and important information about ulcers and other lesions can be obtained by this procedure. Radiologic studies may be useful when endoscopy is not readily available or in the assessment of suspected motility disorders (e.g. gastroparesis). In addition, radiologic examination may be preferred when there are contraindications to safe endoscopy.
3 *Gastric acid secretory studies*. These are useful in the diagnosis of the Zollinger-Ellison syndrome or atrophic gastritis and for determination of completeness of vagotomy. Suspected gastric carcinoma is better diagnosed directly through gastroscopy and biopsy than indirectly through acid secretory studies (achlorhydria). They should not be obtained for the routine diagnosis of uncomplicated duodenal ulcer. There is no convincing evidence that acid studies are useful in determining the type of surgery for duodenal ulcer.

Obstructive and vascular disorders of the small intestine When intestinal problems present as obstructive syndromes, the plain x-ray of the abdomen is the most important diagnostic adjunct to careful physical examination. Patterns of dilatation of individual loops of intestine may be characteristic, as in volvulus or acute pancreatitis; erect and decubitus views will often show fluid levels in the affected segments. Motility disorders of the small intestine (pseudo obstruction) may also present with obstructive symptoms and similar x-ray findings but must be managed medically without surgical intervention. Air under the diaphragm is diagnostic of a perforated viscus; air in the portal vein usually results from intestinal necrosis secondary to mesenteric vascular occlusion. The diagnostic accuracy of the plain x-ray in all types of intestinal obstruction is about 75 percent. In patients with symptoms of incomplete obstruction, the radiographic small-bowel series will often be diagnostic in defining the site and degree of obstruction. Infrequently, in this setting, all conventional x-ray studies are unremarkable. In such cases, the radiologist may perform a small-bowel enteroclysis study by passing a special tube into the proximal jejunum; the rapid instillation of barium through the tube will distend the intestine and often reveal subtle lesions missed by other tests.

Vascular diseases of the small intestine are among the most difficult diseases to diagnose. In chronic mesenteric ischemia, radiographic, endoscopic, and laboratory tests are usually normal. Early in the course of acute mesenteric ischemia, the plain film of the abdomen may be unremarkable despite complaints of severe abdominal pain. In these settings, prompt mesenteric angiography is essential in confirming the diagnosis of vascular disease.

Inflammatory and neoplastic diseases of small and large intestine Patients with these conditions are usually identified by history, physical examination, and careful examination of the stools for exudate and blood. Sigmoidoscopy is valuable in identifying mucosal and neoplastic lesions of the lower 25 cm of the colon. The mucosal surface of the entire colon and terminal ileum can be examined directly and biopsied through the fiberoptic sigmoidoscope or colonoscope. The radiologic examination of the small intestine is highly reliable in identifying the prestenotic and stenotic lesions of Crohn's disease. In the colon a single examination in a well-prepared patient has a diagnostic accuracy of 80 to 85 percent; the addition of air-contrast technique brings the accuracy up over 90 percent, but none of these figures is meaningful if the patient is poorly prepared for the examination. In the demonstration of small polyps the degree of accuracy is understandably not so high, but for polyps larger than 1 cm, which are of greater clinical importance, it is satisfactory. The cecal area is the hardest to examine adequately because of its anatomy; colonoscopy may be preferable. The immunologic assay for the carcinoembryonic antigen has not proved to be specific for colonic cancer; nevertheless, it does contribute to the evaluation of the extent of tumor and to the detection of residual or recurrent disease in postoperative patients.

Peroral biopsy of the small intestine and forceps biopsy of the rectosigmoid are of considerable importance in revealing mucosal disease. Rectal biopsy is an excellent means of demonstrating amyloidosis, schistosomiasis, and amebiasis. Submucosal disease is not seen in these superficial biopsies. Hirschsprung's disease is histologically diagnosed by a deep surgical biopsy of the lower part of the rectum.

Malabsorption syndromes Malabsorption may be suspected on the basis of history and physical examination and is confirmed by examination of the stools. Radiologic examination is of general help in ruling out local lesions and suggesting motor and secretory dysfunction, but it is rarely diagnostic unless an abnormal small-bowel mucosa or fistulas between intestine and stomach are demonstrated.

The tests useful in the diagnosis of malabsorption are discussed in Chap. 237. A simple screening test for excessive fat in the stools can be accomplished by the microscopic examination of a stool specimen stained with Sudan. Chemical analysis of 3-day stool collection for fat, with the patient on a standard diet, is used to establish the diagnosis of steatorrhea. The D-xylose absorption test is about 90 percent accurate in separating mucosal disease from pancreatic insufficiency. Peroral biopsy of the small intestine is of value in the diagnosis of celiac disease, and it may show the less common infiltrations of the mucosa by amyloid or bacterial mucoproteins (Whipple's disease). Leakage of protein into the intestinal lumen may cause hypoproteinemia and can be demonstrated by the recovery in stools of intravenously administered markers such as albumin labeled with iodine or chromium isotopes.

Pancreas The pancreas is difficult to study directly because of its anatomic location and relative inaccessibility. Calcification of the pancreas on a plain abdominal film is highly suggestive of chronic pancreatitis and may be associated with fat malabsorption. Pancreatic exocrine insufficiency can be documented by intubation of the duodenum and collection of pancreatic juice after stimulation with secretin or a test meal. Abdominal ultrasound and CT are the best radiographic means of searching for pancreatic enlargement (see Chaps. 254 and 255). Both techniques may also be used to guide needle biopsies of the pancreas and may provide sufficient diagnostic information to obviate the need for exploratory surgery. The pancreatic duct can be cannulated via the fiberoptic duodenoscope and visualized by the injection of radiographic dye. Visualization of the duct may be helpful in the diagnosis of pancreatic pseudocysts, carcinoma, or chronic pancreatitis.

233 GASTROINTESTINAL ENDOSCOPY

FRED E. SILVERSTEIN

Fiberendoscopes have revolutionized the examination of the gastrointestinal tract. Because of the flexibility of the fiberoptic bundles and because of controllability of the instrument tip, the operator can steer the instrument around multiple bends under visual control. A side channel permits passage of a variety of endoscopic tools such as biopsy forceps, foreign-body forceps, cytology brushes, wash tubes, and electrocautery snares. The viewing window and the light at the instrument's distal end can be washed free of obscuring material. Fluid can be aspirated from hollow organs, and air can be insufflated as needed to improve visualization. A new development is the video endoscope in which a miniature TV camera transmits the image which appears on a TV screen. This system permits storage, analysis, and transmission of the endoscopic images.

The usefulness of fiberendoscopy in diagnosing gastrointestinal disease is well established. Shallow lesions such as erosions or healing ulcers are missed by single-contrast x-ray but not by endoscopy. The brilliant success of polypectomy via the colonoscope has led to the development of other endoscopic techniques which are beginning to replace some invasive surgical techniques; the most significant advances in the future will probably be in this area.

Although esophagogastroduodenoscopy (EGD) is not a procedure for the occasional operator, it should be available in every general hospital. It is a relatively easy procedure to perform technically, but training and continued experience are necessary for optimal diagnostic accuracy. Complications are most frequent when the operator is inexperienced. Before the procedure the competent endoscopist always takes a history and examines the patient. Prior evaluation of cardiac status and clotting mechanisms is also essential.

The more complex procedures such as colonoscopy and endoscopic retrograde cholangiopancreatography (ERCP) require special dexterity, a substantial investment of time for learning, and constant practice to maintain adequate skill; they are probably best accomplished by subspecialists. Colonoscopy, one hopes, will be simplified so that it can be as widely available as esophagogastroduodenoscopy.

UPPER GASTROINTESTINAL ENDOSCOPY Forward-viewing, oblique, and side-viewing instruments may be used for EGD. After a careful explanation of the procedure to the patient, pharyngeal topical anesthesia with viscous lidocaine is followed by intravenous diazepam to the point of mild sedation. With the newer, small-caliber instruments less or no diazepam is needed. The tip of the endoscope is placed at the upper cricopharyngeal sphincter of the esophagus and the patient is encouraged to swallow while gentle pressure is exerted. Small amounts of air are passed through the endoscope to visualize the esophageal lumen. The endoscope is then passed under direct vision into the stomach. The gastric body and antrum are carefully examined. The instrument tip is retroflexed to view the gastric cardia, the fundus, and the whole lesser curvature. The pylorus is traversed, and the first and second portions of the duodenum are visualized. The whole examination is repeated as the instrument is withdrawn. Visualized lesions can be recorded on still photographs, movies, or videotape. Biopsies and brush cytologic examinations can be obtained from suspicious areas.

EGD is a relatively safe procedure in experienced hands. Several large surveys suggest a risk of serious complications during diagnostic EGD of approximately 1 in 800 and a risk of death of approximately 1 in 5000. The risks are higher in emergency procedures and in the elderly or seriously ill. In a survey of patients examined by endoscopy during bleeding, 1 in 200 had serious complications and 1 in 700 died from the procedure. A nationwide survey revealed a morbidity of 0.13 percent and a mortality of 0.004 percent. The main causes of mortality were cardiopulmonary complications and perforations by the instrument. Upper endoscopy is usually substituted for x-ray in the urgent diagnosis of gastrointestinal illness in women who might be pregnant.

Peptic regurgitant esophagitis Esophagitis is one of the commonest benign diseases of the upper gastrointestinal tract (see Chap. 234). Esophageal pain may be confused with cardiac disease, or esophagitis may present as painless blood loss. Because esophagitis usually involves only the superficial mucosa, it cannot be diagnosed by routine single-contrast x-ray. At endoscopy, the diffuse bleeding, linear erosions, friability, and ulcerations of erosive esophagitis are clearly visible. Not every patient with heartburn requires esophagoscopy, but the procedure is indicated if the patient complains of dysphagia, if an x-ray shows a stricture, a mass, or an ulcer, if symptoms persist despite therapy, or if antireflux surgery is contemplated.

The squamous mucosa of the esophagus is far more vulnerable to peptic digestion than is the columnar epithelium of the stomach. Thus, bleeding esophagitis is located on the squamous side of the esophagogastric junction and is most severe in the distal esophagus where the squamous mucosa is most exposed to regurgitated acid and pepsin from the stomach. Discrete peptic ulceration of the esophagus is uncommon.

A short area of esophagitis or a stricture can be seen at levels as high as the arch of the aorta. This is explained by progressive replacement of distal eroded squamous mucosa with metaplastic epithelium, which is more resistant to peptic digestion (Barrett's epithelium). This finding can be documented by biopsy. Such epithelium is more prone to malignant transformation and, therefore, may merit regular surveillance with esophagoscopy and biopsy and/or exfoliative cytology every 12 to 24 months.

Esophagitis may progress to scarring and stricture formation. The endoscopic appearance of a benign stricture is characteristic but not diagnostic because a malignancy can be missed; this should be ruled out before medical treatment is undertaken with dilation and antacids. The whole length of the stricture should therefore be sampled by biopsy and cytologic brushing to rule out cancer, if necessary, at repeat endoscopy after dilation. Endoscopy is often indicated in an esophageal ulcer, with biopsy of the rim of the ulcer to rule out cancer.

Dilations of difficult strictures are best initiated by passing a flexible-tipped guide wire via the side channel of the endoscope through the stricture under direct vision. The endoscope can then be withdrawn over the wire, which serves as a guide for passage of progressively larger metal olives or other dilators through the stricture under fluoroscopic control. A new technique utilizes balloon catheters passed via the endoscope channel or over a guide wire through the stricture. The balloon is inflated under endoscopic and/or fluoroscopic guidance to dilate the stricture.

Peptic ulcer Esophagogastroduodenoscopy is more accurate than upper gastrointestinal x-ray in detecting ulcers. It has been suggested that x-ray be abandoned entirely in favor of endoscopy for detecting ulcers. This makes sense when the source of acute upper gastrointestinal bleeding is sought if urgent surgical intervention is being considered; in such situations, obscuring barium would make endoscopy impossible. However, in the workup of the patient with less pressing ulcer complaints, an upper gastrointestinal x-ray is still often used as the initial diagnostic test. As more radiologists routinely use air contrast to obtain better mucosal detail, diagnostic sensitivity for superficial lesions will increase. The greater expense and discomfort of endoscopy are justified if the x-ray is equivocal, if the ulcer is possibly malignant, if the x-ray is negative but the clinical picture is suggestive of peptic ulceration, or if the patient is about to be operated on for ulcer and there is a need to be sure that an ulcer is present and that other lesions have not been missed. Patients with duodenal ulcers shown by x-ray or with classic ulcer deformities of the duodenal bulb do not require endoscopy for diagnosis if the presenting symptoms are characteristic and if the symptomatic response to strict antiulcer treatment is good. Some feel that screening endoscopy using the new small-diameter endoscopes may be the preferable initial diagnostic approach to the symptomatic patient. These instruments can be passed easily, often without sedation, for rapid and complete upper gastrointestinal examinations. When used in this manner the cost of the endoscopy should be reduced.

There are some situations in which x-ray reveals ulcers missed by endoscopy, e.g., ulcers in hourglass constrictions of the stomach or in small duodenal bulbs incompletely visualized by currently available instruments. Fiberendoscopy is especially useful in visualizing postbulbar ulcers, giant duodenal ulcers, and stomal ulceration after partial gastrectomy, all of which can be missed by x-ray. Endoscopy may be of use in determining the cause of gastric outlet obstruction. In most circumstances, patients with duodenal ulcers do not need follow-up endoscopy to see if the ulcer has healed.

In the enthusiasm for fiberendoscopy one must not forget that visual interpretation of gross pathology is subjective—one observer's ulcer is another's erosion. An erosion is confined to the mucosa and heals without a trace, whereas an ulcer is deeper and usually implies a chronic recurrent disease. Endoscopically, erosions are superficial, small, and multiple; ulcers are deeper and larger and tend to be solitary. In the future it is likely that lesions seen endoscopically will be easily recorded for review on videotape or disk, just as currently all lesions seen fluoroscopically are demonstrated in spot films.

Cancer The endoscopic appearance of upper gastrointestinal cancer may seem obvious, especially if there is a mass growing into the lumen. On the other hand, malignant ulcers, infiltrative carcinomas, or small early carcinomas are frequently impossible to diagnose by their gross appearance. The biopsies obtained with currently available forceps are very small, and deeper lesions can be missed. Only one of multiple biopsies may reveal the cancer. Therefore, it is recommended that six to eight biopsies be taken from the rim of a gastric ulcer. A larger particle of tissue may be removed from a suspicious elevated mucosal lesion with an electrocautery snare or with a large biopsy forceps passed via the large channel of an endoscope, and this may facilitate diagnosis. Experience and skill in choosing the biopsy site improve the accuracy. A cytologic examination of the lavage or brush specimen adds to the diagnostic accuracy in all areas of the upper gastrointestinal tract (see Chap. 236).

It may be impossible to differentiate severe esophagitis from infiltrative cancer by the gross appearance at esophagoscopy. Biopsies from patients with cancer may show only the associated inflammation. Thus, all such lesions should have careful cytologic examination, either by lavage or by brushing. Because chronic inflammation may predispose to esophageal cancer, patients with lye stricture or the stasis esophagitis of achalasia merit esophagoscopy and cytologic examination when they are first seen and when periodically rescreened, or whenever their symptom patterns change.

Radiologic demonstration of healing of a benign-appearing gastric ulcer is very reassuring but not infallible in excluding cancer. A history of ingesting ulcerogenic drugs increases the likelihood of benignancy. Ulcers in such patients are followed to complete healing radiologically or endoscopically after treating the ulcer. Diagnostic accuracy in differentiating benign from malignant gastric ulcer by exfoliative cytologic lavage, endoscopic biopsy, or brush cytology depends on the combined skills of endoscopists, cytologists, and pathologists. Among North American communities accuracy in diagnosing cancer may vary from 70 to 90 percent. Physicians must individually decide which patients should be examined by methods that have proved accurate in their own community, and which patients should be referred to centers with greater resources.

Primary gastric lymphoma can mimic benign gastric ulcer or adenocarcinoma on gastroscopy or x-ray. It can be diagnosed by biopsy or cytology, although the accuracy is not as high as in adenocarcinoma. The 5-year survival for lymphoma is higher than for adenocarcinoma.

If a polypoid lesion of the stomach is covered by mucosa that appears normal by gastroscopy, the likelihood of malignancy is very small. Such lesions are often intramural, extramucosal benign tumors such as leiomyomas or pancreatic rests. Polyps covered by abnormal-appearing mucosa can be benign or malignant. Random biopsy can miss carcinoma within a polyp. If technically feasible, polyps should, therefore, be removed in their entirety by snare cautery for histologic examination. If over 2 cm in diameter, they are more likely to contain cancer (see Chap. 236). Large polyps may require surgical excision.

Ampullary carcinoma may be diagnosed by biopsy and brush cytology during duodenoscopy. Other primary duodenal malignancies are very rare. Extensions from pancreatic or biliary tract cancer are difficult to diagnose because the tumor may not have extended into the mucosa and may therefore not be accessible for endoscopic biopsy or cytologic examination. In these secondary tumors, diagnosis must depend upon some combination of echography, hypotonic duodenography, selective pancreatic angiography, and endoscopic retrograde cholangiopancreatography, with cytologic examination of ductal contents.

Upper gastrointestinal bleeding (see also Chap. 37) Endoscopy within the first 12 to 24 h of an upper gastrointestinal hemorrhage can be very helpful in planning rational therapy by visualizing the bleeding source. Shallow lesions not visible by x-ray may be seen (esophagitis, Mallory-Weiss tear, erosive gastritis, shallow stress ulcer, and telangiectasia). Lesions which are visible by x-ray may not be the source of bleeding. Only endoscopy can determine the actual bleeding site. For example, visualization of a spurting artery which is flooding the stomach indicates massive ongoing bleeding requiring prompt therapeutic intervention. Several studies have shown that the demonstration at endoscopy of any bleeding whatsoever or a nonbleeding vessel in the ulcer base makes rebleeding more likely.

A conservative estimate of the diagnostic accuracy of emergency endoscopy in upper gastrointestinal bleeding is 80 to 85 percent, which is far superior to emergency x-ray examination. Endoscopic diagnosis of bleeding erosive gastritis may be made too frequently when blood from another unsuspected source spreads over the gastric mucosa or when trauma from overly vigorous antecedent lavage creates submucosal ecchymoses. To avoid overdiagnosis of erosive gastritis, portions of the gastric wall should be washed free of blood to determine the true appearance of the underlying gastric mucosa.

Every patient having endoscopy for upper gastrointestinal bleeding merits a complete endoscopic examination of the esophagus, stomach, and duodenum. Finding a potential bleeding lesion is not proof that this is the source of hemorrhage unless active bleeding is seen. Approximately one-half of patients with esophageal varices can be shown endoscopically to be bleeding from another source such as erosive gastritis, duodenal ulcer, or gastric ulcer. Occasionally it is not possible to diagnose the exact lesion which is bleeding, but localizing the area of bleeding can be very helpful; for example, bright red arterial blood may be seen pouring into the stomach from the duodenum when the esophagus and stomach are relatively free of blood.

There are three controversial areas. First, *do all bleeders need endoscopy?* The author feels that endoscopy is indicated in all patients who may require surgery because of continual bleeding or rebleeding. Although 85 percent of upper gastrointestinal bleeders stop spontaneously, it is impossible to predict which ones will; therefore, endoscopy is recommended for most bleeders. Second, *how early should endoscopy be performed in the acutely bleeding patient?* Most studies suggest that the diagnostic accuracy of esophagogastroduodenoscopy remains high for the first 12 to 24 h after the bleeding episode. All would agree that it is desirable to delay endoscopy until vital signs have been stabilized after adequate blood replacement. Upper endoscopy is usually performed during waking hours at a time during the first day of bleeding when the patient's vital signs are stable and when the full endoscopic team is available. Emergency endoscopy at night should be reserved for those patients with continued massive bleeding or rebleeding requiring an immediate decision regarding surgery or other treatment. If the patient is exsanguinating, endoscopy can follow induction of anesthesia just preceding surgery. Thus, the patient's airway is protected by an endotracheal tube. Finally, *does endoscopy affect the clinical outcome?* Current studies suggest that it does not. This may be more a reflection on the inadequacies of medical therapy and the dangers of nonelective surgical treatment of bleeding patients who are severely ill than on the usefulness of more accurate endoscopic detection of the bleeding source. If endoscopic or pharmacologic methods of stopping bleeding prove to be safe and effective in controlled trials, more accurate endoscopic diagnosis may indeed affect the outcome favorably. Endoscopic treatment of bleeding lesions with heater probes, bipolar probes, or lasers (Nd:YAG) is now being studied. The data suggest that these methods are effective and safe and may improve outcome in the bleeding patient.

Emergency endoscopy is not for the inexperienced. It requires considerable technical skill and interpretative experience and the best available instruments.

Other indications Upper endoscopy is usually substituted for x-ray in the urgent diagnosis of gastrointestinal illness in *pregnancy*. Patients with *dysphagia* merit esophagoscopy because the cause is frequently organic and may be missed by x-ray. Dysphagia caused by esophageal spasm or dysrhythmia is best diagnosed by manometry or cineradiography in addition to endoscopy. *Painful swallowing* (odynophagia), especially in immunosuppressed or diabetic patients, may merit esophagoscopy because biopsy and brushings of the involved esophageal wall may reveal monilial, herpetic, or cytomegalic virus infections. Soon after ingestion of a corrosive agent, if there is no indication of wall necrosis, limited and gentle esophagoscopy is useful in evaluating the severity of injury. Many impacted foreign bodies can be removed from the esophagus or stomach with a snare or forceps; sharp foreign bodies are usually best removed by pulling them into the lumen of a rigid tubular esophagoscope or by pulling them into a protective overtube around a fiberoptic endoscope. Careful esophagoscopy after removal of an esophageal foreign body is important to determine whether there is an underlying lesion which caused the impaction (e.g., cancer, benign stricture, peptic esophagitis).

In the postoperative stomach, gastroscopy is especially useful in detecting carcinoma, recurrent ulceration, retrograde intussusception, and stomal stricture. Several European studies indicate a definite threat of carcinoma developing in the gastric stump 10 to 20 years after a Billroth II gastrectomy. The diagnosis of such postoperative carcinomas may require many biopsies of seemingly normal mucosa near the anastomosis. Studies of the natural history of this condition in the United States do not suggest a similar high incidence of postoperative carcinoma.

When the duodenal bulb shows reddening or nodularity, many endoscopists diagnose *duodenitis*. There is little evidence to suggest that this picture is of significance. On the other hand, diffuse and bleeding erosions of the duodenal bulb merit a diagnosis of *erosive duodenitis*, especially after ingestion of gastric irritants such as aspirin; such erosions may also be a precursor of frank ulcerations. A nodular or narrow duodenum will occasionally yield granulomas on biopsy, indicative of Crohn's disease.

ENDOSCOPIC RETROGRADE CHOLANGIOPANCREATOGRAPHY (ERCP) This endoscopic technique involves placing a side-viewing instrument in the descending duodenum. The papilla of Vater is cannulated, contrast medium is injected, and the pancreatic ducts and hepatobiliary tree are visualized radiologically. Skilled operators can visualize 90 to 95 percent of pancreatic ducts and 80 to 85 percent of biliary ducts.

ERCP is performed on an x-ray table. The oropharynx is usually anesthetized with topical lidocaine, and most endoscopists sedate the patient with intravenous diazepam. Atropine and glucagon are given intravenously to induce duodenal hypotonia. The pancreatic duct is usually visualized first and gently filled throughout its entire length with 2 to 5 mL contrast material with constant fluoroscopic monitoring (Fig. 233-1*A*). Injection is continued until the first side branches are seen or until the patient complains of pain. Overfilling is avoided. By insertion of the cannula at a more acute cephalad angle, the common bile duct and the whole biliary tract including the gallbladder are visualized (Fig. 233-1*B*).

At present not all indications for ERCP are clearly established. Those for the hepatobiliary tree are clearer than those for the pancreatic duct. Because ERCP is not without risk, it is justified only to seek an operable lesion or to prevent an unnecessary operation. As therapeutic procedures such as endoscopic papillotomy are being utilized increasingly, the diagnostic ERCP may be performed to determine if endoscopic treatment is indicated. This may be especially relevant in a patient with common duct stones and cholangitis. Asymptomatic amylase elevations occur in 30 to 40 percent of patients after the procedure and are rarely of clinical significance. Pancreatitis occurs in only 1 percent of patients but is usually benign and self-limited. By monitoring the pancreas during injection using a high-resolution TV screen, the force of injection can be limited to avoid filling of pancreatic acini. This probably minimizes the complication of pancreatitis. In a nationwide survey of complications, the morbidity rate was 3 percent and mortality rate 0.2 percent. It is significant that the complication rate was highest for the inexperienced operator (7 percent). The morbidity and mortality rates are substantially lower from large centers with great experience. The main serious complication is retention of nonsterile contrast material proximal to an obstructed duct, causing cholangitis or pancreatic sepsis. Patients suspected of having bile duct obstruction are started on systemic antibiotics prior to the ERCP. Furthermore, if bile duct or pancreatic duct obstruction is first revealed by ERCP, antibiotic coverage is indicated to reduce the incidence of bacteremia; such patients should be drained if possible either with endoscopic therapy (papillotomy, stents, nasobiliary drains, etc.) or surgically within 36 h. No patient should have ERCP unless advance arrangements for possible operation have been made with the patient and a surgical consultant.

Retrograde cholangiography This procedure is especially useful in patients with persistent jaundice the cause of which cannot be established by conventional diagnostic methods. The important differential diagnosis is between "surgical" and "medical" jaundice. When the cause of jaundice is unclear, approximately 15 percent of patients thought to have "medical" jaundice prove to have extrahepatic biliary obstruction requiring surgery, and, conversely, the same percentage of patients thought to have "surgical" jaundice prove to have an open ductal system by ERCP and can be spared unnecessary surgery.

Remediable causes of obstructive jaundice which can be diagnosed by retrograde cholangiography include common duct stones (Fig. 233-1*C*), gallbladder stones, benign strictures, and, occasionally, resectable ductal carcinomas. In jaundiced patients with suspected primary liver disease, such as primary biliary cirrhosis, ERCP can relieve the worry that an operable obstruction is being missed.

In addition to ERCP, there are four other methods of visualizing the biliary tree in the jaundiced patient. Which test to use first depends on the clinical situation, the availability of equipment, and the experience of the specialists using the techniques. The first method is *percutaneous transhepatic cholangiography* (PTC), in which contrast material is injected from the exterior via a "skinny" needle into the intrahepatic bile ducts under fluoroscopic control; success in visualizing the ducts is 90 to 100 percent if the ducts are dilated, but only approximately 66 percent if they are not dilated. PTC is generally safe, but complications do occur (sepsis, bleeding, bile leak, etc.). The morbidity for this procedure is approximately 10 percent; the reported mortality varies from 0.1 to 0.9 percent. The three other methods, which are noninvasive, use *ultrasound*, *computerized tomography* (CT scan), and *PIPIDA scans* (^{99m}Tc-labeled paraisopropyliminodiacetic acid). The first two techniques employ sound waves or x-rays to visualize organs and any stones, cysts, or solid masses within them. They can also be used to determine whether the biliary ducts or gallbladder are enlarged. The PIPIDA scans are used to determine patency of the cystic and common ducts and to study gallbladder emptying after administration of cholecystokinin (CCK).

The relative usefulness of these five tests is not established. Many physicians first try ultrasound or CT scan to see whether the biliary ducts are dilated and to seek the cause of the patient's jaundice (stones, pancreatic mass, etc.). The PIPIDA scan will determine if the cystic duct and bile ducts are patent. Direct visualization is undertaken if the diagnosis is not established, PTC first if the hepatic ducts are dilated, and ERCP if not. Advantages of the endoscopic approach are that the papilla and the pancreatic duct are seen (in addition to the biliary ducts) and that therapy can be performed with papillotomy or drainage when appropriate. In the event of a technical failure or incomplete information resulting from either ERCP or PTC, the other technique is tried. This approach detects most lesions requiring surgical intervention.

ERCP or PTC can also be useful in patients with biliary pain, cholangitis, or impaired liver function after previous biliary surgery. Remediable postoperative lesions such as strictures can be discovered, and their precise anatomy outlined so that reoperation is less difficult.

Retrograde pancreatography Patients with recurrent or chronic pancreatitis may merit retrograde pancreatography to seek a lesion which can be approached surgically, such as localized pancreatitis in the tail or ductal pathology amenable to drainage.

Patients with symptoms, signs, or laboratory findings suggesting pancreatic carcinoma may have pancreatograms suggesting malignancy with a narrowed, encased, or sharply "cutoff" pancreatic duct (Fig. 233-1*D*). Differentiation of such pancreatic ductal findings from benign inflammatory disease can be difficult. Cytologic examination of pancreatic duct contents obtained during ERCP may prove helpful. Unfortunately, most patients with symptomatic pancreatic cancer diagnosed by ERCP are inoperable.

Patients presenting with painless steatorrhea of pancreatic origin may be shown to have a ductal pattern suggesting chronic pancreatitis or pancreatic carcinoma. Pancreatography has not been useful in the study of obscure upper abdominal pain. Pancreatic cysts can be better diagnosed by noninvasive techniques such as ultrasound, and pancreatography should be reserved for those cases where it is desirable to outline the anatomy immediately prior to surgery. Pancreatography alone does not seem promising as a method of screening for early pancreatic carcinoma, although cytologic examination of ductal fluid may prove useful.

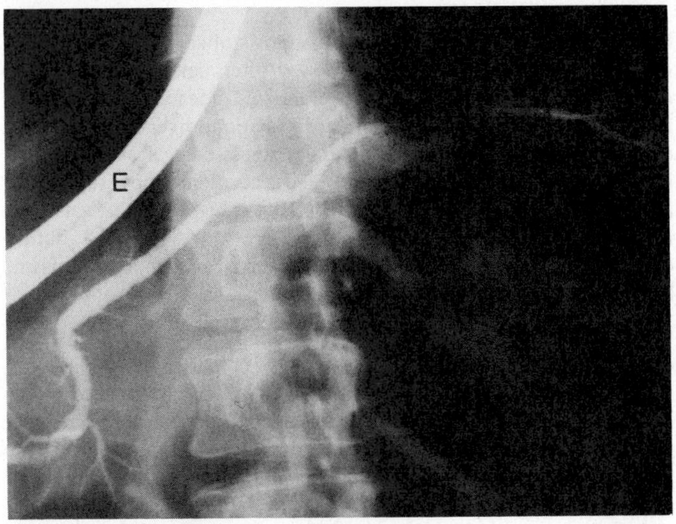

A

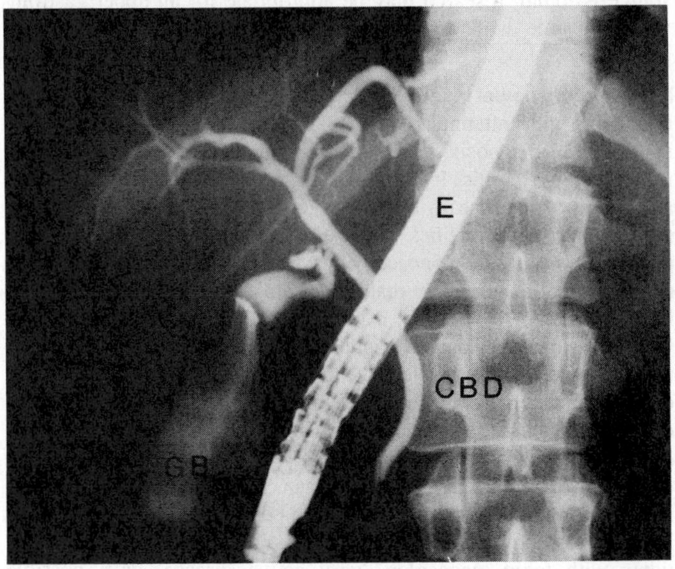

B

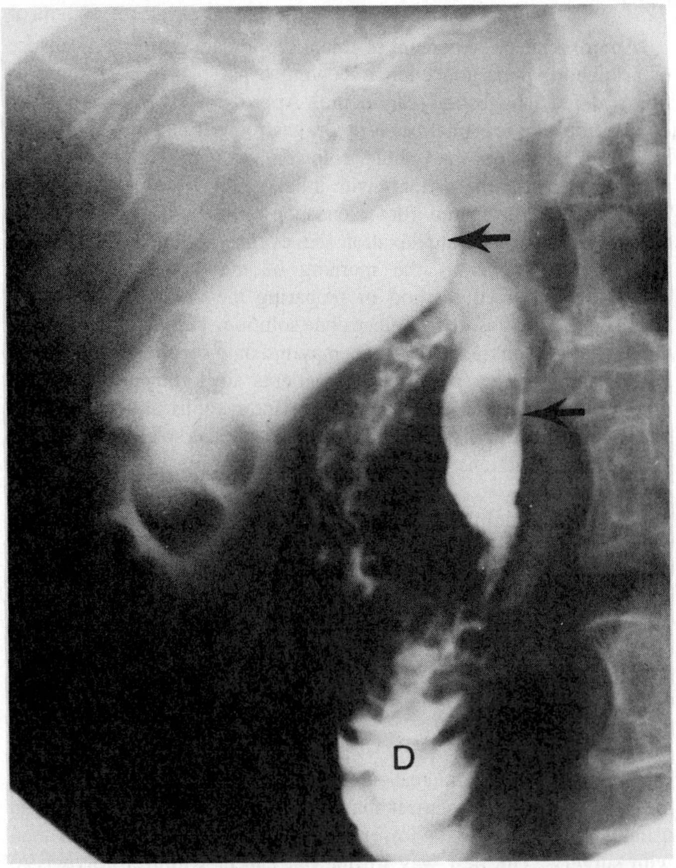

C

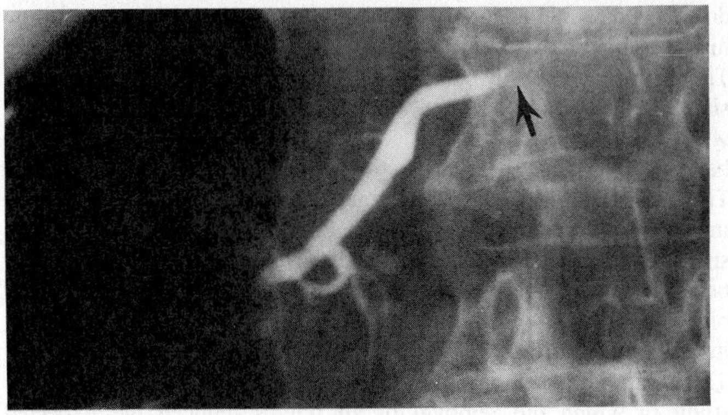

D

FIGURE 233-1 *A. A tapering pancreatic duct of normal caliber is seen and may be compared to the endoscope (E) 1 cm in diameter. B. Normal cholangiogram. The diameter of the common duct (CBD) is normal. The intrahepatic ducts branch normally, and the gallbladder (GB) can be seen. The endoscope (E) is seen in the duodenum. C. Several stones (arrows) can be seen in an obstructed, dilated common duct. The gallbladder also contains several stones. Regurgitated contrast material is seen in the duodenum (D). D. The sharp cutoff (arrow) of the pancreatic duct is caused by a carcinoma of the body of the pancreas. (Courtesy of Dr. Charles Rohrmann.)*

Therapeutic ERCP Successful endoscopic papillotomy of the sphincter of Oddi with extraction of retained stones is possible. An electrosurgical wire attached to the ERCP catheter can be used to cut the sphincter of Vater. Balloon catheters can be used to extract stones which do not pass spontaneously. New devices which mechanically crush or ultrasonically shatter large stones which will not pass spontaneously or with a balloon are being investigated. Certainly this approach is being used increasingly in patients who are poor operative risks. The overall success rate is approximately 90 percent, with a mortality rate of about 0.8 percent and a complication rate of about 7 percent. Complications include bleeding, perforation, pancreatitis, cholangitis, and stone impaction. These results compare favorably with surgery, especially in the high-risk patient with previous biliary surgery. Endoscopic papillotomy may also permit nonoperative biliary drainage via transnasal tubes or stents placed into the common bile duct. Manometry of the sphincter presents certain technical difficulties, but it may yet prove invaluable in the diagnosis of periampullary stenosis.

Other diagnostic techniques Critical comparative studies are needed of the various approaches to biliary tree disorders and to pancreatic diseases (ERCP, PTC, angiography, CT scanning, and ultrasound). The role of magnetic resonance imaging in diseases of the pancreas and biliary tree is yet to be defined. Endoscopic ultrasound may also prove to be a valuable technique to image the intestinal wall and adjacent organs.

COLONOSCOPY The interior of the entire length of the colon from anus to cecum can be visualized by the experienced colonoscopist. This method may prove to be the most significant diagnostic and therapeutic application of fiberoptic endoscopy because it can diagnose potentially curable colonic cancers missed by other techniques and remove potentially precancerous adenomatous polyps.

Approximately 40 percent of colonoscopies are performed because of an abnormal barium enema showing a polyp or a narrowing or filling defect suggesting carcinoma. Approximately 40 percent of colonoscopies are done because of gastrointestinal bleeding. The ability to examine the whole colon is proving valuable in the management of some patients with inflammatory bowel disease.

Patients are prepared for colonoscopy with a liquid diet for 2 days, magnesium citrate laxation the evening before examination, and tap water enemas the morning of the procedure. Another increasingly utilized method of preparing the colon is a total-gut lavage with a nonabsorbable electrolyte solution. This method prepares the patient without laxatives or enemas and only requires a few hours. Immediately before the procedure patients are lightly sedated with intravenous diazepam and meperidine. Intravenous anticholinergics and glucagon are used when needed to relax local spasm. Vasovagal bradycardial reactions can be reversed quickly by intravenous anticholinergics.

The main complications of colonoscopy are hemorrhage and perforation (morbidity rate is 0.5 to 1.3 percent; mortality rate is 0.02 percent). The complication rate for polypectomy is 1 to 2 percent. Diverticular or ischemic disease and prior irradiation make the procedure more difficult and hazardous. The risk of perforation is also increased in the patient with very active colitis, and colonoscopy should be avoided during the acute phase.

Polyps (see also Chap. 239) A polyp seen on barium enema merits colonoscopy for several reasons: It may be an artifact or a cancer, and a second polyp or cancer may have been missed. The polyp can usually be excised, with lower morbidity and mortality rates than with surgery. The best way to rule out cancer within a polyp is to remove it completely for histologic examination. Hyperplastic polyps do not become malignant; colonic polyps which show benign neoplasia histologically may become malignant (tubular and villous adenomas). The risk of neoplastic polyps being cancerous increases with their size. The risk is also higher in villous adenomas. Pedunculated polyps with cancer confined to the mucosa and with an uninvolved stalk can be cured by removal with an electrocautery snare during colonoscopy. Thus, most colonoscopists will remove all polyps more than 0.5 cm in diameter. It is more difficult to know what to do with polyps smaller than 0.5 cm in diameter because more than 50 percent may be adenomatous. A coagulating biopsy technique can be used to both biopsy and destroy even the smallest adenomatous polyp in the hope that the subsequent risk of developing colonic cancer will be reduced. The wisdom of this course of action is suggested by a sigmoidoscopic study in which the removal of all polyps reduced the expected incidence and invasiveness of subsequently developing cancers in the anatomic area screened. Most agree that the patient with adenomatous polyps is more likely to develop another polyp or cancer and therefore merits a regular screening program. The optimal frequency of follow-up examinations after polypectomy is not yet established. The current recommendation is a digital examination and stool test for occult blood yearly. When a polyp is discovered, the entire colon should be examined for synchronous polyps or cancer. This should probably be repeated at 1 year and, if negative, every 3 years thereafter. If stools are positive for occult blood or symptoms develop, immediate evaluation is indicated.

Cancer screening by x-ray All filling defects on barium enema merit evaluation by colonoscopy. If the lesion is a pedunculated polyp, it can be removed for histologic examination; if its appearance suggests a cancer, it can be biopsied and brushed for histologic and cytologic confirmation. When a polyp or a carcinoma is found, the remainder of the colon should be screened for additional polyps and synchronous carcinoma. This avoids multiple colotomies to search for a second lesion and reduces surgical morbidity. Approximately 40 percent of lesions diagnosed as a mass by x-ray are not present on colonoscopy or are found to be due to lesions such as a polyp rather than a cancer.

Narrowing by x-ray An etiologic diagnosis of segmental narrowing may be difficult by x-ray. Colonoscopy often determines the cause of segmental narrowing and differentiates adenocarcinoma from inflammation secondary to ischemia, irradiation, diverticular disease, or Crohn's colitis. Even the most classic "apple-core" lesion indicated by x-ray may be covered by normal mucosa at colonoscopy, suggesting an extrinsic inflammatory lesion. In 10 to 30 percent of patients, narrowed segments present on x-ray are not visualized during colonoscopy, probably because they are areas of temporary spasm. Such findings avoid unnecessary operations.

Chronic bleeding (x-ray and sigmoidoscopy negative) This condition leads to approximately 40 percent of colonoscopies. The x-ray is more likely to miss a lesion when single contrast is used rather than air contrast. The cause of bleeding is found in approximately 40 percent of such patients. The common bleeding sources are adenomatous polyp (20 percent), adenocarcinoma (10 percent), and Crohn's disease (7 percent). Many of these carcinomas are resectable, and this group may benefit most from colonoscopy. If no bleeding source is found, a search may be appropriate for an upper gastrointestinal source with an upper gastrointestinal x-ray and/or upper endoscopy.

Inflammatory bowel disease Colonoscopy is not routinely indicated in patients with inflammatory bowel disease. Colonoscopy may help in the initial diagnosis, especially in differentiating Crohn's colitis from ulcerative colitis. It can aid the surgeon in assessing the activity and extent of the disease before surgery. Colonoscopy can evaluate radiographic abnormalities suggesting cancer, such as strictures, polyps, or masses. Colonoscopy may be indicated in patients with ulcerative colitis of more than 10 years' duration because of the increased risk of carcinoma; it is hoped that repeated colonoscopies will serve to detect these malignancies earlier than x-ray and while the lesions are still curable. The frequency of colonoscopy and/or double-contrast barium enema examination in such patients is not yet established. If an expert pathologist finds "precancer" or "dysplastic" changes in colonic biopsies in a patient with long-standing ulcerative colitis, many consider this to be an indication for colectomy. Preparation for colonoscopy must often be modified for patients with inflammatory bowel disease. Colonoscopy is contraindicated in patients with toxic megacolon, very active disease, or a possible intestinal perforation.

Other indications The flexible sigmoidscope may replace the rigid 25-cm sigmoidoscope for routine screening because it can be passed to 40 to 60 cm with minimal preparation, less discomfort, and a higher diagnostic yield. After segmental colonic resection for carcinoma, colonoscopy may detect early mucosal recurrence and differentiate it from benign anastomotic strictures or bleeding suture granulomas. These patients must also be periodically screened for the development of polyps or additional carcinomas. Colonoscopy is occasionally used during laparotomy to assist the surgeon in ruling out other lesions. The colonoscope can be advanced to the cecum rapidly with the surgeon's assistance, and additional polyps removed without colotomy. The author believes that the best diagnostic approach to acute lower intestinal bleeding is a labeled RBC scan to determine if bleeding is active and to localize the general anatomic area of the source, followed (if active) by selective angiography; this may be useful not only for finding lesions such as angiodysplasia and bleeding diverticula but also for permitting treatment with vasoconstrictors. Endoscopic hemostatic therapy may be useful in some types of bleeding colonic lesions such as angiodysplasia. However, visualizing a bleeding site by colonoscopy may be difficult when there is massive bleeding.

Colonoscopy detects some carriers of the dominant familial polyposis gene before diagnosis by barium enema and sigmoidoscopy. Carcinoma is a great threat in those familial polyposis syndromes which produce many adenomatous polyps (familial polyposis and Gardner's syndrome); in these conditions, polypectomy is useful for diagnosis, but colectomy is the only treatment which prevents development of carcinoma. These patients are also at risk of developing duodenal and periampullary cancer and should probably undergo periodic surveillance with a side-viewing duodenoscope. Peutz-Jeghers syndrome and generalized juvenile polyposis produce mostly hamartomatous polyps and, therefore, have a very much lower incidence of gastrointestinal carcinoma; the cancers that develop in these patients may be related to occasional polyps undergoing adenomatous change or may occur in adjacent colonic mucosa.

Malignant tumors develop in 2 to 3 percent of patients with Peutz-Jeghers syndrome, and they are mostly located in the stomach, duodenum, and the rest of the small intestine. Thus these patients may merit regular upper endoscopy and prophylactic polypectomy.

CONTRAINDICATIONS All types of fiberoptic endoscopy are contraindicated in certain clinical situations, including patients who are uncooperative or combative, who have had an acute myocardial infarction, or who have perforation of the intestine.

CONSCIOUS LAPAROSCOPY The potentials for laparoscopy in conscious patients have not been as fully appreciated in North America as they have been in other countries, where it has been used widely for over 20 years. This procedure has extremely low mortality and morbidity rates in experienced hands. The instrument used for laparoscopy is a stiff tube with a lens system that provides a superb view. Under local anesthesia pneumoperitoneum is gradually induced with air or nitrous oxide.

Much of the exterior of the liver, gallbladder, spleen, peritoneum, diaphragm, and pelvic organs can be clearly visualized. Portions of the colon and small bowel can also be seen. Lesions can be biopsied under direct vision and any resultant bleeding controlled by electrocoagulation. Furthermore, in centers with extensive experience contrast material can be injected into the liver to visualize vascular, lymphatic, and biliary systems.

Laparoscopy may permit one to make a difficult diagnosis without resorting to laparotomy by biopsying localized hepatic disease under direct vision. Laparoscopy can often help differentiate "medical" from "surgical" jaundice and may also enable staging of malignant disease without laparotomy.

REFERENCES

Blackstone MO: *Endoscopic Interpretation.* New York, Raven Press, 1984

Cotton PB, Beales JSM: Endoscopic pancreatography in management of relapsing acute pancreatitis. Br Med J 1:608, 1974

———, Williams CB: *Practical Gastrointestinal Endoscopy.* Oxford, Blackwell, 1982

Fleischer D: Endoscopic therapy of upper gastrointestinal bleeding in humans. Gastroenterology 90:217, 1986

Gilbert DA et al: The national ASGE colonoscopy survey—Analysis of colonoscopic practices and yield. Gastrointest Endosc 30:143, 1984(A)

Haggitt RC et al: Prognostic factors in colorectal carcinomas arising in adenomas: Implications for lesions removed by endoscopic polypectomy. Gastroenterology 89:328, 1985

Koch H: Operative endoscopy. Gastrointest Endosc 24:65, 1977

Peterson WL et al: Routine early endoscopy in upper gastrointestinal tract bleeding: A randomized, controlled trial. N Engl J Med 304:925, 1981

The role of endoscopy in upper gastrointestinal bleeding: Proceedings of the NIH consensus workshop. Dig Dis Sci 26:1s, 1981

Safrany L: Duodenoscopic sphincterotomy and gallstone removal. Gastroenterology 72:330, 1977

Sivak MV (ed): *Gastroenterology Series: Endoscopic Sclerotherapy of Esophageal Varices.* New York, Praeger, 1984

Teague RH et al: Colonoscopy for investigation of unexplained rectal bleeding. Lancet 1:1350, 1978

234 DISEASES OF THE ESOPHAGUS

RAJ K. GOYAL

The two major functions of the esophagus are the transport of the food bolus from the mouth to the stomach and the prevention of retrograde flow of gastrointestinal contents. The transport function is achieved by peristaltic contractions (see Chap. 32). Retrograde flow is prevented by the two esophageal sphincters, which remain closed between swallows and which are functional rather than distinct anatomic entities. The upper esophageal sphincter remains closed by the elastic properties of its wall and by contraction of the cricopharyngeus and inferior pharyngeal constrictor muscles due to continuous neural excitation of the lower motor neurons which innervate these muscles via motor end plates. Many neuromuscular disorders involving these muscles result in reduction in resting sphincter pressure and consequent esophagopharyngeal reflux. In contrast, the lower esophageal sphincter remains closed because of its intrinsic myogenic tone, and a neural pathway, consisting of preganglionic parasympathetic fibers in the vagus nerve and postganglionic myenteric inhibitory neurons, causes its relaxation. The neurotransmitter of preganglionic neurons is acetylcholine and that of postganglionic neurons is vasoactive intestinal peptide (VIP). A reflex increase in the lower sphincter pressure occurs with an increase in intraabdominal pressure and ingestion of a protein meal. Fatty meals, smoking, and beverages with a high xanthine content (tea, coffee, cola) cause a reduction in sphincter pressure. Many hormones and neurotransmitters can modify lower sphincter pressure. Cholinergic muscarinic (M-2 receptor) agonists, alpha-adrenergic agonists, gastrin, pancreatic polypeptide, substance P, and prostaglandin $F_{2\alpha}$ cause contraction; in contrast, ganglionic stimulants, beta-adrenergic agonists, dopamine, cholecystokinin, secretin, VIP, ATP, and adenosine cause relaxation of the sphincter. These effects are mediated by actions on the inhibitory intramural neurons or on the sphincter muscle directly. Effects of many of these agents are pharmacologic rather than physiologic.

SYMPTOMS

DYSPHAGIA See Chap. 32.

ESOPHAGEAL PAIN *Heartburn,* or pyrosis, is characterized by burning retrosternal discomfort that may move up and down the chest like a wave. When severe, it may radiate to the sides of the chest, neck, and angles of the jaw. Heartburn is a characteristic symptom of reflux esophagitis and may be associated with regurgitation or a feeling of warm fluid climbing up the throat. It is aggravated by bending forward, straining, or lying recumbent and is worse after meals. It is relieved by upright posture, by swallowing of saliva or water, or, more reliably, by antacids. Heartburn appears to be produced by heightened mucosal sensitivity and can be reproduced by infusion of dilute (0.1 *N*) hydrochloric acid (Bernstein test) or neutral hyperosmolar solutions into the esophagus.

Odynophagia, or painful swallowing, is characteristic of nonreflux esophagitis, particularly monilial and herpes esophagitis. Odynophagia may also occur with peptic ulcer of the esophagus (Barrett's ulcer), carcinoma with periesophageal involvement, caustic damage of the esophagus, and esophageal perforation. Odynophagia is unusual in uncomplicated reflux esophagitis. Crampy chest pain associated with impaction of the small bowel should be distinguished from odynophagia.

Chest pain other than heartburn and odynophagia occurs when the esophageal muscle contracts with excessive force, for a long duration, and repetitively, as in diffuse esophageal spasm. This may occur spontaneously or during a meal. Chest pain due to periesophageal involvement caused by carcinoma or peptic ulcer may be constant and agonizing. Sometimes different types of esophageal pains exist together in the same patient, and frequently patients are not able to describe the pain accurately enough to allow its classification.

REGURGITATION Regurgitation is the effortless appearance of gastric or esophageal contents in the mouth. In distal esophageal obstruction and stasis, as in achalasia or a large diverticulum, the regurgitated material consists of tasteless mucoid fluid or undigested food. Regurgitation of sour or bitter-tasting material occurs in severe gastroesophageal reflux and is associated with incompetence of both the upper and lower esophageal sphincters. Regurgitation may result in laryngeal aspiration, with spells of coughing and choking that awaken the patient from sleep, and aspiration pneumonia. Water brash is reflex salivary hypersecretion which occurs in response to peptic esophagitis; it should not be confused with regurgitation.

DIAGNOSTIC TESTS

RADIOLOGIC STUDIES Barium swallow with fluoroscopy and esophogram is the most widely used test for diagnosis of esophageal disease and can be used to evaluate both structural and motor disorders. The pharynx is examined to detect stasis of barium in the valleculae and pyriform sinuses and regurgitation of barium into the nose and tracheobronchial tree. Since the pharyngeal phase of swallowing lasts no more than a second, cineradiography may be necessary to permit detection and analysis of abnormalities of pharyngeal function. Spontaneous reflux of barium from the stomach into the esophagus should be sought in patients with suspected reflux esophagitis. Esophageal peristalsis is best studied in the recumbent position since in the upright position the passage of most of the barium occurs by gravity alone. A double-contrast esophagram, obtained by coating the esophageal mucosa with barium and distending the esophageal lumen with air using effervescent granules, is particularly useful in demonstrating mucosal ulcers and early cancers. Figures 234-1 and 234-2 illustrate the radiographic appearance of some esophageal lesions.

ESOPHAGOSCOPY Fiberoptic esophagogastroduodenoscopy is described in Chap. 233. Esophagoscopy is the direct method of establishing the cause of mechanical dysphagia and of identifying mucosal lesions, such as superficial ulcers and esophagitis, which may not be identified by the usual barium swallow. In the presence of marked luminal narrowing, examination can be achieved by using a smaller caliber endoscope, although on occasion a stricture must be dilated prior to a complete endoscopic examination. Transendoscopic biopsies are useful in diagnosing carcinoma, reflux esophagitis, or other mucosal diseases. Obtaining cells by scraping the mucosa with a Teflon brush during endoscopy may enable the cytologist to detect carcinoma missed by mucosal biopsies.

ESOPHAGEAL MOTILITY The study of esophageal motility entails simultaneous recording of pressures from different sites in the esophageal lumen. This is usually done with a train of 3 to 4 water-filled catheters connected to pressure transducers. The assembly is passed by mouth or nose through the esophagus into the stomach and then gradually withdrawn 1 cm at a time until pressures from each centimeter of the esophagus and pharynx are recorded in between and during swallows. The upper and lower esophageal sphincters appear as zones of high pressure which relax on swallowing. The pharynx and esophageal body show peristaltic waves with each swallow.

Esophageal motility studies are very helpful in the diagnosis of achalasia, diffuse esophageal spasm and its variants, scleroderma, and other motor disorders of the esophagus, as well as neuromuscular disorders of the upper esophagus and pharynx (Fig. 234-3) but are of no value in the diagnosis of mechanical dysphagia. In patients with reflux esophagitis, esophageal manometry is useful in quantitating lower esophageal competence and providing information on the status of the esophageal body motor activity. The information obtained by manometry is quantitative and cannot be obtained by barium swallow or endoscopy.

Special tests for the evaluation of reflux esophagitis are described later.

MOTOR DISORDERS

STRIATED MUSCLE Pharyngeal paralysis Pharyngeal paralysis is characterized by dysphagia, nasal regurgitation, and tracheobron-

FIGURE 234-1 *Radiographic appearance of some motor disorders of the pharynx and esophagus. (1) Pharyngeal paralysis with tracheal aspiration (arrow). (2) Cricopharyngeal achalasia. Note the prominent cricopharyngeus which is recognized by its smoothness and location in the posterior wall. (3) Diffuse esophageal spasm. Note typical corkscrew appearance of the lower part of the esophagus. (4) Achalasia showing dilation of esophageal body with air fluid level and closed lower esophageal sphincter. (5) Muscular (contractile) lower esophageal ring. Note a nice symmetric contraction in 5A that has disappeared in 5B obtained during the same examination. (6) Scleroderma esophagus showing dilated esophagus with a stricture in 6A and reflux of barium from the stomach into the esophagus in 6B. (Courtesy of Dr. Harvey Goldstein.)*

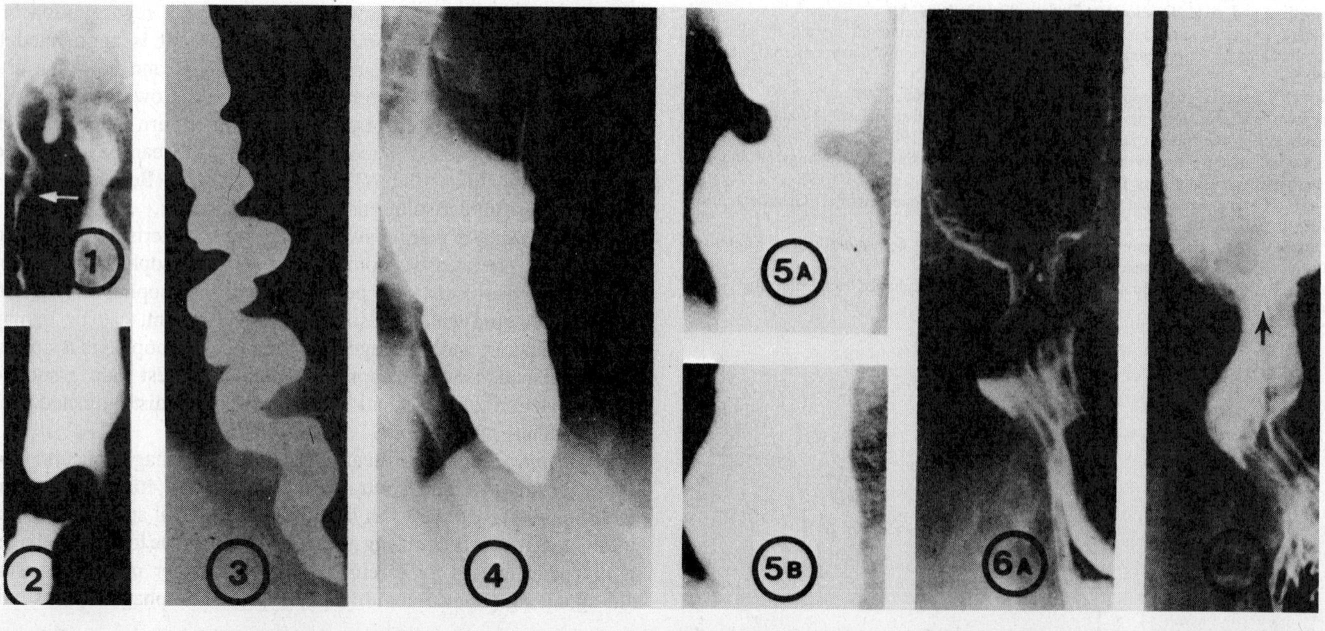

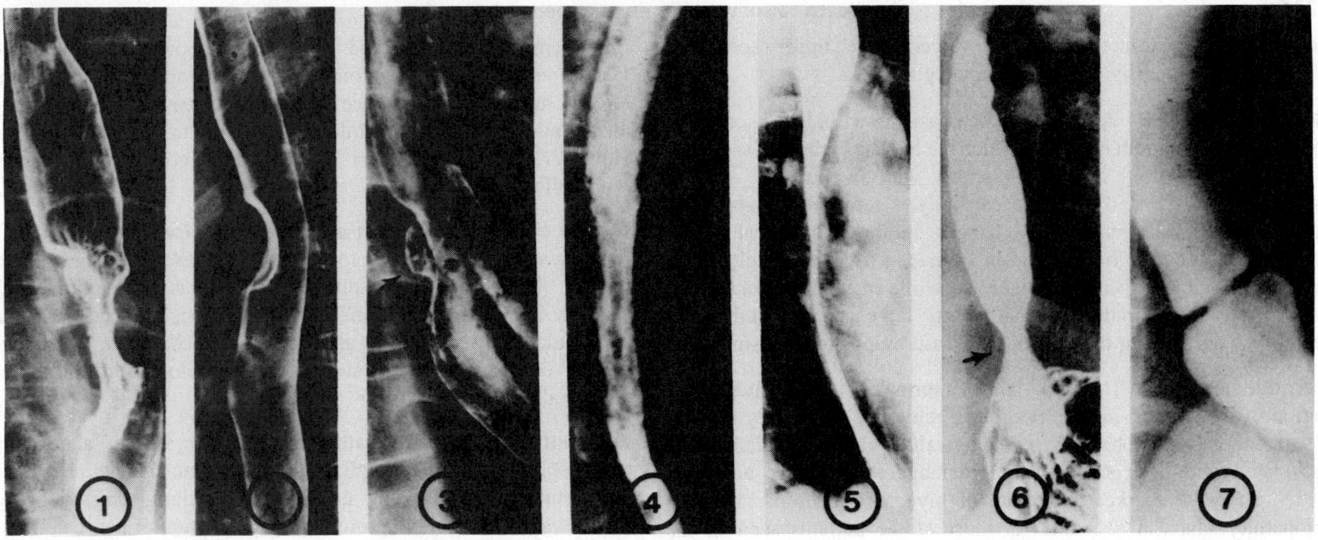

FIGURE 234-2 *Radiographic appearance of selected structural lesions of the esophagus. (1) Carcinoma of the esophagus. Note the typical annular narrowing with overhanging margins and destruction of the mucosa. (2) Leiomyoma of the esophagus. Note the smooth filling defect and right angles of origin from the esophageal wall. (3) Esophageal ulcer in columnar-cell-lined esophagus (Barrett's esophagus). (4) Monilial esophagitis. Note irregular plaquelike filling defects. (5) Long stricture secondary to lye ingestion. (6) Peptic stricture which is short and tubular. Note the associated hiatus hernia. (7) Mucosal lower esophageal mucosal (Schatzki) ring. Note a thin weblike annular constriction at the esophagogastric junction. It is associated with a small hiatal hernia. (Courtesy of Dr. Harvey Goldstein.)*

chial aspiration during swallowing. It occurs in a variety of neuromuscular disorders (see Table 32-2). Some of these disorders may also involve laryngeal and orofacial muscles. When the suprahyoid muscles are also paralyzed, the opening of the upper sphincter with swallowing is also impaired, causing severe dysphagia.

Barium swallow and cineradiography reveal stasis of barium in the valleculae and pyriform sinuses, nasal and tracheobronchial aspiration, and closed upper sphincter (Fig. 234-1). Pharyngeal motility studies demonstrate reduced amplitude of pharyngeal and upper esophageal contractions and reduced basal upper esophageal sphincter pressure without further relaxation on swallowing (Fig. 234-3). Patients with myasthenia gravis and polymyositis respond to treatment for these diseases (see Chap. 358). Dysphagia in patients with cerebrovascular accident improves with time, although not completely. Treatment in most instances is mainly supportive, consisting of nasogastric tube feeding and physiotherapy. Cricopharyngeal myotomy is sometimes performed but its usefulness is unproved. Extensive operative procedures to prevent aspiration are rarely needed. Death is often due to pulmonary complications.

Cricopharyngeal achalasia Failure of the cricopharyngeus to relax on swallowing leads to a contracted cricopharyngeus, which appears as a prominent bar on the posterior wall of the pharynx on barium swallow (Fig. 234-1). A transient cricopharyngeal bar is seen in up to 5 percent of subjects without dysphagia undergoing upper gastrointestinal studies; it can be produced in normal subjects during a Valsalva maneuver. When contraction is persistent, patients may complain of food sticking in their throats. Cricopharyngeal myotomy may be helpful, but it is contraindicated in the presence of gastroesophageal reflux because in such patients this procedure may lead to pharyngeal and pulmonary aspiration.

Globus hystericus A sensation of a constant lump in the throat but with no difficulty during swallowing occurs especially in subjects with emotional disorders, particularly in women. Barium studies are

FIGURE 234-3 *Motility patterns in selected esophageal and pharyngeal disorders. In normal subjects, the upper and lower esophageal sphincters appear as zones of high pressure. With a swallow (indicated by ↑), pressure in the sphincters falls and a contraction wave starts in the pharynx and progresses down the esophagus. In scleroderma, the lower part of the esophagus (smooth muscle) shows reduced amplitude of contractions, which may be peristaltic or simultaneous in onset, and hypotension of the lower sphincter. In achalasia, the lower part of the esophagus shows reduced amplitude of contractions that are simultaneous in onset. In contrast to scleroderma, the lower esophageal sphincter in achalasia is hypertensive and fails to relax in response to a swallow. In diffuse esophageal spasm, the lower part of the esophagus shows simultaneous onset, large amplitude, long duration, repetitive contractions. In polymyositis, the smooth-muscle part of the esophagus is normal. The skeletal muscle part shows reduced amplitude of contractions. The upper esophageal sphincter is hypotensive and may not relax normally on swallowing due to associated weakness of the suprahyoid muscles.*

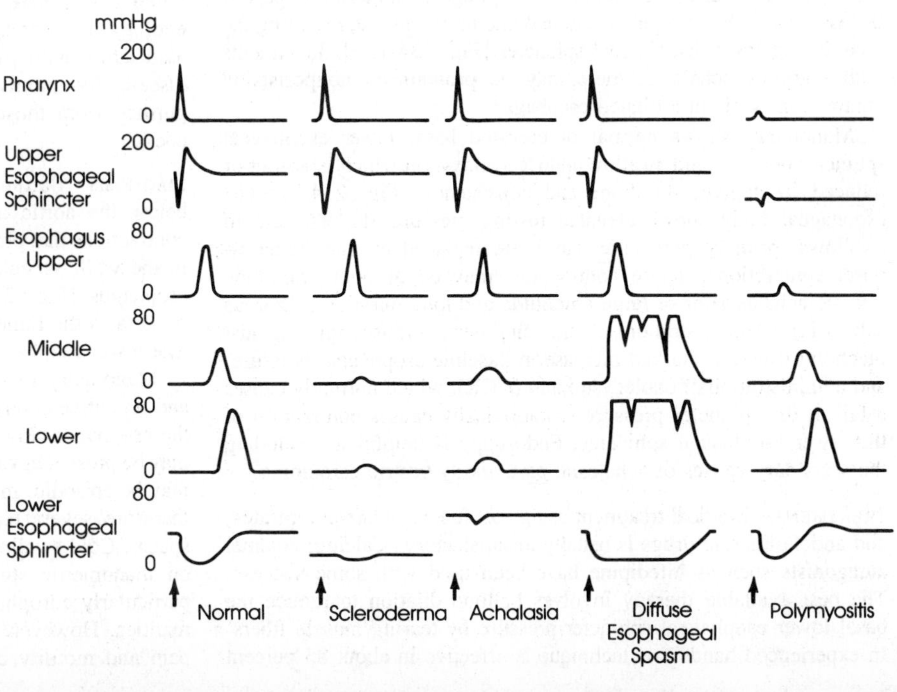

normal, but manometry shows a hypertensive upper sphincter. Treatment is primarily one of reassurance.

SMOOTH MUSCLE Achalasia Achalasia is a motor disorder of the esophageal smooth muscle in which the lower esophageal sphincter is hypertensive, does not relax properly with swallowing, and the normal peristalsis of the esophageal body is replaced by abnormal contractions. Based upon the changes in the esophageal body, achalasia can be of two types: in *classic achalasia* simultaneous contractions of small amplitude occur, while in *vigorous achalasia* contractions are simultaneous in onset, large in amplitude, and repetitive, resembling those seen in diffuse esophageal spasm.

PATHOPHYSIOLOGY The underlying abnormality is defective innervation of the smooth-muscle portion of the esophageal body and the lower esophageal sphincter. Pathologically, vigorous achalasia is associated with less severe neural damage than classic achalasia which shows a marked reduction in myenteric neurons. Primary idiopathic achalasia accounts for most of the patients seen in the United States. Secondary achalasia may be caused by gastric carcinoma infiltrating the esophagus, lymphoma, Chagas' disease, neuropathic chronic intestinal pseudoobstruction syndrome, irradiation, and certain toxins and drugs. Hypertensive or hypercontracting lower esophageal sphincter may be considered as variants of achalasia.

CLINICAL FEATURES Achalasia affects patients of all ages and both sexes. Dysphagia, chest pain, and regurgitation are the main symptoms. Dysphagia occurs early with both liquids and solids and is worsened by emotional stress and hurried eating. Various maneuvers designed to increase intraesophageal pressure, including the Valsalva, may help passage of the bolus into the stomach. Chest pain is more pronounced in vigorous achalasia than in classic achalasia. Regurgitation and pulmonary aspiration occur because of retention of large volumes of saliva and ingested food in the esophagus. The presence of gastroesophageal reflux argues against achalasia, although some of these patients may describe their chest pain as heartburn. The overall course is usually chronic with progressive dysphagia and weight loss over months to years.

DIAGNOSIS Chest x-ray shows absence of the gastric air bubble and sometimes a tubular mediastinal mass beside the aorta. The presence of an air-fluid level in the mediastinum in the upright position represents unpassed food in the esophagus and is characteristic. Barium swallow shows esophageal dilatation, and in advanced cases the esophagus may become sigmoid. On fluoroscopy normal peristalsis is lost in the lower two-thirds of the esophagus. The terminal part of the esophagus shows a persistent beaklike narrowing representing the nonrelaxing lower esophageal sphincter [Fig. 234-1(*2*)]. In patients with vigorous achalasia, there may be pronounced nonperistaltic contractions without a dilated esophagus.

Manometry shows normal or elevated basal lower esophageal sphincter pressure and swallow-induced relaxation which is absent or reduced in degree, duration, and consistency (Fig. 234-3). The esophageal body shows elevated resting pressure. In response to swallows, primary peristaltic waves are replaced by simultaneous-onset contractions. These contractions may be of poor amplitude (classic achalasia) or of large amplitude and long duration (vigorous achalasia). Administration of the cholinergic muscarinic agonist mecholyl causes a marked increase in baseline esophageal pressure, and administration of cholecystokinin (CCK), which normally causes a fall in the sphincter pressure, paradoxically causes contraction of the lower esophageal sphincter. Endoscopy is helpful in excluding the secondary causes of achalasia, particularly gastric carcinoma.

TREATMENT Medical treatment using soft foods, sedatives, nitrates, and anticholinergic drugs is usually unsatisfactory. Calcium channel antagonists such as nifedipine have been used with some success. The best available therapy involves balloon dilation to reduce the basal lower esophageal sphincter pressure by tearing muscle fibers. In experienced hands this technique is effective in about 85 percent of patients. Perforation and bleeding are potential complications. Heller's extramucosal myotomy of the lower sphincter, in which the circular muscle layer is incised, is equally effective. Reflux esophagitis and peptic stricture may follow successful treatment of achalasia. However, this complication is more frequent with myotomy than with balloon dilation.

Diffuse esophageal spasm and related motor disorders Diffuse esophageal spasm is a motor disorder of the esophageal smooth muscle characterized by multiple spontaneous contractions and by swallow-induced contractions that are of simultaneous onset, large amplitude, long duration, and repetitive occurrence. Variants of diffuse esophageal spasm show some but not all of these motor abnormalities.

PATHOPHYSIOLOGY The pathogenesis of the various abnormalities of peristalsis in diffuse esophageal spasm is not known. Histopathologic studies show patchy neural degeneration localized to nerve processes rather than the prominent degeneration of nerve cell bodies seen in achalasia.

Variants of diffuse esophageal spasm, such as large amplitude but peristaltic contractions (sometimes called nutcracker esophagus) or normal amplitude but simultaneous contractions, frequently occur as a primary disease or in association with a variety of diseases as well as emotional stress and aging. Collagen vascular disease, diabetic neuropathy, reflux esophagitis, irradiation esophagitis, esophageal obstruction, and cholinergic and anticholinergic drugs can cause esophageal motor abnormalities. The relationship between reflux esophagitis and motor abnormalities is controversial. Overlapping features of diffuse esophageal spasm and achalasia occur in vigorous achalasia. The variant syndromes are more frequent in clinical practice than classic diffuse esophageal spasm.

CLINICAL FEATURES The symptomatic patient with diffuse spasm or its variants presents with chest pain, dysphagia, or both. Chest pain is particularly marked in patients with esophageal contractions of large amplitude and of long duration. Chest pain usually occurs at rest but may be brought on by swallowing or by emotional stress. The pain is retrosternal; it may radiate to the back, sides of the chest, both arms, or the sides of the jaw and may last for a few seconds to several minutes. It may be acute and severe, mimicking the pain of myocardial ischemia. Dysphagia for solids and liquids may occur with or without chest pain.

Diffuse esophageal spasm must be differentiated from other causes of chest pain, particularly ischemic heart disease with atypical angina. Often a complete cardiac workup is done before the esophageal etiology is seriously considered. The presence of dysphagia in association with pain should point to the esophagus as the site of disease. Symptoms of esophageal spasm should be carefully distinguished from those of reflux esophagitis; sometimes the two may coexist.

DIAGNOSIS Barium swallow shows that normal sequential peristalsis below the aortic arch is replaced by uncoordinated simultaneous contractions that produce the appearance of curling or multiple ripples in the wall, sacculations, and pseudodiverticula—the "corkscrew" esophagus [Fig. 234-1(*3*)]. Sometimes an esophageal contraction obliterates the lumen and barium is pushed away in both directions. The lower esophageal sphincter opens normally.

Manometry reveals the characteristic prolonged large amplitude and repetitive contractions of simultaneous onset in the lower part of the esophagus (Fig. 234-3). Only one or two of these abnormalities may be present in variants of diffuse spasm. Because the abnormalities may be episodic, manometry may be normal at the time of the study; therefore, several techniques are used in attempt to provoke esophageal spasm. Cold swallows produce chest pain but do not produce spasm on manometric studies. Solid boluses and pharmacologic agents, particularly edrophonium, induce both chest pain and motor abnormalities. However, there is a poor correlation between induction of pain and motility changes. Ergonovine may cause coronary artery spasm and should not be used. Overall, the usefulness of pharmacologic provocative tests is limited.

TREATMENT Anticholinergics are usually of limited value because the main nerves that mediate esophageal contractions are noncholinergic. Agents which relax smooth muscle such as sublingual nitroglycerin (0.3 to 0.6 mg) or longer acting agents such as isosorbide dinitrate (2.5 to 10 mg sublingually before meals) and nifedipine (10 to 20 mg before meals) may be helpful in some cases. Esophageal dilation with mercury-filled rubber dilators may produce symptomatic relief as a result of distention of the lower esophagus, but this is largely a placebo effect. Reassurance and tranquilizers are helpful in allaying patients' apprehension. Balloon dilation is sometimes attempted but can be hazardous in inexperienced hands. In severe cases resistant to all therapy, a longitudinal myotomy of esophageal circular muscle is performed; it relieves pain in up to two-thirds of patients.

Scleroderma involving the esophagus The esophageal lesions in systemic sclerosis consist of muscular atrophy of the smooth-muscle portion, with weakness of contraction in the lower two-thirds of the esophageal body and incompetence of the lower esophageal sphincter. The esophageal wall is thin and atrophic with or without areas of patchy fibrosis. Patients present with dysphagia to solids and to liquids in the recumbent position. They may also present with heartburn and regurgitation due to gastroesophageal reflux and esophagitis, which in turn may lead to stricture formation and more pronounced dysphagia. Barium swallow shows dilation and loss of peristaltic contractions in the middle and distal portions of the esophagus. The lower esophageal sphincter is patulous, and gastroesophageal reflux may occur freely (Fig. 234-1). Mucosal changes from esophageal ulceration may be detected, and esophageal stricture may be present. Motility studies show marked reduction in the amplitude of smooth-muscle contractions, which may be peristaltic or nonperistaltic. Lower esophageal sphincter resting pressure is subnormal, but relaxation is normal (Fig. 234-3). Currently, there is no effective treatment for the motor difficulty. Reflux esophagitis and its complications should be treated aggressively as described under reflux esophagitis.

INFLAMMATORY DISORDERS

GASTROESOPHAGEAL REFLUX AND ESOPHAGITIS Reflux esophagitis consists of esophageal mucosal damage resulting from reflux of gastric or intestinal contents into the esophagus. Depending on the causative agent, it is referred to as peptic, bile, or alkaline esophagitis.

Pathophysiology Three considerations involved in the pathophysiology of reflux esophagitis are (1) the pathogenesis of the esophageal reflux episode, (2) the cumulative, or net, esophageal reflux, and (3) the pathogenesis of esophagitis.

Two conditions must be met for a *reflux episode* to occur: the gastrointestinal contents must be "ready" to reflux, and the antireflux mechanism at the lower end of the esophagus must be compromised. Gastrointestinal contents are most likely to reflux (1) when gastric volume is increased (after meals, with pyloric obstruction or gastric stasis syndrome, and in acid hypersecretory states), (2) when the gastric contents are located near the gastroesophageal junction (due to recumbency or bending), and (3) when gastric pressure is increased (with obesity, pregnancy, ascites, or tight binders or girdles).

The normal antireflux mechanisms consist of the lower esophageal sphincter (LES) and the anatomic configuration of the gastroesophageal junction. Reflux occurs only when the LES–gastric pressure gradient is lost. It can be caused by increased intragastric pressure or a transient or sustained decrease in the sphincter tone itself. Most patients with reflux have lower than normal LES pressures. The incompetence of the LES may be primary or secondary. The secondary causes include scleroderma-like diseases, a myopathic type of chronic intestinal pseudoobstruction syndrome, pregnancy, female sex hormones, smoking, smooth-muscle relaxants (such as beta-adrenergics, aminophylline, nitrates, and calcium channel blockers), destruction of the sphincter by surgical resection, myotomy or balloon dilation, and esophagitis. Some patients have normal lower esophageal sphincter pressures but their sphincter relaxes inappropriately, allowing reflux to occur. The importance of the anatomic configuration of the esophagogastric junction is not fully known at present. However, the role of a sliding hiatal hernia in the impairment of the reflux barrier is not felt to be so important as was once thought.

The net or *cumulative esophageal reflux*, i.e., the amount and duration of refluxed material remaining in the esophagus, is dependent on (1) the amount of refluxed material per episode and frequency of episodes, (2) the clearing of the esophagus by gravity and peristaltic contraction, and (3) neutralization by salivary secretion.

Esophagitis is a complication of reflux, and it develops when the mucosal defenses that normally counteract the effect of injurious agents on the esophageal mucosa succumb to the onslaught of the refluxed acid pepsin or bile. *Histologic esophagitis* shows microscopic changes of mucosal infiltration with granulocytes or eosinophils, hyperplasia of basal cells, and elongation of dermal pegs. It can occur with or without endoscopic abnormalities. *Erosive esophagitis* shows endoscopically visible damage to the mucosa in the form of marked redness, friability, bleeding, superficial linear ulcers, and exudates. *Peptic stricture* results from fibrosis that causes constriction of the esophageal lumen. The fibrosis is predominantly submucosal, but it may involve the whole wall. Peptic strictures occur in about 10 percent of patients with reflux esophagitis. Short peptic strictures caused by spontaneous reflux are usually 1 to 3 cm long and are present in the distal esophagus near the squamocolumnar junction (Fig. 234-2). Long and tubular peptic strictures are the result of persistent vomiting or prolonged nasogastric intubation. Replacement of the squamous epithelium of the esophagus by columnar epithelium *(Barrett's esophagus)* may also result from reflux esophagitis. Columnar-cell-lined esophagus may be further complicated by peptic ulcer or peptic stricture high up in the lower or midesophagus, and adenocarcinoma in 2 to 5 percent.

Clinical features Heartburn is the characteristic symptom and is produced by the contact of refluxed material with the inflamed esophageal mucosa. However, this symptom may be absent in some patients. Dysphagia suggests development of peptic stricture. In peptic strictures, the usual history is of several years of heartburn preceding dysphagia. However, in one-third of patients dysphagia may be the presenting symptom. Progressive dysphagia and weight loss may indicate development of adenocarcinoma in Barrett's esophagus. Bleeding occurs due to mucosal erosions or Barrett's ulcer. Reflux in the absence of esophagitis is usually asymptomatic. Severe reflux may reach the pharynx and mouth and result in laryngitis, morning hoarseness, and pulmonary aspiration. Recurrent pulmonary aspiration can cause aspiration pneumonia, pulmonary fibrosis, or chronic asthma.

Diagnosis Evaluation of reflux esophagitis is designed to assess the presence and severity of reflux, nature of refluxant, presence and severity of esophagitis, and pathophysiology of reflux. History, barium swallow, esophagoscopy, mucosal biopsy, esophageal motility, and a variety of special tests are utilized.

The *presence of reflux* is suggested by history. Spontaneous reflux from the stomach into the esophagus on barium examination suggests advanced reflux. Reflux of barium induced by stressful maneuvers is not very helpful, however, because of a high incidence of false-positive and false-negative results. Recently, scintiscan using radiolabeled technetium 99m sulfur colloid has been used to quantitate gastroesophageal reflux. Several tests that utilize the recording of esophageal luminal pH with a small pH electrode have been proposed to detect and quantitate reflux of gastric acid. In these tests the pH electrode is swallowed, positioned in the stomach, gradually withdrawn across the LES, and then fixed at 5 cm above the sphincter. In the standard acid reflux test, a diagnosis of reflux can be made by failure of the pH to rise as the electrode enters the esophagus and by a decrease in esophageal pH with straining maneuvers. Quantitative information on the acid reflux is obtained by long-term (24-h) esophageal pH recording. The pH recordings are helpful only in the evaluation of acid reflux. The presence of bile or alkaline reflux is suggested by the occurrence of reflux symptoms in the absence of gastric acid and by the demonstration of bile in the aspirate of esophageal reflux.

The *presence and complications of reflux esophagitis* are assessed by barium swallow, esophagoscopy, mucosal biopsy, and the Bernstein test. Barium swallow is usually normal in uncomplicated esophagitis but may reveal the complication of stricture or ulcer formation. A high esophageal peptic stricture, deep ulcer, and adenocarcinoma suggest complications of Barrett's esophagus. Uncomplicated Barrett's esophagus is not diagnosed by barium studies. Esophagoscopy may reveal the presence of erosive esophagitis, distal peptic stricture, or columnar-cell-lined lower esophagus with or without a proximally located peptic stricture, ulcer, or adenocarcinoma. Esophagoscopy may be normal in many patients with esophagitis; in such patients mucosal biopsies and Bernstein tests are helpful. The mucosal biopsies should be obtained 5 cm above the LES because in the distal esophagus mucosal changes are quite frequent in normal subjects. False-positive and false-negative results occur in approximately 10 percent of biopsies. Patients with Barrett's esophagus will show columnar mucosa lining the esophagus which may be of gastric fundic, cardiac, or specialized type. The Bernstein test consists of an infusion of solutions of 0.1 *N* HCl and normal saline into the esophagus. It is useful in diagnosing reflux esophagitis which is not endoscopically obvious. In patients with reflux esophagitis, infusion of acid, but not of saline, reproduces the symptoms of heartburn. Infusion of acid in normal subjects produces no symptoms. Reflux esophagitis should be included in the differential diagnosis of chest pain, esophagitis, upper gastrointestinal bleeding, and dysphagia.

The *causative and predisposing factors* are assessed by history, esophageal motility, and esophageal clearance studies. Esophageal motility studies may provide useful quantitative information on the competence of the LES and of esophageal motor function. Barium swallow and scintiscans can be used to study esophageal clearance. An esophageal acid clearance test using a pH electrode quantifies the number of swallows necessary to clear the esophagus of 10 mL of instilled dilute 0.1 *N* HCl.

Full diagnostic evaluation is not necessary in every patient with reflux esophagitis. In transient and mild cases with a clear-cut history of reflux esophagitis, a therapeutic trial may be sufficient. In persistent cases, and in those in whom the diagnosis is not clear, barium swallow, esophagoscopy, and esophageal motility with pH monitoring are indicated.

Treatment The main principle of treatment is neutralization of the offending material (by antacids and H_2-receptor antagonists in peptic esophagitis, and by cholestyramine and aluminum hydroxide in bile esophagitis). In general, management of uncomplicated cases includes weight reduction, sleeping on a bed with elevation of the head of the bed, antacids (80 meq 1 and 3 h after meals), cimetidine (300 mg at bedtime), elimination of factors that increase abdominal pressure, and avoidance of smoking and harmful medications. Patients should avoid fatty foods, coffee, chocolate, alcohol, mint, orange juice, and any other foods they find that exacerbate their symptoms. Anticholinergic drugs should not be used since they may reduce LES pressure and impair esophageal clearance.

In moderate to severe cases, the above measures are more strictly enforced, particularly elevation of the head end of the bed usually by 6 to 8 in. Cimetidine, 300 mg qid, may be added. Long-acting H_2-receptor antagonists, such as ranitidine, may be more convenient to use. In the case of bile esophagitis, cholestyramine or aluminum hydroxide antacid is used. If the patient does not fully respond, metoclopramide (10 mg qid) or bethanecol (25 mg qid) can be prescribed to raise sphincter pressure, hasten gastric emptying, and improve esophageal clearance. Their usefulness, however, is limited. Coating agents such as sucralfate are useful in some cases. Patients with reflux esophagitis with complications such as Barrett's esophagus with or without deep ulcer should be vigorously treated. Patients who have an associated peptic stricture are treated with dilators to relieve dysphagia in addition to vigorous treatment for reflux.

Antireflux surgery (Belsey repair, Nisson's fundoplication, and Hill repair), in which the gastric fundus is wrapped around the esophagus, increases the lower sphincter pressure and should be considered in resistant and complicated cases of reflux esophagitis that do not fully respond to medical therapy and in which there is persistently inadequate lower sphincter pressure but normal peristaltic contractions in the esophageal body.

Close follow-up is indicated in patients with complications of Barrett's esophagus because some of them may develop adenocarcinoma.

VIRAL ESOPHAGITIS (See also Chap. 136) *Herpes simplex virus* may be normally present in saliva and may cause esophagitis in patients who are debilitated and immunosuppressed. These patients complain of the acute onset of odynophagia and dysphagia. Bleeding may occur in severe cases, and systemic manifestations such as fever, chills, and mild leukocytosis may be present. Herpes blisters on the lips provide a clue to the diagnosis. Endoscopy shows vesicles and small, discrete, punched-out superficial ulcerations with or without fibrinous exudate. In later stages of the disease there is diffuse erosive esophagitis caused by enlargement and coalescence of the ulcers. Mucosal cells from biopsy of the edge of an ulcer show ballooning degeneration, ground-glass change in the nuclei with eosinophilic intranuclear inclusions (Cowdry type A), and giant-cell formation. These changes may also be detected in cytologic specimens. Culture of the tissue for herpes simplex virus is required for definitive diagnosis. Examination of serial serum specimens for rising titers of complement-fixing antibodies to herpes simplex type I is helpful in diagnosis. Acyclovir (200 mg qid orally or 5 mg every 8 h intravenously) is the treatment of choice. *Cytomegalovirus* (CMV) can also cause ulcerative esophagitis in immunosuppressed patients. The CMV ulcers usually occur within normal-appearing mucosa. The CMV inclusions have a deeper submucosal location and are best diagnosed on a large biopsy. There is no good treatment for CMV infection.

***CANDIDA* (MONILIAL) ESOPHAGITIS** Many *Candida* species are normal inhabitants of the throat but become pathogenic and produce esophagitis in the setting of malignant neoplasms (particularly lymphoma and leukemia); treatment with immunosuppressive agents, steroids, and broad-spectrum antibiotics; diabetes mellitus; hypoparathyroidism; systemic lupus erythematosus; hemoglobinopathy; and corrosive esophageal injury. Occasionally, monilial esophagitis occurs in the absence of any of the above predisposing factors. Patients may be asymptomatic or complain of odynophagia and dysphagia. Oral thrush or other evidence of mucocutaneous moniliasis may be absent. Systemic invasion with *Monilia* may occur.

Barium swallow may be normal or may show multiple nodular filling defects of various sizes (Fig. 234-2). Large nodular defects may resemble clusters of grapes. Endoscopy shows small yellow-white raised plaques with surrounding erythema in mild disease. In extensive disease, confluent linear and nodular plaques are seen. Diagnosis is made by demonstration of yeast or hyphal forms in the plaques using 10% KOH. Biopsies are not always positive. Culture is helpful in confirming the species and, if needed, the drug sensitivities of the yeast (see Chap. 147).

Nystatin oral suspension (100,000 units per milliliter) in doses of 4 to 6 mL every 4 h) has been used. The current treatment of choice is ketoconazole (200 to 400 mg in a single oral daily dose). In poorly responsive patients, treatment is amphotericin B (10 to 15 mg as intravenous infusion over 6 h, daily for a total dose of 300 to 500 mg).

OTHER TYPES OF ESOPHAGITIS *Irradiation esophagitis* is a common occurrence during radiation treatment for lung, mediastinal, or esophageal carcinoma. The frequency of esophagitis increases with the amount of radiation to the area. Dysphagia and odynophagia are the main symptoms and may last several weeks to several months after the conclusion of therapy. The esophageal mucosa becomes erythematous, edematous, and friable. Superficial erosions coalesce to form larger superficial ulcers. Submucosal fibrosis and degenerative changes in the blood vessels, muscles, and myenteric neurons may be present. The treatment is relief of pain with viscous lidocaine. Esophageal stricture may develop, causing severe dysphagia. Strictures are treated by dilation with rubber dilators. *Corrosive esophagitis* occurs following ingestion of caustic agents, such as strong alkalis, or acids. When severe, corrosive injury may lead to esophageal perforation, bleeding, and death. Healing is usually associated with stricture formation. Caustic strictures are usually long and rigid (Fig. 234-2). They can be dilated by passing a metal dilator of increasing diameter over a guide-wire through the stricture. *Pill-induced esophagitis* is associated with the ingestion of certain pills and now accounts for many cases of errosive esophagitis. Antibiotics account for over half of the patients with pill-induced esophageal injury; the most commonly incriminated has been doxycycline. Other commonly prescribed pills which cause esophageal injury include potassium chloride, ferrous sulfate, quinidine, and various steroidal and nonsteroidal anti-inflammatory agents. *Esophagitis associated with mucocutaneous disease* occurs in epidermolysis bullosa, pemphigoid, Behçet's syndrome, and Stevens-Johnson syndrome. Esophageal involvement in these disorders is indicated by development of odynophagia and dysphagia. Esophageal involvement responds to treatment of primary conditions.

TUMORS OF THE ESOPHAGUS

BENIGN TUMORS Benign tumors of the esophagus account for less than 10 percent of all esophageal tumors. The majority of benign esophageal tumors present as intramural lesions. Among them, leiomyoma accounts for 80 percent, esophageal cysts 10 percent, and all others 10 percent. Benign tumors presenting as an intraluminal mass are rare; almost 80 percent of them are fibrovascular polyps, 10 percent are papillomas, and the rest include all other types. These tumors are frequently asymptomatic, although dysphagia occurs in a few patients when the esophageal lumen is severely compromised. Benign tumors must be distinguished from malignant tumors, although often this distinction cannot be made with certainty prior to surgical removal. Endoscopic mucosal biopsies are not helpful in the diagnosis of submucosal tumors.

MALIGNANT TUMORS The primary malignant tumors of the esophagus are squamous-cell carcinoma (90 percent) and adenocarcinoma (less than 10 percent). Adenocarcinomas usually arise from metaplastic columnar epithelium (Barrett's esophagus) but may rarely arise from esophageal glands. Other uncommon tumors include carcinosarcoma, pseudosarcoma, melanoma, and verrucous squamous-cell carcinoma. In addition, adenocarcinoma of the stomach may spread to the esophagus by direct extension. Local spread from carcinoma of the lung or thyroid is unusual. Metastatic lesions from malignancies of remote organs are rare. Esophageal involvement may occur in up to 25 percent of patients with lymphoma, although symptomatic esophageal involvement occurs in less than 5 percent of these patients.

Squamous-cell carcinoma Squamous-cell carcinoma of the esophagus is the fifth most common cancer in adult males. A unique feature of this tumor is a marked geographic variation with a very high incidence (greater than 35 per 100,000 people per year) in certain regions of China, Iran, and Russia. In the United States the white population is at lower risk than blacks. Throughout the world the incidence increases with age, with males at greater risk than females.

Alcohol and smoking are important predisposing factors in the United States. Esophageal tumors may occur with higher frequency in association with carcinoma of the head and neck, lye strictures, ionizing radiation exposure, achalasia, Plummer-Vinson syndrome, and tylosis, a rare genetic disease in which the skin of the hands and feet is thickened.

CLINICAL FEATURES Progressive dysphagia and weight loss of short duration are characteristic. Dysphagia begins with solid foods and gradually progresses to include semisolids and liquids. In eccentric tumors and those arising from the stomach, dysphagia may be mild and may not occur until late in the disease. Dysphagia is rarely present for more than 1 year. Chest pain occurs as the tumor spreads to periesophageal tissues. Weight loss is usually profound because of anorexia and dysphagia. Bleeding from the tumor is usually slow, but brisk bleeding may occur. Rarely, invasion of the tumor into the aorta causes rapid exsanguination. Pulmonary aspiration, pneumonia, and, rarely, lung abscess can result from esophageal obstruction and aspiration or from tracheoesophageal fistula. Hoarseness may result from recurrent laryngeal nerve involvement. Physical examination is usually not striking except for evidence of recent weight loss. Supraclavicular nodes and an enlarged liver may be found when the tumor has spread to these sites. Signs of pulmonary aspiration may be present. Hypercalcemia may result from tumor production of a parathyroid hormone-like substance.

DIAGNOSIS The disease is usually advanced when the diagnosis is first made, and early detection is unusual. Carcinoma must be excluded by careful workup in all patients with persistent dysphagia and/or weight loss of short duration. Patients with gastric carcinoma involving the terminal esophagus may present with symptoms suggestive of reflux esophagitis, while others may have what appears to be achalasia or diffuse esophageal spasm. Recent development of any such symptoms in subjects over 40 years old should be carefully investigated.

The esophogram is the mainstay of diagnosis. Adequate esophageal distention and multiple views may be needed to diagnose early lesions. Double-contrast studies may also be helpful. An ulcerating lesion should be distinguished from a peptic ulcer in the columnar-cell-lined esophagus. Any esophageal ulcer that occurs without associated columnar-cell-lined esophagus should be considered carcinoma until proved otherwise. An infiltrating lesion may resemble a peptic stricture or may produce a picture resembling achalasia. Polypoid lesions should be distinguished from various benign neoplasms and from other types of carcinoma.

Endoscopy should be performed in all patients to detect suspected cases that may be missed on barium studies and to obtain tissue confirmation of cases that have been diagnosed on x-ray. Multiple biopsies and brush cytologies should be obtained. A thorough examination of the fundus of the stomach by turning the endoscope back on itself is imperative in all cases.

Computerized tomography has been helpful in determining extraesophageal spread to mediastinal structures and paraaortic abdominal lymph nodes.

TREATMENT The prognosis of esophageal carcinoma is poor; the 5-year survival rate is less than 5 percent, regardless of therapy. Curative surgical resection and anastomosis using gastric tube reconstruction and colonic or jejunal interposition is possible particularly in those with disease of the lower third of the esophagus. This is usually combined with radiation therapy [40 to 60 Gy (4000 to 6000 rad)] and/or chemotherapy. In over 60 percent of the patients palliative therapy alone is possible. This may include a surgical bypass procedure or more conservative methods to maintain esophageal luminal patency such as laser curettage, dilation, and sometimes insertion of a prosthesis. These measures are combined with palliative radiation and/or chemotherapy to shrink the tumor.

OTHER ESOPHAGEAL DISORDERS

PHARYNGEAL AND ESOPHAGEAL DIVERTICULA Diverticula are outpouchings of the wall of the esophagus. *Zenker's diverticula* appear in the natural weakness in the posterior hypopharyngeal wall and cause halitosis and regurgitation of saliva and food particles consumed several days previously. When they become large and filled with food, they may compress the esophagus and cause dysphagia or complete obstruction. *Midesophageal diverticula* may be caused by traction from old adhesions or by propulsion associated with esophageal motor abnormalities. *Epiphrenic diverticula* may be associated with achalasia. Small- or medium-sized diverticula and midesophageal and epiphrenic diverticula are usually asymptomatic. *Diffuse intramural diverticulosis* of the esophagus is due to dilation of the deep esophageal glands. This may lead to chronic candidiasis or a stricture high up in the esophagus. These patients may present with dysphagia.

Symptomatic Zenker's diverticula are treated by cricopharyngeal myotomy with or without diverticulectomy. Very large symptomatic esophageal diverticula are removed surgically. When they are associated with motor abnormalities, distal myotomy is performed. Stricture associated with diffuse intramural diverticulosis is treated with rubber dilators.

ESOPHAGEAL WEBS Weblike constrictions of the esophagus are usually congenital but may be acquired. Asymptomatic hypopharyngeal webs are demonstrated in up to 10 percent of normal individuals. When concentric, they cause intermittent dysphagia to solids. Symptomatic hypopharyngeal webs with iron-deficiency anemia in middle-aged women constitute Plummer-Vinson syndrome. The clinical importance of this syndrome is uncertain. Midesophageal webs are rare. Symptomatic webs are treated by rupture of the web with a rubber dilator.

LOWER ESOPHAGEAL RINGS Lower esophageal *mucosal ring* (Schatzki ring) is a thin weblike constriction located at the squamocolumnar mucosal junction at or near the border of the lower esophageal sphincter (Fig. 234-2). It invariably produces dysphagia when the diameter is less than 1.3 cm. The dysphagia to solids is the only symptom and it is usually episodic. Asymptomatic rings may be present in about 10 percent of normal individuals. Lower esophageal ring is one of the common causes of dysphagia. Treatment is simple rupture of the ring with a large-diameter rubber dilator.

Lower esophageal *muscular ring* (contractile ring) is located proximal to the site of mucosal rings and may represent the abnormal uppermost segment of the lower esophageal sphincter. These rings are characterized by a change in size and shape from one time to another (Fig. 234-1). They may also cause dysphagia and should be differentiated from peptic strictures, achalasia, and lower esophageal mucosal rings. They are treated with rubber dilators.

HIATAL HERNIA Hiatal hernia is a herniation of a part of the stomach into the thoracic cavity through the esophageal hiatus in the diaphragm. A *sliding hiatal hernia* is one in which the gastroesophageal junction and fundus of the stomach slide upward. A sliding hernia may result from weakening of the anchors of the gastroesophageal junction to the diaphragm, longitudinal contraction of the esophagus, or increased intraabdominal pressure. Small sliding hernias can be demonstrated commonly during barium studies if intraabdominal pressure is increased. Their incidence increases with age; in the sixth decade of life the prevalence of such hernias is around 60 percent. It is unlikely that a small sliding hiatal hernia by itself produces any clinical symptoms, and its role in the pathogenesis of reflux esophagitis is uncertain.

A *paraesophageal* hernia is one in which the esophagogastric junction remains fixed in its normal location and a pouch of stomach herniates beside the gastroesophageal junction through the esophageal hiatus. A paraesophageal or mixed paraesophageal and sliding hernia may become incarcerated and strangulate. This situation is manifested by acute chest pain, dysphagia, and a mediastinal mass, and requires prompt operative treatment. A herniated gastric pouch may cause dysphagia and may be the site of gastritis and ulceration causing chronic blood loss. A large paraesophageal hernia should be repaired because of a high rate of complications.

ESOPHAGEAL RUPTURE Perforation of the esophagus may be caused by (1) iatrogenic damage from instrumentation of the esophagus or external trauma; (2) increased intraesophageal pressure associated with forceful vomiting or retching (this is also called spontaneous rupture or Boerhaave's syndrome); or (3) diseases of the esophagus such as corrosive ingestion, peptic ulcer, neoplasm, and, rarely, esophagomalacia. The site of perforation is variable and depends on the cause. Instrumental perforation usually occurs in the pharynx or in the lower esophagus. The esophageal perforation often occurs just above the diaphragm in the posterolateral wall.

Esophageal perforation causes severe retrosternal chest pain which may be worsened by swallowing. Free air enters the mediastinum and spreads to neighboring structures and causes palpable subcutaneous emphysema in the neck, mediastinal crackling sounds on auscultation, and pneumothorax. Pleural effusion and hydropneumothorax may ensue, and severe cases are associated with shock. With time, secondary infection supervenes, and mediastinal abscess and pleuropulmonary suppurative complications may develop. Esophageal perforation associated with vomiting usually deposits gastric contents in the mediastinum and causes severe mediastinal complications. On the other hand, instrumental perforation may be mild and free of severe complications.

Spontaneous rupture of the esophagus may mimic myocardial infarction, pancreatitis, or ruptured abdominal viscus. Symptoms of chest pain may be mild, particularly in the elderly. Mediastinal emphysema may develop late. X-ray of the chest shows abnormalities in the majority of patients, and diagnosis is confirmed by swallow of radiopaque contrast material.

Treatment includes esophageal and gastric suction and parenteral broad-spectrum antibiotics. Surgical drainage and repair of the laceration should be performed as soon as possible. In patients with terminal carcinoma, surgical repair may not be feasible, and those with minor instrumental perforations can be treated conservatively. Extensive corrosive damage may require esophageal diversion and subsequent excision of the damaged portion of the esophagus.

MALLORY-WEISS SYNDROME Vomiting and retching may cause a tear that involves only the mucosa and is not transmural. The tear usually involves the gastric mucosa near the squamocolumnar mucosal junction, but it may also involve the esophageal mucosa. Patients present with upper gastrointestinal bleeding which may be severe. Most patients recover with only conservative management, but those with severe arterial bleeding require surgery.

FOREIGN BODIES Foreign bodies may lodge in the cervical esophagus just beyond the upper esophageal sphincter, around the aortic arch, or above the lower esophageal sphincter. Impaction of a bolus of food, particularly a piece of meat or bread, may occur when the esophageal lumen is narrowed due to stricture, carcinoma, or a lower esophageal ring. Acute impaction causes complete inability to swallow and severe chest pain. Both foreign bodies and food boluses may be removed endoscopically. Use of meat tenderizer to facilitate passage of an obstructed meat bolus is to be discouraged because of potential esophageal perforation and aspiration pneumonia.

REFERENCES

CAMERON AJ et al: The incidence of adenocarcinoma in columnar lined (Barrett's) esophagus. N Engl J Med 313:857, 1985

CASTELL DO: Gastroesophageal reflux: Pathogenesis, diagnosis, therapy. Ann Intern Med 97:93, 1982

DEMEESTER TR et al: Esophageal function in patients with angina-like chest pain and normal coronary angiograms. Ann Surg 196:488, 1982

DODDS WJH et al: Mechanism of gastroesophageal reflux in patients with reflux esophagitis. N Engl J Med 307:1547, 1982

FLEISER D, KESSLER F: Endoscopic YAG laser therapy for carcinoma of the esophagus: A new form of palliative treatment. Gastroenterology 85:600, 1983
GELFORD M et al: Isosorbide dinitrate and nifedipine treatment of achalasia: A chemical, manometric and radionuclide evaluation. Gastroenterology 83:963, 1982
GOYAL RK: Disorders of the circopharyngeus muscle. Otolaryngol Clin North Am 17:115, 1984
KELSEN D: Chemotherapy of esophageal cancer. Semin Oncol 11:159, 1984
KIKENDALL JW et al: Pill-induced esophageal injury—case reports and review of the medical literature. Dig Dis Sci 28:174, 1983
LEICHMAN L et al: Properative chemotherapy and radiation therapy for patients with cancer of the esophagus: A potentially curative approach. J Clin Oncol 2:75, 1984
MCDONALD GB et al: Esophageal infections in immunosuppressed patients after marrow transplantation. Gastroenterology 88:1111, 1985
SPECHLER SJ, GOYAL RK: *Barrett's Esophagus: Pathophysiology, Diagnosis and Treatment*. New York, Elsevier, 1985
TRIER JS, BJORKMAN DJ: Esophageal, gastric and intestinal candidiasis. Am J Med 77:39, 1984
VANTRAPPEN G, HELLEMANS J: Treatment of achalasia and related motor disorders. Gastroenterology 79:144, 1980

235 PEPTIC ULCER

JAMES E. McGUIGAN

The term *peptic ulcer* is used to refer to a group of ulcerative disorders of the upper gastrointestinal tract which appear to have in common the participation of acid-pepsin in their pathogenesis. The major forms of peptic ulcer are chronic duodenal and gastric ulcer. The Zollinger-Ellison syndrome, which is caused by gastrin-releasing tumors (gastrinomas), may also be considered a form of peptic ulcer.

Although our present knowledge of the etiology of peptic ulcer is incomplete, information from studies in humans and in experimental animals indicates that acid-pepsin is crucial for development of peptic ulcer. The presence or absence of peptic ulcer is determined by the delicate interplay between aggressive factors (secreted gastric acid and pepsin) and defensive factors (mucosal resistance). Peptic ulcer is produced when the aggressive effects of acid-pepsin dominate the protective effects of gastric or duodenal mucosal resistance. Why do not all humans develop peptic ulcer? The normal capacity of gastric and proximal duodenal mucosa to resist the corrosive effects of acid-pepsin is extraordinary and unique. This resistance to acid-pepsin is not shared by other tissues—hence the susceptibility of the esophageal mucosa to injury when exposed to refluxed gastric juice and the frequent ulceration of the small intestine at the site of surgical attachment to actively secreting gastric mucosa.

Much has been learned concerning the mechanisms regulating gastric secretion and about a variety of factors which appear important in the development of peptic ulcer. Consideration of gastric physiology provides an understanding of some elements responsible for producing peptic ulcer as well as a rational basis for its treatment.

GASTRIC PHYSIOLOGY RELATED TO PEPTIC ULCER

The gastric mucosa possesses an extraordinary capacity to secrete acid. Parietal (oxyntic) cells secrete hydrochloric acid by a process involving oxidative phosphorylation. Parietal cells, located in mucosal glands in the body and fundus of the stomach, can secrete hydrogen ions at a concentration 3 million times that found in blood. Hydrogen ions are secreted into the gastric lumen by a proton pump mechanism involving a specific hydrogen–potassium adenosine triphosphatase (H^+,K^+-ATPase) located on the microvilli of the secretory canaliculi of the parietal cells. The estimated concentration of HCl secreted directly by parietal cells is approximately 160 m*M*. Each secreted hydrogen ion (H^+) is accompanied by a chloride ion (Cl^-). With increased gastric hydrogen ion secretion, there is a reciprocal decrease in sodium ion secretion. For each hydrogen ion secreted into the gastric lumen, one bicarbonate ion (HCO_3^-) is returned via the gastric venous circulation, accounting for the *alkaline tide,* which reflects directly the magnitude of gastric H^+ secretion. Bicarbonate is released from carbonic acid; the latter is generated from carbon dioxide by parietal cell carbonic anhydrase. The two-component hypothesis for secretion of gastric juice proposes that parietal cells secrete pure HCl, which is mixed (in various proportions) with nonparietal cell alkaline secretions, similar in ionic composition to extracellular fluid.

Multiple *chemical, neural,* and *hormonal* factors participate in regulation of gastric acid secretion. Acid secretion is stimulated by gastrin and by cholinergic postganglionic vagal fibers via muscarinic receptors on parietal cells. Gastrin, the most potent known stimulant of gastric acid secretion, is present in cytoplasmic secretory granules in gastrin cells (or G cells) which are interspersed singly or in small clusters among other epithelial cells principally in the mid and deeper portions of the antral pyloric glands. Gastrin, as most, if not all, the gastrointestinal regulatory peptides, is present in multiple molecular forms (Fig. 235-1). The major form of tissue gastrin is heptadecapeptide gastrin (G-17) which contains 17 amino acid residues. Gastrin II is the form of gastrin in which the tyrosyl residue at position 12 is sulfated, and gastrin I is the nonsulfated form. Approximately two-thirds of circulating serum gastrin consists of a larger molecular species of gastrin, namely, "big gastrin," or G-34. This species of gastrin contains 34 amino acids, the carboxyl-terminal 17 of which are identical with heptadecapeptide gastrin and may also be present in sulfated (G-34 II) or nonsulfated (G-34 I) forms. Although G-17 has a shorter half-life than G-34, on a molar basis circulating G-17 is approximately as potent as G-34 in stimulating gastric acid secretion.

More than 90 percent of antral mucosal gastrin is in the form of G-17. Gastrin is also present in duodenal mucosa, the highest concentration being in the most proximal duodenum (approximately 10 percent of the antral concentration). The mucosal concentration of gastrin and the proportion as G-17 decrease with progression down the duodenum. The effects of gastrin and the vagus on gastric acid secretion are intimately related. Vagal stimulation increases gastric acid secretion by (1) directly stimulating parietal cells, (2) stimulating release of gastrin into the circulation, and (3) lowering the parietal cell threshold for response to circulating gastrin concentrations. There is also evidence that certain vagal branches or fibers inhibit gastrin release.

Histamine is present in large concentrations in mast cells in the lamina propria of the parietal cell–containing regions of the gastric mucosa. Histamine-containing mast cells are located in close proximity to parietal cells, with a ratio of one mast cell to every two or three parietal cells. For many years views have differed on the importance of histamine in stimulating gastric acid secretion; some suggested that histamine is the "final common pathway" for cholinergic and

FIGURE 235-1 *Amino acid sequences of selected gastrin peptides, all of which contain the common C-terminal pentapeptide amide. (*Tyrosyl is sulfated in gastrin II and nonsulfated in gastrin I molecules.)*

Big Gastrin (G34)	Glu-Leu-Gly-Pro-Gln-Gly-Pro-Pro-His-Leu-Val-Ala-Asp-Pro-Ser-Lys-Lys--Gln-Gly-Pro-Trp-Leu-Glu-Glu-Glu-Glu-Glu-Ala-Tyr*-Gly-Trp-Met-Asp-Phe-NH_2
Heptadecapeptide Gastrin (G 17)	Glu-Gly-Pro-Trp-Leu-Glu-Glu-Glu-Glu-Glu-Ala-Tyr*-Gly-Trp-Met-Asp-Phe-NH_2
Minigastrin (G 14)	Trp-Leu-Glu-Glu-Glu-Glu-Glu-Ala-Tyr*-Gly-Trp-Met-Asp-Phe-NH_2
C-Terminal Pentapeptide	Gly-Trp-Met-Asp-Phe-NH_2

gastrin stimulation of parietal cell acid secretion, while others were skeptical about any role for histamine in the acid secretory process.

Interest in the role of histamine in acid secretion was renewed by the discovery of H-2-receptor antagonists which competitively inhibit the action of histamine on H-2 receptors (located on gastric parietal, cardiac atrial, and uterine smooth-muscle cells). These drugs exert negligible effect on H-1 receptors, which are readily inhibited by conventional antihistamines. H-2-receptor antagonists (e.g., cimetidine and ranitidine) inhibit both basal acid secretion and secretory responses to feeding, gastrin, histamine, hypoglycemia, and vagal stimulation. Most data support the conclusions that (1) histamine plays an important role in stimulating gastric acid secretion, and that (2) histamine acts in concert with gastrin and cholinergic activity on parietal cells, which bear receptors for histamine, gastrin, and acetylcholine, but that (3) there is still uncertainty as to whether histamine is the final common effector molecule in the stimulation of parietal cell secretion.

Food ingestion is the major physiologic stimulus of gastric acid secretion. Traditionally, gastric acid secretion has been classified into three phases—cephalic, gastric, and intestinal. This classification is of some value in examining the multiple factors which regulate gastric acid secretion. The *cephalic phase* represents the gastric acid secretory response to the sight, smell, taste, and anticipation of food. The *gastric phase* is induced by the presence of food in the stomach. The *intestinal phase* is due to the entry or presence of food within the lumen of the small intestine. Although these three phases are convenient for considering the diverse contributions to gastric acid secretion, each phase is complex and not necessarily due to a single stimulatory control mechanism.

The cephalic phase appears to be mediated primarily by the vagus, which increases gastric acid secretion by stimulation of parietal cells directly and to a lesser extent by stimulating the release of gastrin into the circulation. The gastric phase results from stimulation of chemical and mechanical receptors in the gastric wall by luminal contents. Mechanical distention of the stomach stimulates gastric acid secretion but results in little, if any, gastrin release; this mechanical effect is inhibited by atropine and appears to be mediated by vagal reflexes. Food in the stomach promotes gastric acid secretion by increasing gastrin release, principally due to the *protein* content and the *products* of *protein digestion* contained in the meal; oral glucose and fat cause slight increases in serum gastrin but do not stimulate gastric acid secretion. Food in the proximal small intestine stimulates the intestinal phase of gastric acid secretion. A peptone meal (which contains partially hydrolyzed meat protein) introduced into the small intestine stimulates gastric acid secretion but not gastrin release. It has been proposed that food in the small intestine induces release of an intestinal hormone, presumably a polypeptide, which stimulates gastric acid secretion. This substance is believed to be distinct from gastrin and, unlike gastrin, appears to be degraded substantially during its portal transit through the liver.

Ingestion of both caffeine-containing and caffeine-free *coffee* stimulates gastric acid secretion: both forms of coffee stimulate gastrin release. Ingestion of *ethanol* and ethanol-containing beverages stimulates gastric acid secretion. Specifically, ingestion of 5 and 10% ethanol solutions and 10% bourbon whiskey results in prompt stimulation of gastric acid secretion without increasing gastrin release; however, white wine stimulates both gastric acid secretion and gastrin release. Furthermore, intravenous ethanol stimulates gastric acid secretion, suggesting that both systemic and local mechanisms are involved. Intravenous *calcium* stimulates acid secretion and produces minimal increases in serum gastrin levels. Oral calcium has been reported to stimulate gastric acid secretion directly, i.e., without an increase in serum calcium or gastrin concentrations. Except in patients with gastrinoma, hypercalcemia is usually not associated with acid hypersecretion or increases in serum gastrin.

Inhibition of gastric acid secretion can be produced by several mechanisms. Acid secretion may be inhibited by acid in the stomach or duodenum, by hyperglycemia, or by hypertonic fluids or fat in the duodenum. Reduction of the intragastric pH to 3.0 produces partial inhibition of gastrin release; further reduction to pH 1.5 or below blocks the release of gastrin to almost all stimuli. There is evidence that *somatostatin* is involved in the inhibition of gastrin release produced by acid in the gastric lumen. Somatostatin is present in high concentrations in antral mucosal endocrine cells (D cells) which possess cytoplasmic processes that extend to neighboring gastrin cells. The action of somatostatin in inhibiting gastrin release appears to be mediated by its local (paracrine) effects on gastrin cells. The cytoplasmic processes of somatostatin cells also extend to intimate contact with parietal and other cells in the acid-secreting portions of the stomach. Somatostatin is believed to reduce gastric acid secretion by inhibiting gastrin release and by directly inhibiting parietal cell secretion. Acid in the duodenum also inhibits gastric acid secretion; this may be secondary to stimulating the release of secretin and/or other peptides capable of inhibiting gastric acid secretion. *Secretin* is a linear polypeptide containing 27 amino acids bearing structural similarities to glucagon. Secretin is released from endocrine cells (S cells) in the mucosa of the small intestine in response to mucosal acidification. Fat in the duodenum also inhibits gastric acid secretion; gastric inhibitory peptide (GIP) has been proposed as a candidate for this enterogastrone action; however, this effect for GIP remains to be proved. The mechanisms by which hyperglycemia or intraduodenal hyperosmolality inhibit gastric acid secretion are not known. Additional peptides identified in the mucosa of the gastrointestinal tract which have the capacity to inhibit gastric acid secretion include glucagon-like peptides (e.g., glicentin), vasoactive intestinal peptide (VIP), and urogastrone; the latter appears to be structurally and functionally identical with epidermal growth factor. Vasoactive intestinal peptide, which is located in neurons, is unlikely to inhibit gastric acid secretion as a circulating hormone, since it is inactivated during its portal passage through the liver. The extent to which these peptides contribute to the regulation of gastric acid secretion is not clear.

The proteolytic effects of *pepsins* and the corrosive effects of acid appear to be integral components in the tissue injury which leads to peptic ulceration. Acid catalyzes the cleavage of inactive pepsinogen molecules to active pepsins and also provides the appropriate pH required for pepsin activity. Pepsin activity is substantially reduced above pH 4.0, and these enzymes are irreversibly inactivated at neutral or alkaline pH. There are a variety of pepsinogens and pepsins in gastric juice. Pepsinogens (and their corresponding active pepsins) have been classified by immunochemical techniques as either PG I (pepsinogens 1 through 5) or PG II (pepsinogens 6 and 7). Pepsinogen I is present in chief and mucous cells in the body and fundus of the stomach. Pepsinogen II is located in cells of the pyloric glands, Brunner's glands of the duodenum, mucous cells of the gastric cardiac glands, and the same cells in which PG I is found. Both PG I and PG II are present in plasma, while only PG I can be detected in urine. A high degree of correlation exists between serum concentrations of PG I and maximal gastric acid secretion. In general, agents which stimulate gastric acid secretion also stimulate pepsinogen secretion. Cholinergic action is particularly potent in promoting pepsinogen secretion. Secretin, although it inhibits gastric acid secretion, stimulates pepsinogen secretion.

Parietal cells also secrete *intrinsic factor*. Agents which stimulate gastric acid secretion also lead to secretion of intrinsic factor.

The precise mechanisms whereby the normal stomach and duodenum resist the corrosive effects of acid-pepsin (i.e., *mucosal resistance*) have not been defined. A variety of factors have been proposed as potential contributors to mucosal resistance. Gastric mucus, secreted by gastric mucous cells, is present in solution in gastric juice and as an insoluble mucus gel layer which coats the mucosal surface of the stomach. It has been suggested that *gastric mucus* may play a role in mucosal defense against injury, and thus in preventing peptic ulceration. Mucus secretion is enhanced by mechanical or chemical irritation and by cholinergic stimulation. Gastric mucus is a large polymeric glycoprotein (2×10^6 mol wt) containing four subunits connected by disulfide bridges. Depolymerization of the glycoprotein subunits of mucus, which may be produced by peptic digestion or disruption of disulfide bonds, renders the glycoprotein incapable of forming a viscous gel. When intact, this mucus gel serves as an unstirred layer which permits ionic diffusion but is impermeable to penetration by macromolecules such as pepsin (34,000 mol wt). Bicarbonate ions are secreted by gastric surface epithelial cells (nonparietal cells) and enter the unstirred layer of mucus gel; this mechanism facilitates the development of a microenvironment with a substantial hydrogen ion gradient between the gel opposing the gastrin luminal contents (more acid) and the gel surface facing and in intimate contact with the apical surfaces of gastric mucosal cells (more alkaline). Pepsin secreted into the gastrin lumen is denied reentry by the impermeable mucus gel, thereby potentially protecting the mucosal cells from proteolytic injury. Gastric mucus also contains glycoprotein blood group substances. Approximately three-fourths of the population secrete gastric juice containing these AB(H) substances and those individuals are referred to as *secretors.*

Normally the gastric luminal epithelial cell surfaces and intercellular tight junctions provide an almost completely impermeable barrier to back-diffusion of hydrogen ions from the lumen. This *gastric mucosal barrier* may participate in mucosal resistance to acid-peptic ulceration. This barrier may be interrupted by various agents including bile acids, salicylates, alcohol, and weak organic acids, thus permitting *back-diffusion of hydrogen ions* from the lumen to intra- and intercellular sites. Such back-diffusion may result in cellular injury, release of histamine from mast cells, further stimulation of acid secretion, damage to small blood vessels, mucosal hemorrhage, and superficial ulceration. Interruption of the gastric mucosal barrier may be responsible (at least in part) for the hemorrhagic erosive gastritis associated with salicylate and ethanol ingestion and may also contribute to other forms of gastric mucosal injury.

However, the relationship between the gastric mucosal barrier and mucosal resistance to chronic peptic ulcer has not been completely elucidated. *Decreased mucosal blood flow,* accompanied by back-diffusion of available hydrogen ions, also appears to contribute to gastric mucosal damage. Maintenance of normal mucosal blood flow is an essential component of mucosal resistance to injury. *Prostaglandins* are present in abundant quantities in the gastric mucosa. Various prostaglandins, particularly those of the E series, have been shown to inhibit gastric mucosal injury due to a wide variety of agents. It is possible that endogenous prostaglandins contribute to mucosal resistance and may thereby have a "cytoprotective" function. Mild mucosal injury or irritation may induce prostaglandin synthesis, thereby potentially enhancing mucosal resistance to injury, a concept referred to as *adaptive cytoprotection.*

Other mucosal factors, some of which are genetic, but which have not been clearly defined, apparently contribute to the ability of the gastric mucosa to resist or permit the development of peptic ulceration.

MEASUREMENT OF GASTRIC ACID SECRETION

Since HCl secretion by the stomach appears to be an important factor in the production of peptic ulcer disease, measurement of basal and stimulated gastric acid secretion may be of value in the assessment of peptic ulcer patients. In general, basal and stimulated acid outputs in females are approximately two-thirds to three-fourths those found in males. The range of values for normal subjects is extremely broad and overlaps substantially with those found in patients with duodenal ulcer, gastric ulcer, and even the Zollinger-Ellison syndrome. Mean basal acid output (BAO) in normal males without known ulcer disease is about 1.5 to 2.0 meq/h. In duodenal ulcer patients mean basal acid output averages from 4 to 6 meq/h, again with a wide degree of variation. Patients with gastric ulcer tend to have gastric acid secretory rates which are normal or even slightly less than those of normal subjects.

Measurement of gastric acid output is not helpful in either diagnosing peptic ulcer or excluding it. Thus measuring gastric acid secretion is clearly not necessary in all patients with duodenal ulcer. However, detection of gastric acid hypersecretion is of value when the Zollinger-Ellison syndrome is suspected. Measurement of gastric acid output is useful to detect achlorhydria, as found in patients with pernicious anemia. Since patients with benign gastric ulcer virtually always secrete some acid, pentagastrin-fast achlorhydria in a patient with a gastric ulcer almost always indicates malignancy. Measurement of gastric acid secretion is indicated in the search for the cause of ulcer recurrence after surgery for peptic ulcer.

In order to measure gastric acid output, a radiopaque gastric tube is passed so that its tip is located in the most dependent portion of the stomach. With the patient in a reclining or semirecumbent position on the left side, the position of the tube is verified by fluoroscopy. Gastric contents are aspirated and discarded. Basal gastric acid secretions are then collected in four consecutive 15-min intervals to determine the 1-h basal acid output. Secretion volume and acid concentration (titrated with 0.1 *N* sodium hydroxide to pH 7.0 or calculated by formula from the pH of the aspirated gastric juice) are measured, and acid output is expressed as milliequivalents per hour.

A variety of substances have been used to stimulate maximal acid output (MAO) by the stomach. These have included *histamine, betazole* (Histalog)—a structural analogue of histamine—and *pentagastrin* (Peptavlon). Histamine, the first standard stimulant to be used for gastric acid secretory testing, requires the simultaneous administration of an antihistaminic agent (H-1-receptor antagonist) to inhibit untoward systemic side effects. Betazole possesses fewer undesired side effects of histamine and does not require the concomitant administration of an antihistamine. Pentagastrin (*N-tert*-butyloxycarbonyl-β-Ala-Try-Met-Asp-Phe-NH_2) contains the biologically active carboxyl-terminal tetrapeptide amide portion of the gastrin molecule and is currently the preferred and most commonly used agent to induce maximal acid secretion. Following collection of basal acid secretion gastric juice is collected for four additional consecutive 15-min periods after the subcutaneous injection of pentagastrin (6 μg/kg). The MAO is the expression of the milliequivalents of acid aspirated during the 1 h after pentagastrin administration. Peak acid output (PAO) is calculated by combining the two highest consecutive 15-min acid outputs following pentagastrin injection and multiplying by 2.

DUODENAL ULCER

GENERAL CONSIDERATIONS Duodenal ulcer is a chronic and recurrent disease. The ulcer is usually deep and sharply demarcated. It tends to penetrate through the submucosa and often into the muscularis propria. The ulcer floor contains no intact epithelium and usually consists of a zone of eosinophilic necrosis resting on a base of granulation tissue surrounded by variable amounts of fibrosis. The ulcer bed may be clear or contain either blood or a proteinaceous exudate with entrapped erythrocytes and acute and chronic inflammatory cells. More than 95 percent of duodenal ulcers occur in the first portion of the duodenum, and approximately 90 percent of these are located within 3 cm of the junction of the pyloric and duodenal mucosa. Duodenal ulcers are usually round or oval, but they may be irregular or elliptic. They are usually less than 1 cm in diameter. Rarely, duodenal ulcers may be extremely large (3 to 6 cm in diameter) and may be mistaken radiographically for the entire duodenal bulb. These giant ulcers often escape radiologic detection and are usually identified directly by endoscopy or at surgery or postmortem examination.

The absolute prevalence of duodenal ulcer in the population is not known. Estimates have ranged from 6 to 15 percent. This variation may be related to the populations examined, differences in study design and diagnostic methods (e.g., endoscopy vs. radiological examination), and perhaps to actual changes or differences in frequency of duodenal ulcer disease. The best current estimates suggest that approximately 10 percent of the population has clinical evidence of duodenal ulcer at some time in their lifetime. Duodenal ulcer is slightly more common in males than in females and is three times as frequent as clinically recognized gastric ulcer. During the past 35 years the frequency of duodenal ulcer (and its complications) has been decreasing in the United States and England especially in males. The reason or reasons for this reduction are not known.

Approximately 60 percent of healed duodenal ulcers recur within 1 year and from 80 to 90 percent within 2 years. Although much is now known concerning factors which contribute to the development of duodenal ulcer, we do not completely understand its pathogenesis. Acid secretion by the stomach is required for production of a duodenal ulcer, but the factors which render the acid-secreting subject susceptible to duodenal ulceration are not completely understood. As a group, duodenal ulcer patients secrete more acid than normal; however, from one-half to two-thirds of duodenal ulcer patients have gastric acid secretory rates, both BAO and MAO, within the normal range. Duodenal ulcer patients have been shown to have approximately 1.9 billion parietal cells, with a maximum capacity to secrete approximately 42 meq of gastric acid per hour; this is in contrast to 1.0 billion parietal cells and 22 meq/h for nonduodenal ulcer subjects (mean values). However, variations in both groups are so large that most duodenal ulcer patients fall within the normal range. As a group, duodenal ulcer patients also have comparable increases in gastric secretion of pepsin and in serum pepsinogen I levels. Peptic ulcer is believed to develop when there is an unfavorable balance between gastric acid-pepsin secretion and gastric or duodenal mucosal resistance. In duodenal ulcer disease, the evidence favors the etiologic importance of absolute or, in most instances, relative gastric acid hypersecretion. However, in patients with gastric ulcer, defective mucosal resistance appears to be the major permissive factor.

Fasting *serum gastrin* concentrations are normal in duodenal ulcer patients. However, most studies have shown that in response to a protein-containing meal, more gastrin is released into the circulation in duodenal ulcer patients than in normal subjects. Duodenal ulcer patients also have a greater gastric acid secretory response to gastrin than normal persons. Thus, a given dose of pentagastrin or gastrin produces more acid secretion, and smaller doses of pentagastrin or gastrin are required to achieve the same fraction (50 percent) of the maximal acid secretory response in duodenal ulcer patients than in normal subjects. In addition, in duodenal ulcer patients intragastric acid is less effective in inhibiting both gastrin release and gastric acid secretion. Therefore, although fasting serum gastrin levels are normal in duodenal ulcer patients, gastrin may still play an important role in their often observed acid hypersecretion. Duodenal ulcer patients tend to empty their stomachs more rapidly than nonduodenal ulcer patients. This phenomenon, together with acid hypersecretion, may contribute to greater hydrogen ion concentrations in the first part of the duodenum (the primary location of ulceration) in patients with duodenal ulcer.

Genetic factors appear to be important. Duodenal ulcers are approximately three times as common in first-degree relatives of duodenal ulcer patients when compared with the population at large. Patients with duodenal ulcers have an increased frequency of blood group O and of the nonsecretory status [those who do not secrete AB(H) antigens in their gastric juice], but these associations are weak. An increased incidence of HLA-B5 antigen in white male subjects with duodenal ulcer has also been shown. Elevated serum pepsinogen I (PG I) levels have been found in approximately 50 percent of patients with duodenal ulcer. Increases in serum pepsinogen appear to be inherited as an autosomal dominant trait. Individuals with this trait have a frequency of duodenal ulcer eight times greater than the general population. Thus an elevated PG I level may prove to be a valuable subclinical marker of the duodenal ulcer diathesis in families with this autosomal dominant form of peptic ulcer disease.

Cigarette smoking has been associated with increased duodenal ulcer frequency, decreased responses to therapy, and an increased mortality (from duodenal ulcer). Cigarette smoking does not increase gastric acid secretion. It has been suggested that the increased incidence of duodenal ulcer among cigarette smokers may be secondary to the effects of nicotine or cigarette smoking in inhibiting pancreatic bicarbonate secretion (an endogenous neutralizer of secreted gastric acid) and/or by acceleration of gastric emptying of acid into the duodenum. The incidence of duodenal ulcer has also been reported to be increased in patients with chronic renal failure, alcoholic cirrhosis, renal transplantation, hyperparathyroidism, systemic mastocytosis, and chronic obstructive pulmonary disease. Antibodies to herpes simplex have been reported to be higher in titer and more frequent in serums of patients with duodenal ulcer than in normals.

The importance of *psychological factors* in the pathogenesis of duodenal ulcer remains controversial. Contrary to earlier views, there is no single characteristic duodenal ulcer personality. There is no identifiable difference in frequency of duodenal ulcer among different socioeconomic classes or occupation groups. Chronic anxiety and psychological stress may, however, be factors in exacerbation of ulcer activity.

CLINICAL FEATURES Epigastric pain is the most frequent symptom of duodenal ulcer. The pain is often described as burning or gnawing. Just as frequently, however, the pain may be ill-defined, boring, or aching, or is perceived as abdominal pressure or fullness, or as a sensation of hunger. In approximately 10 percent of patients the pain is located to the right of the midepigastrium. The pain characteristically occurs from 90 min to 3 h after eating. It frequently awakens the patient at night. Pain on awakening before breakfast is sufficiently rare in patients with duodenal ulcer as to challenge the diagnosis. The pain is usually relieved within a few minutes by food or antacids. The severity of pain varies substantially from patient to patient, and symptoms tend to be recurrent and episodic. Duodenal ulcer may recur in the absence of pain. Episodes of pain may persist for periods of several days to weeks or months. Periods of remission may last from weeks to years and are almost always longer than the episodes of pain. In some patients the disease is more aggressive, with frequent persistent symptoms and development of complications. Pain relief (whether with antacids or food) is believed to result from acid neutralization. Ingestion of food leads to a transient partial neutralization of gastric acid, which is followed by gastrin release and resultant stimulation of acid secretion. With subsequent gastric emptying and increasing gastric acid secretion, a sufficiently low pH is achieved that pain results. Acid-induced pain in patients with duodenal ulcer is believed due to (1) acid stimulation of chemical receptors and/or (2) alterations in gastric motility.

Changes in the character of the pain may signal the development of complications. For example, ulcer pain which becomes constant, is no longer relieved by food or antacids, or radiates to the back or either upper quadrant may herald *penetration* of the ulcer (often into the pancreas). Ulcer pain which is accentuated rather than relieved by food, and/or is accompanied by vomiting, often indicates *gastric outlet obstruction*. Abrupt, severe, or generalized abdominal pain is characteristic of free *perforation* into the peritoneal cavity. Weight loss, in the absence of some degree of gastric outlet obstruction, is unusual. Duodenal ulcer may cause acute gastrointestinal *hemorrhage*, with vomiting of blood or coffee-grounds material, or with melena, and the passage of black tarry stools or even frank red blood, if the bleeding is massive.

It is important to emphasize that *many patients with active disease have no ulcer symptoms*. This leads to a significant, although not quantifiable, underestimation of duodenal ulcer frequency and recurrence in the population. Recent studies, especially those using duodenoscopy, indicate that there is poor correlation between ulcer activity, resolution of symptoms, and ulcer healing. Since many duodenal ulcer patients are asymptomatic, the absence of ulcer-type pain does not exclude duodenal ulcer as a potential cause for gastrointestinal hemorrhage or symptoms due to gastric outlet obstruction or abrupt ulcer perforation.

On *physical examination* epigastric tenderness is by far the most frequent abnormal finding. The area of tenderness is usually in the midline, often midway between the umbilicus and the xiphoid process. In 20 to 30 percent of patients the tender area is to the right of the midline. Acute free perforation of the ulcer into the peritoneal cavity often produces a rigid, boardlike abdomen, usually with generalized rebound tenderness. In patients with gastric outlet obstruction caused by a duodenal or pyloric channel ulcer one may find a "succussion splash" due to fluid and air in the distended stomach. Tachycardia or hypotension, in some instances demonstrable only by orthostatic maneuvers, may reflect acute hemorrhage from duodenal ulcer. Cutaneous and mucosal pallor may result from anemia from acute or chronic blood loss.

Only about 5 percent of duodenal ulcers are located distal to the duodenal bulb, and most of these are in the immediate postbulbar portion of the first part of the duodenum. Most postbulbar ulcers are of the common duodenal ulcer variety. However, postbulbar ulceration, when located in or beyond the second portion of the duodenum, suggests the Zollinger-Ellison syndrome. Postbulbar ulcer pain may be located in the right upper quadrant or radiate through to the back. Obstruction and hemorrhage are more frequent with postbulbar ulcers than with those in the duodenal bulb.

The pyloric channel, which is 1 to 2 cm in length, is the narrowest portion of the gastric outlet. Because of their gastric acid secretory characteristics and clinical features, pyloric channel ulcers are classified with duodenal rather than gastric ulcer. Ulcers in this location often produce symptoms similar to those of a duodenal ulcer; however, symptoms due to these tend to be less responsive to food and antacids. In patients with pyloric channel ulcers, food may accentuate rather than relieve ulcer pain and may result in vomiting secondary to partial gastric outlet obstruction. In general, surgery is required more frequently with pyloric channel ulcers than with those in the duodenal bulb.

DIAGNOSIS Epigastric pain readily relieved by food or antacids strongly suggests duodenal ulcer. However, many patients with ulcerlike symptoms may have no evidence of an ulcer even after careful radiographic and endoscopic examination. Barium examination of the upper gastrointestinal tract is of value in identifying duodenal ulcer and is the usual method used to establish the diagnosis. The proportion of ulcers identified radiographically depends on the skill, persistence, enthusiasm, and diagnostic criteria of the radiologist. Using conventional barium contrast techniques, 70 to 80 percent of duodenal ulcers visualized by endoscopy can be identified by x-ray examination. With newer double-contrast barium examinations, it is possible to detect approximately 90 percent of duodenal ulcers. On x-ray the typical duodenal ulcer appears as a discrete crater in the proximal portion of the duodenal bulb. Marked deformity of the duodenal bulb, common in patients with chronic recurrent duodenal ulcer, may make radiographic identification of the ulcer difficult or impossible (Figs. 235-2 and 235-3).

Use of fiberoptic endoscopic examination of the upper gastrointestinal tract has facilitated accurate diagnosis of duodenal ulcer disease. Duodenoscopy is not required for diagnosis of duodenal ulcer when it has been established by barium radiographic examination. Endoscopy may be of great value, however, (1) in detecting suspected duodenal ulcer in the absence of radiographically demonstrable ulcer and in patients with radiographic deformity and uncertainty regarding ulcer activity, (2) in identifying ulcers too small or too superficial to be recognized by x-ray, and (3) in identifying an ulcer as the source of active gastrointestinal hemorrhage. Duodenoscopy also permits direct visualization and photographic documentation of the character of the ulcer, its size, shape, and location, and it may provide a reference basis for the assessment of healing. Endoscopic studies have shown that 85 percent of duodenal ulcers are less than 1 cm in diameter, with approximately 70 percent having a diameter between 0.5 and 1 cm.

Measurement of gastric acid secretion is not necessary in most patients with clinical features of a typical duodenal ulcer. Determination of serum gastrin is recommended in those patients in whom surgery is planned or gastrinoma is suspected.

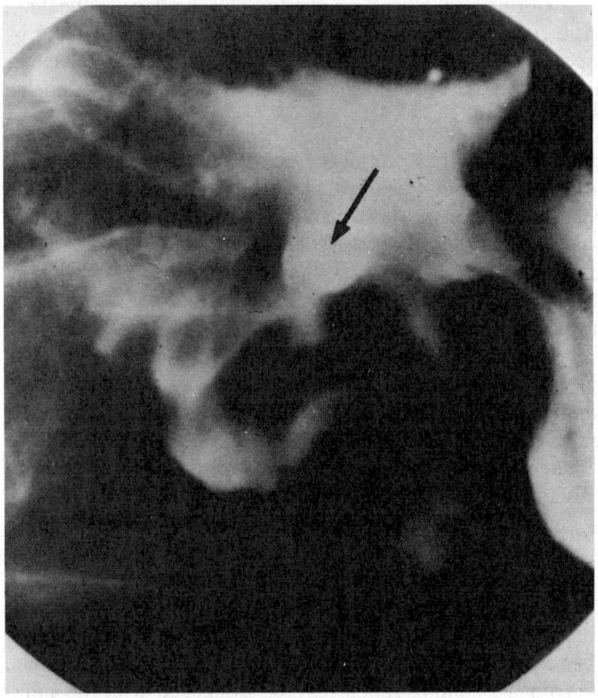

FIGURE 235-2 *Deformed duodenal bulb with ulcer crater.*

MEDICAL TREATMENT Major objectives of therapy are relief of pain and ulcer healing. Prevention of ulcer recurrence and complications are additional objectives. In the past enthusiasm has been expressed for virtually every mode of treatment which has ever been tried for this disease. In many instances conclusions regarding the

FIGURE 235-3 *Distortion of the duodenal bulb with "cloverleaf" deformity.*

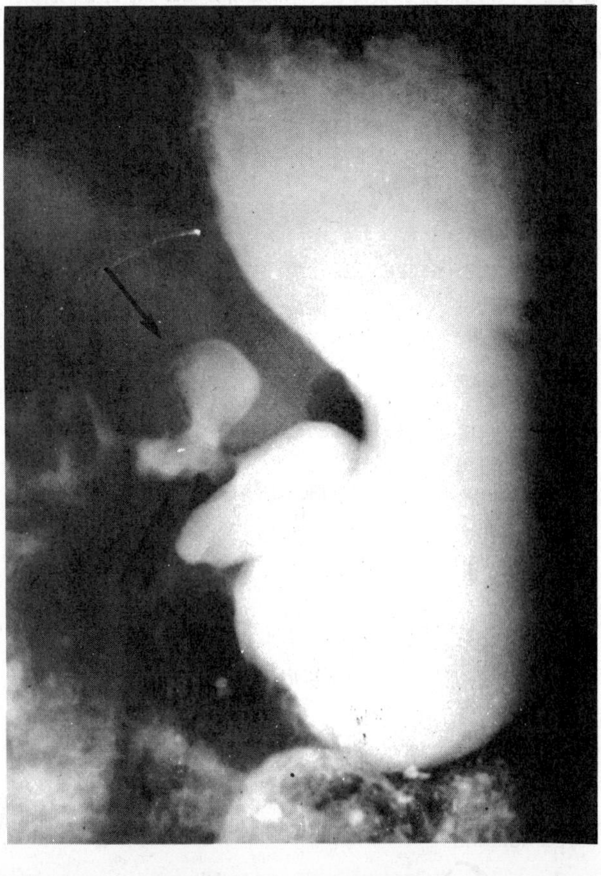

effectiveness of therapy have been obscured by spontaneous healing, an intrinsic component of the natural history of the disease, and by imprecise methods used to assess ulcer activity. Specific agents currently available and recommended for use in treatment of duodenal ulcer are considered below.

Antacids Traditionally, administration of antacids has been the major accepted form of treatment for duodenal ulcer. Studies with endoscopic verification of ulcer activity have established the effectiveness of antacids in accelerating duodenal ulcer healing. Many types of antacids are available and have been used in the treatment of duodenal ulcer. The ideal antacid should be potent in neutralizing acid, inexpensive, not adsorbed from the gastrointestinal tract, and contain negligible amounts of sodium. The ideal antacid should be sufficiently palatable to be readily tolerated with repeated dosage and should be free from side effects. Although the ideal antacid is yet to be developed, a number of preparations are available which can be used in treatment of patients with duodenal ulcer. Individual antacids differ substantially in their capacities to neutralize acid, their sodium contents, their absorption properties, and their potential adverse effects.

Calcium carbonate is a potent and inexpensive antacid. In neutralizing acid, it is converted to calcium chloride in the stomach. Approximately 10 percent of calcium ingested as calcium carbonate is absorbed from the proximal small intestine. Unfortunately, chronic calcium carbonate administration may be associated with the milk-alkali syndrome, producing elevations of serum calcium, phosphate, blood urea nitrogen, creatinine, and bicarbonate. These patients may develop renal calcinosis and progressive renal insufficiency. Calcium carbonate is unique among antacids in that its ingestion is followed by stimulation of gastric acid secretion (a genuine "acid rebound" phenomenon). This is due to the direct action of calcium in stimulating parietal cell acid secretion and, perhaps to a lesser extent, to calcium-mediated stimulation of gastrin release. Because of its potential adverse effects, calcium carbonate is not recommended for use as an antacid for treatment of patients with peptic ulcer.

FIGURE 235-4 *Chemical structures of histamine and the H-2-receptor antagonists cimetidine, ranitidine, and famotidine. Note the imidazole ring shared by histamine and cimetidine but absent in ranitidine and famotidine.*

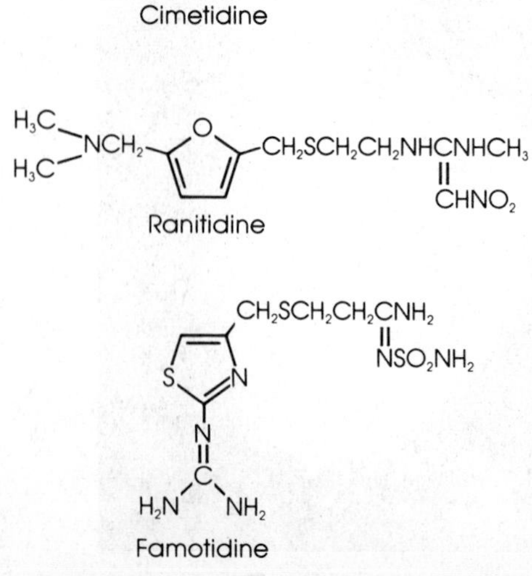

Sodium bicarbonate is a potent, rapidly acting, inexpensive antacid. However, because of its tendency to induce systemic alkalosis and its high sodium content, it should not be used as an antacid in treatment of peptic ulcer.

The most widely used antacid preparations are mixtures of aluminum hydroxide and magnesium hydroxide, in some instances with additional agents. *Aluminum hydroxide* neutralizes hydrochloric acid with the production of aluminum chloride and water. Use of aluminum hydroxide tends to produce constipation. Aluminum binds phosphate within the gut lumen, thereby facilitating its excretion. As a consequence, prolonged and regular use of aluminum hydroxide may induce systemic phosphate depletion with resultant weakness, malaise, and anorexia. This complication is probably restricted to, and must be considered in, patients with a phosphate-deficient diet, e.g., dietary deficiency associated with chronic alcoholism or other states of reduced dietary protein intake.

Magnesium hydroxide is a potent antacid which neutralizes hydrochloric acid to produce magnesium chloride and water. Magnesium hydroxide may produce loosening of the stools. This laxative effect and the constipating effects of aluminum hydroxide can be overcome by using these agents in combination, or by alternating their use. Antacid combinations vary enormously in their capacities to neutralize hydrochloric acid. *Magnesium trisilicate,* which is frequently included in various antacid mixtures, is a slow-acting weak antacid. In general, tablet preparations of magnesium hydroxide–aluminum hydroxide are less potent than their liquid forms.

Acceptance of the crucial role of acid in the pathogenesis of duodenal ulcer provides a rational basis for the use of antacids in treatment of patients with duodenal ulcer. There have been controlled studies on the effects of antacids on duodenal ulcer healing, in which vigorous antacid therapy has been compared with placebo, and ulcer response has been verified by endoscopy. Four weeks of treatment with a potent magnesium and aluminum hydroxide antacid mixture has been shown to increase duodenal ulcer healing. Ulcer healing occurred in 45 percent of patients receiving placebo and in 78 percent of those treated with 30 mL antacid (144 meq) given 1 and 3 h after meals and at bedtime.

H-2-receptor antagonists It has been known for decades that conventional antihistamines, which readily block the actions of histamine on smooth muscle of the gut or bronchi, do not inhibit histamine-stimulated gastric acid secretion. The parietal cell receptor for histamine has been classified as the H-2 receptor and that blocked by classic antihistamines as the H-1 receptor. H-2-receptor antagonists, which are potent inhibitors of basal (unstimulated) and stimulated gastric acid secretion, are the agents which at the present time are most frequently used in the treatment of duodenal ulcer.

The H-2-receptor antagonist *cimetidine* was the first of the agents to be developed and made available for clinical use and is used widely in the treatment of duodenal ulcer. Cimetidine is related structurally to histamine (Fig. 235-4), sharing the same imidazole ring, but bearing an extended side chain which contains a cyanoguanidine group. Cimetidine, at a dose of 300 mg, inhibits basal acid secretion by more than 80 percent and meal-stimulated acid secretion by approximately 70 percent. It strikingly reduces acid secretory responses to histamine, caffeine, insulin, hypoglycemia, and gastrin. Cimetidine has been shown to be more effective than placebo in promoting endoscopically verified duodenal ulcer healing. Its effectiveness in promoting duodenal ulcer healing appears to be comparable to that of vigorous antacid therapy. The oral dose of cimetidine used most commonly for treatment of patients with duodenal ulcer is 300 mg four times daily, with meals and at bedtime. Treatment with 400 mg cimetidine twice each day has also been shown to be effective in treatment of duodenal ulcer. Treatment of active duodenal ulcer with cimetidine is continued for periods from 4 to 8 weeks. Chronic administration of cimetidine, in doses of 400 mg at bedtime or 400 mg twice each day, has been shown to reduce substantially the frequency of duodenal ulcer recurrence during the 12-month period of treatment. Considering the enormous numbers of patients who have been treated with cimetidine, few serious adverse effects have been experienced. Cimetidine administration has been associated with slight and reversible increases in serum transaminase and creatinine levels. Instances of diarrhea, fatigue, and skin rash have also been described. Central nervous system abnormalities (confusion, agitation, coma, disorientation, and seizures) may occur, especially in elderly patients, in those receiving large doses or when there is substantial hepatic/renal functional impairment. Tender gynecomastia may occur especially in patients with the Zollinger-Ellison syndrome, treated with large doses for prolonged periods of time; this is believed to be caused by the weak antiandrogenic effects of cimetidine. Brief increases in serum prolactin have been shown to follow intravenous and oral cimetidine. Cimetidine has been shown to bind to and inhibit the P_{450} cytochrome-mixed oxygenase hepatic enzyme system. As a result, cimetidine may increase blood levels and the duration of action and pharmacologic effects of drugs whose metabolism depends upon this system. These drugs include, among others, phenytoin, chlordiazepoxide, diazepam, warfarin, carbamazepine, and antipyrine. Cimetidine does not interfere with the elimination of benzodiazepines which are eliminated utilizing glucuronide conjugation, for example, lorazepam and oxazepam. Cimetidine also reduces the rate of elimination of lidocaine due to reduced oxidative biotransformation and, perhaps, to reduced hepatic blood flow. Cimetidine may also increase blood levels of theophylline, presumably by inhibition of the terminal oxidase step in its hepatic metabolism.

Ranitidine is a more recently introduced H-2-receptor antagonist which is also commonly used in the treatment of patients with duodenal ulcer. It is a substituted aminomethlyfuran and is structurally unrelated to histamine or cimetidine (Fig. 235-4). On a molar basis, ranitidine is about six times as potent as cimetidine in inhibiting gastric acid secretion. Both cimetidine and ranitidine have similar half-lives of disappearance, approximately 120 min. Ranitidine and cimetidine appear to be comparably effective in accelerating healing of duodenal ulcer. The recommended dose of ranitidine is 150 mg twice each day. It appears to have no antiandrogen properties and exhibits little, if any, inhibitory effect on the cytochrome P_{450} mixed oxygenase enzyme system.

A variety of other H-2-receptor antagonists are under development and evaluation. Among these is *famotidine,* which contains a thiazole ring and is not related structurally to cimetidine or ranitidine (Fig. 235-4). It is not yet available in the United States. Famotidine is an extraordinarily potent H-2-receptor antagonist, being approximately 8 to 10 times as potent as ranitidine in inhibiting gastric acid secretion.

Anticholinergic agents Anticholinergic agents, such as atropine, act by inhibiting the effects of acetylcholine on muscarinic receptors. These agents decrease gastric acid secretion, but not as effectively as H-2-receptor antagonists. Anticholinergics reduce basal gastric acid secretion by approximately 50 percent, histamine- or gastrin-stimulated acid secretion by 40 percent, and postprandial acid secretion by 30 percent. They also delay gastric emptying. Most studies have *not* shown that anticholinergic agents hasten healing or improve symptoms of duodenal ulcer; therefore, they are not recommended as primary therapy for duodenal ulcer. However, anticholinergic agents may prove to be useful when combined in a program of treatment with antacids or H-2-receptor antagonists. Side effects of anticholinergic agents include dryness of mouth, blurring of vision, cardiac arrhythmias, and urinary retention. They should not be used in patients with glaucoma, impaired gastric emptying, or history or symptoms of urinary retention.

There is recent evidence for the existence of two classes of muscarinic cholinergic receptors (M-1 and M-2). *Pirenzepine* appears to be a selective anticholinergic agent in that it is more specific for M-2 receptors. It exhibits greater specificity in inhibiting gastric acid secretion, with fewer side effects than other anticholinergic agents. Pirenzepine, not yet available for use in the United States, has been shown to be effective in the treatment of duodenal ulcer. It may prove to be useful not only as primary therapy but as adjunctive therapy in duodenal ulcer patients.

Coating agents There are several drugs which act neither by neutralization nor by inhibition of gastric acid secretion. Among these is *sucralfate,* a complex polyaluminum hydroxide salt of sucrose sulfate. Its actions are principally local, and it may act in a "cytoprotective" manner. Sucralfate becomes highly polar at acid pH and binds to ulcer tissue for up to 12 h, while relatively little binds to intact gastric or duodenal mucosa. It is believed that adherence of sucralfate to granulation tissue prevents diffusion of hydrochloric acid to the base of the ulcer, thereby potentially protecting it. In addition, sucralfate binds bile acids and pepsin and may therefore reduce their injurious effects on the mucosa. Sucralfate appears to be similar to antacids and H-2-receptor antagonists in its effectiveness in the treatment of duodenal ulcer and in the prevention of duodenal ulcer recurrence. The recommended dose of sucralfate is 1 g 1 h before each meal and at bedtime. It is only minimally absorbed, with less than 5 percent appearing in the urine. *Colloidal bismuth* compounds also aid ulcer healing by forming (in an acid medium) a bismuth-protein coagulant which protects the ulcer from acid-peptic digestion.

Prostaglandins A variety of *prostaglandins,* particularly those of the E series (PGE_1 and PGE_2), are effective in the treatment of duodenal ulcer, with healing rates comparable to those achieved with vigorous antacid therapy and H-2-receptor antagonists. Their action is believed to be twofold: (1) they reduce basal and stimulated gastric acid secretion, and (2) they enhance mucosal resistance to tissue injury (i.e., they are "cytoprotective"). The mechanism, or mechanisms, by which prostaglandins enhance mucosal defense have not been clarified. In addition to their capacity to reduce gastric acid secretion, PGEs (1) stimulate gastric mucus secretion, (2) stimulate gastric and duodenal bicarbonate secretion, (3) maintain gastric mucosal blood flow, (4) maintain the electronegative potential difference of the gastric lumen (compared with the serosa), and (5) stimulate mucosal cellular renewal and regeneration. At present, PGE preparations are not yet available for use in the treatment of duodenal ulcer in the United States.

Diet Many different dietary programs have been recommended and used for treatment of patients with duodenal ulcer. There is no evidence that bland diets reduce gastric acid secretion, promote healing, or relieve symptoms in patients with duodenal ulcer. Similarly soft diets or diets free of spices or fruit juices have not been proved to be of benefit. Traditionally, milk and cream have been prescribed in the treatment of ulcer patients. However, there is no evidence that ulcer healing is benefited by milk and cream diets; in fact, they may contribute to the development of the milk-alkali syndrome.

What dietary measures, if any, should be recommended? Clearly, strict diet control is not necessary. Milk should not be used as a component of treatment for patients with duodenal ulcer. It is reasonable to suggest that if patients experience symptoms after ingestion of certain foods, these should be avoided. A regular diet can be combined with antacids as described below. Because of their effects on gastric secretion it is probably wise for duodenal ulcer patients to avoid coffee, with or without caffeine, as well as other caffeine-containing beverages. It is desirable also to restrict alcohol intake in these patients.

Possible drugs for the future A number of other drugs have been shown in some studies to promote healing of duodenal or gastric ulcer. *Omeprazole,* a specific inhibitor of hydrogen-potassium ATPase of the parietal cells has been shown to be extraordinarily potent in decreasing gastric acid secretion. This drug, which is currently being evaluated clinically, appears to be effective in treatment of patients with common duodenal ulcers and in patients with ulcers associated with gastrinoma (see below). *Sulpiride* is an orthopramide, which is structurally related to metoclopramide, possesses antiemetic and antidepressant properties, and has been used in the treatment of duodenal ulcer patients. *Proglumide,* a derivative of isoglutamic acid, is believed to block gastrin receptors, reduce acid secretion, and increase mucosal resistance.

General therapeutic considerations How does one integrate available information concerning treatment of duodenal ulcer to construct a reasonable therapeutic formulation? Clinical studies have verified the effectiveness of a variety of drugs in the promotion of duodenal ulcer healing. On the basis of present knowledge, there appear to be several alternative effective approaches for the medical treatment of duodenal ulcer—based on the neutralization of gastric acid by frequent use of potent antacids, the inhibition of gastric acid secretion by H-2-receptor antagonists, or the local ''protective'' actions of some of the available agents.

Antacid treatment of duodenal ulcer, when selected, should consist of frequent doses of a potent liquid antacid. However, the minimal or optimal doses of antacids required for duodenal ulcer healing are not precisely known. On the basis of an antacid program which has been shown to be effective, it is recommended that the antacid (100 to 140 meq of neutralizing activity; for most antacids this equals 30 to 60 mL) be given 1 and 3 h after each meal and at bedtime. Such a regimen should be continued for approximately 6 weeks. Symptom recurrence may be treated by shorter periods of therapy, at similar dose levels. When *H-2-receptor antagonist* treatment is selected and when *cimetidine* is used, a 300-mg tablet is recommended with each meal and at bedtime or 400 mg twice daily for 6 to 8 weeks. When *ranitidine* is used, the dose is 150 mg twice daily. The locally acting agent *sucralfate* should be given (1 g) 1 h before each meal and on retiring at night for 6 to 8 weeks. Sucralfate should not be given within 30 min of antacids (before or after) because acid is needed to induce adherence of sucralfate to the ulcer. When anticholinergics are used in conjunction with other drugs, they are administered either once a day at bedtime or four times a day (i.e., before meals and at bedtime).

GASTRIC ULCER

INCIDENCE AND ANATOMIC LOCATION The peak incidence for gastric ulcer is in the sixth decade, approximately 10 years later than for duodenal ulcer. Approximately 55 percent of gastric ulcers occur in males. They are also similar histologically to duodenal ulcers. Characteristically, gastric ulcers are deep and extend beyond the mucosa of the stomach. Almost all benign gastric ulcers are located in the *antrum,* in a zone immediately distal to the junction of the antral mucosa with the acid-secreting mucosa of the body of the stomach. The location of this junction is variable, especially on the lesser gastric curvature. In general, the antrum extends approximately two-thirds of the way up the lesser curvature and one-third of the way up the greater curvature of the stomach. Benign gastric ulcers are rare in the fundus of the stomach. Benign gastric ulcers are almost always accompanied by gastritis and variable amounts of mucosal atrophy involving the antrum. Gastritis may be present or absent with aspirin-associated gastric ulcers; ulcers associated with salicylate ingestion are usually located in the antrum, but they are not confined to the junction of the antral and parietal cell mucosa, as are common gastric ulcers.

ETIOLOGY AND PATHOGENESIS Acid-pepsin appears to be important in the pathogenesis of gastric ulcer. In contrast to duodenal ulcer, however, gastric ulcer patients generally have acid secretory rates which are normal, or even reduced, when compared with nonulcer subjects. Although many patients with gastric ulcer have reduced rates of acid secretion, *true achlorhydria* in response to stimulation *almost never occurs* in patients with *benign* gastric ulcer. Ten to twenty percent of patients with gastric ulcer also have duodenal ulcer disease. Patients with both duodenal and gastric ulcers tend to have acid secretory patterns which parallel those of duodenal ulcer. Patients with pyloric channel ulcers have acid secretory rates and clinical patterns similar to those found with common duodenal ulcer.

Various factors are involved in the pathogenesis of gastric ulcer. Most evidence supports the importance of primary defects in gastric mucosal resistance and/or direct gastric mucosal injury as the most important elements. Serum gastrin levels are increased in some gastric ulcer patients, but these increases are limited to those with gastric acid hyposecretion. Gastric emptying has also been shown to be delayed. It has been suggested that regurgitation of duodenal contents, especially those containing bile, may induce gastric mucosal injury and subsequent gastric ulceration. Gastric ulcer patients have been shown to have increased duodenal-gastric reflux of bile and greater concentrations of bile in their stomachs when compared with nonulcer subjects or duodenal ulcer patients. It has been proposed that bile acids injure the gastric mucosa by interruption of the gastric mucosal barrier with resultant back-diffusion of secreted hydrogen ions. The factors producing duodenal-gastric reflux in gastric ulcer patients have not been clearly established; a defect in pyloric sphincter function has been proposed.

CLINICAL FEATURES As with duodenal ulcer, epigastric pain is the most common symptom. However, this symptom is much less typical and predictable than those in patients with duodenal ulcer. While the pain may be similar to that noted with duodenal ulcers, some gastric ulcer patients experience no relief of pain with eating, and pain may actually be precipitated or accentuated by food. Relief of symptoms with antacids is also less consistent with gastric than with duodenal ulcers. Gastric ulcers tend to heal, but then recur, often in the same location. Recognizable episodes of recurrent gastric ulcer activity are usually less frequent than with duodenal ulcer. The precise incidence of gastric ulcer is not known, since many gastric ulcer patients are asymptomatic. Although duodenal ulcer is identified clinically as more frequent than gastric ulcer, most autopsy studies show an equal or greater proportion of gastric ulcers when compared with duodenal ulcers. This may be due in part to more acute preterminal events but also may reflect the often asymptomatic clinical course of gastric ulcer. While nausea and vomiting almost always indicate gastric outlet obstruction in duodenal ulcer patients, these symptoms may occur in patients with gastric ulcer in the absence of mechanical obstruction. Weight loss occurs in about 40 percent of patients due to anorexia or to food aversion from discomfort produced by eating.

Hemorrhage is a common complication, occurring in approximately 25 percent. Gastric ulcer perforation is less frequent than hemorrhage. Mortality with perforation of gastric ulcers is approximately three times that which occurs with duodenal ulcers. This increased mortality is due only in part to the increased age of gastric ulcer patients. The greater mortality may also be due to uncertainty and delay in diagnosis, as well as to greater soilage of the peritoneum with gastric ulcer perforation. Mortality is also greater in patients with hemorrhage due to gastric ulcer than when associated with duodenal ulcer. Gastric outlet obstruction may develop when ulcers are in the pyloric channel or in the most distal antrum, but it is not a common complication in other parts of the stomach.

DIAGNOSIS The history may be of value in suspecting gastric ulcer, but it is not as characteristic as in duodenal ulcer. The two major methods for diagnosis are barium examination and endoscopy. Gastric ulcer can usually be identified by the standard barium examination with an accuracy that approaches 90 percent. Superficial ulcerations and erosions, however, may escape radiographic identification. Approximately 4 percent of gastric ulcers which appear benign radiographically prove to be malignant (by endoscopic biopsy or at surgery). Both benign and malignant gastric ulcers are more common on the lesser than on the greater curvature (Fig. 235-5). Radiation of gastric mucosal folds from the margin of the ulcer crater suggests a benign lesion. Large gastric ulcers, i.e., those greater than 3 cm in diameter, are more often malignant than smaller ones. An ulcer within a mass, as defined radiographically, also suggests malignancy. Because of false-positive and false-negative errors, radiographic appearance cannot be used as the sole criterion for the benign or malignant nature of a gastric ulcer.

Endoscopic visualization of the ulcer allows one to define its size, location, and, by biopsy, its histologic characteristics. At gastroscopy a total of at least six biopsies should be obtained from the inner

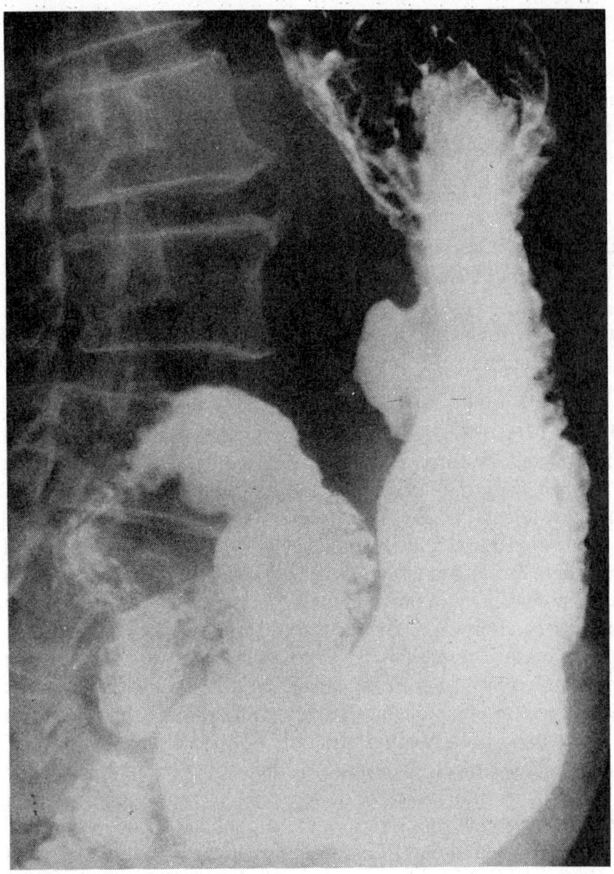

FIGURE 235-5 *Benign lesser curvature gastric ulcer. Note ulceration beyond the projected margins of the stomach and the collar of edema.*

margin of the ulcer and from the ulcer bed. If accurate cytology is available, brushings of the ulcer should be obtained prior to biopsy. By application of combined radiographic, endoscopic, and histologic techniques, distinguishing a malignant from a benign gastric ulcer should be possible with greater than 95 percent confidence.

Gastric ulcer in association with histamine- or pentagastrin-fast achlorhydria, is rare. When it occurs, it almost always indicates that one is dealing with a gastric carcinoma. However, most patients with gastric carcinoma (about two-thirds to three-fourths) are capable of secreting some gastric acid, although it is usually less than normal.

MEDICAL TREATMENT *Antacids* are effective in gastric ulcer treatment. However, since acid hypersecretion is not characteristic of the disease, smaller doses of antacid may be required than for treatment of duodenal ulcer. It is suggested that 15 to 30 mL of a potent liquid antacid be taken 1 and 3 h after meals and at bedtime. *H-2-receptor antagonists* and *sucralfate* are approximately as effective as antacid therapy in the treatment of gastric ulcer. The recommended dosage schedules for these drugs are similar to those in patients with duodenal ulcer. In general, a gastric ulcer tends to heal more slowly than a duodenal ulcer, and the healing response rates are somewhat less than those for a duodenal ulcer.

Anticholinergic agents have been recommended by some physicians. However, because of substantial side effects of anticholinergic drugs, their tendency to reduce gastric emptying, which is already impaired in these patients, the fact that gastric ulcer patients are often older and, therefore, more susceptible to the complications of these agents, and the lack of evidence for their benefit, the use of anticholinergic drugs in gastric ulcer treatment does not appear justified. Some studies suggest that hospitalization and/or cessation of smoking are of benefit in gastric ulcer healing.

Since salicylate ingestion has been associated with the development of gastric ulcers, patients with gastric ulcer should not ingest salicylates. Alcohol, because of its injurious effects on the gastric mucosa, should also be avoided. Milk and cream, as well as bland or homogenized diets, have not been shown to be of value in treatment. In general, it is probably sufficient to recommend that patients take a diet of their own choice. Since coffee (caffeine-containing or caffeine-free) and other caffeine-containing liquids stimulate gastric acid secretion, it may be desirable to omit these beverages.

Carbenoxolone has been used in many countries (but not in the United States) in the treatment of gastric ulcer. This drug is a hydrolytic product of glycyrrhizic acid (derived from licorice) and has been shown to decrease symptoms and increase the rate of gastric ulcer healing. Carbenoxolone does not decrease gastric acid secretion but increases the life span of gastric mucosal epithelial cells and increases the secretion and viscosity of gastric mucus. Carbenoxolone possesses aldosterone-like effects, and thus sodium and water retention tend to occur. It is possible to inhibit the aldosterone-like effects of carbenoxolone by use of aldosterone antagonists; however, the latter also abolish the healing effects of carbenoxolone. Problems with sodium and water retention and the availability of alternative drugs have led to its decreased use.

The failure of gastric ulcer to decrease satisfactorily in size and to heal with medical treatment has been used to suggest gastric malignancy. Benign gastric ulcers should heal completely after 3 months of vigorous therapy. Upper gastrointestinal barium examination or gastroscopy should be performed after 4 weeks of treatment, at which time definite healing should be demonstrable in benign gastric ulcers—the diameter of most ulcers should be reduced by more than 50 percent. If at 4 weeks the ulcer is not reduced in size, malignancy must be suspected and sought for by appropriate biopsies of the ulcer and exfoliative cytology. If the ulcer has not healed completely at 8 weeks, endoscopic examination should be repeated in another month, at which time most benign gastric ulcers should have healed. In general, large gastric ulcers heal more slowly than smaller ones. It is important to continue treatment to endoscopically verify complete ulcer healing. One must be alert, however, to the occasional "healing" of an ulcerating gastric carcinoma with treatment. Apparent complete healing does not assure the benign nature of a gastric ulcer since approximately 70 percent of gastric ulcers eventually found to be malignant will undergo significant healing (albeit usually incomplete) with medical treatment.

COMPLICATIONS AND SURGERY FOR PEPTIC ULCER

Surgery is reserved for patients with complications of peptic ulcer and for those who do not respond to vigorous and attentive medical treatment. Complications include hemorrhage, obstruction, and perforation.

Hemorrhage occurs in approximately 15 to 20 percent of patients with duodenal ulcers; there may be a recurrence of bleeding in about 40 percent of patients with an initial hemorrhage. In most patients hemorrhage from peptic ulcer responds satisfactorily to medical management—including gastric suction and antacid or H-2-receptor antagonist administration.

Free *perforation* into the peritoneal cavity occurs in approximately 6 percent of patients with duodenal ulcer. Five to ten percent of these patients will have had no recognizable ulcer symptoms prior to perforation. Simultaneous hemorrhage occurs in approximately 10 percent of patients with duodenal ulcer perforation; mortality is greatly increased in this group. Duodenal ulcers, especially those located posteriorly, may penetrate into adjacent structures, most often the pancreas—frequently resulting in increased serum amylase levels. Less commonly, duodenal ulcers may penetrate into the liver, biliary tract, or colon.

Gastric outlet *obstruction* occurs in 2 to 4 percent of patients admitted to the hospital with duodenal or pyloric channel ulcers.

Symptoms include abdominal bloating, nausea, vomiting, and weight loss. These patients usually have had ulcer symptoms for many years and often obstructive symptoms for several months.

Failure to respond satisfactorily to medical treatment requires consideration of surgery. The true incidence of lack of ulcer healing with vigorous medical programs is not known; it is clear, however, that most patients with peptic ulcer can be treated successfully without surgery.

Decisions regarding surgery for patients with complications of peptic ulcer must be individualized. Risks of surgery must be balanced with risks of the disease. The patient's discomfort, costs of medical care and hospitalization, and time lost from work must be weighed in relation to the morbidity and possible mortality associated with surgery and anesthesia, risks of recurrent ulcer, and long-term postoperative sequelae. The skill and experience of the surgeon must be weighed as major factors in considering operation.

SURGERY FOR DUODENAL ULCER No single surgical procedure has been accepted universally as the most satisfactory duodenal ulcer operation. At present the most commonly performed surgical procedures are *vagotomy with antrectomy, vagotomy with pyloroplasty, and parietal cell vagotomy* (also referred to as *proximal gastric or superselective vagotomy*) without a gastric drainage procedure. With conventional (truncal) vagotomy and antrectomy, the vagal trunks are transected, the antrum is removed, and gastrointestinal continuity is reestablished by anastomosis of the remaining stomach with the proximal duodenum (Billroth I anastomosis) or with a loop of the jejunum (Billroth II anastomosis). Vagotomy and antrectomy is an effective procedure with a low recurrence rate (approximately 1 percent). Morbidity and mortality with vagotomy and antrectomy are variable, depend upon patient selection and the skill of the surgeon, but are probably slightly greater than with vagotomy and pyloroplasty.

When the procedure of vagotomy and pyloroplasty is selected, pyloroplasty is performed to facilitate gastric drainage after truncal or selective vagotomy. Vagotomy is performed to inhibit vagal stimulation of gastric acid secretion. Vagotomy does not inhibit gastrin release; in fact, release of gastrin is enhanced after vagal interruption. As indicated above, three types of vagotomy are now used in the surgical treatment of duodenal ulcer and pyloric channel ulcer, namely, *truncal vagotomy, selective vagotomy,* and *parietal cell vagotomy.* Pyloroplasty with truncal vagotomy, which is still the most commonly performed method of vagal transection in the United States, is associated with approximately 1 percent mortality. Ulcer recurrence during the 5 years after surgery is about 5 to 8 percent. With selective vagotomy only the branches of the vagus which supply the stomach are transected, preserving the vagal innervation of the other abdominal viscera. Selective vagotomy has been found by some surgeons to result in a more complete vagotomy, less ulcer recurrence, and fewer postvagotomy complications than truncal vagotomy. Parietal cell vagotomy denervates only the acid-secreting portion of the stomach, sparing the branches of the vagus which innervate the antrum, and a gastric drainage procedure is unnecessary. Both immediate and late postoperative complications are less common with parietal cell vagotomy than with truncal vagotomy, and reductions in acid secretion with parietal cell vagotomy are generally comparable with those achieved with truncal or selective vagotomy. Mortality with parietal cell vagotomy is less than 1 percent. Most studies indicate that with experience in the performance of parietal cell vagotomy, recurrence is comparable to that with other forms of vagotomy with pyloroplasty. This procedure, which is being used with increasing frequency, appears to be an effective and safe surgical therapy for duodenal ulcer.

SURGERY FOR GASTRIC ULCER Surgical treatment is required for gastric ulcer patients who do not respond satisfactorily to medical therapy or who develop complications similar to those described for duodenal ulcer. With the available diagnostic accuracy of careful radiographic examination, endoscopy, biopsy of the ulcer margins, and exfoliative cytology, it should rarely be necessary to operate because of a remaining uncertainty regarding the malignant or benign nature of the ulcer. The recommended surgical procedure for the treatment of gastric ulcer is antrectomy with gastroduodenal (Billroth I) anastomosis. It is not necessary to perform a vagotomy when antrectomy is performed for gastric ulcer (not located in the pyloric channel).

CONSEQUENCES AND SYNDROMES AFTER PEPTIC ULCER SURGERY

Modern surgery for peptic ulcer is effective in both the treatment of ulcer complications and in the prevention of ulcer recurrence. However, numerous postoperative sequelae and syndromes may occur.

RECURRENT ULCERATION Recurrent ulceration has been reported in approximately 5 percent of all patients after surgery for peptic ulcer. Approximately 95 percent of these recurrences follow surgery for duodenal ulcer disease. The risk of development of recurrent ulcer is 3 to 10 percent after surgery for duodenal ulcer and approximately 2 percent after gastric ulcer surgery. Recurrence is more common after vagotomy and pyloroplasty and after parietal cell vagotomy than after vagotomy and antrectomy. When ulcers occur after partial gastric resection, the site is usually at the anastomosis or immediately distal to it in the small intestine. Abdominal pain is the most common symptom in patients with a stomal (or marginal) ulcer. The pain is usually epigastric but is often not characteristic of common duodenal ulcer. It is usually, but not always, relieved by meals or antacids and, in general, tends to be more persistent and progressive than that observed with unoperated duodenal ulcer. Hemorrhage or anemia due to blood loss, nausea and vomiting from obstruction, weight loss, or symptoms from perforation may occur. The development of a stomal ulcer after duodenal ulcer surgery usually indicates that an incomplete vagotomy was performed. Inadequate gastric resection, when performed without vagotomy, may also result in stomal ulceration. Additional causes for the development of recurrent ulcer include an excessively long jejunal afferent loop, an inadvertently performed gastroileal or gastrocolic anastomosis, poor gastric drainage, and ingestion of ulcerogenic drugs. Less commonly, a marginal ulcer may be caused by gastrinoma or by acid hypersecretion secondary to retained antrum. If patients with gastrinomas are treated by gastroenterostomy, stomal ulceration is almost inevitable.

Radiographic examination with barium is of limited diagnostic value and identifies only from 50 to 65 percent of stomal ulcerations. Surgical deformity at the anastomotic site may often mimic stomal ulcer in its absence, or conceal it when present. When suspected, endoscopic examination is required to identify stomal ulceration. Medical treatment with antacids is almost always unsatisfactory in patients with stomal ulcer. Cimetidine has been used successfully in inducing healing of recurrent ulcer. The long-term effects of cimetidine on recurrent ulcers and the prevention of their further recurrence remain to be established. Surgery is usually necessary for treatment of ulcer recurrence and it is usually, but not invariably, successful. In patients with recurrent ulcer provocative testing should be performed and measurements made of serum gastrin to identify or exclude gastrinoma (see below).

RECURRENT ULCER DUE TO RETAINED ANTRUM Recurrent ulcers have been described in a small number of patients after antrectomy with gastrojejunostomy (Billroth II anastomosis) in which the antral resection was not complete. In these patients the distal antrum, inadvertently not resected, remains in continuity with the duodenum after surgery. These patients usually develop or continue to have gastric acid hypersecretion due to gastrin release by the residual antral mucosa which is no longer in contact with gastric acid, the normal inhibitor of gastrin release. In these patients fasting serum gastrin levels may be normal to moderately increased. Patients with retained antrum can be distinguished from those with gastrinoma by intravenous injection of secretin with measurements of serum gastrin. Gastrinoma patients exhibit paradoxical increases in serum gastrin, whereas in those with retained antrum, serum gastrin levels decrease after secretin administration (see Table 235-1). These patients can be treated successfully by surgical removal of the remaining antrum.

AFFERENT LOOP SYNDROMES Patients with partial gastric resection with gastrojejunostomy (Billroth II anastomosis) may experience abdominal bloating and pain 20 min to 1 h after eating, frequently followed by nausea and vomiting. The vomitus often contains large amounts of bile. Characteristically, the bloating and abdominal discomfort are relieved by vomiting. This type of afferent loop syndrome, which is uncommon, is believed to be caused by distention of an incompletely draining afferent intestinal loop by pancreatic and biliary secretions which are stimulated by eating. Serum amylase levels may be mildly or moderately increased. Because of partial obstruction it is often difficult to demonstrate the afferent loop by barium meal examination. Treatment is surgical correction of the incomplete afferent loop obstruction, and, in some instances, revision to a gastroduodenal anastomosis.

A second form of afferent loop dysfunction is that due to stasis with bacterial overgrowth within the afferent loop. These patients may exhibit the same characteristics as are found with other forms of small intestinal bacterial overgrowth or blind loop syndromes (see Chap. 237). These include malabsorption, especially of fat and vitamin B_{12}. Correction of the afferent loop bacterial overgrowth syndrome can be accomplished by surgical revision of the afferent loop.

BILE REFLUX GASTRITIS After peptic ulcer surgery a small proportion of patients experience early satiety, abdominal discomfort, and vomiting, which is believed due to reflux of duodenal contents into the stomach. Endoscopic examination usually reveals regurgitated bile in the stomach and diffuse gastritis, often involving the entire gastric remnant. Various terms assigned to this entity include *alkaline reflux gastritis, bile reflux gastritis, duodenogastric reflux,* and *bilious vomiting*. The mechanisms or materials contained in the refluxed intestinal contents accounting for these symptoms have not been defined. Although the term bile reflux gastritis has been used, there is no certainty that regurgitated bile is responsible for the syndrome. Administration of cholestyramine, intended to bind bile acids and facilitate their excretion, has not been of benefit in this disorder. Some surgeons have reported successful treatment of bile reflux gastritis by diversion of duodenal contents from proximity to the stomach with a Roux en Y anastomosis.

DUMPING SYNDROME Following peptic ulcer surgery some patients experience an assortment of vasomotor symptoms after eating. These include palpitation, tachycardia, lightheadedness, diaphoresis, and, less frequently, postural hypotension. Abdominal discomfort and vomiting may also occur. The vasomotor symptoms, referred to as the *early dumping syndrome,* are usually experienced within 30 min after eating and are believed to result from rapid emptying of hyperosmolar gastric contents into the proximal small intestine. This leads to a shift of fluid into the gut lumen and produces intestinal distention and contraction of plasma volume. Additional proposed mechanisms for these symptoms include stimulation of autonomic reflexes secondary to small intestinal distention and/or release of hormones from the gut in response to rapid entry of gastric contents into the duodenum or jejunum.

The *late dumping syndrome* refers to a symptom complex comprising dizziness, lightheadedness, palpitation, diaphoresis, confusion, and, in rare instances, syncope, occurring 90 min to 3 h after eating. The symptoms can often be precipitated by meals rich in simple carbohydrates, especially sucrose. The syndrome appears to be caused by hypoglycemia due to insulin release stimulated by abrupt increases in blood glucose secondary to rapid emptying of sugar-containing meals into the proximal small intestine.

Both forms of the dumping syndrome are treated by dietary measures. These include limitation of simple sugar-containing liquids and solids (sweets), elimination of liquids at mealtime, and frequent small meals. Most patients have not been benefited by surgical procedures such as insertion of reversed jejunal loops and isoperistaltic jejunal interposition.

POSTVAGOTOMY DIARRHEA A significant number of patients experience diarrhea after peptic ulcer surgery, especially with a procedure including truncal vagotomy. Diarrhea usually occurs within 2 h of eating. Although the mechanism is not clear, interruption of vagal fibers to the abdominal viscera appears to play an important role in the production of the diarrhea. The surgical drainage procedure, pyloroplasty or antrectomy, which removes the pyloric regulatory emptying mechanism, may also contribute to the diarrhea. Diarrhea has been estimated to occur in 20 to 30 percent of patients after truncal vagotomy with drainage, in 4 to 20 percent with selective vagotomy and drainage, and in only 1 to 8 percent of those with parietal cell vagotomy (without drainage). Rapid emptying of gastric contents into the small intestine, resulting in increased fluid volume within the intestinal lumen, due to the osmotic action of the meal, may also contribute to the diarrhea.

HEMATOLOGIC COMPLICATIONS Intrinsic factor secreted by gastric parietal cells is necessary for active absorption of vitamin B_{12} by the distal ileum. Patients who have had total gastrectomy invariably will develop malabsorption of vitamin B_{12} and should receive monthly intramuscular injections of vitamin B_{12} (50 to 100 μg indefinitely). Megaloblastic anemia due to vitamin B_{12} deficiency is rare after partial gastric resection; however, reduced serum vitamin B_{12} levels have been observed in about 14 percent of these patients. Even more rarely vitamin B_{12} deficiency may be produced by bacterial overgrowth in a stagnant afferent loop following Billroth II anastomosis. Gastritis in the remaining stomach develops in more than 60 percent of duodenal ulcer patients after vagotomy and antrectomy or vagotomy and pyloroplasty. This may result in decreased vitamin B_{12} absorption. Inasmuch as the stomach secretes intrinsic factor in excess of need by approximately 100 times, peptic ulcer patients treated with partial gastric resection do not develop vitamin B_{12} deficiency secondary to the amount of stomach resected. (In addition, the resected portion of the stomach is almost always principally antrum, which contains few parietal cells.) However, after peptic ulcer surgery patients may develop decreased serum vitamin B_{12} levels due to reduced absorption of food-bound vitamin B_{12}; these patients will often have normal absorption of free vitamin B_{12}, as used in the Schilling test. The precise mechanism for the malabsorption of food-bound vitamin B_{12} is not known. It may be due in part to rapid emptying of gastric contents, with reduced efficiency of intrinsic factor binding of vitamin B_{12}. Anemia after peptic ulcer surgery may also result from deficiency produced by malabsorption of iron or folate. A combined deficiency of vitamin B_{12}, iron, and folate is common in patients with anemia following partial or subtotal gastric resection. Iron deficiency is the

TABLE 235-1 Provocative gastrin tests

	Serum gastrin response (change from basal levels)	
Disorder	After IV secretin injection	After test meal
Zollinger-Ellison (gastrinoma)	Increase (greater than 200 pg/mL)	Little or no increase (increases less than 50%)
Common duodenal ulcer	No change (or slight decrease or slight increase)	Moderate increase (may be slightly more than normal, but less than in gastrin cell hyperplasia)
Antral gastrin cell hyperplasia	Decrease	Striking increase (greater than 200%)
Achlorhydria (e.g., pernicious anemia, chronic gastritis)	Decrease	Moderate increase

most common single hematologic defect after peptic ulcer surgery and may result from either blood loss (e.g., with persistent or recurrent ulcer) or from iron malabsorption. Patients with gastric resection malabsorb dietary iron but have normal absorption of iron salts; therefore they will respond favorably to treatment with therapeutic oral iron preparations. Folate deficiency may result from either reduced dietary intake or impaired folate absorption. Except for the anemia produced by blood loss in association with early recurrent ulcer disease, the development of anemia after peptic ulcer surgery is gradual, usually occurring several years postoperatively.

The nature of the anemia after ulcer surgery should be clarified by determination of the red blood cell morphology and by measurements of serum iron, folate, and vitamin B_{12}. Iron or folate deficiency may be treated by oral replacement. Vitamin B_{12} deficiency should be treated with monthly intramuscular injections of the vitamin.

OSTEOMALACIA AND OSTEOPOROSIS Osteoporosis and osteomalacia may develop after partial or complete gastrectomy but occur rarely after vagotomy and pyloroplasty. Osteomalacia is extremely frequent following gastrojejunostomy or Billroth II anastomosis. These bone changes are believed to result from malabsorption of calcium and vitamin D. Patients may develop bone pain and have pathologic fractures. The incidence of bone fractures in men following gastric resection has been estimated to be almost twice that of control subjects of similar age. Reduced bone density requires years to develop and can be identified by x-ray. Patients with osteomalacia usually have increased levels of serum alkaline phosphatase and may have reduced serum calcium concentrations. These patients should be treated by supplemental oral vitamin D and calcium. In fact, the frequency of osteoporosis and osteomalacia after partial or complete gastrectomy is sufficiently great that treatment with vitamin D and calcium should probably be instituted and continued indefinitely in these patients, especially females, following gastric resection.

GENERAL MALABSORPTION (See Chap. 237) Mild, chemically demonstrable steatorrhea is common in patients after ulcer surgery. Weight loss is more common after partial gastric resection than with vagotomy without resection and occurs in approximately 60 percent of patients in whom a portion of the stomach has been removed. The major cause of weight loss after peptic ulcer surgery is reduced food intake. On a 100-g fat diet, loss of stool fat seldom exceeds 15 g per day (normal individuals, less than 7 g per day). The causes of maldigestion and malabsorption after peptic ulcer surgery include rapid gastric emptying, reduced dispersion of food in the stomach, reduced bile concentrations in the gut lumen, increased rate of transit of the meal through the small intestine, and reduced or delayed pancreatic secretory responses to feeding. Steatorrhea and weight loss, sometimes accompanied by vitamin B_{12} malabsorption, may develop as a result of bacterial overgrowth, especially in patients with afferent loop bacterial stasis. Overt symptoms and other manifestations of malabsorption appearing after surgery for peptic ulcer may also be due to other preexisting conditions, including latent celiac sprue and chronic pancreatitis.

CARCINOMA AFTER PARTIAL GASTRECTOMY Several studies have documented an increased incidence of adenocarcinoma of the stomach in duodenal ulcer patients following partial gastric resection and after vagotomy and drainage without resection. This usually develops 10 or more years after ulcer surgery. The possibility of carcinoma of the stomach should be considered when abdominal symptoms, which may be similar to or distinct from those due to the original ulcer, appear many years after apparently successful surgery.

ZOLLINGER-ELLISON SYNDROME (GASTRINOMA)

In 1955 Zollinger and Ellison described the syndrome which bears their names, i.e., ulcer disease of the upper gastrointestinal tract, marked increases in gastric acid secretion, and nonbeta islet-cell tumors of the pancreas.

ETIOLOGY AND PATHOGENESIS Zollinger and Ellison, in their original description of the syndrome, suggested that the ulcer disease in these patients resulted from liberation of a secretagogue from the islet-cell tumors which accounted for the often enormously increased rates of gastric acid secretion. Their proposal was proved correct when in 1960 extracts of Zollinger-Ellison (Z-E) tumors were shown to stimulate gastric acid secretion. Subsequently, it was found that the pancreatic tumors contained gastrin and that large amounts of this hormone were released into the circulation, producing the pathophysiologic characteristics of the syndrome. These gastrin-containing tumors are, therefore, now referred to as *gastrinomas.* Gastrin has been demonstrated in these tumors by chemical isolation of polypeptides with amino acid compositions and peptide mapping patterns identical with those of human gastrin molecules. In addition, large amounts of gastrin have been demonstrated by radioimmunoassay in gastrinomas and in serums of patients with the Z-E syndrome.

Most gastrinomas are found within the pancreas. Multiple, apparently primary, tumors are common. Pancreatic gastrinomas may be single or multiple and may vary in size from 2 mm to more than 20 cm in diameter. In from one-half to two-thirds of patients multiple gastrinomas are present within the pancreas; however, more than half of these are not identified at surgery. Pancreatic gastrinomas are most common in the body or tail of the pancreas. Approximately 13 percent of patients with this syndrome have tumors in the wall of the proximal duodenum. Gastrinomas have also been located less commonly in other sites, including the hilum of the spleen and very rarely in the stomach. Primary gastrinomas, surrounded by lymphoid tissue, have been found in proximity to the pancreas, proximal duodenum, and spleen. These may be confused with, but are distinct from, metastasis to regional lymph nodes. In rare instances, the Z-E syndrome has resulted from ectopic gastrin-containing tumors, e.g., parathyroid and ovarian adenomas. Many, and when sought for, most, gastrin-secreting islet-cell tumors have been found to contain multiple hormones, which may or may not be released, but are usually clinically silent. These have included adrenocorticotropic hormone, glucagon, insulin, pancreatic polypeptide, and vasoactive intestinal peptide. The absolute frequency of multiple hormones contained in or released by these tumors is not known. Approximately one-third of patients with gastrinomas have increases in serum concentrations of *pancreatic polypeptide.* About two-thirds are histologically or biologically malignant, and about half have spread to the liver when the tumor is identified. Malignant gastrinomas usually grow slowly. From one-half to two-thirds of patients with gastrinomas have metastases, most commonly to regional lymph nodes and liver; spread may also be to peritoneal surfaces, spleen, bone, skin, or mediastinum. Gastrinomas have light-microscopic similarities to carcinoid tumors and may be mistaken for carcinoid tumors, especially when arising from the mucosa of the small intestine or stomach. Pancreatic islet-cell hyperplasia occurs in approximately 10 percent of patients with the Z-E syndrome. Hyperplasia of the islets, accompanying recognizable or unidentified gastrinoma, appears to be an association or a consequence rather than a cause of excess gastrin release, since gastrin is not present in the hyperplastic tissue.

In most gastrinomas approximately 90 to 95 percent of gastrin is in the form of heptadecapeptide gastrin (G-17 or little gastrin), with most of the remainder being big gastrin (G-34). In contrast, approximately two-thirds of circulating gastrin in gastrinoma patients is G-34; most of the remainder of circulating gastrin is G-17. However, smaller amounts of even larger forms of gastrin and smaller gastrin fragments can be detected in the serum. The parietal cell mass is substantially expanded to from three to six times normal, secondary to the trophic effects of gastrin on parietal cells.

In from 20 to 25 percent of patients with the Z-E syndrome, the gastrinoma is a component of the multiple endocrine neoplasia type I (MEN-I) syndrome, an autosomal dominant disorder with a high degree of penetrance and great variability in expressivity. Patients with MEN-I may have hyperplasia, adenomas, or carcinoma involving the parathyroid glands, pancreatic islets, and pituitary: the organs involved are in that order of frequency. Hyperparathyroidism is present in 87 percent of patients with the MEN-I syndrome, and gastrinoma is present in approximately half of these patients (see Chap. 334).

While the true incidence of the Z-E syndrome is not known, estimates are that it accounts for 0.1 to 1 percent of peptic ulcers. The Z-E syndrome may occur at any age, but initial manifestations are most common between ages 30 and 60.

CLINICAL FEATURES From 90 to 95 percent of patients with gastrinomas develop ulceration of the gastrointestinal tract at some point during the course of their disease. Profound gastric hypersecretion is found in most, but not all, patients. Symptoms are often similar to those seen in patients with typical peptic ulcer disease. However, the ulcer symptoms may be more fulminant, progressive, and persistent, and usually respond poorly to usual medical and surgical peptic ulcer treatment programs. The anatomic site of the ulcers in patients with gastrinoma is similar, but not identical, to that of patients with common types of peptic ulcer. About 75 percent of gastrinoma patients have ulcers in the first portion of the duodenum or in the stomach; these are usually single, but may be multiple. When multiple ulcers occur, they are frequently located not only in the first portion of the duodenum, but also in the remainder of the duodenum or even the jejunum. In one large series, 14 percent of the ulcers were found in the duodenum beyond its first portion, and 11 percent in the jejunum. Prompt recurrence of ulcer, often with hemorrhage or perforation, after peptic ulcer surgery without total gastrectomy (in which the Z-E syndrome had not been recognized) is characteristic of gastrinoma.

Diarrhea occurs in about 40 percent of patients, and about 7 percent of patients with gastrinoma may have diarrhea in the absence of ulcer disease. The diarrhea is due to the outpouring of large amounts of hydrochloric acid into the proximal duodenum and can be reduced or eliminated by aspiration of gastric juice. The excessive acid has been shown to reduce the pH within the lumen of the proximal and distal jejunum to as low as 1 and 3.6, respectively. Inflammatory changes may develop in the mucosa of the small intestine, presumably secondary to the injurious effect of the increased amounts of acid and pepsin. Steatorrhea, which is less common than diarrhea, appears to result from inactivation of pancreatic lipase by the large concentration of acid in the proximal small intestine and from decreases in luminal bile acids. The decrease in bile acid concentration of the intraluminal contents is caused by precipitation of the major bile acids at low pH. This leads to impaired micelle formation which, in turn, reduces the intestinal absorption of fatty acids and monoglycerides (see Chap. 237). Vitamin B_{12} malabsorption, not correctable by addition of intrinsic factor, has been detected in some patients with the Z-E syndrome. Although the secretion of intrinsic factor appears normal, the reduced pH within the gut interferes with intrinsic factor mediation of vitamin B_{12} absorption. This can be corrected by neutralization of the intestinal contents. The mechanism by which low pH in the gut interferes with intrinsic factor action is not known.

Diarrhea in patients with gastrinoma is invariably accompanied by gastric acid *hypersecretion*. (This does not occur in patients with common duodenal ulcer with similar rates of hypersecretion of gastric acid; the reason for this difference is not known.) Severe diarrhea is also seen with other nonbeta islet-cell tumors of the pancreas, which are usually associated with *hyposecretion* of gastric acid or even achlorhydria [pancreatic cholera or WDHA (watery diarrhea, hypokalemia, and achlorhydria) syndrome]. In most cases, the pancreatic cholera syndrome appears to be due to tumor release of VIP (see Chaps. 334 and 255).

DIAGNOSIS The presence of a gastrinoma should be suspected in patients with a compatible clinical history, especially in those with evidence of marked acid hypersecretion. Two-thirds of gastrinoma patients have basal gastric acid outputs (BAO) which exceed 15 meq/h. In some instances the basal output may be greater than 100 meq/h. However, as stated earlier, there is substantial overlap in the rates of gastric acid secretion among patients with gastrinoma, duodenal ulcer, and normal subjects. Gastrinoma patients often have basal acid output rates which are greater than 60 percent of those induced by maximal stimulation (MAO). In most normal subjects and duodenal ulcer patients basal acid secretory rates are less than 60 percent of maximal secretion. However, because of frequent patient variations, with exceptions to these guidelines by patients with gastrinomas and common duodenal ulcers, the use of the BAO/MAO ratio is of no value in the certain identification of gastrinoma patients.

Some radiographic features may suggest and support the diagnosis of the Z-E syndrome. Large mucosal folds may be demonstrated in the stomach, duodenum, and, in some instances, the jejunum. The lumen of the stomach and small intestine often contains large amounts of fluid. Radiographic features of most ulcers in these patients, except when they are multiple or distal in location, are similar to the common peptic ulcer. Arteriography is of limited value in identifying patients with gastrinoma; primary tumors or hepatic metastases demonstrated at surgery have been identified in only from 20 to 30 percent of gastrinoma patients. Some reports suggest that computerized axial tomography may be of slightly greater value in identifying primary or metastatic gastrinoma. Endoscopic retrograde pancreaticoduodenography (ERCP) has not proved to be of assistance in the diagnosis or exclusion of pancreatic gastrinomas. A small number of duodenal wall gastrinomas have been identified and confirmed histologically by duodenoscopy.

The diagnosis in a patient with clinical features consistent with the Z-E syndrome depends upon the demonstration of *increased serum gastrin levels* by radioimmunoassay. Fasting serum gastrin levels in normal subjects and patients with typical duodenal ulcer average approximately 40 to 50 pg/mL and usually do not exceed 150 pg/mL. Patients with gastrinoma almost always have fasting serum gastrin levels which are greater than 200 pg/mL and have been reported as high as 450,000 pg/mL. Approximately half of these patients have fasting serum gastrin levels which are less than 1000 pg/mL.

Several provocative tests have been used to evaluate patients with possible gastrinoma, especially in those who do not exhibit pronounced hypergastrinemia (i.e., serum gastrin greater than 1000 pg/mL). These tests utilize the measurement of serum gastrin levels in response to intravenous calcium infusion, secretin injection, or ingestion of a standard test meal (see Table 235-1).

In the *secretin injection test,* secretin (Kabi secretin, 2 units per kilogram) is given intravenously over 30 to 60 s. (Boots secretin is approximately one-sixth as potent as Kabi secretin prepared by the Karolinska Institute, Stockholm. Boots secretin should not be used, since it contains large amounts of gastrin-like material which is immunoreactive with antibodies to gastrin and, therefore, can spuriously increase serum gastrin concentrations.) Gastrin is measured in serum samples obtained before injection of secretin and at 5-min intervals thereafter for 30 min. In normal individuals and patients with common duodenal ulcer, secretin produces either no change or small reductions or small increases in serum gastrin levels. In contrast, in gastrinoma patients intravenous secretin induces substantial increases in serum gastrin. The gastrin levels increase promptly, usually at 5 min, (and virtually always by 10 min), by at least 200 pg/mL. The *calcium infusion test* involves constant 3-h intravenous infusion of calcium gluconate (5 mg calcium per kilogram per hour). Serum samples for gastrin measurements are obtained before and at 30-min intervals for 4 h after initiation of infusion. In gastrinoma patients serum gastrin concentrations usually increase above the basal serum gastrin by at least 50 percent or by more than 400 pg/mL. The third provocative test involves the *feeding of a standard meal;* gastrin is measured in serum samples obtained before the meal and at 15-min intervals for 90 min. In gastrinoma patients peak serum gastrin levels do not increase (or increase minimally) and do not reach values 50 percent greater than fasting levels (see Table 235-1).

The secretin injection test is the provocative test of greatest value in identifying gastrinoma patients. Positive serum gastrin responses to intravenous secretin are detected in more than 95 percent of patients with gastrinoma. Using the criteria suggested, substantial increases in serum gastrin following secretin injection have not been detected in nongastrinoma patients. Exaggerated release of gastrin in response to calcium infusion has been found in more than 80 percent of gastrinoma patients; however, this exaggerated response to calcium infusion has been observed in some nongastrinoma patients with hypergastrinemia (e.g., achlorhydria with or without pernicious anemia). In gastrinoma patients enhanced gastrin release with calcium infusion is not observed in the absence of paradoxical gastrin release in response to secretin. Since the calcium infusion test does not add to the sensitivity or specificity of the secretin injection test and since calcium infusion is potentially more hazardous, it is not recommended as a provocative test in evaluating patients in whom the diagnosis of gastrinoma is considered.

In a very small proportion of duodenal ulcer patients (less than 1 percent), gastric acid hypersecretion may be accompanied by increased serum gastrin levels due to hyperfunction and/or hyperplasia of antral gastrin cells (G cells). These can be distinguished from gastrinoma patients by the secretin and meal stimulation tests. In patients with this antral gastrin cell abnormality, intravenous secretin reduces serum gastrin and ingestion of the test meal leads to striking increases in serum gastrin levels, exceeding the fasting serum gastrin concentration by more than 200 percent.

TREATMENT In general, these patients are resistant to medical treatment regimens and surgical procedures designed for and usually effective in common peptic ulcer. Antacids may produce transient symptomatic relief but seldom induce ulcer healing or sustained relief of symptoms. Incomplete gastric resection (with or without vagotomy or pyloroplasty with vagotomy) is frequently followed by prompt and often fulminant ulcer recurrence. Many patients with gastrinoma have had multiple surgical procedures, particularly when the diagnosis was not established initially. Mortality has been lowest when gastrectomy was performed as the initial surgical procedure. For this reason, when gastric surgery is required in gastrinoma patients, total gastrectomy has been considered the surgical procedure of choice; subtotal gastric resections should not be performed.

The recent development of more effective drugs and more precise diagnostic techniques has substantially altered the therapeutic options available for gastrinoma patients. Patients with the Z-E syndrome due to gastrinoma are highly heterogeneous in respect to their clinical manifestations and extent of disease. The key to management is individualization of treatment.

The *H-2-receptor antagonists* are effective in reducing gastric acid secretion, producing symptom relief and inducing ulcer healing in patients with the Z-E syndrome. *Cimetidine* has been widely and successfully used. Improvement in clinical symptoms, decreases in gastric acid output, and ulcer healing occur in 80 to 85 percent of patients so treated. Administration of cimetidine has been required at 4- to 6-h intervals, with total daily doses usually 2 to 5 times those used in the treatment of common duodenal ulcer. More recently, *ranitidine* has also been effectively used. The increased potency of ranitidine compared with cimetidine has provided a therapeutic advantage because of the large doses required. A further advantage of ranitidine is that it does not produce gynecomastia, a common consequence of large and prolonged doses of cimetidine in male patients with gastrinoma. When instituted, H-2-receptor antagonist therapy must be continued indefinitely, since even its temporary discontinuance is usually followed by ulcer recurrence. The effectiveness of the H-2-receptor antagonist therapy in reducing gastric acid secretion can be assessed by measuring unstimulated gastric acid output for 1 h immediately prior to the next anticipated dose of the drug; the goal is to reduce gastric acid output to less than 10 meq/h. H-2-receptor antagonists are indicated as initial treatment of gastrinoma patients, for prolonged treatment of those patients who are poor candidates for tumor reaction, and in those in whom total gastrectomy is not anticipated.

Clinical trials have also demonstrated even more effective reduction in acid secretion and ulcer healing with omeprazole, a potent hydrogen-potassium ATPase inhibitor. A small number of Z-E patients have been treated effectively with parietal cell vagotomy combined with indefinitely continued treatment with reduced doses of H-2-receptor antagonists.

In selecting the best therapy for the individual patient, the biologic behavior of these turmors and the clinical manifestations in each patient must be taken into consideration. Complete surgical resection of the tumors, when possible, represents optimal treatment in patients with gastrinoma. Successful tumor resection is seldon achieved in gastrinoma patients with MEN-I, because of the overwhelming likelihood of multifocal tumors, frequently with metastasis, at the time of diagnosis. Therapeutic doses of H-2-receptor antagonists are indicated in the period during which the diagnosis is being established, while the location and extent of the tumor are being determined and also as treatment prior to anticipated surgery. At present, H-2-receptor antagonists are certainly indicated for patients who are poor operative candidates, for those who refuse surgery, and for those in whom surgery is not possible. When metastatic or otherwise nonresectable gastrinoma is present, control of the ulcer disease may be achieved in most instances by treatment with H-2-receptor antagonists or by total gastric resection. There is no convincing evidence that tumor progression is influenced by gastrectomy. Patients with progressive invasive gastrinoma may be benefited by streptozotocin and 5-fluorouracil, which may reduce tumor bulk and partially reduce serum gastrin levels.

The most difficult treatment decisions are in those patients in whom the location and extent of the tumor have not been defined. With more general use of gastrin radioimmunoassay, patients with gastrinomas are being detected earlier in the course of their disease. Prior studies indicated that the morbidity and mortality in patients with the Z-E syndrome were largely due to the complications of the severe ulcer disease. However, with earlier diagnosis, effective antiulcer treatment and longer follow-up, more frequent consequences of the invasive properties of malignant gastrinoma are being recognized. Complete surgical removal of gastrinoma, with cure, has been achieved in less than 25 percent of patients with the Z-E syndrome. However, earlier detection, careful examination for tumor in and outside of the pancreas, and use of transhepatic portal venous sampling techniques for gastrin measurement and tumor localization may make it possible to improve upon these results.

STRESS ULCERS AND EROSIONS

A variety of acute ulcerative lesions of the gastrointestinal tract are distinct clinically from chronic peptic ulcer. Among these are the acute upper gastrointestinal erosions and ulcerations which are often observed in patients with shock, burns, sepsis, and severe trauma. These are often referred to as *stress erosions* and *ulcers*. These lesions, which are frequently multiple, are most common in the acid-secreting portion of the stomach, but they may also occur in the antrum and duodenum. Acute stress erosions and ulcerations are usually superficial, with necrosis limited to the mucosa.

These erosions and superficial ulcers are extremely frequent and occur in about 90 percent of patients with massive injuries and burns. The most common clinical finding in patients with acute erosions or ulcerations is painless gastrointestinal hemorrhage. Blood loss is usually minimal but may be substantial. Erosions develop most frequently approximately 24 h after trauma. Small amounts of blood loss may be detected in the first 24 to 48 h after trauma. However, when massive hemorrhage occurs, it is usually more than 2 or 3 days after the acute insult. The diagnosis is best established by upper gastrointestinal endoscopy. The erosive lesions are frequently too superficial to be recognized by barium examination of the upper gastrointestinal tract. Acute ulcerations and erosions should be suspected when there is evidence of upper gastrointestinal bleeding in patients with severe injuries, burns, infections, and shock.

Many theories have been proposed to explain stress-associated acute mucosal ulceration, but the mechanism for the mucosal injury is still not clear. Gastric acid appears to be involved in the production of these acute stress erosions and ulcers, although there is usually no evidence of acid hypersecretion. The lesions cannot be produced in experimental animals in the absence of acid. The two major mechanisms which have been proposed are mucosal ischemia and enhanced back-diffusion of hydrogen ions. Investigation of the gastric mucosal barrier indicates that it is intact after severe burns and injuries. Most evidence supports the conclusion that mucosal ischemia is the most important element in the production of stress erosions and ulceration.

The treatment of acute stress ulcerations and erosions is principally preventive. In high-risk patients the frequency of stress ulcerations can be diminished by the vigorous use of antacids to neutralize gastric contents. While anticholinergics are of no value, there is evidence that inhibition of acid secretion by H-2-receptor antagonists may be effective in prevention of stress ulceration; however, they do not appear as effective as vigorous (every 30 to 60 min) therapy with antacids. When medical therapy fails to arrest bleeding, surgical approaches have varied from pyloroplasty and vagotomy to total gastrectomy.

The term *Cushing's ulcer* has been applied to acute ulceration of the upper gastrointestinal tract associated with intracranial injury or increases in intracranial pressure, e.g., with brain tumors. These ulcers may involve the stomach, proximal duodenum, or esophagus, and frequently lead to hemorrhage or perforation. They do not differ histologically from acute stress ulceration. Treatment includes correction of increased intracranial pressure, when possible, and the usual measures for treatment of acute erosions and ulcerations.

DRUG-ASSOCIATED ULCERS AND EROSIONS

Gastric and duodenal ulcers have been described following administration of many drugs. Salicylate ingestion (specifically aspirin) has been shown to be associated with an increased incidence of gastric ulcer and is a frequent cause of hemorrhagic gastric erosions and gastritis. There is no evidence of an increased frequency of duodenal ulcer among patients treated with salicylates. The specific mechanism by which salicylates induce, or are associated with, gastric ulcer has not been established. However, at least two mechanisms have been proposed. It has been suggested that salicylates contribute to the development of gastric ulcer by mucosal injury induced by interruption of the gastric mucosal barrier, permitting back-diffusion of hydrogen ions and consequent erosive gastritis. An additional mechanism by which salicylates may injure the gastric mucosa is by their capacity to inhibit prostaglandin synthesis, since various prostaglandins have been shown to have cytoprotective properties, by which they prevent damage to the gastric mucosa in response to a variety of agents, including salicylates. Patients with gastric ulcer should avoid salicylates, and many physicians also withhold recommending salicylates in patients with duodenal ulcer. Gastric mucosal injury, similar to that produced by aspirin, has also been observed in patients treated with a variety of nonsteroidal anti-inflammatory agents (e.g., indomethacin, ibuprofen, naproxen, tolmetin, sulindac, piroxicam, diflunisal, fenoprofen). The concerns about aspirin use also apply to these agents.

Administration of corticosteroids has been reported to be associated with development of ulcer disease of the upper gastrointestinal tract. Although for the most part this proposal has been widely accepted, there are no firm data conclusively establishing the association between corticosteroids and gastric or duodenal ulcers. Most controlled studies have failed to demonstrate an increased incidence of ulcers in patients treated with corticosteroids. Most studies have supported an increased incidence of ulcer disease in patients with rheumatoid arthritis: these patients may often be receiving other potentially ulcerogenic drugs, which may account for the apparent increase in ulcer frequency when these patients are treated with corticosteroids. At present a direct association between treatment with corticosteroids and an increased incidence of duodenal or gastric ulcer has not been firmly established.

REFERENCES

BARDHAN KD et al: Double blind comparison of cimetidine and placebo in the maintenance and healing of chronic duodenal ulceration. Gut 20:158, 1979

ELASHOFF JD, GROSSMAN MI: Trends in hospital admissions and death rates for peptic ulcer in the United States from 1970 to 1978. Gastroenterology 78:280, 1980

HOWARD JM et al: Famotidine, a new potent, long-acting histamine H_2-receptor antagonist: Comparison with cimetidine and ranitidine in the treatment of Zollinger-Ellison syndrome. Gastroenterology 88:1026, 1985

ISENBERG JI et al: Increased sensitivity to stimulation of acid secretion by pentagastrin in duodenal ulcer. J Clin Invest 55:330, 1975

KURATA JH et al: Sex differences in peptic ulcer disease. Gastroenterology 88:96, 1985

LAMERS BHW et al: Omeprazole in Zollinger-Ellison syndrome: Effects of a single dose and a long-term treatment in patients resistant to histamine H_2-receptor antagonists. N Engl J Med 310:758, 1984

McGUIGAN JE, TRUDEAU WL: Differences in rates of gastrin release in normal persons and patients with duodenal ulcer. N Engl J Med 288:64, 1973

———, WOLFE MM: The secretin injection test in the diagnosis of gastrinoma. Gastroenterology 79:1324, 1980

MAN WK et al: Histamine and duodenal ulcer: effect of omeprazole on gastric histamine in patients with duodenal ulcer. Gut 27:418, 1986

MARTIN F et al: Comparison of the healing capacities of sucralfate and cimetidine in the short-term treatment of duodenal ulcer: A double blind randomized study. Gastroenterology 82:401, 1982

NYREN O et al: Absence of therapeutic benefit from antacids or cimetidine in non ulcer dyspepsia. N Engl J Med 314:339, 1986

PEURA DA, JOHNSON LF: Cimetidine for prevention and treatment of gastroduodenal lesions in patients in an intensive care unit. Ann Int Med 103:173, 1985

PRIEBE HJ et al: Antacid versus cimetidine in preventing acute gastrointestinal bleeding. N Engl J Med 302:426, 1980

RICHARDSON CT: Sucralfate. Ann Int Med 97:269, 1982

ROBERT A: Cytoprotection by prostaglandins. Gastroenterology 77:761, 1979

TAKEUCHI KD: Role of pH gradient of mucus in protection of gastric mucosa. Gastroenterology 84:331, 1983

WOLFE MM et al: Zollinger-Ellison syndrome associated with persistently normal serum gastrin concentrations. Ann Int Med 103:215, 1985

236 GASTRIC TUMORS, GASTRITIS, AND OTHER GASTRIC DISEASES

WALTER C. MacDONALD / CYRUS E. RUBIN

CANCER

CARCINOMA Throughout the world gastric cancer is one of the most common lethal malignancies. Although its frequency is decreasing in the United States, it still causes about 15,000 deaths each year. Because symptoms in the early, potentially curable phase are often minimal or nonexistent, patients usually seek medical advice too late. Thus, less than 15 percent of patients survive 5 years, despite improved diagnostic and surgical techniques.

Epidemiology Gastric cancer is very common in Japan, in the Central and South American Andes, and in parts of eastern Europe. The children of Japanese who migrated to the United States have a much lower incidence of gastric cancer, suggesting environmental influences on pathogenesis. Gastric cancer has become far less common in the United States, where in the past 50 years its annual mortality has fallen from 25 to 6 per 100,000. A lesser decline is apparent in western Europe and, more recently, even in Japan. When the reasons for this remarkable decline have been elucidated, a giant step will have been made in understanding the pathogenesis of gastric cancer. While the frequency of carcinoma of gastric body and antrum in the United States has declined, carcinoma of the proximal stomach (cardia) has increased from 10 to almost 30 percent of cases. It is uncertain whether this represents a real increase in gastric cardia carcinoma or reflects a change in the incidence of carcinomas extending into the stomach from a primary adenocarcinoma complicating Barrett's columnar-lined esophagus.

Throughout the world, gastric cancer is twice as common in men as in women; it occurs in North America at a mean age of 60 years, with less than 5 percent under 40.

Etiology The cause of gastric cancer is unknown, but diet has been implicated. Gastric cancer can be readily induced in some animals by the oral administration of *N*-methyl-*N*′-nitrosoguanidine. It has been suggested that gastric cancer may be related to the formation of *N*-nitroso compounds by the conversion of ingested nitrates to nitrites, which then interact in the stomach with secondary or tertiary amines. Interestingly, this reaction is inhibited by ascorbic acid. There is also speculation that hypertonic salted, pickled, or smoked foods may be promoting factors in gastric carcinogenesis.

Predisposing factors Gastric cancer is two to four times more common in first-degree relatives of patients with the disease and the concordance rate is greater for identical than dizygotic twins, suggesting a small genetic element in pathogenesis.

Atrophic gastric mucosa, especially when associated with intestinal metaplasia, probably increases the risk of gastric cancer. Such mucosal changes are invariably seen in pernicious anemia, and about 5 percent of these patients develop stomach cancer. Comparison of Japanese and American autopsy results shows that the high-risk Japanese have more extensive atrophic gastritis and intestinal metaplasia than the low-risk Americans. Serial biopsy studies also suggest that persons with atrophic gastritis are more likely to develop gastric cancer than those with normal mucosa. However, atrophic gastritis is common in older people without cancer, and some patients with gastric cancers have no gastritis in the uninvolved portions of the stomach.

Adenomatous gastric polyps either contain adenocarcinoma or are associated with carcinoma elsewhere in the stomach in as many as 30 percent of cases. It is not known whether these uncommon adenomatous polyps contain cancer from the onset or whether they were originally benign. Certainly most gastric cancers do not begin as polyps. Patients with hyperplastic gastric polyps are predisposed to cancer elsewhere in the stomach to a far lesser degree. This predisposition is possibly related to the atrophic gastritis which is regularly seen surrounding both kinds of polyps.

Benign gastric ulcer has not been shown to be a precursor of gastric cancer. Some, but not all, European studies have shown that there is an increased risk of gastric cancer 10 to 20 years after partial gastrectomy for peptic ulcer. In the United States no such risk has been shown.

Pathology Gastric cancers are almost always adenocarcinomas. Gross and microscopic classification of these carcinomas is frequently impossible because many are of mixed pattern. In general, there are five macroscopic types: polypoid, ulcerative, combined ulcerative and infiltrative, diffuse infiltrative (linitis plastica), and superficial spreading. Microscopic classification is particularly difficult and has no prognostic value. Polypoid, ulcerative, and superficial spreading cancers are often less malignant than the infiltrative types. The most important factors in prognosis are the depth of invasion through the gastric wall, the spread to lymph nodes, and the presence of distant metastases.

Gastric cancer spreads by direct extension through the gastric wall to the perigastric tissues. Sometimes direct extension involves the pancreas, colon, or liver. Proximal gastric tumors often involve the esophagus, but distal ones less commonly cross the pylorus into the duodenum. Spread to perigastric nodes is common; nodes in the preaortic area, porta hepatis, and hilum of the spleen are often involved as well. Spread via the thoracic duct can involve the left supraclavicular (Virchow's) lymph nodes. Peritoneal metastases are evident in about 20 percent of patients, but intraabdominal metastases may be confined to the ovary (Krukenberg's tumor) or prerectal pouch (Blumer's shelf). Blood-borne metastases to the liver are apparent in about 30 percent of patients. The lungs, brain, or other organs are involved less often.

Clinical features The history is of little help in distinguishing benign from malignant gastric ulcer because many of the varied symptoms may be seen in both diseases. Approximately 25 percent of patients with cancer have classic ulcer symptoms. The most common presenting complaint, however, is upper abdominal discomfort of insidious onset. This is often mild but varies greatly in severity from a vague, postprandial fullness to a severe, steady pain. Anorexia, often with slight nausea, is very common but is not the usual presenting complaint. Weight loss is observed in at least 50 percent of patients. Nausea and vomiting are particularly prominent with tumors of the pylorus but can occur with advanced disease elsewhere in the stomach. Dysphagia is the major symptom of cardia tumors. Weakness, hematemesis, melena, and alteration in bowel habits are other presenting complaints. Some patients suffer from the symptoms of anemia, or their anemia may be discovered on routine examination. Occasionally an ulcerating carcinoma perforates, and rarely a gastrocolic fistula develops.

The initial symptoms may be related to metastases. These include abdominal distention by malignant ascites; jaundice from biliary tract obstruction by porta hepatis nodes or by intrahepatic metastases; pain from bone involvement; neurologic symptoms secondary to brain or meningeal metastases; and shortness of breath from lung spread. Mechanical bowel obstruction can be secondary to peritoneal metastases, and pelvic symptoms can result from ovarian spread.

The duration of symptoms before patients see a physician is remarkably variable but averages 6 months. Symptoms of several years' duration are not uncommon. Some patients with long-standing functional gastrointestinal complaints may notice a change in their pain pattern. In North America, less than 10 percent of patients with symptoms have early gastric cancer, i.e., disease confined to the mucosa or submucosa. Screening studies in Japan confirm that most patients with early curable gastric cancer are asymptomatic, although some have mild epigastric distress or ulcer symptoms.

An epigastric mass is palpable in only a minority of patients; it is a sign of poor prognosis but does not exclude the possibility of cure. Abdominal tenderness is found in about one-third of patients. Pallor or cachexia may be observed, and occasionally a gastric succussion splash is demonstrable. Physical signs suggesting metastases should be carefully sought because distant metastases that are proved by biopsy or aspiration cytology exclude curative surgery. These include hepatomegaly, jaundice, enlargement of left supraclavicular or scalene nodes, a shelf-like mass anteriorly in the prerectal pouch above the prostate or cervix on rectal examination, an ovarian mass on vaginal or abdominal examination, ascites, an umbilical mass, and skin nodules. A low-grade fever may occur with advanced disease, particularly with liver metastases. Rarely gastric cancer is associated with dermatomyositis, acanthosis nigricans, neuromyopathy, hypoglycemia, or multiple seborrheic keratoses.

Laboratory findings Iron-deficiency anemia because of occult bleeding is found in about two-thirds of patients. Occasionally the cancer is associated with pernicious anemia. Rarely a pancytopenia is caused by bone marrow replacement. A "leukemoid" reaction and disseminated intravascular coagulation are other rare findings. Occult blood is demonstrable in the stools in up to 80 percent of patients if repeated tests are done. Elevation of 5′-nucleotidase suggests the presence of liver metastases, which can be confirmed by liver scan. The serum albumin may be low because of protein leakage from the involved gastric mucosa. Measurement of gastric acid secretion is considered less helpful than in the past. Achlorhydria after stimulation with pentagastrin usually excludes a benign peptic ulcer, but the test is of limited value because most patients with a malignant ulcer secrete some acid. A rise in the carcinoembryonic antigen (CEA) after treatment suggests recurrence of carcinoma, but this test is of little initial diagnostic value.

Diagnosis In North America x-ray of the stomach is still the initial method used for detecting gastric carcinoma. In more than 90 percent of symptomatic patients, skillfully performed, double-contrast x-ray detects gastric abnormalities. In practice, the radiologic differentiation of benign from malignant gastric lesions is accurate in approximately 75 percent of cases. Thus, gastroscopy with biopsy or brush cytology must be used to confirm or exclude a diagnosis of cancer (see Chap. 233). It may be more important to the patient to exclude gastric cancer than to diagnose it because unnecessary emotional trauma and surgical morbidity or mortality can be avoided by definitive diagnosis of benign disease.

The diagnostic accuracy of x-ray is greatest when it is used wisely. Equivocal examinations should always be repeated. The use of double-contrast techniques helps to detect small lesions by improving mucosal detail. The stomach should be distended at some time during every x-ray examination because decreased distensibility may be the only indication of a diffuse infiltrative carcinoma. Although gastric ulcers can be detected fairly easily, it may be impossible to distinguish the benign from the malignant ones. Differential x-ray diagnosis is also difficult when the antrum is narrowed or when mucosal folds are enlarged. Cancer of the proximal stomach invading the neural plexuses of the esophagus may mimic achalasia by x-ray. In cancer of the cardia the x-ray appearance may be considered normal or may be confused with benign mucosal distortion secondary to a hiatus hernia. It is impossible to differentiate adenocarcinoma from lymphoma radiologically. Cancer of the pancreas or colon invading the stomach may be confused with primary gastric neoplasm.

Fiberoptic gastroscopy with biopsy and brush cytology is especially useful for confirming the diagnosis of cancer suspected by x-ray, differentiating cancer from lymphoma, clarifying equivocal radiologic findings, and checking suspicious clinical findings despite negative x-rays. At least six biopsies should be taken from representative areas of a suspected neoplasm; if the tissue is serially sectioned and thoroughly examined by an expert, accuracy in the diagnosis of cancer approaching 95 percent can be achieved. The addition of brush cytology raises the accuracy in detecting cancer even higher but slightly raises the risk of a false diagnosis of cancer. Diffuse infiltrative tumors and recurrent cancers can be impossible to diagnose even by these methods because malignant cells may not be present in the biopsied mucosal layer. Despite improved diagnostic techniques, laparoscopy or laparotomy may be required for diagnosis.

The x-ray demonstration of a benign-appearing gastric ulcer presents special problems. Some physicians feel that gastroscopy is not mandatory if the x-ray features are typically benign, if healing at 6 weeks is complete by x-ray, and if a follow-up x-ray examination several months later is negative. However, many feel that gastroscopic biopsy and brush cytology are required for all patients with a gastric ulcer in order to exclude malignancy, particularly an early, curable gastric cancer. The marked drop in the incidence of malignant gastric ulcers in North America has raised the question whether it is cost-effective to endoscope all patients with gastric ulcer rather than to confine endoscopy to those with a suspicious x-ray or clinical course.

Using x-ray and intragastric photography for mass screening, the Japanese have detected many early, curable cancers of the stomach. In North America, such screening methods are probably not cost-effective because the disease is relatively uncommon. However, special attention must be paid to patients over 40 years of age who are predisposed to gastric cancer because of pernicious anemia, the presence or history of an adenomatous gastric polyp, a family history of gastric cancer, or birth in countries where gastric cancer is common. In addition, one must be certain that all gastric ulcers treated medically are indeed benign.

Treatment Surgical removal of the tumor offers the only chance for cure. A careful evaluation for evidence of distant metastases will avoid unnecessary surgery. Physical examination is supplemented by chest x-ray, liver function tests, and abdominal ultrasound. The use of computerized tomography (CT scan) has increased the accuracy of preoperative staging. Suspected areas of metastasis should be sampled, for example, lymph nodes or liver and pleural or peritoneal effusions. If metastases are suspected but unproved, laparoscopy under local anesthesia with direct biopsy of suspected areas of metastasis is particularly helpful in assessing operability. Cancer of the distal and midstomach is usually treated by subtotal gastrectomy; removal of the regional lymph nodes requires resection of the greater and lesser omentum and sometimes the spleen. Tumors of the proximal stomach are usually treated by distal esophagectomy and proximal gastrectomy. Total gastrectomy is indicated only occasionally. If obstruction is present or if bleeding is a problem, palliative resection may be worthwhile even though the disease is known to be incurable. The operative mortality rate for gastric cancer is still as high as 10 percent in many hospitals.

It is often difficult to assess the reported results of surgical treatment. Careful and standardized descriptions by surgeon and pathologist would facilitate comparison of different series. These should include depth of tumor penetration, extent of lymph node involvement, and presence of distant metastases. More than 80 percent of cancers confined to the mucosa or submucosa are curable, compared with 10 to 20 percent when the tumor extends through the gastric wall. Up to 50 percent survive 5 years after curative resection if the lymph nodes are not involved. Tumor diameter of less than 2 cm and a long history of symptoms are good prognostic signs. However, in North America only 10 to 15 percent survive 5 years after diagnosis. Rarely, patients live for 5 years without treatment or for many years after a palliative resection.

Chemotherapy with 5-fluorouracil (5-FU) causes some tumor regression in about 10 percent of patients. Combination chemotherapy (e.g., 5-FU, doxorubicin, and mitomycin C) induces a response in a higher percentage of patients, but the median survival is still less than 1 year. The effectiveness of adjuvant radiotherapy, or chemotherapy, remains to be proved. Palliative radiotherapy may be useful to control bleeding, to relieve obstruction at the cardia, or to alleviate pain from bone metastases. Other palliative measures include replacement of iron and vitamin B_{12}, dilation of obstructing cardia tumors with or without placement of plastic tubular stents, relief of cardia obstruction by laser therapy, treatment of postgastrectomy problems, and the judicious use of analgesics and antiemetics.

LYMPHOMA Primary gastric lymphomas account for about 5 percent of gastric malignancies although the percentage is higher in referral centers. Most are diffuse large cell (histiocytic) lymphomas or mixed small cell (lymphocytic) and large cell lymphomas; Hodgkin's disease is relatively uncommon, and plasmacytoma is rare. Some gastric lymphomas present a varied histologic picture that defies classification. Gastric involvement secondary to disseminated lymphoma is more common than the primary form. In one large series, one-third of histiocytic lymphomas and one-sixth of lymphosarcomas spread to the stomach. The sexes are affected equally, and the mean age is about 55 years.

The symptoms are indistinguishable from those of gastric ulcer or cancer. Hematemesis and perforation occur more often than with carcinoma. An abdominal mass is palpable in approximately one-third of patients. Approximately half of patients have iron-deficiency anemia, usually with occult blood in the stool.

X-ray studies usually show an abnormality difficult to distinguish from adenocarcinoma. Large rigid folds, multiple ulcers, or duodenal involvement suggest the possibility of lymphoma. The x-ray appearance may also be confused with that of Ménétrier's disease or benign peptic ulcer. The tumor is usually obvious at gastroscopy, but its gross appearance is seldom diagnostic. A preoperative diagnosis can often be made by the combination of endoscopic biopsy and cytologic examination, but even these methods may fail and surgical excision may be required for diagnosis.

A careful search for evidence of disseminated disease should precede treatment and should include chest x-ray, lymphangiography, CT scan, and bone marrow biopsy. Primary gastric lymphoma has most often been treated by a combination of surgical excision and radiotherapy. Usually surgery precedes radiotherapy, but it may be advantageous to shrink large tumor with radiation before attempting to excise them. About 50 percent of patients so treated survive 5 years. Survival is particularly good if the tumor does not penetrate the serosa or involve the perigastric nodes. The role of chemotherapy for primary gastric lymphoma is still not well defined. The tendency of the disease to recur outside the abdomen and the sensitivity of the tumor to available agents have led several groups to recommend adding combination chemotherapy to the initial management. Unresectable gastric lymphoma has a 5-year survival of 25 percent or less. It is now often treated with combination chemotherapy with or without radiotherapy. Newer drug regimens promise to substantially improve the results. The treatment of disseminated lymphoma is discussed in Chap. 79.

LEIOMYOSARCOMA These tumors account for 1 to 3 percent of gastric malignancies. The mean age is about 60 years, and the sexes are affected equally. The tumors are usually large, spherical, and in the upper half of the stomach; they tend to ulcerate and become necrotic in the center. The tumor may spread to the peritoneum or liver but rarely to lymph nodes. Most patients complain of pain. The majority are anemic, and massive bleeding occurs in about one-third. A mass is palpable in more than 50 percent. X-rays show a large, smooth tumor, often with central ulceration and sometimes with a sinus tract to the center of the neoplasm. It is impossible to differentiate leiomyosarcoma by x-ray from benign leiomyoma except that leiomyosarcomas tend to be larger. Though endoscopic biopsy rarely provides a correct preoperative diagnosis, brush cytology of the ulceration may on occasion provide additional information. Treatment is by wide surgical excision if feasible; about 25 to 40 percent of patients are cured. Doxorubicin in combination with various other agents has been used to achieve modest palliation in a minority of patients with advanced disease. Radiotherapy is ineffective.

CARCINOID TUMORS AND OTHER MALIGNANCIES Gastric carcinoids are uncommon. Like carcinoids elsewhere, they may be multiple. As many as 3 percent of patients with pernicious anemia may have gastric carcinoids. Carcinoids are often symptomless but can cause bleeding or epigastric pain. The x-ray appearance is that of a smooth, rounded, sessile filling defect, sometimes with ulceration. About 25 percent are malignant, but only a minority cause the malignant carcinoid syndrome. Small carcinoids can be excised locally; those larger than 2 cm and those that are malignant require partial gastrectomy. The chemotherapy of malignant carcinoids and the treatment of the carcinoid syndrome are described in Chap. 299.

Rare primary gastric malignancies include carcinosarcoma, hemangiopericytoma, neurogenic sarcoma, fibrosarcoma, and liposarcoma. Metastases to the stomach most often originate from generalized lymphoma, lung cancer, breast cancer, or malignant melanoma. Kaposi's sarcoma may involve the stomach, especially in patients with acquired immunodeficiency syndrome (AIDS).

BENIGN TUMORS

EPITHELIAL POLYPS After cancer, benign epithelial polyps are the most common tumors of the stomach (5 to 10 percent). While there is considerable confusion regarding their nomenclature, it is important to remember that 80 to 90 percent of them are not neoplastic and probably never become malignant. The most common nonneoplastic polyp is called *hyperplastic;* it is composed almost completely of normal surface mucous cells and at times of mucus-secreting pyloric glands. The glands are intermingled with smooth-muscle fibers and may be cystic. More than 90 percent of such polyps are less than 1.5 cm in diameter. They may be single or multiple, pedunculated or sessile and can occur in any part of the stomach. They are covered with normal-appearing mucosa and frequently have a superficial ulceration. The mucosa surrounding them often shows nonerosive gastritis or atrophy. Although hyperplastic polyps probably never become malignant, carcinoma elsewhere in the same stomach is somewhat more common than in the general population.

Of epithelial polyps, 10 to 20 percent are composed of benign neoplastic epithelium and are called *adenomas.* In general, they resemble adenomatous polyps of the colon. They are usually larger than 2 cm in diameter and enlarge with time. As many as 40 percent of all adenomatous gastric polyps already contain cancer when first diagnosed and the rest may become malignant. They can be pedunculated but are more often sessile. They are solitary in two-thirds of cases and are covered with abnormal reddened velvety mucosa which may be lobulated or mammillated. Most are located in the antrum. The mucosa surrounding them is usually atrophic, and carcinoma elsewhere in the stomach is common (30 percent or more in various series).

Both hyperplastic and adenomatous polyps occur more frequently in patients over 50 years of age, and 80 percent or more of these patients are achlorhydric. From 6 to 20 percent of patients with pernicious anemia have epithelial polyps. Most are asymptomatic. Occult bleeding is the most frequent symptom and may be associated with vague epigastric distress. Rarely vomiting results from prolapse of a large, pedunculated antral polyp into the duodenum. Radiologically the polyps appear as smooth, rounded, or lobulated filling defects, with or without a stalk. Although those greater than 2 cm in diameter are more likely to be adenomas or polypoid carcinomas, exceptions are not uncommon.

Hyperplastic polyps may have a different gross appearance from adenomas at endoscopy, but one cannot differentiate between the two with certainty even after sampling them by forceps biopsy. To determine the histologic nature of a polyp and to exclude malignancy, the whole lesion is best examined. Most pedunculated or small sessile polyps can be removed with an electrocautery snare during gastroscopy by an experienced endoscopist. Endoscopic removal of larger sessile polyps or those with a broad pedicle may cause severe bleeding. Such lesions can be biopsied endoscopically by removing a sizable superficial portion of the polyp with a coagulating cautery snare. If the lesion is adenomatous, it should be removed surgically because of its malignant potential. Such patients must also be followed regularly with endoscopic and cytologic examinations because of the high risk of cancer in the surrounding mucosa. Partial or even total gastrectomy may eventually be needed.

Diffuse gastric polyposis is a rare and poorly defined condition in which the gastric mucosa is covered with numerous sessile or pedunculated epithelial polyps, most of which are hyperplastic. It is neither practical nor necessary to remove all hyperplastic polyps, but the patient should be endoscoped regularly to detect development of carcinoma in the surrounding epithelium. Multiple gastric adenomas are very rare but may be seen in familial polyposis or Gardner's syndrome and may require gastrectomy. Most of the multiple gastric polyps seen in familial polyposis are made up of benign fundal glands and require no treatment.

Rare hamartomatous gastric polyps are made up of the various benign epithelial cells normally present in the gastric mucosa. They are usually part of two familial polyposis syndromes: Peutz-Jeghers and juvenile polyposis. Twenty-five percent of Peutz-Jeghers cases involve the stomach or duodenum and 2 to 3 percent develop gastric or duodenal carcinoma. Malignant change in gastric juvenile polyposis is either very rare or absent. Cronkhite-Canada syndrome is a rare cause of benign gastric retention polyps composed of dilated cystic glands with markedly edematous stroma.

LEIOMYOMAS AND RARE BENIGN TUMORS Most leiomyomas are tiny and of no clinical significance. Larger ones, usually 3 cm or more in diameter, may cause massive or occult bleeding or epigastric pain. The x-ray appearance is that of a smooth, rounded, sessile filling defect, often with a central ulcer. The gastroscopic appearance is highly suggestive but not diagnostic. Mucosal biopsies are usually too superficial for diagnosis, but brush cytology of the ulcerated area may help rule out leiomyosarcoma. Small symptomatic lesions may be treated by local surgical excision, and larger ones by partial gastrectomy. Other rare benign gastric tumors include lipomas, schwannomas, hemangiomas, lymphangiomas, adenomyomas, and fibromas.

PSEUDOTUMORS A number of gastric conditions other than peptic ulcer simulate neoplasms by x-ray. These include hypertrophic pyloric stenosis; antral gastritis; Ménétrier's disease and other gastric hyperplasias; pseudolymphoma; heterotopic pancreas; gastric eosinophilic granuloma; Crohn's disease; gastric varices; hematoma; deformity after fundoplication (Nissen repair); extrinsic pressure by the liver, pancreas, or spleen; and bezoars or retained food. Often endoscopic evaluation and consideration of the total clinical picture solve these problems, but in rare cases surgical exploration is necessary to exclude malignancy.

GASTRITIS

EROSIVE GASTRITIS Erosive gastritis (also known as hemorrhagic gastritis or multiple gastric erosions) is a frequent cause of upper gastrointestinal bleeding, but it is rarely severe. Erosions may be completely asymptomatic. As detected by endoscopy, multiple bleeding erosions are distributed diffusely throughout the gastric mucosa or are localized to the fundus, body, or antrum. The intervening mucosa may appear reddened and friable, or it may appear normal.

Histologically, the mucosal destruction by erosions does not extend below the muscularis mucosae to involve the more vascular submucosa; characteristically, the mucosal lesions heal completely. At any one time, different erosions can be observed in various stages of evolution and regression. Erosions may occur in flat mucosa or on the crests of small mucosal mounds which may stud the crests of folds. Between erosions there may be areas of surface epithelium depleted of mucus and focal or diffuse extravasation of blood into the lamina propria. Erosions may develop in mucosa that is histologically normal or that shows changes of any histologic type of gastritis. If the process persists, erosions may extend into the submucosa to form acute ulcers (Chap. 235); then bleeding may become severe.

Erosive gastritis can occur for no apparent reason. Many cases, however, are associated with the ingestion of aspirin or nonsteroidal anti-inflammatory drugs (NSAIDs). Because aspirin is not ionized in the acid milieu of the gastric lumen, it is absorbed readily by passive nonionic diffusion. At the neutral intracellular pH within the gastric surface epithelium, aspirin becomes an ionized acid which can destroy the cells and provide an entry point for acid-peptic digestion. When aspirin is given with sodium bicarbonate it does not injure the gastric mucosa because it is ionized and poorly absorbed gastrically. When aspirin is covered with an enteric coating it passes through the stomach and is absorbed in the small bowel. Aspirin and most NSAIDs interfere with prostaglandin synthesis, thus impairing mucosal resistance to injury. NSAIDs such as phenylbutazone or indomethacin are especially associated with erosive gastritis. Acute alcohol ingestion is an important cause of gastric erosions, and portal hypertension is a predisposing factor.

Severe stress secondary to burns, sepsis, trauma, surgery, shock, or respiratory, renal, or liver failure often causes gastric erosions or acute ulcers. Their pathogenesis is poorly understood and probably varies with different predisposing conditions. Alterations in mucosal blood flow may lead to areas of microinfarction with further evolution of the lesion dependent upon acid-peptic digestion. With better intensive care, hyperalimentation, and a strict antacid regimen, erosions in severely stressed patients infrequently progress to ulcers with resultant severe hemorrhage or perforation.

Patients may present with hematemesis and/or melena. Chronic blood loss may occur. Many have no symptoms, but some notice mild epigastric discomfort or nausea. The diagnosis is best made by gastroscopy on the same day as the bleeding episode, because otherwise the lesions may have healed and disappeared. The newer small-caliber screening endoscopes are just slightly bigger than a nasogastric tube and may be passed easily in very sick patients after only pharyngeal anesthesia. Only expert double-contrast x-ray may demonstrate some of these superficial erosions. Presumptive clinical diagnoses of erosive gastritis in patients with upper gastrointestinal bleeding and negative x-rays are often wrong. The source of upper gastrointestinal bleeding is best determined by early esophagogastroduodenoscopy.

The usual measures for restoring circulating blood volume should be undertaken promptly (Chap. 37). Not uncommonly, the bleeding has stopped by the time a tube is passed. If not, lavage of the stomach with iced isotonic saline solution is used, although its efficacy is unproved in all types of upper gastrointestinal bleeding, especially in erosive gastritis. In any event, lavage with noniced saline solution via an Ewald tube may facilitate diagnostic endoscopy by removing some of the obscuring blood. Gravity drainage, *not suction,* should be used for emptying the saline solution from the stomach, lest suction artifacts be produced which are indistinguishable from acute erosions endoscopically.

If bleeding stops, a regimen of hourly antacids and cimetidine or ranitidine is instituted. If bleeding continues, selective infusion of vasopressin into the left gastric artery or embolization may be warranted. In the rare case in which bleeding continues and is life-threatening, one of the erosions may have progressed to a deeper acute ulcer. If this ulcer can be visualized endoscopically, it may be treatable by electrocoagulation or with a heater probe via the endoscope. If this fails, vagotomy and pyloroplasty with oversewing of the bleeding ulcers is the preferred surgical treatment, but it also may not be successful. Very rarely persistent severe bleeding requires total gastrectomy.

NONEROSIVE GASTRITIS This is a *histologic* diagnosis and not a clinically recognizable entity because it probably does not cause symptoms. In fact, histologic evidence of gastritis is frequent in asymptomatic individuals, especially as they get older. Thus, the usual clinical assumption that most nonulcer dyspepsia is caused by "gastritis" is not justified. Similarly, gross endoscopic mucosal appearances of erythema, ecchymoses, petechiae, nodularity, or thickened folds do not necessarily indicate histologic changes. Nonerosive gastritis can *only* be diagnosed by biopsy, and it may or may not be of clinical significance.

The gastric mucosa is divided into two layers: (1) the superficial, nonglandular surface (foveolar) epithelium facing the lumen which is normally replaced every 5 days; and (2) the deeper, glandular layer which is a more stable population of epithelial cells which are replaced very slowly and which have specific functions. These cells include the *parietal cells,* which make HCl and intrinsic factor, the *chief cells* in the fundal glands, which make pepsin, the *pylorocardiac glandular* cells, which make mucus, and the endocrine *G cells* in the pyloric glands, which make gastrin. The patterns of gastritis involve both superficial and glandular areas, and the sequence is one of chronic and/or acute inflammation which may cause glandular destruction and may be followed by regeneration, metaplasia, or loss of glands (atrophy). To the pathologist chronic inflammation means the presence of increased plasma cells and lymphocytes in the lamina propria and acute inflammation means the presence of polymorphonuclear leukocytes. This does not necessarily indicate that the process is clinically chronic or acute, and thus morphologic interpretation may be confusing to clinicians. The probable morphologic sequence is that the superficial layer is first inflamed (superficial gastritis) and that epithelial destruction and inflammation within the surrounding lamina propria then penetrates to the deeper glandular areas (atrophic gastritis) leading finally to loss of glands (gastric atrophy) or replacement by metaplastic glands (intestinal metaplasia or pyloric gland metaplasia of fundal glands).

If one cannot ascribe symptoms to these histologic changes, what indeed is their clinical significance? It is known that chronic atrophic gastritis, gastric atrophy, and intestinal metaplasia occur at a younger age, are more widely distributed in the stomach, and are more frequent in populations with a higher incidence of carcinoma of the body and antrum of the stomach. Perhaps this is the "soil" in which this type of cancer develops more easily. But even in the United States, where this type of gastric cancer is decreasing, such gastric changes with aging are common. What is clinically significant in the United States is a completely normal fundal gland area, free of gastritis, in patients 70 years of age or older. These usually are patients with peptic ulcer disease of the hypersecretory, perhaps hereditary, type who commonly have duodenal ulcers and severe reflux esophagitis. The fundal glands of these patients do not undergo the "normal" gastritic changes of aging. Interestingly, such patients often have antral (pyloric gland) gastritis.

What about the patient with a chronic benign gastric ulcer? These patients have chronic gastritis at the edge of their peptic ulcers and secrete normal or less than normal amounts of HCl. Thus, if endoscopic biopsies of the edge of a gastric ulcer show no gastritis, there is a strong likelihood that the ulcer is not a typical peptic ulcer; rather, it is probably associated with aspirin or NSAID ingestion, and discontinuance of the offending drugs will be curative. Atrophic fundal gland gastritis and/or atrophy is often seen in patients with thyroid disease or idiopathic iron deficiency anemia and is regularly seen in pernicious anemia. Perhaps a common denominator in all of these conditions is an autoimmune destruction of the gastric mucosa, but this hypothesis remains unproven.

Severe fundal gland atrophy is invariably present in pernicious anemia where parietal cells secreting intrinsic factor and HCl are virtually absent. As a result, vitamin B_{12} in food is not absorbed. Serum gastrin levels are high because the uninvolved antrum secretes gastrin continuously in the absence of acid. The pyloric glands are preserved and relatively free of gastritis. Serum antibodies to parietal cells are present in the serum of about 60 percent of persons with atrophic fundal gastritis and in 80 to 90 percent of those with pernicious anemia. Antibodies to intrinsic factor are present in the serum or gastric juice of most patients with pernicious anemia; they are not found in patients with superficial or atrophic gastritis. The relationship between these immunologic findings and the fundal gland atrophy of pernicious anemia is uncertain.

Antral (pyloric gland) gastritis is common in asymptomatic persons. With age, this type of gastritis probably tends to extend proximally and to replace some fundal glands. If peptic ulcer is located in the upper stomach, pyloric gland gastritis may extend far more proximally. Unlike fundal gastritis, in antral gastritis serum gastrin levels tend to be low and there may be antibodies to gastrin-producing cells rather than to parietal cells. It has been postulated that regurgitation of duodenal contents, particularly bile salts, into the stomach causes pyloric gland gastritis. Spiral bacilli have been isolated from some patients, but their significance is uncertain. Occasionally, pyloric gland gastritis is associated with narrowing of the antrum suggestive of malignancy by x-ray; such patients often complain of ulcer-like pain and may, indeed, prove to have ulcers subsequently. At gastroscopy, normal antral motility suggests pliability, and malignancy can usually be excluded. The symptoms often respond to antacids and inhibitors of H-2 receptors.

Ordinarily, nonerosive gastritis requires no treatment, but it is essential to rule out vitamin B_{12} malabsorption in persons who are found to be achlorhydric. If pernicious anemia is proved, it is treated as discussed in Chap. 285. Iron-deficiency anemia should not be attributed to atrophic fundal gland gastritis unless other causes are excluded; it responds to oral iron.

GASTRIC HYPERPLASIAS ("HYPERTROPHIC" GASTRITIS) Hypertrophic gastritis is a histologic misnomer. The individual mucosal epithelial cells are not enlarged (hypertrophic), but there are more of them (hyperplasia), and thus the mucosa is thickened. There are three causes for gastric mucosal hyperplasia: Ménétrier's disease, hypersecretory gastropathy, and Zollinger-Ellison syndrome (gastrinoma; see Chap. 235). Most hyperplastic mucosal conditions produce enlarged gastric folds which may be indistinguishable by x-ray or endoscopy from infiltrative cancer, lymphoma, or a functional abnormality.

Ménétrier's disease The cause of this uncommon type of gastric mucosal hyperplasia is unknown. It is characterized grossly by tortuous enlargement of the gastric mucosal folds resembling cerebral convolutions, and histologically by a thickened mucosa with hyperplasia of mucous cells and loss of most parietal and chief cells. The gastric pits are markedly elongated and tortuous and often exhibit cystic dilatation; these cysts may penetrate through the muscularis mucosae into the submucosa. The lamina propria often contains increased numbers of lymphocytes. Intestinal metaplasia may be present. The mucosal involvement may be localized or diffuse and tends to be most prominent on the greater curvature. The antrum is uninvolved in more than 50 percent of patients. Occasionally the gross appearance suggests diffuse polyposis.

Epigastric pain is the most common complaint. Anorexia, nausea, vomiting, weight loss, or diarrhea are other symptoms. Bleeding is not uncommon because of superficial erosions. Some patients develop a gastric ulcer. Carcinoma may develop rarely. Loss of protein through the mucosa often causes hypoalbuminemia, and sometimes peripheral edema. Widening of tight junctions between surface epithelial cells revealed by electron microscopy may explain the protein loss. The gastric juice contains little or no hydrochloric acid but often excessive mucus. X-ray shows very large folds and sometimes hypomotility. The diagnosis can usually be made from clinical, radiologic, and laboratory data supplemented by gastroscopy (preferably using one of the newer, larger biopsy forceps to get the deeper biopsy needed for diagnosis), and brush cytology to rule out cancer. Occasionally, laparotomy with full-thickness biopsy of the stomach is necessary to establish the diagnosis and to exclude malignancy.

There is no specific treatment, but frequent small meals may give some symptomatic relief. Those with gastric ulcers should receive antacids or H-2 receptor antagonists. A high-protein diet should be given to patients with hypoalbuminemia, but diuretics or intravenous albumin may be necessary for those with severe edema. Treatment with anticholinergic drugs or cimetidine reduces protein loss in some patients. Partial gastrectomy may be helpful for intractable symptoms if the disease is sufficiently well localized. Rarely, total gastrectomy may be necessary. The latter should be deferred as long as possible because spontaneous improvement or complete reversal of chronic disease has been documented.

Hypersecretory gastropathy Patients with this rare syndrome differ from those with classical Ménétrier's disease because the thickened mucosa secretes gastric acid normally or excessively but not at the high rate seen in gastrinoma; furthermore, blood gastrin levels are normal. The mucosa is histologically indistinguishable from that seen in Zollinger's syndrome with an excess of parietal and chief cells. Many of these patients may represent the upper end of the spectrum of increased fundal gland mass seen in patients with duodenal ulcer. Some have a protein-losing gastropathy. Ulcer symptoms may improve after antacids or H-2 receptor inhibitors, but some patients may require surgery. Protein loss, when present, may be difficult to control unless the disease remits spontaneously.

Gastrinoma (Zollinger-Ellison syndrome) This is a fundal gland hyperplasia caused by excessive gastrin secretion by a gastrinoma, usually located in the pancreas. The pathogenesis, clinical features, and treatment are described in the previous chapter on peptic ulcer.

CORROSIVE GASTRITIS The accidental or suicidal ingestion of strong alkali, such as lye, or of acids, such as hydrochloric or carbolic acid, can cause necrosis of the gastric wall, particularly in the prepyloric region. Alkali usually injures the esophagus more severely than the stomach, whereas the reverse tends to occur with acid. The degree of gastric injury varies with the quantity and concentration of irritant ingested and the amount of food present in the stomach. Patients complain of burning of the mouth, throat, and retrosternal area. With gastric injury, there is severe epigastric pain and often vomiting. Perforation, peritonitis, or massive hemorrhage may occur shortly after ingestion of a corrosive agent or may be delayed. Later, scarring may cause esophageal or pyloric stenosis.

If the patient is seen shortly after ingesting a corrosive agent, some clinicians suggest emptying the stomach gently via a small, soft rubber tube. Acid neutralization is not recommended for alkali ingestion because the heat of the ensuing reaction may aggravate the injury. Antacids may be given for acid ingestion after preliminary dilution with milk or water. Intravenous therapy, sedation, analgesia, airway maintenance, and careful observation are instituted. The use of corticosteroids and antibiotics is controversial, but corticosteroids may be helpful if edema threatens the airway and antibiotics may help treat aspiration pneumonia. Visible mouth and pharyngeal burns are not necessarily accompanied by esophageal or gastric injury. Therefore, early, gentle endoscopy with a small-caliber screening endoscope may establish the extent of injury. However, early in the course of acid injury the damage may be missed even endoscopically. If perforation or peritonitis is suspected, laparotomy should be performed and a partial gastrectomy done if full-thickness injury to the wall is found. Surgical treatment may be necessary also for acute massive bleeding or for late obstruction caused by scarring. Parenteral nutrition may be required.

PHLEGMONOUS GASTRITIS This rare condition should be considered when a patient presents with acute upper abdominal pain, signs of peritonitis, fever, purulent ascitic fluid, nausea or vomiting, and a normal serum amylase. It is a bacterial infection of the gastric wall, most often caused by streptococci, although staphylococci, pneumococci, *Escherichia coli,* or gas-forming bacteria can be responsible. Alcoholism, upper respiratory or other infection, peptic ulcer, endoscopic polypectomy, and gastric surgery are predisposing conditions. Vigorous antibiotic therapy should be followed immediately by laparotomy which is both diagnostic and therapeutic. Depending upon the operative findings, drainage or partial gastrectomy should be performed. Without surgery the mortality is nearly 100 percent; with surgery it is approximately 20 percent.

OTHER GASTRIC DISORDERS

ACUTE GASTRIC DILATATION This is an uncommon but serious condition. The use of nasogastric suction has greatly reduced its frequency in the postoperative period. Gastric dilatation may also occur after trauma, the use of body casts, pneumonia, diabetic acidosis, or large doses of anticholinergic drugs. It is a rare complication of many diseases and also may occur for no apparent reason. The patient complains of anorexia and epigastric fullness and often vomits small amounts of fluid. Increasing abdominal distention with tympany, especially in the left hypochondrium, and a succussion splash are demonstrable. Untreated, large volumes of fluid are sequestered in a gastric ''third space'' with resultant sodium and potassium depletion. The patient becomes restless and listless; hypovolemia, tachycardia, reduced urine output, and, finally, shock develop. Aspiration pneumonia may occur. X-ray of the abdomen shows massive gastric distention with an air-fluid level. Continuous nasogastric suction and restoration of fluid and electrolyte balance result in rapid improvement.

ADULT HYPERTROPHIC PYLORIC STENOSIS In this uncommon condition, the pyloric muscle is enlarged because of hypertrophy and possibly hyperplasia of the fibers of the circular layer. Many cases are associated with a peptic ulcer near the pylorus. In others, the pyloric muscle hypertrophy has been attributed to associated antral gastritis or neoplasm. A minority of cases without other gastric disease may be due to unrecognized infantile hypertrophic pyloric stenosis. Most often symptoms of pyloric obstruction such as nausea, vomiting, and epigastric fullness develop in mid-adult life, although occasionally mild symptoms are lifelong. An epigastric mass is not palpable in adults as it is in infants. Barium x-ray studies show a long, narrowed pyloric canal, often with triangular outpouchings within the canal. Gastroscopy shows a narrowed pylorus that is fixed in the open position. Although the diagnosis often appears highly likely from the above studies, an infiltrating cancer may be difficult to exclude without operation. A limited gastric resection is said to give better symptomatic relief than a pyloromyotomy, and in addition it provides an exact histologic diagnosis. The frequently associated juxtapyloric ulcers merit vagotomy.

BEZOARS AND FOREIGN BODIES Conglomerates of food and mucus or phytobezoars composed of vegetable matter sometimes form in the gastric remnant after partial gastrectomy, especially if a vagotomy was also performed. They occur less often after vagotomy and pyloroplasty. Autonomic neuropathy associated with diabetes mellitus is another predisposing condition. Rarely yeast bezoars have been found. Patients complain of anorexia, epigastric fullness, nausea, or vomiting. The diagnosis is often apparent from the barium x-ray examination, but endoscopy may be needed to distinguish the food mass from a neoplasm. The food conglomerate or bezoar can often be removed by vigorous and repeated gastric lavage. Fragmenting the lesion at gastroscopy may facilitate removal by lavage. Some phytobezoars can be partially digested with cellulase and then broken up successfully by lavage. Occasionally surgical removal is necessary. If the mass passes into the small bowel, it can cause obstruction requiring surgery. Treatment with metoclopramide and a low-fiber diet may be tried to prevent recurrence.

Bezoars in the intact stomach are rare. Phytobezoars are most common, a well-known type being the persimmon ball. Trichobezoars are composed of hair. Concretions of inorganic substances such as shellac, asphalt, or calcium carbonate are occasionally seen. Bezoars of the intact stomach often require surgical removal, although nonoperative methods may be successful for phytobezoars. Persimmon balls have responded to treatment with papain and sodium bicarbonate.

Small foreign bodies such as coins, marbles, or even closed safety pins usually pass through the stomach and bowel without difficulty. Elongated, sharp objects such as needles, toothpicks, or open safety pins may hold up at some point and cause obstruction, ulceration, bleeding, abscess, or peritonitis. Occasionally, large objects such as forks or knives are swallowed by emotionally disturbed persons. Patients who have swallowed dangerous objects should be promptly referred to an experienced endoscopist who may elect endoscopic removal, observation, or surgical treatment.

GASTRIC DIVERTICULA These uncommon lesions usually occur just below the cardia on the posterior wall near the lesser curvature. Almost all are asymptomatic and require no treatment. Pain, bleeding, and perforation are rare complications. Surgery should not be undertaken except for severe intractable symptoms that cannot be attributed to another cause. The x-ray appearance is usually diagnostic, but occasionally gastroscopy is needed to distinguish the lesion from a peptic ulcer.

GASTRIC VOLVULUS OR TORSION Rarely the stomach can twist about its longitudinal axis, thus turning itself upside down and obstructing the lower esophagus. The volvulus may be acute but is more often chronic. It tends to be associated with a paraesophageal hernia or eventration of the diaphragm. The stomach can also twist about the vertical axis of the gastrohepatic omentum to produce a torsion rather than a true volvulus. Acute volvulus is associated with severe upper abdominal pain and retching which produces saliva rather than gastric or duodenal contents. Passage of a nasogastric tube beyond the cardia is usually impossible. Plain x-ray films of the abdomen show distention of the stomach; the finding of two separate fluid levels is diagnostic. Acute volvulus may be of short duration and may subside spontaneously or may be associated with strangulation and require emergency surgical treatment. Those with chronic volvulus may be asymptomatic or have intermittent pain, often associated with eating. Severe symptoms may require surgical correction of the volvulus, including repair of an associated paraesophageal hernia, if present.

RARE GASTRIC DISEASES **Pseudolymphoma** This is a localized benign lymphoid hyperplasia of the stomach. Its etiology is unknown, but in some instances it is a reaction to a benign gastric ulcer. Grossly the lesion is usually single and ulcerated. Some lesions are nodular;

others may present as enlarged folds. The x-ray and endoscopic findings may suggest either malignancy or peptic ulcer. There is marked lymphocytic infiltration of the gastric wall which may be transmural. Partial gastrectomy is usually required for diagnosis and treatment. The lesion may be distinguished from true lymphoma by the polyclonal nature of the infiltrate shown by immunohistochemical staining.

Eosinophilic gastroenteritis The antrum may be involved in this condition, which is associated with marked peripheral eosinophilia. The diagnosis can be made by mucosal biopsy, and chronic treatment with small doses of corticosteroids is usually effective.

Inflammatory fibroid polyp This is usually a circumscribed lesion of the antrum and is not associated with peripheral eosinophilia. In the past it has been called *eosinophilic granuloma* but this is a misnomer. It does not respond to corticosteroid treatment and may require excision because of pyloric obstruction or other symptoms.

Gastric granulomas Epithelioid granulomas of the stomach are most commonly caused by Crohn's disease and only rarely are a manifestation of sarcoid or tuberculosis. Some granulomas adjacent to peptic ulcers are foreign-body reactions. Idiopathic isolated granulomas often prove to be due to Crohn's disease or may be a manifestation of immunoglobulin deficiency or of chronic granulomatous disease.

Other specific gastritides Tuberculosis and tertiary syphilis rarely affect the stomach. The diagnosis can sometimes be made from the clinical picture and endoscopic biopsy, but more often operation is needed to exclude malignancy. Appropriate antibiotic therapy is effective. Gastric infections, particularly candidiasis but also cytomegalovirus, herpes simplex, and histoplasmosis, are occasionally seen in immunosuppressed patients. Gastric anisakiasis is a nematode infection of the stomach acquired by eating raw fish. Previously, it was largely confined to Japan, where sashimi (raw fish) is a delicacy. It is now seen occasionally in the United States, where sashimi has become popular.

REFERENCES

ANTONIOLI DA et al: Changes in the location and type of gastric adenocarcinoma. Cancer 50:775, 1982

DIEHL JT et al: Gastric carcinoma—A ten year review. Ann Surg 198:9, 1983

DOMSCHKE S et al Gastroduodenal damage due to drugs, alcohol and smoking. Clin Gastroenterol 13:405, 1984

DWORKEN B et al: Primary gastric lymphoma. Dig Dis Sci 27:986, 1982

GRAHAM DY, SMITH JL: Aspirin and the stomach. Ann Int Med 104:390, 1986

KREUNING J et al: Gastric and duodenal mucosa in "healthy" individuals, an endoscopic and histopathological study of 50 volunteers. J Clin Pathol 31:69, 1978

SHAFER LW et al: The risk of gastric carcinoma after surgical treatment for benign disease. N Engl J Med 309:1210, 1983

WEINSTEIN WM: Gastritis, in *Gastrointestinal Disease*, 3d ed, J Sleisinger and JS Fordtran (eds). Philadelphia, Saunders, 1983

237 DISORDERS OF ABSORPTION

NORTON J. GREENBERGER / KURT J. ISSELBACHER

MECHANISMS OF ABSORPTION

Diseases of the small intestine are frequently accompanied by alterations in intestinal function, and clinically this impaired function is seen as the malabsorption syndrome. In order to obtain a better appreciation of the derangements which occur in the many disorders of intestinal function, the processes of normal absorption will first be reviewed.

It is important to distinguish between digestion and absorption, since an increased loss of nutrients in the stool may be a reflection of a derangement of either process. Digestion involves the breakdown or hydrolysis of nutrients to smaller molecules in order to prepare the ingested substances for absorption, or transport across the intestinal cell. It will be recalled that most of the digestive process is initiated in the stomach by acid and pepsin and is continued in the upper small intestine primarily by the action of pancreatic enzymes such as lipase, amylase, and trypsin. As a result of these digestive actions carbohydrates are broken down to monosaccharides and disaccharides, proteins to peptides and amino acids, and fats to monoglycerides and fatty acids. In the adult it is in this form that nutrients are, to a large extent, transported across the epithelial surface of the intestinal cell.

ANATOMIC AND PHYSIOLOGIC FACTORS The intestine has an enormous surface area. This can be attributed in large part to its length, which in the adult is more than 12 ft, and to the foldings of the surface plicae. At the light microscopic level, the villi of the small intestine provide additional surface area, which is further augmented by the presence of microvilli (approximately 2×10^8 per square centimeter) on the outer, or brush border, region of epithelial cells. Thus the total absorptive area of the small intestine is enormous.

Motility (contractility) of the bowel is an important process which permits nutrients to remain in intimate contact with the intestinal cells and possibly influences the continued movement of the nutrients *into* and along the absorbing channels, such as the lymphatics. Two types of motility aid in this process: the gross motility of the intestine itself and the motility of individual villi. Entrance of the nutrients into the general circulation is achieved via the capillaries into the portal system or via the lacteals into the intestinal lymphatics.

TYPES OF ABSORPTION Four mechanisms have been considered to be important in the transport of substances across the intestinal cell membrane, namely, active transport, passive diffusion, facilitated diffusion, and endocytosis.

Active transport involves the transport of a substance across the cell against an electric or chemical gradient; this process requires energy, is carrier-mediated, and is subject to competitive inhibition. *Passive diffusion* is the opposite of this process; energy is not required, transport is with (rather than against) the electric or chemical gradient, the process is not carrier-mediated, and it does not show properties of competitive inhibition. Thus active transport may be viewed as "uphill" transport, whereas passive diffusion is equivalent to "downhill" transport. *Facilitated diffusion* is similar to passive diffusion except that such a process shows evidence of being carrier-mediated and frequently subject to competitive inhibition.

Endocytosis is a process akin to phagocytosis. By this mechanism nutrients (soluble or particulate) upon entering the cell are surrounded by the components of the outer plasma cell membrane. In the intestinal tract endocytosis occurs in the neonatal period and, contrary to earlier belief, also occurs to a limited extent in the adult organism. While quantitatively limited, it appears to account, for example, for uptake of antigens.

SITES OF ABSORPTION While many substances are absorbed throughout the length of the small intestine, certain nutrients tend to be absorbed more in one region than in others. The proximal intestine is a major area for the absorption of iron, calcium, water-soluble vitamins, and fat (monoglycerides and fatty acids). Sugars are absorbed in the proximal intestine and also the midintestine. While the amino acids appear to be absorbed primarily in the middle of the small intestine, or jejunum, some absorption also occurs in the upper and lower areas. The distal small intestine appears to be the *major* absorptive area for bile salts and vitamin B_{12}. As is emphasized below, this factor is of clinical significance in circumstances where there has been removal or disease of the ileum.

The colon is important for the absorption of water and electrolytes, a process which occurs predominantly in the cecum. Although the rectum is not a usual site for absorption of ingested foodstuffs, drugs introduced by rectum may be absorbed there. Thus drugs introduced by this route, such as salicylates or steroids, may have systemic as well as local effects.

ABSORPTION OF SPECIFIC NUTRIENTS **Carbohydrate absorption** Much of the carbohydrate we ingest is in the form of starch, a complex polysaccharide consisting of many hexose units (attached either in a 1,4 or 1,6 linkage). By the action of salivary and pancreatic amylase, starch is hydrolyzed to oligosaccharides and then to disaccharides (mostly maltose). While monosaccharides such as glucose are readily absorbed, disaccharides are not. Disaccharides are split enzymatically into their component sugars by disaccharidases (or oligosaccharidases) located on or within the microvilli of intestinal epithelial cells. The two types of disaccharidases are β-galactosidases (lactase) and α-glucosidases (sucrase, maltase). By the action of these enzymes, lactose is split into glucose and galactose, sucrose into glucose and fructose, and maltose into two molecules of glucose. The resultant monosaccharides are then transported through the cell into the portal circulation. Most disaccharides are hydrolyzed so rapidly by brush border enzymes that the capacity of the transport mechanism is exceeded and some monosaccharides diffuse back into the intestinal lumen. Lactose, however, is hydrolyzed at a slower rate, and thus lactose hydrolysis is the rate-limiting step in lactose absorption.

Sugars such as glucose and galactose are absorbed by an active transport mechanism. The transport rate of sugars can be related to the substrate concentration by the expression K_t, where K_t stands for the monosaccharide substrate concentration that produces half the maximal transport rate. Published K_t values for glucose transport have varied widely, partly because of failure to consider the unstirred water layer, which constitutes a diffusion barrier for solutes.

Glucose (and galactose) entry into the cell is largely coupled to sodium ions (so-called symport); both sodium and glucose appear to bind to the hexose carrier in the microvillus membrane. Energy is required for the movement of glucose into the cell, which seems largely to come from the sodium pump and the Na^+,K^+-ATPase of the basolateral membrane (see below).

Protein and amino acid absorption Dietary proteins are initially subject to degradation in the stomach by pepsin. However, complete hydrolysis is largely achieved by the action of the pancreatic enzymes trypsin and chymotrypsin as well as by other endopeptidases and exopeptidases such as carboxypeptidase. By these enzymatic processes oligopeptides, dipeptides, and amino acids are formed. Just as there are disaccharidases in mucosal cells to digest disaccharides, there are also oligopeptidases to split small peptides. Dipeptidases are located in the cytoplasm as well as on the microvilli. Dipeptides are absorbed more rapidly than amino acids, and presumably their uptake involves a separate mechanism. Thus, digestion of proteins to amino acids occurs in three locations: intestinal lumen, brush border, and cytoplasm of mucosal cells. As indicated above, contrary to earlier beliefs proteins can also be absorbed by the adult intestine. Although quantitatively limited, protein absorption probably is immunologically significant.

Most naturally occurring amino acids are L-amino acids, and these are subject to a number of different transport processes. *Neutral* amino acids seem to share a common carrier mechanism; thus amino acids such as tryptophan and alanine show competitive inhibition. Among the *dibasic* amino acids which appear to have a distinct transport mechanism are arginine, ornithine, and lysine. The neutral amino acid cystine shares this mechanism. There is also a separate transport system for *glycine* and the *imino acids* proline and hydroxyproline. There is also a transport system for *dicarboxylic* acids such as glutamic and aspartic acids. Therefore, in genetic disorders, such as cystinuria, one will find impaired absorption not only of cystine but also of arginine, ornithine, and lysine. Similarly in Hartnup disease, a defect in the transport of neutral amino acids (especially of tryptophan, phenylalanine, histidine) is found. In these genetic disorders uptake and absorption of dipeptides is normal.

Absorption of amino acids is rapid in the duodenum and jejunum but slow in the ileum. The actual mechanism of the absorption of amino acids by the intestine has not been elucidated. As in the case of carbohydrates, sodium ions appear to be required for the entry of these acids and the energy needed for their concentration within the cell. Some amino acids have affinity for more than one mechanism. For example, glycine may be transported by both the neutral and imino acid transport systems.

Fat absorption (Fig. 237-1) Most of the ingested dietary fats are in the form of long-chain triglycerides. These triglycerides contain both saturated fatty acids (such as palmitic and stearic) and unsaturated fatty acids (such as oleic and linoleic). The particle size of the fat is decreased largely by the churning action of the stomach. The entry of fat into the duodenum plus the presence of acid causes release of secretin and pancreozymin-cholecystokinin, which in turn leads to a stimulation of the flow of bile and pancreatic juice.

ROLE OF PANCREATIC LIPASE The hydrolysis of triglycerides by pancreatic lipase is a complex process involving lipase, colipase, and bile salts. Pancreatic lipase is an enzyme that binds to the oil-water interface of an emulsified triglyceride substrate. The detergent properties of bile salts permit pancreatic lipase to gain access to water-insoluble lipids. One of the important functions of bile salts is to clear the oil-water interface of dietary fat from proteins of exogenous and endogenous origin, thus making it available for pancreatic lipolysis. Colipase, a protein present in pancreatic juice, is also essential for the action of lipase; its function is to anchor the lipase close to the surface of the triglyceride droplet. All three components, i.e., pancreatic lipase, colipase, and bile salts, form a *ternary complex*, which generates lipolytic products that diffuse away from the complex and are absorbed. With colipase present, lipase remains at the interface and forms 2-monoglycerides and fatty acids, which are the major end products of triglyceride hydrolysis. Less than 5 percent of ingested

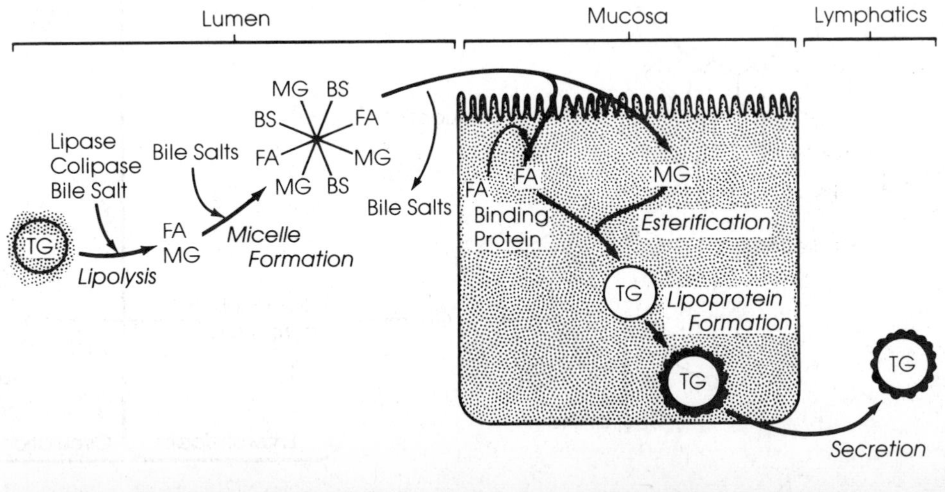

FIGURE 237-1 *Scheme of intestinal digestion, absorption, esterification, and transport of dietary triglycerides. TG = triglycerides; FA = fatty acids; MG = monoglycerides; BS = bile salts.*

fat remains in the form of diglycerides and triglycerides. Without colipase, bile acids would actually wash pancreatic lipase away from the interface, and the hydrolytic rate of triglycerides would be reduced.

ROLE OF BILE SALTS (Fig. 237-2) Bile salts play an important role in the digestion and absorption of fat. They are synthesized in the liver (approximately 200 to 600 mg daily) from cholesterol and excreted in the bile in the form of their glycine or taurine conjugates. In humans the principal bile acids excreted are conjugates of cholic and chenodeoxycholic acid. Bile salts are good detergents, because they have both polar (hydrophilic) and nonpolar (hydrophobic) groups. During digestion the concentration of conjugated bile salts in the lumen is in the range of 5 to 15 μmol/mL, and at these concentrations the bile salts aggregate to form *micelles*. Fatty acids and monoglycerides enter these micelles, forming mixed micelles. An emulsion of triglyceride is turbid; mixed micelles containing bile salts, fatty acids, and monoglycerides are clear solutions. The formation of *mixed micelles* and hence the solubilization of fatty acids and monoglycerides is much more effectively achieved with *conjugated bile salts* at the pH which normally exists in the intestinal lumen (Fig. 237-2).

Most conjugated bile salts are absorbed in the ileum and after entering the portal vein are subject to an enterohepatic circulation. By this process about 90 percent of the conjugated bile salts reaching the ileum is reabsorbed. As a consequence only about 200 to 600 mg bile salts is excreted in the feces per day, while, as part of the enterohepatic circulation, as much as 20 to 30 g bile salts recirculates daily between the liver and intestine. When the enterohepatic circulation is intact, the size of the bile salt pool is largely determined by the frequency of the enterohepatic circulation, i.e., the number of cycles per day (see also Chap. 253). If the ileum is diseased or removed, absorption of bile salts is impaired, and a significant fecal loss of bile salts will occur. As a consequence of this bile salt depletion, the concentration of bile salts in the intestinal lumen will also decrease, leading to further impairment of fat absorption. A similar result will occur if bile salt reabsorption is prevented by chelating agents, such as cholestyramine (see "Regional Enteritis" below).

INTRAMUCOSAL ASPECTS OF FAT ABSORPTION (Fig. 237-1) After the hydrolysis of fatty acids to monoglycerides and their interaction with bile salts to form mixed micelles, the lipids pass through an "unstirred" water layer covering the cell surface. The mixed micelles apparently do not enter the cell, but instead the component fatty acids and monoglycerides are released from the micellar phase and then enter the cell by diffusion. In aqueous duodenal contents, large bile salt mixed micelles saturated with products of lipolysis coexist with larger liquid crystal liposomes of the same lipids saturated with free fatty acids and mixed bile salts. These phases are interconvertible and both may be important in fat digestion and absorption. Upon entry into the mucosal cell, fatty acids may interact with specific binding proteins. The subsequent fate of the intracellular lipid is strongly influenced by the fatty acid chain length. Fatty acids and monoglycerides derived from long-chain triglycerides (i.e., containing C-16 to C-18 fatty acids) are promptly *reesterified to triglycerides* by enzymes of the endoplasmic reticulum. These triglycerides then interact with specific apolipoproteins plus cholesterol and phospholipid to form chylomicrons and very low density lipoproteins. These initially accumulate in the Golgi region of the cell and then are secreted into the lacteals and the intestinal lymph. There are thus four major steps in the absorption of long-chain fatty acids and monoglycerides: (1) mucosal uptake and interaction with binding proteins, (2) reesterification to triglycerides, (3) lipoprotein formation, and (4) secretion into lymph.

By contrast, fatty acids derived from medium-chain triglycerides (i.e., containing C-8 and C-12 fatty acids) are *not reesterified* to any significant extent within the cell and are not incorporated into lipoproteins. Instead, they rapidly enter the portal venous system, where they are transported as fatty acids bound to albumin. The major aspects of fat absorption are summarized in Fig. 237-1.

Absorption of cholesterol and fat-soluble vitamins (A, D, E, K) In addition to contributing significantly to the total-body synthesis of cholesterol, the intestine also plays an active role in the absorption of cholesterol and its esters. Within the lumen, cholesterol esters from the bile and diet are hydrolyzed by a pancreatic esterase. There

FIGURE 237-2 *Scheme of hepatic and intestinal metabolism of bile salts and the enterohepatic circulation (from ileum to liver). Note that bacteria lead to the formation of secondary bile acids; of the latter, only deoxycholic acid is absorbed to any appreciable extent.*

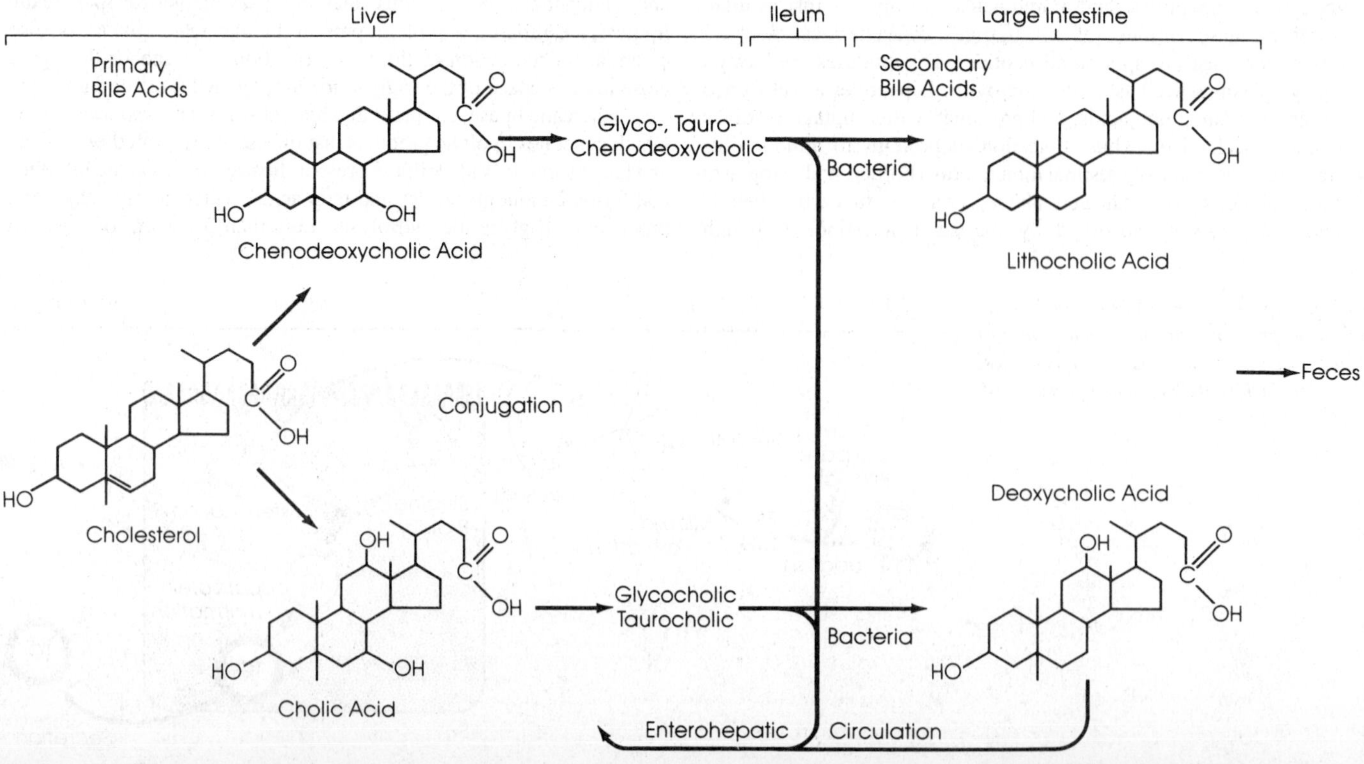

is also a separate cholesterol esterase in the intestinal microvilli, which completes this hydrolysis. As a result, only free cholesterol appears to enter the intestinal cell. However, just as in the case of long-chain fatty acids, much of the cholesterol is reesterified and is then secreted primarily into lymph.

The absorption mechanisms of the fat-soluble vitamins A, D, E, and K are not well understood. The intestine is able to convert β-carotene into vitamin A. The vitamin A thus formed or absorbed from the lumen is esterified in the mucosa primarily with palmitic acid, transported in the chylomicrons of the lymph, and stored as retinol palmitate in the liver. The other lipid-soluble vitamins also appear in lymph chylomicrons, but esterification with fatty acids does not appear to be necessary for their transport.

Water and sodium absorption In spite of extensive investigations the main mechanisms of water and electrolyte transport are not well understood. The mechanisms responsible for fluid absorption differ in the jejunum, ileum, and colon. There are two pathways by which water and ions cross the intestinal mucosa: the paracellular and transcellular pathways. Individual intestinal mucosa cells are joined near their apex by a "tight junction," and ions and water traverse this *paracellular* pathway during absorption and secretion. It is believed that the tight junction pathway contains aqueous-filled channels or pores. Such intercellular spaces are closed in the resting state and dilated during absorption. Considerable evidence has accumulated indicating that pumps and carriers are involved in intestinal water and solute transport. For example, in the ileum, Na^+ enters in exchange for H^+, and Cl^- enters in exchange for HCO_3^-. Sodium entry into the cell also occurs coupled with glucose via the glucose-sodium carrier in the microvillus membrane. Inside the cell, the Na^+ pump located in the basolateral membrane actively transports Na^+ out of the mucosal cell and into the intercellular space. *Transcellular* transport requires passage of ions through two membrane barriers, i.e., the apical brush border plasma membrane and the basolateral membrane. After Na^+ and Cl^- are transported across the brush border membrane into the cell, Na^+ is pumped across the basolateral membrane and Cl^- either follows passively or is also pumped into the intercellular space. The Na^+,K^+-ATPase is present in the basolateral but not in the brush border membrane and is the biochemical mediator of this pump. Bulk water movement obviously influences the movement of Na^+, K^+, and Cl^-. This "solvent drag" effect is explained by two mechanisms: (1) solutes may be caught in a moving stream of water and transported across a membrane, and (2) water movement results in increased concentration of solute on the side of the membrane from which water was transported, which causes solute to diffuse through the direction of flow. Diarrhea can be simply defined as impaired net absorption of water and electrolytes by the small intestine or colon. Some mechanisms producing diarrhea are listed in Table 237-1.

Calcium absorption Calcium is actively transported by the small intestine, and this process is intimately linked to the active form of vitamin D_3, namely, 1,25-dihydroxycholecalciferol. The role of two other intestinal cell proteins, calcium-binding protein and calmodulin, in the absorption of calcium remains unclear.

Iron absorption The formation of soluble iron complexes is important for maintaining intraluminal iron in an absorbable form. Gastric acid facilitates the chelation of inorganic iron with substances such as ascorbic acid, sugars, amino acids, and bile; these macromolecular complexes then remain soluble in the more alkaline duodenum and jejunum. With the average western diet luminal content of the iron intake averages 15 to 25 mg per day; iron absorption averages 0.5 to 1.0 mg per day in men and 1.0 to 2.0 mg per day in women during their reproductive years. A regulatory mechanism for the absorption of inorganic iron appears to exist within the small-intestinal mucosal cells. Iron is actively transported by the small intestine, and the duodenum is the principal site of iron absorption. The absorption of elemental iron in humans and animals involves at least two distinct steps: (1) mucosal uptake of iron from the lumen and (2) mucosal transfer of iron to the plasma. Much of the iron entering the mucosal cell is not transferred to the plasma but remains trapped within the cell and is excreted into the lumen when the cell is shed. Iron lost by this mechanism seems to vary inversely with body iron stores. However, this mucosal regulatory mechanism can be overcome when pharmacologic doses of iron are ingested. Hemoglobin iron is also absorbed by human subjects, depending upon body requirements for iron; the heme is split from globin in the lumen and absorbed as an intact metalloporphyrin. Organic iron in the form of hemoglobin is absorbed more effectively than iron from cereals and vegetables. The absorption of inorganic iron is increased by ascorbic acid. Similarly, the presence of anemia, liver injury, pregnancy, idiopathic hemochromatosis, or a portacaval shunt may result in increased iron absorption. Conversely, the prior ingestion of large doses of iron and the presence in the lumen of phosphates, carbonates, and phytates may lead to decreased absorption of inorganic iron. Impaired absorption of iron is frequent in disorders (such as nontropical sprue) which involve the duodenal mucosa.

Water-soluble vitamins *Vitamin B_{12} absorption* is discussed in Chap. 285. In the case of *folic acid absorption,* it should be emphasized that folates exist in food conjugated with glutamyl peptides. These *polyglutamates* must be deconjugated (by folic deconjugase) to monoglutamates for absorption to occur. Certain drugs (such as oral contraceptives, sulfasalazine, diphenylhydantoin, trimethoprim, and pyrimethamine) inhibit the absorption of dietary folate and hence can cause folate deficiency. Sulfasalazine, for example, competitively inhibits three enzymes important in the intestinal metabolism of folate, i.e., dihydrofolate reductase, methylene tetrahydrofolate reductase, and serine transhydroxymethylase. Thiamine and riboflavin appear to be absorbed by passive diffusion.

TABLE 237-1 Some mechanisms in the production of diarrhea

I Secretory diarrhea
- *A* Secretory agents associated with adenylate cyclase system
  - *1* Enterotoxin-producing bacteria *(Vibrio cholerae, Escherichia coli)*
  - *2* Methylxanthines (caffeine, theophylline)
  - *3* Prostaglandins
  - *4* Vasoactive intestinal peptide (VIP)
  - *5* Dihydroxy bile acids (affect colon primarily; effects seen after ileal resection)
- *B* Secretory agents *not associated* with adenylate cyclase system
  - *1* Glucagon, secretin, cholecystokinin-pancreozymin, serotonin, calcitonin, gastrin inhibitory polypeptide (GIP)
  - *2* Some laxatives* (ricinoleic acid, bisacodyl, phenolphthalein, dioctyl sodium sulfosuccinate)
  - *3* Bacterial enterotoxins *(Shigella, Staphylococcus aureus, Clostridium perfringens)*
- *C* Mucosal injury, altered cell permeability
  - *1* *Salmonella, Shigella,* invasive *E. coli,* gastroenteritis viruses
  - *2* Celiac sprue
  - *3* Inflammatory bowel disease (ulcerative colitis, regional enteritis)
- *D* Neoplasms with or without hormone production
  - *1* Gastrinoma (gastrin)
  - *2* Carcinoid syndrome (serotonin, prostaglandins)
  - *3* Medullary carcinoma of thyroid (calcitonin, prostaglandins)
  - *4* Pancreatic cholera syndrome (? VIP)
  - *5* Villous adenoma

II Osmotic diarrhea
- *A* Impaired carbohydrate absorption
  - *1* Disaccharidase deficiency (lactose or sucrose-isomaltose intolerance)
  - *2* Glucose-galactose malabsorption
- *B* Laxative ingestion or abuse
  - *1* Nonabsorbable osmotically active agents (lactulose, sorbitol, mannitol)
  - *2* Saline purgatives (magnesium phosphate, magnesium hydroxide–containing antacids)
- *C* Postsurgical disorders
  - *1* Vagotomy and pyloroplasty*
  - *2* Gastrojejunostomy* (Billroth I and II)

III Motility disorders
- *A* Laxative abuse*
- *B* Irritable bowel syndrome
- *C* Diverticular disease of the colon
- *D* Diabetic diarrhea with visceral neuropathy

* *Multiple mechanisms involved in production of diarrhea.*

TABLE 237-2 Tests useful in the diagnosis of malabsorptive disorders

Test	Normal values	Typical findings: Malabsorption (nontropical sprue)	Typical findings: Maldigestion (pancreatic insufficiency)	Comment
I Stool studies				
A Quantitative determination of stool fat	<6 g per 24 h; >95% coefficient of fat absorption	>6 g per 24 h	>6 g per 24 h	Best test for establishing presence of steatorrhea
B Fat in stool, %	<6	often <9.5	>9.5	Increased stool fat concentration strongly suggests that steatorrhea is due to pancreatic insufficiency
II Carbohydrate absorption				
A D-Xylose absorption (25-g oral dose)	5-h urinary excretion >4.5 g; peak blood level >30 mg/dL	$\downarrow$	Normal	A good screening test for carbohydrate absorption
III Small-intestine x-rays		Malabsorption pattern	Normal or minimal malabsorption pattern; occasionally pancreatic calcification	Moulage sign and other abnormalities may be present in several disorders (see text)
IV Blood tests				
A Serum calcium	9–11 mg/dL	Frequently $\downarrow$	Usually normal	
B Serum albumin	3.5–5.5 g/dL	Frequently $\downarrow$	Usually normal	Decreased levels of both serum albumin and globulins should raise the question of protein-losing enteropathy
C Serum cholesterol	150–250 mg/dL	$\downarrow$	Frequently $\downarrow$	Usually decreased in disorders associated with significant steatorrhea
D Serum iron	80–150 μg/dL	Frequently $\downarrow$	Normal	Low values may reflect decreased body iron stores
E Serum magnesium	1.2–2.0 meq/liter	Frequently $\downarrow$	Usually normal	
F Serum zinc	12–20 μmol/liter	Frequently $\downarrow$	Usually normal	Decreased levels common in malnutrition, cirrhosis, and malabsorption
G Serum carotenes	>100 IU/dL	$\downarrow$	Usually $\downarrow$	Fairly satisfactory screening tests for malabsorption
H Serum vitamin A	>100 IU/dL	$\downarrow$		
I Prothrombin time	70–100%; 12–15 s	Frequently $\downarrow$	Frequently $\downarrow$	
V Small intestinal mucosal biopsy		Abnormal	Normal	A specific diagnosis can be established in a small number of disorders (see text)
VI Urine tests				
A Vitamin B_{12} absorption	>8% urinary excretion in 48 h	Frequently $\downarrow$	Frequently $\downarrow$	Useful in determining whether vitamin B_{12} malabsorption is due to gastric or small-intestinal disorders
B Urine 5-hydroxyindoleacetic acid (5-HIAA)	2–9 mg per 24 h	$\uparrow$	Normal	Slightly increased level (12–16 mg per 24 h) characteristically found in nontropical sprue
VII Breath tests				
A Breath H_2 (after 50 g lactose)	Minimal breath H_2	May be $\uparrow$	Normal	Secondary to lactase deficiency (see text)
B Breath H_2 (after 10 g lactulose)	Minimal breath H_2	May be normal or $\downarrow$	Normal	Early peak in bacterial overgrowth; can be used to determine intestinal transit time
C Breath $^{14}CO_2$ (after ^{14}C xylose)	Minute amounts $^{14}CO_2$	May be $\downarrow$	Usually normal	Increased in bacterial overgrowth
D Glycocholic acid metabolism (oral glycine-1-[^{14}C]glycocholate)	<1% of dose excreted $^{14}CO_2$ in 4 h	Normal	Normal	Increased $^{14}CO_2$ excretion with bacterial overgrowth or bile acid malabsorption (due to ileal resection or inflammatory disease)
	<4% of dose excreted in stools	Normal	Normal	Increased fecal excretion of ^{14}C in bile acid malabsorption
E [^{14}C]Triolein absorption (breath test)	>3.5% of dose as breath $^{14}CO_2$ per hour	Decreased	Decreased	Correlates well with chemical stool fat; recently introduced test
VIII Miscellaneous				
A Bacteria (culture)	<10^3 organisms per milliliter	Normal	Normal	>10^5 organisms per milliliter indicates bacterial overgrowth
B Secretin test	Volume >1.8 (mL/kg)/h Bicarbonate concentration >80 meq/liter	Normal	Abnormal	See discussion of pancreatic insufficiency in Chaps. 254 and 255
C Bentiromide test	Urine excretion arylamines ≥50%	May be abnormal	Abnormal	See discussion of pancreatic disease in Chaps. 254 and 255

TESTS USEFUL IN THE DIAGNOSIS OF MALABSORPTION Most of the tests useful in the diagnosis of malabsorption indicate the presence of abnormal absorptive or digestive function, and only a few tests may suggest a specific diagnosis. Accordingly, it is frequently necessary to employ a combination of tests to establish a diagnosis. To illustrate the use of various tests, the characteristic findings in nontropical sprue, an example of a primary malabsorptive disorder, and pancreatic insufficiency, an example of impaired digestion, are compared in Table 237-2.

Stool fat The qualitative examination of the stool for undigested muscle fibers, neutral fat, and split fat is a simple and reliable screening test for steatorrhea. The finding of an increased number of muscle fibers indicates impaired intraluminal digestion. Properly performed, the qualitative microscopic examination of a stool specimen with the Sudan III stain is of value and correlates well with the quantitative determination of fecal fat by the Van de Kamer method. The latter remains the most reliable measurement of steatorrhea. A normal fecal fat excretion is less than 6 g for 24 h, or greater than 94 percent coefficient of fat absorption. A fecal fat concentration greater than or equal to 9.5 percent suggests that steatorrhea is due to pancreatic exocrine insufficiency.

Oral [^{14}C]triolein can also be used as an effective test for fat absorption. During the digestive process the triolein is hydrolyzed, and the labeled glycerol is absorbed and metabolized by the liver. The $^{14}CO_2$ produced is exhaled and can then be measured hourly (for 6 h) in the expired air. Normally more than 3.5 percent of the administered label [0.185 MBq (5 μCi)] appears in the breath per hour.

Xylose absorption In the most commonly employed test of carbohydrate absorption, the patient ingests 25 g D-xylose. A 5-h urine xylose excretion of 4.5 g or greater is considered normal. There is some decreased renal excretion with age, and over age sixty-five 3.5 g is the normal value. Low values may be obtained in patients with ascites, intestinal bacterial overgrowth, or renal insufficiency, after administration of certain drugs (e.g., aspirin, indomethacin), and most commonly if the urine collection is incomplete. To obviate difficulties in interpreting the test, it is advisable to determine the blood xylose level 2 h after ingestion of xylose. A blood xylose level of 30 mg/dL or greater indicates normal absorption of D-xylose. An abnormal D-xylose absorption test is found most frequently in disorders affecting the mucosa of the proximal small intestine, such as nontropical and tropical sprue.

Gastrointestinal x-ray studies All patients with malabsorption should have radiographic examinations of the small intestine and, in many cases, of the esophagus, stomach, and colon as well. Occasionally, the latter two examinations may provide important clues to the presence of such disorders as gastroileostomy, scleroderma, Zollinger-Ellison syndrome, ulcerative colitis, and intestinal fistulas. The typical small-bowel radiographic abnormalities in patients with a malabsorption syndrome are a breaking up of the barium column with segmentation, clumping, and coarsening of the mucosal folds. Segmentation or clumping of the barium in a small-bowel loop is often termed a *moulage sign*. Less frequently there is dilatation of the proximal small bowel and loss of a normal mucosal pattern. Collectively, these changes have been referred to as a *malabsorption pattern*. These findings are nonspecific and may be found in several of the disorders listed in Table 237-3. Some representative examples of abnormal small-bowel radiographs are shown in Fig. 237-3.

Small-intestinal biopsy The most commonly used instruments for obtaining peroral biopsy specimens from the small intestine include the Rubin tube, the Crosby, Carey, and Ross-Moore capsules, and the upper gastrointestinal endoscope. Examination of small-bowel biopsy specimens has proved to be of considerable value in the differential diagnosis of malabsorptive disorders. Table 237-3 lists disorders associated with abnormalities in intestinal biopsies, and Fig. 237-4 depicts some illustrative lesions.

Schilling test for vitamin B_{12} absorption The Schilling test is valuable in the differential diagnosis of malabsorption and is frequently carried out in three stages: (1) without intrinsic factor, (2) with intrinsic factor, and (3) after a course of treatment with antibiotics. Since vitamin B_{12} is absorbed primarily in the distal ileum, an abnormal Schilling test may indicate a pathologic condition of the distal small bowel. In disorders affecting the terminal ileum, such as regional enteritis and lymphomas, the first-stage Schilling test is frequently abnormal. The ileal receptor site appears to be damaged in these disorders, and the impaired absorption of B_{12} is not corrected by the addition of intrinsic factor or the use of antibiotics. The Schilling test may also be useful in establishing a diagnosis of abnormal bacterial overgrowth of the small bowel, which may be present in disorders such as blind loop syndrome, scleroderma, and multiple small-bowel diverticula (see below). In the blind loop syndrome, for example, the bacteria can actually take up vitamin B_{12} with resultant impaired absorption of B_{12}. Under these conditions the first-stage Schilling test is frequently abnormal, as is the second stage. After appropriate antibiotic treatment the Schilling test usually returns to normal. Vitamin B_{12} absorption is frequently abnormal in patients with exocrine pancreatic insufficiency (see Chap. 255).

Secretin test The secretin test, secretin pancreozymin test, and intraduodenal perfusion with essential amino acids, which may be useful in establishing a diagnosis of pancreatic insufficiency, are discussed in detail in Chap. 254.

Serum calcium, albumin, cholesterol, magnesium, and iron Abnormal serum calcium, albumin, cholesterol, magnesium, and iron values may be found in several malabsorptive disorders. The primary value of such tests is to suggest that abnormal intestinal absorptive function may be present. These tests are usually of limited value in the *differential diagnosis* of malabsorption, but if abnormal, may be helpful in supporting this diagnosis.

Serum carotenes, vitamin A, and prothrombin time Absorption of the fat-soluble vitamins A, D, K, and E is frequently impaired in patients with steatorrhea. Measurements of serum carotene and vitamin A levels are useful as screening tests for malabsorption. However,

TABLE 237-3 Disorders associated with abnormalities in small-bowel biopsy specimens

I Disorders in which biopsy is of diagnostic value (diffuse lesions)
- *A* Whipple's disease: Lamina propria infiltrated with macrophages containing PAS-positive glycoproteins
- *B* Abetalipoproteinemia: Villus structure normal; epithelial cells vacuolated due to excess fat
- *C* Agammaglobulinemia: Flattened or absent villi; increased lymphocyte infiltration; absence of plasma cells

II Disorders in which biopsy may be of diagnostic value (patchy lesions)
- *A* Intestinal lymphoma: Infiltration of lamina propria and submucosa with malignant cells
- *B* Intestinal lymphangiectasia: Dilated lacteals and lymphatics in lamina propria; clubbed villi
- *C* Eosinophilic enteritis: Diffuse or patchy eosinophilic infiltration in lamina propria and mucosa
- *D* Amyloidosis: Presence of amyloid confirmed by special stains
- *E* Regional enteritis: Noncaseating granulomas
- *F* Parasitic infestations: Parasitic invasion of mucosa; adherence of trophozoites to mucosal surface, as in giardiasis
- *G* Systemic mastocytosis: Mast cell infiltration of lamina propria

III Disorders in which biopsy is abnormal but not diagnostic
- *A* Celiac sprue: Shortened or absent villi; hypertrophied crypts; damaged surface epithelium; mononuclear infiltrate
- *B* "Collagenous" sprue: Indistinguishable from celiac sprue; extensive subepithelial collagen deposition
- *C* Tropical sprue: Lesion similar to celiac sprue with shortened or absent villi; lymphocyte infiltration
- *D* Folate deficiency: Shortened villi; megalocytosis; decreased mitoses in crypts
- *E* Vitamin B_{12} deficiency: Similar to folate deficiency
- *F* Acute radiation enteritis: Similar to folate deficiency
- *G* Systemic scleroderma: Fibrosis around Brunner's glands
- *H* Bacterial overgrowth syndromes: Patchy damage to villi and increased lymphocyte infiltration

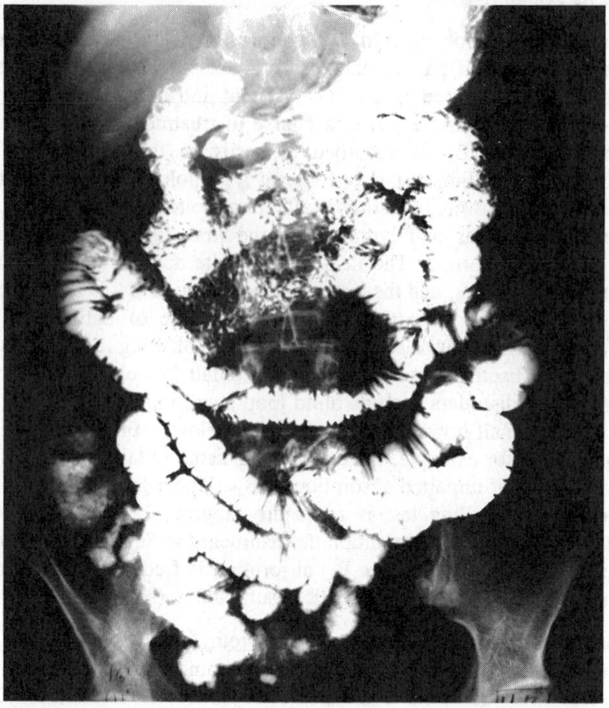

A

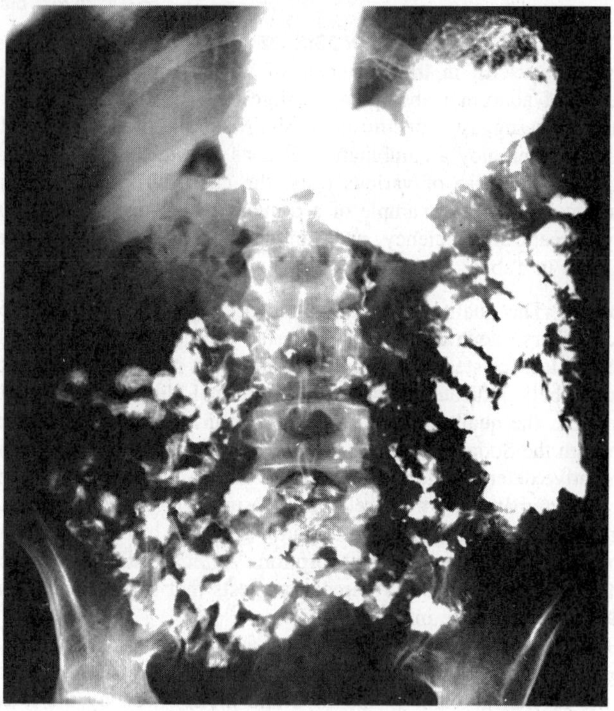

B

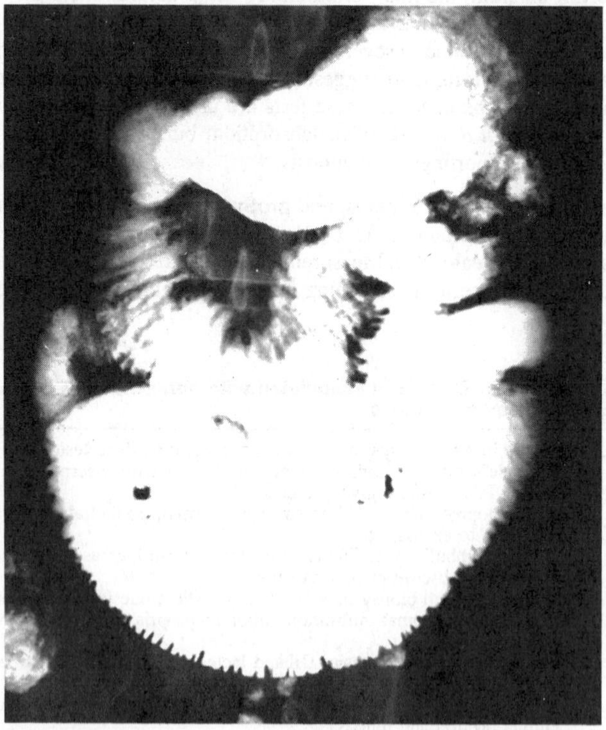

C

FIGURE 237-3 *A. X-ray of a normal small intestine showing good mucosal pattern. B. Intestinal x-ray of a patient with nontropical sprue. Note dilatation of small bowel, lack of mucosal markings, and segmentation and clumping of barium. C. Intestinal x-ray of patient with obstructed lymphatics due to Köhlmeier-Degos disease. Note ''accordion-pleated'' pattern at lower edge of film.*

other tests not only are more sensitive but often give more specific information than the serum carotene and vitamin A levels. The blood prothrombin time is an important test, since patients with malabsorption may present with abnormal bleeding due to vitamin K deficiency. If the decreased prothrombin activity is due to malabsorption, it should be readily correctable with parenteral vitamin K.

Breath tests The bile acid breath test utilizing [^{14}C]cholylglycine is a reasonably reliable screening test for bacterial overgrowth syndromes. Approximately two-thirds of patients with a positive small-bowel culture will have an abnormal bile acid breath test. However, in patients with suspected malabsorption of bile acids the test is rather insensitive without the additional determination of fecal bile acid excretion. The excretion of breath hydrogen after ingestion of lactose is a sensitive, specific, and noninvasive test for detecting lactase deficiency. Lactulose and [^{14}C]xylose breath tests for bacterial overgrowth have also been found helpful.

PATHOPHYSIOLOGIC BASIS FOR SYMPTOMS AND SIGNS IN MALABSORPTIVE DISORDERS The common symptoms and signs found in malabsorptive disorders are listed in Table 237-4. The most frequent symptoms are those of malnutrition, weight loss, and diarrhea. However, in each of the clinical settings listed in Table 237-4, it is important to consider the cause of the malabsorption.

DISORDERS ASSOCIATED WITH MALABSORPTION

(See Table 237-5)

INADEQUATE DIGESTION **Liver and biliary tract disease** It is not generally appreciated that patients with acute or chronic liver disease may develop malabsorption due to impaired intraluminal digestion. Steatorrhea has been described in acute viral hepatitis, chronic extrahepatic biliary tract obstruction, primary biliary cirrhosis, and postnecrotic and nutritional cirrhosis. Absorption of D-xylose and vitamin B_{12} are usually normal, and small-intestinal mucosal biopsy specimens are generally unremarkable. The steatorrhea associated with liver and biliary tract disease is thought to be due to impaired hepatic synthesis or excretion of conjugated bile salts, resulting in impaired formation of micellar lipid. In addition to steatorrhea, patients with liver disease may have impaired absorption of vitamin D and calcium, resulting in severe metabolic bone disease. This is particularly common in patients with primary biliary cirrhosis. Skeletal roentgenograms may show increased porosity of bone, cortical thinning, vertebral compression, and spontaneous pathologic fractures. Patients with alcohol-induced liver disease may also have exocrine pancreatic insufficiency. Accordingly, pancreatic function should be evaluated in patients with liver disease and malabsorption.

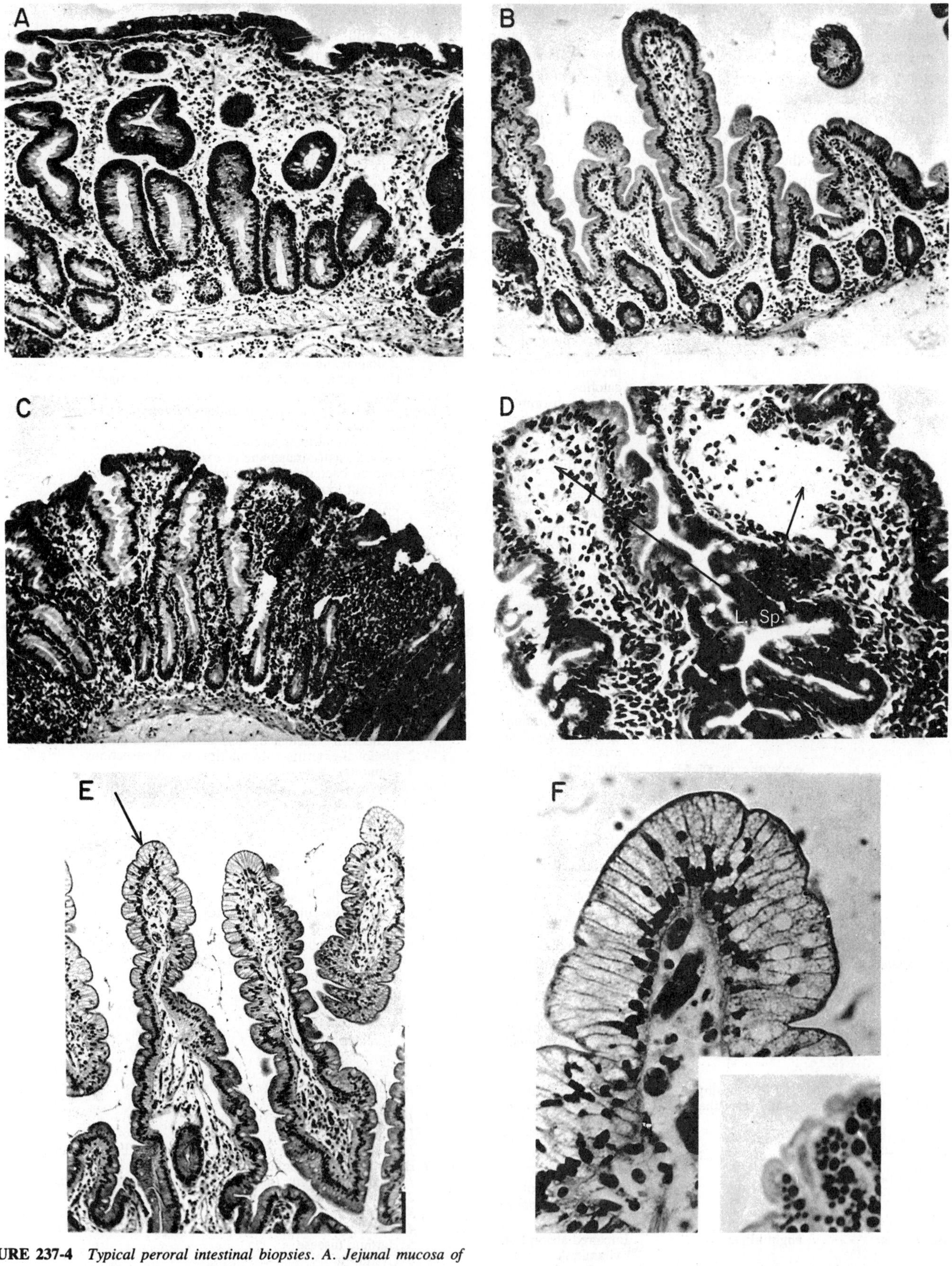

FIGURE 237-4 *Typical peroral intestinal biopsies. A. Jejunal mucosa of patient with nontropical sprue. Note virtual absence of villi, elongated crypts (some are cut in cross section), mononuclear infiltrate, cuboidal instead of columnar epithelium on top of villi (300×). B. Biopsy from the same patient as in A, after 9 months on a gluten-free diet. Note the reappearance of villi with normal-appearing columnar cells and reduction in infiltrate and crypt height (300×). C. Biopsy from patient with agammaglobulinemia. The features bear a striking resemblance to those of nontropical sprue. There is a marked mononuclear infiltration, some of it in aggregates (200×). D. Close-up of villi of patient with protein-losing enteropathy. Tips of villi are broadened and dilated. Lymphatic spaces are present (arrows) (450×). E. Intestinal biopsy from patient with abetalipoproteinemia. The villus tips have a ''lacy'' appearance (arrow) due to retained fat (300×). (This is more apparent at the higher magnification shown in F.) F. High-power micrograph of villus from patient with abetalipoproteinemia. The vacuoles are filled with lipid (750×). Insert shows dark-staining (osmium) lipid droplets in mucosal cells (osmium counterstained with Giemsa; 800×).*

Postgastrectomy malabsorption The presence of a malabsorption syndrome has been documented frequently in patients after subtotal gastrectomy. Steatorrhea is more common with a Billroth II than a Billroth I type of anastomosis. Usually the fat loss is minimal, ranging from 7 to 10 g per 24 h. Patients with gross steatorrhea usually have impaired intraluminal fat digestion due to several factors: (1) With a Billroth II anastomosis the duodenum is bypassed, and there is a decreased entry of stomach contents into the proximal duodenum (i.e., afferent loop). This leads to a decreased stimulus for the release of *secretin* and *cholecystokinin-pancreozymin* from the duodenum and may result in a depressed pancreatic enzyme response. (2) There may be *inadequate mixing* of the pancreatic enzymes and bile salts secreted into the proximal duodenum with the gastric contents entering the jejunum. (3) There may be *stasis* of intestinal contents in the afferent loop, resulting in abnormal bacterial proliferation in the proximal small bowel. This in turn may lead to abnormalities in bile

TABLE 237-4 Pathophysiologic basis for symptoms and signs in malabsorptive disorders

Organ system	Symptom or sign	Pathophysiology
Gastrointestinal	Generalized malnutrition and weight loss	Malabsorption of fat, carbohydrate, and protein → loss of calories
	Diarrhea	Impaired absorption or increased secretion of water and electrolytes; unabsorbed dihydroxy bile acids and fatty acids → decreased absorption of water and electrolytes; excess load of fluid and electrolytes presented to the colon may exceed its absorptive capacity
	Flatus	Bacterial fermentation of unabsorbed carbohydrate
	Glossitis, cheilosis, stomatitis	Deficiency of iron, vitamin B_{12}, folate, and other vitamins
Genitourinary	Nocturia	Delayed absorption of water, hypokalemia
	Azotemia, hypotension	Fluid and electrolyte depletion
	Amenorrhea, ↓ libido	Protein depletion and "caloric starvation" → secondary hypopituitarism
Hematopoietic	Anemia	Impaired absorption of iron, vitamin B_{12}, and folic acid
	Hemorrhagic phenomena	Vitamin K malabsorption → hypoprothrombinemia
Musculoskeletal	Bone pain	Protein depletion → impaired bone formation → osteoporosis Calcium malabsorption → demineralization of bone → osteomalacia
	Osteoarthropathy	Cause uncertain
	Tetany, paresthesias	Calcium malabsorption → hypocalcemia; magnesium malabsorption → hypomagnesemia
	Weakness	Anemia; electrolyte depletion (hypokalemia)
Nervous system	Night blindness	Impaired absorption vitamin A → vitamin A deficiency
	Xerophthalmia	Vitamin A deficiency
	Peripheral neuropathy	Vitamin B_{12}, thiamine deficiency
Skin	Eczema	Cause uncertain
	Purpura	Vitamin K deficiency
	Follicular hyperkeratosis and dermatitis	Deficiency of vitamin A, zinc, essential fatty acids, and other vitamins

TABLE 237-5 Classification of the malabsorption syndromes

I Inadequate digestion
- *A* Postgastrectomy steatorrhea*
- *B* Deficiency or inactivation of pancreatic lipase
  - *1* Exocrine pancreatic insufficiency
    - *a* Chronic pancreatitis
    - *b* Pancreatic carcinoma
    - *c* Cystic fibrosis
    - *d* Pancreatic resection
  - *2* Ulcerogenic tumor of the pancreas (Zollinger-Ellison syndrome, gastrinoma)*

II Reduced intestinal bile salt concentration (with impaired micelle formation)
- *A* Liver disease
  - *1* Parenchymal liver disease
  - *2* Cholestasis (intrahepatic or extrahepatic)
- *B* Abnormal bacterial proliferation in the small bowel
  - *1* Afferent loop stasis
  - *2* Strictures
  - *3* Fistulas
  - *4* Blind loops
  - *5* Multiple diverticula of the small bowel
  - *6* Hypomotility states (diabetes, scleroderma, intestinal pseudoobstruction)
- *C* Interrupted enterohepatic circulation of bile salts
  - *1* Ileal resection
  - *2* Ileal inflammatory disease (regional ileitis)
- *D* Drugs (by sequestration or precipitation of bile salts)
  - *1* Neomycin
  - *2* Calcium carbonate
  - *3* Cholestyramine

III Inadequate absorptive surface
- *A* Intestinal resection or bypass
  - *1* Mesenteric vascular disease with massive intestinal resection
  - *2* Regional enteritis with multiple bowel resections
  - *3* Jejunoileal bypass
- *B* Gastroileostomy (inadvertent)

IV Lymphatic obstruction
- *A* Intestinal lymphangiectasia
- *B* Whipple's disease*
- *C* Lymphoma

V Cardiovascular disorders
- *A* Constrictive pericarditis
- *B* Congestive heart failure
- *C* Mesenteric vascular insufficiency
- *D* Vasculitis

VI Primary mucosal absorptive defects
- *A* Inflammatory or infiltrative disorders
  - *1* Regional enteritis*
  - *2* Amyloidosis
  - *3* Scleroderma*
  - *4* Lymphoma*
  - *5* Radiation enteritis
  - *6* Eosinophilic enteritis
  - *7* Tropical sprue
  - *8* Infectious enteritis (e.g., salmonellosis)
  - *9* Collagenous sprue
  - *10* Nonspecific ulcerative jejunitis
  - *11* Mastocytosis
  - *12* Dermatologic disorders (e.g., dermatitis herpetiformis)
- *B* Biochemical or genetic abnormalities
  - *1* Nontropical sprue (gluten-induced enteropathy); celiac sprue
  - *2* Disaccharidase deficiency
  - *3* Hypogammaglobulinemia
  - *4* Abetalipoproteinemia
  - *5* Hartnup disease
  - *6* Cystinuria
  - *7* Monosaccharide malabsorption

VII Endocrine and metabolic disorders
- *A* Diabetes mellitus*
- *B* Hypoparathyroidism
- *C* Adrenal insufficiency
- *D* Hyperthyroidism
- *E* Ulcerogenic tumor of the pancreas (Zollinger-Ellison syndrome, gastrinoma)*
- *F* Carcinoid syndrome

* *Malabsorption caused by multiple defects.*

salt metabolism (see ''Malabsorption Due to Bacterial Overgrowth of the Small Bowel, Pathophysiology'' below). (4) The presence of maldigestion may lead to *protein depletion,* which in turn may produce further impairment in pancreatic function. (5) The *loss of the reservoir function of the stomach* may result in decreased intestinal transit time. Perhaps the most important factor is rapid gastric emptying, which results in low luminal concentrations of digestive secretions for the first 60 to 80 min after a meal. Such a disorder has been described in patients with subtotal gastrectomy and duodenostomy (Billroth I), gastrojejunostomy (Billroth II), and truncal vagotomy and pyloroplasty (V&P). That gastric emptying rates are somewhat slower in patients with V&P may account for the overall less severe nutritional deficiencies in such patients. In some patients treatment with pancreatic enzymes may lead to significant improvement. Specimens of duodenal or jejunal fluid should be obtained for culture of both aerobic and anaerobic organisms and appropriate antibiotic therapy instituted if there is evidence of abnormal bacterial overgrowth (colony count of greater than 10^7 per milliliter of jejunal fluid). Because the duodenum is the principal site of absorption of iron and calcium, in patients with a Billroth II anastomosis impaired absorption of calcium and iron may also develop. Occult metabolic bone disease occurs frequently in this setting.

INADEQUATE ABSORPTIVE SURFACE (SHORT BOWEL SYNDROME) Extensive intestinal resection often results in the short bowel syndrome. The most common disorders resulting in short bowel syndrome are (1) massive intestinal resection following a vascular insult to the small intestine, (2) regional enteritis with multiple bowel resections, and (3) jejunoileal bypass for morbid obesity. In general, the absorption of nutrients will be influenced by the extent and site of small bowel resected, the presence of the ileocecal valve, and adaptation of the remaining small bowel. Resection of 40 to 50 percent of the small bowel is usually well tolerated, provided the proximal duodenum, the distal half of the ileum, and the ileocecal valve are spared. By contrast, resection of the ileum and the ileocecal valve alone may induce severe diarrhea and malabsorption, even though less than 30 percent of the small intestine is resected.

Several measures are important in the management of short bowel syndrome: (1) The diet should contain at least 2500 kcal and consist primarily of carbohydrate and protein with fat restricted to less than 40 g per day. A fat-restricted diet is effective in reducing diarrhea, presumably because there is decreased production of hydroxy fatty acids from long-chain fats. Such hydroxy fatty acids, in essence, are cathartics and increase net secretion of water and electrolytes by the colon as well as the small bowel. (2) It is often necessary to provide vitamin and mineral supplements, which usually include K^+, Cl^-, Mg^{2+}, Ca^{2+}, trace metals (Zn, Cd, Mn), iron, folate, vitamin B_{12}, other vitamins (A, D, E, K, B_1, B_2, B_6, biotin), and essential fatty acids. (3) Specific drugs (for example, belladonna alkaloids, diphenoxylate, loperamide, and codeine), which decrease intestinal motility and prolong mucosal contact time, are helpful in controlling diarrhea. These agents also decrease ileostomy outputs. (4) A bile salt–sequestering agent such as cholestyramine blunts the effects of bile salts, which stimulate net secretion of water and electrolytes by the colon. (5) Patients with short bowel syndrome may have gastric acid hypersecretion, which is often transient, and which results in dilution of pancreatic secretions as well as inactivation of pancreatic enzymes. Under these conditions, the histamine H-2 receptor antagonist, cimetidine, is useful because it will suppress gastric acid secretion and decrease the volume of fluid entering the proximal small bowel, thus leading to an increased concentration of pancreatic enzymes. In addition, supplemental pancreatic enzyme therapy may be required. (6) A bypassed colon can be used to receive infusions of fluid and electrolytes since a portion of the colon can still absorb 1000 to 1500 mL fluid per day. Finally, (7) total parenteral nutrition is frequently required during the first 6 months after massive intestinal resection until some degree of adaptation has occurred. Such patients may also require long-term parenteral hyperalimentation with a silicone rubber catheter in the superior vena cava, and this can be done at home.

For a discussion of regional enteritis see Chap. 238.

MALABSORPTION DUE TO BACTERIAL OVERGROWTH OF THE SMALL BOWEL The proximal small intestine is usually bacteriologically sterile because of three factors: (1) the acid milieu of the stomach; (2) intestinal peristalsis, which sweeps bacteria to the distal small bowel; and (3) secretion into the lumen of the intestine of immunoglobulins, which may serve as coproantibodies. When bacteria are isolated from the upper small bowel, they are frequently contaminants transported from the mouth and upper respiratory tract, and the colony count rarely exceeds 10^4 per milliliter of jejunal fluid. The major mechanism limiting the growth of bacteria in the small intestine is normal peristalsis. Any disorder leading to impaired intestinal motility may result in abnormal stasis of intestinal contents with ineffective mechanical cleansing of bacteria. This in turn may lead to abnormal bacterial proliferation and malabsorption. Several malabsorptive disorders have been associated with bacterial overgrowth of the small bowel, and these are listed in Table 237-6.

Pathophysiology Bacterial overgrowth may result in changes in bile salt metabolism, and these are believed directly and indirectly to account for the steatorrhea. First, bacteria (especially anaerobic gram-positive bacteria) may lead to the intraluminal deconjugation of bile salts with a consequent production of free bile acids. In contrast to conjugated bile salts, unconjugated bile salts may be absorbed in the proximal small bowel by nonionic diffusion, resulting in decreased intraluminal concentrations of bile salts in the jejunum. Second, the decreased bile salt concentrations, the increase of unconjugated bile salts, and the decrease of the conjugated salts all serve to contribute to impaired intraluminal micelle formation and hence fat malabsorption. In addition to abnormalities in bile salt metabolism, intestinal mucosal lesions have been demonstrated in patients with intestinal stasis. Such lesions are often patchy in distribution, and the histologic appearance ranges in severity from minimal changes in villous architecture to severe lesions with virtual absence of villi. The etiology of these lesions is unclear; possible causes include damage caused by bacterial invasion, bacterial toxins, or metabolic products such as unconjugated bile salts. In this regard, certain bacteria such as *Bacteroides* elaborate proteases which solubilize brush border proteins and destroy disaccharidases such as sucrase and maltase. The impaired absorption of vitamin B_{12} is not related to the disturbed bile salt metabolism but appears to be due to uptake of vitamin B_{12} by microorganisms.

Many of the above abnormalities in bile salt metabolism may be

TABLE 237-6 Causes of intestinal bacterial overgrowth (intestinal colonization)

I Structural abnormalities producing stasis of intestinal contents
- *A* Multiple small-bowel diverticula
- *B* Strictures
  - *1* Regional enteritis*
  - *2* Radiation enteritis*
  - *3* Occlusive vascular disease; vasculitis
- *C* Billroth II subtotal gastrectomy with afferent loop stasis*
- *D* Multiple laparotomies resulting in adhesions and partial small-bowel obstruction

II Fistulas
- *A* Gastrocolic, gastroileal, jejunoileal, jejunocolic

III Motor abnormalities resulting in intestinal hypomotility
- *A* Scleroderma*
- *B* Amyloidosis*
- *C* Diabetes mellitus*
- *D* Hypothyroidism
- *E* Vagotomy
- *F* Intestinal pseudoobstruction (see Table 237-7)

IV Miscellaneous
- *A* Hypogammaglobulinemia*
- *B* Nodular lymphoid hyperplasia
- *C* Pernicious anemia
- *D* Pancreatic insufficiency

V No underlying disorder detected

* *Multiple mechanisms may contribute to malabsorption in these disorders*

reversed by appropriate antibiotic therapy. When such treatment is instituted, unconjugated bile salts in the jejunal fluid decrease, an increase in the micellar lipid phase will occur, and steatorrhea diminishes or disappears. In addition, significant improvement in the absorption of vitamin B_{12} will occur with broad-spectrum antibiotics such as tetracycline.

Clinical manifestations Breath tests, i.e., tests with [^{14}C]-labeled bile acid, [^{14}C]xylose, and lactulose, are useful screening tests for malabsorption syndrome due to abnormal bacterial overgrowth of the small intestine. A definitive diagnosis is established by demonstrating larger numbers of microorganisms (greater than 10^5 per milliliter) and a polymicrobial flora in cultures of duodenal or jejunal fluid. Other clinical features include the following: (1) steatorrhea of a moderate degree, usually in the range of 15 to 30 g fecal fat per 24 h; (2) macrocytic anemia with a megaloblastic bone marrow; (3) impaired absorption of vitamin B_{12} which is not corrected by intrinsic factor; and (4) correction of steatorrhea and impaired vitamin B_{12} absorption by antibiotic therapy. Absorption of D-xylose, peroral small-intestinal biopsy specimens, and other tests of absorptive function (Table 237-2) may be normal in these patients. A single course or intermittent courses (2 to 3 weeks per month) of therapy with antibiotics such as tetracycline, ampicillin, or trimethoprim-sulfamethoxazole are usually given.

Chronic intestinal pseudoobstruction (see also Chap. 239) Chronic intestinal pseudoobstruction is a heterogeneous syndrome with a variety of causes (Table 237-7). Primary or idiopathic intestinal pseudoobstruction is a chronic illness characterized by recurrent episodes of intestinal obstruction in which all known causes of mechanical obstruction and other illnesses known to produce intestinal pseudoobstruction have been excluded. In addition to abnormalities in small-bowel motility, derangements in esophageal, gastric, and colonic motility have also been described. Malabsorption, secondary to stasis of intestinal contents with resultant abnormal bacterial proliferation in the small bowel, is frequently present.

Tropical sprue Tropical sprue is a malabsorptive disorder of unknown cause affecting residents of or visitors to tropical regions. Both epidemic and endemic forms of the disease have been recognized. Tropical sprue may have its onset months or even years after a patient has returned from the tropics. The etiology of the disorder has not been elucidated, but it might well result from one or more of the following: (1) a nutritional deficiency, (2) a transmissible infectious microorganism, and (3) a toxin elaborated by a microorganism or contained in the diet. It is of interest that coliform organisms, shown to produce an enterotoxin causing fluid secretion, have been isolated from the jejunum of tropical sprue patients but not from other patients with bacterial overgrowth of the proximal small bowel. Anorexia, diarrhea, weight loss, symptoms of anemia, sequelae of nutritional deficiency (Table 237-4), and abdominal distention are common findings. Patients are frequently deficient in iron as well as vitamin B_{12} and folate. Laboratory studies usually reveal anemia (megaloblastic in 60 percent of cases) and impaired absorption of fat, xylose, and vitamin B_{12}. Malabsorption of at least two nutrients is considered essential for the diagnosis. Jejunal biopsy classically reveals shortened and thickened villi, increased crypt depth, and increased infiltration of mononuclear cells in the lamina propria and epithelium (Table 237-3). However, these biopsy findings are not specific, and the lesion may be patchy; in addition, interpretation is difficult because "control" biopsies from asymptomatic residents in the same tropical region are often considered abnormal when compared with normal biopsies from patients in temperate zones. Such histologic findings have been termed *tropical jejunitis*. Treatment with vitamin B_{12}, folate, and antibiotics have all been effective in inducing a remission. A short course, i.e., 2 to 4 weeks, of therapy with a sulfonamide or tetracycline is usually given. Occasional patients require more prolonged antibiotic therapy.

TABLE 237-7 Causes of chronic intestinal pseudoobstruction

I Primary: Idiopathic
II Secondary
- *A* Collagen vascular disease
  - *1* Scleroderma
  - *2* Dermatomyositis/polymyositis
  - *3* Systemic lupus erythematosus
- *B* Amyloidosis
- *C* Endocrine disorders
  - *1* Myxedema
  - *2* Diabetes mellitus
- *D* Neurologic diseases
  - *1* Chagas' disease
- *E* Others
  - *1* Jejunoileal bypass
  - *2* Jejunal diverticulosis
  - *3* Drugs (tricyclic antidepressants, clonidine, etc.)

Scleroderma Although there are numerous reports of small-intestinal involvement in scleroderma, frank malabsorption has been reported infrequently. It has been suggested that malabsorption may be due to several factors: (1) lymphatic obstruction; (2) reduced arterial blood supply to the gut; (3) impaired intestinal motility leading to relative stasis of intestinal contents and hence bacterial overgrowth; and (4) involvement of the intestinal wall by the disease. At present there is little evidence to support the first two postulated mechanisms. In some cases abnormal bacterial proliferation in the upper small bowel has been documented, and in these patients antibiotic therapy has resulted in decrease in steatorrhea, gain in weight, and increased absorption of vitamin B_{12}. In the intestinal wall there may also be extensive deposition of collagen, especially in the muscular mucosa, submucosa, and muscularis externa, with significant muscle atrophy. Studies of duodenal myoelectric activity in scleroderma revealed normal slow-wave frequency and propagation velocity but decreased excitability of the bowel to mechanical stimuli such as distention and humoral stimuli such as pentagastrin and secretin. This motor dysfunction may be an important factor in the dilatation, atony, and stasis of intestinal contents in scleroderma.

Malabsorption in the acquired immunodeficiency syndrome Diarrhea and weight loss occur frequently in patients with the acquired immunodeficiency syndrome (AIDS). These symptoms are often due to enteric infections or small-intestinal Kaposi's sarcoma. However, such symptoms can be due to malabsorption, which has been well-documented in patients with AIDS in whom identifiable enteric infections and intestinal involvement with Kaposi's sarcoma have been excluded. The presence of malabsorption in these patients has been documented by steatorrhea and abnormal D-xylose absorption tests. Serum zinc levels may be decreased. In addition, small-bowel biopsy specimens have revealed dense infiltration of mononuclear cells and histiocytes. Microorganisms have also been identified in the mucosa.

DISORDERS ASSOCIATED WITH LYMPHATIC OBSTRUCTION

Whipple's disease This is a rare disorder characterized clinically by arthralgia, abdominal pain, diarrhea, progressive weight loss, dilated lacteals in the bowel wall, and impaired intestinal absorption. Wasting, low-grade fever, increased skin pigmentation, and peripheral lymphadenopathy are frequently present. In addition, central nervous system manifestations including confusion, memory loss, focal cranial nerve signs, nystagmus, and ophthalmoplegia may be present. Laboratory examination usually reveals the presence of steatorrhea, impaired xylose absorption, abnormal small-bowel x-rays, hypoalbuminemia, and anemia. Hypoalbuminemia is due to excessive loss of serum albumin into the gastrointestinal tract as well as impaired synthesis of albumin.

The diagnosis is established by demonstrating the presence in the mucosa of macrophages containing large cytoplasmic granules which give a brilliant magenta stain with the periodic acid Schiff reagent (PAS). Such macrophages may also be seen in other tissues such as lymph nodes, spleen, or liver. The finding of PAS-positive macrophages in the lamina propria is not specific for Whipple's disease, but virtual replacement of most cellular elements in the lamina propria by these macrophages has been seen only in this disorder. In addition to the PAS-positive macrophages, jejunal biopsies frequently show dilated lymphatics and some degree of blunting of the intestinal mucosal villi.

Electron-microscopic studies have revealed the presence of rod-shaped structures (or bacilliform bodies) 0.3 by 1.5 to 2.5 μm within and adjacent to the macrophages in the lamina propria as well as within epithelial cells and polymorphonuclear leukocytes. The ultrastructural features of these bacilliform bodies suggest that they are microorganisms. It is of particular interest that after treatment of the patient with antibiotics the bacilliform bodies decrease or disappear together with a decrease in the number of PAS-positive macrophages. In addition, the reappearance of the bacteria often heralds the onset of a clinical relapse after antibiotics have been withdrawn.

Whipple's disease at one time was thought to be invariably fatal. However, it is now clear that therapy with antibiotics will usually induce a clinical remission. In a few cases there has been complete reversal of the histologic abnormalities in the jejunal mucosa, and some of these cases have been followed for 10 years. Patients with Whipple's disease should be treated with antibiotics such as trimethoprim-sulfamethoxazole for at least 1 year. Treatment with tetracycline alone or penicillin alone is not adequate initial therapy; relapse rates with these drugs are approximately 40 percent. The most important parameter for following the disease and predicting its course is the presence or absence of bacilli in sections of small-bowel biopsies.

Intestinal lymphoma Steatorrhea is a manifestation of *primary* intestinal lymphoma. The disease occurs predominantly in men, and the mean age of onset of symptoms is about 50 years. The diagnosis should be suspected in patients with malabsorption with the following findings: (1) a malabsorption syndrome in which clinical and biopsy features resemble those of nontropical sprue but in which there is an incomplete response to a gluten-free diet, (2) the presence of *abdominal pain* and *fever*, and (3) signs and symptoms of intestinal obstruction. The usual stigmata of generalized lymphoma are frequently absent. Hepatomegaly, splenomegaly, palpable abdominal masses, and peripheral adenopathy are usually not found. Lymphangiography and CT scanning may reveal abnormal intraabdominal nodes. The diagnosis can be established by laparotomy and often may be made by thorough examination of multiple mucosal biopsy specimens obtained perorally. There may be a total absence of villi or lesser degrees of blunting and shortening of the villi. In contrast to nontropical sprue, the lamina propria is usually massively infiltrated with lymphoid cells. Malignancy may be diagnosed by demonstrating lymphoid cells with the cytologic features of malignancy, the presence of reticulum cells outside germinal centers, and infiltration and destruction of crypts by pleomorphic lymphoid cells. Some patients elaborate or secrete a fragment of the heavy chain of IgA immunoglobulins (*α-chain disease*). The latter is probably a variant of intestinal lymphoma.

The mechanism of malabsorption in intestinal lymphoma may be related to several factors: (1) diffuse involvement of the small-intestinal mucosa; (2) involvement of the bowel wall with lymphatic obstruction; and (3) localized stenosis with stasis of intestinal contents and bacterial overgrowth. It should be emphasized that it is often difficult, by clinical and morphologic features alone, to distinguish nontropical sprue from intestinal lymphoma. Indeed, there is evidence to suggest that lymphoma may develop as a late complication of nontropical sprue.

The course of intestinal lymphoma has ranged from 4 months to 4 years from the onset of symptoms. Perforation, bleeding, and intestinal obstruction are common terminal complications. There is insufficient evidence to determine whether radiation therapy, chemotherapy, or localized surgical resection modify the natural course of the disease.

CARDIOVASCULAR DISORDERS Steatorrhea has been described in patients with chronic congestive heart failure, superior mesenteric artery insufficiency, and constrictive pericarditis. Abnormal dilated mucosal lymphatics and excessive enteric loss of protein have been demonstrated in patients with constrictive pericarditis. The mechanism of steatorrhea in patients with chronic heart failure remains uncertain. It might be due to congestion and edema of the mucosa, mucosal hypoxia, or abnormalities in pancreatic function. Although pronounced steatorrhea is uncommon in congestive heart failure, these patients are frequently anorectic, and a low fat intake could mask a latent steatorrhea. Steatorrhea is quite infrequent in patients with vasculitis and is thought to be due to segmental infarction of the small bowel in addition to intestinal ischemia.

DEFECTS IN MUCOSAL FUNCTION

INFLAMMATORY OR INFILTRATIVE DISORDERS **Regional enteritis** The clinical features of regional enteritis are described in Chap. 238. Malabsorption in regional enteritis may result from several factors: (1) interruption of the enterohepatic circulation of bile salts by ileal disease or resection; (2) deconjugation of bile salts due to bacterial overgrowth, in turn related to strictures and/or fistulas; (3) active inflammatory bowel disease causing impaired mucosal cell function; (4) inadequate absorptive surface resulting from intestinal resection or fistulas; and (5) severe protein depletion producing impaired exocrine pancreatic function. Active ileal disease and/or ileal resection resulting in an interrupted enterohepatic circulation of and deficiency of conjugated bile salts appears to be the major factor responsible for steatorrhea as well as impaired absorption of vitamin B_{12}. Small-bowel absorptive function has been correlated with the extent of ileal disease or resection. When the length of ileal dysfunction exceeds 90 to 100 cm, virtually all patients will have steatorrhea and vitamin B_{12} malabsorption. After intestinal resection, the functional capacity of the remaining small bowel will depend on the site and extent of resection as well as the presence of residual inflammatory disease. Massive intestinal resection usually results in impaired absorption of all food constituents. When the malabsorption is due to strictures and blind loops as a result of previous surgical therapy, antibiotic therapy may be helpful, but surgical removal of these areas is usually necessary for long-term improvement. With diffuse inflammatory disease a florid malabsorption syndrome may occur with steatorrhea, hypocalcemia, impaired vitamin B_{12} absorption, and hypoalbuminemia due to increased enteric protein loss. Treatment with sulfasalazine and corticosteroid drugs may be beneficial (see Chap. 238).

After *ileal resection,* patients frequently have bothersome diarrhea. This appears to be due to *interruption of the enterohepatic circulation* whereby increased amounts of bile salts reach the colon, where they interfere with water and electrolyte absorption and thus have a cathartic effect. The *bile salt–induced diarrhea* after ileal resection may respond to treatment with cholestyramine, an exchange resin which binds bile salts and causes them to lose their biochemical effect on the bowel. Patients with ileal resection of less than 100 cm and fecal fat excretion less than 20 g per day show the best symptomatic response to cholestyramine.

Chronic nongranulomatous ulcerative jejunoileitis This disorder is characterized by abdominal pain, weight loss, fever, diarrhea, steatorrhea, hypoalbuminemia, and protein-losing enteropathy. Clinical features mimic those found in both regional enteritis and celiac sprue. Indeed, the intestinal lesion may be indistinguishable from celiac sprue. However, exclusion of gluten from the diet does not result in any benefit. Corticosteroid treatment has resulted in transient improvement, but long-term effects are unpredictable.

Amyloidosis This disorder is discussed in detail in Chap. 259.

Radiation injury to the small bowel Extensive morphologic damage of the small-intestinal mucosa often follows normal or excessive abdominal irradiation. These changes include a decrease in crypt mitoses, marked shortening of the villi, megalocytosis of epithelial cells, and inflammatory cell infiltration of the lamina propria. This may be associated with transient diarrhea and impaired intestinal absorption. However, restoration of normal intestinal architecture is usually complete within 2 weeks after cessation of therapy. Persistent diarrhea and malabsorption may develop shortly after x-ray therapy, or there may be a latent period of several years before the onset of diarrhea. Steatorrhea, ranging from 10 to 40 g per day, has been frequently observed, but impaired absorption of calcium, iron, D-xylose, or vitamin B_{12} is less common. In some patients intestinal strictures due to vasculopathy and ischemia may develop following irradiation, and thus stasis of intestinal contents and abnormal bacterial proliferation may occur. In others, intestinal lymphangiectasia, presumably due to lymphatic obstruction, has been documented. Diarrhea and malabsorption may be refractory to all methods of management. Treatment with antibiotics, pancreatic enzymes, gluten-free diet, adrenal corticosteroids, and opiates has met with but limited success.

Eosinophilic enteritis Eosinophilic gastroenteritis is a disorder of the stomach, small bowel, and colon of unknown etiology characterized by peripheral blood eosinophilia and eosinophilic infiltration of the gut wall but without evidence of vasculitis. The clinical manifestations, usually recurrent, are protean and relate to the site of gastrointestinal tract involvement. Three main patterns have been identified: (1) Predominant mucosal disease manifested by iron-deficiency anemia, hypoalbuminemia due to protein-losing enteropathy, and mild steatorrhea. Patients in this group often present with a malabsorption syndrome and a history of intolerance to specific foods. (2) Predominant muscle layer disease characterized by marked thickening and rigidity of the stomach and proximal small bowel with obstructive symptoms and radiologic features of pyloric narrowing and obstruction. The obstructive form of eosinophilic gastroenteritis accounts for half of the cases reported since 1970. Accordingly, eosinophilic enteritis should be considered in the differential diagnosis of gastric outlet obstruction, diffuse small-bowel disease, and ileocolitis. Indeed, eosinophilic enteritis often mimics regional enteritis. (3) Predominant subserosal disease in which the cardinal manifestation is ascites with marked eosinophilia in the ascitic fluid. Although the above classification based on tissue layer of major involvement is useful in understanding the principal manifestations, it should be emphasized that multiple clinical forms, e.g., ascites (serosal involvement) and obstruction (muscular involvement), also occur.

Previous reports have emphasized food allergy and mucosal features of this disease. However, food sensitivity is related to symptoms in less than 20 percent of patients. In such patients fasting serum IgE levels are often elevated, and challenge with offending foods frequently evokes symptoms of abdominal pain and diarrhea in addition to a marked increase in serum IgE levels. In most patients with eosinophilic enteritis, however, immunologic studies including serum immunoglobulins, serum complement, lymphocyte quantitation, and lymphocyte response to nonspecific mitogens reveal no abnormalities. Thus, both IgE-mediated and IgE-dependent mechanisms may be operative in different patients with eosinophilic gastroenteritis. Several nonreaginic factors influence peripheral blood and tissue eosinophilia. It seems clear that evidence of allergy or food sensitivity is often absent and is not required for the diagnosis of eosinophilic enteritis. In addition, even in patients with food allergies, elimination diets are frequently ineffective and such patients may require prolonged corticosteroid therapy to remain well. Surgical treatment for relief of obstructive symptoms and corticosteroids are the mainstays of therapy.

Dermatitis and malabsorption A malabsorption syndrome, usually mild, has been reported in patients with a variety of dermatologic disorders, including psoriasis, eczematoid dermatitis, and dermatitis herpetiformis. Proximal intestinal mucosal abnormalities are almost invariably found in patients with dermatitis herpetiformis. In one study 21 of 22 patients had lesions ranging in severity from a completely "flat" to an almost normal intestinal mucosa. The mucosal lesions were often patchy in distribution. Clinical and laboratory evidence of significant malabsorption was infrequent, possibly due to the limited length of small intestine involved in this skin disorder. While the skin lesions of dermatitis herpetiformis respond to sulfone, the gut lesions do not. By contrast, in some patients with blunted and flattened intestinal mucosal lesions, and steatorrhea, there may be a striking improvement in villous architecture and regression of steatorrhea after withdrawal of gluten from the diet without improvement in the skin lesions. Further, in patients with dermatitis herpetiformis and a morphologically normal small-intestinal mucosa, administration of a high-gluten diet may result in blunted and flattened mucosal lesions indistinguishable from those of nontropical sprue. As in the latter disease, an increased frequency of HLA-A1 and HLA-B8 are also seen. These observations raise the interesting question as to whether certain patients with dermatitis herpetiformis and a malabsorption syndrome have latent nontropical sprue.

BIOCHEMICAL OR GENETIC ABNORMALITIES Nontropical sprue Nontropical sprue is a disorder characterized by malabsorption, abnormal small-bowel structure, and intolerance to gluten, a protein found in wheat and wheat products. It has been appropriately referred to as *gluten-induced enteropathy*. Celiac disease in children and nontropical sprue of the adult are probably one and the same disorder with the same pathogenesis.

There are insufficient data to provide an accurate estimation of the incidence of nontropical sprue in any population. This is largely because the severity of the disease varies greatly and individuals may have typical mucosal change and yet have no overt symptoms. Seventy percent of the cases in most reported series are women. The incidence in siblings appears to be many times higher than that in the general population, and it has been suggested that sprue may be inherited through a dominant gene of incomplete penetrance. Celiac sprue patients have an increased frequency of serum histocompatibility antigens, particularly of the HLA-B8 and HLA-Dw3 types. The HLA-B8 phenotype has been found in 85 to 90 percent of sprue patients as compared with 20 to 25 percent in normal subjects. The HLA-B8 antigen may be linked to immune response genes which may determine the immunologic recognition of certain substances. It has been suggested that such genetic factors may predispose to immunologic tolerance of dietary proteins such as the peptides in gluten or to the production of pathogenic antigluten antibodies which could result in binding of gluten to epithelial cells with subsequent tissue damage.

PATHOPHYSIOLOGY Gluten and the related substance gliadin are high-molecular-weight proteins found especially in wheat. These proteins, as well as the larger peptide hydrolysis products (containing glutamine), are toxic when administered to patients with sprue in remission. The exact mechanism for this effect is not clear, but two theories have been proposed, namely, a "toxic" and an immunologic theory. One possible mechanism is that patients with sprue lack a specific mucosal peptidase, so that gluten or its larger glutamine-containing peptides are not effectively hydrolyzed to smaller peptides (i.e., dipeptides or amino acids). As a consequence "toxic" peptides might accumulate in the mucosa. It has been demonstrated that patients with sprue in remission will develop steatorrhea and typical mucosal changes when they are given gluten. Similar results will occur with the administration of peptide hydrolysates containing at least eight amino acids with a terminal glutamine residue. It has been shown that when gluten is instilled into the *ileum* of sprue patients, histologic changes begin to occur within hours. This does not occur in the *upper jejunum*, suggesting that the effect is immediate and local rather than systemic. After noxious gluten fractions damage surface absorptive cells, the damaged cells are sloughed rapidly from the mucosal surface into the gut lumen. To compensate for this, cell proliferation increases, crypts hypertrophy, and cell migration is accelerated to replace the damaged and sloughed epithelial cells. This more rapid than normal epithelial cell renewal can be reversed by a gluten-free diet. The intestinal mucosa of patients with sprue shows many enzyme alterations, including decreased levels of disaccharidases, alkaline phosphatase, and peptide hydrolases, as well as impaired ability to digest gluten peptides. However, these abnormalities usually revert toward normal after successful treatment with a gluten-free diet. There is additional evidence supporting the concept of toxicity of gluten and gluten breakdown products in sprue. First, gliadin is toxic to sprue mucosa maintained in organ culture, causing ultrastructural changes and depression of disaccharidase activity. Second, sprue mucosa hydrolyzes a specific fraction of a gliadin digest (i.e., fraction 9) in a defective manner, and fraction 9 is selectively toxic to sprue mucosa. Third, specific fractions of gluten fed to sprue patients cause transient alterations in mucosal histology and depression of disaccharidase activity, but full recovery is observed in 72 h. The rapid onset of these changes and prompt recovery are consistent with a direct toxic effect. Despite intensive study, however, no persistent, specific, or selective peptidase deficiency has been demonstrated.

It has also been suggested that gluten or gluten metabolites may initiate an *immunologic reaction* in the intestinal mucosa. The presence of a mononuclear inflammatory cell infiltrate in the lamina propria of the mucosa, the beneficial response to corticosteroid drugs, the finding of abnormal antibodies to gliadin in the serum of sprue patients, the synthesis of increased amounts of antigliadin antibody by sprue mucosa maintained in organ culture, and the elaboration of lymphokines such as migration inhibitory factor (MIF) by sprue mucosa incubated with gliadin have all been cited as evidence in support of this hypothesis. However, the evidence indicating that an abnormal (immune) mechanism is important in initiating or perpetuating this disease process remains to be determined.

Jejunal biopsy specimens from patients with nontropical sprue usually show a characteristic lesion. There is blunting and flattening of the mucosal surface, with villi either absent or broad and short. The crypts are elongated, and there is generally a dense infiltration of inflammatory cells in the lamina propria. The surface epithelium is altered with a sparse brush border, cuboidal rather than the normal columnar cells, and infiltration of inflammatory cells in the epithelial layer. These changes are usually most severe in the proximal small bowel, presumably because this area of the bowel is exposed to the highest gluten concentration. The typical morphologic changes illustrated in Fig. 237-4 are characteristic of nontropical sprue but are not specific. Similar changes have been described in other conditions, including lymphoma, tropical sprue, and hypogammaglobulinemia associated with malabsorption. Many biochemical abnormalities have been demonstrated in mucosal biopsy specimens from nontropical sprue patients. Impaired esterification of fatty acids to triglycerides, decreased uptake of amino acids, and decreased activity of intestinal disaccharidases (especially lactase) have been well documented. The latter observation may account for the high incidence of milk intolerance in untreated sprue patients or those in relapse. However, the greater abundance of undifferentiated crypt cells may be important, since crypt cells normally have a lower capacity for nutrient uptake than do villus cells.

Since the mucosa is damaged and altered in patients with nontropical sprue, there may be *decreased release of pancreato-tropic hormones* (secretin and cholecystokinin-pancreozymin). This results in decreased stimulation of the pancreas with lower than normal intraluminal levels of pancreatic enzymes in response to a meal. In addition, the gallbladder appears to be resistant to the action of cholecystokinin, resulting in absent or minimal contractions of the gallbladder, in turn leading to sequestration of bile salts in an inert gallbladder. These two defects may result in impaired intraluminal digestion of fat and protein, which will be superimposed on the defect in intestinal transport caused by a damaged mucosa.

Diarrhea is common in sprue patients and is due to a number of factors, including *impaired absorption* of salt and water by duodenum and jejunum, net *secretion* of water and electrolytes by an abnormally permeable jejunal mucosa, and net colonic secretion of water and electrolytes induced by unabsorbed fatty acids and hydroxy fatty acids. However, the distal small intestine in sprue has the ability to adapt to the damage and loss of absorptive capacity in the proximal small intestine. Indeed, increased ileal absorption of sodium, chloride, and water has been demonstrated in sprue patients.

CLINICAL FEATURES Most patients with nontropical sprue will have a typical malabsorption syndrome characterized by weight loss, abdominal distention and bloating, diarrhea, steatorrhea, and abnormal tests of absorptive function. The characteristic alterations in tests of intestinal absorption are outlined in Table 237-2. It should be emphasized, however, that some sprue patients may present with isolated abnormalities which initially do not suggest the diagnosis of nontropical sprue. Thus, a patient may be admitted for investigation of iron-deficiency anemia without apparent blood loss or of abnormal bleeding due to hypoprothrombinemia but may not have diarrhea or overt steatorrhea. Likewise, sprue patients may present with puzzling metabolic bone disease without diarrhea or steatorrhea. Such patients usually complain of bone pain and tenderness and frequently are found to have extensive demineralization of bone, compression deformities, kyphoscoliosis, and Milkman's fractures. Emotional disturbances are common in these patients, and many individuals with a diagnosis of weight loss initially considered related to severe anxiety and depression are subsequently found to have nontropical sprue. In each of the above clinical settings, the diagnosis of sprue should be considered in the differential diagnosis.

Since there is no specific diagnostic test, three criteria should be met in order to establish a definite diagnosis of nontropical sprue: (1) evidence of malabsorption; (2) an abnormal small-bowel (jejunal) biopsy showing blunting and flattening of the villi along with changes in the surface epithelium; and (3) clinical, biochemical, and histologic improvement after institution of a gluten-free diet. In equivocal cases, the patient can be challenged with 30 to 50 g gluten orally, and if this promptly results in increased diarrhea and steatorrhea, the diagnosis of gluten-induced enteropathy is established. It should be emphasized that tests of intestinal absorption may reveal abnormalities which range from very minimal alterations to severe changes. Abnormalities in absorption tests have been shown to correlate reasonably well with the length of small-bowel involvement and to a lesser extent with the severity of the proximal lesion. A possible variant of celiac sprue is *collagenous* sprue. In this disorder small-bowel biopsy specimens characteristically reveal a blunted and flattened mucosa and large masses of eosinophilic hyalin material in the lamina propria. In one study of 349 jejunal biopsy specimens from 145 patients with celiac sprue, 45 (31 percent) showed basement membrane thickening often associated with collagen deposition, but dense collagen deposition was found in only 11 patients. Fatal, unremitting malabsorption developed in four of the latter patients. These observations suggest that collagenous membrane thickening is a fairly frequent finding in jejunal biopsies from patients with sprue but that dense collagen deposits are an unusual feature and may indicate a poor prognosis.

TREATMENT Despite the uncertainties concerned with the diagnosis of nontropical sprue, approximately 80 percent of the patients improve after institution of a *gluten-free diet*. Symptomatic improvement usually occurs within a few weeks, but improvement in tests of absorptive function and small-bowel histologic characteristics may not occur for months. It has been repeatedly demonstrated that strict adherence to a gluten-free diet more consistently results in improvement than does suboptimal gluten restriction. Nevertheless, even with strict diet adherence some cases show little improvement in intestinal histologic features. Patients with nontropical sprue treated with corticosteroids but continuing a normal gluten-containing diet have shown symptomatic improvement as well as improvement in intestinal histology and tests of intestinal absorptive function. The mechanism by which corticosteroids protect the mucosa from the effects of gluten is not clear.

If a patient with nontropical sprue does not respond to a gluten-free diet, other possibilities or complicative factors must be considered:

(1) the diagnosis is incorrect; (2) the patient is not adhering strictly to the diet; (3) there may be another concurrent disease, such as pancreatic insufficiency; (4) the patient may have ulceration of the jejunum or ileum; (5) lactase deficiency may be present with resultant milk intolerance; (6) the patient may have collagenous sprue; or (7) he or she may have developed intestinal lymphoma, a disease which appears to occur more frequently in patients with sprue than in the general population. Finally, it should be emphasized that a small number of patients show a markedly delayed response to a gluten-free diet, with significant improvement occurring only after 24 to 36 months of therapy. Approximately 50 percent of patients with refractory sprue respond to corticosteroids; such patients may also require parenteral hyperalimentation.

Disaccharidase deficiency syndromes As indicated above, the hydrolysis of disaccharides occurs on or within the brush border (microvilli) of intestinal epithelial cells by specific disaccharidases located there. As would be anticipated, both primary (genetic or familial) and secondary (acquired) deficiencies of these disaccharidases have been observed.

LACTASE DEFICIENCY IN THE ADULT Instances of isolated deficiency of mucosal lactase occur; they are associated with symptoms of lactose intolerance. Since lactose is the principal carbohydrate of milk, such individuals show milk intolerance with symptoms of abdominal cramps, bloating or distention, and diarrhea. Similar symptoms will occur following the ingestion of lactose. The symptoms are due to the fact that lactose when not hydrolyzed is not absorbed, and its osmotic effect in the lumen leads to shifts of fluid into the intestinal tract. The pH of the stool will also decrease because of the production of lactic acid and short-chain fatty acids from the fermentation of lactose by colonic bacteria. Although primary intestinal lactase deficiency seems to be hereditary, lactose or milk intolerance may not become clinically evident until puberty or late adolescence. There are significant racial differences in the incidence of this entity. It would appear that about 5 to 15 percent of the adult white population shows intestinal lactase deficiency, but in black Americans, Bantus, and Orientals, the incidence has been reported as high as 80 to 90 percent.

The diagnosis may be suspected when one obtains a history of gastrointestinal symptoms following milk ingestion. It should be emphasized that the ingestion of only moderate amounts of lactose, e.g., 5 to 12 g or the amount contained in 100 to 240 mL milk, often results in symptoms. Bloating, cramps, and flatulence, but not diarrhea, are usually produced with ingestion of small to moderate amounts of lactose. The vast majority of lactose-intolerant patients are aware that they are milk-intolerant and avoid milk. That these symptoms are not due to allergic reactions to the proteins in milk (i.e., milk allergy or hypersensitivity) can be demonstrated by performing a lactose tolerance test. This test consists of administering an oral dose of lactose (usually from 0.75 to 1.5 g per kilogram of body weight) and obtaining serial blood samples for measurements of blood glucose. In a positive test, intestinal symptoms occur, and the blood glucose increases less than 20 mg/dL above the fasting level. However, false-positive and false-negative tests occur in 20 percent of normal subjects because the test is influenced by gastric emptying and glucose metabolism. Measurement of breath hydrogen after ingestion of 50 g lactose is a more sensitive and specific test. The rationale for this test is that hydrogen is released from unabsorbed lactose by colonic bacteria and breath hydrogen excretion subsequently rises. The test is noninvasive and is not influenced by gastric emptying or metabolic factors.

Acquired lactase deficiency is often seen in association with a variety of gastrointestinal diseases, in many of which there is histologic evidence of mucosal damage. The disorders in which lactose intolerance and lactase deficiency may occur include nontropical and tropical sprue, regional enteritis, viral and bacterial infections of the intestinal tract, giardiasis, abetalipoproteinemia, cystic fibrosis, and ulcerative colitis.

DEFICIENCY OF OTHER DISACCHARIDASES Damage to the intestinal mucosa may produce decreased levels of other disaccharidases, such as sucrase-isomaltase, but usually these are not as depressed as lactase, and symptoms of specific intolerance, such as sucrose intolerance, are uncommon. There are instances of primary and apparently hereditary sucrose intolerance, but these always occur in association with sucrase-isomaltase deficiency.

Hypogammaglobulinemia Malabsorption may be associated with hypogammaglobulinemia or agammaglobulinemia. The hypogammaglobulinemia may be of the congenital or the acquired type, with the onset either in childhood or adulthood. When malabsorption has been noted, it has included impaired absorption of fat, D-xylose, and vitamin B_{12}. Peroral intestinal biopsy may reveal changes comparable to those seen in nontropical sprue, but often one finds a more striking mononuclear infiltrate giving a nodular appearance to the mucosa both microscopically and macroscopically. Diarrhea and steatorrhea may precede or follow the development of hypogammaglobulinemia, and these may worsen during infections and subside after the infection is controlled with antibiotics. Intestinal infestation with *Giardia lamblia* is common in hypogammaglobulinemic patients. Meticulous collection and culture of intestinal fluids have revealed excessive numbers of anaerobic bacteria in the small bowel of some patients with hypogammaglobulinemia. However, the relationship between such overgrowth with anaerobes and diarrhea and steatorrhea remains to be clarified. Arthritis, resembling rheumatoid arthritis, and thymoma have also been described in patients with this syndrome. In some patients improvement in diarrhea and malabsorption may occur spontaneously, whereas in others improvement may follow treatment with a gluten-free diet, corticosteroids, antibiotics, injections of gammaglobulin, and cholestyramine. These forms of therapy have not been uniformly successful. Although transient improvement is common, complete cessation of symptoms is distinctly unusual.

The relationship between hypogammaglobulinemia and malabsorption remains obscure. There is no evidence to date indicating that excessive enteric loss of gammaglobulin or alteration of the intestinal microflora occurs, but abnormalities in IgA metabolism may be important in this syndrome. This immunoglobulin is the predominant one in the intestinal mucosa and is found in many exocrine secretions, including tears, saliva, gastric juice, and intestinal juice. A few patients have been described with malabsorption and selective deficiency of IgA.

Abetalipoproteinemia See Chap. 315.

Hartnup disease, cystinuria See Chap. 308.

ENDOCRINE AND METABOLIC DISORDERS **Diabetes mellitus** The occurrence of diarrhea and steatorrhea in patients with diabetes mellitus has been well documented. When steatorrhea accompanies diabetes, it may be due to the presence of (1) exocrine pancreatic insufficiency, (2) coexistent nontropical sprue, (3) abnormal bacterial proliferation in the proximal small bowel, or (4) severe and uncontrolled diabetes per se (e.g., so-called diabetic diarrhea). Patients falling into the first three categories will usually respond in a satisfactory manner to treatment with pancreatic extracts, a gluten-free diet, and antibiotics, respectively. The pathogenesis of diarrhea and steatorrhea in patients in the fourth category remains poorly understood, and the response to various forms of therapy has been quite variable. It has been demonstrated that patients with diabetic diarrhea and steatorrhea may have involvement of the autonomic nervous system with degenerative changes in the sympathetic and parasympathetic nerves and ganglia. In some patients bacterial overgrowth in the stomach and proximal small bowel may occur and contribute to the diarrhea and steatorrhea.

The clinical features in patients with diarrhea and steatorrhea due to diabetes per se seem to be fairly uniform. Diabetes usually develops at a young age and is often severe and difficult to control. There is a distinct predominance of males. Several signs of autonomic neuropathy are usually present, including postural hypotension, anhydrosis, impotence, and bladder irregularities. Peripheral vascular disease and peripheral neuropathy are also common. Gastrointestinal x-rays may show delayed gastric emptying and disordered transit through the small bowel. Peroral small-bowel biopsy specimens are normal. Tests of intestinal absorptive function are normal except for steatorrhea and azotorrhea. There has been no consistent response to therapy with pancreatic extracts, gluten-free diet, or corticosteroids. When bacterial overgrowth is present, broad-spectrum antibiotics may be helpful.

Hypoparathyroidism Steatorrhea has been documented in several patients with idiopathic hypoparathyroidism. In addition to hypocalcemia, impaired absorption of D-xylose and vitamin B_{12}, decreased serum iron values, and abnormal small-intestinal roentgenograms have been demonstrated in some cases. In such patients the serum phosphorus level is elevated (due to the hypoparathyroidism) rather than low (as in primary malabsorption). The cause of malabsorption in this disorder is unclear.

Adrenal insufficiency Although there are few studies on fat excretion in adrenal insufficiency in human beings, malabsorption, especially of fat, appears to occur more frequently than has been generally appreciated. Patients with adrenal insufficiency have been found to have steatorrhea which is corrected by therapy with adrenal corticosteroids.

Hyperthyroidism There are few detailed studies on intestinal absorptive function in patients with hyperthyroidism. Mild to moderate steatorrhea and hypoalbuminemia have been reported, but absorption of D-xylose and vitamin B_{12} is frequently normal. Steatorrhea usually remits after successful treatment of hyperthyroidism. Clinical studies suggest that steatorrhea in hyperthyroidism is not due to any defect of pancreatic, biliary, or small-intestinal mucosal function but is a result of hyperphagia with ingestion of unusually large amounts of fat occurring in association with rapid gastric emptying and intestinal transit.

Ulcerogenic tumor of the pancreas (Zollinger-Ellison syndrome) The clinical features of ulcerogenic tumor of the pancreas are described in Chap. 235. Malabsorption is frequently found in this disease. The acidification and dilution of intestinal contents caused by gastric acid hypersecretion leads to major disturbances in fat digestion and absorption. Impaired formation of micellar lipid due to inactivation of pancreatic lipase is probably the major factor in the production of steatorrhea. Other factors contributing to fat malabsorption in this disorder include (1) precipitation of glycine-conjugated bile salts due to low intraluminal pH, (2) alteration of the intestinal mucosa with ulceration and metaplasia, and (3) impaired fatty acid esterification and chylomicron formation.

Carcinoid syndrome (see Chap. 299) Although diarrhea is common in the carcinoid syndrome, malabsorption with significant steatorrhea is unusual. In many of the cases of carcinoid syndrome with steatorrhea there has been a prior intestinal resection (usually ileal), and in these cases the resection is the important factor in the causation of steatorrhea. However, direct involvement of the bowel wall and mesentery by the carcinoid tumor have been well documented. That abnormalities in serotonin metabolism may also be important is suggested from the decrease in the steatorrhea observed in some of these patients when treated with the antiserotonin drug methysergide. Although side effects may occur, for control of diarrhea and steatorrhea patients may be given a trial of 8 to 12 mg methysergide per day.

PROTEIN-LOSING ENTEROPATHY The gastrointestinal tract has been shown to play a significant role in the metabolism and physiologic degradation of plasma proteins. The exact magnitude of the normal gastrointestinal protein loss in human beings has remained unclear, but studies with labeled albumin have suggested that between 10 and 20 percent of the normal turnover of albumin may be accounted for by enteric protein loss. However, under certain pathologic conditions, excessive gastrointestinal protein loss may develop. An extensive number of disorders have been found to be associated with intestinal protein loss. Some of these are listed in Table 237-8.

Pathophysiology Several mechanisms have been proposed for the passage of plasma proteins across the gastrointestinal mucosa, both normally and in certain disease states. First, plasma proteins may pass into the gastrointestinal tract through an inflamed or ulcerated mucosa and account for the protein loss occasionally seen in regional enteritis and ulcerative colitis. Second, plasma protein loss may occur as a result of disordered mucosal cell structure. For example, patients with nontropical sprue have abnormal villous structure and surface epithelium, and these changes could facilitate the diffusion of plasma protein between the cells. Third, in the presence of increased lymphatic pressure, there may be increased passage of plasma proteins into the lumen via the intercellular spaces of the mucosal epithelium. This might be expected to occur in disorders in which there is granulomatous or neoplastic involvement of lymphatics. Fourth, dilated lymph vessels in the mucosa may rupture through the surface epithelium, discharging their contents into the intestinal lumen. This is thought to be important in the pathogenesis of steatorrhea and hypoproteinemia in patients with idiopathic intestinal lymphangiectasia (see "Intestinal Lymphangiectasia" below).

Several techniques have been developed for the detection and quantitation of gastrointestinal protein loss. In the past these have primarily involved the use of intravenously administered radiolabeled macromolecules such as ^{125}I-labeled serum albumin, $^{51}CrCl_3$, ^{51}Cr-labeled albumin, and indium 111. ^{111}In-labeled transferrin and $^{51}CrCl_3$ (which rapidly become attached to circulating transferrin) are the compounds available commercially for clinical use. After the intravenous administration of 0.93 to 1.11 MBq (25 to 30 μCi) of the labeled compound to normal subjects, between 0.1 and 0.7 percent of the administered radioactivity is recovered in the stool over a 4-day period. Patients with excessive enteric protein loss may excrete from 2 to 40 percent of the injected radioactive label. False-positive results may be obtained if the stool specimen is contaminated with urine. There is also a reliable and sensitive nonisotopic method to measure intestinal protein loss which involves the measurement of α_1-antitrypsin (AT). This serum enzyme, which has the same molecular weight as albumin (50,000), is resistant to proteolysis and when leaked into the intestinal lumen is not degraded. One can easily

TABLE 237-8 Disorders associated with protein-losing enteropathy

I Stomach
- *A* Gastric carcinoma
- *B* Giant hypertrophy of the gastric mucosa
- *C* Atrophic gastritis
- *D* Postgastrectomy syndrome

II Small intestine
- *A* Intestinal lymphangiectasia
- *B* Nontropical sprue
- *C* Tropical sprue
- *D* Regional enteritis
- *E* Whipple's disease
- *F* Lymphoma
- *G* Intestinal tuberculosis
- *H* Acute infectious enteritis
- *I* Scleroderma
- *J* Jejunal diverticulosis
- *K* Allergic gastroenteropathy

III Colon
- *A* Colonic neoplasm
- *B* Ulcerative colitis
- *C* Granulomatous colitis
- *D* Megacolon

IV Heart
- *A* Congestive heart failure
- *B* Constrictive pericarditis
- *C* Interatrial septal defect
- *D* Primary cardiomyopathy

V Miscellaneous
- *A* Esophageal carcinoma
- *B* Gastrocolic fistula
- *C* Agammaglobulinemia
- *D* Nephrosis

measure AT in serum and stool by radial immunodiffusion in order to obtain AT loss in stool (normal loss is less than 2.6 mg per gram of stool) or intestinal clearance of AT (normal is less than 13 mL/day). Results using AT as a marker of intestinal protein loss correlate well with the more cumbersome and costly isotopic methods. Random fecal AT assays can also be used as a simple screening method for enteric protein loss.

The rate of albumin synthesis and degradation can be determined using intravenously administered radioiodinated albumin and measuring the decline in radioactivity in the serum. Such studies carried out in patients with protein-losing enteropathies have demonstrated a reduced circulating (intravascular) and total-body pool of albumin, a normal or increased rate of albumin synthesis, markedly shortened albumin survival, and increased fecal protein loss. Whereas normal subjects catabolize 5 to 10 percent of their intravascular albumin pool each day (the fractional catabolic rate), patients with excessive enteric protein loss may have fractional catabolic rates of 50 to 60 percent.

Studies utilizing radioiodinated immunoglobulins have demonstrated a decreased intravascular globulin pool and increased fractional catabolic rate. However, the synthesis of IgG is usually normal, suggesting that a decreased level of IgG and increased enteric protein loss is not a potent stimulus for IgG synthesis. The increase in fractional catabolic rate is comparable for albumin, IgG, and IgM immunoglobulins, further suggesting that there is bulk loss of plasma proteins into the intestinal tract and not a selective loss of certain proteins. The finding of decreased globulins often is an ancillary aid in excluding renal, cardiac, and hepatic cases of hypoalbuminemia.

Abnormalities in albumin and globulin metabolism in patients with a protein-losing enteropathy may be reversed or diminished within a few months after the institution of appropriate therapy. It is obviously important that a specific etiologic diagnosis should be established in all patients with treatable disorders, who may be expected to have a remission induced by the appropriate therapy for the underlying disease. The intestinal protein loss in patients with nontropical sprue, Whipple's disease, constrictive pericarditis, regional enteritis, ulcerative colitis, and Ménétrier's disease has been ameliorated by therapy appropriate to the underlying disorder.

Intestinal lymphangiectasia PATHOPHYSIOLOGY The disorder intestinal lymphangiectasia is characterized by increased enteric loss of protein, hypoproteinemia, edema, lymphocytopenia, malabsorption, and abnormal dilated lymphatic channels in the small intestine. The high incidence of chylous effusions and abnormal peripheral, retroperitoneal, and thoracic lymphatics indicates that intestinal lymphangiectasia is part of a generalized congenital disorder of the lymphatic system. It has been suggested that the hypoplastic visceral lymphatic channels result in obstruction to lymph flow, with the subsequent development of increased intestinal lymphatic pressure. This in turn may lead to dilated lymphatic vessels throughout the small-bowel wall and mesentery. Hypoproteinemia and steatorrhea are thought to be due to rupture of the dilated lymphatic vessels with discharge of lymph into the bowel lumen. In adults approximately 1500 mL lymph, containing 70 g fat and 50 g albumin, passes through the thoracic duct each day. The leakage of a small amount of this lymph might be expected to result in considerable loss of protein and fat into the intestinal lumen. In addition, absorption of dietary long-chain triglycerides stimulates lymph flow, and this may increase further the retrograde leakage of intestinal lymph into the lumen. Three lines of evidence support the concept of intestinal leakage of lymph in intestinal lymphangiectasia: (1) chylous fluid has been recovered from the duodenum in these patients; (2) retrograde passage of contrast material from retroperitoneal lymphatics into the duodenum and jejunum has been documented; and (3) significant steatorrhea may persist in patients after institution of a completely fat-free diet, suggesting an increased enteric loss of endogenous fat present in lymph.

CLINICAL FEATURES The disease affects primarily children and young adults. All patients have edema, which may be asymmetric because of hypoplastic peripheral lymphatics. Chylous effusions and diarrhea are common symptoms. The primary laboratory finding is hypoproteinemia with decreased serum levels of albumin, immunoglobulins IgG, IgA, and IgM, transferrin, and ceruloplasmin. Despite moderate to severe hypogammaglobulinemia there does not appear to be an increased incidence of pyogenic bacterial infections. In addition, circulating antibody response to challenge with *Brucella* and typhoid antigens is normal. Steatorrhea is usually mild, although in some instances fat loss may be as much as 40 g per day. Some patients have hypocalcemia and impaired absorption of vitamin B_{12}. Lymphocytopenia (due to the loss of lymphocytes in lymph) is common, with lymphocyte counts ranging from 400 to 1000 per milliliter (normal: 1500 to 4000 per milliliter). This is associated with abnormal delayed hypersensitivity, as evidenced by prolonged homograft survival and impaired cutaneous responsiveness to antigens such as mumps and monilia.

Small-bowel roentgenograms are frequently abnormal, showing changes of mucosal edema and a malabsorption pattern. Lymphangiograms may demonstrate hypoplastic peripheral and visceral lymphatics with the absence of groups of retroperitoneal lymph nodes. Specimens of jejunal mucosa characteristically reveal dilated and telangiectatic lymphatic vessels in the lamina propria and submucosa. The villi may be club-shaped because of distortion from grossly dilated lymphatics (Fig. 237-4). Such changes in the intestinal mucosa may be reversed after appropriate therapy. The diagnosis of intestinal lymphangiectasia is therefore established by (1) small-intestinal biopsy and (2) demonstration of increased enteric protein loss using radioactive macromolecules.

TREATMENT A low-fat diet, by decreasing lymph flow, usually results in significant improvement with decreased fecal fat excretion, decreased enteric protein loss, increased serum calcium and albumin levels, and an increased half-life of injected ^{125}I-labeled albumin. Similar results may be obtained by the substitution of medium-chain triglycerides (MCT) for dietary long-chain triglycerides, since MCT are transported as medium-chain fatty acids by the portal vein rather than via the lymph.

REFERENCES

AMENT ME et al: Structure and function of the gastrointestinal tract in primary immunodeficiency syndromes. Medicine (Baltimore) 52:227, 1973

BO-LINN GW et al: Fecal fat concentration in patients with steatorrhea. Gastroenterology 87: 319, 1984

BOND JH, LEVITT MD: Use of breath hydrogen (H_2) in the study of carbohydrate absorption. Am J Dig Dis 22:379, 1977

CALDWELL JH et al: Eosinophilic gastroenteritis with obstruction. Immunological studies of seven patients. Gastroenterology 74:825, 1978

CHUNG YC et al: Protein digestion and absorption in human small intestine. Gastroenterology 76:1415, 1979

COOPER BT et al: Celiac disease and malignancy. Medicine (Baltimore) 59:249, 1980

FLORENT C et al: Intestinal clearance of α_1-antitrypsin: A sensitive method for the detection of protein-losing enteropathy. Gastroenterology 81:777, 1981

GASKIN KJ et al: Colipase and maximally activated pancreatic lipase in normal subjects and patients with steatorrhea. J Clin Invest 69:368, 1982

GRAY GM: Carbohydrate digestion and malabsorption, in *Physiology of the Gastrointestinal Tract*, LR Johnson et al (eds). New York, Raven, 1981

GILLIN JS et al: Malabsorption and mucosal abnormalities of the small intestine in the acquired immunodeficiency syndrome. Ann Intern Med 102:619, 1985

HOWDLE PD et al: Cell-mediated immunity to gluten within the small intestinal mucosa in coeliac disease. Gut 23:115, 1982

KEINATH RD et al: Antibiotic treatment and relapse in Whipple's disease. Long term followup of 88 patients. Gastroenterology 88:1867, 1985

KLIPSTEIN FA: Tropical sprue in travelers and expatriates living abroad. Gastroenterology 80:590, 1981

LOUGHRAN TP et al: T-cell intestinal lymphoma associated with celiac sprue. Ann Int Med 104:44, 1986

MACGREGOR I et al: Gastric emptying of liquid meals and pancreatic and biliary secretion after subtotal gastrectomy or truncal vagotomy and pyloroplasty in man. Gastroenterology 72:195, 1977

NEWCOMER AD et al: Triolein breath test. A sensitive and specific test for fat malabsorption. Gastroenterology 76:6, 1979

PETERS TJ, BJARNASON I: Coeliac syndrome: Biochemical mechanisms and the missing peptidase hypothesis revisited. Gut 25:913, 1984

WESER E et al: Short bowel syndrome. Gastroenterology 77:572, 1979

238 INFLAMMATORY BOWEL DISEASE
Ulcerative colitis and Crohn's disease

ROBERT M. GLICKMAN

DEFINITION *Inflammatory bowel disease* (IBD) is a general term for a group of chronic inflammatory disorders of unknown etiology involving the gastrointestinal tract. Since there are no pathognomonic features or specific diagnostic tests, in a strict sense, these disorders remain diagnoses of exclusion. Their features are sufficiently characteristic, however, to permit accurate diagnosis in the majority of cases. Chronic IBD may be divided into two major groups, chronic nonspecific *ulcerative colitis* and *Crohn's disease*. The original description of the disease by Crohn, Ginzberg, and Oppenheimer in 1932 localized the disease to segments of ileum. However, the same process may involve the buccal mucosa, esophagus, stomach, and duodenum as well as the jejunum and ileum. Crohn's disease of the small bowel is also known as *regional enteritis*. In addition, a similar inflammatory picture may occur in the colon, either alone or with accompanying small-intestinal involvement. In most instances, this form of colitis can be distinguished clinically and pathologically from ulcerative colitis and is also referred to as *Crohn's disease of the colon*. Granulomatous colitis is a less accurate term since only a portion of cases exhibit granulomas. Clinically these disorders are characterized by recurrent inflammatory involvement of intestinal segments with diverse clinical manifestations often resulting in a chronic, unpredictable course.

EPIDEMIOLOGY The epidemiologic and etiologic considerations in ulcerative colitis and Crohn's disease share many features in common and will be discussed together. These diseases are more common in whites than in blacks and orientals with an increased incidence (three- to sixfold) in Jews compared to non-Jews. Both sexes are equally affected.

The incidence and prevalence of the two diseases differ slightly with most studies showing ulcerative colitis to be more common. When analyzed in western Europe and the United States, ulcerative colitis (including ulcerative proctitis) has an incidence of approximately 6 to 8 cases per 100,000 population and an estimated prevalence of approximately 70 to 150 cases per 100,000 population. Estimates of the incidence of Crohn's disease (colonic plus small bowel) are approximately 2 cases per 100,000 population; the prevalence is estimated at 20 to 40 per 100,000 population. Although there is no firm documentation, many believe the incidence of Crohn's disease (especially colonic) to be increasing.

While peak occurrence of both diseases is between ages 15 and 35, it has been reported in every decade of life. A familial incidence of IBD has been recorded with estimates that 2 to 5 percent of persons with Crohn's disease or ulcerative colitis will have one or more relatives affected. There is no specificity, however, for a given form of IBD within a given family. Such epidemiologic clustering of cases could argue for either genetic or common environmental influences on the development of these diseases (see below). It has been suggested that there is a probable hereditary basis for these disorders plus a strong environmental component.

ETIOLOGY AND PATHOGENESIS While the cause of ulcerative colitis and Crohn's disease remains unknown, certain features of these diseases have suggested several areas of possible etiologic importance. These include familial or genetic, infectious, immunologic, and psychological factors.

Inflammatory bowel disease is more common in whites, occurs with an increased frequency in Jews, and exhibits some familial clustering. This suggests that there may be a *genetic* predisposition to the development of the disease. In addition, the disease has been described in monozygotic twins. A search for genetic markers which might be of value in identifying susceptible individuals has not identified any single marker (i.e., histocompatibility antigen) in patients with inflammatory bowel disease.

The chronic inflammatory nature of these diseases has prompted a continuing search for a possible *infectious etiology*. In spite of numerous attempts to find known bacterial, fungal, or viral agents, no etiologic agent has thus far been isolated. Preliminary reports of isolates of cell wall variants of *Pseudomonas* or of transmissible agents producing cytopathic effects in tissue culture have yet to be confirmed. Efforts to produce specific granulomatous tissue reactions with filtrates from Crohn's disease tissue have yielded conflicting and nonreproducible results. As discussed below, many infectious agents can produce *acute* colitis or ileitis; however, there is no evidence that these agents are involved in *chronic* inflammatory bowel disease.

The theory that an *immune* mechanism may be involved is based on the concept that the extraintestinal manifestations which may accompany these disorders (e.g., arthritis, pericholangitis) may represent autoimmune phenomena and that therapeutic agents, such as corticosteroids and azathioprine, may exert their effects via immunosuppressive mechanisms. Patients with inflammatory bowel disease may have *humoral antibodies* to colon cells, bacterial antigens such as *Escherichia coli*, lipopolysaccharide, and foreign proteins such as cow milk protein. In general, the presence and titer of these antibodies does not correlate with disease activity. It is likely that these antigens gain access to immunocompetent cells secondary to epithelial damage. In addition, IBD has been described in association with agammaglobulinemia as well as IgA deficiency, casting further doubt on the pathogenetic role of humoral antibodies. *Immune complexes* have also been invoked to explain extraintestinal manifestations of IBD. While there are well-defined examples of tissue injury resulting from immune complexes, studies utilizing specific detection techniques have failed to demonstrate an increased frequency of immune complexes in patients with IBD.

Associated abnormalities of *cell-mediated immunity* include cutaneous anergy, diminished responsiveness to various mitogenic stimuli, and decreases in the number of peripheral T cells. Since many of these changes may revert to normal when the disease is quiescent, it is likely that they are secondary phenomena. Experimental colitis has been produced in laboratory animals by prior sensitization with dinitrochlorobenzene, suggesting a T-cell–dependent mechanism of tissue injury. It remains to be determined whether the regulation of immune function (e.g., suppressor T cells) is of pathogenic importance in the etiology of IBD. Thus far, none of the altered immunologic findings have been specific for either ulcerative colitis or Crohn's disease.

The *psychological* features of patients with inflammatory bowel disease have also been stressed. It is not uncommon for these diseases to present initially or to flare in association with major psychological stresses such as the loss of a family member. It has been suggested that patients with IBD have a characteristic personality which renders them susceptible to emotional stresses which in turn may precipitate or exacerbate their symptoms. While there is little evidence directly relating possible emotional factors to the etiology of inflammatory bowel disease, there is little doubt that a chronic disease of unknown etiology affecting individuals in the prime of their life often results in feelings of anger, anxiety, and some degree of depression. These reactions are undoubtedly important factors in modifying the course of these diseases and in the response to therapy.

PATHOLOGY In ulcerative colitis there is an inflammatory reaction primarily involving the colonic mucosa. Grossly, the colon appears ulcerated, hyperemic, and usually hemorrhagic (Fig. 238-1). A striking feature of the inflammation is that it is *uniform* and *continuous* with no intervening areas of normal mucosa. The rectum is usually involved (95 percent of cases) and the inflammation extends proximally in a continuous fashion but for a variable distance. When there is involvement of the entire colon, there may be minimal involvement of a few centimeters of the terminal ileum, referred to as "backwash ileitis." This involvement never leads to the thickening and narrowing

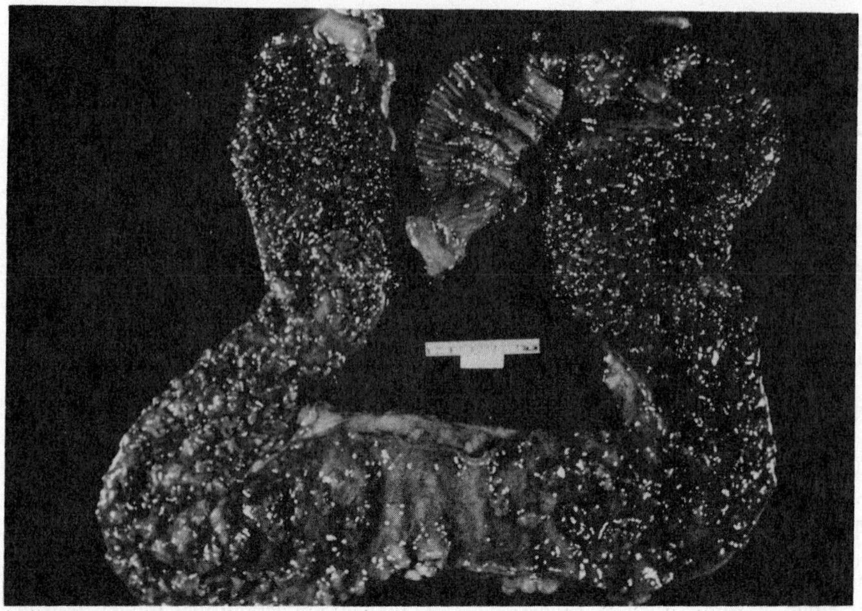

FIGURE 238-1 *Ulcerative colitis. Resected colon with portion of terminal ileum. The specimen showed uniform inflammation, erythema, and hemorrhage and a normal terminal ileum.*

characteristic of Crohn's disease. The surface mucosal cells as well as the crypt epithelium and submucosa are involved in an inflammatory reaction with neutrophilic infiltration (Fig. 238-2*A*). This progresses to epithelial damage with loss of surface epithelial cells resulting in multiple ulcerations. Infiltration of the crypts with neutrophils results in characteristic (but not specific) small crypt abscesses and their eventual destruction. There may also be loss of crypt epithelium with a loss of goblet (mucus-producing) cells and submucosal edema. With repetitive cycles of inflammation, mild submucosal fibrosis develops. Regenerative activity is evidenced by irregular crypt epithelium often showing bifurcation at the base of the crypts. It is important to stress that, unlike Crohn's disease, deeper layers of the bowel beneath the submucosa usually are not involved. In severe ulcerative colitis, as seen with toxic megacolon, the bowel wall may become extremely thin, the mucosa denuded with inflammation extending to the serosa leading to dilatation and subsequent perforation.

Recurrent inflammation may lead to characteristic features of chronicity. Fibrosis and longitudinal retraction result in shortening of the colon. Loss of the normal haustral pattern leads radiologically to a smooth, "lead-pipe" appearance of the colon. Regenerating islands of mucosa surrounded by areas of ulceration and denuded mucosa appear as "polyps" protruding into the lumen of the colon. However, these protrusions are inflammatory in nature and not neoplastic and are therefore called pseudopolyps (Fig. 238-2*B*).

With long-standing ulcerative colitis, the surface epithelium may show features of *dysplasia*. Changes of nuclear and cellular atypia are thought to represent a premalignant change occurring in the setting of long-standing ulcerative colitis. Marked dysplasia in colonic biopsies in the setting of long-standing colitis is associated with a significant risk of a coexistent carcinoma elsewhere in the colon and may influence the decision to advise colectomy.

Crohn's disease, in contrast to ulcerative colitis, is characterized by chronic inflammation extending through *all layers of the intestinal wall* and involving the mesentery as well as regional lymph nodes. Whether or not the small bowel or colon is involved, the basic pathologic process is the same.

The earliest pathologic changes in Crohn's disease are poorly defined since surgery is usually not electively undertaken early in the course of the disease. At laparotomy, the terminal ileum appears hyperemic and boggy, with mesentery and mesenteric lymph nodes swollen and reddened. At this early stage, the bowel wall, although edematous, is usually pliable. While some patients with this initial presentation will subsequently develop typical regional enteritis, a significant number will recover completely. This acute form of ileitis will undoubtedly be shown to have diverse etiologies. Indeed, approximately 80 percent of patients with this presentation have been shown to be infected with *Yersinia enterocolitica,* an organism capable of producing a self-limited, acute inflammatory ileitis.

As the disease progresses, the gross appearance assumes a characteristic picture. The bowel appears greatly thickened and leathery with the lumen narrowed (Fig. 238-3). This characteristic stenosis can occur in any portion of the intestine and may be associated with varying degrees of intestinal obstruction. The mesentery appears greatly thickened, fatty, and often extends over the serosal surface of the bowel in characteristic fingerlike projections. The appearance of the mucosa is variable, depending on the severity and stage of the disease, but may appear relatively normal in sharp contrast to ulcerative colitis. In more advanced cases, the mucosa has a nodular, "cobblestoned" look. This is the result of submucosal thickening and mucosal ulceration, often linear in the long axis of the bowel at the base of mucosal folds. These ulcerations may penetrate into the submucosa and muscularis and coalesce to form intramural channels which become manifested as fistulas and fissures.

There are other morphologic features distinguishing Crohn's disease from ulcerative colitis. In Crohn's disease, the disease is often *discontinuous;* severely involved segments of bowel are separated from each other with intervening segments of apparently normal bowel, producing "skip areas." In approximately 50 percent of Crohn's disease of the colon, the rectum may be spared. In sharp contrast, in ulcerative colitis the involvement is contiguous and the rectum is almost always involved. In addition, in Crohn's disease the transmural inflammatory process, involving serosa and mesentery, also accounts for the characteristic fistula and abscess formation. As a result of serosal inflammation, adjacent loops of small intestine may become adherent and matted together by a fibrinous peritoneal reaction, leading to palpable mass, most often in the right lower quadrant. Fistula formation may occur between adherent loops of intestine, colon, or other adjacent organs such as the bladder or vagina. Fistulous tracts may also lead to the skin or end blindly within the peritoneum or retroperitoneum, surrounded by adherent

FIGURE 238-2 *Colonic biopsies in inflammatory bowel disease. A. Ulcerative colitis. The surface mucosa is destroyed and the submucosa is diffusely infiltrated with polymorphonuclear leukocytes. Crypt abscesses are also present. B. Pseudopolyp. Regenerating island of mucosa with adjacent area of ulceration. C. Ulcerative colitis. Severe dysplasia occurring in long-standing chronic ulcerative colitis. Note atypical changes in the nuclei and marked palisading of nuclei of the crypt epithelium. D. Crohn's disease of the colon. Note the relatively intact mucosa with a solitary granuloma in the lamina propria.*

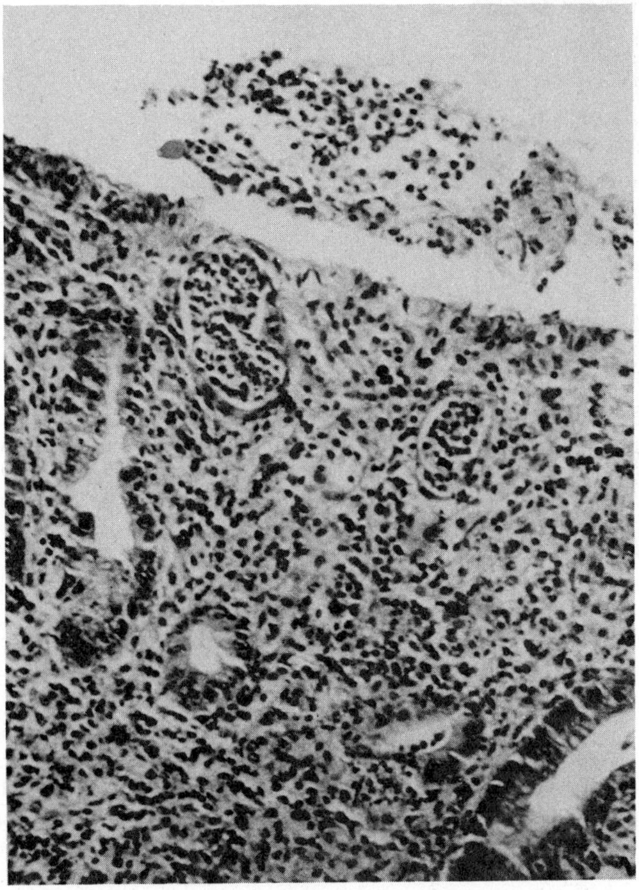

A

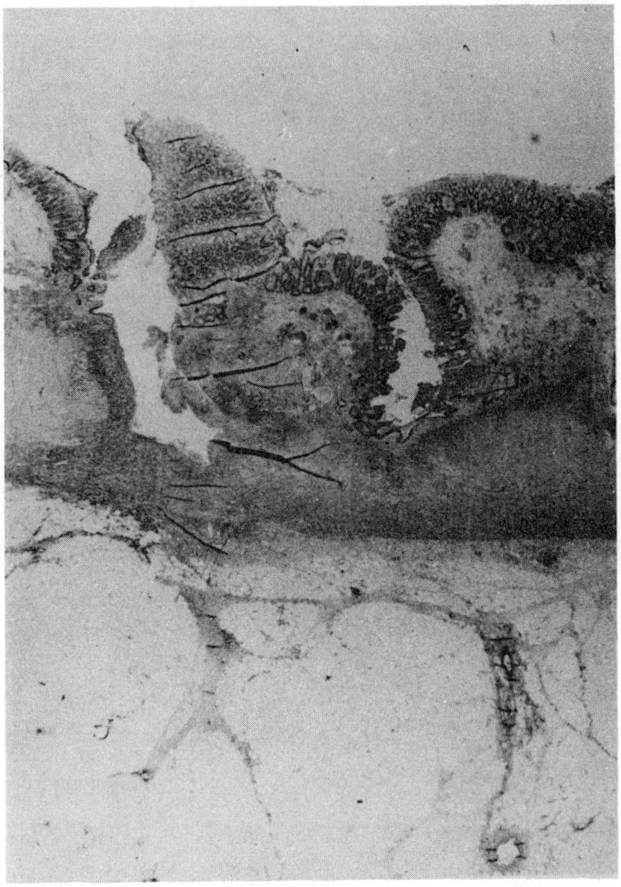

B

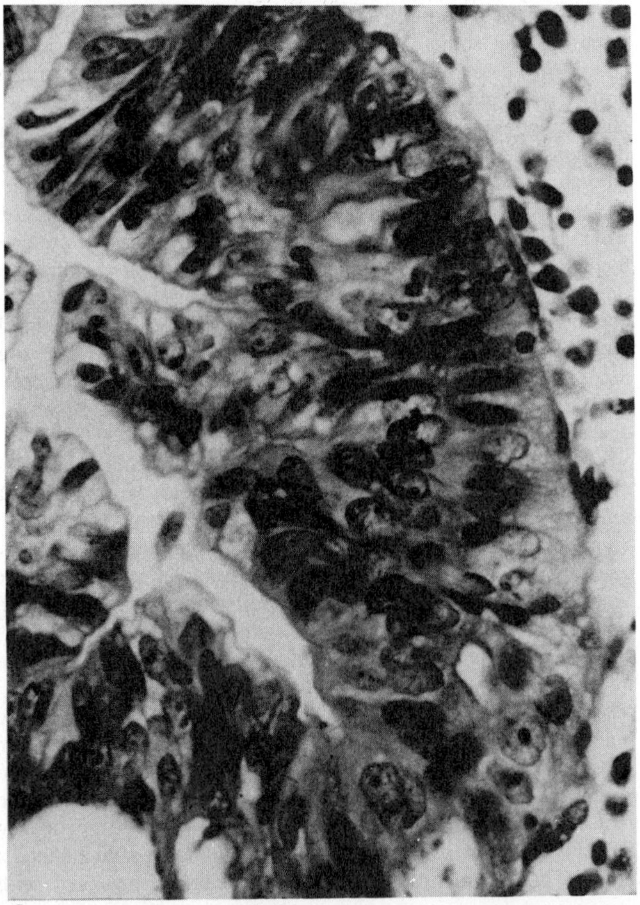

C

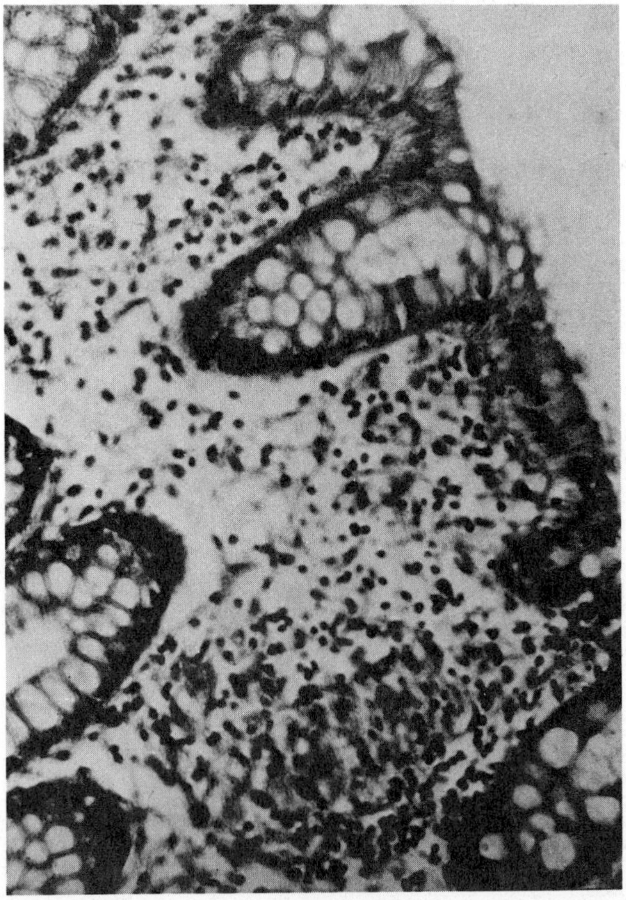

D

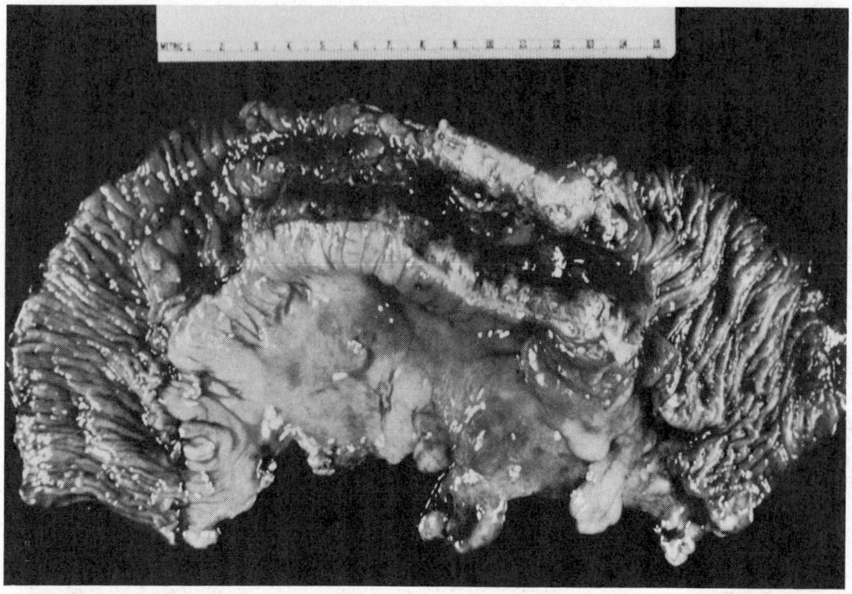

FIGURE 238-3 *Regional enteritis. Resected specimen of terminal ileum demonstrates thickened bowel wall and chronically inflamed mucosa. Note the relatively sharp demarcation of the diseased segment with grossly normal mucosa on either side.*

loops of bowel and inflammatory tissue. Fistula formation is not seen in ulcerative colitis.

Microscopically, granulomas are most helpful in distinguishing Crohn's disease from other forms of inflammatory bowel disease; they do not occur in ulcerative colitis. They may be seen in rectal or colonoscopic biopsies (Fig. 238-2*D*). While granulomas are a helpful finding when present, it is the chronic inflammation involving all layers of the intestinal wall which is most characteristic.

In most series reporting the distribution of Crohn's disease, approximately 30 percent will involve the small intestine (usually the terminal ileum) without colonic disease, 30 percent with only colonic involvement, and 40 percent with ileocolic involvement usually of the ileum and right colon. In a small number of patients (mostly children and adolescents) there may be diffuse and extensive ulceration of the jejunum and ileum.

While there often are sufficient features to permit distinction between ulcerative colitis and Crohn's disease of the colon (Table 238-1), in 10 to 20 percent of cases this distinction may not be possible.

TABLE 238-1 Pathologic and clinical features of IBD

	Ulcerative colitis	Crohn's disease
PATHOLOGIC		
Segmental	0	+ +
Transmural involvement	+/−	+ +
Granulomas	0	+/+ + (50%)
Fibrosis	+	+ +
Fissuring, fistulas	+/−	+ +
Mesenteric fat, lymph node involvement	0	+ +
CLINICAL		
Diarrhea	+ +	+ +
Rectal bleeding	+ +	+
Abdominal pain	+	+ +
Palpable mass	0	+ +
Fistulas	+/−	+ +
Strictures	+	+ +
Small bowel involvement	+/− ("backwash ileitis")	+ +
Rectal involvement	+ + (95%)	+/+ + (50%)
Extracolonic disease	+	+
Toxic megacolon	+	+/−
Recurrence after colectomy	0	+
Malignancy (with long-standing disease)	+	+/−

NOTE: *0 = never; +/− = rare; + = occasional; + + = Frequent, common.*

CLINICAL FEATURES

ULCERATIVE COLITIS The major symptoms of ulcerative colitis are bloody diarrhea and abdominal pain, often with fever and weight loss in more severe cases. With mild disease, there may be one or two semiformed stools containing little blood and with no systemic manifestations. In contrast, the patient with severe disease may have frequent liquid stools containing blood and pus, complain of severe cramps, and demonstrate symptoms and signs of dehydration, anemia, fever, and weight loss. With predominantly rectal involvement, constipation rather than diarrhea may be present, and tenesmus may be a major complaint. On occasion, intestinal symptoms may be overshadowed by fever, weight loss, or one of the extracolonic manifestations of the disease (see below).

The physical findings in ulcerative colitis are usually nonspecific; there may be some abdominal distention or tenderness along the course of the colon. In mild cases, the general physical examination will be normal. Extracolonic manifestations include arthritis, skin changes, or evidence of liver disease. Fever, tachycardia, and postural hypotension are usually associated with more severe disease. The laboratory findings are often nonspecific and usually reflect the degree and severity of bleeding and inflammation. There may be anemia which reflects chronic disease as well as iron deficiency from chronic blood loss. Leukocytosis with a left shift and an elevated sedimentation rate are often seen in the severely ill, febrile patient. Electrolyte abnormalities, especially hypokalemia, reflect the degree of diarrhea. Hypoalbuminemia is common with extensive disease and usually represents luminal protein loss through an ulcerated mucosa. An elevated alkaline phosphatase may indicate associated hepatobiliary disease (see below).

The clinical course of ulcerative colitis is variable. The majority of patients will suffer a relapse within 1 year of the first attack, reflecting the recurrent nature of the disease. There may, however, be prolonged periods of remission with only minimal symptoms. In general, the severity of symptoms reflects the extent of colonic involvement and the intensity of the inflammation. At one end of the spectrum are patients who present with limited involvement of the rectum (ulcerative proctitis) or rectum and sigmoid (ulcerative proctosigmoiditis). Consistent with this limited colonic involvement, the disease is usually mild, with minimal systemic or extracolonic manifestations. The major symptoms are rectal bleeding and tenesmus. Most of these patients, especially those with only rectal involvement, will not develop more extensive disease. In the remainder, the disease may extend proximally with variable involvement. Most patients with ulcerative colitis (perhaps 85 percent) will have mild to moderate disease of an intermittent nature and can be managed without hospitalization. In approximately 15 percent of patients, the disease assumes a more fulminant course, involves the entire colon, and presents with severe bloody diarrhea and systemic signs and symptoms. The patients are at risk to develop toxic dilatation and perforation of the colon (described below) and represent a medical emergency.

CROHN'S DISEASE As discussed above, the basic pathologic features of Crohn's disease are the same whether the disease involves the small bowel or colon. The clinical presentation, however, will largely reflect the anatomic location of the disease and to some degree will predict which complications of the disease may develop. The clinical features of ulcerative colitis and Crohn's disease are compared in Table 238-1.

The major clinical features of Crohn's disease are fever, abdominal pain, diarrhea often without blood, and generalized fatigability. There may be associated weight loss. With *colonic involvement* diarrhea and pain are the most frequent symptoms. Rectal bleeding is distinctly less common than with ulcerative colitis and reflects (1) sparing of the rectum in many patients, and (2) the transmural nature of the disease with only irregular mucosal involvement. There may be associated severe anorectal complications such as fistulas, fissures, and perirectal abscess. Such features may antedate the clinical onset of colitis and should always raise the suspicion of associated Crohn's disease. With recurrent perirectal inflammation the anal canal may be thickened, and perianal fistulas or scarring may be present. With extensive colonic involvement, dilatation of the colon may occur. However, since Crohn's disease often results in a thickened colonic wall, this is less common with Crohn's disease than with ulcerative colitis. Extracolonic manifestations (discussed below), particularly arthritis, are seen more commonly with colonic than with small bowel Crohn's disease (regional enteritis).

With involvement of the *small bowel* there may be additional presenting signs and symptoms. Typically, the disease has its onset in a young adult with a history of fatigue, variable weight loss, right lower quadrant discomfort or pain, and diarrhea. Low-grade fever, anorexia, nausea, and vomiting may also be present. The abdominal pain may be steady and localized to the right lower quadrant or may assume a colicky or crampy pattern, reflecting variable degrees of intestinal stenosis. The diarrhea is often moderate, usually without gross blood; if there is no rectal involvement, tenesmus is absent. Physical examination at this time often reveals right lower quadrant tenderness with an associated fullness or mass reflecting adherent loops of bowel. At this time the patient may have mild anemia, mild to moderate leukocytosis, and an elevated sedimentation rate.

Since acute ileitis may have an abrupt onset with fever, leukocytosis, and right lower quadrant pain, the clinical picture may be indistinguishable from acute appendicitis. The diagnosis can be made only at laparotomy, when the characteristic beefy red terminal ileum, boggy mesenteric fat, and succulent mesenteric lymph nodes indicate that appendicitis alone could not produce this picture.

While the symptoms of diarrhea and abdominal pain will usually alert the clinician to the possibility of regional enteritis, other symptoms may dominate the clinical presentation. In children, and the aged, fever of undetermined origin and unexplained weight loss may be prominent and initially may cause one to suspect underlying malignancy. In some patients, the first manifestation of the disease may be intestinal obstruction; in others the disease may present with fistula formation in the form of perianal sepsis or urinary tract infection resulting from an enterovesical fistula. Similarly, right ureteral obstruction and hydronephrosis may occur due to external compression of the ureter by a right lower quadrant inflammatory mass. On occasion, often in the setting of extensive small-bowel involvement, features of malabsorption may be prominent. These features, along with anorexia and the catabolic effects of the chronic inflammatory process, may combine to produce striking degrees of weight loss.

The complications of the disease are often local, resulting from intestinal inflammation and involvement of adjacent structures.

Intestinal obstruction is a frequent complication, occurring in 20 to 30 percent of patients during the course of the disease. In the initial stages, the obstruction usually is due to the acute inflammation and edema of the involved intestinal segment, usually the terminal ileum. However, as the disease progresses and fibrosis develops, obstruction may be due to a fixed narrowing of the bowel.

Fistula formation is a frequent complication of chronic regional enteritis as well as Crohn's disease of the colon. Fistulas may occur between contiguous segments of intestine; they may also burrow into the retroperitoneal spaces and present as cutaneous fistulas or indolent abscesses. In a significant number of patients, the first indication of the disease may be the presence of persistent rectal fissures, a perirectal abscess, or a rectal fistula. Although uncommon, pneumaturia should raise the suspicion of enterovesical fistula and is often associated with a persistent urinary tract infection.

Since Crohn's disease is a transmural disease with the bowel wall greatly thickened, free *intestinal perforation* is uncommon. In a small number of cases, however, it may be the presenting feature, and the disease is first discovered at the time of laparotomy for a perforated viscus. The passage per rectum of bright red blood should alert one to the possible coexistence of rectal involvement (i.e., ileocolitis). Crohn's disease may also involve the *stomach* and *duodenum*. The involvement is usually of the antrum and/or the first and second portions of the duodenum. Symptoms may include pain mimicking peptic ulcer disease. Later in the course of the disease, chronic scarring may produce gastric outlet or duodenal obstruction.

There are increasing reports of *small-bowel* and *colonic malignancy* developing in the setting of long-standing Crohn's disease. Although the risk of developing malignancy is statistically increased, the complication is uncommon when compared with the frequency of malignancy in ulcerative colitis (see below). As in other chronic inflammatory diseases, patients with long-standing Crohn's disease may rarely develop secondary *amyloidosis*, which may manifest itself with hepatosplenomegaly or significant proteinuria. The presence of extensive ileal disease, resulting in *bile salt malabsorption*, is associated with a decreased bile salt pool and an increased lithogenicity of bile (see Chap. 237). Up to 30 percent of patients with extensive ileal disease will develop gallstones. Also, in the setting of ileal disease and an intact colon there is increased colonic absorption of dietary oxalate with resultant hyperoxaluria and the development of *urinary oxalate stones*. Dehydration due to diarrhea is an additional predisposing factor in renal stone formation.

DIAGNOSIS

The diagnosis of IBD should be entertained in all patients presenting with diarrhea or bloody diarrhea, persistent perianal sepsis, and abdominal pain. There may be atypical presentations such as fever of unexplained origin in the absence of bowel symptoms or with extracolonic manifestations such as arthritis or liver disease antedating or overshadowing the bowel involvement. Since Crohn's disease may also involve the small intestine, it should be considered in the differential diagnosis of all types of malabsorption syndromes, intermittent intestinal obstruction, and abdominal fistulas.

The laboratory examination is usually nonspecific and reflects the extent and severity of the inflammatory reaction. In addition, when Crohn's disease involves the small bowel, laboratory features of malabsorption may be present. There may be a variable degree of anemia, from occult blood loss or the effect of chronic inflammation on the bone marrow. Folate or vitamin B_{12} malabsorption may also contribute to the anemia. While the Schilling test may be abnormal in patients with extensive ileal disease, frank macrocytic anemia due to vitamin B_{12} malabsorption alone is unusual, attesting to the marked efficiency of ileal absorption of the vitamin. When there is significant diarrhea, electrolyte abnormalities (hypokalemia, hypomagnesemia) may be prominent. Hypocalcemia may reflect extensive mucosal involvement and malabsorption of vitamin D. Hypoalbuminemia may result from amino acid malabsorption as well as from protein-losing enteropathy. Variable degrees of steatorrhea may result from bile salt depletion and mucosal damage. Mild abnormalities of liver function (especially an increased serum alkaline phosphatase) may reflect the development of a fatty liver in the malnourished patient or a coexisting pericholangitis. Significant jaundice is unusual. Proteinuria may reflect secondary amyloidosis, a rare complication.

Sigmoidoscopy and *radiologic* studies of the bowel are most important in establishing the diagnosis of inflammatory bowel disease. Sigmoidoscopy must be performed in all patients presenting with chronic diarrhea and in all instances of rectal bleeding. While meticulous air-contrast barium enema examination of the perfectly prepared colon may disclose the earliest mucosal changes in either ulcerative colitis or Crohn's disease (see below), a conventional barium enema examination is often "normal" in early disease. Direct visualization of the colonic mucosa combined with biopsy is the most sensitive way of determining whether rectal inflammation is present. It can often be performed without prior enema preparation in the patient actively having diarrhea. The goal of sigmoidoscopy is to establish *whether* mucosal inflammation is present and not necessarily to determine its full *extent* at the initial examination. Thus, if sigmoidoscopic changes are encountered within the first 8 to 10 cm, it is not necessary to pass the instrument to its full length which may cause discomfort when the bowel is acutely inflamed. In ulcerative colitis, findings include a loss of mucosal vascularity, diffuse erythema, friability of the mucosa, and often an exudate consisting of mucus, blood, and pus. The most characteristic feature is mucosal friability, best demonstrated by lightly wiping the surface of the mucosa with a cotton swab and observing the mucosa for the appearance of diffuse, small bleeding points. Equally characteristic is the uniformity of involvement. Once diseased mucosa is encountered (usually in the rectum), there are no areas of intervening normal mucosa before the proximal extent of the disease is reached. Ulceration is shallow, may be small or confluent, but invariably occurs in segments of active colitis. Rectal biopsy may corroborate mucosal inflammation. With more chronic disease, the mucosa may show a granular appearance and pseudopolyps may be present.

Endoscopic examination of the colon is also of value in the diagnosis of colonic Crohn's disease. The findings are of ulcerations which may be tiny, aphthous erosions or deep, longitudinal fissures. They usually occur in segments of otherwise normal mucosa. Since the mucosa is not uniformly involved, friability and diffuse granularity, which are hallmarks of ulcerative colitis, are not characteristic of Crohn's colitis. Rather a cobblestone appearance, which is a coarse irregularity of the mucosal surface, reflects submucosal inflammation and is characteristic of Crohn's disease. Pseudopolyps, edema, and strictures may be seen in Crohn's colitis as well as in ulcerative colitis. Colonic mucosal biopsy reveals granulomas in 30 to 50 percent of specimens taken from involved areas. Features such as crypt abscesses, infiltration with inflammatory cells, or ulcerations are nonspecific but compatible features. Since skip areas and rectal sparing are characteristic of Crohn's disease, colonoscopy may be superior to sigmoidoscopy in the evaluation of Crohn's disease. Colonoscopic examination is also indicated when Crohn's disease appears only to involve the small bowel. Ileal biopsy may be feasible, and coexisting colonic involvement occurs in a significant number of cases. Perianal inflammatory lesions as well as areas of rectal disease seen at endoscopy will often show granulomatous inflammation. Rectal biopsy of seemingly "uninvolved" areas may also show microscopic evidence of granulomatous inflammation in only 15 percent of patients.

The *radiologic evaluation* of the bowel provides essential information in the diagnosis of IBD. Barium enema, in ulcerative colitis, may reveal the extent of the disease and help define associated features such as stricture, pseudopolyposis, or carcinoma. The earliest features seen in ulcerative colitis are irritability and incomplete filling due to associated inflammation. Fine ulcerations may be seen at this time as serrations along the contour of the bowel producing a hazy

FIGURE 238-4 *Acute ulcerative colitis, air-contrast study. Note the diffuse fine ulceration involving the entire colon producing a fine serration along the contour of the bowel. (Courtesy of Dr R Gold, Columbia Presbyterian Medical Center.)*

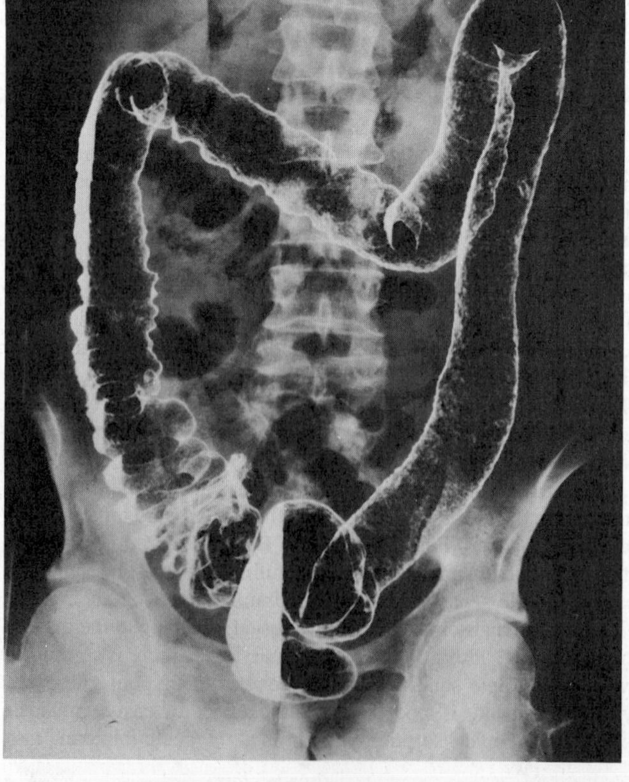

FIGURE 238-5 *Chronic ulcerative colitis. Note the loss of haustrations and the fusiform stricture in the transverse colon. (Courtesy of Dr R Gold, Columbia Presbyterian Medical Center.)*

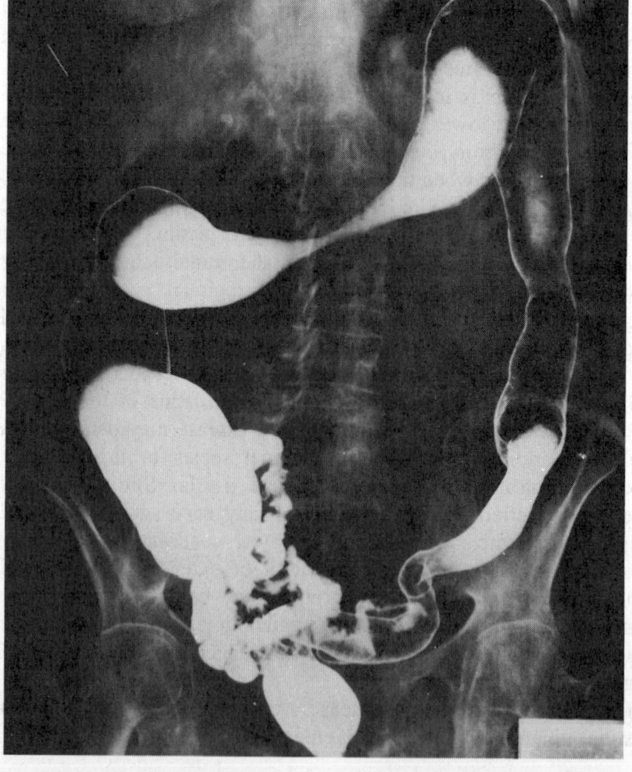

margin (Fig. 238-4). The ulcerations may become deeper and with more fulminant disease produce a grossly ragged and irregular contour. Polypoid defects appear as a result of edematous mucosa between ulcerations. The diffuse pattern of ulceration is best seen on the evacuation film or on air-contrast barium enema. In the chronic stage of the disease (Fig. 238-5), the characteristic features are shortening of the bowel, depression of the flexures, narrowing of the bowel lumen, and rigidity. The bowel has a symmetric, ahaustral, tubular appearance with a decreased mucosal pattern. Although strictures are uncommon, when they occur they have a concentric lumen with fusiform tapering margins. Eccentricity should raise the suspicion of an associated carcinoma.

Barium enema examination in Crohn's disease of the colon has features which usually distinguish it from ulcerative colitis. Features characteristic of Crohn's disease include rectal sparing, the presence of skip lesions, and the finding of small ulcerations occurring on small irregular nodules. The small ulcerations often extend to produce longitudinal ulcers (Fig. 238-6) and transverse fissures which in reality are limited sinus tracts. These may extend into adjacent tissues to produce fistulas. Irregular thickening and fibrosis may lead to stricture formation which may be multiple. In 10 to 15 percent of cases the disease may uniformly involve the entire colon, making differentiation from ulcerative colitis more difficult. Reflux of barium into the terminal ileum during barium enema may reveal characteristic ileal changes of regional enteritis.

When Crohn's disease involves the small intestine, the terminal ileum is most characteristically involved with features similar to colonic involvement. Careful x-ray examination of the small bowel may demonstrate loss of mucosal detail and rigidity of involved segments resulting from submucosal edema or stenosis. The submucosal inflammation may lead to the characteristic radiologic cobblestoned appearance of the mucosa (Fig. 238-7), and fistulous tracts may be seen, especially in the ileocecal area (Fig. 238-8). Involvement of the stomach and duodenum usually appears radiologically as stiffening and infiltration of the mucosa and can mimic an infiltrative tumor. If such an appearance is due to regional enteritis, there is almost always coexistent involvement of either the jejunum or ileum.

While barium studies often provide information on the pattern and extent of inflammatory bowel disease, caution must be exercised in obtaining these studies in the acutely ill patient with severe colitis in whom barium study and the bowel cleansing which precedes it may result in a worsening of the disease and can precipitate toxic dilatation of the colon.

Fiberoptic colonoscopy has added greatly to the diagnosis of colonic inflammatory bowel disease. Areas formerly beyond the reach of the sigmoidoscope can now be directly visualized and biopsy material obtained. Early in the course of colonic inflammation, endoscopic examination and biopsy are the most sensitive techniques to demonstrate mucosal involvement. Polypoid lesions, strictures, and unclear x-ray features can usually be fully defined. Periodic colonoscopic examination and biopsy are being increasingly used in cancer surveillance in patients with long-standing inflammatory bowel disease (see below).

DIFFERENTIAL DIAGNOSIS

Many entities must be considered in the differential diagnosis in IBD. The focus of the differential diagnosis will in large measure be determined by the presenting features of the disease. When *rectal bleeding* is the presenting complaint, a colonic source should be considered. While *hemorrhoids* are commonly found, they must be considered a tentative source of bleeding until sigmoidoscopy and barium enema have eliminated other colonic lesions. Colonic *neoplasms* (carcinoma, adenomatous polyps) may also present with rectal bleeding and can usually be diagnosed by barium enema with subsequent sigmoidoscopic or colonoscopic biopsy. It should be remembered that carcinoma may complicate long-standing colitis. Rectal bleeding from *colonic diverticula* or *arteriovenous malformations* usually present no problem in differential diagnosis since radiologic and endoscopic features of inflammatory bowel disease are absent. *Radiation proctitis,* which may present as a localized area of colitis, is usually found in the setting of pelvic irradiation. The onset may, however, occur at variable (months to years) periods of time after irradiation. Characteristic features on sigmoidoscopy include mucosal atrophy and telangiectasia along with friability and small ulcerations. A colitis sometimes indistinguishable from ulcerative colitis may occur in Behçet's syndrome and is associated with aphthous oral ulceration, uveitis, and urethritis.

Acute colitis may be caused by a variety of *infectious* agents (Chap. 89). Often presenting with bloody diarrhea, infectious colitis may be difficult to distinguish from IBD at initial presentation. A listing of these agents is given in Table 238-2.

Amebiasis may present with bloody diarrhea and at sigmoidoscopy be indistinguishable from idiopathic ulcerative colitis. A history of recent foreign travel or homosexual exposure should always be

FIGURE 238-6 *Crohn's colitis. Air-contrast study.*

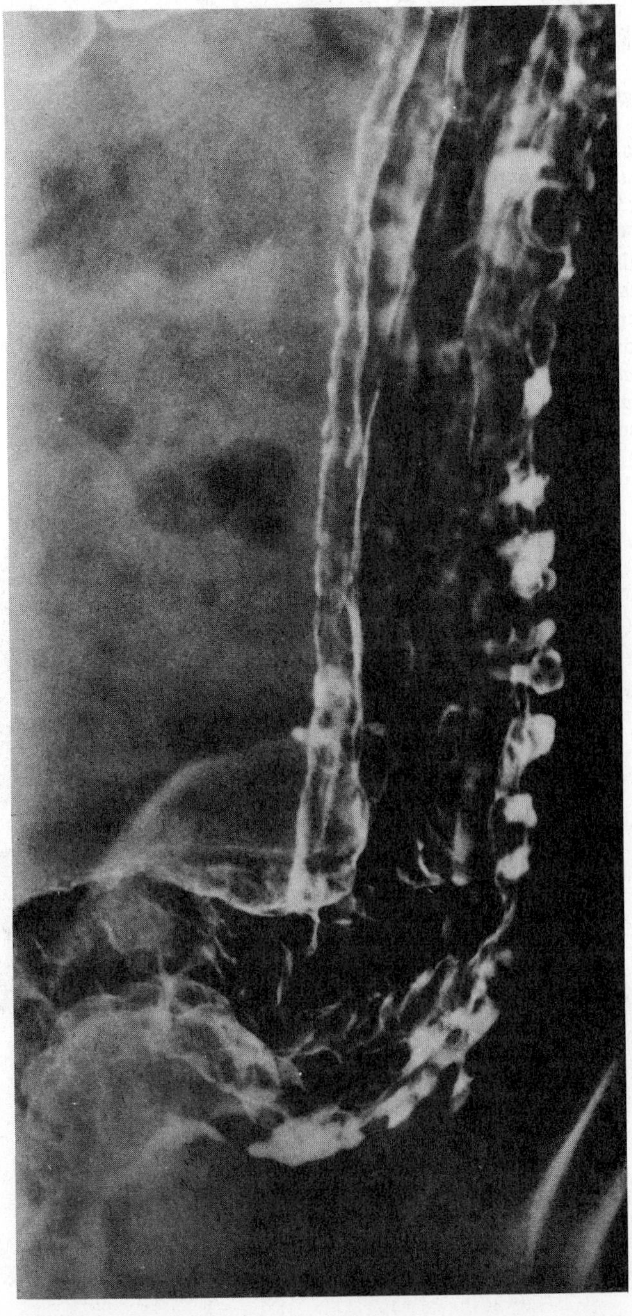

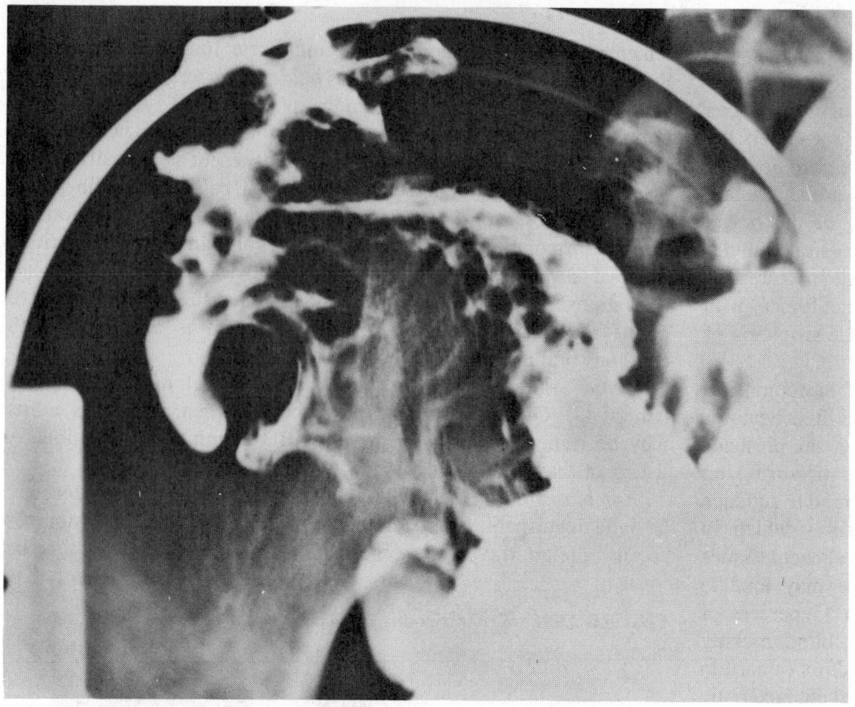

FIGURE 238-7 *Crohn's ileocolitis. Note the nodularity and ulceration of the terminal ileum and the deformity of the cecum.*

sought. Since specific amebicidal therapy is necessary to eradicate this infection and corticosteroids may be detrimental, every effort should be made to exclude this diagnosis in appropriate individuals. Acute *bacillary dysentery* may be caused by *Shigella* and *Salmonella* or *Campylobacter,* all easily diagnosed by stool culture. *Yersinia enterocolitis,* which often presents as acute ileitis, can also produce a self-limited colitis, sometimes with granulomatous reaction. Infectious agents may cause acute proctitis indistinguishable from idiopathic ulcerative proctitis. Such infections, often seen in homosexuals, may be due to *gonorrhea* or *lymphogranuloma venereum* (LGV) as well as *amebiasis.* Recently, in homosexual men, non-LGV strains of *Chlamydia* have been shown to produce a granulomatous proctitis closely resembling Crohn's disease of the rectum.

Pseudomembranous colitis (antibiotic-associated colitis) is caused by a necrolytic toxin elaborated by *Clostridium difficile,* which under certain circumstances proliferates within the bowel. Most often the disease is a result of antibiotic therapy which presumably upsets the normal ecologic balance of the bowel flora permitting *C. difficile* to proliferate. Almost every antibiotic has been implicated, although cases related to the use of vancomycin or aminoglycosides are rare. Most often diarrhea is profuse and watery, although bloody diarrhea occurs in 5 percent of cases. Characteristic lesions are seen on sigmoidoscopy and appear as multiple, discrete yellowish plaques which on biopsy show features of acute inflammation and ulceration with a pseudomembrane of fibrin and necrotic material. On occasion lesions may be beyond reach of the sigmoidoscope and require

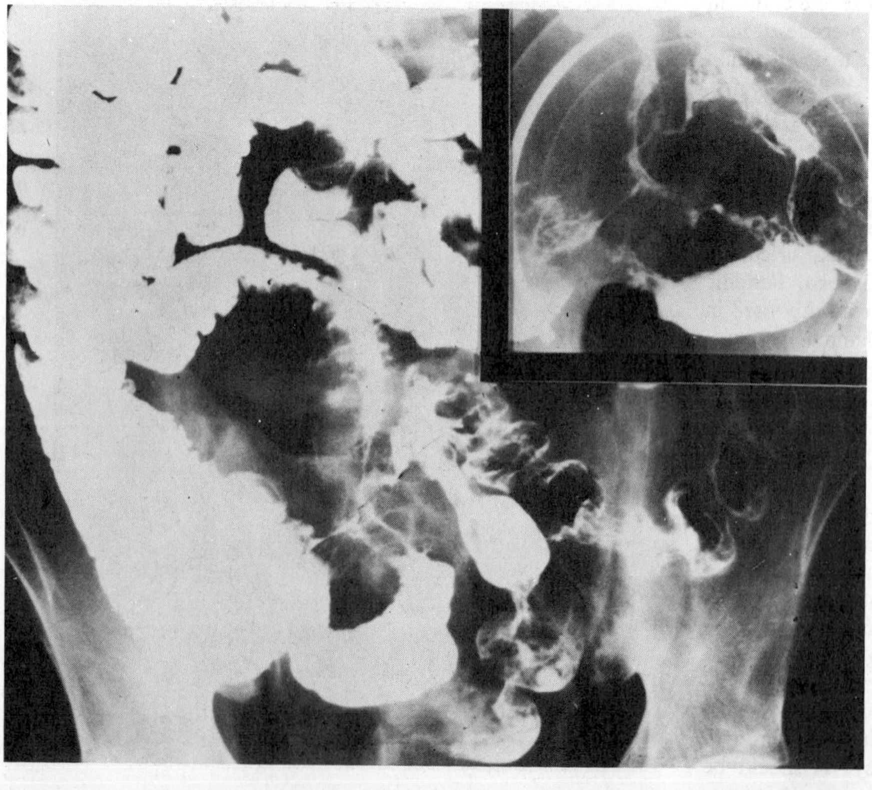

FIGURE 238-8 *Regional enteritis. X-ray showing fistulas between loops of bowel. Insert is a compression film of this area; note fistulas between adjacent loops of bowel.*

TABLE 238-2 Microbiologic causes of colitis

Shigella
Salmonella
Amebiasis
Yersinia
Campylobacter
Lymphogranuloma venereum (LGV)
"Non-LGV" *Chlamydia*
Gonorrhea
Pseudomembranous colitis (*Clostridium difficile* toxin)
Tuberculosis

colonoscopy. Diagnosis is best made by detecting *C. difficile* toxin in the stool. Treatment is either directed at binding the toxin or at eradicating the *C. difficile* organisms. Anion exchange resins such as cholestyramine (4 g PO qid for 5 days) will bind the toxin and may be used in mild cases. Vancomycin (250 mg PO qid for 7 to 14 days) is the treatment of choice for more severely ill patients and should produce clinical improvement within 5 days. Since vancomycin therapy is expensive, alternative therapies have been proposed. Metronidazole (500 mg PO tid) or bacitracin (25,000 units PO qid) have been suggested as alternative therapies. With all forms of therapy, relapse rates (15 to 30 percent) have been observed and may require a subsequent course of therapy to eradicate the organism. On occasion, infectious causes of colitis will be superimposed on ulcerative colitis or Crohn's disease. In this case, once the acute infection has subsided, symptoms and inflammatory mucosal changes may persist, raising the possibility of associated idiopathic IBD. Similar considerations apply to the patient with IBD who uncommonly may develop associated *pseudomembranous* colitis. The finding of *C. difficile* toxin in the stool and subsequent treatment will serve to clarify this presentation.

Abdominal pain in association with rectal bleeding, especially in the older age group, may be due to *ischemic colitis*. Because of an excellent collateral circulation, the rectum is usually spared. Radiologic features are often characteristic.

Inflammatory bowel disease may be difficult to distinguish from functional diarrhea early in the course of disease. The presence of constitutional symptoms such as fatigue, fever, and weight loss, coupled with laboratory features of anemia, elevated erythrocyte sedimentation rate, or occult blood in the stool should alert the clinician to the possibility of IBD. Similarly, finding leukocytes in a stained stool specimen points to an inflammatory basis for the diarrhea. In all cases, stool cultures and parasitologic examination of the stool are required to rule out enteric bacterial pathogens or amebiasis. In the *irritable bowel syndrome* sigmoidoscopy, rectal biopsy, and barium enema examination are all normal.

Once the diagnosis of idiopathic IBD has been established, the distinction between ulcerative colitis and Crohn's disease of the colon is usually possible. Differential diagnostic features are shown in Table 238-1.

With small-intestinal involvement (regional enteritis) the differential diagnosis should include disorders presenting with intraabdominal abscesses, fistulas, intestinal obstruction, and malabsorption. The finding of associated colonic involvement in patients with ileal disease will often serve to distinguish Crohn's disease from other ileal disorders. With diffuse involvement of the jejunum and ileum, regional enteritis must be distinguished from *nongranulomatous ulcerative jejunoileitis*. Abdominal pain and diarrhea are prominent features of this disorder, and weight loss, malabsorption, and hypoproteinemia tend to be more prominent than in regional enteritis. Small-bowel biopsy shows a more diffuse lesion with flattened villi (similar to celiac sprue), infiltration of the lamina propria, and mucosal ulceration. *Abdominal lymphoma* may likewise present with clinical and radiologic features difficult to distinguish from regional enteritis. Hepatosplenomegaly and peripheral adenopathy, when present, are helpful clues, but often disease is confined to the intestine. In such cases, laparotomy is usually required to make the definitive histologic diagnosis.

The advanced presentation of regional enteritis with areas of stenosis and draining fistulas may also be confused with *chronic fungal infection of the bowel,* including actinomycosis, aspergillosis, and blastomycosis. These infections often are seen in debilitated patients with impaired host defenses. Fungal skin tests and examination of fistula drainage and biopsy material for characteristic granules and fungi are helpful in making the diagnosis.

Intestinal tuberculosis characteristically produces stenotic lesions, usually in the terminal ileum, also often involving the contiguous cecum and ascending colon. Unlike regional enteritis, "skip areas" are unusual. Histologically, the granulomatous inflammation seen with *Mycobacterium* tuberculosis may be indistinguishable from regional enteritis; acid-fast stains and cultures are required. Fortunately in western countries primary intestinal tuberculosis is now rare; when intestinal involvement does occur, it invariably is associated with pulmonary tuberculosis.

COMPLICATIONS OF INFLAMMATORY BOWEL DISEASE

The complications of IBD may be classified as local, which are a direct reflection of mucosal inflammation and its extension, or systemic complications (Table 238-3). Local complications of IBD such as fistulas, abscesses, and strictures have been described above. In addition, perforation, toxic dilatation, and the development of carcinoma may complicate both ulcerative colitis and Crohn's disease.

PERFORATION Intestinal perforation can occur in severe ulcerative colitis since with extensive ulceration the bowel wall may become extremely thin. The clinical features are those of acute peritonitis with signs of peritoneal inflammation and the demonstration of free air under the diaphragm on upright film of the abdomen. These are an indication for immediate colectomy.

Toxic dilatation of the colon may occur in Crohn's colitis but is more common in ulcerative colitis. This complication can best be considered as a severe form of ulcerative colitis with the additional feature of colonic dilatation. It is thought that the neuromuscular tone of the bowel is affected by the severe inflammation resulting in dilatation. Injudicious use of hypomotility agents (codeine, diphenoxylate, loperamide, paregoric, anticholinergic agents) to treat diarrhea in the setting of acute colitis can precipitate this complication.

TABLE 238-3 Some systemic complications of inflammatory bowel disease

1 Nutritional and metabolic
- *a* Weight loss, ↓ muscle mass, growth retardation (children)
- *b* Electrolyte deficiency (K^+, Ca^{2+}, Mg^{2+})
- *c* Hypoalbuminemia (↓ nutrition, protein-losing enteropathy)
- *d* Anemia (chronic disease, iron deficiency; rarely folate or vitamin B_{12} deficiency in Crohn's disease)
- *e* Bile salt deficiency with ileal disease (steatorrhea and fat-soluble vitamin deficiency; ↑ colonic oxalate absorption → renal stones; ↑ lithogenicity of bile → gallstones)

2 Musculoskeletal
- *a* Peripheral arthralgia, arthritis
- *b* Ankylosing spondylitis, sacroileitis
- *c* Granulomatous myositis (rare)

3 Hepatobiliary disease
- *a* Fatty liver
- *b* Cholelithiasis
- *c* Pericholangitis, biliary cirrhosis (rare)
- *d* Sclerosing cholangitis
- *e* Bile duct carcinoma
- *f* Chronic active hepatitis and cirrhosis

4 Skin and mucous membrane
- *a* Erythema nodosum
- *b* Pyoderma gangrenosum
- *c* Aphthous stomatitis
- *d* Crohn's disease of buccal mucosa, gingiva, vagina

5 Eye
- Iritis, uveitis, episcleritis

6 Venous thrombosis and thromboembolism (hypercoagulability, dehydration, stasis)

Similarly, cathartic preparation and barium enema examination as well as superimposed hypokalemia may be contributing factors. Clinically, features of severe colitis are present with high fever, tachycardia, volume depletion, electrolyte imbalance, and abdominal pain. On examination, the patient appears toxic, and colonic dilatation may be evident. There is abdominal tenderness and if perforation has already occurred, peritoneal signs are present. Diarrhea may actually decrease markedly due to colonic atony, creating the false impression that the colitis is clinically improved. Plain film of the abdomen will show colonic dilatation with the colonic diameter more than 6 cm. There may be air in the wall of the colon, and irregular, ulcerated islands of mucosa may be silhouetted against the air shadow. While the transverse colon is the most common site of dilatation, this is probably largely positional, since with the patient supine, this is the highest portion of the colon. This presentation of colitis represents a true medical emergency and is associated with a mortality of greater than 30 percent if perforation has occurred. Appropriate therapy is discussed below.

CARCINOMA AND INFLAMMATORY BOWEL DISEASE There is an increased incidence of carcinoma in patients with chronic IBD when compared to the general population, especially in patients who have more extensive mucosal involvement (i.e., pancolitis) and those who have had their disease for extended periods of time. Cumulative risk of cancer rises steadily with the duration of disease. It has been estimated that with pancolitis there is a risk of cancer of 12 percent at 15 years, 23 percent at 20 years, and 42 percent at 24 years. In children, the risk of cancer appears to rise more sharply after the first 10 years of disease, perhaps reflecting the higher incidence of pancolitis in children. Limited involvement of the colon (i.e., proctitis) has a low risk of malignant degeneration. Malignancy developing in Crohn's disease of the colon or small bowel is less well documented, but the incidences of both small- and large-bowel malignancies are increased compared to the general population. The incidence, however, is less than in ulcerative colitis.

The development of colon carcinoma arising in the setting of IBD demonstrates important differences when compared to carcinoma arising in a noncolitic population. Clinically, many of the earlier warning signs of a colonic neoplasm (i.e., rectal bleeding, change in bowel habits) will be difficult to interpret in the setting of colitis. In colitic patients the distribution of carcinomas is more uniform throughout the colon than in noncolitic patients; in the latter the majority of carcinomas are in the rectosigmoid within reach of the sigmoidoscope. In colitis patients the tumors are more often multiple, flat, and infiltrating and appear to have a higher grade of malignancy. There is some evidence to suggest that these features may reflect the younger age at which they occur rather than the associated colitis. Further adding to the difficulty in diagnosis is the frequent occurrence of mucosal irregularities, ulcerations, and pseudopolyps, making a small carcinoma difficult to diagnose radiologically or endoscopically.

Efforts have been directed to devise effective screening procedures to detect carcinoma developing in the setting of IBD. Carcinoembryonic antigen (CEA) may be elevated nonspecifically in ulcerative colitis and therefore is of limited value. Periodic barium enemas and/or sigmoidoscopy or colonoscopy have been suggested, but interpretation is sometimes hampered by abnormalities related to the colitis itself. The addition of colonic mucosal biopsy may add a significant dimension. It was originally suggested that a generalized precancerous lesion may be present in high-risk patients with colitis who either harbor an occult malignancy or who will develop cancer. Subsequent studies of rectal biopsies in patients with long-standing colitis showed that if dysplasia was present, there was approximately a 50 percent chance that an associated malignancy was present in those patients who subsequently came to colectomy. Complicating these findings was the fact that dysplastic changes were only found in rectal biopsies 60 percent of the time, making colonoscopy with multiple biopsies desirable. In addition, in some patients not undergoing colectomy, dysplasia was not a consistent finding on subsequent biopsies. While more information is needed on the prognostic significance and reproducibility of finding dysplastic changes on mucosal biopsy, it seems prudent to examine patients with colonic IBD of greater than 8 to 10 years' duration with colonoscopy and multiple mucosal biopsies at regular intervals. The frequency of such examinations has not been established, with recommendations varying from 6 months to 2 years. If severe dysplasia is found, then confirmation at less than 6-month intervals seems prudent. While most authorities would not advise "prophylactic" colectomy in the patient with long-standing colitis, the finding of severe dysplasia may well identify a subgroup who already harbor an occult carcinoma or who are at high risk of its development. There can be no uniform recommendation for this small group of patients, but many physicians will advise colectomy in this setting.

EXTRAINTESTINAL MANIFESTATIONS OF INFLAMMATORY BOWEL DISEASE

There are a variety of nonintestinal symptoms and signs which may be associated with IBD and occur in both ulcerative colitis and Crohn's disease (Table 238-3). Since some of these manifestations may not coincide with, or may overshadow, the underlying bowel disease, they may on occasion pose difficult diagnostic problems. Their etiology is currently unknown.

Joint manifestations are common in patients with IBD (~25 percent incidence). These may range from arthralgia only to an acute arthritis with painful, swollen joints.

The nondeforming arthritis is mono- or polyarticular and often migratory. Knees, ankles, and wrists are most commonly involved, but any joint may be affected. Joint fluid, if aspirated, reveals findings of an acute arthritis without crystals or evidence of infection. Tests for specific forms of arthritis (rheumatoid factor, antinuclear antibody, and LE factor) are negative. Typically, the arthritis correlates with activity of the underlying bowel disease. Rarely, peripheral arthritis may truly antecede clinical bowel symptoms. Arthritis is more commonly found in patients with colonic than with small-bowel involvement alone (regional enteritis).

In contrast, the central arthritis or ankylosing spondylitis associated with IBD is unrelated to the activity of the underlying bowel disease. It may antedate the bowel disease by years and persist after surgical or medical remission of the disease has been achieved. Symptoms are of low backache and stiffness with eventual limitation of motion. This may be associated with sacroileitis as well. X-rays usually reveal characteristic changes. In contrast to the peripheral arthritis, there is a strong association of HLA-B27 with ankylosing spondylitis, whether or not IBD is present.

Like the peripheral arthritis *skin manifestations* are more common with colonic disease. They occur in about 15 percent of patients, and when present the severity correlates with activity of the bowel disease. *Erythema nodosum* may be seen and heals without scarring. *Pyoderma gangrenosum,* an ulcerating lesion often occurring on the trunk, is relatively painless and may heal with scarring. In the rare patient, the lesion may persist even after colectomy for ulcerative colitis. *Aphthous ulcers* resemble "canker sores" of the mouth, and in approximately 5 to 10 percent of patients they are present during periods of active disease and then resolve. Their etiology is unknown and they are treated symptomatically. *Ocular manifestations* such as episcleritis, recurrent iritis, and uveitis occur in approximately 5 percent of patients and may represent a severe manifestation of the disease. In general, their activity parallels the course of the bowel disease, and the lesions may respond dramatically when colectomy is done for other indications.

Abnormalities of *liver function* are common in IBD. In the severely ill, malnourished patient, mild abnormalities of serum aminotransferases and alkaline phosphatase are often seen and represent nonspecific focal hepatitis or fatty infiltration. Factors favoring fatty infiltration of the liver in the severely ill patient are poor nutrition and often concomitant steroid therapy. The lesion is not progressive and resolves with disease remission. *Pericholangitis* is characterized histologically by portal tract inflammation, some bile ductular proliferation, and concentric fibrosis around bile ductules. Most often, the lesion is clinically insignificant, and its sole manifestation is an elevated serum alkaline phosphatase. It is usually nonprogressive and requires no therapy. Rarely, there may be an apparent progression to cirrhosis of either the postnecrotic or biliary type. Uncommonly, patients with IBD may develop *sclerosing cholangitis* (Chap. 253), a chronic inflammation of unknown etiology involving the extrahepatic and intrahepatic bile ducts which may produce varying degrees of extrahepatic biliary obstruction. Corticosteroids and immunosuppressive therapy are not beneficial. Reversal of the disease after colectomy is an inconsistent result and should not form the sole indication for colectomy. Cholangiocarcinoma, arising in the extrahepatic biliary tree, has an increased incidence in patients with chronic ulcerative colitis. Such patients will present with extrahepatic biliary obstruction which must be distinguished from sclerosing cholangitis. Finally, *chronic active hepatitis* which may progress to *cirrhosis* may be seen in IBD, although the exact relationship between these disorders is unknown. The evaluation and therapy are similar to the disease occurring in noncolitic patients. There is no clear evidence that colectomy influences the course of this form of liver disease.

TREATMENT

In general, the treatment of ulcerative colitis and Crohn's disease shares certain common principles. Initial treatment of all forms of uncomplicated IBD is primarily medical, and the principles of medical therapy are similar. Surgery is reserved for (1) specific complications and (2) intractability of disease. There are certain important differences, however, between ulcerative colitis and Crohn's disease; namely, the response to drug therapy may differ, complications often differ, and the prognosis after surgical therapy is not the same.

ULCERATIVE COLITIS Medical therapy Once the diagnosis is established, the severity of the disease must be assessed. Mild ulcerative colitis, including ulcerative proctitis, can usually be treated on an ambulatory basis. More severe disease, especially at initial presentation, is best treated in a hospital setting. The disease can rapidly worsen, and the course of a given attack cannot be predicted at the outset. The aims of therapy are to control the inflammatory process and replace nutritional losses. A certain degree of improvement usually follows intravenous correction of fluid and electrolyte disturbances. Blood transfusions may be required in severe anemia, especially when there is continued active bleeding. Agents to control diarrhea (diphenoxylate, loperamide, codeine, anticholinergics) should be used with extreme caution for fear of precipitating colonic dilatation and toxic megacolon. The decision to institute specific nutritional replacement therapy will be determined by the nutritional status of the patient and whether a protracted clinical course can be anticipated. In the severely ill patient, even clear liquids orally may stimulate colonic activity, and it is often wise to give the patients nothing by mouth. In this setting, intravenous alimentation, either peripheral or central, has been used as interim nutritional replacement therapy (see Chap. 75). While there is no evidence that intravenous alimentation is effective as primary therapy, it is an important component of a treatment program. In the less severely ill patients able to tolerate fluids by mouth, the use of elemental oral diets may be beneficial providing supplemental nutrition with low fecal volume. While milk is not contraindicated in ulcerative colitis, diarrhea will be exacerbated if there is an associated lactase deficiency.

The principal drugs used in the therapy of ulcerative colitis are the *anti-inflammatory agents, sulfasalazine* (Azulfidine) and *adrenal corticosteroids* or ACTH. Sulfasalazine consists of a sulfonamide (sulfapyridine) moiety chemically bound to a salicylate (5-aminosalicylate); it undergoes bacterial cleavage in the colon. The liberated sulfapyridine is efficiently absorbed and largely excreted in the urine; the liberated 5-aminosalicylate believed to be the active component remains largely in the colon and is excreted in the stool. The salicylate moiety is thought to exert its action through inhibition of prostaglandin synthesis. While most physicians are familiar with the use of sulfasalazine to prevent recurrences of ulcerative colitis, it is less well appreciated that this agent is effective in the therapy of acute ulcerative colitis of mild to moderate severity. Therapeutic doses of 4 to 6 g daily are required. The drug is usually started at a dose of 500 mg bid and then increased daily or every other day by 1 g until the therapeutic dose is achieved.

In the severely ill patient who may not tolerate oral medication and for whom a more rapid time frame of therapy is often desired, initial therapy is begun with corticosteroids or ACTH. While some physicians still prefer ACTH to corticosteroids, these agents appear equally effective when given in equivalent dosages and by comparable routes of administration. The choice is one of individual preference; however, oral prednisone (45 to 60 mg daily) is often employed initially. Alternatively, intravenous ACTH may be given (40 to 60 units) over an 8-h drip infusion. In the severely ill patient, parenteral administration of corticosteroids is preferable to avoid the uncertainty of adequate oral absorption. Improvement is usually noted after 7 to 10 days of such therapy by a reduction in fever, decreased bloody diarrhea, and an improvement in appetite.

After initial improvement low-roughage oral feedings can be resumed. At this point the dose of steroids can be tapered, or if ACTH was used initially, oral prednisone at reduced dosage can be started. There is no specific schedule for tapering corticosteroids. The guiding principle, however, is that once clinical remission is achieved, there is no evidence that chronic steroid administration favorably influences the long-term outlook of the disease or that recurrences can be prevented by chronic steroid therapy. In practice, steroid therapy can be tapered and discontinued over a 2- to 3-month period after discharge. In some patients (10 to 15 percent) efforts to completely eliminate steroids may be associated with a flare of the disease, and low to moderate steroids (10 to 15 mg of prednisone daily) may be required to suppress disease activity. This should not be confused with the prophylactic administration of steroids to patients in remission, but rather represents incompletely responsive disease. Once the acutely ill patient is taking oral feedings, sulfasalazine should be added as described above in a daily dose of 2 g. Controlled trials have shown that this dose of sulfasalazine, when administered chronically to patients with ulcerative colitis, is effective in decreasing the frequency of relapses and should be continued chronically after corticosteroids have been discontinued. Patients with glucose phosphate dehydrogenase deficiency or those exhibiting severe allergic reactions to the drug unfortunately cannot be maintained on it. Patients who exhibit intolerance for the drug (headache, nausea) or mild skin allergic reactions can be "desensitized" by gradually reintroducing the drug in small doses. Sulfasalazine is discontinued for 1 to 2 weeks and then is restarted at a dose of 0.125 to 0.25 g per day for 1 week with a gradual increase by 0.125 g per week to a maintenance dose of 2 g per day.

The use of immunosuppressive therapy with drugs such as azathioprine is less well established in ulcerative colitis. As a single agent in the therapy of acute ulcerative colitis, the drug is ineffective. However, the drug may be added to the regimen at a dose of 1.5 to 2.0 mg/kg when corticosteroids fail or when the steroid dose needed to reduce inflammation is too high. It is desirable to monitor the blood count and observe the patient carefully for infection. Azathioprine may also have a limited role as a "steroid-sparing agent" in the patient with chronic ulcerative colitis who must be maintained on corticosteroids to control disease activity.

Toxic megacolon is a major complication of severe ulcerative colitis which requires rapid, intensive management best carried out jointly by the internist or gastroenterologist and surgeon. Once the diagnosis is established, prompt and vigorous use of intravenous fluids, electrolyte replacement therapy, and blood transfusions are indicated. Because of the fear of perforation and high likelihood that bacteremia and occult perforation have occurred, many physicians will institute broad-spectrum antibiotic coverage after appropriate cultures have been obtained. The patient is given nothing by mouth, and nasogastric suction is often instituted. Full intravenous corticosteroid therapy is also begun. Majority opinion favors an initial period of medical stabilization for the first 24 to 48 h. If significant objective improvement has not occurred and if perforation seems imminent, emergency colectomy should be carried out. While it is certainly true that some patients, under maximal medical therapy, may slowly improve and thus avoid colectomy, the risk of this course of action must be carefully considered. If perforation occurs, mortality rates rise sharply, approaching 50 percent in those who subsequently go on to colectomy.

At the other end of the spectrum is the patient with mild ulcerative colitis, limited to the rectum or rectosigmoid, who is managed on an ambulatory basis. Therapy is initiated with sulfasalazine, 0.5 to 1.0 g four times a day with meals. If rectal symptoms such as tenesmus are prominent, topical steroids in the form of small enemas may produce marked improvement. The equivalent of 100 mg hydrocortisone (20 mg prednisone) in 60 to 100 mL saline is used as a bedtime enema. On occasion the use of steroid foam preparations may be better tolerated in the patient with severe tenesmus. Retention enemas have been shown to deliver medication as far as the descending colon, and absorption of steroid is small (~ 10 to 20 percent). If large doses of rectal steroids are required for control, it is preferable to use oral prednisone at a moderate dosage (20 mg daily).

Psychotherapy The elements of trust and mutual understanding combined with the compassion and expertise of the physician are essential in the therapy of any chronic disease and are particularly important in the long-term management of patients with inflammatory bowel disease. Often these patients are intelligent young adults who are frequently resentful of a disease affecting them during the most productive years. Through the vigorous participation of the physician many patients are able to lead reasonably stable and productive lives. More formal psychiatric assistance may be required in the chronically ill patient, in particular children or adolescents, or in the elderly where severe depressive reactions are common. This is particularly true when colectomy is being advised and in the emotional adjustment which must be made after colectomy.

Pregnancy and ulcerative colitis While many physicians are apprehensive about the management and prognosis of ulcerative colitis in the pregnant patient, the outcome for the patient and the fetus is excellent. In general, the pregnancy is not threatened by coexistent colitis, with no increase in stillbirths or premature deliveries when compared to the general population. When patients with inactive colitis become pregnant, approximately 50 percent may have an exacerbation of their disease with some clustering of these flares during the first trimester and in the postpartum period. The therapy of ulcerative colitis during pregnancy is largely the same as in the nonpregnant patient. Sulfasalazine is used to treat mild to moderate disease since there is no evidence that the drug is harmful to the fetus or leads to increased incidence of fetal malformations. Women with inactive colitis who enter a pregnancy on maintenance sulfasalazine should be continued on the drug. Since sulfapyridine appears in breast milk, in the newborn with unconjugated hyperbilirubinemia from other causes, breast feeding should be discontinued or the drug stopped if the colitis is inactive. In most situations, however, the drug should be continued to protect the mother during the postpartum period from a relapse of disease. Corticosteroids should be used in the same dosage and for the same indications as in the nonpregnant patient.

Thus, it is clear that the patient with colitis can realistically plan to have a family. It is prudent, however, to bring active disease under control before pregnancy is undertaken to ensure the most optimal physical and emotional setting for the pregnancy. Similar conclusions apply to the management of Crohn's disease during pregnancy.

Surgical therapy Approximately 20 to 25 percent of patients with ulcerative colitis will require colectomy during the course of their disease. A major indication for colectomy is failure to respond to intensive medical management. Such patients, although not showing colonic dilatation, may fail to improve after 7 to 10 days of optimal medical therapy. Fever, persistent bloody diarrhea, and severe fatigue may persist, and consideration should be given to semielective colectomy. Elective colectomy may be performed in patients whose disease remains chronically active and who require continuous corticosteroid administration. Such patients are at risk of developing the complications of chronic steroid therapy. After colectomy these patients often feel more energetic and usually gain back weight to their preillness level. As discussed above the patient with long-standing colitis is at high risk for colonic cancer. While most authorities do not advise "prophylactic" colectomy in the patient with quiescent disease, the finding of marked dysplasia on colonoscopic biopsies done as a part of a surveillance program should make the physician think seriously about advising colectomy.

The decision to advise colectomy in other than emergency circumstances is difficult for both patient and physician. Many patients have an understandable reluctance to undergo colectomy and have difficulty in conceptualizing life with an ileostomy. In most metropolitan centers there are ileostomy groups who visit patients preoperatively and can provide answers to many practical questions. It is also desirable for the patient to be visited by a nurse familiar with stoma care to instruct the patient on the practical aspects of handling the ileostomy.

While total proctocolectomy with permanent ileostomy is the procedure of choice for almost all patients undergoing colectomy, several alternative approaches have been suggested. The *continent ileostomy* is an ileal loop reservoir fashioned under the skin with a nipple valve to prevent spilling of ileal contents. Ileal effluent collects in this reservoir which must be emptied with a soft rubber catheter. Only a small stoma is externally visible, thus eliminating an external ileostomy appliance. Problems with this procedure include a failure of continence, irritation of the mucosa of the ileal reservoir from stasis ("pouchitis"), and bacterial overgrowth which may lead to mild malabsorption. Repeat operations are common, and this procedure should only be done by skilled surgeons familiar with the technique. *Ileorectal anastomosis* with *mucosal stripping* of the rectal segment is sometimes done in children who require colectomy. Newer forms of surgical therapy include ileoanal anastomosis with internal reservoirs thus preserving sphincteric function. These approaches are recent and not generally available.

CROHN'S DISEASE The medical management of colonic Crohn's disease is similar in most respects to that of ulcerative colitis. In a multicenter study (National Cooperative Crohn's Disease Study) sulfasalazine was shown to be effective in the therapy of active colonic disease. Corticosteroids also were efficacious but less so than with small-bowel involvement. The indications and dosages of these medications are similar to those for ulcerative colitis. Since in Crohn's disease, intraabdominal sepsis can result from fistula or abscess formation, corticosteroids must be used with caution and constant attention is required to detect evidence of sepsis, which can be masked by these agents. In general, the disease is less explosive in onset, and although toxic dilatation and perforation can occur, they are less common than in ulcerative colitis. The principles of management are the same. Because of the indolent nature of the disease, the response to therapy is often less complete than in ulcerative colitis, and the disease tends to progress despite apparent clinical inactivity. It may be more difficult to achieve a clinical remission and to withdraw steroids completely. As in ulcerative colitis, controlled studies have shown no benefit to continuing steroids after remission since the frequency of recurrence is not altered by prophylactic steroid therapy. Disappointingly, sulfasalazine did not decrease recurrence rates in Crohn's disease.

While response to therapy of the initial attack of Crohn's colitis may be satisfactory, many patients continue to have persistently active disease. This may express itself as progressive weight loss, diarrhea, and deterioration of general health. Perianal disease with predominantly left-sided colonic involvement (fistula formation and perirectal abscesses) may constitute a recurrent problem. In one controlled study, *metronidazole* (20 mg/kg per day in divided dosage) resulted in marked improvement in 10 of 18 patients with chronic perineal fistulas associated with Crohn's disease. It is not clear whether the drug is active because of its antibacterial properties or through another mechanism. It is possible that this drug may prove to be of value in the therapy of the perineal complications of Crohn's disease before surgical therapy is attempted. The role of immunosuppressive therapy such as azathioprine has been controversial in Crohn's disease. The multicenter United States study (National Cooperative Study) found azathioprine to be ineffective as a single agent in the therapy of active Crohn's disease. Yet there have been reports of dramatic improvement in a small percentage of patients when azathioprine (1.5 to 2 mg/kg) is added to a maximal program in the nonresponding patient. Some investigators have found 6-mercaptopurine (the active metabolite of azathioprine) effective in controlling disease activity when added to corticosteroids and sulfasalazine. However, a beneficial response may take 6 to 8 months in some patients.

The management of Crohn's disease of the small intestine (regional enteritis) is similar to that for colonic Crohn's disease, and as noted many patients have concomitant small and large bowel disease. Several additional considerations are pertinent, however. *Intestinal obstruction* is not uncommonly a presenting feature with ileal involvement. Initially, this may be secondary to acute inflammation and will respond to corticosteroids. With recurrent involvement and the development of fibrosis, steroid therapy is less effective and surgical decompression is required. *Nutritional problems* often are more severe with involvement of the small intestine than with colonic involvement alone. Added to the general catabolic nature of the disease may be loss of absorptive surface which may result from progressive involvement or because of surgical resection. Refinements in the technique of parenteral alimentation have made it possible to provide a patient's total daily caloric intake intravenously for a period of weeks or even months (see Chap. 75). Parenteral alimentation has been employed with increasing frequency in the severely ill patient as a means of placing the gastrointestinal tract "at rest" and in preparing the malnourished patient for surgery. With this approach the disease may become quiescent, and the drainage from fistulas may decrease. However, disease activity frequently recurs when oral feedings are resumed. On occasion, prolonged intravenous alimentation, administered at home, may be required when oral feedings are not effective or in children exhibiting severe growth failure associated with Crohn's disease. Most often it is possible to design a dietary program of oral supplementation to nourish the patient adequately.

In patients with extensive small-bowel involvement or in those with a short bowel resulting from extensive intestinal resection, supplementation of electrolytes, minerals, and vitamins will be required. Extensive ileal disease or resection often results in diarrhea induced by bile salts and in malabsorption; cholestyramine may be needed to control the diarrhea and medium-chain triglycerides added to reduce fat malabsorption (see Chap. 237). In patients with stenotic segments of intestine, a low-residue (low-fiber) diet should be recommended. A lactose-free diet should be instituted if there is an associated lactase deficiency. Other dietary modifications have not been shown to have any beneficial effect on the primary disease process. Patients should be encouraged to eat a nutritious, appealing diet of their own choosing. *Surgical therapy* is generally reserved for the complications of Crohn's disease rather than as a primary form of therapy. In contrast to ulcerative colitis, more patients with Crohn's disease will require surgery in the chronic management of the disease. Approximately 70 percent of patients will require at least one operation during the course of their disease. Although each case and situation must be individualized, in general, surgery may be required (1) for persistent or fixed bowel narrowing or obstruction; (2) for symptomatic fistula formation to the bladder, vagina, or skin; (3) for persistent anal fistulas or abscesses; and (4) for intraabdominal abscesses, toxic dilatation of the colon, or perforation. In contrast to ulcerative colitis, where colectomy is curative, in Crohn's disease surgical resection of the small or large intestine is followed by a high rate of recurrence. With resection of segments of small bowel or ileum and reanastomosis a recurrence rate of 50 to 75 percent over a 5-year period is not unusual. Recurrence of disease is invariably proximal to the created anastomosis. When total colectomy and ileostomy are performed for Crohn's disease of the colon without significant small-intestinal involvement, recurrence rates are lower, varying from 10 to 30 percent. Despite these recurrences, most patients do not develop a short bowel syndrome and usually can expect significant improvement. Faced with the possibility of recurrent disease many physicians are reluctant to advise surgery in Crohn's disease, except for the type of clear-cut complications described above. Alternatively, patients with persistently active disease may require chronic maintenance on unacceptably high levels of corticosteroids and with the appreciable risk of steroid side effects. Just as a failure of medical therapy should lead to colectomy in ulcerative colitis, it should be the conclusion in the patient with Crohn's colitis without major small-bowel involvement. While in this setting there is also a definite rate of recurrence, such recurrences are often not disabling. When extensive small-bowel disease is present, surgical therapy is often not feasible and should only be reserved for specific disease complications.

The therapy of Crohn's disease in children presents special problems since normal growth and development may be retarded in the presence of active disease. In addition to conventional drug therapy, intensive nutritional therapy or the judicious use of surgery may be required.

PROGNOSIS

The overall prognosis of IBD has been favorably affected by the use of corticosteroids and sulfasalazine, as well as by supportive techniques such as intravenous alimentation. In *acute* ulcerative colitis these therapeutic modalities can result in a remission in almost 90 percent of patients. The mortality of an initial acute attack is approximately 5 percent. Poor prognostic factors and an increased mortality rate are likely when there is total colonic involvement, when the onset occurs over age 60, and when toxic megacolon develops.

The long-term prognosis of *chronic* ulcerative colitis is more difficult to assess due to the variable and intermittent nature of the disease and improvements in therapy. Left-sided colitis and ulcerative proctitis have a very favorable prognosis and probably no increase in mortality; similarly the long-term prognosis for extensive colitis has improved greatly. Older studies suggested a poor prognosis for extensive colitis, with less than 50 percent of patients surviving 15 years after onset. More recent observations (longest follow-up 11 years) show a 10-year mortality rate of between 5 and 10 percent for severe first attacks (excluding toxic megacolon). Approximately 75 percent of patients will experience relapses, and 20 to 25 percent will require colectomy. The problem of carcinoma developing in the setting of long-standing chronic ulcerative colitis is an important factor in determining the long-term prognosis of ulcerative colitis. As discussed above, periodic surveillance with colonoscopy and multiple biopsies to detect dysplastic changes is indicated to detect a high-risk group for which to advise colectomy.

The prognosis for Crohn's disease is not as favorable as for ulcerative colitis. An exception is *acute regional enteritis,* often discovered during laparotomy for suspected appendicitis; this has an excellent prognosis. More than two-thirds of such patients may show no subsequent evidence of regional enteritis, and this form of acute ileitis may well be due to yersinia infection (see above). Prevailing surgical opinion favors a conservative approach in this situation, and in most instances operative resection is not advised.

In the majority of patients with Crohn's disease the course is chronic and intermittent regardless of the site of involvement. The disease responds less well to medical therapy with time, and over two-thirds of patients develop complications requiring surgery at some point in their disease. In contrast to ulcerative colitis, where mortality appears greatest early in the disease, in Crohn's disease the mortality rate increases with the duration of the disease, and probably ranges from 5 to 10 percent. Most deaths occur from peritonitis and sepsis. As indicated above, following surgery patients with Crohn's disease often have recurrence and relapses. Nevertheless, the therapy of Crohn's disease will result in reasonably stable and productive lives for most Crohn's disease patients.

REFERENCES

General

KIRSNER JB, SHORTER RG (eds): *Inflammatory Bowel Disease*, 2d ed. Philadelphia, Lea & Febiger, 1980

———, ———: Recent developments in "nonspecific" inflammatory bowel disease. N Engl J Med 306:775, 837, 1982

SLEISENGER MH, FORDTRAN JS (eds): *Gastrointestinal Diseases*, 2d ed. Philadelphia, Saunders, 1978

Etiology and diagnostic aspects

BEEKEN WL: Transmissible agents in inflammatory bowel disease. Med Clin North Am 64:1031, 1980

BLASER MJ, RELLER LB: *Campylobacter* enteritis. N Engl J Med 305:1444, 1981

CHAPMAN RW et al: Serum antibodies, ulcerative colitis, and sclerosing cholangitis. Gut 27:86, 1986

GOODMAN MJ et al: The usefulness of rectal biopsy in inflammatory bowel disease. Gastroenterology 72:952, 1977

GREENSTEIN AJ et al: The extraintestinal complications of ulcerative colitis and Crohn's disease: A study of 700 patients. Medicine 55:401, 1976

JESS P: Acute terminal ileitis: A review of recent literature on the relationship to Crohn's disease. Scand J Gastroenterol 16:321, 1981

QUINN TC et al: *Chlamydia trachomatis* proctitis. N Engl J Med 305:195, 1981

TRNKA YM, LAMONT JT: Association of *Clostridium difficile* toxin with symptomatic relapse of chronic inflammatory bowel disease. Gastroenterology 80:693, 1981

VAN TRAPPEN G et al: *Yersinia enteritis* and enterocolitis: Gastroenterological aspects. Gastroenterology 72:220, 1977

Therapy of inflammatory bowel disease

AZAD KHAN AK et al: Optimum dose of sulphasalazine for maintenance treatment in ulcerative colitis. Gut 12:232, 1980

BERNSTEIN LH et al: Healing of perineal Crohn's disease with metronidazole. Gastroenterology 79:357, 1980

FARMER RG et al: Long-term follow-up of patients with Crohn's disease. Relationship between clinical pattern and prognosis. Gastroenterology 88:1818, 1985

GREENSTEEN AJ et al: Reoperation and recurrence in Crohn's colitis and ileocolitis. N Engl J Med 293:658, 1975

GYDE SN et al: Malignancy in Crohn's disease. Gut 21:1024, 1980

KELTS DG et al: Nutritional basis of growth failure in children and adolescents with Crohn's disease. Gastroenterology 76:720, 1979

LENNARD JONES JE et al: Cancer in colitis: Assessment of the individual risk by clinical and histological criteria. Gastroenterology 73:1280, 1977

LOCK MR et al: Recurrence and reoperation for Crohn's disease. N Engl J Med 304:1586, 1981

PEPPERCORN MA: Sulfasalazine. Ann Intern Med 3:377, 1984

PRESENT DH et al: Treatment of Crohn's disease with 6-mercaptopurine. N Engl J Med 302:981, 1980

RIDDELL RH et al: Dysplasia in inflammatory bowel disease. Hum Pathol 14:931, 1983

SUMMERS RW et al: National cooperative Crohn's disease study: Results of drug treatment. Gastroenterology 77:849, 1979

URSING B et al: A comparative study of metronidazole and sulfasalazine for active Crohn's disease. The Cooperative Crohn's Disease Study in Sweden. Gastroenterology 83:550, 1982

239 DISEASES OF THE SMALL AND LARGE INTESTINE

J. THOMAS LaMONT / KURT J. ISSELBACHER

SYMPTOMS OF INTESTINAL DISEASE

SYMPTOMS OF DISEASES OF THE SMALL INTESTINE The major clinical manifestations of small-bowel disease are *motility disturbances*, abdominal *pain* and *distention*, gastrointestinal *bleeding*, and *malabsorption*.

An alteration in the normal propulsive activity of the small intestine is a common manifestation of a variety of diseases. The presentation may be one of decreased motility, such as paralytic ileus resulting from metabolic disturbance or peritonitis, or intestinal obstruction caused by tumors, adhesions, volvulus, or intussusception (Chap. 240). Diarrhea frequently accompanies small-bowel disease (Chap. 36) resulting from direct involvement of the mucosa by inflammatory or infiltrative lesions (sprue, regional enteritis). The associated malabsorption of fat and bile salts is an important factor in the pathogenesis of diarrhea in these conditions (Chaps. 36 and 237).

Abdominal pain due to small-intestinal disease is usually periumbilical or supraumbilical and often poorly localized. With obstruction, pain is classically described as intermittent or colicky. Visceral pain arises from distention or stretching of the intestinal wall, or from inflammation of the overlying parietal peritoneum. As the intestine becomes progressively dilated with loss of muscular tone, the colicky nature of the pain may become less apparent. Acute inflammation of the small intestine which involves the visceral or parietal peritoneum is associated with steady, aching pain, usually located directly over the inflamed area, and may be accompanied by guarding and rebound tenderness if the parietal peritoneum is involved. *Gastrointestinal bleeding* due to small-bowel disease may be detected as occult bleeding or, less commonly, brisk hemorrhage. In general, bleeding from the stomach or small intestine causes black or tarry stool (melena), while bleeding from the colon causes passage of red blood or clots. Obviously, the appearance of blood in the stool depends not only on site of bleeding but also on the rate of the hemorrhage and the rapidity of transit; thus localization of the bleeding site by stool appearance alone may be misleading.

An important clue to the presence of small-bowel disease is the demonstration of malabsorption of fat. With extensive mucosal damage or lymphatic obstruction, the presenting symptoms may relate to any of the features of a malabsorption syndrome or protein-losing enteropathy (Chap. 237) and should direct attention to the small intestine.

SYMPTOMS OF COLONIC DISEASE The major symptoms of colonic disease are *alteration in bowel habit, rectal bleeding*, and *pain*. Alteration in bowel habit implies a change from previous patterns of defecation; hence a detailed history is important. Most normal individuals have one to three movements of well-formed stools each day. *Diarrhea* means the passage of watery or loose stools usually with increased frequency, while *constipation* implies infrequent passage of hard, dry stools; *obstipation* is the absence of spontaneous bowel movements. A persistent change in bowel habit, particularly in older individuals with no previous irregularity, is usually an important early symptom of organic disease of the colon and should never be labeled *functional* unless a thorough diagnostic evaluation is negative. The appearance of the stool may also provide important diagnostic clues. Blood coating the exterior of a formed stool implies a lesion in the anal canal or rectum, while blood admixed with the feces indicates a bleeding source higher in the colon. Brisk hemorrhage from the colon or distal small intestine results in passage of fresh blood, called *hematochezia*. This may appear as fresh blood and clots if the lesion is in the left colon, or darker maroon-colored blood if the bleeding source is in the right colon.

Pain resulting from colonic disease is usually localized to either of the lower abdominal quadrants, as opposed to pain of small-intestinal origin, which is localized to the periumbilical area or higher. Rectal pain is often felt deep in the pelvis, while pain in the anal canal is accurately localized to the perineum. The mechanisms of colonic pain are similar to those in other intestinal viscera (see Chap. 5). Distention from gas or fluid causes crampy or colicky pain from stretching of the muscle layers and resulting contraction or spasm. Pain of this type is often relieved by passage of flatus or stool. Pain may also result if the colonic wall is inflamed or infiltrated by tumor. Acute colonic inflammation which involves the visceral or parietal peritoneum produces sharply localized pain, which may be accompanied by abdominal guarding and rebound tenderness. An important symptom of rectal disease is *tenesmus,* or painful straining at stool, with a sensation of incomplete emptying after defecation. This symptom can be caused by retention of stool in the rectum, by tumors of the rectum which simulate retained stools, or by colonic inflammation.

DIAGNOSTIC PROCEDURES

PHYSICAL EXAMINATION Careful *examination* of the abdomen may disclose a mass or fistula associated with inflammatory or neoplastic disease, localized tenderness, or abdominal distention resulting from ileus or intestinal obstruction. The physical examination and findings in the patient with acute abdominal pain are discussed in Chap. 5.

Thorough examination may also reveal extraintestinal findings associated with small-intestinal diseases. Thus buccal pigmentation or telangiectasia may indicate coexistent small-bowel polyposis or telangiectasia and may clarify episodes of abdominal pain or chronic bleeding. Similarly, evidence of iritis, arthritis, or erythema nodosum may suggest the presence of inflammatory bowel disease.

Perhaps the most important part of the physical examination in the diagnosis of colonic diseases is the *digital rectal examination.* This procedure should never be omitted for reasons of modesty or fear of embarrassment because it is essential in the diagnosis of perianal, sphincteric, and ampullary lesions; prostatic and uterine abnormalities; and even small rectal masses. A metastatic tumor may be felt in the perirectal tissues as a shelf-like deformity (Blumer's shelf), especially anteriorly above the prostate. The fecal material on the glove should be immediately tested with guaiac-impregnated cards for occult blood. Approximately one-half of all rectal carcinomas lie within reach of the index finger, and omission of the rectal examination may delay diagnosis and worsen the prognosis.

STOOL EXAMINATION Abnormal stools constitute important objective evidence of colonic disease. Stools should be examined by the physician as soon as possible after defecation for the presence of visible blood on the surface or within the specimen. A small sample should be tested for occult blood. Microscopic examination of fresh stool is important in the diagnosis of parasitic diseases, particularly in amoebic colitis when motile trophozoites can be seen in fresh, warm stool suspensions. Stool suspensions can also be stained with a drop of methylene blue for polymorphonuclear leukocytes, which indicate the presence of an acute inflammatory exudate characteristic of ulcerative colitis, amoebic colitis, and bacillary dysentery. Fixed and stained slides of stool may also reveal amoebas and other parasites, while stool culture is essential for the diagnosis of bacillary dysentery. Sudan III stain of stool is a useful screening test for steatorrhea.

BARIUM STUDIES The considerable length of the small intestine (some 12 to 22 ft in the adult) makes *radiologic studies* of the small bowel of prime importance and usually forms the basis for the diagnosis of small-bowel diseases. *Small-bowel x-rays* are not usually part of a routine upper gastrointestinal series and must be specifically requested. In view of the length of the small bowel and wide variations in transit time, it is essential to provide the radiologist with as much information as possible, since the precise nature of the problem may determine various technical aspects of the examination. Enteroclysis is a specialized small-bowel barium study during which barium is infused rapidly via a nasogastric tube into the jejunum. This technique allows distention of bowel loops and rapid filling of the entire small intestine, thus avoiding the problems of inadequate distention and poor transit sometimes encountered in routine small-bowel barium studies. Enteroclysis is indicated in patients with suspected small-bowel lesions not visualized by ordinary barium studies.

Barium enema is an extremely accurate diagnostic tool for the identification of structural abnormalities of the colon. A careful study in a well-prepared patient can demonstrate mucosal lesions as small as 0.5 cm. For high-quality resolution of subtle lesions, such as small polyps or early changes of ulcerative colitis, an air-contrast barium enema is useful. In this study the mucosa is outlined by a thin coat of barium, after which air is injected to enhance contrast and outline small lesions. The combined use of the digital examination, stool guaiac test, proctosigmoidoscopy, and barium enema will identify most colonic lesions. However, barium enema does occasionally miss significant tumors or mucosal inflammation. Colonoscopy is often used to complement barium studies or to follow up suspected lesions seen by barium enema. Colonoscopy provides the additional opportunity to biopsy suspicious lesions and to remove smaller polyps.

SIGMOIDOSCOPY Contrary to the general impression, the technique of sigmoidoscopy is not difficult to master, and with practice the discomfort to the patient is minimal. The availability of flexible fiberoptic sigmoidoscopes now makes it possible to examine the lower 40 to 60 cm of the colon, compared to the 25-cm limit of the rigid sigmoidoscope. Flexible sigmoidoscopy is generally less painful than rigid sigmoidoscopy. Because approximately half of all colorectal neoplasms lie in the distal 50 cm of the bowel, sigmoidoscopy is an important diagnostic tool. It should be stressed that a rectal carcinoma can be missed on routine barium enema yet easily visualized and biopsied through the sigmoidoscope. Furthermore, the earliest changes of ulcerative colitis may not be demonstrated radiographically but may be obvious through the sigmoidoscope. Rectal biopsy is easily and painlessly accomplished through the instrument and is associated with minimal morbidity except in the presence of bleeding disorders.

COLONOSCOPY See Chap. 233.

MESENTERIC ANGIOGRAPHY Angiography is helpful in the diagnosis of two conditions: intestinal ischemia and gastrointestinal hemorrhage. Patients suspected of having acute intestinal ischemia from arterial embolus as well as chronic ischemia (intestinal angina) should undergo angiography to locate the site of blockage. Angiography is also very helpful in some patients with acute gastrointestinal blood loss. The success of this technique is related to the rate of blood loss, being most successful when bleeding exceeds 0.5 mL/min.

RADIONUCLIDE BLEEDING SCAN Bleeding from the small or large bowel can be localized in certain circumstances by radionuclide scanning of the abdomen after intravenous injection of technetium 99m sulfur colloid or autologous red cells labeled with the same agent (Fig. 239-1). If the patient is bleeding at a rate of 0.1 to 0.5 mL/min or greater, the location of radioactivity in the abdomen may indicate the source of bleeding. This diagnostic approach usually requires confirmation by another diagnostic modality such as angiography or endoscopy. The radionuclide bleeding scan is noninvasive, a particular advantage in older patients with bleeding from the small bowel or colon. The bleeding scan is not recommended in patients with suspected bleeding from the esophagus, stomach, or duodenum, who are best studied by upper endoscopy.

DISORDERS OF INTESTINAL MOTILITY

A major function of the intestinal tract is to propel the intestinal contents (food, secretions, chyme, feces) from stomach toward anus. Abnormalities of motility comprise the most common intestinal diseases: diverticulosis, megacolon, constipation, and irritable bowel syndrome. Although these conditions share a common abnormality, i.e., dysmotility, their clinical features are quite diverse.

DIVERTICULOSIS Diverticula may be either congenital or acquired and may affect either the small or large intestine. Congenital diverticula are herniations of the entire thickness of intestinal wall, while the more common acquired diverticula consist of herniations of the mucosa through the muscularis, generally at the site of a nutrient artery.

Small-intestinal diverticula Diverticula may occur in any portion of the small intestine; however, with the exception of Meckel's diverticulum, the most common locations are in the duodenum and jejunum. Most often diverticula are asymptomatic and discovered incidentally on upper gastrointestinal x-rays. On occasion, however, they may cause symptoms either because of their anatomic proximity to other structures or rarely from inflammation or bleeding.

Duodenal diverticula arise singly from the medial surface of the second portion of the duodenum. In most patients, they cause no symptoms. Rarely, they may present as acute diverticulitis with abdominal pain, fever, gastrointestinal bleeding or, most rarely, perforation. Adjacent structures, such as the bile or pancreatic ducts, may become involved; cases of common-duct obstruction and pancreatitis have been reported. Jejunal diverticula, while less common, may also be the site of acute inflammation, bleeding, or perforation with resulting abscess or peritonitis.

Multiple jejunal diverticula may be associated with a malabsorption syndrome related to bacterial overgrowth within the diverticula, similar to other situations where intestinal stasis (i.e., blind loops) permits bacterial proliferation. The consequences of bacterial proliferation with resultant mucosal damage, deconjugation of bile salts, and vitamin B_{12} malabsorption are discussed in Chap. 237.

Meckel's diverticulum, a persistent omphalomesenteric duct, is the most frequent congenital anomaly of the digestive tract, occurring in approximately 2 percent of autopsied adults. The diverticulum is wide-mouthed, about 5 cm long, and arises from the antimesenteric border of the ileum, usually within 100 cm of the ileocecal valve. The sac may be lined with normal ileal mucosa (approximately 50 percent) or contain gastric, duodenal, pancreatic, or colonic mucosa. While rarely symptomatic after age 5, Meckel's diverticulum may produce hemorrhage, inflammation, and obstruction in children and teenagers.

Hemorrhage occurs almost exclusively before age 10 and invariably results from peptic ulceration of ileal mucosa adjacent to a Meckel's diverticulum lined with gastric mucosa. The diagnosis may be established by isotope scanning of the abdomen after injection of technetium, which is taken up by the ectopic gastric mucosa in the diverticulum. False-negative and false-positive Meckel's scans are not uncommon; thus other clinical and laboratory features must be carefully assessed before recommending surgery. In older children and young adults inflammation of the diverticulum may mimic acute appendicitis. Mechanical obstruction may also occur if the diverticulum intussuscepts into the lumen of the bowel or twists on a fibrous remnant of the omphalomesenteric duct which extends from the diverticulum to the abdominal wall. The treatment of any of these complications of Meckel's diverticulum is surgical excision.

Colonic diverticula Diverticula of the colon are herniations or saclike protrusions of the mucosa through the muscularis, at the point where a nutrient artery penetrates the muscularis. Diverticula occur most commonly in the sigmoid colon and decrease in frequency in the proximal colon. They increase with age, and the incidence ranges between 20 and 50 percent in western populations over age 50. The exact mechanism for their formation is unknown but may be related to an increase in intraluminal pressure. Thickening of the muscle coat of the colon in most patients with diverticula suggests that herniations of mucosa are caused by increased pressure produced by colonic muscle contractions. The rarity of colonic diverticula in underdeveloped nations in contrast to their frequent occurrence in western countries has led to the speculation that diverticula result from the highly refined western diet, which is deficient in dietary fiber or roughage. It is proposed that such diets result in decreased fecal bulk, narrowing of the colon, and an increase in intraluminal pressure in order to move the smaller fecal mass. The role of dietary fiber in the etiology and treatment of diverticular disease remains to be determined.

Colonic diverticula are usually asymptomatic and are an incidental finding on barium enema performed for other reasons. The major complications of inflammation, both acute and chronic, and hemorrhage occur in only a small percentage of individuals with diverticulosis. Since diverticulosis is quite common in older patients, one must avoid the temptation of attributing symptoms to the diverticula unless other conditions, especially colonic neoplasm, have been excluded.

FIGURE 239-1 *Radionuclide bleeding scan using intravenous injection of technetium-labeled autologous red cells. Ten minutes after injection, a blush appears in the right abdomen over the cecum (arrow). Thirty minutes after injection, the blush has increased in intensity. The cardiac blood pool is noted at the top. Surgery revealed a bleeding diverticulum in the cecum.*

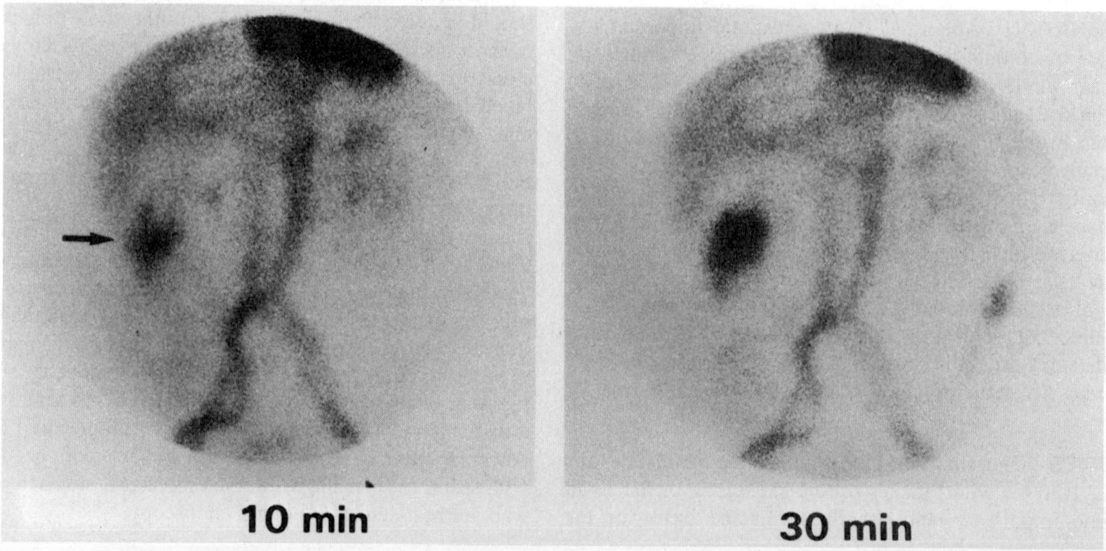

Diverticulitis Inflammation can occur in or around the diverticular sac. The cause of diverticulitis is probably mechanical, related to retention in the diverticula of undigested food residues and bacteria, which may form a hard mass called a *fecalith*. This compromises the blood supply to the thin-walled sac (made up solely of mucosa and serosa) and renders it susceptible to invasion by colonic bacteria. The inflammatory process may vary from a small intramural or pericolic abscess to generalized peritonitis. Some attacks are accompanied by minimal symptoms and seem to heal spontaneously. Studies of resected specimens indicate that most perforations of the diverticular sac are small and result in inflammation of the sac itself and the adjacent serosal surface. Diverticulitis occurs more often in men than women, and three times as often in the left as in the right colon. This suggests that diverticulitis may be related to the higher intraluminal pressures and the more solid fecal material in the sigmoid and descending colon.

Acute diverticulitis is a disease of variable severity characterized by fever, lower abdominal pain, made worse by defecation, and signs of peritoneal irritation—muscle spasm, guarding, rebound tenderness. Rectal examination may reveal a tender mass if the area of inflammation is close to the rectum. Although constipation may not have been noted prior to the onset of the illness, the inflammation around the colon often results in some degree of constipation. Rectal bleeding, usually microscopic, is noted in 25 percent of cases; it is rarely massive. Polymorphonuclear leukocytosis is common. Complications include free perforation, which results in acute peritonitis, sepsis, and shock, particularly in the elderly. The perforation may be walled off by adherent omentum or neighboring structures such as the bladder or small bowel. Abscess formation or fistulas then occur as the inflammatory mass burrows into other organs. Severe pericolitis may cause a dense, fibrous reaction or stricture around the bowel which can be associated with colonic obstruction.

DIFFERENTIAL DIAGNOSIS In the less acute situation differential diagnosis is principally that of a neoplasm in the area of the diverticulosis. Sigmoidoscopy or colonoscopy may show an acutely inflamed mucosa over an apparent extrinsic mass; passing the instrument through the contracted lumen is usually impossible. During the acute phase of diverticulitis, barium enema may be hazardous, since contrast material under pressure may lead to rupture of an inflamed diverticulum and convert a walled-off inflammatory lesion to a free perforation. The examination is usually safe after adequate treatment and healing of the diverticulitis. The radiologic findings on barium enema suggestive of diverticulitis are leakage of barium from a diverticular sac, stricture formation, and the presence of a pericolic inflammatory mass. In many patients, the distortion caused by inflammation prevents a clear distinction between cancer and diverticulitis; surgical excision may be required for accurate diagnosis.

TREATMENT For the mild case without signs of perforation, treatment consists of bed rest, stool softeners, liquid diet, and a wide-spectrum antibiotic such as tetracycline or ampicillin. Repeated attacks of diverticulitis in the same area generally require surgical resection. Severe attacks with acute peritoneal signs, suspected abscess, or perforation require intravenous antibiotics directed against gram-negative anaerobic bacteria, followed by surgical drainage or resection. The usual procedure is a diverting colostomy with resection of the involved colon; reanastomosis is then performed at a second operation.

Painful diverticular disease without diverticulitis Some patients with diverticulosis develop recurrent left lower quadrant colicky pain without clinical or pathologic evidence of acute diverticulitis. They often have bouts of alternating constipation and diarrhea, and the pain may be relieved by defecation or passage of flatus. These features suggest the coexistence of the irritable bowel syndrome (see below). Examination during a bout of pain reveals tenderness of the sigmoid colon, but signs of peritoneal inflammation such as rebound tenderness, muscle guarding, fever, and leukocytosis are absent. Barium enema shows typical diverticula without evidence of inflammation and stricture, plus a ''sawtooth'' irregularity of the lumen reflecting muscle hypertrophy and spasm. In some patients the pain is severe enough to warrant observation in a hospital and restriction of food since feeding aggravates the pain by causing colonic contraction. Anticholinergics, which reduce sigmoid contractions, and mild sedation are usually all that is required. After recovery the patient should be started on a high-residue diet or given a bulk laxative such as hemicellulose, unprocessed bran, or psyllium extract. Surgical excision is usually not indicated unless acute diverticulitis or its complications occur.

Hemorrhage from diverticula Massive hemorrhage from colonic diverticula is one of the commonest causes of hematochezia in patients over age 60. This complication of diverticulosis is caused by erosion of a vessel by a fecalith within the diverticular sac. The bleeding is painless and not accompanied by signs or symptoms of diverticulitis. Most cases of mild or moderate hemorrhage stop spontaneously with bed rest and blood transfusion. Localization of bleeding can be obtained by bleeding scan or angiography. In patients with severe hemorrhage mesenteric angiography can be both diagnostic in localizing the bleeding site and therapeutic since vasoconstrictive drugs or artificial blood clot infused intraarterially can effectively control hemorrhage. The angiographer can direct the surgeon to the area of bleeding if surgery is required for continued or recurrent bleeding. The location of bleeding diverticula demonstrated at angiography on several series has been more commonly in the right colon, particularly the ascending colon, in contrast to the sigmoid colon, where diverticula are more numerous.

MEGACOLON Megacolon, or giant colon, is characterized by massive distention of the colon usually accompanied by severe constipation or obstipation. This condition can be either congenital or acquired and is seen in all age groups. Acute toxic megacolon is a severe complication of chronic ulcerative colitis (see Chap. 238).

Aganglionic megacolon (Hirschsprung's disease) This is a congenital disorder which becomes manifest in early infancy, occurring more frequently in males, and is often familial. These infants have massive abdominal distention, absent bowel movements, and impaired nutrition due to chronic obstruction of the colon. In some individuals with less severe symptoms the disease may not be diagnosed until adolescence or early adulthood. The inability to defecate is caused by the absence of ganglion cells (Meissner's and Auerbach's plexuses) in a small segment of the distal colon, usually near the anus. This aganglionic segment is unable to relax to permit passage of stool, causing the normal colon proximal to it to become greatly dilated. On rectal examination the ampulla is empty of feces and the anal sphincter is normal. Barium enema reveals a narrowed segment in the rectosigmoid area, with massive dilatation above. Diagnosis is made by full-thickness surgical biopsy under anesthesia and demonstration of absent ganglion cells in the diseased segment. In most patients the aganglionic segment is in the rectosigmoid colon; in rare instances the lesion may involve more proximal bowel or even the entire colon. The treatment of choice is surgery which restores normal defecation. The most effective operation is a pull-through procedure in which normally innervated colon is anastomosed to the distal rectum just above the internal sphincter, thus bypassing the contracted aganglionic segment.

Chronic idiopathic megacolon This condition, also called *psychogenic megacolon,* has its onset later in childhood, usually at the time toilet training begins. It is characterized by severe chronic constipation and distention, and in contrast to Hirschsprung's disease, digital examination reveals the rectal ampulla to be invariably distended with feces. Barium enema shows the entire colon to be distended with stools, no narrowed segment is seen, and rectal biopsy discloses the normal complement of ganglion cells in Auerbach's plexus. Treatment is based on education in normal bowel habits, but a long course of enemas or large doses of mineral oil may be required until the patient acquires more normal bowel movements.

Acquired megacolon In Central and South America infection with *Trypanosoma cruzi* (Chagas' disease) can result in destruction of the ganglion cells of the colon, producing a clinical picture similar to congenital megacolon, except that the onset is in adult life rather than childhood. A number of other diseases are associated with megacolon in adults. Patients with schizophrenia or depression, particularly institutionalized patients, may have obstipation and massive colonic dilatation. Severe neurologic disorders including cerebral atrophy, spinal cord injury, and parkinsonism may also cause megacolon. Myxedema, infiltrative diseases such as amyloidosis, and scleroderma can also reduce colonic motility and produce marked colonic distention. Narcotic drugs, particularly morphine and codeine, can cause severe constipation, especially when administered to bedridden patients. Digital rectal examination of adults with acquired megacolon reveals a rectum distended with feces, as opposed to the empty rectum in aganglionic megacolon. Treatment is aimed at the underlying disease as well as the careful use of enemas and cathartics.

INTESTINAL PSEUDOOBSTRUCTION Intestinal pseudoobstruction is an acute or chronic motility disorder characterized by distention or dilatation of the small and large intestine. Abdominal pain, nausea, and vomiting may lead to diagnostic confusion with mechanical obstruction, but as the name of this condition implies, the underlying cause is not obstruction but rather a severe dysmotility resulting in distention. Pseudoobstruction may be primary or secondary and acute or chronic. In primary or idiopathic pseudoobstruction no other contributing condition can be identified, and the motility disorder is attributed to abnormalities of sympathetic innervation or of the muscle layers of the intestine. Secondary pseudoobstruction may result from scleroderma, diabetes, amyloidosis, neurologic diseases, drugs, or sepsis.

Chronic or intermittent secondary pseudoobstruction Numerous medical conditions can cause chronic dilatation of the large and small bowel. Some of these may involve the intestinal smooth muscle such as scleroderma, dermatomyositis, amyloidosis, or muscular dystrophy. Endocrine disorders, including myxedema and diabetes mellitus, may result in chronic distention which in the diabetic results from autonomic visceral neuropathy. Chronic neurologic diseases including Parkinson's disease and stroke may be complicated by chronic pseudoobstruction; in these patients drugs and relative immobility are contributing features. Finally, psychotic patients, (especially those who are institutionalized) may suffer from prolonged megacolon.

The symptoms of chronic secondary pseudoobstruction are chronic or intermittent constipation, crampy abdominal pain, anorexia, and bloating. Gastric distention and disordered swallowing may be present. Abdominal x-rays reveal gaseous distention of the large and small bowel, and occasionally of the stomach. Air fluid levels are unusual and should raise the possibility of mechanical obstruction. Upper gastrointestinal series and barium enema do not reveal specific abnormalities of the intestine such as tumor, stricture, or volvulus. The presence of an autoimmune disorder or endocrinopathy may require confirmation by serologic or blood tests; biopsy may be needed as in amyloidosis or muscular dystrophy.

The treatment of chronic intestinal pseudoobstruction is made difficult due to the complexity and chronicity of the underlying systemic disease. Patients with scleroderma may respond to broad-spectrum antibiotics if intestinal bacterial overgrowth is suspected. Metoclopramide may benefit gastric dysmotility in the diabetic. Discontinuation of psychotropic or anti-Parkinson drugs may occasionally result in improvement. Cathartics and enemas may be required to relieve fecal impaction, and the regular use of stool softeners and a high-fiber diet may help prevent recurrences.

Idiopathic intestinal pseudoobstruction This term encompasses patients with signs and symptoms of pseudoobstruction in whom no systemic disease can be identified. The typical patient has recurrent attacks of abdominal pain and distention with nausea and vomiting. The small intestine is primarily involved, and chronic constipation is much less frequent than in secondary pseudoobstruction. Steatorrhea secondary to bacterial overgrowth of the small intestine is common and may lead to chronic diarrhea and malnutrition. Many patients exhibit abnormalities of motility in the esophagus and urinary bladder, in addition to the small and large intestine. Various defects have been described in patients with this syndrome, including abnormalities of the mesenteric plexus and myopathy of the intestinal and urinary bladder smooth muscle (so-called hollow visceral myopathy). Elevated prostaglandin E levels have been reported in some patients. Treatment of idiopathic pseudoobstruction is unsatisfactory. Surgery to relieve "obstruction" is to be avoided, since the condition is often worsened by abdominal surgery. Medical therapy with metoclopramide and cholinergic agents has been unsuccessful. Nutritional support in the form of low-residue elemental diets or parenteral hyperalimentation may be helpful. Unfortunately the lack of effective therapy and the progressive nature of the illness make the prognosis of idiopathic pseudoobstruction rather unfavorable. Death from malnutrition and steatorrhea are common. The long-term impact of total parenteral nutrition on this disease is not yet clear.

Acute intestinal pseudoobstruction This entity, sometimes referred to as Ogilvie's syndrome, is characterized by acute intestinal dilatation, involving primarily the colon but occasionally also the small intestine. As in other forms of pseudoobstruction, the clinical features are difficult to distinguish from mechanical obstruction. The patient may complain of colicky lower abdominal pain and acute constipation. Examination reveals a distended, tympanitic abdomen, with reduced or absent bowel sounds. Localized tenderness over the distended colon is common, but diffuse abdominal tenderness, rigidity, or rebound tenderness are unusual. Abdominal films reveal massive dilatation of the colon and small intestine, occasionally with the presence of air fluid levels. The cecum, being the most capacious part of the colon, is often massively dilated and tender. The onset of these symptoms usually occurs in patients who have recently undergone severe surgical or medical stress such as major surgery, myocardial infarction, sepsis, or respiratory failure. Patients with acute pseudoobstruction are frequently on a respirator, have received narcotics or sedatives, and have metabolic and electrolyte disturbances.

Management of acute pseudoobstruction requires careful correction of fluid and electrolyte abnormalities, intubation of the stomach or small intestine for decompression, and avoidance of drugs which depress intestinal motility. Barium enema may be hazardous because of the risk of perforating the already dilated bowel. Some authorities recommend cecostomy when the diameter of the colon exceeds 8 cm to avoid ischemic necrosis and perforation. Decompressive colonoscopy is beneficial in some patients. The outcome depends in large part on the prognosis of the associated medical or surgical conditions. Patients who recover from the underlying medical or surgical conditions usually have a return of normal colonic function.

IRRITABLE BOWEL SYNDROME The irritable bowel syndrome (IBS) is the most common gastrointestinal disease in clinical practice, and although not a life-threatening illness, it causes great distress to those afflicted and a feeling of helplessness and frustration for the physician attempting to treat it. The patient with irritable bowel syndrome may present with one of *three clinical variants*. Patients with so-called spastic colitis complain primarily of chronic abdominal pain and constipation. A second group has chronic intermittent watery diarrhea, often without pain. Some patients have both features and complain of alternating constipation and diarrhea.

The basic pathophysiologic abnormality in the irritable bowel syndrome is an alteration of intestinal motility. Patients with the spastic colon variant (pain and constipation) have *increased* resting colonic motility; in contrast, those presenting primarily with diarrhea have *decreased* resting colonic motility. Both groups have an increase in colonic motility after injection of cholinergic drugs or cholecystokinin; motility may also be increased in association with psychological stress. It has been suggested that cholecystokinin may be a normal stimulus of intestinal motility and that the spastic colon may result from an exaggerated response to the normal release of cholecystokinin after eating.

Patients with the irritable bowel syndrome also exhibit an abnormal basic electrical rhythm in the colon, characterized by an increase in 3-cycle-per-minute (cpm) slow-wave activity. It is not certain, however, whether these abnormalities of smooth-muscle contraction are primary or secondary to another underlying abnormality of intestinal neuromuscular function.

Evidence of significant psychological disturbances may be seen in some patients with irritable bowel syndrome. Depression, hysteria, and obsessive-compulsive traits are common, and psychological stress frequently triggers an exacerbation of symptoms. It should be noted, however, that in normal individuals colonic motility is altered by stress. For example, increased intracolonic pressure has been observed in normal volunteers during a stressful interview. This suggests that psychological stress may be a nonspecific trigger of symptoms in the irritable bowel syndrome, as is the case in many other illnesses of diverse etiology.

Clinical features The irritable bowel syndrome is a disease of young or middle-aged adults; female/male ratio is 2:1. The predominant feature is a history of chronic constipation, diarrhea, or both. The typical patient describes watery diarrhea occurring *intermittently* for months or years. The diarrhea is usually worse in the morning upon arising or after breakfast. After the passage of three or four loose stools with excessive mucus the patient may feel well for the remainder of the day. Diarrhea throughout the day or especially nocturnal diarrhea is most unusual. The diarrhea may last for weeks or months and then disappear spontaneously for variable periods of time. Some patients describe "pencil-like" pasty stools rather than diarrhea.

Another typical presentation is that of chronic abdominal pain with constipation, or with alternating constipation and diarrhea. These patients describe intermittent crampy lower abdominal pain, often over the sigmoid colon, which is usually relieved by passage of flatus or stool. The patient may describe excessive bloating which is not discernible to the physician. A variety of other complaints, such as heartburn, excessive bloating, back pain, weakness, faintness, and palpitations, are frequent in patients with irritable bowel syndrome. The pain may occasionally be in the right upper quadrant or midepigastrium, leading to diagnostic confusion with biliary tract or peptic ulcer disease.

Physical examination reveals these patients to be anxious but otherwise normal. During intense pain, the abdomen may be distended, but no visible peristalsis is noted; the abdominal musculature is relaxed, and a tender sigmoid full of feces may be palpated in the left lower quadrant. Characteristically, the rectal ampulla is empty of feces. Sigmoidoscopic examination is usually normal or at most shows a prominent vascular pattern. There may be difficulty in negotiating the rectosigmoid curve at 13 to 15 cm from the anus because of spasm. Large amounts of clear mucus are frequently encountered during the examination.

The *diagnosis* of the irritable colon syndrome is suggested by the chronic intermittent nature of symptoms without obvious signs of physical deterioration, the relation of symptoms to environment or emotional stress, and the exclusion of other conditions. The evaluation should include a careful history, complete physical examination including sigmoidoscopy, stool examination (for occult blood, parasites, and pathogenic bacteria), and in older patients a barium enema. The latter study serves to rule out other lesions since there are no diagnostic x-ray findings for this syndrome, although spasticity of the sigmoid, accentuated haustra, and a tubular appearance to the descending colon may be observed when the patient is symptomatic. Lactase deficiency may masquerade as irritable colon syndrome and should be excluded by a trial of milk restriction, a lactose tolerance test, or a lactose breath hydrogen test (see Chap. 237). Thyrotoxicosis is easily confused with irritable bowel syndrome and should be excluded by appropriate laboratory studies.

Treatment of the irritable colon syndrome requires both skill and patience. It is important that the patient be reassured that this condition normally does not lead to the development of inflammatory bowel disease (i.e., ulcerative colitis) or colonic malignancy. It is also important for both the patient and the physician to realize that the condition is chronic, and while it may be alleviated, it cannot be cured. The patient should be encouraged to adapt to the symptoms so as to minimize their impact on life-style. The physician should not imply that the symptoms are largely emotional or psychological in origin, since this is usually rejected by the patient. It is appropriate, however, to emphasize the relationship between psychological stress and the onset of severity of symptoms, as this may allow the patient to better deal with the disease. After the diagnosis is established, frequent x-rays and endoscopies are not necessary; general physical examinations, hemograms, and stool examinations, however, should be carried out at regular intervals.

Drug treatment is aimed at altering the abnormal colonic motility in this disease. Patients with constipation may respond to an increase in dietary bulk in the form of unprocessed bran or other nonabsorbed bulk laxatives. Mild sedation with phenobarbital or tranquilizers may be indicated, and anticholinergic drugs are useful in some patients. Troublesome diarrhea may respond to diphenoxylate (Lomotil) or paregoric. Unfortunately, no specific drug or dietary regimen affords good relief in all patients, and thus a number of therapeutic maneuvers need to be tried.

CHRONIC CONSTIPATION In Chap. 36 the mechanism of defecation is discussed. Disorders involving the sensory or motor components of this mechanism may arise from destruction of the nerves subserving these functions, from invasion or inflammation of the rectosigmoid itself, or from central nervous system lesions. Most cases of chronic constipation arise from habitual neglect of afferent impulses, failure to initiate defecation, and accumulation of large, dry fecal masses in the rectum. This voluntary suppression of the call to stool may arise during the period of toilet training in childhood, or later in life because of a sense of social impropriety, unaccustomed surroundings, uncomfortable toilet facilities, or illnesses which require confinement to bed. Chronic constipation is much more common in women, with onset typically in late adolescence or early adulthood. As constant distention of the rectum with feces becomes chronic, the patient grows less aware of rectal fullness. Bowel movements become progressively more difficult, and painful hemorrhoids or anal fissures reinforce suppression of the urge to defecate. To avoid these problems, the patient begins the chronic use of laxatives or enemas, without which defecation becomes impossible.

Treatment The physician should make every attempt to educate the patient about the chain of events which has led to chronic constipation. Attempts should be made to alter patterns of many years' duration, and the patient must recognize the importance of responding to, rather than suppressing, the urge to defecate. It is helpful to initiate a routine whereby defecation is attempted at a given time each day. In most individuals the call to stool occurs in the morning after breakfast. Physical exercise such as a brisk walk just before attempts at defecation may be helpful. Patients are instructed to increase dietary bulk with foods rich in fiber, such as green vegetables and unprocessed cereal grains, or by the regular use of bulk laxatives, such as hemicellulose, psyllium extract, and powdered unprocessed bran. The success of such a regimen depends to some extent on the duration of symptoms. Elderly patients with long-standing constipation and reliance on enemas or laxatives are more resistant to these measures than younger patients whose bowel patterns are less established. Moreover, poor muscle tone, reduced physical activity, and increased incidence of other medical conditions make the problem more difficult in the older age group. Bedridden elderly patients often develop severe constipation and even fecal impaction unless preventive measures are taken. This applies not only to patients with previous constipation but also to those with regular bowel movements prior to their confining illness. Regular administration of stool softeners, bulk laxatives, or mild cathartics is necessary until full ambulation and a normal diet are resumed. The onset of fecal impaction in bedridden patients is heralded by a feeling of rectal distention, urgency of defecation, or tenesmus. Occasionally the fecal impaction will result in low-grade chronic obstruction with dilatation and increased fluid content proximal to the impaction; "paradoxical diarrhea" may thus occur as fluid moves past the obstructing fecal mass. This situation will be aggravated if antidiarrheal drugs are given because the underlying constipation will be worsened. The appropriate maneuver is to disimpact the rectum manually or to administer gentle enemas if the impaction is beyond the reach of the finger.

VASCULAR DISORDERS OF THE INTESTINE

Ischemia is the end result of interruption or reduction of the blood supply of the intestine. However the clinical manifestations of intestinal ischemia range from mild chronic symptoms to catastrophic episodes, depending on the segment involved, the degree of involvement, and the rapidity of the process. Thus, the clinician should be aware of a spectrum of intestinal ischemia ranging from mild chronic symptoms to catastrophic episodes. The gut derives its arterial blood supply from the celiac axis and the superior and inferior mesenteric arteries. The small intestine is supplied by the celiac and superior mesenteric arteries; the colon is supplied by branches of the superior and inferior mesenteric arteries. A rich network of anastomotic vessels and the possible development of collateral circulation determine the clinical picture of acute or chronic intestinal arterial insufficiency.

MESENTERIC ISCHEMIA AND INFARCTION Acute small-intestinal ischemia may be classified as *occlusive* or *nonocclusive*. Occlusion may result from arterial thrombus or embolus of the celiac or superior mesenteric arteries, or from venous occlusion in the same distribution. Arterial embolus occurs most commonly in patients with chronic or recurrent atrial fibrillation, artificial heart valves, or valvular heart disease, while arterial thrombosis is associated with extensive atherosclerosis or low cardiac output. Venous occlusion is quite rare and is occasionally seen in women taking oral contraceptives. Approximately two-thirds of patients with mesenteric ischemia do not have a definite occlusion of a major vessel, a condition referred to as *nonocclusive* ischemia. The exact cause of nonocclusive disease is obscure; systemic arterial hypotension, cardiac arrhythmias, prolonged heart failure, digitalis therapy, dehydration, and endotoxemia have been suggested as contributing factors.

The outstanding clinical feature of acute mesenteric ischemia is severe abdominal pain, often colicky and periumbilical at the onset, later becoming diffuse and constant. Vomiting, anorexia, diarrhea, and constipation are also frequent but of little diagnostic help. Examination of the abdomen may reveal tenderness and distention. Bowel sounds are often normal even in the face of severe infarction. Some patients have a surprisingly normal abdominal examination in spite of severe pain. Mild gastrointestinal bleeding is often detected by guaiac examination of stool, but gross hemorrhage is unusual except in ischemic colitis (see below). A typical laboratory finding is a pronounced polymorphonuclear leukocytosis. Late in the course of the disease (24 to 72 h) gangrene of the bowel occurs with diffuse peritonitis, sepsis, and shock. Abdominal plain films in patients with mesenteric ischemia may reveal air fluid levels and distention. Barium study of the small intestine reveals nonspecific dilatation, poor motility, and evidence of thick mucosal folds ("thumbprinting") (Fig. 239-2).

Acute mesenteric ischemia is a grave condition with a high morbidity and mortality. Patients suspected of having acute arterial embolus should undergo immediate celiac and mesenteric angiography to localize the embolus, followed by embolectomy. Restoration of normal circulation may allow complete recovery if performed before irreversible necrosis or gangrene has occurred. Unfortunately infarction and transmural necrosis are frequently found at surgery, necessitating resection. Arterial or venous thrombosis is not generally amenable to surgical removal of the thrombus, and resection of the affected bowel is required. Similarly, patients with nonocclusive ischemia are not candidates for corrective vascular surgery (as major vessels are patent). These individuals often have extensive necrosis of the small or large intestine because of the widespread nature of the ischemic event. The decision to operate on patients with suspected mesenteric ischemia is a difficult one as the typical patient is a poor surgical risk owing to advanced age, dehydration, sepsis, and other serious medical conditions.

Chronic arterial insufficiency may precede acute vascular insufficiency, producing so-called abdominal angina. As in angina pectoris, the pain of chronic mesenteric insufficiency occurs under conditions of increased demand for splanchnic blood flow. The patient complains of intermittent dull or cramping midabdominal pain 15 to 30 min after a meal, lasting for several hours postprandially. Significant weight loss is primarily due to a decreased food intake; however, chronic intestinal ischemia may also produce mucosal damage and malabsorption, which in turn aggravates the weight loss. Since abdominal angina may progress to bowel infarction, serious consideration should be given to performing arteriographic studies to confirm the diagnosis in those patients who are candidates for abdominal vascular surgery. The only definitive treatment is surgical removal of the arterial obstruction or the construction of bypass arterial grafts to the ischemic bowel.

A variety of systemic conditions are associated with *vasculitis* of the large and small arteries supplying the intestine. Most often, these

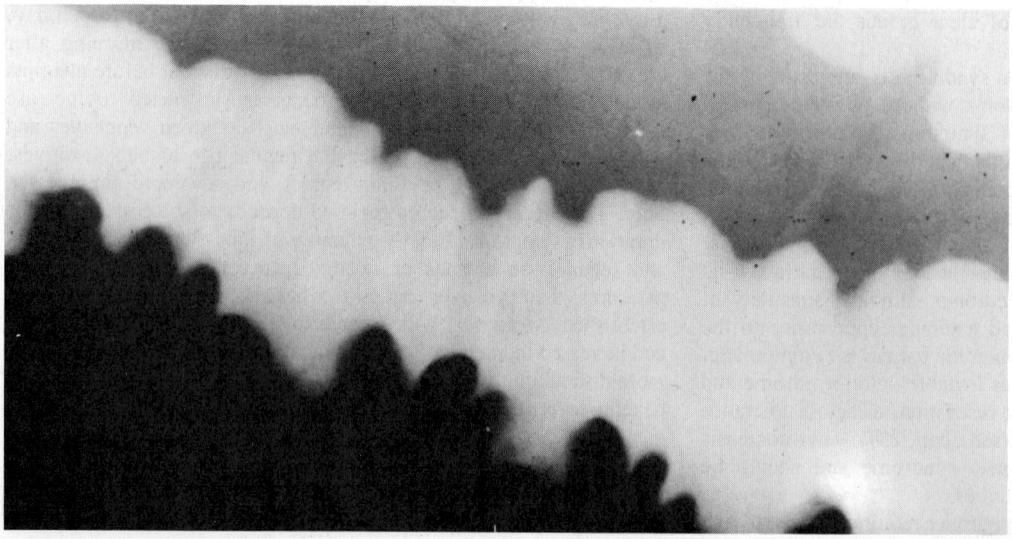

FIGURE 239-2 *Barium enema showing "thumbprinting" or submucosal edema of the inferior margin of the transverse colon, in a patient with acute ischemic colitis.*

disorders can be recognized by the associated extraintestinal manifestations as in polyarteritis nodosa, lupus erythematosus, dermatomyositis, Henoch-Schönlein purpura (allergic vasculitis), and rheumatoid vasculitis. When larger arteries are involved, as in polyarteritis nodosa, the picture of acute intestinal infarction is similar to embolic or atherosclerotic vascular occlusion. Often the involvement of smaller vessels leads to areas of intramural hemorrhage and edema leading to abdominal pain, variable degrees of intestinal obstruction, and bleeding. Barium enema may show "thumbprinting" and "spiculation" due to localized edema, hemorrhage, and ulceration. In many instances, treatment of the underlying disorder may lead to regression of symptoms. If signs of an acute abdomen develop, surgical exploration is usually indicated.

Intramural small-intestinal hemorrhage may occur with vasculitis, trauma, or impaired coagulation, especially in patients receiving anticoagulants. The clinical and radiologic features resemble those seen with vasculitis and local mucosal hemorrhage.

ISCHEMIC COLITIS Ischemia of the colon most often affects the elderly population because of the greater frequency of vascular disease in that group. Ischemic colitis is almost always a nonocclusive disease, that is, obstruction of major arteries is not seen. Shunting of blood away from the mucosa may contribute to this condition, but the mechanism of ischemia is not known.

The clinical picture depends upon the degree of ischemia and the rate of its development. In *acute fulminant ischemic* colitis the major manifestations are severe lower abdominal pain, rectal bleeding, and hypotension. Dilatation of the colon and physical signs of peritonitis are seen in severe cases. Plain abdominal films may reveal thumbprinting from submucosal hemorrhage and edema. Barium enema is hazardous in the acute situation because of the risk of perforation. Sigmoidoscopy or colonoscopy may detect ulcerations, friability, and bulging folds from submucosal hemorrhage. Angiography is not helpful in the management of patients with presumed ischemic colitis since a remedial occlusive lesion is very rarely found. Surgical resection may be required in some patients with fulminant ischemic colitis to remove gangrenous bowel; others with lesser degrees of ischemia may respond to conservative medical management.

Subacute ischemic colitis, the most common clinical variant of ischemic colonic disease, produces lesser degrees of pain and bleeding, often occurring over several days or weeks. The left colon may be involved, but the rectum is usually spared because of collateral blood flow, a distinguishing feature from acute ulcerative colitis. Barium enema reveals edema, cobblestoning, thumbprinting, and occasionally superficial ulceration. Angiography is not indicated as almost all cases are nonocclusive. Occasionally *stricture formation* may follow a bout of ischemic colitis or may present de novo without a history of antecedent pain or bloody diarrhea. Most cases of nonocclusive ischemic colitis resolve in 2 to 4 weeks and do not recur. Surgery is not required except for obstruction secondary to postischemic stricture.

ANGIODYSPLASIA OF THE COLON These are vascular ectasias (not neoplasms) which occur in the right colon of many older individuals and may cause bleeding (see Chap. 37). Angiodysplasia is a degenerative lesion consisting of dilated, distorted, thin-walled vessels lined by vascular endothelium. Grossly these ectasias look similar to spider angiomas of the skin and appear as star-shaped branching vessels in the submucosa measuring from 2 mm to 1 cm in diameter. The lesions are usually multiple and are found primarily in the cecum and ascending colon. Angiodysplasia may result from partial obstruction of the submucosal venous plexus by the tension generated in the cecal wall during muscular contraction.

Cecal angiodysplasia is important because of the likelihood of bleeding, either massively or chronically. In patients over 60 approximately one-quarter of colonic bleeding episodes are secondary to angiodysplasia. The diagnosis requires careful angiography with a demonstration of extravasation of contrast material into the lumen, or by direct visualization of bleeding lesions at colonoscopy. Hemorrhage from angiodysplasia may be controlled by embolization during arteriography or by electrocautery through the colonoscope. Some patients with massive uncontrolled bleeding or multiple sites of angiodysplasia may require right hemicolectomy.

PRIMARY NONSPECIFIC ULCERATION OF THE SMALL INTESTINE

Although the existence of rare solitary and unexplained ulcers of the small intestine has been recognized for many years, a recent increased incidence has suggested vascular factors producing ischemic necrosis of the mucosa in one or more areas of the small bowel. Most of these ulcers occur in patients receiving enteric-coated drugs known to be irritating to the mucosa; the most commonly implicated agent is potassium chloride, given to patients on chronic diuretic therapy. The symptoms are those of abdominal pain and obstruction, rarely with peritonitis and perforation. Surgical excision of the ulcerated or stenotic intestinal segment is generally required.

TUMORS OF THE SMALL INTESTINE

Small-bowel tumors comprise only 3 to 6 percent of gastrointestinal neoplasms. Because of their rarity correct diagnosis is often delayed. Abdominal symptoms are usually vague and poorly defined, and conventional x-ray studies of the upper and lower intestinal tract are usually normal. Small-bowel tumors should be considered in the following situations: (1) recurrent, unexplained episodes of crampy abdominal pain; (2) intermittent bouts of intestinal obstruction, especially in the absence of inflammatory bowel disease or prior abdominal surgery; (3) intussusception in the adult; and (4) evidence of chronic intestinal bleeding in the face of negative conventional x-rays. A careful small-bowel barium study is the diagnostic procedure of choice. The diagnostic accuracy is improved by infusing barium through a nasogastric tube placed in the duodenum (enteroclysis).

BENIGN TUMORS In general, the histology of benign small-bowel tumors is difficult to predict on clinical and radiologic grounds alone. The symptomatology of benign tumors is not distinctive, with pain, obstruction, and hemorrhage being the most frequent symptoms. These tumors are usually discovered in the fifth and sixth decades of life, more often in the distal rather than the proximal small intestine. The most common benign tumors are adenomas, leiomyomas, lipomas, and angiomas.

Adenomas These tumors include those of the islet cells and Brunner's glands as well as polypoid adenomas. *Islet cell adenomas* are occasionally located outside the pancreas, and the associated syndromes are discussed in Chap. 329. *Brunner's gland adenomas* are not truly neoplastic but represent a hypertrophy or hyperplasia of submucosal duodenal glands. These appear as small nodules in the duodenal mucosa. Most often this is an incidental finding on x-ray not associated with any clinical disorder.

Polypoid adenomas Approximately 25 percent of benign small-bowel tumors are polypoid adenomas. They may present as single polypoid lesions or less commonly as papillary villous adenomas. As in the colon, the sessile or papillary form of the tumor is sometimes associated with coexistent carcinoma. Multiple polypoid tumors may occur throughout the small bowel in the Peutz-Jeghers syndrome (Chap. 51) and are usually hamartomas. The malignant potential of these lesions is low.

Leiomyomas These arise from smooth-muscle components of the intestine and are usually intramural lesions affecting the overlying mucosa. Ulceration of the mucosa may cause gastrointestinal hemorrhage of varying severity.

Lipomas These tumors occur with greatest frequency in the distal ileum and at the ileocecal valve. Their radiolucent appearance on x-ray is characteristic. They are usually intramural and asymptomatic but may on occasion be associated with bleeding.

Angiomas While not true neoplasms, these lesions are important because they frequently cause intestinal bleeding. They may take the form of telangiectasia or hemangiomas. Multiple intestinal telangiectasia occurs in a nonhereditary form confined to the gastrointestinal tract or as a part of the hereditary Osler-Rendu-Weber syndrome (Chap. 280). Vascular tumors may also take the form of isolated hemangiomas, most commonly in the jejunum. Angiography, especially during a bout of bleeding, is the procedure of choice in evaluating these lesions.

MALIGNANT TUMORS While not too common, small-bowel malignancies occur in patients with long-standing regional enteritis and celiac sprue with greater frequency than in the general population. In contrast to benign tumors, malignant tumors of the small bowel are frequently associated with fever, weight loss, anorexia, bleeding, and an abdominal mass on physical examination. After ampullary carcinomas [many of which arise from the bile or pancreatic duct (see Chap. 255)], the most frequent small-bowel malignancies are adenocarcinomas, lymphomas, leiomyosarcomas, and carcinoid tumors.

Adenocarcinomas These occur with highest frequency in the distal duodenum and proximal jejunum, where they tend to ulcerate and cause hemorrhage or obstruction. Radiologically, they may be confused with chronic duodenal ulcer disease or Crohn's disease if the patient has long-standing regional enteritis. The diagnosis is best made by endoscopy and biopsy under direct vision.

Leiomyosarcomas Large, bulky tumors, leiomyosarcomas often are greater than 5 cm in diameter and may be palpable on abdominal examination. Bleeding, obstruction, and perforation are the most common manifestations.

LYMPHOMAS Lymphoma of the small bowel is usually of the diffuse non-Hodgkin's type (Chap. 294), with diffuse histiocytic lymphoma comprising the largest group. Lymphoma of the intestine may be primary or secondary; primary intestinal lymphoma indicates that the initial symptoms arise from the intestine even though bone marrow, lymph nodes, and liver may also be involved. Intestinal lymphoma usually involves the jejunum or ileum in the form of localized or nodular mass lesions which narrow the lumen. This results in periumbilical abdominal pain, made worse by eating. Anorexia, weight loss, nausea, and vomiting are common. Intestinal bleeding and abdominal mass lesions are also common in patients with intestinal lymphoma.

Some patients with intestinal lymphoma have diffuse rather than localized or nodular involvement of the small bowel. This type of lymphoma was first described in oriental Jews and Arabs and is referred to as Mediterranean lymphoma. The typical presentation includes chronic diarrhea, malabsorption, and abdominal pain; the clinical findings may be confused initially with infectious diarrhea, Crohn's disease, or sprue. A curious feature in many patients with Mediterranean lymphoma is the presence in the blood and intestinal secretions of an abnormal IgA which contains only alpha-heavy chains and is devoid of light chains. It is suspected that the abnormal alpha chains are produced by plasma cells infiltrating the intestine.

The diagnosis of intestinal lymphoma is often delayed because the patient may initially be suspected of having another disorder, such as peptic ulcer, pancreatitis, Crohn's disease or infectious diarrhea. The diagnosis is suggested by barium studies of the small intestine showing nodular filling defects, irregular strictures, or infiltrated folds. The diagnosis can be confirmed by surgical exploration and resection of involved segments. Intestinal lymphoma may occasionally be diagnosed by peroral intestinal biopsy, but the disease mainly involves the lamina propria and usually requires full-thickness surgical biopsies.

Many authorities recommend staging of the lymphoma by means of bone marrow biopsy, and laparotomy with splenectomy and biopsies of the liver and regional lymph nodes. In patients with localized lymphoma (stage I), surgical excision followed by whole abdominal radiation therapy is recommended. Patients with more advanced lymphoma with lymph node and other organ involvement are best treated with combination chemotherapy, and with radiotherapy for localized recurrences or bulky tumors. The probability of sustained remission or cure is approximately 75 percent in localized disease, but 25 percent or less in patients with widespread lymphoma.

Carcinoid tumors Among the most common epithelial tumors of the small intestine are carcinoid tumors. They arise from argentaffin cells of the crypts of Lieberkühn and are most commonly found from the midduodenum to the transverse colon, areas embryologically derived from the midgut. The appendix is the most common location for gastrointestinal carcinoid, where the tumor is found incidentally at the time of appendectomy. Most intestinal carcinoids are asymptomatic and of low malignant potential, but invasion and metastases may occur and lead to the carcinoid syndrome (see Chap. 299).

TUMORS OF THE LARGE INTESTINE

Neoplasms of the colon, both benign and malignant, are very common in western society. Benign polypoid adenomas of the colon are found at autopsy in about 50 percent of older Americans. While these lesions are generally harmless, it is now recognized that most colon cancers arise in adenomas. Furthermore, recent advances in colonoscopy have made polypectomy a relatively simple procedure. For these reasons, it is important to be familiar with the clinical presentation and management of benign polyps as well as colonic cancers.

COLONIC POLYPS A polyp is defined as a structure arising from the mucosa and projecting into the lumen and is either *neoplastic* or *nonneoplastic*. Neoplastic polyps in turn may be benign (adenomatous polyp) or malignant (polypoid carcinoma). Nonneoplastic polyps include hyperplastic polyps, inflammatory polyps, juvenile polyps, and hamartomas. Although nonneoplastic polyps are more common, most morbidity and mortality are attributed to neoplastic polyps.

Adenomas Single adenomatous polyps are common and increase with age so that about two-thirds of individuals above age 60 will harbor at least one adenoma. Adenomatous polyps occur more commonly in the rectosigmoid colon (80 percent) than in the rest of the colon (20 percent). Adenomas may be pedunculated or sessile. Most of them are silent and are discovered by routine barium enema or screening endoscopy. A few may bleed or cause obstructive symptoms, especially when they are greater than 2 cm in diameter. The major clinical significance of adenomas is that approximately 1 percent become malignant. The size of adenomas correlates with the risk of becoming malignant. Approximately 1 percent of polyps smaller than 1 cm in diameter contain foci of malignant cells, compared to about 50 percent for polyps greater than 2 cm. About 25 percent of patients with polyps will have more than one polyp. The number and size tend to increase with age, as does the risk of malignancy.

Adenomatous polyps of the colon are classified into three histologic types: tubular, tubulovillous, and villous. *Tubular adenomas* are the most common and are generally less than 1 cm in diameter. *Villous adenomas* are less common and are generally larger with approximately 50 to 60 percent over 2 cm in diameter. *Tubulovillous adenomas* are intermediate in size between the smaller tubular and larger villous types, suggesting that some tubular adenomas evolve into villous adenomas.

Villous adenomas tend to be sessile and are much more likely to become malignant; approximately 40 to 60 percent contain foci of carcinoma in situ or frankly invasive carcinoma extending through the lamina propria. Some villous adenomas in the rectosigmoid area may produce rectal bleeding or passage of large amounts of mucus.

Adenomatous polyps are usually diagnosed by detection of occult fecal blood loss in asymptomatic patients being screened for colon cancer. Polyps may also be detected by barium enema examination (Fig. 239-3) or by proctosigmoidoscopy and colonoscopy. Because of their malignant potential *all* colonic adenomatous polyps, but especially those larger than 1 cm in diameter, should be removed in toto via the colonoscope and carefully examined for evidence of malignancy. Removal of all adenomas, even those without malignant change, will reduce the incidence of subsequent colon cancer. Colonoscopic polypectomy is curative if the adenoma removed shows evidence of carcinoma in situ, since metastases from this lesion do not occur. If the carcinoma invades the submucosa of the head of a pedunculated polyp (polyp on a stalk), polypectomy alone is still probably curative. However, if the carcinoma invades the stalk, if the polyp is sessile, or if the carcinoma is undifferentiated, the patient should undergo a standard cancer resection to remove tumor which may have spread beyond the polyp into the wall of the colon or local lymph nodes.

Nonneoplastic colonic polyps Nonneoplastic polyps are a heterogenous group of lesions which occasionally cause rectal bleeding or pain. In contrast to adenomas, which are true neoplasms, these polyps do not undergo malignant change. Therefore, removal of nonneoplastic polyps is required only if they cause bleeding, obstruction, or other symptoms. The most common colonic polyp is the *hyperplastic* polyp, a sessile excrescence usually less than 0.5 cm. These tiny polyps are of no pathologic or clinical significance. Hyperplastic polyps larger than 1 cm in diameter may contain foci of adenoma; thus these larger polyps should be removed colonoscopically. *Juvenile polyps* are hamartomas composed of an excess of lamina propria and dilated cystic glands. They arise during childhood and may bleed or prolapse through the rectum during defecation. They generally do not recur after polypectomy. *Inflammatory polyps* are thought to result from regeneration following injury or inflammation. Histologically these lesions resemble juvenile polyps, but they may occur in other individuals. Sometimes multiple inflammatory polyps may mimic one of the hereditary polyp syndromes.

HEREDITARY POLYP SYNDROMES *Familial colonic polyposis* is a rarer autosomal dominant disorder characterized by the appearance of numerous (often 1000 or more) adenomatous polyps involving the entire colon. Occasional cases with no family history presumably result from a spontaneous mutation. The polyps are not present at birth but appear in childhood and adolescence, giving rise to rectal bleeding or diarrhea. Once this disease is diagnosed, it is imperative that the entire family be screened by sigmoidoscopy and barium enema. The probability of cancer of the colon occurring in affected individuals approaches 100 percent by age 40. Hence, prophylactic colectomy is indicated, usually in late adolescence or early adulthood. Most surgeons prefer total colectomy and ileostomy, while others leave the rectum, which allows the patient to have normal bowel movements. These patients require careful follow-up sigmoidoscopy and removal of all polyps in the rectal stump. However, the rate of carcinoma in the rectal stump is so high that total colectomy is recommended.

Gardner's syndrome refers to the coexistence of multiple colonic and duodenal adenomatous polyps together with benign soft tissue tumors (lipomas, fibromas, sebaceous cysts) and osteomas (particularly of the jaw and skull). In this syndrome the colonic polyps develop later than in multiple colonic polyposis, but the malignant potential is the same and thus colectomy is also recommended. Many patients with Gardner's syndrome have gastric and especially duodenal polyps, and cancer of the duodenum has been reported in some of these individuals.

An entity confused with multiple colonic (adenomatous) polyposis is *juvenile polyposis,* in which multiple hamartomatous polyps occur in the colon or in both large and small bowels. Juvenile colonic polyposis also occurs in kindreds and can cause rectal bleeding or diarrhea, rectal prolapse of the polyp, abdominal pain, and intussusception. Juvenile polyps have no malignant potential and colectomy is not recommended.

The *Peutz-Jeghers syndrome* is characterized by multiple hamartomatous polyps of the entire gastrointestinal tract, associated with melanotic spots on the skin, lips, and buccal mucosa. Although the polyps in this syndrome are most prevalent in the small intestine, colonic polyps may also occur. Several cases of malignant degeneration of duodenal polyps have been reported. Clinical features alone do not allow accurate differentiation of the various hereditary polyp syndromes (see Table 239-1). For this reason, a careful histologic examination of polyps from several areas should always be obtained prior to colectomy in patients with suspected adenomatous polyposis coli.

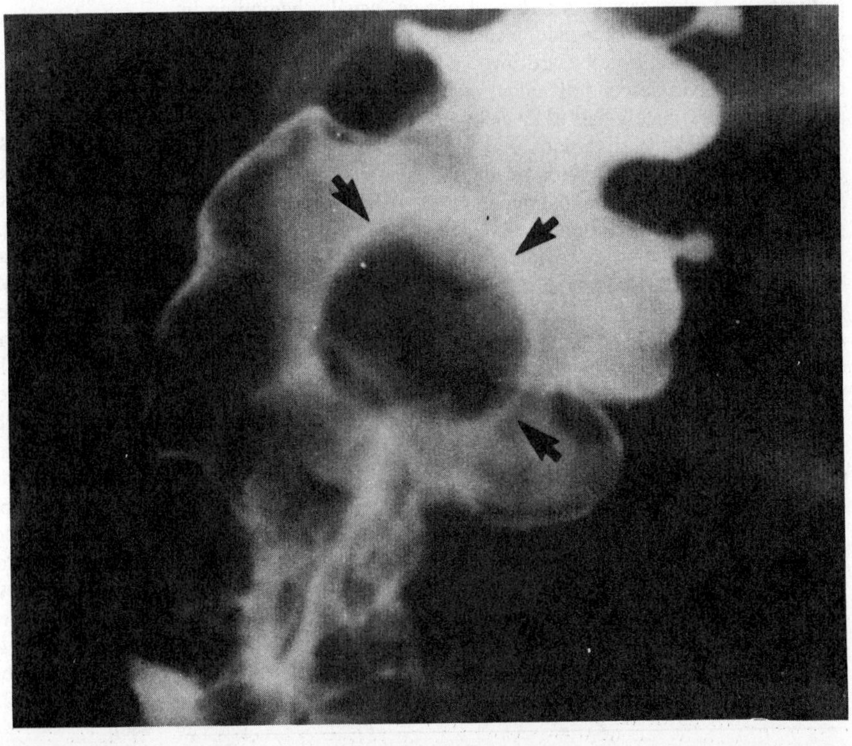

FIGURE 239-3 *Barium enema revealing a 2-cm polyp of the sigmoid colon. Pathologic examination revealed a benign adenoma.*

TABLE 239-1 Hereditable gastrointestinal polyp syndromes

Syndrome	Distribution of polyps	Histologic type	Malignant degeneration	Associated lesions
Familial colonic polyposis	Large intestine	Adenoma	Common	None
Gardner's syndrome	Large intestine and duodenum	Adenoma	Common	Osteomas, fibromas, lipomas, epidermoid cysts
Peutz-Jeghers syndrome	Small and large intestine	Hamartoma	Rare	Mucocutaneous pigmentation
Juvenile polyposis	Small and large intestine	Hamartoma, inflammatory	Absent	None

COLORECTAL CANCER Cancer of the colon and rectum is one of the commonest carcinomas in both males and females, and accounts for about 20 percent of deaths due to malignant disease in the United States. Unfortunately, the death rate for this disease has not changed for the past 40 years and will undoubtedly remain the same until methods for earlier detection and improved treatment are available.

Etiology and risk factors Although the specific cause(s) of colon cancer is unknown, epidemiologic studies suggest that dietary factors may be important. The incidence of colon cancer is much higher in Europe and North America than in the Far East, Africa, and developing nations. Furthermore, migrants from low-incidence areas such as Japan to high-incidence areas such as the United States acquire the higher incidence of the adopted country. It has been suggested that the higher intake of dietary animal fat in western society compared to other countries may account for the excess of colon cancer.

Certain diseases and conditions increase the risk of colon cancer. As noted previously adenomatous polyps of the colon, whether single or multiple, increase the risk of colon cancer. Patients with previous colon polyp or cancer are at higher risk for subsequent development of cancer. It also appears that some women with a history of uterine or breast cancer are at higher risk of developing colon cancer. Ulcerative colitis and to a lesser extent Crohn's colitis are also associated with a higher incidence of colon cancer. The risk in ulcerative colitis is increased in patients with active pancolitis for more than 10 years. Certain families appear to have a much higher incidence of colon cancer, which may affect up to 50 percent or more of family members. However, patients from these high-risk groups account for only 1 percent or less of all colon cancers in the United States. The remainder have no discernible risk factor except age and residence in a high-incidence area.

Pathology Colon cancer is a disease of age, usually beginning in the fourth or fifth decade and increasing steadily thereafter. The cecum and ascending colon are involved in 15 percent; transverse colon, 10 percent; descending colon, rectosigmoid, and rectum in 75 percent. Approximately half of all colorectal cancers are within reach of the 60-cm flexible sigmoidoscope. Colorectal cancers may occur as fungating sessile tumors or as annular constricting lesions; the latter are somewhat more common on the left side, where they produce obstructive symptoms.

Adenocarcinomas of the colon are classified histologically based on degree of differentiation; in general, undifferentiated cancers are more invasive than well-differentiated ones. The presence of mucin-secreting "signet ring" cells indicates a higher likelihood of metastases. The most important prognostic information is the extent of spread of the cancer at the time of diagnosis or surgical removal.

TABLE 239-2 Duke's classification of colorectal cancer

Stage	Pathologic description	Approximate 5-year survival, %
A	Cancer limited to mucosa and submucosa	90
B	Cancer extends into muscularis or serosa	60–75
C	Cancer involves regional lymph nodes	30–40
D	Metastases to liver, bone, lung	5

Colorectal cancers are staged clinically according to the Duke's classification (Table 239-2). When the tumor is confined to the mucosa and submucosa (stage A) or to the colonic wall (stage B), the chance for surgical cure is excellent; spread beyond the wall of the bowel to regional lymph nodes (stage C) or to other organs (stage D) lowers the 5-year survival considerably. Since surgical removal is the only curative therapy currently available, the impact of early diagnosis on survival is obvious.

Clinical features The major symptoms of colon cancer are rectal bleeding, abdominal pain, and change in bowel habit. The clinical presentation in the given patient is related to the size and location of the tumor. Cancers in the cecum and ascending colon are often flat and sessile (Fig. 239-4) and thus remain "silent" because they do not obstruct the lumen. Patients with cecal cancer often present with iron-deficiency anemia and guaiac-positive stool; gross hematochezia is rare. Cancers in the transverse and left colon may grow in an annular fashion (Fig. 239-5), producing symptoms of partial obstruction. The patient typically complains of intermittent crampy pain, often worsened by eating and relieved by passage of gas or feces. Cancer of the rectum or distal sigmoid colon also causes pain which may be confused with diverticulitis. These tumors may also interfere with the normal pattern of defecation, and they can produce diarrhea, constipation, or tenesmus. Rectal bleeding in patients over age 40 should always raise the suspicion of malignancy and should never be attributed to hemorrhoids without further examination. Similarly, unexplained iron-deficiency anemia in older individuals always requires a thorough evaluation for intestinal cancer.

Diagnosis The diagnosis of colon cancer may be suspected by symptoms, such as rectal bleeding, pain, change in bowel habit, weight loss, or anemia. Since colorectal cancer is surgically curable before it has metastasized, delay in diagnosis, on the part of either physician or patient, may seriously lessen the chance of finding a curable lesion.

Evaluation of a patient for colon cancer should include a careful abdominal examination to search for mass lesions or hepatomegaly.

Complications Since it is characteristic for tumors to invade, many tumors of the colon are first diagnosed because of a complication of the original lesion. The tumor may perforate the bowel wall, giving rise to acute peritonitis; may perforate slowly and wall itself off, giving rise to a local inflammatory mass and localized peritonitis; or may invade blood vessels to produce an episode of brisk rectal bleeding. More often, the tumor partially obstructs the bowel lumen for a long period of time, during which the colon proximal to the tumor dilates slowly without dramatic change in symptoms until frank obstruction occurs. This happens most often when the tumor is in the sigmoid, where the stool is driest. Tumors also weaken the colonic wall in such a way that an intussusception may occur, the tumor leading the intussusception. Similarly, fixation of the bowel wall by a tumor may produce a volvulus, which is most frequently seen in the sigmoid colon. Very large and slowly growing tumors may produce symptoms by pressure on neighboring organs such as uterus, bladder, or ureters. Inguinal hernias may become apparent as the first sign of such increased pressure. Fistulas between the colon and pelvic organs should lead to a thorough search for an underlying neoplastic infiltration. Abscesses inside the peritoneal cavity and cellulitis of the abdominal wall secondary to tumor infiltration are occasionally seen.

Treatment The current approach to treatment of colon cancer is primarily surgical. Some surgeons prefer preoperative radiation therapy to prevent metastases, but it has not been convincingly demonstrated that this improves survival. Surgeons generally prefer abdominoperineal resection and colostomy for tumors located below the peritoneal reflection; above this area there is considerably more freedom of choice, depending primarily on the size and extent of the lesion. Even patients with obvious metastases usually benefit from a limited palliative resection, since this will relieve or prevent painful obstruction and hemorrhage. The overall operative mortality for colectomy is about 5 percent, except for emergency resections for perforation or obstruction. The operative mortality is somewhat higher for lesions in the left colon and for tumors which have perforated. Discussion of the complications of surgical therapy and the management of colostomies can be found in surgical texts.

The overall 5-year survival rate for all patients undergoing resection for colonic malignancy is approximately 50 percent. As already noted, surgical cure is possible only when the tumor is confined to the bowel wall. Palliative surgical attempts should not be discouraged because the symptomatic relief they produce may allow the patient to live in comfort for the remaining months of life. Chemotherapy with 5-fluorouracil or other agents is used in patients with metastases to the liver, but temporary improvement is obtained only in 25 percent or less of cases, and overall survival is not significantly affected. Localized radiation therapy for painful liver or bone metastases is occasionally palliative.

ANORECTAL PROBLEMS

HEMORRHOIDS The internal hemorrhoidal plexus of veins is located in the submucosal space above the valves of Morgagni. The anal canal separates it from the external hemorrhoidal venous plexus, but the two spaces communicate under the anal canal, the submucosa of which is attached to underlying tissue to form the interhemorrhoidal depression. Whenever the internal hemorrhoidal plexus is enlarged, there is associated increase in supporting tissue mass, and the resultant venous swelling is called an *internal hemorrhoid*. When veins in the external hemorrhoidal plexus become enlarged or thrombosed, the resultant bluish mass is called an *external hemorrhoid*.

Both types of hemorrhoids are very common and are associated with increased hydrostatic pressure in the portal venous system, such as during pregnancy, straining at stool, or with cirrhosis. When internal hemorrhoids enlarge, pain is not a usual feature until the situation is complicated by thrombosis, infection, or erosion of the overlying mucosal surface. Most persons complain of bright red blood on the toilet tissue or coating the stool, with a feeling of vague anal discomfort. The discomfort is increased when the hemorrhoid enlarges or prolapses through the anus; prolapse is often accompanied by edema and sphincteric spasm. Prolapse, if not treated, usually becomes chronic as the muscularis stays stretched, and the patient complains of constant soiling of underclothing with very little pain. Prolapsed hemorrhoids may become infected or thrombosed; the overlying mucous membrane may bleed profusely as the result of the trauma of defecation.

External hemorrhoids, because they lie under the skin, are quite often painful, particularly if there is a sudden increase in their mass. These episodes result in a tender blue swelling at the anal verge due to thrombosis of a vein in the external plexus and need not be associated with enlargement of the internal veins. Since the thrombus usually lies at the level of the sphincteric muscles, anal spasm often occurs.

The diagnosis of internal and external hemorrhoids is made by inspection, digital examination, and direct vision through the anoscope and proctoscope. Since such lesions are very common, they must not

FIGURE 239-4 *Double-contrast air-barium enema revealing a sessile tumor of the cecum in a patient with iron-deficiency anemia and guaiac-positive stool. The lesion at surgery was a stage B adenocarcinoma.*

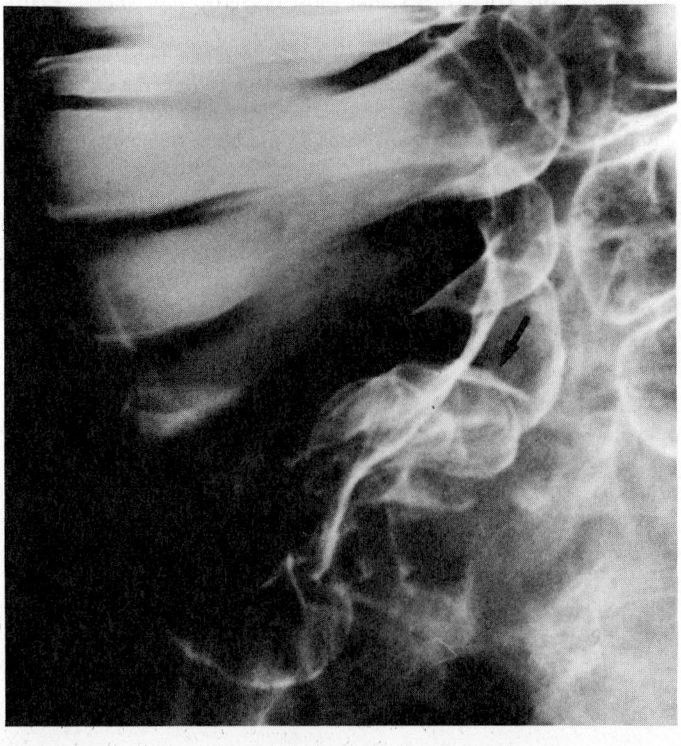

FIGURE 239-5 *Annular, constricting adenocarcinoma of the descending colon. This radiographic appearance is referred to as an "apple-core" lesion and is always highly suspicious of malignancy.*

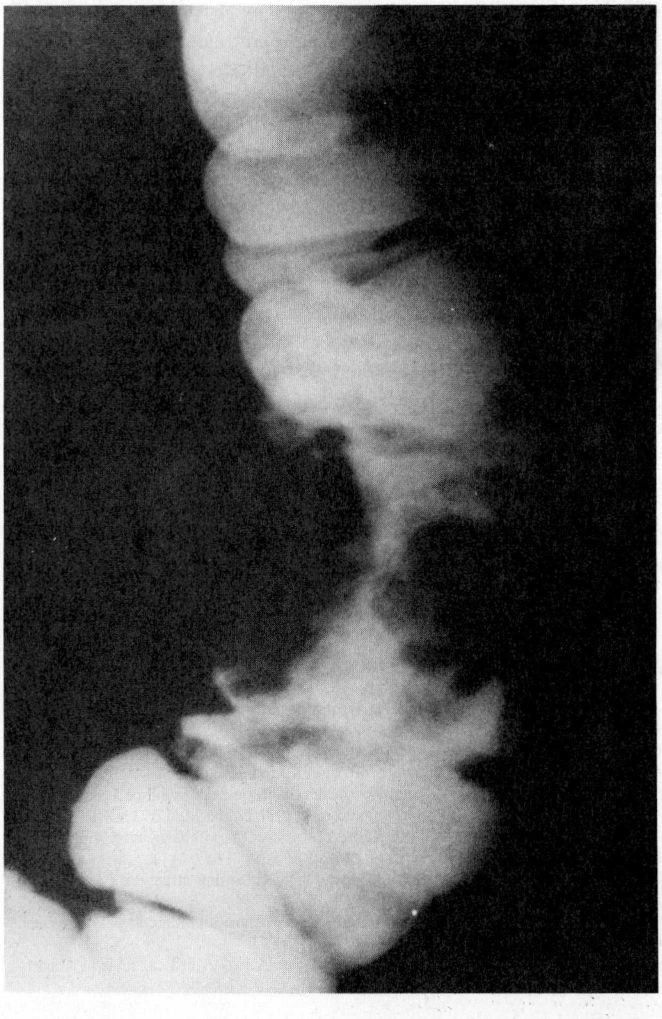

be regarded as the cause of rectal bleeding or chronic hypochromic anemia until a thorough investigation has been made of the more proximal gastrointestinal tract. Acute blood loss can occasionally be attributed to internal hemorrhoids. Chronic anemia in the presence of large but not definitely bleeding hemorrhoids should provoke a search for a polyp, cancer, or ulcer.

Most hemorrhoids respond to conservative therapy such as sitz baths or other forms of moist heat, suppositories, stool softeners, and bed rest. Internal hemorrhoids which remain permanently prolapsed are best treated surgically; milder degrees of prolapse or enlargement with pruritus ani or intermittent bleeding can be successfully handled by banding or injection of sclerosing solutions. External hemorrhoids which become acutely thrombosed are treated by incision, extraction of the clot, and compression of the incised area following clot removal. No surgical procedure should be carried out in the presence of acute inflammation of the anus, ulcerative proctitis, or ulcerative colitis. Both proctoscopy and barium enema should always be performed before a patient is subjected to hemorrhoidectomy.

ANAL INFLAMMATION Perianal inflammatory lesions may be primary or may be associated with inflammatory bowel disease or diverticular disease as mentioned above. Anal *fissures* are superficial erosions of the anal canal which usually heal rapidly with conservative therapy. Anal *ulcers* are more chronic and deep and give symptoms largely as the result of painful spasm of the external anal sphincter during and after defecation. Bleeding may occur with either fissure or ulcer; healing of the ulcer often is associated with a hypertrophied anal papilla and some degrees of anal contracture. *Fistula in ano,* a tract leading from the rectal lumen to the perianal skin, usually results from local crypt abscesses; fewer than 5 percent of such lesions found in medical practice in the United States are due to tuberculosis or cancer. The fistula is a chronically inflamed canal made up of fibrous tissue surrounding granulation tissue, the lumen of which may be difficult to demonstrate. Perirectal *abscesses* often represent the tracking down into the anal area of purulent material escaping from the rectosigmoid; diverticulitis, Crohn's disease, ulcerative colitis, or previous surgery may be the underlying cause. Fistulas between the rectum and vagina or the rectum and bladder represent serious complications of granulomatous, septic, or malignant disorders and require the patient to be hospitalized for definitive diagnostic and therapeutic procedures.

REFERENCES

Disorders of motility

BODE WE et al: Colonoscopic decompression for acute decompression of the colon. Am J Surg 147:243, 1984

LATIMER P et al: Colonic motor and myoelectric activity. Gastroenterology 80:893, 1981

PRESTON DM et al: Positive correlation between symptoms and circulating motilin, pancreatic polypeptide and gastrin concentrations in functional bowel disorders. Gut 26:1059, 1985

SCHUFFLER MD et al: Chronic intestinal pseudo-obstruction. Medicine 60:173, 1981

Intestinal ischemia

ABEL M et al: Ischemic colitis: Comparison of surgical and nonoperative management. Dis Colon Rectum 26:113, 1983

LEVINE D: Intestinal vascular ectasia. Am J Med 76:1151, 1984

MARSHAK RH et al: Ischemia of the colon. Mount Sinai J Med 48:108, 1981

Intestinal neoplasia

BURT RW et al: Upper gastrointestinal polyps in Gardner's syndrome. Gastroenterology 86:295, 1984

DECOSSE JJ: Malignant colorectal polyp. Gut 25:433, 1984

FLETCHER RH: Carcinoembryonic antigen. Ann Int Med 104:66, 1986

LIPKIN M, NEWMARK H: Effect of dietary calcium on colonic epithelial-cell proliferation in subjects at high risk for familial colonic cancer. N Engl J Med 313:1381, 1985

MATUCHANSKY C et al: Malignant lymphoma of the small bowel associated with diffuse nodular lymphoid hyperplasia. N Engl J Med 313:166, 1985

MOORE JR et al: Colorectal cancer: Risk factors and screening strategies. Arch Intern Med 144:1819, 1984

MORSON BC et al: Histopathology and prognosis of malignant colorectal polyps treated by endoscopic polypectomy. Gut 25:437, 1984

SIMON JB: Occult blood screening for colorectal carcinoma. A critical review. Gastroenterology 88:820, 1985

WEINGRAD DN et al: Primary gastrointestinal lymphoma. A 30 year review. Cancer 49:1258, 1982

WELLER IVD: The gay bowel. Gut 26:869, 1985

Other

GILINSKY NH et al: Plasma cell infiltration of the small bowel: Lack of evidence for a non-secretory form of alpha-heavy chain disease. Gut 26:928, 1985

240 ACUTE INTESTINAL OBSTRUCTION

WILLIAM SILEN

ETIOLOGY AND CLASSIFICATION Intestinal obstruction may be *mechanical* or *nonmechanical* (resulting from neuromuscular disturbances which produce either *adynamic* or *dynamic ileus*). The causes of mechanical obstruction of the lumen are conveniently divided into (1) lesions *extrinsic* to the intestine, e.g., adhesive bands, internal and external hernias; (2) lesions *intrinsic* to the wall of the intestine, e.g., diverticulitis, carcinoma, regional enteritis; and (3) obturation of the lumen, e.g., gallstone obstruction, intussusception. From the clinical standpoint, however, it is most useful to consider whether the obstructive mechanism involves the small or large intestine, because the causes, symptoms, and treatment are different (see below). Adhesions and external hernias are the most common causes of obstruction of the small intestine, constituting 70 to 75 percent of cases of this type. Adhesions, however, almost never produce obstruction of the colon, while carcinoma, sigmoid diverticulitis, and volvulus, in that order, are the most common etiologies and together account for about 90 percent of the cases.

Adynamic ileus is probably the most common overall cause of obstruction. Recent studies indicate that the development of this condition is mediated via the hormonal component of the sympathoadrenal system. Adynamic ileus will occur after any peritoneal insult, and its severity and duration will be dependent to some degree on the type of peritoneal injury. Hydrochloric acid, colonic contents, and pancreatic enzymes are among the most irritating substances, whereas blood and urine are less so. Adynamic ileus occurs to some degree after any abdominal operation, and its severity varies directly with the amount of intestinal handling and the length of the operation; it usually lasts 2 to 3 days after most operative procedures. Retroperitoneal hematomas, particularly associated with vertebral fracture, commonly cause severe adynamic ileus, and the latter may occur with other retroperitoneal conditions such as ureteral calculus or severe pyelonephritis. Thoracic diseases including lower-lobe pneumonia, fractured ribs, and myocardial infarction frequently produce adynamic ileus, as do electrolyte disturbances, particularly potassium depletion. Finally intestinal ischemia, whether the result of vascular occlusion or intestinal distention itself, may perpetuate an adynamic ileus. Spastic or dynamic ileus is very uncommon and results from extreme and prolonged contraction of the intestine. It has been observed in heavy metal poisoning, uremia, porphyria, and extensive intestinal ulcerations.

PATHOPHYSIOLOGY Distention of the intestine is caused by the accumulation of gas and fluid proximal to and within the obstructed segment. Seventy to eighty percent of intestinal gas consists of swallowed air, and because this is composed mainly of nitrogen, which is poorly absorbed from the intestinal lumen, removal of air by continuous gastric suction is an important adjunct in the treatment of intestinal distention. The accumulation of fluid proximal to the obstructing mechanism results not only from ingested fluid, swallowed saliva, gastric juice, and biliary and pancreatic secretions but also from interference with normal sodium and water transport. During the first 12 to 24 h of obstruction there is a marked depression of flux from lumen to blood of sodium and consequently water in the distended proximal intestine. After 24 h, there is also movement of sodium and water into the lumen, contributing further to the distention and fluid losses. Intraluminal pressure rises from a normal of 2 to 4 cmH_2O to 8 to 10 cmH_2O. During peristalsis, when simple obstruction or a "closed loop" is present, pressures reach 30 to 60 cmH_2O. Closed-loop obstruction of the small intestine results when the lumen is occluded at two points by a single mechanism such as a hernial ring or adhesive band, thus producing a closed loop whose blood supply is often obstructed at the same time. Strangulation of the loop itself is thus common in association with marked distention proximal to the involved loop. A form of closed-loop obstruction is encountered when complete obstruction of the colon exists in the presence of a competent ileocecal valve (85 percent of individuals). Although the blood supply of the colon is not entrapped within the obstructing mechanism, distention of the cecum is extreme because of its greater diameter (LaPlace's law), and impairment of the intramural blood supply is considerable with consequent gangrene of the cecal wall, usually anteriorly. Necrosis of the small intestine may occur by the same mechanism of interference with intramural blood flow when distention is extreme, but this sequence is uncommon in the small intestine. Once impairment of blood supply occurs, bacterial invasion supervenes and subsequent peritonitis develops. The systemic effects of extreme distention include elevation of the diaphragms with restricted ventilation and subsequent atelectasis. Venous return via the inferior vena cava may also be impaired.

The loss of fluids and electrolytes may be extreme, and unless replacement is prompt, leads to hemoconcentration, hypovolemia, renal insufficiency, shock, and death. Vomiting, accumulation of fluids within the lumen by the mechanisms described above, and the sequestration of fluid into the edematous intestinal wall and peritoneal cavity as a result of impairment of venous return from the intestine all contribute to massive loss of fluid and electrolytes. As soon as significant impedance to venous return is present, the intestine becomes severely congested, and blood begins to seep into the intestinal lumen. Blood loss may reach significant levels when long segments of intestine are involved.

SYMPTOMS *Mechanical small-intestinal obstruction* is characterized by cramping midabdominal pain which tends to be more severe the higher the obstruction. The pain occurs in paroxysms, and the patient is relatively comfortable in the intervals between the pains. Audible borborygmi are often noted by the patient simultaneously with the paroxysms of pain. The pain may become less severe as distention progresses, probably because motility is impaired in the edematous intestine. When strangulation is present, the pain is usually more localized and may be steady and severe without a colicky component, a fact which often causes delay in diagnosis of obstruction. Vomiting is almost invariable, and it is earlier and more profuse the higher the obstruction. The vomitus initially contains bile and mucus and remains as such if the obstruction is high in the intestine. With low ileal obstruction, the vomitus becomes feculent, i.e., orange-brown in color with a foul odor, which results from the overgrowth of bacteria proximal to the obstruction. Singultus is common. Obstipation and failure to pass gas by rectum are invariably present when the obstruction is complete, although some stool and gas may be passed spontaneously or after an enema shortly after onset of the complete obstruction. Diarrhea is occasionally observed in partial obstruction. Blood in the stool is rare, even in the completely obstructed patient, but does occur in cases of intussusception. Other than some minor but inconsistent differences in pain patterns noted above, the symptoms of strangulating obstructions cannot be distinguished from those of nonstrangulating obstructions.

Mechanical colonic obstruction produces colicky abdominal pain similar in quality to that of small-intestinal obstruction but of much lower intensity. Complaints of pain are occasionally absent in stoic elderly patients. Vomiting occurs late, if at all, particularly if the ileocecal valve is competent. Paradoxically, feculent vomitus is very rare. A history of recent alterations in bowel habits and blood in the stool is common because carcinoma and diverticulitis are the most frequent causes. Constipation becomes progressive, and obstipation with failure to pass gas ensues. Acute symptoms may develop over a period of a week.

In *adynamic ileus,* colicky pain is absent, and only discomfort from distention is evident. Vomiting may be frequent but is rarely profuse. It usually consists of gastric contents and bile and is almost never feculent. Complete obstipation may or may not occur. Singultus is very common.

PHYSICAL FINDINGS *Abdominal distention* is the hallmark of all forms of intestinal obstruction. It is least marked in cases of obstruction high in the small intestine and most marked in colonic obstruction. Early in the course of the disease, especially in closed-loop strangulating small-bowel obstruction, distention may be barely perceptible or absent. Tenderness and rigidity are usually minimal; the temperature is rarely above 100°F in nonstrangulating obstruction of the small and large intestine. Contrary to popular belief the same is true of strangulating obstruction until very late in the course of the disease, a fact which has often resulted in unfortunate delay in treatment. Signs and symptoms of shock also occur *very late* in strangulating obstruction. The appearance of shock, tenderness, rigidity, and fever often means that there has been contamination of the peritoneum with infected intestinal content. The presence of a palpable abdominal mass usually signifies a closed-loop strangulating small-bowel obstruction because the tense fluid-filled loop is the palpable lesion. Auscultation may reveal loud high-pitched borborygmi coincident with the colicky pain, but this classic finding is often not present late in strangulating or nonstrangulating obstruction. A quiet abdomen does not eliminate the possibility of obstruction, nor does it necessarily establish the diagnosis of adynamic ileus.

LABORATORY AND X-RAY FINDINGS Leukocytosis, with shift to the left, usually occurs when strangulation is present, but a normal white blood cell count does not exclude strangulation. Elevation of the serum amylase is encountered occasionally in all forms of intestinal obstruction, especially the strangulating variety.

The x-ray is extremely valuable but under certain circumstances may also be misleading. In nonstrangulating complete small-bowel obstruction, x-rays are almost completely reliable. Distention of fluid- and gas-filled loops of small intestine usually arranged in a "step-ladder" pattern with air-fluid levels and an absence or paucity of colonic gas are pathognomonic (Fig. 240-1). These findings, however, are absent in slightly over half the cases of strangulating small-bowel obstruction, especially early in the disease. A general haze due to peritoneal fluid and sometimes a "coffee-bean"-shaped mass are seen in strangulating obstruction. Occasionally the films are normal, but when symptoms are consistent with obstruction of the small intestine, a normal film should suggest strangulation. Roentgenographic differentiation of partial mechanical small-bowel obstruction from adynamic ileus may be impossible since gas is present in both small and large intestine; however, colonic distention is usually more prominent in adynamic ileus. A radiopaque dye given by mouth is useful in making this distinction.

Colonic obstruction with a competent ileocecal valve is easily recognized because distention with gas is mainly confined to the colon. Barium enema, sigmoidoscopy, or colonoscopy, depending upon the suspected site of obstruction, are usually advisable to determine the nature of the lesion except when concomitant perforation is suspected, a rare occurrence. Sigmoidoscopy may be therapeutic in cases of sigmoid volvulus. When the ileocecal valve is incompetent, the films resemble those of partial small-bowel obstruction or adynamic ileus, and barium enema or colonoscopy is necessary to establish the correct diagnosis. Barium given by mouth is perfectly safe when obstruction is in the small intestine since the barium sulfate does not become inspissated in this location. *Barium should never be given by mouth to a patient with possible colonic obstruction* until that possibility has been excluded by barium enema.

PROGNOSIS AND TREATMENT **Small-intestinal obstruction** The overall mortality rate for obstruction of the small intestine is about

10 percent, even under the most optimal conditions. While the mortality rate for nonstrangulating obstruction is as low as 5 to 8 percent, that for strangulating obstruction has been reported to be between 20 and 75 percent. Well over half of the deaths from small-bowel obstruction occur in those with strangulation; however, the latter constitute only one-fourth to one-third of the cases. Careful studies indicate that the clinical, laboratory, and x-ray findings are not reliable in distinguishing strangulating from nonstrangulating obstruction when obstruction is complete. Complete obstruction is suggested when there has been a total cessation in the passage of gas or stool per rectum and when gas is absent in the distal intestine by x-ray. Since strangulating small-bowel obstruction is always complete, operation should always be undertaken in such patients after suitable preparation. Prior to operation, fluid and electrolyte balance should be restored, and decompression instituted by means of a nasogastric tube. Six to eight hours of preparation may be necessary. During this period broad-spectrum antibiotics are indicated if strangulation is felt to be likely, but operation should not be delayed unless there is unequivocal clinical and roentgenographic evidence of resolution of the obstruction during the period of preparation. Attempts to pass a long tube into the small intestine usually fail while putting the patient through uncomfortable unproductive manipulations which delay appropriate fluid replacement and decompression. *There are probably few if any indications for the use of a long intestinal tube.* Procrastination of operation because of improvement in well-being of the patient during resuscitation and gastric decompression usually leads to unnecessary and hazardous delay in proper treatment. Purely nonoperative therapy is safe only in the presence of incomplete obstruction and is best utilized in patients with (1) repeated episodes of partial obstruction, (2) recent postoperative partial obstruction, and (3) partial obstruction following a recent episode of diffuse peritonitis.

Colonic obstruction The mortality rate for colonic obstruction is about 20 percent. As in small-bowel obstruction, nonoperative treatment is contraindicated unless the obstruction is incomplete. Occasionally, but not always, when the obstruction is incomplete, nonoperative therapy may result in sufficient decompression that a definitive operative procedure can be undertaken at a later date. This can usually be accomplished by discontinuation of all oral intake and perhaps by nasogastric suction, although attempts to decompress a *completely* obstructed colon by intubation are almost invariably futile. A long intestinal tube will not decompress an obstructed colon with a competent ileocecal valve. When obstruction is complete, early operation is mandatory, especially when the ileocecal valve is competent; cecal gangrene is likely if the cecal diameter exceeds 10 cm on plain abdominal film. For obstruction on the left side of the colon, the most common site, preliminary operative decompression by cecostomy or transverse colostomy followed by definitive resection of the primary lesion is the treatment of choice. For a lesion of the right or transverse colon, primary resection and anastomosis can safely be performed because distention of the ileum with consequent discrepancy in size and hazard in suture are not present.

FIGURE 240-1 *Acute mechanical obstruction of small intestine (upright film). Note air-fluid levels, marked distention of bowel loops, and absence of colonic gas.*

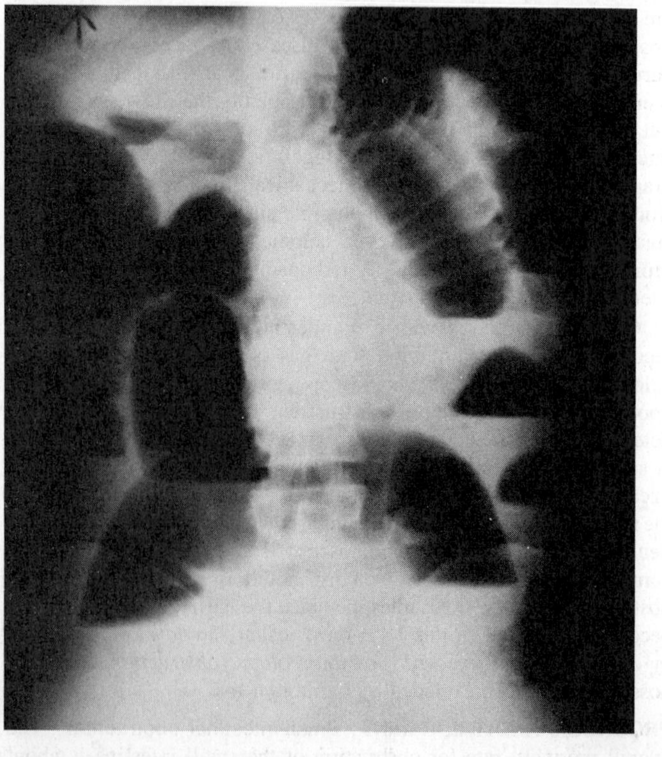

Adynamic ileus This type of ileus usually responds to nonoperative continuous decompression and adequate treatment of the primary disease. The prognosis is usually good. Rarely, adynamic colonic distention may become so great that cecostomy is required if cecal gangrene is feared. Spastic ileus usually responds to treatment of the primary disease.

REFERENCES

Becker WF: Acute adhesive ileus: A study of 412 cases with particular reference to the abuse of tube decompression in treatment. Surg Gynecol Obstet 95:472, 1952

Bulkley GB et al: Intraoperative determination of small intestinal viability following ischemic injury: Prospective controlled trial of two adjuvant methods (Doppler and fluorescein) compared with standard clinical judgement. Ann Surg 193:628, 1981

Cohn I, Atik M: Strangulation obstruction: Closed loop studies. Ann Surg 153:94, 1961

DuBois A et al: Postoperative ileus: Physiopathology, etiology and treatment. Ann Surg 178:781, 1973

Gough IR: Strangulating adhesive small bowel radiographs. Br J Surg 65:431, 1978

Hofsetter SR: Acute adhesive obstruction of the small intestine. Surg Gynec Obstet 152:141, 1981

Jackson BR: The diagnosis of colonic obstruction. Dis Colon Rectum 25:603, 1982

Nolan DJ: Barium examination of the small intestine. Gut 22:682, 1981

Shields R: The absorption and secretion of fluid and electrolytes by the obstructed bowel. Br J Surg 52:774, 1965

Silen W: *Cope's Early Diagnosis of the Acute Abdomen,* 16th ed. London, Oxford, 1983

241 ACUTE APPENDICITIS

WILLIAM SILEN

INCIDENCE AND EPIDEMIOLOGY The maximum incidence of acute appendicitis occurs in the second and third decades of life. While the disease may be encountered at any time of life, it is relatively rare at the extremes of age. Males and females are equally affected except between puberty and age 25, when males predominate in a 3:2 ratio. Perforation is relatively much more common in infancy and in the aged, during which periods mortality rates are highest. The mortality rate has decreased steadily in Europe and the United States from 8.1 per 100,000 of the population in 1941 to less than 1 per 100,000 in 1970. The absolute incidence of the disease also decreased by about 40 percent between 1940 and 1960 but since then has remained unchanged. Although various factors such as changing dietary habits, altered intestinal flora, and better nutrition and intake of vitamins have been suggested to explain the reduced incidence, the exact reasons have not been elucidated. Of interest is that the overall incidence of appendicitis is much lower in underdeveloped countries, especially parts of Africa, and in lower socioeconomic groups.

PATHOGENESIS The primary pathogenetic hallmark has always been thought to be luminal obstruction. While obstruction can be identified by careful examination in 30 to 40 percent of cases, recent studies have shown that ulceration of the mucosa is the initial event in the majority. The causation of the ulceration is unknown, although a viral etiology has been postulated. Whether the inflammatory reaction attendant with ulceration is sufficient to obstruct the tiny appendiceal lumen even transiently is also not clear. Obstruction, when present, is most commonly caused by a fecalith, which results from accumulation and inspissation of fecal matter around vegetable fibers. Enlarged lymphoid follicles associated with viral infections (e.g., measles), inspissated barium, worms (e.g., pinworms, *Ascaris,* and *Taenia*), and tumors (e.g., carcinoid or carcinoma) may also obstruct the lumen. Secretion of mucus distends the organ, which has a capacity of only 0.1 to 0.2 mL, and luminal pressures rise as high as 60 cmH_2O. Luminal bacteria multiply and invade the appendiceal wall as venous engorgement and subsequent arterial compromise result from the high intraluminal pressures. Finally, gangrene and perforation occur. If the process evolves slowly, adjacent organs such as the terminal ileum, cecum, and omentum may wall off the appendiceal area so that a localized abscess will develop, whereas rapid progression of vascular impairment may cause perforation with free access to the peritoneal cavity. Subsequent rupture of primary appendiceal abscesses may produce fistulas between the appendix and bladder, small intestine, sigmoid, or cecum. Occasionally, acute appendicitis may be the first manifestation of Crohn's disease. While chronic infection of the appendix with tuberculosis, amebiasis, and actinomycosis may occur, a useful clinical aphorism states that *chronic appendiceal inflammation is not usually the cause of prolonged abdominal pain of weeks' or months' duration.* In contrast, it is clear that recurrent acute appendicitis does occur, often with complete resolution of inflammation and symptoms between attacks. Recurrent acute appendicitis may become more frequent as antibiotics are dispensed more freely.

CLINICAL MANIFESTATIONS The history and sequence of symptoms are among the most important diagnostic features of appendicitis. The initial symptom is almost invariably *abdominal pain* of the visceral type, resulting from appendiceal contractions or distention of the lumen. It is usually poorly localized in the periumbilical or epigastric regions. There is often an accompanying urge to defecate or pass flatus, neither of which relieves the distress. This visceral pain is mild, often cramping, and rarely catastrophic in nature, usually lasting 4 to 6 h, but may not be noted by stoic individuals or by some patients during sleep. As inflammation spreads to the parietal peritoneal surfaces, the pain becomes somatic, steady, and more severe, aggravated by motion or cough and usually located in the *right lower quadrant. Anorexia* is so frequent that the presence of hunger should arouse serious suspicion of the diagnosis of acute appendicitis. *Nausea* and *vomiting* occur in 50 to 60 percent of cases, but vomiting is rarely profuse and protracted. The development of nausea and vomiting before the onset of pain is extremely rare. Change in bowel habit is of little diagnostic value since any or no alteration may be observed, although the presence of diarrhea caused by an inflamed appendix in juxtaposition to the sigmoid may cause serious diagnostic difficulties. Urinary frequency and dysuria occur if the appendix lies adjacent to the bladder. The typical sequence of symptoms (poorly localized periumbilical pain followed by nausea and vomiting with subsequent shift of pain to the right lower quadrant) occurs in only 50 to 60 percent of patients, and some variations are considered below.

Physical findings vary with time after onset of the illness and according to the location of the appendix, which may be situated deep in the pelvic cul-de-sac, in the right lower quadrant in any relation to the peritoneum, cecum, and small intestine, in the right upper quadrant, or even in the left lower quadrant. *The diagnosis cannot be established unless tenderness can be elicited.* While tenderness is sometimes absent in the early visceral stage of the disease, it ultimately always develops and is found in any location corresponding to the position of the appendix. Abdominal tenderness may be completely absent if a retrocecal or pelvic appendix is present, in which case the sole physical finding may be tenderness in the flank or on rectal or pelvic examination. Percussion, rebound tenderness, and referred rebound tenderness are often, but not invariably, present; they are most likely to be absent early in the illness. Flexion of the right hip and guarded movement by the patient are due to parietal peritoneal involvement. Hyperesthesia of the skin of the right lower quadrant and a positive psoas or obturator sign are often late findings and are rarely of diagnostic value. When the inflamed appendix is in close proximity to the anterior parietal peritoneum, muscular rigidity is present, yet is often minimal early. The temperature is usually normal or slightly elevated (99 to 100.5°F), but a temperature above 101°F should always suggest the presence of perforation. Tachycardia is commensurate with the elevation of the temperature. Rigidity and tenderness become more marked as the disease progresses to perforation and localized or diffuse peritonitis. Distention is rare unless severe diffuse peritonitis has developed. The alleged disappearance of pain and tenderness just prior to perforation is extremely unusual. A mass may develop if localized perforation has occurred but usually will not be detectable before 3 days after onset of the disease. Earlier presence of a mass suggests carcinoma of the cecum or Crohn's disease. Perforation is rare before 24 h after onset of symptoms, but the rate may be as high as 80 percent after 48 h.

Laboratory examination does not establish the diagnosis since the latter is based primarily on clinical grounds. Although moderate leukocytosis of 10,000 to 18,000 cells per cubic millimeter is frequent (with a concomitant shift to immature cells), the absence of leukocytosis does not eliminate the possibility of acute appendicitis. Leukocytosis of greater than 20,000 cells per cubic millimeter should alert the clinician to the probability of perforation. Anemia and blood in the stool suggest a primary diagnosis of carcinoma of the cecum, especially in elderly individuals. The urine may contain a few white or red blood cells without bacteria if the appendix lies close to the right ureter or bladder.

Urinalysis is most useful, however, in excluding genitourinary conditions which may mimic acute appendicitis. X-rays are rarely of value except when an opaque fecalith (5 percent of patients) is observed in the right lower quadrant (especially in children) together with other clinical findings consistent with appendicitis. Consequently there is no routine need to obtain films of the abdomen unless there is a possibility of other conditions such as intestinal obstruction or ureteral calculus. In some cases in which symptoms are either recurrent or more prolonged, a careful barium enema may disclose an extrinsic defect on the medial wall of the cecum or a calcified fecalith.

While the typical historical sequence and physical findings are present in 50 to 60 percent of cases, it is obvious that a wide variety of atypical patterns of disease are encountered, especially at the age extremes and during pregnancy. The 70 to 80 percent incidence of perforation and generalized peritonitis in infants under 2 years of age is dramatic testimony to the importance of the history in the early detection of the disease. Any infant or child with diarrhea, vomiting, and abdominal pain is highly suspect. Fever is much more common in this age group, and abdominal distention is often the only physical finding. In the elderly, pain and tenderness are often obtunded, and thus the diagnosis is frequently delayed. A 30 percent incidence of perforation in patients over 70 attests to the importance of this delay. Elderly patients often present themselves initially with a slightly painful mass (a primary appendiceal abscess), or sometimes appear with adhesive intestinal obstruction 5 or 6 days after a previously undetected perforated appendix. Appendicitis occurs about once in every 1000 pregnancies and is the most common extrauterine condition requiring abdominal operation. The diagnosis may be missed or delayed because of the frequent occurrence of mild abdominal discomfort and nausea and vomiting during pregnancy. During the last trimester when the mortality rate from appendicitis is highest, uterine displacement of the appendix to the right upper quadrant and laterally leads to confusion in diagnosis.

DIFFERENTIAL DIAGNOSIS A listing of the differential diagnoses of acute appendicitis would produce an encyclopedic compendium of all conditions which cause abdominal pain since appendicitis may simulate any of these diseases. Diagnostic accuracy is about 75 to 80 percent for experienced clinicians and must be based solely on the clinical criteria outlined above. It is probably better to err slightly in the direction of overdiagnosis since delay is associated with perforation and increased morbidity and mortality. In unperforated appendicitis the mortality rate is 0.1 percent, little more than that associated with general anesthesia; for perforated appendicitis there is an overall mortality of 3 percent, a figure which increases to 15 percent in the elderly. In doubtful cases 4 to 6 h of observation is always more beneficial than harmful, however. The most common conditions discovered at operation when acute appendicitis is erroneously diagnosed are, in rough order of frequency, mesenteric lymphadenitis, no organic disease, acute pelvic inflammatory disease, ruptured graafian follicle or corpus luteum cyst, and acute gastroenteritis. In addition, acute cholecystitis, perforated ulcer, acute pancreatitis, acute diverticulitis, strangulating intestinal obstruction, ureteral calculus, and pyelonephritis frequently present diagnostic difficulties.

It is useful to consider separately some of the more common and difficult diagnostic possibilities, especially in the female. Differentiation of *pelvic inflammatory disease* from acute appendicitis may be virtually impossible. Gram-negative intracellular diplococci on cervical smear are not pathognomonic unless *Neisseria gonorrhea* can be cultured. Pain on movement of the cervix is not specific and may occur in appendicitis if perforation has occurred or if the appendix lies adjacent to the uterus or adnexa. *Rupture of a graafian follicle* (mittelschmerz) occurs at midcycle with spill of blood and fluid to produce pain and tenderness more diffuse and usually of a less severe degree than in appendicitis. Fever and leukocytosis are usually absent. *Rupture of a corpus luteum cyst* is identical clinically to rupture of a graafian follicle but develops about the time of menstruation. The presence of an adnexal mass and evidence of blood loss help differentiate *ruptured tubal pregnancy*. *Twisted ovarian cyst* and *endometriosis* occasionally are difficult to distinguish from appendicitis.

Acute mesenteric lymphadenitis is the appellation usually given when enlarged, slightly reddened lymph nodes at the root of the mesentery and a normal appendix are encountered at operation in a patient who usually has right lower quadrant tenderness and a somewhat higher temperature than most patients with acute appendicitis. Whether this is a single, discrete entity is unclear since the causative factor is not known. It has been recognized recently that some of these patients have infection with *Yersinia pseudotuberculosis* or *Y. enterocolytica* in which case the diagnosis can be established by culture of the mesenteric nodes or by serologic titers (Chap. 114). The diagnosis is essentially impossible clinically, although retrospectively there often appears to have been more diffuse pain and tenderness. Children seem to be affected more frequently than adults. Operation should be undertaken unless there is rapid resolution of all symptoms and findings. *Acute gastroenteritis* usually causes profuse watery diarrhea, often with nausea and vomiting but without localized findings. Between cramps, the abdomen is completely relaxed. In salmonella gastroenteritis the abdominal findings are similar, although the pain may be more severe and more localized, and fever and chills are common. The occurrence of similar symptoms among other members of the family may be helpful. When the diagnosis of acute pelvic appendicitis with perforation has been missed, gastroenteritis is the most common previous working diagnosis. Persistent abdominal or rectal tenderness should eliminate the diagnosis of gastroenteritis. *Regional enteritis* (Crohn's disease) is usually associated with a more prolonged history, often with previous exacerbations regarded by the patient or physician as episodes of gastroenteritis unless the diagnosis has been established previously. *Meckel's diverticulitis* usually cannot be distinguished from acute appendicitis but is very rare.

TREATMENT Cathartics and frequent enemas should be avoided if appendicitis is under consideration, and antibiotics should not be administered when the diagnosis is in question, as they will only mask the presence or development of perforation. The treatment is early operation and appendectomy as soon as the patient can be prepared. Preparation rarely takes more than 1 to 2 h in early appendicitis but may require 6 to 8 h in cases of severe sepsis and dehydration associated with late perforation. The *only* circumstance in which operation is *not* indicated is the presence of a palpable mass 3 to 5 days after the onset of symptoms. Should operation be undertaken at that time, a phlegmon rather than a definitive abscess will be found, and complications from dissection of such a phlegmon are frequent. Such patients treated with broad-spectrum antibiotics, parenteral fluids, and rest usually show resolution of the mass and symptoms within 1 week. *Interval appendectomy* can and should be done safely 3 months later. Should the mass enlarge or the patient become more toxic, drainage of the abscess is necessary. The complications of subphrenic, pelvic, or other intraabdominal abscesses usually follow perforation with generalized peritonitis and can be avoided by early diagnosis of the disease.

REFERENCES

BOLTON JP: Assessment of the value of the white cell count in management of suspected acute appendicitis. Br J Surg 62:906, 1975

BUSUTTIL RW et al: Effect of prophylactic antibiotics in acute nonperforated appendicitis: A prospective, randomized double-blind clinical study. Ann Surg 194:502, 1981

BUTLER C: Surgical pathology of acute appendicitis. Hum Pathol 12:870, 1981

KOEPSELL TD et al: Factors affecting perforation in acute appendicitis. Surg Gynecol Obstet 153:508, 1981

OWENS BJ III, HAMIT HF: Appendicitis in the elderly. Ann Surg 187:392, 1978

SAKOVER RP, DEL FAVA RL: Frequency of visualization of normal appendix with barium enema examination. Am J Roentgenol Rad Therap Nucl Med 121:312, 1974

THOMAS DR: Conservative management of appendix mass. Surgery 73:677, 1973

VANTRAPPEN G et al.: *Yersinia* enteritis and enterocolitis: Gastroenterological aspects. Gastroenterology 72:220, 1977

242 DISEASES OF THE PERITONEUM AND MESENTERY

KURT J. ISSELBACHER / J. THOMAS LaMONT

ACUTE PERITONITIS Peritonitis is a localized or generalized inflammatory process of the peritoneum that may appear in both acute and chronic forms. In the acute form the motor activity of the intestine is decreased, and the intestinal lumen becomes distended with gas and fluid. Fluid accumulates as a result of failure to reabsorb the 7 or 8 liters normally secreted daily into the lumen and absorbed from the distal small bowel and colon. There is also accumulation of fluid in the peritoneal cavity as well as decreased oral intake. These combined losses can lead to rapid depletion of the plasma volume with impaired cardiac and renal function.

Etiology Peritonitis may be due to entry of bacteria into the peritoneal cavity from a perforation in the gastrointestinal tract or from an external penetrating wound. It may be secondary to severe chemical reactions from the release of pancreatic enzymes, the digestive juices of the upper gastrointestinal tract, or bile as a result of injury or perforation of the intestine or biliary tract. Patients with systemic lupus erythematosus may have bouts of peritonitis during attacks of their disease.

The most common causes of bacterial peritonitis are appendicitis, perforations associated with diverticulitis, peptic ulcer, gangrenous gallbladder, and gangrenous obstruction of the small bowel from adhesive bands, incarcerated hernia, or volvulus. Any lesion leading to the escape of intestinal bacteria may be a source, including a perforating carcinoma, foreign body, and ulcerative colitis. The peritoneal cavity is remarkably resistant to contamination, and unless continuing contamination occurs, the disease process becomes localized. Patients with alcoholic cirrhosis and ascites have an increased susceptibility to spontaneous bacterial peritonitis, usually from enteric pathogens. This complication occurs in the absence of recognizable perforation of a viscus, and may be due to leakage of bacteria through the intestinal wall.

Clinical features These usually consist of increasing abdominal pain, distention, nausea and vomiting, inability to pass feces or flatus, fever, hypotension, tachycardia, thirst, and oliguria. On physical examination the patient appears acutely ill and febrile and has a variable degree of abdominal distention. The abdomen is usually acutely tender and tympanitic, often with rebound tenderness. The location of the pain and tenderness depends on the underlying cause and whether the inflammation is localized or generalized. In *localized* peritonitis, as seen in uncomplicated appendicitis or diverticulitis, the physical findings are limited to the area of inflammation. With widespread peritoneal inflammation there is *generalized* peritonitis with diffuse abdominal tenderness and rebound. Rigidity of the abdominal wall is a common finding in peritonitis and may be localized or generalized.

Peristalsis may be present initially but usually disappears as the illness progresses. Hypotension is common, as is leukocytosis, which often is greater than 20,000 cells per cubic millimeter. Plain abdominal films may reveal dilatation of the large and small bowel with edema of the small-bowel wall as evidenced by the distance between adjacent loops of gas-filled small intestine. Diagnostic paracentesis is sometimes valuable in determining the nature of the exudate as well as whether bacteria can be demonstrated or cultured. Diabetic ketoacidosis, lead colic, gastric crises of syphilis, and acute porphyria may cause severe abdominal symptoms that resemble the picture of acute peritonitis.

GONOCOCCAL PERITONITIS This usually involves an extension of gonococcal infection from a primary focus in the female reproductive tract. The signs of inflammation usually are limited to the pelvis, but there may be findings of a mild generalized peritonitis. Occasionally the patient has right upper quadrant pain and tenderness caused by gonococcal perihepatitis involving the liver capsule and adjacent peritoneum (Fitz-Hugh–Curtis syndrome; see also Chap. 104).

STARCH PERITONITIS An acute granulomatous peritonitis can develop in some patients as a foreign-body reaction to cornstarch used to powder surgical gloves. The clinical picture is that of acute abdominal pain and fever 10 to 30 days after an abdominal operation. The diagnosis can be made by paracentesis and demonstration of starch granules in monocytes. However, most patients are reexplored because of the fear of abscess or bacterial peritonitis, with the finding of foreign-body granuloma studding the peritoneum.

PSEUDOMYXOMA PERITONEI This is a rare condition resulting from rupture of a mucocele of the appendix or of a mucinous ovarian cyst. The abdomen becomes filled with masses of jelly-like material. Occasionally, with removal of the mucocele or the ovarian cyst and most of the myxomatous material, a cure may ensue. In other cases, however, the mucoid material recurs, leading to progressive wasting and eventual death. Colloid carcinoma arising from the stomach or colon with peritoneal implants may resemble pseudomyxoma at laparotomy. The course of this type of highly malignant tumor is one of rapid cachexia and early death. The diagnosis can usually be made by the appearance of many highly malignant cells in the peritoneal implants.

CANCER OF THE PERITONEUM Aside from mesothelioma, which in most patients is caused by previous exposure to asbestos, cancer of the peritoneum is usually secondary to a neoplasm within the abdomen, most commonly of the stomach and ovary. This type of metastatic malignancy is invariably associated with progressive ascites with a high specific gravity and high protein content, often with large numbers of red blood cells or even gross blood. The diagnosis is established by demonstrating malignant cells in the fluid. The clinical progress of this malignant spread can sometimes be arrested by installations of radioactive gold, nitrogen mustard, or chloroquine.

FAMILIAL MEDITERRANEAN FEVER See Chap. 271.

PNEUMATOSIS CYSTOIDES INTESTINALIS This is a condition in which multiple gas-filled blebs or cysts accumulate in the intestinal wall beneath the serosal surface of the bowel. The exact source of the gas has not been explained satisfactorily. In some instances, this disease is associated with specific ulceration of the intestinal mucosa, in particular peptic ulcer with outlet obstruction. Cysts in the wall of the small bowel are seen as an occasional complication of mesenteric vascular occlusion. In the large bowel, these cysts are usually benign, may be seen with a variety of other disorders, and usually disappear in time.

There are no specific physical findings secondary to the pneumatosis, and the diagnosis is made either by x-ray or at laparotomy. Occasionally the subserosal cysts may rupture, resulting in pneumoperitoneum.

CHYLOUS ASCITES This term refers to the accumulation of chyle (intestinal lymph) in the peritoneal cavity. The condition is sometimes associated with chylothorax. The fluid in the peritoneal cavity appears milky or creamy because of the presence of chylomicrons. This fat may be demonstrated microscopically by staining with Sudan III and may be removed by acidification of the fluid followed by extraction with ether. The chyle (lipid) will then go into the ether phase. Many conditions may be associated with the cloudy or milky-appearing peritoneal fluid, so-called pseudochylous ascites. The milky or turbid appearance is usually due to the presence of protein and desquamated cells. The turbidity of this fluid will not be removed with the ether but will clear with addition of alkali.

The causes of chylous ascites include (1) penetrating or nonpenetrating trauma that damages the main duct in the lymphatic system within the abdomen, (2) intestinal obstruction if it is associated with rupture of a major lymphatic channel, (3) congenital lymphangiectasia, (4) malignant disease or tuberculous infection that obstructs the intestinal lymphatics, (5) filariasis, or (6) cirrhosis.

The sudden accumulation of chyle in the peritoneal cavity often results in abdominal pain, signs of peritoneal irritation, and leukocytosis. These symptoms gradually subside, leaving the patient with a distended but nontender, fluid-filled abdomen. Lymphangiography is of value in determining the location of the leak or site of obstruction to the lymphatic channels. The course depends upon the underlying etiologic factors.

MESENTERIC LIPODYSTROPHY This is a rare disorder usually affecting middle-aged women and characterized pathologically by infiltration of the mesentery with lipid-laden macrophages and fibrous tissue. These patients present with ill-defined abdominal pain and occasionally an abdominal mass. The diagnosis is made at laparotomy by demonstration of thick fibrofatty masses at the root of the mesentery with retraction and distortion of the bowel loops.

REFERENCES

HOEFS JC et al: Spontaneous bacterial peritonitis. Hepatology 2:1054, 1982

KIPFER RE et al: Mesenteric lipodystrophy. Ann Intern Med 80:582, 1974

LIMBER GK et al: Pseudomyxoma peritonei. Ann Surg 1978:587, 1973

PRESS OW et al: Evaluation and management of chylous ascites. Ann Intern Med 96:358, 1982

SCHWARTZ SI et al: *Principles of Surgery*, 3d ed. New York, McGraw-Hill, 1979

WARSHAW AL: Diagnosis of starch peritonitis by paracentesis. Lancet 2:1054, 1972

section 2 Hepatobiliary disease

243 APPROACH TO THE PATIENT WITH LIVER DISEASE

KURT J. ISSELBACHER

GENERAL CONSIDERATIONS While disease of the liver or biliary tract may be directly responsible for the symptoms that bring the patient to the physician, examination for nonhepatic complaints may occasionally provide the clues to otherwise asymptomatic or occult hepatobiliary disease. Liver function studies and other diagnostic procedures such as biopsy (as discussed in Chap. 245) are crucial, but much valuable information as to the possible nature and extent of liver disease can be obtained by a carefully elicited history and thorough physical examination.

Importance of clinical history Since laboratory tests often do not establish the specific cause of liver disease, the history is of the greatest significance. *Family history* is important with respect to jaundice, anemia, splenectomy, or cholecystectomy; a positive history may be helpful in diagnosing hemolytic anemia, congenital or familial hyperbilirubinemia, or gallstones. In Wilson's disease (hepatolenticular degeneration), there may be a family history of tremor or neurologic abnormalities. *Occupation* should be reviewed in detail, and *environmental factors* need to be examined. Note should be made of any contact with rats or other animals possibly carrying Weil's disease and of exposure to toxins such as carbon tetrachloride, beryllium, or vinyl chloride. The patient should be asked about travel to other countries, especially to areas where hepatitis may be endemic. Careful questioning regarding alcohol intake is important in most cases. Since the alcoholic often denies or understates the amounts consumed, it is desirable to check the validity of the history with close friends or relatives of the patient.

Contact with jaundiced patients (including intimate or sexual relations) should be noted. If the patient has had any *injections* in the previous 6 months, hepatitis B or non-A, non-B infection may be the underlying disease. Injections include blood tests, blood or plasma transfusions, tattooing, and dental treatment. The patient should be asked about narcotics, hallucinogens, or stimulant *drugs* taken parenterally, as well as about agents taken orally, such as chlorpromazine or estrogen-containing drugs known to affect liver function.

A previous history of indigestion and right upper quadrant pain suggests cholelithiasis or choledocholithiasis. Jaundice following shortly after operation on the biliary tract suggests residual stone, that which occurs within 6 months suggests hepatitis B or posttransfusion hepatitis, and that occurring after 1 or more years may be due to stricture of the common bile duct. Postoperative jaundice may be due to the anesthetic, especially after multiple uses of halothane, or to the impaired hepatic excretory function resulting from relative hypoxemia of liver cells during the operative or postoperative period.

The *onset of the illness* should be noted. The relatively abrupt onset of nausea, anorexia, and aversion to smoking followed by progressive jaundice suggests viral hepatitis. A gradual development of jaundice associated with pruritus suggests cholestasis. Intermittent right upper quadrant abdominal pain followed by cholestatic jaundice points to gallstone disease, while the gradual onset of painless jaundice with weight loss is suggestive of tumor, such as carcinoma of the head of the pancreas. Jaundice associated with fever and chills makes cholangitis and extrahepatic biliary obstruction likely possibilities.

The patient with hepatitis generally feels ill, and dark urine and light stools occur before the appearance of scleral or skin icterus. In cholestatic hepatitis, the patient may feel relatively well and complain only of symptoms due to the obstruction, such as pruritus.

Physical examination Jaundice is looked for in the sclera as well as the skin. Pallor indicative of anemia may be a reflection of hemolysis, cirrhosis, or neoplasm. Significant cachexia, especially of the extremities, may be associated with cancer or active cirrhosis. In the alcoholic, one should look for stigmas of cirrhosis such as parotid gland enlargement, Dupuytren's contracture, gynecomastia, testicular atrophy, and diminished axillary or pubic hair.

The *skin examination* may reveal ecchymoses due to prothrombin deficiency, or purpura due to thrombocytopenia. *Palmar erythema* or *spider angiomas* may reflect acute or chronic liver disease. Spider angiomas are usually found above the umbilicus and especially on the face, neck, shoulders, forearms, and dorsum of the hands. The presence of a few spider angiomas is not abnormal in women, especially during pregnancy. However, their appearance in men is always abnormal and should be carefully searched for. In chronic cholestasis, *scratch marks, finger clubbing,* and *xanthoma* of the eyelids and extensor surfaces of the tendons of the wrists and ankles may be found. A *slate color* to the skin due to increased melanin should suggest the presence of hemochromatosis.

Evaluation of the *mental state* and *neurologic function* is important. Slight deterioration of the intellect and minimal personality changes may suggest hepatocellular disease or the presence of portal-systemic venous shunts, but care must be taken to exclude other causes such as neurologic disease. The presence of flapping tremor of the hands (asterixis) may be found in association with portal-systemic encephalopathy or impending hepatic coma.

Abdominal examination may reveal ascites, which, together with dilatated periumbilical veins, suggests cirrhosis and extensive portal collateral circulation. A very large nodular and rock-hard liver suggests the presence of hepatoma or hepatic metastases. Careful percussion is necessary to evaluate the size of a nonpalpable liver. A small liver may indicate cirrhosis (especially postnecrotic); a small liver which diminishes in size suggests severe hepatitis or massive hepatic necrosis. In the alcoholic, fatty infiltration and cirrhosis often produce a uniform enlargement of the liver. The liver edge is tender in hepatitis, in congestive heart failure, and occasionally in malignant disease and with alcoholism (especially "alcoholic hepatitis").

A palpable and sometimes visibly enlarged gallbladder (Courvoisier's sign) suggests extrahepatic biliary obstruction often due to pancreatic cancer. A tender gallbladder and positive Murphy's sign suggests cholelithiasis or choledocholithiasis. A palpable spleen may indicate hepatitis or cirrhosis; significant splenomegaly may be a reflection of portal hypertension.

Abdominal auscultation may reveal the presence of a venous hum over dilatated collateral veins radiating from the umbilicus, the so-called caput medusae. In advanced cirrhosis this venous hum is virtually diagnostic of significant portal hypertension. A bruit may sometimes be heard over large regenerating nodules in cirrhosis and occasionally over hepatomas and metastatic nodules in the liver. The presence of a friction rub strongly suggests neoplastic disease or a hepatic abscess. A friction rub may occasionally be heard over hepatomas and metastatic liver nodules.

Liver function tests Serum assays for biochemical markers of liver disease are an integral part of the proper evaluation of liver and biliary tract disease. In general, the serum bilirubin is measured to confirm the presence and severity of the jaundice and determine the degree of bilirubin conjugation. Aminotransferase (transaminase) elevations reflect the severity of active hepatocellular damage, and the alkaline phosphatase elevations are found with cholestasis and hepatic infiltrates. Serum albumin and the prothrombin time are determined as indexes of hepatic synthetic function. These and other tests are reviewed in Chaps. 38 and 245.

Diagnostic procedures (see Chap. 245) The further evaluation of patients with hepatobiliary disease should be individualized depending on the history, physical findings, and initial screening laboratory tests. Hepatocellular disease such as hepatitis is often sufficiently clear so that no additional tests are needed. However in severe, chronic, or ambiguous cases, computerized tomography (CT), ultrasound, scintiscans, or liver biopsy may be needed to determine the nature of the liver disease. When hepatic tumors are suspected, CT, ultrasound, or scintiscan may be performed followed by liver biopsy, angiography, or laparoscopy for a more specific diagnosis. When biliary obstruction is suspected, the first examination is usually an ultrasound study to determine the size of the bile ducts, whether gallstones are present, or whether there is the suggestion of a mass in the head of the pancreas. Frequently more information is needed and thus a percutaneous endoscopic cholangiogram or exploratory laparotomy may be performed.

CLASSIFICATION OF LIVER DISEASE The classification of the various types of liver disease has been difficult because in many instances the etiology and pathogenetic mechanism are obscure. As a consequence, one finds an abundance of labels and names applied to hepatic disorders. Some individuals use the term *hepatitis* to imply viral infection, others simply to connote evidence of hepatic inflammation. One finds ambiguity in the use of the words *acute, subacute,* and *chronic*. *Chronicity* should refer to continuing or recurrent disease (i.e., duration). *Activity* should refer to evidence of the presence of perpetuation of liver cell injury; this is most readily identified on biopsy by the degree of hepatocellular necrosis and by serum transaminase elevations.

Because of the difficulties involved in defining the etiology of many types of liver disease, in most instances the process is best defined and described by an examination of the morphologic character of the lesion. Therefore, a *morphologic classification* of liver disease, as outlined in Table 243-1, appears at present more practical than one based on etiology.

TABLE 243-1 Classification of liver disease

- *I* Parenchymal
  - *A* Hepatitis (viral, drug-induced, toxic)
    - *1* Acute
    - *2* Chronic (persistent or active)
  - *B* Cirrhosis
    - *1* Alcoholic (portal, nutritional, Laennec's cirrhosis)
    - *2* Postnecrotic
    - *3* Biliary
    - *4* Hemochromatosis
    - *5* Rare types (e.g., Wilson's disease, galactosemia, cystic fibrosis of pancreas, $alpha_1$-antitrypsin deficiency)
  - *C* Infiltrations
    - *1* Glycogen
    - *2* Fat (neutral fat, cholesterol, gangliosides, cerebrosides)
    - *3* Amyloid
    - *4* Lymphoma, leukemia
    - *5* Granuloma (e.g., sarcoidosis, tuberculosis, idiopathic)
  - *D* Space-occupying lesions
    - *1* Hepatoma, metastatic tumor
    - *2* Abscess (pyogenic, amoebic)
    - *3* Cysts (polycystic disease, *Echinococcus*)
    - *4* Gummas
  - *E* Functional disorders associated with jaundice
    - *1* Gilbert's syndrome
    - *2* Crigler-Najjar syndrome
    - *3* Dubin-Johnson and Rotor syndromes
    - *4* Cholestasis of pregnancy and benign recurrent cholestasis
- *II* Hepatobiliary
  - *A* Extrahepatic biliary obstruction (by stone, stricture, or tumor)
  - *B* Cholangitis
- *III* Vascular
  - *A* Chronic passive congestion and cardiac cirrhosis
  - *B* Hepatic vein thrombosis (Budd-Chiari syndrome)
  - *C* Portal vein thrombosis
  - *D* Pylephlebitis
  - *E* Arteriovenous malformations

REFERENCES

SCHIFF L: *Diseases of the Liver,* 5th ed. Philadelphia, Lippincott, 1982

SHERLOCK S: *Diseases of the Liver and Biliary System,* 7th ed. Philadelphia, Davis, 1985

WRIGHT R et al: *Liver and Biliary Disease,* 2d ed. Philadelphia, Saunders, 1985

244 DERANGEMENTS OF HEPATIC METABOLISM

DANIEL K. PODOLSKY / KURT J. ISSELBACHER

The liver plays a central role in the maintenance of metabolic homeostasis. It is therefore not surprising that the development of clinically important liver disease is accompanied by diverse systemic manifestations of disordered metabolism. The liver has considerable reserve capacity, so minimal or even moderate cell injury may not be reflected by measurable changes in its metabolic function. However, some functions of the liver are more sensitive than others, and a variety of defects may be seen, depending on the nature and extent of the initial insult.

The biochemical functions in which the liver plays a major role include (1) the intermediate metabolism of amino acids and carbohydrates, (2) synthesis and degradation of proteins and glycoproteins, (3) metabolism and degradation of drugs and hormones, and (4) regulation of lipid and cholesterol metabolism. The derangements of these functions are discussed in connection with their occurrence in various forms of parenchymal liver disease. Alterations of bilirubin, bile salt, and porphyrin metabolism are discussed elsewhere (Chaps. 37, 237, 312).

Metabolic derangements are most evident in the patient with advanced liver disease, and the manifestations are similar regardless of the initial etiologic insult. To a varying degree similar abnormalities are observed in patients with severe chronic hepatitis, micronodular cirrhosis, and postnecrotic cirrhosis. Since the many functions of the liver may be affected to varying degrees in individual patients, no single test effectively measures the overall state of liver function. The proper interpretation of liver function tests is discussed in Chap. 245.

CARBOHYDRATE METABOLISM The liver functions to maintain normal levels of blood sugar by a combination of glycogenesis, glycogenolysis, glycolysis, and gluconeogenesis. These pathways are regulated by a number of hormones including insulin, glucagon, growth hormone, and certain catecholamines. Although it has been presumed that exquisite sensitivity of the hepatocytes to insulin is responsible for the uptake of an oral glucose load by the liver, there are also data that have challenged the importance of insulin-mediated glucose uptake by the hepatocyte. In the fasting state, the liver contributes to glucose homeostasis by glycogenolysis and gluconeogenesis in response to hypoinsulinemia and hyperglucagonemia. Maintenance of normal blood glucose levels through gluconeogenesis is ultimately related to catabolism of muscle protein, which provides the neeessary amino acid precursors, especially alanine. In a complementary fashion, in the postprandial state, the liver directs alanine and branched-chain amino acids to the peripheral tissues, where they are then incorporated into muscle protein. These reciprocal pathways form a glucose-alanine shuttle which is modulated by ambient changes in the hormones mentioned above (Fig. 244-1). While it has been presumed that synthesis of glycogen and fatty acid in the postprandial state arises from direct conversion of glucose, there are data to suggest that, in fact, these pathways are *indirect* with products deriving from 3-carbon metabolites of glucose or other gluconeogenic compounds such as lactate, fructose, and alanine.

Abnormalities of glucose homeostasis are common in cirrhosis (Table 244-1). Most frequently hyperglycemia and glucose intolerance are observed. Glucose intolerance is associated with normal or increased levels of plasma insulin (except in patients with hemochromatosis), suggesting that insulin resistance rather than insulin deficiency may be responsible. One of the factors that may play a role in the apparent insulin resistance is an absolute decrease in the liver's ability to metabolize a glucose load because of a decrease in functioning hepatocellular mass. There is also evidence that response to insulin is diminished due to both receptor and postreceptor defects in hepatocytes of patients with cirrhosis. In addition, both hyperinsulinemia and hyperglucagonemia may be present due to decreased hepatic clearance of this hormone resulting from portal-systemic shunting. In patients with hemochromatosis, insulin levels, however, may indeed be low due to pancreatic iron deposition and sometimes concomitant genetic diabetes mellitus. Patients with cirrhosis may also have elevated serum lactate levels reflecting the decreased capacity of the liver to utilize lactate for gluconeogenesis.

Hypoglycemia, although more common in acute fulminant hepatitis, may also be seen with end-stage cirrhosis. Glycogen in the liver accounts for 5 to 7 percent of the normal tissue weight. Because the capacity of the liver to store glycogen is limited (approximately 70 g) and glucose consumption continues at a constant rate (approximately 150 g per day), hepatic glycogen stores are depleted after 1 day of fasting. Hypoglycemia in end-stage cirrhosis may be due to decreased hepatic glycogen stores, diminished glucagon responsiveness, or decreased capacity to synthesize glycogen due to extensive parenchymal destruction.

AMINO ACID AND AMMONIA METABOLISM Through a variety of anabolic and catabolic processes, the liver is the major site of amino acid interconversion. Amino acids utilized for hepatic protein synthesis are derived from dietary protein, metabolic turnover of endogenous protein (primarily from muscle), and direct synthesis in the liver. Most of the amino acids entering the liver via the portal vein are catabolized to urea (except for the branched-chain amino acids leucine, isoleucine, and valine). A lesser amount is released into the general circulation as free amino acids, and these may play an important role in the glucose-alanine cycle mentioned above. In addition, amino acids are utilized for the synthesis of liver intracellular proteins, plasma proteins, and special compounds such as glutathione, glutamine, taurine, carnosine, and creatine. Disruption of normal amino acid metabolism may be reflected in altered plasma amino acid concentrations. In general, levels of aromatic amino acids normally metabolized by the liver (as well as methionine) are elevated, while those of the branched-chain amino acids, largely utilized by skeletal muscle, tend to be normal or depressed. It has been suggested that an alteration in the ratio of these two types of amino acids plays a role in the development of hepatic encephalopathy (see below), but there is not agreement on this concept.

Hepatic catabolism or degradation of amino acids involves two major reactions: transamination and oxidative deamination. Transamination, the process by which the amino group of an amino acid is transferred to a keto acid, is catalyzed by aminotransferases. These enzymes are found in very high amounts in liver but are also present in other tissues, such as kidney, muscle, heart, lung, and brain. Glutamic-oxaloacetic acid transaminase (aspartate aminotransferase, AST) has been studied most extensively, and increased levels are found in the serum secondary to various types of liver injury (e.g., acute viral and drug-induced hepatitis). As a result of transamination, amino acids can enter the citric acid cycle and then function in the intermediary metabolism of carbohydrates and lipids. Most of the nonessential amino acids are also synthesized in the liver by transamination. Oxidative deamination, which results in conversion of amino acids to keto acids (and ammonia), is catalyzed by L-amino-acid oxidase with two exceptions: glycine oxidation is catalyzed by glycine oxidase, and glutamic oxidation is catalyzed by glutamic dehydrogenase. With severe liver damage (e.g., massive hepatic necrosis), utilization of amino acids is impaired, free amino acids in the bloodstream increase, and an "overflow" type of aminoaciduria may occur.

Urea production is intimately related to the metabolic pathways outlined above, providing a means for disposal of ammonia, the toxic product of nitrogen metabolism. Disruption of this process is of particular clinical importance in the patient with severe acute and

FIGURE 244-1 *Carbohydrate-protein exchange between muscle and liver. After an overnight fast there is net release of amino acids by muscle (predominantly alanine and glutamine). These are derived from transamination of pyruvate, degraded amino acids, and glucose. Branched-chain amino acids (BCAA) are particularly important as a source of nitrogen for alanine synthesis. Alanine is utilized for gluconeogenesis by the liver, and urea is formed as a by-product. The main sites of glutamine uptake are the kidney and gut, where it is used for ammonia production and as a possible source of energy, respectively. Following ingestion of dietary protein, skeletal muscle goes into an anabolic phase; there is selective hepatic escape and muscle uptake of dietary BCAA, reduced muscle output of alanine and glutamine, and a reduced rate of hepatic gluconeogenesis. Hepatic tissue protein also goes into an anabolic phase following protein ingestion. (Adapted from A. Tavill, in Wright R et al, eds: Liver and Biliary Disease, 2d ed, Bailliere.)*

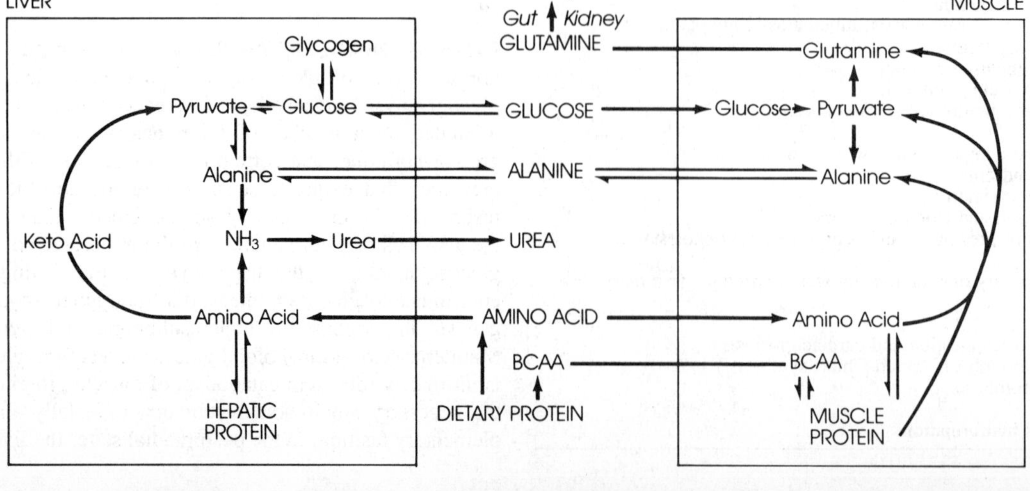

chronic liver disease. The fixation of amino acid–derived NH_3 in the form of urea is carried out via the Krebs-Henseleit cycle. The final step of this cycle, the formation of urea by arginase, is irreversible. In advanced liver disease urea synthesis is often depressed, leading to an accumulation of NH_3, usually with a significant reduction in blood urea nitrogen (BUN), an ominous sign of liver failure. This finding may be obscured by superimposed renal impairment, which often develops in patients with severe hepatic failure. Urea is mostly excreted by the kidney, but approximately 25 percent will diffuse into the intestine where it is converted to NH_3 by bacterial urease. The intestinal production of ammonia also occurs from the bacterial deamination of unabsorbed amino acids and of protein derived from the diet, exfoliated cells, or blood in the gastrointestinal tract.

Gut NH_3 is absorbed and transported to the liver via the portal vein, where it is again converted to urea. The kidney also produces varying amounts of NH_3, largely by the deamination of glutamine. The contributions of the gut and kidney to ammonia synthesis have important implications for the management of the hyperammonemic state frequently seen in patients with advanced liver disease usually in association with portal-systemic shunting of blood.

While the exact chemical mediators of hepatic encephalopathy remain unknown, elevated levels of blood NH_3 generally correlate with the degree of encephalopathy, although approximately 10 percent of such patients have normal levels of blood ammonia. In addition, therapeutic measures that reduce serum NH_3 levels also usually lead to clinical improvement. The several mechanisms known to lead to increased blood NH_3 levels in patients with cirrhosis are illustrated in Fig. 244-2 and include the following: (1) If there is excessive nitrogenous material in the intestine (from bleeding or dietary protein), excessive amounts of NH_3 will be formed by bacterial deamination of amino acids. (2) If renal function declines (as in the hepatorenal syndrome), blood urea nitrogen rises, leading to increased diffusion of urea into the intestinal lumen, where bacterial urease converts it to NH_3. (3) If hepatic function is significantly depressed, diminished urea synthesis may occur with a resultant decrease in the removal of NH_3. (4) If alkalosis (often due to central hyperventilation) and hypokalemia accompany hepatic decompensation, there may be a decrease in the renal availability of H^+ ions; as a result, the NH_3 produced from glutamine by the action of renal glutaminase is permitted to enter the renal vein (rather than being excreted as NH_4^+) leading to increased peripheral blood NH_3 levels. In addition hypokalemia itself leads to increased NH_3 production. (5) If portal hypertension is present and anastomoses exist between the portal vein and systemic venous channels, these portal-systemic shunts will allow NH_3 from the gut to bypass hepatic detoxification, leading to elevated blood NH_3 levels. Thus, with portal-systemic shunting of blood, elevated NH_3 levels may develop even with relatively little hepatocellular dysfunction.

An additional factor important in determining whether a given NH_3 level in the blood will be detrimental to the central nervous system is the blood pH. The more alkaline the pH, the more toxic a given level of NH_3 is likely to be. At 37°C the pK of NH_3 is 8.9; this is close enough to the pH of blood so that minor changes in pH can affect the NH_4^+/NH_3 ratio. Because un-ionized NH_3 crosses membranes more readily than NH_4^+ ions, alkalosis favors the entry of ammonia into the brain (with subsequent changes in cell metabolism) by shifting the equilibrium of the following reaction to the right

$$NH_4^+ + OH^- \rightleftharpoons NH_3 + HOH$$

As a result, alkalosis not only increases peripheral blood NH_3 levels by renal mechanisms but also increases tissue levels by influencing the diffusion of NH_3 across membranes.

TABLE 244-1 Alteration of glucose metabolism in cirrhosis

Factors leading to hyperglycemia:
Decreased hepatic glucose uptake
Decreased hepatic glycogen synthesis
Hepatic resistance to insulin
Portal-systemic glucose shunting
Peripheral insulin resistance
Hormonal abnormalities (serum)
↑ Glucagon
↓ Cortisol
↑ Insulin (↓ in hemochromatosis)
Factors leading to hypoglycemia:
Decreased gluconeogenesis
Decreased hepatic glycogen content
Hepatic resistance to glucagon
Poor oral intake
Hyperinsulinemia secondary to portal-systemic shunting

PROTEIN SYNTHESIS AND DEGRADATION The liver is an important site of protein synthesis and degradation. Although the body muscle mass produces the greatest total amount of protein, the liver has the highest rate of synthesis per gram of tissue. The liver synthesizes not only the proteins it needs, but also and perhaps more importantly it produces numerous export proteins. Among the latter, albumin is the most important; *it is produced at a rate of approximately 12 g per day,* representing 25 percent of total hepatic protein synthesis and half of all exported protein. The average normal half-life of serum albumin is 17 to 20 days. The proportion of hepatocytes carrying out active albumin synthesis varies from 10 to 60 percent depending on the body's requirements. Approximately 60 percent of albumin is found in the extravascular spaces, but plasma albumin is still the most abundant circulating protein. Although albumin secreted by the hepatocytes lacks significant carbohydrate, it may undergo nonenzymatic glycosylation in the circulation as a reflection of ambient serum glucose concentrations.

Albumin contributes significantly to the plasma oncotic pressure. In addition, it is the principal binding and transport protein for numerous substances including some hormones, fatty acids, trace metals, tryptophan, bilirubin, and other organic anions of both endogenous and exogenous origin. Despite the many important functions of albumin, rare individuals with congenital analbuminemia appear to have no major physiologic derangements other than the excessive accumulation of extravascular fluid. While many of the less hydrophobic ligands may be transported in the unbound form, this suggests that other serum proteins may also play a role in binding and transport.

FIGURE 244-2 *Major factors (steps 1 to 4) influencing the level of blood ammonia. In cirrhosis with portal hypertension, venous collaterals allow ammonia to bypass the liver (step 5), permitting the entry of ammonia into the systemic circulation (portal-systemic shunting).*

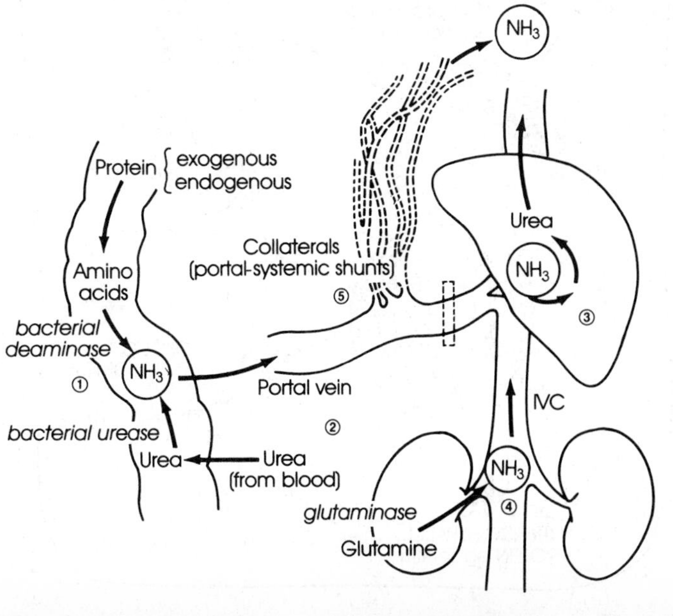

Much has been learned about the mechanisms involved in the synthesis of secretory proteins, especially of albumin (see Fig. 244-3). Polyribosomes bound to the rough endoplasmic reticulum (RER) of the hepatocyte are the principal site of translation of messenger ribonucleic acid (mRNA) coding for export proteins; in contrast proteins destined for intracellular use, such as ferritin, are synthesized on free rather than bound polyribosomes in the cytoplasm. After a short-term fast, there is a decrease in the amount of albumin mRNA associated with the RER; instead more mRNA is found in the cytosol and in a state dissociated from polyribosomes. Albumin, like secretory proteins produced by other organs, appears to be synthesized initially as a larger precursor, preproalbumin. This precursor molecule contains an additional 24 extra amino acid residues on the *N* terminus, referred to as a "signal peptide," which undergoes two sequential cleavages (or "processing"); the molecule is then transported to the Golgi apparatus prior to secretion. The "pre" portion of preproalbumin is cleaved within the RER even before protein synthesis is completed; the "pro" segment is removed within the lumen of the ER. Once synthesis and processing are completed, albumin is transported from the Golgi vesicles to the hepatocyte surface by mechanisms which are unclear but almost certainly involve the microfilaments and microtubule apparatus of the cell. Although the hepatic lymph space of Disse provides a potential avenue for the newly released albumin, most secreted proteins enter the plasma.

Albumin synthesis is subject to a number of regulatory influences. These include the rate of transcription of specific mRNAs and the availability of the substrate tRNA (transfer RNA). At the translational level, the integrity of polyribosomes and their synthetic abilities is modified by factors affecting initiation, elongation, and release of peptides and proteins as well as by the availability of ATP, GTP, and magnesium ions. The rate of albumin synthesis is also influenced by the availability of amino acid precursors, especially tryptophan, the scarcest of the essential amino acids. Indeed in patients with large carcinoid tumors albumin synthesis may decrease precipitously when tryptophan is shunted from albumin production into the pathway leading to 5-hydroxytryptophan (serotonin) synthesis (see Chap. 306). The rate of albumin synthesis is also affected by colloid oncotic pressure with increased production occurring in response to falling oncotic pressure. Finally, hormonal influences on hepatic protein metabolism such as insulin and glucagon are closely integrated with the nutritional factors discussed above.

FIGURE 244-3 *Schematic diagram illustrating major steps in synthesis, processing, and secretion of proteins and glycoproteins by the liver. Ribosomal subunits and mRNA form polysome complexes to initiate protein synthesis. Polyribosomes synthesizing proteins destined for export (e.g., albumin) associate with membranes to form membrane-bound polysomes [i.e., the rough endoplasmic reticulum (RER)]. Synthesis of precursor molecule (e.g., "preproalbumin") occurs and is followed by stepwise proteolytic cleavage and secretion from the cell. Other export proteins (e.g., alpha$_1$ antitrypsin) are first glycosylated in the RER and Golgi prior to secretion. Proteins produced for intracellular use (e.g., ferritin) are synthesized on non-membrane-bound cytosolic polyribosomes and processed by stepwise proteolytic cleavage and secretion from the cell.*

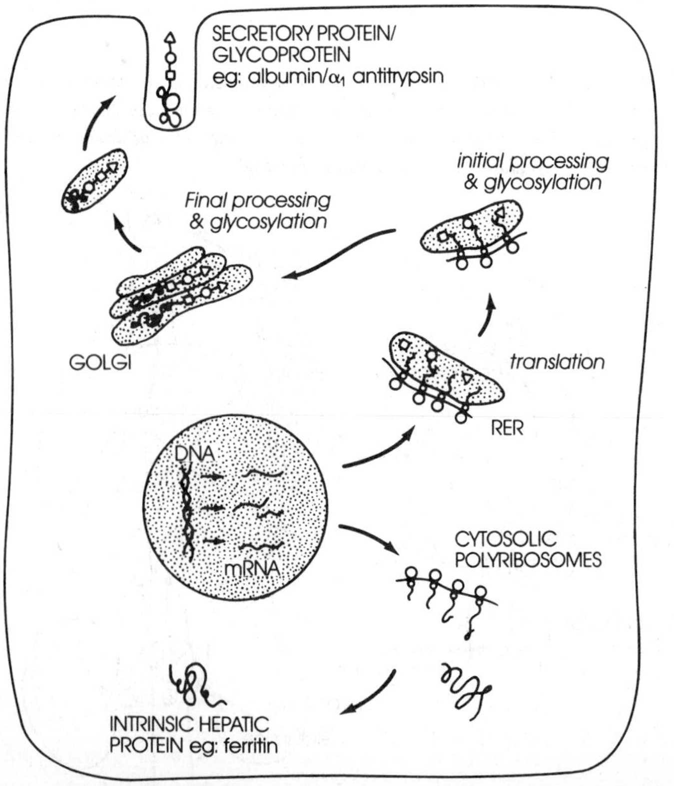

The liver also produces a wide variety of other secretory proteins, most of which have a synthetic pathway and processing procedure similar to albumin (Fig. 244-3). The presence of a *signal peptide,* such as the "prepro" segment of albumin, which is subsequently removed during protein maturation appears to be a general mechanism for orienting proteins in the membranes of the ER and directing them for export rather than for intracellular use or degradation. Most proteins undergo even further modification in the form of sequential *glycosylation* in the RER and Golgi apparatus. The carbohydrate moieties of these glycoproteins appear to be important in determining their site of action and their rate of tissue uptake after secretion. Some of the clinically important secretory glycoproteins include ceruloplasmin, alpha$_1$ antitrypsin, and most other alpha and beta globulins. While the site of albumin catabolism is uncertain, the removal of terminal sialic acid residues after secretion and the resultant exposure of penultimate galactose or *N*-acetylglucosamine residues appears to result in receptor-mediated uptake of "aged" proteins by hepatocytes and Kupffer cells, followed by their subsequent degradation. Reduced amounts of the hepatic receptor for asialoglycoproteins appear to result in elevated serum concentrations of these glycoproteins in patients with severe and chronic liver disease.

One of the clinically most important derangements in protein metabolism is the development of hypoalbuminemia, which results largely from reduced synthetic activity. Decreased synthesis may be caused by a decrease in the number as well as the function of hepatocytes. A decrease in the dietary supply of amino acids can also contribute to deficient synthesis. To some extent the body attempts to compensate for decreased albumin synthesis by reducing the rate of degradation. Attempts to raise the serum albumin level by intravenous infusions are often futile because this compensatory mechanism can be blunted and the decrease in albumin degradation may not occur. The reduced degradation of albumin is not a general phenomenon in chronic liver disease because other proteins such as fibrinogen are degraded more rapidly than normal. The degree of hypoalbuminemia is also augmented in the patient with ascites, in which large amounts of the body's albumin are present in the ascitic fluid. When there is increased hepatic venous pressure (as in postsinusoidal or hepatic vein outflow block), there may be increased hepatic lymph production with extravasation into the peritoneal cavity. In contrast to intestinal lymph, the protein content of hepatic lymph appears to be relatively uninfluenced by ascitic oncotic pressure, most likely reflecting the lack of tight junctions between sinusoidal endothelial cells.

Other proteins produced by the liver include many of the blood-clotting factors: fibrinogen (factor I), prothrombin (factor II), and factors V, VII, IX, and X as well as inhibitors of both coagulation and fibrinolysis. Factors II, VII, IX, and X are vitamin K–responsive and are dependent upon normal intestinal fat absorption. Vitamin K activates an enzyme system in liver endoplasmic reticulum which catalyzes the γ carboxylation of selected glutamyl residues in clotting factor precursors. The γ carboxylation enhances the Ca^{2+} and phospholipid binding capacity of prothrombin and permits its rapid conversion to thrombin in the presence of factors V and X (Chap. 281).

The liver is involved in the process of hemostasis by virtue of both anabolic and catabolic functions. As expected, severe liver disease leads to reduced synthesis of prothrombin, a vitamin K–dependent clotting factor. The presence of malnutrition, the use of broad-spectrum antibiotics, or concomitant impairment of fat absorption due to reduction in intestinal bile salt concentration (e.g., cholestasis) may accentuate hypoprothrombinemia by decreasing the amount of vitamin K that can be absorbed from the intestine. In these situations, prothrombin levels may be at least partially corrected by parenteral vitamin K administration. However, when the coagulopathy results from impaired hepatocellular function and not cholestasis or intestinal factors, exogenous vitamin K is unlikely to correct or improve prothrombin synthesis. The vitamin K–dependent clotting proteins have a substantially shorter serum half-life than albumin; therefore, hypoprothrombinemia usually precedes the development of hypoalbuminemia, especially in the patient with acute hepatocellular disease. In cirrhosis, coagulopathy may be further aggravated by the thrombocytopenia resulting from hypersplenism.

Since the liver is also the site of production of non-vitamin K–dependent clotting factors, severe liver disease injury may lead to decreased plasma concentrations of factor V in addition to factors II, VII, IX, and X. It is unusual for fibrinogen to be reduced significantly, unless there is an associated disseminated intravascular coagulation (DIC). For unclear reasons, the damaged liver may actually produce increased amounts of fibrinogen as well as other proteins collectively designated acute-phase reactants (C-reactive proteins, haptoglobin, ceruloplasmin, and transferrin). The latter are produced both in response to liver injury (e.g., severe chronic active hepatitis) and in association with systemic illnesses such as cancer, rheumatoid arthritis, bacterial infections, burns, and myocardial infarctions. However, while the diseased liver may produce normal or increased amounts of fibrinogen, the molecules themselves may be qualitatively abnormal (i.e., structurally and functionally), reflecting more subtle derangements in protein synthesis. These functionally abnormal fibrinogen molecules may contribute to the altered hemostasis frequently found in patients with chronic liver disease.

DETOXIFICATION MECHANISMS Water-soluble drugs and endogenous substances usually are excreted unchanged in the urine or bile. However, lipid-soluble compounds tend to accumulate in the body and affect cellular processes, unless they are converted to less active compounds or to more water-soluble metabolites which are more easily excreted. Hepatic blood flow, protein binding, and the intrinsic capacity of the liver to eliminate a drug are all primary determinants of hepatic drug clearance. The liver has an important role in the metabolism of many exogenous drugs and endogenous hormones by virtue of several enzyme systems involved in biochemical transformation. The relative importance of these various factors differs depending on how well a drug is extracted by the liver. There are two major types of reactions. The first, *phase I reactions,* result in chemical modification of reactive groups by oxidation, reduction, hydroxylation, sulfoxidation, deamination, dealkylation, or methylation. Such modifications usually involve one of several enzymatic systems, including the mixed function oxidases, cytochromes b_5 and P_{450} (microsomal), and the glutathione *S*-acyltransferases (cytoplasmic). These biochemical reactions usually lead to *inactivation* of drugs such as barbiturates and benzodiazepines. However, *activation* may also occur. For example, cortisone is activated to cortisol and prednisone to prednisolone (both products being more potent than the parent compounds); imipramine, a depressant, is converted to desmethylimipramine, an antidepressant. On the other hand, phase I reactions may convert a nontoxic compound to a toxic one as in the metabolism of isoniazid and acetaminophen. Similarly, some carcinogens may be activated by formation of highly reactive epoxide intermediates in the liver, while other carcinogens may be detoxified.

The enzymes responsible for phase I reactions, especially those involving the cytochrome P_{450} system, can be induced by drugs such as ethanol, barbiturates, haloperidol, and glutethimide. Conversely, hepatic microsomal enzymes may be inhibited by agents such as chloramphenicol, cimetidine, disulfiram, dextropropoxyphene, allopurinol, and, paradoxically, by ethanol. The concomitant administration of two drugs metabolized by the same microsomal enzyme may result in modification, potentiation, or diminution of the pharmacologic efficacy of either or both drugs. Activity of phase I reactions may also change with aging.

Phase II reactions may follow phase I reactions or proceed independently; these involve the conversion of substances to their glucuronide, sulfate, acetyl, taurine, or glycine derivatives, thereby converting lipophilic substances to water-soluble derivatives and permitting their excretion in bile or urine. Conjugation catalyzed by microsomal UDP (uridine diphosphate)-glucuronyltransferases to form glucuronide derivatives is one of the most common phase II reactions. In general, the conjugates are more soluble than the parent compound and are pharmacologically inactive.

An awareness that there may be varying degrees of impairment in the hepatic uptake, detoxification, and excretion of certain drugs is important in the clinical management of patients with chronic liver disease. Portal-systemic shunting of blood may decrease the "first-pass effect" of drugs absorbed from the gut. In cirrhosis, altered intrahepatic hemodynamics due to a disordered liver architecture may also reduce the rates of hepatic drug clearance. Hypoalbuminemia will permit drugs usually bound to albumin to be present in increased concentrations of their unbound form in the circulation and extracellular spaces; this may result in an increased activity of such drugs. Most importantly, a decrease in the amount of function of microsomal enzymes responsible for phase I and phase II reactions will result in slower rates of drug inactivation and elimination. Drugs for which there may be a decreased clearance in patients with liver disease include anticonvulsants (e.g., phenytoin, phenobarbital), anti-inflammatory agents (e.g., acetaminophen, phenylbutazone, corticosteroids), minor tranquilizers, cardioactive drugs (e.g., lidocaine, quinidine, propranolol), and antibiotics (e.g., nafcillin, chloramphenicol, tetracyclines, clindamycin, trimethoprim, rifampin, pyrazinamide). This will lead to decreased dosage requirements and a narrowing of the range between therapeutic and toxic drug levels. In the future, the aminopyrine clearance test may permit an assessment of the degree of impairment of detoxification mechanisms in individual patients. In this test, orally administered $[^{14}C]$aminopyrine is absorbed from the gut and metabolized by the hepatic cytochrome P_{450} system releasing $[^{14}C]O_2$, which is excreted and easily measured in the breath. In hepatocellular disease, the rate of $[^{14}C]O_2$ production will be reduced. Finally, the patient with chronic liver disease may demonstrate alterations in the pharmacologic effects of drugs in addition to or independent of changes in their pharmacokinetics such as an increased central nervous system sensitivity to opiates and other sedatives.

The difficulties in safely administering pharmacologic agents to patients with both acute and chronic liver disease are underscored by the frequency with which administration of benzodiazepines is cited as precipitating hepatic coma. It may be very difficult clinically to determine whether agitation, confusion, and irrational behavior are due to early hepatic encephalopathy or related to the concurrent use of benzodiazepines, opiates, barbiturates, and other depressants. It should be recognized that there is great variation of drug clearance in patients with liver disease; although data on average clearances may provide a reasonable estimate for initial dosages, subsequent adjustments in dose need to be individualized in order to attain the desired plasma drug concentration.

The mechanism by which some agents exert a hepatotoxic effect may involve the same metabolic pathways responsible for normal drug detoxification. The mechanism of acetaminophen toxicity is particularly illustrative. Acetaminophen is metabolized and detoxified by the hepatic mixed-function oxygenase system, but one of the intermediate products is a potent free radical (postulated metabolite

N-acetylimidoquinone) which can inactivate many enzymes and proteins by binding irreversibly to their sulfhydryl groups. Normally this interaction can be prevented by reduced glutathione. In the presence of excessive amounts of the acetaminophen free radical (e.g., from overdosage or underlying liver disease), the glutathione levels of the hepatocytes are readily exhausted and the excess free radicals can lead to inactivation of cellular proteins and produce widespread hepatocellular necrosis. In the case of acetaminophen overdosage, the very early administration of sulfhydryl groups in the form of *N*-acetylcysteine can often prevent this drug-induced liver injury.

HORMONE METABOLISM In addition to its role in the metabolism of diverse pharmacologic agents, the liver is also responsible for inactivation or modification of several endogenous hormones; therefore, chronic liver disease may be accompanied by signs of apparent hormonal imbalance. Some hormones (e.g., insulin and glucagon) are inactivated in the liver by proteolysis or deamination. Thyroxine and triiodothyronine are metabolized in the liver by reactions involving deiodination. Steroid hormones, such as corticosteroids and aldosterone, are first inactivated to their tetrahydro derivative (by reduction of the Δ^4 double bond and the 3-keto group), followed by conjugation, mostly with glucuronic acid. Testosterone is metabolized to the isomeric 17-ketosteroids androsterone and etiocholanolone and excreted in the urine mostly as sulfate conjugates. Estrogens, such as estradiol, may be converted to estriol and estrone and then conjugated with glucuronic acid or sulfate. Abnormalities in estrogen (and testosterone) metabolism are believed to be involved in the development of the spider angiomas, loss of axillary or pubic hair, and testicular atrophy frequently seen in patients with chronic liver disease. In addition, increased portal-systemic shunting of testosterone and androstenedione secondary to portal hypertension may lead to the development of gynecomastia in cirrhotic males due to increased peripheral conversion to estradiol and estrone especially in patients with alcoholic cirrhosis. In patients with alcoholic liver disease, feminization may also be related to the direct toxic effects of alcohol on the gonadal-pituitary-hypothalamic axis which lead to the overall reduction in serum testosterone found in patients with cirrhosis. Similar effects are also seen in patients with hemochromatosis due to deposition of iron in these sites. However, gynecomastia is often lacking in the latter, apparently due to a coincident reduction in plasma concentration of androstenedione a major precursor for estrogen synthesis.

FIGURE 244-4 *Factors in the uptake and esterification of fatty acids to triglyceride by the liver, including the formation and release of triglyceride as lipoprotein. The numbers refer to steps, which, if altered, may result in increased liver triglyceride (i.e., fatty liver).*

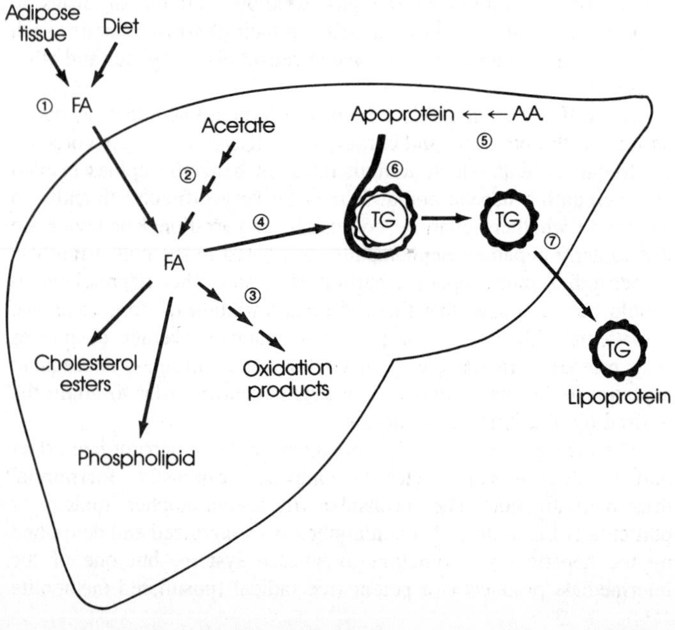

Estrogens also act directly on the liver to impair hepatic secretory activity. Estradiol and related estrogens, such as those present in contraceptive pills, interfere with sodium sulfobromophthalein and bile salt excretion and worsen the preexisting defect in secretion of conjugated bilirubin in patients with Dubin-Johnson syndrome; they may also elevate plasma alkaline phosphatase levels (see Chap. 245). Related steroids such as etiocholanolone and pregnanediol have been shown to stimulate δ-aminolevulinic acid (ALA) synthetase activity leading to increased porphobilinogen excretion. Since these steroids exert these effects only in their unconjugated form, the increased hepatic levels of δ-aminolevulinic acid synthetase in patients with alcoholic cirrhosis may be secondary to the action of gonadal steroids.

LIPID METABOLISM: FATTY ACIDS AND TRIGLYCERIDES Under normal conditions, most of the fatty acids taken up by the liver and esterified to triglyceride are derived from adipose tissue or the diet. Some fatty acids (especially saturated ones) are synthesized in the liver from acetate. The fatty acids may then be converted enzymatically to triglyceride, esterified with cholesterol, incorporated into phospholipids, or oxidized to CO_2 or ketone bodies. Most of the triglyceride is produced for export, but in order to be secreted it must be converted to lipoproteins by combining with relatively specific apoprotein moieties. This emphasizes the importance of protein synthesis for the release and secretion of triglyceride from the liver. It should be noted that the liver plays a major role in regulating lipoprotein levels by virtue of both its degradative and synthetic functions. Thus, the liver is quantitatively the major site of low-density lipoprotein (LDL) catabolism with dual high- and low-affinity receptor-mediated pathways playing a role. In addition chylomicron remnants are removed and degraded by the liver, where their constituents have a number of metabolic effects. The liver is not only the primary site of very low density lipoprotein (VLDL) secretion but also accounts for a major portion of its subsequent degradation by mechanisms similar to that of chylomicron remnant degradation and conversion to LDL via the action of hepatic lipase. The liver may also play a role in high-density lipoprotein (HDL) catabolism. It is noteworthy that with the exception of cholestatic disease (see below), clinically significant alterations in lipoprotein and cholesterol metabolism are usually not found in patients with chronic liver disease.

Studies on the production of fatty liver have shown that singly or in combination, one or more of the steps depicted in Fig. 244-4 may be involved. An increased influx of fatty acids mobilized from adipose tissue due to drugs (e.g., ethanol or corticosteroids) or secondary to diabetic ketosis may lead to a fatty liver. Similarly, increased levels of fatty acids in the liver, either from enhanced fatty acid synthesis or from decreased fatty acid oxidation may lead to increased triglyceride formation. In some instances (e.g., ethanol excess) there may also be increases in the carbohydrate backbone, α-glycerophosphate, involved in fatty acid esterification to triglyceride. Since release of triglyceride involves the formation of lipoproteins, lipid accumulation may occur because of decreased apoprotein synthesis. This appears to be the case in fatty livers seen in patients with protein-calorie malnutrition (kwashiorkor) and due to toxins such as carbon tetrachloride, phosphorus, or ethionine, as well as following excessive doses of antibiotics like tetracycline that can inhibit protein synthesis. Finally, there may be impaired lipoprotein secretion from the liver. Alcohol is perhaps the most common agent leading to a fatty liver, but the mechanism(s) whereby alcohol leads to increased liver triglyceride is not clear. Depending on factors such as dose or duration, alcohol ingestion may affect any of the seven steps shown in Fig. 244-4; however, the primary factor for the production of the alcohol-induced fatty liver remains to be determined. The alterations in the redox state due to excessive accumulation of NADH resulting from oxidation of alcohol may also contribute.

In addition to the changes leading to fatty liver, there are many metabolic alterations which may be found in the blood of patients following the ingestion of large amounts of alcohol. These include, among others, *increased* plasma levels of lactate, proline, urate, and triglycerides and *decreased* plasma levels of glucose, magnesium, phosphate, and triiodothyronine (T_3).

CHOLESTEROL Cholesterol and bile acid synthesis is carried out primarily by the liver. Cholesterol synthesis is subject to a number of metabolic controls, most of them mediated via the rate-limiting biosynthetic enzyme 3-hydroxy-3-methylglutaryl coenzyme A reductase (HMG-CoA reductase). Cholesterol exists either free or combined with fatty acids in the form of cholesterol esters; in the plasma both are found primarily in association with β-lipoproteins. The plasma and liver also contain lecithin–cholesterol acyltransferase (LCAT), an enzyme involved in the conversion of free cholesterol to its esterified form. Since there is exchange of free cholesterol between tissues, changes in plasma cholesterol levels reflect changes in total body cholesterol. However, decreases in plasma cholesterol esters may reflect hepatic damage and impaired hepatic cholesterol esterification.

Severe liver injury often leads to a decrease in *total* serum cholesterol levels, including both free and esterified fractions. This may be due to decreased synthesis of cholesterol and cholesterol esters, decreased apoprotein synthesis, or both. In cholestasis (either intra- or extrahepatic) total serum cholesterol often increases strikingly. Disorders of cholestasis are associated with marked abnormalities of lipoprotein metabolism. In primary biliary cirrhosis there are pronounced elevations in serum free cholesterol and LDL; conversely, serum HDL is reduced and may disappear from the serum in patients with long-standing disease. Similar but less marked changes are seen in other cholestatic conditions.

The increase in serum free cholesterol (and phospholipid) and the concomitant decrease in esterified cholesterol in cholestasis may be related to a decrease in the hepatic production of LCAT. Reduced levels of LCAT are also correlated with the appearance of an abnormal LDL, referred to as lipoprotein X (LP-X). Although LP-X, which has a high content of free cholesterol and triglyceride, was originally thought to be a specific indicator of biliary tract obstruction, it is evident that it appears in any cholestatic condition. While the depressed hepatic production of LCAT may be responsible for altered lipid content and composition of lipoproteins, the factors leading to the overall increase in total serum cholesterol are not clear. In experimental animals, bile duct ligation results in a net increase in hepatic cholesterol synthesis, and in "regurgitation" of bile salts, cholesterol, and LP-X into venous radicals. However, it is difficult to translate these experimental findings to the patient with primary biliary cirrhosis unless any insult to cells lining the biliary canaliculi and ductules can impair the delicate balance of lipid synthesis and removal.

Most of the derangements of hepatic metabolism discussed above are evident only in patients with severe or long-standing liver disease. Indeed, in all but the most severe cases of acute viral hepatitis, hepatic metabolic functions are remarkably well preserved, and in most cases of mild to moderate acute viral hepatitis, it is uncommon to observe clinically important alterations in carbohydrate, protein, and lipid metabolism. However, in the patients with severe or fulminant hepatitis, whether from a viral or toxic agent, the metabolic derangements may be similar to those seen in more chronic disease. For example, in fulminant hepatitis there may be pronounced hypoprothrombinemia and impaired coagulation, hypoalbuminemia, and the relatively acute development of ascites, as well as hyperammonemia and encephalopathy. However, in contrast to patients with cirrhosis, abnormalities in carbohydrate metabolism are more likely to lead to profound hypoglycemia rather than to hyperglycemia. This hypoglycemia appears to reflect both a marked decrease in hepatic glycogen stores as well as diminished glucagon responsiveness. There may also be poor oral intake due to nausea and anorexia together with increased glucose utilization secondary to hyperinsulinemia (due to portal-systemic shunting and decreased insulin degradation).

REFERENCES

CAVALLO-PERIN P et al: Mechanism of insulin resistance in human liver cirrhosis. Evidence of a combined receptor and post-receptor defect. J Clin Invest 75:1659, 1985

COOPER AD: Role of the liver in the degradation of lipoproteins. Gastroenterology 88:192, 1984

FLANNERY DB et al: Current status of hyperammonemic syndromes. Hepatology 2:495, 1982

HOYUMPA AM et al: Hepatic encephalopathy. Gastroenterology 77:803, 1979

KLEG HK et al: Conversion of androgens to estrogens in idiopathic hemochromatosis: Comparison with alcoholic liver disease. J Clin Endocrin Metab 61:1, 1985

ONSTAD GR, ZIEVE L: What determines blood ammonia? Gastroenterology 77:803, 1979

OWEN OE et al: Hepatic, gut and renal substrate flux rates in patients with hepatic cirrhosis. J Clin Invest 68:240, 1981

SHERLOCK S: *Diseases of the Liver and Biliary System,* 7th ed. London, Blackwell, 1985

SMITH AR et al: Alteration in plasma and CSF amino acids, amines and metabolites in hepatic coma. Ann Surg 187:343, 1978

WILLIAMS RC: Drug administration in hepatic disease. N Engl J Med 309:1616, 1983

WRIGHT R et al: *Liver and Biliary Disease.* 2d ed. Philadelphia, Saunders, 1985

245 DIAGNOSTIC PROCEDURES IN LIVER DISEASE

DANIEL K. PODOLSKY / KURT J. ISSELBACHER

The diversity of normal liver functions and their variable disruption by the spectrum of disorders which may affect the liver precludes the use of any single test as a reliable measure of overall liver function. Many disease processes may lead to severe impairment of some liver functions while others remain entirely unaffected. Since no battery of tests is universally applicable, those most appropriate to a given clinical problem must be selected, their potential value and risks considered, and the results interpreted in relation to the clinical findings.

In assessing the severity and course of liver disease, the physician should be guided by several practical principles. The tests selected should (1) assess different parameters of liver function, (2) be used *serially* in order to evaluate the evolution or course of the disease, and (3) be interpreted within the total clinical context, with recognition that any single laboratory test may be fallible.

BLOOD TESTS OF LIVER FUNCTION (See Table 245-1)

Bilirubin Bilirubin metabolism and its assessment are discussed in detail in Chaps. 38 and 246. Spectrophotometric determinations of serum bilirubin in the clinical laboratory measure two pigment fractions: (1) the water-soluble conjugated fraction that gives a *direct reaction* with the diazo reagent and consists largely of conjugated bilirubin (as the mono- and diglucuronide), and (2) the lipid-soluble *indirect-reaction* fraction (total minus direct) that represents primarily

TABLE 245-1 Abnormalities shown by tests of liver function

	Type of liver disease	
Test	Obstructive	Parenchymal
AST and ALT (SGOT and SGPT)	↑	↑–↑↑↑
Alkaline phosphatase	↑↑↑	↑
Albumin	N	↓–↓↓↓
Prothrombin time	N–↑*	↑–↑↑↑
Bilirubin	N–↑↑↑	N–↑↑↑
γ-Glutamyl transpeptidase (GGT)	↑↑↑	N–↑↑↑
5′-Nucleotidase	↑–↑↑↑	N–↑

* *Correctable with parenteral vitamin K if elevated.*
NOTE: *N, normal: ↑, elevated; ↓, decreased.*

unconjugated bilirubin. The serum of normal adults (when measured by the van den Bergh reaction) contains less than 0.25 mg direct-reacting bilirubin per deciliter and 1 mg or less of total bilirubin per deciliter. Studies with high-performance liquid chromatography (HPLC) suggest that even these levels may be artifactually high in normal persons (see Chap. 38).

Conjugated hyperbilirubinemia with elevated direct- and indirect-reacting material indicates impairment of secretion into the bile, while unconjugated hyperbilirubinemia reflects impaired conjugation. The latter is found in a limited number of processes including such nonhepatic conditions as hemolytic anemia and ineffective erythropoiesis (increased pigment load) and a few hepatic disorders, principally Gilbert's syndrome or the relatively rare Crigler-Najjar syndrome. Although measurement of both the direct and total serum bilirubin will determine whether the patient has predominantly unconjugated or conjugated hyperbilirubinemia, this distinction is of limited usefulness since the majority of hepatobiliary disorders lead to conjugated hyperbilirubinemia. Fractionation of serum bilirubin does not distinguish cholestasis due to parenchymal disease from that arising from biliary tract processes.

Bilirubin appears in the urine only after it is converted to a water-soluble form; generally this involves conjugation with polar glucuronide groups which enhance water solubility. Rapid assessment of bilirubinuria is possible using commercially available dipsticks and may be helpful as an initial screening measure. Bilirubinuria occurs with even minimal degrees of jaundice and may be detected before jaundice is evident. Its usefulness is otherwise quite limited. Urobilinogen, a product of lumenal bacterial metabolism of bilirubin, is reabsorbed from the bowel and secreted in the urine. Complete bile duct obstruction blocks excretion of bilirubin into the gut and results in disappearance of urobilinogen from the urine. Assessment of urobilinogen in a freshly collected 2-h urine specimen by the Watson method (normal values 0.2 to 1.2 units) may distinguish biliary tract obstruction from parenchymal dysfunction, but this test has been largely superseded by newer methods.

Serum enzyme assays A number of serum enzymes have been used to distinguish and assess hepatocellular injury and biliary tract dysfunction or obstruction. All have inherent limitations in sensitivity and specificity, and none truly distinguish these processes definitively. Elevations in enzyme activities may also be seen in association with nonhepatic disorders. Nevertheless, with proper and careful interpretation, a number of serum enzymes provide important clinical tools.

AMINOTRANSFERASES (TRANSAMINASES) Assays of many serum enzymes have been proposed as indicators of hepatocellular damage. Of these, aspartate aminotransferase (AST,SGOT) and alanine aminotransferase (ALT,SGPT) activities have proven most useful. These enzymes catalyze the transfer of the γ-amino groups of aspartate and alanine, respectively, to the γ-keto group of ketoglutarate, leading to the formation of oxaloacetic acid and pyruvic acid. In contrast to ALT, which is found primarily in the liver, AST is present in many tissues including heart, skeletal muscle, kidney, and brain and is thus somewhat less specific as an indicator of liver function. The source of serum AST and ALT in the normal person (less than 40 IU) is unclear, and the mechanism responsible for clearance of these enzymes is uncertain. In the hepatocyte, ALT is found exclusively in the cytosol, while different isoenzymes of AST exist in mitochondria and the cytosol. Although elevated serum levels of AST or ALT may be observed in a variety of nonhepatic diseases, notably in myocardial infarction and skeletal muscle disorders, these disorders can usually be clinically distinguished from liver disease. Conversely, uremia may lead to spuriously low aminotransferase values.

Serum AST and ALT are elevated to some extent in nearly all liver disorders. Highest levels are found in association with conditions causing extensive hepatic necrosis, such as severe viral hepatitis, toxin-induced liver injury, or prolonged circulatory collapse. Lesser elevations are encountered in mild acute viral hepatitis as well as in both diffuse and focal chronic liver diseases (e.g., chronic active hepatitis, cirrhosis, and hepatic metastases). However, the absolute levels of aminotransferases correlate poorly with severity of liver injury or prognosis, and serial determinations are usually most helpful. Thus in the patient with massive hepatic necrosis, there may be marked elevations in the early phase (i.e., 24 to 48 h), but by the time the patient is tested 3 to 5 days later the levels may be in the range of 200 to 400 IU. It is noteworthy that in severe alcoholic hepatitis one commonly finds only modest increases in these enzymes (generally less than 300 IU). Minimal elevations of AST and ALT (less than 100 IU) may also be found in association with biliary tract obstruction; higher levels suggest the development of cholangitis with resultant hepatic cell necrosis.

In general AST and ALT levels parallel each other, with one exception. In alcoholic hepatitis the AST/ALT ratio may be greater than 2; this appears to result from a reduction in hepatic ALT content due to a deficiency in the cofactor pyridoxine-5-phosphate.

ALKALINE PHOSPHATASE Human serum contains several forms of alkaline phosphatase, a plasma membrane–derived enzyme of uncertain physiologic function which hydrolyzes synthetic phosphate esters at pH 9. These activities arise from bone, intestine, liver, and placenta. A number of different assays have been developed which utilize different substrates. The most widely used methods are expressed in international units (IU) (normal: 25 to 85 units), Bodansky units (normal: 1.4 to 4.5 units) or King-Armstrong units (normal: 1.5 to 4.5 units).

In the absence of bone disease or pregnancy, elevated levels of alkaline phosphatase activity usually reflect impaired biliary tract function. The increased levels reflect increased synthesis of the enzyme by hepatocytes and biliary tract epithelium rather than regurgitation of enzyme due to obstruction. Bile acids may play a role both by inducing synthesis and by promoting solubilization of the membrane-associated enzyme activity.

Slight to moderate increases in alkaline phosphatase (1 to 2 times normal) occur in many patients with parenchymal liver disorders such as hepatitis and cirrhosis; transient increases may occur in all types of liver disease. However, the most striking increases in alkaline phosphatase (3 to 10 times normal) occur with extrahepatic biliary tract (mechanical) obstruction or with intrahepatic (functional) cholestasis, as in drug-induced cholestasis or primary biliary cirrhosis. Conversely, it is unusual for the serum alkaline phosphatase to remain normal when there is obstructive jaundice, and a normal enzyme level argues strongly against the presence of cholestasis. The alkaline phosphatase is almost always mildly elevated in metastatic or infiltrative liver disease (e.g., leukemia, lymphoma, and sarcoid). The enzyme may be elevated in the presence of incomplete biliary obstruction or when there is obstruction of only one hepatic duct, conditions in which the serum bilirubin is often normal or only slightly elevated. Serum alkaline phosphatase is also elevated in nonhepatic disorders, most notably in some bone disorders (e.g., Paget's disease, osteomalacia, and metastases to bone) and sometimes with malignancy. Occasionally tumors produce an alkaline phosphatase which is identical or similar to the placental form, the so-called Regan isoenzyme.

Although one can usually make a reasonable assessment as to whether an elevation of the alkaline phosphatase is of hepatic or nonhepatic origin, several methods can distinguish the different isoenzymes facilitating resolution of any uncertainty. In contrast to that derived from bone, the hepatic isozyme is stable to treatment with heat (56°C for 15 min) or urea. These enzymes can also be separated by electrophoresis, but this is usually impractical. Parallel determination of serum 5′-nucleotidase activity is also helpful; an increase of both 5′-nucleotidase and alkaline phosphatase is consistent with an hepatobiliary source of the enzyme elevation. Even after correction for age and sex (higher levels being found in the young and in older women), isolated elevations in alkaline phosphatase may occasionally be encountered in adults with no apparent disease.

5′-NUCLEOTIDASE, LEUCINE AMINOPEPTIDASE, AND γ-GLUTAMYLTRANSPEPTIDASE *5′-Nucleotidase* catalyzes the hydrolysis of phosphate from the 5′ position of the pentose component of the nucleotide. Although tissue distribution is widespread, elevations are generally associated with hepatobiliary disease. The principal value of the 5′-nucleotidase measurement is to confirm the hepatic origin of an elevated alkaline phosphatase level in children, pregnant women, or in those settings where coincident bone disease may be present. However, 5′-nucleotidase levels do not always parallel alkaline phosphatase in liver disease, and lack of elevation does not exclude an hepatic source of elevated serum alkaline phosphatase.

Despite a widespread tissue distribution, *leucine aminopeptidase,* a protease which cleaves amino-terminal amino acids from peptides, is significantly elevated only in diseases of the pancreas and hepatobiliary system. There is considerable overlap in values of the peptidase levels found in patients with hepatocellular disease and in those with cholestatic jaundice; thus, in general, its measurement is of little clinical value.

γ-GLUTAMYLTRANSPEPTIDASE (GGT) catalyzes the transfer of the γ-glutamyl group from peptides such as glutathione to other amino acids and may play a role in amino acid transport. It is found throughout the hepatobiliary system as well as in other tissues. In liver disease, GGT correlates with alkaline phosphatase levels and is the most sensitive indicator of biliary tract disease. However, elevations of GGT are nonspecific and may be associated with pancreatic, cardiac, renal, and pulmonary disorders as well as with diabetes and alcoholism. This enzyme may be increased by agents which induce microsomal enzymes, and it has been suggested as a potential marker of alcoholism. However, overall lack of specificity has limited its clinical usefulness.

OTHER ENZYMES Measurement of total serum lactic dehydrogenase (LDH) or its isoenzymes is usually not helpful in diagnosis of liver disease because of this enzyme's nearly ubiquitous body distribution. Moderate LDH elevations are common in acute viral hepatitis, cirrhosis, and metastatic carcinoma to the liver. Biliary tract disease may also produce slight elevations. Numerous other dehydrogenases (e.g., isocitrate dehydrogenase, sorbitol dehydrogenase, and glutamate dehydrogenase) have been used or proposed as markers of liver disease, but none appear to offer significant diagnostic improvement over standard aminotransferase determinations. Elevation of serum ornithine carbamyl transferase (OCT), a urea cycle enzyme present only in liver and intestine, occurs primarily in liver disease, but its lack of association with any specific type of liver disease has limited its diagnostic usefulness also.

Serum proteins Extensive liver injury may lead to *decreased* blood levels of albumin, prothrombin, fibrinogen, and other proteins synthesized exclusively by hepatocytes. In contrast to measurements of serum enzymes, serum protein levels reflect liver synthetic function rather than just cell injury. Three important caveats should be remembered regarding interpretation of serum protein levels: (1) they are neither early nor sensitive indicators of liver disease (because of the extent of hepatic reserve and their half-life, see below), (2) they are of little value in the differential diagnosis of liver disease, and (3) decreases in their serum levels are not specific for liver disease.

ALBUMIN AND GLOBULIN Albumin is quantitatively the most important serum protein synthesized by the liver; the normal serum value ranges from 3.5 to 5 g/dL (see Chap. 244). Albumin has a fairly long half-life (14 to 20 days) with less than 5 percent turnover daily; it is therefore not a good indicator of acute or mild liver injury. Furthermore, there is a substantial reserve of hepatic albumin synthesis; thus, adequate synthesis may continue until there is extensive hepatocellular injury. Serum levels are influenced by a variety of nonhepatic factors, most notably nutritional status, hormonal factors, and plasma oncotic pressure. Routes of degradation in health remain undefined, but nonhepatic conditions may lead to depressed serum albumin levels mainly due to excessive loss despite adequate synthetic function (e.g., nephrotic syndrome or protein-losing enteropathy). Nonetheless, reduction in the serum albumin levels provides an excellent indication of the severity of chronic liver disease. In the patient with ascites, an increased volume of distribution as well as an absolute reduction in protein synthesis may contribute to hypoalbuminemia.

Serum globulins are a heterogeneous group of proteins whose production in a variety of tissues is influenced by a number of factors. Serum globulins (normal: 2 to 3.5 g/dL) include alpha and beta globulins as well as serum immunoglobulins, the latter largely accounting for the gamma fraction. Serum globulins are often diffusely elevated in association with chronic liver disease and in other nonhepatic disorders. In cirrhosis varying degrees of hyperglobulinemia may occur; this may reflect increased stimulation of the peripheral reticuloendothelial compartment due to shunting of antigens past the liver and impaired clearance by hepatic Kupffer cells. Although some have suggested that elevations in different globulin fractions as assessed by electrophoretic or other means may have a differential diagnostic value, this remains a largely unfulfilled promise. Similarly, the albumin/globulin ratio has no physiologic significance.

CLOTTING FACTORS The liver synthesizes six coagulation factors: fibrinogen (factor I), prothrombin (factor II), and factors V, VII, IX, and X. With the exception of factor V, production of functional proteins requires the presence of the cofactor, vitamin K. Because most of these factors are normally present in excess, impaired coagulation is usually seen only in severe liver disease. Abnormalities of these factors can be most efficiently determined by the one-stage *prothrombin time,* which measures the rate of prothrombin conversion to thrombin in the presence of thromboplastin and calcium and requires the integrity of most of the vitamin K–dependent clotting factors (see Chap. 54). Factor VII is the rate-limiting factor in this pathway and thus has the greatest influence on the prothrombin levels. The prothrombin time is dependent on normal hepatic synthesis of clotting factors and sufficient intestinal uptake of vitamin K. Absorption of this fat-soluble vitamin itself requires adequate dietary intake and normal function of intestinal mucosa and biliary secretion. Severe acute or chronic parenchymal liver injury may lead to prolongation of the prothrombin time due to impaired synthesis of the clotting proteins. Because these proteins have a shorter half-life than that of albumin, the prothrombin time may be an earlier indicator than serum albumin of severe liver injury. In both acute and chronic hepatocellular injury, an increase in the prothrombin time serves as an ominous prognostic sign. Because it is a fat-soluble vitamin, prolongation of the prothrombin time may result from vitamin K malabsorption and may occur with cholestasis due either to biliary tract disease or to fat malabsorption (steatorrhea) of any cause (e.g., pancreatic insufficiency). Poor dietary intake, antibiotic therapy, or use of warfarin-type anticoagulants are additional causes of a prolonged prothrombin time, owing to deficiencies of active vitamin K. These processes can be distinguished from hepatic synthetic failure by demonstrating normalization of the prothrombin time (within 24 to 48 h) after parenteral injections of vitamin K. The *partial thromboplastin time,* which reflects the activities of fibrinogen, prothrombin, and factors V, VIII, IX, X, XI, and XII, may also be prolonged in severe liver disease. Clotting functions should be assessed in all patients with liver disease prior to any surgical procedure, including liver biopsy (see Chaps. 54 and 280).

Blood ammonia Ammonia is elevated in the blood of some patients with either acute or chronic liver disease. Although influenced by a number of factors (summarized in Chap. 244), elevations in blood ammonia reflect disruption of the pathways of urea synthesis by which the liver detoxifies amine groups. A markedly elevated blood ammonia usually reflects severe hepatocellular necrosis. Cirrhotic patients, especially those with endogenous or surgically created portal-systemic shunting, often have varying degrees of hyperammonemia and hepatic encephalopathy. However, there is only a rough correlation between blood ammonia levels and the degree of hepatic encephalopathy; some patients will function normally with a twofold elevation, while others will be stuporous at the same concentration. Ammonia levels may increase before the onset of coma; similarly they may return to normal some 48 to 72 h before improvement of the neurologic status.

Serum lipids and lipoproteins and bile acids Abnormalities in serum lipids and lipoproteins are sensitive but nonspecific indicators of liver diseases. Acute parenchymal liver disease is commonly associated with increased plasma triglycerides, decreased cholesterol esters, and abnormal lipoproteins. The absence of alpha and prebeta bands with a concomitant increase in the beta fraction is typical of acute viral hepatitis. Less marked but more persistent abnormalities are found in patients with chronic parenchymal disease reflecting deficiencies in lecithin:cholesterol acyltransferase (LCAT) and hepatic triglyceride lipase. Either intra- or extrahepatic cholestasis may lead to an increase in unesterified cholesterol and in serum phospholipids. Lipoprotein X, a distinctive lipoprotein encountered in cholestasis, consists of equimolar amounts of unesterified cholesterol and lecithin which is regurgitated from the biliary tract. Although characteristically seen in patients with extrahepatic biliary obstruction, lipoprotein X may be found in any cholestatic condition.

Removal of bile acids from portal blood is impaired in liver disease because of parenchymal damage and portal-systemic shunts; there may also be reentry of bile acids into blood from injured hepatocytes or an obstructed biliary tract. Although there are a variety of techniques for measuring serum bile acids, these determinations are not yet of proven value for routine clinical use.

IMMUNOLOGIC AND OTHER TESTS

A number of immunologic derangements may be seen in liver disease. Antimitochondrial antibodies are found in 85 to 90 percent of patients with primary biliary cirrhosis. In this test, serum is incubated with rabbit hepatocytes. The presence of antimitochondrial antibodies can then be assessed after subsequent staining with a fluorescein-tagged second antibody. However, this marker is not entirely specific and is occasionally found in patients with chronic active hepatitis and drug-induced hepatitis. Its primary value is in helping to distinguish primary biliary cirrhosis from extrahepatic biliary obstruction. In chronic active hepatitis the *lupus erythematosus–cell test* (LE-cell test) may be positive, and *antinuclear antibodies* as well as *anti-smooth-muscle antibodies* may be present (see Chap. 262). Alpha-fetoprotein is of value in the diagnosis of hepatoma (see Chap. 250). Measurements of serum $alpha_1$-antitrypsin and ceruloplasmin should be performed in infants with cirrhosis or hepatitis since they may reflect $alpha_1$-antitrypsin deficiency or Wilson's disease, respectively (see Chaps 251 and 311).

RADIOLOGIC AND OTHER IMAGING PROCEDURES

Plain abdominal x-ray and barium studies of the gastrointestinal tract Standard plain films of the upper abdomen and barium studies provide little diagnostic information. The former may permit some estimation of hepatic size and the presence of splenic enlargement or ascites but is of limited value except for the demonstration of calcified lesions (e.g., echinococcal cysts or benign hemangiomas) and the now increasingly uncommon presence of previously administered thorotrast. Barium swallow will demonstrate esophageal varices with reasonable accuracy in patients with portal hypertension, although varices may be better demonstrated endoscopically.

Cholecystography and cholangiography A number of imaging techniques may be used to examine gallbladder function and biliary tract anatomy. *Oral cholecystography* involves assessment of gallbladder opacifiction following overnight oral administration of the dye iopanoic acid, which is normally concentrated in the gallbladder if both intestinal absorption and hepatocellular excretory function are intact. This test may be confounded by a variety of factors (e.g., diarrhea), and as many as 15 percent of normal patients will require a second dose of dye for good visualization. Consequently, the specificity and sensitivity of this test are substantially limited and it has been largely superseded by ultrasonography. *Intravenous cholangiography* requires the administration of dye as an intravenous bolus to visualize the bile ducts and gallbladder. Even mild impairment of liver excretory functions may prevent adequate visualization by this technique, thus limiting its application to the evaluation of patients with serum bilirubin levels below 2.5 to 3 mg/dL. In view of these limitations and a high rate of serious reactions to the contrast dye, this test should no longer be employed.

Ultrasonography has provided an important advance in the noninvasive evaluation of the biliary tree and gallbladder. It is not dependent on liver function and therefore can be used in patients with jaundice. It permits expeditious evaluation of the gallbladder, intra- and extrahepatic bile ducts, and hepatic parenchyma. It is also highly sensitive and specific for the detection of cholelithiasis (>95 percent) or signs of biliary tract obstruction. In the patient with obstructive jaundice, ultrasonography may indicate whether the site of obstruction is in the intra- or extrahepatic ducts. Mass lesions in the head of the pancreas or porta hepatis as well as gallstones may be associated findings that provide clues to the nature of the obstructing lesion. However, successful imaging of the biliary tree and the terminal portion of the common bile duct is confounded by the effects of gas in the overlying intestine in as many as 20 percent of patients. Ultrasonography is discussed in greater detail later in this chapter.

Visualization of the biliary tree by direct injection of radiopaque dye may be accomplished by *percutaneous transhepatic cholangiography (THC)* or by cannulation of the ampulla of Vater during endoscopic retrograde cholangiopancreatography (ERCP). THC involves puncture of the liver with a "skinny" needle which is then advanced under fluoroscopic guidance until ductal opacification is verified by injection of contrast material. With experience and proper precautions, dilated major ducts proximal to an obstructing lesion can be cannulated and visualized in up to 90 percent of cases; normal or small ducts associated with intrahepatic cholestasis are more difficult to demonstrate, but with modern techniques they can be opacified in up to 75 percent of cases.

ERCP with the fiberoptic duodenoscope is another method of demonstrating the bile and pancreatic ducts radiographically. (This is discussed in detail in Chap. 233.) The papilla of Vater is cannulated under direct vision, and contrast material is injected into the biliary and pancreatic ducts. ERCP is particularly useful in jaundiced patients with suspected lesions in the head of the pancreas or ampulla of Vater, since one may also obtain cytologic and histologic evaluation of mass lesions. ERCP does not rely upon dilatation of the bile ducts for success, and since the liver itself is not punctured, there is no risk of bile peritonitis when there is high-grade biliary obstruction. However, acute pancreatitis may result from injection of contrast material into the pancreatic duct, and successful cannulation may not be accomplished in 10 to 15 percent of patients. In most clinical settings THC and ERCP offer equivalent visualization of the biliary tract although particular features of an individual patient may favor one approach. Both techniques also offer the opportunity for therapeutic intervention in the patient with obstructive jaundice following diagnostic evaluation. Decompression of the biliary tree via external drainage or placement of an internal stent may be accomplished following THC. Endoscopic papillotomy may permit passage of common bile duct stones and in some circumstances obviate the need for surgical intervention.

Angiography Improvement in contrast agents and techniques of vascular catheterization has led to increased sophistication in the use of selective angiography in the evaluation of patients with liver disease. Selected cannulation of the hepatic artery or one of its branches is particularly helpful in the assessment of patients with suspected vascular abnormalities (e.g., arteriovenous malformation) and some mass lesions. In some circumstances angiographic features may be nearly diagnostic, as in hemangioma and focal nodular hyperplasia. The technique is especially useful in the preoperative evaluation of patients with isolated mass lesions in whom resection is contemplated. Visualization of the portal venous circulation following arterial injection provides important anatomic information regarding the patency of the portal vein and the direction of portal blood flow and should be a part of the preoperative evalution prior to elective shunt surgery.

Radioisotope liver scans (scintiscans) Hepatic scintiscans are performed by external scanning of the upper abdomen after intravenous injection of gamma-emitting isotopes selectively extracted by the liver. These techniques have limited spatial resolution but are relatively noninvasive and offer particular advantages in some clinical settings. There are basically three types: (1) colloidal scans which depend on uptake of labeled colloid by Kupffer cells, permitting assessment of the liver parenchyma (e.g., ^{99m}Tc-labeled sulfur colloid), (2) the HIDA or PIPIDA scans (^{99m}Tc-labeled, *N*-substituted iminoacetic acids), in which dye is taken up and excreted by hepatocytes into the biliary tree allowing evaluation of biliary tract processes, and (3) the gallium scan in which the radionuclide ^{67}Ga is concentrated in neoplastic and inflammatory cells to a greater extent than in hepatocytes. Because these reagents are concentrated by different cellular components of the liver, they may yield complementary images in various conditions. Hence, a hepatoma or liver abscess will lead to reduced uptake or a "cold spot" on colloid or PIPIDA scans, but to increased uptake or a "hot spot" with gallium.

Colloidal scans with ^{198}Au-labeled gold or ^{99m}Tc-labeled sulfur are the scans most commonly used to assess hepatic parenchyma. Metastatic cancer deposits greater than 2 to 3 cm in diameter may be reliably demonstrated as filling defects. Colloid scans are nearly equivalent to ultrasound in this setting and are most effectively used in conjunction with other liver function tests. However, a distorted lobular architecture, as in cirrhosis, can also result in irregular uptake and produce apparent filling defects.

The HIDA or PIPIDA scans are most useful for assessing patency of the biliary tract since these radionuclides are secreted by hepatocytes into the bile canaliculi. These scans have been used to differentiate intrahepatic from extrahepatic obstruction; in complete biliary obstruction there is failure of the isotope to enter the duodenum, while in intrahepatic cholestasis some isotope will be seen in the lumen of the small bowel. However, clear-cut distinctions may be difficult. These scans are most helpful in the diagnosis of acute cholecystitis, where failure of the nuclide to enter the gallbladder indicates the presence of cystic duct or common bile duct obstruction. Adequate visualization may be accomplished even with moderate hyperbilirubinemia.

Ultrasonography The usefulness of *ultrasound* evaluation of structures in the right upper quadrant continues to increase. Sound waves are generated by a piezoelectric crystal which also serves as a sensitive detector of those waves reflected back from the tissue. This noninvasive technique depends upon the differential reflection of sound waves at tissue interfaces resulting from differences in acoustical impedance. The limits of instrumental resolution continue to improve with gray-scale scanning, while real-time ultrasonography now permits evaluation of some dynamic processes. As mentioned above, ultrasound is the preferred method for imaging the biliary tree and gallbladder. In addition, ultrasound is useful for evaluation of suspected hepatic mass lesions and may resolve deposits as small as 1 to 2 cm. Ultrasound is particularly useful in distinguishing abscesses or cystic structures from solid lesions. However, distinction among solid masses may be difficult, and ultrasound may not reliably differentiate neoplastic (primary hepatocellular or metastatic) from regenerative nodules. In those few patients in whom physical findings are uncertain, particularly in the obese patient, the presence of ascites may be effectively assessed with this modality. This tool may also yield important information about other abdominal structures (e.g., mass in the head of the pancreas). In addition, this imaging technique may be used to facilitate guided "skinny" needle biopsy of isolated hepatic lesions.

Computed tomography and magnetic resonance imaging Computed tomography (CT scan) utilizes a computer to synthesize differences in absorption of a large number of x-rays into a coherent cross-sectional image. Images may be taken with or without prior injection or ingestion of contrast material to highlight vascular or luminal digestive structures. CT scanning is particularly useful in differentiating among intrahepatic fluid collections such as cysts, abscesses, and hematomas, since the fluid density can be determined with relative accuracy. Using the CT scan, the gallbladder, extrahepatic bile ducts, and portal vein as well as a number of solid intraabdominal organs such as pancreas, liver, and spleen may be examined noninvasively with only modest radiation. In contrast to its effect on ultrasound, intestinal gas does not interfere with CT, although paucity of fat sometimes limits resolution in thin patients. CT scanning and ultrasound are often equivalent in their diagnostic yield of mass lesions, gallstones, or obstructive jaundice; in those conditions ultrasound is usually the procedure of choice since it is less expensive and involves no radiation.

Magnetic resonance imaging (MRI) is a technique which depends upon differences in the magnetic properties of molecules within different cell and tissue types based on their effect on the field of a large magnet. This technology offers the opportunity for spatial scanning comparable to that of ultrasound and CT scanning. In particular, it may be helpful in assessing blood flow and portal vein patency. It may also be effective in delineating focal disease processes, e.g., metastases (see Fig. 245-1). The range of applications of MRI is in a state of rapid development and its role relative to other imaging modalities is still evolving.

OTHER DIAGNOSTIC PROCEDURES

Percutaneous needle biopsy of the liver Percutaneous needle biopsy is a safe, simple, and valuable method for the diagnostic evaluation of liver disease. *Diffuse parenchymal disorders* such as cirrhosis, hepatitis, and drug reactions may be diagnosed with remarkable accuracy. In *disseminated focal diseases* (such as granulomas or tumor infiltrates) serial sections may demonstrate characteristic lesions.

Biopsy is performed under local anesthesia, usually with the Menghini (aspiration), Klatskin, or Vim-Silverman (cutting) needle, by either a transpleural or subcostal approach. If the operator is skillful and patients carefully selected, morbidity should be quite low and limited to occasional postbiopsy pain or vasovagal reactions.

Some of the most frequent indications for needle biopsy are (1) unexplained hepatomegaly or hepatosplenomegaly; (2) cholestasis of uncertain cause; (3) persistently abnormal liver function tests; (4) suspected systemic or infiltrative diseases such as sarcoidosis, miliary tuberculosis, or fever of unknown origin; and (5) suspected primary or metastatic liver tumor. Percutaneous liver biopsy may be performed either for diagnostic purposes or to evaluate the extent and severity of a known disease process. However, other new and improved noninvasive diagnostic methods have obviated the need for biopsy in many circumstances, and thus biopsy should be performed only when information from these other techniques is inadequate.

Needle biopsy should not be performed if (1) the patient is unable to cooperate; (2) clinical or laboratory evidence indicates impaired hemostasis (prothrombin time prolonged by 3 s or more over control, thrombocytopenia less than 80,000 to 100,000 platelets per cubic millimeter, or partial thromboplastin time or bleeding time prolonged); (3) there is infection of the right pleural space or septic cholangitis; (4) tense ascites is present, with risk of continued leakage of ascitic

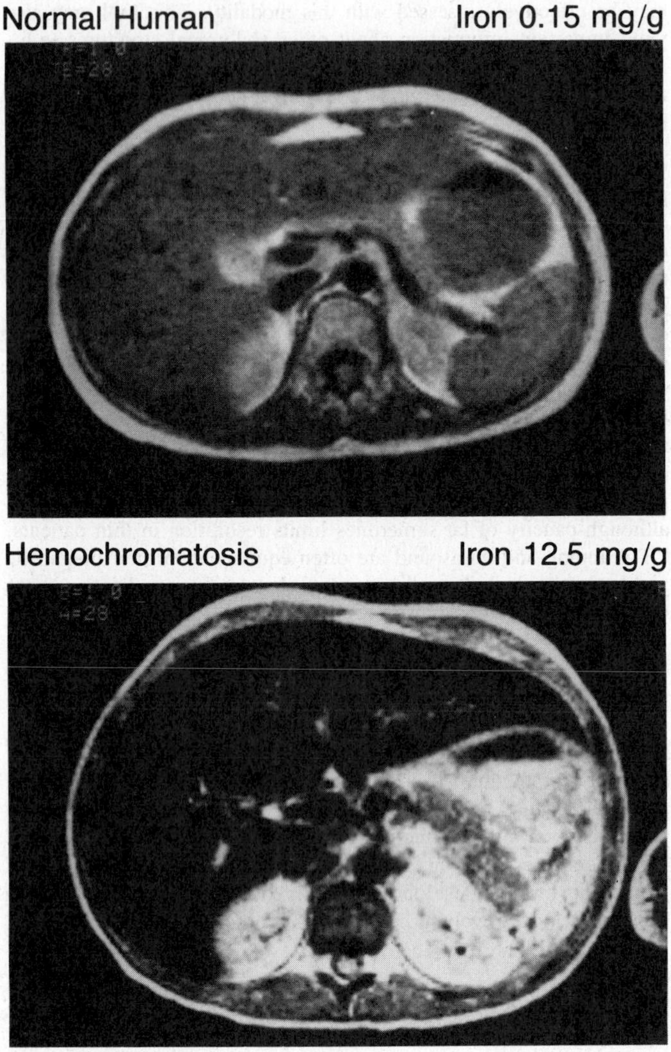

FIGURE 245-1 *Magnetic resonance imaging (MRI) of human liver using spin-echo technique. Upper panel, appearance of normal hepatic parenchyma. Lower panel, alteration in signal in proportion to hepatic iron content. (Courtesy of Dr. David Stark.)*

fluid; (5) compatible blood is not available for transfusion in case of hemorrhage or (6) high-grade biliary obstruction is suspected and there is an increased risk of bile peritonitis. With the increasing use of CT scan and ultrasonography, it is possible to perform "directed" aspiration biopsies of isolated lesions with very thin needles. Aspirated material can be used for cytology (tumors) and culture (abscesses) but is often inadequate for assessment of liver architecture.

Laparoscopy and laparotomy (peritoneoscopy) (see Chap. 233)

REFERENCES

BERK RN JR et al (eds): *Radiology of the Gallbladder and Bile Ducts.* Philadelphia, Saunders, 1983

BRENSILVER HL, KAPLAN MM: Significance of elevated liver alkaline phosphatase in serum. Gastroenterology 68:1556, 1975

FERRUCCI JT JR et al (eds): *Interventional Radiology of the Abdomen,* 2d ed. Baltimore, Williams and Wilkins, 1985

KEMENY MM et al: A projected analysis of laboratory tests and imaging studies to detect hepatic lesions. Ann Surg 195:163, 1982

MAURO MA et al: Hepatobiliary scanning with ^{99m}Tc-PIPIDA in acute cholecystitis. Radiology 142:193, 1982

MOSS, AA et al Hepatic tumors: Magnetic resonance and CT appearance. Radiology 150:191, 1984

ROSALI SB: Enzyme tests in diseases of the liver and hepatobiliary tract, in *The Principles and Practice of Diagnostic Enzymology,* JH Wilkinon (ed). Chicago, Year Book, 1976, pp 303–360

SABESIN SM: Cholestatic lipoproteins—Their pathogenesis and significance. Gastroenterology 83:704, 1982

246 DISTURBANCES OF BILIRUBIN METABOLISM

KURT J. ISSELBACHER

The normal metabolism of bilirubin and the approach to the patient with jaundice have been presented in Chap. 38. With a consideration of these pathways, the disorders of bilirubin metabolism can be divided into four major categories, namely, those due to (1) increased pigment production, (2) reduced hepatic uptake of bilirubin, (3) impaired hepatic conjugation, and (4) decreased excretion of the conjugated pigment from the liver into bile. The first three of these disorders are associated with predominantly unconjugated hyperbilirubinemia. The fourth group, defective excretion, is associated with predominantly conjugated hyperbilirubinemia and bilirubinuria.

DISORDERS CAUSING PREDOMINANTLY UNCONJUGATED HYPERBILIRUBINEMIA

The plasma concentration of unconjugated bilirubin is determined by (1) the rate at which newly synthesized bilirubin enters the plasma (bilirubin turnover) and (2) the rate of removal of bilirubin by the liver (hepatic bilirubin clearance). The latter can result from derangements of hepatic bilirubin uptake, conjugation, or both. Measurements of these variables, although not routinely available, permit a classification of patients into those with *increased bilirubin turnover* (e.g., hemolysis), those with *decreased bilirubin clearance* (e.g., Gilbert's syndrome), and those in whom both mechanisms operate.

OVERPRODUCTION OF BILIRUBIN (INCREASED TURNOVER)

Increased destruction of circulating erythrocytes (intravascular and extravascular hemolysis) In disorders associated with hemolysis, most commonly the hemolytic anemias, the rate of bilirubin production is increased and may even exceed the amount that can be removed by a normal liver. The resulting jaundice is primarily an unconjugated hyperbilirubinemia. There is often also a small increase in the serum conjugated bilirubin (see Chap. 38). If significant anemia or other adverse factors are present (e.g., fever, sepsis, hypoxemia, or vascular collapse), the ability of the liver to handle the pigment load will be compromised, and the degree of jaundice will be greater.

The clinical and diagnostic features of the various hemolytic anemias are described in Chap. 287. The presence of reticulocytosis, shortened red blood cell survival, and increased fecal urobilinogen, in the absence of clinical and laboratory evidence of liver disease, strongly suggest hemolysis and overproduction of bilirubin as the cause of the jaundice. It is obvious, however, that in some cases (e.g., cirrhosis, tumors, and sepsis), hemolysis *plus* deranged liver function may be present. In most cases of uncomplicated hemolytic states, the mean serum bilirubin level will be in the range of 3 to 5 mg/dL; rarely, levels up to 10 mg/dL may be seen.

Jaundice due to increased pigment production may also be seen as a consequence of *tissue infarction* (e.g., pulmonary infarcts) and large *collections of blood in tissues* (e.g., leakage from blood vessels after catheterization studies, rupture of an aortic aneurysm). If hypotension and hypoxemia also supervene, jaundice is usually more pronounced, and the resulting impairment of liver function may also lead to a significant increase in the serum conjugated bilirubin level (see "Postoperative Jaundice" below).

Except in early infancy, elevations of serum unconjugated bilirubin levels are not generally harmful per se, and the prognosis is that of the hemolytic process itself. However, in the neonatal state and infancy, unconjugated bilirubin levels above 20 mg/dL may lead to *kernicterus* due to bilirubin deposition in the lipid-rich basal ganglia (see Chap. 351). Chronic overproduction of bilirubin may result in the formation of gallstones composed predominantly of bilirubin ("pigment stones"). In this situation, all the potential complications of calculus disease of the biliary tract (Chap. 253) may be superimposed on the chronic hemolytic state which produced it.

Increased production of bilirubin from sources other than circulating erythrocytes As indicated in Chap. 38, about 15 to 20 percent of the circulating bilirubin is normally derived from sources other than the destruction of circulating red blood cells. This represents the so-called early-labeled fraction; it includes the synthesis of bilirubin from nonhemoglobin heme in the liver and from hemoglobin heme in the marrow.

In some conditions, jaundice results from an increased destruction of red blood cells or their precursors in the marrow—a process referred to as *ineffective erythropoiesis* (see Chaps. 38 and 53). In patients with thalassemia, pernicious anemia, and congenital erythropoietic porphyria, such an increased rate of formation of the early-labeled bilirubin fraction has been demonstrated. It is possible that some cases of unexplained unconjugated hyperbilirubinemia may be caused by an increased hepatic production of bilirubin from nonhemoglobin heme, but this phenomenon has not yet been demonstrated clinically.

IMPAIRED HEPATIC UPTAKE OF BILIRUBIN Drugs Only a few drugs have been definitely shown to influence the uptake of bilirubin by the liver. Flavaspidic acid, used in the treatment of tapeworm infestation, may cause unconjugated hyperbilirubinemia, as well as impairment of sodium sulfobromophthalein (BSP) clearance, during its administration. The jaundice readily subsides following treatment. Flavaspidic acid competes with bilirubin for binding to ligandin, leading thereby to unconjugated hyperbilirubinemia. The jaundice which may occur with novobiocin and some cholecystographic dyes is also apparently due to an interference in bilirubin uptake.

Gilbert's syndrome Some cases of this syndrome of chronic unconjugated hyperbilirubinemia may be due to a defect in hepatic uptake (as reflected by alteration in BSP kinetics). In most cases, however, a deficiency of bilirubin glucuronyl transferase can be demonstrated. Hence this syndrome is best considered as a defect in bilirubin conjugation (see below).

IMPAIRED BILIRUBIN CONJUGATION (DECREASED ACTIVITY OF BILIRUBIN GLUCURONYL TRANSFERASE) Neonatal jaundice (physiologic jaundice of the newborn) Almost every infant exhibits some transient unconjugated hyperbilirubinemia between the second and fifth days of life. While during gestation the placenta serves to clear bilirubin from the fetus, after birth infants must detoxify the pigments themselves. However, at this stage the hepatic enzyme glucuronyl transferase is still "immature" and inadequate for the task. As a result, unconjugated bilirubinemia develops, usually not exceeding 5 mg/dL. The activity of glucuronyl transferase increases within several days to 2 weeks after birth, and concomitantly the serum bilirubin returns to normal. In the premature infant the glucuronyl transferase activity is less, and the neonatal jaundice may be more pronounced. The "maturation" of the fetal and neonatal liver may be enhanced by treatment of the pregnant mother or the newborn infant with phenobarbital or related drugs. This results in a clear-cut reduction of the degree and duration of unconjugated hyperbilirubinemia in the newborn. In infants with a superimposed hemolytic process (e.g., erythroblastosis), the excessive pigment load leads to more pronounced jaundice, and bilirubin levels may exceed 20 mg/dL. It should be emphasized that neonatal jaundice is not present at the time of delivery; if jaundice is present at birth, other causes must be considered.

The cytoplasmic liver cell protein ligandin binds bilirubin in the hepatocyte and may assist in the transfer of bilirubin to the endoplasmic reticulum for conjugation (Chap. 38). It has been proposed that deficiency of ligandin may contribute to neonatal jaundice.

An additional facet of the "immature" liver is a concomitant defect in the excretion of *conjugated* bilirubin. Rarely this defect persists beyond the time needed for the development of adequate glucuronide conjugation and may explain the occasional presence of conjugated hyperbilirubinemia in infants with erythroblastosis (*inspissated bile syndrome*).

When in the neonatal state unconjugated bilirubin levels approach or exceed 20 mg/dL, the infants may develop and die of *kernicterus* (bilirubin encephalopathy). This condition results from unconjugated bilirubin deposition in the lipid-rich basal ganglia. In the past treatment consisted of exchange transfusions, and albumin infusions were used to increase binding of bilirubin in the circulation and diminish its entry into the brain. The current approach is *phototherapy;* intense illumination of these patients with strong white or blue light leads to the photoisomerization of bilirubin to water-soluble isomers that are rapidly excreted in the bile without the prior need of conjugation.

Hereditary glucuronyl transferase deficiency There are currently three syndromes that fall into this category. As indicated in Table 246-1, they reflect progressive decreases in the activity of glucuronyl transferase and thus may be part of a spectrum, i.e., from minimal deficiency to complete absence of bilirubin glucuronyl transferase.

GILBERT'S SYNDROME Since the original report by Gilbert in 1907, there has been an increased recognition of this benign but chronic disorder characterized by mild, persistent, unconjugated hyperbilirubinemia. The patient usually does not manifest this disorder until after the second decade and is often unaware of the jaundice until it is detected by physical examination or routine laboratory testing. The total serum bilirubin level usually ranges and fluctuates from 1.2 to 3 mg/dL and rarely exceeds 5 mg/dL. With the van den Bergh diazo reaction, less than 20 percent of the bilirubin gives a direct reaction; however, studies using more accurate methods (such as high-pressure liquid chromatography) show that the serum bilirubin in patients with Gilbert's syndrome is almost all unconjugated. Typically the jaundice fluctuates and is exacerbated following prolonged fasting (see below), surgery, fever or infection, and excessive exertion or alcohol ingestion. Liver function tests are normal, and the liver cells usually appear normal by light microscopy.

With the exception of hemolytic anemias, this disorder is probably the most common cause of mild unconjugated hyperbilirubinemia. Detailed studies show these patients to have a partial deficiency of bilirubin glucuronyl transferase. Some patients also manifest decreased bilirubin uptake and increased hemolysis. Decreased glucuronyl transferase alone or together with a decrease in bilirubin uptake appears to account for the observed *decrease in hepatic bilirubin clearance*. A decreased clearance and hepatic uptake of bile salts has also been shown.

Previously Gilbert's syndrome was traditionally defined as mild, chronic, unconjugated hyperbilirubinemia occurring in the absence of hemolysis. However, with the use of radiobilirubin kinetics and erythrocyte half-life studies, at least two forms of Gilbert's syndrome

TABLE 246-1 Hereditary unconjugated hyperbilirubinemias with deficiency of glucuronyl transferase

Features	Mild (Gilbert's syndrome)	Moderate (Crigler-Najjar syndrome type II)	Severe (Crigler-Najjar syndrome type I)
Inheritance	Unclear*	Dominant†	Recessive
Serum bilirubin, mg/dL	1–6	6–20	20–45
Kernicterus	No	Rare	Yes
Conjugated bilirubin in bile	Yes (↑ monoconjugates)	Yes (↑↑ monoconjugates)	No
Response to phenobarbital	Yes	Yes	No
Bilirubin conjugation	↓‡	↓↓	Absent

* *Many cases are without familial incidence.*
† *Variable expressivity.*
‡ *Other defects such as occult hemolysis and ↓ bilirubin uptake may coexist.*

have been described. One group includes patients with decreased bilirubin clearance and *no hemolysis*. A second group includes those who also have *evidence of hemolysis* (often occult) and hence increased bilirubin turnover. The simultaneous presence of both derangements appears to be a chance occurrence of two not uncommon disorders in the same patient and does not imply a causal relationship. There is additional evidence of the heterogeneity of patients with Gilbert's syndrome. Some patients have an increase in hepatocyte lipofuscin and an increase in the smooth endoplasmic reticulum (SER); others show an increase in hepatic lysosomal enzymes.

A feature of Gilbert's syndrome which can be useful diagnostically is the increase in serum bilirubin following prolonged fasting or calorie deprivation. Patients with this disorder, when placed on 300 cal per day for 2 days, will increase their serum bilirubin by 1.5 mg/dL or more, the major increase being in the unconjugated fraction. It appears that a decrease in glucuronyl transferase activity is needed in order to obtain this effect. Patients with hemolysis do not show an increase in serum bilirubin with fasting. As a reflection of the mild decrease in glucuronyl transferase in Gilbert's syndrome (1) serum bilirubin levels will decrease when the enzyme activity is enhanced following phenobarbital administration, and (2) the bile shows a modest increase in monoconjugates of bilirubin (see Table 246-1).

In general, the diagnosis of this benign but not uncommon disorder is made by exclusion. The syndrome is suspected in a patient with low-grade unconjugated hyperbilirubinemia with (1) no systemic symptoms, (2) *no overt* or clinically recognizable hemolysis, (3) normal tests of routine liver function, and (4) a liver biopsy (although usually not necessary) that is normal by light microscopy.

CRIGLER-NAJJAR SYNDROME (TYPES I AND II) This disorder is known to exist in two forms. Type I is the clinically *severe* form (originally described by Crigler and Najjar) and is due to *absence of glucuronyl transferase*. Type II has more *moderate* clinical findings due to *partial deficiency of glucuronyl transferase*. The major differences between the two variants are summarized in Table 246-1.

Type I (Crigler-Najjar) is a rare disorder. Infants develop high unconjugated bilirubin levels in the serum (20 to 45 mg/dL). Absence of the enzyme can be demonstrated in the liver. Routine liver function tests are normal, as is liver histology. Because of the absence of glucuronyl transferase no conjugated bilirubin is formed by the liver; hence no bilirubin is secreted by the liver, and the bile is colorless.

Phototherapy may temporarily and transiently reduce the unconjugated bilirubin level. Phenobarbital has no effect since the enzyme defect is complete and no drug "induction" is therefore possible. Affected infants usually die within the first year of life, although some patients have survived to the second or third decade of life. Death is usually from kernicterus. A strain of rats (Gunn rat) with the type I defect exists and is widely used as an animal model of the Crigler-Najjar syndrome (type I).

Type II patients have a *partial deficiency* of glucuronyl transferase, and their disorder is less severe. Serum unconjugated bilirubin levels are lower (6 to 20 mg/dL), jaundice may not appear until adolescence, and neurologic complications are uncommon. The bile contains variable amounts of conjugated bilirubin with a significant increase in monoconjugates. Phenobarbital is effective in lowering the serum bilirubin level in type II patients. However, the disorder is relatively benign in those patients whose bilirubin is less than 18 to 20 mg/dL.

Acquired deficiency of glucuronyl transferase As with any enzyme, glucuronyl transferase is susceptible to inhibition by a variety of agents, and because of the decreased activity of the enzyme in the neonatal state, such inhibition may be more evident at that time. Neonatal jaundice may be aggravated or prolonged in infants treated with *drugs* such as chloramphenicol or novobiocin, or with *vitamin K*. In some breast-fed infants jaundice has been ascribed to the presence in *breast milk* of pregnane-3β,20α-diol, an inhibitor of glucuronyl transferase. When the infant is removed from the breast, the "breast-milk jaundice" subsides.

Hypothyroidism delays the normal "maturation" of glucuronyl transferase. In cretins, neonatal jaundice may be prolonged for weeks or months. In fact, the presence of prolonged unconjugated hyperbilirubinemia after birth may be a clue to an underlying hypothyroidism.

In the infant, as well as in the adult, *liver cell damage* leads to impairment in glucuronide conjugation as a result of decreased transferase activity. However, since excretion is probably the rate-limiting step in bilirubin metabolism and since this step is always interfered with to a greater extent than conjugation in parenchymal liver disease, the pigment which accumulates in the blood is predominantly conjugated bilirubin.

DISORDERS CAUSING COMBINED CONJUGATED AND UNCONJUGATED HYPERBILIRUBINEMIA

In jaundice due to primary liver disease, the plasma usually exhibits elevated levels of both conjugated and unconjugated bilirubin, and *urine contains bilirubin*. The relative proportions of the two pigments are highly variable. In many familial hepatic abnormalities (described below) and in some forms of liver injury, the jaundice is largely due to increases in conjugated bilirubin. Such a serum pigment pattern is also seen with extrahepatic biliary obstruction. One *cannot differentiate* intrahepatic and extrahepatic causes of jaundice from either the levels or proportions of unconjugated and conjugated bilirubin in serum. Thus the main purpose of the initial fractionation of the serum bilirubin is to distinguish hepatic parenchymal and biliary obstructive disease from the disorders associated with predominantly unconjugated hyperbilirubinemia.

FAMILIAL DEFECTS IN HEPATIC EXCRETORY FUNCTION Dubin-Johnson syndrome This disorder, also called *chronic idiopathic jaundice,* is a benign, autosomally inherited hyperbilirubinemia characterized by the presence of a dark pigment in the centrilobular region of the liver cells. Functionally there exists a *defect in biliary excretion* of bilirubin, cholephilic dyes, and porphyrins. Using the diazo method for measuring bilirubin, the serum pigment in these patients typically has been observed to be in the range of 3 to 15 mg/dL and predominantly of the conjugated type. However, with the newer and more accurate method (alkaline methanolysis and high-pressure liquid chromatography), homozygous patients with the Dubin-Johnson syndrome have been shown to have significant levels of serum *unconjugated bilirubin*. This finding may in part reflect pigment which, after conjugation by the liver, is deconjugated in the hepatobiliary system and refluxed into the plasma. Moreover, the serum contains more diconjugated than monoconjugated bilirubin, just the reverse of what is seen in acquired hepatobiliary disease and Rotor syndrome. This reversed ratio is believed to be characteristic and diagnostic for homozygous patients.

Patients with Dubin-Johnson syndrome may be asymptomatic or have vague constitutional or gastrointestinal symptoms. Not infrequently the liver is slightly enlarged; in about one-fourth of the cases there is mild hepatic tenderness. Oral and intravenous cholangiography fails to visualize the biliary tract. There is typically and characteristically a late rise in the plasma BSP elimination curve at *90 min*. This is caused by the reflux from the liver of the conjugated dye and reflects the defect in the hepatic excretory transport maximum (T_m). It is noteworthy that there is no such secondary rise in plasma when dyes which are not conjugated by the liver are given, such as indocyanine green. When bile salts such as ursodeoxycholic acid are given, these patients show a decreased hepatic uptake and clearance. In the liver the striking feature is the presence of a brown or black pigment in the hepatocytes. Some findings suggest that this unique pigment is "melanin-like"; others indicate it to be a polymer of epinephrin metabolites.

These patients also show an abnormality in coproporphyrin excretion. Normal urine contains mostly coproporphyrin III and small amounts of coproporphyrin I; Dubin-Johnson patients show a reversal of this pattern, i.e., they excrete predominantly coproporphyrin I. Heterozygotes show an intermediate excretory pattern.

There is impaired excretion of many metabolites, including conjugated bilirubin, BSP, and iodinated dyes. Excretion of bile acids, however, is normal. Oral contraceptive agents may accentuate hyperbilirubinemia or may produce jaundice for the first time. Features of cholestasis such as pruritus or steatorrhea are usually lacking, and, specifically, serum alkaline phosphatase levels are *not* elevated. The overall prognosis of the disorder is excellent.

Rotor syndrome This is similar in many respects to the Dubin-Johnson syndrome. However, *there is no pigment in the liver cells,* and the serum conjugated bilirubin has more monoconjugates than diglucuronide conjugates. The gallbladder is usually visualized on cholecystography, and there is an increase in the *total* urinary coproporphyrins but *not* an increased percentage in excretion of coproporphyrin I. The BSP excretion pattern does *not* show a secondary rise at 90 min. The impairment in excretion which is typical of Dubin-Johnson syndrome is not present; instead in most cases of the Rotor syndrome there is impairment of *hepatic storage capacity* (*S*). This rare syndrome is inherited as an autosomal recessive trait and is genetically distinct from Dubin-Johnson syndrome.

Benign familial recurrent cholestasis This is a relatively rare syndrome characterized by recurrent attacks of pruritus and jaundice. During an attack the serum alkaline phosphatase and bile acid levels are markedly elevated, and liver biopsy shows the morphologic features of cholestasis. However, there is no mechanical biliary obstruction, with cholangiography revealing a patent biliary tree. Remissions are the rule, and at such times hepatic function tests and liver morphologic features are usually normal. The cause of the disorder is unknown; cirrhosis does not develop, and the disorder is benign. A congenital origin has been postulated on the basis of the early age of onset and familial incidence.

Recurrent jaundice of pregnancy This form of jaundice is also known as *intrahepatic cholestasis of pregnancy*. During a normal pregnancy some derangements in liver function occur, especially during the last trimester. Usually these consist of slight increases in BSP retention and in serum alkaline phosphatase. This mild increase in alkaline phosphatase during pregnancy is normally of placental rather than of hepatic origin. With a normal pregnancy elevations of serum bilirubin either do not occur or are less than 2 mg/dL.

In a small number of pregnant women an intrahepatic cholestasis may appear. This usually occurs in the third trimester but may develop any time after the seventh week of gestation. The clinical features consist primarily of pruritus and jaundice. Serum bilirubin levels are usually less than 6 mg/dL. The serum alkaline phosphatase and cholesterol levels are elevated significantly, while other liver function tests are only mildly deranged. Histologically the liver shows varying degrees of cholestasis but only a few parenchymal cell changes. The clinical and laboratory abnormalities subside promptly after delivery and are usually normal within 7 to 14 days.

This condition has been seen more frequently in Scandinavia and Europe than in the United States. Since steroid hormones and specifically estrogens can induce changes in hepatic excretory function in normal individuals (see Chap. 244), these patients probably have an increased susceptibility or sensitivity to the hepatic effects of estrogenic and progestational hormones. The intrahepatic cholestasis is usually termed *recurrent,* since the syndrome often (but not always) reappears in subsequent pregnancies. The process is benign and self-limited, and treatment is usually not needed, but cholestyramine administration will diminish the pruritus. This disorder must be distinguished from the many other causes of jaundice not unique to pregnancy, such as viral hepatitis. It must also be distinguished from the idiopathic *acute fatty liver of pregnancy* and the *tetracycline-induced* fatty liver. The latter two conditions are rare, occur in the last trimester, and have a high fatality rate; however, in these disorders there is evidence of diffuse parenchymal damage and not just cholestasis.

ACQUIRED DEFECTS OF HEPATIC EXCRETORY FUNCTION

Drug-induced cholestasis A condition entirely analogous to the intrahepatic cholestasis of pregnancy may occur in some women following the use of oral contraceptive agents. A significant number of individuals using these drugs show mild increases in BSP retention, and even more have decreased BSP excretory capacity as measured by infusion tests. In some, mild cholestatic jaundice may occur, liver function returns to normal when the drugs are withdrawn, and chronic liver disease does not appear to result. It is relevant that one-third of the reported patients with jaundice due to oral contraceptives also have a history of recurrent intrahepatic cholestasis of pregnancy.

The nature of these changes produced by the natural and synthetic female sex hormones is very similar to those resulting from the administration of certain testosterone analogues, especially those with α substitutions at the 17 position of the steroid nucleus. These agents (such as methyltestosterone and norethandrolone) commonly cause BSP retention and less commonly cause jaundice or significant changes in other liver functions. However, unlike the female hormones, these agents have been implicated as a cause of chronic liver disease, especially biliary cirrhosis.

Because of these phenomena, synthetic steroid sex hormones should not be used in patients with liver disease. Conversely, in individuals using these agents the appearance of jaundice or elevations in serum aminotransferase (transaminase) levels or alkaline phosphatase contraindicates their further use. However, mild to moderate increases in BSP retention alone are probably not of clinical significance, although liver function tests should be carried out periodically.

As is discussed in detail in Chap. 247, there are many drugs which may produce not only cholestasis but liver injury resembling acute hepatitis or cholestatic hepatitis. In contrast to the jaundice produced by the steroid hormones, the clinical features are those of fever, rash, arthralgia, and eosinophilia, with the liver showing a pronounced inflammatory reaction. These features suggest that such reactions are *allergic* or *toxic* in nature and therefore differ from the effects caused by the steroid hormones, which probably represent an exaggerated response by the liver to the normal action of these hormones.

Postoperative jaundice The occurrence of postoperative jaundice is a problem of increasing importance. It is perhaps seen more frequently now than in earlier years, because patients are able to undergo more major surgical procedures (i.e., cardiac surgery, repair of ruptured aneurysms) and survive. In approaching this problem the possible pathogenic mechanisms listed in Table 246-2 need to be considered. The patient may have *pigment overload,* especially from blood transfusions (with hemolysis of stored blood), from resorption of blood in extravascular spaces, and less commonly from hemolytic anemia. *Hepatocellular damage* and decreased liver cell function may occur due to concurrent use of hepatotoxic drugs (Chap. 247) or anesthetics such as halothane. Hepatocellular necrosis may follow profound shock; with lesser degrees of hypotension or hypoxemia, morphologic damage may be slight, but significant impairment of

TABLE 246-2 Conditions causing or contributing to postoperative jaundice

I Increased pigment load
- *A* Hemolytic anemia
- *B* Transfusions (especially of stored blood)
- *C* Resorption of hematomas, blood in extravascular spaces

II Impaired hepatocellular function
- *A* Hepatitis-like picture
  - *1* Halothane anesthesia
  - *2* Drugs
  - *3* Shock
  - *4* Infection with hepatitis viruses
- *B* Cholestatic picture
  - *1* Hypotension, hypoxemia
  - *2* Drugs
  - *3* Sepsis

III Extrahepatic obstruction
- *A* Bile duct injury
- *B* Choledocholithiasis

TABLE 246-3 Laboratory features in icteric states

Bilirubin disorder	Serum bilirubin: Unconjugated	Serum bilirubin: Conjugated	Urine bilirubin	Comments
I Overproduction				
A Hemolysis (intra- and extravascular)	↑	N	0	↑ Bilirubin turnover; serum bilirubin rarely exceeds 4 mg/dL
B Ineffective erythropoiesis	↑	N	0	Splenomegaly; normal RBC survival; normoblasts in marrow
II Defective hepatic uptake				
A Some drugs (e.g., flavaspidic acid, novobiocin)	↑	N	0	Normal liver biopsy
B Gilbert's syndrome (some cases)				
III Defective conjugation				
A Neonatal jaundice	↑	Low	0	↓ Glucuronyl transferase; ? ↓ ligandin
B Gilbert's syndrome	↑	Low	0	↓ Glucuronyl transferase and ↓ bilirubin uptake; some may have ↑ hemolysis; bile contains ↑ monoconjugates
C Crigler-Najjar syndrome (types I and II)	↑	Low	0	Type I = absence of transferase Type II = deficiency of transferase; bile contains ↑ ↑ monoconjugates
IV Defective excretion				
A Intrahepatic obstruction				
1 Familial syndromes				
a Dubin-Johnson	↑	↑	+	Abnormal BSP curve, hepatic lipochrome pigment; ↑ urinary coproporphyrin type I
b Rotor	↑	↑		No liver pigment; ↑ total urinary coproporphyrin
2 Drugs (e.g., chloramphenicol, methyltestosterone)	↑	↑	+	↑ Alkaline phosphatase but other function tests usually normal
3 Benign recurrent cholestasis	↑	↑	+	↑ Alkaline phosphatase
4 Recurrent jaundice of pregnancy (third trimester)	↑	↑	+	↑ Alkaline phosphatase; may be reproduced in afflicted subjects by estrogens or progesterone
B Extrahepatic obstruction (tumors, stone, stricture of bile duct)				↑ ↑ Alkaline phosphatase (often > fourfold)
1 Partial	↑	↑	+	
2 Complete	↑	↑	+	
V Hepatocellular disease*				
A Hepatitis	↑	↑	+	Conjugated/total serum bilirubin >50–70%; liver biopsy important for diagnosis
B Cirrhosis: Same as hepatitis	↑	↑		

* *Note that in hepatocellular disease there is generally an interference in all pathways of bilirubin metabolism (i.e., impaired uptake, conjugation, and excretion).*

function may occur. Hence, prior shock or hypotension plus pigment overload may produce significant jaundice. Extensive sepsis can also produce jaundice, often of a cholestatic type. Concurrent renal impairment due to hypotension and hypoxemia may enhance the degree of jaundice because the renal excretion of conjugated bilirubin is decreased. *Extrahepatic obstruction* due to surgical damage or stones needs to be considered, and may be excluded by ultrasound studies.

A form of jaundice referred to as *benign postoperative intrahepatic cholestasis* may be seen. In the typical case the patient has had major and prolonged surgery for a catastrophic event such as a ruptured aortic aneurysm complicated by hypotension and hypoxemia, extensive blood loss into tissues, and massive blood replacement. Jaundice may be noted on the second or third postoperative day, and the serum bilirubin, predominantly conjugated, may reach 20 to 40 mg/dL by the eighth to tenth day. Serum alkaline phosphatase levels may be elevated three- to tenfold. Typically the serum aspartate aminotransferase (AST, SGOT) is only mildly elevated. The liver morphology is striking in that necrosis is not seen, only cholestasis and erythrophagocytosis.

The cause of this type of postoperative cholestatic jaundice is uncertain. However, it probably reflects (1) increased pigment load, (2) decreased liver function due to hypoxemia and hypotension, and (3) decreased renal bilirubin excretion due to varying degrees of tubular necrosis as a result of shock. This diagnostic possibility must be considered in the postoperative patient with marked cholestatic jaundice. The course of the jaundice is self-limited and will subside if the other systemic complications do not predominate and lead to death.

Hepatitis and cirrhosis These disorders, discussed in detail in Chaps. 247 to 249, constitute the *most common disorders associated with jaundice*. As has been stated previously, when the liver cell is damaged, as in viral hepatitis, there is often impairment in all three major hepatic phases of bilirubin metabolism, namely, uptake, conjugation, and excretion. Since the excretory step is the one which is rate-limiting and most readily affected by injury, significant amounts of conjugated bilirubin reenter the systemic circulation. There are also usually lesser increases in the serum unconjugated bilirubin. This phenomenon is probably a reflection of the impaired uptake and conjugation, and is due in part to the shortened life span of red blood cells often found in liver disease. In most patients with hepatitis and cirrhosis, the total serum bilirubin levels tend not to exceed 50 mg/dL, but on rare occasions levels of up to 90 or 95 mg/dL have been described. (For a summary of laboratory features in icteric states, see Table 246-3.)

EXTRAHEPATIC BILIARY OBSTRUCTION Anatomic or mechanical obstruction of the bile ducts is most commonly due to stones, tumors, or strictures. The clinical picture is quite similar to that of intrahepatic cholestasis with pronounced elevations of the serum conjugated bilirubin and alkaline phosphatase levels. Usually, but not always, fever, pain, and chills may be present. In contrast to hepatitis and cirrhosis, the serum bilirubin level often tends to plateau and rarely exceeds levels of 35 mg/dL. The reason for this plateau is not clear but may be related to renal excretion of conjugated bilirubin or alternative pathways of bilirubin catabolism in obstructive jaundice.

REFERENCES

Benign familial recurrent cholestasis

DePagter AGF et al: Familial benign intrahepatic cholestasis. Gastroenterology 71:202, 1976

ENDO T et al: Bile acid metabolism in benign recurrent intrahepatic cholestasis. Gastroenterology 76:1002, 1979

Dubin-Johnson and Rotor syndromes

BERK PD et al: Inborn errors of bilirubin metabolism. Med Clin North Am 59:803, 1975
ROSENTHAL P et al: Homozygous Dubin-Johnson syndrome exhibits a characteristic serum bilirubin pattern. Hepatology 1:540, 1981
SWARTZ HM et al: On the nature and excretion of the hepatic pigment in the Dubin-Johnson syndrome. Gastroenterology 76:958, 1979
WOLKOFF AW et al: Hereditary jaundice and disorders of bilirubin metabolism, in *The Metabolic Basis of Inherited Disease,* 5th ed, JB Stanbury et al (eds). New York, McGraw-Hill, 1983, pp 1385–1420
WOLPERT E et al: Abnormal sulfobromophthalein metabolism in Rotor's syndrome and obligate heterozygotes. N Engl J Med 206:1099, 1977

Glucuronyl transferase deficiency states

BERTHELOT P, DHUMEAUS D: New insights into the classification and mechanisms of hereditary, chronic, non-hemolytic hyperbilirubinemia. Gut 19:474, 1978
DAWSON J et al: Gilbert's syndrome: Evidence of morphologic heterogeneity. Gut 20:848, 1979
FELSHER BF, CARPIO NM: Caloric intake and unconjugated hyperbilirubinemia. Gastroenterology 69:42, 1975
FEVERY J et al: Unconjugated bilirubin and an increased proportion of bilirubin monoconjugates in the bile of patients with Gilbert's syndrome and Crigler-Najjar disease. J Clin Invest 60:970, 1977
OHKUBO H et al: Ursodeoxycholic acid oral tolerance test in patients with constitutional hyperbilirubinemias and effect of phenobarbital. Gastroenterology 81:126, 1981
——— et al: Effects of corticosteroids on bilirubin metabolism in patients with Gilbert's syndrome. Hepatology 1:168, 1981

Postoperative jaundice

KOFF RS: Postoperative jaundice. Med Clin North Am 59:823, 1975
LAMONT JT, ISSELBACHER KJ: Postoperative jaundice, in *Liver and Biliary Disease,* 2d ed, R Wright et al (eds). Philadelphia, Saunders, 1985

247 ACUTE HEPATITIS

JULES L. DIENSTAG / JACK R. WANDS / RAYMOND S. KOFF

ACUTE VIRAL HEPATITIS

Acute viral hepatitis is a systemic infection affecting the liver predominantly. Four categories of viral agents have been implicated: hepatitis A virus (HAV), hepatitis B virus (HBV), non-A, non-B hepatitis agents, and the recently described HBV-associated delta agent. Among these, HAV, HBV, and the delta agent can be distinguished by their antigenic properties, but all four types produce clinically similar illnesses. These range from asymptomatic and inapparent to fulminant and fatal acute infections, on the one hand, and from subclinical persistent infections to rapidly progressive chronic liver disease with cirrhosis and even hepatocellular carcinoma, on the other.

Virology and etiology HEPATITIS A Hepatitis A virus (HAV) is a nonenveloped 27-nm, heat-, acid-, and ether-resistant RNA virus that has been classified as enterovirus type 72 (Fig. 247-1). Its virion is composed of four polypeptides designated VP1 to VP4. Inactivation of viral activity can be achieved by boiling for 1 min, by contact with formaldehyde and chlorine, or by ultraviolet irradiation. All strains of this virus identified to date are immunologically indistinguishable and belong to one serotype. The virus is present in the liver, bile, stools, and blood during the late incubation period and acute preicteric phase of illness. Despite persistence of virus in the liver, viral shedding in feces, viremia, and infectivity diminish rapidly once jaundice becomes apparent. Unlike other hepatitis viruses, hepatitis A virus has been grown in tissue culture. In addition, its genome has been cloned and characterized.

Antibodies to HAV (anti-HAV) can be detected during acute illness when serum aminotransferase activity is elevated and fecal HAV shedding is still occurring. This early antibody response is predominantly of the IgM class and persists for several months. During convalescence, however, anti-HAV of the IgG class becomes the predominant antibody (Fig. 247-2). Therefore, the diagnosis of hepatitis A is made during acute illness by demonstrating high-titer anti-HAV of the IgM class. Following acute illness, anti-HAV of the IgG class remains detectable indefinitely, and patients with serum anti-HAV are immune to reinfection. Indeed, the IgG anti-HAV present in immune globulin preparations accounts for the protection it affords against HAV infection.

HEPATITIS B This viral infection is unique in that concentrations of viral antigen and viral particles in the blood may reach 500 μg/mL and 10 trillion particles per milliliter, respectively. Electron microscopic studies of serum have demonstrated the morphologic appearance of three types of particles (Table 247-1) related to hepatitis B infection (see Fig. 247-1). The most numerous are the 22-nm particles which appear as spherical or long filamentous forms; these are antigenically identical with the outer surface or coat of hepatitis B virus (HBV), and they are thought to represent excess viral coat protein. Outnumbered in serum by a factor of 100 or 1000 to 1 compared to the spheres and tubules are large 42-nm spherical particles, which represent the intact hepatitis B virion. These large particles consist of an outer coat and an inner icosahedral nucleocapsid core measuring 27 nm in diameter. Previous studies have shown that antiserum obtained from hemophiliacs, who had presumably been repeatedly exposed to hepatitis viruses through multiple blood transfusions, would form a precipitin line by diffusion in agar gel with an antigen present in hepatitis serum. This antigen was originally called Australia antigen or hepatitis-associated antigen and is now referred to as hepatitis B surface antigen (HBsAg). The discovery of this antigen provided the first serologic test to distinguish hepatitis B from other types of hepatitis. HBsAg consists primarily of two major polypeptides, one of 24,000 mol wt and its glycosylated counterpart of 28,000 mol wt. A number of different HBsAg subdeterminants have been identified. There is a common group-reactive antigen, *a,* shared by all HBsAg isolates. In addition, HBsAg may contain one of several subtype-specific antigens, namely, *d* or *y, w* or *r,* as well as other more recently characterized specificities. These HBsAg subtypes provide additional epidemiologic markers in evaluating the

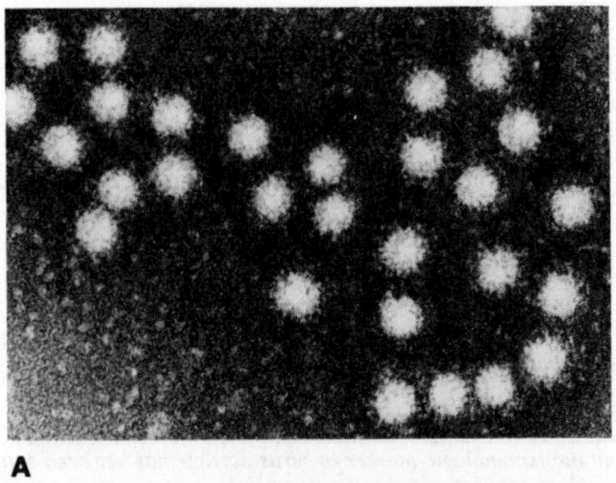

A

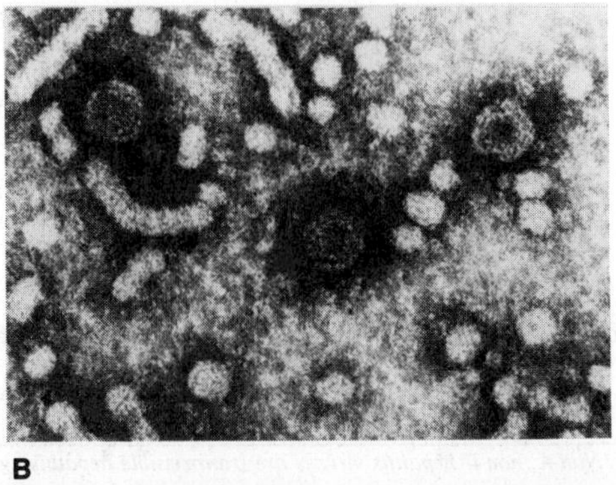

B

FIGURE 247-1 *A. Electron micrograph of 27-nm hepatitis A virus particles purified from stool of a patient with acute hepatitis A virus infection and aggregated by hepatitis A antibody. B. Electron micrograph of concentrated serum from a patient with acute hepatitis B infection, demonstrating the 42-nm virion, tubular forms, and spherical 22-nm particles of hepatitis B surface antigen (132,000×).*

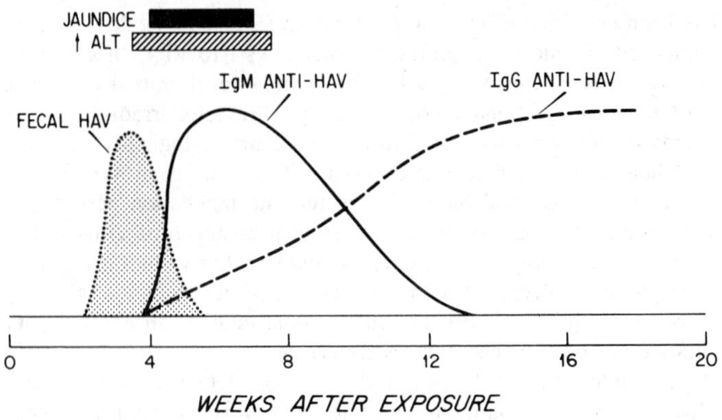

FIGURE 247-2 *Scheme of typical clinical and laboratory features of viral hepatitis type A.*

transmission of hepatitis B infection in that subtypes "breed true." For example, studies of hepatitis outbreaks have shown that index cases and their contacts have identical HBsAg subtypes. Clinical course and outcome, however, are independent of subtype.

The intact 42-nm virion can be disrupted by mild detergents and the 27-nm nucleocapsid core particle isolated. Naked core particles do not circulate in serum. The antigen expressed on the surface of the nucleocapsid core is referred to as hepatitis B core antigen (HBcAg), and the corresponding antibody is anti-HBc. HBcAg does not cross react with HBsAg. A third antigen associated with hepatitis B is hepatitis B e antigen (HBeAg). HBeAg is a soluble, nonparticulate antigen which is found only in HBsAg-positive serum and is immunologically and biochemically distinct from HBsAg and intact HBcAg but appears to be an internal component or degradation product of the core of HBV. HBsAg-positive serum containing HBeAg is more likely to be highly infectious and to be associated with the presence of hepatitis B virions (and DNA polymerase and HBV DNA, see below) than HBeAg-negative or anti-HBe-positive serum. For example, HBsAg carrier mothers who are HBeAg-positive almost invariably transmit hepatitis B infection to their offspring, while HBsAg carrier mothers with anti-HBe rarely infect their offspring.

In every individual with acute hepatitis B infection, HBeAg develops transiently, early in the course of illness, but persistent HBeAg positivity correlates with ongoing viral replication and may be associated with continuing disease actvity in chronic hepatitis; its disappearance may be a harbinger of biochemical improvement and potential resolution of infection. Unfortunately HBeAg is not a sufficiently discriminating marker to support prognostic predictions or to substitute for morphologic evaluation of severity in patients with chronic hepatitis.

Within the nucleocapsid core, in addition to HBeAg, is a predominantly double-stranded, but partially single-stranded, DNA genome measuring 3200 base pairs as well as a DNA polymerase, which directs replication and repair of HBV DNA. In vitro, the polymerase can repair the single-stranded gap and render it double-stranded. Once thought to be unique among viruses, HBV is now recognized as one of a family of animal viruses, hepadnaviruses (hepatotropic DNA viruses), and is classified as hepadnavirus type 1. Viruses similar to HBV infect certain species of woodchucks, ground squirrels, and Pekin ducks, to mention the most carefully characterized. Like HBV, all have the same distinctive three morphologic forms, have counterparts to the virus antigens of HBV, replicate within the liver, contain their own, endogenous DNA polymerase, have partially double-stranded, partially single-stranded genomes, and, for the most part, are associated with acute and chronic hepatitis and hepatocellular carcinoma. Recent evidence suggests that hepadnaviruses rely on replicative strategies typical of retroviruses. Although HBV has not been cultivated in vitro, its genome has been cloned in bacterial, yeast, and mammalian cell vectors and has been completely characterized. Four segments of the genome have been characterized: (1) the pre-S and S gene, which code for HBsAg and several other poorly characterized gene products, including receptors on the HBV surface for polymerized human serum albumin; (2) the C gene, which codes for HBcAg and HBeAg; (3) the P gene, which codes for DNA polymerase; and (4) the X gene, which codes for a recently identified

TABLE 247-1 Nomenclature and features of hepatitis antigens and antibodies

Hepatitis type*	Particle diameter, nm	Description	Antigen	Corresponding antibody	Remarks
A	27	Icosahedral virus particle	Hepatitis A virus (HAV)	Hepatitis A antibody (anti-HAV)	RNA virus; present in stool and serum early in course of hepatitis A
B	42	Intact virion (surface and core); spherical	Hepatitis B surface antigen (HBsAg) Hepatitis B core antigen (HBcAg)	Hepatitis B surface antibody (anti-HBs) Hepatitis B core antibody (anti-HBc)	DNA virus; found in serum
	27	Nucleocapsid core of virion, icosahedral	HBcAg	Anti-HBc	Core contains DNA and DNA polymerase; present in hepatocyte nuclei but not in serum Anti-HBc detected in serum during and after acute infection
	22	Appear as spherical and filamentous forms; both have same antigenic properties as surface of virion; represent excess viral coat material	HBsAg	Anti-HBs	HBsAg detectable in > 90% of patients with acute hepatitis B; found in serum, body fluids, and hepatocyte cytoplasm Anti-HBs appears following B infection; protective antibody
	Nonparticulate	Soluble protein, internal component of nucleocapsid	Hepatitis B e antigen (HBeAg)	Hepatitis B e antibody (Anti-HBe)	HBeAg found in HBsAg-positive serum only, correlates with infectivity and presence of intact virus particles
D	35–37	Hybrid particle with HBsAg coat and delta nucleocapsid core	Hepatitis delta virus (HDV) Hepatitis delta antigen (HDAg)	Hepatitis delta antibody (Anti-HD)	Defective RNA virus, requires helper function of HBV

* *Non-A, non-B hepatitis viruses are transmissible hepatitis agents, but no immunologic marker or virus particle has yet been satisfactorily demonstrated.*

protein seen more frequently in patients with hepatocellular carcinoma but which remains to be further characterized. Not only has the HBV genome been cloned but its gene products have been expressed by recombinant vectors. In addition, the delineation of the gene and amino acid maps of HBV has led to the production in the laboratory of synthetic HBsAg polypeptides.

After infection with HBV, the first virologic marker detectable in serum is HBsAg (Fig. 247-3). Circulating HBsAg precedes elevations of serum aminotransferase activity and clinical symptoms and remains detectable during the entire icteric or symptomatic phase of acute hepatitis B and beyond. In typical cases, HBsAg becomes undetectable 1 to 2 months following the onset of jaundice and rarely persists beyond 6 months. After HBsAg disappears, antibody to HBsAg (anti-HBs) becomes detectable in serum and remains detectable indefinitely thereafter. Because HBcAg is sequestered within an HBsAg coat, HBcAg is not detectable routinely in the serum of patients with HBV infection. On the other hand, antibody to HBcAg (anti-HBc) is readily demonstrable in serum, beginning within the first 1 to 2 weeks after the appearance of HBsAg and preceding detectable levels of anti-HBs by weeks to months. Because variability exists in the time of appearance of anti-HBs following HBV infection, occasionally a gap of several weeks or longer may separate the disappearance of HBsAg and the appearance of anti-HBs. During this "gap" or "window" period, anti-HBc may represent serologic evidence of current or recent HBV infection, and blood containing anti-HBc in the absence of HBsAg and anti-HBs has been implicated in the development of transfusion-associated hepatitis B. In part because the sensitivity of immunoassays for HBsAg and anti-HBs has increased, however, this window period is rarely encountered. In some persons, years after HBV infection, anti-HBc may persist in the circulation longer than anti-HBs. Therefore, isolated anti-HBc does not necessarily indicate active virus replication; most instances of isolated anti-HBc represent hepatitis B infection in the remote past. Distinction between recent and remote HBV infection can be accomplished by determination of the immunoglobulin class of anti-HBc. Anti-HBc of the IgM class (IgM anti-HBc) predominates during the first approximately 6 months after acute infection, whereas IgG anti-HBc is the predominant class of anti-HBc beyond 6 months. Therefore, patients with current or recent acute hepatitis B, including those in the anti-HBc window, have IgM anti-HBc in their serum. In patients who have recovered from hepatitis B in the remote past as well as those with chronic HBV infection, anti-HBc is of the IgG class. Infrequently, in no more than 1 to 5 percent of patients with acute HBV infection, levels of HBsAg are too low to be detected; in such cases, the presence of IgM anti-HBc establishes the diagnosis of acute hepatitis B. Similarly, isolated anti-HBc may occur in the rare patient with chronic hepatitis B whose HBsAg level is below the sensitivity threshold of contemporary immunoassays (a low-level carrier); in such cases, the anti-HBc is of the IgG class. In persons who have recovered from hepatitis B, anti-HBs and anti-HBc persist indefinitely.

The temporal association between the appearance of anti-HBs and resolution of HBV infection as well as the observation that persons with anti-HBs in serum are protected against reinfection with HBV suggest that *anti-HBs is the protective antibody*. Therefore, strategies for prevention of HBV infection are based on providing susceptible persons with circulating anti-HBs (see below).

The other readily detectable hepatitis B virologic marker, HBeAg, appears concurrently with or shortly after HBsAg. Its appearance coincides temporally with high levels of virus replication and reflects the presence of circulating intact virions, DNA polymerase, and HBV DNA, which are not detected routinely in clinical laboratories; in the hepatocyte nucleus, HBV DNA can be detected in free or episomal form. This *replicative* stage of HBV infection is the time of maximal infectivity. In self-limited HBV infections, HBeAg becomes undetectable shortly after peak elevations in aminotransferase activity, before the disappearance of HBsAg, and anti-HBe then becomes detectable, coinciding with a period of relatively lower infectivity (Fig. 247-3). In protracted HBV infection, HBeAg may remain detectable, indicating persistent replicative infection. When HBeAg is absent and anti-HBe present in chronic hepatitis B, infection is usually *nonreplicative*. In this phase of chronic infection, when HBV DNA is demonstrable in hepatocyte nuclei, it tends to be integrated into the host genome.

DELTA HEPATITIS The most recently recognized hepatitis agent, the delta agent hepatitis D virus (HDV), is a defective RNA virus which coinfects with and requires the helper function of HBV for its replication and expression. Slightly smaller than HBV, delta is a 35 to 37 nm virus with a hybrid structure. Its nucleocapsid expresses delta antigen, which bears no antigenic homology with any of the HBV antigens, and contains a small RNA genome that is nonhomologous with HBV DNA. This delta core is "encapsidated" by an outer coat of HBsAg. Thus, delta can only either infect a person simultaneously with HBV or superinfect a person already infected with HBV; when delta infection is transmitted from a donor with one HBsAg subtype to an HBsAg-positive recipient with a different subtype, the delta agent assumes the HBsAg subtype of the recipient, rather than the donor. Because delta relies absolutely on HBV, the duration of delta infection is determined by the duration of and cannot outlast HBV infection. Delta antigen is expressed primarily in hepatocyte nuclei and is occasionally detectable in serum. During acute delta infection, anti-delta of the IgM class predominates; in self-limited infection, anti-delta is low-titer and transient, rarely remaining detectable beyond the clearance of HBsAg and delta antigen. In chronic delta infection, anti-delta circulates in high titer, and both IgM and IgG anti-delta can be detected.

NON-A, NON-B HEPATITIS Sensitive serologic tests for identifying both types A and B hepatitis have led to the identification of hepatitis cases with incubation periods and modes of transmission consistent with an infectious disease but without serologic evidence of hepatitis

FIGURE 247-3 *Scheme of typical clinical and laboratory features of acute viral hepatitis type B.*

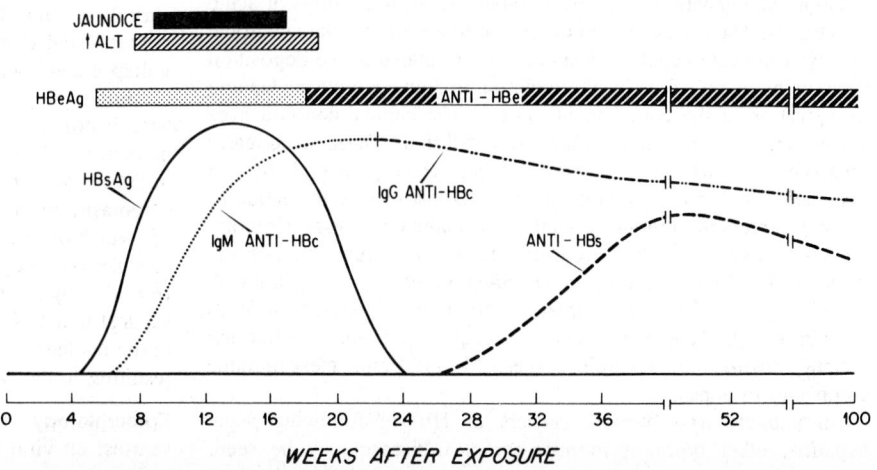

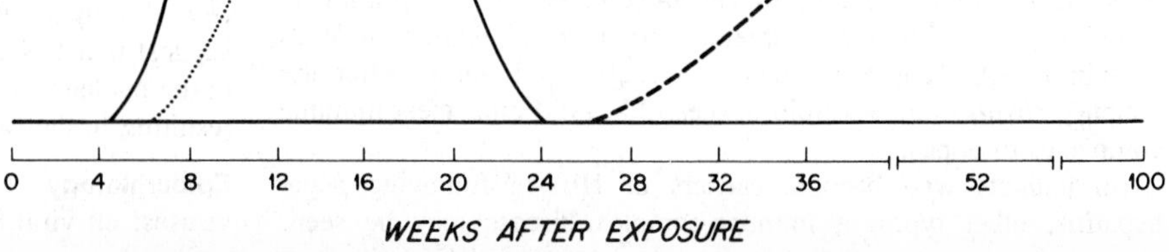

A or B infection. Identified initially among recipients of transfused blood, these cases of so-called non-A, non-B hepatitis have not been associated serologically with Epstein-Barr virus or cytomegalovirus (except in rare instances) or with other viruses known to involve the liver. Although the virus(es) or virus antigens have not been identified definitively, cross-challenge studies in chimpanzees have shown that there are at least two different bloodborne non-A, non-B hepatitis agents. One has been isolated from clotting factor VIII concentrates, is chloroform-sensitive, and induces ultrastructural cytoplasmic tubular changes in hepatocytes. The other has been isolated from clotting factor IX concentrates, is chloroform-resistant, and does not induce cytoplasmic tubular changes in hepatocytes. The latter type appears to be the most frequently encountered after blood transfusion.

In addition, a distinct type of waterborne non-A, non-B hepatitis has been identified in India and Asia (so-called epidemic non-A, non-B hepatitis), which, because of its epidemiologic resemblance to hepatitis A, has been labeled by some "non-A hepatitis." A preliminary report has appeared in which a 27-nm HAV-like virus was detected in stools from patients with epidemic non-A, non-B hepatitis; however, this finding remains to be confirmed.

Acceptable serologic tests to identify antigens and antibodies associated with non-A, non-B hepatitis virus(es) have not been developed. Details of virologic events and humoral immune responses remain to be described.

Pathogenesis While data on the pathogenesis of hepatitis A, non-A, non-B hepatitis, and delta hepatitis are very limited, evidence suggests that the clinical manifestations of and outcomes following acute liver injury associated with HBV infection are determined by the immunologic responses of the host. The existence of asymptomatic hepatitis B carriers with normal liver histology and function suggests that the virus is not directly cytopathic. The facts that lymphoid cells are juxtaposed with necrotic hepatocytes in the livers of patients with liver injury and that patients with defects in cellular immune competence are more likely to remain chronically infected rather than to clear the virus are cited to support the role of cellular immune responses in the pathogenesis of hepatitis B–related liver injury. To date, however, because adequate animal and laboratory models are lacking, support for this hypothesis remains circumstantial. Still, the model that has the most experimental support involves cytolytic T cells sensitized specifically to recognize host and hepatitis B viral antigens on the liver cell surface. Although HBsAg was initially thought to be the most likely viral target antigen on the hepatocyte surface, recent laboratory observations suggest that HBcAg, present on the cell membrane in minute quantities, is the viral target antigen that, with host antigens, invites cytolytic T cells to destroy HBV-infected hepatocytes. Debate does continue, however, over the relative importance of viral and host factors in the pathogenesis of liver injury associated with hepatitis B and its outcome.

Although the mechanism of HBV-induced liver injury remains uncertain, immune complex–mediated tissue damage appears to play a major pathogenetic role in the extrahepatic manifestations of acute hepatitis B. The occasional prodromal serum sickness–like syndrome observed in acute hepatitis B appears to be related to the deposition in tissue blood vessel walls of circulating immune complexes leading to activation of the complement system. The clinical consequences are urticarial rash, angioedema, and arthritis. During the early prodrome of hepatitis B in these patients, HBsAg in high titer in association with small amounts of anti-HBs leads to the formation of soluble, circulating immune complexes (in antigen excess). Complement components in the serum are depressed during the arthritic phase of the illness and are also detectable in the circulating immune complexes. In addition to complement components, these complexes contain HBsAg, anti-HBs, IgG, IgM, IgA, and fibrin. After the patient recovers from the serum sickness–like syndrome, these immune complexes disappear.

In patients who become carriers of HBsAg following acute hepatitis, other types of immune-complex disease may be seen. Glomerulonephritis with the nephrotic syndrome is occasionally observed; HBsAg, immunoglobulin, and C3 deposition has been found in the glomerular basement membrane. While polyarteritis nodosa develops in considerably fewer than 1 percent of patients with hepatitis B, 20 to 30 percent of patients with polyarteritis nodosa have HBsAg in serum. In these patients, the affected small and medium-sized arterioles have been shown to contain HBsAg, immunoglobulins, and complement components.

Pathology The typical morphologic lesions of hepatitis A, B, delta, and non-A, non-B are often similar and consist of panlobular infiltration with mononuclear cells, hepatic cell necrosis, hyperplasia of Kupffer cells, and variable degrees of cholestasis. Hepatic cell regeneration is present, as evidenced by numerous mitotic figures, multinucleated cells, and "rosette" or "pseudoacinar" formation. The mononuclear infiltration consists primarily of small lymphocytes, although plasma cells and eosinophils are occasionally seen. Liver cell damage consists of hepatic cell degeneration and necrosis, cell dropout, ballooning of cells, and acidophilic degeneration of hepatocytes (forming so-called Councilman-like bodies). Large hepatocytes with a ground-glass appearance of the cytoplasm may be seen in chronic but not in acute hepatitis B; these cells have been shown to contain HBsAg and can be identified histochemically with orcein or aldehyde fuchsin. In uncomplicated viral hepatitis, the reticulin framework is preserved.

A more severe histologic lesion, *bridging hepatic necrosis,* also termed *subacute* or *confluent necrosis,* is occasionally observed in some patients with acute hepatitis. "Bridging" between lobules results from large areas of hepatic cell dropout, with collapse of the reticulin framework. Characteristically, the bridge consists of condensed reticulum, inflammatory debris, and degenerating liver cells that span adjacent portal areas, portal to central veins, or central vein to central vein. This lesion has been thought to have prognostic significance; in many of the originally described patients with this lesion, a subacute course terminated in death within several weeks to months, or chronic active hepatitis and postnecrotic cirrhosis developed. More recent investigations have failed to uphold the association between bridging necrosis and such a poor prognosis in patients with acute hepatitis. Although the frequency of bridging may be higher among hospitalized patients with severe acute hepatitis, and although cirrhosis, chronic hepatitis, and even death have been observed in this group, the frequency of bridging necrosis in uncomplicated acute viral hepatitis is probably on the order of 1 to 5 percent. Prospective studies have failed to demonstrate a difference in prognosis between patients with acute hepatitis who have bridging necrosis and those who do not. Therefore, although demonstration of this lesion in patients with chronic hepatitis has prognostic significance (see Chap. 248), its demonstration during acute hepatitis is less meaningful, and liver biopsies to identify this lesion are no longer undertaken routinely in patients with acute hepatitis. In *massive hepatic necrosis* (fulminant hepatitis, acute yellow atrophy), the striking feature at postmortem examination is the finding of a small, shrunken, and soft liver. Histologic examination reveals massive necrosis and dropout of liver cells of most lobules with extensive collapse and condensation of the reticulin framework.

Immunofluorescence and immunoperoxidase antibody studies have been instrumental in localizing HBsAg to the cytoplasm and plasma membrane of infected liver cells. In contrast, HBcAg predominates in the nucleus, but, occasionally, scant amounts are also seen in the cytoplasm and on the cell membrane. Electron-microscopic studies of liver biopsy material have demonstrated the presence of HBsAg particles in the cytoplasm and HBcAg particles in the nucleus of liver cells during hepatitis B infection. These morphologic observations suggest that DNA is synthesized and packaged within core particles in the nucleus, while the surface coat is assembled in the cytoplasm, resulting in the formation of intact hepatitis B virus.

Epidemiology Prior to the availability of serologic tests for hepatitis viruses, all viral hepatitis cases were labeled either as "infectious" or "serum" hepatitis. Modes of transmission overlap, however, and *a clear distinction among the different types of viral hepatitis cannot be made solely on the basis of clinical or epidemiologic features* (Table 247-2). The most accurate means to distinguish the various types of viral hepatitis involves specific serologic testing.

HEPATITIS A *This agent is transmitted almost exclusively by the fecal-oral route.* Spread of HAV is enhanced by poor personal hygiene and overcrowding, and large outbreaks as well as sporadic cases have been traced to contaminated food, water, milk, and shellfish. Intrafamily and intrainstitutional spread are also common. Early epidemiologic observations suggested that there is a predilection for hepatitis A to occur in late fall and early winter. In temperate zones, epidemic waves have been recorded every 5 to 20 years as new segments of nonimmune population appeared; however, in developed countries, the incidence of type A hepatitis has been declining, presumably as a function of improved sanitation, and these cyclic patterns are no longer being observed. No HAV carrier state has been identified after acute type A hepatitis; perpetuation of the virus in nature depends presumably on nonepidemic, inapparent subclinical infection.

In the general population, anti-HAV, an excellent marker for previous HAV infection, increases in prevalence as a function of increasing age and of decreasing socioeconomic status. Serologic evidence of prior hepatitis A infection occurs in about 40 percent of urban populations in the United States, fewer than 5 percent of whom recall having had a symptomatic case of hepatitis. In developing countries, exposure, infection, and subsequent immunity are almost universal in childhood.

HEPATITIS B It has long been recognized that a major route of hepatitis B transmission is percutaneous, but the outmoded designation "serum hepatitis" is an inaccurate label for the epidemiologic spectrum of HBV infection recognized today. As detailed below, most of the hepatitis transmitted by blood transfusion is not caused by HBV; moreover, in approximately half of patients with acute type B hepatitis, there is no history of an identifiable percutaneous exposure. We now recognize that many cases of type B hepatitis result from less obvious modes of nonpercutaneous or covert percutaneous transmission. HBsAg has been identified in almost every body fluid from infected persons—saliva, tears, seminal fluid, cerebrospinal fluid, ascites, breast milk, synovial fluid, gastric juice, pleural fluid and urine and even rarely in feces. Although there is abundant evidence to suggest that feces are not infectious, at least some of these body fluids—most notably semen and saliva—have been shown to be infectious, albeit less so than serum, when administered percutaneously or nonpercutaneously to experimental animals. Among the nonpercutaneous modes of HBV transmission, oral ingestion has been documented as a potential route of exposure but one whose efficiency is quite low. On the other hand, the two nonpercutaneous routes considered to have the greatest impact are intimate (especially sexual) contact and perinatal transmission.

In sub-Saharan Africa, intimate contact among toddlers is considered instrumental in contributing to the maintenance of the high frequency of HBsAg in the population. Perinatal transmission occurs primarily in infants born to HBsAg carrier mothers or mothers with acute hepatitis B during the third trimester of pregnancy or during the early postpartum period. Perinatal transmission is uncommon in North America and western Europe but occurs with great frequency and is the most important mode of HBV perpetuation in the far east and developing countries. Although the precise mode of perinatal transmission is unknown, and although approximately 10 percent of infections may be acquired in utero, epidemiologic evidence suggests that most infections occur approximately at the time of delivery and are not related to breast feeding. Likelihood of perinatal transmission of HBV correlates with the presence of HBeAg; 90 percent of HBeAg-positive mothers but only 10 to 15 percent of anti-HBe-positive mothers transmit HBV infection to their offspring. In most cases, acute infection in the neonate is clinically asymptomatic, but the child is very likely to become an HBsAg carrier.

The more than 200 million HBsAg carriers in the world constitute the main reservoir of hepatitis B in human beings. Serum HBsAg is infrequent (0.1 to 0.5 percent) in normal populations in the United States and western Europe; however, a prevalence of up to 5 to 20 percent has been found in the far east and in some tropical countries, and as high as 30 percent in persons with Down's syndrome, lepromatous leprosy, leukemia, Hodgkin's disease, polyarteritis nodosa, patients with chronic renal disease on hemodialysis, and needle-using drug addicts.

Other groups with high rates of HBV infection include spouses of acutely infected persons, sexually promiscuous persons (especially promiscuous homosexual men), health care workers exposed to blood, persons who require repeated transfusions especially with pooled blood product concentrates (e.g., hemophiliacs), residents and staff of custodial institutions for the mentally retarded, prisoners, and, to a lesser extent, family members of chronically infected patients. In volunteer blood donors, the prevalence of anti-HBs, a reflection of previous HBV infection, ranges from 5 to 10 percent, but the prevalence is higher in lower socioeconomic strata, older age groups, and persons—including those mentioned above—exposed to blood products.

DELTA HEPATITIS Infection with the delta agent has a worldwide distribution, but two epidemiologic patterns exist. In Mediterranean countries (northern Africa, southern Europe, the middle east), delta infection is endemic among those with hepatitis B, and the disease is transmitted predominantly by nonpercutaneous means, especially close personal contact. In nonendemic areas, such as the United States and northern Europe, delta infection is confined to persons exposed frequently to blood and blood products, primarily drug addicts and hemophiliacs. Delta hepatitis can be introduced into a population through drug addicts or by migration of persons from endemic to nonendemic areas. Thus, patterns of population migration

TABLE 247-2 Comparisons of type A, type B, and non-A, non-B hepatitis

Feature	Hepatitis A	Hepatitis B	Non-A, non-B hepatitis
Incubation	15–45 days (mean 30)	30–180 days (mean 60–90)	15–160 (mean 50)
Onset	Acute	Often insidious	Insidious
Age preference	Children, young adults	Any age	Any age but more common in adults
Transmission route:			
Fecal-oral	+ + +	−	Unknown
Other nonpercutaneous*	+/−	+ +	+ +
Percutaneous	+/−	+ + +	+ + +
Severity	Mild	Often severe	Moderate
Prognosis	Generally good	Worse with age, debility	Moderate
Progression to chronicity	None	Occasional (5–10%)	Occasional (10–50%)
Prophylaxis	IG	Standard IG (not documented) HBIG, hepatitis B vaccine	?
Carrier	None	0.1–30%†	Exists but prevalence unknown

* *For example, sexual or maternal-neonatal contact*
† *Varies considerably throughout the world, see text*

and human behavior facilitating percutaneous contact play important roles in the introduction and amplification of delta infection. Occasionally, the migrating epidemiology of delta hepatitis is expressed in explosive outbreaks of severe hepatitis, such as those that have occurred in remote South American villages as well as in urban centers in the United States.

NON-A, NON-B HEPATITIS Routine screening of blood donors for HBsAg and the elimination of commercial blood sources has markedly decreased the incidence of hepatitis B after transfusion, but posttransfusion hepatitis still remains a significant medical problem. The incidence of posttransfusion hepatitis has been reported to be from 0.3 to 9 cases per 1000 units transfused, and the risk of anicteric hepatitis following transfusion is much greater than that of clinical hepatitis with jaundice. The risk of viral hepatitis after transfusion of blood derivatives is dependent on the methods by which these products are processed. The *greatest risk* follows the use of multiple pooled donor products such as concentrates of factors II, VII, VIII, IX, and X. Hepatitis has developed in 20 to 30 percent of individuals receiving these pooled products for the first time. Blood products associated with an *average risk* include whole blood, packed red blood cells, single donor platelets, and plasma. Products such as albumin and immune and hyperimmune globulin, because of prior treatment of these substances by heating to 60°C or by cold ethanol extraction, involve *no risk*. It had been suggested that frozen, glycerol-treated, washed red blood cells may carry a reduced risk of hepatitis, but this has been disproved.

Currently, hepatitis B accounts for only 5 to 10 percent of posttransfusion hepatitis. More of a problem is the occurrence of non-A, non-B hepatitis, which accounts for approximately 90 percent of posttransfusion hepatitis cases following transfusion of voluntarily donated blood prescreened for HBsAg. The fact that non-A, non-B hepatitis is transmitted by transfused blood from asymptomatic donors (Table 247-2) and that it can be transmitted to chimpanzees by blood from patients with chronic hepatitis suggests that there is a carrier state for non-A, non-B hepatitis. Currently, the frequency of posttransfusion non-A, non-B hepatitis approaches 7 to 10 percent of blood recipients, especially recipients of multiple units of blood products. Unfortunately, there is no acceptable serologic screening test to identify non-A, non-B hepatitis agents in blood, and elimination of transfusion-associated non-A, non-B hepatitis will remain an elusive goal until a sensitive, specific test is developed.

In addition to being transmitted by transfusion, non-A, non-B hepatitis cases have been observed in other settings of percutaneous and nonpercutaneous exposure, e.g., intrafamily contact, intravenous drug abuse, occupational contact, nosocomial infection, use of hemodialysis units, and intrainstitutional contact. Special attention is merited by non-A, non-B hepatitis in hemophiliacs, in whom the incubation period may be as brief as 1 to 4 weeks, and in renal transplant recipients, up to 20 percent of whom have chronic liver disease. In the early years after transplantation, the death rate in patients with hepatitis is higher, as a result not of liver failure but of severe infections outside the hepatobiliary tree. However, 5 to 10 years after transplantation complications of chronic liver disease account for increased morbidity and mortality.

The *epidemic form* of non-A, non-B hepatitis identified in India and Asia resembles hepatitis A in its modes of spread. Its distribution has not yet been defined. In western countries, non-A, non-B hepatitis accounts for approximately 15 to 30 percent of sporadic cases of viral hepatitis presenting for medical evaluation. Occurrence of multiple bouts of non-A, non-B hepatitis among drug abusers and hemophiliacs reinforces cross-challenge studies in chimpanzees which suggest that there is more than one non-A, non-B hepatitis agent.

Clinical and laboratory features SYMPTOMS AND SIGNS The *prodromal symptoms* of acute viral hepatitis are systemic and quite variable. Constitutional symptoms of anorexia, nausea and vomiting, fatigue, malaise, arthralgias, myalgias, headache, photophobia, pharyngitis, cough, and coryza may precede the onset of jaundice by 1 to 2 weeks. The nausea, vomiting, and anorexia are frequently associated wth alterations in olfaction and taste. A low-grade fever between 100 and 102°F is more often present in hepatitis A than in non-A, non-B or B, except when hepatitis B is heralded by a serum sickness–like syndrome; rarely, a fever of 103 to 104°F may accompany the constitutional symptoms. Dark urine and clay-colored stools may be noticed by the patient from 1 to 5 days prior to the onset of clinical jaundice.

With the onset of *clinical jaundice* the constitutional prodromal symptoms usually diminish, but in some patients mild weight loss (2.5 to 5 kg) is common and may continue during the entire icteric phase. The liver becomes enlarged and tender and may be associated with right upper quadrant pain and discomfort. Infrequently, patients present with a cholestatic picture, suggesting extrahepatic biliary obstruction. Splenomegaly and cervical adenopathy are present in 10 to 20 percent of patients with acute hepatitis. Rarely, a few spider angiomas appear during the icteric phase and disappear during convalescence. During the *recovery phase,* constitutional symptoms disappear, but usually some liver enlargement and abnormalities in biochemical tests of hepatic function are still evident. The duration of the posticteric phase is variable, ranging from 2 to 12 weeks, and usually is more prolonged in acute hepatitis B and in non-A, non-B hepatitis. Complete clinical and biochemical recovery is to be expected 1 to 2 months after all cases of hepatitis A and 3 to 4 months after the onset of jaundice in three-quarters of uncomplicated cases of hepatitis B and non-A, non-B hepatitis. In the remainder biochemical recovery may be delayed. A substantial proportion of patients with viral hepatitis never become icteric.

Infection with the delta agent (HDV) can occur in the presence of acute or chronic HBV infection; the duration of HBV infection determines the duration of delta infection. When acute delta and HBV infection occur simultaneously, clinical and biochemical features may be indistinguishable from those of HBV infection alone. As opposed to patients with *acute* HBV infection, patients with *chronic* HBV infection can support HDV replication indefinitely. This can happen when acute HDV infection occurs in the presence of a nonresolving acute HBV infection. More commonly, acute HDV infection becomes chronic when it is superimposed on an underlying chronic HBV infection. In such cases, the delta superinfection appears as a clinical exacerbation or an episode resembling acute viral hepatitis in someone already chronically infected with HBV. In the past, events resembling acute hepatitis in a HBV carrier or a patient with chronic hepatitis B were attributed to superimposed non-A, non-B hepatitis or to the natural history of the disease. A proportion of such episodes, however, represent acute superinfection with HDV. Delta superinfection in a patient with chronic hepatitis B often leads to clinical deterioration (see below).

LABORATORY FEATURES The serum aminotransferases, AST and ALT (previously designated SGOT and SGPT) show a variable increase during the prodromal phase of acute viral hepatitis and precede the rise in bilirubin level (see Figs. 247-2 and 247-3). The acute level of these enzymes, however, does not correlate well with the degree of liver cell damage. Peak levels vary from 400 to 4000 IU or more; these levels are usually reached at the time the patient is clinically icteric and progressively diminish during the recovery phase of acute hepatitis. The diagnosis of anicteric hepatitis is difficult and requires a high index of suspicion; it is based on clinical features and on aminotransferase elevations, although mild increases in conjugated bilirubin may also be found.

Jaundice is usually visible in the sclera or skin when the serum bilirubin value exceeds 2.5 mg/dL. When jaundice appears, the serum bilirubin typically rises to levels ranging from 5 to 20 mg/dL. The serum bilirubin may continue to rise despite falling serum aminotransferase levels. In most instances the total bilirubin is equally divided between the conjugated and unconjugated fractions. Bilirubin levels above 20 mg/dL extending and persisting late into the course of viral hepatitis are more likely to be associated with severe disease.

In certain patients with underlying hemolytic anemia, however, such as glucose 6-phosphate dehydrogenase deficiency and sickle cell anemia, high serum bilirubin is common, resulting from superimposed hemolysis. In such patients bilirubin levels greater than 30 mg/dL have been observed and are not necessarily associated with a poor prognosis.

Neutropenia and lymphopenia are transient and are followed by a relative lymphocytosis. Atypical lymphocytes (varying between 2 and 20 percent) are common during the acute phase. These atypical lymphocytes are indistinguishable from those seen in infectious mononucleosis. Measurement of the prothrombin time (PT) is important in patients with acute viral hepatitis, for a prolonged value may reflect a severe synthetic defect, signify extensive hepatocellular necrosis, and indicate a worse prognosis. Occasionally a prolonged PT may occur with only mild increases in the serum bilirubin and aminotransferase levels. Prolonged nausea and vomiting, inadequate carbohydrate intake, and poor hepatic glycogen reserves may contribute to hypoglycemia noted occasionally in patients with severe viral hepatitis. Serum alkaline phosphatase may be normal or only mildly elevated to levels of 80 to 240 IU, while a fall in serum albumin is uncommon in uncomplicated acute viral hepatitis. In some patients mild and transient steatorrhea has been noted as well as slight microscopic hematuria and minimal proteinuria.

A diffuse but mild elevation of the gamma globulin fraction is common during acute viral hepatitis. Serum IgG and IgM are elevated in about one-third of patients during the acute phase of viral hepatitis, but serum IgM elevation is seen more characteristically during acute hepatitis A. During the acute phase of viral hepatitis, antibodies to smooth muscle and other cell constituents may be present, and low titers of rheumatoid factor, antinuclear antibody, and heterophil antibody can also be found occasionally. These antibodies are nonspecific and can also be associated with other viral and systemic diseases. In contrast, virus-specific antibodies, which appear during and after hepatitis virus infection, are serologic markers of diagnostic importance.

As described above, serologic tests are available with which to establish a diagnosis of hepatitis A and B. Tests for fecal or serum HAV are not routinely available. Therefore, a diagnosis of type A hepatitis is based on detection of IgM anti-HAV during acute illness (Fig. 247-2). Rheumatoid factor can give rise to false-positive results in this test.

A diagnosis of HBV infection can usually be made by detection of HBsAg in serum. Infrequently, levels of HBsAg are too low to be detected during acute HBV infection even with the current generation of highly sensitive immunoassays. In such cases, the diagnosis can be established by the presence of IgM anti-HBc. Alternatively, de novo appearance of anti-HBc and anti-HBs during illness and convalescence may support the diagnostic impression.

The titer of HBsAg bears little relation to the severity of clinical disease. Indeed, there is an inverse correlation between the serum concentration of HBsAg and the degree of liver cell damage. Titers are highest in immunosuppressed patients and in normal carriers, lower in chronic liver disease (but higher in chronic persistent than in chronic active hepatitis), and very low in acute fulminant hepatitis. These observations suggest that in hepatitis B the degree of liver cell damage and the clinical course are probably related to variations in the patient's immune response to HBV rather than to the amount of circulating HBsAg.

Another serologic marker which may be of value in patients with hepatitis B is HBeAg. Its principal clinical usefulness is as an indicator of relative infectivity. Because HBeAg is invariably present during early acute hepatitis B, HBeAg testing is indicated primarily during follow-up of chronic infection.

In patients with hepatitis B surface antigenemia of unknown duration, e.g., blood donors whose blood is found to be HBsAg-positive and who are referred to a physician for evaluation, testing for IgM anti-HBc may be useful to distinguish between acute or recent infection (IgM anti-HBc-positive) and chronic HBV infection (IgM anti-HBc-negative, IgG anti-HBc-positive). A false-positive test for IgM anti-HBc may be encountered in patients with high-titer rheumatoid factor.

Anti-HBs is rarely detectable in the presence of HBsAg in patients with *acute* hepatitis B, but 10 to 20 percent of persons with *chronic* HBV infection may harbor low-level anti-HBs. This antibody is directed not against the common group determinant, *a*, but against the heterotypic subtype determinant (e.g., HBsAg of subtype *ad* with anti-HBs of subtype *y*). In most cases, this serologic pattern cannot be attributed to infection with two different HBV subtypes, and the presence of this antibody is not a harbinger of imminent HBsAg clearance. When such antibody is detected, its presence is of no known clinical significance.

After immunization with hepatitis B vaccine, which consists of HBsAg alone, anti-HBs is the only serologic marker to appear. A summary of the commonly encountered serologic patterns of hepatitis B and their interpretations appears in Table 247-3. Tests for the detection of HBV DNA in liver and serum or DNA polymerase in serum are available in a limited number of research laboratories. Like HBeAg, serum HBV DNA and DNA polymerase are indicators of HBV replication, but they are more sensitive. These markers are useful in following the course of HBV replication in patients with chronic hepatitis B receiving experimental antiviral chemotherapy, with interferon for example.

Because there are no reliable serologic tests for non-A, non-B hepatitis, a diagnosis of non-A, non-B hepatitis is made by serologic exclusion of HAV and HBV infection in the setting of a compatible history. A helpful clue is the episodic pattern of aminotransferase elevation seen frequently in non-A, non-B hepatitis. A diagnosis of acute non-A, non-B hepatitis can be made if tests for HBsAg, IgM

TABLE 247-3 Commonly encountered serologic patterns of hepatitis B infection

HBsAg	Anti-HBs	Anti-HBc	HBeAg	Anti-HBe	Interpretation
+	−	IgM	+	−	Acute HBV infection, high infectivity
+	−	IgG	+	−	Chronic HBV infection, high infectivity
+	−	IgG	−	+	Late-acute or chronic HBV infection, low infectivity
+	+	+	+/−	+/−	*1* HBsAg of one subtype and heterotypic anti-HBs (common) *2* Process of seroconversion from HBsAg to anti-HBs (rare)
−	−	IgM	+/−	+/−	*1* Acute HBV infection *2* Anti-HBc window
−	−	IgG	−	+/−	*1* Low-level HBsAg carrier *2* Remote past infection
−	+	IgG	−	+/−	Recovery from HBV infection
−	+	−	−	−	*1* Immunization with HBsAg (after vaccination) *2* Remote past infection (?) *3* False-positive

anti-HBc, and IgM anti-HAV are negative. A diagnosis of non-A, non-B hepatitis may be more difficult to establish in patients with chronic hepatitis who have anti-HBc in their blood. The anti-HBc in such cases will almost invariably be of the IgG class; it represents either HBV infection in the remote past or current HBV infection with low-level virus carriage.

The presence of HDV infection can be identified by demonstrating intrahepatic delta antigen or, more practically, an antidelta seroconversion (a rise in titer of anti-HD or de novo appearance of IgM anti-HD). Circulating HDAg, also diagnostic of acute infection, is detectable only briefly, if at all. Because IgM anti-HD is transient and IgG anti-HD is often undetectable once HBsAg disappears, retrospective serodiagnosis of acute self-limited, simultaneous HBV and HDV infection is difficult.

When a patient presents with acute hepatitis and has HBsAg and anti-HD is the serum, determination of the class of anti-HBc is helpful in establishing the relationship between infection with HBV and HDV. Although IgM anti-HBc does not distinguish *absolutely* between acute and chronic HBV infection, its presence is a reliable indicator of recent infection and its absence a reliable indicator of infection in the remote past. In simultaneous acute HBV and HDV infections, IgM anti-HBc will be detectable, while in acute HDV infection superimposed upon chronic HBV infection, anti-HBc will be of the IgG class.

In the future, tests for the presence of HDV-associated RNA will be useful for determining the presence of ongoing HDV replication and relative infectivity. Currently, probes for this marker are restricted to a limited number of research laboratories.

Liver biopsy is rarely necessary or indicated in acute viral hepatitis, except when there is a question about the diagnosis or when there is clinical evidence suggesting a diagnosis of chronic active hepatitis.

Little agreement exists over routine diagnostic algorithms to be applied in the evaluation of cases of acute viral hepatitis. One potential approach is to test every patient with three serological tests, HBsAg, IgM anti-HAV, and IgM anti-HBc (Table 247-4). The presence of HBsAg, with or without IgM anti-HBc, represents HBV infection. If IgM anti-HBc is present, the HBV infection is considered acute; if IgM anti-HBc is absent, the HBV infection is considered chronic. A diagnosis of acute hepatitis B can be made in the absence of HBsAg when IgM anti-HBc is detectable. A diagnosis of acute hepatitis A is based on the presence of IgM anti-HAV. If IgM anti-HAV coexists with HBsAg, a diagnosis of simultaneous HAV and HBV infections can be made; if IgM anti-HBc (with or without HBsAg) is detectable, the patient has simultaneous acute hepatitis A and B, and if IgM anti-HBc is undetectable, the patient has acute hepatitis A superimposed on chronic HBV infection. Absence of all serologic markers is consistent with a diagnosis of non-A, non-B hepatitis.

TABLE 247-4 Simplified diagnostic approach in patients presenting with acute hepatitis

Test patient's serum for			
HBsAg	IgM anti-HAV	IgM anti-HBc	Diagnostic conclusion
+	−	+	Acute hepatitis B
+	−	−	Chronic hepatitis B
+	+	−	Acute hepatitis A superimposed on chronic hepatitis B
+	+	+	Acute hepatitis A and B
−	+	−	Acute hepatitis A
−	+	+	Acute hepatitis A and B (HBsAg below detectable level)
−	−	+	Acute hepatitis B (HBsAg below detectable level)
−	−	−	Compatible with NANB hepatitis

If a serologic diagnosis of chronic hepatitis B is made, testing for HBeAg and anti-HBe is indicated to evaluate relative infectivity. In patients with hepatitis B, testing for anti-HD is useful under the following circumstances: severe and fulminant cases, severe chronic cases, cases of acute hepatitis-like exacerbations in patients with chronic hepatitis B, persons with frequent percutaneous exposures, and persons from areas where delta infection is endemic.

Prognosis Virtually all previously healthy patients with hepatitis A recover completely from their illness with no clinical sequelae. Similarly in acute hepatitis B, 90 percent of patients have a favorable course and recover completely. There are, however, certain clinical and laboratory features which suggest a more complicated and protracted course. Patients of advanced age and with serious underlying medical disorders such as congestive heart failure, severe anemia, and diabetes mellitus may have a prolonged course and are more likely to experience severe hepatitis. Initial presenting features such as ascites, peripheral edema, and symptoms of hepatic encephalopathy suggest a poorer prognosis. In addition, a prolonged prothrombin time, low serum albumin, hypoglycemia, and very high serum bilirubin values suggest severe hepatocellular disease. Patients with these clinical and laboratory features deserve prompt hospital admission. The case fatality rate in hepatitis A and B is very low (approximately 0.1 percent) but is increased by advanced age and underlying debilitating disorders. Among patients ill enough to be hospitalized for acute hepatitis B, the fatality rate is 1 percent. Non-A, non-B hepatitis occurring after transfusion is less severe during the acute phase than type B hepatitis and is more likely to be anicteric; fatalities are rare, but the precise case fatality rate is not known. In outbreaks of the waterborne type of non-A, non-B hepatitis in India and Asia, the case fatality rate is 10 percent, and pregnant women are at especially high risk. In general, patients with simultaneous acute hepatitis B and delta hepatitis do not experience a higher mortality rate than do patients with acute hepatitis B alone; however, in several recent outbreaks of acute simultaneous HBV and HDV infection among drug addicts, the case fatality rate has approximated 5 percent. In the case of delta superinfection of a person with chronic hepatitis B, the likelihood of fulminant hepatitis and death is increased substantially. Although the case fatality rate for delta hepatitis has not been defined adequately, in outbreaks of severe delta superinfection in isolated populations with a high hepatitis B carrier rate, the mortality rate has been recorded as in excess of 20 percent.

Complications and sequelae During the prodromal phase of acute hepatitis B, a serum sickness–like syndrome characterized by arthralgia or arthritis, rash, angioedema, and rarely hematuria and proteinuria may develop in some patients. This syndrome occurs prior to the onset of clinical jaundice, and these patients are often erroneously diagnosed as having rheumatoid arthritis or other rheumatologic diseases such as systemic lupus erythematosus. This syndrome occurs in about 5 to 10 percent of patients with acute hepatitis B. The diagnosis can be established by measuring serum aminotransferase levels, which are almost invariably elevated, and serum HBsAg.

The most feared complication of viral hepatitis is *fulminant hepatitis* (massive hepatic necrosis); fortunately this is a rare event. This is primarily seen in hepatitis B and delta hepatitis. Hepatitis B accounts for more than 50 percent of fulminant hepatitis cases, a sizeable proportion of which are associated with delta infection. Fulminant hepatitis is seen less frequently in non-A, non-B hepatitis, and only occasionally in hepatitis A. Patients usually present with signs and symptoms of encephalopathy and, in fact, many progress to deep coma. The liver is usually small, and the prothrombin time excessively prolonged. The combination of rapidly shrinking liver size, rapidly rising bilirubin level, and marked prolongation of the prothrombin time, together with clinical signs of confusion, disorientation, somnolence, ascites, and edema, indicates that the patient has hepatic failure with encephalopathy. Cerebral edema is common; brainstem compression, gastrointestinal bleeding, sepsis, respiratory failure, cardiovascular collapse, and renal failure are terminal events.

The mortality is exceedingly high (greater than 80 percent in patients with deep coma), but patients who survive may have a complete biochemical and histologic recovery.

It is particularly important to document the disappearance of HBsAg following apparent clinical recovery from acute hepatitis B. After clinically apparent acute type B hepatitis, approximately 10 percent of patients remain HBsAg-positive for more than 6 months. Half of these individuals may clear the antigen from their circulation during the next several years, but the other 5 percent remain chronically HBsAg-positive. In their serum, anti-HBc is present in high titer; anti-HBs is either undetected or detected at low titer against the opposite subtype specificity of the antigen (see "Laboratory Features" above). These patients may (1) be asymptomatic carriers, (2) have low-grade chronic persistent hepatitis, or (3) have chronic active hepatitis with or without cirrhosis. The likelihood of becoming an HBsAg carrier after acute HBV infection is especially high among neonates, persons with Down's syndrome, chronically hemodialyzed patients, and immunosuppressed patients.

Chronic active hepatitis is a major late complication of acute hepatitis B occurring in approximately 1 to 3 percent of cases (see Chap. 248). Certain clinical and laboratory features suggest progression of acute hepatitis to chronic active hepatitis: (1) lack of complete resolution of clinical symptoms of anorexia, weight loss, and fatigue and the persistence of hepatomegaly; (2) the presence of bridging or multilobular hepatic necrosis on liver biopsy during protracted, severe acute viral hepatitis, (3) failure of the serum aminotransferase, bilirubin, and globulin levels to return to normal within 6 to 12 months following the acute illness; and (4) the continued presence of HBsAg 6 months or more after acute hepatitis, suggesting chronic viral infection of the liver.

Although acute delta hepatitis infection does not increase the likelihood of chronicity of simultaneous acute hepatitis B, delta hepatitis has the potential for contributing to the severity of chronic hepatitis B. Delta hepatitis superinfection can transform asymptomatic or mild chronic hepatitis B into severe, progressive chronic active hepatitis and cirrhosis; it can also accelerate the course of chronic active hepatitis B. Some delta superinfections in patients with chronic hepatitis B lead to fulminant hepatitis. After transfusion-associated acute non-A, non-B hepatitis, as many as 50 percent of patients have abnormal biochemical liver tests for more than a year. In a majority of such patients, liver histology is consistent with chronic active hepatitis. Although many of these patients have no symptoms and a nonprogressive course, ultimately, cirrhosis develops in as many as 20 percent of those with chronic posttransfusion non-A, non-B hepatitis within 10 years of acute illness. The likelihood of chronic hepatitis is only approximately 10 percent after sporadic non-A, non-B hepatitis occurring in the absence of identifiable percutaneous inoculation with blood products or contaminated needles. In contrast, HAV infection does not cause chronic liver disease.

Rare complications of viral hepatitis include pancreatitis, myocarditis, atypical pneumonia, aplastic anemia, transverse myelitis, and peripheral neuropathy. *Carriers* of HBsAg, particularly those infected in infancy or early childhood, appear to have an enhanced risk of hepatocellular carcinoma (see Chap. 250). In children, hepatitis B may rarely present with anicteric hepatitis, a nonpruritic papular rash of the face, buttocks, and limbs, and lymphadenopathy (papular acrodermatitis of childhood or Gianotti-Crosti syndrome).

Differential diagnosis Viral diseases such as infectious mononucleosis; those due to cytomegalovirus, herpes simplex, and coxsackieviruses; and toxoplasmosis may share certain clinical features with viral hepatitis and cause elevation in serum aminotransferase and less commonly in serum bilirubin levels. Tests such as the differential heterophil and serologic tests for these agents may be helpful in the differential diagnosis, if HBsAg, anti-HBc, and IgM anti-HAV determinations are negative. A complete drug history is particularly important, for many drugs can produce a picture of either acute hepatitis or cholestasis (see below). Equally important is a past history of unexplained "repeated episodes" of acute hepatitis. This should alert the physician to the possibility that the underlying disorder is chronic active hepatitis. Alcoholic hepatitis must also be considered, but usually the serum aminotransferase levels are not as markedly elevated and other stigmata of alcoholism may be present. The finding on liver biopsy of fatty infiltration, a neutrophilic inflammatory reaction, and "alcoholic hyalin" would be consistent with alcohol-induced rather than viral liver injury. Because acute hepatitis may present with right upper quadrant abdominal pain, nausea and vomiting, fever, and icterus, it is often confused with acute cholecystitis, common duct stone, or ascending cholangitis. Patients with acute viral hepatitis may tolerate surgery poorly; therefore, it is important to exclude this diagnosis, and a percutaneous liver biopsy may be necessary prior to laparotomy. Viral hepatitis in the elderly is often misdiagnosed as obstructive jaundice resulting from a common duct stone or carcinoma of the pancreas. Because acute hepatitis in the elderly may be quite severe and the operative mortality high, a thorough evaluation including biochemical tests, radiographic studies of the biliary tree, and even liver biopsy may be necessary to exclude primary parenchymal liver disease. Another clinical constellation that may mimic acute hepatitis is right ventricular failure with passive hepatic congestion or hypoperfusion syndromes, such as those associated with shock, severe hypotension, and severe left ventricular failure. Clinical features are usually sufficient to distinguish between the two entities.

Management TREATMENT OF ACUTE ATTACK There is no specific treatment for *typical acute viral hepatitis*. Although hospitalization may be required for clinically severe illness, most patients do not require hospital care. Forced and prolonged bed rest is not essential for full recovery, but many patients will feel better with restricted physical activity. A high-calorie diet is desirable, and because many patients may experience nausea late in the day, the major caloric intake is best tolerated in the morning. Intravenous feeding is necessary in the acute stage if the patient has persistent vomiting and cannot maintain oral intake. Drugs capable of producing adverse reactions such as cholestasis and drugs metabolized by the liver should be avoided. If severe pruritus is present, the use of the bile salt–sequestering resin cholestyramine will usually alleviate this symptom. Corticosteroid therapy has no value in acute viral hepatitis. Even in severe cases associated with *bridging necrosis,* controlled trials have failed to demonstrate the efficacy of steroids. In fact, such therapy may be hazardous.

Physical isolation of patients with hepatitis to a single room and bathroom is rarely necessary except in the case of fecal incontinence for hepatitis A or uncontrolled, voluminous bleeding for hepatitis types B and non-A, non-B. Because most patients hospitalized with hepatitis A excrete little if any HAV, the likelihood of HAV transmission from these patients during their hospitalization is low. Therefore, burdensome enteric precautions are no longer recommended. Although gloves should be worn when the bedpans or fecal material of patients with hepatitis A are handled, these precautions do not represent a departure from sensible procedure for all hospitalized patients. For patients with types B and non-A, non-B hepatitis, emphasis should be placed on blood precautions, i.e., avoiding direct, ungloved hand contact with blood and other body fluids. Enteric precautions for these agents are unnecessary. The importance of simple hygienic precautions, such as hand washing, cannot be overemphasized.

Hospitalized patients may be discharged when there is substantial symptomatic improvement, a significant downward trend in the serum aminotransferase and bilirubin values, and a return to normal of the prothrombin time. Mild aminotransferase elevations should not be considered contraindications to the gradual resumption of normal activity.

In *fulminant hepatitis,* the goal of therapy is to support the patient by maintenance of fluid balance, support of circulation and respiration, control of bleeding, correction of hypoglycemia, and treatment of other complications of the comatose state in anticipation of liver regeneration and repair. Protein intake should be restricted and oral lactulose or neomycin administered. Massive doses of corticosteroids have been administered, but such therapy has been shown in controlled trials to be ineffective. Likewise, exchange transfusion, plasmapheresis, human cross-circulation, porcine liver cross-perfusion, and hemoperfusion have not been proven to enhance survival.

Hazards to medical and paramedical personnel Health care workers exposed frequently to blood, body tissues, and fluids have an increased risk of viral hepatitis, primarily hepatitis B. Approximately 15 percent of health workers have one or more serologic markers of HBV infection, and 1 percent are HBsAg-positive. The risk is higher in surgeons, pathologists, laboratory techologists who process blood specimens, technologists who draw blood and insert intravenous cannulas, hemodialysis staff, and others who perform invasive procedures. Transmission of HBV infection in health care settings, however, appears to be unidirectional, from patients to staff. With rare exceptions, HBsAg-positive health personnel do not increase the risk of HBV infection for their patients. Asymptomatic HBsAg carriers represent the greater risk to health personnel, because there are no readily identifiable clinical features that allow their recognition. Approximately 1 percent of all patients admitted to large metropolitan hospitals are HBsAg-positive, but 90 percent of these are not identified routinely. Patients with a past history of hepatitis or multiple transfusions, patients from countries where hepatitis B is endemic, sexually active homosexual men, intravenous drug abusers, and patients with chronic liver disease, chronic renal failure, polyarteritis nodosa, and Down's syndrome should have routine HBsAg determinations because of the high frequency of the HBsAg carrier state in these groups. If positive, they are potentially infectious, and appropriate precautions should be taken during operative or other acute care procedures. In hemodialysis units, introduction of patient and staff education, routine periodic screening for HBsAg and aminotransferase elevations, and segregation of HBsAg-positive patients from susceptible patients have reduced dramatically the incidence of new HBV infections in both patients and medical personnel.

Prophylaxis Because therapy for viral hepatitis is limited, emphasis is placed on prevention through immunization. The prophylactic approach differs for each of the types of viral hepatitis. In the past, immunoprophylaxis relied exclusively on passive immunization with antibody-containing globulin preparations purified by cold ethanol fractionation from the plasma of hundreds of normal donors. Currently, for hepatitis B, active immunization with a vaccine is available as well.

HEPATITIS A All preparations of immune globulin (IG) contain anti-HAV. Although the titers may vary, all IG preparations appear to have a sufficient antibody concentration to be protective. When administered before exposure or during the early incubation period, IG is effective in preventing clinically apparent type A hepatitis. In some cases, IG does not abort infection but, by attenuating it, renders it inapparent. As a result long-lasting "passive-active" immunity occurs; however, this is now considered to be the exception rather than the rule. For intimate contacts (household, institutional) of persons with hepatitis A, administration of 0.02 mL/kg is recommended as early after exposure as possible; it may be effective even when administered as late as 2 weeks after exposure. Prophylaxis is not necessary for casual contacts (office, factory, school, or hospital) for most elderly persons, who are very likely to be immune, or for those known to have anti-HAV in their serum. In day-care centers for young children, recognition of cases of hepatitis A in children or staff should provide a stimulus for immunoprophylaxis. By the time most common-source outbreaks of type A hepatitis are recognized, however, it is usually too late in the incubation period for IG to be effective; however, prophylaxis may limit the frequency of secondary cases. For travelers to tropical countries, developing countries, and other areas outside of standard tourist routes, IG prophylaxis is recommended. When such travel lasts less than 3 months, 0.02 mL/kg is given; for longer travel or residence in these areas, a dose of 0.06 mL/kg every 4 to 6 months is recommended. Administration of plasma-derived globulin is safe; it has not been associated with transmission of AIDS to recipients, and the AIDS virus, HTLV III, is inactivated by 25 percent alcohol, to which plasma is subjected during the cold ethanol fractionation process. Both live attenuated and genetically engineered hepatitis A vaccines are being developed.

HEPATITIS B Until recently, prevention of hepatitis B was based on *passive* immunoprophylaxis either with standard IG, containing modest levels of anti-HBs, or hepatitis B immune globulin (HBIG), containing high-titer anti-HBs. The efficacy of standard IG has never been established and remains questionable; even the efficacy of HBIG, demonstrated in several clinical trials, has been challenged, and its contribution appears to be in reducing the frequency of clinical *illness,* not in preventing *infection.* Although HBV cannot be cultivated in vitro, a vaccine for *active* immunization has been prepared from purified, noninfectious 22-nm spherical forms of HBsAg derived from the plasma of healthy HBsAg carriers. The vaccine is subjected to three different chemical inactivation steps which, cumulatively, destroy the infectivity of every known virus, including HTLV III. In controlled clinical trials among high-risk persons, this plasma-derived vaccine has been shown to be immunogenic, highly effective in preventing HBV infection, and, despite its unconventional source, very safe. Current recommendations can be divided into those for preexposure and postexposure prophylaxis.

For *preexposure* prophylaxis against hepatitis B in settings of frequent exposure (health workers exposed to blood, hemodialysis patients and staff, residents and staff of custodial institutions for the developmentally handicapped, intravenous drug abusers, promiscuous homosexual men as well as promiscuous heterosexuals, persons such as hemophiliacs who require long-term, high-volume therapy with blood derivatives, household and sexual contacts of HBsAg carriers, and persons living in or traveling extensively in endemic areas), three intramuscular (deltoid, not gluteal) injections of hepatitis B vaccine are recommended at 0, 1, and 6 months. The recommended dose for each injection is 20 μg for immunocompetent adults, 40 μg for immunosuppressed patients (hemodialysis patients, transplant recipients, and oncology patients receiving chemotherapy), and 10 μg for infants and children under the age of 10.

For unvaccinated persons sustaining an exposure to HBV, *postexposure* prophylaxis with a combination of HBIG (for rapid achievement of high-titer circulating anti-HBs) and hepatitis B vaccine (for achievement of long-lasting immunity as well as its apparent efficacy in attenuating clinical illness after exposure) is recommended. For *perinatal* exposure of infants born to HBsAg-positive mothers, a single dose of HBIG, 0.5 mL, should be administered intramuscularly *immediately after birth,* followed by a complete course of three 10 μg injections of hepatitis B vaccine to be started within the first 12 h to 1 week of life. For those experiencing a direct percutaneous inoculation or transmucosal exposure to HBsAg-positive blood or body fluids (e.g., accidental *needle stick* or ingestion), a single intramuscular dose of HBIG, 0.06 mL/kg, administered as soon after exposure as possible, is followed by a complete course of hepatitis B vaccine to begin within the first week. For those exposed by *sexual* contact to a patient with acute hepatitis B, the Immunization Practices Advisory Committee of the United States Public Health Service recommends a single intramuscular dose of HBIG, 0.06 mL/kg, within 14 days of exposure, to be followed by a second HBIG injection or a complete course of hepatitis B vaccine only when HBsAg positivity in the index case persists beyond 3 months. Other authorities, however, recommend a combination of HBIG followed by a complete course of hepatitis B vaccine injections for all sexual contacts of patients with acute hepatitis B, regardless of the duration of HBsAg positivity in the index case. When both HBIG and hepatitis B vaccine are recommended, they may be given at the same time but at separate sites.

DELTA HEPATITIS Infection with the delta hepatitis agent can be prevented by vaccinating susceptible persons with hepatitis B vaccine. No product is available for immunoprophylaxis to prevent delta superinfection in HBsAg carriers; for them, avoidance of percutaneous exposures and limitation of intimate contact with persons who have delta infection are recommended.

NON-A, NON-B HEPATITIS For transfusion-associated non-A, non-B hepatitis, the effectiveness or IG prophylaxis has not been demonstrated consistently and is not recommended. The only effective measure for reducing the frequency of posttransfusion non-A, non-B hepatitis is the elimination of commercially obtained donor blood and reliance exclusively on volunteer blood donors. Studies to test the efficacy of standard IG after needle stick, sexual, or perinatal exposure to non-A, non-B hepatitis have not been done. Because the inoculum is considerably smaller in these settings than that associated with transfusion, and because of its safety and low cost, some authorities do recommend postexposure prophylaxis with a single dose of IG, 0.06 mL/kg (or 0.5 mg for neonatal exposure), in these situations.

TOXIC AND DRUG-INDUCED HEPATITIS

Liver injury may follow the inhalation, ingestion, or parenteral administration of a number of pharmacologic and chemical agents. These include industrial toxins (e.g., carbon tetrachloride, trichloroethylene, and yellow phosphorus), the heat-stable toxic bicyclic octapeptides of certain species of *Amanita* and *Galerina* (hepatotoxic mushroom poisoning), and more commonly, pharmocologic agents used in medical therapy. It is essential that any patient presenting with jaundice or impaired liver function be questioned carefully about exposure to chemicals used in work or at home and drugs taken by prescription or bought "over the counter." In general, two major types of chemical hepatotoxicity have been recognized: (1) direct toxic type and (2) idiosyncratic type.

As shown in Table 247-5, direct toxic hepatitis occurs with predictable regularity in individuals exposed to the offending agent and is dose-dependent. The latent period between exposure and liver injury is usually short (often several hours), although clinical manifestations may be delayed for 24 to 48 h. Agents producing toxic hepatitis are generally systemic poisons or are converted in the liver to toxic metabolites. The direct hepatotoxins result in morphologic abnormalities which are reasonably characteristic and reproducible for each toxin. For example, carbon tetrachloride and trichloroethylene characteristically produce a centrilobular zonal necrosis, whereas yellow phosphorus poisoning typically results in periportal injury. The hepatotoxic octapeptides of *Amanita phalloides* usually produce massive hepatic necrosis. The lethal dose of the toxin is about 10 mg, the amount found in a single deathcap mushroom. Tetracycline, when administered in intravenous doses greater than 1.5 g daily, leads to microvesicular fat deposits in the liver. Liver injury, which is often only one facet of the toxicity produced by the direct hepatotoxins, may go unrecognized until jaundice appears.

In idiosyncratic drug reactions the occurrence of hepatitis is usually infrequent and unpredictable, the response is not dose-dependent, and it may occur at any time during or shortly after exposure to the drug. Extrahepatic manifestations of hypersensitivity, such as rash, arthralgias, fever, leukocytosis, and eosinophilia occur in about one-quarter of patients with idiosyncratic hepatotoxic drug reactions; this observation and the unpredictability of idiosyncratic drug hepatotoxicity contributed to the hypothesis that this category of drug reactions is immunologically mediated. More recent evidence, however, suggests that even idiosyncratic reactions represent direct hepatotoxity but are caused by drug metabolites rather than by the intact compound. Even the prototype of idiosyncratic hepatoxicity reactions, halothane hepatitis, and isoniazid hepatotoxicity, associated frequently with hypersensitivity manifestations, are now recognized to be mediated by toxic metabolites which damage liver cells directly. Currently, idiosyncratic reactions are thought to result from differences in metabolic reactivity to specific agents; host susceptibility is mediated by the kinetics of toxic metabolite generation, which differs among individuals. Idiosyncratic reactions lead to a morphologic pattern that is more variable than those produced by direct toxins; a single agent is often capable of causing a variety of lesions, although certain patterns tend to predominate. Depending on the agent involved, idiosyncratic hepatitis may result in a clinical and morphologic picture indistinguishable from viral hepatitis (e.g., halothane) or may simulate extrahepatic bile duct obstruction clinically with morphologic evidence of cholestasis and minimal hepatocellular damage (e.g., chlorpromazine). Morphologic alterations may also include bridging hepatic necrosis (e.g., methyldopa), or, infrequently, hepatic granulomas (e.g., sulfonamides).

Not all adverse hepatic drug reactions can be classified as either toxic or idiosyncratic in type. For example, oral contraceptives, which combine estrogenic and progestational compounds, may result in impairment of hepatic function and occasionally in jaundice. However, they do not produce necrosis or fatty change, manifestations of hypersensitivity are generally absent, and susceptibility to the development of oral contraceptive–induced cholestasis appears to be genetically determined.

Because drug-induced hepatitis is often a presumptive diagnosis and many other disorders produce a similar clinicopathologic picture, evidence of a causal relationship between the use of a drug and subsequent liver injury may be difficult to establish. The relationship is most convincing for the direct hepatotoxins, which lead to a high frequency of hepatic impairment after a short latent period. Idiosyncratic reactions may be reproduced, in some instances, when rechallenge, after an asymptomatic period, results in a recurrence of signs, symptoms, and morphologic and biochemical abnormalities. Rechallenge, however, is often ethically unfeasible, because severe reactions may occur.

Treatment of toxic and drug-induced hepatic disease is largely supportive, as in acute viral hepatitis. Withdrawal of the suspected agent is indicated at the first sign of an adverse reaction. In the case of the direct toxins, liver involvement should not divert attention from renal or other organ involvement which may also threaten survival.

In Table 247-6, several classes of chemical agents are listed, together with examples of the pattern of liver injury produced by them. Certain drugs appear to be responsible for the development of chronic as well as acute hepatic injury. For example, oxphenisatin, alpha methyldopa, and isoniazid have been associated with chronic active hepatitis, and halothane and methotrexate have been implicated

TABLE 247-5 Some features of toxic and drug-induced hepatic injury

	Direct toxic effect		Idiosyncratic			Other
Features	(Carbon tetrachloride, e.g.)	(Acetaminophen, e.g.)	(Halothane, e.g.)	(Isoniazid, e.g.)	(Chlorpromazine, e.g.)	(Oral contraceptive agents, e.g.)
Predictable and dose-related toxicity	+	+	0	0	0	+
Latent period	Short	Short	Variable	Variable	Variable	Variable
Arthralgia, fever, rash, eosinophilia	0	0	+	0	+	0
Liver morphology	Necrosis, fatty infiltration	Centrilobular necrosis	Similar to viral hepatitis	Similar to viral hepatitis	Cholestasis *with* portal inflammation	Cholestasis *without* portal inflammation

in the development of cirrhosis. A syndrome resembling primary biliary cirrhosis has been described following treatment with chlorpromazine, methyl testosterone, tolbutamide, and other drugs. Portal hypertension in the absence of cirrhosis may result from alterations in hepatic architecture produced by vitamin A or arsenic intoxication, industrial exposure to vinyl chloride, or administration of thorium dioxide. The latter three agents have also been associated with angiosarcoma of the liver. Oral contraceptives have been implicated in the development of hepatic adenoma and, rarely, hepatocellular carcinoma and occlusion of the hepatic vein (Budd-Chiari syndrome). Another unusual lesion, peliosis hepatis (blood cysts of the liver), has been observed in some patients treated with oral contraceptives or anabolic steroids. The existence of these hepatic disorders expands the spectrum of liver injury induced by chemical agents and emphasizes the need for a thorough drug history in all patients with liver dysfunction.

The following are the patterns of adverse hepatic reactions for some prototypic agents.

Acetaminophen hepatotoxicity (direct toxin) Acetaminophen, an analgesic and antipyretic that is available without a prescription, has caused severe centrolobular hepatic necrosis when ingested in large amounts in suicide attempts or accidentally by children. A single dose of 10 to 15 g, occasionally less, may produce clinical evidence of liver injury. Fatal fulminant disease is usually (although not invariably) associated with ingestion of 25 g or more. Blood levels of acetaminophen correlate with the severity of hepatic injury (levels above 300 μg/mL 4 h after ingestion are predictive of the development of severe damage, while levels below 150 μg/mL suggest that hepatic injury is highly unlikely). Nausea, vomiting, diarrhea, abdominal pain, and shock are early manifestations occurring 4 to 12 h after ingestion. Then 24 to 48 h later, when these features are abating, hepatic injury becomes apparent. Maximal abnormalities and hepatic failure may not be evident until 4 to 6 days after ingestion. Renal failure and myocardial injury may be present.

Acetaminophen hepatotoxicity is mediated by a toxic reactive metabolite formed from the parent compound by the cytochrome P450 mixed-function oxidase system of the hepatocyte. This metabolite is detoxified by binding to glutathione. When excessive amounts of the metabolite are formed, glutathione levels in liver fall, and the metabolite is covalently bound to nucleophilic hepatocyte macromolecules. This process is believed to lead to hepatocyte necrosis; the precise sequence and mechanism are unknown. Hepatic injury may be potentiated by prior administration of alcohol or other drugs, by conditions which stimulate the mixed-function oxidase system, or by conditions such as starvation which reduce hepatic glutathione levels.

Treatment of acetaminophen overdosage includes gastric lavage, supportive measures, and oral administration of activated charcoal or cholestyramine to prevent absorption of residual drug. Neither of the latter agents appears to be effective if given more than 30 min after acetaminophen ingestion; if they are used, the stomach lavage should be done before other agents are administered orally. In patients with high acetaminophen blood levels (>200 μg/mL measured at 4 h or >100 μg/mL at 8 h after ingestion) the administration of sulfhydryl compounds (e.g., cysteamine, cysteine, or *N*-acetylcysteine) within 12 h of ingestion appears to reduce the severity of hepatic necrosis. These agents appear to act by providing a reservoir of sulfhydryl groups to bind the toxic metabolites or by stimulating synthesis and repletion of hepatic glutathione. Late administration of sulfhydryl compounds is of uncertain value.

Survivors of acute acetaminophen overdose usually have no evidence of hepatic sequelae. In a few patients prolonged or repeated administration of acetaminophen in therapeutic doses appears to have led to the development of chronic active hepatitis and cirrhosis.

Halothane hepatotoxicity (idiosyncratic reaction) Halothane, a nonexplosive fluorinated hydrocarbon anesthetic agent that is structurally similar to chloroform, has been reported to result in severe hepatic necrosis in a small number of individuals, many of whom have previously been exposed to this agent. The failure to produce similar hepatic lesions in animals, the rarity of hepatic impairment in human beings, and the delayed appearance of hepatic injury suggest that halothane is not a direct hepatotoxin but may be a sensitizing agent. However, manifestations of hypersensitivity are seen in fewer than 25 percent of cases. A genetic predisposition leading to an idiosyncratic metabolic reactivity has been postulated and appears to be the most likely mechanism of halothane hepatotoxicity. Adults (rather than children), obese people, and women appear to be particularly susceptible. Fever, moderate leukocytosis, and eosinophilia may occur in the first week following halothane administration. Jaundice usually is noted 7 to 10 days after exposure but may occur earlier in previously exposed patients. Nausea and vomiting may precede the onset of jaundice. Hepatomegaly is often mild, but liver tenderness is common. The serum aminotransferase levels are elevated. The pathologic changes at autopsy are indistinguishable from massive hepatic necrosis resulting from viral hepatitis. The case fatality rate of halothane hepatitis is not known but may vary from 20 to 40 percent in cases with severe liver involvement. In rare instances cirrhosis has been observed following repeated bouts of halothane hepatitis; however, in most patients who recover, the liver returns to normal. It is strongly suggested that patients in whom unexplained spiking fever, especially delayed fever, or jaundice develops after halothane anesthesia not receive this agent again. Because cross-reactions between halothane and methoxyfluorane have been reported, the latter agent should not be used after halothane reactions.

Methyldopa hepatotoxicity (toxic and idiosyncratic reaction) Minor alterations in liver tests are reported in about 5 percent of patients treated with this antihypertensive agent. These trivial abnormalities typically resolve despite continued drug administration. In less than 1 percent of patients, acute liver injury resembling viral hepatitis, or chronic active hepatitis, or rarely a cholestatic reaction is seen 1 to 20 weeks after methyldopa is started. In 50 percent of cases the interval is shorter than 4 weeks. A prodrome of fever, anorexia, and malaise may be noted for a few days before the onset of jaundice. Rash, lymphadenopathy, arthralgia, and eosinophilia are rare. Serologic markers of autoimmunity are infrequently detected, and fewer than 5 percent of patients have a Coombs-positive hemolytic

TABLE 247-6 Principal alterations of hepatic morphology produced by some commonly used drugs and chemicals

Principal morphologic change	Class of agent	Example
Cholestasis	Anabolic steroid	Methyl testosterone*
	Antithyroid	Methimazole
	Chemotherapeutic	Erythromycin estolate
	Oral contraceptive	Norethynodrel with mestranol
	Oral hypoglycemic	Chlorpropamide
	Tranquilizer	Chlorpromazine*
Fatty liver	Chemotherapeutic	Tetracycline
	Anticonvulsant	Valproic acid (sodium valproate)
Hepatitis	Anesthetic	Halothane†
	Anticonvulsant	Phenytoin
	Antihypertensive	Methyldopa†
	Chemotherapeutic	Isoniazid†
	Diuretic	Chlorothiazide
	Laxative	Oxyphenisatin†
Toxic (necrosis)	Hydrocarbon	Carbon tetrachloride
	Metal	Yellow phosphorus
	Mushroom	*Amanita phalloides*
	Analgesic	Acetaminophen
Granulomas	Anti-inflammatory	Phenylbutazone
	Chemotherapeutic	Sulfonamides
	Xanthine oxidase inhibitor	Allopurinol

* *Rarely associated with primary biliary cirrhosis-like lesion.*
† *Occasionally associated with chronic active hepatitis or bridging hepatic necrosis and cirrhosis.*

anemia. In about 15 percent of patients with methyldopa hepatotoxicity the clinical, biochemical, and histologic features are those of chronic active hepatitis with or without bridging necrosis and macronodular cirrhosis. With discontinuation of the drug, the disorder usually resolves, although progression has been seen in a few patients.

Isoniazid hepatotoxicity (toxic and idiosyncratic reaction) In approximately 10 percent of adults treated with the antituberculosis agent isoniazid, elevated serum aminotransferase levels develop during the first few weeks of therapy; this appears to represent an adaptive response to a toxic metabolite of the drug. Whether or not isoniazid is continued, these values (usually below 200 units) return to normal in a few weeks. In about 1 percent of treated patients, an illness develops which is indistinguishable from viral hepatitis; approximately half of these cases occur within the first 2 months of treatment, while in the remainder, clinical disease may be delayed for many months. Liver biopsy reveals morphologic changes similar to those of viral hepatitis or bridging hepatic necrosis. The disease may be severe, with a case fatality rate of 10 percent. Important liver injury appears to be age-related, increasing substantially in frequency after age 35; the highest frequency is in patients over age 50, the lowest under the age of 20. Fever, rash, eosinophilia, and other manifestations of drug allergy are distinctly unusual. A reactive metabolite of acetylhydrazine, a metabolite of isoniazid, may be responsible for liver injury. A picture resembling chronic active hepatitis has been observed in a few patients.

Sodium valproate hepatotoxicity (toxic and idiosyncratic reaction) Sodium valproate, an anticonvulsant useful in the treatment of petit mal and other seizure disorders, has been associated with the development of severe hepatic toxicity and, rarely, fatalities in both children and adults. Asymptomatic elevations of serum aminotransferase levels have been recognized in as many as 45 percent of treated patients. These "adaptive" changes, however, appear to have no clinical importance, for major hepatotoxicity is not seen in the majority of patients despite continuation of drug therapy. In those rare patients in whom jaundice, encephalopathy, and evidence of hepatic failure are found, examination of liver tissue reveals microvesicular fat and bridging hepatic necrosis predominantly in the centrolobular zone. Bile duct injury may also be apparent. It seems likely that sodium valproate is not directly hepatotoxic but that its metabolite, 4-pentenoic acid, may be responsible for hepatic injury.

Phenytoin hepatotoxicity (idiosyncratic reaction) Phenytoin, diphenylhydantoin, a mainstay in the treatment of seizure disorders, has been associated in rare instances with the development of severe hepatitis-like liver injury leading to fulminant hepatic failure in some instances. In many patients the hepatitis is associated with striking fever, lymphadenopathy, rash (Stevens-Johnson syndrome or exfoliative dermatitis), leukocytosis, and eosinophilia, suggesting an immunologically mediated hypersensitivity mechanism. Despite these observations, there is also evidence that metabolic idiosyncrasy may be responsible for hepatic injury. In the liver, phenytoin is converted by the cytochrome P450 system to metabolites which include the highly reactive electrophilic arene oxides. These metabolites are normally metabolized further by epoxide hydrolases. A defect (genetic or acquired) in epoxide hydrolase activity would permit covalent binding of arene oxides to hepatic macromolecules, thereby leading to hepatic injury. Regardless of the mechanism, hepatic injury is usually manifest within the first 2 months after beginning phenytoin therapy. With the exception of an abundance of eosinophils in the liver, the clinical, biochemical, and histologic picture resembles that of viral hepatitis. In rare instances, bile duct injury may be the salient feature of phenytoin hepatotoxicity with striking features of intrahepatic cholestasis.

Chlorpromazine hepatotoxicity (cholestatic idiosyncratic reaction) In about 1 percent of patients receiving chlorpromazine, intrahepatic cholestasis with jaundice develops after 1 to 4 weeks of treatment. In rare instances, jaundice has been reported after a single exposure. Anicteric reactions are frequent. The onset may be abrupt with fever, rash, arthralgias, lymphadenopathy, nausea, vomiting, and epigastric or right upper quadrant pain. Pruritus may precede the appearance of jaundice, dark urine, and light stools. Eosinophilia with or without mild leukocytosis may be present, and conjugated hyperbilirubinemia, moderately elevated serum alkaline phosphatase, and mildly elevated serum aminotransferase levels (100 to 200 units) are noted. Liver biopsy reveals cholestasis, bile plugs in dilated bile canaliculi, and a dense portal infiltrate of polymorphonuclear, eosinophilic, and mononuclear leukocytes. Occasionally, scattered foci of hepatic parenchymal necrosis may be evident. Jaundice and pruritus usually subside within 4 to 8 weeks following cessation of therapy, without sequelae, and fatalities are rare. Cholestyramine may be of value in relieving severe pruritus. In a small number of patients, jaundice is prolonged for several months to years; rarely, a disorder resembling but distinct from primary biliary cirrhosis may develop.

Erythromycin hepatotoxicity (cholestatic idiosyncratic reaction) The most important adverse effect associated with erythromycin is the infrequent occurrence of a cholestatic reaction. Although most of these reactions have been associated with erythromycin estolate, other erythromycins may also be responsible. The reaction usually begins during the first 2 or 3 weeks of therapy and includes nausea, vomiting, fever, right upper quadrant abdominal pain, jaundice, leukocytosis, and moderately elevated aminotransferase levels. The clinical picture can resemble acute cholecystitis or bacterial cholangitis. Liver biopsy reveals variable cholestasis, portal inflammation comprising lymphocytes, polymorphonuclear leukocytes, and eosinophils, and scattered foci of hepatocyte necrosis. Symptoms and laboratory findings usually subside within a few days of drug withdrawal, and evidence of chronic liver disease has not been found on followup. The precise mechanism remains ill-defined.

Oral contraceptive hepatotoxicity (cholestatic reaction) The administration of oral contraceptive combinations of estrogenic and progestational steroids results in significant bromsulphthalein (BSP) retention in a high proportion of patients, and, to a far lesser extent, elevation of serum alkaline phosphatase. Weeks to months after taking these agents, intrahepatic cholestasis with pruritus and jaundice is noted in a small number of patients. Especially susceptible seem to be patients with recurrent idiopathic jaundice of pregnancy, severe pruritus of pregnancy, or a family history of these disorders. Laboratory studies, with the exception of liver biochemical tests, are normal, and extrahepatic manifestations of hypersensitivity are absent. Liver biopsy reveals cholestasis with bile plugs in dilated canaliculi and striking bilirubin staining of liver cells. In contrast to chlorpromazine-induced cholestasis, portal inflammation is absent. The lesion is reversible on withdrawal of the agent, and sequelae have not been reported. The two steroid components appear to act synergistically on hepatic function, although the estrogen may be primarily responsible. Oral contraceptives are contraindicated in patients with a history of recurrent jaundice of pregnancy. As indicated above, neoplasms of the liver and hepatic vein occlusion have also been associated with oral contraceptive therapy.

17,α-Alkyl-substituted anabolic steroids (cholestatic reaction) In the majority of patients receiving these agents, used mainly in the treatment of bone marrow failure, mild hepatic dysfunction develops. Impaired excretory function is the predominant defect, but the precise mechanism is uncertain. Jaundice, which appears to be dose-related, develops in only a minority of patients and may be the sole clinical manifestation of hepatotoxicity, although anorexia, nausea, and malaise are described in some patients. Pruritus is not a prominent feature. Serum aminotransferase levels are usually under 100 units, and serum alkaline phosphatase levels are normal, mildly elevated, or, in less than 5 percent of patients, three or more times the upper limit of normal. Examination of liver tissue reveals cholestasis without inflammation or necrosis. Hepatic sinusoidal dilatation and peliosis hepatis have been found in a few patients. The cholestatic disorder is usually reversible on cessation of treatment, although fatalities have been linked to peliosis. An association with hepatic adenoma and hepatocellular carcinoma has been reported.

REFERENCES

Viral hepatitis

ALTER HJ (ed): Hepatitis B. Semin Liver Dis 1:1, 1981
——— (ed): Viral hepatitis. Semin Liver Dis 6:1, 1986
DIENSTAG JL, ISSELBACHER KJ: Therapy of acute and chronic hepatitis. Arch Intern Med 141:1419, 1981
———: Non-A, non-B hepatitis. I. Recognition, epidemiology, and clinical features. II. Experimental transmission, putative virus agents and markers, and prevention. Gastroenterology 85:439 and 743, 1983
FAVERO MS et al: Guidelines for the care of patients hospitalized with viral hepatitis. Ann Intern Med 91:872, 1979
GERETY RJ (ed): *Non-A, Non-B Hepatitis*. New York, Academic 1981
——— (ed): *Hepatitis A*. Orlando, Academic, 1984
——— (ed): *Hepatitis B*. Orlando, Academic, 1985
IMMUNIZATION PRACTICES ADVISORY COMMITTEE: Recommendations for protection against viral hepatitis. Ann Intern Med 103:391, 1985
JACOBSON IM, DIENSTAG JL: Viral hepatitis vaccines. Annu Rev Med 36:241, 1985
KOFF RS: Viral hepatitis. New York, Wiley, 1978
LEMON SM: Type A viral hepatitis: New developments in an old disease. N Engl J Med 313:1059, 1985
RIZZETTO M: The delta agent. Hepatology 3:729, 1983
SEEFF LB, HOOFNAGLE JH: Immunoprophylaxis of viral hepatitis. Gastroenterology 77:161, 1979
SEEFF LB, KOFF R: Passive and active immunoprophylaxis of hepatitis B. Gastroenterology 86:958, 1984
SHAFRITZ DA, LIBERMAN HM: The molecular biology of hepatitis B virus. Annu Rev Med 35:219, 1984
SZMUNESS W et al: Hepatitis B vaccine: Demonstration of efficacy in a controlled clinical trial in a high-risk population in the United States. N Engl J Med 303:833, 1980
——— et al (eds): Viral Hepatitis: 1981 International Symposium. Philadelphia, Franklin Institute Press, 1982
THEILMANN L et al: Detection of pre-SI proteins in serum and liver of HBsAg-positive patients: A new marker for hepatitis B virus infection, Hepatology 6:186, 1986
VERME G et al (eds): *Viral Hepatitis and Delta Infection*. New York, Alan R. Liss, 1983
VYAS GN et al (eds): *Viral Hepatitis and Liver Disease*. Orlando, Grune & Stratton, 1984

Drug-induced hepatitis

BLACK M et al: Isoniazid-associated hepatitis in 114 patients. Gastroenterology 69:389, 1975
ISHAK KG, IREY NS: Hepatic injury associated with the phenothiazines: Clinicopathologic and follow-up study of 36 patients. Arch Pathol 93:283, 1972
LUDWIG J, AXELSEN R: Drug effects on the liver: An updated tabular compilation of drugs and drug-related hepatic diseases. Dig Dis Sci 28:651, 1983
MITCHELL JR, JOLLOW DJ: Metabolic activation of drugs to toxic substances. Gastroenterology 68:392, 1975
SHERLOCK S: Hepatic reactions to drugs. Gut 20:634, 1979
ZAFRANI ES et al: Cholestatic and hepatocellular injury associated with erythromycin esters: Report of nine cases. Am J Dig Dis 24:38, 1979
ZIMMERMAN HJ: Hepatotoxicity. New York, Appleton-Century-Crofts, 1978
——— (ed): Drug-induced liver disease. Semin Liver Dis 1:91, 1981
———, ISAK KG: Valproate-induced hepatic injury: Analysis of 23 fatal cases. Hepatology 2:591, 1982

248 CHRONIC HEPATITIS

JACK R. WANDS / RAYMOND S. KOFF / KURT J. ISSELBACHER

Chronic hepatitis refers to three related disorders—chronic persistent hepatitis, chronic lobular hepatitis, and chronic active hepatitis. These are characterized by a combination of hepatocyte necrosis and inflammation of varying severity persisting for more than 6 months. The clinically most important disorder, chronic active hepatitis, may lead to hepatic failure and death or result in the development of cirrhosis and its sequelae. While all three forms of chronic hepatitis share some histopathologic features and appear to be incited by similar etiologic factors, their pathogeneses, clinical presentations, natural histories, prognoses, and therapies are different.

CHRONIC PERSISTENT AND CHRONIC LOBULAR HEPATITIS

Definition and etiology Chronic persistent and chronic lobular hepatitis result from infections with hepatitis B virus (HBV) and non-A, non-B hepatitis virus. Other etiologies may exist but are poorly defined. In general, these are both nonprogressive disorders; hepatic failure is not seen and evolution into cirrhosis is exceedingly rare. Occasionally, however, patients with chronic active hepatitis may be misdiagnosed if they are seen during remission, at which time the histopathologic findings may suggest chronic persistent or chronic lobular hepatitis. Under these circumstances relapses and progression to the more serious underlying chronic active hepatitis may be anticipated. Another exception to the nonprogression of chronic persistent and lobular hepatitis occurs in patients positive to hepatitis B surface antigen (HBsAg), in whom superinfection with delta agent (HDV) may lead to the development of chronic active hepatitis (see Chap. 247).

Pathology In typical chronic persistent hepatitis there is infiltration of the portal areas with mononuclear cells, but there is no erosion of the limiting plate (so-called piecemeal necrosis) or extension of the inflammation into the liver lobule. A "cobblestone" arrangement of liver cells, indicative of hepatic regenerative activity, is a common feature. Minimal fibrosis may be observed, but *cirrhosis is characteristically absent*. In chronic lobular hepatitis, in addition to the portal inflammatory changes, lobular inflammation and focal hepatocellular necrosis are prominent features during clinically active phases. The morphologic features of chronic persistent, lobular, and active hepatitis are compared in Table 248-1.

Clinical and laboratory features Most patients with chronic persistent and/or lobular hepatitis are asymptomatic, although some may complain of anorexia, fatigue, and occasionally of nausea and vomiting. Physical findings are usually normal, but the liver may be slightly enlarged and tender. Laboratory data show mild elevations of aminotransferase and alkaline phosphatase levels and these abnormalities may persist for months to years. During active phases of chronic lobular hepatitis, aminotransferase levels may resemble those seen in acute viral hepatitis.

Management Once the diagnosis of chronic persistent or lobular hepatitis has been established by liver biopsy, no specific therapy is required since such patients generally do not develop fibrosis and cirrhosis. Follow-up examination is recommended every 6 to 12 months until aminotransferase values have returned to normal and to identify the rare patient who may progress to chronic active hepatitis.

CHRONIC ACTIVE HEPATITIS

Definition Chronic active hepatitis is a disorder of diverse etiologies characterized by continuing hepatic necrosis, active inflammation, and fibrosis which may lead to or be accompanied by liver failure, cirrhosis, and death. The prominence of extrahepatic features and seroimmunologic abnormalities has led to the use of a variety of terms to describe this disorder. These terms include autoimmune hepatitis, lupoid hepatitis, subacute hepatitis, and chronic active liver disease. *Chronic active hepatitis* seems to be the most appropriate designation for this clinicopathologic entity, regardless of the etiology and the clinical variations.

Pathology Although chronic active hepatitis may be suspected from the clinical history and the physical findings, *liver biopsy is necessary to establish the diagnosis*. The cardinal histopathologic features observed in the liver include (1) a dense mononuclear and plasma cell infiltration of the portal zones which greatly expands these areas with extension of the inflammatory infiltrate into the liver lobule; (2) destruction of the hepatocytes at the periphery of the lobule (piecemeal necrosis) with erosion of the limiting plate surrounding the portal triads; (3) connective tissue septa extending from the portal zones into the lobule, isolating parenchymal cells into clusters and envel-

TABLE 248-1 Some distinguishing features of chronic persistent, chronic lobular, and chronic active hepatitis

Features	Chronic persistent hepatitis	Chronic lobular hepatitis	Chronic active hepatitis
CLINICAL			
Onset like acute hepatitis	≈70%	≈90%	≈30%
Recurrent acute episodes	Infrequent	Common	Common
Extrahepatic involvement	Rare	Rare	Common
Prognosis	Good	Good	Variable
LIVER HISTOLOGY			
Piecemeal necrosis	Inconstant	Inconstant	Typical
Site of inflammation	Portal	Portal/lobular in active phase	Portal, extending into lobule
Lobular architecture	Preserved	Preserved	Distorted
Fibrosis	Slight	Slight	Common
Progression to cirrhosis	Rare	Rare	Common

oping bile ducts; and (4) evidence of hepatic regeneration with "rosette" formation, thickened liver-cell plates, and regenerative "pseudolobules." This process may be patchy, and individual liver lobules may remain uninvolved. Councilman-like bodies, which represent necrosis of single liver cells, may be seen in the periportal areas. The lesion of bridging hepatic necrosis may be seen in some patients with chronic active hepatitis. This lesion or its more extensive variant, multilobular bridging hepatic necrosis, suggests the presence of severe disease.

There is substantial morphologic evidence that in some instances chronic active hepatitis will progress to or is accompanied by the development of cirrhosis. On liver biopsy, cirrhosis can be demonstrated in 20 to 50 percent of patients, even early in the course of the disease, and at autopsy postnecrotic cirrhosis may be found. It is also possible that many cases of so-called cryptogenic cirrhosis are the result of chronic active hepatitis after inflammation and necrosis have subsided. In other patients fibrosis is not progressive and morphologic evidence of cirrhosis cannot be found.

Etiology Multiple etiologic agents may initiate chronic active hepatitis. Probably the most important and common triggering factors are infection with hepatitis B virus or the non-A, non-B hepatitis viruses. In about one-third of patients the disease begins abruptly following an illness typical of acute viral hepatitis. Persistence of HBsAg in the serum is found in 20 to 30 percent of patients with chronic active hepatitis, suggesting that persistent hepatitis B virus infection may be related to the development of chronic active hepatitis. Many of these HBsAg-positive patients also have positive tests for the hepatitis B e antigen (HBeAg) (see Chap. 247). Superinfection with delta hepatitis agent (HDV) in HBsAg-positive individuals may lead to the development of chronic active hepatitis. Similarly, persistent non-A, non-B hepatitis virus infections may be responsible for cases of chronic active hepatitis following transfusion-associated and sporadic non-A, non-B hepatitis. Drugs are involved in the pathogenesis of some cases. For example, features typical of chronic active hepatitis have been found in some patients in association with the administration of methyldopa. In these patients challenge with methyldopa has led to increased activity of the disease, while discontinuance has resulted in clinical, biochemical, and histologic improvement. Oxyphenisatin, isoniazid, nitrofurantoin, and other drugs have also been incriminated as etiologic agents in patients with chronic active hepatitis. Thus, chemical as well as viral agents may play a role in the production of chronic active hepatitis. The existence of other triggering factors seems likely, but their nature and mechanisms of action remain to be determined.

Immunopathogenesis There is increasing evidence that the progressive parenchymal cell destruction in patients with chronic active hepatitis involves an interaction with the immune system conditioned or controlled by genetic factors. Evidence to support this concept includes the following facts: (1) In the liver the histopathologic lesions are composed predominantly of thymus-derived or T lymphocytes and plasma cells in association with progressive liver cell destruction and replacement by fibrous tissue. (2) A variety of circulating "autoantibodies" are frequently detected, such as anti-smooth-muscle, antimitochondrial, and antithyroid antibodies. (3) The persistence of HBsAg in the serum and the hepatitis B core antigen (HBcAg) in the liver cell following an attack of acute hepatitis B is frequently associated with the development of chronic active or chronic persistent hepatitis. (4) Other "autoimmune" diseases such as thyroiditis, diabetes mellitus, ulcerative colitis, Coombs-positive hemolytic anemia, proliferative glomerulonephritis, and Sjögren's syndrome may be associated with chronic active hepatitis or may occur in relatives of affected patients. (5) Histocompatibility antigens HLA-B1 or -B8 and DRw3 and DRw4 are more prevalent than expected in patients with chronic active hepatitis without HBsAg. (6) Finally, the use of corticosteroids, believed to be effective in a variety of immunologic and autoimmune disorders, is often beneficial in the treatment of severe chronic active hepatitis.

There is increasing evidence that cellular immune reactions may be important in the pathogenesis of chronic active hepatitis. It has been suggested that lymphocytes become sensitized to altered or new antigens present on the surface membranes of hepatocytes. This hypothesis is supported in part by studies demonstrating that circulating and liver-derived lymphocytes may have the capability of causing liver cell damage in vitro.

Humoral immune mechanisms may be responsible for some of the clinical manifestations of chronic active hepatitis. In particular, extrahepatic features such as arthralgias, arthritis, rash, and glomerulonephritis appear to be mediated by the deposition of circulating immune complexes. Furthermore, complement activation, as demonstrated by low serum complement levels, and the presence of complement components in immune complexes suggest that circulating immune complexes may be involved in mediating extrahepatic inflammation and tissue damage.

Clinical features The clinical spectrum of chronic active hepatitis extends from asymptomatic illness at one end to fatal hepatic failure at the other. All age groups are affected. In approximately two-thirds of patients the disease has an *insidious onset* over a period of several weeks to months, or the disease is discovered incidentally, and the duration of the illness is uncertain. In the remainder an abrupt onset similar to that in acute viral hepatitis is seen, but features of chronic active hepatitis usually develop during the ensuing 12 to 24 months. The clinical and laboratory features suggesting progression from acute hepatitis to chronic active hepatitis are discussed in Chap. 247. *Fatigue* is a common symptom. Persistent or recurrent *jaundice* is a common feature in severe disease. Intermittent deepening of jaundice and recurrent symptoms of *malaise, anorexia,* and *low-grade fever,* suggestive of a superimposed acute hepatitis, are common throughout the course of the illness. In some patients complications of cirrhosis, such as ascites, variceal bleeding, encephalopathy, coagulopathy, or hypersplenism, may first bring the patient to medical attention. In others the extrahepatic features dominate the clinical picture, and liver disease is entirely unsuspected. Extrahepatic presenting features may include amenorrhea, bloody diarrhea (due to associated ulcerative colitis), abdominal pain, arthralgia or arthritis, macular or papular eruptions, acne, erythema nodosum, pleurisy, pericarditis, anemia, azotemia, and sicca syndrome (of keratoconjunctivitis and xerostomia). These extrahepatic features and abnormal serologic reactions tend to be more frequent in women than men and in patients without serologic evidence of preceding hepatitis B.

The *course* of chronic active hepatitis is variable, and the disease may persist for long periods without clinically overt liver disease. This appears to be particularly true of chronic active hepatitis associated with hepatitis B or non-A, non-B hepatitis. The condition may occasionally remit into a clinically inactive phase, although continuing hepatocellular necrosis or progression to cirrhosis may also occur. The histologic lesion may reverse itself completely before the development of cirrhosis in some HBsAg-positive patients after their antigenemia has spontaneously cleared or following the loss of HBeAg and the development of anti-HBe. If untreated, the case fatality rate may be high during the first few years of illness, especially in patients with clinically and histologically severe disease. Death usually occurs as a result of liver failure and hepatic coma. Later death is often due to a complication of cirrhosis—variceal hemorrhage or intercurrent infection. Primary hepatocellular carcinoma is an uncommon complication of HBsAg-negative chronic active hepatitis even when the disease has progressed to postnecrotic cirrhosis. This finding is in contrast to long-term HBsAg carriers with chronic active hepatitis and/or cirrhosis in whom the incidence of liver carcinoma is increased (see Chap. 247).

Laboratory findings Liver function tests are invariably abnormal but may not correlate with the clinical severity or histopathologic findings in the individual case. Many patients have normal serum bilirubin, alkaline phosphatase, and globulin levels with only minimial aminotransferase elevations or HBsAg positivity and yet have a liver biopsy consistent with severe chronic active hepatitis. Serum aspartate aminotransferase (SGOT) and alanine aminotransferase (SGPT) levels are increased and fluctuate in the range of 100 to 1000 units in most cases. In severe cases the serum bilirubin is moderately elevated (3 to 10 mg/dL). Mild hypoalbuminemia occurs in patients with active disease or in those with advanced cirrhosis. Serum alkaline phosphatase levels may be moderately elevated or near normal. The prothrombin time is often prolonged, particularly late in the disease or during active phases.

Hypergammaglobulinemia (greater than 2.5 g/dL) is common, particularly in patients with extensive plasma cell infiltration of the liver. A variety of abnormal serologic reactions and circulating autoantibodies are found in chronic active hepatitis. Some of these serologic reactions are nonspecific and may be seen in other viral diseases. Circulating autoantibodies against DNA, IgG, smooth muscle, and mitochrondria support the concept that chronic active hepatitis is indeed a systemic disease. HBsAg may be found in 20 to 30 percent of patients with chronic active hepatitis, more commonly in men than women.

Differential diagnosis Early in the course of chronic active hepatitis the disease may resemble typical *acute viral hepatitis*. However, the persistence of symptoms, including biochemical abnormalities such as elevated serum aminotransferase and bilirubin levels or circulating HBsAg over the ensuing months indicates that a chronic liver disorder is present. The major entities which must be distinguished from chronic active hepatitis are *chronic persistent and lobular hepatitis*. As indicated in Table 248-1, in chronic persistent and lobular hepatitis the onset of the illness frequently resembles acute hepatitis. The aminotransferase enzyme values are variably elevated, and HBsAg may be present in serum. Fatigue, anorexia, malaise, right upper quadrant discomfort, and hepatomegaly may be associated with all three forms of chronic hepatitis. Thus, a definitive diagnosis can only be established by liver biopsy since a *differentiation between chronic active, chronic persistent, and lobular hepatitis cannot be made by clinical and biochemical criteria*. This distinction is important because chronic persistent and lobular hepatitis are not progressive disorders, rarely if ever result in cirrhosis, and require no therapy.

The presence of extrahepatic manifestations in chronic active hepatitis such as pleuritis, arthritis, and arthralgias may cause confusion with *connective tissue disorders* such as rheumatoid arthritis and systemic lupus erythematosus. The existence of clinical and biochemical features suggestive of progressive liver disease clearly distinguishes chronic active hepatitis from these disorders. In adolescence, *Wilson's disease* may present with features of chronic active hepatitis before the neurologic manifestations become apparent; serum ceruloplasmin, serum and urinary copper determination, and measurement of the liver copper levels will establish the diagnosis. Late in the course of chronic active hepatitis some patients may present with *postnecrotic cirrhosis* without evidence of active hepatitis. This lesion, termed cryptogenic cirrhosis, may also represent an end stage of other destructive liver diseases (e.g., primary biliary cirrhosis). *Primary biliary cirrhosis* may share histologic similarities with chronic active hepatitis, particularly early in the disease. However, in primary biliary cirrhosis the prominence of pruritus plus markedly elevated serum alkaline phosphatase and cholesterol levels, the presence of high titers of antimitochondrial antibodies (in contrast to the low levels seen in chronic active hepatitis), and the pattern of histologic progression will usually permit differentiation from chronic active hepatitis.

Management Corticosteroid therapy is the treatment of choice in symptomatic HBsAg-negative and severe chronic active hepatitis. Corticosteroids have been shown to be effective in prolonging survival of these patients during the first few years of illness when the mortality rate is high. A therapeutic response characterized by a complete clinical, biochemical, and histologic remission is to be expected in 60 to 80 percent of patients. Either prednisone or prednisolone therapy should be initiated at a dose of 20 to 40 mg daily. This dose can usually be gradually tapered within 2 to 3 months to 10 to 20 mg daily. The beneficial effects of corticosteroid treatment on the course and prognosis of patients with mild or asymptomatic chronic active hepatitis has not been established.

Improvement of fatigue and anorexia is usually noted within days to several weeks. Biochemical improvement is to be expected over several weeks to months, with a fall in serum bilirubin and globulin levels and a rise in serum albumin. The serum aminotransferase level usually drops promptly, but the absolute value of the aminotransferase *alone* does not appear to be a useful marker of recovery in the individual patient. Histologic improvement, characterized by a decrease in mononuclear infiltration and subsequent improvement in the extent of hepatocellular necrosis, may be delayed for 6 to 24 months. After a favorable clinical and biochemical response, repeat liver biopsy may show features consistent with chronic persistent hepatitis. Despite this histologic improvement, relapses are common when corticosteroids are discontinued.

Reduction of the suppressive corticosteroid doses should be performed cautiously, particularly at lower prednisone levels, since even small decrements in therapy may be associated with clinical worsening, and increasing dosage may be needed for control of spontaneous exacerbation. Unless major complications require discontinuation of corticosteroids, they should be prescribed for at least 12 months or longer in order to reduce the risk of relapse.

Other therapeutic approaches have been used in the treatment of severe chronic active hepatitis, particularly in the elderly and in patients with major side effects from corticosteroids. An initial prednisone dosage of 30 mg, tapered down to 10 to 20 mg, in combination with 50 to 75 mg azathioprine has been demonstrated to be effective; this treatment avoids the adverse effects of high dosage of corticosteroids. However, *azathioprine alone is not effective* in the treatment of chronic active hepatitis. Alternate-day prednisone therapy diminishes steroid side effects but usually does not provide adequate therapy.

Corticosteroids have little if any beneficial effect on the natural course of HBsAg-positive chronic active hepatitis. Treatment of *asymptomatic* HBsAg carriers who only have evidence of chronic active hepatitis on liver biopsy is not justified. In *symptomatic* HBsAg-positive patients with severe chronic active hepatitis, corticosteroids have not been shown to be of value either in short- or long-term therapy. Treatment with interferon and other antiviral agents has been studied, but mixed results have been obtained with respect to a favorable clinical response. Use of such drugs is still experimental.

REFERENCES

BERMAN M et al: The chronic sequelae of non-A, non-B hepatitis. Ann Intern Med 91:1, 1979

CZAJA AJ et al: Laboratory assessment of severe chronic active liver disease during and after corticosteroid therapy. Correlation of serum transaminase and gamma globulin levels with histologic features. Gastroenterology 80:667, 1981

HODGES JR et al: Chronic active hepatitis: The spectrum of disease. Lancet 1:550, 1982

LAM KC et al: Deleterious effect of prednisolone in HBsAg-positive chronic active hepatitis. N Engl J Med 304:380, 1981

MACKAY IR, TAIT BD: HLA associations with autoimmune-type chronic active hepatitis: Identification of B8-DRw3 haplotypes by family studies. Gastroenterology 79:95, 1980

SEEF LB, KOFF RS: Therapy for chronic active hepatitis. Adv Intern Med 29:109, 1984

WEISSBERG JI et al: Survival in chronic hepatitis B. An analysis of 379 patients. Ann Intern Med 101:613, 1984

WELLER IVD et al: Effects of prednisone/azathioprine in chronic hepatitis B viral infection. Gut 23:650, 1982

249 CIRRHOSIS

DANIEL K. PODOLSKY / KURT J. ISSELBACHER

Cirrhosis is a pathologically defined entity which is associated with a spectrum of characteristic clinical manifestations. The cardinal pathologic features reflect irreversible chronic injury of the hepatic parenchyma and include extensive fibrosis in association with the formation of regenerative nodules. These features result from hepatocyte necrosis, collapse of the supporting reticulin network with subsequent connective tissue deposition, distortion of the vascular bed, and nodular regeneration of remaining liver parenchyma. The pathologic process should be viewed as a final common pathway of many types of chronic liver injury. Clinical features of cirrhosis derive from the morphologic alterations and often reflect the severity of hepatic damage rather than the etiology of the underlying liver disease. Loss of functioning hepatocellular mass may lead to jaundice, edema, coagulopathy, and a variety of metabolic abnormalities; fibrosis and distorted vasculature lead to portal hypertension and its sequelae, including gastroesophageal varices and splenomegaly. Ascites and hepatic encephalopathy result from both hepatocellular insufficiency and portal hypertension.

Classification of the various types of cirrhosis based solely on etiology or morphology is unsatisfactory. A single pathologic pattern may result from a variety of insults, while the same insult may produce several morphologic patterns. Nevertheless most types of cirrhosis may be usefully classified by a mixture of etiologically and morphologically defined entities as follows: (1) alcoholic; (2) cryptogenic and postnecrotic; (3) biliary; (4) cardiac; (5) metabolic, inherited, and drug-related; and (6) miscellaneous. This chapter considers first the various types of cirrhosis and then the major clinical complications of chronic liver disease and cirrhosis.

ALCOHOLIC LIVER DISEASE AND CIRRHOSIS

Definition Alcoholic cirrhosis, historically referred to as Laennec's cirrhosis, is the most common type of cirrhosis encountered in North America and many parts of western Europe and South America. It is usually characterized by diffuse fine scarring, fairly uniform loss of liver cells, and small regenerative nodules, and therefore, it is sometimes referred to as micronodular cirrhosis. However, micronodular cirrhosis may also result from other types of liver injury (e.g., following jejunoileal bypass), and thus alcoholic cirrhosis and micronodular cirrhosis are not necessarily synonymous. Conversely alcoholic cirrhosis may progress to macronodular cirrhosis with time.

Alcoholic cirrhosis is only one of many consequences resulting from chronic alcoholic ingestion, and it often accompanies other forms of alcohol-induced liver injury. The three principal alcohol-induced hepatic lesions are designated: (1) alcoholic fatty liver, (2) alcoholic hepatitis, and (3) alcoholic cirrhosis. These morphologic categories are rarely found in a pure form, and features of each may be present to varying degrees in an individual patient.

Etiology Although chronic alcoholism is clearly the major cause of alcoholic cirrhosis, the quantity and duration of drinking necessary to cause cirrhosis remain unclear. The typical alcoholic patient with cirrhosis has had a daily consumption of a pint or more of whiskey, several quarts of wine, or an equivalent amount of beer for at least 10 years. The amount and duration of ethanol ingestion, rather than the type of alcoholic beverage or the pattern of ingestion, appear to be the important determinants of liver injury. In general, the latent period preceding the development of cirrhosis is inversely related to the level of daily alcohol intake. Although rates of ethanol metabolism are under genetic control, no metabolic defect has been identified in cirrhotic patients or their families to suggest a unique "susceptibility" to ethanol or its toxic effects. Although malnutrition per se does not appear to lead to cirrhosis, it is possible that nutritional factors may augment the detrimental effects of chronic alcohol ingestion on the liver. The finding that only 10 to 15 percent of alcoholics develop cirrhosis suggests that other factors may affect the impact of alcohol on the liver. Women appear to be more susceptible to alcohol-induced liver injury, suggesting that hormonal factors may play a role.

Alcoholic fatty liver occurs in most heavy drinkers but is reversible on cessation of alcohol consumption and is not thought to be an inevitable precursor of alcoholic hepatitis or cirrhosis. In contrast, alcoholic hepatitis, an inflammatory lesion characterized by infiltration of the liver with leukocytes, liver cell necrosis, and alcoholic hyaline, is thought to be the major precursor of cirrhosis. Subsequent healing accompanied by fibrosis distorts the normal lobular architecture. Indeed, *deposition of collagen in perivenular spaces* may be the earliest manifestation of the process which ultimately leads to cirrhosis.

Pathology and pathogenesis ALCOHOLIC FATTY LIVER The liver is enlarged, yellow, greasy, and firm. Hepatocytes are distended by large cytoplasmic fat vacuoles which push the hepatocyte nucleus against the cell membrane. Accumulation of fat in the liver of the alcoholic results from the combination of impaired fatty acid oxidation, increased uptake and esterification of fatty acids to form triglycerides, and diminished lipoprotein biosynthesis and secretion.

ALCOHOLIC HEPATITIS Morphologic features include hepatocyte degeneration and necrosis, often with ballooned cells, and an infiltrate of polymorphonuclear leukocytes and lymphocytes. The polymorphonuclear cells may encircle damaged hepatocytes which contain *Mallory bodies,* or *alcoholic hyaline*. These are clumps of perinuclear, deeply eosinophilic material believed to represent aggregated intermediate filaments. Mallory bodies are highly suggestive of, but *not specific* for, alcoholic hepatitis, since morphologically similar material has been seen in association with morbid obesity, jejunoileal bypass surgery, poorly controlled diabetes mellitus, and a variety of other disorders including Wilson's disease and Indian childhood cirrhosis. Deposition of collagen around the central vein and in perisinusoidal areas, often termed central hyaline sclerosis, may be associated with an increased likelihood of progression to cirrhosis.

ALCOHOLIC CIRRHOSIS With continued alcohol intake and destruction of hepatocytes, fibroblasts (including myofibroblasts with contractile properties) appear at the site of injury and stimulate collagen formation. Weblike septa of connective tissue appear in periportal and pericentral zones and eventually connect portal triads and central veins. This fine connective tissue network surrounds small masses of remaining liver cells which regenerate and form nodules. Although regeneration occurs within the small remnants of parenchyma, cell loss generally exceeds replacement. With continuing hepatocyte destruction and collagen depostion, the liver shrinks in size, acquires a nodular appearance, and becomes hard as "end-stage" cirrhosis develops. Although alcoholic cirrhosis is usually a progressive disease, appropriate therapy and strict avoidance of alcohol may arrest the disease at most stages and permit functional improvement.

Clinical features SIGNS AND SYMPTOMS Clinical manifestations of *alcoholic fatty liver* are often minimal or entirely absent, and the disorder may not be recognized unless another illness (frequently alcohol-related) brings the patient to medical attention. Hepatomegaly, at times accompanied by tenderness, may be the only finding. Jaundice, ascites, and edema are only seen with more serious liver injury.

The clinical severity of *alcoholic hepatitis* varies enormously, ranging from asymptomatic or mild illness to fatal hepatic insufficiency. Typically, the clinical features of alcoholic hepatitis resemble those of viral or toxic liver injury. Patients often experience anorexia, nausea and vomiting, malaise, weight loss, abdominal distress, and jaundice. Fever as high as 103°F may be seen in about half of cases. On physical examination, tender hepatomegaly is common, and splenomegaly is found in about one-third of patients. The patient may have cutaneous arterial "spider" angiomas and jaundice. More severe cases may be complicated by ascites, edema, bleeding, and encephalopathy. At the time of initial presentation, the central nervous system findings may be difficult to distinguish from manifestations of concurrent alcohol intoxication or withdrawal (see below).

Although jaundice, ascites, and encephalopathy may subside with abstinence, continued alcohol excess and poor dietary habits usually lead to repeated acute episodes of hepatic decompensation. Some patients die during these acute exacerbations, but most recover after several weeks or months. Even after complete abstinence, clinical recovery may be protracted, and histologic abnormalities can persist up to 6 months or longer. Cholestatic jaundice mimicking biliary tract obstruction may also develop in some cases of acute alcoholic hepatitis.

Alcoholic cirrhosis may also be clinically silent; in fact 10 percent of cases are discovered incidentally at laparotomy or autopsy. In many cases symptoms are insidious in onset, occurring usually after 10 or more years of excessive alcohol use and progressing slowly over subsequent weeks and months. Anorexia and malnutrition lead to weight loss and a reduction in skeletal muscle mass. The patient may experience easy bruising, increasing weakness, and fatigue. Eventually the clinical manifestations of hepatocellular dysfunction and portal hypertension ensue, including progressive jaundice, bleeding from gastroesophageal varices, ascites, and encephalopathy. The abrupt onset of one of these complications may be the first event prompting the patient to seek medical attention. In other cases, cirrhosis first becomes evident when the patient requires treatment of symptoms related to alcoholic hepatitis.

A firm, nodular liver may be an early sign of disease; the liver may be either enlarged, normal, or decreased in size. Other frequent findings include jaundice, palmar erythema, spider angiomas, parotid and lacrimal gland enlargement, clubbing of fingers, splenomegaly, muscle wasting, and ascites with or without peripheral edema. Men may have decreased body hair and/or gynecomastia and testicular atrophy, which, like the cutaneous findings, result from disturbances in hormonal metabolism, including increased peripheral formation of estrogren due to diminished hepatic clearance of the precursor androstenedione. Testicular atrophy may reflect hormonal abnormalities or the toxic effect of alcohol on the testes. In women, signs of virilization or menstrual irregularities may occasionally be encountered. Dupuytren's contractures resulting from fibrosis of the palmar fascia with resulting flexion contracture of the digits are associated with alcoholism but are not specifically related to cirrhosis.

Over a period of 3 to 5 years, the cirrhotic patient typically becomes emaciated, weak, and chronically jaundiced. Ascites and other signs of portal hypertension become increasingly prominent. Most patients with advanced cirrhosis die in hepatic coma, commonly precipitated by hemorrhage from esophageal varices or intercurrent infection. Progressive renal dysfunction often complicates the terminal phase of the illness.

LABORATORY FINDINGS Routine hematologic and biochemical blood tests are usually normal in patients with alcoholic fatty liver, except for minimal elevations of the serum AST [aspartate aminotransferase; serum glutamic oxaloacetic transaminase (SGOT)] level; occasionally alkaline phosphatase and bilirubin levels are also elevated. In more advanced alcoholic liver disease, abnormalities of laboratory tests are more common. Anemia may result from acute and chronic gastrointestinal blood loss, coexistent nutritional deficiency (notably of folic acid and vitamin B_{12}), hypersplenism, and a direct suppressive effect of alcohol on the bone marrow. Hemolytic anemia presumably due to effects of hypercholesterolemia on erythrocyte membranes resulting in unusual spurlike projections (acanthocytosis) has been described in some alcoholics with cirrhosis. Leukocytosis is often present in severe alcoholic hepatitis; however, some patients with this disorder may have leukopenia and thrombocytopenia due to hypersplenism or an inhibitory effect of alcohol on the bone marrow. Mild or pronounced hyperbilirubinemia may be found, usually in association with varying elevations of serum alkaline phosphatase levels. The serum ALT [alanine aminotransferase; serum glutamic pyruric transaminase (SGPT)] is frequently elevated, but levels greater than 300 units are unusual and should prompt one to look for other coincident or complicating factors. In contrast to viral hepatitis, the serum AST is usually disproportionately elevated relative to ALT (AST/ALT ratio > 2). This discrepancy may result from the proportionally greater inhibition of ALT synthesis by ethanol, which may be partially reversed by pyridoxal phosphate.

The serum prothrombin time is frequently prolonged, reflecting reduced synthesis of clotting proteins, most notably the vitamin K–dependent factors (see "Coagulopathy" below). The serum albumin level is usually depressed, while serum globulins are increased. Hypoalbuminemia reflects in part overall impairment in hepatic protein synthesis, while hyperglobulinemia is thought to result from nonspecific stimulation of the reticuloendothelial system. Elevated blood ammonia levels in patients with hepatic encephalopathy reflect diminished hepatic clearance because of impaired liver function and shunting of portal venous blood around the cirrhotic liver into the systemic circulation (see below and Chap. 244).

A variety of metabolic disturbances may be detected. Glucose intolerance due to endogenous insulin resistance may be present; however, clinical diabetes is uncommon. Central hyperventilation may lead to respiratory alkalosis in patients with cirrhosis. *Dietary deficiency* and *increased urinary losses* lead to hypomagnesemia and *hypophosphatemia*. In patients with ascites and dilutional hyponatremia, hypokalemia may occur from increased urinary postassium losses due in part to hyperaldosteronism. Prerenal azotemia is also observed in such patients.

Diagnosis *Alcoholic fatty liver* should be suspected in alcoholic patients with hepatomegaly and normal or minimally deranged liver function tests. Alcoholic fatty liver may be seen in combination with alcoholic hepatitis or established cirrhosis. *Alcoholic hepatitis* should be considered in an alcoholic who has been drinking heavily and demonstrates jaundice, fever, an enlarged, tender liver, or ascites. The clinical impression is often supported by the deranged results of tests of liver function and other laboratory abnormalities described above. Alcoholic hepatitis or fatty liver may be present in association with alcoholic cirrhosis.

Alcoholic cirrhosis should be strongly suspected in patients with a history of prolonged or excessive alcohol intake and physical signs of chronic liver disease. The clinical features and laboratory findings are usually sufficient to provide reasonable indication of the presence and extent of hepatic injury. Although a percutaneous needle biopsy of the liver is not usually necessary to confirm the typical findings of alcoholic hepatitis or cirrhosis, it may be helpful in distinguishing patients with less advanced liver disease from those with cirrhosis and in excluding other forms of liver injury such as viral hepatitis.

Biopsy may also be helpful as a diagnostic tool in evaluating patients with clinical findings suggestive of alcoholic liver disease who deny alcohol intake. In patients with features of cholestasis, ultrasonography may be appropriate to exclude the presence of extrahepatic biliary obstruction. When the clinical status of an otherwise stable cirrhotic patient deteriorates without an obvious explanation, complicating conditions, such as infection, portal vein thrombosis, and hepatocellular carcinoma, should be sought.

Prognosis The patient with an alcoholic fatty liver and no complications has a good prognosis; rapid and complete resolution usually follows cessation of alcohol intake. In patients with alcoholic hepatitis, the presence of marked hyperbilirubinemia (>20 mg/dL), rising serum creatinine, marked prolongation of the prothrombin time (> 1.5 times control), ascites, and encephalopathy are associated with a poor short-term prognosis; the in-hospital mortality in these patients may exceed 50 percent. In milder cases, clinical recovery may be complete, but repeated bouts of alcoholic hepatitis usually lead to irreversible and progressive chronic liver injury. Abstinence from alcohol as well as early and appropriate medical care can decrease long-term morbidity and mortality, and delay or prevent the appearance of further complications. Patients who have had a major complication of cirrhosis and who continue to drink, have a 5-year survival of less than 50 percent. However, those patients who remain abstinent have a substantially better prognosis. In general, overall outlook in patients with advanced liver disease remains poor; most of these patients eventually die as a result of massive variceal hemorrhage and/or profound hepatic encephalopathy.

Treatment Alcoholic hepatitis and cirrhosis are serious illnesses that require long-term medical supervision and careful management. Therapy of the underlying liver disease is largely supportive. Specific treatment is directed at particular complications such as variceal bleeding, ascites, etc. (see below). Some studies suggest that administration of prednisone or prednisolone in moderately large doses may be helpful in patients with severe alcoholic hepatitis and encephalopathy. However, the use of corticosteroids in acute alcoholic hepatitis remains controversial and is not recommended. Other agents, such as propylthiouracil, penicillamine, colchicine, and intravenous infusion of insulin and glucagon have been used experimentally, but their therapeutic efficacy and safety remain to be demonstrated.

In the absence of signs of impending hepatic coma, the patient should be placed on a diet containing at least 1 g protein per kilogram of body weight and 2000 to 3000 kcal per day. Use of diets enriched in branched-chain amino acids has been advocated in patients predisposed to hepatic encephalopathy, but the value of these diets in patients with compensated cirrhosis is unproven. Daily multivitamin supplements should be prescribed, with the addition of large parenteral doses of thiamine in patients with Wernicke-Korsakoff disease (see Chap. 349). The patient should be made to realize that there is no medication that will protect the liver against the effects of further alcohol ingestion. Therefore, alcohol should be absolutely forbidden. An important component of the complete care of such patients is encouragement to become involved in an appropriate alcohol counseling program.

All medicines must be administered with caution in the patient with cirrhosis, especially those eliminated or modified through hepatic metabolism or biliary pathways. In particular, care must be taken to avoid overzealous use of drugs that may directly or indirectly precipitate complications of cirrhosis. For example, vigorous treatment of ascites with diuretics may result in electrolyte abnormalities or hypovolemia which can lead to coma. Similarly, even modest doses of sedative can lead to deepening encephalopathy.

POSTNECROTIC CIRRHOSIS, POSTVIRAL CIRRHOSIS

Definition Postnecrotic cirrhosis represents the final common pathway of many types of advanced liver injury. *Coarsely nodular, posthepatitic,* and *multilobular cirrhosis* are terms synonymous with postnecrotic cirrhosis. The term *cryptogenic cirrhosis* has been used interchangeably with postnecrotic cirrhosis, but this designation should be reserved for those cases in which the etiology of cirrhosis is unknown (approximately 10 percent of all patients with cirrhosis).

Postnecrotic cirrhosis is characterized morphologically by (1) extensive confluent loss of liver cells, (2) stromal collapse and fibrosis resulting in broad bands of connective tissue containing the remains of many portal triads, and (3) irregular nodules of regenerating hepatocytes, varying in size from microscopic to several centimeters in diameter.

Etiology Postnecrotic cirrhosis is a morphologic term referring to a defined stage of advanced chronic liver injury of both specific and unknown (cryptogenic) causes. Epidemiologic and serologic evidence suggests that viral hepatitis (hepatitis B or non-A, non-B) may be an antecedent factor in at least one-fourth of cases of apparently cryptogenic postnecrotic cirrhosis. In areas where hepatitis B virus infection is endemic (e.g., southeast Asia, sub-Saharan Africa), up to 15 percent of the population may acquire the infection in early childhood, and cirrhosis may ultimately develop in one-fourth of these chronic carriers. Although hepatitis B infection is much less prevalent in the United States, it is relatively common among certain high-risk groups (e.g., promiscuous homosexual men, intravenous drug abusers), and contributes to an increased incidence of cirrhosis. In the United States non-A, non-B hepatitis agents appear to account for many cases of cirrhosis following blood transfusions. It is estimated that non-A, non-B hepatitis occurs in up to 10 percent of blood recipients, of whom as many as 5 to 10 percent may ultimately develop postnecrotic cirrhosis. Because reliable serologic markers for non-A, non-B hepatitis are not yet available, the number of cases of postnecrotic cirrhosis attributable to this agent (or agents) is difficult to determine but may be substantial (see Chap. 247). Postnecrotic cirrhosis may also develop in patients with chronic active hepatitis of the autoimmune type (see Chaps. 247 and 248).

Other probable causes of postnecrotic cirrhosis, including drugs and toxins, are listed in Table 249-1. In some instances, advanced alcoholic liver disease and primary biliary cirrhosis may lead to postnecrotic cirrhosis.

TABLE 249-1 Cirrhosis and/or liver disease associated with infectious, metabolic, hereditary, drug-related, and other types of disorders

1 Infectious diseases
- *a* Viral hepatitis [hepatitis B, non-A, non-B, hepatitis D, cytomegalovirus (Chaps. 137, 315, and 319)]
- *b* Toxoplasmosis (Chap 157)
- *c* Schistosomiasis (Chap. 164)
- *d* Ecchinococcus (Chap. 168)
- *e* Brucellosis (Chap. 112)

2 Inherited and metabolic disorders (see also Chap. 251)
- *a* Hemochromatosis (Chap. 310)
- *b* Wilson's disease (Chap. 311)
- *c* $Alpha_1$-antitrypsin deficiency (Chap. 208)
- *d* Galactosemia (Chap. 314)
- *e* Glycogen storage disease (Chap. 313)
- *f* Gaucher's disease (Chap. 316)
- *g* Hereditary fructose intolerance (Chap. 314)
- *h* Hereditary tyrosinemia (Chap. 306)
- *i* Fanconi's syndrome (Chap. 316)

3 Drugs and toxins (Chap. 247)
- *a* Methyldopa
- *b* Methotrexate
- *c* Isoniazid
- *d* Perhexilene maleate
- *e* Oxyphenisatin
- *f* Arsenicals
- *g* Pyrrolidizine alkaloids (venocclusive disease)
- *h* Oral contraceptives (Budd-Chiari)

4 Other or unproven causes
- *a* Sarcoidosis (Chap. 247)
- *b* Graft-versus-host disease
- *c* Chronic inflammatory bowel disease (Chap. 238)
- *d* Cystic fibrosis (Chap. 207)
- *e* Jejunoileal bypass (Chap. 35)
- *f* Diabetes mellitus (Chap. 327)

Pathology The postnecrotic liver is typically shrunken in size, distorted in shape, and composed of nodules of liver cells separated by dense and broad bands of fibrosis. The microscopic picture is consistent with the gross impression: nodules are highly variable in size with large amounts of connective tissue separating the disorganized islands of regenerating parenchyma.

Clinical features In patients with cirrhosis of known etiology in whom there is progression to a postnecrotic stage, the clinical manifestations are an extension of those resulting from the initial disease process. Usually clinical symptoms are related to portal hypertension and its sequelae, such as ascites, splenomegaly, hypersplenism, encephalopathy, and bleeding esophageal varices. The hematologic and liver function abnormalities resemble those seen with other types of cirrhosis. In a few patients with postnecrotic cirrhosis the diagnosis may be made incidentally at operation, at postmortem, or by a needle biopsy of the liver performed to investigate asymptomatic hepatosplenomegaly.

Diagnosis and prognosis Postnecrotic cirrhosis should be suspected in patients with signs and symptoms of cirrhosis or portal hypertension. Needle or operative liver biopsies confirm the diagnosis, although nonuniformity of the pathologic process may result in sampling errors. The diagnosis of cryptogenic cirrhosis is reserved for those patients in whom no known etiology can be demonstrated. About 75 percent of patients have progressive disease despite supportive therapy and die within 1 to 5 years from complications including exsanguinating variceal hemorrhage, hepatic encephalopathy, or superimposed hepatocellular carcinoma.

Treatment Management is usually limited to treatment of the complications of portal hypertension, including control of ascites, avoidance of drugs or excessive protein intake that may induce hepatic coma, and prompt treatment of infections (see below). In patients with asymptomatic cirrhosis, expectant management alone is appropriate. In those patients in whom postnecrotic cirrhosis has developed as a result of a treatable condition, therapy directed at the primary disorder may limit further progression (e.g., Wilson's disease, hemochromatosis).

BILIARY CIRRHOSIS

Biliary cirrhosis results from injury to or prolonged obstruction of either the intrahepatic or extrahepatic biliary system. It is associated with impaired biliary excretion, destruction of hepatic parenchyma, and progressive fibrosis. Primary biliary cirrhosis is characterized by chronic inflammation and fibrous obliteration of intrahepatic bile ductules. Secondary biliary cirrhosis is the result of long-standing obstruction of the larger extrahepatic ducts. Although primary and secondary biliary cirrhosis are separate pathophysiologic entities with respect to the initial insult, many clinical features are similar.

PRIMARY BILIARY CIRRHOSIS **Etiology and pathogenesis** The cause of primary biliary cirrhosis remains unknown. Several observations suggest that a disordered immune response may be involved. Primary biliary cirrhosis is frequently associated with a variety of disorders presumed to be autoimmune in nature, such as the CRST syndrome (calcinosis, Raynaud's phenomenon; sclerodactyly, telangiectasia), the sicca syndrome (dry eyes and dry mouth), autoimmune thyroiditis, and renal tubular acidosis. Most importantly, a circulating IgG antimitochondrial antibody is detected in more than 95 percent of patients with primary biliary cirrhosis and only rarely in other forms of liver disease. In addition, elevated serum levels of IgM and cryoproteins consisting of immune complexes capable of activating the alternate complement pathway are found in 80 to 90 percent of patients. Lymphocytes are prominent in the portal regions and surround damaged bile ducts. These histologic findings resemble those noted in graft-versus-host disease following liver and bone marrow transplantation and suggest that damage to bile ducts may be immunologically mediated, perhaps reflecting a defect in a suppressor cell population.

Pathology Primary biliary cirrhosis is often divided into four stages based on morphologic findings. The earliest recognizable lesion (stage I), termed *chronic nonsuppurative destructive cholangitis*, is a necrotizing inflammatory process of the portal triads. It is characterized by destruction of medium and small bile ducts, a dense infiltrate of acute and chronic inflammatory cells, mild fibrosis, and occasionally bile stasis. At times, periductal granulomas and lymph follicles are found adjacent to affected bile ducts. Subsequently, the inflammatory infiltrate becomes less prominent, the number of bile ducts is reduced, and smaller bile ductules proliferate (stage II). Progression over a period of months to years leads to a decrease in interlobular ducts, loss of liver cells, and expansion of periportal fibrosis into a network of connective tissue scars (stage III). Ultimately, cirrhosis, which may be micronodular or macronodular develops (stage IV).

Clinical features SIGNS AND SYMPTOMS Many patients with primary biliary cirrhosis are asymptomatic, and the disease is initially detected on the basis of elevated serum alkaline phosphatase levels during routine screening. The majority of such patients remain asymptomatic and do not develop progressive liver injury.

Among patients with symptomatic disease 90 percent are women ages 35 to 60. The earliest symptom is usually pruritus, which may be either generalized or limited initially to the palms and soles. After several months or years, jaundice and gradual darkening of the exposed areas of the skin (melanosis) may ensue. Other early clinical manifestations of primary biliary cirrhosis reflect impaired bile excretion. These include steatorrhea and the malabsorption of lipid-soluble vitamins often resulting in easy bruising (vitamin K deficiency), bone pain due to osteomalacia (vitamin D deficiency), occasionally night blindness (vitamin A deficiency), and dermatitis (possibly vitamin E and/or essential fatty acid deficiency). Protracted elevation of serum lipids, especially cholesterol, leads to subcutaneous lipid deposition around the eyes (xanthelasmas) and over joints and tendons (xanthomas). Over a period of months to years, the itching, jaundice, and hyperpigmentation slowly worsen. Eventually signs of hepatocellular failure and portal hypertension develop and ascites appears. Death due to hepatic insufficiency usually occurs within 5 to 10 years after the first signs of the illness and is often precipitated by uncontrolled variceal hemorrhage or infection.

Physical examination may be entirely normal in the early phase of the disease, when patients are asymptomatic or pruritus is the sole complaint. Later there may be jaundice of varying intensity, hyperpigmentation of the exposed skin areas, xanthelasmas and tendinous and planar xanthomas, moderate to striking hepatomegaly, splenomegaly, and clubbing of the fingers. Bone tenderness, signs of vertebral compression, ecchymoses, glossitis, and dermatitis may all be noted. Clinical evidence of the sicca syndrome can be found in as many as 75 percent of patients, and serologic evidence of autoimmune thyroid disease in 25 percent. Other conditions encountered with increased frequency include rheumatoid arthritis, CRST syndrome, scleroderma, pernicious anemia, and renal tubular acidosis.

LABORATORY FINDINGS Primary biliary cirrhosis is increasingly diagnosed at a presymptomatic stage, prompted by the finding of a two- to fivefold elevation of the serum alkaline phosphatase during routine screening. Serum 5′-nucleotidase activity is also elevated. In this setting, serum bilirubin and aminotransferase levels are usually normal, but the diagnosis is supported by a positive antimitochondrial antibody test (titer > 1:40). The latter is both *relatively* specific and sensitive; a positive test is found in over 90 percent of symptomatic patients. As the disease evolves, the serum bilirubin level rises progressively and may reach 30 mg/dL or more in the final stages. Serum aminotransferase values rarely exceed 150 to 200 units. Hyperlipidemia is common, and a striking increase of the serum unesterified cholesterol is often noted. An abnormal serum lipoprotein (lipoprotein X) may be present in primary biliary cirrhosis but is not specific and appears in other cholestatic conditions. A deficiency of bile salts in the intestine leads to moderate steatorrhea and impaired absorption of the fat-soluble vitamins and hypoprothrombinemia. Patients with primary biliary cirrhosis have elevated liver copper levels, but this finding is not specific and is found in all disorders in which there is prolonged cholestasis.

Diagnosis Primary biliary cirrhosis should be considered in middle-aged women with unexplained pruritus or an elevated serum alkaline phosphatase and in whom there may be other clinical or laboratory features of protracted impairment in biliary excretion. Although a positive serum antimitochondrial antibody determination provides important diagnostic evidence, false-positive results do occur, and therefore liver biopsy should be performed to confirm the diagnosis. In most cases the biliary tract should be evaluated to exclude remediable extrahepatic biliary tract obstruction especially in view of the frequent presence of coexisting cholelithiasis.

Treatment There is no specific therapy for primary biliary cirrhosis. Corticosteroids are ineffective and may actually worsen the bone disease. D-Penicillamine has been tried because of its ability to chelate copper and because of its possible antifibrotic and immunomodulating activities. However, the drug appears to be ineffective and has a high incidence of unacceptable side effects. Some have suggested that azathioprine may be helpful in slowing the progression of disease.

Treatment is generally directed toward the relief of symptoms. Although the mechanism of the protracted pruritus is not entirely clear, cholestyramine, an oral bile salt–sequestering resin, may be helpful in doses of 8 to 12 g per day to decrease both the pruritus and the hypercholesterolemia. Steatorrhea can be reduced by a low-fat diet and substituting medium-chain triglycerides for dietary long-chain triglycerides. Fat-soluble vitamins A and K should be given by parenteral injection at regular intervals to prevent or correct night blindness and hypoprothrombinemia, respectively. Zinc supplementation may be necessary if night blindness is refractory to vitamin A therapy. Osteomalacia may be ameliorated by dietary calcium supplements in conjunction with oral vitamin D. In advanced disease, $25(OH)D_3$ or $1,25(OH_2)D_3$ may be preferred to vitamin D since poor hepatic function may limit conversion of vitamin D to the active metabolites. The management of ascites, variceal hemorrhage, and encephalopathy is described below. The role of hepatic transplantation for patients with primary biliary cirrhosis is under study; this may offer the best, and only, hope for survival in patients with end-stage disease.

SECONDARY BILIARY CIRRHOSIS Etiology Secondary biliary cirrhosis results from prolonged partial or total obstruction of the common bile duct or its major branches. In adults, obstruction is most frequently caused by postoperative strictures or gallstones, usually with superimposed infectious cholangitis. Chronic pancreatitis may lead to biliary stricture and secondary cirrhosis. Secondary biliary cirrhosis may also develop in patients with pericholangitis or idiopathic sclerosing cholangitis. Patients with malignant tumors of the common bile duct or pancreas rarely survive long enough to develop secondary biliary cirrhosis. In children, congenital biliary atresia and cystic fibrosis are common causes of secondary biliary cirrhosis. Choledochal cysts if unrecognized may also be a rare cause of secondary biliary cirrhosis.

Pathology and pathogenesis Unrelieved obstruction of the extrahepatic bile ducts leads to (1) bile stasis and focal areas of centrilobular necrosis followed by periportal necrosis, (2) proliferation and dilatation of the portal bile ducts and ductules, (3) sterile or infected cholangitis with accumulation of polymorphonuclear infiltrates around bile ducts, and (4) progressive expansion of portal tracts by edema and fibrosis. Extravasation of bile from ruptured interlobular bile ducts into areas of periportal necrosis leads to the formation of "bile lakes" surrounded by cholesterol-rich pseudoxanthomatous cells. As in other forms of cirrhosis injury is accompanied by regeneration in residual parenchyma. These changes gradually lead to a finely nodular cirrhosis. In general, at least 3 to 12 months is required for biliary obstruction to result in cirrhosis. Relief of the obstruction is frequently accompanied by biochemical and morphologic improvement.

Clinical features SIGNS AND SYMPTOMS The signs and symptoms of secondary biliary cirrhosis are similar to those of primary biliary cirrhosis. Jaundice and pruritus are usually the most prominent features. In addition, fever and/or right upper quadrant pain, reflecting bouts of cholangitis or biliary colic, are typical. The manifestations of portal hypertension are found only in advanced cases.

LABORATORY TESTS Elevation in serum alkaline phosphatase and conjugated hyperbilirubinemia are nearly always present. There is a moderate increase in serum aminotransferases. When the disease is complicated by cholangitis, elevations in aminotransferase levels and leukocytosis are more pronounced. As in primary biliary cirrhosis, there are abnormalities in serum lipids (including the presence of lipoprotein X) and laboratory findings consistent with steatorrhea. However, the antimitochondrial antibody test is usually negative.

Diagnosis Secondary biliary cirrhosis should be considered in any patient with clinical and laboratory evidence of prolonged obstruction to bile flow, especially when there is a history of previous biliary tract surgery or gallstones, bouts of ascending cholangitis, or right upper quadrant pain. Cholangiography (either percutaneous or endoscopic) usually demonstrates the underlying pathologic process. Liver biopsy, although not always necessary from a clinical standpoint, can document the development of cirrhosis.

Treatment Relief of obstruction to bile flow, by either surgical or endoscopic means, is the most important step in the prevention and therapy of secondary biliary cirrhosis. Effective decompression of the biliary tract results in a significant improvement in both symptoms and survival, even in patients with established cirrhosis. When obstruction cannot be relieved, as in sclerosing cholangitis, antibiotics may be helpful acutely in controlling superimposed infection or, when administered on a chronic basis, as prophylactic therapy in suppressing recurring episodes of ascending cholangitis. Without relief of obstruction, there is a steady progression to end-stage cirrhosis and its terminal manifestations.

CARDIAC CIRRHOSIS

Definition Prolonged, severe right-sided congestive heart failure may lead to chronic liver injury and cardiac cirrhosis. The characteristic pathologic features of fibrosis and regenerative nodules distinguish cardiac cirrhosis from both reversible passive congestion of the liver due to acute heart failure and acute hepatocellular necrosis ("ischemic hepatitis" or "shock liver") resulting from systemic hypotension and hypoperfusion of the liver.

Etiology and pathology In right-sided heart failure, retrograde transmission of elevated venous pressure via the inferior vena cava and hepatic veins leads to congestion of the liver. Hepatic sinusoids become dilated and engorged with blood, and the liver becomes tensely swollen. With prolonged passive congestion and ischemia from poor perfusion secondary to reduced cardiac output, necrosis of centrilobular hepatocytes ensues and leads to fibrosis in these central areas. Ultimately centrilobular fibrosis develops with collagen extending outward in a characteristic stellate pattern from the central vein. Gross examination of the liver shows alternating red (congested) and pale (fibrotic) areas, a pattern often referred to as "nutmeg liver." Improvement in management of cardiac disorders, particularly advances in surgical treatment, has reduced the frequency of cardiac cirrhosis.

Clinical features In acute passive congestion, the liver becomes enlarged and tender, and the patient may complain of severe right upper quadrant pain due to stretching of Glisson's capsule. The serum bilirubin is usually only mildly increased and may be predominantly either conjugated or unconjugated. The AST level is mildly elevated but may be transiently very high following a period of marked systemic hypotension (shock liver), when the clinical picture can mimic acute viral or drug-induced hepatitis. The serum albumin and prothrombin are usually normal, but may become abnormal in shock liver or with the development of cirrhosis. In cases of tricuspid insufficiency the liver may be pulsatile, but this finding disappears as cirrhosis develops. With prolonged right-sided heart failure the liver is enlarged, firm, and usually nontender. The signs and symptoms of heart failure usually overshadow the liver disease. Bleeding from esophageal varices is rare, but chronic encephalopathy may be prominent with a waxing and waning course reflecting variations in the severity of right-sided heart failure. Ascites and peripheral edema, often primarily related to the underlying cardiac dysfunction, may be worsened by the superimposed liver disease.

Diagnosis The presence of a firm, enlarged liver with signs of chronic liver disease in a patient with valvular heart disease, constrictive pericarditis, or cor pulmonale of long duration (>10 years) should suggest cardiac cirrhosis. Liver biopsy can confirm the diagnosis but is usually contraindicated because of coagulopathy or ascites. Coexistent chronic heart and liver disease should also raise the possibility of hemochromatosis, amyloidosis, or other infiltrative diseases.

Budd-Chiari syndrome resulting from the occlusion of the hepatic veins or inferior vena cava may be confused with acute congestive hepatomegaly. In this condition the liver is grossly enlarged and tender, and severe intractable ascites is present. However, signs and symptoms of heart failure are notably absent. The most common cause is thrombosis of the hepatic veins, often in the setting of polycythemia rubra vera, myeloproliferative syndromes, paroxysmal nocturnal hemoglobinuria, or other hypercoagulable states; it may also result from invasion of the inferior vena cava by tumor, such as renal cell or primary hepatocellular carcinoma. Idiopathic membranous obstruction of the inferior vena cava is the most common cause of this syndrome in Japan. Hepatic venography or liver biopsy showing centrilobular congestion and sinusoidal dilatation in the absence of right-sided heart failure establishes the diagnosis of Budd-Chiari syndrome. Venocclusive disease affecting the sublobular branches of the hepatic veins and the hepatic venules may result from hepatic irradiation, treatment with some antineoplastic agents, use of oral contraceptives, or ingestion of pyrrolidizine alkaloids present in some herbal teas ("bush tea disease") and can mimic congestive hepatomegaly.

Treatment Prevention or treatment of cardiac cirrhosis depends on the diagnosis and therapy of the underlying cardiovascular disorder. Improvement in cardiac function frequently results in improvement of liver function and stabilization of the liver disease.

METABOLIC, HEREDITARY, DRUG-RELATED, AND OTHER TYPES OF CIRRHOSIS (See Table 249-1). Cirrhosis or hepatitis may result from a wide variety of other processes encompassing the spectrum of etiologic factors listed in Table 249-2. Although some of these disorders have distinctive clinical or morphologic features, the manifestations of cirrhosis are largely independent of the underlying pathogenic mechanism.

TABLE 249-2 Some causes of noncirrhotic hepatic fibrosis

1 Idiopathic portal hypertension (noncirrhotic portal fibrosis, Banti's syndrome); three variants:
a Intrahepatic phlebosclerosis and fibrosis
b Portal and splenic vein sclerosis
c Portal and splenic vein thrombosis
2 Schistosomiasis ("pipe-stem" fibrosis with presinusoidal portal hypertension)
3 Congenital hepatic fibrosis (may be associated with polycystic disease of liver and kidneys)

NONCIRRHOTIC FIBROSIS OF THE LIVER Several diseases, either congenital or acquired, may be associated with localized or generalized hepatic fibrosis. They are distinguished from cirrhosis by the absence of hepatocellular damage and the lack of nodular regenerative activity. The clinical manifestations in such cases are largely secondary to portal hypertension. The different types of these disorders are indicated in Table 294-2; with the exception of schistosomiasis, all these conditions are relatively rare.

MAJOR SEQUELAE OF CIRRHOSIS

The clinical course of patients with advanced cirrhosis is usually complicated by a number of important sequelae which are independent of the etiology of the underlying liver disease. These include portal hypertension and its consequences (i.e., gastroesophageal varices and splenomegaly), ascites, hepatic encephalopathy, spontaneous bacterial peritonitis, hepatorenal syndrome, and hepatocellular carcinoma.

PORTAL HYPERTENSION Definition and pathogenesis Normal pressure in the portal vein is low (10 and 15 cm saline; 7 to 10 mmHg) because vascular resistance in the hepatic sinusoids is minimal. Portal hypertension (>30 cm saline) most commonly results from increased resistance to portal blood flow. Because the portal venous system lacks valves, resistance at any level between the heart and splanchnic vessels results in retrograde transmission of an elevated pressure. Increased resistance can occur at three levels relative to the hepatic sinusoids: (1) presinusoidal, (2) sinusoidal, and (3) postsinusoidal. Obstruction in the *presinusoidal* venous compartment may be anatomically outside of the liver (e.g., portal vein thrombosis) or within the liver itself but at a functional level proximal to the hepatic sinusoids so that the liver parenchyma is not exposed to the elevated venous pressure (e.g., schistosomiasis). *Postsinusoidal* obstruction may also occur outside the liver at the level of the hepatic veins (e.g., Budd-Chiari syndrome), the inferior vena cava, or, less commonly, within the liver (e.g., venocclusive disease in which the central hepatic venules are the primary site of injury). When cirrhosis is complicated by portal hypertension, the increased resistance is usually sinusoidal. While distinctions between pre-, post-, and sinusoidal processes are conceptually appealing, functional resistance to portal flow in a given patient may occur at more than one level. Portal hypertension may also arise from increased blood flow (e.g., massive splenomegaly or arteriovenous fistulas), but the low-outflow resistance of the normal liver makes this a rare clinical problem.

Cirrhosis is the most common cause of portal hypertension in the United States. Clinically significant portal hypertension is present in greater than 60 percent of patients with cirrhosis. *Portal vein obstruction* is the second most common cause; it may be idiopathic or occur in association with cirrhosis, infection, pancreatitis, or abdominal trauma. *Hepatic vein thrombosis* (Budd-Chiari syndrome) and hepatic venocclusive disease are relatively infrequent causes of portal hypertension (see above). Portal vein occlusion may result in massive hematemesis from gastroesophageal varices, but ascites is usually found only when cirrhosis is also present. Noncirrhotic portal fibrosis accounts for only a small number of patients with portal hypertension.

Clinical features The major clinical manifestations of portal hypertension include hemorrhage from gastroesophageal varices, splenomegaly with hypersplenism, ascites, and acute and chronic hepatic encephalopathy. All of these features are related, at least in part, to the development of portal-systemic collateral channels. The absence of valves in the portal venous system facilitates retrograde (hepatofugal) blood flow from the high-pressure portal venous system to the lower-pressure systemic venous circulation. Major sites of collateral flow involve the veins around the rectum (hemorrhoids), cardioesophageal junction (esophagogastric varices), retroperitoneal space, and the falciform ligament of the liver (periumbilical or abdominal wall collaterals). Abdominal wall collaterals appear as tortuous epigastric vessels that radiate from the umbilicus toward the xiphoid and rib margins (caput medusae).

Diagnosis In patients with known liver disease, the development of portal hypertension usually becomes evident by the appearance of splenomegaly, ascites, encephalopathy, and/or esophageal varices. Conversely, the finding of any of these features should lead one to evaluate the patient for the presence of underlying portal hypertension and liver disease. Varices may be documented by either barium swallow or fiberoptic esophagoscopy and lend indirect support to the diagnosis of portal hypertension. Although rarely necessary, portal venous pressure may be measured directly by percutaneous transhepatic ''skinny needle'' catheterization or indirectly through transjugular cannulation of the hepatic veins. Both free and wedged hepatic vein pressure (WHVP) should be measured. While WHVP is elevated in sinusoidal and postsinusoidal portal hypertension including cirrhosis, this measurement is usually normal in presinusoidal portal hypertension. In patients in whom additional information is necessary (e.g., preoperative evaluation before portal-systemic shunt surgery) or percutaneous catheterization is not feasible, mesenteric and hepatic angiography may be helpful. Particular attention should be directed to the venous phase to assess the patency of the portal vein and the direction of portal blood flow.

Treatment Although treatment is usually directed toward a specific complication of portal hypertension, attempts are sometimes made to reduce the pressure in the portal venous system. Surgical decompression procedures have been used for many years to lower portal pressure in patients with bleeding esophageal varices (see below). However, portal-systemic shunt surgery does not result in improved survival rates in patients with cirrhosis. There are also reports that beta-adrenergic receptor blockers, such as propranolol, may reduce portal venous pressure. The efficacy of pharmacologic agents in this setting, however, remains controversial and unproven.

Vigorous treatment of patients with alcoholic hepatitis and cirrhosis, chronic active hepatitis, and other liver diseases may lead to a fall in portal pressure and to a reduction in variceal size. In general, however, portal hypertension due to cirrhosis is not reversible. In selected patients hepatic transplantation may be beneficial (e.g., end-stage primary biliary cirrhosis).

VARICEAL BLEEDING Pathogenesis While vigorous hemorrhage may arise from any portal-systemic venous collaterals, bleeding is most common from varices in the region of the gastroesophageal junction. The factors contributing to bleeding from gastroesophageal varices are not entirely understood but include the degree of portal hypertension and the size of the varices. Esophagitis with erosion of underlying varices does not appear to play an important role.

Clinical features and diagnosis Variceal bleeding often occurs without obvious precipitating factors and usually presents with painless but massive hematemesis with or without melena. Associated signs range from mild postural tachycardia to profound shock, depending on the extent of blood loss and degree of hypovolemia. Because patients with varices may bleed from other gastrointestinal lesions (e.g., peptic ulcer, gastritis), in most cases exclusion of other bleeding sources is important even in patients with prior variceal hemorrhage. Fiberoptic endoscopy is the procedure of choice in evaluating upper gastrointestinal hemorrhage in patients with known or suspected portal hypertension.

Treatment Variceal bleeding is a life-threatening emergency. Prompt estimation and vigorous replacement of blood losses to maintain intravascular volume are essential and take precedence over diagnostic studies and more specific intervention to stop the bleeding. Replacement of clotting factors with fresh frozen plasma is important in patients with coagulopathy. Patients are best managed in an intensive care unit and often require close monitoring of central venous or pulmonary capillary wedge pressures, urine output, and mental status. Only when the patient is hemodynamically stable should attention be directed toward specific diagnostic studies (especially endoscopy) and other therapeutic modalities to prevent further or recurrent bleeding.

About half of all episodes of variceal hemorrhage cease without intervention, although the risk of rebleeding is very high. The medical management of acute variceal hemorrhage includes the use of vasoconstrictors (vasopressin), balloon tamponade, and endoscopic sclerosis of varices (sclerotherapy). Intravenous infusion of *vasopressin* at a rate of 0.1 to 0.9 units per minute results in generalized vasoconstriction leading to diminished blood flow in the portal venous system. Intravenous infusion of vasopressin has been shown to be as effective as selective intraarterial administration. Control of bleeding can be achieved in up to 80 percent of cases, but bleeding recurs in more than half after the vasopressin is tapered and discontinued. Furthermore, a number of serious side effects, including cardiac and gastrointestinal tract ischemia, acute renal failure, and hyponatremia, may be associated with vasopressin therapy. *Balloon tamponade* of the bleeding varices may be accomplished with a triple-lumen (Sengstaken-Blakemore) or four-lumen (Minnesota) tube with esophageal and gastric balloons. After the tube is introduced into the stomach, the gastric balloon is inflated and pulled back into the cardia of the stomach. If bleeding does not stop, the esophageal balloon is inflated for additional tamponade. Careful monitoring for complications such as esophageal rupture is essential. *Endoscopic sclerosis* of esophageal varices may be employed if the above measures are ineffective in controlling bleeding. In this procedure, the varices are injected with one of several sclerosing agents (e.g., sodium morrhuate) via a needle-tipped catheter passed through the endoscope. After initial endoscopic identification of varices as the presumed source of bleeding, such ''sclerotherapy'' controls acute bleeding in up to 90 percent of cases. In addition, repeated sclerotherapy until obliteration of all varices is accomplished should be performed in an effort to prevent recurrent bleeding. While available data support the efficacy of sclerotherapy in controlling bleeding acutely, further studies are needed to define the technique and the overall role of sclerotherapy in the management of variceal bleeding. Transhepatic sclerosis via ''skinny needle'' puncture has also been used in a limited number of centers although its reported efficacy has varied widely. The role of beta-adrenergic blocking agents in reducing the risk of recurrent hemorrhage remains uncertain.

Surgical therapy of portal hypertension and variceal bleeding involves the creation of a portal-systemic shunt to permit decompression of the portal system. Two types of portal systemic shunts have been used: *nonselective shunts* to decompress the entire portal system and *selective shunts* intended to decompress only the varices while maintaining blood flow to the liver itself. Nonselective shunts include end-to-side or side-to-side portacaval and proximal splenorenal anastomoses; selective shunts include the distal splenorenal shunt. Nonselective shunts are more likely to be complicated by encephalopathy than selective shunts. Emergency portal-systemic nonselective shunts may control acute hemorrhage, but such surgery is usually used only as a last resort because early operative mortality is greater than 30 percent. The role of portal-systemic shunt surgery after initial control of bleeding by nonoperative means is also uncertain. Surgically created shunts effectively reduce the risk of recurrent hemorrhage, but the overall mortality of patients undergoing such surgery is comparable to that of unoperated patients. Although patients who have undergone portal-system surgery succumb to recurrent bleeding less commonly than unoperated patients, this improvement is counterbalanced by increased morbidity from encephalopathy and death from progressive liver failure. Prophylactic shunt surgery should not be performed in patients with nonbleeding varices. The relative merits of therapeutic portal-systemic shunt surgery and serial endoscopic sclerotherapy in cirrhotics who have bled from varices remain to be determined. Other surgical procedures (e.g., esophageal transection) have also been advocated for the management of acute variceal bleeding although their efficacy remains unproven.

SPLENOMEGALY Definition and pathogenesis Congestive splenomegaly is common in patients with severe portal hypertension. In rare instances, massive splenomegaly from nonhepatic disease may lead to portal hypertension due to increased blood flow in the splenic vein.

Clinical features Although usually asymptomatic, splenomegaly may be massive and contribute to the thrombocytopenia or pancytopenia of cirrhosis. In the absence of cirrhosis, splenomegaly in association with variceal hemorrhage should suggest the possibility of splenic vein thrombosis.

Treatment Splenomegaly usually requires no specific treatment, although massive enlargement of the spleen may occasionally necessitate splenectomy at the time of shunt surgery. Splenectomy may also be indicated if splenomegaly is the cause rather than the result of portal hypertension. Thrombocytopenia alone is rarely severe enough to necessitate removal of the spleen.

ASCITES Definition Ascites is the accumulation of excess fluid within the peritoneal cavity. It is most frequently encountered in patients with cirrhosis and other forms of severe liver disease, but a number of other disorders may lead to either transudative or exudative ascites (see Chap. 39).

Pathogenesis The accumulation of ascitic fluid represents a state of total-body sodium and water excess, but the event that initiates this imbalance is unclear. Two theories have been proposed (see Fig. 249-1). The "underfilling" theory suggests that the primary abnormality is inappropriate sequestration of fluid within the splanchnic vascular bed due to portal hypertension and a consequent decrease in effective circulating blood volume. According to this theory, an apparent decrease in intravascular volume (underfilling) is sensed by the kidney, which responds by retaining salt and water. The "overflow" theory suggests that the primary abnormality is inappropriate renal retention of salt and water in the absence of volume depletion.

FIGURE 249-1 *Multiple factors involved in development of ascites. Current concepts suggest that initiating factor may be either primary sodium retention ("overflow") or diminished effective intravascular volume ("underfilling").*

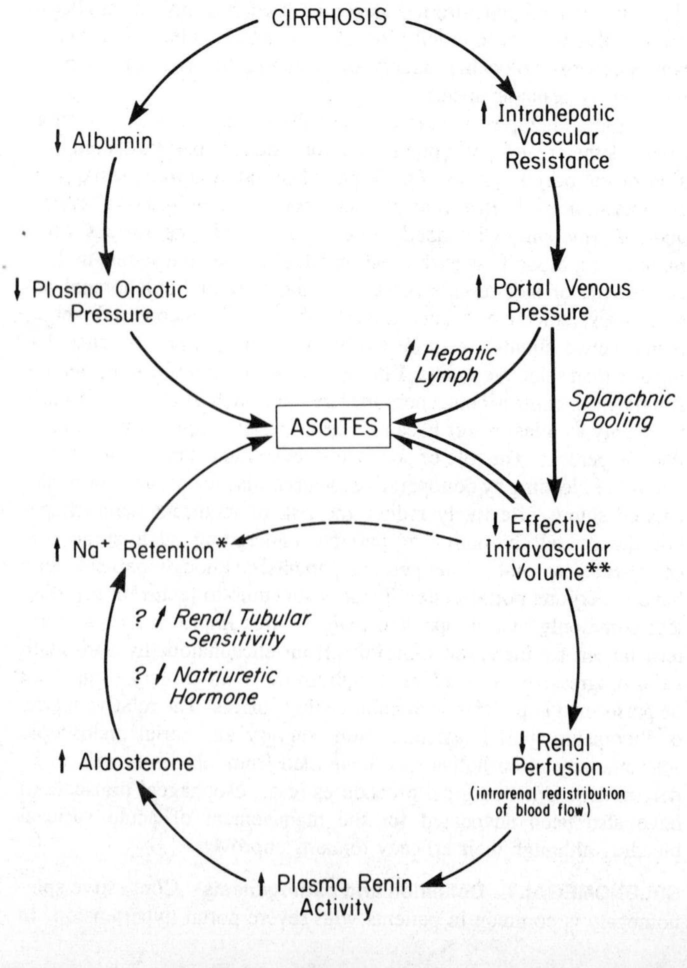

Regardless of the initiating event, a number of factors contribute to accumulation of fluid in the abdominal cavity (see Fig. 249-1). *Portal hypertension* plays an important role in the formation of ascites by raising hydrostatic pressure within the splanchnic capillary bed. *Hypoalbuminemia* and *reduced plasma oncotic pressure* also favor the extravasation of fluid from plasma to peritoneal cavity, and thus ascites is infrequent in patients with cirrhosis unless both portal hypertension and hypoalbuminemia are present. *Hepatic lymph* may weep freely from the surface of the cirrhotic liver due to distortion and obstruction of hepatic sinusoids and lymphatics and contribute to ascites formation. In contrast to the contribution of transudative fluid from the portal vascular bed, hepatic lymph may weep into the peritoneal cavity even in the absence of marked hypoproteinemia because the endothelial lining of the hepatic sinusoids is discontinuous. This mechanism may account for the high protein concentration present in the ascitic fluid of some patients with the Budd-Chiari syndrome.

Renal factors also play an important role in perpetuating ascites. Patients with ascites fail to excrete a water load in a normal fashion. They have increased renal sodium reabsorption by both proximal and distal tubules, the latter due largely to secondary hyperaldosteronism and increased plasma renin activity. Renal vasoconstriction, perhaps resulting from increased serum prostaglandin or catecholamine levels, may also contribute to sodium retention.

Clinical features and diagnosis Usually ascites is first noticed by the patient because of increasing abdominal girth. More pronounced accumulation of fluid may cause shortness of breath because of elevation of the diaphragm. When peritoneal fluid accumulation exceeds 500 mL, ascites may be demonstrated on physical examination by the presence of shifting dullness, a fluid wave, or bulging flanks. Ultrasound examination can detect smaller quantities of ascites and should be performed when physical examination is equivocal. Paracentesis should usually be performed with a small-gauge needle at the time of initial evaluation or at the time of any clinical deterioration of a cirrhotic patient. A small amount of fluid (less than 200 mL) should be obtained and examined for evidence of infection, tumor, or other possible causes and complications of ascites.

Treatment When ascites develops in the setting of severe, acute liver disease, resolution of ascites is likely to follow improvement in liver function. More commonly, ascites develops in patients with stable or steadily worsening liver function. Therapeutic intervention is indicated both to prevent potential complications and to control progressive increase in ascites, which may become pronounced enough to cause physical discomfort. However, overzealous attempts to reduce ascites may deplete the intravascular volume faster than fluid can be mobilized from the ascitic compartment and may precipitate renal failure. Thus, therapy aimed at reducing ascites should be gentle and incremental (see below). The goal is the loss of no more than 1.0 kg daily if both ascites and peripheral edema are present and no more than 0.5 kg daily in patients with ascites alone. To initiate therapy it may be desirable to hospitalize the patient so that daily weights and frequent serum electrolyte levels can be monitored and compliance ensured. Although abdominal girth measurements are frequently used as an index of fluid loss, they tend to be unreliable.

Strict bed rest is often recommended because of improved renal clearance in the supine position. However, salt restriction is the most important cornerstone of therapy. A diet containing 800 mg sodium (2 g NaCl) is often adequate to induce a negative sodium balance and permit diuresis. Response to salt restriction and bed rest alone is more likely to occur if the ascites is of recent onset, the underlying liver disease is reversible, a precipitating factor can be corrected, or the patient has a high urinary sodium excretion (~25 meq per day) and normal renal function. Fluid restriction of approximately 1500 mL per day does little to enhance diuresis but may be necessary to prevent or correct hyponatremia. If sodium restriction alone fails to result in diuresis and weight loss, diuretic therapy should be instituted. Because of the role of hyperaldosteronism in sustaining salt retention, spironolactone or other distal tubular–acting diuretics (triamterene, amiloride) are the drugs of choice. These agents are also preferred because of their gentle action and specific potassium-sparing properties. Spironolactone is initially given in a dose of 25 mg four times a day and increased as needed by 100 mg per day every several days up to a maximum dose of 400 mg daily. An indication of the minimum effective dose of spironolactone may be obtained by monitoring urinary electrolyte concentrations for a rise in sodium and fall in potassium levels reflecting effective competitive inhibition of aldosterone. In some patients, diuresis cannot be initiated despite maximal doses of distal tubule–acting agents (e.g., 400 mg spironolactone) because of avid proximal tubular sodium absorption. When this occurs, more potent and proximally acting diuretics (furosemide, thiazide, or ethacrynic acid) may be added cautiously to the regimen. Spironolactone plus furosemide, 40 or 80 mg daily, is usually sufficient to initiate a diuresis in most patients. However, such aggressive therapy must be used with great caution to avoid plasma volume depletion, azotemia, and hypokalemia which may lead to encephalopathy.

A minority of patients with advanced cirrhosis have "refractory ascites" and fail to respond, despite intensive medical therapy. When this occurs in patients with marked hypoalbuminemia, diuresis may be initiated following cautious intravenous infusion of *salt-poor albumin*. Because of the short half-life of infused albumin, this approach is of short-term benefit and may, in fact, precipitate variceal hemorrhage due to expansion of the intravascular volume. In some patients a side-to-side *portacaval shunt* may result in improvement in ascites although generally these patients are extremely poor surgical risks. Intractable ascites can also be treated with the surgical implantation of a plastic *peritoneovenous shunt* which has a pressure-sensitive, one-way valve allowing ascitic fluid to flow from the abdominal cavity to the superior vena cava. However, the usefulness of this technique is limited by a high rate of complications such as infection, disseminated intravascular coagulation, and thrombosis of the shunt. Although removal of large volumes of ascitic fluid is hazardous, occasionally therapeutic paracentesis of 1 to 2 liters may be needed in patients with massive ascites and pronounced respiratory embarrassment or impending rupture of an umbilical hernia.

SPONTANEOUS BACTERIAL PERITONITIS Patients with ascites and cirrhosis may develop acute bacterial peritonitis without an obvious primary source of infection. Typical features include abrupt onset of fever, chills, generalized abdominal pain, and rebound abdominal tenderness accompanied by cloudy ascitic fluid with a high white cell count and usually positive bacterial cultures. However, the clinical symptoms *may be minimal,* and some patients manifest only worsening jaundice or encephalopathy in the absence of localizing abdominal complaints. The diagnosis is based on careful examination of the ascitic fluid. An ascitic fluid leukocyte count of greater than 500 cells per cubic millimeter or more than 250 polymorphonuclear leukocytes should suggest the possibility of bacterial peritonitis while results of bacterial cultures of ascitic fluid are pending. Empiric therapy with ampicillin and an aminoglycoside or cefotaximene should be initiated when the diagnosis is first suspected because enteric gram-negative bacilli are found in the majority of cases; less frequently the infection is caused by pneumococci and other gram-positive bacteria. Specific antibiotic therapy can be selected once the specific organism is identified. Therapy is usually administered for 10 to 14 days.

HEPATORENAL SYNDROME **Definition and pathogenesis** Hepatorenal syndrome is a serious complication in the patient with cirrhosis and ascites, and is characterized by worsening azotemia with avid sodium retention and oliguria in the absence of identifiable specific causes of renal dysfunction. The exact basis for this syndrome is not clear, but altered renal hemodynamics appear to be involved. The kidneys are structurally intact; urinalysis and pyelography are usually normal. Renal biopsy although rarely needed is also normal, and in fact kidneys from such patients have been successfully used for renal transplantation. There are indications that an imbalance in certain metabolites of arachidonic acid (prostaglandins and thromboxane) may play a pathogenetic role.

Clinical features and diagnosis Worsening azotemia, hyponatremia, progressive oliguria, and hypotension are the hallmarks of the hepatorenal syndrome. This syndrome, which is distinct from prerenal azotemia, may be precipitated by severe gastrointestinal bleeding, sepsis, or overly vigorous attempts at diuresis or paracentesis; it may also occur without an obvious cause. The diagnosis is supported by the demonstration of avid urinary sodium retention. Typically the urine sodium concentration is less than 5 meq per liter, a concentration lower than that generally found in uncomplicated prerenal azotemia. The urinary sediment is unremarkable.

Treatment Treatment is usually unsuccessful. Although some patients with hypotension and decreased plasma volume may respond to infusions of salt-poor albumin, volume expansion must be undertaken with caution to avoid precipitating variceal bleeding. Vasodilator therapy, including intravenous infusion of dopamine, is not effective.

HEPATIC ENCEPHALOPATHY **Definition** Hepatic (portal-systemic) encephalopathy is a complex neuropsychiatric syndrome characterized by disturbances in consciousness and behavior, personality changes, fluctuating neurologic signs, asterixis or "flapping tremor," and distinctive electroencephalographic changes. Encephalopathy may be *acute* and reversible or *chronic* and progressive. In severe cases, irreversible coma and death may occur. Acute episodes may recur with variable frequency.

Pathogenesis The specific cause of hepatic encephalopathy is unknown. The most important factors in the pathogenesis are severe hepatocellular dysfunction and/or intrahepatic and extrahepatic shunting of portal venous blood into the systemic circulation, so that the liver is largely bypassed. As a result of these processes, various toxic substances absorbed from the intestine are not detoxified by the liver and lead to metabolic abnormalities in the central nervous system. Ammonia is the substance most often incriminated in the pathogenesis of encephalopathy. Many, but not all, patients with hepatic encephalopathy have elevated blood ammonia levels, and recovery from encephalopathy is often accompanied by declining blood ammonia levels. Other compounds and metabolites which may contribute to the development of encephalopathy include mercaptans (derived from intestinal metabolism of methionine), short-chain fatty acids, phenol, and gamma-aminobutyric acid (GABA), an inhibitory neurotransmitter. False neurochemical transmitters (e.g., octopamine), resulting in part from alterations in plasma levels of aromatic and branched-chain amino acids, may also play a role. An increase in the permeability of the blood-brain barrier to some of these substances may be an additional factor involved in the pathogenesis of hepatic encephalopathy.

In the patient with otherwise stable cirrhosis, hepatic encephalopathy often follows a clearly identifiable precipitating event (see Table 249-3). Perhaps the most common predisposing factor is *gastrointestinal bleeding,* which leads to an increase in the production of ammonia and other nitrogenous substances which are then absorbed. Similarly, *increased dietary protein* may precipitate encephalopathy as a result of increased production of nitrogenous substances by colonic bacteria. *Electrolyte disturbances,* particularly hypokalemic alkalosis secondary to overzealous use of diuretics, vigorous paracentesis, or vomiting, may precipitate hepatic encephalopathy. Systemic alkalosis causes an increase in the amount of nonionic ammonia (NH_3) relative to ammonium ions (NH_4^+). Only nonionic (uncharged) ammonia readily crosses the blood-brain barrier and accumulates in the central nervous system. Hypokalemia also directly stimulates renal ammonia production. Hypoxia, injudicious use of central nervous system–depressing drugs (e.g., barbiturates, benzodiazepines), and acute infection may trigger or aggravate hepatic encephalopathy, although the mechanisms involved are not clear. Other potential precipitating factors include superimposed acute viral hepatitis, alcoholic hepatitis, extrahepatic bile duct obstruction, surgery, and other coincidental medical complications.

Clinical features and diagnosis Hepatic encephalopathy has protean manifestations, and any neurologic abnormality, including focal deficits, may be encountered. In patients with acute encephalopathy, neurologic deficits are completely reversible upon correction of underlying precipitating factors and/or improvement in liver function, but in patients with chronic encephalopathy the deficits may be irreversible and progressive. Cerebral edema is frequently present and contributes to the clinical picture and overall mortality in patients with both acute and chronic encephalopathy.

The diagnosis of hepatic encephalopathy should be considered when four major factors are present: (1) acute or chronic hepatocellular disease and/or extensive portal-systemic collateral shunts (the latter may be either spontaneous, e.g., secondary to portal hypertension, or surgically created, e.g., portacaval anastomosis); (2) disturbances of awareness and mentation which may progress from forgetfulness and confusion to stupor and finally coma; (3) shifting combinations of neurologic signs, including asterixis, rigidity, hyperreflexia, extensor plantar signs, and rarely, seizures; and (4) a characteristic (but nonspecific) symmetric, high-voltage, slow-wave (2 to 5 per second) pattern on the electroencephalogram. Asterixis (''liver flap,'' ''flapping tremor'') is a nonrhythmic asymmetric lapse in voluntary sustained position of the extremities, head, and trunk. It is best demonstrated by having the patient extend the arms and dorsiflex the hands. Because elicitation of asterixis depends on sustained voluntary muscle contraction, it is not present in the comatose patient. Asterixis is nonspecific and also occurs in patients with other forms of metabolic brain disease. Alterations in personality, mood disturbances, confusion, deterioration in self-care and handwriting, and daytime somnolence are additional clinical features of encephalopathy. *Fetor hepaticus,* a unique musty odor of the breath and urine believed to be due to mercaptans, may be noted in patients with varying stages of hepatic encephalopathy. Some patients may develop spastic paraparesis or *chronic progressive hepatocerebral degeneration,* the latter a clinical variant of hepatic encephalopathy characterized by a slow decline in intellectual function, tremor, cerebellar ataxia, choreoathetosis, and psychiatric symptoms.

Grading or classifying the stages of hepatic encephalopathy is often helpful in following the course of the illness and assessing response to therapy. One useful classification is shown in Table 249-4.

The diagnosis of hepatic encephalopathy is usually one of exclusion. There are no diagnostic liver function test abnormalities, although an elevated serum ammonia level in the appropriate clinical setting is highly suggestive of the diagnosis. Examination of the cerebrospinal fluid is unremarkable, and computerized tomography of the brain shows no characteristic abnormalities. A number of conditions, particularly disorders related to acute and chronic alcoholism, can mimic the clinical features of hepatic encephalopathy. These include acute alcohol intoxication, sedative overdose, delirium tremens, Wernicke's encephalopathy, and Korsakoff's psychosis (see Chap. 349). Subdural hematoma, meningitis, and hypoglycemia or other metabolic encephalopathies must also be considered, especially in patients with alcoholic cirrhosis. In young patients with liver disease and neurologic abnormalities, Wilson's disease should be excluded.

TABLE 249-3 Common precipitants of hepatic encephalopathy

1 Increased nitrogen load
- *a* Gastrointestinal bleeding
- *b* Excess dietary protein
- *c* Azotemia
- *d* Constipation

2 Electrolyte imbalance
- *a* Hypokalemia
- *b* Alkalosis
- *c* Hypoxia
- *d* Hypovolemia

3 Drugs
- *a* Narcotics, tranquilizers, sedatives
- *b* Diuretics (see *2*)

4 Miscellaneous
- *a* Infection
- *b* Surgery
- *c* Superimposed acute liver disease
- *d* Progressive liver disease

Treatment Early recognition and prompt treatment of hepatic encephalopathy are essential. Patients with acute, severe hepatic encephalopathy (stage IV) require the usual supportive measures for the comatose patient. Specific treatment of hepatic encephalopathy is aimed at (1) elimination or treatment of precipitating factors and (2) lowering of blood ammonia (and other toxin) levels by decreasing the absorption of protein and nitrogenous products from the intestine. In the setting of acute gastrointestinal bleeding, blood in the bowel should be promptly evacuated with enemas and laxatives in order to reduce the nitrogen load. Protein should be excluded from the diet, and constipation should be avoided. Ammonia absorption can be decreased by the administration of lactulose, a nonabsorbable disaccharide that acts as an osmotic laxative. Metabolism of lactulose by colonic bacteria may also result in an acid pH that favors conversion of ammonia to the poorly absorbed ammonium ion. In addition lactulose may actually diminish ammonia production through its direct effects on bacterial metabolism. Lactulose syrup can be administered in a dose of 30 to 50 mL every hour until diarrhea occurs; thereafter the dose is adjusted (usually 15 to 30 mL three times daily) so that the patient has two to four soft stools daily. Intestinal ammonia production by bacteria can also be decreased by oral administration of the antibiotic neomycin, at a dose of 0.5 to 1.0 g every 6 h. Although poorly absorbed, neomycin may reach sufficient concentrations in the bloodstream to cause renal toxicity. The use of agents such as levodopa, bromocriptine, keto-analogues of essential amino acids, and intravenous amino acid formulations rich in branched-chain amino acids in the treatment of acute hepatic encephalopathy remain of unproven benefit. Hemoperfusion to remove toxic substances and therapy directed primarily toward coincident cerebral edema in acute encephalopathy are also of unproven value.

Chronic encephalopathy may be effectively controlled by administration of lactulose. Management of patients with chronic encephalopathy should include dietary protein restriction, sometimes to levels as low as 40 g daily, in combination with low doses of lactulose or neomycin. Nephrotoxicity or ototoxicity may be limiting in prolonged usage of neomycin. There are suggestions that vegetable protein may be preferable to animal protein.

OTHER SEQUELAE OF CIRRHOSIS Coagulopathy Patients with cirrhosis often demonstrate a variety of abnormalities in both cellular and humoral clotting function. Thrombocytopenia may result from hypersplenism. In the alcoholic patient, there may be direct bone marrow suppression by ethanol. Diminished protein synthesis may lead to reduced production of fibrinogen (factor I), prothrombin (factor II), and factors V, VII, IX, and X. Reduction in levels of all

TABLE 294-4 Clinical stages of hepatic encephalopathy

Stage	Mental status	Asterixis	EEG
I	Euphoria or depression, mild confusion, slurred speech, disordered sleep	+/−	Usually normal
II	Lethargy, moderate confusion	+	Abnormal
III	Marked confusion, incoherent speech, sleeping but arousable	+	Abnormal
IV	Coma; initially responsive to noxious stimuli, later unresponsive	−	Abnormal

factors except factor V may be worsened by the coincident malabsorption of the fat-soluble cofactor vitamin K due to cholestasis (see Chap. 237). Recent reports have documented the appearance of normal factor VIII levels following liver transplantation in patients with classical hemophilia probably as a result of production by nonhepatocellular components of the donor organ.

Hepatocellular carcinoma (See Chap. 250.)

REFERENCES

Alcoholic and postnecrotic cirrhosis

BARRY RE, MCGIVAN JD: Acetaldehyde alone may initiate hepatocellular damage in acute alcoholic liver disease. Gut 26:1065, 1985
BOROWSKY SA et al: Continued heavy drinking and survival in alcoholic cirrhotics. Gastroenterology 80:1405, 1981
POWELL WJ, KLATSKIN G: Duration of survival in patients with Laennec's cirrhosis. Am J Med 44:406, 1968
SØRENSEN TIA et al: Prospective evaluation of alcohol abuse and alcoholic liver injury in man as predictors of development of cirrhosis. Lancet 2:241, 1984
THEODOSSI A et al: Controlled trial of methylprednisolone therapy in severe acute alcoholic hepatitis. Gut 23:75, 1982
VAN THIEL DH et al: Gastrointestinal and hepatic manifestations of chronic alcoholism. Gastroenterology 81:594, 1981
ZETTERMAN RK, SORRELL MF: Immunologic aspects of alcoholic liver disease. Gastroenterology 81:616, 1981

Biliary cirrhosis

BESWICK DR et al: Asymptomatic primary biliary cirrhosis: A progress report on long-term follow-up and natural history. Gastroenterology 89:267, 1985
CHRISTENSEN E et al: Beneficial effects of azathioprine and predictor of prognosis in primary biliary cirrhosis: Final results of an international trial. Gastroenterology 89:1084, 1985
JAMES O et al: Primary biliary cirrhosis—a revised clinical spectrum. Lancet 1:1278, 1981
NEUBERGER J et al: Double-blind controlled trial of D-penicillamine in patients with primary biliary cirrhosis. Gut 26:114, 1985

Hepatic encephalopathy

ATTERBURY CE et al: Neomycin-sorbitol and lactulose in the treatment of acute portal-systemic encephalopathy. Am J Digest Dis 23:398, 1978
CONN HO et al: Comparison of lactulose and neomycin in the treatment of chronic portal-systemic encephalopathy: A double-blind controlled trial. Gastroenterology 72:573, 1977
DUDLEY FJ et al: Hepatorenal syndrome without avid sodium retention. Hepatology 6:248, 1986
FRASER CL, ARIEFF AI: Hepatic encephalopathy. N Engl J Med 313:865, 1985
JONES EA et al: The neurobiology of hepatic encephalopathy. Hepatology 4:1235, 1984

Portal hypertension and ascites

CELLO JP et al: Endoscopic sclerotherapy versus portacaval shunt in patients with severe cirrhosis and variceal hemorrhage. N Engl J Med 311:1589, 1984
CROSSLEY JR, WILLIAMS R: Spontaneous bacterial peritonitis. Gut 26:325, 1985
EPSTEIN FM: Underfilling versus overflow in hepatic ascites. N Engl J Med 307:1577, 1982
EPSTEIN M: The sodium retention of cirrhosis: A reappraisal. Hepatology 6:312, 1986
LEBREC D et al: The effect of propranolol on portal hypertension in patients with cirrhosis. Hepatology 2:523, 1982
MACDOUGALL BRD et al: Increased long-term survival in variceal haemorrhage using injection sclerotherapy: Results of a controlled trial. Lancet 1:124, 1982
MILLIKAN WJ et al: The Emory prospective randomized trial: Selective versus nonselective shunt to control variceal bleeding. Ann Surg 201:712, 1985
NICHOLLS KM et al: Sodium excretion in advanced cirrhosis: Effect of expansion of central blood volume and suppression of plasma aldosterone. Hepatology 6:235, 1986

250 TUMORS OF THE LIVER

ELLIOT ALPERT / KURT J. ISSELBACHER

PRIMARY CARCINOMA Carcinomas arising within the liver may be of liver cell (*hepatocellular*), bile duct cell (*cholangiocellular*), or mixed origin. Hepatocellular carcinoma (primary liver cell carcinoma) accounts for 80 to 90 percent of liver carcinomas. There is, however, little practical purpose in distinguishing between the two types, since both may be found in different parts of the same tumor and the clinical courses are similar.

Epidemiology and etiology Primary liver cancers account for only 1 to 2 percent of malignant tumors found at autopsy in North and South America and Europe. However, in parts of Africa and Asia they may account for up to 20 to 30 percent of all types of malignancy. Liver cell carcinoma occurs two to four times more frequently in men than in women. The peak incidence occurs in the fifth and sixth decades of life in the United States, but one to two decades earlier in areas with a high prevalence of liver carcinoma. Cirrhosis, usually macronodular or postnecrotic, is found in 60 to 75 percent of autopsied patients with primary liver cell carcinoma in all parts of the world.

There is wide variation in the incidence of hepatocellular carcinoma in different parts of the world, and a number of etiologic factors may be important.

1 *Chronic liver disease* of any etiology appears to predispose to the development of carcinoma. A variety of metabolic, alcoholic, viral, or idiopathic chronic liver diseases can lead to liver cell carcinoma. Alpha$_1$-antitrypsin deficiency and hereditary tyrosinosis, with active liver disease since birth, have a high incidence of developing into carcinoma. In the adult age group, *hemochromatosis* has the highest risk of malignant degeneration, presumably owing to the long duration of the chronic liver inflammation. However, alcoholic and postnecrotic cirrhosis are the most common forms of underlying liver disease in patients with liver carcinoma in the United States.
2 *Viral hepatitis* is endemic in many areas of Africa and Asia. The prevalence of hepatitis B antigenemia in the normal population is 1 to 10 percent in some parts of Africa. In these areas, most patients with hepatocellular carcinoma superimposed on chronic liver disease will have serologic evidence of hepatitis B infection. There is also evidence of the integration of the hepatitis B virus DNA (HBV-DNA) into the genome of liver cells in some patients with prior HB infection, and most patients with long-standing HBV infection including those who have developed a superimposed carcinoma. Therefore, hepatitis B virus infection is an important cause of chronic liver disease and subsequent liver carcinoma in many parts of the world.
3 *Mycotoxins,* metabolites of saprophytic fungi, including certain known hepatic carcinogens (e.g., aflatoxins), are continuously ingested in foodstuffs in small amounts and are found in high concentrations in foods in parts of Africa and Asia, where liver cell carcinoma is found more frequently. Ingested mycotoxins and viral inflammation can act synergistically to increase the risk of malignant hepatocellular transformation.
4 The male predominance in liver cancer and the effect of sex hormones on experimental carcinogenesis suggest that *hormonal factors* may be important. Significantly, hepatocellular carcinoma has been reported in some patients on long-term androgenic therapy.
5 *Iatrogenic factors* include thorium dioxide, an agent widely used for radiologic images for about 20 years until the mid-1950s. Since there is lifelong hepatic storage and virtually no decay of this radioisotope, the liver is exposed to continuous low-level radiation. After a 15- to 20-year latent period, angiosarcoma or chronic liver disease with carcinoma can develop. Long-term use of oral contraceptives rarely leads to development of hepatic cell adenoma, a benign neoplasm, but malignant transformation into carcinoma has been reported.

Clinical features Hepatic cancers may escape clinical recognition during life because they often occur in patients with underlying cirrhosis, and the symptoms and signs may initially suggest a progression of the underlying liver disease. *Hepatomegaly,* with *pain* or *tenderness,* usually moderate in degree and localized to the upper abdomen or the right upper quadrant, is a major complaint in more than half the cases. Other clinical features which should alert the clinician to the diagnosis include a *mass* in the liver, particularly if tender; the presence of a *friction rub* or *bruit* over the liver; and *blood-tinged ascites* (hemoperitoneum) which occurs in about 20 percent of cases. On rare occasions one may find metabolic disturbances such as polycythemia, hypoglycemia, acquired porphyria, hypercalcemia, and dysglobulinemia. Jaundice is characteristic of cholangiocarcinoma but is relatively uncommon in hepatocellular carcinoma in the absence of active liver disease.

Anemia and elevated alkaline phosphatase levels are common laboratory findings. In a patient with cirrhosis, a disproportionately high serum alkaline phosphatase in relation to other abnormal liver function tests is often a clue to an infiltrating or partially obstructing liver carcinoma.

Diagnosis The clinical features outlined above should suggest the possibility of primary liver carcinoma. Liver scintiscans may indicate the presence of one or more hepatic masses but frequently cannot distinguish between regenerating nodules in a cirrhotic liver and primary or metastatic liver tumors. Gallium 67 scans showing hepatocellular uptake in the abnormal area may be more helpful than ^{99m}Tc scans. Ultrasound or CT scans can clearly demonstrate lesions with a density different from normal liver tissue. These two noninvasive techniques also help in directing percutaneous biopsy for definitive diagnosis. Hepatic artery *angiography* may reveal distortion or obstructions of vessels or "tumor blushes" characteristic of neovascularization and usually can define the extent of the tumor and its resectability. Angiography cannot, however, distinguish between types of tumor and may not be able to differentiate benign from malignant solitary tumors.

A unique fetal alpha$_1$ globulin, *alpha fetoprotein* (AFP), is found in the serum of almost all patients with hepatocellular carcinoma. Very high levels, between 500 ng/mL and 5 mg/mL, occur in 70 to 90 percent of patients. The serum AFP may be slightly elevated in about 5 to 10 percent of patients with large hepatic metastases from gastrointestinal tumors, and in about one-third of patients with acute or chronic viral hepatitis, but only rarely to levels over 500 ng/mL in these conditions. Minimally elevated levels of AFP may persist in some patients with chronic hepatitis. AFP is also elevated up to 500 ng/mL in maternal serums during normal pregnancy. Higher levels can occur in maternal serums with fetal distress or death. The detection and persistence of *high levels* of serum AFP (over 500 or 1000 ng/mL) in an adult with liver disease and without an obvious gastrointestinal tract tumor strongly suggest the presence of primary liver carcinoma. Ectopic hormones, such as chorionic gonadotropin, are rarely found. Several variant isoenzymes (including aldolase, alkaline phosphatase, and 5′-nucleotide phosphodiesterase) have been reported in some liver cancer patients and also may be helpful diagnostically when present.

Percutaneous *liver biopsy* can be diagnostic, especially if the biopsy is taken in the area of a palpable nodule or mass localized by ultrasound or CT scans. False negatives may occur in as many as one-fourth of patients if the biopsy is performed in a routine, blind manner with the intercostal approach, and well-differentiated hepatocellular carcinoma may be difficult to diagnose by aspiration cytology or even needle biopsy. Cytologic examination of ascitic fluid is invariably negative for tumor cells. *Laparoscopy* or *laparotomy* with open liver biopsy is often required for diagnosis. This direct approach has the additional advantage of identifying the occasional patient with localized resectable tumor who may be suitable for partial hepatectomy.

Course and management The course of the disease is fatal and usually rapid. Most patients die within 3 to 6 months from gastrointestinal hemorrhage, progressive cachexia, or hepatic failure.

If the patient is young, in good general health, and has no obvious extrahepatic involvement, solitary hepatic lesions may be excised with *partial hepatectomy*, but the 5-year survival rate is low. Persistently high or rising levels of AFP after excision of the tumor are indicative of residual or recurrent tumor. Hepatocellular carcinoma may respond for brief periods to systemic or intraarterial chemotherapy. However, the results are still poor, and further trials of combined drug therapy are in progress. Liver transplantation can now be considered a therapeutic option, but recurrence of tumor and frequent appearance of metastases after transplantation have limited the usefulness of this procedure (see Chap. 252). Aggressive surgery or transplantation may prove to be of value in the treatment of small, localized tumors if diagnosed early or in the slower-growing fibrolamellar type of liver cell carcinoma.

OTHER BENIGN AND MALIGNANT TUMORS These tumors are very rare. Hepatoblastomas are histologically distinct primary malignant tumors of the liver occurring only in infancy and early childhood and characteristically have very high levels of serum AFP. Since they are usually solitary masses, they are more usually resectable and have a higher 5-year survival rate than hepatocellular carcinoma. *Hemangiomas,* the most common of the benign tumors, are usually single and small, but may present as a large hepatic nodule. Percutaneous needle liver biopsy is contraindicated if the diagnosis is suspected because of the danger of hemorrhage. The diagnosis can be made by angiography. Surgical excision is usually not indicated unless the tumors are large and symptomatic or a malignant lesion cannot be excluded. *Hemangioendotheliomas* or *angiosarcomas* are rare malignant vascular tumors. They can be caused by chronic *vinyl chloride* exposure. These rare tumors may also appear 15 to 20 years after the administration of thorium dioxide.

Hepatic adenomas, although quite rare, have been reported with increasing frequency, particularly in women taking oral contraceptives for long periods. These benign neoplasms may regress when the pill is discontinued. Focal nodular hyperplasia, a nonneoplastic hamartoma, may also become more vascular with long-term use of oral contraceptives leading to increased risk of pain or hemorrhage. Other rare tumors include benign cholangiomas, rhabdomyomas, rhabdomyosarcomas, and a number of other benign and malignant tumors arising from various mesenchymal elements. These tumors usually present as a palpable mass in the liver or with intraabdominal hemorrhage. They can be visualized and their extent defined by angiography. Surgical exploration and open biopsy or resection are usually required for definitive diagnosis.

METASTATIC TUMORS Metastatic malignant tumors of the liver are common in clinical practice, ranking second only to cirrhosis as a cause of fatal liver disease. In the United States the incidence of clinically significant metastatic carcinoma is at least 20 times greater than that of primary carcinoma. Hepatic metastases have been reported at autopsy in 30 to 50 percent of patients dying from malignant disease.

Pathogenesis The liver is uniquely vulnerable to invasion by tumor cells. Its size, high rate of blood flow, and double perfusion by hepatic artery and portal vein combine to make it the most common site of metastases except for the lymph nodes. In addition, local tissue factors or endothelial membrane characteristics appear to enhance metastatic implants. Virtually all types of neoplasms except those primary in the brain may metastasize to the liver. The most common primary tumors are those of the gastrointestinal tract, lung, breast, and melanomas. Less common are metastases from tumors of the thyroid, prostate, and skin.

Clinical features Most patients with metastatic malignancy of the liver present with (1) symptoms referable only to the primary tumor, with asymptomatic hepatic involvement discovered in the course of clinical evaluation; (2) nonspecific symptoms of weakness, weight loss, fever, sweating, and loss of appetite; or rarely, with (3) features indicating active hepatic disease, especially abdominal pain, hepatomegaly, or ascites.

Patients with widespread metastatic liver involvement usually have suggestive clinical signs of cancer and hepatic enlargement. Some have localized induration or tenderness, and occasionally a friction rub may be found over tender areas of the liver.

Abnormal liver function tests are frequent but often mild and nonspecific. They reflect the effects of fever and wasting, as well as the infiltrating neoplastic process itself. An increase in serum alkaline phosphatase is the most common and frequently the only abnormality noted. Hypoalbuminemia, anemia, and occasional mild elevation of transaminase levels may also be found with more widespread disease. Greatly elevated serum levels of carcinoembryonic antigen (CEA) are usually found when the metastases are from primary malignancies in the gastrointestinal tract, breast, or lung.

Diagnosis Evidence of metastatic invasion of the liver should be sought actively in any patient with a primary malignancy, especially of the lung, gastrointestinal tract, or breast, before resection of the primary lesion is undertaken. Abnormal liver function tests, particularly an elevated alkaline phosphatase, or demonstration of a mass by liver scintiscan, ultrasound, or CT may provide a presumptive diagnosis. Blind percutaneous needle biopsy of the liver will result in a positive diagnosis in only 60 to 80 percent of cases with established metastases. Serial sectioning of specimens, two or three repeat biopsies, or cytologic examination of biopsy smears may increase the diagnostic yield by 10 to 15 percent. The yield is greatly increased when biopsies are directed by ultrasound or CT or obtained by laparoscopy.

Treatment Most metastatic carcinomas respond poorly to all forms of treatment, which is usually only palliative. Surgical removal of a single large metastasis is rarely feasible. Systemic chemotherapy with combinations of different chemotherapeutic agents briefly may slow tumor growth and reduce symptoms in some patients but does not significantly alter the prognosis. It remains to be determined whether newer drugs or combination chemotherapy eventually will prove to be more effective.

REFERENCES

ALPERT E: Alpha-fetoprotein: Developmental biology and clinical significance, in *Progress in Liver Disease*, vol 5, H Popper, F Schaffner (eds). New York, Grune& Stratton, 1975

BEASLEY RP et al: Hepatocellular carcinoma and hepatitis B virus. Lancet 2:1129, 1981

BRECHOT C et al: Evidence that hepatitis B virus has a role in liver cell carcinoma in alcoholic liver disease. N Engl J Med 306:1384, 1982

LIAW Y-F et al: Early detection of hepatocellular carcinoma in patients with chronic type B hepatitis. A prospective study. Gastroenterology 90:263, 1986

MALT RA: Surgery for hepatic neoplasms. N Engl J Med 313:1591, 1985

MARGOLIS S, HOWEY C: Systemic manifestations of hepatoma. Medicine 51:381, 1972

OKUDA K et al: Prognosis of primary hepatocellular carcinoma. Hepatology 4:13S, 1984

OMATA M et al: Hepatocellular carcinoma in the USA: Etiologic considerations. Localization of hepatitis B antigens. Gastroenterology 76:279, 1979

SHAFRITZ DA et al: Integration of hepatitis B virus DNA into the genome of liver cells in chronic liver disease and hepatocellular carcinoma. N Engl J Med 305:1067, 1981

STARZL T et al: Analysis of liver transplantation. Hepatology 4:47S, 1984

ZAMAN SN et al: Risk factors in development of carcinoma in cirrhosis: Prospective study of 613 patients. Lancet 1:1357, 1985

251 INFILTRATIVE AND METABOLIC DISEASES AFFECTING THE LIVER

KURT J. ISSELBACHER / DANIEL K. PODOLSKY

Many disseminated, systemic, or metabolic diseases involve the liver in a diffuse manner by the infiltration of abnormal cells or the accumulation of chemical substances or metabolites. Chemical accumulation may be extracellular or intracellular and may involve hepatocytes, Kupffer cells, or other elements of the reticuloendothelial system. Although infiltrative diseases may vary widely in their etiology and extrahepatic manifestations, the findings in the liver may be quite similar. Generalized enlargement and firmness of the liver, gradual and nonspecific deterioration of liver function, and, less often, signs of portal hypertension or ascites are typical features of this group of diseases. Differential diagnosis by clinical means may be difficult on occasion, but in patients in whom ancillary clinical findings do not establish the diagnosis, the diffusely infiltrated liver provides an excellent source of tissue for diagnostic purposes.

As discussed in Chap. 58, the tools of molecular biology, especially recombinant DNA probes and restriction fragment length polymorphism will undoubtedly play a significant role in arriving at the molecular basis for many of these disorders. Some diseases will reflect the manifestation of mutant structural genes causing absent or reduced amounts of a gene product (e.g. phenylalanine hydroxylase deficiency leading to classic phenylketonuria), or a structurally *altered* gene which is functionally inactive (e.g., α_1-antitrypsin). In other instances the mutation may affect *gene regulation* as in Menke's syndrome, a rare disorder of zinc metabolism that affects the liver, which appears to result from faulty regulation of metallothionein gene expression.

LIPID INFILTRATIONS

FATTY LIVER Slight to moderate enlargement of the liver due to diffuse infiltration of liver cells by neutral fat (triglyceride) is a common clinical and pathologic finding. Although minimal fatty changes are often transient and have no clinical significance, persistent or extensive fatty infiltration may produce dysfunction and symptoms that require careful evaluation.

Etiology The major causes of fatty liver encountered in clinical practice depend on the age, geographic location, and metabolic-nutritional status of the patient population. *Chronic alcoholism* is the most common cause of fatty liver in this country and in other countries with a high alcohol intake. The severity of fatty involvement is roughly proportional to the duration and degree of alcoholic excess. *Protein malnutrition,* especially in infancy and early childhood, accounts for most cases of severe fatty liver in the tropical zones of Africa, South America, and Asia. The hepatic changes may be associated with other clinical and pathologic features of kwashiorkor. Patients with adult-onset *diabetes mellitus,* especially those who are overweight and are poorly controlled, often have fatty livers. *Obesity* is commonly associated with fatty infiltration of the liver; this recedes as weight reduction occurs. However, *jejunoileal bypass* for surgical treatment of morbid obesity is sometimes associated with severe fatty liver and hepatic failure which may be fatal. In patients with Cushing's syndrome and in those receiving large doses of corticosteroids, fatty infiltration of the liver may occur. In many *chronic illnesses,* especially those complicated by impaired nutrition or malabsorption, increased fat is found in liver cells. For example, patients with ulcerative colitis, chronic pancreatitis, or protracted heart failure frequently have moderately fatty livers at the time of death. Patients maintained on prolonged *intravenous hyperalimentation* may also develop fatty livers.

Acute fatty liver is caused by a number of hepatotoxins and is frequently accompanied by signs and symptoms of liver failure. Carbon tetrachloride intoxication, DDT poisoning, and ingestion of substances containing yellow phosphorus result in severe fatty liver. Acute and prolonged alcohol ingestion may also be considered in this category and may be associated with a rapidly enlarging and fat-laden liver. *Acute fatty liver of pregnancy* is a rare but often fatal condition seen during the third trimester of pregnancy which is characterized by nausea, vomiting, abdominal pain, renal failure, and coma. It should be distinguished from the benign cholestasis more frequently encountered during the third trimester of pregnancy. *Massive tetracycline therapy,* in amounts of 3 to 12 g intravenous, is a rare cause of acute fatty liver and fatal hepatic coma. Other drugs (e.g., valproic acid) have also been associated with the development of a fatty liver.

Pathogenesis The hepatic lipid deposits, which consist largely of triglycerides and lesser amounts of phospholipid and cholesterol, appear as vacuoles of varying size within the cytoplasm of liver cells. In extreme cases, every liver cell is involved, and lipids comprise up to 30 to 40 percent of the total liver weight.

The biochemical mechanisms leading to hepatic triglyceride accumulation are described in Chap. 244. Fatty infiltration has been produced in experimental animals by a variety of toxic agents and drugs, such as alcohol, carbon tetrachloride, and orotic acid. Deficiencies, such as choline deficiency, readily lead to increased fat in the liver in the rat. Many of these factors appear to disrupt synthesis of proteins, including the apoproteins needed for transport of triglycerides out of the liver as lipoproteins. However, with few exceptions experimental studies do not explain the pathogenesis of fatty liver in clinical disease. Moderate doses of ethanol may produce both acute and chronic fatty changes in human subjects, probably by its direct effects on hepatic triglyceride and fatty acid metabolism (Chap. 244). Protein deficiency seems to account for the fatty liver of kwashiorkor, and impaired protein synthesis for the fat accumulation following tetracycline and carbon tetrachloride administration. In diabetes mellitus and in starvation, increased mobilization of fatty acids from adipose tissue may be involved. Fatty infiltration during hyperalimentation appears to be derived from the high concentration of dextrose rather than from any lipid infusions.

Clinical features The signs and symptoms of fatty liver are related to the degree of fat infiltration, the time course of its accumulation, and the underlying cause. The obese or diabetic patient with chronic fatty liver is usually asymptomatic and has only mild tenderness over the enlarged liver. The liver function tests are normal or show mild elevations of alkaline phosphatase, transaminases, or aminotransferases. In contrast, the rapid accumulation of fat seen in the setting of hyperalimentation may lead to marked tenderness, presumably resulting from stretching of Glisson's capsule. Similarly, alcoholic patients with acute fatty liver following a bout of heavy drinking may have right upper quadrant pain and tenderness often with laboratory evidence of cholestasis. The clinical presentation of acute fatty liver of pregnancy or fatty liver from hepatotoxins is similar to that of fulminant hepatic failure arising from any cause, with evidence of hepatic encephalopathy, marked elevations of prothrombin time and transaminases, and variable degrees of jaundice.

Diagnosis The findings of a firm, nontender, and generally enlarged liver with minimal hepatic dysfunction in a patient with chronic alcoholism, malnutrition, poorly controlled diabetes mellitus, or obesity should suggest a fatty liver. When diagnostic uncertainty exists, needle biopsy of the liver will demonstrate the increased fatty content and possibly the underlying primary disorder. In acute fatty liver of pregnancy and in most cases of Reye's syndrome (see below), fat accumulates in small vacuoles (microvesicular fat) rather than in the large cytoplasmic droplets encountered in other disorders. The reason for the morphologic appearance of the fat in these two disorders is unclear.

Treatment Adequate nutritional intake, removal of alcohol or offending toxins, and correction of any associated metabolic disorders usually result in recovery. There is no clinical rationale for the use of lipotropic agents such as choline. When indicated, attention should be directed to abstinence from alcohol, careful control of diabetes, weight loss, or correction of intestinal absorptive defects. In the alcoholic fatty liver there is gradual disappearance of fat from the liver after 4 to 8 weeks of adequate diet and abstinence from alcohol. Similarly, fatty infiltration usually resolves within 2 weeks after discontinuation of parenteral hyperalimentation. However, restitution of intestinal continuity may not prevent progression of disease in patients who have had extensive intestinal bypass surgery.

REYE'S SYNDROME (FATTY LIVER WITH ENCEPHALOPATHY) This acute illness is encountered exclusively in children below 15 years of age. It is characterized clinically by vomiting, and signs of progressive central nervous system damage, signs of hepatic injury, and hypoglycemia. Morphologically there is extensive fatty vacuolization of the liver and renal tubules. The cause is unknown, although viral and toxic agents, especially salicylates, have been implicated. Increased aspirin use and much higher serum salicylate levels in children with this illness than in the general population have been described during outbreaks of Reye's syndrome. However, it seems clear that this illness may also occur in the absence of exposure to salicylates. In fatal cases, the liver is enlarged and yellow with striking diffuse fatty microvacuolization of cells. Peripheral zonal hepatic necrosis has also been present in some cases. Fatty changes of the renal tubular cells, cerebral edema, and neuronal degeneration of the brain are the major extrahepatic changes. Electron microscope studies show structural alterations of mitochondria in liver, brain, and muscle.

The onset usually follows an upper respiratory tract infection, especially influenza or chicken pox. Within 1 to 3 days persistent vomiting occurs, together with stupor, which usually progresses rapidly to generalized convulsions and coma. The liver is enlarged, but *jaundice is characteristically absent or minimal.* Elevations in serum aminotransferases and prothrombin time, hypoglycemia, metabolic acidosis, and elevated serum ammonia levels are the major laboratory findings. The mortality rate in Reye's syndrome is approximately 50 percent. Therapy consists of infusions of glucose and fresh frozen plasma, as well as intravenous mannitol to reduce the cerebral edema. Chronic liver disease has not been reported in survivors.

NIEMANN-PICK DISEASE (See Chap. 316) This rare heritable disorder, of which there are five types, is found mainly in Jewish infants and is characterized by the accumulation of sphingomyelin and cholesterol in reticuloendothelial cells of the liver, spleen, bone marrow, and brain due to deficiency of sphingomyelinase. Hepatomegaly and splenomegaly are present, together with elevations in serum aminotransferase and alkaline phosphatase levels, but jaundice and other evidence of hepatic dysfunction are rare. The liver, which is typically large, yellow, and fatty, shows clusters of lipid-filled, foamy Kupffer cells. Diagnosis is made by lipid analysis of the tissue obtained from bone marrow aspiration.

GAUCHER'S DISEASE (See Chap. 316) Accumulations of large reticuloendothelial cells containing the cerebroside glucosylceramide (Gaucher's cells) in the liver and spleen account for the characteristic moderate to massive hepatosplenomegaly found in patients with the juvenile and adult forms of this disorder. Rarely, ascites or portal hypertension is produced by compression of the intrahepatic vasculature. The diagnosis may be made readily by liver biopsy and demonstration of the Gaucher's cells but should be confirmed by demonstration of a deficiency of the enzyme glucosylceramide β-glucosidase in peripheral leukocytes.

WOLMAN'S AND CHOLESTEROL ESTER STORAGE DISEASES Wolman's disease is a rare and fatal familial lipidosis of infancy producing hepatosplenomegaly and stippled calcification of the adrenal glands. Liver biopsy shows clusters of foam cells (reticuloendothelial cells filled with cholesterol ester and triglycerides), hepatocytes containing fat, and patchy fibrosis. A related but less severe genetic disorder is cholesterol ester storage disease. In this condition there is hypercholesterolemia and accumulation of both cholesterol esters and triglycerides in hepatic lysosomes. Both of these storage disorders are associated with hepatic deficiencies of cholesterol ester hydrolase and triglyceride lipase.

Other rare lipid disorders associated with hepatomegaly and increased fat in the liver include abetalipoproteinemia, Tangier disease, Fabry's disease, and types I and V hyperlipoproteinemia. (See Chap. 315 for details.)

HEPATIC GLYCOGEN ACCUMULATION

DIABETIC GLYCOGENOSIS Hepatic enlargement caused by distention of liver cells with glycogen is present in some poorly controlled diabetic patients and often in juvenile diabetic patients (see Chap 327). More often, however, hepatomegaly is related to fatty infiltration (see above). Ketoacidosis and vigorous insulin therapy may further enhance hepatic enlargement and glycogen deposition. In the absence of cirrhosis, hepatomegaly usually decreases with careful control of the diabetes.

GLYCOGEN STORAGE DISEASE (See Chap. 313) The normal liver contains 1 to 5 percent glycogen (by weight). Except for types V and VII, the liver is involved in all genetically determined glycogen storage diseases. There is disruption of glucose homeostasis due to an inability to mobilize hepatic glycogen stores. In types I, II, and VI hereditary glycogen storage diseases, increased amounts of glycogen (and fat) are found. Types III and IV are associated with derangements of glycogen structure, and cirrhosis may be present. Fasting hypoglycemia is present in all these diseases. Enzymatic and chemical analysis of liver tissue is usually needed for diagnosis.

GALACTOSEMIA

Hepatic changes are common in patients with unrecognized or untreated galactosemia. In early weeks of life fatty infiltration and cholestasis may be noted in acutely ill infants. If the disease goes unrecognized for months or years, cirrhosis may develop. (See also Chap. 314.)

HEPATIC MINERAL ACCUMULATION

WILSON'S DISEASE (See Chap. 311) This rare disease, predominantly of young people, is characterized by cirrhosis, softening and degeneration of the basal ganglia, and pigmentation of the cornea (Kayser-Fleischer rings). Increased copper deposition in the tissues seems to be responsible for the liver and basal ganglia changes. Liver cells are ballooned and show increased glycogen with glycogen vacuolization in the nuclei. The liver shows all grades of changes, from minimal to severe periportal or macronodular cirrhosis.

HEMOCHROMATOSIS (See Chap. 310) This relatively common genetically determined disorder involves accumulation of abnormal amounts of iron due to inappropriate absorption in the intestine. The liver, as a primary site of iron storage, is most directly affected. There is diffuse deposition of excess iron in hepatocytes, in contrast to the characteristic accumulation of iron in the reticuloendothelial compartment typical of secondary iron overload and hemosiderosis. Hepatic iron overload commonly results in hepatomegaly. Although liver function is initially well preserved, if the disease is untreated, progressive impairment is followed by the development of cirrhosis.

OTHER INFILTRATIVE DISEASES

HURLER'S SYNDROME (See Chap. 319) This is an uncommon hereditary disease that is characterized by the widespread tissue deposition of mucopolysaccharide (chondroitin sulfate B and heparin sulfate) in many tissues. The liver is frequently enlarged and firm. Microscopically, Kupffer cells and other macrophages are enlarged and filled with metachromatic granular material. Cirrhosis may be a late complication.

ALPHA$_1$ ANTITRYPSIN DEFICIENCY (See also Chap. 208) Patients with homozygous deficiency of serum alpha$_1$ antitrypsin (α_1-AT) are prone to develop emphysema in adult life. The disease is suggested by the absence of alpha$_1$ globulin on serum electrophoresis (α_1-AT makes up 90 percent of this fraction normally) and confirmed by direct measurement of α_1-AT. The exact phenotype can then be determined by starch electrophoresis. Although there are 16 recognized alleles, only PiZ and PiS are associated with clinical disease. The molecular bases of these altered products have been related to single nucleic acid substitutions, e.g., PiZ is caused by a G (guanine) to A (adenine) transposition which results in a substitution of a glutamic acid for lysine at residue 292 in the α_1-AT protein. Hepatocytes of some patients with this deficiency contain globules positive to the periodic acid Schiff (PAS) reaction. Approximately 10 percent of children with homozygous deficiency (PiZZ phenotype) of α_1-AT will develop significant liver disease including neonatal hepatitis and progressive cirrhosis. It has been suggested that 15 to 20 percent of all chronic liver disease in infancy may be attributed to α_1-AT deficiency. In adults, the most common manifestation of α_1-AT deficiency is asymptomatic cirrhosis, which may progress from a micronodular to a macronodular state and may be complicated by the development of hepatocellular carcinoma. The occurrence of liver disease in these patients is not dependent upon the development of lung disease.

RETICULOENDOTHELIAL DISORDERS (See also Chaps. 55 and 294)

Moderate to massive hepatomegaly and splenomegaly occur frequently in the various types of leukemia and lymphoma. Jaundice, when present, is usually slight and results from hemolysis. Deep and protracted jaundice is distinctly rare and is caused by obstruction of the intrahepatic or extrahepatic bile ducts by tumor. Liver biopsy specimens reveal portal and sinusoidal infiltrates in most cases of leukemia, but the cellular pattern may be mixed and nonspecific. Liver biopsy is diagnostic in only 5 percent of patients with Hodgkin's disease. This percentage is increased in those with advanced disease or splenomegaly. Directed biopsy at laparoscopy or laparotomy is more likely to be positive than "blind" needle biopsy. Nonspecific histologic changes in the liver have been described in patients with lymphoma and may contribute to the abnormal liver function tests.

Myeloid metaplasia and other myeloproliferative disorders associated with extramedullary hematopoiesis produce hepatomegaly which may reach huge proportions, especially following splenectomy. Serum alkaline phosphatase elevations are often found. Ascites and portal hypertension, resulting from diffuse involvement of portal venules and lymphatics, are rare complications.

GRANULOMATOUS INFILTRATIONS

Perhaps as a result of the large population of mononuclear phagocytes, a number of systemic granulomatous diseases involve the liver, including sarcoidosis, miliary tuberculosis, histoplasmosis, brucellosis, schistosomiasis, berylliosis, and drug reactions. In addition, isolated granulomas of no diagnostic importance may be found occasionally in patients with various forms of cirrhosis and hepatitis. The liver infiltrated by granulomas may be slightly enlarged and firm, but hepatic dysfunction is usually limited and manifested only by mild increases in serum alkaline phosphatase and occasionally aminotransferase levels. In a few patients with sarcoidosis or brucellosis, portal hypertension may develop, and extensive postnecrotic scarring or postnecrotic cirrhosis may follow healing of the granulomatous lesions as in schistosomiasis.

Needle biopsy of the liver reveals granulomas and often provides the first definite evidence of a systemic or disseminated granulomatous disease. In patients with sarcoidosis who have neither clinical nor laboratory evidence of hepatic involvement, needle biopsy is positive in about 80 percent of cases. In cases of suspected miliary tuberculosis a portion of the biopsy should be cultured and stained for mycobacteria. The organism can be detected in the majority of cases, particularly when caseating granulomas are present. Serial sections of the biopsy specimen should be examined if granulomas are not apparent. Individual granulomas are rarely specific in their microscopic appearance, and final diagnosis usually requires other clinical, laboratory, or histologic data.

In approximately 20 percent of patients it is not possible to identify a cause for the granulomatous infiltration. When these infiltrates are accompanied by fever of unknown etiology, the diagnosis of granulomatous hepatitis should be considered. This is an uncommon disorder of unknown etiology and is diagnosed by exclusion. While granulomatous hepatitis invariably responds to moderate doses of corticosteroids, relapses are frequent, and such therapy should never be undertaken unless tuberculous disease or other causes of granulomatous infiltration have been excluded. This may include an initial empiric trial of antituberculous therapy.

AMYLOIDOSIS (See also Chap. 259)

Systemic amyloidosis, whether primary and idiopathic, familial, or secondary to chronic inflammatory or neoplastic diseases, often involves the liver. Grossly, the liver infiltrated with amyloid is enlarged and pale and rubbery in consistency. Microscopically, the birefringent amyloid deposits appear as homogeneous waxy material within the space of Disse, often being concentrated in the periportal areas and associated with atrophy of adjacent liver cell plates. Selective involvement of the walls of blood vessels, especially of the hepatic arterioles, may be a striking feature of primary amyloidosis. With this possible exception, however, the hepatic lesions are the same in all forms of amyloidosis and are present in 60 to 90 percent of cases.

An enlarged and firm liver is found in about 60 percent of patients, and ascites occurs in advanced stages of the disease in about 20 percent. Jaundice, portal hypertension, and other signs of chronic liver disease are usually absent. Liver function changes, although frequent, correlate poorly with the extent of liver infiltration. Hypoalbuminemia and elevated serum alkaline phosphatase are common. Hypoalbuminemia, however, may be related to the nephrotic syndrome owing to renal involvement; the prothrombin time is usually normal. The diagnosis is established by biopsy of rectum, skin, liver, or other involved organs and demonstration of the characteristic Congo red–staining deposits by polarizing microscopy.

REFERENCES

BOVE KE: Reye's syndrome, in *Hepatology, A Textbook of Liver Disease,* D Zakim, TD Boyer (eds). Philadelphia, Saunders, 1982, pp 1212–1220

GLENNER GG: Amyloid deposits and amyloidosis. The β-fibrilloses. N Engl J Med 302:1283, 1980

HEUBI JE et al: Grade I Reye's syndrome: Outcome and predictors of progression to deeper coma grades. N Engl J Med 311:1539, 1984

HURWITZ ES et al: Public Health Service Study on Reye's syndrome and medications. N Engl J Med 313:842, 1985

KIDD VJ, WOO SLC: Recombinant DNA probes used to detail genetic disorders of the liver. Hepatology 4:731, 1984

POCKROS PJ et al: Idiopathic fatty liver of pregnancy. Medicine 44:1, 1984

REYNOLDS TB et al: Hepatic granulomas, in *Hepatology, A Textbook of Liver Disease,* D Zakim, TD Boyer (eds). Philadelphia, Saunders, 1982, pp 995–1009

SPECHLER SJ, KOFF RS: Wilson's disease: Diagnostic difficulties in the patient with chronic hepatitis and hyperceruloplasminemia. Gastroenterology 78:103, 1980

STANBURY JB et al: *The Metabolic Basis of Inherited Disease,* 5th ed, New York, McGraw-Hill, 1983

SVEGER T: Liver disease in α_1-antitrypsin deficiency. N Engl J Med 294:1316, 1976

252 LIVER TRANSPLANTATION

RUDI SCHMID

Orthotopic liver transplantation, i.e., replacement of a diseased liver by a healthy organ recovered from a recently brain-dead individual, is surgically difficult, requires a full array of supporting services usually available only in large tertiary medical centers, and carries a considerable operative and postoperative mortality. However, the risk-versus-benefit ratio has improved to an extent where liver transplantation has become a promising approach for selected patients whose liver disease is progressive, life-threatening, and beyond the reach of traditional therapy.

The first orthotopic liver transplantation in a human was performed by Starzl and associates in 1963 at the University of Colorado in Denver, but the survival of this patient and several subsequently transplanted patients was less than 1 month. The following years brought refinements in both surgical technique and postoperative management that improved survival rates, but by 1976 only 24 percent of adults and 33 percent of children who underwent liver transplantation survived for more than 1 year. Until the 1970s, performance of the operation remained almost entirely limited to the Denver center and to another liver transplantation facility established by Calne in 1968 in Cambridge, England. Since 1980, however, the prospect for prolonged survival with good quality of life has improved owing largely to development of better techniques for organ preservation, improvements in surgical techniques including the development of a pump-driven venovenous bypass system, and advances in immunosuppression, particularly the use of cyclosporine in combination with steroids. As a result, a number of transplant centers have been established, and the total number of successful liver transplants exceeded 1000 by mid-1985.

INDICATIONS FOR LIVER TRANSPLANTATION In the absence of absolute or relative contraindications (see below), potential candidates for liver transplantation are children and adults up to age 50 who suffer from severe, irreversible liver disease for which alternative medical or surgical treatments have been exhausted. Timing of the operation is of critical importance; the disease should be in a late enough stage to allow the patient all opportunity for spontaneous stabilization or recovery but early enough to give the surgical procedure a fair chance of success. As a general rule, transplantation should be considered in patients with end-stage liver disease who are experiencing or have experienced life-threatening complications of hepatic failure, whose quality of life has deteriorated to unacceptable levels, or whose liver disease predictably will result in irreversible damage to the central nervous system. The decision to transplant requires the combined judgment of an experienced team of hepatologists, transplant surgeons, anesthesiologists, and specialists in supporting services; the well-informed consent of the patient or the patient's family or authorized representative must also be obtained.

TRANSPLANTATION IN CHILDREN **Biliary atresia** The most common indication for transplantation in children is biliary atresia. Although hepatoportoenterostomy (Kasai procedure) performed in the first 2 months of life may provide substantial albeit transient improvement, the distortion of intrahepatic bile ducts and cirrhosis always are progressive, resulting in eventual hepatic insufficiency and death. It seems advantageous, however, to delay transplantation especially in the first year of life as long as possible to permit the child optimal development.

Metabolic disorders Genetically transmitted diseases associated with progressive liver failure constitute another major indication in children and adolescents. In progressive cirrhosis due to alpha$_1$-antitrypsin deficiency, transplantation results in appearance of the donor alpha$_1$-antitrypsin phenotype and return of the plasma enzyme level toward normal. In Wilson's disease presenting with acute hepatic failure or with progressive neurologic deficiency that is unresponsive to chelation therapy, liver transplantation is the treatment of choice. Improvement in neurologic function and return of plasma ceruloplasmin concentration to normal have been reported. Liver failure in Byler's, Alagille's, and Wolman's disease and in protoporphyria, tyrosinemia, and some types of glycogenosis have been indications for transplantation. In Crigler-Najjar disease type I and in certain hereditary disorders of the urea cycle and of amino acid or lactate-pyruvate metabolism, transplantation may be the only way to prevent impending deterioration of central nervous system function, despite the fact that the replaced liver is structurally normal. Combined heart and liver transplantation yielded dramatic improvement in cardiac function and plasma cholesterol level in a child with homozygous familial hypercholesterolemia. In hereditary oxalosis, improvement has been reported after combined liver and kidney transplantation.

TRANSPLANTATION IN ADULTS **Nonalcoholic cirrhosis** Chronic active hepatitis due to presumed autoimmunity and cirrhosis of nonviral etiology with liver failure are important indications for transplantation. From the mid-1970s to 1985, the actuarial 1-year survival of 275 patients transplanted for these conditions progressively rose from 31 percent to approximately 70 percent.

Primary biliary cirrhosis Because primary biliary cirrhosis has an indolent and often fluctuating course, liver transplantation is indicated only in patients who have progressed to an end stage of the disease or whose quality of life has deteriorated to an unacceptable level. Survival is similar to that in nonalcoholic cirrhosis. In the posttransplantation period, it is often difficult to distinguish between homograft rejection and the recurrence of the original disease because the clinical, laboratory, and histologic features of the two conditions are similar.

Sclerosing cholangitis Transplantation has been successful in patients with primary sclerosing cholangitis or with Caroli's disease in whom surgical drainage procedures failed to prevent progressive deterioration of hepatic function.

Hepatic vein thrombosis Transplantation has been reported in 17 patients with Budd-Chiari syndrome with an actuarial 3-year survival of 60 percent. Because spontaneous recannulization of the obstructed hepatic veins occasionally occurs, the operation should be reserved for patients with progressive hepatic decompensation or irreversible hepatorenal syndrome. It is controversial whether transplantation is indicated for hepatic vein thrombosis associated with polycythemia vera or myeloproliferative disorders.

Hepatobiliary cancer Overall survival of patients who undergo transplantation for primary hepatocellular carcinoma or cholangiocarcinoma is significantly less than that for other categories of liver disease because the majority of patients succumb to disseminated carcinomatosis. Moreover, because the results have improved only slightly in recent years, the proportion of transplanted patients who received homografts for primary liver cancer has progressively decreased since 1980. The most promising approach to primary liver cancer clearly is early detection when the tumor is small and amenable to total resection.

CONTRAINDICATIONS FOR TRANSPLANTATION Absolute contraindications for transplantation include life-threatening systemic diseases; infections; preexisting cardiovascular, pulmonary, or renal disease; metastatic malignancies; portal vein thrombosis; and therapy-resistant arterial hypotension. In alcohol-related liver disease, the outcome of transplantation generally has been disappointing; only 27 out of 819 patients reported up to August 1984 were transplanted for this condition. In patients with advanced alcohol-related cirrhosis who, despite abstinence for at least 6 months and adequate nutritional state, develop hepatic decompensation, transplantation may be contemplated when all other means of therapy have failed; relatively few patients, however, fulfill these qualifications. Patients with chronic viral hepatitis B, particularly those positive for HBsAg and HBeAg, are poor risks for transplantation because the immunosuppression tends to promote recurrence of the infection in the homograft. Information is inadequate to determine whether this also is true in chronic hepatitis B without evidence of active viral replication. In fulminant hepatitis of all etiologies associated with encephalopathy and/or hepatorenal syndrome, results of transplantation generally have been discouraging; this in part may be due to the rapid progression of the disease rendering optimal timing of the operation difficult.

RESULTS OF TRANSPLANTATION **Survival** Since 1983, the survival rate of patients undergoing liver transplantation has steadily improved. In 1985, the overall prospect for 1-year survival was about 70 percent, with children faring slightly better than adults. Of 152 patients who underwent liver transplantation at various centers between January 1980 and April 1983 and who survived the initial three postoperative months, the 3-year survival rate was 79 percent in adults with nonalcoholic cirrhosis and 92 percent in children with biliary atresia; in 102 patients transplanted after April 1983 who survived the initial three postoperative months, 1-year survival rates reached 89 percent in adults and 96 percent in children.

Posttransplantation quality of life In patients who have undergone transplantation for life-threatening chronic liver disease, objective evaluation of the quality of life after surgery inherently is difficult, and reliable information is sparse. Nonetheless, full rehabilitation seems to have been achieved in the majority of those who survived the first three postoperative months and escaped chronic rejection or unmanageable infection. Immunosuppressive medication in reduced doses usually is continued indefinitely. Several women who underwent transplantation and received immunosuppressive therapy have conceived and carried the pregnancy to term without demonstrable damage to the infants.

TECHNICAL AND MANAGEMENT ASPECTS **Surgical techniques** Liver donors commonly are procured from accident victims 2 months to 45 years of age who are brain-dead and without detectable hepatic dysfunction. Cardiovascular and respiratory functions are sustained artificially until the liver can be removed. Prolonged periods of hypotension or hypoxia preclude donation, and compatibility of ABO blood type and organ size are important considerations in donor selection. Multiple-organ procurement (including the liver, heart, and kidneys, but not the pancreas) is technically feasible. Following perfusion with cold electrolyte solution and packing in ice, the donor liver can be preserved for up to 8 h without significant impairment of graft viability.

Removal of the recipient's liver is technically difficult, particularly in the presence of varices or scarring from previous abdominal operations. After the portal vein and inferior vena cava are dissected, a pump-driven bypass system is applied that reroutes blood from the portal vein and inferior vena cava to the superior vena cava, thereby preventing congestion of visceral organs. In implanting the new liver, meticulous attention must be directed to reestablishment of the portal venous and hepatic arterial circulations and to reconstruction of biliary drainage. The latter usually is achieved by anastomosis of the common bile ducts or by choledochojejunostomy to a Roux en Y limb, if the common bile duct of the recipient cannot be used for reconstruction.

A transplant operation requires 8 to 12 h. Because of excessive bleeding associated with portal hypertension and liver failure, large volumes of blood, blood products, and volume expanders may be required during surgery.

POSTOPERATIVE COURSE AND MANAGEMENT **Postoperative complications** Patients who undergo liver transplantation are frequently malnourished, so that attention to multiple organ failure is of primary importance. Because of the fluids administered during surgery, patients may become overloaded during the immediate postoperative period, necessitating continuous monitoring of cardiovascular and pulmonary function. Postoperative jaundice is almost invariable and reflects the large administered pigment load and variable degrees of ischemic or mechanical injury sustained by the liver during harvesting and implantation. Prerenal azotemia, acute kidney injury due to hypotension, or renal toxicity caused by antibiotics or cyclosporine are frequently encountered in the postoperative period and sometimes require dialysis. Other postoperative complications related to technical difficulties include stenosis or leakage of the anastomosed common bile duct, intraperiotoneal hemorrhage, and thrombosis of the reconstructed hepatic artery or of the portal or hepatic vein. Acute upper gastointestinal hemorrhage or unexplained transient hemolytic anemia, with or without thrombocytopenia, may occur.

Bacterial, viral, or fungal infections related to the required immunosuppressive therapy may be life-threatening in the later postoperative period. These infections may involve the biliary tree, liver, upper gastrointestinal tract, or lungs, and they demand early recognition and prompt management. *Candida, Nocardia, Pneumocystis carinii*, and cytomegalovirus are frequent infective agents, but viruses of the herpes group, other mycoses, or gram-negative bacteria may also be pathogens. In most transplant centers, patients routinely are given antibiotic therapy prophylactically.

Immunosuppression The introduction in 1980 of cyclosporine as an immunosuppressive agent contributed substantially to the improvement in transplant survival. The drug depresses both humoral and cell-mediated immunity without affecting rapidly dividing cells in the bone marrow, which may account for the reduced incidence of systemic posttransplantation infection. Unfortunately, cyclosporine causes dose-related renal tubular injury, which usually can be managed by reducing the dose. Other adverse effects of long-term cyclosporine use are hypertension, hyperkalemia, tremor, hirsutism, and hyperplasia of the gums. Because of these side effects, combinations of cyclosporine and prednisone are a preferable regimen for immunosuppressive treatment during the initial postoperative months. For long-term management, renal toxicity may make it necessary to reduce cyclosporine to very low doses, which can be accomplished by adding azathioprine as supplemental immunosuppressive medication. In many centers, cyclosporine treatment is initiated prior to or on the day of surgery and is continued by intravenous route through the operation and the immediate postoperative period until oral administration can be resumed.

Transplant rejection Despite the use of cyclosporine alone or in combination with steroids, homograft rejection still occurs in the majority of patients 1 to 6 weeks after surgery. There appears to be no hepatic counterpart to the "hyperacute" rejection observed after renal transplantation. Early signs suggesting liver rejection are leukocytosis, increase in serum bilirubin level, and rise in aminotransferase activity; these may be followed by fever, tenderness in the right upper abdomen, diarrhea, ascites, and progressive deterioration of hepatic function. Because of the lack of specificity of these manifestations, differential diagnosis between homograft rejection, biliary obstruction, viral hepatitis, and recurrence of the original liver disease frequently is difficult. Radiographic visualization of the biliary tree and/or percutaneous liver biopsy often are helpful in establishing the correct diagnosis. Early morphologic features of rejection characteristically include portal infiltration with small lymphocytes and variable numbers of polymorphonuclear leukocytes, centrolobular bile stasis, selective destruction of small bile ducts associated with polymorphonuclear infiltration, and, at times, endothelial inflammation of portal or central veins and occasionally of hepatic arterioles. These finding are similar to those in graft-versus-host disease and may be indistinguishable from those of primary biliary cirrhosis. As soon as transplant rejection is suspected, it should be treated with intravenous methylprednisolone in repeated boluses; this usually reverses the rejection process. Some centers are also using antilymphocyte antibodies.

Chronic rejection is a relatively rare event that appears to be unrelated to the occurrence of preceding acute rejection episodes. It is associated with progressive cholestasis, bile duct proliferation, focal parenchymal necrosis, mononuclear infiltration, and fibrosis. These morphologic findings may be so similar to those of chronic viral hepatitis that differentiation between the two may be difficult. In some patients with therapy-resistant chronic rejection, retransplantation has yielded encouraging results.

REFERENCES

BUSUTTIL RW, Moderator: Liver transplantation today. Ann Intrn Med 104:377, 1986

NIH CONSENSUS DEVELOPMENT CONFERENCE ON LIVER TRANSPLANTATION: Hepatology 4(suppl):15, 1984

Progress in Liver Transplantation, CH Gips, RAF Krom (eds). Amsterdam, Martinus Nijhoff, 1985.

SCHARSCHMIDT BF: Human liver transplantation: An analysis of 819 patients from 8 centers, in *Recent Advances in Hepatology*, HC Thomas, EA Jones (eds). London, Churchill-Livingstone, 1985, vol 2

253 DISEASES OF THE GALLBLADDER AND BILE DUCTS

MARK S. McPHEE / NORTON J. GREENBERGER

PHYSIOLOGY OF BILE PRODUCTION AND FLOW **Bile secretion and composition** Bile formed in the hepatic lobules is secreted into a complex network of canaliculi, small bile ductules, and larger bile ducts which run with lymphatics and branches of the portal vein and hepatic artery in portal tracts situated between hepatic lobules. These interlobular bile ducts coalesce to form larger septal bile ducts that join to form the right and left hepatic ducts, which in turn unite to form the common hepatic duct. The common hepatic duct is joined by the cystic duct of the gallbladder to form the common bile duct which enters the duodenum (often after joining the main pancreatic duct) through the ampulla of Vater.

Hepatic bile is a pigmented isotonic fluid with an electrolyte composition resembling blood plasma. The electrolyte composition of gallbladder bile differs from that of hepatic bile since most of the inorganic anions, chloride and bicarbonate, have been removed by reabsorption across the basement membrane.

Major components of bile by weight include water (82 percent), bile acids (12 percent), lecithin and other phospholipids (4 percent), and unesterified cholesterol (0.7 percent). Other constituents include conjugated bilirubin, proteins (IgA, by-products of hormones, and other proteins metabolized in the liver), electrolytes, mucus, and, often, drugs and their metabolic by-products.

The total daily basal secretion of hepatic bile is approximately 500 to 600 mL. The metabolic products of hepatocyte uptake and synthesis are secreted into the bile canaliculi, which are lined by microvillus membrane components associated with microfilaments of actin, microtubules, and other contractile elements. Within the hepatocyte, conjugation of many of the bile constituents may occur, while other components of bile such as primary bile acids, lecithin, and some cholesterol are synthesized de novo. Three mechanisms are important in regulating bile flow: (1) active transport of bile acids from hepatocytes into the canaliculi, (2) bile acid–independent ATPase-mediated transport of sodium, and (3) ductular secretion. The last is a secretin-mediated and cyclic AMP–dependent phenomenon which appears to result from the active transport of sodium and bicarbonate into the ductule with resulting passive movement of water across the cell membrane.

The bile acids The primary bile acids, cholic and chenodeoxycholic acids, are synthesized from cholesterol in the liver, conjugated with glycine or taurine, and excreted into the bile. Secondary bile acids, including deoxycholate and lithocholate, are formed in the colon as bacterial metabolites of the primary bile acids. However, lithocholic acid is much less efficiently absorbed from the colon than deoxycholic acid. Other secondary bile acids, found in trace amounts, which include ursodeoxycholic acid (a stereoisomer of chenodeoxycholate) and a variety of other unusual or "aberrant" bile acids, may be produced in increased amounts in patients with chronic cholestatic syndromes. In normal bile, the ratio of glycine to taurine conjugates is about 3:1, while in patients with cholestasis, increased concentrations of sulfate and glucuronide conjugates of bile acids are often found.

Bile acids are detergents which in aqueous solutions and above a critical concentration of about 2 m*M* form molecular aggregates called micelles. Cholesterol alone is poorly soluble in aqueous environments, and its solubility in bile depends upon both the lipid concentration and the relative molar percentages of bile acids and lecithin. Normal ratios of these constituents favor the formation of solubilizing "mixed micelles," while abnormal ratios promote the precipitation of cholesterol crystals in bile.

In addition to facilitating the biliary excretion of cholesterol, bile acids are necessary for the normal intestinal absorption of dietary fats via a micellar transport mechanism (see Chap. 237). Bile acids also serve as a major physiologic driving force for hepatic bile flow and aid in water and electrolyte transport in the small bowel and colon.

Enterohepatic circulation Bile acids are efficiently conserved under normal conditions. Conjugated and unconjugated bile acids are absorbed by *passive diffusion* along the entire gut. Quantitatively much more important for bile salt recirculation, however, is the *active transport* mechanism for conjugated bile acids in the distal ileum (see Chap. 237). The reabsorbed bile acids enter the portal bloodstream and are taken up rapidly by hepatocytes, reconjugated, and resecreted into bile (enterohepatic circulation).

The normal bile acid pool size is approximately 2 to 4 g. During digestion of a meal, the bile acid pool undergoes at least one or more enterohepatic cycles depending upon the size and composition of the meal. Normally the bile acid pool circulates approximately 5 to 10 times daily. Intestinal absorption of the pool is about 95 percent efficient, so that fecal loss of bile acids is in the range of 0.3 to 0.6 g per day. This fecal loss is compensated by an equal daily synthesis of bile acids by the liver, and thus the size of the bile salt pool is maintained. Bile acids returning to the liver suppress de novo hepatic synthesis of primary bile acids from cholesterol by inhibiting the rate-limiting enzyme 7α-hydroxylase. While the loss of bile salts in stool is usually matched by increased hepatic synthesis, the maximum rate of synthesis is approximately 5 g per day, which may be insufficient to replete the bile acid pool size when there is pronounced impairment of intestinal bile salt reabsorption.

Gallbladder and sphincteric functions In the fasting state, the sphincter of Oddi offers a high-pressure zone of resistance to bile flow from the common bile duct into the duodenum. This tonic contraction serves to (1) prevent reflux of duodenal contents into the pancreatic and bile ducts, and (2) promote bile filling of the gallbladder. The major factor controlling the evacuation of the gallbladder is the peptide hormone cholecystokinin, which is released from the duodenal mucosa in response to the ingestion of fats and amino acids. Cholecystokinin produces (1) powerful contraction of the gallbladder, (2) decreased resistance of the sphincter of Oddi, (3) increased hepatic secretion of bile, and thus (4) enhanced flow of biliary contents into the duodenum.

Hepatic bile is "concentrated" within the gallbladder by energy-dependent transmucosal absorption of water and electrolytes. Almost the entire bile acid pool may be sequestered in the gallbladder following an overnight fast for delivery into the duodenum with the first meal of the day. The normal capacity of the gallbladder is 30 to 75 mL of bile.

DISEASES OF THE GALLBLADDER

CONGENITAL ANOMALIES Anomalies of the biliary tract may be found in 10 to 20 percent of the population, including abnormalities in number, size, and shape (e.g., agenesis of the gallbladder, duplications, rudimentary or oversized "giant" gallbladders, and diverticula). Phrygian cap is a clinically innocuous entity in which a partial or complete septum (or fold) separates the fundus from the body. Anomalies of position or suspension are not uncommon and include left-sided gallbladder, intrahepatic gallbladder, retrodisplacement of the gallbladder, and "floating" gallbladder. The latter condition predisposes to acute torsion, volvulus, or herniation of the gallbladder.

GALLSTONES **Pathogenesis of gallstones** Gallstones are quite prevalent in most western countries. In the United States, autopsy series have shown gallstones in at least 20 percent of women and in 8 percent of men over the age of 40. It is estimated that 16 to 20 million persons in the United States have gallstones and that approximately 1 million new cases of cholelithiasis develop each year.

Gallstones are crystalline structures formed by concretion or accretion of normal or abnormal bile constituents. These stones are divided into three major types; cholesterol and mixed stones account for 80 percent of the total, with pigment stones comprising the remaining 20 percent. Mixed and cholesterol gallstones usually contain more than 70 percent cholesterol monohydrate plus an admixture of calcium salts, bile acids and bile pigments, proteins, fatty acids, and phospholipids. Pigment stones are primarily composed of calcium bilirubinate; they contain less than 10 percent cholesterol.

CHOLESTEROL AND MIXED STONES The solubility of cholesterol in bile depends upon the relative molar concentrations of cholesterol, bile acids, and lecithin. These concentrations may be expressed on triangular coordinates as a phase diagram of bile composition (Fig. 253-1). As noted above, cholesterol is relatively water insoluble and normally is kept in solution (in the form of mixed micelles) by bile salts and phospholipids.

The most important mechanism in the formation of lithogenic (stone-forming) bile is increased biliary secretion of cholesterol. This may occur in association with obesity, high-caloric diets, or drugs (e.g., clofibrate) and may result from increased activity of hydroxymethylglutaryl-coenzyme A (HMG-CoA) reductase, the rate-limiting enzyme of hepatic cholesterol synthesis. In some patients, impaired hepatic conversion of cholesterol to bile acids may also occur, resulting in a decrease of the lithogenic cholesterol/bile acid ratio. Lithogenic bile also results from decreased hepatic secretion of bile salts and phospholipids which may follow impaired hepatic synthesis

FIGURE 253-1 *Phase diagram of bile composition. The relative concentrations of cholesterol, bile acids, and lecithin are expressed on triangular coordinates as mole percentages totaling 100 percent. The equilibrium limit of solubility for cholesterol is denoted by the solid line. Hatchmarks indicate the metastable zone, where slow precipitation of cholesterol from supersaturated bile may occur. Point A represents a micellar solution in which cholesterol is solubilized in mixed micelles. Point B, on the equilibrium limit of solubility line, indicates bile saturated with cholesterol. Point C depicts cholesterol supersaturated bile, a composition leading to the precipitation of cholesterol crystals.*

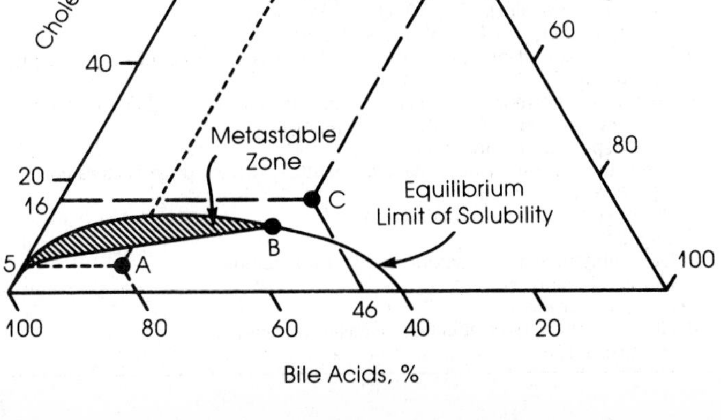

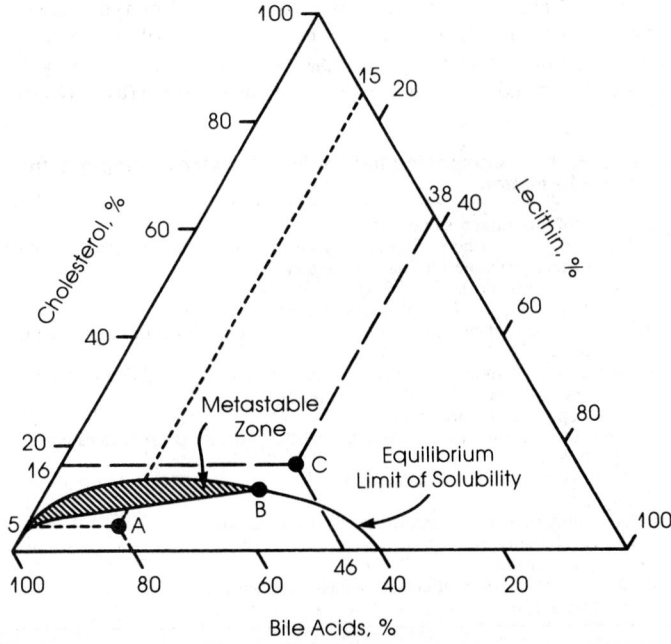

(e.g., rare inborn errors of metabolism such as cerebrotendinous xanthomatosis) or conditions affecting the enterohepatic circulation of these constituents (e.g., prolonged parenteral alimentation or ileal disease or resection). In addition, most patients with gallstones appear to have reduced activity of hepatic cholesterol 7α-hydroxylase, the rate-limiting enzyme for primary bile acid synthesis.

Stone formation in bile supersaturated with cholesterol requires both nucleation and the production of cholesterol monohydrate crystals, which may grow by accretion or concretion to form macroscopic aggregates. In fact, the major difference in supersaturated bile with respect to ability to form cholesterol crystals probably involves the nucleation rather than the crystal growth stage. Gallbladder mucin probably accelerates the nucleation of cholesterol monohydrate crystals and thus may contribute to cholesterol stone formation. Other biliary proteins appear to inhibit cholesterol crystal nucleation in normal human gallbladder bile. The major known predisposing factors to cholesterol stone formation are summarized in Table 253-1.

PIGMENT STONES Gallstones composed largely of calcium bilirubinate are much more common in the orient than in western countries. The presence of increased amounts of unconjugated, insoluble bilirubin in bile results in the precipitation of bilirubin which may aggregate to form pigment stones or may fuse to form the nidus for growth of mixed cholesterol gallstones. In western countries, chronic hemolytic states (with increased conjugated bilirubin in bile) or alcoholic liver disease are associated with an increased incidence of pigment stones. Deconjugation of soluble bilirubin mono- and diglucuronide may be mediated by the enzyme β-glucuronidase, which is sometimes produced when bile is chronically infected by bacteria. Pigment stone formation is especially prominent in Asians and is often associated with infections in the biliary tree (see Table 253-1).

Diagnosis of gallstones Procedures of potential use in the diagnosis of cholelithiasis and other diseases of the gallbladder are detailed in Table 253-2. The plain abdominal film may detect gallstones containing sufficient calcium to be radiopaque (10 to 15 percent of cholesterol and mixed stones and approximately 50 percent of pigment stones). Plain radiography may also be of use in the diagnosis of emphysematous cholecystitis, porcelain gallbladder, limey bile, and gallstone ileus.

Ultrasonography of the gallbladder is very accurate in the identification of cholelithiasis and has several advantages over oral cholecystography (see Fig. 253-2*A*). The gallbladder is easily visualized with the technique, and, in fact, failure to image the gallbladder successfully in a fasting patient correlates well with the presence of underlying gallbladder disease. Stones as small as 2 mm in diameter may be confidently identified provided that firm criteria are used [e.g., acoustic "shadowing" of opacities that are within the gallbladder lumen and that change with the patient's position (by gravity)].

TABLE 253-1 Predisposing factors for cholesterol and pigment gallstone formation

1 Cholesterol and mixed stones
- *a* Demography: northern Europe and North and South America greater than orient; probable familial, hereditary aspects
- *b* Obesity, high-calorie diet (↑ cholesterol output)
- *c* Clofibrate therapy (↑ cholesterol output)
- *d* Malabsorption of bile acids (e.g., ileal disease or resection) (↓ bile salt secretion)
- *e* Female sex hormones: women > men after puberty; oral contraceptives and other estrogens (↓ bile salt secretion)
- *f* Age, especially among males
- *g* Other factors: pregnancy, diabetes mellitus, dietary polyunsaturated fats (↑ cholesterol output)
- *h* Prolonged parenteral alimentation

2 Pigment stones
- *a* Demographic/genetic factors: orient, rural setting
- *b* Chronic hemolysis
- *c* Alcoholic cirrhosis
- *d* Chronic biliary tract infection, parasite infestation
- *e* Increasing age

In major medical centers the false-negative and false-positive rates for ultrasound in gallstone patients are about 2 to 4 percent.

Oral cholecystography (OCG) is a useful procedure for the diagnosis of gallstones but has been largely replaced by ultrasound. False-positive results are rare, but the oral cholecystogram may be falsely negative (when good opacification is achieved) in approximately 5 to 10 percent of patients with gallstones. Factors which may produce nonvisualization of the OCG are summarized in Table 253-2. When these can be excluded, nonvisualization of the gallbladder following a second dose of oral contrast agent is highly correlated with underlying cystic duct obstruction or chronic inflammation of the gallbladder.

Radiopharmaceuticals such as ^{99m}Tc-labeled *N*-substituted iminodiacetic acids (HIDA, DIDA, DISIDA, etc.) are rapidly extracted from the blood and are excreted into the biliary tree in high concentration even in the presence of mild to moderate serum bilirubin elevations. Failure to image the gallbladder in the presence of biliary ductal visualization may indicate cystic duct obstruction, acute or chronic cholecystitis, or surgical absence of the organ. Such scans have their greatest application in the diagnosis of acute cholecystitis.

Symptoms of gallstone disease Gallstones usually produce symptoms by causing inflammation or obstruction following their migration into the cystic duct or common bile duct. The most specific and characteristic symptom of gallstone disease is biliary colic. Obstruction of the cystic duct or common bile duct by a stone produces increased intraluminal pressure and distention of the viscus which cannot be relieved by repetitive biliary contractions. The resultant visceral pain is characteristically a severe, steady aching or pressure in the epigastrium or right upper quadrant of the abdomen with frequent radiation to the interscapular area, right scapula, or shoulder.

Biliary colic begins quite suddenly and may persist with severe intensity for 1 to 4 h, subsiding gradually or rapidly. An episode of biliary pain is sometimes followed by a residual mild ache or soreness in the right upper quadrant which may persist for 24 h or so. Nausea and vomiting frequently accompany episodes of biliary colic, and mild elevations of serum bilirubin (not exceeding 5 mg/dL) occur in 25 percent of patients. Persistence of a high serum bilirubin level suggests common duct stones. Fever or chills (rigors) with biliary colic usually imply an underlying complication, i.e., cholecystitis, pancreatitis, or cholangitis. Complaints of vague epigastric fullness, dyspepsia, eructation, or flatulence, especially following a fatty meal, should not be confused with biliary colic. Such symptoms are frequently elicited from patients with gallstone disease but are not specific for biliary calculi. Biliary colic may be precipitated by eating a fatty meal, by consumption of a large meal following a period of prolonged fasting, or by eating a normal meal.

Natural history of gallstones Gallstone disease discovered in an asymptomatic patient or in a patient whose symptoms are not referable to cholelithiasis is a common clinical problem. The natural history of "silent" or asymptomatic gallstones has occasioned much debate. In contrast to previous reports, a study of predominantly male silent gallstone patients suggests that the cumulative risk for the development of symptoms or complications requiring surgery is relatively low—10 percent at 5 years, 15 percent at 10 years, and 18 percent at 15 years. Patients remaining asymptomatic for 15 years were found to be unlikely to develop symptoms during further follow-up, and most patients who did develop complications from their gallstones experienced *prior* warning symptoms.

Complications requiring cholecystectomy appear to be much more common in gallstone patients who have developed symptoms of biliary colic. Patients found to have gallstones at a young age are more likely to develop symptoms from cholelithiasis than are patients older than 60 years at the time of initial diagnosis. Patients with diabetes mellitus and gallstones may be somewhat more susceptible to septic complications, but the magnitude of risk of septic biliary complications in diabetic patients is incompletely defined. In addition, asymptomatic gallstone patients with nonvisualization of the gall-

TABLE 253-2 Diagnostic evaluation of the gallbladder

Procedure	Diagnostic advantages	Diagnostic limitations	Comment
Plain abdominal x-ray	Low cost Readily available	Relatively low yield ?Contraindicated in pregnancy	Pathognomonic findings in: Calcified gallstones Limey bile, porcelain GB Emphysematous cholecystitis Gallstone ileus
Oral cholecystogram (OCG)	Low cost Readily available Accurate identification of gallstones (90–95%) Identification of GB anomalies, hyperplastic cholecystoses Identification of chronic GB disease after nonvisualization on double dose	?Contraindicated in pregnancy ?Contraindicated with history of reaction to iodinated contrast Nonvisualization with: Serum bilirubin >2–4 mg/dL Failure to ingest or absorb tablets Impaired hepatic excretion Very small stones may be undetected More time consuming than GBUS	Procedure of choice in identification of gallstones if diagnostic limitations prevent GBUS
Gallbladder ultrasound (GBUS)	Rapid Accurate identification of gallstones (>95%) Simultaneous scanning of GB, liver, bile ducts, pancreas "Real-time" scanning allows assessment of GB volume, contractility Not limited by jaundice, pregnancy May detect very small stones	Bowel gas Massive obesity Ascites Recent barium study	Procedure of choice for detection of stones
Radioisotope scans (HIDA, DISIDA, etc.)	Accurate identification of cystic duct obstruction Simultaneous assessment of bile ducts	?Contraindicated in pregnancy Serum bilirubin >6–12 mg/dL Cholecystogram of low resolution	Indicated for confirmation of suspected cholecystitis

bladder on OCG appear to have an increased tendency to develop symptoms and complications.

Treatment of gallstones SURGICAL THERAPY Although the management of "silent" gallstones remains controversial, the risk of developing symptoms or complications requiring surgery is quite small (in the range of 1 to 2 percent per year) in most asymptomatic gallstone patients. Thus, a recommendation for prophylactic cholecystectomy in a patient with gallstones should probably be based on assessment of three factors: (1) the presence of symptoms which are frequent enough or severe enough to interfere with the patient's general routine; (2) the presence of a prior complication of gallstone disease, i.e., history of acute cholecystitis, pancreatitis, gallstone fistula, etc.; or (3) the presence of an underlying condition predisposing the patient to increased risk of gallstone complications (e.g., calcified or porcelain gallbladder, cholesterolosis, adenomyomatosis, nonvisualizing gallbladder on oral cholecystography, and/or a previous attack of acute cholecystitis regardless of current symptomatic status). Patients with very large gallstones (over 2 cm in diameter) and patients having gallstones in a congenitally anomalous gallbladder might also be considered for prophylactic cholecystectomy. Although age under 50 years is a worrisome factor in asymptomatic gallstone patients, few authorities would now recommend routine cholecystectomy in all young patients with silent stones.

MEDICAL THERAPY—GALLSTONE DISSOLUTION Treatment with oral chenodeoxycholic acid (CDCA, chenic acid) or its 7β-epimer, ursodeoxycholic acid (UDCA), to dissolve cholesterol or mixed

FIGURE 253-2 *Examples of ultrasound and radiologic studies of the biliary tract. A. An ultrasound study showing a distended gallbladder containing a single large stone (arrow) which casts an acoustic shadow. B. Endoscopic retrograde cholangiopancreatogram (ERCP) showing normal biliary tract anatomy. In addition to the endoscope and large vertical gallbladder filled with contrast dye, the common hepatic duct (chd), common bile duct (cbd), and pancreatic duct (pd) are shown. The arrow points to the ampulla of Vater. C. Percutaneous transhepatic cholangiogram (PTHC) showing choledocholithiasis. The biliary tract is dilatated and contains multiple radiolucent calculi (small arrows). The dilatation is due to obstruction by a large stone in the distal portion of the duct (large arrow). D. ERCP showing sclerosing cholangitis. The common bile duct is to the right of the endoscope. Following retrograde cholangiography, the common bile duct shows thickening of the wall with a narrow, beaded lumen typical of sclerosing cholangitis.*

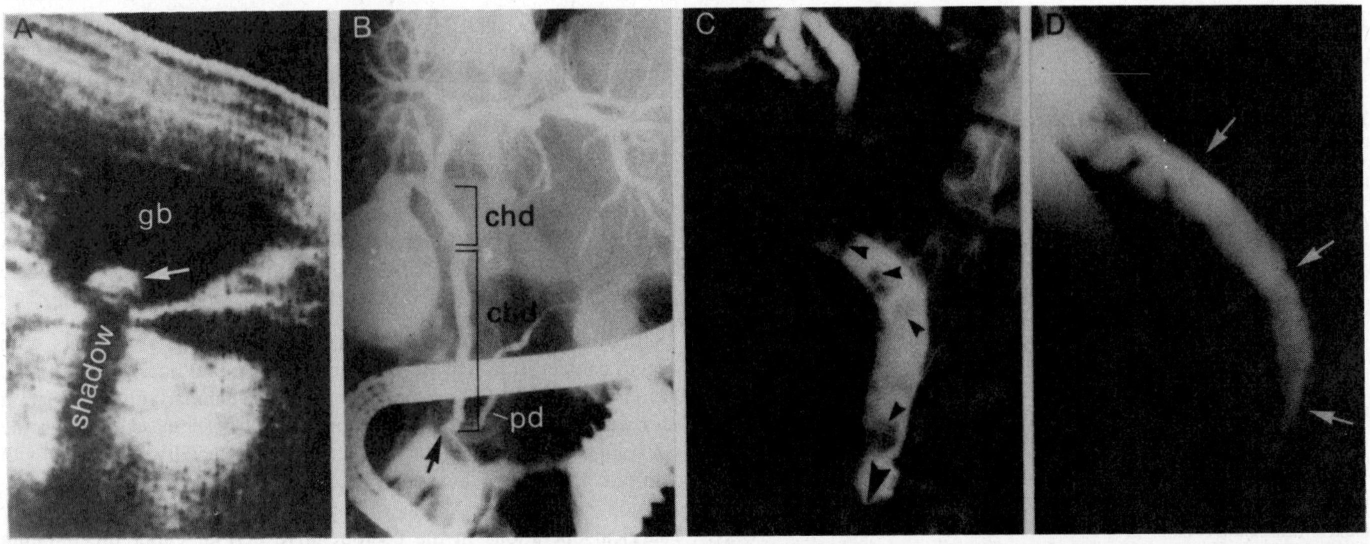

gallstones has resulted in complete or partial dissolution of such stones in approximately 50 to 60 percent of patients with radiolucent gallstones. Biliary secretion of these agents following oral bile acid administration alters the bile acid/cholesterol/lecithin ratio in bile (the lithogenic index). The major therapeutic effect of CDCA, however, is thought to be secondary to a decrease in HMG-CoA reductase activity, which in turn results in decreased hepatic cholesterol synthesis. UDCA administration appears to produce a lamellar liquid crystalline phase in bile which allows dispersion of cholesterol from stones by physical-chemical means.

Oral bile acid therapy is essentially ineffective in dissolving (1) pigment gallstones, which represent approximately 20 percent of radiolucent stones; (2) radiopaque or calcified gallstones; (3) gallstones greater than approximately 1.5 cm in diameter; and (4) gallstones in gallbladders poorly opacified following oral cholecystography. In patients with multiple, small, radiolucent gallstones in a functioning gallbladder, success rates for CDCA therapy of up to 80 percent have been reported if daily doses of 10 to 15 mg/kg of CDCA are used over a 1- to 3-year treatment period. However, lower daily doses of CDCA, i.e., 5 to 10 mg/kg, have resulted in much lower complete dissolution (5 to 15 percent) as well as lower partial dissolution rates (40 percent). Further, some massively obese patients may require doses as high as 20 to 25 mg/kg per day of CDCA to achieve cholesterol desaturation of bile. After successful dissolution of stones and withdrawal of CDCA treatment, *recurrence* of cholelithiasis is likely unless factors initially producing lithogenesis have been altered in the interim. Ultrasound appears to be more sensitive than oral cholecystography in following patients during and after stone dissolution therapy. The results of the U.S. National Cooperative Gallstone Study are summarized in Table 253-3.

Chenodeoxycholic acid therapy is usually associated with self-limited diarrhea in most patients given an optimal therapeutic dose. In addition, approximately 25 percent of patients treated with CDCA acid develop mild (two- to threefold) and transient (less than 6 months) elevations of serum aminotransferase levels. Although hepatic injury has been described, biopsy and liver function studies in humans have shown serious CDCA-related hepatotoxicity in less than 1 to 2 percent of patients.

Ursodeoxycholic acid is therapeutically effective at lower doses (5 to 10 mg/kg per day) than chenodeoxycholic acid and has not been associated with the relatively high incidence of diarrhea and serum aminotransferase elevations seen in CDCA-treated patients. On the other hand, UDCA treatment has been associated with calcification of previously uncalcified gallstones in more than 10 percent of patients.

Direct dissolution of gallstones within a period of hours using methyl tertiary butyl ether or other solvents through percutaneously placed biliary catheters has also been reported. Such solvent dissolution of gallbladder or ductal stones by continuous perfusion appears promising.

TABLE 253-3 Chenodeoxycholic acid (CDCA) and gallstone dissolution

RESULTS OF U.S. NATIONAL COOPERATIVE GALLSTONE STUDY

1 Patients—916 with radiolucent stones, treated 24 months
  a Placebo
  b Low-dose CDCA; 375 mg per day
  c High-dose CDCA; 750 mg per day
2 Results—best with high dose
  a Complete dissolution, 13.5%
  b Partial dissolution, 27.3%; complete plus partial, 40.8%
  c Best results—women, thin patients, small stones
3 Side effects
  a Mild diarrhea
  b Changes in hepatic structure, function; 3% clinically significant liver damage
  c Elevation (10%) of serum LDL cholesterol
4 Recurrence—likely when CDCA stopped

SOURCE: *Schoenfield et al.*

ACUTE AND CHRONIC CHOLECYSTITIS **Acute cholecystitis** Acute inflammation of the gallbladder wall usually follows obstruction of the cystic duct by a stone. Inflammatory response can be evoked by three factors: (1) *mechanical inflammation* produced by increased intraluminal pressure and distention with resulting ischemia of the gallbladder mucosa and wall; (2) *chemical inflammation* caused by the release of lysolecithin (due to the action of phospholipase on lecithin in bile) and other local tissue factors; and (3) *bacterial inflammation*, which may play a role in 50 to 85 percent of patients with acute cholecystitis. The organisms most frequently isolated by culture of gallbladder bile in these patients include *Escherichia coli, Klebsiella* species, group D *Streptococcus, Staphylococcus* species, and *Clostridium* species.

Acute cholecystitis often begins as an attack of biliary colic which progressively worsens. Approximately 60 to 70 percent of patients report having experienced prior attacks which resolved spontaneously. As the episode progresses, however, the pain of acute cholecystitis becomes more generalized in the right upper abdomen. As with biliary colic, the pain of cholecystitis may radiate to the interscapular area, right scapula, or shoulder. Peritoneal signs of inflammation such as increased pain with jarring or on deep respiration may be apparent. The patient is anorectic and often nauseated. Vomiting is relatively common and may produce symptoms and signs of vascular and extracellular volume depletion. Jaundice is unusual early in the course of acute cholecystitis but may occur when edematous inflammatory changes involve the bile ducts and surrounding lymph nodes.

A low-grade fever is characteristically present, but shaking chills or rigors are not uncommon. The right upper quadrant of the abdomen is almost invariably tender to palpation. An enlarged, tense gallbladder is palpable in one-quarter to one-half of patients. Deep inspiration or cough during subcostal palpation of the right upper quadrant usually produces increased pain and inspiratory arrest (Murphy's sign). A light blow delivered to the right subcostal area may elicit a marked increase in pain. Localized rebound tenderness in the right upper quadrant is common, as are abdominal distention and hypoactive bowel sounds from paralytic ileus, but generalized peritoneal signs and abdominal rigidity are usually absent unless perforation has occurred.

The diagnosis of acute cholecystitis is usually made on the basis of a characteristic history and physical examination. The triad of sudden onset of right upper quadrant tenderness, fever, and leukocytosis is highly suggestive. Typically, leukocytosis in the range of 10,000 to 15,000 cells per cubic millimeter with a left shift on differential count is found. The serum bilirubin is mildly elevated (less than 5 mg/dL) in 45 percent of patients, while 25 percent have modest elevations in serum aminotransferases (usually less than a fivefold elevation). The radionuclide (e.g., HIDA) biliary scan may be confirmatory if bile duct imaging is seen without visualization of the gallbladder. Cholecystography by oral or intravenous technique is almost always nonvisualizing.

Approximately 75 percent of patients treated medically have remission of acute symptoms within 2 to 7 days following hospitalization. In 25 percent, however, a complication of acute cholecystitis will occur despite conservative treatment (see below). In this setting, prompt surgical intervention is required. Of the 75 percent of patients with acute cholecystitis who undergo remission of symptoms, approximately one-quarter will experience a recurrence of cholecystitis within 1 year, and 60 percent will have at least one recurrent bout within 6 years. In view of the natural history of the disease, acute cholecystitis is best treated by early surgery whenever possible.

ACALCULOUS CHOLECYSTITIS In 5 to 10 percent of patients with acute cholecystitis, calculi obstructing the cystic duct are not found at surgery. In over 50 percent of such cases an underlying explanation for acalculous inflammation is not found. An increased risk for the development of acalculous cholecystitis is especially associated with serious trauma or burns, with the postpartum period following prolonged labor, and with orthopedic and other nonbiliary major surgical operations in the postoperative period. Other precipitating factors include vasculitis, obstructing adenocarcinoma of the gallbladder, diabetes mellitus, torsion of the gallbladder, "unusual" bacterial infections of the gallbladder (e.g., *Leptospira, Streptococcus, Salmonella,* or *Vibrio cholerae*), and parasitic infestation of the gallbladder. Acalculous cholecystitis may also be seen with a variety of other systemic disease processes (sarcoidosis, cardiovascular disease, tuberculosis, syphilis, actinomycosis, etc.) and may possibly complicate periods of prolonged parenteral hyperalimentation.

Although the clinical manifestations of acalculous cholecystitis are indistinguishable from those of calculous cholecystitis, the setting of acute gallbladder inflammation complicating severe underlying illness is characteristic of acalculous disease. Ultrasound, CT scanning, or radionuclide examinations demonstrating a large, tense, static gallbladder without stones and with evidence of poor emptying over a prolonged period may be diagnostically useful in some cases. The complication rate for acalculous cholecystitis exceeds that for calculous cholecystitis. Successful management of acute acalculous cholecystitis appears to depend primarily upon early diagnosis and surgical intervention with meticulous attention to postoperative care.

EMPHYSEMATOUS CHOLECYSTITIS So-called emphysematous cholecystitis is thought to begin with acute cholecystitis (calculous or acalculous) followed by ischemia or gangrene of the gallbladder wall and infection by gas-producing organisms. Bacteria most frequently cultured in this setting include anaerobes such as *Clostridium welchii,* or *perfringens,* and aerobes such as *E. coli.* This condition occurs most frequently in elderly men and in patients with diabetes mellitus. The clinical manifestations are essentially indistinguishable from those of nongaseous cholecystitis. The diagnosis is usually made on plain abdominal film by the finding of gas within the gallbladder lumen, dissecting within the gallbladder wall to form a gaseous ring, or in the pericholecystic tissues. The morbidity and mortality rates with emphysematous cholecystitis are considerable. Prompt surgical intervention coupled with appropriate antibiotics is mandatory.

Chronic cholecystitis Chronic inflammation of the gallbladder wall is almost always associated with the presence of gallstones and is thought to result from repeated bouts of subacute or acute cholecystitis or from persistent mechanical irritation of the gallbladder wall. The presence of bacteria in the bile occurs in more than one-quarter of patients with chronic cholecystitis. Although the presence of infected bile in a patient with *chronic* cholecystitis undergoing elective cholecystectomy probably adds little to the operative risk, intraoperative Gram's staining and routine culturing of bile has been advocated to identify those patients whose gallbladder is colonized with *Clostridium* species. Appropriate antibiotics intra- and postoperatively are recommended in such patients because colonization with these organisms may be associated with devastating septic complications following surgery. Chronic cholecystitis may remain asymptomatic for years, may progress to symptomatic gallbladder disease or to acute cholecystitis, or may present with one of the complications detailed below.

Complications of cholecystitis EMPYEMA AND HYDROPS Empyema of the gallbladder usually results from progression of acute cholecystitis with persistent cystic duct obstruction to superinfection of the stagnant bile with a pus-forming bacterial organism. The clinical picture resembles that of cholangitis with high fever, severe right upper quadrant pain, marked leukocytosis, and, often, prostration. Empyema of the gallbladder carries a high risk of gram-negative sepsis and/or perforation. Emergency surgical intervention with proper antibiotic coverage is required as soon as the diagnosis is suspected.

Hydrops or mucocele of the gallbladder may also result from prolonged obstruction of the cystic duct, usually by a large solitary calculus. In this instance, the obstructed gallbladder lumen is progressively distended, over a period of time, by mucus (mucocele) or by a clear transudate (hydrops) produced by mucosal epithelial cells. A visible, easily palpable, nontender mass often extending from the right upper quadrant into the right iliac fossa may be found on physical examination. The patient with hydrops of the gallbladder frequently remains asymptomatic, although chronic right upper quadrant pain also may occur. Cholecystectomy is indicated since empyema, perforation, or gangrene may complicate the condition.

GANGRENE AND PERFORATION Gangrene of the gallbladder results from ischemia of the wall and patchy or complete tissue necrosis. Underlying conditions often include marked distention of the gallbladder, vasculitis, diabetes mellitus, empyema, or torsion resulting in arterial occlusion. Gangrene usually predisposes to perforation of the gallbladder, but perforation may also occur in chronic cholecystitis without premonitory warning symptoms. *Localized perforations* are usually contained by the omentum or by adhesions produced by recurrent inflammation of the gallbladder. Bacterial superinfection of the walled-off gallbladder contents results in abscess formation. Most patients are best treated with cholecystectomy, but some seriously ill patients may be managed with cholecystostomy and drainage of the abscess. *Free perforation* is less common but is associated with a mortality rate of approximately 30 percent. Such patients may experience a sudden transient relief of right upper quadrant pain as the distended gallbladder decompresses; this is followed by signs of generalized peritonitis.

FISTULA FORMATION AND GALLSTONE ILEUS *Fistulization* into an adjacent organ adherent to the gallbladder wall may result from inflammation and adhesion formation. Fistulas into the duodenum are most common, followed in frequency by those involving the hepatic flexure of the colon, stomach or jejunum, abdominal wall, and renal pelvis. Clinically "silent" biliary-enteric fistulas occurring as a complication of chronic cholecystitis have been found in up to 5 percent of patients undergoing cholecystectomy. Asymptomatic cholecystoenteric fistulas may sometimes be diagnosed by finding gas in the biliary tree on plain abdominal films. Barium contrast studies or endoscopy of the upper gastrointestinal tract or colon may demonstrate the fistula, but oral cholecystography will almost never result in opacification of either the gallbladder or the fistulous tract. Treatment in the symptomatic patient usually consists of cholecystectomy, common bile duct exploration, and closure of the fistulous tract.

Gallstone ileus refers to mechanical intestinal obstruction resulting from the passage of a large gallstone into the bowel lumen. The stone customarily enters the duodenum through a cholecystoenteric fistula at that level. The site of obstruction by the impacted gallstone is usually at the ileocecal valve, provided that the more proximal small bowel is of normal caliber. The majority of patients do not give a history of either prior biliary tract symptoms or complaints suggestive of acute cholecystitis or fistulization. Large stones over 2.5 cm in diameter are thought to predispose to fistula formation by gradual erosion through the gallbladder fundus. Diagnostic confirmation may occasionally be found on the plain abdominal film (e.g., small-intestinal obstruction with gas in the biliary tree and a calcified, ectopic gallstone) or following an upper gastrointestinal series (cholecystoduodenal fistula with small-bowel obstruction at the ileocecal valve). Early laparotomy is indicated with enterolithotomy and careful palpation of the more proximal small bowel and gallbladder to exclude other stones.

LIMEY (MILK OF CALCIUM) BILE AND PORCELAIN GALLBLADDER Calcium salts may be secreted into the lumen of the gallbladder in sufficient concentration to produce calcium precipitation and diffuse, hazy opacification of bile or a layering effect on plain abdominal roentgenography. This so-called limey bile or milk of calcium bile is usually clinically innocuous, but cholecystectomy is recommended since limey bile most often occurs in an hydropic gallbladder. In the entity called porcelain gallbladder, calcium salt deposition within the wall of a chronically inflamed gallbladder may be detected on the plain abdominal film. Cholecystectomy is advised in all patients with porcelain gallbladder since in a high percentage of cases this finding appears to be associated with the development of carcinoma of the gallbladder.

Treatment of cholecystitis MEDICAL THERAPY Although surgical intervention remains the mainstay of therapy for acute cholecystitis and its complications, a period of in-hospital stabilization may be required before cholecystectomy. Oral intake is eliminated, nasogastric suction is initiated, and extracellular volume depletion and electrolyte abnormalities are repaired. Meperidine or pentazocine are usually employed for analgesia since they may produce less spasm of the sphincter of Oddi than drugs such as morphine. Intravenous antibiotic therapy is usually indicated in patients with severe acute cholecystitis even though bacterial superinfection of bile may not have occurred in the early stages of the inflammatory process. Postoperative complications of wound infection, abscess formation, or sepsis are reduced in antibiotic-treated patients. Effective single-agent antibiotics include ampicillin, cephalosporins, chloramphenicol, or aminoglycosides, but in diabetic or debilitated patients and in those with signs of gram-negative sepsis, combination antibiotic treatment may be preferable (see also Chap. 92).

SURGICAL THERAPY The optimal timing of surgical intervention in patients with acute cholecystitis remains controversial. Urgent (emergency) cholecystectomy or cholecystostomy is probably appropriate in most patients in whom a complication of acute cholecystitis such as empyema, emphysematous cholecystitis, or perforation is suspected or confirmed. In uncomplicated cases of acute cholecystitis up to 30 percent of patients fail to resolve their symptoms on appropriate medical therapy, and progression of the attack or a supervening complication leads to the performance of early operation (within 24 to 72 h). The technical complications of surgery are not increased in patients undergoing early as opposed to delayed cholecystectomy. Delayed surgical intervention is probably best reserved for (1) patients in whom the overall medical condition imposes an unacceptable risk for early surgery, and (2) cases in which the diagnosis of acute cholecystitis is in doubt. Early cholecystectomy is the treatment of choice for most patients with acute cholecystitis. Mortality figures for emergency cholecystectomy in most centers approach 3 percent, while the mortality risk for elective or early cholecystectomy approximates 0.5 percent in patients under age 60. Of course, the operative risks increase with age-related diseases of other organ systems and with the presence of long-term or short-term complications of gallbladder disease. Seriously ill or debilitated patients with cholecystitis may be managed with cholecystostomy and tube drainage of the gallbladder. Elective cholecystectomy may then be done at a later date.

Postcholecystectomy complications Early complications following cholecystectomy include atelectasis and other pulmonary disorders, abscess formation (often subphrenic), external or internal hemorrhage, biliary-enteric fistula, and bile leaks. Jaundice may indicate absorption of bile from an intraabdominal collection following a biliary leak, or mechanical obstruction of the common bile duct by retained calculi, intraductal blood clots, or extrinsic compression. Routine performance of intraoperative cholangiography during cholecystectomy has helped to reduce the incidence of these early complications.

Overall, cholecystectomy is a very successful operation which provides total or near-total relief of presurgical symptoms in 75 to 90 percent of patients. The most common cause of persistent postcholecystectomy symptoms is an overlooked extrabiliary disorder (e.g., reflux esophagitis, peptic ulceration, postgastrectomy syndrome, pancreatitis, or irritable bowel syndrome). In a small percentage of patients, however, a disorder of the extrahepatic bile ducts may result in persistent symptomatology. These so-called postcholecystectomy syndromes may be due to (1) biliary strictures, (2) retained biliary calculi, (3) cystic duct stump syndrome, (4) stenosis or dyskinesia of the sphincter of Oddi, or (5) bile salt–induced diarrhea or gastritis.

CYSTIC DUCT STUMP SYNDROME In the absence of cholangiographically demonstrable retained stones, symptoms resembling biliary colic or cholecystitis in the postcholecystectomy patient have frequently been attributed to disease in a long (> 1 cm) cystic duct remnant (cystic duct stump syndrome). Careful analysis, however, reveals that postcholecystectomy complaints are attributable to other causes in almost all patients in whom the symptom complex was originally thought to result from the existence of a long cystic duct stump. Accordingly, considerable care should be taken to investigate the possible role of other factors in the production of postcholecystectomy symptoms before attributing them to cystic duct stump syndrome.

BILE SALT–INDUCED CATHARSIS AND GASTRITIS Postcholecystectomy patients may develop symptoms and signs of gastritis which has been attributed to duodenogastric reflux of bile. However, firm data linking an increased incidence of bile gastritis with surgical removal of the gallbladder are lacking. Similarly, the occurrence of cholestyramine-responsive diarrhea in a small number of patients following cholecystectomy has been attributed to an alteration of the enterohepatic circulation of bile acids induced or unmasked by removal of the gallbladder.

THE HYPERPLASTIC CHOLECYSTOSES The term *hyperplastic cholecystoses* is used to denote a group of disorders of the gallbladder characterized by excessive proliferation of normal tissue components.

Adenomyomatosis is characterized by a benign proliferation of gallbladder surface epithelium with gland-like formations, extramural sinuses, transverse strictures, and/or fundal nodule ("adenoma" or "adenomyoma") formation. Outpouchings of mucosa termed Rokitansky-Aschoff sinuses may be seen on oral cholecystography in conjunction with hyperconcentration of contrast medium. Characteristic dimpled filling defects may also be seen.

Cholesterolosis is characterized by abnormal deposition of lipid, especially cholesterol esters, in the lamina propria of the gallbladder wall. In its diffuse form ("strawberry gallbladder"), the gallbladder mucosa is brick red and speckled with bright yellow flecks of lipid. The localized form shows solitary or multiple "cholesterol polyps" studding the gallbladder wall. Cholesterol stones of the gallbladder are found in nearly half the cases. Cholecystectomy is indicated in both adenomyomatosis and cholesterolosis when symptomatic or when cholelithiasis is present.

CANCER OF THE GALLBLADDER Most cancers of the gallbladder develop in conjunction with stones rather than polyps. Necropsy series show a prevalence of gallbladder cancer of 0.43 percent, rising to approximately 1 percent in patients with gallstones. In the United States, adenocarcinomas comprise the vast majority of the estimated 6500 new cases of gallbladder cancer diagnosed each year. The female/male ratio is 4:1 and the mean age at diagnosis is approximately 70 years. The clinical presentation is most often one of unremitting right upper quadrant pain associated with weight loss, jaundice, and a palpable right upper quadrant mass. Cholangitis may supervene. The gallbladder is rarely visualized on OCG, and preoperative diagnosis of the condition is rare. Once symptoms have appeared, spread of the tumor outside the gallbladder by direct extension or by lymphatic or hematogenous routes is almost invariable. Over 75 percent of gallbladder carcinomas are unresectable at the time of surgery, the exceptions being tumors discovered incidentally at laparotomy. The 1-year mortality rate for unresectable disease is approximately 95 percent, and only 5 percent of patients survive 5 years or more from the time of diagnosis. Radical operative resection does not appear to improve survival. Results of trials with radiation and chemotherapy of primary gallbladder cancer have also been disappointing (see Chap. 88).

DISEASES OF THE BILE DUCTS

CONGENITAL ANOMALIES **Biliary atresia and hypoplasia** Atretic and hypoplastic lesions of the extrahepatic and major intrahepatic bile ducts are the most common biliary anomalies of clinical relevance encountered in infancy. The clinical picture is one of severe obstructive jaundice during the first month of life, with pale stools. The diagnosis is confirmed by surgical exploration with operative cholangiography. Approximately 10 percent of cases of biliary atresia are treatable with Roux en Y choledochojejunostomy, with the Kasai procedure (hepatic portoenterostomy) being attempted in the remainder in an effort to restore some bile flow. Most patients, even those having successful biliary-enteric anastomoses, eventually develop chronic cholangitis, extensive hepatic fibrosis, and portal hypertension.

Choledochal cysts Cystic dilatation may involve the free portion of the common bile duct, i.e., choledochal cyst, or may present as diverticulum formation in the intraduodenal segment. In the latter situation chronic reflux of pancreatic juice into the biliary tree can produce inflammation and stenosis of the extrahepatic bile ducts leading to cholangitis or biliary obstruction. Because the process may be gradual, approximately 50 percent of patients present with onset of symptoms after age 10. The diagnosis may be made by ultrasound, abdominal computed tomography (CT), or cholangiography. Surgical treatment involves excision of the ''cyst'' and biliary-enteric anastomosis. Patients with choledochal cysts are at increased risk for the subsequent development of cholangiocarcinoma.

Congenital biliary ectasia Cystic dilatation of the intrahepatic bile ducts may involve either the major intrahepatic radicles (Caroli's disease) or the inter- and intralobular ducts (congenital hepatic fibrosis) or both. In Caroli's disease, clinical manifestations include recurrent cholangitis, abscess formation in and around the affected ducts, and, sometimes, gallstone formation within portions of ectatic intrahepatic biliary radicles. The CT scan and cholangiographic patterns are usually diagnostic, and treatment with ongoing antibiotic therapy is usually undertaken in an effort to limit the frequency and severity of recurrent bouts of cholangitis. Progression to secondary biliary cirrhosis with portal hypertension, amyloidosis, extrahepatic biliary obstruction, cholangiocarcinoma, or recurrent episodes of sepsis with hepatic abscess formation is common.

CHOLEDOCHOLITHIASIS Pathophysiology and clinical manifestations Passage of gallstones into the common bile duct occurs in approximately 10 to 15 percent of patients with cholelithiasis. The incidence of common duct stones increases with increasing age of the patient, so that up to 25 percent of elderly patients may have calculi in the common duct at the time of cholecystectomy. Undetected duct stones are left behind in approximately 1 to 5 percent of cholecystectomy patients. The overwhelming majority of bile duct stones are cholesterol or mixed stones formed in the gallbladder which then migrate into the extrahepatic biliary tree through the cystic duct. Primary calculi arising de novo in the ducts are usually pigment stones developing in patients with (1) chronic hemolytic diseases; (2) hepatobiliary parasitism or chronic, recurrent cholangitis; (3) congenital anomalies of the bile ducts (especially Caroli's disease); or (4) dilated, sclerosed, or strictured ducts. Common duct stones may remain asymptomatic for years, may pass spontaneously into the duodenum, or (most often) may present with biliary colic or a complication.

Complications CHOLANGITIS Cholangitis may be acute or chronic, and symptoms result from inflammation which usually requires at least partial obstruction to the flow of bile. Bacteria are present on bile culture in approximately 75 percent of patients with acute cholangitis early in the symptomatic course. The characteristic presentation of acute cholangitis involves biliary colic, jaundice, and spiking fevers with chills (Charcot's triad). Blood cultures are frequently positive and leukocytosis is typical. *Nonsuppurative* acute cholangitis is most common and may respond relatively rapidly to supportive measures and to treatment with antibiotics (see Chap. 92). In *suppurative* acute cholangitis, however, the presence of pus under pressure in a completely obstructed ductal system leads to symptoms of severe toxicity—mental confusion, bacteremia, and septic shock. Response to antibiotics alone in this setting is relatively poor, multiple hepatic abscesses are often present, and the mortality rate approaches 100 percent unless prompt surgical correction of the obstructing lesion and drainage of infected bile is carried out.

OBSTRUCTIVE JAUNDICE Gradual obstruction of the common bile duct over a period of weeks or months usually leads to initial manifestations of jaundice or pruritus without associated symptoms of biliary colic or cholangitis. Painless jaundice may occur in patients with choledocholithiasis, but this manifestation is much more characteristic of biliary obstruction secondary to malignancy of the head of pancreas, bile ducts, or ampulla of Vater.

In patients whose obstruction is secondary to choledocholithiasis, associated chronic calculous cholecystitis is very common and the gallbladder in this setting may be relatively indistensible. The absence of a palpable gallbladder in most patients with biliary obstruction from duct stones is the basis for *Courvoisier's law,* i.e., that the presence of a palpably enlarged gallbladder suggests that the biliary obstruction is secondary to an underlying malignancy rather than to calculous disease. Biliary obstruction causes progressive dilatation of the intrahepatic bile ducts as intrabiliary pressures rise. Hepatic bile flow is suppressed, and regurgitation of conjugated bilirubin into the bloodstream leads to jaundice accompanied by dark urine (bilirubinuria) and light-colored (acholic) stools.

Common bile duct stones should be suspected in any patient with cholecystitis whose serum bilirubin level exceeds 5 mg/dL. The maximum bilirubin level is seldom over 15.0 mg/dL in patients with choledocholithiasis unless concomitant hepatic disease or another factor leading to marked hyperbilirubinemia exists. Serum bilirubin levels of 20mg/dL or more should suggest the possibility of neoplastic obstruction. The serum alkaline phosphatase level is almost always elevated in biliary obstruction. A rise in alkaline phosphatase often precedes clinical jaundice and may be the only abnormality in routine liver function tests. There may be a two- to tenfold elevation of serum aminotransferases, especially in association with acute obstruction. Following relief of the obstructing process, serum aminotransferase elevations usually return rapidly to normal, while the serum bilirubin level may take 1 to 2 weeks to return to normal. The alkaline phosphatase usually falls slowly, lagging behind the decrease in serum bilirubin.

PANCREATITIS The most common associated entity discovered in patients with nonalcoholic acute pancreatitis is biliary tract disease. Biochemical evidence of pancreatic inflammation complicates acute cholecystitis in 15 percent of cases and choledocholithiasis in over 30 percent, and the common factor appears to be the passage of gallstones through the common duct. Coexisting pancreatitis should be suspected in patients with symptoms of cholecystitis who develop (1) back pain or pain to the left of the abdominal midline, (2) prolonged vomiting with paralytic ileus, or (3) a pleural effusion, especially on the left side. Surgical treatment of gallstone disease is usually associated with resolution of the pancreatitis.

SECONDARY BILIARY CIRRHOSIS Secondary biliary cirrhosis may complicate prolonged or intermittent duct obstruction with or without recurrent cholangitis. Although this complication may be seen in patients with choledocholithiasis, it is more common in cases of prolonged obstruction from stricture or neoplasm. Once established, secondary biliary cirrhosis may be progressive even after correction of the obstructing process, and increasingly severe hepatic cirrhosis may lead to portal hypertension or to hepatic failure and death. Prolonged biliary obstruction may also be associated with clinically relevant deficiencies of the fat-soluble vitamins A, D, and K.

Diagnosis and treatment The diagnosis of choledocholithiasis is usually made by cholangiography (see Table 253-4), either preoperatively or intraoperatively at the time of cholecystectomy (see Fig. 255-2*C*). The incidence of coexisting common duct stones in patients with cholelithiasis is relatively high. Operative cholangiography should be performed routinely during surgical procedures on the

TABLE 253-4 Diagnostic evaluation of the bile ducts

Procedure	Diagnostic advantages	Diagnostic limitations	Contraindications	Complications	Comment
Hepatobiliary ultrasound (HBUS)	Rapid Simultaneous scanning of GB, liver, bile ducts, pancreas Accurate identification of dilated bile ducts Not limited by jaundice, pregnancy Guidance for fine-needle biopsy	Bowel gas Massive obesity Ascites Barium Partial bile duct obstruction Poor visualization of distal CBD	None	None	Initial procedure of choice in investigating possible biliary obstruction
Computerized body tomography (CT)	Simultaneous scanning of GB, liver, bile ducts, pancreas Accurate identification of dilated bile ducts, masses Not limited by jaundice, gas, obesity, ascites High-resolution image Guidance for fine-needle biopsy	Extreme cachexia Movement artifact Ileus Partial bile duct obstruction High cost May not be readily available	Pregnancy	Reaction to iodinated contrast, if used	Indicated for evaluation of hepatic or pancreatic masses Procedure of choice in investigating possible biliary obstruction if diagnostic limitations prevent HBUS
Intravenous cholangiogram (IVC)	Noninvasive Readily available	Serum bilirubin >3 mg/dL Misses 40% of common duct stones Poor resolution even with tomography	Pregnancy History of reaction to iodinated contrast	Reaction to iodinated contrast	Few indications unless other cholangiography techniques not available or have failed
Percutaneous transhepatic cholangiogram (PTHC)	Extremely successful when bile ducts dilated Best visualization of proximal biliary tract Possible separate visualization of obstructed left ductal system Bile cytology/culture Percutaneous transhepatic drainage	Nondilated or sclerosed ducts	Pregnancy Uncorrectable coagulopathy Massive ascites ? Hepatic abscess	Bleeding Hemobilia Bile peritonitis Bacteremia, sepsis	Usually, initial cholangiogram of choice when bile ducts are dilated
Endoscopic retrograde cholangiopancreatogram (ERCP)	Simultaneous pancreatography Visualization/biopsy of ampulla and duodenum Best visualization of distal biliary tract Bile or pancreatic cytology Endoscopic sphincterotomy and stone removal ? Biliary manometry Not limited by ascites, coagulopathy, abscess	Gastroduodenal obstruction ? Roux en Y biliary-enteric anastomosis	Pregnancy ? Acute pancreatitis ? Severe cardiopulmonary disease	Pancreatitis Cholangitis, sepsis Infected pancreatic pseudocyst Perforation (rare) Hypoxemia, aspiration	Cholangiogram of choice in: Absence of dilated ducts ? Pancreatic, ampullary or gastroduodenal disease Prior biliary surgery PTHC contraindicated or failed Endoscopic sphincterotomy a treatment possibility

biliary tract. Preoperative indications for common duct exploration include (1) cholangiographic demonstration of ductal stones, (2) jaundice or cholangitis preceding operation, (3) a history of gallstone-related pancreatitis, and (4) cholangiographic evidence of a markedly enlarged common bile duct. Operative indications for exploration of the duct include (1) manual palpation of stones in the common bile duct, (2) positive intraoperative cholangiogram, (3) enlargement of the common bile duct or cystic duct at operation, (4) multiple small stones or "sand" in the gallbladder, and (5) a gallbladder empty of stones at surgery in a patient with previously documented gallstones.

In most cases of choledocholithiasis, the treatment of choice is cholecystectomy with choledocholithotomy and T-tube drainage of the bile ducts. A T-tube cholangiogram is usually performed prior to T-tube removal on or before the tenth postoperative day. Retained calculi seen on T-tube cholangiography may be removed percutaneously by placement of a steerable basket catheter under radiographic guidance through the matured T-tube sinus tract. Endoscopic sphincterotomy followed by spontaneous or basket stone extraction is an additional nonsurgical alternative in the management of patients with common duct stones, especially in elderly or poor-risk patients.

TRAUMA, STRICTURES, AND HEMOBILIA Benign strictures of the extrahepatic bile ducts result from surgical trauma in approximately 95 percent of cases and occur in about 1 in 500 cholecystectomies. Strictures may present with bile leak or abscess formation in the immediate postoperative period or with biliary obstruction or cholangitis as long as 2 years or more following the inciting trauma. The diagnosis is established by percutaneous or endoscopic cholangiography. Successful operative correction by a skillful surgeon with duct-to-bowel anastomosis is usually possible, although mortality rates from surgical complications, recurrent cholangitis, or secondary biliary cirrhosis are high.

Hemobilia may follow traumatic or operative injury to the liver or bile ducts, intraductal rupture of a hepatic abscess or aneurysm of the hepatic artery, biliary or hepatic tumor hemorrhage, or mechanical complications of choledocholithiasis or hepatobiliary parasitism. Diagnostic procedures such as liver biopsy, percutaneous transhepatic cholangiography (PTHC), and transhepatic biliary drainage catheter placement may also be complicated by hemobilia. Patients often present with a classic triad of biliary colic, obstructive jaundice, and melena or occult blood in the stools. The diagnosis is sometimes made by cholangiographic evidence of blood clot in the biliary tree, but selective angiographic verification may be required. Although minor episodes of hemobilia may resolve without operative intervention, surgical ligation of the bleeding vessel is frequently required.

EXTRINSIC COMPRESSION OF THE BILE DUCTS Partial or complete biliary obstruction may sometimes be produced by extrinsic compression of the ducts. The most common cause of this form of obstructive jaundice is carcinoma of the head of the pancreas. Biliary obstruction may also occur as a complication of either acute or chronic pancreatitis or involvement of lymph nodes in the porta hepatis by lymphoma or metastatic carcinoma. The latter should be distinguished from cholestasis resulting from massive replacement of the liver by tumor.

HEPATOBILIARY PARASITISM Infestation of the biliary tract by adult helminths or their ova may produce a chronic, recurrent pyogenic cholangitis with or without multiple hepatic abscesses, ductal stones, or biliary obstruction. This condition is relatively rare but does occur in inhabitants of southern China and elsewhere in southeast Asia. The organisms most commonly involved are trematodes or flukes, including *Clonorchis sinensis, Opisthorchis viverrini* or *felineus,* and *Fasciola hepatica.* The biliary tract may also be involved by intraductal migration of adult *Ascaris lumbricoides* from the duodenum or by intrabiliary rupture of hydatid cysts of the liver produced by *Echinococcus* species. The diagnosis is made by cholangiography and the presence of characteristic ova on stool examination. When obstruction is present, the treatment of choice is laparotomy under antibiotic coverage, with common duct exploration and a biliary drainage procedure. It should be emphasized that in the orient, one also sees cholangiohepatitis associated with pigment lithiasis, which may, in fact, be more common than cholangitis due to parasites.

SCLEROSING CHOLANGITIS Primary or idiopathic sclerosing cholangitis is a disorder characterized by a progressive, inflammatory, sclerosing and obliterative process affecting the extrahepatic and, often, the intrahepatic bile ducts. The lesion may appear as an isolated entity or may occur in association with inflammatory bowel disease, especially ulcerative colitis, or with multifocal fibrosclerosis syndromes such as retroperitoneal, mediastinal, and/or periureteral fibrosis, Riedel's struma, or pseudotumor of the orbit. Secondary sclerosing cholangitis may occur as a long-term complication of choledocholithiasis, cholangiocarcinoma, operative or traumatic biliary injury, or contiguous inflammatory processes.

Patients with sclerosing cholangitis often present with signs and symptoms of chronic or intermittent biliary obstruction: jaundice, pruritus, right upper quadrant abdominal pain, or acute cholangitis. Late in the course, complete biliary obstruction, secondary biliary cirrhosis, hepatic failure, or portal hypertension with bleeding varices may occur. The diagnosis is usually established by finding thickened ducts with narrow, beaded lumina on cholangiography (see Fig. 253-2*D*). Endoscopic retrograde cholangiopancreatogram (ERCP) is probably the cholangiographic technique of choice in suspected cases since intrahepatic ductal involvement may make PTHC difficult or impossible. When a diagnosis of sclerosing cholangitis has been established, a search for associated diseases, especially for chronic inflammatory bowel disease, should be carried out.

Therapy with cholestyramine may help control symptoms of pruritus, and antibiotics are useful when cholangitis complicates the clinical picture. Vitamin D and calcium supplementation may help prevent the loss of bone mass frequently seen in patients with chronic cholestasis. Corticosteroids have not been shown to be efficacious. In cases where complete or high-grade biliary obstruction has occurred, surgical intervention may be appropriate. Efforts at biliary-enteric anastomosis or stent placement may, however, be complicated by recurrent cholangitis and further progression of the stenosing process. The role of colectomy in patients with sclerosing cholangitis complicating chronic ulcerative colitis is uncertain. The prognosis is unfavorable, with a mean survival of 4 to 10 years following the diagnosis, regardless of therapy.

CHOLANGIOCARCINOMA Benign tumors of the extrahepatic bile ducts are extremely rare causes of mechanical biliary obstruction. The majority of these are papillomas, adenomas, or cystadenomas which present with obstructive jaundice or hemobilia. Adenocarcinoma of the extrahepatic ducts is relatively more common. There is a slight male preponderance (60 percent), and the peak age incidence is in the fifth to seventh decades. Apparent predisposing factors include (1) some chronic hepatobiliary parasitic infestations, (2) congential anomalies with ectactic ducts, (3) sclerosing cholangitis and chronic ulcerative colitis, and (4) occupational exposure to possible biliary tract carcinogens (workers in rubber or automotive plants). Cholelithiasis is not clearly associated with cholangiocarcinoma as a predisposing factor. The lesions may be diffuse or nodular; the latter often arise at the confluence of the hepatic ducts (Klatskin tumors).

Patients with cholangiocarcinoma usually present with biliary obstruction, painless jaundice, pruritus, weight loss, and acholic stools. A deep-seated, vaguely localized right upper quadrant pain may be an associated complaint. Hepatomegaly and a palpable, distended gallbladder are frequent accompanying signs. Fever is unusual unless associated with ascending cholangitis. Because the obstructing process is gradual, the cholangiocarcinoma is often far advanced by the time it presents clinically. The diagnosis is most frequently made by cholangiography following ultrasound demonstration of dilated intrahepatic bile ducts. Any focal strictures of the bile ducts should probably be considered malignant until proved otherwise. Long-term palliation of the tumor is possible in some cases when radiation and/or chemotherapy are combined with palliative drainage of the biliary tree.

PAPILLARY STENOSIS AND BILIARY DYSKINESIA Symptoms of biliary colic accompanied by signs of recurrent, intermittent biliary obstruction may occasionally be produced by dysfunction of the sphincter of Oddi. Papillary stenosis is thought to result from acute or chronic inflammation of the papilla of Vater or from glandular hyperplasia of the papillary segment. Criteria for the diagnosis of papillary stenosis are highly debatable, and preoperative identification of the lesion may be extremely difficult except by ERCP with manometric assessment of the sphincter of Oddi. Endoscopic, cholangiographic, and manometric findings during ERCP may suggest the diagnosis. Intraoperative palpation of the ampulla with operative cholangiography, probing of the sphincter, and/or operative manometry may be required for attempted confirmation in strongly suspected cases. Treatment consists of endoscopic or surgical sphincteroplasty to ensure wide patency of the distal portions of both the bile and pancreatic ducts.

Criteria for diagnosing dyskinesia of the sphincter of Oddi are even more controversial than those of papillary stenosis. Proposed mechanisms include spasm of the sphincter, denervation sensitivity resulting in hypertonicity, and abnormalities of the sequencing or frequency rates of sphincteric contraction waves. When thorough evaluation has failed to demonstrate another cause for the pain, and when cholangiographic and manometric criteria suggest a diagnosis of biliary dyskinesia, medical treatment with nitrites or anticholinergics to attempt pharmacologic relaxation of the sphincter has been proposed. Endoscopic sphincterotomy or surgical sphincteroplasty may be indicated in patients who fail to respond to a 2- to 3-week trial of medical therapy.

CARCINOMA OF THE PAPILLA OF VATER The ampulla of Vater may be involved by extension of tumor arising elsewhere in the duodenum or may itself be the primary site of origin of sarcomas, carcinoid tumors, or adenocarcinomas. Papillary adenocarcinomas are associated with slow growth and a more favorable clinical prognosis than diffuse, infiltrative cancers of the ampulla, which are more frequently widely invasive. The presenting clinical manifestation is usually obstructive jaundice. ERCP is probably the preferred diagnostic technique when ampullary carcinoma is suspected, because it allows for direct endoscopic inspection and biopsy of the ampulla as well as for performance of pancreatography to exclude a diagnosis of pancreatic malignancy. Cancer of the papilla is usually treated by wide, often radical, surgical excision. Lymph node or other metastases are present at the time of surgery in approximately 20 percent of cases, and the 5-year survival rate following surgical therapy in this group is only 5 to 10 percent. In the absence of metastases, however, radical pancreaticoduodenectomy (Whipple procedure) is associated with 5-year survival rates as high as 40 percent, and several long-term survivors have been reported.

REFERENCES

BACHRACH WH, HOFMANN AF: Ursodeoxycholic acid in the treatment of cholesterol cholelithiasis. Dig Dis Sci 27:737, 1982

BENNION LJ, GRUNDY SM: Risk factors for the development of cholelithiasis in man. N Engl J Med 299:1161, 1978

BISMUTH H, MALT RA: Carcinoma of the biliary tract. N Engl J Med 301:704, 1979

FERRUCCI JT JR, MUELLER PR: Interventional radiology of the biliary tract. Gastroenterology 82:974, 1982

GRACIE WA, RANSOHOFF DF: The natural history of silent gallstones. The innocent gallstone is not a myth. N Engl J Med 307:798, 1982

HOLZBACH RT et al: Biliary proteins: Unique inhibitors of cholesterol crystal nucleation in human gallbladder bile. J Clin Invest 72:35, 1984

LEVY PF et al: Human gallbladder mucin accelerates nucleation of cholesterol in artifical bile. Gastroenterology 87:270, 1984

MCPHEE MS, SCHAPIRO RH: Biliary obstruction: Current approaches to diagnosis and treatment, in *Update I: Harrison's Principles of Internal Medicine,* KJ Isselbacher et al (eds). New York, McGraw-Hill, 1981, pp 1–22

MESSIN B et al: Does total parenteral nutrition induce gallbladder sludge formation and lithiasis? Gastroenterology 84:1012, 1983

PALME KR, HOFMANN AF: Intraductal monooctanoin for the direct dissolution of bile duct stones: Experience in 343 patients. Gut 27:196, 1986

PARK YH et al: Dissolution of human cholesterol gallstones in simulated chenodeoxycholate-rich and ursodeoxycholate-rich bile: An in vitro study of dissolution rates and mechanisms. Gastroenterology 87:150, 1984

SCHOENFIELD LS et al: Chenodiol (chenodeoxycholic acid) for dissolution of gallstones: The National Cooperative Gallstone Study. A controlled trial of efficacy and safety. Ann Intern Med 95:257, 1981

SHAPERO TF: Discrepancy between ultrasound and oral cholecystography in assessment of gallstone dissolution. Hepalology 2:587, 1982

SOLOWAY RD et al: Pigment gallstones. Gastroenterology 72:167, 1977

WIESNER RH et al: Comparison of clinicopathologic features of primary sclerosing cholangitis and primary biliary cirrhosis. Gastroenterology 88:108, 1985

section 3 Disorders of the pancreas

254 APPROACH TO THE PATIENT WITH PANCREATIC DISEASE

NORTON J. GREENBERGER / PHILLIP P. TOSKES

GENERAL CONSIDERATIONS

Inflammatory disease of the pancreas may be acute or chronic. Although good data exist concerning the frequency of acute pancreatitis (about 5000 new cases per year in the United States with a mortality rate of about 10 percent), the number of patients who suffer with relapsing pancreatitis or chronic pancreatitis is largely undefined. The relative inaccessibility of the pancreas to direct examination and the nonspecificity of the abdominal pain associated with pancreatitis make the diagnosis of pancreatitis difficult and usually dependent on elevation of blood amylase levels. Many patients with chronic pancreatitis do not have elevated blood amylase levels. Some patients with chronic pancreatitis develop signs and symptoms of pancreatic exocrine insufficiency, and thus objective evidence for pancreatic disease can be demonstrated. However, greater than 90 percent of the pancreas must be damaged before maldigestion of fat and protein is manifested. Obviously there is a very large reservoir of pancreatic exocrine function, and the signs and symptoms usually associated with exocrine insufficiency are late manifestations, depending on virtually complete destruction of the gland. Even the secretin stimulation test, which is the most sensitive method of assessing pancreatic exocrine function, is probably abnormal only when greater than 70 percent of exocrine function has been lost. Thus, the number of patients who have subclinical exocrine dysfunction (i.e., less than 90 percent loss of function) is unknown.

The clinical manifestations of acute and chronic pancreatitis and pancreatic insufficiency are protean. Thus, patients may present with hyperlipidemia, vitamin B_{12} malabsorption, hypercalcemia, hypocalcemia, hyperglycemia, ascites, pleural effusions, and chronic abdominal pain with normal amylase levels. Indeed, if the clinician considers pancreatitis as a possible diagnosis only when presented with a patient having classic symptoms (i.e., severe, constant epigastric pain that radiates through to the back, along with an elevated blood amylase level), only a minority of the patients with pancreatitis will be correctly diagnosed.

As emphasized in Chap. 255, the etiologies as well as the clinical manifestations are quite varied. Although it is well appreciated that *pancreatitis* is frequently secondary to alcohol abuse and biliary tract disease, pancreatitis is also caused by drugs, trauma, and viral infections, and is associated with metabolic and connective tissue disorders. In addition, in approximately 25 percent of patients with chronic pancreatitis, the etiology is obscure.

The incidence of *pancreatic cancer* in the United States has increased threefold since 1930. Associations have been made with cigarette smoking, exposure to some industrial carcinogens, and diabetes. The outlook for early diagnosis and effective treatment remains dismal.

Cystic fibrosis is usually considered a disease of childhood. However, an appreciable number of children with this disease reach adulthood because of more effective therapy for pulmonary complications. Eighty-five percent of patients with cystic fibrosis have pancreatic exocrine insufficiency; in some, pancreatic impairment may represent the primary clinical defect. This disease, in which the metabolic defect appears to be related to defective anion permeability, affects many organ systems in addition to the gastrointestinal tract.

TESTS USEFUL IN THE DIAGNOSIS OF PANCREATIC DISEASE

Several tests have proved of value in the evaluation of pancreatic exocrine function. Examples of specific tests and usefulness in the diagnosis of acute and chronic pancreatitis are summarized in Table 254-1.

PANCREATIC ENZYMES IN BODY FLUIDS The serum amylase is widely used as a screening test for acute pancreatitis in the patient with acute abdominal or back pain. A value greater than 150 Somogyi units per deciliter should raise the question of acute pancreatitis. Levels greater than 300 units make the diagnosis more likely, and values greater than three times normal virtually clinch the diagnosis if gut perforation or infarction is excluded. In acute pancreatitis the serum amylase is usually elevated within 24 h and remains so for 1 to 3 days. Levels return to normal within 3 to 5 days unless there is extensive pancreatic necrosis, incomplete ductal obstruction, or pseudocyst formation. Approximately 70 to 75 percent of patients with acute pancreatitis will have an elevated serum amylase. Normal values, however, may occur if (1) there is a delay (2 to 5 days) in obtaining blood samples, (2) the underlying disorder is chronic pancreatitis rather than acute pancreatitis, and (3) hypertriglyceridemia is present. Patients with hypertriglyceridemia and proven pancreatitis

TABLE 254-1 Tests useful in the diagnosis of acute and chronic pancreatitis and pancreatic tumors

Test	Principle	Comment
I Pancreatic enzymes in body fluids		
A Amylase		
1 Serum	Pancreatic inflammation leads to increased enzyme levels	Simple; 20–40% false-negatives and -positives; reliable if test results are two to three times the upper limit of normal
2 Urine	Renal clearance of amylase is increased in acute pancreatitis	May be abnormal when serum levels normal; false-negatives and -positives
3 Amylase/creatinine clearance ratio (C_{am}/C_{cr})	Renal clearance of amylase greater than clearance of creatinine	No more sensitive than the serum amylase; many false-positives
4 Ascitic fluid	Disruption of gland or main pancreatic duct leads to increased amylase concentration	Can establish diagnosis of pancreatitis; false-positives with intestinal obstruction and perforated ulcer
5 Pleural fluid	Exudative pleural effusion with pancreatitis	False-positives with carcinoma of the lung and esophageal perforation
6 Isoenzymes	P isoamylases arise from the pancreas; S isoamylases are from other sources	More sensitive than total serum amylase in diagnosis of acute pancreatitis; useful in identifying nonpancreatic causes of hyperamylasemia
B Serum lipase	Pancreatic inflammation leads to increased enzyme levels	New methods of determination greatly simplified; positive in 70–85% of cases; excellent specificity; normal in nonpancreatic hyperamylasemic conditions
C Serum trypsin-like immunoreactivity (TLI)	Pancreatic inflammation leads to increased levels	*Elevated* in acute pancreatitis and renal failure; *decreased* in chronic pancreatitis *with* steatorrhea; normal in chronic pancreatitis *without* steatorrhea and steatorrhea with normal pancreatic function
D Pancreatic polypeptide (PP)	PP confined almost totally to the pancreas; release stimulated by nutrients and hormones; such release parallels pancreatic enzyme secretion	Basal, meal-simulated, and hormone-(secretin CCK-PZ) stimulated PP levels *decreased* in chronic pancreatitis; fasting PP levels >125 pg/mL argues against chronic pancreatitis and pancreatic cancer
II Studies pertaining to pancreatic structure		
A Radiologic and radionuclide tests		
1 Plain film of the abdomen	Abnormal in acute and chronic pancreatitis	Simple; normal in >50% of both acute and chronic pancreatitis
2 Upper gastrointestinal x-rays	Abnormally thickened duodenal folds; displacement of stomach or widening of duodenal loop suggests a pancreatic mass (inflammatory, neoplastic, cystic)	Simple; frequently normal; largely superseded by US and CT scanning
3 Ultrasonography (US)	Can provide information on edema, inflammation, calcification, pseudocysts, and mass lesions	Simple, noninvasive; sequential studies quite feasible; procedure of choice for diagnosis of pseudocyst
4 Computerized tomography (CT scan)	Permits detailed visualization of pancreas and surrounding structures	Useful in the diagnosis of pancreatic calcification, dilated pancreatic ducts, and pancreatic tumors; may not be able to distinguish between inflammatory and neoplastic mass lesions
5 Selective angiography	Can identify pancreatic neoplasms (1) by sheathing of celiac or superior mesenteric branches by tumor or (2) by tumor staining; displacement of vessels by tumor	Indicated (1) in suspected islet-cell tumors and (2) prior to pancreatic or duodenal resection; most reliable features reflect nonresectable pancreatic cancer
6 Endoscopic retrograde cholangiopancreatography (ERCP)	Cannulation of pancreatic and common bile duct permits visualization of pancreatic-biliary ductal system	Provides diagnostic data in 60–85% of cases; differentiation of chronic pancreatitis from pancreatic carcinoma may be difficult
B Pancreatic biopsy with US or CT guidance	Percutaneous biopsy with skinny needle and localization of lesion by US	High diagnostic yield; laparotomy avoided; requires special technical skills
III Tests of exocrine pancreatic function		
A Direct stimulation of the pancreas with analysis of duodenal contents		
1 Secretin-pancreozymin (CCK-PZ) test	Secretin leads to increased output of pancreatic juice and HCO_3^-; CCK-PZ leads to increased output of pancreatic enzymes; pancreatic secretory response related to functional mass of pancreatic tissue	Sensitive enough to detect occult disease; involves duodenal intubation and fluoroscopy; poorly defined normal enzyme response; overlap in chronic pancreatitis; large secretory reserve capacity of the pancreas
B Indirect stimulation of pancreas with measurement of pancreatic enzymes		
1 Lundh test meal	Test meal (fat, carbohydrate, and protein) causes increased release of CCK-PZ, which causes increased enzyme output; trypsin concentration measured	Useful in pancreatic exocrine insufficiency; false-negatives with delayed gastric emptying; false-positives in primary mucosal disease of the gut and choledocholithiasis; does not measure secretory capacity
2 Benzoyl-tyrosyl-*p*-aminobenzoic (Bz-Ty-PABA, bentiromide) test	Synthetic peptide (Bz-Ty-PABA) specifically cleaved by chymotrypsin, liberating PABA which is absorbed and PABA metabolite excreted in the urine	Simple and reliable test of pancreatic exocrine function
C Measurement of intraluminal digestion products		
1 Microscopic examination of stool for undigested meat fibers and fat	Lack of proteolytic and lipolytic enzymes causes decreased digestion of meat fibers and triglycerides	Simple, reliable; not sensitive enough to detect milder cases of pancreatic insufficiency
2 Quantitative stool fat determination	Lack of lipolytic enzymes brings about impaired fat digestion	Reliable, reference standard for defining severity of malabsorption; does not distinguish between maldigestion and malabsorption
3 Fecal fat concentration	Patients with pancreatic exocrine insufficiency have less severe diarrhea than patients with gastrointestinal disease	Values ≥9.5% in a patient with steatorrhea ≥20 g/day suggest pancreatic insufficiency as the cause of fat malabsorption

TABLE 254-1 Tests useful in the diagnosis of acute and chronic pancreatitis and pancreatic tumors *(continued)*

Test	Principle	Comment
4 Fecal nitrogen	Lack of proteolytic enzymes leads to imparied protein digestion, causing increase in stool nitrogen	Does not distinguish between maldigestion and malabsorption; low sensitivity
D Measurement of pancreatic enzymes in feces		
1 Chymotrypsin	Pancreatic secretion of proteolytic enzymes	May be useful in cystic fibrosis; tedious; 10% false-positives and false-negatives

have been found to have spuriously low levels of amylase activity presumably because of a circulating amylase inhibitor; serial dilutions of plasma will frequently correct this abnormality and permit identification of hyperamylasemia. Importantly, serum lipase and urinary amylase levels are usually abnormal in this setting, thus facilitating the diagnosis of acute pancreatitis.

The serum amylase is often elevated in other conditions (Table 254-2), in part because the enzyme is found in many organs in addition to the pancreas (salivary glands, liver, small intestine, kidney, fallopian tube) and can be produced by various tumors (carcinoma of the lung, esophagus, and ovary). Isoenzymes of amylase fall into two general categories, those arising from the pancreas (P isoamylases) and those from nonpancreatic sources (S isoamylases). The measurement of serum isoamylases is of clinical importance. Isoamylase analysis of normal serum shows that about 35 to 45 percent of the amylase is of pancreatic origin. For example, in patients with acute pancreatitis, the total serum amylase returns to normal more rapidly than pancreatic isoamylase. Thus, in patients seen after the first day, the pancreatic isoamylase is a more sensitive indicator of pancreatitis than the total serum amylase. In addition, in certain conditions, such as the postoperative state, acute alcohol intoxication, and diabetic ketoacidosis, it had been assumed that elevations in serum amylase indicated acute pancreatitis. However, the elevation of serum amylase in such conditions has been shown

TABLE 254-2 Causes of hyperamylasemia and hyperamylasuria

I Pancreatic disease
- *A* Pancreatitis
  - *1* Acute
  - *2* Chronic: ductal obstruction
  - *3* Complications of pancreatitis
    - *a* Pancreatic pseudocyst
    - *b* Pancreatogenous ascites
    - *c* Pancreatic abscess
- *B* Pancreatic trauma
- *C* Pancreatic carcinoma

II Nonpancreatic disorders
- *A* Renal insufficiency
- *B* Salivary gland lesions
  - *1* Mumps
  - *2* Calculus
  - *3* Irradiation sialadenitis
  - *4* Maxillofacial surgery
- *C* "Tumor" hyperamylasemia
  - *1* Carcinoma of the lung
  - *2* Carcinoma of the esophagus
  - *3* Ovarian carcinoma
- *D* Macroamylasemia
- *E* Burns
- *F* Diabetic ketoacidosis
- *G* Pregnancy
- *H* Renal transplantation
- *I* Cerebral trauma
- *J* Drugs: morphine

III Other abdominal disorders
- *A* Biliary tract disease: cholecystitis, choledocholithiasis
- *B* Intraabdominal disease
  - *1* Perforated or penetrating peptic ulcer
  - *2* Intestinal obstruction or infarction
  - *3* Ruptured ectopic pregnancy
  - *4* Peritonitis
  - *5* Aortic aneurysm
  - *6* Chronic liver disease
  - *7* Postoperative hyperamylasemia

SOURCE: *After WB Salt II, S Schenker, Medicine 55:269, 1976.*

to actually be of the S type. The general availability of a simple assay that employs a protein which selectively inhibits nonpancreatic amylase has led to more widespread use of isoamylase determinations.

Urine amylase is increased in acute pancreatitis and may be elevated for 7 to 10 days after serum values have returned to normal. The finding that the renal clearance of amylase is increased in acute pancreatitis has led to the suggestion that the amylase/creatinine clearance ratio (C_{am}/C_{cr}) may be a more sensitive and specific test for the diagnosis of acute pancreatitis.

However, experience with the C_{am}/C_{cr} has demonstrated that it is no more sensitive than the serum amylase. In addition, the specificity of the C_{am}/C_{cr} has been seriously questioned because the ratio is also increased in a number of other disorders, e.g., diabetic ketoacidosis, burns, pancreatic neoplasms, renal failure, and the postoperative state. The mechanism of increased renal amylase clearance in acute pancreatitis is secondary to a reversible renal tubular defect which results in decreased amylase reabsorption.

Elevation of ascitic fluid amylase occurs in acute pancreatitis as well as (1) in pancreatogenous ascites due to disruption of the main pancreatic duct of a leaking pseudocyst and (2) in other abdominal disorders which simulate pancreatitis (e.g., intestinal obstruction, intestinal infarction, and perforated peptic ulcer). Elevation of pleural fluid amylase occurs in acute pancreatitis, chronic pancreatitis, carcinoma of the lung, and esophageal perforation.

In the past, serum lipase levels were not frequently performed because of methodological problems. However, newer methods are now available and development of automated lipase assays should lead to their routine use and obviate present reliance on total amylase measurements in the diagnosis of acute pancreatitis. In two representative studies, lipase determinations exhibited good *sensitivity* and excellent *specificity;* lipase levels were elevated in 70 to 85 percent of patients with acute pancreatitis and the specificity was 99 percent. An obvious advantage of the lipase assay is that this enzyme is normal in several disorders associated with hyperamylasemia (e.g., macroamylasemia, diabetic ketoacidosis, renal failure, salivary gland lesions).

Assay for trypsinogen (or trypsin-like immunoreactivity) has a theoretical advantage over amylase and lipase determinations in that the pancreas is the only organ that contains this enzyme. The test appears to be useful in the diagnosis of both acute and chronic pancreatitis. Sensitivity and specificity are comparable to amylase and lipase determinations. Since trypsinogen is also excreted by the kidney, elevated values are found in renal failure.

A recent study evaluated the sensitivity and specificity of five assays used to diagnose acute pancreatitis: two amylase assays, one lipase, one trypsinlike immunoreactivity (TLI), and one pancreatic isoamylase. The data obtained show that (1) if the best cutoff level is used, all assays have similar specificities and suggest that (2) total serum amylase is as good an indicator of acute pancreatitis as any of the others. However, inherent in many such studies is the problem that the recognition and diagnosis of acute pancreatitis hinges upon the finding of an elevated serum amylase. The question arises as to whether any diagnostic test result can be proved superior to the total serum amylase level if hyperamylasemia is required for the diagnosis. In other studies, when "objective" confirmation of the clinical diagnosis of pancreatitis was required (ultrasonography, CT, laparotomy), the sensitivity of the serum amylase has been as low as 68 percent. With these limitations in mind, the recommended screening tests for acute pancreatitis are *total serum amylase and serum lipase activities*. Serum amylase values greater than two to three times normal are highly specific.

STUDIES PERTAINING TO PANCREATIC STRUCTURE Radiologic tests Plain films of the abdomen provide useful information in 30 to 50 percent of patients with acute pancreatitis. The most frequent abnormalities include (1) a localized ileus usually involving the jejunum ("sentinel loop"); (2) a generalized ileus with air-fluid levels; (3) the "colon cutoff sign," which results from isolated distention of the transverse colon; (4) duodenal distention with air-fluid levels; and (5) a mass, which is frequently a pseudocyst. In chronic pancreatitis, an important radiographic finding is pancreatic calcification, which characteristically is localized adjacent to and superimposed on the second lumbar vertebra (see Fig. 255-1).

Upper gastrointestinal x-rays may reveal displacement of the stomach by the retroperitoneal mass (see Fig. 255-2*A*) or widening and effacement of the duodenal C loop, which also suggests the presence of a pancreatic mass that could be an inflammatory, cystic, or neoplastic process. The use of hypotonic duodenography or good-quality air-contrast studies increases the diagnostic yield of upper gastrointestinal x-rays in patients with carcinoma of the head of the pancreas.

Ultrasonography (echography) can provide important information in patients with acute pancreatitis, chronic pancreatitis, pancreatic calcification, pseudocyst, and pancreatic carcinoma. It is the procedure of choice in the evaluation of the patient with acute pancreatitis. Echographic appearances can indicate the presence of edema, inflammation, and calcification (not obvious on plain films of the abdomen), as well as pseudocysts, mass lesions, and gallstones (see Figs. 255-1 to 255-3). In acute pancreatitis the pancreas is characteristically enlarged. In pancreatic pseudocyst the usual appearance is that of an echo-free, smooth, round fluid collection. Pancreatic carcinoma distorts the usual landmarks, and mass lesions greater than 3.0 cm are usually detected as localized, echo-free solid lesions. Ultrasound is often the initial investigation for most patients with suspected pancreatic disease. However, obesity, excess small- and large-bowel gas, and recently performed barium-contrast examinations can interfere with ultrasound studies, which are often technically unsatisfactory.

Computerized tomography (CT scan) is the best imaging study for initial evaluation of a suspected chronic pancreatic disorder. It is especially useful in the detection of pancreatic tumors, fluid-containing lesions such as pseudocysts and abscesses, and calcium deposits. Most lesions are characterized by (1) enlargement of the pancreatic outline, (2) distortion of the pancreatic contour, or (3) fluid-containing lesions that have different attenuation coefficients than normal pancreas. However, it is occasionally difficult to distinguish between inflammatory and neoplastic lesions. Oral water-soluble contrast agents may be used to opacify the stomach and duodenum during CT scans; this permits more precise delineation of various organs as well as mass lesions.

Selective catheterization of the celiac and superior mesenteric arteries combined with superselective catheterization of others such as the hepatic, splenic, and gastroduodenal arteries permits visualization of the pancreas and detection of pancreatic neoplasms and pseudocysts. Pancreatic neoplasms can be identified by the sheathing of blood vessels by a mass lesion (see Fig. 255-3). Hormone-producing pancreatic tumors are especially likely to exhibit increased vascularity and tumor staining. Angiographic abnormalities are noted in many patients with pancreatic carcinoma but are uncommon in patients without pancreatic disease. Angiography complements ultrasonography and endoscopic retrograde cholangiopancreatography (ERCP) in the study of a patient with a suspected pancreatic lesion and may be carried out if ERCP is either unsuccessful or nondiagnostic.

Endoscopic retrograde cholangiopancreatography ERCP may provide useful information on the status of the pancreatic ductal system and thus aid in the differential diagnosis of pancreatic disease (see Figs. 255-2 and 255-3). Pancreatic carcinoma is characterized by stenosis or obstruction of either the pancreatic duct or common bile duct; both ductal systems are often abnormal. In chronic pancreatitis ERCP abnormalities include (1) luminal narrowing; (2) irregularities in the ductal system with stenosis, dilatation, sacculation, and ectasia; and (3) blockage of the pancreatic duct by calcium deposits. Differentiation from carcinoma may be difficult because of similar overlapping features, i.e., ductal stenosis and irregularity. Elevated serum amylase levels following ERCP have been reported in 25 to 75 percent of patients, but clinical pancreatitis is uncommon. In a series of 300 patients pancreatitis occurred in only five patients following ERCP.

Pancreatic biopsy with radiologic guidance Percutaneous aspiration biopsy of the pancreas under ultrasound or CT guidance can provide a definitive diagnosis of pancreatic neoplasms.

TESTS OF EXOCRINE PANCREATIC FUNCTION (See Table 254-1)

Pancreatic function tests can be divided into the following categories:

1 Direct stimulation of the pancreas by intravenous infusion of secretin or secretin plus cholecystokinin (CCK) followed by collection and measurement of duodenal contents
2 Indirect stimulation of the pancreas utilizing nutrients or amino acids, fatty acids, and synthetic peptides followed by assay of proteolytic, lipolytic, and amylolytic enzymes
3 Study of *intraluminal digestion products* such as undigested meat fibers, stool fat, and fecal nitrogen
4 Measurement of fecal pancreatic enzymes such as chymotrypsin

The secretin test, used to detect diffuse pancreatic disease, is based on the physiologic principle that the pancreatic secretory response is directly related to the functional mass of pancreatic tissue. In the standard assay, secretin is given intravenously in a dose of 1 clinical unit (CU) per kilogram, either as a bolus or continuous infusion. Obviously, results will vary with the secretin preparation used, dose, mode of administration, and completeness of collection of duodenal contents. Normal values for the standard secretin test are (1) volume output >2.0 mL/kg, (2) bicarbonate (HCO_3^-) concentration >80 meq per liter, and (3) HCO_3^- output >10 meq in 30 min. The most reproducible measurement having the highest level of discrimination between normal subjects and patients with chronic pancreatitis appears to be the maximal bicarbonate concentration.

The *combined secretin-CCK test* permits measurement of pancreatic amylase, lipase, trypsin, and chymotrypsin. Although there is overlap in the distribution of enzyme output in normal subjects and patients with pancreatitis, markedly decreased enzyme outputs suggest advanced damage and destruction of acinar cells. With frank exocrine pancreatic insufficiency there is usually an overall reduction in both HCO_3^- concentration and output of several enzymes. However, with lesser degrees of pancreatic damage there may be a dissociation between HCO_3^- concentration and enzyme output. There may also be a dissociation between the results of the secretin test and other tests of absorptive function. For example, patients with chronic pancreatitis often have abnormally low outputs of HCO_3^- after secretin but have normal fecal fat excretion. Thus, the secretin test measures the secretory capacity of ductular epithelium, while fecal fat excretion indirectly reflects intraluminal lipolytic activity. Steatorrhea does not occur until intraluminal levels of lipase are markedly reduced, underscoring the fact that only small amounts of enzymes are necessary for intraluminal digestive activities. An abnormal secretin test should suggest only that chronic pancreatic damage is present; it will not consistently distinguish between chronic pancreatitis and pancreatic carcinoma.

Another test of exocrine pancreatic function, which indirectly reflects intraluminal chymotrypsin activity, has been evaluated in patients with pancreatic disease. This test (the *tripeptide hydrolysis test*) utilizes a synthetic peptide, *N*-benzoyl-L-tyrosyl-*p*-aminobenzoic acid (Bz-Ty-PABA), that is specifically cleaved by chymotrypsin to Bz-Ty and PABA. Normally, after oral administration, the peptide reaches the small intestine, where it is hydrolyzed by chymotrypsin with the liberation of PABA, which is rapidly absorbed and excreted in the urine. Results in several hundred patients with chronic pancreatitis and other disorders indicate that PABA excretion is significantly lower in chronic pancreatitis compared with controls. The overall sensitivity and specificity of the test remains to be determined.

Measurement of *intraluminal digestion products,* i.e., undigested muscle fibers, stool fat, and fecal nitrogen, is discussed in Chap. 237. Measurement of chymotrypsin in stool reflects pancreatic output of this proteolytic enzyme. Decreased chymotrypsin activity in stool has been reported in patients with chronic pancreatitis and cystic fibrosis. However, normal values may occur in patients with pancreatic insufficiency, and false-positive results have been reported in up to 10 percent of normal individuals.

Tests useful in the diagnosis of exocrine pancreatic insufficiency and the differential diagnosis of malabsorption are also discussed in Chaps. 237 and 255.

255 DISEASES OF THE PANCREAS

NORTON J. GREENBERGER / PHILLIP P. TOSKES / KURT J. ISSELBACHER

BIOCHEMISTRY AND PHYSIOLOGY OF PANCREATIC EXOCRINE SECRETION

GENERAL CONSIDERATIONS The pancreas secretes 1500 to 3000 mL isosmotic alkaline (pH > 8.0) fluid per day containing about 20 enzymes and zymogens. The pancreatic secretions provide the enzymes needed to effect the major digestive activity of the gastrointestinal tract and provide an optimum pH for the function of these enzymes.

REGULATION OF PANCREATIC SECRETION Hormonal and neural mechanisms The exocrine pancreas is under both hormonal and neural control, with hormonal control being of primary importance. *Gastric acid* is the stimulus for the release of secretin, a peptide with 27 amino acids. Sensitive radioimmunoassay studies for secretin suggest that the pH threshold for the release of secretin from the duodenum and jejunum is 4.5. Secretin stimulates the secretion of pancreatic juice rich in *water and electrolytes.* Release of cholecystokinin-pancreozymin (CCK-PZ) from duodenum and jejunum is largely produced by long-chain fatty acids, certain essential amino acids (tryptophan, phenylalanine, valine, methionine), and acid itself. CCK-PZ (a peptide with 33 amino acids) evokes an *enzyme-rich secretion from the pancreas.* Gastrin, although it shares an identical terminal tetrapeptide with CCK-PZ, is a weak stimulus for pancreatic enzyme output. The *parasympathetic nervous system* (via the vagus) exerts some control over pancreatic secretion. Part of this is mediated by the release of gastrin, and part is secondary to a direct effect of acetylcholine on the pancreatic acinar cell. In addition, vagal stimulation effects release of vasoactive intestinal peptide (VIP), a secretin agonist. Vagal control of pancreatic secretion seems to be most important following a truncal vagotomy, but even in such patients severe maldigestion does not ensue. Bile salts also stimulate pancreatic secretion, thereby integrating the functions of the biliary tract, pancreas, and small intestine.

Pancreatic secretion at the cellular level There appear to be two functionally distinct pathways by which secretagogues can stimulate pancreatic secretion. Studies with isolated pancreatic acinar cells indicate that secretin, VIP, and cholera toxin interact with receptors on the acinar cell, leading to an increase in cellular cyclic adenosine monophosphate (cyclic AMP). CCK-PZ, acetylcholine, gastrin, and various other peptides (e.g., bombesin, caerulein) react with other receptors on the acinar cell to cause an increased turnover of phosphatidylinositol and the release of membrane calcium and induce changes in the electrical properties of the pancreatic acinar cell surface and junctional membranes. When a secretagogue that increases cyclic AMP is added to a secretagogue that increases calcium outflux, potentiation of enzyme secretion occurs.

WATER AND ELECTROLYTE SECRETION Although sodium, potassium, chloride, calcium, zinc, phosphate, and sulfate are found within pancreatic secretion, *bicarbonate is the ion of primary physiologic importance.* In the acini and in the ducts, secretin causes the cells to add water and bicarbonate to the fluid. In the ducts an exchange occurs between bicarbonate and chloride. There is a good correlation between the maximal bicarbonate output after stimulation with secretin and the pancreatic mass. The bicarbonate output of 120 to 300 meq per day helps neutralize gastric acid production and creates the appropriate pH for the activity of the pancreatic enzymes.

ENZYME SECRETION The pancreas secretes amylolytic, lipolytic, and proteolytic enzymes. Amylolytic enzymes such as amylase hydrolyze starch to oligosaccharides and to the disaccharide maltose. The *lipolytic enzymes* include lipase, phospholipase A, and cholesterol esterase. Bile salts *inhibit* lipase, but colipase, another constituent of pancreatic secretion, binds to lipase and prevents this inhibition. Bile salts *activate* phospholipase A and cholesterol esterase. *Proteolytic enzymes* include *endopeptidases* (trypsin, chymotrypsin), which act on the internal peptide bonds of proteins and polypeptides; exopeptidases (carboxypeptidases, aminopeptidases), which act on the free carboxyl terminal end and free amino terminal end of peptides, respectively; and elastase. The proteolytic enzymes are secreted as inactive precursors (zymogens). Ribonucleases (deoxyribonucleases, ribonuclease) are also secreted. *Enterokinase,* an enzyme found within the duodenal mucosa, cleaves the lysine-isoleucine bond of trypsinogen to form trypsin. Trypsin then activates the other proteolytic zymogens in a cascade phenomenon. All pancreatic enzymes have pH optima in the alkaline range.

AUTOPROTECTION OF THE PANCREAS Autodigestion of the pancreas is prevented by the packaging of proteases in precursor form and by the synthesis of protease inhibitors. These protease inhibitors are found within the acinar cell, the pancreatic secretions, and the $alpha_1$- and $alpha_2$-globulin fractions of plasma.

EXOCRINE-ENDOCRINE RELATIONSHIPS Pancreatic glucagon (29 amino acid residues) has a high degree of structural similarity to secretin. It decreases volume and enzyme secretion by the pancreas but not bicarbonate secretion. Glucose, in large concentrations, may also inhibit pancreatic exocrine secretion. The choleretic and insulinotropic effects of secretin are shared by glucagon.

ACUTE PANCREATITIS

GENERAL CONSIDERATIONS Pancreatic inflammatory disease may be classified as follows: (1) acute pancreatitis, and (2) chronic pancreatitis. This classification is based primarily on clinical criteria with the obvious difference between the acute and chronic varieties; restoration of normal function occurs in the former and permanent residual damage occurs in the latter. The pathologic spectrum of acute pancreatitis varies from *edematous pancreatitis,* which is usually a mild and self-limited disorder, to *necrotizing pancreatitis,* in which the degree of pancreatic necrosis correlates with the severity of the attack and its systemic manifestations. The term *hemorrhagic pancreatitis* is less meaningful in a clinical sense because variable amounts of interstitial hemorrhage can be found in pancreatitis as well as in other disorders such as pancreatic trauma, pancreatic carcinoma, and severe congestive heart failure.

The incidence of pancreatitis varies in different countries and depends upon etiologic factors, e.g., alcohol, gallstones, metabolic factors, and drugs (Table 255-1). In the United States, for example, acute pancreatitis is related to alcohol ingestion more commonly than to gallstones; in England the opposite obtains. Epidemiologic data based on autopsy data indicate that in the United States the overall prevalence of acute pancreatitis is approximately 0.5 percent. An upward trend has been noted in the crude death rate from 1.0 per 100,000 in 1955 to 1.3 in 1965.

ETIOLOGY AND PATHOGENESIS There are many causative factors in the pathogenesis of acute pancreatitis (Table 255-1), but the mechanisms by which these conditions trigger pancreatic inflammation have not been identified. Alcoholic patients with pancreatitis may represent a special subset, since most alcoholics do not develop pancreatitis. The list of identifiable causes is growing, and it is likely that pancreatitis related to viral infections and drugs is more common than heretofore recognized.

Autodigestion is one pathogenetic theory which proposes that proteolytic enzymes (e.g., trypsinogen, chymotrypsinogen, proelastase, and phospholipase A) are activated within the pancreas rather than in the intestinal lumen. A variety of factors (such as endotoxins, exotoxins, viral infections, ischemia, anoxia, and direct trauma) are believed to activate these proenzymes. Activated proteolytic enzymes, especially trypsin, not only digest pancreatic and peripancreatic tissues but also can activate other enzymes such as elastase and phospholipase. The active enzymes then digest cellular membranes and cause proteolysis, edema, interstitial hemorrhage, vascular damage, coagulation necrosis, fat necrosis, and parenchymal cell necrosis. Cellular injury and death result in the liberation of activated enzymes. In addition, activation and release of bradykinin peptides and vasoactive substances (e.g., histamine) are believed to produce vasodilatation, increased vascular permeability, and edema. There is thus a cascade of events culminating in the development of acute necrotizing pancreatitis.

The autodigestion theory has largely eclipsed two older theories. The "common channel" theory holds that such an anatomic arrangement facilitates reflux of bile into the pancreatic duct, and this results in activation of pancreatic enzymes. (Actually, a common channel with free communication between the common bile duct and main pancreatic duct is infrequently encountered.) The second theory is that obstruction and hypersecretion are pivotal in the development of pancreatitis. Obstruction of the main pancreatic duct, however, produces pancreatic edema but not pancreatitis.

A third hypothesis to explain the intrapancreatic activation of zymogens is that they become activated by *lysosomal hydrolases* within the pancreatic acinar cell itself. In two different types of experimental pancreatitis, it has been demonstrated that digestive enzymes and lysosomal hydrolases become admixed; as a result the former can be activated within the acinar cell by the latter. Importantly, lysosomal enzymes such as cathepsin B can activate trypsinogen, and trypsin can activate the other protease precursors.

CLINICAL FEATURES *Abdominal pain* is the major symptom of acute pancreatitis. Pain may vary from a mild and tolerable discomfort to severe, constant, and incapacitating distress. Characteristically, the pain which is steady and boring in character is located in the epigastrium and periumbilical region and often radiates to the back as well as to the chest, flanks, and lower abdomen. The pain is frequently more intense when the patient is supine, and patients often obtain relief by sitting with the trunk flexed and knees drawn up. Nausea, vomiting, and abdominal distention due to gastric and intestinal hypomotility and chemical peritonitis are also frequent complaints.

Physical examination frequently reveals a distressed and anxious patient. Low-grade fever, tachycardia, and hypotension are fairly common. Shock is not unusual and may result from (1) hypovolemia secondary to exudation of blood and plasma proteins into the retroperitoneal space, i.e., a "retroperitoneal burn"; (2) increased formation and release of kinin peptides which cause vasodilatation and increased vascular permeability; (3) systemic effects of proteolytic and lipolytic enzymes released into the circulation; and (4) impairment of myocardial contractility by kinins and other poorly characterized peptides. Jaundice occurs infrequently; when present it usually is due to edema of the head of the pancreas with compression of the intrapancreatic portion of the common bile duct. Erythematous skin nodules due to subcutaneous fat necrosis may occur. In 10 to 20 percent of patients there are pulmonary findings, including basilar rales, atelectasis, and pleural effusion, the latter most frequently left-sided. Abdominal tenderness and muscle rigidity are present to a variable degree, but compared with the intense pain, these signs may be unimpressive. Bowel sounds are usually diminished or absent. A pancreatic pseudocyst may be palpable in the upper abdomen. A faint blue discoloration around the umbilicus (Cullen's sign) may occur as the result of hemoperitoneum, and a blue-red-purple or green-brown discoloration of the flanks (Turner's sign) reflects tissue catabolism of hemoglobin. The latter two findings, which are uncommon, indicate the presence of a severe necrotizing pancreatitis.

LABORATORY DATA The diagnosis of acute pancreatitis is usually established by the presence of an increased serum amylase. Values

TABLE 255-1 Causes of acute pancreatitis

I Alcohol ingestion (acute and chronic alcoholism)
II Biliary tract disease (gallstones)
III Postoperative (abdominal, nonabdominal)
IV Post-endoscopic retrograde cholangiopancreatography (ERCP)
V Trauma (especially blunt abdominal type)
VI Metabolic
- *A* Hypertriglyceridemia
- *B* Hypercalcemia, e.g., hyperparathyroidism
- *C* Renal failure
- *D* After renal transplantation*
- *E* Acute fatty liver of pregnancy†

VII Hereditary pancreatitis
VIII Infections
- *A* Mumps
- *B* Viral hepatitis
- *C* Other viral infections (coxsackievirus, echovirus)
- *D* Ascariasis
- *E* Mycoplasma

IX Drug-associated
- *A* Definite association
  - *1* Azathioprine
  - *2* Sulfonamides
  - *3* Thiazide diuretics
  - *4* Furosemide
  - *5* Estrogens (oral contraceptives)
  - *6* Tetracycline
  - *7* Valproic acid
- *B* Probable association
  - *1* Chlorthalidone
  - *2* Ethacrynic acid
  - *3* Procainamide
  - *4* Iatrogenic hypercalcemia
  - *5* L-Asparaginase

X Connective tissue disorders with vasculitis
- *A* Systemic lupus erythematosus
- *B* Necrotizing angiitis
- *C* Thrombotic thrombocytopenic purpura

XI Penetrating peptic ulcer
XII Obstruction of the ampulla of Vater
- *A* Regional enteritis
- *B* Duodenal diverticulum

XIII Pancreas divisum
XIV Recurrent bouts of acute pancreatitis without obvious cause
- *A* Consider
  - *1* Occult disease of the biliary tree or pancreatic ducts
  - *2* Drugs
  - *3* Hypertriglyceridemia
  - *4* Pancreas divisum

XV Other

* *Pancreatitis occurs in 3 percent of renal transplant patients and is due to many factors including surgery, hypercalcemia, drugs (corticosteroids, azathioprine, L-asparaginase, diuretics), and viral infections.*
† *Pancreatitis also occurs in otherwise uncomplicated pregnancy and is most often associated with cholelithiasis.*

elevated two- to threefold above normal virtually clinch the diagnosis if overt salivary gland disease and gut perforation or infarction are excluded. However, there appears to be no definite correlation between the severity of pancreatitis and the degree of serum amylase elevation. After 48 to 72 h, even with continuing evidence of pancreatitis, total serum amylase values tend to return to normal. Importantly, pancreatic isoamylase and lipase levels may remain elevated for 7 to 14 days. It will be recalled that amylase elevations in serum and urine occur in many conditions other than pancreatitis (see Table 254-2). The urine amylase C_{am}/C_{cr} ratio is usually elevated in patients with severe pancreatitis; this ratio usually is not increased in patients with normal serum. Serum lipase activity increases in parallel with amylase activity, and measurement of both enzymes increases the diagnostic yield. An elevated serum lipase is virtually diagnostic of acute pancreatitis; the test is especially helpful in patients with nonpancreatic causes of hyperamylasemia (see Table 254-4). Markedly increased levels of peritoneal or pleural fluid amylase (>5000 units per deciliter) are also helpful, if present, in establishing the diagnosis.

Leukocytosis (15,000 to 20,000 leukocytes per cubic millimeter) occurs frequently. More severe cases may show hemoconcentration with hematocrit values exceeding 50 percent because of loss of plasma into the retroperitoneal space and peritoneal cavity. *Hyperglycemia* is common and is due to multiple factors that include decreased insulin release, increased glucagon release, and increased output of adrenal glucocorticoids and catecholamines. *Hypocalcemia* occurs in approximately 25 percent of cases and its pathogenesis is incompletely understood. While earlier studies suggested that the parathyroid gland response to a decrease in serum calcium is impaired, subsequent observations have failed to confirm this. Intraperitoneal saponification of calcium by fatty acids in areas of fat necrosis occurs as well as increased plasma levels of glucagon and calcitonin, but it is felt that these abnormalities do not adequately explain the hypocalcemia. *Hyperbilirubinemia* (serum bilirubin > 4.0 mg/dL) occurs in approximately 10 percent of patients. However, jaundice is transient and serum bilirubin levels return to normal in 4 to 7 days. Serum alkaline phosphatase and aspartate aminotransferase (SGOT) levels are also transiently elevated and parallel serum bilirubin values. When markedly elevated (i.e., >500 units), serum lactic dehydrogenase (LDH) levels suggest a poor prognosis. Serum albumin is decreased to ≤3.0 g/dL in about 10 percent of cases and is associated with more severe pancreatitis and an increased mortality rate (Table 255-2). Methemalbumin, a circulating heme metabolite attached to albumin, has been considered as a useful index of severe necrotizing pancreatitis. Its usefulness, however, has been limited by its nonspecificity for pancreatitis (it occurs, for example, in abdominal trauma, bone fractures, soft-tissue trauma, and retroperitoneal hematoma) and its absence in the majority of cases of severe necrotizing pancreatitis. *Hypertriglyceridemia* occurs in 15 to 20 percent of cases, and serum amylase levels in such patients are often spuriously normal (see Chap. 254). Most patients with hypertriglyceridemia and pancreatitis, when subsequently examined, show evidence of an underlying derangement in lipid metabolism which probably antedated the pancreatitis. Approximately 25 percent of patients have *hypoxemia* (arterial $P_{O_2} \leq 60$ mmHg), which may herald the onset of adult respiratory distress syndrome. Finally, the electrocardiogram is occasionally abnormal in acute pancreatitis with ST-segment and T-wave abnormalities simulating myocardial ischemia.

Radiologic studies useful in the diagnosis of acute pancreatitis are listed in Table 254-1 and discussed in Chap. 254. Although one or more of the abnormalities are found in over 50 percent of patients, the findings are inconstant and nonspecific. The chief value of conventional x-rays [chest; kidney, ureter, and bladder (KUB)] in acute pancreatitis is to help exclude other diagnoses, especially a perforated viscus. Upper gastrointestinal tract x-rays have been superseded by ultrasonography and CT scanning. A computerized tomography (CT) scan may confirm the clinical impression of acute pancreatitis even in the face of normal serum amylase levels. Sonography and radionuclide scanning (PIPIDA, HIDA) are useful in acute pancreatitis to evaluate the gallbladder and biliary tree.

TABLE 255-2 Factors adversely influencing survival in acute pancreatitis*

I Risk factors identifiable upon admission to hospital
- *A* Increasing age
- *B* Hypotension
- *C* Abnormal pulmonary findings
- *D* Abdominal mass
- *E* Hemorrhagic or discolored peritoneal fluid
- *F* Increased serum LDH levels
- *G* Leukocytosis
- *H* Hyperglycemia
- *I* First attack of pancreatitis

II Risk factors identifiable during initial 48 h of hospitalization
- *A* Fall in hematocrit > 10 percent with hydration and/or hematocrit < 30 percent
- *B* Necessity for massive fluid and colloid replacement
- *C* Hypocalcemia
- *D* Hypoxemia with or without adult respiratory distress syndrome
- *E* Hypoalbuminemia
- *F* Azotemia

* *Increased mortality with three or more risk factors.*

DIAGNOSIS Any severe acute pain in the abdomen or back should suggest acute pancreatitis. The diagnosis is usually entertained when a patient with a possible predisposition to pancreatitis presents with severe and constant abdominal pain, nausea, emesis, fever, tachycardia, and abnormal findings on abdominal examination. Laboratory studies frequently reveal leukocytosis, abnormal x-rays of the abdomen and chest, hypocalcemia, and hyperglycemia. The diagnosis is usually confirmed by finding an elevated serum amylase and/or lipase. Obviously, not all the above features have to be present for the diagnosis to be established.

The *differential diagnosis* should include consideration of the following disorders: (1) perforated viscus, especially peptic ulcer; (2) acute cholecystitis and biliary colic; (3) acute intestinal obstruction; (4) mesenteric vascular occlusion; (5) renal colic; (6) myocardial infarction; (7) dissecting aortic aneurysm; (8) connective tissue disorders with vasculitis; (9) pneumonia; and (10) diabetic ketoacidosis. A penetrating duodenal ulcer can usually be identified by upper gastrointestinal x-rays and/or endoscopy. A perforated duodenal ulcer is readily diagnosed by the presence of free intraperitoneal air. It may be difficult to differentiate acute cholecystitis from acute pancreatitis since an elevated serum amylase may be found in both disorders. Pain of biliary tract origin is more right-sided and gradual in onset, and ileus is usually absent; sonography and radionuclide scanning are helpful in establishing the diagnosis of cholelithiasis and cholecystitis. Intestinal obstruction due to mechanical factors can be differentiated from pancreatitis by the history of colicky pain, findings on abdominal examination, and x-rays of the abdomen showing characteristic changes of mechanical obstruction. Acute mesenteric vascular occlusion is usually evident in elderly debilitated patients with brisk leukocytosis, abdominal distention, and bloody diarrhea, in whom paracentesis shows sanguinous fluid and arteriography shows vascular occlusion. Serum as well as peritoneal fluid amylase levels are increased, however, in patients with intestinal infarction. Systemic lupus erythematosus and polyarteritis nodosa may be confused with pancreatitis, especially since pancreatitis may develop as a complication of those diseases. Diabetic ketoacidosis is often accompanied by abdominal pain and elevated total serum amylase levels, thus closely mimicking acute pancreatitis. However, the serum lipase and pancreatic isoamylase are not elevated in diabetic ketoacidosis.

COURSE OF THE DISEASE AND COMPLICATIONS There is an increased mortality rate with three or more risk factors identifiable either at the time of admission to hospital or during the initial 48 h of hospitalization (see Table 255-2). It is important to identify the patient with acute pancreatitis with an increased risk of dying. In one large series such a subgroup was characterized by at least three of the following features: (1) respiratory failure requiring intubation, (2) shock, (3) massive colloid replacement, and (4) serum calcium < 8.0 mg/dL. The survival rate was only 29 percent in the patients treated with medical measures but increased to 64 percent with operative treatment. In another series the mortality rate was 0.9 percent in patients with zero to two factors, 16 percent in patients with three to four factors, and 40 percent with five to six factors present. The high mortality of such severely ill patients, despite maximal medical treatment, suggests that alternative therapeutic approaches such as peritoneal lavage or early surgical intervention merit broader consideration.

The local and systemic complications of acute pancreatitis are listed in Table 255-3. Patients frequently develop an inflammatory mass in the first 2 to 3 weeks after pancreatitis. These may be phlegmons, abscesses, or pseudocysts (see below). Systemic complications include pulmonary, cardiovascular, hematologic, renal, metabolic, and central nervous system abnormalities. Pancreatitis, hypertriglyceridemia, and alcoholism constitute a triad in which cause and effect remain incompletely understood. However, several reasonable conclusions can be drawn. First, hypertriglyceridemia can precede and apparently cause the development of pancreatitis. Second, the vast majority (>80 percent) of patients with acute pancreatitis do not have hypertriglyceridemia. Third, almost all patients with pancreatitis and hypertriglyceridemia are *either* alcoholics who have been drinking shortly before the onset of pancreatitis *or* patients with preexistent hypertriglyceridemia. Fourth, many of the patients with this triad have persistent hypertriglyceridemia after recovery from pancreatitis and abstention from alcohol. Finally, patients with a deficiency of apolipoprotein CII have an increased incidence of pancreatitis; apolipoprotein CII activates lipoprotein lipase, which is important in clearing chylomicrons from the bloodstream.

Purtscher's retinopathy, a relatively unusual complication, refers to the sudden and severe loss of vision in patients with acute pancreatitis. It is characterized by a peculiar funduscopic appearance with cotton-wool spots and hemorrhages confined to an area limited by the optic disk and macula; it is believed to be due to posterior retinal artery occlusion with aggregated granulocytes.

TREATMENT In most patients (approximately 85 to 90 percent) with acute pancreatitis, the disease is self-limited and subsides spontaneously, usually within 3 to 7 days after treatment is instituted. Medical therapy is aimed at reducing pancreatic secretion and, in essence, "putting the pancreas at rest." Conventional measures include (1) analgesics for pain, (2) intravenous fluids and colloids to maintain normal intravascular volume, (3) no oral alimentation, and (4) nasogastric suction to decrease gastrin release from the stomach and prevent gastric contents from entering the duodenum. Recent controlled trials, however, have shown that nasogastric suction offers no clear-cut advantages in the treatment of mild to moderately severe acute pancreatitis. Its use, therefore, must be considered elective rather than mandatory.

Anticholinergic drugs have previously been considered standard therapy in patients with acute pancreatitis, the rationale being to blunt stimulation of the pancreas. However, there are no controlled trials demonstrating that anticholinergic drugs are superior to placebo. Moreover, anticholinergics may make it difficult to determine whether tachycardia, decreased urine output, bowel hypomotility, need for additional fluid replacement, and signs of toxicity are due to the drugs or to a worsening of the pancreatitis. Accordingly, their use is not recommended. Although antibiotics have been used in the treatment of acute pancreatitis, three recent randomized prospective trials have shown no benefit from the use of antibiotics in acute pancreatitis of mild to moderate severity. However, because secondary infection of necrotic pancreatic tissue (phlegmon, abscess, pseudocyst) or obstructed biliary passages (ascending cholangitis, complicating choledocholithiasis) contributes to much of the late mortality, appropriate *antibiotic therapy of established infection* is obviously quite important. Previous reports suggested that glucagon was useful in acute pancreatitis, but controlled trials have not provided convincing evidence of effectiveness. Similarly, aprotinin (Trasylol) and cimetidine have not proved effective.

The patient with mild to moderate pancreatitis usually requires treatment with intravenous fluids, fasting, and possibly nasogastric suction for 2 to 4 days. A clear liquid diet is frequently started on the third to sixth day and a regular diet by the fifth to seventh day. The patient with unremitting *fulminant pancreatitis* usually requires inordinate amounts of fluid and close attention to complications such as cardiovascular collapse and respiratory insufficiency. Removal of toxic pancreatic exudate from the peritoneal cavity may alter the course of this lethal situation. This can be accomplished by either *peritoneal lavage* via a percutaneous dialysis catheter or *laparotomy* with wide sump drainage. One study has suggested that a 3-day regimen of therapeutic lavage with a conventional peritoneal dialysis solution does not influence the outcome of an attack of severe idiopathic acute pancreatitis. However, occasionally a dramatic response occurs if lavage is accomplished early in an attack of alcohol-induced pancreatitis. If peritoneal lavage does not halt the patient's deterioration, laparotomy should be considered. The use of parenteral nutrition makes it possible to give nutritional support to patients with severe, acute, or protracted pancreatitis who are unable

TABLE 255-3 Complications of acute pancreatitis

I Local
- *A* Pancreatic phlegmon
- *B* Pancreatic abscess
- *C* Pancreatic pseudocyst
  - *1* Pain
  - *2* Rupture
  - *3* Hemorrhage
  - *4* Infection
  - *5* Obstruction of gastrointestinal tract (stomach, duodenum, colon)
- *D* Pancreatic ascites
  - *1* Disruption of main pancreatic duct
  - *2* Leaking pseudocyst
- *E* Involvement of contiguous organs by necrotizing pancreatitis
  - *1* Massive intraperitoneal hemorrhage
  - *2* Thrombosis of blood vessels
  - *3* Bowel infarction
- *F* Obstructive jaundice

II Systemic
- *A* Pulmonary
  - *1* Pleural effusion
  - *2* Atelectasis
  - *3* Mediastinal abscess
  - *4* Pneumonitis
  - *5* Adult respiratory distress syndrome
- *B* Cardiovascular
  - *1* Hypotension
    - *a* Hypovolemia
    - *b* Hypoalbuminemia
  - *2* Sudden death
  - *3* Nonspecific ST-T changes in electrocardiogram simulating myocardial infarction
  - *4* Pericardial effusion
- *C* Hematologic
  - *1* Disseminated intravascular coagulation (DIC)
- *D* Gastrointestinal hemorrhage*
  - *1* Peptic ulcer disease
  - *2* Erosive gastritis
  - *3* Hemorrhagic pancreatic necrosis with erosion into major blood vessels
  - *4* Portal vein thrombosis, variceal hemorrhage
- *E* Renal
  - *1* Oliguria
  - *2* Azotemia
  - *3* Renal artery and/or renal vein thrombosis
- *F* Metabolic
  - *1* Hyperglycemia
  - *2* Hypertriglyceridemia
  - *3* Hypocalcemia
  - *4* Encephalopathy
  - *5* Sudden blindness (Purtscher's retinopathy)
- *G* Central nervous system
  - *1* Psychosis
  - *2* Fat emboli
- *H* Fat necrosis
  - *1* Subcutaneous tissues (erythematous nodules)
  - *2* Bone
  - *3* Miscellaneous (mediastinum, pleura, nervous system)

* *Aggravated by coagulation abnormalities (DIC).*

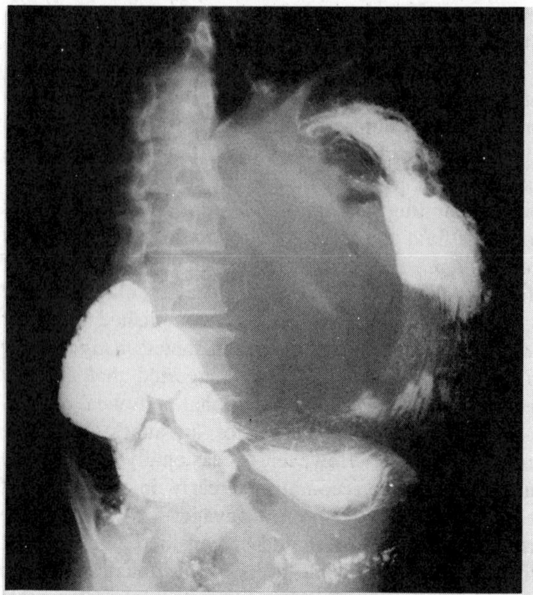

A

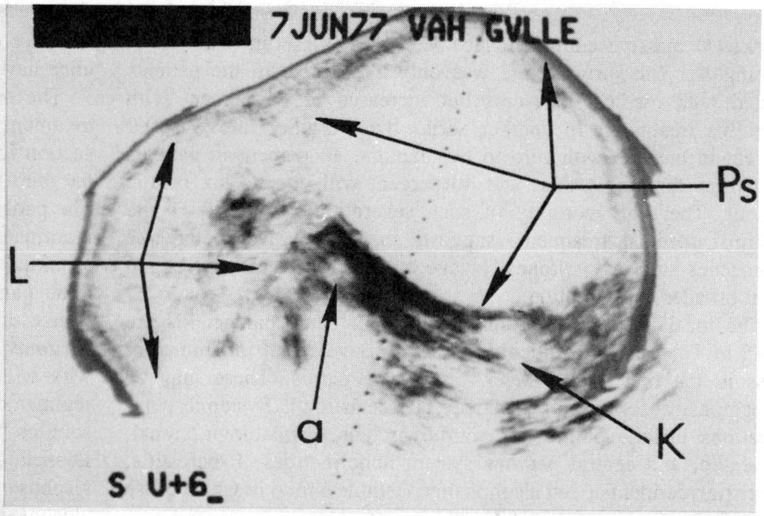

B

FIGURE 255-1 *Pseudocyst of the pancreas. A. Upper gastrointestinal x-ray showing displacement of stomach by pseudocyst. B. Sonogram showing pseudocyst (Ps), K = kidney, a = aorta, L = liver. C. CT scan showing pseudocyst (arrow) compressing left kidney.*

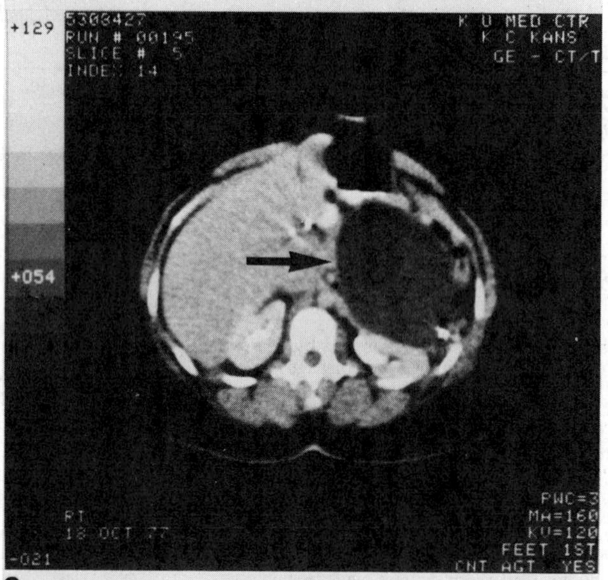

C

to eat normally. Finally, patients with gallstone-induced pancreatitis may improve dramatically if papillotomy is carried out within the first 36 h of the attack.

PANCREATIC PHLEGMON, ABSCESS, AND PSEUDOCYST The *phlegmon* is a solid mass of swollen, inflamed pancreas often containing patchy areas of necrosis; it may be present for 1 to 2 weeks. This prolonged inflammatory process should not be confused with a pseudocyst, a differentiation which is usually accomplished by sonography. Occasionally, extensive areas of pancreatic necrosis develop in phlegmons and require incision and drainage. Phlegmons may also be secondarily infected, resulting in abscess formation. The latter occurs in 5 to 10 percent of patients with acute pancreatitis. Severe pancreatitis with the presence of three or more risk factors, postoperative pancreatitis, early oral feeding, early laparotomy, and perhaps injudicious use of antibiotics predispose to the development of pancreatic abscess. Pancreatic abscess may also develop because of communication of a pseudocyst with the colon, after inadequate surgical drainage of a pseudocyst, or after needling of a pseudocyst. The characteristic signs of abscess are fever, leukocytosis, ileus, and rapid deterioration in a patient initially recovering from pancreatitis. However, the only manifestations may be persistent fever and signs of continuing pancreatic inflammation. Drainage of pancreatic abscesses by nonsurgical percutaneous catheter techniques, using CT guidance, has been only moderately successful (resolution in 50 to 60 percent of patients). Accordingly, laparotomy with radical sump drainage and possibly resection of necrotic tissue is usually required because the mortality rate for undrained pancreatic abscess approaches 100 percent. Multiple abscesses are common and reoperation is frequently required.

Pseudocysts of the pancreas are collections of tissue, fluid, debris, pancreatic enzymes, and blood, which develop over a period of 1 to 4 weeks after the onset of acute pancreatitis. In contrast to true cysts, pseudocysts do not have epithelial lining and the walls consist of necrotic tissue, granulation tissue, and fibrous tissue. Disruption of the pancreatic ductal system is common. However, the subsequent course of this disruption varies widely, namely, from spontaneous healing to continuous leakage of pancreatic juice causing tense ascites. Pseudocysts are preceded by pancreatitis in 90 percent of cases and by trauma in 10 percent. Approximately 85 percent are located in the body or tail of the pancreas and 15 percent in the head. Some patients have two or more pseudocysts. Abdominal pain, with or without radiation to the back, is the usual presenting complaint. A palpable, tender mass may be found in the middle or left upper abdomen. The serum amylase is elevated in 75 percent of patients some time during their illness and may fluctuate markedly.

Pseudocysts often displace some portion of the gastrointestinal tract on x-ray examination in 75 percent of cases (Fig. 255-1). Sonography, however, is reliable in detecting pseudocysts and should be the initial diagnostic procedure in a patient suspected of having a pseudocyst (Fig. 255-1). Sonography also permits differentiation between an edematous and an inflamed pancreas (pancreatic phlegmon), which can give rise to a palpable mass and an actual pseudocyst. Furthermore, serial ultrasound studies will indicate whether a pseudocyst has resolved. CT scanning complements the use of ultrasound in the diagnosis of pancreatic pseudocyst (Fig. 255-2), especially when it is infected.

The management of pseudocysts is compromised by incomplete knowledge of the natural history of this disorder. In earlier studies utilizing sonography, pseudocysts resolved in 20 to 30 percent of patients; however, the time frequency of this is not clear. In others, serious complications may occur such as (1) pain caused by expansion of the lesion and pressure on other viscera, (2) rupture, (3) hemorrhage, and (4) abscess. Rupture of a pancreatic pseudocyst is a particularly serious complication. Shock almost always supervenes and mortality rates range from 14 percent if the rupture is not associated with hemorrhage to over 60 percent if hemorrhage has occurred. Rupture and hemorrhage are the prime causes of mortality in pancreatic pseudocyst. A triad of findings, e.g., increase in size of the mass, localized bruit over the mass, and a sudden decrease in hemoglobin and hematocrit levels without obvious signs of external blood loss should alert one to the diagnosis of hemorrhage from a pseudocyst. Thus, in pseudocyst patients who are stable and uncomplicated, and in whom serial ultrasound studies show a decreasing pseudocyst, conservative therapy is indicated. Conversely, patients with a pseudocyst which is expanding and which is complicated by rupture, hemorrhage, and abscess should be operated on. Needle aspiration of pseudocysts present for longer than 6 months results in permanent resolution in approximately 25 percent of patients; the remainder require surgical therapy. Therapy consists of internal or external drainage of the cyst. Prolonged observation of a nonresolving pancreatic pseudocyst exposes the patient to increased risks which exceed those of elective surgery.

PANCREATIC ASCITES AND PANCREATIC PLEURAL EFFUSIONS

Pancreatic ascites is usually due to disruption of the main pancreatic duct, often associated with an internal fistula between the duct and the peritoneal cavity or a leaking pseudocyst (see also Chap. 39). The diagnosis of pancreatic ascites is suggested in a patient with an elevated serum amylase who also has increased levels of albumin (>3.0 g/dL) and amylase in the ascitic fluid. In addition, endoscopic retrograde cholangiopancreatography (ERCP) will often demonstrate passage of contrast material from a major pancreatic duct or a pseudocyst into the peritoneal cavity. As many as 15 percent of patients with pseudocysts have concurrent pancreatic ascites. The differential diagnosis should include intraperitoneal carcinomatosis, tuberculous peritonitis, constrictive pericarditis, and Budd-Chiari syndrome.

If the pancreatic duct disruption is posterior, an internal fistula may develop between the pancreatic duct and pleural space producing a pleural effusion, which is usually left-sided and often massive. This often requires thoracentesis or chest tube drainage.

Treatment usually involves placing the patient on nasogastric solution and parenteral alimentation to decrease pancreatic secretion. In addition, paracentesis is performed to keep the peritoneal cavity free of fluid and, it is hoped, effect sealing of the leak. If ascites continues to recur after 2 to 3 weeks of medical management, the

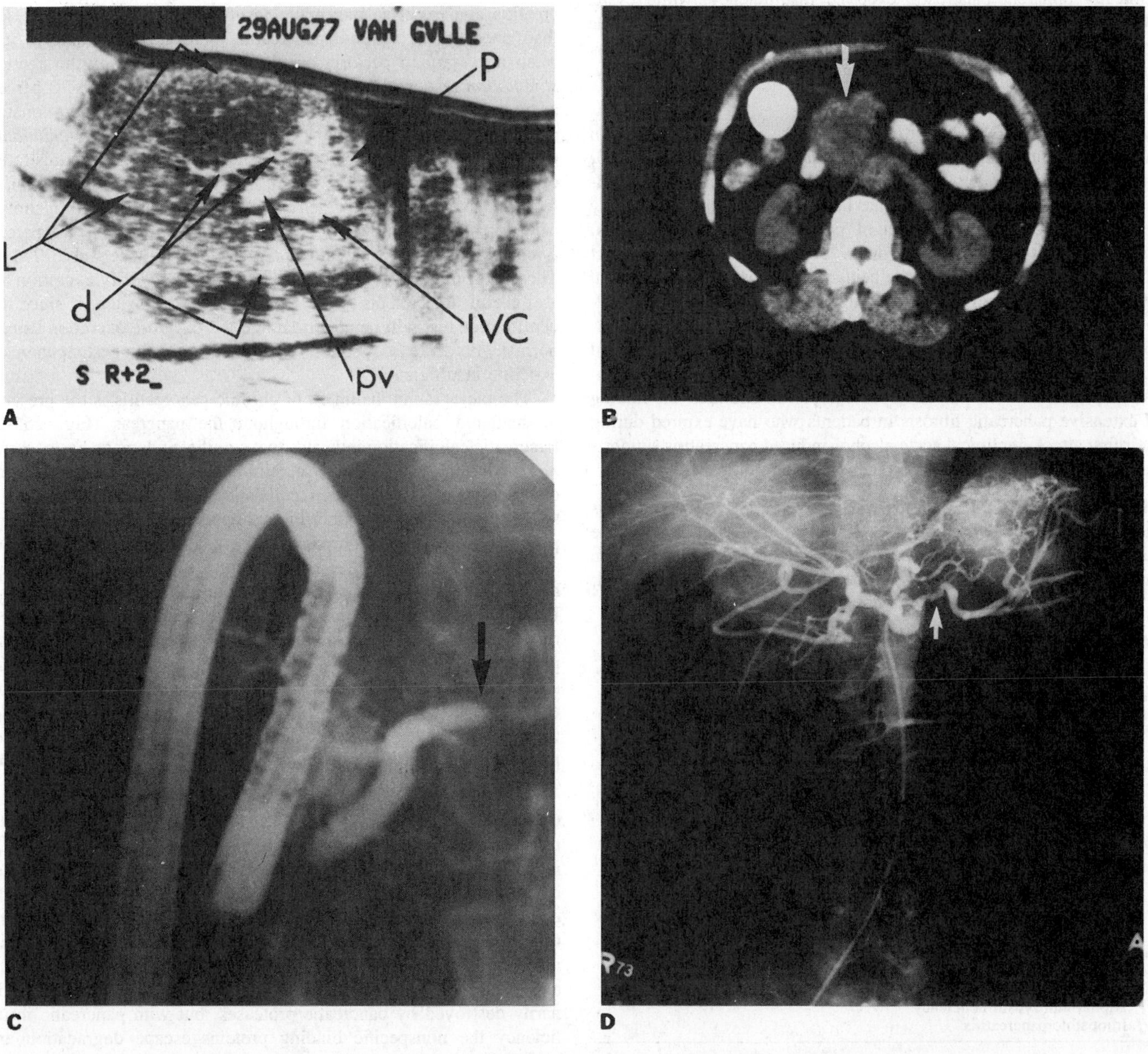

FIGURE 255-2 *Carcinoma of the pancreas. A. Sonogram showing pancreatic carcinoma (P), dilated intrahepatic bile ducts (d), dilated portal vein (pv), and inferior vena cava (IVC). B. CT scan showing pancreatic carcinoma (arrow). C. ERCP showing abrupt cut off of the duct of Wirsung (arrow). D. Arteriogram showing sheathing of splenic artery by tumor encasement (arrow).*

patient should be operated on following pancreatography to define the anatomy of the abnormal duct.

CHRONIC PANCREATITIS AND PANCREATIC EXOCRINE INSUFFICIENCY

GENERAL AND ETIOLOGIC CONSIDERATIONS Chronic inflammatory disease of the pancreas may present as episodes of acute inflammation superimposed upon a previously injured pancreas or as chronic damage with persistent pain or malabsorption. The causes of relapsing chronic pancreatitis are similar to those of acute pancreatitis (Table 255-2), except that frequently the cause is an appreciable incidence of cases of undetermined origin. In addition, the pancreatitis associated with gallstones is predominantly acute or relapsing acute in nature. A cholecystectomy is almost always performed in patients after the first or second attack of gallstone-associated pancreatitis. Patients with chronic pancreatitis may present with persistent abdominal pain, with or without steatorrhea, and some may present with steatorrhea and no pain.

Patients with chronic pancreatitis who develop extensive destruction of the pancreas (i.e., less than 10 percent of exocrine function remaining) will demonstrate steatorrhea and azotorrhea. In the adult in the United States, alcoholism is the most common cause of clinically apparent pancreatic exocrine insufficiency, while cystic fibrosis is the most frequent cause in children. In other parts of the world, severe protein calorie malnutrition is a common etiology. Table 255-4 lists other causes of pancreatic exocrine insufficiency, but they are relatively uncommon.

PATHOPHYSIOLOGY Unfortunately, the events that initiate an inflammatory process within the pancreas are still not well understood, and the many hypotheses will not be reviewed. In the case of alcohol-induced pancreatitis, however, it has been suggested that the primary defect may be the precipitation of protein (inspissated enzymes) within the ducts. The resulting ductal obstruction can lead to duct dilatation, diffuse atrophy of the acinar cells, fibrosis, and eventual calcification of some of the protein plugs. While patients with alcohol-induced pancreatitis generally consume large amounts of alcohol, some consume very little (i.e., 50 g or less per day). Thus, prolonged consumption of "socially acceptable" amounts of alcohol is compatible with the development of pancreatitis. In addition, the finding of extensive pancreatic fibrosis in patients who have expired during their first attack of clinical acute alcohol-induced pancreatitis supports the concept that such patients already have chronic pancreatitis.

CLINICAL FEATURES Patients with relapsing chronic pancreatitis may present with symptoms identical with those found in acute pancreatitis, but their pain may be continuous or intermittent, or pain may be absent. The pathogenesis of this pain is poorly understood.

TABLE 255-4 Causes of pancreatic exocrine insufficiency

I	Alcohol, chronic alcoholism
II	Cystic fibrosis
III	Severe protein calorie malnutrition with hypoalbuminemia
IV	Pancreatic and duodenal neoplasms
V	Pancreatic resection
VI	Gastric surgery
	A Subtotal gastrectomy with Billroth II anastomosis
	B Subtotal gastrectomy with Billroth I anastomosis
	C Truncal vagotomy and pyloroplasty
VII	Gastrinoma (Zollinger-Ellison syndrome)
VIII	Hereditary pancreatitis
IX	Traumatic pancreatitis
X	Hemochromatosis
XI	Shwachman's syndrome (pancreatic insufficiency and bone marrow dysfunction)
XII	Trypsinogen deficiency
XIII	Enterokinase deficiency
XIV	Isolated deficiencies of amylase, lipase, or proteases
XV	Alpha$_1$-antitrypsin deficiency
XVI	Idiopathic pancreatitis

Although the classic description is that of epigastric pain radiating through the back, the pain pattern is often atypical. The pain may be maximal in the right or left upper quadrants in the back or diffuse throughout the upper abdomen; it may even be referred to the anterior chest or flank. Characteristically, the pain is persistent, deep-seated, and unresponsive to antacids. It often is increased by alcohol and ingestion of heavy meals (especially foods rich in fat). Often the pain is so severe as to require the frequent use of narcotics.

Weight loss, abnormal stools, and other signs of symptoms suggestive of malabsorption (see Table 237-5) are common in chronic pancreatitis. However, clinically apparent deficiencies of fat-soluble vitamins are surprisingly rare. The physical findings in these patients are usually not impressive such that there is a disparity between the severity of the abdominal pain and the paucity of physical signs (save some abdominal tenderness and mild temperature elevation).

DIAGNOSTIC EVALUATION (See Chap. 254) In contrast to patients with relapsing acute pancreatitis, the serum amylase and lipase levels are usually not elevated. Elevations of the serum bilirubin and alkaline phosphatase may indicate cholestasis secondary to chronic inflammation around the common bile duct (Fig. 255-3). Many patients demonstrate impaired glucose tolerance, and some may have an elevated fasting blood glucose level.

The classic triad of pancreatic calcification, steatorrhea, and diabetes mellitus usually establishes the diagnosis of chronic pancreatitis and exocrine pancreatic insufficiency but is found in less than one-third of chronic pancreatitis patients. Accordingly, it is often necessary to perform an intubation test such as the *secretin stimulation test,* which usually becomes abnormal when 70 percent or more of pancreatic exocrine function has been lost. Approximately 40 percent of patients with chronic pancreatitis have *cobalamin (vitamin B_{12}) malabsorption* which is corrected by the administration of oral pancreatic enzymes. There is usually a marked excretion of fecal fat (see Chap. 237), which can be reduced with the administration of oral pancreatic enzymes. A fecal fat concentration $\geq$9.5 percent is characteristic of pancreatogenous steatorrhea (see Table 254-1). The bentiromide test (Chap. 254) and D-xylose urinary excretion test are useful in patients with "pancreatic steatorrhea," since the bentiromide test will be abnormal and the D-xylose excretion usually normal. A decreased serum trypsin strongly suggests pancreatic exocrine insufficiency.

The radiographic hallmark of chronic pancreatitis is the presence of scattered calcification throughout the pancreas (Fig. 255-3). Pancreatic calcification indicates that significant damage has occurred and obviates the need for the secretin test. Alcohol by far is the most common cause of pancreatic calcification, but it may also be seen in severe protein calorie malnutrition, hyperparathyroidism, hereditary pancreatitis, posttraumatic pancreatitis, and islet-cell tumors.

Special techniques such as sonography, CT scanning, and ERCP have added new dimensions to the diagnosis of pancreatic disease. In addition to excluding pseudocysts and pancreatic cancer, sonography may show calcification or dilated ducts associated with chronic pancreatitis (Fig. 255-3). Similar benefits can be derived from CT scans, but the availability and lower cost make sonography preferable at present. ERCP is the only nonoperative technique which provides a direct view of the pancreatic duct. In patients with alcohol-induced pancreatitis, ERCP may reveal a pseudocyst missed by sonography or CT scan.

COMPLICATIONS OF CHRONIC PANCREATITIS The complications of chronic pancreatitis are protean. *Cobalamin (vitamin B_{12}) malabsorption* occurs in 40 percent of patients with alcohol-induced chronic pancreatitis and in virtually all with cystic fibrosis. The cobalamin malabsorption is consistently corrected by the administration of pancreatic enzymes (containing proteases). The cobalamin malabsorption may be due to excessive binding of cobalamin by nonintrinsic factor cobalamin-binding proteins. The latter are ordinarily destroyed by pancreatic proteases, but with pancreatic insufficiency the nonspecific binding proteins escape degradation and compete with intrinsic factor for cobalamin binding. Although the majority of patients show *impaired glucose tolerance,* the development of diabetic ketoacidosis and coma is uncommon. Similarly, end organ damage (retinopathy, neuropathy, nephropathy) is also uncommon, and the appearance of these complications should raise the question of concomitant genetic diabetes mellitus. A nondiabetic retinopathy, peripheral in location and secondary to vitamin A and/or zinc deficiency, is common in these patients. High amylase-containing *effusions* occur within the pleura, pericardium, or peritoneum. *Gastrointestinal bleeding* may occur from a peptic ulcer, gastritis, a pseudocyst eroding into the duodenum, or from ruptured varices secondary to splenic vein thrombosis due to inflammation of the tail of the pancreas. *Icterus* may occur, owing to either edema of the head of the pancreas compressing the common bile duct or chronic cholestasis secondary to chronic inflammatory reaction around the intrapancreatic portion of the common bile duct (Fig. 255-3). This chronic obstruction may lead to cholangitis and ultimately biliary cirrhosis. *Subcutaneous fat necrosis* may appear as tender red nodules on the lower extremities. *Bone pain* may be secondary to intramedullary fat necrosis. Inflammation of the large and small joints of the upper and lower extremities may occur. The incidence of pancreatic carcinoma is probably increased. Perhaps the most common and troublesome complication is addiction to narcotics.

TREATMENT AND APPROACH TO MANAGEMENT Therapy for patients with chronic pancreatitis is directed to two major problems, namely, pain and malabsorption. Patients with intermittent attacks of pain are essentially treated like those with acute pancreatitis (see above). Patients with severe and persistent pain should avoid alcohol completely and avoid large meals rich in fat. Since the pain is often severe enough to require frequent use of narcotics (and hence addiction), a number of surgical procedures have been developed for pain relief. ERCP allows the surgeon to plan the operative approach. If there is a stricture of the pancreatic duct, then a *local resection* may ameliorate the pain. Unfortunately isolated localized strictures are not common. In most patients with alcohol-induced disease, the pancreas is diffusely involved and surgically correctible localized ductal disease is rare. When there is primary ductal obstruction, side-to-side pancreaticojejunostomy may provide effective pain palliation. In some of these patients, however, pain relief can be achieved only by resecting 50 to 95 percent of the gland. Although pain relief is achieved in three-quarters of these patients, they tend to develop

FIGURE 255-3 *Radiologic abnormalities in chronic pancreatitis. A. Pancreatic calcification (arrows) and stenosis (tapering) of the intrapancreatic portion of the common bile duct demonstrated by percutaneous transhepatic cholangiography. B. Pancreatic calcification (Ca) demonstrated by sonography. gb = gallbladder; K = kidney; a = aorta. C. Pancreatic calcification (vertical arrows) and dilated pancreatic duct (horizontal arrow) demonstrated by CT scan. D. Endoscopic retrograde cholangiopancreatogram shows grossly dilated pancreatic ducts (arrows) in a patient with long-standing pancreatitis.*

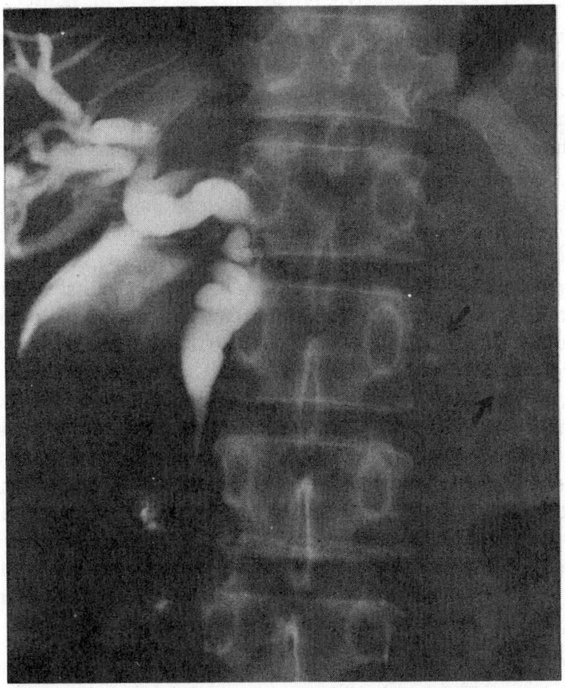

A

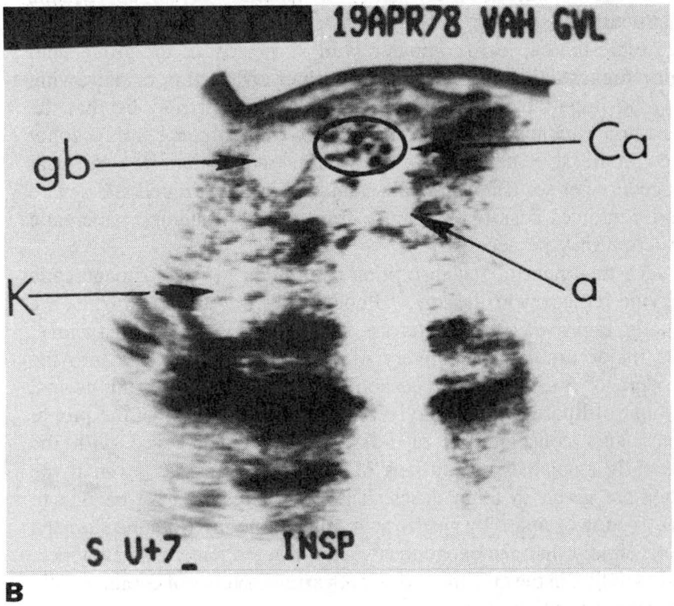

B

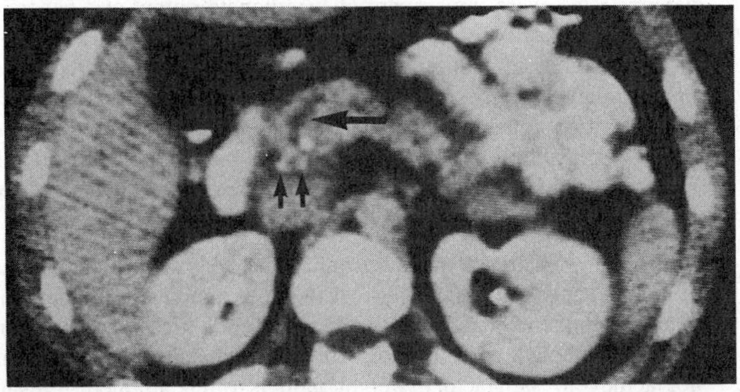

C

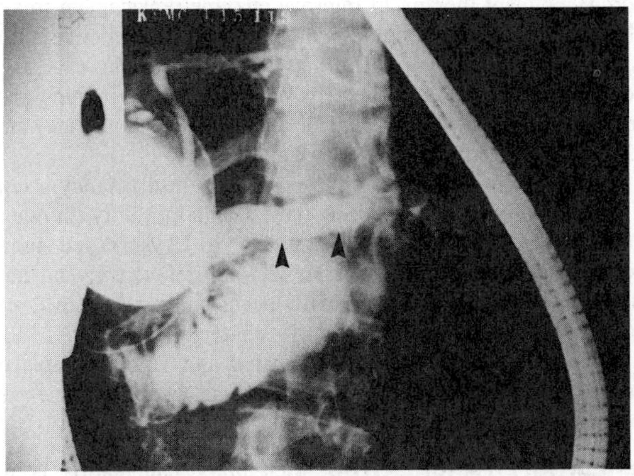

D

pancreatic endocrine and exocrine insufficiency. It is important to screen the patients carefully, for such radical surgery is contraindicated in those who are severely depressed or suicidal or continue to drink. Procedures such as sphincteroplasty, splanchnicectomy and celiac ganglionectomy, and nerve blocks usually bring only temporary relief and are not recommended.

Large doses of pancreatic extract (see below) seem to ameliorate and even abort the pain in some patients with chronic pancreatitis. These clinical observations seem to fit in with data in experimental animals which demonstrate a negative feedback regulation for pancreatic exocrine secretion controlled by the amount of proteases within the lumen of the proximal small intestine. It seems reasonable to approach the patient with severe persistent or continuous abdominal pain thought to be secondary to chronic pancreatitis in the following manner. After other causes of abdominal pain (peptic ulcer, gallstones, etc.) have been appropriately excluded, a pancreatic *sonogram* should be done. If no mass is found, a *secretin test* may be performed, since with chronic pancreatitis and pain this test usually will be abnormal. If the secretin test is abnormal (i.e., decreased bicarbonate concentration or volume output), a 3- to 4-week *trial of pancreatic enzymes* is appropriate. Three to eight capsules or tablets are taken at meals and at bedtime. If no relief is obtained, and especially if the volume secreted during the secretin test is very low, ERCP should be performed. If a pseudocyst or a localized ductal obstruction is found, appropriate surgery should be considered. A provocative study from South Africa questions the significance of the relationship of dilated ducts and/or strictures to pain. The finding of an appreciable obstruction or stricture in 65 percent of the patients who were pain-free more than 1 year, compared with 79 percent of the group with pain, suggests that factors other than duct obstruction or narrowing may be important in the pathogenesis of pain. It may be that the most important factors in the relief of pain are abstinence from alcohol and progressive pancreatic dysfunction rather than the surgical procedure per se. If no surgically remedial lesion is found and severe pain continues despite abstinence from alcohol, subtotal pancreatic resection may be necessary.

The treatment of malabsorption rests upon the use of pancreatic enzyme replacement therapy. Although diarrhea and steatorrhea are usually improved, the results are frequently less than satisfactory. The major problem is delivery of enough active enzyme into the duodenum. Steatorrhea can be abolished if 10 percent of the normal amount of lipase could be delivered into the duodenum at the proper time. This concentration of lipase cannot be achieved with the presently available preparations of pancreatic enzymes, even if the latter are given in large doses. These poor results may be due to inactivation of lipase by gastric acid, food emptying from the stomach more rapidly than the exogenously administered pancreatic enzymes, and variation in the enzyme activity of various batches of commercially available pancreatic extracts.

For the usual patient three to eight tablets or capsules of a potent enzyme preparation should be administered with meals. Some patients require adjuvant therapy to improve enzyme replacement treatment. Although initially cimetidine was considered an effective adjuvant, studies have failed to confirm this. Sodium bicarbonate (1.3 g with meals) is effective and inexpensive. Antacids containing calcium carbonate or magnesium hydroxide are not effective and may actually result in increased steatorrhea.

Patients with severe exocrine pancreatic insufficiency secondary to alcohol who continue to drink have a high mortality (in one series 50 percent were dead when followed for 5 to 12 years) and significant morbidity (weight loss, lassitude, vitamin deficiency, and narcotic addiction). Those with pain usually do not have steatorrhea and are approached as described above. If steatorrhea develops, the pain usually abates. If abstinence is pursued and vigorous replacement therapy is utilized for the maldigestion-malabsorption, the patients do reasonably well.

HEREDITARY PANCREATITIS Hereditary pancreatitis is a rare disease similar to chronic pancreatitis except for an early age of onset and evidence of hereditary factors (involving an autosomal dominant gene with incomplete penetrance). These patients have recurring attacks of severe abdominal pain which may last from a few days to a few weeks. The serum amylase and lipase levels may be elevated during acute attacks. Patients frequently develop pancreatic calcification, diabetes mellitus, and steatorrhea, and in addition, they have an increased incidence of pancreatic carcinoma. Abdominal complaints in relatives of patients with hereditary pancreatitis should raise the question of pancreatic disease.

CYSTIC FIBROSIS (See also Chap. 207)

GENERAL CONSIDERATIONS Cystic fibrosis is the most common hereditary lethal disease in white children. It is transmitted as an autosomal recessive trait, with a prevalence of 1 per 1500 to 2500 births and with approximately 1 in 20 whites being heterozygous for the condition. Patients with cystic fibrosis have defective anion permeability of the mucus-producing exocrine glands in the bronchi, pancreas, liver, and intestine. The decrease in bicarbonate output when pancreatic secretion is stimulated leads to defective water flow and hyperconcentration of protein. However, the basic metabolic defect is unknown. This disease is no longer one of childhood and adolescence. With improvement in the therapy of patients with cystic fibrosis, an increasing number reach adulthood. Twenty-five years ago the mean survival was only 1 year; now, 50 percent of patients may survive to at least 25 years of age.

CLINICAL FEATURES Although the triad of recurrent pulmonary infections, maldigestion-malabsorption, and an abnormal sweat test are characteristic, patients are frequently seen without these classic manifestations. Approximately 85 percent of patients with cystic fibrosis have impairment of pancreatic exocrine function. Steatorrhea is often marked and accompanied by deficiencies of fat-soluble vitamins (e.g., low prothrombin levels). A small number of patients may have recurrent pancreatitis with abdominal pain and elevated amylase levels. Biliary cirrhosis develops in 5 to 10 percent. Approximately 15 percent of patients may develop intestinal obstruction at birth because of the thick, tenacious intestinal secretions. Similarly, children or adults may develop small- or large-bowel obstruction, ileocolic intussusception, cecal or sigmoid volvulus, rectal impaction, and rectal prolapse. Cobalamin and bile acid malabsorption are common but correctable by oral pancreatic extract. Cobalamin deficiency is rare, perhaps due to the almost universal administration of pancreatic extract to these patients beginning at an early age. The incidence of gallstones is increased. Although frank diabetes is uncommon, glucose intolerance may be present in 40 percent of patients. Nearly all males have aspermia because of a failure in development of the vas deferens, epididymis, and seminal vesicles.

DIAGNOSIS A properly performed and interpreted sweat test (quantitative pilocarpine iontophoresis) is essential for the diagnosis of cystic fibrosis. In almost all patients the sweat chloride is greater than 60 meq per liter. Secretin or CCK-PZ tests will usually demonstrate severe impairment of bicarbonate output and pancreatic enzymes, respectively. The bentiromide test (Chap. 254) is usually abnormal, and, in addition, may be used to assess the effectiveness of pancreatic enzyme replacement therapy. Recent studies indicate that elevation of serum trypsin levels within the first few weeks of life is diagnostic of cystic fibrosis and thus may serve as an effective screening test. However, as the disease progresses and frank pancreatic insufficiency develops, serum trypsin levels will be decreased.

THERAPY Treatment includes antibiotics for recurrent pulmonary infections, inhalation and physical therapy, pancreatic extracts, and vitamin supplementation, as well as psychological and emotional support. Although complete correction of fat malabsorption is usually not achieved, satisfactory weight gain is often attained. Elevated blood and urine uric acid levels may occur in children taking excessive doses of pancreatic enzymes, but this is reversible with reduction in dosage and has not been observed with the newer enteric-coated preparations.

CANCER OF THE PANCREAS

GENERAL CONSIDERATIONS Carcinoma of the pancreas is now the fourth commonest cancer causing death in the United States; only cancer of the lung, colon, and breast occur more frequently. It accounts for 10 percent of all tumors of digestive organs and over 20,000 deaths per year. The incidence has increased 300 percent since 1930 to approximately 11 per 100,000 population. The disease is more common in males than females (1.5:1), and the peak incidence is between the ages of 60 to 70. Although the etiologic factors in most cases are not known, incidence of carcinoma of the pancreas is 2.0 to 2.5 times greater in *smokers* than in nonsmokers, and about 2 times greater in patients with *diabetes mellitus*. Epidemiologic evidence suggests that a high-fat diet and certain occupational chemical exposures (e.g., β-naphthylamine) increase the risk of pancreatic cancer. Some reports have also suggested an association between heavy coffee intake and increased risk of pancreatic cancer, but whether a true causal relationship exists is questionable. The tumors are usually adenocarcinomas arising from ductal epithelium. The head of the pancreas is involved in about 65 percent, the body and tail in 30 percent, and the tail alone in 5 percent. At the time of diagnosis the tumor is confined to the pancreas in only 15 percent of patients; 25 percent demonstrate local invasion or regional lymph node spread, and the remaining 60 percent exhibit distinct metastases.

CLINICAL FEATURES Weight loss, abdominal pain, anorexia, and jaundice are the classic symptoms. Nausea, weakness and fatigue, vomiting, diarrhea, dyspepsia, and back pain are also fairly common. The weight loss in carcinoma is extensive (average total loss about 25 lb) and is not fully explained by anorexia and maldigestion. The weight loss in patients with lesions in the body and tail, in whom malabsorption should be minimal, is often as pronounced as when the carcinoma is in the head of the pancreas.

Pain occurs at some time in the course of the disease in 75 to 90 percent of patients. With tumors of the head of the pancreas, the pain is likely to be in the epigastrium and right upper quadrant; with lesions in the body of the pancreas, pain often localizes in the midline, whereas with lesions in the tail, pain may be referred to the left upper quadrant. Abdominal pain may be vague or may be a steady dull, aching, or boring pain often radiating through to the back. Severe and unrelenting pain suggests extension into the retroperitoneal area with invasion of the neural plexus around the celiac axis ganglion.

Jaundice occurs some time in the course of the disease in 80 to 90 percent of patients with carcinoma of the head, and in 10 to 40 percent in patients with tumors of the body and tail. When it occurs it is progressive and accompanied by pruritus. Both constipation and diarrhea have been cited as the predominant alteration of bowel habits. Emotional disturbances frequently occur in cancer of the pancreas and may take the form of insomnia, restlessness, rage, anxiety, depression, suicidal tendencies, and a sense of impending doom.

Physical examination frequently reveals evidence of weight loss, jaundice, and enlarged liver and abdominal tenderness. Although the gallbladder is usually enlarged, it is palpable in only 15 to 40 percent of cases (Courvoisier's sign). The finding of an enlarged gallbladder in a jaundiced patient without biliary colic should suggest malignant obstruction of the extrahepatic biliary tree. Splenomegaly may result from compression, invasion, and thrombosis of the portal venous system, especially the splenic vein. Erosion of the duodenal mucosa may cause occult or frank gastrointestinal bleeding. In carcinoma of the body and tail, an abdominal mass can be felt in 40 to 50 percent of patients; hepatomegaly is less common than in tumors of the head of the pancreas, and obvious hepatic enlargement should suggest hepatic metastasis. An important physical finding is an abdominal bruit which is usually heard in the periumbilical area and left upper quadrant, and this is due to invasion and/or compression of the splenic artery by tumor. Thrombophlebitis occurs in approximately 10 percent of patients and is more common with the tumors of the body or tail of the pancreas. In acinar-cell carcinomas, which are uncommon, tender subcutaneous nodules due to subcutaneous fat necrosis and polyarthralgia occur.

The diagnosis of pancreatic carcinoma should be suspected in patients past the age of 50 who present with any of the following findings: (1) unexplained weight loss greater than 10 percent of normal body weight; (2) unexplained upper abdominal pain, especially with a negative upper gastrointestinal tract workup; (3) unexplained back pain; (4) an attack of pancreatitis without an obvious cause; (5) stigmata of exocrine pancreatic insufficiency without an obvious cause; (6) sudden onset of diabetes mellitus without a predisposing cause such as obesity or family history; and (7) jaundice with obstructive features. Carcinoma of the hepatic duct bifurcation, of the ampulla of Vater, and of the duodenum also need to be considered in the differential diagnosis, but these all occur quite infrequently.

LABORATORY FINDINGS Laboratory data are only occasionally helpful in suggesting the diagnosis of pancreatic carcinoma. The serum amylase and lipase values are abnormal in only 10 percent of cases. About 20 percent of patients have fasting hyperglycemia or glycosuria. Anemia, which occurs in one-third of patients, and occult blood in the stool, which occurs in one-half of patients, are usually due to erosion of the duodenal mucosa by tumor. Although the stools may have a greasy or pultaceous consistency, frank steatorrhea occurs in only about 10 percent of patients. Carcinoma of the head of the pancreas with bile duct obstruction is accompanied by hyperbilirubinemia and clay-colored stools. By contrast, the blood, urine, and feces in patients with carcinoma of the body and tail of the pancreas are often normal. The serum alkaline phosphatase is usually elevated in patients with jaundice (and may antedate the hyperbilirubinemia). It is elevated in about 35 percent of cases without jaundice.

DIAGNOSTIC PROCEDURES Although standard gastrointestinal x-rays may suggest the presence of carcinoma of the head of the pancreas, the tumor is usually of considerable size before it distorts the duodenal mucosa and the configuration of the duodenal loop. Thus, only 50 percent of patients with carcinoma of the head of the pancreas have an abnormal examination. The frequency of abnormal exams is even lower with lesions in the body and tail of the pancreas.

Ultrasound is valuable in the diagnosis of pancreatic carcinoma, especially as an initial screening procedure; abnormalities are found in 70 to 90 percent of patients with pancreatic carcinoma. Sonography is most likely to be positive if the tumor is over 2 cm in diameter and lies in the head or body of the pancreas; lesions in the body and tail of the pancreas are more difficult to recognize.

CT scanning is frequently abnormal in pancreatic carcinoma; in most series of proved cases, CT scans detected the lesion in over 80 percent. In 5 to 15 percent of patients with proven pancreatic carcinoma the CT scan shows only generalized pancreatic enlargement suggestive of pancreatitis rather than malignancy. False-positive results have also been reported in about 5 to 10 percent of cases where no tumor was found at laparotomy. CT scanning has some advantages over ultrasound, such as better definition of the body and tail of the pancreas as well as contiguous organs, but the cost is greater. Selective and superselective angiography is of definite value in some patients. Advantages of angiography include (1) detection of carcinoma in the body and tail of the pancreas by observing vessel sheathing (Fig. 255-2), vessel displacement, and vascular occlusion; (2) detection of metastatic spread to the liver; and (3) assessment of the degree of involvement of huge pancreatic vessels which may be an important consideration preoperatively. When the arteriogram is positive, about 85 percent of patients can be expected to have pancreatic cancer; however, false-negatives occur in about 15 percent of patients.

ERCP may be diagnostic in 75 to 85 percent of cases. The

characteristic findings are stenosis or obstruction of either the pancreatic or the common bile duct; both duct systems are abnormal in over half the cases. The differentiation, however, between carcinoma and chronic pancreatitis by ERCP can be quite difficult if both diseases are present. False-negative results with ERCP are quite low (less than 5 percent) and usually occur with acinar-cell rather than ductal carcinoma. Finally, *percutaneous aspiration biopsy of the pancreas* under ultrasonic or CT guidance is a procedure which can provide a definitive diagnosis and may obviate surgical exploration.

Tests of exocrine pancreatic function with duodenal intubation and analysis of duodenal contents are abnormal in approximately 80 percent of cases. However, pancreatic function tests do not permit discrimination between pancreatic carcinoma and chronic pancreatitis. Cytologic examination of pancreatic fluid obtained after secretin-cholecystokinin stimulation has not been found reliable enough to diagnose pancreatic cancer. Of the many serologic markers available, none have proved useful in detecting asymptomatic patients with pancreatic cancer.

To summarize, if pancreatic carcinoma is suspected, the first test should be either ultrasound or CT scan. If an abnormality is noted, the next test should be ERCP. If ERCP is nondiagnostic or unsuccessful, selective angiography should be considered. At present, pancreatic function tests, radionuclide pancreatic scintigraphy, and measurement of tumor markers are of limited value in the workup of a patient with suspected pancreatic cancer.

It should be emphasized that patients with carcinoma of the pancreas are frequently investigated for several months before a diagnosis is established. Even laparotomy may not provide a definitive diagnosis because chronic pancreatitis may produce a hard mass in the head of the pancreas indistinguishable from carcinoma by palpation. Furthermore, biopsy of such a mass may not show neoplastic tissue and reveal only evidence of pancreatitis because the carcinoma is often surrounded by edematous, inflamed, and fibrotic tissue, e.g., changes of chronic pancreatitis.

TREATMENT AND COURSE When the diagnosis is confirmed at laparotomy, the tumor is usually inoperable. The resectability rate in most series is only about 15 to 20 percent. If the tumor is localized and has not spread to portal lymph nodes, and is not fixed to other structures (e.g., portal vein, superior mesenteric vein, and common bile duct), the lesion should be considered resectable. Resection under these circumstances offers an opportunity for palliation, although survival does not appear to be prolonged. In many patients, just palliative bypass of biliary tract obstruction should be performed. Importantly, the mortality rate with a Whipple procedure (pancreatoduodenal resection) is about 20 percent in most series. The median survival is 6 months from the time of diagnosis. Approximately 10 percent of patients survive 1 year, and in most reported series, the 5-year survival rate is a dismal 1 to 2 percent. Multicenter studies on patients with inoperable pancreatic cancer suggest that either high-dose small-volume radiation therapy or multidrug chemotherapy (fluorouracil, cyclophosphamide, methotrexate, and vincristine followed by fluorouracil and mitomycin for maintenance) prolong survival in 15 to 30 percent of patients.

PANCREATIC ENDOCRINE TUMORS

Pancreatic endocrine tumors are summarized in Table 255-5 and discussed in Chap. 329.

OTHER CONDITIONS

ANNULAR PANCREAS When there is a failure in communication of the ventral and dorsal anlage of the pancreas, a ring of pancreatic tissue encircles the duodenum. Such an annular pancreas may cause intestinal obstruction in the neonate or the adult. Symptoms of postprandial fullness, epigastric pain, nausea, and vomiting may be present for years before the diagnosis is entertained. The radiographic findings are symmetric dilatation of the proximal duodenum with bulging of the recesses on either side of the annular band, effacement of the duodenal mucosa without destruction of the mucosa, accentuation of the findings in the right anterior oblique position, and the lack of change on repeated examinations. The differential diagnosis should include duodenal webs, tumors of the pancreas or duodenum, postbulbar peptic ulcer, regional enteritis, and adhesions. Patients

TABLE 255-5 Pancreatic endocrine tumors

Syndrome	Hormone(s) produced	Primary hormone effects	Pathologic features	Clinical features
Zollinger-Ellison	Gastrin	Gastric acid hypersecretion with basal acid outputs usually >15 meq/h	Delta-cell islet tumors; 10% aberrant (duodenal); 60% malignant	Severe peptic ulcer disease often refractory to therapy; ectopic ulcers; diarrhea; multiple endocrine adenomas (parathyroid, pituitary, adrenal, thyroid)
Insulinoma	Insulin	Hypoglycemia with inappropriately increased serum insulin levels	Beta-cell islet tumors; 80–90% benign	Hypoglycemic symptoms
Glucagonoma	Glucagon; pancreatic polypeptide	Hyperglucagonemia → glucose intolerance	Alpha-cell islet tumors; 60% malignant	Slow-growing pancreatic tumor; hyperglycemia; bullous and eczematoid dermatitis, weight loss; anemia; gastric and intestinal motor abnormalities
Somatostatinoma	Somatostatin; pancreatic polypeptide	Somatostatin inhibits insulin, gastrin and pancreatic enzyme secretion; decreased bile flow	Delta-cell islet tumor	Pancreatic tumor; diarrhea; steatorrhea; gallstones; diabetes mellitus; anemia
Pancreatic cholera	Vasoactive intestinal peptide (VIP) ? Gastric inhibitory polypeptide ? Prostaglandin E ? Pancreatic peptide	Net secretion of salt and water by gut	? Delta-cell tumor; >50% malignant	Pancreatic tumor with severe watery diarrhea; flushing; weight loss; hypokalemia; hypercalcemia; hypochlorhydria; hyperglycemia; inordinate fecal water and electrolyte losses
Carcinoid	Serotonin; prostaglandins	Altered gut motility; diarrhea	Enterochromaffin cells; non-beta-cell islet tumors	Carcinoid syndrome with flushing; wheezing; diarrhea; alcohol intolerance; hepatomegaly

with annular pancreas have an increased incidence of pancreatitis and peptic ulcer. Because of these and other potential complications, the treatment is surgical even though the condition has been present for years. Retrocolic duodenojejunostomy is the procedure of choice, although some surgeons advocate Billroth II gastrectomy, gastroenterostomy, and vagotomy.

PANCREAS DIVISUM Pancreas divisum occurs when the embryologic ventral and dorsal parts of the pancreas fail to fuse so that pancreatic drainage is accomplished mainly through the accessory papilla (Fig. 255-4). This condition should be thought of not only in patients with recurrent pancreatitis without obvious cause, but also in patients who develop pancreatitis after ingesting small amounts of alcohol, and in patients having ERCP who complain of abdominal pain immediately following the injection of small amounts of contrast material (due to overdistention of the small duct of Wirsung). Since the accessory papilla in the duct of Santorini is too small to accept total pancreatic secretion, obstructive pain and pancreatitis may result. Up to 25 percent of patients with unexplained attacks of acute pancreatitis are associated with pancreas divisum. Accordingly, patients with pancreas divisum and symptoms or signs of pancreatic disease usually have some stenosis of the orifice of the duct of Santorini. The appropriate therapy for this condition is still being defined.

MACROAMYLASEMIA Macroamylasemia is a condition whereby amylase is circulating in the blood in a polymer form too large to be easily excreted by the kidney. The patient with this condition will demonstrate an elevated serum amylase value, a low urinary amylase, and a C_{am}/C_{cr} of less than 1 percent. The presence of macroamylase can be documented by chromatography of the serum. The prevalence of macroamylasemia is 1.5 percent of the nonalcoholic general adult hospital population. Usually macroamylasemia is an incidental finding and is not related to disease of the pancreas or other organs. It is important to be aware of this condition so that patients with macroamylasemia will not be needlessly evaluated and treated for pancreatic disease.

REFERENCES

BRADLEY EL et al: The natural history of pancreatic pseudocysts: A unified concept of management. Am J Surg 137:135, 1979

COTTON PB: Cogenital anomaly of pancreas divisum as a cause of obstructive pain and pancreatitis. Gut 21:105, 1980

FRIESEN SR: Tumors of the endocrine pancreas. N Engl J Med 306:580, 1982

GARDNER JD, JENSEN RT: Gastrointestinal peptides: The basis of action at the cellular level, in *Recent Progress in Hormone Research,* vol 39. New York, Academic, 1983

JACOBSON DG et al: Trypsin-like immunoreactivity as a test for pancreatic insufficiency. N Engl J Med 310:1307, 1984

KOLARS JC et al: Comparison of serum amylase, pancreatic isoamylase and lipase in patients with hyperamylasemia. Dig Dis Sci 29:289, 1984

KOPELMAN H et al: Pancreatic fluid secretion and protein hyperconcentration in cystic fibrosis. N Engl J Med 312:329, 1985

MALLORY A, KERN F: Drug-induced pancreatitis. A critical review. Gastroenterology 78:813, 1980

MALT RA: Treatment of pancreatic cancer. JAMA 250:1433, 1983

FIGURE 255-4 *Illustration of the pancreatic ducts and typical ERCP of pancreas divisum. A. Diagram of the ventral and dorsal structures of the pancreas: (1) duct of Santorini; (2) pancreatic duct from the dorsal analogue; (3) pancreatic duct from the ventral analogue; (4) duct of Wirsung; and (5) common bile duct. B. ERCP showing filling only of the ventral component of the pancreatic duct and the common bile duct (CBD) from cannulization of the duct of Wirsung. Failure to fill the pancreatic duct of the body and tail of the pancreas is diagnostic of ventral pancreas or pancreas divisum. E = endoscope.*

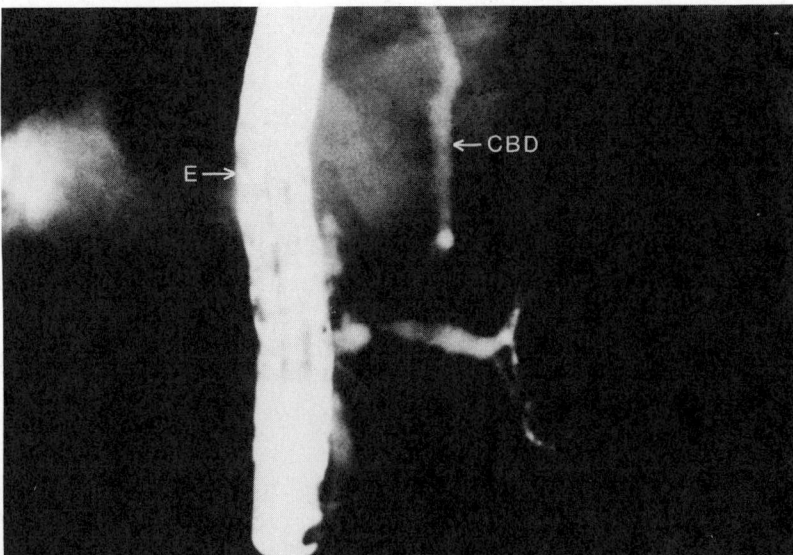

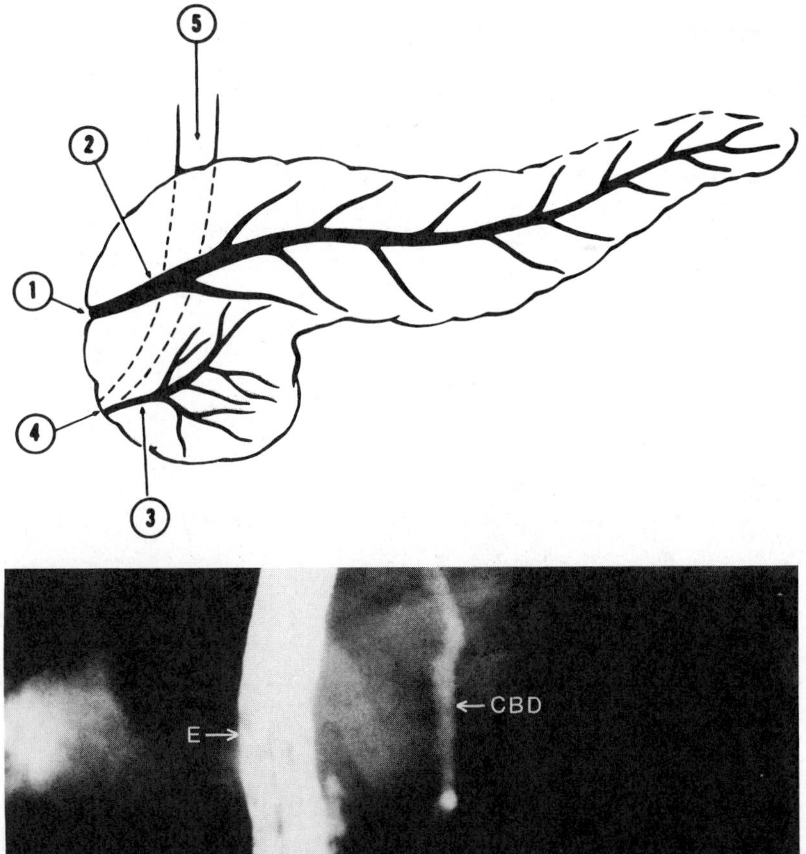

A

B

MAYER DA et al: Controlled clinical trial of peritoneal lavage for the treatment of severe acute pancreatitis. N Engl J Med 312:399, 1985

NIEDERAU C, GRENDELL JH: Diagnosis of chronic pancreatitis. Gastroenterology 88:1973, 1985

RANSON JH-C: Risk factors in acute pancreatitis. Hosp Pract 20:69, 1985

SCHWACHMAN H et al: Cystic fibrosis: A new outlook: 70 patients above 25 years of age. Medicine 56:129, 1977

SLAFF J et al: Protease specific suppression of pancreatic exocrine secretion. Gastroenterology 87:44, 1984

SOLOMON TE: Regulation of pancreatic secretion. Clin Gastroenterol 13:657, 1984

STEER ML et al: Pancreatitis. The role of lysosomes. Dig Dis Sci 29:934, 1984

STEINBERG WM et al: Comparison of sensitivity and specificity of CA19-9 and carcinoembryonic antigen assays in detecting cancer of the pancreas. Gastroenterology 90:343, 1986

——— et al: Diagnostic assays in acute pancreatitis. Ann Int Med 102:576. 1985

TOSKES PP, GREENBERGER NJ: Acute and chronic pancreatitis. DM vol 24, 1983

VAN DYKE JA et al: Pancreatic imaging. Ann Intern Med 102:212, 1985

PART EIGHT DISORDERS OF THE IMMUNE SYSTEM, CONNECTIVE TISSUE, AND JOINTS

section 1 Disorders of the immune system

256 IMMUNE DEFICIENCY DISEASES

MAX D. COOPER / ALEXANDER R. LAWTON III

INTRODUCTION Immunologic functions are mediated by two developmentally independent, but functionally interacting, families of lymphocytes. The activities of B and T lymphocytes, and their products, in host defense are closely integrated with the functions of other cells of the reticuloendothelial system. Macrophages, dendritic cells, and the Langerhans' cells in the skin play an important role in the trapping and presentation of antigens to T and B cells to initiate the immune response. Macrophages also become effector cells, especially when activated by products of lymphocytes. The scavenger activity of polymorphonuclear leukocytes is directed and made specific by antibodies in concert with products of the complement system (see Chap. 62). Natural killer (NK) cells, a recently recognized population of granular lymphocytes, may spontaneously kill tumor and virus-infected cells, activities that are enhanced by the interferon products of immune and inflammatory cells. Killing by NK cells can also be targeted by IgG antibodies for which NK cells have cell-surface receptors. The interaction of basophils and tissue mast cells with IgE antibodies in causation of immediate hypersensitivity is discussed in Chap. 260. Consideration of these interrelationships is an important part of the analysis of patients with suspected immune deficiency.

CLINICAL DISEASE FEATURES COMMON TO IMMUNE DEFICIENCY Immunodeficiency syndromes, whether congenital, spontaneously acquired, or iatrogenic, are characterized by unusual susceptibility to infection and, sometimes, to autoimmune disease and lymphoreticular malignancies. The types of infection often provide the first clue to the nature of the immunologic defect.

Patients with defects in humoral immunity have recurrent or chronic sinopulmonary infection, meningitis, and bacteremia, most commonly caused by pyogenic bacteria such as *Haemophilus influenzae, Streptococcus pneumoniae,* and staphylococci. The same pathogens tend to infect patients with normal immune responses, but with either neutropenia or a deficiency of the pivotal third component of complement (C3), suggesting that a tripartite collaboration involving antibody, complement, and phagocytes exists as the chief mechanism of host defense against pyogenic organisms. Binding of antibody to the bacterial surface causes activation of the complement system. One cleavage product of activated C3 serves as a chemotactic factor for polymorphonuclear leukocytes. Activated C3b fixed to bacterial surfaces facilitates phagocytosis by interaction with C3b receptors on neutrophils.

Agammaglobulinemic patients in whom cell-mediated immunity is intact have an interesting response to viral infections. The clinical course of primary infection with viruses such as varicella zoster or rubeola, unless complicated by bacterial infection, does not differ significantly from that of the normal host. However, long-lasting immunity may not develop, and as a result multiple bouts of chickenpox and measles may occur. Such observations suggest that intact T cells may be sufficient for control of established viral infections, while antibodies play an important role in limiting the initial dissemination of virus and in providing long-lasting protection. Exceptions to this generalization are becoming more widely recognized. Agammaglobulinemic patients fail to clear hepatitis B virus from their circulation and have a progressive, and often fatal, course. Poliomyelitis has occurred following live-virus vaccination in some patients. Chronic encephalitis, which may progress over a period of months to years, is being observed with apparently increasing frequency. Echoviruses and adenoviruses have been isolated from brain, spinal fluid, or other sites in such patients; in others no agent has been detected. Immunologic injury resulting from a partial and ineffective immune response may contribute as much to the pathogenesis of these diseases as the direct effects of the viruses.

The occurrence of unusual serious infection, for example, *H. influenzae* meningitis in an older child or adult, warrants consideration of humoral immune deficiency. Bacterial infections in certain sites may also suggest this possibility. Chronic otitis media occurs frequently in patients with hypogammaglobulinemia, and is significant because of its relative rarity in normal adults. Pansinusitis, although almost invariably present in immunoglobulin deficiency, is a less helpful finding because it is not rare in apparently normal people. Bacterial infections of the skin or urinary tract are less frequent problems in hypogammaglobulinemic patients.

Infestation with the intestinal parasite *Giardia lamblia* is a frequent enough cause of diarrhea in antibody-deficient patients to warrant diagnostic duodenal aspiration and intestinal biopsy when the organism cannot be demonstrated in the stool.

Abnormalities of cell-mediated immunity predispose to *disseminated virus infections,* particularly with latent viruses such as herpes simplex (see Chap. 136), varicella zoster (see Chap. 135), and cytomegalovirus (see Chap. 137). In addition, patients so affected almost invariably develop mucocutaneous candidiasis and frequently acquire widely disseminated fungal infections. Pneumonia caused by the protozoan *Pneumocystis carinii* is also common (see Chap. 158).

T-cell deficiency is probably always accompanied by some abnormality of antibody responses (see Fig. 256-1), although this may not be reflected by hypogammaglobulinemia. This may explain in part why patients with primary T-cell defects are also subject to overwhelming bacterial infection.

The most severe form of immune deficiency occurs in individuals, often infants, who lack both cell-mediated and humoral immune functions. They are susceptible to the whole range of infectious agents including organisms not ordinarily considered pathogenic. Multiple infections with viruses, bacteria, and fungi occur, often simultaneously. Because donor lymphocytes cannot be rejected by the recipients, blood transfusions can produce fatal graft-versus-host disease.

DIFFERENTIATION OF T AND B CELLS The functional deficits which occur in both congenital and acquired immunodeficiencies are usefully viewed as being caused by defects at various points along the differentiation pathways of immunocompetent cells. For this reason certain features of the development and differentiation of T and B cells that are especially relevant to the analysis of immunodeficiency are briefly presented here; Chap. 62 provides a general account of their roles in cellular and humoral immunity.

A subpopulation of hematopoietic stem cells may become restricted to lymphoid differentiation prior to migration to the thymus, where T cells are generated, or to the fetal liver and adult bone marrow, where B-cell development begins (Fig. 256-1). A major function of central lymphoid tissues is to generate the clonal diversity characteristic of the immune system. Each T or B lymphocyte is induced to express surface receptor molecules of a unique specificity for antigen. The receptors of B lymphocytes are immunoglobulin molecules which are formed by paired heavy and light chains of either κ or λ type. The heavy chain gene loci are on the long arm of chromosome 14; the 5′-3′ order of these is V_H (variable), D (diversity), and J_H (joining) minigene families followed by the C_H (constant region) genes, C_μ, C_δ, $C_{\gamma3}$, $C_{\gamma1}$, $C_{\alpha1}$, $C_{\gamma2}$, $C_{\gamma4}$, C_ϵ, and $C_{\alpha2}$. The κ gene family, consisting of V_κ, J_κ, and C_κ genes, is located on chromosome 2, and the homologous λ gene loci on chromosome 22.

The T-cell receptors are related cell surface molecules with antigen-binding specificity. The T-cell receptor is composed of two polypeptide chains, presently called α and β. The β-chain family is located on chromosome 7, and consists of V_β, D_β, J_β, and C_β minigene loci. The α-chain family on chromosome 14 similarly consists of a series of V_α, D_α, J_α, and C_α genes.

The genetic strategy for creating functional gene complexes encoding antigen receptors is similar for T and B cells. For example,

FIGURE 256-1 *Differentiation of lymphoid cells is accompanied by acquisition and loss of specific cell-surface antigens as well as morphologic and functional changes. Some antigens are expressed as stem cells, differentiate within the thymus, and are shared by all mature T cells; commercially available monoclonal antibodies to such pan-T-cell antigens include T3 and Leu 4. T6, the human counterpart to the mouse thymic leukemia (TL) antigen, is expressed only by thymocytes. Within the thymus, cells acquiring helper-inducer functions selectively lose the T8 (Leu 2) antigen, while T4 (Leu 3) antigen is lost by cells destined to serve cytotoxic and suppressor functions. HLA-DR antigens are expressed by all cells of the B lineage, up to and including some plasma cells. T cells, in contrast, express HLA-DR only when they have been activated. These differentiation antigens serve as useful markers for evaluation of disorders of development and function of T and B cells. Failure to develop T and B cells may result from defective stem cells or from inborn metabolic errors affecting both cell types. Rarely, other hematopoietic cell lines are also absent. Absence of either T or B cells suggests malfunction of central lymphoid tissues, including the thymus and the fetal liver–bone marrow complex. B-cell deficiency may result from failure to generate pre-B cells from their stem cell precursors or from failure of pre-B cells to give rise to their B-lymphocyte progeny. Similarly, differentiation may be arrested at several levels within the T-cell lineage; arrests at the thymocyte level and failure to develop the helper-inducer subset have been observed in immunodeficient patients. Agammaglobulinemia and deficiencies of some T-cell functions may occur despite the presence of normal numbers of B or T cells in the circulation. Failure of B lymphocytes to differentiate to plasma cells can be due to intrinsic cellular abnormalities or to faulty T-cell regulation.*

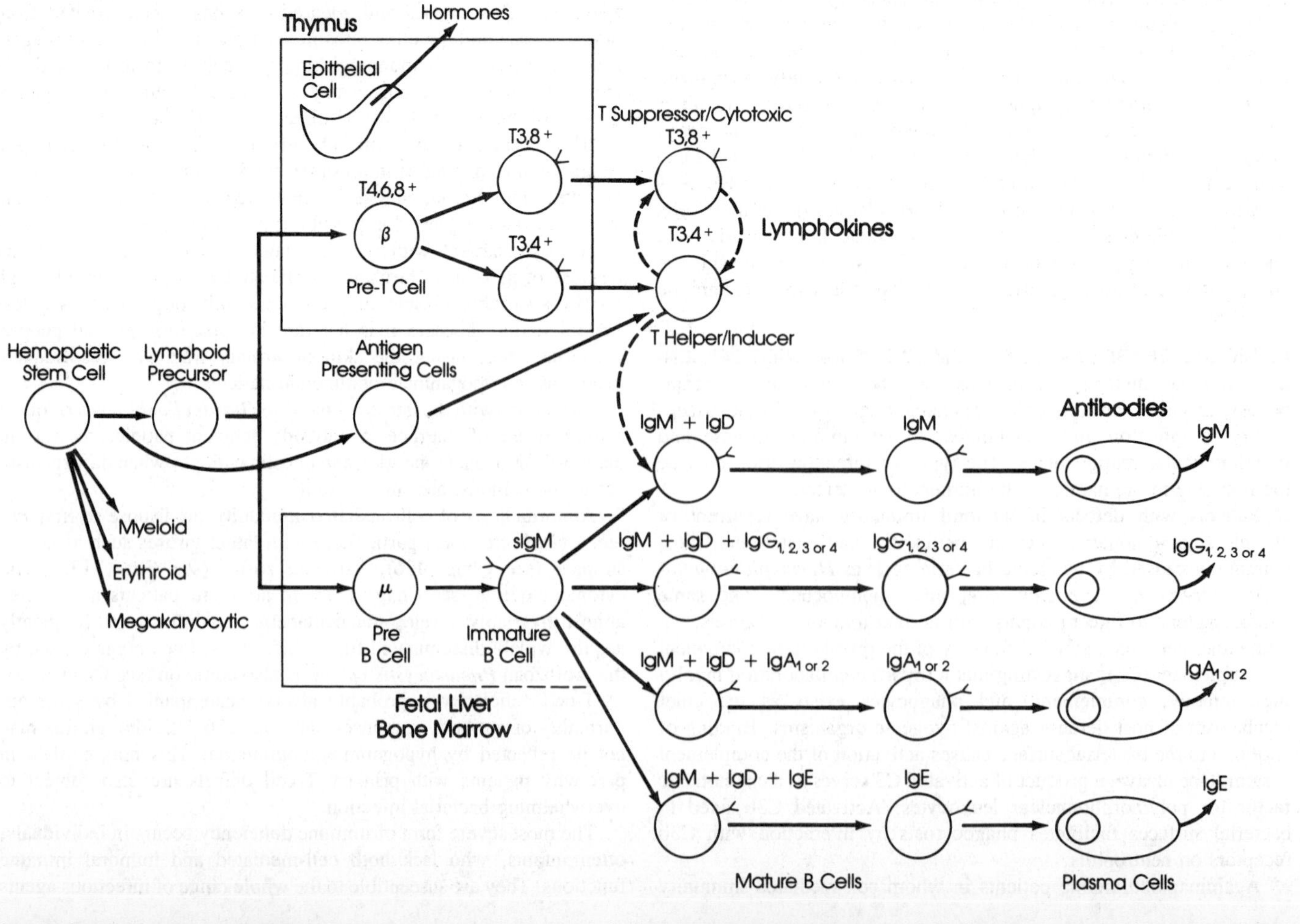

a productive V region gene of the immunoglobulin heavy chain is formed by rearrangement of one each of the V_H, D, and J_H genes and deletion of the intervening DNA to generate a contiguous coding structure which is then transcribed together with the nearest C_H gene. Functional light chain genes are formed by a V-J rearrangement in either the κ or λ gene loci. The V_β gene is similarly composed of a rearranged set of V_β, D_β, and J_β genes to form a contiguous coding structure, which the T cell then transcribes along with the nearest C_β gene. Because there are many different V, D, and J genes, they can be put together in various combinations to encode a large number of receptor molecules having different antigen-binding specificities.

Generation of clonal diversity requires cellular proliferation, such that each of the different receptor specificities encoded in the genome comes to be uniquely expressed by individual cells. A clone consists of all cells that express the identical antigen-binding receptors. Estimates for the total number of B-cell clones usually vary between 10 and 100 million. T-cell clonal diversity is also extensive, but may be less than that of the B-cell population. The process of clonal development is independent of antigen and reflects a genetically programmed sequence of differentiation analogous to that of primary erythropoiesis or myelopoiesis. This phase, termed *primary differentiation,* begins early in human fetal development but probably continues into adult life.

The most primitive morphologically identifiable cell in the B lineage is called a pre-B cell. These cells have undergone a productive V_HDJ_H rearrangement and express cytoplasmic μ chains (the heavy chain of IgM). Since light chain gene rearrangements have not yet occurred at this stage, pre-B cells lack the membrane-bound immunoglobulin receptors which characterize B lymphocytes. Pre-B cells are first generated in fetal liver and are produced exclusively in bone marrow of adults. Pre-B cells proliferate rapidly and, after undergoing a productive rearrangement of light chain VJ genes, spawn immature B lymphocytes which express surface IgM receptors and divide rarely. Young B lymphocytes differ from their more mature counterparts in an important physiologic characteristic; they are highly susceptible to inactivation when their receptors bind antigen. This phenomenon almost certainly is one important mechanism for the development of tolerance to self-antigens.

The developmental sequence for expression of diverse immunoglobulin classes by human B lymphocytes begins with expression of IgM. The expression of IgD on IgM-bearing cells occurs later. Lymphocytes committed to synthesis of IgG, IgA, and IgE are all derived from IgM-bearing precursors through a genetic switch mechanism. Each of the heavy chain constant region genes except C_δ is preceded by a switch region composed of repetitive nucleotide sequences. The heavy chain class switch is accomplished by splicing of the switch region of μ with the switch region in front of the downstream heavy chain gene to be expressed next.

T cells also appear to undergo sequential rearrangements of the minigene families encoding their antigen receptors. Initially, pre-T cells beginning development along this differentiation pathway in the thymus rearrange one each of the V_β, D_β, and J_β genes prior to the expression of a complete β chain. At a later differentiation stage, similar rearrangements occur in the α-chain gene family, and then the completed antigen receptor molecule of one α chain and one β chain is expressed on the cell surface of an immature T cell.

The expression of a group of differentiation antigens, defined by their reactivity with monoclonal antibodies, has become a powerful tool in elucidating developmental relationships of both T and B lymphocytes (Fig. 256-1). All immunocompetent T cells express T3 or Leu 4 molecules, which form a functional complex with the antigen receptor molecules on the cell surface. Of major clinical importance is the demarcation of two independent sets of T lymphocytes. T cells bearing the T4 or Leu 3 markers constitute approximately 70 percent of total T cells and function as helper-inducer cells, necessary for expression of effector functions of both T and B cells. $T8^+$ (or Leu 2^+) lymphocytes, constituting 20 to 30 percent of circulating T cells, are responsible for suppression of immune responses and mediate cytotoxic reactions. Developmental arrests or failure of function of one or the other of these T-cell subsets may be responsible for immunodeficiency or autoimmune diseases.

In addition to generating T cells, the thymus apparently secretes hormonal products which regulate cellular maturation in peripheral lymphoid tissues. These hormones have been called *thymosin* or *thymopoietin;* deficiencies of these factors have been implicated in some immunodeficiencies.

The events designated *secondary differentiation* follow stimulation of specific clones of lymphocytes by antigen. These processes are synonymous with the immune response (see Chap. 62). Particularly important in consideration of immunodeficiencies are the collaborative interactions among macrophages, T cells, and B cells. B lymphocytes can proliferate in response to thymus-dependent antigens without the help of T cells, and may differentiate to IgM-secreting plasma cells when stimulated by thymus-independent antigens such as polysaccharides. However, production of normal quantities of antibodies, particularly those of the IgA and IgG classes, requires the collaboration of T cells.

Differentiation of T or B cells may be arrested at either the primary or secondary stages. Reflecting the complex cellular interactions involved in immune responses and the pivotal role played by T lymphocytes, immune deficiencies primarily involving T cells are usually also associated with abnormal B-cell function. Conversely, immunodeficiencies manifested primarily by inability to produce antibodies may be caused by T-cell defects not associated with abnormal cell-mediated immunity.

EVALUATION OF IMMUNODEFICIENT PATIENTS Many of the laboratory assays used for precise evaluation of immunologic functions in humans are available only in specialized centers; nevertheless, most immunodeficiencies may be diagnosed by thoughtful use of tests available in most clinical laboratories. Table 256-1 presents a résumé of laboratory investigations roughly in order of increasing complexity.

A careful history will usually indicate whether the major problem involves the antibody-complement-phagocyte system or cell-mediated immunity. A history of a normal response to smallpox vaccination or of contact dermatitis due to poison ivy suggests intact cellular immunity. Lymphopenia and the absence of palpable lymph nodes may be important findings. However, patients with profound immunodeficiency may have diffuse lymphoid hyperplasia.

Humoral immunity With rare exceptions, deficiency of humoral immunity is accompanied by diminished serum concentration of one or more classes of immunoglobulin. Normal values vary with age, and adult concentrations of IgM (100 mg/dL) are reached at about 1 year, of IgG (1000 mg/dL) at 5 to 6 years, and of IgA (200 mg/dL) at puberty (see Chap. 62). Also, the wide range of values among normal adults creates difficulty in defining the lower limits of normal. Reasonable estimates for low normal values are 40 mg/dL for IgM, 500 mg/dL for IgG, and 50 mg/dL for IgA. In the presence of borderline hypogammaglobulinemia, assessing the patient's capacity to produce specific antibodies becomes particularly important. Most hospital laboratories can measure isohemagglutinins, anti-streptolysin O, and "febrile agglutinins." Typhoid H and O agglutinins can be measured before and after immunization with standard typhoid vaccine. Many state public health laboratories can perform titrations for antibodies to common viral agents.

Since antibody deficiency may be mimicked clinically by deficiency of complement components, measurement of total hemolytic complement (CH_{50}) should be a part of the evaluation of host defense. Measurement of C3 alone is inadequate for screening, since deficiencies of both early and late complement components may predispose to bacterial infection (see Chap. 62). Estimation of numbers of circulating B lymphocytes has been of great value in determining the pathogenesis of certain types of immune deficiency. B lymphocytes are identified by the presence of membrane-bound immunoglobulins; additional markers include HLA-DR antigens, receptors for aggregated

IgG (Fc receptor), receptors for the third component of complement (C3 receptor), and receptors which specifically bind the Epstein-Barr virus. Following activation, B cells also express receptors for soluble growth and differentiation-promoting factors that are made by T cells. Most of these molecules on the B-cell surface can be identified and enumerated by specific monoclonal antibodies.

Pokeweed mitogen (PWM), an extract of the plant *Phytolacca americana,* has the capacity to induce B lymphocytes in culture to proliferate and differentiate to plasma cells. This activity requires the presence of T lymphocytes, which also proliferate in response to PWM. Thus, this assay can measure not only the capacity of B lymphocytes to differentiate but also the "helper" or "suppressor" function of patients' T lymphocytes.

TABLE 256-1 Laboratory evaluation of host defense defects

I Preliminary screen*
- *A* Complete blood count with differential smear
- *B* Quantitative immunoglobulin levels

II Readily available studies†
- *A* B-cell function
  - *1* Natural or commonly acquired antibodies: isohemagglutinins, "febrile" agglutinins, antibodies to common viruses (rubella, rubeola, influenza) and toxins (diphtheria, tetanus)
  - *2* Response to immunization (typhoid, polio, diphtheria-tetanus vaccines)
- *B* T-cell function
  - *1* Skin tests (PPD, *Candida, Trichophyton,* histoplasmin), tetanus toxoid (1:100 dilution)
  - *2* Chest x-ray (thymus shadow in infants, thymoma in adults)
- *C* Complement
  - *1* C3
  - *2* CH_{50} (total hemolytic complement)
- *D* Phagocyte function
  - *1* Reduction of nitroblue tetrazolium
  - *2* Inflammatory skin window (Rebuck)
  - *3* Bacteria phagocytic and bactericidal indexes

III In-depth investigation
- *A* B cell
  - *1* Pre-B cell examination in bone marrow samples
  - *2* B-lymphocyte membrane markers: IgM, IgD, IgG, IgA; receptors for aggregated IgG (Fc receptor), C3, Epstein-Barr virus; antigens detected by anti-B antibodies
  - *3* Induction of B-lymphocyte differentiation in vitro stimulated by pokeweed mitogen, Epstein-Barr virus, or other polyclonal B-cell activators
  - *4* Kinetics and immunoglobulin class of antibody produced in response to specific primary and secondary immunization
  - *5* Measurement of IgG subclasses and κ/λ ratio
  - *6* Histologic and immunofluorescent examination of biopsy specimens (intestinal mucosa, lymph node, bone marrow)
- *B* T cell
  - *1* Surface markers: binding of sheep erythrocytes (E rosettes), reactivity with monoclonal antibodies recognizing all T cells and the helper and suppressor subsets
  - *2* In vitro correlates of delayed hypersensitivity
    - *a* Proliferative response to mitogens: phytohemagglutinin, concanavalin A–specific antigens (PPD, *Candida*); allogeneic cells (one-way mixed lymphocyte response)
    - *b* Quantification of lymphokines (migration inhibitory factor, etc.)
    - *c* Induction of killer cells by stimulation with allogeneic lymphocytes
  - *3* Measurement of thymus hormones
  - *4* Assays for T-cell "helper" function using supernatants of antigen-activated T cells or T cells plus PWM or antigens to trigger B-lymphocyte differentiation
  - *5* Skin graft rejection
- *C* Phagocytes and complement
  - *1* Chemotactic response in vitro
  - *2* Bactericidal function
  - *3* Classic and alternative complement components
- *D* Natural killer cells
  - *1* Enumeration with monoclonal antibodies
  - *2* Functional assay using appropriate target cells
- *E* Miscellaneous
  - *1* Lymphocytotoxic antibodies
  - *2* Measurement of adenosine deaminase and purine nucleoside phosphorylase enzyme activities

* *Together with a history and physical examination, these tests will identify more than 95 percent of patients with primary immunodeficiencies.*

† *These assays are generally available in either hospitals or state public health laboratories. With rare exceptions, information gained from tests in categories I and II is sufficient to diagnose and treat those immunodeficiencies amenable to conventional treatment with gamma globulin or plasma.*

Cellular immunity Human T lymphocytes may be enumerated by their expression of surface molecules which can bind sheep erythrocytes, forming what are called *E rosettes.* The normal function of these receptors is unknown, but they are not related to the antigen-specificity of T cells. The monoclonal antibodies T11 and Leu 5 recognize the sheep erythrocyte sites on human T cells and may soon supplant the E-rosette test. Other monoclonal antibodies which recognize all peripheral T cells (T3 and Leu 4) and distinguish the helper-inducer subset ($T4^+$, Leu 3^+) from cytotoxic-suppressor T cells ($T8^+$, Leu 2^+) are also commercially available.

T-lymphocyte function can be measured in vivo by delayed hypersensitivity skin testing, using a variety of antigens to which the majority of older children and adults have been sensitized. The most generally useful skin test antigen is a 1:100 dilution of tetanus toxoid injected intradermally, since almost all individuals will have been sensitized. Purified protein derivative (PPD), histoplasmin, mumps antigen, and extracts of *Candida* or *Trichophyton* may also be used.

T-lymphocyte function may be estimated in vitro by the capacity of cells to proliferate in response to antigens to which the patient has been sensitized, to lymphocytes from an unrelated donor, or to the T-cell mitogens, which include phytohemagglutinin, concanavalin A, and pokeweed mitogen. The response is usually quantified by measurement of incorporation of radioactive thymidine into newly synthesized DNA. It is also possible to measure the production of lymphokines by activated T cells. Finally, the ability of T cells activated in mixed lymphocyte culture to lyse target cells can be measured.

The capacity of T lymphocytes from immunologically normal persons to be activated in vitro with antigens or mitogens may be markedly diminished by acute febrile illness, treatment with corticosteroids, or stress. Caution should be exercised in interpreting abnormal results in these circumstances.

CLASSIFICATION Primary immunodeficiencies may be either congenital or acquired, and are currently classified according to mode of inheritance and whether the defect involves T cells, B cells, or both. Unfortunately, the best current classification, established by an expert committee of the World Health Organization, still places the majority of immunodeficiency diseases in an ill-defined category called *common varied immunodeficiency.* In general, this classification will be followed in the following discussion, which emphasizes three related concepts; first, that immunodeficiencies are most logically viewed as defects of cellular differentiation; second, that these defects may involve either primary development of T or B cells or the antigen-dependent phase of their differentiation; and third, that defects of secondary B-cell differentiation may in some instances reflect T-cell abnormalities resulting from faulty T-B collaboration.

Secondary immunodeficiencies are those not caused by intrinsic abnormalities in development or function of T and B cells. The best known of these is the acquired immunodeficiency disease (AIDS) which may follow infection with the human lymphotropic virus HTLV III (see Chap. 257). Other examples are immune deficiency associated with malnutrition, protein-losing enteropathy, and intestinal lymphangiectasia. Also considered secondary are immunodeficiencies resulting from hypercatabolic states such as occur in myotonic dystrophy, immunodeficiency associated with lymphoreticular malignancy, and immunodeficiency resulting from treatment with x-rays, antilymphocyte serum, or cytotoxic drugs.

Incidence As a group, the immunodeficiency syndromes discussed in this chapter are relatively common. Isolated IgA deficiency occurs in approximately 1 in 600 individuals; no other specific category approaches this frequency, but the cumulative total is not insignificant. The incidence of diagnosed immunodeficiency diseases is clearly a function of the awareness of physicians in a community. An epidemic of immunodeficiency diseases commonly follows the addition of a clinical immunologist to a medical center staff.

The more severe forms of primary immunodeficiency have their onset early in life and all too frequently result in death during childhood. Immunodeficiencies may be acquired at any age, however, and a substantial number of patients with congenital hypogammaglobulinemia survive to middle age or beyond. In a referral center for patients with immunodeficiency diseases, approximately two-thirds of the immunodeficient patients under care are adults. Improved methods of diagnosis and treatment can be expected to increase this ratio in the future.

Severe combined immunodeficiency (SCID) This syndrome is characterized by gross functional impairment of both humoral and cell-mediated immunity. It is usually congenital, may be inherited either as an X-linked or autosomal recessive defect, or may occur sporadically. Affected infants rarely survive beyond 1 year without treatment. This syndrome has been associated with a diversity of defects in development of immunocompetent cells, some of which may be related to specific enzymatic abnormalities.

The classic example of SCID, *Swiss-type agammaglobulinemia,* is characterized by severe lymphopenia involving both T and B cells, and is inherited with an autosomal recessive pattern. Rarely, other hematopoietic cell lines fail to develop in a variant form of SCID called *reticular dysgenesia*. The cellular defect in these forms of SCID logically rests with the precursor common to both T and B cells. The immunologic defects in a few of these patients have been repaired following transplantation of fetal liver as a source of stem cells, confirming the hypothesis that they have a thymus and bursa equivalent capable of supporting T- and B-cell differentiation of normal stem cells. About half of patients with autosomal recessive SCID are deficient in an enzyme involved in purine metabolism, adenosine deaminase (ADA). These patients have varying degrees of lymphopenia, T cells usually being more deficient than B cells. Studies of the pathophysiologic relationship of ADA deficiency to abortive lymphoid differentiation suggest that intracellular accumulation of adenosine and deoxyadenosine triphosphate, by inhibiting ribonucleotide reductase enzymes, interferes with DNA synthesis. Improvement of both clinical status and immunologic function has occurred in some but not all patients treated with a source of exogenous ADA.

SCID may also occur with an X-linked inheritance pattern. Affected boys may not have severe lymphopenia; some have had normal numbers of B lymphocytes with few or no circulating T lymphocytes. This developmental pattern (which may also occur with autosomal recessive inheritance) suggests the possibility of a faulty thymus epithelium. Mononuclear cells from bone marrow of such patients have been induced to express T-cell characteristics by coculture on normal thymus epithelium or by treatment with thymus hormones.

The SCID syndrome may occur as a consequence of more subtle defects of T-cell maturation. In one patient, circulating T cells present in normal numbers had the phenotypic markers of cortical thymocytes (Fig. 256-1) and lacked functions of mature T cells. Other patients have a selective deficiency of $T4^+$, Leu 3^+ helper T cells.

Patients with SCID with and without ADA deficiency have been successfully treated by transplantation of histocompatible bone marrow from sibling donors. The same treatment has been used in children and adults with leukemia or aplastic anemia (see Chap. 291) following purposeful destruction of the immune system by irradiation and cytotoxic drugs. Other modes of treatment, including fetal liver and thymus transplants, have been successful in restoring immunocompetence, but as yet there are only short-term survivors. Treatment of these patients should probably be attempted only in centers with a strong research interest in this problem. It is crucial that these patients be recognized early and not be given blood transfusions which may cause fatal graft-versus-host disease.

T-cell immunodeficiency Reflecting the diversity of T-cell functions, abnormalities of T-cell development may be responsible for a wide spectrum of immune deficiencies including severe combined immunodeficiency, apparently isolated defects in cell-mediated immunity, and syndromes presenting as antibody deficiency with apparently normal cell-mediated immunity. These defects may be acquired (see Chap. 257) as well as congenital. Until recently, laboratory assays of T-lymphocyte function were limited to correlates of cell-mediated immunity; no means were available for studying T-cell regulatory functions. Quantification of T-cell subsets and of their growth factor receptors using monoclonal antibodies, accompanied by functional measurements of helper, suppressor, and cytotoxic activity, are expanding the spectrum of immunodeficiencies primarily related to T-cell abnormalities. The recent identification of the T-cell receptor genes and the availability of these DNA probes for studies of immunodeficient patients will also allow more precise definition of T-cell disorders, the numbers of which will increase with the use of more sophisticated tools for T-cell analysis.

DI GEORGE'S SYNDROME This is the classic example of isolated T-cell deficiency and results from maldevelopment of organs derived embryologically from the interaction between neural crest mesenchyme and epithelial elements of the third and fourth pharyngeal pouches. Affected infants usually present with congenital cardiac defects, particularly those involving the great vessels, hypocalcemic tetany due to failure of parathyroid development, and absence of a normal thymus. Associated abnormalities may include abnormal ears, shortened philtrum, and hypertelorism. Serum immunoglobulin concentrations are frequently normal, but antibody responses, particularly of IgG and IgA isotypes, are usually impaired. Lymphocyte counts may be near normal, but virtually all the lymphocytes are B cells. Carefully performed autopsies have often revealed a tiny, histologically normal thymus, usually in an ectopic location. With time, a few patients developed functional T cells. Several patients with Di George's syndrome transplanted with fetal thymus have developed immunocompetent T cells of host origin. However, it is difficult to be certain whether long-term improvement is the result of a small thymus gland in an ectopic location or due to grafted thymus epithelium.

Children lacking the congenital anomalies associated with Di George's syndrome may present with severe impairment of cell-mediated immunity. Some have normal or even increased immunoglobulin levels, while others have selective deficiencies of one or more immunoglobulin classes. Specific antibody responses are usually impaired even in patients with normal concentrations of immunoglobulins. This ill-defined entity has been called the *Nezelof's syndrome*.

Inherited deficiency of the enzyme purine nucleoside phosphorylase (PNP) is associated with an often severe and selective deficiency of T-lymphocyte function. This enzyme functions in the same purine salvage pathway as ADA; toxic effects of its deficiency may be related to intracellular accumulation of deoxyguanosine triphosphate (GTP).

A few patients with isolated T-cell deficiency have been treated with fetal thymus grafts or thymic humoral factors. Some have shown improvement in numbers of circulating T cells, in vitro reactivity to mitogens, and clinical condition, while others have had no change in status.

ATAXIA-TELANGIECTASIA This is an autosomal recessive genetic disorder characterized by cerebellar ataxia, oculocutaneous telangiectasia, and immunodeficiency. Onset of truncal ataxia usually occurs in infancy and is progressive. Immunodeficiency is clinically manifest by recurrent and chronic sinopulmonary infection leading to bronchiectasis. However, not all patients have immunodeficiency. The two most frequent causes of death are chronic pulmonary disease and malignancy. Lymphomas are most common, although carcinomas have also occurred.

The immunologic abnormalities seem to be related to maldevelopment of the thymus. If found at all, the thymus in autopsied patients has been markedly hypoplastic and similar in appearance to an embryonic thymus. Patients' lymphocytes frequently respond poorly to T-cell mitogens in vitro. Cutaneous anergy and delayed rejection of skin grafts are common. Although the number and class distribution of B lymphocytes are usually normal, most patients are deficient in serum IgE and IgA, and a smaller number have reduced serum levels of IgG, particularly of the IgG2, IgG4 subclasses. IgM and IgD are usually normal.

There is circumstantial evidence that ataxia-telangiectasia may involve a generalized defect in cellular differentiation related to the defects in DNA repair mechanisms which have been identified in these patients. Cultured cells from these patients are highly susceptible to radiation-induced chromosomal damage. Defective DNA repair mechanisms may account for the high incidence of malignancies in these patients. Ovarian agenesis also occurs frequently. Persistence of very high serum levels of oncofetal proteins, including alphafetoprotein and carcinoembryonic antigen, may be of diagnostic value.

Only symptomatic treatment is available. Unless a severe IgG deficiency is present, therapy with gamma globulin is not indicated. Unusual sensitivity to x-irradiation should be kept in mind in planning therapy for patients who develop cancer.

Immunoglobulin deficiency syndromes X-LINKED AGAMMAGLOBULINEMIA This syndrome was long thought to represent a central failure of development of all elements of the B-cell lineage. Recent evidence has modified this concept. Affected males have very few immunoglobulin-bearing B lymphocytes in their circulation and lack primary and secondary lymphoid follicles. However, pre-B cells are found in normal frequency in their bone marrow. This developmental block contrasts with earlier and later arrests in B-cell differentiation characterizing other immunodeficiencies (see below and Fig. 256-1). Patients usually have a substantial number of small mononuclear cells bearing receptors for aggregated immunoglobulin and C3. Although resembling B lymphocytes, these cells have been shown to have markers characteristic of the monocyte line and to lack the B-lymphocyte specific surface antigen(s) and receptors for Epstein-Barr virus. A few patients with well-documented X-linked agammaglobulinemia have had a normal number of B lymphocytes, suggesting that there may be two distinct forms of this disease.

Agammaglobulinemia is a misnomer, as most patients with this and other forms of severe panhypogammaglobulinemia synthesize some immunoglobulins. Within the same family some affected males have had substantial levels of IgM, IgG, and IgA, while others have been nearly agammaglobulinemic. All these patients were markedly deficient in circulating B lymphocytes. This observation suggests that the few B lymphocytes which are generated are fully capable of differentiating to plasma cells and secreting immunoglobulins. A form of arthritis with some of the features of rheumatoid disease occurs in some of these patients and may remit following treatment with gamma globulin. Mycoplasma organisms are sometimes the cause of arthritis in hypogammaglobulinemic patients. Chronic encephalitis, of proven or presumed viral etiology, appears to be an increasingly frequent terminal complication. Some of these patients have also had an associated dermatomyositis.

TRANSIENT HYPOGAMMAGLOBULINEMIA OF INFANCY This is a reversible syndrome in which normal physiologic hypogammaglobulinemia of infancy is unusually prolonged and severe. IgG levels of normal-term infants commonly drop to levels of 300 to 400 mg/dL between 3 and 6 months of age as maternally derived IgG is catabolized; levels subsequently rise reflecting the infants' increased synthetic capacity. In transient hypogammaglobulinemia, the rate of synthesis of IgM, IgG, and IgA remains low for long periods. Reduced numbers of $T4^+$ helper T cells have recently been reported in infants with this condition.

ISOLATED DEFICIENCY OF IgA This is by far the most commonly encountered immunodeficiency, occurring with a frequency of approximately 1 in 600 individuals of European origin. With rare exceptions, IgA1 and IgA2 subclasses are deficient in both serum and mucous secretions. Many adults with isolated IgA deficiency do not seem to have unusual problems with infection. Nevertheless, this condition is not benign. A substantial proportion of IgA-deficient individuals develop precipitating antibodies to IgA. These patients may have severe anaphylactic reactions when transfused with normal blood from a blood bank.

As a group, individuals with IgA deficiency have an increased number of respiratory infections of varying severity, and a few have had severe pulmonary disease such as bronchiectasis. Chronic diarrheal disease also occurs. The incidence of asthma and other atopic diseases among IgA-deficient patients is high, and, conversely, the incidence of IgA deficiency among atopic children has been found to be 20 to 40 times that in the normal population. In one study it was found that combined deficiency of IgE and IgA (or IgE deficiency alone) did not predispose to recurrent respiratory infections, while IgA-deficient patients with normal or elevated IgE had recurrent sinopulmonary disease. Selective reductions in the IgG2 and IgG4 subclasses have also been associated with increased infections in IgA-deficient individuals. IgA deficiency is also significantly associated with autoimmune diseases such as rheumatoid arthritis and systemic lupus erythematosus.

IgA deficiency may be familial, but no single pattern of inheritance has been encountered consistently. It has occurred in association with congenital intrauterine infections, such as toxoplasmosis, rubella, and cytomegalovirus infection. Several patients with abnormalities of chromosome 18 have had isolated IgA deficiency. Most commonly, the syndrome appears as a sporadic defect. It may be transient or acquired late in life.

The pathogenesis of IgA deficiency, whether genetic or caused by environmental insult, involves a block in terminal differentiation of B lymphocytes. Virtually all patients have detectable IgA-bearing B lymphocytes, although their numbers may be reduced. In normal children and adults, B lymphocytes bearing IgA have only that immunoglobulin class on their surface, while in IgA-deficient patients and normal neonates, IgA-bearing lymphocytes also bear surface IgM. This immature phenotype is associated in most patients with failure of their cultured lymphocytes to secrete IgA when stimulated by pokeweed mitogen. Selective T-cell suppression of IgA responses has been described in some patients, and a variety of other, usually mild, defects of T-cell function in others. While there is as yet no generally accepted pathogenic mechanism, suspicion remains high that many of these patients have a primary defect in regulatory T-cell function.

Treatment of IgA deficiency is symptomatic. IgA cannot be effectively replaced by exogenous gamma globulin or plasma, and use of either would increase the risk of development of antibodies to IgA. IgA-deficient patients in need of transfusion should be screened for the presence of antibodies to IgA, and ideally should be given blood only from IgA-deficient donors. All patients known to be IgA-deficient should be warned of the risk of severe transfusion reactions which may occur following infusion of only a few milliliters of blood.

X-LINKED IMMUNODEFICIENCY WITH INCREASED LEVELS OF IgM This is a specific syndrome only because of its inheritance pattern. IgG levels are usually very low, and IgA low or undetectable, while IgD levels may be high. The clinical patterns of infection are similar to those occurring with other hypogammaglobulinemic states. The number and distribution of B lymphocytes bearing IgM, IgG, and IgA have been normal, suggesting that this type of immunodeficiency may also involve a block in terminal differentiation of B lymphocytes. Neutropenia often occurs in affected males and can increase their vulnerability to infections.

ISOLATED DEFICIENCY OF IgM This syndrome has been reported rarely in this country but was detected frequently in a British population. Approximately 20 percent of these patients were asymptomatic while 60 percent had severe recurrent infections, often with bacteremia. Pneumococcal pneumonia and meningitis have often been noted in IgM-deficient patients. Other associated conditions included gastrointestinal disease, atopy, splenomegaly, and development of malignancy. The condition was frequently familial, and was four times more common in males than females. The number of circulating B lymphocytes has varied from very low to normal.

COMMON VARIED IMMUNODEFICIENCY This represents a heterogeneous group of syndromes which may be congenital or acquired, sporadic or familial, and which occur in both males and females. These patients have in common the clinical manifestations of antibody deficiency associated with panhypogammaglobulinemia, with deficiency of IgG and IgA, or rarely, with selective IgG deficiency.

A small subpopulation of these patients have reduced numbers of circulating B lymphocytes, suggesting a central failure of development of this cell line. The remainder have normal numbers of B lymphocytes, although these may have an immature phenotype. In the few patients studied, B lymphocytes capable of binding specific antigens were present, and these increased in frequency following immunization. Consistent with the evidence that B lymphocytes in these patients are able to recognize antigens and proliferate but fail to differentiate to plasma cells is the fairly common finding of lymphoid hyperplasia, including splenomegaly and nodular lymphoid hyperplasia of the gut.

In agammaglobulinemic patients having B lymphocytes, the pathogenesis of immune deficiency must involve the failure of these cells to differentiate to plasma cells. By use of assays capable of measuring B-lymphocyte differentiation to plasma cells in vitro, four major types of defect have been tentatively identified. First, and most common, is an intrinsic abnormality of B lymphocytes. B lymphocytes from these patients can be activated via their immunoglobulin receptors to express functional receptors for T cell–derived growth factors, but they fail to differentiate into immunoglobulin-secreting plasma cells even when provided with differentiation factors from normal T cells. Second, there is evidence that in some patients the T cells, or their products, may actively suppress terminal differentiation of autologous or normal B lymphocytes. The increase in suppressor activity could be either a primary or secondary abnormality; the latter could explain the increase in T-cell suppressor activity in patients with abnormal B lymphocytes and others in whom B lymphocytes are congenitally absent. Third, quantitative deficiency of helper T-cell function has been observed in some patients, usually also in association with defective B-cell function. This functional defect may or may not be associated with reduced numbers of $T4^+$ cells. Finally, in rare instances, plasma cells may produce abnormal immunoglobulins which are degraded in the cytoplasm.

Patients with common varied immunodeficiency may present with signs and symptoms highly suggestive of lymphoid malignancy, including fever, weight loss, splenomegaly, generalized lymphadenopathy, and lymphocytosis. Routine histologic examination of lymphoid tissues usually reveals germinal center hyperplasia which may be difficult to distinguish from nodular lymphoma (see Chap. 294). Demonstration of a normal distribution of immunoglobulin isotypes and light chain classes on circulating and tissue B lymphocytes can serve to distinguish these patients from those having a monoclonal B-cell malignancy with secondary hypogammaglobulinemia. Treatment of several patients with gamma globulin has resulted in relief of symptoms and reversal of lymphoid hyperplasia.

IMMUNODEFICIENCY WITH THYMOMA Recognition of the association of hypogammaglobulinemia with spindle cell thymoma provided one of the early clues as to the role of the thymus in immunobiology. Although T-cell numbers and cell-mediated immunity are frequently intact, several abnormalities have been identified. Patients' lymphoid cells suppress differentiation of normal B lymphocytes in the pokeweed mitogen assay and may also suppress development of erythroid precursors. The suppressor activity is mediated by the subset of lymphocytes bearing receptors for IgG, which are found in increased numbers. It is presently uncertain as to whether the suppressor cells are T cells or NK cells. These patients are very deficient in circulating B lymphocytes, frequently have eosinopenia, and may develop erythroid aplasia. Failure to produce B lymphocytes has been traced to the stem-cell level, since pre-B cells could not be found in their bone marrow. The relationship between the thymoma, T-cell, or NK dysfunction, and apparent abnormalities of hematopoietic stem cells remains conjectural.

WISKOTT-ALDRICH SYNDROME This is an X-linked genetic disease characterized by eczema, thrombocytopenia, and repeated infections. Affected boys often present with bleeding in infancy. Most do not survive childhood, dying of complications of bleeding, infection, or lymphoreticular malignancy. The immunologic defects in this disease are well characterized but poorly understood. Serum concentrations of IgM are usually decreased, while IgA and IgG are normal and IgE is frequently increased. However, synthetic rates for all three classes may be elevated, indicating a significant element of hypercatabolism. The number and class distribution of B lymphocytes usually have been normal. Functionally, these boys are consistently unable to make antibodies to polysaccharide antigens normally; responses to protein antigens are often not impaired. While most patients acquire a diminished number of T cells, serial appraisal of affected males suggests that the T-cell defects are secondary. They frequently become anergic, and their T cells do not respond normally to challenge with ubiquitous antigens. The nature of the primary defect is still unknown.

Transplantation of histocompatible bone marrow from a sibling donor has corrected both hematologic and immunologic abnormalities in several patients. In patients lacking a suitable donor, splenectomy may improve platelet counts and reduce the risk of serious hemorrhage. Because of the increased risk of pneumococcal bacteremia, splenectomized patients should probably receive prophylactic penicillin.

Miscellaneous immunodeficiency syndromes Infection with *Candida albicans* is the almost universal accompaniment of severe deficiencies in cell-mediated immunity. The syndrome of *chronic mucocutaneous candidiasis* is different because superficial candidiasis is usually the only major manifestation of immunodeficiency. These patients rarely develop systemic infection with *Candida* or other fungal agents and are not unusually susceptible to virus or bacterial disease. The syndrome is often congenital and may be associated with single or multiple endocrinopathies as well as iron deficiency. Treatment of associated conditions may lead to improvement or even cure of *Candida* infection.

No uniformity of immunologic defects has been identified in these patients, although defects of antibody formation have been detected occasionally. Humoral immunity, including ability to make specific anti-*Candida* antibodies, is usually normal. Many patients are anergic, some to a variety of antigens and some only to *Candida;* anergy in some patients has been related to inability of their lymphocytes to produce migration inhibition factor.

Results of treatment with antifungal agents, such as amphotericin B, have been variable but generally not encouraging. In some patients, intensive treatment with amphotericin B coupled with surgical removal of infected nails has led to sustained improvement. Ketoconazole, an oral antifungal agent, is reported to be quite effective.

IMMUNODEFICIENCY ASSOCIATED WITH SERUM LYMPHOCYTOTOXINS This syndrome has been reported in a few patients with recurrent bacterial and fungal infections. Most have had fluctuating lymphopenia. Both cellular immunity and specific antibody responses were impaired, although immunoglobulin levels were usually normal. Antibodies specific for B-cell antigens have also been reported as a cause of selective elimination of B cells and resultant hypogammaglobulinemia.

IMBALANCES OF IgG SUBCLASSES Some patients with repeated infections and only moderately decreased serum IgG levels may have a selective deficiency of one or more of the four IgG subclasses. A few such patients appeared to benefit from administration of gamma globulin; others do well without antibody replacement therapy. K *light chain deficiency* has also been reported in association with recurrent infections, and doubtless many more subtle gaps in antibody diversity, which may be clinically significant, will be elucidated.

X-LINKED LYMPHOPROLIFERATIVE SYNDROME This is an X-linked recessive disease in which there appears to be a selective impairment in immune elimination of Epstein-Barr virus (EBV). Infectious mononucleosis in affected males may have a fulminant and fatal outcome, may be associated with development of B-cell malignancies, or may result in acquired hypogammaglobulinemia, aplastic anemia, or agranulocytosis. Antibodies to EBV have been detected in some patients but are often absent in the face of infection. Generation of cytotoxic T cells appears to be the primary mechanism of control of EBV infection in normal persons, and natural killer cells may also play a role in eliminating EBV-infected B cells. While a reduction of natural-killer-cell activity has been noted, the nature of the defect which prevents a normal response to EBV in patients with the X-linked lymphoproliferative syndrome has not been defined.

Metabolic abnormalities associated with immunodeficiency The relation of deficiencies of the purine salvage enzymes, adenosine deaminase and purine nucleoside phosphorylase, to immunodeficiency was discussed earlier. Other inherited metabolic defects should be briefly mentioned because of their potential importance in understanding the molecular basis of immunologic function. Inherited *deficiency of transcobalamin II,* the serum carrier molecule responsible for transport of vitamin B_{12} to tissues, was associated with failure of immunoglobulin production as well as megaloblastic anemia, leukopenia, thrombocytopenia, and severe malabsorption. All abnormalities were reversed by administration of pharmacologic doses of vitamin B_{12}. The syndrome of *acrodermatitis enteropathica* includes severe desquamating skin lesions, intractable diarrhea, bizarre neurologic symptoms, variable combined immunodeficiency, and an often fatal outcome. This disease is apparently caused by an inborn error of metabolism resulting in malabsorption of dietary zinc, and can be effectively treated by parenteral or large oral doses of zinc. Similar disease manifestations have occurred in mice and cattle with different inherited defects leading to zinc malabsorption. Zinc deficiency might in part account for the immunodeficiency which accompanies severe malnutrition.

TREATMENT OF IMMUNODEFICIENCIES Treatment of immunodeficiency diseases involving severe abnormalities of T-cell function, with or without hypogammaglobulinemia, is currently limited in effectiveness and extremely complicated. Experimental approaches, including transplantation of bone marrow, fetal liver, and thymus, were mentioned in preceding sections. Also under investigation is the use of thymic hormones and of pharmacologic agents which may correct defects in lymphoid function caused by inherited metabolic disorders. The increasing availability of purified gamma interferon, T-cell growth factors, and other biologically active mediators promises to be important in the therapy of certain immunologic disorders. Genetic engineering also holds promise for future therapy of certain genetic defects of the immune system.

Replacement therapy with human gamma globulin should be used in patients who have recurrent bacterial infections and are deficient in IgG. Maintenance of serum IgG levels between 100 and 300 mg/dL is sufficient to prevent most overwhelming infections, although chronic sinusitis, otitis media, and bronchitis often persist. These serum levels usually can be achieved by intramuscular injection of IgG, 100 mg/kg, at monthly intervals, following a loading dose of twice this amount given over a period of several days. Forty milliliters of 16% gamma globulin, given in two or more sites at one time, is about the maximum tolerable in adults. Immunoglobulin preparations suitable for intravenous administration are now available, and provide a needed alternative mode of antibody replacement therapy. The primary advantage of intravenous gamma globulin is that higher amounts of antibodies can be given with less discomfort. In patients with mild to moderate IgG deficiency (300 to 400 mg/dL), the decision to treat must be based on clinical symptoms and on failure to respond to antigenic challenge, because injection of gamma globulin at the recommended doses will not significantly elevate serum IgG levels. Gamma globulin treatment is of no value in patients with deficiencies of immunoglobulins other than IgG. This form of treatment is not benign. Some patients may develop symptoms of diaphoresis, tachycardia, and hypotension immediately following injections. This reaction is thought to be mediated by aggregates of IgG in the gamma globulin preparation, but why it develops after years of treatment in some patients, and never in others has not been adequately explained. Most patients intolerant of intramuscular gamma globulin injections can be treated successfully with intravenous preparations of gamma globulin or plasma.

Infusion of fresh plasma, 10 to 20 mL/kg at intervals of 3 to 4 weeks, has the advantages of being less painful and of replacing IgM and IgA as well as IgG; however, both IgM and IgA have a half-life of only a few days. The major disadvantage of plasma is the risk of transmitting hepatitis, which is particularly devastating in immunodeficient patients. This risk can be minimized by use of selected donors, usually family members, carefully screened for the absence of HTLV and hepatitis virus infections.

Use of plasma or gamma globulin selected on the basis of a high titer of antibodies to a particular agent may be indicated in certain situations. For example, antibodies to the causative echovirus may dramatically improve encephalitis in immunodeficient patients.

Therapy with exogenous IgG usually does not prevent chronic sinopulmonary infection and its all too frequent progression to pulmonary fibrosis and bronchiectasis. Therefore, maintenance of good pulmonary toilet with regular postural drainage is an especially important part of patient management. The principles of antibiotic therapy are not different in these than other patients, except that the index of suspicion of bacterial infection should remain very high.

REFERENCES

CHANDRA RK et al: Immunodeficiency: Report of a WHO scientific group. WHO Tech Rep 630, 1978

MEISCHER PA, MÜLLER-EBERHARD HJ (eds): *Seminars in Immunopathology,* vol 1: *Immunodeficiency Diseases.* Berlin, Springer-Verlag, 1978

MÖLLER G (ed): T-cell receptors and genes. Immunol Rev 81:1, 1984

REINHERZ EL et al: Abnormalities of T cell maturation and regulation in human beings with immunodeficiency disorders. J Clin Invest 68:699, 1981

ROSEN FS et al: The primary immunodeficiencies. N Engl J Med 311:235, 300, 1984

STIEHM ER, FULGINITI VA (eds): *Immunologic Disorders in Infants and Children,* 2d ed. Philadelphia, Saunders, 1979

STITES DP et al: *Basic and Clinical Immunology,* 5th ed. Los Gatos, Calif, Lange, 1984

WEDGWOOD RJ et al (eds): *Primary Immunodeficiency Diseases, Birth Defects,* Original Article Series, vol XIX. Sunderland, Mass, The National Foundation–March of Dimes, Sinauer Associations, 1983

257 THE ACQUIRED IMMUNODEFICIENCY SYNDROME (AIDS)

ANTHONY S. FAUCI / H. CLIFFORD LANE

DEFINITION The acquired immunodeficiency syndrome (AIDS) was originally defined empirically by the Centers for Disease Control (CDC) as the presence of a reliably diagnosed disease that is at least moderately indicative of an underlying defect in cell-mediated immunity. Typical examples of such diseases are Kaposi's sarcoma in an individual less than 60 years old or a life-threatening opportunistic infection such as *Pneumocystis carinii* pneumonia. These disorders must occur in the absence of known causes of underlying immune defects, such as iatrogenic immunosuppression or malignant neoplasms. This surveillance definition was used for national reporting and was formulated prior to the recognition of human T lymphotropic virus type III (HTLV III) or lymphadenopathy-associated virus (LAV) as the etiologic agent of the disease. Since tests for HTLV III/LAV antibody and virus are now available, the CDC has refined the case definition. The diagnosis is now excluded if tests for serum antibody to HTLV III/LAV are negative, all other types of HTLV III/LAV tests are negative, and the number of thymus-derived (T) helper lymphocytes is normal. Furthermore, in the absence of a classic opportunistic disease required by the original case definition, in the presence of a positive serologic or virologic test for HTLV III/LAV, any of the following diseases are considered indicative of AIDS: disseminated histoplasmosis; isosporosis causing chronic diarrhea; bronchial or pulmonary candidiasis; non-Hodgkin's (lymphocytic) lymphoma of high-grade pathologic type and of B-cell or unknown immunologic phenotype; and Kaposi's sarcoma diagnosed by biopsy in patients who are 60 years old or older when diagnosed. In addition, in the absence of opportunistic diseases required by the original case definition, a histologically confirmed diagnosis of chronic lymphoid interstitial pneumonitis in a child under 13 years of age is considered indicative of AIDS unless tests for HTLV III/LAV are negative. Finally, patients who have a lymphoreticular malignancy diagnosed more than 3 months after the diagnosis of an opportunistic disease used as a marker for AIDS were previously excluded as AIDS cases based on the presumption that the malignancy could have accounted for the immunosuppression which led to the opportunistic disease. Such patients are now included as having AIDS if they are seropositive for HTLV III/LAV.

ETIOLOGY AIDS is caused by the human retrovirus HTLV III/LAV (see Chap. 293). This is truly a novel virus which has never before been identified. The virus is a human retrovirus which is lymphocytotropic and selectively infects human T lymphocytes of the helper/inducer subset which is designated by the T4 or Leu 3 phenotypic markers. This tropism is similar to that of HTLV I, which is the cause of adult T-cell leukemia/lymphoma (see Chaps. 293 and 294). However, HTLV I causes malignant proliferation of the T4 subset of lymphocytes, while HTLV III causes a cytopathic effect on these cells. The nucleotide sequence of HTLV III differs from that of HTLV I or HTLV II, which has been implicated in hairy-cell leukemia (see Chap. 292). It is, however, quite similar to the lentivirus group of retroviruses, particularly the visna virus which causes a demyelinating disease in sheep.

INCIDENCE AND PREVALENCE AIDS did not exist in the United States until the late 1970s. In the summer of 1981 the CDC announced the unexplained occurrence of *Pneumocystis carinii* pneumonia in previously healthy male homosexuals in Los Angeles and Kaposi's sarcoma in 26 previously healthy male homosexuals in New York and Los Angeles. Since that time, the number of cases has increased geometrically. By mid-1986, approximately 22,000 cases had been reported in the United States. The incidence of the disease has doubled approximately every 12 months. By 1990 over 100,000 cases are anticipated in the United States. The disease will almost certainly evolve into a global epidemic. It is occurring with an increased frequency in several countries in Europe as well as in other continents, particularly Africa, where at least several thousand cases have occurred in central Africa.

Sexual contact is the major mode of transmission of the AIDS retrovirus. Transmission can also occur via blood or blood products as in individuals who share contaminated needles for intravenous drug abuse or individuals who receive blood transfusions or blood products for replacement therapy. Mothers may transmit the virus perinatally to their infants.

Among the adult cases reported in the United States, 73 percent have occurred among homosexual or bisexual men. The highest numbers of cases have been reported from New York City, San Francisco, and Los Angeles, which reflects the high concentration of male homosexuals in these cities. However, the number of cases in other areas of the United States is increasing, and the disease is seen in virtually every state. The next largest number of cases in the United States is found among intravenous drug abusers, who constitute approximately 17 percent of the total cases. Approximately 1 percent of cases occur in hemophiliacs with no history of other risk factors. These individuals are exposed to the AIDS retrovirus by virtue of the large amounts of factor VIII concentrates which they receive intravenously as replacement for deficient clotting factors. An additional 2 percent of cases occur among nonhemophiliacs who have received blood or blood products usually associated with surgery. Approximately 1 percent of cases have occurred in the heterosexual partners of individuals with AIDS or at risk for AIDS. Approximately 7 percent of adult patients fall into none of the above risk categories. For a significant proportion of these patients, there was not sufficient information to allow classification, usually because the patients died before they could be interviewed. Also included among these 7 percent of patients are Haitian immigrants to the United States who have no history of homosexuality or intravenous drug abuse. It is very likely that the disease has been transmitted among these individuals by heterosexual contact, similar to the situation in Zaire, where the male-to-female ratio for AIDS is approximately equal. In this regard, there are cases reported in the United States among men who have no apparent risk factor except heterosexual promiscuity, usually involving contacts with prostitutes who may also be intravenous drug abusers and hence be at risk for exposure to the AIDS retrovirus. This observation coupled with the reported infection of their sexual partners by male intravenous drug abusers and hemophiliacs raises the possibility of further heterosexual spread of AIDS in the United States among individuals not in the established risk groups. However, while the number of cases of AIDS apparently transmitted by heterosexual contact has increased over the years since AIDS was recognized, the relative proportion of these cases compared to the total number of cases has remained constant. It is possible that cofactors which contribute to the establishment of infection and/or disease in the risk groups are not usually present in the general population in the United States, and for this reason, an increase in the proportion of cases among heterosexuals has not occurred in the United States as in Zaire. There is no indication that the virus can be spread by insects, such as the bite of a mosquito.

There are at least 200 cases of pediatric AIDS (children less than 13 years old) reported in the United States and probably hundreds more who have been infected with the AIDS retrovirus but have not developed the full-blown disease. The vast majority of these children were born of parents with AIDS or at increased risk for AIDS. It is highly likely that these children were infected with the AIDS retrovirus in utero or perinatally. Most of the remainder were hemophiliacs or transfusion recipients.

All epidemiologic data strongly indicate that the AIDS retrovirus is not spread via casual contact. Large seroepidemiologic studies in the United States have shown that thousands of health care workers who are in close daily contact with AIDS patients have not developed AIDS or immunologic abnormalities, or seroconverted to anti-HTLV III antibody positivity. However, a few of the hundreds of health care workers who have been exposed to the virus by penetrating injuries and who are not in an established risk group have been found to have antibodies to HTLV III/LAV. Except for sexual transmission, there is no evidence that the virus is spread among family members living in the same household with AIDS patients. In contrast, the prevalence of infection with the AIDS retrovirus in the established risk groups is extraordinarily high. At least 65 percent of male homosexuals attending a clinic in San Francisco for sexually transmitted diseases were antibody-positive; 87 percent of intravenous drug abusers in New York City and 72 percent of asymptomatic persons with hemophilia A were antibody-positive. In contrast, less than 0.1 percent of the general blood donor pool has been confirmed as antibody-positive. It is estimated that at least 10 percent of asymptomatic individuals and up to 25 percent of symptomatic individuals (see definition of AIDS-related complex below) who are antibody-positive will develop full-blown AIDS within 3 years.

PATHOPHYSIOLOGY AND IMMUNOPATHOGENESIS The hallmark of AIDS is a profound defect in cell-mediated immunity which leads to severe opportunistic infections and Kaposi's sarcoma as well as certain lymphoid malignancies. The underlying cause of the immune defect is quite specific. HTLV III/LAV selectively infects the helper/inducer (T4 or Leu 3) subset of T lymphocytes resulting in a cytopathic effect; lymphopenia ensues, predominantly at the expense of the T4 cell. The suppressor/cytotoxic T lymphocyte defined by the T8 or Leu 2 phenotypic marker is either normal in number or slightly increased or decreased, generally resulting in a marked decrease in the T4/T8 ratio within the peripheral blood T-cell compartment. In addition to the quantitative deficiency in the T4 subset, there is also a qualitative or functional defect in this subset. This is particularly evident in the subset of T4 cells which are responsible for antigen recognition and responsiveness; this particular T4 subset is selectively defective early in the course of the disease.

Since the T4 subset of lymphocytes is responsible for the induction or orchestration of virtually the entire immune response, the selective defect in this subset results in global defects in a number of components of immunity which depend at least in part on inductive signals from the T4 cell. These include defects in natural killer cells, virus-specific cytotoxic T cells, B cells, and monocytes. In addition to defects in chemotaxis, secretion of interleukin 1 (IL-1), and certain cytotoxic functions, monocytes also show a defect in ability to present antigen to T cells. The mechanisms of these defects are unclear at present; however, they may relate to the fact that under certain circumstances both B cells and monocytes may be susceptible to infection with HTLV III/LAV in vitro. It has also been demonstrated that HTLV III/LAV can directly activate B cells without infecting them. This may explain in part the observation that B cells from patients with AIDS are polyclonally activated in vivo. There is a gradation of degree of immunologic dysfunction among the various subsets of AIDS patients. Those patients with Kaposi's sarcoma alone tend to have more competent immune systems compared to those who present with opportunistic infections.

It is unclear what mechanisms are responsible for the development of Kaposi's sarcoma in certain patients with AIDS. Kaposi's sarcoma occurs with a much greater frequency in homosexuals with AIDS than in AIDS patients in the other risk groups. In addition, certain opportunistic infections such as *Pneumocystis carinii* pneumonia and *Mycobacterium avium-intracellulare* occur with a much greater frequency in AIDS patients than in individuals who are immunosuppressed for other reasons. On the other hand, certain infections such as nocardiosis and listeriosis are very rare in AIDS patients despite their relatively frequent occurrence in other immunosuppressed patients. The reasons for these discrepancies are unclear, but likely reflect the selectivity and specificity of the immune defect in AIDS.

HTLV III/LAV has been demonstrated in the brain, which might explain the neuropsychiatric abnormalities which have been noted in many infected patients (see below). Virus has also been isolated from semen, saliva, plasma, tears, and cerebrospinal fluid.

CLINICAL MANIFESTATIONS Infection with HTLV III/LAV results in a spectrum of clinical illnesses. On the one hand, patients may have one or more of the secondary complications of the immune defect thereby fulfilling the criteria for the surveillance definition of AIDS as indicated above. On the other hand, there are a larger number of individuals who have been infected with HTLV III/LAV who are symptomatic, but who do not fulfill the empiric criteria for the full-blown disease. These patients may have fever, weight loss, diarrhea, fatigue, night sweats, lymphadenopathy, and immunologic abnormalities. This constellation of signs and symptoms in the context of HTLV III/LAV infection has been termed the *AIDS-related complex (ARC)*. It is estimated that approximately 25 percent of patients with ARC will develop full-blown disease within 3 years. Nonetheless ARC itself may be a very serious disease. A substantial number of patients have died from the wasting syndrome of ARC without it ever evolving to full-blown AIDS according to the surveillance definition.

An acute illness occurring 3 to 6 weeks after primary infection with HTLV III/LAV infection has been documented in a few patients. It is characterized by fevers, rigors, arthralgias, myalgias, maculopapular rash, urticaria, abdominal cramps, and diarrhea. The symptoms lasted 2 to 3 weeks and resolved spontaneously. Seroversion occurred 8 to 12 weeks after presumed exposure.

Patients with the full-blown syndrome demonstrate one of a number of patterns of disease. Approximately 50 percent of patients develop *Pneumocystis carinii* pneumonia in the absence of Kaposi's sarcoma, and approximately 27 percent develop Kaposi's sarcoma without *Pneumocystis carinii* pneumonia. Less than 10 percent develop both *Pneumocystis carinii* pneumonia and Kaposi's sarcoma. Not infrequently, an individual patient will have more than one opportunistic infection simultaneously. An increasing number of patients are being recognized with lymphoid neoplasms, which are felt to be secondary to the underlying immune defect. The clinical manifestations in any given patient usually reflect closely the type and location of the opportunistic infection or the anatomic distribution of the neoplastic process.

Patients with *Pneumocystis carinii* pneumonia may present with typical findings of the disease such as fever, dyspnea, and hypoxia. However, in contrast to the more classic presentation of *Pneumocystis carinii* pneumonia in non-AIDS immunosuppressed patients in whom the onset is usually abrupt and explosive, patients with AIDS often have a more indolent presentation with symptoms gradually accelerating over weeks prior to establishment of the diagnosis. Because of the usual copiousness of microorganisms, the diagnosis can generally be made by bronchoscopy with histochemical staining of material from transbronchial biopsy or bronchial lavage. This is in contrast to *Pneumocystis carinii* pneumonia in non-AIDS patients in whom thoracotomy and lung biopsy are often required to establish the diagnosis.

Cytomegalovirus (CMV) infections are extremely common in AIDS patients and appear as fever and disseminated organ system involvement. Of particular note is CMV chorioretinitis, which results in serious visual impairment and may eventuate in complete blindness. CMV enteritis may result in intractable diarrhea. Herpes simplex virus may cause serious mucocutaneous disease in AIDS patients, with perianal involvement being typical. Candida albicans is an extremely common infection in AIDS patients and is usually manifest as oral thrush or esophagitis. *Mycobacterium avium-intracellulare* infections generally occur in AIDS patients as smoldering infections and rarely are primarily responsible for the death of the patient despite the fact that there is no effective treatment. *Mycobacterium tuberculosis* is a common opportunistic infection associated with AIDS in Haiti, in Haitians in the United States, and in Zaire, but is rarely seen in the general AIDS patient population in the United States. This discrepancy is likely due to the prevalence of this infection in these populations in general. *Cryptococcus neoformans* infection occurs as meningitis or as disseminated disease. *Toxoplasma gondii* infections may occur as chorioretinitis or more commonly as intracerebral mass lesions. Pediatric patients with AIDS have a much higher incidence of bacterial infections than do adults with the syndrome. In adults, common bacterial infections are not considered part of the spectrum of opportunistic infections.

Persistent diarrhea is extremely common in AIDS as well as in ARC. Diarrheal syndromes have been demonstrated to occur as a result of CMV enteritis, secondary to infection with the coccidial protozoon cryptosporidium (Chap. 161), secondary to Kaposi's sarcoma in the gastrointestinal tract, or secondary to other intestinal parasites. However, a substantial number of patients with AIDS develop intractable diarrhea and malabsorption for which no underlying cause can be identified.

Severe neuropsychiatric disease characterized by a wide range of neurologic findings, including acute or chronic meningitis and progressive dementia in the presence or absence of localizing signs, occurs in approximately one-third of patients with AIDS. In certain patients, this can be attributed to infections of the central nervous system with organisms such *Cryptococcus neoformans, Toxoplasma gondii,* or CMV. In others, neoplasms such as primary lymphoma of the brain or Kaposi's sarcoma have been identified. However, in many patients no underlying cause of the central nervous system syndrome can be ascertained, and on histopathologic examination, multifocal leukoencephalopathy may or may not be present. Since it has been shown that HTLV III/LAV can infect brain tissue and since

HTLV III nucleic acid has been identified in the brain tissue of AIDS patients, it is likely that neuropsychiatric syndromes directly related to HTLV III/LAV infection of the brain are occurring in at least a portion of AIDS patients. A small number of patients who are HTLV III/LAV antibody–positive have developed neuropsychiatric disease in the absence of other manifestations of full-blown AIDS, indicating that the virus can infect and cause disease in the brain early on prior to the development of other clinical manifestations of infection.

Many patients with AIDS develop a hypercatabolic wasting syndrome that does not appear to be related to the other manifestations of their disease such as opportunistic infections or Kaposi's sarcoma. In the majority of patients, no underlying cause of the syndrome is identified; however, in others the findings may be explained by unrecognized disseminated CMV or *Mycobacterium avium-intracellulare* infections.

Kaposi's sarcoma is a neoplasm manifested primarily by multiple vascular nodules in the skin and other organs. The disease is multifocal with a course ranging from indolent, with only skin manifestations, to fulminating, with extensive visceral involvement. The pattern of Kaposi's sarcoma in AIDS patients differs significantly from that of patients in nonepidemic groups such as elderly men in the United States and Europe and organ transplant recipients who are iatrogenically immunosuppressed. In the latter groups, the disease is generally indolent, and extracutaneous involvement occurs in only 10 percent of patients. In children and young adults with Kaposi's sarcoma in central Africa, there is a 20 percent incidence of extracutaneous spread of disease. In contrast, extracutaneous involvement of Kaposi's sarcoma is seen in over 70 percent of AIDS patients with this neoplasm. Although any organ system can be involved in the disseminated form of the disease, lymph nodes, gastrointestinal tract, and lungs are most commonly involved. Pulmonary involvement often leads to severe diffusing capacity abnormalities and may result in massive pulmonary hemorrhage. Patients with Kaposi's sarcoma of the oral mucous membranes may have extensive, but clinically undetectable, involvement of the remainder of the gastrointestinal tract.

In addition to AIDS, ARC, and neurologic abnormalities, there is increasing evidence that infection with HTLV III/LAV can be associated with a number of other disorders such as lymphomas, certain carcinomas, lymphoid interstitial pneumonitis, and immune-mediated thrombocytopenia (Chap. 293).

DIAGNOSIS The diagnosis of full-blown AIDS relies on the presence of the empirically defined secondary complications of the underlying immune defect as described above. A highly sensitive and readily available enzyme-linked immunosorbent assay (ELISA) exists for detection of antibodies against HTLV III/LAV. Western blot analysis, which establishes the specificity of the immunologic reaction between the antibodies and the viral encoded proteins, can be used to confirm the ELISA findings, when necessary. Presence of antibodies to the retrovirus does not indicate that an individual has AIDS or even will develop AIDS. It merely indicates that the individual has been exposed to and/or infected with the AIDS retrovirus. Infection can be documented further by isolation of the virus from peripheral blood lymphocytes or other body materials. Here again, isolation of the virus does not indicate that the patient has AIDS unless the other clinical criteria are present. Given the fact that the virus can be isolated from the lymphocytes of a high percentage of patients who are antibody-positive and who do not have AIDS, it must be presumed that such individuals are capable of transmitting the virus.

The common denominator of AIDS is the immunologic profile described above. The presence of lymphopenia with a selective deficiency of the T4 subset of lymphocytes further substantiates the diagnosis in an individual with the characteristic clinical features. However, immunologic abnormalities may be seen in certain individuals within the high-risk groups, particularly male homosexuals, and this does not mean that the person has AIDS or is even infected with HTLV III/LAV. For example, certain viral infections such as CMV and Epstein-Barr virus (EBV) cause reversal of the T4/T8 lymphocyte ratio. However, this is usually due to a relative increase in number of the T8 subset and not to a decrease in the T4 subset as is the case in AIDS.

TREATMENT AND PROGNOSIS Treatment of AIDS takes three forms: treatment of the secondary complications of the disease, i.e., the opportunistic infections and neoplasms; treatment of the HTLV III/LAV infection; and enhancement or reconstitution of the defective immune system.

Radiation therapy has been successful in the transient palliation of localized Kaposi's sarcoma. Extensive extremity or truncal disease and visceral disease have not shown substantial clinical responses to radiation. However, the use of alpha interferon or single-agent chemotherapy or combination chemotherapy has met with some success in the treatment of advanced disease and some clinical improvement has occurred. Nonetheless, it has not been demonstrated that successful treatment and remission of Kaposi's sarcoma significantly affects survival of patients with AIDS. A major difficulty with the use of chemotherapy is the resulting compounding of an already markedly immunosuppressed state and the increase in risk of opportunistic infections.

Several of the opportunistic infections in AIDS such as *Pneumocystis carinii* pneumonia (Chap. 158), toxoplasmosis (Chap. 157), candidiasis (Chap. 146), cryptococcosis (Chap. 146), herpes simplex (Chap. 136), and *Mycobacterium tuberculosis* (Chap. 119) can be treated with available antimicrobial agents; however, all have a high rate of recurrence. Of note is the fact that although *Pneumocystis carinii* pneumonia in AIDS generally responds to trimethoprim-sulfamethoxasole or pentamidine isethionate, therapy beyond the standard 2 weeks may often be required to eradicate the organisms. Because of the high rate of recurrence of disease, *Toxoplasma gondii* in AIDS patients may need to be treated for life with pyrimethamine-sulfadiazine. In addition, continuous treatment or prophylaxis for other infections may be required.

Substantial but transient success in the treatment of CMV disease in AIDS, particularly the retinitis, has been observed with the use of 9-(1,3-dihydroxy-2-propoxymethyl) guanine (DHPG) (Chap. 137). There is no effective treatment for *Mycobacterium avium-intracellulare* and EBV infections or for cryptosporidiosis.

A number of agents have been demonstrated to have activity in vitro against HTLV III/LAV, predominantly by inhibiting reverse transcriptase activity of the virus. One of these is suramin, which has been used successfully as an antiparasitic agent for the treatment of onchocerciasis and trypanosomiasis (Chaps. 156 and 163). HPA-23, ribavirin, and 3′-azido-3′-deoxythymidine are also agents with demonstrated anti-HTLV III/LAV activity. Phase I clinical trials have demonstrated that several of these agents also inhibit the AIDS retrovirus in vivo in that the virus cannot be isolated from the patient during and immediately after treatment with these agents. However, a clinical effect on the syndrome has not been demonstrated, perhaps because of persistence of undetected virus and/or the irreversibility of the immune defect, or inadequate duration of treatment.

A number of attempts at immune reconstitution have been undertaken. These have included bone marrow transplantation, especially between identical twins when one of the pair has AIDS; infusion of histocompatible lymphocytes; and the administration of soluble immune mediators such as IL-2 and the interferons. Although partial reconstitution of the immune response has been noted in some cases, it has been invariably temporary. Clearly, the virus must be suppressed if immune reconstitution is to be successful or else the reconstituted immune response will also succumb to the cytopathic effect of the causative retrovirus. The greatest hope for cure of the disease lies in the combination of antiretroviral therapy and immunologic reconstitution.

Since the causative virus has been isolated and cloned, vaccine development is being actively pursued.

There have been no reports of spontaneous reversal of the immune defect in AIDS. The typical clinical pattern is one of recurrent bouts of opportunistic infections with or without progressive Kaposi's sarcoma leading ultimately to the death of the patient. The overall mortality of AIDS is approximately 50 percent. However, the long-range mortality of patients with the full-blown disease is likely to approach 100 percent since there are few long-term (5-year) survivors of the disease.

REFERENCES

BARRÉ-SINOUSSI E et al: Isolation of a T-lymphotropic retrovirus from a patient at risk for acquired immune deficiency syndrome. Science 220:868, 1983

CURRAN JW et al: The epidemiology of AIDS: Current status and future prospects. Science 229:1352, 1985

FAUCI AS et al: Acquired immunodeficiency syndrome: Epidemiologic, clinical, immunologic, and therapeutic considerations. Ann Intern Med 100:92, 1984

——— et al: The acquired immunodeficiency syndrome: An update. Ann Intern Med 102:800, 1985

GALLIN JI, FAUCI AS (eds): *Advances in Host Defense Mechanisms*, Vol V: *Acquired Immunodeficiency Syndrome (AIDS)*. New York, Raven, 1985

GALLO RC et al: Frequent detection and isolation of cytopathic retrovirus (HTLV III) from patients with AIDS and at risk for AIDS. Science 224:500, 1984

GOTTLIEB MS et al: The acquired immunodeficiency syndrome. Ann Intern Med 99:208, 1983

HO DD et al: Primary human T-lymphotropic virus type III infection. Ann Intern Med 103:880, 1985

JAFFE HW et al: The acquired immunodeficiency syndrome in a cohort of homosexual men: A six year follow-up study. Ann Intern Med 103:210, 1985

LANE HC et al: Abnormalities of B-cell activation and immunoregulation in patients with the acquired immunodeficiency syndrome. N Engl J Med 309:453, 1983

——— et al: Qualitative analysis of immune function in patients with the acquired immunodeficiency syndrome. N Engl J Med 313:79, 1985

SELIK RM et al: Acquired immune deficiency syndrome (AIDS) trends in the United States, 1978–1982. Am J Med 76:493, 1984

258 PLASMA CELL DISORDERS

DAN L. LONGO / SAMUEL BRODER

GENERAL PRINCIPLES The plasma cell disorders are monoclonal neoplasms related to each other by virtue of their development from common progenitors in the B-lymphocyte lineage. Multiple myeloma, Waldenström's macroglobulinemia, primary amyloidosis, and the heavy chain diseases comprise this group and may be designated by a variety of synonyms such as monoclonal gammopathies, paraproteinemias, plasma cell dyscrasias, and dysproteinemias. A schema for the normal development of B lymphocytes is depicted in Fig. 258-1. Mature B lymphocytes bear surface immunoglobulin molecules of both M and G heavy chain isotypes with both isotypes having identical idiotypes (variable regions). Under normal circumstances, maturation to antibody-secreting plasma cells is stimulated by exposure to the antigen for which the surface immunoglobulin is specific; however, in the plasma cell disorders the control over this process is lost. The clinical manifestations of all the plasma cell disorders relate to the expansion of the neoplastic cells, to the secretion of cell products (immunoglobulin molecules or subunits, lymphokines), and to some extent to the host's response to the tumor.

There are three categories of structural variations among immunoglobulin molecules that form antigenic determinants, and these are used to classify immunoglobulins (Chap. 62). *Isotypes* are those determinants that distinguish among the main classes of antibodies of a given species and are the same in all normal individuals of that species. Therefore, isotypic determinants are by definition recognized by antibodies from a distinct species (heterologous serums) but not by antibodies from the same species (homologous serums). There are five chain isotypes (M, G, A, D, E) and two light chain isotypes (kappa, lambda). *Allotypes* are distinct determinants that reflect regular small differences between individuals of the same species in the amino acid sequences of otherwise similar immunoglobulins. These differences are determined by allelic genes, and by definition they are detected by antibodies made in the same species. *Idiotypes* are the third category of antigenic determinants. They are unique to the molecules produced by a given clone of antibody-producing cells. Idiotypes are formed by the unique structure of the antigen binding portion of the molecule.

Antibody molecules (see Fig. 258-2) are composed of two heavy (mol wt ~ 50,000) and two light (mol wt ~ 25,000) chains (Chap. 62). Each chain has a constant portion (limited amino acid sequence variability) and a variable region (extensive sequence variability). The light and heavy chains are linked by disulfide bonds and are aligned so their variable regions are adjacent to one another. This

FIGURE 258-1 *Schematic representation of the pathway of differentiation of normal B cells. CALLA, B1, B2, B4, Ia, PC-1, and sIg (surface immunoglobulin) are cell markers used to distinguish discrete stages of development. Terminal transferase (TdT) is a cellular enzyme. The stage of differentiation arrest for each lymphoproliferative disorder is shown. The following abbreviations are used: ALL, acute lymphoblastic leukemia; DWDL, diffuse well-differentiated lymphocytic lymphoma; CLL, chronic lymphocytic leukemia; NPDL, nodular poorly differentiated lymphocytic lymphoma; DPDL, diffuse poorly differentiated lymphocytic lymphoma; DHL, diffuse histiocytic or large-cell lymphoma.*

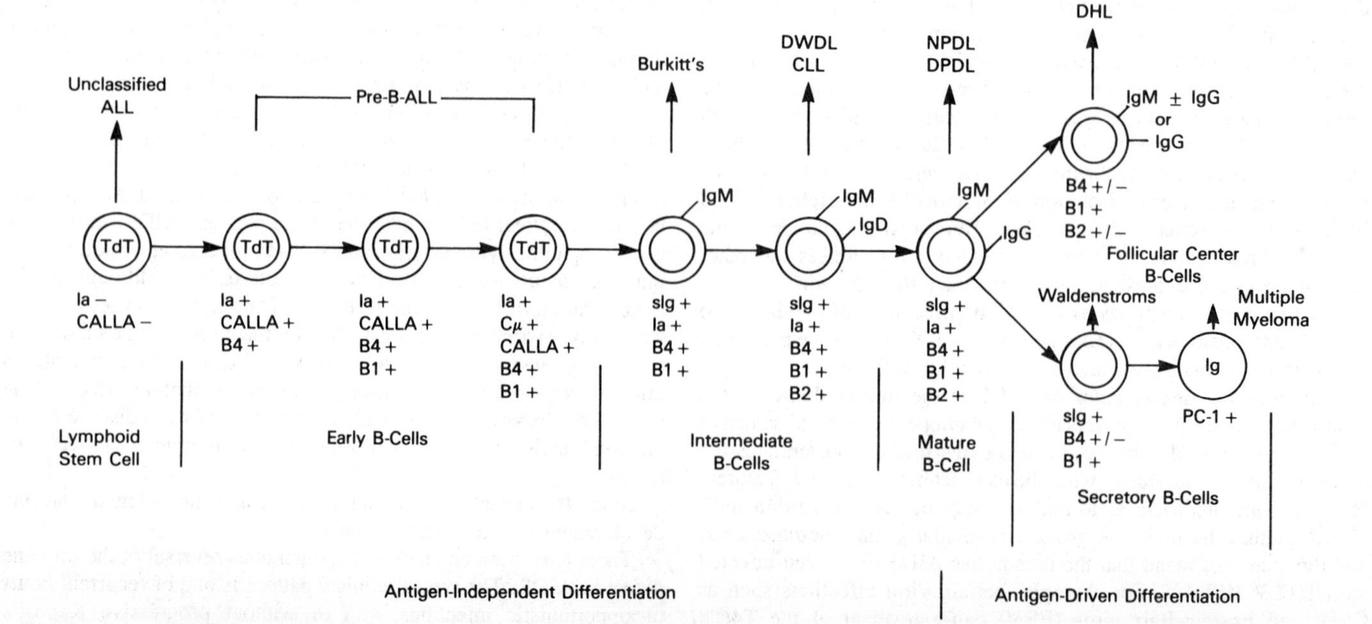

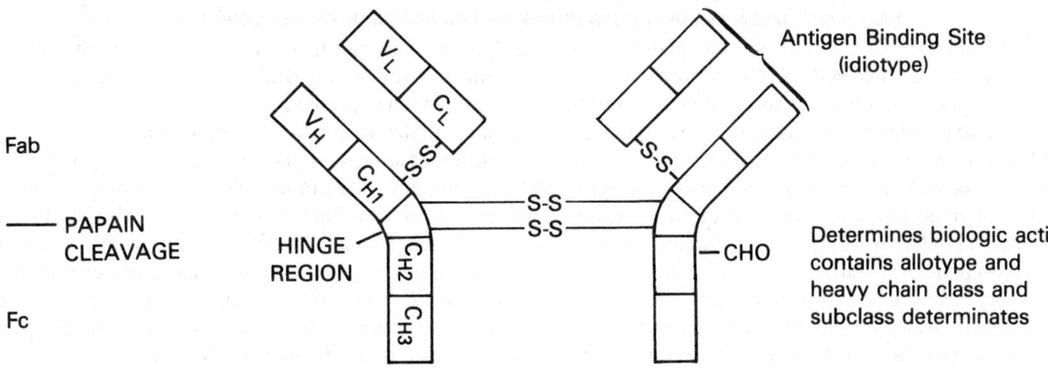

FIGURE 258-2 *Schematic depiction of an IgG molecule. Each molecule consists of two heavy and two light chains linked by disulfide bonds. There are two types of light chains, kappa (genes on chromosome 2) and lambda (chromosome 22), each containing two domains. There are 10 types of heavy chains: 4 types of G (G_1 to G_4), 2 of A (A_1, A_2), 2 of M (M_1, M_2), and 1 each of D and E (all on chromosome 14), each with four domains. A domain is 100 to 110 amino acids in length. Within each domain is an intrachain disulfide bond that produces a loop. V_H (variable domain of the heavy chain) and V_L (variable domain of the light chain) form an antigen binding site whose unique determinants form an idiotype. Immunoglobulins of the same isotype (e.g., $IgG_1\kappa$) differ between individuals. The determinants that distinguish them are called allotypic determinants and are located on C_L (constant domain of the light chain) and C_{H2} (second constant domain of the heavy chain). C_{H2} is also the main site of glycosylation (CHO) and complement binding. Papain cleaves the molecule into antigen-binding (Fab) and crystallizable (Fc) components. The portion of the heavy chain in an Fab fragment is called the Fd piece. Fc receptors on cells bind to the C_{H3} domain. IgM and IgA occur as polymers and each unit of two heavy and two light chains is connected by a J (joining) chain. The heavy chain isotypes determine the function of the antibody.*

variable region forms the antigen recognition site of the antibody molecule; its unique structural features form a particular set of determinants called idiotypes that are reliable markers for a particular clone of cells because each antibody is formed and secreted by a single clone. Each chain is specified by distinct genes, synthesized separately, and assembled into an intact antibody molecule after translation (see Fig. 258-3). Because of the mechanics of the gene rearrangements necessary to specify the immunoglobulin variable regions (VDJ joining for the heavy chain, VJ joining for the light chain; see Fig. 258-3), a particular clone rearranges only one of the two chromosomes to produce an immunoglobulin molecule of only one light chain isotype and only one allotype (allelic exclusion). After exposure to antigen, the variable region may become associated with a new heavy chain isotype (class switch). Each clone of cells performs these sequential gene arrangements in a unique way. This results in each clone producing a unique immunoglobulin molecule. In most cells, light chains are synthesized in slight excess, are secreted as free light chains by plasma cells, and are cleared by the kidney, but less than 10 mg of such light chains is excreted per day.

Electrophoretic analysis of components of the serum proteins permits determination of the amount of antibody in the serum (Fig. 258-4). The variety of immunoglobulins move heterogeneously in an electric field and form a broad peak in the gamma region. The gamma globulin region of the electrophoretic pattern is increased in the serum of patients and animals with plasma cell tumors. There is a sharp spike in this region called an M component (M for monoclonal). The antibody must be present at a concentration of at least 0.5 g/dL to be detectable. This corresponds to approximately 10^9 cells producing the antibody. Confirmation that such an M component is truly monoclonal relies on the use of immunoelectrophoresis that shows a single light and heavy chain type. Hence, immunoelectrophoresis and electrophoresis provide qualitative and quantitative assessment of the M component, respectively. Once the presence of an M component has been confirmed, electrophoresis provides the more practical information for managing patients with monoclonal gammopathies. In a given patient, the amount of M component in the serum is a reliable measure of the tumor burden. This makes the M component an excellent tumor marker; yet it is not specific enough to be used

FIGURE 258-3 *Schematic diagram of the organization and translocation of immunoglobulin genes. Immunoglobulin heavy chains are encoded by four distinct genetic elements, variable (Igh-V), diversity (Igh-D), joining (Igh-J), and constant (Igh-C) genes. The variable region of the immunoglobulin heavy chain is encoded by the V, D, and J genes. The same variable region may be associated with any of the 10 heavy chain constant region genes. In the germline genome (all cells except B cells) the V, D, and J genes are widely separated and there are numerous forms of each. Once a cell becomes committed to B-cell differentiation, a single V gene and a single D gene translocate to a single J gene, and the intervening genetic material is excised. This is called VDJ joining. The newly formed VDJ gene is transcribed into a single message along with either an M or D isotype C gene. Upon exposure to antigen, another rearrangement may occur so that the VDJ gene may be associated with a G, A or E isotype C gene. In light chain genes, there appear to be no D genes, and thus, light chain variable regions are formed by VJ joining.*

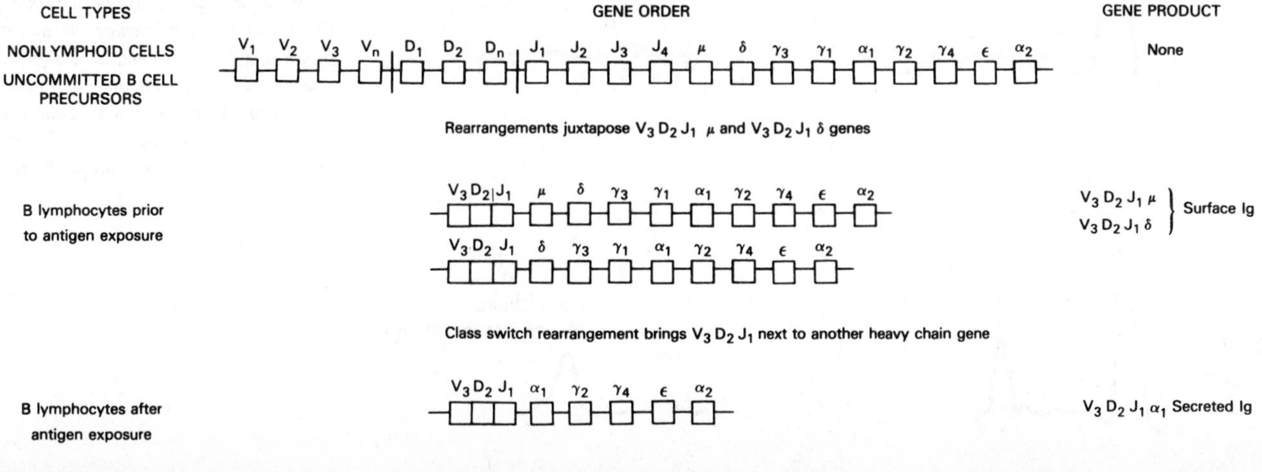

to screen asymptomatic patients. In addition to the plasma cell disorders, M components may be detected in other lymphoid neoplasms such as chronic lymphocytic leukemia and lymphomas of B- or T-cell origin; nonlymphoid neoplasms such as chronic myelogenous leukemia, breast and colon cancer; a variety of nonneoplastic conditions such as cirrhosis, sarcoidosis, parasitic diseases, Gaucher's disease, and pyoderma gangrenosum; and a number of autoimmune conditions, including rheumatoid arthritis and cold agglutinin disease. The nature of the M component is variable. It may be an intact antibody molecule of any heavy chain subclass, or it may be an altered antibody or fragment. Isolated light or heavy chains may be produced. In some plasma cell tumors such as extramedullary or solitary bone plasmacytomas, less than a third of patients will have an M component. In about 20 percent of myelomas, only light chains are produced. The frequency of myelomas of a particular heavy chain class is roughly proportional to the serum concentration, so that IgG myelomas are more common than IgA and IgD myelomas. In some cases, the antigen specificity of the monoclonal antibody is known.

MULTIPLE MYELOMA Definition Multiple myeloma represents a malignant proliferation of plasma cells. The terms multiple myeloma and myeloma may be used interchangeably. The disease results from the uncontrolled proliferation of plasma cells derived from a single clone. The tumor, its products, and the host response to it result in a number of organ dysfunctions and symptoms of bone pain or fracture, renal failure, susceptibility to infection, anemia, hypercalcemia, and occasionally clotting abnormalities, neurologic symptoms, and vascular manifestations of hyperviscosity.

Etiology The etiology of myeloma is not known. Myeloma was found to occur with increased frequency in those exposed to the radiation of nuclear warheads in World War II after a 20-year latency. Although there is no direct evidence implicating oncogenes in human myeloma, the observations on c-*myc* and b-*lym* oncogenes in Burkitt's lymphoma, the high incidence of chromosomal translocations in human B-cell tumors, and the role of type C RNA viruses in murine plasmacytoma formation suggest that cells of the B-cell lineage may be susceptible to growth deregulation by such stimuli. The murine plasmacytoma models are particularly interesting in that there is evidence that the induction of plasmacytomas may require exposure to foreign antigens as well as a cellular event. This suggests that chronic antigenic stimulation may play a role in the transformation of a particular B-cell clone. There is also some evidence for a genetic predisposition to myeloma in humans. Patients with myeloma have a significantly higher incidence of expressing the Glm(x) heavy chain allotype marker, and there is a weak but significant linkage dysequilibrium that shows the HLA-B5 determinant being expressed more commonly than expected in myeloma patients. There is the possibility that the neoplastic event in myeloma may involve cells earlier in B-cell differentiation than the plasma cell. Circulating B cells bearing surface immunoglobulin that share the idiotype of the M component are present in myeloma patients. It is possible that the malignant clone escapes normal control mechanisms at a pre-plasma cell stage of differentiation and the chronic exposure to a particular antigenic stimulus drives the cell to terminal differentiation. It remains difficult to distinguish benign from malignant plasma cells on the basis of morphologic criteria in all but a few cases.

Incidence and prevalence Myeloma is primarily a disease of the elderly and increases in incidence with age. The median age at diagnosis is 64 years. The disease is rare under age 40. The yearly incidence is around 3 per 100,000 and remarkably similar in a variety of countries throughout the world. Males are slightly more commonly affected than females and blacks have nearly twice the incidence of whites. In the age group over 25 years of age the incidence is 30 per 100,000.

Pathogenesis and clinical manifestations (Table 258-1) Bone pain is the most common symptom in myeloma and is present in nearly 70 percent of patients. The pain usually involves the back and ribs, and unlike the pain of metastatic carcinoma which often is worse at night, the pain of myeloma is precipitated by movement. Persistent localized pain in a patient with myeloma usually signifies a pathologic fracture. The bone lesions of myeloma are caused by the proliferation of the tumor cells and the activation of osteoclasts which destroy the bone. The osteoclasts respond to osteoclast activating factor (OAF) made by the myeloma cells; however, production of this factor stops following administration of corticosteroids. The bone lesions are lytic in nature and are rarely associated with osteoblastic new bone formation; therefore, radioisotopic bone scanning is less useful in diagnosis than plain radiography. The bony lysis results in substantial mobilization of calcium from bone, and serious acute and chronic complications of hypercalcemia may dominate the clinical picture (see below). Localized bone lesions may expand to the point that mass lesions may be palpated, especially on the skull (Fig. 258-5), clavicles, and sternum, and the collapse of vertebrae may lead to symptoms of spinal cord compression.

The next most common clinical problem in patients with myeloma is susceptibility to bacterial infections. The most common infections are pneumonias and pyelonephritis, and the most frequent pathogens

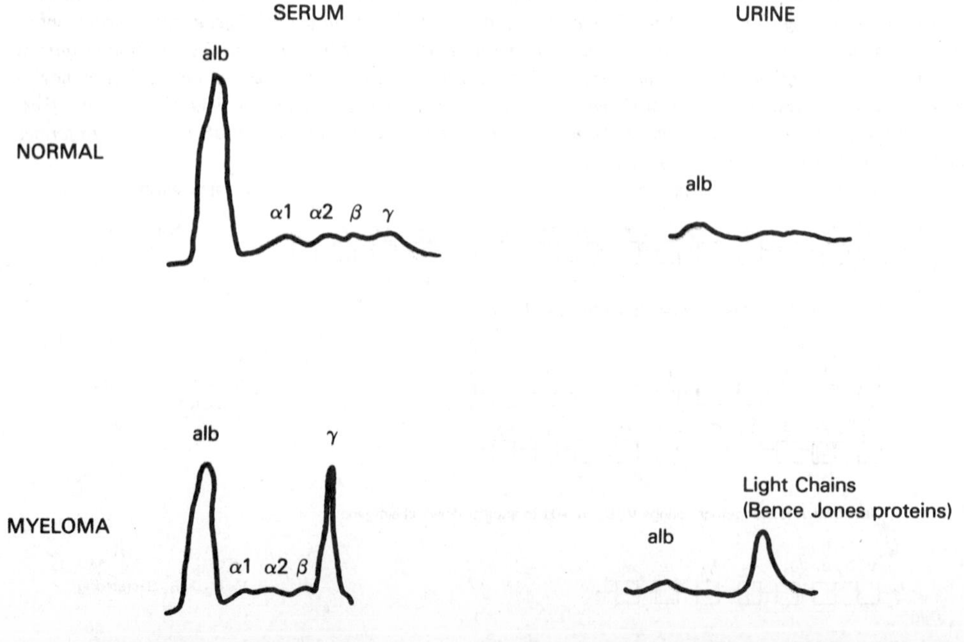

FIGURE 258-4 *Representative electrophoretic patterns of serum and urine. The upper panel illustrates the normal pattern of serum and urine protein on electrophoresis. Since there are many different immunoglobulins in the serum, their differing mobilities in an electric field produce a broad peak. The lower panel illustrates the patterns of serum and urine proteins in a patient with myeloma. The predominance of a product of a single cell is reflected by a "church spire" sharp peak. The presence of free light chains in the urine is reflected in a peak, as well.*

are *Streptococcus pneumoniae*, *Staphylococcus aureus*, and *Klebsiella pneumoniae* in the lungs and *Escherichia coli* and other gram-negative organisms in the urinary tract (Chap. 84). In about 25 percent of patients recurrent infections are the presenting features, and over 75 percent of patients will have a serious infection at some time in their course. The susceptibility to infection has several contributing causes. First, patients with myeloma have diffuse hypogammaglobulinemia if the M component is excluded. The hypogammaglobulinemia is related to both decreased production and increased destruction of normal antibodies. Moreover, some patients generate a population of circulating regulatory cells in response to their myeloma that can suppress normal antibody synthesis. In the case of IgG myeloma, normal IgG antibodies are broken down more rapidly than normal because the catabolic rate for IgG antibodies varies directly with the serum concentration. The large M component results in fractional catabolic rates of 8 to 16 percent instead of the normal 2 percent. These patients have very poor antibody responses, especially to polysaccharide antigens such as those on bacterial cell walls. Such responses are normally T-cell-independent. Most measures of T-cell function in myeloma are normal. Granulocyte migration is not as rapid as normal in patients with myeloma, probably the result of a product of the tumor. All of these factors contribute to the immune deficiency of these patients.

Renal failure occurs in nearly 25 percent of myeloma patients, and some renal pathology is noted in over half. There are many contributing factors. Hypercalcemia is the most common cause of renal failure. Glomerular deposits of amyloid, hyperuricemia, recurrent infections, and occasional infiltration of the kidney by myeloma cells all may contribute to renal dysfunction. However, tubular damage associated with the excretion of light chains is almost always present. Normally, light chains are filtered, reabsorbed in the tubules and catabolized. With the increase in amount of light chains presented to the tubule, the tubular cells become overloaded with these proteins, and tubular damage results either directly from light chain toxic effects or indirectly from the release of intracellular lysosomal enzymes. The earliest manifestation of this tubular damage is the adult Fanconi syndrome with increased loss of glucose, amino acids, and defects in the ability of the kidney to acidify and concentrate the urine. The proteinuria is not accompanied by hypertension, and the protein is nearly all light chains. Generally, there is very little albumin in the urine because glomerular function is usually normal. When the glomeruli are involved, the proteinuria is nonselective. Patients with myeloma also have a decreased anion gap [i.e., sodium minus (chloride plus bicarbonate)] because the M component is cationic, resulting in retention of chloride. This is often accompanied by hyponatremia that is felt to be artificial (pseudohyponatremia) because each volume of serum has less water as a result of the increased protein.

Anemia occurs in about 80 percent of myeloma patients. It is usually normocytic and normochromic and related both to the replacement of normal marrow by expanding tumor cells and to the inhibition of hematopoiesis by factors made by the tumor. In addition, mild hemolysis may contribute to the anemia. A larger than expected fraction of patients may have megaloblastic anemia due to either folate or vitamin B_{12} deficiency. Granulocytopenia and thrombocytopenia are very rare. Clotting abnormalities may be seen due to the failure of antibody-coated platelets to function properly or to the interaction of the M component with clotting factors I, II, V, VII, or VIII. Raynaud's phenomenon and impaired circulation may result if the M component forms cryoglobulins, and hyperviscosity syndromes may develop depending on the physical properties of the M component (most common with IgM, IgG3, and IgA paraproteins).

Although neurologic symptoms occur in a minority of patients, they may have many causes. Hypercalcemia may produce lethargy, weakness, depression, and confusion. Hyperviscosity may lead to headache, fatigue, visual disturbances, and retinopathy. Bony damage and collapse may lead to cord compression, radicular pain, and loss of bowel and bladder control. Infiltration of peripheral nerves by amyloid can be a cause of carpal tunnel syndrome and other sensorimotor mono- and polyneuropathies.

Diagnosis and staging The classic triad of myeloma is marrow plasmacytosis (>10 percent), lytic bone lesions, and a serum and/or urine M component. The diagnosis may be made in the absence of bone lesions if the plasmacytosis is associated with a progressive increase in the M component over time or if extramedullary mass lesions develop. There are two important variants of myeloma,

TABLE 258-1 Pathogenesis and clinical manifestations of multiple myeloma

Clinical finding	Underlying cause	Pathogenic mechanism
Hypercalcemia, pathologic fractures, cord compression, lytic bone lesions, osteoporosis, bone pain	Skeletal destruction	Tumor expansion; production of osteoclast activating factor (OAF) by tumor cells
Renal failure	Light chain proteinuria, hypercalcemia, urate nephropathy, amyloid glomerulopathy (rare)	Toxic effects of tumor products; light chains, OAF, DNA breakdown products:
	Pyelonephritis	Hypogammaglobulinemia
Anemia	Myelophthisis, decreased production, increased destruction	Tumor expansion; production of inhibitory factors and autoantibodies by tumor cells
Infection	Hypogammaglobulinemia, decreased neutrophil migration	Decreased production due to tumor-induced suppression; increased IgG catabolism
Neurologic symptoms	Hyperviscosity, cryoglobulins, amyloid deposits	Products of tumor; properties of M component; light chains; OAF
	Hypercalcemia, cord compression	
Bleeding	Interference with clotting factors, amyloid damage of endothelium, platelet dysfunction	Products of tumor; antibodies to clotting factors; light chains; antibody coating of platelets
Mass lesions		Tumor expansion

FIGURE 258-5 *Bony lesions in multiple myeloma. The skull demonstrates the typical "punched out" lesions characteristic of multiple myeloma. The lesion represents a purely osteolytic lesion with little or no osteoblastic activity. (Courtesy of Dr. Geraldine Schechter.)*

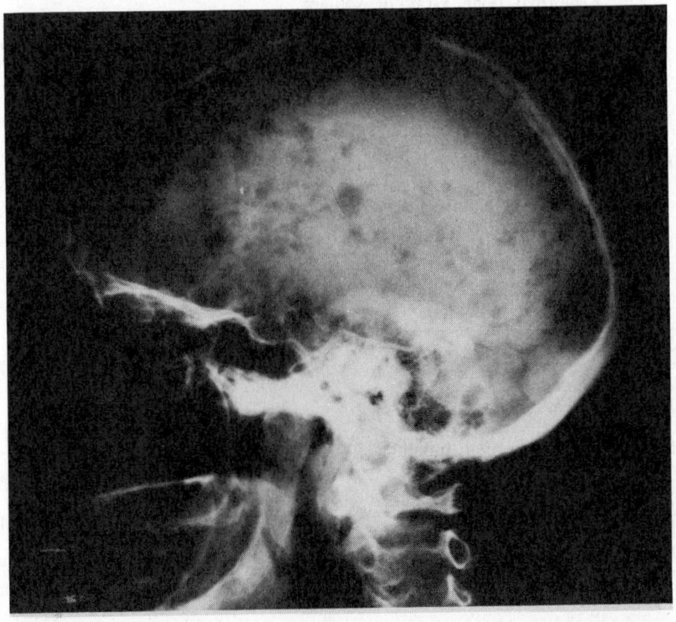

solitary bone plasmacytoma and extramedullary plasmacytoma. These lesions are associated with an M component in less than 30 percent of the cases, they may affect younger individuals, and both are associated with median survivals of 10 or more years. Solitary bone plasmacytoma is a single lytic bone lesion without marrow plasmacytosis. Extramedullary plasmacytomas usually involve the submucosal lymphoid tissue of the nasopharynx or paranasal sinuses without marrow plasmacytosis. Both tumors are highly responsive to local radiation therapy. If an M component is present, it should disappear after treatment. Solitary bone plasmacytomas may recur in other bony sites or evolve into myeloma. Extramedullary plasmacytomas rarely recur or progress.

The most difficult differential diagnosis in patients with myeloma involves their separation from people with benign monoclonal gammopathies or monoclonal gammopathies of uncertain significance (MGUS). MGUS is vastly more common than myeloma, occurring in 1 percent of the population over age 50 and in 3 percent over age 70. Patients with MGUS usually have M components less than 2 g/dL, no urinary Bence Jones protein, less than 5 percent marrow plasmacytosis, and no anemia, renal failure, lytic bone lesions, or hypercalcemia. When bone marrow cells are exposed to radioactive thymidine in order to quantitate dividing cells, patients with MGUS always have a labeling index less than 1 percent and patients with myeloma always have a labeling index greater than 1 percent. Other discriminators include plasma cell acid phosphatase and β-glucuronidase, both of which are low in MGUS patients, and the salmon calcitonin stimulation test, which is positive only in patients with active ongoing bone destruction. Only about 11 percent of patients with MGUS go on to develop myeloma.

Typically, patients with MGUS require no therapy. A number of other diseases may produce M components, including other B-cell neoplasms (especially chronic lymphocytic leukemia and malignant lymphomas), other types of cancer (Hodgkin's disease, chronic myelogenous leukemia, breast and colon cancer), Gaucher's disease, biliary tract diseases like hepatitis and cirrhosis, collagen vascular diseases, chronic infections, and myasthenia gravis. A very rare skin disease known as lichen myxedematosus or papular mucinosis is associated with a monoclonal gammopathy. Highly cationic IgGλ is deposited in the dermis of patients with this disease. It is unclear whether this organ specificity reflects the specificity of the antibody for some antigenic component of the dermis.

TABLE 258-2 Myeloma staging system

Stage	Criteria	Estimated tumor burden (× 10^{12} cells/m^2)
I	All of the following: *1* Hemoglobin >10g/dL *2* Serum calcium <12 mg/dL *3* Normal bone x-ray or solitary lesion *4* Low M-component production *a* IgG level <5 g/dL *b* IgA level <3 g/dL *c* Urine light chain <4 g/24 h	<0.6 (low)
II	Fitting neither I nor III	0.6–1.20 (intermediate)
III	One or more of the following: *1* Hemoglobin <8.5 g/dL *2* Serum calcium >12 mg/dL *3* Advanced lytic bone lesions *4* High M-component production *a* IgG level >7 g/dL *b* IgA level >5 g/dL *c* Urine light chains >12 g/24 h	>1.20 (high)

Subclassification

A Serum creatinine <2 mg/dL
B Serum creatinine >2 mg/dL

Stage	Median survival, months
IA	61
IIA,B	55
IIIA	30
IIIB	15

The clinical evaluation of patients with myeloma includes a careful physical examination searching for tender bones and masses. It is paradoxic that only a small minority of patients have an enlargement of the spleen and lymph nodes, the physiologic sites of antibody production. Chest and bone radiographs may reveal lytic lesions. A complete blood count with differential may reveal anemia. Very rare patients may have plasma cell leukemia with more than 2000 plasma cells per cubic millimeter. This may be seen in disproportionate frequency (~12 percent) in IgD myelomas. Serum calcium, urea nitrogen, creatinine, and uric acid may be elevated. Protein electrophoresis and measurement of serum immunoglobulins are useful for detecting and characterizing M spikes. Electrophoresis of a 24-h urine specimen with immunologic typing of any M component is necessary. Serum alkaline phosphatase is usually normal even with extensive bone involvement because of the absence of osteoblastic activity. It is also important to quantitate serum beta$_2$ microglobulin (see below).

The serum M component will be IgG in 53 percent of patients, IgA in 25 percent, IgD in 1 percent, and 20 percent of patients will have only light chains in serum and urine. Dipsticks for detecting proteinuria are not reliable at identifying light chains, and the heat test for detecting Bence Jones protein is falsely negative in about 50 percent of patients with light chain myeloma. Fewer than 1 percent of patients have no identifiable M component, and these are usually light chain myelomas in which renal catabolism has made them undetectable in the urine. About two-thirds of patients with serum M components also have urinary light chains. The light chain isotype may have an impact on survival. Patients secreting lambda light chains have a significantly shorter overall survival than those secreting kappa light chains. It is not clear whether this is due to some genetically important determinant of cell proliferation or because lambda light chains are more likely to cause renal damage and form amyloid than are kappa light chains. The heavy chain isotype may have an impact on patient management as well. About half of patients with IgM paraproteins develop hyperviscosity compared to only 2 to 4 percent of patients with IgA and IgG M components. Among IgG myelomas, it is the IgG3 subclass that has the highest tendency to form both concentration- and temperature-dependent aggregates, leading to hyperviscosity and cold agglutination at lower serum concentrations.

The staging system for patients with myeloma is a functional system for predicting survival and is based on a variety of clinical and laboratory tests, unlike the anatomic staging systems for solid tumors. Details of the staging system are given in Table 258-2. Based upon the hemoglobin, calcium, M component, and degree of skeletal involvement, the total-body tumor burden is estimated to be low (stage I, <0.6 × 10^{12} cells per square meter), intermediate (stage II, 0.6 to 1.2 × 10^{12} cells per square meter), or high (stage III, >1.2 × 10^{12} cells per square meter), and the stages are further subdivided on the basis of renal function (A if serum creatinine <2 mg/dL, B if >2). Patients in stage IA have a median survival of more than 5 years and those in stage IIIB about 15 months. Serum beta$_2$ microglobulin [an 11,000-mol wt protein with homologies with the constant region of immunoglobulins that occurs together with the class I major histocompatibility antigens (HLA-A, -B, -C) on the surface of every cell] is the single most powerful predictor of survival and can substitute for staging. Patients with beta$_2$ microglobulin levels less than 6 μg/mL have a median survival of 52 months and those with levels higher than 6 μg/mL only 26 months. It is also felt that once the diagnosis of myeloma is firm, histologic features of atypia may also exert an influence on prognosis.

Treatment and course About 10 percent of patients with myeloma will have an indolent course demonstrating only very slow progression of disease over many years. Such patients rarely require antitumor therapy. Patients with solitary bone plasmacytomas and extramedullary plasmacytomas may be expected to enjoy prolonged, disease-free survival after local radiation therapy to a dose of around 40 Gy. There is a low incidence of occult marrow involvement in patients with solitary bone plasmacytoma. Such patients are usually detected because their serum M component falls slowly or disappears initially only to return after a few months. These patients respond well to systemic chemotherapy.

The vast majority of patients with myeloma require therapeutic intervention. In general, such therapy is of two sorts: systemic chemotherapy to control the progression of myeloma and symptomatic supportive care to prevent serious morbidity from the complications of the disease. All patients with stage II or III disease and stage I patients exhibiting Bence Jones proteinuria, progressive lytic bone lesions, vertebral compression fractures, recurrent infections, or rising serum M component should be treated with systemic combination chemotherapy. Although there are no reported cases of long-term disease-free survival (i.e., cured patients), there is no doubt that therapy can prolong and improve the quality of life in myeloma.

The standard treatment has consisted of intermittent pulses of an alkylating agent [L-phenylalanine mustard (L-PAM, melphalan), cyclophosphamide, or chlorambucil] and prednisone administered for 4 to 7 days every 4 to 6 weeks. The alkylating agents appear to be roughly equally active, but resistance to one agent is often accompanied by resistance to the others. The usual doses are as follows: melphalan, 8 mg/m^2 per day; cyclophosphamide, 200 mg/m^2 per day; chlorambucil, 8 mg/m^2 per day; prednisone, 25 to 60 mg/m^2 per day. Because of their near equivalence in antitumor efficacy, we favor cyclophosphamide because it is less toxic to the marrow stem cell compartment and results in a lower incidence of acute myelodysplastic syndromes than do the other alkylating agents. Doses may need adjustment based on marrow tolerance. Patients responding to therapy generally have a prompt and gratifying reduction in bone pain, hypercalcemia, and anemia, and often have fewer infections. The serum M component lags substantially behind the symptomatic improvement, often taking 4 to 6 weeks to fall. This fall depends upon the rate of tumor kill and the fractional catabolic rate of immunoglobulin, which in turn depends upon the serum concentration (for IgG). Light chain excretion, with a functional half-life of approximately 6 h, may fall within the first week of treatment. However, since urine light chain levels may relate to renal tubular function, they are not a reliable measure of tumor cell kill. Calculations of tumor cell kill are made by extrapolation of the serum M-component level and rely heavily on the assumption that every tumor cell produces immunoglobulin at a constant rate. The data on which this assumption is based are reasonable, but recently it has been possible to alter the rate of immunoglobulin production of a myeloma in vitro with calcium channel blockers, a finding that may have clinical utility, for example, in patients with hyperviscosity. Thus, it is possible that a treatment might affect immunoglobulin production without killing the tumor cell, a situation that would result in an overestimation of the antitumor effects of the treatment if current criteria for response were applied. About 60 percent of patients will achieve at least a 75 percent reduction in serum M-component level and tumor cell mass in response to an alkylating agent and prednisone. Although this is a tumor reduction of less than one log, clinical responses may last many months. Efforts to improve the fraction of patients responding and the degree of response have involved adding other active chemotherapeutic agents to the treatment program. Patients with more advanced disease may benefit most from such approach, but such therapy is experimental at this time.

The ideal duration of therapy has not been determined. Most physicians treat every 4 to 6 weeks for 1 or 2 years. Cessation of therapy is followed by relapse, usually within a year. Retreatment may be associated with a second response in up to 80 percent of patients. Maintenance therapy may prolong the duration of response, but no study has demonstrated this to result in prolonged survival. The regrowth rate of the tumor during relapse accelerates with each relapse. Patients primarily resistant to initial therapy have a median survival of less than a year.

About 15 percent of patients die within the first 3 months after diagnosis, and subsequently the death rate is about 15 percent per year. The disease usually follows a chronic course for 2 to 5 years before developing an acute terminal phase usually marked by the development of pancytopenia with a cellular marrow that is refractory to treatment. Widespread organ infiltration by myeloma cells occurs and survival is less than 6 months. About 46 percent of patients die in the chronic phase of disease from progressive myeloma (16 percent) and renal failure (10 percent), sepsis (14 percent), or both (6 percent). Death in the acute terminal phase (26 percent) is chiefly from progressive myeloma (13 percent) and sepsis (9 percent). Five percent of patients die of acute leukemia, myeloblastic or monocytic, and although it has been debated that this is related to the primary disease, it appears more likely to be the result of chronic therapy with alkylating agents. Nearly 23 percent of patients die of myocardial infarction, chronic lung disease, diabetes, or strokes, all intercurrent illnesses related more to the age of the patient group than the tumor.

Supportive care directed at the anticipated complications of the disease may be as important as primary antitumor therapy. The hypercalcemia generally responds well to corticosteroid therapy, hydration, and natriuresis. Dichloromethane diphosphonate has also been shown to reduce osteoclastic bone resorption. Treatments aimed at strengthening the skeleton, like fluorides, calcium, and vitamin D with or without androgens, have been suggested but are not of proven efficacy. Iatrogenic worsening of renal function may be prevented by the use of allopurinol during chemotherapy to avoid urate nephropathy and by maintaining a high fluid intake to help excrete light chains and calcium. In the event of acute renal failure, plasmapheresis is approximately 10 times more effective at clearing light chains than peritoneal dialysis, and acutely reducing the protein load may result in functional improvement. Urinary tract infections should be watched for and treated early. Chronic dialysis probably should not be initiated in patients who have failed to respond to antitumor therapy. Plasmapheresis may be the treatment of choice for hyperviscosity syndromes. Although the pneumococcus is a dreaded pathogen in myeloma patients, they do not respond to pneumococcal polysaccharide vaccines. The advent of intravenous gamma globulin preparations raises some hope that prophylactic administration may prevent some serious infections, but this has not been tested. Chronic oral antibiotic prophylaxis is probably not warranted. Patients developing neurologic symptoms in the lower extremities, severe localized back pain, or problems with bowel and bladder control may need emergency myelography and radiation therapy for palliation. Most bone lesions respond to analgesics and chemotherapy, but certain painful lesions may respond most promptly to localized radiation. The chronic anemia may respond to hematinics (iron, folate, cobalamin) and some have responded to androgens. The pathogenesis of the anemia should be established and specific therapy instituted, where possible.

WALDENSTRÖM'S MACROGLOBULINEMIA In 1948, Waldenström described a malignancy of lymphoplasmacytoid cells that secreted IgM. In contrast to myeloma, the disease was associated with lymphadenopathy and hepatosplenomegaly, but the major clinical manifestation was the hyperviscosity syndrome. The disease resembles the related diseases chronic lymphocytic leukemia, myeloma, and lymphocytic lymphoma. Waldenström's macroglobulinemia and IgM myeloma both follow a similar clinical course. The diagnosis of IgM myeloma is usually reserved for patients with lytic bone lesions and is important only because of the hazard of pathologic fractures.

The etiology of macroglobulinemia is unknown. The disease is similar to myeloma in being slightly more common in men and occurring with increased incidence with age (median, 64 years). There have been reports that the IgM in some patients with macroglobulinemia may have specificity for myelin-associated glycoprotein

(MAG), a protein that has been associated with demyelinating disease of the peripheral nervous system and may be lost earlier and to a greater extent than the better known myelin basic protein in patients with multiple sclerosis. There is a surface antigen on natural killer cells that is cross-reactive with the MAG, and coincidentally, natural killer cells are decreased in multiple sclerosis. Sometimes patients with macroglobulinemia develop a peripheral neuropathy before the appearance of the neoplasm. There is speculation that the whole process begins with a viral infection that may elicit an antibody response that cross-reacts with a normal tissue component.

Like myeloma, the disease involves the bone marrow, but unlike myeloma, it does not cause bone lesions or hypercalcemia. Like myeloma, a serum M component is present in the serum in excess of 3 g/dL, but unlike myeloma, the size of the IgM paraprotein results in little renal excretion and only around 20 percent of patients excrete light chains. Therefore, renal disease is not common. The light chain isotype is kappa in 80 percent of the cases. Patients present with weakness, fatigue, and recurrent infections, similar to myeloma patients, but epistaxis, visual disturbances, and neurologic symptoms like peripheral neuropathy, dizziness, headache, and transient paresis are much more common in macroglobulinemia. Physical examination reveals adenopathy and hepatosplenomegaly, and ophthalmoscopic examination may reveal vascular segmentation and dilatation of the retinal veins characteristic of hyperviscosity states. Patients may have a normocytic, normochromic anemia, but rouleaux formation and a positive Coombs' test are much more common than in myeloma. Malignant lymphocytes are usually present in the peripheral blood. About 10 percent of macroglobulins are cryoglobulins. These are pure M components and are not the mixed cryoglobulins seen in rheumatoid arthritis and other autoimmune diseases. Mixed cryoglobulins are composed of IgM or IgA complexed with IgG, for which they are specific. In both cases, Raynaud's phenomenon and serious vascular symptoms precipitated by the cold may occur, but mixed cryoglobulins are not associated with malignancy. Patients suspected of having a cryoglobulin based on history and physical examination should have their blood drawn into a warm syringe to avoid errors in quantitating the cryoglobulin.

Control of serious hyperviscosity symptoms like an altered state of consciousness or paresis can be achieved acutely by plasmapheresis because 80 percent of the IgM paraprotein is intravascular. Aside from this, management is identical to that of myeloma. About 80 percent of patients respond to chemotherapy and their median survival is over 3 years. The absence of other serious organ toxicities results in a longer life span of patients with macroglobulinemia compared to those with myeloma.

HEAVY CHAIN DISEASES The heavy chain diseases are rare lymphoplasmacytic malignancies. Their clinical manifestations vary with the heavy chain isotype. They secrete a defective heavy chain that usually has an intact Fc fragment and a deletion in the Fd region. Gamma, alpha, and mu heavy chain diseases have been described, but no reports of delta or epsilon heavy chain diseases have appeared. Molecular biologic analysis of these tumors has revealed structural genetic defects that may account for the aberrant chain secreted.

Gamma heavy chain disease (Franklin's disease) This disease affects people of widely different age groups and countries of origin. It is characterized by lymphadenopathy, fever, anemia, malaise, hepatosplenomegaly, and weakness. Its most distinctive symptom is palatal edema, resulting from node involvement of Waldeyer's ring, and this may progress to produce respiratory compromise. The diagnosis depends upon the demonstration of an anomalous serum M component (often <2 g/dL) that reacts with anti-IgG but not anti-light chain reagents. Most of the paraproteins have been of the $gamma_1$ subclass, but other subclasses have been seen. The patients may have thrombocytopenia, eosinophilia, and nondiagnostic bone marrow. Patients usually have a rapid downhill course and die of infection; however, some patients have survived 5 years with chemotherapy.

Alpha heavy chain disease (Seligmann's disease) This is the commonest of the heavy chain diseases. It is closely related to a malignancy known as Mediterranean lymphoma, a disease that affects young people in parts of the world such as the Mediterranean, Asia, and South America in which intestinal parasites are common. The disease is characterized by an infiltration of the lamina propria of the small intestine with lymphoplasmacytoid cells that secrete truncated alpha chains. Demonstrating alpha heavy chains is difficult because the alpha chains tend to polymerize and appear as a smear instead of a sharp peak on electrophoretic profiles. Light chains are absent from serum and urine. The patients present with chronic diarrhea, weight loss, and malabsorption and have extensive mesenteric and paraaortic adenopathy. Respiratory tract involvement occurs rarely. Patients may vary widely in their clinical course. Some may develop diffuse aggressive histologies of malignant lymphoma. Chemotherapy may produce long-term remissions. Rare patients appear to have responded to antibiotic therapy, raising the question of the etiologic role of antigenic stimulation perhaps by some chronic intestinal infection.

Mu heavy chain disease The secretion of isolated mu heavy chains into the serum appears to occur in a very rare subset of patients with chronic lymphocytic leukemia. The only features that may distinguish patients with mu heavy chain disease are the presence of vacuoles in the malignant lymphocytes and the excretion of kappa light chains in the urine. The diagnosis requires ultracentrifugation or gel filtration to confirm the nonreactivity of the paraprotein with the light chain reagents because some intact macroglobulins fail to interact with these serums. The tumor cells seem to have a defect in the assembly of light and heavy chains because they appear to contain both in their cytoplasm. There is no evidence that such patients should be treated differently from other patients with chronic lymphocytic leukemia.

PRIMARY AMYLOIDOSIS Amyloidosis is a systemic illness resulting from the deposition of polymerized immunoglobulin light chain fragments in organs and tissues. The light chains are arranged in a beta pleated-sheet configuration, appear as homogeneous pink-staining material on light microscopy of hematoxylin-eosin–stained tissue sections, and are identified specifically by their green birefringence under polarized light when tissue secretions are stained with Congo red. The amyloid fibrils are labeled AL in immunocytic amyloidosis because they are composed of light chains. The fibrils of secondary or reactive amyloidosis, which is seen in chronic or acute recurrent infections, and chronic inflammatory diseases like rheumatoid arthritis, are called AA or amyloid A protein. This protein is unrelated to immunoglobulin and is thought to be a fragment of a larger protein called serum amyloid A (SAA) protein.

Immunocytic amyloidosis occurs in about 15 to 20 percent of patients with myeloma and is related to lambda light chains twice as frequently as kappa light chains. About 20 percent of amyloidosis patients have myeloma, and the remainder have monoclonal gammopathies of another origin or even agammaglobulinemia (such patients may produce light chains but not intact immunoglobulins). Even when no underlying diagnosis is apparent, the patient will be found to have a light chain in the urine, a serum M component, or marrow plasmacytosis. Not all light chains are capable of forming amyloid, but the structural features that are prerequisite are not known.

The pathophysiology of amyloidosis is that of organ infiltration. It produces stiffness where there should be flexibility, creates barriers where there should be free flow, and distorts size where there should be fit. The stiffness is particularly damaging to the heart, lungs, blood vessels, and both smooth and skeletal muscle. The barrier effect results in malabsorption in the gastrointestinal tract, renal glomerular dysfunction, cardiac and peripheral nerve conduction defects, and limitation of joint range of motion. The enlarged tongue and narrowed carpal tunnel result in functional compromise. The patient with amyloidosis may have congestive heart failure resistant to the usual therapeutic measures, nephrotic syndrome and nonselective proteinuria from glomerular damage, a bleeding tendency in the skin and gastrointestinal tract from vascular endothelial damage, diarrhea and malabsorption from alterations in the coordinated contraction of intestinal smooth muscle and mucosal infiltration, and orthostatic hypotension and peripheral neuropathies from nerve infiltration. Patients may present with peripheral edema, weakness, paresthesias, light-headedness, and shortness of breath. In addition to the findings of myeloma, they may have hepatomegaly, the "shoulder pad" sign from shoulder muscle infiltration, and the "raccoon sign," i.e. periorbital hemorrhage. The diagnosis depends upon demonstrating amyloid on tissue biopsy. The safest reliable biopsy site is the rectal mucosa, which is diagnostic in about 75 percent of cases. Skin, tongue, or gingival biopsy may yield a diagnosis in most of the remaining cases. Endomyocardial biopsies have been advocated by those experienced in this approach. Biopsies and surgical procedures are generally associated with a greater than normal risk of significant bleeding. Renal and heart failure are the leading causes of death, and the median survival is about a year. Treating amyloidosis patients with therapy which is effective in myeloma has been disappointing. Colchicine and penicillamine have not been found to be effective. Once deposited, it is rare for amyloid to regress.

REFERENCES

Bergsagel DE et al: The chemotherapy of plasma cell myeloma and the incidence of acute leukemia. N Engl J Med 301:743, 1979

Broder SB et al: Impaired synthesis of polyclonal (non-paraprotein) immunoglobulins by circulating lymphocytes from patients with multiple myeloma. N Engl J Med 293:887, 1975

Durie BGM et al: Pretreatment tumor mass, cell kinetics and prognosis in multiple myeloma. Blood 55:364, 1980

Frangione B, Franklin EC: Heavy-chain diseases: Clinical features and molecular significance of the disordered immunoglobulin structure. Semin Hematol 10:53, 1973

Kyle RA: Monoclonal gammopathy of undetermined significance. Natural history in 241 cases. Am J Med 64:814, 1978

———, Greipp PR: Amyloidosis (AL), clinical and laboratory features in 229 cases. Mayo Clin Proc 58:665, 1983

MacKenzie MR, Fudenberg HH: Macroglobulinemia: An analysis of 40 patients. Blood 39:874, 1972

Rosner F, Grunwald HW: Simultaneous occurrence of multiple myeloma and acute myeloblastic leukemia: Fact or myth? Am J Med 76:891, 1984

Salmon SE et al: Alternating combination chemotherapy and levamisole improves survival in multiple myeloma: A Southwest Oncology Group study. J Clin Oncol 1:453, 1983

Seligmann M: Alpha chain disease: Immunoglobulin abnormalities, pathogenesis and current concepts. Br J Cancer 31:356, 1975

259 AMYLOIDOSIS

ALAN S. COHEN

DEFINITION AND CLASSIFICATION Amyloidosis may be defined as the extracellular deposition of the fibrous protein amyloid in one or more sites of the body. This protein has unique ultrastructural, x-ray diffraction, and biochemical characteristics. It can be deposited locally where it has no clinical consequences or may involve virtually any organ system of the body leading to severe pathophysiologic changes, or the disease may fall between these two extremes. The natural history of amyloidosis is poorly understood, and the clinical diagnosis is often not made until the disease is far advanced. The following classification is clinically the most useful: (1) primary (AL type) amyloidosis (no evidence for preexisting or coexisting disease); (2) amyloid associated with multiple myeloma; (also AL type); (3) secondary or reactive (AA type) amyloidosis associated with chronic infectious diseases (e.g., osteomyelitis, tuberculosis, leprosy) or chronic inflammatory diseases (e.g., rheumatoid arthritis and ankylosing spondylitis); (4) heredofamilial amyloidosis, the amyloidosis associated with familial Mediterranean fever (AA type) and a variety of neuropathic (AF prealbumin type), renal, cardiovascular, and other syndromes; (5) local amyloidosis (local, often tumorlike, deposits which occur in isolated organs without evidence of systemic involvement); and (6) amyloidosis associated with aging, especially in the heart and in the brain.

PATHOLOGY AND STRUCTURE Amyloid is amorphous, eosinophilic, hyaline, extracellular, and ubiquitous in distribution. The involved organs may have a rubbery, firm consistency and a waxy, pink or gray appearance. Organ enlargement, especially of the liver, kidney, spleen, and heart, may be prominent.

Microscopically, amyloid stains pink with the hematoxylin-eosin stain and shows metachromasia with crystal violet. The Congo red stain imparts a unique green birefringence when sections are viewed in the polarizing microscope. This is the single most useful procedure for establishing the presence of amyloid. Amyloid deposits may be focal in almost any area of the body but are most often perivascular.

The heart may show focal or diffuse interstitial deposits in the myocardium, endocardium, or pericardium. In the aged heart, the atrium is usually focally involved or there may occur more diffuse lesions of the atria and ventricles. In the kidney, the glomerulus is primarily affected, although interstitial, peritubular, and vascular amyloid occur. In early lesions, small nodular or diffuse deposits appear near the basement membrane and, as the disease progresses, the glomerulus may be massively laden with amyloid, and its capillary bed will be occluded. In the gastrointestinal tract, there may be perivascular deposits only, or irregular or diffuse deposits may be found in the submucosa, in the muscularis mucosa, or subserosa. The amyloid may appear at any level or portion of the gastrointestinal tract including the gallbladder and pancreas. In the nervous system, amyloid has been described along peripheral nerves, in autonomic ganglia, and in senile plaques, in neurofibrillary tangles, as well as blood vessels ("congophilic angiopathy") of the central nervous system. It may be found in any portion of the orbit including the vitreous humor and cornea. In summary, there is virtually no area of the body that is spared. This ubiquitous distribution elicits a wide variety of clinical symptoms and signs.

All types of human amyloid consist of fine, nonbranching rigid fibrils that in tissue sections measure approximately 100 Å in diameter. The amyloid fibrils are usually seen earliest in the mesangial cell in the kidney and Kupffer cell in the liver. Isolated amyloid fibrils have a delicate, thin, nonbranching fibrous character. The individual fibril (or filament) has a diameter of about 70 Å and tends to aggregate laterally. Each fibril (filament) has subunit protofibrils of 30 to 35 Å diameter.

A second component, the plasma component or pentagonal unit (P component) with a different ultrastructure, x-ray diffraction pattern, and chemical characteristics, has also been isolated from amyloid and is identical with a serum alpha globulin. It has many similarities to C-reactive protein, but it does not behave as a classic acute phase protein. It is not responsible for the characteristic tinctorial properties or ultrastructure of amyloid.

BIOCHEMISTRY OF AMYLOID FIBRILS The bulk of amyloid deposits consists of fibrils. Purified amyloid derived from the fibril is a protein. The chemical composition of the different clinical forms of amyloid are distinct and allow for more precise diagnosis (Table 259-1). The homology of the fibril of primary and myeloma amyloid to the *N*-terminal region of the variable fragment of an immunoglobulin light chain and subsequently, in a limited number of cases, to a homogeneous light polypeptide chain, has been demonstrated. These light chain–related proteins range in size from about 5000 to 25,000 daltons and are now termed amyloid light chain (AL) or AL_{κ} or AL_{λ} (Table 259-1). Amino acid sequence analysis indicates that most primary amyloid proteins contain the *N*-terminal amino acid residue identical to the variable regions of the light chain (Asp-Ile-Gln-Ser-Pro-Ser-Ser-Leu- . . .).

Another protein that is unrelated to any known immunoglobulin has been described in the secondary amyloid deposits. This protein, amyloid A (AA) protein, can be isolated from the amyloid of patients with secondary amyloidosis and from that associated with familial

TABLE 259-1 Classification of amyloid

Biochemical type	Clinical form	Comment
AL	*1* Primary amyloid *2* Multiple myeloma–associated amyloid	Homologous to *N*-terminal residue of variable region of κ or λ light chain (or rarely whole chain). Varied molecular weight.
AA	*1* Secondary (reactive) amyloid *2* Amyloid of familial Meditarranean fever	Serum protein SAA is putative precursor; Arg-Ser-Phe-Phe-Ser sequence to 76 amino acids.
$AF_{prealbumin}$	*1* Familial amyloid polyneuropathy (Japanese, Swedish, Portuguese)	Most with single amino acid subsitution of methionine for valine at position 30; probably other variants exist.
AE_{mct}	*1* Amyloid-associated medullary carcinoma of thyroid	Probable calcitonin precursor; may be true of other endocrine-related forms of amyloid.
AS_c	*1* Senile cardiac	May be prealbumin.
AP	*1* P component	Distinct from amyloid fibril; found in all systemic forms. Serum SAP is the precursor.

Mediterranean fever. It is a unique protein with a molecular weight of about 8500 daltons made up of 76 amino acid residues arranged in a single chain, and an amino acid sequence beginning with Arg-Ser-Phe. . . . Some heterogeneity has been demonstrated (i.e., AAs of different molecular weights).

Antiserums to alkali-degraded amyloid fibrils of the AA protein have detected an antigenically related serum component, SAA. Amino acid analysis, peptide maps, and sequence studies suggest that AA protein is an amino terminal fragment of SAA and is derived from it by proteolysis. SAA behaves as an acute phase reactant and is elevated in infection and inflammation. In addition, SAA is elevated in amyloid-resistant animals suggesting that the appearance of amyloid is not solely determined by the level of SAA. SAA associates with the HDL_3 subclass of serum lipoproteins and is often referred to as apoSAA. In human beings there are two major isotypes of SAA, and four minor variants have been described. An SAA inducing factor (now known to be interleukin 1) has been shown to be released from stimulated macrophages and to cause the release of SAA from hepatocytes, the site of SAA synthesis. SAA appears to suppress antibody response, suggesting that it might act as an immune regulator. Heterogeneity of SAAs has also been recognized.

Familial amyloid polyneuropathy (FAP) is a dominant hereditary disease affecting kinships originating in Portugal, Japan, Sweden, and elsewhere. A 14,000-dalton protein has been isolated from the tissues of patients from each of the above-noted geographically distributed kinships. Immunologic and amino acid sequence analysis has identified it as prealbumin, the first association of this molecule with a disease. It has also been shown that there is a single amino acid substitution, methionine for valine at position 30 in the prealbumin isolated from the amyloid. Data suggest that other variants may also exist.

In addition, a prothyrocalcitonin has been isolated from the amyloid of medullary carcinoma of the thyroid. It has been suggested that the amyloid associated with other endocrine organs is also made up of a prehormone or preprohormone precursor.

P component of amyloid In addition to the characteristic fibrils described above, a second component, the P component, has been noted in most amyloid deposits. P component (AP) has been recognized by electron microscopy as a pentagonal-shaped structured unit having an outside diameter of about 90 Å and an inside diameter of about 40 Å. On immunoelectrophoresis it migrates as an alpha globulin, and it possesses antigenic identity with a constituent of normal human plasma (SAP). The amino acid sequence is distinct from that of the amyloid fibrils. Its pentagonal ultrastructure is similar to C-reactive protein (CRP), but the latter is one-half the molecular weight of AP and has other well-defined differences despite a 50 to 60 percent homology on amino acid sequence. AP binds to amyloid fibrils in a calcium-dependent fashion.

IMMUNOBIOLOGY OF AMYLOID The etiology and pathogenesis of amyloidosis are unknown. Electron-microscopic autoradiographic studies have revealed high concentrations of fibrils adjacent to reticuloendothelial cells.

Endotoxin stimulation of macrophages has been shown to produce a mediator (interleukin 1) that stimulates hepatic cells, now recognized as a major source of SAA synthesis, to produce SAA. Other studies suggest that SAA is partially degraded by monocyte or leukocyte surface enzymes to form tissue AA. The other form of amyloid (AL) is probably produced by the partial degradation of immunoglobulins by macrophages.

An excess antigenic stimulus has been shown to induce amyloid in animals. However, the basic conditions for the experimental induction of amyloidosis have not been clearly defined. Marked depression of T cells with maintenance of normal or hyperactive B-cell function has been described. These findings suggest that disturbances in immunoregulatory mechanisms may be an important step in the pathogenesis of amyloid disease. A transferable amyloid enhancing factor (AEF) that can be isolated from the spleens of experimental animals has also been identified.

CLINICAL MANIFESTATIONS The clinical manifestations of amyloidosis are varied and depend entirely on the area of the body which is involved.

Kidney Renal involvement may consist of mild proteinuria or frank nephrosis. In some cases, the urinary sediment may show only a few red blood cells. The renal lesion is usually not reversible and in time leads to progressive azotemia and death. The prognosis does not appear to be related to the degree of the proteinuria; when azotemia finally develops, the prognosis is grave. In one series the mean survival of patients with renal amyloid from the time of biopsy was 29 months, but in a few cases there was presumptive evidence of regression of the renal amyloid. Hypertension is rare except in long-standing amyloidosis. Renal tubular acidosis or renal vein thrombosis may occur. Localized accumulation of amyloid may be noted in the ureter, bladder, or other parts of the genitourinary tract.

Liver While hepatic involvement is common, liver function abnormalities are minimal and occur late in the disease. The two tests most useful in indicating hepatic amyloid are the Bromsulphalein (BSP) extraction and serum alkaline phosphatase activity. Liver scans produce variable and nonspecific results. Portal hypertension occurs but is uncommon. Intrahepatic cholestasis has been noted in about 5 percent of patients with AL (primary) amyloidosis. In a series of 38 patients in whom liver tissue was available for examination, all 38 had some amyloid present, irrespective of the type of amyloidosis (primary or secondary), and contrary to previous notions, parenchymal amyloid was more extensive in the AL cases. Amyloidosis of the spleen characteristically is not associated with leukopenia and anemia.

Heart Cardiac manifestations consist primarily of congestive failure and cardiomegaly (with or without murmurs) and a variety of arrhythmias. Although the cardiac manifestations reflect predominantly diffuse myocardial amyloid, the endocardium, valves, and pericardium may be involved as well. Pericarditis with effusion is rare, although the differential diagnosis of constrictive pericarditis versus restrictive cardiomyopathy frequently arises. Echocardiography has demonstrated symmetric thickening of the left ventricular wall, hypokinesia and decreased systolic thickening of the interventricular septum and left ventricular posterior wall, and left ventricular cavities of small to normal size. Two-dimensional echocardiography is said to produce the characteristic findings of thickened right and left ventricles, a normal left ventricular cavity, and especially a diffuse hyperrefractile "granular sparkling" appearance. Hearts which are heavily infiltrated with amyloid may or may not show an enlarged silhouette. Fluoroscopy usually shows decreased mobility of the ventricular wall; angiographic studies usually demonstrate thickened ventricular wall, decreased ventricular mobility, and absence of rapid ventricular filling in early diastole. Cardiac amyloidosis can present as intractable heart failure. Electrocardiographic abnormalities include a low-voltage QRS complex and abnormalities in atrioventricular and intraventricular conduction, often resulting in varying degrees of heart block. Owing to their propensity to develop conduction defects and arrhythmias, patients with cardiac amyloidosis appear to be especially sensitive to digitalis, and this drug should be used with caution.

Skin Involvement of the skin is one of the most characteristic manifestations of so-called primary amyloidosis. The lesions may consist of slightly raised, waxy papules or plaques which usually are clustered in the folds of the axillae, anal, or inguinal regions, the face and neck, or mucosal areas such as ear or tongue. The lesions are seldom pruritic. Involvement of the skin or mucosa may not be apparent clinically but may be disclosed by biopsy. Gentle rubbing of the skin may induce bleeding into the skin, leading to purpura. Cutaneous involvement also can occur in secondary amyloidosis; in one series it was found in 42 percent of such patients, in 55 percent of a group of patients with primary disease, and in all 11 patients with hereditary amyloid neuropathy.

Gastrointestinal tract Gastrointestinal symptoms are common in amyloidosis. They may result from direct involvement of the gastrointestinal tract at any level or from infiltration of the autonomic nervous system with amyloid. The symptoms include those of obstruction, ulceration, malabsorption, hemorrhage, protein loss, and diarrhea. Infiltration of the tongue occasionally leads to macroglossia. When not enlarged, the tongue may become stiffened and firm to palpation. While infiltration of the tongue is characteristic of primary amyloidosis or amyloidosis accompanying multiple myeloma, it is occasionally seen in the secondary form of the disease.

Gastrointestinal bleeding may occur from any of a number of sites, notably the esophagus, stomach, or large intestine, and may be severe. Amyloid infiltration of the esophagus may lead to an incompetent or nonrelaxing lower esophageal sphincter, nonspecific motility disorders of the esophageal body, or rarely achalasia. Small-bowel lesions may lead to clinical and x-ray changes of obstruction. A malabsorption syndrome is seen at times. Amyloidosis may develop in association with other entities involving the gastrointestinal tract, especially tuberculosis, granulomatous enteritis, lymphoma, and Whipple's disease; differentiation of these conditions, which give rise to secondary amyloidosis, from diffuse primary amyloidosis of the small bowel may be difficult. Similarly, amyloidosis of the stomach may closely mimic gastric carcinoma, with obstruction, achlorhydria, and the radiologic appearance of tumor masses.

Nervous system Neurologic manifestations may include peripheral neuropathy, postural hypotension, inability to sweat, Adie's pupil, hoarseness, and sphincter incompetence. These manifestations are especially prominent in the heredofamilial amyloidoses. The cranial nerves are generally spared except for those involving the pupillary reflexes. Amyloid occurs in the central nervous system as a component of senile plaques, neurofibrillary tangles, and in blood vessels ("congophilic angiopathy"). The protein concentration in the cerebral spinal fluid may be increased. Infiltrates of the cornea or vitreous body may be present in hereditary amyloid syndromes. Certain of these syndromes are characterized by a bilateral scalloping appearance of the pupil. Amyloid may infiltrate the thyroid or other endocrine glands but rarely causes endocrine dysfunction. Local amyloid deposits almost invariably accompany medullary carcinoma of the thyroid. Amyloid infiltration of muscle may lead to a pseudomyopathy.

Joints Amyloid can directly involve articular structures by its presence in the synovial membrane and synovial fluid or in the articular cartilage. Amyloid arthritis can mimic a number of rheumatic diseases because it can present as a symmetric arthritis of small joints with nodules, morning stiffness, and fatigue. Most patients with amyloid arthropathy eventually are found to have multiple myeloma. The synovial fluid usually has a low white blood cell count, a good to fair mucin clot, a predominance of mononuclear cells, and no crystals. Studies of surgical specimens suggest a significant incidence of amyloid in cartilage, capsule, and synovium in osteoarthritis.

Respiratory system The nasal sinuses, larynx, and trachea may be involved by accumulations of amyloid which block the ducts, in the case of the sinuses, or the air passages. Amyloidosis of the lung involves the bronchi and alveolar septa diffusely. The lower respiratory tract is affected most frequently in primary amyloidosis and in the disease associated with dysproteinemia. Pulmonary symptoms attributable to amyloid are present in about 30 percent of these patients and in some are the most serious manifestations of the disease. In secondary amyloidosis, pulmonary disease is a frequent histopathologic accompaniment but seldom gives rise to clinically significant symptoms. Amyloid may also be localized in the bronchi or pulmonary parenchyma and may resemble a neoplasm. In these cases, local excision should be attempted and, when successful, may be followed by prolonged remissions.

Hematopoietic system Hematologic changes may include fibrinogenopenia, increased fibrinolysis, and selective deficiency of clotting factors. Deficient factor X seems to be due to nonspecific calcium-dependent binding to the polyanionic amyloid fibrils. Splenectomy in the patient with such a factor-X deficiency can relieve the deficiency and the associated bleeding disorder.

HEREDOFAMILIAL AMYLOIDOSIS There is no generally accepted nosology for the heredofamilial amyloid syndromes. Some reports emphasize the site of predominant organ involvement as neuropathic, nephropathic, or cardiopathic amyloidosis, while others stress the genetic aspects. To date, virtually all analyses of pedigrees have shown that, with one major exception, the mode of inheritance is autosomal dominant. The exception is amyloidosis of familial Mediterranean fever, which is inherited as an autosomal recessive disorder and is an AA type of amyloid. The recognizable clinical patterns still form the basis for classification, although serum abnormalities (decreased serum prealbumin in several types of familial amyloid polyneuropathy) have been reported. Table 259-2 proposes a tentative

TABLE 259-2 Familial amyloid

Types	Forms
Familial amyloid polyneuropathy	
Type I Portuguese (Andrade)	*1* Portuguese *2* Swedish *3* Japanese *4* Greek *5* English *6* German
Type II Indiana (Rukavina)	*1* Swiss *2* German
Type III Iowa (Van Allen) (possibly same as type I)	*1* Scottish-English-Irish *2* Spanish
Type IV Cranial neuropathy and corneal lattice dystrophy (Meretoja)	*1* Finnish *2* Danish *3* Dutch
Familial oculoleptomeningeal amyloid	*1* German *2* Dutch *3* Japanese
Hereditary cerebral amyloid with hemorrhage	*1* Icelandic
Familial nephropathy	
Type I Familial Mediterranean fever (Heller)(recessive)	*1* Sephardic Jewish *2* Armenian *3* Turkish *4* Arab
Type II Fever and abdominal pain	*1* Swedish *2* Sicilian
Type III Urticaria, deafness, renal disease	
Familial cardiopathy	
Type I Progressive heart failure	*1* Danish
Type II Hereditary atrial standstill	*1* Mexican-American

classification and is based largely on the major site of organ involvement, in addition to genetic data and ethnic background.

The heredofamilial amyloidoses include a group primarily involving the nervous system. Among these are lower limb neuropathy [familial amyloid polyneuropathy (FAP)], first described in Portugal, which has a poor prognosis and is characterized by progressively severe neuropathy including marked autonomic nervous system involvement. This variety also has been described in Japan, Sweden, and in families of Greek and of Swedish origin in the United States. In some of these individuals, bilateral "scalloped" pupils are pathognomonic of the disease. The second type of neuropathy has been found in families of Swiss origin in Indiana and of German origin in Maryland. It is a milder disease and is often associated with a carpal tunnel syndrome and vitreous opacities. A more severe variety of generalized neuropathy associated with renal amyloidosis has been described in Iowa in a family of English-Irish-Scottish ancestry.

Several types of severe familial renal disease in association with amyloid have been described. Possibly the most remarkable is familial Mediterranean fever (FMF), a disorder subdivided into phenotype I, with irregularly occurring fever and abdominal, chest, or joint pain, preceding or accompanying renal amyloid, and phenotype II, in which amyloidosis is the first or only manifestation of the disease (Chap. 271). Colchicine treatment prevents attacks of FMF and appears to prevent subsequent deposition of amyloid as well. Sporadically, other hereditary forms of renal amyloidosis have been described, including the curious association of urticaria, deafness, and renal amyloid.

Severe familial amyloid heart disease has been described in a Danish family, and familial persistent atrial standstill with amyloid in a family of Mexican-American origin. Hereditary cerebral amyloid with hemorrhage in an Icelandic family appears to be due to gamma trace protein deposits and is associated with decreased gamma trace proteins in the cerebrospinal fluid. Miscellaneous hereditary amyloid syndromes include hereditary multiple endocrine neoplasms type II (including medullary carcinoma of the thyroid with amyloid) as well as others listed in Table 259-2.

DIAGNOSIS The specific diagnosis of amyloidosis depends upon obtaining a tissue specimen by biopsy and the demonstration of amyloid with appropriate stains. First, of course, the disease must be suspected. When a patient with a chronic disorder predisposing to amyloid such as rheumatoid arthritis, tuberculosis, paraplegia, multiple myeloma, bronchiectasis, or leprosy develops hepatomegaly, splenomegaly, malabsorption, cardiac disease, or, most importantly, proteinuria, amyloid should come to mind. In addition, in any heredofamilial syndromes, especially those which have a dominant autosomal mode of inheritance and are characterized by peripheral neuropathy, nephropathy, or cardiopathy, the diagnosis of amyloid should be considered. Finally, primary systemic amyloid should be considered in any individual with a diffuse noninflammatory infiltrative disease involving either mesenchymal tissues—blood vessels, heart, gastrointestinal tract—or parenchymal tissues—kidney, liver, spleen, adrenal.

When the diagnosis is suspected, it is good practice to perform an abdominal subcutaneous fat pad aspirate or a rectal biopsy. If there is a specific reason for not carrying out these procedures, other sites including skin, gums, or the suspected organ—kidney, liver—may be biopsied. All tissues obtained must be stained with Congo red and examined in the polarizing microscope for green birefringence. A modified potassium permanganate stain will allow reasonably accurate differentiation of the AA type from AL amyloid. In the former, pretreatment with permanganate, followed by the standard Congo red stain, abolishes the green birefringence (i.e., the tissue is permanganate-sensitive). The AL and AF prealbumin types are permanganate-resistant.

In order to establish the relationship of immunoglobulin-related amyloid to multiple myeloma, electrophoretic and immunoelectrophoretic studies on serum or urine should be performed when the biopsy reveals amyloid deposition. Most of these patients will have only relatively small paraprotein components and only a few will have frank multiple myeloma. The therapeutic implications of these findings are discussed in greater detail in Chap. 258.

PROGNOSIS AND TREATMENT The course of amyloidosis is difficult to document since dating the time of origin of the disease is rarely possible. When amyloidosis develops in patients with rheumatoid arthritis, it seldom becomes evident when the arthritis is less than 2 years in duration. The mean duration of arthritis before amyloidosis was detected was 16 years in one series. When amyloidosis develops in patients with multiple myeloma, manifestations leading to initial hospitalization are more apt to be related to amyloid disease than to myeloma. In these cases prognosis is very poor, and life expectancy is usually less than 6 months.

Instances have been reported of amyloidosis accompanying treatable infections, such as osteomyelitis, in which at least partial remission has occurred following treatment of the primary disease. There have been similar experiences following successful treatment of tuberculosis or drainage of chronic empyema. However, many such reports are not substantiated by biopsy proof of resorption.

Generalized amyloidosis is usually a slowly progressive disease and leads to death in several years, but it may have a better prognosis than was suspected in the past. The average survival in most large series is 1 to 4 years, but a number of individuals with amyloid have been followed 5 to 10 years and longer.

The major cause of death is renal failure. Sudden death, presumably due to arrhythmias, is also quite common. Occasionally, gastrointestinal hemorrhage, respiratory failure, intractable heart failure, and superimposed infections are the terminal events.

There is no specific therapy for any variety of amyloidosis. Rational therapy should be directed at (1) decreasing chronic antigenic stimuli that produce amyloid, (2) inhibition of the synthesis and extracellular deposition of amyloid fibrils, and (3) promoting lysis or mobilization of existing amyloid deposits.

A variety of agents have been used to treat amyloidosis. Proof of their efficacy is not available. The finding that a portion of the immunoglobulin light chain is incorporated in the amyloid of patients with primary amyloidosis and its presumed synthesis by plasma cells has led to the use of alkylating agents. However, these agents cause bone marrow depression, and there are reports of acute leukemia developing in amyloidosis patients receiving melphalan. Moreover, there is experimental evidence that immunosuppressive agents may enhance the deposition of preexisting amyloid. Hence, conservative and supportive measures provide the mainstay of management. It is important to provide these patients with a more optimistic outlook.

Two patients with severe renal amyloidosis and azotemia were subjected to bilateral nephrectomy and renal transplantation followed by immune therapy. One patient died of infection 5 months after surgery. The donor kidney showed no evidence of amyloidosis. The second patient achieved a 10-year clinical remission after receiving a transplanted kidney. Notwithstanding the hazards of operating upon patients with systemic amyloidosis who may have cardiac involvement, carefully selected azotemic patients could benefit from transplantation.

Colchicine has been shown to be effective in preventing acute attacks in patients with FMF, and two groups of investigators independently have reported the inhibition of amyloid deposition in the mouse model by colchicine. It is conceivable, therefore, that colchicine is effective in blocking amyloid deposition. One large preliminary study has shown it to be effective in prolonging life in primary (AL) amyloidosis using a life-table survivorship analysis. However, the exact mechanism of its action is unknown, and no controlled human clinical study has been reported. The role of dimethylsulfoxide (DMSO) in the treatment of amyloid is also under investigation.

REFERENCES

COHEN AS: Amyloidosis. N Engl J Med 277:522, 1967

———, SKINNER M: Diagnosis of amyloidosis, in *Laboratory Diagnostic Procedures in the Rheumatic Diseases*, 3d ed, AS Cohen (ed). Orlando, Fla, Grune & Stratton, 1985

——— et al: Amyloid proteins, precursors, mediator, and enhancer, Lab Invest 48:1, 1983

GLENNER GG et al: Amyloid fibril proteins: Proof of homology with immunoglobulin light chains. Science 172:1150, 1971

——— et al: *Amyloid and Amyloidosis*. New York, Excerpta Medica, 1980

KYLE RA, GREIPP PR: Amyloidosis (AL): Clinical and laboratory features in 229 cases. Mayo Clin Proc 58:665, 1983

section 2 Disorders of immune-mediated injury

260 DISEASES OF IMMEDIATE TYPE HYPERSENSITIVITY

K. FRANK AUSTEN

The term *atopic allergy* implies a familial tendency to manifest alone or in combination such conditions as asthma, rhinitis, urticaria, and eczematous dermatitis (atopic dermatitis). However, individuals without an atopic background may also develop hypersensitivity reactions, particularly urticaria and anaphylaxis, associated with the same class of antibody, IgE, found in atopic individuals. The designation *diseases of immediate type hypersensitivity* presents a more suitable framework than the broad term *allergy* or the restrictive definition of atopy.

The fixation of IgE to human basophils has been demonstrated by radioautography and electron microscopy and to intraepithelial and perivenular mast cells in tonsils, adenoids, and nasal polyps of humans by immunofluorescence. IgE-dependent mediator generation and release also occur in the mast cells of human lung slices, nasal polyps, or skin and have been observed in those tissues most involved in diseases of immediate type hypersensitivity.

Studies with purified rat peritoneal mast cells have indicated that the IgE receptor is transmembrane-linked to adenylate cyclase and that stereospecific receptor perturbation generates second messenger cyclic 3′,5′-adenosine monophosphate (cyclic AMP). Cyclic AMP then activates cytoplasmic cyclic AMP–dependent protein kinase, which presumably acts to phosphorylate cell proteins, thereby continuing the biochemical sequence of the coupled activation-secretion response. A parallel membrane response to stereospecific IgE receptor perturbation involves the formation of calcium ion channels with augmented ion influx and the activation of phospholipases. Phospholipases then cleave membrane phospholipids to generate lysophospholipids or diacylglycerol which, being fusogenic, may facilitate the fusion of the secretory granule perigranular membrane with the cell membrane, a step which releases the membrane-free granule containing the preformed or primary mediators of mast cell effects. The arachidonic acid, generated simultaneously by phospholipase action, is processed oxidatively into secondary mediators of the prostaglandin (Fig. 260-1) and leukotriene (Fig. 260-2) classes. The secretory granule of the human mast cell has a crystalline structure, unlike mast cells of lower species, and IgE-dependent cell activation can be characterized morphologically by solubilization and swelling

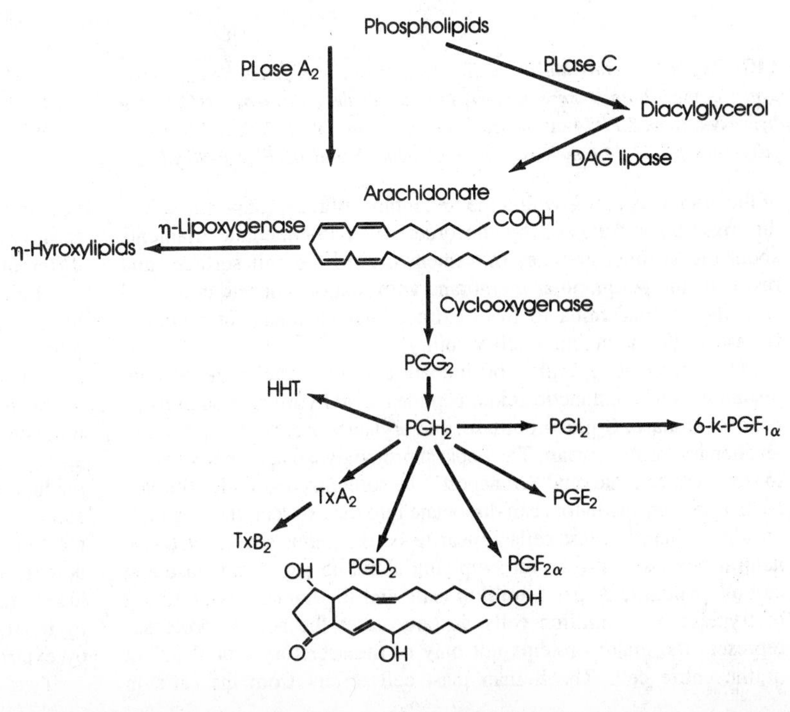

FIGURE 260-1 *Metabolism of phospholipids to arachidonic acid and cyclooxygenase-derived products. Cleavage of arachidonic acid from membrane phospholipids during cellular activation proceeds either by the action of phospholipase A_2 (PLase A_2) or by the sequential action of phospholipase C (PLase C) and diacylglycerol lipase (DAG lipase). Biosynthesis of prostaglandins is depicted with the structure of PGD_2, which is the predominant product from mast cells via the terminal action of a PGD_2 synthetase. η-Lipoxygenase, family of monolipoxygenases; PGG_2, PGH_2, PGI_2, PGE_2, $PGF_{2\alpha}$, PGD_2, prostaglandins G_2, H_2, I_2, E_2, $F_{2\alpha}$, and D_2, respectively; TxA_2, TxB_2, thromboxane A_2 and B_2, respectively; 6-k-$PGF_{1\alpha}$, 6-keto-prostaglandin $F_{1\alpha}$; HHT, 12-hydroxy-heptadecatrienoic acid. [Modified from Schwartz and Austen,* Immunological Diseases, *4th ed (in press).]*

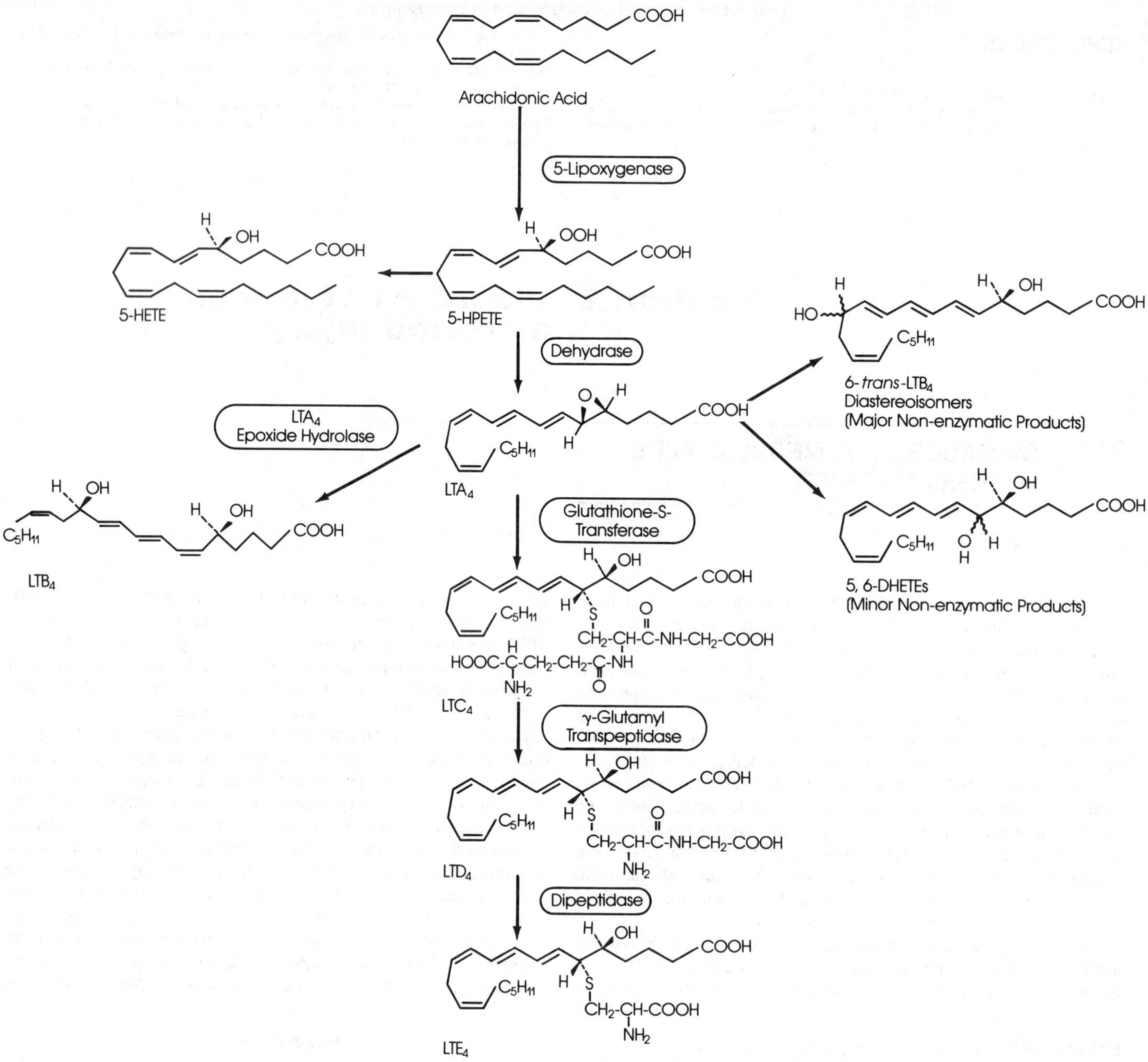

FIGURE 260-2 *Biosynthetic pathways of leukotriene generation. The enzymes of the 5-lipoxygenase pathway are specifically indicated. 5-HETE, 5S-hydroxy-6-*trans*-8,11,14-*cis*-eicosatetraenoic acid; 5-HPETE, 5S-hydroperoxy-6-*trans*-8,11,14-*cis*-eicosatetraenoic acid; 5,6-diHETE, 5,6-dihydroxy-eicosatetraenoic acid; LTA_4, LTB_4, LTC_4, LTD_4, LTE_4, leukotrienes A_4, B_4, C_4, D_4, and E_4, respectively. (Modified from Lewis and Austen, J Clin Invest 73:889, 1984.)*

of the granule contents within the first minute of receptor perturbation; this reaction is followed by the ordering of intermediate filaments about the swollen granule, movement toward the cell surface, and fusion of the perigranular membrane with that of other granules and with the plasmalemma to form extracellular channels for mediator release while maintaining cell viability.

The secretory granules of human and rat mast cells contain histamine; eosinophilactic acidic peptides; acid hydrolases such as β-hexosaminidase, β-glucuronidase, and arylsulfatase; neutral protease; and heparin proteoglycan. The heparin proteoglycan apparently serves to store, concentrate, and "transport" the solubilized granule complex so that primary mediators can dissociate into the extracellular channels by ion exchange. Mast cells appear to be the major source of tissue neutral protease with the rat supplying about 45 μg of chymase and carboxypeptidase A per 1 million cells and the human about 15 μg of tryptase per 1 million cells; in both cases the neutral proteases represent the major proteins not only of the secretory granules, but of the entire cell. The human mast cell differs from the rat's in having about one-tenth the histamine and heparin content, in lacking serotonin, and in containing a physicochemically and functionally different neutral protease.

Human mast cells that have been enzymatically dispersed from lung fragments and concentrated by differential centrifugation and purified rat and murine peritoneal mast cells respond to receptor perturbation by generation of prostaglandin D_2 (PGD_2) in preference to the leukotrienes. However, the remarkable vasoactive and spasmogenic potency of the leukotriene products in human skin and airways in vivo, compared to histamine, prostaglandins, and other mediators, indicates that this class of compounds represents an additional important group of mediators in immediate hypersensitivity reactions. Leukotrienes C_4 and D_4 (LTC_4, LTD_4) are 10^3 times more potent and leukotriene E_4 (LTE_4) is ten times more potent than histamine in impairing airflow in normal subjects when administered by inhalation and assessed in terms of effects on peripheral airways by expiratory flow initiated at 30 percent of vital capacity.

Two subclasses of mast cells have been recognized in terms of histochemical staining characteristics, a connective tissue mast cell distributed to perivenular sites and serosal surfaces and a mucosal mast cell localized primarily to gastrointestinal and bronchial intraepithelial sites. At present the connective tissue mast cell is defined chemically by the presence of heparin proteoglycan in the secretory granule and the mucosal mast cell by a nonheparin (oversulfated chondroitin sulfate) proteoglycan and by a dependence on a T lymphocyte–derived interleukin for proliferation in vivo or in vitro. In addition there is evidence from studies of rodent mast cells that the heparin mast cell subclass preferentially metabolizes arachidonic acid to PGD_2, whereas the non-heparin-containing mast cell yields predominantly LTC_4 and comparable amounts of LTB_4 and PGD_2. Thus, the mast cells, bearing specific recognition units in the form of IgE Fc receptors and positioned at mucosal surfaces and in tissues about venules, are redistributed to portals of entry for foreign substances and can respond in the sensitized host directly and in sequence to alter the microenvironment. A local increase in venular permeability would represent the action of preformed mediators such as histamine and newly generated mediators such as PGD_2 and the sulfidopeptide leukotrienes and would introduce plasma proteins such as those of the complement system and specific antibody. Phagocytic cells would be attracted by chemotactic peptides released from the secretory granule and by the newly generated lipid chemotactic mediator, LTB_4. Local and subclinical regulation of the tissue microenvironment would represent an initial and homeostatic physiologic response, while an intense or continuous stimulus would result in inflammation and tissue injury which could be either beneficial or detrimental (hypersensitivity) depending upon the appropriateness of the immunologic specificity (Fig. 260-3).

Consideration of the mechanism of immediate type hypersensitivity diseases in the human has focused largely on the IgE-dependent recognition of otherwise nontoxic substances. Support for this thesis has come from the finding that clinical atopic allergy is associated with elevated total levels of IgE and in some instances with an immune response that is specifically linked to the histocompatibility locus. Populations of allergic whites have a significantly higher total serum level of IgE than nonallergic individuals, and highly atopic persons with asthma have significantly higher serum levels of IgE than those with fewer allergic manifestations. IgE distribution in families is consistent with the dominant inheritance of the low IgE phenotype. As a result of the action of a single IgE regulator gene the majority of family members would have elevated IgE levels as a possible basis for their atopic state. The association between HLA histocompatibility type and the immediate hypersensitivity response has been noted in persons of the low IgE phenotype who were studied with highly purified allergens, generally of small size. Such presumptive evidence of immune response (Ir) genes by linkage disequilibrium, that is, the association of the hypersensitivity response with a particular histocompatibility haplotype, represents an additional element in the polygenic atopic allergic state. Nonetheless, all the studies taken together, both of families and of populations, seem to indicate that the genetically determined elevated IgE levels found in about three-fourths of atopic allergic subjects exert the predominant influence on most specific IgE responses. It is also likely that diseases of immediate type hypersensitivity may occur because of deficient intracellular controls of mediator generation or release, or both, or that the extracellular controls directed against mediator inactivation may be impaired.

ANAPHYLAXIS Definition The life-threatening anaphylactic response of a sensitized human appears within minutes after administration of specific antigen and is manifested by respiratory distress often followed by vascular collapse, or shock without antecedent respiratory difficulty. Cutaneous manifestations exemplified by pruritus and urticaria with or without angioedema are characteristic of such systemic anaphylactic reactions. Gastrointestinal manifestations include nausea, vomiting, crampy abdominal pain, and diarrhea.

Predisposing factors and etiology There is no convincing evidence that age, sex, race, occupation, or geographic location predisposes a human to anaphylaxis except through exposure to some immunogen. According to most studies, atopy does not predispose individuals to penicillin anaphylaxis.

The materials capable of eliciting the systemic anaphylactic reaction in the human include the following: heterologous proteins in the form of antiserum, hormones, enzymes, Hymenoptera venom, pollen extracts, and foods; polysaccharides such as iron dextran; and most commonly diagnostic agents and drugs such as antibiotics and even vitamins. The diagnostic and therapeutic agents are generally of low molecular weight and are considered to function as haptens which form immunogenic conjugates with host proteins. The conjugating hapten may be the parent compound, a nonenzymatically derived storage product, or a metabolite formed in the host.

Pathophysiology and manifestations Individuals differ in the time of appearance of perception of symptoms and signs, but the hallmark

FIGURE 260-3 *Schematic role for mediators in IgE-dependent reactions.*

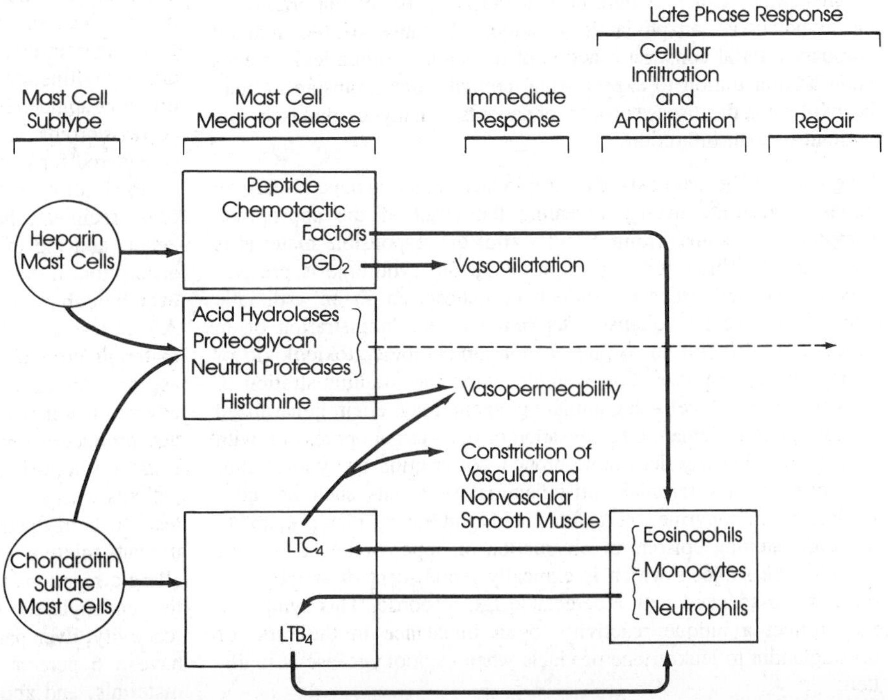

of the anaphylactic reaction is the onset of some manifestation within seconds to minutes after introduction of the antigen, generally by injection or less commonly by ingestion. There may be upper or lower airway obstruction or both. Laryngeal edema may be experienced as a "lump" in the throat, hoarseness, or stridor, while bronchial obstruction is associated with a feeling of tightness in the chest or audible wheezing. A particularly characteristic feature is the eruption of well-circumscribed, discrete cutaneous wheals with erythematous, raised, serpiginous borders and blanched centers. These urticarial eruptions are intensely pruritic and may be localized or distributed. They may coalesce to form giant hives, and seldom persist beyond 48 h. A localized, nonpitting, deeper edematous cutaneous process, angioedema, may also be present. It may be asymptomatic or cause a burning or stinging sensation.

In fatal cases with clinical bronchial obstruction, the lungs show marked hyperinflation on gross and microscopic examination. The microscopic findings in the bronchi, however, are limited to luminal secretions, peribronchial congestion, submucosal edema, and eosinophilic infiltration, and the acute emphysema is attributed to intractable bronchospasm which subsides with death. The angioedema resulting in death by mechanical obstruction occurs in the epiglottis and larynx, but the process is also evident in the hypopharynx and to some extent the trachea; on microscopic examination there is wide separation of the collagen fibers and the glandular elements; vascular congestion and eosinophilic infiltration are also present. Patients dying of vascular collapse without antecedent hypoxia from respiratory insufficiency have visceral congestion but no major shift in the distribution of blood volume. The associated electrocardiographic abnormalities, with or without infarction, noted in some patients could reflect a primary cardiac event or be secondary to a critical reduction in plasma volume.

The angioedematous and urticarial manifestations of the anaphylactic syndrome have been attributed to release of endogenous histamine. A role for the sulfidopeptide leukotrienes in altering pulmonary mechanics by causing marked bronchiolar constriction seems likely. Vascular collapse without respiratory distress in response to experimental challenge with the sting of a hymenopteran was associated not only with marked and prolonged elevations in blood histamine but also with evidence of intravascular coagulation and kinin generation. Based upon the findings that patients with systemic mastocytosis and episodic hypotension proceeding to vascular collapse excrete large amounts of PGD_2 in addition to histamine and are controlled by administration of a nonsteroidal agent but not by antihistamines alone, it may be that PGD_2 is also of importance in the hypotensive anaphylactic reactions. Because of the marked coronary arterial constrictor action of the sulfidopeptide leukotrienes upon administration to experimental animals, these substances may be involved in the disease process of patients with myocardial ischemia without or with infarction.

Diagnosis The diagnosis of an anaphylactic reaction depends largely upon an accurate history revealing the onset of the appropriate symptoms and signs within minutes after the responsible material is encountered. When only a portion of the full syndrome is present, such as isolated urticaria, sudden bronchospasm in an asthmatic patient, or vascular collapse after intravenous administration of an agent, it is difficult to exclude a nonimmunologic, toxicologic or idiosyncratic, response. For example, intravenous administration of a chemical mast cell–degranulating agent may elicit generalized urticaria, angioedema, and a sensation of retrosternal oppression with or without clinically detectable bronchoconstriction or hypotension. Furthermore, nonsteroidal anti-inflammatory agents such as indomethacin, aminopyrine, mefenamic acid, and aspirin may precipitate a life-threatening episode of obstruction of upper or lower airways in asthmatic subjects which is clinically reminiscent of anaphylaxis but is not associated with a detectable IgE response. This syndrome may reflect a unique reactivity to an imbalance in the ratio of prostaglandin to leukotriene products when cyclooxygenase is inhibited.

The presence of a labile reagin (IgE) in the heart blood of a patient dying of systemic anaphylaxis has been demonstrated at postmortem by passive transfer of the serum intradermally into a normal recipient, followed in 24 h by antigen challenge into the same site, with subsequent development of a wheal and flare, the Prausnitz-Küstner reaction. Indeed, such a reagin can be transiently identified in the serum of most patients who develop systemic anaphylaxis to a variety of different agents. In order to avoid the hazards of transferring hepatitis to the recipient in the Prausnitz-Küstner reaction, it is preferable to employ the less sensitive monkey recipient or a human leukocyte suspension enriched with basophils for subsequent antigen challenge. It is presumed that the activity responsible for most cases of systemic anaphylaxis resides with the IgE class, since the Prausnitz-Küstner activity in the serums of patients with systemic reactions to Hymenoptera venom or human seminal plasma protein can be removed by IgE immunosorbent columns. Furthermore, radioimmunoassays have demonstrated specific IgE antibodies in patients with anaphylactic reactions to insulin and to parathormone, but such approaches require purified antigens. In the transfusion anaphylactic reaction which occurs in patients with IgA deficiency, the responsible specificity resides in IgG anti-IgA rather than in IgE; the mechanism of the reaction is presumed to be complement activation with secondary mast cell participation.

Treatment and prevention Early recognition of an anaphylactic reaction is mandatory, since death occurs within minutes to hours after the first symptoms. Mild symptoms such as pruritus and urticaria can be controlled by administration of 0.2 to 0.5 mL of 1:1000 epinephrine subcutaneously, with repeated doses as required at 3-min intervals for a severe reaction. If the antigenic material was injected into an extremity, the rate of absorption may be reduced by prompt application of a tourniquet proximal to the reaction site, administration of 0.2 mL of 1:1000 epinephrine into the site, and removal without compression of an insect stinger, if present. An intravenous infusion should be initiated to provide a route for administration of epinephrine, diluted 1:50,000, volume expanders, and vasopressor agents if intractable hypotension occurs. Epinephrine most likely acts to reverse the action of mediators on target tissues, and its early administration appears critical. When epinephrine fails to control the situation, hypoxia due to airway obstruction or related to a cardiac arrhythmia, or both, must be considered. Oxygen via a nasal catheter or intermittent positive pressure breathing of oxygen with 0.5 mL isoproterenol diluted 1:200 in saline may be helpful, but either endotracheal intubation or a tracheostomy is mandatory if progressive hypoxia exists. Ancillary agents such as the antihistamine diphenhydramine, 50 to 80 mg intramuscularly or intravenously, and aminophylline, 0.25 to 0.5 g intravenously, are appropriate for urticaria-angioedema and bronchospasm, respectively. Intravenous corticosteroids are not effective for the acute event but may be considered for persistent bronchospasm and hypotension.

Prevention of anaphylaxis must take into account the sensitivity of the recipient, the dose and character of the diagnostic or therapeutic agent, and the effect of the route of administration on the rate of absorption. If there is a definite history of a past anaphylactic reaction, even though mild, it is advisable to select another agent or procedure. A skin test should be performed before the administration of certain materials producing a high incidence of anaphylactic reactions, such as horse serum or allergenic extracts, or when the nature of the past adverse reaction is unknown. Since even a skin or conjunctival test can produce a serious reaction, a scratch test should precede these tests in a high-risk situation. With regard to penicillin, two-thirds of patients with a positive reaction history and positive intradermal skin tests to benzylpenicilloyl-polylysine (BPL) and/or the minor determinant mixture (MDM) of benzylpenicillin products experience allergic reactions with treatment, and these are almost uniformly of the anaphylactic type in those patients with minor determinant reactivity. Even patients without a history of previous clinical reactions have a 6 percent incidence of positive skin tests to the two test materials, and about 3 per 1000 with a negative history experience anaphylaxis with therapy with a mortality of about 1 per 100,000. The value of skin testing is both to permit therapy with the agent in question when the risk does not exist and to emphasize the hazards where the sensitivity is confirmed. In the event that an agent must be used despite a positive history, a positive skin test, or both, the following precautionary measures should be taken. An intravenous infusion should be started, with intubation equipment and a tracheostomy set at hand; the material should be given intradermally, then subcutaneously, and then intramuscularly in increasing doses at 20- to 30-min intervals so that the initial dose by the next route does not exceed the final dose by the previous route. It is difficult to be certain that the mediator-containing cells have been exhausted, and therapeutic use of the agent may be accompanied by untoward consequences. It may be critical to give the therapeutic agent at regular intervals to prevent the reestablishment of a sensitized cell pool of large size. A different form of protection involves the development of blocking antibody of the IgG class which is protective against Hymenoptera venom–induced anaphylaxis by interacting with antigen so that less reaches the sensitized tissue mast cells; to be effective this immunotherapy requires the use of specific or cross-reacting Hymenoptera venom rather than whole-insect-body extracts.

URTICARIA AND ANGIOEDEMA Definition Urticaria and angioedema may appear separately or together as cutaneous manifestations of localized nonpitting edema; a similar process may occur at mucosal surfaces of the upper respiratory or gastrointestinal tract. *Urticaria* involves only the superficial portion of the dermis presenting as well-circumscribed wheals with erythematous raised serpiginous borders with blanched centers which may coalesce to become giant wheals. *Angioedema* is a well-demarcated localized edema involving the deeper layers of the skin including the subcutaneous tissue. Recurrent episodes of urticaria and/or angioedema of less than 6 weeks' duration are considered acute, while attacks persisting beyond this period are designated chronic.

Predisposing factors and etiology The occurrence of urticaria and angioedema is probably more frequent than usually described because of the evanescent, self-limited nature of such eruptions, which seldom require medical attention when limited to the skin. Although persons in any age group may experience acute or chronic urticaria and/or angioedema, these lesions increase in frequency after adolescence, with the highest incidence occurring in persons in the third decade of life; indeed, one survey of college students indicated that some 15 to 20 percent had experienced a pruritic wheal reaction.

The classification of urticaria/angioedema presented in Table 260-1 focuses on the different mechanisms for eliciting clinical disease. Only the IgE-dependent and the IgG-mediated reactions in IgA-deficient persons should be considered immediate hypersensitivity. However, the other mechanisms are important for differential diagnosis, and most cases of chronic urticaria are idiopathic. The appearance of urticaria and angioedema in atopic persons in the absence of a specific exposure is attributed to the atopic diathesis and implies an IgE mechanism. Urticaria and/or angioedema occurring during the appropriate season in patients with seasonal respiratory allergy or as a result of exposure to animals or molds is attributed to inhalation of pollens, animal dander, and mold spores, respectively. However, urticaria and angioedema secondary to inhalation are relatively uncommon compared with ingestion of fresh fruits, shellfish, chocolate, nuts, tomatoes, and various drugs, including penicillin-contaminated milk products, which may elicit not only the anaphylactic syndrome with prominent gastrointestinal complaints but also chronic urticaria. Additional etiologies include physical stimuli such as cold, solar rays, exercise, and mechanical irritation (dermographism). Angioedema without urticaria occurs with $C\bar{1}$ inhibitor ($C\bar{1}$INH) deficiency that can be inborn as an autosomal dominant characteristic or can be acquired in association with lymphoproliferative disorders. The urticaria and angioedema associated with classical serum sickness or with idiopathic cutaneous necrotizing angiitis is believed to be an immune-complex disease when hypocomplementemia is a concomitant. The idiosyncratic drug reactions to mast cell granule-releasing agents and to nonsteroidal anti-inflammatory drugs can be systemic, resembling anaphylaxis, or limited to cutaneous sites.

Pathophysiology and manifestations Urticarial eruptions are distinctly pruritic, involve any area of the body from the scalp to the soles of the feet, and appear in crops of 24- to 72-h duration with old lesions fading as new ones appear. The most common sites are the extremities, external genitalia, and face, particularly the region of the eyes and lips. Although self-limited in duration, angioedema of the upper respiratory tract may be life-threatening due to laryngeal obstruction, while gastrointestinal involvement may present with abdominal colic, with or without nausea and vomiting, and may precipitate unnecessary surgical intervention. No residual discoloration occurs with either urticaria or angioedema unless there is an underlying process leading to superimposed extravasation of erythrocytes.

The pathology of urticaria and angioedema is usually characterized by massive edema of the dermis in urticaria, and the subcutaneous tissue as well as dermis in angioedema. Collagen bundles in affected areas are widely separated, and the venules are sometimes dilated. The perivenular infiltrate may consist of lymphocytes, eosinophils, and neutrophils that are present in varying combination and number throughout the dermis. Allergen-induced wheal and flare reactions are characterized by mast cell degranulation and an accumulation of eosinophils over hours to days. The elicitation of a wheal and flare response upon injection of the relevant allergen into a patient with urticaria and/or angioedema, or into a site in a normal recipient prepared with serum from the patient, the Prausnitz-Küstner reaction, indicates an IgE-dependent, mast cell–mediated reaction.

Perhaps the best-studied example of mast cell–mediated urticaria and angioedema is *cold urticaria*. Acquired cold urticaria is a disorder in which patients exposed to cold experience an urticarial eruption that may evolve into angioedema and be associated with syncope. Cryoglobulins, cryofibrinogens, cold agglutinins, or hemolysins may be recognized, but not in the majority of patients. The finding in a number of patients of a serum factor, characterized as being of the IgE class, that is capable of transferring the cold urticaria reaction to a skin site of a normal recipient has focused attention upon the mast cell in this condition. Immersion of an extremity in an ice bath precipitates angioedema of the distal portion with urticaria at the air interface within minutes of the challenge. Histologic studies reveal marked mast cell degranulation with associated edema of the dermis and subcutaneous tissues. The venous effluent of the cold-challenged and angioedematous extremity reveals a marked rise in plasma content of histamine, low-molecular-weight eosinophilotactic activity, and high-molecular-weight neutrophil chemotactic activity which are presumably of mast cell origin, whereas the venous effluent of the contralateral normal extremity contains none of these mediators. Elevations of plasma histamine with biopsy-proven mast cell degranulation have also been demonstrated with systemic attacks of *cholin-*

TABLE 260-1 Classification of urticaria with angioedema

1 IgE-dependent
- *a* Atopic diathesis
- *b* Specific antigen sensitivity (pollens, foods, drugs, fungi, molds, Hymenoptera venom, helminths)
- *c* Physical: dermographism; cold; light; cholinergic; vibratory; exercise-related

2 Complement-mediated urticaria
- *a* Hereditary angioedema
- *b* Acquired angioedema with lymphoproliferative disorders
- *c* Necrotizing vasculitis
- *d* Serum sickness
- *e* Reactions to blood products

3 Nonimmunologic urticaria
- *a* Direct mast cell–releasing agents: opiates; antibiotics; curare, D-tubocurarine; radiocontrast media
- *b* Agents which presumably alter arachidonic acid metabolism: aspirin and nonsteroidal anti-inflammatory agents; azo dyes and benzoates

4 Idiopathic urticaria

ergic urticaria and *exercise-induced erythema-angioedema* precipitated experimentally by exercise on a treadmill while wearing a wet suit.

Diagnosis The rapid onset and self-limited nature of urticarial and angioedematous eruptions are distinguishing features. Additional characteristics are the occurrence of the urticarial crops in various stages of evolution and the asymmetric distribution of the angioedema. Urticaria and/or angioedema involving IgE-dependent mechanisms are often appreciated by historical considerations implicating specific allergens, by seasonal incidence, by exposure to certain environments, or by physical stimuli such as cold, exercise, sunlight (solar urticaria), or trauma (dermographism). Direct reproduction of the lesion with physical stimuli is particularly valuable because it so often establishes the cause of the lesion. The diagnosis can be confirmed by careful testing with the putative foreign substance to determine if a local wheal and flare results, and by passive transfer of such a reaction with serum of the patient to a skin site in a normal recipient, the Prausnitz-Küstner phenomenon. Passive transfer to the skin of a nonhuman primate or in vitro to human basophils may also be attempted. IgE-mediated urticaria and/or angioedema may or may not be associated with an elevation of total IgE or with peripheral eosinophilia. Fever, leukocytosis, or an elevated sedimentation rate are characteristically absent.

The classification of urticarial and angioedematous states noted in Table 260-1 in terms of possible mechanisms necessarily includes some differential diagnostic points. Hypocomplementemia is not observed in IgE-mediated mast cell disease and can reflect either an acquired abnormality generally attributed to the formation of immune complexes or a genetic deficiency of C$\bar{1}$INH. Chronic recurrent urticaria, generally in females, associated with arthralgias, an elevated sedimentation rate, and normo- or hypocomplementemia suggests an underlying cutaneous necrotizing angiitis. Confirmation depends upon a biopsy which reveals cellular infiltration, nuclear debris, and fibrinoid necrosis of the venules.

Hereditary angioedema is an autosomal dominant state associated with the absence of functional C$\bar{1}$INH. The diagnosis is suggested not only by family history but also by the lack of urticarial lesions, the prominence of recurrent gastrointestinal attacks of colic, and episodes of laryngeal edema. Laboratory diagnosis depends upon demonstrating the antigenic lack of C$\bar{1}$INH in most kindreds, but some kindreds have an antigenically intact nonfunctional protein and require a functional assay to establish the diagnosis. The natural substrates of uninhibited C$\bar{1}$, C4, and C2 are chronically depleted but fall further during attacks due to the activation of additional C1 to C$\bar{1}$. An acquired form of C$\bar{1}$INH deficiency, associated with lymphoproliferative disorders, has the same clinical manifestations and differs in the lack of a familial element; in the reduction of C1/C$\bar{1}$ as well as C$\bar{1}$INH, C4, and C2; and in the presence of an anti-idiotypic antibody to the monoclonal immunoglobulin expressed on the B cells.

Urticaria and angioedema must be differentiated from contact sensitivity, an acute vesicular eruption that progresses to chronic thickening of the skin with continued allergenic exposure. They must also be differentiated from atopic dermatitis, a condition that may present as erythema, edema, papules, vesiculation, and oozing proceeding to a subacute and chronic stage in which vesiculation is less marked or absent, and in which scaling, fissuring, and lichenification predominate in a distribution that characteristically involves the flexor surfaces. In cutaneous mastocytosis the reddish-brown macules and papules, characteristic of urticaria pigmentosa, urticate with pruritus upon trauma, and in systemic mastocytosis, without or with urticaria pigmentosa, there is an episodic systemic flushing with or without urticaria but no angioedema.

Prevention and treatment Identification of the etiologic factor(s) and their elimination provide the most satisfactory therapeutic program; this approach is feasible to varying degrees with IgE-mediated reactions to allergens or physical stimuli. Topically applied steroids are of no benefit in the management of urticaria and/or angioedema, and while systemic steroids have no general value, they are helpful in an occasional patient with necrotizing cutaneous angiitis, pressure urticaria, or even ordinary urticaria and angioedema. Antihistamines of the H1 class and sympathomimetic agents often provide symptomatic relief; cyproheptadine, hydroxyzine, and a combination of H1 and H2 antihistamines are held to be even more beneficial. The therapy of inborn C$\bar{1}$INH deficiency has been simplified by the finding that attenuated androgens correct the biochemical defect and afford prophylactic protection. Since the affected individuals are heterozygous, with the depletion of C$\bar{1}$INH being due to a combination of deficient synthesis and excessive utilization of the normal gene product, the efficacy of the attenuated androgens is attributed to production by the normal gene of an amount of functional C$\bar{1}$INH sufficient to contain the spontaneous activation of C1 to C$\bar{1}$. Since the use of such agents for children and pregnant women is not yet accepted, the antifibrinolytic agent ϵ-aminocaproic acid may be used occasionally to control spontaneous attacks or for preoperative prophylaxis in some patients.

ALLERGIC RHINITIS

Definition Allergic rhinitis is characterized by sneezing, rhinorrhea, obstruction of the nasal passages, conjunctival and pharyngeal itching, and lacrimation. Although commonly seasonal because of its relation to airborne pollens, other patterns and etiologies occur. The use of the term "hay fever" to describe seasonal allergic rhinitis is a common convention but is literally inappropriate because the symptom complex is neither produced by hay nor associated with fever.

Predisposing factors and etiology Allergic rhinitis generally presents in atopic individuals, that is, in persons with a family history of a similar or related symptom complex and a personal history of collateral allergy expressed as eczematous dermatitis, urticaria, and/or asthma (see Chap. 202). Symptoms generally appear before the fourth decade of life and tend to diminish gradually with aging, although complete spontaneous remissions are uncommon. A relatively small number of weeds which depend upon wind rather than insects for cross-pollination, as well as certain grasses and trees, produce sufficient quantities of pollen suitable for wide distribution by air currents to elicit seasonal allergic rhinitis. The dates of pollination of these species generally vary little from year to year in a particular locale but may be quite different in another climate. Molds, which are widespread in nature because they occur in soil or decaying organic matter, may propagate spores in a pattern dependent upon climatic conditions. Perennial allergic rhinitis occurs in response to allergens that are present throughout the year such as in desquamating epithelium in animal dander, the processed materials or chemicals utilized in an industrial setting, or the dust accumulating at work or at home. Dust has a diverse content including mites, and many patients with perennial rhinitis are sensitive only to house dust. Moreover, in many patients with perennial rhinitis, no clear-cut allergen can be demonstrated. The ability of allergens to cause rhinitis rather than lower respiratory symptoms may be attributed to their size, 10 to 100 μm, and retention within the nose. However, even when the allergen penetrates to the lower respiratory tract, whether it elicits a bronchoconstrictor response resulting from mediator release depends on the presence of chronically hyperirritable airways.

Pathophysiology and manifestations Episodic rhinorrhea, sneezing, and obstruction of the nasal passages with lacrimation and pruritus of the conjunctiva, nasal mucosa, and oropharynx are the hallmarks of allergic rhinitis. The nasal mucosa is pale and boggy, but the nares are not reddened or excoriated. The conjunctiva may be congested and edematous; the pharynx is generally unremarkable but may appear injected. Swelling of the turbinates and mucous membranes with obstruction of the sinus ostia and eustachian tubes precipitates secondary infections of the sinuses and middle ear, respectively, commonly in perennial but rarely in seasonal disease. Nasal polyps often arise concurrently with edema and/or infection within the sinuses and increase obstructive symptoms.

The nose presents a large mucosal surface area through the folds of the turbinates and serves to adjust the temperature and moisture content of inhaled air and to filter out particulate materials. The convoluted nasal passages readily filter out particles above 10 μm in size by impingement in a mucous blanket at bends in their course; ciliary action then moves the entrapped particles toward the pharynx. Entrapment of pollen and digestion of the outer coat by mucosal enzymes such as lysozymes release protein allergens generally of 10,000 to 40,000 molecular weight. Although the initial interaction occurs between the allergen and intraepithelial mast cells sensitized with specific IgE, the bulk of the mast cells are located beneath the mucosal surface and are recruited secondarily. During the symptomatic season when the mucosa are already swollen and hyperemic, there is enhanced adverse reactivity to the seasonal pollen as well as to antigenically unrelated pollens for which there is underlying hypersensitivity. This priming effect is attributed to improved penetration of the allergens to the deeper perivenular mast cells. Biopsy specimens of nasal mucosa during an episodic allergic reaction show profound submucosal edema with infiltration predominantly by eosinophils, although some neutrophil polymorphonuclear leukocytes are present. Polyps, a feature in perennial rhinitis, are mucosal protrusions containing chiefly edema fluid with variable degrees of eosinophilic infiltration.

The mucosal surface fluid contains not only IgA that is present preferentially because of its secretory piece, but also IgE, which apparently arrives by diffusion from plasma cells distributed in proximity to mucosal surfaces. IgE fixes to mucosal and submucosal mast cells, and the intensity of the clinical response to inhaled allergens is quantitatively related to the naturally occurring or experimentally defined pollen dose. Specific IgE is distributed not only to tissue mast cells but also to circulating basophilic leukocytes; patients with more severe clinical disease have basophils which release histamine in response to lesser concentrations of allergen in vitro than do cells from patients with milder disease. Human nasal polyps from ragweed-sensitive patients release histamine, eosinophilotactic peptides, and spasmogenic leukotrienes upon challenge with ragweed allergen in vitro. In sensitive individuals, the introduction of allergen into the nose is associated with sneezing, "stuffiness," and discharge, and the fluid contains histamine, PGD_2, and leukotrienes. Thus, the mast cells of nasal polyp tissue, and of the nasal mucosa and submucosa, generate and release mediators through IgE-dependent reactions which are capable of producing tissue edema and eosinophilic infiltration.

Diagnosis The diagnosis of seasonal allergic rhinitis depends largely upon an accurate history of occurrence coincident with the pollination of the offending weeds, grasses, or trees. The continuous character of perennial allergic rhinitis due to contamination of the home or place of work makes historical analysis difficult, but there may be a variability in symptoms that can be related to animal exposure or work habits. Patients with perennial rhinitis commonly develop the problem in adult life, are more often women than men, and manifest nasal polyps and thickening of the sinus membranes by x-ray. The term *vasomotor rhinitis* designates a symptom complex resembling perennial allergic rhinitis without an established allergic basis. Other entities to be excluded are exposure to irritants, upper respiratory infection, pregnancy with prominent nasal mucosal edema, prolonged topical use of alpha-adrenergic agents in the form of nose drops, and the use of certain therapeutic agents such as rauwolfia. Nasal polyps are a characteristic of perennial allergic rhinitis and are often associated with sinus infection.

The nasal secretions of allergic patients are rich in eosinophils, and peripheral eosinophilia with elevations in relation to clinical exacerbations is a common feature. Local or systemic neutrophilia implies infection. Total serum IgE is frequently elevated, but the demonstration of immunologic specificity for IgE is critical to an etiologic diagnosis. Some normal individuals will exhibit a wheal and flare skin response to intracutaneous inoculation of high concentrations of common airborne allergens. The diagnosis rests not only on the skin test alone, but also on the correlation of the clinical history with skin reactivity to concentrations of allergen selected by controlled testing. This provides the best balance of selectivity with specificity. Scratch tests with food allergens are unreliable, while intracutaneous testing may be dangerous, and elimination diets are the best approach to the diagnosis. Regardless of method of testing, food allergy is uncommon as a significant cause of allergic rhinitis.

Although standard radioimmunodiffusion techniques can be used to screen for patients with markedly elevated levels of IgE, their sensitivity of less than 1000 ng/mL is insufficient to detect the elevations in most atopic allergic patients. A commonly employed technique, sensitive to about 50 ng/mL, is known as the competitive radioimmunosorbent test (RIST). In this procedure, the IgE of the serum competes with radiolabeled IgE for solid-phase-bound anti-IgE; the displacement of radiolabeled IgE is compared to a standard curve to yield the IgE concentration of the serum. Other assays, such as the noncompetitive RIST, in which the anti-IgE immunosorbent is exposed to a series of standard IgE preparations before introducing the unknown, and double antibody radioimmunoprecipitin test (RIP), have greater sensitivity and reproducibility, respectively, and, like the competitive RIST, establish a normal geometric mean serum IgE for nonallergic whites of less than 120 ng/mL. Even more useful is the measurement of specific anti-IgE in serum by its binding to a solid-phase allergen and quantitation by the subsequent uptake of radiolabeled anti-IgE. This radioallergosorbent technique (RAST) correlates satisfactorily with the bioassay of specific IgE by skin test or histamine release from peripheral blood leukocytes and is convenient for the patients; however, it requires defined allergens and full standardization. Further, neither the immunochemical nor bioassay detection of a previous immune response to a foreign material mandates a therapeutic intervention, unless there is relevant concomitant evidence of a significant clinical problem.

Prevention and treatment Avoidance of exposure to the offending allergen is the most effective means of controlling allergic diseases; removal of pets from the home to avoid animal danders, utilization of air filtration devices to minimize the concentrations of airborne pollens, travel to nonpollinating areas during the critical periods, and even a change of domicile to eliminate a mold spore problem may be necessary. *Immunotherapy,* often termed *hyposensitization,* consists of repeated subcutaneous injections of gradually increasing concentrations of the allergen(s) considered to be specifically responsible for the symptom complex. Controlled studies in ragweed and grass allergic rhinitis have established that patients are partially relieved of their symptoms by such treatments applied over a period of years. Improvement appears to be dose-related, and the end point is based either on severe adverse local or systemic reactions to the allergen injection or on satisfactory relief of symptoms. The immunologic characteristics of a response include a rise in antibodies of the IgG class, a small increase in specific IgE early in the treatment course followed by a plateau or decline, and a decline in the percentage of histamine released from peripheral blood basophilic leukocytes challenged with a fixed concentration of the allergen. The antibodies of the IgG class might well reduce or neutralize the quantity of allergen available for interaction with the tissue mast cells but, more importantly, could modify the seasonal booster response in specific IgE synthesis. None of the individual parameters of the response to immunotherapy correlates well with the assessments of clinical efficacy, suggesting that benefit is derived from a complex of effects. Immunotherapy should be reserved for clearly documented seasonal diseases that cannot be managed with drugs because of their side effects.

Management with pharmacologic agents offers a diverse approach. Antihistamines are the only specific end-organ antagonists available for control of a mast cell–derived reaction and are limited to competition with but one mediator. Nonetheless, antihistamines are very effective for some patients, and the side effects such as drowsiness and gastrointestinal distress, which limit the dosage of a particular preparation, can sometimes be circumvented by use of an agent of different structure. An orally active agent with alpha-adrenergic activity is often employed for its decongestant effects and to partially counteract the drowsiness produced by antihistamines. Topical administration of alpha-adrenergic agents may be helpful but has the immediate disadvantage of rebound vasodilatation, and prolonged usage may produce a chronic rhinitis. The topically active steroids of the beclomethasone class ameliorate symptoms of both seasonal and perennial rhinitis without detectable adrenal suppression and represent a major advance in therapy. Cromolyn sodium inhaled nasally has also given encouraging prophylactic results and is of particular merit because it acts to prevent mast-cell activation.

REFERENCES

AUSTEN KF: Biologic implications of the structural and functional characteristics of the chemical mediators of immediate-type hypersensitivity. The Harvey Lectures, Series 73, 1977–1978, p 93

CAULFIELD JP et al: Secretion in dissociated human pulmonary mast cells. Evidence for solubilization of granule contents before discharge. J Cell Biol 85:299, 1980

CRETICOS PS et al: Peptide leukotriene release after antigen challenge in patients sensitive to ragweed. N Engl J Med 310:1626, 1984

GREEN GR et al: Evaluation of penicillin hypersensitivity: Value of clinical history and skin testing with penicilloyl-polylysine and penicillin G. J Allerg Clin Immunol 60:339, 1977

KALINER M et al: Immunologic release of chemical mediators from human nasal polyps. N Engl J Med 289:277, 1973

LEWIS RA, AUSTEN KF: The biologically active leukotrienes: Biosynthesis, metabolism, receptors, functions, and pharmacology. J Clin Invest 73:889, 1984

MARSH DG et al: Genetics of the human immune response to allergens. J Allerg Clin Immunol 65:322, 1980

SCHWARTZ LB, AUSTEN KF: The mast cells and mediators of immediate hypersensitivity, in *Immunological Diseases*, 4th ed, M Samter et al (eds). Boston, Little, Brown (in press)

SOTER NA et al: Urticaria and arthralgias as manifestations of necrotizing angiitis (vasculitis). J Invest Dermatol 63:485, 1974

———: Release of mast cell mediators and alterations in lung function in patients with cholinergic urticaria. N Engl J Med 302:604, 1980

261 IMMUNE-COMPLEX DISEASES

THOMAS J. LAWLEY / MICHAEL M. FRANK

DEFINITION The term immune-complex disease refers to a group of diseases thought to be mediated by the deposition of immune complexes in specific organ or tissue sites including the glomerulus of the kidney and blood vessel walls. In general these immune deposits are thought to arise from antigen-antibody complexes formed in the circulation. Once deposited in tissues the complexes activate a variety of potent soluble mediators of inflammation, such as the complement proteins, causing an influx of polymorphonuclear neutrophils and monocytes. These activated cells release toxic products of oxygen metabolism as well as various proteases and other enzymes, ultimately causing tissue damage. While the specific etiology of these diseases is variable, they share a common pathophysiology. The clinical features of these diseases are quite diverse, ranging from mild cutaneous eruptions to severe organ involvement with pericarditis, glomerulonephritis, and vasculitis.

PATHOPHYSIOLOGY The introduction of foreign or noxious materials into an individual is often followed by an immune response. Specific antibody produced in the course of this response binds to antigen, forming immune complexes. In general, these complexes are phagocytosed and destroyed by macrophages of the reticuloendothelial system. However, at times these complexes are deposited in tissues, causing inflammation and tissue damage. In recent years, there has been a concerted effort to understand the mechanisms underlying this damage.

The biologic activity of the complexes has been studied in detail. It has been shown that the isotype of antibody affects biologic activity. Thus IgG- and IgM-containing complexes activate the classic complement pathway, and IgA-containing complexes may activate the alternative complement pathway. In contrast, IgE complexes are capable of mediating the degranulation of mast cells by a noncytotoxic, complement-independent mechanism.

The size of the circulating immune complexes is an important parameter of toxicity. In general the larger (>19 S) complexes cause more tissue damage than do smaller complexes. The size is related to the concentration and molar ratio of antibody and antigen, as well as to the avidity of the antibody for the antigen. The ratio of antigen to antibody may range from antibody excess through antigen-antibody equivalence to antigen excess. In antibody excess, antigen valences are saturated and in general the complexes are small. Under conditions of antigen excess, antibody-combining sites are saturated, chances for lattice formation are limited, and again the complexes are small. At equivalence or mild antigen excess, lattice formation is facilitated and large complexes can form. Immune complexes formed at moderate antigen excess are thought to be most pathogenic, perhaps because they are most efficient at activating the various mediator systems like the complement cascade.

Net charge of antigen and antibody also appears to be important in determining the pathophysiologic effect of the complexes. It has been shown that positively charged immune complexes tend to deposit in renal glomeruli, while complexes containing similar antigen with neutral charge tend to penetrate glomeruli slowly. This is presumably due to the fact that the glomerulus presents a negatively charged surface to the circulation. Similarly, there is a relationship between the degree of binding of immune complexes to the basement membrane of skin which is also negatively charged and the degree of positive charge of the complexes.

The first human disease in which circulating immune complexes were thought to play a pathogenic role was serum sickness. In their classic monograph "Die Serumkrankheit," Clemens von Pirquet and Bela Schick described in great detail their experiences with the use of horse antidiphtheria toxin in children. They found that a reproducible reaction pattern occurred 8 to 13 days following the subcutaneous injection of horse serum protein. The patients developed fever, malaise, cutaneous eruptions, arthralgias, leukopenia, lymphadenopathy, and albuminuria. The authors suggested that this reaction pattern was caused by the interaction of host antibody, formed in the 8 days following the injection of the horse serum, with horse serum protein. They believed that this interaction led to the deposition of antigen-antibody complexes in tissue with resulting tissue damage, but the technology necessary to pursue this hypothesis was not available.

Numerous large retrospective studies of human serum sickness confirmed the observations of von Pirquet and Schick, but it was not until the studies of Germuth and Dixon that evidence for the role of circulating immune complexes in serum sickness was obtained. These investigators utilized rabbit models of serum sickness.

In the acute serum sickness model, the injection of antigen is followed by a period of intravascular equilibration and then by intravascular-extravascular equilibration lasting several days. The equilibration period is followed by a progressive decline in the level of antigen in the circulation, representing the normal degradation of the injected serum protein. Following this period of decay, there is a sudden acceleration in the clearance of the antigen from the circulation, usually beginning at about 7 to 8 days. The period of rapid decline in the level of antigen in the circulation is due to the development of an immune response in the recipient animal. This results in the formation of antigen-antibody complexes and subsequent clearance of the complexes from the circulation by the cells of the reticuloendothelial system (RES) (Fig. 261-1). During the period in which the complexes are being formed in the circulation, there is a fall in the animal's serum complement levels. At this time pathologic changes occur in large arteries, renal glomeruli, joints, and cardiac vessels. The glomerulonephritis noted during this period has been studied extensively. It is characterized by swelling of the endothelial cells and marked proteinuria with little hematuria; an infiltrate of monocytes but very few granulocytes is found in the renal glomeruli. Immunofluorescence studies have shown that antigen, host immunoglobulin, and C3 are deposited along the glomerular basement membrane in a typical granular pattern. On electron-microscopic examination of kidney sections, few abnormalities are seen except swelling of endothelial cells. Late in the reaction subepithelial deposits of electron-dense material are noted in some animals; however, at this time fluorescent antibody examination is negative for immunglobulin and complement in the glomeruli. The deposits may represent immunologically altered immunoglobulin or complement.

There is also a very high incidence of arteritis in the coronary artery outflow tract and at branching points of the aorta in the acute serum sickness model. The arteritis is characterized by marked intimal proliferation of endothelium. Polymorphonuclear neutrophils enter the site of intimal proliferation. This is followed by degradation of the internal elastic lamina and adventitia with resulting fibrinoid necrosis of the vessel. On immunofluorescence microscopy, host immunoglobulin, antigen, and C3 are found roughly in the region of the internal elastic lamina, but these immunoreactive materials are rapidly removed and are gone in several days. It has been suggested that the polymorphonuclear neutrophils present in the lesions phagocytize these complexes. In contrast to the findings in glomerulonephritis, materials which decrease complement activity or inhibit the polymorphonuclear response diminish or block the development of arteritis.

At the time of the development of serum sickness in this animal model, there are high-molecular-weight immune complexes in the circulation; the animals that become sick regularly have complexes that are greater than 19 S in their sedimentation characteristics. Acute serum sickness is present only as long as these circulating immune complexes persist and resolves rapidly once the antigen is cleared from the circulation and the immune complexes are gone.

It is possible to induce chronic glomerulonephritis in animals by the repeated intravenous injection of antigen. The dose of antigen injected is critical to the development of the disease. Antigen excess must be produced after each antigen administration, and immune complexes must circulate in the animals. These animals develop glomerulonephritis but not the arteritis characteristic of acute serum sickness.

Other animal models of immune-complex disease closely resemble systemic lupus erythematosus. The most widely studied and best characterized is the disease which occurs spontaneously in the F_1 hybrid of New Zealand black (NZB) and New Zealand white (NZW) mice. These animals develop antibodies to nucleic acids including double-stranded DNA and have decreased numbers of suppressor T cells. They also develop circulating immune complexes and an immune-complex–mediated glomerulonephritis which eventuates in renal insufficiency and death. Direct immunofluorescence microscopy of the kidneys in these animals reveals deposits of DNA, antibodies to DNA, and C3 in the glomerular basement membrane. The female NZB-NZW mice develop these changes before the males, and this sex difference may be related to a switch in the class of antibodies to DNA from IgM to IgG that occurs much earlier in the females than in the males.

Over the years a great deal of attention has been paid to the fate of immune complexes in animal models. Injection of antigens into immunized animals is followed by the deposition of the antigen in the liver, spleen, and lung, all elements of the RES. Detailed studies have examined the fate of preformed immune complexes of carefully determined size in a variety of animals. In general, the findings of these studies have paralleled those reported in the animal models of serum sickness. The larger complexes are rapidly removed from the circulation, and complexes which are greater than 19 S in their sedimentation characteristics are removed so rapidly by the liver that they persist in the circulation for only a matter of minutes. The major factor appearing to govern the rate of clearance of these large preformed complexes from the circulation is the rate of hepatic blood flow. In some studies complement activation by complexes is also important in their metabolism, and injected complexes go through a complex series of processing steps. Large lattice-size complexes appear to be dissociated by complement into smaller entities. Following injection, complexes containing complement components become associated with cells with complement receptors. Human erythrocytes have complement receptors, and these cells appear to be particularly important in the processing of complexes. It is believed that complement-coated complexes associate with complement receptors on red cell surfaces and the complexes are stripped from these cells as they course through the sinusoids of the liver. They are then metabolized. Fc receptors for IgG also play a prominent role in the removal of IgG-containing immune complexes from the circulation, and any manipulation that affects the interaction of Fc receptors and the Fc fragment of IgG in the complexes predisposes to failure to clear the complexes and to tissue deposition. It is possible to measure RES Fc receptor functional activity in patients and normal individuals by intravenously injecting IgG-sensitized autologous radiolabeled erythrocytes and then monitoring the rate of disappearance of these immune particles from the bloodstream. In those diseases with tissue deposition of immune complexes there tends to be an associated RES Fc receptor defect and delayed clearance of the antibody sensitized cells from the circulation.

DETECTION OF CIRCULATING IMMUNE COMPLEXES Many different assays are available for the detection of soluble immune complexes in various biologic fluids. Although these assays vary in their sensitivity and reproducibility, they have expanded our understanding of circulating immune complexes and their role in various disease states. In general, early tests for the detection of circulating

FIGURE 261-1 *The rabbit model of acute serum sickness. Radiolabeled antigen is injected at day 0. After a period of equilibration of antigen between the intravascular and extravascular space, there is progressive elimination of antigen from the circulation. With the onset of the animal's immune response there is rapid elimination of antigen from the circulation. Coincident with the phase of rapid elimination is the appearance of antigen-antibody complexes in the circulation and a fall in serum complement. Complete antigen clearance is associated with the appearance of free antibody in the circulation. At the time when antigen-antibody complexes are seen in the circulation, immunopathologic findings are maximal.*

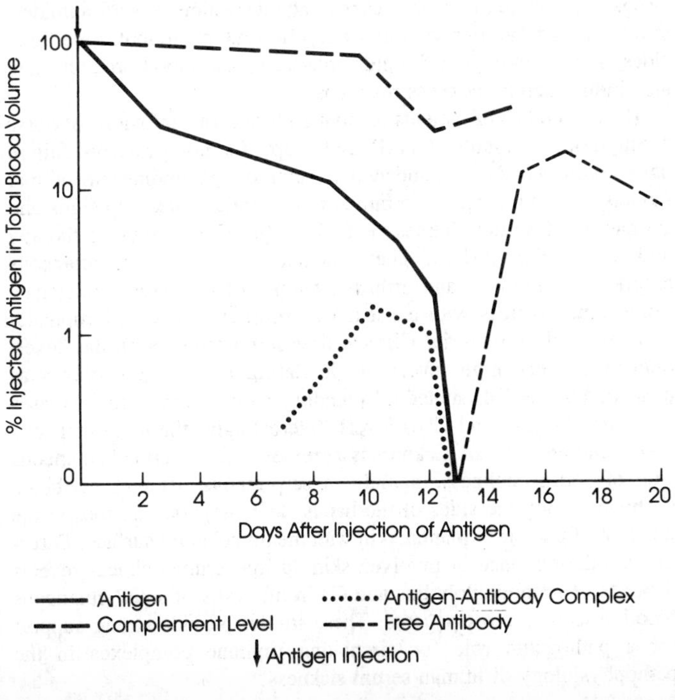

immune complexes relied on physical characteristics of the immune complexes, such as their high molecular weight or cold insolubility. These rather insensitive techniques have been replaced by assays for immunologic components or biologic activities of immune complexes. Although there are now sensitive radioimmunoassays for the detection of circulating immune complexes containing IgG, IgM, and IgA, these tests are not antigen-specific. In fact, in most cases in which circulating immune complexes are demonstrable, the component antigen(s) is (are) unknown. As with most laboratory tests, immune-complex assays may be influenced by other factors. Anticoagulants, endotoxin, and free DNA as well as immunoglobulin aggregates formed after the sample is obtained may result in false-positive results. The impact of these factors can be reduced by the selection of immune-complex assays that are unaffected by these variables and the use of two or more different assays in situations in which critical evaluation of circulating immune complexes is desired. Several of the most sensitive and commonly used immune-complex assays will be described briefly: (1) C1q binding or solid-phase radioassays. C1q is a subcomponent of the first component of complement and will bind to immune complexes containing IgG subclasses 1 to 3 or IgM via noncovalent attachment to a specific site on the Fc portion of immunoglobulin. (2) Raji cell assays. Raji cells are a lymphoblastoid cell line with cell surface receptors for complement, especially C3. The assays are based on the ability of circulating immune complexes which contain bound complement components in their lattices to bind to the surface of the Raji cells via the complement receptors. The bound complexes are easily detected. (3) Conglutinin assays. Conglutinin is a 750,000-dalton nonimmunoglobulin protein found in certain bovine serums that will bind to a cleavage fragment of human C3 known as iC3b. Immune complexes containing iC3b will bind to conglutinin attached to a solid-phase substrate and can be detected.

SERUM SICKNESS Drug hypersensitivity reactions are the most common cause of serum sickness today. Commonly occurring signs and symptoms of serum sickness include fever, cutaneous eruptions (morbilliform and/or urticarial), arthralgias, lymphadenopathy, and albuminuria. Less common manifestations are arthritis, nephritis, neuropathy, and vasculitis. The time required for primary sensitization to an offending agent is approximately 1 to 3 weeks. However, clinical manifestations may develop within 12 to 36 h if there is a history of a previous immunizing exposure. Drug-induced serum sickness usually abates within days after withdrawal of the causative agent. Reactions may persist for longer intervals, particularly if repository or long-acting agents are responsible for the problem. Drugs responsible for serum sickness include penicillin, sulfonamides, thiouracils, hydantoins, *p*-aminosalicyclic acid, phenylbutazone, thiazides, and streptomycin. Foreign antiserums and blood products may also induce serum sickness reactions.

Recent studies of patients receiving intravenous infusions of horse antithymocyte globulin (ATG) as therapy for bone marrow failure have confirmed and expanded the immunologic findings in animal models of serum sickness in humans. The patients develop signs and symptoms of serum sickness 8 to 13 days after beginning therapy with ATG (Fig. 261-2). These include fever; malaise; cutaneous eruptions; arthralgias and arthritis, mainly of the large joints; gastrointestinal distress with nausea, vomiting, and melena; lymphadenopathy, and proteinuria. Clinical disease coincides with the development of very high levels of circulating immune complexes as measured by the ^{125}I-labeled C1q binding assay and marked decreases in serum C3, C4, and CH_{50} levels. Interestingly, the first cutaneous manifestation of serum sickness is a previously undescribed cutaneous sign of serum sickness, namely, a serpiginous band of erythema occurring along the sides of the hands, feet, fingers, and toes at the junction of palmar or plantar skin with the dorsolateral surface. Direct immunofluorescence of involved skin during serum sickness reveals deposits of immunoglobulins and C3 in the walls of small cutaneous blood vessels in most patients. These studies provide strong support for a pathogenic role for circulating immune complexes in the pathophysiology of human serum sickness.

SYSTEMIC LUPUS ERYTHEMATOSUS Systemic lupus erythematosus (SLE) is a multisystem disease associated with a number of immunologic abnormalities including the production of autoantibodies, hypergammaglobulinemia, suppressor T-cell abnormalities, decreased levels of serum complement, and increased levels of circulating immune complexes. Immune complexes are thought to play a critical role in the pathophysiology of SLE. Early evidence for the role of circulating immune complexes in SLE included the finding by direct immunofluorescence of glomerular deposits of immunoglobulin, complement, and DNA in kidney biopsies. Mixed IgM-IgG cryoglobulins were found in the serums of a substantial number of SLE patients, and when the antibody specificity of these cryoprecipitates was examined, reactivity was found against single- and double-stranded DNA as well as ribonucleoprotein. Utilizing the newer, more sensitive assays, circulating immune complexes have been found in a high percentage of patients with SLE. An explanation for the continued circulation of immune complexes in patients with SLE has been provided by the demonstration of defective function of the reticuloendothelial system (RES) in these patients. Patients with SLE have been shown to have delayed clearance of autologous red blood cells coated with IgG from the circulation, suggesting an impaired function of RES Fc-IgG receptors. The prolonged RES clearance in these patients was found to be correlated with increased levels of circulating immune complexes as measured by the C1q binding assay and with clinical disease activity. Studies in these same patients after their disease improved with treatment revealed a significant correlation between clinical improvement, improvement of Fc-mediated clearance, and decreased levels of circulating immune complexes. Individuals with SLE also have decreased numbers of C3b receptors on their erythrocytes. Whether the decreased number of receptors is primary or secondary remains to be established. Nonetheless, abnormalities of both Fc-IgG and C3b receptors which are responsible for phagocytosis of circulating immune complexes are present in patients with SLE.

VASCULITIS There is strong circumstantial evidence for the role of circulating immune complexes in the various forms of hypersensitivity or necrotizing vasculitis. Features of the classic "palpable purpura" of cutaneous necrotizing vasculitis closely resemble the clinical, histopathologic and immunopathologic features of the Arthus reaction. The Arthus reaction is a model for immune-complex–mediated vascular damage in which antigen is injected intradermally into an animal which possesses circulating antibody against that antigen. In both vasculitis and the Arthus reaction, deposits of immunoglobulin and complement are found in the walls of blood vessels in early lesions. The histopathology of both consists of infiltrates of polymorphonuclear neutrophils, leukocytoclasis, endothelial cell damage and necrosis, hemorrhage, and perivascular deposits of fibrin. Electron microscopy of lesions of cutaneous necrotizing vasculitis reveals subendothelial electron-dense deposits compatible with immune complexes. The available evidence indicates the presence of immune complexes at the site of tissue damage in necrotizing vasculitis. In accord with these findings is the demonstration of circulating immune complexes in a high percentage of patients with this disease.

LABORATORY FINDINGS In theory the essential feature of immune-complex disease would be the finding of circulating immune complexes. In practice there is great variability from disease to disease in the frequency of positive immune-complex assays. In some diseases such as SLE there is a high frequency of positive immune-complex assays. In others like membranoproliferative glomerulonephritis the frequency of positive assays is much lower. Part of the reason for this has to do with the stage of disease under study. In some cases immunologic phenomena are responsible for the initiation of the disease and the initial tissue insult. However, subsequent injury is caused by scarring, inflammation, and repair mechanisms that result in more extensive tissue damage. Thus, disease progression may occur at a time when immunologic injury is no longer occurring. A second reason for the failure to detect circulating immune complexes in diseases thought to be mediated by them has to do with technical difficulties in the measurement of such complexes. There are many types of assays for immune complexes. Most are indirect and rely on a biologic or biochemical property of the complexes such as the binding of complement components. The pattern of positive reaction clearly varies from disease to disease. Clearly each assay recognizes a different type of complex with maximal efficiency. Since multiple assays are rarely performed on one specimen, complexes, although present, may not be detected. Finally, although a disease is classified as immune-complex–related because of the finding of immune deposits in affected tissues or because of the similarity of pathologic findings to animal models, the disease may not be actually caused by circulating immune complexes. For example, antibody may be formed to a tissue component, bind to it in a tissue site, and induce damage. Such is thought to be the case in Goodpasture's disease. For all of these reasons assays for the detection of circulating immune complexes are generally used only for research purposes and are rarely critical for diagnosis or patient management.

Examination of tissues using immunofluorescent techniques to detect immune deposits is also of great interest in establishing the diagnosis of immune-complex disease. Immune complexes deposited in tissues may be evanescent. For example, in cutaneous vasculitis, lesions must be biopsied within 12 h of their appearance. Although helpful in diagnosis and in establishing pathogenesis, testing for immune deposits in tissue is rarely required for diagnosis.

Another test commonly used to infer the presence of immune complexes is the measurement of serum complement. Decreased levels are taken to indicate the presence of complexes. In fact, it has been suggested that the levels of serum C4 and C3 are the most sensitive indexes of disease activity in SLE. However, the correlation between disease activity and complement levels is rough at best, and some patients with active SLE may have relatively normal complement levels for several reasons. The normal range of complement component levels is wide, and a given patient may have depressed levels with serum concentrations falling from high normal levels to low normal levels. In general complement components act as acute phase reactants, and the lowering of serum complement may be masked by increased synthesis. Moreover, under many circumstances activation of complement may mediate profound pathophysiologic effects, although few molecules of complement are actually involved. For example, complement binding to red cells may be responsible for much of the red cell destruction that occurs with ABO mismatched transfusions; yet serum complement levels may be unchanged because too few molecules are used in erythrocyte destruction to detect a fall in titer. Finally, all types of complexes do not activate complement in the

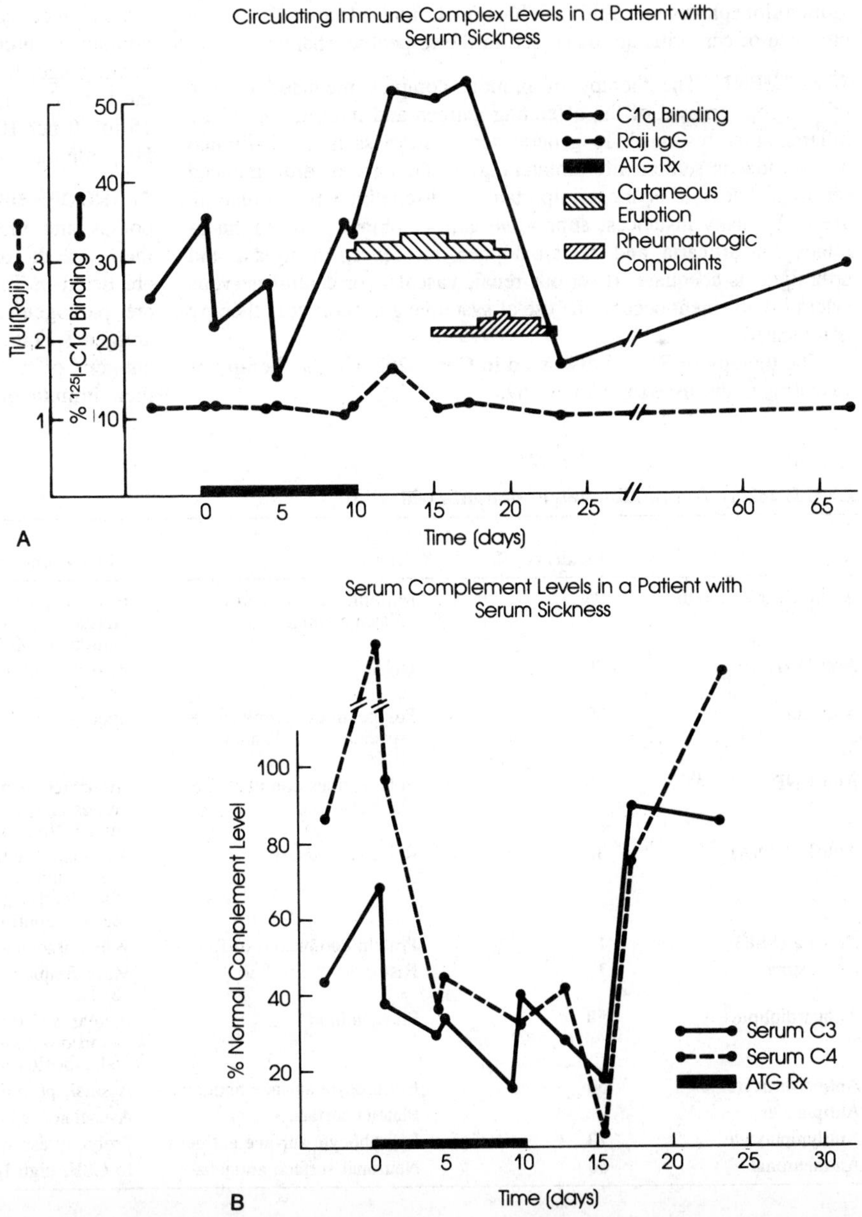

FIGURE 261-2 *Serum sickness in human beings. Horse antithymocyte globulin was injected into patients with aplastic anemia daily for 10 days. After the fifth day of injection, C1q binding activity begins to rise (A). At the same time there is a dramatic fall in plasma levels of C3 and C4 and onset of clinical symptoms (B).*

same way. Massive antigen release from red cells occurring during the course of vivax malaria infection leads to the rapid formation of antigen-antibody complexes in the circulation. For unknown reasons these complexes only interact with the early components of the classic complement pathway, while C3 and the later complement components are not recruited. Thus, if one measures levels of C3, no fall in titer is noted, although complexes are present and massive complement activation has taken place. The complexes formed in SLE activate optimally the classic pathway; presumably those involved in IgA glomerulonephritis activate the alternative pathway. Therefore, the complement test chosen for examination may be important.

Other tests may suggest indirectly the presence of immune-complex disease. For example, a finding of mixed IgG-IgM cryoprecipitates suggests the presence of immune complexes. The presence of antinuclear antibodies suggests autoimmunity, as does the presence of a number of tissue-component-specific antibodies. Similarly the presence of specific antigen such as hepatitis B surface antigen in the circulation together with appropriate clinical symptoms may suggest an immune-complex disease. Most patients with active immune-complex–mediated disease have an elevated erythrocyte sedimentation rate, although this is not invariably the case. Patients with Takayasu's arteritis may have a normal erythrocyte sedimentation rate during the later phases of the evolution of lesions where most pathology is caused by scarring, fibrosis, and repair within vessel walls. Finally, specific laboratory tests such as red cell casts in the urine in glomerulonephritis or mild cerebrospinal fluid pleocytosis in the presence of cerebritis are discussed in the respective chapters.

TREATMENT The therapy of immune-complex–mediated disease relies upon removal of the offending antigen and interruption of the inflammatory response. In general serum sickness is a self-limited disease that is seldom life-threatening. In the case of drug-induced serum sickness it is most important to discontinue the offending agent. In many instances, supportive care combined with antihistamines for urticaria and acetaminophen for fever, myalgias, and arthralgias is adequate. If serious renal, vascular, or central nervous sytem involvement occurs, the use of systemic glucocorticoid therapy is indicated.

The therapy of SLE is discussed in Chap. 262 and the therapy of vasculitis is discussed in Chap. 269.

REFERENCES

Cochrane CB, Koffler D: Immune complex disease in experimental animals and man. Adv Immunol 16:185, 1963

Dixon F: The role of antigen-antibody complexes in disease. Harvey Lect 52:21, 1963

Frank MM et al: Immunoglobulin G Fc receptor mediated clearance in autoimmune diseases. Ann Intern Med 98:206, 1983

Germuth FC Jr.: A comparative histologic and immunologic study in rabbits of induced hypersensitivity of the serum sickness type. J Exp Med 97:257, 1953

Lawley TJ et al: A prospective clinical and immunologic analysis of patients with serum sickness. N Engl J Med 311:1407, 1984

Mannik M, Arend WP: Fate of preformed immune complexes in rabbits and rhesus monkeys. J Exp Med 134:19s, 1971

von Pirquet C, Schick B: Serum sickness. Baltimore, Williams & Wilkins, 1951

Theofilopoulos AN, Dixon FJ: The biology and detection of immune complexes. Adv Immunol 28:89, 1979

262 SYSTEMIC LUPUS ERYTHEMATOSUS

BEVRA HANNAHS HAHN

DEFINITION AND PREVALENCE Systemic lupus erythematosus (SLE) is a disease of unknown etiology in which tissues and cells are damaged by deposition of pathogenic autoantibodies and immune complexes. Ninety percent of cases occur in women, usually of child-bearing age, but children, men, and the elderly can be affected. In the United States, the prevalence of SLE in urban areas varies from 15 to 50 per 100,000; it is more common in blacks than in whites. Hispanic and Asian populations also are susceptible.

PATHOGENESIS AND ETIOLOGY Production of pathogenic antibodies and immune complexes, coupled with failure to suppress them, are the basic abnormalities underlying SLE. These antibodies are listed in Table 262-1. Not all antibodies or immune complexes are pathogenic. Some antibodies cause disease because of their antigen specificity. Examples are antibodies to erythrocyte surface antigens or to coagulation factors. Others cause disease because of their immunoglobulin (Ig) isotype, ability to fix complement (C′),

TABLE 262-1 Autoantibodies in patients with SLE

	Incidence, %	Antigen detected	Clinical importance
Antinuclear antibodies	95	Multiple nuclear and cytoplasmic antigens	Human cell line substrates are more sensitive than standard murine tissues. A repeatedly negative test on both makes SLE diagnosis unlikely. Multiple antibodies are detected.
Anti-DNA	70	DNA	Anti-dsDNA is relatively disease-specific; anti-ssDNA is not. Associated with nephritis and clinical activity.
Anti-Sm	30	Polypeptides complexed to 6 species of small nuclear RNA	Specific for SLE.
Anti-RNP	40	Polypeptides complexed to U1RNA	High titer seen in syndromes with features of polymyositis, scleroderma, lupus and mixed connective tissue disease. If present in SLE without anti-DNA, risk for nephritis is low.
Anti-Ro (SSA)	30	RNA polymerase	Associated with Sjögren's syndrome, DR3 haplotype, subacute cutaneous lupus, complement deficiencies, ANA-negative lupus, lupus in the elderly, neonatal lupus, congenital heart block in infants. Can cause nephritis.
Anti-La (SSB)	10	Protein complexed to RNAs	When associated with anti-Ro, risk for nephritis is low.
Antihistone	70	Histones	More frequent in drug-induced LE (95 percent) than in spontaneous SLE.
Anticardiolipin	50	Phospholipid	Increases risk for venous or arterial thrombosis and for spontaneous abortion. Associated with prolonged PTT (lupus anticoagulant) and false-positive VDRL.
Antierythrocyte	60	Erythrocyte surface antigens	A small proportion of these patients develop overt hemolysis.
Antiplatelet	–	Platelet surface	Associated with thrombocytopenia.
Antilymphocyte	70	Lymphocyte surface antigens	Probably associated with leukopenia and abnormal T-cell function.
Antineuronal	60	Neuronal surface antigens	In CSF, high IgG titers correlate with diffuse but not focal CNS lupus.

tissue avidity, and/or electric charge. For example, complement-fixing cationic antibodies bind to the polyanions in glomerular basement membrane, fix complement, and cause tissue damage.

The pathogenesis of SLE includes genetic, environmental, and sex hormonal factors; abnormal humoral and cellular immune responses; and inadequate clearing of antibodies and immune complexes. Genetic predisposition is indicated by high concordance for clinical disease in monozygotic but not dizygotic twins, a 10 percent frequency of patients with more than one affected individual in the family, a significantly increased frequency of the MB1/MT1 HLA haplotype (and of HLA-DR2 and -DR3 in some studies), and the fact that 6 percent of SLE patients have inherited deficiencies of complement components, especially C2. Viruses have been suspected as etiologic agents but this is not proven. Phospholipids in cell walls of enteric bacteria may act as polyclonal B-cell activators or antigens to elicit antibodies cross-reactive with the ribose phosphate backbone in DNA. In some patients, exposure to ultraviolet light causes disease flare-ups, probably by altering the antigenicity of DNA or the composition of dermal-epidermal junctions. Sex hormonal influences contribute to the pathogenesis of SLE. In general, estrogen enhances and testosterone reduces antibody responses. Men and women with SLE have increased hydroxylation of estrogen and estrone to 16α-hydroxyestrone, producing prolonged estrogenic stimulation. The ultimate outcome of all these factors is B-cell hyperactivity, accompanied by multiple abnormalities in immunoregulation. For example, quantities of T helper/inducer and T suppressor/cytotoxic cells are diminished during periods of disease activity, and many functions are abnormal, including their ability to suppress anti-DNA synthesis or to participate in direct and antibody-mediated cytotoxicity. Ability of T cells to secrete interleukins is suppressed, and abnormal interferon is produced by macrophages. Failure to suppress antibodies also results from abnormalities in the humoral idiotype–anti-idiotype network. Finally, immune complexes are cleared more slowly than normal, related in part to both inherited and acquired deficiencies of complement receptors (CR1) on cell surfaces.

Clinical manifestations of the disease are determined by which antibody subpopulations and immune complexes are present in the patients' repertoire, which organs, cells, or cell products are their targets, and which patients have the ability to correct these abnormalities.

CLINICAL MANIFESTATIONS At its onset, SLE may involve only one organ system, with additional manifestations occurring later, or may be multisystemic. Clinical manifestations are listed in Table 262-2. Autoantibodies are usually (but not always) detectable on the patient's initial visit. Disease severity varies from mild and intermittent to persistent and ultimately fatal. Most patients experience exacerbations interspersed with periods of relative quiescence. Fewer than 10 percent have long-lasting symptom-free remissions. *Systemic symptoms* are usually prominent and include fatigue, malaise, fever, anorexia, weight loss, and nausea.

Musculoskeletal Almost all SLE patients experience arthralgias and myalgias; most develop arthritis. Pain is often out of proportion to physical findings, which include symmetric fusiform swelling of joints [most frequently proximal interphalangeal (PIP) and metacarpophalangeal (MCP) joints of the hands, wrists, and knees], diffuse puffiness of hands and feet, and tenosynovitis. Joint deformities are unusual, although 10 percent of patients develop swan neck deformities and ulnar drift at the MCP joints. Erosions are rare, but subcutaneous nodules over the elbows and fingers occur. Myopathy can be inflammatory and related to active disease, or iatrogenic, secondary to hypokalemia or direct damage caused by glucocorticoids or hydroxychloroquine. Ischemic necrosis of bone also causes "joint" pain and is a common cause of hip and shoulder pain in these patients.

Cutaneous The *malar ("butterfly") rash* is a fixed erythematous rash, flat or raised, over the cheeks and bridge of the nose, often involving the chin and ears. It is usually exacerbated by ultraviolet light. Scarring is absent, but telangiectasias may develop. A more diffuse maculopapular rash, predominant in sun-exposed areas, is also common. Its presence usually indicates disease flare-up. Loss of scalp hair (which often heralds a flare-up) is usually patchy but can be extensive; the hair will regrow, except in discoid lupus erythematosus (DLE). *Vasculitic skin lesions* include subcutaneous nodules, ulcers (usually on the legs), purpura, and infarcts of skin or digits. *DLE lesions* occur in some patients with SLE and can be disfiguring. They are circular with an erythematous rim, raised, and scaly with follicular plugging and telangiectasia. Central scarring produces depigmentation and permanent loss of appendages. They

TABLE 262-2 Clinical manifestations of SLE

	Percent of patients positive during course of disease
Systemic	95
Fatigue, malaise, fever, anorexia, nausea, weight loss	95
Musculoskeletal	95
Arthralgias/myalgias	95
Nonerosive polyarthritis*	60
Hand deformities	10
Myopathy/myositis	40/5
Ischemic necrosis of bone	15
Cutaneous	80
Malar rash*	50
Discoid rash*	15
Photosensitivity*	40
Oral ulcers*	40
Other rashes—maculopapular, urticarial, bullous, subacute cutaneous lupus	40
Alopecia	40
Vasculitis	20
Panniculitis	5
Hematologic	85
Anemia (of chronic disease)	70
Hemolytic anemia } *	10
Leukopenia (<4000/mm^3) } *	65
Lymphopenia (<1500/mm^3) } *	50
Thrombocytopenia (<100,000/mm^3) } *	15
Circulating anticoagulant	10–20
Splenomegaly	15
Lymphadenopathy	20
Neurologic	60
Organic brain syndromes	35
Psychosis } *	10
Seizures } *	20
Other CNS (see text)	15
Peripheral neuropathy	15
Cardiopulmonary	60
Pleurisy } *	50
Pericarditis } *	30
Myocarditis	10
Endocarditis (Libman-Sacks)	10
Pleural effusions	30
Lupus pneumonitis	10
Interstitial fibrosis	5
Pulmonary hypertension	<5
ARDS/hemorrhage	<5
Renal	50
Proteinuria >500 mg/24 h } *	50
Cellular casts } *	50
Nephrotic syndrome	25
Renal failure	5–10
Gastrointestinal	45
Nonspecific (anorexia, nausea, mild pain,	30
diarrhea)	5
Vasculitis—with bleeding or perforation	<5
Ascites	40
Abnormal liver enzymes	15
Thrombosis	15
Venous	10
Arterial	5
Ocular	15
Retina vasculitis	5
Conjunctivitis/episcleritis	10
Sicca syndrome	15

* *In addition to two positive laboratory tests [positive ANA plus one or more of (1) positive LE cells, (2) anti-dsDNA, (3) anti-Sm, or (4) false-positive VDRL], a combination of these clinical and laboratory manifestations totalling four meet American Rheumatism Association criteria for classifying patients in SLE. Bracketed features count as one, even if more than one are present, e.g., leukopenia plus thrombocytopenia = one criterion.*

occur over the scalp, external ears, face, and sun exposed areas of the arms, back, and chest. Only 5 percent of individuals with DLE progress to SLE; however 20 percent of SLE patients have DLE lesions. Less frequent SLE skin lesions include urticaria, periorbital edema, bullae, erythema multiforme, lichen-planus–like lesions, and panniculitis (''lupus profundus'').

Patients with *subacute cutaneous lupus* (SCLE) are a distinct subset with recurring extensive skin lesions. Arthritis and fatigue are frequent; central nervous system and renal involvement are not. Some patients are antinuclear antibody (ANA)–negative. The majority have antibodies to Ro (SS-A) or to single-stranded (ss) DNA and carry the HLA-DR3 phenotype. The skin lesions are photosensitive polycyclic annular or papulosquamous psoriasiform over the arms, trunk, and face; they become hypopigmented but not scarred.

Mucous membrane lesions are usually small, shallow, painless ulcers in the mouth (usually over the palate) and nose.

Renal manifestations Although almost all patients with SLE have deposits of immunoglobulin in glomeruli, only one-half have clinical nephritis, defined by persistent proteinuria. At presentation, most patients are asymptomatic (unless already uremic) except for those with edema of the nephrotic syndrome. Urinalysis shows hematuria, cylindruria, and proteinuria. As discussed under ''Pathology'' (see below), most patients with mesangial or mild focal glomerulonephritis do not develop deterioration of renal function. In patients with more severe, active, or chronic lesions, renal failure is a major cause of death. Since mild lesions may not require aggressive therapy with glucocorticoids and/or cytotoxic drugs, whereas severe lesions do, renal biopsy may provide information that will affect therapeutic decisions over the subsequent several months. Patients with deteriorating renal function and active urine sediment also require prompt, aggressive therapy; biopsy is not necessary unless they fail to respond. However, patients with a high proportion of sclerotic glomeruli on biopsy (usually with a serum creatinine >3 mg/100 mL) are unlikely to respond to immunosuppressive therapy. In these cases, dialysis or transplantation should be planned. Patients with persistently abnormal urinalyses associated with high titers of antibodies to double-stranded (ds) DNA and hypocomplementemia are also at risk for severe nephritis; kidney biopsy is useful in these cases if the results are likely to have an impact on therapeutic decisions.

Nervous system Any region of the brain can be involved in SLE, as can the meninges, spinal cord, and cranial and peripheral nerves. Central nervous system (CNS) events may be isolated, single, or multiple, but usually occur in the setting of active disease in other systems. Mild mental dysfunction is the most frequent manifestation. Seizures are frequent and may be grand mal, petit mal, or focal. Other manifestations include psychosis, organic brain syndromes, headache (including migraine), focal infarcts with resultant deficits, extrapyramidal disorders, cerebellar dysfunction, hypothalamic dysfunction with inappropriate ADH secretion, pseudotumor cerebri, subarachnoid hemmorrhage, aseptic meningitis, transverse myelitis with paraplegia or quadriplegia, optic neuritis, cranial nerve palsies, and peripheral sensorimotor neuropathy resulting either in mononeuritis multiplex or glove-and-stocking deficit. Depression and anxiety are frequent.

The laboratory diagnosis of CNS disease can be difficult. Abnormal electroencephalograms are found in about 70 percent of patients and usually show diffuse slowing or focal abnormalities. The cerebrospinal fluid (CSF) shows elevated protein levels in 50 percent and an elevated number of mononuclear cells in 30 percent of patients. Lumbar puncture should be performed whenever CNS symptoms could result from infection, especially in patients receiving immunosuppressive therapy. Brain scans (including CAT), nuclear magnetic resonance imaging, and angiograms are most likely to be positive when focal neurologic deficits are present, and are less helpful in cases with diffuse, nonfocal manifestations. Standard laboratory measures of disease activity (Table 262-3) often do not correlate with neurologic manifestations. Neurologic problems usually improve (with the exception of deficits related to infarcts) with therapy and/or time; recurrences are common.

TABLE 262-3 Laboratory manifestations of SLE

Tests which help *confirm the clinical diagnosis and predict severity*	Tests which may be helpful in *following the clinical course**
Relatively specific for SLE:	Titer of anti-dsDNA
Anti-dsDNA	Serum complement levels
Anti-Sm	Westergren erythrocyte sedimentation rate
Not specific:	Hematocrit
ANA (most sensitive)	Leukocyte count
CH_{50}, C3, C4	Platelet count
Anti-Ro	Urinalysis
Direct Coombs' test	Serum creatinine
VDRL	
PTT	
Anticardiolipin	
Hematocrit	
Leukocyte count	
Platelet count	
Urinalysis	
Serum creatinine	

* *For each patient, the pattern of laboratory abnormalities (if any) associated with a disease flare-up should be established and only those tests used as adjunct to clinical assessments.*

Vascular Thrombosis in capillaries, in small vessels, and in medium-sized veins and arteries can be a major problem. Although vasculitis may play a role, there is increasing evidence that antibodies against phospholipids (anticardiolipin) may initiate clotting. These antibodies may be the ''lupus anticoagulant.'' In addition, degenerative vascular changes associated with years of immune-complex deposition in vessel walls may predispose to symptomatic coronary artery disease in relatively young individuals with SLE. Anticoagulation with warfarin sodium is usually effective in reducing recurrences of venous clots; it is unclear whether any therapies reduce the incidence of arterial clotting.

Hematologic abnormalities The lupus anticoagulant usually binds to phospholipids in the prothrombin activator complex. It prolongs the partial thromboplastin time; an abnormality not corrected by addition of normal plasma. Three clinical sequelae may be associated with it. First, some patients experience repeated episodes of either venous or arterial clotting; these are often serious, especially if associated with pulmonary emboli, strokes, or occlusion of major arteries. Second, if the anticoagulant is associated with thrombocytopenia or hypoprothrombinemia, significant bleeding can occur. Third, in the absence of clotting or bleeding disorders, it may be a benign laboratory abnormality; biopsies and surgery can be performed without increased risk of bleeding. Antibodies to clotting factors (VIII, IX) are also associated with bleeding. Bleeding syndromes usually respond to glucocorticoids.

Anemia of chronic disease occurs in most patients during periods of disease activity. Frank hemolysis occurs in a small proportion of those with positive Coombs' tests; that syndrome is usually responsive to high-dose glucocorticoids. Splenectomy is sometimes effective in steroid-resistant patients.

Leukopenia is common and usually reflects lymphopenia. In general, it is not associated with recurrent infections and does not require treatment.

Mild thrombocytopenia is common. Severe thrombocytopenia with bleeding and purpura occurs in 5 percent of patients and should be treated with high-dose glucocorticoids. If the platelet count has not risen to a safe range in 5 to 14 days, splenectomy should be considered.

Cardiopulmonary Pericardial pain is the most frequent symptom of cardiac lupus; pericardial effusions also occur. Tamponade has been reported and constrictive pericarditis occurs, but is rare. Myocarditis can cause arrhythmias and/or cardiac failure. Endocarditis of the Libman-Sacks verrucous type, a diagnosis made at autopsy, is usually not clinically significant; however, it can cause aortic or mitral regurgitation. Rarely, myocardial infarcts result from vasculitis of the coronary arteries; more often they are associated with degenerative arterial disease.

Pleurisy and pleural effusions are common manifestations of SLE. Lupus pneumonitis causes recurrent episodes of fever, dyspnea, and cough; x-rays show infiltrates which come and go over a period of days or weeks, and/or areas of platelike atelectasis; this syndrome responds to glucocorticoids. However, *the most common cause of pulmonary infiltrates in patients with SLE is infection.* Interstitial pneumonitis leading to fibrosis occurs in a small proportion of patients; the inflammatory phase may respond to treatment, while the fibrosis does not. Occasionally, patients develop pulmonary hypertension. Infrequent but often fatal pulmonary manifestations include adult respiratory distress syndrome (ARDS) and massive intraalveolar hemorrhage.

Gastrointestinal Nonspecific gastrointestinal symptoms are common, but vasculitis of the intestine is the most dangerous manifestation. It causes acute or subacute crampy pain, vomiting, and diarrhea and leads to intestinal perforation and death in almost one-half of the affected patients. Vasculitis is usually present simultaneously in other systems. Another gastrointestinal manifestation of SLE is a pseudoobstruction picture in which patients present with acute crampy abdominal pain; x-rays show dilated loops of small bowel which may be edematous. Surgery should be avoided unless true obstruction is present. Patients generally respond to glucocorticoid therapy. Acute pancreatitis occurs and can be severe; it may result from glucocorticoid therapy or from active SLE. Elevated serum levels of liver enzymes, especially transaminases, are common in patients with active SLE, but are not associated with significant hepatic damage; they return to normal as the disease is treated.

Ocular The most important ocular manifestation of SLE is retinal vasculitis with infarcts; blindness can develop over a period of days. Examination of the retina shows areas of sheathed, narrow arterioles, and cytoid bodies (white exudates) adjacent to vessels. Other ocular abnormalities include conjunctivitis, episcleritis, and optic neuritis. The sicca syndrome is frequent.

PATHOLOGY **Cutaneous lesions** Acute systemic, discoid (DLE) and subacute cutaneous LE skin lesions show similar histopathology. Characteristic changes include degeneration of the basal layer of the epidermis with disruption of the dermal-epidermal junction (DEJ), and scattered mononuclear cell infiltrates around vessels and appendages in the upper dermis. In DLE follicular plugging and hyperkeratosis are prominent. Deposits of Ig and C′ are seen in the DEJ in 80 to 100 percent of lesional and 50 percent of nonlesional skin in patients with active disease; the proportions are lower during remissions. Active subacute cutaneous lesions are positive for deposits of Ig and C′ only 50 percent of the time. Ig deposition in the DEJ *is not specific* for *LE*. Vasculitic lesions usually show leuocytoclastic angiitis.

Renal lesions Most renal lesions are caused by in situ immune-complex formation or by deposition of circulating immune complexes. In mild nephritis, histology shows either no changes or proliferation confined to the mesangium. Ig deposits are found solely in the mesangium; in this setting the prognosis is good and renal failure is rare. If Ig and C′ extend outside the mesangium into capillary loops, the prognosis worsens. Associated glomerular histologic changes in ascending order of severity are (1) focal proliferative, (2) membranoproliferative, or (3) diffuse proliferative (see Chap. 224). Membranous changes without proliferation occur but are not common. In addition to those histologic categories, *active disease* and *increased risk of progression to renal failure* are associated with glomerular necrosis, epithelial crescents, hyaline thrombi, or leukocyte infiltrates and with mononuclear cell infiltrates in the tubular interstitium or necrotizing vasculitis. In addition, measures of *chronicity* are important, as they are associated with a *high incidence of renal failure*. They include glomerular sclerosis, fibrous crescents, interstitial fibrosis, and tubular atrophy. Focal proliferative and membranous changes are associated with an 85 percent 5-year survival; diffuse proliferative glomerulonephritis is associated with 70 percent 5-year survival. Progression from focal to diffuse lesions can occur.

Laboratory manifestations The presence of characteristic antibodies (Table 262-1) confirms the diagnosis of SLE. Antinuclear antibodies (ANA) are the best screening test. If the test substrate is living human nuclei as in WIL-2 or HEP-2 cells from tissue culture, more than 95 percent of lupus patients will have positive tests. The more frequently used rodent liver or kidney does not detect as wide a range of ANA or anticytoplasmic antibodies; approximately 85 percent of SLE serums are positive on those substrates. A positive ANA is not specific for SLE; ANA occur (usually in low titer) in some normal individuals; the frequency increases with aging. Furthermore, other autoimmune diseases, acute viral infections, and chronic inflammatory processes may cause ANA positivity. Therefore, a positive ANA supports a diagnosis of SLE but *is not specific;* a negative ANA makes the diagnosis unlikely, but not impossible. Antibodies to dsDNA and to Sm are relatively specific for SLE; other autoantibodies listed in Table 262-1 are not. High serum levels of ANA and anti-DNA and low levels of complement usually reflect disease activity, especially in patients with nephritis. Serum levels of cryoglobulins or other immune complexes occasionally correlate with disease activity. Total functional hemolytic complement (CH_{50}) levels are the most sensitive measure of complement activation but also are the most subject to laboratory error. Quantitative levels of C3 and C4 are widely available. Very low levels of CH_{50} with normal levels of C3 suggest inherited deficiency of a complement component.

Hematologic abnormalities are common and include anemia (usually normochromic, normocytic, but occasionally hemolytic), leukopenia, lymphopenia, and thrombocytopenia. In some patients elevation of the Westergren erythrocyte sedimentation rate correlates with disease activity.

Urinalysis and serum creatinine should be measured periodically in patients with SLE. When active nephritis is present, the urinalysis usually shows proteinuria, microscopic hematuria, and cellular or granular casts. Renal biopsy is indicated when results would influence therapeutic decisions (see discussion under "Clinical Manifestations").

Other tests which may be abnormal in SLE include false-positive tests for syphilis and abnormal coagulation tests, especially a prolonged partial thromboplastin time. Both are related to antibodies to cardiolipin, discussed under "Clinical Manifestations." Rheumatoid factors are present in 30 to 50 percent of patients.

The tests which are useful for diagnosis and for following the clinical course of patients with SLE are listed in Table 262-3.

Pregnancy Since SLE is predominantly a disease of young women, pregnancy is a frequent occurrence. Fertility rates are normal in patients with SLE, but the rate of spontaneous abortion and stillbirths is high (30 to 50 percent), especially in women with lupus anticoagulant and/or antibodies to cardiolipin. There may be increased flare-ups of SLE during the first trimester (SLE may begin during pregnancy) and especially during the first 6 weeks postpartum. If severe renal or cardiac disease are absent and SLE is controlled, many patients complete pregnancy safely and deliver normal infants. Glucocorticoids are inactivated by placental enzymes and do not cause fetal abnormalities except for low birth weights. Neonatal lupus (related to the presence of anti-Ro in maternal serum) occurs in infants but is rare; two syndromes are seen—a transient DLE-like rash and congenital heart block.

DIFFERENTIAL DIAGNOSIS The American Rheumatism Association has developed diagnostic criteria for SLE. Manifestations which are included are indicated by asterisks in Table 262-2. Any four of those in addition to two characteristic autoantibodies establish the diagnosis of definite SLE. Disease confined to one or two systems may be more difficult to classify. The disorders with which SLE can be confused include rheumatoid arthritis; skin disorders such as urticaria, erythema multiforme, rosacea, lichen planus; neurologic disorders such as idiopathic epilepsy or multiple sclerosis; hematologic disorders such as idiopathic thrombocytopenic purpura; and psychiatric disorders. In these cases, the physician may wish to delay a diagnosis of SLE until additional manifestations appear. It may also be difficult to distinguish SLE from other autoimmune disorders such as dermatomyositis and overlap syndromes. Some authorities classify patients with features of SLE, rheumatoid arthritis, polymyositis, and scleroderma, accompanied by high titers of anti-RNP, as "mixed connective tissue disease" (Chap. 265) and report a low incidence of nephritis and CNS disease and a high incidence of pulmonary disease and evolution into scleroderma. It is impossible to classify some patients into a definite category; therapy should be directed toward the dominant manifestations. The possibility of drug-induced lupus should always be ruled out.

Drug-induced lupus Several drugs can cause a syndrome resembling SLE in individuals without any obvious predisposition to the disease. The most common offender is procainamide, which induces ANA in 50 to 75 percent of individuals within a few months; 20 percent of patients receiving the drug develop clinical drug-induced LE. Hydralazine induces ANA in 25 to 30 percent of individuals, and lupus-like symptoms in 10 percent. Both procainamide and hydralazine-induced lupus occur more commonly in women, are uncommon in blacks, and are more likely to occur in individuals who acetylate the drug slowly; this is especially true for hydralazine. The clinical syndrome consists of polyarthralgias and systemic symptoms in most patients. Polyarthritis occurs in 25 to 50 percent, and pleuropericarditis in 30 percent, of patients with hydralazine and 50 percent of patients with procainamide-induced lupus. Other manifestations typical of idiopathic SLE are unusual, including nephritis and CNS involvement. All patients with drug-induced lupus are ANA-positive; most have antibodies to histones. Antibodies to dsDNA and hypocomplementemia are rarely present—a helpful point in distinguishing drug-induced from idiopathic lupus. Anemia, leukopenia, lupus anticoagulant, thrombocytopenia, cryoglobulins, rheumatoid factors, false-positive VDRL, and positive direct Coombs' tests can occur. The initial therapeutic approach should be discontinuance of the suspect drug; most patients improve in days or a few weeks. In patients with severe symptoms, a short course (2 to 10 weeks) of glucocorticoids is indicated. Clinical symptoms rarely persist more than 6 months; ANA may remain positive for years. Other drugs which infrequently induce lupus-like illnesses include isoniazid, chlorpromazine, *d*-penicillamine, practolol, methyldopa, oral contraceptives, and possibly hydantoins and ethosuximide. Most lupus-inducing drugs can be used safely in patients with idiopathic lupus if there are no suitable alternatives.

Prognosis The overall survival in patients with SLE is approximately 71 percent over 10 years. Patients with severe involvement of the brain, lungs, heart, or kidney have the worst outcomes in terms of survival and disability. Infections and renal failure are the leading causes of death.

TREATMENT There is no cure for SLE. Complete remissions occur but are rare, so patient and physician should plan to control acute, severe flare-ups and to develop maintenance therapies in which symptoms are suppressed to an acceptable level, usually at the cost of some drug side effects. From 20 to 30 percent of SLE patients have mild disease with no life-threatening manifestations. However, their disease may be disabling because of pain and fatigue. These patients should be managed without glucocorticoids. Arthralgias, arthritis, myalgias, fever, and mild serositis may improve on nonsteroidal anti-inflammatory drugs (NSAID) including salicylates. However, some NSAID toxicities are especially frequent in SLE patients (hepatitis, aseptic meningitis, and renal impairment). The dermatitides of SLE (including DLE), and occasionally lupus arthritis, may respond to antimalarials. Doses of 400 mg of hydroxychloroquine daily are associated with improvement of skin lesions in a few weeks in patients destined to respond. Side effects include retinal toxicity, rash, myopathy, and neuropathy. Regular ophthalmologic examinations should be performed at least every 6-months, since retinal toxicity is related to cumulative dose. Other therapies for skin rash include use of sunscreens (an SPF rating of 15 or higher is recommended) to prevent rashes, and of topical or intralesional glucocorticoids if rashes develop. Systemic glucocorticoids should be reserved for patients with disabling, severe lesions.

Life-threatening and severely disabling manifestations of SLE are treated with high doses of *glucocorticoids* (1 to 2 mg/kg per day). When the disease is active, glucocorticoids should be given in divided doses every 8 to 12 h. After the disease has been controlled for several days, doses should be consolidated to one morning dose; thereafter, the daily dose should be tapered as rapidly as clinical disease permits. Ideally, patients should be slowly converted to alternate-day therapy with a single morning dose of a short-acting glucocorticoid (prednisone, prednisolone, methylprednisolone) to minimize side effects. However, the disease may flare-up on alternate days, in which case the lowest single daily dose which suppresses symptoms and major organ damage should be used. Undesirable side effects of chronic glucocorticoid therapy include cushingoid habitus, weight gain, hypertension, infection, capillary fragility, acne, hirsutism, accelerated osteoporosis, ischemic necrosis of bone, cataracts, glaucoma, diabetes mellitus, myopathy, hypokalemia, irregular menses, irritability, insomnia, and psychosis. Prednisone doses of 15 mg daily (or less) given before the hour of noon usually do not suppress the hypothalamic pituitary axis. Side effects can be partially minimized by being alert for them; hyperglycemia, hypertension, edema, and hypokalemia should be treated. Infections should be identified early and treated promptly. Immunizations with influenza and pneumococcal vaccines are safe and generally effective in patients with stable disease. Supplemental calcium (1000 to 1500 mg daily) with vitamin D (50,000 units weekly) in carefully selected patients (normal 24-h urine calcium, normal serum calcium, ambulatory) receiving stable doses of glucocorticoids may help maintain bone mass. Some acutely ill lupus patients, including those with diffuse nephritis, have been treated with 3 to 5 days of 1000-mg intravenous "pulses" of methylprednisolone, followed by maintenance daily or alternate-day glucocorticoids. It is unclear whether there are any special advantages or toxicities to this regimen.

The use of *cytotoxic agents* (azathioprine, chlorambucil, cyclophosphamide) in SLE is somewhat controversial. Their use in lupus nephritis is probably associated with a lower rate of renal failure and fewer disease flare-ups, and permits faster tapering to low maintenance doses of glucocorticoids. Undesirable side effects include bone marrow suppression, irreversible gonadal failure (in approximately 30 percent of patients), hepatotoxicity (azathioprine), bladder toxicity (cyclophosphamide), and an increased risk for malignancies. If a lupus patient has life-threatening disease unresponsive to glucocorticoids, or requires an unacceptably high maintenance dose of glucocorticoids, it is appropriate to consider cytotoxic drugs. Azathioprine is the least toxic; it may be given in a dose of 2 to 3 mg/kg per day orally. Cyclophosphamide is the most effective and the most toxic. Intravenous pulse doses (10 to 15 mg/kg) given once every 4 weeks have less urinary bladder toxicity and more rapid onset of action (5 to 15 days) than daily oral doses, but bone marrow suppression can be severe. Cyclophosphamide can also be used in daily oral doses (1.5 to 2.5 mg/kg per day), or in combination with low doses of azathioprine (0.5 to 1 mg/kg per day of each). After disease activity has been controlled for several months, tapering of cytotoxic agents and attempts to discontinue them are appropriate.

Several experimental therapies for SLE are being studied, including plasmapheresis, total-lymph node irradiation, cyclosporine, and sex hormone therapy.

Patients with nephrotic syndrome often maintain stable renal function in spite of persistent edema and hypoalbuminemia; hypertension is usually a concomitant problem. Such patients should be treated with 3 to 6 months of high-dose glucocorticoid therapy; if proteinuria does not diminish, the drug should be tapered and discontinued and treatment directed toward control of hypertension and hyperlipidemia.

It is appropriate in patients with end-stage nephritis to plan for dialysis or transplantation; their survival is similar to that of patients with other immune nephritides.

In the subsets of patients with SLE who do not have progressive, severe disease, patients should be informed that although SLE is a chronic, potentially serious disease, some patients can lead relatively normal lives if their disease is appropriately managed.

REFERENCES

AUSTIN HA III et al: Prognostic factors in lupus nephritis. Am J Med 75:382, 1983

CARETTE S et al: Controlled studies of oral immunosuppressive drugs in lupus nephritis. Ann Intern Med 99:1, 1983

GINZLER E et al: A multi-center study of outcome in systemic lupus erythematosus. I. Entry variables as predictors of prognosis. Arthritis Rheum 25:601, 1982

ROTHFIELD N: Systemic lupus erythematosus: Clinical aspects and treatment, in *Arthritis and Allied Conditions*, 10th ed, DJ McCarty (ed), Philadelphia, Lea & Febiger, 1985, chap 61, pp 911–935

STEINBERG AD et al: Systemic lupus erythematosus: Insights from animal models. Ann Intern Med 100:714, 1984

STEVENS MB, HAHN BH: Therapy of systemic lupus erythematosus. Bull Rheum Dis 32:35, 1982

Systemic lupus erythematosus, GRV Hughes (ed). Clin Rheum Dis 8:1, 1982

TAN EM: Systemic lupus erythematosus: Immunological aspects, in *Arthritis and Allied Conditions*, 10th ed, DJ McCarty (ed), Philadelphia, Lea & Febiger, 1985, chap 62, pp 936–941

——— et al: The 1982 revised criteria for the classification of systemic lupus erythematosus. Arthritis Rheum 25:1271, 1982

TSOKAS GC, BALOW JE: Cellular immune responses in systemic lupus erythematosus. Prog Allergy 35:93, 1984

263 RHEUMATOID ARTHRITIS

PETER E. LIPSKY

Rheumatoid arthritis (RA) is a chronic, multisystem disease of unknown etiology. Although there are a variety of systemic manifestations, the characteristic feature of RA is persistent inflammatory synovitis, usually involving peripheral joints in a symmetric distribution. The potential of the synovial inflammation to cause cartilage destruction and bone erosions and subsequently joint deformities is the hallmark of the disease. Despite its destructive potential, the course of RA can be quite variable. Some patients may experience only a mild oligoarticular illness of brief duration with minimal joint damage, while others will have a relentless progressive polyarthritis with marked joint deformity. Most patients will experience an intermediate course.

EPIDEMIOLOGY The prevalence of definite RA is approximately 1 percent of the population (range 0.3 to 2.1 percent); women are affected approximately three times more often than men. The prevalence increases with age, and sex differences diminish in the older age group. RA is seen throughout the world and affects all races. The onset is most frequent during the fourth and fifth decade of life, with 80 percent of all patients developing the disease between the ages of 35 and 50.

Family studies indicate a genetic predisposition. For example, severe RA is found at approximately four times the expected rate in first-degree relatives of individuals with seropositive disease. Moreover, 30 percent of monozygous twins are concordant for RA, whereas only 5 percent of dizygous twins are concordant. The role of genetic influences in the etiology of RA was established by the demonstration of an association with the class II major histocompatibility gene complex antigen, HLA-DR4. As many as 70 percent of whites or Japanese with classic or definite RA express HLA-DR4 compared with 28 percent of control individuals. An association with HLA-DR4 has also been noted in blacks, Latin Americans, and Chippewa Indians, although the incidence of HLA-DR4 positivity in individuals with RA in these groups is not as great as in whites. In a number of groups, including Ashkenazi Jews, non-Ashkenazi Jews, Asian Indians, and Yakima Indians, there is no association between the development of RA and HLA-DR4. It was thought initially that HLA-DR4 was associated with seropositive RA, but not with the development of rheumatoid factor in normal people. Recent studies however, have suggested that HLA-DR4 may be associated with severe erosive disease especially in younger women rather than with seropositive disease. No association with HLA-DR4 has been found in individuals with nonerosive RA independent of the occurrence of rheumatoid factor. The explanation for the association of HLA-DR4 and RA remains obscure, although the relationship of the class II histocompatibility gene complex products to immune response genes has suggested that these determinants may play a role in controlling the immunopathogenesis of RA.

There appears to be a genetic predisposition for the development of certain toxic reactions induced by drugs used to treat RA. For example, the presence of the HLA-DR3 allele is highly associated with the development of side effects to gold therapy, including proteinuria, thrombocytopenia, and perhaps skin rash. Similarly, the presence of this allele appears to predispose to the development of proteinuria following therapy with D-penicillamine.

CLINICAL MANIFESTATIONS Onset Characteristically, RA is a chronic polyarthritis. In approximately two-thirds of patients, it begins insidiously with fatigue, anorexia, generalized weakness, and vague musculoskeletal symptoms until the appearance of synovitis becomes apparent. This prodrome may persist for weeks or months and defy diagnosis. Specific symptoms usually appear gradually as several joints, especially those of the hands, wrists, knees, and feet, become affected in a symmetric fashion. In approximately 10 percent of individuals, the onset is more acute with a rapid development of polyarthritis often accompanied by constitutional symptoms including fever, lymphadenopathy, and splenomegaly. In approximately one-third of patients, symptoms may initially be confined to one or a few joints. Although the pattern of joint involvement may remain asymmetric in a few patients, a symmetric pattern is more typical.

Signs and symptoms of articular disease Pain, swelling, and tenderness may initially be poorly localized to the joints. Pain in affected joints, aggravated by movement, is the most common manifestation of established RA. It corresponds in pattern to the joint involvement but does not always correlate with the degree of apparent inflammation. Generalized stiffness is frequent and is usually greatest after periods of inactivity. Morning stiffness of greater than 1-h duration is an almost invariable feature of inflammatory arthritis and serves to distinguish it from various noninflammatory joint disorders. The length and intensity of the stiffness can be used as a crude assessment of disease activity. The majority of patients will experience constitutional symptoms such as weakness, easy fatigability, anorexia, and weight loss. Although fever to 40°C occurs on occasion, temperature elevation in excess of 38°C is unusual and suggests the presence of an intercurrent problem such as infection.

Clinically, synovial inflammation causes swelling, tenderness, and limitation of motion. Warmth is usually evident on examination, especially of large joints such as the knee, but erythema is infrequent. Pain originates predominantly from the joint capsule, which is abundantly supplied with pain fibers and is markedly sensitive to stretching or distention. Joint swelling results from accumulation of synovial fluid, hypertrophy of the synovium, and thickening of the joint capsule. Initially, motion is limited by pain. The inflamed joint is usually held in flexion to maximize joint volume and minimize distention of the capsule. Later, fibrous, bony ankylosis, or soft tissue contractures lead to fixed deformities.

Although inflammation can affect any diarthrodial joint, RA most often causes symmetric arthritis with characteristic involvement of certain specific joints such as the proximal interphalangeal and metacarpophalangeal joints. The distal interphalangeal joints are rarely involved. Synovitis of the wrist joints is a nearly uniform feature of RA and may lead to limitation of motion, deformity, and median nerve entrapment (carpal tunnel syndrome). Synovitis of the elbow joint often leads to flexion contractures that may develop early in the disease. The knee joint is commonly involved with synovial hypertrophy, chronic effusion, and frequently ligamentous laxity. Pain and swelling behind the knee may be caused by extension of inflamed synovium into the popliteal space (Baker's cyst). Arthritis in the forefoot, ankles, and subtalar joints can produce severe pain with ambulation as well as a number of deformities. Axial involvement is usually limited to the upper cervical spine. Involvement of the lumbar spine is not seen, and lower back pain cannot be ascribed to rheumatoid inflammation. On occasion, inflammation from the synovial joints and bursae of the upper cervical spine leads to atlantoaxial subluxation. This usually presents as pain in the occiput but on rare occasions may lead to compression of the spinal cord.

With persistent inflammation, a variety of characteristic deformities develop. These can be attributed to a number of pathologic events including laxity of supporting soft tissue structures from destruction or weakening of ligaments, tendons, and the joint capsule; cartilage destruction; muscle imbalance; and unopposed physical forces associated with the use of affected joints. Characteristic deformities of the hand include (1) radial deviation at the wrist with ulnar deviation of the digits often with palmar subluxation of the proximal phalanges ("Z" deformity); (2) hyperextension of the proximal interphalangeal joints, with compensatory flexion of the distal interphalangeal joints (swan neck deformity); (3) flexion deformity of the proximal interphalangeal joints and extension of the distal interphalangeal joints (boutonnière deformity); and (4) hyperextension of the first interphalangeal joint and flexion of the first metacarpophalangeal joint with a consequent loss of thumb mobility and pinch. Typical deformities may also develop in the feet, including eversion at the hindfoot (subtalar joint), plantar subluxation of the metatarsal heads, widening of the forefoot, hallux valgus, and lateral deviation and dorsal subluxation of the toes.

Extraarticular manifestations RA is a systemic disease with a variety of extraarticular manifestations. Although these occur frequently, not all of them have clinical significance. However, on occasion, they may be the major evidence of disease activity and source of morbidity and require management per se. As a rule, these manifestations take place in individuals with high titers of rheumatoid factors.

Rheumatoid nodules develop in 20 to 30 percent of persons with RA. They are usually found on periarticular structures, extensor surfaces, or other areas subjected to mechanical pressure, but they can develop elsewhere including the pleura and meninges. Common locations include the olecranon bursa, the proximal ulna, the Achilles tendon, and the occiput. Nodules vary in size and consistency and are rarely symptomatic, but on occasion they break down as a result of trauma or become infected. They are found almost invariably in individuals with circulating rheumatoid factor.

Clinical weakness and atrophy of skeletal muscle are common. Muscle atrophy may be evident within weeks of the onset of RA and usually is most apparent in musculature approximating affected joints. Muscle biopsy may show type II fiber atrophy and muscle fiber necrosis with or without a mononuclear cell infiltrate.

Rheumatoid vasculitis which can affect nearly any organ system is seen in patients with severe RA and high titers of circulating rheumatoid factor. In its most aggressive form, rheumatoid vasculitis can cause polyneuropathy and mononeuritis multiplex, cutaneous ulceration and dermal necrosis, digital gangrene, and visceral infarction. While such widespread vasculitis is very rare, more limited forms are not uncommon, especially in white patients with high titers of rheumatoid factor. Neurovascular disease presenting either as a mild distal sensory neuropathy or as mononeuritis multiplex may be the only signs of vasculitis. Cutaneous vasculitis usually presents as crops of small brown spots in the nail beds, nail folds, and digital pulp. Larger ischemic ulcers, especially in the lower extremity, may also develop. Myocardial infarction secondary to rheumatoid vasculitis has been reported as has vasculitic involvement of lungs, bowel, liver, spleen, pancreas, lymph nodes, and testes. Renal vasculitis is rare.

Pleuropulmonary manifestations, which are more commonly observed in men, include pleural disease, interstitial fibrosis, pleuropulmonary nodules, pneumonitis, and arteritis. Evidence of pleuritis is found commonly at autopsy, but symptomatic disease during life is infrequent. Typically, the pleural fluid contains very low levels of glucose in the absence of infection. Pleural fluid complement is also low compared with the serum level when these are related to the total protein concentration. Pulmonary fibrosis can produce impairment of the diffusing capacity of the lung. Pulmonary nodules may appear singly or in clusters. When they appear in individuals with pneumoconiosis, a diffuse nodular fibrotic process (Caplan's syndrome) may develop. On occasion, pulmonary nodules may cavitate and produce a pneumothorax or bronchopleural fistula. Rarely pulmonary hypertension secondary to obliteration of the pulmonary vasculature occurs. In addition to pleuropulmonary disease, upper airway obstruction from cricoarytenoid arthritis or laryngeal nodules may develop.

Clinically apparent heart disease attributed to the rheumatoid process is rare, but evidence of asymptomatic pericarditis is found at autopsy in 50 percent of cases. Pericardial fluid has a low glucose level and is frequently associated with the occurrence of pleural effusion. Although pericarditis is usually asymptomatic, on rare occasions death has occurred from tamponade. Chronic constrictive pericarditis may also occur.

RA tends to spare the central nervous system directly, although vasculitis can cause peripheral neuropathy. *Neurologic manifestations* may also result from atlantoaxial or midcervical spine subluxations. Nerve entrapment secondary to proliferative synovitis or joint deformities may produce neuropathies of median, ulnar, radial (interosseus branch), or anterior tibial nerves.

The rheumatoid process involves the *eye* in less than 1 percent of patients. Affected individuals usually have long-standing disease and nodules. The two principal manifestations are episcleritis, which is usually mild and transient, and scleritis, which involves the deeper coats of the eye and is a more serious inflammatory condition. Histologically, the lesion is similar to a rheumatoid nodule and may result in thinning and perforation of the globe (scleromalacia perforans). Fifteen to twenty percent of persons with RA may develop Sjögren's syndrome with attendant keratoconjunctivitis sicca.

Felty's syndrome consists of chronic RA, splenomegaly, neutropenia, and on occasion anemia and thrombocytopenia. It is most common in individuals with long-standing disease. These patients frequently have high titers of rheumatoid factor, subcutaneous nodules, and other manifestations of systemic rheumatoid disease. Circulating immune complexes are often present, and evidence of complement consumption may be seen. Felty's syndrome may develop after joint inflammation has regressed. The leukopenia is a selective neutropenia with polymorphonuclear leukocyte counts of less than 1500 per cubic millimeter, and sometimes less than 1000 per cubic millimeter. Bone marrow examination usually reveals moderate hypercellularity with a paucity of mature neutrophils. However, the bone marrow may be normal, hyperactive, or hypoactive; maturation arrest may be seen. Hypersplenism has been proposed as one of the causes of leukopenia, but splenomegaly is not invariably found and splenectomy does not always correct the abnormality. Excessive margination of granulocytes caused by antibodies to these cells, complement activation, or binding of immune complexes may contribute to granulocytopenia. Patients with Felty's syndrome have increased frequency of infections usually associated with neutropenia. The cause of the increased susceptibility to infection is related to the defective function of polymorphonuclear leukocytes as well as the decreased number of cells.

Osteoporosis secondary to rheumatoid involvement is common and may be aggravated by corticosteroid therapy and immobilization. Osteopenia involves both juxtaarticular bone and long bones distant from involved joints.

LABORATORY FINDINGS No tests are specific for diagnosing RA. However, rheumatoid factors, which are autoantibodies reactive with IgG, are found in more than two-thirds of adults with the disease. Widely utilized tests largely detect IgM rheumatoid factors. Although rheumatoid factors are found in less than 5 percent of healthy persons, they are not specific for RA. The frequency of rheumatoid factor in the general population increases with age, and 10 to 20 percent of individuals over 65 years old have a positive test. In addition, a number of conditions besides RA are associated with the presence of rheumatoid factor. These include systemic lupus erythematosus, Sjögren's syndrome, chronic liver disease, sarcoidosis, interstitial pulmonary fibrosis, infectious mononucleosis, hepatitis B, tuberculosis, leprosy, syphilis, subacute bacterial endocarditis, visceral leishmaniasis, schistosomiasis, and malaria. In addition, rheumatoid factor may appear transiently in normal individuals after vaccination or transfusion and may also be found in relatives of individuals with RA.

The presence of rheumatoid factor does not establish the diagnosis of RA but can be of prognostic significance because patients with high titers tend to have more severe and progressive disease with extraarticular manifestations. Rheumatoid factor is uniformly found in patients with nodules or vasculitis. Less than one-third of unselected patients with a positive test for rheumatoid factor will be found to have RA. The test is not useful as a screening procedure but can be employed to confirm a diagnosis in individuals with a suggestive clinical presentation and, if present in high titer, to designate patients at risk for severe systemic disease.

Normochromic, normocytic anemia is frequently present in active RA. It is thought to reflect ineffective erythropoiesis; large stores of iron are found in the bone marrow. In general, anemia and thrombocytosis correlate with disease activity. The white blood cell count is usually normal, but a mild leukocytosis may be present. Leukopenia may also exist without the full-blown picture of Felty's syndrome. Eosinophilia, when present, usually reflects severe systemic disease.

The erythrocyte sedimentation rate is increased in nearly all patients with active RA. A variety of other acute phase reactants including ceruloplasmin and C-reactive protein are also elevated, and generally such elevations correlate with disease activity and the likelihood of progressive joint damage.

Synovial fluid analysis confirms the presence of inflammatory arthritis, although none of the findings is specific. The fluid is usually turbid, with reduced viscosity, increased protein content, and a slightly decreased or normal glucose concentration. The white cell count varies between 5 and 50,000 per cubic millimeter; polymorphonuclear leukocytes predominate. Total hemolytic complement, C3, and C4 are markedly diminished in synovial fluid relative to total protein concentration as a result of activation of the classic complement pathway by locally produced immune complexes.

When monoclonal antibodies specific for T-lymphocyte subsets are used to examine peripheral blood mononuclear cells of patients with RA, those with active disease are found to have an increased ratio of T4:T8 (helper-inducer/suppressor-cytotoxic) cells. In addition, an increased number of circulating T cells express class II major histocompatibility gene complex products (HLA-DR), an indication of T-cell activation. This finding is most frequent in patients with active joint disease.

RADIOGRAPHIC EVALUATION Early in the disease, roentgenograms of the affected joints are usually not helpful in establishing a diagnosis. They reveal only that which is apparent from physical examination, namely evidence of soft tissue swelling and joint effusion. As the disease progresses, abnormalities become more pronounced, but none of the radiographic findings are diagnostic of RA. The diagnosis, however, is supported by a characteristic pattern of abnormalities including the tendency toward symmetric involvement. Juxtaarticular osteopenia may become apparent within weeks of onset. Loss of articular cartilage and bone erosions develop after months of sustained activity. The primary value of radiography is to determine the extent of cartilage destruction and bone erosion produced by the disease, particularly when one is considering therapy with disease-modifying drugs or surgical intervention.

CLINICAL COURSE AND PROGNOSIS The course of RA is quite variable and difficult to predict in an individual patient. Five years after the onset of RA, evidence of disease activity may be found in as few as one-third of all patients. However, RA can cause significant social and financial disadvantages in those patients with persistently active disease. Most patients experience persistent but fluctuating disease activity, accompanied by a variable degree of joint deformity. Approximately 15 percent have a short-lived inflammatory process that remits without major deformity, whereas 10 percent experience relentlessly progressive disease leading to marked deformity and disability.

Several features of patients with RA appear to have prognostic significance. Remissions of disease activity are most likely to occur during the first year. White females tend to have more persistent synovitis and progressively erosive disease than males. Persons who present with high titers of rheumatoid factor, C-reactive protein, and haptoglobin also have a worse prognosis, as do individuals with subcutaneous nodules or radiographic evidence of erosions at the time of initial evaluation. Although sustained disease activity of more than 1 year's duration portends a poor outcome, the rate of progression of joint abnormalities is not constant; the greatest progression takes place during the first 6 years of disease and at a much slower rate thereafter.

The median life expectancy of persons with RA is shortened by 3 to 7 years. Of the 2.5-fold increase in mortality rate, RA itself is a contributing feature in 15 to 25 percent. The increased mortality rate seems to be limited to patients with more severe articular disease and can be attributed largely to infection and gastrointestinal bleeding. Drug therapy may also play a role in the increased mortality rate seen in these individuals.

DIAGNOSIS The diagnosis of RA is easily made in persons with typical established disease. In a majority of patients, the disease assumes its characteristic clinical features within 1 to 2 years of onset. The typical picture of bilateral symmetric inflammatory polyarthritis involving small and large joints in both the upper and lower extremities with sparing of the axial skeleton except the cervical spine suggests the diagnosis. Constitutional features indicative of the inflammatory nature of the disease, such as morning stiffness, support the diagnosis. Demonstration of subcutaneous nodules is a helpful diagnostic feature. Additionally, the presence of rheumatoid factor, inflammatory synovial fluid with increased numbers of polymorphonuclear leukocytes, and radiographic findings of juxtaarticular bone demineralization and erosions of the affected joints substantiate the diagnosis.

The diagnosis is somewhat more difficult early in the course when only constitutional symptoms or intermittent arthralgias or arthritis in an asymmetric distribution may be present. A period of observation may be necessary before the diagnosis can be established. A definitive diagnosis of RA depends predominantly on characteristic clinical features and the exclusion of other inflammatory processes. The isolated finding of a positive test for rheumatoid factor or an elevated erythrocyte sedimentation rate, especially in an older person with joint pains, should not itself be used as evidence of RA.

The American Rheumatism Association has developed criteria for the diagnosis of RA (Table 263-1). The presence of seven of these criteria establishes the diagnosis of classic RA, whereas five criteria indicate definite RA, and three, probable RA. Although these criteria were developed as a means of disease classification for epidemiologic purposes, they are useful as guidelines for establishing the diagnosis. Failure to meet these criteria, however, especially during the early stages of the disease, does not exclude the diagnosis.

PATHOLOGY AND PATHOGENESIS Microvascular injury and an increase in the number of synovial lining cells appear to be the earliest lesions of RA. The nature of the insult causing this response is not known. Subsequently, an increased number of synovial lining cells is seen along with perivascular infiltration with mononuclear cells. As the process continues, the synovium becomes edematous and protrudes into the joint cavity as villus projections.

Light-microscopic examination discloses a characteristic constellation of features which include hyperplasia and hypertrophy of the synovial lining cells, focal or segmental vascular changes, and infiltration with mononuclear cells often collected into aggregates or follicles around small blood vessels. The mononuclear cell collections are variable in composition and size. The predominant infiltrating cell is the T lymphocyte. T4 (helper-inducer) cells predominate over T8 (suppressor-cytotoxic) cells and are frequently found in close proximity to HLA-DR–positive macrophages. Although this pathologic picture is typical of RA, it can also be seen in a variety of other chronic inflammatory arthritides.

Although the etiologic stimuli have not been identified, established rheumatoid synovitis is characterized by persistent immunologic activity. The infiltrating T cells express activation antigens such as HLA-DR and produce a variety of lymphokines such as interleukin 2, γ-interferon, macrophage migration inhibition factor, monocyte chemotactic factor, and leukocyte migration inhibition factor which have been isolated from rheumatoid synovial fluid. Evidence of B-cell activation can also be found in the inflamed synovium, and plasma cells producing immunoglobulin and rheumatoid factor are characteristic features of rheumatoid synovitis. Large numbers of macrophages are also found in rheumatoid synovium. In addition, the macrophage-derived cytokine interleukin 1 can be found in rheumatoid synovial fluid. This factor has a wide spectrum of activities both within and outside the immune system and may explain some of the local and systemic manifestations of RA.

These findings have suggested that the propagation of RA is an immunologically mediated event, although the original initiating stimulus has not been characterized. One view is that the inflammatory process in the tissue is driven by the T4 helper-inducer cells infiltrating the synovium. Evidence for this includes (1) the predominance of T4 cells in the synovium; (2) the local production of lymphokines by these infiltrating T cells; and (3) amelioration of the disease by removal of T cells by thoracic duct drainage or suppression of their function by total lymphoid irradiation. Since T lymphocytes produce a variety of cytokines that promote B-cell proliferation and differentiation into antibody-forming cells, T-cell activation may also promote local B-cell stimulation. The resultant production of immunoglobulin and rheumatoid factor can lead to immune-complex formation with consequent complement activation and exacerbation of the inflammatory process by the production of anaphylatoxins and chemotactic factors. The tissue inflammation is reminiscent of delayed-type hypersensitivity reactions occurring in response to soluble antigens or microorganisms. It is, however, unclear whether this represents a response to a persistent exogenous antigen or to altered autoantigens such as collagen, or immunoglobulin. Alternatively, it could represent persistent responsiveness to activated autologous cells such as might occur as a result of Epstein-Barr virus infection. Also, the persistent inflammation could result from deranged immunoregulatory mechanisms.

Overriding the chronic inflammation in the synovial tissue is an acute inflammatory process in the synovial fluid. The exudative synovial fluid contains a large number of polymorphonuclear leukocytes and relatively few mononuclear cells. A number of mechanisms play a role in stimulating the exudation of synovial fluid. Locally produced immune complexes can activate complement and generate anaphylatoxins and chemotactic factors. Local production by mononuclear phagocytes of factors such as interleukin 1 and leukotriene B4, which can act as powerful chemotactic attractants, may also play a role in the emigration of polymorphonuclear leukocytes. In addition, vasoactive mediators such as histamine produced by mast cells may also facilitate the exudation of inflammatory cells into the synovial fluid. Once in the synovial fluid, the polymorphonuclear leukocytes can ingest immune complexes with the resultant production of reactive oxygen metabolites and other inflammatory mediators, further adding to the inflammatory milieu. The production of large amounts of cyclooxygenase and lipoxygenase pathway products of arachidonic acid metabolism by cells in the synovial fluid and tissue further accentuate the signs and symptoms of inflammation.

The precise mechanism by which bone and cartilage destruction occurs has not been completely resolved. The majority of destruction occurs in juxtaposition to the inflamed synovium or pannus that spreads to cover the articular cartilage. This vascular granulation tissue is composed of proliferating fibroblasts, small blood vessels, and a variable number of mononuclear cells. The macrophage-derived cytokine interleukin 1 may play an important role by stimulating the cells of the pannus to release collagenase and other neutral proteases. Cytokines such as interleukin 1 or catabolin may also activate chondrocytes in situ, stimulating them to produce proteolytic enzymes that can degrade cartilage locally. In addition, other mechanisms may contribute to the local demineralization of bone, including the production of osteoclast activating factor by activated T cells and prostaglandin E_2 by fibroblasts and macrophages.

TREATMENT General principles Since the etiology of RA is unknown and the pathogenesis speculative, therapy remains empirical. None of the therapeutic interventions are curative, and, therefore, all must be viewed as palliative, aimed at relieving the signs and symptoms of the disease. The various therapies employed are directed at nonspecific suppression of the inflammatory process in the hope of ameliorating symptoms and preventing progressive damage to articular structures.

Management of patients with RA involves an interdisciplinary approach which attempts to deal with the various problems that these individuals have with functional as well as psychosocial interactions. A variety of physical therapies may be useful in decreasing the symptoms of RA. Rest ameliorates symptoms and can be an important component of the total therapeutic program. In addition, splinting to reduce unwanted motion of inflamed joints may be useful. Exercise directed at maintaining muscle strength and joint mobility without exacerbating joint inflammation is also an important aspect of the therapeutic regimen. A variety of orthotic devices can be helpful in supporting and aligning deformed joints to reduce pain and improve function.

Medical management of RA involves two general approaches. The first is the use of aspirin and other nonsteroidal anti-inflammatory drugs, simple analgesics, and if necessary, low-dose glucocorticoids to control the symptoms and signs of the local inflammatory process. These agents are rapidly effective at mitigating signs and symptoms, but they appear to exert little effect on the progression of the disease. A second group of drugs includes a variety of agents that have been

TABLE 263-1 American Rheumatism Association criteria for the diagnosis of rheumatoid arthritis*

1	Morning stiffness
2	Pain on motion or tenderness in at least one joint
3	Swelling (soft tissue thickening or fluid) in at least one joint
4	Swelling of at least one other joint
5	Symmetric joint swelling
6	Subcutaneous nodules
7	Radiologic changes typical of RA
8	Demonstration of "rheumatoid factor" in serum
9	Poor mucin precipitate from synovial fluid
10	Characteristic histologic changes in synovium
11	Characteristic histologic changes in nodules

* *Criteria 1 to 5 must be continuous for at least 6 weeks. Criteria 2 to 6 must be observed by a physician. The presence of seven or more criteria indicates classic disease; five to six criteria indicate definite disease; three to four criteria indicate probable disease.*

classified as the disease-modifying drugs and the cytotoxic immununosuppressive drugs. These agents appear to have the capacity to modify the course of the disease and to slow its progress in some patients.

A number of experimental approaches such as total lymphoid irradiation or lymphoplasmapheresis have also been used to treat RA. Although some show potential for ameliorating disease, none has been shown to be a safe and cost-effective way to treat patients on a long-term basis. A variety of nontraditional approaches have also been claimed to be effective in treating RA, including diets, plant and animal extracts, vaccines, hormones, and topical preparations of various sorts. Many of these are costly and none has been shown to be effective. However, belief in their efficacy ensures their continued use by some patients.

Nonsteroidal anti-inflammatory drugs Besides aspirin, there are now several additional nonsteroidal anti-inflammatory drugs available to treat RA. These include fenoprofen, ibuprofen, indomethacin, naproxen, meclofenamate, piroxicam, sulindac, and tolmetin. As a result of the capacity of these agents to block the activity of the enzyme cyclooxygenase and therefore the production of prostaglandins, prostacycline, and thromboxanes, they have analgesic, anti-inflammatory, and antipyretic properties. These agents are all associated with a wide spectrum of toxic side effects. Some, such as gastric irritation, azotemia, platelet dysfunction, and exacerbation of allergic rhinitis and asthma, are related to the inhibition of cyclooxygenase activity, while a variety of others such as rash, liver function abnormalities, and bone marrow depression may not be. Elderly patients on diuretics may be at higher risk for certain toxic effects. None of the nonsteroidal anti-inflammatory drugs has been shown to be more effective than aspirin in the treatment of RA. However, these nonaspirin drugs are associated with a lower incidence of gastrointestinal intolerance. None of the newer nonsteroidal anti-inflammatory drugs appears to show significant therapeutic advantages over the other available agents. In addition, there is no consistent advantage of any of these newer agents over the others with respect to the incidence or severity of toxic manifestations.

Disease-modifying drugs Clinical experience has delineated a number of agents that appear to have the capacity to alter the course of RA. This group of agents includes gold compounds, D-penicillamine, and the antimalarials. In practice, these agents share a number of characteristics. They exert minimal direct nonspecific anti-inflammatory or analgesic effects, and therefore nonsteroidal anti-inflammatory drugs must be continued during their administration, except in a few cases when true remissions are induced with them. The appearance of benefit from disease-modifying drug therapy is usually delayed for weeks or months. As many as two-thirds of patients develop some clinical improvement as a result of therapy with any of these agents, although the induction of true remissions is unusual. In addition to clinical improvement, there is frequently an improvement in serologic evidence of disease activity, and titers of rheumatoid factor and the erythrocyte sedimentation rate frequently decline as a result of therapy. Despite this, there is only a small body of evidence to support the conclusion that disease-modifying drugs actually retard the development of bone erosions or facilitate their healing.

Each of these drugs is associated with considerable toxicity, and therefore, careful patient monitoring is necessary. Which disease-modifying drug should be the drug of first choice remains controversial, and trials have failed to demonstrate a consistent advantage of one over the other. Toxicity of the various agents thus becomes important in determining the drug of first choice. Failure to respond or development of toxicity to one agent does not preclude responsiveness to another. For example, a similar percentage of RA patients who have failed to respond to gold will respond to D-pencillamine when this agent is administered as the initial disease-modifying drug. No characteristic features of patients have emerged that predict responsiveness to a disease-modifying drug. Guidelines for the use of these drugs are given in Table 263-2.

Glucocorticoid therapy Although systemic glucocorticoid therapy can provide effective symptomatic therapy in patients with RA, these drugs should be avoided if possible because they do not alter the course of the disease and the potential toxicity of long-term therapy is substantial. Low-dose (less than 7.5 mg per day) prednisone has been advocated as useful additive therapy to control symptoms, but trials have not confirmed its efficacy and even low-dose therapy may promote osteoporosis.

Cytotoxic immunosuppressive therapy The cytotoxic immunosuppressive drugs azathioprine and cyclophosphamide have been shown to be effective in the treatment of RA and to exert therapeutic effects that are similar to the disease-modifying drugs. However, these agents are no more effective than the disease-modifying drugs. Moreover, they cause a variety of toxic side effects, and cyclophosphamide appears to predispose the patient to the development of malignant neoplasms. Therefore, these drugs have been reserved for patients who have clearly failed therapy with disease-modifying drugs. On occasion, extraarticular disease such as rheumatoid vasculitis may require cytotoxic immunosuppressive therapy.

Intermittent low-dose methotrexate, a folic acid antagonist, also may be useful in the treatment of RA. Although methotrexate appears to be effective, as many as 20 percent of treated patients develop liver function abnormalities. The long-term significance of these abnormalities has not been elucidated.

Surgery Surgery plays a role in the management of patients with severely damaged joints. Although arthroplasties and total joint replacements can be done on a number of joints, the most successful procedures are carried out on hips and knees. Realistic goals of these procedures are relief of pain, correction of deformity, and modest functional improvement. Reconstructive hand surgery may lead to cosmetic improvement, although functional benefit is marginal. Open or arthroscopic synovectomy may be useful in some patients with persistent monarthritis, especially of the knee. In addition, early tenosynovectomy of the wrist may prevent tendon rupture.

TABLE 263-2 Major disease-modifying drugs: Guide to therapy

	Hydroxychloroquine	Auranofin (oral gold)	Gold sodium thiomalate and gold thioglucose (intramuscular gold)	D-Penicillamine
Administration	<6.5 mg/kg per day	3 mg twice daily	50 mg per week loading → 1 g total; then taper to 50 mg per month	250 mg per day on empty stomach; increase daily dose by 250 mg every 3 months; maximum, 1 g per day
Major toxicity	Retinopathy	Rash, diarrhea; thrombocytopenia, granulocytopenia, and proteinuria rarely seen	Rash, thrombocytopenia, granulocytopenia, proteinuria	Rash, gastrointestinal intolerance, proteinuria, thrombocytopenia, granulocytopenia
Precautions	Ophthalmologic examination every 6 months	CBC, platelet count, urinalysis monthly, prescriptions should be nonrenewable	CBC, platelet count, urinalysis before each injection	CBC, platelet count, urinalysis every 2 weeks × 6 months, then every month

Approach to the patient with RA At the onset of disease it is difficult to predict the natural history of an individual patient's illness. Therefore, the usual approach is to attempt to alleviate the patient's symptoms with nonsteroidal anti-inflammatory drugs. The major reason to delay more definitive therapy is the possibility that a spontaneous remission will occur. Moreover, since the disease-modifying drugs are potentially toxic and not universally effective, enthusiasm for their use is muted when a natural remission is still a possibility.

At some time during most patient's course, the possibility of initiating disease-modifying drug therapy is entertained. With aggressive disease this might occur sooner, often within 3 to 6 months of disease onset, while in patients with more indolent disease, smoldering activity may not require such therapy for many years. The development of bone erosions or radiographic evidence of cartilage loss is clear-cut evidence of the destructive potential of the inflammatory process and indicates the need for disease-modifying drug therapy. The other indications such as persistent pain, joint swelling, or functional impairment are much more subjective, however. The decision to begin use of a disease-modifying drug requires careful monitoring of joint swelling and functional activity, as well as an understanding of the patient's pain tolerance and expectation of therapy. In this setting, the fully informed patient must play an active role in the decision to begin disease-modifying drug therapy, after careful review of the therapeutic and toxic potential of the various drugs.

If a patient responds to a disease-modifying drug, therapy is continued with careful monitoring to avoid toxicity. All disease-modifying drugs provide a suppressive effect and therefore require prolonged administration. Even with successful therapy, local injection of glucocorticoids may be necessary to diminish inflammation that may persist in a limited number of joints. In addition, nonsteroidal anti-inflammatory drugs may be necessary to mitigate symptoms. Even after inflammation has totally resolved, symptoms from loss of cartilage and supervening degenerative joint disease or deformities may require additional treatment. Surgery may also be necessary to relieve pain or diminish the functional impairment secondary to deformity. Only when patients have persistent inflammatory disease or severe extraarticular manifestations is the use of cytotoxic immunosuppressive drugs or experimental procedures justified.

REFERENCES

BURMESTER GR et al: Identification of three major synovial lining cell populations by monoclonal antibodies directed to Ia antigens and antigens associated with monocytes/macrophages and fibroblasts. Scand J Immunol 17:69, 1983

DECKER JL et al: Rheumatoid arthritis: Evolving concepts of pathogenesis and treatment. Ann Intern Med 101:810, 1984

FEIGENBAUM SL et al: Prognosis in rheumatoid arthritis: A longitudinal study of newly diagnosed younger adult patients. Am J Med 66:377, 1979

HARRIS JR ED: Rheumatoid arthritis: The clinical spectrum, in *Textbook of Rheumatology*, WN Kelley et al (eds). Philadelphia, Saunders, 1981, pp 928–963

HOCHBERG MC: Adult and juvenile rheumatoid arthritis: Current epidemiologic concepts. Epidemiol Rev 3:27, 1981

HURD ER: Extra-articular manifestations of rheumatoid arthritis. Semin Arthritis Rheum 8:151, 1979

KURASAKA M, ZIFF M: Immunoelectron microscopic study of the distribution of T-cell subsets in rheumatoid synovium. J Exp Med 158:1191, 1983

LEGRAND L et al: HLA-DR genotype risks in seropositive rheumatoid arthritis. Am J Hum Genet 36:690, 1984

LIANG MH et al: Costs and outcomes in rheumatoid arthritis and osteoarthritis. Arthritis Rheum 27:522, 1984

LINDBLAD S et al: Phenotypic characterization of synovial tissue cells in situ in different types of synovitis. Arthritis Rheum 26:1321, 1983

LIPSKY PE: Remission-inducing therapy in rheumatoid arthritis. Am J Med 74(4B):40, 1983

MITCHELL DM, FRIES JF: An analysis of the American Rheumatism Association criteria for rheumatoid arthritis. Arthritis Rheum 25:481, 1982

POULTER LW et al: The involvement of interdigitating (antigen-presenting) cells in the pathogenesis of rheumatoid arthritis. Clin Exp Immunol 51:247, 1983

ROTHSCHILD B, MASI AT: Pathogenesis of rheumatoid arthritis: A vascular hypothesis. Semin Arthritis Rheum 12:11, 1982

UTSINGER PD et al (eds): *Rheumatoid Arthritis*. Philadelphia, Lippincott, 1985

VANDENBROUCKE JP et al: Survival and cause of death in rheumatoid arthritis: A 25 year prospective follow-up. J Rheum 11:158, 1984

YOUNG A et al: Association of HLA-DR4/DW4 and DR2/DW2 with radiologic changes in a prospective study of patients with rheumatoid arthritis. Preferential relationship with HLA-DW rather than HLA-DR specificities. Arthritis Rheum 27:20, 1984

ZVAIFLER NJ: The immunopathology of joint inflammation in rheumatoid arthritis. Adv Immunol 16:265, 1973

264 PROGRESSIVE SYSTEMIC SCLEROSIS (DIFFUSE SCLERODERMA)

BRUCE C. GILLILAND

Progressive systemic sclerosis (PSS) is a multisystem disorder characterized by inflammatory, vascular, and fibrotic changes of the skin (scleroderma) and a variety of internal organs, most notably the gastrointestinal tract, lungs, heart, and kidney. The course, extent of involvement, and severity of disease varies greatly among patients. In some patients, skin changes restricted to the distal extremities may be present for many years before visceral involvement becomes apparent, while in others widespread skin changes and visceral disease develop rapidly over a few years. Visceral disease may also occur in the absence of skin involvement. The disease is not always progressive, and skin changes may actually return to near normal after many years. Survival is determined by the severity of visceral disease involving especially the heart, lungs, and/or kidneys.

ETIOLOGY AND PATHOGENESIS This disease has a worldwide distribution but is apparently rare in Asia, especially among the Chinese, Indians, and Malaysians. The onset of disease is usually in the third to fifth decades, and women are affected four times as often as men. The etiology and pathogenesis of PSS are not known, and the role of heredity has not been clarified. Several examples of familial PSS have been reported. The increased fibrosis in the skin and other organ systems is considered to be due to overproduction of normal collagen. The amount of collagen synthesized by individual fibroblasts is increased compared to appropriate controls. Studies have suggested an abnormal regulation of connective tissue synthesis, degradation, or both.

The primary event in systemic sclerosis is postulated to be endothelial cell injury in blood vessels ranging from small arteries to capillaries. The cause of this endothelial damage is not known, but a serum cytotoxic factor, a serine protease, has been identified in some patients with systemic sclerosis. In small arteries, disruption of endothelial cells leads to platelet aggregation, myointimal cell proliferation, and fibrosis resulting in narrowing, decreased distensibility, and obliteration of the vessels. Elevated plasma levels of von Willebrand factor and antigen in PSS patients reflect endothelial cell damage. The binding of von Willebrand factor to the exposed subendothelium permits adhesion and subsequent aggregation of platelets. Activated platelets release vascular permeability factors and procoagulant factors. Increased vascular permeability from endothelial cell damage produces interstitial edema, fibroblast stimulation, and eventually fibrosis in the surrounding tissue. Thus, the early phase of systemic sclerosis is characterized by target organ edema followed later by fibrosis. The number of capillaries in the skin is reduced by this fibrotic process; the remaining capillaries dilate and proliferate to become visible telangiectatic lesions.

Both humoral and cell-mediated immune phenomena are present in patients with PSS. Hypergammaglobulinemia and antinuclear antibodies are frequent findings. Antibodies have also been demonstrated to the cell membrane of fibroblasts as well as to type I and type IV collagen. The pathogenic role of these various autoantibodies is not known. Perivascular cell infiltrates are found in early skin lesions of PSS. These infiltrates contain T cells, plasma cells, and macrophages. In chronic lesions, fibroblasts and histiocytes predominate. Evaluation of the T-cell population in involved skin utilizing monoclonal antibodies shows an increased T4/T8 ratio due to decreased number of T8 cells. A similar T4/T8 ratio is found in the peripheral blood of some patients with PSS. Soluble extracts from normal and scleroderma skin stimulate lymphocytes from PSS patients as measured by the macrophage migration inhibition test. Peripheral blood lymphocytes from PSS patients have also been shown to be cytotoxic to fibroblasts in cell cultures. It is speculated that T cells sensitized to altered endothelial antigens or other skin tissue antigens elaborate lymphokines which attract and activate monocytes-macrophages. Monokines from stimulated monocytes-macrophages damage endothelium and diffuse into the interstitium to stimulate fibroblasts. In support of cell-mediated immunity playing a role in the pathogenesis of PSS is the appearance of scleroderma-like lesions in patients with graft-versus-host disease following marrow transplantation, a condition known to be mediated by cell-mediated events.

Chromosomal abnormalities have been noted in greater than 90 percent of PSS patients. These acquired abnormalities include chromatid breaks, acentric fragments, and ring chromosomes, and are found in approximately 30 percent of mitotic cells. A chromosomal breakage factor has been found in the serum of PSS patients. The significance of these chromosomal abnormalities is unknown.

Occupational hazards have been associated with the development of PSS. The occurrence of PSS in coal and gold miners appears to be more common than in nonminers, suggesting that silica dust may be a predisposing factor. Workers exposed to polyvinyl chloride may develop Raynaud's phenomenon, acroosteolysis, and scleroderma-like skin lesions. Nail-fold capillary abnormalities similar to those observed in PSS are also present. In addition, these workers also developed hepatic fibrosis and angiosarcoma. Extensive sclerosis of the dermis and subcutaneous tissue has been noted in patients receiving pentazocine, a nonnarcotic analgesic agent. Bleomycin, an anticancer agent, produces fibrotic skin nodules, linear hyperpigmentation, alopecia, gangrene of fingers, and pulmonary fibrosis affecting mainly the lower lobes. Absence of Raynaud's phenomenon and sparing of the face and distal extremities distinguish this entity from PSS.

PATHOLOGY In the skin, a thin epidermis overlies compact bundles of collagen which lie parallel to the epidermis. Fingerlike projections of collagen extend from the dermis into the subcutaneous tissue and bind the skin to the underlying tissue. Dermal appendages are atrophied, and rete pegs are lost. Increased numbers of lymphocytes identified as mostly T cells may be present at the border of skin lesions.

In the lower two-thirds of the esophagus, the histologic findings consist of a thin mucosa and increased collagen in the lamina propria, submucosa, and serosa. The degree of fibrosis is less than in the skin. Atrophy of the muscularis in the esophagus and throughout the involved portions of the gastrointestinal tract is more prominent than the amount of fibrotic replacement of muscle. Ulceration of the mucosa is often present and may be due to either PSS or superimposed peptic esophagitis. Striated muscles in the upper one-third of the esophagus are relatively spared. Similar changes may be found throughout the gastrointestinal tract, especially in the second and third portions of the duodenum, jejunum, and large intestine. Atrophy of the muscularis of the large intestine may lead to the development of large-mouth diverticula. In the later stages of the disease, the involved portions of the gastrointestinal tract become dilated. Infiltration of lymphocytes and plasma cells in the lamina propria is also present.

With pulmonary involvement, diffuse interstitial fibrosis, thickening of the alveolar membrane, and peribronchial fibrosis are observed. Bronchiolar epithelial proliferation accompanies the pulmonary fibrosis. Rupture of septa produces small cysts and areas of bullous emphysema. Small pulmonary arteries and arterioles show intimal thickening, fragmentation of the elastica, and muscular hypertrophy; this may occur without interstitial pulmonary fibrosis and produce pulmonary hypertension.

The synovium in patients with PSS and arthritis is similar to that seen in early rheumatoid arthritis and shows edema with infiltration of lymphocytes and plasma cells. A characteristic finding is a thick layer of fibrin overlying and within the synovium. Later in the disease the synovium may become fibrotic. Fibrinous deposits appear on the surfaces of tendon sheaths and in the overlying fascia, and may lead to audible creaking over moving tendons.

Histologic features of muscle involvement consist of interstitial and perivascular lymphocytic infiltrations, degeneration of muscle fibers, and interstitial fibrosis. Arterioles may be thickened, and capillaries may be decreased in number.

In the heart, myocardial interstitial fibrosis replaces myocardial fibers. Fibrosis also involves the conduction system, leading to atrioventricular conduction defects and arrhythmias. The wall of smaller coronary arteries may be thickened, and lymphocytic infiltration is seen. Fibrinous pericarditis and pericardial effusions are found in some patients.

Renal involvement is found in over half the patients and consists of intimal hyperplasia of the interlobular arteries, fibrinoid necrosis of the afferent arterioles, including the glomerular tuft, and thickening of the glomerular basement membrane. These lesions result in cortical infarctions and glomerulosclerosis. The renal pathologic change is often indistinguishable from that observed in malignant hypertension. Renal vascular lesions, however, may be present in the absence of hypertension. Angiographic renal studies in patients with PSS may show constriction of the intralobular arteries, a finding that simulates the vasospasm of the digital arteries observed in Raynaud's phenomenon. Along with Raynaud's phenomenon, induced by cooling, a decrease in renal blood flow has been observed. These studies are of interest because three-quarters of the deaths from renal involvement in PSS have been shown to occur in the fall and winter.

Primary liver involvement is not common, but diffuse cirrhosis, intrahepatic cholestasis, and chronic passive congestion occur occasionally. Fibrosis of the thyroid may develop. Thickening of the periodontal membrane with replacement of the lamina dura is demonstrated radiographically as widening of the periodontal space and rarely causes loosening of the teeth.

Small arterial and arteriolar lesions are found in many tissues; they consist of concentric acellular thickening of the intima with narrowing or occlusion of the lumen. These lesions are found in the digital arteries and arterioles in patients with PSS and Raynaud's phenomenon. Vascular abnormalities have been described in the lung, skin, kidney, muscle, gastrointestinal tract, pancreas, synovium, vasa vasorum, and the central nervous system. Arteritis with fibrinoid necrosis and infiltration by mononuclear cells of all three layers is occasionally observed.

CLINICAL MANIFESTATIONS PSS usually begins insidiously; the first symptom is frequently Raynaud's phenomenon. Raynaud's phenomenon is defined as episodic vasoconstriction of arteries and arterioles of the fingers, toes, and sometimes the face which is brought on by cold or emotional stimuli. Patients may experience triphasic color changes consisting of pallor, cyanosis, and rubor, occurring usually in this order. Raynaud's phenomenon should be considered when the patient experiences any one or combinations of these changes. Pallor and cyanosis are most often associated with numbness and coldness of the fingers, and rubor with pain and tingling. Raynaud's phenomenon may precede the skin changes by months or even years. Raynaud's phenomenon occurs in 90 percent of patients with the skin changes of scleroderma. The fingers and hands in the early stages are swollen. Subsequently the skin becomes firm, thickened, and leathery in appearance, and tightly bound to the underlying subcutaneous tissue. The skin changes spread to involve the arms, face, chest, abdomen, and back. The lower extremities are relatively spared. The taut skin over the fingers gradually limits full extension, and may lead to fixed flexion contractures. Ulcers may appear on the fingertips and over bony prominences and may become infected. The soft tissue of the fingertips is lost, and in some instances the bone of terminal phalanges is resorbed. The skin may become darkly pigmented even without exposure to the sun; areas of depigmentation and numerous telangiectatic mats often appear on the skin. The skin becomes dry and coarse, and hair is lost. Examination of nail folds with a wide-angle microscope or an ophthalmoscope shows initially disorganization of the capillary bed followed later by a decrease in the number of capillary loops and dilatation of the remaining loops. In some patients, calcific deposits develop in the subcutaneous and periarticular tissue. The overlying skin may break down, with draining of calcific material. Involvement of the face results in the loss of normal skin wrinkles, loss of facial expression, and inability to open the mouth fully. In disease of many years' duration, the hidebound skin may soften and become pliable, but will usually remain atrophic.

The coexistence of *c*alcinosis, *R*aynaud's phenomenon, *e*sophageal hypomotility, *s*clerodactyly, and *t*elangiectasia has been termed the CREST syndrome and initially was considered a benign form of PSS. Patients may have skin changes of PSS limited to the distal extremities for many years. However, some of these patients have subsequently developed visceral and more extensive cutaneous lesions of PSS. Pulmonary hypertension may occur any time during the course.

More than half the patients with PSS complain of pain, swelling, and stiffness of the fingers and knees. A symmetric polyarthritis, resembling rheumatoid arthritis, may be seen. In more advanced stages of the disease, leathery crepitation can be palpated over moving joints, especially the knee. Extensive fibrotic thickening of the tendon sheaths in the wrist can produce a carpal tunnel syndrome. Acute myositis with proximal muscle weakness and enzyme elevation occurs in PSS and is indistinguishable from polymyositis. Patients also develop a distinctive indolent myopathy characterized by mild muscle weakness with few laboratory abnormalities.

Symptoms attributable to esophageal involvement, which are present in more than 50 percent of patients, include epigastric fullness, burning pain in the epigastric or retrosternal regions, and regurgitation of gastric contents. These symptoms, most noticeable when the patient is lying flat or bending over, are due to the reduced tone of the gastroesophageal sphincter and to dilatation of the distal esophagus. Peptic esophagitis frequently occurs and may lead to strictures and narrowing of the lower esophagus. However, it seldom results in bleeding. Dysphagia, particularly of solid foods, may occur independent of other esophageal symptoms and is caused by the loss of esophageal motility due to neuromuscular dysfunction. Manometry or cineradiography reveals decreased amplitude or disappearance of peristaltic waves in the lower two-thirds of the esophagus. A closer correlation exists between this finding and Raynaud's phenomenon than with cutaneous manifestations of PSS. Later in the course of the illness, dilatation and atony of the lower portion of the esophagus as well as reflux are seen. With gastric involvement, barium studies show dilatation, atony, and delayed gastric emptying.

Symptoms referable to involvement of the small intestine by PSS include bloating and abdominal pain and may suggest intestinal obstruction or paralytic ileus. Malabsorption syndrome with weight loss, steatorrhea, and anemia also occurs secondary to obliteration of the lymphatics by fibrosis or in some patients due to bacterial overgrowth in the atonic intestine. Involvement of the large intestine may cause chronic constipation and fecal impaction with episodes of bowel obstruction. Roentgenographic features of the second and third portions of the duodenum and of the jejunum include dilatation, loss of the usual feathery pattern, and delayed disappearance of barium. Pneumatosis intestinalis, which occasionally occurs in PSS, is seen as radiolucent cysts or linear streaks within the wall of the small intestine. Benign pneumoperitoneum may result from the rupture of these cysts. Barium studies of the large intestine may show dilatation, atony, and large-mouth diverticula. Some patients may have gastrointestinal PSS with little or no cutaneous or other organ involvement. Hypothyroidism occurs in a few patients with PSS, particularly in those with long-standing cutaneous disease. Fibrosis of the thyroid gland was found in 14 percent of PSS patients at autopsy.

Patients with pulmonary fibrosis often complain of a dry cough and exertional dyspnea; however, shortness of breath as a presenting complaint is unusual. Bilateral basilar rales may be present. Though pleural involvement is not infrequent at postmortem, symptoms of pleurisy are unusual. Restriction of chest movement may rarely occur with extensive skin involvement of the thorax. Additional pulmonary problems result from aspiration pneumonia secondary to esophageal malfunction. Superimposed bacterial or viral pneumonia may be a serious complication in patients with pulmonary fibrosis. Malignant alveolar or bronchiolar cell neoplasms have been reported in some patients with PSS and pulmonary fibrosis. However, no other association of PSS with malignancy has been shown. Pulmonary function test results are abnormal even in early disease and show a low diffusion capacity and a low P_{O_2} on exercise. Roentgenograms of the chest may show a pattern of linear densities, mottling, and honeycombing. These changes are more evident in the lower two-thirds of the lungs. Patients may develop pulmonary arterial hypertension without significant interstitial fibrosis, presumably secondary to the proliferative vascular lesion of PSS involving pulmonary arteries and arterioles. These patients complain of shortness of breath, and on physical examination they have an accentuated pulmonic second heart sound, a fixed split second heart sound, and the systolic murmur of pulmonary artery dilatation. Electrocardiographic evidence of pulmonary hypertension may also be present.

Cardiac involvement by PSS often goes clinically unrecognized; however, varying degrees of heart block and arrhythmias may be seen. Cardiomyopathy attributable to diffuse myocardial fibrosis may also occur. Other cardiac manifestations may be secondary to pulmonary disease and hypertension. Left ventricular failure develops more frequently than cor pulmonale, even with the presence of pulmonary fibrosis. Acute and chronic pericarditis may develop and occasionally produce tamponade. Cardiac involvement is the cause of death in 15 percent of PSS patients.

Renal failure is the leading cause of death in PSS, accounting for almost half of the deaths. The onset of renal involvement is frequently within 3 years of the diagnosis of PSS. Renal failure, however, can present abruptly at any time in an apparently stable patient and is fatal unless treated. Acute renal failure can develop in association with malignant hypertension or in a setting of mild chronic hypertension. Proteinuria, an abnormal urine sediment, hypertension, azotemia, and microangiopathic hemolytic anemia are clinical features associated with progressive renal disease. It is difficult to predict the patient who will develop renal failure. One indicator of impending renal failure is microangiopathic anemia, which may appear several weeks before renal failure. The presence of chronic pericardial effusion may also be associated with subsequent renal failure.

LABORATORY FINDINGS The erythrocyte sedimentation rate may be elevated. Hypoproliferative anemia related to chronic inflammation is the most common cause of anemia in PSS. Anemia may also be caused by iron deficiency secondary to gastrointestinal bleeding. Bacterial overgrowth due to atony of the small bowel may lead to vitamin B_{12} and/or folic acid–deficiency anemia. Microangiopathic hemolytic anemia is most often associated with renal involvement and is caused by the presence of fibrin deposition in the renal arterioles. Hypergammaglobulinemia, with elevated levels mainly of IgG, is found in approximately half the patients. Rheumatoid factor, in low titer, is present in 25 percent of patients. Antinuclear antibodies (ANA) are reported in 33 to 96 percent depending on the tissue substrate used in the test. Utilizing a cultured human laryngeal carcinoma cell line (HEp-2), 96 percent of PSS patients are found to be ANA-positive. Specific antinuclear antibodies include antibodies to nucleolar antigens, nuclear ribonucleoprotein (RNP), centromere, and Scl-70 (an extractable nonhistone nuclear protein, 70,000 daltons). Anti-Scl-70 is relatively specific for PSS but is found in only 20 percent of patients. Antibodies reacting with the centromeric region of metaphase chromosomes are found in most patients meeting the criteria for CREST syndrome, less often in patients with diffuse PSS, and in a few patients with only Raynaud's phenomenon. Anticentromere antibodies rarely occur in other connective tissue disorders.

DIAGNOSIS The diagnosis of PSS presents no difficulty in the presence of Raynaud's phenomenon, with typical skin lesions and visceral involvement. PSS should always be included in the differential diagnosis of patients with Raynaud's phenomenon. Other causes of Raynaud's phenomenon include thoracic outlet (scalenus anticus and cervical rib) syndromes, shoulder-hand syndrome, trauma (jackhammer or vibratory machine operators), previous cold injury, vinyl chloride exposure, and circulating cryoglobulins or cold agglutinins. Linear scleroderma and morphea are localized forms of PSS and may be associated with Raynaud's phenomenon and hypergammaglobulinemia. PSS may initially be confused with rheumatoid arthritis, systemic lupus erythematosus, or polymyositis when articular or muscle involvement is prominent early in the disease. PSS without cutaneous involvement should be considered in patients with unexplained pulmonary fibrosis, pulmonary hypertension, cardiomyopathies, heart block, dysphagia, or malabsorption syndrome. Several conditions have scleroderma-like features but lack the visceral involvement. Scleredema (scleredema adultorum of Buschke) occurs predominantly in children and is characterized by painless edematous induration involving the face, scalp, neck, trunk, and proximal portions of the extremities. Involvement of the hands and feet usually does not occur. Scleredema may be associated with previous streptococcal infection and is usually self-limited, resolving in 6 to 12 months. Histology reveals accumulation of mucopolysaccharides in the dermis and skeletal muscle. A rare entity, scleromyxedema (lichen myxedematosus), is manifested by yellowish or pale-red papules in association with diffuse skin thickening which may involve the face and hands. Acid mucopolysaccharide deposits are found in the dermis. Monoclonal IgG may be detected in some of these patients. Primary amyloidosis may involve the skin of the extremities and face diffusely to give the appearance of scleroderma. Biopsy will clearly differentiate these entities.

Diffuse fasciitis with eosinophilia A scleroderma-like syndrome consisting of fasciitis, myositis, eosinophilia, and hypergammaglobulinemia has been recognized. Patients usually do not have Raynaud's phenomenon or develop sclerodactyly. Systemic involvement seldom occurs. Several patients with eosinophilic fasciitis have been reported to have aplastic anemia; however, the significance of the association is not understood. Patients develop tenderness and swelling of the extremities with the onset of symptoms often related to strenuous physical exertion. The trunk and neck can also be involved. In affected areas, the skin is thickened with a cobblestone or puckered appearance. Full-thickness biopsy consisting of skin, fascia, and superficial muscle shows perivascular infiltration of histiocytes, eosinophils, lymphocytes, and plasma cells in the dermis, subcutaneous fat and fascia, and underlying muscle. Improvement has been noted with administration of glucocorticoids, but spontaneous improvement has also been recorded.

PROGNOSIS In the majority of patients PSS is characterized by a prolonged, relentless course of progressive skin and/or visceral involvement. In some patients remissions occur, including partial improvement of the skin, and the disease progresses slowly; 80 percent of one group of patients were alive 2 years after onset of symptoms, and 20 percent were alive 10 years after onset. Patients with mainly skin involvement have a more gradual and favorable course than those with visceral disease, involving especially the heart, kidneys, and lungs. Among whites the prognosis is worse in males than in females, and worse in patients whose onset of disease occurs after 45 years of age. The disease tends to be more severe in black females. Death occurs most often from cardiac, renal, and pulmonary involvement.

TREATMENT Effectiveness of drug therapy in PSS is difficult to evaluate because of the variable course and severity of the disease. Many drugs have been used in the treatment of PSS without any consistent or prolonged benefit. In uncontrolled studies D-penicillamine has been reported to reduce skin thickening and prevent development of significant organ involvement. Antiplatelet therapy may play a role in the treatment of PSS since the biologic products of platelets affect blood vessels. Low doses of aspirin block the formation of thromboxane A_2, a powerful vasoconstrictor and platelet aggregator. In addition, dipyridamole 200 to 400 mg in divided daily doses also decreases platelet adhesion to damaged vessel walls. Reports of beneficial effects of colchicine or chlorambucil have not been documented in controlled studies. Even though no drug or combination of drugs has been proved to stop this disease, management directed at the involved organ systems may prolong life and improve the quality of life.

The management of Raynaud's phenomenon is directed at control of vasospasm. It is important to prevent periods of vasospasm since the resulting ischemia may be a further stimulant for vascular fibrosis and eventual obliteration. Patients should be advised to dress warmly and wear mittens and socks, not to smoke, to remove causes of external stress, and to avoid drugs such as amphetamine and ergotamine. Warmth of the central body induces peripheral vasodilation. Drugs that block sympathetic vasoconstriction, such as reserpine, guanethidine, α-methyldopa, phenoxybenzamine, and prazosin may be useful in the treatment of Raynaud's phenomenon, but their side effects often curtail extended use. Nifedipine and other calcium channel blockers are sometimes effective in alleviating Raynaud's phenomenon. The dose of nifedipine is 10 to 20 mg tid. Techniques of biofeedback have also been used with variable success for teaching patients to control the temperature of their hands. Surgical sympathectomy usually provides only temporary improvement, and it, along with other forms of therapy, does not prevent progression of the vascular lesion. The response to any therapy for Raynaud's phenomenon is limited by the degree of existing structural narrowing of digital arteries.

Numerous drugs have been claimed to soften the hidebound skin, but documentation in controlled studies is lacking. These drugs include D-penicillamine, colchicine, *p*-aminobenzoic acid, vitamin E, and dimethyl sulfoxide (DMSO). Dryness of the skin may be reduced by avoiding frequent use of detergent soaps and by applying regularly hydrophilic ointments and bath oils. Regular exercise helps to maintain flexibility of extremities and pliability of skin. Massaging the skin several times a day may also be beneficial. Skin ulcers should be kept clean by soaking or by surgical or chemical debridement. Sympatholytic drugs or local nitroglycerine paste may be beneficial in promoting healing. Infected ulcers can usually be treated with topical antibiotics.

Patients with reflux esophagitis are treated with small frequent meals, antacids between meals, and elevation of the head of the bed. Patients should be advised not to lie down for a few hours after a meal, and to avoid coffee, tea, and chocolate, which reduce the pressure of the lower esophageal sphincter. Cimetidine or ranitidine may be beneficial in some patients. Patients with dysphagia should be instructed to chew their food thoroughly and wash it down with fluids. Malabsorption syndrome due to duodenal hypomotility and bacterial overgrowth may improve with intermittent use of appropriate antibiotics. Stool softeners and mild laxatives are usually adequate for the constipation due to involvement of the colon.

Acute myositis is usually responsive to glucocorticoids; these drugs should not be used for the indolent form of muscle disease of PSS. Articular symptoms are treated with aspirin or other nonsteroidal anti-inflammatory agents.

The pulmonary fibrosis of PSS is not reversible, and therefore the treatment is directed at symptoms or complications. Pulmonary infection requires prompt treatment with antibiotics. Hypoxia necessitates giving low concentrations of oxygen. The role of glucocorticoids in preventing progression of interstitial lung disease is not clear.

Recognition of early renal failure is important in order to preserve remaining function. Renal involvement is usually accompanied by hypertension, but occasional patients may be normotensive. Since most patients have increased renin, drugs that block the renin-angiotensin pathway may be effective in stabilizing or reversing renal failure, as well as lowering the blood pressure. These drugs include propranolol, clonidine, and minoxidil. Another effective drug in treating the renal failure of PSS is captopril, which is an inhibitor of angiotensin converting enzyme. Dialysis may be required in patients with progressive renal failure.

Patients with cardiac failure require careful monitoring of digitalis and diuretic administration. Pericardial effusions may also improve with diuretics. Care should be taken to avoid overdiuresis which may lead to decreased effective plasma volume, decreased cardiac output, and renal failure.

REFERENCES

LeRoy EC: Scleroderma (systemic sclerosis), in *Textbook of Rheumatology*, 2d ed, WN Kelley et al (eds). Philadelphia, Saunders, 1985, pp 1183–1205

Maricq HR et al: Diagnostic potential of in vivo capillary microscopy in scleroderma and related disorders. Arthritis Rheum 23:183, 1980

Shulman LE: Diffuse fasciitis with eosinophilia: A new syndrome. Arthritis Rheum 20:S205, 1977

Whiteside TL et al: Suppressor cell function and T lymphocyte subpopulations in peripheral blood of patients with progressive systemic sclerosis. Arthritis Rheum 26:841, 1983

265 MIXED CONNECTIVE TISSUE DISEASE

GORDON C. SHARP

DEFINITION Mixed connective tissue disease (MCTD) is a syndrome characterized by a combination of clinical features similar to those of systemic lupus erythematosus (SLE), scleroderma, polymyositis, and rheumatoid arthritis and unusually high titers of circulating antibody to a nuclear ribonucleoprotein (RNP) antigen.

ETIOLOGY, PATHOGENESIS, AND PATHOLOGY The etiologic and pathogenic mechanisms of MCTD remain unknown, but a number of clues point to the involvement of immune aberrations: (1) persistence of extremely high titers of antibody to nuclear RNP and a marked polyclonal hypergammaglobulinemia indicative of B-cell hyperactivity; (2) a suppressor T-cell defect; (3) circulating immune complexes during active disease; (4) deposition of IgG, IgM, and complement within vascular walls and along sarcolemmal and glomerular basement membranes; and (5) widespread lymphocytic and plasma cell infiltration of numerous tissues. One of the chief underlying pathologic findings in some adults and children with MCTD is a proliferative intimal and/or medial vascular lesion resulting in narrowing of the lumen of large vessels (e.g., pulmonary, renal, and coronary vessels and aorta) and of small arterioles of many organs. Such lesions in the lungs may contribute to pulmonary hypertension and abnormalities of pulmonary function.

CLINICAL MANIFESTATIONS The age range in published reports of MCTD is from 4 to 80 years, with a mean of 37 years. Approximately 80 percent of patients have been female. Typical clinical features include Raynaud's phenomenon, polyarthritis, swollen hands or sclerodactyly, esophageal dysfunction, pulmonary involvement, and inflammatory myopathy. Malar rash, alopecia, lymphadenopathy, and cardiac and renal disease are less frequent manifestations.

Cutaneous manifestations of MCTD include the swollen, sausage-like appearance of the fingers, nonscarring alopecia, lupus-like rashes, heliotrope eyelids, erythematous patches over the knuckles, periungual telangiectasia, and "squared" telangiectasia over the hands and face. Scleroderma-like changes may be present but only occasionally become extensive.

Musculoskeletal abnormalities occur in most patients. Arthritis is usually nondeforming but may resemble rheumatoid arthritis. Proximal muscle weakness is frequent and may be severe. Serum levels of creatine phosphokinase and aldolase are often markedly elevated, electromyograms are typical of inflammatory myopathy, and biopsies show degeneration of muscle fibers and interstitial and perivascular infiltrates of lymphocytes and plasma cells.

Esophageal dysfunction has been demonstrated in 80 percent of all patients, including 70 percent of asymptomatic patients. Characteristic abnormalities include reduced upper and lower esophageal sphincter pressures and decreased amplitude of peristalsis in the distal two-thirds of the esophagus.

Pulmonary involvement occurs in 85 percent of patients with MCTD but may be clinically silent until far advanced. The most common clinical finding is exertional dyspnea, followed by pleuritic pain and bibasilar rales. Reduced diffusing capacity for carbon monoxide is the most frequent functional abnormality.

Cardiac disease is less common than pulmonary involvement in adults with MCTD but may be more frequent in children. Pericarditis is the most common cardiac finding; other findings have included mitral valve prolapse, myocarditis, congestive heart failure, and aortic insufficiency.

Renal disease in children and adults with MCTD has a combined prevalence of about 28 percent. Progressive renal failure is uncommon, and clinical and histologic findings suggest that vascular lesions may represent a more serious problem than immune complex nephritis in MCTD.

Other less frequent clinical manifestations include fever, lymphadenopathy, neurologic abnormalities, Sjögren's syndrome, hepatosplenomegaly, and intestinal involvement similar to that seen in scleroderma.

LABORATORY FINDINGS Almost all patients have positive fluorescent antinuclear antibody tests at high titers (usually greater than 1:1000) with a speckled pattern and very high titers of antibodies directed against the ribonuclease-sensitive nuclear RNP component of extractable nuclear antigen (ENA). Elevated anti–native DNA antibody titers and antibodies to the ribonuclease-resistant Sm component of ENA are uncommon in MCTD; their presence is usually associated with a severe flare-up of lupus-like features. Rheumatoid factor is found, often at very high titers, in over half of the patients. Diffuse hypergammaglobulinemia is frequently noted and may be elevated to a level of 5 g/dL. A mild to moderate reduction in serum complement levels occurs in about 30 percent of patients. Other less frequent laboratory findings include leukopenia, anemia, and thrombocytopenia (mainly in children).

DIAGNOSIS The diagnosis of MCTD is based on a combination of typical overlapping clinical findings and high titers of circulating antibody to nuclear RNP antigen. In some patients, all the clinical manifestations may be present on initial evaluation. However, as clinicians have become more aware of the syndrome and tests for RNP antibody are being performed more frequently, MCTD is being recognized in an earlier phase in patients presenting with minimal symptoms (e.g., Raynaud's phenomenon, arthralgias, myalgias, and swollen hands). In some this mild "undifferentiated connective tissue disease" syndrome may persist for years, but a recent prospective, long-term study showed that the majority of patients with high titers of RNP antibodies and limited clinical manifestations ultimately developed signs and symptoms consistent with a diagnosis of MCTD.

TREATMENT AND PROGNOSIS Lacking controlled studies, specific treatment recommendations for MCTD are based on anecdotal information. Salicylates, other nonsteroidal anti-inflammatory agents, hydroxychloroquine, vasodilators, and/or low doses of corticosteroids are used to treat mild disease. In general, mild disease is quite responsive to low-dose corticosteroids. If the disease is more severe and significantly involves major organ systems, higher doses of corticosteroids (e.g., 1 mg/kg per day of prednisone) are usually required. As with SLE, a cytotoxic agent may be added in steroid-resistant or -dependent cases. However, the efficacy of this latter therapeutic regimen has not been substantiated by controlled clinical trials. The prognosis for MCTD is generally similar to that of SLE and somewhat better than for scleroderma.

REFERENCES

Grant KC et al: Mixed connective tissue disease—a subset with sequential clinical and laboratory features. J Rheumatol 8:587, 1981

Sharp GC, Singsen BH: Mixed connective tissue disease, in *Arthritis and Allied Conditions*, 10th ed., DJ McCarty (ed). Philadelphia, Lea & Febiger, 1985, chap 64

Sullivan WD et al: A prospective evaluation emphasizing pulmonary involvement in patients with mixed connective tissue disease. Medicine 63:92, 1984

266 SJÖGREN'S SYNDROME

H. CLIFFORD LANE / ANTHONY S. FAUCI

DEFINITION Sjögren's syndrome is an immunologic disorder characterized by progressive destruction of the exocrine glands leading to mucosal and conjunctival dryness (sicca syndrome) accompanied by a variety of autoimmune phenomena. The disease can occur either by itself, in which case it is referred to as primary Sjögren's syndrome, or in association with other autoimmune diseases (see Chaps. 262 and 263), in which case it is referred to as secondary Sjögren's syndrome. In addition, some authors have divided the disease into two forms: glandular, when the only clinical manifestations are within the exocrine system, and extraglandular, when other tissues are involved as well.

INCIDENCE AND PREVALENCE The disease predominantly affects women in the third or fourth decades of life. Although precise incidence figures are not known, it has been suggested that Sjögren's syndrome is the second most common rheumatologic disease in the United States. Up to 30 percent of patients with rheumatoid arthritis, 10 percent of patients with systemic lupus erythematosus, and 1 percent of patients with scleroderma have been reported as having secondary Sjögren's syndrome. Immunogenetic predisposition appears to play an important role in the incidence of Sjögren's syndrome. The frequency of the HLA-B8, the HLA-DRw3, and the MT-2 histocompatibility antigens is significantly increased in patients with primary Sjögren's syndrome.

PATHOPHYSIOLOGY AND IMMUNOPATHOGENESIS The two main mechanisms of tissue destruction in Sjögren's syndrome are lymphocytic infiltration and immune-complex deposition. In addition, approximately 10 percent of these patients develop a lymphoproliferative process known as *pseudolymphoma*. This disorder has many histologic features of lymphoma but is associated clinically with a benign course.

Virtually any organ system of the body may be affected in the patient with Sjögren's syndrome. The disease process is most striking in the salivary glands, where there is a progressive mononuclear cell infiltrate which generally leads to complete scarring. Renal disease may result from a lymphocytic interstitial nephritis or an immune-complex glomerulonephritis. Pulmonary involvement is most frequently due to interstitial pneumonitis caused by an infiltration of mononuclear cells, although discrete mass lesions due to pseudolymphoma may occur. Patients with Sjögren's syndrome may also develop an immune-complex vasculitis, at times associated with cryoglobulinemia. Thromboangiitis obliterans has also been seen, usually in patients with preexisting Raynaud's phenomena. Both the peripheral and the central nervous system manifestations of this disease are felt to be due to blood vessel inflammation.

Patients with Sjögren's syndrome exhibit two main types of immunoregulatory defects. The first of these is an abnormally active cellular immune system. This is evident by the intense inflammatory mononuclear cell infiltrates seen in the salivary glands of these patients. These infiltrates are made up predominantly of activated T cells; however, activated B lymphocytes can be detected as well. These mononuclear cell infiltrates are responsible for many of the clinical manifestations of Sjögren's syndrome, including the profound dryness of conjunctival and mucosal surfaces, interstitial nephritis, interstitial pneumonitis, and meningoencephalitis. The second immunoregulatory defect seen in patients with Sjögren's syndrome is oligoclonal B-cell activation. This results in hypergammaglobulinemia, oligoclonal spikes on protein electrophoresis, elevated levels of circulating immune complexes, and the production of autoantibodies. Among the autoantibodies seen are rheumatoid factor, SSA (anti-Ro), and SSB (anti-La). While the precise clinical significance of these and other serologic markers is unclear, it does appear that most patients with the more serious systemic manifestations of Sjögren's syndrome are SSA-positive.

CLINICAL MANIFESTATIONS AND LABORATORY ABNORMALITIES The most common clinical manifestations of Sjögren's syndrome are keratoconjunctivitis sicca and xerostomia. Patients often complain initially of a gritty sensation in the eyes or severe dryness of the mouth. Mucosal dryness may extend into the upper airway, in which case patients may complain of a persistent cough or hoarseness which is worse in cold weather. Corneal dryness may be so severe as to result in corneal ulcerations.

Renal involvement is seen in approximately 40 percent of patients with primary Sjögren's syndrome. This generally presents clinically as a mild interstitial nephritis which may result in renal tubular acidosis. This form of kidney disease rarely leads to chronic renal failure; however, it may be associated with a 50 percent reduction in creatinine clearance. A minority of patients with renal disease demonstrate an immune-complex glomerulonephritis. This is seen usually in the context of systemic vasculitis.

Twenty-five percent of patients with primary Sjögren's syndrome develop vasculitis (Chap. 269). This usually takes the form of a cutaneous palpable purpura or hypersensitivity vasculitis of the lower extremities. Patients with Sjögren's syndrome may also develop a severe, systemic vasculitis. This is often seen in the setting of cryoglobulinemia and may result in fever, skin rash, and bowel infarction. The vasculitic syndromes seen in patients with Sjögren's syndrome are generally episodic rather than chronic.

A variety of neurologic conditions have been described in patients with Sjögren's syndrome. The most common nervous system presentation is that of a sensory polyneuropathy and/or mononeuritis multiplex. Central nervous system involvement has been reported in this illness and may be focal or diffuse in its presentation. Patients have also been noted to develop a diffuse proximal myositis.

Pulmonary involvement generally takes the form of an interstitial pneumonitis which is usually of little clinical significance. Pulmonary mass lesions may occur which may be infectious, inflammatory, or neoplastic.

Approximately 10 percent of patients with Sjögren's syndrome develop pseudolymphoma. This unusual lymphoproliferative disorder may present as lymphadenopathy, parotid gland enlargement, or pulmonary nodules. Approximately 10 percent of the Sjögren's syndrome patients with pseudolymphoma may go on to develop a lymphocytic (non-Hodgkin's) lymphoma.

Autoimmune thyroid disease resembling Hashimoto's thyroiditis is a common accompaniment of Sjögren's syndrome. Approximately 50 percent of patients with Sjögren's syndrome have some evidence of biochemical hypothyroidism, and 10 percent of patients require thyroid supplement.

Pregnant women with anti-Ro (SSA) antibodies are at an increased risk of delivering infants with cardiac conduction defects. Thus, pregnancies need to be carefully monitored in this group of patients.

A variety of laboratory abnormalities may be seen in patients with Sjögren's syndrome. Among the serologic and hematologic abnormalities are elevated levels of circulating immune complexes, autoantibodies, leukopenia, thrombocytosis, and an elevation in the erythrocyte sedimentation rate. In addition, patients often have a high urine pH.

While the presence of these abnormalities may increase one's level of suspicion of a diagnosis of Sjögren's syndrome, they are not diagnostic by themselves.

DIAGNOSIS A diagnosis of Sjögren's syndrome is made when the triad of keratoconjunctivitis sicca, xerostomia, and mononuclear cell infiltration of the salivary gland is noted. This latter finding is made by a lower lip biopsy. The differential diagnosis of Sjögren's syndrome includes sarcoidosis, lymphoma, primary amyloidosis, and graft-versus-host disease.

TREATMENT AND PROGNOSIS Treatment is geared toward symptomatic relief of mucosal dryness, and includes artificial tears, ophthalmologic lubricating ointments, nasal sprays of normal saline, moisturizing skin lotions, and frequent sips of water. There is currently no effective treatment for the ongoing exocrine gland destruction. Corticosteroids have been used with varying degrees of success in the management of glomerulonephritis, interstitial pneumonitis, and pseudolymphoma. They have not proved to be effective in the management of the cutaneous vasculitis. Patients with systemic vasculitis associated with cryoglobulinemia may benefit from brief courses of immunosuppressive therapy (Chap. 269). It should be stressed that this form of systemic vasculitis is episodic, and therefore, in contrast to most forms of systemic necrotizing vasculitis, does not require chronic immunosuppressive therapy. Therapy of pseudolymphoma should be reserved for those cases in which vital organ function is threatened. Due to the fact that there is some suggestion that cytotoxic therapy may predispose to the transition from pseudolymphoma to true lymphoma, this form of immunosuppressive therapy should be reserved for potentially life-threatening situations.

The overall prognosis for patients with Sjögren's syndrome is quite good. Patients with secondary Sjögren's syndrome generally have less severe manifestations of Sjögren's than those with the primary form. Patients with primary disease are best managed with ocular and mucosal lubricants, attention to oral hygiene, frequent monitoring of thyroid function, and the reassurance that their disease, while a substantial source of morbidity, generally does not shorten life.

REFERENCES

ALEXANDER EL et al: Neurologic complications of primary Sjögren's syndrome. Medicine 61:247, 1982

FOX RI et al: Primary Sjögren's syndrome: Clinical and immunopathologic features. Semin Arthritis Rheum 14:77, 1984

MOUTSOPOULOS HM et al: Sjögren's syndrome: Current issues. Ann Intern Med 92:212, 1980

PAVLIDIS NA et al: The clinical picture of primary Sjögren's syndrome: A retrospective study. J Rheumatol 9:685, 1982

267 ANKYLOSING SPONDYLITIS

BRUCE C. GILLILAND

Ankylosing spondylitis, a disease that has been called by many names, including rheumatoid spondylitis and Marie-Strümpell disease, is a chronic and usually progressive inflammatory disease involving the articulations of the spine and adjacent soft tissues. The sacroiliac joints are always affected. Involvement of the hip and shoulder joints commonly occurs; peripheral joints are affected less frequently. The disease predominantly affects young men and begins most often in the third decade. A high association has been found between this disorder and the histocompatibility antigen HLA-B27. The clinical features of this disease are distinctly different from those of rheumatoid arthritis. The etiology is not known.

EPIDEMIOLOGY Ankylosing spondylitis is found throughout the world. In the white population, the prevalence in men is 0.5 to 4 per 1000 and in women 0.05 to 0.5 per 1000, depending on the criteria employed.

Hereditary factors play an important role in the development of ankylosing spondylitis. Histocompatibility typing has revealed the presence of HLA-B27 antigen in 88 to 96 percent of spondylitic patients, while in the normal white population 7 percent have this antigen. In blacks, HLA-B27 occurs less frequently, which may account for the lower prevalence of this disease among them.

HLA-B27 is inherited in a mendelian fashion, and HLA-B27 is found in 50 percent of first-degree relatives of those spondylitic patients who are positive for HLA-B27. Within the group of relatives, 20 percent have either symptomatic or asymptomatic spondylitis. Ankylosing spondylitis is seen occasionally in patients who are negative for HLA-B27, indicating that other genetic or environmental factors are necessary for the development of the disease.

Several diseases that possess clinical features in common with ankylosing spondylitis also occur more frequently in patients with the HLA-B27 antigen. These disorders include Reiter's syndrome, psoriatic spondyloarthritis, *Yersinia* arthritis, spondyloarthritis of inflammatory bowel disease, and acute anterior uveitis. The role of HLA-B27 antigen in the pathogenesis of these disorders is not known. The currently favored hypothesis is that the HLA-B27 antigen, because of a close association with the immune response genes, is only a marker distinguishing a group of individuals whose immune response to an as yet undefined infectious agent leads to one of the HLA-B27–associated forms of arthritis.

PATHOLOGY The earliest histopathologic changes usually occur in the sacroiliac joints but may start anywhere in the spine. The disease usually progresses up the spine, and occasionally segments will be skipped.

Synovitis of the involved diarthrodial joints of the spine (apophyseal and costovertebral joints) and of the sacroiliac, hip, shoulder, and peripheral joints resembles that of rheumatoid arthritis. Synovial hyperplasia and focal accumulation of lymphoid and plasma cells are seen histologically. Bony erosions and cartilage destruction ensue, followed later by fibrosis and bony ankylosis. In cartilaginous joints (intervertebral disks, manubriosternal, and symphysis pubis), granulation tissue invades the fibrocartilage, and adjacent bone is replaced later by fibrosis and ossification.

Occasionally, fibrous tissue invades the vertebral body to produce a radiolucent cyst which may be confused with an infectious process. Erosions at the anterior corners of the vertebral bodies destroy their normal anterior concavity and give the vertebrae a square appearance on lateral radiographs. Ossification of the outer layers of the annulus fibrosus at its lateral margins produces the syndesmophytes and "bamboo spine" observed radiographically. Ossification also involves the anterior portion of the annulus fibrosus and occasionally the inner aspect of the anterior longitudinal ligament. The radiographic appearance of the ossification at the anterior disk margins has led to the misconception that only the anterior longitudinal ligament is involved. In ankylosing spondylitis, a common site of inflammation is at the insertion of ligaments, tendons, and capsules into bone. Inflammation at these sites is termed *enthesitis*. The site where a ligament or tendon inserts into bone is the enthesis. The disease process is referred to as enthesopathy, which is common to the spondylarthropathies (ankylosing spondylitis, Reiter's disease, psoriatic arthritis). Bony erosions and new bone formation follow at these sites, most notably at the spinous processes, greater trochanters, pelvic bones, and heels.

Focal medial necrosis at the root of the aorta causes dilatation of the aortic ring. The aortic cusps may be shortened and thickened but are not fused. These processes lead to aortic valve incompetence. Fibrous tissue may enter the membranous septum and invade the atrioventricular bundle, resulting in conduction defects.

MANIFESTATIONS The disease occurs most commonly between the ages of 15 and 40 years and rarely after age 50. The initial symptoms are low back pain and stiffness, often worse in the early morning. Stiffness of the low back may last for several hours after the patient gets out of bed in the morning and also occurs after periods of inactivity during the day. Pain in the hips, buttocks, and shoulders is often present. Nocturnal back pain may force the patient to walk around in an attempt to gain relief. In approximately 10 percent of patients, early symptoms resemble sciatica, with pain in the buttocks and in back of the thighs. The pain may alternate from side to side and seldom radiates below the knee. Abnormal findings on neurologic examination are unusual. Patients may have the simultaneous onset of peripheral arthritis and back pain; however, peripheral arthritis uncommonly precedes back symptoms in adults. Peripheral arthritis, other than in the hips or shoulders, is relatively infrequent, and residual damage of these joints occurs infrequently. Hip disease occurs in approximately 30 percent of patients and may be a major cause of disability. Severe involvement early in the disease may result in ankylosis of the hip. Hip involvement, on the other hand, may lead to arthritis indistinguishable from osteoarthritis of the hip. Occasionally, patients may experience anterior chest pain from thoracic skeletal involvement which may mimic angina pectoris. Pleuritic chest pain may occur on deep breathing due to inflammation at the insertion of the costosternal and costovertebral muscles. Other causes of chest pain are involvement of the manubriosternal and sternoclavicular joints. Radicular pain from the spine may radiate to the abdomen, suggesting visceral disease. Atlantoaxial subluxation and spinal cord compression occur less commonly than in rheumatoid arthritis. Patients with fused cervical spines are especially susceptible to fractures of the neck on falling.

Aortic valve incompetence is present in 3 percent of patients and may result in severe aortic regurgitation, requiring surgical repair. Conduction abnormalities include varying degrees of heart block and left bundle branch block. The conduction defects are more apt to appear in patients with aortic valve incompetence, but they may exist alone. Some patients require implantation of a pacemaker.

Acute anterior uveitis is observed in 20 to 30 percent of patients and may be recurrent. Occasionally, this may be the presenting symptom, calling attention to the diagnosis of ankylosing spondylitis. Amyloidosis is found in a small number of patients at autopsy and is a cause of uremia in this disease. Bilateral upper lobe fibrosis is a recognized late manifestation of ankylosing spondylitis and may mimic tuberculosis. Patients develop chronic productive cough and dyspnea. The disease may progress to dense fibrosis, and death can result from massive hemoptysis.

The constitutional symptoms are usually mild at the onset and throughout the disease, but in a few patients with severe disease, fatigue, anemia, fever, and weight loss may be present.

Symptoms may be persistent or intermittent for months or years with the typical deformities usually evolving after 10 years or more of disease. In some patients ankylosis of the spine may progress with little or no pain. The degree of spinal involvement varies among patients, ranging from only sacroiliac joint involvement to complete ankylosis of the spine. Once ankylosis of joints occurs, pain usually disappears.

The *cauda equina syndrome* is a rare complication appearing usually in patients with long-standing and apparently inactive disease. The cause of this syndrome is unclear but may be the result of previous arachnoiditis or ischemia. Symptoms result from the involvement of the lumbosacral nerve roots and include buttock or leg pain, lower extremity weakness, and loss of bladder and rectal sphincter control. Loss of sensation occurs in the saddle area, posterior thighs, and lateral aspects of the feet. The deep tendon reflexes are diminished. Myelography shows posterior diverticula along the lumbar nerve root sheets or throughout the entire dural sac, when the study is done with the patient in the supine position. Neurologic manifestations are usually slowly progressive. Adequate treatment is not available.

Physical findings early in the disease may be minimal. Tenderness over the sacroiliac joints can be elicited by direct palpation or percussion, or by maneuvers that stress the joint. Tenderness may also be present over the costosternal joints, spinous processes, iliac crests, ischial tuberosities, greater trochanters, and heels. The lumbar spine will show loss of the normal lordosis and paraspinal muscle spasm. The anterior flexion of the lumbar spine is measured by the Schober test. With the patient standing erect, the skin is marked over the fifth lumbar vertebra and two additional points, 10 cm above and 5 cm below the first mark. The patient is instructed to bend over as far as possible, and the distance between the upper and lower mark is measured. The difference between the original measurement of 15 cm and the measurement with full flexion is calculated and should be 5.0 cm or more in patients below the age of 50 years. Serial measurements in a given patient will reflect the progression of spine involvement. No distraction of such skin marks is seen in a patient with an ankylosed spine. Costovertebral involvement is best measured by chest expansion. The more advanced changes of spondylitis are easily recognized by the rigid spine, often fused in varying degrees of flexion, which may be quite pronounced in the thoracic region of the spine.

LABORATORY FINDINGS The erythrocyte sedimentation rate (ESR) is elevated in the majority of cases, but its level poorly reflects fluctuations of disease activity, and the ESR is normal in 20 percent of patients with mild disease. A mild hypoproliferative anemia may be present during severe active disease. Tests for rheumatoid factor are negative even when peripheral joint disease is present. Mild to moderate elevations of the spinal fluid protein level may be present in active spondylitis. Synovial fluid from peripheral joints usually shows a moderate neutrophilic leukocytosis.

At the onset of symptoms the radiographs of the sacroiliac joints and the spine are often normal and may remain so for variable periods of time, depending on the rate of progression of the disease. Radiographs of the sacroiliac joints in early disease show blurring of the margins, irregular subchondral erosions, and patchy sclerosis. These changes are initially more pronounced in the lower third of the joint. Both sacroiliac joints are characteristically involved, but findings may first appear on one side. With progression, sclerosis becomes more marked, the joint space is lost, and later osteoporosis appears. Similar changes are observed in other articulations of the axial skeleton, including the symphysis pubis and apophyseal joints. At points of tendon insertions (e.g., pelvis, os calcis) the adjacent bone shows erosions, sclerosis, and fluffy new bone formation. Lateral films of the os calcis may show bony spurs at the site of attachment for the Achilles tendon and for the plantar fascia.

Radiographs of the spine in early phases of the disease may show straightening of the lumbar spine and squaring of the lumbar and lower thoracic vertebrae. With progression, syndesmophytes appear along the lateral and anterior surfaces of the intervertebral disks and bridge adjacent vertebrae. They are characteristically present on both lateral sides of the intervertebral disk at any given level and usually arise from the margin of the vertebral body. The widespread distribution of syndesmophytes in advanced disease produces the picture of the "bamboo spine." Syndesmophytes must be differentiated from the osteophytes observed in degenerative joint disease. The syndesmophyte extends vertically from the adjacent vertebral margins along the outer aspect of the intervertebral disk, while the osteophyte projects horizontally before curving to form an intervertebral bridge.

DIAGNOSIS A patient with ankylosing spondylitis in the advanced stage is easily recognized by the characteristic bent-over posture, rigid spine, exaggerated dorsal kyphosis, and waddling gait. When peripheral arthritis is present in the early stages of ankylosing spondylitis, confusion with rheumatoid arthritis may occur. Ankylosing spondylitis is predominantly a disease of young men, but the disease also exists in women in a milder form. HLA-B27 antigen is usually present, rheumatoid factor tests are negative, and rheumatoid nodules are not found. Radiographs of the spine show bilateral sacroiliitis and syndesmophytes, which are features not seen in adult rheumatoid arthritis. Ankylosing spondylitis in children often presents as a peripheral arthritis and, therefore, may be initially diagnosed as juvenile rheumatoid arthritis. Hip, sacroiliac, and spine involvement along with attacks of acute anterior uveitis eventually point to the diagnosis of spondylitis. Older boys are most often affected. HLA-B27 is usually present in these children in contrast to juvenile rheumatoid arthritis in which the prevalence of this antigen does not differ from normal persons.

Differentiation from other diseases with spondylitis early in the course may be difficult. Since the spondylitis is indistinguishable from that associated with ulcerative colitis and regional enteritis and may antedate the bowel disease by months or years, symptoms and signs of intestinal disease should always be sought. The spondylitis with Reiter's syndrome and psoriatic arthritis have common radiographic features, but differ from ankylosing spondylitis in having a greater tendency for syndesmophytes to appear at only one lateral margin of the intervertebral disk at any given level and to arise beyond the margin of the vertebral body. The distribution of syndesmophytes is more random, and the degree of spinal involvement is usually less than in ankylosing spondylitis. Other clinical features of Reiter's syndrome and psoriatic arthritis allow for easy separation of these diseases from ankylosing spondylitis. Diffuse idiopathic skeletal hyperostosis (DISH, or Forestier's disease with extra spinal involvement) is distinguished from ankylosing spondylitis by the lack of apophyseal and sacroiliac joint involvement and by its more frequent occurrence in men over 50. Laminated new bone formation involves the anterior and lateral spinal ligaments most prominently in the middle to lower thoracic regions, particularly on the right side, and resembles the dripping of candle wax. The radiologic findings of sacroiliitis are distinguished from osteitis condensans ilii by the finding of sclerosis on only the ilial side of the joint and the preservation of the joint space in the latter. Sciatica of ankylosing spondylitis can be differentiated from that of disk disease, since it may alternate from side to side, the pain seldom radiates below the knee, and neurologic signs are usually absent. Malignancies should be considered in both youngsters and older patients with symptoms of back pain.

TREATMENT The goal of therapy is to prevent or minimize the deformities of the spine inherent in this disease. With minimal spine deformity, patients may be able to continue working and living in a reasonably normal fashion if hip disease is not severe. Patients should be instructed to maintain an erect posture whether walking, standing, or sitting. They should be encouraged to sleep in a prone position or, if this is not possible, in a supine position on a flat firm mattress using a small pillow or none at all. Breathing exercises should be encouraged.

Drugs will not halt the progression of the disease, but they provide adequate relief to permit maintenance of posture. Indomethacin is effective in maintenance doses of 75 to 150 mg per day. Salicylates or other nonsteroidal anti-inflammatory drugs may be effective. Phenylbutazone in a dose of 200 to 300 mg per day is also effective but because of its potential to cause aplastic anemia, its use is recommended only after all other nonsteroidal anti-inflammatory drugs have failed. Therapy should be discontinued when symptoms abate. Gold and chloroquine have not been beneficial. Any benefit from glucocorticoids is outweighed by their side effects. Iritis can usually be treated with intraocular steroids. No effective therapy is available for the lung fibrosis occurring in patients with ankylosing spondylitis.

Surgical correction of extreme flexion deformities of the spine by wedge resection and refusion in an improved position may be helpful in selected patients. The potential danger of spinal cord damage and the long convalescent period should be carefully considered before advising surgery. Patients with crippling hip disease may benefit from total hip replacement.

REFERENCES

CALIN A: Ankylosing spondylitis, in *Textbook of Rheumatology*, 2d ed, WN Kelley et al (eds). Philadelphia, Saunders, 1985, pp 993–1007

——— et al: Genetic differences between B27-positive patients with ankylosing spondylitis and B27-positive health controls. Arthritis Rheum Dec:1460, 1983

RESNICK D, NIWAYAMA G: Diffuse idiopathic skeletal hyperostosis (DISH), in *Diagnosis of Bone and Joint Disorders*, D Resnick, G Niwayama (eds). Philadelphia, Saunders, 1981, pp 1416–1452

———, ———: Ankylosing spondylitis, in *Diagnosis of Bone and Joint Disorders*, D Resnick, G Niwayama (eds). Philadelphia, Saunders, 1981, pp 1040–1102

268 REITER'S SYNDROME AND BEHÇET'S SYNDROME

HARALAMPOS M. MOUTSOPOULOS

REITER'S SYNDROME Reiter's syndrome was originally described as a triad of arthritis, conjunctivitis, and urethritis. Today, the presence of seronegative, oligoarticular, asymmetric arthritis with urethritis and/or cervicitis has been proposed as sufficient manifestations for the diagnosis of the syndrome.

Prevalence, pathogenesis, and pathology Two clinical forms of Reiter's syndrome are recognized: the postvenereal and the postdysenteric (epidemic). The latter is also called "reactive arthritis." Postvenereal Reiter's syndrome prevails in North America and western Europe, whereas in developing countries, the postdysenteric form appears to be more common.

The exact prevalence of the syndrome is not known. Reiter's syndrome is the most common cause of arthritis in young men, and there is a striking correlation between the disease prevalence and the frequency of the HLA-B27 alloantigen in a given population. The syndrome develops in 1 to 3 percent of males with nongonococcal urethritis, in 2 to 3 percent of patients with bacillary dysentery, and in 20 percent of individuals with the HLA-B27 antigen. In contrast to 10 percent of normal controls, up to 90 percent of Reiter's syndrome patients are HLA-B27–positive. The postvenereal disease is less common in females. The postdysenteric form affects both sexes equally. In children and in the elderly, the syndrome almost always follows dysentery.

The cause and pathogenesis of Reiter's syndrome remain speculative. It is recognized, however, that an infectious process of the urogenital tract or the gut coupled with a specific genetic background in some patients can trigger the development of Reiter's syndrome. Through epidemiologic and serologic studies, *Chlamydia trachomatis* and a *Mycoplasma (Ureoplasma urealyticum)* have been implicated as the most common agents associated with the postvenereal Reiter's syndrome, while *Shigella dysenteriae* and *S. flexneri*, *Salmonella enteritidis*, *Yersinia enterocolitica*, and *Campylobacter jejuni* have been proposed as the responsible microorganisms for the postdysenteric Reiter's syndrome.

This syndrome lacks a specific histopathologic lesion. The histologic changes of an affected synovial membrane vary with the clinical activity and duration of the process. In acute arthritis of a few weeks' duration, the synovial membrane shows hyperemia with an infiltrate consisting primarily of polymorphonuclear leukocytes. In patients with long-standing arthritis, the histologic lesion is indistinguishable from that seen in rheumatoid arthritis. The histology of the skin lesion, which is termed keratoderma blenorrhagica, is similar to pustular psoriasis.

Clinical features The syndrome usually begins with urethritis followed by conjunctivitis and rheumatologic findings. Urethritis can be observed in both forms of the syndrome.

The urethral discharge is intermittent and, in most cases, moderate in amount, serous, and asymptomatic. Infrequently, it is profuse, purulent, and blood-stained. Other rare urologic problems include prostatitis, urethral strictures, seminal vasculitis, cystitis, and urethral stenosis.

The conjunctivitis is usually minimal and lasts for only a few days or weeks. Infrequently, the conjunctivitis is symptomatic, presenting with "red eyes," burning, itching, and profuse purulent discharge. Rarely, nongranulomatous anterior uveitis, symptomatic superficial keratitis, posterior uveitis, and optic neuritis are present.

Rheumatologic manifestations include arthritis, tenosynovitis, dactylitis, and plantar fasciitis. Arthritis is usually acute, asymmetric, oligoarticular, involving predominantly the joints of the lower extremities; knees, ankles, metatarsophalangeal, and toe interphalangeal joints are affected in both types of Reiter's syndrome. The acute arthritis is accompanied by malaise and fever. The joints are warm, erythematous, and painful. Plantar fasciitis and Achilles tendonitis are common. The duration of the acute episode ranges from a few days to several months. Relapses are frequent and may be precipated by sexual exposure followed by urethritis. Permanent foot abnormalities include calcaneal spurs, pes cavus or planus and dorsiflexion, and tibular deviation of the toes at the metatarsophalangeal joints. Sacroiliitis occurs in Reiter's patients. However, the precise frequency of spondylitis in these patients has not been estimated.

Mucocutaneous lesions are common and appear in the mouth, on the glans penis, the palms, and the soles. Superficial oral mucosal and glans penile lesions are painless and found in approximately one-third of the patients. Keratoderma blenorrhagica, which consists of crusted scaling papules, occurs in up to 30 percent of postvenereal Reiter's syndrome patients, but not in the postdysenteric syndrome patients. These papules appear mainly on the palms, soles, and glans penis, but occasionally may be found on the limbs, trunk, scalp, and scrotum. Accumulation of subungual cornified material occurs in patients with or without keratoderma blenorrhagica. This material lifts the nail plate. Pitting of the nails does not occur, distinguishing this lesion from psoriatic arthritis.

Uncommon manifestations of Reiter's syndrome include pleuropericarditis, aortic regurgitation, neurologic manifestations, and secondary amyloidosis.

Long-term follow-up studies have shown that one-third of patients with Reiter's syndrome have recurrent or sustained disease, while about 15 to 25 percent develop permanent disability. Chronic heel involvement appears to be an early sign of poor prognosis.

Laboratory manifestations There are no specific tests for the syndrome. Mild anemia of chronic disease, leukocytosis, elevated erythrocyte sedimentation rate, and C-reactive protein levels are common. Synovial fluid analysis is also nondiagnostic. The fluid is inflammatory with polymorphonuclear leukocytosis and high complement levels. Rheumatoid factors and antinuclear antibodies are negative.

Roentgenograms in the acute phase are not helpful, revealing only soft tissue edema. In chronic cases, bony erosions and joint space narrowing can be seen. Periosteal bone apposition along the shaft adjacent to the involved joint is frequently seen and is suggestive of Reiter's syndrome. Calcaneal spurs appear late in the disease. In case of ileosacral joint involvement, one or both joints may show irregularity, sclerosis, and fusion.

Diagnosis and differential diagnosis According to the preliminary criteria introduced by the American Rheumatism Association, the presence of asymmetric, seronegative oligoarthritis of 1 month's duration in combination with nonspecific urethritis or cervicitis is sufficient for the diagnosis of Reiter's syndrome with a specificity of around 80 percent. The bases for the differential diagnosis from gonococcal and psoriatic arthritis are presented in Table 268-1.

Treatment Treatment of Reiter's syndrome is empirical and aimed at relieving symptoms. Patient education, reassurance, and physical therapy are of paramount importance.

Acute arthritis is treated with analgesics and nonsteroidal anti-inflammatory drugs such as indomethacin (100 to 150 mg per day).

Systemic corticosteroids must be avoided because they can aggravate the cutaneous manifestations. However, local administration can be helpful for persistent monarthritis, fasciitis, and tendonitis. In cases of chronic destructive arthritis, cytotoxic drugs like methotrexate or azathioprine may be beneficial. The use of antibiotics remains controversial. It is clear that they do not have any direct effects on arthritis. Conjunctivitis and oral lesions usually do not require any treatment. Uveitis is treated with corticosteroids, either topical, periocular, or systemic, depending on the severity of the inflammation.

BEHÇET'S SYNDROME Behçet's syndrome is a multisystem disorder presenting with recurrent oral and genital ulcerations as well as uveitis often leading to blindness.

Prevalence, pathogenesis, and pathology The disease has a worldwide distribution. The prevalence of Behçet's syndrome ranges from 1:1000 in Japan to 1:500,000 in North America and Europe. In the Mediterranean countries the prevalence might be higher. It affects mainly young adults.

The etiology and pathogenesis of this syndrome remain obscure. Bacteria and viruses have been suggested as the causative agents but without convincing proof. Today, Behçet's syndrome is considered an autoimmune disease because of the common denominator of vasculitis in most patients. Circulating autoantibodies to human oral mucous membrane and immune complexes are found in approximately 50 percent of the cases. Familial occurrence has been reported, and in patients from eastern Mediterranean countries and Japan, the disease appears to be linked to HLA-B5 and HLA-DR5 alloantigens.

Clinical features The recurrent aphthous ulcerations are a sine qua non for the diagnosis. The ulcers are usually painful with a diameter ranging from 2 to 10 mm. They can be shallow or deep with a central yellowish necrotic base, appear singly or in crops, and are located on the lips, gums, buccal mucosa, tongue, tonsils, and larynx. The ulcers persist for 1 to 2 weeks and subside without leaving scars. The genital ulcers resemble the oral ones in both appearance and course. Vaginal ulcers are usually painless and may be detected during routine pelvic examination. Painful genital ulcers may occur on the external genitalia.

Skin involvement includes folliculitis, erythema nodosum, and an acnelike exanthem. Severe dermal vasculitis is an infrequent event. Nonspecific skin inflammatory reactivity to any scratches, needle pricks, and intradermal saline injection (pathergy test) is a common and specific manifestation in Japanese and eastern Mediterranean patients.

Eye involvement is the most dreaded complication in that it can occasionally progress rapidly to blindness. The eye disease is usually

TABLE 268-1 Differences between Reiter's syndrome (RS), gonococcal arthritis (GA), and psoriatic arthritis (PA)

	RS	GA	PA
Conjunctivitis	+	−	+
Uveitis	+	+	−
Gonococcus culture	±	±	−
Sacroiliitis	±	−	±
Stomatitis	+	−	−
Balanitis	+	−	−
Keratoderma blenorrhagica	+	−	±
Arthritis	Lower extremities	Upper extremities	Upper extremities
Response to penicillin	−	+	−
HLA-B27	80%	10%	20–50%
Course	Recurrent	Acute	Chronic

present at the onset but also may develop within the first few years. In addition to iritis, posterior uveitis, retinal vessel occlusions, and optic neuritis can be seen in some cases of the syndrome. Hypopyon uveitis, which is considered the hallmark of Behçet's syndrome, is in fact a rare manifestation.

The arthritis of Behçet's syndrome is not deforming and affects the knees and ankles.

Superficial or deep peripheral vein thrombosis is seen in one-fourth of the patients. Pulmonary emboli, however, appear to be an exceptionally rare complication. The superior vena cava is obstructed occasionally, producing a dramatic clinical picture. Arterial involvement occurs infrequently and presents with aortitis or peripheral arterial aneurysm and arterial thrombosis.

The prevalence of central nervous system involvement differs geographically. High figures are quoted from northern Europe and the United States. The most common lesions are benign intracranial hypertension, a multiple sclerosis–like picture, and pyramidal involvement. Psychiatric disturbances are frequent.

Gastrointestinal involvement is reported in patients from Japan and include mucosal ulcerations of the gut.

Laboratory findings are nonspecific indexes of inflammation such as leukocytosis, elevated erythrocyte sedimentation rate as well as C-reactive protein levels, and antibodies to human oral mucosa.

Prognosis and treatment The severity of the syndrome usually abates with time; male sex and younger age at onset seem to predispose for severe illness. Apart from the cases with neurologic complications, the life expectancy seems to be normal and the only serious complication is blindness.

Treatment of Behçet's syndrome is symptomatic and empirical. Mucous membrane involvement may respond to topical corticosteroids, while the serious manifestations of Behçet's syndrome, i.e., uveitis and central nervous system involvement, require systemic corticosteroid therapy (prednisone, 1 mg/kg per day) and/or cytotoxic agents (chlorambucil, 0.1 mg/kg per day; azathioprine, 1 to 2 mg/kg per day; or cyclophosphamide, 1 to 2 mg/kg per day). There are early reports of the beneficial use of cyclosporin A in the uveitis of Behçet's syndrome. The arthritis responds to rest and analgesics. Thrombophlebitis is treated with aspirin, 500 mg per day, and dipyridamol, 250 mg per day.

REFERENCES

CALIN A, FRIES JF: An "experimental" epidemic of Reiter's syndrome revisited: Follow-up evidence of genetic and environmental factors. Arthritis Rheum 84:564, 1976

KEAT A: Reiter's syndrome and reactive arthritis in perspective. N Engl J Med 309:1606, 1983

MARTIN DH et al: *Chlamydia trachomatis* infections in men with Reiter's syndrome. Ann Intern Med 100:207, 1984

O'DUFFY JD et al: Behçet's disease: Report of 10 cases, 3 with new manifestations. Ann Intern Med 75:561, 1971

SHIMIZU T et al: Behçet's disease (Behçet's syndrome). Semin Arthritis Rheum 8:223, 1979

WILLKENS RF et al: Reiter's syndrome. Evaluation of preliminary criteria for definite disease. Arthritis Rheum 24:844, 1981

YAZICI H, MOUTSOPOULOS HM: Behçet's disease, in *Current Therapy in Allergy and Immunology*, LM Lichtenstein, AS Fauci (eds). Philadelphia, Decker, 1985

269 THE VASCULITIS SYNDROMES

ANTHONY S. FAUCI

DEFINITION Vasculitis is a clinicopathologic process characterized by inflammation of and damage to blood vessels. The vessel lumen is usually compromised, and this is associated with ischemia of the tissues supplied by the involved vessel. A broad and heterogeneous group of syndromes may result from this process since any type, size, and location of blood vessel may be involved. Vasculitis and its consequences may be the primary or sole manifestation of a disease; alternatively, vasculitis may be a secondary component of another primary disease. Vasculitis may be confined to a single organ such as the skin, or it may simultaneously involve several organ systems.

PATHOPHYSIOLOGY AND PATHOGENESIS Generally, most of the vasculitic syndromes are assumed to be mediated at least in part by immunopathogenic mechanisms. However, evidence to this effect is for the most part indirect. Deposition of immune complexes in tissues (see Chap. 261) is the most widely accepted pathogenic mechanism of vasculitis. Nonetheless, the causal role of immune complexes has not been clearly established in most of the vasculitic syndromes. Circulating immune complexes need not result in deposition of the complexes in blood vessels with ensuing vasculitis, and many patients with active vasculitis do not have demonstrable circulating or deposited immune complexes. This situation may result from an inadequacy of the techniques for detecting certain types of immune complexes or from the rapidity with which complexes may be cleared from the circulation. The actual antigen contained in the immune complex has only rarely been identified in vasculitic syndromes. In this regard, hepatitis B antigen has been identified in both the circulating and deposited immune complexes in a subset of patients with systemic vasculitis, most notably within the polyarteritis nodosa group (see below).

The mechanisms of tissue damage in immune-complex–mediated vasculitis resemble those described for serum sickness (Chap. 261). In this model, antigen-antibody complexes are formed in antigen excess and are deposited in vessel walls whose permeability has been increased by vasoactive amines from platelets or from mast cells which have released their intracellular contents as a result of IgE-triggered mechanisms. The deposition of complexes results in activation of complement components, particularly C5a which is strongly chemotactic for neutrophils. These cells then infiltrate the vessel wall, phagocytose the immune complexes, and regurgitate their intracytoplasmic enzymes which damage the vessel wall. As the process becomes subacute or chronic, mononuclear cells infiltrate the vessel wall. The common denominator of the resulting syndrome is compromise of the vessel lumen with ischemic changes in the tissues supplied by the involved vessel.

In addition to the classic immune-complex–mediated mechanisms of vasculitis, other immunopathogenic mechanisms may be involved in damage to vessels. The most prominent of these is cell-mediated immune injury as reflected in the histopathologic feature of granulomatous vasculitis. However, immune complexes themselves may induce granulomatous responses, and the presence of granulomas in or around blood vessels may be indicative of immune-complex mechanisms, delayed hypersensitivity or cell-mediated immune responses, or both. Other mechanisms such as direct cellular cytotoxicity or antibody directed against vessel components or antibody-dependent cellular cytotoxicity have been suggested in certain types of vessel damage. However, there is no convincing evidence to support their contribution to the pathogenesis of any of the recognized vasculitic syndromes.

It is unclear why certain individuals develop vasculitis in response to certain antigenic stimuli whereas others do not. However, it is likely that a number of factors are involved in the ultimate expression of a vasculitic syndrome. These include the genetic predisposition, the regulatory mechanisms associated with immune response to certain antigens, and the ability of the reticuloendothelial system to clear circulating complexes from the blood. The size and physicochemical properties of immune complexes, the relative degree of turbulence of blood flow, the intravascular hydrostatic pressure in different vessels, and the preexisting integrity of the vessel endothelium likely explain why only certain types of immune complexes cause vasculitis and why the vasculitic process is selective for only certain vessels in individual patients.

CLASSIFICATION OF VASCULITIC SYNDROMES A major feature of the vasculitic syndromes as a group is the fact that there is a great deal of heterogeneity at the same time as there is considerable overlap among them. This has led to both difficulty and confusion with regard to the categorization of these diseases. The classification scheme listed in Table 269-1 takes into account this heterogeneity and overlap, and will serve as a matrix to emphasize the fact that certain syndromes are predominantly systemic in nature and almost invariably lead to irreversible organ system dysfunction and even death if untreated, while others are usually localized to the skin and rarely result in irreversible dysfunction of vital organs. The distinguishing and overlapping features of the diseases listed in Table 269-1, which justify this classification scheme, will be discussed below.

SYSTEMIC NECROTIZING VASCULITIS

CLASSIC POLYARTERITIS NODOSA **Definition** Polyarteritis nodosa (PAN) in its classic form was described in 1866 by Kussmaul and Maier. It is a multisystem, necrotizing vasculitis of small- and medium-sized muscular arteries in which involvement of the renal and visceral arteries is characteristic. Classic PAN does not involve pulmonary arteries, although bronchial vessels may be involved; granulomas, significant eosinophilia, and an allergic diathesis are not part of the classic syndrome.

Incidence and prevalence It is difficult to establish an accurate incidence of this disease because of the fact that many reports of PAN actually have included diseases other than the classic syndrome. It is clearly an uncommon, but not a rare, disease. The mean age at onset is 45 years and the male to female ratio is 2.5:1.

Pathophysiology and pathogenesis The vascular lesion in classic PAN is a necrotizing inflammation of small- and medium-sized muscular arteries. The lesions are segmental and tend to involve bifurcations and branchings of arteries. They may spread circumferentially to involve adjacent veins. However, involvement of venules is not seen in classic PAN, and if present, suggest the polyangiitis overlap syndrome (see below). In the acute stages of disease, polymorphonuclear neutrophils infiltrate all layers of the vessel wall and perivascular areas, which results in intimal proliferation and degeneration of the vessel wall. Mononuclear cells infiltrate the area as the lesions progress to the subacute and chronic stages. Fibrinoid necrosis of the vessels ensues with compromise of the lumen, thrombosis, infarction of the tissues supplied by the involved vessel, and, in some cases, hemorrhage. As the lesions heal, there is collagen deposition, which may lead to further occlusion of the vessel lumen. Aneurysmal dilatations up to 1 cm in size along the involved arteries are characteristic of classic PAN. Granulomas and substantial eosinophilia with eosinophilic tissue infiltrations are not characteristically found and suggest allergic angiitis and granulomatosis (see below).

Multiple organ systems are involved, and the clinicopathologic findings reflect the degree and location of vessel involvement and the resulting ischemic changes (Table 269-2). As mentioned above, pulmonary arteries are not involved in classic PAN, and bronchial artery involvement is uncommon. The pathology in the kidney is predominantly that of arteritis; however, glomerulitis occurs in up to 30 percent of patients. In patients with significant hypertension, typical pathologic features of glomerulosclerosis may be seen alone or superimposed on lesions of glomerulonephritis. In addition, pathologic sequelae of hypertension may be found elsewhere in the body.

The presence of hepatitis B antigenemia in approximately 30 percent of patients with systemic vasculitis, particularly of the classic PAN type, together with the isolation of circulating immune complexes composed of hepatitis B antigen and immunoglobulin, as well as the demonstration by immunofluorescence of hepatitis B antigen, IgM, and complement in the blood vessel walls, strongly suggest the role of immunologic phenomena in the pathogenesis of this disease.

Clinical and laboratory manifestations Nonspecific signs and symptoms are the hallmarks of classic PAN. Fever, weight loss, and malaise are present in over one-half of cases. Patients usually present with vague symptoms such as weakness, malaise, headache, abdominal pain, and myalgias. Specific complaints related to the vascular involvement within a particular organ system may also dominate the presenting clinical picture as well as the entire course of the illness (Table 269-3). Renal involvement most commonly manifests as ischemic changes in the glomeruli; however, glomerulonephritis is seen in approximately 30 percent of patients. Hypertension may be related to both the renal polyarteritis as well as the glomerulitis and may dominate the clinical picture. Classic PAN may involve any organ system; the clinical manifestations related to specific organ system involvement are listed in Table 269-3.

There are no diagnostic serologic tests for classic PAN. In over 75 percent of patients the leukocyte count is elevated with a predominance of neutrophils. Eosinophilia is only rarely seen and, when present at high levels, suggests the diagnosis of allergic angiitis and granulomatosis. The anemia of chronic disease may be seen, and an elevated erythrocyte sedimentation rate (ESR) is invariably present. Other common laboratory findings reflect the particular organ involved. Hypergammaglobulinemia may be present, and up to 30 percent of patients have a positive test for hepatitis B surface antigen. Arteriograms may demonstrate characteristic abnormalities such as

TABLE 269-1 Classification of the vasculitic syndromes

Systemic necrotizing vasculitis
Classic polyarteritis nodosa
Allergic angiitis and granulomatosis of Churg-Strauss
Polyangiitis overlap syndrome
Hypersensitivity vasculitis
Exogenous stimuli proved or suspected
Henoch-Schönlein purpura
Serum sickness and serum sickness–like reactions
Other drug-induced vasculitides
Vasculitis associated with infectious diseases
Endogenous antigens likely involved
Vasculitis associated with neoplasms
Vasculitis associated with connective tissue diseases
Vasculitis associated with other underlying diseases
Vasculitis associated with congenital deficiencies of the complement system
Wegener's granulomatosis
Giant cell arteritis
Temporal arteritis
Takayasu's arteritis
Other vasculitic syndromes
Mucocutanous lymph node syndrome (Kawasaki's disease)
Isolated central nervous system vasculitis
Thromboangiitis obliterans (Buerger's disease)
Miscellaneous vasculitides

TABLE 269-2 Organ system involvement at autopsy in classic PAN

Organ system	Percent
Kidney	85
Heart	76
Liver	62
Gastrointestinal tract:	51
Jejunum	37
Ileum	27
Mesentery	24
Colon	20
Duodenum	10
Gallbladder	10
Rectosigmoid	10
Appendix	7
Muscle	39
Pancreas	35
Testes	33
Peripheral nerves	32
Central nervous system	27
Skin	20

SOURCE: *Cupps and Fauci, 1981, p 32.*

aneurysms in the small- and medium-sized muscular arteries of the kidneys and abdominal viscera.

Diagnosis The diagnosis of classic PAN is based on the demonstration of characteristic findings of vasculitis on biopsy material of involved organs. In the absence of easily accessible tissue for biopsy, the angiographic demonstration of involved vessels, particularly in the form of aneurysms of small- and medium-sized arteries in the renal, hepatic, and visceral vasculature, is sufficient to make the diagnosis. Aneurysms of vessels are not pathognomonic of classic PAN; furthermore, aneurysms need not always be present, and angiographic findings may be limited to stenotic segments and obliteration of vessels. Biopsy of symptomatic organs such as nodular skin lesions, painful testes, and muscle groups provides the highest diagnostic yields, while blind biopsy of asymptomatic organs is frequently negative. In cases associated with hepatitis B antigenemia, the demonstration of circulating hepatitis B antigen serves as important circumstantial evidence in support of the diagnosis.

Treatment and prognosis The prognosis of untreated classic PAN is extremely poor. The usual clinical course is characterized either by fulminant deterioration or by relentless progression associated with intermittent acute flare-ups. Death usually results from renal failure; from gastrointestinal complications, particularly bowel infarcts and perforation; and from cardiovascular causes. Intractable hypertension often compounds dysfunction in other organ systems such as the kidneys, heart, and central nervous system leading to additional late morbidity and mortality. The 5-year survival rate of untreated patients has been reported to be 13 percent, while corticosteroid treatment may increase this figure to over 40 percent. Extremely favorable therapeutic results have been reported in classic PAN with the combination of prednisone, 1 mg/kg per day, and cyclophosphamide, 2 mg/kg per day (see section of Wegener's granulomatosis for a detailed description of this therapeutic regimen). This regimen has been reported to result in up to a 90 percent long-term remission rate even following the discontinuation of therapy. Isolated reports have indicated favorable therapeutic responses in classic PAN using plasmapheresis together with corticosteroids and cytotoxic agents.

ALLERGIC ANGIITIS AND GRANULOMATOSIS (CHURG-STRAUSS DISEASE) **Definition** Allergic angiitis and granulomatosis was described in 1951 by Churg and Strauss and is a disease characterized by granulomatous vasculitis of multiple organ systems, particularly the lung. It is similar in many respects to classic PAN except that the former has a high frequency of lung involvement, vasculitis of blood vessels of various types or sizes including veins and venules, intra- and extravascular granuloma formation together with eosinophilic tissue infiltration, and a strong association with severe asthma and peripheral eosinophilia.

TABLE 269-3 Clinical manifestations related to organ system involvement in classic PAN

Organ system	Percent incidence	Clinical manifestations
Renal	60	Renal failure, hypertension
Musculoskeletal	64	Arthritis, arthralgia, myalgia
Peripheral nervous system	51	Peripheral neuropathy, mononeuritis multiplex
Gastrointestinal tract	44	Abdominal pain, nausea and vomiting, bleeding, bowel infarction and perforation, cholecystitis, hepatic infarction, pancreatic infarction
Skin	43	Rash, purpura, nodules, cutaneous infarcts, livedo reticularis
Cardiac	36	Congestive heart failure, myocardial infarction, pericarditis
Genitourinary	25	Testicular, ovarian, or epididymal pain
Central nervous system	23	Cerebral vascular accident, altered mental status, seizure

SOURCE: *Cupps and Fauci, 1981, p 29.*

Incidence and prevalence Allergic angiitis and granulomatosis is an uncommon disease whose exact incidence, similar to classic PAN, is difficult to determine due to the grouping of multiple types of vasculitic syndromes in many reported series. The disease can occur at any age with the possible exception of infants. The mean age of onset is 44 years with a male to female ratio of 1.3:1.

Pathophysiology and pathogenesis The vasculitis which is characteristic of allergic angiitis and granulomatosis is similar to that of classic PAN (see above) with certain notable exceptions. In addition to small- and medium-sized muscular arteries, capillaries, veins, and venules can be involved in the former disease. The characteristic histopathologic features of allergic angiitis and granulomatosis are granulomatous reactions that may be present in the tissues or even within the walls of the vessels themselves. These are usually associated with infiltration of the tissues with eosinophils. This process can occur in any organ in the body; however, in sharp contrast to classic PAN, lung involvement is predominant, with skin, cardiovascular system, kidney, peripheral nervous system, and gastrointestinal tract also commonly involved. Although the precise pathogenesis of this disease is uncertain, its strong association with asthma, its clinicopathologic manifestations which strongly suggest hypersensitivity phenomena, and its close similarity to classic PAN point to aberrant immunologic phenomena.

Clinical and laboratory manifestations Patients with allergic angiitis and granulomatosis exhibit nonspecific manifestations such as fever, malaise, anorexia, and weight loss similar to patients with classic PAN. In contrast to the latter disease, the pulmonary findings in allergic angiitis and granulomatosis clearly dominate the clinical picture with severe asthmatic attacks and the presence of pulmonary infiltrates. Skin lesions occur in approximately 70 percent of patients and include nonthrombocytopenic purpura in addition to cutaneous and subcutaneous nodules. Apart from the characteristic pulmonary findings, the multisystem involvement in this disease is quite similar to that of classic PAN (see above); an important exception is the fact that the renal disease in allergic angiitis and granulomatosis is less common and generally less severe than that of classic PAN.

The characteristic laboratory finding in virtually all patients with allergic angiitis and granulomatosis is a striking eosinophilia which reaches levels greater than 1000 cells per cubic millimeter in more than 80 percent of patients. The other laboratory findings are similar to those of classic PAN and reflect the organ systems involved.

Diagnosis Similar to classic PAN, the diagnosis of allergic angiitis and granulomatosis is made by biopsy, demonstrating vasculitis in a patient with the characteristic clinical manifestations. The biopsy findings are distinctive in the latter disease in that granulomatous vasculitis with eosinophilic tissue involvement together with peripheral eosinophilia are typical. Furthermore, pulmonary involvement is extremely common and is usually manifested by severe asthma associated with pulmonary infiltrates that may be fleeting in nature.

Treatment and prognosis The prognosis of untreated allergic angiitis and granulomatosis is poor with a reported 5-year survival of 25 percent. Unlike classic PAN, the cause of death is more likely to be related to pulmonary and cardiac disease as opposed to renal or gastrointestinal involvement. Corticosteroid therapy has been reported to increase the 5-year survival to more than 50 percent. In corticosteroid failures or in patients who present with fulminant multisystem disease, the treatment of choice is a combined regimen of cyclophosphamide and alternate-day prednisone which has resulted in a high rate of complete remission similar to the experience with classic PAN (see above).

POLYANGIITIS OVERLAP SYNDROME Many patients with systemic necrotizing vasculitis manifest clinicopathologic characteristics which overlap both classic PAN and allergic angiitis and granulomatosis and also show features of the hypersensitivity small vessel group of vasculitides (see below). This subgroup has been referred to as the ''polyangiitis overlap syndrome'' and is part of the major grouping of systemic necrotizing vasculitis. It is clear that this entity does exist, and it has been designated with a distinct classification in order to avoid confusion in attempting to fit such overlap syndromes into one or other of the more classic vasculitic syndromes. This subgroup is truly a systemic vasculitis with the same potential for resulting in irreversible organ system dysfunction as the other systemic necrotizing vasculitides. The diagnostic and therapeutic considerations as well as the prognosis for this subgroup are the same as those for classic PAN and allergic angiitis and granulomatosis.

HYPERSENSITIVITY VASCULITIS

DEFINITION The term hypersensitivity vasculitis has been used to designate a heterogeneous group of disorders which are characterized by a vasculitic syndrome presumed to be associated with a hypersensitivity reaction following exposure to an antigen such as an infectious agent, a drug, or other foreign or endogenous substances. The common denominator of this group of diseases is the involvement of small vessels. Although any organ can be involved with this type of vasculitis, skin involvement generally dominates the clinical picture and the extracutaneous involvement is usually much less severe than that of the systemic vasculitides. There are multiple subgroups within the larger category of hypersensitivity vasculitis.

INCIDENCE AND PREVALENCE Although the exact incidence of this group of vasculitic syndromes is uncertain, it is clearly more common than the systemic necrotizing vasculitis group. The disease can occur at any age and in both sexes; however, different subgroups have a higher incidence in certain age groups and some are more common in males than females, or vice versa.

PATHOPHYSIOLOGY AND PATHOGENESIS The typical histopathologic feature of the hypersensitivity vasculitides is the presence of vasculitis of small vessels. Postcapillary venules are the most commonly involved vessels; capillaries and arterioles may be involved less frequently. This vasculitis is characterized by a leukocytoclasis which refers to the nuclear debris remaining from the neutrophils which have infiltrated in and around the vessels during the acute stages. In the subacute or chronic stages, mononuclear cells predominate; in certain subgroups, eosinophilic infiltration is seen. Erythrocytes often extravasate from the involved vessels, leading to palpable purpura.

Immune-complex deposition is generally considered to be the immunopathogenic mechanism of this type of vasculitis; however, formal proof that this is the case has not been established for all subgroups (see above). The hypersensitivity vasculitides can be broken down into two major categories depending on the type of putative antigen involved in the hypersensitivity reaction. In the originally described group, the antigen was foreign to the host, i.e., a drug, microbe, or foreign protein. In the second category, the antigen is felt to be endogenous to the host. Examples of these are the ''self'' proteins such as DNA or immunoglobulin which form immune complexes with their respective antibodies and lead to vasculitic complications in systemic lupus erythematosus and rheumatoid arthritis, respectively; other examples are the tumor antigens which form immune complexes with antibody and lead to vasculitis associated with certain neoplasms.

CLINICAL AND LABORATORY MANIFESTATIONS The hallmark of the broad group of hypersensitivity vasculitides is the predominance of skin involvement. Skin lesions may appear typically as palpable purpura; however, other cutaneous manifestations of the vasculitis may occur, including macules, papules, vesicles, bullae, subcutaneous nodules, ulcers, as well as recurrent or chronic urticaria. Despite the fact that skin lesions predominate, other organ systems may be involved to varying degrees and the extent to which this occurs may define a relatively distinct subgroup. Even in patients with isolated cutaneous involvement, the disease may be characterized by systemic signs and symptoms such as fever, malaise, myalgia, and anorexia. The skin lesions may be pruritic or even quite painful with a burning or stinging sensation. Lesions most commonly occur in the lower extremities in ambulatory patients or in the sacral area in bedridden patients due to the effects of hydrostatic forces on the postcapillary venules. Edema may accompany certain lesions, and hyperpigmentation often occurs in areas of recurrent or chronic lesions.

There are no specific laboratory tests which are diagnostic of hypersensitivity vasculitis. A mild leukocytosis with or without eosinophilia is characteristic as is an elevated ESR. Cryoglobulins and rheumatoid factor may be seen in certain cases, and serum complement levels follow no definite pattern. Laboratory abnormalities related to specific organ dysfunction reflect the involvement of these organs in the particular syndrome in question.

Henoch-Schönlein purpura The most distinctive subgroup of the hypersensitivity vasculitides is Henoch-Schönlein purpura, also referred to as anaphylactoid purpura, which is characterized by palpable purpura, most commonly distributed over the buttocks and lower extremities; arthralgias; gastrointestinal signs and symptoms; and glomerulonephritis. The disease is usually seen in children; however, individuals of any age may be affected. It has a remarkable tendency to resolve and recur several times over a period of weeks or months, usually ending in spontaneous resolution. A small percentage of patients progress to chronic disease. A number of antigens have been implicated in the immunopathogenesis of this disease, including infectious agents, drugs, certain foods, insect bites, and immunizations. IgA is the antibody class most often seen in the immune complexes of these patients. The typical palpable purpura is seen in virtually all patients; most patients develop polyarthralgias in the absence of frank arthritis. Gastrointestinal involvement, which is seen in almost 70 percent of pediatric patients, is characterized by colicky abdominal pain usually associated with nausea, vomiting, diarrhea, or constipation, which is frequently accompanied by the passage of blood and mucus per rectum; bowel intussusception may occur rarely. The renal involvement is usually characterized by a mild glomerulitis leading to hematuria with red blood cell casts (see also Chap. 224). Most patients recover completely and some do not require therapy. When corticosteroid therapy is required, it is usually administered as 1 mg/kg per day of prednisone and tapered according to the clinical response.

Serum sickness and serum sickness–like reactions These reactions are characterized by the occurrence of fever, urticaria, polyarthralgias, and lymphadenopathy 7 to 10 days after primary exposure and 2 to 4 days after secondary exposure to a heterologous protein (classic serum sickness) or a nonprotein drug such as penicillin or sulfa (serum sickness–like reaction). Most of the manifestations are not due to a vasculitis; however, occasional patients will have typical cutaneous venulitis which may progress rarely to a systemic vasculitis. This disorder is discussed in detail in Chap. 261.

Vasculitis associated with other underlying primary diseases A number of diseases have vasculitis as a secondary manifestation of the underlying primary process. Foremost among these are the connective tissue diseases, particularly systemic lupus erythematosus (Chap. 262), rheumatoid arthritis (Chap. 263), and Sjörgen's syndrome (Chap. 266). The most common form of vasculitis in these conditions is the small vessel venulitis isolated to the skin and clinically indistinguishable from the hypersensitivity vasculitides noted in response to an exogenous antigen. However, certain patients may develop a fulminant systemic necrotizing vasculitis indistinguishable from the polyarteritis nodosa group. Cryoglobulinemia may be seen in a number of the diverse vasculitic syndromes. Essential mixed cryoglobulinemia may present as a typical hypersensitivity vasculitis confined to the skin. However, typically it is associated with glomerulonephritis, arthralgias, hepatosplenomegaly, and lymphadenopathy in addition to skin involvement. The cryoglobulins usually consist of cryoprecipitable IgM rheumatoid factor directed against normal endogenous IgG.

Vasculitis can be associated with certain malignancies, particularly lymphoid or reticuloendothelial neoplasms. Leukocytoclastic venulitis confined to the skin is the most common finding; however, widespread systemic vasculitis may occur. Of particular note is the association of hairy-cell leukemia (Chap. 292) with classic PAN.

A leukocytoclastic vasculitis predominantly involving the skin with occasional involvement of other organ systems may be a minor component of many other diseases. These include subacute bacterial endocarditis, chronic Epstein-Barr virus infection, chronic active hepatitis, ulcerative colitis, congenital deficiencies of various complement components, retroperitoneal fibrosis, and primary biliary cirrhosis. Association of hypersensitivity vasculitis with $alpha_1$ antitrypsin deficiency, intestinal bypass surgery, and relapsing polychondritis have been reported.

DIAGNOSIS The diagnosis of hypersensitivity vasculitis is made by the demonstration of vasculitis on biopsy. Given the predominance of cutaneous involvement, biopsy material is generally readily available. Patients who present with what appears to be isolated cutaneous vasculitis should undergo a systemic (usually noninvasive) workup of other organ systems since skin involvement is often the presenting feature of systemic vasculitis.

TREATMENT AND PROGNOSIS Most cases of hypersensitivity vasculitis resolve spontaneously, and others, such as Henoch-Schönlein purpura, remit and relapse before finally remitting completely. In those patients in whom persistent cutaneous disease evolves or in whom extracutaneous organ system involvement occurs, a variety of therapeutic regimens have been tried with variable results. In general, the treatment of this type of vasculitis has not been satisfactory. This is in contrast to the systemic necrotizing vasculitis group (see above) and Wegener's granulomatosis (see below) which generally are much more serious diseases than hypersensitivity vasculitis, but usually respond dramatically to the combination of prednisone and cyclophosphamide. Fortunately, since the disease is generally limited to the skin, this lack of consistent response to therapy usually does not lead to a life-threatening situation. When an antigenic stimulus is recognized as the precipitating factor in the vasculitis, it should be removed; if this is a microbe, appropriate antimicrobial therapy should be instituted. If the vasculitis is associated with another underlying disease, treatment of the latter often results in resolution of the former. In situations where disease is apparently self-limited, no therapy, except possibly symptomatic therapy, is indicated. When disease persists or results in progressive organ system dysfunction such as renal failure in Henoch-Schönlein purpura, corticosteroid therapy should be instituted, usually as prednisone, 1 mg/kg per day, in a regimen aimed at rapid tapering where possible, either directly to discontinuation or by conversion to an alternate-day regimen followed by ultimate discontinuation. In cases that prove refractory to corticosteroids in which irreversible organ system dysfunction is likely, a trial of a cytotoxic agent such as cyclophosphamide in the regimen described above for systemic vasculitis is warranted. Patients with chronic vasculitis isolated to cutaneous venules rarely respond dramatically to any therapeutic regimen, and cytotoxic agents should be used only as a last resort in these patients. Plasmapheresis has been used with some success in fulminant cases.

WEGENER'S GRANULOMATOSIS

DEFINITION Wegener's granulomatosis is a distinct clinicopathologic entity characterized by granulomatous vasculitis of the upper and lower respiratory tracts together with glomerulonephritis. In addition, variable degrees of disseminated vasculitis involving both small arteries and veins may occur.

INCIDENCE AND PREVALENCE Wegener's granulomatosis is an uncommon disease whose true incidence is difficult to determine. It is extremely rare in blacks compared to whites; the male to female ratio is 1.3:1. The disease can be seen at any age but is infrequent among preadolescents; the mean age of onset is approximately 40 years. The disease has been reported to be associated with an increased prevalence of HLA-B8 and HLA-DR2.

PATHOPHYSIOLOGY AND PATHOGENESIS The histopathologic hallmarks of Wegener's granulomatosis are necrotizing vasculitis of small arteries and veins together with granuloma formation which may be either intravascular or extravascular. Lung involvement typically appears as multiple, bilateral, nodular cavity infiltrates which on biopsy almost invariably reveal the typical necrotizing granulomatous vasculitis. Endobronchial disease either in its active form or as a result of fibrous scarring may lead to obstruction with atelectasis. Upper airway lesions, particularly those in the sinuses and nasopharynx, typically reveal inflammation, necrosis, and granuloma formation with or without vasculitis.

It its earliest form, renal involvement is characterized by a focal and segmental glomerulitis which may evolve into a rapidly progressive crescentic glomerulonephritis. Granuloma formation is only rarely seen on renal biopsy. In addition to the classic triad of upper and lower respiratory tracts and kidney disease, virtually any organ can be involved with vasculitis, granuloma, or both.

The immunopathogenesis of this disease is unclear, although the involvement of upper airways and lung suggests an aberrant hypersensitivity response to an exogenous or even endogenous antigen that enters through or resides in the upper airway. The demonstration of circulating and deposited immune complexes in certain patients together with granulomatous reactivity suggests either an overlap of delayed hypersensitivity and immune-complex–mediated mechanisms or a granulomatous response to the immune complexes themselves.

CLINICAL AND LABORATORY MANIFESTATIONS A typical patient presents with severe upper respiratory tract findings such as paranasal sinus pain and drainage, and purulent or bloody nasal discharge with or without nasal mucosal ulceration. Nasal septal perforation may follow, leading to saddle nose deformity. Serous otitis media may occur as a result of eustachian tube blockage.

Pulmonary involvement may be manifested as asymptomatic infiltrates or may be clinically expressed as cough, hemoptysis, dyspnea, and chest discomfort. It is present in approximately 95 percent of patients.

Eye involvement (60 percent of patients) may range from a mild conjunctivitis to episcleritis, scleritis, granulomatous sclerouveitis, ciliary vessel vasculitis, and retroorbital mass lesions leading to proptosis.

Skin lesions (45 percent of patients) appear as papules, vesicles, palpable purpura, ulcers, or subcutaneous nodules; biopsy reveals vasculitis, granuloma, or both. Cardiac involvement (12 percent of patients) manifests as pericarditis, coronary vasculitis, or, rarely, cardiomyopathy. Nervous system manifestations (22 percent of patients) include cranial neuritis, mononeuritis multiplex, or, rarely, cerebral vasculitis and/or granuloma.

Renal disease (85 percent of patients) generally dominates the clinical picture and, if left untreated, accounts directly or indirectly for most of the mortality in this disease. Although it may smolder in some cases as a mild glomerulitis with proteinuria, hematuria, and red blood cell casts, it is clear that once clinically detectable renal functional impairment occurs, rapidly progressive renal failure usually ensues unless appropriate treatment is instituted.

While the disease is active, most patients have nonspecific symptoms and signs such as malaise, weakness, arthralgias, anorexia, and weight loss. Fever may indicate activity of the underlying disease, but more often reflects secondary infection, usually of the upper airway.

Characteristic laboratory findings include a markedly elevated ESR, mild anemia and leukocytosis, mild hypergammaglobulinemia, particularly of the IgA class, and mildly elevated rheumatoid factor. Thrombocytosis may be seen as an acute phase reactant; hypocomplementemia is not seen despite the presence of circulating immune complexes.

DIAGNOSIS The diagnosis of Wegener's granulomatosis is a clinicopathologic one made by the demonstration of necrotizing granulomatous vasculitis on biopsy of appropriate tissue in a patient with the clinical findings of upper and lower respiratory tract disease together with evidence of glomerulonephritis. Pulmonary tissue, preferably obtained by open thoracotomy, offers the highest diagnostic yield, almost invariably revealing granulomatous vasculitis. Biopsy of upper airway tissue usually reveals granulomatous inflammation with necrosis but may not show vasculitis. Renal biopsy confirms the presence of glomerulonephritis.

In its typical presentation, the classic clinicopathologic complex of Wegener's granulomatosis usually provides ready differentiation from other disorders. However, if all of the typical features are not present at once, it needs to be differentiated from the other vasculitides, particularly allergic angiitis and granulomatosis, Goodpasture's syndrome (Chap. 224), tumors of the upper airway or lung, and infectious or noninfectious granulomatous diseases. Of particular note is the differentiation from idiopathic midline granuloma (see Chap. 272) which frequently erodes through the skin of the face, a feature never seen in Wegener's granulomatosis.

Of particular importance in the differential diagnosis is a disease called *lymphomatoid granulomatosis*. It is characterized by lung, skin, central nervous system, and kidney involvement in which atypical lymphocytoid and plasmacytoid cells infiltrate tissue in an angioinvasive manner. In this regard, it clearly differs from Wegener's granulomatosis in that it is not an inflammatory vasculitis in the classic sense, but an infiltration of vessels with atypical mononuclear cells; granuloma may be present in involved tissues. Approximately 50 percent of patients develop a true malignant lymphoma.

TREATMENT AND PROGNOSIS Wegener's granulomatosis was formerly universally fatal, usually within a few months after the onset of clinically apparent renal disease. Corticosteroids alone led to some symptomatic improvement with little effect on the ultimate course of the disease. It has been well established that the treatment of choice in this disease is cyclophosphamide given in doses of 2 mg/kg per day orally. The leukocyte count should be closely monitored during therapy and the dosage adjusted in order to maintain the count above 3000 per cubic millimeter, which generally maintains the neutrophil count at approximately 1500 per cubic millimeter. With this approach, clinical remission can usually be induced and maintained without causing severe leukopenia with its associated risk of infection. Cyclophosphamide should be continued for 1 year following the induction of complete remission and gradually tapered and discontinued thereafter. Patients who cannot tolerate cyclophosphamide or who develop serious toxicity such as severe cystitis may be treated with azathioprine in similar doses.

At the initiation of therapy, corticosteroids should be administered together with cyclophosphamide. This can be given as prednisone, 1 mg/kg per day initially (for the first month of therapy) as a daily regimen with gradual conversion to an alternate-day schedule followed by tapering and discontinuation after approximately 6 months.

Using the above regimen, the prognosis of this disease is excellent and long-term remission is achieved in over 90 percent of patients. A number of patients who developed irreversible renal failure, but who achieved subsequent remission on appropriate therapy, have undergone successful renal transplantation.

TEMPORAL ARTERITIS

DEFINITION Temporal arteritis, also referred to as cranial or giant cell arteritis, is an inflammation of medium- and large-sized arteries. It characteristically involves one or more branches of the carotid artery, particularly the temporal artery, hence the name cranial or temporal arteritis. However, it is a systemic disease and can involve arteries in multiple locations.

INCIDENCE AND PREVALENCE Temporal arteritis is an uncommon disease estimated to occur in 24 per 100,000 people. It is a disease of the elderly, occurring almost exclusively in individuals older than 55 years; however, well-documented cases have occurred in patients 40 years old or younger. It is more common in women than in men and is rare in blacks. Familial aggregation of this disease has been reported as has an increased prevalence of HLA-DR4.

PATHOPHYSIOLOGY AND PATHOGENESIS Although the temporal artery is most frequently involved in this disease, patients often have a systemic vasculitis of multiple medium- and large-sized arteries which may go undetected. Histopathologically, the disease is a panarteritis with inflammatory mononuclear cell infiltrates within the vessel wall with frequent giant cell formation. There is proliferation of the intima and fragmentation of the internal elastic lamina. Pathophysiologic findings in organs result from the ischemia related to the involved vessels. Immunopathogenic mechanisms, particularly cell-mediated immunity, are felt to be involved in this disease, although the etiology is entirely unknown.

CLINICAL AND LABORATORY MANIFESTATIONS The disease is characterized clinically by the classic complex of fever, anemia, high ESR, and headaches in an elderly patient. Other manifestations include malaise, fatigue, anorexia, weight loss, sweats, and arthralgias. Temporal arteritis is closely associated with the polymyalgia rheumatica syndrome, which is characterized by stiffness, aching, and pain in the muscles of the neck, shoulders, lower back, hips, and thighs.

In patients with involvement of the temporal artery, headache is the predominant symptom and may be associated with a tender, thickened, or nodular artery which may pulsate early in the disease but may become occluded later. Scalp pain and claudication of the jaw and tongue may occur. A well-recognized and dreaded complication of temporal arteritis, particularly in untreated patients, is ocular involvement due primarily to ischemic optic neuritis, which may lead to serious visual symptoms, even sudden blindness in some patients. However, most patients have complaints relating to the head or eyes for months before objective eye involvement. Claudication of the extremities, strokes, myocardial infarctions, aortic aneurysms and dissections, and infarctions of visceral organs have been reported.

Characteristic laboratory findings in addition to the elevated ESR include a normochromic or slightly hypochromic anemia. Liver function abnormalities are common, particularly increased alkaline phosphatase levels. Increased levels of IgG and complement have been reported as have increased levels of circulating immune complexes.

DIAGNOSIS The diagnosis of temporal arteritis and its associated clinicopathologic syndrome can often be made clinically by the demonstration of the classic picture of fever, anemia, and high ESR with or without symptoms of polymyalgia rheumatica in an elderly patient. The diagnosis is confirmed by biopsy of the temporal artery. Since involvement of the vessel may be segmental, the diagnosis may be missed on routine biopsy. Dramatic response to a trial of corticosteroid therapy can confirm the diagnosis.

TREATMENT AND PROGNOSIS Temporal arteritis and its associated symptoms are exquisitely sensitive to corticosteroid therapy. Treatment should begin with prednisone, 40 to 60 mg per day followed by a gradual tapering to a maintenance dose of 7.5 to 10 mg per day. When ocular signs and symptoms occur, it is important that therapy be initiated or adjusted to control them. Because of the possibility of relapse, therapy should be continued for at least 1 to 2 years. The prognosis is generally good, and most patients achieve complete remission that is often maintained after withdrawal of therapy.

TAKAYASU'S ARTERITIS

DEFINITION Takayasu's arteritis is an inflammatory and stenotic disease of medium- and large-sized arteries characterized by a strong predilection for the aortic arch and its branches. For this reason, it is often referred to as the aortic arch syndrome.

INCIDENCE AND PREVALENCE Takayasu's arteritis is an uncommon disease, much less common than temporal arteritis. It is most prevalent in adolescent girls and young women. Although it is more common in the Orient, it is neither racially nor geographically restricted. An association of the disease has been described with HLA-DR2, MB1 in Japan and HLA-DR4, MB3 in the United States.

PATHOPHYSIOLOGY AND PATHOGENESIS The disease involves medium- and large-sized arteries with a strong predilection for the aortic arch and its branches; the pulmonary artery may also be involved. The most commonly affected arteries seen by angiography are the subclavians, followed by the aortic arch, ascending aorta, carotids, and femorals. The involvement of the major branches of the aorta is much more marked at their origin than distally. Partial renal artery occlusion with resulting hypertension is common. The disease is a panarteritis with inflammatory mononuclear cell infiltrates and occasionally giant cells. There is marked intimal proliferation and fibrosis, scarring and vascularization of the media, and disruption and degeneration of the elastic lamina. Narrowing of the lumen occurs with or without thrombosis. The vasa vasorum are frequently involved. Pathologic changes in various organs reflect the compromise of blood flow through the involved vessels.

Immunopathogenic mechanisms, the precise nature of which is uncertain, are suspected in this disease.

CLINICAL AND LABORATORY MANIFESTATIONS Takayasu's arteritis is a systemic disease with generalized as well as local symptoms. The generalized symptoms include malaise, fever, night sweats, arthralgias, anorexia, and weight loss which may occur months before vessel involvement is apparent. These symptoms may merge into those related to pain over the involved vessels followed by symptoms of ischemia in organs supplied by the compromised vessels. Pulses are commonly absent in the involved vessels, particularly the subclavian artery. Aortic regurgitation may occur; hypertension is seen in almost 50 percent of cases. Cardiomegaly and cardiac failure secondary to aortic or pulmonary hypertension occur commonly; the coronary arteries themselves are rarely involved. Carotid artery involvement leads to a variety of central nervous system signs and symptoms with over one-half of patients experiencing syncopal episodes; ocular signs and symptoms are present in 60 percent of patients.

The clinical course may be fulminant, may progress gradually, or may stabilize. Complications are related to the distribution of the involved vessels. Death usually occurs from congestive heart failure or cerebrovascular accidents.

Characteristic laboratory findings include an elevated ESR, mild anemia, leukocytosis, and elevated immunoglobulin levels. Angiography of involved vessels reveals the characteristic stenotic or occluded vessels.

DIAGNOSIS The diagnosis of Takayasu's arteritis should be suspected strongly in a young woman who develops a decrease or absence of peripheral pulses, discrepancies in blood pressure, and arterial bruits. The diagnosis is confirmed by the characteristic pattern on arteriography which includes irregular vessel walls, stenosis, poststenotic dilatation, aneurysm formation, occlusion, and evidence of increased collateral circulation. Histopathologic demonstration of inflamed vessels adds confirmatory data; however, tissue is rarely readily available for examination.

TREATMENT AND PROGNOSIS The course of the disease is variable, and spontaneous remissions may occur. However, it is generally considered to be progressive and fatal within a few years. Although corticosteroid therapy in doses of 40 to 60 mg prednisone per day alleviates symptoms, there are no convincing studies which indicate that they alone increase survival. However, recent studies suggest that corticosteroid therapy can induce remissions in a high percentage of individuals and when combined with reconstructive surgery on severely involved vessels, can remarkably improve survival. A few patients who were refractory to corticosteroid therapy responded favorably to cyclophosphamide, 2 mg/kg per day. However, long-term studies will be needed to confirm this.

MUCOCUTANEOUS LYMPH NODE SYNDROME (KAWASAKI'S DISEASE)

Mucocutaneous lymph node syndrome is an acute, febrile, multisystem disease of children. Patients show characteristic findings in the mucous membranes and skin together with lymphadenopathy (see also Chap. 49). Although the disease is generally benign and self-limited, it is associated with coronary artery aneurysms in 17 to 31 percent of cases, with an overall case fatality rate of 0.5 to 2.8 percent. These complications usually occur between the third and fourth week of illness during the convalescent stage. Vasculitis of the coronary arteries is seen in almost all of the fatal cases which have been autopsied. There is typical intimal proliferation and infiltration of the vessel wall with mononuclear cells. Beadlike aneurysms and thromboses may be seen along the artery. Most investigators agree that many of the cases of PAN formerly reported in children were actually arteritic complications of unrecognized mucocutaneous lymph node syndrome. Other manifestations include pericarditis, myocarditis, myocardial ischemia and infarction, and cardiomegaly.

Apart from the up to 2.8 percent of patients who develop fatal complications, the prognosis of this disease for uneventful recovery is excellent. The treatment of choice is aspirin during the acute and convalescent phases of the disease; this has been reported to result in a decrease in the incidence of cardiac complications.

ISOLATED VASCULITIS OF THE CENTRAL NERVOUS SYSTEM

Isolated vasculitis of the central nervous system is an uncommon clinicopathologic entity characterized by vasculitis restricted to the vessels of the central nervous system without other apparent systemic vasculitis. Although the arteriole is most commonly affected, vessels of any size can be involved. The inflammatory process is usually composed of mononuclear cell infiltrates with or without granuloma formation. Cases have been associated with Hodgkin's disease and varicella-zoster infections; however, in several cases no underlying disease process has been identified.

Patients may present with severe headaches, altered mental function, and focal neurologic defects. Systemic symptoms are generally absent. Devastating neurologic abnormalities may occur depending on the extent of vessel involvement. The diagnosis is generally made by demonstration of characteristic vessel abnormalities on arteriography and confirmed by biopsy of the brain parenchyma and leptomeninges. The prognosis of this disease is poor; however, some reports indicate that corticosteroid therapy alone or together with cyclophosphamide in steroid-resistant patients administered as described above for the systemic vasculitides has induced sustained clinical remissions in a small number of patients.

THROMBOANGIITIS OBLITERANS (BUERGER'S DISEASE)

Thromboangiitis obliterans is an inflammatory occlusive peripheral vascular disease of unknown etiology which affects arteries and veins. Thrombosis of the vessels is likely the primary event, and so this disease is not a classic vasculitis. However, it is considered among the vasculitides because of the intense inflammatory response within the thrombus and the fact that there is often a vasculitis of the vasa vasorum in the arterial wall. The disease is discussed in detail in Chap. 198.

MISCELLANEOUS VASCULITIDES

A variety of disorders, many of which are uncommon, are characterized by varying degrees of inflammatory responses involving blood vessels. *Behçet's syndrome* is a clinicopathologic entity characterized by recurrent episodes of oral and genital ulcers, iritis, and cutaneous lesions. The underlying pathologic lesion is a leukocytoclastic venulitis, although vessels of any size and in any organ can be involved. This disorder is described in detail in Chap. 268.

Cogan's syndrome is a disease characterized by nonsyphilitic interstitial keratitis together with vestibuloauditory symptoms. It may be associated with a systemic vasculitis involving vessels of different sizes as well as the aortic valve.

Erythema nodosum is a common disease which is recognized as a hypersensitivity manifestation of a number of other disorders. It is a painful nodular process of the dermis and subcutaneous tissues. However, histopathologically, there is a vasculitis of small venules (see Chap. 48).

Erythema elevatum diutinum is a rare, chronic skin disorder of unknown etiology characterized by persistent red, purple, and yellowish papules, plaques, and nodules usually distributed symmetrically over the extensor surface of the limbs which on biopsy demonstrate a leukocytoclastic venulitis together with a marked dermal inflammatory infiltrate. The disease responds dramatically to dapsone therapy.

Eales' disease is a retinal vasculitis which predominantly affects males in the second and third decade of life and which produces a syndrome of recurrent hemorrhages into the retina and vitreous.

REFERENCES

Alarcon-Segovia D: The necrotizing vasculitides. Med Clin North Am 61:240, 1977

Christian CL, Sergent JS; Vasculitic syndromes: Clinical and experimental models. Am J Med 61:385, 1976

Cupps TR, Fauci AS: *The Vasculitides*. Philadelphia, Saunders, 1981

——— et al: Chronic, recurrent small-vessel cutaneous vasculitis. Clinical experience in 13 patients. JAMA 247:1994, 1982

——— et al: Isolated angiitis of the central nervous system. Prospective diagnostic and therapeutic experience. Am J Med 74:97, 1983

Fauci AS: Vasculitis, in *Clinical Immunology*, CW Parker (ed). Philadelphia, Saunders, 1980, pp 475–519

———: Vasculitis. J Allergy Clin Immunol 72:211, 1983

——— et al: The spectrum of vasculitis. Clinical, pathologic, immunologic, and therapeutic considerations. Ann Intern Med 89:660, 1978

——— et al: Wegener's granulomatosis: Prospective clinical and therapeutic experience with 85 patients for 21 years. Ann Intern Med 98:76, 1983

Leavitt RY, Fauci AS: Polyangiitis overlap syndrome. Am J Med, 1986

Shelhamer JH et al: Takayasu's arteritis and its therapy. Ann Intern Med 103:121, 1985

Zeek PM: Periarteritis nodosa and other forms of necrotizing angiitis. N Engl J Med 148:764, 1953

270 SARCOIDOSIS

RONALD G. CRYSTAL

DEFINITION Sarcoidosis is a chronic, multisystem disorder of unknown etiology characterized in affected organs by an accumulation of lymphocytes and mononuclear phagocytes, noncaseating epithelioid granulomas, and derangements of the normal tissue architecture. Although there are usually skin anergy and depressed cellular immune processes in the blood, sarcoidosis is characterized at the sites of disease by exaggerated helper T-lymphocyte immune processes. All parts of the body can be affected, but the organ most frequently affected is the lung. Involvement of the skin, eye, and lymph nodes is also common. The disease can be acute and self-limiting, but in many individuals it is chronic, waxing and waning over many years.

ETIOLOGY The etiology of sarcoidosis is unknown. A variety of infectious and noninfectious agents have been implicated, but there is no proof that any one agent is responsible. It is likely that there is no specific etiologic agent but that the disease results from an abnormal immune response (acquired, inherited, or both) to many different antigens.

INCIDENCE AND PREVALENCE Sarcoidosis is a relatively common disease affecting individuals of both sexes and almost all ages, races, and geographic locations. Females appear to be slightly more susceptible than males. Cases of sarcoid have been described in all of the major races and the disease is found throughout the world. It has been suggested that sarcoid is more common in certain geographic areas such as the southeastern part of the United States but when case-matched controls have been used, these geographic differences are less convincing. The prevalence of sarcoidosis is from 10 to 40 per 100,000 in the United States and Europe. In the United States, the majority of patients are black, with a ratio of blacks to whites ranging from 10:1 to 17:1. In Europe, however, the disease affects mostly whites. There is a remarkable diversity of the prevalence of sarcoidosis among certain ethnic and racial groups. For example, in Irish females living in London it is 200 per 100,000. In contrast, the disease is very rare among Canadian Indians, New Zealand Maoris, and Southeast Asians.

Most patients present with sarcoidosis between the ages of 20 and 40, but it can occur in children and in the elderly. Several hundred kindred groups with familial sarcoidosis have been described, and the disease has been observed in twins, more commonly in monozygotic than in dizygotic pairs. There have also been several instances of husband-wife pairs identified, arguing for some environmental factors in the pathogenesis of the disease. Although the histocompatibility locus HLA-B8 has been suggested to confer certain responses to sarcoidosis, no clear patterns in any HLA locus have emerged. Unlike many diseases in which the lung is involved, sarcoidosis is less common in smokers than in nonsmokers.

PATHOPHYSIOLOGY AND IMMUNOPATHOGENESIS The first manifestation of the disease is an accumulation of mononuclear inflammatory cells, mostly T-helper lymphocytes and mononuclear phagocytes, in affected organs. This inflammatory process is followed by the formation of granulomas, aggregates of macrophages and their progeny, epithelioid cells, and multinucleated giant cells. The typical sarcoid granuloma is a compact structure composed of an aggregate of mononuclear phagocytes surrounded by a rim of T-helper lymphocytes and, sometimes, B lymphocytes. The overall structure is relatively discrete and is interspersed with fine collagen fibrils, presumably remnants of the underlying connective tissue matrix. The giant cells within the granuloma can be of the Langhans' or foreign-body variety and often contain inclusions such as Schaumann bodies (conch-like structures), asteroid bodies (stellate-like structures), and residual bodies (refractile calcium-containing inclusions).

Together, the accumulated T cells, mononuclear phagocytes, and granulomas represent the active disease. Other than the fact that they take up space and thus modify the local architecture, there is no evidence that the mononuclear inflammatory cells either alone or in the granuloma injure the affected organ by releasing mediators that damage the normal parenchymal cells or the extracellular matrix. Rather, organ dysfunction in sarcoid results from the fact that the accumulated inflammatory cells distort the architecture of the affected tissue; if a sufficient number of structures vital to the function of the tissue are involved, the disease becomes clinically apparent in that organ. Thus, while autopy series show that, to some extent, sarcoidosis involves most organs in the majority of patients, the disease manifests clinically only in organs where it affects function (such as the lung and eye) or in organs where it is readily observed (such as the skin or, by x-ray, the hilar nodes). For example, in the lung the inflammatory cells and granulomas distort the walls of the alveoli, bronchi, and blood vessels (Fig. 270-1*A*), thus altering the intimate relationships between air and blood necessary for normal gas exchange; this is sensed by the individual as dyspnea. In contrast, most individuals with sarcoidosis have granulomatous mononuclear cell inflammation in the liver but usually do not have symptoms or functional derangements referable to that organ, likely because the disease process does not modify the local structures sufficiently to affect function.

If the disease is suppressed, either spontaneously or with therapy, the mononuclear inflammation is reduced in intensity and the number of granulomas is reduced. The granulomas resolve either by dispersion of the cells or by centripetal proliferation of fibroblasts from the periphery of the granuloma inward, to form a scar which eventually disappears. In chronic cases, the mononuclear cell inflammation persists for years. If the intensity of the inflammation is sufficiently high for a sufficiently long period, the derangements to the affected tissues result in extensive damage, the development of fibrosis, and permanent loss of organ function.

All available evidence suggests that active sarcoidosis results from an aberrant immune response to a variety of antigens, in which the process of T-lymphocyte triggering, proliferation, and activation is skewed in the direction of helper T-lymphocyte processes (Fig. 270-1*B*). The result is an undamped helper T-cell response, and thus the accumulation of large numbers of activated T cells in the affected organs. Since the activated helper T lymphocyte releases mediators that attract and activate mononuclear phagocytes, it is likely that the process of granuloma formation is a secondary phenomen which is a consequence of the exaggerated T-helper cell process. In this context, the current hypotheses of the cause of sarcoidosis, not mutually exclusive, include: (1) the disease is caused by a class of antigens, nonself or self, that trigger only the helper T-cell arm of the immune response; (2) the disease results from an inadequate suppressor arm of the immune response, such that helper T-cell processes cannot be shut down in a normal fashion; or (3) the disease results from inherited (and/or acquired) differences in immune response genes, such that the response to a variety of antigens is an uncontrolled, helper T-cell process.

Independent of the inciting agent(s) or the reason why there is an undamped helper T-cell response, there is a general understanding of the processes responsible for the maintenance of the inflammation and the development of the granuloma. The T-helper lymphocytes

FIGURE 270-1 *Pathogenesis of sarcoidosis. A. Histologic abnormalities. The normal alveolar wall (left) and the alveolar wall in active sarcoidosis (right), which is distorted by the accumulated T-helper lymphocytes, alveolar macrophages, and macrophages aggregated into granulomas, are illustrated. There is mild damage to alveolar epithelial and endothelial cells. B. The exaggerated T-helper lymphocyte processes in affected organs result in the accumulation of T-helper cells, macrophages, and macrophages aggregated into granulomas. The triggering signal for the T-helper cells is unknown; it is assumed to be a variety of antigens. The immune response is skewed to produce activated T-helper cells that release interleukin 2, which drives the accumulation of more T-helper cells. The activated T-helper cells also release monocyte chemotactic factor and interferon-gamma, mediators that contribute to the recruitment and activation of monocytes and hence to granuloma formation.*

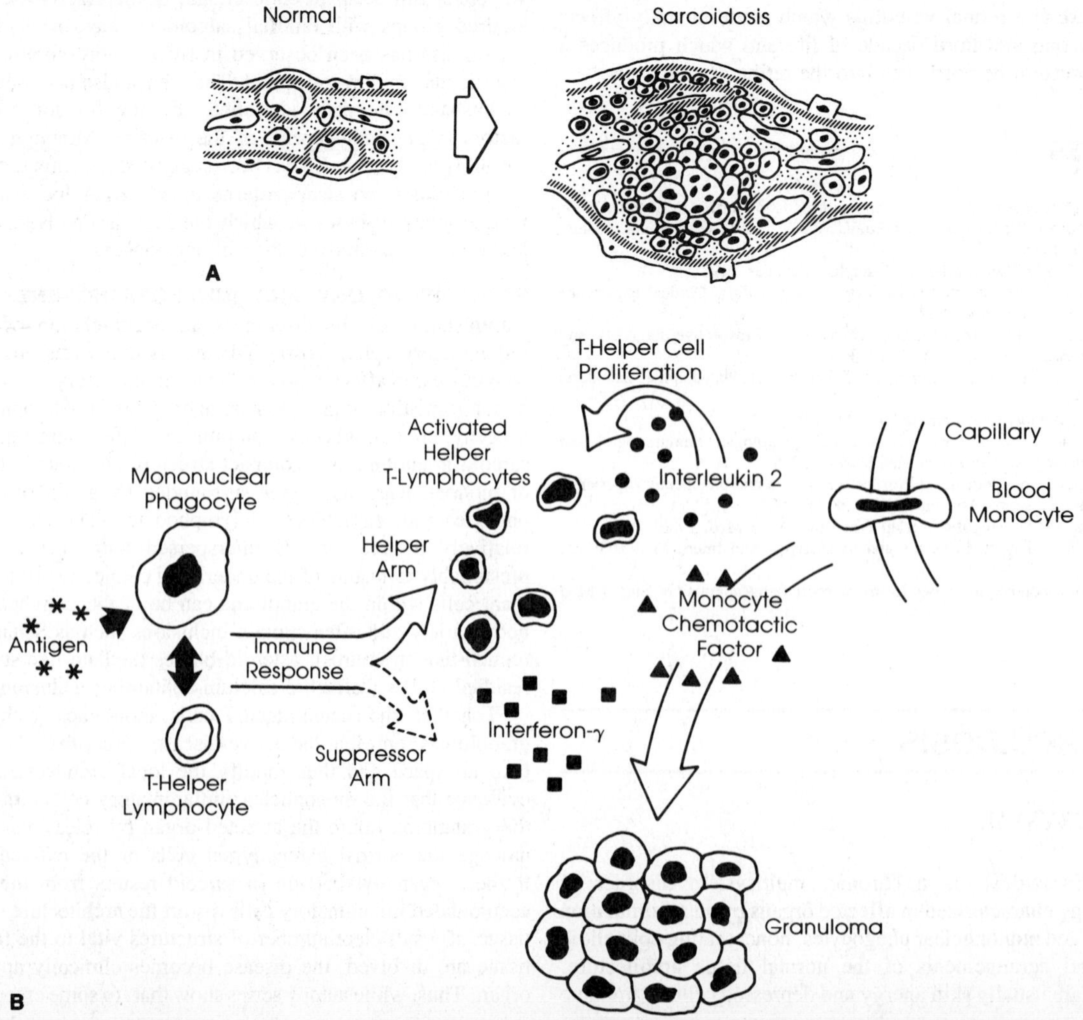

accumulate at the sites of disease because they proliferate in these sites at an exaggerated rate. This T-cell proliferation is maintained by the spontaneous release of interleukin 2 (IL-2), the T-cell growth factor, by activated T-helper cells in the local milieu. In this regard, sarcoidosis is a remarkable example of compartmentalization of the immune system and a dramatic illustration of why disease activity of sarcoidosis cannot be assessed by evaluating the immune system only in the blood. Whereas the T-helper cells in the involved organs are releasing IL-2 and proliferating at an enhanced rate, the T cells in other sites, such as blood, are quiescent. Furthermore, while there is a marked enhancement of the number of T-helper cells at the sites of disease, the numbers of T-helper cells in the blood are normal or slightly reduced. In this regard, in the involved organs, the ratio of T-helper to T-suppressor cells may be as high as 10:1 compared to the ratio of 2:1 found in normal tissues or in the blood of affected individuals.

In addition to driving other T-helper cells in the affected organs to proliferate, the T-helper cells at the sites of disease are activated and release mediators that both recruit and activate mononuclear phagocytes. The T-helper cells accomplish this by releasing a variety of mediators (lymphokines) including monocyte chemotactic factor, a protein capable of recruiting blood monocytes to the local milieu of the activated T cells, and gamma interferon, a protein that, among its many actions, activates mononuclear phagocytes. Together, these mediators recruit blood monocytes to the affected organs and activate them, providing the building blocks for the formation of the granuloma.

In addition to these aberrant cellular immune processes, active sarcoid is also characterized by hyperglobulinemia. Included among the immunoglobulins are antibodies against a variety of infectious agents as well as IgM anti-T-cell antibodies; there is no evidence that they play a role in the pathogenesis of the disease, and they are thought to result from the nonspecific polyclonal stimulation of B cells by the activated T cells at the site of disease.

If the damage in the affected organs is sufficiently extensive so that the remaining parenchymal cells cannot reestablish the normal tissue architecture, the usual result is fibrosis, the proliferation of mesenchymal cells and deposition of their connective tissue products. The current concepts relating to this process are described in Chap. 209.

CLINICAL MANIFESTATIONS Sarcoidosis is a systemic disease, and thus the clinical manifestations may be generalized or focused on one or more organs. However, because the lung is almost always involved, most patients have symptoms referable to the respiratory system. Independent of the site, the clinical manifestations of the disease relate directly to the exaggerated T-helper cell–mononuclear phagocyte granulomatous inflammatory process itself, or to the sequela resulting from the permanent damage caused by this process.

Sarcoidosis is occasionally discovered in a completely asymptomatic individual, but more commonly it presents abruptly over 1 to 2 weeks or the affected individual develops symptoms insidiously over several months. Independent of the mode of presentation, about 75 percent of all cases present when the individual is less than 40 years of age.

The asymptomatic form is usually detected by a routine examination, such as a chest film. In the United States, this represents about 10 to 20 percent of all cases, but in countries where chest films are mandatory in preemployment screening programs, the proportion of asymptomatic patients is higher.

So-called acute or subacute sarcoidosis develops abruptly over a period of a few weeks and represents 20 to 40 percent of all cases. These individuals usually have constitutional symptoms such as fever, fatigue, malaise, anorexia, or weight loss. These symptoms are usually mild, but in approximately 25 percent of these acute cases, the constitutional complaints are extensive. Many have respiratory symptoms, including cough, dyspnea, or a vague retrosternal chest discomfort. Two syndromes have been identified in the acute group. Löfgren's syndrome, frequent in Scandinavian, Irish, and Puerto Rican females, includes the complex of erythema nodosum and x-ray findings of bilateral hilar adenopathy, often accompanied by joint symptoms. The Heerfordt-Waldenstrom syndrome describes individuals with fever, parotid enlargement, anterior uveitis, and facial nerve palsy.

The insidious form of sarcoidosis develops over months and is associated usually with respiratory complaints without constitutional symptoms. About 10 percent of these individuals have symptoms referable to organs other than the lung. It is the individuals who present with the insidious form of sarcoidosis that most commonly go on to develop chronic sarcoidosis, with permanent damage to the lung and other organs.

Despite the fact that sarcoidosis is a systemic disease and some evidence of inflammation can be detected in most organs in the majority of patients, sarcoidosis is important clinically because of the pulmonary abnormalities and, to a lesser extent, lymph node, skin, and eye involvement. Far less commonly, other organs are involved significantly.

Lung Of individuals with sarcoidosis, 90 percent have an abnormal chest x-ray at some time during their course. Overall, approximately 50 percent develop permanent pulmonary abnormalities and 10 to 20 percent have progressive fibrosis of the lung parenchyma. Sarcoidosis of the lung is primarily an interstitial lung disease (see Chap. 209) in which the inflammatory process involves the alveoli, small bronchi, and small blood vessels. These individuals typically have symptoms of dyspnea, particularly with exercise, and a dry cough. Physical examination reveals dry rales. Hemoptysis is rare, as is production of sputum. Occasionally, the large airways are involved to a degree sufficient to cause dysfunction. Distal atelectasis can result from endobronchial sarcoidosis or from external compression from enlarged intrathoracic nodes. Rarely, wheezing is heard, incorrectly suggesting asthma. Large-vessel pulmonary granulomatous arteritis is common, but it rarely causes major problems. If it dominates the pulmonary lesions, it is sometimes called "necrotizing sarcoidal granulomatosis." The pleura is involved in 1 to 5 percent of cases, almost always manifesting as a unilatereal pleural effusion with characteristics of an exudate containing lymphocytes. The effusions usually clear within a few weeks, but chronic pleural thickening can result. Pneumothorax is very rare.

Lymph nodes Lymphadenopathy is very common in sarcoidosis. Intrathoracic nodes are enlarged in 75 to 90 percent of all patients; usually this involves the hilar nodes, but the paratracheal nodes are commonly involved. Less frequently, there is enlargement of subcarinal, anterior mediastinal, or posterior mediastinal nodes. Peripheral lymphadenopathy is very common, particularly involving the cervical, axillary, epitrochlear, and inguinal nodes. The nodes in the retroperitoneal area and in the mesenteric chain can also enlarge. All of these nodes are nonadherent, with a firm, rubbery texture. Palpation causes no pain. Unlike nodes in tuberculosis, the nodes do not ulcerate. The lymphadenopathy rarely causes a problem for the affected individual; however, if it is massive, it can be disfiguring and can impinge on other organs and lead to functional impairment.

Skin Sarcoidosis involves the skin in about 25 percent of cases. The most common lesions are erythema nodosum, plaques, maculopapular eruptions, subcutaneous nodules, and lupus pernio. Erythema nodosum, comprising bilateral, tender red nodules on the anterior surface of the legs, is not specific for sarcoidosis but is common, particularly in acute sarcoidosis, in combination with systemic symptoms and polyarthralgias. The plaques are purple, indolent lesions, often raised, and usually occur on the face, buttocks, and extremities. The maculopapular eruptions occur on the face around the eyes and nose, on the back, and on the extremities. These are elevated lesions less than 1 cm in diameter with a flat, waxy top. Subcutaneous nodules are most common on the trunk and extremities. Lupus pernio is characterized by indurated blue-purple, swollen, shiny lesions on the nose, cheeks, lips, ears, fingers, and knees. The lesions on the tip of the nose cause a bulbous appearance, sometimes associated with varicosities. The nasal mucosa is usually involved, and underlying bone can be destroyed. Sarcoidosis can also involve old surgical scars and tattoos. Although it may be disfiguring, cutaneous sarcoidosis rarely causes major problems.

Eye Eye involvement occurs in approximately 25 percent of patients with sarcoidosis and it can cause blindness. The usual lesions involve the uveal tract, iris, ciliary body, and choroid. Of those cases with eye involvement, approximately 75 percent have anterior uveitis and 25 to 35 percent have posterior uveitis. There is blurred vision, tearing, and photophobia. The uveitis can develop rapidly and may clear spontaneously over a 6- to 12-month period. It can also develop insidiously and be chronic. Conjunctival involvement is also common, usually with small, yellow nodules. When the lacrimal gland is involved, a keratoconjunctivitis sicca syndrome, with dry, sore eyes, can result.

Upper respiratory tract The nasal mucosa is involved in up to 20 percent of patients, usually presenting with nasal stuffiness. Any of the structures of the mouth can be involved, particularly the tonsils. Sarcoidosis involves the larynx in about 5 percent of cases. The epiglottis and areas around the true vocal cords are usually involved, but the cords themselves are not. These individuals are usually hoarse and they have dyspnea, wheezing, and stridor; complete obstruction can occur.

Bone marrow and spleen Sarcoidosis of the marrow is reported in 15 to 40 percent of cases, but it rarely causes hematologic abnormalities other than a mild anemia and occasionally thrombocytopenia. Although splenomegaly occurs in only 5 to 10 percent of patients, celiac angiography or splenic biopsy reveals involvement in 50 to 60 percent of cases. The presentation and complications of splenomegaly in sarcoidosis are similar to those of splenomegaly in general.

Liver Although liver biopsy reveals liver involvement in 60 to 90 percent of cases, usually it is not important clinically. Sarcoidosis involves generally the periportal areas. Approximately 20 to 30 percent have hepatomegaly and/or biochemical evidence of liver involvement. Usually these changes reflect a cholestatic pattern and include an elevated alkaline phosphatase level; the bilirubin and aminotransferases are only mildly elevated, and jaundice is rare. Rarely, portal hypertension can occur, as can intrahepatic cholestasis with cirrhosis.

Kidney Clinically apparent primary renal involvement in sarcoidosis is rare, although tubular, glomerular, and renal artery disease have been reported. More commonly, but still in only 1 to 2 percent of all cases, there is a disorder of calcium metabolism with hypercalcinuria, with or without hypercalcemia. If chronic, nephrocalcinosis and nephrolithiasis can result. It is believed that the calcium abnormalities are associated with enhanced calcium absorption in the gut, which is related to an abnormally high level of circulating 1,25-dihydroxyvitamin D.

Nervous system All components of the nervous system can be involved in sarcoidosis. Neurologic findings are observed in about 5 percent of patients. Seventh nerve involvement with unilateral facial paralysis is most common. It occurs suddenly and is usually transient. Other common manifestations of neurosarcoid include optic nerve dysfunction, papilledema, palate dysfunction, hearing abnormalities, hypothalamic and pituitary abnormalities, chronic meningitis, and occasionally, space-occupying lesions. Psychiatric disturbances have been described, and seizures can occur. Rarely, multiple lesions which mimic multiple sclerosis, spinal cord abnormalities, and peripheral neuropathy can occur.

Musculoskeletal system The bones, joints, and/or muscles can be involved in sarcoidosis. Bone lesions are observed in 5 percent of patients and include variable-sized cysts in areas of expanded bone, well-defined round punched-out lesions, or lattice-like changes. Hand and foot bones are the common sites, but most bones can be involved. Occasionally, the bone lesions are tender and painful. Joint involvement is more common, with an incidence of 25 to 50 percent in known cases of sarcoidosis. Arthralgias and frank arthritis occur mostly in large joints; they can be migratory and are usually transient, but then can be chronic and result in deformities. Although muscle biopsy frequently demonstrates granulomatous inflammation, muscle dysfunction is rare. However, nodules, polymyositis, and chronic myopathy have been described.

Heart Approximately 5 percent of patients have significant heart involvement, with clinical evidence of cardiac dysfunction. Left ventricular wall involvement is common. Arrhythmias are frequent, and serious conduction disturbances, including complete heart block, can occur. Papillary muscle dysfunction, pericarditis, and congestive heart failure are also observed. Cor pulmonale secondary to chronic pulmonary fibrosis may occur but is uncommon.

Endocrine and reproductive system The hypothalamic-pituitary axis is the part of the endocrine system most commonly involved; this usually presents as diabetes insipidus. Anterior pituitary dysfunction is also seen, manifesting as a deficiency in one or more pituitary hormones. Complete hypopituitarism is rare. Much less frequently, sarcoidosis can cause primary dysfunction of other endocrine glands. Adrenal cortical involvement resulting in Addison's syndrome has been described. Involvement of the reproductive organs occurs, but infertility is rare. Pregnancy is rarely affected by sarcoidosis, and patients with sarcoidosis who become pregnant usually improve during pregnancy. However, the disease may flare post partum; presumably this variation results from fluctuations in endogenous corticosteroid production.

Exocrine glands Parotid enlargement is a classic feature of sarcoidosis, but clinically apparent parotid involvement occurs in less than 10 percent of patients. Bilateral involvement is the rule. The gland is usually nontender, firm, and smooth. Xerostomia can occur; other exocrine glands are affected only rarely.

Gastrointestinal tract Although sarcoidosis involvement of the gastrointestinal tract is found occasionally at autopsy, it rarely has clinical importance. Occasionally, patients have esophageal or gastric symptoms.

COMPLICATIONS The respiratory tract abnormalities cause most of the morbidity and mortality associated with sarcoidosis. The major problems are those characteristic of interstitial lung disease (see Chap. 209), particularly dyspnea and insufficient oxygen delivery to vital organs. Respiratory failure with carbon dioxide retention is rare. In some patients, lung destruction results in formation of bullae that may harbor mycetomas, which are usually aspergillomas; erosion into the parenchyma can result in massive bleeding. The most common complications apart from the lung are associated with the eye; however, with therapy blindness is rare. Complications of other organs include a gamut of abnormalities. The most serious are central nervous system lesions or cardiac involvement leading to congestive heart failure or sudden death.

LABORATORY ABNORMALITIES Abnormalities in the blood include lymphocytopenia, an occasional mild eosinophilia, an increased erythrocyte sedimentation rate, hyperglobulinemia, and an elevated level of angiotensin-converting enzyme. Hypercalcemia is rare. Other serum abnormalities relate to involvement of specific organs such as liver, kidney, or endocrine glands.

Because the lung is involved so commonly, the routine chest film is almost always abnormal (Fig. 270-2*A*). The three classic x-ray patterns of pulmonary sarcoidosis are type I—bilateral hilar adenopathy with no parenchymal abnormalities; type II—bilateral hilar adenopathy with diffuse parenchymal changes; and type III—diffuse parenchymal changes without hilar adenopathy. The type III pattern is sometimes split into two categories with films that show fibrosis and upper lobe retraction classified separately. Although patients with type I x-rays tend to have the acute, reversible form of the disease while those with types II and III often have the chronic, progressive disease, these patterns do not represent the ''stages'' of sarcoidosis. Except for epidemiologic purposes, this x-ray categorization is mostly of historic interest. The hilar adenopathy is almost always bilateral, but unilateral node enlargement can be seen. Nodes are also common in the paratracheal region. The diffuse parenchymal changes are typically reticulonodular infiltrates, but an acinar pattern is observed occasionally. Large nodules, similar to those of metastatic disease, are unusual but can occur. When there is massive fibrosis, the hila are pulled upward and there are conglomerate masses in the mid-lung zones. Some of the unusual chest x-ray findings in sarcoidosis include ''egg shell'' calcification of hilar nodes, pleural effusions, cavitation, atelectasis, pulmonary hypertension, pneumothorax, and cardiomegaly.

The lung function abnormalities of sarcoidosis are typical for interstitial lung disease (see Chap. 209) and include decreased lung volumes and diffusing capacity with a normal ratio of the forced expiratory volume in 1 s to the forced vital capacity. Occasionally there is evidence of airflow limitation. There is usually mild hypoxemia and a mild, compensated hypocarbia.

The gallium 67 lung scan is usually abnormal, showing a pattern of diffuse uptake. If present, enlarged nodes are detected in these scans, as is inflammation in a variety of extrathoracic sites that usually have no clinical importance (Fig. 270-2*B*). Bronchoalveolar lavage demonstrates typically an increased proportion of lymphocytes, most of which are activated helper T lymphocytes. The remainder of the cells are mostly alveolar macrophages. In patients with significant fibrosis, a small number of neutrophils are also found. Eosinophils are rare.

The other laboratory features of sarcoidosis depend on the specific organ involved.

DIAGNOSIS For a typical case, the diagnosis of sarcoidosis is made by a combination of clinical, radiographic, and histologic findings. In a young adult with constitutional complaints, respiratory symptoms, erythema nodosum, blurred vision, and bilateral hilar adenopathy, the diagnosis is almost always sarcoidosis. Commonly, however, the findings are more subtle. Furthermore, because sarcoidosis can occur in almost any place in the body, like tuberculosis or syphilis, it can be confused with many other disorders. In this context, the differential diagnosis of sarcoidosis must cover a wide range. However, it is confused most commonly with disorders characterized also by a mononuclear cell granulomatous inflammatory process, such as the mycobacterial and fungal disorders.

The chest x-ray cannot be used as the sole criterion for the diagnosis of sarcoidosis. While the finding of bilateral hilar adenopathy is the hallmark of this disease, a similar pattern can be found in lymphoma, tuberculosis, coccidioidomycosis, brucellosis, and bronchogenic carcinoma.

Whether or not the presentation is ''classic,'' biopsy evidence of a mononuclear-cell granulomatous inflammatory process is mandatory

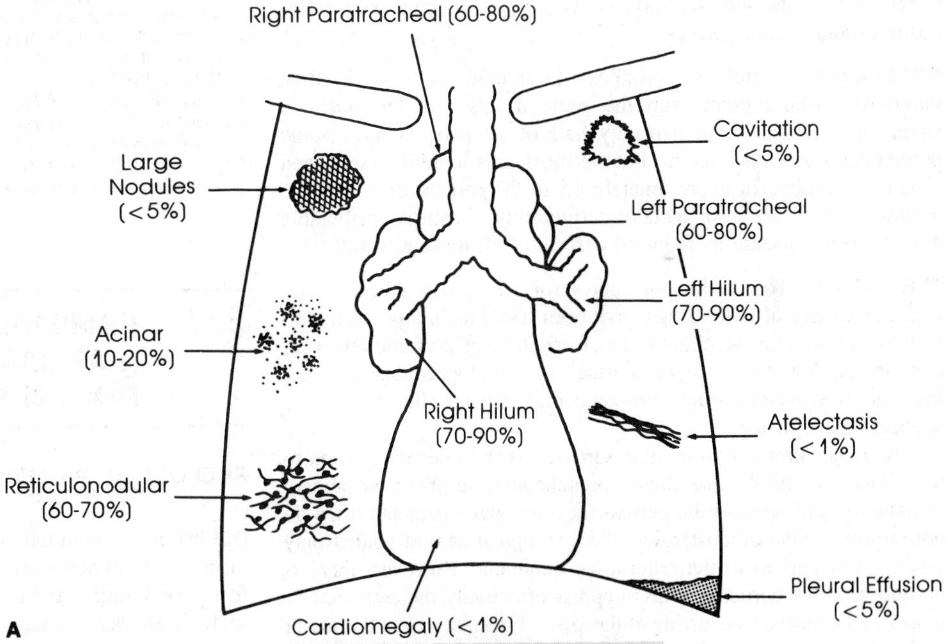

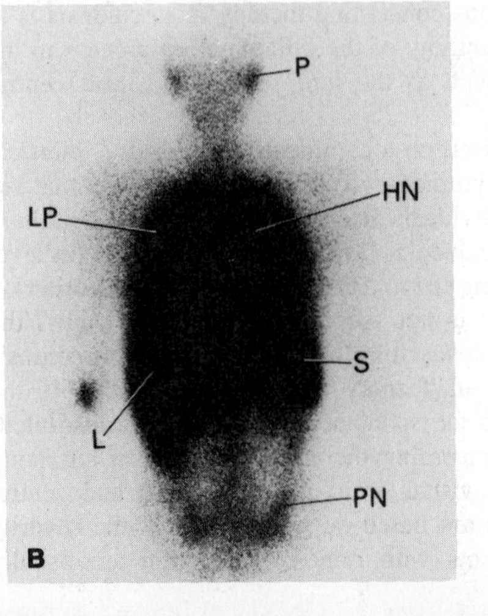

FIGURE 270-2 *Common laboratory findings of sarcoidosis. A. Schematic view of the abnormal findings on the chest x-ray. Shown are changes observed with the average frequency of occurrence. B. Typical gallium 67 scan of an individual with active sarcoidosis. The isotope has accumulated in the lung parenchyma (LP), liver (L), spleen (S), parotid (P), hilar nodes (HN), and pelvic nodes (PN).*

in order to make a definitive diagnosis of sarcoidosis. Because the lung is involved so frequently, it is the most common site to be biopsied, usually through a fiberoptic bronchoscope. Less common, but acceptable, sites for biopsy are the hilar nodes (by mediastinoscopy), the skin, conjunctiva, or lip. Rarely, the spleen, intraabdominal nodes, muscle, parotid or other salivary glands, upper respiratory tract, or the heart are biopsied for diagnostic purposes. At any of these sites, the findings must include the typical noncaseating granulomas. However, although histologic evidence is mandatory for a definitive diagnosis of sarcoidosis, the histologic findings are not sufficiently specific to make the diagnosis by themselves, as noncaseating granulomas are found in a number of other diseases, including infections and malignancy. Furthermore, although the liver or scalene nodes often reveal "positive" biopsies in cases of sarcoidosis, noncaseating granulomas from other causes are so frequent in these sites that they are not considered acceptable sites for establishing the diagnosis.

The presence of skin anergy is typical but not diagnostic of sarcoidosis. The Kveim-Siltzbach skin test, the intradermal injection of a heat-treated suspension of a sarcoidosis spleen extract which is biopsied 4 to 6 weeks later, yields sarcoidosis-like lesions in 70 to 80 percent of individuals with sarcoidosis with less than 5 percent false-positives. However, the material is not available for general use, and with the widespread use of the transbronchial biopsy to obtain lung parenchyma for diagnostic purposes, the Kveim-Siltzbach test is now only of historic interest.

No blood findings are diagnostic of the disease. Angiotensin-converting enzyme is elevated in the serum in approximately two-thirds of patients with sarcoidosis, but there are numerous false-positives and false-negatives.

PROGNOSIS Overall, the prognosis in sarcoidosis is good. Most individuals who present with the acute disease are left with no significant sequela. Approximately half of all patients have some permanent organ dysfunction, but for most, this is mild, stable, and progresses rarely. In approximately 15 to 20 percent of cases, the disease remains active or recurs intermittently. Death is attributable directly to the disease in about 10 percent of all those affected.

TREATMENT The therapy of choice for sarcoidosis is corticosteroids. A variety of other drugs have been tried, including indomethacin, oxyphenbutazone, chloroquine, methotrexate, *p*-aminobenzoate, allopurinol, levamisole, cyclosporine, and cyclophosphamide, but there is no evidence, apart from anecdotal, uncontrolled reports, to support their efficacy.

The major problem in treating sarcoidosis is in deciding when to treat. Because the disease clears spontaneously in about 50 percent of patients, and because the permanent organ derangements often do not improve with corticosteroids, there is a great deal of controversy among clinicians as to the criteria for treatment. However, there is no question that corticosteroids suppress effectively the activated T-helper cell processes occurring at the sites of disease. Thus the major problem in making decisions concerning therapy in sarcoidosis is to determine the extent and activity of the inflammatory process in the organs at greatest risk, such as the lung, eye, heart, and central nervous system.

For the lung, this is based on a combination of history, physical findings, chest x-ray, and pulmonary function tests. Centers that see large numbers of these individuals also use criteria based on gallium 67 lung scans and bronchoalveolar lavage findings. The serum level of the angiotensin-converting enzyme has been suggested as a criterion for disease activity, but it is not specific for the lung. Unless the respiratory impairment is devastating, active pulmonary sarcoidosis is observed usually without therapy for 2 to 3 months; if the inflammation does not subside spontaneously, therapy is instituted. For the eye, decisions concerning therapy are based on slit lamp examination and tests for visual acuity. For the heart and central nervous system, decisions are based on an estimate of the severity of the involvement; patients with minor dysfunction are usually observed, while patients with significant cardiac or neurologic abnormalities are treated. Usually, it is not necessary to treat the systemic symptoms, but occasionally the extent of the fevers, fatigue, and/or weight loss will necessitate therapy.

The usual therapy for sarcoidosis is prednisone, 1 mg/kg, for 4 to 6 weeks followed by a slow taper over 2 to 3 months. This is repeated if the disease again becomes active. Alternate-day therapy is used by some clinicians, but there is no evidence that it is any better or avoids complications in these patients. High-dose bolus intravenous corticosteroids are used occasionally, but are probably not as effective as oral therapy. Inhaled corticosteroids are not efficacious. Mild ocular disease responds usually to local therapy but suppression of the uveitis often requires systemic corticosteroids.

REFERENCES

Chretien J et al (eds): *Ninth International Conference on Sarcoidosis and Other Granulomatous Disorders*. Paris, Pergamon, 1981

Crystal RG et al: Interstitial lung disease of unknown etiology: Disorders characterized by chronic inflammation of the lower respiratory tract. N Engl J Med 310:154, 235, 1984

——— et al: Pulmonary sarcoidosis: A disease characterized and perpetuated by activated lung T-lymphocytes. Ann Intern Med 94:73, 1981

Fanburg BL (ed): *Sarcoidosis and Other Granulomatous Diseases of the Lung*. New York, Marcel Dekker, 1983

Fraser RG, Pare JAP: *Diagnosis of Diseases of the Chest*. Philadelphia, Saunders, 1979, vol 3, p 1658

Hunninghake GW et al: Maintenance of granuloma formation in pulmonary sarcoidosis by T-lymphocytes within the lung. N Engl J Med 302:594, 1980

Mitchell DN et al: Sarcoidosis: Histopathologic definition and clinical diagnosis. J Clin Pathol 30:395, 1977

Pinkston P et al: Spontaneous release of interleukin-2 by lung T-lymphocytes in active pulmonary sarcoidosis. N Engl J Med 308:793, 1983

Robinson BWS et al: Gamma interferon is spontaneously released by alveolar macrophages and lung T-lymphocytes in patients with pulmonary sarcoidosis. J Clin Invest 75:1488, 1985

Sharma OP: *Sarcoidosis: Clinical Management*. London, Butterworths, 1984

Siltzbach LE (ed): *Seventh International Conference on Sarcoidosis and Other Granulomatous Disorders*. New York, NY Acad Sci, 1976

Venet A et al: Enhanced alveolar macrophage-mediated antigen-induced T-lymphocyte proliferation in sarcoidosis. J Clin Invest 75:293, 1985

271 FAMILIAL MEDITERRANEAN FEVER (FAMILIAL PAROXYSMAL POLYSEROSITIS)

SHELDON M. WOLFF

DEFINITION Familial Mediterranean fever (FMF) is an inherited disorder of unknown etiology, characterized by recurrent episodes of fever, peritonitis, and/or pleuritis. Arthritis, skin lesions, and amyloidosis are seen in some patients.

TERMINOLOGY The variety of names given to FMF has led to confusion concerning its clinical features. None of the names, including FMF, is completely satisfactory. Such terms as *periodic disease, periodic peritonitis, la maladie périodique* are inaccurate because the disease often is not cyclical. *Benign paroxysmal peritonitis* is inappropriate because many of the patients have involvement of serosal surfaces other than the peritoneum, and some die of amyloidosis. *Familial paroxysmal polyserositis* is an acceptable alternative for the term *familial Mediterranean fever*.

ETHNOLOGY AND GENETICS FMF occurs predominantly in patients of non-Ashkenazi (Sephardic) Jewish, Armenian, and Arabic ancestry. However, the disease is not restricted to these groups, and has been seen in patients of Italian, Ashkenazi Jewish, and Anglo-Saxon descent as well as others.

The best studies of the genetics of FMF have been done in Israel, where the disease appears to be inherited as an autosomal recessive.

Nevertheless, approximately 50 percent of patients give no family history of the disease. Consanguinity among the parents of FMF patients is as high as 20 percent, a figure which may be an underestimate because most patients came from very inbred ethnic groups. Approximately 60 percent of patients are male.

ETIOLOGY Although numerous pathogenetic mechanisms have been suggested, the etiology of FMF is unknown. Fever and inflammation are such prominent signs that frequent attempts have been made to implicate infectious agents and/or their products. However, extensive studies utilizing modern microbiologic and serologic techniques have failed to implicate these or any other specific infectious agents.

It has been reported that FMF is due to an allergy or to hypersensitivity, but such hypersensitive states have not been substantiated. There is no firm evidence favoring an autoimmune etiology.

It has been suggested that FMF may be a pathologic exaggeration of normal periodic temperature rhythmicity. However, extensive studies of temperature and other circadian rhythms in FMF patients have failed to demonstrate alterations from normal.

Because many FMF patients note that certain emotional or environmental changes may have profound effects on the frequency with which episodes of their disease occur, a psychosomatic basis has been suggested for the illness. There is no question that most patients eventually have transient or even permanent psychological alterations, which probably reflect their reaction to a chronic recurring illness that is forever threatening their social, economic, and personal well-being, but there is no evidence for a functional etiology for FMF.

The demonstration that FMF is inherited as an autosomal recessive disorder has led to the thesis that it is another inborn error of metabolism. Despite extensive studies, no such error has been found. Reported instances of excessive urinary excretion of porphyrins in FMF are probably examples of true porphyria and not FMF.

It has been reported that blood levels of unconjugated etiocholanolone were elevated during fever in six patients with FMF. Subsequent studies, however, showed no correlation between levels of etiocholanolone and fever.

PATHOLOGY Despite the striking clinical manifestations during an acute attack of FMF, no specific pathologic alterations have been found. At laparotomy, only acute peritoneal inflammation in which the exudate contains a predominance of polymorphonuclear leukocytes is found to be present. A disproportionately large number of male patients develop gallbladder disease with and without cholelithiasis, but extensive histopathologic examination has failed to reveal any specific pathologic changes. Pleural and joint inflammation are also nonspecific.

In the amyloidosis which accompanies FMF, amyloid is deposited in the intima and media of the arterioles, the subendothelial region of venules, the glomeruli, and the spleen. Aside from their vessels, the heart and liver are uninvolved.

MANIFESTATIONS In the majority of patients, the symptoms of FMF begin between the ages of 5 and 15, although attacks sometimes commence during infancy, and onset has occurred as late as age 52. The duration and frequency of attacks vary greatly in the same patient, and there is no set rhythm or periodicity to their occurrence. The usual acute episode lasts 24 to 48 h, but some may be prolonged for 7 to 10 days. The attacks range in frequency from twice weekly to once a year, but 2 to 4 weeks is the commonest interval. Spontaneous remissions lasting years have been seen. In the majority of cases, pregnancy is associated with an absence of acute episodes, and many patients note less frequent attacks in the summer than in the winter. There may be a decrease in the severity and frequency of the attacks with age or with development of amyloidosis.

Fever Fever is a cardinal manifestation of FMF and is present during most but not all attacks. Rarely, fever may be present without serositis. The temperature may be preceded by a chill and will peak in 12 to 24 h. Defervescence is often accompanied by diaphoresis. The fever ranges from 38.5 to 40°C but is quite variable.

Abdominal pain Abdominal pain occurs in more than 95 percent of patients, and may vary in severity in the same patient. Minor premonitory discomfort may precede an acute episode by 24 to 48 h. The pain usually starts in one quadrant and then spreads to involve the whole abdomen. The initial site is usually very tender. Tenderness may remain localized with referred pain in other areas, and there may be radiation to the back. There may be splinting of the chest and pain in one or both shoulders, typical of diaphragmatic irritation. Nausea and vomiting sometimes occur. The abdomen is usually distended, and may become rigid with decreased or absent bowel sounds. On x-ray, the wall of the small intestine may appear edematous, transit of barium is slowed, and fluid levels may be seen. Because the manifestations of an acute abdominal attack can simulate those of a perforated viscus so closely, patients should be advised to have an elective appendectomy between attacks so that acute appendicitis will not obfuscate the picture at a later date. An abdominal operation may precipitate an acute attack of FMF which may be confused with other postoperative complications.

Chest pain Most patients with abdominal attacks have referred chest pain at one time or another, and 75 percent also develop acute pleuritic pain with or without abdominal symptoms. In 30 percent, the attacks of pleuritis precede the onset of abdominal attacks by varying periods of time, and a small number of patients never develop abdominal attacks. Chest pain is usually unilateral and is associated with diminished breath sounds, a friction rub, or a transient pleural effusion.

Joint pain In Israel, 75 percent of patients report at least one episode of acute arthritis. Arthritis can be distinct from abdominal or pleural attacks, can be acute or, rarely, chronic, and may involve one or several joints. Effusions are common and the large joints are involved most frequently. Radiologic findings are nonspecific. Despite careful search, frank arthritis rarely has been seen in the United States. Some patients have a history of rheumatic fever–like illness in childhood, but in a large series of patients, including 30 from the Middle East, acute arthritis was not observed. Mild arthralgia is common during acute attacks but is nonspecific.

Skin manifestations Skin involvement is reported by 25 to 35 percent of patients. These lesions consist of painful, erythematous areas of swelling from 5 to 20 cm in diameter, usually located on the lower legs, the medial malleolus, or the dorsum of the foot. They may occur without abdominal or pleural pain and subside within 24 to 48 h.

Other signs and symptoms Involvement of other serosal membranes has been reported, but pericarditis is rare, and it is probable that descriptions of recurrent meningitis have been diseases other than FMF. Hematuria, splenomegaly, and small white dots called *colloid bodies* in the ocular fundus are among the findings of questionable significance. Rarely migraine-like headaches accompany acute abdominal attacks, and some patients have become somewhat irrational or show extreme emotional lability during attacks. Whether these are primary manifestations of FMF or secondary effects of pain and fever is not known.

Complications A serious complication of FMF is drug addiction or habituation, and obviously efforts should be made to avoid use of narcotics. Depression and lack of motivation are common, and patients with FMF require considerable encouragement and support. A striking number of patients in one American series have developed gallbladder disease.

Amyloidosis has been reported in Israel, North Africa, and elsewhere in the Middle East, but there have been only rare reported instances of amyloidosis complicating FMF in the United States. These findings are even more striking because there are probably as many known FMF patients in the United States as in Israel. These differences are unexplained and suggest that environmental or nutritional, as well as genetic, factors may play a role in the development of amyloidosis in FMF.

LABORATORY FINDINGS There is no specific diagnostic test. Polymorphonuclear leukocytosis ranging from 15,000 to 30,000 cells per cubic millimeter is almost invariable during acute attacks. The erythrocyte sedimentation rate is elevated during attacks but returns to normal between attacks. Plasma fibrinogen, serum haptoglobin, ceruloplasmin, and C-reactive protein increase during the episodes. Plasma lipids are normal, and there are no consistent abnormalities of hepatic or renal function. When amyloidosis is present, laboratory findings are typical of a nephrotic syndrome followed by renal insufficiency. Electrocardiographic and electroencephalographic changes are inconstant and nonspecific.

DIAGNOSIS When the typical acute attacks of FMF occur in an individual of appropriate ethnic background who has a family history of FMF, the diagnosis is easy. When a patient is seen for the first time, a variety of other febrile illnesses must be excluded by appropriate study or observation. These include acute appendicitis, acute pancreatitis, porphyria, cholecystitis, intestinal obstruction, and other major abdominal catastrophes.

Some of the inherited forms of the hyperlipidemias may mimic the clinical picture of FMF, but lipid analysis will eliminate them from consideration. The patient with FMF is not immune to other diseases, and when an attack differs from the usual pattern or is more prolonged, consideration should be given to other diagnostic possibilities. The pleural form of the disease is sometimes difficult to differentiate from acute pulmonary infection or infarction, but the rapid disappearance of signs and symptoms resolves the problem. The joint manifestations may be more prolonged than other forms of FMF, and differentiation from septic arthritis, gout, and acute rheumatoid disease may be necessary. The erythema is sometimes difficult to differentiate from superficial thrombophlebitis or cellulitis.

Whether or not the patient is of the appropriate ethnic group, the most difficult diagnostic problem in FMF is the patient who presents with fever alone. In this situation, an extensive diagnostic workup for fever of unknown origin may be required. Fortunately, such patients are rare, and all eventually develop serosal involvement. Until specific diagnostic tests for FMF are available, patients with recurrent fever but without signs of inflammation of one of the serosal membranes should not be categorized as having FMF.

PROGNOSIS Despite the severity of the symptoms during some acute attacks, most patients are remarkably free of any debilitation during the intervals between attacks. With encouragement and an understanding of their disease, most FMF patients lead fairly normal lives. The greatest hazard to patients is prolonged periods of hospitalization due to erroneous diagnoses or failure to understand the disease. In the United States, the prognosis of patients with FMF does not seem to be different from that of patients with other chronic nonfatal illnesses. Death usually results from causes unrelated to the underlying disease.

The complication of amyloidosis in Israel, parts of North Africa, Turkey, and other parts of the Middle East makes the prognosis quite different from that in America. In the past, approximately 25 percent of FMF patients in Israel were known to have amyloidosis, and this complication usually led to death. However, there is now evidence to suggest that the widespread use of colchicine has resulted in dramatically decreasing the incidence of amyloidosis.

TREATMENT Among the therapies tried have been antibiotics, hormones (including estrogens and adrenal corticosteroids), antipyretic drugs, immunotherapy, psychotherapy, elimination and low-fat diets, chloroquine, and phenylbutazone. When carefully studied and followed up, none of these therapies proved effective.

During the past 14 years, the outlook of patients with FMF has been altered dramatically. Goldfinger reported in 1972 that the prophylactic use of colchicine in five patients dramatically reduced the number of attacks. Subsequently, controlled trials in the United States and Israel have shown that chronic administration of colchicine will greatly reduce the number of acute attacks of FMF. It is recommended that 0.6 mg colchicine be taken by mouth three times a day. Patients often develop gastrointestinal side effects with this dose, however, in which case the dose should be reduced to 0.6 mg taken twice a day. Although an occasional patient will respond to 0.6 mg taken only once a day, this amount is less likely to be beneficial. Most but not all FMF patients will respond favorably to colchicine prophylaxis.

Since colchicine is known to occasionally result in nondisjunction of chromosomes and in azospermia, patients who are attempting to have children should be advised to withhold the drug during the time of conception. In some patients, intermittent therapy may be beneficial. The patient should take 0.6 mg colchicine by mouth every hour for 4 h, then every 2 h for 4 h, and every 12 h thereafter for 48 h. The colchicine should be given at the first premonitory sign of an attack. If both acute and prophylactic colchicine therapy fail, supportive therapy is all that can be offered. Except for unusual circumstances, narcotics should not be given to FMF patients.

The mechanism of colchicine's action against acute attacks of FMF is unknown. It is postulated that it may work by preventing the normal cellular response to inflammation. There are strong suggestions that as colchicine therapy becomes more widespread, the incidence of amyloidosis is decreasing.

REFERENCES

DINARELLO CA et al: Colchicine therapy for familial Mediterranean fever. A double-blind trial. N Engl J Med 291:934, 1974

MEYERHOFF J: Familial Mediterranean fever: Report of a large family, review of the literature, and discussion of the frequency of amyloidosis. Medicine 59:66, 1980

SCHWABE AD, PETERS RS: Familial Mediterranean fever in Armenians. Analysis of 100 cases. Medicine 53:453, 1974

WRIGHT DG et al: Efficiency of intermittent colchicine therapy in familial Mediterranean fever. Ann Intern Med 86:162, 1977

ZEMER D et al: Colchicine in the prevention and treatment of the amyloidosis of familial Mediterranean fever. N Engl J Med 314:1001, 1986

272 MIDLINE GRANULOMA

SHELDON M. WOLFF

DEFINITION Midline granuloma is an uncommon disease characterized by localized inflammation, destruction, and often mutilation of the tissues of the upper respiratory tract and face. This condition has also been referred to as *lethal midline granuloma, malignant granuloma,* and *granuloma gangrenescens,* none of which is an appropriate term.

ETIOLOGY The etiology of midline granuloma is unknown. In view of the intense granulomatous inflammation, the disease is thought to represent a localized hypersensitivity reaction which leads to tissue destruction and mutilation. However, the responsible antigen(s) is unknown, and there is no immunologic evidence supporting this hypothesis. A variety of microorganisms have been considered as possible causative agents, but detailed microbiologic investigations have failed to detect the consistent presence of pathogenic organisms. In view of the clinical and pathologic features of the illness as well as the fact that some upper-airway tumors can elicit a similar intense inflammatory response, some authors have suggested a neoplastic basis for midline granuloma. However, when malignant tissue (usually of a lymphomatous nature) is found in the lesions, the diagnosis of midline granuloma is no longer tenable.

PATHOLOGY The most characteristic pathologic finding is acute or chronic inflammation with necrosis. Superimposed pyogenic infection of the involved tissues, including the sinuses, may contribute to nonspecific histologic findings. The pathologic hallmark, noncaseating granulomas, with or without giant cells, may be obscured by the inflammatory reaction, but when present this is strong evidence in favor of the diagnosis. Primary vasculitis is seen rarely; when it occurs, a search for other causes, most notably Wegener's granulomatosis, should be made. The presence of malignant cells makes the diagnosis of midline granuloma unacceptable. Until an etiology is established, the diagnosis of midline granuloma will rest on the characteristic clinical features outlined below.

CLINICAL FEATURES The disease may occur at any age, but the majority of patients are in the fifth and sixth decades. It is more common in women than men and has been reported in all races. Many patients report recurrent "sinus" problems, and some have histories of allergic rhinitis, although the significance of these features is unknown.

The major symptoms are usually related to the nose. Patients frequently complain of nasal stuffiness and occasionally of discharge. The first symptom in a smaller percentage of patients relates to ulceration of the mucosa of the nose, the buccal mucosa, or the gums. This has led to loosening of the teeth, and dentists are often first consulted by these patients. Rarely, patients will present first with eye findings related to conjunctival inflammation or even ulceration. Although the progression of symptoms in some patients may be slow, all too often the disease steadily, and sometimes rapidly, progresses. The characteristic symptoms of nasal discharge, difficulty in breathing through the nose, and pain over the sinuses, nose, or eye become more prominent with time. Once ulceration begins, the disease often progresses rapidly. The ulcers frequently involve the nasal septum and will lead to the characteristic septal perforation and a saddlenose deformity. The majority of patients develop ulceration and eventually perforations of the soft and hard palates. Untreated, the disease can lead to massive destruction and mutilation of the tissues involved, including the skin of the face and the eyes. Frequently, the necrotic tissue becomes infected, and systemic symptoms such as fever and anorexia appear. The destructive lesions can become very malodorous. The disease extends to involve local tissues and does not progress below the neck; if this happens, other diseases should be considered. As the necrotic process progresses and involves vital organs, patients may lose sight in the affected eye, experience dysphagia, and have difficulty in speech. Although spontaneous temporary remissions have been reported, untreated midline granuloma is fatal. The progression of the disease can be rapidly accelerated by surgical procedures in the affected areas. The patient usually dies from secondary infection, although erosion by the process into a major blood vessel or penetration into the central nervous system with superimposed meningitis can also cause death.

Aside from the granulomatous inflammation, necrosis, and destruction, no other specific clinical or pathologic findings are associated with midline granuloma. Occasionally, with superimposed infection, local lymphadenopathy may be noted, but it is not characteristic of the disease per se.

LABORATORY FINDINGS With progression of the disease, a variety of nonspecific abnormalities may be noted. These changes are characteristic of inflammatory processes in general or of secondary infections. For example, mild anemia, leukocytosis, elevated sedimentation rate, and hyperglobulinemia are common in these patients. Radiographic examination reveals pansinusitis, and as the disease advances, destruction of bone in the involved areas is characteristic.

DIFFERENTIAL DIAGNOSIS The diagnosis of midline granuloma is made by finding the characteristic histologic lesions in biopsies of the affected tissues. When the specimens show only inflammatory tissue, a presumptive diagnosis of midline granuloma can be made only when the characteristic clinical picture is present and other diseases with similar presentation have been excluded. The diagnosis of Wegener's granulomatosis is ruled out by the absence of vasculitis in the biopsy specimens and the localized nature of midline granuloma (i.e., no pulmonary or renal involvement). In addition, Wegener's granulomatosis rarely, if ever, causes erosion through facial tissues. It is often difficult to differentiate true midline granuloma from neoplasms of the upper airways such as malignant reticulosis and certain lymphomas. These may be clinically similar to midline granuloma and are often associated with granulomatous inflammation. Careful examination of generous biopsy material as well as concomitant workup for disseminated neoplasm often provides the clinicopathologic distinction. Other diseases to be excluded by appropriate laboratory techniques are histoplasmosis, blastomycosis, coccidioidomycosis, leprosy, tuberculosis, syphilis, mucocutaneous leishmaniasis, rhinoscleroma, and pseudotumor of the orbit.

TREATMENT The complications of midline granuloma such as superimposed infections can be treated specifically. Although adrenal corticosteroids are often used in the therapy of midline granuloma, they are of no value and probably are contraindicated if infection is present. Sporadic reports of therapy with cytotoxic agents are difficult to interpret, since some of the patients reported clearly had lymphoma or Wegener's granulomatosis, diseases where such agents are of definite value. Surgical removal of the involved tissue has been attempted but is useless and may, in fact, cause rapid progression of the disease.

The treatment of choice is radiotherapy to the local lesion. Although low dosages [10,000 mGy (1000 rads) and below] have been reported to be effective, many patients relapse after such therapy. Radiotherapy should be given in a dose of 50,000 mGy (5000 rads) to the involved areas. Where such a regimen is employed, long-lasting remissions (more than 15 years) and possible cures have been achieved. Following irradiation and after an appropriate period to allow for tissue healing (usually 1 year), reconstructive and plastic surgery, which may be of enormous cosmetic and functional value, can be undertaken.

REFERENCES

FAUCI AS et al: Radiation therapy of midline granuloma. Ann Intern Med 84:140, 1976

FECHNER RE, LAMPPIN DW: Midline malignant reticulosis. Arch Otolaryngol 95:467, 1972

section 3 Disorders of the joints

273 APPROACH TO DISORDERS OF THE JOINTS AND MUSCULOSKELETAL DISORDERS

JOHN J. CUSH / PETER E. LIPSKY

Musculoskeletal complaints account for nearly 10 percent of all outpatient evaluations in general medical practice. In the United States, musculoskeletal disorders are among the leading causes of disability and absenteeism from work. Many of the musculoskeletal complaints that cause patients to seek medical attention are related to self-limited conditions requiring minimal evaluation and only symptomatic therapy and reassurance. However, others with similar symptoms may require additional laboratory testing to confirm a suspected diagnosis or document the extent and nature of the pathologic process. The initial goal of the clinician is to diagnose accurately and provide timely therapy while avoiding excessive diagnostic testing and unnecessary treatment.

Individuals with musculoskeletal complaints should be evaluated in a uniform, logical manner with a thorough history, a comprehensive physical examination, and appropriate laboratory testing. With such an approach and an understanding of the pathophysiologic processes underlying musculoskeletal complaints, an adequate diagnosis can be made in 90 percent of individuals. Approximately 10 percent of patients will not fit immediately into an established diagnostic category. Moreover, many musculoskeletal disorders resemble each other at the outset and may take months or even years to evolve fully into a specific recognizable syndrome. Such knowledge should temper the desire to establish a definitive diagnosis at the first encounter.

A paramount objective during the initial encounter is to determine whether the condition requires additional evaluation or immediate therapy. To make this decision, a knowledge of the particular anatomic sites of involvement (articular, periarticular, or extraarticular) and the nature of the pathologic processes (inflammatory or noninflammatory) is important (Table 273-1). Information derived from the patient's symptoms and signs allows the clinician to narrow the diagnostic considerations and assess the need for therapeutic intervention, immediate diagnostic testing, or continued observation over a period of time.

TABLE 273-1 Musculoskeletal disorders

- *I* Tissue involvement
  - *A* Articular
    - *1* Synovium
    - *2* Articular cartilage
    - *3* Juxtaarticular bone
    - *4* Other—menisci, capsule
  - *B* Periarticular
    - *1* Ligaments
    - *2* Tendons
    - *3* Bursae
  - *C* Extraarticular
    - *1* Muscle
    - *2* Fascia
    - *3* Bone
    - *4* Nerve
    - *5* Skin and subcutaneous tissue
- *II* Pathologic processes
  - *A* Inflammatory
    - *1* Infectious
    - *2* Crystal-induced
    - *3* Immunologic
    - *4* Reactive
    - *5* Idiopathic
  - *B* Noninflammatory
    - *1* Traumatic
    - *2* Mechanical or degenerative
    - *3* Neoplastic
    - *4* Functional
    - *5* Other

MUSCULOSKELETAL DISORDERS: HISTORIC FEATURES Historic features of the disorder are important in establishing the nature and extent of the pathologic process and may also provide important clues to the diagnosis. Aspects of the patient profile including age, sex, race, and family history can provide important information. Certain diagnoses are more frequent in different age groups. Systemic lupus erythematosus and Reiter's syndrome occur more frequently in the young, while fibrositis is most frequent in middle age and osteoarthritis and polymyalgia rheumatica are more prevalent among the elderly. Diagnostic clustering is also evident when *sex* and *race* are considered. Gout and the spondyloarthropathies are more common in men, whereas rheumatoid arthritis and fibrositis are more frequent in women. Racial predilections are noted with disorders such as polymyalgia rheumatica (whites) and sarcoidosis (blacks). *Familial aggregation* may be seen in disorders such as ankylosing spondylitis, gout, rheumatoid arthritis, and Heberden's nodes of osteoarthritis.

Features of the clinical presentation also provide important diagnostic clues. The *mode of onset* is characteristically acute in infection or gout, while osteoarthritis and fibrositis may have more indolent presentations. The length of time the patient has had signs and symptoms alters the diagnostic considerations. Thus, the signs and symptoms of the arthritis associated with hepatitis B virus infection may be identical with those of rheumatoid arthritis, but rarely persist beyond 2 weeks.

Precipitating events such as trauma, drug administration, or antecedent illnesses should be sought. The *number and pattern* of involved structures often provide useful information. Disorders such as trauma and gout are typically focal, whereas others, such as polymyositis and fibrositis, involve more than a single site. Rheumatoid arthritis tends to be symmetric, whereas the spondyloarthropathies are asymmetric. The upper extremities are frequently involved in rheumatoid arthritis, while lower extremity arthritis is characteristic of gout at its onset. Involvement of the axial skeleton is common in ankylosing spondylitis but is infrequent in rheumatoid arthritis with the notable exception of the cervical spine. The *chronology and evolution* of the patient's complaints may also be useful in suggesting diagnostic categories. Chronic (osteoarthritis), intermittent (gout), migratory (rheumatic fever), and additive (Reiter's syndrome) patterns are suggestive of certain disease processes.

Associated features outside the musculoskeletal systems may also provide useful diagnostic information. A variety of musculoskeletal disorders may be associated with systemic features such as fever (systemic lupus erythematosus, infection), rash (systemic lupus erythematosus, Reiter's syndrome, rheumatic fever), or morning stiffness (inflammatory arthritis). In addition, some are associated with involvement of other organs including ocular (Reiter's syndrome), gastrointestinal (scleroderma, inflammatory bowel disease), genitourinary (Reiter's syndrome, gonococcemia), or neurologic involvement (rheumatoid arthritis, vasculitis).

PHYSICAL EXAMINATION The goal of the physical examination is to document the structures involved, the nature of the disorder, the extent and functional consequences of the process, and the presence of systemic manifestations. A knowledge of topographic anatomy is necessary to identify the primary site(s) of involvement and differentiate between articular, periarticular, and extraarticular disease. The musculoskeletal evaluation is largely dependent on careful inspection, palpation, and a variety of physical maneuvers to elicit diagnostic signs.

Examination of involved and uninvolved joints will determine the absence or presence of *warmth, erythema,* or *swelling*. The examination should distinguish true articular swelling caused by synovial effusion or synovial proliferation from periarticular involvement which usually extends beyond the normal joint margins. Synovial effusion can be distinguished from synovial hypertrophy or bony hypertrophy by palpation. Bursal effusions (i.e., olecranon, prepatellar) overlie bony prominences and are fluctuant with sharply defined borders. Joint *stability* can be assessed by palpation and by the application of manual stress. Subluxation or dislocation, which may be secondary to traumatic, mechanical, or inflammatory causes, can be assessed by inspection and palpation. Joint *volume* can be assessed by palpation. Distention of the articular capsule by various processes causes pain. The patient will attempt to minimize the pain by maintaining the joint in the position of greatest volume and least intraarticular pressure, usually flexion. Clinically, this may be reflected as obvious swelling, voluntary or eventually fixed flexion deformities, or diminished range of motion, especially on extension when joint volumes are decreased. Active and passive *range of motion* should be assessed in all planes and is best quantified by a goniometer with contralateral comparison. Joint *crepitus* may be felt during these maneuvers and may be prominent in degenerative disorders. Limitation of motion is frequently caused by effusion, pain, deformity, or contracture. Contractures may be an indication of antecedent synovial inflammation. Joint *deformity* usually indicates a long-standing pathologic process. Deformities may result from ligament destruction, soft tissue contracture, bony enlargement, ankylosis, erosive disease, or subluxation. Examination of the musculature will document strength and the presence of atrophy, and also will elicit pain or spasm.

ADDITIONAL INVESTIGATIONS The vast majority of musculoskeletal disorders can be easily diagnosed by a complete history and physical examination. However, in a number of circumstances, additional investigations may be required to establish the diagnosis or confirm a suspected etiology. A number of features indicate the need for additional evaluation. Patients with *acute monarticular* conditions require additional evaluation, as do those who present with *traumatic* or *inflammatory* conditions or those with *neurologic changes* or *systemic manifestations* of serious disease. Finally individuals with *chronic (>6 weeks)* symptoms, even of minor severity, are candidates for additional evaluation. The extent and nature of the additional investigation should be dictated by the pattern of the involvement and suspected pathologic process. Broad batteries of diagnostic tests and radiographic procedures are rarely a useful or cost-effective means to establish a diagnosis.

Besides a complete blood count including a white blood cell and differential count, the routine evaluation should include a determination of the erythrocyte sedimentation rate, which can be useful in discriminating inflammatory from noninflammatory musculoskeletal disorders. A radiographic evaluation is indicated when there is a history of prior trauma, suspected chronic infection, progressive disability, monarticular involvement, or when therapeutic alterations are considered. Early in most inflammatory disorders radiographs are rarely helpful in establishing a diagnosis and often reveal only soft tissue swelling and juxtaarticular demineralization. As the disease progresses, calcification (soft tissue, cartilage, or bone), joint space narrowing, erosions, bony ankylosis, new bone formation (sclerosis, osteophytes, or periostitis), or subchondral cysts can be demonstrated.

Synovial fluid aspiration and analysis is always indicated in acute monarthritis or when a septic or crystal-induced arthropathy is suspected. Synovial fluid can be classified according to its appearance, cell count, glucose level, and viscosity. Noninflammatory synovial fluid is clear, amber-colored, with a white blood cell count of <3000 cells per cubic millimeter and a mononuclear cell predominance. The glucose and viscosity are normal. Such effusions are typical of osteoarthritis and trauma. Inflammatory fluid is turbid and yellow with an increased white cell count (3000 to 50,000 cells per cubic millimeter) and a polymorphonuclear leukocyte predominance. The protein is elevated, the glucose is normal or low, and the viscosity is poor. Such effusions are found in rheumatoid arthritis, gout, other inflammatory arthritides, and occasionally septic arthritis. Infectious fluid is turbid and opaque, with a white cell count >50,000 cells per cubic millimeter, and a polymorphonuclear leukocyte predominance. The protein is elevated, the glucose is low, and viscosity is poor. Such effusions are typical of septic arthritis but may rarely occur with sterile arthritides such as rheumatoid arthritis. Additionally, hemorrhagic synovial fluid may be seen with hemarthrosis or trauma. Synovial fluid should be analyzed immediately for crystals using a polarizing microscope. Monosodium urate, seen in gouty effusions, appears as long, needle-shaped, negatively birefringent, usually intracellular crystals, whereas calcium pyrophosphate dihydrate found in chondrocalcinosis and pseudogout is usually seen as short, rhomboid-shaped, positively birefringent crystals. When infection is suspected, synovial fluid should be Gram-stained and cultured appropriately. Whenever gonococcal arthritis is suspected, immediate plating out of the fluid on appropriate culture media is indicated. It should be noted that on occasion both crystal-induced arthritis and infection may occur in the same joint.

Serologic tests for rheumatoid factor (antibodies to IgG), antinuclear antibodies, complement levels or antistreptolysin O titers should only be carried out when there is clinical evidence to suggest a specific diagnosis.

EVALUATION OF THE ELDERLY FOR RHEUMATIC DISEASES Musculoskeletal disorders in geriatric patients are often not diagnosed since complaints in the elderly may be insidious in onset and chronic in nature. In addition, older individuals frequently possess multiple interactive variables, including other medical conditions and therapies that may obscure the nature of the problem. This is compounded by the diminished reliability of laboratory testing in the elderly, owing to the wider range of nonpathologic serologic variability, including elevated erythrocyte sedimentation rates and low titers of rheumatoid factor or antinuclear antibodies. Although nearly all rheumatic disorders can afflict the elderly, certain diseases and drug-induced disorders are more common in this age group (Table 273-2). The elderly should be approached in the same uniform manner used for all patients with musculoskeletal complaints, with additional inquiry to exclude common geriatric musculoskeletal disorders. An emphasis on identifying intercurrent medical conditions and therapies is extemely important. Drug-induced lupus erythematosus, gout, and chronic salicylate toxicity all are more common in the elderly. The physical examination should emphasize coexistent disease that may influence subsequent diagnosis and treatment.

TABLE 273-2 Common musculoskeletal disorders in the elderly

I	Inflammatory
	Polymyalgia rheumatica
	Temporal (giant cell) arteritis
	Gout
	Calcium pyrophosphate dihydrate deposition disease
II	Mechanical
	Degenerative joint disease
	Spinal stenosis
III	Metabolic
	Osteoporosis
	Myxedema
	Paget's disease
IV	Associated with neoplastic disease
	Carcinomatous arthropathy or neuromyopathy
	Dermatomyositis
	Hypertrophic osteoarthropathy
V	Drug-induced
	Diuretics (gout)
	Drug-induced lupus
	Corticosteroids (osteopenia, myopathy)

REFERENCES

BLUESTONE R: The patient who hurts all over: Practical approach to diagnosis and management. Postgrad Med 72:71, 1982

FRIES JF, MITCHELL DM: Joint pain or arthritis. JAMA 235:199, 1976

GATTER RA: *Practical Handbook of Joint Fluid Analysis*. Philadelphia, Lea & Febiger, 1984

HALL H: Examination of the patient with low back pain. Bull Rheum Dis 33:1, 1983

HUGHES GRV: Auto antibodies in lupus and its variants: Experience in 1000 patients. Lancet 289:339, 1984

POLLEY HF, HUNDER GG: *Rheumatologic Interviewing and Physical Examination of the Joints*. Philadelphia, Saunders, 1978

STEVENS MB: Rheumatic disease: An overview of geriatric problems. Geriatrics 38:67, 1983

TAN EM: Antinuclear antibodies in diagnosis and management. Hosp Pract 18:79, 1983

WILSON FC: Principles of diagnosis and treatment of musculoskeletal trauma, in *The Musculoskeletal System: Basic Processes and Disorders*, FC Wilson (ed). Philadelphia, Lippincott, 1983, pp 270–274

274 DEGENERATIVE JOINT DISEASE

BRUCE C. GILLILAND

Degenerative joint disease (osteoarthritis), is the most common form of arthritis and affects almost all joints, especially weight-bearing and frequently used joints. The disorder is characterized by progressive deterioration and loss of articular cartilage accompanied by proliferation of new bone and soft tissue in and around the involved joint. Osteoarthritis is divided into a primary or idiopathic form in which no underlying predisposing factor(s) are apparent and into a secondary form in which a predisposing cause such as previous trauma, congenital abnormality, or metabolic disorder is present.

EPIDEMIOLOGY Osteoarthritis affects both men and women, being slightly more frequent in men before the age of 45 and in women after age 55. The prevalence of osteoarthritis increases with age and is almost universal in individuals over the age of 75. Osteoarthritis is found in all races. The placement of stress on joints is thought to be a factor in the development of osteoarthritis. For example, osteoarthritis of shoulders and knees is more frequent in coal miners, presumably because of stress placed on these joints during work. On the other hand, studies have shown no increase in osteoarthritis in runners or in persons performing heavy physical work. Hereditary factors also appear to play a role in some forms of osteoarthritis. Heberden's nodes are twice as frequent in mothers and three times more frequent in sisters of the affected individual. The inheritance of Heberden's nodes appears to involve a single autosomal dominant gene.

PATHOGENESIS Articular cartilage together with subchondral bone, joint capsule, and muscle absorb the energy of weight bearing. Normal articular cartilage is compressible and elastic and able to lubricate its surfaces under high-pressure loads, providing smooth and almost frictionless movement. The materials which give cartilage these properties are primarily collagen, proteoglycans, and hyaluronic acid. The form and tensile strength of cartilage is due to collagen. The type of collagen in articular cartilage is type II, which is unique to joints. The other major component of cartilage is proteoglycan. The proteolglycan molecule is composed of glucosaminoglycans, chondroitin sulfate, and keratin sulfate, which extend from a protein core in a configuration that has been likened to a bottle brush. Most of the proteoglycan molecules exist in aggregates in which individual molecules are noncovalently linked to a long chain of hyaluronic acid. The large aggregates of proteoglycans are extremely hydrophilic and bind most of the water present in cartilage. Water represents approximately 70 percent of the total weight of articular cartilage. The large hydrophilic proteoglycan aggregates are interwoven and constrained within the network of collagen fibers, giving cartilage the property of resiliency.

Normal articular cartilage undergoes continuous internal remodeling. Chondrocytes secrete collagen and proteoglycans as well as enzymes that degrade matrix. Enzymes include cathepsin D, neutral proteases, and collagenase. A substance named catabolin, which is released from mononuclear cells in synovium, stimulates chondrocytes to produce enzymes that degrade cartilage matrix. The degradative process is kept under control by small proteins that inhibit these enzymes secreted by cells in synovium. Chondrocytes in normal cartilage are metabolically active but do not synthesize DNA or divide unless their microenvironment is altered.

The initiating event in primary osteoarthritis that leads to stimulation of chondrocytes and the changes in cartilage is not known. The first event may be microfractures of subchondral bone which occur from repeated impact loading. The healing of these fractures results in stiff and thickened subchondral bone which poorly absorbs the energy of weight bearing. Chondrocytes in articular cartilage therefore are subjected to increased pressure, which stimulates cell division and synthesis of DNA, collagen, and proteoglycans as well as degradative enzymes. Others have suggested that the initial changes occur in cartilage, leading to loss of cartilage resiliency. Microfractures of subchondral bone occur as a consequence of decreased cartilage compressibility. Initially, in the development of osteoarthritis, the reparative process is able to keep pace with degradation. Eventually, the degradative process predominates, resulting in loss of cartilage.

Inflammation plays a role in the pathogenesis of osteoarthritis. Breakdown products of cartilage stimulate the release of collagenase and other hydrolytic enzymes from cells in the synovium. The finding of immunoglobulin and complement in the superficial layer of cartilage suggests that immune complexes may induce an inflammatory response. Hydroxyapatite, calcium pyrophosphate crystals, or both are often found in the synovial fluid. These crystals have been proposed as a possible factor in the production or exacerbation of osteoarthritis.

PATHOLOGY In the early stages of osteoarthritis, cartilage shows fissuring and pitting which progress to focal erosions. Cartilage is disrupted along the planes of collagen fibrils, resulting in flaking, fibrillation, and eventually denuded areas. The proteoglycan and water content of cartilage is decreased in proportion to the severity of the disease. Clusters of chrondrocytes are observed followed later by a decreased number of cells. Subchondral bone shows osteoblastic and osteoclastic activity resulting eventually in a thickened, dense bony plate. The development of this ivory-like bone is termed *eburnation*. Subchondral cysts represent focal areas of necrosis and may also develop from the penetration of synovial fluid through microfractures in the bone. New bone proliferation at the joint margins forms osteophytes (spurs) which are covered by a layer of articular cartilage. The synovium is thickened by an increase of lining cells and a mild to moderate infiltration of lymphocytes, plasma cells, and occasional multinucleated giant cells. Fibrotic thickening of the joint capsule and ligaments is present.

CLINICAL FEATURES The clinical manifestations are usually limited to one or a few joints. Osteoarthritis can also be more generalized, suggesting a systemic form of arthritis. Symptoms usually begin insidiously in the form of a deep, aching, poorly localized pain occurring with use of the involved joint and relieved by rest. Stiffness of the affected joint(s) occurs in the morning and after periods of inactivity during the day, usually lasting 15 min or less. Joint pain, which may be due to the absence of protective splinting of the joint and/or to increased intraosseous venous pressure frequently awakens the patient at night. Patients may experience joint pain with changes in the weather. Crepitus may occur with joint movement due to loss of cartilage and joint surface irregularities. The involved joint may give way on weight bearing. Subsequently, joint motion becomes limited, and subluxation and deformity of joints appear. Flares of acute arthritis may occur in involved joints from trauma or crystal-induced synovitis due to either calcium pyrophosphate or hydroxyapatite crystals.

The most common finding in primary osteoarthritis is *Heberden's nodes,* which usually appear after age 45 (see Fig. 274-1). They usually develop slowly over months or years in association with osteoarthritis of the distal interphalangeal joints. Heberden's nodes are firm enlargements appearing on the dorsomedial and dorsolateral aspect of the distal interphalangeal joint, and are composed of bone covered by cartilage. Similar enlargements at the proximal interphalangeal joint are called *Bouchard's nodes.* Gelatinous cysts may precede the development of Heberden's nodes. These cysts initially communicate with the distal interphalangeal joint, but may lose their connection later. Heberden's and Bouchard's nodes usually develop with little or no pain, but in some patients may be associated with pain, paresthesias, erythema, and swelling.

Osteoarthritis of interphalangeal joints of the hands causes symptoms of pain, swelling, and stiffness. Nodes develop at the joint margins along with flexor and lateral deviation of fingers. When ankylosis develops, joints become asymptomatic. A syndrome termed erosive osteoarthritis is characterized by recurrent episodes of acute inflammation and progressive destruction of the interphalangeal joints. Middle-aged women are most often affected.

Primary generalized osteoarthritis is characterized by involvement of three or more joints or group of joints. The proximal interphalangeal joints are considered as one group and the distal interphalangeal joints as another. This form of osteoarthritis also appears most often in middle-aged women and involves distal and proximal interphalangeal joints of hands, first carpometacarpal joint, knees, hips, and first metatarsophalangeal joint. The spine may also be involved. The joints may be episodically warm and swollen and the erythrocyte sedimentation rate mildly elevated.

Osteoarthritis of the hip is more common in men than women and is often initially unilateral. The opposite side will eventually be affected in approximately 20 percent of patients. It has been estimated that 80 percent of cases are secondary to an underlying congenital or developmental abnormality. These abnormalities include hip dysplasia, slipped capital femoral epiphysis, and Legg-Calvé-Perthes disease. Avascular necrosis related to deep-water diving, glucocorticoid therapy, alcohol, or sickle cell disease leads to collapse of the femoral head and severe osteoarthritis. The pain of hip disease is felt in the groin or inguinal area. Hip pain may also be experienced over the greater trochanter, in the buttock, or down the anterior and inner thigh. In some patients, involvement may manifest as pain in the distal thigh or knee since the obturator nerve and its branches supply both hip and knee. Patients may limp as the disease progresses and complain of difficulty in rising from a sitting position. On examination, internal rotation is limited initially, followed by decreased extension, adduction, and flexion. Adduction and/or flexion contractures may lead to a functional shortening of the leg on the involved side, causing the patient to walk with a shuffling gait.

Osteoarthritis of the knee involves the medial, lateral, and/or patellofemoral compartments. Pain may be diffuse or localized to a compartment and is aggravated by motion. Stiffness occurs after periods of inactivity. The knee may lock due to a loose body or give way suddenly because of a pain reflex. Small joint effusions are often present. With progression, ligamentous laxity, limitation of motion, and flexion contractures subsequently develop. Chondromalacia patellae is a clinical syndrome occurring in adolescents and young adults, being more common in women. The cartilage on the undersurface becomes softened, fibrillated, and eroded. The changes are indistinguishable from early osteoarthritis but usually do not progress. The lesion is thought to result from trauma or abnormal forces on the patella from lateral displacement of the patella as it moves through the shallow groove between the femoral condyles.

Osteoarthritis of the first carpometacarpal joint causes pain and tenderness at the base of the thumb. Enlargement and radial subluxation give the hand a squared appearance. Osteoarthritis also involves the scaphotrapezoid joint. The first metatarsophalangeal joint is another common site for osteoarthritis.

Osteoarthritis of the spine affects the intervertebral disks, apophyseal joints, and paraspinal ligaments. In the neck, the joints of Luschka (uncovertebral joints) may also be affected. The term *spondylosis* is preferred by some for disease of the intervertebral disks while disease in the apophyseal joints is considered true osteoarthritis. Cervical spine involvement produces localized pain or pain referred to the interscapular region, occiput, shoulder, and arm, depending upon the level of involvement. Compression of the spinal cord by posteriorly protruding disk or osteophytes as well as occlusion of the anterior spinal artery by a herniated disk will cause long tract signs. A congenitally narrowed cervical spinal cord may contribute to cord compression. Osteophytes extending from the joint of Luschka may impinge on the vertebral arteries producing symptoms of basilar artery insufficiency. Symptoms include vertigo, nystagmus, diplopia, scotomas, tinnitus, and ataxia. Symptoms are usually intermittent and related to position of the head. Osteoarthritis of the thoracic spine is less common. Costovertebral joints may be affected. Neoplasm, infection, or osteoporosis should be considered in the differential diagnosis of thoracic spine pain. Symptoms of lumbar spine involvement include localized pain and stiffness and radicular pain radiating into the buttocks and legs depending on the level of disease (see Chaps. 7, 353).

Lumbar stenosis causes cord compression, affecting older-age patients. Posterior vertebral osteophytes impinge on the cord particularly in those persons who have congenitally narrowed spinal canals. Symptoms develop gradually and include bilateral paresthesias and weakness of lower extremities. Symptoms may be induced by hyperextension of the lumbar spine and relieved by flexion. Lumbar

FIGURE 274-1 *Osteoarthritis. A. Heberden's nodes of the distal interphalangeal joints and Bouchard's nodes of the proximal interphalangeal joints are present. The carpometacarpal joint is radially subluxed giving the hand a squared appearance. There is also angulation of the distal and proximal interphalangeal joints. B. Radiograph of the second, third, and fourth proximal and distal interphalangeal joints. Loss of joint space, osteophytes, and subchondral sclerosis and cysts are evident.*

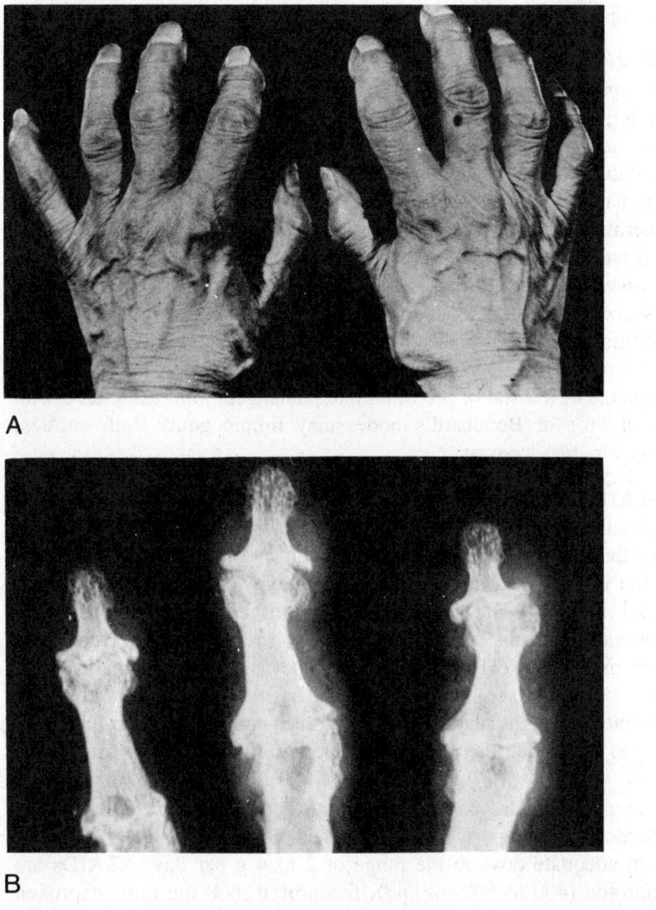

A

B

stenosis is differentiated from vascular insufficiency by these positional symptoms and by the presence of weakness and paresthesia. Laminectomy may be required if symptoms and signs persist or progress.

Secondary osteoarthritis may be due to traumatic, systemic, or congenital disorders. The arthritis may be unilateral, appear at an earlier age, and involve joints that are not commonly observed in primary osteoarthritis. Previous trauma to a joint, resulting, for example, in a torn knee meniscus or ligamentous instability leads to joint surface incongruity and subsequent osteoarthritis. Joint damage caused by septic arthritis or noninfectious inflammatory arthritis, for example, rheumatoid arthritis, also predisposes the involved joint(s) to osteoarthritis. Neuropathic joint disease (Charcot's joint) is a severe form of osteoarthritis associated with loss of pain sensation, proprioception, or both (see Chap. 278). Joint hypermobility syndromes, either inherited or idiopathic, may be associated with early onset of osteoarthritis. Metabolic disorders associated with osteoarthritis include hemochromatosis, Wilson's disease, calcium pyrophosphate deposition disease, Paget's disease, and ochronosis (alkaptonuria). Acromegaly and hyperparathyroidism are also associated with osteoarthritis.

LABORATORY AND RADIOGRAPHIC FINDINGS Routine laboratory work is normal in patients with primary osteoarthritis. The erythrocyte sedimentation rate is usually normal, but may be mildly elevated in patients with primary generalized or erosive osteoarthritis. The synovial fluid is straw colored and has good viscosity. The leukocyte count is usually less than 2000 per cubic millimeter with the majority of cells being mononuclear. Elevated leukocyte counts are found during acute episodes of calcium pyrophosphate deposition disease associated with osteoarthritis. Calcium pyrophosphate and/or hydroxyapatite crystals may be found in some synovial fluids (see Chap. 275). Radiographs of the involved joints are initially normal, but as the disease progresses, joint space narrowing, subchondral bone sclerosis (eburnation), and osteophytes are observed. Erosions are found on the joint surfaces in association with sclerosis of subchondral bone, and bony ankylosis may be present. Radiographic findings may not correlate with clinical symptoms.

DIAGNOSIS Osteoarthritis can usually be distinguished from other arthropathies by the pattern of joint involvement (especially in the hands), normal laboratory tests, low leukocyte counts in synovial fluid, and characteristic radiographic findings. The erythrocyte sedimentation rate is usually normal for the age of the patient, and rheumatoid factor and antinuclear antibody tests are negative. Primary generalized and erosive osteoarthritis may have inflammatory features suggesting a systemic arthritis such as rheumatoid arthritis. The involvement of distal and proximal interphalangeal joints and the absence of wrist disease in osteoarthritis differs from rheumatoid arthritis, in which metacarpophalangeal, proximal interphalangeal, and wrist joints are characteristically affected. Painful swelling and erythema of a distal or proximal interphalangeal joint associated with Heberden's or Bouchard's nodes may mimic gout. Both entities, however, may coexist.

TREATMENT The goals of treatment are to decrease pain and maintain and improve function. Management of osteoarthritis requires coordinating the patient's care which at various times in the course of the disease may involve physical therapy, occupational therapy, social services, and orthopedics. Patient education is extremely important. Patients should be advised to protect the involved joints from overuse. Weight reduction is important in those patients with back, hip, and knee involvement. The use of a cane also reduces the amount of weight placed on an involved joint. Isometric exercises help to strengthen the muscles around a joint and thereby protect the joint.

In symptomatic patients, salicylates or other nonsteroidal anti-inflammatory drugs (NSAIDs) are used. Salicylates should be given in an adequate dose in the range of 2 to 4 g per day. NSAIDs are ibuprofen (400 to 600 mg qid), fenoprofen (600 mg qid), naproxen (250 to 500 mg bid), diflunisal (500 mg bid), indomethacin (25 to 50 mg tid), tolmetin (200 to 400 mg qid), sulindac (200 mg bid), meclofenamate (50 mg qid), and piroxicam (10 to 20 mg once a day). The NSAIDs share several similar side effects, including gastrointestinal bleeding and sodium retention (see Chap. 263). Drugs that are primarily analgesic, such as acetaminophen or propoxyphene, may also be beneficial at times. Phenylbutazone, because of the increased risk of agranulocytosis, should only be used after all other NSAIDs have been found to be ineffective. If given, the physician and patient should be well aware of its toxicity and the need for only short-term usage.

Intraarticular steroid injections may be very effective in reducing pain and swelling. They should be used judicially in weight-bearing joints and limited to no more than three injections per year. Injection of glucocorticoids into the juxtaarticular soft tissue may benefit some patients. Orthopedic surgery may provide patients with improved pain relief and function. Osteotomy of the knee will correct a valgus or varus deformity and improve weight distribution within the knee. Replacement of the hip with a prosthetic joint has been one of the most dramatic forms of surgery for patients with osteoarthritis. Total knee replacements also have been helpful in some patients, although not nearly as successful as the total hip. Debridement, removal of loose bodies, and placement of partial prostheses are other procedures that may benefit individual patients. Splinting of a joint for short periods of time, for example, the carpometacarpal joint of the thumb, often alleviates pain. Hot packs, ultrasound, and other physical therapy modalities also provide pain reduction and improvement of joint motion.

REFERENCES

BLAND JH, COOPER SM: Osteoarthritis: A review of the cell biology involved and evidence for reversibility: Management rationally related to known genesis and pathophysiology. Semin Arthritis Rheum 14:106, 1984

BRANDT KD: Pathogenesis of osteoarthritis in *Textbook of Rheumatology*, WN Kelley et al (eds). Philadelphia, Saunders, 1985, chap 88, pp 1417–1431

———: Osteoarthritis: Clinical patterns and pathology in *Textbook of Rheumatology*, WN Kelley et al (eds). Philadelphia, Saunders, 1985, chap 89, pp 1432–1448

GIBILISCO PA et al: Synovial fluid crystals in osteoarthritis. Arthritis Rheum 28:511, 1985

HOWELL DS: Etiopathogenesis of osteoarthritis, in *Osteoarthritis: Diagnosis and Management*, RW Moskowitz et al (eds). Philadelphia, Saunders, 1984, chap 7, pp 129–146

PAINE KWT et al: Clinical features of lumbar spinal stenosis. Clin Orthop 115:77, 1976

WARD J, SAMUELSON CO: Nonsteroidal anti-inflammatory drugs, in *Update II: Harrison's Principles of Internal Medicine*, KJ Isselbacher et al (eds). New York, McGraw-Hill, 1982, pp 91–110

275 CALCIUM PYROPHOSPHATE (PSEUDOGOUT) AND CALCIUM HYDROXYAPATITE DEPOSITION DISEASES

BRUCE C. GILLILAND

The deposition of calcium pyrophosphate dihydrate crystals in the joint is referred to as *calcium pyrophosphate deposition disease* (CPDD) and is characterized by acute and chronic inflammatory joint disease, usually affecting older individuals. The acute or subacute form of this arthritis is called *pseudogout,* but this term is also used as a synonym for CPDD. The calcium deposits in articular cartilage (chondrocalcinosis) are detected radiographically in most patients with CPDD. Knee and other large joints are the most frequent sites of involvement.

In *hydroxyapatite arthropathy,* arthritis is induced by deposition of calcium hydroxyapatite crystals. Differential diagnosis is based on crystal identification.

EPIDEMIOLOGY, PATHOGENESIS, AND PATHOLOGY CPDD occurs in persons of either sex, usually over age 50; its prevalence increases sharply with age. Approximately one symptomatic CPDD patient is observed for every two to three patients with gouty arthritis. An indication of the prevalence of chondrocalcinosis comes from autopsy studies, which have shown that approximately 3 to 5 percent of the adult population have calcium pyrophosphate dihydrate deposits in the knee joints.

CPDD is classified into three groups: a hereditary type, CPDD associated with metabolic disease, and idiopathic CPDD. Reports of hereditary CPDD have come from outside the United States; this disease occurs in individuals in the fourth to sixth decade. Sometimes it is severe, crippling, and involves many joints. Another form of familial disease is oligoarticular and affects older patients.

CPDD appears to have a definite association with primary hyperparathyroidism and hemochromatosis. CPDD has been reported in up to approximately 40 percent of patients with both of these disorders. Other associated metabolic disorders include hypophosphatasia, hypomagnesemia, hypothyroidism, gout, ochronosis, and Wilson's disease. In hypothyroidism, acute arthritis attacks usually occur only after treatment with thyroid hormone. The relationship of these disorders to the pathogenesis of chondrocalcinosis is unknown; furthermore, the association of some of them with chondrocalcinosis may not be greater than with osteoarthritis alone. In general, CPDD has a close association with degenerative joint disease.

Levels of inorganic pyrophosphate are elevated in the synovial fluid of many patients with CPDD but are also elevated in patients with osteoarthritis without evident chondrocalcinosis. Elevated levels of inorganic pyrophosphate most likely reflect increased metabolic activity of cartilage. The concentrations of calcium and pyrophosphate ions in joint fluid do not exceed their solubility product, and therefore it is unlikely that crystals form within synovial fluid. The initial site of crystal formation is believed to be in articular cartilage; however, the mechanism has not been elucidated. It is not yet clear whether idiopathic CPDD is a primary event or a secondary effect of osteoarthritis. Some investigators have suggested that mineral formation is a consequence of disturbed cartilage metabolism occurring in osteoarthritis.

The crystals in synovial fluid are believed to be shed from crystals in the cartilage. Several mechanisms have been postulated for the release of crystals from cartilage into the joint fluid. Lowering of either calcium or pyrophosphate ions in synovial fluid may result in the shedding of crystals from cartilage into synovial fluid. This hypothesis is supported by two observations: (1) lowering of the concentration of ionized calcium in joint fluid brings on an acute attack of crystal-induced arthritis, and (2) acute attacks of arthritis are associated with illness in which blood calcium concentrations decrease. Crystals may also enter the joint fluid as a consequence of mechanical disruption of cartilage secondary to microfractures of subchondral bone. The occurrence of acute attacks following trauma supports this concept. Another proposed mechanism is the release of crystals resulting from degradation of the cartilage matrix by enzymes. This mechanism may explain the occurrence of pseudogout superimposed on infectious arthritis, gout, or osteoarthritis. The finding of calcium pyrophosphate crystals may sometimes be the result and not the primary cause of joint inflammation.

The presence of calcium pyrophosphate crystals in the synovial fluid leads to an inflammatory response. Acute arthritis can be induced experimentally by the injection of calcium pyrophosphate crystals into a normal joint. Phagocytosis of the crystals by polymorphonuclear leukocytes leads to release of lysosomal enzymes and a chemotactant for leukocytes.

The *pathologic changes* in the joint involve deposits of calcium pyrophosphate dihydrate crystals in the joint capsule, synovium, tendons, and ligaments, in the midzonal area of articular hyaline cartilage, and diffusely in fibrocartilage. The menisci of the knee are a common site of crystal deposition. Crystals can be seen at the margin of degenerating cartilage and surrounding the lacunae of chondrocytes; this site is considered the earliest detectable lesion. The deposition of crystals varies from microcrystalline aggregates to large masses intermixed with fibrous tissue. Crystals may also be observed in normal-appearing cartilage.

The synovium in acute arthritis is edematous, with numerous polymorphonuclear leukocytes. In chronic arthritis, mononuclear cell infiltration and fibroblastic proliferation are present; crystals are rarely observed.

CLINICAL MANIFESTATIONS Several patterns of joint involvement are recognized in calcium pyrophosphate deposition disease. Acute attacks occur in approximately 25 percent of patients, and this clinical picture is commonly called *pseudogout.* The onset of the acute attack of pseudogout is rapid, and it reaches a peak usually in 12 to 36 h. The involved joint is erythematous, swollen, warm, and painful. The acute attack is usually confined to a single joint, but in some patients involvement of other joints may follow in rapid progression. The knee is by far the most frequent site of acute arthritis, but attacks occur in the ankles, wrists, elbows, hips, and cervical and lumbar spine. As in gout, the metatarsophalangeal joint of the great toe may be a site of involvement. Furthermore, attacks may be provoked by trauma, surgery, or medical illness. The acute arthritis is usually intermittent, and the same joint is often involved in subsequent attacks. The acute episode usually subsides in 1 to 2 weeks. Between attacks the involved joint appears relatively normal. Most patients have radiographic evidence of chondrocalcinosis.

Approximately 5 percent of patients with calcium pyrophosphate deposition disease have what is termed *pseudorheumatoid disease,* which is characterized by multiple joint involvement with subacute attacks lasting several weeks to several months. The attacks affect one or several joints, then move on to involve other joints. Patients may complain of morning stiffness and fatigue. Synovial proliferation, limitation of joint motion, and flexion deformities can develop. Rheumatoid arthritis and CPDD may coexist.

Another group, predominantly middle-aged and elderly women and representing half the patients with calcium pyrophosphate deposition disease, has a chronic form of the disease. Progressive degenerative joint changes occur in multiple joints. The knees are the most frequently involved, followed by the wrists, metacarpophalangeal joints, hips, shoulders, elbows, and ankles. The joint involvement is usually symmetric, and flexion contractures may develop. Approximately one-half of the patients with this form of the disease experience intermittent acute attacks. Another group of patients has typical articular chondrocalcinosis without any symptoms. Finally, CPDD may resemble neuropathic arthropathy; in these patients a severe oligo- or polyarticular destructive arthropathy is seen without neurologic deficits. Calcium pyrophosphate deposits, however, are also seen in neuropathic arthropathies.

DIAGNOSIS The microscopic examination of *synovial fluid* in an acute attack shows large numbers of polymorphonuclear leukocytes. Calcium pyrophosphate dihydrate crystals are frequently found extracellularly and in polymorphonuclear leukocytes. In chronic arthritis, the crystals are observed less frequently and are most often extracellular. With polarized light, the crystals appear as short blunt rods, rhomboids, and cuboids. They have weakly positive birefringence under compensated polarized light, in contrast to the strongly negative birefringence of sodium urate crystals. The diagnosis is made by finding typical crystals under compensated polarized light and is supported by radiographic evidence of chondrocalcinosis.

Radiographically, calcifications in articular hyaline cartilage appear as fine linear densities parallel to and separated from the underlying subchondral bone surface. Sites commonly involved are the knee, wrist, elbow, hip, and glenohumeral joints. Calcifications in fibrocartilage usually appear as thick and irregular densities within the central portion of the joint cavity. Common sites of fibrocartilage involvement include the menisci of the knee, triangular cartilage of the wrist, symphysis pubis, and the annulus fibrosis of the intervertebral disk. Calcifications in tendons are thin and linear, affecting most often the Achilles, supraspinatus, and triceps tendons. Calcification in the synovium has a cloudy appearance. Evidence for chondrocalcinosis can usually be obtained with radiographs of the knees, wrists, and symphysis pubis. Radiographs of the joints in chronic CPDD are similar to those in osteoarthritis, showing sclerosis of the subchondral bone, joint space narrowing, and subchondral cysts. The latter are often larger and more numerous than in osteoarthritis.

Gout and septic arthritis are the main considerations in the *differential diagnosis* of the acute arthritis. Gout and pseudogout are frequently indistinguishable clinically, and the diagnosis depends on the identification of their characteristic crystals under compensated polarized light. Both crystals occasionally have been found together in the synovial fluid of patients with typical radiographic articular calcifications of chondrocalcinosis. Bacterial smears and cultures should be performed on synovial fluid in all patients with an acute monarticular arthritis even if crystals are present, since crystals may be shed into synovial fluid during septic arthritis. The symptoms of osteoarthritis and chronic CPDD are very similar, and radiographic evidence for both is often present. The role played by each is difficult to determine. Features that may distinguish CPDD from osteoarthritis are the involvement in CPDD of non-weight-bearing joints such as the elbows, wrists, and shoulders and the rapid progression of joint destruction. Pseudogout should be considered when intermittent attacks of acute arthritis occur in a patient presumed to have osteoarthritis. The finding of a chronic effusion in patients with symptoms of osteoarthritis also suggests the possibility of pseudogout. The diagnosis should not be made only on the radiographic findings of intraarticular calcific deposits; it depends also on the identification of the characteristic crystals, since other forms of inflammatory arthritis may affect the same joints. Attacks of pseudogout may occur in patients without radiographic evidence of chondrocalcinosis, requiring a careful search for calcium pyrophosphate dihydrate crystals in any case of acute arthritis, especially in older patients. On the other hand, radiographic evidence of calcific deposits is found not infrequently in the knees of elderly patients who have no joint symptoms. Intraarticular calcifications and joint inflammation may be caused by deposition of calcium hydroxyapatite crystals. Hydroxyapatite arthropathy tends to affect one or only a few joints, while chronic CPDD may be more generalized. Intraarticular calcifications in hydroxyapatite arthropathy tend to have a more diffuse and amorphous pattern than that in CPDD. Differential diagnosis requires identification of the respective crystals. The arthritis of hemochromatosis and CPDD may be difficult to distinguish, since both affect the metacarpophalangeal joints, especially the second and third, and have similar changes on x-ray.

TREATMENT Indomethacin, 75 to 150 mg per day, or other nonsteroidal anti-inflammatory drugs (NSAIDs) are usually effective and should be given for approximately 10 to 14 days. Aspiration of the synovial fluid, followed by intraarticular injection of glucocorticosteroids, also may be effective. Results of treatment with colchicine are variable, but this drug may be useful in those patients who require parenteral therapy. In chronic arthritis, salicylates or the newer NSAIDs may give symptomatic relief. The deposition of calcium pyrophosphate crystals in articular tissues cannot be prevented or reversed.

HYDROXYAPATITE ARTHROPATHY Crystal-induced arthritis is also observed with calcium hydroxyapatite crystals. This arthritis has been mainly described in the knee and shoulder. A group of elderly women who were studied in Milwaukee, Wisconsin, were found to have glenohumeral osteoarthritis, rotator cuff defects, joint effusions with few cells, and the presence of calcium hydroxyapatite crystals in the fluid. This constellation of findings was termed "Milwaukee shoulder." The joint fluid of these and other patients studied subsequently also contained collagenase, neutral proteases, and particulate collagen, types I, II, and III. Similar findings have been noted in synovial fluid of involved knees. Hydroxyapatite and calcium pyrophospate crystals have been found together in synovial fluid in some patients, suggesting that both crystals may be involved in the inflammatory process. Diagnosis is based on crystal identification. Hydroxyapatite crystals cannot be recognized by light microscopy because of their small size (0.1 to 1 μm in length). Electron-microscopic or x-ray diffraction studies are required for the accurate diagnosis of this crystal. Alizarin red S staining can be used as a screening test to detect calcium components in synovial fluid. Radiographic changes are as described above for CPDD. Treatment consists of administration of a nonsteroidal anti-inflammatory drug, repeated joint aspiration, and rest of the affected joint.

REFERENCES

HALVERSON PB et al: Milwaukee shoulder syndrome: Eleven additional cases with involvement of the knee in seven (basic calcium phosphate crystal deposition disease). Semin Arthritis Rheum 14(1):36, 1984

HOWELL DS: Diseases due to the deposition of calcium pyrophosphate and hydroxyapatite, in *Textbook of Rheumatology*, WN Kelley et al (eds). Philadelphia, Saunders, 1985, chap 87, pp 1398–1416

MCCARTHY DJ: Pseudogout and pyrophosphate metabolism, in *Advances in Internal Medicine*, GH Stollerman (ed). Chicago, Year Book, 1980, pp 363–390

PAUL H et al: Alizarin red S staining as a screening test to detect calcium compounds in synovial fluid. Arthritis Rheum 26:191, 1983

RESNICK D, NIWAYAMA G: Calcium pyrophosphate dihydrate (CPDD) crystal deposition disease, in *Diagnosis of Bone and Joint Disorders*, D Resnick, G Niwayama (eds). Philadelphia, Saunders, 1981, chap 44, pp 1520–1574

276 PSORIATIC ARTHRITIS AND ARTHRITIS ASSOCIATED WITH GASTROINTESTINAL DISEASES

BRUCE C. GILLILAND

PSORIATIC ARTHRITIS The prevalence of arthritis in patients with psoriasis is higher than that found in the general population, even when degenerative joint disease and rheumatoid arthritis are excluded. Arthritis related to psoriasis occurs in approximately 5 percent of patients with skin disease.

The *etiology* and *pathogenesis* of psoriatic arthritis are not known; however, studies showing aggregation of psoriatic arthritis in first-degree relatives of psoriatic patients suggest that hereditary factors may play a role. Approximately 50 percent of psoriatic patients with spondylitis have the HLA-B27 antigen. The presence of HLA-B27 apparently does not predispose to peripheral arthritis in psoriatic patients.

The age of onset of psoriatic arthritis is usually in the third or fourth decade, and the sex ratio is approximately equal. Psoriasis usually precedes the onset of arthritis by months or years. In approximately 15 percent of patients, the arthritis precedes the skin lesions. Simultaneous onset of arthritis and skin lesions is uncommon, but arthritis and nail abnormalities often begin together. In general, the prognosis of psoriatic arthritis is more favorable than that of rheumatoid arthritis, except in patients with the severe destructive form of psoriatic arthritis (arthritis mutilans). The course of psoriatic arthritis in most patients is mild, intermittent, and affects only a few joints. Spontaneous remission may occur.

Several patterns of joint involvement are observed in psoriatic arthritis. Approximately 70 percent of patients will have an asymmetric oligoarticular arthritis involving two or three joints at a time. The proximal joints of the hands and feet are frequently affected. "Sausage" digits are also present as seen in Reiter's syndrome. Another pattern observed in about 15 percent of patients consists of a symmetric polyarthritis similar to rheumatoid arthritis. The rheumatoid factor test in these patients is negative. Patients with psoriasis and symmetric polyarthritis who have rheumatoid factor are considered to have coexistent rheumatoid arthritis and psoriasis. Another pattern of arthritis found in approximately 10 percent of patients has prominantly distal interphalangeal joint involvement. The adjacent nail usually has changes of psoriasis. A very few patients have a pattern of disease referred to as "arthritis mutilans," which is characterized by a severe destructive and deforming polyarthritis. These patients have ankylosis of joints, dissolution of bone, and "telescoping" of fingers. In addition, they may have ankylosis of the spine.

Approximately 20 percent of patients with psoriatic arthritis have spine involvement in the form of sacroiliitis and/or spondylitis, which in some patients may be asymptomatic and evident only on x-ray. The spondylitis tends to be more asymmetric than in ankylosing spondylitis and may occur even in the absence of peripheral arthritis.

The peripheral joints in psoriatic arthritis are warm, swollen, and tender. Flexion contractures and ankylosis of joints may occur, with long periods of persistent joint inflammation. No definite correlation exists between the degree of skin involvement and joint disease, but in some patients the activity of both tends to be parallel. A closer temporal relationship has been found between psoriatic nail lesions and arthritis than between the skin lesions and arthritis. Psoriatic nail changes include onycholysis, pits, and ridges.

Laboratory abnormalities include hypoproliferative anemia and an elevated erythrocyte sedimentation rate. Tests for rheumatoid factor are negative. Hyperuricemia is observed in 10 to 20 percent of patients, similar to uncomplicated psoriasis, and reflects the severity of skin involvement. Synovial fluid and biopsy findings are those of nonspecific inflammation.

Several *radiographic* features are characteristic of psoriatic arthritis. These include severe destruction of isolated joints, osteolysis, bony ankylosis, whittling of the tufts of the terminal phalanges, and the "pencil-in-cup" deformity, which is most commonly observed in the joints of the fingers and toes. Whittling of the distal end of the middle phalanx produces the "pencil" which projects into a widened, cuplike erosion in the joint surface of the terminal phalanx. Bony absorption of phalanges produces the opera-glass deformity of the hands (telescoped fingers). The radiographic findings in spondylitis associated with psoriatic arthritis are similar to those found in spondylitis with Reiter's syndrome (Chap. 268).

The *diagnosis* of psoriatic arthritis is suggested by the presence of an inflammatory arthritis in a patient with typical skin or nail lesions of psoriasis. Skin lesions may be quite small and hidden in the scalp, intergluteal fold, or umbilicus. The asymmetry of joint involvement, negative test for rheumatoid factor, and the absence of rheumatoid nodules help to distinguish psoriatic arthritis from rheumatoid arthritis. Psoriatic arthritis presenting as monarticular arthritis or asymmetric oligoarthritis may be differentiated from Reiter's syndrome by the chronic nature of the skin lesions, the absence of urethritis and conjunctivitis, and the rarity of mucous membrane lesions. At times, however, differentiation of these two diseases may not be possible. Psoriatic arthritis presenting as an acute arthritis in a toe or finger may be mistaken for gouty arthritis especially in the presence of hyperuricemia due to psoriatic skin disease. The appearance of the joint also may suggest septic arthritis. These diagnostic considerations are easily excluded by examining synovial fluid for sodium urate crystals and for microorganisms with appropriate cultures. Development of acute Heberden's nodes may be confused with psoriatic arthritis, but other features such as Bouchard's nodes at the proximal interphalangeal joints, involvement of the first carpometacarpal joint, and a normal erythrocyte sedimentation rate (ESR) point to the diagnosis of primary osteoarthritis. Fungal disease of the toenails may be mistaken for psoriatic nails; the distinction may require examination of nail scrapings for mycelia.

In the *treatment* of psoriatic arthritis, patient education and physical and occupational therapy are all important. Aspirin or other nonsteroidal anti-inflammatory drugs are recommended initially. Intraarticular injection of glucocorticoids may be of value in patients with few joints involved, but should be limited to three injections per year for any one joint. In patients with more progressive and severe peripheral arthritis, gold salts may be indicated and have resulted in clinical improvement in greater than 50 percent of patients in some studies. Methotrexate has been shown to be beneficial for both the skin and joint disease of psoriasis but because of its potential serious liver toxicity, should be used only in patients with severe psoriatic disease. The most widely used regimen of methotrexate is three oral doses 12 h apart once a week beginning with three 2.5-mg doses (7.5 mg) and with the maximum being three 5-mg doses (15 mg) per week. Patients should have a complete blood count, blood urea nitrogen, creatinine, and liver function tests done monthly. This drug should be used cautiously, if at all, in patients with creatinine greater than 2.0 mg/dL since the risk of toxicity greatly increases. Cirrhosis of the liver is a major concern. It is seldom seen before a total dose of 1.5 g. Alcohol abusers and patients with underlying liver disease should not be given methotrexate. Some have recommended that a liver biopsy be obtained before treatment and then annually. However, its value in identifying patients at risk for cirrhosis is not proven. Other immunosuppressive agents, azathioprine or 6-mercaptopurine, have been reported to be beneficial. Gold, methotrexate, and other immunosuppressive agents should only be given under the supervision of experienced clinician. Adequate control of skin disease may lead to improvement of the joint disease in an occasional patient.

ARTHRITIS ASSOCIATED WITH GASTROINTESTINAL DISEASES

Inflammatory bowel disease The articular manifestations of ulcerative colitis and regional enteritis (Crohn's disease, granulomatous colitis) are similar and will be discussed together. Two patterns of joint involvement may be distinguished: arthritis of peripheral joints and spondylitis. The frequency of peripheral arthritis in regional enteritis is approximately 20 percent and in ulcerative colitis, 10 percent. The frequency of spondylitis in both bowel disorders is 4 percent.

The peripheral arthritis of inflammatory bowel disease (IBD) most commonly begins between the ages of 25 and 45 years and affects both sexes equally. Arthritis usually follows the onset of colitis by 6 months to several years, but uncommonly the onset of both may coincide or the arthritis may precede colitis. Arthritis is more frequent in ulcerative colitis patients who have pseudopolyps or perianal disease and also is more common with extensive colitis than disease limited to the rectum. In regional enteritis, arthritis is more frequent in patients with colon disease and less common with disease limited to the small bowel. Patients with aphthous stomatitis, erythema nodosum, or uveitis are likely also to have arthritis. These extraintestinal manifestations often flare up with exacerbation of colitis.

The typical attack of arthritis presents acutely, reaching a peak within 24 h, and often affects a single joint in the lower extremity. Involvement of other joints, without definite symmetry, may follow over the next few days. Usually fewer than four joints are involved during an episode. The involved joint is usually red, swollen, and painful. The knee and ankle are most frequently affected, followed by the proximal interphalangeal, elbow, shoulder, and wrist joints. The arthritis usually subsides within several weeks, but occasionally lasts for months. Complete resolution without residual damage is the general rule. Some patients may experience only migratory arthralgias as evidence of an attack.

Spondylitis with IBD is indistinguishable from ankylosing spondylitis. However, the usual male preponderance observed in ankylosing spondylitis is not seen in patients with IBD and spondylitis. The onset of spondylitis antedates IBD in approximately one-third of patients. The HLA-B27 antigen is found in approximately 70 percent of these patients. In some patients, spondylitis and bowel disease may have a nearly simultaneous onset, while in others spondylitis follows the onset of colitis. Spondylitis usually progresses regardless of remission of the bowel disease or colectomy. The disease may progress to complete ankylosis of the spine.

Radiographic evidence of sacroiliitis without symptoms is found in patients with IBD, the prevalence ranging from 4 to 15 percent.

The majority of these patients will probably not become symptomatic or progress to ankylosing spondylitis. In this group of patients the prevalence of HLA-B27 is not increased.

Radiographs of involved peripheral joints usually are normal except for soft tissue swelling. An occasional patient with recurrent or persistent disease will show small bony erosions and joint space narrowing. Films of the spine show changes indistinguishable from those of ankylosing spondylitis.

The peripheral white blood cell count, anemia, and erythrocyte sedimentation rate usually reflect the intestinal disease. Tests for rheumatoid factor are negative. Synovial fluid shows a moderate leukocytosis, in the range of 10,000 cells per cubic millimeter, consisting predominantly of polymorphonuclear leukocytes.

Treatment should be directed primarily at the underlying IBD. Joint symptoms can usually be managed with salicylates or other nonsteroidal anti-inflammatory drugs. Glucocorticoids used for control of colitis and extraintestinal manifestations, such as erythema nodosum, may lead to suppression of arthritis. Colectomy or systemic glucocorticoids are not indicated for treatment of the arthritis alone. Physical therapy is directed toward maintenance of posture in spondylitis and prevention of contractures in the peripheral form of arthritis.

Intestinal bypass arthritis Approximately one-third of patients with jejunocolic and a somewhat smaller percentage of patients with jejunoileal bypass develop arthritic manifestations which occur from several weeks to years following the surgery. These consist of recurrent episodes of migratory polyarthralgia, polyarthritis, and, sometimes, tenosynovitis. Episodes last from a few days to a few weeks. Some patients may experience persistent arthritis for months. The knees, ankles, wrists, and shoulders are most commonly affected. Neck and back symptoms may also occur. Joint damage usually does not occur. However, in some patients with persistent arthritis, erosions of the joint margins have been described. The arthritis may be accompanied by vasculitic skin lesions which can be urticarial, pustular, or nodular. Raynaud's phenomenon also occurs in some of these patients.

Examination of synovial fluid has shown a mild leukocytosis with polymorphonuclear white cells predominating. Circulating immune complexes and cryoglobulins are found in the serum of many bypass patients with arthritis. Immunoglobulins, complement, and antibodies to *Escherichia coli* and other bacteria have been identified in cryoglobulins from these patients.

The pathogenesis of bypass arthritis and vasculitis is postulated to be mediated by immune complexes. Bacterial growth in the blind loop of the intestine leads to absorption of bacterial antigens, and subsequent development of antibodies to these antigens results in formation of immune complexes.

The definitive treatment of bypass arthritis is reconnecting the bowel. When this is not possible, treatment with tetracycline or other appropriate antibiotics to reduce the bacterial growth in the blind loop has produced clinical improvement. Aspirin or other nonsteroidal anti-inflammatory drugs may help to control symptoms. Arthritis and vasculitis are also suppressed with systemic glucocorticoids in most patients.

Whipple's disease Whipple's disease (intestinal lipodystrophy) is a rare disorder affecting predominantly middle-aged males and is characterized by arthritis, serositis, diarrhea, malabsorption, weight loss, skin hyperpigmentation, and lymphadenopathy. The diagnosis is confirmed by the identification of periodic acid Schiff (PAS) staining of bacilliform structures intercellularly or as inclusions in foamy macrophages. Electron microscopy has demonstrated rod-shaped organisms in the lamina propria of the small intestine. The PAS-staining material is thought to consist of partially degraded bacteria. PAS-staining granules can also be seen in abdominal and peripheral lymph nodes and in other tissues.

Arthritis occurs in approximately two-thirds of the patients and usually precedes the appearance of intestinal symptoms by months or years. With the onset of intestinal symptoms, the arthritis may subside. The joint disease involves predominantly peripheral joints, affecting knees and ankles most commonly, followed by fingers, hips, shoulders, elbows, and wrists. It is typically acute, migratory, and transient, lasts only a few days, and causes no permanent joint damage. Long, irregular periods of remission are common. Joints may be quite tender and erythematous. Arthritis may be chronic in other patients. Some patients with peripheral joint involvement have radiographic changes in the sacroiliac joints similar to those of ankylosing spondylitis. Synovial fluid analysis has shown leukocyte counts ranging from 450 to 36,000 per cubic millimeter with 30 to 95 percent neutrophils. Synovial fluid, however, may only show a mild monocytosis without characteristic foamy macrophages. PAS-positive macrophages have been seen in synovial biopsy tissue. This disease, including the joint manifestations, responds well to therapy with penicillin, 1.2 million units, and streptomycin, 1 g daily for 2 weeks, followed by tetracycline, 1 g daily for 1 year. Relapse while on tetracycline requires administration again of penicillin and streptomycin. Glucocorticoids may be necessary in addition to antimicrobials in severely ill patients but are not indicated for the treatment of arthritis alone. Salicylates or other nonsteroidol anti-inflammatory drugs may be helpful in controlling joint symptoms.

REFERENCES

ARNETT FC: HLA and the spondylarthropathies, in *Spondylarthropathies*. New York, Grune & Stratton, 1984, chap 15, pp 297–321

CALIN A: Diagnosis and treatment—HLA-B27: To type or not to type? Ann Intern Med 92:208, 1980

———: Reiter's syndrome, in *Textbook of Rheumatology*, WN Kelley et al (eds). Philadelphia, Saunders, 1985, chap 65, pp 1007–1020

GOOD AE, UTSINGER PD: Enteropathic arthritis, in *Textbook of Rheumatology*, 2d ed, WN Kelley et al (eds). Philadelphia, Saunders, 1985, chap 67, pp 1031–1041

KAMMER GM et al: Psoriatic arthritis: A clinical, immunologic and HLA study of 100 patients. Semin Arthritis Rheum 9:75, 1979

WRIGHT V: Psoriatic arthritis, in *Textbook of Rheumatology*, 2d ed, WN Kelley et al (eds). Philadelphia, Saunders, 1985, chap 166, pp 1021–1031

277 INFECTIOUS ARTHRITIS

BRUCE C. GILLILAND / ROBERT G. PETERSDORF

ACUTE BACTERIAL ARTHRITIS Septic arthritis is a serious medical problem requiring prompt recognition and appropriate treatment to avoid permanent joint damage. All ages are affected.

Etiology and Pathogenesis Bacteria most often infect the joint during an episode of bacteremia. A source of bacteremia can be identified in the majority of patients. Because the synovium is very vascular and does not have a limiting basement membrane, bacteria can enter the joint freely. Host factors, however, must be important since joint infection is not a common sequel of bacteremic episodes. Certain bacteria, such as *Neisseria gonorrhoeae* and *Staphylococcus aureus*, have a propensity to infect a joint during bacteremia. Joint sepsis may also result from a penetrating wound, direct extension of adjacent osteomyelitis, arthroscopy, intraarticular steroid injection, or prosthetic joint surgery.

An increased susceptibility to joint infection occurs in patients with diabetes, cancer, hypogammaglobulinemia, or chronic liver disease, and in those receiving corticosteroids or immunosuppressive drugs. Patients with chronic alcoholism are more prone to develop infections in general, and bacterial arthritis in particular. In addition, joints previously damaged by trauma or by chronic arthritis, especially rheumatoid arthritis, are more susceptible to infections.

Pathology The synovium in the early stages of infection is edematous and infiltrated by neutrophils. An effusion with many neutrophils forms rapidly. Enzymes released from neutrophils or synovial cells destroy articular cartilage, subchondral bone, and joint capsule. Increased intraarticular pressure also contributes to joint damage. Small abscesses appear in the synovium and subchondral bone, and necrotic debris collects in the joint space. During healing, proliferation of fibroblasts may lead to ankylosis.

Acute *bacterial arthritis* is caused by many different types of bacteria; the ones most commonly encountered are *N. gonorrhoeae, S. aureus, Streptococcus pneumoniae, Streptococcus pyogenes, Haemophilus influenzae,* and gram-negative bacilli (*Escherichia coli, Salmonella, Pseudomonas* spp.). Septic arthritis due to *H. influenzae* occurs mostly in neonates. *S. aureus* is the most common nongonococcal infecting agent in adults. Joint sepsis with gram-negative bacilli tends to occur in patients with underlying infection of the urinary, biliary, or intestinal tract, in patients with impaired resistance to infection, and in intravenous drug abusers. Osteomyelitis is also a feature of infections with gram-negative bacilli, and joint infection is a common sequel. Patients with *Salmonella* arthritis often have evidence of underlying osteomyelitis. Infectious arthritis of the spine is most often caused by staphylococci. Brucellosis, tuberculosis, and *Salmonella* also preferentially involve the spine.

Manifestations The onset of bacterial arthritis usually occurs over several days and is accompanied by fever. Shaking chills are uncommon. One or a few joints may be involved. The affected joint is warm, erythematous, swollen, and painful; however, these signs may be less marked in elderly patients or in patients receiving corticosteroids or immunosuppressive drugs. Marked guarding of the joint and muscle spasms are common. The knee is involved in approximately one-half of the cases. Other commonly involved joints include hips, shoulders, wrists, ankles, and elbows. Sternoclavicular and sacroiliac joints are affected less often; however, predilection of these two joints for septic arthritis has been observed in intravenous drug abusers. The articulations of the spine or any peripheral joint may be a site of infection. In the spine, infection involves the vertebral body and adjacent intervertebral disk space, and may extend to the adjacent apophyseal joint. Localized tenderness and spasm of the paraspinal or psoas muscles are often present. The diagnosis of septic arthritis of the hip is often delayed, because swelling of this joint is not readily detected. Pain from the hip may be felt in the groin, buttock, or lateral upper thigh, or referred to the anterior knee. The thigh is usually held in adduction, flexion, and internal rotation. In some instances, the thigh becomes edematous and swelling appears in the anterior groin.

Laboratory and x-ray findings Aspiration and examination of joint fluid should be performed immediately in any patient suspected of having a septic joint. The needle should not be inserted into the joint through an overlying area of cellulitis or an infected bursa. The appearance of synovial fluid in infectious arthritis is usually cloudy or grossly purulent. The white blood cell count ranges from 10,000 to greater than 100,000 per cubic millimeter, and more than 90 percent of the cells are neutrophils. The peripheral blood often shows a leukocytosis; however, the leukocyte count may be normal. The concentration of glucose in the joint cavity is often less than 50 percent of a simultaneous blood sugar reading when obtained at least 6 h after a meal, or after cessation of intravenous glucose infusions to allow equilibrium of glucose between blood and synovial fluid. In some patients with gonococcal arthritis, the reduction of synovial fluid glucose may be less marked. Gram's stain frequently reveals microorganisms in patients with nongonococcal infections. Blood and synovial fluid should be cultured for aerobes and anaerobes. Cultures of the synovial fluid and blood should be performed even if Gram's stain is negative. Radiographs of the joint early in infection show soft tissue swelling and distention of the joint capsule, and later show juxtaarticular osteoporosis, periosteal elevation, joint space narrowing due to cartilage destruction, and bony erosions on the articular surface. Radiographic evidence of coexisting osteomyelitis may be present. In the spine, radiographic changes may not be seen for several months. The first changes consist of narrowing of the involved disk space or vertebra and proliferation of bone at the vertebral margins. Subsequently, lytic lesions appear in the vertebra and may extend to the disk space. During healing adjacent vertebrae may become fused. Radioisotope scanning techniques utilizing technetium polyphosphonate or gallium may be useful in distinguishing whether the site of the infection is cellulitis, osteomyelitis, or septic arthritis. Both types of scan are positive in septic arthritis and osteomyelitis, but only the gallium scan is positive in cellulitis. Radioisotope scans may point to infection in such joints as hip, shoulder, spine, and sacroiliac. A positive scan, however, is not specific for infection, since other causes of inflammatory joint disease as well as degenerative joint disease will give a positive scan.

Diagnosis The diagnosis of acute bacterial arthritis can be made by finding microorganisms on Gram's stain of synovial fluid or in synovial tissue, and is confirmed by a positive culture. With involvement of the spine or sacroiliac joint, needle biopsy or open surgical biopsy may be required to obtain tissue for examination and culture. The possibility of infectious arthritis should be entertained in a patient with fever and unilateral sacroiliac or back pain. Other forms of acute arthritis may be mistaken for infectious arthritis. These include gout, pseudogout, Reiter's syndrome, psoriatic arthritis, peripheral arthritis of inflammatory bowel disease, and rheumatic fever. These disorders usually are not associated with chills, high fever, and marked leukocytosis. Crystal deposits of sodium urate or calcium pyrophosphate may be found in fluid of a septic joint, and may have played a role in predisposing this joint to infection. On the other hand, the enzymes of the inflammatory process of infectious arthritis may have released into the joint fluid preexisting crystal deposits from synovial tissue or cartilage, a process referred to as "enzymatic strip mining." In patients with rheumatoid arthritis who develop chills and fever and have one or two joints disproportionately more inflamed than others, superimposed infectious arthritis in those joints should be carefully excluded by examination and culture of synovial fluid.

Infection of a bursa or juxtaarticular soft tissue and skin should be distinguished from infectious arthritis. Bursae and tendon sheaths become infected with the same types of microorganisms that invade joints. Care must be taken not to infect a bursa or joint by passing a needle through an overlying area of cellulitis.

Treatment Septic arthritis requires prompt treatment with appropriate antibiotics. The preferred antibiotic regimens for the more common organisms are given in the chapters dealing with these organisms as well as in Chap. 88, which summarizes the properties of each antibiotic. When no organisms are seen on Gram's stain, the patient should be given a penicillinase-resistant penicillin and gentamicin until culture and sensitivities dictate the appropriate antibiotic. Bactericidal levels of antibiotics are achieved with systemic administration; therefore, direct administration of an antibiotic into the joint is not necessary and may in itself produce a chemical synovitis. During treatment, bactericidal assays of synovial fluid may be performed to ensure that therapeutic levels of antibiotic have been achieved. Drainage, recommended when the joint is tightly distended or when the fluid contains a high neutrophil count, reduces pressure and removes pus that generates proteolytic enzymes. Needle aspiration, during which the joint cavity can be irrigated with sterile saline to enhance removal of inflammatory substances, usually provides adequate drainage. The frequency of aspiration depends on the amount of fluid and the cell count of that which reaccumulates. Aspiration ordinarily is necessary only during the first few days of treatment. Open surgical drainage is usually not indicated except in septic arthritis of the hip or in a joint with chronic suppuration and loculated pus. Splinting of the affected joint may make the patient more comfortable and reduce the degree of flexion deformity. Passive range of motion should be performed once pain has decreased, followed later by active exercises to restore mobility and strength. A severely damaged weight-bearing joint may require bony fusion.

GONOCOCCAL ARTHRITIS (See Chap. 104) Gonococcal arthritis is the most common cause of arthritis in young adults, especially women. Pregnancy and menstruation are predisposing factors for bacteremia and arthritis. Patients with homozygous deficiency of a terminal complement component (C5 to C8) or those with low levels due to excessive complement consumption are also more susceptible to disseminated *Neisseria* infections, since these organisms are killed by complement-mediated cell lysis requiring the terminal complement components.

Patients with gonococcal arthritis may present with fever, chills, skin lesions, and polyarthritis. The polyarthritis usually evolves in a few days to a monarticular septic arthritis. The clinical picture, however, is quite variable, and some patients present with monarticular septic arthritis and few if any systemic manifestations. The leukocyte count in synovial fluid may not be as high as in nongonococcal infections, but usually is above 50,000 cells per cubic millimeter. Diagnosis is confirmed by positive cultures of blood, synovial fluid, or skin lesion. Cultures of synovial fluid, however, are positive in less than half the cases and blood cultures in less than 20 percent. Skin lesions are usually sterile. The diagnosis is often assumed when culture of cervix, urethra, or throat is positive for gonococcus. Arthritis usually responds to antibiotic therapy. The gonococcal organisms associated with disseminated infection are usually very sensitive to penicillin.

TUBERCULOUS ARTHRITIS (See also Chap. 119) Tuberculous arthritis is a chronic destructive form of septic arthritis caused by *Mycobacterium tuberculosis*. Approximately 1 percent of patients with tuberculosis have skeletal involvement. Many patients with skeletal tuberculosis do not have evidence for active or even inactive pulmonary disease. Tuberculous arthritis occurs more frequently in nonwhites and men, and tends to involve an older population of patients, in their fifth and sixth decades. Tuberculous arthritis, however, can occur at any age.

The most frequently involved joints are the spine, hips, knees, sacroiliac, wrists, and ankles. In the spine (Pott's disease) the infection begins in the margins of the vertebral bodies and extends into the adjacent disk space. Destruction of bone leads to vertebral collapse and angulation of the spine resulting in kyphosis or gibbus. Extension of the infection into the paraspinal muscles produces a cold abscess which can spread up or down the spine or along the rib and eventually point in the groin, neck, chest wall, or sternum. Cord compression may cause paraplegia, and extension into the meninges results in tuberculous meningitis. A rare complication is the formation of a mycotic aneurysm by the erosion of a cold abscess into the aorta. Common clinical manifestations of spinal involvement are back pain, muscle spasm, local tenderness, kyphosis, and referred pain from spinal nerve root compression.

Peripheral or axial joints are infected by direct hematogenous spread or by extension from a tuberculous process in the adjacent bone. A combination of arthritis and osteomyelitis often occurs in skeletal tuberculosis. The tuberculous process produces synovitis with the formation of a pannus of granulation tissue over the articular cartilage. Destruction of articular cartilage initially occurs at the joint margins and gradually progresses. The rate of destruction is slower than in other acute infectious bacterial arthritis. The subchondral bone is involved and areas of necrosis develop. The joint infection can extend to the juxtaarticular soft tissues to produce a cold abscess and eventually a sinus tract.

Tuberculous arthritis has an insidious onset and is usually monarticular, and hips and knees are the most commonly affected peripheral joints. A low-grade fever and night sweats may be present, but most patients do not have prominent constitutional symptoms. The affected peripheral joint is swollen, warm, and tender and has a decreased range of motion. Erythema is minimal, and pain is initially mild. The hypertrophied synovium gives the joint a boggy, doughy feeling. Muscle atrophy, spasm, and contracture of the affected extremity occur. Tenosynovitis of the flexor tendon sheaths of the wrist may compress the median nerve and produce a carpal tunnel syndrome.

The synovial fluid white cell count is usually greater than 10,000 per cubic millimeter, with polymorphonuclear cells predominating. The tubercle bacilli are seen on smears of synovial fluid in approximately 20 percent of patients but are more likely to be found on biopsy of synovial tissue.

Radiographs of peripheral joints in early disease show joint capsule distention and juxtaarticular osteoporosis. Bony erosions at the joint margin, subchondral bone destruction, and joint space narrowing are observed later in the disease. Films of the spine show destruction of the vertebral body, vertebral collapse, and loss of intervertebral disk space.

The diagnosis of tuberculous arthritis is made by demonstrating tubercle bacilli in synovial fluid or tissue by smear, histology, or culture. The tuberculin skin test is almost always positive. Anergy may occur in advanced disease, old age, or severe malnutrition.

Nontuberculous (atypical) mycobacteria (see Chap. 121) (e.g., *M. kansasii, M. marinum, M. intracellulare*) can also cause septic arthritis and infect bursae and tendons. Microorganisms usually reach the joint by hematogenous spread but also can be introduced into the bone or joint by direct inoculation. Involvement of the tendon sheaths in the hand and wrist often occurs and may result in a carpal tunnel syndrome. Peripheral joint involvement is similar to that in tuberculosis. The correct diagnosis depends on a positive culture from synovial or bursal fluid or tissue. Treatment of tuberculosis and nontuberculous mycobacterial infections is described in Chaps. 119 and 121.

MYCOTIC, SYPHILITIC, AND VIRAL ARTHRITIS **Mycotic arthritis** The systemic mycoses (coccidioidomycosis, histoplasmosis, blastomycosis, cryptococcosis, candidiasis, and sporotrichosis) may involve bone and joints. In the primary phase of coccidioidomycosis, a transient polyarthritis, lasting up to 1 month, may occur in association with erythema nodosum (desert arthritis), but no residual joint damage ensues. However, with chronic disseminated disease, arthritis may occur alone or secondary to adjacent bone infection. The arthritis is usually monarticular, affects the knee predominantly, and leads in time to joint destruction. Sporotrichosis arthritis occurs in two distinct clinical forms: in the unifocal form, one or a few joints are chronically affected; while in the multifocal form, multiple joints, skin, and other tissues are involved. Progressive joint damage ensues in the absence of treatment. Young infants receiving parenteral nutrition or patients receiving glucocorticosteroids or immunosuppressive or antibiotic drugs are at risk for *Candida* infections which can involve joints. In other mycotic diseases, joint involvement is infrequent.

Actinomycosis infection due to an anaerobic bacteria-like obligate parasite may involve the spine. The diagnosis of fungal arthritis is established by the identification of the organisms in synovial fluid or in a biopsy specimen. Treatment with amphotericin B is usually successful; however, surgical debridement may be necessary. Penicillin is the drug of choice for actinomycosis.

Syphilitic arthritis This form of arthritis (see Chap. 122) occurs in congenital, secondary, or tertiary syphilis. During the first year of life, congenital syphilis may produce an osteochondritis in the juxtaepiphyseal region which results in the breakdown of bone and articular cartilage (Parrot's pseudoparalysis). At puberty, congenital disease may cause a synovitis which most commonly involves the knees and elbows (Clutton's joints). The joint is often red, swollen, and tender, but pain may be minimal. Synovial fluid shows a leukocytosis, predominantly lymphocytes.

In secondary syphilis, transient polyarthritis and polyarthralgia occur. Gummatous involvement of the synovium may occur in tertiary syphilis and most often involves the larger joints.

In addition to direct involvement of the joint, syphilis also produces a neuropathic joint (Charcot's joint).

The proper diagnosis of the joint disease can be established only after the correct diagnosis of syphilis. A positive serologic test for syphilis is not diagnostic, since biologic false-positive tests may occur in rheumatic diseases such as systemic lupus erythematosus.

Viral arthritis A self-limited polyarthritis may be a manifestation of several viral diseases. Three viral infections especially are accompanied by significant arthritis: rubella, type B hepatitis, and arboviruses not found in the western hemisphere (chikungunya and o'nyong-nyong in Africa, and Ross River arthritis in Australia). Other viral infections with arthritis include mumps, infectious mononucleosis, varicella, and adenoviral infections.

Rubella infection (see Chap. 133) may present with a polyarthritis, usually involving the fingers, wrists, and knees symmetrically. The arthritis is seen most often in young adults, especially women. Arthritis is also observed in children and young adults after vaccination with live, attenuated rubella vaccine, and is similar to that observed with natural disease. The onset of arthritis coincides with or shortly follows the appearance of the rash. The arthritis lasts up to 2 weeks or occasionally a month. In a few patients, the arthritis may be recurrent for months to years. Permanent joint damage does not usually occur even with chronic disease. Joint effusions are usually small, and synovial fluid shows mild leukocytosis with either lymphoctyes or neutrophils predominating. Rheumatoid factor tests may be positive.

Arthritis is a relatively common manifestation of type B hepatitis (serum hepatitis). It is often accompanied by a rash, may precede the onset of clinical jaundice by a few days to 2 weeks, or coincide with the appearance of jaundice. Jaundice may not appear in some patients with arthritis; however, liver function tests are abnormal in such patients. The rash is most often urticarial, but can be macular, papular, or petechial. The onset of arthritis is usually abrupt, with symmetric involvement of both small and large joints. The most commonly involved joints are the fingers, followed by the knee, shoulder, ankle, elbow, and wrist. The arthritis can also be asymmetric or migratory. Permanent joint damage does not occur. Synovial fluid shows a varying degree of leukocytosis with polymorphonuclear cells. Rheumatoid factor tests usually are negative.

Serum and joint fluid complement levels are usually low during arthritis. Serum complement level returns to normal with the appearance of overt liver disease. Hepatitis B antigen (Australia antigen, hepatitis-associated antigen) can usually be detected in both serum and joint fluid during the prodromal period of hepatitis. The synovitis is thought to be induced by immune complexes consisting of viral antigens and their antibodies.

LYME DISEASE Lyme disease is a multisystem disorder caused by a spirochete transmitted by the bite of *Ixodes dammini* or related ticks. The spirochete has been recovered from skin lesions, blood, and cerebrospinal fluid. The disease is characterized by skin lesions and neurologic and cardiac abnormalities and arthritis. It is described in detail in Chap. 127.

REFERENCES

GOLDENBERG DL, REED JI: Bacterial arthritis. N Engl J Med 312:764, 1985

HOFFMAN GS: Mycobacterial and fungal infections of bones and joints, in *Textbook of Rheumatology*, WN Kelley et al (eds). Philadelphia, Saunders, 1985, pp 1527–1540

JOHNSTON YE et al: Lyme arthritis: Spirochetes found in synovial microangiopathic lesions. Am J Pathol 118:26, 1985

SCHNITZER TJ: Viral arthritis, in *Textbook of Rheumatology*, WN Kelley et al (eds), Philadelphia, Saunders, 1985, pp 1540–1556

STEERE AC, MALAWISTA SE: Lyme disease, in *Textbook of Rheumatology*, WN Kelley et al (eds). Philadelphia, Saunders, 1985, pp 1557–1563

278 MISCELLANEOUS ARTHRITIDES AND EXTRAARTICULAR RHEUMATISM

BRUCE C. GILLILAND

NEUROPATHIC JOINT DISEASE Neuropathic joint disease (Charcot's joint) is a severe form of osteoarthritis associated with loss of pain sensation, proprioception, or both. In addition, normal muscular reflexes which modulate joint movement are decreased. Without these protective mechanisms, joints are subjected to repeated trauma, resulting in progressive cartilage damage. The distribution of joint involvement depends on the underlying neurologic disorder. In tabes dorsalis, knees, hips, and ankles are most commonly affected; in syringomyelia, the glenohumeral joint, elbow, and wrist; and in diabetes mellitus, the tarsal and tarsometatarsal joints. Resorption of metatarsals and phalanges is also seen in diabetic patients. In children, neuropathic joint disease is caused by congenital indifference to pain or meningomyelocele. Neuropathic joint disease is also observed in patients with amyloidosis and leprosy or following repeated intraarticular glucocorticoid injections. The mechanism of injury in this situation is thought to be an analgesic effect of steroids leading to overuse of a previously damaged joint which results in accelerated cartilage deterioration.

Neuropathic joint disease usually begins in a single joint and then progresses to involve other joints, depending on the underlying neurologic disorder. The involved joint progressively becomes enlarged from bony overgrowth and synovial effusion. Loose bodies may be palpated in the joint cavity. Joint instability, subluxation, and crepitus occur as the disease progresses. Charcot's joints may develop rapidly, and a totally disorganized joint with multiple bony fragments may evolve in a patient within weeks or days. The amount of pain experienced by the patient is less than would be anticipated based on the degree of joint involvement. Patients may experience sudden joint pain from intraarticular fractures of osteophytes or condyles. Initially, radiographs show early features of osteoarthritis followed subsequently by marked destructive and hypertrophic changes. Large, bizarre-shaped osteophytes and intraarticular bone fragments are observed. The radiographic findings of the diabetic Charcot's foot may be difficult to distinguish from those of osteomyelitis. Osteomyelitis is often suspected when the diabetic patient has an infected cutaneous ulcer on the foot. The Charcot's joint radiographically shows osteopenia, sharp cortical margins, and severe disruption and disorganization of the midtarsal and tarsometatarsal joints. In osteomyelitis, the bone margins are indistinct. The synovial fluid is usually noninflammatory, may be bloody or xanthochromic, and may contain fragments of synovium, cartilage, and/or bone.

The primary focus of treatment is to provide stabilization of the joint. Treatment of the underlying disorder, even if successful, usually does not alter the joint disease. Braces and splints are helpful. Their use requires close surveillance since patients may be unable to appreciate pressure from a poorly adjusted brace. Fusion of a very unstable joint may improve function, but nonunion is frequent especially when immobilization of the joint is inadequate.

RELAPSING POLYCHONDRITIS Relapsing polychrondritis is an inflammatory disorder of unknown etiology affecting cartilaginous structures as well as the cardiovascular system, eyes, and ears. The onset is usually between 40 and 60 years of age and the disorder occurs predominantly in whites. No familial tendency is apparent, and both sexes are equally affected.

Histologically, the cartilage matrix has decreased basophilic staining indicating a loss of glucosaminoglycans. Lymphocytes and plasma cells are found at the edge of cartilage destruction. Granulation tissue invades degenerating cartilage followed by fibrosis. Both humoral and cell-mediated immunity are considered to be operative in tissue damage.

The cartilage of the ears and nose is involved in 80 to 90 percent of patients. The patient may experience the sudden onset of pain, tenderness, and swelling of the cartilaginous portion of the ear. Prolonged or recurrent episodes lead to floppy ears and saddle deformity of the nose. Swelling may narrow the external auditory meatus, interfering with hearing. The eustachian tube may also be closed off, leading to otitis media. Arteritis of the internal auditory artery and its cochlear branch produces hearing loss, vertigo, ataxia, nausea, and vomiting.

Eye manifestations include conjunctivitis, episcleritis, scleritis, and iritis. Oral and/or genital ulcerations may occur. Patients also may experience an episodic nondeforming polyarthritis which lasts a few days to several weeks and involves both large and small peripheral joints. Synovial fluid is noninflammatory. Destruction of the cartilage in the larynx and trachea leads to hoarseness and stridor and may necessitate tracheostomy. Respiratory insufficiency and recurrent pulmonary infections develop because of collapse of the supporting bronchial cartilage rings. Aortic regurgitation occurs in 25 percent of patients, predominantly men, and is due to progressive dilatation of the aortic ring or to destruction of the valve cusps. Other heart valves can be affected. Vasculitis of either medium or large vessels may lead to aneurysm formation and thrombosis. Focal proliferative glomerulonephritis may occur, and in some patients may dominate the clinical picture. The clinical course is highly variable. The prognosis usually depends on the extent of pulmonary and cardiac involvement.

A mild leukocytosis and a normocytic, normochromic anemia may be present. The erythrocyte sedimentation rate is usually elevated. Rheumatoid factor and antinuclear antibody tests may be positive, and circulating immune complexes have been identified in some patients. Radiographs may show calcifications in the cartilage of the nose, larynx, and trachea. Bronchography and computed tomography can be used to demonstrate tracheal stenosis and bronchial narrowing.

The diagnosis is based on the recognition of the typical clinical features. Biopsy of involved cartilage from the ear, nose, or respiratory tract will confirm the diagnosis but is only necessary when clinical features are not typical. Polychondritis may be associated with a variety of connective tissue disorders including systemic vasculitis (Wegener's granulomatosis, Takayasu's arteritis), rheumatoid arthritis, or systemic lupus erythematosus. The connective tissue disorder usually precedes polychrondritis by months to years. It is not clear whether this association represents two separate disorders which coexist or whether the polychrondritis is a manifestation of one of these connective tissue disorders.

Prednisone in a dose of 40 to 60 mg per day is often effective in suppressing disease activity and is tapered gradually once the disease is controlled. If not controlled by steroids, cyclophosphamide or azathioprine may be beneficial.

HYPERTROPHIC OSTEOARTHROPATHY Hypertrophic osteoarthropathy is characterized by the presence of periosteal new bone formation, clubbing of the digits, and arthritis. In adults, this syndrome is seen almost always in its secondary form associated with a pulmonary neoplasm; rarely, it is seen with chronic lung or liver disease. In children, it occurs in association with a variety of congenital heart, lung, and liver conditions. Idiopathic and familial forms also occur in which no underlying associated disorder can be found.

In hypertrophic osteoarthropathy, the periosteum is elevated. Mononuclear cell infiltration is present in the adjacent soft tissue. New bone is deposited beneath the periosteum while at the same time endosteal bone is resorbed. These changes occur primarily at the distal ends of metacarpals, metatarsals, and the long bones. Occasionally, scapulas, clavicles, ribs, and pelvic bones are also affected. Proliferation of connective tissue occurs in the nail bed and soft tissue of the volar pad of the digits, giving the distal phalanges a clubbed appearance. The small blood vessels are dilated and thickened. The number of arteriovenous anastomoses in the soft tissue of the digits is increased. The synovium of involved joints is edematous and may contain a mild infiltration of lymphocytes and plasma cells.

The etiology of hypertrophic osteoarthropathy is unknown. Stimulation of the vagal neural arc is suggested by the reversal of this syndrome by vagotomy. Furthermore, disorders associated frequently with clubbing have in common sites of involvement innervated in part by the vagus. A circulating vasodilator, hormones, or immune complexes have also been proposed as etiologic factors.

While hypertrophic osteoarthropathy is usually associated with clubbing, it can occur alone either in primary or secondary forms. Primary clubbing occurs in familial and idiopathic forms. Secondary clubbing is most often associated with chronic bronchitis, diffuse infiltrative diseases of the lung, and bacterial endocarditis, and usually has a more rapid onset than primary clubbing.

The syndrome of hypertrophic osteoarthropathy is less common, occurring most often in association with bronchogenic carcinoma and is also observed with the disorders mentioned above. It occurs rarely with metastases to the lung or with pleural tumors. The frequent occurrence of hypertrophic osteoarthropathy with pulmonary disorders has led to this syndrome being referred to as hypertrophic pulmonary osteoarthropathy. The number of cases associated with chronic pulmonary infections has declined markedly with early diagnosis and effective antibiotic therapy.

Hyperthyroidism may occasionally be associated with clubbing and periostitis of the bones of the hands and feet. The condition is referred to as *thyroid acropachy*. Periostitis is asymptomatic and occurs in the midshaft and diaphyseal portion of the metacarpal and phalangeal bones. The long bones of the extremities are seldom affected.

Familial hypertrophic osteoarthropathy, also referred to as *pachydermoperiostosis,* usually begins insidiously during puberty and is characterized by thickening of the skin of the face, scalp, and extremities along with features of hypertrophic osteoarthropathy. The skin of the face and scalp is greasy, and excessive sweating of the palms and soles occurs. The distal extremities are enlarged due to proliferation of new bone and connective tissue. The disorder is inherited as an autosomal dominant with variable expression.

The onset of hypertrophic osteoarthropathy is often insidious and may precede clinical features of the associated disorder by months. The onset is more rapid than in the idiopathic syndrome or clubbing alone. Patients may experience burning pain or deep aching in the distal extremities which is aggravated by dependency and relieved by elevation of the affected limbs. Joint manifestations vary from arthralgias to severe pain and swelling, most often affecting metacarpophalangeal and metatarsophalangeal joints, wrists, ankles, and knees. The skin over the distal extremities may be warm, erythematous, and edematous. Pressure applied over the distal ends of the forearms and legs may be quite painful. Clubbing of digits is manifested by widening of the fingertips, enlargement of the distal volar pads, convexity of the nail, and loss of the normal 15° angle between the nail and cuticle. The nails and surrounding skin become shiny. Nails become brittle and grow more rapidly.

The laboratory abnormalities reflect the underlying disorder. The synovial fluid of involved joints has less than 500 predominantly mononuclear white cells per cubic millimeter. Radiographs show periosteal thickening with new bone formation along the shaft of long bones at their distal ends. The ends of the distal phalanges show hypertrophic changes and in more advanced cases, osteolysis. Radionuclide studies show pericortical linear uptake along the shafts of long bones which may be present in advance of any x-ray changes.

The treatment of hypertrophic osteoarthropathy is to identify the associated disorder and treat it appropriately. Symptoms and signs of hypertrophic osteoarthropathy may disappear completely with removal or effective chemotherapy of a tumor or with antibiotic therapy and drainage of a chronic pulmonary infection. Vagotomy or percutaneous block of the vagus nerve may be beneficial in some patients. Aspirin, other nonsteroidal inflammatory drugs, or analgesics may help control symptoms of hypertrophic osteoarthropathy.

FIBROSITIS Fibrositis is a commonly encountered disorder characterized by pain, aching, and stiffness of the trunk and extremities and the presence of a number of specific tender sites. The disorder is more common in women between the ages of 25 and 45 years. The etiology is unknown, but may be produced or exacerbated by a sleep disturbance. Symptoms of fibrositis were produced in normal subjects by disturbing normal slow wave sleep with a buzzer without awakening them.

Symptoms are generalized aching and stiffness, often referred to muscle and bony prominences. Patients may feel that their joints are swollen; however, joint examination is normal. Patients complain of exhaustion and wake up tired. They also awake frequently at night and have difficulty falling asleep. Patients often attribute their lack of a refreshing night's sleep to pain. Some complain of urinary frequency and a sensation of bladder fullness. Irritable bowel syndrome has been associated with fibrositis.

The characteristic physical feature is the demonstration of specific tender sites or trigger points, which are exquisitely more tender than adjacent areas. The patient may suddenly jump or withdraw when the site is palpated. The sites of tenderness are remarkably constant in location. Common sites of tenderness are over the midpoint of the upper fold of the trapezius, lateral epicondyles, supraspinatus, lower cervical spine, lumbar spine, posterior iliac spine, costochondral junctions, especially the second, gluteus maximus, and medial fat pad of the knee. Skinfold tenderness may be present, particularly over the upper scapular region. Tender subcutaneous nodules may be felt in these regions. Nodules in similar location are present in normal persons but are not tender.

The diagnosis of fibrositis is made by recognizing the clinical manifestations. The joint and muscle examination is normal, and there are no laboratory abnormalties. The disease must be distinguished from polymyositis, in which weakness occurs and muscle enzyme levels are elevated, and from polymyalgia rheumatica, in which pain and an elevated sedimentation rate are present.

Patients should be informed that they have a treatable condition which is not a crippling, deforming, or degenerative process. Salicylates or other nonsteroidal anti-inflammatory drugs along with a benzodiazepine at bedtime may help. The sleep disturbance may improve with the use of tricyclic agents such as amitriptyline or imipramine. These drugs are more effective if taken early in the evening instead of at bedtime. Local measures such as heat, massage, injection of trigger points with corticosteroids or lidocaine, or acupuncture may help to relieve pain. Fibrositis can occur in patients with rheumatoid arthritis or other connective tissue diseases and should be treated appropriately.

PSYCHOGENIC RHEUMATISM Patients may experience severe joint pain involving a few to several joints without physical findings of arthritis. These patients are often convinced that they have rheumatoid arthritis or systemic lupus erythematosus. This disorder is recognized by the inconsistencies, exaggerations, and emotional lability of the patient during the history and physical examination. Laboratory studies are normal. Organic disease needs to be excluded, which requires seeing the patient at intervals. This condition also needs to be distinguished from fibrositis. Anti-inflammatory or other drugs are not helpful.

CARPAL TUNNEL SYNDROME Carpal tunnel syndrome is an entrapment neuropathy of the median nerve at the wrist producing paresthesias and weakness in the hands. The syndrome is caused by pressure on the median nerve where it passes in company with the flexor tendons of the fingers through the tunnel formed by carpal bones and the transverse carpal ligament.

Compression of the median nerve is produced by any process that encroaches on the carpal tunnel. Localized tenosynovitis of the flexor tendons of the fingers is a frequent cause of carpal tunnel syndrome, particularly in middle-aged women. Premenstrual edema or edema occurring in pregnancy may also cause these symptoms. Symptoms can be precipitated by activities which require repeated flexion, pronation, and supination of the wrist, for example, sewing, driving, and operating computers. Other causes of carpal tunnel syndrome include trauma, tuberculosis, rheumatoid arthritis, gout, acromegaly, hypothyroidism, and amyloidosis.

Patients experience numbness or paresthesias of the palmar surface of the thumb, index, middle, and radial half of the ring finger. Numbness or paresthesias of the whole hand may occur. Pain may be referred to the forearm and less commonly to the shoulder and neck regions. Pain or tingling of the fingers often occurs at night and is relieved by shaking the hand. Weakness and atrophy of the thenar muscles usually appear later and can occur without significant sensory symptoms.

Thenar muscle weakness is manifested by decreased strength of abduction, opposition, and flexion of the thumb. On examination, symptoms of paresthesia or pain in the fingers may be reproduced by percussion over the volar surface of the wrist (Tinel's sign) or by full flexion of the wrist for over 1 min (Phalen's maneuver). Decreased touch or hyperpathia to pinprick may be demonstrated over the fingers supplied by the median nerve. Nerve conduction studies of the median nerve show delayed latency across the wrist, confirming the diagnosis.

Treatment of patients with only sensory symptoms and minor nerve conduction abnormalities consists of wrist splints to be worn mainly at night, anti-inflammatory drugs, and local injection of steroids. If symptoms persist or motor abnormalities are present, surgical decompression of the carpal tunnel with release of the transverse carpal ligament and debridement is indicated.

REFLEX SYMPATHETIC DYSTROPHY SYNDROME The reflex sympathetic dystrophy syndrome (RSDS) is characterized by pain and tenderness usually of a distal extremity accompanied by signs and symptoms of vasomotor instability, trophic skin changes, and the rapid development of bony demineralization. A precipitating event can be identified in two-thirds of the cases. These include local trauma, myocardial infarction, strokes, and peripheral nerve injuries. RSDS is observed most often in individuals over the age of 50, reflecting the frequency of the underlying disorder. The sex distribution is equal. An entire hand or foot is usually affected. Occasionally, RSDS will involve an isolated site such as the patella, hip, or one or two rays of a foot or hand. The contralateral side may be affected in up to 50 percent of patients, and subclinical disease may be present in virtually all patients.

The first clinical manifestation of RSDS is pain and swelling of a distal extremity which develops weeks to months following the precipitating event. The pain is of a burning quality (causalgia). The involved extremity is warm, edematous, and tender especially around joints. Increased sweating and hair growth are observed. Later in the course, the skin becomes thin, shiny, and cool. Flexion contractures of the fingers develop, and thickening of the palmar fascia results in a Dupuytren's contracture. The shoulder on the involved side frequently becomes painful and restricted in motion (shoulder-hand syndrome).

The course of RSDS is divided into three overlapping phases. The first phase, which lasts 3 to 6 months, is characterized by pain, swelling, warmth, and sweating of the involved extremity, followed later by a cool shiny skin in the second phase. In the third phase, the skin and subcutaneous tissue become atrophic, and irreversible flexion contractures of the hand or foot develop. Fluctuation occurs between the first two phases during which time the disorder is potentially reversible if treated.

The laboratory abnormalities are those of the associated disorder. Radiographs of the involved distal extremity demonstrate mottled osteopenia referred to as Sudeck's atrophy. Later in the course, diffuse osteopenia develops. Similar changes, however, are observed in an immobilized limb following a fracture or paralysis. Bone scans with radionuclides show increased uptake in periarticular bone on the involved side. Uptake may also be increased on the contralateral side indicating subclinical involvement.

Early recognition and treatment are important to prevent permanent disability. Appropriate mobilization of the patient following a myocardial infarction, stroke, or injury may help to prevent this syndrome. Pain should be properly controlled. Application of heat or cold along with exercises are useful. Sympathetic nerve block may be effective and if it is, can be followed by surgical sympathectomy. The response, however, may not be sustained. A short course of high-dose prednisone in conjunction with physical therapy has been beneficial in some patients. Prednisone is started at 60 mg for 4 days and gradually tapered over a 3-week period.

TSIETZE'S SYNDROME Tsietze's syndrome is manifested by painful swelling of one or more costochondral articulations. Age of onset is usually before 40, and both sexes are equally affected. Most patients have only one joint involved, usually the second or third costochondral joint. The onset of anterior chest pain may be sudden or gradual. The pain may radiate to the arms or shoulder and is aggravated by sneezing, coughing, deep inspirations, or twisting motions of the chest. The term *costochondritis* is often used interchangeably with Tsietze's syndrome, but some restrict the former term to pain of the costochondral articulations without swelling. This disorder is observed in patients over age 40, tends to affect the third, fourth, and fifth costochondral joints, and occurs more often in women. Both syndromes may mimic cardiac or upper abdominal causes of pain. Rheumatoid arthritis, ankylosing spondylitis, or Reiter's syndrome may involve costochondral joints but are distinguished easily by their clinical features. Other skeletal causes of anterior chest wall pain are xyphodynia and the slipping rib syndome, which usually involves the tenth rib. Analgesics, anti-inflammatory drugs, or local steroid injections usually relieve symptoms.

MUSCULOSKELETAL DISORDERS ASSOCIATED WITH HYPERLIPIDEMIA Patients with familial hypercholesterolemia (type II hyperlipidemia) may experience a recurrent transient migratory arthritis involving the proximal interphalangeal joints, knees, ankles, wrists, shoulders, or elbows. Achilles tendinitis may also be present. The onset of arthritis is sudden and lasts approximately 48 h in each affected joint. The episodes of arthritis are of approximately 1-week duration, and several attacks occur a year without residual joint deformity. Patients may also have tendinous xanthomas in the Achilles, patellar, and extensor tendons of the hands and feet, and tuberous xanthomas over the elbows, knees, or buttocks. A mild inflammatory arthritis affecting a few peripheral joints in an asymmetric pattern has been observed in a few patients with familial hypertriglyceridemia (type IV hyperlipidemia). Large juxtaarticular bone cysts have been noted in a few patients. The cause of arthritis in both groups of patients is not known. Analgesics or anti-inflammatory drugs provide relief of symptoms.

PERIARTICULAR DISORDERS **Bursitis** Bursitis is inflammation of a bursa, which is a thin-walled sac lined with synovial tissue. The function of the bursa is to facilitate movement of tendons and muscles over bony prominences. Excessive frictional forces, trauma, systemic disease (e.g., rheumatoid arthritis, gout), or infection may cause bursitis. Subacromial bursitis (subdeltoid bursitis) is the most common form of bursitis. Another is trochanteric bursitis, which involves the bursa around the insertion of the gluteus medius to the greater trochanter of the femur. Patients experience pain over the lateral aspect of the hip and upper thigh and are tender over the posterior aspect of the greater trochanter. External rotation and resisted abduction of the hip elicit pain. Olecranon bursitis occurs over the posterior elbow, and when the area is acutely inflamed, infection should be excluded. Achilles bursitis involves the bursa located above the insertion of the tendon to the calcaneus and results from wearing tight shoes. Ischial bursitis (weaver's bottom) affects the bursa separating the gluteus medius from the ischial tuberosity and develops from prolonged sitting on hard surfaces. Anserine bursitis is an inflammation of the sartorius bursa over the medial side of the tibia just below the knee and is manifested by pain on climbing stairs. Tenderness is present over the insertion of the conjoint tendon of the sartorius, gracilis, and semitendinosus. Prepatellar bursitis (housemaid's knee) occurs over the patellar tendon and is caused by kneeling on hard surfaces. Treatment of bursitis consists of prevention of the aggravating condition, rest of the involved part, a nonsteroidal anti-inflammatory drug, and local steroid injection.

Rotator cuff tendinitis Tendinitis of the rotator cuff is the major cause of a painful shoulder. Of the tendons forming the rotator cuff, the supraspinatus tendon is most often affected, probably because of its repeated impingement between the acromion and humeral head as well as its reduced blood supply occurring with abduction of the arm. The process evolves through inflammation, fibrosis, and tears of the tendon. Symptoms usually occur after injury or overuse, particularly in individuals over age 40. Patients complain of a dull aching in the shoulder that may interfere with sleep. Severe pain is experienced when the arm is actively abducted into an overhead position. Tenderness is present over the lateral aspect of the humeral head just below the acromion. Nonsteroidal anti-inflammatory drugs, local steroid injection, and physical therapy may relieve symptoms.

Patients may tear the supraspinatus tendon acutely by falling on an outstretched arm or lifting a heavy object. Symptoms are pain, along with weakness of abduction and external rotation of the shoulder. Atrophy of the supraspinatus muscles develops. The diagnosis is established by arthrogram. Surgical repair may be necessary in patients who fail to respond to conservative measures.

Calcific tendinitis This is characterized by deposition of calcium salts, primarily hydroxyapatite, within a tendon. The exact mechanism for calcification is not known but may be due to ischemia or degeneration of the tendon. The supraspinatus tendon is most often affected because of its frequent impingement and reduced blood supply when the arm is abducted. It usually develops after age 40. Calcification within the tendon may evoke acute inflammation, producing sudden and severe pain in the shoulder. Tendon calcification, however, may be asymptomatic or not related to the patient's symptoms.

Bicipital tendinitis and rupture Bicipital tendinitis, or tenosynovitis, is produced by friction on the tendon of the long head of the biceps as it passes through the bicipital groove. When the inflammation is acute, patients experience anterior shoulder pain which radiates down the biceps into the forearm. Abduction and internal rotation of the arm are painful and limited. The bicipital groove is very tender to palpation. Pain may be elicited along the course of the tendon by resisting supination of the forearm with the elbow at 90° (Yergason's supination sign). Acute rupture of the tendon may occur with vigorous exercise of the arm and is often painful. In a young patient, it should be repaired surgically. Rupture of the tendon in an older person may be associated with little or no pain and is recognized by the presence of persistent swelling of the biceps (''Popeye'' muscle). Surgery is usually not necessary in this setting.

Adhesive capsulitis Often referred to as ''frozen shoulder,'' adhesive capsulitis is characterized by pain and restricted movement of the shoulder usually in the absence of intrinsic shoulder disease. Adhesive capsulitis, however, may follow bursitis or tendinitis of the shoulder or be associated with systemic disorders such as chronic pulmonary disease, myocardial infarction, and diabetes mellitus. Prolonged immobility of the arm contributes to the development of adhesive capsulitis, and reflex sympathetic distrophy is thought to be a pathogenic factor. The capsule of the shoulder is thickened, and a mild chronic inflammatory infiltrate and fibrosis may be present.

Adhesive capsulitis occurs more commonly in women after age 50. Pain and stiffness usually develop gradually over several months to a year, but may progress rapidly in some patients. Pain may interfere with sleep. The shoulder is tender to palpation, and both active and passive movement are restricted. Radiograph of the shoulder shows osteopenia. The diagnosis is confirmed by arthrogram, in that only a limited amount of contrast material, usually less than 15 mL, can be injected under pressure into the shoulder joint.

The majority of patients improve spontaneously 12 to 18 months after the onset of disease, but some may have permanent restriction of movement. Early mobilization of the arm following an injury to the shoulder may prevent the development of this disease. Slow but forceful injection of contrast material into the joint may lyse adhesions and stretch the capsule, resulting in improvement of shoulder motion. Manipulation under anesthesia may be helpful in some patients. Once established, therapy may have little effect on the natural course of the disease. Local injections of corticosteroids, nonsteroidal anti-inflammatory drugs, and physical therapy may provide relief of symptoms.

TUMORS OF JOINTS Primary tumors and tumorlike disorders of synovium are uncommon but should be considered in the differential diagnosis of monarticular joint disease. In addition, metastases to bone and primary bone tumors adjacent to a joint may produce joint symptoms.

Pigmented villonodular synovitis is characterized by exuberant proliferation of synovial cells usually involving a single joint. It occurs most often in young adults and affects both sexes equally. The etiology of this disorder is unknown.

The synovium is a brownish color and has numerous large, fingerlike villi which fuse to form pedunculated nodules. There is marked hyperplasia of synovial cells within the stroma of the villi. Hemosiderin granules and lipids are found in the cytoplasm of macrophages and in the interstitial tissue. Multinucleated giant cells may be present. The proliferative synovium grows into the subsynovial tissue and invades adjacent cartilage and bone.

The clinical picture of pigmented villonodular synovitis is characterized by the insidious onset of swelling and pain in one joint, most commonly the knee. Other joints affected include the hips, ankles, calcaneocuboid joints, elbows, and small joints of the fingers or toes. The disease may also involve the common flexor sheath of the hand. Symptoms may be mild, intermittent, and present for years before the patient seeks medical attention. Radiographs may show joint space narrowing, erosions, and subchondral cysts. The joint fluid contains blood and is dark-red or almost black in color. Lipid containing macrophages may be present in the fluid. The joint fluid may be clear if hemorrhages have not occurred.

The treatment of pigmented villonodular synovitis is complete synovectomy. With incomplete synovectomy, the villondular synovitis recurs, and the rate of tissue growth may be faster than occurred originally. Irradiation of the involved joint has been successful in some patients.

Synovial chondromatosis is a disorder characterized by multiple focal metaplastic growths of normal-appearing cartilage in the synovium or tendon sheath. Segments of cartilage break loose and continue to grow as loose bodies. When calcification and ossification of loose bodies occur, the disorder is referred to as synovial osteochondromatosis. The disorder is usually monarticular and affects young to middle-aged individuals. The knee is most often involved followed by hip, elbow, and shoulder. Symptoms are pain, swelling, and decreased motion of the joint. Radiographs may show several rounded calcifications within the joint cavity. Treatment is synovectomy; however, the tumor may recur.

Hemangiomas occur in synovium and in tendon sheaths. The knee is affected most commonly. Recurrent episodes of joint swelling and pain usually begin in childhood. The joint fluid is bloody. Treatment is excision of the lesion. *Lipomas* occur most often in the knee, originating in the subsynovial fat on either side of the patellar tendon. Lipomas also appear in tendon sheaths of the hands, wrists, feet, and ankles.

Synovial sarcoma (malignant synovioma) is a neoplasm of connective origin arising from tissue adjacent to large joints and seldom from the joint itself. It occurs most often in young adults and is more common in men. The tumor presents as a slowly growing mass near a joint, without much pain. The tumor spreads along tissue planes. The most common site of visceral metastasis is lung. The diagnosis is made by biopsy. Treatment is wide resection of the tumor including adjacent muscle and regional lymph nodes. Amputation of the involved distal extremity may be required. Chemotherapy may be beneficial in some patients with metastatic disease.

Synovial chondrosarcoma may arise in the synovium, tendon sheath, or bursa and is very rare. Treatment is radical excision or amputation.

REFERENCES

ALTMAN RD, TENENBAUM J: Hypertrophic osteoarthropathy, in *Textbook of Rheumatology*, WN Kelley et al (eds). Philadelphia, Saunders, 1985, chap 103, pp 1594–1603

HERMAN JH: Polychondritis, in *Textbook of Rheumatology*, WN Kelley et al (eds). Philadelphia, Saunders, 1985, chap 91, pp 1458–1467

KOZIN F et al: The reflex sympathetic dystrophy syndrome (RSDS). III. Scintigraphic studies, further evidence for the therapeutic efficacy of systemic corticosteroids, and proposed diagnostic criteria. Am J Med 70:23, 1982

MYERS BW et al: Pigmented villonodular synovitis and tenosynovitis: A clinical epidemiologic study of 166 cases and literature review. Medicine 59:223, 1980

NEER CS II: Impingement lesions. Clin Orthop 173:70, 1983

RODNAN GP: Neuropathic joint disease (Charcot joints), in *Arthritis and Allied Conditions*, 9th ed, DJ McCarty (ed). Philadelphia, Lea & Febiger, 1979, chap 58, pp 892–904

ROONEY PJ et al: Transient polyarthritis associated with familial hyperbetalipoproteinemia. Q J Med 47:249, 1978

SCHILLER AL: Tumors and tumor-like lesions involving joints, in *Textbook of Rheumatology*, WN Kelley et al (eds). Philadelphia, Saunders, 1985, chap 108, pp 1711–1732

SCHUMACHER HR JR: Articular manifestations of hypertrophic pulmonary osteoarthropathy in bronchogenic carcinoma: A clinical and pathological study. Arthritis Rheum 19:629, 1976

THORNHILL TS: The painful shoulder, in *Textbook of Rheumatology*, WN Kelley et al (eds). Philadelphia, Saunders, 1985, chap 29, pp 435–448

YUNUS M et al: Primary fibromyalgia (fibrositis): Clinical study of 50 patients with matched normal controls. Semin Arthritis Rheum 11:151, 1981

PART NINE HEMATOLOGY AND ONCOLOGY

section 1 Clotting disorders

279 DISORDERS OF THE PLATELET AND VESSEL WALL

ROBERT I. HANDIN

Patients with platelet or vessel wall disorders usually bleed into superficial sites such as the skin, mucous membranes, genitourinary tract, and gastrointestinal tract. Bleeding begins immediately after trauma and either responds to simple measures like pressure and packing or requires therapy with corticosteroids, plasma fractions, or platelet concentrates. The most common platelet/vessel wall disorders are (1) various forms of thrombocytopenia, (2) von Willebrand's disease, and (3) drug-induced platelet dysfunction. This chapter reviews the diagnosis and treatment of quantitative and qualitative platelet disorders as well as vessel wall defects which cause bleeding. The physiology of normal hemostasis and the cardinal manifestations of bleeding from the primary hemostatic disorders have been reviewed in Chap. 54.

PLATELET PRODUCTION AND KINETICS Platelets arise from the fragmentation of megakaryocytes, which are very large, polyploid bone marrow cells produced by several cycles of chromosomal duplication without cytoplasmic division. After leaving the marrow space, approximately one-third of the platelets are sequestered in the spleen, while the other two-thirds circulates for 7 to 10 days. Normally, only a small fraction of the platelet mass is consumed in the process of hemostasis, so that most platelets circulate until they become senescent and are removed by phagocytic cells. The normal blood platelet count is maintained between 150,000 and 450,000 per cubic millimeter. Although the regulatory signals are not well-defined, a decrease in platelet mass stimulates an increase in the number, size, and ploidy of megakaryocytes releasing additional platelets into the circulation.

The platelet count varies during the menstrual cycle, rising following ovulation and falling at the onset of menses. It is also influenced by the patient's nutritional state and can be decreased in severe iron, folic acid, or vitamin B_{12} deficiency. Platelets are *acute phase reactants* and patients with systemic inflammation, tumors, bleeding, and mild iron deficiency may have an increased platelet count, a benign condition called *secondary or reactive thrombocytosis*. In contrast, the increase in platelet count that is characteristic of the myeloproliferative disorders such as polycythemia vera, chronic myelogenous leukemia, myeloid metaplasia, and essential thrombocytosis can cause either severe bleeding or thrombosis.

MECHANISM OF THROMBOCYTOPENIA Thrombocytopenia is caused by one of three mechanisms—decreased bone marrow production, increased splenic sequestration, or accelerated destruction of platelets. In order to determine the etiology of thrombocytopenia, each patient should have a careful examination of the peripheral blood film, an assessment of marrow morphology by examination of an aspirate or biopsy, and an estimate of splenic size by bedside palpation. A scheme for classifying patients with thrombocytopenia based on these clinical observations and laboratory tests is outlined in Fig. 279-1.

Impaired production Disorders that injure stem cells or prevent their proliferation in marrow frequently cause thrombocytopenia. They usually affect multiple hematopoietic cell lines so that throm-

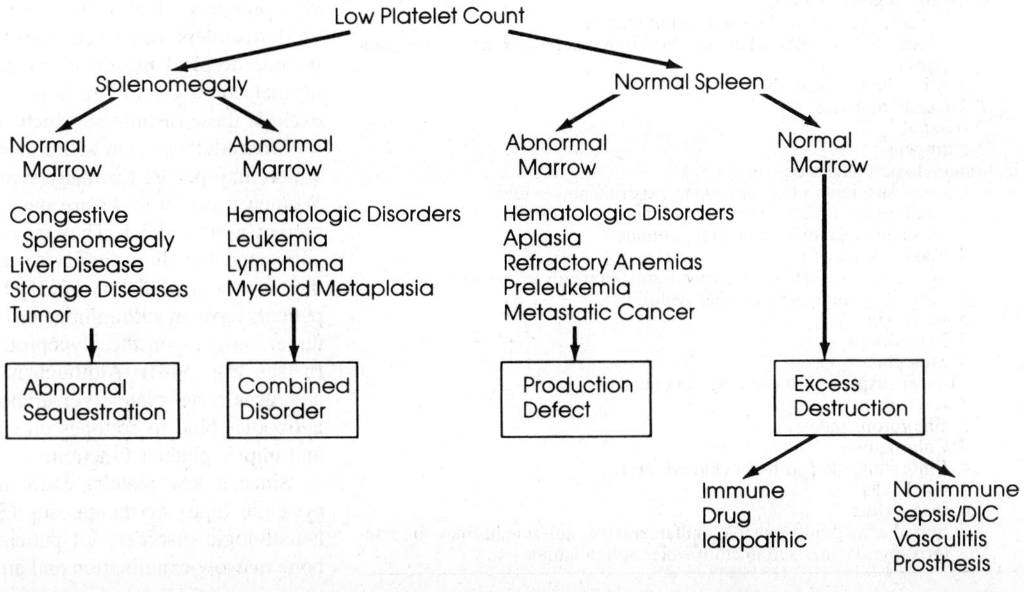

FIGURE 279-1 *The clinical evaluation of patients with thrombocytopenia [Modified from RI Handin, in W Beck (ed). Hematology, 4th ed, MIT Press, Cambridge, Mass., 1985.]*

bocytopenia is accompanied by varying degrees of anemia and leukopenia. Diagnosis of a platelet production defect is readily established by examination of a bone marrow aspirate or biopsy, which should show a reduced number of megakaryocytes. The most common causes of decreased platelet production are marrow aplasia, fibrosis, or infiltration with malignant cells; these produce highly characteristic marrow abnormalities. Occasionally, thrombocytopenia is the presenting laboratory abnormality in these disorders. Cytotoxic drugs, which are frequently used in cancer chemotherapy, impair megakaryocyte proliferation and maturation and frequently cause thrombocytopenia. There are also rare marrow disorders like congenital amegakaryocytic hypoplasia and thrombocytopenia with absent radii (TAR syndrome), which selectively decrease megakaryocyte production.

Splenic sequestration Since one-third of the platelet mass is normally sequestered in the spleen, splenectomy will increase the platelet count by 30 percent. In contrast, when the spleen enlarges, the fraction of sequestered platelets increases, lowering the platelet count. The most common causes of splenomegaly are portal hypertension secondary to liver disease, splenic infiltration with tumor cells in myeloproliferative or lymphoproliferative disorders, or with macrophages in storage disorders like Gaucher's disease. Isolated splenomegaly is rare and, in most patients, splenomegaly is accompanied by other clinical manifestations of the underlying disease. Many patients with leukemia, lymphoma, or a myeloproliferative syndrome have both marrow infiltration and splenomegaly and develop thrombocytopenia from a combination of impaired marrow production and splenic sequestration of platelets.

Accelerated destruction Abnormal vessels, fibrin thrombi, or intravascular prostheses can all shorten platelet survival and cause *nonimmunologic thrombocytopenia*. For example, thrombocytopenia is common in patients with vasculitis, the hemolytic uremic syndrome, thrombotic thrombocytopenic purpura (TTP), as a manifestation of disseminated intravascular coagulation (DIC), and in patients with prosthetic cardiac valves. In addition, platelets coated with antibody, immune complexes, or complement are rapidly cleared by mononuclear phagocytes in the spleen or other tissues inducing *immunologic thrombocytopenia*. The most common causes of immune thrombocytopenia are viral infections, drugs, and a chronic autoimmune disorder referred to as idiopathic thrombocytopenic purpura (ITP). These patients do not usually have splenomegaly and have an active bone marrow with an increased number of megakaryocytes.

TABLE 279-1 Drugs implicated in thrombocytopenia

I Suppression of platelet production
- *A* Myelosuppressive drugs
  - *1* Severe: cytosine arabinoside, daunorubicin
  - *2* Moderate: cyclophosphamide, busulfan, methotrexate, 6-mercaptopurine
  - *3* Mild: vinca alkaloids
- *B* Thiazide diuretics
- *C* Ethanol
- *D* Estrogens

II Immunologic platelet destruction
- *A* Clinical suspicion plus convincing experimental evidence
  - *1* Antibiotics: sulfathiazole, novobiocin, *p*-aminosalicylate
  - *2* Cinchona alkaloids: quinidine, quinine
  - *3* Foods: beans
  - *4* Sedatives, hypnotics, anticonvulsants: apronalide, carbamazepine
  - *5* Arsenical drugs used to treat syphilis
  - *6* Digitoxin
  - *7* Methyldopa
  - *8* Stibophen
- *B* Clinical suspicion (major drugs implicated)
  - *1* Aspirin
  - *2* Chlorpropamide
  - *3* Chloroquine
  - *4* Chlorothiazide and hydrochlorothiazide
  - *5* Gold salts
  - *6* Insecticides
  - *7* Sulfadiazine, sulfisoxazole, sulfamerazine, sulfamethazine, sulfamethoxypyridazine, sulfamethoxazole, sulfatolamide

DRUG-INDUCED THROMBOCYTOPENIA Many common drugs can cause thrombocytopenia (see Table 279-1). As previously mentioned, some chemotherapeutic agents are cytotoxic and depress megakaryocyte production. Ingestion of large quantities of alcohol has a similar marrow-depressing effect leading to transient thrombocytopenia, which is particularly common in binge drinkers. Thiazide diuretics, which are commonly used to treat hypertension or congestive heart failure, impair megakaryocyte production and can produce mild thrombocytopenia (50,000 to 100,000 per cubic millimeter), which may persist for several months after the drug is discontinued.

Most drugs induce thrombocytopenia by eliciting an immune response in which the platelet is an innocent bystander. The platelet is damaged by complement activation following the formation of drug-antibody complexes. Current laboratory tests can identify the causative agent in 10 percent of patients with clinical evidence of drug-induced thrombocytopenia. The best proof of a drug-induced etiology is a prompt rise in the platelet count when the suspected drug is discontinued. Patients with immune-mediated platelet destruction may also have a secondary increase in megakaryocyte number without other marrow abnormalities.

Although most patients recover within 7 to 10 days and do not require therapy, occasional patients with platelet counts below 10,000 to 20,000 per cubic millimeter have severe hemorrhage and may require temporary support with corticosteroids, plasmapheresis, or platelet transfusions while waiting for the platelet count to rise. A patient who has recovered from drug-induced immune thrombocytopenia should be instructed to avoid the offending drug in the future since only minute amounts of drug are needed to set up subsequent immune reactions. Certain drugs like diphenylhydantoin and gold salts may induce prolonged thrombocytopenia, since the drugs are cleared from body storage depots quite slowly.

IDIOPATHIC THROMBOCYTOPENIC PURPURA (ITP) The immune thrombocytopenias can be classified on the basis of the pathologic mechanism, the inciting agent, or the duration of the illness. The explosive onset of severe thrombocytopenia following recovery from a viral exanthem or upper respiratory illness is common in children and accounts for 90 percent of the pediatric cases of immune thrombocytopenia. This syndrome is usually called *acute idiopathic thrombocytopenic purpura* (Acute ITP). Of these patients, 60 percent recover in 4 to 6 weeks and over 90 percent recover within 3 to 6 months. Transient immune thrombocytopenia also complicates some cases of infectious mononucleosis, acute toxoplasmosis, or cytomegalovirus infection and can be part of the prodromal phase of viral hepatitis. Acute ITP is rare in adults and accounts for less than 10 percent of postpubertal patients with immune thrombocytopenia. Acute ITP is caused by immune complexes containing viral antigens which bind to platelet Fc receptors or by antibodies produced against viral antigens which cross react with the platelet. In addition to the viral disorders described above, the differential diagnosis should include atypical presentations of aplastic anemia, acute leukemias, or metastatic tumor. A bone marrow examination is essential to exclude these disorders, which can occasionally mimic acute ITP.

Most adults present with a more indolent form of thrombocytopenia which may persist for many years and is referred to as *chronic ITP*. Women aged 20 to 40 are most commonly afflicted and outnumber men by a ratio of 3:1. They may present with an abrupt fall in platelet count and bleeding similar to patients with acute ITP. More often they have a prior history of easy bruising or menometrorrhagia. These patients have an autoimmune disorder with antibodies directed against target antigens on the glycoprotein IIb-IIIa complex or glycoprotein Ib (see Fig. 54-2). Although most antibodies function as opsonins and accelerate platelet clearance by phagocytic cells, occasional antibodies bind to epitopes on critical regions of these glycoproteins and impair platelet function.

Since a low platelet count may be the initial manifestation of systemic lupus erythematosus (SLE) or the first sign of a primary hematologic disorder, all patients with chronic ITP should have a bone marrow examination and an antinuclear antibody determination.

In addition, patients with hepatic or splenic enlargement, lymphadenopathy, or atypical lymphocytes should have serologic studies for hepatitis, cytomegalovirus, Epstein-Barr virus, toxoplasma, and HTLV III.

Treatment of patients with ITP must be planned taking into account the age of the patient, the severity of the illness, and the suspected natural history. Although adults have a higher incidence of intracranial bleeding than children, specific therapy may not be necessary unless the platelet count is under 20,000 per cubic millimeter or there is extensive bleeding. Hemorrhage in patients with either acute or chronic ITP can usually be controlled with corticosteroids but, in rare cases, may require plasmapheresis to reduce the antibody or immune complex level, or temporary phagocytic blockade with intravenous gamma globulin. Emergency splenectomy is usually reserved for patients with chronic ITP who are desperately ill and have not responded to any medical measures to improve hemostasis.

Symptomatic patients with chronic ITP are usually placed on corticosteroids. In one standard regimen, 60 mg of prednisone is administered for 2 to 4 weeks and rapidly decreased over another week. Approximately 50 percent of patients with chronic ITP will normalize their platelet count on these high doses of prednisone. However, the majority will have a fall in platelet count following steroid withdrawal. Patients with chronic ITP who fail to maintain a normal platelet count after 2 to 3 weeks of steroids are eligible for elective splenectomy. These steroid-responsive but steroid-dependent patients are very likely to respond to splenectomy, and 70 percent will have a normal platelet count within 1 week after surgery. Some patients who do not respond to corticosteroids may still respond to splenectomy.

Patients who are still thrombocytopenic after steroid therapy or splenectomy or who relapse months to years after initial therapy have received a variety of immunosuppressive drugs including azathioprine, cyclophosphamide, vincristine, and vinblastine. More recently danazol, an impeded androgen, has been used with some success. Although each of these drugs may be beneficial, it is important to use some restraint as they have serious side effects. If a patient is not bleeding and maintains a platelet count over 20,000 per cubic millimeter consideration should be given to withholding therapy since there are many patients with severe chronic thrombocytopenia who have lived with their disease for two or three decades.

VON WILLEBRAND'S DISEASE Von Willebrand's disease (vWD) is the most common inherited bleeding disorder and may occur in as many as 1 in 800 to 1000 individuals. The von Willebrand's factor (vWF) is a heterogeneous multimeric plasma glycoprotein with two major functions. It facilitates platelet adhesion under conditions of high shear stress by forming a bridge between platelet membrane receptors and the vascular subendothelium; it also serves as the plasma carrier for factor VIII, the antihemophilic factor, a critical blood coagulation protein. The normal plasma vWF level is 10 μg/mL. The vWF activity is distributed among a series of plasma multimers with estimated molecular weights ranging from 400,000 to over 20 million. A single large vWF precursor subunit is synthesized in endothelial cells and megakaryocytes, where it is cleaved and assembled into the disulfide-linked multimers present in plasma and the vascular subendothelium. A modest reduction in plasma vWF concentration, or a selective loss in the high-molecular-weight multimers, decreases platelet adhesion and causes clinical bleeding.

Although vWD is heterogeneous, there are certain clinical features which are common to all the syndromes. With one exception (type III disease), all forms are inherited as autosomal dominant traits. In mild cases, bleeding occurs only after surgery or trauma. More severely affected patients have spontaneous epistaxis or oral mucosal, gastrointestinal, or genitourinary bleeding. The laboratory findings are variable. The most diagnostic pattern is the combination of (1) a prolonged bleeding time, (2) a reduction in plasma vWF concentration, (3) a parallel reduction in ristocetin cofactor activity, and (4) reduced factor VIII activity. The variability in laboratory tests is related both to the heterogeneous nature of the defects in vWD and the fact that vWF synthesis or release is increased by central nervous disorders, systemic inflammation, or pregnancy. Since vWD is an autosomal dominant disorder, some vWF is produced by the remaining normal allele. Thus, patients with mild defects may have laboratory values that fluctuate over time and may occasionally be within the normal range.

Although vWF cDNA has been cloned and the gene localized to chromosome 12, there is no information regarding the molecular genetics of the von Willebrand syndromes. There are three major types of vWD. Patients with *type I disease,* the most common abnormality, have a mild to moderate decrease in plasma vWF. In the milder cases, although hemostasis is clearly impaired, the vWF level is just below the lower limit of normal (50 percent activity, or 5 μg/mL). In type I disease there is a parallel decrease in vWF antigen, factor VIII activity, and ristocetin cofactor activity, with a normal spectrum of multimers detected by sodium dodecyl sulfate–agarose (SDS-agarose) gel electrophoresis.

The variant forms of vWD (*type II disease*), which are much less common, are characterized by normal or near-normal levels of dysfunctional protein. Patients with the *type IIa variant* of vWD have a deficiency in the high-molecular-weight forms of vWF multimer detected by SDS-agarose electrophoresis. This is due either to an inability to assemble the high-molecular-weight multimers or to a premature catabolism after they leave the endothelial cell and enter the circulation. The quantity of vWF antigen and the amount of associated factor VIII are usually normal. In the *type IIb variant,* there is also a loss in high-molecular-weight multimers. However, in type IIb cases, it is due to the inappropriate binding of vWF to platelets. This forms intravascular platelet aggregates which are rapidly cleared from the circulation causing mild, cyclic thrombocytopenia. Levels of vWF antigen and factor VIII usually remain normal.

Approximately 1 in 1 million individuals have a very severe form of vWD that is phenotypically recessive (*type III disease*). Type III patients are usually the offspring of two parents with mild type I disease. They may actually inherit a different abnormality from each parent (a doubly heterozygous state) or be homozygous for a single defect. Type III patients have severe mucosal bleeding, no detectable vWF antigen or activity, and may have sufficiently low factor VIII levels to have occasional hemarthroses like mild hemophiliacs.

Appropriate therapy of vWD depends on the symptoms and the underlying type of disease. There are two therapeutic options. One involves the use of cryoprecipitate, which is a plasma fraction enriched in vWF and is appropriate treatment for all the inherited forms of vWD. During surgery or after major trauma, patients should receive ten bags of cryoprecipitate. This regimen should be continued twice daily for 48 to 72 h to ensure optimal hemostasis. Minor bleeding episodes such as prolonged epistaxis or severe menorrhagia may respond to a single transfusion of cryoprecipitate. Recurrent menorrhagia, a major problem for women with severe vWD, can be effectively treated with oral contraceptive agents that suppress menses.

A second therapeutic option is the use of 1-desamino-8-D-arginine vasopressin (DDAVP), a vasopressin analogue which has minimal blood pressure–elevating and fluid-retaining properties and raises the plasma vWF level in normal individuals and patients with mild vWD. Patients with type I disease are the best candidates for DDAVP therapy. However, they must be tested for an adequate response prior to anticipated surgery, and vWF levels must be closely monitored during therapy since the patient may develop tachyphylaxis when therapy is continued for more than 48 h. DDAVP should not be given to patients with vWD variants, since it does not improve multimer pattern or hemostasis in type IIa patients, and it may actually worsen the defect or cause thrombotic complications in type IIb patients, since it increases the number of platelet-vWF aggregates and the degree of thrombocytopenia.

Although most cases of vWD are inherited, there are acquired forms of vWD caused by antibodies which block vWF function or by lymphoid or other tumors which selectively adsorb vWF multimers onto their surfaces. Anti-vWF antibodies have developed in patients with severe vWD following multiple transfusions, as well as in patients with autoimmune and lymphoproliferative disorders. Adsorption of vWF to tumor surfaces has been documented in patients with Waldenstrom's macroglobulinemia and Wilm's tumor and inferred in other patients with lymphoma. Treatment of acquired vWD should focus on controlling the underlying disease, since cryoprecipitate and DDAVP are usually not effective and the disorder can be fatal.

PLATELET MEMBRANE DEFECTS Receptors which modulate platelet adhesion and aggregation are located on the two major platelet surface glycoproteins. As previously discussed (see Chap. 54), vWF facilitates platelet adhesion by binding to glycoprotein Ib, while fibrinogen links platelets into aggregates via sites on the glycoprotein IIb-IIIa complex. There are two rare but well-defined platelet defects characterized by the loss of these glycoprotein receptors. Patients with the *Bernard-Soulier syndrome* have markedly reduced platelet adhesion and cannot bind vWF to their platelets owing to a deficiency in glycoprotein Ib. They also have reduced levels of several other membrane proteins, mild thrombocytopenia, and extremely large, lymphocytoid platelets. Platelets from patients with *Glanzmann's disease* or *thrombasthenia* are missing or markedly deficient in the glycoprotein IIb-IIIa complex. Their platelets do not bind fibrinogen and cannot form aggregates. The platelets undergo shape change and secretion and are of normal size.

Both of these disorders are inherited as autosomal recessive traits and are characterized by markedly impaired hemostasis and lifelong episodes of severe mucosal hemorrhage. In keeping with the selective nature of the defects, Bernard-Soulier platelets react normally to all stimuli except ristocetin. In contrast, thrombasthenic platelets adhere normally and will agglutinate with ristocetin but will not aggregate with any of the agonists which require fibrinogen binding, such as adenosine diphosphate (ADP), thrombin, or epinephrine.

The only effective therapy for hemorrhagic episodes in these two disorders is transfusion with normal platelets. This is usually effective, although alloimmunization will eventually limit the lifespan of infused platelets. In addition, a few patients have developed inhibitor antibodies with specificity for the missing protein. These antibodies bind to the protein which is expressed on the transfused normal platelets and impair their function.

PLATELET RELEASE DEFECTS The most common mild bleeding disorders arise from the ingestion of nonsteroidal anti-inflammatory drugs (NSAIDS) which inhibit platelet production of thromboxane A_2, an important mediator of platelet secretion and aggregation (see Figs. 54-3, 54-4). These drugs inhibit platelet cyclooxygenase, which converts arachidonic acid to a labile endoperoxide intermediate that is critical for thromboxane formation. Aspirin is the most potent agent, since it irreversibly acetylates the platelet enzyme; a single dose impairs hemostasis for 5 to 7 days. The other agents are competitive and reversible inhibitors with more transient effects. Blocking thromboxane A_2 synthesis partially inhibits platelet release and aggregation with weak agonists such as ADP and epinephrine and produces a mild hemostatic defect.

Patients generally have minimal symptoms such as easy bruising, and bleeding is usually confined to the skin. Occasional patients will have prolonged oozing after surgery, particularly with procedures involving mucous membranes such as periodontal, oral, or reconstructive plastic surgery. Not surprisingly, the antiplatelet effect of drugs like aspirin is more dramatic when they are administered to patients with underlying defects like vWD or hemophilia. Patients with drug-induced cyclooxygenase deficiency have a prolonged bleeding time, and their platelets fail to aggregate when incubated with arachidonic acid, epinephrine, or low doses of ADP. Platelet responses to collagen and thrombin are impaired at low doses but normal at higher doses. Symptomatic patients should be encouraged to use drugs like acetaminophen which do not impair platelet function. Although most cases of cyclooxygenase deficiency are drug-induced, occasional patients have inherited disorders in platelet cyclooxygenase activity which impair thromboxane production or receptor level defects which prevent platelets from responding to thromboxane A_2.

STORAGE POOL DEFECTS Platelet granules have considerable amounts of adenine nucleotides, calcium, and adhesive glycoproteins like thrombospondin, fibronectin, and vWF, all of which promote platelet adhesion and aggregation. Thus, it is not surprising that patients with defective platelet granules have a mild bleeding disorder. Platelet storage pool defects may be inherited as an isolated disorder or be part of systemic granule packaging defects such as oculocutaneous albinism or the Chediak-Higashi syndrome. Clinically, these patients cannot be distinguished from those with other functional platelet disorders since they all have easy bruising, mucosal bleeding, and a prolonged bleeding time. They can be differentiated from patients with the cyclooxygenase defects since their platelets will usually aggregate in response to arachidonic acid. In addition, their platelets have decreased levels of specific granule constituents like ADP and serotonin and abnormalities in granule morphology that are best visualized by electron microscopy.

Occasionally, patients with acute and chronic leukemia or one of the myeloproliferative disorders develop an acquired storage pool disorder due to dysplastic megakaryocyte development. In addition, patients with liver disease and some patients with systemic lupus or other immune complex–mediated disorders may have circulating platelets which have degranulated prematurely. Platelet degranulation and a transient storage pool disorder have also been described following prolonged cardiopulmonary bypass.

VESSEL WALL DISORDERS Bleeding from vascular disorders (nonthrombocytopenic purpura) is usually mild and confined to the skin and mucous membranes. The pathogenesis of bleeding is poorly defined in many of the syndromes, and classical tests of hemostasis, including the bleeding time and tests of platelet function, are usually normal. Vascular purpura arises from damage to capillary endothelium, abnormalities in the vascular subendothelial matrix or extravascular connective tissues which support blood vessels, or from the formation of abnormal blood vessels. There are also several idiopathic disorders which involve the vessel wall and which can cause more severe bleeding and organ dysfunction.

Thrombotic thrombocytopenic purpura Thrombotic thrombocytopenic purpura (TTP) is a fulminant, often lethal disorder that may be initiated by endothelial injury and subsequent release of vWF and other procoagulant materials from the endothelial cell. In addition, some patients with TTP have a unique circulating protein which induces platelet aggregation. Characteristic findings include the microvascular deposition of hyaline thrombi which stain for fibrin, thrombocytopenia, microangiopathic hemolytic anemia, fever, renal failure, fluctuating levels of consciousness, and evanescent focal neurologic deficits. The presence of hyaline thrombi in arterioles, capillaries, and venules without any inflammatory changes in the vessel wall is diagnostic. Gingival biopsies are positive in 30 to 40 percent of patients, and marrow biopsies are occasionally helpful. The presence of a severe Coombs negative hemolytic anemia, coupled with thrombocytopenia, and minimal activation of the coagulation system help to confirm the clinical suspicion of TTP. This disorder should be distinguished from vasculitis and systemic lupus erythematosus, which can predispose patients to TTP and ITP. Levels of platelet-associated IgG and complement are usually normal in TTP.

The treatment of acute TTP has changed radically in the past few years. The use of steroids and heparin or emergency splenectomy have been abandoned, and the enthusiasm for antiplatelet therapy has diminished. Increasingly, treatment has involved the use of exchange transfusion or intensive plasmapheresis coupled with infusion of fresh frozen plasma. With this therapeutic approach, the overall mortality has been markedly reduced, and over half the patients with TTP are recovering from this formerly fatal disorder. Most patients surviving the acute illness recover completely with no residual renal or neurologic disease. Occasional patients with a chronic relapsing form of TTP require maintenance plasmapheresis and plasma infusion, and a few patients are only controlled with corticosteroids.

Hemolytic-uremic syndrome Hemolytic-uremic syndrome (HUS) is a disease of infancy and early childhood which closely resembles TTP. Patients present with fever, thrombocytopenia, microangiopathic hemolytic anemia, hypertension, and varying degrees of acute renal failure. In many cases, onset is preceded by a minor febrile or viral illness, and an infectious or immune complex–mediated etiology has been proposed. As in TTP, there is no evidence of disseminated intravascular coagulation. In contrast to TTP, the disorder remains localized to the kidney where hyaline thrombi are seen in the afferent aterioles and glomerular capillaries. Such thrombi are not present in other vessels, and neurologic symptoms, other than those associated with uremia, are uncommon. There is no effective therapy; however, with dialysis for acute renal failure, the initial mortality is only 5 percent. Between 10 and 50 percent of patients are left with some chronic renal impairment.

Henoch-Schönlein purpura Henoch-Schönlein or anaphylactoid purpura is a distinct, self-limited type of vasculitis which occurs in children and young adults. Patients have an acute inflammatory reaction in capillaries, mesangial tissues, and small arterioles which leads to increased vascular permeability, exudation, and hemorrhage. Vessel lesions contain IgA and complement components. The syndrome may be preceded by an upper respiratory infection or streptococcal pharyngitis or be associated with food or drug allergies. Patients develop a purpuric or urticarial rash on the extensor surface of the arms and legs and on the buttocks; they also have polyarthralgias or arthritis, colicky abdominal pain, and hematuria from focal glomerulonephritis. Despite the hemorrhagic features, all coagulation tests are normal. A small number of patients may develop fatal acute renal failure, and 5 to 10 percent develop chronic nephritis. Corticosteroids provide symptomatic relief of the joint and abdominal pains but do not alter the course of the illness.

Metabolic and inflammatory disorders A number of acute febrile illnesses cause capillary fragility and skin bleeding. Immune complexes containing viral antigens, or the viruses themselves, may damage endothelial cells. In addition, certain pathogens such as the rickettsiae which cause Rocky Mountain spotted fever replicate in endothelial cells and damage them. Thrombocytopenia is also a frequent finding in acute infectious disorders and may contribute to skin bleeding. In addition, whenever the platelet count falls below 10,000 per cubic millimeter gaps which develop between endothelial cells allow the diapedesis of red cells into the dermis leading to the formation of petechiae. Drugs such as the sulfonamides, penicillin, and allopurinol may cause vascular inflammation resulting in maculopapular or urticarial rashes. Some of these mechanisms are additive, and drug reactions in thrombocytopenic individuals cause an intensely hemorrhagic rash.

Occasionally, patients with diffuse polyclonal hyperglobulinemia will develop purpuric lesions on the lower limbs—a benign condition referred to as *hyperglobulinemic purpura.* Vascular purpura may occur in patients with various monoclonal plasma protein abnormalities including Waldenstrom's macroglobulinemia, multiple myeloma, and cryoglobulinemia. These proteins markedly increase serum viscosity and may impair blood flow through capillaries. Thus, retinal hemorrhage, central nervous system dysfunction, and skin necrosis have all been described in these syndromes due to the marked elevation in viscosity. In addition, the globulins may impair platelet aggregation and adhesion and interfere with fibrin polymerization. Patients with mixed cryoglobulinemia develop a more extensive maculopapular lesion due to immune complex–mediated damage to the vessel wall. The mixed cryoglobulinemia (usually IgG and anti-IgG) may be associated with arthalgias, diffuse weakness, and unexplained nephritis. Plasmapheresis will temporarily lower the level of globulins, remove immune complexes, and improve symptoms in these patients. However, long-term management must include control of the underlying disease which produces the abnormal globulins or immune complexes.

Patients with *scurvy* (vitamin C deficiency) develop painful episodes of perifollicular skin bleeding as well as bleeding into muscles and, occasionally, into the gastrointestinal and genitourinary tracts. The diagnosis is confirmed by the presence of hyperkeratosis of skin, gum swelling, and low levels of the vitamin in leukocytes. Vitamin C–deficient patients have markedly defective collagen synthesis, since ascorbic acid is needed to synthesize hydroxyproline, an essential constituent of collagen. Patients with *Cushing's syndrome,* which is characterized by excess production of glucocorticoids, or patients on large doses of corticosteroids develop generalized protein wasting and may show skin bleeding or easy bruising due to atrophy of the supporting connective tissue around blood vessels. Aging causes a similar atrophy of perivascular connective tissue on the extensor surface of the hands and arms, leading to "senile purpura." These patients develop dark purple, irregularly shaped hemorrhagic areas due to abnormal skin mobility which tears small blood vessels.

Patients with inherited disorders of the connective tissue matrix such as *Marfan's syndrome, Ehlers-Danlos syndrome,* and *pseudoxanthoma elasticum* also have easy bruising. In addition to having fragile skin vessels and easy bruising, patients with Ehlers-Danlos syndrome may develop aneurysms in intraabdominal vessels and apoplectic rupture and hemorrhage due to defects in the vascular collagen network. Primary vascular abnormalities can also lead to bleeding. Patients with *Osler-Rendu-Weber disease* (hereditary hemorrhagic telangiectasia), an inherited autosomal dominant disorder, have frequent episodes of nasal and gastrointestinal bleeding from abnormal telangiectatic capillaries; patients with *angiodysplasia* of the colon have increased incidence of gastrointestinal bleeding. In the *Kasabach-Merritt syndrome* patients may have very extensive and progressively enlarging vascular malformations which may involve large portions of their extremities. Bleeding is secondary to disseminated intravascular coagulation triggered by stagnant blood flow through the tortuous abnormal vessels.

REFERENCES

GEORGE JN et al: Molecular defects in interactions of platelets with the vessel wall. N Engl J Med 311:1084, 1984

HOLMBERG L et al: Platelet aggregation induced by 1-desamino-8-D-arginine vasopressin (DDAVP) in type IIb von Willebrand's disease. N Eng J Med 309:816, 1983

KING DJ, KELTON JG: Heparin-associated thrombocytopenia. Ann Intern Med 100:535, 1984

KITCHENS CS: The purpuric disorders. Semin Thromb Hemost 10:173, 1984

LIND SE: Prolonged bleeding time. Am J Med 77:305, 1984

MCMILLAN R: Chronic idiopathic thrombocytopenic purpura. N Eng J Med 304:1135, 1982

MOAKE JL et al: Unusually large plasma factor VIII: von Willebrand's factor multimers in chronic relapsing thrombotic thrombocytopenia purpura. N Eng J Med 307:1432, 1982

VON SCHACKY C, WEBER PC: Metabolism and effects on platelet function of the purified eicosapentaenoic and docosahexaenoic acids in humans. J Clin Invest 76:2446, 1985

ZIMMERMAN TS, RUGGIERI ZM: von Willebrand's disease. Prog Hemost Thromb 6:203, 1983

280 COAGULATION DISORDERS

ROBERT I. HANDIN

Patients with congenital plasma coagulation defects characteristically bleed into muscles, joints, and body cavities, hours or days after an injury. The *inherited* plasma coagulation disorders result from rare defects in single coagulation proteins, with the two X-linked disorders, factors VIII and IX deficiency, accounting for almost all of the known congenital coagulation defects. These patients merit special attention since they may have severe bleeding and chronic disability and require specialized medical therapy. With the exception of factor XIII deficiency, each of the known disorders prolongs either the prothrombin time (PT) or partial thromboplastin time (PTT), the two important screening laboratory tests. If they are abnormal, quantitative assays of specific coagulation proteins are then carried out using PT or PTT tests with plasma from congenitally deficient individuals as substrate. The corrective effect of varying concentrations of patient plasma is measured and expressed as a percentage of a normal pooled plasma standard. The interval range for most coagulation factors is from 50 to 150 percent of this average value, and the minimal level of most individual factors needed for adequate hemostasis is 25 percent.

Acquired coagulation disorders are both more frequent and more complex, arising from deficiencies of multiple coagulation proteins and simultaneously affecting both primary and secondary hemostasis. The most common acquired hemorrhagic disorders are (1) disseminated intravascular coagulation, (2) the hemorrhagic diathesis of liver disease, and (3) vitamin K deficiency and complications of anticoagulant therapy. This chapter reviews the diagnosis, natural history, and therapy of congenital and acquired disorders of secondary hemostasis or plasma coagulation. The physiology of normal hemostasis and the cardinal manifestations of hemorrhagic and thrombotic disorders are described in Chap. 54.

FACTOR VIII DEFICIENCY—HEMOPHILIA A Pathogenesis and clinical manifestations The antihemophilic factor (AHF) or factor VIII coagulant protein is a large (265,000-dalton), single-chain protein which regulates the activation of factor X by proteases generated in the intrinsic coagulation pathway (see Figs. 54-5, 54-6). It is synthesized in liver parenchymal and endothelial cells and circulates complexed to the von Willebrand protein (vWF). Previous efforts to purify and characterize the factor VIII molecule were limited by its low concentration (10 ng/mL) and susceptibility to proteolysis. However, the cloning and sequencing of complementary DNA (cDNA) encoding the factor VIII molecule and the mapping of the factor VIII gene on the X chromosome have provided the first detailed picture of its structure and have resulted in improved methods for carrier detection and prenatal diagnosis.

One in 10,000 males is born with a deficiency or dysfunction of the factor VIII molecule. The resulting disorder, hemophilia A, is characterized by bleeding into soft tissues, muscles, and weight-bearing joints. Although normal hemostasis requires 25 percent factor VIII activity, symptomatic patients usually have factor VIII levels below 5 percent, with a close correlation between the clinical severity of hemophilia and plasma AHF level. Patients with <1 percent factor VIII activity have *severe* disease; they bleed frequently even without discernible trauma. Patients with levels between 1 and 5 percent have *moderate* disease with less frequent bleeding episodes. Those with levels over 5 percent have *mild* disease with infrequent bleeding that is usually secondary to trauma. Occasional patients with factor VIII levels as high as 25 percent are discovered when they bleed after major trauma or surgery, although the vast majority of patients with hemophilia A have factor VIII levels below 5 percent.

Hemophilic bleeding occurs hours or days after injury, can involve any organ, and, if untreated, may continue for days or weeks. This can result in large collections of partially clotted blood putting pressure on adjacent normal tissues and can cause necrosis of muscle (compartment syndromes), venous congestion (pseudophlebitis), or ischemic damage to nerves. For example, hemophiliacs often develop femoral neuropathy due to pressure from an unsuspected retroperitoneal hematoma. They can also develop large calcified masses of blood and inflammatory tissue that are mistaken for soft tissue sarcomas (pseudotumor syndrome).

Patients with severe hemophilia are usually diagnosed shortly after birth because of an extensive cephalhematoma or profuse bleeding at circumcision. However, patients with moderate disease may not bleed until they begin to walk or crawl, and mild hemophiliacs may not be diagnosed until they are adolescents or young adults. Typically, a hemophiliac patient presents with pain followed by swelling in a weight-bearing joint, like the hip, knee, or ankle. The presence of blood in the joint (hemarthrosis) causes synovial inflammation, and repetitive bleeding erodes articular cartilage and causes osteoarthritis, articular fibrosis, joint ankylosis, and eventually muscle atrophy. Although bleeding may occur into any joint, after a joint has been damaged it may become a site for subsequent bleeding episodes.

Hematuria, in the absence of any genitourinary pathology, is also common. It is usually self-limited and may not require specific therapy. The most feared complications of hemophilia are oropharyngeal and central nervous system bleeding. Patients with oropharyngeal bleeding may require emergency intubation to maintain an adequate airway. Central nervous system bleeding can occur without antecedent trauma or without evidence of a specific lesion.

Therapy There are several tenets regarding the treatment of bleeding in hemophiliac patients: (1) Symptoms often precede objective evidence of bleeding. (2) Signs of bleeding may not appear until several days after well-documented trauma. Physicians caring for these patients have learned to rely on their patients to inform them of early symptoms, usually pain, and to begin treatment at that time. Early treatment is more effective, less costly, and can be lifesaving. (3) It is critical to avoid the use of aspirin or aspirin-containing drugs which impair platelet function and may cause severe hemorrhage.

Plasma products enriched in factor VIII have revolutionized the care of hemophilia patients, reduced the degree of orthopedic deformity, and permitted virtually any form of elective and emergency surgery. The widespread use of factor VIII concentrates has also produced serious complications including viral hepatitis, chronic liver disease, and the acquired immunodeficiency syndrome (AIDS). The standard therapeutic products are cryoprecipitate and factor VIII concentrate. *Cryoprecipitate,* which contains about half the factor VIII activity of fresh frozen plasma in one-tenth the original volume, is simple to prepare and is produced in hospital or regional blood banks. It must be stored frozen and is thawed and pooled prior to administration. However, most patients utilize partially purified *factor VIII concentrate* prepared from multiple donors and supplied as a lyophilized powder. It can be refrigerated and reconstituted just prior to use. Each unit of factor VIII, which is the amount present in 1 mL of normal plasma, will raise the plasma level of the recipient by 2 percent per kilogram of body weight. Factor VIII has a half-life of 8 to 12 h, making it necessary to infuse it continuously or at least twice daily to sustain a chosen factor VIII level. In patients with mild hemophilia an alternative to the use of plasma products is DDAVP (1-desamino-8-D-arginine vasopressin) which transiently increases the factor VIII level.

An uncomplicated episode of soft tissue bleeding, or an early hemarthrosis, can be treated with one infusion of cryoprecipitate or factor VIII concentrate, raising the factor VIII level to 15 or 20 percent. A more extensive hemarthrosis or retroperitoneal bleeding requires twice-daily or continuous infusions in order to keep the factor VIII level between 25 and 50 percent for at least 72 h. Life-threatening bleeding into the central nervous system or major surgery may require therapy for 2 weeks with levels kept at a minimum of 50 percent of normal. In addition to the prompt infusion of factor VIII–enriched plasma products, patients need skilled orthopedic care with immobilization of inflamed joints to promote healing and to prevent contractures, and physical therapy to strengthen muscles and maintain joint mobility. Prior to surgery every patient should be screened for the presence of an inhibitor to factor VIII.

Patients with hemophilia who do not have an inhibitor should receive factor VIII infusions just prior to surgery and will require daily monitoring so that the factor VIII level is maintained above 50 percent for 10 to 14 days after surgery. When patients undergo joint replacement or other major orthopedic surgery, therapy should be continued for 3 weeks. This permits adequate wound healing and the institution of necessary joint mobilization and physical therapy.

Hemophiliacs also require treatment prior to dental procedures. Filling of a carious tooth can be managed by a single infusion of cryoprecipitate or factor VIII concentrate coupled with the administration of 4 to 6 g of ε-aminocaproic acid (EACA) four times daily for 72 to 96 h after the dental procedure. EACA is a potent antifibrinolytic agent which will inhibit plasminogen activators present in oral secretions and stabilize clot formation in oral tissue. For major oral and periodontal surgery and extractions of permanent teeth, patients should be hospitalized and treated with factor VIII. Therapy should begin just prior to surgery and be continued for a minimum of 48 to 72 h.

Many centers have organized home care programs so that patients can administer their own factor VIII infusions with the onset of symptoms. Occasional patients with very frequent bleeding receive regularly scheduled infusions. However, the expense and inconvenience usually limit the use of "prophylactic" infusions. Concern regarding transmission of AIDS has complicated therapy of hemophilia. Some patients are reluctant to treat themselves, and many centers have returned to the use of cryoprecipitate to limit donor exposure. Recently, a commercial heating process has been introduced which appears to inactivate the AIDS-associated retrovirus, HTLV III, without destroying factor VIII activity, and all hemophilia centers now use heat-treated material.

Complications Most hemophiliacs have had multiple episodes of hepatitis, and a majority have elevated hepatocellular enzyme levels and abnormalities on liver biopsy. Ten to twenty percent of hemophiliacs also have hepatosplenomegaly, and a small number develop chronic active or persistent hepatitis or cirrhosis. Recently, a few patients with hemophilia and end-stage liver disease have received liver transplants with cure of both diseases. Along with homosexuals and intravenous drug abusers, hemophiliacs are at high risk for AIDS since they frequently receive blood products. Hemophiliacs also present with the full range of AIDS-related syndromes including diffuse lymphadenopathy and immune thrombocytopenia.

Despite frequent bleeding, severe iron-deficiency anemia is uncommon since most of the bleeding is internal and iron is effectively recycled. Mild iron deficiency from chronic epistaxis or gastrointestinal bleeding has been noted in some hemophiliacs. In addition, after receiving large doses of factor VIII concentrate, some patients develop a mild Coombs'-positive hemolytic anemia due to anti-A and anti-B antibody present in commercial concentrates which bind to red cells and cause hemolysis.

Following multiple transfusions, between 10 and 20 percent of patients with severe hemophilia develop inhibitors to factor VIII. Inhibitors are, generally, IgG antibodies which rapidly neutralize factor VIII activity and prevent effective transfusion therapy. There are two types of inhibitors which have different biologic characteristics and lead to different clinical presentations. Patients with type I inhibitors have a typical anamnestic response in that they raise their antibody titer after exposure to factor VIII. Patients with a type II inhibitor have a low antibody titer which cannot be stimulated by factor VIII infusion. Patients with the type I inhibitor should not receive factor VIII. In an emergency, control of bleeding may require intensive plasmapheresis, or infusion of prothrombin complex concentrates which contain trace quantities of activated coagulation factors and can bypass the block in coagulation produced by the inhibitor. Patients with low-titer type II antibodies may respond to higher than normal doses of factor VIII.

Genetic counseling and carrier detection Until recently, carrier detection required biologic and immunologic assays which compared the ratio of factor VIII to vWF (von Willebrand factor) protein and were predictive in only 70 to 80 percent of cases. It is now possible to trace the defective allele in some families by examining the inheritance of restriction fragment length polymorphisms (RFLPs) linked to the factor VIII gene. In addition, certain families have been identified with specific mutations and deletions in the factor VIII gene that can be detected by restriction enzyme digestion of their DNA. Previously, prenatal diagnosis required sampling fetal blood for coagulant activity. Now, in families with an identifiable RFLP linked to the gene or a gene deletion or rearrangement, precise diagnosis is possible early in pregnancy from either chorionic villus biopsy or amniocentesis.

Most women carriers of hemophilia produce sufficient factor VIII for normal hemostasis from the factor VIII allele on their normal X chromosome. However, occasional hemophilia carriers will have factor VIII levels far below 50 percent due to random inactivation of normal X chromosomes in tissue producing factor VIII. These symptomatic carriers may bleed with major surgery or occasionally with menses. Rarely, true female hemophiliacs arise from consanguinity within families with hemophilia, or from concomitant Turner's syndrome or XO mosaicism in a carrier female.

FACTOR IX DEFICIENCY—HEMOPHILIA B Factor IX is a single-chain 55,000-dalton proenzyme which is converted to an active protease (IXa) by factor XIa. Factor IXa then activates factor X in conjunction with activated factor VIII. Factor IX is one of a group of six proteins, synthesized in the liver, which require vitamin K for biologic activity. As previously discussed (see Chap. 54), vitamin K serves as cofactor for a unique posttranslational modification which inserts a second carboxyl group onto certain glutamic acid residues on factor IX. This modification permits calcium binding and adsorption onto phospholipid surfaces. Factor IX cDNA has been cloned, the gene mapped on the X chromosome, linked RFLPs identified, and several patients with deletions and mutations in the IX gene have been discovered.

Factor IX deficiency or dysfunction (hemophilia B, Christmas disease) occurs in 1 in 100,000 male births. Accurate laboratory diagnosis is critical, since it is clinically indistinguishable from factor VIII deficiency (hemophilia A) but requires treatment with a different plasma fraction. Either fresh frozen plasma or a plasma fraction enriched in the prothrombin complex proteins is used. In addition to the expected complications of hepatitis, chronic liver disease, and AIDS, the therapy of factor IX deficiency has a special hazard. Trace quantities of activated coagulation factors in prothrombin complex concentrates may activate the coagulation system and cause thrombosis and embolism. This is particularly common in immobilized surgical patients and patients with liver disease. As a result, some centers have returned to fresh frozen plasma for factor IX–deficient surgical patients; others have recommended the addition of small doses of heparin to the concentrate to activate antithrombin III during the infusion and reduce hypercoagulability.

FACTOR XI DEFICIENCY Factor XI is a 160,000-dalton, dimeric protein which is activated via the intrinsic coagulation pathway. It is converted to an active protease (XIa) by factor XIIa, in conjunction with high-molecular-weight kininogen and kallikrein (see Figs. 54-4 and 54-5). Factor XI deficiency is inherited as an autosomal recessive trait and is especially common in Ashkenazi Jews. In contrast to factors VIII and IX deficiency, the correlation between factor level and propensity to bleed is not as precise, and there is minimal spontaneous bleeding and hemarthroses are rare. Many patients with factor XI deficiency present with posttraumatic bleeding or with bleeding in the perioperative period, and occasional factor XI–deficient women have menorrhagia. Daily infusions of fresh frozen plasma are sufficient since the half-life of factor XI is approximately 24 h.

OTHER FACTOR DEFICIENCIES Deficiencies in factors V, VII, X, and prothrombin (factor II) are all exceedingly rare autosomal recessive disorders. Although spontaneous or posttraumatic musculoskeletal bleeding or menorrhagia can occur with these deficiencies, hemarthroses are uncommon. Fresh frozen plasma is the appropriate therapy, although prothrombin concentrates may be employed for patients with severe prothrombin or factors VII or X deficiency so long as the risks of hepatitis and thrombosis are recognized.

Defects in the contact activation pathway involving Hageman factor (factor XII), high-molecular-weight kininogen, and prekallikrein cause laboratory abnormalities but no clinical bleeding. Despite dramatic prolongation of the PTT, which is often greater than 100 s, deficient individuals have normal hemostasis and can undergo major surgery without plasma replacement therapy. It is important to

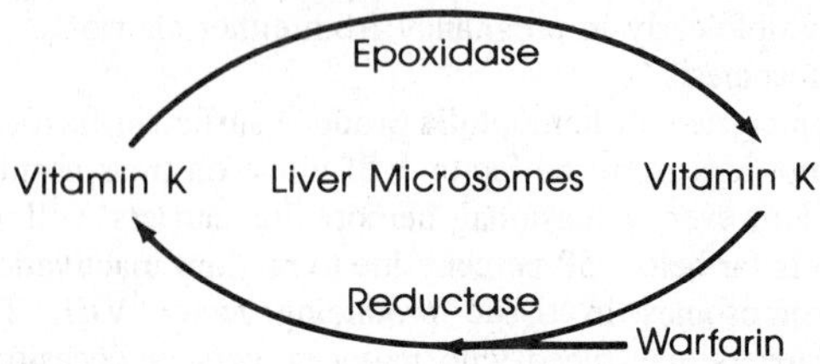

FIGURE 280-1 *The mechanism of action of vitamin K, which is a cofactor in the formation of di,γ-carboxyglutamic acid residues on coagulation proteins, is depicted. Vitamin K is converted to an epoxide in liver microsomes. The epoxide is the active form and is reduced back to vitamin K by a liver membrane reductase. Warfarin blocks the action of the reductase and competitively inhibits the effects of vitamin K.*

recognize and diagnose these disorders since the patients should neither be inappropriately treated with plasma nor denied indicated surgery on the basis of these laboratory abnormalities.

AFIBRINOGENEMIA AND DYSFIBRINOGENEMIA Fibrinogen is a 340,000-dalton dimeric molecule made up of two sets of three covalently linked polypeptide chains. Thrombin sequentially cleaves fibrinopeptides A and B from the α and β chains of fibrinogen to produce fibrin monomer, which then polymerizes to form a fibrin clot. Although fibrinogen is needed for platelet aggregation and fibrin formation, severe fibrinogen deficiency, paradoxically, does not usually cause serious bleeding except after surgery. Patients with afibrinogenemia, who have no detectable fibrinogen in plasma or platelets, may have infrequent, mild spontaneous bleeding episodes. Preliminary genetic analyses do not show any deletion or structural changes in the genes encoding the α, β, and γ chains of fibrinogen despite the total absence of plasma fibrinogen.

Fibrinogen is an abundant plasma protein (250 mg/dL) that has been purified and completely sequenced. Mutations have been identified which alter the release of fibrinopeptides from the α and β chains of fibrinogen, the rate of polymerization of fibrin monomers, and the sites for fibrin cross-linking. These dysfibrinogenemias are almost always inherited as autosomal dominant traits, so that patients have approximately equal concentrations of normal and mutant fibrinogen in their plasma. Patients with dysfibrinogenemia have a slightly prolonged PT and PTT, a prolonged thrombin time, and a disparity between the quantity of fibrinogen measured with functional and immunologic assays. Despite these abnormalities most patients have no symptoms while other patients have moderate bleeding. A few dysfibrinogenemias induce a hypercoagulable state and increase the risk of thrombosis, and others have been associated with an increased incidence of abortion (see Chap. 281).

TABLE 280-1 Etiologic factors and disorders causing disseminated intravascular coagulation

Liberation of tissue factors	Obstetrical syndromes—abruptio placentae, amniotic fluid embolism, retain dead fetus, second trimester abortion
	Hemolysis
	Neoplasms, particularly mucinous adenocarcinomas, acute promyelocytic leukemia
	Intravascular hemolysis
	Fat embolism
	Tissue damage—burns, frostbite, head injury, gunshot wounds
Endothelial damage	Aortic aneurysm
	Hemolytic uremic syndrome
	Acute glomerulonephritis
	Rocky Mountain spotted fever
Vascular malformation and decreased blood flow	Kasabach-Merritt syndrome
Infections	Bacterial: staphylococci, streptococci pneumococci, meningococci, gram-negative bacilli
	Viral: arboviruses, varicella, variola, rubella
	Parasitic: malaria, kala-azar
	Rickettsial: Rocky Mountain spotted fever
	Mycotic: acute histoplasmosis

SOURCE: *Modified from RI Handin, RD Rosenberg, in Hematology, 4th ed, WS Beck (ed), Cambridge, MA, MIT Press, 1985.*

FACTOR XIII DEFICIENCY AND DEFECTIVE FIBRIN CROSS-LINKING Factor XIII is a transglutaminase which stabilizes fibrin clots by forming ε-amino-γ-glutamyl cross-links between adjacent α and γ chains of fibrin. Factor XIII deficiency is an extremely rare inherited syndrome with only a few hundred documented cases. Patients usually bleed in the neonatal period from their umbilical stump or circumcision. In addition to hemorrhage, these patients may have poor wound healing, a high incidence of infertility among males and abortion among affected females, and a high incidence of intracerebral hemorrhage. These observations suggest that the enzyme may be important in other physiologic and pathologic processes beyond hemostasis, including placental implantation, spermatogenesis, and wound healing. Several drugs, including isoniazid, may bind to cross-linking sites on fibrinogen and mimic factor XIII deficiency by blocking enzyme activity. Normal hemostasis requires only 1 percent of normal enzyme activity, which can be achieved with small amounts of fresh frozen plasma.

VITAMIN K DEFICIENCY Vitamin K is a fat-soluble vitamin which plays a critical role in hemostasis. Dietary vitamin K is absorbed in the small intestine and stored in the liver. The vitamin is also synthesized by endogenous bacterial flora resident in the small intestine and colon; however, there is controversy regarding the quantity of endogenous vitamin K that is absorbed from the large intestine. Following absorption and transport, vitamin K is converted to an active epoxide in liver microsomes and serves as a cofactor in the enzymatic carboxylation of glutamic acid residues on prothrombin complex proteins (Fig. 280-1).

There are three major causes of vitamin K deficiency—inadequate dietary intake, intestinal malabsorption, and loss of storage sites due to hepatocellular disease. Neonatal vitamin K deficiency, which causes hemorrhagic disease of the newborn, has disappeared from western countries with the routine administration of vitamin K to all newborn infants. Although there is, theoretically, a 30-day store of vitamin K in the normal liver, acutely ill patients can become deficient within 7 to 10 days. Acute vitamin K deficiency is particularly common in patients recovering from biliary tract surgery who have no dietary intake of vitamin K, have T-tube drainage of bile, and are on broad-spectrum antibiotics, especially the newer cephalosporins. Vitamin K deficiency is also seen in chronic liver disease, particularly primary biliary cirrhosis, and in some malabsorption states (see Chaps. 237 and 249).

With the onset of vitamin K deficiency, plasma levels of the prothrombin complex proteins (factors II, VII, IX, X; protein C and protein S) decrease. Factor VII, which has the shortest half-life, decreases first. Thus, patients with mild vitamin K deficiency may have a prolonged PT and a normal PTT. Later, as the levels of the other factors fall, the PTT also becomes prolonged. Parenteral administration of 10 mg of vitamin K rapidly restores vitamin K levels in the liver and permits normal production of prothrombin complex proteins with 8 to 10 h. Severe hemorrhage can be treated with fresh frozen plasma, which immediately corrects the hemostatic defect. If the cause of vitamin K deficiency cannot be eliminated, patients may need monthly injections. Purified prothrombin complex concentrates should be avoided as they can cause thrombosis in patients with liver disease and will expose patients to an increased risk of hepatitis.

DISSEMINATED INTRAVASCULAR COAGULATION Disseminated intravascular coagulation (DIC) may be an explosive and life-threatening bleeding disorder. Although there is a long list of diseases complicated by DIC, it is most frequently associated with obstetrical catastrophes, disseminated malignancy, massive trauma, and bacterial sepsis (Table 280-1). In each case, a tentative triggering mechanism has been identified. For example, tumors and traumatized or necrotic tissue release materials resembling tissue factor into the circulation, while endotoxin from gram-negative bacteria activates several steps in the coagulation cascade. These potent thrombogenic stimuli cause the deposition of small thrombi and emboli throughout the microvasculature. This early thrombotic phase of DIC is then followed by a phase of secondary fibrinolysis. Continued fibrin formation and fibrinolysis leads to hemorrhage from the depletion of coagulation proteins and platelets and the antihemostatic effects of fibrin degradation products (see Fig. 280-2).

The clinical presentation varies with the stage and severity of the syndrome. Most patients have extensive skin and mucous membrane bleeding and hemorrhage from multiple sites—usually surgical incisions, venipuncture, or catheter sites. Less often, patients present with peripheral acrocyanosis, thrombosis, and pregangrenous changes in digits, genitalia, and nose—areas where blood flow is markedly reduced by vasospasm or microthrombi. Occasional patients, particularly those with chronic DIC secondary to malignancy, have laboratory abnormalities without any evidence of thrombosis or hemorrhage.

The laboratory manifestations include thrombocytopenia and the presence of schistocytes or fragmented red blood cells which arise from cell trapping and damage within fibrin thrombi; prolonged PT, PTT, and thrombin time and a reduced fibrinogen level from depletion of coagulation proteins; and elevated fibrin degradation products (FDPs) from intense secondary fibrinolysis. The cardinal manifestation of DIC, which correlates most closely with bleeding, is the plasma fibrinogen level.

Treatment DIC can cause life-threatening hemorrhage and requires prompt treatment. This should include (1) an attempt to correct any reversible cause of DIC; (2) measures to control the major symptom, either bleeding or thrombosis, and (3) a prophylactic regimen to prevent recurrence in cases of chronic DIC. Treatment will vary with the clinical presentation. In patients with an obstetric complication like abruptio placentae or acute bacterial sepsis, the underlying disorder is easy to correct, and prompt delivery of the fetus and placenta or treatment with appropriate antibiotics will reverse the DIC syndrome. In patients with a metastatic tumor causing DIC, control of the primary disease may not be possible and long-term prophylaxis may be necessary.

Patients with bleeding as a major symptom should receive fresh frozen plasma and cryoprecipitate to replace depleted clotting factors and platelet concentrates to correct thrombocytopenia. Those with acrocyanosis and incipient gangrene or thrombosis need immediate anticoagulation with intravenous heparin. The use of heparin in the treatment of bleeding is still controversial, although it is a logical way to reduce thrombin generation and prevent further consumption of clotting proteins. It should be reserved for patients with thrombosis or those rare patients who continue to bleed despite vigorous treatment with plasma and platelets.

Patients with mild DIC, who may not be symptomatic, may begin to bleed following stresses such as surgery or chemotherapy. For example, mild DIC, without clinical bleeding, can be documented during saline- or prostaglandin-induced midtrimester abortions. Prophylactic treatment of patients with heparin may prevent progression of the DIC syndrome and has been used in the treatment of patients with acute promyelocytic leukemia and in some patients with a retained dead fetus who require surgical extraction. Chronic DIC does not respond to oral warfarin anticoagulants, but it can be controlled with long-term heparin infusion. Occasional patients with indolent tumors and severe DIC have been maintained on heparin administered by intermittent subcutaneous injection or continuous infusion with portable pumps.

Despite our detailed understanding of the pathophysiology of DIC and a vigorous approach to therapy, there is little evidence that its treatment will change the natural history of the underlying disorder. Therapy will only stabilize the patient, prevent exsanguination or massive thrombosis, and permit institution of definitive therapy.

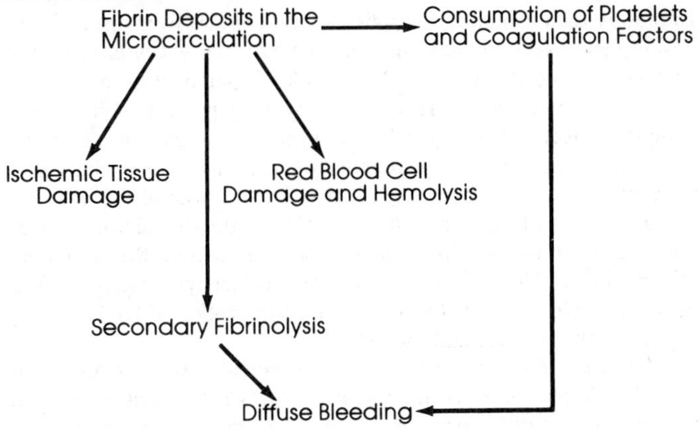

FIGURE 280-2 *The pathophysiology of disseminated intravascular coagulation (DIC). Shown are the interactions between coagulation and fibrinolytic pathways which result in bleeding in patients with DIC.*

COAGULATION DISORDERS IN LIVER DISEASE Since the liver plays a central role in the synthesis and metabolism of coagulation proteins, liver dysfunction is frequently accompanied by a hemostatic defect. The major causes of hemorrhage in patients with liver disease are outlined in Table 280-2. It is important to recognize that bleeding is usually due to an anatomic lesion, which is then exacerbated by the hemostatic defect. Most patients bleed from complications of portal hypertension such as esophageal varices, or from gastritis and peptic ulceration of the gastrointestinal tract. Portal hypertension also causes splenomegaly, with splenic sequestration of platelets and thrombocytopenia, which contributes to the hemostatic defect (see Chap. 249).

Patients with hepatocellular liver disease cannot store vitamin K optimally and may have some degree of vitamin K deficiency. Cholestasis, which is a frequent feature of liver disease, impairs vitamin K absorption and further decreases liver vitamin K stores. Patients also may have decreased production of other coagulation proteins including fibrinogen and factor V. The liver also produces inhibitors of coagulation such as antithrombin III, proteins C and S and is the clearance site for activated coagulation factors and fibrinolytic enzymes. Thus, patients with liver disease are both "hypercoagulable" and predisposed to developing DIC and may develop systemic fibrinolysis. For these reasons coagulation defects in advanced liver failure are often difficult to distinguish from those of DIC.

Each patient with hemorrhage and liver disease should have a PT, PTT, platelet count, and fibrinogen determination, although it is not always possible to determine the major hemostatic abnormality from a single set of laboratory values. It is helpful to have previous

TABLE 280-2 Causes of bleeding in liver disease

I Anatomic factors
- *A* Portal hypertension
  - *1* Varices
  - *2* Splenomegaly and secondary thrombocytopenia
- *B* Peptic ulceration
- *C* Gastritis

II Hepatic function abnormalities
- *A* Decreased synthesis of procoagulant systems: fibrinogen, prothrombin, factors V, VII, IX, X, XI
- *B* Decreased synthesis of coagulation inhibitors: protein C, protein S, antithrombin III
- *C* Impaired absorption and metabolism of vitamin K
- *D* Failure to clear activated coagulation proteins leading to
  - *1* Disseminated intravascular coagulation
  - *2* Systemic fibrinolysis

III Complications of therapy
- *A* Dilution of platelets and coagulation proteins from massive transfusions
- *B* Infusion of activated coagulation proteins in prothrombin complex concentrates
- *C* Bleeding from heparin; thrombosis from ϵ-aminocaproic acid (EACA)

laboratory data available for patients with chronic liver disease who develop an acute complication. Most patients present with moderate prolongation of the PT and PTT, mild thrombocytopenia, and a normal fibrinogen level. However, they may present with a more complex defect combining defective synthesis, abnormal clearance, and active consumption of coagulation proteins. Since vitamin K deficiency is so common, it is advisable to administer a single parenteral dose of vitamin K after initial laboratory studies have been obtained, even though this may only partially correct the laboratory abnormalities. The presence of severe thrombocytopenia or a low fibrinogen level suggests the additional complication of DIC and may require further studies and therapy.

The safest replacement therapy for a patient with liver disease is fresh frozen plasma since it supplies all known coagulation factors. However, even this form of therapy has drawbacks since large quantities of plasma may precipitate hepatic encephalopathy and cause fluid and sodium overload. Prothrombin complex concentrates should be avoided since they only replace the vitamin K–dependent factors, may be contaminated with hepatitis and AIDS virus, and contain trace quantities of activated coagulation proteins. Similarly, fibrinogen concentrates or cryoprecipitate, which are rich in factor VIII and fibrinogen should not be used without additional fresh frozen plasma. Anticoagulation with heparin has been advocated to control DIC, but this is particularly hazardous and not recommended in cirrhosis since heparin is metabolized erratically and may thus lead to severe bleeding.

FIBRINOLYTIC DEFECTS Bleeding can also occur from defects in the fibrinolytic system. Patients with $alpha_2$ plasmin inhibitor deficiency have excess fibrinolysis when it is triggered by fibrin deposition after trauma or surgery and so may experience recurrent hemorrhage. Patients with cirrhosis have an impaired clearance of tissue plasminogen activator and systemic fibrinolysis which may contribute to their hemorrhagic defect. Rarely, patients with tumors such as metastatic prostatic carcinoma may develop diffuse bleeding from primary fibrinolysis rather than DIC. Clues to the diagnosis include a disproportionately low fibrinogen with a relatively normal PT and PTT and the presence of a normal or nearly normal platelet count. However, at times it is difficult or impossible to differentiate primary fibrinolysis from the secondary fibrinolysis accompanying DIC. Patients with clearly established primary fibrinolysis should not receive heparin; they do require plasma therapy and, occasionally, fibrinolytic inhibitors like EACA. However, EACA should not be given to patients suspected of having DIC unless they are also receiving heparin, since EACA can cause massive, often fatal, thrombosis in a patient with DIC.

CIRCULATING ANTICOAGULANTS Circulating anticoagulants, or inhibitors, are usually IgG antibodies which interfere with coagulation reactions. Specific inhibitors inactivate individual coagulation proteins and may cause severe hemorrhage. As discussed above, they arise in 15 to 20 percent of patients with factor VIII or IX deficiency who have received plasma infusions. Specific inhibitors also occur in previously normal individuals. Although the most common target protein is factor VIII, inhibitors have been described with a specificity for each of the coagulation proteins. Anti-factor VIII antibodies in nonhemophiliacs are seen in postpartum females, in patients on various drugs, as part of the spectrum of autoantibodies in systemic lupus erythematosus patients, and in normal elderly individuals. *Nonspecific* (lupuslike) inhibitors prolong coagulation tests by binding to phospholipids; they do not perturb hemostasis in vivo, unless associated with thrombocytopenia or prothrombin deficiency. While they are most often encountered in patients with systemic lupus erythematosus, nonspecific inhibitors have also been noted in patients with many other disorders and also in otherwise normal individuals.

The critical laboratory feature, which identifies the presence of either type of inhibitor, is the failure of normal plasma to correct a prolonged PT, PTT, or both. Plasma from patients with a specific inhibitor will progressively inactivate a coagulation protein and thus prolong whichever of these screening tests require the participation of that clotting factor. This effect persists after dilution. Nonspecific inhibitors immediately prolong the PT and PTT and, at low dilution, block multiple coagulation reactions. However, these effects can be overcome by altering the quantity or type of phospholipid or by diluting the plasma.

Hemorrhage in patients with specific inhibitors may require treatment with massive plasma or concentrate infusion, the use of activated prothrombin complex concentrates to bypass the antibodies against factors VIII or IX, and plasmapheresis or exchange transfusion to lower antibody titer. Chronic immunosuppressive regimens have been sometimes employed, and have been particularly useful in otherwise normal elderly individuals with an acquired factor VIII antibody. Many patients lose their antibody and recover within 6 to 12 months, although the acute mortality rate from uncontrollable bleeding may approach 10 percent. Patients with nonspecific anticoagulants have normal hemostasis and do not require any therapy, unless they are concomitantly thrombocytopenic or prothrombin deficient. There is some evidence that nonspecific anticoagulants may also predispose patients to thrombosis and are associated with habitual abortions in some women.

REFERENCES

GIDDINGS JC, PEAKE IR: Laboratory support in the diagnosis of coagulation disorders. Clin Haematol 14:571, 1985

KASPER CK, DIETRICH SL: Comprehensive management of haemophilia. Clin Haematol 14:489, 1985

LAWN R: The molecular genetics of hemophilia. Sci Am 254:48, 1986

MAMMEN E: Congenital coagulation disorders. Semin Thromb Hemost 9:1, 1983

SHAPIRO SS, TIAGARAJAN P: Lupus anticoagulants. Prog Hemost Thromb 6:263, 1982

WHITE GC II et al: Factor VIII inhibitors: A clinical overview. Am J Hematol 13:335, 1982

281 INHERITED THROMBOTIC DISORDERS AND ANTITHROMBOTIC THERAPY

ROBERT I. HANDIN

Venous and arterial thrombosis and embolism are common medical disorders which have been recognized for over 100 years. Although risk factors such as atherosclerotic vascular disease, congestive heart failure, malignancy, and immobility predispose patients to thrombosis, specific coagulation defects have not yet been identified in most patients with thromboembolism. Several inherited deficiencies of coagulation inhibitors or abnormalities of coagulation proteins have now been described which induce a hypercoagulable or prethrombotic state and predispose patients to thrombosis. These disorders merit special attention since they affect young people, cause recurrent episodes of thromboembolism, and may involve multiple members of a single family. An understanding of the biochemical basis of thromboembolism is also important, since anticoagulant and antithrombotic regimes are based on the premise that modifying critical coagulation reactions will reduce the incidence of thrombosis. This chapter reviews both the inherited prethrombotic disorders and the use and complications of anticoagulant and antithrombotic therapy.

INHERITED PRETHROMBOTIC DISORDERS As previously discussed (see Chap. 54), coagulation is carefully regulated by a series of inhibitors which limit thrombin generation and fibrin formation and by the fibrinolytic system which effectively removes fibrin thrombi (see Figs. 54-5 and 54-7). Inherited defects of the natural coagulation inhibitors (i.e., antithrombin, protein C, and protein S), abnormalities in the fibrinolytic system, and certain dysfibrinogenemias predispose patients to thrombosis (see Table 281-1). Although they are an important and rapidly expanding group of disorders, they account for less than 10 percent of patients with recurrent thromboembolism. The known disorders are all inherited as autosomal dominant traits, so that heterozygous individuals, who have a 50 percent reduction in protein concentration or a mixture of mutant and normal molecules, will have an increased risk of thrombosis. These patients all have similar clinical presentations with a strong family history of thrombosis, episodes of recurrent venous thromboembolism, and symptoms by their early twenties. Any patient with this distinctive history should be tested for the molecular abnormalities described below.

TABLE 281-1 Inherited prethrombotic disorders

Antithrombin III deficiency and dysfunction
Protein C deficiency
Protein S deficiency
Dysplasminogenemia
Dysfibrinogenemia
Defective release of plasminogen activator
Diminished venous content of plasminogen activator
Heparin cofactor II deficiency

ANTITHROMBIN DEFICIENCY Antithrombin III complexes with activated coagulation proteins and blocks their biologic activity (see Fig. 54-5). The rate of this reaction is enhanced by heparin-like molecules within the vessel wall or on endothelial cells. Plasma antithrombin III content varies from 5 to 15 μg/mL (50 to 150 percent), with values only slightly below normal increasing the risk of thrombosis. For optimal screening, it is important to assess both the antithrombin III concentration by immunoassay and the plasma antithrombin and heparin cofactor activity with functional assays. The most common defect is mild (heterozygous) antithrombin deficiency, which occurs in 1 out of 2000 individuals. In addition, dysfunctional antithrombin molecules, with mutations affecting either the serine protease–binding site or the heparin-binding site, or activation of inhibitor by heparin have been described. Some investigators have suggested that another molecule called heparin cofactor II may also be a clinically important thrombin inhibitor. In fact, some patients have been described who are heparin cofactor II–deficient.

Patients with antithrombin deficiency who develop acute thrombosis or embolism can be treated with intravenous heparin, since there is usually sufficient normal antithrombin to act as a heparin cofactor. Following their first episode of thromboembolism, patients should be placed on oral anticoagulants for life to prevent recurrent thrombosis. Family studies should be conducted when an antithrombin-deficient individual is discovered, since up to one-half the members of a kindred group may be affected. Asymptomatic individuals with antithrombin deficiency should receive prophylactic anticoagulation with heparin or plasma infusions to raise their antithrombin level prior to medical or surgical procedures which may increase their risk of thrombosis. Chronic oral anticoagulation is not recommended until patients have a clinical thrombotic episode.

DEFICIENCIES OF PROTEINS C AND S Protein C is a vitamin K–dependent hepatic protein which binds to the endothelial cell surface protein thrombomodulin and is converted to an active protease by thrombin (Fig. 54-5). Activated protein C, in conjunction with protein S, proteolyzes factors Va and VIIIa, which shuts off fibrin formation. Activated protein C may also stimulate fibrinolysis and accelerate clot lysis. Deficiencies of proteins C and S are autosomal dominant disorders which may be more common than antithrombin deficiency and may cause identical problems—recurrent venous thrombosis and pulmonary embolism. No dysfunctional molecules have as yet been definitely identified in patients with thrombosis. However, protein S activity may be reduced when there is an excess of C4b binding protein.

Heterozygous patients with acute thrombosis and moderate protein C or S deficiency should be heparinized and then placed on oral anticoagulants. There are, however, two potential problems with the use of coumarin anticoagulants in these patients. First, these vitamin K antagonists (see Fig. 280-1 and Fig. 54-5), which lower the level of the procoagulant factors II, VII, IX, and X, may also reduce the concentration of proteins C and S and nullify the described antithrombotic effect. In addition, there are patients with coumarin-induced skin necrosis who have protein C deficiency, suggesting that this defect may predispose patients to a rare but serious complication of oral anticoagulants.

Homozygous protein C deficiency, which is very rare, can cause fulminant intravascular coagulation in the neonatal period. Patients with homozygous protein C deficiency may require periodic plasma infusions rather than oral anticoagulants to prevent recurrent intravascular coagulation and thrombosis.

DYSFIBRINOGENEMIAS AND FIBRINOLYTIC DEFECTS Several families have been described with recurrent venous thrombosis and embolism due to defects in fibrinogen or plasminogen or with decreased synthesis or release of tissue plasminogen activator. While the majority of dysfibrinogenemias cause bleeding, one variant, fibrinogen New York, is characterized by excessively rapid release of fibrinopeptides and recurrent thromboembolism. Patients with this disorder as well as those with an abnormal plasminogen which resists activation by streptokinase and urokinase have been successfully treated with heparin and oral anticoagulants. Defects in tissue plasminogen activator content or release have not been completely characterized. One group of patients with recurrent venous thrombosis and embolism failed to increase venous blood fibrinolytic activity when challenged with local ischemia or physical exercise. The other group had impaired fibrinolytic activity in extracts prepared from biopsied veins. The recent cloning of cDNA for tissue plasminogen activator (TPA) and the availability of immunoassays for TPA should facilitate more detailed studies of this class of defects.

ANTICOAGULANT AND FIBRINOLYTIC THERAPY Anticoagulation with heparin, followed by treatment with oral vitamin K antagonists, has become the standard treatment for acute venous thrombosis and pulmonary embolism. In addition, chronic oral anticoagulation is used to prevent cerebral arterial embolism from cardiac sources such as mural thrombi, atrial thrombi, a stenotic mitral valve, or from an atherosclerotic, partially stenosed carotid or vertebral artery. Anticoagulants are also used, but less successfully, to treat peripheral or mesenteric arterial thrombosis. These agents retard fibrin deposition on established thrombi and prevent the formation of new thrombi. The induction of a fibrinolytic state by the infusion of recombinant TPA or pharmacologic agents such as streptokinase (SK) and urokinase (UK) has become an accepted mode of therapy for some thromboembolic disorders. This approach has been advocated for some patients with massive pulmonary embolism and circulatory instability and to restore the patency of acutely occluded peripheral and coronary arteries.

ACUTE ANTICOAGULATION WITH HEPARIN Heparin is a naturally occurring mucopolysaccharide polymer which has tetrasaccharide sequences that bind to and activate antithrombin III. It is an extremely potent anticoagulant which can dramatically reduce thrombin generation and fibrin formation in patients with acute venous and arterial thrombosis or embolism. Heparin is usually administered by continuous intravenous infusion at a rate sufficient to raise the partial thromboplastic time (PTT) to 1.5 to 2 times the control value. This usually requires 1000 U.S.P. units per hour and is continued for 7 to 10 days while patients are begun on oral anticoagulants. Alternatives include the administration of 5000 U.S.P. units four times a day either subcutaneously or intravenously. Long-term heparin administration via portable external or implantable pumps is occasionally needed for patients with recurrent thromboembolism that is refractory to oral anticoagulants, for pregnant women with thromboembolism, and for patients with chronic disseminated intravascular coagulation (DIC). Lower doses of heparin (5000 units every 12 h) have also been used to prevent deep venous thrombosis in high-risk surgical and medical patients.

The major complication of heparin therapy is bleeding—especially from surgical sites and into the retroperitoneum. It is important to avoid aspirin or aspirin-containing drugs, which impair platelet function, and to avoid intramuscular injections in these patients. Heparin's anticoagulant effect can be rapidly reversed by the administration of protamine sulfate. However, in most cases this is not necessary and reduction or omission of heparin will improve hemostasis and stop bleeding. Thrombocytopenia occurs in about 10 percent of heparin recipients; it can occasionally be very severe and be accompanied by intravascular platelet agglutination and arterial thrombosis. Recognition of this rare complication—thrombocytopenia and paradoxical thrombosis—is critical, since discontinuing heparin can reverse the syndrome and may be lifesaving. Heparin administration for longer than 2 months carries a risk of osteoporosis and osteomalacia.

CHRONIC ORAL ANTICOAGULATION The coumarin group of anticoagulants, which includes drugs like warfarin and dicumarol, prevents the reduction of vitamin K epoxides in the liver microsomes and induces a state analogous to vitamin K deficiency (see Fig. 280-1). They slow thrombin generation and clot formation by impairing the biologic activity of the prothrombin complex proteins and are frequently used to prevent the recurrence of venous thrombosis and pulmonary embolism. Although regimens employing loading doses of drug have been advocated, the simplest way to induce anticoagulation is to administer a single dose of a coumarin compound and monitor the prothrombin time (PT) until the desired prolongation is achieved. For example, treatment can be initiated with 5 to 10 mg per day of warfarin or equivalent, with the goal of prolonging the PT to 1.5 to 2 times the control value. Although the PT may reach this value after a few days of therapy, effective anticoagulation, with stable reduction of all the prothrombin complex proteins, requires at least 1 week of coumarin administration. Most patients require a daily maintainence dose of 2.5 to 7.5 mg of warfarin to remain anticoagulated.

Although warfarin anticoagulants reduce the recurrence of deep venous thrombosis and pulmonary or cerebral embolism, they also cause bleeding. Any patient who takes oral anticoagulants requires frequent monitoring of the PT. Despite the most careful management, frequent fluctuations in PT can occur. Various drugs which alter liver microsomal metabolism of coumarins or compete for albumin binding sites can increase or decrease the biologic potency of a given warfarin dose (Table 281-2).

TABLE 281-2 Effect of drugs and metabolic changes on oral anticoagulant potency

I Factors leading to enhanced potency and increased prothrombin time
- *A* Reduced coumarin clearance
  - *1* Disulfiram (Antabuse)
  - *2* Metronidazole (Flagyl)
  - *3* Trimethoprim-sulfamethoxazole (Bactrim, Septra)
- *B* Reduced albumin binding
  - *1* Phenylbutazone
- C Additive hemostatic effect of certain drugs or disorders
  - *1* Aspirin
  - *2* Heparin
  - *3* Liver disease
  - *4* Thrombocytopenia
  - *5* Vitamin K deficiency
- *D* Increased turnover of vitamin K
  - *1* Clofibrate
  - 2 Hypermetabolism (e.g., hyperthyroidism)

II Factors leading to diminished potency and decreased prothrombin time
- *A* Accelerated coumarin clearance—induction of hepatic metabolizing enzymes
  - *1* Barbiturates
  - 2 Rifampin
- *B* Reduced absorption
  - *1* Cholestyramine
- *C* Impaired metabolism
  - *1* Genetic coumarin resistance

There is a direct relationship between the duration of anticoagulation and the risk of recurrent thrombosis. Although recommendations vary somewhat, most patients with a single uncomplicated thromboembolic event will have derived maximal benefit after 3 to 6 months of anticoagulation. It is estimated that 10 percent of patients on an oral anticoagulant for 1 year will have a serious complication requiring medical supervision, and 0.5 to 1 percent may have a fatal hemorrhagic event despite the most careful medical management. The anticoagulant effect of coumarins can be reversed by infusion of fresh frozen plasma or by the administration of vitamin K. In many cases, reduction or omission of several doses will improve hemostasis and stop hemorrhage. Despite the risk of bleeding, many patients with prosthetic heart valves, tight mitral stenosis, cardiomyopathy, chronic congestive heart failure, recurrent atrial fibrillation or with an inherited prethrombotic disorder will require lifelong anticoagulation.

One devastating complication of oral anticoagulation is hemorrhagic skin necrosis which in the past was thought to represent an allergic reaction. As previously discussed, several studies have found that patients with this complication are deficient in protein C, which may be the predisposing factor. There are some patients who have an inherited trait associated with coumarin resistance; they may require extemely high doses to get an anticoagulant effect. Psychologically disturbed patients may surreptitiously ingest coumarin and present with unexplained bleeding and a prolonged PT. Plasma coumarin levels can be measured by a quantitative spectrofluorometric assay to confirm such ingestion.

FIBRINOLYTIC THERAPY Fibrinolysis, an important part of the hemostatic process, is initiated by the release of TPA from endothelial cells. TPA preferentially activates plasminogen when it is adsorbed to fibrin clots; this helps to localize the lytic process to sites containing fibrin thrombi. Although fibrinolysis begins immediately after vascular injury, clot lysis and vessel recanalization may not be complete for 7 to 10 days. As previously discussed, this pathway is important for normal hemostasis since defects in the fibrinolytic pathway can predispose patients either to hemorrhage or to recurrent thrombosis. In addition, pharmacologic activators like SK and UK are used to accelerate clot lysis in patients with massive pulmonary embolism, acute arterial and coronary thrombosis, and peripheral venous thrombosis.

SK is a bacterial enzyme, and UK is a product of renal tubular epithelial cells. In contrast to TPA, these agents cannot discriminate between free and fibrin-bound plasminogen; when they are used for localized clot lysis, they produce hypofibrinogemenia and a systemic lytic state. SK is an indirect activator which forms an equimolar complex with plasminogen. Following the binding of SK, plasminogen develops proteolytic activity which activates additional plasminogen molecules and intiates fibrinolysis. In contrast, UK (like TPA) has intrinsic proteolytic activity and can directly convert plasminogen to plasmin. The major complication of fibrinolytic therapy is hemorrhage due to severe hypofibrinogenemia and intense systemic fibrinolysis. Such lytic therapy is not recommended for patients with recent surgery, indwelling cannulas or a history of neurologic lesions or gastrointestinal bleeding.

Fibrinolytic therapy is recommended for patients with massive pulmonary emboli complicated by hypotension, severe hypoxemia, and strain of the right side of the heart. In addition, fibrinolytic agents have been successfully administered to patients with acute peripheral arterial embolism and to patients with extensive iliofemoral thrombophlebitis. In the case of SK, one usually administers a total loading dose of 250,000 units; with UK one gives a loading dose of 4400 units per kilogram of body weight over 10 to 30 min. This will induce an intense lytic state as evidenced by a drop in fibrinogen, a prolongation of the thrombin time, and a prolongation of the euglobulin lysis time—a measure of fibrinolytic activity, predominantly the presence of plasminogen activator activity. After the initial loading dose, hourly doses of 100,000 units of SK or 4400 units of UK per kilogram of body weight are continued for 24 to 72 h. At the desired time, the lytic state is reversed by discontinuing UK or SK, and heparinizing the patient for 7 to 10 days. Heparin can be started 6 h after the fibrinolytic agent has been stopped. To maximize the likelihood of success, fibrinolytic therapy should be initiated as soon as possible after the onset of thrombosis or embolism.

Fibrinolytic therapy is also gaining favor among cardiologists since there is evidence that prompt institution of intracoronary lytic therapy with broad-spectrum agents such as SK or UK or systemic administration of a fibrin-specific agent like TPA may restore coronary arterial patency and reduce myocardial damage following acute coronary occlusion. It has been suggested that TPA, which is now produced by recombinant DNA techniques, may be a more useful pharmacologic agent than SK or UK since, in theory, it should lyse fibrin clots without causing systemic fibrinolysis and bleeding. As more experience is gained with TPA, it is apparent that some systemic lysis occurs with doses needed to lyse localized thrombi. In addition, TPA cannot discriminate between pathologic (and therefore undesirable) thrombi and vitally important hemostatic plugs, since both contain fibrin and may coexist in the same patient. Until more definitive results are obtained, TPA should be considered an important but experimental form of fibrinolytic therapy.

REFERENCES

Clouse LJ, Comp PC: The regulation of hemostasis: The protein C system. N Engl J Med 314:1298, 1986

Hirsh J: Effectiveness of anticoagulants. Semin Thromb Hemost 12:21, 1986

Laffel GL, Braunwald E: Thrombolytic therapy: A new strategy for the treatment of acute myocardial infarction. N Engl J Med 311:710, 770, 1984

Levine MN, Hirsh J: Hemorrhagic complications of anticoagulant therapy. Semin Thromb Hemost 12L:39, 1986

Rosenberg RD, Rosenberg JS: Natural anticoagulant mechanisms. J Clin Invest 74:1, 1984

Schafer AI: The hypercoagulable states. Ann Int Med 102:814, 1985

American College of Physicians, Health and Public Policy Committee: Thrombolysis for evolving myocardial infarction. Ann Int Med 103:463, 1985

Winter JH et al: Familial antithrombin III deficiency. Q J Med 51:373, 1982

282 BLOOD GROUPS AND BLOOD TRANSFUSION

ELOISE R. GIBLETT

BLOOD GROUP ANTIGENS AND ANTIBODIES

INTRODUCTION Human red blood cell membranes contain over 300 different antigenic determinants, the molecular structure of which is dictated by genes at an unknown number of chromosomal loci. The term *blood group* is applied to any well-defined system of red blood cell antigens controlled by a locus having a variable number of allelic genes, such as *A, B,* and *O* in the ABO system. Twenty-one blood group systems are currently recognized. The term *blood type* refers to the antigen phenotype, which is the serologic expression of the inherited blood group genes.

Alloantibodies specific for the blood group antigens may occur "naturally" (i.e., in the absence of known stimulus by foreign red blood cells) or in response to transfusion or pregnancy. Naturally occurring antibodies tend to be IgM molecules, and many of them (notably excepting anti-A and anti-B) react poorly at body temperature but readily agglutinate red blood cells at 5 to 20°C. Antibodies formed in response to exposure to another person's red blood cells or soluble blood group substances initially belong to the IgM class but usually change to the IgG class within a few weeks or months. In general, these "immune" antibodies react best at body temperature, and special laboratory procedures are required for their detection.

BLOOD GROUP SYSTEMS **ABO system: Genes and antigens** There are four major allelic genes in this system: A^1, A^2, B, and O. The locus for these alleles is on the long arm of chromosome 9. The actual products of the first three genes are glycosyltransferases which select specific sugars, *N*-acetyl-D-galactosamine (GalNAc) by the A^1 and A^2 transferases and D-galactose (Gal) by the *B* transferase, attaching them by alpha-linkage to short (oligo) saccharide chains. These chains comprise the carbohydrate moiety of glycolipid and glycoprotein molecules on the red blood cells or in other tissues and fluids. Although the A^1 and A^2 transferases perform the same function, they have different rate constants, so people who inherit an A^1 gene have more A-reactive sites than those with an A^2 gene. The *O* gene product is a protein which cross-reacts immunologically with the *A* and *B* transferase molecules but has no detectable enzyme activity; thus it is functionally "silent."

Nearly all individuals produce "naturally occurring" antibodies against the A or B antigens not present on their own red blood cells, as shown in Table 282-1. This fact is used as the basis for confirming the red blood cell type. Most of the major phenotypes represent more than one genotype. In the absence of family studies, it is possible to infer the genotype from only three phenotypes: A_1B, A_2B, and O. In routine practice, the ABO type is determined by testing the red blood cells with anti-A and anti-B and by testing the serum against A, B, and O red blood cells. Under special circumstances, a further distinction between A and AB types is made by using anti-A_1, an antiserum prepared by absorbing anti-A typing serum with A_2 red blood cells. The remaining unabsorbed antibodies have A_1 specificity, reacting with A_1 and A_1B, but not with A_2 and A_2B cells. (Alternatively, anti-A_1 is prepared as a lectin from extracts of certain seeds.) The frequencies of the various phenotypes in two American blood donor populations are also given in Table 282-1.

Red blood cells of types O and A_2 have large amounts of another antigen, called H, which is the immediate precursor to A and B. H specificity depends on the presence of a fucose (Fuc) residue attached to the oligosaccharides by a transferase that is the product of a very common gene called *H*. (The H and ABO loci are not genetically linked.) In very rare individuals who fail to inherit an *H* gene from either parent (i.e., they are homozygous for its allele, *h*), the *H* transferase is not made, and the H-determining fucose is not attached. This prevents the addition of specific sugars by the *A* and *B* transferases. As a result, even if an *A* or *B* gene has been inherited, the red blood cells are not agglutinated by anti-A, anti-B, or anti-H, while the serum contains all three antibodies. When a patient requiring transfusion has this so-called O_h (or Bombay) phenotype, special arrangements are necessary to obtain blood of the same rare type from a source such as the Red Cross.

About 80 percent of people are either homozygous or heterozygous for the "secretor," or *Se*, gene, which has no effect on the formation of antigens intrinsic to red blood cells but which activates the *H* gene to produce its fucosyltransferase in secretory tissues. Homozygotes for the apparently inactive allele *se* are called *nonsecretors* because their secretory cells do not produce a very weakly reactive *H* transferase, so their body fluids virtually lack H, A, and B antigen activities.

Antibodies in ABO system Red blood cells of newborn infants have a decreased number of H, A, and B reactive sites, and their plasma normally contains very little anti-A or anti-B. This finding is due to the fact that fetal immunoglobulin production is minimal, while most of the anti-A and anti-B produced in the mother are IgM molecules which cannot cross the placenta. However, in some type O adults, the anti-A, anti-B, and anti-AB (a cross-reacting antibody sometimes called anti-C) are of the IgG class. For this reason, ABO hemolytic disease of the newborn usually occurs in A (or B) infants of O mothers.

It is not acceptable medical practice to transfuse A, B, or AB blood into patients whose red blood cells lack the corresponding antigens, since their plasma contains incompatible antibodies. However, it is acceptable to give A or B blood (preferably as packed red

TABLE 282-1 Blood types of the ABO system (including Hh)

Genotype*	Phenotype	Antigens on red blood cells†	Antibodies in serum‡	Phenotype frequencies in Americans, % — Western European descent	African descent
A^1A^1, A^1A^2, A^1O	A_1	A_1, (H)	Anti-B (anti-H)	35	23
A^2A^2, A^2O	A_2	A_2, H	Anti-B (anti-A_1)	10	6
BB, *BO*	B	B, (H)	Anti-A, -A_1	8	17
A^1B	A_1B	A, A_1, B	(Anti-H)	3	3
A^2B	A_2B	A, B, H	(Anti-A_1)	1	1
OO	O	H	Anti-A, -A_1 Anti-B	43	50
hh	O_h	None	Anti-A, -A_1 Anti-B Anti-H	Very rare	Very rare

* *In all types except the last, the H allele is present as HH or Hh.*
† *(H) indicates occasional presence of weakly reacting H antigen.*
‡ *Antibodies in parentheses are, if present, weak cold agglutinins.*
SOURCE: *Race and Sanger.*

blood cells) to AB recipients, or to give O packed red blood cells (*not* whole blood, except in severe emergencies) to patients of type A, B, or AB when the transfusion requirement exceeds the supply of type-specific blood. Although antibodies with A_1 specificity frequently occur in the plasma of A_2 and A_2B subjects, they are almost always weak cold agglutinins. Therefore, if anti-A_1 has been identified in a transfusion patient, it can be ignored unless it reacts in vitro with A_1 red blood cells at 37°C.

Lewis system Antigens in the Lewis system are not produced by red blood cells but are taken up as glycosphingolipid molecules from the surrounding plasma. About 80 percent of western Europeans are either homozygous or heterozygous for the *Le* gene. The other 20 percent are homozygous for its presumably inactive allele, *le*. There are two well-defined Lewis antigenic determinants, Le^a and Le^b, both of which are structurally related to the H, A, and B antigens. The *Le* gene product, like the *H* gene product, is a fucosyltransferase, but it attaches fucose to a different sugar (*N*-acetyl-D-glucosamine instead of D-galactose) in the oligosaccharide chains. The Le^a determinant is a monofucosyl structure which lacks the fucose attached by the *H* transferase. The Le^b determinant has two fucose residues placed there by the *H* and *Le* transferases, in that order.

Anti-Le^a and anti-Le^b are fairly common naturally occurring antibodies, produced mainly by subjects of phenotype O, Le(a−b−). Nearly all examples of these antibodies are of the IgM class, so they rarely, if ever, can cross the placenta during pregnancy. Were they to do so, destruction of the infant's red blood cells would be highly unlikely, since the Lewis glycosphingolipids are very poorly developed during fetal life.

Lewis antibodies (particularly anti-Le^a) are complement-binders; anti-Le^a is rarely the cause of a transfusion reaction with intravascular hemolysis. However, the plasma of Le(a+) donors usually contains enough soluble Le^a antigen to neutralize the patient's anti-Le^a before it can attack the vulnerable red blood cells. Nevertheless, patients whose plasma contains an anti-Le^a that strongly hemolyzes Le(a+) red blood cells or agglutinates them at temperatures above 30°C should be given blood from either Le(a−b+) or Le(a−b−) donors. Anti-Le^b is virtually never a transfusion hazard.

P system Several structurally related antigens are considered together under the heading of a single system called P. As in the ABO and Lewis systems, the gene products are glycosyltransferases, attaching either D-galactose, *N*-acetyl-D-galactosamine, or *N*-acetyl-D-glucosamine to glycosphingolipids on the red blood cell membrane. P_1 and P, the major antigenic determinants, were previously thought to represent the expression of two allelic genes at the same locus, analogous to A^1 and A^2 in the ABO system. However, these two antigens represent quite different sugar sequences, and the genetic interpretation is complex.

Anti-P_1, which occurs frequently, almost never causes red blood cell destruction—the exceptions being those rare examples which react strongly with P_1 red blood cells in vitro at 37°C. In patients with paroxysmal cold hemoglobinuria, the so-called Donath-Landsteiner autoantibodies frequently react with globoside, a very common red blood cell glycosphingolipid with P specificity.

I system The I and i antigenic determinants are structurally heterogeneous, biochemically related to the H, A, B, Le, and P antigens. Most people inherit a gene associated with I antigen production, but the red blood cells of newborn infants react very weakly with anti-I and strongly with anti-i. A gradual reversal occurs during the first year or two, representing the development of I antigen in association with branching of carbohydrate chains on the cell membrane. In patients with certain kinds of "marrow stress," particularly thalassemia and hypoplastic anemia, red blood cell I activity increases.

Anti-I is a common antibody, frequently found as a weak cold agglutinin of no clinical concern. In patients with the cold type of autoimmune hemolytic anemia, autoantibodies usually have anti-I or anti-I plus i specificity, and most of them belong to the IgM class (see Chap. 287). Anti-i production is associated mainly with lymphoid cell diseases, especially infectious mononucleosis and lymphosarcoma. A patient already having a "marrow-stressing" disorder such as thalassemia may develop an intense autoimmune hemolytic anemia due to anti-i. When transfusions are required, finding compatible blood poses no problem, since the red blood cells of most adults are i-negative. Even patients with strong cold-reacting anti-I antibodies are usually not difficult to transfuse safely if they are kept warm during the infusion. However, since anti-I often fixes complement, washed red cells may be preferable for transfusion to prevent exposure to additional complement components.

MNS system Closely linked genes on chromosome 4 determine the MN and Ss antigens, respectively. There are four inherited haplotypes: MS, Ms, NS, and Ns. Glycophorin A carries M and N specificity, while S and s are on glycophorin B. Absence of these sialoglycoproteins is associated with rare phenotypes such as En(a-), S^u, and M^k, but there are no accompanying hematologic abnormalities.

Anti-M and anti-N are usually naturally occurring IgM agglutinins with little capability of destroying red blood cells. Patients on long-term renal dialysis tend to form anti-N as either an auto- or alloantibody. These N-specific autoantibodies have no hemolytic potential, but they are alleged to cause rejection of kidneys kept refrigerated before transplantation.

Formation of anti-S or anti-s usually requires the stimulus of transfusion or pregnancy, and accordingly these antibodies often belong to the IgG class. A third antibody, anti-U, behaves serologically somewhat like anti-S plus anti-s, being formed in sensitized black subjects whose red blood cells have the S^u phenotype lacking S and

TABLE 282-2 Rh alleles, their antigenic determinants, and frequencies

Allele	Associated antigenic determinants* R-S	W	Approximate allele frequencies in Americans† Western European descent	African descent	Oriental descent
R^1	D, C, e	Rh_o, rh′, hr″	0.45	0.10	0.55
r	c, e	hr′, hr″	0.37	0.15	0.10
R^2	D, c, E	Rh_o, hr′, rh″	0.14	0.10	0.35
R^o	D, c, e	Rh_o, hr′, hr″	0.02	0.60	Low
r''	c, E	hr′, rh″	0.01	Low	Low
r'	C, e	rh′, hr″	0.01	Low	
R^z	D, C, E	Rh_o, rh′, rh″	Low	Low	Low
r^y	C, E	rh′, rh″	Low	Low	Low

* *R-S = Race and Sanger; W = Wiener (see references).*
† *Low frequency means less than 0.01. Individuals of African descent have other alleles not listed here, thus accounting for failure of their frequencies to total 1.0.*

s antigens. All three of these antibodies can hemolyze incompatible red blood cells in vivo, but they are readily detectable by adequate compatibility testing.

Rh system The Rh locus is on chromosome 1. Rh antigenic determinants may be dependent on interaction between red blood cell membrane protein and phospholipid molecules. Many Rh phenotypes have been described serologically, but the underlying biochemical genetics is unknown. It is convenient to envision a stretch of nucleotides at the Rh locus which dictates the structure of a set of three antithetical determinants: C or c, E or e, and D or d (the latter having no corresponding antibody and therefore being simply the absence of D). These sets are inherited from each parent as a haplotype, such as CDe, cde, cDE, and so forth. This nomenclature, used by Race and Sanger, is compared with the alternative nomenclature of Wiener in Table 282-2, which also gives the approximate frequencies of the corresponding alleles in Americans of western European, African, and Oriental origins.

The D(Rh_o) antigen is by far the most immunogenic of this or any other blood group system (except for those previously described systems in which the formation of antibodies does not depend on exposure to foreign red blood cells). About 15 percent of Caucasians lack the D(Rh_o) antigen and are Rh-negative. When transfused only once with Rh-positive blood, these Rh-negative persons have about a 50 percent chance of forming anti-D(Rh_o) antibodies, which could cause destruction of any subsequently transfused Rh-positive red blood cells. For this reason, Rh-negative patients are always given Rh-negative blood except when the transfusion requirements of a male or postmenopausal female exceed the available supply. Giving Rh-positive blood to Rh-negative premenopausal females is a very serious matter, because, unless adequate amounts of Rh immunoglobulin are given to prevent immunization, any subsequent pregnancy with an Rh-positive infant will almost always stimulate a secondary immune response, resulting in hemolytic disease of the newborn.

The Rh antigens C, c, E, and e are considerably less immunogenic than D, and it is impractical to match these antigens in donors and recipients. Of course, when previously sensitized patients form the corresponding antibodies, it is necessary to find donor blood lacking the specific antigens. The difficulty of this search varies. For example, about 20 percent of the population lack the c antigen and thus are compatible donors for a patient whose plasma contains anti-c. However, only 2 percent lack the e antigen, so patients with anti-e pose serious problems, especially when large amounts of blood are required. Blood banks often maintain donor calling lists or frozen red blood cells for use in such cases.

A large proportion of patients with acquired hemolytic anemia of the warm type have IgG autoantibodies which react with one or more Rh-associated antigens. In some instances, the specificity is clear-cut (for example, anti-e), but more often the antibodies react with all red blood cells except those of the rare type known as Rh_{null}. These cells lack all known Rh antigens, and the cell membrane is defective, reinforcing the belief that in normal red blood cells, molecules bearing the Rh determinants are an intrinsic part of the membrane protein structure.

Kidd, Kell, Duffy, and Lutheran systems The major antigens of these four clinically important systems and their average phenotype frequencies in Americans of western European and African origins are presented in Table 282-3 along with the frequencies of S and s in the MNS system. Anti-K and anti-Fy^a are frequently encountered antibodies capable of marked alloimmune red blood cell destruction. Even more dangerous are the antibodies in the Kidd system, anti-Jk^a

TABLE 282-3 The major antigens and phenotypes in five clinically important blood group systems (excepting ABO and Rh)*

System	Major antigens	Phenotypes	Approximate phenotype frequencies in Americans, %† Western European descent	African descent
Kidd	Jk^a Jk^b	Jk(a+b−)	26	55
		Jk(a−b+)	24	7
		Jk(a+b+)	50	38
Kell	K, k, Js^a	K−k+Js(a−)	91	83
		K−k+Js(a+)	Low	15
		K+k−Js(a−)	Low	Low
		K+k+Js(a−)	9	2
		K+k+Js(a+)	Low	Low
Duffy	Fy^a, Fy^b	Fy(a+b−)	18	10
		Fy(a−b+)	33	20
		Fy(a+b+)	49	2
		Fy(a−b−)	Low	68
Lutheran	Lu^a, Lu^b	Lu(a+b−)	Low	Low
		Lu(a−b+)	92	97
		Lu(a+b+)	8	3
(MN) Ss	S, s	S−s+	47	65
		S+s−	10	9
		S+s+	43	24
		S−s−	Low	2

* *See Tables 282-1 and 282-2 for information about ABO and Rh types.*
† *Low means less than 1 percent.*
SOURCE: *ER Giblett,* Genetic Markers in Human Blood, *Philadelphia, Davis, 1969.*

and anti-Jk[b], which are notoriously difficult to detect. Whenever a patient has a hemolytic transfusion reaction after transfusion of blood found to be compatible by the usual laboratory tests, the most likely cause is anti-Jk[a]. Antibodies in the Lutheran system have only rarely been reported to cause red blood cell destruction.

Other blood group antigens Many other red blood cell antigens have been described. The Xg[a] antigen is of considerable importance, since its locus is on the X chromosome. Other antigens are of clinical interest because they occur on the red blood cells of 95 percent or more of most populations, making it difficult to find compatible blood when their antibodies are present in patients requiring transfusion. Many of these antibodies have little ability to destroy red blood cells, even though they consist of IgG molecules and react in vitro at 37°C. Included in this category are most examples of anti-Sd[a] (Sid), anti-Yt[a] (Cartwright), anti-Yk[a] (York), and many others. Nevertheless, both caution and experience are necessary when considering the transfusion of serologically incompatible blood, particularly when the antibodies react in vitro at body temperature. Antibodies with Chido (Ch[a]) and Rodgers (Rg[a]) specificity are incapable of causing hemolysis. Their respective antigenic determinants are located on the C4d fragment of the fourth component of complement and are thereby taken up from the plasma by red cells.

BIOLOGIC SIGNIFICANCE OF BLOOD GROUPS Immune reactions The relationship of blood group antigens and antibodies to alloimmune red blood cell destruction has been briefly discussed in the previous sections. Because antigens in the ABO system are present in other tissues, they play a role in determining *histocompatibility,* so that transplantation of ABO-incompatible kidneys and other organs carries a risk of rejection (see Chap. 221). However, successful grafting of ABO-incompatible bone marrow is possible when the patient is immunosuppressed and either given exchange transfusions of plasma compatible with the donor's red blood cells or the patient's own plasma is passed over a column containing oligosaccharides with A and/or B specificity.

Infertility and early fetal loss Both of these effects have been ascribed to ABO incompatibility, although in some instances the data are of marginal significance. Nevertheless, many population geneticists believe that this factor plays a significant role in the processes of natural selection.

Disease-related phenotype changes A and, to a lesser extent, B determinants are subject to certain biochemical changes, such as those caused by bacterial glycosidases and other enzymes. As a result, the red blood cells may develop new specificities, becoming either "polyagglutinable" or having "pseudo-B" characteristics. Another acquired alteration in ABO type occurs in some patients with acute myelocytic leukemia whose original type is A_1 or B. This change in phenotype, with partial or complete loss of agglutinability by anti-A or anti-B, can be a diagnostic aid in the early hypoplastic phase of leukemia. The changes in Ii specificity associated with "marrow stress" are described above (see "I System").

Other disease relationships The incidence of certain diseases is related to blood type. For example, type O "nonsecretors" have about twice the incidence of duodenal ulcer than do secretors of types A or B. On the other hand, type A carries a higher incidence of tumors of salivary glands, stomach, and pancreas than does type O. Persons with the rare Rh_{null} type, whose red cells lack all the Rh antigens, have some degree of increased hemolysis, as do people with the McLeod phenotype. McLeod red blood cells react only weakly with antibodies against antigens of the autosomally controlled Kell system, and they lack Kx, a very common X-linked antigen. Some boys with the X-linked form of chronic granulomatous disease have the McLeod phenotype and others do not. In both instances, the Kx antigen, also a normal granulocyte component, is not detectable on these cells. Individuals (mainly of African origin) who lack both Fy[a] and Fy[b]—the major antigens in the Duffy system—are protected against infestation by the malarial parasite, *Plasmodium vivax,* presumably because Fy[a] and Fy[b] act as specific recognition or acceptor sites for the merozoites.

Chromosome mapping Blood genetic markers, including the red and white blood cell allotypes as well as the plasma and blood cell enzyme phenotypes, are very useful for mapping the human chromosomes. Some of these markers are genetically linked to loci for genes causing metabolic diseases, and, as more markers are identified, it will be increasingly possible to predict the development of inherited malfunctions from specimens obtained in utero or from newborn infants. For example, the secretor gene locus is closely linked to the locus of the gene causing myotonic dystrophy, and a determination of the secretor status of a baby at risk can be used to predict the likelihood of its developing this disease, since both characters are inherited as autosomal dominants.

Medicolegal applications When the red blood cell antigens are combined with the other genetic markers in blood, the probability of distinguishing one person from another is about 2 million to 1. This high degree of individuality promotes the usefulness of genetic markers for ruling out paternity, maternity, and monozygosity in nearly all cases where those relationships do not exist.

BLOOD TRANSFUSION

INTRODUCTION Considerable morbidity and, to a lesser extent, mortality are associated with blood transfusion therapy. Responsible medical practice dictates that physicians have sufficient background information to make soundly reasoned judgments concerning the risks as well as the benefits of this procedure. They must decide not only what blood components (if any) are indicated but also what quantities are needed.

WHOLE BLOOD A unit of whole blood consists of approximately 450 mL blood collected into a plastic bag containing 63 mL of either citrate-phosphate-dextrose (CPD) or citrate-phosphate-dextrose–adenine (CPD-A) solution as anticoagulant and preservative. Blood collected in CPD has a refrigerated storage life of only 3 weeks, while CPD-A blood may be kept 5 weeks. At the end of these periods, about 70 to 80 percent of red blood cells are still viable, white blood cells and platelets are nonviable, and clotting factors V and VIII have low levels of activity. The storage time for packed red blood cells harvested from blood collected in CPD can be increased to 49 days by the addition of preservative solutions that contain mannitol.

Virtually the only reason to transfuse whole blood is to restore blood volume lost through recent hemorrhage, as with gastrointestinal bleeding, major surgery, or trauma. For assessing blood loss, routine laboratory tests are misleading for several hours after hemorrhage. Both hemoglobin and hematocrit measurements reflect the ratio of red blood cell mass to blood volume, rather than indicating the total circulating red blood cells. Since the compensatory vasoconstriction evoked by hemorrhage initially prevents extravascular fluids from replacing intravascular fluid loss, both laboratory measurements may be falsely high. Clinically, postural hypotension provides a warning that blood transfusion may be required. Pallor, syncope, tachycardia, thirst, and air hunger are useful indicators of massive blood loss (i.e., 1500 mL or more in adults), sometimes requiring immediate transfusion of type O red blood cells that have not been cross-matched. In less severe cases, maintaining the blood volume with saline or plasma expanders provides time for accurate blood typing and compatibility testing.

During surgery, blood loss can be measured quite accurately, and there is a tendency to "keep up" or even to "stay ahead" of lost volume by transfusion. Such practices lead to unwarranted use of blood with its attendant hazards. In most adult subjects, blood loss of 500 mL is easily tolerated, being equivalent to the amount given by a blood donor. Judicious use of crystalloid infusions is frequently all that is required to circumvent blood transfusion, even with blood losses up to a liter. In modern medicine, ordering ''fresh'' blood at any time is not acceptable practice, since proper component therapy is both safer and more scientifically based.

PACKED RED BLOOD CELLS The preparation of packed red blood cells from whole blood involves sedimentation or centrifugation followed by removal of plasma into a satellite bag, all in a closed system. Such packed cells have the same storage periods as whole blood. Removal of the plasma provides protection against circulatory overload as well as against excessive loads of sodium, potassium, citrate, ammonia, and antibodies (particularly anti-A) which might be harmful to the patient. Furthermore, the removed plasma can be used for preparing such products as cryoprecipitate, albumin, and immunoglobulins.

In the absence of recent blood loss, most transfusions are given to patients who need replacement of oxygen-carrying capacity. Packed red blood cells are much preferred to whole blood for this purpose, since the plasma serves no useful purpose and may be detrimental, especially in hypervolemic subjects. Diagnoses most frequently associated with the need for packed red blood cells fall into two major categories of anemia, hypoplastic and hemolytic.

Red blood cell hypoplasia Chronic bone marrow depression may, under favorable circumstances, be treated by bone marrow transplantation (see Chap. 291). However, many patients either have no access to a marrow donor or are unsuitable candidates. The red blood cell mass of these patients can be maintained at functional levels for long periods, provided they do not develop multiple antibodies against red blood cell antigens. These patients are in general more liable to become immunologically refractory to platelets and white blood cells than to red blood cells. Patients whose red blood cell hypoplasia is secondary to marrow invasion by malignancy and/or to various chemo- or radiotherapeutic agents also require red blood cell transfusions. Again, sensitization to transfused platelets and white blood cells creates a greater problem than red blood cell immunization.

Hemolytic anemia In severe cases of inherited nonimmune hemolysis due to intrinsic red blood cell defects (e.g., sickle cell anemia, thalassemia, or severe deficiencies of glucose 6-phosphate dehydrogenase), the only hope of maintaining oxygen-carrying capacity through a crisis is the careful use of red blood cell transfusion. Patients with other forms of nonimmune hemolysis or ineffective erythropoiesis (e.g., vitamin B_{12}, folate, or iron deficiencies) are candidates for transfusion only if they are severely anemic and if the cause cannot be corrected by specific replacement therapy. Whenever any infusion is given to a patient with severe anemia, the possibility of precipitating heart failure must be circumvented by careful monitoring.

Patients with autoimmune hemolytic anemia are not good candidates for red blood cell transfusion. Not only are they liable to develop new alloantibodies, but they may have already formed such antibodies as the result of earlier transfusion or pregnancy. In the presence of circulating *auto*antibodies, alloantibodies are often difficult to detect, and transfused red blood cells may be rapidly destroyed. Consultation with a blood transfusion expert is desirable in cases where severe anemia with hypoxemia or cardiac failure poses an immediate threat to life.

PLATELETS Platelet concentrates are prepared by centrifugation of platelet-rich plasma to yield about 5×10^{10} platelets from each donor unit. More porous plastic bags and gentle agitation facilitate gas transport across the container walls during storage at room temperature. A continuous supply of oxygen maintains aerobic platelet metabolism and prevents harmful drops in pH due to lactic acid production and CO_2 retention. These factors permit platelet storage for up to 7 days with posttransfusion survivals of 6 to 7 days. In adult thrombocytopenic patients without consumptive coagulopathy or platelet-specific antibodies, 1 unit of platelet concentrate raises the platelet count by about 10,000 per microliter.

Patients with idiopathic thrombocytopenic purpura produce autoantibodies which react with all human platelets (see Chap. 279), and therefore derive little or no benefit from platelet transfusion. Similarly, in patients with thrombocytopenia due to a consumptive coagulopathy (as in infection or metastatic malignancy) the usefulness of platelet therapy is limited, unless its purpose is to keep the patient from bleeding while the primary cause is being treated.

The most rational use of platelets is to control bleeding in patients either with a temporary loss of platelets not due to immunity (e.g., massive blood replacement, prolonged surgery) or with suppressed platelet production (leukemia, lymphoma, treatment with radio- or chemotherapy). Since platelets are very immunogenic, and typing and cross-matching techniques are not yet practical, this blood component should not be given in the absence of clear indication. Most nonbleeding patients with platelet counts above 10,000 per microliter can maintain adequate hemostasis. Patients in the immediate postoperative period may need to have their platelet counts elevated to as high as 100,000 per microliter. In other bleeding situations, a platelet count of 50,000 per microliter or more suggests other causes for hemorrhage, especially if there is no recent history of ingestion of aspirin or other drugs that interfere with platelet function, which would be reflected by a prolonged bleeding time. The effectiveness of platelet transfusion is assessed by comparing the platelet count before the infusion with counts obtained about 1 and 24 h later.

Choice of blood type Ideally, donors of platelets should have the same ABO and Rh types as the patient, since it is impossible to remove all red blood cells and plasma from the platelet concentrate. When it is necessary to use O donors for A, B, or AB recipients, the plasma may contain sufficient anti-A (or anti-B) to destroy some of the patient's red blood cells. Although this possibility is small, it deserves consideration in children or in adults receiving large numbers of platelet concentrates. When platelets of A, B, or AB donors are given to patients of unlike ABO type, the posttransfusion platelet increment may be somewhat diminished, although this is rarely a major problem. However, it is important that the number of red blood cells in such ABO-incompatible preparations be kept as small as possible.

Since some red blood cells are inevitably present in platelet concentrates, Rh-negative patients should receive platelets from Rh-negative donors whenever feasible, particularly if there is a possibility of subsequent pregnancy. However, lack of platelets from Rh-negative donors should not preclude transfusing Rh-positive donor platelets in a life-threatening situation. Patients who have the potential of becoming mothers can be protected against Rh alloimmunization by an injection of Rh immunoglobulin, about 20 μg for each milliliter of Rh-positive red blood cells present in the infusion. In other Rh-negative patients given platelets from Rh-positive donors, Rh-antibody formation can be expected to occur with a high frequency, but these antibodies do not interfere with the survival of subsequently transfused Rh-positive donor platelets, since they do not themselves contain Rh antigens.

Refractory state Patients who receive random donor platelets on more than one or two occasions frequently develop alloantibodies with either HLA or platelet antigen specificities. Such refractory patients can often be maintained with concentrates prepared by plateletpheresis from family members or HLA-compatible community pheresis donors. Failure to achieve a good response to histocompatible platelets suggests the presence of platelet-specific alloantibodies, nonimmune causes of platelet refractoriness, or hypersplenism.

WHITE BLOOD CELL TRANSFUSIONS Since it is now possible with platelet transfusions to control bleeding in many patients with hematologic malignancies, hemorrhage has been supplanted by infection as the most frequent cause of death. In general, neutrophil transfusion therapy should be considered in patients with severe neutropenia who have documented bacterial infections not responsive to appropriate antibiotic therapy. A course of neutrophil support usually consists of daily transfusion of 10 to 30 $\times 10^9$ neutrophils, obtained from normal donors by leukapheresis. Problems of maintaining patients for long periods in this way are even more difficult than those associated with platelets. Neutrophils have a very short life span in the bloodstream, and many questions remain unanswered about the best dosage schedules, the feasibility of neutrophil storage, the efficacy of neutrophils for fungal infections, and the recognition and management of alloimmunization. Hazards include alloimmunization to HLA and other antigens, pulmonary damage and other transfusion reactions, as well as transmission of infection, particularly cytomegalovirus, to immunosuppressed recipients.

PLASMA COMPONENT THERAPY Fresh frozen plasma and cryoprecipitate are major blood component preparations because they are necessary for the care of patients with coagulation disorders. Plasma can be used for expanding intravascular volume, but it carries the risk of viral transmission. Commercially prepared albumin solutions are preferable as volume expanders, as they have been heated to inactivate viruses. They are useful in special cases, such as nephrosis, certain gastroenteropathies, and severe malnutrition. Immunoglobulin preparations are also commercially made, including specific hyperimmune globulin for preventing the development of certain infectious diseases and for blocking the immune response to Rh antigen.

PLASMAPHERESIS The introduction of cell separators has made plasmapheresis a simple procedure wherein as much as one to two plasma volumes may be exchanged in 1 to 3 h. The procedure has generally been used to reduce the plasma concentration of proteins, lipids, protein-bound hormones or toxins, antibodies, antigens, or immune complexes. While the number of different diseases that have been managed by this procedure is considerable, there are only a few in which the role of plasmapheresis is generally accepted. Even then, there is controversy regarding the frequency and volume of exchange as well as the nature of replacement fluids.

The most established indication is symptomatic hyperviscosity syndrome; plasmapheresis in this setting reproducibly results in clinical improvement. Plasmapheresis can also be used successfully in selected patients with myasthenia gravis, Goodpasture's syndrome, thrombotic thrombocytopenic purpura, and immune-complex-mediated vasculitis.

COMPLICATIONS OF BLOOD TRANSFUSION Transfusion reactions are classified as immune or nonimmune. The immunologically mediated reactions may be directed against red or white blood cells, platelets, or at least one of the immunoglobulins, IgA. Other less well defined hypersensitivity reactions also occur. The major nonimmune reactions are due to circulatory overload, massive transfusion, or transmission of an infectious agent.

Immunologically mediated reactions Hemolysis due to red blood cell alloantibodies may occur within the circulation or extravascularly. The very rapid cell destruction associated with *intravascular hemolysis* is usually due to incompatibility within the ABO system, since both anti-A and anti-B fix complement, regardless of whether they are IgM or IgG molecules. Other possibilities to consider are anti-Jk^a, anti-Fy^a, and anti-Le^a. Rh antibodies are only rarely associated with hemoglobinemia. Symptoms include restlessness, anxiety, flushing, chest or lumbar pain, tachypnea, tachycardia, and nausea, followed by the typical findings of shock and renal failure. In comatose or anesthetized patients, the first sign of danger is often oozing of blood from the mucous membranes or operative site, due to intravascular coagulation.

Extravascular hemolysis is most commonly caused by antibodies of the Rh system, but several other antibodies, especially of the Kell, Duffy, and Kidd systems, are among the offenders. The clinical manifestations are usually milder, consisting of malaise and fever. Shock and renal complications rarely occur. Some patients have delayed reactions in which the transfused red blood cells have normal survival initially, but about a week later they are rapidly destroyed in the reticuloendothelial system. Such delayed reactions are commonly due to an anamnestic rise in antibodies previously stimulated by transfusion or pregnancy. Rarely, patients are found to have destroyed all the transfused cells in the absence of demonstrable antibodies.

LABORATORY INVESTIGATION Of first importance in the investigation of a hemolytic transfusion reaction is a careful check on the identity of both the donor and the recipient, since clerical errors, especially mistakes in identity, are most frequently involved. Then the necessary steps include demonstrating that red blood cell destruction has occurred, investigating its cause, and determining the status of the patient's renal and coagulation mechanisms.

With recent *intravascular* lysis, the hemoglobin level is elevated in both plasma and urine (blood must be drawn cautiously to avoid red blood cell rupture). Also, depending on the number of red blood cells destroyed, there may be methemalbuminemia accompanied by marked reduction of serum haptoglobin and hemopexin. (Measuring the latter two substances is rarely necessary, and to be meaningful, both tests require knowledge of the pretransfusion levels for comparison.) The best indicator of *extravascular* lysis is a rise in unconjugated bilirubin, accompanied by failure of the hematocrit to reach the expected posttransfusion level.

Having a *pretransfusion* specimen of the patient's blood is very helpful, so that determination of both donor and recipient blood types can be repeated, along with the compatibility test. If antibodies are detected, this pretransfusion specimen is also valuable for determining specificity, aided by knowledge of the full antigen composition, since alloantibodies are formed only against antigens not present on the patient's own cells. The *posttransfusion* specimen may not contain the offending antibodies, since they could have been completely absorbed by the donor's incompatible red blood cells. However, it is desirable to examine the red blood cells in the posttransfusion sample, both microscopically for agglutinates and by the direct antiglobulin (Coombs) test. A positive result usually means that some of the donor's red blood cells, coated by the patient's antibodies, were still present when the blood was drawn. But it is also possible that the *donor's* plasma contained antibodies, missed during the donor screening procedure, which reacted with the red blood cells of the patient. Thus, if the direct antiglobulin test on the posttransfusion specimen is positive, the plasma of both donor and recipient should be examined for the responsible antibodies. In the absence of ABO incompatibility, significant destruction of a patient's red blood cells by a donor's alloantibodies is distinctly rare. More typically, the antibody-coated red blood cells survive well in vivo, but their presence can lead to a misdiagnosis of acquired hemolytic anemia.

TREATMENT The care of patients with extravascular hemolysis should be conservative, avoiding additional transfusion unless the patient's life is otherwise threatened. Intravascular hemolysis is a far greater hazard, since shock and renal failure can occur. Immediate treatment with an osmotic diuretic is indicated unless acute tubular necrosis has already occurred. Renal blood flow can be increased with appropriate agents, shock controlled symptomatically, and disseminated intravascular coagulation treated appropriately. Management of the coagulopathy is discussed in Chap. 281, and treatment of renal shutdown in Chap. 219.

In the absence of red blood cell destruction, most febrile reactions can be ascribed to immunity against white blood cell, platelet, or plasma antigens. Further laboratory workup is required only when the reaction is unusually severe. For example, patients with antibodies against IgA molecules sometimes undergo severe shock upon exposure to the blood of other human subjects. Such individuals must be transfused only with blood that lacks IgA or with repeatedly washed red blood cells. Patients with antibodies against white blood cells or platelets can usually be given packed red blood cells from which the buffy layer has been removed after centrifugation or by filtration. Some centers use frozen and thawed red blood cells for transfusing patients sensitized to white blood cells, or to retard the occurrence of such sensitization in candidates for bone marrow transplantation. However, in patients who are candidates for renal transplantation, prior transfusions with white cell–containing products are often associated with improved prognosis—especially if the blood donor is subsequently used as the kidney donor.

Nonimmune transfusion reactions Included in this category are circulatory overload, adverse effects of massive transfusion, infections, metabolic shock, air and fat embolisms, thrombophlebitis, and siderosis. The first three are by far the most common.

CIRCULATORY OVERLOAD Patients with renal or cardiac insufficiency are liable to develop circulatory failure and pulmonary edema with even modest amounts of intravenous infusion. Infants are also vulnerable, since their vasculature does not accommodate rapidly to infusions. The onset may be immediate or delayed for up to 24 h after transfusion, with dyspnea and chest pain progressing to the full-blown picture of pulmonary edema. Susceptible patients should be transfused in a sitting position, with the rate of red blood cell flow not exceeding 2 mL/min, depending on body size and degree of impairment. A rise in central venous pressure heralds the danger of administering more red blood cells unless they are exchanged with whole blood removed from the patient.

MASSIVE TRANSFUSION When the amount of stored blood transfused to bleeding patients exceeds the amount of their normal blood volume, complications can include hyperkalemia, ammonia and citrate toxicity, and dilutional coagulopathy, which is most commonly associated with thrombocytopenia. Platelet concentrates are frequently indicated for this condition, while fresh frozen plasma is only rarely useful. If the factor 8 level or fibrinogen content is low, concentrates such as cryoprecipitate should be considered.

INFECTION Many diseases, such as hepatitis, cytomegalovirus infection, syphilis, malaria, toxoplasmosis, brucellosis, and the acquired immunodeficiency syndrome (AIDS) can be transmitted by transfusion. In addition, blood that becomes infected during handling and storage can cause very severe shock, owing to toxic bacterial metabolites. Testing donated blood for evidence of transmissible infection is increasingly important to reduce transfusion risks. Tests for hepatitis B virus and syphilis, as well as for the antibody to HTLV III (the AIDS-associated virus), are now routinely performed on all donor units. No tests for non-A, non-B hepatitis are available. Immunocompromised patients, including low birthweight neonates, are candidates to receive blood found negative for the cytomegalovirus antibody. To reduce the risk of AIDS transmission, patients at high risk for the disease are asked to defer serving as donors. In addition, all blood is tested for the antibody using an ELISA technique. Confirmatory tests, such as the western blot technique, are performed before the donor is informed of a positive result, but blood found positive by the ELISA test is discarded.

REFERENCES

ANSTEE DJ: The blood group MNSs-active sialoglycoproteins. Semin Hematol 18:13, 1981

CASH JD: Blood replacement therapy, in *Haemostasis and Thrombosis*, AL Bloom, DP Thomas (eds). Edinburgh, Churchill Livingston, 1981, pp 473–490

GIBLETT ER: Blood group alloantibodies: An assessment of some laboratory practices. Transfusion 17:299, 1977

HAKOMORI S: Blood group ABH and Ii antigens of human erythrocytes: Chemistry, polymorphism and their developmental change. Semin Hematol 18:39, 1981

MARSH WL: Molecular defects associated with the McLeod blood group phenotype, in *Blood Groups and Other Red Cell Surface Markers in Health and Disease*, C Salmon (ed). New York, Masson, 1982

MCKUSICK VA: Human gene map, in *Genetic Maps, 1984*, SJ O'Brien (ed). New York, Cold Spring Harbor Laboratory, 1984, pp 417–446

MOHN JF et al (eds): *Human Blood Groups*. New York, Karger, 1977

MOLLISON PL: *Blood Transfusion in Clinical Medicine*, 7th ed. Philadelphia, Lippincott, 1983

MOURANT AE et al: *The Distribution of the Human Blood Groups and Other Biochemical Polymorphisms*, 2d ed. New York, Oxford University Press, 1975

PETZ LD, SWISHER SN (eds): *Clinical Practice of Blood Transfusion*. New York, Churchill Livingston, 1981

Provisional public health service interagency recommendations for screening donated blood and plasma for antibody to the virus causing acquired immunodeficiency syndrome. Morb Mort Week Rep 34:1, 1985

RACE RR, SANGER R: *Blood Groups in Man*, 6th ed. Oxford, Blackwell, 1975

SLICHTER SJ: Controversies in platelet transfusion therapy. Ann Rev Med 31:509, 1980

WATKINS WM: Biochemistry and genetics of the ABO, Lewis, and P blood group systems, in *Advances in Human Genetics*, H Harris, K Hirschhorn (eds). New York, Plenum, 1980, vol 10, pp 1–136, 379–385

section 2 Disorders of the hematopoietic system

283 PATHOPHYSIOLOGY OF THE ANEMIAS

H. FRANKLIN BUNN

There is a large and coherent body of information on the birth, life, and death of red cells. A thorough familiarity with erythropoiesis and erythrocyte structure and function is necessary to understand the pathogenesis of the various anemias as well as to develop an orderly approach to diagnosis and management. Conversely, investigation of specific red cell disorders has provided unique insights into normal erythroid physiology.

RED CELL PRODUCTION Red cells are derived from an undifferentiated progenitor cell in the bone marrow called the *pluripotent stem cell* (Fig. 283-1). A stem cell is one which is capable of both self-renewal and differentiation. *Pluripotent* implies that granulocytes, monocytes, and platelets also evolve from this ancestor cell. The pluripotent stem cell has the morphologic characteristics of a mature lymphocyte. The control of proliferation into differentiated cell lines is poorly understood. Experiments have been hampered by difficulty in isolating early red cell precursors from the bone marrow. However, considerable advances have been made in culturing erythroid progenitor cells in vitro. As Fig. 283-1 shows, the most primitive erythroid progenitor which has been cultured from both bone marrow and peripheral blood is called the *erythroid burst-forming unit* (BFU_e). After 10 to 15 days in tissue culture it produces a large colony of recognizable red cell precursors. The BFU_e is responsive to high doses of the erythroid-promoting hormone erythropoietin, which acts synergistically with other growth factors which are derived from lymphocytes and monocytes. A more mature cell, the *erythroid colony-forming unit* (CFU_e), produces a smaller clone of erythroid cells after 4 to 7 days in culture and is very sensitive to erythropoietin. Various other factors such as catecholamines, steroids, thyroid hormone, growth hormone, and cyclic nucleotides may also influence erythropoiesis. Well-designed experiments involving incubation of uniform cell populations with purified growth factors should provide considerably more information about the mechanisms underlying the

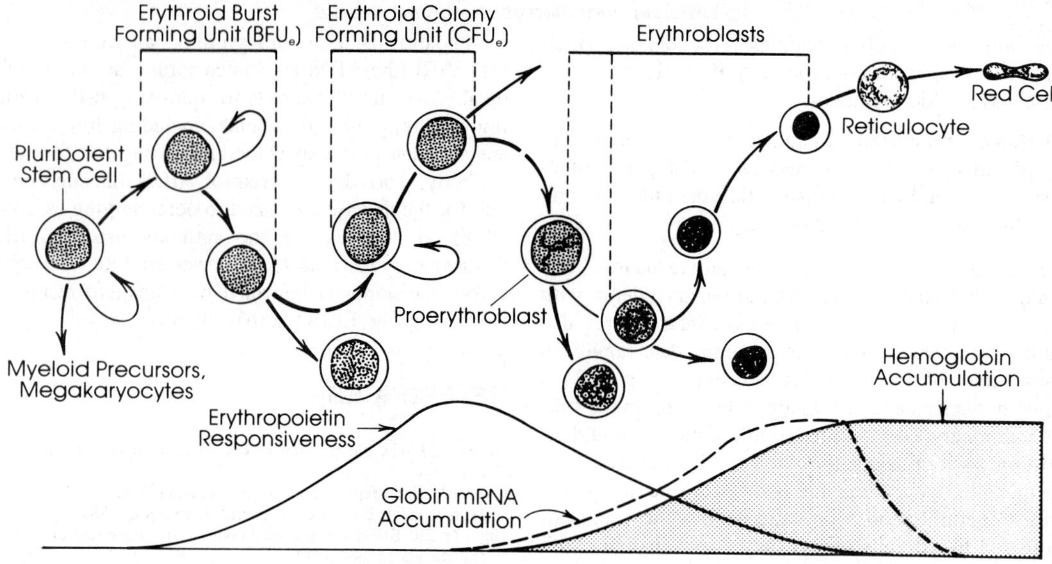

FIGURE 283-1 *Differentiation and morphologic maturation of erythroid cells. Erythroid cells are derived from pluripotent stem cells shown on left. Under the influence of erythropoietin, erythroid stem cells ($BFU_e \rightarrow CFU_e$) differentiate into proerythroblasts, the earliest recognizable red blood cell precursors in the bone marrow. During further maturation, globin mRNA accumulates, directing the cell to synthesize hemoglobin.*

differentiation and maturation of erythroid cells, as well as insights into certain disorders of erythropoiesis.

Erythropoietin, a glycoprotein having a molecular weight of about 36,000, has been purified to homogeneity. The cloning of the erythropoietin gene has made possible the synthesis of large amounts of biologically active hormone. Erythropoietin is produced primarily by the kidneys in response to hypoxic stimuli. The purification of erythropoietin has permitted the development of a radioimmunoassay which is more accurate and sensitive than conventional bioassays. Reliable measurements of erythropoietin will have a number of diagnostic applications and will also provide new information about the pathogenesis of several types of anemias.

Erythropoietin probably interacts with specific receptors on the surfaces of committed erythroid stem cells, inducing them to differentiate into pronormoblasts, the earliest red cell precursor that can be recognized on examination of the bone marrow. In addition, erythropoietin acts on later red cell precursors, stimulating hemoglobin synthesis. Normally the transition from the proerythroblast to the most mature normoblast involves three or four cell divisions over a 4-day period (Fig. 283-1). During this time, the nucleus becomes smaller, and an increasing amount of hemoglobin is produced in the cytoplasm. Following the last division, the pyknotic nucleus is removed from the normoblast, forming the reticulocyte which stays in the bone marrow for 2.5 to 3 days. The reticulocyte is then released into the general circulation, where it remains for another 24 h before it loses its mitochondria and ribosomes and assumes the morphologic appearance of a mature red cell.

Erythroid precursor cells ranging from the pronormoblast to the reticulocyte possess a specific surface receptor for the iron-transferrin complex, enabling them to incorporate sufficient iron for hemoglobin production (Fig. 238-2). The use of a radioactive iron label such as ^{59}Fe permits a quantitative assessment of erythropoiesis. From the rate at which injected ^{59}Fe-labeled transferrin disappears from the plasma, plasma iron turnover can be calculated. This parameter is generally proportional to the total developing erythroid cell mass. Normally, about 80 percent of ^{59}Fe bound to plasma transferrin goes to erythroid cells in the marrow (Fig. 284-3*B*). After 4 to 6 days the labeled iron reappears in circulating erythrocytes. The extent to which

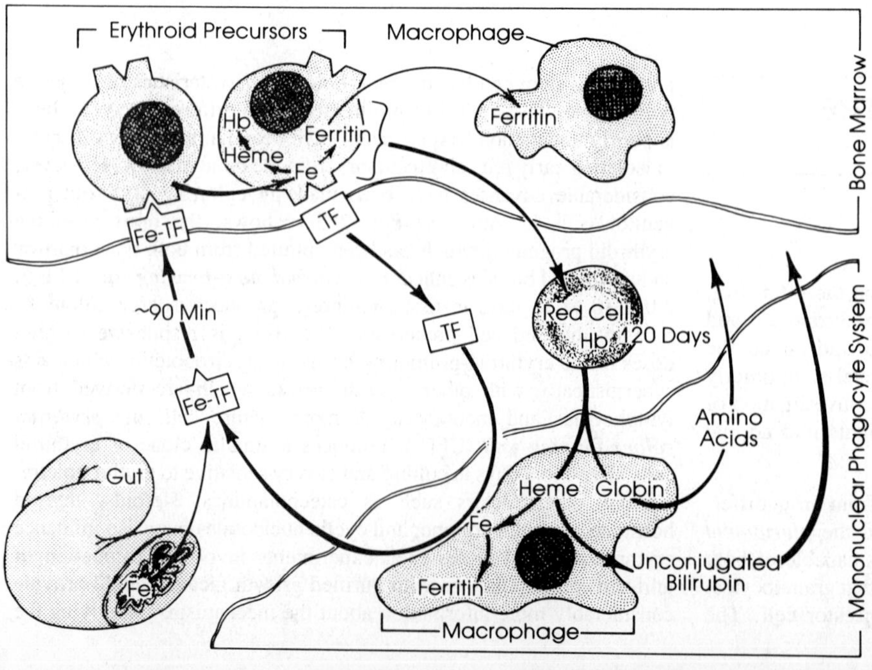

FIGURE 283-2 *Erythrocyte production, circulation, and destruction. Circulating iron-bound transferrin (TF) is bound to specific receptors on the surface of red blood cell precursors in the marrow. Most of this iron is incorporated into hemoglobin; the remainder is stored as ferritin. Following maturation of the erythroid precursor, the nucleus is shed and the red blood cell emerges from the marrow into the plasma where it circulates for approximately 120 days. The senescent red blood cell is taken up by the mononuclear phagocyte system and is destroyed. The heme iron is initially incorporated into ferritin. This storage iron is available for transport to the marrow via transferrin.*

circulating red cells acquire the label provides an index of the efficiency or effectiveness of erythropoiesis.

The normal marrow is capable of increasing its red cell production to about three to five times the normal rate within a week or two following maximal stimulation. In chronic hemolytic anemias, erythropoiesis may increase five- to sevenfold. As the erythroid marrow expands, fat is replaced by erythroid cells, and formerly inactive or "yellow" marrow becomes active or "red."

HEMOGLOBIN BIOSYNTHESIS Erythroid cell development involves the production of hemoglobin-containing cells. About 98 percent of the protein in the cytoplasm of circulating red cells is hemoglobin. This protein is a tetramer composed of two pairs of polypeptide chains designated α, β, γ, and δ, each of which is covalently linked to a heme group. The synthesis of a particular globin subunit is directed by a corresponding gene inherited from each parent. As shown in Fig. 283-1, there is a marked amplification in the transcription of globin chain mRNA during the development of proerythroblasts.

In the red cells of normal adults, hemoglobin A ($\alpha_2\beta_2$) composes about 97 percent of the total hemoglobin. The remaining 3 percent is primarily hemoglobin A_2 ($\alpha_2\delta_2$). As discussed in Chap. 288, this minor component is increased in patients with β thalassemia. Fetal hemoglobin (HbF or $\alpha_2\gamma_2$) usually accounts for less than 1 percent of total hemoglobin in normal adult red cells. HbF is localized to 1 to 7 percent of red cells. In contrast, it is the main hemoglobin component of fetal red cells. During the last 3 months of gestation, γ-chain synthesis switches to β-chain synthesis. However, in certain types of congenital hemolytic anemias such as the β thalassemias and sickle cell anemia, the production of γ chains (and therefore of HbF) persists. In addition, increased levels of HbF may also be encountered in certain acquired anemias in which there is disordered red cell proliferation.

Normally α- and β-chain synthesis in erythroid precursors is evenly balanced. In contrast, the thalassemias (Chap. 288) are characterized by imbalance in globin chain synthesis.

The synthesis of *heme* in red cell precursors is closely matched to globin chain production. As shown in Fig. 283-3 the initial and rate-limiting step is the condensation of succinyl coenzyme A (CoA) and glycine to form δ-aminolevulinic acid. This reaction, which takes place in mitochondria, requires that glycine be activated by pyridoxal phosphate. Accordingly, patients with sideroblastic anemia in whom heme synthesis is usually defective may sometimes respond to pyridoxine therapy (Chap. 284). The next steps of heme synthesis take place in the cytosol. Two molecules of δ-aminolevulinic acid condense to form a ring structure, prophobilinogen. This colorless pyrrole is elevated in acute intermittent porphyria and can be detected in urine by the Watson-Schwartz test. The subsequent steps in prophyrin synthesis are also shown in Fig. 283-3. The last three reactions take place in mitochondria. Iron is inserted into protoporphyrin IX to form heme. In iron deficiency, as well as in lead poisoning, increased levels of protoporphyrin can be detected in red cells. Disorders of porphyrin synthesis and metabolism are discussed in Chap. 312.

HEMOGLOBIN STRUCTURE AND FUNCTION The primary role of red cells is to transport oxygen from lungs to tissues and to transport carbon dioxide in the reverse direction. Both of these functions are assumed by hemoglobin. The three-dimensional structure of human hemoglobin has been determined from x-ray crystallographic analysis. The important functional properties of hemoglobin such as heme-heme interaction, the pH dependency of oxygen affinity (the Bohr

FIGURE 283-3 *The biosynthesis of heme. The following abbreviations are used: CoA, coenzyme A; GTP, guanosine triphosphate; GDP, guanosine diphosphate; Pi, inorganic phosphorus; GSH, glutathione; Δ-ALA-DH, Δ-aminolevulinate dehydrase; UIS, uroporphyrinogen I synthetase; UIII CoS, uroporphyrinogen III cosynthetase; UD, uroporphyrinogen decarboxylase; CO, coproporphyrinogen oxidase; HS, heme synthetase; A, acetate; P, proportionate; M, methyl; V, vinyl. Enzymatic steps that occur in mitochondria are shown.*

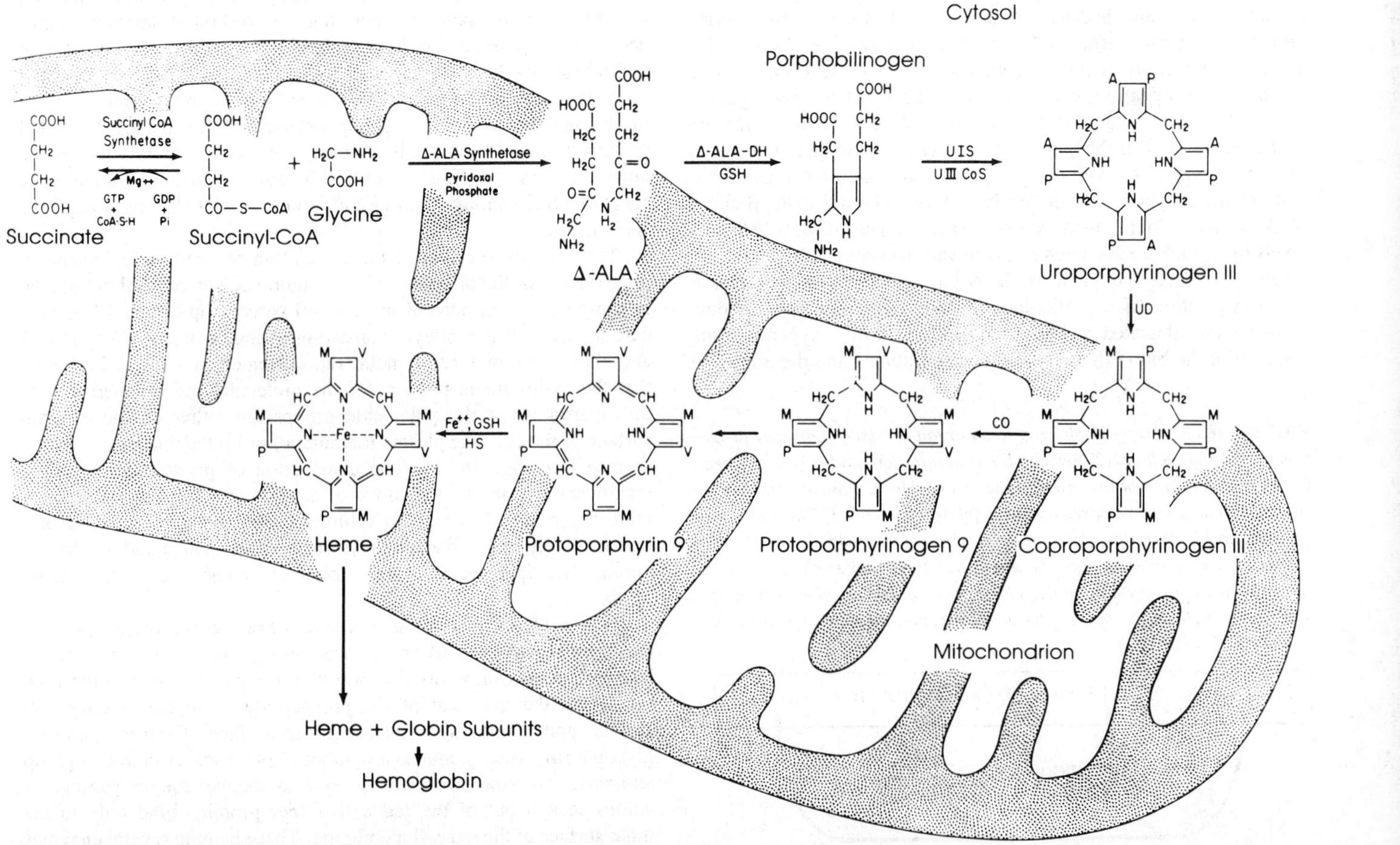

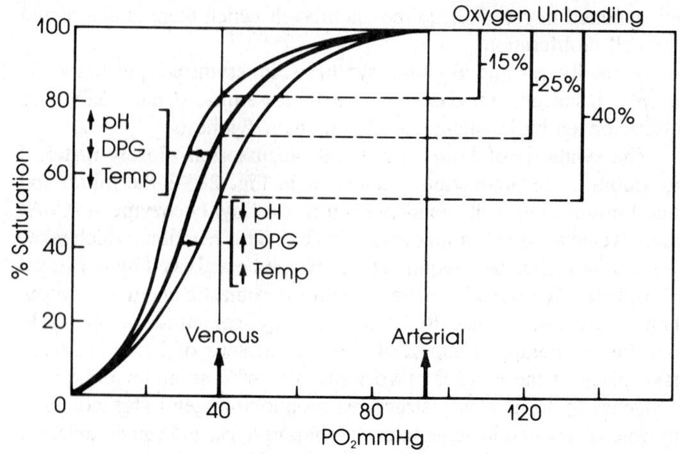

FIGURE 283-4 *The oxyhemoglobin dissociation curve of normal blood. The major factors influencing the position of the curve are pH, temperature, and the intracellular concentration of 2,3-DPG. An increase in plasma pH or a decrease in temperature and 2,3-DPG causes an increase in oxygen affinity (shift to the left) and a relative decrease in oxygen unloading when going from an arterial P_{O_2} of 95 mmHg to a venous P_{O_2} of 40 mmHg. Conversely, a decrease in pH or an increase in temperature and 2,3-DPG causes a decrease in oxygen affinity (shift to the right) and a relative increase in oxygen unloading.*

effect), and the interaction with 2,3-diphosphoglycerate can now be understood on a stereochemical basis. This structural information has also been useful in explaining the abnormal functional properties of a number of human hemoglobin variants which are associated with clinical and hematologic manifestations (see Chap. 288).

During the circulation through the lungs, hemoglobin becomes almost fully saturated with oxygen (1.34 mL O_2 per gram of hemoglobin). As red cells perfuse the capillary beds, oxygen is extracted. Efficient unloading of oxygen at relatively high oxygen tensions is possible because of the sigmoid shape of the oxygen dissociation curve (heme-heme interaction) (see Fig. 283-4). The affinity of hemoglobin for oxygen is modified by three intracellular cofactors: hydrogen ion, carbon dioxide, and 2,3-diphosphoglycerate (2,3-DPG). Increasing concentrations of each of these three effectors results in a "shift to the right" in the oxygen dissociation curve. In human red cells, 2,3-DPG appears to be an important regulator of hemoglobin function. One molecule of 2,3-DPG binds to the β chains of deoxyhemoglobin, thereby decreasing oxygen affinity. Elevated levels of 2,3-DPG have been noted in various states of hypoxia. The resulting decrease in oxygen affinity permits enhanced oxygen release. The oxygenation of a particular organ or tissue depends on three main factors (depicted in Fig. 283-5): blood flow, oxygen-carrying capacity of the blood (hemoglobin concentration), and the affinity of

FIGURE 283-5 *Oxygen delivered to an organ or tissue is directly proportional to (1) blood flow, (2) hemoglobin concentration, and (3) the difference in oxygen saturation of the arterial and venous blood. Patients with various types of hypoxia may compensate in the following ways: (1) The distribution of blood flow is altered to maintain oxygenation of vital organs; total cardiac output increases when hypoxia is severe. (2) Increased erythropoietin production stimulates erythropoiesis. (3) Oxygen unloading is enhanced by a shift to the right in the oxygen dissociation curve, mediated by an increase in red cell 2,3-DPG.*

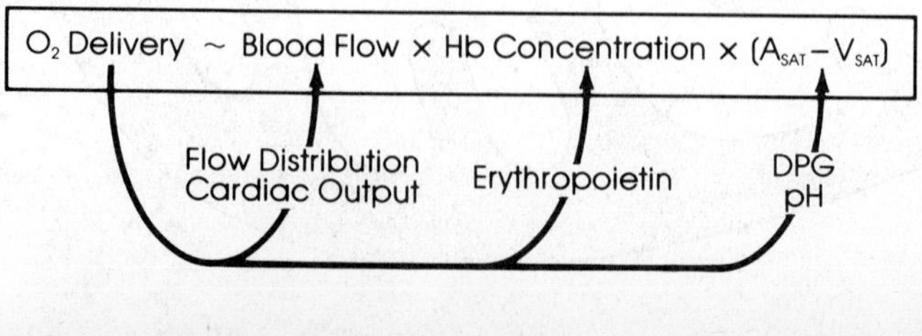

the hemoglobin for oxygen. Patients with a primary abnormality of one of these three factors depend on adjustments in one or both of the other two in order to maintain optimal tissue oxygenation. For example, patients with anemia have two available modes of compensation: enhanced blood flow and decreased oxygen affinity, mediated by increased levels of 2,3-DPG. Conversely, individuals with a hemoglobin variant having increased oxygen affinity have a primary defect in oxygen unloading. As discussed in Chap. 288, such patients compensate by developing secondary erythrocytosis.

RED BLOOD CELL METABOLISM As the red cell emerges from the bone marrow, it loses its nucleus, ribosomes, and mitochondria and therefore all capability for cell division, protein synthesis, and oxidative phosphorylation. Compared with other cells, the erythrocyte has a rather simple scheme of intermediary metabolism. Glucose is virtually the only fuel utilized by the red cell. It readily enters the red cell by facilitated diffusion and is then converted to glucose 6-phosphate. There are two major pathways available for glucose 6-phosphate (Fig. 287-2). About 80 to 90 percent of this intermediate is converted to lactate by means of the glycolytic (or Embden-Meyerhof) pathway. Two moles of adenosine triphosphate (ATP) are generated for every mole of glucose that is metabolized. The intracellular mediator of hemoglobin function, 2,3-diphosphoglycerate, is synthesized in a side reaction shown in Fig. 287-2. About 10 percent of intracellular glucose 6-phosphate undergoes oxidation by means of the hexose-monophosphate shunt. This pathway maintains glutathione in the reduced form, thereby protecting sulfhydryl groups in hemoglobin and the red cell membrane from oxidation by peroxides and superoxide as well as by certain drugs and toxins. Such oxidant stress can compromise red cell function and viability in patients with a deficiency in glucose 6-phosphate dehydrogenase, the first enzymatic step in the hexose-monophosphate shunt (see Chap. 287). Less commonly, individuals may have a deficiency in one of the enzymes of the glycolytic pathway or in one of the other enzymes of the hexose-monophosphate shunt.

The red cell has rather modest metabolic obligations in keeping with its simplified structure. A significant portion of the ATP generated by glycolysis is spent in operating the sodium-potassium pump, necessary to preserve the ionic milieu in the cytoplasm and prevent colloid osmotic lysis. In addition, some metabolic energy is expended on maintenance and repair of the red cell membrane. Certain proteins in the membrane become phosphorylated by means of ATP and protein kinases, but the physiologic significance of this process is not yet understood. Finally, a small amount of metabolic currency is spent on maintaining hemoglobin iron atoms in the reduced form (Fe^{2+}).

The 120-day survival of the circulating red cell is dependent on preservation of the pliability of its membrane. The red cell membrane is composed of 50 percent protein, 40 percent lipid, and 10 percent carbohydrate. It is a bilayer consisting of molecules of phospholipid and cholesterol in a 1.2:1 molar ratio oriented in a stacked array so that the hydrophobic portions of the molecules are oriented toward the interior while the polar side groups are either on the external surface of the cell (the plasma membrane) or on the inner cytoplasmic surface (see Fig. 283-6). The distribution of phospholipids differs significantly in the two portions of the bilayer. The outer surface is relatively rich in lecithin and sphingomyelin while the inner surface has relatively more phosphatidyl serine and phosphatidyl ethanolamine. The lipids on the outer surface exchange freely with plasma lipids.

The red cell membrane contains about eight major proteins (depicted in Fig. 283-6) and a large number of minor components. These proteins can be divided into two groups. A few span the lipid bilayer so that one end of the polypeptide is on the external cell surface and the other is on the inner surface. Examples include glycophorin, which contains a number of polysaccharide blood group antigens, and band 3, which serves as a channel for the passage of anions in and out of the red cell. Other proteins bind only to the inner surface of the red cell membrane. These include several enzymes

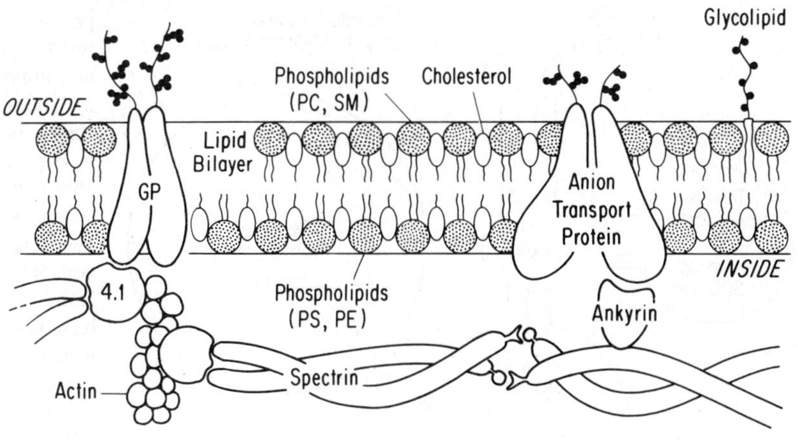

FIGURE 283-6 *Diagram of a cross section of the red blood cell membrane. Spectrin, actin, and protein 4.1 form a meshwork which laminates the inner surface of the membrane. In contrast, other proteins such as the glycophorins (GP) and the anion transport protein traverse the lipid bilayer. Long polysaccharide chains are covalently attached to these proteins on the outer surface of the cell and also to glycolipid. The protein ankyrin forms a bridge between spectrin and a fraction of the anion transport proteins. Protein 4.1 binds to GP. Phospholipids in the lipid bilayer include phosphatidylcholine (PC) and sphingomyelin (SM), which are located primarily on the outer surface of the membrane, and phosphatidyl serine (PS) and phosphatidyl ethanolamine (PE), which are located primarily on the inner surface of the membrane.*

as well as structural proteins such as spectrin and actin, which interact to form a meshwork that laminates the cytoplasmic surface of the membrane.

It is likely that the physiologic demise of 120-day-old red cells is due to a loss of membrane flexibility preventing them from negotiating the narrow-bore channels of the microcirculation, including the sinusoids of the spleen. The factors responsible for red cell senescence are poorly understood. Experimental evidence indicates that deterioration of the red cell's metabolic machinery, sufficient to deplete it of ATP, can cause the cell to become spiculated (ecchinocytic) and lose its normal pliability. Depletion of ATP disrupts the spectrin and actin meshwork lining the inner membrane surface, resulting in aggregation of these proteins. Other factors such as enhanced rigidity and, perhaps, coating with immunoglobulin may also contribute to the recognition of the senescent red cell by the mononuclear phagocyte system. In contrast to normal red cells, there is a large and well-documented body of information on the mechanisms responsible for red cell destruction in various hemolytic anemias. These are discussed in Chap. 287.

Once the senescent red cell is sequestered (Fig. 283-2), hemoglobin is readily catabolized. Amino acids are released by proteolytic digestion and subsequently metabolized. The heme group is catabolized by a microsomal oxidizing system. The porphyrin ring is converted to bile pigments which are excreted almost quantitatively by the liver. One mole of carbon monoxide is formed per mole of heme that is broken down. Endogenous carbon monoxide production correlates directly with erythroid cell destruction. As Fig. 283-2 shows, the iron that is released during heme catabolism is initially incorporated into the storage protein ferritin, but it is eventually transported to marrow erythroid precursors by transferrin, the plasma iron–binding protein.

If red cell production is disordered, there may be significant destruction of erythroid cells within the bone marrow. A number of anemias are chararcterized by *ineffective erythropoiesis,* particularly those in which erythroid maturation is morphologically abnormal and the circulating red cells are abnormal in size. Examples discussed in detail elsewhere include megaloblastic anemias, sideroblastic anemias, and β thalassemia major. Such disorders are characterized by erythroid hyperplasia in the bone marrow and rapid uptake of labeled iron into the marrow but a low recovery of the labeled iron in circulating red cells. Endogenous carbon monoxide production and plasma levels of unconjugated bilirubin are generally elevated in ineffective erythropoiesis.

REFERENCES

BABIOR BM, STOSSEL TP: *Hematology: A Pathophysiological Approach.* New York, Churchill Livingston, 1984

BECK WS (ed): *Hematology,* 4th ed. Boston, MIT Press, 1985

BENNETT V: The membrane skeleton of human erythrocytes and its implications for more complex cells. Ann Rev Biochem 54:273, 1985

BUNN HF, FORGET BG: *Hemoglobin: Molecular, Genetic and Clinical Aspects.* Philadelphia, Saunders, 1986

COHEN CM: The molecular organization of the red cell membrane skeleton. Semin Hematol 20:141, 1983

CROSBY WH: Red cell mass: Its precursors and perturbations. Hosp Pract 15:2, 71, 1980

EAVES AC, EAVES CJ: Erythropoiesis in culture. Clin Haematol 13:371, 1984

ERSLEV AJ, GABUZDA TG: *Pathophysiology of Blood,* 3 ed. Philadelphia, Saunders, 1985

FINCH CA: Erythropoiesis, erythropoietin and iron. Blood 60:1241, 1982

FRIED W, MORLEY C: Update on erythropoietin. Int J Art Org 8:79, 1985

WILLIAMS WJ et al (ed): *Hematology,* 2 ed. New York, McGraw-Hill, 1983

284 ANEMIAS OF IRON DEFICIENCY AND IRON OVERLOAD

ANDREW I. SCHAFER / H. FRANKLIN BUNN

Among the transition metals that are essential to life, iron is the most abundant and important, being used in a broad repertoire of biochemical reactions. When complexed with porphyrin and inserted into an appropriate protein, iron not only binds oxygen reversibly but also participates in a number of vital oxidation-reduction reactions. Since inorganic iron is highly toxic, specific processes have evolved for its assimilation, transport, and storage. Under normal circumstances iron homeostasis is precisely maintained but can go awry in a variety of clinical settings, leading either to iron deficiency or iron overload.

IRON METABOLISM

The amount of iron obtained from the diet must replace the obligatory losses from the skin and gastrointestinal and genitourinary tracts; these losses generally do not exceed 1 mg daily in the adult male or nonmenstruating female. Additional iron requirements due to menstrual blood loss vary greatly but average about 0.5 mg daily. The amount of iron present in the diet, about 10 to 20 mg daily in the United States, greatly exceeds that required to meet physiologic demands. Thus, the widespread prevalence of iron deficiency is due in part to the inefficient absorption of dietary iron. Heme iron is better absorbed than is nonheme iron. Unfortunately, the diet of most of the population of the world is virtually devoid of meats and hence of heme iron. Even in the more developed countries, only 5 to 10 percent of the iron in the diet is absorbed.

ABSORPTION Because there is no major physiologic route for the excretion of iron, body iron content normally is largely determined by its absorption. Iron is absorbed mainly in the duodenum and proximal jejunum. The absorption of nonheme iron is modified by several factors in the diet and in gastrointestinal secretions. Iron-binding anions in food, such as ethylenediaminetetraacetic acid (EDTA), which is used as a preservative in a number of foodstuffs, tannates (contained in tea), carbonates, oxalates, and phosphates all

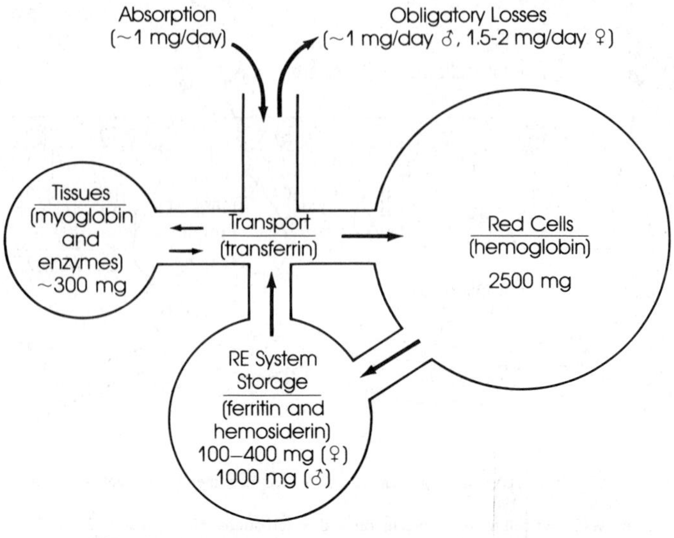

FIGURE 284-1 *The distribution of iron in normal adults and internal iron kinetics. Bold arrows indicate major pathways of iron movement.*

inhibit iron absorption. Medicinal antacids, such as magnesium trisilicate, and clay may also impair iron absorption. In contrast, other substances in the diet, including ascorbic acid, citric acid, amino acids, and sugars, enhance iron absorption. Gastric secretions and hydrochloric acid facilitate nonheme iron absorption by poorly understood mechanisms which probably involve the stabilization of ionic iron, thereby preventing its precipitation as insoluble ferric hydroxide. Most of these dietary and secretory factors do not affect the absorption of heme iron, which is taken up by the mucosal cells as the intact metalloporphyrin.

Intestinal iron absorption depends on both the amount and bioavailability of dietary iron and is controlled by the gut mucosal "setting" which is responsive to the state of body iron stores. The amount of iron entering the mucosal cell and passing into the portal circulation is regulated to maintain a normal body iron content. The signals which determine this "mucosal intelligence" are largely unknown. However, when the demand for iron is increased by depletion of body reserves due to growth spurts, pregnancy, or menstrual and pathologic hemorrhage, the efficiency of iron absorption can increase to about 10 to 20 percent. Conversely, when excessive body stores of iron are present, intestinal iron absorption is markedly reduced.

DISTRIBUTION The distribution of iron in normal adults is shown in Fig. 284-1. Most of the body iron is found in red cells as the iron porphyrin complex of hemoglobin. Smaller quantities of iron are utilized in various tissues in the form of myoglobin as well as heme and nonheme enzymes. Excess iron is stored in the body as ferritin and hemosiderin. The iron in ferritin is enclosed within a protein shell, apoferritin, which can take up Fe^{2+} and oxidize it so that Fe^{3+} is deposited within the iron core. The synthesis of apoferritin is stimulated by iron. Small quantities of ferritin can be measured in serum. Under normal conditions there is a close correlation between serum ferritin concentration and body iron stores, with serum ferritin concentration of 1 μg/L equivalent to 10 mg of storage iron. Hemosiderin is a degraded form of ferritin in which the molecules have lost part of their protein shell and have aggregated. Most storage iron is normally present as ferritin, but an increasing proportion is present as hemosiderin as iron overload progresses. Storage iron is distributed primarily in mononuclear phagocyte cells of the spleen, liver, and bone marrow and in hepatic parenchymal cells. Exchange of iron between these communicating tissue compartments is effected by the carrier plasma protein transferrin, a beta globulin synthesized in the liver.

FIGURE 284-2 *Serum iron and iron-binding capacity in various disorders.*

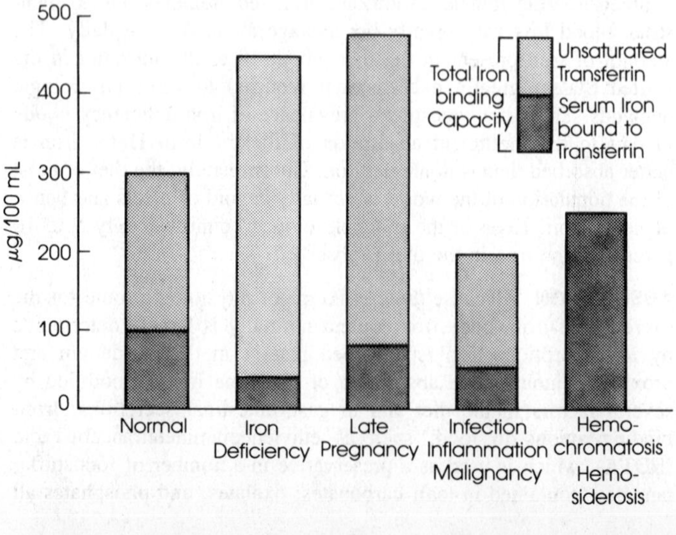

TRANSPORT The major destination of plasma transferrin–bound iron is the erythron, where immature red cell precursors assimilate the iron for hemoglobin synthesis. A much smaller amount of transferrin iron is delivered to other sites, particularly the parenchymal cells of the liver. Transferrin has two iron-binding sites. Diferric transferrin is more effective in donating iron to the developing erythron than is monoferric iron. When transferrin iron saturation is increased, tissue iron uptake is increased. Virtually no iron is deposited in mononuclear phagocyte cells from the plasma transferrin pool. These cells derive most of their iron from the phagocytosis of senescent red cells. Following phagocytosis, the iron is liberated from the porphyrin ring by heme oxygenase and is either released to the plasma to be bound by transferrin or is stored in the form of ferritin and hemosiderin. Therefore, the passage of iron through the mononuclear phagocyte system is unidirectional (see Fig. 284-1). Iron metabolism is characterized by conservation of body iron, so that the iron of hemoglobin degradation is continually reutilized for erythropoiesis. Storage iron is readily mobilized in response to increased demand by the erythron, but chronic infection, inflammation, or malignancy can interfere with the release of iron from mononuclear phagocyte stores.

LABORATORY EVALUATION In the laboratory assessment of body iron status, the most direct and sensitive tests involve *examination of tissues for iron content*. Depletion of bone marrow iron stores is the earliest stage in the development of iron deficiency and can be detected by the absence of Prussian blue–stainable iron in an aspirate of bone marrow. Histochemical assessment of increased bone marrow iron does not correlate as well with body iron stores in disorders of transfusional iron overload, and it is an unreliable index of iron overload in idiopathic hemochromatosis. The most sensitive test of iron loading in hemochromatosis (Chap. 310) is quantitative measurement of liver iron content in a liver biopsy specimen. Computerized tomography can show increased density of the liver.

Measurement of *serum iron and total iron-binding capacity* (or transferrin) is useful in the diagnosis of both iron deficiency and overload states (Fig. 284-2). The degree to which transferrin is saturated with iron represents a reliable indicator of iron supply to the developing red cell. Transferrin is normally about 20 to 45 percent saturated. The serum iron is characteristically decreased both in iron deficiency and in association with chronic disorders; however, in the latter the iron-binding capacity is generally also decreased to maintain a transferrin saturation of over 15 percent, while in the former it is usually increased so that transferrin saturation falls below 10 percent. In hypoproliferative and iron-overload states, serum iron is elevated and transferrin saturation may approach 100 percent. A disadvantage of this test is that serum iron (and hence transferrin saturation) is subject to pronounced diurnal and day-to-day variations.

Assay of *serum ferritin* correlates closely with total-body iron stores. The "normal range" of serum ferritin is not clearly established since it depends on age and sex; however, serum ferritin concentrations of 15 to 300 μg/L can be generally considered to be normal in adults. The finding of a low ferritin level is diagnostic of iron deficiency and obviates the need to perform bone marrow aspiration for the purpose of assessing stainable iron. Measurement of serum ferritin is also useful in detecting and determining the degree of iron overload, although it may underestimate iron stores in some patients with early hemochromatosis. The serum ferritin level depends not only on tissue iron stores but also on the rate of release of ferritin from the tissues. Therefore, in cases of extensive tissue damage, as may occur in patients with inflammation, liver disease, and certain malignancies, the ferritin level is usually elevated in the absence of iron overload and may be normal in the presence of coexisting iron deficiency.

Ferrokinetics *Ferrokinetic studies,* using tracer amounts of a radioactive isotope of iron, provide a more dynamic laboratory assessment of iron supply to the marrow and erythropoiesis in general than do the static methods described above. Radioactive iron (^{59}Fe) is injected intravenously and binds readily to plasma transferrin. From serial samples of the peripheral blood following injection the plasma iron turnover can be determined as well as the subsequent incorporation of iron into the hemoglobin of circulating red cells. In normal subjects, injected radioiron disappears rapidly and exponentially from plasma, with a half-time of 60 to 90 min. Figure 284-3*A* shows the linear clearance of plasma radioiron when it is plotted semilogarithmically. Plasma iron turnover (PIT) is the measure of the absolute amount of iron released from plasma transferrin per unit of time and is calculated from the rate of disappearance of iron label from the plasma, the plasma iron content, and the plasma volume. In normal individuals 30 to 40 mg of iron leaves the plasma daily. The PIT reflects the rate of *total* erythropoiesis. The *effectiveness* of erythropoiesis is indicated by the extent that the iron label is incorporated into hemoglobin in circulating red cells (Fig. 284-3*B*). In about a week, red cells normally accumulate 80 to 90 percent of the injected dose of radioiron.

In conditions of severe bone marrow failure (hypoplastic anemias) plasma iron clearance is slow, PIT is decreased, and there is very little incorporation of ^{59}Fe into hemoglobin. In iron deficiency, ^{59}Fe is removed from plasma more rapidly than normal and is almost entirely utilized by the hemoglobin of newly formed red cells. A similar pattern of ferrokinetics is seen in polycythemia vera, which is characterized by increased effective erythropoiesis. In hemolytic states, radioiron is rapidly cleared from the plasma and rapidly appears in circulating red cells, but because of the premature removal of red cells from the circulation, the apparent maximal recovery is less than normal. In disorders of hemoglobin synthesis, such as thalassemia and the sideroblastic anemias, plasma iron clearance is likewise rapid and PIT is increased; however, because of ineffective erythropoiesis, red cell radioiron utilization is low. A similar ferrokinetic profile is seen in megaloblastic anemias and myeloid metaplasia, which are likewise characterized by ineffective erythropoiesis.

IRON-DEFICIENCY ANEMIA

When the supply of iron to the bone marrow falls short of that required for the production of red blood cells, anemia will ensue. Iron deficiency is the most common cause of anemia throughout the world. This condition is particularly prevalent in tropical areas where the dietary intake of meat is low and where infestation with hookworm is endemic. In the United States, about 20 percent of women in the childbearing age group are iron-deficient, while the overall prevalence in adult males is about 2 percent.

ETIOLOGY The development of iron deficiency depends upon one or more of the following factors: (1) increased requirements, (2) inadequate dietary intake, (3) decreased intestinal absorption, and (4) blood loss. Accordingly, certain groups of individuals can be readily identified to be at increased risk for developing iron deficiency.

Increased requirements for iron occur during the growth spurts of infancy and adolescence and during pregnancy. Up to 10 percent of pre-school-age children in the United States are iron-deficient, with a peak incidence at 1 to 2 years of age. The increased demand for iron during infancy is not adequately met by a diet rich in milk and cereals and poor in meat and vegetables. The iron content of such a diet is low, and assimilation may be further impaired by the presence of iron-binding anions, particularly phosphates. Accordingly, an infant's diet should be supplemented with iron. During adolescence, iron intake also may be compromised owing to irregular dietary habits and the current predilection for "junk food." During pregnancy the growing fetus usurps about 500 mg of iron from the mother, even if she is already iron-deficient. The daily iron requirement increases about threefold during pregnancy. Currently, the vast majority of pregnant women who seek medical attention are routinely given prophylactic treatment with iron salts. Among pregnant women who do not receive adequate antenatal care, the incidence of iron deficiency exceeds 50 percent.

Inadequate intake of iron is prevalent in certain parts of the world where diets are low in animal proteins. The low iron content of the diets of infants and adolescents is mentioned above. Among indigent and elderly individuals, iron intake is often suboptimal, owing to a combination of economic constraints, poor dentition, and apathy.

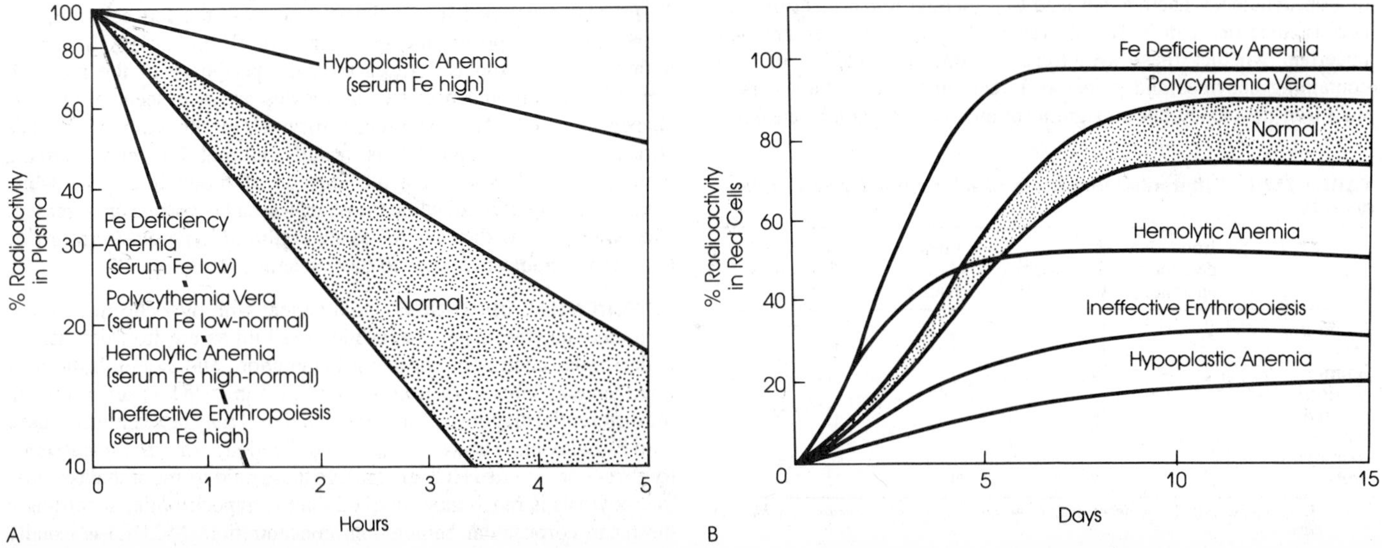

FIGURE 284-3 *Ferrokinetics in normal subjects and patients with disorders of erythropoiesis. A. Plasma radioiron clearance. B. Red cell radioiron utilization.*

Decreased absorption of iron can occur in many clinical settings. After partial or total gastrectomy, the assimilation of dietary iron is impaired, owing primarily to increased motility and bypass of the proximal intestine, which is the primary site of iron absorption. Achlorhydria also contributes to decreased iron absorption. Patients with chronic diarrhea or intestinal malabsorption may also develop iron deficiency, particularly if the duodenum and proximal jejunum are involved. Sometimes iron-deficiency anemia is a harbinger of nontropical (celiac) sprue.

Blood loss is by far the most important cause of iron deficiency in adults. Among women in the childbearing age group, menstrual blood loss is responsible for most cases of iron deficiency. Women who take estrogen-progesterone birth control pills tend to have reduced menstrual blood loss, whereas those with intrauterine devices have increased menstrual blood flow.

Gastrointestinal blood loss is the primary cause of iron deficiency among adult males but must be carefully considered in any iron-deficient patient. The testing of stool for occult blood is an indispensable part of the evaluation of all patients with iron deficiency or unexplained anemia. Since gastrointestinal bleeding can be intermittent, it may be necessary to test multiple specimens over an extended time span. The most common causes of gastrointestinal blood loss are peptic ulcer, hiatus hernia, diverticulosis, and cancer. Hemorrhoids and salicylate ingestion are often responsible for the presence of occult blood in the stool but rarely cause significant blood loss. In about 15 percent of patients with documented gastrointestinal bleeding, no source can be determined, even after extensive radiologic and endoscopic investigation. In tropical areas parasitic infestations, particularly hookworm, are a major cause of blood loss. Occasionally, as in patients with hereditary telangiectasia or in those with a bleeding diathesis, gastrointestinal bleeding arises from multiple sites. Thrombocytopenia, qualitative platelet disorders, and von Willebrand's disease are more apt to cause gastrointestinal bleeding than are deficiencies of the soluble coagulation factors.

Regular blood donors undergo a progressive depletion of iron reserves, and menstruating female donors in particular may develop frank iron-deficient erythropoiesis. The prevalence of iron depletion increases progressively with the rate of donations.

In rare patients, iron deficiency may be caused by impaired incorporation of transferrin-bound iron by erythroid precursors. This may be a congenital condition or it may be acquired with the development of autoantibodies to transferrin receptors.

CLINICAL FINDINGS Because iron deficiency usually develops insidiously, anemic patients are often relatively free of symptoms. In general, the signs and symptoms of iron-deficiency anemia are shared by other anemias of comparable severity (Chap. 53). Weakness, fatigue, lassitude, palpitations, and lightheadedness are common complaints. Subtle behavioral changes may occur. Even mild degrees of iron deficiency anemia can lead to a marked impairment of work performance that can be rapidly reversed by iron replacement. It is uncertain whether these symptoms are due to depletion of iron-containing enzymes and cofactors in certain tissues. Many persons with iron deficiency but no significant anemia complain of weakness and fatigue, but such nonspecific symptoms are difficult to evaluate. Iron deficiency is sometimes associated with pica, a desire to gnaw on solid substances. Patients develop a craving for clay (geophagia), cornstarch (amylophagia), or ice (pagophagia). This peculiar symptom subsides when iron deficiency is corrected. Iron deficiency may also be associated with a variety of gastrointestinal symptoms. Following severe and prolonged deficiency, patients sometimes develop dysphagia owing to thin membranous webs at the postcricoid area (Plummer-Vinson syndrome). More commonly, iron-deficient patients develop a variety of less specific gastrointestinal symptoms, such as anorexia, nausea, eructation, and constipation, but it is uncertain whether these complaints are caused by iron deficiency per se. Those with prolonged iron deficiency often have achlorhydria and gastric atrophy. Menorrhagia is a common symptom in iron-deficient women. Gastric atrophy and menorrhagia may contribute toward the development of iron deficiency rather than being sequelae.

Physical findings may include pallor, tachycardia, and a "hemic" flow murmur, signs shared by patients with other types of anemia. Those with prolonged iron deficiency often have dry, brittle, and ridged nails which occasionally assume a concave surface (koilonychia). The epithelium at the edges of the lips may be cracked (angular stomatitis), and the tongue may become atrophic and even tender (glossitis). The spleen is seldom enlarged. The nonhematologic manifestations of iron deficiency, such as koilonychia, angular stomatitis, glossitis, and esophageal webs, are rarely encountered nowadays, probably because iron deficiency is more readily diagnosed and more promptly treated than in earlier times.

TABLE 284-1 Differential diagnosis of microcytic hypochromic anemia

	Iron-deficiency anemia	β-Thalassemia trait	Anemia of chronic disease	Sideroblastic anemia
Serum iron	↓	N	↓	↑
TIBC	↑	N	↓	N
Serum ferritin	↓	N	↑	↑
Red cell protoporphyrin	↑	N	↑	↑ or N
HbA_2	↓	↑	N	↓

NOTE: ↑ = *increased;* ↓ = *decreased; N = normal; TIBC = serum iron binding capacity.*

LABORATORY FINDINGS A variety of laboratory tests can be used to assess varying degrees of iron deficiency. The development of iron deficiency progresses in an orderly sequence of events, each of which correlates with clinical laboratory abnormalities. *Storage iron depletion* occurs first, during which iron reserves are lost without compromise of the iron supply for erythropoiesis. At this stage, a bone marrow aspirate stained with Prussian blue will show markedly reduced or absent deposits of iron in macrophages. This finding is accompanied by a decrease in the level of serum ferritin. The next stage is *iron-deficient erythropoiesis,* during which the erythroid iron supply is reduced without the development of anemia. The iron-binding capacity of the serum (TIBC) first rises, followed by a drop in serum iron. As a result, the fractional saturation of transferrin falls markedly. The circulating red cells become microcytic and hypochromic. This is accompanied by an increase in free erythrocyte protoporphyrin (FEP). Protoporphyrin IX accumulates in the red cell because there is insufficient iron to convert it to heme (see Fig. 283-3). The fluorometric assay of FEP is a reliable and cost-effective way of screening large groups of individuals such as schoolchildren for iron deficiency. The final stage is the development of *iron-deficiency anemia.*

In well-developed iron-deficiency anemia, the red cells become more severely hypochromic and microcytic (Fig. A5-4). Often, only a thin rim of cytoplasm appears on the periphery of the red cell. Small fragments and bizarre poikilocytes are also seen. Such misshapen red cells have shortened survival in the circulation. The percentage of reticulocytes is usually normal but may increase temporarily following an acute episode of blood loss. The white count is usually normal, while the platelet count is normal or increased. The bone marrow displays moderate erythroid hyperplasia. Many of the late normoblasts appear to have scanty cytoplasm.

DIFFERENTIAL DIAGNOSIS In a patient with hypochromic microcytic anemia, the major diagnostic possibilities are iron deficiency, thalassemia, anemia of chronic inflammation, and sideroblastic anemia. Several laboratory tests (shown in Table 284-1) are useful in the differential diagnosis. Mild iron deficiency may be readily confused with β-thalassemia trait or with the two-deletion forms of α thalassemia ($\alpha-/\alpha-$ or $--/\alpha\alpha$) (Chap. 288). In these mild forms of thalassemia, microcytosis is much more marked than is hypochromia; accordingly the mean corpuscular hemoglobin concentration (MCHC) is usually normal. The red cell size distribution is more uniform than that in iron deficiency. Target cells and basophilic stippling are more prominent in thalassemia than in iron deficiency. Hemoglobin A_2 is elevated in β-thalassemia trait and decreased in iron deficiency and α thalassemia. β-Thalassemia trait may be masked by the finding of a normal level of hemoglobin A_2 if the patient has coexisting iron deficiency. The serum iron is normal or elevated in the thalassemias and decreased in both iron deficiency and in the anemia of chronic disease. However, as Fig. 284-2 shows, the transferrin level is also decreased in the latter. The laboratory tests shown in Table 284-1 are not very helpful in determining whether a patient with a chronic inflammatory disease, such as rheumatoid arthritis, has become iron-deficient. The finding of a low serum ferritin level or absent iron stores in a bone marrow aspirate would be diagnostic of iron deficiency. A trial of iron therapy may be necessary to settle the issue. The diagnosis of sideroblastic anemia rests on the demonstration of ringed sideroblasts in the bone marrow. These patients often have a population of hypochromic microcytic red cells, even though the red cell indexes are usually normal.

TREATMENT Iron-deficiency anemia responds very effectively to iron therapy. However, an equally important part of management is to elicit and, if possible, correct the cause of the iron deficiency. Unless the patient has a clear-cut history of menorrhagia or bleeding from an obvious local site such as prolonged epistaxis or hemorrhoids, the gastrointestinal tract must be evaluated with appropriate radiologic and endoscopic studies.

Among the many iron preparations available, ferrous sulfate taken by mouth is the simplest and preferred treatment for most patients. The addition of extraneous minerals (copper, molybdenum) or vitamins or the addition of slow-release forms adds to the cost of the preparation but adds little to its efficacy. In some prenatal multivitamin preparations, calcium carbonate and magnesium oxide may actually interfere with the absorption of the iron. Most patients respond well to ferrous sulfate, 300 mg (60 mg elemental iron) three times daily. Absorption is somewhat enhanced if the iron is administered between meals. Conversely, patients experience less gastric distress if the iron is taken with meals. Some patients tolerate therapy better if it is begun with only one tablet per day and gradually increased over several days. About 15 percent of orally administered iron is absorbed during the first 3 weeks of therapy. Thereafter, absorption decreases, averaging about 5 percent. Treatment for at least 6 months is needed in most cases if body stores are to be replenished.

The response to treatment is generally very satisfactory. A peak reticulocytosis is generally seen at about day 10 with a gradual increase in hemoglobin and correction of red cell indexes.

Failure to respond to therapy usually means that (1) the diagnosis was incorrect; (2) the patient has failed to take the prescribed iron; (3) blood loss has exceeded the buildup of hemoglobin; (4) erythropoiesis has been suppressed by infection, inflammation, or tumor; or (5) the iron has not been properly absorbed.

Parenteral therapy is rarely required. When iron is absorbed poorly, as in some patients who have undergone gastrectomy or those with proximal intestinal disease, particularly celiac sprue, iron-dextran complex may be given intramuscularly. The first dose should be limited to 50 mg because severe reactions sometimes occur. By repeated injections, a total of 1.5 to 2.0 g may be given in this way. Although more likely to produce an adverse reaction, intravenous administration is also possible in patients who cannot tolerate intramuscular injections. The iron-dextran solution can be given by direct infusion, or it can be diluted in about 20 mL sterile saline solution and administered by intravenous drip. One or two drops should be given intravenously, and then, if no untoward symptoms develop in the next 5 min, 500 mg is infused slowly. With intravenous iron-dextran complex, the total replacement dose of iron can be infused at one time. The total amount of parenteral iron that should be given is based on the calculated deficit in red blood cell mass, plus an additional 1000 mg to replenish iron stores. Transfusion of blood is seldom indicated, unless the patient has evidence of cardiovascular compromise, such as congestive heart failure or coronary or cerebral ischemia.

IRON-LOADING ANEMIAS

Dependence on multiple blood transfusions by some patients with acquired or congenital anemias can lead to a state of generalized iron overload. One unit of blood contains about 200 to 250 mg iron. Therefore, in a patient with failure of bone marrow erythroid activity who requires about 4 units of blood every month, at least 20 g of elemental iron can be expected to accumulate within 2 years; this is enough iron to produce clinical symptoms in some patients with idiopathic hemochromatosis. Hyperabsorption of dietary iron in idiopathic hemochromatosis (Chap. 310), in which excess iron is distributed predominantly in parenchymal cells, leads to earlier signs of clinical organ damage than does transfusional iron loading, in which excess iron initially is deposited in the mononuclear phagocyte system. However, most patients who have received more than 100 units of blood exhibit evidence of organ damage in a pattern which resembles that observed in idiopathic hemochromatosis. The most common clinical manifestations of iron overload include hyperpigmentation of the skin, abnormal liver function and cirrhosis, diabetes mellitus, anterior pituitary insufficiency manifesting as hypogonadism, adrenal insufficiency or hypothyroidism, and cardiomyopathy manifesting as congestive heart failure, arrhythmias, or conduction disturbances.

In anemias associated with ineffective erythropoiesis, transfusional iron overload is compounded by excessive intestinal iron absorption. The importance of this factor is exemplified by patients with sideroblastic anemia or thalassemia intermedia who can develop advanced hemochromatosis even in the absence of transfusions. The mechanisms responsible for the inappropriate hyperabsorption of dietary iron in patients with ineffective erythropoiesis are unknown, but iron absorption can be reduced if the anemia is corrected and erythropoiesis is suppressed by transfusion. Thalassemia is discussed in Chap. 288.

SIDEROBLASTIC ANEMIA Sideroblastic anemia consists of a group of disorders of diverse etiologies (Table 284-2) characterized by ringed sideroblasts in the nucleated red cell population of the bone marrow. Ringed sideroblasts are normoblasts which contain iron deposits within mitochondria. The partial or complete rings of Prussian blue–staining granules are produced by the perinuclear distribution of these iron-laden mitochondria. A number of metabolic abnormalities has been noted in the sideroblastic anemias, including defects in one or more of the enzymatic steps in heme synthesis. Since the initial and terminal steps in heme porphyrin synthesis are localized in the mitochondria, it is difficult to determine whether such abnormalities are the cause or the result of mitochondrial iron loading. In addition to the presence of ringed sideroblasts in the bone marrow, these disorders share certain other characteristics: a population of microcytic and hypochromic red cells in the peripheral smear due to defective heme synthesis; bone marrow erythroid hyperplasia as a result of ineffective erythropoiesis; increased levels of red cell porphyrins; and marked increase in the serum iron and transferrin saturation often accompanied by evidence of generalized iron overload.

Hereditary sideroblastic anemia may be either X-linked or autosomal recessive and is often pyridoxine-responsive. Severe anemia is usually first noted in young adulthood, although the age of detection

TABLE 284-2 The sideroblastic anemias

1 Hereditary or congenital sideroblastic anemias
2 Acquired sideroblastic anemias
- *a* Associated with drugs and toxins (e.g., alcohol, lead, isoniazid, chloramphenicol)
- *b* Associated with neoplastic and inflammatory disease (e.g., carcinoma, leukemia, myeloproliferative disorders, Hodgkin's disease, other lymphomas, myeloma, rheumatoid arthritis)
- *c* Idiopathic refractory sideroblastic anemia

may vary greatly even within a single kindred. Large doses of vitamin B_6 result in at least a partial correction of the anemia in patients with hereditary pyridoxine-responsive sideroblastic anemia. The genetic lesion may affect the first and rate-limiting enzyme of porphyrin synthesis, δ-aminolevulinic acid synthetase (ALA-S), either directly or through metabolism of its essential cofactor, pyridoxal 5′-phosphate.

A variety of drugs and toxins can cause a reversible sideroblastic anemia which usually resolves following removal of the offending agent. These include isoniazid (INH) and alcohol, which cause abnormalities in pyridoxine metabolism, and lead, which interferes with several reactions in the pathway of heme synthesis. Sideroblastic anemia occurs in about 30 percent of hospitalized alcoholics; ringed sideroblasts in the bone marrow disappear within several days after cessation of alcohol ingestion. Sideroblastic changes in the bone marrows of alcoholics usually occur in the setting of coexisting malnutrition and folate deficiency. Secondary sideroblastic anemia has also been observed occasionally in association with a variety of inflammatory, neoplastic, and preleukemic states; in these disorders the clinical picture is dominated by the underlying illness.

Sideroblastic anemia is a common form of refractory anemia in older patients in whom other associated diseases, drugs, or toxins cannot be identified. Many of these patients have an indolent course and die of nonhematologic causes. However, some patients become transfusion-dependent and develop complications of iron overload. Unlike the other types of sideroblastic anemia, this can be a preleukemic disorder which is frequently associated with chromosomal abnormalities and transforms into acute nonlymphocytic leukemia in approximately 10 percent of cases.

TREATMENT In cases of secondary sideroblastic anemia, withdrawal of the offending drug or toxin or treatment of the underlying disease is usually beneficial. Patients with acquired idiopathic sideroblastic anemia rarely respond to pyridoxine, although a 2- to 3-month trial of this vitamin in a dose of 200 mg daily should be attempted. A trial of androgens, in a regimen similar to that used in aplastic anemia, may ameliorate the anemia in some cases. In idiopathic refractory sideroblastic anemia, therapy is usually supportive. Many patients require frequent blood transfusions, and measures to reduce transfusional iron loading are required.

While phlebotomy is the most effective treatment for hemochromatosis, in anemic patients with transfusional iron overload, in whom phlebotomy is precluded, elimination of excess iron can be achieved only with iron-chelating agents. Deferoxamine is presently the only clinically effective iron chelator available. Deferoxamine-chelated iron is excreted primarily in the urine and to a lesser extent in the stool. Because the drug is not well absorbed when given orally and has a short half-life, it should be administered by continuous parenteral infusion. Deferoxamine can be administered to ambulatory patients by means of a subcutaneous infusion delivered by a portable pump. Doses are generally 1.5 to 2.5 g daily, infused over 16 to 24 h; however, there is considerable individual variation, and the optimal regimen should be established for individual patients. Adverse effects from deferoxamine are unusual. Patients may develop cataracts after long-term use, and periodic slit-lamp eye examinations are indicated in patients on chronic therapy. Local erythema and discomfort at the subcutaneous injection site can usually be prevented by the addition of hydrocortisone to the deferoxamine solution. Hypersensitivity reactions occur rarely.

Oral ascorbic acid supplementation may markedly enhance the iron-chelating efficiency of deferoxamine, presumably by liberating more free intracellular iron which becomes available for chelation. However, increased amounts of free iron may also damage cells by generating free oxygen radicals. This may be manifested clinically by cardiac irritability or congestive heart failure. Therefore, the administration of ascorbic acid to patients with iron overload may be hazardous.

Manipulation of blood transfusions to selectively infuse young red cells (neocytes), and thereby prolong the interval between transfusions, is a promising measure for the avoidance of iron overload in transfusion-dependent patients, but its application to adult patients has not been established.

REFERENCES

Bothwell TH et al: *Iron Metabolism in Man*. Oxford, Blackwell Scientific, 1979

Bottomley SS: Sideroblastic anaemia. Clin Haematol 11:389, 1982

Cook JD: Clinical evaluation of iron deficiency. Semin Hematol 19:6, 1982

Crosby WH: Current concepts in nutrition: Who needs iron? N Engl J Med 297:543, 1977

Dallman PR: Manifestations of iron deficiency. Semin Hematol 19:19, 1982

Finch CA, Huebers H: Perspectives in iron metabolism. N Engl J Med 360:1520, 1982

Huebers HA, Finch CA: Transferrin: Physiologic behavior and clinical implications. Blood 64:763, 1984

Lanzkowsky P: Problems in diagnosis of iron deficiency anemia. Pediatr Ann 14:618, 622, 627, 1985

Schafer AI: Iron overload, in *Current Hematology*. New York, Wiley, 1981 vol 1, chap 5

Schwartz S et al: Chromosome abnormalities in acquired idiopathic sideroblastic anemia with subsequent leukemic transformation. Cancer Genet Cytogenet 19:291, 1986

Worwood M: Iron and hemochromatosis. J Inherited Metab Dis 6(Suppl 1):63, 1983

285 MEGALOBLASTIC ANEMIAS

BERNARD M. BABIOR / H. FRANKLIN BUNN

The megaloblastic anemias are disorders caused by impaired deoxyribonucleic acid (DNA) synthesis. Cells primarily affected are those having a relatively rapid turnover, especially hematopoietic precursors and gastrointestinal epithelial cells. Cell division is sluggish, but cytoplasmic development progresses normally, so megaloblastic cells tend to be large, with an increased ratio of ribonucleic acid (RNA) to DNA. Megaloblastic erythroid cells tend to be destroyed in the marrow in excessive numbers, an abnormality termed *ineffective erythropoiesis* (Chaps. 53 and 283).

Most megaloblastic anemias are due to a deficiency of vitamin B_{12} and/or folic acid. The various clinical entities associated with megaloblastic anemia are listed in Table 285-1. This classification is easier to comprehend if the physiologic and biochemical principles discussed below are kept in mind.

PHYSIOLOGIC CONSIDERATIONS

FOLIC ACID Folic acid is the common name for pteroylmonoglutamic acid. It is synthesized by many different plants and bacteria. Fruits and vegetables constitute the primary dietary source of the vitamin. Some forms of dietary folic acid are labile and may be destroyed by cooking. The minimum daily requirement is normally about 50 μg but may be increased severalfold during periods of enhanced metabolic demand such as pregnancy.

The assimilation of adequate amounts of folic acid is dependent on the nature of the diet and its means of preparation. Folates in various foodstuffs are largely conjugated to polyglutamic acid. This highly polar side chain impairs the intestinal absorption of the vitamin. However, conjugases (γ-glutamyl carboxypeptidases) in the lumen of the gut convert polyglutamates to mono- and diglutamates, which are readily absorbed in the proximal jejunum.

There are binding proteins in plasma for folates, but their physiologic significance is unclear. Plasma folate is primarily in the form of N^5-methyltetrahydrofolate, a monoglutamate. N^5-Methyltetrahydrofolate is transported into cells by a carrier which is specific for the tetrahydro forms of the vitamin. Once in the cell, the folate is reconverted to the polyglutamate form, after removal of the N^5-methyl group in a vitamin B_{12}–requiring reaction (see below). The polyglutamate form may be useful for retention of folate by the cell.

Normal individuals have about 5 to 20 mg folic acid in various body stores, half in the liver. In light of the minimum daily

TABLE 285-1 Classification of the megaloblastic anemias

- *I* Vitamin B_{12} deficiency
  - *A* Inadequate intake: vegetarians (rare)
  - *B* Malabsorption
    - *1* Inadequate production of intrinsic factor (IF)
      - *a* Pernicious anemia
      - *b* Gastrectomy
      - *c* Congenital absence or functional abnormality of IF (rare)
    - *2* Disorders of terminal ileum
      - *a* Tropical sprue
      - *b* Nontropical sprue
      - *c* Regional enteritis
      - *d* Intestinal resection
      - *e* Neoplasms and granulomatous disorders (rare)
      - *f* Selective vitamin B_{12} malabsorption (Imerslund's syndrome) (rare)
    - *3* Competition for vitamin B_{12}
      - *a* Fish tapeworm
      - *b* Bacteria: blind loop syndrome
    - *4* Drugs: *p*-Aminosalicylic acid, colchicine, neomycin
  - *C* Other
    - *1* Nitrous oxide
    - *2* Transcobalamin II deficiency (rare)
- *II* Folic acid deficiency
  - *A* Inadequate intake: Unbalanced diet (common in alcoholics, teenagers, some infants)
  - *B* Increased requirements
    - *1* Pregnancy
    - *2* Infancy
    - *3* Malignancy
    - *4* Increased hematopoiesis (chronic hemolytic anemias)
    - *5* Chronic exfoliative skin disorders
    - *6* Hemodialysis
  - *C* Malabsorption
    - *1* Tropical sprue
    - *2* Nontropical sprue
    - *3* Drugs: Phenytoin, barbiturates, (?) ethanol
  - *D* Impaired metabolism
    - *1* Inhibitors of dihydrofolate reductase: Methotrexate, pyrimethamine, triamterene, pentamidine, etc.
    - *2* Alcohol
    - *3* Rare enzyme deficiencies: Formiminotransferase, dihydrofolate reductase, others
- *III* Other causes
  - *A* Drugs which impair DNA metabolism
    - *1* Purine antagonists: 6-mercaptopurine, azathioprine, etc.
    - *2* Pyrimidine antagonists: 5-fluorouracil, cytosine arabinoside, etc.
    - *3* Others: Procarbazine, hydroxyurea
  - *B* Metabolic disorders (rare)
    - *1* Hereditary orotic aciduria
    - *2* Others
  - *C* Megaloblastic anemia of unknown etiology
    - *1* Refractory megaloblastic anemia
    - *2* Di Guglielmo's syndrome*
    - *3* Congenital dyserythropoietic anemia

* *A form of acute nonlymphocytic leukemia with atypical, dysplastic changes in erythroid series.*

requirement, it is not surprising that a deficiency will occur within months if dietary intake or intestinal absorption is curtailed.

VITAMIN B_{12} This vitamin is a complex organometallic compound in which a cobalt atom is situated within a corrin ring, a structure similar to the porphyrin from which heme is formed (Fig. 283-3). As with heme, both δ-aminolevulinic acid and porphobilinogen are precursors in the biosynthesis of vitamin B_{12}. However, unlike heme, vitamin B_{12} cannot be synthesized in the human body and must be supplied in the diet. The only dietary source of vitamin B_{12} is animal products: meat and dairy foods. The minimum daily requirement for vitamin B_{12} is about 2.5 μg.

During gastric digestion, vitamin B_{12} in food is released and forms a stable complex with gastric R binder, one of a group of closely related glycoproteins of unknown function which are found in secretions (e.g., saliva, milk, gastric juice, bile), phagocytes, and plasma. On entering the duodenum, the vitamin B_{12}–R binder complex is digested, releasing the vitamin B_{12}, which then binds to intrinsic factor (IF). This glycoprotein of molecular weight 50,000 is produced by the parietal cells of the stomach. The secretion of intrinsic factor generally parallels that of hydrochloric acid. The vitamin B_{12}–IF complex is resistant to proteolytic digestion and travels to the distal ileum, where specific receptors on the mucosal brush border bind the vitamin B_{12}–IF complex, thereby enabling the vitamin to be absorbed. Thus, intrinsic factor serves as a cell-directed carrier protein. Vitamin B_{12} is transferred from the ileal receptor across the mucosa to the capillary circulation where it binds initially to another transport protein, transcobalamin II (TC II). The vitamin B_{12}–TC II complex is rapidly taken up by the liver, the bone marrow, and other cells. Normally, about 2 mg vitamin B_{12} is stored in the liver, and another 2 mg is stored elsewhere in the body. In view of the minimum daily requirement, about 3 to 6 years would be required for a normal individual to become deficient in vitamin B_{12} if absorption were to cease abruptly.

Although TC II is the acceptor for newly absorbed vitamin B_{12}, most circulating vitamin B_{12} is bound to transcobalamin I (TC I), a glycoprotein closely related to gastric R binder. TC I appears to be derived in part from leukocytes. The paradox that most circulating vitamin B_{12} is bound to TC I rather than TC II, even though TC II receives all the vitamin B_{12} which is absorbed by the intestine, is explained by the fact that vitamin B_{12} bound to TC II is rapidly cleared from the blood ($t_{1/2}$ about 1 h), while clearance of vitamin B_{12} bound to TC I requires many days. The function of TC I is unknown.

BIOCHEMICAL CONSIDERATIONS

FOLATE The *prime function* of this vitamin is to transfer one-carbon moieties such as methyl and formyl groups to various organic compounds (see Fig. 285-1). The source of these one-carbon moieties is usually serine, which reacts with tetrahydrofolate to produce glycine and $N^{5,10}$-methylenetetrahydrofolate. An alternative source is formiminoglutamic acid, an intermediate in histidine catabolism, which gives up its formimino group to tetrahydrofolate to yield N^5-formiminotetrahydrofolate and glutamic acid. These derivatives provide entry into an interconvertible donor pool consisting of tetrahydrofolate derivatives carrying various one-carbon moieties (see Fig. 285-1). The constituents of this pool can donate their one-carbon moieties to appropriate acceptor compounds to form metabolic intermediates which are ultimately converted to building blocks used in the synthesis of biologic macromolecules. The most important building blocks are (1) purines, in which the C-2 and C-8 atoms are introduced in folate-dependent reactions; (2) deoxythymidylate monophosphate (dTMP), synthesized from $N^{5,10}$-methylenetetrahydrofolate and deoxyuridylate monophosphate (dUMP); and (3) methionine, formed by the transfer of a methyl group from N^5-methyltetrahydrofolate to homocysteine. Vitamin B_{12} is also required for the formation of methionine from homocysteine (see below).

In all but one of the one-carbon transfer reactions, tetrahydrofolate is produced. It can immediately accept a one-carbon moiety and reenter the donor pool. The single exception is the thymidylate

FIGURE 285-1 *Scheme of folate metabolism.*

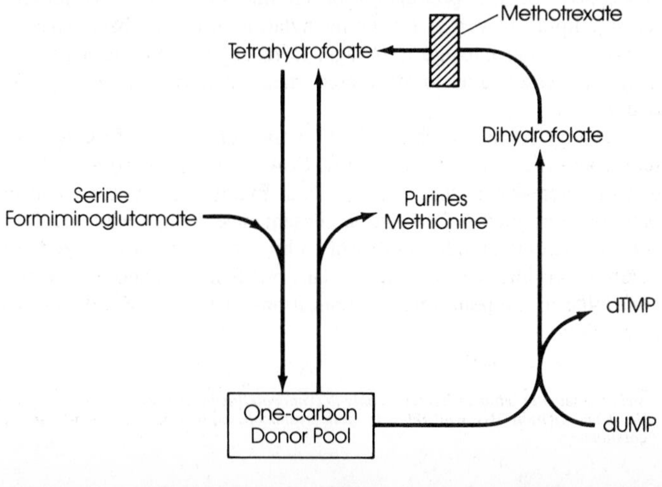

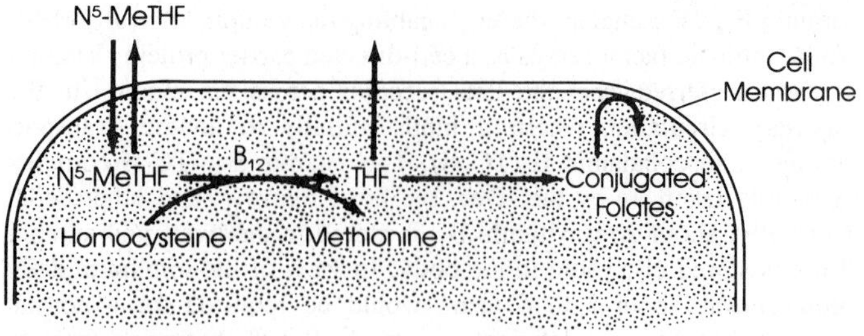

FIGURE 285-2 *Diagram showing the interrelationship between vitamin B_{12} (methylcobalamin) and folate metabolism within the cell.*

synthetase reaction (dUMP → dTMP), in which dihydrofolate is the product (Fig. 285-1). This must be reduced to tetrahydrofolate by the enzyme dihydrofolate reductase before it can reenter the donor pool. A number of drugs are able to inhibit dihydrofolate reductase, thereby diverting folate from the donor pool and producing what amounts to a state of folate deficiency in the face of normal tissue folate concentrations.

VITAMIN B_{12} In humans there are two metabolically active forms of vitamin B_{12}, identified by the alkyl group attached to the sixth coordination position of the cobalt atom: methylcobalamin and adenosylcobalamin. The vitamin preparation which is used therapeutically is cyanocobalamin. Cyanocobalamin has no known physiologic role and must be converted to a biologically active form before it can be used by tissues.[1]

Methylcobalamin is an essential cofactor in the conversion of homocysteine to methionine (Fig. 285-2). When this reaction is impaired, folate metabolism is deranged, and it is this derangement which is thought to underlie the defect in DNA synthesis and the megaloblastic maturation pattern in patients who are deficient in vitamin B_{12} (see Fig. 285-2). What appears to happen in vitamin B_{12} deficiency is that the unconjugated N^5-methyltetrahydrofolate newly taken from the bloodstream cannot be converted to other forms of tetrahydrofolate by methyl transfer. This is the so-called folate trap hypothesis. Since N^5-methyltetrahydrofolate is a poor substrate for the conjugating enzyme (this has been shown in rats but has not yet been demonstrated in humans), it largely remains in the unconjugated form and slowly leaks from the cell. Tissue folate deficiency therefore develops, and this results in megaloblastic hematopoiesis. This hypothesis explains the fact that tissue folate stores in vitamin B_{12} deficiency are substantially reduced, with a disproportionate reduction in conjugated as compared with unconjugated folates, despite normal or supranormal serum folate levels. It also explains why large doses of folate can produce a partial hematologic remission in patients with vitamin B_{12} deficiency.

Impairment in the conversion of homocysteine to methionine may also be partly responsible for the neurologic complications of vitamin B_{12} deficiency (see below). The methionine formed in this reaction is needed for the production of choline and choline-containing phospholipids as well as for the methylation of myelin basic protein. Nervous system damage is thought to result from interference with these processes due to decreased methionine production in B_{12} deficiency.

Adenosylcobalamin is required for the conversion of methylmalonyl coenzyme A (CoA) to succinyl CoA. Lack of this cofactor leads to large increases in the tissue levels of methylmalonyl CoA and its precursor, propionyl CoA. As a consequence, nonphysiologic fatty acids containing an odd number of carbon atoms are synthesized and incorporated into neuronal lipids. This biochemical abnormality may contribute to the neurologic complications of vitamin B_{12} deficiency (see below).

[1] *Strictly speaking, vitamin B_{12} refers only to cyanocobalamin. However, in this chapter, the term* vitamin B_{12} *will refer to both cyanocobalamin and biologically active cobalamins.*

CLINICAL DISORDERS

CLASSIFICATION OF MEGALOBLASTIC ANEMIAS The etiology of megaloblastic anemia varies in different parts of the world. In temperate zones, folate deficiency in alcoholics and pernicious anemia are the common types of megaloblastic anemias. In certain areas close to the equator, tropical sprue is endemic and an important cause. In Scandinavia, megaloblastic anemia is sometimes secondary to infestation by the fish tapeworm *Diphyllobothrium latum*.

The dietary intake of vitamin B_{12} is more than adequate for the body's requirements, except in true vegetarians (individuals who live on a purely vegetable diet) and their breast-fed infants. Thus, deficiency of vitamin B_{12} is almost always due to malabsorption. As explained in the section above, the absorption of vitamin B_{12} depends upon a specific binding protein produced in the stomach and uptake by a specific receptor in the mucosa of the distal ileum. Accordingly, several steps in this process can go awry and lead to malabsorption. These are listed in Table 285-1. In contrast, the dietary intake of folic acid is marginal in many parts of the world. Furthermore, since the body's stores of folate are relatively low, folic acid deficiency can arise rather suddenly during periods of decreased dietary intake or increased metabolic demand. Finally, folic acid deficiency may be due to malabsorption. Often two or more of these factors coexist in a given patient.

Combined deficiencies of vitamin B_{12} and folic acid are not uncommon. Patients with tropical sprue are often deficient in both vitamins. The biochemical lesion that results in megaloblastic maturation of bone marrow cells also causes structural and functional abnormalities of the rapidly proliferating epithelial cells of the intestinal mucosa. Thus, severe deficiency of one vitamin can lead to malabsorption of the other. Furthermore, as discussed above, a deficiency of vitamin B_{12} causes a secondary reduction in cellular folic acid.

Finally, megaloblastic anemias may occasionally be induced by factors unrelated to a vitamin deficiency. Most such cases are caused by one or more of the many drugs which interfere with DNA synthesis. Less commonly, megaloblastic maturation is encountered in certain acquired defects of hematopoietic stem cells. Rarest of all are specific congenital enzyme deficiencies in which megaloblastic anemia is characteristically encountered.

VITAMIN B_{12} DEFICIENCY There are many conditions in which vitamin B_{12} deficiency may develop. Although each has its own characteristic manifestations, certain clinical features are common to all. These clinical features involve the blood, the gastrointestinal tract, and the nervous system.

The hematologic manifestations are almost entirely the result of anemia although very rarely purpura may appear, due to thrombocytopenia. Symptoms of anemia may include weakness, lightheadedness, vertigo, and tinnitus, as well as palpitations, angina, and the symptoms of congestive failure. On physical examination, the patient with florid vitamin B_{12} deficiency is pale, with slightly icteric skin and eyes. The pulse is rapid, and the heart may be enlarged; auscultation will reveal a systolic flow murmur. The spleen and liver may be somewhat enlarged. There may be a slight fever.

The gastrointestinal manifestations reflect the effect of vitamin B_{12} deficiency on the rapidly turning over gastrointestinal epithelium. The patient sometimes complains of a sore tongue, which on inspection will be smooth and beefy red. Anorexia with moderate weight loss may also be evident, possibly accompanied by diarrhea and other gastrointestinal symptoms. These latter manifestations may be in part caused by megaloblastosis of the small intestinal epithelium, which results in malabsorption.

The neurologic manifestations are the most worrisome of all, because they often fail to remit completely on treatment. They begin pathologically with demyelination, followed by axonal degeneration and eventual neuronal death; the final stage, of course, is irreversible. Sites of involvement include peripheral nerves, the spinal cord, where the posterior and lateral columns undergo demyelination, and the cerebrum itself. Signs and symptoms include numbness and paresthesias in the extremities (the earliest neurologic manifestations), weakness, ataxia, and poor finger coordination. There may be sphincter disturbances. Reflexes may be diminished or increased. The Romberg and Babinski signs may be positive, and position sense and vibration sense are usually diminished. Disturbances of mentation will vary from mild irritability and forgetfulness to severe dementia or frank psychosis. It should be emphasized that occasionally *neurologic disease may occur in a patient with a normal hematocrit.*

In the usual patient, in whom hematologic problems predominate, the blood and bone marrow show characteristic megaloblastic changes which are described under "Diagnosis" below. The anemia may be very severe—hematocrits of 15 to 20 are not infrequent—but is surprisingly well tolerated by the patient because it develops so slowly.

Pernicious anemia The most common cause of vitamin B_{12} deficiency in temperate climates is pernicious anemia, in which intrinsic factor secretion ceases owing to atrophy of the gastric mucosa. It is most frequently seen in individuals of northern European descent and is much less common in southern Europeans, blacks, and Orientals. Men and women are equally affected. It is a disease of the elderly, the average patient presenting near age 60; it is rare under 30, although typical pernicious anemia can be seen in children under 10 (juvenile pernicious anemia). Inherited conditions in which a histologically normal stomach secretes either an abnormal intrinsic factor or none at all will cause vitamin B_{12} deficiency which appears in infancy or early childhood.

On the basis of incomplete evidence, pernicious anemia is currently thought to be caused by an autoimmune reaction against gastric parietal cells. There is considerable evidence for immunologic abnormalities in pernicious anemia. The incidence of pernicious anemia is substantially increased in patients with other diseases thought to be of immunologic origin, including Graves' disease, myxedema, thyroiditis, idiopathic adrenocortical insufficiency, vitiligo, and hypoparathyroidism. Patients with pernicious anemia also have abnormal circulating antibodies related to their disease: 90 percent have antiparietal cell antibody while 60 percent have anti-intrinsic factor antibody. Antiparietal cell antibody is also found in 50 percent of patients with gastric atrophy without pernicious anemia as well as in 10 to 15 percent of an unselected patient population, but anti-intrinsic factor antibody is usually absent from these patients. Relatives of patients with pernicious anemia show an increased incidence of the disease, and even clinically unaffected relatives may have anti-intrinsic factor antibody in their serum. A final point supporting an immunologic basis for pernicious anemia is the fact that corticosteroids have been reported to reverse the disease both pathologically and clinically.

The destruction of parietal cells in pernicious anemia is thought to be mediated by the cellular immune system. Humoral factors such as anti-intrinsic factor antibody probably have little role in the pathogenesis of the disease, a view supported by the observation that pernicious anemia is unusually common in patients with agammaglobulinemia.

Pathologically, the most characteristic finding in pernicious anemia is gastric atrophy which involves only the acid- and pepsin-secreting portion of the stomach; the antrum is spared. Other pathologic changes, which are secondary to the deficiency of vitamin B_{12}, include megaloblastoid alterations in the gastric and intestinal epithelium and the neurologic changes described above. The abnormalities in the gastric epithelium are evident as cellular atypia in gastric cytology specimens, a finding which must be carefully distinguished from the cytologic abnormalities seen in gastric malignancy.

The *clinical manifestations* are primarily those of vitamin B_{12} deficiency, as described above. The disease is of insidious onset and progresses slowly. An additional physical finding is the tendency of patients with pernicious anemia to be fair-haired or prematurely gray. Laboratory examination will reveal hypergastrinemia and pentagastrin-fast achlorhydria as well as the hematologic and other laboratory abnormalities discussed below in "Diagnosis."

Through appropriate replacement therapy, patients with pernicious anemia should experience complete and lifelong correction of all abnormalities which are due to vitamin B_{12} deficiency, except to the extent that irreversible changes in the nervous system may have occurred prior to treatment. These patients, however, are unusually subject to gastric polyps and have about twice the normal incidence of cancer of the stomach. In view of the latter complication, patients should be followed with frequent stool guaiac examinations together with further diagnostic studies when indicated.

Postgastrectomy Following total gastrectomy or extensive damage to gastric mucosa as, for example, by ingestion of corrosive agents, megaloblastic anemia may develop because the source of intrinsic factor has been removed. In such patients the absorption of orally administered vitamin B_{12} is impaired. Megaloblastic anemia may also follow partial gastrectomy, but the incidence is lower than after total gastrectomy, in which vitamin B_{12} malabsorption occurs in 100 percent of patients. The cause of vitamin B_{12} deficiency after partial gastrectomy may be intestinal overgrowth of bacteria, but it does not always respond to antibiotics.

Intestinal organisms The macrocytic anemia seen in association with intestinal strictures, diverticula, anastomoses, and "blind loops" may be attributed to colonization of the small intestine by large masses of bacteria which divert vitamin B_{12} from the host. Steatorrhea may also be seen under these circumstances, because bile salt metabolism is disturbed when the intestine is heavily colonized with bacteria. Hematologic responses have been observed after administration of oral antibiotics such as tetracycline and ampicillin.

Megaloblastic anemia is seen, in Scandinavia especially, in persons harboring the tapeworm *D. latum*. The anemia has been attributed to competition by the worm for vitamin B_{12}. Destruction of the worm eliminates the problem.

Ileal abnormalities Vitamin B_{12} deficiency is commonly found in tropical sprue, while it is an unusual complication of nontropical sprue (gluten-sensitive enteropathy; see Chap. 237). Virtually any disorder which compromises the absorptive capacity of the distal ileum can result in vitamin B_{12} deficiency. Specific entities include regional enteritis, Whipple's disease, and tuberculosis. Segmental involvement of the distal ileum by disease can cause megaloblastic anemia without any other manifestations of intestinal malabsorption such as steatorrhea. Vitamin B_{12} malabsorption is also seen after ileal resection. The Zollinger-Ellison syndrome (intense gastric hyperacidity due to a gastrin-secreting tumor) may cause vitamin B_{12} malabsorption by acidifying the small intestine. This will retard the transfer of the vitamin from R binder to intrinsic factor and will impair the binding of the vitamin B_{12}–IF complex to the ileal receptors. Chronic pancreatitis may also cause vitamin B_{12} malabsorption by impairing the transfer of the vitamin from R binder to intrinsic factor. This abnormality can be detected by tests of vitamin B_{12} absorption (see below, Schilling test), but it is invariably mild and never causes clinical vitamin B_{12} deficiency. Finally, there is a rare congenital disorder, described by Imerslund, in which a selective defect in vitamin B_{12} absorption is accompanied by proteinuria.

FOLIC ACID DEFICIENCY Patients with folic acid deficiency are more apt to be malnourished than those with vitamin B_{12} deficiency. Accordingly, they are likely to appear wasted. The gastrointestinal manifestations are similar to, but may be more widespread and more severe than those of, pernicious anemia. Diarrhea is often present, and cheilosis and glossitis are also encountered. However, in contrast to vitamin B_{12} deficiency, neurologic abnormalities do not occur.

The hematologic manifestations of folic acid deficiency are the same as those of vitamin B_{12} deficiency. Folic acid deficiency can generally be attributed to one or more of the following factors: increased demand for folate, inadequate intake, and malabsorption.

Inadequate intake Folic acid malnutrition is commonly encountered among a number of groups. Alcoholics frequently become folate-deficient because their main source of caloric intake is in the form of alcoholic beverages. Distilled spirits are virtually devoid of folic acid, while beer and wine do not contain enough of the vitamin to satisfy the daily requirement. In addition, alcohol may interfere with folate metabolism. Narcotic addicts are also prone to become folate-deficient because of malnutrition. Many indigent and elderly individuals who subsist primarily on canned foods or "tea and toast" and occasional teenagers whose diet consists of soft drinks and potato chips develop folate deficiency.

Increased demand Tissues with a relatively high rate of cell division such as the bone marrow or gut mucosa have a large requirement for folate. Therefore, patients with chronic hemolytic anemias or other causes of very active erythropoiesis may become deficient if their high folate requirement is not met by dietary intake. Likewise, a pregnant woman may become deficient in folic acid because of the high demand of the developing fetus. Folate deficiency may also occur during the growth spurts of infancy and adolescence.

Malabsorption Folic acid deficiency is a common accompaniment of tropical sprue. Both the gastrointestinal symptoms and malabsorption are improved by the administration of either folic acid or antibiotics by mouth. Patients with nontropical sprue (gluten-sensitive enteropathy) may also develop significant folic acid deficiency which parallels other parameters of malabsorption. Similarly, alcohol-related folate deficiency may be due in part to malabsorption. In addition, other primary small-bowel disorders are sometimes associated with vitamin deficiency. These entities are all discussed in Chap. 237.

DRUGS Next to deficiency of folate or vitamin B_{12}, the most common cause of megaloblastic anemia is drug ingestion. Drugs which cause megaloblastic anemia do so by interfering with DNA synthesis, either directly or by antagonizing the action of folate. They can be classified as follows:

1 *Direct inhibitors of DNA synthesis.* The drugs in this category are used in the treatment of malignancy. Their efficacy depends on their ability to disrupt DNA synthesis. They include purine analogues (6-thioguanine, azathioprine, 6-mercaptopurine), pyrimidine analogues (5-fluorouracil, cytosine arabinoside), and certain other drugs which interfere with DNA synthesis by a variety of mechanisms (hydroxyurea, procarbazine).
2 *Folate antagonists.* The most toxic of these is methotrexate, an exceedingly powerful inhibitor of dihydrofolate reductase which is used in the treatment of certain malignancies. Much less toxic, but still capable of inducing a megaloblastic anemia, are several weak dihydrofolate reductase inhibitors which are used to treat a variety of nonmalignant conditions. These include pentamidine, trimethoprine, triamterene, and pyrimethamine.

   The megaloblastic changes in methotrexate poisoning appear to result from the following sequence of events. In methotrexate-poisoned cells, the methylation of dUMP to dTMP is grossly impaired. As a consequence, the phosphorylation of dUMP to dUTP, normally a very minor reaction, becomes a major route of dUMP metabolism. The capacity of a highly specific dUTP pyrophosphatase to degrade dUTP back to dUMP is exceeded under these conditions, and dUTP accumulates in the cell. This dUTP is incorporated into newly synthesized DNA, because DNA polymerase cannot distinguish between dUTP and the closely related normal substrate, dTTP. As a result, defective strands of DNA are produced in which T is partly replaced by U. The U-containing regions of these defective strands are recognized by a specific repair system, which excises them and attempts to replace them with normal DNA. In methotrexate-poisoned cells, however, there is so much dUTP and so little dTTP that the new DNA is also likely to be defective. It is this futile cycle of faulty replication, error excision, faulty repair, etc., which explains the megaloblastic pattern of DNA synthesis in methotrexate-poisoned cells. The megaloblastic changes in folate and vitamin B_{12} deficiency might have a similar biochemical origin.
3 *Nitrous oxide.* Nitrous oxide inhalation causes the destruction of endogenous vitamin B_{12}. As ordinarily used, this anesthetic does not destroy enough of the vitamin to cause clinical manifestations. Repeated or protracted exposure, however, may lead to a megaloblastic anemia. Fatal megaloblastic anemia has been reported in patients with tetanus who were given nitrous oxide continuously for weeks.
4 *Others.* A number of drugs antagonize folate by mechanisms which are poorly understood but are thought to involve an effect on absorption of the vitamin by the intestine. In this category are certain anticonvulsants [phenytoin (Dilantin), primidone (Mysoline)] and phenobarbital (Luminal). Megaloblastic anemia induced by these agents is mild.

OTHER Hereditary Megaloblastic anemia may be seen in several hereditary disorders. It is a regular feature of orotic aciduria, a defect in pyrimidine metabolism which is also characterized by retarded growth and development as well as the excretion of large amounts of orotic acid, and which is due to a deficiency of orotidylic decarboxylase and phosphorylase. Megaloblastic anemia has been reported in a single case of the Lesch-Nyhan syndrome, a condition resulting from a deficiency of hypoxanthine-guanine phosphoribosyltransferase whose clinical manifestations include gout, mental retardation, and self-mutilation. It has also been described in methylmalonic aciduria due to a defect in the biosynthesis of the two metabolically active alkyl cobalamins, though it is not seen in methylmalonic aciduria due to methylmalonyl CoA mutase deficiency. Congenital folate malabsorption causes megaloblastic anemia, accompanied by ataxia and mental retardation. Megaloblastic anemia has been reported to accompany the congenital deficiency of other folate-metabolizing enzymes including formiminotransferase, dihydrofolate reductase, and N^5-methyltetrahydrofolate reductase. These deficiencies are less well documented than is congenital folate malabsorption. Megaloblastic changes as well as multinuclearity of red blood cell precursors are seen in the marrow of certain patients with congenital dyserythropoietic anemia, a group of inherited disorders characterized by mild to moderate anemia presenting at any age and pursuing a benign course.

Transcobalamin II deficiency, as well as the congenital abnormalities in vitamin B_{12} absorption described previously, causes pronounced deficiencies in vitamin B_{12} in infancy or early childhood, with all the accompanying manifestations. Megaloblastic anemia is not seen in hereditary transcobalamin I deficiency.

Acquired idiopathic anemia Some patients with acquired sideroblastic anemia and other forms of refractory anemia show megaloblastic erythropoiesis. Megaloblastic changes are restricted to the red blood cell series; large granulocyte precursors and giant metamyelocytes are not seen (see below). Both are associated with an increased incidence of acute leukemia.

Megaloblastic changes are seen in erythremic myelosis and acute erythroleukemia (di Guglielmo) where red blood cell precursors are prominently involved. Here, the marrow is characterized by bizarre erythroid maturation, with multinuclearity and multipolar mitotic figures in the red blood cell precursors. Erythremic myelosis is discussed further in Chap. 292.

DIAGNOSIS The finding of significant macrocytosis [mean corpuscular volume (MCV) > 96 fl] suggests the presence of a megaloblastic anemia. Other causes of macrocytosis include hemolysis, liver disease, alcoholism, hypothyroidism, and aplastic anemia. If the macrocytosis is marked (MCV > 110 fl), the patient is much more likely to have a megaloblastic anemia. The reticulocyte count is low, and the leukocyte and platelet count may also be decreased, particularly in severely anemic patients. The blood smear (Fig. A5-2) demonstrates marked anisocytosis and poikilocytosis, together with macroovalocytes which are large, oval, fully hemoglobinized erythrocytes typical of megaloblastic anemias. There is some basophilic stippling, and an occasional nucleated red blood cell may be seen. In the white blood cell series, the neutrophils show hypersegmentation of the nucleus. This is such a typical finding that a single cell with a nucleus of six lobes or more should raise the immediate suspicion of a megaloblastic anemia. A rare myelocyte may also be seen. Bizarre, misshapen platelets are also observed. The bone marrow examination is very helpful in the diagnosis of megaloblastic anemia. The marrow is hypercellular with a decreased myeloid/erythroid ratio and abundant stainable iron. Red blood cell precursors are abnormally large and have nuclei that appear much less mature than would be expected from the development of the cytoplasm (nuclear-cytoplasmic asynchrony). The nuclear chromatin is more dispersed than it should be and consequently stains less intensely than normal. To the extent that it is aggregated, it condenses in a peculiar fenestrated pattern which is very characteristic of megaloblastic erythropoiesis. Abnormal mitoses may be seen. Granulocyte precursors are also affected, many being larger than normal, including giant bands and metamyelocytes. Megakaryocytes are decreased and show abnormal morphology.

Megaloblastic anemias are characterized by ineffective erythropoiesis (Chaps. 283 and 284). In a severely megaloblastic patient as many as 90 percent of the red blood cell precursors may be destroyed before they are released into the bloodstream, compared with 10 to 15 percent in the normal subject. Enhanced intramedullary destruction of erythroblasts results in an increase in unconjugated bilirubin and lactic acid dehydrogenase (isoenzyme 1) in plasma. Abnormalities in iron kinetics also attest to the presence of ineffective erythropoiesis, with increased iron turnover but low incorporation of labeled iron into circulating red blood cells.

In evaluating a patient with megaloblastic anemia, it is important to determine whether there is a specific vitamin deficiency by measuring serum B_{12} and folate levels. At one time the assay for B_{12} was unreliable, giving false-normal values in B_{12} deficiency because of its inability to distinguish authentic B_{12} from biologically inactive B_{12} analogues present in serum. Within the past few years, however, this problem with the B_{12} assay has been corrected.

The normal range of vitamin B_{12} in serum is 200 to 900 pg/mL; values less than 100 pg/mL indicate clinically significant deficiency. The normal serum concentration of folic acid ranges from 6 to 20 ng/mL; values of 4 ng/mL or less are generally considered to be diagnostic of folate deficiency. Unlike serum vitamin B_{12}, serum folate levels may reflect recent alterations in dietary intake. Measurement of red blood cell folate occasionally provides useful information since it is not subject to short-term fluctuations in folate intake and is, therefore, a better index of tissue folate stores than serum folate.

A test which is occasionally used in the diagnosis of megaloblastic anemia is the deoxyuridine (dU) suppression test. This test is based on the observation that the uptake of tritiated thymidine by bone marrow cells, suppressed sharply (10 times or more) by deoxyuridine under normal circumstances, is affected to a much smaller extent in megaloblastic anemia. The abnormality in deoxyuridine suppression is probably related in some way to alterations in nucleotide pool sizes in megaloblastic cells.

Once vitamin B_{12} deficiency has been established, its pathogenesis can be delineated by means of a Schilling test. A patient is given radioactive vitamin B_{12} by mouth followed shortly thereafter by an intramuscular injection of unlabeled vitamin B_{12}. The proportion of the administered radioactivity excreted in the urine during the next 24 h provides an accurate measure of absorption of vitamin B_{12}, assuming that a complete urine sample has been collected. Since vitamin B_{12} deficiency is almost always due to malabsorption (Table 285-1), this first stage of the Schilling test should be abnormal. The patient is then given labeled vitamin B_{12} bound to intrinsic factor. Absorption of the vitamin will now approach normal if the patient has pernicious anemia or some other type of intrinsic factor deficiency. If vitamin B_{12} absorption is still decreased, the patient may have bacterial overgrowth (blind loop syndrome) or ileal disease (including an ileal absorptive defect secondary to the B_{12} deficiency itself). Vitamin B_{12} malabsorption due to bacterial overgrowth can frequently be corrected by the administration of antibiotics. The Schilling test can provide equally reliable information after the patient has had adequate therapy with parenteral vitamin B_{12}.

TREATMENT

VITAMIN B_{12} DEFICIENCY Apart from specific therapy related to the underlying disorder (e.g., antibiotics for intestinal overgrowth with bacteria), the mainstay of treatment for B_{12} deficiency is replacement therapy. Since the defect is one of absorption, replacement should be administered parenterally, specifically in the form of intramuscular cyanocobalamin. (If intramuscular administration is contraindicated or refused, vitamin B_{12} deficiency can be managed by oral replacement therapy, but at doses of 300 to 1000 μg daily, it is an exceedingly expensive mode of treatment which requires very close medical supervision to avoid relapse.) Treatment should be started with 100 μg vitamin B_{12} per day for a week. The frequency of administration of the vitamin may then be decreased, the goal being to give a total of 2000 μg during the first 6 weeks. The patient may then be placed on 100 μg cyanocobalamin intramuscularly every month, a regimen that must be maintained for the rest of the patient's life. If necessary, larger doses may be given at less frequent intervals (e.g., 1 mg every 2 to 4 months), but the risk of relapse is substantially greater than if the vitamin is given monthly.

The response to treatment is gratifying. Shortly after treatment is begun, and several days before a hematologic response is evident in the peripheral blood, the patient will experience an increase in strength and an improved sense of well-being. Marrow morphology begins to revert toward normal within a few hours after treatment is initiated. Reticulocytosis begins 4 to 5 days after therapy is started and peaks at about day 7 (Fig. 285-3), with subsequent remission of the anemia over the next several weeks. If a reticulocytosis does not occur, or if it is less brisk than expected from the level of the hematocrit, a search should be made for other factors contributing to the anemia (e.g., infection, coexisting folate deficiency, or hypothyroidism). The sudden development of hypokalemia and salt retention may occur early in the course of therapy; usually these are of no consequence, but occasionally they may represent clinical problems.

In most cases, replacement therapy is all that is needed for the treatment of vitamin B_{12} deficiency. Occasionally, however, a patient with a severe anemia will have such a precarious cardiovascular status that emergency transfusion is necessary. This must be done with great care, since it is very easy to precipitate florid congestive failure in such patients by fluid overload. Blood must be administered slowly in the form of packed cells, with very close observation, giving as an initial dose no more than 100 mL. This small volume will frequently be enough to ameliorate the cardiovascular problems sufficiently that further therapy can be restricted to vitamin B_{12} replacement. If necessary, blood may be administered by exchanging patient blood (mostly plasma) for packed cells.

With lifelong treatment, patients should experience no further manifestations of B_{12} deficiency. As previously stated, neurologic symptoms may not be fully corrected even by optimal therapy. The potential for late development of gastric carcinoma in pernicious anemia necessitates careful follow-up of the patient.

FOLATE DEFICIENCY Like vitamin B_{12} deficiency, folate deficiency is treated by replacement therapy. The usual dose of folate is 1 mg per day, by mouth, but higher doses (up to 5 mg per day) may be required for folate deficiency due to malabsorption. Parenteral folate is rarely necessary. The hematologic response is similar to that seen after replacement therapy for vitamin B_{12} deficiency—that is, a brisk reticulocytosis after about 4 days, followed by correction of the anemia over the next 1 to 2 months. The duration of therapy depends on the basis of the deficiency state. Patients with a continuously

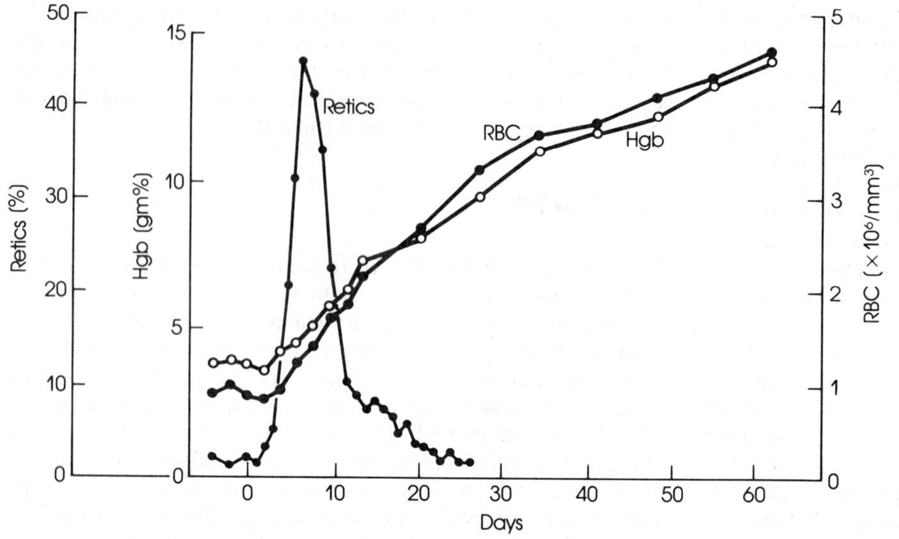

FIGURE 285-3 *Hematologic response of a patient with pernicious anemia to an intramuscular injection of 100 μg vitamin B_{12} on day 0. (From A Erslev, TG Gabuzda, Pathophysiology of Blood, Philadelphia, Saunders, 1975.)*

increased requirement (such as patients with hemolytic anemia) or those with malabsorption or chronic malnutrition should continue to receive oral folic acid indefinitely. In addition, the patient should be encouraged to maintain an optimal diet containing adequate amounts of folate.

Folate, particularly in large doses, can correct the megaloblastic anemia of vitamin B_{12} deficiency without altering the neurologic abnormalities. The neurologic manifestations may even be aggravated by folate therapy. Vitamin B_{12} deficiency can thus be masked in patients who for one reason or another are taking large doses of folate. For this reason, a hematologic response to folate must never be used to rule out vitamin B_{12} deficiency in a given patient; vitamin B_{12} deficiency can be excluded only by appropriate laboratory evaluation.

OTHER CAUSES OF MEGALOBLASTIC ANEMIA Megaloblastic anemia due to drugs can be treated, if necessary, by reducing the dose of the drug or eliminating it altogether. The effects of folate antagonists which inhibit dihydrofolate reductase can be counteracted by folinic acid (citrovorum factor) in a dose of 100 to 200 mg per day. Since folinic acid is a derivative of tetrahydrofolate, it circumvents the block in folate metabolism imposed by dihydrofolate reductase inhibitors, replenishing the tissues with a form of folate which can directly enter the one-carbon donor pool.

Certain of the congenital megaloblastic anemia–producing enzyme deficiencies can be treated by appropriate specific therapeutic regimens. The anemia of orotic aciduria is corrected by uridine, and the anemia in one case of Lesch-Nyhan syndrome responded to adenine. Both congenital folate malabsorption and homocystinuria have been treated successfully with oral folate, the former with very large doses (40 mg per day). Transcobalamin II deficiency can be treated with cyanocobalamin, but the vitamin has to be administered parenterally in very large doses so that it can enter cells by mass action without the aid of TC II.

For the megaloblastic forms of sideroblastic anemia, pyridoxine in pharmacologic doses (as high as 300 mg per day) should be tried. A few patients will respond to this therapy. Simple supportive measures are all that appear to be in order for treatment of refractory megaloblastic anemia. Acute erythroleukemia (di Guglielmo's disease) is usually treated like other types of acute nonlymphocytic leukemia (see Chap. 292).

REFERENCES

Allen RH: The plasma transport of vitamin B_{12}. Br J Haematol 36:153, 1976
Beck WS: The megaloblastic anemias, in *Hematology*, WJ Williams et al (eds). New York, McGraw-Hill, 1983
Borch K: Epidemiologic, clinicopathologic, and economic aspects of gastroscopic screening of patients with pernicious anemia. Scand J Gastroenterol 21:21, 1986
Chanarin I et al: Cobalamin folate interactions: A critical review. Blood 66:474, 1985
Eriksson S et al: Pernicious anemia as a risk factor in gastric cancer: The extent of the problem. Acta Med Scand 210:481. 1981
Lawson DH et al: Early mortality in the megaloblastic anemias. Q J Med 41:1, 1972
Lindenbaum J: Status of laboratory testing in the diagnosis of megaloblastic anemia. Blood 61:624, 1983
———: Aspects of vitamin B_{12} and folate metabolism in malabsorption syndromes. Am J Med 67:1037, 1979
———: Folate and vitamin B_{12} deficiencies in alcoholism. Semin Hematol 17:119, 1980
Rosenberg LE: Disorders of propionate and methylmalonate metabolism, in *Metabolic Basis of Inherited Disease*, JB Stanbury et al (eds). New York, McGraw-Hill, 1983
Scott JM, Weir DG: Drug induced megaloblastic change. Clin Haematol 9:587, 1980

286 ANEMIA ASSOCIATED WITH CHRONIC DISORDERS

H. FRANKLIN BUNN

Among the most commonly encountered anemias are those that accompany a variety of chronic underlying diseases. They can be corrected only if the primary condition is reversible. As shown in Table 286-1, these anemias can be subdivided into several groups. Those associated with chronic inflammation are characterized by an abnormality in iron metabolism.

ANEMIA OF CHRONIC INFLAMMATION

CLINICAL FEATURES Patients who have a chronic systemic inflammatory disorder persisting more than a month usually develop a mild or moderate anemia. The extent of the anemia is roughly proportional to the duration and severity of the inflammatory process. These disorders include chronic infections such as subacute infective endocarditis, osteomyelitis, lung abscess, tuberculosis, and pyelonephritis. Among noninfectious causes of anemia of chronic inflammation, the most common is rheumatoid arthritis. Other noninfectious inflammatory disorders often associated with chronic anemia include systemic lupus erythematosus, vasculitides (such as temporal arteritis), sarcoidosis, regional enteritis, and tissue injury such as fractures.

This kind of anemia is also commonly encountered in neoplastic disorders, including Hodgkin's disease and a variety of solid tumors such as carcinoma of the lung and breast. Other factors may contribute to the development of more severe anemia in cancer patients. In those with gastrointestinal cancer, blood loss can be the predominant factor. Chronic gastrointestinal bleeding will lead to iron deficiency. Furthermore, cancer patients may develop progressive anemia if the bone marrow is invaded with tumor cells. Myelophthisic anemia is discussed in Chap. 290. Cancer patients are often malnourished and may develop folate deficiency. Rarely, patients with disseminated malignancy develop severe traumatic hemolytic anemia (Chap. 287). Finally, suppression of hematopoiesis by chemotherapeutic agents or radiation therapy may aggravate anemia.

HEMATOLOGIC FEATURES Hemoglobin values generally range between 9 and 11 g/dL. A hemoglobin level less than 8 g/dL indicates the presence of one or more of the aggravating factors mentioned above. Although this group of anemias is generally classified as normocytic-normochromic, red blood cells are often slightly microcytic. The mean corpuscular hemoglobin concentration is about 32 g/dL (normal $\cong$ 34 g/dL). Examination of the bone marrow reveals normal erythroid maturation. However, the red blood cell precursors have less stainable iron than normal (i.e., fewer sideroblasts), while the macrophages in the marrow usually contain increased amounts of iron. Myeloid hyperplasia and an increase in plasma cells are often seen in chronic infections.

The reticulocyte count is usually normal ($<$3 percent). Careful measurement of red blood cell survival generally reveals moderately shortened erythrocyte life span. Cross-transfusion studies point to an extracorpuscular mechanism, probably hyperplasia of the mononuclear-phagocyte system. There is seldom any other evidence of significant hemolysis. However, in certain chronic infections such as subacute infective endocarditis and miliary tuberculosis, splenomegaly can contribute to further shortening of the red blood cell life span, thereby increasing the severity of the anemia. In this setting spherocytes are often seen on the blood smear.

Serum iron is characteristically subnormal in this group of anemias, but in contrast to iron deficiency, the total transferrin level is also reduced (see Fig. 284-2). The fractional saturation of transferrin is lower than normal. The serum iron falls within hours or days following the onset of the inflammation, whereas several weeks elapse before the transferrin level falls. Serum ferritin is increased in patients with inflammatory disorders. Certain other plasma proteins are characteristically elevated in chronic inflammation, probably under the stimulus of interleukin 1, a protein hormone released by activated macrophages. These "phase reactants" include gamma globulin, the third component of complement, haptoglobin, alpha$_1$ antitrypsin, orosomucoid, and fibrinogen. The latter is usually not measured since protein electrophoresis is routinely done on serum rather than plasma. Elevation of these proteins is responsible for the increased rate of red blood cell sedimentation which is so commonly observed.

It is often difficult to detect iron deficiency in a patient with chronic inflammation. The serum iron is low, and red blood cell protoporphyrin is increased in both conditions. When iron deficiency is superimposed on a chronic inflammatory state, the serum ferritin falls and transferrin level rises, usually to within normal limits. Under such circumstances, the amount of storage iron in the bone marrow is unpredictable. This problem is commonly encountered in patients with rheumatoid arthritis who may have developed iron deficiency owing to gastrointestinal blood loss. Because of this diagnostic uncertainty, it is often prudent to give such a patient a trial of iron and ascertain whether the hemoglobin level increases. However, it is important to avoid prolonged administration of iron unless a true deficiency state persists.

PATHOGENESIS The anemia of chronic inflammation is primarily due to defective red blood cell production and failure to compensate for the slightly decreased red blood cell life span. The subnormal amounts of iron in erythroblasts, in spite of an abundance of storage iron, suggests a defect in the transfer of iron to the developing erythroid cells. The cells that are formed are somewhat "iron deficient," and therefore tend to be small and pale. As in true iron deficiency, increased red blood cell protoporphyrin reflects the reduced availability of iron for heme synthesis. This defect can be quantitated by iron kinetic studies. If radioactive iron bound to transferrin is administered, there is normal uptake into erythroblasts and incorporation into circulating red cells. In contrast, if hemoglobin labeled with radioactive iron is injected, the incorporation of label into circulating red cells is only half normal. The hyperplastic mononuclear phagocyte system which is responsible for decreased survival of circulating red cells probably traps the hemoglobin iron and prevents its transfer to the bone marrow. The macrophages' increased avidity for iron may be due to one of the actions of interluekin 1, i.e., release of lactoferrin from neutrophils. The iron-binding protein lactoferrin captures free iron and rapidly transfers it to macrophages.

The modest suppression of red blood cell production is caused in part by decreased availability of iron. In addition, erythropoietin levels tend to be lower than expected for the degree of anemia. However, erythropoietin levels are not as low as in the anemia of renal failure (see below) and probably do not play a significant role in the pathogenesis of the anemia.

MANAGEMENT The anemia of chronic inflammation is not responsive to hematinic agents such as iron, folic acid, or vitamin B_{12}. Since the anemia is seldom severe, blood transfusion is rarely indicated. Efforts should be directed toward correcting the underlying disorder. In addition, if the anemia is more severe than expected, it is essential to search for other factors such as blood loss or drug-induced myelosuppression that could contribute to the reduction of red blood cell mass.

ANEMIA OF UREMIA

Anemia almost always accompanies the uremic syndrome (Chap. 220). Although the hemoglobin level is highly variable among uremic patients, the severity of the anemia is roughly proportional to the degree of azotemia. The etiology of the renal failure usually has little bearing on the extent of anemia. However, for any level of serum creatinine patients with polycystic disease tend to be less anemic than those with other types of renal disease. In contrast to anemias associated with other chronic disorders discussed in this chapter, the anemia of uremia can be very severe, with hemoglobin levels as low as 4 g/dL. However, patients often tolerate such marked anemia fairly well. This is largely due to compensatory adjustments such as redistribution of blood flow and a decrease in the oxygen affinity of the blood (see Chap. 53).

The anemia of uremia is normochromic and normocytic. Examination of the bone marrow seldom reveals any abnormalities. Red blood cell morphology is usually normal. In about one-third of patients, so-called burr cells are seen in the peripheral blood smear. These red blood cells have a characteristic evenly scalloped border (see Fig. A5-9). Neither the degree of anemia nor the red blood cell life span is influenced by the presence of burr cells. In most patients the reticulocyte count is normal and the red blood cell survival is only modestly decreased. Thus the low red blood cell mass is due to decreased red blood cell production. The primary basis for this defect is that the diseased kidneys are unable to secrete adequate amounts of erythropoietin. Plasma erythropoietin levels are lower than those of nonuremic patients with a comparable degree of anemia. Erythropoiesis is further impaired but not abolished in patients who have undergone bilateral nephrectomy. In addition, red blood cell production may be suppressed by the accumulation of substances that are normally cleared by the kidneys. Iron kinetic measurements reveal impaired incorporation of iron into circulating red blood cells. Thus, it is likely that the anemia is due in part to ineffective erythropoiesis

TABLE 286-1 Anemias secondary to chronic systemic diseases

1 Anemia of chronic inflammation
- *a* Infection
- *b* Connective tissue disorders, etc.
- *c* Malignancy

2 Anemia of uremia
3 Anemia due to endocrine failure
4 Anemia of liver disease

(see Chap. 283). Improvement in the rate of utilization of iron by the bone marrow has been noted following hemodialysis.

A small minority of uremic patients, particularly those with advanced disease, have brisk hemolysis. Red blood cell survival studies indicate that the hemolysis is due to extracorpuscular factors. Both metabolic and mechanical factors contribute to the hemolysis. Some patients may acquire a defect in the hexose monophosphate shunt which renders the red blood cell vulnerable to the formation of Heinz bodies (see Chap. 287). The hemolysis can be aggravated by oxidant drugs or oxidant compounds such as chloramine in the dialysis bath. If the renal failure is due to thrombotic thrombocytopenic purpura or hemolytic-uremic syndrome, patients will have a severe form of microangiopathic hemolytic anemia, with characteristic abnormalities of red blood cell morphology (see Chap. 287).

Treatment of the anemia of uremia should focus on an attempt to reverse the renal failure. The anemia may be modestly improved following hemodialysis. A prompt and dramatic correction of the anemia follows successful renal transplantation. Occasionally, polycythemia may be encountered following the renal engraftment, and may be a harbinger of impending rejection. In those patients who are not candidates for renal transplantation the administration of androgens has proved effective in stimulating erythropoiesis, particularly in patients who have not undergone bilateral nephrectomy. The recent development of synthetic erythropoietin offers the hope of definitive therapy in the near future.

It is important to be aware of other factors that may aggravate the anemia of renal disease. Uremic patients have a propensity to hemorrhage, owing to a qualitative defect in platelet function. Thus, gastrointestinal blood loss is commonly encountered. Furthermore a small but significant amount of blood loss occurs during hemodialysis. For these reasons some uremic patients become iron deficient. Folic acid deficiency may also occur, owing to the poor nutrition of many patients or to the loss of this vitamin during dialysis.

ANEMIA SECONDARY TO ENDOCRINE FAILURE

A number of hormones, including thyroxine, glucocorticoids, testosterone, and growth hormone are known to affect proliferation of human erythroid cells in vitro. Therefore it is not surprising that a mild to moderate normochromic-normocytic anemia generally accompanies a number of endocrine deficiency states, including hypothyroidism, Addison's disease, hypogonadism, and panhypopituitarism. It is possible that the anemias associated with hypothyroidism and hypopituitarism are related to the decreased need for oxygen transport, since oxygen consumption is reduced when thyroid hormone or growth hormone is lacking.

The anemia of *myxedema* is usually normocytic. Red blood cell life span is normal and erythropoiesis is effective. A minority of patients have macrocytic red blood cells which can usually be attributed to either folic acid or B_{12} deficiency. Patients with myxedema have an increased incidence of pernicious anemia. Hypothyroid patients, particularly females with menorrhagia, often develop iron deficiency and a microcytic anemia. Because the plasma volume may be reduced along with the red blood cell mass, the anemia of hypothyroidism may be masked. Since the signs and symptoms of myxedema are sometimes elusive, this diagnosis should be considered in the evaluation of any patient with unexplained anemia.

The anemia of *Addison's disease* is also masked by a decrease in plasma volume. Untreated patients have an average hemoglobin level of about 13 g/dL. Upon hormone replacement, the plasma volume is rapidly reconstituted and the hemoglobin level falls to 80 percent of its pretreatment value. With continued therapy, the red blood cell mass returns to normal.

Testosterone has a physiologic influence on red blood cell mass. During passage through adolescence the mean hemoglobin level of males increases from 13 to 15 g/dL. Eunuchoid males generally have a mild decrease in hemoglobin, averaging 13 g/dL. Pituitary dysfunction or ablation is associated with a mild normochromic normocytic anemia as well as occasional leukopenia.

The anemias secondary to endocrine failure are all readily corrected when adequate hormone replacement is given.

ANEMIA OF LIVER DISEASE

Patients with chronic liver disease, regardless of etiology, usually have a mild to moderate anemia which is normocytic or slightly macrocytic. An increased plasma volume may artificially lower the hematocrit and make the anemia seem worse than it is. Red blood cell morphology is normal, except for the presence of target cells (see Fig. A5-3) and occasional stomatocytes, which have increased membrane surface area owing to increased deposits of cholesterol and phospholipid. The bone marrow is usually normal. Erythropoiesis fails to compensate for a moderate shortening of red blood cell life span. The anemia persists as long as hepatic function is defective, but it may be corrected if normal hepatic function can be restored.

The situation is much more complex in patients with *alcoholic liver disease*. Many factors can contribute to the development of anemia. Alcohol is a direct suppressor of erythropoiesis. In alcoholics who have continued to drink up to the time of clinical evaluation, the bone marrow often reveals vacuoles in the cytoplasm of red and white blood cell precursors. In addition, ringed sideroblasts may be observed, particularly in patients who are malnourished. In alcoholics there is often suboptimal intake of dietary folic acid and impairment of folate utilization. Furthermore, alcoholics commonly develop significant hemorrhage from gastritis, esophageal varices, or duodenal ulcer, which contributes to the anemia. The risk of gastrointestinal blood loss is further increased by the presence of thrombocytopenia or deficiencies in soluble clotting factors. Although alcoholics usually have increased iron stores, they may become iron-deficient after prolonged gastrointestinal bleeding. Rarely patients with alcoholic cirrhosis develop a severe hemolytic anemia accompanied by the appearance of rigid red blood cells with irregular borders called acanthocytes or "spur" cells (see Fig. A5-8). This entity is discussed in detail in Chap. 287. In addition, alcoholics may acquire a defect in the erythrocyte hexose monophosphate shunt, similar to that encountered in patients with uremia.

REFERENCES

Budman DR, Steinberg AD: Hematologic aspects of systemic lupus erythematosus. Ann Intern Med 86:220, 1977

Colman D, Herbert V: Hematologic complications of alcoholism: Overview. Semin Hematol 17:164, 1980

Eschbach JW, Adamson J: Anemia of end-stage renal disease. Kideny Int 28:1, 1985

Lee GR: The anemia of chronic disease. Semin Hematol 20:61, 1983

Mowat AG: Hematologic abnormalities in rheumatoid arthritis. Semin Arthritis Rheum 1:195, 1972

Neff MS et al: A comparison of androgens for anemia in patients on hemodialysis. N Engl J Med 304:871, 1981

———: Anemia in chronic renal failure. Acta Endocrinol 271(Suppl):80, 1985

Orrego H et al: Interrelation of the hypermetabolic state, necrosis, anemia and cell enlargement as determinants of severity of alcoholic liver disease. Acta Med Scand 703(Suppl):81, 1985

287 HEMOLYTIC ANEMIAS

RICHARD A. COOPER / H. FRANKLIN BUNN

Red blood cells undergo premature destruction by two general mechanisms. First, red blood cells may lyse in the circulation and release their contents directly into the plasma. Intravascular hemolysis may be caused by trauma to the red blood cell, by fixation of complement to the red blood cell, or by exogenous toxins. Second, and more commonly, red blood cells are taken up by macrophages in the spleen and liver (mononuclear-phagocyte system), where they are destroyed and digested (extravascular lysis). The mononuclear-phagocyte system clears the cells from the circulation under two general conditions: first, the presence of surface abnormalities such as bound immunoglobulin for which macrophages have specific receptors; second, the presence of physical characteristics that limit the deformability of red blood cells, thereby impeding their ability to traverse the fine filtering system of the spleen.

The discoid shape of red blood cells favors deformability, providing a surface area that is 60 to 70 percent in excess of the minimum that is necessary to encompass the content of the cell. Deformability is determined by three independent variables: (1) the viscoelastic properties of the red blood cell membrane, (2) the ratio of surface area to volume, and (3) the intracellular concentration of hemoglobin or the aggregation of hemoglobin into polymers or precipitates.

One or more of these factors play a role in the pathogenesis of the various hemolytic anemias that are described in this chapter. A classification of these anemias is shown in Table 287-1. A number of clinical and laboratory features are shared by various types of hemolytic anemia. Patients with congenital hemolysis often have lifelong anemia and may have a positive family history. Splenomegaly is seen in most chronic hemolytic anemias, both congenital and acquired. Patients with significant red blood cell turnover may be icteric, owing to an increase in unconjugated bilirubin.

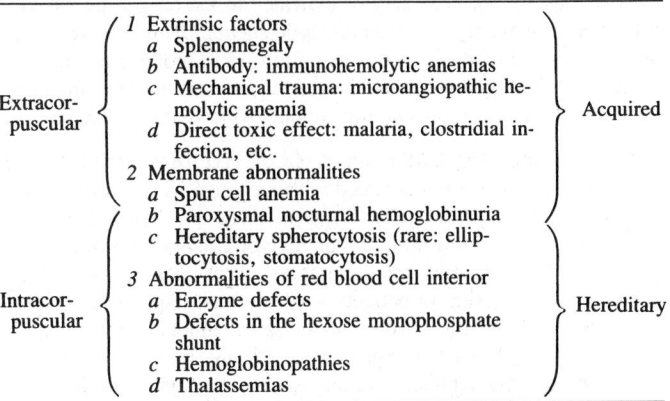

TABLE 287-1 Hemolytic anemias

Extracorpuscular	*1* Extrinsic factors	Acquired
Extracorpuscular	*a* Splenomegaly	Acquired
Extracorpuscular	*b* Antibody: immunohemolytic anemias	Acquired
Extracorpuscular	*c* Mechanical trauma: microangiopathic hemolytic anemia	Acquired
Extracorpuscular	*d* Direct toxic effect: malaria, clostridial infection, etc.	Acquired
Extracorpuscular	*2* Membrane abnormalities	Acquired
Extracorpuscular	*a* Spur cell anemia	Acquired
Intracorpuscular	*b* Paroxysmal nocturnal hemoglobinuria	Acquired
Intracorpuscular	*c* Hereditary spherocytosis (rare: elliptocytosis, stomatocytosis)	Hereditary
Intracorpuscular	*3* Abnormalities of red blood cell interior	Hereditary
Intracorpuscular	*a* Enzyme defects	Hereditary
Intracorpuscular	*b* Defects in the hexose monophosphate shunt	Hereditary
Intracorpuscular	*c* Hemoglobinopathies	Hereditary
Intracorpuscular	*d* Thalassemias	Hereditary

LABORATORY EVALUATION OF HEMOLYSIS

The reticulocyte count is the single most useful test in the initial evaluation (Table 287-2). Patients with hemolytic anemia generally have a brisk reticulocytosis. The bone marrow predictably reveals erythroid hyperplasia. Since it seldom provides useful additional information, a bone marrow examination is generally not indicated in the evaluation of a patient with hemolytic anemia, unless an associated disorder such as lymphoma is suspected.

A number of serum tests are useful in establishing the presence of hemolysis (see Table 287-2), most importantly, the measurement of bilirubin, a tetrapyrrole formed from the oxidative catabolism of heme. *Unconjugated* or *"indirect" bilirubin* circulates in the plasma in transit from the mononuclear-phagocyte system to the liver where it is conjugated. When measured accurately, unconjugated bilirubin is a reliable guide to the presence of increased heme catabolism and is usually elevated in patients with hemolysis. The serum level of conjugated or "direct" bilirubin is normal unless the patient has associated hepatic or biliary dysfunction. Unconjugated bilirubin is also increased in patients with ineffective erythropoiesis, a condition in which there is enhanced destruction of red cell precursors within the bone marrow. Since circulating unconjugated bilirubin is tightly bound to albumin, it does not pass through renal glomeruli. Thus, patients with hemolytic anemia have acholuric jaundice, whereas the hyperbilirubinemia of liver disease is associated with bilirubin in the urine.

Other serum tests are also useful in the assessment of hemolysis. *Haptoglobin* is an alpha globulin which is present in high concentration (~100 mg/dL) in the plasma (and serum). It binds specifically and tightly to the protein (globin) in hemoglobin. The hemoglobin-haptoglobin complex is cleared within minutes by the mononuclear-phagocyte system, while free haptoglobin has a long circulation time ($t_{1/2}$ = 4 days). Thus, patients with significant hemolysis, either intravascular or extravascular, have low or absent levels of serum haptoglobin. Haptoglobin synthesis is decreased in patients with hepatocellular disease. Conversely, synthesis is enhanced in inflammatory states. Haptoglobin, like alpha$_1$ antitrypsin, orosomucoid, and the third component of complement are acute phase reactants. These facts must be considered in the interpretation of serum haptoglobin. *Hemopexin* is a plasma beta globulin which binds specifically to heme. It becomes depleted in patients with moderate and severe hemolysis. In addition to that bound by hemopexin, some of the heme from circulating free hemoglobin is transferred to albumin, resulting in the formation of *methemalbumin*. This complex is encountered only in severe intravascular hemolysis. Plasma hemoglobin is increased in proportion to the degree of hemolysis, but may be falsely elevated owing to lysis of red cells in vitro.

Once the haptoglobin binding capacity of the plasma is exceeded, free hemoglobin permeates renal glomeruli, primarily as $\alpha\beta$ dimers with a molecular weight of 32,000. This filtered hemoglobin is reabsorbed by the proximal tubule, where it is catabolized in situ, and the heme iron is incorporated into storage proteins (ferritin and hemosiderin). The presence of hemosiderin in the urine, detected by staining the sediment with Prussian blue, indicates that a significant amount of circulating free hemoglobin has been filtered by the kidneys. When the absorptive capacity of the tubular cells is exceeded, hemoglobinuria ensues. The presence of hemoglobinuria indicates severe intravascular hemolysis. Sometimes the clinician is faced with the dilemma of whether benzidine-positive heme pigment in the urine is hemoglobin or myoglobin. The easiest way to distinguish between these alternatives is to examine an anticoagulated blood specimen after centrifiguration. Because of its higher molecular weight, hemoglobin has lower glomerular permeability than myoglobin and is less rapidly cleared by the kidneys. The plasma of patients with hemoglobinuria has a reddish-brown color. Conversely, patients with myoglobinuria have normal-appearing plasma.

Tagging red cells with an appropriate isotopic label provides the most direct and precise measure of cell survival. The most commonly used label is sodium [^{51}Cr]chromate. Since it does not bind irreversibly to red cells, the measured survival of normal red cells ($t_{1/2}$ = 26 to

TABLE 287-2 Laboratory evaluation of hemolysis

	Moderate hemolysis (RBC life span 20–40 days)	Severe hemolysis (RBC life span 5–20 days)
HEMATOLOGIC		
Routine blood film	Polychromatophilia	Polychromatophilia
Reticulocyte count	↑	↑ ↑
Bone marrow examination	Erythroid hyperplasia	Erythroid hyperplasia
PLASMA OR SERUM		
Bilirubin	↑ Unconjugated	↑ Unconjugated
Haptoglobin	↓, absent	Absent
Hemopexin	Normal, ↓	↓, absent
Plasma hemoglobin	↑	↑ ↑
Lactate dehydrogenase	↑ (variable)	↑ ↑ (variable)
Methemalbumin	0	+ *
URINE		
Bilirubin	0	0
Urobilinogen	Variable	Variable
Hemosiderin	0	+
Hemoglobin	0	+ *

* *Intravascular hemolysis.*

32 days) is shorter than the true red cell survival ($t_{1/2} \simeq$ 60 days). Such studies are not necessary or indicated in the diagnostic workup of the majority of patients with hemolytic anemia. However, scanning with a collumnated detector can be employed to monitor the sequestration of ^{51}Cr-tagged red cells in the liver and spleen. This approach is sometimes useful in evaluating patients for possible splenectomy.

RED CELL MORPHOLOGY AS A CLUE TO DIAGNOSIS Most hemolytic disorders are associated with a change in the morphologic appearance of red blood cells. Some of these are depicted in Atlas 5. Spherocytes are the most common morphologic abnormality in hemolytic diseases, and small numbers occur in many disorders. They are most striking in patients with hereditary spherocytosis and in patients with warm antibody-induced immunohemolytic disease (Figs. A5-10 and A5-11). Spherocytes are the hallmark of splenic conditioning. Fragmented red blood cells suggest traumatic injury of the red cell including valve hemolysis or one of the microangiopathic hemolytic anemias such as thrombotic thrombocytopenic purpura (Fig. A5-7), hemolytic uremic syndrome, or disseminated intravascular coagulation. Target-shaped red blood cells which are well filled with hemoglobin occur in patients with hemoglobin C. They are prevalent in sickle cell anemia, where they were first described, and they are found in patients with the underhydrated form of hereditary stomatocytosis. The most common cause of target cells is liver disease (Fig. A5-3). Target cells which are deficient in hemoglobin (hypochromic) are the hallmark of the thalassemia syndromes (Fig. A5-5).

Spiculated red blood cells often cause confusion because of the frequency with which they are induced as an artifact during the preparation of a blood smear. Under these conditions, they are particularly frequent at the edges of the smear. When surrounded by otherwise normal-appearing red blood cells, spiculated red blood cells can be a clue to diagnosis. They occur, usually in small numbers, in conjunction with uremia or following splenectomy even in the absence of an underlying red blood cell disorder. Bizarrely spiculated red blood cells (acanthocytes) occur in the rare condition abetalipoproteinemia (Chap. 315) and in anorexia nervosa; however, in each of these instances minimal hemolysis is present. As discussed below, acanthocytes are a striking feature of spur-cell anemia (Fig. A5-8).

Permanently sickled, crescent-shaped red blood cells (Fig. A5-6) are the hallmark of sickle cell anemia (see Chap. 288). Boat-shaped red cells are a clue to the double heterozygous state of hemoglobin SC disease (see Chap. 288). The presence of both crescent-shaped cells and hypochromic target cells on the same smear is suggestive of the doubly heterozygous state, sickle cell–β thalassemia (see Chap. 288).

While in no case can the peripheral blood smear be totally diagnostic, in many it is a low-cost, important clue to the diagnosis. In addition to red blood cell morphology, a large battery of specific diagnostic tests are available for determining the etiology of the various hemolytic anemias. These are discussed in broad outline in Chap. 53 (Table 53-1) and in detail in this chapter.

EXTRINSIC CAUSES OF HEMOLYSIS

SPLENOMEGALY The spleen is particularly efficient in trapping and destroying red blood cells which have minimal defects, often so mild as to be undetectable by in vitro techniques. This unique ability of the spleen to filter mildly damaged red blood cells results from its unusual vascular anatomy. Almost all the blood circulating through the spleen flows rapidly from arterioles in the white pulp to sinuses in the spleen's red pulp, and then on into the venous system. In contrast, a small portion of splenic blood flow (normally 1 to 2 percent) leaves the arterioles of the white pulp to enter a nonendothelialized portion of the spleen. In this sense, it is extravascular, although the entire spleen may be considered as a specialized part of the vascular system. This blood passes into the "marginal zone" of the lymphatic white pulp. Although the cells which occupy this zone are not phagocytic, they serve as a mechanical filter hindering the progress of severely damaged red blood cells. As red blood cells leave this zone and enter the red pulp, they flow into narrow cords which end blindly but which communicate with sinuses through small openings between the lining cells of the sinuses. These openings, averaging 3 μm in diameter, test the ability of red blood cells to undergo a deformation of shape. Red blood cells which do not pass the stringent test imposed upon them by the spleen filter are engulfed by phagocytic cells and destroyed.

The normal spleen poses no threat to normal red blood cells. However, splenomegaly exaggerates the adverse conditions to which red blood cells are exposed. Splenic enlargement may be considered in three broad categories. In the first are infiltrative disease (such as myeloproliferative disorders, Chap. 289), lymphomas (Chap. 294), and storage diseases (such as Gaucher's disease, Chap. 316). In the second are systemic inflammatory diseases leading to splenic hypertrophy. In the third are diseases which cause congestive splenomegaly. Hemolysis may occur whenever the spleen is enlarged. Its occurrence is least predictable in infiltrative diseases of the spleen where substantial splenomegaly may exist with no apparent hemolysis. Inflammatory and congestive splenomegaly are commonly associated with mild to moderate shortening of red blood cell survival.

RED CELL ANTIBODIES Immune hemolysis in the adult may be induced by three general types of antibodies:

1 Alloantibodies acquired by blood transfusions or pregnancies and directed against transfused red blood cells (Chap. 282).
2 Antibodies reactive at body temperature and directed against the patient's own red blood cells (Table 287-3).
3 Antibodies reactive in the cold and directed against the patient's own red blood cells (Table 287-3).

Coombs' antiglobulin test is the major tool for diagnosing these disorders. This test relies on the ability of antibodies prepared in animals and directed against specific human serum proteins to agglutinate red blood cells if these human serum proteins are present on the red blood cell surface. The serum proteins of particular interest are IgG and C3. The ability of anti-IgG or anti-C3 antiserums to agglutinate the patient's red blood cells is referred to as the *direct Coombs test.* At times it is advantageous to know whether there is antibody in the serum of patients which is reactive against other human red blood cells. This is important in cross matching prior to blood transfusion (Chap. 282), and it is of prognostic significance in patients with warm-antibody hemolytic anemia. To determine this, an *indirect Coombs test* is performed by incubating normal ABO- and Rh-compatible red blood cells with the patient's serum and subsequently performing a direct Coombs test on these incubated red cells.

"Warm" antibodies Antibodies which react at body temperature are usually of the IgG class, although occasionally they are IgA. They induce a pattern of hemolysis which affects both the patient's own cells and normal transfused cells. This acquired syndrome is frequently designated *autoimmune hemolytic anemia.* In recent years, as a number of drugs which induce this clinical syndrome have become recognized, attention has focused on the exogenous factors which may underlie the formation of these red blood cell antibodies, and the expression *immunohemolytic anemia* is preferred.

CLINICAL MANIFESTATIONS Warm-antibody immunohemolytic anemia occurs at all ages but is most common in adults, particularly women and older individuals. In approximately one-fourth of patients this disorder occurs as a complication of an underlying disease affecting the immune system, especially chronic lymphocytic leukemia, non-Hodgkin's lymphoma, and systemic lupus erythematosus (SLE). Occasionally, immunohemolytic anemia is seen in patients with advanced, active Hodgkin's disease. Case reports link it to a variety of nonlymphoid neoplasms.

The presentation and course of immunohemolytic anemia are quite variable. In its mildest form, the only manifestation is a positive direct Coombs test. In this instance, insufficient antibody is present on the red blood cell surface to permit the reticuloendothelial system to recognize the cell as abnormal. This is particularly common in SLE. A large fraction of patients with immunohemolytic anemia have a chronic mild anemia and splenomegaly. The direct Coombs test is positive for IgG but seldom for C3, and the indirect Coombs test is negative. In other cases this disorder may be more severe, with hemoglobin levels less than 7.0 g/dL and reticulocyte counts of 30 percent and higher. Spherocytosis is usually marked (Fig. A5-11). Coombs' test is positive for IgG and frequently for C3 as well. Large quantities of antibody are present not only on the patient's red blood cells but also in the patient's serum as demonstrated by the indirect Coombs test. Thrombocytopenia may also be present. The coexistence of immune destruction of red blood cells and platelets is referred to as *Evans' syndrome,* a disorder in which separate antibodies are directed against platelets and red blood cells. In its most severe form, immunohemolytic anemia presents with fulminant, overwhelming hemolysis associated with hemoglobinemia, hemoglobinuria, and shock, a syndrome which may be fatal.

Associated findings include hyperbilirubinemia, decreased or absent haptoglobin levels, and occasionally hepatomegaly. Fever and abdominal pain occur in some patients. Venous thrombosis occurs commonly, the most frequent site being the deep veins of the legs, but thrombosis of mesenteric and portal veins has also been reported. Arterial thromboses occur as well.

PATHOGENESIS Little is known about the origin of red blood cell antibodies in the immunohemolytic anemias. Much more information exists concerning the mechanism of destruction of red blood cells coated with IgG antibodies. Although spherocytosis is often a prominent feature of hemolysis in vivo, the simple exposure of normal red blood cells to IgG antibodies does not lead to spherocytosis in vitro. However, human red blood cells coated with IgG antibodies are bound to the surface of monocytes or splenic macrophages and undergo a spherical transformation. The ability to cause this red blood cell–leukocyte interaction is greatest with IgG of subclasses 1 and 3 (the most common subclasses). It is not shared by IgM or IgA. However, C3 on the red blood cell surface also promotes this cell-cell interaction, but binding may be more transient because of the ability of the plasma C3 inactivator to release bound cells. Indeed, IgG and C3 behave in a synergistic fashion in this regard, accounting for the more severe hemolytic disease in patients in whom both IgG and C3 are present on the red blood cell surface. The slow flow compartment of the spleen is particularly efficient in trapping red blood cells which are coated with IgG antibodies, and the spleen is the major site of red blood cell destruction in this disorder.

THERAPY AND PROGNOSIS In the initial evaluation of the patient, it is important to rule out drugs which are known to cause immunohemolytic anemia. This topic is discussed below.

Patients having a mild degree of hemolysis usually do not require therapy. In those with clinically significant hemolysis, initial therapy consists of corticosteroids (e.g., prednisone, 1.0 mg/kg per day). A rise in hemoglobin is frequently noted within 3 or 4 days and occurs in most patients within 1 week. Prednisone is continued until the hemoglobin level has risen to normal values, and thereafter it is tapered slowly over the course of several months. More than 75 percent of patients will achieve a significant and sustained reduction in hemolysis; however, in half of these patients the disease will relapse either during the period of steroid tapering or following the cessation of steroid therapy. Steroids appear to have two modes of action: an immediate effect due to inhibition of the clearance of IgG-coated red blood cells by the mononuclear phagocyte system, and a later effect due to steroid-induced inhibition of antibody synthesis.

Patients with severe anemia may require blood transfusions. Because the antibody in this disease is a "panagglutinin," reacting with all normal donor cells, the usual cross matching is impossible. The goal in selecting blood for transfusion is to avoid administering red cells with antigens to which patients have previously been sensitized and which are known to be associated with complement lysis and intravascular hemolysis. In addition to A and B, Kell, Kidd (Jk^a), and Duffy (Fy) account for almost all examples of this type of hemolysis. A common procedure is to adsorb the panagglutinin present in patient's serum using the patient's own red cells from which antibody has previously been eluted. Serum freed of autoantibody in this way can then be tested for the presence of alloantibody to specific donor blood groups. ABO-compatible red cells matched in this fashion are administered slowly with attention paid to the possibility of an immediate-type transfusion reaction.

Splenectomy is the second line of therapy in this disorder. It is recommended for patients who cannot tolerate steroid therapy, in whom steroid therapy has been insufficient to control the disease process, or in whom a normal hematologic status can be maintained only with excessive doses of steroids. When red blood cells are labeled with chromium, their site of destruction can be determined. In 75 percent of patients, the spleen is the dominant site, whereas the liver predominates in the remaining patients. However, this test is not generally useful for selecting those patients who would respond to splenectomy. Rather, a favorable response to splenectomy is obtained in approximately two-thirds of patients in whom a splenic pattern of localization is found and in approximately one-third of patients in whom it is not found. Therefore, splenectomy must be undertaken on clinical grounds alone. To provide prophylaxis against pneumococcal infection, a risk in splenectomized individuals, patients should be immunized with polyvalent pneumococcal antiserum.

In recent years, patients who have been refractory to steroid therapy and to splenectomy have been treated with immunosuppressive drugs. The greatest experience is with azathioprine (Imuran) and cyclophosphamide (Cytoxan). A variable success rate has been reported with each.

In the majority of patients, this disease is controlled by steroid therapy alone, by splenectomy, or by a combination. In most of the remaining patients, a partial degree of control is achieved. Fatalities occur among three categories: first, rare patients with overwhelming hemolysis in whom death is directly attributable to anemia; second, those with major thrombotic events coincident with active hemolysis; third, those whose host defenses are impaired by corticosteroids, splenectomy, and/or immunosuppressives. In patients in whom immunohemolysis develops as a complication of an underlying disorder, the prognosis is dominated by that of the primary disease.

Immunohemolytic anemia secondary to drugs Drugs which have been directly related to immunohemolytic anemia are of three kinds, as distinguished by their three mechanisms of actions: (1) Drugs, such as α-methyldopa (Chap. 196), which induce a disorder identical almost in every respect to the warm-antibody immunohemolytic anemia described above. (2) Drugs of the penicillin type which can become associated with the red blood cell surface and induce the formation of an antibody directed against the red blood cell–drug complex. (3) Drugs, such as quinidine, that form a complex with plasma proteins to which an antibody forms; this drug–plasma protein–antibody complex settles out on red blood cells or platelets to involve them in a destructive process on an "innocent bystander" basis.

TABLE 287-3 Hemolysis due to antibodies

I Warm-antibody immunohemolytic anemia
- *A* Idiopathic
- *B* Lymphomas: Chronic lymphocytic leukemia, non-Hodgkin's lymphomas, Hodgkin's disease (infrequent)
- *C* Systemic lupus erythematosus
- *D* Tumors (rare)
- *E* Drugs
  - *1* α-Methyldopa type
  - *2* Penicillin type (hapten)
  - *3* Quinidine type (innocent bystander)

II Cold-antibody immunohemolytic anemia
- *A* Cold agglutinin disease
  - *1* Acute: Mycoplasma infection, infectious mononucleosis
  - *2* Chronic: Idiopathic, lymphoma
- *B* Paroxysmal cold hemoglobinuria

α-METHYLDOPA-TYPE ANTIBODIES A positive direct Coombs test is observed in up to 10 percent of patients receiving α-methyldopa therapy in a dose of 2.0 g daily. A small minority of these patients develop spherocytosis and hemolysis, often of severe degree. This "autoimmune" disorder may be triggered by a deficiency of suppressor T lymphocytes. Two distinctive features are that the indirect Coombs test is positive in almost all patients with hemolysis and that the red cells are coated with IgG but not C3. The IgG antibody is directed against the Rh complex as it is in most patients with idiopathic immunohemolytic anemia due to IgG. Hemolysis decreases over the course of several weeks after cessation of drug therapy, although the direct Coombs test may remain positive for more than 1 year.

PENICILLIN (HAPTEN)-INDUCED IMMUNOHEMOLYSIS An antibody directed against "penicillinized" red blood cells induces hemolysis in patients receiving large, intravenous doses of penicillin and penicillin-type antibiotics (e.g., 15 to 20 million units of penicillin per day, or 12 to 15 g oxacillin per day). Hemolysis usually begins 7 to 14 days after the start of penicillin therapy and is associated with spherocytosis and hyperbilirubinemia. The patient's red blood cells are Coombs-positive for IgG during the period of penicillin therapy. An indirect Coombs test can be demonstrated with the patient's serum using normal red blood cells "penicillinized" in vitro. Hemolysis ceases abruptly when penicillin therapy is stopped, although the serum antibody can be demonstrated for many weeks.

INNOCENT BYSTANDER IMMUNOHEMOLYSIS Innocent bystander antibodies may be of either the IgG or IgM class, and the antigen-antibody complexes which adhere to the red blood cell surface are capable of fixing complement. The drug-antibody complex dissociates from the red blood cell, leaving only C3 to be detected by Coombs' test. The pattern of hemolysis may be primarily extravascular red blood cell destruction, or it may be intravascular hemolysis due to complement lysis with hemoglobinemia, hemoglobinuria, and acute renal failure. This is an uncommon form of hemolysis despite the fact that the drugs associated with it are in very common usage. They include quinine and quinidine, isoniazid, sulfonamides, phenacetin, stibophen, *p*-aminosalicylic acid, dipyrone, and various insecticides.

Immune hemolysis due to cold-reactive antibodies Antibodies which are reactive in the cold induce hemolysis under two general conditions. First, in cold agglutinin disease IgM antibodies, usually reactive with the I antigen, occur spontaneously, in the course of a lymphoproliferative disease or as a complication of infectious mononucleosis or mycoplasma pneumonia. Second, in paroxysmal cold hemoglobinuria, antibodies of the IgG class (Donath-Landsteiner) occur spontaneously or as a complication of certain viral diseases or of syphilis.

COLD AGGLUTININ DISEASE *Clinical manifestations.* Agglutination of red blood cells by IgM cold agglutinins is most profound at very low temperatures, and disagglutination occurs quickly upon warming. In most patients agglutination ceases at 32°C. The fixation of complement is a warm-reactive process. Therefore, patients may have very high titers of cold agglutinins as measured at low temperatures, but these antibodies may be inefficient in fixing complement to the cell surface and totally unable to induce agglutination at temperatures achieved in the bloodstream. Most cold agglutinins cause little or no shortening of red blood cell survival.

In mycoplasma pneumonia, cold agglutinins are very common, whereas only the occasional patient will have significant hemolysis about 5 to 10 days after recovery from the infection. Spherocytes may be seen occasionally, but the red blood cell morphology is usually normal. The antibody is directed against the I antigen, and the entire process is self-limited.

The cold agglutinin in infectious mononucleosis is most frequently directed against the i antigen, an antigen accessible on the surface of fetal red blood cells but not adult red blood cells. Therefore, this cold agglutinin is of serologic interest, but rarely induces hemolysis in humans. Antibody directed against the I antigen and complex antibodies involving both antigens have also been reported, with hemolysis.

A chronic form of cold-induced hemolysis occurs in patients de novo or in association with lymphoid neoplasms. It most commonly affects individuals in their seventh or eighth decades. The clinical manifestations relate to hemolysis and less commonly to agglutination of red blood cells in capillaries in those portions of the body exposed to low temperature, causing acrocyanosis. Gangrene is uncommon. Hemoglobin levels are usually above 10 g/dL and rarely below 7 g. Reticulocytes are fewer in number than might be anticipated, presumably because of the selective destruction of young cells (including reticulocytes) in this disorder.

In most patients with cold agglutinin disease, the antibody titer is very high (e.g., 1:10,000) at 4°C and very low (e.g., 1:16) at 37°C. In some patients the antibody shows a flatter thermal spectrum with a moderately high titer at 4°C (e.g., 1:320) and a readily demonstrable titer at 37°C (e.g., 1:64). Hemolysis tends to be more severe in this latter group. The Coombs test demonstrates the presence of C3 on the red blood cell surface, but IgM (which is responsible for the C3 coating of red cells) is not found.

Pathogenesis. The etiology of the antibody is unknown. It appears to exert its hemolytic effect not through agglutination per se but rather by the fixation of C3 to the red blood cell surface. The liver is particularly efficient at detecting red blood cells coated with C3 in the form of C3b and clearing them from the circulation. A plasma enzyme, C3 inactivator, is capable of cleaving C3b into a small fragment (C3c) which leaves the cell surface and reenters the plasma, and C3d, which adheres to the red blood cell surface where it is recognized as C3 in Coombs' test but not as C3 by the mononuclear phagocyte system. The presence of C3d on the red blood cell surface decreases the ability of IgM anti-I to begin anew the complement sequence and thereby reestablish C3b on the red cell surface. Because of this, red blood cells that have survived in the circulation for a period of time have become "protected," while the younger red blood cells are in greater jeopardy.

Therapy. The cutaneous manifestations of this disorder are best treated by maintaining the patient in a warm environment. Because transfusion of normal blood presents to the patient a large number of red blood cells which have not previously been exposed to the cold agglutinin and are therefore not "protected," transfusion may be associated with an acceleration of the hemolytic process. Splenectomy is usually not of value in this disorder. Corticosteroids are of limited value, although patients with the panthermal variety of cold agglutinin disease may respond favorably to this therapy. Chlorambucil and cyclophosphamide are the most commonly employed agents in those patients in whom therapy is indicated. Although some patients have experienced a dramatic improvement, the effectiveness of this therapy is usually marginal.

Cold agglutinin disease tends to be chronic and unremitting. The overall prognosis is dominated by the underlying lymphoproliferative disease, if present. In those patients in whom cold agglutinin disease appears to arise spontaneously, lymphoproliferative disease may become apparent after several years.

PAROXYSMAL COLD HEMOGLOBINURIA (PCH) Now a rare disorder, PCH was more frequent at a time when tertiary syphilis was more prevalent. It results from the formation of the Donath-Landsteiner antibody, an IgG antibody which is directed against the P antigen complex and which can induce complement-mediated lysis. Attacks are precipitated by exposure to cold and are associated with hemoglobinemia and hemoglobinuria, chills and fever, back, leg, and abdominal pain, headache, and malaise. Recovery from the acute episode is prompt, and between episodes patients are asymptomatic. When this syndrome accompanies acute viral infections (e.g., measles and mumps), it is self-limited. When secondary to syphilis, it responds favorably to specific therapy for this disorder. No specific therapy exists for idiopathic cases. Despite the severity of individual episodes, the natural history of this disease extends over many years.

TRAUMA IN THE CIRCULATION Mechanical trauma can cause hemolysis in three ways: (1) when red blood cells flow through small vessels over the surface of bony prominences and are subject to external impact during various physical activities; (2) when they flow across a pressure gradient created by an abnormal heart valve or valve prosthesis and are disrupted by a shear stress; and (3) when the deposition of fibrin in the microvasculature exposes them to a physical impediment that fragments them (Table 287-4).

External impact Hemoglobinemia and hemoglobinuria have been observed in individuals who have undergone a prolonged march or a prolonged jog, most typically on a hard surface and while wearing thin-soled shoes. The role of direct external trauma in this process has been demonstrated by the fact that hemolysis can be prevented by the insertion of a soft inner sole in the runner's shoes. Similar types of hemolysis have been described following karate and the playing of bongo drums. No abnormality of red blood cell morphology has been demonstrated, even during the acute episode, and no underlying red blood cell abnormality has been uncovered. A large percentage of individuals will develop hemoglobinemia and hemoglobinuria when exposed to the conditions described above. As a result of muscle damage that occurs during some of these activities, myoglobinuria commonly occurs, but renal function is preserved. No specific therapy is required.

Cardiac hemolysis Hemolysis associated with fragmented red blood cells (Fig. A5-7) occurs in approximately 10 percent of patients with artificial aortic valve prostheses. This incidence is somewhat greater with valves having stellite rather than silastic occluders, greater with small valves as compared with larger valves, and greater when valves are cloth-covered or when there is a paravalvular leak with increased flow across the prosthesis. Traumatic hemolysis is much less common in recipients of porcine valves. Severe hemolysis may occur after repair of ostium primum or endocardial cushion defects with a prosthetic patch. Mitral valve prostheses have also been associated with hemolysis, but since the pressure gradient across these is lower than across aortic prostheses, the incidence is lower. A moderately shortened red blood cell survival with little or no anemia occurs in some patients with severe calcific aortic stenosis. Indeed, almost any intracardiac lesion which alters hemodynamics may lead to some shortening of red blood cell survival. In addition, traumatic hemolysis has been observed in patients who have undergone aortofemoral bypass.

CLINICAL MANIFESTATIONS In severe cases hemoglobin levels fall to 5.0 to 7.0 g/dL with reticulocytosis, fragmented red blood cells in the peripheral blood, depressed haptoglobin, elevated serum lactic dehydrogenase, and hemoglobinemia and hemoglobinuria. Iron loss (as hemoglobin or hemosiderin) in the urine may lead to iron deficiency. Direct Coombs test may rarely become positive.

PATHOGENESIS A number of factors combine to cause the fragmentation and destruction of red blood cells in this disorder. Direct mechanical trauma of red blood cells at the time of seating of the occluder of the prosthetic valve, the deposition of fibrin across disrupted attachment points, but probably most important, the shear stress resulting from turbulent blood flow may all result in the fragmentation of red blood cells. The last explains the higher incidence of hemolysis in patients who have a paravalvular leak and therefore greater velocity of blood flow across the aortic orifice during systole.

THERAPY AND PROGNOSIS Iron deficiency should be corrected by the administration of oral iron. The elevated hemoglobin which results may permit a decrease in the cardiac output and a slowing of the hemolytic rate. Limitation in physical activity also lessens the hemolytic rate. When these measures fail, any paravalvular leak must be repaired or the prosthetic valve replaced.

Deposition of fibrin in the microvasculature Fibrin becomes deposited in the microvasculature where it traps platelets and fragments red blood cells, under three general conditions: (1) abnormalities of the vessel wall in recognized disorders, such as malignant hypertension, eclampsia, rejection of a renal allograft, disseminated cancer, and hemangiomas; (2) two potentially fatal syndromes of unknown etiology, thrombotic thrombocytopenic purpura and the hemolytic uremic syndrome; and (3) disseminated intravascular coagulation.

ABNORMALITIES OF THE VESSEL WALL The degree of hemolysis induced by this family of disorders is usually quite mild, although the number of fragments in the peripheral blood may be striking. In occasional patients, thrombocytopenia may be severe. In each case, therapy is best directed at the primary disease. Thus, reversal of renal graft rejection, treatment of malignant hypertension and eclampsia, control of cancer, etc., lead to a cessation of the hemolytic process. The relative importance of the primary vascular abnormality and of the deposition of fibrin in causing hemolysis is unclear.

Thrombotic thrombocytopenic purpura (TTP) This disease of unknown etiology affects individuals of all ages but primarily young adults, more often women.

CLINICAL MANIFESTATIONS Hemolysis is a striking feature of this disease. Anemia occurs in association with fragmented red blood cells, nucleated red cells in the peripheral blood, an elevated reticulocyte count, and thrombocytopenia of varying degree. Platelet counts range from 5000 to 100,000 per cubic millimeter. Jaundice is common, and petechiae may be present, although usually to a less striking degree than in idiopathic thrombocytopenic purpura (ITP). Tests of coagulation, such as the prothrombin time, partial thromboplastin time, fibrinogen concentration, and the level of fibrinogen split products, are usually normal or only mildly abnormal. If the coagulation tests indicate disseminated intravascular coagulation, the diagnosis of TTP is doubtful. Erythroid hyperplasia and an increased number of megakaryocytes are present in the bone marrow. The life span of platelets is decreased to hours, and no site of organ localization of destroyed platelets is observed. A positive antinuclear antibody (ANA) is obtained in approximately 20 percent of patients. Some patients experience significant bleeding of uterine, gastrointestinal, or other origin, but severe bleeding is not common. Fever is present in almost all patients, and many experience nonspecific constitutional symptoms such as nausea, abdominal pain, and arthralgias. The spleen and liver may be palpable.

The course of TTP spans days to weeks in most patients, but occasionally continues for months. As the disease progresses, the brain and kidneys become progressively involved, and their dysfunction is the ultimate cause of death in the majority of patients. Proteinuria and a moderate elevation of blood urea nitrogen may be found on initial presentation, and there is a continued rise in blood urea nitrogen and a fall in urine output as the disease progresses. Neurologic symptoms evolve in more than 90 percent of patients

TABLE 287-4 Disturbances of the formed elements of blood secondary to intravascular trauma

Etiology	Fragments	Hemolysis	Thrombocytopenia
Impact: march hemoglobinuria, etc.	0	+	0
Cardiac (turbulence):			
Aortic valve prosthesis	+ + + +	+ + + +	0
Ostium primum repair	+ + + +	+ + + +	0
Mitral valve prosthesis	+ +	+ +	0
Calcific aortic stenoses	+	±	0
Vessel disease: Malignant hypertension, Eclampsia, Renal graft rejection, Hemangiomas, Immune disease (scleroderma)	+ + +	+	+
Thrombotic thrombocytopenic purpura	+ + + +	+ + + +	+ + + +
Hemolytic uremic syndrome	+ + + +	+ + + +	+ + + +
Disseminated intravascular coagulation	+ +	±	+ + + +

whose disease terminates in death. Initially, there may be changes in mental status such as confusion, delirium, or altered states of consciousness. Focal findings include seizures, hemiparesis, aphasia, and visual field defects. These neurologic symptoms may fluctuate and terminate in coma. Involvement of myocardial blood vessels may be a cause of sudden death in some patients.

PATHOGENESIS The etiology of TTP is unknown. Arterioles are filled with hyalin material, presumably fibrin and platelets, and similar material may be seen beneath the endothelium of otherwise uninvolved vessels. Immunofluorescence studies have shown the presence of immunoglobulin and complement in arterioles. Microaneurysms of arterioles are often present. Controversy exists concerning the specificity of these changes, some authorities noting them in the hemolytic uremic syndrome and in disseminated intravascular coagulation. An association with systemic lupus erythematosus (SLE), scleroderma, and Sjögren's syndrome suggests an immunologic etiology.

DIAGNOSIS The combination of hemolytic anemia with fragmented and nucleated red blood cells, thrombocytopenia, fever, neurologic disorders, and renal dysfunction is virtually pathognomonic of TTP. The diagnosis is further supported by the finding of normal coagulation tests, although occasional patients have an isolated abnormality of coagulation. Although they are not usually required for diagnosis, biopsies of skin and muscle, gingiva, lymph node, or bone marrow will frequently reveal the pathologic abnormalities described above. TTP should be considered in every patient in whom the diagnosis of ITP or Evans' syndrome (ITP plus immunohemolytic anemia) is made. The finding of fragmented red blood cells in the peripheral blood is particularly helpful in this regard. Because the clinical course can fluctuate widely, therapy is difficult to evaluate.

THERAPY AND PROGNOSIS Until recently, this disease was almost universally fatal. A large number of therapeutic modalities have been attempted with variable success. These include corticosteroids, plasma exchange, splenectomy, and antiplatelet drugs. Patients are initially treated with high doses of corticosteroids (100 to 1000 mg prednisone per day). However, additional therapy is indicated once the diagnosis has been established. The most consistent improvement (60 to 75 percent) has been noted with exchange transfusion or plasmapheresis. In most patients plasmapheresis is as effective as exchange transfusion. In others the response may depend upon the infusion of plasma. Splenectomy is also effective, but with a lower frequency of response and with additional risk in these critically ill patients. The benefit of antiplatelet drugs (dipyridamole, sulfinpyrazone, dextran, aspirin) is unclear, but they are commonly used together with the therapeutic measures described above. Aspirin may increase the risk of bleeding and should be employed with caution. Vincristine may be effective in otherwise refractory patients. In addition, rare responses to heparin infusion have been reported. Because of the ever-present risk of sudden death, therapy should be instituted promptly. Even deep coma is not a contraindication to therapy since full neurologic recovery is the rule in patients responding to therapy. If treatment is instituted early in the disease, remission occurs in approximately two-thirds of patients. Relapses have been noted in approximately 10 percent of patients but are usually responsive to therapeutic intervention.

Hemolytic uremic syndrome The hemolytic uremic syndrome is a disorder usually encountered in young children with laboratory features similar to those of TTP. Often the patient has a prodrome of a viral-like illness. Less commonly, the disorder appears to be familial. Patients present with acute hemolytic anemia, thrombocytopenic purpura, and acute oliguric renal failure. Most patients have either hemoglobinuria or anuria. Unlike TTP, neurologic manifestations are uncommon. The peripheral blood findings, coagulation tests, and pathologic changes on biopsy specimens are usually indistinguishable from those of TTP. Patients are treated with dialysis and transfusions. The efficacy of corticosteroids, dextran, and heparin is uncertain. The mortality in children ranges from 5 to 20 percent, but is considerably higher in adults. A disorder resembling the hemolytic-uremic syndrome has recently been described in adults treated with the antineoplastic drug mitomycin C, usually in combination with other drugs.

Disseminated intravascular coagulation (DIC) Red blood cell fragmentation in the microvasculature (microangiopathic hemolytic anemia) is seen in about one-third of patients with DIC (Chap. 281). The degree of hemolysis is much less in DIC than in either TTP or the hemolytic uremic syndrome, and anemia with reticulocytosis and nucleated red blood cells is distinctly rare.

DIRECT TOXIC EFFECTS A variety of infections may be associated with severe hemolysis. The microorganisms in bartonellosis (Chap. 116) and malaria (Chap. 154) directly parasitize red blood cells. Babesiosis (Chap. 159) also may cause a mild to moderate hemolytic anemia by direct parasitization of red blood cells.

Other infectious organisms exert their damaging effects on red blood cells indirectly. The most striking is that resulting from septicemia with *Clostridium welchii* (Chap. 101). The phospholipase produced by this organism is capable of cleaving the phosphoryl bond of lecithin thereby lysing human red blood cells. A mild, transient hemolysis frequently accompanies bacteremia with diverse organisms such as pneumococci, staphylococci, and *Escherichia coli.*

Hemolysis may result from the direct action of snake and spider venoms on the red blood cell. Although cobra venom is directly lytic in vitro, the clinical disease induced by the bite of the cobra is one of moderate hemolysis associated with spherocytosis. Spider bites are known to induce acute intravascular hemolysis associated with spherocytosis. It is thought that the brown recluse spider which inhabits the central and southern portions of the United States and portions of South America is responsible. The hemolytic disease continues for several days up to 1 week.

Copper has a direct hemolytic effect on red blood cells. Hemolysis has been observed following exposure of individuals to copper salts (such as during hemodialysis). In addition, the transient episodes of hemolysis observed in patients with Wilson's disease are probably due to copper toxicity.

The red blood cell membrane is unstable at temperatures above 49°C due to denaturation of the cytoskeletal protein, spectrin. When studied in vitro, the red blood cell undergoes a process of budding, cleavage, and resealing above this temperature. The same process is observed in individuals who have suffered extensive burns. These patients have prominent spherocytosis as well as hemoglobinemia and sometimes hemoglobinuria.

MEMBRANE ABNORMALITIES

ACQUIRED DISORDERS OF THE MEMBRANE There are two well-defined acquired disorders of the red blood cell membrane: spur cell anemia and paroxysmal nocturnal hemoglobinuria (PNH).

Spur cell anemia Hemolytic anemia with bizarre-shaped red blood cells occurs in some patients with severe hepatocellular disease. Most patients with spur cell anemia have advanced Laennec's cirrhosis. This hemolytic disorder is observed in approximately 5 percent of patients with manifestations of severe cirrhosis, such as ascites, jaundice, and hepatic encephalopathy. Spur cell anemia has also been reported in neonatal hepatitis.

CLINICAL MANIFESTATIONS Anemia is moderate to severe, with hematocrit levels ranging from 16 to 30 percent. Thus, the anemia is more severe than is observed in otherwise uncomplicated cirrhosis, in which hematocrit levels are rarely below 28 percent, unless there is accompanying folic acid deficiency, blood loss, iron deficiency, etc. (Chap. 286). Splenomegaly is a constant feature, and the spleen is generally more prominent than in patients who have cirrhosis but who do not have spur cell anemia. Jaundice is also a constant feature, and hepatic encephalopathy is common. Other tests of liver function are similar to values obtained in most patients with severe cirrhosis, although there is a tendency to longer prothrombin times. Chromium half-survival times of red blood cells are decreased to as short as 6 days (normal being 26 to 32 days), and red cell destruction is localized to the spleen. Normal transfused red blood cells have a survival similar to that of the patient's own red blood cells. Red blood cells are irregularly shaped with multiple spicules, and a small number of bizarre-shaped fragments are commonly seen on peripheral blood smears (see Fig. A5-8). Reticulocytes range from 5 to 15 percent.

PATHOGENESIS The surface membrane of spur cells contains 50 to 70 percent excess cholesterol, but its total phospholipid content is normal. In this way, spur cells are distinct from the more usual target red blood cells in liver disease, which possess an excess of both cholesterol and phospholipid. Cholesterol out of proportion of phospholipid decreases the fluidity of the spur cell membrane, and cell deformability is also decreased. Normal red blood cells acquire the spur abnormality when incubated in serum from affected patients. This results from the presence in serum of an abnormal low-density lipoprotein with an increased mole ratio of free (unesterified) cholesterol to phospholipid. Thus, red blood cells in spur cell anemia may be considered to be "innocent bystanders." These rigid, cholesterol-laden red blood cells are detected by the filtering system of the spleen, aided by congestive splenomegaly in cirrhosis. In contrast to circulating spur cells, normal red blood cells which have acquired cholesterol in vitro have an increased surface area and a decreased osmotic fragility, and they have a regular pattern of spicule deformity. This is also true in vivo for normal red blood cells during their initial 24 h in the circulation. However, during continued circulation in vivo in the presence of the spleen, cholesterol-rich spur cells lose surface area and transform to the irregular pattern of spiculation associated with acanthocytes (see "Red Blood Cell Morphology" above). This process of membrane "conditioning" by the spleen continues, and the cell is destroyed in the spleen.

DIAGNOSIS Increasing anemia in a patient with chronic cirrhosis most commonly results from blood loss, folic acid deficiency, or iron deficiency. The hemolytic rate may increase transiently during periods of acute fatty liver. The combination of an elevated reticulocyte count and elevated bilirubin in the presence of the characteristic morphologic abnormality on peripheral blood smear is diagnostic. Red blood cells of similar morphologic appearance are seen in patients with abetalipoproteinemia. However, these individuals have a minimal amount of hemolysis.

Spur cells and acanthocytes must be distinguished from regularly scalloped, crenated red blood cells (echinocytes). These are a frequent artifact on blood smears, and they are present in some patients with uremia ("burr cells") (Fig. A5-9). Small, dense crenated spheres (spheroechinocytes) are sometimes seen in congenital nonspherocytic hemolytic anemia due to enzyme deficiencies in the Embden-Meyerhof pathway.

TREATMENT Since normal red blood cells acquire the spur abnormality when transfused into patients with this form of anemia, transfusion therapy is of limited benefit. Attempts to influence red blood cell cholesterol by the use of various lipid-lowering agents have thus far been unsuccessful. Splenectomy has been reported to prevent both the conditioning of red blood cells in the spleen and their premature destruction. However, splenectomy carries a high risk in patients with severe liver disease complicated by portal hypertension and coagulation defects, and it must be reserved for selected patients in whom hemolysis is a major clinical problem and who appear to be relatively good surgical risks.

PROGNOSIS In most patients spur cell anemia occurs during the late stages of cirrhosis, and more than 90 percent of patients succumb to their underlying liver disease within 1 year of the diagnosis of spur cell anemia.

Paroxysmal nocturnal hemoglobinuria (PNH) This condition is distinctive among hemolytic disorders in humans because it is an intracorpuscular defect acquired at the stem cell level. It occurs primarily in young adults.

CLINICAL MANIFESTATIONS Anemia is of exceedingly variable degree with hematocrit values of 20 percent and lower in occasional patients and normal values in others. Mild granulocytopenia and thrombocytopenia are commonly present. Although regarded as a classic feature of this disease, gross hemoglobinuria is present only intermittently in most patients, and never occurs in some. Hemosiderinuria is usually present. Other features of diagnostic significance are a low leukocyte alkaline phosphatase and a low red blood cell acetylcholinesterase. Red blood cells are normochromic and normocytic unless iron deficiency has occurred from the chronic loss of iron in the urine. The diagnosis is established by a positive acid hemolysis test or sucrose lysis test, both of which demonstrate the enhanced sensitivity of PNH red blood cells to complement (see below). Venous thromboses are a common complication of this disorder, and they have been reported in peripheral veins as well as in mesenteric, hepatic, portal, and cerebral veins. Thromboses are a common cause of death in patients severely affected with PNH. A second manifestation, possibly related to thromboses in small veins, is the occurrence of back and abdominal pain similar in character to that which occurs in sickle cell anemia. Headache has also been reported. Since the widespread use of the sucrose lysis test, many patients have been discovered with mild, chronic disease.

PATHOGENESIS The underlying abnormality which affects red blood cells, granulocytes, and platelets in PNH is an inordinate sensitivity to complement. This may be demonstrated in vitro using a complement-fixing antibody. PNH red blood cells fix more C1 than normal red cells per unit of antibody present, and this C1 promotes more C3 fixation per molecule of C1 than is seen with normal red cells. However, antibody is not necessary for the lysis of red blood cells in PNH. Rather, C3 is readily fixed to the red blood cell surface by means of the alternate (properdin) pathway. Careful analytic procedures have demonstrated two and in some cases three separate populations of red blood cells with varying sensitivities to complement in patients with PNH. The clinical manifestations relate directly to the proportion of the red blood cells produced that are most sensitive to complement. Although platelets share with red blood cells this sensitivity to complement, platelet survival is normal in PNH. However, a functional modification of platelets induced by complement may underlie the thrombotic complications of this disease. The increased sensitivity of red blood cells to complement has been demonstrated to result from the lack of a red cell membrane regulatory protein, decay-accelerating factor (DAF), which is partially responsible for the rapid conversion of C3b to the inactive C3d.

Since it affects granulocytes, platelets, and red blood cells but not lymphocytes, this defect is thought to occur because of an acquired change in the pluripotent stem cell which generates these cells. In this respect it is similar to both acute myelogenous leukemia and the myeloproliferative syndromes, disorders which appear to affect the stem cells responsible for platelet, granulocyte, and red blood cell production. Both acute myelogenous leukemia and PNH may be secondary manifestations of a primary bone marrow injury that is manifested initially as aplastic anemia. Moreover, a number of patients with PNH have subsequently developed acute myelogenous leukemia. The red blood cell abnormality characteristic of PNH (complement sensitivity) occurs to a mild degree in some patients with aplastic anemia and in some with myelofibrosis, further linking this series of bone marrow disorders. The precise mechanism has not been identified. It appears likely that PNH results from a somatic mutation in the marrow stem cell pool. The phenotypic representation of this presumed mutation is not known.

DIAGNOSIS As indicated above, PNH is commonly undiagnosed for a period of months to years. The classic manifestation of gross hemoglobinuria may be present only intermittently, and an awareness of its presence may be obtained only by repeated questioning of the patient. In some patients, a chronic hemolytic process occurs without gross hemoglobinuria. Therefore, diagnoses such as refractory anemia, hemolytic anemia of unknown etiology, and pancytopenia are common in patients subsequently proven to have PNH. A decreased leukocyte alkaline phosphatase is a clue to the diagnosis, and the presence of hemosiderin in the urine sediment is strongly suggestive. Hemosiderinuria may occur with intravascular hemolysis of any etiology. However, only a few disorders in humans result in intravascular hemolysis. These are PNH, paroxysmal cold hemoglobinuria, hemolytic transfusion reaction, traumatic hemolysis, and hemolysis due to lysins (snake venom, *C. welchii* bacteremia) or to extensive acute burns. The acid hemolysis test is also positive in the rare congenital disorder hereditary erythrocytic multinuclearity with positive acidified-serum test (HEMPAS). In this latter disorder, complement sensitivity results from an inordinate fixation of C4 molecules per molecule of C1. Since this sensitivity exists in the classic (antibody-mediated) pathway but not in the alternate (properdin) pathway, spontaneous fixation of complement with lysis in vivo is not a feature of the HEMPAS disorder.

It should be noted that chromium survival studies often produce information which is confusing in PNH. This results from the bi- or trimodal population of red blood cells. The cells most sensitive to complement have a very short survival, and they account for a minority of circulating red blood cells, whereas the cells less sensitive to complement have a more normal survival and account for the majority of circulating cells. Thus, the chromium survival is longer than might be anticipated from other measures of hemoglobin turnover.

TREATMENT Transfusion therapy is useful in PNH not only for raising the hemoglobin level but also for suppressing the marrow production of red blood cells during episodes of sustained hemoglobinuria or of sustained painful crisis. The transfusion of blood prior to surgery may reduce the incidence of postoperative thrombotic complications. For reasons that are still unclear, whole blood transfusions frequently cause an exacerbation of the hemolytic process. This can be prevented by using washed red blood cells rather than whole blood.

Therapy with androgens frequently results in a rise of hemoglobin level. Adrenocortical steroids may also be effective in reducing the rate of hemolysis.

Because of iron loss in the urine, iron deficiency is common. An exacerbation of hemolysis often follows the administration of iron because of the formation of a large number of young red blood cells, many of which are sensitive to complement. This may be minimized by suppressing the bone marrow with transfusions.

Splenectomy has been undertaken in some patients with the hope of decreasing the hemolytic rate and the transfusion requirement. However, because of the limited therapeutic benefit and the high risk attendant upon surgery in patients with PNH, splenectomy cannot be recommended.

Anticoagulation with coumarin-type drugs may have some benefit in preventing thromboses, particularly in the postsurgical patient. On the other hand, therapy with heparin has been noted to cause an increased amount of hemolysis in some patients with PNH, and caution must be exercised when using this drug.

PROGNOSIS Most patients with classic PNH have a life expectancy of less than 10 years, although some survive for much longer. A series of 17 patients surviving more than 20 years has been compiled by questioning hematologists nationally. In more than one-third of these patients, there had been an amelioration of disease symptoms, and in two patients PNH was totally quiescent. The major morbidity relates to venous thromboses. Despite the overwhelming degree of iron deposition in the kidney, death from renal failure is rare. The prognosis is uncertain in patients in whom the manifestations of PNH are more subtle and in whom the diagnosis was made because of the widespread use of the sucrose lysis test. Some patients may lead a normal life.

FIGURE 287-1 *Osmotic fragility of red blood cells in hereditary spherocytosis. When the spleen is present, a small subpopulation of cells which are "conditioned" in the spleen form the fragile "tail" of the osmotic fragility curve. After splenectomy a single population exists which is more osmotically fragile than normal.*

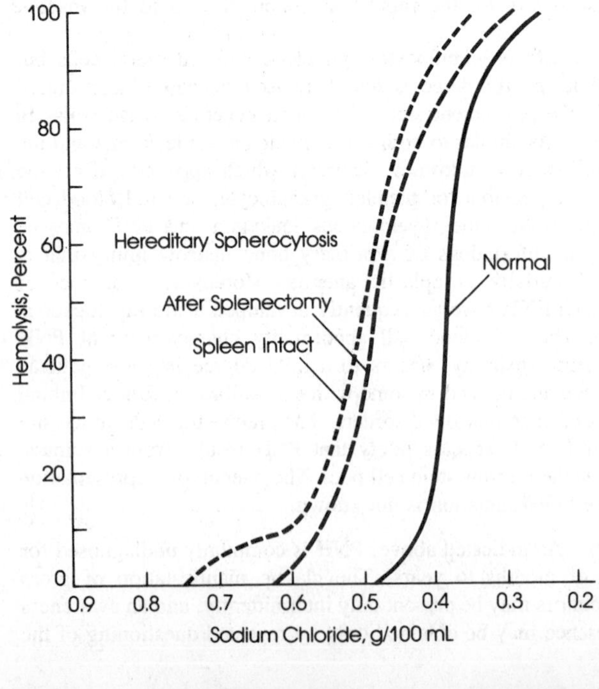

CONGENITAL ABNORMALITIES OF THE RED CELL MEMBRANE

There are four types of inherited abnormalities of the red cell membrane: hereditary spherocytosis, hereditary elliptocytosis, hereditary pyropoikilocytosis, and hereditary stomatocytosis. Each syndrome may represent a group of disorders with a differing structural basis. The molecular pathogenesis of these disorders has not been completely defined.

Hereditary spherocytosis This is a disease of autosomal dominant inheritance in which intrinsically abnormal red blood cells are destroyed in the presence of an otherwise normal spleen. Its incidence is approximately 1:4500. In 20 percent of patients the absence of hematologic abnormalities in family members suggests that a spontaneous mutation has occurred. The disorder is sometimes clinically apparent in early infancy, but often escapes detection until adult life.

CLINICAL MANIFESTATIONS The major clinical features of hereditary spherocytosis are anemia, splenomegaly, and jaundice. The prominence of the latter finding accounts for its prior designation "congenital hemolytic jaundice" and is due to an increased concentration of unconjugated (indirect-reacting) bilirubin in plasma. Jaundice may be intermittent and tends to be less pronounced in early childhood. Because of the increased bile pigment production, gallstones of pigment type are common, even in childhood. Compensatory normoblastic hyperplasia of the bone marrow occurs with the extension of red marrow into the midshafts of long bones and occasionally with extramedullary erythropoiesis, at times leading to the formation of paravertebral masses visible on chest x-ray. Because the bone marrow's capacity to increase erythropoiesis by six- to tenfold exceeds the usual rate of hemolysis in this disease, anemia is usually mild or moderate and may even be absent in an otherwise healthy individual. Compensation may be temporarily interrupted by episodes of erythroid hypoplasia precipitated by infections, often of a minor nature. Splenomegaly is a constant feature of hereditary spherocytosis. The hemolytic rate may increase transiently during systemic infections which induce further splenic enlargement. Chronic leg ulcers, similar to those observed in sickle cell anemia, occasionally occur.

The characteristic erythrocyte abnormality is the spherocyte (Fig. A5-10). The mean corpuscular volume (MCV) is usually normal or slightly decreased, and the mean corpuscular hemoglobin concentration (MCHC) is increased to 35 to 38 g/dL. Spheroidicity may be quantitatively assessed in terms of osmotic fragility (Fig. 287-1). Because spherocytes have a decreased surface area per unit volume, they lyse more readily when exposed to solutions of low salt concentration. On microscopic examination spherocytes are usually detected even when present in very small numbers. However, they will ordinarily not influence the osmotic fragility test unless they constitute more than 1 or 2 percent of the total cell population. A prominent increase in the osmotic fragility of red blood cells following sterile incubation of whole blood for 24 h at 37°C is also characteristic of hereditary spherocytosis. The autohemolysis test is an extension of this latter procedure and measures the amount of spontaneous hemolysis occurring after 48 h of sterile incubation. In hereditary spherocytosis about 10 to 50 percent of the red blood cells are lysed (versus less than 4 percent of normal red blood cells). Autohemolysis of these red blood cells is largely prevented by the addition of glucose prior to incubation.

PATHOGENESIS Although not well understood, the molecular abnormality in hereditary spherocytosis involves the proteins of the cytoskeleton. Nearly all patients have a significant deficiency of spectrin (see Fig. 283-6) which correlates with the severity of the anemia. The spheroidal contour and rigid structure of the red blood cells impede their passage through the spleen. There, the red blood cells are exposed to an environment in which their increased metabolic rate cannot be sustained. The first injury imposed upon them by the spleen is a further loss of surface membrane "conditioning," which produces a subpopulation of hyperspheroidal red blood cells in the peripheral blood. These are subsequently destroyed in the spleen. The intracorpuscular nature of the red blood cell defect in hereditary spherocytosis is demonstrated by a diminished life span of the patient's red cells in normal subjects when the spleen is present and a normal survival of normal cells transfused into patients with hereditary spherocytosis.

DIAGNOSIS Hereditary spherocytosis must be distinguished from the spherocytic hemolytic anemias associated with red blood cell antibodies. The family history is helpful, when present. The diagnosis of immune spherocytosis is usually readily established by a positive direct Coombs test. Spherocytes, often in considerable numbers, are seen in association with hemolysis induced by splenomegaly in patients with cirrhosis or chronic infections, and a few spherocytes are seen in the course of a wide variety of hemolytic disorders, particularly glucose 6-phosphate dehydrogenase deficiency.

TREATMENT AND PROGNOSIS Splenectomy reliably corrects the anemia, although the red blood cell defect persists. The operative risk is low. Red blood cell survival after splenectomy is normal or nearly so. Rare relapses have been reported and are probably attributable to postoperative growth of splenic autotransplants or to hyperplasia of secondary spleens which were overlooked at operation. Because of the potential for gallstones and for episodes of bone marrow hypoplasia or hemolytic crises, splenectomy should be performed in most individuals with hereditary spherocytosis, even those with mild anemia. Splenectomy in children should be postponed until the age of 4 years, if possible, although it may be performed at any age. Beyond age 3, severe infections following splenectomy in hereditary spherocytosis are rare. Nonetheless, polyvalent pneumococcal vaccine should be administered to all patients who are to undergo splenectomy. Because of the increased requirement for folic acid in patients with hemolysis, they sometimes become deficient in this vitamin. Therapy with folic acid may result in an increased hemoglobin level.

Hereditary elliptocytosis and hereditary pyropoikilocytosis Red blood cells of oval or elliptic shape are normally found in birds, reptiles, camels, and llamas; however, they occur in appreciable numbers in humans only in *hereditary elliptocytosis,* a disorder which is transmitted as an autosomal dominant and affects 1 per 4000 to 5000 of the population, a frequency similar to that of hereditary spherocytosis. It is also referred to as *hereditary ovalocytosis*. Less commonly, homozygotes have been encountered with an absence of a red cell membrane protein (band 4.1) that is important in stabilizing the interaction of spectrin and actin in the cytoskeleton (see Fig. 283-6).

The great majority of patients manifest only mild hemolysis, with hemoglobin levels above 12 g/dL, reticulocytes less than 4 percent, depressed haptoglobin levels, and red blood cell survivals within or just under the normal range. In 10 to 15 percent of patients the rate of hemolysis is substantially increased with chromium half-survival times of red blood cells as short as 5 days and reticulocytes ranging to 20 percent. Hemoglobin levels rarely fall below 9 to 10 g/dL. Red blood cell destruction occurs predominantly in the spleen, which is enlarged in patients with overt hemolysis, and hemolysis is corrected by splenectomy.

In both the anemic and nonanemic varieties of this disorder the red blood cells are normochromic and normocytic. At least 25 percent and, more commonly, greater than 75 percent of red blood cells are elliptic, with an axial ratio (width/length) of less than 0.78. Patients with hemolysis frequently have microovalocytes, bizarre-shaped red blood cells, and red cell fragments, and these increase in number following splenectomy. The degree of hemolysis does not correlate with the percentage of elliptocytes. Osmotic fragility is usually normal but may be increased in patients with overt hemolysis. The pathogenesis of the red blood cell defect probably involves abnormalities of assembly of spectrin subunits.

Hereditary pyropoikilocytosis (HPP) is thought to be related to hereditary elliptocytosis, since both have been reported in the same family. HPP is a rare disorder characterized by bizarre-shaped, microcytic red cells which undergo disruption at temperatures of 44 to 45°C (in contrast to the normal thermal instability at 49°C). This results from an abnormality of spectrin structure. Hemolysis, which is usually severe, is recognized in childhood and is partially responsive to splenectomy.

Hereditary stomatocytosis Stomatocytes are red blood cells having a slit-like central zone of pallor on dried smears. The syndrome of hereditary hemolytic anemia and stomatocytic red blood cells is inherited in an autosomal dominant pattern. It may represent a number of discrete entities. Two major red blood cell defects have been delineated in this syndrome. First, the red blood cells have an increased permeability to sodium and potassium, which is compensated for by an increased active transport of these cations. Second, red cells have an increased surface area associated with an increase in membrane lipid content, particularly phosphatidylcholine. In some patients, the red blood cell is swollen with an excess of ions and water and a decreased mean corpuscular hemoglobin concentration (overhydrated stomatocytes, "hydrocytosis"); in other patients the red cell is shrunken with a decreased ion and water content and an increased mean corpuscular hemoglobin concentration (dehydrated stomatocytes, "desiccytosis"). Those patients in whom the red blood cells are overhydrated have true stomatocytes on dried smears. Dehydrated stomatocytes assume the morphology of target cells on dried smears. In both instances, red blood cells are cup- or bowl-shaped when examined in wet preparation. Osmotic fragility is increased in overhydrated stomatocytes and decreased in underhydrated stomatocytes. Autohemolysis is increased and is corrected by glucose.

Most patients have splenomegaly and mild anemia. Splenectomy decreases but does not totally correct the hemolytic process. Its indications are similar to those for hereditary spherocytosis.

DISORDERS OF THE INTERIOR OF THE RED CELL

RED CELL ENZYME DEFECTS During its maturation, the red blood cell loses its nucleus, ribosomes, and mitochondria and thus its capability for protein synthesis and oxidative phosphorylation. The mature circulating red blood cell has a relatively simple pattern of intermediary metabolism (Fig. 287-2) in keeping with its modest metabolic obligations. As discussed in Chap. 283, some ATP must be generated from the Embden-Meyerhof pathway to drive the cation pump which maintains the ionic milieu within the red blood cell. Smaller amounts of energy are needed for the preservation of hemoglobin iron in the ferrous (Fe^{2+}) state, and perhaps for the renewal of the lipids in the red blood cell membrane. About 10 percent of the glucose consumed by the red blood cell is metabolized via the hexose-monophosphate shunt (Fig. 287-2). This pathway protects both hemoglobin and the membrane from exogenous oxidants including certain drugs.

Studies of red blood cell enzyme defects have provided valuable information on the metabolic control of normal erythrocytes. Figure 287-2 shows a large number of recognized specific enzyme deficiency states affecting the glycolytic pathway or the hexose-monophosphate shunt. Many of these enzyme abnormalities appear to be restricted to red blood cells. The long life span of the red blood cell and its inability to synthesize proteins pose a challenge to the stability of its enzymes. Therefore, a mutation resulting in decreased stability will be expressed more readily in the red blood cell compared with other tissues.

Defects in the Embden-Meyerhof pathway Deficiencies of most of the enzymes of the Embden-Meyerhof (or glycolytic) pathway have been reported. In general, all these enzymopathies have similar pathophysiologic and clinical features. Patients present with a congenital nonspherocytic hemolytic anemia of variable severity. The red blood cells are often relatively deficient in ATP, considering their young age. As a result, there is an increased leak of potassium ion from inside these cells. Abnormalities in red blood cell morphology (see below) indicate that the red cell membrane is secondarily affected by the enzyme defect. These red blood cells are apt to be rigid and thus more readily sequestered by the mononuclear-phagocyte system.

Some of these glycolytic enzyme deficiencies such as pyruvate kinase (PK) deficiency and hexokinase deficiency are localized to the red blood cell. There is no apparent metabolic abnormality in leukocytes or other cells that have been studied. In other disorders, the enzyme deficiency is more widespread. Glucose phosphate isomerase deficiency and phosphoglycerate kinase deficiency also involve leukocytes, although affected individuals have no apparent abnormalities of white blood cell function. Individuals with deficiency of triose phosphate isomerase have decreased levels of enzyme in leukocytes, muscle cells, and central nervous system fluid. Furthermore, they have a progressive neurologic disorder. Some patients with phosphofructokinase deficiency have a myopathy.

Among the reported defects of glycolytic enzymes, about 95 percent are due to PK deficiency and about 4 percent are due to glucose phosphate isomerase deficiency. The remainder shown in Fig. 287-2 are extremely rare. Most have been encountered in isolated families. There is considerable variability in the clinical manifestations

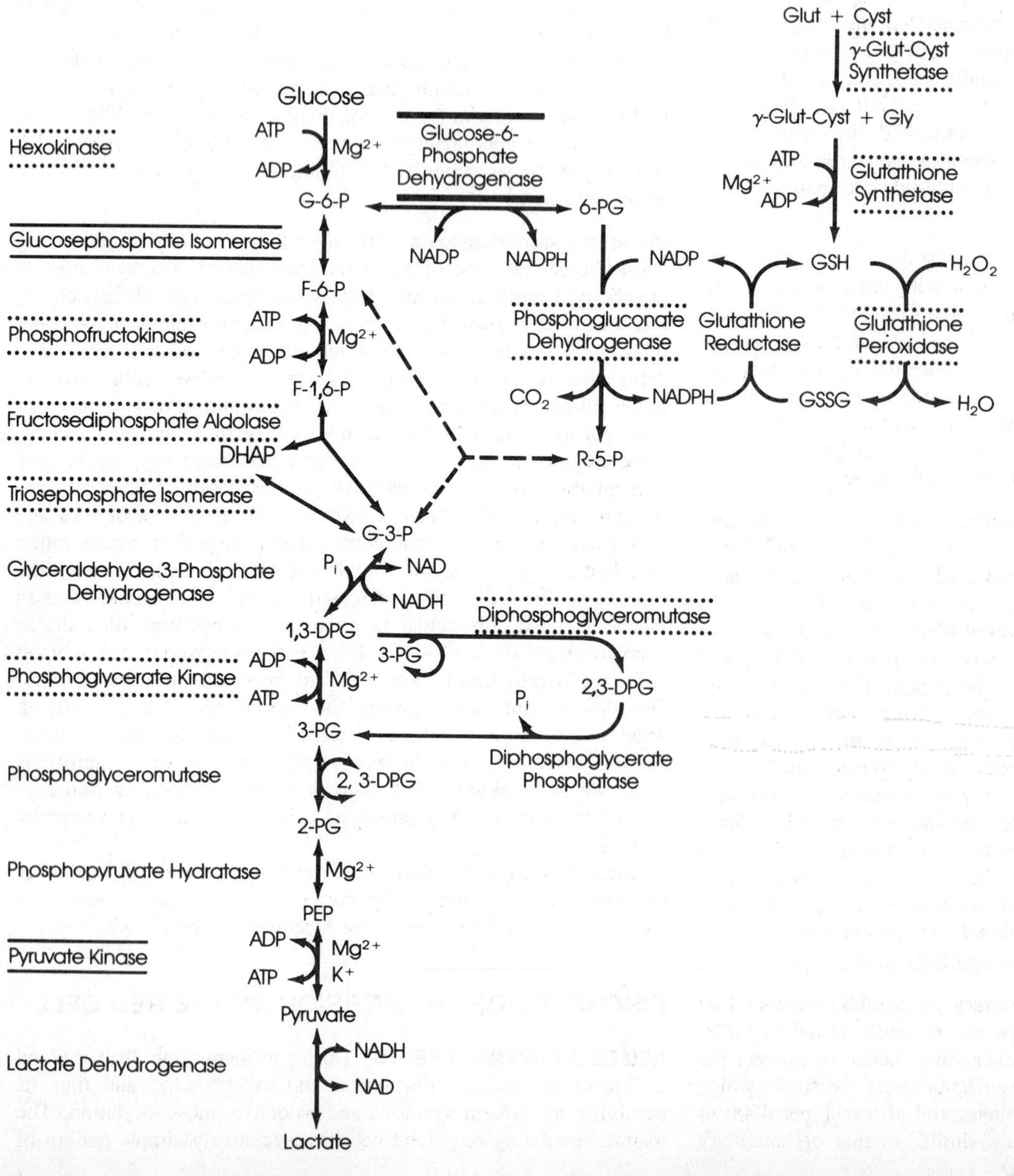

FIGURE 287-2 *Metabolic pathways in the red blood cell. The glycolytic pathway is outlined vertically from glucose to lactate. The pentose phosphate pathway is shown on the right. Known enzyme deficiency states are shown. Bold solid lines denote common states, light solid lines less common ones, and dotted lines rare ones. (From WN Valentine, Semin Hematol 8:309, 1971.)*

and laboratory findings among reported cases of PK deficiency. This is probably due to the fact that a number of different PK variants have been reported. This heterogeneity probably also applies to the other less common glycolytic enzyme defects. Accordingly, the clinical manifestations of these disorders are quite variable.

GENETICS Most of the glycolytic enzyme defects are inherited in an autosomal recessive pattern. Thus, the parents of affected patients are heterozygotes. Heterozygotes generally possess half-normal levels of enzyme activity which are more than adequate for normal metabolic function. Thus, these individuals are entirely asymptomatic. Since the gene frequency for this group of enzymopathies is low, it is not surprising that true homozygotes are often the offspring of a consanguineous mating. Alternatively, affected individuals may be double heterozygotes, inheriting an abnormal allele from each parent. Phosphoglycerate kinase deficiency is inherited as a sex-linked disorder. Affected males have a severe hemolytic anemia while female carriers may have a mild hemolytic process.

CLINICAL MANIFESTATIONS Patients with severe hemolysis usually present during early childhood with anemia, icterus, and splenomegaly. Other stigmata of chronic hemolysis are occasionally seen. Occasionally, siblings are similarly affected.

LABORATORY FINDINGS Patients have a normocytic (or slightly macrocytic) normochromic anemia with reticulocytosis. In those with PK deficiency, bizarre erythrocytes are noted on the peripheral smear with large numbers of spiculated red blood cells. Spherocytes are usually infrequent or absent. Hence, the term *congenital nonspherocytic hemolytic anemia* has been applied to these disorders. Unlike hereditary spherocytosis, the osmotic fragility of freshly drawn blood is usually normal. Incubation brings out an osmotically fragile population of red blood cells.

The diagnosis of this group of anemias depends upon specific enzymatic assays. An abnormality in enzyme kinetics may be demonstrated. In addition, differences in electrophoretic mobility, pH optimum, or heat stability may be noted. This information is useful in documenting heterogeneity among enzyme variants.

TREATMENT Most patients do not require therapy. Those with severe hemolysis should be given a daily supplement of folic acid (1 mg per day). Blood transfusions may be necessary during a hypoplastic crisis. Patients with PK deficiency may be benefited by splenectomy. Because of their enzymatic defect, the younger cells (reticulocytes) depend on mitochondrial respiration rather than glycolysis for maintenance of ATP. However, in the hypoxic environment of the spleen, aerobic metabolism is curtailed and the ATP-depleted cells are destroyed in situ. It is of interest that following splenectomy patients with PK deficiency often have a marked increase in circulating reticulocytes. Patients with deficiency of glucose phosphate isomerase may also be improved by splenectomy. There is not sufficient information to indicate whether this operation would help individuals with other glycolytic enzymopathies.

Defects in the hexose-monophosphate shunt The normal red blood cell is well endowed to protect itself against oxidant stress. Upon exposure to an offending drug or toxin, the amount of glucose that is metabolized via the hexose-monophosphate shunt is increased severalfold. In this way reduced glutathione is regenerated, protecting the sulfhydryl groups of hemoglobin and the red blood cell membrane from oxidation. Individuals with an inherited defect in the hexose-monophosphate shunt are unable to maintain an adequate level of reduced glutathione in their red blood cells. As a result, hemoglobin sulfhydryl groups become oxidized, and the hemoglobin tends to precipitate within the red blood cell forming Heinz bodies.

Among the congenital shunt defects, by far the most common is *G6PD deficiency*. It affects millions of people throughout the world. Like the glycolytic enzymopathies, there is considerable genetic heterogeneity among affected individuals. Indeed, over 250 variants of G6PD have been described. In contrast to the hemoglobin variants (Chap. 288) abnormalities in primary structure have been established in only a few of the G6PD variants. The remainder are presumed to have abnormal structure because of differences in electrophoretic mobility, enzyme kinetics, pH optimum, and heat stability. Like many of the hemoglobin variants, some G6PD mutants were discovered by chance and are not associated with any significant functional abnormalities. The normal or ''wild'' form of G6PD is designated by type B. About 20 percent of blacks have a G6PD (designated A+) which differs electrophoretically but is functionally normal. Among the clinically significant G6PD variants, the most common is the so-called A− type encountered primarily in blacks who originated from central Africa. The A− G6PD has the same electrophoretic mobility as the A+ type, but it is unstable and has abnormal kinetic properties. Like the HbS gene, the A− type of G6PD may confer protection against malaria. This variant is found in about 15 percent of black males in the United States. A second relatively common G6PD variant is encountered among peoples of the eastern Mediterranean area, particularly Sephardic Jews. A third relatively common variant occurs in the Chinese.

The G6PD gene is located on the X chromosome. Thus the deficiency state is a sex-linked trait. Affected males (hemizygotes) inherit the abnormal gene from their mothers who are usually carriers (heterozygotes). Because of inactivation of one of the two X chromosomes (Lyon hypothesis, see Chap. 57), the heterozygote has two populations of red blood cells: normal and deficient in G6PD. Most female carriers are asymptomatic. Those who happen to have a high proportion of deficient cells resemble the male hemizygotes.

G6PD activity normally declines about 50 percent during the 120-day life span of the red blood cell. This decay is moderately accelerated in A− red blood cells and markedly so in red blood cells containing the Mediterranean variant. Individuals with the A− variant may have a slightly shortened red blood cell survival, but they are not anemic. Clinical problems arise only when the affected individual is subjected to some type of environmental stress. Most often, hemolytic episodes are triggered by viral and bacterial infections. The mechanism for this is unknown. Drugs or toxins which pose an oxidant threat to the red blood cell by serving as oxidation-reduction catalysts also cause hemolysis in individuals deficient in G6PD (see Table 287-5). Of these, sulfa drugs, antimalarials, and nitrofurantoin are most commonly incriminated. Although aspirin is frequently mentioned as a likely offender, it has no deleterious effect in A− individuals. Occasionally, accidental ingestion of toxic compounds such as naphthalene (found in moth balls) can cause severe hemolysis. Finally, metabolic acidosis can precipitate an episode of hemolysis in subjects deficient in G6PD.

CLINICAL AND LABORATORY FEATURES The patient may experience an acute hemolytic crisis within hours of exposure to the oxidant stress. In severe cases, hemoglobinuria and peripheral vascular collapse can develop. Since only the older population of red blood cells is rapidly destroyed, the hemolytic crisis is usually self-limited, even if the exposure to the oxidant continues. Among black males with the A− variant, the red cell mass decreases by a maximum of 25 to 30 percent. During the period of acute hemolysis, a rapid drop in hematocrit is accompanied by a rise in plasma hemoglobin and unconjugated bilirubin and a decrease in plasma haptoglobin. The oxidation of hemoglobin leads to the formation of Heinz bodies visualized by means of a supravital stain such as crystal violet. However, Heinz bodies are usually not seen after the first day or so,

TABLE 287-5 Drugs causing hemolysis in subjects deficient in G6PD

Antimalarials: Primaquine, pamaquine, chloroquine, dapsone
Sulfonamides: Sulfanilamide, sulfasoxazole, etc.
Nitrofurantoin
Analgesics: Phenacetin, acetanilid
Miscellaneous: Vitamin K (water-soluble form), probenecid, methylene blue, *p*-aminosalicylic acid, nalidixic acid, quinine,* quinidine,* chloramphenicol*

* *Not known to cause hemolysis in blacks with A− type G6PD.*

since these inclusions are readily removed by the spleen. Their removal leads to the formation of "bite cells," red cells which have lost a peripheral portion of the cell. Multiple bites cause the formation of fragments. Small numbers of spherocytes may also be present.

Individuals with the *Mediterranean type G6PD* have a more unstable enzyme and, therefore, a much lower overall enzyme activity than blacks with the A− variant. As a result, they have more severe clinical manifestations. Some have a chronic hemolytic anemia, even in the absence of any exposure to oxidants. A minority of patients are exquisitely sensitive to fava beans and will develop a fulminant hemolytic crisis following exposure. Sensitivity to *Vicia fava* is a poorly understood phenomenon that appears to be determined by a separate gene. Favism is not encountered in blacks with the A− variant. Individuals with the Mediterranean variant sometimes have a temporary episode of hemolysis during the newborn period.

The *diagnosis* of G6PD deficiency should be considered in any individual, particularly a black male, who experiences an acute hemolytic episode. The patient should be thoroughly questioned about possible exposure to oxidant agents. A number of screening tests are available to establish the diagnosis. However, since the deficiency occurs primarily in older red blood cells, a false-negative test may be seen during a hemolytic episode when there is a high proportion of young red blood cells. It may be necessary to repeat these diagnostic tests after the patient has recovered. Unusual features in the case should prompt further investigation including a more complete and specific characterization of the enzyme.

TREATMENT Since hemolysis in patients deficient in A− G6PD is usually self-limited, no specific treatment is necessary. Splenectomy does not appear to be of benefit to Mediterranean patients with chronic hemolysis. Blood transfusions are rarely indicated. If a patient develops a severe hemolytic episode with hemoglobinuria, maintaining adequate urine output is important.

Attention should be directed toward the *prevention* of hemolytic episodes. Infections ought to be treated promptly. Subjects deficient in G6PD should be warned about risks posed by oxidant drugs and fava beans. Any black patient about to be given an oxidant drug should be screened for G6PD deficiency.

OTHER DEFECTS OF THE HEXOSE-MONOPHOSPHATE SHUNT A few kindreds have been found to have congenital deficiency in red blood cell glutathione due to a defect in either of the two enzymes responsible for the synthesis of this tripeptide. Affected individuals have a hemolytic anemia with Heinz bodies that is aggravated by oxidant drugs. Deficiency of glutathione reductase has been reported, but its relationship to clinically significant hemolysis is not well established. Sometimes the deficiency state can be corrected by the administration of riboflavin (5 mg per day). There are also isolated reports of deficiencies of glutathione peroxidase and 6-phosphogluconate dehydrogenase, but, again, their association with hemolysis is uncertain.

Other enzyme defects Hemolytic anemia may sometimes be caused by abnormalities in enzymes of nucleotide metabolism. A growing number of individuals with pyrimidine 5′-nucleotidase deficiency have been encountered. Their red cells have marked basophilic stippling. Hemolytic anemia has also been noted in individuals whose red blood cells have supranormal levels of adenosine deaminase and relatively low levels of ATP.

HEMOGLOBINOPATHIES The sickling disorders constitute an important form of congenital hemolytic anemia. Less commonly, hemolysis may be due to the inheritance of an unstable hemoglobin variant. These disorders of hemoglobin are discussed in Chap. 288.

REFERENCES

ANTMAN KH et al: Microangiopathic hemolytic anemia and cancer: A review. Medicine 58:377, 1979

BEUTLER E: Red cell enzyme defects as nondiseases and as diseases. Blood 54:1, 1979

BUKOWSKI RM et al: Therapy of thrombotic thrombocytopenic purpura: An overview. Semin Throm Hemo 7:1, 1981

COOPER RA: Abnormalities of cell-membrane fluidity in the pathogenesis of disease. N Engl J Med 297:371, 1977

———: Hemolytic syndromes and red cell membrane abnormalities in liver disease. Semin Hematol 17:103, 1980

MIWA S, FUJII H: Molecular aspects of erythroenzymopathies associated with hereditary hemolytic anemias. Am J Hemat 19:293, 1985

PALEK J, LUX SE: Red cell membrane skeletal defects in hereditary and acquired hemolytic anemias. Semin Hematol 20:189, 1983

PANGBURN et al: Paroxysmal nocturnal hemoglobinuria: Deficiency in factor H-like functions of the abnormal erythrocytes. J Exp Med 157:1971, 1983

PETZ LD, GARRATTY G: *Acquired Immune Hemolytic Anemias*. New York, Churchill Livingstone, 1980

PISCIOTTA AV: Thrombotic thrombocytopenic purpura. Ann Intern Med 92:249, 1980

ROSSE WF: Autoimmune hemolytic anemia. Hosp Prac 20:105, 1985

———, PARKER CG: Paroxysmal nocturnal hemoglobinuria. Clin Haematol 14:105, 1985

SCHRIER SL (ed): The red blood cell membrane. Clin Haematol 14:1, 1985

VALENTINE WN et al: Hemolytic anemias and erythrocyte enzymopathies. Ann Intern Med 103:245, 1985

288 DISORDERS OF HEMOGLOBIN

H. FRANKLIN BUNN

In 1910, Herrick described a medical student from Jamaica who had a hemolytic anemia in conjunction with elongated "sickled" red blood cells. Subsequently, it was shown that all the red blood cells of such patients assume a classic holly leaf or sickle shape following deoxygenation of the blood. In 1949, Itano and Pauling discovered the association of sickle cell anemia with an electrophoretically abnormal hemoglobin. Eight years later, Ingram demonstrated that this hemoglobin (designated Hb S) differed from normal Hb A by the substitution of valine for glutamic acid at the sixth position of the β chain. Since then, over 400 structurally different human hemoglobin variants have been discovered in widely scattered parts of the world. Generally, a new hemoglobin is named after the place where it is first encountered. No more than a third of these mutant hemoglobins are associated with significant clinical manifestations. The remainder have been discovered by serendipity or as a result of large population surveys. All told, the hemoglobinopathies have taught us many valuable lessons in such diverse areas as the mechanisms of hemolysis, the pathophysiology of oxygen transport, the stereochemistry of hemoglobin function, and the genetic bases of protein synthesis.

This chapter focuses on the clinically significant variants. In addition, disorders of the biosynthesis of globin (the thalassemias) and methemoglobinemia are discussed.

GENETIC CONSIDERATIONS The synthesis of each of the subunits of hemoglobin (α, β, γ, δ, ε, ζ) is governed by separate genes. The ε and ζ subunits are found only in embryonic hemoglobin. Normal individuals inherit two β-chain genes (one from each parent), four α-chain genes, and four γ-chain genes. The ε-, γ-, δ-, and β-chain genes occupy adjacent loci on chromosome 11 (see Fig. 288-1). The ζ and α genes are located on chromosome 16. The structure and function of normal hemoglobin ($\alpha_2\beta_2$) are discussed in Chap. 283. The inheritance of abnormal hemoglobins follows classic mendelian genetics. If two parents are heterozygous for a hemoglobin variant such as Hb S, statistically one-quarter of the offspring will be SS homozygotes, another quarter will be normal (AA genotype), and half will have sickle trait (AS). The commonly encountered hemoglobinopathies such as S, C, and E are β-chain variants. Occasionally, an individual inherits two different β-chain variants, one from each parent. Hemoglobin SC disease is an example of such a double heterozygous state. Genes for β thalassemia are located on the β-chain structural gene. Accordingly, an individual can inherit from one parent (and pass on to a child) either β thalassemia or a β-chain variant, but not both. Among the hemoglobinopathies associated with sickling (described below), only the homozygous state (Hb SS) or double heterozygous state (Sβ thalassemia or SC) has important

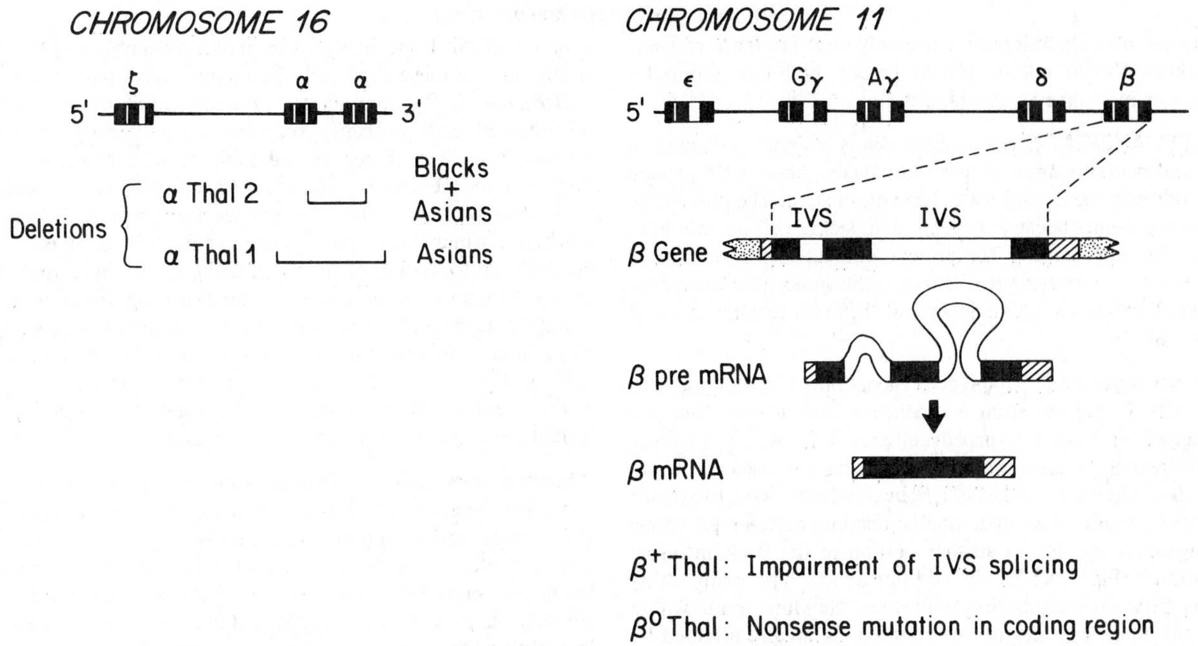

FIGURE 288-1 *Diagram of human globin genes. Left: The α-globin gene complex includes the embryonic ζ gene as well as two α genes. In the vast majority of individuals with α thalassemia 2 (α−) one α gene is deleted owing to a nonhomologous crossover between adjacent α genes. In α thalassemia 1 (− −) both α genes are deleted. Right: The β-globin gene complex includes the embryonic ϵ gene, two fetal genes ($^G\gamma$ and $^A\gamma$), the δ gene, and the β gene. Below is a diagram of the β gene showing the coding regions (■), the intervening segments (IVS, □) and the flanking regions (▨) that are transcribed into mRNA, shown below. Most cases of β^+ thalassemia in Mediterranean individuals involve a base substitution causing partial impairment of splicing of an IVS. Most cases of β^0 thalassemia in Mediterraneans involve a base substitution that creates either a stop codon or a frame shift.*

clinical manifestations. In contrast, the unstable variants and those having abnormal oxygen-binding properties are encountered only in heterozygotes. In many cases, the homozygous state would be incompatible with life.

About 90 percent of these abnormal hemoglobins are single amino acid replacements, due to a single base substitution in the corresponding triplet codon. The structural information accumulated on human mutant hemoglobins has provided ample verification of the fidelity of the genetic code. Other genetic mechanisms must be invoked to explain the structure of a few interesting hemoglobin variants. The Lepore hemoglobins have arisen because of nonhomologous crossover between the adjacent δ- and β-chain genes, giving rise to a fusion subunit in which the *N*-terminal end has the amino acid sequence of the δ chain and the *C*-terminal end has the sequence of the β chain (see Fig. 288-1). Some of the unstable hemoglobins have deletions of one or more residues in sequence within a subunit. Finally there are a few variants which have elongated subunits (e.g., Hb Constant Spring). These have arisen either because of a base substitution in the termination codon or because of a frame shift which puts the termination codon out of phase.

CLINICAL CLASSIFICATION The clinically significant hemoglobin variants are classified in Table 288-1. By far the most important and prevalent type of hemoglobinopathy is due to the presence of sickle hemoglobin, either in the homozygous state or in conjunction with another type of hemoglobin abnormality. The inheritance of an unstable hemoglobin variant may give rise to congenital hemolytic anemia associated with the presence of inclusions of precipitated hemoglobin within the red blood cells (Heinz bodies). Finally, hemoglobin variants may have abnormal functional or spectral properties, resulting in familial erythrocytosis or familial cyanosis.

SICKLE SYNDROMES

SICKLE CELL TRAIT About 8 percent of black Americans are heterozygous for Hb S. The gene frequency is highest in central Africa, particularly in regions where malaria is endemic. In some parts of Nigeria, over 30 percent of the population has sickle trait. The gene has persisted because heterozygotes gain slight protection against falciparum malaria. This is an example of balanced polymorphism.

The diagnosis of sickle trait or any of the other sickle syndromes depends upon the demonstration of sickling under reduced oxygen tension. In the widely used sickle preparation, sickled cells can be visualized microscopically after the addition of an oxygen-consuming reagent such as metabisulfite. Many clinical laboratories prefer a solubility test which depends on the fact that deoxyhemoglobin S has a low solubility at high ionic strength. These tests are reasonably specific for Hb S although some of the unstable variants may give a false-positive solubility test. Therefore, if one of these screening tests is positive, hemoglobin electrophoresis should be performed. Individuals with sickle trait usually have about 35 to 40 percent Hb S and 55 to 60 percent Hb A.

Hemoglobin S heterozygotes have minimal clinical problems. Their overall life expectancy and frequency of hospitalization are no different from those of a comparable group of individuals with hemoglobin A. AS red blood cells require a much lower oxygen tension for sickling than SS red cells. Accordingly, individuals with sickle trait may develop sickle cell crises only if they become severely hypoxic. They may occasionally sustain a splenic infarct. As discussed below, the renal medulla is particularly susceptible to sickling. Many AS individuals have impaired ability to form concentrated urine, and a few have recurrent episodes of painless hematuria as a result of medullary infarction. Infarction due to sickling has been encountered

TABLE 288-1 Clinically important hemoglobin variants

I Sickle syndromes
- *A* Sickle cell trait (AS)
- *B* Sickle cell anemia (SS)
- *C* Double heterozygous states: Sickle β thalassemia, sickle C disease (SC), sickle D disease (SD)

II Unstable hemoglobin variants: congenital Heinz body hemolytic anemia
III Variants with high oxygen affinity: familial erythrocytosis
IV M hemoglobins: familial cyanosis (see Table 288-3)

in other organs in sickle trait but is extremely rare. For these reasons, AS individuals should not be placed in any high-risk group for employment or insurance considerations.

SICKLE CELL ANEMIA Sickle cell anemia is a significant cause of morbidity and mortality among black individuals. About 0.15 percent of black children in the United States have the disease. The prevalence is lower among adults because patients with sickle cell anemia have a decreased life expectancy. The protean clinical manifestations of this disorder can all be attributed to a specific molecular lesion: the substitution of valine for glutamic acid at the sixth residue of the β chain (Fig. 288-2).

Molecular pathogenesis Upon deoxygenation, a red blood cell containing Hb S changes from a biconcave disk to an elongated crescent-shaped or "sickle"-shaped cell (see Fig. A5-6). Electron micrographs reveal the presence of fibers having a diameter of about 20 nm. Each sickle fiber consists of a helical polymer with 14 strands The polymer is stabilized by hydrophobic bonding between β6 valine and a complementary site on another portion of the β chain on an adjacent strand (Fig. 288-2). In addition, there are many other interactions between neighboring molecules. Sickling, both within the intact red blood cell and in free solution, is greatly affected by the presence of non-S hemoglobin. Hb A participates more readily than Hb F in copolymerization with Hb S.

Cellular pathogenesis As discussed in Chap. 283, the ability of red blood cells to traverse the microcirculation depends in large part on their pliability. As a red blood cell sickles, it becomes rigid, and, as a result, may obstruct capillary blood flow. The deoxygenation of blood from patients with sickle cell disease is associated with a marked increase in viscosity. It is likely that obstruction to flow leads to local tissue hypoxia. As a result, further deoxygenation takes place, leading to further sickling. This vicious cycle may result in the amplification of microscopic obstruction into a larger area of infarction. The oxygen-dependent sickle cycle is ordinarily reversible. However, the membrane of SS red blood cells may become sufficiently damaged so that the cells lose potassium and water, leading to the formation of irreversibly sickled forms. In these cells, the characteristic sickle shape persists even after they are exposed to ambient oxygen tension at room temperature and can readily be seen on examination of Wright-stained blood films (see Fig. A5-6). The proportion of irreversibly sickled cells varies considerably among homozygous sicklers and is not correlated with clinical severity. Hemoglobin F is distributed unevenly among red blood cells of SS patients, and composes between 2 and 20 percent of the total hemoglobin (the remainder is almost entirely Hb S). Since Hb F inhibits the polymerization of Hb S, those cells that are relatively rich in Hb F are protected from sickling, whereas those cells that have relatively small amounts of Hb F are likely to become irreversibly sickled. It is not surprising that these rigid cells are readily culled from the circulation and destroyed. The continuous formation and destruction of irreversibly sickled cells probably contributes significantly to the severe hemolytic anemia shared by all patients with sickle cell anemia. Furthermore, these rigid cells may initiate small-vessel occlusions.

Factors such as acidosis or increased erythrocyte 2,3-diphosphoglycerate, which lower the oxygen affinity of red blood cells, will enhance the formation of deoxyhemoglobin and, therefore, promote intracellular polymerization and eventual sickling. In addition, sickling is highly dependent on hemoglobin concentration. Any pathophysiologic process which tends to pull water out of sickle red blood cells will greatly increase their tendency to sickle. Thus, the hypertonic environment of the renal medulla can cause local sickling and the formation of papillary infarcts, even in individuals with sickle trait.

Clinical manifestations Patients with homozygous sickle cell anemia have a variety of clinical problems broadly outlined in Table 288-2. Signs and symptoms usually do not appear until after the sixth month of life, at which time most of the Hb F has been replaced by Hb S. Among the *constitutional* manifestations of sickle cell anemia are delay of growth and development and a general failure to thrive. In addition, these patients have an increased tendency to develop serious infections, particularly due to pneumococcus. SS patients have marked impairment of splenic function, preventing effective clearance of circulating bacteria. With the passage of time, the organ sustains recurrent infarcts and eventually becomes a nubbin of fibrous tissue.

ANEMIA SS homozygotes have a severe hemolytic anemia with hematocrit values between 18 and 30 percent. The destruction of red blood cells is independent of cell age. The mean red blood cell survival is about 10 to 15 days. Those cells having relatively low levels of Hb F have a shorter life span, in part due to a greater chance of becoming irreversibly sickled. As a result of accelerated red blood cell breakdown, patients with sickle cell disease have characteristic clinical and laboratory findings discussed in Chap. 283. Even though hemolysis is primarily extravascular, plasma haptoglobin is generally low or absent, and plasma hemoglobin levels are moderately elevated.

The anemia becomes increasingly severe if erythropoiesis is suppressed. There are two main causes of "aplastic crises"—infection and folic acid deficiency. As discussed in Chap. 286, infection brings about a transient reduction in red blood cell production. In particular, parvovirus causes an abrupt suppression of erythropoiesis. In SS patients with severe ongoing hemolysis, this usually results in a rapid drop in hematocrit (Table 288-2).

VASOOCCLUSIVE PHENOMENA The morbidity and mortality of sickle cell disease are due primarily to recurrent vasoocclusive phenomena.

FIGURE 288-2 *Polymerization of sickle hemoglobin. When the red cell (A) is deoxygenated, deoxyhemoglobin S aggregates to form domains of elongated rodlike polymers (B). In most cells these fibers align and distort the cell into the classic sickle shape (C). The individual Hb S molecules form a closely packed polymer consisting of 14 strands having a helical configuration (D). A close-up of the contacts between a pair of aligned strands (E) shows the abnormal β6 valine forming a hydrophobic contact with an acceptor site on the β chain of a molecule on the adjacent strand.*

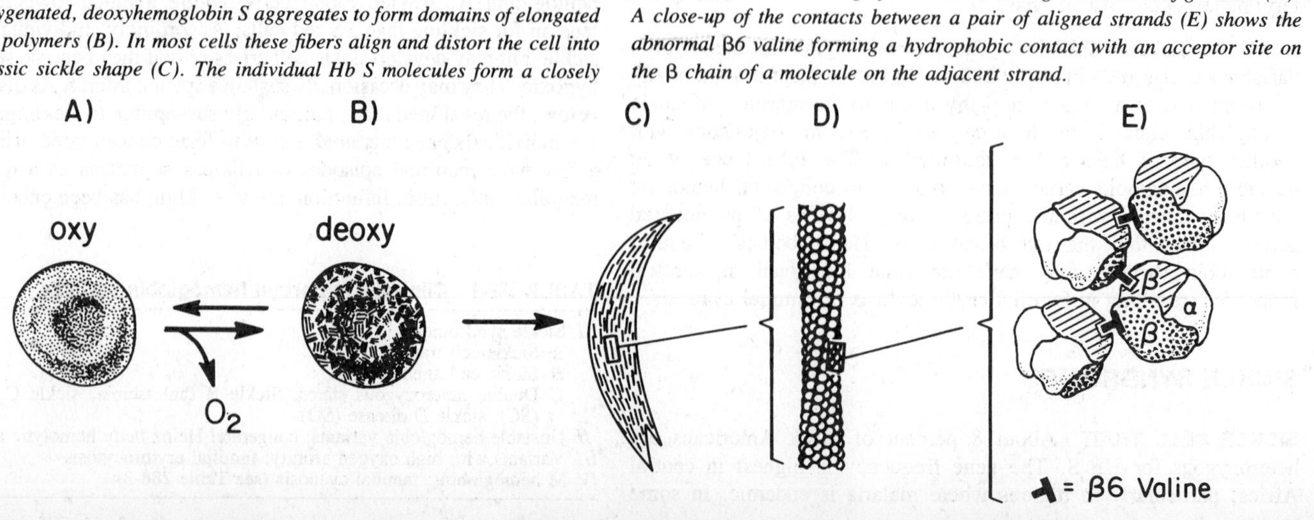

As shown in Table 288-2, these can be divided into two groups. Throughout their lives, SS patients are plagued by recurrent *painful crises*. These episodes may appear with explosive suddenness and attack various parts of the body, particularly the abdomen, chest, and joints. About a third of painful crises are preceded by a viral or bacterial infection (Table 288-2). The frequency of painful crises is highly variable. A given patient may have months or even years without a crisis and then have a cluster of frequent severe attacks. In some individuals, crises occur more frequently in cold weather, perhaps precipitated by reflex vasospasm. In others, crises come more often in warm weather, during times when patients are likely to become dehydrated. It is often difficult to distinguish between painful sickle crisis and some other type of acute process such as biliary colic, appendicitis, or a perforated viscus. Many patients have undergone exploration because they were considered to have an acute surgical problem. Patients having abdominal sickle crises usually have normal bowel sounds and no rebound tenderness. If the abdominal pain is due to sickling, the surgeon usually finds no gross evidence of infarction or ischemia.

SS homozygotes frequently develop attacks of acute pleuritic chest pain with fever. Although the initial chest x-ray is often unremarkable, an infiltrate may evolve. The important differential is between pneumonitis and pulmonary infarction. Culture and Gram's stain of the sputum will be helpful in establishing the presence of pneumonia. In these patients, pulmonary infarctions are much more likely due to thrombosis in situ than to emboli. Occasionally, pulmonary infarcts become secondarily infected.

When a sickle crisis is localized in the extremities, it may mimic osteomyelitis or an acute arthritis such as gout or rheumatoid arthritis. Patients commonly develop acute synovitis with joint effusion. Examination of the joint fluid is helpful in this differential diagnosis. If the effusion is due to sickling, the fluid will be clear and yellow, with a low white blood cell count (100 to 1000 mononuclear cells per cubic millimeter) and an absence of crystals or bacteria. Synovial biopsy may show sickled red blood cells in the lumen of small vessels.

Sickle crises may occasionally involve the central nervous system. Patients can present with a seizure, stroke, or coma. Although such crises are frequently reversible, they may be fatal.

CHRONIC ORGAN DAMAGE By the time that patients reach adulthood, there is often objective evidence of anatomic or functional damage to various tissues, due to the cumulative effect of recurrent vasoocclusive episodes. Almost any organ may be involved, but most commonly the lungs, kidneys, liver, skeleton, and skin.

Cardiopulmonary. Impairment of pulmonary function is a common complication of sickle cell disease. Resting arterial P_{O_2} is usually reduced in part because of intrapulmonary arterial-venous shunting. Since SS red blood cells have decreased oxygen affinity, arterial blood will be significantly undersaturated, leading to an increased tendency for red cells to sickle when they reach the peripheral circulation. SS homozygotes frequently develop congestive heart failure. The chronic severe anemia and hypoxemia impose a sustained burden on the heart. Most patients have a systolic ejection murmur as a result of their hyperdynamic circulation. Even though more oxygen is extracted by the myocardium than any other tissue, SS patients rarely develop myocardial infarction.

Hepatobiliary. Like other patients with congenital hemolytic anemia, those with sickle cell anemia have icterus and an increased tendency to form gallstones. It is often difficult to distinguish between the abdominal pain of acute cholecystitis and that due to a sickle crisis. Jaundice deepens markedly if a patient develops choledocholithiasis, and bilirubin levels as high as 50 mg/dL have been reported. As a rule, cholecystectomy is not recommended unless gallstones cause symptoms. In addition, patients with sickle cell anemia may develop hepatic infarcts which occasionally become infected, resulting in abscess formation. If a significant portion of hepatic parenchyma becomes infarcted, fibrosis and deterioration of liver function may result, with deepening of jaundice.

Genitourinary (see also Chaps. 224 and 227). The hypertonic and acidic environment of the renal medulla promotes sickling, resulting in microinfarcts. Virtually all patients have isosthenuria. The inability to form concentrated urine increases the risk of significant dehydration. In addition, like those with sickle trait or SC disease, SS homozygotes may develop significant and prolonged painless hematuria as a result of papillary infarcts. Hematuria may be so extensive that iron deficiency develops. ε-Aminocaproic acid has proved to be effective in severe cases but must be used with caution since it may prevent the lysis of clots in the renal pelvis.

A small number of patients develop frank renal failure, sometimes following the nephrotic syndrome. The pathogenesis of the glomerular lesions is not well understood. Mild nitrogen retention is commonly encountered, accompanied by moderate hyperuricemia. However, patients rarely have uric acid nephropathy or gout. Male patients with sickle cell anemia occasionally develop priapism (spontaneous and painful engorgement of the penis). This distressing complication occurs with about equal frequency in prepubertal and postpubertal patients, although the latter are more difficult to treat and may develop impotence following the acute episode. Patients should be treated conservatively with sedation, analgesia, and intravenous fluids. The administration of packed red blood cells may also be effective. Surgical intervention is rarely indicated.

Skeletal. Like other patients with congenital hemolytic anemia, patients with sickle cell anemia demonstrate radiologic abnormalities due to the expansion of red marrow. However, the development of bony infarcts results in more characteristic x-ray abnormalities. The biconcave or "fishmouth" vertebrae are pathognomonic of sickle cell disease. Skeletal infarction generally leads to increased bony trabeculation and sclerosis. Aseptic necrosis of the head of the femur is particularly common in patients with sickle cell disease and can lead to considerable disability. Like infarcts in other organs, bony infarctions are more likely to become infected. In patients who develop osteomyelitis, salmonella is a frequent pathogen.

Ocular. A variety of ocular abnormalities are encountered in patients with SS and SC disease. These include retinal infarcts, peripheral vessel disease, arteriovenous anomalies, vitreous hemorrhage, retinitis proliferans, and retinal detachment. In addition, when viewed with a strong magnifying lens, angulated and "corkscrew" vessels can be seen in the bulbar conjunctiva. The major ocular complications are more commonly encountered in SC and Sβ thalassemia patients than in SS patients. The early diagnosis of retinal lesions in sickle disease is important since retinal detachment may be prevented by appropriate therapy.

Skin. Chronic skin ulcers often occur in the distal lower extremities. The lesions appear to be commoner in patients with more severe anemia. Ankle ulcers have also been encountered in rare patients with other types of congenital hemolytic anemia. This complication is more commonly seen in tropical areas. Ankle ulcers generally respond to conservative management, such as elevation of the leg, maintenance of strict cleanliness, and application of a mild chemical debriding agent such as Dakin's solution. The weekly application of Unna boots has been effective. In patients with refractory ulcers, a hypertransfusion regimen is probably indicated. Skin grafting should be undertaken only after all other measures have failed.

Neurologic. A variety of central nervous system manifestations

TABLE 288-2 Clinical manifestations of sickle cell anemia

I Constitutional
- *A* Impaired growth and development
- *B* Increased susceptibility to infection

II Vasoocclusive
- *A* Microinfarcts → Painful crises
- *B* Macroinfarcts → Organ damage

III Anemia
- *A* Severe hemolysis
- *B* Aplastic crises

may be encountered in sickle cell anemia. Although cerebral thrombosis is the principal neurologic complication, SS patients also have an increased incidence of subarachnoid hemorrhage. A patient has about a 25 percent chance of developing some type of neurologic complication during a lifetime. Hemiplegia is encountered more frequently than coma, convulsions, or visual disturbances. Patients generally make a full recovery, particularly from their first cerebral vascular accident. Preliminary studies in children indicate that a hypertransfusion program is beneficial to those who have sustained a major neurologic complication.

Diagnosis The diagnosis of sickle cell anemia should be considered in any black patient with a hemolytic anemia. The history of painful crises, arthropathy, ankle ulcers, etc., can be very helpful. If a patient has a relatively mild form of the disease, the diagnosis may not have been made during childhood. A number of laboratory tests are useful in distinguishing sickle cell anemia from other hemoglobinopathies. Examination of the peripheral blood smear reveals normochromic normocytic red blood cells, many of which appear as targets. The presence of irreversibly sickled forms is very helpful (see Fig. A5-6). In addition, the presence of Howell-Jolly bodies, siderocytes, and occasional normoblasts suggests the absence of effective splenic function. A positive test for sickling, such as the metabisulfite preparation or the solubility test, indicates the presence of Hb S but does not distinguish between SS, AS, and double heterozygotes (SThal, SC). Hemoglobin electrophoresis is necessary to establish the diagnosis. Patients with homozygous sickle cell anemia have about 2 to 20 percent Hb F and 2 to 4 percent Hb A_2. The remainder is Hb S. No Hb A is detected unless the patient has been transfused within the past 4 months. Patients with sickle β thalassemia will have hypochromic microcytic red blood cells, fewer irreversibly sickled forms, and a variable proportion of Hb A (0 to 30 percent). SC diseases can be readily diagnosed by hemoglobin electrophoresis. In hemoglobin SD disease, the two hemoglobin variants comigrate during conventional electrophoresis at pH 8.6 but can be separated by agar gel electrophoresis at pH 6.0.

Treatment Understanding the molecular pathogenesis of sickling has not yet led to an effective form of therapy. A large array of antisickling regimens has been proposed, but thus far none has stood the test of time. Recent investigation has focused on drugs that alter cell division and thereby increase the proportion of F cells. Currently accepted management of sickle cell anemia is primarily supportive and conservative. Since patients with sickle cell anemia are at increased risk of developing infections, many of which trigger painful and aplastic crises, it is very important to detect infection early and give appropriate antibiotics promptly. Malaria prophylaxis should be administered in endemic areas. The development of pneumococcal sepsis in children may be prevented by the administration of the polyvalent vaccine.

The anemia of sickle cell disease increases markedly if the patient becomes deficient in folic acid. Since these patients have a continuous increased requirement for folic acid, it is reasonable to maintain them on a daily oral supplement. Testosterone increases the red blood cell mass in patients with sickle cell anemia. However, the potential risk of hepatotoxicity, and of priapism in males, limits its utility.

Painful crises should be treated promptly with adequate analgesia and hydration. Some patients feel that their crises can be aborted if treated early. Therefore, it is expedient to give patients a supply of an analgesic such as codeine which can be taken at home. However, these patients are at risk of becoming addicted to opiates. Oxygen should be administered during acute pain crisis if the patient has arterial hypoxemia.

Blood transfusions play a limited role in the management of sickle cell anemia. Between crises, patients tolerate anemia quite well and do not derive much subjective benefit from transfusions. However, partial replacement of the patients' red blood cells by transfused red cells (hypertransfusion) may be an effective way of preventing vasoocclusive crises. In order to lower the viscosity of the patient's blood significantly, it is necessary that over 50 percent of the patient's red blood cells be of donor origin. Hypertransfusion is a reasonable approach to getting a patient through a limited period of risk such as surgery. However, the problems of isoimmunization, iron overload, and hepatitis dictate against its widespread use.

Prevention Genetic counseling can play an important role in the prevention of sickle cell anemia. Parents who are both AS heterozygotes should be informed that there is a 25 percent chance that their offspring will be homozygous. The antenatal diagnosis of sickle cell anemia can be made in the second trimester of pregnancy by obtaining fetal cells from the amniotic fluid and analyzing the DNA following digestion with a restriction endonuclease that recognizes the β6 valine mutation. If it is established that the fetus is an SS homozygote, the parents may decide to interrupt the pregnancy.

Prognosis The clinical course of patients with sickle cell anemia is highly variable. Many assessments of prognosis that have appeared in the literature have been unduly pessimistic. During the past 30 years there has been considerable improvement in the care of patients with sickle cell anemia. An increasing number of patients are surviving into adulthood and even bearing offspring. There has also been a decline in the mortality of SS mothers during pregnancy and childbirth. However, in underdeveloped nations, the mortality in sickle cell anemia remains very high.

No single clinical or laboratory finding is a consistent predictor of prognosis in sickle cell disease. Although those patients who have relatively high amounts of Hb F tend to have milder clinical manifestations, this relationship is of no prognostic value in any given patient. Considerable variation in the severity of sickle cell disease has been reported among different ethnic and geographical groups. A group of Shi Arabs from Saudi Arabia has been found to have a benign form of sickle cell anemia with very high levels of Hb F (15 to 30 percent). A mild type of sickle cell anemia has also been seen among the Veddoids of India. SS patients with coexisting α thalassemia have less severe hemolysis but do not appear to have a significant reduction in vasoocclusive phenomena.

SICKLE β THALASSEMIA This disease is highly variable in its clinical severity and complications. It is commonly encountered in people from the Mediterranean countries as well as those from central Africa. Sickle β thalassemia tends to be milder in blacks, just as homozygous β thalassemia is much less severe in blacks than in the Mediterranean populations. Patients have a congenital hemolytic anemia of variable severity, accompanied by splenomegaly in about 70 percent of cases. They may have all the various types of vasoocclusive phenomena described above for homozygous sickle cell anemia. However, painful crises are generally less frequent and less severe.

Examination of the blood film reveals hypochromic microcytic red blood cells, with polychromatophilia, target cells, stippling, and rare fixed sickle forms. The electrophoretic pattern shows from 60 to 90 percent Hb S and 10 to 30 percent Hb F. Hemoglobin A will be about 10 to 30 percent if the β-thalassemia gene is capable of producing some β^A chains (β^+ thalassemia, see below). In patients who have sickle β^0 thalassemia, no Hb A will be present, and therefore the disorder may be difficult to distinguish from homozygous sickle cell anemia. Hemoglobin A_2 is moderately elevated in sickle β thalassemia, but it is difficult to measure this minor component accurately in the presence of Hb S. Sickle β^0 thalassemia is significantly more severe than sickle β^+ thalassemia. Occasional patients may derive benefit from splenectomy if the spleen is sequestering a significant amount of red blood cells.

SICKLE C DISEASE Although the gene frequency for Hb C (β6 Glu→Lys) is only one-fourth that for Hb S, the prevalence of SC disease among adults is almost as high as SS disease since the former group of patients has a nearly normal life expectancy. These individuals have a mild to moderate hemolytic anemia, usually accompanied by splenomegaly. On peripheral blood smears, target cells and occasional plump sickled forms are seen. Hemoglobin electrophoresis reveals 50 percent Hb S, 50 percent Hb C. Hemoglobin S copolymerizes with Hb C to the same extent as with Hb A. The increased tendency of SC red cells to sickle, compared with sickle trait cells, can be explained by two phenomena: increased intracellular hemoglobin concentration and significantly higher percent Hb S. Patients with SC disease may occasionally have painful crises or organ infarcts. They are at particular risk of developing ocular complications described above, including proliferative retinopathy and retinal detachment. In addition, patients with SC disease are at relatively high risk of developing hematuria from renal medullary infarcts and avascular necrosis of the femoral head. Pregnant women with SC disease have a high rate of complications during pregnancy. Individuals with an electrophoretic pattern suggestive of Hb SC disease but with more severe clinical manifestations are likely to be double heterozygotes for Hb S and Hb O Arab (β121 Glu→Lys).

SICKLE D DISEASE A number of hemoglobins comigrate with Hb S on routine electrophoresis. The most commonly encountered variant is Hb D Los Angeles (β121 Glu→Gln). Hemoglobins S and D can be separated by special electrophoretic methods. The diagnosis of Hb SD disease is suggested by the demonstration of a positive sickle cell preparation in only one of the patient's two parents. SD double heterozygotes have moderately severe anemia.

HOMOZYGOUS Hb C DISEASE Patients have a mild congenital hemolytic anemia accompanied by splenomegaly. Hemoglobin C has a tendency to form intracellular crystals, particularly if red blood cells are suspended in a hypertonic medium. The intracellular hemoglobin concentration is markedly increased owing to loss of potassium and water from the cytoplasm. As a result, the blood film reveals striking target cells. Red blood cell osmotic fragility is decreased. Patients rarely develop significant complications. No specific therapy is indicated.

UNSTABLE HEMOGLOBIN VARIANTS

In the early 1950s several patients in England were found to have congenital nonspherocytic hemolytic anemia associated with inclusions of precipitated hemoglobin (Heinz bodies) within red blood cells. The presence of an abnormal hemoglobin was suspected by the fact that a precipitate was formed when the patients' hemolysates were gently heated. Currently, over 90 different unstable hemoglobin variants have been identified. The great majority are single amino acid substitutions in the β chain. A few are due to deletion of one or more amino acids within the β chain. Patients present with a hemolytic anemia of variable degree. Severe cases are usually detected in late infancy or early childhood and have jaundice, splenomegaly, and dark-colored urine. An autosomal dominant mode of inheritance can usually be established, although about a fifth of the cases appear to be spontaneous mutants.

Pathogenesis These hemoglobin variants have structural alterations at sites in the molecule that drastically affect its stability and solubility. Many involve an amino acid substitution in the portion of the subunit where heme is inserted. In such instances, the heme may be displaced from the heme pocket. As a result, the abnormal hemoglobin has decreased solubility and forms an intracellular precipitate (Heinz body). Red blood cells which contain this type of inclusion are recognized by the mononuclear phagocyte system and are either cleansed of their intracellular debris (pitting) or destroyed. The displaced heme moiety is aberrantly catabolized, forming dipyrroles, such as mesobilifuscin, instead of bilirubin. Pigmenturia is probably due to the excretion of these dipyrroles. The degree of instability of these hemoglobin variants and, therefore, the extent of hemolysis vary considerably. In some, such as Hb Zürich, an additional oxidant stress, such as the ingestion of certain drugs, is required for significant hemolysis. In contrast, patients with Hb Hammersmith have continuous and marked red blood cell breakdown. The degree of anemia is influenced not only by the severity of the hemolysis but also by the ability of the blood to unload oxygen. Thus, patients having unstable variants with increased oxygen affinity, such as Hb Köln, may have a near-normal hemoglobin level, i.e., compensated hemolysis.

Diagnosis The red blood cell morphology is somewhat variable. Often, patients with a functioning spleen have normal-appearing red blood cells. Slight hypochromia and basophilic stippling are not uncommon. The blood may have to be incubated in order to bring out Heinz bodies. In some cases, red blood cells appear as if a bite had been taken from a margin. It is tempting to speculate that at this site a Heinz body had been pitted. Following splenectomy, red blood cells appear much more abnormal, and Heinz bodies are larger and more numerous.

The diagnosis of a congenital Heinz body hemolytic anemia is established by the following laboratory tests and results:

1 *Hemoglobin electrophoresis* will often reveal an abnormal component, usually composing less than 30 percent of the total.
2 *Heinz bodies* can be demonstrated by incubating a freshly drawn sample of blood with a supravital stain.
3 A significant *precipitate* is formed when the hemolysate is incubated at 50°C, or in the presence of 17% isopropanol.
4 The unstable hemoglobins often have an abnormal *oxygen dissociation curve.*

If these tests are negative in a patient with congenital nonspherocytic hemolytic anemia, a defect of the membrane or one of the red blood cell enzymes is likely.

Treatment The treatment of congenital Heinz body hemolytic anemia is primarily supportive. Anemia is rarely severe enough to warrant blood transfusion. Oxidant drugs should be avoided. Like others with chronic hemolysis, these patients have an increased requirement for folic acid. Those with severe hemolysis often benefit from prophylactic folate therapy. The red blood cell mass may fall during a period of bone marrow suppression, such as that resulting from folate deficiency or acute infection. Although patients with severe hemolysis may benefit from splenectomy, this operation is not curative. Because of the risk of bacterial sepsis in infants and young children who have been splenectomized, this treatment should be postponed until the child is over 4 years old. The diagnostic tests cited above become more abnormal following splenectomy. For this reason, in some cases the diagnosis may not be definitely established until after the operation.

STABLE VARIANTS HAVING ABNORMAL OXYGEN AFFINITY

In 1966 certain members of a large family were discovered to have erythrocytosis in association with an electrophoretically abnormal hemoglobin, Hb Chesapeake, which had a very high affinity for oxygen. Since then, more than 40 other stable high-affinity hemoglobin variants have been encountered in families with erythrocytosis. Their structural alterations tend to be at sites which influence hemoglobin's functional behavior. As a result of the hemoglobin's increased oxygen affinity, oxygen unloading to tissues is decreased, and there is an erythropoietin-mediated stimulus to erythropoiesis. This disorder is manifested in the heterozygous state and follows an autosomal codominant pattern of inheritance. Hematocrit levels are rarely high enough to cause a significant increase in blood viscosity. Thus, affected individuals are generally asymptomatic and lack any pertinent physical findings other than a ruddy complexion. The diagnosis should be suspected in all patients with unexplained erythrocytosis, particularly when other family members are similarly affected, and can be established by the demonstration of increased oxygen affinity of the whole blood. About two-thirds of the high-affinity variants can be readily separated from Hb A by electrophoresis. No treatment is indicated. The patient should be reassured that the disorder is benign.

Hemoglobin variants having a marked decrease in oxygen affinity cause one form of familial cyanosis (Table 288-3). Because of the abnormality of hemoglobin function, arterial blood is partially unsaturated despite normal oxygen tension. Thus, the cyanosis is due to increased levels of deoxyhemoglobin in the blood. Except for this cosmetic problem, affected individuals have no other clinical manifestations. Blood values are otherwise normal.

METHEMOGLOBINEMIA

Oxygen transport depends on the maintenance of intracellular hemoglobin in the reduced (Fe^{2+}) state. When hemoglobin is oxidized to methemoglobin, the heme iron becomes Fe^{3+} and is incapable of binding oxygen. Normal red cells contain less than 1 percent methemoglobin. A small amount of hemoglobin autooxidizes as red cells circulate. This process probably occurs by the dissociation of the superoxide anion from oxyhemoglobin:

$$Hb^{2+}O_2 \rightarrow Hb^{3+} + O_2^-$$

Normally, the methemoglobin that is formed is reduced by the following reaction:

$$Hb^{3+} + \text{RedCyt } b_5 \rightarrow Hb^{2+} + \text{OxCyt } b_5$$

Reduced cytochrome b_5 (RedCyt b_5) is regenerated by the enzyme cytochrome b_5 reductase (methemoglobin reductase):

$$\text{OxCyt } b_5 + \text{NADH} \xrightarrow[\text{reductase}]{\text{Cytochrome } b_5} \text{RedCyt } b_5 + \text{NAD}$$

Hereditary methemoglobinemia is due either to the presence of one of the M hemoglobins or to the deficiency of the enzyme cytochrome b_5 reductase (Table 288-3). These inherited disorders are clinically mild, while the induction of methemoglobinemia by drugs or toxins can be life-threatening.

If methemoglobin exceeds 1.5 g/dL (10 percent of the total hemoglobin), affected individuals will have clinically obvious cyanosis. The color of the skin is indistinguishable from the much commoner cyanosis due to impairment of oxygen saturation that may occur in pulmonary and cardiac disorders (Table 288-3). With higher amounts of methemoglobin, patients become symptomatic. At a methemoglobin level of about 35 percent, the affected individual experiences headache, weakness, and breathlessness. Levels in excess of 80 percent are usually incompatible with life.

The toxicity of methemoglobinemia can be readily explained in terms of hemoglobin function. The fact that a certain proportion of the heme moieties is no longer able to bind oxygen is not a serious physiologic handicap per se. A proportion of 30 percent methemoglobin is much more deleterious than a 30 percent decrement in red cell mass, because the oxidized hemes have a profound effect on the remaining functional hemes in the hemoglobin tetramer. The conformation of methemoglobin (like that of carboxyhemoglobin) is very similar to that of oxyhemoglobin. Thus, a partially oxidized hemoglobin tetramer has the same tertiary and quaternary structure as a molecule which is comparably oxygenated. In each case, the affinity of the remaining hemes for oxygen is increased. For this reason, methemoglobinemia (as well as carbon monoxide) causes a "shift to the left" of the oxyhemoglobin dissociation curve and, consequently, impaired unloading of oxygen to tissues.

TABLE 288-3 Differential diagnosis of cyanosis

I Decreased oxygenation of hemoglobin (↑ deoxyhemoglobin)
- *A* Reduced arterial oxygen tension (common)
  - *1* Pulmonary disease
  - *2* Cardiac right-to-left shunt
- *B* Hemoglobin variant having decreased oxygen affinity (rare)

II Methemoglobinemia (rare)
- *A* Hereditary
  - *1* M hemoglobins
  - *2* Cytochrome b_5 reductase deficiency
- *B* Acquired
  - *1* Nitrites and nitrates: sodium nitrite, amyl nitrite, nitroglycerin, nitroprusside, silver nitrate
  - *2* Aniline dyes
  - *3* Acetanilid and phenacetin
  - *4* Sulfonamides
  - *5* Other: lidocaine, chlorate, phenazopyridine

M Hemoglobins Five hemoglobin variants have abnormal absorbance spectra, owing to the oxidation of the heme iron in the affected subunit. They involve amino acid substitutions of residues responsible for the binding of the heme iron to the globin. These so-called M hemoglobins (Table 288-3) result in a rare form of congenital and familial cyanosis. Individuals with the α-chain variants Hb M Boston and Hb M Iwate are cyanotic at birth, while cyanosis does not appear in those with the β-chain variants (Hb M Saskatoon, Hb M Hyde Park, and Hb M Milwaukee) until about 4 to 6 months of age, when fetal hemoglobin has been replaced by adult hemoglobin. As with the unstable and high-affinity variants, an autosomal codominant inheritance pattern is found. Except for cyanosis, patients are asymptomatic.

CYTOCHROME b_5 REDUCTASE (METHEMOGLOBIN REDUCTASE) DEFICIENCY This condition is inherited in an autosomal recessive pattern. The enzyme is a flavoprotein having properties similar to those of liver microsomal cytochrome b_5 reductase. The soluble erythrocyte enzyme is formed by cleavage of a hydrophobic tail from the microsomal enzyme.

Individuals with cytochrome b_5 reductase deficiency have lifelong cyanosis of variable degree, depending on the level of methemoglobin, but usually have no associated symptoms or other physical findings. Some may have mild polycythemia owing to increased oxygen affinity. Others have been noted to be mentally retarded. Untreated individuals usually have 15 to 30 percent methemoglobin. Methemoglobin levels are higher in the older population of red cells because the activity of the abnormal enzyme declines markedly with red cell age. There appears to be considerable heterogeneity in the variant enzymes from different families, as shown by differences in their electrophoretic mobility and kinetic parameters. In these ways, cytochrome b_5 reductase deficiency resembles glucose 6-phosphate dehydrogenase deficiency (Chap. 287).

ACQUIRED METHEMOGLOBINEMIA This disorder is generally due to exposure to certain drugs or toxins. Compounds which can cause clinically significant methemoglobinemia are listed in Table 288-3. Some agents such as nitrite and chlorate oxidize the heme iron directly. Others such as sulfa drugs and aniline must undergo biochemical transformation before they cause methemoglobinemia. Few drugs currently in use cause significant methemoglobinemia, unless the individual is unusually susceptible. Exposure to local anesthetics such as procaine and to nitroprusside occasionally causes severe methemoglobinemia. As might be expected, individuals heterozygous for methemoglobin reductase deficiency are much more likely than normal individuals to develop clinically apparent methemoglobinemia after exposure to an oxidant stress. Thus, the extent of methemoglobinemia depends not only on the dose of the toxic agent but also on the susceptibility of the exposed individual.

DIAGNOSIS Methemoglobinemia should be considered in any cyanotic patient with no evidence of heart or lung disease. If the cyanosis is due to decreased oxygen saturation, a blood specimen will change from a purple to a red color upon mixing with air. In contrast, a blood specimen from a methemoglobinemic individual remains a chocolate brown color irrespective of exposure to air. Methemoglobinemia can be documented by spectroscopic examination of the hemolysate. Individuals with hereditary methemoglobinemia will have lower levels than patients symptomatic from acquired methemoglobinemia. Patients who have ingested an oxidant drug may have an additional hemoglobin derivative called sulfhemoglobin in which the protoporphyrin has been chemically modified. Sulfhemoglobinemia tends to cause cyanosis even more readily than methemoglobinemia. Unlike methemoglobin, the absorbance of sulfhemoglobin at 620 to 630 nm is not decreased by the addition of cyanide. The M hemoglobins have characteristic spectral abnormalities which differ from those obtained when normal Hb A is partially oxidized. Furthermore, these hemoglobin variants can be detected by hemoglobin electrophoresis.

Treatment In individuals with methemoglobin reductase deficiency, the oral administration of methylene blue (100 to 300 mg per day) or ascorbic acid (300 to 500 mg per day) will result in a marked reduction in the level of methemoglobin. The purpose of treatment is primarily cosmetic. Severe toxic methemoglobinemia is treated by the intravenous administration of methylene blue (2 mg/kg, repeat if needed). Within an hour, the methemoglobin level is usually reduced by at least 50 percent. Treatment is neither necessary nor possible in individuals having Hb M.

THALASSEMIAS

The thalassemias are a diverse group of congenital disorders in which there is a defect in the synthesis of one (or more) of the subunits of hemoglobin. As a result of decreased production of hemoglobin, the red blood cells are microcytic and hypochromic (Table 53-2). The thalassemias involve a spectrum ranging from subtle morphologic abnormalities to life-threatening disease. In contrast to the qualitative hemoglobin abnormalities listed in Table 288-1, the thalassemias are quantitative abnormalities of subunit synthesis. Thus, the β chains of patients with β thalassemia have normal structure but are produced in reduced and sometimes undetectable amounts. Conversely, patients with α thalassemia have impaired production of α chains. The reduction in globin chain synthesis can be demonstrated in vitro by incubating reticulocytes with labeled amino acids and determining the incorporation of radioactivity into globin subunits (Table 288-4). Most forms of thalassemia can be identified from the information summarized in Table 288-4. Occasionally, establishing a definitive diagnosis requires measurement of globin chain synthesis or analysis of globin gene structure.

α THALASSEMIA As mentioned at the beginning of this chapter, normal individuals inherit two α-chain genes from each parent. The great majority of cases of α thalassemia can be explained by deletions of α-chain genes, owing to nonhomologous crossover (Fig. 288-1). Specific gene deletions can be identified by analysis of patients' DNA following digestion by restriction endonucleases. The clinical manifestations of α thalassemia depend upon the number of genes deleted (Table 288-4). In the silent carrier state, heterozygous α thalassemia 2 (α−/αα), one of the four genes is deleted. Affected individuals have no hematologic abnormalities. Individuals with deletion of two of the four α-chain genes (α-thalassemia trait) have either homozygous α thalassemia 2 (α−/α−) or heterozygous α thalassemia 1 (−−/αα). They have microcytic and slightly hypochromic red blood cells but no significant hemolysis or anemia. Hemoglobin electrophoresis is normal except for a decreased amount of Hb A_2. Deletion of three α-chain genes (−−/α−) produces a well-compensated hemolytic state with microcytic hypochromic red blood cells including many target cells. Intracellular inclusions or Heinz bodies are formed by the precipitation of Hb H, a tetramer composed of β chains which accumulates because of the marked impairment of α-chain synthesis. The most severe form of α thalassemia, hydrops fetalis, is usually due to deletion of all four α-chain genes. The affected fetus has red blood cells containing only Hb Barts, a tetramer composed of γ chains. This condition is incompatible with life, since oxygen transport depends upon the presence of heterotetramers such as $\alpha_2\beta_2$ and $\alpha_2\gamma_2$. In orientals both the α− and the −− haplotypes are relatively common; thus both Hb H disease and hydrops fetalis are frequently encountered. In contrast, blacks commonly have the α− haplotype (gene frequency ≅ 0.15) but rarely have the −− haploptype. Therefore Hb H disease is very rare in blacks and hydrops fetalis has not been reported. Homozygous α thalassemia 2 is encountered in about 2 percent of blacks and is therefore a relatively common cause of microcytosis in an individual who is otherwise healthy and not iron-deficient.

The elongated α-chain variant Hb Constant Spring, commonly encountered among southeast Asians, also has an α-thalassemia phenotype, and when inherited with the −− haplotype can cause Hb H disease.

β THALASSEMIA Since individuals inherit only one β-chain gene from each parent, affected individuals are either heterozygotes, homozygotes, or double heterozygotes. The gene frequency for β thalassemia approaches 0.1 in southern Italy and certain Mediterranean islands. β Thalassemia is also encountered quite commonly in central Africa, Asia, the south Pacific, and certain parts of India. Statistically, one-quarter of the offspring of two heterozygotes (β-thalassemia trait) will have the homozygous state: β thalassemia major or Cooley's anemia. An individual may inherit a β-thalassemia gene from one parent and a β-chain structural variant from the other (Fig. 288-1). Sickle β thalassemia (discussed above) is a commonly encountered example of such a double heterozygous state.

The molecular pathogenesis of the β thalassemias is more complex and heterogeneous than that of α thalassemia. In contrast to α thalassemia, gene deletion is an uncommon cause of β thalassemia. Among the recognized types of β-gene deletion, an entity known as "pancellular hereditary persistence of fetal hemoglobin" has minimal clinical manifestations owing to efficient synthesis of γ chains on the chromosome in which the β and δ genes are deleted. Hemoglobin Lepore is a fusion protein formed from a nonhomologous crossover between the δ and β genes resulting in the absence of normal β-chain synthesis and therefore a β-thalassemia phenotype (Fig. 288-1). In the great majority of cases of β thalassemia, restriction endonuclease maps reveal no gross abnormalities of the β-globin

TABLE 288-4 Classification of the thalassemias

Diagnosis	Globin chain synthesis in reticulocytes	RBC morphology	Hb electrophoresis	Clinical severity
α Thalassemia:	α/β*			
Silent carrier (α−/αα)	0.9	Normal	Normal, ↓ A_2	0
α-thalassemia trait [(α−/α−) or (−−/αα)]	0.7	↓ MCV†	Normal, ↓ A_2	0
Hb H disease (−−/α−)	0.3	↓ MCV Heinz bodies, targets	↑ Hb H (β_4) (10–15%)	2+
Hydrops fetalis (−−/−−)	0	↑ ↑ Nucleated RBC	↑ ↑ Hb Barts (γ_4)	4+
β thalassemia:	β/α*			
Heterozygous	0.5	↓ MCV, stippling	↑ A_2 (± ↑ HbF)	0 to +
Homozygous (or double heterozygous)	0–0.3	↓ MCV, hypochromic Nucleated RBC, targets bizarre shapes	↑ ↑ HbF	4+ (major) 2−3+ (intermedia)

* *Normal = 1.*
† *MCV = mean corpuscular volume.*

gene complex. Nevertheless, there are several steps in β-globin synthesis that could go awry and lead to a thalassemic phenotype. A number of cases involve mutations in or near one of the intervening sequences of the β-globin gene, leading to errors in the processing of mRNA. Often β^A chains are made but in reduced amounts (β^+ thalassemia) (see Fig. 288-1). Others have nonsense mutations in the coding region, causing premature termination of β-globin chains. This is the most common cause of β^0 thalassemia (Fig. 288-1).

Cellular pathogenesis As a result of imbalance in globin chain synthesis, the β thalassemias have varying degrees of ineffective erythropoiesis (Chap. 283) and hemolysis. In β thalassemia major there is a marked relative excess of α-chain production. Free α chains have decreased solubility and will form insoluble aggregates or inclusions within red blood cell precursors in the bone marrow. Like congenital Heinz body hemolytic anemia due to unstable hemoglobin variants, the inclusion bodies in thalassemia bring about abnormalities in membrane permeability as well as entrapment and destruction of red blood cells by the macrophages in the mononuclear phagoycte system. As a result, β thalassemia is characterized by both intramedullary erythroid destruction and also a shortening of the life span of circulating red blood cells that emerge from the bone marrow. Thus, these patients have the characteristic parameters of both ineffective erythropoiesis (increased plasma iron turnover, decreased incorporation of iron into red blood cells) and peripheral hemolysis. Because these red blood cells are under double jeopardy, there is an enormous compensatory stimulus to erythropoiesis, resulting both in expansion of the red marrow and in extramedullary hematopoiesis in the liver and spleen. Chain imbalance in β thalassemia is attenuated to a variable degree by the "compensatory" synthesis of γ chains which are able to combine with excess free α chains and form a stable tetramer (Hb F). Patients with Cooley's anemia who have a relatively high rate of γ-chain production have a less severe clinical course. Individuals with β thalassemia minor have absent or very mild ineffective erythropoiesis and hemolysis, detectable in some patients by a slight elevation in fecal urobilinogen and a modest shortening of the red blood cell life span.

In the α thalassemias a relative excess production of non-α chains can be detected, leading to the formation of Hb Barts (γ_4) in the newborn and young infant. Children and adults with deletion of 3 α-globin genes usually have Hb H (β_4). In contrast to the α-chain inclusions found in β thalassemia, the Heinz bodies due to Hb H are more stable and develop in mature circulating red blood cells. As a result, Hb H disease is primarily a hemolytic disorder without a significant amount of ineffective erythropoiesis.

β thalassemia minor This common entity, also referred to as *β-thalassemia trait,* is rarely associated with significant clinical manifestations. The diagnosis is generally made in patients being evaluated for mild anemia or in follow-up of abnormalities found on routine blood studies. Most individuals with β-thalassemia trait escape diagnosis. About one-fifth of affected individuals have splenomegaly. Icterus is occasionally noted, particularly in those individuals who also have Gilbert's disease, another common and benign congenital disorder (Chap. 246).

In otherwise healthy individuals with β-thalassemia trait, the mean hemoglobin level is about 15 percent lower than in normal persons of the same age and sex; the red blood cell count is usually elevated, and the cells are microcytic. Indeed, at any level of hematocrit, patients with β thalassemia minor have more marked microcytosis than those with iron deficiency. In contrast, the mean corpuscular hemoglobin concentration is normal. In addition to microcytosis, examination of the blood film reveals occasional target cells, cigar-shaped cells, and a moderate amount of basophilic stippling; the reticulocyte count is normal. Special isotope techniques are required to demonstrate a slightly reduced red blood cell life span. The red blood cells have decreased osmotic fragility. Serum iron is normal unless the patient also happens to be iron-deficient. Hemoglobin electrophoresis is very useful in establishing the diagnosis of β thalassemia minor. Most affected individuals will have a twofold increase in Hb A_2 (5 percent versus normal of 2.5 percent). In contrast, Hb A_2 is subnormal in α thalassemia, iron deficiency, and sideroblastic anemias. Patients with β-thalassemia trait who become iron-deficient usually have a "normal" level of Hb A_2 which increases to above normal after correction of the deficiency. Almost half of individuals with β thalassemia minor also have moderate elevation of Hb F (2 to 5 percent). In the less common state, δβ thalassemia, in which there is a deletion of the adjacent δ and β chain genes, Hb A_2 levels will be normal or decreased, but Hb F is increased (5 to 15 percent).

No treatment is indicated for individuals with β-thalassemia trait. They should be reassured that they do not have a serious hematologic problem. The genetic implications of thalassemia should be explained, particularly to those of childbearing age. Many individuals have been given long-term iron treatment on the mistaken impression that they had iron-deficiency anemia. These patients may gradually develop clinically significant siderosis. Establishing the diagnosis of β thalassemia minor should prevent such inappropriate therapy.

β thalassemia major Also termed Cooley's anemia, this is probably the most severe form of congenital hemolytic anemia. Clinical manifestations generally appear after the first 4 to 6 months of life when the switch from γ-chain to β-chain production usually occurs. Patients develop a severe anemia with a hematocrit of less than 20 unless they are supported by transfusions. Accordingly, patients have all the signs and symptoms associated with severe anemia. In addition, they have findings related to severe intramedullary and peripheral hemolysis and to iron overload. Patients with β thalassemia major often have marked wasting and appear malnourished. Children have slow rates of growth and development. In adolescents, the onset and development of secondary sex characteristics are delayed. Patients have a peculiar skin color due to a combination of icterus, pallor, and increased melanin deposition. They usually have skeletal abnormalities, secondary to expansion of the erythroid marrow. Enlargement of the malar bones may give the characteristic "chipmunk" facies or cause malocclusion of the jaw. Patients invariably have cardiomegaly which may be accompanied by signs of congestive heart failure. Marked hepatomegaly and splenomegaly are always found in these patients.

The *diagnosis* of β thalassemia major should be considered in any patient with a severe hemolytic anemia and hypochromic microcytic red blood cells. Examination of the peripheral blood smear reveals marked variations in the size and shape of red blood cells, including many target cells as well as teardrop and cigar-shaped cells (Plate 9-5). Normoblasts are usually seen, particularly if the patient has undergone splenectomy. Hemoglobin electrophoresis shows the presence of large amounts of Hb F and variable amounts of Hb A. In patients who are homozygous for β^0 thalassemia, no Hb A can be detected. Hemoglobin A_2 is usually increased about twofold, although it can be normal in β thalassemia major.

Patients with β thalassemia major have a short life expectancy. It is unusual for a patient with the most severe form of the disease to survive into adulthood. Most patients have such severe anemia that they are dependent upon transfusions. The chronic administration of large amounts of blood along with an inappropriate increase in iron absorption from the gastrointestinal tract inevitably leads to clinically significant hemosiderosis. As a result of iron overload, these patients develop abnormalities in cardiac, endocrine, and hepatic function. The combination of chronic hypoxia and myocardial siderosis leads to cardiac arrhythmias, congestive failure, and ultimately death.

Homozygotes who survive into adulthood are likely to have a less severe form of the disease, designated as *β thalassemia intermedia.* There are several genetic subtypes which are associated with less severe clinical manifestations: (1) β thalassemia with unusually high levels of Hb F synthesis, (2) δβ thalassemia in which there is absence of δ-chain as well as β-chain synthesis, and (3) the presence of α thalassemia in combination with homozygous β thalassemia, leading to more balanced subunit synthesis. A milder clinical course is also seen in individuals who are doubly heterozygous for β thalassemia and hereditary persistence of Hb F. Patients with the above genotypes usually have moderately severe anemia, but do not require transfusions.

Treatment of β thalassemia major is primarily supportive. The obvious benefits of transfusion therapy are partially offset by the risk of iron overload, hepatitis, and alloimmunization. Despite these problems, children with Cooley's anemia fare better if their hemoglobin is maintained at greater than 9 g/dL. In view of the increased demands of the hyperplastic marrow, it is reasonable to maintain these patients on a daily supplement of folic acid. Since splenic sequestration contributes to shortened red blood cell survival, many patients derive some benefit from splenectomy. The prevention and treatment of iron overload is a continuing concern in these patients. Transfusion of young low-density red blood cells, "neocytes," reduces the rate of iron accumulation. Continuous subcutaneous injection of desferrioxamine permits the mobilization and excretion of significant amounts of iron and, when administered over a prolonged period, can prevent or retard the development of chronic iron toxicity.

Considerations of genetic counseling and antenatal diagnosis are as relevant in the *prevention* of β thalassemia major as they are for sickle cell anemia (see above). Because of linkages between β thalassemias and restriction enzyme polymorphisms, prenatal diagnosis can often be made by DNA analysis of amniotic fluid cells. However, in some cases it is necessary to take the risk of obtaining fetal red blood cells for globin chain synthesis measurements.

REFERENCES

ALTER BP: Advances in the prenatal diagnosis of hematologic diseases. Blood 64:329, 1984

BENZ ES, FORGET BG: The thalassemia syndromes: Models for the molecular analysis of human disease. Ann Rev Med 33:363, 1982

BUNN HF, FORGET BG: *Hemoglobin: Molecular, Genetic and Clinical Aspects.* Philadelphia, Saunders, 1986

CASTLE WB: From man to molecule and back to mankind. Semin Hematol 13:159, 1976

CHARACHE S: Advances in the understanding of sickle cell anemia. Hosp Pract 21:173, 182, 1986

JAFFE EF: Methemoglobinemia. Clin Hematol 10:99, 1981

KAN YW: Thalassemia: Molecular mechanism and detection. Am J Hum Genet 38:4, 1986

LEY TJ, NIENHUIS AW: Induction of Hb F synthesis in patients with β thalassemia. Ann Rev Med 36:485, 1985

NIENHUIS AW et al: Advances in thalassemia research. Blood 63:738, 1984

NOGUCHI CT, SCHECHTER AN: The intracellular polymerization of sickle hemoglobin and its relevance to sickle cell disease. Blood 58:1057, 1981

POWARS DR: Natural history of sickle cell disease: The first ten years. Semin Hematol 12:267, 1975

SCHECHTER AN, BUNN HF: What determines severity in sickle cell disease. N Engl J Med 306:295, 1982

SERJEANT GR: *The Clinical Features of Sickle Cell Disease.* New York, American Elsevier, 1986

WEATHERALL DJ, CLEGG JB: *The Thalassemia Syndromes.* Oxford, Blackwell, 1982

289 THE MYELOPROLIFERATIVE DISEASES

JOHN W. ADAMSON

DEFINITION The myeloproliferative diseases are neoplasms of the multipotent hematopoietic stem cell. They include chronic myelogenous leukemia (CML), polycythemia vera (PV), agnogenic myeloid metaplasia with myelofibrosis (AMM/MF), and essential thrombocytosis (ET). In addition to their common stem cell origin, other features are shared which occasionally lead to a blurring between the various disorders. However, apparent transitions from one disorder to another are uncommon. With the exception of CML, the diseases tend to run a chronic course over many years.

The stem cell origin and clonal nature of these diseases have been shown through cytogenetic analyses and through studies in female patients who are heterozygous for glucose 6-phosphate dehydrogenase (G6PD). Consistent with the stem cell origin and neoplastic nature of these diseases a single G6PD enzyme is found in peripheral blood granulocytes, platelets, red cells, and monocytes in patients who have been shown to be G6PD heterozygotes by analysis of skin fibroblasts. In at least some patients, the level of stem cell involvement includes a progenitor capable of giving rise to lymphocytes, as well. In patients with characteristic cytogenetic abnormalities, abnormal metaphases may be found in precursors of platelets, red cells, and granulocytes. These findings indicate that the diseases arise as clonal expansions of single transformed stem cells. At the time of diagnosis, virtually all of the myeloid cells of the blood are derived from the neoplastic clone.

CHRONIC MYELOGENOUS LEUKEMIA

DEFINITION AND ETIOLOGY CML is characterized by marked splenomegaly and the production of increased numbers of granulocytes, particularly neutrophils. The disorder is associated with a characteristic chromosomal abnormality (see below) and runs a generally mild course until it transforms to a frankly leukemic (blastic) phase. No specific etiologic agent can usually be identified; however, an increased incidence of CML in atomic bomb survivors has been noted. CML occurs at any age, but the peak incidence occurs in the third and fourth decades. The sexes are affected equally.

PATHOPHYSIOLOGY AND SYMPTOMATOLOGY The natural course of CML can be divided into a chronic and a blastic or acute phase. The chronic phase of CML is characterized by an excessive proliferation and accumulation of granulocytes and their precursors in the marrow and blood. Typically, the white blood cell count is markedly elevated, often exceeding 200,000 per cubic millimeter. At this stage, myeloblasts are less than 5 percent of the cells in the marrow and blood. The diagnosis often is made because of incidental laboratory tests which reveal an elevated white blood count, or because a patient complains of left upper quadrant discomfort due to an enlarged spleen. About 20 percent of cases are diagnosed on the basis of an elevated blood count in the absence of symptoms. In the majority, however, the signs and symptoms of the disease are related to the expanded myeloid mass in the marrow and spleen. Presenting symptoms are related to splenomegaly, anemia, or hypermetabolism manifested by weight loss and fever. Arthralgias may be severe. Lymphadenopathy is rare in this phase. Thrombohemorrhagic complications such as excessive bleeding, either spontaneously or with surgical or dental procedures, are found occasionally. Ninety percent of patients have palpable splenomegaly.

During the course of the chronic phase of CML the disease transforms to the more malignant blastic phase. After the first 6 to 12 months following diagnosis, the rate of transformation to the blastic phase is about 25 percent of the remaining patients per year and over 85 percent of patients with CML will eventually die in this phase. Occasionally, patients may present in the blastic phase of the disease. The chronic phase may be restored if such patients respond successfully to chemotherapy. There is no single test which predicts precisely when a patient's disease will transform to the blastic phase, but certain features associated with early transformation include the degree of leukocytosis, the presence of an excessively large liver and spleen, the percentage of immature cells in the marrow, and the presence of large numbers of eosinophils or basophils. Overall survival for patients from the time of diagnosis averages $3\frac{1}{2}$ years.

The blastic phase of CML represents an evolution in the disease from hyperplasia of mature marrow elements of the marrow to increased numbers of blasts and promyelocytes. Half of the patients progress to blast crisis through an "accelerated" phase characterized by progressively increasing leukocytosis, thrombocytosis or thrombocytopenia, and splenomegaly, which are refractory to previously effective drugs. In some patients, the transition to a state resembling acute myelogenous leukemia may take only a few weeks. A minority of patients will present with or develop extramedullary tumors, usually in lymph nodes or skin, or osteolytic bone lesions. Meningeal leukemia is rare.

The blastic phase may be lymphoid or myeloid in origin. One-third of cases have characteristics of lymphoblasts including the enzyme terminal deoxynucleotidyl transferase (TdT), a DNA-synthesizing enzyme associated with acute lymphoblastic leukemia and normal thymic lymphocytes, as well as the common acute lymphoblastic leukemia antigen (CALLA). This is consistent with the known level of stem cell involvement in the original disease. Lymphoid blast crisis in some patients is associated with arrested rearrangements of the immunoglobulin genes typical of pre-B cells. Myeloid blast crisis resembles acute myelogenous leukemia, but a few patients will have a basophilic or erythroleukemic conversion from the chronic phase of the disease. The latter, and the fact that the blasts may react positively with monoclonal antibodies to erythroid- or megakaryocyte-associated antigens, emphasize the diversity of this phase and the stem cell nature of the disease. Auer rods are virtually never seen in the myeloblasts of CML in blastic phase.

LABORATORY FINDINGS Table 289-1 summarizes the distinguishing laboratory features of the various myeloproliferative diseases. The most prominent laboratory finding in CML is the leukocytosis. Unlike the finding in leukemoid reactions, there is generally a bimodal distribution of neutrophils in the blood with a peak of mature polymorphonuclear neutrophils (PMNs) and a second peak of myelocytes or metamyelocytes. Platelet morphology is more normal than in the other myeloproliferative disorders, and in vitro platelet function, as marked by aggregation in the presence of agents such as epinephrine, is also generally normal. Basophilia, typical of all of the myeloproliferative disorders, may be prominent. A number of unique biochemical abnormalities are also found. Accompanying the leukocytosis of CML is a marked elevation of serum vitamin B_{12} levels, as well as an increased serum vitamin B_{12}–binding capacity. This is due to excessive serum levels of transcobalamin I, a glycoprotein of alpha globulin electrophoretic mobility. A vitamin B_{12}–binding protein with similar properties has been shown to be produced by mature normal and leukemic granulocytes in vitro. Elevated levels in the serum of patients with CML are probably derived from the turnover of the increased granulocytic mass. The high levels of vitamin B_{12}, as well as the increased serum binding capacity, return toward normal with treatment of the disease. Leukocyte alkaline phosphatase, an enzyme in granulocytes, is markedly reduced in the granulocytes of nearly all patients with CML. However, with infection or steroid administration, the level of the enzyme in granulocytes may rise to the normal range. The levels of the enzyme may also return toward normal with successful therapy of the disease and reduction of the white cell count. The only other hematologic disorder with low or absent leukocyte alkaline phosphatase is paroxysmal nocturnal hemoglobinuria. The marrow as well as the spleen of patients with CML may contain glycolipid-laden phagocytes which resemble Gaucher cells. Hyperuricemia related to the increased cell turnover may occur in all the myeloproliferative diseases prior to therapy and can be exacerbated by treatment. The mature granulocyte in CML is a cell that is functionally normal with respect to phagocytosis and bactericidal activity. Granulocyte kinetics in CML have been studied with isotope-labeling techniques, and there is clear evidence for increased production of mature granulocytes. The numbers of primitive myeloid progenitors (colony-forming cells) in the marrow and blood of patients with CML are also increased. This includes both committed erythroid as well as granulocytic progenitors, and their numbers in the blood may be 10,000 times the normal number.

CYTOGENETICS More than 95 percent of patients with CML have a unique and characteristic chromosome marker in metaphases of marrow—the Philadelphia chromosome (Ph^1). This chromosomal abnormality represents a reciprocal translocation of genetic material between the long arms of chromosome 22 and chromosome 9. This particularly interesting chromosomal rearrangement involves break points near two cellular proto-oncogenes, c-*abl* on chromosome 9 and c-*sis* on chromosome 22. The proto-oncogene c-*sis* is the cellular homologue of the simian sarcoma virus oncogene and encodes sequences for platelet-derived growth factor (PDGF). The proto-oncogene c-*abl* is translocated to a specific region of chromosome 22, the breakpoint cluster region (*bcr*). As a result, a fusion gene product of *bcr/abl* is formed which has tyrosine kinase activity and may have a role in the development or persistence of the disease. This chromosome abnormality persists throughout the course of the disease, in remission and relapse, and is unaffected by the usual therapies. It is present in virtually all metaphases of granulocytic, megakaryocytic, and erythroid precursors but not in traditionally prepared lymphocyte preparations or skin fibroblasts. In addition to the Ph^1 chromosome, the blastic phase of CML is often associated with the acquisition of other chromosomal abnormalities, such as aneuploidy, which reflect the more malignant character of this phase of the disease. Double Ph^1 chromosomes also may be seen. Less than 5 percent of patients with clinically typical CML lack the Ph^1 chromosome. These patients are generally younger and have a more rapidly progressive clinical course. Although considered with CML, this disease is probably a distinct myeloproliferative disorder.

While the Ph^1 chromosome is a consistent feature of CML, there is evidence, using other cell markers such as G6PD, that the appearance of the chromosomal abnormality is not the primary event in the acquisition of the disease. Thus, some lymphocyte populations which appear by G6PD analysis to be clonally derived lack the Ph^1 chromosome. These and other results suggest a multistep pathogenesis in CML with the acquisition of the Ph^1 chromosome as a secondary event.

DIAGNOSIS CML which presents with splenomegaly, a markedly elevated white cell count, a low leukocyte alkaline phosphatase, and the Ph^1 chromosome is an easy diagnosis. Atypical presentations must be differentiated from leukemoid reactions associated with infections or neoplasms. In the latter, the leukocyte alkaline phosphatase is usually elevated and the Ph^1 chromosome is absent. A closely related myeloproliferative disorder is agnogenic myeloid metaplasia (AMM/MF) (see below). This disease usually presents with marked myelofibrosis and splenomegaly. The white blood cell count and platelet count may be elevated, but leukocyte alkaline phosphatase is normal or increased and the Ph^1 chromosome is absent. Among the myeloproliferative diseases, the serum vitamin B_{12} level cannot be used as a differential diagnostic test in patients with elevated white cell counts.

THERAPY Chronic phase CML can be controlled by a number of alkylating agents such as busulfan, cyclophosphamide, or melphalan. Splenic irradiation is not as effective as chemotherapy for control of the disease. The most commonly used drug is busulfan. It may be administered on an intermittent schedule or on a continuous daily basis with approximately the same results. The most serious compli-

TABLE 289-1 The myeloproliferative diseases

Disease	Hematocrit	White blood cell count	Platelet count	Splenomegaly	Leukocyte alkaline phosphatase	Marrow fibrosis	Ph^1 chromosome
CML	Normal or ↓	↑↑↑	↑ to ↓	+++	↓ to 0	±	+
PV	↑↑	↑	↑	+	↑↑	±	0
AMM/MF	↓	↑ to ↓	↑ to ↓	+++	↑ or normal	+++	0
ET	Normal	Normal	↑↑↑	+	↑ or normal	±	0

cation of busulfan therapy is prolonged myelosuppression. Occasionally, remission of the disease for periods in excess of 1 year may follow a single course of treatment. The principal side effects include increased skin pigmentation resembling adrenal insufficiency and, rarely, pulmonary or retroperitoneal fibrosis. An initial daily oral dose of 4 to 8 mg will reduce the white cell count to less than 20,000 per cubic millimeter in 2 to 3 weeks. The dose of busulfan should be reduced progressively, roughly in proportion to the reduction in white blood cell count. Patients achieve an excellent hematologic remission, with return of blood counts to normal and reduction in organomegaly. The Ph[1] chromosome remains, however. A true remission of the disease does not occur; rather, the proliferating granulocyte mass is reduced to the point where immature cells disappear from the peripheral blood. Furthermore, neither conventional therapy nor high-dose combination chemotherapy designed to eradicate the Ph[1]-positive clone significantly prolongs survival. Encouraging results with interferon have been reported, but more extensive trials with this or similar agents will be necessary.

Splenectomy has little place in the primary management of CML but may be reserved for those patients with evidence of hypersplenism or repeated painful splenic infarctions or for the rare instance in which prolonged thrombocytopenia follows busulfan therapy. Splenectomy in the chronic phase of CML does not prolong survival or delay the onset of blastic transformation.

Acceleration of the disease is reflected by progressive refractoriness to chemotherapy, increased leukocytosis with a larger proportion of immature forms, thrombocytosis, and increasing splenomegaly. Prior to blastic transformation, the drug hydroxyurea can effectively control the proliferative aspects of the disease. The dose ranges from 1 to 3 g per day by mouth. The blastic phase of CML is refractory to most drug regimens, but short-lived remissions in about 20 percent of cases have been obtained with the use of vincristine and prednisone or other intensive combination chemotherapy programs useful in the treatment of acute leukemia (see Chap. 292). There is a correlation between the appearance of TdT in the blast cells and the response to vincristine and prednisone, drugs commonly used for acute lymphoblastic leukemia in childhood. However, the correlation is not perfect, and therapy for the blastic phase should begin with vincristine and prednisone, regardless of the presence or absence of TdT or the morphology of the blasts. Hydroxyurea may be used here, as well, to suppress the proliferation of blasts; however, meaningful remissions are rarely, if ever, obtained and patients die of infection or bleeding. Symptomatic extramedullary myeloblastic tumors can be controlled with local radiation therapy.

It has been demonstrated that eradication of Ph[1]-positive cells can be achieved in the majority of chronic phase patients treated with intensive chemotherapy and radiation and transplanted with bone marrow from an identical twin or sibling compatible for human histocompatibility leukocyte antigens (HLA). Analysis of patients receiving bone marrow transplantation suggests that the best results are obtained in patients transplanted in chronic phase within the first year of diagnosis. Long-term disease-free survival in good-risk transplant patients is approximately 70 percent, although late relapses have been reported with reappearance of the Ph[1] chromosome. Progressively poorer results with higher relapse rates are obtained in patients when they are transplanted in the accelerated or blastic phase of the disease.

POLYCYTHEMIA VERA

DEFINITION AND ETIOLOGY Polycythemia vera (PV) is characterized by splenomegaly and an increased production of all myeloid elements; however, the disease is generally dominated by an elevated hemoglobin concentration. PV is gradual in onset and runs a chronic but usually slowly progressive course.

The disease generally begins in late middle life and is slightly more common in males. Only rarely is PV found in children or multiple members of a single family. The disease is relatively uncommon in Blacks and occurs with increased frequency in Jews of European extraction.

PATHOPHYSIOLOGY AND SYMPTOMATOLOGY None of the recognized physiologic mechanisms of increased red blood cell production is present in PV. The disease must be distinguished from secondary forms of polycythemia, in which an elevated hemoglobin concentration results from increased erythropoietin production. Secondary polycythemia may arise through hypoxia or occasionally may be found with certain neoplasms. PV is also distinct from spurious (relative) polycythemia, which results from a decrease in the plasma volume rather than a true increase in red blood cell mass. Also, secondary causes of polycythemia are not associated with splenic enlargement or increased leukocytes and platelets, which are typical of PV.

In PV there is a unique relationship of erythropoietin to red blood cell production. As opposed to the findings in secondary forms of polycythemia, urine and serum levels of erythropoietin in patients with PV are substantially reduced or absent. Presumably, erythropoietin production is suppressed by the elevated hemoglobin concentration, since phlebotomy results in a rise in both erythropoietin excretion and red blood cell production (provided that there is no deficiency in iron). This demonstrates the marrow's ability to respond to humoral regulation.

In cell culture, marrow from patients with PV forms colonies of hemoglobin-synthesizing cells in the absence of added erythropoietin. This is rarely the case with marrow cells from normal persons or from patients with secondary polycythemia. A reduced production of erythropoietin, the appearance of "endogenous" erythroid colonies in marrow cultures, and the clonal origin from the pluripotent hematopoietic stem cell indicate that hematopoiesis in PV is not regulated by the usual mechanisms.

PV produces symptoms associated with increased blood volume and blood viscosity. The hemoglobin concentration, hematocrit, and total blood volume may become markedly elevated, a consequence of the sharply increased red blood cell mass. The plasma volume is usually normal but may be increased. Associated with the expanded blood volume is a consistently elevated increase in cardiac output and a less uniform, but significant, increase in cardiac index. Reduction of the hematocrit and blood volume by phlebotomy leads to a reduction in the stroke volume and cardiac output in these patients and generally to an improvement in exercise tolerance. The increased cardiac output occurs in association with an increase in blood viscosity and, presumably, in vascular resistance associated with the elevated hematocrit.

Complaints related to the increased viscosity and/or decreased cerebral perfusion include headache, dizziness, vertigo, a sense of fullness of the head, rushing in the ears, visual alterations (scotomas, double vision, or blurred vision), tinnitus, syncope, and even chorea. Peripheral vascular symptoms of both arterial and venous insufficiency are common; in one large series, more than 35 percent of patients gave a history of some thrombotic or hemorrhagic event during the course of their disease. The risk of thrombosis may be increased by the accelerated atherosclerosis in this disease. Bleeding is common and comes most often from the nose or from peptic ulcer disease. Intramuscular hemorrhages and bruising also are seen. The tendency to increased bleeding may be due to the distended vasculature resulting from the increased blood volume. However, intrinsic platelet dysfunction also may contribute to bleeding, particularly from the gastrointestinal tract. The incidence of peptic ulcer disease is estimated to be four to five times higher in patients with PV than it is in the general population, although the reasons are unclear.

Late in the disease, the spleen may become greatly enlarged, producing symptoms of early satiety, a sense of abdominal fullness, and pleuritic chest or left upper quadrant pain secondary to capsular stretching or infarction. Pruritus, particularly after bathing, is reported frequently and may be disabling. Occasionally, urticaria is seen.

The increased cellular proliferation seen with PV results in hyperuricemia in 25 to 30 percent of patients and may be associated with formation of urate stones and uric acid nephropathy.

LABORATORY FINDINGS The most prominent laboratory feature is the elevated hemoglobin concentration. Unless altered by iron deficiency, the red blood cells are normochromic and normocytic. Polychromasia is frequently seen, and nucleated red blood cells may be found in the later stages of the disease. These findings represent cells released from extramedullary sites of hematopoiesis or reflect damage to marrow stroma due to fibrosis. The erythrocyte sedimentation rate is frequently very low (0 to 3 mm/h).

The white cell count is elevated in two-thirds of patients and is usually in the range of 15,000 to 25,000 per cubic millimeter but may be as high as 60,000 per cubic millimeter. An increase in the absolute basophil count (to more than 100 per cubic millimeter) is found in about 70 percent of patients. The leukocyte alkaline phosphatase is increased in more than 80 percent of cases. Serum vitamin B_{12} levels vary and are increased in about one-third of the patients; however, the binding capacity is increased in as many as 75 percent. In addition to increased transcobalamin I, transcobalamin III is also increased.

Thrombocytosis is seen in over half of all patients with PV. In vitro studies of platelet function demonstrate defective platelet adhesiveness and impaired secondary release of adenosine diphosphate (ADP) in response to epinephrine. These are poorly correlated with the bleeding time, and the contribution of these functional abnormalities to the thrombotic and hemorrhagic events in patients with PV is uncertain. Abnormal liver function studies, including an elevated alkaline phosphatase, may occur if there is massive hepatomegaly.

Splenomegaly occurs in 75 percent of patients but is usually not as marked as in CML or AMM/MF. Splenomegaly persists even when the elevated hemoglobin concentration has been reduced by repeated phlebotomies. Microscopic examination of the spleen reveals multiple foci of extramedullary hematopoiesis and fibrosis. The follicular pattern of the organ is retained, unlike the loss of normal architectural structure observed in CML. Foci of extramedullary hematopoiesis also may be found in the liver.

Bone marrow examination shows either erythroid hyperplasia or panhyperplasia without distinctive morphologic features. There is increased megakaryocyte nuclear ploidy in the face of thrombocytosis. This pattern of platelet regulation is different from that observed in the reactive thrombocytosis associated with inflammation or neoplasia, where megakaryocyte nuclear ploidy is inversely related to the peripheral platelet count. As PV progresses, fibrosis may appear in central areas of the marrow, and scanning techniques will demonstrate expansion of hematopoietic tissue to more peripheral skeletal sites.

Cytogenetic abnormalities, including trisomy 1, 8, or 9 and 20q−, have been reported in about 10 percent of untreated patients. Prior treatment with myelosuppressive agents or radioactive phosphorus (^{32}P) appears to increase the incidence of such abnormalities.

DIAGNOSIS The plethoric patient with pancytosis and splenomegaly, and without evidence of chronic cardiac or pulmonary disease, presents few diagnostic problems. However, it is more common to see patients with PV who have less than the full clinical disease or in whom an elevated hemoglobin or hematocrit has been discovered at the time of routine laboratory evaluation. Under these circumstances, it is important that the diagnosis of PV be made with certainty in order to direct therapeutic efforts appropriately.

First, there is little statistical likelihood that hematocrits consistently near or greater than 60 percent represent a simple decrease in plasma volume. When hematocrit levels are in the range of 50 to 55 percent, however, the likelihood of true erythrocytosis is reduced to about 50 percent and the red blood cell mass should be determined directly by isotope dilution using ^{51}Cr-labeled autologous red blood cells. While the plasma volume may be calculated indirectly from the red blood cell mass, it is preferable to measure this compartment independently using a second label. The results for red blood cell mass are best expressed as a function of the lean body mass, which may be estimated from the patient's height and weight. If the results of such a study are equivocal, the clinical findings must establish whether the patient has a true increase in red blood cell production or else the patient should be restudied at a later time.

The patient who presents with a hematocrit or hemoglobin in the high normal range, microcytosis, leukocytosis, and iron deficiency should be considered as possibly having PV. Evaluation of red and white blood cell morphology, basophil count, and platelet morphology should be carried out to make certain that this is not a patient with PV who has bled.

While measurements of red blood cell mass distinguish spurious from true erythrocytosis, the results do not distinguish between the various forms of polycythemia. If the diagnosis is uncertain, additional indexes which may be helpful include the absolute basophil count, the leukocyte alkaline phosphatase score, and results of radioisotope scanning to quantitate spleen size. This last is particularly useful in obese individuals or patients in whom the spleen is enlarged but not palpable.

If the diagnosis of PV remains obscure, an intravenous pyelogram or abdominal CT scan should be obtained to exclude hypernephroma or other renal pathology which might result in increased erythropoietin production. Arterial blood gas measurements should be obtained, including carboxyhemoglobin levels if the patient is a smoker. Perhaps 20 percent of patients with PV may have a hemoglobin oxygen saturation below 92 percent, but almost all will have a saturation equal to or greater than 88 percent. This modest impairment of oxygen loading may be due to decreased diffusing capacity of the lung, possibly triggered by repeated episodes of thromboembolism or thrombosis in situ.

When the diagnosis is not clear following routine investigation, measurement of serum levels or of urinary excretion of erythropoietin may be helpful. Patients with PV excrete little or no measurable erythropoietin, whereas patients with secondary forms of polycythemia excrete at least normal and frequently elevated amounts. Measurements of serum erythropoietin may be performed using a bioassay or a radioimmunoassay. Other types of immunologic assays are not helpful. In vitro growth characteristics of bone marrow cells from patients with PV suggest that such determinations may be useful in diagnosis, but experience with these tests is limited.

COURSE AND PROGNOSIS The course of PV has been a subject of disagreement, some observers believing that later complications are hastened by myelosuppressive therapy. About 15 to 20 percent of patients will progress to marrow fibrosis, marked splenomegaly, and anemia; one view holds that if patients live long enough, all will enter this so-called spent phase of the disease. However, the majority of patients die of vascular complications of their disease or of unrelated causes. Although the incidence is low, there is a statistically significant association of second hematologic neoplasms in patients with PV; these include lymphocytic and histiocytic lymphomas and multiple myeloma. Of patients with PV, 1 to 2 percent experience transformation into acute leukemia even without prior radiation or chemotherapy.

THERAPY Optimal therapy of PV remains unsettled. The median survival has been extended to 10 to 12 years with phlebotomy alone, while patients receiving no therapy at all survive only 2 years. However, neither myelosuppressive therapy nor phlebotomy holds a clear advantage for survival. For many years after its introduction in 1940, ^{32}P was the therapy of choice. However, a retrospective analysis of a large number of cases suggested that ^{32}P increased the incidence of acute leukemia to nearly 15 percent while not clearly enhancing survival over other forms of therapy. In order to resolve the major questions regarding the most effective therapy, the incidence of complicating factors, and the prognostic implication of certain features such as thrombocytosis or cytogenetic abnormalities, the International

Polycythemia Vera Study Group was established. This group prospectively assigned patients who met strict diagnostic criteria into three treatment programs at random: ^{32}P therapy augmented by phlebotomy, myelosuppressive therapy plus phlebotomy, and phlebotomy alone. Analysis of the survival curves demonstrated similar survivals for the various treatment groups until the seventh year after randomization. At that point, patients treated with alkylating agents had poorer survival. The findings indicated that those patients in the phlebotomy-only group suffered from increased risk of death due to hemorrhage or thrombosis within the first four years, while leukemia and other neoplasms were more prevalent later in the course of the patients treated with chemotherapy or ^{32}P. However, a simultaneous European cooperative therapy trial did not demonstrate increased leukemia in patients treated with chemotherapy, and the survival in those patients was superior to that of patients treated with phlebotomy alone.

Despite the controversy, certain therapeutic tenets meet with agreement. Phlebotomy is safe, can be done repeatedly, and is preferred in individuals with mild disease, young patients, or those with polycythemia of uncertain etiology. Myelosuppression is best in patients with extreme symptomatic thrombocytosis, rapidly enlarging spleen, or symptoms of hypermetabolism. It may also spare elderly patients the symptoms associated with phlebotomy. Regardless of eventual decisions involving therapy, phlebotomy should be used initially to reduce the red blood cell mass and blood volume. The end point of phlebotomy therapy should be a hematocrit or hemoglobin value in the low-normal range. This form of treatment may lead to prolonged clinical remission. Iron should not be given if phlebotomy is the primary mode of therapy. Phlebotomy is especially important if a patient with PV must undergo emergency surgery, since intra- and postoperative morbidity and mortality are four to five times greater in uncontrolled as opposed to controlled (phlebotomized) patients. Under these circumstances, the red blood cell mass should be reduced acutely by exchange phlebotomies and the blood replaced with a suitable plasma expander. This will prevent the vascular instability associated with too rapid a reduction in total blood volume.

Marrow suppression may be achieved by radiation or chemotherapy. The administration of ^{32}P is easy, provides long, trouble-free remissions in most cases, and successfully reduces the morbidity associated with the disease. The regimen recommended by the International Polycythemia Vera Study Group consists of the intravenous administration initially of 85.2 MBq of ^{32}P per square meter of body surface area. The patient is then followed for a period of 3 months and retreated at that time, as needed, with a dose 25 percent greater than that given originally. This program may be repeated 3 months later but is rarely required. Remissions may last 6 to 24 months, during which time the patient is often symptom-free. This ^{32}P therapy may be repeated if relapse occurs. Exposure to ^{32}P increases the incidence of leukemia in patients with PV, and the risk of leukemic transformation may be related to the cumulative dose of isotope.

Suppression of marrow function with chemotherapy has been common during the last 15 years. Effective drugs include melphalan, busulfan, and chlorambucil. Busulfan, in doses of 4 to 6 mg per day orally, reduces the white blood cell and platelet counts, but suppression may be unpredictable and prolonged and the drug is relatively less effective in suppressing erythropoiesis. Moreover, continued use of this drug may lead to pulmonary fibrosis and a syndrome resembling adrenal insufficiency. Chlorambucil, originally employed in the prospective treatment trial by the International Polycythemia Vera Study Group, resulted in a high incidence (over 10 percent) of acute leukemia, and the study group has recommended against the routine use of this or other alkylating agents in this disease. Currently, no form of treatment is clearly better than any other in terms of patient survival, but management with ^{32}P may be simpler. Hydroxyurea, a drug active in the DNA synthetic phase of the cell cycle and not known to be leukemogenic, is currently being evaluated. Hydroxyurea given orally in doses of 1 to 3 g per day may control symptoms of hypermetabolism and the elevated leukocyte and platelet counts, but phlebotomy is generally required for adequate control of the red cell mass.

Other symptoms associated with PV may be managed conservatively. In the case of pruritus, cyproheptadine, 12 to 16 mg per day, may be effective. Allopurinol in doses of 300 mg per day will reduce serum uric acid. Symptomatic splenomegaly is usually improved with treatment, although splenectomy may be indicated in rare instances.

AGNOGENIC MYELOID METAPLASIA/MYELOFIBROSIS

DEFINITION AND ETIOLOGY AMM/MF is characterized by the tendency of the neoplastic stem cells to lodge and grow in multiple sites outside the marrow. Typically, there is progressive splenomegaly, the gradual replacement of marrow elements by fibrosis, progressive anemia, and variable changes in the number of granulocytes and platelets. The disease begins in late middle life and is gradual in onset, chronic, and progressive. Males and females are equally involved, and there is only rare familial occurrence.

While erythrocytes, granulocytes, and platelets are members of a single neoplastic clone, the fibrosis is reactive and not part of the abnormal clone. AMM is an integral part of the disease and is seen early in its course. There is no evidence that AMM arises in compensation for replacement of the marrow by fibrous tissue.

PATHOPHYSIOLOGY AND SYMPTOMATOLOGY AMM/MF presents most commonly with vague constitutional symptoms associated with anemia, such as fatigue, weakness, and anorexia, or with splenomegaly. An enlarged spleen is seen in virtually all patients; however, the disease progresses slowly and splenomegaly may be present for years prior to diagnosis. The enlargement may become so extensive as to produce symptoms of pain, abdominal fullness, and dyspnea. Hepatomegaly occurs in more than 50 percent of patients and also may become massive, but enlargement of the liver due to AMM does not occur in the absence of splenomegaly. Petechiae are found in 20 percent of patients as a result of thrombocytopenia, and a history of bleeding is obtained in 10 percent. Less common findings include lymphadenopathy, jaundice, ascites, and bone pain. Weight loss, fever, sweating, and extremity pain may occur occasionally and are associated with a hypermetabolic state. The increased cellular turnover results in hyperuricemia in 25 to 30 percent of patients.

LABORATORY FINDINGS The blood counts of patients with AMM/MF are variable. Mild anemia is observed in over one-half of the patients at the time of diagnosis and progresses during the course of the disease. Eventually, almost all patients become anemic. The recognized mechanisms leading to anemia include ineffective erythropoiesis, increased splenic pooling of red cells, and a decrease in red blood cell survival. Low serum folate and megaloblastic maturation may contribute. The peripheral blood smear usually shows dramatic changes in red cell and platelet morphology. Basophilic stippling is prominent and bizarre red cell shapes, including teardrop poikilocytes, fragmented cells, and nucleated red cells, are common, as are giant platelet forms.

An elevation in the white blood cell count is found in about 50 percent of patients, and values as high as 50,000 per cubic millimeter may be seen. However, 20 percent of patients are leukopenic, with white blood cell counts less than 4000 per cubic millimeter. Generally, there is a shift toward immature forms in granulocyte maturation, and circulating blast forms may be found. The appearance of these cells does not imply a bad prognosis. An increase in the absolute basophil count may be observed in 25 percent of patients. The leukocyte alkaline phosphatase activity is elevated in about half the patients, the remainder being equally distributed between having normal or low values. Serum vitamin B_{12} levels are normal or slightly elevated, as are vitamin B_{12}-binding proteins. These values usually do not approach those seen with CML.

A normal or elevated platelet count is frequently found early in the course of the disease, but thrombocytopenia eventually develops in most patients, owing to ineffective production and splenic pooling. The circulating platelets vary considerably in size and shape, and megakaryocyte nuclei may be found on the peripheral blood smear. In vitro studies of platelet function reflect defective platelet adhesiveness and impaired secondary release of ADP in response to epinephrine. Abnormal liver function tests, including elevated bilirubin and alkaline phosphatase, may be associated with massive hepatomegaly.

The spleen may become massive. There are multiple foci of extramedullary hematopoiesis on pathologic examination, but the normal follicular architecture of the spleen is maintained. Other organs which may be involved include the kidneys, lymph nodes, adrenal glands, and lungs. Bone marrow examination early in the course of the disease reveals a hypercellular marrow in about 20 percent of patients and may be difficult to distinguish from PV. Special stains of the marrow reveal increased reticulin deposition. However, a minority of patients develops obvious patchy collagen fibrosis separating areas of hyperplastic marrow, or diffuse fibrosis with osteosclerosis. Megakaryocytes may be preserved remarkably well in the areas of fibrosis. One hypothesis to account for the marrow fibrosis is that neoplastic megakaryoblasts and megakaryocytes release growth factors, such as PDGF, which stimulate fibroblasts or other connective tissue cells to synthesize collagen or reticulin. This is also consistent with the fact that successful bone marrow transplantation leads to the reversal of established fibrosis.

The fibrosis and osteosclerosis of the marrow generally correlate with one another and also with the degree of splenomegaly. However, there is no clear relationship between the histopathology of the marrow and the peripheral blood counts. In 40 to 50 percent of patients, the appearance of marrow sclerosis is reflected on x-ray examination by increased bone density involving particularly the axial skeleton and proximal long bones. These x-ray changes result from thickened cortical bone and the loss of medullary spaces due to increased and thickened bony trabeculae.

No unique cytogenetic abnormalities have been described in AMM/MF; however, certain nonrandom abnormalities, including monosomy 7 and trisomy 9, have been found. Reports of the Ph^1 chromosome in this disorder probably reflect examples of atypical CML.

DIAGNOSIS A bone marrow biopsy is essential to the evaluation of this disease, and without it the diagnosis cannot be made with certainty. This disorder may be difficult to distinguish from other myeloproliferative diseases.

In CML the white blood cell count is usually greater than 20,000 per cubic millimeter, while in AMM/MF it is generally 10,000 to 20,000 per cubic millimeter. Leukocyte alkaline phosphatase is usually lower in CML, and this determination may be useful in distinguishing between the two disorders. Fibrosis of the marrow is found in only 10 to 15 percent of patients with CML and is usually present only as a preterminal event; osteosclerosis is almost never seen. In the absence of the Ph^1 chromosome, however, the distinction between these diseases is occasionally difficult.

The separation of PV and essential thrombocytosis (ET) from AMM/MF occasionally is troublesome because all may present with thrombocytosis, splenomegaly, leukocytosis, and anemia. However, ET generally is not associated with advanced fibrosis. The most difficult distinction is between AMM/MF and the late stages of PV, and attempts to separate them are probably unwarranted. Approximately 15 to 25 percent of patients with PV progress to advanced marrow fibrosis and marked splenomegaly. It is impossible to be certain that a patient with typical AMM/MF did not initially have PV. Postpolycythemia myeloid metaplasia with myelofibrosis has a poorer prognosis.

Secondary causes of myelofibrosis include metastatic carcinoma, leukemia and lymphomas, tuberculosis, Gaucher's disease, Paget's disease, and exposure to toxins such as benzene or to x-rays. These associations are usually not difficult to distinguish from AMM/MF.

THERAPY There is no definitive therapy for this disorder, and no treatment has been shown to affect life span favorably. Anemia is treated with transfusions as required. Androgens may be administered to improve the anemia, although they are helpful in less than half of the cases. Oxymetholone (2 to 4 mg/kg per day) or fluoxymesterone may be given, particularly if there is marked ineffective erythropoiesis. Corticosteroids may enhance the response to androgens but alone are not helpful. Myelosuppressive therapy is only occasionally indicated, but it may be used to control painful splenomegaly or marked thrombocytosis. Chlorambucil or melphalan may be employed, but other blood elements may be depressed and the period of remission is relatively short (4 to 5 months). External radiation to the spleen will reduce its size, but the effects are transient and therapy may lead to severe pancytopenia. Allopurinol may be given to reduce a high uric acid level.

The role of splenectomy in the treatment of AMM/MF is controversial. Late in the course of the disease the hazards of removing a massively enlarged organ are considerable, and intraoperative mortality and postoperative complications, particularly thrombosis and infection, are frequent. Some clinicians have advocated early removal of the spleen, as soon as the diagnosis is made, believing that this will reduce later complications and make management easier. This is unlikely. The only clear indications for splenectomy are hemolysis, severe thrombocytopenia, and intractable symptoms related to spleen size.

COURSE AND PROGNOSIS AMM/MF generally follows a prolonged course, with a median survival of 4 to 5 years from the time of diagnosis; 25 percent of patients may live 15 years. Anemia occurs eventually in most patients, and many will require transfusions. Complicating features of the disease include gout or other problems related to hyperuricemia and symptoms related to the enlarging spleen. Portal hypertension may be seen due to hepatic fibrosis, hepatic vein thrombosis, or the markedly increased blood flow through the spleen. Clinically evident bleeding occurs in about 25 percent, and it is important for thrombocytopenic patients to avoid drugs such as aspirin or nonsteroidal anti-inflammatory agents which further impair platelet function. While the degree of splenomegaly appears to be of no prognostic importance, a platelet count of less than 100,000 per cubic millimeter, hemoglobin of less than 10 g/dL, and hepatomegaly are associated with poorer survival.

The major causes of death include infection, congestive heart failure, renal failure, portal hypertension, and hemorrhage. Transformation to acute leukemia occurs in 5 to 10 percent of patients and may be related to radiation or chemotherapy. A particularly fulminant variant of AMM/MF, known as acute myelofibrosis, is characterized by rapid progression of fibrosis and pancytopenia without splenic enlargement. Death due to marrow failure usually occurs within 1 year of diagnosis. This disorder is now more correctly recognized as acute megakaryoblastic leukemia.

ESSENTIAL THROMBOCYTOSIS

DEFINITION AND ETIOLOGY Essential thrombocytosis (ET) is dominated clinically by a markedly elevated platelet count which is invariably above 400,000 per cubic millimeter and which may reach levels of 3 to 4 million per cubic millimeter. The disease closely resembles PV and AMM/MF. Although an elevated platelet count is the dominant laboratory feature, all cell lines are involved in the expansion of the neoplastic clone.

As opposed to secondary forms of thrombocytosis, which arise in response to inflammation, acute bleeding, iron deficiency, or neoplasms, ET represents the overproduction of platelets in the absence of a recognizable stimulus. However, no specific etiologic agent has been implicated. In cultures of bone marrow cells from patients with

ET, colonies of megakaryocytes from megakaryocytic progenitors often form in the absence of added stimulus. This does not happen with marrow cell cultures from normal individuals or patients with secondary thrombocytosis.

PATHOPHYSIOLOGY AND SYMPTOMATOLOGY Symptoms associated with ET are linked to the platelet dysfunction and perhaps to platelet aggregation in the microvasculature of the central nervous system. Patients with ET may present with erythromelalgia, venous or arterial thromboses, or spontaneous bleeding. This may be seen as easy bruisability, unusual bleeding following minor dental procedures or other surgery, or large-vessel bleeding into soft tissues or muscles in the absence of a history of trauma. The first clue may be such a hemorrhagic or thrombotic episode. Transient ischemic attacks or even frank strokes may occur in patients with markedly elevated platelet counts. In general, there is a correlation between symptomatology and platelet counts in patients with this disease. However, the correlation is imperfect and individual patients will manifest symptoms at different platelet levels.

LABORATORY FINDINGS The most prominent laboratory feature is the elevated platelet count. Examination of the peripheral blood smear reveals platelets of markedly different morphology with many large forms and forms which appear hypogranular. In vitro platelet function tests typically reveal an abnormality in platelet aggregation in response to epinephrine, collagen, or ADP. The epinephrine defect is the most characteristic. These in vitro aggregation abnormalities do not correlate with the history of bleeding or thrombosis or with a prolonged bleeding time. Splenomegaly is seen in a large number of patients with this disease but is generally modest, and the spleen does not achieve the size observed in CML or AMM/MF. Bone marrow examination reveals large numbers of hyperploid megakaryocytes and, with disease progression, there may be evidence of fibrosis. This is rarely as marked as in AMM/MF.

DIAGNOSIS A markedly elevated platelet count with typical platelet morphology in the absence of a cause for secondary thrombocytosis is generally sufficient to make the diagnosis. Confirmation may be obtained by in vitro platelet function tests, measurement of bleeding time, or the association of splenomegaly. Cytogenetic abnormalities are uncommon with this disease. A useful feature is the matching of megakaryocyte size to platelet number on examination of a marrow aspirate and biopsy. Secondary thrombocytosis is associated with increased numbers of megakaryocytes which are of generally small diameter and lower ploidy. In ET, the elevated platelet number is associated with increased numbers of large, hyperploid megakaryocytes.

COURSE AND PROGNOSIS The median survival of patients with ET is not well-defined. A prospective study evaluating therapy in this disease is being conducted by the Polycythemia Vera Study Group. It is anticipated that survival will be at least as good as for those patients with PV and possibly better. Complications of the disease, such as hemorrhage or fatal thrombosis, represent the terminal event in the majority of cases. In less than 10 percent of cases does the disease transform to a more aggressive or frankly leukemic phase. If this does occur, aggressive chemotherapy is rarely effective.

THERAPY The indications for therapy in ET are unsettled and the effect of therapy in prolonging survival has not been quantitated. However, there is agreement that patients with symptomatic thrombocytosis who have had bleeding or thrombotic episodes should be treated. Previous therapy has employed alkylating agents such as busulfan or chlorambucil. However, because of the concern that these drugs may result in or enhance the likelihood of leukemic transformation, therapy with hydroxyurea is being evaluated. The available data suggest good control of the disease, but the overall effect on survival cannot be judged as yet. If patients are symptomatic at a particular platelet count, their counts should be maintained well below that level through the use of myelosuppression. Alkylating agents or ^{32}P may be used if hydroxyurea becomes ineffective. Treatment of acute events such as thrombosis or hemorrhage in an uncontrolled or previously undiagnosed patient with ET should be by emergent plateletpheresis. Although it appears anomalous, the use of aspirin and dipyridamole may prove useful in preventing symptoms in some patients with ET.

REFERENCES

Adamson JW, Fialkow PJ: Pathogenesis of the myeloproliferative syndromes. Brit J Haematol 38:299, 1978

Berk PD et al: Increased incidence of acute leukemia in polycythemia vera associated with chlorambucil therapy. N Engl J Med 304:441, 1981

Champlin RE, Golde DW: Chronic myelogenous leukemia (CML): Recent advances. Blood 65:1039, 1985

Golde DW et al: Polycythemia: Mechanisms and management. Ann Intern Med 95:71, 1981

Jacobson RJ et al: Agnogenic myeloid metaplasia: A clonal proliferation of hematopoietic stem cells with secondary myelofibrosis. Blood 51:189, 1978

Polycythemia vera: An update I and II. In *Seminars in Hematology*, vol. 23, PA Miescher, ER Jaffe (eds). Orlando, Grune & Stratton, Nos. 2 (April) and 3 (July), 1986

Silverstein MK: Primary thrombocythemia, in *Hematology*, WJ Williams et al (eds). New York, McGraw-Hill, 1983, pp 218–222

Stam K et al: Evidence of a new chimeric *bcr/abl* mRNA in patients with chronic myelocytic leukemia and the Philadelphia chromosome. N Engl J Med 313:1429, 1985

Talpaz M et al: Hematologic remission and cytogenetic improvement induced by recombinant human interferon alpha-a in chronic myelogenous leukemia. N Engl J Med 314:1065, 1986

Thomas ED et al: Marrow transplantation for the treatment of chronic myelogenous leukemia. Ann Intern Med 104:155, 1986

290 BONE MARROW FAILURE: APLASTIC ANEMIA AND OTHER PRIMARY BONE MARROW DISORDERS

JOEL M. RAPPEPORT / H. FRANKLIN BUNN

An important group of anemias is caused by primary disorders of the bone marrow which impair the formation of erythropoietic precursors. The term *aplastic anemia* should be restricted to conditions in which an acellular or markedly hypocellular bone marrow results in pancytopenia (anemia, neutropenia, and thrombocytopenia). Rare patients develop selective aplasia of only erythroid cells (*pure red blood cell aplasia*). Alternatively, in *myelophthisic anemia,* erythropoiesis is suppressed because the marrow is infiltrated with tumor, granulomas, or fibrosis. The pathophysiology, differential diagnosis, and treatment of these entities are discussed in this chapter.

APLASTIC ANEMIA

ETIOLOGY Aplastic anemia is thought to be due to injury or destruction of a common pluripotential stem cell affecting all subsequent cell populations. The diverse factors associated with the development of aplastic anemia are listed in Table 290-1. In approximately half of the cases of aplastic anemia in the United States, no etiologic agent is identifiable, although this figure may vary with the vigor with which an agent is sought. In other areas of the world where a larger percentage of the population may be exposed to toxins such as insecticides and benzenes in uncontrolled dose, the percentage of idiopathic cases is probably smaller.

Congenital causes Fanconi's anemia, the most common type of constitutional aplastic anemia, is an autosomal recessively inherited disease usually appearing in childhood. This disorder is often associated with multiple congenital somatic anomalies, including hypoplasia or other malformations of the kidney, hyperpigmentation of the skin, and bony abnormalities, particularly hypoplastic or absent thumbs or radii. Many patients have chromosomal abnormalities owing to a defect in DNA repair. Patients who survive the complications of progressive marrow failure are at high risk of developing leukemia. Other syndromes associated with bone marrow failure include dyskeratosis congenita as well as constitutional predisposition to aplasia without the stigmata of Fanconi's anemia.

Immune causes A number of clinical observations have led to the concept that a significant proportion of cases of aplastic anemia may be mediated by immunologic mechanisms. These include autologous recovery following immunosuppressive preparation for marrow grafting, failure of hematopoietic reconstitution in some patients following marrow transplantation from identical twin donors in the absence of immunosuppression, and the identification of antibodies which inhibit the growth of hematopoietic cells in culture. A variety of in vitro culture techniques have also supported the concept of a cellular autoimmune process in some patients with aplasia. However, in any given case the identification of an immune process may be difficult.

Drugs and toxins Multiple and seemingly unrelated drugs and chemical agents have been incriminated as etiologic agents in aplastic anemia. The association varies from a predictable dose-related aplasia to idiosyncratic reactions unrelated to dose.

The agents which in an adequate dose will predictably produce bone marrow depression are the antineoplastic and immunosuppressive drugs along with ionizing radiation. The degree of aplasia is dose related but may vary from individual to individual. These drugs include folic acid antagonists, alkylating agents, the anthracyclines, the nitrosoureas as well as purine and pyrimidine analogues. The effects of combination chemotherapy may be additive. Withdrawal of the drug usually permits recovery of the marrow elements, although irreversible aplasia is occasionally noted. Marrow aplasia may also be induced by therapeutic x-rays or, less commonly, by acute exposure from a laboratory or industrial accident. The severity of aplasia is dependent upon the dose and rate of the exposure as well as the extent of marrow irradiated.

Benzene derivatives have been associated with multiple hematologic abnormalities including aplastic anemia. Safety regulations in the United States control industrial exposure but not the domestic use of benzene-containing products. Benzene-induced marrow aplasia may be reversible, although mild abnormalities such as macrocytosis may persist.

Chloramphenicol, a commonly used broad-spectrum antibiotic, is associated with two forms of bone marrow toxicity. The more common effect upon the bone marrow is a reversible dose-related suppression of erythroid and, on occasion, granulocytic and megakaryocytic precursors. This condition is characterized by a transient anemia, associated with a drop in reticulocytes and elevation of serum iron. The bone marrow is normocellular with vacuolization of the cytoplasm of early erythroid and occasionally granulocytic precursors. This bone marrow suppression is related to the dose and duration of administration of chloramphenicol. Similar features are seen much more commonly in some patients who have ingested large amounts of alcohol.

The more serious form of bone marrow failure associated with chloramphenicol is an "idiosyncratic" reaction. This nitrobenzene compound has been the single most commonly incriminated drug in cases of aplastic anemia. These patients develop severe pancytopenia and often irreversible, fatal marrow aplasia. This complication occurs in approximately 1 in 50,000 patients who take the drug. The development of aplastic anemia seems to be unrelated to dose or duration of administration. Marrow aplasia cannot be anticipated or prevented by hematologic monitoring, since it may appear long after cessation of the drug. Unfortunately, many cases of fatal aplastic anemia have occurred in patients who received chloramphenicol for trivial or dubious reasons. Therefore, this antibiotic should not be used when there are reasonable alternatives.

Other unrelated chemicals and drugs may be responsible for the development of aplastic anemia. These agents can be placed into two classes: those in which a number of associations have been reported and, therefore, a definite toxic potential has been established, and those in which only a few reported cases exist and, therefore, only a possibility of toxic potential exists at present. The establishment of these relationships is often further confused by the fact that many of the patients have taken multiple drugs. Those agents in which a definite potential toxicity exists are shown in Table 290-1.

Infectious hepatitis A number of cases of aplastic anemia have been reported following infectious hepatitis. The antecedent hepatitis is not distinguished by its severity, and the aplastic anemia commonly appears as the hepatitis resolves. Aplasia has usually followed non-A, non-B hepatitis but on occasion has been associated with types A and B. The aplasia tends to be severe and frequently has a fatal outcome. Other viruses, including Epstein-Barr virus, have been implicated in aplastic anemia. Many cases of so-called "idiopathic aplastic anemia" are preceded by a benign-appearing viral respiratory illness. Parvovirus selectively infects erythroblasts and therefore acutely aggravates anemia in patients with hemolysis (Chap. 287).

Aplastic anemia has also been reported in association with a number of other illnesses (Table 290-1). The clinical and laboratory findings associated with paroxysmal nocturnal hemoglobinuria may accompany or precede the development of aplasia. Aplastic anemia that develops during pregnancy may remit following delivery of the fetus.

TABLE 290-1 Causes of pancytopenia

I Aplastic anemia
- *A* Idiopathic anemias
- *B* Constitutional anemias (Fanconi's anemia)
- *C* Chemical and physical agents
  - *1* Dose-related: benzene, ionizing irradiation, alkylating agents, antimetabolites (folic acid antagonists, purine and pyrimidine analogues), mitotic inhibitors, anthracyclines, inorganic arsenicals
  - *2* Idiosyncratic: chloramphenicol, phenylbutazone, sulfa drugs, methylphenylethylhydantoin, gold compounds, organic arsenicals, insecticides
- *D* Immunologically mediated aplasia
- *E* Other associations: hepatitis, other viral infections, systemic lupus erythematosus, diffuse eosinophilic faciitis

II Pancytopenia with normal or increased bone marrow cellularity
- *A* Myelodysplastic syndromes (Chap. 292)
- *B* Hypersplenism (Chap. 55)
- *C* Vitamin B_{12} and folate deficiencies (Chap. 285)

III Paroxysmal nocturnal hemoglobinuria (Chap. 287)

IV Bone marrow replacement
- *A* Hematologic malignancies (Chaps. 292 to 294)
- *B* Nonhematologic metastatic tumor
- *C* Storage cell disorders (Chap. 316)
- *D* Osteopetrosis (Chap. 339)
- *E* Myelofibrosis (Chap. 289)

CLINICAL MANIFESTATIONS The onset of aplastic anemia is usually insidious. Initial presenting symptoms include mild progressive weakness and fatigue attributable to the anemia and/or hemorrhage from the skin, nose, gums, vagina, or gastrointestinal tract due to the thrombocytopenia. The bleeding is usually mild, but occasionally retinal or central nervous system hemorrhage may be the initial mode of presentation. Although the patient may be severely neutropenic, it is less common for the initial presentation to be a bacterial infection.

Physical examination generally reveals pallor. Petechiae or ecchymoses may be noted in the skin, mucous membranes, the conjunctivae, and fundi. Lymphadenopathy and hepatosplenomegaly are notably absent. Fever may be present, but despite the presence of an infection, the usual signs of inflammation may be absent because of neutropenia.

The *course* of the disease is generally determined by the severity of the aplasia, rather than by the etiology. Mild disease can progress to a more severe disorder. Conversely, complete recovery or partial recovery of one or more cell lines may develop. It is important to obtain an accurate assessment of the degree of aplasia. Severe aplasia is defined as marked pancytopenia with at least two of the following criteria: granulocytes fewer than 500 per cubic millimeter, platelets fewer than 20,000 per cubic millimeter, or anemia with corrected reticulocyte count less than 1 percent. The bone marrow is markedly hypoplastic and depleted of hematopoietic cells. Patients with severe disease have a high risk of dying from bleeding and/or infections in a matter of months, while patients with a milder form of the disease may live for years. The clinical course of the disease is affected primarily by infections and by the nature and location of bleeding. Although infections may not dominate the clinical picture initially, they assume greater importance with the passage of time. Because of the need for multiple red blood cell and platelet transfusions, over a period of time one may encounter the sequelae of hemosiderosis and/or hepatitis. Other clinical manifestations may be due to side effects from the administration of corticosteriods and androgens. Even those patients who recover may have mild thrombocytopenia and persistent macrocytosis for many years.

LABORATORY DIAGNOSIS The diagnosis of aplastic anemia and the assessment of its relative severity depend upon a thorough laboratory evaluation. The peripheral blood usually shows pancytopenia. The absolute granulocyte count is low, or becomes progressively depressed during the illness. The red blood cells are normochromic and normocytic or mildly macrocytic reflecting stress erythropoiesis, and the reticulocyte count is very low or zero. Since the incidence of serious bleeding and/or infection correlates with the degree of thrombocytopenia or neutropenia, these values must be determined initially and followed serially. A bone marrow aspirate may yield a "dry tap," but a bone marrow biopsy will reveal a severely hypocellular or aplastic marrow with replacement by fat. There is usually a severe depression of megakaryocytes and myeloid cells and a marked but relatively less severe depression of the erythroid precursors.

The serum iron concentration is elevated, and the iron-binding capacity is normal. There is no evidence of increased red blood cell destruction. As predicted from the nature of this disease, plasma iron clearance is prolonged, and incorporation of iron into red blood cells is markedly decreased.

DIFFERENTIAL DIAGNOSIS The diagnosis of aplastic anemia implies the exclusion of the other causes of pancytopenia that are listed in Table 290-1. Splenomegaly and/or lymphadenopathy argue strongly against aplastic anemia. Malignant and nonmalignant invasion of the bone marrow must be excluded by microscopic examination of the marrow. Paroxysmal nocturnal hemoglobinuria and systemic lupus erythematosus should be ruled out by appropriate tests including the sugar water and acid hemolysis tests. Vitamin B_{12} and folate deficiencies can be excluded by serum assays and morphologic changes. Pancytopenia rarely may be secondary to various infections. Before aplastic anemia can be classified as idiopathic, a careful history must exclude exposure to all known and suspected agents. In our complex society, all patients are exposed to potentially toxic agents in their environment. Nevertheless this difficulty should not discourage a careful and extensive search for a cause.

TREATMENT The management of aplastic anemia has become one of the most challenging aspects of modern medicine, requiring a diligent multidisciplinary team of care givers in a well-equipped tertiary care center. For patients with mild aplasia, every effort should be made to do as little as possible except to remove possible etiologic agents in expectation of spontaneous recovery. As noted below, androgens may be of value in mild aplasia. Patients with severe aplasia should be considered for a bone marrow transplantation, if a suitable donor is available. The efficacy of this treatment with complete correction of the hematopoietic defect has been most clearly demonstrated in younger patients (Chap. 291).

Supportive care Regardless of the therapy chosen, the mainstay of treatment is good supportive care. The first and most immediate step is the removal of any suspected etiologic agent. If the disease is mild at presentation, no further supportive care need be instituted, unless there is a subsequent further deterioration. If a severe neutropenia exists (polymorphonuclear leukocytes fewer than 500 per cubic millimeter), the patient should be shielded from potential infections. Prophylactic systemic antibiotics should not be utilized. Intramuscular injections should be minimized and, if necessary, should be administered with care. Established infections should be treated vigorously with specific antibiotics, and fever of undetermined etiology may, after appropriate evaluation, call for broad-spectrum antibiotic coverage until a specific diagnosis is established. Menstruating females should be placed on suppressive doses of birth control pills.

TRANSFUSIONS These should be used *judiciously* and restricted to appropriate component therapy, since future therapy and ultimate survival may be affected by transfusions. Red blood cells should be administered to maintain the well-being of the patient rather than to establish a certain hemoglobin level. Transfusions pose significant risks such as risk of hepatitis, hemosiderosis, and sensitization to both red blood cell antigens and transplantation antigens. Platelet transfusions should be administered in the face of serious hemorrhage. Some groups employ prophylactic transfusions when the platelet count is lower than 20,000 per cubic millimeter. Others fearful of the development of resistance to future transfusions administer platelets only when faced with hemorrhage. Responses to platelet transfusions may be blunted by the presence of infection. Over a period of time many patients will develop immune resistance to subsequent transfusion at which time HLA-compatible platelet transfusions may be useful (Chap. 282). Should a bone marrow transplant be considered, family members should be avoided as a source of blood products, since the patient may develop antibodies to minor transplantation antigens. Leukocyte transfusions are not administered prophylactically. However, white blood cell infusions may be of value in patients with documented gram-negative infections and severe neutropenia who have failed to respond to antimicrobial therapy.

Marrow-stimulating agents Although patients with mild aplasia sometimes respond to androgens, and a few appear to be androgen-dependent, those with severe aplasia are unresponsive. Patients with mild aplasia should be treated with androgens as the initial mode of therapy. The most widely used drugs at present are oxymetholone, fluoxymesterone, and nandrolone decanoate. Responses may occur 3 to 6 months after the initiation of therapy.

Immunosuppressive agents Increasing clinical and laboratory evidence suggests that 40 to 50 percent of patients will have a complete or partial response to immunosuppressive therapy. The specificity and mechanism of this therapy is as yet undefined. The most commonly administered therapy is animal antiserums directed against human lymphocytes and thymocytes. The effectiveness as well as the dose and duration of administration of these heterogeneous serums is variable from batch to batch as are the not inconsequential side effects. Although very high doses of adrenal corticosteroids may yield similar responses, these agents increase the predisposition to opportunistic infections.

In general, splenectomy has no role in the management of aplastic anemia.

Bone marrow transplantation (see Chap. 291)

OTHER PRIMARY BONE MARROW DISORDERS

PURE RED CELL APLASIA Pure red cell aplasia involves a selective failure in the production of erythroid elements in the bone marrow. Granulopoiesis and megakaryocytopoiesis remain normal. Patients have a normochromic normocytic anemia with normal granulocyte count and platelet count. Severe reticulocytopenia exists, and the bone marrow is characterized by a virtual absence of any erythroid precursors in the face of otherwise normal cellular elements. An increase in lymphocytes may be seen in the marrow.

Constitutional red cell aplasia Blackfan-Diamond syndrome, a rare chronic constitutional red blood cell aplasia, may appear in infants from the time of birth to the age of 2 years. Twenty-five percent of patients have minor congenital anomalies. The disorder is of unknown etiology.

Acquired red cell aplasia The rare acquired form of pure red blood cell aplasia is seen predominantly in middle-aged adults. About one-third of patients have thymomas. Five percent of all patients with thymomas have pure red blood cell aplasia. The association between thymoma and myasthenia gravis is somewhat stronger. In many patients both with and without thymomas, erythropoiesis is inhibited by a complement-fixing IgG immunoglobulin which has selective cytotoxicity for marrow erythroblasts. A much smaller group of patients has been noted to have an inhibitor against erythropoietin. Occasionally, pure red cell aplasia is encountered in a patient with non-Hodgkins lymphoma.

TREATMENT Since these patients have virtually no endogenous red blood cell production, they are totally dependent on red blood cell transfusion. If thymic enlargement is noted, a thymectomy may induce a remission in approximately 50 percent of patients. If the thymus is normal, thymectomy is of no benefit. Patients without thymoma or those with an unsuccessful thymectomy should receive a combination of corticosteroids and an immunosuppressive agent such as cyclophosphamide. Treatment often results in both prolonged clinical remission and disappearance of the inhibitor.

MYELOPHTHISIC ANEMIA Infiltration of the bone marrow with tumor, fibrosis, or granulomas can result in the development of a severe anemia. Tumor may be derived from cell lines indigenous to the bone marrow, as in leukemia, lymphoma, or myeloma, or the marrow may be invaded by metastatic deposits of solid tumor, usually carcinoma. Among the solid tumors most frequently associated with myelophthisic anemia are carcinoma of the breast, stomach, prostate, lung, and thyroid. Hepatomegaly and splenomegaly may develop in this setting, along with marrow fibrosis.

A myelophthisic anemia may accompany the development of fibrosis in the bone marrow, usually in association with myeloid metaplasia. This entity is discussed in Chap. 289. Granulomatous involvement of the bone marrow is usually due to advanced tuberculosis. Primary lipid storage disorders, such as Gaucher's disease and Niemann-Pick disease, occasionally produce a myelophthisic anemia, and the rare disorder osteopetrosis, or marble bone disease, may also give a similar hematologic picture.

The invasion of the bone marrow by tumor or granulomas impairs both erythropoiesis and thrombopoiesis. In contrast, neutrophil production is generally normal or increased. It is unlikely that the anemia and thrombocytopenia are due merely to "crowding" of the bone marrow space by extrinsic cells. Myelophthisis also causes a distortion of the microcirculation of the marrow, with premature release of immature cells.

Myelophthisis usually results in a severe normochromic normocytic anemia. A variety of misshapen erythrocytes are noted, particularly teardrop cells and fragmented cells with some basophilic stippling. In addition, normoblasts are usually seen in the peripheral blood. The reticulocyte percentage is often slightly increased (4 to 7 percent). However, when corrected for the anemia and the premature release from the bone marrow, the absolute reticulocyte count is actually reduced and reflects a decrease in red blood cell production. While thrombocytopenia is usually present, the white blood cell count is often elevated, with a marked shift to the left in the differential count. The combination of immature myeloid cells and normoblasts in the peripheral blood constitutes the "leukoerythroblastic" morphology so characteristic of myelophthisic anemia. Striking abnormalities are usually seen on examination of the bone marrow. Often an aspirate yields a "dry tap" owing to the infiltration of the marrow with abnormal tissue. Marrow biopsy is more likely to be diagnostic, revealing leukemia, lymphoma, or foci of metastatic tumors or granulomas. However, marrow involvement is often segmental, so that the primary pathologic process may be missed on a single biopsy.

Treatment Treatment consists of attempts to reverse the primary pathologic process. Disseminated tumors of the breast or prostate may respond remarkably well to appropriate hormonal therapy. It is particularly important to search for the presence of tuberculosis, since this disease is readily treatable. More often, however, the disease is not amenable to therapy, and supportive measures, such as blood transfusions, must be employed.

REFERENCES

ANASETTI C et al: Marrow transplantation for severe aplastic anemia. Long-term outcome in fifty "untransfused" patients. Ann Intern Med 104:461, 1986

CAMITTA BM et al: Aplastic anemia: Pathogenesis, diagnosis, treatment and prognosis. N Engl J Med 306:645, 1982

CLARK DA et al: Studies on pure red cell aplasia. XI. Results of immunosuppressive treatment of 37 patients. Blood 63:277, 1984

ELLMAN L: Bone marrow biopsy in the evaluation of lymphoma, carcinoma and granulomatous disease. Am J Med 60:1, 1976

HUMPHRIES RK, YOUNG N: Aplastic anemia and stem cell biology, in *Aplastic Anemia*. New York, AR Liss, 1984

KRANTZ SB, DESSYPRIS EN: Pure red cell aplasia, in *Hematopoietic Stem Cells*, DW Golde and F Takaka (eds). New York, Dekker, 1985

RAPPEPORT JM, NATHAN DG: Acquired aplastic anemia: Pathophysiology and treatment. Adv Intern Med 27:547, 1982

SPECK B et al: Treatment of severe aplastic anemia. Exp Hematol 14:126, 1986

WILLIAMS DM et al: Drug induced aplastic anemia. Semin Hematol 10:195, 1973

291 BONE MARROW TRANSPLANTATION

E. DONNALL THOMAS

SELECTION OF THE PATIENT Marrow transplantation is a rational therapeutic option only if the patient's disease involves the marrow or if hazard to the normal marrow is the limiting factor in aggressive treatment of a disease. A marrow transplant involves a transplant not only of the donor myeloid, erythroid, and megakaryocytic systems but also of the donor lymphoid and macrophage systems. The rationale is illustrated by the three types of disease for which marrow transplantation has been widely utilized:

1 *Genetic disease*. For immunologic deficiency diseases, the objective is to replace the recipient's genetically defective lymphoid system with the normal lymphoid system of the donor. For genetic diseases such as thalassemia major, the abnormal marrow must be destroyed and replaced by normal marrow.
2 *Aplastic anemia*. Regardless of etiology, the disease process results in loss of the marrow, and the objective is to replace the defective organ with a normal functioning organ.
3 *Acute leukemia*. For leukemia (and other hematologic malignancies) the objective is the complete destruction of the leukemic cell population and, unavoidably, normal marrow cells by intensive chemoradiotherapy with restoration of normal marrow function by the transplanted marrow.

TYPES OF TRANSPLANTS A *syngeneic* graft describes a graft in which donor and recipient are genetically identical, i.e., identical twins. An *allogeneic* graft is one in which donor and recipient are of different genetic origins. A *chimera* is an individual whose body contains living, proliferating cells of different genetic origin. An *autologous* marrow graft refers to the removal of a patient's marrow, administration of chemo- and/or radiotherapy, and then return of the patient's own marrow.

SELECTION OF THE DONOR The donor must be in good health, and the donor, or an appropriate advocate, must be capable of giving informed consent. The principal risk is the anesthesia. Beyond these considerations, selection of the donor is largely determined by histocompatibility testing. Red blood cell incompatibility is not a barrier to marrow transplantation.

Histocompatibility typing (see Chap. 63) The HLA region is composed of a series of closely linked genetic loci on chromosome 6. The array of antigens encoded by this region on a chromosome is known as a haplotype. Each individual has two haplotypes, one inherited from each parent. The antigens encoded at HLA-A, HLA-B, and HLA-C are detected on lymphocytes by serologic techniques in a microcytotoxicity assay and those at HLA-D by the mixed leukocyte culture. Loci within the D region can now be recognized serologically by typing of B lymphocytes. These closely linked genetic loci, each with a large number of known alleles, make the HLA region the most complex genetic polymorphism yet described. Despite this complexity, within a family there can be only four haplotypes. Therefore, for a given patient, each sibling has one chance in four of being HLA-identical with the patient. The most widely used transplants are those between HLA-identical siblings.

PREPARATION OF THE PATIENT Infants with severe combined immunologic deficiency are conditioned to accept a transplant by the nature of their disease. All other patients are immunologically competent, to a greater or lesser degree, and are able to reject the marrow graft unless prepared with some form of immunosuppressive therapy. An immunosuppressive regimen commonly used for patients with aplastic anemia uses large doses of cyclophosphamide. Preparation of the patient with leukemia involves high-dose chemoradiotherapy for immunosuppression and to kill leukemic cells. A commonly used regimen involves cyclophosphamide followed by total-body irradiation (TBI). Approximately 10 gray (Gy) must be used for immunosuppression sufficient to permit consistent engraftment of marrow even though only 4 to 5 Gy will cause lethal marrow injury. Patients with genetic disease of the marrow may be prepared with busulfan or dimethyl busulfan to destroy the abnormal marrow along with cyclophosphamide for immunosuppression.

Marrow aspiration and infusion The pelvic bones are the most readily accessible sites for procurement, although marrow may be obtained from the sternum, ribs, or, in the case of children, the tibia. In the operating room and under general or spinal anesthesia multiple marrow aspirations are performed on the iliac crests. For adult donors, the volume of the mixture of blood and marrow cells is from 500 to 800 mL. As each aspiration is performed, the marrow is mixed with heparin and tissue culture medium. When the collection is completed, the marrow is passed through stainless steel screens to break up particles. It is then given to the recipient by intravenous infusion. The marrow stem cells pass through the lungs and subsequent growth and reconstitution of the marrow is confined almost exclusively to the medullary cavities.

Support for the patient without marrow function Usually 2 to 4 weeks are required before the transplanted marrow starts to produce the critical formed elements of the peripheral blood. Supportive care is crucial for survival. The patient should be cared for using the most effective available isolation facilities. Platelet transfusions are usually unnecessary at levels above 20,000 per cubic millimeter (see Chap. 279). Below that level, they should be used until values above 20,000 are sustained, especially if there is any evidence of bleeding. If the patient becomes refractory to random donor platelets, the use of platelets from HLA-matched unrelated donors may be necessary. Aspirin, and other drugs that depress platelet function, should be avoided. Routine use of prophylactic granulocyte transfusions is controversial and impractical. Granulocyte transfusions (see Chaps. 56 and 84) may be indicated for therapy of any significant infection in a granulocytopenic patient. Packed red blood cells should be given as needed to control symptoms of anemia, usually to keep the hematocrit above 25 percent. All blood products should be irradiated with 1.5 Gy to inactivate lymphocytes that might cause a graft-versus-host reaction.

Since infection is an ever-present danger, bacteriologic cultures should be obtained frequently. Onset of significant fever (38.5°C) should arouse a strong suspicion of infection in the granulocytopenic patient. Fever with clinical signs of bacteremia or fever sustained more than 24 h is an indication for starting systemic antibacterial therapy even if cultures are negative. Initial therapy usually includes an aminoglycoside active against *Pseudomonas* (gentamicin, tobramycin, amikacin) and carbenicillin or ticarcillin with additional antibiotics added as indicated by culture results (see Chaps. 84 and 88). Subsequently, if cultures are negative but fever persists, therapy with a combination of trimethoprim and sulfamethoxazole or with amphotericin may be considered. Once broad-spectrum antibiotic therapy has been initiated, it should be continued until the granulocyte count rises above 200 per cubic millimeter even if clinical signs of infection disappear.

Many patients coming to marrow transplantation have had inadequate nutrition because of their disease or the efforts to treat it. The preparation for marrow grafting results in nausea, vomiting, and mucositis which results in poor oral intake for at least several weeks. A Hickman modification of the Broviac catheter is installed routinely. The catheter makes it possible to administer hyperalimentation, medications, and blood products and is also used for drawing blood samples. Although some catheters are removed because of infection or suspected infection, about 90 percent of the patients have the catheter in place for approximately 3 months, the period of time when it is needed.

ENGRAFTMENT AND PROOF OF ENGRAFTMENT Engraftment is signaled by a rise in granulocytes and platelets and the reappearance of reticulocytes. The median time required to reach a granulocyte count of 1000 per cubic millimeter is 26 days. The rise in platelet count usually occurs a week or two later.

Proof of engraftment depends upon use of cytogenetics, blood genetic markers, and/or restriction enzyme fragment length polymorphisms to distinguish donor from host cells. The regenerating marrow is usually entirely of host type. Occasional patients show persistence of some host cells for a few weeks. Rare patients have an increasing number of host cells, and eventually the marrow is repopulated by host cells.

COMPLICATIONS FOLLOWING ENGRAFTMENT The complications that may follow successful marrow engraftment are (1) graft rejection, a problem primarily occurring in patients with aplastic anemia; (2) infection, including early bacterial infections or later opportunistic infections such as cytomegalovirus interstitial pneumonia; (3) acute graft-versus-host disease (GVHD), the result of the immunologic reaction of the engrafted lymphoid elements against tissues of the recipient; (4) chronic GVHD; (5) recurrence of leukemia; and (6) miscellaneous complications such as hemorrhagic cystitis, cardiomyopathy, cataract formation, venocclusive liver disease, leukoencephalopathy, and sterility.

CLINICAL RESULTS OF MARROW TRANSPLANTATION Immunodeficiency diseases Despite the rarity of these disorders, these patients are unique in that immunosuppressive therapy is not necessary to condition the patient to accept a graft, and because some myeloid function is usually present, rapid marrow engraftment is not essential. One such patient was the first to be transplanted from an HLA-identical sibling and some 100 similar patients have been successfully reconstituted in the intervening 15 years.

Genetically determined hematologic diseases Marrow grafts have now been reported for Kostmann's syndrome, chronic granulomatous disease, Chédiak-Higashi syndrome, Blackfan-Diamond syndrome, congenital aplastic anemia, and sickle cell disease (one patient, transplanted because of leukemia). Of particular interest is marrow transplantation for thalassemia major. Thalassemia major is a significant cause of death in children in many parts of the world. In developed countries, therapy with transfusions and chelating agents can prolong life for one to three decades but at great expense. In 1981, a patient with thalassemia major was prepared with dimethyl busulfan and cyclophosphamide and given a marrow graft from an HLA-identical older sister who did not have the thalassemia trait. There was prompt resolution of laboratory and clinical evidence of thalassemia, and the patient's growth and development have been normal. Since then, some 80 marrow transplants for thalassemia major have been reviewed. Approximately 10 percent of the children died of complications of marrow grafting and 15 percent regenerated their own marrow and again developed thalassemia major. Seventy-five percent of the patients appear to be cured of the disease although some 10 to 15 percent of the cured patients are under treatment for chronic GVHD. These results indicate that marrow grafting can cure genetically determined hematopoietic disorders which, at present, cannot be cured in any other way. Gene transfer for therapy of these diseases is an exciting possibility currently under investigation in many laboratories.

Transplantation for severe aplastic anemia (see Chap. 290) Because of the poor prognosis on conventional therapy, patients with severe aplastic anemia are logical candidates for marrow transplantation.

HLA-IDENTICAL SIBLING DONORS Patients with severe aplastic anemia must be prepared for engraftment with immunosuppressive therapy. The most widely used regimen is cyclophosphamide 50 mg/kg on each of 4 days followed 36 h later by donor marrow. The first two successful transplants were reported in 1972, and these recipients are alive and well 14 years later.

For ethical reasons the initial marrow transplants were carried out in patients who had failed to benefit from conventional therapy. As a consequence these end-stage patients had already received multiple transfusions, and many were severely infected at the time of transplantation. One-third of the patients rejected the graft, and the long-term survival of these end-stage patients was 40 to 50 percent.

Studies of marrow transplantation in dogs showed that blood transfusions could sensitize an intended marrow transplant recipient, resulting in rejection of the marrow graft. Accordingly, patients with severe aplastic anemia were identified early in the course of the disease so that marrow transplantation could be carried out before blood transfusions were given. The long-term survival of these patients has been approximately 80 percent. Therefore, patients with severe aplastic anemia and their families should have tissue typing performed immediately upon diagnosis. If a suitable donor can be identified, marrow transplantation should be carried out promptly before transfusions become necessary.

However, many patients with severe aplastic anemia present to the physician with bleeding and/or infection, and transfusions must be given as an urgent medical necessity. Therefore, marrow transplant teams are investigating other preparative regimens designed to prevent graft rejection and to improve survival. These include procarbazine and antithymocyte globulin administered before the standard cyclophosphamide regimen, cyclophosphamide followed by 3-Gy TBI, a cyclophosphamide regimen followed by 8-Gy TBI with shielding of the lung to 4 Gy, and the use of cyclophosphamide followed by 7.5 Gy of total-nodal irradiation. Another regimen is based on the fact that patients given a smaller number of marrow cells have had an increased probability of graft rejection. Since it was not practical to get more marrow cells from the donor, peripheral blood mononuclear cells have been used as an added source of donor cells. The standard cyclophosphamide regimen was administered followed by the marrow transplant. Then, on each of 3 to 5 days following marrow transplantation, buffy coat white blood cells were collected from 4 units of donor blood by a leukapheresis technique and administered intravenously to the recipient without in vitro irradiation. For patients who have been transfused, these modified regimens have largely solved the problem of graft rejection. Reported long-term survival ranges from 50 to 75 percent.

IDENTICAL TWIN DONORS Aplastic anemia is not a common disease, and to find a patient with it who has an identical twin is even more uncommon. Nevertheless, a number of transplants have been carried out for severe aplastic anemia using an identical twin as the marrow donor. In some patients the simple intravenous infusion of marrow without any immunosuppressive treatment resulted in recovery. These results reinforce the concept that aplastic anemia is due to an acquired abnormality of the stem cell which can be corrected by transplantation of normal syngeneic stem cells. However, some patients did not recover after simple intravenous marrow infusion. These patients were then treated with the cyclophosphamide regimen and given a second infusion of marrow from the twin which resulted in complete hematopoietic reconstitution. The results suggest that some cases may be due to an immune mechanism or abnormal regulators of cell growth. Whatever the mechanism, the rare patient with aplastic anemia who has a genetically identical twin has a 90 percent chance of being cured with marrow transplantation.

Transplantation for acute leukemia Acute leukemia (see Chap. 292) has served as a prototype malignant disease of the marrow for treatment by intensive chemoradiotherapy and marrow transplantation. Almost all regimens used for preparing leukemic patients for marrow transplantation have employed supralethal TBI. This has been done for several reasons: (1) much of the laboratory experience with marrow transplantation in animals has used supralethal TBI; (2) irradiation is an effective means of eradicating leukemic cells; (3) irradiation penetrates to the so-called privileged sites where leukemic cells may be inaccessible to chemotherapeutic agents; and (4) irradiation is a powerful immunosuppressive agent.

ACUTE LEUKEMIA IN RELAPSE USING HLA-IDENTICAL SIBLING DONORS For ethical reasons, marrow transplantation was initially attempted only in patients with acute leukemia in relapse after combination chemotherapy. These end-stage patients were poor candidates for any therapeutic procedure because they usually presented with a heavy body burden of leukemic cells, were usually granulocytopenic and thrombocytopenic, and often already infected with antibiotic-resistant bacteria and fungi. In early studies 10-Gy total-body irradiation was given in preparation for grafting. Then an attempt was made to kill more leukemic cells by giving cyclophosphamide a few days before administration of TBI and the marrow transplant. For these end-stage patients there were many deaths related to advanced illness at the time of transplantation, graft-versus-host disease, opportunistic infections, or recurrence of leukemia. An analysis of survival shows that 10 percent of these patients are long-term survivors with the leading patients now 14 years postgrafting. It appears that these patients, on no maintenance chemotherapy, are cured of their disease. Marrow transplant teams have utilized several different chemoradiotherapy preparative regimens for end-stage patients, but the long-term survival rate remains at 5 to 15 percent.

ACUTE LYMPHOBLASTIC LEUKEMIA (ALL) IN REMISSION USING HLA-IDENTICAL SIBLING DONORS The fact that some patients in the end stages of acute leukemia could apparently be cured led to transplantation earlier in the course of disease. Many patients with ALL, particularly children in the "good-risk" category, can be cured by combination chemotherapy, but once marrow relapse has occurred, long-term survival is rare. Therefore, the decision was made to transplant patients in the second or subsequent remission. It was recognized that some of these patients would be lost early to transplant complications, but this risk seemed acceptable if some patients could, in fact, be cured. Most marrow transplant teams are reporting long-term survival and apparent cure of 25 to 40 percent of these patients. Recurrent leukemia is a major problem. These recurrences, in host-type cells, show that the preparative regimen was often ineffective in eradicating the residual leukemic cell population.

ACUTE NONLYMPHOBLASTIC LEUKEMIA (ANL) IN REMISSION USING HLA-IDENTICAL SIBLING DONORS In contrast to patients with ALL, patients with ANL in first remission are known to have a poor prognosis. With combination chemotherapy the median duration of the first remission in most reported series is approximately 12 to 15 months, and only 20 percent of the patients are alive at 5 years after initial chemotherapy. Therefore, a study of marrow transplantation in these patients in first remission was considered to be ethically acceptable. In an initial series of 19 consecutive patients transplanted in first remission, 11 (58 percent) are in continued disease-free remission 6 to 9 years after grafting. Several hundred such transplants have now been carried out with various transplant teams reporting 45 to 70 percent long-term survival.

PATIENTS WITH CHRONIC GRANULOCYTIC LEUKEMIA (CGL) The term *chronic* is inappropriate in describing the clinical course of patients with CGL. The conversion to blast crisis and death occurs at a fairly constant rate, and the median survival in most series of patients is approximately 30 to 40 months (see Chap. 289). Although a small fraction of patients may live for a long time in the chronic phase, in general, the outlook for most patients with CGL is quite grim. When blast crisis appears, therapy is usually ineffective. A subset of patients whose blasts appear to be more like lymphoblasts (terminal transferase-positive) and with a hypodiploid number of chromosomes may respond for a period of a few months to treatment with vincristine and prednisone.

Marrow transplantation from HLA-identical donors has been carried out in patients with CGL in blast crisis. As expected from the experience with acute leukemia in relapse, there were many deaths. However, 10 to 20 percent of these patients are long-term survivors without the Philadelphia chromosome and appear to be cured.

A study of marrow transplantation during the chronic phase of the disease for patients with an identical twin to serve as marrow donor was initiated. The twin donors were clinically and hematologically normal. After preparation with cyclophosphamide and irradiation, a complete hematologic and cytogenetic remission was induced in 11 of 12 patients. One patient relapsed 30 months after transplantation and died of leukemia at 51 months. Two others have relapsed into the chronic phase. The other eight patients are clinically and cytogenetically normal 5 to 9 years after transplantation. These results of syngeneic marrow transplantation, indicating that the Philadelphia chromosome–positive leukemic clone can be eliminated, suggested that it may be reasonable to carry out marrow transplantation in the chronic phase of CGL utilizing allogeneic donors. Seven marrow transplant teams have now reported HLA-identical grafts in approximately 200 patients in the chronic phase of CGL. Long-term survival ranges from 50 to 70 percent and absence of the Philadelphia chromosome indicates cure in the majority of these patients.

PATIENTS WITH ACUTE LEUKEMIA USING DONORS OTHER THAN HLA-IDENTICAL SIBLINGS The general experience in the United States has been that only one-third of the patients with acute leukemia will have an HLA-identical sibling, but the majority of patients will not. Therefore, a cautious exploration of the use of other donors has been initiated by several marrow transplant teams. One such study involved marrow transplantation in family member donor-recipient pairs in which one of the HLA haplotypes was genetically identical and the other haplotype phenotypically identical for one or more of the HLA loci. The results of these transplants when donor and recipient are mismatched at only one locus are quite similar to the results using an HLA-identical sibling donor. The outcome is largely a function of the stage of the disease in which the transplant was carried out. The incidence of acute GVHD was greater, but the causes of death were not significantly different. There are too few patients to permit an analysis according to the family relationship of the donor or according to the HLA locus involved in the mismatch.

Serologic HLA typing makes it technically possible to find a suitably matched unrelated donor, at least for patients with the more common HLA haplotypes, given a large panel of potential donors whose HLA types have been determined. A few transplants using unrelated donors have been reported. Some have been successful, but others have failed because of GVHD. These results indicate the feasibility of utilizing unrelated donors for marrow transplantation.

Autologous marrow transplantation The technique for procuring and cryopreserving marrow has been established for 20 years. The patient's own marrow can be cryopreserved during intensive chemoradiotherapy and then returned to the patient in order to avoid subsequent lethal marrow aplasia. The concept is attractive because use of the patient's own marrow avoids the risk of GVHD. The following points are pertinent in considering autologous marrow transplantation: (1) The patient's marrow should not be contaminated with malignant cells. (2) Autologous marrow is of value only in protecting the patient against lethal hematopoietic toxicity. If the regimen of chemoradiotherapy involves lethal toxicity to other organ systems, autologous marrow will not be of benefit. (3) The tumor being treated must show a dose-response curve such that supralethal chemoradiotherapy can be expected to result in a significantly enhanced antitumor response. Unfortunately, with currently available agents, only a few tumors appear to fall into this category. (4) The protocol must be designed so that the role of autologous marrow can be demonstrated. In animals it is feasible to administer "supralethal" therapy and to demonstrate that animals given syngeneic marrow will survive while those not given marrow will die. For obvious reasons, this kind of controlled experiment cannot be done in humans. Failure to recognize these four principles accounts for much of the current uncertainty about the value of autologous marrow transplantation in the treatment of patients with malignant disease.

Nevertheless, the potential use of autologous marrow is the subject of a new wave of interest and some results are encouraging. The tumors that might be expected to show a significant improvement in response to high-dose chemoradiotherapy include the leukemias, Hodgkin's disease, non-Hodgkin's lymphoma, small cell cancer of the lung, breast cancer, testicular tumors, and ovarian tumors. Techniques being explored for removal of tumor cells from the marrow include physical separation, destruction by chemotherapeutic agents, and destruction by monoclonal antibodies. Several transplant centers are conducting studies of the utility of cryopreserved autologous marrow, and all have reported successful hematopoietic reconstitution in most patients. It is too early to evaluate the clinical impact of these studies on the course of the several diseases.

IMMUNOLOGIC ASPECTS OF MARROW TRANSPLANTATION Marrow graft rejection "Marrow graft rejection" describes a phenomenon in which the transplanted marrow graft begins to function, but after a few days or weeks, the peripheral blood counts suddenly drop and marrow biopsy shows the marrow to be devoid of myeloid elements. Immunologically mediated marrow graft rejection is usually a consequence of sensitization by transfusions. In addition, inadequate immunosuppressive therapy before grafting may facilitate marrow graft rejection. Marrow graft rejection is a common problem in patients with aplastic anemia, but is very uncommon in patients with leukemia, which may be due to several factors: (1) Transfusions are usually given to leukemic patients while they are receiving antileukemic chemotherapy which is also immunosuppressive. This chemotherapy may prevent sensitization to transplantation antigens contained in blood products. (2) Leukemia may damage the lymphoid system so that the disease process itself interferes with sensitization. And (3) leukemic patients receive a more intensive immunosuppressive regimen before grafting.

Marrow graft failure may be due to causes other than immunologic mechanisms. With a solid organ, such as the kidney, histologic proof of graft rejection is easily obtained, but such proof usually cannot be obtained with a marrow graft since the myeloid marrow simply disappears. Other possible mechanisms of graft failure include (1) defective or inadequate numbers of "stem cells" in the donor marrow; (2) defective microenvironment in the marrow recipient; (3) allogeneic resistance not associated with HLA; and (4) susceptibility of the donor marrow to the same etiologic mechanism(s) responsible for the original disease process.

Acute graft-versus-host disease (GVHD) A "wasting disease" or "runt disease" was described many years ago in newborn mice or in rodents exposed to lethal TBI and given infusions of allogeneic hematopoietic cells. These observations were later confirmed for other species, including humans, and were recognized to be due to an immunologic reaction of engrafted lymphoid cells, presumably T cells, against the tissues of the host. This graft-versus-host reaction and its consequences, referred to as GVHD, is one of the major complications of marrow transplantation in humans. In patients given a marrow graft from an HLA-identical sibling and postgrafting immunosuppression, approximately one-half develop moderate to severe GVHD.

Acute GVHD in humans usually involves the skin, gastrointestinal tract, and/or the liver. A skin rash is usually the first sign of GVHD. Intestinal involvement results in diarrhea and may progress to abdominal pain and ileus. Liver disease is characterized by rises of bilirubin, serum glutamic oxaloacetic transaminase, and alkaline phosphatase. Severe immunologic deficiency accompanies GVHD, and death from infection is frequent.

Since GVHD is immunologically mediated, efforts to prevent its development have involved the use of immunosuppressive therapy. Of the many agents studied, methotrexate and cyclophosphamide were found to be useful. A standard regimen consists of methotrexate, 15 mg/m^2 on day 1 postgrafting and 10 mg/m^2 on days 3, 6, 11, and 18, and weekly thereafter through day 102. An alternative consists of cyclophosphamide, 7.5 mg/kg for five doses on alternate days, beginning on the first day after marrow grafting followed by additional doses at irregular intervals. Despite these regimens, acute GVHD remains a serious problem.

Cyclosporine has been shown to be a potent new immunosuppressive agent. It is particularly valuable in organ grafts such as kidney, heart, and liver. Randomized trials have been carried out to compare cyclosporine with methotrexate post grafting for their effectiveness in preventing acute GVHD. These trials have not shown a difference in patient survival between the two regimens. However, cyclosporine is useful because it does not cause mucositis as methotrexate does, and it does not suppress the marrow graft so that effective marrow function is evident approximately 1 week earlier. Cyclosporine is nephrotoxic, and marrow graft recipients often receive other nephrotoxic agents such as amphotericin for suspected fungal infection. Creatinine level and serum cyclosporine level must be monitored carefully with prompt reduction of dosage if renal function is threatened.

A number of studies have been carried out in an effort to treat acute GVHD once it becomes established. Recipients of HLA-identical marrow have been treated with rabbit or goat antithymocyte globulin with improvement in some patients. In a clinical trial, without untreated controls because of ethical considerations, prednisone, horse antithymocyte globulin, and cyclosporine gave equivalent results in the treatment of established human GVHD. Despite these efforts, about one-third of the patients who develop moderate to severe GVHD will die with this complication. It is clear that the treatment of acute GVHD is unsatisfactory and that new approaches in preventing or treating GVHD must be found.

Experiments are underway designed to eliminate from the marrow inoculum the T cells believed to be responsible for GVHD while retaining hematopoietic stem cells. One approach involves treatment of the donor marrow with lectins for agglutination and separation of the T cells. Monoclonal antibodies that react with human T cells or subsets of T cells are being used in conjunction with complement, or are bound to toxins, such as the A chain of ricin, to create an immunotoxin. The preliminary results of these studies indicate a reduction in the incidence and severity of GVHD. However, the incidence of graft failure is significantly increased. The nature of the graft failure is under investigation.

Chronic GVHD Chronic GVHD occurs in approximately one-fourth of those recipients of marrow from an HLA-identical sibling who survive beyond 100 days. The manifestations include skin disease, keratoconjunctivitis, buccal mucositis, esophageal strictures, small- and large-intestinal involvement, pulmonary insufficiency, chronic liver disease, and generalized wasting. Histologically, the disease resembles the systemic collagen vascular diseases, especially morphea and lupus erythematosus profundus. Chronic GVHD may be associated with recurrent and occasionally fatal bacterial infections.

Initial efforts to treat chronic GVHD with short courses of antithymocyte globulin or prolonged treatment with prednisone were ineffective. Recently, treatment with prednisone and either procarbazine, cyclophosphamide, or azathioprine has resulted in recovery of about 80 percent of the patients, although treatment may be required for 1 or even 2 years. Twenty percent continue to have problems which may be disabling, and cyclosporine and steroids are being tried for the refractory patients.

Recovery of immunologic function Almost all patients given a marrow transplant from an HLA-identical sibling develop a functional graft with adequate levels of circulating granulocytes and platelets. Nevertheless, particularly in the first 3 months after grafting, these patients are susceptible to a wide variety of opportunistic infections. Approximately one-third of patients develop an interstitial pneumonia, and cytomegalovirus can be demonstrated in approximately one-half of these pneumonias. The mortality rate is approximately 80 percent. The high incidence of infection is the result of a very slow return of immunologic function, which may be made worse by GVHD and by efforts to prevent or treat GVHD. Fortunately, by the end of the first year after grafting, most patients have recovered immunologically and are able to lead normal lives without an increased incidence of infection.

Tolerance The long-term healthy human recipients of allogeneic marrow transplants are true chimeras. Their myeloid, lymphoid, and monocyte-macrophage systems are entirely made up of cells of donor origin. Clearly, these donor cells in the recipient are "tolerant" of the hosts' tissues. Studies of tolerance constitute a fascinating story in immunobiology, but a clear understanding of the state of tolerance has not emerged. At least three mechanisms may be operative, including classical central tolerance, tolerance maintained by "blocking factors," and tolerance related to the presence of "suppressor" cells.

The effect of age The success of allogeneic marrow grafting is inversely proportional to the age of the recipient. For example, for patients transplanted in first remission of ANL, long-term survival for those under age 20 is approximately 75 percent and for patients aged 30 to 50, 40 percent. The most apparent explanation for this difference is the increased incidence and severity of GVHD in older patients. Most marrow transplant centers do not transplant patients over the age of 50. These age restrictions do not apply to syngeneic transplants since these patients do not have GVHD, although patients over the age of 50 do not tolerate intensive treatment as well as younger patients.

RECURRENT LEUKEMIA AFTER GRAFTING **Frequency of recurrence of leukemia** For patients with leukemia transplanted in relapse or in second remission, an actuarial analysis shows a rather constant rate of recurrence of leukemia in the first year, a decreasing rate in the second year, and few recurrences thereafter. If there were no other causes of death, approximately 35 percent of the patients would be cured, while 65 percent would be destined to relapse. However, only about 25 percent of patients with ANL transplanted in first remission subsequently relapse. It is evident that recurrent leukemia after grafting is a major problem for patients transplanted in relapse or in second or subsequent remission. The low incidence of recurrent leukemia for those patients transplanted in the first remission may be explained by the presence of only a very small number of residual leukemic cells at the time of transplant and/or by the possibility that the leukemic cells of patients in first remission may not as yet have acquired resistance to therapeutic agents.

Nature of recurrent leukemia Blood genetic makers, cytogenetic techniques, and restriction enzyme fragment length polymorphisms can be used to identify the donor or host origin of the leukemic cells in patients who relapse after marrow transplantation. In the vast majority of patients the recurrent leukemia is in host-type cells. However, 10 cases have now been reported in which the recurrent leukemic cells were shown to be of donor origin. The mechanism of donor-cell transformation is unknown. However, in three cases a lymphoblastic lymphoma occurred in donor cells. The presence of Epstein-Barr virus genomes indicated transformation by this virus.

Graft-versus-leukemia In recipients of allogeneic marrow grafts, evidence supporting the existence of a graft-versus-leukemia effect has been difficult to obtain because of the large number of deaths from other causes among patients with severe GVHD. Sophisticated statistical methods have shown that the relative relapse rate for patients transplanted in relapse or for ALL in second remission was 2.5 times greater in recipients without GVHD than in those with GVHD. Recipients of allogeneic marrow who did not develop GVHD had approximately the same relapse rate as recipients of syngeneic marrow, indicating that subclinical GVHD did not reduce the relapse rate.

SOME GENERALIZATIONS ABOUT MARROW TRANSPLANTATION Because of the complexity of the marrow grafting regimens, transplantation should be undertaken only by teams with all of the resources needed to ensure an optimal result. The number of such teams has increased rapidly over the past few years.

Marrow transplantation is obviously an expensive undertaking, primarily because of hospital costs, but cost has been reduced appreciably by transplantation earlier in the course of the disease when the patient is in relatively good condition. Three centers (UCLA, Children's Orthopedic Medical Center of Seattle, and the Royal Marsden Hospital) have carried out cost analysis studies comparing marrow transplantation with combination therapy and have found marrow transplantation to be less expensive than current chemotherapy regimens.

The ethical problems of exposing a patient and donor to the marrow transplant regimen and the risk of death in the first 1 to 3 months after grafting have limited the use of marrow transplantation. However, the demonstration of better long-term survival rates with marrow transplantation compared to conventional therapy for several diseases and the cure of some diseases not cured by conventional therapy should alleviate the ethical concern. Extension of this form of therapy to other malignant diseases and to a variety of genetic disorders is being reported, and the current rapid rate of progress may soon make a much broader application of marrow grafting a reality.

REFERENCES

Appelbaum FR et al: Treatment of aplastic anemia by bone marrow transplantation in identical twins. Blood 55:1033, 1980

Beatty PG et al: Marrow transplantation from donors other than HLA genotypically identical siblings: The immunogenetics of acute graft versus host disease, in *Histocompatibility Testing 1984*, ED Albert et al (eds). New York, Springer-Verlag, 1984, p 670

Blume KG et al: Bone-marrow ablation and allogeneic marrow transplantation in acute leukemia: Clinical candidacy and outcome. N Engl J Med 302:1041, 1980

Bortin MM, Rimm AA for the Advisory Committee of the International Bone Marrow Transplant Registry: Severe combined immunodeficiency disease: Characterization of the disease and results of transplantation. JAMA 238:591, 1977

Fefer A et al: Treatment of chronic granulocytic leukemia with chemoradiotherapy and transplantation of marrow from identical twins. N Engl J Med 306:63, 1982

Martin P et al: Effects of in vitro depletion of T cells in HLA-identical allogeneic marrow grafts. Blood (in press)

Meyers JD, Thomas ED: Infection complicating bone marrow transplantation, in *Clinical Approach to Infection in the Immunocompromised Host*, RH Rubin, LS Young (eds). New York, Plenum, 1981, p 507

O'Reilly RJ: Allogeneic bone marrow transplantation: Current status and future directions. Blood 62:941, 1983

Powles RL et al: The curability of acute leukaemia, in *Topical Reviews of Haematology*, S Roath (ed). London, Wright & Sons, 1980, p 186

Rappeport JM et al: Application of bone marrow transplantation in genetic diseases. Clin Haematol 12:755, 1983

Schubach WH et al: A monoclonal immunoblastic sarcoma in donor cells bearing Epstein-Barr virus genomes following allogeneic marrow grafting for acute lymphoblastic leukemia. Blood 60:180, 1982

Shields AF et al: Adenovirus infections in patients undergoing bone-marrow transplantation. N Engl J Med 312:529, 1985

Storb R et al: Marrow transplantation for aplastic anemia. Semin Hematol 21:27, 1984

Sullivan KM et al: Chronic graft-versus-host disease in 52 patients: Adverse natural course and successful treatment with combination immunosuppression. Blood 57:267, 1981

Thomas ED et al: Bone-marrow transplantation. N Engl J Med 292:832, 895, 1975

———: Marrow transplantation for malignant diseases (Karnofsky Memorial Lecture). J Clin Oncol 1:517, 1983

——— et al: Marrow transplantation for thalassemia. Lancet 2:227, 1982

Weiden PL et al: Antileukemic effect of graft-versus-host disease in human recipients of allogeneic-marrow grafts. N Engl J Med 300:1068, 1979

292 THE LEUKEMIAS

RICHARD CHAMPLIN / DAVID W. GOLDE

The leukemias are a heterogeneous group of neoplasms arising from the malignant transformation of hematopoietic (blood-forming) cells. Leukemic cells proliferate primarily in the bone marrow and lymphoid tissues where they interfere with normal hematopoiesis and immunity. Ultimately they emigrate into the peripheral blood and infiltrate other tissues.

Leukemias are classified according to the cell types primarily involved (*myeloid* or *lymphoid*) and as *acute* or *chronic* based upon the natural history of the disease. Acute leukemias have a rapid clinical course, resulting in death within a matter of months without effective treatment, whereas chronic leukemias have a more prolonged natural history. This chapter will cover acute lymphocytic leukemia (ALL), acute myelogenous leukemia (AML), chronic lymphocytic leukemia (CLL), and hairy-cell leukemia. Chronic myelogenous leukemia (CML) is discussed in Chap. 289.

ETIOLOGY The cause of leukemia is not known in most patients, although both genetic and environmental factors may be important. There is a high concordance rate among identical twins if acute leukemia develops in the first year of life, and families with an excessive incidence of leukemia have been identified. Acute leukemia occurs with an increased frequency in a variety of congenital disorders, including Down's, Bloom's, Klinefelter's, Fanconi's, and the Wiskott-Aldrich syndromes.

Environmental factors are also known to play a role in the etiology of leukemia. Ionizing radiation causes leukemia in experimental animals, and there is a clear relationship between such exposure and the development of leukemia in humans. For example, individuals with occupational exposure, patients receiving radiation therapy, or Japanese survivors of the atomic bomb explosions have a predictable and dose-related increased incidence of leukemia. Radiation exposure increases the risk of developing CML, AML, and possibly ALL, but there is no known relationship to CLL or to hairy-cell leukemia. Chemicals such as benzene and other aromatic hydrocarbons have also been associated with the development of AML.

While leukemias induced by retroviruses (RNA viruses) have been studied in laboratory animals for many years, it was not until very recently that a viral etiology was established for a form of human leukemia. A unique human retrovirus, referred to as human T-cell leukemia virus (HTLV) (see Chap. 293) has been isolated from the cells of patients with adult T-cell leukemia (ATL), an aggressive malignancy composed of mature T-lymphoid cells. There is overwhelming evidence that HTLV I causes ATL in many parts of the world. The disease is endemic in southwestern Japan and parts of the Caribbean and central Africa. Except for the HTLV family, no other virus has been causally associated with the more common human acute and chronic leukemias.

INCIDENCE AND PREVALENCE The incidence of all leukemias is approximately 13 per 100,000 people per year, and the age-related incidence of the various forms of leukemia is shown in Fig. 292-1. The incidence of both acute and chronic leukemias is somewhat higher in men than in women. Acute lymphoblastic leukemia is primarily a disease of children and young adults, whereas AML

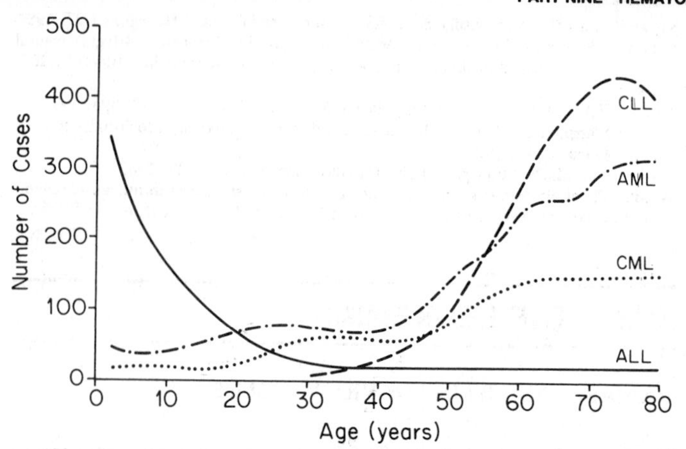

FIGURE 292-1 *Age-related incidence of various forms of leukemia: ALL = acute lymphoblastic leukemia, AML = acute myelogenous leukemia, CLL = chronic lymphocytic leukemia, CML = chronic myelogenous leukemia. (From Surveillance and Mortality Data 1973–1977, U.S. Department of Health and Human Resources.)*

occurs primarily in adults. Chronic lymphocytic leukemia and hairy-cell leukemia tend to occur in the elderly.

There have been several epidemiologic reports of case clustering of leukemias within communities and even in successive occupants of the same house. The bulk of evidence, however, indicates that the common forms of acute and chronic leukemias are not contagious and the incidence of leukemia is not increased among close contacts, such as marital partners or in the offspring of women who develop leukemia during pregnancy. The clear exception, ATL, is caused by HTLV I; in this type of leukemia there is evidence of passage of virus from infected to uninfected individuals.

PATHOPHYSIOLOGY Acute leukemia is characterized by proliferation of immature myeloid or lymphoid cells. The leukemia arises following malignant transformation of a single hematopoietic or lymphoid progenitor, followed by cellular replication and expansion of the transformed clone. A fundamental characteristic of the malignant cells in acute leukemia is their failure to mature beyond the myeloblast or promyelocyte level in AML and the lymphoblast level in ALL. Leukemic cells accumulate in the bone marrow due both to excessive proliferation and to a defect in terminal differentiation. The failure to mature to nonreplicating end cells is the primary reason for the accumulation of leukemic cells in AML. The leukemic cells proliferate primarily in the bone marrow, circulate in the blood, and may infiltrate into other tissues such as lymph nodes, liver, spleen, skin, viscera, and the central nervous system.

The mechanism of neoplastic transformation producing leukemia is poorly understood but involves a fundamental alteration of DNA conferring hereditable malignant characteristics to the transformed cell and its progeny. The neoplastic phenotype can be induced in nonmalignant cells in vitro by transfer (transfection) of DNA from the leukemic cells. In animals, leukemias can be induced by retroviruses which either carry a transforming gene (viral oncogene) or integrate into specific sites in DNA causing activation of cellular proto-oncogenes (insertional mutagenesis). The role of oncogenes in the pathogenesis of neoplasia is discussed in Chap. 59. With sensitive techniques, clonal cytogenetic abnormalities can be detected in most patients with acute and chronic leukemias. A wide range of cytogenetic abnormalities is associated with the various forms of leukemias, and distinctive nonrandom chromosomal abnormalities are associated with AML, ALL, and CLL, as shown in Table 292-1. Chromosomal rearrangements in leukemic cells may alter the structure or regulation of cellular oncogenes, producing quantitative or qualitative changes in their gene products, which may play a role in initiating or maintaining the leukemic state. Most data suggest the development of leukemia is a multistep process. In many cases, acute leukemia develops in patients with a preexisting myelodysplastic or myeloproliferative disorder.

The pathophysiology of bone marrow failure in leukemia is complex. Pancytopenia is typically present and results at least in part from physical replacement of the normal precursor cells by leukemic cells. Some patients with acute leukemia and pancytopenia have a hypocellular bone marrow indicating that marrow failure is not simply due to overcrowding by leukemic cells. Leukemic cells may directly inhibit normal hematopoiesis via cell-mediated or humoral mechanisms. Alternatively, leukemic cells may occupy critical niches in the bone marrow (stromal) microenvironment and interfere with normal cellular interactions. Normal hematopoietic stem cells do remain in the bone marrow and are capable of proliferating and restoring hematopoiesis following effective antileukemic treatment.

TABLE 292-1 Chromosomal abnormalities associated with acute leukemias

Abnormalities	Leukemia subtype	Relative prognosis
AML		
t(8;21)	M2 (myelocytic)	Good
+8	M1, M2, M4, M5	—
t(15;17)	M3 (promyelocytic)	Good if remission is achieved
t(9;11)	M5(monocytic)	Poor
inv 16	AML usually M4 with eosinophilia	Good
t(6;9)	AML with basophilia	—
5q−, −5, −7	AML following preleukemic syndrome or treatment-related leukemia	Poor
Ph[1], t(9;22)	Occasionally present in M1, M2, M4, M5, M6; must distinguish from CML blast crisis	Poor
ALL		
Hyperdiploidy	L1, L2	Good
6 q−	L1, L2	Good
14q+	L1, L2	—
t(8;14)	L3 (B cell)	Poor
Ph[1], t(9;22)	L1, L2	Poor
t(4;11)	L2 (or M4 form AML)	Poor
CLL		
+12	B-cell type	Good
+12, 14 q+	B-cell type	Poor
+12, + other abnormalities	B-cell type	Poor
t(11;14)	B-cell type	Poor

ACUTE LEUKEMIAS—ACUTE LYMPHOCYTIC LEUKEMIA (ALL) AND ACUTE MYELOGENOUS LEUKEMIA (AML)

PATHOLOGY AND CLASSIFICATION The diagnosis of acute leukemia requires the demonstration of leukemic cells in the bone marrow, peripheral blood, or extramedullary tissues. The bone marrow is typically hypercellular with a monomorphic infiltration of leukemic blasts and a marked reduction in normal bone marrow elements. It is critical to distinguish ALL from AML since these two diseases differ in natural history, prognosis, and response to various therapeutic agents.

Acute lymphocytic leukemia can be identified and classified on the basis of morphology and immunologic phenotype related to the stage of lymphoid differentiation. The leukemic lymphoblasts in ALL are typically smaller than myeloblasts (10 to 15 μm in diameter) and often have only a thin rim of agranular cytoplasm. The nucleus may be round or convoluted (see Fig. A5-24). Three morphologic subtypes have been described in the French-American-British classification: L1 cells are small and homogeneous with a regular nuclear membrane and a small nucleolus. L2 cells are larger and have a lower nuclear-cytoplasmic ratio with more pleomorphic size and shape. L2 cells typically have one or more prominent nucleoli. The L3 form of ALL is uncommon, occurring in less than 5 percent of cases; the leukemic cells in this variant contain large vesicular nuclei with basophilic, often vacuolated cytoplasm. L3 cells have a high mitotic index and represent the leukemic form of Burkitt's lymphoma.

Leukemic lymphoblasts in more than 90 percent of patients with ALL contain a nuclear enzyme *terminal deoxynucleotidal transferase* (TdT) which is only rarely present in AML cells. The functional role of this enzyme is not known. TdT is normally found in 1 percent of normal bone marrow cells and is present in immature T and B lymphocytes; it is absent in mature lymphocytes, hairy-cell leukemia, and CLL. The leukemic cells from approximately half of patients with ALL react with the periodic acid Schiff stain showing blocklike inclusions of glycogen. Lymphoblasts do not contain granulocytic or monocytic lysosomal enzymes and therefore do not react with cytochemical stains for peroxidase, Sudan black, and nonspecific esterase.

Several forms of ALL can be defined based upon immunologic phenotype. Approximately 60 percent of cases are termed *common ALL;* the cells are TdT-positive and have the common ALL antigen (CALLA) but do not express surface membrane immunoglobulin or T-cell antigens. These cells are usually derived from precursors of the B-cell lineage, as they may express immature B-cell antigens and have immunoglobulin gene rearrangements. CALLA is not a leukemia-specific antigen since it is present on immature lymphoid cells including approximately 1 percent of cells in the normal bone marrow. About 20 percent of cases of ALL are of the *T-cell type,* where the T lymphoblasts express the E-rosette receptor or other T-lymphocyte-related antigens; these cells are TdT-positive, usually CALLA-negative, and stain positively for acid phosphatase. T-cell ALL typically occurs in adolescent males and is frequently associated with a high leukocyte count and an anterior mediastinal mass. Less than 5 percent of cases of ALL are *B-cell type.* The cells in this variant produce a monoclonal immunoglobulin which is bound to the surface membrane and have L3 morphology. In B-cell ALL, the cells are usually negative for TdT and contain the t(8;14) chromosomal abnormality characteristic of Burkitt's lymphoma. Approximately 15 percent of cases of ALL are termed *null cell type* because the cells do not elaborate CALLA or T- or B-cell antigens.

The leukemic cells in AML are 12 to 20 μm in diameter, larger than lymphoblasts, and have a lower nuclear-cytoplasmic ratio. The leukemic myeloblasts typically have discrete nuclear chromatin and multiple nucleoli. The presence of Auer rods, abnormal primary granules, in the cytoplasm of leukemic cells is diagnostic of AML; these inclusions are present in 10 to 20 percent of patients with AML (see Fig. A5-22). Dysplastic morphologic abnormalities may be prominent in residual granulocytic, erythroid, and megakaryocytic cells. Cytochemical stains are often helpful in distinguishing AML from ALL and in classifying the pathologic subtypes of AML. Myeloperoxidase, α-naphthyl-AS-D-chloracetate esterase, and Sudan black are primarily present in cells undergoing granulocytic differentiation. Nonspecific esterase (α-naphthyl butyrate esterase) stains cells of the monocyte-macrophage lineage. A number of cell surface antigens present in AML cells have also been described. These stains and markers, however, may be negative in leukemias of undifferentiated cells.

A collaborative French-American-British group has divided AML into seven pathologic subtypes based upon the degree of differentiation and maturation of the predominant cells toward granulocytes, monocytes, erythrocytes, or megakaryocytes. The characteristics of each subtype are summarized in Table 292-2. There are only subtle differences in the clinical features of each subtype. Patients with the acute promyelocytic subtype (M3) typically present with disseminated intravascular coagulation (DIC) induced by thromboplastic material released by the leukemic cells; DIC is usually present at the time of diagnosis and may be markedly exacerbated during chemotherapy. Acute myelomonocytic leukemia (M4) and acute monocytic leukemia (M5) are more likely than other subtypes to have extramedullary involvement of the skin, gingiva, central nervous system, and other tissues.

It is often difficult to distinguish the undifferentiated form of AML (M1) from the L2 form of ALL by morphology alone. In these cases additional studies including cytochemical stains and analysis of myeloid and lymphoid antigens are required. Electron microscopy may be helpful in some cases to demonstrate small numbers of promyelocytic granules in cells that appear undifferentiated by light microscopy.

The cellular blood elements are derived from pluripotent and committed hematopoietic stem cells which reside in the bone marrow.

TABLE 292-2 Morphologic subtypes of AML

			Reactivity with special strains		
Subtype	% of AML	Morphology	Peroxidase Sudan black	Nonspecific esterase	PAS*
M1 Acute undifferentiated leukemia	20	Few if any azurophilic granules	+/−	+/−	−
M2 AML with differentiation	30	Blasts with promyelocytic granules, Auer rods may be present	+ + +	+/−	+
M3 Promyelocytic leukemia	5	Hypergranular promyelocytes often with multiple Auer rods per cell	+ + +	+	+
M4 Acute myelomonocytic leukemia	30	Monocytoid-appearing cells in peripheral blood associated with serum lysozyme	+ +	+ + +	+ +/+
M5 Acute monocytic leukemia	10	Two subtypes identified: (a) undifferenitated; (b) differentiated associated with serum lysozyme	+/−	+ + +	+ +/+
M6 Acute erythroleukemia	5	Predominance of erythroblasts and markedly dysplastic erythroid precursors	−	−	+ +
M7 Acute megakaryocytic leukemia	5	Undifferentiated blasts react with antiplatelet antibodies and contain platelet peroxidase	−	+/−	+

* *Periodic acid Schiff.*

Leukemic transformation may occur in cells at several levels of differentiation. In some patients with AML who are heterozygous for glucose 6-phosphate dehydrogenase (G6PD) isoenzymes, the granulocytes, macrophages, erythrocytes, and megakaryocytes all contain the single G6PD isoenzyme present in the leukemic cells, suggesting that these cells are derived from the malignant clone and that leukemic transformation involved a pluripotent stem cell. In other AML patients, only granulocytes and/or macrophages appear monoclonal, and in these patients, transformation may have occurred at the level of the committed granulocytic-macrophage progenitor. Some patients appear to have a *biphenotypic acute leukemia*. In these patients, subpopulations of malignant cells contain both myeloid and lymphoid markers. These cells may represent leukemias of primitive pluripotent stem cells, or more likely they result from aberrant gene expression in a transformed myeloid or lymphoid progenitor.

Some patients develop AML after a preleukemic syndrome. The preleukemic and myelodysplastic syndromes are a heterogeneous group of disorders, and the nomenclature describing them is confusing and poorly standardized. These syndromes generally occur in middle-aged or elderly patients. Sometimes included under the heading of myelodysplastic syndromes are refractory anemia with excessive blasts, chronic myelomonocytic leukemia, and acquired idiopathic sideroblastic anemia. The term *preleukemia* should be reserved to refer to a recognizable syndrome of hematopoietic dysfunction that typically precedes the classic findings of AML. This syndrome is usually characterized by a picture of ineffective hematopoiesis with anemia, thrombocytopenia, and sometimes granulocytopenia associated with a hypercellular, dysplastic bone marrow. In preleukemia, the leukemic clone is already established, and usually there is progressive impairment of hematopoiesis and accumulation of blasts. Megaloblastic hematopoiesis is common, and folate or vitamin B_{12} deficiency must be ruled out. Cytogenetic abnormalities are frequent; the most common chromosomal abnormalities are 5q−, −5, −7, and trisomy 8. When 5q− exists as the sole abnormality, the patient usually presents with refractory anemia associated with mild thrombocytosis. Many patients with preleukemic or myelodysplastic syndromes never develop overt AML but die from complications of bone marrow failure. Smoldering AML refers to a syndrome in which the diagnostic features of acute leukemia are present, but the disease follows an indolent or subacute course. This disorder also tends to occur in elderly patients.

CLINICAL AND LABORATORY FEATURES Acute lymphocytic leukemia (ALL) and AML share many clinical features. In the majority of patients, the initial symptoms of acute leukemia are present for less than 3 months. A preleukemic syndrome can be identified in approximately 25 percent of patients with AML; in these patients, anemia and other cytopenias are usually present for months to years preceding the development of overt leukemia.

Patients with ALL and AML may present with pancytopenia without circulating blasts, with a normal leukocyte count, or with marked leukocytosis. Leukostasis due to occlusion of the microcirculation by leukemic blast cells can lead to hypoperfusion of vital tissues, most commonly lung and brain. Leukostasis becomes increasingly common when the number of circulating blasts exceeds 100×10^9 per liter. Patients may complain of manifestations of anemia such as pallor, easy fatigability, and dyspnea on mild exertion. The metabolic activity of large numbers of blasts can lead to artifactual results in laboratory tests, especially glucose and potassium concentrations and arterial blood gas analysis.

Bleeding is a major problem in patients with acute leukemia and is primarily related to thrombocytopenia. Coagulation defects may also be present. In some patients, megakaryocytes are derived from the leukemic clone and produce platelets with abnormal function. Petechiae and easy bruisability are common. Hemorrhage becomes increasingly common when the platelet count is less than 20×10^9 per liter, typically occurring from oral (particularly gingiva) and gastrointestinal mucous membranes. Spontaneous bleeding involving the central nervous system, lungs, or other viscera may also occur.

Infection is a frequent complication of acute leukemia. The incidence of infection is inversely related to the number of circulating granulocytes and becomes a major risk in patients with granulocyte counts less than 0.5×10^9 per liter. Granulocytes derived from leukemic progenitors may also function abnormally, further compromising host defenses. The leukemia and its treatment cause a breakdown of mucosal barriers, and systemic infections usually develop from organisms colonizing the skin, throat, and gastrointestinal tract. Common sites of infections in patients with acute leukemia include the skin, gingiva, perirectal tissues, lung, and urinary tract. Septicemia often occurs without an apparent source. Gram-negative bacteria, gram-positive cocci, and *Candida* species are frequent pathogens.

Hepatomegaly and splenomegaly due to leukemic infiltration are present in approximately one-half to three-fourths of patients with ALL and a minority of patients with AML. This visceral involvement can produce symptoms of nausea, abdominal fullness, or early satiety. Lymphadenopathy is more common in ALL than in AML. An anterior mediastinal mass is usually present in patients with the T-cell variant of ALL, and rarely occurs in other forms of ALL or in AML. Acute leukemia may infiltrate into extramedullary tissues such as the skin, lung, eye, nasopharynx, or kidneys. Testicular involvement is particularly common in males with ALL. Soft tissue masses of leukemic cells, "chloromas," can develop in any location. Occasionally, extramedullary leukemia can precede detectable involvement in the bone marrow.

Symptoms related to the expanding malignant cell mass, such as bone pain and sternal tenderness, occur in approximately half of patients with acute leukemia; osteolytic lesions are rare. Renal abnormalities can develop as a result of leukemic infiltration, ureteral obstruction by uric acid stones or enlarged lymph nodes, urate nephropathy, or from infectious or hemorrhagic complications. Gastrointestinal symptoms of early satiety, distention, and constipation may result from organomegaly or from leukemic infiltration or bleeding into the bowel and other viscera.

In acute leukemia, the neoplastic cells may infiltrate into the subarachnoid space, causing leukemic meningitis or direct involvement of the brain or spinal cord parenchyma. Neurologic involvement can only rarely be demonstrated at the time of diagnosis, but the central nervous system is a frequent site of relapse, particularly in patients with ALL. The first symptoms of leukemic meningitis are usually headache and nausea. Papilledema, cranial nerve palsies, seizures, and altered mentation develop with disease progression. Cytocentrifuge preparations of cerebrospinal fluid (CSF) characteristically reveal leukemic blast cells, the CSF protein concentration is increased, and the glucose reduced.

Patients with acute leukemia often develop metabolic abnormalities. Hyponatremia and hypokalemia are common due to renal tubular abnormalities induced by lysozyme or other products of the leukemic cells. The serum lactic acid dehydrogenase (LDH) level may be increased. Hyperuricemia may be present due to accelerated turnover of cells with increased purine release, and lactic acidosis rarely occurs in patients with a large burden of leukemic cells.

TREATMENT OF ACUTE LEUKEMIA: GENERAL CONSIDERATIONS The growth of leukemic cells follows a Gompertzian growth curve with near exponential growth at a lower cell mass and progressive slowing of the growth rate at higher leukemic cell burdens. The leukemic mass is usually between 10^{11} to 10^{12} cells at the time of diagnosis. Chemotherapeutic agents produce a fractional cell kill, that is, a percentage of tumor cells (not an absolute number) is killed with each course of treatment. Most chemotherapeutic regimens employed for acute leukemias are probably capable of a 3 to 5 log kill, resulting in the elimination of 99.9 to 99.999 percent of the leukemia cells. Another potential effect of some chemotherapeutic drugs is to induce differentiation and maturation of the leukemic cells to mature nonproliferating cells. When the leukemia cell mass is reduced below approximately 10^9 cells, leukemia can no longer be detected in the blood or bone marrow, and the patient appears to be in complete remission. The clinical criteria for complete remission include (1) less than 5 percent blasts in the bone marrow and absence of leukemic cells in the peripheral blood, (2) the restoration of normal peripheral blood counts, and (3) the absence of physical findings attributable to extramedullary involvement of the leukemia. If no further treatment is given, however, the residual clonogenic leukemic cells will proliferate, leading to relapse.

The treatment of acute leukemia is divided into distinct phases. *Remission induction chemotherapy* is the most critical phase. Intensive systemic chemotherapy is administered with the goal of reducing the leukemic cell mass below the level of detection. After remission is achieved, additional systemic chemotherapy must be given to further reduce the leukemic cell mass and, ideally, eradicate the leukemia. Intensive chemotherapy administered immediately following remission induction is referred to as *consolidation* or *early intensification* treatment. Lower dose chemotherapy that is generally continued over several years is referred to as *maintenance treatment*. Intensive chemotherapy administered more than 6 months after remission induction is termed *late intensification*. Another aspect of treatment involves local chemotherapy or radiation to frequent sites of relapse which are considered to be sanctury sites, such as the central nervous system where systemic treatment may fail to eradicate the disease. The value of these forms of treatment for ALL and AML will be discussed separately.

Supportive care The supportive care of patients with pancytopenia is a critical aspect of the treatment of acute leukemia. This primarily involves the appropriate administration of blood products and management of infections.

Adequate levels of hemoglobin can usually be maintained with transfusions of packed red blood cells. An adequate number of circulating platelets can initially be attained by transfusions of platelets from unselected donors, but some transfused patients eventually develop antiplatelet antibodies which shorten platelet survival and render the patient unresponsive to further platelet transfusions. Patients who fail to respond to transfusions of platelets from unselected donors may respond to platelets from an HLA-identical donor. The risk of spontaneous hemorrhage is directly related to the degree of thrombocytopenia. It is generally advisable to transfuse platelets to maintain the platelet count above 20×10^9 per liter. Also, uterine bleeding should be minimized in menstruating women with thrombocytopenia by administering an anovulatory agent.

The potential therapeutic benefit of granulocyte transfusions has been extensively studied in patients receiving treatment for acute leukemia. Most data indicate that survival is not improved by granulocyte transfusions either to prevent infections or to treat documented infections, and that their routine use cannot be recommended. The major limitations in the use of granulocyte transfusions are the current technical difficulty in collecting sufficient numbers of granulocytes from normal donors and the adverse effects associated with their transfusion such as fever, leukoagglutination, pulmonary infiltrates, and transmission of cytomegalovirus (CMV) and other infections.

The prevention and treatment of infections is of critical importance in the management of patients with acute leukemia. Since most infections are caused by organisms colonizing the skin and gastrointestinal tract, a variety of approaches have been evaluated to suppress the endogenous flora in these sites. Most centers recommend the use of face masks, careful hand washing, oral nonabsorbable antibiotics, and reverse isolation for granulocytopenic patients. The development of bacterial and fungal infections may be delayed or avoided by these measures.

Granulocytopenic patients who develop fever or other signs of infection require prompt evaluation and treatment. Fever is usually due to a bacterial, fungal, or viral infection. Gram-negative sepsis is common in this setting and may be rapidly fatal. Granulocytopenic patients with unexplained fever or overt infections should be evaluated and receive empiric treatment for a presumed bacterial infection until a definitive diagnosis can be established. A combination of broad-spectrum antibiotics, such as an aminoglycoside or a third-generation cephalosporin in combination with a semisynthetic penicillin, should be employed and modified when the results of bacterial and fungal cultures are available. Systemic fungal infections are also common in granulocytopenic patients with leukemia and should be suspected in patients who fail to respond to antibiotic or who respond and develop recurrent fever. Definitive diagnosis of fungal infections may be difficult, and a therapeutic trial of amphotericin B is often indicated. The problem of infections in the immunocompromised host is discussed in Chap. 84.

TREATMENT OF ACUTE LYMPHOBLASTIC LEUKEMIA The treatment of ALL is one of the major successes in modern oncology. Forty years ago the disease was uniformly fatal and had a median survival of only 3 months. With current therapy, more than 50 percent of children with ALL achieve long-term remissions and probable cure. Adults and high-risk subgroups of children with ALL do not have a good prognosis, and long-term remissions are only achieved in a minority of patients. Therapy for ALL consists of three phases: (1) remission induction chemotherapy (2) central nervous system prophylaxis, and (3) continuation (maintenance) chemotherapy.

The goal of remission induction chemotherapy is to eliminate all clinical signs and morphologic evidence of leukemia, as well as to restore normal bone marrow function. The intensity of treatment is important, because the duration of remission is prolonged by reducing the leukemic cell burden to the smallest possible fraction.

The combination of vincristine and prednisone plus either L-asparaginase or daunorubicin induces complete remissions in over 90 percent of children with ALL within 4 weeks. Some patients with persistent leukemia may achieve remission with 2 to 4 additional weeks of treatment with the same or alternate drugs. Failure to achieve remission can be attributed primarily to the development of drug resistance, severe infections, or central nervous system (CNS) leukemia.

In patients who achieve remission, local prophylactic treatment to the CNS is required to prevent leukemic meningitis. The rationale for this treatment is based on the hypothesis that circulating leukemic cells infiltrate into the CNS and cerebrospinal fluid early in the course of the disease. Since the drugs used in remission induction in ALL penetrate poorly into the cerebrospinal fluid, these leukemic cells are sheltered from the effects of systemic chemotherapy. Over the ensuing months these cells may proliferate, producing overt leukemic meningitis. Leukemic meningitis is the initial site of relapse in up to two-thirds of patients with ALL who do not receive prophylactic therapy. Prophylactic treatment to the CNS, instituted immediately after remission induction, has been successful in dramatically reducing the incidence of CNS relapse. Most centers employ 24-Gy (2400-rad) whole-brain radiation in combination with intrathecal methotrexate. Cranial irradiation does produce subtle abnormalities in neurologic function, particularly in young children, and there is considerable interest in evaluating lower-dose radiotherapy regimens or alternative methods of CNS treatment. Preliminary data suggest that the combination of intrathecal and high-dose systemic methotrexate may provide adequate prophylactic treatment to the CNS.

Since patients in remission still harbor leukemia cells, further systemic treatment is required to prevent or delay leukemic relapse. The optimal approach to continuation therapy involves the administration of combination chemotherapy given in doses approaching maximal tolerance. As a rule, the drugs that are effective in inducing remission in ALL have not been useful in maintenance chemotherapy. The combination of 6-mercaptopurine and methotrexate is the most frequently employed maintenance regimen, but more intensive consolidation and maintenance regimens are required for adult patients and children with poor prognostic features.

The optimal duration of maintenance chemotherapy is unknown. Many patients can discontinue chemotherapy after 2 to 3 years and remain in long-term remission. Up to one-quarter of patients will relapse, however, after maintenance therapy is discontinued. It is not known whether maintenace therapy given for more than 3 years will further reduce the likelihood of relapse. Since there is currently no method to reliably detect small numbers of residual leukemic cells, there is no objective means to determine when therapy can be safely discontinued.

Complications of therapy for ALL Chemotherapy-induced myelosuppression and immunosuppression are inevitable side effects of the treatment for ALL. The chemotherapy directed toward the leukemic lymphoblasts also affects normal T and B lymphocytes, resulting in lymphocytopenia and immunodeficiency. Peripheral blood B cells generally recover to normal levels within several months after treatment is discontinued, but T-cell numbers and function may remain depressed for up to 1 year. *Pneumocystis carinii* pneumonia can occur while patients are in remission; trimethoprim-sulfamethoxazole prophylaxis is effective in preventing this complication. Growth in children is somewhat retarded during the administration of chemotherapy. Catch-up growth generally occurs once therapy is discontinued, and most children ultimately attain normal height and weight. Sterility may result from treatment with most chemotherapeutic agents and irradiation. Gonadal function may recover after a prolonged interval. The gonads in prepubertal patients are relatively resistant to the effects of chemotherapy, and most patients undergo normal puberty after therapy is discontinued.

Prognosis in ALL The two factors most affecting prognosis are age and the leukocyte count at the time of diagnosis. Children between the ages of 3 and 9 years with white blood counts less than 10×10^9 per liter have the best prognosis; 50 to 70 percent achieve long-term survival and probable cure with current treatment. Older patients and those with higher leukocyte counts have a poorer prognosis. Fewer than 20 percent of adults with ALL are long-term survivors in most series, and it is uncertain whether the maintenance therapy which is effective in children is of benefit for adults. Males have a worse prognosis than females, due in part to the problem of testicular relapse. In children, patients with the L1 morphologic subtype have a better prognosis than the L2 form, but this is probably not true in adults. Patients with T-cell ALL tend to have a poorer prognosis than the common ALL (CALLA) subgroup. These patients are generally older and present with a high white blood count, and it is uncertain if T-cell type, per se, is an independent poor prognostic factor. The B-cell (L3) variant of ALL has the worst prognosis.

Chromosomal abnormalities provide independent prognostic information. Approximately one-half of the patients with ALL have detectable cytogenetic abnormalities, including hypodiploidy, pseudodiploidy, or hyperdiploidy. A number of nonrandom chromosomal abnormalities are associated with ALL. Approximately 10 percent of patients with ALL have the Philadelphia (Ph^1) chromosome, an abnormality typical of chronic myelogenous leukemia. Associated with ALL, and possibly with hybrid (biphenotypic) leukemias, is t(4;11). Patients with pseudodiploidy, particularly t(4;11) and t(9;22), have a poor prognosis, while patients with hyperdiploidy have a better prognosis.

Remission and survival rates in adult patients with ALL (those over 15 years of age) are significantly lower than for children with the same disease. Remission induction rates in adults and high-risk children are generally between 50 to 70 percent following treatment with vincristine, prednisone, and daunorubicin; the median duration of remission is 10 to 12 months, and the 5-year survival rate is 10 to 30 percent with standard maintenance chemotherapy. Several centers have reported improved results with more intensive, multiple-drug consolidation and maintenance programs, but the optimal therapy for high-risk forms of ALL is uncertain.

Treatment of recurrent ALL Leukemia may recur either in the bone marrow or in extramedullary sites. Patients who relapse while receiving maintenance therapy have a very poor prognosis with little possibility of a long-term second remission. Combination chemotherapy with a three- or four-drug regimen including vincristine, prednisone, L-asparaginase, and/or daunorubicin results in a second remission in 50 to 70 percent of these patients. Remission duration, however, is usually brief, and subsequent relapse is inevitable. Patients who relapse after discontinuation of maintenance therapy have a better prognosis. Second remissions can be induced in about 90 percent of these patients. Although most will relapse again, some have achieved long-term survival. These patients should probably have CNS prophylaxis repeated to prevent recurrent disease in this extramedullary site.

Meningeal leukemia is the most common site of extramedullary relapse in patients with ALL. Cranial irradiation plus intrathecal methotrexate alone or in combination with cytarabine is the standard therapy for CNS leukemia. Testicular relapse is common in male patients with ALL and may occur during or after cessation of maintenance therapy. The treatment of choice is irradiation of the affected testicle. Patients with extramedullary relapse involving the CNS, testes, or other tissues are at very high risk for subsequent relapse in the bone marrow. Systemic reinduction therapy is indicated and may prevent generalized relapse of ALL.

TREATMENT OF ACUTE MYELOGENOUS LEUKEMIA The initial goal in the treatment of AML is to induce a complete hematologic remission. The drugs active in AML have little selectivity for leukemic cells over their normal bone marrow counterparts. Induction of severe myelosuppression is necessary in order to achieve a complete remission. The two most active drugs are cytarabine and daunorubicin. The combination of these agents with or without 6-thioguanine results in a complete remission rate of 60 to 80 percent. If residual leukemia is present 2 to 4 weeks after chemotherapy, the treatment is repeated. Patients who fail to enter remission with this approach have a poor prognosis.

Patients with AML who achieve complete remission still have a substantial number of residual leukemic cells. Further therapy is required to reduce and hopefully to eradicate these occult leukemia cells. The benefits of available forms of consolidation and maintenance treatment are controversial. The best results have been achieved in patients receiving one to three intensive cycles of consolidation chemotherapy using agents such as daunorubicin, cytarabine, 6-thioguanine, 5-azacitidine, and amsacrine. Median remission duration varies from 9 months to 2 years in most series. Ten to thirty percent of patients survive over 5 years free of disease, and most of these patients are probably cured. Better results have been reported in preliminary studies using very intensive consolidation regimens, including high-dose cytarabine alone or in combination with other drugs. The results of these studies suggest a benefit for patients receiving consolidation treatment when compared to historical controls, but these observations remain to be confirmed in prospectively controlled clinical trials.

Although some uncontrolled studies suggested that maintenace therapy with lower doses of these same agents or late intensification treatment improved remission duration, recent prospective controlled studies reported no benefit for patients receiving this form of treatment. Current data suggest that the major benefit in therapy is achieved with intensive induction and consolidation treatment.

Most patients who achieve complete remission will ultimately relapse. At that point, the disease is usually much less responsive to therapy; only a minority of patients achieve a brief second remission, and median survival is 3 to 6 months.

Central nervous system leukemia in AML occurs in 10 to 20 percent of patients at some point in their disease, and most commonly develops in patients with monocytic (M5) or myelomonocytic (M4) subtypes. Unlike ALL, the CNS is rarely an isolated site of relapse in AML; CNS involvement usually occurs in the setting of systemic relapse. This may not be a biologically important leukemic sanctuary in patients with AML, and prophylactic treatment to the CNS has not improved remission duration or survival. Patients who develop meningeal leukemia are treated with cranial irradiation and intrathecal chemotherapy with cytarabine and/or methotrexate.

Prognostic factors in AML Chromosomal abnormalities in AML are of prognostic value; patients with abnormalities such as t(8;21), t(15;17), or inv 16 tend to have a relatively good prognosis, while −5, −7, t(9;22), and complex chromosomal abnormalities are associated with a poor prognosis.

Age is a major prognostic factor in many series; elderly patients (over 70 years of age) are less likely to achieve complete remission. This group also tolerates intensive therapy poorly and is more difficult to support through the complications of pancytopenia. In addition, elderly patients are more likely to have leukemic cells with poor-risk chromosomal abnormalities such as −7, −5 and are more likely to have a defined preleukemic syndrome. However, elderly patients who do achieve remission have a similar remission duration and survival as younger patients. Since the major factor influencing survival is the achievement of complete remission, intensive chemotherapy should be administered to most elderly patients.

The leukemic subtype is of limited prognostic significance. Acute promyelocytic leukemia (M3) is typically associated with disseminated intravascular coagulation, and fatal CNS hemorrhage is a common complication during remission induction chemotherapy for this type of leukemia. Prophylactic heparin therapy is generally indicated during induction treatment to suppress DIC and prevent hemorrhagic complications. Patients with promyelocytic leukemia who do achieve remission appear to have a greater chance of long-term survival than other subgroups. Patients with monocytic or myelomonocytic leukemia may have a poorer prognosis than the M1 to M3 subgroups.

Patients with preleukemia evolving into AML or smoldering leukemia respond poorly to chemotherapy; less than half of these patients achieve complete remission. Such patients also tend to have prolonged bone marrow aplasia following treatment and often succumb to complications of pancytopenia. Patients who do achieve remission have a similar remission duration as patients with de novo AML, and intensive induction therapy is usually indicated. No treatment has been consistently effective during the preleukemic phase, and chemotherapy should be withheld until progressive overt leukemia develops. Low-dose cytarabine has been reported to be successful in selected patients with preleukemia or smoldering AML; this therapy will transiently worsen cytopenias, and responses tend to be brief. An innovative approach to therapy for preleukemia involves agents such as retinoic acid which induce cellular diferentiation. A small number of patients with preleukemia have had improvement in peripheral blood counts with retinoic acid therapy, but it is uncertain whether progression to overt leukemia is delayed or if survival is improved. Patients who develop acute leukemia after a preexisting myeloproliferative disorder or paroxysmal nocturnal hemoglobinuria also have a poor prognosis.

Patients who receive cytotoxic chemotherapy with or without concomitant extensive radiation therapy have an increased risk of developing AML. Secondary or treatment-related leukemia is most commonly associated with prolonged therapy with alkylating agents, nitrosoureas, or procarbazine, and has been seen primarily in patients with Hodgkin's disease, multiple myeloma, and ovarian carcinoma. Almost all of the patients with treatment-related AML have chromosomal abnormalities, usually hypodiploidy with −5 and/or −7. These patients typically develop a preleukemic syndrome with pancytopenia several months before overt AML is recognized. They respond poorly to chemotherapy, and despite treatment, median survival is only 3 months after development of AML.

Other factors such as white blood and platelet counts, LDH level, and the presence of fever and hemorrhage have been reported to have prognostic importance. The impact of each of these variables is uncertain.

IMMUNOTHERAPY FOR ACUTE LEUKEMIAS Immunotherapy has been reported to be capable of suppressing small numbers of tumor cells in experimental animals. As such, immunotherapy has been evaluated to prevent leukemic relapse from the residual leukemic cells remaining after induction treatment in patients with ALL and AML. Unfortunately, clinical trials with nonspecific immune potentiating agents such as bacillus Calmette-Guérin (BCG), *Corynebacterium parvum*, or levamisole have not shown any benefit in prolonging the duration of remission. There are no convincing data to support the use of currently available immunotherapy in patients with either ALL or AML.

BONE MARROW TRANSPLANTATION FOR ACUTE LEUKEMIAS

Bone marrow transplantation from an identical twin or an HLA-identical sibling donor is effective treatment for both ALL and AML. The objective of this approach is to administer very high doses of chemotherapy alone or with total-body irradiation, and then to rescue the patient from severe myelosuppression by the transplantation of bone marrow from a normal donor. In addition, the transplantation of allogenic bone marrow may confer an immune-mediated graft-versus-leukemia effect. The current results with bone marrow transplantation are summarized in Table 292-3. Bone marrow transplantation is discussed in detail in Chap. 291.

Allogeneic bone marrow transplantation is associated with substantial risks. Approximately one-third of patients transplanted for leukemia will die from transplant-related complications including graft-versus-host disease, interstitial pneumonitis, and opportunistic infections. Most centers limit the use of bone marrow transplantation to patients under 45 years of age, since older patients generally have a poor outcome. Reports from several centers indicate that 10 to 15 percent of otherwise end-stage patients with refractory leukemia have achieved long-term disease-free survival and probable cure following bone marrow transplantation. Although only a small proportion of patients in this category benefit, the results compare favorably to those obtained with other forms of treatment.

These survival figures are substantially improved when bone marrow transplantation is performed during remission, the burden of leukemic cells is low, and the patients are in relatively good general condition. Because many patients with ALL can achieve a prolonged initial remission with chemotherapy, bone marrow transplantation has generally been reserved for patients in second remission; in this group 30 to 60 percent have achieved prolonged survival with marrow transplantation. It is uncertain whether patients with high-risk forms of ALL should receive marrow transplants in first complete remission.

Approximately 30 percent of patients with AML transplanted in early relapse or second remission have achieved long-term survival. There is controversy whether patients with AML should receive allogenic bone marrow transplantation or postremission chemotherapy while in first complete remission. Over 500 marrow transplants have been reported in this setting. It is clear that the risk of recurrent leukemia is lower following bone marrow transplantation than with postremission chemotherapy; however, bone marrow transplantation is more likely to be associated with fatal treatment complications. Overall 3- to 5-year survival is 40 to 60 percent with bone marrow transplantation compared with 10 to 50 percent survival achieved with optimal chemotherapy. Patient age appears to be a major prognostic factor with bone marrow transplantation; the best results have been reported in children and young adults. Although young patients probably have better results with bone marrow transplantation

TABLE 292-3 Representative results of bone marrow transplantation (BMT) compared with conventional chemotherapy for AML and ALL

	Survival >3 Years, %	
	BMT	Chemotherapy
ALL		
First remission	30–60	20–70*
Second remission	30–50	<10
Third remission or relapse	10–20	0
AML		
First remission	40–60	10–50
Second remission or early relapse	30	<10
Third remission or relapse	10–20	0

* *Best results in children with low white blood count.*

than with chemotherapy, it is uncertain whether this is true for patients over 30 years of age. One major limitation of bone marrow transplantation as a general therapeutic approach is that only a minority of patients are currently eligible; most patients are either too old to be considered or lack an HLA-identical donor.

Autologous bone marrow transplantation has been evaluated in patients with acute leukemia who lack a histocompatible donor for allogeneic transplantation. With this therapy, remission bone marrow is collected and cryopreserved. The patient may then receive intensive chemoradiotherapy followed by reinfusion of the cryopreserved bone marrow. Since remission bone marrow is likely to contain small numbers of residual leukemic cells, the bone marrow has usually been treated with antileukemic monoclonal antibodies or chemotherapy prior to cryopreservation. Selected patients with ALL and AML transplanted in first or second remission have achieved prolonged survival, but further studies are required to critically assess the efficacy of autologous marrow transplantation for acute leukemia.

SUMMARY AND FUTURE DIRECTIONS IN ACUTE LEUKEMIA Effective induction chemotherapy capable of inducing remission in most patients with ALL and AML is now available, but long-term survival has been achieved in only a minority of patients. In the next decade, the focus of clinical research should be toward measures to prolong the duration of remission. Innovative methods of consolidation treatment with intensive chemotherapy or high-dose chemoradiotherapy and bone marrow transplantation must be evaluated for their effect on remission duration and survival. It will also be important to develop effective but less toxic approaches for favorable prognostic groups such as children with low-risk forms of ALL to improve the quality of life in long-term survivors. Innovative new therapies are required for poor-risk groups, particularly the elderly and patients with preleukemic syndromes.

Sensitive techniques to detect residual leukemia during morphologic complete remission must also be developed to help guide the intensity and duration of treatment. Most importantly, new and effective drugs are required with selectivity toward leukemic cells which would spare the host from morbidity and mortality attendant to the currently available agents.

CHRONIC LYMPHOCYTIC LEUKEMIA

Chronic lymphocytic leukemia (CLL) is a hematologic neoplasm characterized by the accumulation of mature-appearing lymphocytes in the peripheral blood associated with infiltration of the bone marrow, spleen, and lymph nodes. The disease is uncommon before the fourth decade of life and is usually seen in patients over 50 years of age. It is the most common form of chronic leukemia in the United States but is rare in Orientals. CLL is more frequent in males than females.

CLL represents a clonal expansion of neoplastic B lymphocytes in more than 95 percent of cases. These cells commonly have trisomy 12 alone or with additional chromosomal abnormalities. Clonality has also been demonstrated by expression of a single light chain (kappa or lambda) or immunoglobulin idiotype specificity. In less than 5 percent of cases, CLL may be due to an expansion of T lymphocytes. An unusual type of T-cell CLL is seen in patients with ataxia-telangiectasia and is often associated with a translocation of genetic material between the number 14 chromosomes (t14;14).

The diagnosis of CLL can usually be made on the basis of physical examination and a review of the peripheral blood smear. Leukocytosis is present, and the malignant cells characteristically appear as morphologically normal small lymphocytes (see Fig. A5-23). They have markers of B lymphocytes. In most cases a monoclonal immunoglobulin can be demonstrated on the cell surface, although immunofluorescent staining is usually weak. Monoclonal surface IgM with or without IgD is characteristically present, and a small amount of this IgM paraprotein can often be detected in the serum with sensitive techniques. The CLL cells also have receptors for the Fc portion of IgG, and complement receptors may or may not be present. Most patients develop some degree of hypogammaglobulinemia. Approximately 5 percent of patients have the T-cell form of CLL. The neoplastic cells form rosettes with sheep erythrocytes and contain other T-cell surface markers. T-cell CLL cannot usually be distinguished from B-cell CLL morphologically.

It is important to distinguish early CLL from reactive lymphocytosis in asymptomatic patients. In reactive lymphocytosis, the cells are polyclonal and predominantly T lymphocytes, whereas in CLL they are usually B cells. The demonstration of monoclonal surface membrane immunoglobulin unambiguously defines a B-cell lymphocytosis as neoplastic. T-cell CLL must be distinguished from Sézary syndrome where the cells have a characteristic lobulated nucleus and there is extensive skin involvement. T-cell CLL also must be distinguished from adult T-cell leukemia (ATL). Prolymphocytic leukemia is a CLL variant seen in older people and is characterized by massive splenomegaly, usually in the absence of lymphadenopathy. The neoplastic cell in prolymphocytic leukemia usually is of B-cell origin. It is larger than that seen in CLL and has a prominent nucleolus. Prolymphocytic leukemia is typically associated with very high white counts (in excess of 200×10^9 per liter) and a poor response to therapy. Lymphosarcoma cell leukemia represents a leukemic phase of lymphocytic lymphoma and is typically an aggressive disease (Chap. 294). The cellular morphology is suggestive of an acute rather than a chronic leukemia. Monoclonal immunoglobulin is usually easily detected on these cells, and the fluorescent staining is bright, often with spontaneous capping. Hairy-cell leukemia is distinguished on the basis of the typical cellular morphology and the presence of tartrate-resistant acid phosphatase in the hairy cells. Waldenström's macroglobulinemia is differentiated from CLL on the basis of bone marrow morphology and lower white blood cell counts, and the secretion of a large amount of a monoclonal IgM paraprotein.

CLINICAL FEATURES The clinical features of CLL are very different from acute leukemia. In more than 25 percent of patients with CLL, the disorder is discovered as an incidental finding. The common practice of ordering routine complete blood counts in adults has led to an earlier diagnosis of CLL in asymptomatic patients. The signs and symptoms of CLL usually relate to tissue infiltration, peripheral blood cytopenias, or immunosuppression. Patients may present with symptoms of anemia, lymph node enlargement, or intercurrent infection. Splenomegaly seldom leads to symptoms, and the liver is minimally enlarged in only about half of patients.

The white cell count ranges between 15×10^9 and 200×10^9 per liter, with a preponderance of mature-appearing lymphocytes. There is little correlation between the leukocyte count and symptomatology. Patients with advanced disease may present with anemia, granulocytopenia, and thrombocytopenia resulting from bone marrow infiltration by the leukemic cells. About 20 percent of patients develop a Coombs-positive autoimmune hemolytic anemia during the course of their disease. Occasionally, autoimmune thrombocytopenia may occur. Rarely, CLL evolves into an aggressive lymphocytic lymphoma referred to as *Richter's syndrome*, which is believed to be due to a clonal evolution of the original leukemia.

TREATMENT The therapeutic objectives in CLL differ sharply from those for the acute leukemias. The available drugs and radiation therapies are incapable of eradicating the leukemia and producing true complete remissions. Current therapy is effective to reduce the lymphocyte count and lymphadenopathy and to palliate symptoms produced by the leukemia. There is little evidence, however, that survival is substantially affected.

Although a number of prognostic classifications of CLL have been suggested, the new international classification appears most useful (Table 292–4). Prognosis correlates well with stage of disease; however, the rate of progression of patients from one stage to another is highly variable. Patients with stage A disease, in which the disease is limited to lymphocytosis alone or lymphocytosis plus limited lymphadenopathy, have a good prognosis. Median survival exceeds 7 years; these patients usually require no treatment. Patients with

TABLE 292-4 International workshop on CLL staging classification

Stage	Description	Median survival, years
A	Lymphocytosis with clinical involvement of fewer than 3 lymph node groups*; no anemia or thrombocytopenia	>10
B	More than 3 lymph node groups* involved	5
C	Anemia or thrombocytopenia regardless of number of lymph node groups involved	2

* *Lymph node groups—cervical, axillary, inguinal, liver, spleen.*

more substantial lymphadenopathy and hepatosplenomegaly (stage B) have an intermediate prognosis with a median survival of approximately 5 years. Patients with anemia or thrombocytopenia (stage C) have a worse prognosis with a median survival of less than 2 years.

The indications for therapy in CLL include hemolytic anemia, important cytopenias, disfiguring lymphadenopathy, symptomatic organomegaly, or marked systemic symptoms. When treatment is required, the cornerstone of therapy is usually an alkylating agent. Chlorambucil is the most frequently prescribed drug for CLL at a recommended daily dose of 0.1 to 0.2 mg/kg per day. The chlorambucil dose is generally reduced and the drug is eventually stopped when the lymphocyte count falls below 20×10^9 per liter. The drug may also be given in pulses every 3 to 6 weeks, or continuously in low daily doses. Cyclophosphamide appears to be as effective as chlorambucil in the treatment of CLL. Maintenance therapy has no definite value, and continuing alkylating agent therapy may increase the risk of future development of AML.

Glucocorticosteroids are useful for CLL in special circumstances. These drugs do not have a prominent lympholytic effect in CLL and are therefore not effective as primary therapy. Glucocorticosteroids are useful, however, in the treatment of associated Coombs-positive hemolytic anemia or immune thrombocytopenia, and may be transiently effective in treating patients with pancytopenia and the "packed marrow" syndrome. Glucocorticosteroids have important side effects, including a predisposition to opportunistic infection. In more advanced CLL, combination chemotherapy may be useful. Regimens that include an alkylating agent, vincristine, and prednisone are often employed. Splenectomy may be indicated in patients with hypersplenism, refractory hemolytic anemia, or thrombocytopenia. Radiation therapy may occasionally be useful for control of localized disease, and total-body radiation has rarely been useful in palliating end-stage disease. In preliminary trials, interferon does not appear to be effective in this disease, although agents such as deoxycoformycin, an adenosine deaminase inhibitor, are promising.

Hypogammaglobulinemia is common in patients with CLL, and life-threatening infectious complications may occur. Intramuscular injections of gamma globulin have not been effective, but it is uncertain whether the recently developed intravenous immunoglobulin preparations will be useful in preventing infections in these patients.

HAIRY-CELL LEUKEMIA

Hairy-cell leukemia is a lymphoid neoplasm characterized by peripheral blood cytopenias, splenomegaly, and morphologically typical malignant cells in the blood and bone marrow. The disease superficially resembles CLL but has distinct clinical features and requires different therapy. Hairy-cell leukemia is usually seen in patients over 40 years of age, and there is a very definite male preponderance. Originally, this disorder was thought to account for about 2 percent of all leukemias; however, the disease is now recognized with increased frequency, and many large series have been reported. Hairy-cell leukemia has been reported to occur worldwide.

The disease was originally referred to as leukemic reticuloendotheliosis; however, the term hairy-cell leukemia is now widely accepted because it is descriptive of the characteristic cytoplasmic projections seen on the leukemic cell. The disorder is due to expansion of neoplastic B lymphocytes which often produce monoclonal immunoglobulin; however, rare T-cell variants have been reported. The etiology of hairy-cell leukemia is unknown; a single case of T-cell hairy-cell leukemia has been reported, from which a unique species of human T-cell leukemia virus (HTLV II) was recovered.

CLINICAL FEATURES AND PATHOLOGY Patients with hairy-cell leukemia usually present with symptoms due to splenomegaly, infection caused by impaired host defense, or vasculitis. Many asymptomatic patients are detected on routine complete blood counts. More than three-quarters of patients will have palpable splenomegaly and, in some cases, splenic involvement is massive. Lymphadenopathy is rare, and substantial hepatomegaly is uncommon at the time of diagnosis, although infiltration of the portal triads by hairy cells is often seen microscopically. Occasionally bone lesions may cause symptoms of hip pain. Approximately 30 percent of patients with hairy-cell leukemia have an associated vasculitis-like disorder. Common manifestations include erythema nodosum and cutaneous nodules due to perivasculitis. Visceral involvement similar to polyarteritis nodosa may occur.

Moderate pancytopenia is usually present at diagnosis. The leukocyte count is normal or low, and characteristic hairy cells are seen in the peripheral blood. These cells are about 15 to 20 μm in diameter and have an eccentrically placed nucleus with characteristic foamy cytoplasm. Cytoplasmic projections may be seen on smear, but they are best appreciated by phase microscopy. These cells stain positively for tartrate-resistant acid phosphatase (TRAP), which is a cytochemical stain for the isoenzyme 5 of acid phosphatase. Bone marrow aspiration is seldom successful because of reticulin fibrosis. The biopsy typically shows replacement of the normal architecture by mononuclear cells that are not packed together but maintain spaces between the intercellular contacts. Splenic histology is typical, consisting of mononuclear cell infiltration of the red pulp and engorgement of the sinuses.

Hairy-cell leukemia must be distinguished from chronic lymphocytic leukemia, Waldenström's macroglobulinemia, and acute leukemia. Some patients with hairy-cell leukemia present with a hypocellular bone marrow which may be misdiagnosed as aplastic anemia. The diagnosis depends on identifying the characteristic cells in the bone marrow and peripheral blood.

TREATMENT OF HAIRY-CELL LEUKEMIA The course of hairy-cell leukemia can be quite indolent; however, there is a wide spectrum of severity and rate of progression of the disease among patients. Approximately one-quarter of patients present without significant cytopenias and without other complications of the disease; these patients require no immediate treatment. They should be followed at intervals and closely observed for infections. Infection is the primary cause of death in patients with hairy-cell leukemia. Common infections include *Legionella* pneumonitis, toxoplasmosis, tuberculosis, and atypical mycobacterial disease, nocardiosis, and pyogenic infections. Patients probably benefit from pneumococcal vaccination. Any significant fever should be thoroughly evaluated and aggressively treated with antibiotics. Since *Legionella* pneumonitis is relatively common in these patients, high-dose erythromycin should usually be administered to patients with pulmonary infiltrates.

Therapy directed at the leukemia is indicated in patients presenting with marked pancytopenia, a history of infections, massive splenomegaly, or a rapid rate of disease progression. The cornerstone of therapy is splenectomy, which appears to ameliorate the disease in a majority of patients. The role of splenectomy in patients with no splenic enlargement is uncertain. Patients with progressive disease following splenectomy or those in whom splenectomy is contraindicated should be treated with α-interferon. Interferon is an experimental drug which has recently been shown to be effective in hairy-cell leukemia. Virtually all treated patients have responded to α-interferon.

Patients requiring interferon therapy should be referred to research centers specializing in such treatment. Glucocorticosteroids are not effective in hairy-cell leukemia, and they are potentially dangerous because they further predispose these patients to infections. Short courses of glucocorticosteroids may be useful, however, in controlling the vasculitis or autoimmune manifestations that are often associated with the disease. Chemotherapy with alkylating agents or other myelotoxic drugs is hazardous in patients with hairy-cell leukemia because of poor bone marrow reserve. The adenosine deaminase inhibitor deoxycoformycin has been shown to be useful for selected patients. Aggressive chemotherapy may be tried when other therapeutic interventions have failed, and there is anecdotal information that some patients respond to treatment with lithium and androgens. Bone marrow transplantation has also been successful in a small number of patients with advanced hairy-cell leukemia.

The prognosis in hairy-cell leukemia is variable, and published series are outdated because of the recent improvements in diagnosis and treatment. At least 50 percent of patients will survive more than 8 years from diagnosis, and this prognosis should improve further with the application of new treatments and better supportive care.

SELECTED REFERENCES

General

GALE RP (ed): *Leukemia Treatment.* Boston, Blackwell, 1986

———, GOLDE DW (eds): *Leukemia: Recent Advances in Biology and Treatment.* New York, Alan R Liss Inc., 1985

GOLDE DW, TAKAKU E (eds): *Hematopoietic Stem Cells.* New York, Marcel Dekker Inc, 1985

GUNZ FW, HENDERSON ES (eds): *Leukemia,* 4th ed. New York, Grune & Stratton, 1983

ROWLEY JD: Biological implications of consistent chromosome rearrangements in leukemia and lymphoma. Cancer Res 44:3159, 1984

WONG-STAAL F, GALLO RC: The family of human T-lymphotropic leukemia viruses: HTLV-I as the cause of adult T cell leukemia and HTLV-III as the cause of acquired immunodeficiency syndrome. Blood 65:253, 1985

YUNIS JJ: The chromosomal basis of human neoplasia. Science 221:227, 1983

Acute leukemias

BENNETT JM et al: Proposals for the classification of the acute leukaemias. Br J Haematol 33:451, 1976

BENNETT JM et al: Criteria for the diagnosis of acute leukemia of megakaryocytic lineage. Ann Intern Med 103:460, 1085

CHAMPLIN RE, GALE RP: Role of bone marrow transplantation in the treatment of hematologic malignancies and solid tumors: Critical review of syngeneic, autologous, and allogeneic transplants. Cancer Treat Rep 68:145, 1984

ALL

JACOBS AD, GALE RP: Recent advances in the biology and treatment of acute lymphoblastic leukemia in adults. N Engl J Med 311:1219, 1984

JOHNSON FL et al: A comparison of marrow transplantation with chemotherapy for children with acute lymphoblastic leukemia in second or subsequent remission. N Engl J Med 305:846, 1981

MAUER AM: Therapy of acute lymphoblastic leukemia in childhood. Blood 56:1, 1980

RITZ J et al: Autologous bone marrow transplantation in CALLA-positive acute lymphoblastic leukemia after in vitro treatment with J5 monoclonal antibody and complement. Lancet 2:60, 1982

SHAUER P et al: Treatment of acute lymphoblastic leukemia in adults; results of the L-10 and L-10M protocols. J Clin Oncol 1:462, 1983

AML

APPELBAUM FR et al: Bone marrow transplantation or chemotherapy after remission induction for adults with acute nonlymphoblastic leukemia. Ann Intern Med 101:581, 1984

CHAMPLIN RE et al: Treatment of acute myelogenous leukemia: A prospective controlled trial of bone marrow transplantation versus consolidation chemotherapy. Ann Intern Med 102:285–291, 1985

——— et al: Prolonged survival in acute myelogenous leukaemia without maintenance chemotherapy. Lancet 1:894, 1984

FIALKOW PJ et al: Acute nonlymphocytic leukemia: Heterogeneity of stem cell origin. Blood 57:1068, 1981

FOON KA et al: The role of immunotherapy in acute myelogenous leukemia. Arch Intern Med 143:1726, 1983

GALE RP: Progress in acute myelogenous leukemia. Ann Intern Med 101:702, 1984

———, CHAMPLIN RE: How does bone marrow transplantation cure leukaemia? Lancet 2:28, 1984

GREENBERG PL: The smoldering myeloid leukemic states: Clinical and biologic features. Blood 61:1035, 1983

HERZIG RH et al: High-dose cytosine arabinoside therapy for refractory leukemia. Blood 62:361, 1983

KOEFFLER HP: Induction of differentiation of human acute myelogenous leukemia cells: Therapeutic implications. Blood 62:709, 1983

WEINSTEIN HJ et al: Chemotherapy for acute myelogenous leukemia in children and adults: VAPA update. Blood 62:315, 1983

WISCH JS et al: Response of preleukemic syndromes to continuous infusion of low-dose cytandine. N Engl J Med 309:599, 1983

Chronic lymphocytic leukemia

BINET J-L et al: Chronic lymphocytic leukaemia: Proposals for a revised prognostic staging system. Br J Haematol 48:365, 1981

CALIGARIS-CAPPIO F, JANOSSY G: Surface markers in chronic lymphoid leukemias of B cell type. Semin Hematol 22:1, 1985

FOON K GALE RP: Chronic lymphocytic leukemia: Recent advances in biology and treatment. Ann Intern Med 101:120, 1985

HAN T et al: Prognostic importance of cytogenetic abnormalities in patients with chronic lymphocytic leukemia. N Engl J Med 310:288, 1984

Hairy-cell leukemia

GOLOMB HM (ed): Hairy cell leukemia. Semin Oncol 11, 1984

——— et al: Hairy cell leukemia: A five year update on seventy-one patients. Ann Intern Med 99:485, 1983

JACOBS AD et al: Recombinant alpha-2 interferon for hairy-cell leukemia. Blood 65:1017, 1985

QUESADA JR et al: Alpha interferon for induction of remission in hairy-cell leukemia. N Engl J Med 310:15, 1984

section 3 Neoplastic diseases

293 THE HUMAN T-LYMPHOTROPIC VIRUSES

ROBERT C. GALLO / ANTHONY S. FAUCI

BIOLOGY OF THE RETROVIRUSES Retroviruses were first isolated from chickens at the beginning of this century. In the 1950s the first mammalian retroviruses were isolated from mice with leukemia, and these are now known to be associated with malignancies in many species and with some nonmalignant disorders. Retroviruses may be subdivided according to the types of disease they cause: malignant, nonmalignant, both malignant and nonmalignant, and nonpathogenic. Nonpathogenic retroviruses are often transmitted in the germ line as normal genetic mendelian elements, a unique feature of this class of viruses, i.e., endogenous retroviruses. An example of a retrovirus causing malignant and nonmalignant disease is feline leukemia virus (FeLV), which can cause T-cell leukemia but more frequently causes a disorder mimicking the acquired immunodeficiency syndrome (AIDS) of human beings (see Chap. 257). Retroviruses of a class that causes nonmalignant disease, e.g., encephalitis, other neurologic abnormalities, arthritis, and lung disease, are the slow-acting lentiretroviruses. Lentiretroviruses occur in ungulates, in human beings (human T-lymphotropic virus type III [HTLV III]), and in nonhuman primates (simian T-lymphotropic virus type III [STLV III]).

Retroviruses are enveloped, bud from cell membranes, and contain an electron-dense, central core structure surrounding a viral RNA genome. The *sine qua non* of a retrovirus is the DNA polymerase, known as reverse transcriptase (RT), which is complexed to the RNA in the viral core and catalyzes the transcription of the RNA genome into a DNA form (the provirus). The DNA form usually migrates from the cytoplasm to the nucleus and then, after becoming a double-stranded circular form, integrates into the host cell DNA, where the viral genes may remain for the lifetime of the cell (Fig. 293-1). Because the provirus is duplicated with the cell DNA during the S phase of the cell cycle, the viral genes are passed to daughter cells. Therefore, infection of an organism is generally lifelong. When the provirus is expressed, viral RNA and proteins are found in the cell cytoplasm and assembled at the cell membrane, where budding and release of the viruses completes the virus's life cycle. Sometimes deletions of the provirus occur, and this may be followed by the acquisition of host cellular sequences by normal or abnormal processing of RNA. As a consequence, the virus subsequently formed with these newly acquired nucleotide sequences acquires some properties that differ from the original virus.

Structural features of the retroviral genome determine the molecular mechanism by which these viruses alter a cell. The most common are the chronic leukemia viruses which contain only the three essential genes for virus replication: *gag, pol,* and *env* (Fig. 293-2) (see Chap. 59). *Gag* codes for the viral internal structural proteins, *pol* codes for RT, and *env* codes for the glycoprotein envelope of the virus. The properties of the envelope have a major influence on the kind of cell the virus can infect, and production of antibodies against the envelope is one of the essential features sought for in a vaccine. The viral genes are flanked at each end by nucleotide sequences called *long terminal repeats* (LTR), which contain regulatory elements that influence the expression of the viral genes and sometimes of nearby cellular genes. The LTRs contain the signals determining proviral integration into the host cell DNA and form the terminals of the integrated proviral sequence. Some examples of chronic leukemia viruses are FeLV, mouse leukemia virus, and avian leukosis virus (ALV). These viruses replicate extensively in the host prior to the induction of leukemia. There is evidence that they cause leukemia by integration into a specific region of a chromosome so that the associated LTRs act to promote continual expression of a cellular gene involved in growth. The best example of this *cis* mechanism is in chickens, where the LTR of ALV promotes expression of a cellular oncogene believed to be the first step in the induction of leukemia by this virus. Since integration by retroviruses is random, a high rate of replication favors the chance of integration into regions sufficiently near the cellular oncogene to enable the LTR to activate this gene. This may explain the apparent need for extensive virus replication prior to the development of malignancy.

When retroviruses acquire through genetic recombination a host cell gene which rapidly transforms cells and induces acute malignancies, the virus is often called an acute leukemia or sarcoma virus, and the gene is called a viral *onc* gene (Fig. 293-2) (see Chaps. 58 and 59). Viruses with *onc* genes are rare, have never been identified in humans, and are of interest in animals chiefly for investigating neoplastic transformation rather than as causes of naturally occurring

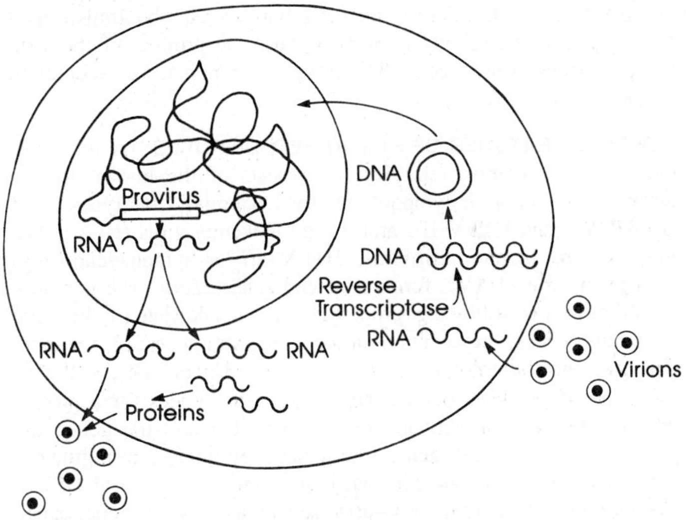

FIGURE 293-1 *Life cycle of a retrovirus. Intact virions are endocytosed via a specific cellular receptor. The uncoated viral single-stranded RNA is then transcribed into double-stranded DNA, enters the cell nucleus, and integrates into the host genome. The DNA provirus in some conditions is unexpressed. In other cases it is transcribed, giving rise to viral RNA encoding viral proteins and to genome-length viral RNA molecules which then reassemble with viral proteins to make complete virions. These progeny are released by budding from the cell membrane.*

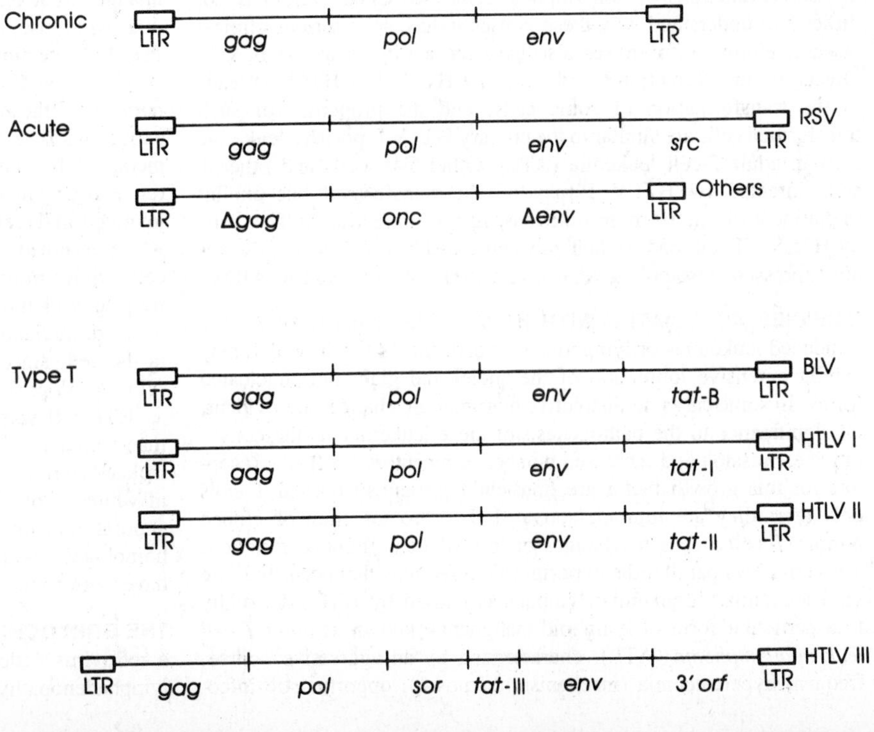

FIGURE 293-2 *Genetic structure and proposed classification of retroviruses.* gag, *core proteins;* pol, *reverse transcriptase;* env, *envelope; LTR, long terminal repeat;* gag, env, *incomplete genes;* src, *one of the* onc *genes; BLV, bovine leukemia virus;* tat, *transacting transcriptional activator gene;* sor, *short open reading frame;* 3′ orf, *3′ open reading frame. The latter two are genes in HTLV III of unknown function.*

cancer. Every cell infected by these viruses can be transformed (giving rise to polyclonal tumors) because the product of the viral *onc* gene transforms directly. Therefore, a common site of integration is not needed.

GENERAL FEATURES OF HUMAN RETROVIRUSES A third category, transactivation retroviruses, consists of the known human retroviruses, human T-lymphotropic (or leukemia) virus types I and II (HTLV I and HTLV II), and bovine leukemia virus (BLV). The third known human retrovirus, HTLV III or lymphadenopathy-associated virus (LAV), forms a special subcategory. The genomes of all have the following properties: (1) in addition to the viral replication genes, they contain one or more extra genes; (2) the extra gene(s) is not homologous to mammalian cell gene, i.e., is not an *onc* gene; (3) at least one of these extra genes codes for a protein which is involved in activating expression of other viral genes and probably of certain cell genes (presumably by binding to regulatory enhancer elements in the cell which are similar to the viral LTRs). The biologic effects of these viruses are mediated by this gene, called *transacting transcriptional activator* or *tat*. Since *tat* codes for a nuclear protein which can activate other genes, these viruses do not need to integrate in a special region to induce disease. This may explain why extensive virus replication is not essential for them to cause neoplastic or nonneoplastic disease. A similar phenomemon is seen in bovine lymphoma induced by BLV. HTLV III not only contains the three genes for virus replication and a *tat* gene but also contains at least two other genes of undefined function.

HTLV I and HTLV II are similar in structure, HTLV III differs in its mature form, containing a highly condensed cylindrical core. HTLV I, the first human retrovirus to be identified, was isolated in 1978 from a man with an aggressive T-cell malignancy. Techniques for virus detection were based on the use of reverse transcriptase as a "footprint" of a retrovirus, since this assay can be much more sensitive than electron microscopy. In addition, the necessary prerequisite for the growth of the target T lymphocytes, which allow virus replication, was fulfilled with the discovery of T-cell growth factor, now called interleukin 2 (IL-2). This same basic technique was used for the isolation of the virus that causes AIDS.

A striking feature of all known human retroviruses is their tropism for the T4$^+$ helper lymphocyte. Although other cells can be infected, this helper T cell is preferentially infected in vitro by all three types of human retroviruses and the diseases caused by them almost always involve this cell. Since the T4$^+$ cell regulates many immune functions and some functions of nonlymphoid cells (see Chap. 62), it is not difficult to understand why these viruses induce such serious clinical disease. Human retroviruses also have the ability to mimic in vivo effects in vitro. Infection of T4$^+$ cells by HTLV I or HTLV II leads to the transformation of some cells, and the properties of such transformed cells are similar to the primary HTLV I–positive leukemic cells in adult T-cell leukemia (ATL). Other T4$^+$ cells and other T cells infected by HTLV I may not be transformed but exhibit impairment of one or more functions. In vitro infection of T4$^+$ cells by HTLV III can lead to their premature death when the viral genes are expressed, resembling what is assumed to be the case in AIDS.

DISEASES ASSOCIATED WITH HTLV I The majority of HTLV I–induced leukemias or lymphomas involve the T4$^+$ cell, which may exhibit extensive lobulation of the nuclei and giant multinucleated forms. In some cases no distinctive morphologic changes are evident. Of significance to the pathogenesis of these leukemias is the constitutive expression and increased number of receptors for IL-2. Receptors for this growth factor are transiently present in normal T cells only after they are immune-activated. In vitro infection of cloned normal T cells leads to changes or loss of their immune function. These findings parallel the opportunistic infections that occur in these viral leukemias. Leukemias/lymphomas caused by HTLV I usually fit a particular form of lymphoid malignancy known as *adult T-cell leukemia/lymphoma* (ATL), characterized by an aggressive course, frequent hypercalcemia (mechanism unknown), opportunistic infection, and, in over half the cases, leukemic skin infiltrates (see Chap. 294).

HTLV I may also be involved in T4-cell leukemias/lymphomas that exhibit a more chronic course (15 to 20 percent of cases) and have other features differing from ATL. These may be indistinguishable pathologically or clinically from T-cell chronic lymphocytic leukemia (CLL), diffuse histiocytic lymphoma, large and mixed cell lymphomas, and mycosis fungoides or Sézary leukemias. In the United States only a small percentage of these diseases are HTLV I–positive, whereas close to 100 percent of ATL cases are virus-positive. In areas of the world where HTLV I is endemic, some B-cell lymphoid malignancies and certain other cancers are associated with HTLV I infection more frequently than expected from the prevalence of the virus in the general population. In contrast to virus-positive T-cell leukemias where the viral genes are integrated into the DNA of the leukemic cell, HTLV I was not found in the DNA of these B-cell tumors. Instead, the virus was found in the normal T cells of these patients. The malignant B cells in this disorder make a single type of antibody directed against a protein of HTLV I. Therefore, the B-cell tumors may arise in part by an indirect effect of HTLV I, i.e., by chronic antigenic stimulation combined with diminished T-cell immune surveillance, thereby increasing the chance for a neoplastic transformation in the expanding B-cell compartment.

ORIGIN AND EPIDEMIOLOGY OF HTLV I Although HTLV I was originally discovered in two sporadic cases of T-cell malignancies in blacks in the United States and although the first clusters of this disease were found in Japanese and later in Caribbean-born blacks, the virus likely originated in Africa for the following reasons: (1) it is widely distributed throughout Africa, (2) in the Americas and Europe, ATL occurs chiefly in people with African ancestry, and (3) a closely related virus (STLV I) has been found in African old world monkeys. HTLV I is also prevalent in the two small southwestern islands of Japan, Kyushu and Shikoku, where it may have been brought by Africans in the sixteenth century. The geographic distribution of HTLV I is relatively restricted, e.g., less than 1 percent of whites in the United States and Europe are infected, and the virus is unusual in most of Asia. Thus, it was not complicated to establish an epidemiologic link of this virus to the diseases caused. Transmission is by intimate contact, by blood or blood products, and by infection of the developing fetus in utero. It has been speculated that the virus may also be transmitted by insect vectors, but there are no data bearing on this important question. Because of increase in travel, changes in sexual habits, drug abuse (blood-contaminated needles), and wide use of blood and blood products, the prevalence of HTLV I infection may be increasing.

Upon infection of T cells with HTLV I or HTLV II a small number of these cells become immortalized, losing their need for exogenous IL-2 to maintain growth. This phenomenon appears to be mediated by the *tat* gene product, which is believed to bind to regulatory elements of T cells which activate the expression of gene(s) involved in T-cell proliferation. One such gene is the IL-2 receptor, which, as noted earlier, is constitutively expressed in these transformed cells. Since cells other than T4 can be infected, the reason for the frequency of transformation of the T4$^+$ cell is unclear. The maintenance of malignancy is believed to require additional genetic changes in the cell, since the HTLV I genes are usually not expressed after ATL develops.

HTLV II was originally isolated from a cell line derived from a man with a T-cell variant of hairy-cell leukemia. The virus was again isolated from two more cases of chronic forms of T-cell malignancies in whites. Considerable details exist on the nature of the HTLV-II genome and on its in vitro effects (it is overall about 50 percent homologous with HTLV I), and a few major biologic differences have been found between the two viruses.

THE ETIOLOGIC AGENT OF AIDS The etiologic agent of AIDS is a retrovirus called HTLV III. Other designations for the virus are lymphadenopathy-associated virus (LAV) and AIDS-associated retrovirus (ARV). The pathogenesis of the syndrome relates to the infection of the T4+ inducer/helper subset of lymphocytes with the virus, leading to the premature death of these critical cells. The resulting immune defect predisposes the patient to overwhelming opportunistic infections and certain malignancies. For a detailed description of AIDS, see Chap. 257.

OTHER HTLV III–ASSOCIATED DISEASES In addition to full-blown AIDS, with its opportunistic infections and increased incidence of Kaposi's sarcoma, and to the AIDS-related complex of disease (Chap. 257), infection with HTLV III/LAV can also be associated with other diseases. The virus can infect the brain and lead to severe neuropsychiatric abnormalities. A lymphoid interstitial pneumonitis has been associated with HTLV III/LAV infection. AIDS patients have an increased incidence of certain B-cell lymphomas. Furthermore, the incidence of Hodgkin's disease and certain carcinomas (cloacogenic squamous-cell carcinoma and head and neck tumors) may be increased in patients with HTLV III/LAV infection. The reason for the increase in these malignancies is not understood. HTLV III/LAV is not the direct cause because viral sequences are not found in the DNA from the majority of tumor cells. For the B-cell lymphomas, the mechanism may be similar to the indirect role described above for HTLV I. HTLV III/LAV infection may also cause autoimmune thrombocytopenia and congenital abnormalities.

THE CYTOPATHIC EFFECT OF HTLV III/LAV ON T4+ CELLS Infection of T4+ cells by HTLV III/LAV leads to the premature death of these cells, and there is evidence that one or more genes of HTLV III/LAV leads to T4-cell death upon transfection of the DNA provirus into these cells. It is impossible to induce a productive viral infection of T4+ cells in vitro unless the T cells are immune-activated. The activated, infected T cells appear to go through the same process of cell gene expression as do uninfected cells, except that the viral genes are eventually expressed. When this occurs, a higher percentage of the cells than normal terminally differentiate, and the rate of terminal differentiation is faster than that in the uninfected T cells. This process may involve the *tat*-III gene (Fig. 293-2). Expression of this gene may in turn activate an extremely high level of transcription of another viral gene or of cellular genes that augment terminal differentiation.

HETEROGENEITY OF HTLV III/LAV Molecular analysis of various HTLV III/LAV isolates reveals variation of nucleotide sequences of certain parts of the genome, especially in the envelope gene. Detailed analysis of different isolates indicates that there is a continuum from very closely related isolates (1 to 2 percent variation) to those that vary more than 5 percent. Variation develops after successive infections and does not occur during prolonged tissue culture, suggesting that these changes occur during transcription of the viral RNA genome to the DNA form and/or during the recombinational process when the DNA provirus integrates into the host cell DNA. RTs are DNA polymerases that tend to be error prone. The RT of HTLV III/LAV may be particularly error prone. It may be that variation in other parts of the viral genome leads to noninfectious particles.

PREVENTION AND TREATMENT OF HTLV III/LAV INFECTION There are three special problems in the prevention and treatment of HTLV III/LAV infection: (1) T cells are the principal cells involved in protection against a virus, and these are the cells destroyed by the virus. If infection occurs by cell-cell contact, there may be little one can do to augment defense against the virus. (2) The envelope heterogeneity among different HTLV III/LAV isolates presents a problem, but the nucleotide sequences of the envelope of several isolates have been recently compared and analysis reveals that there are conserved areas of the envelope gene, some of which should be immunogenic. It is conceptually feasible, therefore, to develop a vaccine to induce protective antibodies. (3) Since infection may mean integration of the viral genes into the DNA of the infected cell and these are transmitted to progeny cells, infection with HTLV III/LAV is likely lifelong. More than one million people in the United States are known to be infected by HTLV III/LAV. Avoidance of other infections which could activate already infected T cells, promoting both their death and spread of virus, is important. Antiviral compounds are being developed, including those which utilize RT inhibitors and agents that interact with the viral envelope. Other approaches result from structural-functional studies of the viral genome, e.g., inhibitors of *tat*-III gene expression or function. Treatment will probably have to be lifelong, and to avoid toxicity and reduce the chances for viral resistance, it may be necessary to use a combination of compounds with different mechanisms of action. Another approach would be to kill infected cells. Hypothetically, if this could be achieved for all infected cells, a cure could be effected. However, this may not be possible with human retroviruses because most infected cells do not express viral proteins and hence would not be distinguishable from uninfected cells.

HTLV III/LAV is a new infection of humans with severe and often fatal consequences. Like HTLV I (and probably HTLV II), it is likely that HTLV III/LAV entered African humans from African green monkeys or related primates directly or through intermediary vectors and subsequently spread to other regions. Also similar to HTLV I is its mode of transmission, T4 tropism, in vitro mimicry of the disease, and presence of the *tat* gene. Unlike HTLV I or HTLV II, the AIDS virus contains at least two additional genes, has strong cytopathic effects, has greater structural similarities to the lentiretroviruses, and is generally more infectious.

REFERENCES

BALTIMORE D: RNA-dependent DNA polymerase in virions of RNA tumor viruses. Nature 226:1209, 1970

BRODER S, GALLO RC: A pathogenic retrovirus (HTLV-III) linked to AIDS. N Engl J Med 311:1292, 1984

Cold Spring Harbor Symposia on Quantitative Biology, vol 39: *Biology of Tumor Viruses*. Cold Spring Harbor, New York, Cold Spring Harbor, 1975

GALLO RC: Introduction: Human T-lymphotropic retroviruses, in *Human T-Cell Leukemia/Lymphoma Virus*, RC Gallo et al (eds). Cold Spring Harbor, New York, Cold Spring Harbor, 1984, pp 1–8

GROSS L: *Oncogenic Viruses*, 3d ed. Oxford, Pergamon Press, 1983

HAHN BH et al: Genomic diversity of the acquired immune deficiency syndrome virus HTLV-II: Different viruses exhibit greatest divergence in their envelope genes. Proc Natl Acad Sci USA 83:4813, 1985

ROBERT-GUROFF M et al: T-cell growth factor, in *Growth and Maturation Factors*, G Guroff (ed). New York, Wiley, 1984, vol 2, pp 267–308

SAXINGER WC, GALLO RC: Human T-cell growth factor (TCGF): Its discovery, properties and some basic and applied uses in the long term propagation of human mature T-cells, in *Human Cancer Immunology*, B Serou, CL Rosenfeld (eds). Amsterdam, North-Holland, 1981, pp 463–568

SHAW GM et al: Human T-cell leukemia virus: Its discovery and role in leukemogenesis and immunosuppression, in *Advances in Internal Medicine*, GH Stollerman et al (eds). Chicago, Year Book, 1984, vol 30, pp 1–27

TEMIN HM, MIZUTANI S: RNA-directed DNA polymerase in virions of Rous sarcoma virus. Nature 226:1211, 1970

WONG-STAAL F, GALLO RC: The family of human T-lymphotropic leukemia and HTLV-III as the cause of acquired immunodeficiency syndrome. Blood 65:253, 1985

———: Human T lymphotropic retrovirus. Nature 317:395, 1985

294 HODGKIN'S DISEASE AND THE LYMPHOCYTIC LYMPHOMAS

VINCENT T. DeVITA, JR. / JOHN E. ULTMANN

DEFINITION The lymphomas should be considered tumors of the immune system. They include tumors of lymphocytes and Hodgkin's disease. They rarely include tumors thought to be derived from histiocytes. While they have been referred to as Hodgkin's disease and the non-Hodgkin's lymphomas, more sophisticated diagnostic tools can precisely delineate the subcategories of disease. The old terminology should be abandoned.

EPIDEMIOLOGY About 34,000 new cases of lymphoma were diagnosed in 1985; 40 percent of these were Hodgkin's disease. The most common lymphocytic lymphomas are those of follicular morphology followed by diffuse large-cell lymphomas, each constituting about 40 percent of the remaining cases. Because of the young average age of the population (32 years for Hodgkin's disease and 42 for the other adult lymphomas), the toll in person-years of life lost because of deaths from lymphomas ranks them fourth among cancers in terms of economic impact. Although the incidence of lymphomas is increasing each year, mortality is falling because of improvements in treatment. In Hodgkin's disease, survival has improved markedly since 1970, and national mortality has fallen 58 percent since 1973. In diffuse large cell lymphomas, national 5-year survival rates have improved from less than 5 percent to over 40 percent in the past decade.

Worldwide, there are differences in the prevalence of lymphomas. In the United States, Hodgkin's disease has a bimodal age-specific incidence rate, one mode occurring at ages 15 to 35 years and the second above 50. A disproportionate number of patients in the first modal peak have the nodular sclerosing variety of Hodgkin's disease. The first peak is absent in Japan. Hodgkin's disease in children under 10 years is seen much more frequently in underdeveloped countries and, when it is observed, the histologic varieties and stages are characteristic of more advanced disease in the United States. These observations and the occasional report of clusters of Hodgkin's disease suggest environmental and/or genetic influences operating on the development of these diseases. Following reports of several clusters of Hodgkin's disease in the United States, population-based studies using the cancer registries of Connecticut and California indicated that these reported clusters probably occurred by chance alone. Medical personnel who specialize in the care of patients with lymphoma do not seem to have a higher incidence of these diseases than do others. An excellent epidemiologic study, however, has made a strong case for the hypothesis that Hodgkin's disease may be a rare manifestation of a common infection. Factors that increase the risk of early exposure to infections, such as large family size or multiple families per dwelling, decrease the risk of Hodgkin's disease. The data also suggest that different risk factors are involved for Hodgkin's disease among the young and in the old. These data may explain several curious epidemiologic associations, such as the absence of the early peak in Japan. Some of the lymphocytic lymphomas have unique epidemiologic characteristics. Burkitt's lymphoma occurs characteristically in children of central Africa, although a small number of cases have been reported in this country, but with a different clinical presentation. Abdominal lymphomas with associated production of heavy chains of immunoglobulin occur in the Mediterranean region but are rarely seen in other parts of the world.

TABLE 294-1 Cellular origins of malignant lymphomas

Neoplasms of B-cell origin	Neoplasms of T-cell origin	Neoplasms of histiocytic/reticulum cell origin
Chronic lymphocytic leukemia (98%)	Chronic lymphocytic leukemia (2%)	Malignant histiocytosis (histiocytic medullary reticulosis)
Small lymphocytic (well-differentiated lymphoma)	Mycosis fungoides/ Sézary syndrome	Monocytic leukemia
Lymphocytic lymphoma, intermediate and/or small cleaved cell type	Diffuse aggressive lymphomas of adults (25%) Mixed cell type Large cell, immunoblastic	Large cell lymphomas (<5%) Hodgkin's disease
Follicular lymphomas	Adult T-cell leukemia/lymphoma	
Diffuse aggressive lymphomas of adults (65%) Mixed cell type Large cell type Large cell immunoblastic Small noncleaved cell	Antiocentric lymphomas (lymphomatoid granulomatosis) (polymorphic reticulosis)	
Burkitt's (small noncleaved cell) lymphoma		
Acute lymphocytic leukemia (70%)	Acute lymphocytic leukemia (25%)	
Lymphoblastic lymphomas (10%)	Lymphoblastic lymphomas (85%)	

SITE OF ORIGIN OF THE LYMPHOMAS The lymphomas arise in the lymph nodes or in the lymphoid tissues of parenchymal organs such as the gut, lung, or skin. Ninety percent of cases of Hodgkin's disease originate in lymph nodes; 10 percent are of extranodal origin. In the lymphocytic lymphomas, the tissues of the parenchymal organs are more often involved; 60 percent of these lymphomas originate in the nodes and 40 percent are of extranodal origin.

Phenotype With the availability of more specific antiserums, the lymphomas can be classified by their cells of origin (Table 294-1). Sixty-five percent of lymphomas of lymphocyte origin derive from a monoclonal population of B cells and as many as 30 to 40 percent from T cells. With DNA probes to the immunoglobulin gene and the β-chain T-cell receptors, the lineage of most lymphoid tumors can now be precisely delineated. In some series as many as 10 percent of tumors have been found to be bicloval. Only a few appear to be true derivatives of tissue histiocytes despite the morphologic similarity of some malignant lymphomas to these cells. It is also possible to relate B-cell tumors to functional subsets of B-cell populations. Follicular lymphomas are derived from the proliferative site of the B-cell system, the lymphoid follicle, while the diffuse small lymphocytic lymphomas relate to the secretory compartment of the medullary cords. B-cell lymphomas are recognized by the demonstration of monoclonal surface immunoglobulin or, if absent, by immunoglobulin gene rearrangement using specific DNA probes. Lymphomas of T-cell origin are less common in the United States than in other parts of the world. Approximately 15 to 35 percent of diffuse large cell lymphomas are of T-cell origin and are referred to as peripheral T-cell lymphomas, in contrast to the immature T-cell lymphomas of thymic origin, such as lymphoblastic lymphoma of adolescence and childhood. They are identified by their characteristic rosetting with sheep red blood cells and T cell–specific monoclonal antibodies. In some cases the phenotypic expression of the T cell is matched by functional capabilities. In mycosis fungoides/Sézary syndrome, which is a peripheral T-cell lymphoma, a helper cell phenotype and comparable function has been identified. While many monoclonal antibodies have been developed that allow characterization of T cells, a smaller number are available that recognize antigens specific for B cells. The monoclonal antibody with the broadest activity is anti-B1, a pan-B cell antibody. Another commonly used monoclonal antibody, J5, was at first thought to react exclusively with common acute lymphoblastic leukemia antigen (CALLA). Further studies have shown that this antigen is expressed in many B-cell malignancies, including most follicular lymphomas and Burkitt's lymphoma. The origin of the Hodgkin's disease (HD) cell may be the antigen-presenting interdigitating reticulum cell found in the paracortex regions of lymph nodes. Sternberg-Reed cells in culture and their mononuclear variants have Fc and C3 receptors and Ia antigens. They do not synthesize immunoglobulins, are not phagocytic, and lack diffuse activity for nonspecific esterase and acid phosphatase, all characteristics that support an origin from antigen-presenting cells. Sternberg-Reed cells, even in paraffin sections, stain with the monoclonal antibody anti-Leu M1, which also stains interdigitating reticulum cells after neuraminidase digestion, and rosette with T cells. Anti-Leu M1 does not react with morphologically similar T cells. A monoclonal antibody Ki1 prepared against HD cell lines also reacts with HD cells in frozen sections of involved nodes but has also been found to react with antigens on the surface of some large cell lymphomas of B-cell origin. Several monoclonal antibodies are available that detect the common leukocyte antigen, expressed on all normal lymphoreticular cells. These antibodies can be useful in distinguishing carcinomas and sarcomas from malignant lymphomas.

ETIOLOGY There is clear evidence that viruses are the cause of lymphomas in rodents, birds, cats, and cows. Such a relationship has now been demonstrated in humans for the first time by American and Japanese investigators who isolated a unique retrovirus from patients with mycosis fungoides in the United States and acute T-cell lymphomas in Japan. The latter disease is a relatively new syndrome rarely found in the United States but common in Japan and in blacks from the Caribbean. This class of virus has been termed human T-cell leukemia/lymphoma virus (HTLV). There is reason to believe that other lymphomas of humans may be due to viruses of the HTLV class. Cases of diffuse immunoblastic lymphoma have been reported in patients with acquired immunodeficiency syndrome (AIDS). While HTLV viruses thus far identified are T cell–trophic in humans, a distantly related virus, the bovine lymphoma/leukemia virus, causes a B-cell lymphoma in cows and HTLV-like viruses have been isolated from cells of human B-cell lymphomas. With new technology to grow lymphoma cells in long-term culture, the viral association with human lymphomas is undergoing reexamination. A virus may be related to the causation of Hodgkin's disease, in which the immune defect that accompanies the disease is in T cells and could result from an infection from a T cell–trophic virus. There is also a strong association between the Epstein-Barr DNA virus (EBV) and the rare lymphoma described by Burkitt in east Africa (anti-EBV antibodies appear in serum of patients, and complementary DNA appears in the human genome of Burkitt's cells), but the association is less strong in Burkitt's lymphomas diagnosed in the United States. In addition, in large series of patients with infectious mononucleosis, a disease caused by the Epstein-Barr virus, after long follow-up a small but consistent increase in the incidence of lymphomas has been noted compared to controls who have not had infectious mononucleosis. A lymphomatous disease of chickens, Marek's disease, is known to be caused by another herpes-like DNA virus and can now be prevented by vaccination.

A hereditary influence on the incidence of lymphomas is suggested by their higher incidence in patients with inherited immunologic deficiency diseases and by a slightly increased incidence in families of patients with immunologic disorders. In one study, a significantly increased incidence of Hodgkin's disease was noted in siblings of the index case, particularly in siblings of the same sex. A slight increase in incidence of lymphomas has been noted in large series of patients with collagen-vascular diseases compared with the general population adjusted for age. This increased incidence approached 10 percent in patients with long-standing Sjögren's syndrome, who tend to develop diffuse lymphomas or immunoblastic sarcomas.

Lymphoma-like syndromes have been found in patients who take phenytoin. Although in most cases the disease regresses when the patient stops taking the drug, a significant fraction proceed to develop frank lymphoma of several different varieties, including Hodgkin's disease. Such observations suggest that the drug is acting on patients with an inherited tendency to develop the disease. Patients who are chronically immunosuppressed, particularly those who have received renal or heart transplants or have AIDS, have a higher incidence of diffuse large cell lymphomas and immunoblastic lymphomas (often of the brain).

Cytogenetics of lymphomas The cells of Hodgkin's disease have been shown to be aneuploid although no specific chromosomal abnormality has been identified. In contrast, almost all of the lymphocytic lymphomas have nonrandom chromosomal abnormalities, usually translocations involving chromosome 14 (8;14, 11;14, and 14;18). The first translocation was described in Burkitt's lymphoma, where a portion of the 8 chromosome is translocated to chromosome 14. This translocation brings the c-*myc* oncogene, on chromosome 8, in close proximity to the promoter sequence of the heavy chain gene and results in the constitutive expression of c-*myc*. Other, less common translocations (8;2, 8;22), bring the same gene under the control of the κ and λ light chain promoter, respectively. The 14;11 and 14;18 translocations are common in the follicular lymphomas, and two previously undescribed genes, which may be lymphoma-specific oncogenes, have been identified on chromosomes 11 and 18 (called BCL 1 and BCL 2) in close proximity to the breakpoint. The breakpoints of these translocations have now been cloned, and specific DNA probes have been made that should serve as diagnostic tools to identify lymphocytes that have the specific chromosomal abnormality.

HODGKIN'S DISEASE

NATURAL HISTORY AND CLINICAL MANIFESTATIONS There are two theories about the origin and spread of Hodgkin's disease. Careful mapping of sites involved by tumor suggest that the disease is unifocal in origin and spreads initially by involving contiguous lymph node areas. This hypothesis has two flaws—the high degree of involvement of retroperitoneal lymph and left cervical nodes without intervening mediastinal involvement and the common involvement of the spleen, which has no afferent lymphatics. Kaplan has proposed that retroperitoneal lymph nodes are involved by retrograde spread through the thoracic duct due to obstructing cervical nodes. This explanation is difficult to accept because almost total occlusion of the duct's flow would be required. Smithers has proposed an alternative hypothesis, referred to as "the susceptibility hypothesis." He suggests that the malignant Hodgkin's cell freely circulates but grows only in preferential sites, giving the appearance of contiguous spread; this theory is supported by the finding of early involvement of the spleen with tumor. The fact that this multifocal disease can be cured by irradiation, a local form of treatment, seems improbable if one accepts Smithers' proposal, but a possible explanation may be that preferential sites of involvement are destroyed by irradiation, thereby limiting future growth of the tumor.

Hodgkin's disease usually presents either with asymptomatic, discrete, painless, rubbery enlargement of lymph nodes or with symptoms of fever, night sweats, weight loss, and sometimes pruritus associated with adenopathy. Asymptomatic adenopathy may be noted by the patient or by the doctor on routine physical examination. Often mediastinal adenopathy is noted on a routine chest x-ray or a film taken because the patient has a dry, nonproductive cough. These presentations are more common in young people, and such patients often have the nodular sclerosing variety of the disease. Other, usually older, patients present with fever and night sweats or both, followed by increasing malaise and weight loss. Whereas superficial adenopathy is present in most such patients at some time in the course of the disease, in some cases, the enlarging lymph nodes are located exclusively in the abdomen, and these patients often present to the physician with a differential diagnosis of fever of undetermined origin. When diagnosed, they are usually found to have the lymphocyte-depleted variety of Hodgkin's disease.

The fever in Hodgkin's disease is usually remittent. While commonly discussed, a cyclical pattern of fever, called Pel-Ebstein fever, which is characterized by several days or weeks of fever, alternating with afebrile periods, is rarely observed. Fever, night sweats, and weight loss (referred to as B symptoms) have been found to correlate with a poorer prognosis in Hodgkin's disease than the absence of symptoms. The prognostic significance of pruritus is uncertain. It rarely occurs in the absence of fever and/or night sweats and has been dropped as a staging criterion indicating the presence of more advanced disease. Alcohol-induced pain in Hodgkin's disease is uncommon but has been reported to coincide with heavy eosinophilic infiltration at the sites involved by tumor. If alcohol-associated pain occurs, it may serve to direct the physician's attention to a site of involvement which can be biopsied. Occasionally a patient with Hodgkin's disease will present with obstruction of the superior vena cava as the first symptom. Sudden spinal cord compression can be a presenting complaint in patients with Hodgkin's disease but is usually a complication of progressing disease in a patient with known disease.

Asymptomatic patients may have their adenopathy for extended periods of time with waxing and waning of lymph node size. Old x-ray films, in retrospect, may reveal that evidence of mediastinal widening had been present for several years. Slow progression of the disease, usually by extension to contiguous lymph node areas, occurs, especially in the nodular sclerosing variety of the disease. With the invasion of the hilar lymph nodes, the gateway to the lungs, the tumor mass may invade the pulmonary parenchyma. At some point in the progression of the disease, blood vessel invasion may occur. Vascular invasion can be easily demonstrated in biopsy specimens of lymphoid tissue stained with Weigert's stain, especially in patients with more advanced histologic subtypes. Unsuspected involvement of the spleen, an organ which has no afferent lymphatics, suggests that vascular invasion and circulation of the malignant cell may be a common occurrence, even in patients with apparently localized disease. Later, with further progression of disease and clear evidence of vascular invasion, the bone marrow, liver, and other viscera become involved. Symptoms, if they were not present initially, appear as the volume of tumor increases, and if the patient is not successfully treated, cachexia and widespread involvement of visceral organs by tumor occurs, infections complicate the course, and the patient dies. Patients symptomatic at the outset seem to have disease which progresses more rapidly, have smaller-sized but more widespread lymphadenopathy, and more often have the lymphocyte-depleted or mixed cellularity varieties of Hodgkin's disease. Bone and visceral involvement occurs earlier in such patients. Bone lesions are often osteoblastic, and the "ivory" vertebra is characteristic of Hodgkin's disease. Bone pain is common, but pathologic fractures are rare.

DIFFERENTIAL DIAGNOSIS Adenopathy in young people occurs more often as a result of infectious diseases with symptoms of fever, headache, or pharyngitis, and is often due to infectious mononucleosis, viral syndromes, or infection by *Toxoplasma gondii*. In older patients, cervical adenopathy may occur as a result of local spread of head and neck cancers. A good rule is that any lymph node of 1 cm or greater in diameter which does not show signs of regression after 6 weeks of observation should be biopsied.

Mediastinal and hilar adenopathy should be distinguished from sarcoidosis, which is almost always panhilar, erythema nodosum, and primary tuberculosis, which, although unilateral like Hodgkin's disease, is almost always accompanied by a resolving pulmonary infection and usually does not cause mediastinal lymph node enlargement. In older patients, the differential diagnosis includes primary tumors of the lung and mediastinum, specifically oat cell and epidermoid carcinomas. Reactive mediastinitis and hilar adenopathy from histoplasmosis can be confused with lymphoma, particularly in regions where histoplasmosis is endemic, since it occurs in otherwise asymptomatic young people. Histoplasma mediastinitis usually involves the esophagus and should be suspected by obtaining a history of difficulty in swallowing; the diagnosis is confirmed by an abnormal esophagogram or node calcification. Biopsy may be complicated by hemorrhage. Hodgkin's disease presenting as "fever of undetermined origin" may remain undiagnosed despite extensive investigations until an exploratory celiotomy is done.

TABLE 294-2 Evolution of histopathologic classification of Hodgkin's disease*

Jackson-Parker (1947)	Lukes-Butler (1966)	Rye classification (1966)
Paragranuloma	Lymphocytic and/or histiocytic *1* Nodular *2* Diffuse	Lymphocytic predominance
	Nodular sclerosis	Nodular sclerosis
Granuloma	Mixed	Mixed cellularity
	Diffuse fibrosis	Lymphocytic depletion
Sarcoma	Reticular	

* *The current classification by Lukes et al. provides greater prognostic information than the old Jackson-Parker classification by virtue of identifying those patients whose tissue shows intense fibrosis in nodules.*

DIAGNOSIS AND PATHOLOGY The diagnosis and classification of a lymphoma can be made only by biopsy and histopathologic examination under a light microscope. Needle aspiration of lymph nodes, while it may suggest the diagnosis, does not yield sufficient tissue to classify lymphoma accurately, and the error rate is high. Needle aspiration, however, may be useful to distinguish recurrent disease from reactive hyperplasia and to supply tissue samples for analysis of gene rearrangements characteristic of lymphomas of B- and T-cell origin. Even experienced pathologists, using fixed sections of lymph nodes, disagree on classification of 25 percent of cases and on whether the resected tissue shows evidence of malignancy in as many as 6 percent of cases. Frozen section material should not be used alone when lymphoma is suspected because slightly crushed normal lymphoid tissue in frozen sections mimics malignancy. Frozen sections, however, can now be used with a panel of monoclonal antibodies to phenotype lymphocytic lymphomas.

Hodgkin's disease is unique among cancers because the tumor observed by the physician contains largely normal tissue, reactive lymphocytes, plasma cells, and the fibrous stroma of the lymph node and only a scattering of the characteristic malignant cell of Hodgkin's disease, the Sternberg-Reed cell. In the absence of Sternberg-Reed cells, the diagnosis of Hodgkin's disease should rarely be made, although the presence of such a cell by itself is not pathognomonic of the disease, since cells simulating Sternberg-Reed cells have been found in patients with infectious mononucleosis and breast cancer. The presence of the mononuclear variety of the Sternberg-Reed cell, which has a large eosinophilic nucleolus, is sufficient to demonstrate Hodgkin's disease involving the liver or bone marrow in a patient known to have Hodgkin's disease elsewhere; however, the finding of mononuclear Sternberg-Reed cells is not sufficient for the diagnosis of the primary tumor itself.

On the basis of histologic classification and knowledge of the rates of spread of tumor, the likelihood that an apparently localized lesion will be disseminated can often be predicted. The histologic classification by Lukes and Butler used for Hodgkin's disease is shown in Table 294-2, along with the older Jackson-Parker classification. The original, more complete version of the Lukes and Butler classification was modified at the Rye Staging Conference to include the four major histologic subgroups shown in the right column of Table 294-2.

IMMUNOLOGIC ABNORMALITIES In the 1950s, patients with Hodgkin's disease were shown to have a higher incidence of cutaneous anergy to a battery of intradermal skin tests than did normal controls. In most studies, the immunologic defect has been shown to have no influence on the prognosis within a given clinical stage, when modern therapy is used. This is an important observation because it indicates that immunosuppressive chemotherapy has no adverse effect, even when the patients are already immunosuppressed by their disease, as long as it effectively eradicates the malignant cell, an observation that pertains to other cancers as well.

The functional T-lymphocyte defect can now be detected even in patients with very early stage I Hodgkin's disease, if dose-response curves are done with topical dinitrochlorobenzene (DNCB) and with lymphocyte response to phytohemagglutinin (PHA) in vitro. These data show that a T-cell defect is always a concomitant of Hodgkin's disease. Following successful treatment with chemotherapy or radiation therapy, a permanent immunologic defect, both in number and function of T lymphocytes, remains even in patients who have been free of tumor for many years; this does not occur in other lymphoma patients cured with the same treatments. Antibody production is normal in most patients with Hodgkin's disease, but antibody production can be influenced by therapy. Combined multidrug chemotherapy and radiotherapy, especially in patients who have undergone splenectomy, have been shown to diminish the primary response to capsular antigens of *Haemophilus influenzae* type B. This may lead to a higher incidence of sepsis with *H. influenzae* and other encapsulated pathogens and accounts for the failure of pneumococcal vaccines to prevent infection in treated patients after splenectomy. While no firm data exist, vaccination with pneumococcal vaccine prior to staging and treatment should be considered if patients will undergo splenectomy.

HEMATOLOGIC ABNORMALITIES A moderate, normochromic, normocytic anemia associated with low serum iron and low iron-binding capacity, but normal or increased iron stores in the bone marrow, may be present in patients with Hodgkin's disease. This profile is similar to that found in other patients with malignancy. A Coombs-positive hemolytic anemia occurs in less than 1 percent of patients with advanced disease. The erythrocyte sedimentation rate (ESR) is usually rapid and serves as a useful test to follow disease activity; however, it has limited sensitivity and returns to normal when residual disease is still present. It can be useful in monitoring patients who are in remission to determine the early evidence of recurrence. Extensive radiation therapy may cause the ESR to be elevated for as long as 1 year after treatment without evidence of recurrent tumor. Numerous more complicated and usually more expensive laboratory tests of disease activity have not been shown to be superior to the ESR. A moderate to marked leukemoid reaction is common in Hodgkin's disease, particularly in symptomatic patients. White blood cell counts as high as 67,000 per deciliter, a level which can easily be confused with the level found in chronic granulocytic leukemia, may be seen. The leukemoid reaction disappears with successful treatment. Mild peripheral eosinophilia is not uncommon especially in patients with pruritus. Absolute lymphocytopenia (<1000 cells per cubic millimeter) usually occurs in patients with more advanced disease.

Marrow aspiration has not yielded results comparable to those obtained by biopsy, probably because of the fibrosis and granuloma formation in the marrow of patients with Hodgkin's disease. On smear or section, the myeloid/erythroid ratio may be increased, and marrow eosinophilia is common; neither is sufficient to diagnose marrow involvement by tumor. Involvement of the marrow by tumor is demonstrated by finding either classic Sternberg-Reed cells or their mononuclear variant, distributed focally or diffusely throughout the bone marrow. Marrow involvement is often associated with reticular fibrosis, which sometimes obscures the architecture of the marrow. In a patient with known Hodgkin's disease, intense marrow fibrosis, even in the absence of the characteristic malignant cells, is strong evidence of tumor in the bone marrow. Surprisingly, effective treatment by chemotherapy often leads to total resolution of marrow fibrosis in patients who achieve remission.

SELECTED CLINICAL PROBLEMS Infections are common in patients with Hodgkin's disease. Those who have progressive tumor usually die of the complications of bone marrow failure, bacteremia, or disseminated fungal infections. Diffuse pulmonary infiltrates may appear in patients who are in remission between cycles of chemotherapy due to infection with the protozoan *Pneumocystis carinii*, a disease now so commonly reported in patients with AIDS. The first cases of pneumonia caused by the protozoan *P. carinii* were reported in adults under these circumstances and subsequently in children with leukemia. In rodents, the appearance of this infection between cycles of treatment seems to be related to a rebound inflammatory response to the growing organism. Patients with Hodgkin's disease are prone to develop cryptococcosis, either in the form of meningitis or as a primary pulmonary infiltrate with or without meningitis. Herpes zoster (shingles) occurs in 10 percent of treated Hodgkin's patients and in 20 percent of treated patients who have had a splenectomy. Most patients who develop herpes zoster have a few scattered papules outside the involved dermatome; this minimal evidence of spread usually does not require systemic treatment.

Cord compression is the most serious acute complication caused by growing tumor masses and is usually seen in patients with progressive tumor who have failed primary treatment. It can be caused by vertebral body involvement with collapse, which is easily seen on x-ray or bone scan, or by invasion of the epidural space from retroperitoneal lymph nodes with compression of the cord or compression of the vascular supply to the cord. Computerized tomograph (CT) scanning can be useful in detecting encroachment on the spinal cord from the retroperitoneal area. Selective electromyography is a useful way to detect regional denervation, but a myelogram is usually needed to confirm the diagnosis. Tumor masses can also obstruct the superior vena cava. This may occur as a presenting syndrome or late in the course of the disease when the diagnosis is obvious.

STAGING The staging classification developed for Hodgkin's disease and used for all lymphomas is shown in Table 294-3. Accurate staging of Hodgkin's patients is vital for planning long-term management. The primary physician must take a detailed history, do a thorough physical examination, and seek evidence of systemic symptoms such as fever, night sweats, and weight loss. Weight loss of 10 percent or greater, with no attempt at dieting, usually indicates serious disease in this young population. Soaking night sweats can occur in anxious patients, and a history of sweats preceding knowledge of the diagnosis should be sought carefully. Every lymph node area of the body should be examined carefully, and the presence or absence of enlargement noted for future reference; the size, shape, and consistency should be recorded. Reactive hyperplasia is a cause for lymph node enlargement around the lymph nodes involved with tumor, especially in the neck region; the largest lymph nodes in a group should be marked for biopsy. These may be less accessible to the surgeon, who should be urged nonetheless to seek them out. Nodes in areas other than the primary site, that might change the patient's stage from local to generalized disease, should be biopsied at the same time. Unfortunately, internists are prone to omit examination of the oro- and nasopharynx by indirect laryngoscopy. Such

TABLE 294-3 Staging classification for lymphomas

Stage	Definition
I	Involvement of a single lymph node region (I) or of a single extralymphatic organ or site (I_E).
II	Involvement of two or more lymph node regions on the same side of the diaphragm (II) or localized involvement of an extralymphatic organ or site and of one or more lymph node regions on the same side of the diaphragm (II_E).
III	Involvement of lymph node regions on both sides of the diaphragm (III), which may also be accompanied by involvement of the spleen (III_S) or by localized involvement of an extralymphatic organ or site (III_E) or both (III_{SE}).
III_1	Involvement limited to the lymphatic structures in the upper abdomen, that is, spleen, or splenic, celiac, or hepatic portal nodes, or any combination of these.
III_2	Involvement of lower abdominal nodes, that is, paraaortic, iliac, or mesenteric nodes, with or without involvement of the splenic, celiac, or hepatic portal nodes.
IV	Diffuse or disseminated involvement of one or more extralymphatic organs or tissues, with or without associated lymph node involvement.

NOTE: *E = extralymphatic site; S = splenic involvement. The presence of fever, night sweats, and/or unexplained loss of 10 percent of body weight in the 6 months preceding admission is denoted by the suffix letter B. The letter A indicates the absence of these symptoms. Biopsy-documented involvement of stage IV sites is also denoted by letter suffixes; marrow = M+; lung = L+; liver = H+; pleura = P+; bone = O+; skin and subcutaneous tissue = D+.*

examination is essential to uncovering Waldeyer's ring involvement by lymphoma, although this finding is more common in the lymphocytic lymphomas than in Hodgkin's disease. Epitrochlear nodes are also more likely to indicate a lymphocytic lymphoma. The size of the liver and spleen should be noted. In Hodgkin's disease, palpable splenomegaly is significant because, in most cases, it indicates more generalized disease. The procedures required for staging patients with Hodgkin's disease under various circumstances are shown in Tables 294-3 to 294-6.

Radiologic examination should include a routine chest film. When any evidence of disease is noted on this x-ray, whole-chest CT scanning is performed to identify the extent of mediastinal or hilar adenopathy or evidence of contiguous invasion of the lung from the hilar nodes. Lower extremity lymphogram should always be done unless medically contraindicated. On occasion, the lymphogram will not fill high retroperitoneal lymph nodes. CT scans and ultrasound have been shown to be effective in delineating the status of the retroperitoneal lymph nodes in these upper node regions and should supplement lymphography. Bone involvement can be assessed using the lymphogram films in most cases. Symptomatic patients should have a separate skeletal survey and/or bone scan. The latter is the more sensitive test for identifying bone lesions.

Routine blood counts, ESR, urinalysis, liver function studies, and renal function studies are all necessary parts of the medical workup, but by themselves do not provide information about the extent of Hodgkin's disease or specific organ involvement. Liver function abnormalities, in particular, are poor indicators of Hodgkin's involvement of the liver but are helpful in ruling out the presence of other complicating illnesses. Bone marrow biopsy, not aspiration, should be done in all symptomatic patients with Hodgkin's disease and in those asymptomatic patients with evidence of generalized adenopathy and in patients who are undergoing staging laparotomy. Asymptomatic patients who have disease clinically localized above the diaphragm, that is, whose lymphography, CT scan, and sonogram are found to be negative, rarely have bone marrow involvement, and the biopsy can be omitted in such cases.

In 1968, a group of investigators at Stanford University introduced routine staging laparotomy as a research tool to evaluate the extent of Hodgkin's disease, to define its mode of spread, and to determine the implications of such information for therapy. In one-third of patients with normal-sized spleens, Hodgkin's disease was found in the spleen removed at surgery; conversely, in those patients with clinically enlarged spleens, up to 25 percent had no evidence of tumor in the spleen but appeared instead to have reactive hyperplasia. Splenic enlargement due to involvement by HD has been linked to liver involvement. The liver is rarely involved when splenic involvement is not associated with splenomegaly (<0.5 percent). Liver involvement is present in as many as 28 percent of patients with positive lymphograms and enlarged spleens. The Stanford data also showed that the lymphogram is an accurate test to detect lymph node involvement by tumor. Only 15 percent of patients with positive lymphograms are found to have normal lymph node biopsies at surgery. Even in these patients, an explanation may be found in the reactive lymphoid hyperplasia normally found adjacent to tumor.

Staging laparotomy should not be considered a routine concomitant of staging. Knowledge of the type of treatment to be used by the radiotherapist or medical oncologist, for the variety of stages of Hodgkin's disease, should be known *in advance* of a decision to operate, since general treatment strategy may markedly influence the decision to perform a staging laparotomy. When it is performed, the laparotomy should always be complete and include at least two needle biopsies of each lobe of the liver, a wedge biopsy of edge of the right lobe of the liver and biopsies of other suspicious areas in the liver, splenectomy, and biopsy of selected lymph nodes in the retroperitoneal area, marked on the lymphogram prior to the operation. A postoperative film should confirm that the proper lymph nodes were removed. Nodes in the porta hepatis should also be biopsied and in female patients in the reproductive period the ovaries should be moved laterally or centrally to avoid the major part of the radiation ports. The spleen should be sectioned in 0.3-cm slices and, if tumor is found, the number of nodules enumerated. Determining whether or not the liver is involved with tumor can have a major influence on the selection of therapy and obviate the need for splenectomy or examination of the retroperitoneum. Laparoscopy has been shown to be a useful alternative approach to laparotomy in staging abdominal disease. Results from laparotomy may change the stage in as many as 35 percent of patients. It should be emphasized that the change of stage following laparotomy infrequently results in a change in the plan of therapy, especially if chemotherapy is to be used alone or in combination with radiotherapy. Nationwide, the mortality from staging laparotomy in Hodgkin's disease is 1.5 percent, with a complication rate of approximatley 12 percent. However, mortality rates up to 6.6 percent and morbidity rates of greater than 25 percent have been reported from institutions where laparotomies are done infrequently. In some stages and types of Hodgkin's disease, the operative mortality may exceed the expected death rate at 5 years from the disease itself. Splenectomy itself has not been shown to have a beneficial side effect either in the delivery or outcome or radiotherapy or combination chemotherapy.

The Ann Arbor Conference on Staging of Hodgkin's Disease recommended that results of staging should be reported using both the clinical stage (CS, i.e., all tests leading up to invasive studies) and the final pathologic stage (PS), which includes the results of invasive tests such as liver biopsy, peritoneoscopy, and laparotomy. This was recommended to ensure that investigators, using different staging approaches, could make comparisons of the results of therapy based on the clinical stage of the patient.

TABLE 294-4 Staging the lymphomas: Required evaluative procedures

1 Adequate surgical biopsy, reviewed by an experienced hematologist
2 A detailed history recording the absence or presence of and duration of fever, unexplained sweating and its severity, unexplained pruritus, and unexplained weight loss
3 A careful and detailed physical examination; special attention to all node-bearing areas, including Waldeyer's ring (indirect laryngoscopy), and determination of size of liver and spleen
4 Necessary laboratory procedures:
  a Complete blood count, including an erythrocyte sedimentation rate
  b Serum alkaline phosphatase
  c Evaluation of renal function
  d Evaluation of liver function
5 Radiologic studies
  a Chest roentgenogram (posteroanterior and lateral)
  b Bilateral lymphogram of lower extremities
  c CT scan of abdomen, with or without ultrasonography
  d Views of skeletal system to include thoracic and lumbar vertebrae, the pelvis, proximal extremities, and any area of bone tenderness

TABLE 294-5 Staging the lymphomas: Procedures required under certain conditions

1 Whole-chest CT scan if any abnormality is noted or suspected on routine chest roentgenogram
2 Bone marrow *biopsy* (needle or surgical) in the presence of
  a An elevated alkaline phosphatase
  b Unexplained anemia or other blood count depression
  c Other evidence of bone disease (scan or x-ray)
  d Disease of stage III or greater
3 Exploratory laparotomy and splenectomy, if management decisions will depend on the identification of abdominal disease

TABLE 294-6 Staging the lymphomas: Useful ancillary procedures

1 Skeletal scintigrams*
2 Hepatic and splenic scintigrams*
3 Gallium whole-body scans*
4 Serum chemistries to include serum calcium and uric acid for overall management of patient

* *Cannot be used as evidence of Hodgkin's disease without biopsy confirmation.*

TREATMENT More than 70 percent of all patients with Hodgkin's disease are now curable using either radiotherapy or combination chemotherapy, or both. Because of the stringent requirements for shielding and field piecing, the radiotherapy used for Hodgkin's disease is the most difficult treatment a radiation therapist performs. The treatment of Hodgkin's disease by radiotherapy requires extensive experience with more than a few patients a year and adequate equipment. A linear accelerator, preferably a 4- to 8-MeV model is the preferred instrument. Kilovoltage equipment is inadequate and should no longer be used. Cobalt 60 equipment can be used, but is associated with an increase in side effects from greater scatter of the radiotherapy beam.

Current drug treatment programs require precise metering of doses using a sliding scale for increases and decreases of dosage, based on nadir blood counts and blood counts determined the day a new cycle is to begin. Consistently safe delivery of chemotherapy requires experience in treating the disease and using the drugs, and therefore, should not be attempted by anyone not expert in the field. Inexperienced physicians will often use reduced doses, omit drugs, and use improper sequencing and disrupted schedules, all of which have been shown to diminish the chance of cure.

Although highly successful, treatment of Hodgkin's disease is still in transition. Clinical trials are in progress to develop and study ways to make both drugs and radiation treatment safer, to further facilitate their general use, and to evaluate the role of each alone and together in various stages and histologic subtypes. Some general principles have, however, emerged. At the present time, the best approach to treatment is to use either radiotherapy or combination chemotherapy alone in the appropriate stage. Studies comparing both types of treatment used together to each used alone have shown that patients who relapse after radiotherapy can be retreated successfully with combination chemotherapy with survival results equivalent to those obtained in previously untreated patients of the same stage and histologic subtype. This means that patients cured by radiotherapy alone can be spared exposure to drugs and those patients treated with radiotherapy who relapse have a second chance for cure. Interpretation of results of radiotherapy of localized disease is complicated by the fact that with the success of combination chemotherapy, patients who are inadequately treated with radiotherapy can be salvaged by chemotherapy. Until the results are in, less-than-standard radiotherapy should not be given intentionally just because of the potential for salvage by chemotherapy of those patients who fail this treatment. Studies are now underway to determine the effectiveness of chemotherapy alone in patients with early stages of disease.

The role of radiotherapy as a supplement to drug treatment of stages III and IV disease is also experimental. Such an approach has not yet been proved to be superior to chemotherapy alone and runs the risk of increasing the rate of late complications. Adding full-dose radiotherapy to combination chemotherapy has not proved useful in any study so far. Interesting results have been reported from low-dose radiotherapy given to organs involved with tumors between cycles of chemotherapy.

The dose of radiotherapy is important, because the risk of relapse in a treated field is inversely proportional to dose, falling to about 1 percent at 44 Gy (4400 rad). Because of the sharpness of the field edge with minimal scatter achieved by a linear accelerator, the large fields required to treat Hodgkin's disease can be given with less toxicity to the bone marrow and less scatter to uninvolved but susceptible essential organs. In spite of shielding and sharp field edges, scatter to the entire lung fields is often in the range of 2 Gy (200 rad), and similar scatter doses are routinely received by the testes if the lower abdomen is irradiated, even when extensive shielding is used.

Three types of radiation fields are used for all lymphomas. Involved-field (IF) radiotherapy treats only the tumor mass with a minimal margin of normal tissue. Mantle-field irradiation gives radiation treatment to the cervical, axillary, mediastinal, and upper paraaortic nodes, as well as preauricular nodes, usually as one field. When used in this way, it is referred to as extended-field (EF) radiotherapy. The "inverted-Y" field is used to irradiate the retroperitoneal lymph nodes as a single field, and when used with the mantle field, is referred to as total-nodal irradiation (TNI). Actually, TNI is a misnomer since many lymph nodes are outside the usual TNI fields; total-axial lymph node irradiation (TANI) is a more accurate designation. Critical to applying these treatments is the shielding of the spinal cord at the field match sites, the cervical region, and the heart. Field overlap can result in delivery of sufficient radiation to the spine to cause radiation myelitis.

There is little role for single-agent chemotherapy as the primary treatment in patients with advanced disease unless they are medically infirm for reasons other than Hodgkin's disease. The four-drug program with the acronym MOPP [nitrogen *m*ustard, vincristine (*O*ncovin), *p*rednisone, and *p*rocarbazine] has emerged as the standard treatment program for stages III and IV Hodgkin's disease. Through the use of the MOPP combination program, 80 percent of patients with advanced stages can achieve complete remissions; 63 percent of patients at risk for 20 years have remained free of their disease after remission was induced with only six cycles of treatment. Most patients who relapse do so in the first 4 years of follow-up. Numerous variations on the MOPP program using similar drugs to diminish toxicity without sacrificing results have not proved superior, but can be used under special circumstances. A detailed review of these programs is to be found in DeVita et al. Non-cross-resistant drug combinations are now available and are being tested along with MOPP treatment to determine whether alternating cycles of non-cross-resistant drug combinations are superior to combining drug combinations with radiation therapy in patients with advanced disease. The combination ABVD (*A*driamycin, *b*leomycin, *v*inblastine, and *d*acarbazine) may be as effective as MOPP. Its use in alternating cycles with MOPP is under study. A new approach using hybrid half-cycles of MOPP and Adriamycin, bleomycin, and vinblastine (MOPP-ABV) shows early promise. Other combinations of old and new single drugs are also used to salvage those patients who relapse after MOPP-induced remission, or who fail to achieve remission.

Many variables influence the outcome of patients within a given stage. These include the presence or absence of symptoms and the various histologic subtypes in the treatment groups. Symptoms adversely affect prognosis since they generally indicate a greater volume of tumor as well as rapidity of spread. Volume is a clinical variable that is difficult to assess in current staging classifications. However, a large mediastinal mass, occurrence of more than four splenic nodules, and PS III_2 are poor prognostic factors. Histology is also important. The nodular sclerosing variety of Hodgkin's disease favorably influences the prognosis of patients treated by radiotherapy alone. The selection of treatment for patients presenting with a large mediastinal mass, contiguous involvement of the lung (E), more than four splenic nodules, CS III, or PS III_2 is not settled, and these patients are often considered for combined-modality therapy.

Use of specific radiation treatment approaches INVOLVED-FIELD RADIOTHERAPY Patients with single-node involvement in the high right neck, especially those who have lymphocyte-predominant Hodgkin's disease, do not require a laparotomy, since they rarely have splenic or retroperitoneal lymph node involvement by tumor and can be rendered free of disease for extended periods 95 percent of the time when treated with 35 to 40 Gy (3500 to 4000 rad) to the involved field.

EXTENDED-FIELD RADIOTHERAPY Patients with CS IA and IIA, with nodular sclerosing or mixed cellular Hodgkin's disease, limited to lymph node areas above the diaphragm, can be rendered free of disease more than 90 percent of the time for periods extending beyond a decade, by EF radiotherapy alone, without the need for laparotomy. However, the normal-sized spleen needs to be included in the EF port. Those patients who present with single sites of involvement in the groin should be treated with EF radiotherapy (in this case the inverted-Y field) rather than IF radiotherapy. Some assessment of the status of the liver should also be made in such patients, either by laparoscopy or laparotomy.

TOTAL-AXIAL LYMPH NODE RADIOTHERAPY (TANI) TANI has provided results superior to EF or mantle-field radiotherapy when relapse-free survival is the major criterion of effectiveness. TANI includes a splenic port and should not be used in patients with enlarged spleens. All symptomatic patients with localized disease (CS and PS IB and IIB), if they are to receive radiotherapy alone, should receive TANI, even if a laparotomy demonstrated no evidence of disease below the diaphragm, since there is evidence that withholding radiation therapy to retroperitoneal nodes is not safe in patients with negative random lymph node biopsies. Laparotomy is therefore unnecessary in most of these cases. The type of radiotherapy to be given for supradiaphragmatic CS and PS IIA mixed-cellularity and lymphocyte-predominant Hodgkin's disease is debatable. Equivalent results are achievable with TANI in clinically staged patients and EF in patients staged by laparotomy.

Patients with large mediastinal masses If the mediastinum is involved with Hodgkin's disease and the mass exceeds one-third of the diameter of the chest on a posteroanterior (PA) film, the control rate by radiotherapy alone in patients with stage II disease is poor. Some evidence exists to suggest that survival of relapsing patients is not compromised because they can be salvaged with chemotherapy, but the weight of evidence now favors the use of combination chemotherapy and radiotherapy in these patients as the primary treatment. One of two sequences can be used: radiotherapy first with a shrinking field to minimize lung damage, or chemotherapy first to shrink the mass. Combination chemotherapy alone may prove sufficient, but this point is presently under study. It is suggested by the fact that in some series patients with stages III *and* IV disease and massive mediastinal disease do as well with chemotherapy alone as those patients with advanced disease but without massive mediastinal involvement.

Combination chemotherapy Stage IIIA responds well to MOPP or variants of MOPP chemotherapy; recent studies report a superior remission rate and fewer relapses over a decade of follow-up compared to the use of TANI alone, and the results equal those from the use of TANI and combination chemotherapy together. Several studies clearly show that patients with CS and PS IIIB Hodgkin's disease have a better chance of relapse-free survival with MOPP chemotherapy than with TANI and that the addition of full doses of radiotherapy to chemotherapy does not appear to provide much benefit. An exception may be found in patients with nodular sclerosing stage IIIB Hodgkin's disease, with bulky tumor, especially in the mediastinum. These patients may profit from the combined use of MOPP and TANI radiotherapy.

All patients with stage IV disease are best treated with MOPP chemotherapy or other drug combinations that have been equally effective in producing relapse-free survivals beyond 5 years with no treatment beyond the initial induction cycles. Remission rate and duration are not influenced by specific organs involved with tumor. A patient with bone marrow involvement by Hodgkin's disease should receive full doses of chemotherapy and can expect the same frequency and duration of remission as those patients who have liver or lung involvement. Other drug combinations such as ABVD may be useful in patients who fail the MOPP chemotherapy program. It has been shown to produce a significant fraction of durable complete remissions in MOPP treatment failures. When a patient has failed treatment with both MOPP and ABVD, the greater side effects produced by combinations of drugs must be weighed more carefully against the use of single-agent treatment as palliation. Because of the lack of durability of remissions achieved after resistance has developed to the first two trials of combination drug treatment, cure by standard chemotherapy alone is no longer a reasonable expectation. Under these circumstances, it is sometimes helpful to return to the use of single-agent chemotherapy, including drugs used in previous combinations, but given in a different dose or by a new schedule. For example, patients with advancing MOPP-resistant Hodgkin's disease may still respond to daily oral procarbazine or intermittent large doses of alkylating agents.

Some institutions are investigating the use of high-dose chemotherapy and total-body irradiation in conjunction with autologous bone marrow transplantation in patients who have failed primary chemotherapy. Some long-term remissions have been realized. Clinical trails with biologicals are also under study. Monoclonal antibody therapy with anti-Ki1 antibody armed with alpha-emitting isotopes hold great promise.

Side effects Acute side effects of radiotherapy are nausea and vomiting, marrow suppression, and gastrointestinal ulceration. All of these are troublesome but usually subside shortly after radiation therapy is terminated. After completion of radiotherapy, the more serious side effects, radiation myelitis, pneumonitis, and rarely pericarditis may occur 6 weeks to several months following completion of therapy. Late complications include fibrosis of soft tissue and lungs within the radiation field, coronary artery disease, persistent bone marrow fibrosis, and pancytopenia, as well as an increased incidence of tumors within the treated field.

With chemotherapy, marrow suppression is the most life-threatening acute side effect. It should be monitored carefully, and drug doses adjusted using sliding scales provided in publications reporting the results of treatment. Nausea, vomiting, and alopecia are the most troublesome complications of drug therapy to patients. Delta-9-tetrahydrocannabinol and metaclopramide have been shown to be useful in ameliorating nausea and vomiting associated with cancer chemotherapy. Most patients respond to emotional support and reassurance from their physicians that the symptoms are temporary, hair grows back, and they will return to normal post treatment. Sterility, more commonly seen in males, is a consequence of chemotherapy. The effective use of drugs requires experience; it is unacceptable to give smaller or widely spaced doses of chemotherapy, both of which adversely affect the probability of cure, because of convenience or to avoid nausea and vomiting, especially if the patient is not fully aware of the consequences of altering the treatment.

In combined treatment with radiation and chemotherapy, particularly in patients with early disease, one of the late complications is an increased incidence of acute myelocytic leukemia. The actuarial incidence is 5 to 7 percent at 10 years following completion of therapy. An increased incidence of lymphocytic lymphoma following combined-modality treatment has also been reported. While such a risk may be acceptable in patients who would otherwise have died without treatment, it may not be acceptable in patients who might have been effectively treated with either chemotherapy or radiotherapy alone.

THE LYMPHOCYTIC LYMPHOMAS

This group of diseases, like Hodgkin's disease, have their origin in lymphoreticular tissue. There are differences among them in the cell of origin, age distribution, presentation, stage at onset, complications, and response to therapy. They encompass a wide spectrum of disorders, ranging from Burkitt's lymphoma in children in Africa to follicular and diffuse lymphomas in adults. Lymphocytic lymphoma is the correct designation, not non-Hodgkin's lymphomas. The majority of cases of lymphocytic lymphomas are monoclonal B-cell neoplasms (see Table 294-1).

CLINICAL FEATURES The lymphocytic lymphomas usually present as painless, localized, or generalized enlargements of lymph nodes with or without hepatosplenomegaly and not infrequently as an abdominal mass. Involvement of Waldeyer's ring is more common in lymphocytic lymphomas than in Hodgkin's disease and is often associated with gastrointestinal involvement. A discrete lesion or multiple lesions of the lung, bone, gastrointestinal system, skin, or other parenchymal sites may be the presenting feature. The systemic symptoms described for Hodgkin's disease are less common in patients with lymphocytic lymphomas, but their presence is also thought to influence the prognosis negatively. In the follicular lymphomas, the lymphadenopathy may have been present for a long period of time; often a previous lymph node biopsy may have been interpreted as "atypical" or "hyperplastic." Review of such material by a hematopathologist at a later time and comparison with a second biopsy often reveals that a lymphoma was present from the start.

DIFFERENTIAL DIAGNOSIS The differential diagnosis of lymphocytic lymphomas as a cause of adenopathy is similar to that of Hodgkin's disease. Since the average age of the population is a decade and a half older than for Hodgkin's disease, other malignancies are more likely prospects in the differential diagnosis.

DIAGNOSIS AND PATHOLOGY The diagnosis of a lymphocytic lymphoma is made by histopathologic examination of biopsy material usually obtained from lymph nodes; diagnosis and classification of material obtained from other sites may be more difficult. This is a most important step because, in contrast to Hodgkin's disease, selection of therapy depends on the histologic type more than the stage of disease. The histologic classification proposed by Rappaport has been generally employed because it was reproducible and useful in predicting prognosis (Table 294-7). Familiarity with this system is important since it has been employed in the majority of clinical trials. In addition to the Rappaport classification, six other classifications have been proposed, leading to considerable confusion. The National Cancer Institute sponsored a study to develop a "Working Formulation for Clinical Usage" that amalgamates the best of each classification system. This classification is now used widely and will be used throughout this chapter with the Rappaport classification given in brackets when necessary. The basic approach in the Working Formulation is similar to that of Rappaport in dividing lymphocytic lymphomas on the basis of follicular or diffuse patterns and cytologic composition. Immunologic terminology is not used, but correlations with immunologic phenotypes, when established, are easily drawn. In addition, the Formulation divides the lymphocytic lymphomas into three grades: low, intermediate, and high, depending on the aggressiveness of their growth behavior; low-grade lymphomas are more indolent and high-grade the most aggressive. Utilizing this system makes cross-correlations between studies easier. Most older data, however, have been reported in the Rappaport system and when specific studies are cited, the terminology in those studies will be used.

The presence of a follicular or a diffuse pattern in the nodal architecture is a most influential prognostic factor. Follicular lymphomas tend to follow a more indolent course than those with a diffuse pattern of equivalent cytologic appearance. The pace of evolution and response to treatment within the follicular variety is also influenced by the cytologic features of the cells within the follicles—slower for small cleaved cells and more rapid for large cells. The diffuse lymphomas are clinically more aggressive than the follicular lymphomas, except for the small lymphocytic lymphoma, which resembles chronic lymphocytic leukemia and follows a chronic course. At the time of initial clinical staging, 40 percent of patients with diffuse large cell lymphomas appear to have regional disease, although if treated only locally, the relapse rate is high (see below). In contrast, patients with follicular, predominantly small cleaved cell lymphomas show a propensity for widespread dissemination, easily demonstrated with routine tests, and for a pattern of continuous, late recurrence extending over a period of 5 to 10 years.

IMMUNOLOGIC ABNORMALITIES Immune function is less affected in lymphocytic lymphomas than in Hodgkin's patients, although a defect in delayed hypersensitivity reactions can be found in patients with intermediate- and high-grade lymphomas such as diffuse large cell lymphoma. Skin reactivity and phytohemagglutinin response in follicular, predominantly small cleaved cell lymphoma are sometimes depressed but usually only in association with advanced tumor. A defect in humoral immune function can be demonstrated more frequently in patients with diffuse small lymphocytic lymphomas than with Hodgkin's disease and is manifest as a monoclonal gammopathy or hypogammaglobulinemia.

STAGING The stage of disease must be determined prior to treatment after the confirmation of the histologic diagnosis. The extent of clinical evaluation is guided by histologic subtype and the type of therapy proposed for a particular patient. The staging classification developed for Hodgkin's disease (Ann Arbor Staging Classification, Table 294-3) is used in lymphocytic lymphomas as well; however, the sequence of staging procedures differs because extralymphatic presentations occur more frequently in lymphocytic lymphomas than in Hodgkin's disease. Further, since many approach stages II, III, and IV disease therapeutically in a similar manner, utilizing systemic therapy with or without radiotherapy, this distinction may be far less relevant. For those occasional patients who, after clinical staging, still appear to have localized disease (less than 10 percent of all lymphocytic lymphoma patients) and are considered eligible for radiotherapy alone, extensive staging, even employing laparotomy, may be justified. For the remainder, documentation of advanced disease is usually quite simple, with few or no invasive tests indicated. In those whose age or general medical problems limit therapy to local palliation with radiotherapy or systemic treatment with a single drug, even fewer invasive staging procedures are indicated. Thus, surgical staging should never be considered a routine procedure in patients with lymphocytic lymphomas. The major task of staging is to determine whether the patient has limited nodal or extranodal (E) disease, which is radiocurable (stage I or contiguous stage II), or disseminated disease, which requires systemic therapy (discontiguous stage II or stages III and IV).

Because the histologic patterns correlate well with specific disease patterns, response to therapy, and prognosis, the histologic diagnosis

TABLE 294-7

Working formulation	Rappaport terminology
LOW-GRADE	
A Malignant lymphoma, small lymphocytic, consistent with chronic lymphocytic leukemia; plasmacytoid	Diffuse well-differentiated lymphocytic (DWDL)
B Malignant lymphoma, follicular, predominantly small cleaved cell; diffuse areas, sclerosis	Nodular poorly differentiated lymphocytic (NPDL)
C Malignant lymphoma, follicular, mixed, small cleaved and large cell; diffuse areas, sclerosis	Nodular mixed lymphocytic histiocytic (NML)
INTERMEDIATE-GRADE	
D Malignant lymphoma, follicular, predominantly large cell; diffuse areas, sclerosis	Nodular histiocytic (NHL)
E Malignant lymphoma, diffuse small cleaved cell	Diffuse poorly differentiated lymphocytic (DPDL)
F Malignant lymphoma, diffuse mixed, small and large cell; sclerosis, epithelioid cell component	Diffuse mixed lymphocytic-histiocytic (DML)
G Malignant lymphoma, diffuse large cell; cleaved cell, noncleaved cell, sclerosis	Diffuse histiocytic (DHL)
HIGH-GRADE	
H Malignant lymphoma, large cell, immunoblastic; plasmacytoid, clear cell, polymorphous, epithelioid cell component	Diffuse histiocytic (DHL)
I Malignant lymphoma, lymphoblastic; convoluted cell, nonconvoluted cell	Diffuse lymphoblastic
J Malignant lymphoma small noncleaved cell; Burkitt's follicular areas	Diffuse undifferentiated (DUL)

can be used to determine the appropriate staging procedures needed to choose the appropriate treatment strategy for a particular patient. For example, 80 percent of patients with a follicular pattern have a histopathologic diagnosis of follicular, predominantly small cleaved cell [nodular, poorly differentiated lymphoma (NPDL)] or follicular mixed, small cleaved and large cell lymphoma [nodular mixed lymphoma (NML)], and 80 to 90 percent of these patients will be in stages III and IV after clinical staging and simple needle biopsy techniques. Early in the patient's staging evaluation, only diagnostic studies that have a low morbidity and a high probability of disclosing advanced disease should be employed. Lymphograms, bone marrow biopsies, and liver biopsy meet these requirements and can usually obviate the need for staging laparotomy. Approximately 90 percent of patients with follicular and 60 to 70 percent with diffuse lymphocytic lymphomas have positive lymphograms. For patients with positive lymphograms, the incidence of spleen, liver, and/or bone marrow involvement is high (90 percent); in contrast, in patients with negative lymphograms, such involvement is 10 percent or less. Bone marrow aspirates are inadequate for diagnosis, and bilateral posterior iliac crest biopsies are recommended. In low-grade lymphomas, follicular or diffuse, the incidence of bone marrow involvement is at least 50 to 60 percent, even though there is usually no evidence of peripheral blood count abnormalities.

Search for liver involvement should be pursued if the bone marrow biopsies prove to be negative and if the therapeutic plan is to treat the patient with less than a systemic approach. Nondirected percutaneous biopsies detect 20 percent of cases with liver involvement, peritoneoscopy-directed multiple biopsies detect an additional 20 to 30 percent of cases, and finally, if no evidence of stage IV disease has been shown after these procedures, and if it is important to detect microscopic liver involvement, liver biopsies at laparotomy detect the remaining 50 percent of cases. Liver involvement occurs in 65 percent of cases with low-grade lymphomas, whether the architecture is nodular or diffuse. In contrast are the findings in patients diagnosed as having intermediate- or high-grade lymphomas of the diffuse large cell variety. Some 20 percent of patients with diffuse large cell disease appear to be in clinical stage I after clinical staging and may be candidates for megavoltage radiotherapy alone; in such patients, laparotomy is advisable to ensure that patients are truly stage I since radiotherapy alone for stage II disease is inferior to radiotherapy with chemotherapy or chemotherapy alone. Extranodal presentations in Waldeyer's ring and extralymphatic local presentations in bone, brain, testes, or other sites are more frequent in high-grade large cell lymphomas than in low-grade lymphoma.

TYPES OF LYMPHOCYTIC LYMPHOMAS Follicular, predominantly small cleaved cell [nodular poorly differentiated lymphocytic type (NPDL)] This is the most common follicular lymphoma and presents a more uniform clinical picture than the other follicular types. The disease afflicts adults, usually over the age of 40, and is very rare in children, though instances below the age of 15 are known. Follicular, small cleaved cell lymphomas are usually asymptomatic at the onset and are characterized by painless adenopathy in the cervical, axillary, inguinal, and femoral regions. In some patients, large abdominal masses of retroperitoneal or mesenteric lymph nodes cause acute gastrointestinal problems, including obstruction, hemorrhage, and intussusception. Some patients present with ureteral obstruction and consequent renal failure. Even though the patient may notice only one or several enlarged lymph nodes, examination and stu with lymphography or other tests usually reveals widespread, often symmetric, lymphadenopathy. In some patients, the lymph node enlargement may have been present for several years but is so gradual or fluctuating that patients were not sufficiently concerned to seek medical attention. The spleen is often enlarged but rarely produces symptoms at the onset of the disease. Later in the course of the disease, it may become considerably larger and result in local symptoms and significant hypersplenism. Involvement of the lymphoid tissue in Walu yer's ring is much more common than in Hodgkin's disease. Epitrochlear and popliteal adenopathy usually indicates the disease is a low-grade lymphocytic lymphoma. Lymphoid masses may result in chylous pleural effusions and/or ascites presumably because of lymphatic obstruction. It is extremely rare for the central nervous system to become involved, though peripheral nerve compression and epidural tumor masses may develop. The peripheral blood picture is usually normal at the onset of the disease, but careful examination of the blood smear may reveal typical notched or cleft, so-called buttock cells, thought to be characteristic, but not diagnostic of follicular lymphomas. Ordinary bone marrow aspirations are usually normal. However, study of the bone marrow by the needle or open biopsy technique will reveal bone marrow involvement with the cells located in the paratrabecular area of the marrow (in contrast to the centrally placed normal lymphoid follicles) in up to 85 percent of patients with low-grade, follicular lymphoma, even at the onset of the disease.

The clinical course of follicular lymphoma is variable, and affected by the cytologic appearance of cells within the follicles. In some it is indolent, and lymphadenopathy may have been present for years prior to the diagnosis, and may be well tolerated for 5 years or more after the diagnosis is established. In other patients the tempo of the disease is accelerated from the start, and such patients may experience early difficulties that require prompt therapy. It is also now clear that follicular low-grade lymphomas evolve in time to high-grade diffuse large cell lymphomas. In all cases the disease is malignant, however, and though there may be spontaneous regression of lymphadenopathy, in rare cases, in the majority of patients clinical problems appear within the first year after diagnosis, especially in those who show evidence of a mixture of large and small cells in the follicles. When the disease accelerates, lymph node masses grow rapidly, often in localized or asymmetric locations. They cause serious local problems and are less responsive to treatment which was previously effective. Fever, night sweats, and weight loss may appear. Involvement of the nonlymphoid organs and tissues occurs. If biopsy is repeated when the tempo of clinical progression increases, the histologic picture commonly shows a change in cytology to larger, less differentiated cells with a persistent follicular pattern or effacement of the nodal architecture with diffuse large cells. Clinical evolution of this type occurs in 60 percent of all cases of low-grade follicular, small cleaved lymphomas. Autopsy studies of such patients reveal that fewer than 10 percent of patients whose initial diagnosis was NPDL have evidence of a follicular pattern at the time of death.

Low-grade follicular, mixed small cleaved and large cell [nodular mixed lymphoma (NML)] There are many similarities between follicular, small cleaved lymphoma and the less frequently occurring follicular, mixed small cleaved and large cell lymphoma. The latter differs in overall prognosis, frequency of initial bone marrow involvement, and type and location of lymph node enlargement. The difference may relate to the lessened propensity of large, blastic-type lymphocytes to migrate. Bone marrow involvement at the onset is less common, and unusual large abdominal masses may be seen more often. In contrast to the predominantly small cleaved lymphomas, combination chemotherapy has been found to yield a significant percentage of complete remissions with long-term disease-free intervals, suggesting cure.

Intermediate-grade follicular, predominantly large cell lymphomas [nodular "histiocytic" (NH) lymphomas] This group of intermediate-grade lymphomas generally is considered together with the diffuse large cell lymphomas since the course and prognosis are unlike those of the low-grade follicular lymphomas. The cells in this lymphoma are large and poorly differentiated, indicating a more aggressive growth pattern although follicle structure is preserved.

Diffuse lymphomas The diffuse lymphocytic lymphomas consist of a number of diseases with variable presentation and clinical evolution. Low-grade small lymphocytic lymphoma is generally considered the most indolent lymphocytic lymphoma and in its outcome is usually indistinguishable from chronic lymphocytic leukemia. The low-grade diffuse small cleaved cell lymphoma (DPDL) presents and behaves like the follicular variant. When the patient is first seen, the disease usually is disseminated to all lymph node areas, the liver, spleen, and bone marrow. The incidence of bone marrow and liver involvement is over 50 percent. Low-grade diffuse small cleaved lymphoma is not generally curable by chemotherapy. In contrast, intermediate- and high-grade diffuse and mixed cell lymphomas (diffuse histiocytic lymphomas of Rappaport) often present with localized lymph node enlargement, or local extralymphatic manifestations. The lymph nodes are most prominently located in the neck or in abdominal masses. Presentations in the gastrointestinal tract, bone, thyroid, testes, brain, and the lymph node tissue of Waldeyer's ring also occur frequently. The bone marrow is involved initially in less than 10 percent of the patients and is not commonly involved, even late in the course of the disease. In 20 percent of the patients, even after extensive diagnostic efforts, the disease is found to be relatively localized. Diffuse large cell lymphoma is, however, highly invasive locally, and involvement of peripheral nerves, epidural tumors, compression of the vena cava or airways, and destruction of the osseous tissue occur during the course of the disease. The skin, liver, kidneys, lung, and even the brain may be involved. Occasionally bone marrow invasion results in the appearance of large undifferentiated cells in the peripheral blood.

Truly localized diffuse large cell lymphoma may be curable by megavoltage radiotherapy. In some studies, over 70 percent 5-year actuarial disease-free survival has been achieved in patients with true stage I disease, of whom 75 percent will have 5-year actuarial disease-free survival.

The diffuse lymphoblastic lymphomas of T-cell origin and Burkitt's and diffuse undifferentiated non-Burkitt's lymphomas that occur in children, adolescents, and young adults must be separated from those that occur in the older age groups because of differences in clinical patterns and in response to therapy. Several unique clinical pathologic entities have been recognized.

High-grade diffuse lymphocytic lymphomas (lymphoblastic lymphoma) These tumors constitute about 30 percent of all childhood lymphocytic lymphomas and 5 to 10 percent of lymphocytic lymphomas in adolescents and adults. Males predominate in this group. The characteristic presentation is supradiaphragmatic with cervical, supraclavicular, or axillary lymph nodes; in half the cases, a massive anterior mediastinal mass is found. Pleural effusions may occur. Some patients may present with inguinal nodes or with disease in extranodal sites (breast, gonads, long bones, skin, etc.). Initially, the blood and bone marrow may not be involved but a leukemia-like picture is inevitable if the disease is not successfully treated. The tumors are composed of convoluted or nonconvoluted lymphocytes, but all are associated with T-cell characteristics. Following a 2- to 3-month period, 30 to 50 percent of cases develop acute leukemia cytologically identical with common acute lymphocytic leukemia of childhood. Central nervous system involvement occurs frequently. These T-cell tumors of children and young adults are also cytologically distinct from the B-cell Burkitt's and undifferentiated non-Burkitt's lymphomas. Patients identified by clinical and histopathologic criteria as having lymphoblastic lymphoma require only minimal staging procedures since all stages require chemotherapy. Newer combination chemotherapy, together with central nervous system prophylaxis have recently improved results to the extent that half of all patients may have long disease-free survival (see Table 294-8).

Burkitt's lymphoma Burkitt first described this diffuse lymphoma of follicular center B cells in children in Africa. It has unique clinical and epidemiologic features. Although found worldwide, Burkitt's lymphoma is endemic in certain areas of east Africa and New Guinea. In endemic regions, serologic evidence of infection with Epstein-Barr virus has been documented repeatedly. It is associated with specific cytogenetic abnormalities (see "Cytogenetics").

The disease appears to predominate in males (the male/female ratio in Africa is 8:5; in America it is 2:1). The median age at onset in African children is 7 years, whereas in American children it is 11 years. In its typical African form, the disease presents primarily as an extralymphatic tumor arising in the bones of the jaw. In addition, there appears to be a predilection for spread to the abdominal viscera, particularly the ovaries, as well as the breasts and meninges. Bone marrow involvement occurs but is not common; leukemia is seen infrequently. In American children, bony tumors of the jaw are less frequent, and abdominal or pelvic sites, particularly in the gastrointestinal tract, are involved with tumor at the time of presentation. Bone marrow and/or cerebrospinal fluid involvement occurs eventually in one-third of patients.

The diagnosis is made by recognition of the clinical picture and the characteristic histologic and cytochemical findings. The tumor is very responsive to chemotherapy. Response to therapy depends on stage and tumor volume. Regardless of stage, all patients are now treated with combination chemotherapy, and long-term complete remissions occur without maintenance therapy in half of all cases and in 90 percent of patients with minimal tumor masses in one site.

TREATMENT Treatment approaches to the lymphocytic lymphomas have undergone considerable change in the past decade. Various treatments, including regional radiotherapy, total-lymphoid irradiation, single-drug chemotherapy, combination chemotherapy, and combinations of both modalities have been tested. Treatment strategies based on clinical stage and pathologic classification have been developed. These strategies address three issues: (1) Most localized lymphomas with the exception of pathologic stage I large cell lymphoma are *not* cured by radiotherapy alone; thus an attempt to cure by radiotherapy must be planned with ports which will not harm bone marrow function often required later to administer effective chemotherapy. (2) The treatment of low-grade (follicular) lymphomas is controversial. Although current research focuses on curability with initial aggressive treatment versus no initial treatment, present data dictate a conservative approach with treatment only as required by

TABLE 294-8 Primary chemotherapy of advanced stages of diffuse aggressive lymphomas

Regimen	Number of patients	Percent complete remissions	Percent disease-free at 2 years	Comments
ProMACE-MOPP*	79	74	65	—
M-BACOD†	101	72	59	—
COP-BLAM‡	33	73	—	Average follow-up < 2 years
CHOP-HOAP-Bleo-IM VP-16§	56	100 (stages 1–III) 66 (stage IV)	93 (stages I–III) 55 (stage IV)	—
APO¶	21	95	58	For lymphoblastic lymphomas
Modified LSA_2-L_2	15	73	64	For lymphoblastic lymphomas

* *ProMACE-MOPP = prednisone, methotrexate, Adriamycin, cyclophosphamide, epipodophyllotoxin (VP-16); nitrogen mustard, Oncovin (vincristine), procarbazine, and prednisone in altering cycles.*
† *M-BACOD = methotrexate, bleomycin, Adriamycin, cyclophosphamide, Oncovin, and dexamethasone.*
‡ *COP-BLAM = cyclophosphamide, Oncovin, prednisone, bleomycin, Adriamycin, and Matulane (procarbazine).*
§ *CHOP-HOAP-Bleo-IM VP-16 = CHOP = cyclophosphamide, hydroxydaunorubicin (Adriamycin), Oncovin, prednisone; HOAP = hydroxydaunorubicin, Oncovin, arabinosyl cytosine, prednisone, bleomycin; IM VP-16 = iphosphamide, methotrexate, VP-116.*
¶ *APO and LSA_2-L_2 are acronyms for cyclical ten-drug combinations reviewed in detail in Blaney et al.*

symptoms. (3) There is no controversy regarding an aggressive approach to attempt to *cure* the intermediate- and high-grade lymphomas using third-generation drug combinations.

Involved-field (IF) radiotherapy The principles of delivery of effective radiotherapy described for Hodgkin's disease pertain for lymphocytic lymphomas when irradiation is selected as the primary treatment with curative intent. The effectiveness of regional radiotherapy alone depends largely on the histologic type of lymphoma. For follicular lymphomas following treatment with 44 Gy (4400 rad), the local recurrence rate in the treated field is close to zero but the occurrence of distant relapse is continuous at 10 to 15 percent per year of treated cases. The local recurrence rate (21 to 37 percent) for patients with large cell lymphoma does not appear to be dose-related for doses between 25 and 65 Gy (2500 and 6500 rad). Local control with radiotherapy translates into long-term disease-free survival in 60 to 80 percent of patients with laparotomy staged PS I but in only 30 percent with pathologic stage II disease.

Chemotherapy For the follicular variety of the lymphomas, three treatment options are available; no treatment initially, treatment with a single drug, or treatment with combinations of drugs. Even when patients with indolent disease are carefully selected, most will require treatment within 12 to 24 months.

When chemotherapy first became available for the treatment of cancer, the most responsive tumors were the lymphomas, and continuous oral single-agent chemotherapy evolved initially as the treatment of choice. Two well-established facts now dictate the aggressive use of combination chemotherapy when treatment does become necessary, as the initial treatment for patients with advanced follicular lymphocytic lymphoma. First, modern combination chemotherapy induces a greater fraction of complete remissions in the first year of treatment than does single-agent chemotherapy. Second, patients who attain a complete remission survive longer than those patients who achieve partial responses; therefore the therapy that induces the greatest fraction of complete remissions is always the superior choice, provided toxicity is not too severe. Continuous chlorambucil, the single-agent most often used in the past, is frequently associated with development of bone marrow aplasia, a side effect which is not noted when intermittent cyclical combination chemotherapy is used. Once older forms of chemotherapy of patients with low-grade follicular lymphomas is discontinued, the rate of relapse tends to be persistent at 10 to 15 percent per year, as in patients with localized disease. While maintenance drug treatment of patients with low-grade follicular lymphomas prolongs the duration of initial remissions, it is not generally recommended, since it has not been shown to prolong survival when compared with intermittent reinduction of remission. With the uncertainty over whether more aggressive newer approaches to drug treatment or the use of biologicals such as anti-idiotypic monoclonal antibodies will control low-grade lymphomas, and the certainty that continuous oral alkylating agents or older drug combinations of cyclophosphamide, vincristine, and prednisone (CVP) alone or combined with Adriamycin (CHOP) will not, the decision to start chemotherapy should not be taken lightly. Recent studies, employing κ-λ analyses to detect circulating monoclonal B cells, have shown a high incidence (90 to 100 percent) of monoclonal B cells in the blood of lymphoma patients prior to therapy, regardless of histologic subtype. In patients with low-grade follicular (nodular) lymphomas in complete remission for longer than 18 months, 16 to 25 percent showed circulating monoclonal B cells. This contrasts sharply with the fact that no circulating B cells were found in 14 patients with intermediate- or high-grade lymphomas in complete remission. These laboratory findings offer an explanation for the persistent relapse rate in the low-grade lymphomas in contrast to the curability of intermediate- and high-grade lymphomas and serve as a rationale for clinical trials of initial intensive chemotherapy. Presently most patients with low-grade follicular lymphoma should be entered into clinical trials comparing more intensive initial chemotherapy, which shows some promising early results, to expectant management using intensive chemotherapy only where necessary. In either case, when chemotherapy is offered, combinations of the type shown in Table 294-8 are preferred to older programs. Recently, high-dose 5-day pulses of chlorambucil have produced a complete remission rate and relapse-free survival equivalent to combination chemotherapy and are under evaluation.

The situation is clearly different for patients with the low- and intermediate-grade follicular mixed cell lymphomas (NML) and follicular large cell (nodular histiocytic lymphoma). Here studies have shown that combination chemotherapy is clearly more effective than single agents. At the National Cancer Institute, patients achieved complete remission in 75 percent of cases. In contrast to patients with follicular, predominantly small cleaved lymphomas (NPDL), these patients remain in complete remission for periods up to 10 years after therapy is discontinued, and the relapse rate diminishes after 2 years.

Selection and results of treatment in patients who have diffuse lymphomas again depends, in a major way, on the cytologic characteristics of the individual tumor cell. Patients with low-grade small lymphocytic lymphomas have a long, indolent course that waxes and wanes in a manner similar to the course of patients with chronic lymphocytic leukemia. Conservative single-agent treatment, usually with chlorambucil or cyclophosphamide, employed only when disease progression dictates its use, is the treatment of choice. For patients with advanced stages of intermediate-grade diffuse small cleaved cell lymphomas, the approach should be similar to that for follicular predominantly small cleaved cell types and treatment is the same.

Intermediate- and high-grade diffuse lymphomas such as diffuse large cell, diffuse mixed cell, immunoblastic, and diffuse small noncleaved cell have been known to be highly curable diseases since 1974, and the treatment of choice is one of several third-generation drug combinations shown in Table 294-8. In these lymphomas, the poor differentiation of the cellular component that leads to the more aggressive clinical behavior apparently makes the tumor cells more vulnerable to the cytocidal effects of chemotherapy. Complete remissions in patients with these poorly differentiated diffuse lymphomas are possible in up to 80 percent of treated patients. Failure to achieve a complete remission in these patients is associated with an extremely short survival time, usually 6 months to 2 years. Relapses rarely occur in patients who have been in remission for more than 2 years after therapy is discontinued. In some studies, relapse-free survival has been reported to extend for more than 15 years beyond the end of drug treatment. Patients with the diffuse lymphomas who achieve a complete remission do not benefit from maintenance therapy.

Combined modality treatment of lymphocytic lymphomas Involved-field radiotherapy with combination chemotherapy (RT + CT) has been shown to be superior to radiotherapy (RT) alone in stage II intermediate- and high-grade lymphomas in several United States and European centers. For stage I intermediate- and high-grade lymphoma, radiotherapy can be used alone. There appears to be no significant improvement, however, in relapse-free survival for patients with low-grade lymphomas of the follicular variety treated with chemotherapy in addition to radiotherapy.

Whole-body radiotherapy (WBR) This modality has been employed for the management of patients with low-grade lymphocytic lymphomas in stages III and IV. The 56 percent complete remission rate achieved is similar to that obtained in parallel studies using various older drug regimens. This approach is prone to long-term complications. Moreover, the difficulty in retreatment of relapse with drugs dictates the use of WBR only when other treatments have failed.

Biological therapy of lymphocytic lymphomas For the past decade, numerous studies have been carried out to determine the role of nonspecific immunotherapy in the management of lymphocytic lymphoma. A controlled study shows that combination chemotherapy combined with bacillus Calmette-Guérin (BCG) vaccination produced a slightly better overall survival than the use of that particular combination chemotherapy alone. While this observation is of some interest, other drug programs alone now produce superior results and BCG use is not recommended for any patients with lymphoma. In recent years, interest has been heightened with the use of pure biologicals to treat lymphomas. Early positive results using crude interferon preparations in low-grade, follicular, small cleaved cell lymphomas have been confirmed using purified recombinant alpha interferon. A significant fraction of patients will achieve complete remission that can be maintained for periods of 1 year or more. More aggressive varieties of the disease do not respond well. Interferon can be used as an alternative to chemotherapy as an early treatment in indolent lymphoma, but its use is complicated by the requirement for continuous parenteral administration, and side effects such as extreme fatigue, fever, and leukopenia—in addition to the uncertainty over long-term benefit. Thus its exact role in patient management is not clear.

Interesting results have been obtained using monoclonal antibodies to the idiotypic protein unique to each monoclonal B-cell line in patients with B-cell lymphomas. Although many patients have been treated, only one completely durable remission has been reported. Resistance to this therapy develops because of biclonal lymphoma cell populations now recognized by immunoglobulin gene rearrangement, and the ability of point mutations to alter the idiotypic target. Further studies are underway to exploit labeling of monoclonal antibodies with radioisotopes. Monoclonal antibodies to T cell–specific antigens have been used in T-cell lymphomas with transient responses.

Bone marrow transplantation Studies are in progress utilizing autologous bone marrow transplantation coupled with very intensive chemotherapy and/or total-body irradiation in patients with lymphocytic lymphomas. This approach is reserved for patients who have failed chemotherapy. Autologous marrow is generally harvested after a second chemotherapy remission has been achieved, and purge of lymphoma cells from the marrow is accomplished using monoclonal antibodies to the specific cell type (anti-B1 antibodies for B-cell lymphomas, or T cell–specific antibodies for T-cell lymphomas) or chemicals such as 4-hydroperoxycyclophosphamide and/or phototherapy with hematoporphyrins. After further very high dose chemotherapy and/or total-body irradiation, the marrow is reinfused. Interesting results have been achieved in small series sufficient to warrant using this approach in clinical trials in follicular lymphoma patients with an accelerated course or who have failed chemotherapy and in patients with diffuse large cell lymphomas in their first relapse.

NEWLY RECOGNIZED LEUKEMIA/LYMPHOMA SYNDROMES

Acute T-cell leukemia/lymphomas Acute T-cell leukemia/lymphomas (ATL) is a relatively newly recognized syndrome caused by a unique T cell–trophic human retrovirus, HTLV I. The syndrome was originally described in southwest Japan, where it is endemic, and has since been identified in the Caribbean and the southeast United States. It is characterized by highly pleomorphic and polylobulated cells in the peripheral blood (65 percent of cases). Generalized adenopathy, hepatosplenomegaly, cutaneous involvement, hypercalcemia, and lytic bone lesions also occur associated with secretion of osteoclast activating factor. ATL is a neoplasm of the postthymic T cell which expresses a helper cell phenotype T4+ T8−, but functionally, in vitro, the cells behave as suppressor cells. The course is rapidly progressive, and although combination chemotherapy of the types used in diffuse large cell lymphomas produces remissions, they are usually temporary, and experience is limited to a few patients. ATL deserves to be recognized as a separate entity in the high-grade lymphoma category in the Working Formulation. It is likely that in the past a few such cases were classified as high-grade, diffuse large cell immunoblastic lymphomas.

Histiocytic medullary reticulosis (HMR) HMR, also called malignant histiocytosis, is a rare, usually rapidly progressive systemic disease characterized by abrupt onset, fever, progressive pancytopenia, splenomegaly, and mild lymphadenopathy. It is a malignancy of true histiocytes of the reticuloendothelial system. The malignant cells exhibit phagocytic activity of erythrocytes and leukocytes associated with progressive pancytopenia. Occasional long-term remissions have been observed with high doses of the alkylating agent cyclophosphamide.

Angioimmunoblastic lymphadenopathy with dysproteinemia (AILD) Angioimmunoblastic lymphadenopathy is a lymphoma-like, systemic disorder characterized by acute onset, generalized lymphadenopathy, hepatomegaly, splenomegaly, and severe constitutional symptoms including fever, sweats, and weight loss. Pruritus and skin rashes may be present. These clinical features closely mimic many of the presenting symptoms and signs of advanced Hodgkin's disease and of the other lymphomas. The disorder occurs in adults (age 28 to 92, median 62). In half the patients, a generalized pruritic maculopapular rash precedes the onset of the other signs and symptoms by weeks or a few months. In some patients, ingestion of drugs, including penicillin or other antibiotics, phenytoin, sulfonamide, halothane, methyldopa, and aspirin, antedates the onset of the disease. AILD is not considered a histologically malignant disease but rather an extreme form of hypersensitivity (hyperimmune) reaction. Some have considered this a clinical example of a graft-versus-host reaction. A proliferation of B cells and a profound deficiency of T cells have been demonstrated. The laboratory data show anemia, which in one-quarter of the cases is due to Coombs-positive hemolytic anemia. A majority of the patients have a polyclonal hypergammaglobulinemia. Leukocytosis and eosinophilia may be present.

Characteristic lesions are found in biopsy specimens of lymph nodes and consist of alterations of nodal architecture or complete effacement with a pleomorphic cellular proliferation in which immunoblasts, lymphocytes, and plasma cells predominate. In addition, vascular proliferation and prominent eosinophilic interstitial material are seen. The changes in the liver, spleen, and bone marrow do not have the diagnostic specificity of the lesions seen in the lymph nodes.

The course of AILD is usually fulminant. Some patients (approximately 25 percent) appear to have a long survival (20 to 45 months) with or without small doses of corticosteroids and do not require intensive chemotherapy. Others (25 percent), although requiring intensive cytotoxic chemotherapy, nevertheless have a long survival (28 to 67 months). A third group of patients (50 percent of cases) have a rapid course (1 to 20 months) terminating in death, regardless of the therapeutic approach employed. Many patients die of overwhelming infections often with pneumonia due to *Pseudomonas* and other gram-negative organisms, *Pneumocystis carinii,* cytomegalovirus, or mycoses. Acute hepatic failure or acute renal failure have also been reported to occur as terminal events.

The correct treatment of AILD has not been devised. Treatment should be initiated with corticosteroids. If there is no response, a combination chemotherapy regimen effective in lymphomas has been advocated. Radiotherapy may be employed for control of local problems. In view of the high failure rate of cytotoxic drugs, brief use of corticosteroids has been recommended to diminish the hyperimmune response along with levamisole to stimulate T-cell function.

COMPLICATIONS OF HODGKIN'S DISEASE AND LYMPHOCYTIC LYMPHOMAS

The complications of lymphoma may be due to progressive enlargement of lymph nodes, involvement of parenchymal organs, and hematologic, metabolic, or immunologic abnormalities. Complications may also result from therapy.

Progressive lymph node enlargement causes compression or obstruction of surrounding structures such as vascular structures (superior vena cava syndrome), airway, esophagus, urinary tract, or gastrointestinal tract. Serious complications may ensue depending on the site affected. Direct infiltration of the lymphoma from involved mediastinal lymph nodes into the parenchyma of the lung, pleura, pericardium, and heart may occur. Infiltration from retroperitoneal lymph nodes through lymphatic channels leads to involvement of the gastrointestinal tract and may result in ulceration, perforation, hemorrhage, intussusception, or malabsorption. Jaundice may be caused by obstruction of the biliary duct by portal lymph nodes or by infiltration of the liver secondary to hematogenous spread.

Central nervous system involvement may occur by direct extension of tumor from the mediastinum or retroperitoneum to the spinal canal. Symptoms of cord compression which are produced in this way occur more frequently in Hodgkin's disease than in the lymphocytic lymphomas and, in the latter, most often in the diffuse large cell lymphomas. Cranial nerves and brain may be affected by Hodgkin's disease and the lymphocytic lymphomas. Occasionally, lymphomatous meningitis may occur, and lymphoma cells, high protein, and low glucose appear in the spinal fluid. In diffuse large cell lymphomas with demonstrated bone marrow involvement, meningeal carcinomatosis occurs with sufficiently high frequency to recommend prophylactic therapy, although this complication has diminished with the more modern chemotherapy programs. More rarely, bizarre neurologic manifestations may occur without demonstrable direct involvement by lymphoma. Progressive multifocal leukoencephalopathy, subacute cerebellar degeneration, myelopathy, and neuropathy have been described. Occasionally, polymyositis may occur. The differential diagnosis of these central and peripheral nervous system complications includes bacterial and viral meningitis, herpes zoster, and drug toxicity, particularly with the vinca alkaloids.

The lung may be involved by direct extension from the mediastinal-hilar lymph nodes or by hematogenous spread. In the lymphocyte-predominant type of Hodgkin's disease and in follicular lymphomas the lungs are rarely involved; in contrast, nodular sclerosis–type Hodgkin's disease with hilar node involvement frequently involves the lung. Pneumonia is a frequent complication of treatment and constitutes the major differential diagnostic problem. Bleomycin, methotrexate, and other drugs may cause pulmonary manifestations and must be considered in the differential diagnosis of lung disease.

Skin involvement occurs as part of hematogenous dissemination of the lymphoma, especially in the newly described acute T-cell lymphoma syndrome. A number of nonspecific skin lesions also occur in lymphoma, including excoriations secondary to pruritus, urticaria, erythema multiforme, erythema nodosum, exfoliative dermatitis, and dermatomyositis.

Bone marrow involvement occurs most frequently in low-grade lymphomas (50 to 60 percent) but less frequently in intermediate- or high-grade lymphomas (10 percent). In Hodgkin's disease, initial bone marrow involvement is rare; it is seen most often in patients with symptoms (B category) and in patients with the lymphocyte-depleted subtype. Anemia, neutropenia, and thrombocytopenia are the consequences of bone marrow replacement but usually only occur late in the course of the disease; however, these conditions may also be caused by hypersplenism, immunologic mechanisms, blood loss, or complications of therapy.

Hematologic complications occur frequently. Anemia may be caused by blood loss secondary to gastrointestinal infiltration and ulceration or nonspecific lesions, malabsorption of iron or folate, bone marrow infiltration by lymphoma, or hemolysis. Coombs-positive hemolytic anemia is seen most often with diffuse low-grade lymphomas; it occurs less frequently with diffuse large cell lymphomas or in the follicular lymphomas and Hodgkin's disease. Chronic illness and radiotherapy or chemotherapy result in diminished or ineffective erythropoiesis. Changes in white blood cell counts are frequent. The leukemic phase of lymphoma is seen most frequently in the low-grade lymphomas; rarely, in the intermediate- or high-grade lymphomas. Leukopenia in an untreated patient suggests hypersplenism. In the patient undergoing therapy, leukopenia is usually due to the therapy. Thrombocytosis occurs occasionally in Hodgkin's disease and lymphocytic lymphoma. Frequently following staging splenectomy, the platelet count rises briefly. More often, thrombocytopenia occurs because of bone marrow replacement by lymphoma, hypersplenism, or therapy.

Metabolic abnormalities may occur as a consequence of the lymphoma or of therapy. Hyperuricemia is seen in patients with large volume of lymphoma. Effective therapy with rapid reduction of the tissue mass may exacerbate the hyperuricemia and lead to a decrease in renal function or acute renal failure and infrequently to gouty arthritis. Hydration and administration of allopurinol can prevent these complications.

Hypercalcemia occurs in less than 10 percent of cases and is usually related to bone destruction. It is seen most frequently in diffuse large cell lymphoma and Hodgkin's disease of the lymphocytic-depletion and mixed cellularity varieties. Occasionally, the hypercalcemia may be due to release of a parathyroid-like substance. It is a common concomitant of the rare syndrome of acute T-cell lymphoma caused by the human retrovirus HTLV I. In this disease, it appears to be due to tumor release of lymphokines and osteoclast activating factor rather than direct bone invasion. Hypercalcemia requires prompt and appropriate treatment to lower the serum calcium level and specific therapy appropriate for the management of the lymphoma.

Serum protein abnormalities occur frequently. Particularly in Hodgkin's disease, but also in lymphocytic lymphomas, the $alpha_1$, $alpha_2$, and beta fractions of globulins may be increased. The $alpha_2$ increase in Hodgkin's disease has been shown to be due to increases in haptoglobin and ceruloplasmin. Polyclonal gamma globulin elevation is seen in 40 percent of patients with Hodgkin's disease; it is less frequent in lymphocytic lymphoma. Paraproteinemia may occur in lymphocytic lymphoma, especially in low-grade diffuse types and occasionally in Hodgkin's disease. Hypogammaglobulinemia may precede the onset of some low-grade diffuse lymphomas, occurs eventually in 60 percent of patients, but is seen less frequently in advanced Hodgkin's disease. Antibody production is usually decreased in response to both primary and recall challenge.

Complications of treatment include radiation damage associated with therapy of specific sites, toxicity due to chemotherapeutic agents, sterility, and second malignancies. Chemotherapy with multidrug regimens leads to some decrease in ovarian or testicular function in most patients. Amenorrhea, inability to conceive, or hypo- or aspermia may result; however, in those patients who have achieved a complete remission and are off all chemotherapy, these functions may return.

Second malignancies, particularly nonlymphocytic acute leukemias, have been reported to occur in patients with Hodgkin's disease and lymphocytic lymphomas treated with radiation alone, combination chemotherapy alone, or with both modalities. The incidence is estimated to be 1 to 8 percent of cases, with time of onset 1.2 to 19 years and a mean interval of 7 years following initial therapy. Hypoplastic or aplastic bone marrow may antedate the occurrence of frank leukemia. In the preleukemic phase, chromosome analysis employing chromosome banding techniques has demonstrated a high incidence of abnormalities in chromosomes 5, 8, and 7.

REFERENCES

BLAYNEY DW et al: The human T-cell leukemia/lymphoma virus (HTLV) defines a distinct clinical entity. Blood 62(2):401, 1982

BLOOMFIELD CD et al (eds): Proceedings of the Symposium on Contemporary Issues in Hodgkin's Disease: Biology, Staging and Treatment. San Francisco, California, September 9–12, 1981. Cancer Treat Rep 66(4):601, 1982

——— et al: Nonrandom chromosome abnormalities in lymphoma. Cancer Res 43:2975, 1983

DEVITA VT: The consequences of the chemotherapy of Hodgkin's disease (10th David A. Karnofsky Memorial Lecture). Cancer 47(1):1, 1981

——— et al: Hodgkin's disease and the non-Hodgkin's lymphomas, in *Cancer: Principles and Practice of Oncology*, 2d ed, VT DeVita et al (eds). Philadelphia, Lippincott, 1985, pp 1623–1697

FISHER RI et al: Advances in the treatment of diffuse aggressive lymphoma, in *UT M.D. Anderson Clinical Conference on Cancer*, vol. 27, RJ Ford et al (eds). New York, Raven, 1984, pp 377–390

GOLOMB HM (ed): Non-Hodgkin's lymphoma. Semin Oncol 7(3):221, 1980

HORNING SJ, ROSENBERG SA: The natural history of initially untreated low-grade non-Hodgkin's lymphomas. N Engl J Med 311(23):1471, 1984

KAPLAN HS: Hodgkin's Disease, 2d ed. Cambridge, Harvard University, 1980
LONGO DL et al: What is so good about the "good prognosis" lymphomas? in *Recent Advances in Clinical Oncology No 1*, CS Williams et al (eds). New York, Churchill Livingstone, 1982, pp 223–231
ROSENBERG SA, KAPLAN HS (eds): *Malignant Lymphomas: Etiology, Immunology, Pathology, Treatment*, vol 3: *Bristol-Myers Cancer Symposia*. New York, Academic, 1982, pp 1–682
——— et al: National Cancer Institute sponsored study of classifications of non-Hodgkin's lymphomas. Cancer 49:2112, 1982
SMITH BR et al: Circulating monoclonal B lymphocytes in non-Hodgkin's lymphoma. N Engl J Med 311:1476, 1984
VOKES EE et al: Long-term survival of patients with localized diffuse histiocytic lymphoma. J Clin Oncol 3:1309, 1985

295 BREAST CANCER

JANE E. HENNEY / VINCENT T. DeVITA, JR.

Breast cancer is a major public health problem in the western hemisphere. In 1985, in the United States, 119,000 women and approximately 1000 men were diagnosed as having this disease. Until it was surpassed by lung cancer, it had been the most common cause of cancer death in women and accounted for 38,400 deaths each year in the United States.

RISK FACTORS: ETIOLOGY AND EPIDEMIOLOGY In the United States, no woman is at such a low risk from breast cancer that she can be excluded from education and screening programs appropriate for her age. Even if no risk factors are present, one woman of every 11 develops this disease.

At risk for the development of breast cancer (in decreasing order) is the woman whose mother had bilateral breast cancer diagnosed prior to menopause, the woman with a first-degree relative who developed bilateral or unilateral breast cancer but was postmenopausal, the woman older than 50 who is nulliparous or whose first parity occurred after age 30, the woman with a history of chronic breast disease, particularly epithelial hyperplasia, the woman exposed to ionizing radiation of more than 0.5 Gy (50 rad) during adolescence, and finally the woman who is obese.

Except for a plateau at age 50, the risk of breast cancer increases with age. Early menstruation, late menopause (after 55) and/or irregularity in the menstrual cycle also increase a woman's chances of developing breast cancer. Artificial menopause before age 35 confers some degree of protection; such women have only one-third the risk of developing breast cancer of those who undergo natural menopause. Women who bear their first child before age 18 have one-third the risk of those who bear their first child after age 30. The older primiparas, however, are at slightly higher risk of developing breast cancer than women who are nulliparous.

With respect to the familial association of breast cancer, the cause is not understood, although a gene that is transmitted in an autosomal dominant manner through either maternal or paternal line has been described in rare families. This particular gene is felt to have wide distribution but low penetrance. The allele that increases the susceptibility for this penetrance may be linked to the glutamic pyruvate transaminase locus.

The breast is one of the most susceptible organs to the effects of ionizing radiation. Exposure of the breast to ionizing radiation is a major risk enhancer for the development of malignancy. Data which support these observations are derived from studies of survivors of the bombings at Hiroshima and Nagasaki and women who have undergone radiation therapy, as well as those who have had multiple fluoroscopies during pneumothorax treatment for tuberculosis. The dose-effect relationship appears to be linear with an increased risk present in women who have received as small a dose as 0.5 Gy. There also appears to be an additional risk for those women who are exposed to radiation during adolescence. Fractionated or intermittent dosing does not appear to diminish this risk, nor does time since exposure, even after 45 years. The interval between exposure and the appearance of breast cancer is likely mediated by many factors including the age of the woman and related hormonal factors.

The occurrence of breast cancer varies greatly among different geographic areas and is influenced markedly by migration patterns. For example, Asian women living in eastern countries are at low risk for developing breast cancer. Yet Asian women whose ancestors migrated to Hawaii or the continental United States develop breast cancer at rates observed in populations native to these areas. Although no etiologic hypothesis has been established unequivocally, dietary factors (high fat intake and obesity) may be a main cause of the differing incidences by affecting the metabolism of estrogens which act as promoters of tumor growth.

The incidence of breast cancer varies among racial groups within the United States; it is highest in whites, intermediate in blacks, and lowest in American Indians in New Mexico and Filipinos in Hawaii. The extent to which different dietary habits may influence these variations in incidence rates has not been well studied.

High doses of diethylstilbestrol have been implicated in the development of breast cancer and benign uterine tumors. However, estrogens in conventional doses do not cause an increased incidence of breast cancer, and estrogen with added progesterone therapy may afford some protection for the postmenopausal woman with no prior history of breast cancer. Similarly, oral contraceptives of the combination type have no associated risk for the development of breast cancer and may confer some degree of protection.

Hair dyes and other chemicals frequently used by women have been shown to be mutagenic but their role in the etiology of breast cancer has not been established.

Because of the relatively low incidence of breast cancer in males, its epidemiology and etiology have been largely unexplored. It is known, however, that males with altered estrogen metabolism, gynecomastia, and/or Klinefelter's syndrome, or who have testicular damage or atrophy from mumps orchitis, injury, or aging, are at greatest risk.

NATURAL HISTORY AND PROGNOSTIC FACTORS One important characteristic of breast cancer is multicentricity, that is, in approximately 13 percent of patients with breast cancer, microscopic foci of invasive and noninvasive tumor can be detected in quadrants of the breast other than that in which the dominant primary lesion is discovered. The clinical significance of such nondominant lesions is unclear; it is unusual for multiple cancers in a single breast to become clinically overt or for bilateral cancers to occur synchronously. In women over 70 who have died from other causes, the incidence of clinically inapparent intraductal carcinoma is 19 times the reported incidence of breast cancer. Whether these cancers are controlled by the body's own defense mechanisms because they represent a low tumor burden or undergo regression for other reasons, such as removal of a dominant primary, has not been elucidated. Data linking invasion of lymph nodes to the presence of receptors for the basement membrane protein laminen suggest that multiple steps may be involved in the development of a fully invasive and metastasizing cancer; such events may not have occurred in nondominant microscopic foci. This observation of multicentricity has been central to the debate about the extent of treatment necessary for breast cancer with local modalities. Long-term follow-up of the women who were treated with segmental mastectomy only in a trial comparing this approach to segmental mastectomy and radiation therapy conducted by the National Surgical Adjuvant Breast Project (NSABP) should provide an answer to the clinical relevance of multicentricity in breast cancer (see "Surgical Options" below).

The size of the primary tumor, a clinical predictor of outcome, can be determined easily by palpation combined with mammography. Tumors less than 2 cm in size are generally associated with the most favorable outcome. Tumor size is also correlated with the likelihood of axillary lymph node involvement, another prognostic indicator. Lesions <1.5 cm are less likely to have nodal metastases (38 percent) than are large lesions (≥ 5.5 cm), which have metastasized to axillary lymph nodes 70 percent of the time. A correlation also exists between increased tumor size and the presence of four or more positive axillary lymph nodes.

Establishing whether there is nodal involvement and the number of axillary nodes involved is critical (Table 295-1). In those patients with no histologic involvement of axillary nodes, an 83 percent rate of 5-year disease-free survival has been found; those with one to three positive nodes have a 50 percent disease-free, 5-year survival rate. Those patients with four or more positive nodes have a 21 percent disease-free survival at 5 years. Further analysis indicates that the group with four or more positive nodes should be split because there is a 25 percent greater disease-free survival or 18 percent overall survival) in those with four to six positive nodes than in those with 13 or more positive nodes. In contrast to measuring the size of the primary, the physical examination of the axillary nodes is an inaccurate predictor of histologic involvement. In approximately 25 percent of cases examined, when axillary nodes are palpable, histologic evidence of disease is not found. Likewise, in 30 percent of cases in which axillary nodes are not palpable, histologic involvement with tumor is discovered. Axillary involvement can be assessed accurately only by surgically removing the nodes.

In addition to the size of the tumor and the number of positive axillary nodes, an important prognostic factor is the presence or absence of the estrogen receptor (ER) and the progesterone receptor (PR). Unlike the size of tumor, receptor content is not predictive of the degree of axillary nodal involvement. The ER is capable of binding and transferring the steroid molecule into nuclei to exert specific hormonal functions. The PR production in breast cancer cells is likely an end product in the pathway regulated by estrogens and involving the ER. The degree of ER binding capacity is expressed in femtomoles per milligram of cytosol protein. Values above 10 are positive, 3 to 10 intermediate, and less than 3 negative. The degree of positivity is proportional to the degree of cellular differentiation and subtype and is also a measure of potential responsiveness of the tumor to hormonal manipulation. The ER expression tends to increase with the age of the patient while PR shows no such relationship to age. Women who have ER levels in the positive range have a more favorable prognosis than those whose ER is either in the intermediate or negative range. Observations from women who have more advanced disease indicate that approximately 60 percent of patients who are ER-positive respond to hormonal manipulation while fewer than 10 percent of patients who are ER-negative respond to hormonal therapy.

Other factors which are predictive of outcome of breast cancer are the patient's age and menopausal status. The group found to be most likely to have a favorable outcome are those postmenopausal women whose primary cancer is less than 2 cm and positive for ER, and who have no evidence of spread to the axillary lymph nodes.

SCREENING In order to detect earlier clinical stages of breast cancer (Table 295-2), which confer a more favorable outcome, major emphasis is being placed on screening large asymptomatic populations for breast cancer. Ninety percent of breast masses are found by the patient either accidentally or during deliberate self-examination. The remaining 10 percent are discovered during examination by health professionals or by mass screening techniques such as mammography.

The Health Insurance Plan of New York evaluated mammography as a screening tool in 62,000 patients; their screening included physical examination as well. A 10-year follow-up period showed a 30 percent reduction in mortality for women 50 or older who had been screened compared to a control group. The risk/benefit ratio involved in exposing large populations of asymptomatic women to ionizing radiation has been widely debated. High-quality mammograms can be performed which expose the patient to radiation doses which do not exceed 0.01 Gy. In general, annual mammograms are recommended for asymptomatic women over 50, with annual mammograms of women from 40 to 49 who are considered to be at high risk. This high-risk group is defined as those who have had prior breast cancer or have a mother or sibling with the disease. Regardless of the age, a patient with a palpable breast mass or other symptom suggestive of breast cancer should have a biopsy. Mammography prior to biopsy is not required, but it can provide supplemental preoperative information to the surgeon. Other screening techniques such as thermography pose a lesser risk to the patient but are not considered sufficiently accurate to be used as the sole screening tool. In addition, ultrasound and computerized tomography (CT) are currently being evaluated as screening techniques.

TABLE 295-1 Disease-free survival related to lymph node status

Axillary node status	Percent surviving disease-free	
	5 years	10 years
Negative	82	76
Positive:	35	24
1–3 nodes	50	35
≥ 4 nodes	21	11

SOURCE: *National Surgical Adjuvant Breast Project.*

TABLE 295-2 Breast cancer clinical stage and prognosis

Stage	American Joint Committee staging	Approximate frequency of stage at presentation, %	Approximate 5-year survival, %
I	Primary tumor <2 cm; nodes, if palpable, not felt to contain metastases; no distant metastases	55–70	80
II	Primary tumor >2 cm and <5 cm; nodes, if palpable, not fixed; no distant metastases evident	20–25	65
III	Tumor >5 cm or fixed to chest wall or skin invasion present; supraclavicular nodes palpable; no distant metastases evident	10	40
IV	Distant metastases	10	10

PATHOLOGY The anatomic units of the female breast are the small, medium, and large ducts. Tumors can arise from any of these structures, but carcinoma of the breast most frequently arises in a large duct. In 70 to 75 percent of cases, no distinctive histologic structure can be distinguished and these infiltrating duct carcinomas are designated NOS (not otherwise specified). In spite of the small size of the primary, these cancers frequently metastasize to axillary lymph nodes and their prognosis is the worst of all breast cancer types. To palpation these lesions are firm, and a fibrotic response within the tumor is characteristic. Lobular invasive, medullary, and colloid or mucinous tumors of the breast are generally seen in their pure form but can appear in combinations and make up 20 percent of all breast cancers.

Lobular carcinoma makes up approximately 5 percent of breast cancers and arises in the small end ducts. This carcinoma may be either invasive, with tumor extending beyond the duct in which it arises, or noninvasive. In the noninvasive form, carcinoma in situ, the anaplastic cells are contained within the lobules. In the invasive form the tumor extends beyond the lobule or end duct from which it arises. This type of lobular carcinoma has a poor prognosis.

Medullary carcinoma comprises 5 to 7 percent of all breast cancers. Unlike intraductal carcinomas, these tumors are well-circumscribed and often attain large size but are not as likely to infiltrate, and patients generally have a good prognosis. Another slow-growing invasive carcinoma that reaches large, bulky proportion is the colloid carcinoma, a mucinous-producing tumor which comprises 3 to 5 percent of breast cancers. The tumor occurs in older women (over the age of 70) and has a tendency to occur in areas readily accessible to palpation.

Rare histologic types of breast cancer with a favorable outcome are tubular, adenocystic, and secretory carcinoma. The latter occurs primarily in children and adolescents. Tumors with unfavorable rare histologies are squamous metaplasia and carcinomas with sarcomatoid, osseous, or chondrometaplastic elements; these tend to be quite large when discovered. Other significant histologic forms of breast cancer are inflammatory breast cancer and Paget's disease.

Inflammatory breast carcinoma presents with a unique clinical picture in which much of the skin overlying the breast becomes erythematous and thickened. The diagnosis must be confirmed pathologically. Biopsies of the erythematous areas of the breast as well as normal-appearing skin will reveal undifferentiated cancer cells in the subdermal lymphatics. In Paget's disease, the nipple epithelium contains nests of tumor cells, but the tumor may be either intraductal or of the invasive duct type. The prognosis is related to the histologic type of the tumor.

Staging following the histologic confirmation of breast cancer using both the clinical and surgical staging systems illustrated in Table 295-2 is essential. In addition, receptor status should be determined for establishing the patient's prognosis and prescribing an appropriate form of treatment. Frequently, metastases to distant sites occur early and metastatic spread follows no predictable pattern. The axillary lymph nodes, liver, bones, skin, and lungs are the most common sites of metastases while the adrenal glands, kidneys, ovaries, spleen, and thyroid are less frequently involved.

DIAGNOSIS In 70 to 80 percent of cases, the patient presents with a hard, circumscribed mass in the breast. If this mass is fixed to skin or deep muscle, or if there is edema of the skin or retraction of the nipple, cancer is almost a certainty. However, 75 percent of all breast lumps are benign. Breast cancer presents most frequently (in 45 percent of cases) in the upper outer quadrant of the breast; it is present in the central or subareolar portion of the breast in 25 percent of cases, in the upper inner quadrant in 15 percent of cases, and in the lower inner quadrant in only 5 percent of cases. A mobile mass with well-defined margins in a woman under 30 is much more likely to be a fibroadenoma, a benign condition. On rare occasions, infectious mastitis may be mistaken for adenoma.

Once a well-defined breast mass has been detected, a complete history and physical examination should be followed by a biopsy or needle aspiration. A breast mass is an indication for biopsy regardless of the results of mammography. There is no necessity for the biopsy and definitive surgical treatment to be undertaken as a single operative procedure. Prior custom was to perform the initial biopsy while the patient was under general anesthesia, examine a frozen section of the tissue, and proceed with a radical mastectomy if the biopsy was positive. Biopsy can be done using local anesthesia and the interval between diagnostic biopsy and definitive surgery or radiation therapy provides a period during which metastatic disease can be ruled out and the physician can discuss all of the options for further management with the patient. In the workup for metastatic disease, the patient should be questioned and examined thoroughly for signs and symptoms of bone pain, neurologic deficit, or behavioral changes which would indicate the need to search for distant metastases. However, routine scanning of the bones in patients who are asymptomatic has not proved to be cost-effective. Likewise, radioisotopic or CT scans of the liver and brain should be undertaken only in patients with abnormal physical findings or liver function studies.

Two infrequent but nonetheless important clinical presentations of breast cancer are *inflammatory breast carcinoma* and *Paget's disease*, which have been briefly described above. With inflammatory breast disease there is increased local temperature, redness, and a visible erysipeloid margin; the entire breast is often indurated and firm to hard. This particular type of breast cancer implies systemic disease; axillary and supraclavicular node involvement and distant metastases are invariably present and require an initial systemic rather than surgical approach. Patients with inflammatory breast cancer have had an extremely poor prognosis. Results of combination chemotherapy as the initial treatment appear promising. In Paget's disease eczematoid changes in the nipple, including itching, burning, oozing, and bleeding, occur over a relatively long period and a mass can be palpated in two-thirds of patients. The prognosis is related to the treatment of the disease.

Extremely rare, but clinically distinctive, is *cystosarcoma phyllodes,* a form of sarcoma which can arise from a fibroadenoma. This tumor presents as a warm, tender, cystic mass. In the presence of a breast mass, a bloody discharge from the nipple is usually a classic sign of cancer. However, *intraductal papilloma,* a benign lesion, is associated with a bloody discharge from the nipple, without a palpable mass. These tumors are generally exceedingly small but can be located by noting the area which, when palpated, results in bleeding from the nipple. Infrequently, sarcomas, or nonepithelial malignancies, including fibrosarcomas, lymphomas, liposarcomas, and hemangiosarcomas, may be associated with breast masses.

Inflammatory lesions Mammary duct ectasia is a benign condition, usually seen in elderly women with atrophic breasts, in which the mammary ducts in or just beneath the nipple become dilated and filled with cellular debris and lipid-containing material. Intermittent pain and local inflammatory changes may be present, and because a discharge, at times bloody, and retraction of the nipple may occur, this condition must be differentiated from carcinoma. Excision of the nipple is usually indicated.

Fat necrosis is a common occurrence following trauma that may be so slight as to have not been noticed. It presents as a painful lump usually associated with some ecchymosis and may be followed by local atrophy and dimpling of the skin, at which stage biopsy must be performed to distinguish it from carcinoma.

Thrombosis of the thoracoepigastric veins and sclerosing subcutaneous phlebitis (Mondor's disease) occur after trauma or for no apparent reason and are manifested by the appearance of long cord-like structures, initially tender, in the outer half of the breast, frequently extending up into the axilla or down toward the epigastrium. They may persist for up to a year, but no treatment is indicated.

Sarcoid may very rarely involve the skin of the chest, and secondary amyloidosis may involve the breast tissue itself. Eosinophilic granuloma may occur in the submammary folds.

Fibrocystic disease With each menstrual cycle there is a recurring biphasic stimulation, first of proliferation of breast tissue by estrogens, then of alveolar secretory activity by progesterone, followed by a period of involution. In most women these changes are of such slight degree as to cause few if any clinical symptoms. Not infrequently, however, inflammatory changes may precede each menses, with tenderness, engorgement, and increasing nodularity of the breasts. This is more often seen in nulliparous women and may subside after childbearing and lactation. Suspected cysts in the breast may be aspirated safely in the office with local anesthesia if biopsy is done promptly in any of the following circumstances: (1) no fluid is obtained; (2) the cyst fluid is grossly bloody; (3) the mass does not completely disappear with aspiration; and (4) the fluid reaccumulates during succeeding days. Cytologic examinations of cyst aspirates are of little value if negative.

In the later years of reproductive life the continued recurrent stimulation and involution of the breasts in the course of each menstrual cycle may result in diffuse and nodular fibrosis and the formation of cysts of varying sizes, called chronic cystic mastitis. This condition may simulate carcinoma but is usually distinguishable by the fact that it is intermittently painful and may subside to some extent following menstruation. Nevertheless, carcinoma may coexist and be masked by the diffuse nodularity of the cystic disease.

Moreover, the incidence of mammary carcinoma is greater in patients with fibrocystic disease of the breasts, and it is unwise to delay biopsy of suspicious areas in the hope that they may subside by the end of the next menstrual cycle.

LOCAL MANAGEMENT OF BREAST CANCER (STAGE I AND STAGE II) Background Until a decade ago, the radical mastectomy, which involves removal of the breast, both the major and minor pectoralis muscles, ipsilateral axillary lymph nodes, and, in the medial lesions, the ipsilateral supraclavicular and mediastinal lymph chains, was considered the sole therapeutic option for breast cancer. This treatment was based on the rationale that breast cancer begins as a single focus of disease which, after a considerable period of time, will spread in an orderly fashion from the breast to the axillary nodes and from there into the systemic channels of the blood and lymphatic systems. With this underlying assumption, treatment was targeted at arresting the spread of tumor by removing the primary breast tumor and the surrounding tissue en bloc.

Data from many studies have changed the conceptual underpinnings for such radical therapy. Breast cancer is now appreciated to be a disease which is localized for only a brief period and then disseminates into the circulatory and lymphatic channels early in its course. The current emphasis in the management of breast cancer is removal of the primary site of tumor with the minimum disfigurement necessary to gain local control by surgical or radiation therapy and control of the distant microscopic foci of disease with adjuvant systemic therapy. No single procedure can be recommended as ideal for all patients. It is estimated that annually approximately 50,000 women in the United States have breast cancer masses of 4 cm or less in diameter and are eligible for breast-preserving therapy.

Surgical options The radical mastectomy described previously not only confers no increased benefit in terms of survival, but often, because of the removal of the pectoralis minor, results in edema of the arm and a shallow, shrunken chest which make fitting a prosthesis difficult. Various other surgical options attain survival outcomes similar to those in patients treated with the radical mastectomy while obtaining a more acceptable cosmetic result. The radical mastectomy is occasionally useful in patients with locally invasive tumors.

If the surgical option selected includes removal of a breast, many forms of external prosthesis are available, but they are often clumsy and uncomfortable. Alternatively, reconstructive surgical techniques are available. The nature and timing of the procedure should be tailored to the requirements of the patient.

The modified radical mastectomy is the most common primary surgical treatment for breast cancer in this country. This operation differs from the radical mastectomy in that the pectoralis muscles are spared but an axillary dissection is done en bloc. Women with little breast tissue often favor complete removal of the breast with subequent reconstruction since the amount of tissue removed even in the more conservative procedures such as the quadrantectomy or segmental resection can result in a distorted-appearing breast.

The total or simple mastectomy is an operation in which the breast is removed but the pectoralis muscles are not excised, and the axillary lymph nodes are removed through a separate incision. In comparative clinical trials conducted by NSABP, this operation produced survival benefits similar to that of the radical mastectomy.Total or simple mastectomy without axillary dissection is generally not recommended because an informed judgment regarding the necessity for further adjuvant therapy cannot be made without this information.

The segmental mastectomy (lumpectomy) and the tylectomy involve removal of the primary tumor and a minimal amount of surrounding tissue. Both operative procedures are aimed at preserving most of the breast. These procedures are appropriate for women who have small lesions, <2 cm, located in the periphery of the breast, and who have ample breast tissue remaining so that the desired aesthetic effect can be achieved. The segmental mastectomy has been evaluated in a randomized prospective clinical study. Patients eligible for a segmental mastectomy were randomized into three groups; one group received the segmental mastectomy, the second the segmental mastectomy plus radiation to the breast, and the third a total mastectomy. In all patients entered in this trial, an axillary dissection was performed and chemotherapy given to those with nodes positive for tumor.

After five years, the results indicate that segmental mastectomy followed by breast irradiation in all patients plus adjuvant chemotherapy given to those with positive nodes is acceptable therapy for tumors of 4 cm or less when margins of resected specimens are tumor-free. In fact, in this group the overall survival was better than overall survival after total mastectomy.

A quadrantectomy is the removal of the breast quadrant in which the primary occurs along with the overlying skin and the fascia of the pectoralis major. In this study no difference was observed in the 9-year survival rate of two groups of women with breast cancer, one that had been treated by a radical mastectomy and the other by quadrantectomy plus axillary dissection coupled with radiotherapy. Local control of disease in those treated with the less-extensive surgical procedures was not markedly different from patients treated with radical mastectomy, and when local recurrences did occur, they could be treated effectively with further surgery or irradiation.

Radiation therapy Other nonsurgical means of achieving local-regional control of tumor, such as radiation therapy, have been under investigation for over 50 years. A study by United States investigators has evaluated a selected group of women with stages I and II breast cancer. This group of 357 women received local treatment consisting of external beam radiation therapy utilizing tangential and nodal fields to deliver 44 to 50 Gy (2 Gy daily, four to five times per week) plus a booster dose of 10 to 20 Gy from either an external beam or radium implants. At 6 years, the rate of local control of tumor is similar to that of the historical controls who underwent extensive surgical treatment.

However, a subgroup of patients at increased risk of local recurrence when treated by radiation therapy has been defined. The histologic features include poor nuclear grade, extensive mitoses, and intraductal carcinoma in the primary tumor and adjacent tissue. While the breast remains intact in those women who received primary radiation therapy, this procedure can cause fibrosis and hardening of the affected breast and the shrinkage caused by this technique may result in an asymmetric appearance in the patient with small breasts. This treatment modality also raises the possibility of tumor induction in the irradiated area; data in patients who had received postoperative radiation suggest that this risk is slight. Whether the primary breast cancer is treated with surgery or radiation, sampling of the ipsilateral axillary lymph nodes should be undertaken to ascertain whether any nodes are positive for carcinoma, indicating the need for further therapy.

ADJUVANT THERAPY OF BREAST CANCER Background Because only 80 percent of patients with stage I disease and 65 percent of those with stage II disease (Table 295-2) attained a 5-year survival following surgery, clinicians began to investigate other modalities such as postoperative radiation and hormonal manipulation in an effort to improve these results. Radiation therapy was aimed at achieving survival by increasing local-regional control of tumor, while hormonal manipulation by means of prophylactic castration was designed to reach deposits of tumor that had already undergone systemic dissemination. Neither of these modalities has improved the overall survival of treated patients. Radiation proved ineffective because it could only affect local disease. Hormonal manipulation failed as well, probably because it was not applied selectively to only those patients who were ER-positive, a technology that was not available at the time. Animal experiments with chemotherapeutic agents suggested these drugs administered systemically might be effective in patients with micrometastatic breast cancer.

Selected adjuvant chemotherapy trials Two prospective randomized studies of the efficacy of postoperative chemotherapy were initiated first by the NSABP in 1972 and then by the Cancer Institute of Milan, Italy in 1973. The first group of investigators studied the agent melphalan (L-phenylalanine mustard or L-PAM) versus placebo, the second studied a combination of cyclophosphamide, methotrexate, and 5-fluorouracil (CMF). After nearly a decade of follow-up, both studies demonstrate a statistically significant improved relapse-free survival, particularly for patients with one to three positive nodes. Not only was adjuvant therapy successful in preventing distant recurrence of disease but local-regional control was similar to that achieved in women who received postoperative radiation therapy.

Subsequent sequential studies completed by the NSABP group included a combination of melphalan and 5-FU compared to melphalan alone. The two-drug combination proved superior to the single agent not only in those patients under 50 but also in those patients over 50 with four or more positive lymph nodes in whom a 40 percent reduction in mortality was observed at 5 years. The third study was a comparison of the two-drug combination to a three-drug combination of melphalan, 5-FU, and methotrexate. This three-drug combination showed no distinct advantage over two drugs. However, in a fourth study, tamoxifen—an antiestrogen—was substituted for methotrexate and compared to the two-drug combination. A significant improvement in relapse-free survival and overall survival was noted. This improvement was largely attributable to improved results in patients older than 50 with four or more positive nodes. Five additional studies are still in progress.

Numerous other clinical trials were initiated by other investigators. During the fall of 1985, a review of all randomized trials (approximately 100) comparing adjuvant therapy with either antiestrogen therapy or cytotoxic chemotherapy to untreated controls was sponsored by the United Kingdom Breast Cancer Trials Coordinating Subcommittee. This analysis indicated a significant reduction in mortality among those women receiving either form of therapy, but the reduction was greatest in premenopausal women who received cytotoxic chemotherapy, for the most part CMF or slight variations of CMF. Systemic adjuvant chemotherapy produced not only significant reductions in early mortality in women with breast cancer under the age of 50 but was also effective in the postmenopausal group. In postmenopausal women, antiestrogens alone also produced a significant reduction in early mortality. A consensus development conference held at the National Institutes of Health concluded that all women with positive nodes should receive some sort of adjuvant treatment, preferably in a clinical trial designed to define better regimens. Another piece of confirmatory evidence of the effectiveness of adjuvant chemotherapy is the change in age-specific breast cancer mortality rates among white females in the United States. From 1976 to 1981, a 20 percent decline in mortality in women below age 50 occurred. Mortality has always been closely linked to nulliparity rates of women between the ages of 20 and 25. Because nulliparity was high in the early 1960s due to increased use of birth control agents, an increase in mortality in this cohort of women would have been predicted. This first-time divergence in mortality and nulliparity trends suggest that the major influences on decreasing mortality in premenopausal women between 1976 and 1981 was the widespread use of adjuvant chemotherapy. It has been estimated that wide application of adjuvant therapy could save approximately 5000 lives a year in the United States.

Investigators at the Cancer Institute of Milan have suggested that a dose-response effect may be responsible for the less promising results in postmenopausal patients. When they reviewed those patients who had received 85 percent of the planned dose, 77 percent had a relapse-free survival at 5 years. However, the patients who received only 65 percent of the planned dose had only a 48 percent rate of relapse-free survival, a result no different from the controls. An analysis of dose intensity of the drug regimens used as adjuvant treatment showed that there is a direct correlation between dose intensity and relapse-free survival at 3 years. These data suggest that adjuvant chemotherapy should be administered early and used as aggressively as possible to ensure the most favorable results. Short courses of chemotherapy may be as effective and are certainly tolerated better than longer ones. The Milan group has demonstrated that 6 months of therapy provides similar results to treatment of women for 12 months.

Selecting adjuvant chemotherapy CMF for 6 to 12 months' duration has been studied extensively and is probably the most commonly used combination. Although other combinations of drugs have yielded similar results, the combination of drugs that appears most promising in postmenopausal patients is a modification of CMFVP (cyclophosphamide, methotrexate, 5-fluorouracil, vincristine, and prednisone). Although each patient's clinical situation must be considered individually, those recommended for adjuvant chemotherapy are stage II (node-positive) premenopausal patients and stage II postmenopausal patients who are ER- and PR-negative. Adjuvant therapy is not commonly recommended for stage I (node-negative) patients. These patients, however, should be considered candidates for clinical trials. One of the most profound predictors of outcome is that of nuclear grade. This characteristic exceeds other major prognostic factors such as tumor stage, menopausal status, or estrogen receptor status in predicting aggressiveness of tumor as measured by disease-free interval or survival. Prospective studies of the future will likely test the utility of this index for selection of patients for treatment.

Side effects of chemotherapy Acute side effects of adjuvant therapy such as malaise, nausea, and vomiting are common. Nausea and vomiting can often be relieved by the administration of phenothiazines prior to and during treatment. Alopecia must be anticipated and can be minimized by cooling the scalp with a cap specifically designed for this purpose, 30 min prior to, during, and 30 min after the administration of chemotherapy. The long-term side effects of adjuvant therapy have not yet been fully delineated, but the adverse long-term effects appear to be low. Analyses of 8483 women entered into NSABP trials indicate only 36 patients (0.4 percent) developed leukemia and 7 (0.1 percent) a myeloproliferative syndrome. The cumulative risk of leukemia before or after the development of metastatic disease or a second primary tumor was 0.27 percent at 10 years. Cardiotoxicity from anthracycline-containing combinations should be watched for. Clearly, long-term follow-up will continue to be required to elucidate the risk/benefit ratio of each adjuvant regimen.

Adjuvant radiotherapy Postoperative radiotherapy, a common practice in the past, is effective only in decreasing the rate of local-regional recurrence. If a patient has four or more positive nodes, the local-regional recurrence rates range from 15 to 25 percent. If one to three nodes are positive, 5 to 10 percent of patients develop local-regional recurrence. If the nodes are negative, only 2 to 8 percent develop recurrence. Radiation delivered postoperatively can reduce the overall local-regional recurrence rate to less than 5 percent but does not increase overall survival. Patients who have received adjuvant chemotherapy have an incidence of local-regional recurrence similar to that observed in women treated with local-regional radiation therapy and have the additional benefit of longer survival. Should a patient who has received adjuvant chemotherapy develop a local-regional recurrence, radiation therapy is effective in controlling the lesion in 60 to 70 percent.

Postoperative radiotherapy should only be considered if clinically apparent tumor remains following surgery, if the tumor is >5 cm, or if the histologic type is undifferentiated or inflammatory.

Adjuvant hormone therapy Prior attempts to evaluate hormonal manipulation as an adjuvant therapy were done without the benefit of the assay for the ER protein and were, for the most part, inconclusive. One trial, however, has yielded positive findings. After 10 years of follow-up, an improvement in overall survival was observed in those stage II premenopausal patients whose ovaries were ablated by radiation (20 Gy in five daily fractions) plus prednisone (7.5 mg per day) after surgery and postoperative regional radiation. The survival rate for women in this treatment group was 77 percent, in contrast to a survival rate of 61 percent in women who received only primary surgery and a postoperative regimen of radiation. Evaluation of the antiestrogens, such as tamoxifen, as adjuvant therapy is limited. A worldwide analysis conducted in Bethesda, Maryland, in September 1985 did indicate a highly significant benefit in reduction of mortality in postmenopausal women who received tamoxifen as adjuvant therapy. The reduction in mortality was slightly superior in postmenopausal women who received adjuvant combination chemotherapy. Women most likely to benefit from the addition of an antiestrogen to a chemotherapy combination are ER-positive and postmenopausal, and women with the greatest tumor burden (i.e., a primary >3 cm and/or four or more nodes involved). Which combination of drugs should be used in addition to antiestrogen therapy and what the duration of antiestrogen treatment (continuous versus 1 to 2 years) should be are under study, although administration of antiestrogens for at least 2 years appears to be the treatment of choice at present.

MANAGEMENT OF DISSEMINATED BREAST CANCER While fewer than 10 percent of patients present with stage IV breast cancer, approximately one-third to one-half of all breast cancer patients treated with surgery or radiation alone will eventually have recurrence of the disease. Therefore, it is important to document the extent and location, ER status, and rate of progress of the cancer since it is useful in determining a patient's prognosis and in selecting the proper approach to management if metastases appear. Once systemic disease has occurred, nearly half of the patients with metastatic disease will respond to chemotherapy, one-third with complete remissions. While survival has improved, the duration of response is generally limited to 6 months to 1 year.

Hormone receptors and hormonal management Conventional forms of hormonal manipulation are aimed at abolishing estrogen or estrogen precursors. In the majority of patients the initial ER determination remains unchanged and the ER values of the primary and metastatic sites are similar. A woman who has changed menopausal status since the original ER determination is the most likely candidate to have changed ER status from negative to positive or vice versa. Although on a statistical basis women who are ER-positive are more likely to respond to estrogen deprivation, in any given patient, the absence or presence of ER should not totally influence the choice of therapy. Certainly patients with absent estrogen receptors may respond to estrogen deprivation therapy, and those with receptors present may not. If, at the time of relapse, tissue for ER evaluation is not obtainable, the therapeutic plan should consider the results from earlier evaluation of breast tissue. Even if the ER status of a patient is unknown, a 30 percent response rate of approximately 12 to 18 months' duration has been observed after either additive or ablative hormonal manipulation. In the absence of ER data, clinical findings which predict a favorable response to hormonal manipulation are postmenopausal status, a disease-free interval longer than 2 years, metastases which are confined to the soft tissue or bones, and a prior positive response to hormone therapy. In general, the response to hormone therapy is not rapid, but 90 percent of those patients who are going to respond do so within an 8-week period. Hypercalcemia may develop during hormone therapy (see "Hypercalcemia" below) and may indicate a favorable response. The x-ray picture created by bone lesions which are responding favorably to hormone treatment, i.e., a healing osteoblastic lesion, can easily be confused with tumor progression.

ANTIESTROGENS These estrogen analogues are the hormonal treatment of choice; they bind to the ER, are translocated like estrogens with the receptor into the cell's nucleus, and block the action of estrogens. Tamoxifen, 10 mg twice daily, is considered the antiestrogen of choice. Although sixty percent of patients who are ER-positive respond to antiestrogens, patients with visceral metastases, especially hepatic lesions, are the least likely to respond. Common side effects of tamoxifen are mild nausea, vomiting, and, occasionally, hot flashes. Corneal opacities and retinal degeneration have been observed only rarely at normal dose levels.

MEDICAL ADRENALECTOMY/AMINOGLUTETHIMIDE Women who are postmenopausal should be considered for such therapy to reduce estrogen production. Approximately half the patients who had previously been hormone-sensitive respond to this treatment. Medical adrenalectomy using aminoglutethimide (AG) is an alternative to surgical adrenalectomy for ablating adrenal function, reducing estrogen production by inhibiting adrenal androgen synthesis, and thereby depleting the substrate for aromatization to estrogen. While achieving the same response rate as surgical ablation (a procedure that is now rarely indicated), the drug can be withdrawn should the treatment fail without the patient's being rendered permanently hypoadrenal. The recommended dosage of AG is 250 mg every 6 h. Hydrocortisone 20 to 40 mg per day is administered to mimic glucocorticoid administration and to prevent the reflex ACTH rise (see Chap. 325). Hydrocortisone is preferred to dexamethasone because this drug's metabolism is accelerated by AG, thereby reducing availability of the steroid. Side effects of AG include lethargy, rash, transient ataxia, and dizziness; most of these are acute and transient.

Hormones ESTROGEN If a patient is no longer responding to tamoxifen or AG, one hormonal approach to be considered is the use of estrogen. Estrogens such as diethylstilbestrol, 15 mg daily, or ethinyl estradiol, 3 mg daily, are most effective in postmenopausal women with soft-tissue and slowly progressive visceral metastases. Acute side effects include nausea, vomiting, and uterine bleeding, which can be controlled with cyclic administration of progesterone.

ANDROGENS Androgens can be considered for some premenopausal patients, but their greatest utility is in the postmenopausal patient with bony metastases.

Surgical approaches The advent of antiestrogens and aminoglutethimide has diminished the use of surgical procedures such as castration, adrenalectomy, or hypophysectomy.

CASTRATION Premenopausal females who relapse after having achieved a response to tamoxifen and other hormonal manipulations and who have no evidence of hepatic metastases or lymphatic spread to the lungs may be candidates for castration. The response rate to this procedure in ER-positive women is 50 percent, while 20 percent of men respond. The average duration of such a response is 15 to 18 months.

SURGICAL ADRENALECTOMY/HYPOPHYSECTOMY If, after having responded to antiestrogen therapy and/or castration, a premenopausal patient develops recurrent tumor, hypophysectomy should be considered. Surgical adrenalectomy is appropriate only for the rare patient who cannot comply with the medical adrenalectomy regimen.

Chemotherapy Patients who have failed or exhausted prior hormonal manipulation, or who are ER-negative, and those with visceral disease that is progressing rapidly should be considered for chemotherapy. Single-agent chemotherapy with drugs such as 5-fluorouracil, methotrexate, doxorubicin, or cyclophosphamide produces partial responses in 20 to 40 percent of patients. While the overall response rates to doxorubicin hydrochloride and cyclophosphamide may approach that of some combination programs, the responses are usually only partial. Overall response rates of the common drug combinations are illustrated in Table 295-3 and range from 50 to 75 percent, with 15 to 20 percent of patients achieving a complete response with a fraction remaining disease-free. Combination chemotherapy is therefore the treatment of choice in patients with metastatic disease. The "Cooper regimen," CMFVP, was originally reported to attain a response rate of 90 percent with nearly all responses being complete. However, numerous clinical trials using these same drugs in a variety of schedules have attained an overall response rate of 40 percent and only 10 to 20 percent of patients achieved a complete response. An analysis of the relative dose intensity of these drug combinations compared to the Cooper regimen shows a decreased dose intensity that correlates with the lower response rate. Other combinations of drugs show similar results. The median duration of response of patients who achieve a complete remission is 1 year, while for those who have partial regression of tumor it is 6 to 9 months. Should the patient initially respond to chemotherapy and then fail, subsequent chemotherapy regimens produce responses of brief duration in 25 to 40 percent of cases. The high relapse rate and diminished sensitivity to second-line chemotherapy are strong indicators of cells which have become or were inherently resistant. Experimental approaches, including monoclonal antibodies, in a protocol setting should be considered for these patients. At some cancer centers, high-dose chemotherapy and autologous bone marrow transplantation have yielded a significant number of complete responses in previously treated patients.

Clinical predictors of a favorable response to chemotherapy include a disease-free interval of more than 2 years and pre- or perimenopausal status. All sites of metastatic disease are not equally responsive to chemotherapy; metastases to soft tissue, such as skin and lymph modes, are most responsive; visceral sites of metastases show intermediate responsiveness, and bone lesions are least likely to respond to chemotherapy, although pain relief often results.

Selecting an appropriate combination depends primarily on two factors: the patient's prior exposure to drugs in the adjuvant setting, and a medical history which would contraindicate the use of specific drugs in combination. Patients exposed to melphalan in the adjuvant setting can respond to a non-cross-resistant drug or drug combination such as doxorubicin or CMF if metastases occur. Patients exposed previously to CMF remain responsive to doxorubicin-containing combinations, but are unlikely to respond to standard doses of single-agent alkylating therapy once combination therapy has failed. Such regimens should be considered for the patient with a prior history of congestive heart failure only if the patient has failed to respond to non-anthracycline-containing combinations. A maximum total dose of 550 mg per square meter of body surface should be used in all patients who receive doxorubicin.

MANAGEMENT OF COMPLICATIONS DUE TO BREAST CANCER

Skeletal system Painful and destructive lesions of the skeleton often occur in breast cancer patients with advanced disease. Bone scans are the most sensitive test for detecting early signs of metastatic disease but have not proved to be cost effective in asymptomatic patients. When following a patient, x-rays of sites which become symptomatic are appropriate. Bone-scanning is required only if x-rays are negative.

Limited field irradiation is effective for palliation of pain. The extent of disease, the patient's requirements for narcotics, and the overall health status should be carefully evaluated before radiation for pain relief is recommended. Preventing fractures of weight-bearing bones can also be accomplished by limited field irradiation. Total dosage in this instance is generally 20 to 40 Gy over 3 to 4 weeks. If the site of involvement is a weight-bearing bone and if the lesion is approximately 2.5 cm or larger, stabilization by internal fixation or, in some cases, replacement of the femoral head should be considered.

If the patient complains of back pain, a careful neurologic examination should be carried out and, if the findings are equivocal, a CT scan and occasionally a myelogram should be performed to rule out compression of the spinal cord due to pathologic fracture of a vertebra or epidural involvement by tumor. Prevention of paralysis is preferable to treatment after the fact.

Hypercalcemia Elevated levels of calcium occur in breast cancer patients for many reasons. Skeletal metastases which result in destruction of bone can result in hypercalcemia, but the severity of the hypercalcemia does not necessarily correlate with the extent of bone destruction. A response to hormonal therapy, dehydration, and immobilization because of increased bone reabsorption of calcium, as well as use of long-term prednisone can also cause hypercalcemia in breast cancer patients.

The severity of symptoms dictates the urgency and measures that should be employed to treat the hypercalcemia. The more common symptoms—nausea, vomiting, anorexia, lethargy, confusion, stupor, and eventually coma—may be confused with side effects due to

TABLE 295-3 Commonly used combination chemotherapies for the treatment of breast cancer

Combination	Dose and schedule*	Overall response rate, %	Complete response rate, %
CMFVP:		50–90	10–20
Cyclophosphamide	80 mg/m² PO daily		
Methotrexate	20 mg/m² IV weekly × 8 weeks		
5-Fluorouracil	500 mg/m² IV weekly		
Vincristine	1.0 mg/m² IV weekly × 4–5 weeks		
Prednisone	30 mg/m² PO daily × 15 (then taper)		
CMFP (repeat every 4 weeks):		65	26
Cyclophosphamide	100 mg/m² PO days 1–14		
Methotrexate	60 mg/m² IV days 1 & 8		
5-Fluorouracil	700 mg/m² IV days 1 & 8		
Prednisone	40 mg/m² PO days 1 & 14		
CMF (repeat every 4 weeks):		50	15
Cyclophosphamide	100 mg/m² PO days 1–14		
Methotrexate	30–40 mg/m² IV days 1 & 8		
5-Fluorouracil	600 mg/m² IV days 1 & 8		
CAF (repeat every 4 weeks):		80	18
Cyclophosphamide	100 mg/m² PO days 1–14		
Doxorubicin	40 mg/m² IV day 1		
5-Fluorouracil	400 mg/m² IV days 1 & 8		
AC (repeat cycle every 3–4 weeks):		80	12
Doxorubicin	40 mg/m² IV day 1		
Cyclophosphamide	200 mg/m² PO days 3–6		

* *These are doses appropriate to a patient whose marrow is not compromised and must be adjusted according to a sliding scale if marrow, hepatic, or renal functions are abnormal.*

therapy or with a terminal state of cancer. In patients who are relatively asymptomatic or have only mild elevation of calcium, administration of fluids and/or diuretics such as furosemide, as well as increasing the patient's level of activity, may be sufficient. If hypercalcemia is due to additive hormonal agents, glucocorticoids (40 to 100 mg of prednisone or its equivalent in divided doses) are recommended. In patients with hypercalcemia, substitutes should be found for medications such as thiazide, antacids which contain calcium, and lithium, which also tends to increase the serum calcium level. Dose adjustments should be made in drugs like digoxin which are dependent on calcium for their action. In breast cancer as in other malignancies, treatment of the tumor is the most effective means to control complications such as hypercalcemia. Because effects of such treatment take days to weeks, it may be necessary to administer plicamycin (mithramycin) 25 μg per kilogram of body weight as a rapid intravenous infusion to achieve a lowering of calcium levels in the more severe cases. This drug usually acts to lower serum calcium within 48 h of administration, and the effect may last for a week or more. If, however, it has not had the desired effect within that period, a similar dose (not to exceed two doses per week) should be given. These dosages of plicamycin rarely cause toxic side effects.

Central nervous system Changes in behavior or evidence of cranial or peripheral neurologic deficit should raise the possibility of brain or spinal involvement. A thorough neurologic examination, CT scan, and lumbar puncture should be undertaken and, if lesions can be localized, whole-brain radiotherapy is generally the treatment of choice. If metastases appear to be solitary, the possibility of surgical removal followed by cranial radiotherapy should be considered. Cytologic examination should be carried out on the spinal fluid as well as culture for opportunistic infections. If leptomeningeal metastases are observed, intrathecal administration of methotrexate is recommended.

Eye Breast cancer is the most common cause of retro- or intraorbital metastases. Visual impairment with or without proptosis in the breast cancer patient is an indication for further evaluation. Intraorbital metastases can be revealed by careful fundoscopic examination, but retroorbital metastases require evaluation by CT scan.

REFERENCES

BONADONNA G et al: Adjuvant CFM chemotherapy inoperable breast cancer: Ten years later. Lancet 1:976, 1985

Consensus Conference. Adjuvant chemotherapy for breast cancer. JAMA 254(24):3461, 1985

FISHER B et al: A summary of findings from NSABP trials of adjuvant therapy, in *Adjuvant Therapy of Cancer IV*, S. Jones et al (eds). New York, Grune & Stratton, 1984, p 185

———: Five-year results of a randomized clinical trial comparing total mastectomy and segmental mastectomy with or without radiation in the treatment of breast cancer. N Engl J Med 312:665, 1985

———: Ten-year results of a randomized clinical trial comparing radical mastectomy and total mastectomy with or without radiation. N Engl J Med 312:674, 1985

HARRIS J et al: The role of radiation therapy in the primary treatment of carcinoma of the breast. Semin Oncol 5:403, 1978

——— et al: Cancer of the breast, in *Cancer: Principles and Practices in Oncology*, VT DeVita et al (eds). New York, Lippincott, 1985, p 1119

MILLER A et al: The epidemiology and etiology of breast cancer. N Engl J Med 303:1246, 1980

Review of mortality results in randomized trials in early breast cancer, editorial. Lancet 2:1205, 1984

SANTEN R et al: A randomized trial comparing surgical adrenalectomy with aminoglutethimide plus hydrocortisone in women with advanced breast cancer. N Engl J Med 305:545, 1981

SORACE R et al: The management of nonmetastatic locally advanced breast cancer using primary induction chemotherapy with hormonal synchronization followed by radiation therapy with or without debulking surgery. World J Surg (in press)

296 CARCINOMA OF THE OVARY

FRED J. HENDLER

The occurrence rate of ovarian cancer is relatively low, only 1.5 percent, and it is only the seventh most common cause of cancer in women. However, cancer of the ovary is the leading cause of death from gynecologic malignancies and the fourth most common cause of cancer-related death among women. Survival is excellent with early stage disease and poor when extensive disease is present. The apparent discrepancy between incidence and survival reflects the fact that most women at diagnosis have extensive disease. The high death rate associated with advanced disease has led to the development of aggressive multimodal therapy encompassing surgery, radiation, and/or chemotherapy. As a result, survival in patients with advanced disease has improved, and some advanced ovarian carcinomas may be cured.

INCIDENCE AND EPIDEMIOLOGY

Each year 18,500 new cases are diagnosed, and about 11,500 women die in the United States from ovarian cancer (Table 296-1). The disease is responsible for a fifth of all pathologically documented ovarian masses and is the most frequent ovarian mass detected in postmenopausal women. The peak incidence is in the sixth and seventh decades, with the disease eventually affecting 1 in 70 women. The incidence and death rate have remained fairly constant during the past 20 years, namely 14 and 9, respectively, per 100,000 women per year.

The epidemiology varies with histologic cell type. In the United States ovarian germ cell tumors are more frequent in young nonwhite women, and epithelial tumors are more common among postmenopausal white women. The epidemiology of epithelial tumors is similar to that of breast cancer. The highest incidence of ovarian cancer is in the western industrialized countries, and the lowest incidence is in Japan and the Mediterranean countries. The rate of ovarian cancer is increased in Japanese immigrants to the United States and in their descendants, suggesting that environmental factors are important epidemiologic variables. Hormones may also influence the incidence. Risk is higher in nulliparous women, women who have difficulty conceiving, and women with fewer pregnancies. However, no conclusive data link birth control pills or exogenous estrogen administration with an increased incidence. Familial ovarian cancer is not as common as familial breast cancer. Genetic disorders that affect the intestinal epithelium, such as Peutz-Jeghers syndrome, are associated with a five- to tenfold increased risk. Some chromosomal abnormalities (pure gonadal dysgenesis of the 46,XY type and mixed gonadal dysgenesis of the 46,XY/45,X type) are associated with an increased incidence of gonadoblastomas, while others (gonadal dysgenesis of the 46,XX and 45,X types) are not associated with ovarian malignancies (see Chap. 333). Chromosomal changes have been described in ovarian cancer tissue, but these appear to be acquired defects.

TABLE 296-1 Incidence and death rate of invasive gynecologic cancer

Tissue	Incidence, per year	Deaths, per year
Ovarian	18,500	11,600
Cervix, invasive	15,000	6,800
Uterine corpus and endometrium	37,000	2,900
Other	4,400	1,100

SOURCE: *Modified from the National Cancer Institute's Surveillance, Epidemiology, and End Results Program (1977–1981).*

HISTOLOGIC CLASSIFICATION

Tumors can arise from all of the component cells of the ovary—epithelial, germinal, and stromal (Table 296-2). They may be benign, have a borderline malignancy (i.e., have some but not all the features of malignancy), or be truly neoplastic. Even in the neoplastic category, many gradations exist. The histologic grade of the tumor is based on the most aggressive cytologic and histologic pattern that is identified. Approximately 85 percent of ovarian carcinomas are of epithelial origin, derived from the coelomic epithelium or mesothelium from the embryonal gonadal ridge. The remaining 15 percent encompass a wide variety of cell types. In most, the tissue of origin can be identified, and, when more than one cell type is present, tumors are classified by the predominant cell type.

EPITHELIAL TUMORS

CLINICAL FEATURES AND DIAGNOSIS Tumors derived from epithelial cells represent 85 percent of ovarian carcinoma. These malignancies most frequently occur in peri- or postmenopausal women. Frequently, the symptoms at presentation are nonspecific and usually include abdominal pain, increasing abdominal girth, and/or dysfunctional uterine bleeding. The symptoms have often been present for long periods and have been ignored. Thus, 75 percent of these tumors are widely disseminated at diagnosis. When the tumors are detected in premenopausal women they may be more limited because menstrual abnormalities are associated with an earlier diagnosis.

Epithelial ovarian malignancies are rarely confined to one ovary and may be multifocal. Dissemination may occur early with small primary tumors. In limited disease, the tumors are confined to the ovaries and pelvic tissue. With extensive disease, the mode of spread is by diffuse peritoneal implantation of serosal surfaces and metastasis to regional lymphatics. The inferior surface of the right diaphragm is a frequent site for extrapelvic metastases. Hematogenous metastases are infrequent at the time of diagnosis. Careful examination of the entire abdominal cavity and retroperitoneal lymph nodes is required for accurate staging. Development of ascites with advanced disease is due to increased exudation and to blockage of diaphragmatic lymphatics.

PROGNOSTIC FACTORS **Tumor stage** A staging classification for all ovarian cancer was developed by the International Federation of Gynecology and Obstetrics (FIGO) in 1969. Tumor stage for epithelial carcinomas correlates the extent of disease with prognosis (Table 296-3). With a thorough and systematic diagnostic staging evaluation, many patients previously designated as stage I are now shown to have stage III disease. Similarly, malignant peritoneal washings in the presence of limited disease (stages Ic and IIc) probably indicate extensive disease outside the true pelvis, and such tumors should now be viewed as stage III. In short, many patients with apparent Ib, Ic, and IIc disease, when carefully staged, are at least stage III, and the prevalence of IIa and IIb disease has thereby been reduced. Apparently, only 20 to 30 percent of patients have limited ovarian cancer at presentation. By separating patients with previously unrecognized advanced disease, the prognosis in stages I and II has apparently improved to projected cure rates of approximately 80 percent and 60 percent, respectively. In addition, the prognosis of patients with stage II disease has improved because patients with less bulky disease have been added to this stage. These stage shifts have no effect on true prognosis. Nevertheless, the staging system has documented the importance of the tumor burden to the prognosis. Furthermore, modern chemotherapy has altered the natural history of ovarian cancer, prolonging the time to relapse. As a result, 5-year survical may no longer be synonymous with cure.

Tumor burden Confined disease, although bulky, has a better prognosis than does disease of similar total burden that is diffusely distributed. Survival is better for stage Ia than for Ic, and survival for stage IIa is better than for IIb or IIc. When extensive disease is present (stages III or IV), survival correlates with the tumor burden at presentation and with the minimal residual tumor burden following surgical debulking (Table 296-4).

Histologic grade and cell type The histologic grade of the tumor is an important prognostic factor. Histologic grading systems are applied to tumors with proliferative activity (not borderline malignancies) and are based on the ability of tumors to form papillary structures and glands and on the degree of cellular atypia (Broder's classification). The histologic grade correlates with survival (Fig.

TABLE 296-2 Primary ovarian neoplasms

Cell type	Incidence, percent
I Epithelial cell	85
A Serous	
B Mucinous	
C Endometrioid	
D Mesonephroid (clear cell)	
E Brenner	
F Undifferentiated	
G Carcinosarcoma	
II Stromal cell	<10
A Granulosa	
B Thecoma	
C Arrhenoblastoma	
D Sertoli	
E Gynandroblastoma	
F Lipoid	
III Germ cell	<5
A Teratoma	
1 Not otherwise specified	
2 Dermoid cyst	
3 Struma ovarii	
B Teratocarcinoma	
C Dysgerminoma	
D Embryonal carcinoma	
E Endodermal sinus	
F Choriocarcinoma	
G Gonadoblastoma	
H Mixed tumors	
IV Mesenchymal cell	2

TABLE 296-3 Pathologic staging of ovarian cancer

Stage	Extent of disease	Incidence, percent	Projected 5-year survival, percent
I	Involvement of ovaries only	15	80
a	Limited to one ovary, no ascites		
b	Both ovaries involved, no ascites		
c	Ia or Ib with ascites and/or malignant cells in peritoneal washings		
II	Ovarian involvement and extension into true pelvis	10	60
a	Extension or metastasis to uterus and/or tubes		
b	Extension to other pelvic tissues		
c	IIa or IIb with ascites and/or malignant cells in peritoneal washings		
III	Ovarian involvement with extension and/or metastasis into abdominal cavity including metastic implantation on the peritoneal surfaces of the liver and diaphragm and the serosal surface of the bowel	70	40
IV	Ovarian involvement with distant metastasis; pleural effusions must contain malignant cells; liver involvement must be parenchymal	5	0

TABLE 296-4 Five-year survival with respect to residual tumor size in stage III ovarian cancer

Tumor size, cm	Number of patients	Survival, percent: Two years	Survival, percent: Five years
0	31	80	63
0–1	84	70	41
1–2	46	49	15
3–6	144	28	8
7	309	16	3

SOURCE: *Smith and Day, 1979*

296-1). Well-differentiated tumors (lower histologic grades) have a better prognosis than do poorly differentiated tumors (higher histologic grades). The tumors with higher histologic grade are usually stages III and IV at presentation and respond poorly to radiation and/or chemotherapy.

The histologic cell type similarly appears to be an important prognostic factor (Fig. 296-1). Mucinous and endometrial tumors with good prognosis can be distinguished from those with moderately poor prognosis, such as serous tumors, and from those more-undifferentiated carcinomas with poor prognosis.

Biologic markers Alpha fetoprotein and human chorionic gonadotropin (hCG) are useful tumor markers in germ cell tumors but not in epithelial carcinoma of the ovary. Carcinoembryonic antigen is often detectable in patients with epithelial cell tumors who have ascites and/or liver involvement, but it does not fluctuate consistently with tumor burden. Using a monoclonal antibody (OC125), a mucin-like glycoprotein (CA125) can be detected in normal coelomic epithelium, in normal müllerian duct cells, and in serum in about 80 percent of patients with epithelial ovarian malignancies. CA125 is also present in serum from some patients with other adenocarcinomas, in some subjects with melanomas, and in some women who do not have carcinoma. The antigen level correlates with the extent of disease and fluctuates with therapy; it may be useful in quantitating tumor burden and documenting responses to therapy.

FIGURE 296-1 *Prognosis factors in carcinomas of the ovary. (From K. Sigurdsson et al. Reprinted with permission.)*

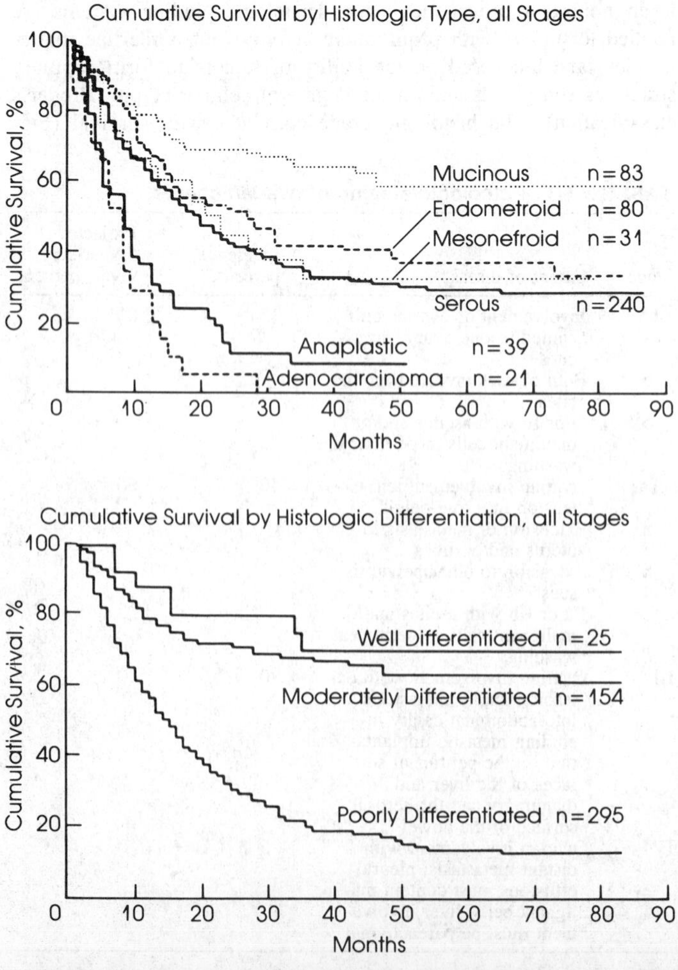

STAGING EVALUATION A standard schema for evaluating suspected ovarian cancer is outlined in Table 296-5. Noninvasive diagnostic studies are of limited usefulness in detecting minimal abdominal involvement but are helpful in designing the surgical procedure.

The usual approach to staging an ovarian mass is to proceed directly to surgery once the diagnosis is suspected (Table 296-5). Paracentesis preoperatively is contraindicated in patients with ascites and a pelvic mass unless there is concern that the patient is infected. Once an epithelial cancer is diagnosed, the surgery should include (1) bilateral salpingo-oophorectomy, (2) hysterectomy, (3) omentectomy, (4) inspection and biopsy of the liver, diaphragmatic surfaces, and peritoneal gutters, and (5) cytologic examination of abdominal fluid and washings. Attempts should be made to remove all residual disease. When patients with bulk disease present following a diagnostic procedure, an aggressive surgical procedure should be undertaken. When patients present following an incomplete staging procedure with no clinical evidence of residual or bulk disease, peritoneoscopy should be performed; if disease is present a second, more complete surgical procedure is indicated for complete staging and debulking.

THERAPEUTIC CONSIDERATIONS Stage I Stage I disease is adequately treated by a bilateral salpingo-oophorectomy and total abdominal hysterectomy done in the context of a staging procedure (Table 296-5). When the tumor is a borderline grade malignancy (approximately 25 percent of the stage I disease) and the patient is premenopausal and desires to have children, removal of the involved ovary and biopsy of the contralateral ovary may be adequate therapy. However, if the lesion is frankly malignant, if tumor involves both ovaries (Ib), or if ascites is present (Ic) a complete staging procedure should be performed. The prognosis for stage I disease treated with surgery alone may be as high as 90 percent for 5-year survival. Postoperative therapy has not been shown to be beneficial.

Stage II With a careful staging procedure less than 10 percent of epithelial tumors are stage II. Survival at 5 years may approach 60 percent. The standard approach is to treat stage II patients with postoperative radiation and/or chemotherapy. Clinical trials evaluating the benefits of postoperative therapy in stage II disease are ongoing.

Stages III and IV At least 70 percent of patients with ovarian carcinoma present with advanced disease. Multiagent chemotherapy may result in improved survival if the total measurable tumor mass is reduced to less than 2 cm in diameter prior to chemotherapy. Reduction of the tumor mass to a diameter between 0.5 and 1.5 cm may be associated with additional survival benefits. When the tumor

TABLE 296-5 Evaluation of epithelial ovarian carcinoma

A Staging evaluation:
- *1* History and physical examination
- *2* Ultrasound and/or computerized tomography of entire abdomen, including liver
- *3* Chest x-ray
- *4* Surgery
  - *a* Bilateral salpingo-oophorectomy
  - *b* Infracolic omentectomy, inspection of small bowel
  - *c* Periaortic node sampling
  - *d* Biopsy of liver, diaphragm, peritoneal gutters
  - *e* Peritoneal surface washing for cytologic examination

B Pathologic evaluation:
- *1* Review of all tissue and peritoneal fluid blocks by at least two independent observers
- *2* Determination of histologic type
- *3* Determination of histologic grade
- *4* Review by ovarian cancer referral center

bulk is reduced to microscopic disease, some patients may be cured. If a complete remission is not achieved, cytoreductive surgery may prolong survival but not alter the cure rate.

Chemotherapy in advanced ovarian cancer has improved the 5-year survival to between 20 and 30 percent and altered the natural history of the disease. It can palliate and probably cure some patients with advanced disease. The chemotherapeutic regimens induce approximately a 60 percent complete clinical response rate, and 30 percent of patients attain a pathologic complete remission. About 20 percent of tumors of stages III and IV, typically histologic grade IV, do not respond. The most effective drugs are cisplatin, doxorubicin, alkylating agents (cyclophosphamide, melphalan, and chlorambucil), and hexamethylmelamine. Cisplatin-containing multiagent regimens appear to be most effective, but an ideal drug regimen has not yet been developed (Table 296-6). Thus, patients with stages III and IV disease should be entered into cooperative group clinical trails.

To achieve complete remissions in patients with residual disease following cytoreductive surgery and chemotherapy, many modes of therapy have been evaluated. Radiation therapy can reduce mass disease in stages III and IV patients and has a role in the treatment of advanced disease. Furthermore, radiation therapy following cytoreductive surgery and multiagent chemotherapy may increase the remission rate in patients with bulk residual disease but has not improved survival or cure rates. Intraperitoneal administration of chemotherapeutic or radioactive agents requires further evaluation. Selection of appropriate chemotherapeutic agents in an assay utilizing cloned tumor cells can aid in the management of a fraction (10 percent) of patients who fail conventional treatment.

STROMAL TUMORS

Stromal tumors constitute only a tenth of ovarian malignancies but account for most of the hormone-secreting tumors. The majority have either masculinizing or feminizing effects, and the severity of the clinical syndrome is dependent in part on the patient's age (see Chaps. 46 and 331). Tumors that secrete hormones have a better prognosis because the tumors are relatively well-differentiated and because of the earlier clinical awareness that is associated with the hormonal effects. Feminizing tumors of the granulosa-theca-cell variety are readily detected in prepubescent children because of the resultant precocious puberty, with breast development and uterine bleeding, and in postmenopausal women as a result of dysfunctional uterine bleeding. However, in the reproductive years these tumors are usually insidious since menstrual irregularities are often disregarded. Androgen-secreting tumors, which include arrhenoblastoma, lipoid and hilar cell tumors, adrenal-rest tumors, and gynandroblastomas, are more readily diagnosed because of the hirsutism and virilization (see Chap. 46). The endocrine syndromes may be caused by secretions of a steroid hormone that acts directly as an estrogen or an androgen (e.g., estradiol synthesis by granulosa cell tumors, testosterone synthesis by arrhenoblastomas), by secretion of a hormone that must be converted peripherally to active androgens or estrogens (e.g., androstenedione by thecomas), or by secretion of a peptide hormone that induces the synthesis of steroid hormones by uninvolved ovarian tissue (e.g., hCG by germ cell tumors).

As a result of the endocrine abnormalities, stromal tumors are detected at earlier stages than are epithelial tumors. Prospective clinical studies on the response to therapy are not available, but the prognosis for a given tumor stage appears to be no different than that of epithelial tumors (Table 296-3). When stromal tumors are confined to one ovary in reproductive or prepubescent women, a conservative approach is warranted. Removal of the involved ovary with a biopsy of the contralateral ovary may be adequate and will maintain ovarian and reproductive function without jeopardizing survival. Since chemotherapy and radiation therapy have no significant benefit in these tumors, extensive disease and late recurrences are often managed by surgical debulking.

GERM CELL TUMORS

Germ cell tumors comprise less than 5 percent of ovarian malignancies, occur in young women, and have a higher incidence in blacks than in whites. They are usually unilateral with metastases to regional lymph nodes, hematogenous spread to the lungs, and direct extension to other pelvic organs. Peritoneal implantation and ascites are rare. Tumors that contain yolk sac epithelium produce alpha fetoprotein, and those with syncytiotrophoblasts produce hCG. These tumor markers make it possible to monitor the disease status and response to therapy. High levels of hCG are associated with feminizing syndromes and with hyperthyroidism because of structural similarities of the hCG alpha chain with alpha chains of follicle-stimulating hormone and thyroid-stimulating hormone (see Chap. 303). Hyperthyroidism also occurs in struma ovarii which are derived from specialized thyroid tissue within teratomas. Struma carcinoid tumors can arise from argentaffin tissue in teratomas, although carcinoid syndrome is more frequently associated with metatasis to the ovary from a primary intestinal tumor than from strumal carcinoid. Pure choriocarcinoma of the ovary is rare and is due to a primary ovarian gestation, to metastasis from a choriocarcinoma of the uterus, or to direct germ cell derivation. Most commonly, elements of choriocarcinoma are observed as a component of a mixed germ cell tumor.

When germ cell tumors are clinically stage I, surgical removal of the involved ovary, biopsy of the contralateral ovary, and a limited node dissection should be performed. However, these tumors tend to be disseminated at presentation. They are responsive to multiagent chemotherapy and poorly controlled by surgery and radiation therapy. Mot patients with disseminated germ cell tumors have been treated primarily with vincristine, actinomycin D, and cyclophosphamide. However, cisplatin-containing chemotherapeutic regimens that are effective in testicular cancer appear to be similarly effective in ovarian germ cell tumors (see Chap. 297).

REFERENCES

BAST RC et al: A radioimmunoassay using a monoclonal antibody to monitor the course of epithelial ovarian cancer. N Engl J Med 309:883, 1983

BEREK JS et al: Survival of patients following secondary cytoreductive surgery in ovarian cancer. Obstet Gynecol 61:189, 1983

DECKER DG: Mayo Clinic experience with epithelial ovarian cancer. Clin Obstet Gynecol 10:337, 1981

DEMBO AJ: Radiation therapy in the management of ovarian cancer. Clin Obstet Gynecol 10:261, 1983

TABLE 296-6 Responses to combination chemotherapy in advanced ovarian carcinoma

Regimen*	Investigators	No. of patients	Overall responses, percent	Complete responses, percent	Pathologic complete responses, percent
Hexa-CAF	Young, 1978	40	75	—	33
H-CAP	Greco, 1981	46	96	76	30
CHAD	Vogl, 1983	26	92	42	22
PAC	Ehrlich, 1983	56	79	41	18
CHEX-UP	Young, 1984	51	75	41	20

* *Hexa-CAF: altretamine, cyclophosphamide, methotrexate, 5-fluorouracil; H-CAP: altretamine, cyclophosphamide, doxorubicin, cisplatin; CHAD: cyclophosphamide, altretamine, doxorubicin, cisplatin; PAC: cisplatin, doxorubicin, cyclophosphamide; CHEX-UP: cyclophosphamide, altretamine, 5-fluorouracil, cisplatin.*

FUKS A et al: The multimodal approach to the treatment of stage IV ovarian cancer. Int J Radiat Oncol Biol Phys 8:903, 1982
GRIFFITHS CT et al: Role of cytoreductive surgical treatment in the management of advanced ovarian cancer. Cancer Treat Rep 63:235, 1979
HACKER NF et al: Primary cytoreductive surgery for epithelial ovarian cancer. Obstet Gynecol 61:413, 1983
LONGO DL, YOUNG RC: The natural history and treatment of ovarian cancer. Ann Rev Med 32:475, 1981
KATZ ME et al: Epithelial carcinoma of the ovary: Current strategies. Ann Intern Med 95:98, 1981
OZOLS RF et al: Advanced ovarian cancer—correlation of histologic grade with response to therapy. Cancer 45:572, 1980
——— et al: Phase I and pharmacologic studies of adriamycin administered intraperitoneally to patients with ovarian cancer. Cancer Res 42:4265, 1983
SIGURDSSON K et al: Prognostic factors in malignant epithelial tumors. Gynecol Oncol 15:370, 1983
SMITH JP, DAY TG: Review of ovarian cancer at The University of Texas System Cancer Center, M.D. Anderson Hospital and Tumor Institute. Am J Obstet Gynecol 135:984, 1979
SORBE B et al: Importance of histologic grading in the prognosis of epithelial ovarian carcinoma. Obstet Gynecol 59:576, 1982
WHARTON JT, HENSON J: Surgery for common epithelial tumors of the ovary. Cancer 48:582, 1981
YOUNG RC: Ovarian carcinoma. Semin Oncol 9:209, 1984
——— et al: Staging laparotomy in early ovarian cancer. JAMA 250:3072, 1983
——— et al: Cancer of the ovary, in *Cancer Principles and Practice of Oncology*, VT DeVita, Jr. et al (eds). Philadelphia, Lippincott, 1985, pp 1083–1117

297 TESTICULAR CANCER

MARC B. GARNICK

Carcinoma of the testis is a disease that serves as a model of a curable, solid neoplasm. Patients with localized forms of germinal cell cancer have a high cure rate when treated either with surgery or radiation therapy, and the advanced, metastatic forms, which in the past were almost universally fatal, are now also potentially curable. In 1977 testicular cancer was the third leading cause of cancer death in men between the ages of 15 and 34, but by 1981 the disease was no longer among the top five causes of cancer death in the same age group. The multidisciplinary principles and strategies that evolved for the management of patients with advanced testicular cancer are now being applied to other cancers.

Approximately 5000 new cases are diagnosed annually. The incidence in blacks is substantially lower than in whites. There is a peak frequency in early childhood and a larger peak incidence between 20 and 35 years. The disease is uncommon after age 40. A lesion suggestive of testicular neoplasm in a patient over the age of 50 should suggest a lymphoma rather than primary germinal cell carcinoma. This is especially true if there is bilateral involvement of the testes.

Several factors are known to predispose to development of testicular tumor. Men with a history of cryptorchid (undescended) testes have a several-fold increased risk, intraabdominal testes being more at risk than high inguinal testes. Both the cryptorchid testis itself and the contralateral normally descended testis are at risk, suggesting that some underlying testicular defect may predispose both to maldescent and to tumor development. Although the effectiveness of orchiopexy in reducing risk is not established, it is generally agreed that a high inguinal testis should be brought into the scrotum so that it can be followed carefully. Abdominal testes that cannot be treated in this manner should probably be removed. Other predisposing factors include a prior history of mumps orchitis, inguinal hernia in childhood, and a history of prior testicular cancer in the contralateral testis. In the majority of cases no predisposing factor can be identified.

CLINICAL FEATURES AND DIAGNOSIS The manifestations of testicular cancer range from an asymptomatic nodule or swelling detected while performing testicular self-examination to dyspnea secondary to massive pulmonary metastases. Most testicular cancers are diagnosed because of symptoms related to the testes, but significant delay in making a diagnosis is common and is the result of oversight by physicians and by patients. Most testicular cancers occur in men under age 40, and the public should be educated to the need to seek prompt medical advice for any change in previously normal testes, including the presence of a mass, a feeling of heaviness, pain, swelling, or any other unusual findings. Other causes of testicular masses include hydrocele, epididymitis, spermatocele, and orchitis, but to reduce delay in reaching a diagnosis, physicians should consider any testicular mass to be malignant until proven otherwise. Testicular pain occurs in many men with testicular neoplasms (for example, due to associated torsion or epididymitis) and hence does not rule out cancer.

Back or abdominal pain secondary to retroperitoneal adenopathy, weight loss, dyspnea secondary to pulmonary metastases, gynecomastia, supraclavicular lymphadenopathy, and urinary obstruction may also be present at diagnosis.

A testicular ultrasound can aid in establishing the presence of a testicular parenchymal abnormality. Once the diagnosis of a testicular neoplasm in suspected, a blood sample should be set aside, prior to orchiectomy, for subsequent determination of the tumor marker glycoproteins, alpha fetoprotein (AFP) and human chorionic gonadotropin (hCG). The correct operative approach is a high radical inguinal orchiectomy. A transscrotal biopsy of the testis or a transscrotal orchiectomy should never be performed if the diagnosis of testicular cancer is likely. Because the lymphatic drainage of the testis (to the retroperitoneal lymphatics between L1 and L3) differs from that of the scrotum (to superficial and deep inguinal groin nodes), a scrotal incision in the presence of a testicular cancer may predispose to the development of local recurrences and metastases to the inguinal lymphatics. This rarely, if ever, happens if a radical, high inguinal orchiectomy is performed.

CLASSIFICATION AND PATHOLOGY The most widely used classification of testicular tumors is that of Mostofi and is based on the cell type from which the tumor is derived, namely germinal or stromal (Leydig and Sertoli) cells (Table 297-1). Germinal cell tumors, the most common of these tumors and the focus of this chapter, can be subdivided into seminomas and nonseminomas. Seminomas are characterized by large cells with clear cytoplasm in a delicate fibrovascular stroma infiltrated with lymphocytes. Indeed, the granulomatous reaction around the tumor can be so intense as to suggest a graft-versus-host reaction. These tumors account for about half of all testicular neoplasms and can be divided into typical, spermatocytic, and anaplastic varieties. Germinal cell tumors of the nonseminoma type can be divided into embryonal cell tumors (yolk sac tumors), teratomas, and choriocarcinomas. Embryonal carcinomas are common in children and resemble embryonal carcinomas of the ovary. Choriocarcinomas contain syncytiotrophoblastic cells. Teratomas contain at least two types of germinal cell layers and in childhood are second in frequency to embryonal tumor. Mixed tumors that contain combinations of germinal cell types account for 40 percent of germinal

TABLE 297-1 Classification of testicular tumors

I Germinal cell tumors (95%)
- *A* Single cell tumors
  - *1* Seminomas
  - *2* Nonseminomas
    - *a* Embryonal cell tumors (yolk sac tumors)
    - *b* Teratomas
    - *c* Choriocarcinomas
- *B* Combination tumors

II Tumors of gonadal stroma (1–2%)
- *A* Leydig cell
- *B* Sertoli cell
- *C* Primitive gonadal structures

III Gonadoblastoma: germinal cell + stomal cell

SOURCE: *After FK Mostofi, Cancer 45:1735, 1980.*

cell tumors; the biology of such tumors is usually determined by the least differentiated (most malignant) elements. All four types of germinal cell tumors can also originate in extragonadal sites, most commonly the mediastinum or brain. Such extragonadal tumors are presumed to arise either from aberrant migration of germinal cells during embryogenesis or, alternatively, from some common precursor stem cell line that gives rise to the germinal cells, the thymus, and the pineal.

From the clinical standpoint, the critical distinction is between *seminomas* and *nonseminomas*, based upon the histopathology of the orchiectomy specimen. The former must be in pure form; the latter may either be a mixed cancer with both seminomatous and nonseminomatous components or a pure form of a nonseminoma, such as embryonal cell carcinoma, teratoma, or choriocarcinoma. The term *teratocarcinoma* generally refers to a mixed nonseminomatous cancer consisting of teratoma and embryonal cell cancer.

The distinction between seminoma and nonseminoma is important because the staging evaluation and subsequent management in the two differ as a consequence of the relative radioresponsiveness of seminomas compared to the radioresistance of nonseminomas. Radiation therapy to the lymphatics of the abdomen and/or chest is the mainstay of therapy in patients with pure seminoma but is rarely utilized in patients with nonseminoma. In addition, seminomas usually spread via the regional lymphatics to the retroperitoneal nodes of the abdomen and/or to the mediastinal and supraclavicular lymph nodes before gaining access to other visceral structures. Pulmonary and other hematogenous metastases are more common in patients with nonseminomas than in patients with seminomas. In advanced disease patients with nonseminoma may have pulmonary, hepatic, central nervous system, and, rarely, osseous metastases during the course in addition to lymphatic metastases in the retroperitoneum.

BIOLOGIC TUMOR MARKERS Germinal cell cancers of the testis often secrete biologic tumor markers that can be detected in the peripheral blood (see Chap. 303). Following orchiectomy, the presence of such markers in blood reflects the presence of metastatic disease. Such assays can also be valuable in monitoring therapy (marker levels fall with disease regression and increase with disease progression), and elevated levels in blood may predate the detection of new clinical or radiologic metastatic disease by weeks to months. The two most common markers are AFP and hCG. AFP is commonly secreted by embryonal cell cancer: its biologic half-life is approximately 6 days. AFP is not produced by pure seminoma, and its detection implies the presence of nonseminomatous elements, either in the primary lesion itself or in the metastatic site, even when the primary orchiectomy specimen is thought to be a pure seminoma. hCG is secreted by syncytiotrophoblastic giant cells present most commonly in choriocarcinomas; such giant cells may be present in embryonal cell components and occasionally in so-called pure seminomas. The biologic half-life of hCG is approximately 24 h. hCG may be biologically active, and hCG-enhanced secretion of estrogen by the testis is the cause of gynecomastia in such patients (see Chap. 332).

Clinicopathologic correlations can be drawn from immunohistochemical staining of primary testis cancers for AFP and hCG. Pure seminomas usually stain negatively for both AFP and hCG. Approximately 5 percent of pure seminomas may stain positively for hCG, helping to explain the clinical situation of a patient with a pure seminoma and an elevated hCG value. These patients often have syncytiotrophoblastic giant cells within the primary lesion. Nonseminomatous components, such as embryonal cell carcinoma, stain for AFP, and choriocarcinomas stain positively for hCG. Teratomas usually stain for neither AFP nor hCG.

STAGING EVALUATION The function of staging is to determine whether or not the cancer is localized to the testis or to regional lymphatics or is widely disseminated. Such information is necessary to determine if disease is amenable to local or regional therapy. If the disease is disseminated at presentation, the initial staging evaluation serves as a baseline in assessing subsequent response. Since the approach to staging and management is dictated by the pathologic diagnosis of the orchiectomy specimen, the appropriate evaluation will be outlined for each.

Pure seminoma The routine workup involves careful physical examination, an abdominal-pelvic computerized tomographic (CT) scan to determine the presence of retroperitoneal adenopathy or visceral involvement, a chest x-ray with or without lung tomography, measurement of routine chemistries, and assessment of the biologic markers (AFP and hCG). In most cases, the biologic markers are undetectable. If AFP is elevated, the patient should be treated as having a nonseminoma, even though the pathologic interpretation is pure seminoma.

The portals for radiation therapy for pure seminomas were traditionally determined on the basis of bipedal lymphangiography. However, the necessity of lymphangiography for such purposes is less imperative today because computerized tomographic scanning may provide similar information.

If plasma hCG is elevated in a patient with a diagnosis of pure seminoma, a search should be made for syncytiotrophoblastic giant cells. Otherwise, there may be some uncertainty of whether occult foci of nonseminomatous components are responsible for the hCG production. Also, if the physical or radiographic examinations fail to reveal any evidence of metastatic disease and the hCG is elevated before orchiectomy, it is necessary to follow the level of hCG sequentially. If the marker does not decline as predicted by its biologic half-life, the presence of occult metastatic cancer should be considered.

Nonseminoma The staging evaluation outlined for the seminoma is employed for the patient with a nonseminomatous germinal cell tumor of the testis. On the basis of these noninvasive staging studies, patients can be categorized as having stage I, early stage II, advanced stage II, or stage III disease. Patients with stage I disease have no clinical, radiographic, or marker evidence of tumor presence beyond the confines of the testis. Patients with early stage II have nonpalpable, small, retroperitoneal adenopathy on computerized tomographic scans, usually measuring <4 to 5 cm. Advanced stage II is defined as retroperitoneal lymphadenopathy measuring >5 cm on CT scan or palpable retroperitoneal adenopathy with disease limited to lymphatics below the diaphragm. Stage III disease includes visceral involvement below the diaphragm (e.g., liver or bowel) or above the diaphragm (e.g., lung or supraclavicular lymphadenopathy). Furthermore, patients with stage III disease can be further subdivided according to anatomic location of disease and disease bulk. Stage III disease of "minimal" to "moderate" risk involves supraclavicular lymphadenopathy (stage IIIA), gynecomastia $\pm$ elevated biologic markers (IIIB1), or more than five pulmonary lesions, none of which is >2 cm in greatest diameter (IIIB2). More advanced forms of stage III disease include pulmonary involvement with mediastinal or hilar lesions, positive pleural effusion or pulmonary metastases greater than 2 cm, palpable abdominal mass, ureteral displacement or hydronephrosis (IIIB4), and hepatic, gastrointestinal, central nervous system, bone, or vena caval involvement (IIIB5).

Conceptually, patients with testicular cancer can be categorized pathologically as having either *seminoma* or *nonseminoma* and staged as having either "early" or "advanced" disease. Patients with *early* disease would be considered to have stage I and early stage II disease, while patients with *advanced* disease have advanced stage II or any form of stage III disease. This formulation allows rational decision making for nearly all categories of disease.

TREATMENT MODALITIES ACCORDING TO HISTOLOGY AND STAGE (Table 297-2) **Early seminoma** These patients have either a normal abdominal CT scan or retroperitoneal lymphadenopathy measuring less than 5 cm in greatest diameter. Most such patients are treated with abdominal radiotherapy, delivering 30 Gy (3000 rad) to the subdiaphragmatic lymph nodes and ipsilateral groin and a 6-Gy (600-rad) boost in areas of known disease. Although prophylactic medias-

TABLE 297-2 Testicular cancer: General approach to management*

	Seminoma	Nonseminoma
Stage I	XRT	RPLND or orchiectomy alone/observation
Early stage II	XRT	RPLND ± Chemo[a] or Chemo[a]
Advanced stage II Stage III	Chemo[a]	Chemo[a] ± TRS ± Chemo[b]

* *XRT = radiation therapy, delivered to subdiaphragmatic lymphatics [30 Gy (3000 rad)]; RPLND = retroperitoneal lymph node dissection; chemo[a] = combination chemotherapy (see Table 297-3); TRS = tumor-reductive surgery; chemo[b] = additional chemotherapy given if surgical specimen reveals viable cancer.*

tinal and supraclavicular radiation therapy was used in the past, this practice is generally not employed today. When treated with radiation following orchiectomy, patients with clinical stage I have a 95 to 97 percent cure rate, and patients with early stage II disease have an 85 to 90 percent survival rate.

Advanced seminoma In the past, patients with large retroperitoneal masses or mediastinal involvement were often treated with radiation therapy to fields including the subdiaphragmatic lymph nodes, whole abdomen, mediastinum, and supraclavicular nodes; however, survival rates were only 40 to 70 percent. If these patients subsequently suffered a relapse in an area outside the radiation therapy field, the ability to administer myelosuppressive combination chemotherapy was diminished and was associated with drug-related morbidity. Today, most patients with advanced forms of seminoma are treated initially with combination chemotherapy that includes cisplatin. Substantial tumor shrinkage occurs in the majority of patients. However, the proper management for partially regressed retroperitoneal masses following chemotherapy is controversial. Some patients are treated with postchemotherapy radiation to areas of bulk disease, and, in rare instances, debulking of residual tumor masses is undertaken. However, residual masses following chemotherapy may continue to shrink after therapy is discontinued. Nonetheless, one treatment strategy allows for cisplatin-combination chemotherapy to be given over a span of 12 to 14 weeks. Patients are then restaged; decisions regarding further chemotherapy, radiation therapy, or surgery are then made.

Stage I nonseminoma Patients with stage I nonseminoma are routinely treated with a retroperitoneal lymph node dissection (RPLND), using either a transabdominal or a thoracoabdominal approach. The rationale for this operation is based upon the inexact data generated from the noninvasive staging evaluation of the retroperitoneal lymphatics. The false-negative rate of abdominal CT scans in patients with clinical stage I is 35 to 50 percent., Thus, surgical removal of the retroperitoneal lymph nodes not only serves as therapy but also determines the need for possible additional therapy. If microscopic disease is detected and surgically removed, an 85 to 90 percent cure rate can be expected following RPLND.

Stage II nonseminoma The optimal management of patients with retroperitoneal lymphadenopathy measuring between 2 and 5 cm on the CT scan is controversial. While RPLND may be curative, a relapse rate of 30 to 45 percent can be expected. If relapse occurs after RPLND, combination chemotherapy can be administered, or chemotherapy may sometimes be given as an adjuvant to RPLND. Alternatively, combination chemotherapy can be given prior to RPLND. If complete resolution of disease is achieved following chemotherapy, RPLND would not be performed, obviating the need for the operation in this subset of patients.

Advanced stage (bulky stage II or stage III) nonseminoma Testicular cancer has been responsive to varying antineoplastic agents of differing mechanisms of action. The early encouraging results using chlorambucil, methotrexate, and actinomycin D were followed by the more successful programs of vinblastine and bleomycin. The introduction of cisplatin was associated with further improvement in both the response rate and duration of response of advanced testicular cancer. Cisplatin-containing programs are in nearly universal use today, either with vinblastine and bleomycin (PVB) or the combination of cisplatin with vinblastine, actinomycin D, bleomycin, and cyclophosphamide (VAB program) (Table 297-3). The use of these agents is associated with complete remission in as many as 80 to 85 percent of patients with advanced nonseminomatous germ cell cancer.

Following such therapy, patients are then restaged (with physical, radiographic, and biochemical examinations) to assess the response of areas which previously contained disease and to determine the need for additional therapy. Large abdominal masses may undergo astonishing regression. Pulmonary nodules often resolve completely, and biologic markers frequently return to normal after 12 weeks of such chemotherapy. If after chemotherapy, a residual abdominal or pulmonary mass persists in the setting of normal levels of plasma markers, surgical removal of the mass(es) should be undertaken. Table 297-4 outlines current recommendations. Preoperatively, it is difficult to determine the nature of such residual masses. Approximately 20 percent contain residual, viable cancer; 40 percent contain fibrosis, necrosis, or hemorrhage, and an additional 40 percent demonstrate the phenomenon of "teratomatous transformation." The latter is thought to result either from chemotherapy-induced differentiation of the primary mass into a teratoma or from the selective elimination of the more malignant elements of the mass but persistence of residual teratomatous components. If either fibrosis, hemorrhage, or teratoma is found following chemotherapy, additional postsurgical chemotherapy is usually not indicated. If, however, residual cancer is demonstrated, additional cisplatin combination chemotherapy is required.

If biologic markers are persistently positive following remission induction chemotherapy, additional chemotherapy is also indicated. "Tumor-reductive" surgery should not be attempted until biologic markers return to normal. Some patients experience complete resolution of physical, radiographic, and biochemical marker abnormalities

TABLE 297-3 Commonly used chemotherapy programs for advanced testicular cancer

PVB		
Vinblastine	0.15 mg/kg body weight per day	IV days 1, 2
Bleomycin	30 mg	IV days 1, 8, 15
Cisplatin	20 mg/m² surface area per day	IV days 1–5
Repeat cycles q 21 days × 4 cycles.		
VAB-6		
Cyclophosphamide	600 mg/m² surface area	IV day 1
Bleomycin	30 mg bolus	IV day 1, then
	20 mg/m² surface area/day	IV* days 1–3†
Actinomycin D	1 mg/m² surface area	IV day 1
Vinblastine	4 mg/m² surface area	IV day 1
Cisplatin	120 mg/m² surface area	IV day 4
Repeat cycles 21–28 days × 3–5 cycles.		

* *Continuous intravenous infusion.*
† *Bleomycin omitted after cycle 2.*

TABLE 297-4 Advanced testicular cancer, nonseminoma: Approach to management after initial chemotherapy

Biologic "markers"*	Radiographic abnormalities	Therapeutic choice
Positive	Present or absent	Additional chemotherapy†
Normal	Present	TRS‡ ± chemotherapy§
Normal	Absent	Observation

* *Alpha fetoprotein and human chorionic gonadotropin.*
† *Chemotherapy with a "second-line" program, with attempts to "normalize" biologic markers.*
‡ *Tumor-reductive surgery.*
§ *Additional chemotherapy determined by presence of "viable" cancer in surgical specimen. Chemotherapy withheld if surgical specimen contains only fibrosis or teratoma.*

after cisplatin-containing chemotherapy and may require no additional chemotherapy or surgery following their program of chemotherapy.

All patients with testicular cancer, regardless of pathology or stage, require meticulous follow-up with monthly physical exams, chest x-rays, and assessment of markers for 18 to 24 months. The frequency of these tests can be decreased in the third or fourth year following diagnosis. The goal is to detect relapse when the tumor burden is minimal. Most relapses from testicular cancer occur within the first 2 years following diagnosis, but late relapses do occur.

Approximately 85 percent of patients with advanced nonseminomatous testicular cancer have a complete remission and are potentially cured (Fig. 297-1), and the relapse rate from a complete remission status is low. However, certain subsets of patients with "high-risk" forms of advanced disease have a lower complete remission, a low cure rate, and a high relapse rate. Such patients require different treatment strategies. These include patients with extragonadal presentations (e.g., with extensive nonseminomatous germinal cell cancer in the anterior mediastinum or brain, but with normal testes), or patients with high levels of biologic markers in serum, such as high hCG titers (usually >5000 mIU/mL). Alterations in the duration of therapy and doses of chemotherapy are being tested in hopes of improving treatment results in this "high-risk" population.

Testicular cancer which is refractory to PVB or VAB-6 programs may sometimes respond to the addition of the epipodophyllotoxin derivative, etoposide. The combination of cisplatin with etoposide will cause a second remission, which may be durable, in approximately 25 to 30 percent of patients.

SIDE EFFECTS OF THERAPY **Radiation therapy and surgery** Infertility can result both from radiation therapy and RPLND. Because these modalities are generally reserved for the management of early stage patients, a full discussion with patients about the potential loss of fertility is appropriate. Although of questionable benefit, the possiblity of sperm banking should be considered prior to the initiation of either definitive radiation therapy for early stage seminomas or RPLND for early stage nonseminomas. Modifications in the surgical technique of RPLND (limited dissection) may decrease the incidence of fertility loss and ejaculatory disturbances.

Combination chemotherapy When standard cisplatin-vinblastine-bleomycin programs are employed, the major side effects are myelosuppression, potential for nephrotoxicity, nausea and vomiting, weight loss, anemia, ileus, pulmonary toxicity, ototoxicity, peripheral neuropathy, Raynaud's phenomenon, alopecia, hypomagnesemia, and stomatitis. Infertility is usual during therapy, although fertility may return years after completion of therapy. The use of the chemotherapy programs requires skill on the part of the treating physician and should not be attempted by the occasional user. With proper expertise these side effects can often be minimized.

Bleomycin is known to cause pulmonary toxicity (see Chap. 203), and special precautions must be taken in patients who have received bleomycin and are scheduled for a surgical procedure. The acute respiratory distress syndrome has occurred in some and is thought to be related to excessive fluid overload and high inspired oxygen concentration (FIO_2) during the operative procedure. Current recommendations now call for the FIO_2 to be maintained at ≤24 percent and for patients to be kept in a hypovolemic or euvolemic state in the perioperative period. Such measures seem to minimize the postoperative pulmonary complications.

ORCHIECTOMY ALONE FOR CLINICAL STAGE I DISEASE Because combination chemotherapy with or without tumor-reductive surgery can cure 80 to 85 percent of patients with advanced disease, the possibility of orchiectomy alone for stage I patients has gained support. Treatment with chemotherapy (or radiation therapy) is instituted if relapse occurs. Such an approach prevents RPLND or radiation therapy from being performed in the 60 to 70 percent of patients who have negative nodes and are already cured by the orchiectomy. Patients who do relapse can nearly always be treated successfully with chemotherapy at the time of first relapse, assuming patient compliance. However, patients selected for an orchiectomy-only policy must satisfy strict criteria relating to the clinical stage of disease, pathologic interpretation of the primary lesion, and willingness to undergo meticulous follow-up.

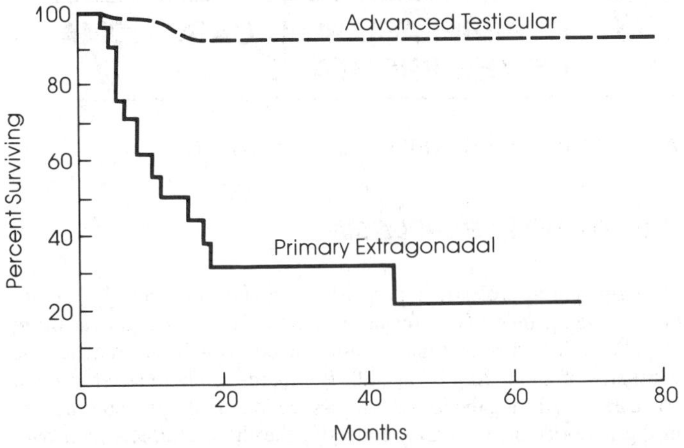

FIGURE 297-1 *Survival curves of patients with advanced primary testicular nonseminoma and extragonadal germinal cell cancer treated at the Dana Farber Institute and Brigham and Women's Hospital, Boston. Relapses are unusual in the primary testicular patients after 2 years following diagnosis. In contrast, extragonadal patients have a lower survival rate, and many continue to relapse years after the original diagnosis. (Adapted from MB Garnick et al, JAMA 250:1733, 1983.)*

THE EXTRAGONADAL GERMINAL CELL SYNDROME Patients with extragonadal germinal cell tumors may present with a large anterior mediastinal mass, central nervous system abnormalities, or retroperitoneal disease. The response to therapy is generally lower when compared to primary testicular cancer, justifying the need for more intensive therapy. However, a proportion of these patients may be cured when treated with chemotherapy and tumor-reductive surgery. In addition, patients with "undifferentiated" cancer of the mediastinum or retroperitoneum may have an unrecognized form of extragonadal germinal cell cancer. Biologic markers and immunohistochemical staining of the biopsy material for AFP or hCG may provide useful clues. If positive, these patients should be treated as if they have potentially curable advanced testicular cancer.

REFERENCES

BOSL GJ: Treatment of germ cell tumors at Memorial Sloan-Kettering Cancer Center: 1960 to present, in *Genitourinary Cancer: Contemporary Issues in Clinical Oncology*, vol 5, MB Garnick (ed). New York, Churchill Livingstone, 1985

EINHORN EH (ed): *Testicular Tumors: Management and Treatment*. New York, Masson, 1980

———, DONOHUE JP: Cis-diamminedichloroplatinum, vinblastine, and bleomycin combination chemotherapy in disseminated testicular cancer. Ann Intern Med 87:293, 1977

GARNICK MB: Advanced testicular cancer: Treatment choices in the "land of plenty" (editorial). J Clin Oncol 3:294, 1985

——— et al: The treatment and surgical staging of testicular and primary extragonadal germ cell cancer. JAMA 250:1733, 1983

HAINSWORTH JD et al: Advanced extragonadal germ-cell tumors. Ann Intern Med 97:7, 1982

———, GRECO FA: Testicular germ cell neoplasms. Am J Med 75:817, 1983

LOEHRER PJ, EINHORN LH: Management of testicular cancer, in *Harrison's Principles of Internal Medicine Update VI*, RG Petersdorf et al (eds). New York, McGraw-Hill, 1985

PECKHAM MJ et al: Orchiectomy alone for stage I testicular nonseminoma. Br J Urol 55:754, 1983

POTTERN LM et al: Testicular cancer risk among young men: Role of cryptorchidism and inguinal hernia. J Natl Cancer Inst 74:377, 1985

298 HYPERPLASIA AND CARCINOMA OF THE PROSTATE

ARTHUR I. SAGALOWSKY / JEAN D. WILSON

PROSTATIC HYPERPLASIA

Development of prostatic hyperplasia is an almost universal phenomenon in aging men. The prostate weighs only a few grams at birth; at puberty it undergoes androgen-mediated growth and reaches the adult size of about 20 g by age 20. It remains stable in size for about 25 years, and during the fifth decade a second growth spurt commences in the majority of men. Consequently, the disease affects men over the age of 45 and increases in frequency with age so that by the eighth decade more than 90 percent of men have prostatic hyperplasia at autopsy. Because of refinements in prostatic surgery, the disorder is not a major cause of death, but it is a leading cause of morbidity in elderly men. The prostate surrounds the urethra, and any enlargement is a potential cause of urinary tract obstruction; indeed, prostatic hyperplasia is the most common cause of obstruction to urinary outflow in men. Overall, about 10 percent of men at some time require prostatic surgery to relieve urinary tract obstructions. The disorder occurs in all populations but is less common in the orient. The mean age for development of symptomatic disease is about 65 years for whites and about 60 years for blacks. It is probable that prostatic hyperplasia does not predispose to the development of prostatic cancer.

PATHOGENESIS Unlike the pubertal growth spurt which involves the gland diffusely, prostatic hyperplasia begins in the periurethral region as a localized proliferation and progresses to compress the remaining normal gland. Histologically, the hyperplastic tissue is nodular and composed of varying amounts of glandular epithelium, stroma, and smooth-muscle elements. The hyperplastic process can compress and obstruct the urethra; rarely, the hyperplastic gland grows posteriorly to obstruct the rectum and cause constipation.

The pathogenesis is not well-understood, but two necessary features for the process are aging and the presence of testes; whether the testes play a direct or permissive role is not known, but the active androgen that mediates prostatic growth at all ages is dihydrotestosterone, which is formed within the prostate from plasma testosterone (see Chap. 330). In the castrated dog, hormonal therapy that increases dihydrotestosterone levels in the prostate causes prostatic enlargement comparable to that seen in spontaneous canine prostatic hyperplasia. Estradiol levels in men increase with age (absolutely or relative to testosterone levels), and in dogs estrogen acts synergistically with dihydrotestosterone to induce prostatic growth by enhancing the amount of androgen receptor protein in the tissue. Consequently, the role of aging in the development of prostatic hyperplasia in men would be explained if dihydrotestosterone is the mediator of the hyperplasia and if estradiol augments dihydrotestosterone action.

DIAGNOSIS Urethral obstruction results from the elongation, tortuosity, and compression of the posterior urethra, but there is no straightforward relationship between obstruction and prostatic size; indeed, severe obstruction can occur when the hyperplasia does not exceed the size of the normal gland. Early symptoms can be minimal because compensatory hypertrophy of the detrusor musculature of the bladder is capable of compensating for the increased resistance to urine flow. With increasing obstruction, diminution in the caliber and force of the urinary stream, hesitancy in initiating voiding, postvoiding dribbling, the sensation of incomplete emptying, and on occasion, urinary retention supervene. These *obstructive* symptoms must be distinguished from *irritative* symptoms such as dysuria, frequency, and urgency that can result from inflammatory, infectious, or neoplastic causes. As the amount of residual urine increases, nocturia, overflow urinary incontinence, and a mass in the lower abdomen may develop. Eventually, the manifestations of chronic urinary retention and obstruction supervene, or acute urinary retention can be precipitated by infection, the ingestion of tranquilizing drugs, or alcohol. On occasion, significant obstruction can be compensated to the extent that symptoms are minimal or absent, and patients present with obstructive uropathy.

The prostate is palpated during digital rectal examination with attention to size, consistency, and shape. Hyperplasia commonly produces a smooth, firm, elastic enlargement, recognizing that obstruction can occur in the absence of abnormalities on rectal examination. Ultrasonography with a rectal probe allows a quantitative estimate of prostate size but ordinarily provides no information beyond that provided by rectal examination. An intravenous pyelogram with postvoiding film will document the degree of upper urinary tract obstruction and the extent of bladder emptying. To evaluate vesicle neck obstruction, cystourethroscopy is indicated. Measurement of urine flow rate and/or residual urine volume is recommended to document the degree of obstruction to outflow. More detailed urodynamic evaluation is occasionally required to rule out other causes of voiding dysfunction such as neurogenic bladder.

TREATMENT The treatment is surgical, and when surgery is indicated, transurethral prostatectomy is the usual procedure of choice. In the case of massive glands, open prostatectomy may be employed using either retropubic, suprapubic, or perineal approaches. Because the majority of men above age 60 have some degree of prostatic hyperplasia, the presence of the disorder is not an indication for treatment. Indications for surgery include decrease in urine flow of sufficient magnitude to cause men to seek relief, persistent residual urine, acute urinary retention due to obstruction with no reversible precipitating cause, and hydronephrosis. In men who lack definite indications for prostatectomy, it is advisable that they be examined periodically to determine the natural history of the process; many patients who receive no therapy experience no progression in symptoms over many years.

PROSTATIC CARCINOMA

Cancer of the prostate is the second most common malignancy in men and is the third most common cause of cancer death in men older than age 55 (after carcinomas of the lung and colon). In 1980 there were some 66,000 newly diagnosed cases and 21,500 deaths from the disorder in the United States. Only about a third of cases identified at autopsy are manifest clinically. The disease is rare before age 50, and the incidence increases with advancing age.

The frequency varies in different parts of the world. In terms of age-adjusted mortality rates, the United States has 14 deaths per 100,000 men per year compared to 22 for Sweden and 2 for Japan. However, Japanese immigrants to the United States develop prostatic cancer at a frequency similar to the rest of the men in this country, suggesting that an environmental factor is the principal cause for population differences. The disease is more common among black men than white men in the United States; the reason for this difference is not known.

CLASSIFICATION Some carcinomas of the prostate are slow-growing and may persist for long periods without causing significant symptoms, whereas others behave aggressively. It is not known whether tumors can become more malignant with time. Insight into the natural history of a given tumor is provided by careful histopathologic grading of the lesion combined with surgical evaluation of the pelvic lymph nodes.

Histologic grading Over 95 percent of prostatic cancers are adenocarcinomas that arise in the prostatic acini. Adenocarcinoma may begin anywhere in the prostate but has a predilection for the periphery. The tumors are frequently multifocal. Variability in cellular size, nuclear and nucleolar shape, glandular differentiation, and the content of acid phosphatase and mucin may occur within a single specimen, but the most poorly differentiated area of tumor (i.e., the area with the highest histologic grade) appears to determine its biologic behavior. In the Gleason grading scheme the dominant and any other glandular histologic patterns are independently assigned numbers from 1 to 5 (best- to least-differentiated), and these numbers are summed to give a total score of 2 to 10 for each tumor. Such grading is reproducible and correlates with the course of the disease and with patient survival.

The remainder of prostatic cancers are comprised of squamous-cell and transitional-cell carcinomas that arise in the prostatic ducts, carcinoma of the prostatic utricle (a müllerian duct remnant), carcinosarcomas that arise in the mesenchymal elements of the gland, and occasional metastic tumors (usually carcinoma of the lung, melanoma, or lymphoma). These tumors will not be considered further.

Surgical staging Adenocarcinoma of the prostate may spread by three routes: direct extension, the lymphatics, and the bloodstream. The prostatic capsule is a natural boundary against growth of tumor into adjacent structures, but direct extension occurs upward into the seminal vesicles and bladder floor. Lymphatic spread can best be assessed by surgical exploration; the frequency with which it occurs correlates with the size and the histologic grade of the tumor. Only about one-tenth of tumors with a grade of less than 5 have lymph node involvement, while more than 70 percent of tumors with a Gleason grade of 9 or 10 have coexisting lymphatic invasion at the time of diagnosis. The route of lymphatic spread (in decreasing order) is to obturator, internal iliac, common iliac, presacral, and paraaortic nodes. Hematogenous metastases occur to bone (pelvis > lumbar vertebrae > thoracic vertebrae > ribs) more frequently than to viscera (lung > liver > adrenal gland). Diffuse pulmonary involvement is infrequent.

The standard staging scheme is that of Whitmore. Stage A represents cancer not detectable by rectal examination but found in a surgical specimen obtained during operation for prostatic hyperplasia or at autopsy. Stage A is subdivided into two groups: stage A_1, in which well-differentiated tumor is present in only a few transurethral chips from one lobe; and stage A_2, in which involvement is more diffuse. Stage B disease is palpable but confined to the prostate. Stage B_1 disease is a single nodule involving only one lobe and surrounded by tissue that is normal to palpation; stage B_2 involves the gland more diffusely. In stage C, palpable tumor extends beyond the prostate, but there are no distant metastases. In stage D, metastatic disease is present. Stage D_1 refers to involvement of pelvic nodes only with no other metastases, whereas in the D_2 category metastatic disease is more widespread. Any of the lower stages (A, B, or C) may progress directly to stage D. Failure to include pelvic lymphadenectomy in the staging process results in marked underestimation of the frequency of lymph node metastases; for example, about one-fifth of tumors tentatively classified as A_2 solely on the basis of prostate pathology actually constitute stage D disease when appropriate surgical staging is performed. The frequency with which early hematogenous metastases are missed with the current staging procedures is uncertain.

DIAGNOSIS Symptoms and signs Both early and advanced carcinoma of the prostate may be asymptomatic at the time of diagnosis, and more than 80 percent of patients have stage C or D disease at the time of diagnosis. In symptomatic subjects common presenting complaints (in descending order) include dysuria, difficulty in voiding, increased urinary frequency, complete urinary retention, back or hip pain, and hematuria. A high index of suspicion should be entertained in all men over age 40 with dysuria, frequency, or difficulty in voiding in the absence of mechanical urethral obstruction.

Palpation of the prostate is the best predictor for the diagnosis of all stages of disease other than stage A. Indeed, the importance of the rectal examination in the routine physical examination of men cannot be stressed too strongly. The posterior surfaces of the lateral lobes, where carcinoma begins most often, are easily palpable on digital rectal examination. Carcinoma characteristically is hard, nodular, and irregular, but induration may be due to fibrous areas in benign prostatic hyperplasia, to focal infarcts, or to calculi as well as to tumor. The midline furrow between the lateral lobes may be obscured by either benign or malignant enlargement. Local extraprostatic extension of tumor into the seminal vesicles can also be detected by rectal exam. Scrotal and/or lower extremity lymphedema secondary to infiltration of pelvic lymph nodes are manifestations of extensive disease.

When a transrectal probe is used for pelvic sonography, carcinoma is manifested by asymmetric densities within the prostate. The procedure is not a sensitive means of establishing a diagnosis but is useful for documenting the degree of extension of the tumor into bladder and seminal vesicles. Computerized tomography (CT) of the prostate may also be helpful in defining the extent of tumor and locating nodes for aspiration needle biopsy.

Biopsy Biopsy of the prostate is essential for establishing the diagnosis and is indicated when a palpable abnormality is detected or when lower urinary tract symptoms occur in men who have no know cause of obstruction. Core-needle biopsy may be performed transperineally or transrectally with less risk of bacterial contamination with the former and more precise sampling with the latter. Fine-needle aspiration cytology offers immediate diagnosis with minimal patient discomfort and morbidity. Open perineal biopsy is performed infrequently because it carries risk of at least temporary impotence and is a more extensive surgical procedure. Transurethral biopsy is also used infrequently because most early lesions are in the peripheral regions of the gland.

Biochemical markers Several biochemical markers provide ancillary information in diagnosing prostatic cancer. Elevated serum acid phosphatase is present in some localized disease, more commonly with bony metastases. However, no technique of assay for the enzyme (including counterimmune electrophoresis and radioimmunoassay) is sufficiently specific or sensitive for use in screening, and the major application of the assay is in following the progress of the disease. Likewise, none of the other biochemical markers studied—bone marrow acid phosphatase, hydroxyproline, cholesterol, isoleucine, glycine, aspartic acid, glutamic acid, methionine, or spermidine—has sufficiently high specificity or sensitivity for routine screening.

Assessment of metastic disease Bony metastases from prostatic carcinoma usually contain both osteoblastic and osteolytic components. The bony pelvis and lumbar vertebrae are involved most often, and metastases also occur in thoracic vertebrae, ribs, skull, and long bones. Skeletal survey has a low sensitivity of detection because a significant portion of bone must be involved to permit detection on a routine x-ray. Bone scans using radionuclides such as technetium 99 are more sensitive, but the specificity is not high because positive scans may occur in any metabolically hyperactive bone; this includes sites of inflammation, healing fractures, osteoarthritis, and Paget's disease. Therefore, when a positive radionuclide scan is obtained during an initial survey for bone metastases, the presence of other lesions must be excluded by conventional radiography of the affected site. Radionuclide bone scans are also useful for monitoring progression and response to therapy.

Surgical staging is the common modality for assessing lymph node involvement and determining therapy. The procedure usually includes removal of the external iliac, internal iliac, and obturator lymph node chains and is either performed by itself or in conjunction with prostatic surgery or implantation of radioactive beads. In some centers the initial procedure is either lymphangiography or pelvic computerized tomography (CT) scan, followed when positive by confirmatory thin-needle biopsy of the affected lymph nodes. When the CT scan or the lymphangiogram is negative, however, operative staging is mandatory.

TREATMENT Surgery Total prostatoseminovesiculectomy is the oldest treatment for carcinoma of the prostate. Radical perineal prostatectomy allows an easier vesicourethral anastomosis and less bleeding, while radical retropubic prostatectomy affords access to the pelvic lymph nodes. In experienced hands both procedures have a low risk of urinary incontinence (~ 1 percent for radical perineal and 1 to 4 percent for radical retropubic prostatectomy). Formerly both operations caused impotence in most patients. Improvements in surgical technique for the retropubic procedure allow preservation of the neurovascular supply to the corpora cavernosa and preservation of potency in the majority of patients without compromising the thoroughness of the operation.

Radical prostatectomy is not indicated for stage A_1 cancer, since this disease is cured definitively by the simple prostatectomy at which the diagnosis is made. The role of radical prostatectomy in stage A_2 is unsettled. However, true stage A_2 disease in which pelvic nodes show no evidence of metastases may behave aggressively and be benefited by radical surgery, particularly when the neoplasm is anaplastic. Indeed, 5- and 10-year survivals equivalent to those of age-matched controls have been reported following such treatment for stage A_2 disease.

Radical prostatectomy has its clearest indication in stage B disease. Nearly all of the apparent surgical cures in this stage are in men who have 1- to 2-cm nodules involving only one lobe of the prostate (e.g., stage B_1), a group comprising only 5 percent of prostatic carcinoma patients. In addition, subjects with true stage B_2 disease may also be appropriate candidates for radical prostatectomy.

The effectiveness of radical prostatectomy for stage C disease is less certain. Morbidity rates from local pelvic symptoms, bladder outlet obstruction, hematuria, and ureteral obstruction may be decreased by radical prostatectomy in stage C disease, but controlled studies comparing morbidity rates after surgery with those following other therapies are lacking. Radical prostatectomy has no place in the treatment of stage D disease, and lymph node removal has no therapeutic benefit. Therefore, other means of therapy should be tried.

Radiation Radiation therapy was developed as a primary treatment in prostatic carcinoma because of a desire to avoid the impotence and occasional incontinence that followed radical prostatectomy. In most series, approximately 60 to 70 Gy (6000 to 7000 rad) are administered to the prostate over 6 weeks by a variety of delivery patterns. Radiation to the pelvic nodes may or may not be performed. Acute proctitis and urethritis are common side effects but are usually controllable by local measures and adjustments in radiation therapy. Chronic complications after full courses of external beam radiation include impotence in 30 to 60 percent; chronic proctitis in 10 to 15 percent; and occasional rectal stricture, rectal fistula, or rectal bleeding. It is not clear whether external beam radiation actually eradicates prostatic carcinoma, because many patients in whom progression of the tumor is slowed or halted have persistent tumor on rebiopsy, and the biologic potential of these persistent tumors is not clear.

The largest series on external beam radiation for prostatic cancer is that of Bagshaw; a variety of delivery techniques and doses were utilized in nearly 1300 patients, many of whom had received prior hormone manipulation. There was about 50 percent 10-year survival in stages A and B and a mean 10-year survival of 30 percent in stage C. The 5-year survival in stage D patients who received radiation to the pelvis as well was 58 percent. Several smaller studies have reported responses that in the aggregate are similar. The best results are obtained when the tumors are less than 2 cm in size at the time of therapy. There appears to be no consistent correlation between tumor grade and radiosensitivity.

Focal external beam radiation may be pallative for bone pain due to metastases. The duration of relief is variable. Radiation is less effective for alleviating ureteral obstruction secondary to metastatic tumor because the time lag for a successful response may be 6 to 8 weeks.

Interstitial radiation involves retropubic implantation of seeds of ^{125}I. This treatment avoids major extirpative surgery and provides a concentrated delivery of radiation to the target tissue. Successful ^{125}I implantation requires a well-defined primary tumor with a diameter less than 5 cm, a tumor volume less than 30 to 40 mL, and uniform distribution of ^{125}I seeds throughout the prostate. In the initial reports, 5-year survival following staging pelvic lymphadenectomy and retropubic implantation of ^{125}I seeds was comparable to survival rates after other forms of treatment, but the incidence of tumor progression is higher. Potency is preserved in more than 90 percent, and early complications are fewer and less severe than those after external beam radiation.

In summary, except for impotence following external beam radiation, serious morbidity is infrequent following either form of radiation therapy. Practical considerations make ^{125}I seed implantation most suited to stage B_1 disease. The long-term efficacy of either form of radiation as compared to radical prostatectomy for treatment of localized carcinoma (stages A_2, B_1, and B_2) is not clear, but current data suggest that radiotherapy may be less curative than radical prostatectomy.

Androgen deprivation Since growth of the normal prostate is dependent upon testicular androgens (see Chap. 330), it was logical to try androgen deprivation for treatment of prostatic cancer. Androgen deprivation can be achieved in four ways: (1) surgical extirpation of the glands that synthesize androgens (castration and adrenalectomy), (2) inhibition of pituitary gonadotropin (and/or adrenocorticotropic hormone, ACTH) production [estrogen therapy, hypophysectomy, or treatment with luteinizing hormone–releasing hormone (LHRH) analogues such as leuprolide or buserelin], (3) inhibition of androgen synthesis by the testes and adrenals (aminoglutethimide), and (4) inhibition of androgen binding to its receptor protein (cyproterone or flutamide).

The common means of achieving androgen deprivation at the clinical level are castration and estrogen therapy. Since testicular secretion accounts for more than 95 percent of testosterone production, bilateral orchiectomy results in a decline of plasma levels from approximately 5 ng/mL to 0.3 to 0.5 ng/mL. Estrogens such as diethylstilbestrol are potent inhibitors of the release from the pituitary gland of luteinizing hormone, the gonadotropin that regulates testosterone production, and consequently its administration also causes a fall in plasma testosterone to castration levels. Maximum depression of plasma testosterone is achieved with 3 mg of diethylstilbestrol per day. Other estrogens (conjugated estrogens, ethinyl estradiol, diethylstilbestrol diphosphate) are no more effective in lowering plasma testosterone than is diethylstilbestrol. Luteinizing hormone–releasing hormone analogues also inhibit leuteinizing hormone secretion and lower plasma testosterone levels.

Androgen depletion beyond that achieved by surgical castration, estrogen administration, or ACTH analogues can be accomplished by adrenalectomy. Since adrenal androgen production is under the control of ACTH, the adrenal sources of androgen can also be eliminated by hypophysectomy. The alternative to surgical ablation is the induction of a medical adrenalectomy and/or castration with drugs that inhibit the synthesis and/or binding of androgen to its cytoplasmic receptor protein. While these ancillary surgical and medical means have theoretical benefits for enhancing androgen deprivation, their usefulness in treating prostatic cancer is not established.

Androgen deprivation therapy utilizing bilateral orchiectomy, diethylstilbestrol therapy, or combined orchiectomy plus diethylstilbestrol was a standard form of treatment for carcinoma of the prostate for many years, based largely upon clinical reports comparing treatment groups with historical controls. Subsequently, the role of such therapy was assessed in three controlled prospective studies conducted by the Veterans Administration Cooperative Urological Research Group. These studies failed to establish the effectiveness of high-dose diethylstilbestrol or orchiectomy, alone or in combination, in enhancing survival in any stage of prostatic cancer. (Low-dose diethylstilbestrol, 1 mg per day, may decrease deaths from cancer; since this dosage does not uniformly suppress testosterone levels, the drug may work by means other than or in addition to inhibiting testosterone formation.)

A prospective, randomized multicenter trial comparing an LHRH analogue to 3 mg diethylstilbestrol per day for metastatic prostate cancer suggests equivalent response rates and patient survival in the two groups at 1 year. Cardiovascular complications were fewer in the LHRH analogue group. Whether the duration of response with LHRH analogue therapy will be equal to that with orchiectomy or estrogen is not known.

Even when there is no beneficial effect upon survival, androgen deprivation causes decreased bone pain in two-thirds of symptomatic stage D patients. Whether androgen deprivation therapy should be administered early (asymptomatic phase) or late (symptomatic phase) in stage D disease is unsettled.

Chemotherapy The age group at greatest risk for prostatic cancer has poor tolerance for chemotherapy. This feature, coupled with the variable course of the disease, makes it difficult to determine the effectiveness of such therapy. However, several comprehensive trials utilizing chemotherapy have been undertaken in stage D disease following relapse after hormonal treatment, a situation in which mean survival time is only 7 to 8 months. The agents studied most extensively are estramustine phosphate, prednimustine, and cisplatin; more limited trials have been conducted with 5-fluorouracil, melphalan, and hydroxyurea. Complete response is rare, and only one-tenth of stage D patients have an objective partial response. In other trials combinations of chemotherapeutic agents have been tested in stage D disease, most commonly estramustine phosphate plus prednimustine or cyclophosphamide plus another agent. Complete response is again rare, and only one-fourth of patients or fewer show any objective improvement. For progressive, symptomatic stage D prostatic cancer, endocrine ablation therapy should be undertaken first, but chemotherapeutic agents may provide some benefit when such patients relapse.

REFERENCES

Benign prostatic hyperplasia

HORTON R, COFFEY DS: *Benign Prostatic Hyperplasia*, Washington, DC, US Department of Health Education, and Welfare, in press, 1986

WALSH PC: Benign prostatic hyperplasia, in *Campbell's Urology*, PC Walsh et al (eds). Philadelphia, Saunders, 1986, p 1248–1267

WILSON JD: The pathogenesis of prostatic hyperplasia. Am J Med 68:745, 1980

Carcinoma of the prostate

BAGSHAW MA: External radiation therapy of carcinoma of the prostate. Cancer 45:1912, 1980

BYAR DP, CORLE DK: VACURG randomized trial of radical prostatectomy for Stages I and II prostate cancer. Urology 17(4) (Suppl):7, 1981

CATALONA WJ, SCOTT WW: Carcinoma of the prostate, in *Campbell's Urololgy*, PC Walsh et al (eds). Philadelphia, Saunders, 1985

GUINAN P et al: The accuracy of the rectal examination in the diagnosis of prostatic carcinoma. N Engl J Med 303:499, 1980

HERR HW: Iodine 125 implantation in the management of localized prostatic carcinoma. Urol Clin North Am 7:605, 1980

JEWETT HJ: Radical perineal prostatectomy for palpable clinically localized, non-obstructive cancer. Experience at the Johns Hopkins Hospital, 1909–1963. J Urol 124: 492, 1980

KLEIN LA: Prostatic carcinoma. N Engl J Med 300:824, 1979

MURPHY GP et al: Current status of classification and staging of prostate cancer. Cancer 45:1889, 1980

SAGALOWSKY AI, WILSON JD: Carcinoma of the prostate: The therapeutic dilemma, in *Update IV: Harrison's Principles of Internal Medicine*, KJ Isselbacher et al (eds.) New York, McGraw-Hill, 1982

SCHMIDT JD: Chemotherapy of hormone-resistant stage D prostatic cancer. J Urol 123:797, 1980

STAMEY TA: Cancer of the prostate. An analysis of some important contributions and dilemmas. 1982 Monographs in Urology 3:67, 1983

WALSH PC: Physiologic basis for hormonal therapy in carcinoma of the prostate. Urol Clin N Am 2:125, 1975

——— et al: Radical surgery for prostatic cancer. Cancer 45:1906, 1980

299 CARCINOID SYNDROME

JOHN A. OATES / L. JACKSON ROBERTS II

The association of carcinoid tumors with cutaneous flushes, telangiectasia, diarrhea, cardiac valvular lesions, and bronchial constriction suggested that the peripheral manifestations are mediated by release of one or more biologically active agents by the tumor. Serotonin was the first such agent to be discovered, and overproduction of this amine is the most consistent biochemical indicator of the carcinoid syndrome. Serotonin, however, is not the sole mediator of the symptoms. These tumors may elaborate additional indoles and chemically unrelated agents including vasoactive peptides and histamine. Furthermore, unidentified substances may participate in the flushing. Within the broad classification of carcinoid tumors there is great diversity in the substances produced and in the mechanisms for their storage and release. Accordingly, there is a varied spectrum of clinical manifestations.

THE TUMOR Carcinoid tumors are slowly growing neoplasms of enterochromaffin cells. The metastatic tumors associated with carcinoid syndrome usually arise from small primary tumors in the ileum. The syndrome is also produced by neoplasms arising from the remainder of the small intestine, from organs derived from the embryonic foregut (e.g., bronchus, stomach, pancreas, and thyroid), and from ovarian or testicular teratomas.

Carcinoid tumors have an unusual proclivity for metastasis to the liver and may involve this organ extensively, with minimal metastatic disease elsewhere. Extrahepatic metastases occur in bone, where they are often osteoblastic, and in lung, pancreas, spleen, ovaries, adrenals, and other organs.

Primary carcinoid tumors of the appendix are common, but they rarely metastasize. Those from the large intestine may metastasize but almost never exhibit endocrine effects.

The usual carcinoid tumor arising from the ileum has the histologic pattern of dense nests of cells with uniform size and nuclear appearance. Histochemically, they typically exhibit an argentaffin reaction in which the cells convert a silver salt to metallic silver. A positive argentaffin reaction is not required for the diagnosis, however, and carcinoid tumors arising from organs of the embryonic foregut usually contain few if any argentaffin cells. Tumors from these organs also have a broad histologic spectrum, which in the lung ranges from typical bronchial carcinoid to a form indistinguishable from oat cell carcinoma. Ultrastructural examination of carcinoid tumors reveals electron-dense secretion granules.

CLINICAL FEATURES Unlike most metastatic neoplasms, carcinoid tumors have an unusually slow rate of growth; many patients survive for 5 to 10 years after the disease is recognized. For much of the duration of the illness, morbidity may result largely from the endocrine function of the tumor. Death results from cardiac or hepatic failure and from complications associated with tumor growth.

Vasomotor paroxysms The most common clinical feature is cutaneous *flushing*. The typical flush is erythematous and involves the head and neck (blush area). The color may change from red to violaceous to pallor during its course. Prolonged flushing attacks may be associated with lacrimation and periorbital edema. The systemic effects of the flush are variable. It may be accompanied by tachycardia, and the blood pressure may fall or not change. A rise in blood pressure during flushing is rare, and carcinoid syndrome is not a cause of sustained hypertension.

Flushing may be provoked by excitement, exertion, eating, and ethanol ingestion. In addition, the administration of pentagastrin and beta-adrenoceptor agonists such as epinephrine can trigger episodes of vasodilatation; as the hemodynamic changes associated with such pharmacologically induced attacks may be severe, these drugs should be administered with great caution.

Telangiectasia In addition to paroxysms of cutaneous vasodilatation, some patients also develop purple telangiectasia, primarily on the face and neck and most marked in the malar area.

Gastrointestinal symptoms Intestinal hypermotility with borborygmi, cramping, and explosive diarrhea may accompany the episodic flushes. Chronic diarrhea is more common and may have a secretory component. When this is severe, malabsorption may occur.

Cardiac manifestations There is a unique deposition of fibrous tissue on the endocardium of the valvular cusps and cardiac chambers. It occurs primarily in the right side of the heart but may involve the left side to a minimal degree. The plaque-like thickening of the endocardium is composed of smooth-muscle cells embedded in a stroma rich in mucopolysaccharides, collagen, and microfibrils and does not penetrate the internal elastic membrane. Distortion of the valve cusps, chordae tendineae, and papillary muscles interferes with valvular function in the right side of the heart and may lead to regurgitation, stenosis, or combined functional lesions. The fibrosing process tends to produce incompetence at the tricuspid valve and stenosis of the smaller pulmonary orifice, a deleterious hemodynamic combination. A high cardiac output, with its attendant imposition on cardiac function, may be due either to a continuing release of a vasodilator or to excessive flow in the metastatic tumors.

Pulmonary symptoms Bronchoconstriction is a less common feature of the syndrome, but it may be severe. It is usually most pronounced during flushing attacks.

General In addition to the endocrine effects, the tumors themselves may cause intestinal obstruction or bleeding. Necrosis of intestinal or hepatic tumor masses may produce abdominal pain, tenderness, fever, and leukocytosis. Hepatomegaly from the metastatic disease is usually present with the syndrome. Extensive metastatic involvement of the liver by these slowly growing tumors may occur before the liver function test results become abnormal. Rarely, a tumor-associated myasthenia accompanies the carcinoid syndrome.

FIGURE 299-1 *Metabolic pathway of serotonin.*

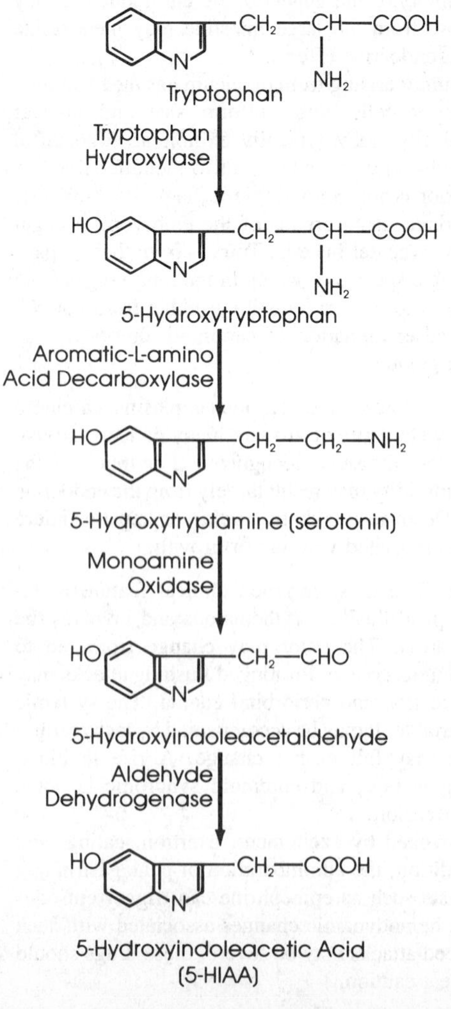

ENDOCRINE FUNCTION OF THE TUMORS The most constant biochemical characteristic of carcinoid tumors is the presence of tryptophan hydroxylase, which catalyzes the formation of 5-hydroxytryptophan (5-HTP) from tryptophan (Fig. 299-1). Most tumors also contain the enzyme aromatic L-amino acid decarboxylase, which catalyzes the formation of 5-hydroxytryptamine (serotonin). Carcinoids from the stomach and from other organs derived from the embryonic foregut, however, are frequently deficient in this decarboxylase and release 5-HTP from the tumor. Following its release from the tumor, serotonin is inactivated primarily by the enzyme monoamine oxidase; uptake into platelets also contributes to removal of free serotonin from blood. Monoamine oxidase oxidizes serotonin to 5-hydroxyindoleacetaldehyde, which is rapidly converted to 5-hydroxyindoleacetic acid (5-HIAA) by aldehyde dehydrogenase. This acid is rapidly excreted in the urine, and almost all circulating serotonin can be accounted for as urinary 5-HIAA. Carcinoid tumors vary widely in their capacity to store serotonin, with concentrations of the amine in tumors ranging from a few micrograms per gram to 3 mg/g. The concentration in the tumor appears unrelated to the rate of synthesis of serotonin as reflected by urinary 5-HIAA. Generally, tumors from the ileum have a higher storage capacity for serotonin than do tumors from organs of the embryonic foregut.

Peptides in the class of tachykinins have been found in the tumors and blood of patients with carcinoid syndrome. There are numerous vasodilator peptides in the tachykinin group, including the undecapeptide substance P, and the specific structure(s) associated with the tachykinins in carcinoid syndrome has not been classified.

Bradykinin, also a vasodilator peptide, is released during flushes in some, but not all, cases of carcinoid syndrome. Accordingly, it is not likely to be the principal agent causing flushing.

Some carcinoid tumors, particularly those of gastric origin, produce and release excessive amounts of histamine. This can be detected by an increased excretion of this amine in the urine. In such patients, the release of histamine from the tumors is responsible for the episodic vasodilatation with flushing, tachycardia, and hypotension.

Carcinoid syndrome has been associated with hyperadrenocorticism in a number of instances. This results from ectopic production of adrenocorticotropic hormone or of a corticotropin-releasing factor by the tumors, which usually originate from sites other than the ileum (bronchus, pancreas, ovary, and stomach) (see Chap. 303 and Chap. 321).

In a few cases, ''multiple endocrine adenomas'' have been seen in conjunction with carcinoids arising from organs of the embryonic foregut. The associated tumors have included parathyroid adenomas and pancreatic tumors, producing Zollinger-Ellison syndrome (see Chap. 334).

Neoplasms of foregut origin with histologic features resembling carcinoids may produce excessive amounts of gastrin, insulin, calcitonin, glucagon, corticotropin, growth hormone, a growth hormone–releasing factor, and vasoactive intestinal polypeptide without exhibiting the usual features of carcinoid syndrome. These carcinoid tumors probably share a common embryologic origin with those producing carcinoid syndrome.

PATHOPHYSIOLOGY Serotonin contributes to those aspects of the syndrome related to intestinal hypermotility, and the fibrous deposits on the endocardium may result from increased levels of circulating serotonin.

A secondary effect of serotonin overproduction occurs when a large fraction of dietary tryptophan is shunted into the hydroxylation pathway, leaving less tryptophan available for the formation of nicotinic acid and protein. When urinary excretion of 5-HIAA exceeds

200 to 300 mg daily, low levels of plasma tryptophan and evidence of nicotinamide deficiency are seen (see Chap. 76).

Mechanism of the flush Although the flushes of patients with gastric carcinoids that secrete histamine can be attributed to this amine, the mechanism of the flush in the more typical carcinoid syndrome has not yet been elucidated. Current evidence suggests that serotonin is not the mediator of the flush.

Release of the flush-provoking substance(s) can be triggered by catecholamines, and this probably accounts for the association of flushing with excitement and emotional stimuli. For experimental induction of flushing, injection of isoproterenol in amounts of as little as 0.5 μg may be effective. Pentagastrin in doses as small as 0.25 μg also can trigger flushing, an action that may explain the provocation of flushes by eating in some patients. Flushing episodes can be blocked by somatostatin, probably by inhibition of the release of the vasodilator substance(s).

DIAGNOSIS With its full constellation of clinical features, carcinoid syndrome is easily recognized. The diagnosis also must be considered when any one of its features is present. The diagnostic hallmark is *overproduction of 5-hydroxyindoles* with *increased urinary excretion of 5-hydroxyindoleacetic acid.* Normally, excretion of 5-HIAA does not exceed 9 mg daily. Ingestion of foods containing serotonin may complicate the biochemical diagnosis of carcinoid syndrome; walnuts and bananas contain enough serotonin to produce elevated urinary excretion of 5-HIAA after their ingestion. Some drugs also interfere with the analysis of urinary 5-HIAA; cough syrups containing guaiacolate cause falsely elevated values, and phenothiazines interfere with the colorimetric test. When dietary 5-hydroxyindoles are excluded, a urinary excretion of more than 25 mg 5-HIAA daily is diagnostic of carcinoid. Elevations in the range of 9 to 25 mg may be seen with carcinoid syndrome, nontropical sprue, or acute intestinal obstruction.

Measurement of *serotonin in blood or platelets* is of less diagnostic value than assay of the major metabolite of serotonin in the urine.

Measurement of an increased concentration of *serotonin in tumor tissue* is a useful and sometimes necessary supplement to histologic examination. A portion of suspected tumor should always be frozen for serotonin analysis (see Table 299-1).

Differential diagnosis Attacks of flushing in a patient with normal urinary excretion of 5-HIAA raises other diagnostic possibilities. Disorders associated with systemic mastocyte activation, including mastocytosis, produce flushing, hypotension, and even syncope and are a consideration when 5-HIAA excretion is not elevated. Flushing also occurs in the postmenopausal state and in conjunction with other tumors, particularly medullary carcinoma of the thyroid.

VARIANTS OF THE SYNDROME The origin of the tumor influences the biologically active substances produced and their storage and release. Carcinoid tumors arising from organs derived from the embryonic foregut (bronchus, stomach, and pancreas) tend to differ from those arising distal to the midduodenum (midgut). The typical carcinoid syndrome usually results from tumors of midgut origin, which almost invariably secrete serotonin with little or no 5-HTP. Tumor serotonin content is likely to be high, and the tumor usually contains dense nests of argentaffin-positive cells.

In contrast, tumors arising from the embryonic foregut contain fewer argentaffin cells, have lower serotonin content, and may secrete 5-HTP. Hyperadrenocorticism and multiple endocrine adenomas are more likely to be associated with this group.

In addition to the general characteristics of the foregut group, certain clinical and biochemical features have been associated with gastric and bronchial carcinoids. Patients with gastric carcinoids frequently exhibit unique flushing which begins as a bright-red patchy erythema with sharply delineated serpentine borders; these patches tend to coalesce as the blush heightens. Food ingestion is especially likely to produce flushes. The tumors usually are deficient in decarboxylase enzyme and secrete 5-HTP; histamine secretion is also common, as is a high incidence of peptic ulcers. Diarrhea and heart lesions are not prominent features in the patients who secrete largely 5-HTP from the tumor without much preformed serotonin.

When the carcinoid tumor arises from the bronchus, attacks of flushing tend to be prolonged and severe and may be associated with periorbital edema, excessive lacrimation and salivation, hypotension, tachycardia, anxiety, and tremulousness. Nausea, vomiting, explosive diarrhea, and bronchoconstriction may progress to a severe degree. This group is distinctive in that the severe flushes often can be prevented by glucocorticoids, and chlorpromazine may relieve the symptoms.

TREATMENT Treatment of the carcinoid syndrome is directed toward (1) reducing tumor mass by surgical and/or chemotherapeutic approaches and (2) relief of humorally mediated symptoms.

Recognition of the carcinoid syndrome has led to complete surgical cure of a few patients with tumors arising in ovarian or testicular teratomas or in the bronchus. By releasing their secretions directly into the systemic circulation, tumors from these locations can produce the syndrome before metastatic disease occurs. As the humoral substances released by tumors draining into the portal circulation are largely metabolized by the liver, tumors arising in this location produce the syndrome only after metastasis, usually to the liver. Because of the relatively slow growth of carcinoid tumors, palliative resection of hepatic metastases may be beneficial in selected cases. Resection of large isolated hepatic metastases has led to relief of the symptoms of carcinoid syndrome and reduction in urinary 5-HIAA excretion for periods of several years. In some cases with multiple metastases, removal of as much as a hepatic lobe may be considered when the metastases are located primarily in the portion of the liver to be resected, as indicated by arteriography, radionuclide scanning of the liver, ultrasonography, computerized tomography or inspection of the hepatic surface at surgical exploration.

In patients with diffuse metastatic disease involving both lobes of the liver, reduction of tumor mass and control of symptoms has been accomplished by surgical ligation or percutaneous embolization of the hepatic artery. Experience with these approaches, however, is limited, and further studies are required to define efficacy and associated complications.

There is no universally effective chemotherapeutic regimen, and none will eradicate carcinoid tumors. Palliation has been achieved in some patients with 5-fluorouracil, cyclophosphamide, streptozotocin, doxorubicin, and methotrexate, used singly or in combination. Objective response rates to chemotherapy are low, the average duration of remission is usually less than 1 year, and associated toxicity of drug therapy is high. An occasional patient may respond to 5-fluorouracil alone with minimal toxicity. Initial doses of chemotherapeutic agents should be low in patients with 5-HIAA levels over 150 mg per day or florid manifestations of the carcinoid syndrome, because rapid lysis of tumor may result in massive mediator release (''carcinoid crisis''). Radiation therapy can be effective in the treatment of symptomatic metastases, e.g., bone. The antiestrogen tamoxifen and leukocyte interferon have been tried in a few patients.

Pharmacologic therapy directed at the humoral mediators of the

TABLE 299-1 Outline of diagnostic approach to a patient with suspected carcinoid syndrome

1 Quantitative determination of 24-h urinary excretion of 5-HIAA (5-hydroxyindoleacetic acid).
2 When elevated 5-HIAA confirms carcinoid syndrome, curable ovarian, testicular, or bronchial primary tumors should be sought.
3 Consideration of possible treatment of the syndrome by surgical resection of hepatic metastases requires
  a Assessment of the location and character of hepatic metastases with computerized tomography, scintillation scanning of the liver, arteriography, and ultrasonography.
  b Evaluation of hepatic and cardiac function.
  c A search for extrahepatic metastases in bone and other sites.
4 In patients with substantial diarrhea, possible malabsorption of nutrients should be investigated.

syndrome may be useful. When the flush is associated with release of histamine, as may be the case with gastric carcinoids, combined treatment with an H-1 antagonist (e.g., diphenhydramine) and an H-2 antagonist (cimetidine or ranitidine) will block the vasodilator action of histamine. Diarrhea should be treated symptomatically if possible, e.g., with loperamide. Treatment with serotonin antagonists such as cyproheptadine and methysergide can also be helpful in controlling diarrhea. Prolonged therapy with methysergide, however, can produce retroperitoneal fibrosis. Blockade of serotonin synthesis with the tryptophan hydroxylase inhibitor *p*-chlorophenylalanine (an experimental drug) also ameliorates the diarrhea. Somatostatin (also an experimental agent) decreases flushing, diarrhea, and bronchoconstriction and may contribute to the management of episodes with massive mediator release or "carcinoid crisis." The prevention of severe flushing by glucocorticoids and amelioration of the syndrome by phenothiazines are limited largely to patients with tumors arising from the bronchus and other organs derived from the embryonic foregut.

There are no known means to reverse or halt the progression of endocardial fibrosis. Surgical replacement of damaged cardiac valves is associated with technical problems because of the marked fibrosis of the endocardium.

In patients with urinary 5-HIAA levels about 100 mg per day supplemental niacin therapy prevents the development of pellagra.

Hypotensive episodes should not be treated with catecholamines; by stimulating the release of vasoactive substances from the tumor, norepinephrine, epinephrine, and other agents with adrenergic activity can exaggerate and prolong the circulatory disturbance. If hypotension requires therapy, volume expansion or methoxamine infusion is the preferred approach.

REFERENCES

MARTIN JK et al: Surgical treatment of functioning metastatic carcinoid tumors. Arch Surg 118:537, 1983

MELIA WM et al: Use of arterial devascularization and cytotoxic drugs in 30 patients with the carcinoid syndrome. Br J Cancer 46:331, 1982

MOERTEL CG, HANLEY JA: Combination chemotherapy trials in metastatic carcinoid tumor and malignant carcinoid syndrome. Cancer Clin Trials 2:327, 1979

OATES JA, BUTLER TC: Pharmacologic and endocrine aspects of carcinoid syndrome. Adv Pharmacol 5:109, 1967

SJOERDSMA A et al: A clinical, physiologic and biochemical study of patients with malignant carcinoid. Am J Med 20:520, 1956

SKRABANEK P et al: Substance P in ovarian carcinoid. J Clin Pathol 33:160, 1980

300 CUTANEOUS MANIFESTATIONS OF INTERNAL MALIGNANCY

HARLEY A. HAYNES

One of the most satisfying aspects of dermatologic diagnosis is the detection of previously unknown malignant disease in a treatable stage by recognition of an apparently irrelevant alteration of the skin as a clue to the presence of the neoplasm. Although less satisfying, the recognition of the probability of a neoplastic disease may be of great assistance in clarifying a difficult diagnostic problem, even if the neoplasm should be untreatable when discovered. Sometimes these skin changes are induced directly by infiltration of the neoplasm into the skin, but more often they are induced indirectly by a variety of mechanisms.

This chapter is an attempt to classify the wide range of skin signs of internal malignancy in a logical fashion (Table 300-1). Since the types of skin alterations and the number of neoplasms are extremely large, grouping of the alterations by pathogenetic mechanisms was selected. There remains a substantial idiopathic category; the entities therein will be grouped by pathogenesis when this becomes understood. The skin alterations induced by neoplasms of the endocrine organs are not included here as they generally are the alterations one would expect from excess or deficiency of the hormone in question and are mentioned in the appropriate chapters.

SKIN INFILTRATION BY AN INTERNAL MALIGNANCY

METASTASES FROM CARCINOMA Cutaneous metastases of malignant lesions occur in 3 to 5 percent of patients with metastatic disease. These lesions may provide the first indication of recurrence

TABLE 300-1 Classification of skin signs of internal malignancy

I Skin infiltration by an internal malignancy
- *A* Metastatic: lymphatic, hematogenous, or by surgical implantation
  - *1* Carcinoma
  - *2* Leukemia
- *B* Metastatic: intraepidermal
  - *1* Paget's disease of the breast
  - *2* Extramammary Paget's disease
- *C* Autochthonous or metastatic (?)
  - *1* Lymphoma
  - *2* Malignant histiocytosis

II Skin changes due to exposure to a carcinogen that also induces internal malignancy
- *A* Arsenical keratoses
- *B* Bowen's disease

III Skin malignancies associated with increased risk of separate primary internal malignancy
- *A* Bowen's disease
- *B* Kaposi's sarcoma
- *C* Any skin malignancy (??)

IV Skin changes due to metabolic products of malignancies
- *A* Malignant carcinoid syndrome
- *B* Addisonian hyperpigmentation with Cushing's syndrome, from carcinomas producing MSH- and ACTH-like peptides
- *C* Generalized dermal melanosis (slate gray), from malignant melanoma
- *D* Nodular fat necrosis, due to lipases from pancreatic carcinoma
- *E* Raynaud's syndrome with cryoproteinemia, from multiple myeloma
- *F* Amyloidosis, from multiple myeloma
- *G* Necrolytic migrating erythema, from functioning glucagonoma
- *H* Porphyria cutanea tarda secondary to primary hepatoma

V Skin changes due to functional disturbances in other systems induced by nonendocrine malignancies
- *A* Jaundice, obstructive
- *B* Addisonian hyperpigmentation from adrenal infiltration by a tumor
- *C* Purpura, thrombocytopenic
- *D* Pallor, from anemia
- *E* Herpes zoster
- *F* Herpes simplex, severe, protracted, recurrent
- *G* Pyoderma, recurrent
- *H* Delayed hypersensitivity, exaggerated to mosquito bites

VI Skin changes, idiopathic
- *A* Changes frequently related to internal malignancy
  - *1* Dermatomyositis, adult-onset
  - *2* Acanthosis nigricans
  - *3* Thrombophlebitis, migratory
  - *4* Ichthyosis, adult-onset
  - *5* Alopecia mucinosa, adult
  - *6* Pachydermoperiostosis, acquired
  - *7* Hypertrichosis lanugosa, acquired ("malignant down")
  - *8* Erythema gyratum repens
- *B* Changes occasionally related to internal malignancy
  - *1* Pruritus, without causative skin lesions
  - *2* Clubbing, with and without hypertrophic osteoarthropathy
  - *3* Erythroderma
  - *4* Normolipemic xanthomatosis
  - *5* Erythema multiforme
  - *6* Urticaria and erythema perstans
  - *7* Pyoderma gangrenosum, atypical and acute febrile neutrophilic dermatosis
  - *8* Bullous disease (bullous pemphigoid and dermatitis herpetiformis)
  - *9* Seborrheic keratoses, multiple, sudden onset (sign of Leser-Trelat)
  - *10* Dermatoses, bizarre

VII Heritable diseases with skin manifestations and the propensity to develop internal malignancy (see Table 300-2)

in a patient with a known primary tumor or may be the presenting lesions of a hitherto unsuspected tumor. Typical skin metastases are dermal nodules, varying from skin color to purple, which are more easily felt than seen and are very firm to the touch; they ulcerate rarely. Metastases from renal and thyroid carcinomas may be pulsatile and have a bruit. Breast carcinomas may produce an erysipelas-like appearance on the chest. The location of skin metastases may give a clue to the origin of the primary tumor. The abdominal wall is the most common site in both sexes for lesions initially presenting as metastases. In this situation, the primary sites are usually the lung, stomach, or kidney in men, and the ovary in women. In women with metastases on the chest wall, the most likely primary site is the breast. Other skin areas that tend to be involved by metastases are the scalp, from lung, kidney, or breast; the chest, in men, from lung; the back, from lung or breast; the extremities, from malignant melanomas; and the face, from oropharyngeal carcinomas. Histologic examination of a skin metastasis may reveal the identity of the primary tumor.

METASTASES FROM LEUKEMIA Leukemic deposits in skin are more common in myelomonocytic leukemia than in lymphocytic or granulocytic leukemias (Chap. 292). Firm papules or nodules ranging in color from pink to purple are the usual lesions, although ulcerations may develop. If thrombocytopenia is present, purpura often occurs in the nodules. Leukemic infiltrates may develop in recent scars, in traumatized areas, and in lesions of herpes zoster and herpes simplex. Cytologic examination of "touch" preparations from the cut surface of a nodule more readily identifies the cell type than does examination of histologic sections. The only clinically pathognomonic lesion of any of the leukemias is chloroma, named for its green color, which is due to myeloperoxidase in the cells of acute granulocytic leukemia. In addition to specific leukemic cell infiltrates, a variety of lesions occur that are nonspecific on biopsy.

INTRAEPIDERMAL METASTASES: PAGET'S DISEASE *Paget's disease of the nipple* and areola is an uncommon but well-known skin sign of underlying intraductal carcinoma of the breast. The primary ductal carcinoma extends upward within the epithelium of the mammary ducts and into the epidermis, where it causes the skin lesion. The clinical appearance is that of an eczematous, weeping, crusted, or scaly lesion resembling atopic eczema or contact dermatitis. Paget's disease is unaffected by topical corticosteroids, in contrast to the responsiveness of eczema. Therefore, any such "eczematous" lesions that fail to respond to treatment must be biopsied. The histopathologic appearance of Paget's disease is diagnostic; the presence in the epidermis of clear cells containing mucopolysaccharides is apparent.

Extramammary Paget's disease is a similar eczematous-appearing lesion occurring on the pubis, perineum, thighs, or genitalia. It is related usually to underlying apocrine or eccrine sweat gland carcinoma but occasionally to rectal or urethral adenocarcinoma. Occasionally, a primary malignant origin cannot be found. The histopathologic appearance of extramammary Paget's disease of apocrine gland origin is identical to that of Paget's disease of the breast, which is an apocrine gland. Special staining of the mucopolysaccharides will permit differentiation between Paget's disease of cloacogenic and apocrine gland origin.

LYMPHOMA Lymphomatous deposits in the skin secondary to an internal lymphoma are seen most often in histiocytic lymphoma and lymphoblastic lymphoma. Such cutaneous deposits are rare in Hodgkin's disease. Mycosis fungoides, the most frequent lymphomatous skin disorder, is discussed in Chap. 301. Lymphoma lesions in the skin are dermal or subcutaneous nodules that typically have a purple or red-brown color. The lesions usually are covered by relatively normal intact epidermis. Skin infiltrates may be the initial manifestations or may appear at any time in the course of the disease. Biopsy of these lesions is necessary to establish the correct diagnosis. The nonspecific skin changes in lymphoma are discussed below.

MALIGNANT HISTIOCYTOSIS In the Letterer-Siwe, Schüller-Christian disease complex, a variety of skin lesions may occur: (1) scaly papules or vesicles with or without purpura on trunk or scalp; (2) pruritic seborrheic or eczematous lesions in intertriginous areas that do not respond to local treatment for the benign conditions; (3) petechiae due to perivascular infiltrates, thrombocytopenia, or both; (4) scaly or exudative eruptions of the scalp; and (5) xanthomas, usually late in the course. When there is lack of response to local therapy, directed at presumptive diaper dermatitis, seborrheic dermatitis, moniliasis, or intertrigo, early biopsy of these various lesions should be done and is usually diagnostic if histiocytosis is present. Skin lesions may be the presenting sign and may lead to the correct diagnosis, or they may appear late in the course of the disease if it is not controlled.

SKIN CHANGES DUE TO EXPOSURE TO A CARCINOGEN THAT ALSO INDUCES INTERNAL MALIGNANCY

ARSENICAL KERATOSES Inorganic arsenicals are the only well-recognized carcinogens which cause both skin and visceral malignancies. These salts were widely used in medicine a few decades ago for the treatment of a large variety of disorders, such as arthritis, asthma, and psoriasis, and were also used as herbicides in agriculture. Arsenic contamination of drinking water occurs in many parts of the world. Exposure may therefore be intentional and known or accidental and wholly unsuspected. Multiple, discrete, hard hyperkeratotic wartlike lesions, termed *arsenical keratoses,* on the palms and soles occur characteristically in patients a decade or more after exposure to arsenic. These lesions are similar to actinic or solar keratoses in that they are premalignant lesions, but they have a very low incidence of malignancy. The histopathologic changes produced by these two types of keratosis also are similar.

BOWEN'S DISEASE Squamous-cell carcinoma of the skin in situ is known as Bowen's disease. The lesions are single or multiple sharply defined plaques that are slightly thickened and brownish red and have a varying amount of scale. At times the lesions of Bowen's disease resemble eczema or psoriasis but fail to respond to local therapy. Such lesions must be biopsied. Arsenical exposure is definitely the cause of many cases of Bowen's disease and may be the cause of nearly all. The lesions are easily treated by surgical excision or by various methods of local destruction. Although about 5 percent become invasive, less than 2 percent metastasize. More important is the recognition of the fact that the patient is at significant risk of developing carcinomas of the respiratory, genitourinary, and gastrointestinal systems. This risk is especially high in patients in whom Bowen's disease develops on skin that is not usually exposed to sunlight. Thorough examinations to detect visceral neoplasia must be performed at intervals, as the average latent period between the onset of Bowen's disease and the development of visceral neoplasia is more than 8 years. Even without a history or stigmata of arsenical exposure, there is an increased risk of visceral neoplasms in patients with this condition.

SKIN MALIGNANCIES ASSOCIATED WITH INCREASED RISK OF SEPARATE PRIMARY INTERNAL MALIGNANCY

BOWEN'S DISEASE See preceding section.

KAPOSI'S SARCOMA Initially Kaposi's sarcoma may be a multiple, autochthonous, reactive, lymphoreticular and endothelial cell proliferation rather than a neoplasm. It usually behaves in an indolent fashion, although frank, aggressive, sarcomatous change develops in a small percentage of patients. The lesions begin on the feet or ankles, then may progress proximally and also be found on the hands and arms. Extracutaneous lesions are most frequently seen in the gastrointestinal tract, where bleeding is the major complication. The respiratory tract is the second most frequently involved extracutaneous site. Generally these extracutaneous lesions are not clinically significant, unless frankly sarcomatous. There is a marked genetic predisposition to the disease among Jews, Italians, and the Bantus in the Congo. A pronounced male predominance of 9:1 has been noted. The skin lesions of Kaposi's sarcoma are rather distinctive dark blue or purple-brown nodules or plaques, primarily located on the distal extremities. The color is due to the vascular nature of the lesions and the chronic extravasation of erythrocytes, resulting in hemosiderin deposition. Almost invariably, chronic lymphedema is associated with, and at times precedes, the lesions. Lymphoma and leukemia are associated in about 10 percent of cases in the western hemisphere, but not in the eastern. The histopathologic picture is sufficiently characteristic for confirmation of the clinical diagnosis. For the average case, very conservative therapy, such as elastic support hose to reduce edema and low-dose x-ray treatment of symptomatic skin lesions, is all that is required. Chemotherapy should be considered only in the presence of clinically significant visceral lesions or aggressive sarcomatous behavior.

In recent years Kaposi's sarcoma has been described with increasing frequency in homosexual males. This type of Kaposi's sarcoma is quite aggressive and occurs in association with suppressor T-cell-induced immunologic suppression and HTLV infection in approximately one-third of patients with AIDS. Immunosuppression and HTLV III infection have also been identified in the Zaire African type of Kaposi's sarcoma. Therapeutic immunosuppression with prednisone and azathioprine for renal transplants also has been reported to result in the development of Kaposi's sarcoma in genetically predisposed individuals. Thus, the mechanism in AIDS and in therapeutic immunosuppression is similar.

ANY SKIN MALIGNANCY Neoplasia of the skin of any type may be an indication of increased risk of visceral neoplasia, but the exact relationship is difficult to ascertain because of the high incidence of skin malignancies.

SKIN CHANGES DUE TO METABOLIC PRODUCTS ASSOCIATED WITH MALIGNANCIES

MALIGNANT CARCINOID SYNDROME The hallmark of the syndrome (Chap. 299) is the sudden onset of bright red flushing of the skin, especially of the face, neck, and upper part of the chest.

ADDISONIAN HYPERPIGMENTATION WITH CUSHING'S SYNDROME (See Chap. 325) Some nonendocrine tumors, particularly oat cell carcinoma of the lung, secrete polypeptide hormones. The most commonly observed syndrome is Addisonian hyperpigmentation with Cushing's syndrome. Intense hyperpigmentation combined with proximal muscle weakness, hypertension, diabetes mellitus, edema, and confusion are typical features. Hypokalemic alkalosis and elevated serum cortisol levels are more frequent findings than are the usual physical signs of Cushing's disease. The syndrome is caused by the production of adrenocorticotropic hormone and β-melanocyte-stimulating hormone by the tumor.

GENERALIZED DERMAL MELANOSIS (SLATE GRAY) In some patients with widespread metastases from malignant melanoma, metabolic precursors of melanin enter the circulation and are deposited in all tissues, where they become oxidized to melanin. Excretion of these intermediates results in urine that turns black upon exposure to air. Inasmuch as most of the visible melanin in this type of melanosis is in the dermis, the Tyndall effect causes the skin to look gray or blue-black rather than brown.

NODULAR FAT NECROSIS The syndrome of tender subcutaneous nodules, fever, eosinophilia, and polyarthritis of the small joints is produced by pancreatic adenocarcinoma as well as by pancreatitis. In this syndrome, the subcutaneous nodules are various shades of red and may undergo central necrosis with discharge of oily material. The increased circulating levels of lipase and other pancreatic enzymes are probably responsible for the syndrome. The histopathologic picture of the nodules usually permits the diagnosis of pancreatic fat necrosis but does not permit differentiation of benign from malignant etiology.

RAYNAUD'S PHENOMENON (See Chap. 198) The production of cryoglobulins in patients with myeloma may cause Raynaud's phenomena. Such an etiology should be especially suspected when the syndrome is atypical, appears in men, or begins in individuals over 50 years of age.

SYSTEMIC AMYLOIDOSIS From 10 to 20 percent of patients with multiple myeloma develop amyloidosis (Chap. 259). The characteristic presentation resembles "primary" amyloidosis and includes macroglossia, extraordinarily easy bruising, and, occasionally, yellowish papules or plaques visible in the skin. All organs may be affected. The purpura appears to result from vascular fragility as a consequence of deposition of amyloid. Purpura may often be induced by gentle stroking or pinching of apparently normal skin, particularly the eyelids and body folds. When the skin lesions of amyloidosis are isolated rather than scattered diffusely, the etiology is unlikely to be systemic. Such local skin amyloidosis is not rare and must be differentiated from systemic amyloidosis.

NECROLYTIC MIGRATING ERYTHEMA The glucagonoma syndrome includes a characteristic dermatitis, somewhat resembling chronic mucocutaneous candidiasis and acrodermatitis enteropathica. The skin lesions are often most severe on the lower abdomen, groin, and perineum and about the mouth. Their morphology consists of vesicles or bullae with a migrating erythematous, scaly margin. There is a tendency to heal centrally. A red, smooth, painful tongue is common (see Chap. 329).

PORPHYRIA CUTANEA TARDA The cutaneous manifestations of porphyria cutanea tarda include hyperpigmentation (especially on the dorsum of the hands in sun-exposed areas), blisters, erosions, superficial scars with milia as a result of minimal trauma, periorbital erythema, hypertrichosis, and occasionally sclerodermoid changes in exposed skin. Patients do not generally note photosensitivity. Most patients with porphyria cutanea tarda have hepatic dysfunction; a few cases have been reported secondary to primary hepatoma.

SKIN CHANGES DUE TO FUNCTIONAL DISTURBANCES IN OTHER SYSTEMS INDUCED BY NONENDOCRINE MALIGNANCIES

See Table 300-1.

IDIOPATHIC SKIN SIGNS OF INTERNAL MALIGNANCY

SIGNS FREQUENTLY RELATED TO INTERNAL MALIGNANCY

Dermatomyositis (see Chap. 370) Adults with dermatomyositis have an associated malignancy in at least 15 percent of cases, the association being slightly higher in men than in women. The skin changes may be either subtle and transient initially or widespread, persistent, and rapid in onset. Transient, blotchy, red or violaceous areas, with or without fine scaling, may be incorrectly diagnosed as contact dermatitis, eczema, or seborrheic dermatitis. When the initial lesions are sudden in onset and marked on the face, neck, and other sun-exposed areas, a photosensitivity dermatitis or contact dermatitis may be simulated. Indeed, photosensitivity is frequently noted in dermatomyositis. Later, telangiectasia develops in the lesions, and often edema and telangiectasia of the malar area or the eyelids may result in the violaceous (heliotrope) color. Linear telangiectasia adjacent to the cuticles on the nail folds within areas of periungual erythema are usually seen, as in systemic lupus erythematosus. Accentuation of cutaneous lesions over the joints on the dorsum of the hands, as well as over large joints, is often noted.

Acanthosis nigricans This skin sign is a highly significant marker of probable malignant disease when it develops in adults. The clinical problem is to differentiate between the different types of acanthosis nigricans, all of which look the same clinically and histopathologically. The lesions typically involve the axilla, groin, umbilicus, and nipples, but more extensive lesions may occur. The epidermis shows brown to black hyperpigmentation in areas of multiple confluent papillomas, resulting in a velvety elevation of the surface of the epidermis. Pruritus is sometimes present. The histopathologic appearance of the lesions confirms the diagnosis of acanthosis nigricans but does not permit differentiation between the various types. It is the history, the family history, and the physical examination which provide the most helpful data in classifying the type of acanthosis nigricans. Lesions present at birth or developing in childhood or at puberty are genetically determined and not related to malignancy. Obese individuals may develop intertriginous acanthosis nigricans without underlying disease. Various endocrinopathies, particularly Cushing's syndrome, acromegaly, and Stein-Leventhal syndrome, may be associated with acanthosis nigricans. When these conditions are absent and acanthosis nigricans develops in an adult, an underlying malignancy will be associated in most of the cases. Adenocarcinomas are the usual type of malignancy, and 60 percent of these are gastric (Chap. 236). Occasionally an undifferentiated or squamous-cell carcinoma or a lymphoma is the associated neoplasm. Though the course of the acanthosis nigricans in two-thirds of cases tends to parallel the course of the neoplasm, including remission with cure, intervals as long as 6 years between the skin lesion and the onset of the malignancy have been observed. If no benign explanation can be found for acanthosis nigricans in an adult, periodic efforts to locate a neoplasm are mandatory.

Migratory thrombophlebitis Superficial and multiple deep venous thromboses, not readily explained by the usual causes, are likely to be associated with a malignancy, usually pancreatic carcinoma (Chap. 255). Involvement of atypical sites, such as upper extremities, should also alert the physician to this possible association. An involved area may resolve in a few days. Pulmonary embolism is not a frequent complication. The migratory thrombophlebitis may precede detection of the neoplasm by several months. Unfortunately, the neoplasms associated with recurrent phlebitis tend to be inoperable.

Ichthyosis The development of ichthyosis in adults having no personal or family history of the disorder is very likely to be associated with lymphoma (usually Hodgkin's disease), although occasionally other types of malignancy have been reported. Hypothyroidism can result in similar skin changes. The skin appears dry, and the stratum corneum cracks to produce rhomboidal scales with flaky edges. Hyperkeratosis of the palms and soles may occur as well. The histopathologic changes are epidermal atrophy and hyperkeratosis, but they do not distinguish ichthyosis as a manifestation of malignancy from certain hereditary types. Although the association of this ichthyosiform alteration with lymphoma is strong, only a small number of cases have been reported.

Alopecia mucinosa Dermal papules, often with follicular accentuation and usually with hair loss in affected areas, are the typical findings. Usually this disorder is benign and self-limited, especially in patients under 40 and with a small number of lesions. In patients over 40 and when there are multiple infiltrated plaques with alopecia, the lesions are likely to represent a lymphoma with associated follicular mucinosis. However, alopecia mucinosa may develop before the lymphoma can be diagnosed in a certain number of patients.

Pachydermoperiostosis This term describes hypertrophic osteoarthropathy combined with acromegaloid features (Chap. 322). Thickening of the skin of the hands, forearms, and legs, as well as marked accentuation of facial folds, is typical. When the scalp is involved, the skin is reduplicated and furrowed (cutis verticis gyrata). A familial form of the disorder occurs and is unrelated to malignant disease. The acquired form usually occurs in men over 40 years of age who have bronchogenic carcinoma. Some acquired cases are associated with pulmonary infections, congenital heart disease, and hepatic disease.

Hypertrichosis lanugosa This sign is quite rare but so striking in its appearance and in its association with internal malignancy that it deserves discussion. A congenital form, often familiarly known as "dog face" or "monkey face," is inherited as an autosomal dominant trait and has no association with malignancy. Acquired hypertrichosis of lanugo hair type in adults has been associated with malignant disease. The associated neoplasms have been carcinomas of the breast, urinary bladder, lung, gallbladder, colon, and rectum. The hypertrichosis in this condition is composed of extremely fine, silky, and lightly pigmented hairs of the lanugo type. This hair growth is most apparent on the face and ears but may occur on the trunk and extremities. Care must be taken to differentiate this lanugo hair growth from adult-type hair growth in women with disorders of androgen excess and in either sex with porphyria cutanea tarda, erythropoietic porphyria (Chap. 52), and phenytoin administration.

Erythema gyratum repens See "Urticaria" below.

SIGNS OCCASIONALLY RELATED TO INTERNAL MALIGNANCY

Pruritus Since pruritus is one of the major symptoms expressed in the skin (Chap. 50), obviously most causes of pruritus are not related to malignant disease. Yet pruritus may be a significant symptom in up to 30 percent of patients with Hodgkin's disease. Other lymphomas are less frequently associated with pruritus, excepting mycosis fungoides, in which pruritus is almost universal. Occasionally carcinomas of the lung, stomach, colon, breast, or prostate are associated with pruritus. In such patients the pruritus usually is not limited to a small discrete area. An association with malignancy should be considered in any patient in whom pruritus cannot be explained by the finding of a metabolic cause (Chap. 50) or a local skin disease, aside from excoriations, which could explain it. Hodgkin's disease is the most likely malignancy in patients in their teens through the thirties. In the elderly, xerosis (dry skin) is common and presents a tempting explanation of pruritus. However, if decreased frequency of bathing and the use of emollients do not eliminate the pruritus, then a malignant disease must be considered. The pruritus of malignant disease will cease upon successful therapy of the malignancy.

Clubbing This alteration of the fingers and toes may sometimes be a manifestation of tumors arising either intrathoracically or metastatic to the thorax (Chap. 213).

Erythroderma This dramatic reaction of the skin is a response to a variety of stimuli (Chap. 48). Approximately 8 percent of persons with generalized erythroderma are patients with lymphoma, particularly mycosis fungoides, or leukemia. Only occasionally is erythroderma a manifestation of a carcinoma. In patients with erythroderma due to mycosis fungoides, atypical cells are present in the skin and a skin biopsy will often be diagnostic. In erythroderma related to other types of lymphoma, leukemia, or carcinoma, there is not usually a definable infiltration of the skin by the atypical cells, and the diagnosis must be made from the blood smear, the bone marrow, involved lymph nodes, or other such tissue. In such cases, this erythroderma syndrome may represent an expression of a hypersensitivity reaction to tumor products. The course of the erythroderma parallels the response of the malignant disease to therapy, but it may precede the detection of the malignancy by a year or more, making repeated diagnostic investigations necessary.

Normolipemic xanthomatosis Malignant diseases of the reticuloendothelial system have been reported in approximately one-half the reported cases of normolipemic plane xanthomatosis. Multiple myeloma is the most frequent type of associated malignant process, but several cases of lymphoma and malignant histiocytosis have been reported. Lesions are yellow to yellow-brown, flat or slightly elevated plaques. There is marked variation in size, and the lesions may be sharply demarcated or may have indistinct borders. The eyelids, sides of the neck, and upper trunk are favored sites, but lesions may appear on any portion of the body. The histopathologic appearance of these xanthomas does not differ from that of clinically similar lesions not associated with malignant disease.

Erythema multiforme (see Chap. 48) This skin reaction occasionally occurs days to weeks after deep radiation therapy of internal malignant disease, perhaps representing a hypersensitivity reaction to components of tumor tissue. Erythema multiforme is also occasionally reported as an apparent manifestation of a lymphoma, leukemia, or carcinoma, in the absence of radiation therapy. The number of cases which are related to malignant disease is a very small fraction of the total number. The skin reaction tends to resolve spontaneously even in the presence of persistent malignant disease.

Urticaria (see Chap. 48) This frequent skin reaction is an uncommon manifestation of malignant disease. A cause-effect relationship is difficult to establish unless a clear effect on the urticaria results from therapy of the associated condition. In a few patients with chronic urticaria in whom investigation disclosed a malignant disease, removal of the malignant process was associated with remission of the urticaria. Variants of urticaria present with wheal-like lesions that persist for days to months in the same site, possibly slowly changing position to form annular, arcuate, polycyclic, concentric, or other patterns. This reaction pattern is often classified under the heading of *erythema perstans*. One clinically spectacular but rare syndrome is known as *erythema gyratum repens*, in which concentric, arcuate lesions look like the grain of a soft wood. Only a few cases have been reported, but all were associated with a malignant disease, and in several the skin reaction cleared after successful treatment of the malignancy. These urticarial cutaneous vascular reactions are presumed to represent a hypersensitivity reaction to some component of the malignant disease.

Pyoderma gangrenosum, atypical (neutrophilic dermatosis) Various myeloproliferative disorders have been found in association with pyoderma gangrenosum. Myelogenous and myeloblastic leukemia, myeloma, myeloid metaplasia, monoclonal gammopathy, and polycythemia have been so described. The lesions begin as papules,

TABLE 300-2 Heritable diseases with skin manifestations and propensity to develop internal malignancy

Disorder	Skin signs	Alterations of other systems	Predominant malignancy
DOMINANT INHERITANCE			
Multiple hamartoma syndrome (Cowden's disease)	Acral verrucous papules, trichilemmomas of face, fibromas of oral mucosa	Multiple hamartomas: Lipomas, hemangiomas, fibrocystic disease of breast, thyroid adenomas, neuromas	Thyroid carcinoma, breast carcinoma
Gardner's syndrome	Epidermal cysts, sebaceous cysts, dermoid tumors, lipomas, fibromas	Polyposis of colon, osteomas	Colonic adenocarcinomas (very high incidence, unless colectomy done)
Multiple mucosal neuromas	Neuromas on eyelids, lips, tongue, nasal or laryngeal mucosae	Parathyroid adenomas, hypertension	Pheochromocytoma, medullary carcinoma of thyroid (high incidence)
Neurofibromatosis (Recklinghausen's)	Neurofibromas, café au lait spots, axillary "freckles," giant nevi	Acoustic and spinal neuromas, meningiomas, osseous fibrous dysplasia	Malignant neurilemmoma (5% incidence), pheochromocytoma (uncommon), astrocytoma, glioma (uncommon)
Nevoid basal-cell carcinoma syndrome	Multiple basal-cell carcinomas, epidermoid cysts, "pits" on palms and soles	Jaw cysts, rib and vertebral abnormalities, short metacarpals, ovarian fibromas, hypertelorism	Medulloblastoma, fibrosarcoma of jaw (low incidence)
Palmar-plantar hyperkeratosis (tylosis)	Hyperkeratosis of palms and soles (usually onset after age 10)	None	Esophageal carcinoma (95% incidence)
Peutz-Jeghers syndrome	Pigmented macules on lips, oral mucosa, digits	Intestinal polyposis (predominantly small intestine)	Gastric, duodenal, and colonic adenocarcinomas (low incidence)
Tuberous sclerosis	Hypopigmented macules, shagreen patches, adenoma sebaceum, subungual fibromas	Epilepsy, mental retardation, hamartomas in brain, kidneys, heart	Astrocytomas, glioblastomas (low incidence)
AUTOSOMAL RECESSIVE INHERITANCE			
Ataxia-telangiectasia	Telangiectasia: neck, malar, antecubital fossae, popliteal fossae, ears	Cerebellar ataxia, sinopulmonary infections, IgA deficiency, ± IgE deficiency	Lymphoma, leukemia (10% incidence)
Bloom's syndrome	Telangiectasia of sun-exposed skin, photosensitivity	Short stature, fine features, dolichocephaly	Leukemia (high incidence)
Chédiak-Higashi syndrome	Dilution of skin and hair color, recurrent pyoderma, giant melanosomes	Recurrent infections, azurophilic leukocytic inclusions, nystagmus, iris translucence, photophobia, pancytopenia	Lymphoma (high incidence)
Fanconi's anemia	Patchy hyperpigmentation	Bone anomalies, chromosomal aberrations	Leukemia (high incidence)
Werner's syndrome (adult progeria)	Premature aging, scleroderma-like changes, graying hair and baldness, leg ulcers	Arteriosclerosis, cataracts	Sarcoma, meningiomas (10% incidence)
SEX-LINKED RECESSIVE INHERITANCE			
Bruton's sex-linked agammaglobulinemia	Recurrent infections	Recurrent infections, agammaglobulinemia	Leukemia, lymphoma (5% incidence)
Dyskeratosis congenita	Reticulate hyperpigmentation, leukoplakia of mucosae, loss of nails, hyperkeratosis of palms and soles, atrophy of skin of extensor surfaces	Pancytopenia	Carcinomas (high incidence), leukemia (occasional)
Wiscott-Aldrich syndrome	Eczematous dermatitis, petechiae–purpura, recurrent pyoderma	Decreased IgM, thrombocytopenia	Leukemia, lymphoma (10% incidence)

nodules, or bullae and progress rapidly to central necrosis and ulceration with an epithelial rim of violaceous hue, undermined edge, and occasionally peripheral bulla formation. The lesions are quite often tender. Bacterial cultures and skin biopsy should be done to evaluate possible sepsis, vasculitis, or leukemia cutis. In pyoderma gangrenosum the biopsy is not diagnostic, but there is a neutrophilic dermal infiltrate with varying degrees of tissue necrosis. Another neutrophilic dermatosis with pustules and/or areas resembling cellulitis (Sweet's syndrome) has also been associated with myeloproliferative disease. The atypical pyoderma gangrenosum and Sweet's syndrome have occurred simultaneously, suggesting they are related neutrophilic dermatoses.

Bullous disease Blistering disorders of various types may occur as a manifestation of malignant disease. The most common type is the subepidermal bullous disease known as *bullous pemphigoid* (Chap. 48). This disorder usually occurs in the elderly and may affect any of or all the skin and mucosal surfaces. Although there appears not to be an increased incidence of malignant disease in such patients, this point is not proved. Removal of a neoplasm has been associated with remission of the dermatosis in a few cases. Another bullous reaction which should cause the physician to think of the possibility of a malignant disease is *dermatitis herpetiformis*. The disease is characterized by intensely pruritic, grouped vesicles which tend to be symmetrically distributed on the extensor surfaces of the limbs and over the scalp, buttocks, and back. Any patient over 40 or 50 years of age who has a dermatitis herpetiformis–like disorder which is atypical and which does not respond well to sulfone or sulfapyridine therapy should be suspected of having an occult malignant process. This situation is distinctly uncommon.

Seborrheic keratoses, multiple, sudden-onset This cutaneous lesion (sign of Leser-Trelat) is a rare occurrence, while seborrheic keratoses are very common. The suspicion of any paraneoplastic significance should be reserved for the very sudden appearance of unusually large numbers of seborrheic keratoses and/or a rapid increase in their size. This syndrome can occur along with acanthosis nigricans and may be related. No consistent tumor type has been associated with the sign of Leser-Trelat.

Dermatoses, bizarre From time to time patients present very strange skin reactions, difficult to identify, and are discovered to have a malignant process. Some of these patients appear to have a cutaneous vasculitis, but this eventually is recognized to be a lymphoma. The variety of such skin reactions is great and cannot be clearly defined. The major importance of including this category is to alert the physician to the possibility of occult malignancy in a patient who presents an unusual, or atypical, or bizarre skin reaction.

HERITABLE DISORDERS WITH SKIN MANIFESTATIONS AND THE PROPENSITY TO DEVELOP INTERNAL MALIGNANCY

The role of heredity in neoplasia is interesting and complex. At times congenital immunologic deficiency states predispose to malignancy, as does acquired immune deficiency. In other cases the relationship between the hereditary condition and neoplasia is unclear. Both types are listed here to increase the awareness of the association. The list is not complete but has been selected to include the most significant syndromes. The manifestations in the skin and other organ systems, as well as the predominant type of malignancy, are presented in Table 300-2. The reader should refer to specific discussion of these entities for more complete information.

REFERENCES

Barnes BE: Dermatomyositis and malignancy: A review of the literature. Ann Intern Med 84:68, 1976

Callen JP: Skin signs of internal malignancy, in *Cutaneous Aspects of Internal Disease*, JP Callen (ed). Chicago, Year Book, 1981, pp 207–222

———, Headington J: Bowen's and non-Bowen's squamous intraepidermal neoplasia of the skin. Relationship to internal malignancy. Arch Dermatol 116:422, 1980

Caughman W et al: Neutrophilic dermatoses of myeloproliferative disorders. J Am Acad Dermatol 9:751, 1983

Crocker AC: The histiocytosis syndromes, in *Dermatology in General Medicine*, 3d ed, TB Fitzpatrick et al (eds). New York, McGraw-Hill, 1987

DiGiovanna JJ, Safai B: Kaposi's sarcoma: Retrospective study of 90 cases with particular emphasis on the familial occurrence, ethnic background, and prevalence of other diseases. Am J Med 71:779, 1981

Friedman-Kien AE, Green JB: The acquired immune-deficiency syndrome, in *Update V, Harrison's Principles of Internal Medicine*, RG Petersdorf et al (eds). New York, McGraw-Hill, 1984

Kahan RS et al: Necrolytic migratory erythema. Distinctive dermatosis of the glucagonoma syndrome. Arch Dermatol 113:792, 1977

Lewis SJ et al: Atypical pyoderma gangreenosum with leukemia. JAMA 239:935, 1978

McLean DJ, Haynes HA: Cutaneous manifestations associated with malignant internal disease, in *Dermatology in General Medicine*, 3d ed, TB Fitzpatrick et al (eds). New York, McGraw-Hill, 1987

Minna JD, Bunn PA Jr: Paraneoplastic syndromes, in *Cancer, Principles and Practice of Oncology*, VT DeVita Jr, et al (ed). Philadelphia, Lippincott, 1985, pp 1823–1842

Rigel DS, Jacobs MI: Malignant acanthosis nigricans: A review. J Dermatol Surg Oncol 6:923, 1980

Stone SP, Schroeter AL: Bullous pemphigoid and associated malignant neoplasms. Arch Dermatol 111:991, 1975

301 PRIMARY CANCER OF THE SKIN

HARLEY A. HAYNES

Carcinoma of the skin is the most common carcinoma occurring in white individuals. Inasmuch as the lesions can be seen with the naked eye when they are in an early stage, the potential for cure is well over 90 percent. Although not responsible for all carcinomas of the skin, chronic exposure to ultraviolet radiation of the sunburn wavelengths (290 to 320 nm) in individuals not protected by intense melanin pigmentation is the most important single etiologic factor (Chap. 52). Hence, most of these cancers occur on areas of the skin that remain uncovered when the individual is fully clothed. As discussed in Chap. 52, genetic factors markedly mediate this tendency for carcinogenesis. Heritable diseases such as albinism, xeroderma pigmentosum, and the nevoid–basal-cell carcinoma syndrome are less common conditions associated with a greater risk of skin cancer. The routine local use of effective sun-screen preparations by individuals at risk can undoubtedly reduce tumor incidence. Chemical carcinogens, especially inorganic arsenicals and certain organic hydrocarbons, are separate and additional causes of skin cancers, particularly of the squamous-cell variety. Chemical and ultraviolet (UV) carcinogenesis may share some mechanisms as UV radiation is both an initiator and a promotor of carcinoma of the skin. Ionizing radiation, including x-rays, grenz rays, and gamma rays, is also carcinogenic. As with other organ systems, the skin is predisposed to the development of malignant lesions in immunologic deficiency states, such as those associated with lymphoma or immunosuppressive therapy. In fact, there is increasing evidence that UV radiation of the skin is in itself immunosuppressive by several mechanisms: (1) destruction of lymphocyte-activating Ia antigens on the surface of lymphoid cells, (2) impairment of antigen-processing function, (3) induction of suppressor lymphocytes that prevent the rejection of UV-induced tumors in mice, and (4) depletion from the epidermis of functional Langerhans cells, the bone marrow–derived dendritic cells which serve as the sentinel cells for contact dermatitis and other types of delayed hypersensitivity. Although any of the cell types in the skin may give rise to malignant neoplasms, the most common are basal cell and squamous cell carcinomas.

BASAL CELL CARCINOMA Basal cell carcinoma accounts for over 75 percent of all skin cancers. These carcinomas arise from the epidermis, cytologically resemble the normal basal cells, and show little tendency to undergo the usual differentiation into squamous cells which produce keratin. Although these tumors very rarely metastasize, they are locally invasive and, if neglected, may invade widely and deeply into underlying structures, including nerves, bone, and brain. Like most cancers these tumors are remarkably painless in their course. This lack of symptoms often leads to prolonged neglect of a lesion. The typical basal cell carcinoma is a noninflamed, smooth, waxy nodule that appears translucent, usually has numerous telangiectatic vessels visible near the surface, and may have variable amounts of melanin pigment in the form of small dots. Such nodules often ulcerate and form a crust. This ulceration may reepithelialize, causing the patient to assume that the nodule is resolving. Basal cell carcinomas may take many other forms, including subtle infiltrating lesions that do not produce elevated nodules, as well as fibrosing lesions resembling cicatrices. Biopsy for confirmation of the diagnosis should be routine. The patient with one basal cell carcinoma is likely to have others, either at the same time or in following years. Some patients come to the physician with a dozen or more concurrent primary basal cell carcinomas. Although there is no visible premalignant lesion that precedes a basal cell carcinoma, the lesion is usually seen in patients who manifest the stigmata of skin damage from sunlight (or x-rays). Treatment is selected according to the size, depth, type, and location of the lesion; the age, gender, and complexion of the patient; and the particular abilities of the physician. If a simple excision will suffice, there is no other procedure that can equal the cosmetic result. Curettage and electrodesiccation for small lesions give a cure rate of more than 95 percent in experienced hands, as does x-ray treatment. Cryosurgery with liquid nitrogen seems to give cure rates similar to those of curettage and electrodesiccation and often yields a better cosmetic result. The specialized technique of microscopically controlled serial shave excision (Mohs' technique) gives the highest cure rate known (about 99 percent) and is recommended for difficult or recurrent lesions not manageable by the usual forms of therapy. Local chemotherapy with 5-fluorouracil is not recommended as routine treatment of basal cell carcinomas, but may have a role in the treatment of multiple superficial lesions. Immunotherapy is investigational.

Education of the patient as to the role of UV radiation and strategies to reduce future such exposure by proper clothing, avoidance of noonday sun, and regular use of potent sunscreens with a sun protection factor (SPF) of 15 is important. Physician follow-up at 6- to 12-month intervals for 5 years following each new carcinoma of the skin is desirable. Recurrences of treated basal cell carcinomas occur within 5 years in 97 percent of recurrent lesions and will be seen in 3 to 5 percent of all treated lesions. More importantly, the patient with a previous carcinoma of the skin is at high risk for the development of additional such lesions.

SQUAMOUS CELL CARCINOMA Squamous cell carcinoma also arises from the epidermis but shows significant squamous differentiation and usually keratin production. These tumors have a variable tendency to metastasize, depending upon their size, extent of invasion, location, and whether they arise from a premalignant lesion, a burn scar, a chronic inflammatory condition, or from apparently normal skin. The typical squamous cell carcinoma is a painless, firm, red nodule or plaque with visible scales on the surface. Ulceration and crusting may occur. Relatively undifferentiated lesions that do not produce much keratin may fail to show noticeable scaling on the surface. In contrast to the basal cell variety, squamous cell carcinomas most commonly arise from preexisting *actinic* or *solar keratoses.* These premalignant keratoses are scaly, rough, red plaques that occur in chronically sun-damaged skin. Although very few of these keratoses progress to carcinoma, most squamous cell carcinomas on exposed skin do arise from such keratoses. This type of squamous cell carcinoma has the lowest frequency of metastasis (under 2 percent). However, because of the potential of malignant change in solar keratoses, which though small is real, it seems prudent to remove them, especially in younger patients. At present, the local application of 5-fluorouracil (1 to 5%) in cream or lotion seems to be the most effective method and one that generally produces no scarring. Cryosurgery with liquid nitrogen is also effective, but carries a higher risk of scarring. Squamous cell carcinomas arising from mucous membranes, mucocutaneous junctions, burn scars, chronic ulcers, or sinus tracts or from apparently normal skin have a much higher tendency to metastasize. An in situ stage of cutaneous squamous cell carcinoma is known as Bowen's disease (Chap. 300). Although some of these in situ lesions are the result of chronic sun damage, a significant proportion occurs in patients who had received inorganic arsenic preparations either accidentally or for medicinal purposes a decade or more before. In these patients there is also an increased risk of carcinomas of the respiratory, genitourinary, and gastrointestinal systems.

Patients with squamous cell carcinoma must be examined carefully for the presence of metastases so that therapy may be appropriate. In the absence of metastases, therapy of the local lesion may generally be as indicated for basal cell carcinoma, with preference for surgical excision or x-irradiation in view of the potential for metastasis. Extensive local or metastatic lesions may benefit from systemic chemotherapy, sometimes via local perfusion.

Patients with squamous cell carcinoma should be instructed in methods of reducing their UV radiation exposure, and should be followed for a minimum of 5 years to check for local recurrence, additional new primary lesions, and the infrequent development of metastatic disease.

MYCOSIS FUNGOIDES LYMPHOMA *Lymphoma of the skin* may be a primary or secondary manifestation of various types of lymphoma. Histiocytic lymphoma and lymphoblastic lymphoma may occasionally begin with only skin lesions, but Hodgkin's disease rarely does so. The most common lymphoma of the skin is *mycosis fungoides,* which always begins with cutaneous lesions, usually with no evidence of visceral infiltration for several years. The initial lesions may be clinically confused with eczema, contact dermatitis, or psoriasis, and the biopsy may not be diagnostic. Later, more typical patches of infiltrated skin develop, often with a tendency for central clearing or an arciform or polycyclic arrangement. At this point, the biopsy may be diagnostic. In some patients, diffuse exfoliative erythroderma develops, and there may be circulating mycosis fungoides cells in the blood, at times causing diagnostic confusion with chronic lymphocytic leukemia. The skin biopsy may resolve the confusion if it is sufficiently characteristic, as may electron microscopy of the atypical cells, which are quite distinct in mycosis fungoides. The atypical cells found in the skin appear to be the same cells found in the blood or in visceral infiltrates. These cells have been identified as thymus-dependent lymphocytes and are usually of the helper/inducer type as determined by the monoclonal antibody technique. In blood smears these cells resemble large lymphocytes with scant cytoplasm and folded nuclei. In routine tissue sections these cells sometimes look like lymphocytes and sometimes like reticulum cells with the characteristic infolded nucleus. Electron-microscopic examination shows the nucleus of this cell to be highly irregular, convoluted, lobulated, and drawn into narrow threads and ribbons. At some point in time, most patients develop larger tumors as well. Although any of the viscera may be affected, disability from internal involvement usually does not occur until quite late in the course of the disease. For a patient with the early stage of the disease, the prognosis is for survival for several decades. Once the histologic diagnosis of mycosis fungoides is confirmed, the median survival for all patients is 5 years. Patients with skin tumors, ulceration, or lymphatic involvement have a median survival of 30 months.

Treatment is best planned so as to not restrict unnecessarily the future options of therapy. Topical applications of dilute, nonvesicant concentrations of mechlorethamine are often very effective for months or even years. Photochemotherapy with psoralens and long-wave UV radiation (PUVA) is often helpful (see Chap. 300). Selected lesions can be treated with grenz rays. Whole-skin electron beam treatment may be given without hematologic suppression, since the voltage is regulated to control the depth of penetration of electrons. The use of orthovoltage x-irradiation of multiple sites should be carefully restricted, so as not to compromise the marrow or complicate further therapy with electron beam. Electron beam followed by topical mechlorethamine is probably the most effective therapy for disease limited to cutaneous plaques. Systemic chemotherapy with agents such as methotrexate, cyclophosphamide, vinca alkaloids, procarbazine, chlorambucil, steroids, and combinations of these agents often can cause dramatic objective regression of disease but has not yet been proved to prolong life expectancy. Even though most patients at necropsy are found to have infiltrates in various viscera, early systemic chemotherapy has not been found advantageous, as a rule, perhaps because of the adverse effect of such therapy on the clinically very apparent resistance of the host to this lymphoma. In fact, this lymphoma was the first human malignancy to regularly show regression of lesions that were challenged locally with delayed hypersensitivity reactions.

REFERENCES

BURN PA JR et al: Prospective staging evaluation of patients with cutaneous T-cell lymphomas: Demonstration of a high frequency of extracutaneous dissemination. Ann Intern Med 93:223, 1980

EDELSON RL: Cutaneous T-cell lymphoma (mycosis fungoides, Sézary syndrome, and related presentations), in *Update: Dermatology in General Medicine,* TB Fitzpatrick et al (eds). New York, McGraw-Hill, 1983, pp 143–158

FITZPATRICK TB et al (eds): Neoplasms of the dermis, in *Dermatology in General Medicine,* 3d ed. New York, McGraw-Hill, 1987

GRANSTEIN RD, SOBER AJ: Current concepts in ultraviolet carcinogenesis. Proc Soc Exp Biol Med 170:115, 1982

HAYNES HA et al: Cancers of the skin, in *Cancer, Principles and Practice of Oncology,* 2d ed, VT DeVita Jr et al: (eds). Philadelphia, Lippincott, 1985

HONIGSMANN H et al: Photochemotherapy for cutaneous T-cell lymphoma. A follow-up study. J Am Acad Dermatol 10:238, 1984

MCDONALD CJ, BERTINO JR: Treatment of mycosis fungoides lymphoma—effectiveness of infusions of methotrexate followed by oral citrovorum factor. Cancer Treat Rep 62:1009, 1978

PRICE NM et al: Ointment-based mechlorethamine treatment for mycosis fungoides. Cancer 52:2214, 1983

302 MALIGNANT MELANOMA OF THE SKIN

THOMAS B. FITZPATRICK / ARTHUR J. SOBER / MARTIN C. MIHM, JR.

Primary malignant melanoma of the skin is the leading cause of death from all diseases arising in the skin, and the detection of early lesions must be the task of every physician, regardless of specialty. At every occasion when the entire cutaneous surface can be viewed, a careful search for suspicious pigmented lesions should be made.

Pigmented moles are among the most common growths on the skin, and yet cancer involving pigment cells (i.e., malignant melanoma) is relatively uncommon, constituting about 2 percent of all cancers. There has been a disturbing increase in the incidence of primary melanoma of the skin. The rate has doubled in the past 10 years, possibly due to increased "weekend" exposure to sunlight, especially among persons in professional and managerial positions. During 1985, 22,000 cutaneous melanomas are estimated for the population of the United States. Primary cutaneous malignant melanoma, moreover, does not respond or responds only poorly to chemotherapy or radiation therapy, and, so far, hope for survival has been based on surgical excision during the very early primary stages before deep invasion occurs. The problem for the physician, therefore, is to recognize early primary malignant melanoma and also those precancerous lesions that will develop into malignant melanoma among the large number of pigmented lesions that occur on the skin.

Primary malignant melanoma of the skin, even in the early stages, is now considered relatively easy to detect by clinical examination alone. In the past, the clinical description of primary cutaneous malignant melanoma was presented incompletely. Physicians and patients were told to have concern only for those pigmented lesions that showed changes in growth pattern or color or were bleeding or ulcerated—criteria indicating deep invasion in the skin and, usually, a poor prognosis.

Follow-up study of more than 1100 patients with primary melanoma has provided evidence indicating that a primary cutaneous melanoma may exist in a "silent," intraepidermal, preinvasive form for several years. These early "silent" primary malignant melanomas, even when 3 to 4 mm in size, can be recognized by certain simple criteria, which are delineated below.

Two criteria, *variegation of color* and *irregular border* often with a "notch," are so characteristic of primary cutaneous malignant melanoma that histologic examination is advised when they are present. The important colors that are signs of primary malignant melanoma *include shades of red, white, or blue* and the shades resulting from their mixture with brown or black. Furthermore, a lesion may be uniformly colored, e.g., *bluish black or bluish red.*

The diagnostic significance of various shades of brown or black, or both, in pigmented primary cutaneous malignant melanoma has been stressed in the past. It is, however, the diagnostic significance of the various shades of red, white, or blue, or all three mixed with brown or black, that requires emphasis. Of the colors present in pigmented primary cutaneous malignant melanomas, shades of blue (bluish red, bluish gray, and bluish black) are the most significant in the diagnosis. Variegation in the pigment pattern with unevenness and disarray is another important sign. *Examination with a magnifying lens and bright lighting* may assist greatly in recognizing the diagnostic feature of melanoma (Table 302-1).

Before 1967, malignant melanoma was considered a single morphologic entity with a uniformly grave prognosis. Later histopathologic investigations, especially by Clark, McGovern, Mihm, and colleagues, have permitted a new approach to the classification of primary human cutaneous malignant melanomas, based on the correlation of the clinical and histologic features with prognosis. Four types of primary malignant melanoma have been delineated (Table 302-2) and have been placed in two groups, depending on the presence or absence of an adjacent intraepidermal component around the tumor nodule:

Malignant melanoma with adjacent intraepidermal component:

1 Superficial spreading melanoma
2 Lentigo maligna melanoma
3 Acral lentiginous melanoma

Malignant melanoma without an adjacent intraepidermal component:

4 Nodular melanoma

It should be emphasized that lentigo maligna melanoma and superficial spreading melanoma may exist for several years in the preinvasive stage. Hence, early diagnosis of malignant melanoma of the skin makes excision of the identified lesions possible before deep invasion has occurred. The survival rate of malignant melanoma is related to the level of invasion of the tumor or the thickness of the primary tumor expressed in millimeters (see Table 302-3). These levels of invasion have been classified on the basis of anatomic structure as follows:

TABLE 302-1 Indications for excision or diagnostic biopsy of pigmented lesions

I History
  A Change in size or color, bleeding
  B Symptoms
    1 Itching (25%)
    2 Tenderness
  C Congenital, raised pigmented lesions
II Lesion characteristics
  A Color
    1 Uniform blue or gray
    2 Variegated: blue, gray, white, red, mixed with brown or black
    3 Variegation in pigment pattern
  B Border: irregular, often with a notch
  C Surface: irregular

TABLE 302-2 Clinical features of malignant melanoma

Type	Site	Average age at diagnosis, years	Duration of known existence, years	
Superficial spreading melanoma	Any site (more common on upper back and in women on lower legs)	40–50	1–7	Shades of brown and black mixed with bluish red (violaceous), bluish black, reddish brown, and often whitish pink, and the border of lesion is at least in part visibly and/or palpably elevated
Lentigo maligna melanoma	Exposed surfaces usually, and particularly malar region of cheek and temple	70	5–20* or longer	In flat portions, shades of brown and black predominant, but whitish gray occasionally present; in nodules, shades of reddish brown, bluish gray, bluish black
Acral lentiginous melanoma	Palm, sole, nailbed, mucous membrane	64	1–10	In flat portions, dark brown predominantly; in raised lesions (plaques), brown-black or blue-black color predominantly
Nodular melanoma	Any site	40–50	Months to less than 5 years	Reddish blue (purple) or bluish black, either uniform in color or mixed with brown or black

* *During much of this time the precursor stage, lentigo maligna, is actively confined to the epidermis.*

Level 1: Intraepidermal melanocytic atypism, a level recognized for purposes of research. Patients with this finding are at present labeled with the diagnosis melanoma in situ by some pathologists and severely atypical intraepidermal melanocytic hyperplasia by others.
Level 2: Tumor invading the papillary layer but not extending to the reticular layer.
Level 3: Tumor filling and expanding the papillary layer but not invading the reticular layer.
Level 4: Tumor penetrating into the reticular layer of the dermis.
Level 5: Tumor invading the subcutaneous fat.

When thickness of the primary tumor is determined by measuring the vertical thickness with a light microscope fitted with an ocular micrometer, tumors measuring less than 0.85 mm in thickness have a uniformly favorable outcome, while patients with tumors greater than 3.65 mm are at high risk for recurrent disease and death. At the present time, the determination of prognosis by thickness is the most practical (see Table 302-3 for survival by thickness).

Suspicious lesions require biopsy, which will confirm the benign or malignant nature of the lesion. Simple excisional biopsy with narrow margins is the procedure of choice, but trephine (punch) or incisional biopsies are also acceptable depending on the situation and the experience of the physician performing the procedure. Table 302-1 lists the indications for biopsy of cutaneous lesions.

TABLE 302-3 Summary data on malignant melanoma of skin

I Incidence: 2% of all cancers (excluding nonmelanoma skin cancer)
- *A* Annual incidence rates (United States) for 1985: 22,000
- *B* Increasing with time (Connecticut Registry)
  - *1* 1935–1939: 1.2/10^5/year
  - *2* 1965–1969: 4.8/10^5/year
  - *3* 1976–1977: 7.2/10^5/year
  - *4* 1979–1980: 9/10^5/year
- *C* Latitude-dependent crude incidence rates:
  - *1* Northern United States (Connecticut):9/10^5/year
  - 2 Southern United States (Arizona):26/10^5/year

II Frequency for type of melanoma
- *A* Superficial spreading: 70%
- *B* Nodular: 16%
- *C* Lentigo maligna melanoma: 5%
- *D* Unclassified (includes acral lentiginous type): 10%

III Five-year survival
- *A* Stage III (distant metastases): <10%
- *B* Stage II (regional lymph nodes clinically enlarged): 30%
- *C* Stage I (clinically localized disease): 85%
  - *1* Based on level of invasion
    - *a* Level 2: 99%
    - *b* Level 3: 95%
    - *c* Level 4: 75%
    - *d* Level 5: 39%
  - 2 Based on thickness of primary tumor
    - *a* <0.85 mm: 99%
    - *b* 0.85–1.69 mm: 94%
    - *c* 1.70–3.60 mm: 78%
    - *d* ≥3.65 mm: 42%

Treatment of malignant melanoma at the present is primarily by surgical excision of the primary lesion; there is no agreement as to whether prophylactic lymph node dissection affects the course of the disease. Data of Breslow and Macht suggest that limited excision may be effective for thin (≤0.75 mm) lesions. We have been recommending surgical margins of 1.5 cm for tumors smaller than 0.85 mm and margins of up to 3 cm for tumors greater than 0.85 mm. Elective lymph node dissection is considered when the tumor drains to only one lymph node group in patients with primary tumors thicker than 1.7 to 2.0 mm. Age, patient preference, and convictions of the surgeon are also factors which are weighed in the decision to perform elective nodal dissection. No benefit from dissection has mostly been shown in randomized trials. However, retrospective or nonrandomized prospective trials show a small benefit in survival favoring patients who have received node dissection. Surgery for lentigo maligna melanoma is less aggressive; the recommendation is for surgical margins of 1 cm and lymph node dissection only if therapeutically indicated.

In the past few years, considerable interest has been directed toward the factors that influence both the development of primary malignant melanomas of the skin and also the rate and degree of dissemination of the tumor. The possibility that there is a population with a high risk for the development of these melanomas is being studied. It is suspected that persons, both male and female, who have poor tolerance to sunlight and who develop sunburn on short exposures and who tan poorly have a higher incidence of malignant melanoma (Table 302-3). Risk for melanoma is increased by having had blistering sunburns in childhood or adolescence. It has recently been demonstrated that within countries an inverse relationship exists between melanoma incidence and latitude. For example, incidence rates of 9 per 100,000 per year in Connecticut can be contrasted to rates greater than 20 per 100,000 per year in the white population of the southwestern United States.

Families have been studied in the members of which malignant melanomas have aggregated. Many of these family members appear to have a type of nevus which resembles clinically miniature early superficial spreading melanomas. These lesions, termed *dysplastic nevi,* may be a genetically determined precursor lesion for malignant melanomas. The dysplastic nevus also occurs sporadically in patients with malignant melanoma and is currently thought to be the associated precursor lesion in up to 40 percent of cases. (For clinical illustrations of dysplastic nevi, see Greene et al.) Patients with large congenital melanocytic nevi are also at recognized higher risk for melanoma development in these lesions.

Several well recognized patterns of spread are observed for cutaneous melanoma. The most frequent pathway of spread is up the lymphatic channels within the skin to produce satellite, intransit, and regional nodal metastases. This pattern of recurrence tends to occur earlier than the second pattern of spread—hematogenous, blood-borne metastases to distant sites (cutaneous and/or visceral). Preferential visceral sites include liver, lung, bone, and brain, and perhaps half of the deaths from melanoma can now be attributed to central nervous system metastases.

Currently about 80 to 90 percent of patients present with clinical stage I disease (localized disease). Work-up for dissemination should include a detailed history and physical examination and a chest x-ray. Other studies should be obtained (scans, other biopsies, liver function tests) if there is a suggestion of disease at a location other than the primary site. Follow-up involves careful evaluation of the operative sites for local recurrence, palpation of the skin for intransit or disseminated intracutaneous metastases, palpation of lymph node areas, palpation of viscera, and a complete cutaneous examination to look for second primary tumors.

Only a few factors are presently known to influence the dissemination of melanoma. Incidence of melanoma by sex is equal, but the death rate is higher among men. When multifactorial analyses are performed, the primary tumor site appears to be important in outcome. Torso lesions have a worse prognosis than lower extremity lesions. The most common site for melanoma in males is the torso. The immune status of the patient is another factor under investigation. The possibility that immunologic factors are involved in the course of malignant melanoma is suggested by the high rate of spontaneous regressions of melanoma, by the long periods of freedom from the time of excision of the primary lesion to the development of metastases, and by the improved prognosis of those lesions in which on histologic examination a marked lymphocytic response is found. Both cellular and hormonal immunities to melanoma cells have been demonstrated by in vitro techniques.

The management of metastatic disease presents real problems since chemo- and immunotherapeutic techniques are ineffective in the majority of patients. The most effective single agent, dacarbazine (dimethyltriazenoimidazole carboxamide or DTIC), induces a partial remission in only 20 percent and complete responses in less than 5 percent of cases. Remissions are usually of only a few months duration. Many experimental chemotherapeutic combinations are now undergoing clinical trial. At the present time the best strategy in the management of melanoma is early recognition, which will prevent the development of metastases.

The physician examining a patient with many pigmented lesions should recognize the features that are highly suggestive of primary melanoma of the skin and indicate that the lesion be removed, or, if it is very large, at least biopsied (see Table 302-1). If these early lesions can be detected and excised, the 5-year survival rate of patients with malignant melanoma should approach 90 to 95 percent.

REFERENCES

Balch CM et al: Tumor thickness as a guide to surgical management of clinical stage I melanoma patients. Cancer 43:883, 1979

———, Milton GW: *Cutaneous Melanoma*. Philadelphia, Lippincott, 1985

Breslow A, Macht SD: Optimum size of resection margin for thin cutaneous melanoma. Surg Gynecol Obstet 145:691, 1977

Day CL Jr et al: The natural breakpoints for primary tumor thickness in clinical stage I melanoma. N Engl J Med 305:1155, 1981

———: Prognostic factors for melanoma patients with lesions 0.76 through 1.69 mm in thickness: An appraisal of thin level IV lesions. Ann Surg 195:30, 1982

Greene MH et al: Acquired precursors of cutaneous malignant melanoma: The familial dysplastic nevus syndrome. N Engl J Med 312:91, 1985

Mihm MC Jr et al: Early detection of primary cutaneous malignant melanoma: Color atlas. N Engl J Med 289:989, 1973

Reimer RR et al: Precursor lesions in familial melanoma. JAMA 239:744, 1978

Sober AJ et al: Early recognition of cutaneous melanoma. JAMA 242:2795, 1979

———: Primary melanoma of the skin: Recognition and management. J Am Acad Dermatol 2:179, 1980

———: Primary melanoma of the skin: Recognition of precursor lesions and estimation of prognosis in stage I, in *Update: Dermatology in General Medicine*, TB Fitzpatrick et al (eds). New York, McGraw-Hill, 1983

Veronesi U et al: Inefficacy of immediate node dissection in stage I melanoma of the limbs. N Engl J Med 297:627, 1977

303 ENDOCRINE MANIFESTATIONS OF NEOPLASIA

LAWRENCE A. FROHMAN

Hormone secretion by tumors derived from nonendocrine tissue has been recognized for more than 50 years. Initially, the majority of reported cases were associated with hypoglycemia and hypercalcemia, but the term *ectopic hormone secretion* was first used in relation to Cushing's syndrome caused by adrenocorticotropic hormone (ACTH) secretion from a variety of tumors. The spectrum of ectopic hormone secretion is now expanded as a result of increased clinical awareness and the availability of more sophisticated and sensitive assay techniques. However, the use of the term *ectopic* in this regard has been questioned with the recognition that hormones once believed to be tissue-specific may have widespread sites of production, i.e., gonadotropins are produced by the normal gonad and intestine, thyrotropin-releasing hormone (TRH) and ACTH by the pancreas, and somatostatin by the kidney and thyroid C cells. Nevertheless, the original term serves to distinguish tumor-associated hormone production from syndromes due to excess secretion of the major and characteristic hormone of a particular endocrine tissue.

THEORIES OF ECTOPIC HORMONE SECRETION Several possible pathogenetic mechanisms have been proposed to explain ectopic hormone secretion. The "sponge" theory assumed a selective update of the circulating hormone by tumor tissue with subsequent release upon tumor cell death. This concept was abandoned, however, after the demonstration of arteriovenous differences of hormones across tumor vascular beds and of hormone biosynthesis by tumor preparation in vitro. The theory that random mutations resulted in abnormal DNA sequences and gene products was also discounted when it became apparent that the production of ectopic hormones by tumors is not random, i.e., that certain tumors produce specific endocrinopathies. A third theory, that of gene derepression, proposed that regions of the genome not normally expressed become active and are transcribed in tumors presumably as a result of loss of a normal suppressive mechanism during neoplastic transformation; in fact, however, there is no overall increase in gene transcription (derepression) in neoplastic cells. Two other explanations have also been proposed: *cellular dedifferentiation*, a theory that neoplastic cells revert to a more primitive level and again produce peptide hormones that were produced normally at an earlier developmental stage, and *arrested differentiation*, whereby hormone secretion is due to persistence of a function present during development because of a failure (arrest) of the developmental process. Arguments against these theories include an absence of evidence that cells can retrace their pathways of differentiation or that incompletely differentiated cells routinely secrete the hormone in question. The pathogenesis of ectopic hormone secretion is thus unclear.

CRITERIA FOR DIAGNOSIS Criteria for the diagnosis of ectopic hormone secretion have changed as more sophisticated laboratory methodology has made it possible to recognize clinically inapparent cases (Table 303-1). Although many of these criteria cannot be

TABLE 303-1 Criteria for establishing the diagnosis of ectopic hormone secretion

1. Association of a nonendocrine neoplasm with a syndrome attributable to excessive hormone secretion or with inappropriately elevated plasma and/or urine hormone levels
2. Failure of plasma and/or urine hormone levels to respond to normal homeostatic suppression
3. Exclusion of other possible causal mechanisms for hormone hypersecretion
4. Reduction in hormone levels after tumor-specific therapy
5. Arteriovenous step-up gradients across tumor
6. Demonstration of hormone in tumor tissue
7. Biosynthesis and/or secretion of hormone by tumor tissue in vitro
8. Demonstration in the tumor of hormone-specific messenger RNA by cell-free translation or by hybridization with cDNA

satisfied in individual cases, the majority have been fulfilled in the commonly recognized syndromes.

TUMOR TYPES ASSOCIATED WITH ECTOPIC HORMONE SECRETION Ectopic secretion of hormones is associated with a large variety of tumors. Although original reports of these syndromes described primarily lung carcinomas, carcinoids, thymomas, and fibrosarcomas, virtually all tumor types have the potential of hormone secretion. Nevertheless, the frequency of occurrence of ectopic hormone secretion among various tumor types is not random. The tumors most frequently associated with clinically recognized ectopic hormone production are small cell lung carcinomas, carcinoids, and pancreatic islet tumors. Carcinoid tumors are generally found in the lung or in the gastrointestinal tract. Gastrointestinal carcinoids may be present in either the foregut or the hindgut, though it is primarily those in the former location that are hormonally active and tend to be malignant. In the lung these tumors are usually endobronchial and may remain undetected for long periods of time. There are many morphologic similarities between bronchial carcinoid tumors and small cell carcinoma of the lung. Indeed, the two types may have a common cell of origin, namely the Kulchitsky cell, a bronchial mucosal cell that has been called a neuroendocrine cell of the lung because of its peptide-containing granules observed on electron microscopy. Bombesin (gastrin-releasing peptide) or a bombesin-like peptide is present in Kulchitsky cells during fetal life and is the most frequent peptide produced by small cell carcinoma of the lung. Ectopic hormone secretion is also associated with other types of lung tumors, most commonly the squamous type of bronchogenic carcinomas.

In the 1960s Pearse proposed the theory that certain hormone-secreting cells are components of a "diffuse neuroendocrine system". Such cells were originally considered to be of neural crest or neuroectodermal origin, and were designated APUD (amine precursor uptake and decarboxylation) cells on the basis of their ability to decarboxylate precursors of biogenic amines. Later it was discovered that many of these cells also produce the enzyme neuron-specific enolase. A corollary of the APUD theory was that tumors derived from APUD cells had the capability of hormone secretion. At present, there is doubt concerning the validity of the APUD theory on several grounds. First, all APUD cells are not of neuroectodermal origin. Second, the APUD function of these cells is not inherently linked with peptide hormone production, and third, some ectopic hormone-secreting tumors do not possess APUD characteristics. Nevertheless, the association of particular tumor types with the secretion of certain hormones is useful in evaluating these syndromes.

CHARACTERIZATION OF ECTOPIC HORMONES **Type of hormone secreted** Of the four classes of hormones—steroids, monoamines, substituted amino acids, and peptides/proteins—only the latter are secreted ectopically. Although the explanation is not known with certainty, the ectopic production of peptide/protein hormones may require less complicated derangements in cell metabolism. For example, an oncogene containing an initiator or inducer of gene transcription may be responsible for the expression of a gene coding for a peptide hormone. In contrast, the synthesis of steroids, thyroid hormones, or monoamines requires multiple enzymatic steps and specifically targeted translocation of the precursor molecules through various cell compartments. The likelihood that this degree of cell specialization would occur as a consequence of neoplastic change is much less than the possibility that a process (protein synthesis) common to all cells might be initiated aberrantly.

Ectopic secretion of nearly all peptide hormones has been reported. These hormones may be grouped according to their usual site of origin (Table 303-2). The first group of hormones, common to the central nervous system and gastrointestinal tract, are most frequently secreted by carcinoids, small cell lung carcinomas, and pancreatic islet tumors. The second group, normally produced by the fetoplacental unit and/or the anterior pituitary, tends to be produced by gastrointestinal, hepatic, adrenal, and gonadal tumors. The third group, which includes insulin-like growth factors and parathyroid hormone–like factors, tends to be produced by mesenchymal, hepatic, genitourinary, and squamous cell lung tumors. In addition to the hormones listed, other humoral factors are believed responsible for tumor-associated syndromes such as hypertrophic osteoarthropathy, polyneuropathy, hypophosphatemic osteomalacia, and anorexia.

Relation to naturally secreted hormones The primary amino acid sequences of all ectopically secreted hormones analyzed to date are identical to those of the native hormones. However, other differences in structure between ectopically secreted and native hormones can occur as a result of incomplete or abnormal processing of the precursor hormone. Several abnormal forms of ectopic hormones have been defined: (1) large-molecular-weight species due to incomplete enzymatic cleavage of the precursor; (2) small-molecular-weight fragments due to unregulated intracellular processing; and (3) altered glycosylation species (microheterogeneity) due either to failed cleavage of carbohydrate residues during postribosomal hormone processing (glycosylated ACTH) or failure of normal glycosylation (the glycosylated alpha subunit common to the gonadotropins and TSH). The usual consequence is a hormone variant with diminished or aberrant biologic activity. If modification of hormone structure is sufficient to cause loss of all biologic activity, ectopic secretion is not accompanied by clinical manifestations. Even if a neoplastic cell can synthesize and store a biologically active hormone, a syndrome of hormone excess may not result if an intact secretory mechanism is absent. The frequency with which either an inactive hormone is synthesized or an active hormone is synthesized but not secreted is probably greater than that of classical ectopic hormone secretion since only a small percentage of tumors that contain ectopic hormones cause clinically recognizable syndromes.

Other considerations Hormones may be secreted by both benign and malignant tumors. Although hormone secretion normally requires a high level of cellular differentiation, an incompletely differentiated tumor may still be able to secrete some hormone. For example, the process of granule formation and hormone storage is not generally expressed by hormone-secreting tumors; consequently the concentration of hormone in the tumor is usually low compared to that in endocrine glands. Overall hormone secretion per unit weight is also less and, as a result, considerable tumor mass is usually present before ectopic hormone secretion is clinically apparent. One notable exception is the relatively benign, highly differentiated neoplasm, usually a carcinoid or pancreatic islet tumor, that contains and secretes hormone at a level comparable to that of normal endocrine tissue and that is sufficiently small to escape detection for long periods.

Many tumors produce multiple hormones. In some this is due to the existence of a common precursor for multiple hormones, e.g., ACTH, lipotropins, melanocyte-stimulating hormones (MSHs), and endorphins are all derived from a single precursor, proopiomelanocortin (POMC), and both vasoactive intestinal peptide (VIP) and peptide histidyl-methionine (PHM) are encoded in a single precursor. In other instances multiple hormones are produced in the absence of common precursors, e.g., production of ACTH, calcitonin, and somatostatin by medullary thyroid carcinoma and by small cell carcinoma of the lung. In some tumors separate cells secrete individual hormones, whereas in others multiple hormones are produced by the same cell. Furthermore, variation may occur in cell lines cloned from such tumors, suggesting that gene expression may change with succeeding generations of tumor cells.

FREQUENCY The frequency of ectopic hormone secretion varies with the criteria used for its definition. The most frequently encountered syndromes are those of ACTH hypersecretion, hypercalcemia, and organic hypoglycemia. Ectopic ACTH secretion occurs in approximately 15 to 20 percent of patients with Cushing's syndrome. Thus, consideration of this diagnosis is of great importance. Similarly, nearly half of patients with hypercalcemia unrelated to volume depletion, excess ingestion of vitamin D, or sarcoidosis have a malignancy rather than hyperparathyroidism, and of these about 70

TABLE 303-2 Spectrum of ectopic hormone production

Group/hormone	Tumor type: Common	Tumor type: Infrequent
1 Neuroendocrine-gastrointestinal		
a ACTH, β-lipotropin, endorphins, MSHs, enkephalins	Lung carcinoma (small cell) Thymoma Pancreatic islet tumors Carcinoid Thyroid medullary carcinoma Pheochromocytoma Parotid tumor Prostatic carcinoma Renal carcinoma	Squamous cell, adenocarcinoma, and large cell carcinoma of the lung Breast carcinoma Colonic carcinoma Gallbladder tumors Testicular carcinoma Uterine carcinoma Laryngeal carcinoma Plasmacytoma
b Vasopressin, oxytocin, neurophysin	Lung carcinoma (small cell, anaplastic, adenocarcinoma) Carcinoid	Pancreatic carcinoma Duodenal carcinoma
c Corticotropin-releasing factor	Lung carcinoma (small cell) Carcinoid	Pituitary gangliocytoma
d Growth hormone–releasing factor	Carcinoid Pancreatic islet adenoma Lung carcinoma (small cell)	Adrenocortical adenoma Neurofibroma Endometrial carcinoma Pheochromocytoma Pituitary gangliocytoma
e Somatostatin	Lung carcinoma (small cell) Carcinoid Pheochromocytoma	
f Calcitonin	Lung carcinoma (small cell) Carcinoid	Breast carcinoma
g Gastrin	Lung carcinoma (small cell)	Ovarian carcinoma
h Vasoactive intestinal peptide	Lung carcinoma (small cell) Pancreatic islet tumors	
i Insulin		Gastric carcinoma Lung carcinoma Carcinoid
j Glucagon		Lung carcinoma Carcinoid
k Gastrin-releasing peptide (Bombesin)	Lung carcinoma Carcinoid	
2 Fetoplacental and/or anterior pituitary		
a Chorionic gonadotropin (and subunits)	Lung carcinoma Gastric carcinoma Ovarian carcinoma Adeno- and islet cell carcinoma of the pancreas Hepatoma	Testicular carcinoma Ovarian carcinoma Adrenocortical carcinoma Breast carcinoma Bladder carcinoma Melanoma Carcinoid
b Placental lactogen	Lung carcinoma (small cell)	Lymphoma Pheochromocytoma Hepatoma
c Growth hormone		Lung carcinoma (large cell) Carcinoid Pancreatic islet tumor
d Prolactin		Lung carcinoma Renal carcinoma
3 Others		
a Tissue growth factors (somatomedins)	Mesenchymal tumors (i.e., fibrosarcoma) Hepatoma Adrenocortical carcinoma Pancreatic/bile duct carcinoma	Lung carcinoma Ovarian carcinoma Neuroblastoma Wilms's tumor
b Erythropoietin	Cerebellar hemangioblastoma Uterine fibroma Renal carcinoma	Adrenocortical carcinoma Hepatoma Pheochromocytoma
c Parathyroid hormone, osteoclast-activating factor, and humoral hypercalcemic factor of malignancy	Renal carcinoma Lung carcinoma (squamous) Hepatoma	GI tract tumors Parotid tumors Genitourinary tract tumors Melanoma Lymphoma

percent have a humoral hypercalcemic factor that is not parathyroid hormone but has parathyroid hormone–like biologic activity. In contrast, hypoglycemia due to ectopic production of an insulin-like growth factor is infrequent in patients suspected of having an insulinoma, and ectopic growth hormone–releasing factor (GRH) secretion is a rare (<1 percent) cause of acromegaly.

CONSEQUENCES OF ECTOPIC HORMONE SECRETION The consequences of ectopic hormone secretion may be of greater significance than the tumor itself. This is particularly true for patients with benign ACTH- or gastrin-producing tumors in whom fulminant Cushing's syndrome or bleeding peptic ulceration may be life-threatening. In others, the hormone may cause medical problems that shorten the life span beyond that attributable to the tumor itself, i.e., severe hypercalcemia, hyponatremia, or hypoglycemia.

The symptoms of ectopic hormone secretion may be the presenting manifestations of the neoplasm or occur late in the course of the disease. The rapidity of onset of the clinical features of hormone hypersecretion affects the frequency with which the syndrome is recognized. For example, excessive secretion of ACTH or vasopressin is clinically evident within weeks or months; thus, a fully developed syndrome can be associated with rapidly growing malignant tumors as well as with benign tumors. In contrast, acromegaly due to ectopic GRH secretion typically requires years to become apparent and therefore is observed only when caused by slowly growing malignant neoplasms. Ectopic hormone secretion, once established, does not necessarily persist for as long as the tumor is present. Hormone secretion may cease or decline to clinically insignificant levels either spontaneously or in response to radiation or chemotherapy. With tumor relapse, hormone secretion usually, but not invariably, recurs.

In addition to effects on the host, ectopic hormone secretion has numerous important biologic implications. Since tumor-secreted factors that exhibit biologic effects are unlikely to be unique substances, their identification and characterization can assist in the search for the naturally occurring (eutopic) peptide. For example, tumor-secreted GRH was the source for the purification, isolation, and structural characterization of hypothalamic GRH. Relatively little attention has been given to possible effects of ectopically secreted hormones on the growth or survival of the tumor.

DIAGNOSIS Occasionally, the clinical manifestations of ectopic hormone secretion are so distinctive that they suggest the diagnosis before any hormone measurements have been performed. The development of gynecomastia in the absence of associated diseases such as cirrhosis or testicular failure may suggest the presence of ectopic gonadotropin secretion, while Cushing's syndrome and increased pigmentation or severe muscle weakness (due to hypokalemia) point to ectopic ACTH secretion.

More commonly, however, clinical manifestations of hormone excess are subtle or absent. In such instances basal levels of hormones, e.g., ACTH, may be elevated out of proportion to the biologic effects observed. This may be the result of ACTH precursor molecules that have little or no biologic activity. Identification of these hormonal forms can be accomplished by molecular sieve chromatography or by multiple, site-specific radioimmunoassays. Similarly, disproportionate elevations of hCG may reflect the presence of the glycoprotein alpha subunit, which is biologically inactive but exhibits cross-reactivity in some radioimmunoassays. A specific alpha-subunit assay is used to confirm the diagnosis.

In other instances the diagnosis of ectopic hormone secretion may be suggested by finding suppressed levels of hormones that are subject to feedback inhibition. Low or undetectable levels of insulin or parathyroid hormone in the presence of hypoglycemia or hypercalcemia are suggestive of tumors that secrete an insulin-like growth factor or a humoral hypercalcemic factor of malignancy, respectively.

Alterations in normal feedback regulation may also provide clues that elevated circulating hormone levels are derived from ectopic sources. Patients with ectopic ACTH production do not respond to suppression by glucocorticoids (presumably because of the absence of glucocorticoid receptors in the tumor tissue), an observation that helps distinguish them from patients with pituitary-dependent Cushing's disease. Apparent suppression of ACTH, which has been noted in several case reports, could be explained by intermittent secretion of ACTH by the tumor (an uncommon and poorly understood phenomenon of ectopic hormone secretion) or by the coproduction of corticotropin-releasing factor.

If the diagnosis is still in doubt, or if the source of ectopic secretion is unknown, differential venous catheterization, often with fluoroscopic control, may be an effective means of locating the tumor. As long as the tumor is actually secreting hormone at the time of study, a step-up gradient in the concentration of the hormone is of value in tumor localization and/or a search for metastases.

THERAPY Primary treatment of ectopic hormone–secreting tumors should be directed, if possible, toward removal of the tumor. Measurement of circulating hormone levels can serve as a marker for completeness of tumor excision or of the effect of radiation and chemotherapy for tumors considered inoperable, i.e., small cell carcinoma of the lung. In addition recurrence of tumor may be heralded by reappearance of elevated hormone levels prior to clinical evidence of the tumor mass. However, occasional tumors may not secrete hormones at the time of recurrence, so that one cannot rely entirely on hormone measurements as a marker of tumor activity.

Frequently, the tumor cannot be removed or is already metastatic at the time of diagnosis. In such cases, two other approaches are available for eliminating the effects of ectopic hormone secretion. Pharmacologic agents may be used to inhibit hormone release. Somatostatin and a long-acting somatostatin analogue have been used effectively in inhibiting gastrin secretion, VIP secretion, and the clinical symptoms of the carcinoid syndrome. This drug is being investigated in the United States at the time of this writing.

The other approach involves blocking the action of the hormone when its secretion cannot be altered. Pharmacologic agents may interfere with hormone effects on target tissues. Examples include (1) demeclocycline to inhibit vasopressin action on the renal tubule in the syndrome of inappropriate antidiuretic hormone (SIADH) associated with malignancy, and (2) aminoglutethimide amd metyrapone and/or mitotane to inhibit adrenal steroidogenesis in the ectopic ACTH syndrome. Alternatively, surgical removal of the target tissue may avoid life-threatening complications and permit relatively symptom-free long-term survival if the tumor itself is benign or is slowly growing. Examples include adrenalectomy for the ectopic ACTH syndrome and gastrectomy for recurrent gastrointestinal bleeding caused by gastrin-producing tumors. This form of therapy will be used with decreasing frequency as newer and more specific pharmacologic agents become available.

ECTOPIC HORMONES AS MARKERS FOR NEOPLASIA With the initial recognition of ectopic hormone secretion it was hoped that by measuring these hormones a generally applicable means of screening for clinically silent tumors would become available. As knowledge of the spectrum of ectopic hormone secretion has increased, however, this hope has faded. The list of hormones that are secreted ectopically has lengthened to the point that cost considerations preclude the use of this form of screening. Even if the number of hormones were not as extensive, the limited correlation of tumor site and type with secretion of specific hormones means that an extensive workup to localize the tumor would still be necessary. Screening programs, when performed, have yielded relatively few positive results. Moreover evidence is lacking that earlier diagnosis, as a result of such procedures, reduces subsequent morbidity or mortality. Consequently, screening for ectopic hormone production is not part of routine cancer detection programs.

REFERENCES

BAYLIN SB, MENDELSOHN G: Ectopic (inappropriate) hormone production by tumors: Mechanisms involved and the biological and clinical implications. Endocr Rev 1:45, 1980

FROHMAN LA: Ectopic hormone production by tumors: Growth hormone-releasing factor, in *Neuroendocrine Perspectives,* EE Muller et al (eds). Amsterdam, Elsevier, 1984 vol 3

HANSEN M et al: Diagnostic and therapeutic implications of ectopic hormone production in small cell carcinoma of the lung. Thorax 35:101, 1980

HEITZ PU et al: Ectopic hormone production by endocrine tumors: Localization of hormones at the cellular level by immunocytochemistry. Cancer 48:2029, 1981

IMURA H: Ectopic hormone production viewed as an abnormality in regulation of gene expression. Adv Cancer Res 33:39, 1980

LOKICH JJ: The frequency and clinical biology of the ectopic hormone syndromes of small carcinoma. Cancer 50:2111, 1982

MUNDY GR et al: The hypercalcemia of cancer. Clinical implications and pathogenetic mechanisms. N Engl J Med 310:1718, 1984

ODELL WD, WOLFSEN AR: Humoral syndromes associated with cancer: Ectopic hormone production. Prog Clin Cancer 8:57, 1982

ORTH D: Ectopic hormone production, in *Endocrinology and Metabolism,* P Felig et al (eds). New York, McGraw-Hill, 1981

SORENSEN GS: Hormone production by cultures of small cell carcinoma of lung. Cancer 47:1289, 1981

STEVENS RE, MOORE GE: Inadequacy of APUD concept in explaining production of peptide hormones by tumours. Lancet 1:118, 1983

304 NEUROLOGIC MANIFESTATIONS OF SYSTEMIC NEOPLASIA

KARI STEFANSSON / BARRY G.W. ARNASON

INTRODUCTION Neurologic disorders commonly complicate systemic neoplasia. Tumors metastasize to brain with distressing frequency. Radiation treatment in doses exceeding 4500 rad may cause delayed necrosis of central nervous tissue secondary to occlusion of small- or intermediate-sized blood vessels. Chemotherapy of cancer may also be followed by nervous system damage; intrathecal methotrexate enhances radiosensitivity and can cause central nervous system necrosis directly, and cytosine arabinoside and 5-fluorouracil treatment may cause cerebellar damage. Many anticancer drugs cause peripheral neuropathy, and vincristine invariably does so. Opportunistic infections of the nervous system may also complicate cancer in persons immunosuppressed by the tumor or its treatment. When tumors damage vital organs, metabolic derangements may follow, and these too may compromise nervous system function (see Chap. 345).

In addition to the above, systemic tumors may occasionally be complicated by neurologic disorders not ascribable to invasion or compression of nervous tissue by tumor, to drugs used in cancer treatment, to infection, or to metabolic disturbance. Such neurologic disorders are termed paraneoplastic syndromes. Those that are currently recognized are summarized in Table 304-1.

TABLE 304-1 Remote effects of cancer on the nervous system

Site	Evolution	Clinical features	Cancer	Pathology
BRAIN				
Limbic encephalitis	Weeks to months	Confusional state followed by loss of retentive memory and dementia; anxiety, depression, and agitation common early in course	Oat cell tumor of lung	Neuronal loss in medial temporal lobe and other parts of limbic system; perivascular and meningeal infiltration
Photoreceptor degeneration	Months	Visual loss progressing to blindness	Oat cell tumor, rarely cervical cancer	Loss of rods and cones with retinal infiltration of mononuclear cells
CEREBELLUM AND BRAINSTEM				
Subacute cortical cerebellar degeneration	Weeks to months	Cerebellar ataxia Dysarthria	Oat cell tumor, ovarian and breast cancer, Hodgkin's disease	Loss of Purkinje cells with perivascular and leptomeningeal lymphocytic infiltration
Opsoclonus-myoclonus	Weeks	Dancing eyes, myoclonic jerks, cerebellar ataxia, (in children)	Neuroblastoma	Loss of Purkinje cells
Bulbar encephalitis	Days to weeks	Nystagmus, diplopia, vertigo, ataxia, (in adults)	Lung tumor	Neuronal loss in pons and medulla, mononuclear infiltration
SPINAL CORD				
Necrotizing myelopathy	Hours, days, or weeks	Paraplegia or quadriplegia with sensory loss and bladder dysfunction	Oat cell tumor, lymphomas	Severe necrosis of white and gray matter
Subacute motor neuronopathy	Weeks or months	Flaccid weakness and muscle atrophy; legs affected more than arms	Non-Hodgkin's lymphoma	Degeneration and loss of anterior horn cells
ROOT AND PERIPHERAL NERVE				
Subacute sensory neuronopathy	Weeks or months	Severe sensory loss with areflexia; often precedes the discovery of the malignant tumor	Oat cell tumor, other lung tumors	Degeneration and loss of neurons in dorsal root ganglia; infiltration with mononuclear cells
Acute polyneuritis (Guillain-Barré syndrome)	Days to weeks	Ascending weakness with minimal sensory findings	Hodgkin's disease	Segmental demyelination; inflammatory infiltration of peripheral nerves
Sensory motor neuropathy	Weeks to months	Distal motor and sensory loss; distal reflex loss	Oat cell tumor	Segmental demyelination, Wallerian degeneration
Peripheral neuropathy associated with monoclonal gammopathy	Weeks to months	Heterogeneous group; some predominantly sensory, others motor	Proliferative disorders of plasma cells and B lymphocytes	Segmental demyelination or axonal degeneration
Neuropathy with insulinoma	Weeks to months	Weakness, without sensory loss	Insulinoma	Axonal degeneration
NEUROMUSCULAR JUNCTION				
Myasthenia gravis	Weeks to months	Weakness, fatigability, normal sensory findings, normal reflexes	Thymoma, breast cancer, gastric cancer	Destruction of motor end plate and postsynaptic junctional folds
Eaton-Lambert syndrome	Weeks to months	Weakness, fatigability proximal leg muscles	Oat cell tumor	Abnormalities of presynaptic membrane of myoneural junction
MUSCLE				
Polymyositis	Months to years	Proximal muscle weakness, tender muscles, arrhythmias, heart failure	Breast, ovarian, lung cancer, lymphomas	Degeneration of muscle fibers with mononuclear cellular infiltration

Three of these paraneoplastic syndromes are considered elsewhere and need only be mentioned briefly here: *myasthenia gravis,* which in 10 percent of cases occurs against a background of thymoma (see Chap. 358); *acute idiopathic polyradiculoneuropathy* (Guillain-Barré syndrome), the incidence of which is increased in Hodgkin's disease (see Chap. 355); and *polymyositis,* which in older people is associated with an increased probability of neoplasm in the breast, ovary, lung, or lymphoid tissue (see Chap. 356). All three occur far more often in the absence of cancer than in its presence, indicating that neoplasia, while favoring these complications, cannot be their sole cause. Even though the link to cancer is tighter in several other paraneoplastic syndromes, cases in which no cancer can be found, even at autopsy, have been reported, and all probably occur in the absence of cancer. More than one paraneoplastic complication may occur simultaneously in the same individual, and the histopathology of the various syndromes overlap. All may precede the detection of a tumor by months to years, and all can develop at any time during its course.

The paraneoplastic syndromes pose difficult diagnostic problems, and other complications that plague cancer patients (e.g., metastasis, infections, drug toxicity) must be excluded before the definitive diagnosis can be made. This is particularly important since the paraneoplastic syndromes are less likely to respond to therapeutic intervention than are the other problems.

NEUROMUSCULAR DISORDERS Eaton-Lambert syndrome (see also Chap. 358) The syndrome is characterized by weakness and fatigability, primarily of the muscles of the pelvic girdle and thighs. It occurs often in conjunction with dry mouth, impotence, aching thighs, peripheral paresthesias, and diminished or absent tendon reflexes. The tensilon test may be weakly positive. Electromyograms show a pathognomonic increase in amplitude on repetitive stimulation at high rates. Electron-microscopic studies show characteristic abnormalities of the presynaptic membrane of the myoneural junction.

The basic physiologic defect in Eaton-Lambert syndrome is a failure of quantal release of acetylcholine from the terminal axons of motor neurons although quantum, when released, is normal. There is reason to believe that Eaton-Lambert syndrome, like myasthenia gravis, may be caused by autoantibodies. Mice injected with serum IgG from patients develop the electrophysiologic and electron-microscopic characteristics of the Eaton-Lambert syndrome. The syndrome is associated with cancer in 70 percent of cases; half of these are small cell cancers of the lung. The prognosis for the tumor itself is remarkably favorable; patient survival for a small cell cancer of the lung in the presence of Eaton-Lambert syndrome averages 4 years versus less than 2 years in its absence. The tumor mass is often remarkably small, and may be found only at autopsy.

Eaton-Lambert syndrome patients without cancer have a significant increase over expected values in the frequency of the HLA-B8 and HLA-DR3 histocompatibility alleles. It appears that humoral immunity plays a major role in the pathogenesis of Eaton-Lambert syndrome and that immunogenetic factors influence propensity to develop the syndrome in noncancer cases.

Tumor removal often brings about some relief from Eaton-Lambert syndrome; spontaneous remissions also occur both in tumor and nontumor cases. Guanidine hydrochloride, a drug that facilitates acetylcholine release, may give symptomatic relief. Plasmapheresis and immunosuppressive medications may be beneficial, in keeping with the proposed autoimmune nature of the disease.

Sensorimotor polyneuropathy The most common paraneoplastic syndrome is a combined sensorimotor symmetric distal polyneuropathy characterized by weakness, sensory loss, and absence of distal tendon reflexes. Pathologic studies show segmental demyelination in most examined cases, but Wallerian degeneration can also occur. The clinical features are indistinguishable from those seen in other forms of sensorimotor neuropathy. Since the etiology of the disorder is unknown in one-third to one-half of patients who present with polyneuropathy without cancer, it is uncertain what role the tumor has when present in the evolution of the clinical syndrome. The distal polyneuropathy associated with cancer is refractory to treatment with vitamins, and does not usually improve, even after removal of the tumor. Most commonly associated with the distal polyneuropathy are tumors arising in the lung (oat cell), breast, stomach, and thymus, and rarely Hodgkin's disease and multiple myeloma.

Subacute sensory neuronopathy (Chap. 355) The clinical characteristics include profound sensory loss, most often developing over a period of weeks although sometimes more slowly. Muscle strength is relatively preserved. Numbness, paresthesias, dysesthesias, and pain begin distally in the extremities and spread proximally. The legs are affected more severely than the arms. Loss of position sense of the feet invariably leads to profound gait ataxia. Deep tendon reflexes are diminished or absent. Patients with subacute sensory neuronopathy often have signs and symptoms that indicate dysfunction of the central nervous system, particularly of the brainstem and cerebral cortex. Most patients have lymphocytosis and an increased concentration of protein in the cerebrospinal fluid (CSF).

The main histopathologic findings occur in the dorsal root ganglia with loss of neurons, reactive proliferation of supporting satellite cells, and infiltration by lymphocytes and macrophages. It is not uncommon to find inflammatory cell infiltrates elsewhere in the neuraxis. Small cell cancer of the lung has been the underlying neoplasm in half the reported cases; most of the remainder have been accompanied by other types of lung tumors. The onset of the neuronopathy has preceded detection of the tumor by an interval of 1 year or more in better than half the cases.

Attempts to culture viruses from dorsal root ganglia of patients with subacute sensory neuronopathy have been unsuccessful. Patients with the disorder often have IgG in their serum that reacts with neurons in dorsal root ganglia, spinal cord, and brain. It has been postulated, but not proven, that these antibodies play a role in the pathogenesis of the neuronopathy. Disease progression sometimes ceases with tumor resection.

Subacute motor neuropathy of lymphomas This syndrome is characterized by subacute progressive lower motor neuron weakness, more pronounced in legs than arms with sparing of the bulbar musculature. A small proportion of patients complain of sensory symptoms, but sensory signs are absent. The neuropathy is rarely severe enough to disable the patient. It does at times precede the detection of the lymphoma and can appear at any time during its course. In most cases it resolves or stabilizes after a few months to a year. The course of the neuropathy is independent of the course of the underlying lymphoma. The CSF is usually normal. Patients with subacute motor neuropathy are remarkably sensitive to the neurotoxic effects of vinca alkaloids, and therefore their neuropathic problems may fluctuate with treatment of the underlying lymphoma.

Autopsies of a few cases have revealed degeneration and loss of anterior horn cells and to a lesser extent loss of cells in Clarke's column and the intermediolateral column of the spinal cord. Areas of demyelination and reactive gliosis are seen in the white matter. There is demyelination of anterior spinal roots accompanied by reactive proliferation of Schwann cells. A rare Schwann cell has a peculiar hyperchromatic giant nucleus. Striated muscles in involved areas show neurogenic atrophy. The etiology and pathogenesis of subacute motor neuropathy are unknown; it has been postulated that it may be caused by a viral infection, but no direct evidence supports this hypothesis. There is no effective treatment for subacute motor neuropathy.

Peripheral neuropathies accompanying plasma cell dyscrasias Peripheral neuropathy is common among patients suffering from plasma cell dyscrasias. In prospective studies, for example, 13 percent of patients with multiple myeloma suffer from clinical peripheral neuropathies and between 40 and 60 percent have slowed nerve conduction velocities and/or histopathologic changes in peripheral nerves. Fifty percent of patients with sclerosing myeloma and 25 percent of patients with Waldenström's macroglobulinemia have peripheral neuropathies. Viewed from another perspective, 10 percent of patients with chronic peripheral neuropathies not readily ascribed to other causes have plasma cell dyscrasias. Because the neuropathies that accompany plasma cell dyscrasias are highly pleomorphic in their clinical features, a search for plasma cell dyscrasias is warranted in any patient with chronic peripheral neuropathy of unknown origin. The clinical course is usually independent of that of the underlying plasma cell dyscrasia. There is no reliable treatment, but plasmapheresis is said to be beneficial in some cases.

Two distinct neuropathic syndromes have emerged from the heterogeneous group of neuropathies that accompany plasma cell dyscrasias.

DISTAL SENSORIMOTOR NEUROPATHY IN PATIENTS WITH WALDENSTRÖM'S MACROGLOBULINEMIA. The peripheral neuropathy is usually a slowly evolving distal sensorimotor neuropathy without significant pain or autonomic involvement. Nerve conduction velocities are considerably slowed. Cerebrospinal fluid is acellular and the protein concentration is normal. The histopathology of the sural nerves is characterized by evidence of demyelination and remyelination with relative sparing of axons and by deposition of monoclonal IgM on the myelin. Electron microscopy shows a characteristic increase in the distance between the major dense lines of the outermost lamellae of some myelin sheaths, a change not described in other human diseases.

The monoclonal IgM in the serum of patients with this syndrome binds to an epitope(s) shared by myelin-associated glycoprotein, a minor component of both central and peripheral myelin, and to a glycolipid and several low-molecular-weight proteins confined to peripheral nerves. Preliminary work indicates that this monoclonal IgM can induce demyelination in peripheral nerves of animals. It is likely, therefore, that the monoclonal IgM plays a direct role in the pathogenesis of the neuropathy.

PERIPHERAL NEUROPATHY IN PATIENTS WITH OSTEOSCLEROTIC MYELOMA. The neuropathy is a symmetric, predominantly motor neuropathy that can lead to profound weakness of the extremities within months or years. There may be some involvement of all sensory modalities, but pain and autonomic dysfunction are rare. Thirty percent of patients develop papilledema. A small proportion of patients with osteosclerotic myeloma also have one or more of the following; hypogonadism, gynecomastia, hyperpigmentation, hypertrichosis, hyperhidrosis, effusions into body cavities, hepatosplenomegaly, generalized lymphadenopathy, and clubbing. Most of these patients have been Japanese but several cases have also been reported in the United States and in Europe. Nerve conduction velocities are moderately to severely slowed, and CSF contains an increased concentration of protein.

Nerve biopsies show a mixture of axonal degeneration and segmental demyelination. No monoclonal immunoglobulin is found within nerves. Only 60 percent of patients with osteosclerotic myeloma have circulating monoclonal immunoglobulins, and antineural antibodies have not been found in their sera. When a monoclonal gammopathy is detected, it is of IgG or IgA class. It is probable that the pathogenesis of this neuropathy differs from that accompanying Waldenström's macroglobulinema. The peripheral neuropathies of sclerotic myeloma respond poorly to chemotherapy; radiation of the sclerotic bone lesion, which may be small and solitary, is sometimes followed by significant relief.

Peripheral neuropathy associated with insulinomas. This rare syndrome is characterized by acute or subacute loss of strength of all extremities. The arms are usually weaker than the legs. Weakness is followed by atrophy but fasciculations are rare. Although sensory complaints are prominent, minimal sensory signs are found. There is mild to moderate slowing of nerve conduction and electromyograms show denervation. The cerebrospinal fluid is normal. Removal of the insulinoma may be followed by a considerable recovery of strength; apart from this no treatment is known for this neuropathy.

CENTRAL NERVOUS SYSTEM DISORDERS

SPINAL CORD DISORDERS Necrotizing myelopathy Necrosis of the spinal cord occurs rarely on a background of cancer. The clinical syndrome is one of severe, acute, or subacute transverse myelopathy. Necrosis begins most often in the thoracic region and progresses both rostrally and caudally until the greater part of the vertical extent of the spinal cord is destroyed. Occasionally, it begins as a Brown-Séquard syndrome (see Chap. 353) which evolves into paraplegia or quadriplegia. Protein concentration and the cell count in the cerebrospinal fluid may be increased. Myelography sometimes shows swelling of the cord, as in other acute myelopathies. An identical syndrome occurs in the absence of cancer.

The basic histologic lesion is necrosis of both gray and white matter with relative sparing of the periphery of the cord. In some cases necrotic lesions have been found in cerebral cortex and brainstem in addition to spinal cord.

One-third of tumor-associated cases occur in patients with lymphoma, another one-third in patients with lung tumors, and the remaining one-third in patients with other neoplasms. Necrotizing myelopathy may present months to years before the neoplasm becomes detectable and may also appear after the patient's tumor has been cured. There is no effective treatment.

CEREBELLUM AND BRAINSTEM Subacute cortical cerebellar degeneration This condition presents as a subacute progressive cerebellar ataxia which can stabilize after a few weeks or months. The patient may be rendered quite helpless. Half have upper motor neuron signs, mental disturbances are frequent, and 10 percent become deaf. Most patients have an increased number of lymphocytes and an elevation of protein in the cerebrospinal fluid. Cerebellar atrophy is often evident on computerized tomography or magnetic resonance imaging a few weeks after onset of the disease. This condition may account for up to 50 percent of patients with nonfamilial idiopathic cerebellar degeneration of late onset (over 45 years of age).

The histopathology is characterized by loss of Purkinje and granule cells and by thinning of the molecular layer. Frequently there are perivascular and leptomeningeal lymphocytic infiltrates in the cerebellum and elsewhere in the neuraxis. Occasionally there is also loss of anterior horn cells and of neurons in the dorsal root ganglia.

Subacute cortical cerebellar degeneration occurs in association with various neoplasms, but half the reported cases have been associated with small cell carcinoma of the lung. Other cases have been described with ovarian and breast cancer, and with Hodgkin's disease and other tumors. There are reports of patients who have developed subacute cerebellar degeneration up to a year before their tumor was diagnosed. Attempts to culture viruses from the cerebellum of affected individuals have been unsuccessful. Several reports have appeared describing antineural antibodies in the serum of patients with subacute cerebellar degeneration, and it has been proposed that these antibodies may play a role in the pathogenesis of the syndrome; this hypothesis has not been proven. There is no effective treatment for the condition; tumor resection may arrest progression in some patients.

Opsoclonus-myoclonus Patients with opsoclonus-myoclonus suffer from rapid and irregular involuntary movements of the eyes and limbs. The condition has consequently been called the "dancing eyes–dancing feet syndrome." Most patients with opsoclonus-myoclonus have normal cerebrospinal fluid although lymphocytosis and an increased concentration of immunoglobulins may occur. Elevation of serum immunoglobulins has also been reported in a few cases.

Most cases occur in children, and half of the childhood cases accompany a well-differentiated neuroblastoma. Although neuroblastomas are secretory tumors, the secretion (of catecholamines) is less conspicuous in cases of neuroblastoma accompanied by opsoclonus-myoclonus than in those that are not associated with the condition. Opsoclonus-myoclonus can occur in adults with neoplasms other than neuroblastoma, and a similar syndrome has been described in both children and adults following upper respiratory and gastrointestinal illnesses. As with other paraneoplastic entities, opsoclonus-myoclonus may occur months to years before the tumor is recognized.

The histopathology of active childhood opsoclonus-myoclonus has yet to be described, but two reports of the histopathology of opsoclonus-myoclonus in adults indicate that the lesions resemble those that cause subacute cerebellar degeneration. Why children with neuroblastomas are prone to develop the clinical syndrome of opsoclonus-myoclonus while adults with other neoplasms (small cell cancer, ovarian cancer, breast cancer, etc.) and the same histologic lesions are more likely to develop subacute cerebellar ataxia is not understood. Successful treatment of the underlying neoplasm by resection and/or radiation has resulted in relief from opsoclonus-myoclonus in some patients. Glucocorticosteroid treatment is frequently effective. Children who recover from opsoclonus-myoclonus often have residual mild mental retardation.

Bulbar encephalitis. Brainstem symptoms and signs including diplopia, vertigo, nystagmus, dysarthria, and dysphagia may rarely develop insidiously or subacutely in patients with cancer, usually of the lung. Neuronal loss in the pons and medulla and perivascular infiltration are present. The cause is unknown, and no effective treatment has been found.

Limbic encephalitis. Limbic encephalitis usually presents as an agitated confusional state followed by a loss of retentive memory. The clinical picture is similar to herpes simplex encephalitis, but there is no concomitant rise in titer of antiherpes antibody, and the disease evolves more slowly. The cerebrospinal fluid often contains mononuclear cells, and the protein concentration is elevated. The histopathology is marked by a loss of neurons in the medial aspect of the temporal lobes and by perivascular and leptomeningeal infiltration with lymphocytes and phagocytes. There is also reactive astrocytosis in the involved brain areas. Similar histopathology is seen in the cerebellum in half of the cases. Most reported instances have occurred in association with small cell cancer of the lung. There is no effective treatment.

PHOTORECEPTOR DEGENERATION Patients with neoplasms arising outside of the nervous system can lose vision due to direct compression by metastases to the leptomeninges or choroid, or indirectly due to increased cerebrospinal fluid pressure from intracranial metastases. Radiation damage to the eyes or visual pathways can also cause loss of vision. Paraneoplastic photoreceptor degeneration presents yet another mechanism whereby the cancer patient may lose vision. It is a rare condition that presents with a gradual and painless loss of vision progressing to blindness. Electroretinograms are abnormal, and the cerebrospinal fluid may show pleocytosis. There is loss of rods and cones, and the retina is infiltrated by lymphocytes and macrophages. Reported cases have occurred in association with lung tumors or cervical cancer. Antiretinal antibodies have been found in the serum of patients with photoreceptor degeneration, but their role in the pathogenesis of the syndrome is unknown. There is no effective treatment for paraneoplastic photoreceptor degeneration.

Several other neurologic disorders have been reported in the past as occurring with increased frequency in patients with various neoplasms. These include optic neuritis, thalamic degeneration, and amyotrophic lateral sclerosis. Most of these reports have been anecdotal, and it is likely that the association of cancer with these neurologic problems is coincidental.

REFERENCES

Arnason BGW: Paraneoplastic syndromes of muscle, nerve and brain: Immunological considerations, in *Clinical Neuroimmunology*, FC Rose (ed). Oxford, Blackwell, 1979

Graus F et al: Sensory neuronopathy and small cell lung cancer. Am J Med 80:45, 1986

Greenlee JE, Brashear HR: Antibodies to cerebellar Purkinje cells in patients with paraneoplastic cerebellar degeneration and ovarian carcinoma. Ann Neurol 14:609, 1983

Grunwald GB et al: Autoimmune basis for visual paraneoplastic syndrome in patients with small-cell lung carcinoma. Lancet 1:65, 1985

Henson RA, Urich H: *Cancer and the Nervous System*. Oxford, Blackwell, 1982

Jaeckle KA et al: Autoimmune response of patients with paraneoplastic cerebellar degeneration to a Purkinje cell cytoplasmic protein antigen. Ann Neurol 18:592, 1985

Jaspan JB et al: Hypoglycemic peripheral neuropathy in association with insulinoma: Implication of glycopenia rather than hyperinsulinism. Medicine 61:33, 1982

Kelly JJ et al: The spectrum of peripheral neuropathy in myeloma. Neurology 31:24, 1981

Kinsbourne M: Myoclonic encephalopathy of infants. J Neurol Neurosourg Psych 25:271, 1962

Mancall EL, Rosales RK: Necrotizing myelopathy associated with visceral carcinoma. Brain 87:639, 1964

Prior C et al: Action of Lambert-Eaton myasthenic syndrome IgG at mouse motor nerve terminals. Ann Neurol 17:587, 1985

Shy M et al: Specificity of human IgM M-proteins that bind to myelin associated glycoprotein: Peptide mapping, deglycosylation and competitive binding studies. J Immunol 133(5):2509, 1984

Zeromski J: Immunological findings of sensory carcinomatous neuropathy: Application of peroxidase labeled antibody. Clin Exp Immunol 6:663, 1970

PART TEN ENDOCRINOLOGY AND METABOLISM

section 1 Disorders of metabolism

305 OVERVIEW OF INHERITED METABOLIC DISEASES

LEON E. ROSENBERG

GENE-ENVIRONMENT INTERACTION Metabolism comprises all the processes by which living matter is built up (anabolism) or broken down (catabolism). These processes begin with the earliest chemical reactions leading to the formation of the sperm and egg; continue throughout fertilization, growth, maturation, and senescence; and end inexorably with the death of cell, tissue, organ, and finally the individual. Metabolic processes are controlled by two integrated inputs: the *genes,* which delimit the capacity of any given cell (and pari passu of any organism), and the *environment,* which determines how those genes will be expressed. It follows that all metabolic disorders result from some disturbance in the interaction between genetic and environmental factors, and, in the strictest sense, that no metabolic disorder can be classified as either purely *inherited* or *acquired.* When we have little or no information about the genetic determinants of a disease, as in susceptibility to tuberculosis or to traumatic fractures of bones, we think of the condition as acquired. Conversely, when a metabolic disorder is due to a primary abnormality of a specific protein (and hence to a mutation of a specific gene) and when this abnormality is inherited as a simple mendelian trait (as in acute intermittent porphyria or phenylketonuria), we consider the metabolic derangement inherited. In fact, neither acute intermittent porphyria nor phenylketonuria would be significant clinically were it not for precipitating and modifying factors in the environment (drugs and hormones in porphyria; dietary phenylalanine in phenylketonuria). Appreciation of this gene-environment continuum is of more than nosologic interest. Identification of genes controlling susceptibility to tuberculosis would enable us to identify individuals and groups at risk, and additional information about age-related dietary phenylalanine requirements would permit more effective nutritional treatment of phenylketonuria.

CHARACTER OF INBORN ERRORS Literally hundreds of inherited metabolic diseases or, as they were originally designated by Garrod, ''inborn errors of metabolism,'' are now recognized, and new ones continue to be described at a rapid rate. As a group, these conditions affect all phases of metabolism and have contributed enormously to the understanding of normal metabolic pathways. They share only the two common features mentioned earlier: each is inherited as a simple mendelian trait, and each has been traced (or is attributed) to a functional abnormality of a specific protein. In other ways the conditions are diverse. Most are inherited as autosomal recessive traits, implying that a double dose of the mutant gene is required for the disorder to be phenotypically manifest (see Chap. 57); others are inherited as X-linked or autosomal dominant traits. Some have an incidence as high as 1:500 (familial hypercholesterolemia); others have an incidence as low as 1:1,000,000 (alcaptonuria). Some demonstrate prominent racial or ethnic clustering (sickle cell anemia, thalassemia, Tay-Sachs disease), and others appear to be uniformly distributed in races and groups. Some produce clinical manifestations at birth (or even before), others only in adult life (or not at all). Some are uniformly lethal regardless of treatment; others are compatible with a normal life span and health.

LEVELS OF UNDERSTANDING Since the clinical and chemical abnormalities observed with a given inherited metabolic disease reflect the mutation of a specific gene, it is theoretically possible to understand each inborn error at four levels: the gene, the protein coded for by the gene, the metabolic step at which the protein works, and the clinical or chemical phenotype produced by abnormalities at that step. A number of defects in globin-chain synthesis (the thalassemias and hemoglobinopathies) have been explored at each of these levels (see Chap. 288). In hemoglobin S disease (sickle cell anemia), for example, the specific nucleotide base change in the structural gene for β globin and the precise amino acid substitution in the β-globin polypeptide have been identified. Furthermore, physicochemical studies with hemoglobin S have shown why this mutant protein has a tendency to gel in the deoxygenated state and form the tactoids that distort the erythrocyte and lead to the hyperviscosity, sludging, tissue infarction, and hemolysis characteristic of this disorder. Until recently, information at the level of the gene was available only for disorders of globin-chain synthesis. The development of recombinant DNA technology has led to an explosive increase in the number of human genes that have been cloned and isolated (see Chap. 58) and in the number of inherited disorders understood at the level of the gene. This list now includes loci coding for such proteins as α_1-antitrypsin, argininosuccinate synthetase, collagen, growth hormone, hypoxanthine-guanine phosphoribosyltransferase, insulin, ornithine transcarbamylase, and phenylalanine hydroxylase. For many loci, however, understanding stops at the level of the gene product and, even there, is incomplete. For example, in the ''classic'' form of galactosemia, galactose 1-phosphate uridyltransferase activity is markedly deficient; this deficiency leads to accumulation of galactose and galactose 1-phosphate, which results in serious hepatic and central nervous system dysfunction. However, we know little about the molecular nature of the transferase deficiency or the means by which metabolite accumulation leads to cirrhosis and mental retardation. In other instances, such as Wilson's disease or cystinosis, the particular protein whose function is deranged is unknown, although it is recognized that copper and cystine, respectively, accumulate in tissues of affected patients. In the case of Huntington's disease we still have no biochemical ''handle'' with which to confront its therapeutic, diagnostic, and prognostic dilemmas, but a genetic marker of the disease has been identified (see Chap. 58).

PROTEINS AS GENE PRODUCTS

SPECTRUM OF MUTANT PROTEINS Genes and messenger RNAs are polymers of nucleic acids often referred to as "informational macromolecules." Along similar lines proteins and polypeptides can be called "functional macromolecules." These polymers of amino acids convert the informational potential of genes and messengers into chemical and physiologic work. Proteins are ubiquitous. They are a vital constituent of the membranes that separate tissues, cells, and organelles from one another. In the blood, lymph, and cerebrospinal fluid they maintain osmotic pressure and selectively bind and transport a large number of small molecules. As enzymes and hormones, whether extracellular or intracellular, they catalyze or regulate reactions that allow anabolic and catabolic pathways to proceed. Proteins display almost limitless variation in size, shape, and function. Molecular weights vary from a few hundred for the pituitary hormone-releasing factors to more than a million for gamma macroglobulin. Some are monomeric; others are oligomers of two, three, four, or more like or unlike polypeptide chains. Some are globular while others are helical; still others have both globular and helical regions. Some have metal ions as prosthetic groups or cofactors, while others require organic constituents for activity. Each, however, owes its unique structural features and functional specificity to a single feature—the primary amino acid sequence. Since this primary sequence is dependent on the nucleotide sequence of the gene and messenger RNA that codes for the polypeptide, inherited variations in protein structure or function are the visible expression of gene mutation. Mutations occur in all genes, and hence variation must occur in all proteins. Some variants are detected easily because they lead to obvious chemical or clinical disturbance. Others are detected with great difficulty, either because they produce early lethality or because they are clinically or chemically silent.

In general, mutations responsible for inherited metabolic disorders affect the structural genes that code for the *primary structure* of the protein (see Chap. 57). Single codon changes usually lead to single amino acid substitutions and are referred to as *missense* mutations. Other point mutations (those leading to inappropriately placed terminator codons) as well as deletions and insertions (of codons, segments, or entire genes) result in absence of the gene product or one so incomplete or distorted as to be essentially functionless. Alternatively, mutations can modify the *rate* at which a protein is made. Such rate control may be exerted either by modifying control genes or by changing codons in structural genes in a way that leads to accelerated or retarded transcription or translation. Finally, mutations can influence the posttranslational modification of proteins. Since most proteins destined for secretion, for membrane insertion, or for transport to organelles such as lysosomes or mitochondria are synthesized as precursors which must be processed, trimmed, or glycosylated as part of their delivery system, mutations can alter such "traffic." Hyperproinsulinemia and I-cell disease are examples of defective processing of secretory and lysosomal proteins, respectively.

Inborn errors have been described for all types of proteins. Enzymatic defects that produce a block in an anabolic or catabolic pathway were the first to be recognized. Hundreds of examples of this type of defect are known (see subsequent chapters), and new enzymatic deficiencies are described at a rate of about 10 per year. Inborn errors of transport affecting gut and kidney may selectively impair transmembrane movement of sugars, amino acids, phosphate, vitamins, or water (see Chap. 308). Disorders like cystinuria or glycosuria reflect deficiency of specific membrane carrier proteins required for transepithelial movement of dibasic amino acids or glucose, respectively. Other transport defects lead to abnormal binding of hormones to membrane receptors as in vasopressin-resistant diabetes insipidus or of protein-ligand complexes as in the cell surface receptor defect for low-density lipoprotein in familial hypercholesterolemia (see Chap. 315). Still other mutations alter circulating proteins rather than membrane or intracellular constituents. Analbuminemia, transcobalamin II deficiency, and abetalipoproteinemia are examples of such deficiencies.

FUNCTIONAL DERANGEMENTS **Increased activity** Simply put, metabolic disorders can be thought of as resulting from too much or too little of a specific protein (or of that protein's activity). Variant forms of glucose 6-phosphate dehydrogenase (G6PD), pseudocholinesterase, and phosphoribosylpyrophosphate synthetase have been described in which enzyme activity is *increased.* In these instances, mutations result in an increase in intracellular enzyme content because either the mutant protein is synthesized more rapidly than normal or it is degraded more slowly. In acute intermittent porphyria and familial hypercholesterolemia, rate-controlling enzymes are increased as well (see Chaps. 312 and 315). In the latter disorders, however, enzyme overactivity is a secondary event, reflecting impaired feedback regulation produced by other primary genetic disturbances.

Decreased activity Most inborn errors are associated with decreased activity (or content) of a protein. The deficiency may be *virtually complete* (as in the classic forms of phenylketonuria and galactosemia) or *partial* (as in the benign variants of those disorders). It should be emphasized that complete loss of enzyme activity cannot be equated with complete absence of a protein. For example, in classic galactosemia, no galactose 1-phosphate uridyltransferase activity can be detected in tissues of affected patients, but such tissues contain a protein that cross-reacts with antibody to the native transferase molecule. Numerous examples of cross-reacting material positive (CRM^+) abnormalities are recognized. They indicate that the mutation has resulted in the synthesis of a protein that has lost catalytic activity but retains antigenic specificity. Other metabolic disorders characterized by complete enzyme deficiency such as muscle phosphorylase deficiency or von Willebrand's disease are CRM^-, implying either that no protein is made or that the gene product is so altered that both catalytic and antigenic functions have been lost.

Most inborn errors are characterized by partial, rather than complete, loss of activity. Such partial deficiency may result from several different mechanisms. First, it may reflect a reduced rate of synthesis of normal or abnormal enzyme molecules. Second, it may result from accelerated destruction of a structurally altered enzyme. Third, reduced activity may reflect reduced affinity of the active enzyme for substrate or cofactor. Fourth, for oligomeric enzymes, reduced activity can result from impaired interaction of identical or nonidentical subunits. Fifth, for those enzymes in which more than a single isoenzyme exists in a tissue, reduced activity can reflect isolated loss of one form of the enzyme. Examples of each of these mechanisms exist among inherited metabolic disorders. Moreover, the same phenotypic manifestations can result from different mechanisms. For example, some G6PD variants exhibit increased lability, others abnormal affinity for substrate, and still others impaired oligomer formation. These abnormalities result from different structural alterations in a single polypeptide chain.

CONSEQUENCES OF TRANSPORT OR ENZYMATIC DEFECTS

The effect of a given genetic alteration on cellular metabolism and clinical status depends on the role that the mutant protein plays and the severity of the defect. As mentioned earlier, most inborn errors are the result of intracellular enzymatic defects or of membrane transport abnormalities. Since these kinds of mutations are discussed repeatedly in the following chapters, it is appropriate to summarize the possible consequences of inherited transport or enzyme defects. The model reaction sequence shown in Fig. 305-1 is used for illustrative purposes. A, B, C, D, F, and G are substrates or products of a series of enzymatic reactions; T_A, E_{AB}, E_{BC}, and E_{CD} refer to specific transport systems or enzymes catalyzing specific reactions in this sequence. The major pathway involves the conversion of A to

D via intermediates B and C. F and G are products of an alternate metabolic pathway. The arrow from D to E_{AB} represents negative feedback control of the first enzyme in the pathway by the final product of the sequence. Where possible, examples of specific inborn errors that illustrate specific consequences of transport or enzyme defects will be cited.

PRECURSOR DEFICIENCY If T_A, the receptor or carrier system that transports A into the cell, is defective, the intracellular concentration of A may be so low that E_{AB} will not be saturated with its substrate. This could slow the entire reaction sequence and result in inadequate formation of B, C, and D. In Hartnup's disease (see Chap. 308), intestinal transport of tryptophan is defective. This transport defect has important chemical and clinical consequences, since tryptophan is converted to nicotinamide intracellularly. Patients with this disorder may exhibit cerebellar ataxia and temporary or permanent dementia due to nicotinamide deficiency if they do not receive supplements of niacin in the diet. Similarly, patients with inherited defects in intestinal absorption of vitamin B_{12} develop megaloblastic anemia unless the vitamin is supplied parenterally. Precursor or substrate deficiency may also occur if the defect involves a circulating protein that transports substance A in the blood and carries it to the cell surface.

PRECURSOR ACCUMULATION Let us next consider the effect of reduced activity of one of the intracellular enzymes (E_{AB}, E_{BC}, or E_{CD}). Such a defect might lead to intracellular and extracellular accumulation of the immediate or remote precursors of the reaction. If E_{AB} is defective, only A will accumulate. Such a result is illustrated by the marked increase in lysosomal glucocerebroside content in Gaucher's disease (see Chap. 316) and of blood galactose concentration in galactokinase deficiency (see Chap. 314). Defects of E_{BC} may result in accumulation of A as well as B, and a defect of E_{CD} could lead to the pileup of A, B, and C. In homocystinuria due to cystathionine synthase deficiency, methionine, a remote precursor, accumulates, as does homocystine, the immediate precursor of the blocked reaction (see Chap. 306).

ALTERNATE PATHWAY UTILIZATION If the conversion of A to B is impaired by deficiency of E_{AB}, not only will A accumulate, but the usually minor, alternate pathway to F and G may become prominent. Phenylketonuria represents an excellent example of this phenomenon. The absence of phenylalanine hydroxylase activity leads to gross overproduction and excretion of phenylpyruvic, phenylacetic, and phenyllactic acids, compounds not usually detectable in blood or urine (see Chap. 306). Such alternate pathway augmentation may have important physiologic significance if the products of the alternate pathway interfere with cell processes when present in more than minute concentrations.

FIGURE 305-1 *Schematic representation of metabolic pathway including transport system, enzymes, alternate route, and feedback regulation. (From Rosenberg.)*

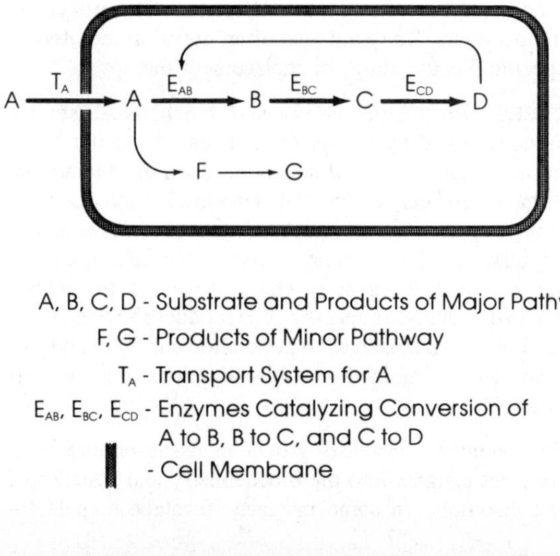

PRODUCT DEFICIT If D is the physiologically active product of the hypothetical reaction sequence, a block at any of the steps from A to D results in inadequate synthesis of D. The formation of thyroxine in the thyroid gland proceeds through just such a series of reactions, involving first the transport of iodide into the gland and then its subsequent oxidation and organification. Several enzymatic defects lead to goitrous cretinism due to impaired synthesis of thyroxine. Similarly, in some patients with congenital adrenal hyperplasia due to a defect in hydroxylation on carbon 21 of the steroid nucleus, aldosterone production is impaired, leading to renal salt wasting and hyponatremic crises. Deficient synthesis of product may cause overproduction of precursors, as in acute intermittent porphyria, because of loss of feedback control ($D \rightarrow E_{AB}$).

PRODUCT EXCESS As shown in Fig. 305-1, the end product of the reaction sequence D is presumed to regulate the activity of E_{AB}, the first enzyme in this biosynthetic pathway. Several inborn errors demonstrate abnormalities in feedback regulation, but the biochemical events involved are not well understood. In some patients with primary gout, urate is overproduced, presumably because the first enzyme in the purine pathway is defective and does not respond to its normal feedback inhibitors, hypoxanthine and adenine. Abnormal feedback control occurs in the congenital adrenal hyperplasias and congenital goitrous cretinism as well, presumably by different chemical mechanisms. In these disorders the formation or release of adrenocorticotropic hormone (ACTH) and thyroid-stimulating hormone (TSH), respectively, is not impeded by their usual ''servo'' regulators, cortisol and thyroxine, resulting in hyperplasia and functional disturbances in the two target glands.

Faulty feedback control is not the only mechanism capable of producing product excess. In those disorders characterized by enzyme excess, such as hyperuricemia resulting from increased phosphoribosylpyrophosphate (PRPP) synthetase activity (see Chap. 309), product excess is a consequence of a primary acceleration in conversion of precursor to product.

GENETIC HETEROGENEITY

A given abnormal phenotype may be produced by more than one genotype. This genetic heterogeneity is ubiquitous and important. Clinically, an appreciation of genetic heterogeneity has important implications for diagnosis, treatment, and counseling. Elucidation of the mechanisms of heterogeneity is also imperative for understanding the ways in which the human genome can be modified. As noted in Table 305-1, heterogeneity has been discerned using three approaches: clinical, biochemical, and genetic.

TABLE 305-1 Methods of demonstrating genetic heterogeneity

1 Clinical analysis	
	a Age of onset
	b Severity
	c Specific features
2 Biochemical analysis	
	a Constituents of blood, urine, and cerebrospinal fluid
	b Enzymatic activity
	c Protein characterization
	d DNA-RNA or DNA-DNA hybridization
3 Genetic analysis	
	a Chance matings
	b Mode of inheritance
	c Manifestations in heterozygotes
	d Linkage relationships
	e Complementation in mixed cells or heterokaryons

CLINICAL EVIDENCE In the absence of independent biochemical or genetic information, it is often impossible to determine whether subtle variations in clinical expression of a given metabolic disorder in affected individuals reflect the presence of different mutations or result from modification of an identical mutation by other genetic and environmental influences. However, information gleaned from biochemical techniques may support the clinical evidence of heterogeneity. For example, patients with juvenile Gaucher's disease probably have an earlier age of onset and a more rapid downhill course than do those with adult Gaucher's disease because the mutant glucocerebrosidase in the former group is distinct from and retains less catalytic activity than that in cells from the latter (see Chap. 316). It follows that tissue glucocerebroside content will increase more rapidly if glucocerebrosidase activity is 3 percent of normal than if it is 15 percent of normal. Similarly, the reason that patients with Hunter's disease do not have corneal clouding, whereas patients with the phenotypically similar Hurler's disease do, almost certainly depends on the different enzymatic dysfunctions in the two disorders: iduronate sulfatase deficiency in Hunter's, α-L-iduronidase deficiency in Hurler's.

BIOCHEMICAL TECHNIQUES More often, heterogeneity is first defined through chemical or biochemical assays. Such assays vary in design and complexity—from identification of compounds in blood, urine, or cerebrospinal fluid to molecular hybridization analyses. Illustrative examples of disorders shown to be heterogeneous by each of the four kinds of biochemical assays are noted in Table 305-1. For example, the "ketotic hyperglycinemia" syndrome, characterized by episodic ketoacidosis, protein intolerance, and hyperglycinemia, was shown by chemical analyses of blood and urine to be a feature of several different disturbances of organic acid metabolism—α-methylacetoacetic acidemia, propionic acidemia, and methylmalonic acidemia. Patients from different families with "congenital, nonspherocytic hemolytic anemia" were found to have deficiencies in different glycolytic enzymes in the erythrocyte. The nature of the heterogeneity in patients with G_{M2} gangliosidosis did not become apparent until the lysosomal hexoseaminidases were subdivided into A and B isoenzymes whose activities could be measured individually in patients with Tay-Sachs or Sandhoff's disease. Another approach is directed at the gene rather than the gene product. Molecular hybridization experiments employing DNA and RNA provided the evidence for two general categories of β-thalassemia: β^0, characterized by the apparent absence of β-globin mRNA, and β^+, characterized by reduced but detectable amounts of β-globin mRNA. As gene probes for more and more human loci become available, we can anticipate a sharp increase in the use of DNA-DNA hybridization analysis as a means of identifying heterogeneity. Such techniques have already been useful in defining heterogeneity in α- and β-thalassemia, Lesch-Nyhan syndrome, phenlyketonuria, and ornithine transcarbamylase deficiency.

GENETIC METHODS Genetic methods have also been important in demonstrating heterogeneity (Table 305-1). One of the earliest and most convincing evidences of such heterogeneity came from the chance mating of two individuals each affected with autosomal recessively inherited nerve deafness. None of their progeny was deaf, demonstrating conclusively that the mutations that produced deafness in the parents were different and likely nonallelic. In several instances heterogeneity was suggested by different modes of inheritance of phenotypically similar (or identical) disorders. For example, Hunter's and Hurler's diseases were differentiated early because the former is inherited as an X-linked trait, the latter as an autosomal recessive. Similarly, at least three forms of spastic diplegia are now recognized: one inherited as an autosomal dominant, a second as an autosomal recessive, and a third as an X-linked trait. In a few instances heterogeneity was first appreciated by studying obligate heterozygotes for a recessive phenotype. For example, cystinuria was shown to be heterogeneous by the observation that all obligate heterozygotes in some families excreted increased amounts of cystine and lysine, whereas in other pedigrees urinary findings in obligate heterozygotes were normal. A fourth genetic tool that has revealed heterogeneity is linkage analysis. Through this type of investigation hereditary elliptocytosis was divided into two forms—one closely linked to the Rh blood group locus, the other not. Finally, heterogeneity has been demonstrated by complementation analyses. The general strategy of such studies is simple. Cultured fibroblasts from two affected individuals are cocultivated in the same dish or are fused into heterokaryons. If the abnormal phenotype expressed in both cell strains remains in the mixed culture, the defect in the two patients is assumed to be identical; if correction occurs in the mixed culture, the defects in the original strains must be different. This approach has been used to define heterogeneity in a wide variety of disorders, including the mucopolysaccharidoses, the G_{M2} gangliosidoses, the methylmalonic acidemias, the propionic acidemias, xeroderma pigmentosum, and branched-chain ketoaciduria. Theoretically, positive complementation tests could reflect either of two general mechanisms: intergenic complementation, in which two different loci are involved, or interallelic complementation, in which two different mutations at the same locus are mutally corrective. The majority of positive complementation tests probably reflects the intergenic mechanism.

COMPOUND HETEROZYGOTES Some individuals with a given metabolic disorder are "compound heterozygotes" rather than true homozygotes. Compound heterozygotes are individuals who have received a different mutant allele at a given locus from each parent rather than identical mutant alleles. Patients with hemoglobin SC disease were the first compound heterozygotes identified, having inherited the gene for hemoglobin S from one parent and that for hemoglobin C from the other. These individuals have a double dose of a mutation for β-globin-chain synthesis and thus make no normal β chains. They are clinically and chemically distinct from true SS or CC homozygotes. Compound heterozygotes have also been identified in patients with cystinuria, iminoglycinuria, galactose 1-phosphate uridyltransferase deficiency, L-iduronidase deficiency, methylmalonyl-CoA mutase deficiency, and cystathionine synthetase deficiency. Some, but not all, compound heterozygotes are as severely affected as true homozygotes, depending on the nature of the mutant alleles inherited.

DIAGNOSTIC TECHNIQUES AND TARGETS

PHYSIOLOGIC FLUIDS Most of the early information concerning the inborn errors and their mode of detection came from chemical studies of blood or urine. Such chemical determinations identified specific biochemical abnormalities and provided the clues in many instances for enzymatic studies that clarified the specific defect involved. They also allowed large populations to be screened for specific disorders, thereby facilitating the detection of affected subjects prior to the onset of overt clinical problems. The use of screening tests in blood and urine has allowed the detection of heterozygous carriers for many disorders. They are also often useful in monitoring the effects of specific dietary, drug, or replacement therapy.

TISSUE ANALYSES Enzymatic assays and biochemical studies using human tissue obtained by biopsy have revealed specific enzymatic defects in more than a hundred metabolic diseases. Membrane transport defects have also been demonstrated in vitro in such disorders as hereditary spherocytosis, cystinuria, and the glucose-galactose malabsorption syndrome. These assays have often identified the biochemical and genetic heterogeneity characteristic of the inborn errors, in addition to documenting specific gene product abnormalities. Tissue studies do not lend themselves to population surveys and have the greatest impact when combined with investigations of abnormalities in blood and urine.

CELL CULTURE Human fibroblasts grown in tissue culture have also yielded important insights into the biochemistry and genetics of inborn metabolic disorders. In some instances (acatalasia, galactosemia, glucose 6-phosphate dehydrogenase deficiency, glycogen storage disease type II, branched-chain ketoaciduria, and orotic aciduria), enzymatic defects initially described in other tissues were confirmed in cultured fibroblasts. In citrullinemia and Refsum's disease, specific enzymatic defects were first demonstrated in fibroblasts, while in the Lesch-Nyhan syndrome defective hypoxanthine-guanine phosphoribosyl transferase activity was demonstrated coincidently in erythrocytes, leukocytes, and cultured fibroblasts. Abnormalities found in cells from heterozygous carriers have also been of significance. For example, the study in obligate heterozygotes of several X-linked traits provided evidence confirming the validity of the Lyon hypothesis.

DNA ANALYSIS Use of DNA-DNA blot hybridization techniques for diagnosis of inherited metabolic disorders constitutes one of the most powerful applications of recombinant DNA technology to medicine (see Chap. 58). This approach, often referred to as "Southern blotting," employs DNA isolated from such accessible tissues as peripheral blood leukocytes, cultured fibroblasts, or amniotic fluid cells. The DNA, after being "cut" with restriction endonucleases and sized by gel electrophoresis, is reacted with labeled gene probes specific for particular loci (and, therefore, for particular disorders). When the precise molecular defect responsible for a disorder is known, as in sickle cell disease or the Z variant of α_1-antitrypsin, disease-precise oligonucleotide probes can be employed. In other instances, diagnosis can be accomplished by taking advantage of *restriction fragment length polymorphisms* (RFLP) that segregate in families and constitute useful linkage markers for disease detection (see Chap. 58). Such RFLPs have been employed in detection of Huntington's disease, phenylketonuria, citrullinemia, Lesch-Nyhan syndrome, and ornithine transcarbamylase deficiency.

HETEROZYGOTE DETECTION The detection of heterozygous carriers contributes to the study of inborn errors in two important ways. First, such detection provides the most convincing evidence for a recessive mode of inheritance of a disorder, whether the mutation is autosomal or X-linked. Second, the identification of heterozygous carriers in a single pedigree provides valuable information for counseling family members. In those diseases in which clinical manifestations may be observed in the carriers (i.e., in dominantly inherited conditions such as acute intermittent porphyria or familial hypercholesterolemia) heterozygote detection has direct clinical relevance.

Identification of heterozygotes can be made by many of the methods employed for the recognition of defects in affected subjects. In a few instances, blood or urine screening techniques may be sufficient to detect carriers. Enzymatic assays using blood cells or serum have been helpful in other conditions. In some disorders blood or urine analyses fail to discriminate between normal subjects and heterozygous carriers, but carriers can be detected after administration of oral or parenteral loads of the metabolic precursor involved in the chemical defect. Thus, heterozygotes for galactosemia and phenylketonuria respond to oral loads of galactose and phenylalanine, respectively, with higher plasma concentrations of these substances than observed in normal subjects. Carriers for a number of diseases have been detected by enzymatic assays or phenotypic appearance of cells in biopsy material. Finally, DNA-DNA hybridization techniques are being used frequently for carrier detection and, importantly, for carrier exclusion. These techniques for carrier detection have usually been worked out and utilized in one laboratory or, in some instances, a few centers. Because of their complexity, they have not been employed for carrier detection in large populations.

PRENATAL DETECTION There is now considerable interest in the detection of genetic diseases in utero (see Chap. 58). More than 50 inherited metabolic disorders have been identified by chemical examination of amniotic fluid or enzymatic assays on amniotic fluid cells. The largest group of disorders so detected are those mucopolysaccharide or lipid storage diseases due to deficiency of particular lysosomal hydrolases, but disorders of amino acid, organic acid, carbohydrate, and purine metabolism have been identified as well. A few inborn errors have been diagnosed by examination of fetal blood obtained by placental puncture or under fetoscopic control. Sickle cell anemia, β-thalassemia, and hemophilia have been detected in this way. Whereas the above techniques examine gene products or metabolites, diagnosis of other disorders are being accomplished using DNA-DNA blot hybridization techniques. These techniques hold great promise because they can be used on cells such as cultured amniotic fluid cells that contain, but do not express, the genes for many highly differentiated functions including globin and polypeptide hormone synthesis. DNA-DNA blot hybridization has been used prenatally to detect phenylketonuria, α_1-antitrypsin deficiency, hemophilia, sickle cell anemia, thalassemia, and ornithine transcarbamylase deficiency.

GENETIC SCREENING

Genetic screening is the search in a population for persons possessing genotypes that are known to be associated with or to predispose to disease in the individuals or their descendants. As a research tool, screening can define the incidence of a particular genotype in the population and can be used to search for polymorphisms. In the context of discussion of inherited metabolic diseases, however, screening has two important applications: early identification of at-risk patients with treatable disease prior to onset of clinical symptoms and identification of at-risk couples who may benefit from appropriate genetic counseling. A prototypic example of the former application is neonatal screening for phenylketonuria. The features of this screening application include a relatively common disease (about 1:10,000 in whites) with serious clinical consequences (severe mental retardation); evidence that institution of dietary phenylalanine restriction by age 30 days can return blood phenylalanine concentrations to values commensurate with normal or near normal development; and a simple, sensitive, and specific assay that can be performed in the neonatal period. More than 90 percent of neonates in North America and western Europe are screened for phenylketonuria using the bacterial inhibition assay. The human and monetary savings of this screening program have been enormous and have prompted extension to neonatal detection of other treatable diseases such as galactosemia, hypothyroidism, and homocystinuria. Such "secondary" prevention emphasizes the interaction between environment and heredity and raises no serious ethical problems.

That statement, however, cannot be made with regard to the other screening application—identification of couples at risk for having offspring with untreatable (or nearly untreatable) disorders. The prototype is Tay-Sachs disease in Ashkenazi Jews. When two Ashkenazim marry, there is a 1:900 chance that both individuals are carriers for the Tay-Sachs gene. Theoretically, if all Ashkenazim were screened before marriage, if all pregnancies in at-risk couples were monitored by prenatal diagnosis, and if all affected fetuses were aborted, the incidence of Tay-Sachs disease could be decreased to zero. However, mandatory screening is not possible, and compliance for voluntary testing is poor. Education, motivation, and effective follow-up are crucial to the success of such a venture. Similar programs have been mounted in the black community, where 1:100 couples are at risk for having children with sickle cell anemia. Early programs were not only ineffective but indeed counterproductive, owing to inadequate pretesting educational programs, misunderstanding about the difference between sickle trait and sickle cell disease, and penalties for diagnosis levied by employers and insurance companies. This debacle points out the importance of ethical and social issues in such screening programs.

TREATMENT

Effective therapy is available for many inherited metabolic disorders, particularly those in which the biochemical abnormalities have been defined. As more is learned about the mutations responsible for specific disorders and about the chemical consequences of the mutations, other inborn errors will surely be controlled or modified by specific therapeutic programs. Two potential levels of treatment exist: the first is directed to means by which the basic genotype of the affected subject can be altered; the second aims to manipulate the environment so as to mitigate the harmful effect of the mutant phenotype. Successful therapy of the inborn errors has, thus far, been achieved only at the latter level. Although there is great interest in the possibility of genotypic alteration in humans, clinical application remains only a hope.

Several prerequisites are necessary for successful therapy at the phenotypic level. The correct diagnosis must be established. Some inborn errors such as phenylketonuria have harmless phenocopies that produce transient but similar biochemical abnormalities in the newborn. Whereas a low-phenylalanine diet mitigates the central nervous system complications of true phenylketonuria, such a diet may have catastrophic effects on the growth and development of a newborn with transient hyperphenylalaninemia due to delayed maturation of phenylalanine hydroxylase. Next, the physician must be convinced that the disorder is harmful and requires therapy. As stated earlier, some inborn errors such as pentosuria or iminoglycinuria do not appear to cause any significant clinical pathology and require no treatment. Finally, any therapeutic program must be continually scrutinized for evidence of harmful effects as well as for documentation of beneficial effects of therapy. These may be difficult parameters to dissociate. Penicillamine is an effective drug in Wilson's disease because of its ability to chelate copper; it is also efficacious in solubilizing and preventing the formation of cystine stones in cystinuria. Unfortunately, penicillamine also causes untoward effects that limit its usefulness and demand careful medical follow-up.

MODALITIES EMPLOYED Phenotypic modification has been approached in many ways, depending on the nature of the defect and the timing of its deleterious effects. Both medical and surgical modalities have been employed, the range and experience with the former far exceeding those with the latter. Five medical modalities have been used and will be described briefly.

Avoidance For several disorders, clinical consequences can be mitigated or forestalled entirely by avoiding exposure to particular environmental influences. For example, the hemolytic episodes in patients with G6PD deficiency can be modified significantly by avoiding exposure to such drugs as primaquine or sulfonamides and to such foods as fava beans. Similarly, the prolonged apnea that occurs after succinylcholine administration in individuals deficient in pseudocholinesterase activity will not occur if this anesthetic is not used. Avoiding barbiturates and many other drugs in acute intermittent porphyria and avoidance of tobacco smoke and other noxious fumes in alpha$_1$-antitrypsin deficiency are examples of this approach.

Restriction There are numerous disorders in which the phenotypic abnormalities result from the accumulation of a specific substrate or its metabolic by-products. Such disorders may respond to restriction of intake of the injurious substrate or its precursors, providing that the substrate is essential in the dietary sense and thus cannot be manufactured by the organism. Phenylketonuria, branched-chain ketoaciduria, homocystinuria, galactosemia, essential fructosuria, and Refsum's disease are examples of inborn errors that have been effectively treated in this way. Similarly, patients with the glucose-galactose malabsorption syndrome who develop profound diarrhea when fed lactose-containing foods do well if their source of dietary carbohydrate is changed. In contrast, dietary restriction is of no value in hyperprolinemia, hydroxyprolinemia, or citrullinemia, because these amino acids are synthesized extensively de novo. Even in those conditions in which dietary restriction is of value, there may be uncertainty about the needed duration of such restriction. The injurious effects of excess phenylalanine, galactose, or branched-chain amino acids or keto acids may be limited to the early years of life when brain development and organization are proceeding at a maximal rate. If this is so, it should be possible to modify or even discontinue dietary restrictions after a given age. More experience is needed before meaningful recommendations can be made.

Replacement Many disorders caused by the failure to make a specific protein or small-molecular-weight product have responded dramatically to replacement therapy. Hemophilia and agammaglobulinemia are examples of inborn errors that respond to parenteral protein replacement. These disorders are amenable to such replacement because the proteins involved normally circulate in abundance. In most instances, however, the missing protein or enzyme is confined to some intracellular organelle and is present in very small amounts. Replacement therapy in these instances may be difficult or impossible for three reasons: first, because large amounts of the protein are difficult to purify or synthesize; second, because mere parenteral administration of the protein will not ensure its delivery to that portion of the cell in which it is required; and third, because the protein may initiate unfavorable immunologic reactions. Despite these drawbacks, attempts along these lines continue to be made. For example, pure human glucocerebrosidase has been administered intravenously to a few patients with Gaucher's disease. Tissue glucocerebroside content fell modestly in these patients, suggesting that some enzyme was being taken up by cells and was active intracellularly, for a brief interval. As we learn more about the mechanisms by which proteins are targeted to different cellular organelles, such replacement strategies may become more effective.

The clinical stigmata of a disorder may be related not to the protein whose synthesis is defective but rather to the product of the blocked pathway. Cortisol synthesis is blocked in several variants of congenital adrenal hyperplasia, and replacement therapy with this steroid produces dramatic improvement. Similarly, administration of thyroid hormone and uridine reverses the serious clinical disturbances in familial goitrous cretinism and orotic aciduria, respectively.

Supplementation Some metabolic disorders respond clinically and/or chemically to supplementary amounts of specific vitamins. Infants with seizures controlled only by supraphysiologic amounts of pyridoxine provided the first evidence for this phenomenon. Now more than 20 different disorders are known to respond to supplements of a single vitamin. Most of these disorders are caused by primary enzymatic disturbances that result in impaired affinity for cofactor. Others are caused by primary abnormalities in the pathway of coenzyme or metabolite synthesis from vitamin precursors. Several disorders responsive to cobalamin (vitamin B_{12}), folate, or vitamin D fall in this category. Long-term experience with such vitamin supplements is limited.

Drug administration Clinical disturbances in several inherited metabolic disorders result from deposition of a specific substance in one or more tissues. Successful treatment of these conditions may be achieved by enhancing the excretion of the stored chemical or by preventing its formation. Copper deposition in Wilson's disease can be controlled by drugs such as penicillamine, which chelates copper and enhances its urinary excretion. The excretion of iron in hemochromatosis is augmented by phlebotomy and by the administration of deferoxamine. Penicillamine is also effective in solubilizing cystine calculi in cystinuria by reacting with cystine to form the more soluble cysteine-penicillamine disulfide. In this instance, the amount of cystine excreted is not changed, but its chemical form is altered in a therapeutically advantageous fashion. Uric acid deposition in gout responds both to drugs that enhance its excretion, such as sulfinpyrazone and probenecid, and to metabolic inhibitors like allopurinol that inhibit uric acid biosynthesis.

Surgical intervention The use of surgery is restricted to a few conditions, such as gout, cystinuria, and oxalosis, in which nephrolithotomy or ureterolithotomy may provide important symptomatic relief while other programs of therapy are initiated. Several reports indicate that tissue transplants may be beneficial in some diseases. Thus, kidney transplants have been undertaken in cystinosis, hyperoxaluria, and Fabry's disease. Here the aim is restoration of renal function in conditions which produce progressive, and ultimately lethal, renal injury. Results have been variable. In hyperoxaluria, the transplanted kidney has been destroyed by oxalate deposition. In cystinosis, this has not occurred. A second, and different, goal of transplantation involves restitution of normal function. Thus, in combined immune deficiency, administration of fetal liver cells or thymocytes has produced clinical improvement. Similar beneficial results of bone marrow transplantation have been reported in other immune deficiency diseases and in β-thalassemia. In the future, spleen transplantation may provide lasting benefit to patients with hemophilia or agammaglobulinemia by providing a constant source of antihemophilic globulin or gamma globulin, respectively. Likewise, hepatic transplantation has been used successfully to cure Wilson's disease, tyrosinemia, and the homozygous form of familial hypercholesterolemia. This modality will surely be tried in other inborn errors as its morbidity and mortality fall to the range where risk-benefit assessment favors its application in conditions such as glycogen storage disease, branched-chain ketoaciduria, and disorders of urea cycle enzymes.

REFERENCES

HARRIS H: *The Principles of Human Biochemical Genetics,* 3d ed. Amsterdam, North-Holland, 1980

ROSENBERG LE: Inborn errors of metabolism, in *Metabolic Control and Disease,* 8th ed, PK Bondy, LE Rosenberg (eds). Philadelphia, Saunders, 1980, pp 73–102

STANBURY JB et al: Inborn errors of metabolism in the 1980s, in *The Metabolic Basis of Inherited Disease,* 5th ed, JB Stanbury et al (eds). New York, McGraw-Hill, 1983, pp 3–59

306 INHERITED DISORDERS OF AMINO ACID METABOLISM

LEON E. ROSENBERG

All polypeptides and proteins are polymers of 20 different amino acids. Eight of these, referred to as *essential,* cannot be synthesized by humans and must be obtained from dietary sources. The others are formed endogenously. Although most of the body's amino acids are "tied up" in proteins, small intracellular pools of *free* amino acids are in equilibrium with extracellular reservoirs in plasma, cerebrospinal fluid, and the lumina of the gut and kidney. Physiologically, amino acids are more than mere "building blocks." Some (glycine, γ-aminobutyric acid) are neurotransmitters. Others (phenylalanine, tyrosine, tryptophan, glycine) are precursors of hormones, coenzymes, pigments, purines, or pyrimidines. Each has a unique degradative pathway by which its nitrogen and carbon components are used for the synthesis of other amino acids, carbohydrates, and lipids.

Current concepts of inherited metabolic diseases are based to a considerable degree on investigations of amino acid disorders. More than 70 inherited aminoacidopathies are now known, the catabolic defects (approximately 60) discussed in this and the following chapter far outnumbering the transport abnormalities (approximately 10) considered in Chap. 308. Each of these disorders is rare—the incidences range from 1 in 10,000 for phenylketonuria to 1 in 200,000 for alkaptonuria. Collectively, however, they occur in perhaps 1 in 500 to 1 in 1000 live births.

The salient features of inherited disorders of amino acid catabolism are summarized in Table 306-1. In general, these disorders are named for the compound which accumulates to highest concentration in blood (*-emias*) or urine (*-urias*). For many conditions the parent amino acid is found in excess; for others, products in the catabolic pathway accumulate. Which process takes place depends, of course, on the site of the enzymatic block, the reversibility of the reactions proximal to the lesion, and the existence of alternate pathways of metabolic "run-off." For some amino acids, such as the sulfur-containing or branched-chain molecules, defects at nearly each step in the catabolic pathway have been described. For others numerous gaps in our knowledge remain. Biochemical and genetic heterogeneity are common among the aminoacidopathies. Four distinct forms of hyperphenylalaninemia, three variants of homocystinuria, and five types of methylmalonic acidemia are recognized—variants of both chemical and clinical interest.

The manifestations of these conditions differ widely (Table 306-1). Some, such as sarcosinemia or hyperprolinemia, appear to produce no clinical consequences. At the other extreme, complete deficiency of ornithine transcarbamylase or of branched-chain keto acid dehydrogenase causes neonatal death in the untreated patient. Central nervous system dysfunction, in the form of developmental retardation, seizures, alterations in sensorium, or behavioral disturbances, occurs in more than half of the disorders. Protein-induced vomiting, neurologic dysfunction, and hyperammonemia occur in many disorders of urea cycle intermediates. Metabolic ketoacidosis often accompanied by hyperammonemia is a frequent presenting finding in the disorders of branched-chain amino acid metabolism. Occasional disorders produce focal tissue or organ involvement such as liver disease, renal failure, cutaneous abnormalities, or ocular lesions.

The clinical manifestations in many of these conditions can be prevented or mitigated if diagnosis is achieved early and appropriate treatment (i.e., dietary protein or amino acid restriction or vitamin supplementation) is instituted promptly. For this reason, aminoacidopathies are screened for in mass newborn surveys which analyze blood or urine with an array of chemical and microbiologic techniques. Once a presumptive diagnosis is made, confirmation can be provided by direct enzyme assay on extracts of leukocytes, erythrocytes, cultured fibroblasts, or liver or by DNA-DNA hybridization studies. The latter approach has been used to diagnose and characterize phenylketonuria, ornithine transcarbamylase deficiency, citrullinemia, and propionic acidemia. As additional genes are cloned, DNA-based analysis will become more common. Several disorders (cystinosis, branched-chain ketoaciduria, propionic acidemia, methylmalonic acidemia, phenylketonuria, ornithine transcarbamylase deficiency, citrullinemia, and argininosuccinic aciduria) have been diagnosed in utero by chemical analysis or by DNA-DNA blot hybridization on cultured amniotic fluid cells. The remainder of this and the subsequent chapter are focused on selected disorders that illustrate the problems posed by aminoacidopathies.

THE HYPERPHENYLALANINEMIAS

DEFINITION The hyperphenylalaninemias (Table 306-1), result from impaired conversion of phenylalanine to tyrosine. The most important is phenylketonuria, which is characterized by an increased concentration of phenylalanine in blood, increased concentrations of phenylalanine and its by-products (notably phenylpyruvate, phenylacetate, phenyllactate, and phenylacetylglutamine) in urine, and severe mental retardation.

ETIOLOGY AND PATHOGENESIS Each of the hyperphenylalaninemias results from reduced activity of the enzyme complex called *phenylalanine hydroxylase.* This system is found in appreciable amounts only in liver and kidney. Phenylalanine and molecular oxygen are substrates for the enzyme which requires a reduced pteridine, tetrahydrobiopterin, as a cofactor. Tyrosine and dihydrobiopterin are the products of this catalytic system, the latter being reconverted to tetrahydrobiopterin by a second enzyme, dihydropteridine reductase. In classic phenylketonuria, activity of the hydroxylase apoenzyme is almost totally deficient but the hydroxylase gene is present and not grossly rearranged or deleted. Benign hyperphenylalaninemia results from a less complete deficiency, whereas transient hyperphenylalaninemia (sometimes called transient phenylketonuria)

TABLE 306-1 Inherited disorders of amino acid catabolism

Amino acid(s) affected	Disorder or condition	Enzyme defect	Clinical manifestations*: Mental retardation	Neuropsychiatric dysfunction	Protein intolerance	Metabolic ketoacidosis
AROMATIC—HETEROCYCLIC						
Phenylalanine	Classic phenylketonuria	Phenylalanine hydroxylase	+	+	–	–
	Benign hyperphenylalaninemia	Phenylalanine hydroxylase	–	–	–	–
	Transient hyperphenylalaninemia	Phenylalanine hydroxylase	–	–	–	–
	Variant phenylketonuria	Dihydropteridine reductase	+	+	–	–
	Variant phenylketonuria	Dihydrobiopterin synthetase (?)	+	+	–	–
Tyrosine	Hypertyrosinemia	Tyrosine aminotransferase (cytosol)	+	–	–	–
	Tyrosinosis	Tyrosine aminotransferase (?)	–	–	–	–
	Hereditary tyrosinemia	Unknown	–	–		–
	Alkaptonuria	Homogentisic acid oxidase	–	–	–	–
	Albinism (oculocutaneous)	Tyrosinase	–	–	–	–
	Albinism (ocular)	Unknown	–	–	–	–
Tryptophan	Tryptophanuria	Unknown	+	+	–	–
	Xanthurenic aciduria	Kynureninase	?	–	–	–
Histidine	Histidinemia	Histidine-ammonia lyase	±	±	–	–
	Urocanic aciduria	Urocanase	+	+	–	–
	Formiminoglutamic aciduria	Formiminotransferase	?	+	–	–
GLYCINE-IMINO ACIDS						
Glycine	Hyperglycinemia	Glycine cleavage	+	+	–	–
	Sarcosinemia	Sarcosine dehydrogenase	–	–	–	–
	Hyperoxaluria (type I)	α-Ketoglutarate: glyoxylate carboligase	–	–	–	–
	Hyperoxaluria (type II)	D-Glyceric acid dehydrogenase	–	–	–	–
Imino acids	Hyperprolinemia (type I)	Proline oxidase	–	–	–	–
	Hyperprolinemia (type II)	Δ′-Pyrroline dehydrogenase	–	–	–	–
	Hyperhydroxyprolinemia	Hydroxyproline reductase	–	–	–	–
	Iminopeptiduria	Prolidase	+	–	–	–
SULFUR-CONTAINING						
Methionine	Hypermethioninemia	Methionine adenosyltransferase	–	–	–	–
Homocystine	Homocystinuria	Cystathionine β-synthase	±	±	–	–
	Homocystinuria	5,10-Methylenetetrahydrofolate reductase	±	±	–	–
	Homocystinuria and methylmalonic acidemia (cbl C, D, E)‡	Cobalamin (vitamin B_{12}) reductase (cytosol) (?)	±	±	–	–
Cystathionine	Cystathioninuria	Cystathionase	±	–	–	–
Cystine	Cystinosis	Unknown	–	–	–	–
S-Sulfo-L-cysteine	*S*-Sulfo-L-cysteine, sulfite, and thiosulfaturia	Sulfite oxidase	+	+	–	–
CATIONIC						
Lysine	Hyperlysinemia (type I)	Lysine dehydrogenase	–	+	+	–
	Hyperlysinemia (type II)	Lysine: α-ketoglutarate reductase	±	±	–	–
	Saccharopinuria	Saccharopine dehydrogenase	–	–	–	–
	Hydroxylysinemia	Unknown	+	–	–	–
	Pipecolic acidemia	Unknown	+	+	–	–
	α-Ketoadipic aciduria	α-Ketoadipic acid decarboxylase	±	±	–	–
	Glutaric aciduria (type I)	Glutaryl CoA dehydrogenase	–	+	–	–
	Glutaric aciduria (type II)	Medium-chain acyl CoA dehydrogenase (?)	–	+	–	–
Ornithine	Hyperornithinemia (type I)	Ornithine decarboxylase	+	+	+	–
	Hyperornithinemia (type II)	Ornithine aminotransferase	–	–	–	–
UREA CYCLE						
Carbamyl-phosphate	Hyperammonemia (type I)	Carbamylphosphate synthetase I	+	+	+	–
N-acetylglutamate	Hyperammonemia (type IA)	*N*-acetylglutamate synthetase	?	+	+	–

* *+, regularly present; ±, sometimes present; –, absent; ?, uncertain; all designations refer to manifestations in untreated disorder.*
† *AR, autosomal recessive; XL, X-linked; (AR), probably autosomal recessive.*
‡ *Designations in parentheses refer to complementation groups assigned by genetic analysis with cultured cells.*

Ammonia intoxication	Other	Inheritance pattern†
–	Hypopigmented skin and hair, eczema	AR
–		AR
–		(AR)
–		(AR)
–		(AR)
–	Palmar keratosis, corneal dystrophy	(AR)
–	Myasthenia gravis	?
–	Cirrhosis, hepatic failure, renal tubular dysfunction	AR
–	Ochronosis, arthritis	AR
–	Hypopigmentation of hair, skin, and optic fundus	AR
–	Hypopigmentation of optic fundus	XL
–	Photosensitive skin rash	AR
–		?
–	Hearing and speech deficit	AR
–		?
–		(AR)
–		AR
–		AR
–	Renal failure	AR
–	Calcium oxalate nephrolithiasis, renal failure	AR
–		AR
–		AR
–		AR
–	Crusting erythematous, ecchymotic dermatitis	AR
–		?
–	Dislocated lenses, osteoporosis, thrombotic vascular disease	AR
–		(AR)
–	Megaloblastic anemia	(AR)
–		AR
–	Fanconi syndrome, renal failure, photophobia	AR
–	Dislocated lenses	AR
+		?
–		AR
–		?
–		(AR)
–	Hepatomegaly, dysplastic optic disks	?
–		?
–		AR
–	Hypoglycemia	?
+		(AR)
–	Gyrate atrophy of choroid and retina	AR
+		AR
+		XL

(Table continues next page)

is caused by a delayed maturation of the hydroxylase apoenzyme. In two variants of phenylketonuria, however, persistently impaired hydroxylating activity results not from abnormality in the apohydroxylase but from a lack of tetrahydrobiopterin. The tetrahydrobiopterin deficiency has two distinct metabolic bases: a block in the pathway by which biopterin is synthesized from its precursors or deficiency of dihydropteridine reductase, the enzyme that regenerates tetrahydrobiopterin from dihydrobiopterin.

As a group the hyperphenylalaninemias occur in about 1 in 10,000 births. Classic phenylketonuria, which accounts for nearly half of these, is an autosomal recessive trait and is widely distributed among whites and Orientals. It is rare in blacks. Phenylalanine hydroxylase activity in obligate heterozygotes is less than normal but higher than it is in homozygotes. Heterozygous carriers are clinically well but usually have slightly increased phenylalanine concentrations in plasma. The other hyperphenylalaninemias also appear to be inherited as autosomal recessive traits.

Phenylalanine accumulation in blood and urine and reduced tyrosine formation are direct consequences of the impaired hydroxylation. In untreated phenylketonuria and in its tetrahydrobiopterin-deficient variants, plasma concentrations of phenylalanine become sufficiently high (greater than 20 mg/dL) to activate alternate pathways of metabolism and lead to formation of phenylpyruvate, phenylacetate, phenyllactate, and other derivatives that are rapidly cleared by the kidney and excreted in urine. Plasma concentrations of several other amino acids are moderately reduced, probably secondary to inhibition of gastrointestinal absorption or impairment of renal tubular reabsorption by the excess phenylalanine in body fluids. The severe brain damage appears to be related to several consequences of phenylalanine accumulation: deprivation of other amino acids required for protein synthesis, impaired polyribosome formation or stabilization, reduced myelin synthesis, and inadequate formation of norepinephrine and serotonin. Phenylalanine is a competitive inhibitor of tyrosinase, a key enzyme in the pathway of melanin synthesis. This block plus reduced availability of the melanin precursor, tyrosine, accounts for the hypopigmentation of hair and skin.

CLINICAL MANIFESTATIONS No abnormalities are apparent at birth. Untreated children with classic phenylketonuria fail to attain early developmental milestones and demonstrate progressive impairment of cerebral function. Most require chronic institutionalization within a few years of birth because of the hyperactivity and seizures that accompany the severe mental retardation. Electroencephalogram abnormalities, "mousy" odor of skin, hair, and urine (due to phenylacetate accumulation), and a tendency to hypopigmentation and eczema complete the devastating clinical picture. In contrast, children who are detected at birth and treated promptly show none of these abnormalities. Children with transient hyperphenylalaninemia or with the benign variant are not at risk for any of the clinical consequences seen in untreated classic phenylketonuria. Those children with tetrahydrobiopterin deficiency, however, are the most unfortunate. Seizures appear early, followed by progressive cerebral and basal ganglia dysfunction (rigidity, chorea, spasms, hypotonia). Each has succumbed to secondary infection within a few years despite early diagnosis and standard treatment.

Occasionally, women with untreated classic phenylketonuria have reached adulthood and had children. More than 90 percent of the offspring are markedly retarded, and many exhibit other congenital anomalies such as microcephaly, growth retardation, and congenital heart defects. Since these children are heterozygous, not homozygous for the phenylketonuria mutation, the clinical manifestations must be attributed to damage produced by the elevated maternal concentrations of phenylalanine to which they have been exposed in utero.

DIAGNOSIS Plasma phenylalanine concentrations may be normal at birth in all the hyperphenylalaninemias but rise rapidly after institution of protein feedings and are usually abnormal by day 4. Since diagnosis and initiation of dietary treatment of classic phenylketonuria must be completed before the child is 30 days of age if

TABLE 306-1 Inherited disorders of amino acid catabolism *(continued)*

Amino acid(s) affected	Disorder or condition	Enzyme defect	Clinical manifestations*: Mental retardation	Neuropsychiatric dysfunction	Protein intolerance	Metabolic ketoacidosis
UREA CYCLE *(continued)*						
Ornithine	Hyperammonemia (type II)	Ornithine transcarbamylase	±	+	+	−
Citrulline	Citrullinemia	Argininosuccinate synthetase	+	+	+	−
Argininosuccinic acid	Argininosuccinic aciduria	Argininosuccinase	+	+	+	−
Arginine	Argininemia	Arginase	+	+	+	−
BRANCHED-CHAIN						
Valine	Hypervalinemia	Valine aminotransferase	+	+	+	−
Leucine, isoleucine	Hyperleucine-isoleucinemia	Leucine-isoleucine aminotransferase	+	+	+	−
Valine, leucine, isoleucine	Classic branched-chain ketoaciduria	Branched-chain ketoacid dehydrogenase	+	+	+	
	Intermittent branched-chain ketoaciduria	Branched-chain ketoacid dehydrogenase	±	−	+	+
Leucine	Isovaleric acidemia	Isovaleryl CoA dehydrogenase	±	±	+	+
	β-Methylcrotonyl glycinuria	β-Methylcrotonyl CoA carboxylase	+	+	−	+
	β-Hydroxy-β-methylglutaric aciduria	β-Hydroxy-β-methylglutaryl CoA lyase	−	+	+	+
Isoleucine, valine	α-Methylacetoacetic aciduria	β-Ketothiolase	±	±	+	+
	Propionic acidemia (pcc A, B, C)‡	Propionyl CoA carboxylase	±	±	+	+
	Propionic acidemia (bio)‡	Holocarboxylase synthetase; biotinidase	+	±	+	+
	Methylmalonic acidemia (mut)‡	Methylmalonyl CoA mutase	±	±	+	+
	Methylmalonic acidemia (cbl A)‡	Cobalamin (vitamin B_{12}) reductase (mitochondrial) (?)	±	±	+	+
	Methylmalonic acidemia (cbl B)‡	Cobalamin (vitamin B_{12}): ATP adenosyltransferase	±	±	+	+
DICARBOXYLIC						
Glutamic acid	Glutathionemia	γ-Glutamyl-transpeptidase	+	−	−	−
5-Oxoprolinuria	Glutathione synthetase	±	±	±		

* +, *regularly present;* ±, *sometimes present;* −, *absent;* ?, *uncertain; all designations refer to manifestations in untreated disorder.*
† *AR, autosomal recessive; XL, X-linked; (AR), probably autosomal recessive.*
‡ *Designations in parentheses refer to complementation groups.*

developmental retardation is to be prevented, most newborns in North America and Europe are screened by determinations of blood phenylalanine concentration using the Guthrie bacterial inhibition assay. Infants with abnormal values are followed up with more quantitative fluorometric or chromatographic assays. In classic phenylketonuria and in tetrahydrobiopterin deficiency, values greater than 20 mg/dL are regularly observed. In transient or benign hyperphenylalaninemia concentrations are usually lower but above control values of less than 1 mg/dL. Distinction of classic phenylketonuria from its benign variants depends on following serial plasma phenylalanine concentrations as a function of age and dietary restriction. In transient hyperphenylalaninemia plasma values return to normal within 3 to 4 months. In benign hyperphenylalaninemia dietary restriction produces a more profound fall in plasma phenylalanine than that observed in classic phenylketonuria. Deficiency of tetrahydrobiopterin must be considered in any child with hyperphenylalaninemia who develops progressive neurologic impairment despite prompt diagnosis and dietary treatment. Diagnostic confirmation of these variants, which account for 1 to 5 percent of phenylketonuric children, can be achieved by enzyme assay on cultured fibroblasts. Of potentially greater therapeutic value, however, is the observation that administration of oral tetrahydrobiopterin loads can distinguish children with classic phenylketonuria (who show no chemical response) from those with tetrahydrobiopterin deficiency (who exhibit a sharp fall in plasma phenylalanine). Prenatal diagnosis of classic phenylketonuria is now feasible using restriction length polymorphisms identified by DNA-DNA blot hybridization.

TREATMENT Classic phenylketonuria is the first inherited metabolic disease in which it was demonstrated that mitigating the accumulation of the offending metabolite prevented the clinical abnormalities. This is accomplished by a special diet in which the bulk of protein is replaced by an artificial amino acid mixture low in phenylalanine. By supplementing this formula with a small amount of natural foods, an amount of dietary phenylalanine is provided that is sufficient for normal growth but is insufficient to produce markedly increased quantities of phenylalanine in blood. Ordinarily, plasma phenylalanine concentrations are maintained between 3 and 12 mg/dL.

Until it is determined whether dietary treatment can be terminated safely at any age, dietary restriction in classic phenylketonuria should be continued indefinitely. The transient and benign forms of hyperphenylalaninemia do not require long-term dietary restriction. As mentioned earlier, children with tetrahydrobiopterin deficiency deteriorate despite dietary phenylalanine restriction; efficacy of pteridine cofactor replacement is under study.

THE HOMOCYSTINURIAS

The homocystinurias are three biochemically and clinically distinct disorders (Table 306-1), each characterized by increased concentration of the sulfur-containing amino acid, homocystine, in blood and urine. The most common form results from reduced activity of cystathionine β-synthase, an enzyme in the transsulfuration pathway by which methionine is converted to cysteine. The two other forms are the

Ammonia intoxication	Other	Inheritance pattern†
+		AR
+		AR
+		AR
+		
−		?
−		?
−	"Maple syrup" odor	AR
−		AR
±	"Sweaty feet" odor	AR
−	"Cat's urine" odor	AR
−		?
+		AR
+		AR
−		?
+		AR
+		AR
+		AR
−		?
−		AR

result of impaired conversion of homocysteine to methionine, a reaction catalyzed by homocysteine:methyltetrahydrofolate methyltransferase and two essential cofactors methyltetrahydrofolate and methylcobalamin (methyl–vitamin B_{12}). Depending on the underlying disorder, some patients with each of the homocystinurias show chemical and, in some instances, clinical improvement following administration of specific vitamin supplements (pyridoxine, folate, or cobalamin).

CYSTATHIONINE β-SYNTHASE DEFICIENCY Definition Deficiency of this enzyme leads to increased concentrations of methionine and homocystine in body fluids and to decreased concentrations of cysteine and cystine. The clinical hallmark is dislocated optic lenses. Mental retardation, osteoporosis, and thrombotic vascular disease are frequent.

Etiology and pathogenesis The sulfur atom of the essential amino acid methionine is transferred ultimately to cysteine by a series of reactions designated as the transsulfuration pathway. In one of these steps, homocysteine condenses with serine to form cystathionine. This reaction is catalyzed by the pyridoxal phosphate–dependent enzyme, cystathionine β-synthase. More than 600 patients have been described with deficiency of this enzyme. The condition is common in Ireland (1 in 40,000 births) but rare elsewhere (less than 1 in 200,000 births).

Homocysteine and methionine accumulate in cells and body fluids; cysteine synthesis is impaired, resulting in reduced concentrations of this amino acid and its disulfide form, cystine. In approximately half of patients synthase activity in liver, brain, leukocytes, and cultured fibroblasts is undetectable. In the remaining patients, tissues retain 1 to 5 percent of normal activity, and this residual activity can often be stimulated by pyridoxine supplementation. Heterozygous carriers of this autosomal recessive trait show no reproducible chemical abnormalities in body fluids but have reduced tissue synthase activity.

Homocysteine interferes with the normal cross-linking of collagen, an effect that likely plays an important role in the ocular, skeletal, and vascular complications. Altered collagen in the suspensory ligament of the optic lens and in bone matrix may account for the dislocated lenses and osteoporosis. Similarly, interference with normal ground substance metabolism in vascular walls may predispose to the arterial and venous thrombotic diathesis. Recurrent cerebrovascular accidents secondary to thrombotic disease may account for the mental retardation, but direct chemical effects on cerebral cell metabolism have not been excluded.

Clinical manifestations More than 80 percent of homozygotes for complete synthase deficiency have dislocated optic lenses. This abnormality usually appears by 3 to 4 years of age and often results in acute glaucoma as well as impaired visual acuity. Mental retardation occurs in about half of such patients, often accompanied by ill-defined behavioral disturbances. Osteoporosis is a common radiologic finding (seen in 64 percent of patients by age 15) but rarely causes clinical disease. Life-threatening vascular complications, probably initiated by damage to vascular endothelium, are the major cause of morbidity and mortality. Occlusion of coronary, renal, and cerebral arteries with attendant tissue infarction can occur during the first decade of life. Nearly one-quarter of patients die of vascular disease before age 30. These vascular complications seem to be exacerbated by angiographic procedures. Importantly, pyridoxine-responsive patients have milder clinical manifestations in all regards. Heterozygous carriers for synthase deficiency (about 1 in 70 in the population) may be at increased risk for premature peripheral and cerebral occlusive vascular disease.

Diagnosis The cyanide-nitroprusside test is a simple way of demonstrating increased excretion of sulfhydryl-containing compounds in urine. Since cystine and *S*-sulfocysteine also give a positive test, other disorders of sulfur metabolism must be excluded, but this is usually possible on clinical grounds. Distinction of cystathionine β-synthase deficiency from other causes of homocystinuria can usually be accomplished by measurements of plasma methionine, which tend to be increased in synthase-deficient patients and normal or low in those with impaired methionine formation (see below). Diagnostic confirmation depends on measurements of synthase activity in tissue extracts. Heterozygotes can be identified by measurement of peak serum homocystine after an oral methionine load and by measurement of tissue synthase activity.

Treatment As with classic phenylketonuria, effective treatment depends on early diagnosis. A few infants diagnosed in the newborn period have been treated successfully with methionine-restricted, cystine-supplemented diets. Their clinical course has, thus far, been benign compared with that of untreated affected siblings. In approximately half of patients, oral supplements of pyridoxine (25 to 500 mg per day) produce a fall in plasma and urinary methionine and homocystine and an increase in cystine concentration in body fluids. This effect probably reflects a modest increase in synthase activity in cells of patients in whom the enzymatic defect is characterized by either reduced affinity for cofactor or accelerated degradation of mutant enzyme. Since such vitamin supplementation is simple and apparently harmless, it should be tried in all patients. There are no reports of the effect of pyridoxine supplementation therapy that has been initiated soon after birth. Similarly, there are no data regarding pyridoxine supplements in heterozygous carriers.

5,10-METHYLENETETRAHYDROFOLATE REDUCTASE DEFICIENCY Definition In this form of homocystinuria, methionine concentrations in body fluids are normal or decreased because deficiency of 5,10-methylenetetrahydrofolate reductase leads to impaired synthesis of 5-methyltetrahydrofolate, a cofactor in the enzymatic formation of methionine from homocysteine. Central nervous system dysfunction occurs in most patients.

Etiology and pathogenesis 5-Methyltetrahydrofolate:homocysteine methyltransferase catalyzes the conversion of homocysteine to methionine. The methyl group transferred in this reaction comes from 5-methyltetrahydrofolate, which is converted to tetrahydrofolate in the process. 5-Methyltetrahydrofolate, in turn, is synthesized enzymatically from 5,10-methylenetetrahydrofolate by another enzyme, 5,10-methylenetetrahydrofolate reductase. Thus, reductase activity controls both methionine synthesis and tetrahydrofolate generation. This series of reactions is critical to normal DNA and RNA synthesis. A primary defect in the reductase activity results, secondarily, in deficient methyltransferase activity and impaired conversion of homocysteine to methionine. Methionine deficiency and impaired nucleic acid synthesis may contribute to the central nervous system dysfunction. The disorder appears to be inherited as an autosomal recessive trait.

Clinical manifestations Fewer than 10 children with homocystinuria due to reductase deficiency have been reported. The most severely affected have presented with profound developmental retardation and cerebral atrophy early in life. Others manifested behavioral disturbances (catatonia) during the second decade or mild retardation. Presumably the severity of the clinical manifestations reflects the severity of the reductase deficiency.

Diagnosis and treatment The combination of increased concentrations of homocystine in body fluids with normal or decreased concentrations of methionine should suggest this entity. Serum folate concentrations are low in some patients. Confirmation requires direct reductase assays in tissue extracts (brain, liver, cultured fibroblasts). Although therapeutic experience is limited, one teenage girl with a catatonic psychosis responded dramatically, both chemically and clinically, to folate supplements (5 to 10 mg per day). When the folate was withdrawn, behavior worsened. This observation suggests that early diagnosis followed by folate supplementation may forestall neurologic or psychiatric disturbances.

DEFICIENCY OF COBALAMIN (VITAMIN B_{12}) COENZYME SYNTHESIS Definition This form of homocystinuria also reflects impaired conversion of homocysteine to methionine. The primary defect is in the synthesis of methylcobalamin, a cobalamin (vitamin B_{12}) coenzyme required by methyltetrahydrofolate:homocysteine methyltransferase. Methylmalonic acid accumulates in body fluids as well because synthesis of a second coenzyme, adenosylcobalamin, required for isomerization of methylmalonyl coenzyme A (CoA) to succinyl CoA is also impaired.

Etiology and pathogenesis As with 5,10-methylenetetrahydrofolate reductase deficiency, this disorder impairs remethylation of homocysteine. The primary defect concerns deficient synthesis of cobalamin coenzymes. Since methylcobalamin is required for methyl-group transfer from methyltetrahydrofolate to homocysteine, impaired cobalamin metabolism leads to deficient methyltransferase activity. The defect responsible for impaired synthesis of methylcobalamin involves some early step in lysosomal or cytosolic activation of the vitamin precursor. Somatic cell genetic studies indicate that three distinct lesions can cause deficient coenzyme formation, each of which appears to be inherited as an autosomal recessive trait.

Clinical manifestations The first reported patient died of infection at age 6 weeks following severely arrested development. Clinical manifestations in the other affected children vary: two had megaloblastic anemia and pancytopenia; three had significant spinocerebellar neurologic impairment; one exhibited little clinical abnormality.

Diagnosis and treatment Homocystinuria, hypomethioninemia, and methylmalonic aciduria are the chemical hallmarks. These findings may also be present in juvenile- or adult-onset pernicious anemia in which intestinal cobalamin absorption is impaired. Measurement of serum cobalamin concentrations, low in pernicious anemia and normal in patients with defective conversion of cobalamin vitamin to coenzymes, helps in the differential diagnosis. Definitive diagnosis depends on demonstrating impaired coenzyme synthesis in cultured cells. Treatment of affected children with cobalamin supplements (1 to 2 mg per day) shows promise: homocystine and methylmalonate excretion fall to near normal values; the hematologic and neurologic deficits have also lessened to a variable degree.

REFERENCES

BOERS GHJ et al: Heterozygosity for homocystinuria in premature peripheral and cerebral occlusive arterial disease. N Engl J Med 313:709, 1985

MCKUSICK VA: Homocystinuria, in *Heritable Disorders of Connective Tissue*, 4th ed. St. Louis, Mosby, 1972, pp 224–281

MUDD SH, LEVY HL: Disorders of transsulfuration, in *The Metabolic Basis of Inherited Disease*, 5th ed, JB Stanbury et al (eds). New York, McGraw-Hill, 1983, pp 552–559

——— et al: Natural history of homocystinuria due to cystathionine β-synthase deficiency. Am J Hum Genet 37:709, 1985

ROSENBERG LE, SCRIVER CR: Disorders of amino acid metabolism, in *Metabolic Control and Disease*, 8th ed, PK Bondy, LE Rosenberg (eds). Philadelphia, Saunders 1980, pp 583–776

SCRIVER CR, CLOW CL: Phenylketonuria: Epitome of human biochemical genetics. N Engl J Med 303:1336, 1394, 1980

WOO SLC et al: Cloned human phenylalanine hydroxylase gene allows prenatal diagnosis and carrier detection of classical phenylketonuria. Nature 306:151, 1983

307 STORAGE DISEASES OF AMINO ACID METABOLISM

LEON E. ROSENBERG

A number of inherited metabolic disorders are characterized by deposition or storage of particular metabolites in tissues. In most, storage reflects impaired degradation of the substance in question; in others, the mechanism is unknown. Many storage diseases involve large molecules such as glycogen, sphingolipids, mucolipids, cholesterol esters, and mucopolysaccharides (see Chaps. 313, 315, and 316); in others, metals such as iron and copper are deposited (see Chaps. 310 and 311). Finally, there is a group of storage diseases in which relatively small organic molecules are deposited. These include gout (see Chap. 309) and a group of disorders of amino acid metabolism.

ALKAPTONURIA

DEFINITION Alkaptonuria is a rare disorder of tyrosine catabolism. Deficiency of the enzyme homogentisic acid oxidase leads to excretion of large amounts of homogentisic acid in urine and to accumulation of oxidized homogentisic acid pigment in connective tissues (ochronosis). After many years ochronosis produces a distinctive form of degenerative arthritis.

ETIOLOGY AND PATHOGENESIS Homogentisic acid is an intermediate in the catabolism of tyrosine to fumarate and acetoacetate. Activity of homogentisic acid oxidase, the enzyme that catalyzes the opening of the phenolic ring yielding maleylacetoacetic acid, is deficient in liver and kidney of patients with alkaptonuria, and homogentisic acid accumulates in cells and body fluids. Patients have minimally increased concentrations of homogentisic acid in blood because it is rapidly cleared by the kidney. As much as 3 to 7 g homogentisic acid may be excreted in the urine per day, but this is of little pathophysiologic significance. However, homogentisic acid and its oxidized polymers bind to collagen, leading to the progressive deposition of a gray to bluish-black pigment. The mechanism(s) by which degenerative changes develop in cartilage, intervertebral disk, and other connective tissues is unknown but may involve direct chemical irritation or an impairment of normal connective tissue metabolism.

Alkaptonuria was the first human disease shown to be inherited as an autosomal recessive trait. Affected homozygotes occur with a frequency around 1 in 200,000. Heterozygous carriers are clinically well and excrete no homogentisic acid in urine, even after loading doses of tyrosine.

CLINICAL MANIFESTATIONS Alkaptonuria may go unrecognized until middle life when degenerative joint disease develops in the majority. Prior to this time the tendency of the patient's urine to darken on standing may go unnoticed, as may slight discoloration of the sclerae and ears. The latter manifestations are generally the earliest external evidence of the disorder and develop after age 20 to 30. Foci of gray-brown scleral pigment and generalized darkening of the concha, antihelix, and, finally, helix of the ear are typical. Ear cartilages may be irregular and thickened. *Ochronotic arthritis* is heralded by pain, stiffness, and some limitation of motion of the hips, knees, and shoulders. Intermittent periods of acute arthritis, which may resemble rheumatoid arthritis, occur, but small joints are usually spared. Limitation of motion and ankylosis of the lumbosacral spine are common late manifestations. Pigmentation of heart valves, larynx, tympanic membranes, and skin occurs, and occasional patients develop pigmented renal or prostatic calculi. An increased incidence of degenerative cardiovascular disease may occur in older patients.

DIAGNOSIS A patient whose urine darkens to blackness on standing must be suspected of having alkaptonuria, but because of modern plumbing conditions this finding is not often observed. The diagnosis is usually made from the triad of degenerative arthritis, ochronotic pigmentation, and urine which turns black upon alkalinization. Homogentisic acid in urine may be identified presumptively by other tests: upon addition of ferric chloride, a purple-black color is observed; treatment with Benedict's reagent yields a brown color; addition of a saturated silver nitrate solution produces an immediate black color. These screening tests can be confirmed by chromatographic, enzymatic, or spectrophotometric determinations of homogentisic acid. X-rays of the lumbar spine are virtually pathognomonic. They show degeneration and dense calcification of the intervertebral disks and narrowing of the intervertebral spaces.

TREATMENT There is no specific treatment for ochronotic arthritis. Joint manifestations might be mitigated if homogentisic acid accumulation and deposition could be curbed by dietary restriction of phenylalanine and tyrosine, but the long course of the disease has discouraged such therapeutic attempts. Since ascorbic acid impedes oxidation and polymerization of homogentisic acid in vitro, its use has been suggested as a possible means of decreasing pigment formation and deposition. The efficacy of this form of treatment has not been established. Symptomatic treatment is similar to that for osteoarthritis (Chap. 274).

CYSTINOSIS

DEFINITION Cystinosis is a rare disorder characterized by the intralysosomal accumulation of free cystine in body tissues. This results in the appearance of cystine crystals in the cornea, conjunctiva, bone marrow, lymph nodes, leukocytes, and internal organs. Three variants have been identified: an infantile (nephropathic) form leading to the Fanconi syndrome and renal insufficiency in the first decade; a juvenile (intermediate) form in which renal disease becomes manifest during the second decade; and an adult (benign) form characterized by deposition of cystine in the cornea but not in the kidney.

ETIOLOGY AND PATHOGENESIS The basic defect in cystinosis involves impaired efflux of cystine from lysosomes rather than an abnormality in cystine catabolism. Lysosomal cystine efflux is an active, ATP-dependent process. The cystine content of tissues may be more than 100 times normal in the infantile form, more than 30 times normal in the adult form. Intracellular cystine appears to be located in lysosomes and does not exchange with other intracellular or extracellular pools of this amino acid. Neither plasma nor urinary concentrations of cystine are particularly elevated.

The extent of cystine crystal deposition varies from patient to patient, depending on the form of the disease and on the methods used to prepare pathologic specimens. Cystine accumulation in the kidney causes renal insufficiency in the infantile and juvenile forms. The kidneys are pale and shrunken, the capsule is adherent, and the corticomedullary junction is obscured. Microscopically, nephron organization is interrupted, glomeruli are hyalinized, connective tissue is increased, and the normal epithelium of the tubules is replaced by cuboidal cells. Narrowing and shortening of the proximal tubule produces the swan neck deformity that is characteristic of but not specific for cystinosis. Patchy depigmentation and degeneration of the peripheral retina occurs in the infantile and juvenile forms. Cystine crystals may also be deposited in the ocular conjunctiva or uvea.

Each form of cystinosis appears to be inherited as an autosomal recessive trait. Obligate heterozygotes have intracellular cystine contents intermediate between those of normal persons and affected patients but are free of clinical abnormalities.

CLINICAL MANIFESTATIONS In the infantile form abnormalities are usually apparent by 4 to 6 months of age. Growth retardation, vomiting, fever, vitamin D–resistant rickets, polyuria, dehydration, and metabolic acidosis are prominent. Generalized proximal tubular dysfunction (the Fanconi syndrome) leads to hyperphosphaturia and hypophosphatemia, renal glycosuria, generalized aminoaciduria, hypouricemia, and often hypokalemia. Pyelonephritis may contribute, along with interstitial fibrosis, to progressive glomerular insufficiency. Death due to uremia or intercurrent infection usually occurs before age 10. Ocular manifestations are prominent. Photophobia is usually demonstrable within the first few years of life due to cystine deposits in the cornea, and retinal degeneration may appear even earlier.

In contrast, patients with the adult form manifest only ocular abnormalities. Photophobia, headache, and burning or itching of the eyes are major complaints. Glomerular and tubular function and the integrity of the retina are preserved. The findings in the juvenile variant fall between these extremes. These patients have both ocular and renal manifestations, but the latter do not become significant until the second decade. The renal lesion, albeit milder than that seen in the infantile form, eventually leads to renal insufficiency.

DIAGNOSIS Cystinosis must be considered in any child with vitamin D–resistant rickets, the Fanconi syndrome, or glomerular insufficiency. Hexagonal or rectangular cystine crystals can be detected in the cornea (by slit-lamp examination), in leukocytes from peripheral blood or bone marrow, or in biopsies of rectal mucosa. Diagnosis can be confirmed by quantification of cystine in peripheral blood leukocytes or cultured fibroblasts. The infantile form has been diagnosed prenatally by the demonstration of increased cystine content in cultured amniotic fluid cells.

TREATMENT The adult form is benign and requires no treatment. Symptomatic treatment of renal disease in the infantile or juvenile form of cystinosis does not differ from that of other forms of chronic renal insufficiency: maintenance of adequate fluid intake to prevent dehydration; correction of the metabolic acidosis; and ingestion of supplementary calcium, phosphate, and vitamin D to heal the rickets. Such measures are effective in maintaining growth, development, and well-being in affected children for a time. Two types of more specific therapy have been attempted without much success. Cystine-restricted diets have not prevented progression of renal disease. Likewise, the use of sulfhydryl reagents (penicillamine, dimercaprol) and reducing agents (vitamin C) have yielded no long-term benefit.

The most promising form of therapy for nephropathic cystinosis is renal transplantation. More than 20 affected children with end-stage renal disease have been so treated. Those patients who tolerated the procedure and did not develop immunologic problems have shown return of kidney function toward normal. The transplanted kidneys have not developed the functional abnormalities typical of cystinosis (i.e., the Fanconi syndrome or glomerular insufficiency). They may, however, reaccumulate some cystine, apparently owing to migration of interstitial or mesangial cells from the host. This experience justifies offering renal transplantation to patients with terminal renal failure.

PRIMARY HYPEROXALURIA

DEFINITION Primary hyperoxaluria is the designation for two rare disorders characterized by chronic excessive urinary excretion of oxalic acid and by calcium oxalate nephrolithiasis and nephrocalcinosis. Typically, patients with both forms develop renal insufficiency early in life and die of uremia. At postmortem examination, calcium oxalate deposits are widespread in renal and extrarenal tissues, a condition referred to as *oxalosis*.

ETIOLOGY AND PATHOGENESIS The metabolic basis for the primary hyperoxalurias involves pathways of glyoxylate metabolism. In type I hyperoxaluria, urinary excretion of oxalate and of the oxidized and reduced forms of glyoxylate is increased. The excessive synthesis of these substances results from a block in an alternate route of glyoxylate metabolism. Activity of α-ketoglutarate:glyoxylate carboligase, which catalyzes the formation of α-hydroxy-β-ketoadipic acid, is reduced in liver, kidney, and spleen. The resulting expansion of the glyoxylate pool leads to enhanced oxidation of glyoxylate to oxalate and to enhanced reduction of glyoxylate to glycolate. Each of these 2-carbon acids is then excreted in excess in the urine. In type II hyperoxaluria, L-glyceric acid is excreted in excess along with oxalate. In this condition, activity of D-glyceric acid dehydrogenase, which catalyzes the reduction of hydroxypyruvate to D-glyceric acid in the catabolic pathway of serine metabolism, is absent in leukocytes (and presumably other tissues). The accumulated hydroxypyruvate is instead reduced by lactic dehydrogenase to the L-isomer of glycerate, which is excreted in the urine. The reduction of hydroxypyruvate is coupled in some way to the oxidation of glyoxylate to oxalate, thus causing the formation of increased oxalate. Both disorders appear to be inherited as autosomal recessive traits. Heterozygotes are asymptomatic.

The pathogenesis of stone formation, nephrocalcinosis, and oxalosis relates directly to the insolubility of calcium oxalate. Extrarenal deposits of oxalate are prominent in the heart, walls of arteries and veins, male urogenital tract, and bone.

CLINICAL MANIFESTATIONS Nephrolithiasis and oxalosis may be manifest during the first year of life. Most patients experience renal colic or hematuria between ages 2 and 10 and succumb to uremia before age 20. With the onset of uremia, patients may develop severe peripheral arterial spasm and necrosis with resulting vascular insufficiency. Oxalate excretion falls as renal failure worsens. In patients with delayed onset of symptoms, survival to age 50 or 60 has been reported, despite recurrent nephrolithiasis.

DIAGNOSIS Oxalate excretion in normal children or adults is less than 60 mg per 1.73 square meters of surface area per day. Patients with type I or type II hyperoxaluria generally excrete two to four times this amount. Distinction between the two types of primary hyperoxaluria depends on measurements of the other organic acids that identify them: glycolic acid in type I and L-glyceric acid in type II. Since patients with pyridoxine deficiency or chronic ileal disease may excrete excessive amounts of oxalate, these conditions must be excluded.

TREATMENT There is no satisfactory treatment. Urinary oxalate concentration can be transiently reduced by increasing the urinary flow rate. Large doses of pyridoxine (100 mg per day) may reduce urinary oxalate, but long-term effects are not dramatic. A diet high in phosphate content seems to reduce the frequency of attacks of renal colic, but oxalate excretion is unaffected. Finally, after renal transplantation renal function is lost because of calcium oxalate deposition in the transplanted kidney.

REFERENCES

GAHL WA: Cystine transport is defective in isolated leukocyte lysosomes from patients with cystinosis. Science 217:1263, 1982

JONAS AJ: ATP-dependent lysosomal efflux is defective in cystinosis. J Biol Chem 257:12185, 1982

LADU NB: Alcaptonuria, in *The Metabolic Basis of Inherited Disease,* 4th ed, JB Stanbury et al (eds). New York, McGraw-Hill, 1978, pp 268–282

SCHNEIDER JA, SCHULMAN, JD: Cystinosis, in *The Metabolic Basis of Inherited Disease,* 5th ed, JB Stanbury et al (eds). New York, McGraw-Hill, 1983, pp 1844–1866

WILLIAMS HE, SMITH LH JR: Primary hyperoxaluria, in *The Metabolic Basis of Inherited Disease,* 5th ed, JB Stanbury et al (eds). New York, McGraw-Hill, 1983, pp 204–228

308 INHERITED DEFECTS OF MEMBRANE TRANSPORT

LEON E. ROSENBERG / ELIZABETH M. SHORT

The passage of certain molecules across plasma cell membranes depends on specific transport systems that owe their specificity to membrane receptor and "carrier" proteins. These membrane constituents recognize individual molecules or structurally related substances and catalyze their transmembrane movement by mechanisms poorly understood. The disorders considered in this chapter have three features in common: each is characterized by a specific defect in the transport of one or more compounds; each is inherited as a dominant or recessive trait, implying that a single genetic locus is involved; and each is presumed to reflect a primary alteration in a specific membrane protein. Many of these defects have been well characterized physiologically, but in none has the putative mutant transport protein been isolated.

More than 20 inherited disorders of membrane transport have been described in humans (Table 308-1). Most affect the gut and/or kidney only. Numerous classes of substrates are represented, including amino acids, sugars, cations, anions, vitamins, and water. Some are discussed elsewhere in this text. Those impairing the transport of amino acids, hexoses, urate, and chloride are discussed here as examples of the abnormalities encountered.

DISORDERS OF AMINO ACID TRANSPORT

As noted in Table 308-1, 10 disorders of amino acid transport have been described. Five of these (cystinuria, dibasicaminoaciduria, Hartnup disease, iminoglycinuria, and dicarboxylicaminoaciduria) show transport abnormalities for structurally related amino acids, thereby implying the existence of group-specific membrane receptors or carriers. With the exception of iminoglycinuria and dicarboxylicaminoaciduria, these defects have important clinical consequences. The remaining five disorders affect the transport of only one amino acid, implying the existence of substrate-specific transport systems. Each of these conditions affects transport in the kidney, gut, or both; none has been shown to alter transport in other tissues.

CYSTINURIA Definition Cystinuria is the most common inborn error of amino acid transport. It is characterized by excessive urinary excretion of the dibasic amino acids: lysine, arginine, ornithine, and cystine. This aminoaciduria results from impaired tubular reabsorption of these amino acids. A similar transport defect exists in the intestinal mucosa. Because cystine is the least soluble of the naturally occurring amino acids, its overexcretion predisposes to the formation of renal, ureteral, and bladder calculi. Such calculi are responsible for the signs and symptoms of the disorder.

Etiology and pathogenesis Massive excretion of cystine and the other dibasic amino acids occurs only in classic cystinuria. The disorder, inherited as an autosomal recessive trait, is believed to result from alterations in a membrane carrier protein essential for transport of this group of amino acids in the apical brush border of proximal renal tubule and small intestinal cells. The putative protein has a greater affinity for ornithine and arginine than for lysine and cystine. Although the renal clearance of all four amino acids is increased in homozygotes, the presence of some residual transport capacity for these compounds plus the existence of three other disorders marked by selective excretion of members of this group (dibasicaminoaciduria, hypercystinuria, lysinuria) argues for the existence of at least three discrete renal transport systems for these amino acids: one for each amino acid alone; one shared by lysine, arginine, and ornithine; and one for all four amino acids.

Whereas urinary excretion patterns and renal clearance abnormalities in all homozygotes are similar, evidence for three allelic variants has come from studies of intestinal transport in homozygotes and of urinary excretion in obligate heterozygotes. Type I homozygotes lack mediated intestinal transport of cystine, lysine, arginine, and ornithine; heterozygotes have normal urinary amino acid excretion patterns. Type II homozygotes lack mediated lysine transport in the gut but retain some capacity for cystine transport; heterozygotes have moderately increased urinary excretion of each of the four amino acids. Type III homozygotes retain some capacity for mediated intestinal transport of the four involved substrates; heterozygotes have modestly increased urinary lysine and cystine.

Clinical manifestations Cystinuria is among the most common inborn errors, homozygotes occurring with a frequency of 1 in 10,000 to 1 in 15,000 in many ethnic groups. Two-thirds of adults with cystinuria are type I homozygotes. Cystine stones account for 1 to 2 percent of all urinary tract calculi. The maximum solubility of cystine in the physiologic urinary pH range of 4.5 to 7.0 is about 300 mg per liter. Since affected homozygotes regularly excrete 600 to 1800 mg per day, crystalluria and calculus formation are a constant threat. Cystine stone formation usually becomes manifest in the second or third decade but may occur in the first year of life. Symptoms and signs are those typical of urolithiasis: hematuria, flank pain, renal colic, obstructive uropathy, and infection. Recurrent urolithiasis may lead to progressive renal insufficiency.

Diagnosis The presence of cystine in a urinary tract stone is pathognomonic of cystinuria. However, since 50 percent of the stones excreted by cystinuric subjects are of mixed composition and since as many as 10 percent may contain *no* detectable cystine, a urinary nitroprusside test should be done on all patients with urolithiasis to exclude this diagnosis. The nitroprusside test is also positive (appearance of a cherry red color) in some heterozygotes for cystinuria, in patients with hypercystinuria, homocystinuria, and cysteine β-mercaptolactate disulfiduria, and in the presence of acetone in the urine. When cystine content exceeds 250 mg per liter, cystine crystals may be seen in the sediment of acidified, concentrated, chilled urine. These hexagonal crystals are pathognomonic of cystine overexcretion in patients not taking sulfonamides.

Diagnostic confirmation of cystinuria depends upon the demonstration of the characteristic amino acid excretion pattern in the urine. Selective excretion of cystine, lysine, arginine, and ornithine can be demonstrated by paper chromatography or electrophoresis, and quantitative determinations can be made by column chromatography. Quantitation is important for differentiating some heterozygotes from homozygotes and documenting the reduction of free cystine excretion during therapy.

Treatment Medical management is aimed at reducing the concentration of cystine in urine. The most important treatment is maintenance of a large urine volume. Fluid ingestion in excess of 4 liters per day is essential, and 5 to 7 liters per day is optimal. Urinary cystine excretion should measure less than 250 to 300 mg per liter. The daily fluid ingestion necessary to maintain this dilution of excreted cystine should be spaced over the waking hours, with one-quarter to one-third of the total volume ingested at bedtime. Stones can be prevented and even dissolved by such hydration. It must be made clear to the cystinuric subject that water is a drug. Solubility of cystine rises sharply in urine above pH 7.5, and urinary alkalinization can be therapeutic in some situations. Vigorous administration of sodium bicarbonate, acetazolamide, and polycitrates is required to maintain a persistently alkaline pH, but this measure introduces the danger of inducing formation of other "alkaline" stones (calcium oxalate, calcium phosphate, magnesium ammonium phosphate) and even of producing nephrocalcinosis.

Another treatment involves administration of penicillamine which undergoes sulfhydryl-disulfide exchange with cystine to form the mixed disulfide of penicillamine and cysteine. Since this disulfide is more than 50 times as soluble as cystine, penicillamine (in doses of 1 to 3 g per day) has the capacity to reduce free cystine excretion markedly, thereby preventing new stone formation and promoting dissolution of existing calculi. Unfortunately, allergic manifestations include acute serum sickness, agranulocytosis, pancytopenia, immune glomerulitis, and the Goodpasture syndrome. Thus, its use should be reserved for patients who fail to respond to hydration alone or who are in a high-risk category (one remaining kidney, renal insufficiency). Those patients unable to tolerate penicillamine may benefit from α-mercaptopropionylglycine, an experimental drug whose mechanism of action is similar to that of penicillamine but whose structure, and hence toxicity, is different. When medical management fails, urologic surgery is required. An occasional patient may require renal transplantation because of renal failure.

DIBASICAMINOACIDURIA Families have been described in which affected members have a defect in renal tubular reabsorption of lysine, arginine, and ornithine but *not* of cystine. The disorder almost surely reflects mutations in the genes coding for a renal transport protein used by the three dibasic amino acids only. Two variants have been observed, each apparently inherited as an autosomal recessive trait. Manifestations are related to the losses of ornithine, arginine, and perhaps lysine.

In the common form of dibasicaminoaciduria (type II), also known as lysinuric protein intolerance, homozygotes show defective intestinal transport of dibasic amino acids as well as exaggerated renal losses. The transport defect may affect renal basolateral rather than luminal membrane transport. A defect in hepatic cell uptake of these substances has also been proposed. Affected patients present in childhood with hepatosplenomegaly, protein intolerance, and episodic ammonia intoxication. Plasma concentrations of lysine, arginine, and ornithine are reduced. The clinical findings have been attributed to hyperammonemia resulting from insufficient amounts of arginine and ornithine to maintain proper function of the urea cycle. Treatment includes dietary protein restriction and supplementation with citrulline, a neutral amino acid that has unimpaired intestinal and hepatic transport, that when metabolized to arginine and ornithine fuels the urea cycle. With 2.0 to 3.0 g of oral citrulline daily, dietary protein intake can be increased and growth improved in pediatric patients. Obligate heterozygotes are healthy and show no excess urinary loss of dibasic amino acids.

Type I dibasicaminoaciduria has been described in only one homozygote. She was moderately mentally retarded but had no clear history of protein intolerance or hyperammonemia. Her urinary losses of dibasic amino acids were not as great as those seen in type II homozygotes. The condition was distinguished from type II by the presence of modest excesses of dibasic amino acids in urine of both asymptomatic parents. Other pedigrees containing asymptomatic heterozygotes have been identified by urinary screening programs. Type I disease may involve a renal luminal membrane transport defect.

TABLE 308-1 Genetic disorders of membrane transport

Class of substance and disorder	Individual substrates	Tissues manifesting transport defect	Proposed molecular basis of defect	Major clinical manifestations	Mode of inheritance	Location of discussion
AMINO ACIDS						
Classic cystinuria	Cystine, lysine, arginine, ornithine	Proximal renal tubule, jejunal mucosa	Mutation of shared dibasic-cystine transport protein	Cystine nephrolithiasis	Autosomal recessive	Chap. 308
Dibasicaminoaciduria	Lysine, arginine, ornithine	Proximal renal tubule, jejunal mucosa	Mutation of dibasic transport protein	Type I: Moderate retardation Type II: Protein intolerance, hyperammonemia, retardation	Autosomal recessive	Chap. 308
Hypercystinuria	Cystine	Proximal renal tubule	Mutation of cystine transport protein	Some risk of cystine nephrolithiasis	Autosomal recessive	Chap. 308
Lysinuria	Lysine	Proximal renal tubule, jejunal mucosa	Mutation of lysine transport protein	Seizures, physical and mental retardation	Possible autosomal recessive	Chap. 308
Hartnup disease	Neutral amino acids	Proximal renal tubule, jejunal mucosa	Mutation of shared neutral amino acid transport protein	Constant neutral aminoaciduria, intermittent symptoms of pellagra	Autosomal recessive	Chap. 308
Tryptophan malabsorption	Tryptophan	Jejunal mucosa	Mutation of tryptophan transport protein	Indoluria, ?hypercalcemia, ?nephrocalcinosis	Probable autosomal recessive	Chap. 308
Methionine malabsorption	Methionine	Jejunal mucosa	Mutation of methionine transport protein	α-Hydroxybutyric-aciduria, white hair, mental retardation, convulsions, hyperpneic attacks, edema	Probable autosomal recessive	Chap. 308
Histidinuria	Histidine	Proximal renal tubule, jejunal mucosa	Mutation of histidine transport protein	Mental retardation	Autosomal recessive	Chap. 308
Iminoglycinuria	Glycine, proline, hydroxyproline	Proximal renal tubule, jejunal mucosa	Mutation of shared glycine–imino acid transport protein	None	Autosomal recessive	Chap. 308
Dicarboxylic-aminoaciduria	Glutamic acid, aspartic acid	Proximal renal tubule, jejunal mucosa	Mutation of shared dicarboxylic amino acid transport protein	None	Probable autosomal recessive	Chap. 308
HEXOSES						
Renal glycosuria	D-Glucose	Proximal renal tubule	Mutation of D-glucose transport protein	Glycosuria with normal blood glucose	Autosomal recessive	Chap. 308
Glucose-galactose malabsorption	D-Glucose D-Galactose	Jejunal mucosa, proximal renal tubule	Mutation of shared glucose-galactose transport protein	Watery diarrhea on feeding glucose, lactose, sucrose, or galactose	Autosomal recessive	Chaps. 237, 308
LIPIDS						
Familial hypercholesterolemia	Cholesterol	Fibroblasts, lymphoid lines, leukocytes	Mutation of membrane LDL–cholesterol receptor protein	Hypercholesterolemia, tendon xanthomas, arcus corneae, coronary artery atherosclerosis	Autosomal dominant	Chap. 315
URATE						
Hypouricemia	Uric acid	Proximal renal tubule	Mutation of urate transport protein	Hypouricemia, hyperuricosuria, ?hypercalcinuria	Autosomal recessive	Chap. 308
ANIONS						
Familial hypophosphatemic rickets	Inorganic phosphate	Proximal renal tubule, jejunal mucosa	Mutation of inorganic phosphate transport protein	Hypophosphatemia, phosphaturia, phosphatopenic rickets/osteomalacia	X-linked dominant	Chap. 337
Congenital chloridorrhea	Chloride	Ileal and colonic mucosa	Mutation of Cl^-/HCO_3^- exchange pump carrier protein	Hydramnios, watery diarrhea, elevated fecal chloride, achloriduria, metabolic alkalosis with volume depletion, hyperaldosteronism	Autosomal recessive	Chaps. 237, 308

TABLE 308-1 Genetic disorders of membrane transport *(continued)*

Class of substance and disorder	Individual substrates	Tissues manifesting transport defect	Proposed molecular basis of defect	Major clinical manifestations	Mode of inheritance	Location of discussion
ANIONS *(continued)*						
Familial goiter	Inorganic iodide	Thyroid gland, salivary gland, gastric mucosa	Mutation of iodide transport protein	Congenital hypothyroidism (cretinism), goiter	Probable autosomal recessive	Chap. 324
CATIONS						
Distal renal tubular acidosis (type I—gradient)	Hydrogen ion	Distal renal tubule	Mutation of distal tubule H^+ pump carrier protein	Hyperchloremic acidosis, hypokalemia, acquired nephrocalcinosis, and hypercalcinuria	Autosomal dominant	Chap. 228
Proximal renal tubular acidosis (type II—HCO_3^- wasting)	Hydrogen ion	Proximal renal tubule	Mutation of proximal tubule H^+ pump carrier protein	Hyperchloremic acidosis, bicarbonate wasting	Probable autosomal recessive	Chap. 228
Menkes' disease	Copper	Duodenal and jejunal intestinal cells	Possible serosal transport protein or intracellular transport defect	Severe mental retardation, pili torti (kinky hair), typical facies, arterial tortuosity, excess Wormian bones, thermal instability	X-linked recessive	Chaps. 77, 319
Hereditary Spherocytosis Elliptocytosis Ovalocytosis Stomatocytosis	Sodium	Red blood cell (RBC) membranes	Mutation of membrane structure (? lipid or protein) resulting in increased sodium permeability	Increased RBC fragility resulting in variable degrees of hemolytic anemia, splenomegaly, and jaundice; RBC shape respectively spherocytic, elliptocytic, ovalocytic, or stomatocytic (target-shaped)	Each of these diseases of RBC morphology is a separately inherited autosomal dominant	Chap. 287
WATER						
Nephrogenic diabetes insipidus (AVP-resistant)	Water	Distal renal tubule	Lack of activation of AVP-responsive luminal membrane adenylate cyclase, possible defect in receptor or enzyme protein	Polyuria, polydipsia, hyposthenuria	X-linked recessive	Chap. 228
VITAMINS						
Juvenile pernicious anemia	Cobalamin (vitamin B_{12})	Ileal mucosa	Mutation of receptor for intrinsic factor–cobalamin complex	Megaloblastic anemia	Autosomal recessive	Chap. 285
Folate malabsorption	Folic acid	Small bowel	Mutation of folate transport protein	Megaloblastic anemia	Autosomal recessive	Chap. 285
Multiple carboxylase deficiency (type II)	Biotin	Small bowel	Mutation of biotin transport protein	Ketoacidosis, alopecia, eczematoid eruption	Undefined	

HARTNUP DISEASE Pellagra-like skin lesions, variable neurologic manifestations, and aminoaciduria for the monoaminomonocarboxylic amino acids with neutral or aromatic side chains characterize Hartnup disease. Alanine, serine, threonine, valine, leucine, isoleucine, phenylalanine, tyrosine, tryptophan, glutamine, asparagine, and histidine are excreted in urine in quantities 5 to 10 times normal, and intestinal transport for these same amino acids is defective. The clinical manifestations result from nutritional deficiency of the essential amino acid tryptophan, caused by the combination of intestinal malabsorption and renal loss. Disease manifestations are episodic, related, at least in part, to metabolic demands for tryptophan.

The major pathway of tryptophan metabolism leads to the synthesis of niacin and nicotinamide-adenine dinucleotide (NAD). This pathway supplies about 50 percent of daily niacin needs. In patients with Hartnup disease, the renal and intestinal transport defect for tryptophan leads to niacin deficiency. The transport defect likely reflects abnormalities of a group-specific system for neutral amino acids. Some residual reabsorptive capacity persists for each involved amino acid. This suggests that they are transported by other carrier systems as well, a conclusion supported by the identification of patients with substrate-specific transport errors for tryptophan, methionine, and histidine.

Hartnup disease is inherited as an autosomal recessive trait. Homozygotes occur with a frequency of about 1 in 16,000 births. Heterozygotes exhibit no clinical or chemical abnormalities.

Pellagra is the clinical syndrome produced by dietary niacin deficiency, and its clinical features are those that characterize Hartnup disease (see Chap. 76). The diagnosis should be suspected in any patient with pellagra without a history of dietary niacin deficiency. The neurologic and psychiatric manifestations range from attacks of cerebellar ataxia to mild emotional lability to frank delirium and usually accompany exacerbations of the erythematous, eczematoid skin rash. Fever, sunlight, stress, and sulfonamide therapy provoke clinical relapses. Diagnosis is made by detection of the neutral aminoaciduria that does not occur in dietary niacin deficiency. Treatment is directed at niacin repletion and includes a high-protein diet and daily nicotinamide supplementation (50 to 250 mg).

IMINOGLYCINURIA This trait is characterized by excessive urinary excretion of glycine and the imino acids proline and hydroxyproline. Homozygotes for this autosomal recessive disorder occur with a frequency of about 1 in 16,000. The exaggerated renal clearance of glycine, proline, and hydroxyproline reflects a defect in the tubular transport system shared by these three compounds. An intestinal transport defect may also be present. This suggests that more than one mutation may lead to persistent iminoglycinuria, a thesis corroborated by the demonstration that obligate heterozygotes from some but not all families manifest glycinuria. No consistent clinical abnormalities have been reported in homozygotes, who are usually detected by urinary amino acid screening programs. Individuals with iminoglycinuria should be reassured as to the benign nature of the disturbance.

DICARBOXYLICAMINOACIDURIA Selective urinary loss and exaggerated endogenous renal clearance of glutamic and aspartic acids have been described in two unrelated children. Intestinal absorption of these dicarboxylic amino acids was impaired in one. This patient suffered from recurrent hypoglycemia; the other was asymptomatic.

SUBSTRATE-SPECIFIC DEFECTS IN AMINO ACID TRANSPORT Rare pedigrees exist in which individuals have defective renal tubular reabsorption and/or impaired intestinal absorption of a single free amino acid. These disorders, each apparently inherited as an autosomal recessive trait, suggest that transport of amino acids is catalyzed by substrate-specific as well as group-specific transport mechanisms.

Hypercystinuria Two siblings exhibited modest cystinuria without excessive urinary excretion of lysine, arginine, or ornithine. Fractional tubular reabsorption of cystine was reduced to about 80 percent of the filtered load, and up to 250 mg per day was excreted in the urine. Neither showed any abnormality in intestinal absorption of cystine. Both were clinically well, although the cystine excretion places them at risk for cystine urolithiasis. Urinary cystine excretion by the parents was normal.

Lysinuria A child with selective impairment of renal tubular reabsorption of lysine has been described. Endogenous lysine clearance was increased; intestinal transport was impaired; plasma lysine was reduced. Mental and growth retardation and seizures were present. A lysine-supplemented diet stimulated growth. Urinary lysine excretion was normal in the parents.

Histidinuria Two siblings, each with mental retardation, exhibited a renal transport defect for histidine only. Urinary loss of histidine approached 40 to 50 percent of the filtered load, and an intestinal transport defect for histidine was also present. The clinically normal parents had normal urinary excretion but a modest defect in intestinal absorption of histidine. In two additional cases of isolated histidinuria myoclonic seizures occurred.

Methionine malabsorption Single children from two pedigrees have shown an intestinal transport defect for methionine. One may have had a renal transport defect as well. This disorder was detected because of urinary excretion of α-hydroxybutyric acid, a by-product of the intestinal bacterial breakdown of the unabsorbed methionine. This compound, which gives an odor resembling malt or dried celery to the urine, appears to be responsible for the white hair, attacks of hyperpnea, convulsions, edema, and mental retardation. Treatment of one of these children with a methionine-restricted diet caused improvement in all clinical manifestations.

Tryptophan malabsorption An isolated defect in intestinal absorption of tryptophan has been described in two siblings. The renal tubular reabsorption of tryptophan was normal. A variety of indoles were excreted in stool and urine. These compounds result from chemical degradation of unabsorbed tryptophan by intestinal bacteria and may be present in patients with Hartnup disease as well. Because of concomitant renal disease, hydrolytic enzymes were released into the urine, acted upon the indoles found there, and led to the formation of a blue pigment, indigotin. This sequence of events earned this condition the sobriquet "blue-diaper syndrome." No pellagra-like symptoms were described. The mother also excreted indole compounds, suggesting that she is a carrier of this trait.

DISORDERS OF HEXOSE TRANSPORT

Nondiabetic melituria occurs in a number of conditions. Pentoses, hexoses, heptoses, and disaccharides have been identified in the urine; all except sucrose yield a positive test for reducing substances. Some melliturias result from diffuse renal injury, others from ingestion of nonmetabolizable sugars. In still others the sugars accumulate in blood owing to deficient activity of catabolizing enzyme systems and "spill" into the urine. Only among the hexoses have specific inherited disorders of sugar transport been identified. The existence of renal glycosuria and intestinal glucose-galactose malabsorption as heritable, autosomal recessive disorders points to the existence of at least two specific carrier proteins for hexoses in human jejunal and renal brush border membranes: one for glucose and one shared by glucose and galactose.

RENAL GLYCOSURIA To avoid confusion with diabetes mellitus, Marble's criteria for the diagnosis of renal glycosuria should be followed: (1) glycosuria in the absence of hyperglycemia, (2) constant glycosuria with little fluctuation related to diet, (3) normal (or slightly flat) oral glucose tolerance test, (4) identification of urinary reducing substance as glucose, and (5) normal storage and utilization of carbohydrates. The Fanconi syndrome, in which renal glycosuria occurs as part of generalized proximal tubular dysfunction, should also be excluded. The incidence is less than 1 in 500. The condition is benign, but occasionally glycosuria may be great enough to cause polyuria and polydipsia. Even more rarely, dehydration or ketosis may develop under conditions of stress such as pregnancy or starvation.

In normal persons glucose is present in the glomerular filtrate at a concentration equal to that in plasma water and is reabsorbed throughout the proximal renal tubule by a sodium-dependent, phlorizin-inhibitable transport process. Reabsorptive capacity exceeds normal plasma glucose concentration. Thus, glucose does not appear in the urine until the threshold for reabsorption is reached. The plasma concentration at which filtered glucose begins to escape proximal tubular reabsorption is 200 to 240 mg/dL. Maximal renal reabsorptive capacity is exceeded at a filtered load of 325 ± 36 mg/min per 1.73 square meters of body surface area, and this value is defined as the tubular maximum for glucose (TmG).

Two patterns of glycosuria are recognized: type A characterized by a reduced tubular maximum reabsorptive capacity and type B showing a reduced threshold for glycosuria, an increased "splay" in the titration curve, and a normal TmG. Marked renal glycosuria occurs in individuals homozygous for either of these recessively inherited mutations and in genetic compounds for these presumably allelic mutations. Modest reduction in renal threshold or TmG is present in obligate heterozygotes in some pedigrees; modest glycosuria occurs in such family members when plasma glucose is elevated. The gene responsible for renal glycosuria segregates with the human histocompatibility leukocyte antigen (HLA) haplotype suggesting its location on chromosome 6. No linkage disequilibrium was observed, and no specific HLA antigens have been associated with renal glycosuria.

GLUCOSE-GALACTOSE MALABSORPTION In this condition, infants develop a profuse, watery diarrhea when fed milk or foods containing lactose, sucrose, glucose, or galactose. Fructose or carbohydrate-free formulas are well tolerated. A specific defect in intestinal absorption of glucose and galactose can be demonstrated by oral tolerance tests that produce little or no increase in plasma glucose or galactose. Treatment with a glucose- and galactose-free diet leads to resolution of symptoms in childhood. Although the basic transport defect is present throughout life, most patients show an improved tolerance for glucose and galactose with age.

Active D-glucose and D-galactose transport is absent in affected children, and intermediate transport capacity is present in their parents. These findings confirm the specificity and the autosomal recessive inheritance of the disorder.

A number of these patients have renal glycosuria at normal plasma glucose concentrations. Renal titration studies generally demonstrate a reduced threshold for glucose reabsorption (type B renal glycosuria) with a normal TmG. Urinary glucose loss is not as severe as in isolated renal glycosuria. This finding suggests the presence of multiple glucose transport proteins in the kidney. One, responsible for the bulk of glucose reabsorption and specific for glucose only, is affected in renal glycosuria; another, shared by glucose and galactose and responsible for transporting less of the filtered load of glucose, is affected in glucose-galactose malabsorption. Either the former is not present in intestinal mucosa, or the shared system is more important in that tissue. In both disorders transport of sugars in all other tested tissues is normal, reflecting the multiplicity and tissue specificity of membrane transport proteins.

DEFECTIVE URATE TRANSPORT: HYPOURICEMIA

Individuals with a selective defect in renal tubular reabsorption of sodium urate have marked hypouricemia. Since little serum urate is bound to plasma proteins, failure to reabsorb filtered urate results in a serum urate ranging from 0.2 to 1.8 mg/dL. Moderate uricosuria is present, and half of patients have renal calculi.

Renal urate clearance normally averages 15 percent of glomerular filtration rate, and the excreted urate is composed both of filtered urate that has escaped reabsorption and secreted urate. Subjects with isolated hypouricemia have urate clearances averaging from 33 to 85 percent of the filtration rate; in some, urate clearance exceeds the glomerular filtration rate. Studies with probenecid, which blocks tubular reabsorption of urate, and pyrazinamide, which blocks tubular secretion, reveal that six of the eight families described have a presecretory urate reabsorptive defect, and two have defective transport affecting the entire tubule. In four families hypercalciuria due to enhanced intestinal calcium absorption is also present, but in others only uricosuria has been demonstrated. The defect is inherited as an autosomal recessive trait. Urate transport has not been studied in nonrenal tissue or in obligate heterozygotes. The defect is presumed to reflect mutation of one or both of the proximal renal tubular membrane proteins that transport sodium urate. The findings in these families support the hypothesis that renal urate reabsorption is controlled by more than one transport protein.

DEFECTIVE ANION TRANSPORT: CHLORIDORRHEA

This rare, autosomal recessive disease results from impairment of active transport of chloride in the ileum and colon. Absence of the chloride-bicarbonate ion exchange "pump" causes profound symptoms even before birth (polyhydramnios and absence of meconium). Massive watery diarrhea is apparent from the first days of life. This fluid loss, with its attendant impairment of electrolyte homeostasis, is life-threatening. A hypokalemic, hypochloremic, hyponatremic metabolic alkalosis develops with dehydration and secondary hyperaldosteronism. Fecal fluid contains an excess of chloride ion over the sum of the accompanying cations, sodium and potassium. Fecal chloride concentration always exceeds 90 mmol per liter when volume and serum electrolyte disturbances are corrected, and this chloridorrhea is diagnostic. Renal chloride transport is normal. Decreased urine chloride results from the kidney's attempts to conserve salt and water.

Treatment requires adequate, life-long repletion of electrolyte and fluid losses, since no way has yet been found to mitigate the transport disorder. Exact replacement of water, sodium chloride, and potassium chloride can prevent the growth and psychomotor retardation and the development of progressive renal damage. The renal lesion, with hyalinized glomeruli, juxtaglomerular hyperplasia, calcifications, and arteriolar changes, is probably a result of chronic volume depletion. Treatment of hyperreninemia and hypokalemia with prostaglandin inhibitors may reduce renal damage but does not alter intestinal symptoms or the need for chronic sodium chloride repletion.

REFERENCES

DEMARCHI S et al: Close genetic linkage between HLA and renal glycosuria. Am J Nephrol 4:280, 1984

ELSAS LJ, ROSENBERG LE: Renal glycosuria, in *Strauss and Welt's Diseases of the Kidney,* 3d ed, LE Earley, CW Gottschalk (eds). Boston, Little, Brown, 1979, pp 1021–1028

HOLMBERG C, PERHEENTUPA J: Congenital chloride diarrhoea (CCD), in *Population Structure and Genetic Disorders,* AW Erikson et al (eds). New York, Academic, 1980, pp 596–599

KAMOUN PP et al: Renal histidinuria. J Inherited Metab Dis 4:217, 1981

RAJANTIE J et al: Lysinuric protein intolerance: A 2-year trial of dietary supplementation therapy with citrulline and lysine. J Pediatr 97:927, 1980

RAJANTIE J et al: Lysinuric protein intolerance: Basolateral transport defect in renal tubuli. J Clin Invest 67:1078, 1981

ROSENBERG LE: Intestinal hexose transport in familial glucose-galactose malabsorption, in *Membranes and Disease,* L Bolis et al (eds). New York, Raven Press, 1976, pp 253–262

———, SCRIVER CR: Disorders of amino acid metabolism, in *Metabolic Control and Disease,* 8th ed, PK Bondy, LE Rosenberg (eds). Philadelphia, Saunders, 1980, pp 616–645

SEGAL S, THIER SO: Cystinuria, in *The Metabolic Basis of Inherited Disease,* 5th ed, JB Stanbury et al (eds). New York, McGraw-Hill, 1983, pp 1774–1791

SHORT EM, ROSENBERG LE: Renal aminoaciduria, in *Strauss and Welt's Diseases of the Kidney,* 3d ed, LE Earley, CW Gottschalk (eds). Boston, Little, Brown, 1979, pp 975–1020

WEITZ R, SPERLING O: Hereditary renal hypouricemia: Isolated tubular defect of urate reabsorption. J Pediatr 96:850, 1980

309 GOUT AND OTHER DISORDERS OF PURINE METABOLISM

WILLIAM N. KELLEY / THOMAS D. PALELLA

Gout is a term representing a heterogeneous group of diseases, which in their full development are manifested by (1) an increase in the serum urate concentration; (2) recurrent attacks of a characteristic acute arthritis, in which crystals of monosodium urate monohydrate are demonstrable in leukocytes of synovial fluid; (3) aggregated deposits of monosodium urate monohydrate (tophi) chiefly in and around the joints of the extremities and sometimes leading to severe crippling and deformity; (4) renal disease involving interstitial tissues and blood vessels; and (5) uric acid nephrolithiasis. These may occur singly or in combination.

PREVALENCE AND EPIDEMIOLOGY The serum urate value is elevated in an absolute sense when it exceeds the limit of solubility of monosodium urate in serum. At 37°C the saturation value of urate in plasma is about 7.0 mg/dL; a value above this represents supersaturation in a physicochemical sense. The serum urate concentration is relatively elevated when it exceeds the upper limit of an arbitrary normal range, usually defined as the mean serum urate value plus 2 standard deviations in a healthy population matched for age and sex. In most studies the upper limit is about 7.0 mg/dL in men and 6.0 mg/dL in women. In epidemiologic terms a serum urate value in excess of 7.0 mg/dL carries an increased risk of gouty arthritis or renal stones.

Sex and age influence urate levels. In both boys and girls the serum urate concentration before puberty averages approximately 3.6 mg/dL. After puberty, levels increase in boys more than in girls. Values in men reach a plateau in the early twenties and are essentially stable thereafter. Values in women are constant from age 20 through 40, but with menopause the values rise and approach or equal those in men. These age and sex differences are thought to be related to differences in the renal clearance of urate, perhaps influenced by the levels of estrogens and androgens. Certain physiologic variables such as height, body weight, creatinine, blood urea nitrogen, serum creatinine, and blood pressure correlate with serum urate concentration. Other factors, including warm ambient temperature, alcohol intake, high social status, and achievement or intelligence also appear to correlate with a higher serum urate concentration.

Hyperuricemia by one or more of the above definitions is present in 2 to 18 percent of the population. In one hospitalized group, 13 percent of adult men exhibited a serum urate concentration in excess of 7.0 mg/dL.

The incidence and prevalence of gout are less than those of hyperuricemia. In most of the western world the incidence of gout ranges from 0.20 to 0.35 per 1000, resulting in an overall prevalence of 0.13 to 0.37 percent of the population. The prevalence relates both to the degree of elevation of the serum urate and to the duration over which this elevation is sustained. Gout is therefore primarily a disease of adult men, and only about 5 percent of cases occur in women; it occurs rarely in the prepubertal child of either sex. The usual form is uncommon before the third decade, and the peak incidence is in the fifth decade.

INHERITANCE In the United States a family history of gout is obtained in 6 to 18 percent of gouty subjects, and figures as high as 75 percent are noted after persistent questioning. A precise definition of the inheritance of gout is complicated by the environmental factors that alter the serum urate concentration. In addition, the identification of several specific causes of gout indicates that the disorder is the common clinical manifestation of a heterogeneous group of diseases. Accordingly, analysis of the inheritance of hyperuricemia and gout in the population or even within families is difficult. Two specific enzymatic causes of gout, hypoxanthine-guanine phosphoribosyltransferase deficiency and 5-phosphoribosyl-1-pyrophosphate (PRPP) synthetase overactivity, are X-linked. In other families the inheritance is consistent with an autosomal dominant mode. More commonly, genetic studies suggest multifactorial inheritance.

CLINICAL FEATURES The full natural history of gout comprises four stages: asymptomatic hyperuricemia, acute gouty arthritis, intercritical gout, and chronic tophaceous gout. Nephrolithiasis may occur in any stage but the first.

Asymptomatic hyperuricemia Asymptomatic hyperuricemia is that stage in which the serum urate level is raised but arthritic symptoms, tophi, or uric acid stones have not yet appeared. In men vulnerable to classic gout, hyperuricemia begins at puberty, whereas in women at risk hyperuricemia is usually delayed until menopause. In contrast, patients with certain of the enzyme defects to be described later may be hyperuricemic from birth. While asymptomatic hyperuricemia may last throughout the lifetime with no recognizable consequences, the tendency toward acute gouty arthritis increases as a function of the level and the duration of hyperuricemia. The risk of nephrolithiasis also increases as serum urate values increase and correlates with the magnitude of uric acid excretion. While virtually all gouty subjects are hyperuricemic, only about 5 percent of hyperuricemics ever develop gout.

The phase of asymptomatic hyperuricemia ends with the first attack of gouty arthritis or nephrolithiasis. In most, gout comes before stone, usually after at least 20 to 30 years of sustained hyperuricemia. However, between 10 and 40 percent of gouty subjects have renal colic prior to the first episode of arthritis.

Acute gouty arthritis The primary manifestation of acute gout is exquisitely painful arthritis, at first usually monoarticular and associated with few constitutional symptoms but later often polyarticular and accompanied by fever. Estimates vary as to the percentage of patients in whom the initial gouty episode is polyarticular. Some authors' estimates are as high as 40 percent, and the majority of reports range from 3 to 14 percent. Attacks last a variable but limited period of time and are separated by asymptomatic intervals. In at least half the initial attack occurs in the first metatarsal phalangeal joint. Ultimately, 90 percent of patients experience an acute attack in the great toe (podagra).

Acute gouty arthritis is predominantly a disease of the lower extremities. The more distal the site of involvement the more typical are the attacks. Following the toe in order of frequency as sites of initial involvement are the insteps, ankles, heels, knees, wrists, fingers, and elbows. Acute attacks in the shoulder, hips, spine, sacroiliac, sternoclavicular, and mandibular joints are rare except in patients with established, severe disease. Gouty bursitis also occurs, the prepatellar and olecranon bursae being the most commonly involved sites. The patient may report trivial episodes of pain, often described as "twinges," preceding the first dramatic gouty attack. More commonly, the initial attack is unheralded and explosive. Often, the major attack begins at night, is exquisitely painful with inflamed joints, and may be triggered by a specific event such as trauma, alcohol ingestion, certain drugs, dietary excess, or surgery. The pain reaches peak intensity within several hours, and the associated signs of inflammation progress. The inflammatory response is typically so intense as to suggest pyogenic arthritis. Systemic signs may include fever, leukocytosis, and an elevated sedimentation rate. It is difficult to improve upon Sydenham's classic description:

The victim goes to bed and sleeps in good health. About two o'clock in the morning he is awakened by a severe pain in the great toe; more rarely in the heel, ankle or instep. This pain is like that of a dislocation, and yet the parts feel as if cold water were poured over them. Then follow chills and shivers, and a little fever. The pain, which was at first moderate, becomes more intense. With its intensity the chills and shivers increase. After a time this comes to its height, accommodating itself to the bones and ligaments of the tarsus and metatarsus. Now it is a violent stretching and tearing of the ligaments—now it is a gnawing pain and now a pressure and tightening. So exquisite and lively meanwhile is the feeling of the part affected, that it cannot bear the weight of bedclothes nor the jar of a person walking in the room. The night is passed in torture, sleeplessness, turning of the part affected, and perpetual change of posture; the tossing about of the body being as incessant as the pain of the tortured joint, and being worse as the fit comes on. Hence the vain effort by change of posture, both in the body and the limb affected, to obtain an abatement of the pain.

The initial gouty episode indicates the serum urate concentration has been sufficiently elevated for a long enough period of time to result in tissue deposition of substantial amounts of urate.

Intercritical period The attack of gout may last only a day or two or up to several weeks but characteristically subsides spontaneously. No sequelae ensue, and resolution is complete. An asymptomatic phase termed the *intercritical period* then commences. The patient is totally free of symptoms during this stage, a feature that is diagnostically important. While approximately 7 percent never have a second attack, approximately 60 percent experience a recurrence within 1 year. However, the intercritical period may last up to 10 years and is terminated by successive attacks each of which may last longer and resolve less completely than its predecessors. Later attacks tend to be polyarticular, more severe, more prolonged, and associated with fever. In this stage gout may be difficult to differentiate from

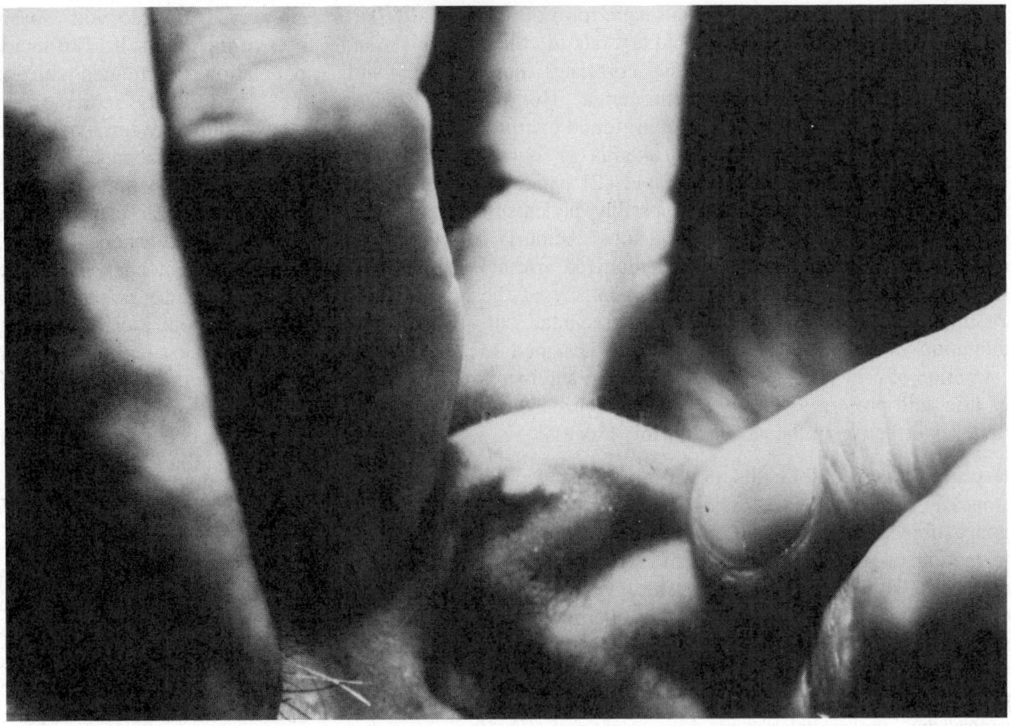

FIGURE 309-1 *Tophus of the helix of the ear adjacent to the auricular tubercle.*

other types of polyarticular arthritis such as rheumatoid arthritis. Rare patients progress directly from the initial acute attack to chronic polyarticular disease with no remissions.

Tophi and chronic gouty arthritis In the untreated patient the rate of urate production exceeds the rate of urate disposition. As a result, the urate pool expands, and crystal deposits of monosodium urate eventually appear in cartilage, synovial membranes, tendons, and soft tissues. The rate of formation of these tophaceous deposits is a function of the degree and duration of hyperuricemia and of the severity of renal disease. The classic, but by no means the most common, location of a tophus is the helix or antihelix of the ear (Fig. 309-1). Tophi also commonly occur along the ulnar surface of the forearm, as saccular distensions of the olecranon bursae (Fig. 309-2), as enlargements of the Achilles tendon, or at other pressure points. Patients with the most severe tophi, interestingly, often have sparing of the helix and antihelix of the ear.

Tophi are difficult to differentiate from rheumatoid nodules and other types of subcutaneous nodules. They may ulcerate and exude chalky or pasty material rich in monosodium urate crystals. In contrast to other subcutaneous nodules, tophi are rarely transient although they may resolve slowly in response to treatment of hyperuricemia. Documentation of monosodium urate crystals by polarizing microscopy of an aspirate establishes the nodule in question as a tophus. It is rare for a tophus to become infected. Patients with severe tophaceous disease appear to have milder and less frequent attacks of acute gouty arthritis than do nontophaceous subjects. Chronic tophaceous gout rarely occurs prior to the onset of gouty arthritis.

Effective therapy alters the natural history of the disease. Since the advent of effective antihyperuricemic therapy, only a minority of patients develop visible tophi, permanent joint changes, or chronic symptoms.

Nephropathy Some renal dysfunction occurs in up to 90 percent of subjects with gouty arthritis. Prior to the advent of chronic hemodialysis, renal failure accounted for 17 to 25 percent of deaths in the gouty population. The initial manifestation of renal involvement may be albuminuria or isosthenuria. If the patient presents in an advanced stage of renal failure it may be difficult to determine whether renal failure is a consequence of hyperuricemia or hyperuricemia is the result of renal disease.

Several types of parenchymal renal damage have been described. The first, urate nephropathy, has been attributed to the deposition of monosodium urate crystals in the renal interstitial tissue. The second, obstructive uropathy, is due to the formation of uric acid crystals in the collecting tubules, renal pelvis, or ureter, with resulting blockage of urine flow.

There is considerable controversy over the pathogenesis of urate nephropathy. While crystals of monosodium urate have been demonstrated in the interstitium of kidneys from some gouty subjects, such crystals are not present in the kidneys of most people with gout. Conversely, renal interstitial urate deposition occurs in the absence of gout, although the clinical significance of such deposition is unclear. Unidentified factors may participate in the formation of urate deposits in the kidney. Further, there is a close correlation between the development of renal disease and the presence of hypertension in patients with gout. It is frequently not clear whether the hypertension causes the renal disease or the gouty renal disease is the cause of the hypertension.

FIGURE 309-2 *Effusions of olecranon bursae of patient with gout. Note also the cutaneous deposits of urate and the minimal inflammatory response.*

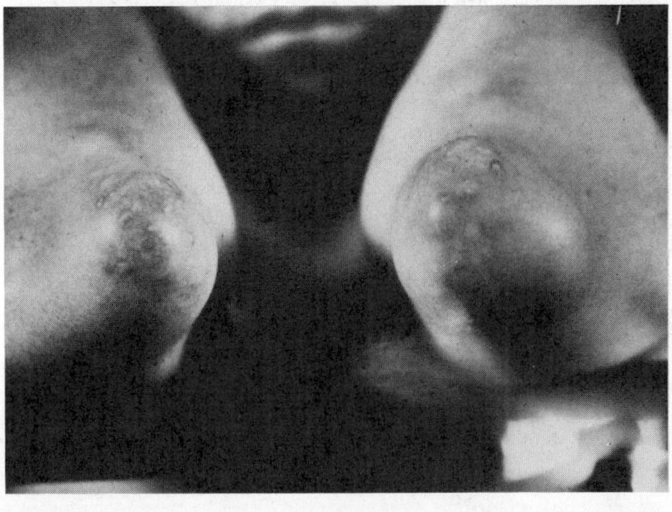

Acute obstructive uropathy is a severe form of acute renal failure due to the precipitation of uric acid crystals in collecting ducts and ureters. Renal failure in this setting correlates more strongly with hyperuricaciduria than with hyperuricemia. This condition occurs most commonly in (1) patients with profound overproduction of uric acid, particularly subjects with leukemia or lymphoma who are subjected to aggressive chemotherapy, (2) patients with gout and marked hyperuricaciduria, and (3) (possibly) patients following severe exercise, rhabdomyolysis, or convulsions. Aciduria favors the formation of the relatively insoluble nonionized uric acid and, hence, may contribute to crystal precipitation in any of these conditions. Postmortem studies reveal intraluminal precipitates of uric acid with dilatation of proximal tubules. Therapy designed to decrease the formation of uric acid, accelerate urine flow, and increase the fraction of uric acid present as the more soluble ionized form, monosodium urate, is effective in the reversal of this process.

Nephrolithiasis While the prevalence of subjects with uric acid stones in the United States is about 0.01 percent, the prevalence in gouty subjects ranges from 10 to 25 percent. The major factor favoring formation of uric acid stones is the increased urinary excretion of uric acid. Hyperuricaciduria may be due to primary gout, inborn errors of metabolism resulting in the overproduction of uric acid, myeloproliferative disease, and other neoplastic disorders. When the urinary uric acid exceeds 1100 mg per day, the incidence reaches 50 percent. There is also correlation with increasing serum urate concentrations, the prevalence reaching approximately 50 percent at a serum urate value of 13 mg/dL or above. Other factors contributing to the formation of uric acid stones include (1) undue acidity of the urine, (2) increased urine concentration, and (3) (perhaps) abnormalities of urinary constituents that affect the solubility of uric acid itself.

Gouty subjects also have an increased frequency of calcium-containing stones; the occurrence in gout is 1 to 3 percent, while that in the general population is about 0.1 percent. While the mechanisms for this association are unclear, there is a high frequency of hyperuricemia and hyperuricaciduria in patients seen because of calcium stones. Uric acid crystals may serve as a nidus for calcium stone formation.

Associated conditions Obesity, hypertriglyceridemia, and hypertension are common. The hypertriglyceridemia of primary gout is strongly associated with obesity or alcohol ingestion and not with hyperuricemia itself. The incidence of hypertension in the nongouty population is correlated with age, sex, and obesity; when these factors are appropriately scored, there appears to be little or no direct relationship between hyperuricemia and hypertension. The increased frequency of diabetes is also probably related to factors such as age and obesity and not to hyperuricemia itself. Finally, the increased incidence of atherosclerosis has been attributed to the concomitant obesity, hypertension, diabetes, and hypertriglyceridemia.

Independent analysis of these variables suggests that obesity is most important. Hyperuricemia in the obese subject appears to be related to both increased production and reduced excretion of uric acid. Chronic alcohol ingestion also results in both overproduction and underexcretion of uric acid.

Rheumatoid arthritis, systemic lupus erythematosus, and amyloidosis rarely coexist with gout. The reasons for these negative associations are not known.

Acute gout should be suspected in any patient presenting with the sudden onset of monoarthritis, particularly in a distal joint of the lower extremity. Synovial aspiration should be performed in all such patients. The diagnosis of gout is established with certainty upon demonstration of monosodium urate crystals in leukocytes of synovial fluid from the involved joint by compensated polarized light microscopy (Fig. 309-3). The crystals are typically needle-shaped and negatively birefringent. Such crystals can be identified in synovial fluid of over 95 percent of patients with acute gouty arthritis. Failure to demonstrate urate crystals in synovial fluid after careful search under appropriate conditions makes the diagnosis unlikely. The presence of intracellular urate crystals establishes the diagnosis but does not exclude the possibility that another type of arthropathy is present concurrently.

Infection or pseudogout (calcium pyrophosphate dihydrate deposition) may coexist with gout. A Gram stain of the synovial fluid should be examined, and cultures should be obtained to exclude coexistent infection. Calcium pyrophosphate dihydrate is weakly positively birefringent and is more rectangular than monosodium urate. With polarized light microscopy, the crystals are easily differentiated. Synovial aspiration need not be repeated with subsequent episodes unless an alternative diagnosis is being considered.

During asymptomatic intercritical periods, synovial aspiration may still be helpful. Extracellular urate crystals can be found in more than two-thirds of aspirates from the first metatarsophalangeal joints of asymptomatic gouty patients Less than 5 percent of hyperuricemic patients without gout have such crystals.

Synovial fluid analysis may also be helpful in other ways. The total leukocyte count may range from 1000 to more than 70,000 per milliliter. The predominant cell type is the polymorphonuclear leukocyte. As with other inflammatory fluids, the mucin clot is fair to poor. The concentrations of glucose and uric acid are the same as in serum.

In the patient in whom synovial fluid cannot be obtained or in whom intracellular crystals cannot be demonstrated, a presumptive diagnosis of gout can be seriously entertained if the patient has (1) hyperuricemia, (2) the classic clinical features described above, and (3) a dramatic response to colchicine. In the absence of crystals or this highly suggestive triad, the diagnosis of gout should be considered tentative. A dramatic therapeutic response to colchicine is strongly suggestive of the diagnosis of gouty arthritis but is not pathognomonic by itself.

Acute gouty arthritis must be differentiated from other causes of monoarticular and polyarticular arthritis. A common initial presentation in the gouty patient is podagra, but many conditions mimic the painful, swollen big toe characteristic of the disease. These include soft tissue infection, pyogenic arthritis, inflamed bunions, local trauma, rheumatoid arthritis, degenerative arthritis with acute inflammation, acute sarcoidosis, psoriatic arthritis, pseudogout, acute calcific tendonitis, palindromic rheumatism, Reiter's disease, and sporotrichosis. Rarely, confusion may be caused by cellulitis, gon-

FIGURE 309-3 *Crystals of monosodium urate monohydrate in joint aspirate.*

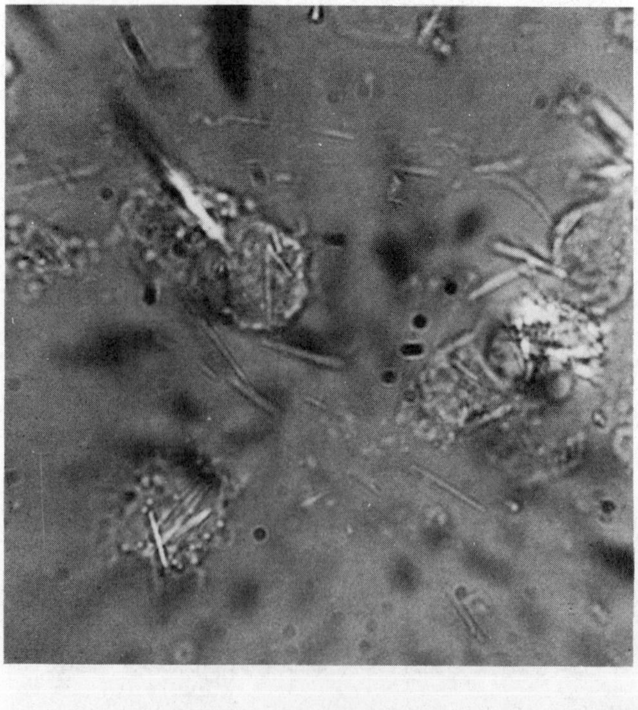

orrhea, fibrosis of the sole and heel, hematoma, and subacute bacterial endocarditis with embolization or suppurative arthritis. Gouty involvement of other joints such as the knee must also be differentiated from acute rheumatic fever, serum sickness, hemarthrosis, and the peripheral joint involvement of ankylosing spondylitis or inflammatory bowel disease.

Chronic gouty arthritis must be differentiated from rheumatoid arthritis, inflammatory osteoarthritis, psoriatic arthritis, enteropathic arthritis, and the peripheral arthritis associated with the spondyloarthropathies. A history of antecedent, self-limited monoarticular arthritis, the presence of tophi, typical radiographic changes, and the demonstration of hyperuricemia add support to the diagnosis of chronic gout. Chronic gout can be similar to other inflammatory arthropathies. The existence of effective therapy for gout justifies a vigorous workup to establish or exclude this diagnosis.

PATHOPHYSIOLOGY OF HYPERURICEMIA Classification The biochemical hallmark and prerequisite of gout is hyperuricemia. The concentration of uric acid in body fluids is determined by the balance between rates of production and elimination. Uric acid is formed by oxidation of purine bases, which may be exogenous or endogenous in origin. About two-thirds of uric acid is excreted into the urine (300 to 600 mg per day), and approximately one-third is excreted into the gastrointestinal tract, where it is ultimately destroyed by bacteria. Hyperuricemia may be due to an excessive rate of uric acid production, a decrease in the renal excretion of uric acid, or a combination of both events.

Hyperuricemia and gout may be classified as metabolic or renal (Table 309-1). In those patients with hyperuricemia of metabolic origin, there is an increased production of uric acid, whereas in those with hyperuricemia of renal origin, decreased renal excretion of uric acid causes the hyperuricemia. The distinction between metabolic and renal origins of hyperuricemia is not always clear-cut. A large number of gouty subjects have evidence of both mechanisms when thoroughly investigated. In such cases, the dominant component—renal or metabolic—directs classification. In the classification used here *primary* refers to those cases in which gout or hyperuricemia is the central manifestation of the disease, namely, gout that is neither secondary to another acquired disorder nor a subordinate manifestation of an inborn error that leads initially to a major disease unlike gout. While some cases of primary gout have a defined genetic basis, others do not. *Secondary* hyperuricemia or gout refers to those cases which develop in the course of another disease or as a consequence of drugs.

Overproduction of uric acid Overproducers of uric acid by definition excrete in excess of 600 mg per day after a 5-day period of dietary purine restriction; such patients probably represent less than 10 percent of the gouty population. In these patients there is an acceleration in the rate of purine biosynthesis de novo or an increased turnover of purines. Understanding the basic mechanisms responsible for these abnormalities requires an understanding of purine metabolism (Fig. 309-4).

The purine nucleotides, adenylic acid (AMP), inosinic acid (IMP), and guanylic acid (GMP), are the end products of purine biosynthesis. They can be synthesized in one of two ways: either directly from the purine bases, e.g., guanine to GMP, hypoxanthine to IMP, and adenine to AMP; or they may be synthesized de novo, beginning with nonpurine precursors and progressing through a series of steps to the formation of IMP, which is the common intermediate purine nucleotide. IMP can be converted either to AMP or to GMP. Once the purine nucleotides are formed, they are utilized for the synthesis of nucleic acids, adenosine triphosphate (ATP), cyclic AMP, cyclic GMP, and certain cofactors.

The various purine components are degraded to the purine nucleotide monophosphates. GMP is degraded via guanosine, guanine, and xanthine to uric acid. IMP is degraded through inosine, hypoxanthine, and xanthine to uric acid. AMP can be deaminated to IMP and further catabolized through inosine to uric acid, or it may be degraded to inosine by an alternate pathway with the intermediate formation of adenosine.

While the purine pathway is regulated in a complex manner, the intracellular concentration of 5-phosphoribosyl-1-pyrophosphate (PRPP) appears to be a major determinant of the rate of synthesis of uric acid in humans. Generally, when the concentration of PRPP in the cell is elevated, uric acid synthesis is elevated; when the concentration of PRPP is reduced, the synthesis of uric acid is also reduced. Although exceptions are recognized, this concept is applicable to most situations.

Overproduction of uric acid in a small minority of adult gouty subjects occurs as either a primary or a secondary manifestation of an inborn error in metabolism. Hyperuricemia and gout occur as a primary manifestation of partial hypoxanthine-guanine phosphoribosyltransferase deficiency (reaction 2, Fig. 309-4) and of PRPP synthetase superactivity (reaction 3, Fig. 309-4). In the Lesch-Nyhan syndrome, the virtually complete deficiency of hypoxanthine-guanine phosphoribosyltransferase results in secondary hyperuricemia. These important inborn errors are discussed more fully below.

These two inborn errors of purine metabolism, hypoxanthine-guanine phosphoribosyltransferase deficiency and PRPP synthetase overactivity, account for less than 15 percent of all patients with primary hyperuricemia associated with an overproduction of uric acid. The cause of the overproduction in the majority of patients has not been defined.

There are numerous causes of secondary hyperuricemia associated with an increased production of uric acid. In some, the increased excretion of uric acid is related, as it is in primary gout, to an accelerated rate of purine biosynthesis de novo. Patients with glucose 6-phosphatase deficiency (type I glycogen storage disease) uniformly

TABLE 309-1 Classification of hyperuricemia and gout

Type	Metabolic disturbance	Inheritance
Metabolic (10%):		
Primary		
Molecular defects undefined	Not established	Polygenic
Associated with specific enzyme defects		
PRPP synthetase variants, increased activity	Overproduction of PRPP and of uric acid	X-linked
Hypoxanthine-guanine phosphoribosyltransferase deficiency, partial	Overproduction of uric acid, increased purine biosynthesis de novo driven by surplus PRPP	X-linked
Secondary		
Associated with increased purine biosynthesis de novo		
Glucose 6-phosphatase deficiency or absence	Overproduction plus underexcretion of uric acid; glycogen storage disease, type I (von Gierke)	Autosomal recessive
Hypoxanthine-guanine phosphoribosyltransferase deficiency, "virtually complete"	Overproduction of uric acid; Lesch-Nyhan syndrome	X-linked
Associated with increased nucleic acid turnover	Overproduction of uric acid	
Renal (90%):		
Primary		
Secondary		

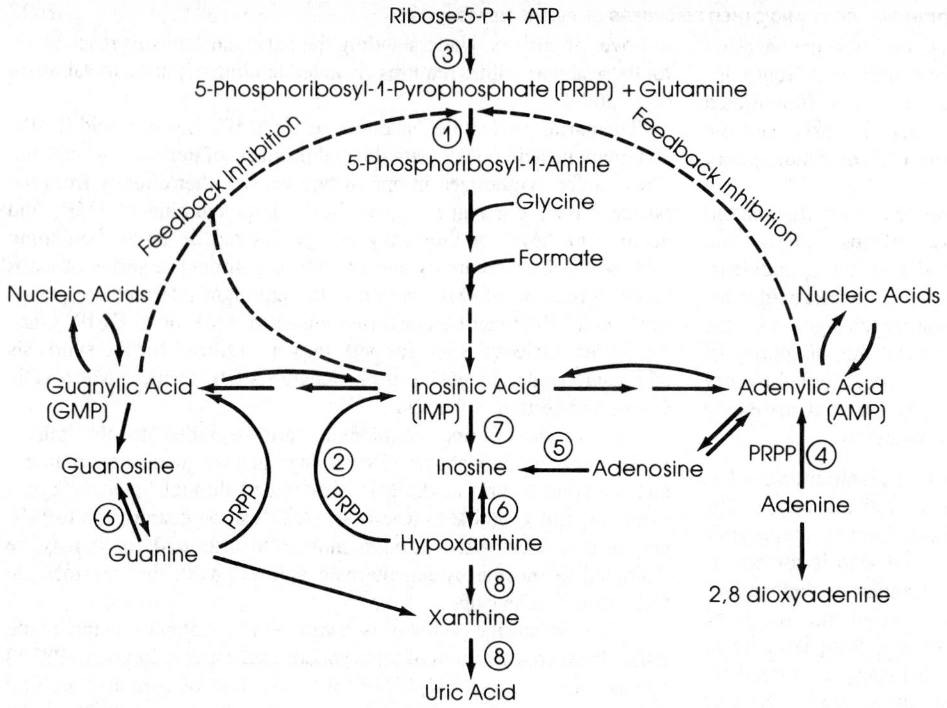

FIGURE 309-4 *Outline of purine metabolism: (1) amidophosphoribosyltransferase; (2) hypoxanthine-guanine phosphoribosyltransferase; (3) PRPP synthetase; (4) adenine phosphoribosyltransferase; (5) adenosine deaminase; (6) purine nucleoside phosphorylase; (7) 5′-nucleotidase; (8) xanthine oxidase.*

exhibit an increased production of uric acid as well as an accelerated rate of purine biosynthesis de novo (see Chap. 313). Overproduction of uric acid in patients with this enzyme defect is multifactorial. An accelerated rate of de novo purine synthesis may be due in part to accelerated synthesis of PRPP. Additionally, accelerated degradation of purine nucleotides contributes to an increased rate of uric acid excretion. Both of these mechanisms are due to the deficiency of glucose as an energy source, and the production of uric acid can be decreased by the sustained correction of hypoglycemia in this disorder.

FIGURE 309-5 *Rate of uric acid excretion at various plasma urate levels in nongouty (solid symbols) and gouty (open symbols) subjects. Large symbols represent mean values; small symbols represent individual data of a few mean values selected to illustrate the degree of scatter within groups. Studies were conducted under basal conditions, after RNA feeding, and after infusions of lithium urate. (From Wyngaarden. Reproduced by permission of Academic Press.)*

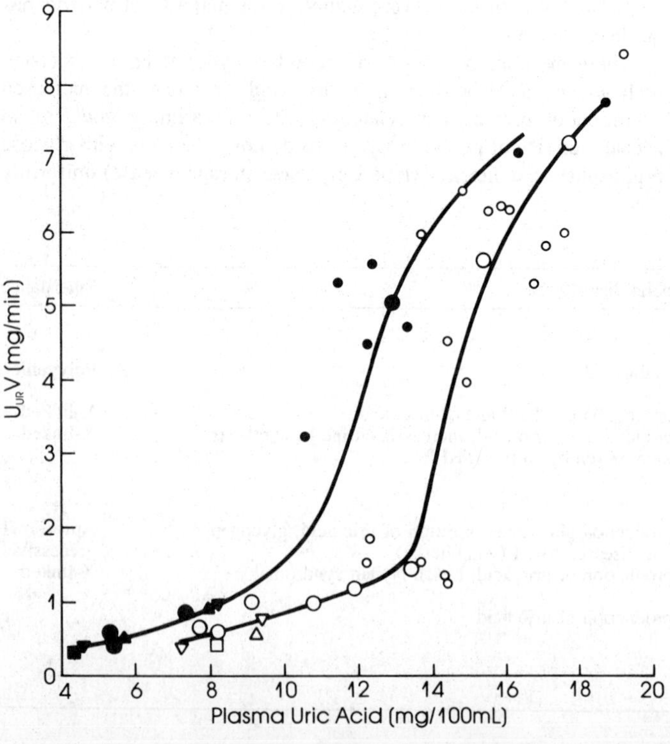

In the majority of patients with secondary hyperuricemia due to an overproduction of uric acid, the predominant abnormality appears to be an increased turnover of nucleic acids. A number of diseases, including the myeloproliferative and lymphoproliferative disorders, multiple myeloma, secondary polycythemia, pernicious anemia, certain hemoglobinopathies, thalassemia, other hemolytic anemias, infectious mononucleosis, and some carcinomas, may be associated with increased marrow activity or increased cell turnover at other sites and an associated increased turnover of nucleic acids. The increased turnover in nucleic acids leads in turn to hyperuricemia, hyperuricaciduria, and a compensatory increase in the rate of purine biosynthesis de novo.

Reduced excretion A large proportion of gouty subjects require a plasma urate value 1 to 2 mg/dL higher than normal subjects to achieve a given rate of uric acid excretion (Fig. 309-5). This abnormality is most prominent in the gouty subject with a normal production of uric acid and is not present in most subjects with overproduction of uric acid.

The excretion of urate is dependent on glomerular filtration, tubular reabsorption, and tubular secretion. Uric acid appears to be completely filtered at the glomerulus and reabsorbed in the proximal tubule (i.e., presecretory reabsorption). Uric acid secretion then occurs in a subsequent segment of the proximal tubule, and partial reabsorption takes place at a second reabsorptive site in the distal portion of the proximal tubule (i.e., postsecretory reabsorption). While some uric acid reabsorption may also occur in the ascending limb of the loop of Henle and in the collecting duct, these latter two sites are thought to be quantitatively less important. Attempts to define further the location and nature of these latter sites and to quantify their contribution to uric acid transport in normal humans or in various disease states have been largely unrewarding.

Theoretically, the altered renal excretion of uric acid exhibited by most patients with gout could be due to (1) reduced filtration of uric acid, (2) enhanced reabsorption, or (3) decreased secretion. No unequivocal data establish any one of these mechanisms as the basic defect, and it is likely that all three are operative within the gouty population.

Numerous secondary causes of hyperuricemia and gout can also be attributed to a decrease in the renal excretion of uric acid. A reduction in the glomerular filtration rate leads to a decrease in the filtered load of uric acid and thus to hyperuricemia; patients with renal disease are hyperuricemic on this basis. Other factors, such as decreased secretion of uric acid, have been postulated in patients with some types of renal disease (e.g., polycystic kidney disease and lead nephropathy). Gout is a rare complication of the secondary hyperuricemia due to renal disease.

Diuretic therapy is one of the most important causes of secondary hyperuricemia. Diuretic-induced volume depletion leads to enhanced tubular reabsorption of uric acid as well as decreased uric acid filtration. Decreased secretion of uric acid may also be a mechanism in diuretic-induced hyperuricemia. A number of other drugs lead to hyperuricemia by undefined renal mechanisms; these agents include low-dose aspirin, pyrazinamide, nicotinic acid, ethambutol, and ethanol.

Impaired renal excretion of uric acid is thought to be an important mechanism for the hyperuricemia associated with several disease states. Volume depletion may be important in patients with hyperuricemia associated with adrenal insufficiency and nephrogenic diabetes insipidus. In some situations hyperuricemia has been attributed to competitive inhibition of uric acid secretion by excess organic acids thought to be secreted by the same renal tubular mechanism responsible for uric acid secretion. Examples include starvation (ketosis and free fatty acids), alcoholic ketosis, diabetic ketoacidosis, maple syrup urine disease, and lactic acidosis of any cause. Hyperuricemia in conditions such as hyperparathyroidism, hypoparathyroidism, pseudohypoparathyroidism, and hypothyroidism may also have a renal basis, but the mechanism is unclear.

PATHOGENESIS OF ACUTE GOUTY ARTHRITIS The events leading to the initial crystallization of monosodium urate in a joint after an average of 30 years of asymptomatic hyperuricemia are not completely understood. Sustained hyperuricemia leads eventually to the development of microtophi in the synovial lining cells and perhaps to an accumulation in cartilage of monosodium urate on proteoglycans that have a high affinity for urate. By one of several mechanisms, probably including trauma with disruption of the microtophi and increased turnover of the cartilage proteoglycans, there is an episodic release of urate crystals into the synovial fluid. Other factors, such as a lower temperature in the joint space or an unequal reabsorption of water and urate from the synovial fluid, may accelerate urate precipitation.

A sufficient amount of crystals in the joint space triggers the acute attack by a process that appears to include (1) phagocytosis of the crystals by leukocytes with the rapid release of a chemotactic protein from the leukocytes, (2) activation of the kallikrein system, (3) activation of complement with the consequent formation of the chemotactic complement components, and (4) the ultimate urate-mediated disruption of lysosomes within the leukocytes, leading to destruction of white blood cells and release of lysosomal products into the synovial fluid. While progress in the understanding of acute gouty arthritis has occurred, questions about factors responsible for spontaneous resolution of the acute attack and the effect of colchicine remain to be answered.

TREATMENT The therapeutic aims in gout are (1) to terminate the acute attack as promptly and gently as possible; (2) to prevent recurrences of acute gouty arthritis; (3) to prevent or reverse complications of the disease resulting from deposition of monosodium urate crystals in joints, kidneys, and other sites; (4) to prevent or reverse associated features such as obesity, hypertriglyceridemia, or hypertension; and (5) to prevent formation of uric acid kidney stones.

Treatment of the acute gouty attack Acute gouty arthritis is treated with an anti-inflammatory agent. Colchicine is the drug most frequently employed. Standard therapy involves administration of 0.5 mg each hour or 1.0 mg every 2 h by mouth until one of three things occurs: (1) the patient improves, (2) gastrointestinal side effects develop, or (3) a maximum of 6 mg is taken without relief. Colchicine is most effective if therapy is begun shortly after the onset of symptoms. Over 75 percent of patients with gout show major improvement in symptoms within the first 12 h of treatment. However, as many as 80 percent of patients are unable to tolerate an optimal dose because of gastrointestinal side effects, which may precede or coincide with clinical improvement. Orally administered colchicine results in peak plasma levels in approximately 2 h. Consequently, it has been suggested that 1.0 mg every 2 h is less likely to lead to the accumulation of toxic levels before the onset of therapeutic effect. However, since therapeutic benefit relates to colchicine levels within leukocytes rather than plasma levels, the efficacy of this regimen requires further evaluation.

Intravenous administration of colchicine eliminates gastrointestinal side effects and provides a more rapid response. Colchicine levels become high in leukocytes, remain constant for 24 h, and are detectable for over 10 days after a single intravenous infusion. As an initial dose 2 mg should be given intravenously, followed by two additional doses of 1 mg at 6-h intervals if needed. Special care must be taken in the intravenous administration of colchicine. The drug is irritative and can lead to severe pain and necrosis if allowed to extravasate to surrounding tissues. It is important to make certain that the intravenous route is secure and that the drug is diluted with 5 to 10 volumes of normal saline solution and infused over a period of no less than 5 min. Colchicine by either oral or parenteral route may cause bone marrow depression, alopecia, hepatocellular failure, mental depression, seizures, ascending paralysis, respiratory depression, and death. Toxic effects are more likely in patients with hepatic, bone marrow, or renal disease and in those subjects on maintenance colchicine. The dosage should be reduced for these individuals, and the drug should not be used in neutropenic patients.

Other anti-inflammatory agents, including indomethacin, phenylbutazone, naproxen, and fenoprofen, are also effective in the treatment of acute gouty arthritis. Indomethacin may be given at a dose of 75 mg orally, followed by 50 mg every 6 h and continued at that dose for 24 h after relief is obtained. The drug is then tapered to 50 mg every 8 h for three doses and then to 25 mg every 8 h for three doses. Side effects of indomethacin include gastrointestinal toxicity, sodium retention, and complaints referable to the central nervous system. While the incidence of side effects may be as high as 60 percent in patients taking the doses described above, the drug is generally better tolerated than colchicine and probably is the treatment of choice in the patient with a well-established diagnosis of acute gouty arthritis. To improve the therapeutic response and thus diminish morbidity of the disease, the patient may be instructed to begin therapy with an anti-inflammatory agent at the first twinge of an acute attack. Uricosuric drugs and allopurinol have no role in the treatment of the acute gouty attack.

Systemic or locally administered (i.e., intraarticular) glucocorticoids are useful in treating acute gout particularly when colchicine and nonsteroidal anti-inflammatory drugs are contraindicated or ineffective. When given systemically, moderate doses should be administered either by the oral or intravenous route for several days at most before the drug is rapidly tapered and discontinued. An isolated monoarthritis or bursitis can be terminated within 24 or 36 h by the intraarticular instillation of a long-acting steroid preparation (e.g., triamcinolone hexacetonide, 15 to 30 mg). This is particularly useful when standard drug regimens are not practical.

Prophylaxis Once the acute episode has resolved, a number of measures can reduce the likelihood of recurrence: (1) the institution of prophylactic daily colchicine or indomethacin, (2) controlled weight reduction for the obese patient, (3) avoidance of known precipitating factors such as heavy alcohol consumption or a diet rich in purines, and (4) the institution of antihyperuricemic therapy.

The administration of small daily doses of colchicine is effective prophylaxis against further acute attacks. A program of 1 to 2 mg colchicine a day is successful in about three-fourths of patients with gout and fails completely in only about 5 percent. In addition, this program is safe and essentially free of side effects. However, unless serum urate is maintained at normal levels, the patient is spared only acute arthritis and may develop other manifestations of gout. Maintenance colchicine therapy is particularly helpful during the first year or two after institution of antihyperuricemic drugs.

Prevention or reversal of the deposition of monosodium urate in tissues Antihyperuricemic agents are effective in reducing serum urate concentration and should be used in patients with (1) one or more attacks of acute gouty arthritis, (2) one or more tophi, and (3) uric acid nephrolithiasis. The aim of antihyperuricemic therapy is to maintain the serum urate below 7.0 mg/dL, the minimal concentration at which urate saturates the extracellular fluid. Reduction to these levels may be achieved by use of drugs that increase the renal excretion of uric acid or decrease uric acid production. Antihyperuricemic drugs generally do not have anti-inflammatory properties. Uricosuric agents reduce serum urate by enhancing the renal excretion. While a large number of drugs exhibit this property, the most effective agents available in the United States are probenecid and sulfinpyrazone. Probenecid is usually started in doses of 250 mg twice a day; it is increased over a period of several weeks to the dose necessary to achieve effective reversal of the hyperuricemia. A total dose of 1 g per day is appropriate for half of patients; the maximum dose should not exceed 3.0 g per day. Because the half-life is 6 to 12 h, it should be given in two to four evenly spaced doses per day. Hypersensitivity, skin rash, and gastrointestinal complaints are the major side effects. Although serious toxicity is rare, side effects may cause up to a third of the patients to discontinue probenecid.

Sulfinpyrazone is a metabolite of phenylbutazone with no anti-inflammatory activity. The drug is usually started at a dose of 50 mg twice a day and gradually increased to a maintenance level of 300 to 400 mg per day given in three or four divided doses. The maximum effective daily dose is 800 mg. Side effects are similar to those with probenecid, although the incidence of bone marrow toxicity may be higher. Approximately a fourth of patients stop the drug for one reason or another.

Probenecid and sulfinpyrazone are effective in most patients with hyperuricemia and gout. In addition to intolerance, failures can result from poor patient compliance, concomitant salicylate ingestion, or impaired renal function. Aspirin at any dose blocks the uricosuric effect of probenecid and sulfinpyrazone. These agents begin to lose effectiveness as the creatinine clearance falls below 80 mL/min and are ineffective when clearance reaches 30 mL/min.

During the negative urate balance induced by uricosuric therapy, the serum urate value drops and urinary uric acid excretion is elevated above pretreatment levels. With continuation of therapy excess urate is mobilized and eliminated, the serum urate falls, and uric acid excretion returns essentially to pretreatment levels. The transient increase in uric acid excretion, which usually lasts for only a few days, may lead to the development of renal calculi in a tenth of patients so treated. To avoid this complication uricosuric agents should be started at low doses and gradually increased as described. Maintaining an ample urine flow with adequate hydration and alkalinizing the urine with oral sodium bicarbonate alone or in combination with acetazolamide reduce the likelihood of stone formation. The ideal candidate for uricosuric agents is under 60 and has normal renal function, uric acid excretion of less than 700 mg per day on a general diet, and no history of renal stones.

Hyperuricemia may also be controlled by allopurinol, a drug that decreases uric acid synthesis. Allopurinol inhibits xanthine oxidase (reaction 8, Fig. 309-4), the enzyme that catalyzes the oxidation of hypoxanthine to xanthine and xanthine to uric acid. While allopurinol has a half-life in vivo of only 2 to 3 h, it is metabolized largely to oxipurinol, which also is an effective inhibitor of xanthine oxidase and has a half-life ranging from 18 to 30 h. In most patients 300 mg per day is an effective antihyperuricemic dose. Because of the long half-life of the major metabolite the drug may be administered once a day. Since oxipurinol is largely excreted in the urine, its half-life is prolonged in patients with renal insufficiency. The dose of allopurinol should, therefore, be reduced by half in patients with significant renal dysfunction.

Significant side effects of allopurinol include gastrointestinal distress, skin rashes, fever, toxic epidermal necrolysis, alopecia, bone marrow suppression, hepatitis, jaundice, and vasculitis. The overall incidence of side effects is about 20 percent; they are more common in the presence of renal insufficiency. In only 5 percent of patients the side effects are sufficient to force discontinuation of the drug. Important drug-drug interactions involving allopurinol include prolongation of the half-lives of mercaptopurine and azathioprine and enhancement of the toxicity of cyclophosphamide.

Specific indications for choosing allopurinol over a uricosuric drug include (1) an increased urinary uric acid excretion (greater than 700 mg per day on a general diet), (2) impairment of renal function with a creatinine clearance less than 80 mL/min, (3) tophaceous gout regardless of renal function, (4) uric acid nephrolithiasis, and (5) gout not controlled by uricosuric agents because of ineffectiveness or intolerance. Allopurinol and a uricosuric drug may be used simultaneously in the rare patient who cannot be controlled by a single medication. Such combination therapy requires no modification in the dosage of either agent and usually results in further lowering of the serum urate concentration.

Acute gouty arthritis may occur whenever there is a rapid and substantial change in the serum urate concentration. Thus, the initiation of antihyperuricemic therapy with any agent may precipitate acute gouty arthritis. In addition, recurrent attacks may occur for a year or longer when large tophaceous deposits are present, even if hyperuricemia is controlled. For these reasons, it is prudent to begin prophylactic therapy with colchicine prior to initiation of antihyperuricemic drugs and to continue it until the serum urate is controlled for at least a year or until all tophi have resolved. Patients should be warned of the possibility of flare-up during the early phase of therapy. While it is not necessary in most gouty patients, strict dietary purine restriction should be instituted in patients with severe tophaceous gout and/or renal failure.

Prevention and treatment of acute uric acid nephropathy Immediate and vigorous therapy is essential for acute uric acid nephropathy. The first step is to increase urine flow by vigorous hydration coupled with administration of a potent diuretic such as furosemide. The urine should be alkalinized to achieve conversion of uric acid to the more soluble monosodium urate. Alkalinization can be accomplished by the administration of sodium bicarbonate alone or in combination with acetazolamide. Allopurinol should also be administered to reduce uric acid formation. The initial dose in this setting should be 8 mg per kilogram of body weight per day given as a single daily dose. The dose should be decreased after 3 or 4 days to 100 to 200 mg per day if renal insufficiency persists. Treatment for uric acid kidney stones is similar to that for acute uric acid nephropathy. In most cases allopurinol combined only with high fluid intake is effective.

WORKUP OF THE HYPERURICEMIC PATIENT Evaluation of the patient with hyperuricemia is directed toward (1) defining the cause of the hyperuricemia (which may disclose an important disease other than gout), (2) assessing the presence and extent of damage to tissues and organs, and (3) identifying associated abnormalities. From a practical standpoint these inquiries are pursued simultaneously, since decisions about the significance of hyperuricemia and about therapy depend on the answers to all of these.

The most important single test in the hyperuricemic patient is analysis of the urine for uric acid. If a history of stone disease is present, a flat plate of the abdomen and intravenous pyelogram may be indicated. If a renal stone is recovered, analysis for uric acid and other constituents is useful. If joint disease is present, synovial fluid analysis and x-rays of the involved joints are helpful. If there is a history of exposure to lead, measurement of urinary lead excretion after an infusion of calcium edetate may be useful in documenting the presence of gout due to lead exposure. In cases where the patient appears to be an overproducer, measurement of erythrocyte hypoxanthine-guanine phosphoribosyltransferase and PRPP synthetase levels may be indicated.

Management of asymptomatic hyperuricemia There is considerable controversy about the indications for therapy of the patient with asymptomatic hyperuricemia. Generally, treatment should be withheld unless the patient (1) becomes symptomatic; (2) has a strong family history for gout, nephrolithiasis, or renal failure; or (3) excretes large quantities of uric acid (greater than 1100 mg per day).

OTHER DISORDERS OF PURINE METABOLISM ASSOCIATED WITH HYPERURICEMIA AND GOUT **Hypoxanthine-guanine phosphoribosyltransferase deficiency states** Hypoxanthine-guanine phosphoribosyltransferase catalyzes the conversion of hypoxanthine to inosinic acid and guanine to guanosinic acid (reaction 2, Fig. 309-4). PRPP serves as the phosphoribosyl donor. The deficiency of hypoxanthine-guanine phosphoribosyltransferase leads to decreased consumption of PRPP which accumulates to higher than normal levels. The excess PRPP accelerates de novo purine biosynthesis and consequently increases uric acid production.

The Lesch-Nyhan syndrome is an X-linked disorder. The characteristic biochemical abnormality is a profound deficiency of the enzyme hypoxanthine-guanine phosphoribosyltransferase (reaction 2, Fig. 309-4). Affected patients have hyperuricemia and a profound overproduction of uric acid. In addition, they have a bizarre neurologic disorder characterized by self-mutilation, choreoathetosis, spasticity, and retardation of growth and mental function. The incidence is estimated at 1:100,000 births.

From 0.5 to 1.0 percent of adult gouty subjects with overproduction of uric acid have a partial deficiency of hypoxanthine-guanine phosphoribosyltransferase. These patients typically have the onset of gouty arthritis at a young age (15 to 30 years), a high incidence of uric acid stones (75 percent), and the occasional occurrence of mild neurologic dysfunction characterized by dysarthria, hyperreflexia, incoordination, and/or mental retardation. This disease is inherited as an X-linked trait so that men are affected through carrier females.

The enzyme whose deficiency results in these disorders, hypoxanthine-guanine phosphoribosyltransferase, is of considerable interest in genetics. With the possible exception of the globin gene family, the hypoxanthine-guanine phosphoribosyltransferase locus is the single most studied human gene.

Human hypoxanthine-guanine phosphoribosyltransferase has been purified to homogeneity, and its amino acid sequence has been determined. The normal enzyme has a native subunit molecular weight of 24,470 and consists of 217 amino acid residues. The normal enzyme is a tetramer with four identical subunits. Four variant forms of hypoxanthine-guanine phosphoribosyltransferase from deficient patients have been sequenced as well (Table 309-2). In each a single amino acid substitution leads to either a catalytically incompetent protein or decreased steady-state concentrations of hypoxanthine-guanine phosphoribosyltransferase as a result of diminished synthesis or accelerated degradation of the mutant protein.

The DNA sequence complementary to messenger RNA (mRNA) encoding hypoxanthine-guanine phosphoribosyltransferase has been cloned and sequenced as well. As a molecular probe, this cDNA sequence has been used to identify carrier status in a female at risk for whom conventional carrier detection techniques were not successful. The human gene has been transferred to mice via retroviral vector–infected bone marrow transplantation. Expression of the human hypoxanthine-guanine phosphoribosyltransferase in mice so treated has been conclusively demonstrated. A transgenic strain of mice has also recently been established in which the human enzyme is expressed with a tissue distribution characteristic of humans.

The associated biochemical abnormalities leading to the devastating neurologic consequences of the Lesch-Nyhan syndrome are incompletely understood. Evidence obtained from postmortem examination of brains from subjects with the Lesch-Nyhan syndrome indicates a specific defect in the central dopaminergic pathways, particularly those found in the basal ganglia and nucleus accumbens. Corroborating in vivo evidence is emerging from positron emission tomography (PET) studies of subjects deficient in hypoxanthine-guanine phosphoribosyltransferase. A defect in the metabolism of 2′-fluorodeoxyglucose in the caudate nuclei is present in the majority of subjects studied with this technique. The relationships between dopaminergic nervous system abnormalities and the aberrant metabolism of purines remain unknown.

The hyperuricemia resulting from partial or complete deficiency of hypoxanthine-guanine phosphoribosyltransferase can be successfully controlled with allopurinol, an inhibitor of xanthine oxidase. A few patients have developed xanthine stones with such therapy, but in the majority the renal stones and gout are effectively treated. No specific therapy exists for the neurologic abnormalities in the Lesch-Nyhan syndrome.

PRPP synthetase variants Several families are described in which there is increased activity of the enzyme PRPP synthetase (reaction 3, Fig. 309-4). The mutant enzymes, of which three different types are recognized, all exhibit increased activity, resulting in increased intracellular concentrations of PRPP, accelerated purine biosynthesis, and elevated excretion of uric acid. The inheritance pattern in this disease is also X-linked. These patients, like those with partial hypoxanthine-guanine phosphoribosyltransferase deficiency, generally develop gout in the second or third decade and have a high incidence of uric acid stones. Several kindred have been described in which nerve deafness is associated with PRPP synthetase overactivity groups.

OTHER DISORDERS OF PURINE METABOLISM **Adenine phosphoribosyltransferase deficiency** Adenine phosphoribosyltransferase catalyzes the conversion of adenine to AMP (reaction 4, Fig. 309-4). The first subjects described with a deficiency of this enzyme were heterozygous for deficiency of the enzyme and had no associated disease. It subsequently became apparent that heterozygosity for this deficiency is common, perhaps as frequent as 1:100. A homozygous deficiency of this enzyme has now been described in 11 patients with a history of renal stones composed of 2,8-dioxyadenine. Because of chemical similarity, 2,8-dioxyadenine may be confused with uric acid, and in each of these patients an incorrect diagnosis of uric acid nephrolithiasis was made initially.

Adenosine deaminase deficiency and purine nucleoside phosphorylase deficiency See Chap. 256.

TABLE 309-2 Structural and functional abnormalities in mutant forms of human hypoxanthine-guanine phosphoribosyltransferase

		Mutation		Functional abnormalities			
						Michaelis constants	
Mutant enzyme	Clinical presentation	Amino acid substition	Position	Intracellular concentration	Maximal velocity	Hypoxanthine	PRPP
$HPRT_{Toronto}$	Gout	Arg→Gly	50	Decreased	Normal	Normal	Normal
$HPRT_{London}$	Gout	Ser→Leu	109	Decreased	Normal	↑ 5-fold	Normal
$HPRT_{Ann\ Arbor}$	Nephrolithiasis	ND	ND	Decreased	Normal	Normal	Normal
$HPRT_{Munich}$	Gout	Ser→Arg	103	Normal	↓ 20-fold	↑ 100-fold	Normal
$HPRT_{Kinston}$	Lesch-Nyhan Syndrome	Asp→Asn	193	Normal	Normal	↑ 200-fold	↑ 200-fold

NOTES: *PRPP denotes 5-phosphoribosyl-1-pyrophosphate; Arg, arginine; Gly, glycine; Ser, serine; Leu, leucine; Asn, asparagine; Asp, aspartic acid; ND, not determined; →, is replaced by.*
SOURCE: *Wilson et al.*

Xanthine oxidase deficiency Xanthine oxidase catalyzes the oxidation of hypoxanthine to xanthine, xanthine to uric acid, and adenine to 2,8-dioxyadenine (reaction 8, Fig. 309-4). Xanthinuria, the first inborn error of purine metabolism to be defined at the enzyme level, is due to a deficiency of xanthine oxidase. As a result, affected patients with xanthinuria have hypouricemia and hypouricaciduria as well as an increased urinary excretion of the oxypurines, hypoxanthine, and xanthine. Half are asymptomatic and a third have urinary xanthine stones. Several patients have been noted to have a myopathy. Three patients have been reported with polyarthritis, which may represent a crystal-induced synovitis. Precipitation of xanthine is thought to be the important factor in the development of each of these clinical manifestations.

Four patients have been described with combined congenital deficiencies of xanthine oxidase and sulfate oxidase. The clinical presentation is dominated by the serious neurologic abnormalities in the neonatal period seen in isolated sulfate oxidase deficiency. Although deficiency of a molybdate cofactor required by both enzymes has been postulated as the primary abnormality, therapy with ammonium molybdate has little effect on the neurologic manifestation. An acquired disorder mimicking combined xanthine oxidase and sulfate oxidase deficiency has been described in a patient on chronic total parenteral nutrition. Therapy with oral ammonium molybdate successfully restored enzymatic function and resulted in clinical resolution.

Myoadenylate deaminase deficiency Myoadenylate deaminase is an isozyme of adenylate deaminase found only in skeletal muscle. This enzyme catalyzes the conversion of adenylate (AMP) to inosinic acid (IMP). This reaction is a component of the purine nucleotide cycle and is probably important in the maintenance of energy production and utilization in skeletal muscle.

Deficiency of this enzyme is limited to skeletal muscle. The majority of deficient patients demonstrate exercise-induced myalgias, muscle cramps, and fatigue. Approximately one-third report weakness even in the absence of exercise. A few patients are apparently asymptomatic.

The disorder typically presents in childhood or adolescence. The clinical manifestations are those of a metabolic myopathy. Creatine kinase is elevated in less than half of subjects. Electromyograms and routine histology of muscle biopsies show nonspecific abnormalities. Presumptive evidence of adenylate deaminase deficiency can be obtained from performance of an ischemic forearm exercise test. Ammonia production is reduced in deficient patients since AMP deamination is blocked. The diagnosis must be confirmed by actual assay of AMP deaminase activity in a skeletal muscle biopsy since reduced ammonia production with exercise occurs in other myopathies. The disorder is slowly progressive, leading to mild disability in most cases. No specific therapy has been shown to be effective.

Adenylosuccinase deficiency Subjects deficient in adenylosuccinase are mentally retarded and often autistic. Additional neurologic abnormalities include seizures, psychomotor retardation, and other movement disorders. Urinary excretion of succinylamino-imidazole carboxamide riboside (SAICAR) and succinyladenosine is elevated. Diagnosis depends upon demonstration of partial or complete absence of enzyme activity in liver, kidney, or skeletal muscle. Lymphocytes and fibroblasts show a partial deficiency. The prognosis is not known, and no specific therapy exists.

REFERENCES

KELLEY WN: Crystal-induced arthropathies, in *The Clinics in Rheumatic Diseases*. Philadelphia, Saunders, 1977, vol 3, pp 1–171

———, FOX IH: Gout and related disorders of purine metabolism, in *Textbook of Rheumatology*, WN Kelley et al (eds). Philadelphia, Saunders, 1985, pp 1359–1397

———, HOLMES EW: Antihyperuricemic drugs, in *Textbook of Rheumatology*, WN Kelley et al (eds). Philadelphia, Saunders, 1985, pp 857–870

——— et al: Hypoxanthine-guanine phosphoribosyltransferase deficiency in gout. Ann Intern Med, 70:155, 1969

PALELLA TD, KELLEY WN: Purine and deoxypurine metabolism, in *Textbook of Rheumatology*, WN Kelley et al (eds). Philadelphia, Saunders, 1985, p 337

SEEGMILLER JE: Diseases of purine and pyrimidine metabolism, in *Duncan's Diseases of Metabolism*, 8th ed, PK Bondy, LE Rosenberg (eds). Philadelphia, Saunders, 1980, p 777

TALBOTT JH, YU TF: *Gout and Uric Acid Metabolism*. New York, Grune & Stratton, 1976

WILSON JM et al: Hypoxanthine-guanine phosphoribosyltransferase deficiency: The molecular basis of the clinical syndromes. N Engl J Med 309:900, 1983

WYNGAARDEN JB: Gout, in *Advances in Metabolic Disorders*, R Levine and R Luft (eds). New York, Academic, 1965, vol 2, pp 2–78

———, KELLEY WN: *Gout and Hyperuricemia*. New York, Grune & Stratton, 1976

———, ———: Gout, in *The Metabolic Basis of Inherited Diseases*, 5th ed, JB Stanbury et al (eds). New York, McGraw-Hill, 1983

310 HEMOCHROMATOSIS

LAWRIE W. POWELL / KURT J. ISSELBACHER

DEFINITION Hemochromatosis is an iron-storage disorder in which an inappropriate increase in intestinal iron absorption results in deposition of iron with eventual tissue damage and functional insufficiency of the organs involved, especially the liver, pancreas, heart, and pituitary. In 1889, von Recklinghausen named the disease *hemochromatosis* and the iron-storage pigment *hemosiderin* because he believed that the pigment was derived from the blood. The terms *hemosiderosis* or *siderosis* are often used to describe the presence of stainable iron in tissues, but quantitative measurement of tissue iron is necessary for accurate assessment of body iron status (see below and Chap. 284). *Hemochromatosis* implies progressive and massive iron overload leading to fibrosis and organ failure. Although there is debate about definitions, it seems logical to use the following terminology: (1) *genetic hemochromatosis*—the inherited disease now known to be associated with an abnormal iron-loading gene tightly linked to the A locus of the HLA complex on chromosome 6, (2) *acquired hemochromatosis*—iron overload with tissue injury arising secondarily to other disease, usually thalassemia or sideroblastic anemia. It should be emphasized, however, that in these acquired iron-loading disorders massive iron deposits in parenchymal tissues can lead to the same clinical and pathologic features that are seen in genetic hemochromatosis.

The metabolic defect leading to increased iron absorption in hemochromatosis is unknown. The genetic disease can now be recognized during its early stages when the iron overload is of lesser degree and organ damage is minimal. At this stage the disease is best referred to as *latent* or *precirrhotic hemochromatosis* (see Fig. 310-1).

PREVALENCE Genetic hemochromatosis is not as rare as previously believed. In white Anglo-Saxon populations the gene frequency is approximately 5 percent, the disease (homozygote) frequency is 0.3 percent, and the carrier (heterozygote) frequency is 10 percent. However, expression of the disease is modified by several factors, especially blood loss associated with menstruation and pregnancies in women. The disease is observed 5 to 10 times more frequently in males than in females. Nearly 70 percent of patients develop their first symptoms between ages 40 and 60. The disease is rarely clinically evident below age 20, although with family screening (see below) asymptomatic subjects with iron overload can be identified, including young menstruating women.

PATHOGENESIS Normally the body iron content of 3 to 4 g is maintained such that intestinal mucosal absorption of iron is equal to loss. This amount is approximately 1 mg per day in men and 1.5 mg per day in menstruating women. In hemochromatosis mucosal absorption is inappropriate to body needs, amounting to 4 mg per day or more. The resulting progressive accumulation of iron is reflected in an early elevation in the plasma iron and an increased saturation of transferrin. In advanced disease, the body may contain over 20 g iron. This excess iron is deposited mainly in parenchymal cells of

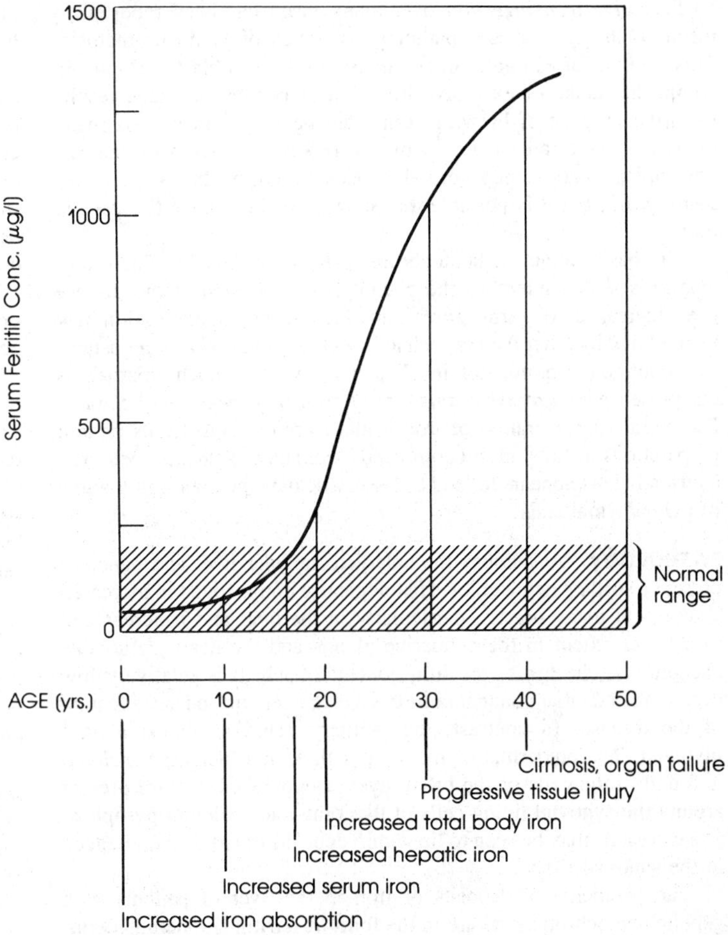

FIGURE 310-1 *Sequence of events in genetic hemochromatosis and their correlation with the serum ferritin concentration. Increased iron absorption is present throughout life. Overt, symptomatic disease usually develops between ages 40 and 60, but latent precirrhotic disease can be detected long before this.*

the liver, pancreas, and heart. Iron in the liver and pancreas increases 50 to 100 times; in the heart, 5 to 25 times; in the spleen, kidney, and skin, about 5 times. Tissue injury may result from disruption of iron-laden lysosomes and lipid peroxidation of subcellular organelles by excess iron. The demonstration of an association between hemochromatosis and the histocompatibility antigens HLA-A3, HLA-B14, and HLA-B7 has confirmed the genetic basis for the disease. The mode of inheritance is autosomal recessive, with homozygotes usually developing severe iron overload and symptomatic disease and heterozygotes developing only minor derangements in iron metabolism without progressive iron overload or clinical evidence of the disease.

Gross parenchymal iron overload leading to *acquired* hemochromatosis occurs in association with chronic disorders of erythropoiesis, particularly in those with a defect in hemoglobin synthesis and ineffective erythropoiesis such as sideroblastic anemia and thalassemia. In this group of disorders the absorption of iron is increased, and these patients are also frequently treated with iron and blood transfusions. Porphyria cutanea tarda, a disorder characterized by a defect in porphyrin biosynthesis (Chap. 312), is also sometimes associated with excessive parenchymal iron deposits; however, the magnitude of the iron load is usually insufficient to produce tissue damage.

Alcoholic subjects with chronic liver disease may show evidence of increased tissue iron stores. They can be divided into two groups. The first group comprises patients who have a mild to moderate increase in stainable hepatic iron but relatively normal body iron stores. These patients have alcoholic liver disease (usually cirrhosis) but not hemochromatosis. The reason for the increased iron may be related in part to cell necrosis and uptake of iron released from adjacent Kupffer and parenchymal cells. The second (less common) group of alcoholic subjects with increased hepatic iron have gross iron deposition and increased body iron stores and are usually found to have genetic hemochromatosis with or without superimposed alcoholic liver disease. Hemochromatosis occurring in a heavy drinker may be distinguished from alcoholic liver disease by two means: (1) by measurement of hepatic iron concentration (see below and Table 310-1) and (2) by studying relatives for evidence of the disease, including HLA typing of family members.

TABLE 310-1 Representative iron values in normal subjects, patients with hemochromatosis, and patients with alcoholic liver disease

Determination	Normal	Symptomatic hemochromatosis	Homozygotes with early, asymptomatic hemochromatosis	Alcoholic liver disease
Plasma iron, μg/dL	50–150	180–300	Usually elevated	Often elevated
Total iron-binding capacity, μg/dL	250–370	200–300	200–300	250–370
Percent transferrin saturation, μg/dL	22–46	50–100	50–100	22–60
Serum ferritin, ng/mL	10–200	900–6000	200–500	10–500
Urinary iron,* mg/24 h	0–2	9–23	2–5	Usually < 5
Liver iron, μg/100 mg dry wt	30–140	600–1800	200–400	30–200

* *After intramuscular administration of 0.5 g deferoxamine.*

Excessive iron ingestion over many years has been reported to result in the clinical and pathologic features of hemochromatosis. This occurs, for example, in certain South African blacks (Bantu) in whom the intake of excessive iron in an alcoholic beverage results from the practice of brewing fermented beverages in vessels made of iron. There are a few isolated reports of hemochromatosis developing in apparently normal subjects taking medicinal iron over many years, but it is possible that such individuals have the genetic trait.

The basic defect in hemochromatosis is not known. Therefore, diagnosis is dependent on the phenotypic expression of the disease (i.e., increased body iron stores), and the phenotypic expression may be modified by other factors such as blood loss and oral iron ingestion. The common denominator in all patients with hemochromatosis is the presence of *excessive amounts of iron in parenchymal tissues.* Parenteral administration of iron in the form of transfusions or iron preparations results in predominantly *reticuloendothelial cell* iron overload. This appears to lead to less tissue damage than iron loading of parenchymal cells.

PATHOLOGY At autopsy the enlarged, nodular liver and pancreas present a striking ochre color. Histologically iron is found in increased amounts in many organs, particularly in the liver and pancreas and to a lesser extent in the endocrine glands and the heart. A notable exception is the testis, the iron content of which is relatively low despite the fact that gonadal failure is a characteristic and early feature of the disease. In contrast, the pituitary gland is almost always involved. The epidermis of the skin is thin, and increased *melanin* is found in the cells of the basal layer. Deposits of iron are present around the synovial lining cells of the joints, and calcium pyrophosphate crystals may be seen to lie within deposits of calcium embedded in the synovial tissue.

The parenchymal deposits of iron in the liver of patients with genetic hemochromatosis are in the form of ferritin and hemosiderin. In the early stages, these deposits are found in the periportal parenchymal cells, especially within lysosomes in the pericanalicular cytoplasm of the hepatocytes. This stage progresses to perilobular fibrosis and deposition of iron in bile duct epithelium, Kupffer cells, and fibrous septa. Inflammatory cells are few in contrast to prominent proliferation of bile ductules. Wedge biopsy specimens show a characteristic pattern of fibrosis with dense fibrous septa surrounding groups of lobules somewhat analogous to the pattern in chronic biliary disease. In the advanced stage, a macronodular or mixed macro- and micronodular cirrhosis develops.

CLINICAL MANIFESTATIONS The symptoms and signs of hemochromatosis include skin pigmentation, diabetes, liver and cardiac impairment, arthropathy, and hypogonadism. The initial symptoms most frequently encountered are weakness, lassitude, weight loss, change in skin color, abdominal pain, loss of libido, and symptoms related to the onset of diabetes. Hepatomegaly, pigmentation, spider angiomas, splenomegaly, arthropathy, ascites, cardiac arrhythmias, congestive heart failure, loss of body hair, testicular atrophy, and jaundice are the most prominent physical signs in the fully established disease.

The *liver* is usually the first organ to be affected, and hepatomegaly is present in more than 95 percent of symptomatic cases. Hepatic enlargement may exist in the absence of symptoms or in the presence of normal liver function tests. Indeed, over half the patients with symptomatic hemochromatosis have little or no laboratory evidence of functional impairment of the liver, in spite of hepatomegaly and fibrosis. Loss of body hair, palmar erythema, testicular atrophy, and gynecomastia are common. Manifestations of portal hypertension and esophageal varices occur less commonly than in Laennec's cirrhosis. Splenomegaly is present in approximately half the symptomatic cases. Hepatocellular carcinoma develops in about 30 percent. The incidence of this complication increases with age and is now the most common cause of death in treated patients. However, it appears to occur only in cirrhotic patients; hence the importance of early diagnosis and therapy.

Excessive *skin pigmentation* is present in about 90 percent of symptomatic patients at the time the diagnosis is established. The melanin deposition in the skin usually gives rise to bronzing. The characteristic metallic gray hue is believed to result from the presence of increased melanin or both melanin and iron in the dermis. Pigmentation usually is diffuse and generalized, but frequently it is deeper on the face, neck, extensor aspects of the lower forearms, dorsa of the hands, lower legs, genital regions, and in scars. In only 10 to 15 percent of cases is there demonstrable pigmentation of the oral mucosa. Pigmentation of the hard palate and retina has been described.

Diabetes mellitus occurs in about 65 percent of patients and is more likely to develop in patients with a family history of diabetes. The presence of a family history of diabetes and direct damage to the pancreas by iron deposition both may contribute to the development of diabetes in hemochromatosis. The management of the diabetes is similar to that of idiopathic diabetes mellitus except for a higher incidence of insulin resistance and of fat atrophy. Late degenerative sequelae are the same as in diabetes mellitus.

Arthropathy develops in 25 to 50 percent of patients. It most commonly occurs after the age of 50 but may occur at any time in the course of the disease, even as a first manifestation or long after therapy. The small joints of the hands, especially the second and third metacarpophalangeal joints, are usually the first joints to be involved. A progressive polyarthritis involving wrists, hips, and knees may ensue. Acute brief attacks of synovitis may occur, associated with deposition of calcium pyrophosphate (chondrocalcinosis or pseudogout), chiefly in the knees. Roentgenologic manifestations consist of cystic changes of sclerosis of the subchondral bones, loss of articular cartilage with narrowing of the joint space, diffuse demineralization, hypertrophic bone proliferation, and calcification of the synovium. The mechanism of these abnormalities and their relationship to iron metabolism are not known.

Cardiac involvement is the presenting manifestation in about 15 percent of patients. The most common cardiac manifestation, congestive heart failure, is observed in about 10 percent of young adults with the disease. Symptoms of congestive failure may develop suddenly, with rapid progression to death if untreated. The heart is diffusely enlarged, and such cases may be misdiagnosed as idiopathic cardiomyopathy if other overt manifestations are absent. A variety of cardiac arrhythmias may be present, particularly supraventricular beats and paroxysmal tachyarrhythmias. Atrial flutter, atrial fibrillation, and varying degrees of atrioventricular block have also been described.

Loss of libido and *testicular atrophy* are common. The former may antedate the other clinical manifestations of the disease. Testicular atrophy is usually due to the decreased production of gonadotropins associated with impaired hypothalamic-pituitary function due to iron deposition. Adrenal insufficiency, hypothyroidism, and hypoparathyroidism have been described but are rare.

DIAGNOSIS The association of (1) hepatomegaly, (2) skin pigmentation, (3) diabetes mellitus, (4) heart disease, (5) arthritis, and (6) evidence of hypogonadism should suggest the diagnosis of hemochromatosis. However, a parenchymal iron overload of comparatively short duration or modest degree may exist without any of these clinical manifestations, or with only some of them [e.g., in young subjects (see Fig. 310-1)]. Therefore, the diagnosis should be considered in any patient with unexplained hepatomegaly, idiopathic cardiomyopathy, abnormal skin pigmentation, loss of libido, diabetes, or arthritis.

The history should be particularly detailed in regard to disease in other members of the family, alcohol ingestion, iron intake, and the ingestion of large doses of ascorbic acid which promotes iron absorption. The blood should be examined for evidence of anemia and abnormal erythropoiesis to rule out iron loading secondary to a hematologic disorder. Confirmation of the presence of liver, pancreatic, cardiac, and joint disease should be obtained by physical examination, roentgenologic examination, and routine function tests of these organs. It then remains to be demonstrated that there is an increase in total body iron stores and, in particular, an increased parenchymal iron concentration associated with tissue damage.

The methods available for the demonstration of excessive parenchymal iron stores include (1) measurement of serum iron, (2) determination of percent saturation of transferrin, (3) estimation of chelatable iron stores using the agent deferoxamine, (4) measurement of serum ferritin concentration, (5) liver biopsy (Table 310-1), and (6) computerized tomography. Each has its inherent advantages and limitations. The serum iron level and percent saturation of transferrin are elevated early in the course of the disease, but their specificity is reduced by relatively high false-positive and false-negative rates. In particular, an increased serum iron concentration may be present in patients with alcoholic liver disease without iron overload; in this situation, however, the iron-binding capacity is usually not decreased as in hemochromatosis (Table 310-1).

The serum ferritin concentration is usually a good index of body iron stores, whether they are decreased or increased. In untreated patients with hemochromatosis, the serum ferritin level is greatly increased (Fig. 310-1 and Table 310-1). This test is also useful as a noninvasive screening test for the diagnosis of early disease, since it is usually abnormal before there is any morphologic evidence of liver damage and the ferritin concentration correlates with the magnitude of body iron stores. It has, therefore, generally replaced the more cumbersome screening tests involving measurement of urinary iron excretion. However, in patients with inflammation and hepatocellular necrosis serum ferritin levels may be elevated out of proportion to body iron stores due to increased rate of release from tissues. Also, some families have been reported in whom serum ferritin levels in symptomatic relatives are normal despite increased iron stores; the reason for this finding is unclear, but it would appear to be unusual. In clinical practice, the *combined measurements* of the (1) serum iron concentration, (2) percent transferrin saturation, and (3) serum ferritin level provide the simplest and most reliable screening test for hemochromatosis, including the precirrhotic phase of the disease. If any of these tests are abnormal, liver biopsy should be performed since it is the *definitive* test for the diagnosis of hemochromatosis. It permits histochemical estimation of tissue iron, measurement of hepatic iron concentration, and assessment of the extent of tissue damage. Computerizd tomography shows increased density of the liver due to iron deposition. However, dual-energy scanning and experienced personnel are required, and the lower limits for accurate detection of increased tissue iron are unclear.

It is of particular importance to examine family members at risk when the diagnosis of hemochromatosis is established. Asymptomatic as well as symptomatic family members with the disease will usually have an increase in plasma iron, a decrease in total iron-binding capacity, an increased saturation of transferrin, and an increased or increasing serum ferritin concentration. These changes occur even before the iron stores are greatly increased (see Fig. 310-1). A liver biopsy should then be performed, since it is imperative to establish the diagnosis and begin therapy before tissue damage occurs. HLA typing may be helpful in evaluating families with the disease. Affected siblings usually have both HLA haplotypes identical with those of the proband, and where children of a proband are affected, a homozygous-heterozygous mating probably occurred.

The distinction between hemochromatosis and alcoholic cirrhosis associated with increased tissue iron is discussed above. It is usually not difficult if measurement of liver iron concentration is made, and the deferoxamine excretion test can provide additional diagnostic information (Table 310-1).

TREATMENT The therapy of genetic hemochromatosis involves the removal of the excess body iron and supportive treatment of damaged organs.

Iron is best removed from the body by weekly or twice weekly phlebotomy of 500 mL. Although there is an initial modest decline in the volume of packed red blood cells to about 35 mL/dL, the level stabilizes after several weeks. The plasma iron concentration remains increased until the available iron stores are depleted. The plasma ferritin concentration falls progressively, reflecting the gradual decrease in body iron stores. Since one 500-mL unit of blood contains from 200 to 250 mg iron and about 25 g iron must be removed, 2 or 3 years of weekly phlebotomy are usually required. When the plasma iron and ferritin levels become normal, phlebotomies are performed at such time intervals as are required to maintain a plasma iron concentration of less than 150 μg/dL. Usually one phlebotomy every 3 months will suffice. The adequacy of the therapy may be evaluated at any time by measuring the plasma iron, the percentage of saturation of transferrin with iron, or the serum ferritin concentration. These measurements become abnormal promptly with iron reaccumulation.

Chelating agents such as deferoxamine, when given parenterally, remove 10 to 20 mg iron per day, less than half that mobilized by one weekly phlebotomy. Phlebotomy is also generally a less expensive, more convenient, and safer treatment for patients with genetic hemochromatosis, but chelating agents are indicated when anemia or hypoproteinemia is severe enough to preclude phlebotomy. Subcutaneous infusions of deferoxamine using a portable slow pump are most effective.

The management of the hepatic failure, cardiac failure, and diabetes differs little from conventional management of these conditions. Loss of libido and change in secondary sex characteristics are partially relieved by testosterone therapy or gonadotropin therapy.

PROGNOSIS The principal causes of death in *untreated* patients are cardiac failure (30 percent), hepatocellular failure or portal hypertension (25 percent), and hepatocellular carcinoma (30 percent).

Life expectancy of symptomatic patients is extended to an average of more than 8 years by removal of the excessive stores of iron and maintenance of these stores at near-normal levels. The 5-year survival rate with therapy is increased from 33 to 89 percent. With removal of iron by repeated phlebotomy, the liver and spleen decrease in size, liver function studies return to normal, pigmentation of skin decreases, and cardiac failure is reversed. Carbohydrate tolerance improves in about 40 percent. Removal of excess iron has little or no effect on hypogonadism or arthropathy. The fibrosis in the liver may decrease, but cirrhosis is irreversible. Hepatocellular carcinoma occurs as a late sequela in about one-third of the patients despite adequate iron removal. The apparent increase in its incidence in treated patients is probably related to their increased life span. This complication does not appear to develop if the disease is treated in the precirrhotic stage. Hence, the importance of family screening and early therapy cannot be emphasized too strongly. Asymptomatic subjects who are detected by family studies should have phlebotomy therapy if iron stores are moderately to severely increased. Screening for increasing iron stores at appropriate intervals is also important. With this approach most manifestations of the disease can be prevented. Indeed, the life expectancy of such treated precirrhotic patients appears to be similar to that of the normal population.

REFERENCES

BASSETT ML et al: HLA typing in idiopathic hemochromatosis: Distinction between homozygotes and heterozygotes with biochemical expression. Hepatology 1:120, 1981

——— et al: Diagnosis of hemochromatosis in young subjects: Predictive accuracy of biochemical screening tests. Gastroenterology 87:628, 1984

BOTHWELL TH et al: *Iron Metabolism in Man*. Oxford, Blackwell, 1979

EDWARDS CQ et al: Hereditary hemochromatosis. N Engl J Med 297:7, 1977

MILDER MS et al: Idiopathic hemochromatosis, an interim report. Medicine 59:1, 34, 1980

POWELL LW, KERR JFR: The pathology of liver in hemochromatosis, in *Pathobiology Annual*, H Joacim (ed). New York, Appleton-Century-Crofts, 1975

SIMON M et al: Idiopathic hemochromatosis: Demonstration of recessive transmission and early detection by family HLA typing. N Engl J Med 297:1017, 1977

311 WILSON'S DISEASE

I. HERBERT SCHEINBERG

Wilson's disease is an autosomal recessive abnormality in the hepatic excretion of copper that results in toxic accumulations of the metal in liver, brain, and other organs. The disease occurs in populations of every ethnic and geographic origin and has a worldwide prevalence of about 1 in 30,000. Deficiency of the plasma copper protein ceruloplasmin is a characteristic feature.

NATURAL HISTORY Normal babies have low levels of plasma ceruloplasmin and high concentrations of hepatic copper. During the first year of life ceruloplasmin values rise, and hepatic copper concentrations fall to normal adult levels. In contrast, serum ceruloplasmin changes very little in homozygotes for the Wilson's disease gene, and the concentration of hepatic copper remains elevated. However, clinical manifestations of copper excess are rare before age 6, and one-half of untreated patients remain asymptomatic through adolescence.

Wilson's disease presents with hepatic involvement in about one-half of patients. The toxic effects of copper in the liver may be manifest as acute hepatitis, cirrhosis of the liver, or asymptomatic hepatosplenomegaly. The acute hepatitis is similar to viral hepatitis, can be mistaken for infectious mononucleosis, and may evolve in three different ways. The first is a fulminant, sometimes lethal disease characterized by jaundice, malaise, and at times ascites, hypoalbuminemia, and elevated levels of liver enzymes in plasma. In the acute phase sufficient copper may be released into plasma to cause a hemolytic anemia. The disease may not be diagnosed until autopsy or until the diagnosis in a younger sibling leads to copper analysis of preserved tissues. Second, parenchymal liver disease may develop insidiously and result in a clinical and histologic picture indistinguishable from chronic active hepatitis. Third, patients may apparently recover from the hepatitis, although cirrhosis always develops. Years or decades may elapse with no sign or symptom of disease. In these patients the past history of an episode of hepatitis can be overlooked unless they are questioned carefully or unless the cirrhosis becomes clinically manifest.

More frequently, the copper-induced hepatic disease evolves to cirrhosis without any recognized hepatitis. In these patients the initial manifestations are extrahepatic. Neurologic or psychiatric disturbances are the first clinical signs in most of this group and are always accompanied by Kayser-Fleischer rings (Fig. A4-16). These green or golden deposits of copper in Descemet's membrane of the cornea do not interfere with vision but indicate that hepatic copper has been released and has caused the brain damage. Rarely Kayser-Fleischer rings may be accompanied by sunflower cataracts. If a patient with frank neurologic or psychiatric disease does not have Kayser-Fleischer rings when examined by a trained observer using a slit lamp, the diagnosis of Wilson's disease can be excluded.

The primary neurologic manifestations are those of a movement disorder, particularly resting and intention tremors. Spasticity, rigidity, chorea, drooling, dysphagia, and dysarthria are common. Babinski responses and absent abdominal reflexes are occasionally noted; sensory changes never occur. Psychiatric disturbances, in part due to the toxic effects of copper on the brain and in part to the reactions to a life-threatening disease, are present in most patients with symptomatic disease. Syndromes indistinguishable from schizophrenia, manic-depressive psychoses, and classic neuroses may occur, and some bizarre behavioral disturbances defy classification. Improvement in the psychiatric state can occur with pharmacologic reduction of the copper excess, but psychotherapy is often also required.

In occasional patients the clinical onset reflects neither a hepatic nor a central nervous system disturbance. For example, primary or secondary amenorrhea may be the first evidence of disease in some young women; in others, repeated spontaneous abortions may result from excess free copper in intrauterine secretions. Routine ophthalmologic examination in patients without symptomatic liver or neurologic disease occasionally reveals Kayser-Fleischer rings, leading to the diagnosis.

PATHOGENESIS The metabolic defect in Wilson's disease is an inability to maintain a near-zero balance of copper. Excess copper accumulates possibly because hepatic lysosomes lack the normal mechanism to excrete into bile the copper that has been catabolically cleaved from ceruloplasmin. This may cause deficiency of ceruloplasmin since a stoichiometric excess of copper inhibits the formation of ceruloplasmin from apoceruloplasmin and copper. The capacity of hepatocytes to store copper is eventually exceeded, and release into blood and uptake in extrahepatic sites occurs (Table 311-1).

Under normal circumstances essentially all tissue copper is present as the prosthetic element of copper proteins such as cytochrome oxidase, tyrosinase, superoxide dismutase, and ceruloplasmin. There is normally little or no free (non-protein-bound) copper. In Wilson's disease more copper is present than can be bound by specific copper proteins; such copper is as toxic as excess iron, zinc, mercury, or lead. Toxicity of these cations is probably effected in large degree by pathologic combinations with proteins that ordinarily do not contain metal.

The pathologic consequences of the accumulated copper occur first in the liver. Abnormal fat and glycogen deposits are the earliest findings by light microscopy (Fig. 311-1). With electron microscopy mitochondrial abnormalities are observed early and appear to be specific for Wilson's disease (Fig. 311-2). Later, necrosis, inflammation, fibrosis, bile duct proliferation, and cirrhosis occur. Abnormalities in liver chemistries develop later than the histologic changes.

Death can occur from the effects of copper toxicosis in the central nervous system with little or no evidence of liver dysfunction, but significant liver disease usually becomes apparent sometime during the course. Patients with prolonged survival always show hepatic cirrhosis.

In the brain the excess copper is distributed ubiquitously. Necrosis of neurons with cavitation may be preceded by the appearance of Opalski and Alzheimer type II cells; however, neither is specific for Wilson's disease.

Increased copper in the kidney produces little if any structural change and commonly does not alter renal function. Hematuria,

TABLE 311-1 Summary of analytic data in patients with Wilson's disease, heterozygous carriers, and control subjects

	Serum ceruloplasmin			Hepatic copper concentration		
Group	No. of patients	Range, mg/dL	Mean ± SD, mg/dL	No. of patients	Range, μg/g dry weight	Mean ± SD, μg/g dry weight
Wilson's disease:						
Asymptomatic	31	0–19.5	3.6±5.3	36	152–1828	983.5±368
Symptomatic	84	0–43.0	5.9±7.1	33	94–1360	588.3±304
Heterozygous carriers	95*	1–50.1	28.4±8.5	14	39–213	117.0±51
Normal subjects	180	18.5–65.9	30.7±3.5	16	20–45	31.5±6.8

* *71 parents of patients with Wilson's disease and 24 children, each of whom had one parent with Wilson's disease.*
SOURCE: *Sternlieb and Scheinberg, 1968.*

proteinuria, the Fanconi syndrome, and renal tubular acidosis occur rarely. Pathologic effects in other organs and tissues are minor.

DIAGNOSIS The diagnosis is easy—*provided it is suspected.* Wilson's disease should be considered in any patient under the age of 40 with an unexplained disorder of the central nervous system, signs or symptoms of chronic active hepatitis, unexplained persistent elevations of serum transaminase, hemolytic anemia in the presence of hepatitis, or unexplained cirrhosis, or in any patient who has a relative with Wilson's disease.

The diagnosis is confirmed in suspected cases by the demonstration either of (1) a serum concentration of ceruloplasmin less than 20 mg/dL and Kayser-Fleischer rings, or (2) a serum ceruloplasmin less than 20 mg/dL and a concentration of copper in a liver biopsy sample greater than 250 μg per gram of dry weight. Most patients also excrete more than 100 μg copper per day in urine and exhibit histologic abnormalities on liver biopsy.

About 5 percent of patients have a serum concentration of ceruloplasmin greater than 20 mg/dL, and some patients with other hepatic disorders have elevated hepatic copper levels and Kayser-Fleischer rings. In either circumstance measurement of the ability to incorporate radioactive copper into ceruloplasmin is useful as a discriminating test. Even in the presence of a normal concentration of ceruloplasmin, patients with Wilson's disease incorporate little or no isotope into the protein, while patients with other liver disorders and elevated hepatic copper incorporate the isotope normally.

TREATMENT Treatment consists of removing the deposits of copper as rapidly as possible and should be instituted once the diagnosis is secure whether the patient is ill or asymptomatic. The drug of choice is D-penicillamine. It is administered orally in an initial dose of 1 g daily, usually in divided doses before meals and at bedtime. Since penicillamine has an antipyridoxine effect in animals, 25 mg per day of vitamin B_6 is also given. Effectiveness of therapy should be assayed chemically and clinically. Initially, the 24-h urinary excretion of copper should increase fivefold or more over the pretreatment level, and 1 to 3 mg copper per day may be excreted during the first months of therapy.

White blood cell and platelet counts, urinalysis, and body temperature should be monitored several times weekly for the first month of therapy and at intervals thereafter. Sensitivity to penicillamine usually appears within the first 14 days of treatment and may cause rash, fever, leukopenia, thrombocytopenia, lymphadenopathy, or proteinuria. Discontinuation of treatment is required if sensitivity develops. Therapy can often be resumed if the drug is reinstituted in small and gradually increasing dosage, although reactions are less likely to recur if 20 mg of prednisone is given daily for the first 2 weeks of penicillamine treatment and subsequently gradually discontinued. Reactions requiring a desensitizing regimen may recur several times before penicillamine can be administered without a steroid.

Lifelong treatment is required. Inadequate treatment or interruption of therapy causes relapse that may be irreversible. Reinstitution of penicillamine after temporary interruption of therapy may be accompanied by the appearance or reappearance of sensitivity reactions. At any time—even after years of uneventful administration—granulocytopenia (or agranulocytosis), thrombocytopenia, the nephrotic syndrome, Goodpasture's syndrome, systemic lupus erythematosus, severe arthralgias, or myasthenia gravis may supervene. Toxicity is sometimes dose-related, and reduction of the dose to a level that is therapeutically effective but nontoxic may be possible. Continued low dosage of steroids may control penicillamine-associated lupus or arthralgias. After temporary interruption of the drug in patients with the nephrotic syndrome, it is sometimes possible to reinstitute therapy without recurrence of proteinuria. However, although irreversible intolerance to D-penicillamine is rare, the toxicity may be such that

FIGURE 311-1 *Fatty changes, glycogen deposits, and cellular infiltrates in a hematoxylin and eosin–stained section of liver from an asymptomatic boy with Wilson's disease.*

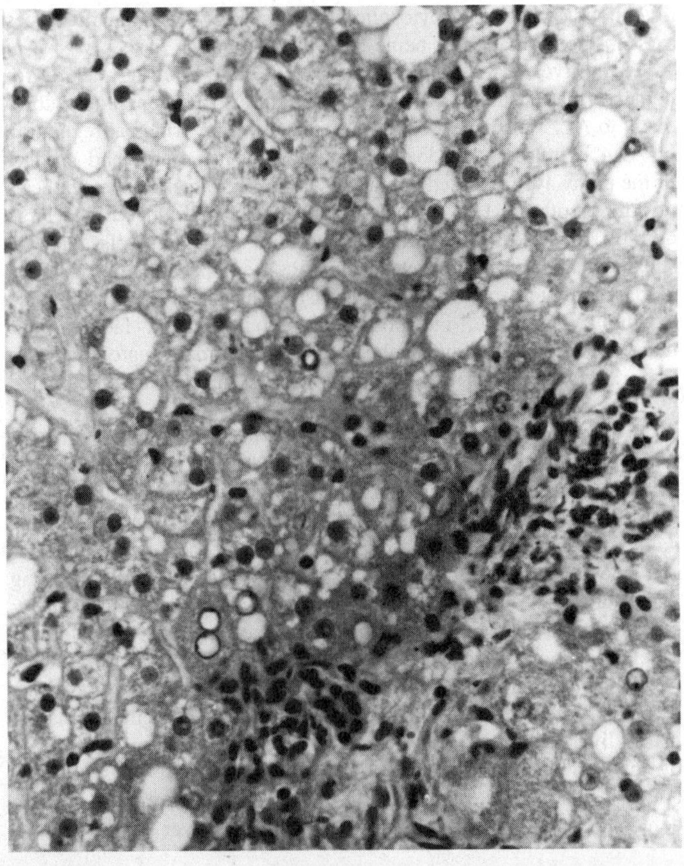

FIGURE 311-2 *Electron micrograph of a liver biopsy sample from a 6-year-old asymptomatic boy. There are prominent vacuoles, containing granular material, in mitochondria (M). P, peroxisome; PM, plasma membrane.*

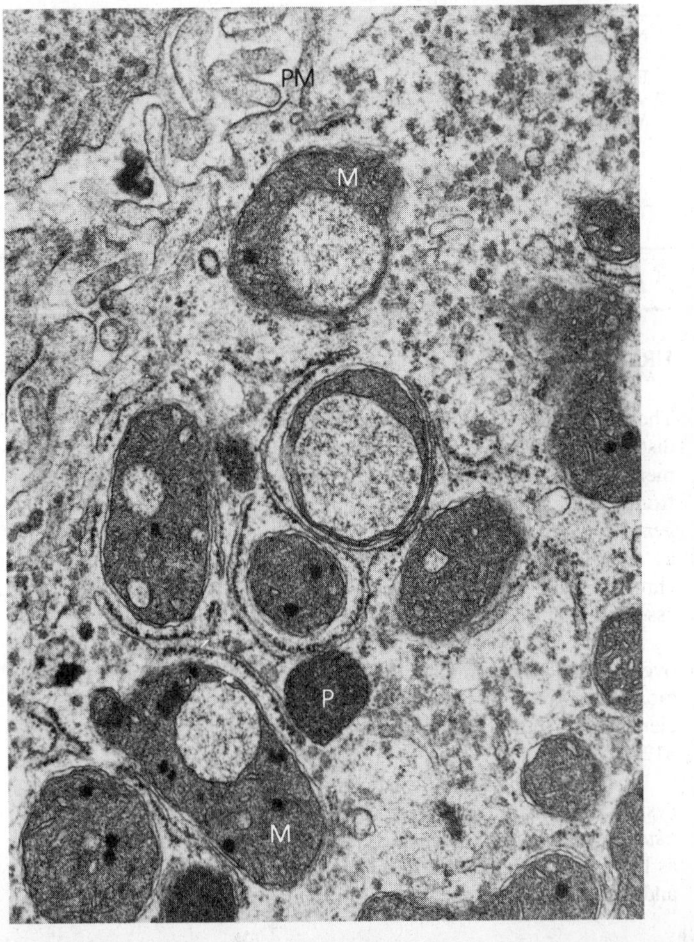

the drug must be withdrawn permanently. The lifelong administration of dimercaprol by injection is impractical, and the only other alternative mode of therapy is trientine.

After therapy with penicillamine has been successfully instituted, the patient should be seen indefinitely at 1- to 3-month intervals to detect drug toxicity and to manage the disease. Physical examination, including relevant neurologic assessment and inspection of the corneas with a slit lamp, and the patient's own evaluation provide the best indicators of the efficacy of treatment. Serial determinations of serum transaminase levels, albumin, and bilirubin are useful in following the course of liver function. Lack of clinical improvement or worsening of the disease may be due to irreversible damage present before therapy was begun, poor compliance, or inadequate dosage of penicillamine. Quantitative determinations of urinary copper excretion and of free copper in serum (total serum copper minus ceruloplasmin-bound copper) can help determine which is the case. After treatment for long periods, the level of urinary copper should be lower than at the onset of therapy, and rarely exceeds 1.5 mg per day. Even more helpful, the concentration of free serum copper is generally less than 10 μg/dL in the adequately treated patient. After a patient has remained asymptomatic with no laboratory evidence of liver dysfunction for a year and in patients with minimal residual disease that has not changed, the dose of penicillamine may be reduced to 0.75 g per day.

Treatment of more than 100 asymptomatic patients with a confirmed diagnosis has established that continued administration of D-penicillamine can prevent virtually every manifestation of this disease.

REFERENCES

SCHEINBERG IH, STERNLIEB I: Wilson's disease, in *Major Problems in Internal Medicine*. Philadelphia, Saunders, 1984, vol XXIII

STERNLIEB I: Evolution of the hepatic lesion in Wilson's disease (hepatolenticular degeneration), in *Progress in Liver Diseases*, H Popper et al (eds). New York, Grune & Stratton, 1972, vol IV, pp 511–526

———, SCHEINBERG IH: Prevention of Wilson's disease in asymptomatic patients. N Engl J Med 278:352, 1968

———, ———: Chronic hepatitis as a first manifestation of Wilson's disease. Ann Intern Med 76:59, 1972

WALSHE JM: Wilson's disease (hepatolenticular degeneration), in *Handbook of Clinical Neurology*, PJ Vinken et al (eds). New York, American Elsevier, 1976, vol 27

312 PORPHYRIAS

URS A. MEYER

The porphyrias are disorders associated with inherited or acquired disturbances in heme biosynthesis. Porphyrins are tetrapyrrole pigments that serve as intermediates in this pathway and are formed from the precursors δ-aminolevulinic acid (ALA) and porphobilinogen. Heme, the ferrous iron complex of protoporphyrin IX, functions as a prosthetic group for hemoproteins such as hemoglobin, cytochromes, catalase, and tryptophan oxygenase. Heme biosynthesis is essential to life and is operative in all aerobic cells.

Each of the porphyrias is characterized by a unique pattern of overproduction, accumulation, and excretion of intermediates of heme biosynthesis. These patterns are the metabolic expression of deficiencies of specific enzymes of the heme biosynthetic pathway (Table 312-1, Fig. 312-1).

The main clinical manifestations are intermittent attacks of nervous system dysfunction and/or sensitivity of the skin to sunlight. The *neurologic syndrome* is characteristically precipitated by drugs such as barbiturates and results in abdominal pain, peripheral neuropathy, and mental disturbance. The neuropsychiatric symptoms occur only in those porphyrias in which there is great overproduction of the porphyrin precursors ALA and porphobilinogen. The pathogenesis of the neurologic lesion is unclear. The *skin photosensitivity* is related directly to increased porphyrin accumulation, although the lesions differ among the different disorders. The photosensitivity is due to the photodynamic action of porphyrins and is probably mediated through the formation of singlet-oxygen with consequent destructive processes such as the peroxidation of lipids in the membranes of lysosomes. The dominantly inherited human porphyrias exhibit variable expressivity. Only the biochemical or enzymatic abnormalities may be apparent. Such latent disease may occur as a phase or persist throughout life, or manifestations can be precipitated by factors such as drugs, hormones, or liver disease.

CLASSIFICATION The porphyrias are usually divided into two main groups, erythropoietic and hepatic, according to the two major sites of heme synthesis where the error of metabolism is expressed (Table 312-1). The only pure erythropoietic form of porphyria is the rare *congenital erythropoietic porphyria* (CEP). In *protoporphyria* (PP) porphyrins accumulate in both erythropoietic and hepatic tissue. In *intermittent acute porphyria* (IAP), *hereditary coproporphyria* (HCP), and *variegate porphyria* (VP), dominantly inherited enzyme deficiencies impair heme biosynthesis predominantly in the liver, apparently without affecting hemoglobin formation. *Porphyria cutanea tarda* (PCT) was previously considered to be an acquired hepatic porphyria. However most if not all patients with this disease have been found to have hereditary deficiency of uroporphyrinogen decarboxylase. Acquired porphyria resembling PCT occurs in individuals exposed to polychlorinated hydrocarbons and in association with hepatic tumors. Poisoning with lead also produces abnormalities in porphyrin and heme synthesis (see Chap. 172). Small increases in urinary excretion of porphyrins or precursors and accumulation of porphyrins in erythrocytes may accompany numerous clinical conditions; these secondary phenomena do not produce symptoms or signs of porphyria.

BIOCHEMICAL CONSIDERATIONS The sequence of reactions that leads from the substrates glycine and succinyl coenzyme A to ALA, porphobilinogen (PBG), and finally heme is mediated by four mitochondrial and four cytosolic enzymes (Fig. 312-2). Differences exist in the regulation of heme biosynthesis among tissues.

In the liver ALA synthase catalyzes the rate-limiting reaction for heme formation under physiologic conditions. The enzymes subsequent to ALA synthase are present in excess. The principal regulation of ALA synthase is feedback repression by heme, the end product of the pathway. Increased demands for heme are met by the synthesis of ALA synthase. Hepatic ALA synthase can be induced by a large number of lipid-soluble drugs, steroids, and chemicals that are substrates and inducers of cytochrome P_{450} hemoproteins, the terminal oxidases in microsomal drug metabolism. This induction is modulated by multiple genetic, metabolic, and environmental factors. The interdependence of heme synthesis and microsomal drug oxidation is important in some hepatic porphyrias where symptoms are precipitated by these drugs.

In the bone marrow ALA synthase is also rate-limiting in cells with fully expressed heme synthesis, but little is known of the role of the enzyme in heme synthesis during division, differentiation, and maturation of erythroid cells. With maturation of erythroid cells the nuclei and mitochondria are extruded, and the mitochondrial enzymes of heme synthesis disappear, while the cytosolic enzymes catalyzing the reactions between ALA and coproporphyrinogen persist. Therefore, erythrocytes can be used for the diagnosis of porphyrias due to a defect in a cytosolic enzyme.

Control of heme synthesis differs in bone marrow and liver. The level of ALA synthase is the major determinant of heme formation in the liver, while heme synthesis in the bone marrow is triggered by the complex process of erythroid differentiation. These considerations probably explain the different manifestations of enzyme defects of heme synthesis in erythroid cells and liver.

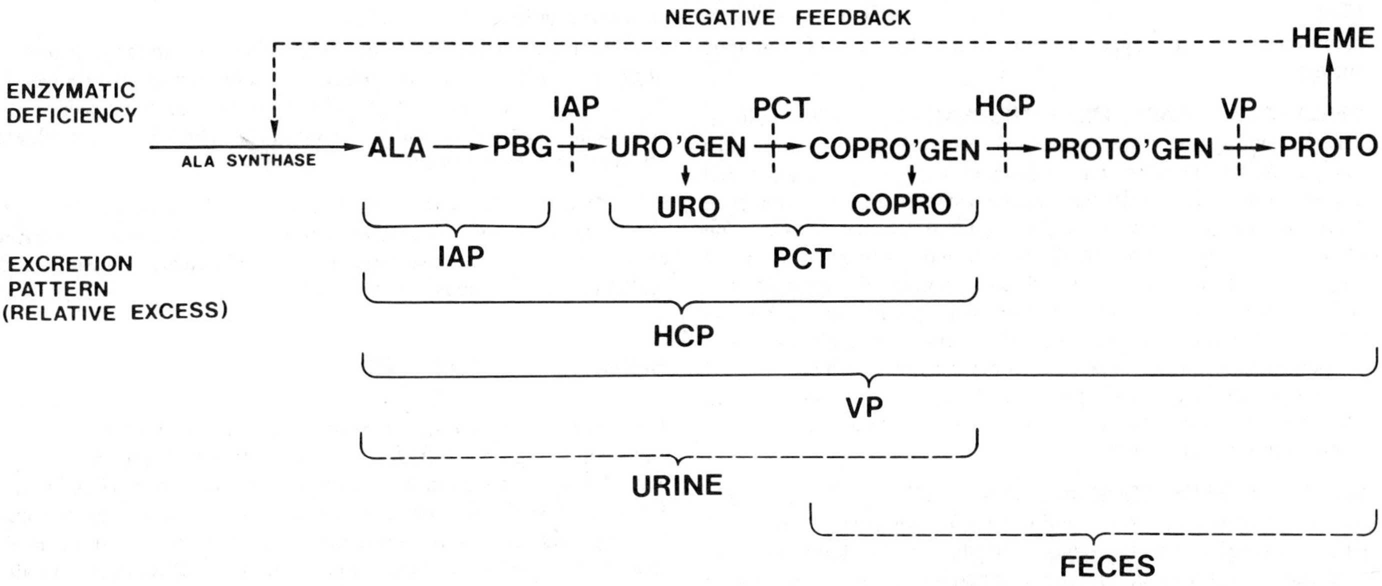

FIGURE 312-1 *Patterns of urinary porphyrin and porphyrin precursor excretion in the hepatic porphyrias in relation to the enzymatic deficiency in the pathway of heme biosynthesis. Intermediates of the pathway excreted excessively during the acute phase of each of the hepatic porphyrias are within the respective brackets. (ALA, δ-aminolevulinic acid; PBG, porphobilinogen; URO'GEN, uroporphyrinogen; COPRO'GEN, coproporphyrinogen; PROTO'GEN, protoporphyrinogen; PROTO, protoporphyrin; IAP, intermittent acute porphyria; PCT, porphyria cutanea tarda; HCP, hereditary coproporphyria; VP, variegate porphyria.)*

The porphyrinogens serve as intermediates between porphobilinogen and protoporphyrin. Porphyrinogens are colorless and nonfluorescent. With the exception of protoporphyrin porphyrins are byproducts that have escaped from the biosynthetic path by irreversible oxidation of the corresponding porphyrinogen. Porphyrins do not possess physiologic function but are responsible, through their pigment and fluorescent properties, for the spectacular appearance of urine and erythrocytes in some patients.

The arrangement of two substituent side chains on the pyrrole ring of porphyrins determines the structural isomer types, numbered I to IV. In nature only types I and III have been identified, and only type III serves as substrate for the terminal steps of the pathway leading to protoporphyrin IX and heme. The catabolism of heme does not lead to porphyrins but to noncyclic tetrapyrroles referred to as *bile pigments*.

CONGENITAL ERYTHROPOIETIC PORPHYRIA

DEFINITION Congenital erythropoietic porphyria (CEP; Günther's disease, congenital photosensitive porphyria, erythropoietic uroporphyria) is a rare, recessively inherited defect that causes chronic

TABLE 312-1 Characteristics of the porphyrias

	Erythropoietic porphyria	Hepatic porphyrias				Erythrohepatic porphyria
	Congenital erythropoietic porphyria (CEP)	Intermittent acute porphyria (IAP)	Hereditary coproporphyria (HCP)	Variegate porphyria (VP)	Porphyria cutanea tarda (PCT)	Protoporphyria (PP)
Enzyme deficiency	Porphobilinogen deaminase and/or uroporphyrinogen III cosynthase (?)	Porphobilinogen deaminase	Coproporphyrinogen oxidase	Protoporphyrinogen oxidase	Uroporphyrinogen decarboxylase	Ferrochelatase
Inheritance	Autosomal recessive	Autosomal dominant	Autosomal dominant	Autosomal dominant	Autosomal dominant	Autosomal dominant
Metabolic expression	Erythroid cells	Liver	Liver	Liver	Liver	Erythroid cells and liver
Signs and symptoms:						
Photosensitive cutaneous lesions	Yes	No	Infrequent	Yes	Yes	Yes
Attacks of abdominal pain, neuropsychiatric syndrome	No	Yes	Yes	Yes	No	No
Laboratory abnormalities:						
Red blood cells:						
Uroporphyrin	+ + +	N	N	N	N	N
Coproporphyrin	+ +	N	N	N	N	+
Protoporphyrin	(+)	N	N	N	N	+ + +
Urine:						
δ-Aminolevulinic acid	N	(+ + +)	(+ + +)	(+ + +)	N	N
Porphobilinogen	N	(+ + +)	(+ + +)	(+ + +)	N	N
Uroporphyrin	+ + +	+ +	+	+	+ + +	N
Coproporphyrin	+ +	N	+ +	+ +	+	(+)
Feces:						
Coproporphyrin	+	N	+ + +	+	(+)	(+)
Protoporphyrin	+	N	+	+ + +	N	+ +

NOTE: *N, normal; +, increased levels or excretion; + +, moderately increased; + + +, markedly increased; (+), increased in some patients only; (+ + +), frequently increased only during acute attacks.*

photosensitivity with severe, mutilating skin lesions and hemolytic anemia.

GENETICS, INCIDENCE, AND PATHOGENESIS Affected individuals are homozygous for an autosomal recessive gene; heterozygotes rarely have demonstrable abnormalities in porphyrin metabolism and appear normal. The underlying enzyme abnormality has not been elucidated but may involve a functional imbalance between the activities of porphobilinogen deaminase and uroporphyrinogen III cosynthase. The defect is expressed solely in maturing erythroid cells and results in massive overproduction of uroporphyrinogen I while the production of uroporphyrinogen III is normal or slightly increased. Uroporphyrinogen I cannot be used for heme synthesis but is converted to coproporphyrinogen I. Uroporphyrin I, coproporphyrinogen I, and coproporphyrin I accumulate in tissues and are excreted in excess amounts in urine and feces.

CLINICAL PRESENTATION AND DIAGNOSIS Porphyrins accumulate in affected individuals during fetal development. Excretion of pink or red urine usually begins at or shortly after birth, whereas cutaneous photosensitivity, intermittent hemolysis, and splenomegaly may be manifested later. Hypertrichosis and red discoloration of the teeth and bones are common. Death may occur in childhood. With longer survival, severe scarring and mutilation occur, mostly affecting fingers, nose, and ears. The urine contains high concentrations of uroporphyrin I, coproporphyrin, and porphyrins with seven, six, five, and three carboxyl groups, whereas the excretion of ALA and PBG is normal. Large amounts of coproporphyrin I are found in the feces. Normoblasts, reticulocytes, and erythrocytes contain large quantities of uroporphyrin I and lower concentrations of coproporphyrinogen I. Normoblasts and reticulocytes exhibit intense red fluorescence. In accordance with the normal excretion of ALA and PBG, neurologic disturbance does not occur.

TREATMENT Exposure to sunlight should be avoided. In some cases, splenectomy has ameliorated hemolytic anemia, porphyrin excretion, and photosensitivity. The use of hematin infusions and oral β-carotene remains experimental.

HEPATIC PORPHYRIAS

Three hepatic porphyrias, intermittent acute porphyria (IAP), hereditary coproporphyria (HCP), and variegate porphyria (VP), have many features in common. All are transmitted as autosomal dominants. Acute attacks of a life-threatening neurologic syndrome are precipitated by a variety of drugs, hormones, and other agents. During acute attacks increased urinary excretion of ALA and PBG occurs in all, but the patterns of porphyrins in urine and feces differ (Fig. 312-1).

INTERMITTENT ACUTE PORPHYRIA Definition Intermittent acute porphyria [IAP, acute intermittent porphyria (AIP), pyrroloporphyria] is characterized by recurrent attacks of neurologic and psychiatric dysfunction. Photosensitivity does not occur. The primary defect is in porphobilinogen deaminase.

Genetics, incidence, and pathogenesis IAP is an autosomal dominant trait with variable expressivity. The frequency of the abnormal

FIGURE 312-2 *Outline of heme biosynthesis. (ALA, δ-aminolevulinic acid; PBG, porphobilinogen; URO'GEN, uroporphyrinogen.)*

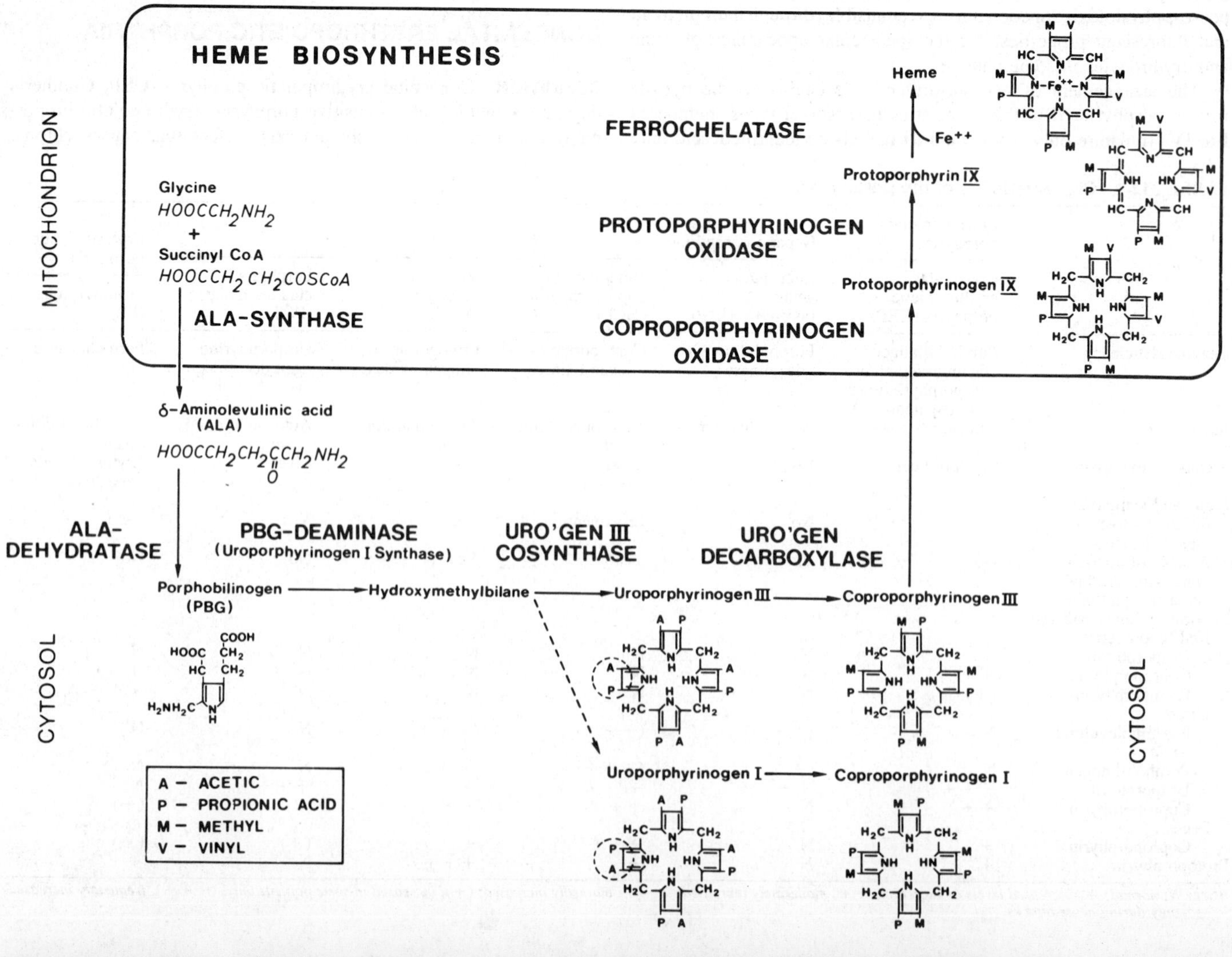

gene is estimated to be between 1 in 10,000 and 1 in 50,000, but in certain regions the incidence may be higher. Homozygous cases have not been observed. The defect consists of a partial (50 percent) deficiency of porphobilinogen deaminase, the enzyme that converts PBG to uroporphyrinogen I. More than one mechanism at the gene level can cause this deficiency, the most common mutation resulting in a decreased amount of immunoreactive enzyme protein. In the liver a partial deficiency of the enzyme leads to increased activity and/or inducibility of ALA synthase by drugs and other factors and, consequently, to increased formation and urinary excretion of ALA and PBG. Preformed porphyrins do not accumulate, and, therefore, cutaneous photosensitivity does not occur. Decreased porphobilinogen deaminase activity is present in liver, erythrocytes, cultured skin fibroblasts, lymphocytes, and amniotic cells of patients with IAP. Thus, the enzymatic defect is present, albeit metabolically unexpressed, in tissues other than liver. Deficiency of the enzyme does not necessarily result in clinical manifestations of acute porphyria without additional acquired factors, and only a third or less of individuals with the genetic defect ever experience an attack of porphyria. The relation between the genetic defect and the neurologic lesions is unknown.

Clinical presentation and diagnosis Symptoms rarely occur before puberty. Abdominal pain is frequently the initial and most prominent symptom of the porphyric attack. It may be moderate or severe, colicky, localized or generalized; radiation to the back or loins may occur. The pain probably results from autonomic neuropathy causing disturbed gastrointestinal motility with alternate areas of spasm and dilatation. The abdomen is usually soft, and tenderness is not marked. Because it is often accompanied by fever and leukocytosis, the acute porphyric attack can mimic any inflammatory abdominal disease. Severe vomiting and persistent constipation are common. Neurologic manifestations and mental disturbance are variable. Peripheral nerves, the autonomic nervous system, brainstem, cranial nerves, or cerebral function may be involved. Sinus tachycardia and labile hypertension with postural hypotension, urinary retention, and excessive sweating are frequent. Hypertension and tachycardia correlate with increased excretion of catecholamines. Peripheral neuropathy is predominantly motor, but sensory components may be present. Deep tendon reflexes are diminished or absent. Neuritic pain in the extremities, areas of hypesthesia and paresthesia, and foot and wrist drop are typical. Paraplegia or complete flaccid quadriplegia may ensue. In the past, respiratory paralysis was a leading cause of death. Cranial nerve involvement may lead to optic nerve atrophy, ophthalmoplegia, and dysphagia. With more severe CNS involvement, delirium, coma, and seizures occur. Although the neuropathy is reversible to a surprising degree, residual paresis may last for years following an acute attack. Many patients have a long history of vague nervousness, emotional instability, and functional disturbances. Signs of mental disturbance occur in one-third, and an organic brain syndrome with restlessness, disorientation, and visual hallucinations may supervene. Hyponatremia can be severe. Multiple mechanisms (including gastrointestinal loss of sodium, imprudent fluid therapy, and a sodium-losing nephropathy related to a toxic effect of ALA) have been implicated, but the major mechanism appears to be inappropriate release of antidiuretic hormone. Hypomagnesemia may be severe enough to cause tetany.

Acute attacks may last from days to months and vary in frequency and severity. In periods of remission symptoms may be slight or completely absent. Clinical (and biochemical) manifestations may be precipitated by usual therapeutic doses of barbiturates, anticonvulsants, estrogens, contraceptives, or alcohol. All these drugs are oxidized by hemoproteins of the cytochrome P_{450} system. Impaired hepatic metabolism of some of these drugs can occur during acute attacks. In some women, exacerbations correlate with the menstrual cycle, and latent porphyria may become manifest late in pregnancy or shortly after delivery. Prolonged periods of decreased caloric intake (fasting) and infections may also provoke attacks.

Laboratory findings Excessive excretion of ALA and PBG in the urine is characteristic during acute attacks and does not differentiate IAP from HCP and VP. The levels do not correlate with the severity of the symptoms. The qualitative determination of porphobilinogen in the urine by the Watson-Schwartz or the Hoesch test is a simple and valuable screening aid for the diagnosis of an acute attack in IAP, HCP, and VP. These tests are almost always positive during episodes of neuropsychiatric dysfunction but are positive only when the concentration of PBG in the urine is three to five times the upper limit of normal; as a consequence, both assays may be negative in latent cases and in patients in whom urinary excretion of PBG becomes normal following recovery from an acute attack. In these instances urinary ALA and PBG excretion should be measured quantitatively by chromatographic methods. In latent IAP with normal excretion of ALA and PBG, diagnosis is possible by measuring the activity of porphobilinogen deaminase in erythrocytes, lymphocytes, or cultured skin fibroblasts. However, there is an overlap between the activities of the enzyme in erythrocytes from normals and patients with IAP, and definite diagnosis is not always possible.

In IAP the porphyrin precursors ALA and PBG are excreted in increased amounts, consistent with the enzymatic defect. Freshly passed urine is, therefore, usually colorless and contains little preformed uro- or coproporphyrin. The urine may darken on standing because PBG polymerizes spontaneously to uroporphyrin and porphobilin, a dark-brown pigment of unknown structure. However, some patients have enough nonenzymatically formed pigments to impart a dark-red appearance to freshly voided urine. The fecal porphyrin concentration is usually normal.

Conventional liver function tests are normal except for increased Bromsulphalein (BSP) retention. A moderate reduction in red blood cell mass and blood volume or a transient normochromic, normocytic anemia are the only hematologic disturbances. Metabolic abnormalities during acute attacks include hypercholesterolemia with increased low-density lipoprotein levels, increased serum thyroxine (without hyperthyroidism), impaired glucose tolerance, and defective 5α-reduction of testosterone in liver. The relationship of these abnormalities to the genetic defect is unknown.

Treatment The treatment of the acute attack is identical in IAP, HCP, and VP. Some acute attacks seemingly can be aborted by administration of large quantities (500 g per day) of carbohydrates (glucose effect), although no objective study of the efficacy of this therapy has been performed. Intravenous administration of glucose at a rate of 20 g/h is recommended. If the patient does not improve within 48 h of continued glucose infusion or if neuropsychiatric symptoms progress, intravenous infusion of hematin (4 mg per kilogram of body weight infused over 10 to 15 min every 12 h for 3 to 6 days) should be tried. Hematin is commercially available (Panhematin) as lyophilized powder; solutions are prepared immediately before infusion. Complications of hematin treatment with the recommended doses seem to be exceedingly rare. Thrombophlebitis at the site of infusion, a coagulopathy (manifested by thrombocytopenia, prolonged prothrombin time, abnormal partial thromboplastin time, and hypofibrinogenemia), and hemolysis have been reported rarely. Both hematin and glucose prevent the induction of hepatic ALA-synthase in experimental animals, and both may reverse the biochemical abnormalities and cause improvement within 48 h. Supportive treatment with careful monitoring of fluid and electrolytes is important to prevent and/or correct hyponatremia, hypomagnesemia, and azotemia. Tachycardia and hypertension should be treated with beta-adrenergic blocking drugs. A list of agents considered to be "safe" or "probably safe" in patients with latent and acute IAP, HCP, and VP is given in Table 312-2. Acute attacks carry a substantial risk of fatality if the diagnosis is delayed and neurologic lesions progress. Complete recovery occurs in the majority, but neurologic deficits may require months or years to resolve. The most important measure in the management is prevention of acute attacks by instructing the patient to avoid provocative factors, such as drugs, gonadal steroids, alcohol excess, and deliberate fasting.

TABLE 312-2 Drugs considered to be safe (or probably safe) in patients with intermittent acute porphyria, hereditary coproporphyria, and variegate porphyria

Analgesics:
- Salicylates, ibuprofen
- Morphine and related opiates (meperidine)

Antibiotics:
- Penicillins, cephalosporins,
- Methenamide mandelate, aminoglycosides

Psychoactive drugs:
- Phenothiazines (chlorpromazine)

Antihistamines:
- Diphenhydramine

Antihypertensives:
- Guanethidine
- Propranolol
- Reserpine, thiazides

Miscellaneous:
- Atropine
- Neostigmine
- Propanidid
- Procaine
- Succinylcholine
- Ether
- Nitrous oxide
- Corticosteroids
- Oxazepam
- Chlordiazepoxide
- Insulin
- Heparin

HEREDITARY COPROPORPHYRIA Definition and genetics Hereditary coproporphyria (HCP) is a hepatic porphyria characterized by attacks of neuropsychiatric dysfunction identical with those of IAP and VP. In addition, photosensitivity occurs in some. The primary genetic defect is a partial deficiency of coproporphyrinogen oxidase. The disease is inherited as an autosomal dominant trait. The incidence of HCP is uncertain since the majority of affected individuals remain asymptomatic.

Pathogenesis and clinical picture HCP is characterized by the excretion of large amounts of coproporphyrin III, mainly in feces but also in urine. Excretion of ALA and PBG is increased during acute attacks (positive Watson-Schwartz or Hoesch test) but usually returns to normal during remission. Acute attacks are indistinguishable from those of IAP and VP and are precipitated by the same factors. Skin photosensitivity occurs in approximately one-third of patients with overt disease. Its onset is frequently associated with intercurrent hepatic disease. A partial deficiency of coproporphyrinogen oxidase can be demonstrated in leukocytes and cultured skin fibroblasts.

Treatment Treatment is identical with that described for IAP.

VARIEGATE PORPHYRIA Definition Variegate porphyria (VP; South African genetic porphyria) is characterized both by acute attacks of neuropsychiatric dysfunction and by chronic skin sensitivity to sunlight and to mechanical trauma. The primary enzymatic lesion in heme biosynthesis is a partial deficiency of protoporphyrinogen oxidase.

Genetics, incidence, and pathogenesis VP is inherited as an autosomal dominant trait. The disease is particularly common among the white population of South Africa, where its incidence is estimated at 1 in 400, and many cases have been identified as descendants of a woman who emigrated to Cape Town from the Netherlands in 1688. Elsewhere the disease is less frequent, but VP has been recognized in many countries. The defect leads to the excretion of large amounts of protoporphyrin in bile and feces (with lesser increases in the fecal excretion of coproporphyrin) and to increased urinary excretion of ALA, PBG, and coproporphyrin during acute attacks.

Clinical presentation and diagnosis Overt cases with VP usually present in the second or third decade. The features include acute attacks of abdominal pain and neuropsychiatric symptoms, coupled with photocutaneous lesions. Neurologic and cutaneous manifestations may occur simultaneously or at different times. Most South African patients have cutaneous involvement, consisting of dermal abrasions, superficial erosions, and blister formation after trivial mechanical trauma. The mechanical fragility usually is limited to light-exposed parts of the skin. The lesions often leave depigmented or pigmented scars. Secondary infection may delay healing. Hyperpigmentation of the face and hands is common, and women often have hirsutism. The skin lesions are indistinguishable from those of porphyria cutanea tarda (PCT). Severe exacerbations of the cutaneous lesions may be associated with intercurrent hepatic disease, presumably related to decreased fecal excretion and a concomitant increase in the urinary excretion of porphyrins. Acute attacks of neuropsychiatric dysfunction are indistinguishable from those of IAP and HCP and are precipitated by the same factors. The characteristic chemical finding in VP is the continuous excretion of large amounts of proto- and coproporphyrin, even when clinical manifestations are minimal or absent. The levels of protoporphyrin exceed those of coproporphyrin, the reverse of the situation in HCP. Urinary excretion of ALA, PBG, and porphyrins is either normal or moderately increased in asymptomatic patients or those who have only skin symptoms. During acute attacks the urinary excretion of ALA and PBG is increased (positive Watson-Schwartz or Hoesch test), and there also is increased urinary excretion of coproporphyrin and uroporphyrin. Erythrocyte porphyrins are normal, allowing distinction from protoporphyria.

Treatment Prophylactic measures and treatment of the acute attack with glucose and possibly hematin infusions are the same as for IAP and HCP, although the experience with hematin in VP is limited. Avoidance of exposure to direct sunlight and use of protective clothing (gloves, hats) are advocated. The prognosis is similar to or better than that of patients with IAP.

PORPHYRIA CUTANEA TARDA Definition Porphyria cutanea tarda (PCT; symptomatic cutaneous hepatic porphyria, symptomatic porphyria) is the most common form of porphyria. The disease is characterized by chronic skin lesions, the frequent presence of hepatic disease (and hepatic siderosis), and a distinct pattern of urinary excretion of porphyrins. The disorder is probably caused by an inherited or acquired deficiency of hepatic uroporphyrinogen decarboxylase. Neurologic manifestations are absent.

Genetics, incidence, and pathogenesis PCT was considered to be an acquired disorder because of its sporadic (and usually nonfamilial) occurrence late in life and its common association with alcoholic liver disease and hepatic siderosis.

The incidence of the disease is not established, but PCT is frequent where both alcoholism and iron overload are common, as among the Bantus in South Africa. PCT can be a familial disease, inherited in an autosomal dominant fashion with variable expressivity (familial PCT). The inherited defect consists of a partial decrease of demonstrable uroporphyrinogen decarboxylase activity in liver, erythrocytes, and cultured fibroblasts; clinically and chemically latent carriers of the defect have been identified. In sporadic PCT a partial deficiency of uroporphyrinogen decarboxylase is found only in liver. It is unknown if this is a consequence of a genetic or acquired (toxic) mechanism. Deficiency (of whatever etiology) in uroporphyrinogen decarboxylase, which catalyzes the conversion of uroporphyrinogen to coproporphyrinogen, leads to a disturbance of hepatic heme synthesis and consequent skin photosensitivity only in the presence of additional factors such as iron overload, usually in association with liver disease and the prolonged administration of estrogens. The mechanism by which iron overload and hormones cause clinical expression of latent PCT is unknown. In contrast to IAP, HCP, and VP, the enzymatic defect in PCT does not result in altered regulation of the hepatic heme synthetic pathway, and ALA synthase activity remains normal or only minimally increased even in overt cases. This probably accounts for the absence of acute neuropsychiatric attacks, the usually normal urinary ALA and PBG, and the lack of sensitivity to drugs such as barbiturates.

Clinical presentation and diagnosis Photosensitivity is the only major manifestation. The skin lesions are indistinguishable from those in VP. Skin symptoms usually begin insidiously, most often in men aged 40 to 60, and consist of enhanced facial pigmentation, increased fragility to trauma, erythema, and vesicular and ulcerative lesions. Sclerodermatous changes and increased hair on the forehead, malar region, or forearms are common.

Liver disease, frequently related to alcohol, is common, and hepatic siderosis is an almost constant finding, although the degree of iron deposition is variable and rarely severe. Spontaneous remission may occur. Occasionally, estrogens (including contraceptive pills) or known hepatotoxic drugs precipitate the clinical disease. The incidence of diabetes mellitus is increased in PCT, and association with systemic lupus erythematosus and other autoimmune syndromes has been noted.

The excretion in urine of uroporphyrin and, to a lesser extent, coproporphyrin is increased. The urine may be pink or brown. The excretion of ALA and PBG in urine is usually normal (negative Watson-Schwartz or Hoesch test). Although uroporphyrin is the major porphyrin in the urine, intermediary porphyrins (particularly hepta-carboxylic porphyrin) are also found. Increases in fecal porphyrins are less marked and usually restricted to the coproporphyrin fraction. The diagnosis is established by the combined presence of skin photosensitivity, liver disease, increased urinary uroporphyrin excretion, the lack of an increase in porphyrin precursors (ALA, PBG), and absence of a history of neuropsychiatric attacks.

Toxic acquired porphyria resembling PCT can occur in individuals accidentally exposed to hexachlorobenzene, polychlorinated biphenyls, tetrachlorodibenzo-*p*-dioxin (TCDD), and other polychlorinated hydrocarbons. Moreover, several instances of PCT in association with benign or malignant primary tumors of the liver have been observed.

Treatment Abstinence in alcoholic patients usually leads to improvement of PCT. Removal of hepatic iron by repeated phlebotomy may lead to long-lasting remissions: 400 mL of blood (or the equivalent amount of erythrocytes) is removed weekly or less frequently with careful monitoring of the hemoglobin and plasma protein levels. For patients unable to tolerate phlebotomy, the administration of small doses of chloroquine (125 mg twice weekly) apparently removes uroporphyrins from the liver and has produced remissions. However, chloroquine carries the risk of hepatotoxicity. Chelation therapy with desferoxamine is another alternative to remove iron. Topical sunscreens and oral carotenoids are not effective in protecting against the skin lesions of PCT.

PROTOPORPHYRIA

DEFINITION Protoporphyria (PP; erythropoietic protoporphyria, erythrohepatic protoporphyria), a disorder in which mild skin photosensitivity is associated with high concentrations of protoporphyrin in erythrocytes, is due to a deficiency of ferrochelatase. Protoporphyrin may also accumulate in the liver.

GENETICS, INCIDENCE, AND PATHOGENESIS PP is inherited as an autosomal dominant trait with variable expressivity. Activity of ferrochelatase, the mitochondrial enzyme that catalyzes the incorporation of ferrous iron into protoporphyrin, is deficient in bone marrow, peripheral blood, liver, and cultured skin fibroblasts. This deficiency results in the excessive accumulation of protoporphyrin in late normoblasts, reticulocytes, and young erythrocytes; protoporphyrin leaks into the plasma from erythrocytes as they age. Photosensitivity is mediated by protoporphyrin in plasma and skin and is evoked by visible light (380 to 560 nm). Skin photosensitivity shows seasonal variability. The liver participates in excess porphyrin production in some patients or, alternatively, may take up protoporphyrin from plasma. Many carriers of the defect remain clinically (and chemically) asymptomatic, and diagnosis may be possible only through enzymatic studies.

CLINICAL PRESENTATION AND DIAGNOSIS Mild photosensitivity usually begins in childhood. Exposure to sunlight is followed by pruritus, erythema, and occasional edema (solar urticaria). The lesions subside over hours or days without scarring. Cutaneous manifestations may occur only after prolonged exposure to sunlight; alternatively, the initial skin lesions may progress to a chronic eczematous phase (solar eczema). There is no abnormal mechanical fragility or blister formation in skin as is characteristic for VP and PCT. Erythrodontia, hypertrichosis, and hyperpigmentation are absent. Attacks of neuropsychiatric dysfunction do not occur.

PP is generally benign, but may be associated with abnormalities of liver, biliary tract, or blood. The incidence of cholelithiasis is increased, and the gallstones contain protoporphyrin. Liver disease due to massive deposition of protoporphyrin may rarely progress to fatal cirrhosis. All patients therefore should have routine evaluation of liver function. Mild anemia is common.

PP is diagnosed by the detection of high concentrations of protoporphyrin in erythrocytes. Large numbers of red-fluorescing erythrocytes are seen by fluorescent microscopy. Protoporphyrin may also be elevated in plasma and feces, while urinary porphyrins, ALA, and PBG are usually normal.

TREATMENT Topical sunscreens usually are ineffective. Orally administered β-carotene (usually as a mixture of β-carotene and canthaxanthine) substantially improves the tolerance to sunlight. Serum carotene levels should be maintained between 600 and 800 μg/dL.

REFERENCES

BONKOWSKY KL, SCHADY W: Neurologic manifestations of acute porphyria. Semin Liver Dis 2:108, 1982
DEAN G: *The Porphyrias*, 2d ed. London, Pitman Medical Publishing Company, 1972
DELEO VA et al: Erythropoietic protoporphyria: 10 years' experience. Am J Med 60:8, 1976
ELDER GH: The porphyrias: Clinical chemistry, diagnosis and methodology. Clin Haematol 9:371, 1980
KAPPAS A et al: The porphyrias, in *The Metabolic Basis of Inherited Disease*, 5th ed, JB Stanbury et al (eds). New York, McGraw-Hill, 1983
PIERACH CA: Hematin therapy for the porphyric attack. Semin Liver Dis 2:125, 1982

313 THE GLYCOGEN STORAGE DISEASES

ARTHUR L. BEAUDET

The glycogen storage diseases are a group of genetic disorders involving the pathways for storage of carbohydrate as glycogen and for its utilization to maintain blood sugar and to provide energy. Some forms are not associated with actual increases in glycogen content in tissues.

Glycogen is a highly branched polymer of glucose with the majority of residues in 1,4 linkage and with 7 to 10 percent of residues in 1,6 linkage. The treelike structure undergoes addition and removal of residues at its periphera. Glycogen molecules have molecular weights of many millions, and molecules may aggregate to form structures recognizable by electron microscopy. Liver generally contains less than 70 mg glycogen per gram of tissue, and muscle usually contains less than 15 mg/g, but these levels fluctuate as a consequence of feeding and hormonal stimuli. Abnormalities of glycogen structure can result either from decreased or increased branching.

The metabolic pathways involved in glycogen synthesis and breakdown are outlined in Fig. 313-1. These pathways differ among tissues; for example, certain reactions are active in liver but trivial or absent in muscle, and some enzyme functions are encoded by

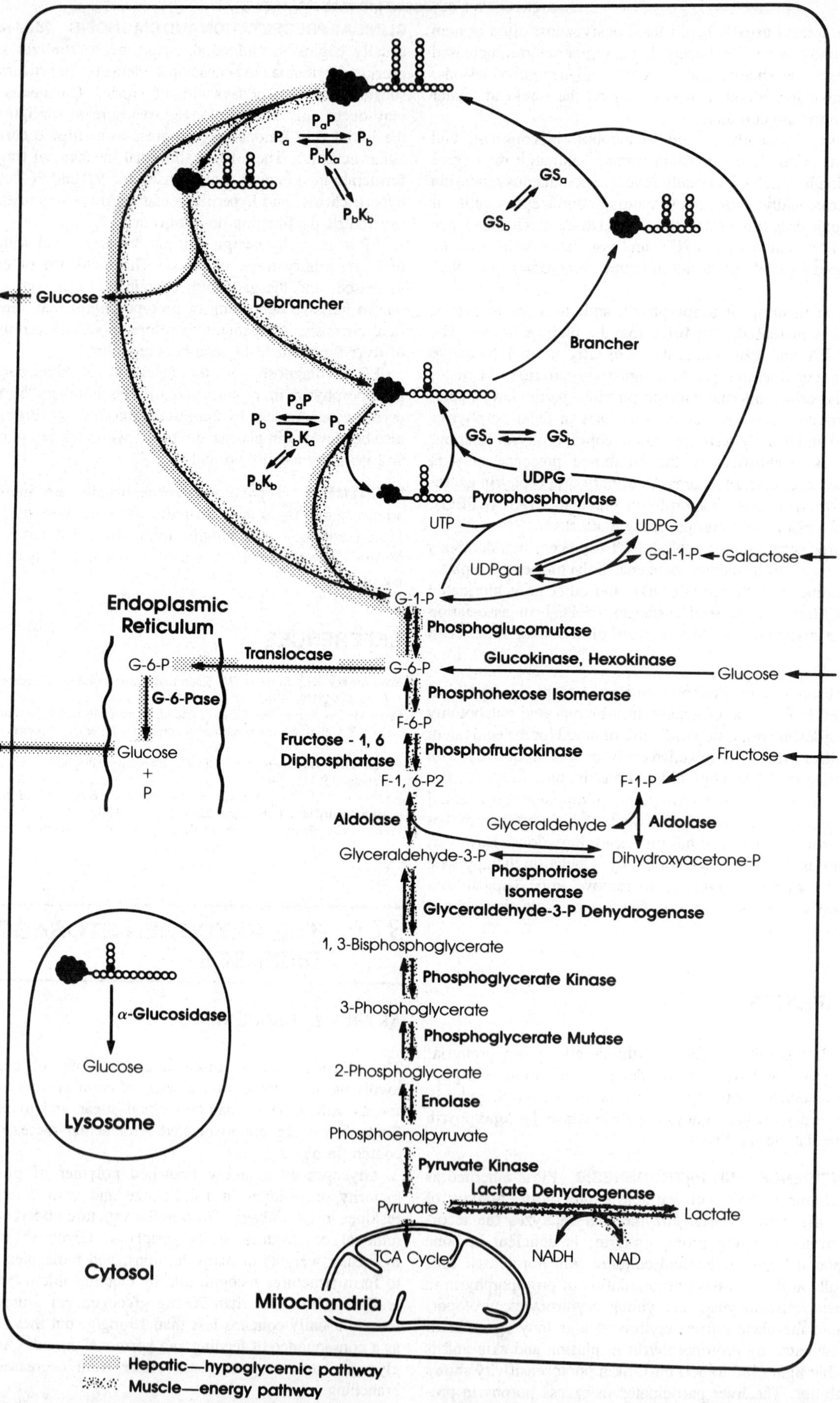

FIGURE 313-1 *Metabolic pathways related to glycogen storage disease. A hypothetical composite cell is shown depicting both hepatic and muscle pathways. The shaded areas depict pathways that are blocked in the hepatic-hypoglycemic diseases or in the muscle-energy diseases. Nonstandard abbreviations are as follows:* GS_a, *active glycogen synthase;* GS_b, *inactive glycogen synthase;* P_a, *active phosphorylase;* P_b, *inactive phosphorylase;* P_aP, *phosphorylase a phosphatase;* P_bK_a, *active phosphorylase b kinase;* P_bK_b, *inactive phosphorylase b kinase.*

different genes in muscle and liver. Plasma glucose enters the cell and is phosphorylated by glucokinase or hexokinase. The former enzyme is found in liver where it accomplishes the majority of phosphorylation of glucose, while multiple hexokinases are distributed more widely in tissues. Glucose 6-phosphate (G6P) is converted to glucose 1-phosphate (G1P) in a reversible reaction catalyzed by phosphoglucomutase. Uridine diphosphate glucose (UDPG) is synthesized from G1P and UTP by UDPG pyrophosphorylase. Genetic deficiency has not been documented for any of the hepatic enzymes. Glycogen is then elongated by the addition from UDPG of individual glucose residues to an existing polymer. This reaction is catalyzed by glycogen synthase, which exists in an active dephosphorylated form and in an inactive phosphorylated form. Synthesis of a normally branched glycogen structure also requires the action of a branching enzyme (1,4-α-glucan:1,4-α-glucan 6-glucosyltransferase) which transfers a 1,4-linked oligosaccharide to a 1,6-linkage position.

Glucose is mobilized from glycogen by a complex group of enzyme reactions. Glycogen is acted upon directly by the active form of phosphorylase, phosphorylase *a*, to remove individual glucose units and yield G1P. Phosphorylase is encoded by different gene products in muscle and in liver. In both tissues, the enzyme can exist in an active phosphorylated form and in an inactive dephosphorylated form. Phosphorylase is a dimer of identical subunits, and both forms of the enzyme are subject to complex allosteric regulation. The inactive phosphorylase *b* is converted to the active form by phosphorylase *b* kinase. Phosphorylase *b* kinase also exists in an active phosphorylated form and in an inactive dephosphorylated form. Phosphorylase *b* kinase is composed of four nonidentical subunits $(\alpha,\beta,\gamma,\delta)_4$, and the δ chain is identical with the calcium-binding protein calmodulin. The rate of glucose mobilization by this system is regulated by a cascade of kinase reactions, including cyclic AMP–dependent protein kinase. Epinephrine and glucagon act to increase blood sugar via this cascade system by activation of phosphorylase and simultaneous inactivation of glycogen synthase. Glycogen also is acted upon directly by a debranching enzyme which carries out the debranching process by first transferring an oligosaccharide from a branch point to leave a single 1,6-linked glucose residue and then hydrolyzing the 1,6 linkage. Thus, the debrancher enzyme has both glucan transferase activity (oligo-1,4 → 1,4-transferase) and a glucosidase (amylo-1,6-glucosidase) activity and yields a single residue of glucose for each branch point removed. The G1P generated by phosphorylase, as mentioned above, must be further metabolized to G6P by phosphoglucomutase. In the liver G6P is transported by a specific translocase to the inner surface of the endoplasmic reticulum for hydrolysis by glucose 6-phosphatase. Glucose is then free to exit the hepatic cell to maintain blood levels. Many genetic deficiencies occur in the enzymes required for the conversion of glycogen to free glucose in the liver, and these cause the hepatic-hypoglycemic forms of glycogen storage disease.

If glycogen is used as a direct energy source, as in muscle, G6P and G1P must enter the pathways for glycolysis. Again, numerous enzymes are required in muscle for proper breakdown of glycogen and entry into the glycolytic pathway and tricarboxylic acid cycle. The enzymatic steps known to be associated with genetic deficiency states in muscle include muscle phosphorylase, debranching enzyme, muscle phosphofructokinase (PFK), and probably muscle phosphoglycerate mutase (PGAM) and lactate dehydrogenase (LDH) M subunit.

The lysomal enzyme α-glucosidase, which is structurally and metabolically separate from the above-described pathways, is capable of degrading both 1,4 and 1,6 linkages in glycogen to give free glucose. This enzyme has widespread distribution in tissues, but its deficiency affects primarily skeletal and cardiac muscle.

CLASSIFICATION The clinical manifestations, diagnostic criteria, and therapy for glycogen storage diseases can be formulated in terms of the metabolic pathway outlined above (Table 313-1). According to this schema, two broad categories of disease can be delineated—those with a *hepatic-hypoglycemic* pathophysiology and those with a *muscle-energy* pathophysiology. Diseases with individualized pathophysiology also occur. It is suggested that disorders be designated by the specific protein deficiency, i.e., glucose 6-phosphatase deficiency. Although the roman numeral designations for types I through VII are in widespread use, numbering for higher types is confused and is to be avoided. Eponyms are of historical interest.

The hepatic-hypoglycemic disorders include glucose 6-phosphatase deficiency (type Ia), G6P microsomal translocase deficiency (type Ib), debrancher enzyme deficiency (type III), hepatic phosphorylase deficiency (type VI), and phosphorylase *b* kinase deficiency. Within this group, a distinction can be made between those disorders in which G6P and its metabolites are likely to be elevated (types Ia and Ib) and those disorders where G6P and related metabolites are likely to be decreased. This explains why increased glycolysis and lactic acidosis occur in types Ia and Ib disease but not in other forms of hepatic-hypoglycemic disease. Likewise, types Ia and Ib disease are distinct because gluconeogenesis, galactose, and fructose cannot contribute effectively to maintenance of blood sugar, in contrast to the other forms of hepatic-hypoglycemic disease. The glycemic response to epinephrine or glucagon tends to be blunted in the hepatic-hypoglycemic disorders. Dietary therapy with frequent feeding is a rational approach to the hepatic-hypoglycemic disorders and is tailored to reduce protein and to eliminate sources of galactose and fructose in types Ia and Ib disease.

The muscle-energy disorders include muscle phosphorylase deficiency (type V), phosphofructokinase deficiency (type VII) phosphoglycerate mutase deficiency, and LDH M-subunit deficiency. The clinical picture is one of muscle pain, myoglobinuria, and elevation of muscle enzymes in serum following vigorous exercise. The interruption of the pathway from glycogen to lactate with the accompanying failure to oxidize NADH is the unifying theme in these disorders. The failure of blood lactate to increase in response to exercise is a useful diagnostic test for the muscle-energy deficiency disorders. Debrancher enzyme deficiency constitutes an overlap syndrome; it presents primarily as a hepatic-hypoglycemic disorder, and the glucose released by phosphorylase appears to be sufficient to prevent myoglobinuria but not to prevent skeletal myopathy and weakness.

Two other disorders are best considered individually. Deficiency of lysosomal α-glucosidase is a lysosomal storage disease without major impact on either carbohydrate metabolism or maintenance of blood sugar (see Chap. 316). The major pathologic process in branching enzyme deficiency is a severe hepatic cirrhosis, possibly due to the harmful effects of the abnormal glycogen that accumulates. Glycogen content is generally normal, and the ability to maintain a normal blood sugar is not impaired.

HEPATIC-HYPOGLYCEMIC DISEASES **Glucose 6-phosphatase deficiency, type Ia** CLINICAL FEATURES Glucose 6-phosphatase deficiency, or von Gierke disease, is an autosomal recessive genetic disorder with an incidence of 1 in 100,000 to 400,000. The disorder is usually manifested during the first 12 months of life by symptomatic hypoglycemia or by the recognition of hepatomegaly. Occasional patients experience hypoglycemia in the immediate neonatal period, and rare patients never have hypoglycemia. Characteristic findings include a full-cheeked, rounded facial appearance; a protuberant abdomen due to marked hepatomegaly; and thin extremities. Hyperlipidemia may cause eruptive xanthomas and lipemia retinalis. Splenomegaly is usually mild or absent, although massive enlargement of the left lobe of the liver may be mistaken for enlargement of the spleen. Growth is usually normal for the first few months of life; growth retardation then supervenes, and adolescence is delayed. Mental development is usually normal except for injury from hypoglycemia.

The characteristic profound symptomatic hypoglycemia may be associated with blood glucose levels below 15 mg/dL. Liver enzymes are mildly elevated if at all. The presence of lactic acidosis is helpful in diagnosing this disorder, although blood lactate may be normal in the fed state in young infants. However, these patients are relatively

TABLE 313-1 Glycogen storage diseases

Type	Basic defect*	Clinical findings	Laboratory	Diagnosis	Treatment	Comments
DISORDERS WITH HEPATIC-HYPOGLYCEMIC PATHOPHYSIOLOGY						
Ia von Gierke	Glucose 6-phosphatase deficiency	Hypoglycemia, hepatomegaly, bleeding diathesis, short stature, delayed adolescence, hepatic adenomas, enlarged kidneys	Increased lactate, cholesterol, triglyceride, and uric acid	Enzyme assay on liver or intestine, increased glycogen with normal structure in liver	Frequent feeding, nighttime tube feeding, 60–70% carbohydrate, restrict sucrose and lactose, bicarbonate and allopurinol as needed	Common, severe, autosomal recessive
Ib	G6P microsomal translocase deficiency	As for Ia with addition of neutropenia and recurrent infection	As for Ia	Enzyme assay on liver with and without detergent	As for Ia	Rare, severe, autosomal recessive
III Cori	Debrancher enzyme deficiency	Hypoglycemia, hepatomegaly, some short stature and delayed adolescence, mild myopathy worsening in some adults	Normal lactate and uric acid; increased cholesterol, triglyceride, and SGOT	Enzyme assay on liver, muscle, or fibroblasts; leukocytes variable; increased glycogen with abnormal structure in liver and muscle	Frequent feeding, nighttime tube feeding, 50% carbohydrate and 15–20% protein	Common, intermediate severity, some hepatic fibrosis
VI Hers	Hepatic phosphorylase deficiency	Hepatomegaly, variable hypoglycemia	Minimal changes, ? hyperlipidemia	Enzyme assay on liver, increased hepatic glycogen with normal structure	Dietary therapy as for type III, often little treatment required	Rare and poorly characterized; ? autosomal recessive
Formerly VIb, VIII, or IX	Hepatic phosphorylase *b* kinase deficiency	Hepatomegaly, variable hypoglycemia, occasional findings in heterozygous females	Minimal changes	Enzyme assay on leukocytes, fibroblasts, or liver; increased hepatic glycogen with normal structure	Dietary therapy as for type III, often little treatment required	Very mild but may be fairly common, X-linked
DISORDERS WITH MUSCLE-ENERGY PATHOPHYSIOLOGY						
V McArdle	Muscle phosphorylase deficiency	Pain, cramps, and myoglobinuria on strenuous exercise	Increased CPK with episodes, deficient lactate production with ischemic exercise test	Muscle enzyme assay, increased muscle glycogen with normal structure	Avoid exercise, glucose or fructose before exercise	Some clearly autosomal recessive, male preponderance
VII	Muscle phosphofructokinase deficiency	As for type V, mild hemolytic anemia	As for type V	Muscle enzyme assay, increased muscle glycogen with normal structure	As for type V	Rare, autosomal recessive
	Muscle phosphoglycerate mutase deficiency	As for type V	As for Type V	Muscle enzyme assay, normal glycogen content	? As for type V	Based on one affected male
	LDH-M subunit deficiency	As for type V	Increased CPK with episodes; pyruvate but not lactate rises with ischemic exercise test	LDH isozymes on serum, erythrocytes or leukocytes; enzyme assay on muscle; ? glycogen content normal	? As for type V	Based on sibship of 3 males and 1 female affected
DISORDERS WITH INDIVIDUAL PATHOPHYSIOLOGY						
II Pompe	Lysosomal α-glucosidase deficiency	*Infantile:* hypotonia, muscle weakness, cardiac enlargement and failure, enlarged tongue, fatal early; *juvenile:* progressive skeletal muscle weakness; *adult:* progressive skeletal muscle weakness, pulmonary insufficiency presentation	Increased CPK, no hypoglycemia	Enzymes assay on muscle or fibroblasts, enzyme assay on leukocytes possible but pitfalls are serious	No effective treatment	Common, autosomal recessive, prenatal diagnosis available and widely utilized in infantile
IV Andersen	Brancher enzyme deficiency	Infantile failure to thrive, cirrhosis and liver failure, extreme hypotonia and weakness in some, fatal early	No hypoglycemia, changes of liver disease	Enzyme assay on liver, muscle, leukocytes, or fibroblasts; glycogen content not remarkable but structure abnormal	No effective treatment	Very rare, autosomal recessive

* *These defects provide the preferred nomenclature for the diseases.*

resistant to development of ketosis. Hyperlipidemia is frequent and involves elevation of both cholesterol and triglycerides. Hypertriglyceridemia can be extreme with levels as high as 5000 to 6000 mg/dL. Hyperuricemia due both to decreased renal excretion and increased production is frequent and often becomes more severe after adolescence. The rise in plasma glucose following administration of epinephrine or glucagon is impaired, as is the rise in blood glucose following administration of galactose by mouth. Renal enlargement can be demonstrated by radiologic or sonographic techniques. Mild renal tubular dysfunction or the Fanconi syndrome may occur. Moderate anemia is usually due to recurrent nosebleeds and chronic acidosis but may become severe after prolonged acidosis. A bleeding diathesis is due to a platelet dysfunction.

Once type Ia disease is suspected clinically, the diagnosis is established by liver biopsy. The diagnosis is suggested by lactic acidosis, an abnormal galactose tolerance test, or renal enlargement. Proper handling of biopsy material should be arranged to distinguish types Ia and Ib. Sufficient material for enzyme assay may be obtained by needle biopsy provided the bleeding time is normal, or alternatively, open liver biopsy provides more tissue for analysis. Microscopic examination of liver reveals increased glycogen in cytoplasm and nuclei; lipid vacuoles in hepatocytes are prominent, and fibrosis is usually absent.

The hypoglycemia and lactic acid acidosis may be life-threatening. Other troublesome features include short stature, delayed adolescence, and hyperuricemia. During adult years uric acid nephropathy and hepatic adenomata may develop. The latter lesions are often large and either palpable or demonstrable by radioisotopic scan. There is a significant risk of malignant degeneration, often during the third decade, and subjects who live long enough are probably at increased risk for atherosclerosis.

TREATMENT The mainstay of management is frequent feeding. The most widely used approach in children has been the combination of frequent daytime feeding by mouth and continuous nighttime feeding by nasogastric tube (see Chap. 74). The regimen should include approximately 60 percent carbohydrate, and no significant portion of carbohydrate should come from sources containing galactose or fructose, which cannot be utilized effectively to maintain blood sugar. The ability of a family to carry out such a program is a significant variable, but in some instances the metabolic abnormalities and the rate of growth have improved substantially. Raw cornstarch feeding provides a convenient, economical, and palatable source of slowly digested glucose polymer, and cornstarch therapy may become the primary dietary treatment for this disease. Optimal management requires a team attentive to the dietary and psychosocial needs of patient and family. Control of elevated plasma urate may require the addition of allopurinol. This regimen provides a reasonably optimistic short-term prognosis, but it is not known whether the long-term risks of hepatic malignancy and atherosclerosis are ameliorated. Portacaval anastomosis was previously used in the management of some forms of glycogen storage disease, but the enthusiasm for the procedure has declined. Prenatal diagnosis is not possible at present.

G6P microsomal translocase deficiency, type Ib G6P microsomal translocase deficiency, historically referred to as *pseudo type I,* has an incidence of perhaps one-tenth or less that of type Ia. The term *microsomal translocase* describes the capacity to transport G6P into the endoplasmic reticulum. The clinical features are similar to those in type Ia, but unique features include neutropenia, impaired neutrophil migration, and recurrent pyogenic infections; in general, type Ib is more severe than Ia. Laboratory findings, responses to tolerance tests, and management are similar in the two disorders.

Type Ib disease was initially distinguished from type Ia by the presence of normal glucose 6-phosphatase activity on assay of biopsy tissue in the presence of detergent. However, glucose 6-phosphatase activity is low in type Ib disease when fresh tissue is homogenized and assayed in the absence of detergent. These results have been interpreted to imply a genetic deficiency of a microsomal glucose 6-phosphate transport system as a primary defect in type Ib glycogen storage disease. The cause for the neutropenia and abnormal neutrophil migration is unknown, although the disease suggests a role for G6P transport in these cells.

Debrancher deficiency, type III CLINICAL FEATURES Debrancher enzyme deficiency, also known historically as Cori disease, is an autosomal recessive disorder and is one of the more frequent forms of glycogen storage diseases, occurring with a particularly high frequency in North African Jews. Symptomatic disease in the newborn period is unusual, and patients usually present with hypoglycemia or hepatomegaly during the first year of life. The physical findings are similar to those in type Ia, except that splenomegaly is more prominent, but the clinical course tends to be less severe. The skeletal myopathy is usually mild or insignificant in childhood but may be disabling and progressive in adults. Some patients with myopathy are first diagnosed as adults because the features in childhood were mild and overlooked.

Fasting hypoglycemia occurs in about 80 percent of patients. The glucose response after glucagon or epinephrine is abnormal in the fasting state but may be normal shortly after eating since the terminal glucose residues in glycogen can be mobilized. The galactose tolerance test is usually normal. Ketosis is prominent, and blood lactate is normal. Serum transaminase is elevated, and further increases may occur with minor illnesses. Blood cholesterol and triglyceride are elevated in about two-thirds. Hyperuricemia is rare.

Two diagnostic modalities are used to establish the diagnosis—analysis of glycogen and measurement of debranching enzyme in tissue samples. The glycogen content of red blood cells and liver is increased in almost all, whereas glycogen content of muscle is increased only in some. Documentation of abnormal structure of glycogen with the use of spectrophotometric techniques is a more consistent finding than the increase in glycogen content. The establishment of the diagnosis by enzymatic assay is complicated both by methodologic problems and what is believed to be genetic heterogeneity. Both debrancher functions—the glucan transferase activity and glucosidase activity—are believed to reside in a single polypeptide, but as many as six subtypes of the disease may occur. While the diagnosis can be made in some patients using red cells, leukocytes, or fibroblasts, it is generally preferable to document the abnormal glycogen structure and the enzyme deficiency directly in biopsy material from liver or muscle. The pathologic findings in liver are similar to those in type Ia except for less lipid deposition and more prominent fibrous septae.

In regard to growth retardation and abdominal protuberance, the course is one of progressive improvement following adolescence, so that the adult appearance may be normal and hypoglycemia is less frequent. Liver tumors are not reported, and there is no information regarding the long-term risks of hyperlipidemia. The fraction of adult patients who develop a debilitating myopathy is probably low. Affected patients have had children.

TREATMENT Frequent feeding is also the mainstay of therapy for type III in childhood. Gluconeogenesis is normal, and as described above patients can ingest galactose, fructose, or protein to help maintain blood glucose. Thus, dietary therapy can include a larger percentage of calories as protein, but carbohydrate intake should be 40 to 50 percent of the total. An evening feeding is often sufficient to avoid hypoglycemia, but nighttime nasogastric tube feeding or cornstarch therapy may be required in severely affected children. Attempts to lower blood lipids using dietary means are desirable. Prenatal diagnosis is possible.

Hepatic phosphorylase deficiency, type VI The diagnosis of hepatic phosphorylase deficiency, or Hers disease, was previously applied to a diverse group of patients with reduced hepatic phosphorylase levels due to a variety of causes but is now limited to patients in whom deficiency of hepatic phosphorylase is the primary defect. This nosologic difficulty is a consequence of the fact that phosphorylase exists in both active and inactive forms, and many factors may inhibit the activation of the enzyme secondarily. Consequently, diagnosis requires documentation that phosphorylase is absent and that the phosphorylase *b* kinase responsible for its activation is normal. The disorder is probably due to an autosomal recessive mutation.

Most patients have features similar to those in type III but in a milder form. The diagnosis is suspected because of hepatomegaly or hypoglycemia, and patients generally respond to dietary management similar to that employed in type III disease.

Phosphorylase *b* kinase deficiency Phosphorylase *b* kinase deficiency, now known to be a separate entity, was previously included in the type VI category. Various authors have designated this disorder as type VIa, type VIII, or type IX, but it is best termed *phosphorylase b kinase deficiency*. The best characterized form of the disorder is the X-linked variety, but there is potential for genetic heterogeneity, since the enzyme is composed of four nonidentical subunits. This disorder is relatively benign and is manifested in affected males by hepatomegaly, occasional fasting hypoglycemia, and some growth retardation, all of which tend to resolve spontaneously at the time of adolescence. Mild hepatomegaly may occur in female heterozygotes. The diagnosis can be established by specific enzyme assay of leukocytes, cultured skin fibroblasts, or liver. Muscle phosphorylase *b* kinase is believed to be normal in this condition. Dietary management similar to that employed in type III can be employed for hypoglycemia or growth retardation. It is possible that this condition is relatively common and passes undiagnosed. Healthy adults with a history of abdominal protuberance in childhood are often identified during family studies of patients with this condition.

MUSCLE-ENERGY DISEASES (See also Chap. 357) In recognizing the various glycogen storage diseases that affect muscle, the *ischemic exercise test* is of particular use in the initial evaluation. A blood pressure cuff is inflated above arterial pressure, and the ischemic hand is exercised to maximum effort. The pressure cuff is released, and blood is drawn from the other arm at 2, 5, 10, 20, and 30 min for assay of lactate and pyruvate, muscle enzymes, and myoglobin.

Myophosphorylase deficiency, type V Myophosphorylase deficiency, or McArdle disease, is uncommon. Symptoms of pain and cramps after exercise usually develop during the second or third decade. A history of myoglobinuria is present in most, and on occasion myoglobinuria can cause renal failure. Affected individuals are otherwise healthy, without evidence of hepatic, cardiac, or metabolic disturbance. Performance of an ischemic exercise test usually causes painful cramping, which is helpful diagnostically. In addition, blood lactate does not rise whereas serum creatine phosphokinase is elevated after strenuous exercise.

The diagnosis is established by documentation of elevated glycogen content and reduced phosphorylase activity in biopsied muscle tissue. The glycogen is usually deposited in subsarcolemmal regions of the muscle. The gene for human myophosphorylase has been cloned and is located on chromosome 11, in keeping with the autosomal recessive nature of the disease. There is an excess of male patients, which may be due to better ascertainment in males, genetic heterogeneity, or other factors. A fatal infantile form of hypotonia in association with myophosphorylase deficiency also has been described.

Management of myophosphorylase deficiency requires the avoidance of strenuous exercise. Glucose or fructose ingestion prior to exercise can reduce symptoms.

Muscle phosphofructokinase deficiency, type VII There are two genetically distinct forms of phosphofructokinase. Activity in muscle is due to a distinct muscle isoenzyme, whereas activity in red cells is due both to a red cell isoenzyme and to the muscle form of the enzyme. A small number of families have been identified with deficiency of the muscle isoenzyme. Symptoms similar to those in myophosphorylase deficiency were present with pain and cramps, myoglobinuria, and elevated muscle enzymes in serum after strenuous exercise. Lactate production was impaired, and a mild nonspherocytic hemolytic anemia was present. Other patients have the anemia but no muscle symptoms; the latter phenomenon might be due to a qualitatively abnormal, unstable enzyme that rapidly disappears from the anucleate red cell but is replaced effectively in muscle cells and consequently prevents muscle symptoms.

Other muscle-energy diseases A group of even rarer familial metabolic disorders must be considered in the differential diagnosis of patients with myoglobinuria and elevated muscle enzymes in serum after exercise. These include phosphoglycerate mutase deficiency, LDH M-subunit deficiency, and carnitine palmityl transferase deficiency. (Older reports of phosphoglucomutase deficiency and phosphohexoseisomerase deficiency seem inconclusive by current standards.) When myophosphorylase, phosphofructokinase, or phosphoglycerate mutase are deficient, neither lactate nor pyruvate rises following exercise, whereas in deficiency of LDH M subunit there is a rise in pyruvate in the face of a failure of lactate production. Carnitine palmityl transferase deficiency is a disorder of lipid metabolism and is discussed in Chap. 329. Definitive diagnosis of these disorders must be established by enzyme assay of muscle tissue. Some patients with this clinical presentation have none of the above-mentioned enzyme deficiencies, and identification of other defects in muscle metabolism is likely in the future.

DISORDERS WITH INDIVIDUAL PATHOPHYSIOLOGY α-Glucosidase deficiency, type II Alpha-glucosidase deficiency, or Pompe disease, is a lysosomal storage disease, and the pathophysiology is discussed in Chap. 316. The incidence is not known but may exceed 1 in 100,000. The disorder is not associated with hypoglycemia, ketosis, or other abnormalities of intermediary metabolism.

The infantile form presents within the first 6 months of life and may be manifested at birth. Clinical features include skeletal muscle hypotonia and weakness, massive cardiac enlargement, enlargement of the tongue, and varying degrees of hepatomegaly. Muscle enzymes such as creatine phosphokinase and aldolase are usually elevated, and the ECG may show large QRS complexes and a shortened PR interval. Motor weakness and developmental delay may be present. Death occurs in the first 2 to 3 years in most cases due to the cardiac involvement.

The juvenile form has features suggestive of a progressive form of muscular dystrophy. These patients have gait abnormalities but no cardiac symptoms. Plasma creatine phosphokinase and aldolase are elevated, and the length of survival is variable. An even milder adult form presents as skeletal muscle weakness in the third to the fifth decade. Again, cardiac symptoms are absent, and serum muscle enzymes are elevated. Some patients have respiratory failure due to involvement of the muscles of respiration and are often misdiagnosed as having some form of muscular dystrophy.

Vacuolization of muscle and increased glycogen content are demonstrable on muscle biopsy. Electron-microscopic studies demonstrate membrane-bound vacuoles containing glycogen, a finding strongly suggestive of the disorder. Excessive glycogen is also found in other tissues including liver and central nervous system, particularly in the anterior horn cells of the spinal cord. Specific diagnosis is made by enzyme assay in biopsy material from muscle or liver or in cultured skin fibroblasts. In general, some residual enzyme activity is present in patients with the adult form of disease, but the exact level is not of prognostic significance. Prenatal diagnosis is reliable and has been used extensively for the infantile form. Various forms of enzyme infusion therapy have been tried but are ineffective.

Brancher deficiency, type IV Brancher enzyme deficiency, or Andersen disease, is a rare, autosomal recessive disorder. Features in infants include hepatomegaly, failure to thrive, and hypotonia in the first few months of life with subsequent development of progressive cirrhosis. In other patients the predominant feature is cardiac involvement and/or extreme hypotonia similar to that observed in spinal muscular atrophy and anterior horn cell degeneration. Death occurs within the first 2 or 3 years.

The symptoms are thought to be related primarily to the abnormal glycogen structure that results from a generalized deficiency of brancher enzyme. The presence of long outer chains on the glycogen molecules has led to the designation of the disease as amylopectinosis. The laboratory findings are generally those associated with severe liver disease except that hypoglycemia usually does not occur. The absence of hypoglycemia and the presence of normal glycogen content in the liver make the diagnosis difficult to establish. The diagnosis is suggested by finding abnormally structured glycogen in biopsy material and is established by direct assay of the enzyme in liver, leukocytes, or cultured skin fibroblasts. No effective treatment is known, but prenatal diagnosis is possible using cultured amniotic cells.

Other possible disorders of glycogen metabolism Deficiency of glycogen synthase has been reported in a small number of families. Affected patients usually have fasting hypoglycemia, seizures, and some degree of mental impairment. The presence of some hepatic glycogen, the increase in plasma glucose in response to glucagon or galactose, and the known lability of the activation system for glycogen synthase have all led to skepticism as to whether such a disorder actually exists. This syndrome may be confused with ketotic hypoglycemia of childhood (see Chap. 329).

There are also reports of more than one enzyme defect in the same patient and of different enzyme defects among siblings. Many of these reports may be related to difficulties inherent in measuring enzymes of glycogen metabolism in human pathologic tissue. At present no specific syndrome of multiple primary enzyme deficiency is documented.

REFERENCES

CHEN Y-T et al: Cornstarch therapy in type I glycogen-storage disease. N Engl J Med 310:171, 1984

FERNANDES J: Hepatic glycogen storage diseases, in *The Treatment of Inherited Metabolic Disease,* DN Raine (ed). New York, American Elsevier, 1974

GREENE HL et al: Type I glycogen storage disease: A metabolic basis for advances in treatment. Adv Pediatr 26:63, 1979

HOWELL RR, WILLIAMS JC: The glycogen storage diseases, in *The Metabolic Basis of Inherited Disease,* 5th ed, JB Stanbury et al (eds). New York, McGraw-Hill, 1983, pp 141–166

314 GALACTOSEMIA, GALACTOKINASE DEFICIENCY, AND OTHER RARE DISORDERS OF CARBOHYDRATE METABOLISM

KURT J. ISSELBACHER

DEFINITION Galactosemia refers to either of two inborn errors of galactose metabolism. *"Classic" galactosemia* is due to the deficiency of galactose 1-phosphate uridyl transferase (GALT) and is typically associated with cataract formation, mental retardation, and cirrhosis. The second disorder, *galactokinase deficiency,* leads primarily to cataract formation.

PATHOGENESIS Lactose, the main carbohydrate in milk, is a disaccharide containing galactose and glucose; when ingested it is hydrolyzed by intestinal lactase. Normally the absorbed galactose is converted to glucose in the liver. The first reaction in this pathway is the phosphorylation of galactose to galactose 1-phosphate by galactokinase (specified by a gene on chromosome 17):

$$\text{Galactose} + \text{ATP} \xrightarrow{\text{galactokinase}} \text{galactose 1-phosphate}$$

The next step involves the conversion of galactose 1-phosphate to glucose 1-phosphate by GALT, the gene for which is on chromosome 9:

$$\text{Galactose 1-phosphate} + \text{UDP-glucose} \xrightarrow{\text{GALT}} \text{UDP-galactose} + \text{glucose 1-phosphate}$$

The UDP sugars can be reversibly interconverted by an epimerase reaction:

$$\text{UDP-galactose} \longleftrightarrow \text{UDP-glucose}$$

Galactose can also be metabolized by alternate pathways. It can be converted (reduced) in the presence of NADPH (or NADH) to galactitol (dulcitol) by aldose reductase. It can also be oxidized to a limited extent by galactose dehydrogenase, leading to the formation of galactonic acid, xyulose, and CO_2. These pathways account for limited galactose metabolism in patients with galactosemia.

In galactokinase deficiency, galactose accumulates in the blood and tissues. In the lens galactose is converted by aldose reductase to galactitol, a sugar to which the lens is impermeable. As a consequence, excessive hydration occurs which, together with a decrease in glutathione in the lens, leads to cataract formation.

In classic galactosemia, GALT deficiency results in tissue accumulation of galactose 1-phosphate and galactose. As in galactokinase deficiency, cataracts develop secondary to galactitol accumulation in the lens. It is assumed that the cirrhosis and mental retardation of classic galactosemia are related to increased amounts of galactose 1-phosphate in these tissues. Elevated blood galactose levels may lead to a decreased hepatic output of glucose and hence to hypoglycemia. In the kidney and intestine accumulation of galactose and galactose 1-phosphate appears to lead to an inhibition of amino acid transport. In some women ovarian malfunction develops in association with hypergonadotrophic hypogonadism; the pathogenesis is unclear.

Both galactokinase and GALT deficiencies are transmitted as autosomal recessive traits. Heterozygotes for these disorders have half-normal enzyme levels but are asymptomatic. Maternal deficiency of galactokinase, together with lactose intake during pregnancy, may contribute to cataract formation during fetal development. However, not all persons with half-normal GALT enzymes in their cells are carriers of classic galactosemia. Some individuals homozygous for another gene, called the *Duarte variant,* normally have half-normal GALT levels and are asymptomatic. This group can be differentiated from classic galactosemia heterozygotes on the basis of the electrophoretic properties of the mutant enzyme. In both galactokinase deficiency and classic galactosemia there is a functional deficiency or absence of the involved enzyme. Classic galactosemia is due to a structural gene mutation, and the altered enzyme (GALT) protein does not function normally. Other clinical variants with altered enzyme electrophoretic mobility have been described.

The incidence of classic galactosemia is about 1 per 80,000 births in the white population. Approximately 0.8 to 1.3 percent of the population are heterozygotes for the galactosemia (GALT) gene, and about 10 percent carry the Duarte variant. During screening of newborns for galactosemia the most frequent cause of an abnormal result is compound heterozygosity for the Duarte variant and for classic galactosemia in which GALT levels are about 17 percent of normal. Such individuals are clinically asymptomatic.

CLINICAL FEATURES Symptoms of classic galactosemia usually begin within days to weeks after birth. The infant usually is reluctant to ingest breast milk or milk formulas, develops vomiting, shows poor nutrition, and fails to thrive. Jaundice, hepatomegaly, and evidence of liver disease may develop. Cataracts are usually not present at birth but develop gradually over weeks to months. Mental retardation becomes evident after 6 to 12 months. Infants with classic galactosemia are subject to bacterial sepsis (especially with *Escherichia coli*), and this may be the leading cause of death in the neonatal period. The only consistent feature of galactokinase deficiency is cataract formation.

DIAGNOSIS Galactokinase deficiency should be suspected in infants or children with cataract formation who have non-glucose-reducing substances in the urine. The diagnosis is made by demonstrating the deficiency of galactokinase in red blood cells.

TABLE 314-1 Some other disorders of carbohydrate metabolism

Disorder	Metabolic defect	Manifestations
Hereditary fructose intolerance	Deficiency of fructose-l-phosphate aldolase leads to accumulation of fructose-1-PO_4 in tissues.	Liver disease, renal tubular damage, and hypoglycemia.
Fructose 1,6-diphosphatase deficiency	Deficiency of the enzyme prevents gluconeogenesis from its normal precursors, lactate, glycerol, and alanine. Thus, maintenance of blood sugar is dependent upon exogenous glucose.	Lactic acidosis leads to hyperventilation, somnolence, and coma, usually with hypoglycemia and ketosis.

Classic galactosemia must be considered when one or more of the clinical features described above are found. If the patient is ingesting milk, reducing sugar is present in the urine but gives a negative glucose oxidase reaction (i.e., is not glucose) and is identified as galactose by other techniques, such as chromatography. If the child is vomiting, has a poor food intake, or is on intravenous glucose feedings, galactose may not be present in the urine. The definitive diagnosis is made by demonstrating a lack or deficiency of red cell GALT by one of several techniques. The disease can also be diagnosed prenatally by enzyme studies on culture amniocentesis cells or by demonstrating increased galactitol in amniotic fluid.

In the neonatal period galactosemia needs to be differentiated from primary liver disease. With liver damage, galactose removal from the blood is impaired, and elevated blood galactose levels and galactosuria may be present. However, GALT levels are normal in patients with liver damage.

TREATMENT The treatment of galactosemia consists of the removal of galactose-containing foods from the diet, especially milk. Milk substitutes such as Nutramigen are often used. Although soybean preparations contain polysaccharide-bound galactose, they appear to be well tolerated because the bound galactose is not readily liberated. In general, the red cell levels of galactose 1-phosphate are not increased in affected infants fed soybean formulas.

The institution of a galactose-free diet usually leads to a dramatic improvement in all clinical features except for mental retardation. Patients should be kept on galactose-free diets indefinitely or at least until they have attained adequate physical and neurologic development.

OTHER DISORDERS OF CARBOHYDRATE METABOLISM Features of hereditary fructose intolerance and fructose 1,6-diphosphatase deficiency, two autosomal recessive disorders of fructose metabolism that lead to hypoglycemia, are summarized in Table 314-1 (also see Chaps. 313 and 329).

REFERENCES

ALLEN TJ et al: Evidence of galactosemia in utero. Lancet 1:603, 1980

BURMAN D et al (eds): *Inborn Errors of Carbohydrate Metabolism*. Lancaster, MTP Press, 1979

GITZELMANN R et al: Galactose metabolism in a patient with hereditary galactokinase deficiency. Eur J Clin Invest 4:79, 1974

——— et al: Essential fructosuria, heredity fructose intolerance, and fructose 1,6-diphosphatase deficiency, in *The Metabolic Basis of Inherited Disease*, 5th ed, JB Stanbury et al (eds). New York, McGraw-Hill, 1983, p 118

SCHWARTZ HP et al: Galactose intolerance in individuals with double heterozygosity for Duarte variant and galactosemia. J Pediatr 100:704, 1982

SEGAL S: Disorders of galactose metabolism, in *The Metabolic Basis of Inherited Disease*, 5th ed, JB Stanbury et al (eds). New York, McGraw-Hill, 1982, p 167

315 THE HYPERLIPOPROTEINEMIAS AND OTHER DISORDERS OF LIPID METABOLISM

MICHAEL S. BROWN / JOSEPH L. GOLDSTEIN

The *hyperlipoproteinemias* are disturbances of lipid transport that result from accelerated synthesis or retarded degradation of lipoproteins that transport cholesterol and triglycerides through plasma. Elevated plasma lipoprotein levels are important clinically because they can cause two life-threatening diseases: atherosclerosis and pancreatitis. A reduction in plasma lipoprotein-cholesterol levels, achieved by diet and drugs, reduces the risk of myocardial infarction in subjects with hyperlipoproteinemia. Some hyperlipoproteinemias are the direct result of *primary* defects in the synthesis or degradation of lipoprotein particles. Other hyperlipoproteinemias are *secondary*, that is, the elevated plasma lipoprotein level occurs as part of a constellation of abnormalities caused by an underlying disorder in a related metabolic system, such as thyroid hormone deficiency or insulin deficiency. The primary hyperlipoproteinemias can be divided into two broad categories: (1) *single-gene disorders* that are transmitted by simple dominant or recessive mechanisms and (2) *multifactorial disorders* with complex inheritance patterns in which multiple variant genes, each having a subtle effect, interact with environmental factors to produce varying degrees of hyperlipoproteinemia in members of a family.

ROLE OF LIPOPROTEINS IN LIPID TRANSPORT The lipoproteins are globular particles of high molecular weight that transport nonpolar lipids (primarily *triglycerides* and *cholesteryl esters*) through the plasma. A general model for the structure of a lipoprotein particle is shown in Fig. 315-1. Each lipoprotein particle contains a nonpolar *core,* in which many molecules of hydrophobic lipid are packed to form an oil droplet. This hydrophobic core, which accounts for most of the mass of the particle, consists of triglycerides and cholesteryl esters in varying proportions. Surrounding the core is a polar *surface coat* of phospholipids that stabilize the lipoprotein particle so that it can remain in solution in the plasma. In addition to phospholipids, the polar coat contains small amounts of unesterified cholesterol. Each lipoprotein particle also contains specific proteins (termed *apoproteins*) that are exposed at the surface. The apoproteins bind to specific enzymes or transport proteins on cell membranes, thus directing the lipoprotein to its sites of metabolism.

Table 315-1 describes the characteristics of the five major classes of lipoproteins that normally circulate in human plasma. These lipoprotein classes differ in the composition of the nonpolar lipids in the core; in the composition of the apoproteins; and in density, size, and electrophoretic mobility.

Lipid transport: The exogenous pathway Figure 315-2 shows the pathways by which lipoproteins transport lipids in plasma. The largest amounts of lipoproteins are involved in the transport of dietary fat, which amounts to more than 100 g triglyceride and about 1 g cholesterol per day. Within intestinal epithelial cells, dietary triglycerides and cholesterol are incorporated into large lipoprotein particles called *chylomicrons*. The chylomicrons are secreted into the intestinal lymph and pass into the general circulation for transport to the capillaries of adipose tissue and skeletal muscle, where they adhere to binding sites on the capillary walls. While bound to these endothelial surfaces, the chylomicrons are exposed to the enzyme *lipoprotein lipase*. The chylomicrons contain an apoprotein, apoprotein CII, that activates the lipase, liberating free fatty acids and monoglycerides (Fig. 315-3). The fatty acids pass through the endothelial cells and enter the underlying adipocytes or muscle cells, where they are either reesterified to triglycerides or oxidized.

After the core triglycerides have been removed, the remainder of the chylomicron dissociates from the capillary endothelium and

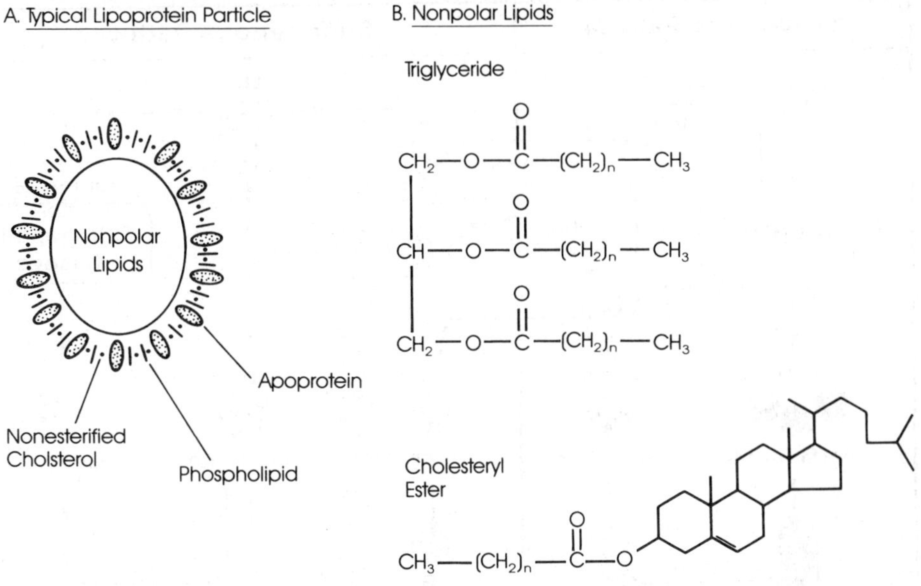

FIGURE 315-1 *A. Diagrammatic representation of the structure of a typical plasma lipoprotein particle. The core of the spherical lipoprotein particle is composed of two nonpolar lipids, triglyceride and cholesteryl ester, which are present in different lipoproteins in varying amounts. The nonpolar core is surrounded by a surface coat composed primarily of phospholipids. Apoproteins are exposed at the surface and extend into the core. Variable amounts of unesterified cholesterol are interdigitated with the phospholipids of the surface coat. The qualitative composition of each of the five major classes of lipoprotein particles in human plasma is summarized in Table 315-1. B. Structures of the two nonpolar lipids, triglyceride and cholesteryl ester. In order for these nonpolar lipids to be assimilated into tissues, the ester bonds between the fatty acids and either glycerol (triglycerides) or cholesterol (cholesteryl esters) must be broken by lipoprotein lipase and the lysosomal cholesterol esterase, respectively.*

reenters the circulation. It has now been transformed into a particle that is relatively poor in triglyceride and enriched in cholesteryl esters. It has also undergone an exchange of apoproteins with other plasma lipoproteins. The net result is the conversion of the chylomicron to a *chylomicron remnant particle,* enriched in cholesteryl esters and apoproteins B48 and E. This remnant travels to the liver, where it is taken up with great efficiency. This uptake is mediated by the binding of apoprotein E to specific receptors, called *chylomicron remnant receptors,* on the surface of the hepatocytes. The surface-bound remnants are taken into the cell and degraded within lysosomes by a process called receptor-mediated endocytosis (Fig. 315-3). The overall result of the chylomicron transport process is to deliver dietary triglyceride to adipose tissue and cholesterol to the liver.

Some of the cholesterol that reaches the liver is converted to bile acids, which are excreted into the intestine to act as detergents and facilitate the absorption of dietary fat. In addition, some cholesterol is excreted into the bile without metabolism to bile acids. The liver also distributes cholesterol to other tissues by the endogenous pathway, which is discussed below.

Lipid transport: The endogenous pathway Triglyceride synthesis in the liver is enhanced when the diet contains excess carbohydrates. The liver converts the carbohydrate to fatty acids, esterifies the fatty acids with glycerol to form triglycerides, and secretes the triglyceride into the bloodstream in the core of *very low density lipoprotein (VLDL).* The VLDL particles are relatively large, carry 5 to 10 times more triglycerides than cholesteryl esters, and contain a form of apoprotein B, designated B100, that differs from the apoprotein B48 of chylomicrons (Table 315-1).

The VLDL particles are transported to tissue capillaries, where they interact with the same lipoprotein lipase enzyme that catabolizes chylomicrons. The core triglycerides of the VLDL are hydrolyzed, and the fatty acids are used for triglyceride synthesis within adipose tissue. The remnants generated from the action of lipoprotein-lipase on VLDL are designated *intermediate-density lipoprotein (IDL).* A portion of the IDL particles are catabolized by the liver through binding to receptors called *low-density lipoprotein (LDL) receptors,* which are distinct from the chylomicron remnant receptors. The remaining IDL remain in plasma, where they undergo a further transformation in which nearly all the residual triglycerides are removed. During this conversion, all the apoproteins are removed from the particle with the exception of apoprotein B100. The result is the transformation of the IDL particle into cholesterol-rich LDL. The core of LDL is composed almost entirely of cholesteryl esters, and the surface coat contains only one apoprotein, apoprotein B100. In humans a relatively high fraction of IDL escapes hepatic uptake, and consequently humans have relatively high circulating levels of LDL. Indeed, about three-fourths of the total cholesterol in normal human plasma is contained within LDL particles.

One function of LDL is to supply cholesterol to a variety of extrahepatic parenchymal cells, such as adrenal cortical cells, lymphocytes, muscle cells, and renal cells. These cells have *LDL receptors* localized on the cell surface. LDL that binds to this receptor is taken up by receptor-mediated endocytosis and digested by lysosomes within the cells (Fig. 315-3). The cholesteryl esters of LDL are hydrolyzed by a lysosomal cholesteryl esterase (acid lipase), and the liberated cholesterol is used both for membrane synthesis and as a precursor for steroid hormone synthesis. Like extrahepatic tissues, the liver also has abundant LDL receptors; it uses the LDL-cholesterol for synthesis of bile acids and for generation of free cholesterol, which is secreted into the bile. In humans 70 to 80 percent of LDL is removed from the plasma each day by the LDL receptor pathway. The remainder is degraded by a scavenger cell system in phagocytic cells in the reticuloendothelial system. In contrast to the receptor-mediated pathway for LDL degradation, the scavenger cell pathway is thought to function solely to degrade LDL when the lipoprotein

TABLE 315-1 Characteristics of the major classes of lipoproteins in human plasma

Lipoprotein class	Major lipids	Apoproteins	Density, g/mL	Diameter, Å	Electrophoretic mobility
Chylomicrons and remnants	Dietary triglycerides	AI, AII, B48, CI, CII, CIII, E	<1.006	800–5000	Remains at origin
VLDL	Endogenous triglycerides	B48, CI, CII, CIII, E	<1.006	300–800	Pre-β
IDL	Cholesteryl esters, triglycerides	B100, CIII, E	<1.019	250–350	Slow pre-β
LDL	Cholesteryl esters	B100	1.019–1.063	180–280	β
HDL	Cholesteryl esters	AI, AII	1.063–1.210	50–120	α

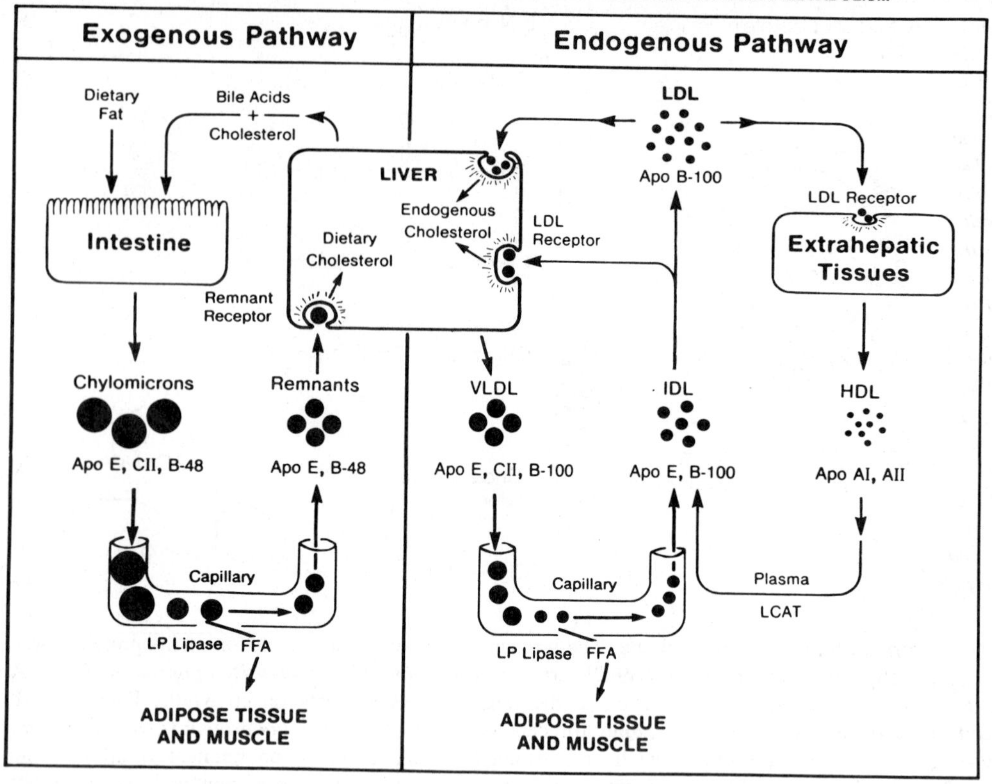

FIGURE 315-2 *Model for plasma triglyceride and cholesterol transport in humans. The details of this model are described in the text. VLDL, very low density lipoprotein; IDL, intermediate-density lipoprotein; LDL, low-density lipoprotein; HDL, high-density lipoprotein; LCAT, lecithin:cholesterol acyltransferase; LP lipase, lipoprotein lipase; FFA, free fatty acids. The major apoprotein for each class of lipoproteins is shown. Other apoproteins are also present, and these are listed in Table 315-1.*

reaches high concentrations in plasma rather than to supply cholesterol to cells.

As the membranes of parenchymal and scavenger cells undergo turnover and as cells die and are renewed, unesterified cholesterol is released into plasma, where it binds initially to *high-density lipoprotein* (*HDL*). This unesterified cholesterol is then coupled to a fatty acid in an esterification reaction catalyzed by the plasma enzyme *lecithin:cholesterol acyltransferase* (*LCAT*). The cholesteryl esters that are formed on the surface of HDL are transferred to VLDL and eventually appear in LDL. This establishes a cycle by which LDL delivers cholesterol to extrahepatic cells and by which cholesterol is returned to LDL from extrahepatic cells via HDL. Most of the cholesterol released from extrahepatic tissues is transported to the liver for excretion in the bile.

DIAGNOSIS OF HYPERLIPOPROTEINEMIA A variety of diseases cause elevations in the concentrations of one or more lipoprotein classes in plasma. In general, these abnormalities are detected by the finding of an elevated concentration of triglycerides or cholesterol in fasting plasma, a condition called *hyperlipidemia*. The value for plasma cholesterol represents the total cholesterol, which includes both cholesteryl esters and unesterified cholesterol. The plasma cholesterol and triglyceride levels provide information regarding the nature of the lipoprotein particle that is increased. An isolated elevation in plasma triglycerides indicates that the concentrations of chylomicrons or VLDL are increased. On the other hand, an isolated elevation of plasma cholesterol nearly always indicates that the concentration of LDL is increased. Frequently, both triglycerides and cholesterol are elevated. Such a combined abnormality may be produced by a marked elevation in chylomicrons or VLDL, in which case the ratio of triglyceride to cholesterol in plasma will be greater than 5:1. Alternatively, there may be an elevation of both VLDL and LDL, in which case the triglyceride/cholesterol ratio in plasma is usually less than 5:1.

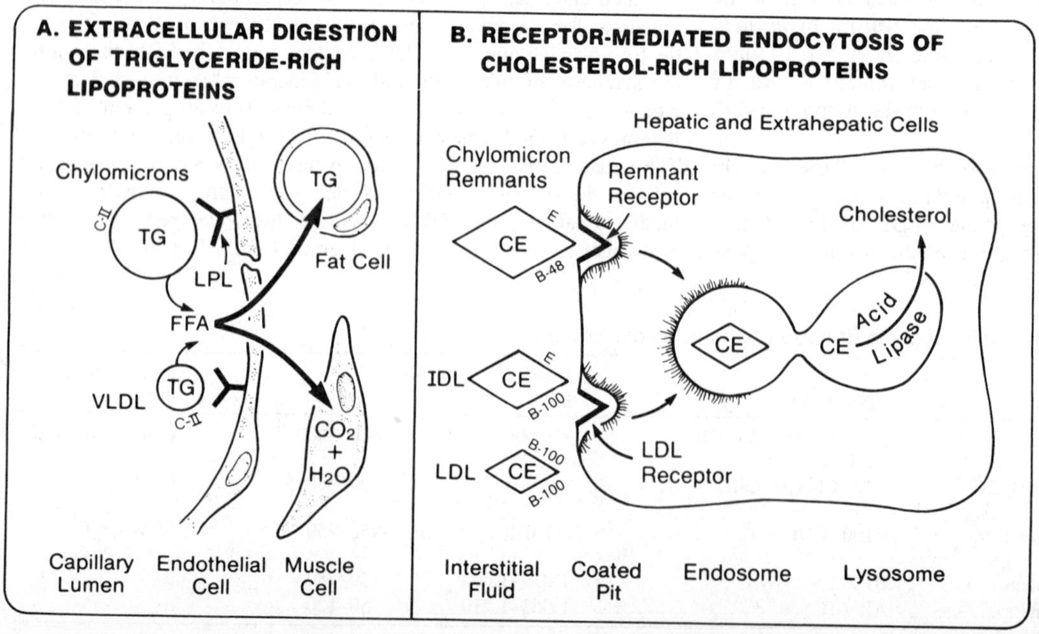

FIGURE 315-3 *Comparison of the mechanisms by which triglyceride-rich lipoproteins and cholesterol-rich lipoproteins deliver their core lipids to target tissues. Triglycerides are hydrolyzed by an extracellular enzyme (LPL) that is attached to endothelial cells and operates at the endothelial surface. Cholesteryl esters are hydrolyzed by an intracellular enzyme, acid lipase, that is located in lysosomes and cleaves the esters that enter cells via receptor-mediated endocytosis. TG, triglycerides; LPL, lipoprotein lipase; VLDL, very low density lipoproteins; CE, cholesteryl esters; IDL, intermediate-density lipoproteins; LDL, low-density lipoproteins; FFA, free fatty acid. The apoproteins responsible for the interactions (CII, B, and E) are indicated.*

TABLE 315-2 Patterns of lipoprotein elevation in plasma (lipoprotein types)

Lipoprotein pattern	Major elevation in plasma: Lipoprotein	Lipid
Type 1	Chylomicrons	Triglycerides
Type 2a	LDL	Cholesterol
Type 2b	LDL and VLDL	Cholesterol and triglycerides
Type 3	Remnants	Triglycerides and cholesterol
Type 4	VLDL	Triglycerides
Type 5	VLDL and chylomicrons	Triglycerides and cholesterol

The definition of hyperlipoproteinemia is arbitrary because plasma lipid and lipoprotein levels exhibit a bell-shaped distribution in the population, without clear separation between normal and abnormal values. Since lipoprotein concentrations are influenced by diet and other environmental factors, standards must be established for the population under consideration. Usually, arbitrary statistical limits of normal concentrations are selected, based on the examination of a large number of healthy-appearing subjects of different ages. The usual cut-off limit is the upper 5 to 10 percent of values (i.e., the 90th to 95th percentile values). However, analysis of blood lipid levels in individuals from industrialized and more agrarian cultures indicates that lipid and lipoprotein concentrations that are "normal" in a statistical sense are not necessarily healthy. As a working rule, significant hyperlipoproteinemia is considered to be present in any individual below the age of 20 whose total plasma cholesterol level exceeds 190 mg/dL or whose triglyceride level exceeds 140 mg/dL. In individuals above the age of 20, significant hyperlipoproteinemia exists whenever the plasma cholesterol level exceeds 220 mg/dL or the triglyceride level exceeds 200 mg/dL.

The various combinations of elevated lipoproteins that occur in disease states have been divided into six lipoprotein types or patterns (Table 315-2). Most of the lipoprotein types can be caused by several different genetic diseases (Table 315-3); conversely, some genetic diseases can produce more than one lipoprotein type. In addition, each of the abnormal lipoprotein types can occur as a secondary consequence of another metabolic disease (Table 315-4). Hence, the lipoprotein type must be considered a shorthand notation to describe an abnormal lipoprotein pattern in plasma and not a designation of a specific disease.

Ordinarily, the simple measurement of plasma lipid levels, coupled with a clinical assessment, is sufficient to classify the type of lipoprotein abnormality present (Table 315-2). Occasionally, paper electrophoresis of the plasma is useful either when an elevation in remnant particles is suspected (type 3 lipoprotein pattern giving a "broad beta" band on electrophoresis) or when chylomicronemia is a possibility (type 1 pattern). On occasion, HDL levels are measured, since high levels of this lipoprotein class are statistically associated with a decreased risk of myocardial infarction (see Chap. 195). The level of HDL can be estimated in clinical laboratories using standardized lipoprotein separation techniques, but the value of such measurement for predicting the occurrence of myocardial infarction in the individual patient has not been established.

PRIMARY HYPERLIPOPROTEINEMIAS RESULTING FROM SINGLE-GENE MUTATIONS

FAMILIAL LIPOPROTEIN LIPASE DEFICIENCY This rare autosomal recessive disorder is attributable to the absence or marked reduction in the activity of the enzyme lipoprotein lipase. This deficiency leads to a metabolic block in the metabolism of chylomicrons, causing these lipoproteins to accumulate to massive levels in plasma.

Clinical features The disease usually presents in infancy or childhood with recurrent attacks of abdominal pain. The pain is caused by pancreatitis occurring as a consequence of the massive elevation of chylomicrons in plasma. Affected individuals intermittently develop eruptive xanthomas, small yellowish papules, frequently surrounded by an erythematous base, that appear predominantly on the buttocks and other pressure-sensitive surfaces. The xanthomas are caused by the deposition of large amounts of chylomicron triglycerides in cutaneous histiocytes. Triglycerides are also deposited in phagocytes of the reticuloendothelial system, producing hepatomegaly, splenomegaly, and foam cell infiltration of the bone marrow. When the level of chylomicrons in the blood is massively elevated (i.e., plasma triglyceride level greater than 2000 mg/dL), the blood appears pale and creamy and is said to be *lipemic*. When viewed with the ophthalmoscope, the retina is pale, and the retinal vessels are white, producing the appearance of lipemia retinalis. Despite the massive elevation of plasma triglycerides, accelerated atherosclerosis does not occur.

Pathogenesis Affected individuals are homozygous for a mutation that prevents normal expression of lipoprotein lipase activity. The primary genetic defect appears to involve the structure of the enzyme itself; the activator of lipoprotein lipase, apoprotein CII, is present in normal amounts. The parents are obligate heterozygotes for the lipoprotein lipase defect, but they are clinically normal. As a result of the deficiency of lipoprotein lipase in homozygotes, chylomicrons cannot be metabolized normally, and the level of chylomicrons in

TABLE 315-3 Characteristics of the primary hyperlipoproteinemias resulting from single-gene mutations

Genetic disorder	Primary biochemical defect	Plasma lipoprotein elevation	Lipoprotein pattern	Typical clinical findings: Xanthomas	Pancreatitis	Premature atherosclerosis	Lipoprotein pattern in affected relatives
Familial lipoprotein lipase deficiency	Deficiency of lipoprotein lipase	Chylomicrons	1	Eruptive	+		1
Familial apoprotein CII deficiency	Deficiency of apoprotein CII	Chylomicrons and VLDL	1 or 5		+		1 or 5
Familial type 3 hyperlipoproteinemia	Abnormal apoprotein E of VLDL	Chylomicrons and IDL	3	Xanthelasma; tuberous; palmar creases		+	3, 2a, 2b, or 4
Familial hypercholesterolemia	Deficiency of LDL receptor	LDL	2a (rarely 2b)	Xanthelasma; tendon		+	2a (rarely 2b)
Familial hypertriglyceridemia	Unknown	VLDL (rarely chylomicrons)	4 (rarely 5)	(Eruptive)	(+)	+	4 (rarely 5)
Multiple lipoprotein-type hyperlipidemia (familial combined hyperlipidemia)	Unknown	LDL and VLDL	2a, 2b, or 4 (rarely 5)			+	2a, 2b, or 4 (rarely 5)

TABLE 315-4 Clinical disorders associated with secondary hyperlipoproteinemia

Underlying disorder	Plasma lipoprotein elevation: Chylomicrons	IDL	VLDL	LDL	Lipoprotein type	Proposed mechanism for hyperlipoproteinemia	Associated abnormality of carbohydrate metabolism
ENDOCRINE AND METABOLIC							
Diabetes mellitus	+		+ + +		4 (rarely 5)	Increased secretion of VLDL Decreased catabolism of VLDL and chylomicrons due to reduced lipoprotein lipase activity	Insulin deficiency or resistance
von Gierke's disease (glycogen storage disease, type I)	+		+ + +		4 (rarely 5)	Increased secretion of VLDL Decreased catabolism of VLDL and chylomicrons due to reduced lipoprotein lipase activity	Hypoglycemia with decreased insulin secretion
Lipodystrophies (congenital and acquired forms)			+ +		4	Increased secretion of VLDL	Insulin resistance
Cushing's syndrome			+	+ +	2a or 2b	Increased secretion of VLDL with conversion to LDL	Insulin resistance
Sexual ateliotic dwarfism (isolated growth hormone deficiency)			+ +	+ +	2b	Increased secretion of VLDL with conversion to LDL	Insulin deficiency or resistance
Acromegaly			+		4	Increased secretion of VLDL	Insulin resistance
Hypothyroidism		+		+ + +	2a (rarely 3)	Decreased catabolism of VLDL and IDL	
Anorexia nervosa				+ +	2a	Reduced biliary excretion of cholesterol and bile acids	
Werner's syndrome				+ +	2a	Unknown	Insulin resistance
Acute intermittent porphyria				+ +	2a	Unknown	
DRUG-INDUCED							
Alcohol	+		+ + +		4 (rarely 5)	Increased secretion of VLDL in individuals genetically predisposed to hypertriglyceridemia	
Oral contraceptives	+		+ + +		4 (rarely 5)	Increased secretion of VLDL in individuals genetically predisposed to hypertriglyceridemia	Insulin resistance
Glucocorticoids			+	+ +	2a or 2b	Increased secretion of VLDL with conversion to LDL	Insulin resistance

the blood rises to high levels after a fat meal. In normal individuals chylomicrons disappear from the blood after a 12-h fast. However, in affected patients high levels of chylomicrons are found in the plasma even after several days of fasting or ingestion of a fat-free diet.

The circulating chylomicrons inflame the pancreas when they pass through its capillaries. Within the capillary lumen in the pancreas, chylomicrons are exposed to small amounts of pancreatic lipase that leaks from the tissue. Partial hydrolysis of the triglycerides and phospholipids of the chylomicron produces toxic products, including fatty acids and lysolecithin, that break down tissue membranes, produce further leakage of lipase from the pancreatic acinar cells, and eventually cause fulminant pancreatitis.

Diagnosis The diagnosis of familial lipoprotein lipase deficiency is suggested by the finding of lipemic plasma in a young individual who has been fasting for at least 12 h. This lipemic plasma, when collected in the presence of EDTA, has a characteristic appearance after it has incubated overnight in a refrigerator at 4°C. A white layer of cream (which consists of chylomicrons) appears at the top of the tube. The layer beneath the cream is clear. The diagnosis of familial lipoprotein lipase deficiency is supported by the finding of a type 1 pattern on lipoprotein electrophoresis. It is confirmed by the demonstration that lipoprotein lipase levels in plasma fail to increase following the infusion of heparin. In normal individuals, intravenous heparin releases lipoprotein lipase from its binding sites within the capillary endothelium, and increased amounts of enzyme can then be assayed in the plasma. Gel electrophoresis of VLDL apoproteins in patients with lipoprotein lipase deficiency shows a normal amount of activator apoprotein CII, thus distinguishing these patients from those with the related disorder, familial apoprotein CII deficiency (see below).

Treatment The symptoms and signs of the disease recede when the patient is placed on a fat-free diet. Every attempt should be made to maintain the fasting plasma triglyceride level below 1000 mg/dL to prevent pancreatitis. It has been found empirically that the chronic fat intake in affected adults must be less than 20 g per day to prevent symptomatic hyperlipemia. Since medium-chain triglycerides are not incorporated into chylomicrons, they have been employed to help achieve normal caloric intake. The diet should be supplemented with fat-soluble vitamins.

TABLE 315-4 Clinical disorders associated with secondary hyperlipoproteinemia *(continued)*

Underlying disorder	Plasma lipoprotein elevation: Chylomicrons	IDL	VLDL	LDL	Lipoprotein type	Proposed mechanism for hyperlipoproteinemia	Associated abnormality of carbohydrate metabolism
RENAL							
Uremia			+ + +		4	Decreased catabolism of VLDL due to reduced lipoprotein lipase activity	Insulin resistance
Nephrotic syndrome			+ +	+ + +	2a or 2b	Increased secretion of VLDL Direct secretion of LDL from liver Decreased catabolism of VLDL and LDL	
HEPATIC							
Primary biliary cirrhosis and extrahepatic biliary obstruction					↑ Cholesterol ↑ Phospholipids ↑ Lipoprotein X	Diversion of biliary cholesterol and phospholipids into bloodstream	
Acute hepatitis (nonfulminant)			+ + +		4	Decreased hepatic secretion of lecithin: cholesterol acyltransferase (LCAT)	
Hepatoma				+ +	2a	Lack of feedback inhibition of hepatic cholesterol synthesis by dietary cholesterol	
IMMUNOLOGIC							
Systemic lupus erythematosis	+ +				1	Presence of IgG or IgM that binds heparin, thereby decreasing activity of lipoprotein lipase	
Monoclonal gammopathies (myeloma, macroglobulinemia, lymphoma)	+ +	+ +	+ +		3 or 4	Presence of IgG or IgM that forms immune complex with chylomicron remnants and/or VLDL, thereby decreasing their catabolism	
STRESS-INDUCED							
Emotional stress, acute myocardial infarction, extensive burns, acute gram-negative sepsis			+ +		4	Increased secretion and decreased catabolism of VLDL	

FAMILIAL APOPROTEIN CII DEFICIENCY This rare autosomal recessive disorder is due to the absence of apoprotein CII, an essential cofactor for lipoprotein lipase. Deficiency of this peptide creates a functional lipoprotein lipase deficiency, thus producing a syndrome that is similar but not identical to familial lipoprotein lipase deficiency (see above). Because of the apoprotein CII deficiency, lipoprotein lipase is not activated, and its two substrate lipoproteins, chylomicrons and VLDL, accumulate in the blood, thus causing hypertriglyceridemia (type 1 or type 5 lipoprotein pattern). The disorder is diagnosed in children or adults on the basis of recurrent attacks of pancreatitis or by milky plasma detected by chance. The diagnosis is made by showing an absence of apoprotein CII on gel electrophoresis of VLDL apoproteins. Transfusion of normal plasma (which contains abundant apoprotein CII) into the patient is followed by a dramatic fall in plasma triglyceride levels. Heterozygotes, who have 50 percent reduction in apoprotein CII levels, may exhibit slightly elevated triglyceride concentrations but do not have pancreatitis. Treatment involves use of a fat-restricted diet throughout life. In case of severe pancreatitis, transfusion of one or two units of normal plasma is helpful. As compared with patients with familial lipoprotein lipase deficiency, subjects with homozygous apoprotein CII deficiency are generally detected at a later age, accumulate more VLDL in their plasma, and rarely show cutaneous eruptive xanthomas. The reason for these clinical differences is not known.

FAMILIAL TYPE 3 HYPERLIPOPROTEINEMIA This is an inherited disorder in which the plasma concentrations of both cholesterol and triglycerides are elevated owing to the accumulation in plasma of remnant-like particles derived from the partial catabolism of VLDL. Also called familial dysbetalipoproteinemia, the disorder is transmitted by a single-gene mechanism, but its expression appears to require the presence of contributory environmental and/or genetic factors (discussed below).

Clinical features Affected individuals characteristically do not manifest hyperlipidemia or any clinical feature of the disease until after age 20. A unique clinical feature is the occurrence of two types of cutaneous xanthomas: xanthoma striata palmaris, which appear as orange or yellow discolorations of the palmar and digital creases, and tuberous or tuberoeruptive xanthomas, which are bulbous cutaneous xanthomas that may vary from pea to lemon size. The tuberous xanthomas are characteristically located over the elbows and knees. Xanthelasmas of the eyelids also occur but are not unique to this disorder (see "Familial Hypercholesterolemia" below).

Severe and fulminant atherosclerosis involves the coronary arteries, the internal carotids, and the abdominal aorta and its branches. The sequelae include premature myocardial infarctions, strokes, intermittent claudication, and gangrene of the lower extremities. Patients who develop clinical manifestations of this disorder often have hypothyroidism, obesity, or diabetes mellitus as aggravating factors.

Pathogenesis The hyperlipidemia is caused by the accumulation of large lipoprotein particles that contain both triglycerides and cholesteryl esters. These particles consist of chylomicron remnants produced from the catabolism of chylomicrons and IDL produced from the catabolism of VLDL through the action of lipoprotein lipase. In normal subjects, chylomicron remnant particles are rapidly taken up by the liver, and hence they are barely detectable in plasma. A portion of the IDL is also taken up by the liver while the rest is converted to LDL. In patients with type 3 hyperlipoproteinemia the uptake of IDL and chylomicron remnants by the liver is blocked, and these lipoproteins accumulate to high levels in plasma and tissues, producing xanthomas and atherosclerosis.

The mutation responsible for this disease involves the gene that encodes the structure of apoprotein E, a protein normally found in IDL and chylomicron remnants. This protein binds with very high affinity to both the chylomicron remnant receptor and the LDL receptor. Apoprotein E thus mediates the rapid uptake for both chylomicron remnants and IDL by the liver. The gene for apoprotein E is polymorphic in the population. There are three common alleles, designated E^2, E^3, and E^4, with approximate frequencies of 0.12, 0.75, and 0.13 in the population. Each allele specifies a distinctive form of apoprotein E that can be detected by isoelectric focusing. The three alleles create six genotypes: E^2/E^2, E^3/E^3, E^4/E^4, E^2/E^3, E^2/E^4, and E^3/E^4. Type 3 hyperlipoproteinemia occurs only in individuals who are homozygous for the E^2 allele (genotype, E^2/E^2). The protein produced by the E^2 allele is defective in its ability to bind to the liver receptors that mediate uptake of chylomicron remnants and IDL, as a result of which these particles accumulate in plasma.

The frequency of the E^2/E^2 genotype in the population is about 1 in 100. Yet the frequency of type 3 hyperlipoproteinemia is only about 1 in 10,000. Thus, only 1 percent of the individuals having genotype E^2/E^2 have symptomatic disease. It seems that most homozygotes for the E^2 allele are somehow able to compensate for the abnormal apoprotein E, because other apoproteins such as apoproteins B48 and B100 can also mediate binding to liver receptors, albeit less efficiently than apoprotein E. Familial type 3 hyperlipoproteinemia occurs only in those individuals who are homozygous for the E^2 allele and who are also unable to compensate for the abnormal function of the E protein. The inability to compensate may be caused by the independent inheritance of another defect in lipoprotein metabolism, such as familial hypercholesterolemia or multiple lipoprotein–type hyperlipoproteinemia (see below). When an individual is a heterozygote for one of these dominant diseases and is also homozygous for the E^2 allele, he or she expresses the syndrome of type 3 hyperlipoproteinemia. The expression of hyperlipoproteinemia is also brought out when an individual of genotype E^2/E^2 develops hypothyroidism, diabetes mellitus, or obesity. It should be emphasized that heterozygotes for the E^2 allele never show the clinical syndrome of familial type 3 hyperlipoproteinemia.

Diagnosis The diagnosis is suggested by the finding of palmar or tuberous xanthomas in a patient with elevated plasma levels of both cholesterol and triglyceride. Approximately 80 percent of symptomatic patients exhibit these xanthomas. The diagnosis is also suggested when a moderate elevation in the plasma concentration of both cholesterol and triglyceride occurs in such a way that the absolute concentrations of cholesterol and triglyceride are nearly equal (e.g., the plasma cholesterol and triglyceride level are both about 300 mg/dL). However, this finding does not always hold true and becomes especially unreliable when the disease is in severe exacerbation, in which case the plasma triglyceride tends to rise higher than the cholesterol.

The diagnosis is supported by the finding of a so-called broad beta band on lipoprotein electrophoresis (type 3 pattern). This appearance results from the presence of chylomicron remnants and IDL. The diagnosis can be established in specialized laboratories by two procedures. First, the plasma can be subjected to ultracentrifugation, and the chemical composition of the VLDL fraction can be measured. In affected patients, the VLDL fraction contains IDL and chylomicron remnants that have a relatively high ratio of cholesterol to triglyceride. Second, the diagnosis can be confirmed by the finding of homozygosity for the E^2 allele on isoelectric focusing of the proteins extracted from the remnant particles.

Treatment A vigorous search for occult hypothyroidism should be made, including measurement of plasma thyroid stimulating hormone (TSH) levels. If hypothyroidism exists, levothyroxine should be instituted. Patients who have hypothyroidism show a dramatic lowering of lipid levels with treatment. In addition, attempts should be made to control obesity and diabetes mellitus through diet and insulin treatment. If these measures are not successful, patients with type 3 hyperlipoproteinemia should be treated with clofibrate. Affected patients usually show a dramatic and sustained reduction in plasma lipid levels when treated with this drug.

FAMILIAL HYPERCHOLESTEROLEMIA This common autosomal dominant disorder affects approximately 1 in every 500 persons. It is caused by a mutation in the gene for the LDL receptor. Heterozygotes manifest a two- to threefold elevation in the concentration of total plasma cholesterol which is attributable to an elevation in the level of LDL. Patients with two mutant LDL receptor genes (called familial hypercholesterolemia homozygotes) have six- to eightfold elevations in plasma LDL-cholesterol levels.

Clinical features Heterozygotes with familial hypercholesterolemia can be diagnosed at birth because their umbilical cord blood contains a two- to threefold increase in the concentration of LDL and hence a similar increase in total cholesterol. The elevated levels of plasma LDL persist throughout life, but symptoms typically do not develop until the third or fourth decade. The most important feature is the occurrence of premature and accelerated coronary atherosclerosis. Myocardial infarctions begin to occur in affected men in the third decade and peak in the fourth and fifth decades. By age 60, approximately 85 percent have experienced a myocardial infarction. In women the incidence of myocardial infarction is also increased, but the mean age of onset is delayed 10 years as compared with men. Heterozygotes for this disorder constitute about 5 percent of all patients who have a myocardial infarction.

Xanthomas of the tendons constitute the second major clinical manifestation of the heterozygous state. These xanthomas are nodular swellings that typically involve the Achilles and other tendons about the knee, elbow, and dorsum of the hand. They are formed by the deposition of LDL-derived cholesteryl esters in tissue macrophages. The macrophages are swollen with lipid droplets and form foam cells. Cholesterol is also deposited in the soft tissue of the eyelid, producing xanthelasma, and within the cornea, producing arcus corneae. Whereas tendon xanthomas are essentially diagnostic of familial hypercholesterolemia, xanthelasma and arcus corneae also occur in many adults with normal plasma lipid levels. The incidence of tendon xanthomas in familial hypercholesterolemia increases with age, and up to 75 percent of heterozygotes display this sign. The absence of tendon xanthomas does not rule out familial hypercholesterolemia.

Approximately 1 in 1 million persons in the general population inherits two copies of the familial hypercholesterolemia gene and is a homozygote for the disorder. These individuals have marked elevations in the plasma level of LDL from birth. A unique type of planar cutaneous xanthoma is often present at birth and always develops within the first 6 years of life. These xanthomas are raised, yellow, plaque-like lesions at points of cutaneous trauma, such as the knees, elbows, and buttocks. Xanthomas are almost always present in the interdigital webs of the hands, particularly between the thumb and index finger. Tendon xanthomas, arcus corneae, and xanthelasma are also characteristic. Coronary artery atherosclerosis frequently has its clinical onset before age 10, and myocardial infarction has been reported as early as 18 months of age. In addition, cholesterol deposition in the aortic valve may produce symptomatic aortic stenosis. Homozygotes usually succumb to the complications of myocardial infarction before age 20.

Obesity and diabetes mellitus do not occur with increased frequency in familial hypercholesterolemia. A slender body habitus is the rule.

Pathogenesis The primary defect resides in the gene for the LDL receptor. Studies of cultured cells suggest that at least 12 mutant alleles occur at this locus. These mutant alleles can be grouped into three classes. The most common, designated receptor-negative, specifies a gene product that is nonfunctional. The second most frequent mutant, designated receptor-defective, produces a receptor that has 1 to 10 percent of normal LDL binding activity. The third type, designated internalization-defective, produces a receptor that binds LDL normally but is unable to transport the receptor-bound lipoprotein into the cell. This rare allele produces the so-called internalization defect.

Phenotypic homozygotes possess two mutant alleles at the LDL receptor locus, and hence their cells show a total or near-total inability to bind or take up LDL. Heterozygotes have one normal allele and one mutant allele at the LDL receptor locus, and hence their cells are able to bind and take up LDL at approximately half the normal rate.

Because of the reduction in LDL receptor activity, LDL catabolism is blocked, and the level of LDL in plasma rises in a manner that is inversely proportional to the reduction in LDL receptors. In addition to the impaired catabolism of LDL, LDL production is increased in homozygotes. Enhanced production of LDL has been attributed to the lack of an LDL receptor on liver cells. The liver fails to remove IDL from the plasma normally, with the result than an increased amount of IDL is converted to LDL. This overproduction of LDL, together with its inefficient catabolism, accounts for the high concentrations in affected patients. The elevated LDL levels cause an increase in the uptake of LDL by scavenger cells, which accumulate at various sites in the body, producing xanthomas.

The accelerated coronary atherosclerosis in familial hypercholesterolemia also results from the high LDL levels, which lead to an enhanced infiltration of LDL into the artery wall following episodes of endothelial damage. The large amounts of LDL that penetrate the artery wall cannot be cleared from the interstitial space by the scavenger cells, and atherosclerosis ultimately results. High LDL levels may also act to accelerate platelet aggregation at sites of endothelial injury, thereby enhancing the growth of the atherosclerotic plaque (see Chap. 195).

Diagnosis The diagnosis of heterozygous familial hypercholesterolemia is suggested by the finding of an isolated elevation of plasma cholesterol, with a normal concentration of plasma triglycerides. Such an isolated elevation in plasma cholesterol is usually due to an elevation in the plasma concentration of LDL alone (type 2a pattern). However, most individuals in the general population with type 2a hyperlipoproteinemia do not have familial hypercholesterolemia. Rather, they have a form of polygenic hypercholesterolemia that puts them on the upper end of the bell-shaped curve for the general population (see "Polygenic Hypercholesterolemia" below). Type 2a hyperlipoproteinemia is also caused by multiple lipoprotein-type hyperlipidemia (discussed below). In addition, a variety of metabolic disorders, including hypothyroidism and nephrotic syndrome, can cause type 2a hyperlipoproteinemia (Table 315-4).

Among individuals who have a type 2a lipoprotein pattern, those with heterozygous familial hypercholesterolemia can be distinguished from those with polygenic hypercholesterolemia and multiple lipoprotein-type hyperlipidemia on several grounds. (1) In familial hypercholesterolemia the plasma cholesterol level tends to be higher. A plasma cholesterol level in the range of 350 to 400 mg/dL is more suggestive of heterozygous familial hypercholesterolemia than of the other disorders. However, many patients with heterozygous familial hypercholesterolemia have cholesterol levels of 285 to 350 mg/dL, a range in which the other disorders cannot be excluded. (2) The occurrence of tendon xanthomas virtually establishes the diagnosis of familial hypercholesterolemia, since such xanthomas usually do not occur in patients with other forms of hyperlipidemia. (3) In cases in which the diagnosis is in doubt, other family members should be surveyed. In familial hypercholesterolemia half of the first-degree relatives show an elevated plasma cholesterol level. Hypercholesterolemia in relatives is particularly informative when it occurs in children, since elevated levels of cholesterol in childhood are characteristic of familial hypercholesterolemia but not of the other disorders.

Approximately 10 percent of heterozygotes with familial hypercholesterolemia have a concomitant elevation in plasma triglyceride levels (type 2b pattern). In these cases, the disease is difficult to differentiate from multiple lipoprotein-type hyperlipidemia. The finding of a tendon xanthoma or a hypercholesterolemic child in the family establishes the diagnosis of familial hypercholesterolemia.

The diagnosis of homozygous familial hypercholesterolemia ordinarily affords no problem, providing the physician is familiar with the clinical picture. Most patients are first seen by dermatologists in childhood because of the cutaneous xanthomas. Occasionally, the presentation is delayed until the onset of angina pectoris or until the child suffers a syncopal episode owing to the xanthomatous aortic stenosis. The finding of a cholesterol level greater than 600 mg/dL with normal triglyceride values in a nonjaundiced child is highly suggestive of the diagnosis. Both parents should have elevated cholesterol levels and other features of heterozygous familial hypercholesterolemia.

In specialized laboratories the diagnosis of both heterozygous and homozygous familial hypercholesterolemia can be made by direct measurement of the number of LDL receptors on cultured skin fibroblasts or freshly isolated blood lymphocytes. Homozygous familial hypercholesterolemia has been diagnosed in utero by the absence of LDL receptors on cultured amniotic fluid cells. The mutant genes for the LDL receptor can also be visualized directly in genomic DNA from affected individuals by using restriction enzyme digests and so-called southern blots (see Chap. 58).

Treatment Inasmuch as the atherosclerosis in this disorder is a consequence of the long-standing elevation in plasma LDL levels, every effort should be made to lower the plasma LDL level into the normal range. Patients should be placed on a diet that is low in cholesterol, low in saturated fats, and high in polyunsaturated fats. This generally means the avoidance of milk, butter, cheese, chocolate, shellfish, and fatty meats and the addition of polyunsaturated cooking oils such as corn oil and safflower oil. With such a diet heterozygotes usually show a 10 to 15 percent drop in plasma cholesterol level.

Bile acid–binding resins, such as cholestyramine, should be added to the regimen when dietary therapy fails to lower the cholesterol levels to the normal range. These resins trap the bile acids excreted by the liver into the intestine and prevent their reabsorption. The liver responds to bile acid depletion by converting additional cholesterol into bile acids. This leads to an enhanced production of LDL receptors by the liver, which in turn lowers the plasma level of LDL. Unfortunately, affected subjects also respond to bile acid depletion by enhancing cholesterol synthesis in the liver, and this compensatory response ultimately limits the long-term success of bile acid sequestrant therapy. With the combination of diet and bile acid–binding resins, the extent of reduction in plasma cholesterol level usually is in the range of 15 to 20 percent in heterozygotes. The addition of nicotinic acid may help to block the compensatory increase in hepatic cholesterol synthesis, thus allowing a further lowering of the cholesterol. Major side effects of bile acid–binding resins include gastrointestinal bloating, cramps, and constipation. The major side effect of nicotinic acid is hepatotoxicity; it also produces flushing and headaches in most patients. Probucol has also been used for the treatment of familial hypercholesterolemia. Its mechanism of action is unknown.

A new class of experimental drugs shows great promise for treatment of hypercholesterolemia. These drugs inhibit 3-hydroxy-3-methylglutaryl coenzyme A reductase, an enzyme in the cholesterol biosynthetic pathway. When cholesterol synthesis is inhibited, the production of LDL is diminished and the clearance of LDL by the liver is enhanced as a result of an increased production of LDL receptors. These two effects combine to lower plasma LDL levels by 30 to 50 percent. The HMG CoA reductase inhibitors are even more effective when given together with a bile acid binding resin such as cholestyramine. One of the inhibitors, mevinolin, is undergoing clinical trial.

Heterozygotes often show a moderate to marked lowering of plasma cholesterol level in response to the creation of an intestinal anastomosis that bypasses the ileum. This operation has the same functional effect as bile acid–binding resins, i.e., it accelerates the loss of bile acids in the stool. In certain patients in whom drug therapy is not tolerated, the creation of an ileal bypass may be indicated.

Homozygotes tend to be more resistant to treatment, probably because they are unable to increase production of LDL receptors. In general, combination therapy consisting of diet, a bile acid–binding resin, and nicotinic acid has little effect. Ileal bypass is uniformly ineffective. Several children have responded to surgical creation of a portacaval anastomosis. However, this procedure is still experimental. The use of a continuous-flow blood cell centrifuge to perform plasma exchanges at monthly intervals lowers the cholesterol in all homozygotes. After each plasma exchange, the plasma cholesterol level drops to about 300 mg/dL and then gradually rises over the ensuing 4 weeks to the pretreatment level. If facilities are available, plasma exchange is the treatment of choice for homozygotes. One child has been treated with liver transplantation, which provided LDL receptors and lowered LDL levels by 80 percent.

FAMILIAL HYPERTRIGLYCERIDEMIA This is a common autosomal dominant disorder in which the concentration of VLDL is elevated in the plasma, causing hypertriglyceridemia.

Clinical features Affected individuals do not usually express hypertriglyceridemia until puberty or early adulthood. Thereafter, the fasting plasma triglyceride level tends to be moderately elevated in the range of 200 to 500 mg/dL (type 4 lipoprotein pattern). The typical patient exhibits the clinical triad of obesity, hyperglycemia, and hyperinsulinemia. Hypertension and hyperuricemia are also frequent.

The incidence of atherosclerosis is increased. In one study affected patients constituted 6 percent of all individuals with myocardial infarction. However, it has not been established that the hypertriglyceridemia per se causes the increased atherosclerosis. As discussed above, many patients with this disease have diabetes, obesity, and hypertension. Each of these disorders by itself may predispose to atherosclerosis. Xanthomas are not a characteristic feature of familial hypertriglyceridemia.

Affected patients ordinarily have mild to moderate hypertriglyceridemia but may develop a severe exacerbation when exposed to a variety of precipitating factors. These include poorly controlled diabetes mellitus, excessive consumption of alcohol, ingestion of birth control pills containing estrogen, and the development of hypothyroidism. In response to any of these stimuli, the plasma triglyceride level can rise to more than 1000 mg/dL. During exacerbations such patients develop *mixed hyperlipidemia;* that is, they show an elevation in the concentration of both VLDL and chylomicrons (type 5 lipoprotein pattern). Whenever the concentration of chylomicrons rises to high levels, patients are predisposed to the formation of eruptive xanthomas and the development of pancreatitis. With treatment of the exacerbating condition, the chylomicron-like particles disappear from plasma, and the concentration of triglycerides returns to the moderately elevated basal condition.

In certain families some patients exhibit a severe mixed hyperlipidemia, even in the absence of known exacerbating factors. This is the so-called familial type 5 hyperlipidemia. Other individuals in the same family may have only the mild form of the disease with moderate hypertriglyceridemia and no hyperchylomicronemia (type 4 pattern).

Pathogenesis Familial hypertriglyceridemia is transmitted as an autosomal dominant trait, implying a mutation in a single gene. However, the nature of the mutant gene and the mechanism by which it produces hypertriglyceridemia have not been identified. It is likely that the disorder is genetically heterogeneous; that is, the hypertriglyceridemia phenotype in different families may result from different mutations.

Some patients with familial hypertriglyceridemia seem to have an underlying defect in the ability to catabolize the triglycerides of VLDL. When VLDL production rates become elevated due to obesity or diabetes, they are unable to increase the catabolism of VLDL proportionately, and hypertriglyceridemia results. The reason for this defect in catabolism is not apparent. Lipoprotein lipase activity increases normally in plasma after the administration of heparin, and no abnormalities of lipoprotein structure have been identified.

The increased prevalence of diabetes and obesity in this syndrome is believed to be fortuitous, owing to the fact that both conditions tend to increase VLDL production and hence to exacerbate hypertriglyceridemia. In family studies, one can find relatives who have diabetes without hypertriglyceridemia and relatives who have hypertriglyceridemia without diabetes, indicating that the two are inherited by independent mechanisms. When an individual inherits the gene(s) for diabetes as well as the gene for hypertriglyceridemia, the hypertriglyceridemia is more severe, and such a person is more apt to come to medical attention. Similarly, an individual with familial hypertriglyceridemia who has a normal weight usually has mild hypertriglyceridemia and is less likely to come to medical attention. However, if obesity develops, the hypertriglyceridemia worsens, and a diagnosis is more likely to be made.

Diagnosis A moderate elevation in the plasma triglyceride level, together with a normal cholesterol level, raises the possibility of familial hypertriglyceridemia. In most patients, the plasma is clear to somewhat cloudy on inspection. Chylomicrons typically are not found at the top of the plasma after overnight refrigeration. Electrophoresis of the plasma reveals an increase in the pre-β fraction (type 4 lipoprotein pattern). As mentioned above, an occasional patient exhibits severe hypertriglyceridemia with an elevation in both chylomicrons and VLDL. In this case, a cream layer develops on top (chylomicrons) and a cloudy infranatant (VLDL) is present after overnight storage of plasma in the refrigerator (type 5 lipoprotein pattern).

Given an individual who has an elevation in VLDL levels with or without an elevation in chylomicrons, there is no simple test to determine whether this subject has familial hypertriglyceridemia or hypertriglyceridemia due to some other genetic or acquired cause, such as multiple lipoprotein-type hyperlipidemia or sporadic hypertriglyceridemia. In a typical case of familial hypertriglyceridemia, half of the first-degree relatives have hypertriglyceridemia and no relatives have isolated hypercholesterolemia. Measurement of plasma lipid levels in children is not helpful inasmuch as the disease is typically not manifest until the time of puberty.

Treatment Attempts should be made to control all the exacerbating conditions. Caloric restriction is required in the obese subject. The dietary content of saturated fat should also be limited. Alcohol and oral contraceptives should be avoided. Diabetes mellitus, if present, should be treated vigorously. Thyroid function should be checked, and hypothyroidism treated if found. If the above measures fail, some patients respond to the administration of nicotinic acid or gemfibrozil. The mechanism of action of neither drug is well defined. Patients with severe hypertriglyceridemia frequently show a dramatic response to a fish oil diet.

MULTIPLE LIPOPROTEIN-TYPE HYPERLIPIDEMIA This common disorder, which is also called familial combined hyperlipidemia, is inherited as an autosomal dominant trait. Affected individuals in a single family characteristically show one of three different lipoprotein patterns: hypercholesterolemia (type 2a), hypertriglyceridemia (type 4), or both hypercholesterolemia and hypertriglyceridemia (type 2b).

Clinical features Hyperlipidemia is not present in childhood. Elevations in the plasma cholesterol and/or triglyceride level appear at puberty and continue throughout life. The lipid elevations tend to be mild and vary from time to time so that affected individuals may have a mildly elevated cholesterol level at one examination and/or a mildly elevated triglyceride level at another time. Xanthomas are not a feature. However, premature atherosclerosis occurs, and the incidence of myocardial infarction in middle age is elevated in affected women as well as men.

Patients usually have a strong family history of premature coronary artery disease. This disorder is found in about 10 percent of all patients who have a myocardial infarction. The frequency of obesity, hyperuricemia, and glucose intolerance is increased in affected individuals, especially those with hypertriglyceridemia. However, this association is not as striking as in familial hypertriglyceridemia.

Pathogenesis The disease is transmitted within families as an autosomal dominant trait, implying a mutation in a single gene. Family studies show that about half of the first-degree relatives of an affected individual have hyperlipidemia. However, blood lipid levels are variable among affected individuals in the same family as well as in the same individual at different times. About one-third of hyperlipidemic relatives have hypercholesterolemia (type 2a lipoprotein pattern), one-third hypertriglyceridemia (type 4), and one-third both hypercholesterolemia and hypertriglyceridemia (type 2b). In most affected relatives the plasma lipid levels tend to be just above the 95th percentile for the population and to dip into the normal range intermittently.

While the extent (if any) of the genetic heterogeneity and the nature of the underlying biochemical mechanisms are not known, affected individuals may have an elevated rate of secretion of VLDL by the liver. Depending on the interplay of factors governing the efficiency of conversion of VLDL to LDL and the efficiency of catabolism of LDL, this overproduction of VLDL may manifest itself alternatively as an elevation in plasma VLDL levels (hypertriglyceridemia), an elevation in LDL levels (hypercholesterolemia), or both. The hyperlipidemia is worsened by diabetes, alcoholism, and hypothyroidism.

Diagnosis No clinical or laboratory methods exist by which to determine whether an individual with hyperlipidemia has the multiple lipoprotein-type disorder. The 2a, 2b, and 4 lipoprotein patterns can each occur in patients with several other diseases (see Tables 315-3 and 315-4). However, this disorder should be suspected in any individual whose hyperlipoproteinemia is mild and whose lipoprotein type changes with time. The diagnosis is supported by the finding of multiple abnormal lipoprotein types in relatives. The diagnosis can be ruled out by the finding of tendon xanthomas in the patient or the patient's relatives or by the finding of hypercholesterolemia in a relative under the age of 10 years.

Treatment Therapy should be directed at the predominant lipid elevated at the time of examination. General measures such as weight reduction, restriction of dietary saturated fat and cholesterol, and avoidance of alcohol and oral contraceptives are useful. Triglyceride elevations may respond to nicotinic acid or gemfibrozil. When only the cholesterol level is elevated, a bile acid–binding resin should be given. However, in some individuals the lowering of cholesterol levels with such a drug is accompanied by an increase in triglyceride levels.

PRIMARY HYPERLIPOPROTEINEMIAS OF UNKNOWN ETIOLOGY

POLYGENIC HYPERCHOLESTEROLEMIA By definition, 5 percent of individuals in the general population have LDL-cholesterol levels that exceed the 95th percentile and therefore have hypercholesterolemia (type 2a or type 2b lipoprotein patterns). On the average, among every 20 such hypercholesterolemic persons, 1 person has the heterozygous form of familial hypercholesterolemia, and 2 have multiple lipoprotein-type hyperlipidemia. The remaining 17 have a form of hypercholesterolemia, designated polygenic hypercholesterolemia, that owes its origin not to a single mutant gene but rather to a complex interaction of multiple genetic and environmental factors.

Most of the factors that place an individual in the upper part of the bell-shaped curve for cholesterol levels are not known. It is likely that subtle genetic differences exist among people with regard to many processes governing cholesterol metabolism. For example, among normal people there may be genetic polymorphisms in the proteins that govern the rates of intestinal cholesterol absorption, bile acid synthesis, cholesterol synthesis, and LDL synthesis or catabolism. Certain unfavorable combinations of these mildly altered proteins, coupled with an environmental challenge, such as a diet high in cholesterol or saturated fat, may raise the plasma cholesterol level.

Clinically, polygenic hypercholesterolemia can be distinguished from familial hypercholesterolemia and multiple lipoprotein-type hyperlipidemia in two ways: (1) family studies (hyperlipidemia is present in no more than 10 percent of first-degree relatives in polygenic hypercholesterolemia in contrast to 50 percent in the other two disorders) and (2) examination for tendon xanthomas (absent in both polygenic hypercholesterolemia and multiple lipoprotein-type hyperlipidemia but present in about 75 percent of adult heterozygotes with familial hypercholesterolemia).

Certain patients with polygenic hypercholesterolemia respond to dietary restriction of saturated fat and cholesterol. Other patients require drug therapy. Probucol is sometimes effective in this latter group. Cholestyramine with or without nicotinic acid may also be used.

SPORADIC HYPERTRIGLYCERIDEMIA In addition to the forms of primary hypertriglyceridemia that show familial aggregation, endogenous hypertriglyceridemia with or without hyperchylomicronemia is sometimes seen in individuals whose relatives do not manifest hyperlipidemia. For purposes of classification, this disorder is called sporadic hypertriglyceridemia. Affected patients comprise a heterogeneous group. Some would undoubtedly be classified under one of the genetic disorders described above if a larger number of relatives were available for lipid measurements. Other than an absence of hyperlipidemic relatives, patients with sporadic hypertriglyceridemia cannot be distinguished clinically from patients with the single-gene forms of primary hypertriglyceridemia. Inasmuch as patients with sporadic hypertriglyceridemia may develop hyperchylomicronemia and pancreatitis, they should be treated with diet and drugs as in the familial disease.

FAMILIAL HYPERALPHALIPOPROTEINEMIA This entity is characterized by elevated plasma levels of HDL, also called alpha lipoprotein. The plasma levels of LDL, VLDL, and triglycerides are normal. The elevated HDL causes a slight elevation in the total plasma cholesterol level. Although a selective elevation in plasma HDL cholesterol can be observed in individuals after exposure to chlorinated hydrocarbon pesticides, in alcoholism and after administration of estrogen, most cases of hyperalphalipoproteinemia have a genetic basis. In some families, hyperalphalipoproteinemia is inherited as an autosomal dominant trait, while in others a multifactorial or polygenic basis is suspected. Individual subjects with familial hyperalphalipoproteinemia show no distinctive clinical features.

Hyperalphalipoproteinemia is associated with a slightly increased longevity and an apparent protection against myocardial infarction.

The mechanism for the increase in plasma HDL levels in this disorder has not been determined.

SECONDARY HYPERLIPOPROTEINEMIAS

A variety of clinical disorders produce secondary hyperlipoproteinemias. These are summarized in Table 315-4. The most frequently encountered forms of secondary hyperlipoproteinemia occur in association with diabetes mellitus, consumption of alcohol, and ingestion of oral contraceptives.

DIABETES MELLITUS Three distinct patterns of hypertriglyceridemia occur in patients with diabetes mellitus. Classic "diabetic hyperlipemia" consists of a massive elevation in the plasma triglyceride level that occurs in patients who have suffered from insulin deficiency or insulin resistance for many weeks or months. Such insulin-deprived patients develop a progressive increase in concentration of plasma VLDL and eventually of chylomicrons as well. Triglyceride levels as high as 25,000 mg/dL are seen. Eruptive xanthomas, lipemia retinalis, and hepatomegaly can occur. Ketosis is frequently present, but severe acidosis is not characteristic. This form of massive hyperlipemia is seen only in partial insulin deficiency. Patients with this form of diabetic hyperlipidemia usually respond to a fat-free diet and to the administration of insulin, although triglyceride levels may not return entirely to normal.

The second type of hypertriglyceridemia in diabetics is associated with acute ketoacidosis. Such patients usually exhibit a mild hyperlipidemia with elevations of VLDL but not chylomicrons. On occasion, however, marked elevations of triglyceride are seen with lipemia retinalis. In this case both VLDL and chylomicrons are present.

The third type of hypertriglyceridemia is a mild to moderate elevation in plasma VLDL that persists even when patients appear to be adequately treated for their diabetes. This chronic triglyceride elevation generally occurs in patients who are obese. Inasmuch as most patients with well-controlled diabetes have normal plasma triglyceride levels, the occasional patient with persistent hypertriglyceridemia is likely to have an underlying familial hyperlipoproteinemic disorder. Indeed, family studies indicate that many of these patients have inherited the trait for familial hypertriglyceridemia in a pattern independent of the inheritance of diabetes mellitus.

The insulin deficiency or insulin resistance of diabetes produces a high VLDL level by two mechanisms. With acute insulin deprivation there is an increase in VLDL secretion from the liver as a secondary response to the increased mobilization of free fatty acids from adipose tissue. As the state of insulin deprivation becomes prolonged, the rate of removal of VLDL and chylomicrons from the circulation declines because lipoprotein lipase activity becomes diminished.

ALCOHOL CONSUMPTION In any individual the daily consumption of large amounts of ethanol can produce a mild, asymptomatic elevation in the plasma triglyceride level due to an elevation of VLDL. However, in a subgroup ethanol ingestion regularly produces massive and clinically significant hyperlipidemia with elevations in both VLDL and chylomicrons (type 5 lipoprotein pattern). In most of this group, the VLDL level remains mildly elevated (type 4 lipoprotein pattern), even in the basal state after recovery from the severe alcoholic hyperlipidemia. This suggests that these individuals have a form of familial hypertriglyceridemia or multiple lipoprotein-type hyperlipidemia that is exacerbated and converted to a type 5 pattern by the ethanol ingestion.

Ethanol elevates the plasma triglyceride level primarily because it inhibits fatty acid oxidation and enhances fatty acid synthesis in the liver. The excess fatty acids are esterified to triglyceride. Some of this excess triglyceride accumulates in the liver, producing the characteristic enlarged fatty liver of alcoholics. The remainder of the

TABLE 315-5 Rare autosomal recessive disorders of lipid metabolism

Disorder	Typical age of onset	Plasma lipid abnormality	Major clinical manifestations	Pathogenesis	Treatment
Abetalipoproteinemia	Early childhood	Cholesterol, ~50 mg/dL; triglycerides, <10 mg/dL	Malabsorption of fat, ataxia, neuropathy, retinitis pigmentosa, acanthocytosis	Defective synthesis of apoprotein B leads to absence of chylomicrons, VLDL, and LDL in plasma	Vitamin E
Tangier disease	Childhood	Cholesterol, 40 to 125 mg/dL; triglycerides, normal to slightly elevated	Large orange tonsils, corneal opacities, relapsing polyneuropathy No premature atherosclerosis	Absence of HDL from plasma leads to generation of abnormal chylomicron remnants, which are taken up and stored as cholesteryl esters in phagocytic cells	None
Lecithin:cholesterol acyltransferase (LCAT) deficiency	Young adult	Total plasma cholesterol level variable with marked decrease in esterified cholesterol and increase in unesterified cholesterol; elevated VLDL level; structure of all lipoproteins is abnormal	Corneal opacities, hemolytic anemia, renal insufficiency, premature atherosclerosis	Decreased LCAT activity in plasma leads to accumulation of excess unesterified cholesterol in plasma and body tissues	Fat-restricted diet, kidney transplantation
Cerebrotendinous xanthomatosis	Young adult	None	Progressive cerebellar ataxia, dementia and spinal cord paresis, subnormal intelligence, tendon xanthomas, cataracts	Defective synthesis of primary bile acids in liver leads to increased hepatic synthesis of cholesterol and cholestanol, which accumulate in brain, tendons, and other tissues	None
Sitosterolemia	Childhood	Elevated levels of plant sterols in plasma, elevated or normal levels of cholesterol, normal triglyceride levels	Tendon xanthomas	Increased intestinal absorption of dietary sitosterol and other plant sterols with accumulation in plasma and tendons	Diet low in plant sterols

newly formed triglyceride is secreted into plasma, resulting in an increased secretion of VLDL. In those who develop massive alcoholic hyperlipidemia, there appears to be a partial defect in the catabolism of these VLDL particles. As the concentration of VLDL increases, the lipoprotein begins to compete with chylomicrons for hydrolysis by lipoprotein lipase, and the plasma concentration of chylomicrons also rises.

In severe alcoholic hyperlipidemia, eruptive xanthomas and lipemia retinalis are frequent. The most serious complication, pancreatitis, may be difficult to diagnose, since elevated triglyceride levels can interfere with the estimation of serum amylase. There is no evidence to indicate that pancreatitis can cause hyperlipidemia; rather the hyperlipidemia is the cause of the pancreatitis.

Plasma from patients with alcoholic hyperlipidemia is creamy in appearance. If a blood sample is drawn in calcium edetate and the plasma placed in the refrigerator at 4°C overnight, the chylomicrons float to the top, and the infranatant layer is turbid, owing to the combined elevation of VLDL and chylomicrons (type 5 pattern).

ORAL CONTRACEPTIVES The ingestion of estrogen-containing birth control pills causes an increase in the VLDL secretion rate from the liver. In most women the catabolism of VLDL also increases, so that the overall increase in plasma triglyceride level is modest. However, in women who have an underlying genetic disorder (such as familial hypertriglyceridemia or multiple lipoprotein-type hyperlipidemia) the plasma VLDL-triglyceride level can increase markedly, and hyperchylomicronemia can develop when estrogen-containing medications are taken. These women generally have mild hypertriglyceridemia prior to the institution of oral contraceptive therapy, and they presumably are unable to increase VLDL catabolism in response to the stimulation of VLDL production. The elevated VLDL prevents the normal catabolism of chylomicrons by lipoprotein lipase, and secondary hyperchylomicronemia ensues. When the latter develops, severe pancreatitis can occur.

Ingestion of oral contraceptives may be a risk factor in promoting thromboembolic disease in young women, especially those with preexisting hypercholesterolemia. Thus, it is important to measure the plasma cholesterol and triglyceride levels prior to the institution of birth control therapy. The finding of hyperlipidemia is a contraindication to the use of these drugs.

RARE DISORDERS OF LIPID METABOLISM

Table 315-5 summarizes the clinical and pathophysiologic features of five rare autosomal recessive disorders of lipid metabolism. In two—abetalipoproteinemia and Tangier disease—the major effect of the abnormality is to cause a decrease in lipid levels in plasma. In two—cerebrotendinous xanthomatosis and sitosterolemia—the major effect of the inborn error is to cause an accumulation of unusual sterols in tissues. In LCAT deficiency, the underlying mutation produces both an abnormal pattern of lipoproteins in plasma and an accumulation of unesterified cholesterol in tissues.

REFERENCES

BILHEIMER DW: Treatment of hyperlipidemia, in *Harrison's Principles of Internal Medicine, Update VI,* RG Petersdorf et al (eds). New York, McGraw-Hill, 1985, p 215

BROWN MS, GOLDSTEIN JL: How LDL receptors influence cholesterol and atherosclerosis. Sci Am 251:58, 1984

———, ———: Drugs used in the treatment of hyperlipoproteinemias, in *The Pharmacological Basis of Therapeutics,* 7th ed, AG Gilman et al (eds). New York, Macmillan, 1986, pp 827–845

CONNOR WE et al: Reduction of plasma lipids, lipoproteins and apoproteins by dietary fish oils in patients with hypertriglyceridemia. N Engl J Med 312:1210, 1985

GOLDSTEIN JL, BROWN MS: Familial hypercholesterolemia, in *The Metabolic Basis of Inherited Disease,* 5th ed, JB Stanbury et al (eds). New York, McGraw-Hill, 1983, pp 672–712

MAHLEY RW, ANGELIN B: Type III hyperlipoproteinemia: Recent insights into the genetic defect of familial dysbetalipoproteinemia. Adv Intern Med 29:385, 1984

NIKKILA E: Familial lipoprotein lipase deficiency and related disorders of chylomicron metabolism, in *The Metabolic Basis of Inherited Disease,* 5th ed, JB Stanbury et al (eds). New York, McGraw-Hill, 1983, pp 622–642

STANBURY JB et al (eds): *The Metabolic Basis of Inherited Disease,* 5th ed. New York, McGraw-Hill, 1983

316 LYSOSOMAL STORAGE DISEASES

ARTHUR L. BEAUDET

GENERAL FEATURES

DEFINITION Lysosomes are cytoplasmic organelles that enclose an acidic environment containing numerous enzymes capable of hydrolyzing most biologic macromolecules (Fig. 316-1). Primary lysosomes, the original bodies derived from the Golgi apparatus, may fuse with other membrane-bound vesicles to form secondary lysosomes. Secondary lysosomes contain material derived from outside the cell through endocytosis or material from within the cell through autophagy. A major function of the lysosome is degradation of used macromolecules related to normal turnover and tissue remodeling. Studies of the metabolism of vitamin B_{12}, lipoproteins, peptide hormones, and growth factors indicate that the lysosome is also important in the uptake of molecules through the process of adsorptive endocytosis. The initial cellular vacuole resulting from adsorptive endocytosis is the receptosome, or endosome, and this vacuole fuses with lysosomes. The lysosomal enzymes are glycoproteins which are synthesized within the endoplasmic reticulum. The initial products of protein synthesis undergo extensive modification including proteolytic cleavage, addition of complex oligosaccharides, synthesis of recognition markers (mannose 6-phosphate in some instances), and compartmentalization into primary lysosomes. These processes occur in the endoplasmic reticulum, in the Golgi apparatus, and probably in the primary, if not secondary, lysosomes as well.

The concept of lysosomal storage diseases arose from the studies of type II (Pompe) glycogen storage disease. The demonstration of lysosomal accumulation of glycogen as the result of α-glucosidase deficiency and data from other disorders led Hers to define an inborn lysosomal disease as one in which (1) a single lysosomal enzyme is deficient and (2) abnormal deposits (of substrate) are present within vacuoles related to lysosomes. This definition can be modified to include single-gene defects affecting one or more lysosomal enzymes and thus encompass disorders such as the mucolipidoses and multiple sulfatase deficiency. The concept also can be expanded to include the deficiency of other proteins necessary for lysosomal function such as sphingolipid activator proteins. Biochemical and genetic evidence indicates that these activator proteins are essential for hydrolysis of some substrates.

The lysosomal storage diseases include most of the lipid storage disorders, the mucopolysaccharidoses, the mucolipidoses, glycoprotein storage diseases, and others, as indicated in Table 316-1. The enzyme deficiencies have an autosomal recessive basis with the exception of Hunter's mucopolysaccharidosis II (MPS II), which is X-linked recessive, and Fabry's disease, which is X-linked with frequent manifestations in females. The target organs are determined by the usual sites of degradation for a macromolecule. For example, cerebral white matter is affected in patients with defects in degradation of myelin, hepatosplenomegaly develops in those with defects in degradation of glycolipids from red cell stroma, and generalized tissue involvement may occur in patients with defects in the degradation of ubiquitous mucopolysaccharides. The accumulated material often causes visceromegaly or macrocephaly, but secondary atrophy also can occur, particularly in brain or muscle. In simple terms, the symptoms appear to be due to damage from stored material, but exactly how this causes cell death or dysfunction often is unclear.

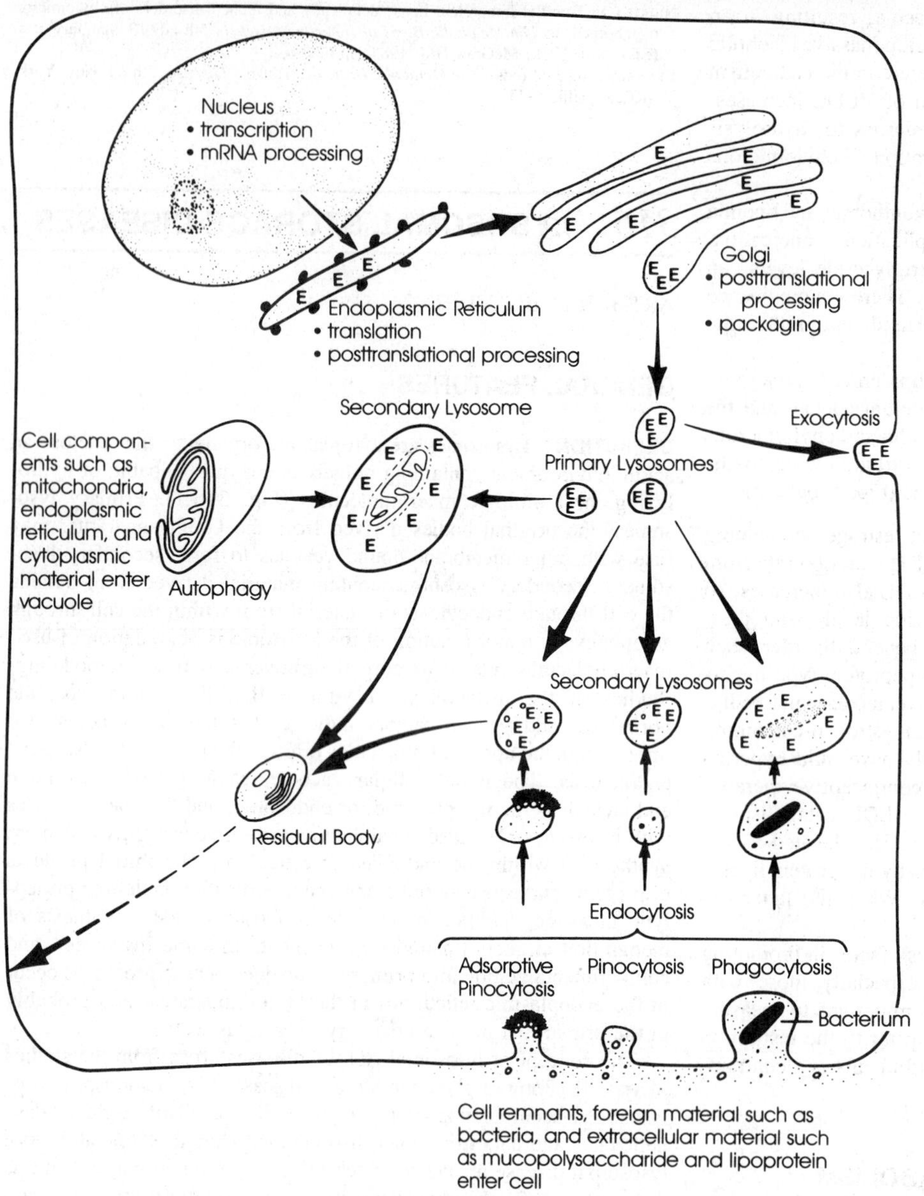

FIGURE 316-1 *Biology of lysosomes. E represents lysosomal enzymes, including precursor forms. Lysosomal enzymes are synthesized in the endoplasmic reticulum and then undergo posttranslational processing that allows packaging into the primary lysosomes. The primary lysosomes can then undergo any of the several fates outlined.*

All the disorders are progressive, and many are fatal in childhood or adolescence. Definitive diagnosis is accomplished best by specific enzyme assays on serum, leukocytes, or cultured skin fibroblasts, selecting the appropriate tests on clinical grounds. There is extensive phenotypic variation within disorders with infantile, juvenile, and adult forms of many entities. In addition, varying combinations of visceral, skeletal, and neurologic involvement can occur within a single enzyme disorder.

DIAGNOSIS A lysosomal storage disease is usually suspected on the basis of progressive neurologic dysfunction, visceromegaly, skeletal dysostosis, or some more specific finding, as outlined in Table 316-1. Progressive or degenerative disease is the hallmark of these disorders. The superimposition of degeneration upon normal childhood development results in a slowing of progress prior to loss of previously acquired abilities. The history should focus on the course of childhood development, neurologic symptoms, including seizures and visual or auditory impairment, the course of physical growth, and more specific findings such as coarsening facies, corneal clouding, exaggerated startle response, abdominal distention, joint pain, joint stiffness, hernias, and recurrent infection. The family history may reveal similarly affected siblings or consanguinity in autosomal recessive disease or other affected male family members in X-linked disorders. Ethnic background may be helpful because several lipid storage diseases are more frequent in Ashkenazi Jews and mannosidosis and aspartylglucosaminuria may occur with increased frequency in Scandinavian populations. The juvenile form of sialidosis is frequent in the Japanese.

On physical examination the head circumference may be enlarged. Gigantism occurs early in the course of some mucopolysaccharidoses and glycoprotein storage diseases, while short stature is a later finding in many disorders. Ophthalmologic examination should include slit-lamp and careful funduscopic examination. Enlargement of the tongue, coarsening of the facies, and hepatosplenomegaly may occur. Skeletal findings may include gibbus deformity, broadening of the long bones, and joint stiffness. Cutaneous findings are rare except in fucosidosis, sialidosis, Fabry's disease, and Hunter's disease. Careful neurologic examination should attempt to distinguish the extent of involvement of gray matter, white matter, and peripheral nerves. Preliminary diagnostic studies should include examination of the peripheral blood smear for vacuolated or granulated leukocytes, urinary spot test for mucopolysaccharide, and radiologic bone survey. The preferred method of diagnosis is to use the above information to select specific enzyme assays in serum, leukocytes, or cultured skin fibroblasts. If a mucopolysaccharide screening test is positive or if clinical findings are suggestive, quantitative mucopolysaccharide analysis can be carried out. If a specific diagnosis is not readily established, biopsy of skin, bone marrow, rectal mucosa, liver, peripheral nerve, conjunctiva, or other tissue for light and electron microscopy can be helpful. Electron-microscopic findings can direct one toward or away from the general category of lysosomal storage diseases based on the presence or absence of engorged lysosomes. Again, enzyme assay is the proper method for diagnosis of the standard disorders. When significant evidence favors a lysosomal storage disease but no enzyme deficiency is demonstrable, chemical analysis of biopsy tissue from liver or brain may be an appropriate research starting point.

HETEROGENEITY There is extensive clinical and biochemical heterogeneity within the lysosomal storage diseases. The biochemical genetic principles underlying this heterogeneity are reviewed in Chaps. 57 and 305. In general, a structural gene for lysosomal enzyme produces products which undergo posttranslational modification to become glycoproteins, often resulting in a series of electrophoretic variants, or isozymes. These isozymes may hydrolyze one or a variety of substrates, and the substrate specificity of particular isozymes may vary. Differences in substrate specificity also arise from the occurrence of similar but genetically distinct enzymes, for example, the β-galactosidases. Mutations within a gene may totally eliminate or reduce enzyme activity, alter the ability of the enzyme to undergo posttranslational modification, or alter the activity of the enzyme for specific substrates.

In most instances different mutations within the structural genes for lysosomal enzymes account for varying degrees of severity from individual to individual as well as for the diverse combinations of visceral, skeletal, neurologic, ocular, and other manifestations. The heterogeneity is increased further by the recessive nature of most of the conditions in that each affected individual must have two mutant genes at the same locus. The exact mutation may vary in the two copies of the gene, making the patient a genetic compound heterozygote. In this instance either one or both genes may encode some form of residual enzyme activity for one or more substrates. Patients with intermediate clinical phenotypes with mucopolysaccharidosis type I (MPS I) have been cited as likely examples of compound heterozygotes. At a molecular level the majority of lysosomal storage disease patients might prove to be compound heterozygotes. Although it is useful to characterize clinical phenotypes as infantile, juvenile, adult, neuropathic, or nonneuropathic, the existence of different mutant alleles and of genetic compounds provides an explanation for those occasional patients who appear aberrant or intermediate as compared with the usual phenotype. Another type of heterogeneity is illustrated by MPS III A, B, C, and D, which are very similar disorders caused by different gene defects. Thus, biochemical heterogeneity can underlie apparent clinical homogeneity.

Further complexity results from the fact that certain enzyme activities are derived from complexes of nonidentical subunits. As a consequence, different mutations can cause deficiency of the same enzyme, as for example, hexosaminidase A deficiency in Tay-Sachs and Sandhoff's diseases, and can explain multiple enzyme deficiencies due to a single-gene defect as in Sandhoff's disease. Genetic disorders involving the posttranslational modification of lysosomal enzymes and general defects in the integrity and function of the lysosome may also cause lysosomal storage diseases. The mucolipidoses II and III represent situations in which a single-gene defect alters the ability of a number of lysosomal enzymes to enter the lysosome. Thus, mutations outside the structural genes for the enzymes themselves can account for further heterogeneity. Better biochemical understanding of the identity, subunit structure, posttranslational processing, and substrate specificities of lysosomal enzymes should provide further insight into phenotypic and genotypic heterogeneity.

Clinical diagnosis is facilitated but also somewhat complicated by the widespread use of synthetic substrates for measuring lysosomal enzyme activities. These substrates often measure a group of related activities attributable to different enzymes. Thus, the activity of β-galactosidase using an artificial substrate may represent the sum of various β-galactosidases encoded by different structural genes and having different substrate specificities. Clinical reliability generally is achieved by manipulating in vitro conditions to reflect that enzyme activity whose deficiency is characteristic of a clinical disorder. Genetic heterogeneity has, however, resulted in individuals with a mutant enzyme that either hydrolyzes the natural substrate and not the artificial substrate, or vice versa. This is exemplified by the normal individuals who have hexosaminidase A deficiency using artificial substrate and by patients with Tay-Sachs disease who have substantial levels of hexosaminidase A activity with artificial substrates. The presence or absence of disease correlates with ability to hydrolyze the natural G_{M2} ganglioside substrate. These phenomena have considerable significance for identification of affected patients, for heterozygote screening, and for prenatal diagnosis. They indicate the need to go beyond artificial substrate enzyme assays if normal results occur in the face of overwhelming clinical, electron-microscopic, or chemical evidence of a storage disease.

MANAGEMENT AND PREVENTION Specific therapy is not effective in lysosomal storage diseases at present, and care is largely symptomatic. The relentless, progressive course in many instances represents a tragic burden. Transplantation is effective in reversing the renal failure that commonly occurs in Fabry's disease, and splenectomy frequently is helpful in adult Gaucher's disease. Considerable attention has been focused on enzyme replacement for lysosomal storage diseases using organ or fibroblast transplantation or the infusion of either plasma, leukocytes, purified enzyme itself, or enzyme trapped in erythrocytes or liposomes. Although these approaches offer promise for treatment of manifestations outside the central nervous system, they are not of proven efficacy. The most distressing aspects of lysosomal storage diseases involve the central nervous system, where the blood-brain barrier presents an additional obstacle to the development of effective enzyme replacement therapy.

Genetic counseling is important in the management of these disorders. All the lysosomal storage diseases in which the specific enzyme deficiency is known either have been or presumably could be diagnosed in utero, since lysosomal enzyme activities appear to be expressed in cultured amniotic fluid cells as well as in cultured skin fibroblasts. Prenatal diagnosis can also be made using chorionic villus biopsy. Although the incidence of miscarriage after this procedure may be slightly higher, the possibility of earlier diagnosis is very attractive to families with high genetic risks. Heterozygote detection in close relatives is sometimes possible, although it can be difficult to achieve adequate statistical confidence for such determinations. Heterozygote detection is further complicated by random inactivation of X chromosomes in 46,XX carriers of X-linked diseases, but counseling of females at risk in such families should be pursued vigorously. More effective approaches to prevention require identification of heterozygous couples prior to the birth of an affected offspring. The feasibility of this approach has been demonstrated by heterozygote testing programs for Tay-Sachs disease. Such programs could result in a decreased frequency of these disorders through extensive testing and appropriate reproductive decisions on the part of the rare couples at risk for having affected offspring; the high frequency of the heterozygous state in Ashkenazi Jews and favorable biochemical aspects of carrier detection for Tay-Sachs disease have facilitated this program. Efficient, accurate heterozygote detection methods would be needed to apply this approach to other diseases and to populations with lower heterozygote frequencies. Even under optimal conditions genetic variants might cause false-positive or false-negative results in any screening process.

CLONING OF LYSOSOMAL ENZYME GENES The cloning of DNAs that encode several lysosomal enzymes has been reported, and the majority of these genes will be cloned eventually. These developments should increase the understanding of the biochemistry and genetics for the lysosomal disorders, although clinical diagnosis and prenatal diagnosis are not likely to be altered significantly. The major hope would be that availability of the cloned genes might allow for some form of gene replacement therapy.

TABLE 316-1 Summary of lysosomal storage diseases

Disorder	Heterogeneity (onset)	Enzyme deficiency	Stored material	Neurologic
G_{M1} gangliosidosis	Infantile (birth) Juvenile (6–20 mo) Adult	β-Galactosidase	G_{M1} ganglioside Glycoproteins Keratan sulfate	Mental retardation, seizures, blindness; later in juvenile form, variable in adults
Tay-Sachs and variants, G_{M2} gangliosidosis	Infantile (3–6 mo) Juvenile Adult forms	Hexosaminidase A	G_{M2} ganglioside	Mental retardation, seizures, blindness; later in juvenile form
Sandhoff, G_{M2} gangliosidosis	Infantile (3–6 mo)	Hexosaminidase A and B	G_{M2} ganglioside Globoside	Mental retardation, seizures, blindness
G_{M2} gangliosidosis, AB variant	Findings similar to Tay-Sachs except primary defect is a ganglioside activator protein.			
Krabbe, galactosylceramide lipidosis	Infantile (2–6 mo) Late onset	Galactosylceramide β-Galactosidase	↑ Galactoscerebroside/sulfatide ratio	Mental retardation, leukodystrophy; variable in late onset
Metachromatic leukodystrophy, sulfatide lipidosis	Late infantile (1–4 yr) Juvenile (4–20 yr) Adult	Arylsulfatase A (cerebroside sulfatase)	Galactosyl sulfatides	Mental retardation, leukodystrophy, psychosis and dementia in adults
Sphingolipid activator protein 1 deficiency	Findings similar to metachromatic leukodystrophy except primary defect is activator protein.			
Niemann-Pick, sphingomyelin lipidosis	Infantile neuropathic (1–4 mo) Late onset neuropathic Visceral	Sphingomyelinase ? Specific isozymes in some	Sphingomyelin	Mental retardation, ataxia, and seizures in neuropathic forms
Gaucher, glucosylceramide lipidosis	Infantile (1–12 mo) Juvenile (2–6 yr) Adult	β-Glucocerebrosidase	Glucosylceramide	Mental retardation; spastic, later flaccid, ataxia in juvenile; no neurologic symptoms in adult form
Fabry, trihexosyl ceramidosis	Hemizygous males Heterozygous females	α-Galactosidase A	Trihexosylceramide	Painful neuropathy
Acid lipase deficiency	Infantile Wolman's disease (0–3 mo) Late onset cholesteryl ester storage disease (CESD)	Acid lipase	Cholesteryl ester Triglyceride	Mental retardation but mild related to growth failure in Wolman; none in CESD
Farber, ceramide deficiency	Infantile (0–4 mo) Rare juvenile	Ceramidase	Ceramide	Occasional mental retardation, but may be secondary to somatic features
Pompe, glycogen storage type II	Infantile (0–6 mo) Juvenile Adult	Acid maltase (α-1,4- and 1,6-glucosidase)	Glycogen	Probably normal mentally
Acid phosphatase deficiency	Infantile (0–3 mo)	Acid phosphatase	Not characterized	Mental retardation
Fucosidosis	Infantile (3–12 mo) Juvenile	α-Fucosidase	Glycopeptides Glycolipids Oligosaccharides	Mental retardation

* *AR = autosomal recessive.*

Liver and/or spleen enlargement	Skeletal dysplasia	Ophthalmic	Hematologic	Genetics	Unique manifestations	References
+ + + + Less in juvenile, variable in adult	+ + + + Variable in juvenile and adult forms	Cherry-red spot in 50% of infantile; corneal clouding variable but more in adults	Foam cells Vacuolated lymphocytes	AR*	Coarse facies, edema, macroglossia, mucopolysacchariduria; early blindness in infantile, milder in juvenile; in adults often spondyloepiphyseal dysplasia +/− mucopolysacchariduria	Hers and Van Hoof, chap 12 Stanbury et al, chap 46 Ho et al
0	0	Cherry-red spot in infantile form, rare in juvenile	0	AR	Macrocephaly, hyperacusis in infantile; increased in Ashkenazi Jews	Hers and Van Hoof, chap 13 Stanbury et al, chap 46 Ho et al
0	0	Cherry-red spot	0	AR	Macrocephaly, hyperacusis, visceral histiocytosis	Hers and Van Hoof, chap 14 Stanbury et al, chap 46 Ho et al
0	0	Optic atrophy	0	AR	Extreme irritability, ↑ CSF protein, fever, globoid cell neuropathology	Hers and Van Hoof, chap 17 Stanbury et al, chap 43 Ho et al
0	0	Optic atrophy, less in juvenile and adult forms	0	AR	↑ CSF protein and early gait abnormalities in late infantile; peripheral neuropathy	Hers and Van Hoof, chap 18 Stanbury et al, chap 44
+ + + + Less prominent in late onset forms	0	Macular degeneration and cherry-red spot in neuropathic forms	Distinctive foam cell Vacuolated lymphocytes	AR	Pulmonary infiltrates, brownish skin, infantile neuronopathic form increased in Ashkenazi Jews, sea-blue histiocytes	Hers and Van Hoof, chap 19 Stanbury et al, chap 41
+ + + + Hypersplenism common	+ +	Usually normal	Distinctive foam cell	AR	Adult form includes ↑ acid phosphatase, pathologic fractures; Ashkenazi Jewish predilection	Hers and Van Hoof, chap 16 Stanbury et al, chap 42 Ho et al
0	0	Corneal dystrophy, vascular lesions, cataracts	0	X-linked dominant	Cutaneous angiokeratoma, vascular thromboses, hypohidrosis	Hers and Van Hoof, chap 15 Stanbury et al, chap 45 Ho et al
+ + +	0	0	Foam cells Vacuolated lymphocytes	AR	Adrenal calcification, anemia, vomiting and poor growth in Wolman; hepatic fibrosis and ↑ blood cholesterol in CESD	Hers and Van Hoof, chap 20 Stanbury et al, chap 39
+/−	?	Mild macular degeneration	0	AR	Arthropathy—subcutaneous, periarticular and visceral nodules (lipogranulomatosis); ↑ CSF protein	Hers and Van Hoof, chap 24 Stanbury et al, chap 40 Ho et al
Mild hepatomegaly	0	0	0	AR	Lethal skeletal and cardiac myopathy in infantile; primarily skeletal myopathy in adults	See chap 313 Hers and Van Hoof, chap 7 Stanbury et al, chap 6
+ +	0	0	0	AR?	Lethal disorders described in two families	Hers and Van Hoof, chap 21 Hirschhorn and Weissmann
+ +	+ +	0	Vacuolated lymphocytes Foam cells	AR	Coarse facies, increased sweat electrolytes, angiokeratoma in juvenile	Hers and Van Hoof, chap 11 Ho et al Stanbury et al, chap 38

(Table continues next page)

TABLE 316-1 Summary of lysosomal storage diseases *(continued)*

Disorder	Heterogeneity (onset)	Enzyme deficiency	Stored material	Neurologic
Mannosidosis	Infantile (6–18 mo) Milder form	α-Mannosidase	Oligosaccharides	Mental retardation
Aspartylglucosaminuria	Young adult onset	Aspartylglucosamine amidase	Aspartylglucosamine Glycopeptides	Mental retardation
Mucopolysaccharidosis IH and IS	Infantile Hurler (6–12 mo) Intermediate Adult Scheie	α-Iduronidase	Dermatan sulfate Heparan sulfate	Mental retardation, absent in Scheie
Hunter, mucopolysaccharidosis II	Severe infantile (6–12 mo) Mild juvenile	Iduronosulfate sulfatase	Dermatan sulfate Heparan sulfate	Mental retardation, less in mild form
Sanfilippo A, mucopolysaccharidosis III A	Late infantile (1–4 yr)	Heparan *N*-sulfatase (sulfamidase)	Heparan sulfate	Severe mental retardation
Sanfilippo B, mucopolysaccharidosis III B		*N*-Acetyl-α-glucosaminidase		
Sanfilippo C, mucopolysaccharidosis III C		Acetyl-CoA:α-glucosaminide *N*-acetyltransferase		
Sanfilippo D, mucopolysaccharidosis III D		*N*-Acetylglucosamine 6-sulfate sulfatase		
Morquio, mucopolysaccharidosis IV	Some variation	*N*-Acetylgalactosamine 6-sulfate sulfatase	Keratan sulfate	0
Maroteaux-Lamy, mucopolysaccharidosis VI	Variation in severity and cardiovascular involvement	*N*-Acetylhexosamine 4-sulfate sulfatase (arylsulfatase B)	Dermatan sulfate	0
β-Glucuronidase deficiency, mucopolysaccharidosis VII	Few patients; infantile to adult forms	β-Glucuronidase	Dermatan sulfate ? Heparan sulfate	Mental retardation ? absent in some adults
Multiple sulfatase deficiency	Late infantile (1–4 yr)	Arylsulfatases A, B, and C Other sulfatases	Sulfatides Mucopolysaccharides	Mental retardation
Sialidosis	Congenital, infantile, juvenile, cherry-red spot myoclonus	Glycoprotein neuraminidase (sialidase)	Sialyloligosaccharides	Mental retardation, myoclonus
Mucolipidosis II, I cell disease	Infantile (0–3 mo)	UDP-*N*-acetylglucosamine (GlcNAc):glycoprotein GlcNAc1-phosphotransferase	Glycoproteins Glycolipids	Mental retardation
Mucolipidosis III, pseudo-Hurler polydystrophy	Late infantile (>2 yr)		Glycoproteins Glycolipids	Mild mental retardation
Mucolipidosis VI	Infantile	? Ganglioside neuraminidase	? Multiple	Mental retardation
Neuronal ceroid lipofuscinoses	Late infantile Juvenile Adult	Unknown	"Ceroid" "Lipofuscin"	Mental retardation, dementia variable in adults, seizures

SPECIFIC DISORDERS

SPHINGOLIPIDOSES G_{M1} gangliosidosis G_{M1} gangliosidosis is due to deficiency of β-galactosidase. Prominent features of the infantile form are the presence of abnormalities at or near birth, developmental delay, seizures, coarse facies, edema, hepatosplenomegaly, macroglossia, ocular cherry-red spot, and a distinctive mucopolysaccharidosis-like dysostosis multiplex. Death usually occurs in the first or second year of life. The juvenile form is characterized by a later onset, survival to the latter half of the first decade, neurologic impairment and seizures, and milder skeletal and ocular findings. In the adult form, spondyloepiphyseal dysplasia similar to that in MPS IV, corneal clouding and normal intelligence are common. Joint pain and limitation of motion, particularly at the hips, can be disabling in these patients. Prominent spasticity and ataxia with mild bony abnormalities may be present. A high index of suspicion is necessary

Liver and/or spleen enlargement	Skeletal dysplasia	Ophthalmic	Hematologic	Genetics	Unique manifestations	References
+ + +	+ +	Cataracts, corneal clouding	Vacuolated lymphocytes Granulated neutrophils	AR	Coarse facies, enlarged tongue	Hers and Van Hoof, chap 11 Stanbury et al, chap 38
0	+ +	Lens opacities	Vacuolated lymphocytes	AR	Coarse facies, detectable by urine amino acid analysis	Hers and Van Hoof, chap 24 Stanbury et al, chap 38
+ + +	+ + + +	Corneal clouding	Granulated lymphocytes	AR	Coarse facies, cardiovascular involvement, joint stiffness	Hers and Van Hoof, chaps 8 and 9 Stanbury et al, chap 36 McKusick
+ + +	+ + + +	Retinal degeneration, no significant corneal clouding	Granulated lymphocytes	X-linked	Coarse facies, cardiovascular involvement, joint stiffness	
+	+	0	Granulated lymphocytes	AR	Mild coarsening of facies	
+	Severe, distinctive	Corneal clouding	Granulated neutrophils	AR	Severe deformity, odontoid hypoplasia, aortic regurgitation	
+ +	+ + + +	Corneal clouding	Granulated neutrophils and lymphocytes	AR	Mild coarsening of facies, joint stiffness, valvular heart disease	
+ + +	+ + +	Corneal clouding	Granulated neutrophils	AR	Coarse facies, ↑ vascular involvement	
+	MPS features	Retinal degeneration	Vacuolated and granulated cells	AR	Icthyosis, combined MPS and metachromatic leukodystrophy phenotype	Hers and Van Hoof, chaps 8 and 18 Stanbury et al, chap 44
+ + Less in late form	+ + Less or absent in late form	Cherry-red spot	Vacuolated lymphocytes	AR	MPS phenotype in all but cherry-red spot myoclonus	Hers and Van Hoof, chap 8 Stanbury et al, chap 38
0/+	+ + + +	Corneal clouding	Vacuolated and granulated neutrophils	AR	Coarse facies, inclusions in cultured fibroblasts, normal mucopolysacchariduria	Hers and Van Hoof, chap 8 Stanbury et al, chap 37
0	+ + +	Corneal clouding	Vacuolated plasma cells	AR	Coarse facies, inclusions in cultured fibroblasts, joint contractures, valvular heart disease, normal mucopolysacchariduria	
0	0	Corneal clouding, retinal degeneration	0	AR	Diagnosis based on electron microscopy; ? Ashkenazi Jewish predilection	Stanbury et al, chap 37
0	0	Optic atrophy, macular degeneration, retinitis pigmentosa	Vacuolated lymphocytes Granulated neutrophils	AR AR	Electron microscopy helpful, degree of genetic heterogeneity unknown	Hers and Van Hoof, chap 23

to recognize the diverse phenotypes caused by β-galactosidase deficiency in juvenile and adult patients, since almost any combination of skeletal, ocular, neurologic, and visceral findings can occur. Isozymes of β-galactosidase occur, and the diversity of phenotypes is due to different mutations in the same structural gene. All forms of G_{M1} gangliosidosis have an autosomal recessive inheritance. There is no ethnic predilection. The frequency of the disease is low, with fewer than 50 patients reported for any given phenotype. Some patients originally reported to have β-galactosidase deficiency were subsequently shown to have combined deficiency of neuraminidase and β-galactosidase.

G_{M2} gangliosidosis Tay-Sachs disease is a relatively common inborn error of metabolism with thousands of documented cases. Although it is clinically very similar to Sandhoff's disease, the two are genetically distinct with deficiency of hexosaminidase A in the former and hexosaminidase A and B in the latter. An additional disorder, called the AB variant of G_{M2} gangliosidosis, occurs with normal hexosaminidase A and B activity. This variant is due to a deficiency of a protein factor (activator) necessary for activity of the enzyme against natural substrate. The presenting features are similar in all of the infantile disorders and include a developmental delay beginning in the third to sixth month with subsequent, rapidly progressive neurologic deterioration. Macrocephaly, seizures, retinal cherry-red spot, and an augmented startle response to sound suggest the diagnosis. The diagnosis is confirmed by enzyme assay. Most juvenile-onset patients with hexosaminidase deficiency present with dementia, seizures, and ocular findings, and some have an atypical spinocerebellar degeneration. Some juvenile and adult patients have presented with clinical features of spinal muscular atrophy.

Sandhoff's disease is nonallelic with Tay-Sachs disease, whereas the juvenile forms of hexosaminidase deficiency are usually allelic with Tay-Sachs disease. Tay-Sachs disease is the most frequent form of hexosaminidase deficiency, the risk being about 100 times higher in Ashkenazi Jews than in other ethnic groups. All forms of G_{M2} gangliosidosis are autosomal recessive. Hexosaminidase B is composed of β subunits whose structural locus is on chromosome 5, while hexosaminidase A is composed of α and β subunits with the structural locus for the α subunit on chromosome 15. Thus there is a defect in the α subunit in Tay-Sachs disease and in the β subunit in Sandhoff's disease.

Although no specific therapy is available, extensive programs for heterozygote detection to prevent Tay-Sachs disease have been carried out throughout the world. As of 1982, more than 400,000 people had been tested, and more than 15,000 heterozygotes and 333 couples at risk for Tay-Sachs in their offspring had been identified. Six hundred sixty-seven pregnancies had been monitored by prenatal diagnosis because of a previous affected child, and 391 pregnancies had been monitored based on results of carrier screening by 1982.

LEUKODYSTROPHIES Krabbe's galactosylceramide lipidosis or globoid cell leukodystrophy is an infantile disease due to deficiency of galactosylceramide β-galactosidase. The disorder is characterized by onset at 2 to 6 months of age, with irritability, hyperesthesia, hypersensitivity to external stimuli, unexplained fever, optic atrophy, and sometimes seizures. Spinal fluid protein is usually increased. Initially there is hypertonicity and increased deep tendon reflexes with progression to a hypotonic state. Rapid neurologic deterioration and death occur within 1 to 2 years of onset. Premortem diagnosis is accomplished by enzyme assay. The presence of globoid cells on neuropathologic examination is characteristic and possibly specific for this enzyme deficiency. Galactosylceramide β-galactosidase functions in the degradation of sulfatides derived from myelin. Myelin synthesis is so impaired by tissue damage that the absolute amount of the galactocerebroside substrate is usually not increased in postmortem tissue. Galactosylceramide β-galactosidase is genetically distinct from the β-galactosidase that is deficient in G_{M1} gangliosidosis.

Krabbe's disease is relatively rare, with about 150 reported cases. It has an autosomal recessive genetic basis and is present in all ethnic groups with a possible increased frequency in the Scandinavian countries. Although no specific therapy is available, prenatal diagnosis has been accomplished.

Deficiency of arylsulfatase A (cerebroside sulfatase) is the basis of metachromatic leukodystrophy, a lipid storage disease with a frequency of 1 in 40,000. The age of onset is later than that in Tay-Sachs disease or Krabbe's disease. Patients develop the ability to walk and frequently present with gait abnormalities in the second to fourth year of life. Initially the patients may be hypotonic with decreased deep tendon reflexes, the latter reflecting peripheral nerve involvement. The disease progresses over the first decade to include ataxia, increased muscle tone, decorticate or decerebrate posturing, and eventual loss of all contact with surroundings. Duration of survival depends on nursing care and support such as nasogastric or gastrostomy feeding.

Although some diagnostic studies have been performed on urine, leukocytes or fibroblasts are preferable for diagnostic enzyme assay. Changes demonstrable on metachromatic staining of nerve tissue are nonspecific and not an adequate substitute for enzyme assay. Rare patients with a juvenile form of metachromatic leukodystrophy have the onset between 4 and 20 years of age and a slower progression. The adult form deserves special mention as an example of the difficulties presented by subtle, slowly progressive forms of lysosomal storage diseases. The onset is in the second to fifth decade with a slowly progressive dementia. Emotional difficulties, motor dysfunction, and indistinct speech are often present. Even though conduction velocity in peripheral nerves is usually diminished, the deep tendon reflexes are often increased. Typical premortem diagnoses include organic dementia, schizophrenia, and multiple sclerosis; a correct premortem diagnosis is made rarely.

Arylsulfatase A is routinely measured using artificial substrate, and complexities involving low levels of activity in normal individuals and moderate levels of residual activity in symptomatic patients have been described. Heterogeneity involving mutations in multiple components of the cerebroside sulfatase activity may exist, but the majority of patients probably have simple allelic disorders on an autosomal recessive basis. A few patients with a phenotype similar to metachromatic leukodystrophy have been shown to have deficiency of a sphingolipid activator protein. Arylsulfatase A deficiency also occurs in multiple sulfatase deficiency discussed below.

NIEMANN-PICK DISEASE Niemann-Pick disease is a sphingomyelin lipidosis. In type A and B disease, there is a clear deficiency of sphingomyelinase, an enzyme that hydrolyzes sphingomyelin to yield ceramide and phosphorylcholine. The most common disorder, Niemann-Pick A, begins shortly after birth with hepatosplenomegaly, failure to thrive, and neurologic impairment. Retinal cherry-red spots occur, but seizures and hypersplenism are rare. The diagnosis can be made by recognition of the distinctive Niemann-Pick cell in the bone marrow but should be confirmed by enzyme assay. Niemann-Pick B disease is a relatively benign disorder with hepatosplenomegaly, sphingomyelinase deficiency, and sometimes pulmonary infiltrates; but there is no neurologic involvement. Niemann-Pick C disease is characterized by sphingomyelin lipidosis, progressive neurologic deterioration in childhood, and substantial or normal sphingomyelinase activity. Niemann-Pick D disease resembles type C but is separated primarily on the basis of occurrence in a Nova Scotian population. Niemann-Pick E disease causes visceral sphingomyelin lipidosis without neurologic involvement and without sphingomyelinase deficiency. The biochemical basis for Niemann-Pick types C, D, and E is not understood. Many patients described with the sea-blue histiocyte syndrome may have had sphingomyelinase deficiency; other patients with the sea-blue histiocyte syndrome may have defects not yet characterized.

GAUCHER'S DISEASE Gaucher's disease is a glucosylceramide lipidosis caused by deficiency of glucosylceramidase. An infantile form is characterized by early onset, marked hepatosplenomegaly, and severe neurologic progression to early death. A juvenile form with milder neurologic involvement exists. The adult form of the disease may be the most common lysosomal storage disease. Patients with juvenile and adult Gaucher's disease have been observed within the same family but not within the same sibships, suggesting that these are allelic disorders.

All forms of Gaucher's disease have an autosomal recessive genetic basis. The adult disorder is about 30 times more frequent in Ashkenazi Jews, with an incidence in this group of about 1 in 2500 births. Although commonly termed "adult Gaucher's disease," this variant frequently has its onset in childhood. Absence of neurologic involvement is the criterion for inclusion in this category. Adult Gaucher's disease is one of the lysosomal storage diseases most likely to present in the practice of internal medicine, although patients may be diagnosed at almost any age. The clinical presentation is usually either the incidental discovery of splenomegaly or the occurrence of thrombocytopenia secondary to hypersplenism. In addition, bone pain or pathologic fractures may occur including aseptic necrosis of the femoral heads and vertebral collapse. Bone pain with fever has been described as pseudoosteomyelitis. Pulmonary infiltrates, pulmonary hypertension, and moderate hepatic dysfunction may be present. Serum acid phosphatase is characteristically elevated. A distinctive storage cell occurs in the bone marrow in all forms of Gaucher's disease, but enzyme assay should be performed because the Gaucher cell may also be found in patients with granulocytic leukemia and myeloma.

The clinical course is variable; pulmonary involvement may lead to early death, but in many patients life span is not shortened. Bleeding secondary to thrombocytopenia frequently responds to splenectomy. Bone marrow transplantation may be considered in the face of life-threatening complications from the disease. Because of the frequency of the disease and the lack of neurologic involvement, the adult form of Gaucher's disease is particularly worthy of efforts to develop enzyme replacement therapy.

FABRY'S DISEASE Fabry's disease involves the accumulation of a trihexoside, galactosylgalactosylglucosylceramide, due to deficiency of α-galactosidase A. The disorder is X-linked, and the most severe symptoms are in affected males. Fabry's disease usually presents during adulthood. If symptoms occur during childhood, they are likely to take the form of a painful neuropathy. During adolescence and early adulthood, patients often experience hypohidrosis, and a history of heat stroke during military training is frequent. A characteristic corneal dystrophy allows for diagnosis by the astute ophthalmologist, but the patients rarely have visual complaints. Frequently the disease is diagnosed only after development of progressive renal impairment in the third to fifth decade. Vascular thromboses may occur even in childhood. Death most often results from renal failure, typically in the fourth or fifth decade. Heterozygous females are affected more mildly. Corneal dystrophy is the most frequent finding, but all other manifestations may be seen also. Life expectancy is greater in women, although fatal complications can occur rarely.

Therapeutic intervention of several types may be helpful. Counseling regarding the risks of hypohidrosis is important. Painful neuropathy frequently responds to administration of phenytoin. Renal failure can be treated by chronic dialysis, and the patients are acceptable candidates for transplantation since the donor kidney will not be impaired by the disease. The disease in the future might be amenable to enzyme replacement therapy, since the central nervous system is spared.

ACID LIPASE DEFICIENCY Acid lipase deficiency is the basis for two disorders with different phenotypic features. Wolman's disease is a severe disorder of early onset, with prominent hepatosplenomegaly, anemia, vomiting, failure to thrive, and characteristic adrenal calcification. Neurologic involvement is minimal compared with the severe somatic handicap. Cholesteryl ester storage disease is a rare disorder with mild phenotypic features by comparison. The most constant features are hepatosplenomegaly and increased plasma cholesterol. Hepatic fibrosis, esophageal varices, and poor growth have occurred. One reported sibship may represent an intermediate phenotype, since two females died at 7 and 9 years of age with unexplained acute hepatic failure, and a third sibling developed adrenal calcification and pulmonary hypertension early in life. Tissues from patients with acid lipase deficiency demonstrate inability to hydrolyze triglycerides as well as cholesteryl esters. Possibly a single enzyme hydrolyzes multiple substrates, but the subunit structure and hydrolytic capacities of various lysosomal lipases are not well studied. Deficiency of acid lipase results in impairment of low-density lipoprotein degradation as described in Chap. 315 and may be associated with premature atherosclerosis. Both Wolman's and cholesteryl ester storage diseases have an autosomal recessive basis.

GLYCOPROTEIN STORAGE DISORDERS Fucosidosis, mannosidosis, and aspartylglucosaminuria are rare, autosomal recessive disorders involving hydrolases that degrade polysaccharide linkages. Glycolipids as well as glycoproteins are accumulated in fucosidosis. All are characterized by neurologic impairment and varying somatic involvements, as outlined in Table 316-1. Fucosidosis and mannosidosis are most often lethal disorders in childhood, while aspartylglucosaminuria presents as a late-onset lysosomal storage disease with prominent mental retardation and a prolonged course. Abnormal sweat electrolytes and cutaneous angiokeratomas are distinctive in fucosidosis, and an unusual cartwheel-type cataract occurs in mannosidosis. Aspartylglucosaminuria is remarkable in that urinary amino acid analysis is diagnostic with an increase of aspartylglucosamine; it is more frequent in the Finnish population. Sialidosis encompasses a group of phenotypes associated with glycoprotein neuraminidase (sialidase) deficiency. The phenotypes include an adult cherry-red spot myoclonus syndrome, infantile and juvenile presentations with mucopolysaccharidosis-like phenotypes, and a congenital presentation with hydrops fetalis. Many patients previously classified as having mucolipidosis I have been proven to have mannosidosis or sialidosis. Some patients with sialidosis have β-galactosidase deficiency as well as neuraminidase deficiency. The molecular basis for the combined β-galactosidase and neuraminidase deficiency is uncertain, but a defect in a "protective protein" has been proposed. Each of the glycoprotein storage diseases can be diagnosed by appropriate enzyme assay.

MUCOPOLYSACCHARIDOSIS (MPS) The mucopolysaccharidoses represent a broad spectrum of disorders due to deficiencies of one of a group of enzymes which degrade three classes of mucopolysaccharides: heparan sulfate, dermatan sulfate, and keratan sulfate. The general MPS phenotype includes coarse facies, corneal clouding, hepatosplenomegaly, joint stiffness, hernias, dysostosis multiplex, mucopolysaccharide excretion in the urine, and metachromatic staining in peripheral leukocytes and bone marrow. Various components of the MPS phenotype are also found in the mucolipidoses, glycoprotein storage disorders, and other lysosomal storage diseases. Detailed clinical and radiologic evaluation and identification of the type of MPS excreted in the urine help to narrow the diagnostic possibilities. Definitive diagnosis requires assay of specific enzymes in various tissues such as cultured skin fibroblasts.

Hurler's or MPS IH disorder is the prototype MPS. Virtually all the components of the phenotype mentioned above are present and expressed in a severe degree. Nasal congestion and grossly visible corneal clouding are early features. Excessive growth during the first year of life is followed by poor growth late in the course. Radiologic features include enlargement of the sella turcica with a distinctive "shoe-shaped" fossa, broadening and shortening of the long bones, and hypoplasia and beaking of the vertebrae in the lumbar area. The vertebral beaking gives rise to an accentuated kyphosis or gibbus deformity. Death occurs within the first decade; postmortem findings include hydrocephalus and cardiovascular disease with occlusion of the coronary arteries. The biochemical defect is α-iduronidase deficiency with accumulation of heparan sulfate and dermatan sulfate.

MPS IS, or Scheie's syndrome, a clinically distinct disorder with childhood onset but adult survival, is characterized by joint stiffness, corneal clouding, aortic regurgitation, and usually normal intelligence. Surprisingly, this much milder disorder is also the result of α-iduronidase deficiency; it is allelic with Hurler's syndrome, as shown by lack of cross-correction of enzyme activity in cocultures of skin fibroblasts. Phenotypes occur that are clearly intermediate between Hurler's and Scheie's syndromes. It is believed that patients with an intermediate phenotype represent genetic compounds with one Hurler's allele and one Scheie's allele. Although genetic compounds must occur, in any one case their existence is difficult to distinguish from still other mutations of intermediate severity.

Hunter's, or MPS II, syndrome is distinguishable from Hurler's phenotype by the absence of gross corneal clouding and the X-linked recessive inheritance. The infantile form resembles the Hurler's disease phenotype, and a milder form allows survival into adulthood.

The severe and mild forms may be allelic, since both are X-linked and share the same enzyme deficiency (iduronosulfate sulfatase).

Sanfilippo's mucopolysaccharidoses (MPS IIIA, IIIB, IIIC, and IIID) are distinguished by the accumulation of heparan sulfate without dermatan or keratan sulfate and by the marked central nervous system involvement with milder somatic involvement. Sanfilippo's mucopolysaccharidosis usually is diagnosed in the evaluation of mental retardation in childhood. Because the somatic features of this MPS are mild, the condition can be overlooked in the evaluation of an apparently isolated central nervous system problem. Death usually occurs during the second or third decade. The MPS III disorders are approximate genocopies. That is, four different enzyme deficiencies give rise to relatively indistinguishable clinical phenotypes with the same storage product. The four MPS III disorders can be diagnosed and distinguished by enzyme assay (Table 316-1).

Morquio's or MPS IV syndrome is distinguished by the absence of mental retardation and the presence of a distinctive bony dystrophy which can be classified as a spondyloepiphyseal dysplasia. Marked hypoplasia of the odontoid process can cause cervical dislocation and usually leads to some degree of spinal cord compression. Aortic regurgitation is frequent. The deficiency of *N*-acetylgalactosamine 6-sulfate sulfatase is the basis for this condition. Bone changes somewhat suggestive of Morquio's syndrome may also occur in β-galactosidase deficiency and in other forms of spondyloepiphyseal dysplasia. Maroteaux-Lamy's or MPS VI disorder is characterized by prominent osseous involvement, corneal clouding, and normal intellect. Allelic forms with variable severity but the same deficiency of arylsulfatase B (*N*-acetylhexosamine 4-sulfate sulfatase) have been described. MPS VII, or β-glucuronidase deficiency, has been described in only a few patients with a rather complete MPS phenotype. Extreme variability from a lethal infantile form to a mild adult disease occurs.

MULTIPLE SULFATASE DEFICIENCY Multiple sulfatase deficiency is a unique disorder, which, although autosomal recessive, is characterized by deficiency of five or more cellular sulfatases. Arylsulfatase A, arylsulfatase B, other mucopolysaccharide sulfatases, and a nonlysosomal steroid sulfatase are deficient in this condition. The clinical picture combines features of metachromatic leukodystrophy, an MPS phenotype, and ichthyosis. The last feature presumably relates to the steroid sulfatase deficiency which also occurs as an isolated X-linked enzyme deficiency characterized by abnormal parturition and ichthyosis. Biochemical studies of this condition should provide further insight into biochemical and clinical genetic heterogeneity.

MUCOLIPIDOSES Mucolipidosis is a general term for lysosomal storage diseases involving some combination of MPS, glycoprotein, oligosaccharide, and glycolipids. The category of mucolipidosis I probably can be abandoned since most or all of these patients actually have a specific glycoprotein storage disease.

Mucolipidosis II, or I-cell disease, is an early onset disorder with mental retardation and an MPS phenotype. The distinctive features are striking inclusions in cultured skin fibroblasts and markedly elevated serum levels of lysosomal enzymes. The disorder has an autosomal recessive basis and is now known to represent a defect in the posttranslational processing of lysosomal enzymes. Mucolipidosis III, or pseudo-Hurler's polydystrophy, is a milder disorder with many aspects of the MPS phenotype, particularly dysostosis multiplex. The disorder presents in the first decade with joint stiffness, the diagnosis of rheumatoid arthritis often being considered. The major handicaps are progressive physical disabilities, particularly claw hand deformity and hip dysplasia. Mild mental retardation is common. Aortic and/or mitral valvular disease is routinely present, although often not functionally significant. Survival into adult life with possible stabilization of the condition is characteristic, with greater disability in males than in females. Inclusions in cultured skin fibroblasts and elevation of serum lysosomal enzymes are essentially identical with the findings in mucolipidosis II, suggesting that these are allelic disorders. The primary defect in mucolipidosis II and III is deficiency of UDP-*N*-acetylglucosamine (GLcNAc):glycoprotein GLcNAc 1-phosphotransferase, an enzyme involved in posttranslational synthesis of the oligosaccharide portion of the lysosomal enzymes.

Mucolipidosis IV is a disorder with mental retardation, corneal clouding, and retinal degeneration without other somatic features. Diagnosis has been made primarily on electron-microscopic findings. A small number of patients, all of Ashkenazi Jewish origin, have been described. The disorder may be due to deficiency of a neuraminidase which is active against ganglioside substrates.

NEURONAL CEROID LIPOFUSCINOSES The neuronal ceroid lipofuscinosis disorders include a wide clinical spectrum with onset in childhood, juvenile, or adult periods. It is uncertain if these disorders are true lysosomal storage diseases, indeed whether single or multiple biochemical genetic disorders are present. The clinical features include central nervous system deterioration with cerebral atrophy, usually commensurate with degree of impairment. Seizures, particularly myoclonic jerks, are prominent. Ocular involvement with optic atrophy, retinitis pigmentosa, and macular degeneration is present in the infantile and juvenile disorders but often absent in adult forms. Autosomal recessive inheritance is likely in most instances. The neuropathologic findings form the basis of the descriptive term for the disease. Electron microscopy demonstrates abnormal inclusions within lysosomes throughout a wide variety of tissues, despite the rather isolated neurologic clinical involvement. The presence of curvilinear bodies, electron-dense material, and fingerprint profiles on electron microscopy of white blood cells, liver biopsy, or muscle biopsy can be helpful diagnostically.

OTHER LYSOSOMAL STORAGE DISEASES Glycogen storage disease type II (Pompe's disease) is the prototype lysosomal storage disease. The predominant clinical features of skeletal and cardiac myopathy are described in Chap. 313. Acid phosphatase deficiency and Farber's lipogranulomatosis are included in Table 316-1. Lactosyl ceramidosis appears to represent a variant of Niemann-Pick disease; in vitro hydrolysis of lactosyl ceramide is accomplished by those enzymes that are deficient in G_{M1} gangliosidosis or in Krabbe's disease, depending upon the in vitro conditions used. Reports of *N*-acetylglucosamine 6-sulfate sulfatase deficiency causing a type VIII mucopolysaccharidosis may be incorrect. Adrenoleukodystrophy is a distinct X-linked disorder with accumulation of long-chain fatty acid cholesteryl esters in tissues, but it may not represent a lysosomal storage disease. The recognition of females with the Hunter's MPS II phenotype and identical enzyme deficiency has raised the possibility of an autosomal recessive form of Hunter's syndrome. Such could occur if the enzyme in question had nonidentical subunits coded for by one autosomal and one X-linked gene or if regulatory genetic elements were invoked. On the other hand phenotypic manifestations in females could be caused by a variety of X-chromosome aberrations. One family has been described with G_{M3} gangliosidosis. This is not a lysosomal storage disease but does possibly represent a defect in ganglioside synthesis. The clinical features are similar to those seen in lysosomal storage diseases, but inconsistencies between siblings leave the question of whether this is a unique genetic disorder. Other neurodegenerative diseases may eventually become classifiable as lysosomal storage diseases. Disorders such as juvenile dystonic lipidosis, neuroaxonal dystrophy, Hallervorden-Spatz disease, Pelizaeus-Merzbacher disease, and other candidates exist. In addition, it is not unusual to identify patients with distinctive clinical features suggestive of lipidosis, mucolipidosis, or mucopolysaccharidosis, in which none of the present biochemically identifiable disorders can be identified. For these reasons, the number of distinct lysosomal storage diseases is likely to continue to increase.

REFERENCES

HERS HG, VAN HOOF F (eds): *Lysosomes and Storage Diseases*. New York, Academic, 1973

HIRSCHHORN R, WEISSMANN G: Genetic disorders of lysosomes, in *Progress in Medical Genetics*, AG Steinberg et al (eds). Philadelphia, Saunders, 1976, vol 1

HO MW et al: Glycosphingolipid hydrolases: Properties and molecular genetics. Mol Cell Biochem 17:125, 1977

MCKUSICK VA: *Heritable Disorders of Connective Tissue*, 4th ed. St Louis, Mosby, 1972

STANBURY JB et al (eds): *The Metabolic Basis of Inherited Disease*, 5th ed. New York, McGraw-Hill, 1983

WARNER TG, O'BRIEN JS: Genetic defects in glycoprotein metabolism. Ann Rev Genet 17:395, 1983

317 OBESITY

JERROLD M. OLEFSKY

The ability to store food energy as fat provides survival value when the food supply is scarce or sporadic. Unlike glycogen or protein, triglyceride does not require water or electrolytes for storage purposes and can be retained essentially as pure fat; 1 g adipose tissue yields close to the full theoretical equivalent of 9 kcal. Because of the efficient storage of energy in adipose tissue, an individual of normal weight can survive up to 2 months of total starvation. However, western society is generally not characterized by periodic or insufficient food supply but rather by constant and abundant food. As a consequence, the ability to store fat all too frequently is of negative survival value because of overconsumption and the resulting obesity.

DEFINITION AND INCIDENCE Obesity can most easily be assessed in terms of height and weight. One way is to relate weight to an average range for height and age. This measure of *relative weight* can lead to an underestimation of the incidence of obesity, since in the United States the "average" individual is somewhat obese. Tables of *ideal* and *desirable* weight are based on actuarial estimates of what is consistent with normal life expectancy. Such tables are more useful if adjusted for differences in body build. An alternative method of estimating obesity is the *body mass index* or *BMI* [(body weight in kg) divided by (height in meters)^2]. For adults ages 20 to 29, the 85th percentile for BMI is 27.8 for males and 27.3 for females. Although relative weight and BMI correlate with the degree of adiposity, excess poundage can be either lean or fat tissue. For example, heavily muscled individuals would be considered obese with these measurements. Nevertheless, such assessments correlate fairly well with the risk of adverse effects on health and longevity. More precise assessment of obesity can be made with measurements of body density or with isotopic dilution methods, but these are unsuitable for routine use. Alternatively anthropometry can be utilized for assessing the degree of adiposity. Assessment of skin-fold thickness over various areas of the body together with height, weight, and age can be used to assess the degree of adiposity. Triceps and subscapular skin folds are most commonly employed (see Chap. 71). From a health standpoint, certain patterns of obesity may be less desirable than others. Fat deposition about the waist and flank, as evidenced by a high ratio of waist to hip circumference, is associated with a greater health risk than fat deposition at the hips.

The term *obesity* implies an excess of adipose tissue, but the meaning of excess is hard to define. Aesthetic considerations aside, obesity can best be viewed as any degree of excess adiposity that imparts a health risk. This cutoff between normal and obese can only be approximated. The Framingham Study demonstrated that a 20 percent excess over desirable weight imparted a health risk. A National Institutes of Health consensus panel on obesity agreed with this definition and concluded that a 20 percent increase in relative weight or a BMI above the 85th percentile for young adults constitutes a health risk; by use of these criteria 20 to 30 percent of adult men and 30 to 40 percent of adult women are obese. Significant health risks at lower levels of obesity can occur in the presence of diabetes, hypertension, heart disease, or other associated risk factors.

ETIOLOGY When caloric intake exceeds expenditure, the excess calories are stored in adipose tissue, and if this net positive caloric balance is prolonged, obesity results, i.e., there are two components to weight balance, and an abnormality on either side (intake or expenditure) can lead to obesity.

The regulation of eating behavior is incompletely understood. To some extent, appetite is controlled by discrete areas in the hypothalamus: a feeding center in the ventrolateral nucleus of the hypothalamus (VLH) and a satiety center in the ventromedial hypothalamus (VMH). The cerebral cortex receives positive signals from the feeding center that stimulate eating (Fig. 317-1), and the satiety center modulates this process by sending inhibitory impulses to the feeding center. In animals destruction of the feeding center results in decreased food intake, and destruction of the satiety center leads to overeating and obesity. Several regulatory processes may influence these hypothalamic centers. The satiety center may be activated by the increases in plasma glucose and/or insulin that follow a meal. It is of interest in this regard that the VMH contains insulin receptors and is insulin-sensitive. Meal-induced gastric distention is another possible inhibitory factor. The total adipose tissue mass may also influence the activity of the hypothalamic centers; i.e., there is a relatively fixed "set point" for body adiposity. An elevated set point may account for the frequent recidivism in obese patients who have lost weight. How the "set point" is established and how the hypothalamus senses total fat stores are unknown. Glycerol release from fat cells and ascending neural impulses may be signals of adipose tissue size. Additionally, the hypothalamic centers are sensitive to catecholamines, and beta-adrenergic stimulation inhibits eating behavior. This provides at least one rationale for the anorexiant effects of amphetamines.

Ultimately, the cerebral cortex controls eating behavior, and impulses from the feeding center to the cerebral cortex are only one input. Psychological, social, and genetic factors also influence food intake. In many obese subjects these influences are overriding; indeed, obese subjects usually respond to external signals such as time of day, social setting, and smell or taste of food to a greater extent than do persons of normal weight.

Although overeating is the usual cause of obesity, other factors may participate. Daily caloric needs range between 31 and 35 kcal per kilogram of body weight; this figure is higher in active and lower in sedentary individuals. Physical activity clearly modulates overall caloric balance, and obese individuals tend to be less active. This

FIGURE 317-1 *The regulation of eating. The ventromedial satiety center is considered to be inhibitory, and the ventrolateral feeding center stimulatory. See text for discussion.*

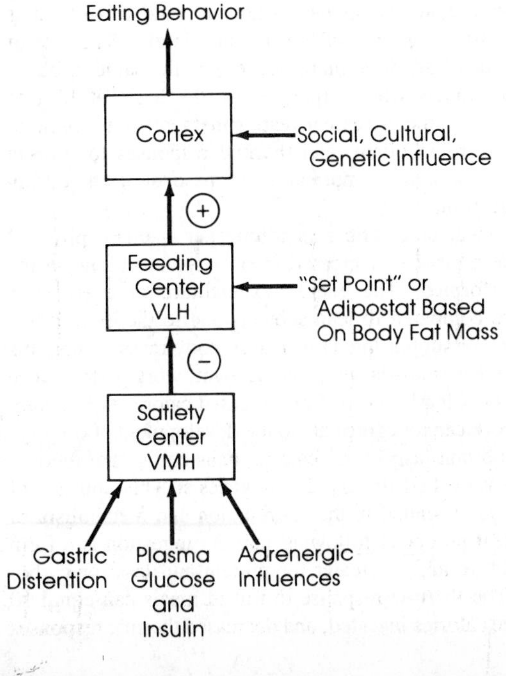

can be a contributory factor in the maintenance of excess weight, but decreased physical activity is unlikely to be an important cause of major weight gain in the most obese subjects. Rather, obesity leads to inactivity. The modest increase in weight that often accompanies the middle years may be related more directly to diminished physical activity. Injury or illness may lead to chronic restricted activity and predispose to weight gain unless caloric intake is appropriately curtailed. Perhaps the greatest factor tending to diminish the output side of the equation is simply a sedentary life-style.

Decreased caloric expenditure and a metabolic abnormality associated with overefficient caloric utilization have also been postulated to be involved in the pathogenesis of obesity. With rare exceptions major metabolic abnormalities have not been detected in obese individuals, although subtle defects may be undetected. There are three major components to overall energy expenditure: resting metabolic rate, exercise-induced thermogenesis, and the thermic response to food.

The resting metabolic rate accounts for 60 to 75 percent of daily caloric expenditure and is measured in a thermoneutral environment while the subject is at rest following an overnight fast and several hours after any significant physical activity. The resting metabolic rate should be expressed as a function of fat-free body weight (by subtracting the subject's total adipose mass from body weight), since triglyceride mass is metabolically inert. When expressed in this way, the resting metabolic rate is normal in most obese subjects. However, a distinction must be made between static obesity and the actual process of gaining weight. When normal subjects consume hypercaloric diets, less weight is gained than would be predicted on the basis of the excess calories ingested. This effect is most marked when carbohydrate is consumed and disappears when the excess calories consist of fat. Thus, humans can apparently partially adapt to chronic excessive carbohydrate and protein intake, and this protective effect attenuates the weight gain. Part of this adaptive response is related to an increase in thermogenesis manifested as an increase in the resting metabolic rate. The mechanism of adaptive thermogenesis is unknown, but overeating of carbohydrate or mixed nutrients leads to increased plasma levels of triiodothyronine (T_3) and decreased levels of reverse T_3 (rT_3). A converse effect is seen in starvation with decreased T_3 and increased rT_3 levels. The conversion of thyroxine to T_3 occurs largely in the liver; excess food may induce adaptive thermogenesis by increasing the concentration of T_3 relative to that of T_4 and rT_3. Increased central or peripheral sympathetic outflow leading to increased catecholamine-induced caloric utilization and increased heat production may also play a role in the thermogenic response to overnutrition. Adaptive thermogenesis can lead to a 10 to 15 percent increase in resting metabolic rate, and this effect is seen after a 2- to 3-week period of hypercaloric intake. The rate of onset and the degree of adaptive thermogenesis is the same in obese and nonobese individuals when expressed on the basis of fat-free body mass. Specifically, the increase in resting metabolic rate, changes in thyroid hormone metabolism, and thermic responses to infused catecholamines are similar in normal and obese subjects during periods of overnutrition.

Work performance, or caloric expenditure per standard physical work load, can be normal or increased in obesity depending on the kind of work performed. The energy expenditure of exercise is increased in obese compared to lean subjects due to the extra effort involved in moving or supporting an increased body mass. When this effect of increased body mass is taken into account, work performance is normal in obesity. Clearly, normal or increased caloric expenditure during physical work cannot contribute to the development of obesity.

The third important aspect of caloric balance is the thermic response to food, so-called dietary thermogenesis. This consists of the heat, or energy, expended in the assimilation and metabolism of foodstuffs. The heat produced following nutrient ingestion is a form of caloric expenditure and is greater for protein and less for carbohydrate and fat. The thermic response to mixed meals can equal 10 to 15 percent of the calories ingested, and decreased thermic responses have been described in human obesity. This difference may be due to altered flux rates through different pathways of intermediary metabolism, with more energy-efficient pathways such as those leading to caloric storage being favored in obesity. As an example, the rate of glucose utilization is related to the extent of the thermic response to carbohydrate-containing meals, and small decreases in the thermic response to food may be due to insulin resistance and decreased glucose disposal in obese subjects. It is clear that small differences in caloric utilization maintained over years can lead to a significant net positive caloric balance. However, while it is tempting to postulate that this decreased thermic response may contribute to obesity, the published comparisons have been made between normal persons and subjects who are already obese. Thus, the obesity-associated changes in thermic response to food may be secondary to the obese state rather than a primary abnormality. More importantly, differences in the thermic response to meals between the obese and nonobese are at most in the range of 30 to 50 kcal per day. Such minor differences can easily be counterbalanced by minor decreases in food intake and/or increases in exercise-induced thermogenesis. Since such compensation does not occur, it seems more probable that obesity is the result of impaired coupling between caloric intake and expenditure.

Another potential regulatory process in the control of adipose tissue mass involves adipose tissue lipoprotein lipase (ATLPL). This enzyme is synthesized within adipocytes, secreted into the extracellular space, and attached to the luminal surface of nearby endothelial cells. At this location ATLPL hydrolyzes fatty acids from the triglycerides of circulating triglyceride-rich lipoproteins. The released fatty acids are taken up by adipocytes, converted to triglycerides, and stored. Thus, ATLPL participates in the storage of excess fat calories in adipose tissue. The *lipoprotein lipase hypothesis* holds that in some obese states excessive levels of this enzyme induce obesity by causing preferential deposition of fat calories in adipose tissue. In support of this hypothesis, ATLPL levels are increased in obese rodents and humans. More importantly, levels of this enzyme do not return to normal following weight reduction. This latter finding is of particular interest since it is one of the few characteristics of the obese state that is not corrected by weight reduction and could explain the propensity of obese patients to regain lost weight.

Certain types of obesity in animals have clear-cut genetic causes, but the role of genetic influences in most human obesity is difficult to evaluate because of confounding social and cultural factors.

SECONDARY OBESITY **Hypothyroidism** Obesity can result from hypothyroidism because of decreased caloric needs. However, only a minority of hypothyroid patients are truly obese, and an even smaller proportion of obese patients are hypothyroid. Indiscriminate use of thyroid hormone in the treatment of obesity is to be deplored and should never be instituted in the absence of documentation of decreased thyroid function.

Cushing's disease Cushing's disease is a rare cause of obesity. Hyperadrenocorticism elicits a typical pattern of obesity with predominantly centripetal fat stores, characteristic rounded or moon facies, and cervical or supraclavicular fat deposits.

Insulinoma Hyperinsulinemia, secondary to an insulinoma, can occasionally cause obesity, presumably because of increased caloric intake secondary to recurrent hypoglycemia. Most patients with islet-cell tumors and hypoglycemia are not obese.

Hypothalamic disorders Froehlich's syndrome in boys is characterized by obesity and hypogonadotrophic hypogonadism with other variable features such as diabetes insipidus, visual impairment, and mental retardation. The anterior pituitary is usually normal, and the syndrome is thought to be the result of hypothalamic dysfunction. This syndrome likely includes a number of overlapping disorders having in common hypothalamic lesion that leads to overeating and to hypogonadotrophism. Occasionally pituitary tumors are present (as in Froehlich's original case) which may physically impair the hypothalamus.

Other rare causes of obesity include the Laurence-Moon-Biedl syndrome characterized by retinitis pigmentosa, mental retardation, skull deformities, polydactyly and syndactyly, and the Prader-Willi syndrome which is associated with hypotonia, mental retardation, and a predilection for diabetes mellitus. Both of these disorders also feature obesity and hypogonadism that are thought to be hypothalamic in origin.

PATHOLOGIC SEQUELAE Increased adipose tissue stores are deposited subcutaneously, around all internal organs, throughout the omentum, and in the intramuscular spaces. Obese individuals also have an expansion of lean body mass as evidenced by increased size of the kidneys, heart, liver, and skeletal muscle mass. Fatty livers are common in extreme obesity.

Adipocyte size and number Attempts have been made to classify obese individuals on the basis of the relative degree of adipocyte hypertrophy versus hyperplasia. This classification scheme was generated as the result of experimental data indicating that in several rodent species and in humans the capacity to increase adipocyte number exists for only a limited period in early life and perhaps at the time of puberty. Thus, prior to reaching adulthood the ability to increase the number of adipocytes declines, and after this time expansion of adipose tissue mass is accompanied primarily by an increase in fat-cell size. Individuals with severe obesity have both increased adipocyte size and number, and those with the greatest degree of adipocyte hyperplasia have a strong tendency toward onset of obesity early in life. Patients having mild to moderate obesity show predominantly adipocyte hypertrophy, and the onset is usually during adult life. Weight reduction leads to a decrease in adipocyte size with no change in cell number. The above observations led to the concept of the existence of a ''critical period'' in early life when final adipocyte number is determined and after which cell number cannot be changed. This formulation implies that alterations in adipocyte number can only be induced during this critical period. However, the concept of a strictly defined critical period for hyperplasia of the adipocytes is only partially correct. When severe obesity is induced in adult rats, both adipocyte number and cell size increase. Adipocyte hypercellularity also occurs in some patients with adult-onset obesity.

Thus while substantial overnutrition at any stage of life can lead to hypertrophy of individual existing adipocytes, there are periods during childhood and adolescence when overnutrition has an enhanced ability to induce the development of new adipocytes. Furthermore, even in adult life, if the degree of overnutrition is sufficient to induce existing adipocytes to enlarge to some limiting size, then new adipocytes will form. Whether this latter population of cells represents new cell formation or simply the filling with lipid of previously undetectable preadipocytes formed earlier in life is not known. Regardless of the cause or time of development of increased adiposity (adipocyte hypertrophy with or without hyperplasia), subsequent weight reduction only leads to a decrease in the size of existing adipocytes and not a decrease in adipocyte number. Thus, once a given complement of adipocytes is attained, this number is fixed and cannot be reduced.

METABOLIC SEQUELAE Obesity has a profound impact on diabetes mellitus and on various hyperlipoproteinemic states primarily through its influences on insulin secretion and insulin sensitivity.

Hyperinsulinemia: Insulin resistance Increased insulin secretion is a common feature of obesity. It occurs in the basal state and in response to a wide variety of insulinogenic agents. A correlation exists between the degree of obesity and the magnitude of the hyperinsulinemia—particularly the basal insulin levels. Some obese patients exhibit hyperglycemia or frank diabetes in the face of hyperinsulinemia. The combination of hyper- or euglycemia and hyperinsulinemia indicates an insulin-resistant state, and decreased hypoglycemic responses to insulin are common in obese humans and animals. Insulin resistance could be due to an abnormal beta-cell product, circulating insulin antagonists, or tissue insulin insensitivity. Since abnormal islet secretory products or circulating antagonists have not been identified, it is thought that the insulin resistance of obesity is primarily due to tissue insensitivity. The initial step in the cellular action of insulin involves binding to cell surface receptors in target tissues. Cells from obese animals and humans contain decreased numbers of insulin receptors, and this decrease doubtless plays a role in the insulin resistance. However, other factors participate. The enlarged adipocytes of obese rats have both a decrease in insulin receptors and an even greater defect in the capacity to metabolize glucose, suggesting a major biochemical abnormality distal to the receptor mechanism. A similar postreceptor defect presumably exists in other insulin target tissues such as muscle and liver. In the obese human insulin resistance is due to a combination of receptor and postreceptor defects in insulin action. In those obese patients with the mildest degree of hyperinsulinemia and insulin resistance, the decrease in insulin action is predominantly due to a decreased number of insulin receptors. As the insulin-resistance state worsens, a postreceptor defect emerges, and in obese subjects with the most severe degree of insulin resistance, the postreceptor defect is the predominant abnormality.

Diabetes mellitus (see also Chap. 327) Although only a minority of obese patients are diabetic, the converse is not the case. Non-insulin-dependent, or type II, diabetes comprises about 90 percent of the diabetic population in the United States, and 80 to 90 percent of type II diabetics are obese. Obesity is an important contributory factor to the diabetes in these patients, predominantly through its influences on insulin resistance. Obesity exacerbates the diabetic state, and in many cases diabetes can be ameliorated by weight reduction.

Hyperlipoproteinemia (see also Chap. 315) Most plasma cholesterol circulates in the low-density lipoprotein (LDL) fraction, and, in the fasting state, very low density lipoproteins (VLDL) contain most of the circulating triglyceride. The association between obesity and elevated LDL levels is modest at best, especially when the relationship is corrected for factors such as age. Total body cholesterol is increased in obesity, but this is mainly accounted for by adipose tissue cholesterol stores. Cholesterol turnover may be increased, leading to increased biliary excretion of cholesterol. This may contribute to the increased incidence of gallstone formation. Obesity has a more pronounced effect on VLDL metabolism. Hypertriglyceridemia is frequent, and the degree of obesity correlates with the level of hypertriglyceridemia. The increased triglyceride levels are due to increased hepatic VLDL production with no defect in the removal of VLDL from plasma. As discussed above, plasma insulin levels are elevated, particularly in the portal venous blood. Hyperinsulinemia can promote increased hepatic VLDL synthesis and secretion. In addition, increased plasma free fatty acid (FFA) turnover exists in obesity, and FFA extraction by the liver provides an important precursor for hepatic triglyceride synthesis. Thus, the hypertriglyceridemia in obesity may be secondary to increased hepatic VLDL secretion due to hyperinsulinemia and augmented FFA availability.

MANIFESTATIONS AND COMPLICATIONS Gross obesity produces mechanical and physical stresses that aggravate or cause a number of disorders including osteoarthritis (especially the hips) and sciatica. Varicose veins, thromboembolism, ventral and hiatal hernias, and cholelithiasis are also more common.

Hypertension In significantly obese persons, use of the standard size blood pressure cuff leads to erroneously high readings; an oversize cuff should always be used. A strong association between hypertension and obesity is observed even when accurate measurements are obtained. The mechanism by which obesity causes hypertension is uncertain, but peripheral vascular resistance is usually normal while blood volume is increased. Weight loss leads to reductions in systemic blood pressure independent of changes in sodium balance.

Hypoventilation syndrome (Pickwickian syndrome) The obesity-hypoventilation syndrome is a heterogeneous group of disorders with differing clinical manifestations. The hypersomnolence that can occur in obesity is a manifestation of nighttime sleep apnea. In these individuals, once sleep begins, upper airway obstruction leads to hypoxemia and hypercapnia, causing arousal with return of normal respiration. Many such episodes occur each night, leading to chronic sleep deprivation and daytime somnolence. The combination of the obese habitus plus sleep-induced relaxation of the pharyngeal musculature is believed to be the cause of the intermittent upper airway obstruction. Occasionally such episodes are life-threatening (causing serious cardiac arrhythmias) and require long-term tracheostomy therapy. Chronic daytime hypoventilation is usually not as severe as that occurring during sleep and may be due to abnormalities of the respiratory control centers. Patients with hypoventilation display blunted ventilatory responses to hypercapnia and hypoxia and often develop hypercapnia and hypoxemia due to decreased basal ventilation; in addition, ventilation-perfusion mismatch may result from mechanical factors. In severe cases polycythemia, pulmonary hypertension, and cor pulmonale can result. Weight reduction will reverse these abnormalities if instituted before permanent cardiac damage develops. Some obese patients with sleep apnea and hypersomnolence do not have daytime hypoventilation and have normal ventilatory responses to hypoxia and hypercapnia. Progestational agents have been used therapeutically in the obesity-hypoventilation syndrome since they stimulate the ventilatory response to hypercapnia and hypoxia in normal subjects. Medroxyprogesterone increases ventilation and improves heart failure and erythrocytosis in these patients, although obstructive sleep apnea continues.

Adrenal function Although Cushing's disease can usually be distinguished from simple obesity on clinical grounds, laboratory testing is occasionally necessary. This can lead to confusion since 24-h urinary 17-hydroxycorticoid excretion is often elevated in obesity. Less commonly, plasma cortisol levels are also increased. Corticosteroid levels are usually suppressible with dexamethasone in obesity, but occasionally suppression is incomplete, rendering the diagnosis difficult (also see Chap. 325).

Growth hormone Secretory responses of growth hormone to a variety of stimuli such as hypoglycemia, exercise, and arginine infusion are reduced, and the starvation-induced rise in plasma growth hormone levels is attenuated.

Atherosclerosis Obesity is a risk factor for the development of coronary artery disease and stroke. Most of the risk is mediated through the associated hypertension, hyperlipoproteinemia, and diabetes. Nevertheless, even when these abnormalities are factored out, an additional, smaller risk can be ascribed to obesity per se.

TREATMENT Amelioration of hyperinsulinemia, insulin resistance, diabetes, hypertension, and hyperlipidemia can occur following weight loss. These changes are significant and enduring provided the weight loss is maintained. During weight loss all adipose tissue depots diminish proportionately. Sometimes generalized loss does not produce the attractive cosmetic effects desired. Many techniques have been proposed to effect selective adipose tissue reduction over particular regions of the body, but none is effective.

Methods of weight reduction In instances where obesity is secondary, the appropriate therapy is to treat the underlying disease. Most of the time the difficult problem of primary weight reduction must be undertaken.

Diet Caloric restriction is the cornerstone of weight reduction. From the standpoint of patient and physician this is a frustrating and demanding undertaking. The basic principles are simple. If caloric intake is less than caloric expenditure, stored calories, predominantly in the form of fat, will be consumed. In general, a deficit of 7700 kcal leads to loss of about 1 kg fat. By estimating the patient's daily caloric needs (approximately 30 to 35 kcal per kilogram of body weight) one can calculate the daily deficit necessary to achieve a given rate of weight loss.

Dietary restriction can range from total starvation to mild caloric deprivation, and these approaches will be discussed separately. Dietary recommendations are most effective when they are specific and geared to the patient's life-style. A dietitian or a similarly trained health professional should interview each patient and estimate average daily caloric intake, identify food preferences, and characterize the eating patterns. The amount of calories to be consumed on the restricted diet should be carefully explained in terms of quantities of specific foodstuffs. Frequently, the therapist must balance the degree of restriction against potential noncompliance. The more restrictive the diet, the more rapid the weight loss, but this often leads to a greater rate of nonadherence. It is preferable to design a diet with which the patient is comfortable and that produces a modest but steady weight loss.

Schemes for weight reduction have become a multimillion-dollar business in the United States, and there are almost as many diets as there are therapists. Each proponent claims that the presence or absence of certain foodstuffs is desirable for more effective weight loss. However, little evidence exists to support the claim that calorie for calorie one hypocaloric diet will lead to a greater weight loss than another. The relationship between the patient and the therapist, plus patient education and encouragement, are more important to success than are the specific dietary constituents. The major virtue of "fad" diets is that patients are usually motivated to try them, at least initially, and patient cooperation is often better. Provided a particular diet is not harmful, probably the best course for the therapist is to maintain flexibility in the treatment program. Nevertheless, diets markedly deficient in any major class of foodstuff are to be avoided. For example, whole-food diets that are exceedingly low in carbohydrate are by nature high in fat and, depending on the type and quantity of fat ingested, may lead to hypercholesterolemia. The major virtue of a low-carbohydrate diet is the attendant ketosis (ketone bodies have a central anorexant effect). This provides part of the rationale for the widely touted liquid or powdered protein diets. These diets have been dubbed "protein-sparing modified fasts," and claims have been made that they allow drastic long-term caloric restriction without inducing negative nitrogen balance. These claims have not been substantiated, nor has it been shown that the diets lead to a greater degree of tissue weight loss than mixed diets of equal caloric value. Basically a calorie is a calorie whether it comes from protein, carbohydrate, or fat. Furthermore, deaths have been reported in otherwise healthy individuals participating in such long-term dietary programs, even under medical supervision. This has been attributed to the fact that some of these diets contain mostly protein of low biologic value. Other very low calorie diets involve formula preparations containing 350 to 800 kcal per day, with 40 to 80 g of high-quality protein. The remaining calories consist of carbohydrate and fat. Vitamin and micronutrient supplements are incorporated in the formula or provided as an added supplement. Such very low calorie diets lead to relatively rapid weight loss but should not be taken continuously as the sole caloric source for more than 6 weeks. In the absence of coexisting diseases such as gout, renal insufficiency, cardiac arrhythmias, etc., such diets are safe when taken under medical supervision.

Prior to therapy it is wise to warn patients that when caloric restriction is started there is usually a marked initial weight loss, in large part due to fluid loss, but that such rapid rates of loss will not persist. Likewise, positive shifts in fluid balance can sometimes mask loss of adipose mass, a fact that can sometimes be demonstrated to the patient's satisfaction by recording skin-fold thickness at periodic intervals.

Total-starvation diets have been advocated for the treatment of obesity; provided gout, renal insufficiency, and ketosis-prone diabetes are not present, short-term (2- to 3-day) fasts are usually well tolerated. Ketonemia and hyperuricemia regularly develop during starvation but rarely lead to acidosis or gout. Because of these potential complications, total fasting should be carried out only under medical supervision. Probably the major usefulness of total fasting is as a motivational aid at the beginning of a dietary program or when weight loss has stopped. Even though much of the weight loss during short-term fasting represents fluid, this weight loss can be encouraging to frustrated patients and motivate them to improve compliance with the long-term weight reduction program.

The major problem in the treatment of obesity is not weight reduction but maintenance of the reduced weight. Provided the therapist works hard and long enough, most motivated patients can eventually lose weight. Unfortunately, only the rare patient maintains the weight loss permanently. Obesity is an eating disorder, and the underlying mechanisms are not reversed by limiting food intake.

Behavior modification In recognition of the problems involved, the techniques of behavior modification have been devised to treat abnormal patterns of eating behavior. Many studies demonstrate that obese individuals respond less well than normal individuals to internal cues that regulate eating behavior such as gastric contractions, fear, and previous food ingestion. Conversely, obese subjects overrespond to external cues such as taste, smell, food attractiveness, food abundance, and the ease of obtaining food. Given the fact that the obese individual is unusually susceptible to external stimuli, food intake may be altered by changing the pattern and nature of these external cues, and this is the major premise underlying the behavior modification approach to weight reduction.

Behavior modification begins with a detailed individual history of the patient's eating patterns with respect to time of day, length of eating period, place of ingestion (restaurant, dining table, standing in front of open refrigerator), simultaneous activities (watching television, reading, idleness), emotional state, companions (relatives, friends, or alone), and finally the kinds and quantities of foods ingested. Once this detailed record is obtained, the therapist and patient can design specific behavioral changes aimed at disrupting or aborting recurring behavior patterns which initiate or prolong abnormal eating activity. As examples: if a patient eats in response to certain emotional states, then other activities can be substituted when the patient perceives such a state; if the patient snacks frequently from readily available food storage areas (refrigerators, cookie jars, etc.), then he or she is encouraged to eat only while sitting down at a table with a fixed place setting; if eating frequently occurs while watching television alone, then efforts to avoid this activity can be initiated. Many other examples of specific and general interventions could be given. Results with behavior modification techniques indicate that many patients can maintain long-term weight reduction providing the new behavior patterns are truly "learned."

Exercise Exercise has a place in any weight reduction program. However, the importance of exercise in terms of caloric balance must be clearly understood. Even moderate daily exercise would not lead to a large enough increase in caloric expenditure to alter significantly the initial rate of weight reduction (Table 317-1). This does not mean exercise is unimportant in weight reduction, since even modest increases in caloric expenditure can lead to large long-term differences in caloric balance, provided exercise is performed on a regular basis. For example, a daily increase in caloric expenditure of 300 kcal over a period of 4 months could lead to a 4.5-kg weight loss. More importantly, incorporation of regular exercise into the overall weight reduction program improves the chances that the patient will maintain the weight loss.

Drugs Two classes of drugs are frequently used in the treatment of obesity: anorexants and thyroid hormone supplements. The addition of L-thyroxine or triiodothyronine to a weight reduction program is of no benefit. These drugs are ineffective in promoting adipose tissue loss and, if anything, accentuate lean tissue loss and cause negative nitrogen balance. In susceptible individuals, cardiotoxicity may occur. Thus, unless clear-cut hypothyroidism is present, thyroid supplementation has no role in the treatment of obesity.

The major anorexants are amphetamine-like agents that presumably exert their effect at the level of the hypothalamus. They probably have a modest effect in promoting short-term weight loss in some individuals. However, they are effective only for short periods, and problems of habituation, addiction, and generalized drug abuse limit their usefulness. Two anorexants, diethylpropion and fenfluramine, may be less addictive and, therefore, somewhat more useful. However, none of these agents treats the underlying eating disorder, and they are of little use in maintenance of weight reduction.

Injections of human chorionic gonadotropin (hCG) have been tried as an adjunct to weight reduction, but no evidence exists to indicate

TABLE 317-1 Energy equivalents of food calories expressed in minutes of activity

		Activity				
Food	Calories, kcal	Walking*	Riding bicycle†	Swimming‡	Running§	Reclining¶
Apple, large	101	19	12	9	5	78
Bacon, 2 strips	96	18	12	9	5	74
Beer, 1 glass	114	22	14	10	6	88
Bread and butter	78	15	10	7	4	60
Carbonated beverage, 1 glass	106	20	13	9	5	82
Carrot, raw	42	8	5	4	2	32
Cheese, cottage, 1 tbsp	27	5	3	2	1	21
Chicken, fried, ½ breast	232	45	28	21	12	178
Cookie, chocolate chip	51	10	6	5	3	39
Egg, fried	110	21	13	10	6	85
Ham, 2 slices	167	32	20	15	9	128
Ice cream, ⅙ qt	193	37	24	17	10	148
Mayonnaise, 1 tbsp	92	18	11	8	5	71
Milk, skim, 1 glass	81	16	10	7	4	62
Milk shake	421	81	51	38	22	324
Orange, medium	68	13	8	6	4	52
Pancake with syrup	124	24	15	11	6	
Peas, green, ½ cup	56	11	7	5	3	43
Pizza, cheese, ⅛	180	35	22	16	9	138
Potato chips, 1 serving	108	21	13	10	6	83
Sandwiches:						
Hamburger	350	67	43	31	18	269
Tuna fish salad	278	53	34	25	14	214
Sherbet, ⅙ qt	177	34	22	16	9	136

* *Energy cost of walking for 70-kg individual = 5.2 kcal/min at 3.5 mph.*
† *Energy cost of riding bicycle = 8.2 kcal/min.*
‡ *Energy cost of swimming = 11.2 kcal/min.*
§ *Energy cost of running = 19.4 kcal/min.*
¶ *Energy cost of reclining = 1.3 kcal/min.*

a beneficial effect. The primary effectiveness of the hCG-diet program is due to the calorically restricted diet, frequent physician contact, and placebo effects. Comparable weight loss is achieved if saline injections are substituted for hCG, suggesting a placebo or physiologic effect of the act of parenteral injection.

Jejunoileal shunt Small-bowel bypass is an effective means of achieving weight reduction in morbidly obese patients. However, it is an experimental procedure and should be attempted only in institutions where a trained team is committed to regular, systematic, and long-term follow-up.

The most common operative procedures involve end-to-end or end-to-side anastomosis of about 38 cm of proximal jejunum to 10 cm of terminal ileum. Weight loss is initially rapid, reaching a plateau at 18 to 24 months. While all patients lose weight, few return to ideal weight. The mean weight loss is about 30 to 50 percent of initial excess weight, leaving patients still about 50 percent overweight once a steady state is reached. Although some degree of malabsorption occurs, the major portion of the weight loss is due to decreased food intake.

Most teams performing this surgery select patients who are at least 50 kg overweight and in whom adequate attempts at medical management have failed repeatedly. Because of postoperative morbidity, older patients (>50 years) and psychologically unstable individuals are usually excluded.

The overall surgical mortality ranges from 0.5 to 7.8 percent with an average of around 4 percent. Mortality is inversely related to the experience of the surgical team. The major postoperative morbidity is related to wound infection and thromboembolism. The common serious medical complications are cirrhosis and hepatic failure, nephrolithiasis, electrolyte imbalances, cholelithiasis, and arthritis (Table 317-2). Severe liver disease probably occurs in 5 percent of patients, and milder degrees of hepatic dysfunction are more common. The long-range implications of mild hepatic abnormalities are unknown. Possible causes of liver damage following small-bowel bypass include (1) protein and particularly essential amino acid deficiency, (2) accumulation of hepatotoxic, secondary bile salts, and (3) release of unknown toxic substances from the excluded bowel. Hypokalemia is most likely secondary to diarrhea. Persistent deficiency of calcium and magnesium can result from malabsorption and must be treated with appropriate replacement. Transient depression of plasma 25-hydroxyvitamin D levels may also contribute to abnormal mineral metabolism. Nephrolithiasis occurs in up to 30 percent of patients and is due to hyperoxaluria secondary to calcium malabsorption. It can be treated by calcium supplements and a low oxalate intake. Migratory polyarthritis occurs in up to 6 percent of patients and may be due to circulating immune complexes. This operation is now rarely performed, in part due to the decision of many insurance companies not to render compensation for this procedure.

TABLE 317-2 Complications of bypass surgery

Complication	Percentage
EARLY	
Perioperative mortality	2–6
Thromboembolic disease	1–5
Wound infection	2–5
Renal failure	3
Severe nausea, vomiting	3
Wound dehiscence	1–3
LATE	
Urinary calculi	3–10
Severe electrolyte imbalance	5–8
Acute cholecystitis	0–5
Progressive liver disease	2–4
Intestinal obstruction	2
Peptic ulcer	1–2
Osteoporosis	?
Tuberculosis	1
MINOR	
Diarrhea	100
Weakness	80
Hypokalemia	80
Hypoproteinemia	50
Vomiting	50
Thirst	50
Hypocalcemia	30
Arthralgias	15
Incisional hernias	3
Hyperuricemia	<10
Anemias	<10

Gastric surgery Gastroplasty establishes a small upper gastric remnant connected to a larger lower gastric pouch by a narrow 1- to 1.5-cm channel. Gastric bypass excludes the lower 90 percent of the stomach pouch and maintains intestinal continuity of the upper 10 percent via a retrocolic gastrojejunostomy. Both of these procedures cause patients to limit food intake by delaying gastric emptying and providing a small gastric reservoir so that fullness is experienced after a small meal. Weight loss with these procedures is comparable with that achieved with small-bowel bypass operations but without the complications related to malabsorption, diarrhea, and hepatic dysfunction. The procedure can be reversed if a decision to restore normal anatomy is made at a later time. For these reasons, gastroplasty is frequently performed for the surgical treatment of morbid obesity, especially since the number of intestinal bypass procedures has decreased.

SUMMARY For most patients obesity is an eating disorder, and a major hope for effective long-term treatment of this disease lies in understanding the causes of overeating. No single etiology explains all cases, and different causes exist for different individuals. At present a variety of techniques are available to effect initial weight loss. Unfortunately, initial weight loss is not the real therapeutic goal. Rather, the problem is that most obese patients eventually regain their weight. An effective means to sustain weight loss is the major challenge in the treatment of obesity today. The technique of behavioral modification, when professionally and rigorously applied, is the best tool for this task. As information develops concerning the hypothalamic "set point," or *adipostat*, and the factors that regulate it, other therapies may emerge that will effect long-term correction of abnormal eating patterns.

REFERENCES

ASSIMACOPOULOS-JEANNET F, JEANRENAUD B: The hormonal and metabolic basis of experimental obesity. Clin Endocrinol Metab 5:337, 1976

BRAY GA: Current status of intestinal bypass surgery in the treatment of obesity. Diabetes 26:1072, 1977

FOSTER DW: Eating disorders: Obesity and anorexia nervosa, in *Williams Textbook of Endocrinology,* 7th ed, JD Wilson, DW Foster (eds). Philadelphia, Saunders, 1985, p 1081

HASHIM SA, PORIKOS K: Food intake behavior in man: Implications for treatment of obesity. Clin Endocrinol Metab 5:503, 1976

HENRY RR et al: Metabolic consequences of very low calorie diet therapy in obese non-insulin dependent diabetic and non-diabetic subjects. Diabetes 35:155, 1986

HORTON ES, DANFORTH E JR: Energy metabolism and obesity, in *Diabetes Mellitus and Obesity,* SJ Bleicher, BN Brodoff (eds). Baltimore, Williams & Wilkins, 1981, p 261

KOLTERMAN OG et al: Mechanisms of insulin resistance in human obesity. Evidence for receptor and postreceptor defects. J Clin Invest 65:1272, 1980

MANN GV: The influence of obesity on health. N Engl J Med 291:226, 1974

NATIONAL INSTITUTES OF HEALTH CONSENSUS DEVELOPMENT PANEL ON THE HEALTH IMPLICATIONS OF OBESITY: Health implications of obesity. Ann Intern Med 103:147, 1985

OLEFSKY JM et al: Insulin action and insulin resistance in obesity and non-insulin dependent, type II diabetes mellitus. Am J Physiol 243:E15, 1982

SALANS L: The obesities, in *Endocrinology and Metabolism,* P Felig et al (eds). New York, McGraw-Hill, 1981, p 891

WOO R et al: Regulation of energy balance, in *Annual Review of Nutrition,* vol 5. Palo Alto, Annual Reviews Inc, 1985, pp 411–433

318 THE LIPODYSTROPHIES AND OTHER RARE DISORDERS OF ADIPOSE TISSUE

DANIEL W. FOSTER

This chapter is concerned with abnormalities in adipose tissue. The disorders are rare, the pathophysiology is frequently not clear, and only clinical descriptions can be given.

THE LIPODYSTROPHIES

The lipodystrophies are characterized by generalized or partial loss of body fat and metabolic abnormalities, including insulin resistance, hyperglycemia, and hypertriglyceridemia. A classification is shown in Table 318-1. In *generalized lipodystrophy* essentially all body fat is lost, while in *partial lipodystrophy* fat atrophy is limited. The common acquired form of partial lipodystrophy ordinarily involves half the body, usually the upper segment. Dominantly transmitted partial lipodystrophy tends to spare the face. One variant is associated with eye and tooth malformations, the Rieger anomaly. *Localized lipodystrophy* may be either inflammatory or noninflammatory. The best-studied syndrome is *centrifugal lipodystrophy* in which fat atrophy begins in the groins or axillae of children under the age of 3 and spreads centrally to involve the entire abdomen. The edge of the lesion is red and scaly with an inflammatory infiltrate demonstrable on histologic examination. Fat atrophy usually disappears spontaneously when the patient is around 13 years of age.

GENERALIZED LIPODYSTROPHY Generalized lipodystrophy (also called lipoatrophic diabetes) may be either congenital or acquired. The congenital form is transmitted as an autosomal recessive trait. Males and females are equally affected. Rates of parental consanguinity are high. Loss of fat is usually obvious at birth, but the rest of the clinical picture may not appear until later (up to 30 years). The acquired disease often develops after some other illness. Measles, chicken pox, whooping cough, or infectious mononucleosis are common precipitating events, but hypothyroidism, hyperthyroidism, and pregnancy have been implicated. Some cases begin with the appearance of painful nodular swellings of adipose tissue resembling acute panniculitis (see below). The congenital and acquired forms are similar in clinical manifestations (Table 318-2).

Fat atrophy Loss of body fat is the characteristic feature. In congenital cases the skin of the face is tightly drawn over the bony structures, and the entire body is devoid of adipose tissue. Rarely, a small amount of breast fat remains. In the acquired form the face may be spared, but all other fat disappears. Adipose tissue cells can be identified microscopically, but they contain no triglyceride stores. Paradoxically the liver is engorged with fat, and the reticuloendothelial system contains lipid-laden macrophages (foam cells). The cause of the fat atrophy is not known. Fat-mobilizing polypeptides have been reported in the urine of patients with generalized lipodystrophy, but their role in the disease is uncertain.

A candidate molecule for the induction of lipodystrophy is a compound similar to cachectin (tumor necrosis factor), which has powerful inhibitory effects on lipoprotein lipase and results in fat depletion and hypertriglyceridemia when injected into animals. Lipoprotein lipase activity is low in generalized lipodystrophy, as would be predicted if a cachectin-like inducer were the cause. Hepatic lipase is not impaired. Since triglyceride content of the adipocyte is the result of a balance between fat synthesis and fat breakdown, an alternative mechanism might involve activation of the hormone-sensitive lipase that catalyzes hydrolysis of triglycerides in the fat cell. For example, a defect in a natural inhibitor of the lipase, such as adenosine, could result in enhanced response to physiologic (nonelevated) concentrations of lipolytic hormones. Release of free fatty acids into plasma following norepinephrine infusion is impaired, but this may simply reflect the depleted triglyceride stores.

Although an inducing molecule could act as a circulating hormone in generalized lipodystrophy, such an etiology is unlikely in partial lipodystrophy where autotransplantation of adipocytes from an affected area to a nonaffected site resulted in reaccumulation of fat, and reverse transplantation from normal to affected site resulted in fat atrophy. An autocrine or paracrine function may be involved. In the former a cellular product would act on the cell of origin while in the latter a cellular product would act on adjacent cells, but in neither case would the putative inducer of lipodystrophy enter the circulation to act as a typical hormone.

Growth and maturation Linear growth is accelerated in the first few years of life in the congenital disorder and in acquired disease that begins early in childhood. Epiphyses close early, however, so that the final height is usually normal. True muscular hypertrophy is present, and patients may have an acromegalic appearance with coarse facial features and large hands and feet. The ears tend to be prominent in the congenital form. Many viscera are enlarged, and generalized lymphadenopathy may be present. The cause of the growth disorder is not known. Levels of growth hormone and insulin-like growth factor I (IGF-I/SM-C) are normal or low. Insulin-like growth factor II has not been systematically assessed. One possibility is that abnormal growth and pseudoacromegaly are due to high concentrations of insulin in plasma secondary to insulin resistance (see below). The elevated insulin might cross-react with the IGF-I/SM-C receptor in muscle and cartilage and promote growth via this mechanism.

Liver Enlargement of the liver causes protuberance of the abdomen. Fatty liver may progress to cirrhosis, especially in the acquired disorder. Several patients have died from bleeding esophageal varices. Splenomegaly does not occur in the absence of portal hypertension.

Kidneys The kidneys are usually enlarged. Subjects with the acquired disorder may have proteinuria and the nephrotic syndrome, although not as frequently as in partial lipodystrophy. Moderate hypertension is common.

Genitalia The external genitalia (penis and testes in males, clitoris and labia majora in females) are usually hypertrophied in congenital disease. In women polycystic ovaries are common, resulting in the clinical picture of Stein-Leventhal syndrome. The cause of the genital abnormalities is not known. Systematic investigation of gonadotropin, estrogen, and androgen metabolism has not been carried out.

Skin Acanthosis nigricans is present in most. Hypertrichosis of face, neck, trunk, and limbs is frequent. Scalp hair is usually thick and curly, particularly early in life.

Central nervous system Mental retardation is present in about half the congenital cases. Dilatation of the third ventricle and basal cisterns has been demonstrated by pneumoencephalography. Central nervous system involvement appears to be less marked in the acquired disease, although two patients had astrocytomas arising in the floor of the third ventricle. Few patients have been examined with computerized tomography or magnetic resonance imaging.

TABLE 318-1 The lipodystrophies

1 Generalized lipodystrophy
- *a* Congenital (familial or sporadic)
- *b* Acquired (sporadic)

2 Partial lipodystrophy
- *a* Common (sporadic)
- *b* Dominant (familial)
  - (*1*) Limb and trunk
  - (*2*) With Rieger anomaly

3 Localized lipodystrophy
- *a* Inflammatory
- *b* Noninflammatory

TABLE 318-2 Characteristics of the lipodystrophies

Finding	Congenital general	Acquired general	Acquired partial	Dominant partial
Inheritance	Autosomal recessive	Sporadic	Usually sporadic	Autosomal dominant
Age of onset	Infancy	Childhood to adult	Childhood to adult	Puberty
Sex incidence	Males and females equal	Female preponderance	Female preponderance	Female preponderance
Lipoatrophy	Face, trunk, limbs	Face, trunk, limbs	Face, upper trunk, upper limbs	Trunk and limbs
Liver involvement	+	++	Rare	0
Renal disease	+	+	++	0
Insulin resistance	+	+	+	+
Hyperglycemia	+	+	+	+
Hypertriglyceridemia	+	+	+	+
Acanthosis nigricans	+	+	Rare	+
Genital hypertrophy	+	+	Rare	+
Bone age	Accelerated	Normal to accelerated	Normal	Normal

Other abnormalities Bones tend to be sclerotic in generalized lipodystrophy, and cystic angiomatosis may be present. Cardiomegaly is common, but heart failure appears to be rare. Goiter is frequent. The associated abnormalities in generalized lipodystrophy are summarized in Table 318-3.

Metabolic and endocrine abnormalities Three major metabolic disturbances are characteristic.

1 *Severe insulin resistance with hyperglycemia.* Insulin resistance may be mild or severe. Insulin and C-peptide concentrations are relatively or absolutely elevated, and response to exogenous insulin is impaired. Resistance is due to several causes, and affected siblings may exhibit different mechanisms. Increased insulin clearance, decreased number of insulin receptors, diminished affinity of the receptor for insulin, and postreceptor defects have all been reported. Insulin in the plasma of affected subjects is biologically active. Although glucagon levels are high (indicating insulin resistance in the alpha cell of the islets of Langerhans) and free fatty acid concentrations are elevated, ketoacidosis is unusual. One patient had recurrent epidoses of metabolic acidosis considered to be ketoacidosis, but concentrations of acetoacetate and β-hydroxybutyrate were characteristic of fasting ketosis, not ketoacidosis; presumably lactate or other organic acids were involved.

   Ketoacidosis may be infrequent because insulin resistance spares liver and skeletal muscle (or is less severe); glycogen levels in the liver are high (insulin stimulates glycogen synthesis), and branched-chain amino acids fall normally in response to injected insulin. Elevated insulin levels in portal vein plasma would counteract the actions of glucagon in the insulin-responsive hepatocyte. This would prevent activation of the ketone body synthesis in liver and assure utilization of incoming fatty acids for triglyceride synthesis and production of very low density lipoproteins. The elevated long-chain fatty acids in the plasma are of dietary origin and fall toward normal with restriction of dietary fat. The diabetes mellitus accompanying lipodystrophy appears to be typical apart from insulin resistance, including the propensity to develop late degenerative complications.

2 *Hypertriglyceridemia with accumulation of both chylomicrons and very low density lipoproteins in the blood.* Eruptive xanthomas, lipemia retinalis, and recurrent pancreatitis may be seen. Although lipoprotein lipase is low, as noted, and there is a defect in disposal of triglycerides in the atrophied fat tissue, the major cause for the hypertriglyceridemia is overproduction of very low density lipoproteins (VLDL) in the liver. This overproduction is probably driven by the elevated free fatty acids in blood since dietary fat restriction results in a fall of VLDL production rates toward normal. Hyperinsulinemia may contribute by enhancing hepatic fat synthesis.

3 *A hypermetabolic state with normal thyroid function.* Basal metabolic rates are usually elevated although thyroid hormone values (thyroxine, triiodothyronine, reverse triiodothyronine) are normal. Patients do not gain weight with excessive caloric intake, indicating a facile capacity to waste calories as heat. Food intakes as high as 5000 kcal per day are not unusual. One 16-month-old child ate 2400 kcal/day. Following thyroidectomy in one patient, the basal metabolic rate decreased but did not return to normal; symptoms and signs of hypothyroidism supervened requiring treatment with thyroid hormone despite continued high metabolic rates. It thus seems clear that hypermetabolism is not due to hyperthyroidism. There is also no evidence of mitochondrial disease. Abnormal dietary thermogenesis is the likely cause of the increased metabolic rate. Metabolic rates are increased by fat, carbohydrate, and protein in the diet, but protein is the most important. There is no evidence for adrenal medullary dysfunction.

Course and treatment Patients with generalized lipodystrophy may die at an early age. Hepatic failure, hemorrhage from esophageal varices, and renal failure are common causes of death. Despite the almost constant hypertriglyceridemia, symptomatic coronary artery disease is rare. There is no specific treatment for lipodystrophy, although moderate caloric and fat restriction (sufficient to maintain weight) is generally recommended. Medium-chain triglyceride supplementation has been reported to be of benefit. Pimozide therapy, hypophysectomy, and plasmapheresis are ineffective.

ACQUIRED PARTIAL LIPODYSTROPHY This is the most common of the lipodystrophies and usually affects women. Fat atrophy occurs in the upper half of the body, including the face, but spares the lower extremities. Rarely the lower half of the body is affected, leaving the upper torso intact. Occasionally the lesion affects only one side. The other anatomic features of generalized lipodystrophy are usually absent, and liver disease is unusual. Proteinuria, with or without the nephrotic syndrome, occurs more frequently than in other forms. The complement system is abnormal, and C3 levels tend to be low. C3 nephritic factor, a polyclonal IgG immunoglobulin that interacts with alternative pathway convertase to augment C3 activation, is present in serum. C3 levels may be low in unaffected first-degree relatives, but C3 nephritic factor is absent. Complement abnormalities disappeared after renal transplantation in one subject. Dermatomyositis and Sjögren's syndrome may occur. Rarely partial lipodystrophy progresses to the generalized form of the disease.

LIPODYSTROPHY WITH DOMINANT TRANSMISSION This variant is characterized by fat atrophy of the limbs and trunk with sparing of the face, which may actually be rounded. The neck may also be exempt. The disease usually begins at puberty but may not appear until middle age. Males are rarely affected. In families with the Rieger anomaly onset tends to be in infancy. Insulin resistance and hyperglycemia are usual, and severe hypertriglyceridemia with eruptive xanthoma may occur. The labia majora are hypertrophied, and polycystic ovaries may be seen. Acanthosis nigricans is usually present. Liver and renal disease do not occur.

TABLE 318-3 Accompanying abnormalities of lipodystrophy

Bone	Sclerosis, cystic angiomatosis
Brain	Mental retardation, third ventricle dilatation
Genitalia	Clitoromegaly, polycystic ovaries, penile hypertrophy
Heart	Cardiomegaly
Kidneys	Hypertrophy without renal failure
Liver	Hepatomegaly, fatty liver, cirrhosis, hepatic failure
Lymph nodes	Generalized lymphadenopathy
Skin	Acanthosis nigricans, hypertrichosis
Thyroid	Goiter, euthyroid state

MULTIPLE SYMMETRIC LIPOMATOSIS

Multiple symmetric lipomatosis, a disease found predominantly in men, is characterized by formation of multiple nonencapsulated lipomas in various areas. Two patterns of distribution are noted. In the *type I* variant, lipomas are primarily in the nape of the neck and in the supraclavicular and deltoid regions, resulting in an extraordinary bull-necked appearance (*Madelung collar*). Extension into the mediastinum may produce obstruction of the trachea or vena cava. Fat over the remainder of the body appears normal. In the *type II* pattern, lipomas are not localized to the neck but extend down over the body giving the appearance of simple obesity. Correct diagnosis requires recognition that the fat masses are symmetric and that the distal arms and legs are spared. Deep lipomatosis is absent in type II disease, and vena caval and tracheal compression do not occur.

Multiple symmetric lipomatosis may occur sporadically or in families. Autosomal dominant transmission has been postulated in the latter. Alcoholism is common. Coexisting folate deficiency, macrocytic anemia, and abnormal liver function may be due to alcohol and not lipomatosis. Neuropathy, which may be sensory, motor, or autonomic, is prominent, and neuropathic foot ulcers may be present.

Metabolic abnormalities include hyperuricemia, hypertriglyceridemia (VLDL, chylomicrons) and, paradoxically, an elevation of high-density lipoproteins (HDL) as well. Diabetes has not been reported, although hyperinsulinism may be present. A few patients have had renal tubular acidosis.

The cause of multiple symmetric lipomatosis is not known. The fat cells are slightly smaller than normal, suggesting hyperplasia. Isolated adipocytes appear to have a marked increase in lipoprotein lipase activity and a defect in adrenergic lipolysis. Lipolytic response to cyclic AMP is intact, suggesting an abnormality at the hormone receptor/adenylate cyclase unit. The biochemical abnormalities are not present in all cases.

There is no treatment except for surgical removal of lipomas that cause compression. They may also be removed for cosmetic reasons.

MEDIASTINO-ABDOMINAL LIPOMATOSIS

This syndrome may be a variant of multiple symmetric lipomatosis. The features include (1) exertional dyspnea due to compression of airways by lipomas of the mediastinum, (2) massive enlargement of the abdomen (pseudoascites) due to intraperitoneal and retroperitoneal fat, and (3) abnormal glucose tolerance or diabetes mellitus. The metabolic abnormalities and enzymic changes in adipocytes are identical with those in multiple symmetric lipomatosis except that HDL levels are not elevated.

ACUTE PANNICULITIS (NODULAR FAT NECROSIS)

The appearance of single or multiple crops of tender nodules in subcutaneous fat with a histologic picture of fat-cell necrosis, infiltration of inflammatory cells, and development of fat-filled macrophages (foam cells) is the hallmark of acute panniculitis. The nodules range in size from 0.5 to 10 cm and may be firm or fluctuant. They are usually, but not always, tender. On occasion they drain an oily solution, and suppuration may occur. Individual lesions last from 1 to 8 weeks before disappearing, and a pigmented depressed area may be left at the involved site. While some patients have only nodular panniculitis, which may or may not be relapsing, others develop fever, abnormal liver function, involvement of the bone marrow with leukemoid response, bleeding tendencies, nodular pulmonary lesions, and evidence of pancreatic disease with elevated plasma amylase and lipase levels. In the past this constellation of findings was called *Weber-Christian disease*. However, since painful or nonpainful panniculitis may result from a variety of conditions, Weber-Christian disease is not a specific entity, and the term should probably be abandoned.

It is not possible to develop a firm classification of acute panniculitis since the lesions may appear in sporadic fashion with many conditions. One classification system is given in Table 318-4.

Panniculitis without systemic disease is usually due to trauma (sometimes factitiously induced) or cold. For example, in equestrian cold panniculitis the lesions appear in the outer thighs of persons riding horseback for several hours in icy weather. One variant, subcutaneous fat necrosis of the newborn, may be due to a combination of obstetric trauma and hypothermia.

Panniculitis with systemic disease can be divided into several large categories. Collagen vascular disease is a frequent cause, although few patients with connective tissue disorders develop this complication. Lupus is probably most common, and scleroderma is second. About 2 to 3 percent of patients with lupus have nodular fat necrosis; it is more common in discoid lupus than in the systemic variant. Lymphomas and histiocytosis represent a second category. Cytophagic histiocytic panniculitis, an illness characterized by severe hemorrhagic diathesis and high mortality rates, may occur in association with lymphoma or as a separate disease. Deficiencies of α_1-antitrypsin have been found in a number of patients with acute panniculitis. It is postulated that the α_1-antitrypsin deficiency predisposes to panniculitis secondary to trauma and induces a hyperactive immune response. Severe pancreatic disease may also cause acute panniculitis. One distinct syndrome has been called *disseminated fat necrosis* and is described below. Finally, panniculitis may be associated with generalized lipodystrophy, especially the acquired type.

Acute panniculitis can be diagnosed only histologically. Once the lesion is identified a search for the cause must be made. If systemic symptoms are present and the course is rapidly downhill, the primary differential diagnosis is between collagen vascular disease, lymphoproliferative disorder, and pancreatitis or pancreatic cancer. Milder cases raise the possibility of α_1-antitrypsin deficiency.

Treatment is unsatisfactory, but steroids and immunosuppression may be tried.

DISSEMINATED FAT NECROSIS

Disseminated fat necrosis (also called metastatic fat necrosis) is a syndrome in which patients with pancreatitis (two-thirds) or carcinoma of the pancreas (one-third) develop lesions that appear to be similar to or identical with nodular panniculitis. The fat necrosis has a predilection for periarticular sites. Fever is almost invariably present. Arthritis occurs in about 60 percent of cases and may be severe, resulting in destruction of the joint. Often there are sinus tracts running from the site of subcutaneous fat necrosis into the joint space, leading to deposition of necrotic material. Lytic bone lesions may underlie the site of fat necrosis. Polyserositis and vasculitis may be present. Since complement levels are low and immunofluorescent staining shows deposition of complement and IgG, the syndrome resembles, in some respects, lupus-associated panniculitis. Serologic studies for lupus have not been systematically carried out. Antinuclear antibody (ANA) and rheumatoid factor were negative in one patient.

Disseminated fat necrosis may be due to release of pancreatic enzymes into blood or lymph, and these enzymes may initiate fat necrosis at distal sites. Presumably free fatty acids released by pancreatic lipase and phospholipase A, both of which may be elevated in serum, induce tissue necrosis, with trypsin playing an ancillary role. Necrosis in pericardial, subpleural, and subcutaneous fat can be produced by ligation of pancreatic ducts, and amylase and lipase

TABLE 318-4 Causes of panniculitis

1 Panniculitis without systemic disease
- *a* Trauma
- *b* Cold
- *c* Subcutaneous fat necrosis of the newborn

2 Panniculitis with systemic disease
- *a* Connective tissue disorders (lupus erythematosus, scleroderma)
- *b* Lymphoproliferative disease (lymphoma, histocytosis)
- *c* α_1-Antitrypsin deficiency
- *d* Pancreatic disease (cancer, pancreatitis)
- *e* Generalized lipodystrophy

levels may be elevated in pleural, pericardial, and ascitic fluid. These enzymes have also been found in fluid aspirated from subcutaneous nodules. A fistula developed between a pancreatic pseudocyst and the portal vein in one patient; shortly thereafter nodular fat necrosis appeared over most of the body. On the other hand an immune mechanism may be causal, given that polyserositis is common and that low complement levels and vasculitis may be present. The meaning of the eosinophilia that frequently accompanies disseminated fat necrosis is not known.

Mortality rates are high (even in the absence of pancreatic carcinoma), and death may occur in weeks to months. No treatment is known. Infusion of the protease inhibitor aprotinin appeared to have beneficial effects in one patient.

ADIPOSIS DOLOROSA

Adiposis dolorosa (Dercum's disease) is characterized by painful circumscribed adipose tissue deposits in subcutaneous tissues of the extremities and of other parts of the body. Juxtaarticular areas, particularly the knees, are the most common sites. Lesions vary from 0.5 to 5.0 cm. Pain and paresthesias may occur spontaneously or result from pressure. Affected subjects are frequently women (30:1). They are usually obese. The syndrome is associated with weakness, fatigue, emotional instability, and occasional dementia and rarely begins until after menopause. Most cases are sporadic, but familial occurrence has been noted with a presumed dominant inheritance. Multiple associations have been reported, but they are probably chance phenomena. Autopsy reports from early in the century suggested abnormalities of the pituitary and other endocrine glands, but modern endocrinologic evaluations have not been undertaken.

Biopsy of affected sites may show no abnormalities, but granulomas with giant cell formations are usually seen. Fat necrosis is rare, thus separating the condition from acute panniculitis.

Treatment is unsatisfactory, although intravenous lidocaine has apparently provided relief in two cases.

REFERENCES

Lipodystrophy

Aarskog D et al: Autosomal dominant partial lipodystrophy associated with Rieger anomaly, short stature, and insulinopenic diabetes. Am J Med Genet 15:29, 1983

Beutler B et al: Purification of cachectin, a lipoprotein lipase-suppressing hormone secreted by endotoxin-induced raw 264.7 cells. J Exp Med 161:984, 1985

Dunnigan MG et al: Familial lipoatrophic diabetes with dominant transmission: A new syndrome. Q J Med 43:33, 1974

Franklin B et al: Very low-density lipoprotein metabolism in an unusual case of lipoatrophic diabetes. Metabolism 33:814, 1984

Lillystone D, West RJ: Lipodystrophy of limbs associated with insulin resistance Arch Dis Child 50:737, 1975

Seip M: Generalized lipodystrophy, in *Ergebnisse der Inneren Medizin und Kind kunde*, P Frick et al (eds). Berlin, Springer Verlag, 1971, pp 59–95

Soler NG et al: Lipoatrophic diabetes: Endocrine dysfunction and the response to control of hypertriglyceridemia. Metabolism 31:19, 1982

Wachslicht-Rodbard H et al: Heterogeneity of the insulin-receptor interaction in lipoatrophic diabetes. J Clin Endocrinol Metab 52:416, 1981

Wilson DE et al: Eucaloric substitution of medium chain triglycerides for dietary long chain fatty acids in acquired total lipodystrophy: Effects on hyperlipoproteinemia and endogenous insulin resistance. J Clin Endocrinol Metab 57:517, 1983

Multiple symmetric lipomatosis

Enzi G: Multiple symmetric lipomatosis: An updated clinical report. Medicine 63:56, 1984

Mediastino-abdominal lipomatosis

Enzi G et al: Mediastino-abdominal lipomatosis: Deep accumulation of fat mimicking a respiratory disease and ascites. Clinical aspects and metabolic studies *in vitro*. Q J Med 53:453, 1984

Acute panniculitis

Aronson IK et al: Panniculitis associated with cutaneous T-cell lymphoma and cytophagocytic histiocytosis. Br J Dermatol 112:87, 1985

Bleumink E, Klokke HA: Protease-inhibitor deficiencies in a patient with Weber-Christian panniculitis. Arch Dermatol 120:936, 1984

Winkelmann RK: Panniculitis in connective tissue disease. Arch Dermatol 119:336, 1983

Disseminated fat necrosis

Phillips MR Jr et al: Inflammatory arthritis and subcutaneous fat necrosis associated with acute and chronic pancreatitis. Arthritis Rheum 23:355, 1980

Wilson HA et al: Pancreatitis with arthropathy and subcutaneous fat necrosis. Evidence for the pathogenicity of lipolytic enzymes. Arthritis Rheum 26:121, 1983

Adiposis dolorosa

Atkinson RL: Intravenous lidocaine for the treatment of intractable pain of adiposis dolorosa. Int J Obes 6:351, 1982

319 HERITABLE DISORDERS OF CONNECTIVE TISSUE

DARWIN J. PROCKOP

Heritable disorders of connective tissues are among the most common genetic diseases. The most general in their manifestations are osteogenesis imperfecta (OI), Ehlers-Danlos syndrome (EDS), and Marfan's syndrome.

The usual classification of OI, EDS, and Marfan's syndrome is based on the work of McKusick, who analyzed signs, symptoms, and pathologic changes in a large number of patients. Such an attempt to classify the diseases is complicated by their heterogeneity. For example, some families lack one or more of the cardinal features of a disease. Other families have features characteristic of two or three different diseases. Heterogeneity may also exist among members of the same family. For example, some individuals from one family can have joint dislocations characteristic of EDS, other members can have increased brittleness of bone characteristic of OI, and still others with the same gene defect can be asymptomatic. Because of these problems, classifications based upon clinical features will eventually be replaced by analyses based upon molecular defects in specific genes.

ORGANIZATION AND CHEMICAL COMPOSITION OF CONNECTIVE TISSUES Connective tissues are loosely defined as the extracellular components that provide the structural support of the body and bind together its cells, organs, and tissues. The major connective tissues are bone, skin, tendons, ligaments, and cartilage. The term is also applied to blood vessels and to synovial spaces and fluids. Indeed, all organs and tissues contain connective tissue in the form of membranes and septa.

Connective tissues contain large amounts of fluid in the form of a filtrate of blood that includes about half the body albumin. Most connective tissues are filled with, or surrounded by, fibrils or fibers of collagen (Table 319-1). Most connective tissues also contain proteoglycans.

To a degree, the differences among connective tissues are due to subtle differences in the size and orientation of collagen fibrils. In tendons collagen fibrils are packed into thick, parallel bundles of fibers. In skin the collagen fibrils are oriented more randomly. In bone, the fibrils are organized into an orderly architecture around the haversian canals that is made rigid by the presence of hydroxyapatite. The principal collagen of tendons, skin, and bone, type I collagen, comprises two polypeptide chains that are the products of different structural genes. The differences among these tissues are in large part due to differences in how the structural genes for type I collagen are expressed, namely, how much collagen is synthesized, the thickness and length of the fibrils formed, and how the fibrils are oriented.

Some of the differences among connective tissues reflect the presence of tissue- or organ-specific gene products. Bone contains proteins that have a critical role in the mineralization of the collagen. Aorta contains elastin and an associated microfibrillar protein, several different types of collagen, and other components. The basal lamina found beneath all epithelial and endothelial cells contains type IV collagen and other tisse-specific macromolecules. Skin and several other connective tissues contain small amounts of additional kinds of collagen.

BIOSYNTHESIS OF CONNECTIVE TISSUE The synthesis of connective tissues involves the self-assembly of molecular subunits of the correct size, shape, and surface properties. In the case of collagen, the molecule is a long, thin rod comprising three α-polypeptide chains wrapped into a rigid, ropelike structure (Fig. 319-1). Each α chain has a simple, repetitive amino acid sequence in which glycine (Gly) appears as every third amino acid. Since each α chain has about 1000 amino acids, the amino acid sequence of each α chain can be designed as $(\text{-Gly-X-Y-})_{333}$, where X and Y represent amino acids other than glycine. It is essential that every third amino acid be glycine, the smallest amino acid, since this residue must fit in a sterically restricted space where the three chains of the triple helix come together. Two of the α chains in type I collagen are identical and are called α1(I). One has a slightly different amino acid sequence and is called α2(I). Some collagens contain three identical α chains whereas others contain three different α chains. Sequences in the α chains in which the X position is occupied by proline or the Y position is occupied by hydroxyproline give rigidity to the molecule and hold it in the triple-helical conformation. The hydrophobic and charged amino acids in the X and Y positions appear as clusters on the surface of the molecule and define the manner in which one molecule spontaneously binds to other molecules to form the cylindrical arrays characteristic of every collagen fibril (Fig. 319-1).

The simplicity of the structure and function of the collagen molecule is in contrast to the complexity of its synthesis (Fig. 319-1). The protein is first assembled as a precursor called procollagen, which has a mass about 1.5 times that of the collagen molecule. The additional mass is due to amino acid sequences at both the *N* terminus and *C* terminus of the procollagen molecule. To generate collagen fibrils, the *N*-terminal propeptides must be cleaved by a specific *N*-proteinase, and the *C*-terminal propeptides must be cleaved by a specific *C*-proteinase. As the proα chains of procollagen are assembled on ribosomes, they pass into the cisternae of the rough endoplasmic reticulum. Hydrophobic "signal peptides" at the *N* terminus are cleaved, and a series of additional posttranslational reactions begin. Proline residues in the Y position are converted to hydroxyproline by a specific hydroxylase requiring ascorbic acid. Lysine residues in the Y position are similarly hydroxylated to hydroxylysine by another hydroxylase requiring ascorbic acid. The requirement for ascorbic acid by the two hydroxylases probably explains why wounds fail to heal in scurvy (see Chap. 76). Many of the hydroxylysine residues are further modified by glycosylation with galactose or with galactose and glucose. A large mannose-rich oligosaccharide is added to the *C*-terminal propeptide of each chain. The *C*-terminal propeptides associate and become disulfide-linked. When each proα chain acquires a critical level of about 100 hydroxyproline residues, the protein spontaneously folds into a triple-helical conformation. Once the protein is folded, it is processed to collagen by *N*-proteinase and *C*-proteinase.

The fibrils formed by the self-assembly of the collagen molecule have considerable tensile strength, and the strength is increased by cross-linking reactions that form covalent bonds between α chains in one molecule and the α chains in adjacent molecules. The first step in cross-linking is oxidation by the enzyme lysyl oxidase of amino groups on lysine or hydroxylysine residues to form aldehydes; the aldehydes then interact to form stable covalent bonds.

The collagen fibrils and fibers in tissues other than bone are stable throughout most of adult life and turn over only with marked starvation or tissue wastage. However, fibroblasts, synovial cells, and other cells can produce collagenases that cleave the collagen molecule at a point about three-quarters of the distance from its *N* terminus and thereby trigger further degradation of collagen fibrils and fibers by additional proteinases. In bone, there is continual degradation and resynthesis of collagen fibrils as part of bone remodeling. In summary, the assembly and maintenance of collagen fibrils in tissues require the coordinated expression of a series of genes whose products are required in the posttranslational assembly of collagen fibrils or are involved in the metabolic turnover of collagen.

The assembly of type I collagen fibrils is similar to that for type II collagen fibrils in cartilage and the type III collagen fibrils in aorta and skin. Assembly of nonfibrillar collagens such as the type IV of basement membranes does not involve cleavage of globular domains at the ends of the molecules. Instead, these domains participate in the self-assembly of the monomers into interlocking networks. Elastin

TABLE 319-1 Constituents of connective tissue in various tissues

Connective tissue	Known constituents	Approximate amounts (% dry wt)	Characteristics
Skin (dermis), ligaments, tendons	Type I collagen	80	Bundles of fibers of high tensile strength
	Type III collagen	5 to 15	Thin fibrils
	Type IV collagen, laminin, entactin, nidogen	<5	In basal laminae under epithelium and in blood vessels
	Types V to VII	<5	Distributions and functions unclear
	Fibronectin	<5	Associated with collagen fibers and cell surfaces
	Proteoglycans*	0.5	Provides resiliency
	Hyaluronate	0.5	Provides resiliency
Bone (demineralized)	Type I collagen	90	Complex organization of fibrils
	Type V collagen	1 to 2	Function unclear
	Proteoglycans	1	Function unclear
	Sialoproteins	1	Function unclear
	Osteonectin	2 to 3	Role in ossification
	Osteocalcin	1	Probable role in ossification
	α_2-Glycoprotein	1	Possible role in ossification
Aorta	Type I collagen	20 to 40	
	Type III collagen	20 to 40	Thin fibrils
	Elastin, microfibrillar protein	20 to 40	Amorphous, elastic fibrils
	Type IV collagen, laminin, entactin, nidogen	<5	In basal lamina
	Types V and VI collagens	<2	Functions unclear
	Proteoglycans	<3	Mucopolysaccharides, mainly chondroitin sulfate and dermatan sulfate; heparan sulfate in basal lamina
Cartilage	Type II collagen	40 to 50	Thin fibrils
	Types IX and X collagen	5 to 25	Possible role in maturation
	Proteoglycans	15 to 50	Provides resiliency
	Hyaluronate	0.5 to 2	Provides resiliency

* *Proteoglycan structures are incompletely defined. About five different protein cores have been identified, and each has one or more kind of mucopolysaccharides attached. Major mucopolysaccharides of skin and tendon are dermatan sulfate and chondroitin 4-sulfate; of aorta, chondroitin 4-sulfate and dermatan sulfate; of cartilage, chondroitin 4-sulfate, chondroitin 6-sulfate, and keratan sulfate. Basal lamina contains heparan sulfate.*

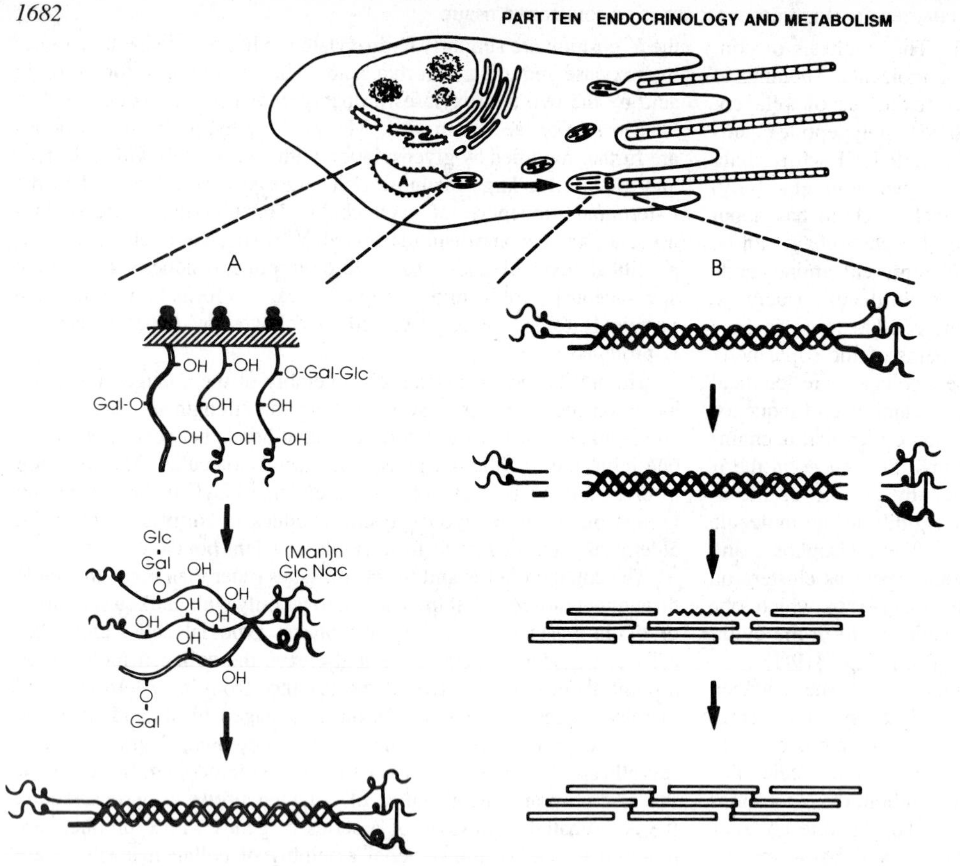

FIGURE 319-1 *Schematic representation of synthesis of a type I collagen fibril by a fibroblast. A. Intracellular steps in the assembly of the procollagen molecule. Hydroxylations and glycosylations of the proα chains begin soon after the* N *termini pass into the cisterni of the rough endoplasmic reticulum and continue after the three chains associate through their* C-*propeptides and become disulfide-linked. B. Cleavage of procollagen to collagen, self-assembly of the collagen molecule into quarter-staggered fibrils, and cross-linking of the molecules in the fibrils. Cleavage of the propeptides may occur within crypts of the fibroblast, as shown here, or some distance from the cell. (Reproduced with permission from Prockop and Kivirikko.)*

fibers are also assembled by a similar pathway. The elastin monomer, however, is a single polypeptide chain without a defined three-dimensional structure, and it self-assembles into amorphous elastic fibers.

Proteoglycan synthesis is similar to collagen synthesis in that it begins with assembly of a polypeptide chain, called the protein core, in the cisternae of the rough endoplasmic reticulum, and the protein core undergoes modification by addition of sugar residues and sulfate that generate large mucopolysaccharide side chains on the protein core. After secretion into the extracellular space, the core protein with its mucopolysaccharide side chains binds to a link protein and then to a long chain of hyaluronic acid to form the mature proteoglycan with a molecular weight of several millions.

The assembly of bone follows the same principles as that for other connective tissues (see also Chap. 335). The first step is deposition of osteoid tissue that consists largely of type I collagen (Fig. 319-1). Mineralization of the osteoid occurs by steps that are still incompletely defined; specific proteins such as osteonectin bind to specific sites on the collagen fibril and then chelate calcium to initiate mineralization.

FIGURE 319-2 *Approximate locations of mutations in the structure of type I procollagen. EDS denotes the Ehlers-Danlos syndrome, OI, osteogenesis imperfecta; and MS, Marfan's syndrome. Other symbols: proα1^S, mutation giving rise to a shortened proα1 chain; proα2^S, mutation giving rise to a shortened proα2 chain; proα1^{cys}, mutation introducing a cysteine residue; proα$^{c\text{-}man}$, mutation introducing excess mannose into one or both proα chains; proα2^X, unknown structural mutation that prevents cleavage of the chain by* N-*proteinase; proα2^L, mutation giving rise to a lengthened proα2 chain; proα2^{CX}, mutation altering the structure of the* C-*terminal propeptide of the proα2 chain. Roman numerals indicate specific type of EDS or OI as discussed in text. Exons where specific deletions occur are indicated with the exons being numbered from the 3′ end to the 5′ end of the gene. Other deletions are defined in terms of the approximate number of amino acids deleted from the chain. The symbol aa 988 indicates that the glycine residue in amino acid position 988 of the α1 chain is replaced by cysteine. As discussed in the text, the proα2^L mutation involves insertion of 38 base pairs into an intervening sequence and was found in a patient with atypical Marfan's syndrome. Proα2$^{S\text{-}100\ aas}$ refers to an apparent deletion of about 100 amino acids in a variant of type II osteogenesis imperfecta. (Modified and reproduced with permission from Prockop and Kivirikko.)*

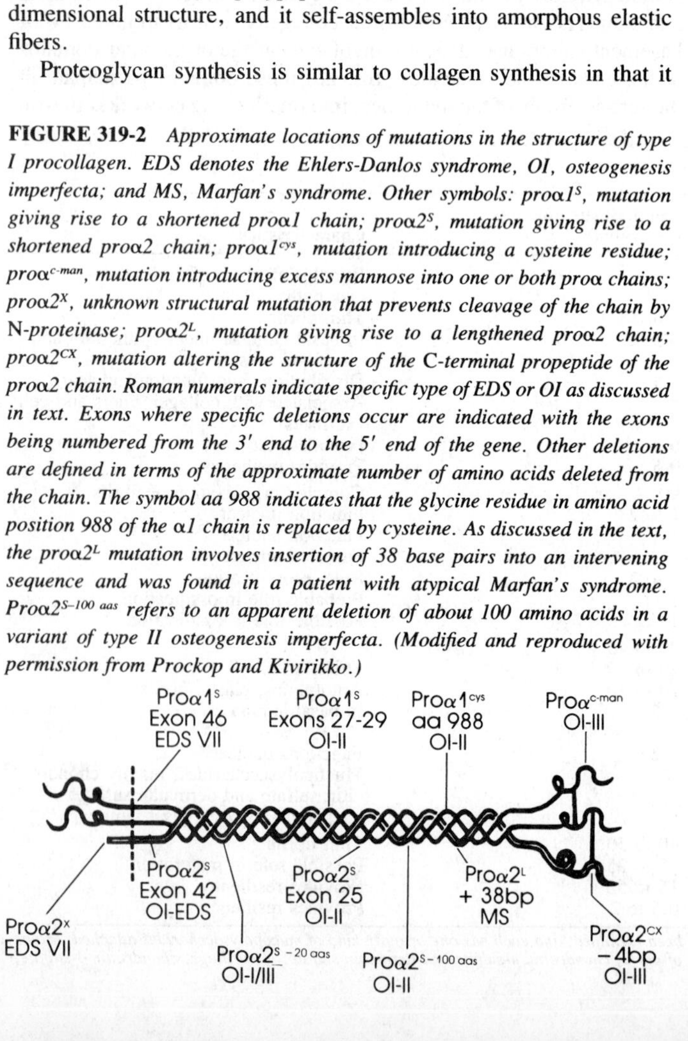

CONSEQUENCES FOR HERITABLE DISEASES Our understanding of the chemistry and biochemistry of connective tissues is incomplete but nevertheless provides insight into the clinical features of heritable diseases of connective tissue. For example, it explains why many of the diseases are systemic in their manifestations. Since all type I collagen is synthesized from the same two structural genes, any mutation in these genes must be expressed in all the tissues containing type I collagen. Tissue or organ specificity of the diseases can be explained by either of two major mechanisms. One is that the diseases are produced by mutations in genes expressed in only one or two connective tissues. For example, patients with the type IV form of Ehlers-Danlos syndrome have mutations in genes for the type III procollagen, and the symptoms are confined to skin, aorta, and intestine—tissues rich in type III collagen. A second reason for tissue specificity of the diseases is more subtle. Different regions of collagen molecules have different biologic functions. In the case of type I collagen, removal of the *N*-terminal propeptides is necessary for assembly of large collagen fibrils and fibers in ligaments and tendons. If the *N*-propeptides are incompletely cleaved, the protein self-assembles into thin fibrils. Hence, patients with mutations in type I procollagen genes that prevent efficient cleavage of the *N*-propeptides suffer primarily from dislocations of hips and other large joints. They rarely have fractures, because assembly of thick fibrils of type I

TABLE 319-2 Classification of osteogenesis imperfecta (OI) based on clinical manifestations and mode of inheritance as proposed by Sillence

Type	Bone fragility	Blue sclerae	Abnormal dentition	Hearing loss	Inheritance*
I	Mild	Present	Absent in IA, present in IB	Present in some	AD
II	Extreme	Present	Present in some	Unknown	AR or S
III	Severe	Bluish at birth	Present in some	Low incidence	AR
IV	Variable	Absent	Absent in IVA, present in IVB	Low incidence	AD

* *AD, autosomal dominant; AR, autosomal recessive; S, sporadic.*

collagen appears to be less important for the normal function of bone than for normal joint ligaments. In contrast, patients with mutations altering the structure of other regions of the type I procollagen molecule may have primary manifestations in bone.

The current information about the chemistry of matrix also provides insight into the heterogeneity of signs and symptoms in patients with identical gene defects. The expression of a collagen or proteoglycan gene depends on coordinated expression of genes for posttranslational enzymes and on the expression of genes for other components of the same matrix. Therefore, the ultimate effect of a given mutation on the functional properties of a complex structure such as bone or a large blood vessel is influenced by differences in the ''genetic background'' among individuals, namely, differences in the expression of a large family of other genes whose products influence the same structure. The manifestations must also be subject to other factors that influence connective tissues such as exercise, trauma, nutrition, and hormonal changes. Hence, there is broad scope for variable manifestations in patients with the same defect.

DEFINITION OF THE MOLECULAR DEFECTS Defining the defect in patients with heritable disorders of connective tissue requires an intensive research effort (Fig. 319-2). One reason is that no two unrelated patients have the same molecular defects even when the clinical manifestations appear identical. Another is that the proteins and proteoglycans in connective tissues are large molecules that are difficult to solubilize and obtain in pure form. Also, in many patients the defect causes synthesis of an abnormal protein that is rapidly degraded. Therefore, it is difficult to establish which gene product is at fault by analysis of tissues. Still another reason is that the genes for matrix components are large. In the case of type I procollagen, the gene for the proα1(I) chain contains 18,000 base pairs, and the gene for the proα2(I) chain contains 38,000 base pairs. Each of these genes has about 50 exons, most of which have a very similar structure. With the recombinant DNA technologies currently available, locating a mutation of one or more bases in a collagen gene is a formidable challenge. However, newer technologies will probably overcome most of these problems.

OSTEOGENESIS IMPERFECTA

General features The term osteogenesis imperfecta (OI) is used for heritable defects that make bones brittle (Fig. 319-3). The diagnosis is made by excluding other heritable defects or environmental factors that produce osteopenia or osteoporosis and by establishing that the mutation is expressed in more than one connective tissue. The increased fragility of bone is usually associated with blue sclerae, hearing loss, abnormalities of dentition, or a combination of these features (Table 319-2). The presence of blue sclerae and fractures early in life is usually sufficient to establish the diagnosis. Also, fractures together with the characteristic dental abnormalities (dentinogenesis imperfecta) are sufficient for a diagnosis. Some consider brittleness of bone associated with early hearing loss in the patient or members of the same family as diagnostic, and others make the diagnosis on the basis of fragile bones that cannot be attributed to environmental facts such as physical inactivity or malnutrition or to any other heritable syndromes, such as the skeletal dysplasias (Table 319-3). Since some individuals from families with OI do not develop fractures until after menopause, mild forms of OI may not be distinguishable from postmenopausal osteoporosis. Some individuals with osteoporosis may be heterozygous carriers for gene defects that produce OI in homozygotes. Therefore, it may prove useful to include postmenopausal osteoporosis in the same spectrum of diseases as OI.

The most common classification scheme for OI is the one developed by Sillence (Table 319-2). Type I disease has a frequency of about 1:30,000. It is a mild to moderately severe disorder that is inherited as an autosomal dominant trait and is associated with blue sclerae. Type II is the most severe form of the disease. Types III and IV OI are intermediate in severity between types I and II.

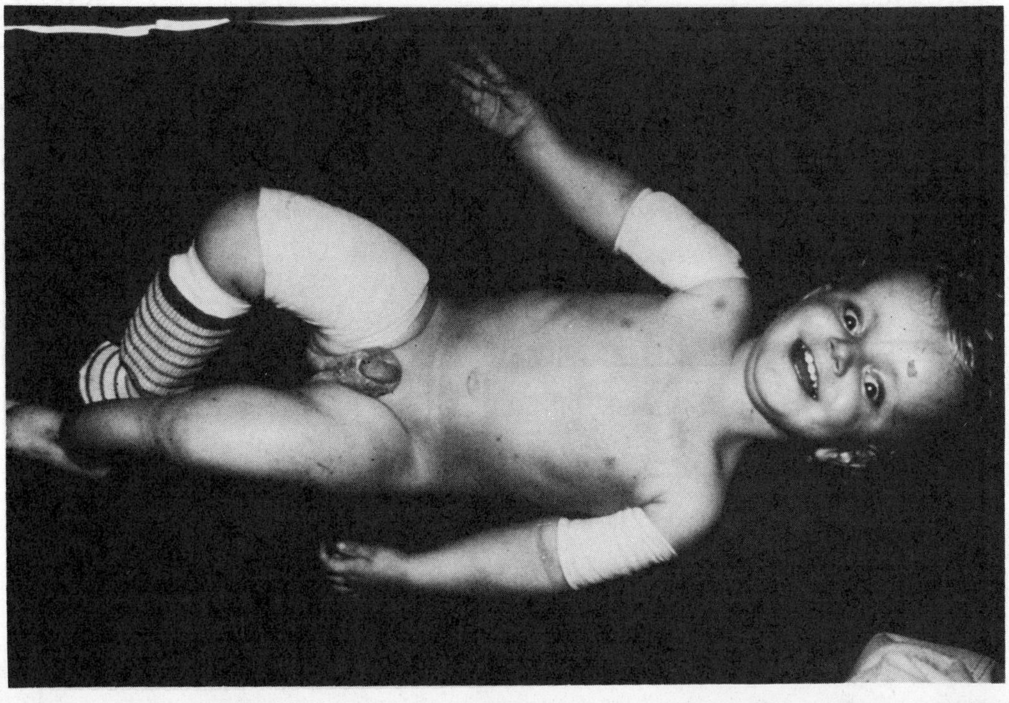

FIGURE 319-3 *A 21-month-old boy with type III OI. Child has had multiple fractures of arms and legs. He is homozygous for a four-base-pair deletion in the genes for proα2(I) chains that changes the sequence of the last 33 amino acids in these proteins. Therefore, the proα2(I) chains do not associate with proα1(I) chains, and the only type I procollagens formed are trimers of proα1(I) chains that have a partially unfolded C-terminal region. (Reproduced with permission from Nicholls et al.)*

TABLE 319-3 Partial differential diagnosis of OI

Age	Diagnosis	Distinguishing features
At birth	Hypophosphatasia	Unmineralized skull
	Achondrogenesis	Unmineralized vertebrae
	Thanatophoric dwarfism	H-shaped vertebrae
	Asphyxiating thoracic dystrophy	Cylindrical thorax
	Achondroplasia	Large head, short, tubular bones
Infancy	Battered child syndrome	Skull and rib fractures more common
	Immobilization osteogenesis	
	Scurvy	
	Congenital syphilis	
Childhood	Idiopathic juvenile osteogenesis	Prepubertal and self-limiting
	Homocystinuria	Marfanoid appearance and mental deficiency
	Celiac disease	Steatorrhea, anemia
	Adrenal cortical tumor	
	Corticosteroid therapy	

SOURCE: *Modified from Smith et al., p. 126*

Skeletal changes In type I OI the fragility of bones may be so marked as to limit physical activity or so mild that individuals may be unaware of any debility. In type II OI, bones and other connective tissues are so fragile that death occurs in utero, during delivery, or within a few weeks after birth. In types III and IV disease, multiple fractures resulting from minor physical stress can lead to a stunting of growth and to skeletal abnormalities. Many patients have an increase in fractures during childhood, a decrease after puberty, and then an increase with pregnancy and after menopause. Severe kyphoscoliosis may cause respiratory impairment and predispose to pulmonary infections. Bone density is decreased in unfractured bone, but there is no consensus about specific morphologic changes. The general impression is that the repair of fractures is normal. The skull of some patients with relatively mild symptoms has a mottled appearance, apparently because of small islands of ossification.

Ocular changes The sclerae can vary in color from normal to a slightly bluish or slate color to a bright blue. The blueness is caused by a thinness or transparency of the collagen fibers of the sclera that allows the choroid layer to be seen. Some patients also have other ocular changes. Blue sclerae can be an inherited trait in some families without any evidence of increased bone fragility.

Dentinogenesis imperfecta The enamel of the lamina dura is relatively normal, but the teeth have an amber, yellowish-brown or translucent bluish-gray color because of improper deposition of dentine. The deciduous teeth are usually smaller than normal whereas the permanent teeth are bell-shaped and constricted at the base. Indistinguishable tooth defects can be inherited independently of OI.

Presenile hearing loss The deafness usually begins in the second decade of life or later. It arises from impaired transmission through the middle ear as far as the footplate of the stapes. The histologic features include deficient ossification, persistence of cartilage areas normally ossified, and calcified strial deposits.

Associated features Many patients and families show involvement of other connective tissues. Some patients show skin and joint changes indistinguishable from those of EDS (see below). A few patients have cardiovascular manifestations such as aortic regurgitation, floppy mitral valves, mitral incompetence, and fragility of large blood vessels. Hypermetabolic states can occur with elevated serum thyroxine levels, hyperthermia, and excessive sweating. In mild forms of OI, the associated features can be the presenting symptom.

Mode of inheritance The type I form of OI has an autosomal dominant mode of inheritance with variable expressivity so that apparent skipping of a generation may occur. In the lethal type II variant, the inheritance may be autosomal recessive, but in the few cases of type II OI in which the genetic defect has been defined new mutations are involved. The mode of inheritance is a primary criterion for distinguishing type III from type IV (Table 319-2), but it may be difficult to distinguish recessive inheritance from a new autosomal dominant mutation.

Molecular defects Because most of the affected tissues are rich in type I collagen, most forms of the disease are believed to be caused by mutations in the structural genes for the protein, in genes for its posttranslational processing, or in genes regulating its expression. Mutations in the genes for type I procollagen have now been identified in four variants of type II OI. One variant had a deletion mutation in one allele for the proα1(I) gene (Fig. 319-4*A*). The deletion removed three exons but did not interfere with the transcription of the gene. As a result, the proα1(I) chain was 84 amino acids shorter than normal. The mutation was lethal because the shortened proα1(I) chain associated with normal proα1(I) and proα2(I) chains (Fig. 319-4*B*). The shortening in the proα1(I) chain prevented molecules from folding in the triple-helical conformation. As a result, most of the procollagen remained nonhelical and was rapidly degraded in a process that has been referred to as "protein suicide" or negative complementarity (Fig. 319-4*B*). In a second lethal type II variant,

FIGURE 319-4 *Schematic representation of the molecular defect in a patient with type II OI. A. Schematic representation of the gene deletion. As indicated, the human proα1(I) gene is about 18,000 base pairs long and contains about 50 exons (vertical dark bars). The deletion removed three exons containing 252 base pairs of coding sequences. B. Scheme of "protein" suicide or negative complementarity. Shortened proα1(I) chains were synthesized, and they associated with and became disulfide-bonded to normal proα chains. Procollagen molecules containing one or two shortened proα1(I) chains did not fold into a triple helix at 37°C and were degraded. Hence, a sporadic homozygous defect reduced the amount of functional procollagen by about 75 percent. (Modified from and reproduced with permission from Prockop and Kivirikko.)*

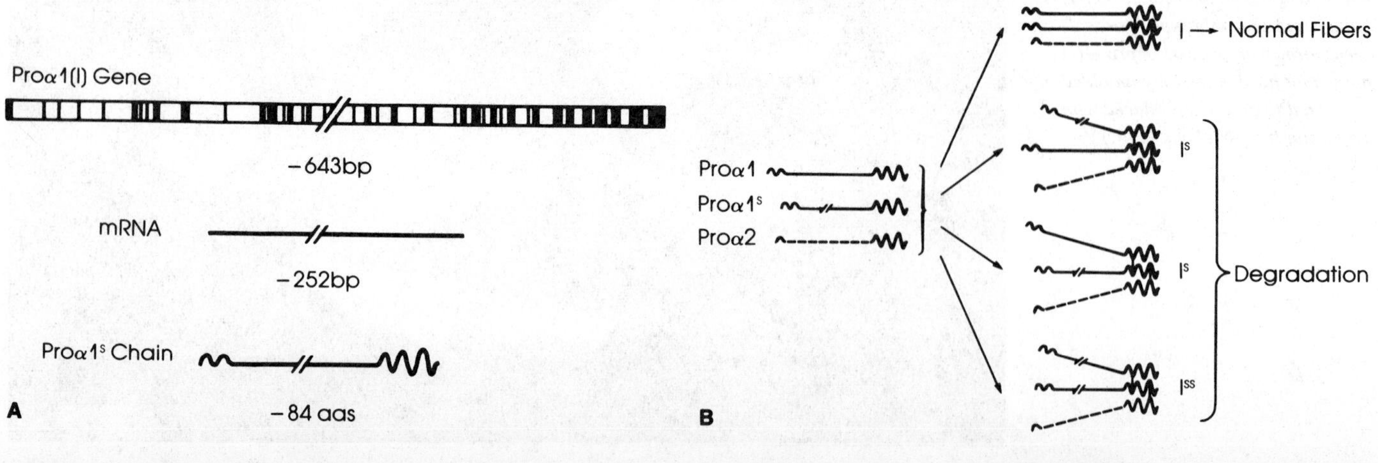

the mutation led to the synthesis of a proα2(I) chain that was about 20 amino acids shorter than normal. The other allele was nonfunctioning, and therefore all the proα2 chains were shortened. In a third type II variant, a deletion mutation in an allele for proα2(I) chains caused the synthesis of proα2 chains that were shortened by about 100 amino acids. In a fourth type II variant, a single-base substitution introduced a cysteine residue instead of a glycine residue in the α1(I) chain and thereby disrupted the triple-helical conformation of the protein.

Mutations in genes for type I procollagen have also been detected in two variants of type III. In one, the mutation was a four-base-pair deletion that produced a change in the reading frame for the last 33 amino acids of the proα2(I) chain. The patient was homozygous for the defect, and none of the proα2(I) chains were incorporated in procollagen molecules. Instead, the type I procollagen consisted of a trimer of proα1(I) chains. The trimer of proα1(I) chains was triple-helical but unstable. The parents, who were third cousins, were heterozygous for the same mutation and had osteoporosis while in their thirties. In another type III variant, a structural alteration in the *C*-terminal propeptide caused increased mannose in the *C*-propeptides. In a patient who had some manifestations of the type I disorder and some of type II, proα2(I) chains were shortened by about 100 amino acids.

These data suggest several generalizations about mutations in collagen genes. One is that a mutation that causes synthesis of an abnormal protein can be more deleterious than a nonfunctioning allele. Another is that mutations that give rise to shortened polypeptide chains may be more frequent than in other gene systems. Nevertheless, the molecular defects in most patients with OI have not been identified. Many may be RNA-splicing mutations or single-base mutations that are difficult to detect in genes as large as those for type I procollagen. Other variants of OI may be due to mutations in other genes whose expression is required for the assembly and maintenance of bone and other connective tissues.

Diagnosis Diagnosis is difficult in patients who lack the cardinal features of the disease and is probably often missed. Other conditions that produce brittle bones in infancy and childhood must be considered (Table 319-3). In a third of patients, abnormal proα can be identified by polyacrylamide gel electrophoresis of type I procollagen synthesized by cultured skin fibroblasts. In most instances, the altered migration reflects posttranslational modification and does not define the exact nature of the mutation or the type of OI.

Treatment No convincing data have been presented that OI can be effectively treated. Patients with mild forms may need little treatment after fractures decrease at the age of 15 to 20 years, but they may need special attention during pregnancy or after menopause when fractures again increase. More severely affected children require a comprehensive program of physical therapy, surgical management of fractures and skeletal deformities, vocational education, and emotional support for the patients and their parents. Many patients appear to be unusually intelligent and have successful careers in spite of severe deformities. A program for orthotic management developed by Bleck is a useful guide. Many of the fractures are minimally displaced and have little soft tissue swelling. Therefore, they can be treated with minimal support or traction for a week or two followed by a light cast. If fractures are relatively painless, physical therapy can be initiated early. There is controversy over correcting limb deformities with steel rods inserted into long bones. The rationale for the procedure is that correcting deformities during childhood may make it possible to align the limbs adequately for walking during adulthood.

Genetic counseling may be difficult in families with types II, III, and IV because of uncertainty about the mode of inheritance. OI has been identified in fetuses as early as 20 weeks of pregnancy with x-rays and sonography. In the few families in which the precise gene defect has been defined, DNA can be analyzed for prenatal diagnosis in the research laboratories that have studied the defects. Restriction fragment length polymorphisms have been identified for the type I procollagen genes and may be useful for prenatal diagnosis. Cultured amniotic fluid cells synthesize collagen, but it appears impractical to use such cultures to detect mutations.

EHLERS-DANLOS SYNDROME

General features The Ehlers-Danlos syndrome (EDS) describes a group of heritable disorders characterized by hypermobile joints and abnormalities of skin (Fig. 319-5). Beighton initially identified five types of EDS (Table 319-4). Type I is the classical, severe form of the disease with both joint hypermobility and characteristically velvety and hyperextensible skin. Type II is similar to type I but milder. In type III joint hypermobility is more prominent than the skin changes. Type IV is characterized by a striking thinness of skin and a

FIGURE 319-5 *Schematic of the skin and joint changes in EDS. Girl in upper right has type VIIB EDS with dislocations of both hips that were not corrected by surgery. (Reproduced with permission from Prockop and Guzman, Hosp Prac, 12(12):61, 1977.)*

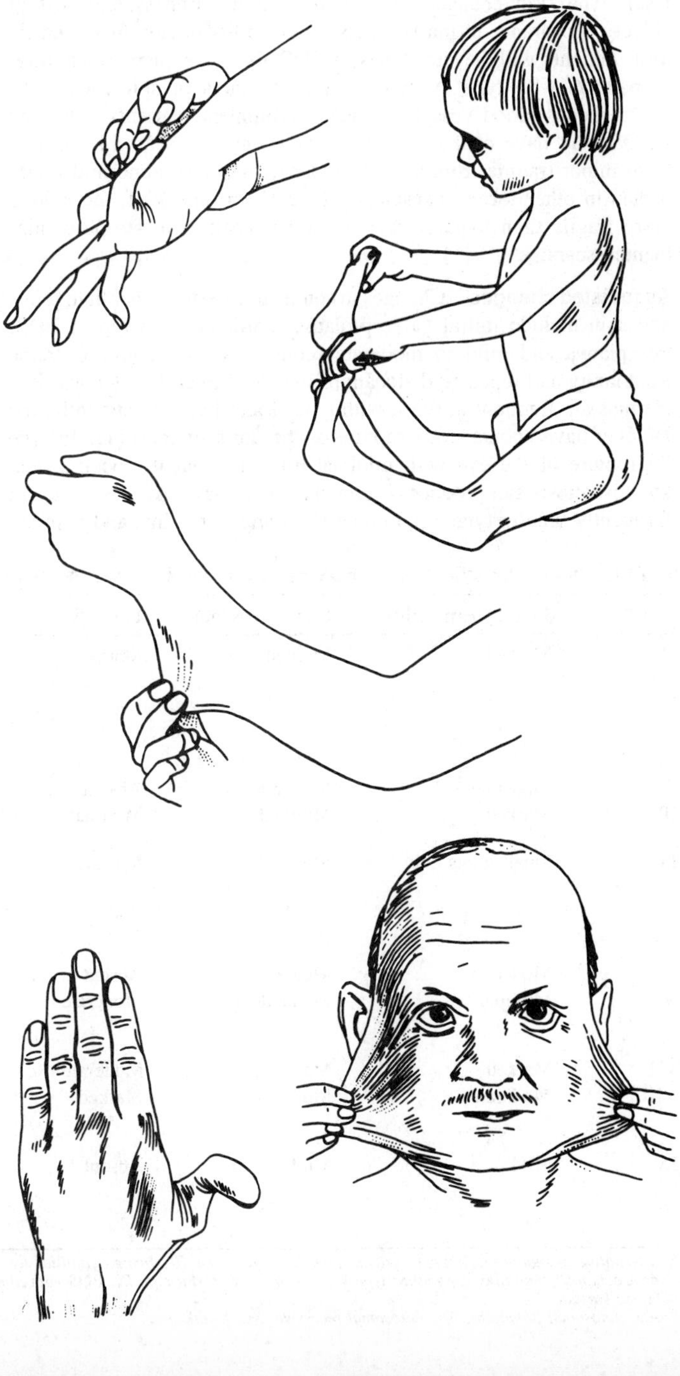

predisposition to sudden death from rupture of large blood vessels or the large bowel. Type V is similar to type II but characterized by X-linked inheritance.

The additional types VI, VII, and IX were defined because of the presence of biochemical defects and phenotypes that did not fit into the types defined by Beighton. However, not all patients with these phenotypes have the molecular defect initially used to establish the classification. Type VIII was identified by the presence of generalized periodontitis together with moderate joint and skin changes. Many patients and families cannot be assigned to any of the nine defined types of EDS.

Ligaments and joint changes Laxity and hypermobility of joints can vary from mild changes to those that are severe enough to produce unreducible dislocations of hips and other joints. In milder forms, patients learn to reduce dislocations themselves or to avoid them by limiting physical activity. In more severe forms, surgical repair is required. Some patients have progressive difficulty with increasing age, but severe joint laxity can be compatible with a normal life span.

Skin The skin changes vary from a slight thinness and soft or velvety appearance to marked hyperextensibility or skin that is easily torn. Patients with several types of EDS also have easy bruisability. In patients with type IV EDS marked thinness of skin makes the subcutaneous blood vessels unusually prominent. Patients with type I EDS may have characteristic "cigarette-paper" scars of the skin from minor trauma. Similar but milder evidence of abnormal repair occurs in other forms, particularly type V. In type VIII, the skin is more fragile than hyperextensible, and it heals with atrophic, pigmented scars.

Associated changes Changes in connective tissues other than joints and skin include mitral valve prolapse, particularly in type I EDS. Pes planus and mild to moderate scoliosis are common. Extreme joint laxity and repeated dislocations may lead to early osteoarthritis. Hernias are frequent in those with types I and IX. Patients with type IV may have spontaneous rupture of the aorta or intestine. In type VI rupture of the eye with minimal trauma frequently occurs, and kyphoscoliosis can produce respiratory impairment. Also, sclerae are frequently blue in type VI. In type IX changes in joints and skin are minimal. This type is primarily defined by the presence of abnormalities in copper metabolism and includes diseases previously classified as X-linked cutis laxa, X-linked EDS, and Menkes's syndrome. Patients frequently have bladder diverticuli that can rupture, hernias, skeletal abnormalities that include characteristic occipital horns, and laxity of skin. In the variants formerly defined as cutis laxa, skin laxity is the most prominent finding and results in an appearance of premature senescence. These patients frequently develop pulmonary emphysema and pulmonary stenosis.

Molecular defects The molecular defects in the type I, type II, and type III variants of EDS are unknown. Electron microscopy of the skin from some patients has shown an unusual morphology of collagen fibers, but similar types of collagen fibrils are occasionally seen in normal skin.

Patients with the type IV variant appear to have a defect either in the synthesis or the structure of type III collagen. This is consistent with the fact that they are prone to spontaneous rupture of the aorta and intestines, tissues that are rich in type III collagen. In one variant of type IV EDS, the defect involves synthesis of structurally abnormal proα(III) chains. The abnormal proα(III) chains were incorporated into molecules of type III procollagen in an equal stoichiometry with normal proα(III) chains so that most of the type III procollagen molecules contained one or more abnormal proα(III) chains. These molecules underwent "protein suicide" or negative complementarity, so that the skin contained no detectable type III collagen. In other variants of type IV EDS, the synthesis or secretion of type III procollagen is defective.

Type VI EDS was first characterized in two sisters by the fact that their collagen contained a decreased amount of hydroxylysine secondary to a deficiency of lysyl hydroxylase; a similar enzyme deficiency has been detected in other patients. Some patients with the clinical features of type VI EDS, however, do not have deficiency of lysyl hydroxylase.

Type VII EDS was first identified as a defect in the conversion of procollagen to collagen in patients with joint hypermobility and joint dislocations. At the molecular level, two kinds of genetic changes produce this disease. One, defined as type VIIA, is a deficiency of procollagen *N*-proteinase, the enzyme that removes the *N*-terminal peptide from type I procollagen. This form is inherited

TABLE 319-4 Classification of EDS based on clinical manifestations and mode of inheritance

Type*	Joint hypermobility	Skin extensibility	Fragility	Bruisability	Other manifestations	Inheritance†
I	Marked	Marked	Marked	Marked	Skin characteristically soft, velvety; cigarette-paper scars; hernias; varicose veins; premature birth because rupture of fetal membranes	AD
II	Moderate	Moderate	Absent	Moderate	Milder than type I	AD
III	Marked	Minimal	Minimal	Minimal	Joint dislocations with minimal changes in skin	
IV	Small joints only	Minimal	Marked	Marked	Rupture of large arteries and bowel; thin skin with prominent venous network; characteristic facies in some	AD or AR
V	Moderate	Moderate	Absent	Moderate	Similar to type II	XL
VI	Minimal	Moderate	Moderate	Moderate	Similar to type II; intramuscular hemorrhage or keratoconus in some	XL
VII	Marked	Moderate	Moderate	Moderate	Multiple dislocations	AR or AD
VIII	Moderate	Moderate	Marked	Moderate	Advanced periodontitis; atrophic pigmented scars of skin	AD
IX	Mild	Mild	Absent	Absent	Bladder diverticuli with spontaneous rupture; hernias; skeletal abnormalities; skin laxity	XL

* *Alternative designations; type I, gravis; type II, mitis; type III, benign familial hypermobility; type IV, ecchymotic or aortic; type V, X-linked; type VI, ocular; type VII, arthrochalosis multiplex congenita; type VIII, periodontal form; type IX, EDS with abnormal copper metabolism, Menkes's steely-hair syndrome (some variants) and cutis laxa (some variants).*

† *AD, autosomal dominant; AR, autosomal recessive; XL, X-linked.*

as an autosomal recessive trait. The second form, defined as type VIIB, involves a series of different mutations that make the type I procollagen resistant to cleavage by *N*-proteinase. The enzyme requires a protein substrate in a native conformation, and it will not cleave type I procollagen that has an abnormal conformation. The change in amino acid sequences of the proα chains of type I procollagen can be located as much as 90 amino acids away from the site at which the enzyme cleaves the protein. In both type VIIA and type VIIB variants, the persistence of the *N*-propeptide on the molecule causes the formation of fibrils that are unusually thin. As discussed above, such thin fibrils can provide a scaffolding for bone but do not provide the necessary tensile strength for ligaments and joint capsules.

A defect in copper metabolism is present in most patients studied with type IX EDS (see Chap. 77). Low levels of serum copper and serum ceruloplasmin are accompanied by marked elevation of copper within cells. The molecular defects in some patients appear to be linked to synthesis of a diffusable factor involved either in regulation of the metallothionein gene or in some other aspect of copper metabolism.

Diagnosis Diagnosis is still based primarily on clinical evaluation of patients. Biochemical assays for known defects in EDS are still difficult and time-consuming. In type IV variants, incubation of cultured skin fibroblasts with radioactive proline or glycine followed by gel electrophoresis of the newly synthesized proteins will usually demonstrate a defect in the synthesis or secretion of type III procollagen. The approach is not currently applicable to prenatal diagnosis. A protocol for observing both the secretion and the rate of processing of type I procollagen in cultures of skin fibroblasts provides a simple method of identifying deficiencies of procollagen *N*-proteinase and structural mutations that prevent cleavage of the *N*-propeptide. It should therefore be useful in the diagnosis of both type VIIA and type VIIB EDS. However, some patients with OI are also positive by this assay. In patients suspected of having type IX EDS, the assignment to this general category can be confirmed by assays of copper and ceruloplasmin in serum and in fibroblast cultures. Specific DNA tests should soon be available for families in which the exact mutations in type I genes have been defined. Also, it is likely that restriction fragment length polymorphisms will be applicable for prenatal diagnosis in families with severe forms of EDS (see also Chap. 58).

Treatment There are no specific treatments for the disease. Surgical repair and tightening of the joint ligament require careful evaluation of individual patients since the ligaments frequently will not hold sutures. The cardiovascular status should be evaluated in all patients, particularly those suspected of having type IV. Patients with bruisability should be evaluated for specific bleeding disorders, but such tests are usually negative.

MARFAN'S SYNDROME

Diagnosis Marfan's syndrome is defined on the basis of characteristic changes in three connective tissue systems: the skeleton, the eyes, and the cardiovascular system (Fig. 319-6). The disease is inherited as an autosomal dominant trait, and 15 to 30 percent of cases may be due to new mutations. ''Skipped generations'' due to variable expressivity is relatively common. Also, the typical marfanoid habitus, lens dislocations, and cardiovascular abnormalities can each be inherited independently in some families. Therefore, the diagnosis is usually not made unless at least one member of a family has characteristic changes in at least two of the three connective tissue systems.

Skeletal changes Patients are unusually tall compared to other members of the same family and have unusually long limbs. The ratio of the upper segment (top of head to top of pubic ramus) to the lower segment (top of pubic ramus to floor) is usually 2 standard deviations below mean for age, race, and sex. The patients usually have long and slender fingers and toes (called arachnodactyly or dolichostenomelia), but these are difficult to evaluate objectively.

Because of longitudinal overgrowth of the ribs, many patients have chest deformities, including depression (pectus excavatum), protrusion (pectus carinatum), or marked asymmetry. Scoliosis is usually present, often accompanied by kyphosis.

Patients fall into three categories in terms of joint mobility. Most have moderate hypermobility of most joints. Some have marked hypermobility similar to that in EDS, but a few have exceptionally tight joints with contractures of hands and fingers. The group with the latter disorder, which is known as contractual arachnodactyly, appears to be less prone to cardiovascular problems.

Cardiovascular changes Mitral valve prolapse and aortic dilatation are common. Dilatation of the aorta begins in the root and is usually progressive so that dissection and rupture are common. Echocardiography is particularly helpful in evaluation.

Ocular changes The characteristic finding is subluxation of the lens (ectopia lentis), usually in an upward direction. The lens dislocation, however, may be detectable only by slit lamp examination. Displacement of the lens into the anterior chamber may cause glaucoma, but glaucoma is more frequent after surgical removal of the lens. The axial length of the globe is greater than normal, predisposing to myopia and retinal detachment.

Associated changes Striae may occur over the shoulders and buttocks. Otherwise the skin is normal. A number of patients develop

FIGURE 319-6 *A 16-year-old boy with Marfan's syndrome. Manifestations include dislocated lens; long, thin face; long fingers (arachnodactyly) and extremities (dolichostenomelia); and inward displacement of the sternum (pectus excavatum). (Courtesy of JG Hall.)*

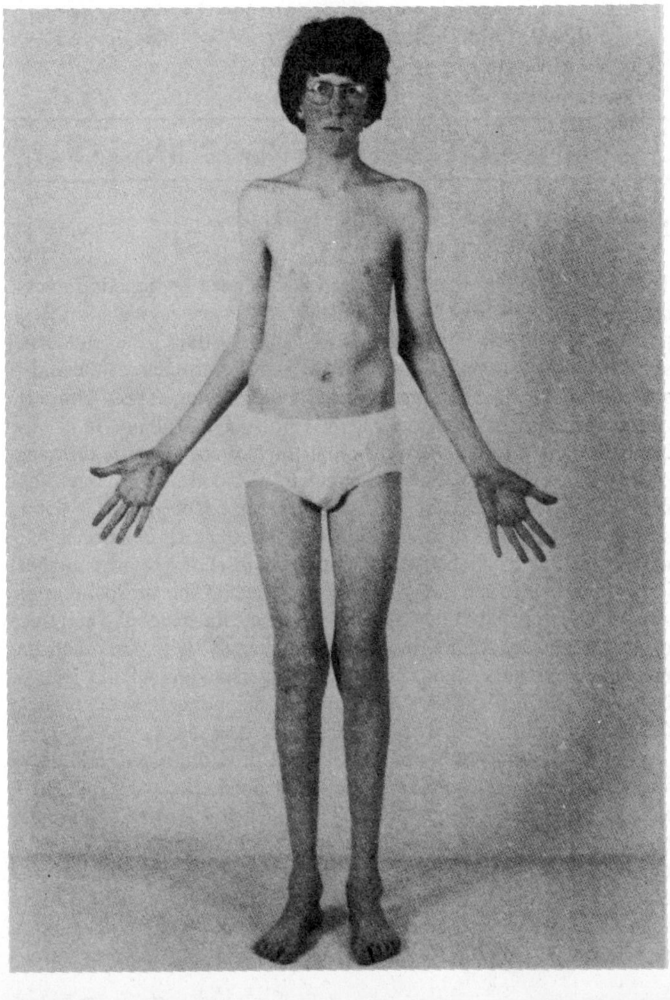

spontaneous pneumothorax. High-arched palate and high pedal arches are frequent.

Diagnosis The diagnosis is easiest to establish if the patient or members of the family have objective evidence of subluxed lenses, aortic dilatation, and severe kyphoscoliosis or chest deformities. The diagnosis is frequently made if ectopia lentis and an aneurysm of the ascending aorta are present without evidence of a Marfan habitus or a positive family history. All patients in whom the diagnosis is suspected should have a slip lamp examination and an echocardiogram. Also, homocystinuria (Table 319-3) should be ruled out by a negative cyanide-nitroprusside test for disulfides in the urine. Patients with types I, II, and III EDS may have ectopia lentis but lack the Marfan habitus and have characteristic skin changes not present in Marfan's syndrome.

Treatment As with other heritable disorders of connective tissue, there is no established treatment. Several investigators have recommended use of propranolol to delay or prevent the severe aortic complications, but the therapy is unproven. Surgical replacement of the aorta, aortic valve, and mitral valve has been undertaken in a number of patients.

The scoliosis tends to be progressive and should be treated by mechanical bracing and physical therapy if greater than 20° or by surgery if it continues to progress and becomes greater than 45°. Estrogen to induce menarche has been tried in girls with progressive scoliosis, but the results are inconclusive.

The subluxated lens rarely requires surgical removal, but patients should be followed closely for signs of retinal detachment.

Counseling is based on a 50 percent probability of passing on the defective gene. Because of the heterogeneity of the disease, offspring may be more or less severely affected than their parents. Women should be advised that the cardiovascular risk of pregnancy is high.

REFERENCES

BLECK EE: Non-operative treatment of osteogenesis imperfecta: Orthotic and mobility management. Clin Orthop 159:115, 1981

BYERS PH et al: Ehlers-Danlos syndrome, in *Principles and Practice of Medical Genetics*, vol 2, AEH Emery, DL Rimoin (eds). New York, Churchill Livingston, 1983, p 36

MCKUSICK VA: *Heritable Disorders of Connective Tissue*, 4th ed. St. Louis, Mosby, 1972

PROCKOP JD, KIVIRIKKO KI: Heritable diseases of collagen. N Engl J Med 311:376, 1984

PYERITZ RE: Marfan syndrome, in *Principles and Practice of Medical Genetics*, vol 2, AEH Emery DL Rimoin (eds). New York, Churchill Livingston, 1983, p 57

SILLENCE DO: Osteogenesis imperfecta: An expanding panorama of variance. Clin Orthop 191:11, 1981

———: Disorders of bone density, volume and mineralization, in *Principles and Practice of Medical Genetics*, vol 2, AEH Emery, DL Rimoin (eds). New York, Churchill Livingston, 1983, p 736

SMITH R et al: *The Brittle Bone Syndrome: Osteogenesis Imperfecta*. London, Butterworths, 1983

UITTO J, BAUER EA: Diseases associated with collagen abnormalities, in *Collagen in Health and Disease*, JB Weiss, MID Jayson (eds). New York, Churchill Livingston, 1982, p 289

section 2 Endocrinology

320 PRINCIPLES OF ENDOCRINOLOGY

JEAN D. WILSON

The functional capacities of cells are determined by genetic factors, but the rates of the metabolic pathways in cells are regulated in large part by two interlocking and coordinated systems, the endocrine system and the nervous system. As originally formulated, these two systems were considered distinct, information being carried either by neural impulses or by chemical mediators in the blood. It is now clear that this conception is incomplete. Not only may neurotransmitters such as norepinephrine circulate in blood as hormones, but neural impulses have major effects on the release of chemical mediators such as testosterone and insulin. This interlocking relationship is most apparent in the hypothalamus, which serves as the highest integrative center for the two systems. Hence, one neuroendocrine system has evolved to integrate and coordinate the metabolic activities of the organism. Endocrinology deals largely with the chemical mediators in this system, but proper understanding of the role of hormones requires knowledge of both the autonomic nervous system (Chap. 66) and the metabolic capacities of cells.

The formulation of endocrinology has been blurred in additional ways. The term *hormone* was originally applied to substances that are secreted into the circulation and act as chemical effectors in other tissues. However, the capacity to form such chemical mediators is not limited to so-called endocrine organs. Some hormones such as angiotensins II and III are formed in the bloodstream itself. Others such as testosterone in women and dihydrotestosterone and estradiol in men are in part secreted and in part formed in peripheral tissues from circulating precursors, so-called prohormones. Still other chemical mediators circulate only in restricted compartments such as the hypothalamic-pituitary portal system and do not reach the systemic circulation in appreciable quantities. Finally, certain hormones such as insulin, dihydrotestosterone, and thyrotropin-releasing hormone (TRH) have paracrine actions in the same tissues in which they are formed and exert different actions at distal sites. Therefore, the action as well as the origins should be considered when deciding whether or not a given effector should be classified as a hormone.

BIOCHEMISTRY Synthesis The mammalian hormones, now recognized to be more than 60 in number, fall into three major categories—peptides or peptide derivatives, steroids, and amines—and are synthesized in one of two ways. In the case of peptide hormones, genes code for messenger RNA, which is then translated into protein precursors. These proteins undergo posttranslational cleavage (preproparathyroid hormone → proparathyroid hormone → parathyroid hormone and proinsulin → insulin) and/or processing (thyroglobulin → thyroxine → triiodothyronine) to form the active hormone recognized by the target tissue. The distinct feature of peptide hormones is that one (or a few) genes code for the amino acid sequence of the peptide while other genes are responsible for the alteration of the peptide to its final form. In the case of peptide hormones with subunits, the different subunits may either be derived from a single precursor (insulin) or from separate precursors [luteinizing hormone (LH)]. Furthermore, the same peptide hormone (somatostatin) can be formed from different prohormones encoded by distinct genes, and individual prohormones such as pro-opiomelanocortin can be metabolized to different hormones in different cells, depending on the complement of processing enzymes in the cell in question (see Chap. 69). Peptide hormones can also be formed ectopically in malignancies of nonendocrine origin such as carcinoma of the lung (see Chap. 303).

In the case of steroid hormones the fundamental precursor—cholesterol (for most steroid hormones) or 7-dehydrocholesterol (for vitamin D metabolites)—undergoes a series of enzymatic transformations to form the final products. At least six enzymes (or enzyme complexes) and consequently six or more genes are required to transform cholesterol to estradiol. Because of the number of enzymes required the synthesis of steroids from cholesterol is unusual in malignancies of nonendocrine tissues. However, many tissues that cannot form steroid hormones de novo from cholesterol do contain enzymes that convert circulating steroids to other hormones, for example, the conversions of androgens to estrogens by trophoblastic tumors and the conversion of progesterone to deoxycorticosterone by the kidney.

The amine hormones are synthesized by a similar series of reactions to those involved in steroid hormone synthesis except that the precursors are amino acids. For example, tyrosine is the precursor for epinephrine and norepinephrine (see Chap. 66).

Storage Most tissues that synthesize hormones have a limited capacity to store the completed product. For example, the normal adult testes contain only about one-sixth of the quantity of testosterone needed for daily turnover, and consequently the testicular pool turns over several times to provide the normal daily output of hormone. Even when tissues have special storage organelles for hormone, the amount of hormone stored is usually limited: the insulin granules in the pancreatic beta cell ordinarily contain amounts of insulin sufficient only for short-term, reserve needs, whereas nerve endings may contain a several-day supply of norepinephrine. The limited capacity to store hormones is a chemical consequence of their unsuitability for incorporation into any of the three main storage compartments of the body (lipids, glycogen, or protein). For example, most steroid hormones are too polar to be stored in large quantities in lipid compartments, and peptide and amine hormones are unsuitable for incorporation into proteins. As a consequence of these factors the body pools of most hormones tend to be small. The major exceptions to this rule are those instances in which the precursor forms of hormone can be stored either as protein or in neutral lipid compartments; the normal thyroid gland contains the equivalent of a 2-week supply of thyroid hormones in the form of the protein thyroglobulin, and the precursor and intermediate forms of vitamin D can be stored in considerable quantity in hepatic lipid.

Release The biochemical mechanisms involved in the release process are poorly understood. In some instances they are thought to involve conversion of insoluble to soluble derivatives (proteolysis of thyroglobulin to thyroid hormones). In others, release is due to exocytosis of storage granules (insulin, glucagon, prolactin, growth hormone). Finally, release may involve passive diffusion of newly synthesized molecules such as steroid hormones down activity gradients into plasma; under this circumstance the rate of hormone release may be determined in part by the rate of blood flow to the tissue.

Because of the limited capacity for storage, most hormones are released into plasma as a reflection of the rates of formation. The pituitary trophic hormones [LH, adrenocorticotropin (ACTH) thyrotropin (TSH)] act in their target tissues to influence rates of both hormone synthesis and release. Even when peptide hormones are stored in granules, initial release of the stored material is followed by an enhanced rate of synthesis (as, for instance, the two-phase release of insulin induced by glucose infusion). For some hormones, major diurnal, sleep-related, developmental, and neural factors influence hormone release; again it is assumed that in most of these instances synthesis and release are tightly linked.

In many instances, the regulation of hormone release on a short-term basis is poorly understood. Some hormones are released in a pulsatile fashion with bursts of secretion occurring in a repetitive pattern; whether this intermittent release is a function of alterations in synthetic rates, alterations in blood flow, or other mechanisms is uncertain. While the physiologic significance of pulsatile release is not fully understood, changes in frequency or in amplitude of the release pattern may have profound effects on hormone function; i.e., the pulsatile administration of luteinizing hormone–releasing hormone (LHRH) stimulates the release of LH by the pituitary whereas the constant infusion of the same amount of hormone per unit time has the opposite effect. Furthermore, changes in frequency or amplitude of hormone release may characterize specific disease states; loss of the diurnal rhythm of cortisol release is characteristic of the early phase of Cushing's disease.

Transport Hormones are transported via lymph, blood, and extracellular fluids from sites of synthesis to sites of cellular action and ultimately of metabolic inactivation and degradation. The plasma is probably a passive diluent for most peptide and amine hormones but provides specific proteins for binding and transport of certain steroid and thyroid hormones. The generalization can be made that the more insoluble a hormone in water, the more important the role of transport proteins. No transport protein yet characterized is exclusive; for example, testosterone can be transported both by a specific binding protein [testosterone-binding globulin (TeBG)] and by albumin; thyroxine can be transported both by prealbumin and by thyroxine-binding globulin (TBG). Protein-bound hormone (HP) cannot enter most cellular compartments and serves as a reservoir from which free hormone (H) is liberated in sufficient quantities for diffusion into intracellular compartments:

$$H + P \rightleftharpoons HP$$

Distribution of bound and free hormone in plasma is determined by the amount of hormone, the amount of binding protein, and the binding affinity of hormone for the protein. However, in the intact organism the effective level of free hormone is influenced by additional factors. When the rate of dissociation of a hormone from a binding protein is rapid (more rapid than the capillary transit time for a specific organ), then the functional free fraction in vivo is also influenced by capillary transit time and membrane permeability.

Understanding the relation between free and bound hormone is essential for assessment of endocrine function. First, the free (dialyzable) fraction in vitro is generally less than the actual free fraction available for transport in vivo; this is because the portion of hormone bound to weak binding proteins such as albumin (in contrast to that portion bound to specific, high-affinity binding proteins) rapidly dissociates from the albumin as the free fraction diffuses from the capillary; consequently the albumin-bound hormone may function in vivo as a free fraction. Under many conditions, measurement of the dialyzable fraction does provide a useful index of the in vivo apparent free fraction. However, in hypoalbuminemic states, the in vitro free (dialyzable) fraction may increase when the in vivo free hormone level is diminished. In addition, in those tissue compartments such as liver in which proteins including hormone-transport protein complexes are cleared (in contrast to the situation in peripheral tissues in which only the free hormone enters the cell) free hormone levels have lesser effects on hormone uptake by the tissue.

Second, the net distribution of hormones between plasma and tissue is a function of the balance between tissue binding proteins and plasma binding proteins. Therefore, levels of true or apparent free hormone do not reflect the amounts of hormone within cells.

Third, only the free hormone interacts with peripheral cells and participates in the regulatory feedback mechanisms that control the rates of hormone synthesis. As a consequence, changes in the amount of transport protein alone cannot cause endocrine pathology in the steady state, provided the remainder of the endocrine feedback loop is intact. For example, profound elevations or decreases in TBG (either because of genetic or other factors) are both compatible with a euthyroid state. To illustrate, a sudden increase in TBG lowers the level of free (dialyzable) hormone and of the amount bound to albumin; as a consequence TSH secretion increases, and the output of thyroxine by the thyroid is increased *until* TBG is again saturated so that the level of free hormone returns to the normal range, at which time TSH levels and thyroid hormone secretion also return to normal. Likewise, a decrease in TBG temporarily increases the level of free hormone, and TSH secretion and thyroxine output fall until the free level returns to normal. To summarize, a change in the amount of a specific, high-affinity binding protein can cause profound alterations in hormone levels but by itself cannot cause either a steady-state hormone excess or deficiency, provided the regulatory feedback mechanisms that control hormone synthesis are intact. However, alteration of the amount of a binding protein may cause endocrine pathology in those instances in which hormone formation is not regulated by ordinary feedback control mechanisms. For example, testosterone production in women is not regulated directly by testosterone levels, and alterations in TeBG levels in women may alter the steady state levels of free testosterone.

Degradation and turnover The plasma level (PL) of any hormone is dependent on two factors—the secretion rate (SR) of the hormone and the rates of metabolism and excretion, the so-called metabolic clearance rate (MCR):

$$PL = \frac{SR}{MCR} \quad \text{or} \quad SR = MCR \times PL$$

Metabolic clearance of hormones is accomplished by several mechanisms. Only small fractions of hormones are excreted intact in urine or bile. Degradation and inactivation of the hormone can take place in target tissues, in nontarget tissues such as liver and kidneys, or in both target and nontarget tissues. In many instances hormone metabolism facilitates excretion by rendering the hormone soluble in urine or bile. Peptide hormones are in general inactivated by proteases, largely in target tissues. Thyroid hormones are deiodinated, deaminated, and deconjugated primarily by the liver. Steroid hormones are reduced, hydroxylated, and converted into glucuronide and sulfate conjugates. On occasion biliary conjugates may be hydrolyzed in the gastrointestinal tract and reabsorbed into the circulation. The degradative mechanisms for different hormones have one common feature, namely, that alternative pathways exist for the catabolism of all hormones described to date.

Because of the nature of the feedback control of hormone secretion, changes in rates of hormone degradation alone do not cause endocrine pathology, provided the feedback loops that regulate synthesis are intact. For example, in severe liver disease and in myxedema, the degradation of glucocorticoids by the liver is impaired; as a consequence the turnover of cortisol slows, but the plasma level does not rise because secretion of ACTH is inhibited. Thus, a normal level of free hormone is maintained by decreasing the rate of cortisol secretion. The opposite is the case when glucocorticoid degradation is enhanced (as in thyrotoxicosis); in this situation cortisol secretion rises to keep the level of the hormone normal.

Although changes in rates of hormone degradation alone do not result in hormone deficit or excess, such changes may cause profound alterations in endocrine pharmacology. Thus, ordinary doses of glucocorticoids may cause the Cushing syndrome in patients with myxedema or liver disease, and consequently glucocorticoid dosage must be reduced in both conditions. Likewise, doses of glucocorticoids may have to be increased in the presence of hyperthyroidism. In addition, the development of hyperthyroidism in a patient with inadequate adrenal reserve might precipitate an adrenal crisis by accelerating the rate of glucocorticoid catabolism. Thus, in circumstances in which the normal servomechanisms that regulate hormone synthesis are either circumvented or inoperative, changes in rates of hormone degradation may aggravate or cause pathology.

REGULATION OF HORMONE PRODUCTION As stated above, fluctuations of hormone levels in the normal person are determined primarily by changes in rates of production. A unifying feature of all endocrine systems is the fact that the production of most hormones is regulated directly or indirectly by the metabolic activity of the hormone itself. This regulation is accomplished through a series of negative feedback loops (Fig. 320-1). In some cases a fairly constant blood level of hormone is required, and some sensing device must exist to monitor either the hormone level itself or some related function such as plasma osmolality, blood glucose, plasma calcium, or body sodium content. For example, hormones produced in response to pituitary trophic hormones (cortisol, thyroxine, gonadal steroids) feed back on the hypothalamic-pituitary system to regulate their own rates of secretion. Similarly, parathyroid hormone and insulin are secreted in response to feedback signals from serum calcium and glucose levels, respectively. Feedback systems are generally more complex than this description indicates, sometimes operating indirectly by several steps; in those instances in which the hormone itself acts as the direct regulator of feedback (testosterone on the pituitary), the effect is mediated by the same cellular machinery by which the action of the hormone is accomplished in other target tissues.

Both negative and positive feedback can occur; an example of positive feedback is the stimulation of LH release by estradiol prior to ovulation. Nonhormonal and environmental factors may alter either positive or negative feedback control mechanisms or the response to such control.

A usual feature of the feedback systems is rapidity of action; indeed, most respond within minutes or hours to varying metabolic demands to maintain homeostatic control within a narrow range. The main exceptions relate to gametogenesis in the ovary and testis (see Chaps. 330 and 331). In both instances, a complex differentiative process is involved. The steady-state operation of these systems is such that sperm production tends to be relatively constant from day to day whereas ovulation is cyclic. However, spermatogenesis requires approximately a month to complete so that changes in FSH levels may not result in altered rates of sperm production for long periods.

The fact that the secretion of hormones is under regulatory control has several important clinical implications. First, the clinical significance of plasma levels of hormones may be interpretable only if the appropriate regulatory factors are taken into account (Fig. 320-2). The meaning of a borderline low testosterone value may become clear only when LH is measured simultaneously; likewise, plasma insulin and parathyroid hormone levels may be interpretable only in conjunction with simultaneous measurements of plasma glucose and calcium, respectively. Second, the finding of simultaneous elevations of hormone pairs (or hormone-regulatory factor pairs) in the absence of signs of hormone excess suggests the presence of a hormone-resistance state. For example, simultaneous elevation of plasma glucose and insulin is characteristic of insulin resistance; simultaneous elevation of LH and testosterone suggests androgen resistance, etc. Third, insight into the regulatory control of hormone secretion is the basis for the various dynamic tests of hormone reserve and hormone secretion.

FIGURE 320-1 *Feedback control of an endocrine organ such as the adrenal, thyroid, or gonads by the pituitary.*

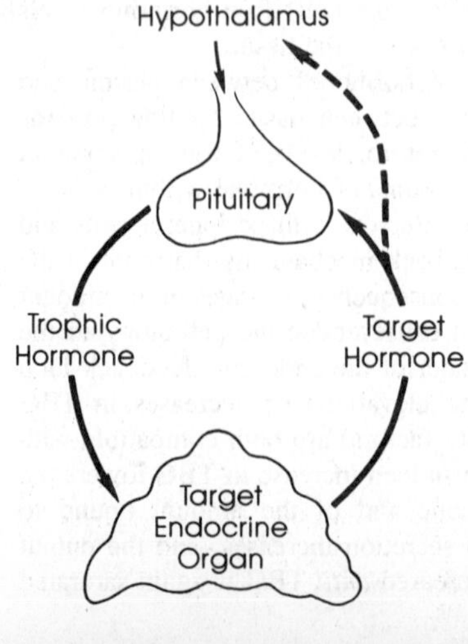

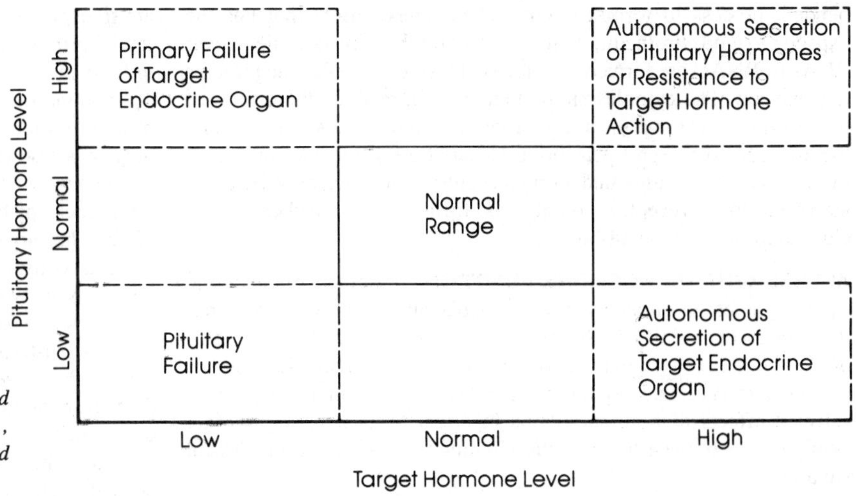

FIGURE 320-2 *Relation between target hormone level and trophic hormone level in normal and disease states (e.g., TSH and thyroid hormones, ACTH and cortisol, LH and testosterone).*

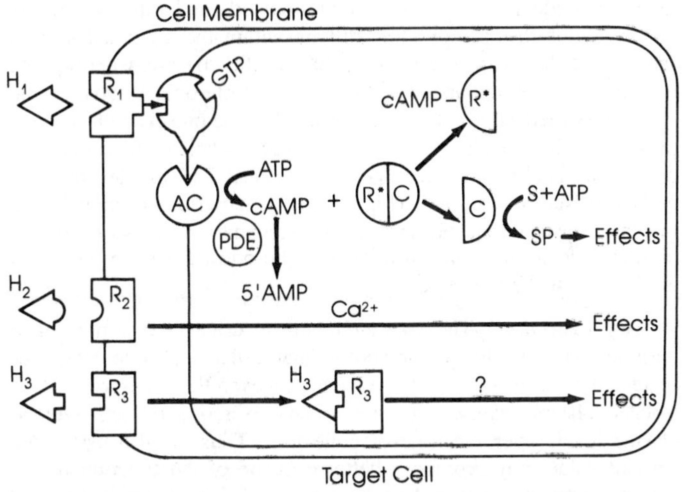

FIGURE 320-3 *Schema of action of hormones with cell surface receptors. H = hormone; R = receptor; C = catalytic subunit of protein kinase; R* = cAMP-binding subunit of protein kinase; cAMP = cyclic AMP; AC = adenylate cyclase; S = substrate; SP = phosphorylated substrate; PDE = phosphodiesterase.*

MECHANISMS OF HORMONE ACTION The first step in hormone action is the interaction of the hormone with specific macromolecules in the cell, so-called hormone receptors either on the plasma membrane of the cell surface or in the cell cytoplasm.

Hormones with cell surface receptors The hormones of the first type bind to surface receptors localized on the plasma membrane (Fig. 320-3). At least three categories of plasma membrane–hormone interaction can be distinguished. In the first category (H_1 in Fig. 320-3) the hormone-receptor complex on the cell surfaces causes the production of a so-called second messenger, cyclic adenosine 3′,5′-monophosphate (cAMP), and the subsequent actions of the hormone are mediated by cAMP (for details see Chap. 67). This mechanism applies to several protein hormones and to the biogenic amines. In the second category (H_2 in Fig. 320-3) the cell surface receptor causes the production or release of other second messengers, for example, calcium. This mechanism applies to certain neurotransmitters and TRH. The precise mechanism of calcium release and action in such systems is not known; the latter may involve binding of calcium to the enzyme-regulating protein calmodulin. In the third category (H_3 in Fig. 320-3) the cell surface receptor–hormone complex is internalized within the cell, but the subsequent events have not been defined. A hormone of the last category is insulin (see Chap. 327).

The best understood of these systems is that in which cAMP serves as the second messenger (Fig. 320-3). Cellular concentration of cAMP is controlled by two enzymes with opposite activities. Adenylate cyclase (AC), localized in the plasma membrane, converts adenosine triphosphate (ATP) into cAMP. Phosphodiesterase (PDE), found largely in the cell cytosol, inactivates cAMP by converting it to 5′-adenosine monophosphate (5′-AMP). Hormones (H_1) that act at the cell surface form a reversible complex with specialized membrane protein receptors (R_1). These proteins bind the hormone with high affinity but limited capacity. The formation of the hormone-receptor complex causes stimulation of the adenylate cyclase. The H_1R_1 complex binds the N subunit of the adenylate cyclase (a protein that also binds GTP) and activates the catalytic subunit of the enzyme AC, thus stimulating cAMP synthesis. Phosphorylating enzymes—known as protein kinases—appear to play an important role in the overall process; these kinases (RC) are composed of catalytic (C) and regulatory (R) subunits. Binding of cAMP to R frees C and allows phosphorylation of various proteins (S) with consequent activation or inactivation.

Hormones with intracellular receptors Steroid and thyroid hormones are transported in plasma bound to carrier proteins (Fig. 320-4). The protein-bound hormones (HP) are in dynamic equilibrium with small amounts of free hormones (H) that diffuse by a passive mechanism into cells where they act by fundamentally different mechanisms than do the peptide hormones. In most instances the principal form of the hormone secreted into plasma (cortisol, progesterone, aldosterone, estradiol) undergoes no further metabolism within the cell and is responsible for hormone action within the target cell. Other hormones (thyroxine, testosterone) undergo chemical conversion to more active forms (triiodothyronine and dihydrotestosterone).

H binds to specific receptor proteins (R) in the cytoplasm to form a hormone-receptor complex (HR). The hormone-receptor complex undergoes transformation by a poorly understood, temperature-de-

FIGURE 320-4 *Mechanism of action of hormones with intracellular receptors. H = hormone; P = plasma transport protein; R = receptor; R* = activated receptor; mRNA = messenger RNA.*

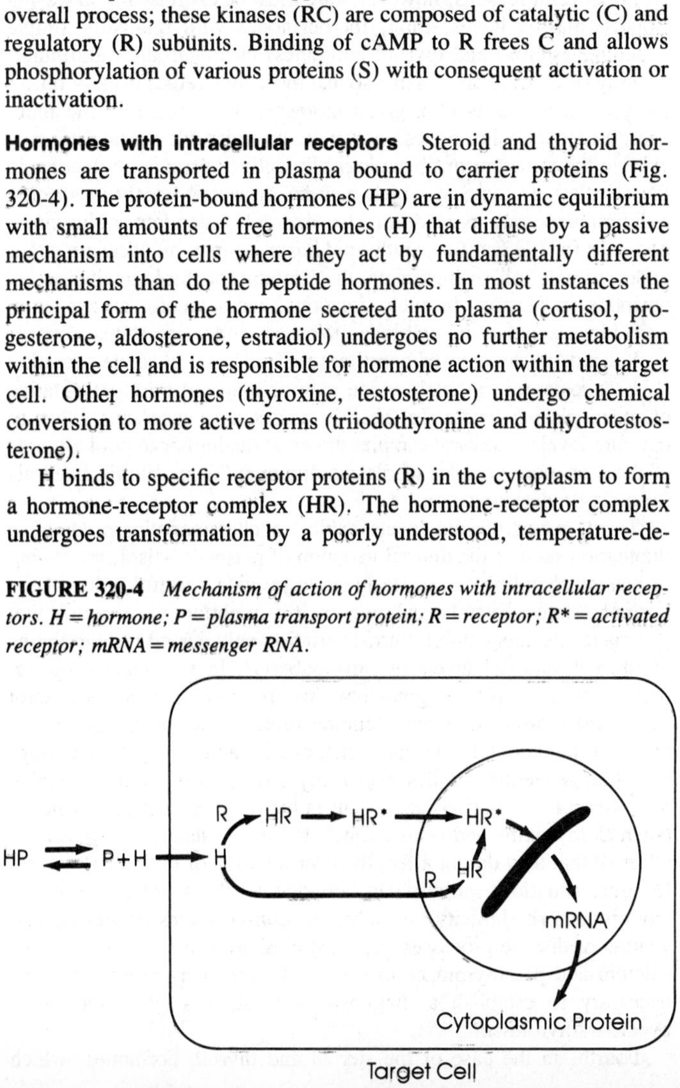

pendent process to form an activated complex (HR*) that has the capacity to bind chromatin. As the result of this binding new messenger RNAs (mRNAs) are formed, and the synthesis of cytoplasmic proteins is enhanced. The cytoplasmic proteins in turn mediate the effects of the hormone. In some instances (triiodothyronine and some steroids) the unoccupied receptor proteins are located predominantly in nuclei; in such cases the unbound hormone enters the nucleus where the active hormone-receptor complex is formed and attaches to the chromatin in a similar fashion.

ASSESSMENT OF HORMONE FUNCTION In practice endocrine status is assessed either by measuring plasma levels of a hormone, the urinary excretion of a hormone or of some metabolite, the rates of secretion of hormones into the circulation, dynamic tests of hormone reserve and regulation, the levels of hormone receptors, selected effects of hormone action in target tissues, or appropriate combinations of these tests. Each technique is useful in certain clinical situations.

Plasma levels The plasma levels of steroid and thyroid hormones range between 1 n*M* and 1 μ*M*, while those of peptide hormones are generally in the range of 1 p*M* to 0.1 n*M*. The application of modern chemical, chromatographic, radioreceptor, and radioimmunoassay techniques for the assessment of plasma constituents in low concentrations constitutes one of the significant advances of modern medicine and has transformed endocrinology to a more quantitative discipline. In the case of hormones whose plasma levels are relatively constant from moment to moment and day to day (thyroxine and triiodothyronine), the measurement of isolated plasma levels alone provides a reliable assessment of the hormone status in most clinical situations.

For several reasons, however, care must be exercised in assessing isolated plasma levels. First, for hormones with relatively simple structures (steroid and thyroid hormones) chemical and radioimmunoassay techniques are reliable so that measured values usually reflect the plasma levels as of a given moment. In the case of the more complex peptide hormones, however, considerable variability may exist in the structure of physiologically active hormone molecules in the circulation, some of which may be measured poorly in specific radioimmunoassay procedures; for example, standard radioimmunoassays for LH and for parathyroid hormone may on occasion either underestimate or overestimate the amount of biologically active hormone in plasma. In such situations, radioreceptor assays or in vitro bioassays may be employed to assess endocrine status.

Second, in the case of hormones that undergo pulsatile secretion (LH, testosterone) a single value may or may not be representative of mean plasma levels. In these instances it is necessary either to measure levels in several samples drawn at random or to pool aliquots of three or more samples of plasma drawn at 20- to 30-min intervals for a single determination.

Third, when plasma levels exhibit a characteristic, predictable fluctuation such as the diurnal variation of plasma cortisol, the timing of plasma sampling can be designed to provide a useful index of the hormone status. Even here, however, it is important to recognize that plasma levels may exhibit diurnal variation only during certain phases of life (plasma LH levels in early puberty). In women appropriate interpretation of plasma gonadotropins, progesterone, and estradiol during the reproductive years requires reference to the corresponding phase of the ovulatory and menstrual cycles, and it may be necessary to obtain sequential studies over many days to provide interpretable data. Seasonal variations also occur in the levels of certain hormones (such as thyroxine and testosterone), but these changes are generally so small that they do not affect the interpretation of individual values. In some situations variation in hormone levels is not the result of any obvious rhythmicity but rather the consequences of waxing and waning of disease processes; repeated measurements of cortisol or of calcium and parathyroid hormone levels over many months may be necessary to establish a diagnosis of Cushing's syndrome or of hyperparathyroidism.

Fourth, in the case of the steroid and thyroid hormones, which are transported in plasma largely bound to proteins, measurement of total hormone concentration provides an index of endocrine status *only* to the extent that it allows a deduction of the level of the free or unbound hormone. Indeed, direct measurements of the free levels of these hormones (usually 1 percent or less of the total) can be done only in a few labs. Since the amount of free hormone is a function of the amount and the affinity of binding of transport proteins and the amount of hormone, the total hormone level reflects the amount of free hormone only as long as the amount of binding protein(s) remains constant or fluctuates only within narrow limits. In those instances in which the level of binding protein is increased (TBG and TeBG in pregnancy) or decreased [hereditary decreases in TBG and corticosteroid-binding globulin (CBG)] it is essential to utilize some other assessment of the amount of binding protein to allow deduction of the free hormone level (T_3 resin uptake for TBG or direct measurement of TBG, TeBG, or CBG).

Fifth, the range of plasma levels of most hormones within the normal population is broad. As a consequence, the level of a hormone in an individual may be halved or doubled (and thus be grossly abnormal for that person) but still be within the so-called normal range. For this reason it is frequently useful to assess appropriate hormone pairs simultaneously (LH and testosterone, thyroxine and TSH); a borderline low testosterone level in the presence of elevated plasma LH is indicative of testicular failure, whereas the same level of testosterone in the presence of a normal LH implies that the endocrine status is normal (Fig. 320-2). Likewise, in women with increased testosterone production and secondary decrease in TeBG, plasma testosterone concentration may be normal despite increased production of the hormone.

Urinary excretion The measurement of urinary excretion of a hormone or a hormone metabolite that reflects plasma levels or secretory rates offers certain advantages over the measurement of isolated plasma levels, e.g., the urinary excretion reflects average plasma levels over the time of collection. Thus, a 24-h urine free cortisol value may provide a better estimate of the function of the adrenal cortex than isolated measurements of plasma cortisol. Again, however, certain limitations of the use of urinary measurements must be kept in mind. (1) Creatinine determinations should be done routinely to document the adequacy of the urine collection. Women excrete on average about 1 g, and men about 1.8 g per day. Day-to-day variation should not exceed 20 percent. (2) The excretion of individual metabolites may not reflect changes in hormone secretion under all conditions. For example, the formation of the 18-oxo derivative of aldosterone may be influenced by drugs that do not alter secretion or plasma levels of the hormone. (3) Urine values are obviously meaningless for those hormones (thyroxine, triiodothyronine) excreted into bile. Of more importance is the fact that peptide hormones such as gonadotropins may be metabolized differently in different individuals prior to excretion into the urine so that establishment of the range of normal is difficult. (4) Hormones from more than one source may be excreted as common metabolites; urinary 17-ketosteroids are derived from both adrenal and gonadal androgens, and consequently their measurement is of little value in assessing testicular androgen production in men. (5) Changes in renal function may influence rates of hormone excretion into urine. Such changes can in part be corrected by measurement of urine creatinine, but in the case of metabolites or conjugates formed in the kidney itself excretion patterns may be distorted out of proportion to the decrease in creatinine clearance.

Secretion and production rates The measurement of the actual secretion rate of a hormone circumvents most problems inherent in measurement of plasma levels and urinary excretion. Such measurements involve the administration of radioactive hormone and measuring the dilution that such a hormone undergoes as a consequence of mixture with endogenously secreted, nonradioactive hormones over a given period of time. In practice the plasma hormone itself or a unique metabolite of the hormone from urine is isolated, purified to radiochemical homogeneity, and used to calculate the amount of the hormone secreted during the time of study. In the case of hormones formed principally in peripheral tissues (estradiol and dihydrotestosterone in men, triiodothyronine in both sexes) radioactive precursors can be administered, and the rates of conversion to the metabolites in question can be measured for assessment of overall production rates. Alternatively, as described above, clearance rates of hormones can be measured and, together with mean plasma levels, used to estimate secretion rates. Unfortunately, these various techniques are complex and expensive to perform, require use of radioactive isotopes, and can be done in only a few centers.

Dynamic tests of hormone reserve and regulation When hypo- or hyperfunction is severe, measurement of the level of hormone in blood or urine may be satisfactory for making a diagnosis, particularly when the tests demonstrate appropriate feedback relationships; e.g., low plasma testosterone coupled with high plasma LH indicates primary testicular failure. In less clear-cut instances, however, stimulation tests are useful in establishing the significance of borderline low values. Likewise, suppression tests are used to document the presence of hyperfunction of endocrine systems. All such dynamic tests are designed to take advantage of the known feedback control mechanisms for various hormones (Fig. 320-1).

Two types of stimulation tests are in common usage. In one, endogenous hormone production or action is blocked (cortisol production by metyrapone, estradiol action by clomiphene), and the capacity of the pituitary to respond by increasing endogenous production of the trophic hormone and/or the capacity of the target tissue to respond are then assessed; ideally such tests measure the integrity of an entire hypothalamic–pituitary–target tissue loop. In the other type of stimulation test, the trophic hormone itself is administered under some standardized regimen, and the capacity of the target tissue to respond is determined (cortisol levels before and after ACTH administration). Stimulation tests are particularly useful in four situations: (1) assessing hormone status when precise quantification of plasma levels is difficult or imperfect (ACTH), (2) assessing endocrine status when static tests are borderline low, (3) distinguishing primary from secondary (pituitary) causes of endocrine failure, and (4) assessing gonadal reserve in prepubertal patients in whom plasma gonadotropins and gonadal steroids are difficult to interpret.

Suppression tests are useful for the diagnosis of hyperfunction because the hyperfunctioning gland by definition does not operate under normal control mechanisms. Suppression can either be quantitatively or qualitatively abnormal. For example, the feedback control of the pituitary may be reset to respond to high levels of the suppressing hormone (pituitary ACTH secretion in Cushing's disease), or secretion can be autonomous (ACTH secretion by carcinoma of the lung). In principle, the feedback regulator is administered, and the capacity of the secretion of the hormone to be inhibited is assessed for the endocrine system in question (change in ^{131}I uptake after administration of thyroid hormones, change in cortisol secretion after the administration of potent exogenous glucocorticoids, suppressibility of plasma growth hormone by glucose).

The clinical usefulness of dynamic tests of endocrine function is limited by the fact that they are altered by a multitude of secondary factors. Age, coexisting disease states, and concurrent drug regimens all interact to influence responsiveness and hence to limit the specificity of such tests.

Hormone receptors and antibodies The measurement of hormone receptors in biopsy material from target tissues or in fibroblasts propagated from biopsy material is useful—for example, in the diagnosis of partial hormone-resistance states such as rickets due to vitamin D resistance, hyperglycemia and hyperinsulinemia associated with insulin resistance, and male pseudohermaphroditism due to androgen resistance. Likewise, under selected conditions measurement of antibodies to hormones (such as antibodies to thyroid hormones that can cause hypothyroidism) or antibodies to target tissues (adrenal gland, gonads, thyroid) may be essential for the assessment of endocrine status. With certain exceptions (antibodies to thyroid tissue) these tests are not widely available.

Tissue effects The ideal hormone test perhaps is the measurement of the peripheral end result of hormone action in the target tissues for the hormone. For example, demonstration of the capacity to concentrate urine maximally following water restriction indicates that the hypothalamic control mechanisms are intact, that the posterior pituitary has a normal capacity to secrete vasopressin, that the vasopressin receptor is intact, and that the postreceptor effector mechanisms for the hormone are operative. Optimally such a test assesses the function of the entire pathway of hormone secretion and action. In practice, many such tests are imperfect. For example, even though vasopressin secretion is normal, intrinsic renal disease can result in a fixed low urine osmolality and thus distort the interpretation of the functional test of vasopressin action. In other instances the tests are difficult to perform and subject both to artifact and to influences from diverse parameters (for example, the metabolic rate is increased by fever even when thyroid function is normal). For these reasons, the identification of additional specific tissue markers for hormone action would be very useful.

CLINICAL SYNDROMES Endocrinopathy can result from hormone deficiency, hormone excess, or resistance to hormone action, and abnormalities in more than one endocrine system commonly coexist in the same individual.

Deficiency states With few exceptions (calcitonin) hormone deficiency results in pathologic manifestations. The study of clinical disorders that result from hormone deficiency or absence played an important role in the evolution of endocrinology as a discipline. Such studies were followed by attempts to extract the responsible hormone from normal endocrine tissues, characterize its chemical nature (and ultimately synthesize it), and administer the hormone to replace the deficit. The routine treatment of hypothyroidism by the administration of thyroid hormone is probably as successful as any therapeutic measure in medicine. Because clinical deficiency states can be induced in experimental animals by appropriate destruction or removal of the endocrine organ, an enormous amount is known about the pathophysiology of the deficiency states (diabetes mellitus, pituitary and adrenal insufficiency, hypothyroidism, and hypogonadism).

The nature of the destructive processes involved in the failure of the endocrine organs is also understood in many instances; these include infections (adrenal insufficiency due to tuberculosis), infarction (postpartum pituitary failure) and tissue death of other causes (diabetes secondary to pancreatitis), tumors (chromophobe adenomas of the pituitary), autoimmune processes (Hashimoto's thyroiditis), dietary inadequacy (hypothyroidism due to iodine deficiency), and hereditary defects (pituitary dwarfism). In certain forms of diabetes mellitus, the cause may be a hereditary predisposition that renders the pancreas subject to destruction by several mechanisms (see Chap. 327). In other endocrine-deficiency diseases the etiology of the defect is unidentified (ordinary myxedema and congenital anorchia).

Hormone excess With few exceptions (testosterone in men, progesterone in men and women) hormone excess causes pathologic effects. Four general types of hormone excess are recognized. In one, the hormone is overproduced by the gland that is the usual site of its production (hyperthyroidism, acromegaly, Cushing's disease); such excess production results from failure or circumvention of the feedback control mechanisms that regulate production of the hormone in the normal state, but the underlying mechanism is often obscure because animal models for the diseases are rare. The second type of hormone excess results when a hormone is produced by a tissue (usually malignant) that ordinarily is not a major endocrine organ (for example, ACTH production in oat cell carcinoma of the lung, thyroid hormone secretion by struma ovarii). Such hormone-excess states have been described for many hormones (see Chap. 303). A third type of hormone-excess state involves the overproduction of hormones in peripheral tissues from circulating precursors; for example, overproduction of estrogen in liver disease because of diversion of the precursor androstenedione from its usual sites of catabolism in the liver to sites of extraglandular estrogen formation. Finally, hormone excess all too commonly results from iatrogenic causes; for example, the complications resulting from glucocorticoid therapy constitute a major clinical problem (see Chap. 325).

Excess of a given hormone may result from more than one cause. Thyrotoxicosis can result from overproduction of hormone by the thyroid as a result of overproduction of TSH (rare), from stimulation by extrapituitary thyroid-stimulating factors, from autonomous thyroid hyperfunction; from leakage of preformed hormone from the thyroid due to an inflammatory injury; or from excess hormone from sources other than the thyroid itself, as in thyroid hormone overdosage or struma ovarii (see Chap. 324). The unraveling of the cause of specific hormone-excess states can be one of the most challenging problems of clinical endocrinology.

Production of abnormal hormones In some instances abnormal hormones can cause endocrine disease. One form of diabetes mellitus is the result of a single-gene mutation that results in the production of an abnormal insulin molecule that is ineffective because of defective binding to the insulin receptor. In other cases, hormone precursors or incompletely processed peptide hormones may be released into the circulation, as is common in so-called ectopic hormone production of neoplasia (see Chap. 303). Alternatively, immunoglobulins may bind to hormone receptors and thus exert hormonal actions, for example, the thyroid-stimulating immunoglobulins in hyperthyroidism (Chap. 324) or the antibodies to the insulin receptor that have some insulin-like actions (Chap. 327).

Hormone resistance The concept that an endocrinopathy could result because the tissues cannot respond to normal (or increased) levels of a hormone evolved from the deduction that pseudohypoparathyroidism is due to peripheral resistance to the action of parathyroid hormone (see Chaps. 67 and 336). This concept has had far-reaching implications. First, the concept of hormone resistance has served as a major stimulus for the study of how hormones act within cells. Second, more and more forms of hormone resistance have been identified so that diseases are now recognized to result from resistance to most hormones. Such hormone resistance is frequently due to hereditary causes. Third, hormone resistance can be due to a variety of causes, including defects in receptors and in postreceptor effector mechanisms for hormones, development of antibodies to hormones or hormone receptors, and the absence of target cells. Fourth, abnormalities of receptors are now implicated in the pathogenesis of diseases outside the endocrine domain, such as myasthenia gravis and familial hypercholesterolemia.

A common feature of hormone-resistance states is the coexistence of a normal or *elevated* level of the hormone in the circulation with evidence of deficient hormone action (Fig. 320-1). This feature is a consequence of the fact that most hormones are under regulatory feedback control, and failure of hormone action usually leads to increased hormone production.

However, hormone resistance does not necessarily involve equally all target tissues for the hormone. For example, selective resistance to thyroid hormone can be restricted to the pituitary itself, and in one form of androgen resistance androgen action is more severely impaired in the testis than in other target tissues. Elucidation of the pathogenesis of these selective defects will doubtlessly provide insight into the factors that determine the nature of "target tissues" for hormones.

Diseases affecting multiple endocrine systems The fact that disorders can affect more than one endocrine system has been known since the description of panhypopituitarism in the nineteenth century. Such disorders encompass diverse etiologies including autoimmunity (autoimmune polyglandular dysfunction, or Schmidt's syndrome), receptor abnormalities (gonadotropin and thyrotropin resistance in pseudohypoparathyroidism), tumors (multiple endocrine neoplasia, or MEN), and hereditary disorders of unknown etiology (lipodystrophies) (see Chap. 334). They may include both hypo- and hyperfunctioning states, and some clinical syndromes may occur in the context of more than one polyendocrine state (pheochromocytoma in MEN II and MEN III, diabetes mellitus in Schmidt's syndrome and in lipodystrophy).

Because each endocrinopathy in such a constellation can also occur alone, all endocrine patients must be approached with a high index of suspicion for abnormalities of multiple systems. This is of particular importance because treatment of one condition may cause worsening of another (surgical procedures such as thyroidectomy can cause worsening of unrecognized pheochromocytoma) and because in certain of the familial syndromes it is mandatory to make systematic searches for the disease in potentially affected family members.

REFERENCES

CLARK JH et al: Mechanisms of steroid hormone action, in *Williams' Textbook of Endocrinology*, 7th ed, JD Wilson, DW Foster (eds). Philadelphia, Saunders, 1985, pp 33–75

GILMAN AG: Guanine nucleotide-binding regulatory proteins and dual control of adenylate cyclase. J Clin Invest 73:1, 1984

GORDEN P, WEINTRAUB BD: Radioreceptor and other functional hormone assays, in *Williams' Textbook of Endocrinology*, 7th ed, JD Wilson, DW Foster (eds). Philadelphia, Saunders, 1985, pp 133–146

HABENER JF: Genetic control of hormone formation, in *Willimas' Textbook of Endocrinology*, 7th ed, JD Wilson, DW Foster (eds). Philadelphia, Saunders, 1985, pp 9–32

KRIEGER DT, ASCHOFF J: Endocrine and other biological rhythms, in *Endocrinology*, vol 3, LJ DeGroot et al (eds). New York, Grune & Stratton, 1979, pp 2079–2109

PARDRIDGE WM: Transport of protein-bound hormones into tissues in vivo. Endocr Rev 2:103, 1981

ROTH J, GRUNFELD C: Mechanism of action of peptide hormones and catecholamines, in *Williams' Textbook of Endocrinology*, 7th ed, JD Wilson, DW Foster (eds). Philadelphia, Saunders, pp 76–122

VERHOEVEN GFM, WILSON JD: The syndromes of primary hormone resistance. Metabolism 28:253, 1979

YALOW RS: Radioimmunoassay of hormones, in *Williams' Textbook of Endocrinology*, 7th ed, JD Wilson, DW Foster (eds). Philadelphia, Saunders, 1985, pp 123–132

321 NEUROENDOCRINE REGULATION AND DISEASES OF THE ANTERIOR PITUITARY AND HYPOTHALAMUS

GILBERT H. DANIELS / JOSEPH B. MARTIN

The pituitary, appropriately titled the master gland, produces six major hormones and stores an additional two hormones. Growth hormone (GH) regulates growth and has important influences on intermediary metabolism (see Chap. 322). Prolactin (PRL) is necessary for lactation. Luteinizing hormone (LH) and follicle-stimulating hormone (FSH) control the gonads in men and women. Thyroid-stimulating hormone (TSH, thyrotropin) controls the function of the thyroid gland. Adrenocorticotropic hormone (ACTH) is responsible for controlling glucocorticoid function of the adrenal cortex. These hormones are all synthesized in the anterior pituitary. Antidiuretic hormone (AVP, arginine vasopressin) and oxytocin are produced in neurons of the hypothalamus and stored in the posterior lobe of the pituitary (see Chap. 323). AVP controls water conservation by the kidneys; oxytocin is necessary for milk let-down during lactation (Fig. 321-1).

An important feedback relationship exists between the anterior pituitary and its three target glands—the gonads, the adrenal cortex, and the thyroid. When the gonads fail or are removed the concentrations of LH and FSH rise, a condition known as primary hypogonadism. When the adrenal cortex is removed or destroyed, primary adrenal insufficiency (or Addison's disease) results, and the serum ACTH concentration increases. Thyroid failure results in the characteristic TSH rise of primary hypothyroidism.

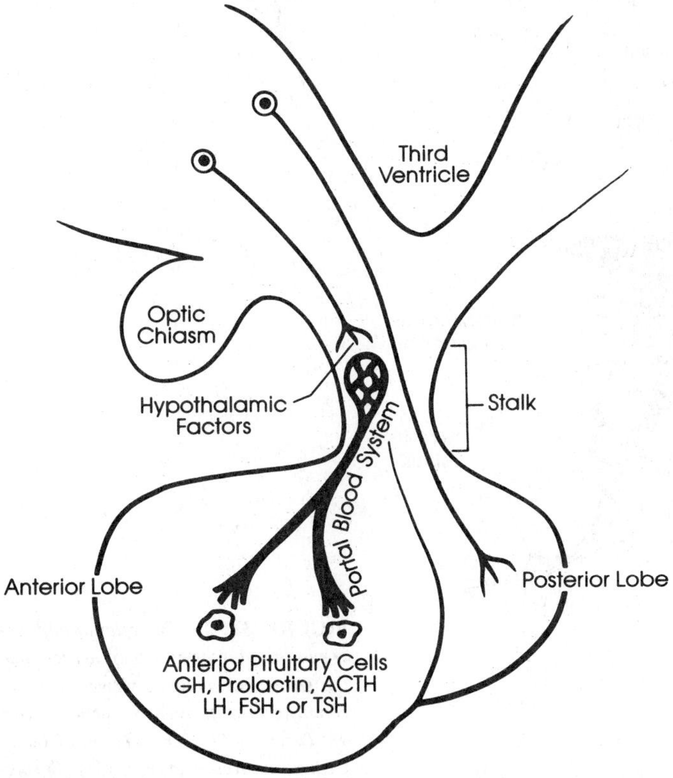

FIGURE 321-1 *The relationship between the hypothalamus and pituitary. See text for details.*

When the pituitary gland is removed or destroyed, loss of the trophic hormones results in secondary hypogonadism, adrenal insufficiency, or hypothyroidism. Growth hormone and prolactin function are also lost. AVP and oxytocin function are not affected by destruction of the pituitary provided their site of origin in the hypothalamus is not disturbed.

The pituitary is in turn under the control of the hypothalamus, which produces a number of chemical mediators. These hormones are synthesized in the hypothalamus and enter the portal vascular system which carries them through the pituitary stalk to the anterior lobe (Fig. 321-1). Interruption of the pituitary stalk is followed by reduction in the release of GH, LH, FSH, TSH, and ACTH from the anterior pituitary. This implies that stimulatory influences from the hypothalamus are necessary for release of these hormones. In contrast, the level of prolactin rises after interruption of the stalk, implying a normal tonic inhibitory hypothalamic influence on prolactin secretion. The rise in prolactin secretion also provides evidence that stalk section does not lead to pituitary destruction. If the stalk section is not performed at too high a level, AVP and oxytocin release continue principally from axons that terminate in the median eminence of the hypothalamus. With hypothalamic ablation, the levels of GH, LH, FSH, TSH, ACTH, AVP, and oxytocin fall, whereas prolactin levels increase (Fig. 321-1).

Most hypothalamic factors that control secretion of the pituitary hormones are peptides (Table 321-1). Growth hormone–releasing hormone (GRH) is the dominant influence on GH release; in addition, somatostatin acts as an inhibitory hormone for GH release. Although LH and FSH levels vary independently in physiologic states, a single releasing hormone [luteinizing hormone–releasing hormone (LHRH), also called gonadotropin-releasing hormone (GnRH)] plays a major role in controlling their release. Thyrotropin-releasing hormone (TRH) controls TSH release and may also influence prolactin release, and corticotropin releasing hormone (CRH) controls ACTH release. In addition, dopamine acts as the prolactin inhibitory factor (PIF).

Pituitary tumors may lead to hormonal over- or underproduction or may cause mechanical problems by impinging on neighboring structures. The most common hormones produced by pituitary tumors are prolactin and GH, the two hormones that lack simple end-organ feedback inhibitory loops. Prolactin excess leads to galactorrhea and/or hypogonadism; GH excess leads to gigantism and acromegaly. ACTH-secreting tumors produce Cushing's disease. TSH-secreting tumors are rare causes of hyperthyroidism. Gonadotropin-secreting tumors are paradoxically most often associated with hypogonadism. Large pituitary tumors may cause partial or complete hypopituitarism by compression of the adjacent normal gland or pituitary stalk and are associated with visual field disturbances due to compression of the optic chiasm with other neurologic disturbances caused by invasion of cavernous sinuses or cranial fossae.

Hypothalamic disease may cause hypopituitarism with the exception that secretion of prolactin may be increased. AVP deficiency leading to diabetes insipidus is virtually diagnostic of hypothalamic disease or of high interruption of the pituitary stalk. Disturbances of thirst, temperature regulation, appetite, and blood pressure may occur with hypothalamic disorders as well. Large hypothalamic masses may lead to visual field disturbances, obstruction of the third ventricle, and invasion of surrounding brain tissue.

ANATOMY AND EMBRYOLOGY

The pituitary gland (hypophysis) sits within the sella turcica ("Turkish saddle") of the sphenoid bone at the base of the skull and is composed principally of the anterior (adenohypophysis) and posterior lobes (neurohypophysis). The intermediate lobe is rudimentary in humans. The normal pituitary gland weighs between 0.5 and 0.9 g.

The pituitary is separated from the brain by the diaphragma sella, an extension of the dura mater, and from the sphenoid sinus anteriorly and inferiorly by a thin layer of bone. The lateral walls of the sella abut on the cavernous sinuses, which contain the internal carotid arteries and cranial nerves III, IV, V, and VI. The optic chiasm is slightly anterior to the pituitary stalk, just above the diaphragma sella. Thus, tumors of the pituitary may lead to visual field defects, to cranial nerve palsies, or to invasion of the sphenoid sinus (Figs. 321-2 and 321-3).

The hypothalamus extends anteriorly to the margin of the optic chiasm and posteriorly to include the mammillary bodies. Superiorly, the hypothalamic sulcus of the third ventricle separates the thalamus from the hypothalamus. The rounded inferior base of the hypothalamus

TABLE 321-1 Anterior pituitary and hypophysiotrophic hormones

	Hypophysiotrophic hormones	
Pituitary hormone	Name	Structure
Thyrotropin (TSH)	Thyrotropin-releasing hormone (TRH)	Tripeptide
Adrenocorticotropin (ACTH)	Corticotropin-releasing hormone (CRH)	41 Amino acids
Luteinizing hormone (LH)	Luteinizing hormone–releasing hormone (LHRH)	Decapeptide
Follicle-stimulating hormone (FSH)	LHRH	Decapeptide
Growth hormone (GH)	Growth hormone–releasing hormone (GRH)	44 Amino acids
	Growth hormone release–inhibiting hormone* (somatostatin, GIH)	14 Amino acids
Prolactin	Prolactin release–inhibiting factor (PIF)	Dopamine
	Prolactin-releasing factor (PRF)†	Peptide ? Vasoactive intestinal polypeptide (VIP)

* *Somatostatin also inhibits TRH-stimulated TSH release*
† *TRH stimulates prolactin release*

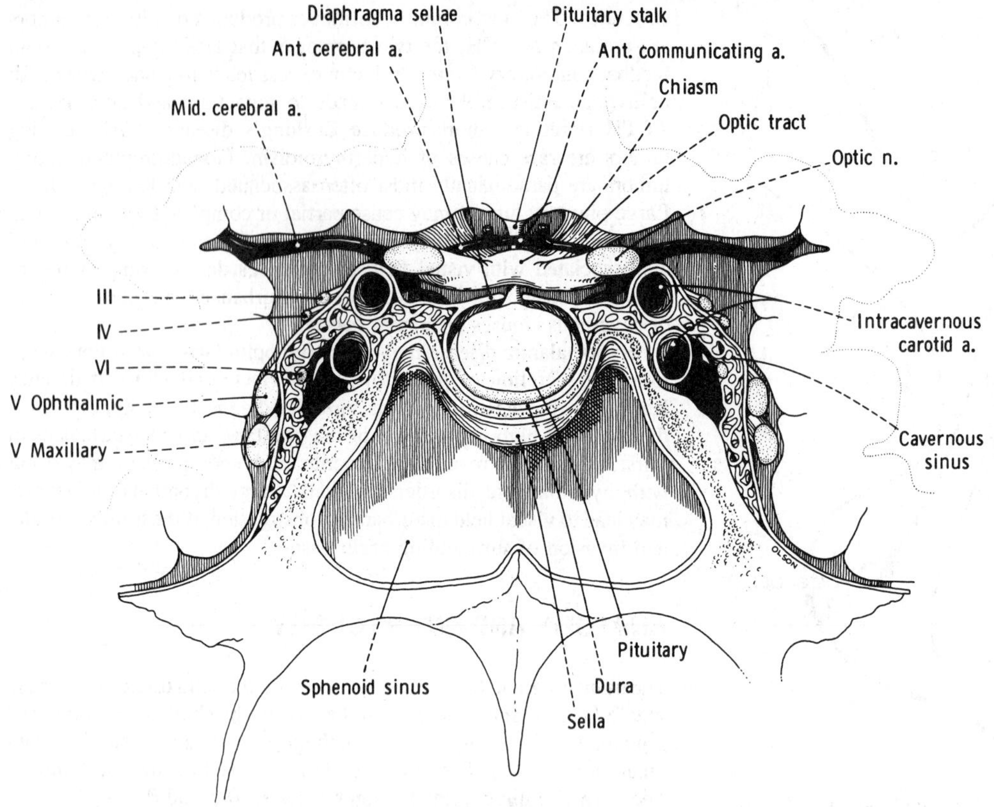

FIGURE 321-2 *The relationship between the pituitary, cranial nerves, and the cavernous sinus as viewed in a coronal section through the sella. (From JA Taren in RC Schneider et al (eds). Correlative Neurosurgery, 3d ed, Springfield, Ill., Charles C Thomas, 1982.)*

forms the tuber cinereum. The central portion of the base (termed the infundibulum or median eminence) is formed by the floor of the third ventricle (Fig. 321-3) and continues inferiorly to form the pituitary stalk. The releasing factors are synthesized in neurons that are located along the margins of the third ventricle and that project fibers which terminate in the median eminence adjacent to the portal capillaries.

The cell bodies of the supraoptic and paraventricular nuclei of the hypothalamus produce vasopressin and oxytocin, which travel down nerve axons in the supraopticohypophysial and paraventriculohypophysial nerve tracts to reach the posterior lobe.

The communication between the hypothalamus and the anterior pituitary is chemical rather than physical. Releasing factors produced by hypothalamic neurons reach the anterior pituitary via the portal system to stimulate or inhibit hormone production. Some of the vasopressin-containing neurons also terminate in the median eminence, and vasopressin can stimulate release of ACTH and GH.

The anterior pituitary has the highest blood flow of any tissue in the body [0.8 (mL/g)/min]. The blood supply reaches the anterior pituitary by a circuitous route through the hypothalamus. Two derivatives of the internal carotid arteries, the superior hypophysial arteries (SHA), branch in the subarachnoid space around the pituitary

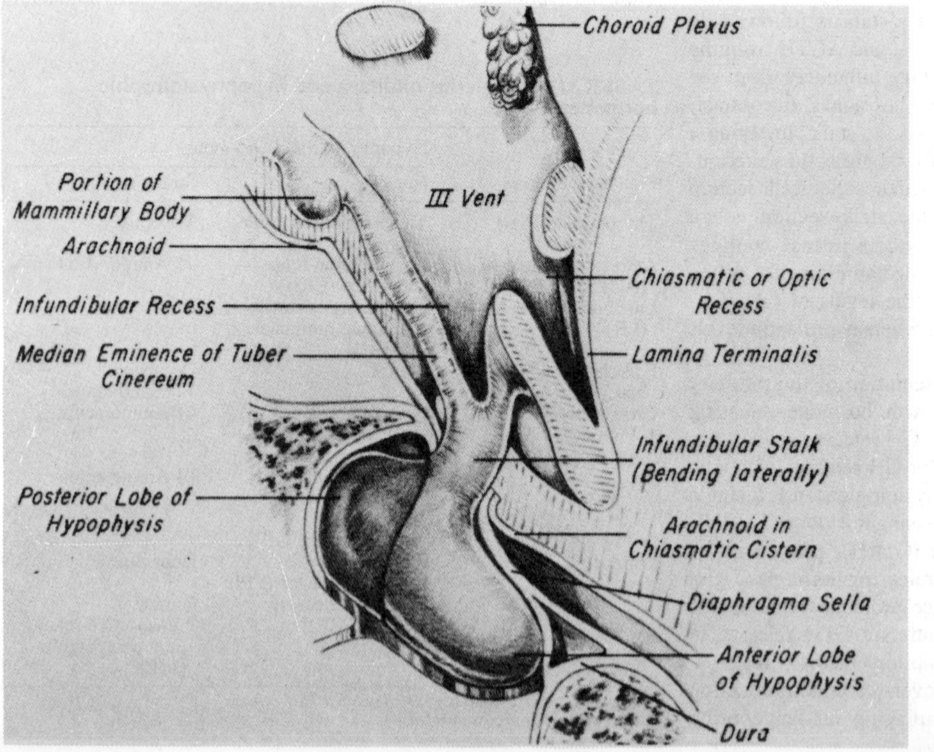

FIGURE 321-3 *Sagittal view of the human hypothalamic-pituitary unit, demonstrating the anatomic relationships between optic chiasm and pituitary stalk. (From Reichlin in Post et al.)*

stalk and terminate in the capillary network of the median eminence. These capillaries have a fenestrated endothelium which allows easy access to the hypothalamic releasing hormones. Transport of substances from the capillaries to the median eminence is also facilitated because the median eminence lies outside the blood-brain barrier. The capillaries then coalesce to form 6 to 10 straight veins known as the hypothalamic-pituitary portal circulation. These veins constitute the main direct blood supply to the anterior lobe and supply it with nutrients as well as information from the hypothalamus. A minor arterial blood supply to the anterior lobe comes from the trabecular branches of the SHA. The posterior pituitary is supplied entirely by blood from the inferior hypophysial arteries.

The anterior lobe of the pituitary is formed predominantly from the lateral proliferation of Rathke's pouch, an embryologic outpouching from the floor of the primitive oral cavity. Rathke's pouch is met by a diverticulum extending downward from the floor of the third ventricle, which forms the posterior lobe.

Rathke's pouch is closed off by proliferation of the anterior and posterior lobe and forms a thin residual cleft in the gland (Rathke's cleft). This small cleft may persist as a cyst lined with cuboidal or columnar epithelium. Since the pituitary gland rotates as it grows, these cysts usually lie in a position superior to the pituitary gland. The further growth and proliferation of these cysts can give rise to craniopharyngiomas, tumors that generally occupy a suprasellar position. Development of the sphenoid bone separates the pituitary from the oral cavity. Remnants of the pituitary, known as pharyngeal pituitaries, occasionally persist within or below the sphenoid bone. These remnants may produce pituitary hormones and occasionally develop into pituitary tumors.

Five distinct cell types in the anterior pituitary secrete six different hormones: lactotrophs (prolactin), somatotrophs (GH), gonadotrophs (LH and FSH), thyrotrophs (TSH), and corticotrophs (ACTH).

PROLACTIN

PHYSIOLOGY The lactotrophs constitute 10 to 25 percent of the normal pituitary and increase to 70 percent of the gland during pregnancy. The prolactin gene on chromosome 6 codes for a precursor molecule that is larger than the circulating hormone. The predominant form of the processed hormone contains 198 amino acids (23,000 mol wt) in a single polypeptide chain containing three intrachain disulfide bonds. Higher-molecular-weight forms of prolactin, up to 100,000 mol wt, (''big'' and ''big-big'' prolactin) may be present in small amounts in the circulation of normal persons and in larger amounts in patients with pituitary adenomas; these molecules react in prolactin immunoassays but do not have normal biologic potency.

Prolactin is essential for lactation. Receptors for the hormone are present in human breast and gonads, whereas in other animals they are found in a variety of tissues. Prolactin is an important promoter of breast cancer in rodents; a similar connection has not been established in human breast cancer (see Chap 295).

During pregnancy increasing placental estrogen production stimulates the growth and replication of the pituitary lactotrophs and causes increased prolactin secretion. The pituitary doubles in size during a normal pregnancy and returns to normal after delivery. Prolactin secretion during pregnancy prepares the breast for postpartum lactation. Estrogen inhibits prolactin action at the breast, so that lactation does not occur until estrogen levels decline post partum.

Prolactin levels rise in the fetus beginning at about 25 weeks, probably owing to maternal estrogen transfer and stimulation of the fetal pituitary. The level falls rapidly after delivery, reaching a nadir by 2 to 4 weeks post partum. High concentrations of prolactin are present in amniotic fluid, although the origin and functional significance are unknown.

Under normal circumstances, prolactin secretion by the anterior pituitary is restrained by the hypothalamus. With hypothalamic destruction or pituitary stalk section, prolactin secretion increases and serum concentrations rise. The hypothalamic inhibitory factor for prolactin appears to be dopamine, although peptide inhibitory factors have been described. The arcuate nucleus of the hypothalamus is the primary hypothalamic site of dopamine synthesis; dopamine travels down axons to nerve terminals in the median eminence where it is released (tuberoinfundibular dopamine system). Dopamine enters the portal circulation and reaches the anterior pituitary to inhibit prolactin release. The intravenous administration of dopamine (2 μg/min per kilogram of body weight) or the oral administration of dopamine precursors (e.g., levodopa) or dopamine agonists (e.g., bromocriptine) inhibits prolactin release. Increased blood prolactin appears to increase hypothalamic dopamine production, which in turn partially inhibits prolactin release via a ''short'' feedback loop.

The prolactin rise during suckling appears to require a prolactin-releasing factor, which has not yet been conclusively identified. Vasoactive intestinal peptide (VIP) may be responsible, as it is a potent stimulator of prolactin release. Suckling-induced prolactin rise is blocked by serotonin antagonists, such as methysergide, which suggests an influence of serotonin on prolactin release. TRH is also a potent stimulator of prolactin release; indeed the lowest dose of TRH capable of stimulating TSH stimulates prolactin release as well. However, TSH and prolactin release are under independent control in most physiologic states; lactation does not lead to TSH elevation, and primary hypothyroidism is rarely associated with prolactin excess.

Prolactin concentrations rise during sleep, a phenomenon which requires the input of higher centers into the hypothalamus. Stress-related prolactin release can be blocked by opiate antagonists such as naloxone and is probably mediated by endogenous opioids. Morphine can stimulate prolactin release, which may contribute to the amenorrhea that occurs with narcotic addiction, but basal prolactin secretion is not influenced by opiate antagonists.

HYPERPROLACTINEMIA Clinical features Prolactin excess (hyperprolactinemia) is associated with hypogonadism and/or galactorrhea and may be an important clue to the presence of a pituitary adenoma or hypothalamic disease. Of women with amenorrhea, 10 to 40 percent have hyperprolactinemia, and as many as one-third of women with amenorrhea and galactorrhea have prolactin-secreting pituitary tumors.

The hypogonadism associated with hyperprolactinemia appears to be due to inhibition of hypothalamic release of LHRH, resulting in a decrease in LH and FSH secretion. This functional hypogonadism can be regarded, in part, as a physiologic mechanism since breast feeding causes decreased fertility and delayed resumption of menses. In general, the higher the plasma prolactin, the greater the likelihood of amenorrhea. Milder degrees of hyperprolactinemia in women cause irregular menses or infertility due to a shortened luteal phase. The estrogen deficiency associated with hyperprolactinemia may lead to osteoporosis.

Prolactin excess in men can cause impotence and infertility. In some series 8 percent of men with impotence and 5 percent of men with infertility have hyperprolactinemia. With prolactin elevation, FSH and LH levels in men also decline, and serum testosterone is often low.

Galactorrhea, defined as milk production in a patient who is not postpartum, is present in 30 to 90 percent of hyperprolactinemic women (see Chap. 332). The variation in incidence reflects, in part, variation in the intensity with which clinicians search for this finding. Galactorrhea may occur without hyperprolactinemia, particularly in parous women. However, galactorrhea is often an important clue to prolactin excess; when galactorrhea is coupled with amenorrhea, hyperprolactinemia is present in 75 percent of patients. Hyperprolactinemia in men rarely causes gynecomastia or galactorrhea (see Chap. 332).

Differential diagnosis Prolactin excess has several causes: (1) autonomous production (pituitary adenomas), (2) decreased dopamine or dopamine inhibitory action (e.g., due to hypothalamic disease or drugs that block dopamine synthesis or release or inhibit dopamine action), (3) stimuli that overcome the normal dopaminergic inhibition (e.g., estrogens, possibly hypothyroidism), and (4) decreased clearance of prolactin (renal failure). No single suppression test can separate physiologic from pharmacologic or pathologic causes of hyperprolactinemia (Table 321-2).

Prolactin concentrations are slightly higher (<20 ng/mL) in women than in men (<15 ng/mL). During pregnancy, prolactin concentrations begin to increase during the second trimester and peak at term; maximal values are 100 to 300 ng/mL, usually less than 200 ng/mL. A pregnancy test is mandatory in all patients with hyperprolactinemic amenorrhea, as it is with amenorrhea alone. The mean prolactin concentration declines post partum but rises with each suckling episode. Gradually, over several months, basal and suckling-stimulated prolactin concentrations diminish; by 4 to 6 months post partum, basal prolactin levels are normal, and the suckling-induced rise is absent despite continued nursing.

A careful drug history should be obtained in hyperprolactinemic patients. Dopamine-blocking drugs (e.g., phenothiazines, butyrophenones, metoclopramide) and dopamine-depleting drugs (e.g., methyldopa and reserpine) are important causes of hyperprolactinemia. Prolactin concentrations are rarely greater than 100 ng/mL with these agents, provided renal failure is not present. Although high-dose estrogens cause hyperprolactinemia, oral contraceptives containing low doses of estrogen do not.

End-stage renal failure is associated with elevated serum prolactin in 70 to 90 percent of women and 25 to 60 percent of men. This contributes to hypogonadism in some patients with renal failure. Both decreased prolactin clearance and increased prolactin secretion may contribute to this elevation. The increased prolactin in cirrhosis has not been adequately explained.

Severe primary hypothyroidism may cause a mildly elevated serum prolactin concentration, either due to elevated TRH levels or due to decreased dopaminergic tone. Since primary hypothyroidism may also cause enlargment of the sella turcica, mimicking a pituitary adenoma, thyroid function tests are essential in all patients with elevated serum prolactin. Rarely, primary adrenal insufficiency causes reversible serum prolactin elevation.

TABLE 321-2 Causes of hyperprolactinemia

I Physiologic states
- *A* Pregnancy
- *B* Nursing (early)
- *C* "Stress"
- *D* Sleep
- *E* Nipple stimulation

II Drugs
- *A* Dopamine receptor antagonists
  - *1* Phenothiazines
  - *2* Butyrophenones
  - *3* Thioxanthenes
  - *4* Metoclopramide
- *B* Dopamine-depleting agents
  - *1* Methyldopa
  - *2* Reserpine
- *C* Estrogens
- *D* Opiates

III Disease states
- *A* Pituitary tumors
  - *1* Prolactinomas
  - *2* Adenomas secreting GH and prolactin
  - *3* Adenomas secreting ACTH and prolactin (Nelson's syndrome and Cushing's disease)
  - *4* Nonfunctioning chromophobe adenomas with pituitary stalk compression
- *B* Hypothalamic and pituitary stalk disease
  - *1* Granulomatous diseases especially sarcoidosis
  - *2* Craniopharyngiomas and other tumors
  - *3* Cranial irradiation
  - *4* Stalk section
  - *5* Empty sella
  - *6* Vascular abnormalities including aneurysm
- *C* Primary hypothyroidism
- *D* Chronic renal failure
- *E* Cirrhosis
- *F* Chest wall trauma (including surgery, *herpes zoster*)

If a hyperprolactinemic patient is not pregnant, postpartum, cirrhotic, on medications, hypothyroid, or in renal failure, that patient is likely to have disease of the pituitary or hypothalamus. Ectopic production of prolactin by nonpituitary tumors occurs rarely if at all. Diseases of the hypothalamus or pituitary stalk cause moderate prolactin elevation (usually less than 150 ng/mL). Hyperprolactinemia occurs in 20 to 50 percent of patients with hypothalamic tumors.

Prolactin-secreting pituitary adenomas (prolactinomas) may either be small tumors within the parenchyma of the gland (so called microadenomas) or cause enlargement of the pituitary gland (macroadenomas). Large, nonfunctioning pituitary adenomas may also cause modest prolactin elevation as a result of stalk compression and a consequent impedence of delivery of dopamine to the gland. Acromegalics (25 to 45 percent) and patients with Nelson's syndrome (postadrenalectomy pituitary tumors in Cushing's disease) commonly also have elevated serum prolactin. Hyperprolactinemia is less common in untreated Cushing's disease.

Laboratory evaluation Serum prolactin levels should be measured in all patients with hypogonadism or galactorrhea. If basal prolactin concentration is elevated, further evaluation is warranted after establishing that minimal prolactin elevations (e.g., less than 30 ng/mL) are not stress-related. Although there is no simple test to distinguish the various causes of hyperprolactinemia, a serum prolactin level of over 300 ng/mL is diagnostic of a pituitary adenoma; a serum prolactin of over 100 ng/mL in a nonpregnant patient is usually caused by a pituitary adenoma. Administration of dopamine agonists, such as bromocriptine, lowers prolactin regardless of the etiology and, therefore, is not useful as a differential test (Fig. 321-4). Prolactin stimulation tests do not distinguish among the various etiologies of hyperprolactinemia. For example, the majority of patients with prolactinomas have only a minimal or no rise in prolactin in response to TRH, as compared to the normal rise of 200 percent or more and the intermediate response (usually a doubling at serum prolactin) in patients with hypothalamic disease and those on dopamine-blocking agents. Unfortunately, the response to TRH is too variable to be useful in individual patients.

All patients with unexplained hyperprolactinemia require contrast-enhanced computerized tomography (CT) scanning of the hypothalamus and pituitary or magnetic resonance imaging (MRI) of this area. Pituitary macroadenomas are easily visualized on CT scans, but microadenomas (<10 mm) may be more difficult to delineate. When no radiologic abnormalities are found the disorder is designated "idiopathic hyperprolactinemia," although it is recognized that a small microadenoma may still be present. Sella tomography is not a useful screening test for small pituitary adenomas because of the high prevalence of false-positive and false-negative results.

Microprolactinomas do not cause hypopituitarism (except for hypogonadism). If a small pituitary lesion is seen in a patient with hypopituitarism and hyperprolactinemia, sarcoidosis or other lesions involving the pituitary stalk should be suspected, rather than a microprolactinoma. In patients with macroprolactinomas or hypothalamic lesions, evaluation of pituitary function and formal visual field examinations are essential.

Prolactinomas PATHOLOGY Prolactinomas are the most common type of functional pituitary adenomas. Small unsuspected microadenomas are found in 15 to 25 percent of unselected autopsies; 40 percent of these small tumors contain prolactin by immunologic staining techniques, but the percentage that actually secrete prolactin is unknown. About 70 percent of macroadenomas previously thought to be nonfunctioning are, in fact, prolactinomas. Prolactin-secreting pituitary carcinomas are rare.

Prolactinoma size correlates with hormonal output; in general, the larger the tumor, the higher the prolactin levels. Large pituitary tumors with modest prolactin elevation (50 to 100 ng/mL) are not true prolactinomas and differ in their biologic behavior. Microprolactinomas cause only hyperprolactinemia and hypogonadotropism, whereas macroprolactinomas may influence other pituitary hormones and cause headaches, visual field disturbances, and other structural problems.

CLINICAL PRESENTATION Microprolactinomas are more common than macroprolactinomas, and 90 percent of patients with microprolactinomas are women. In contrast, 60 percent of patients with macroprolactinomas are men. Irregular menses, amenorrhea, and galactorrhea are likely to result in early diagnosis, and this probably explains the preponderance of microadenomas in women. Sexual dysfunction occurs in most men with prolactinomas, but this is the presenting complaint in 15 percent or less. Although delay in seeking medical help probably explains the larger tumors in men, more aggressive tumor behavior in men has not been excluded.

Estrogens promote the growth of lactotrophs, but an etiologic role has not been established for oral contraceptives in the pathogenesis of prolactinomas. Many women with prolactinomas first develop galactorrhea while on oral contraceptives or develop amenorrhea when the drug is discontinued. Some of these women may have been started on oral contraceptives for irregular menses that were the consequence of a prolactinoma. Although amenorrhea after discontinuing oral contraceptives is rare (about 2 percent), about one-third of patients with postpill amenorrhea have prolactinomas. Development of galactorrhea in a woman on oral contraceptives mandates a prolactin determination. About 5 to 7 percent of prolactinoma patients have never menstruated (primary amenorrhea), making this an important treatable cause of primary amenorrhea. Prolactinomas may grow during pregnancy, and 15 percent of prolactinoma patients are first diagnosed in the postpartum period.

Women with prolactinomas who desire pregnancy need special consideration. Medical treatment of patients with microprolactinomas results in uneventful pregnancies 95 to 98 percent of the time; the remainder may develop headaches or visual field disturbances due to tumor enlargement that rarely requires therapy. Asymptomatic enlargement of microprolactinomas, as ascertained by radiologic studies, occurs in about 5 percent. With macroprolactinomas, the complications of tumor growth during pregnancy are more common. Symptomatic tumor enlargement occurs in about 15 percent of these patients, although individual series report complications in up to 35 percent. The majority of patients who develop symptoms do so during the first trimester.

In prolactinoma patients, the effect of pregnancy on prolactin secretion is variable. A further rise in prolactin during pregnancy may not occur even in some patients in whom tumor growth occurs. Prolactin concentrations should be measured periodically throughout pregnancy in women with prolactinomas. If marked prolactin rise occurs (greater than 300 to 400 ng/dL), then postpartum prolactin is usually greater than the prepartum level, and tumor growth is likely. Patients with stable or declining prolactin concentrations during pregnancy may have lower prolactin concentrations after pregnancy than before. In such patients infarction or involution of the adenomas may have occurred during pregnancy.

The therapy of prolactinomas is influenced by the natural history of the disorder. Although large pituitary adenomas must begin as small tumors, most microadenomas do not progress to macroadenomas. Knowledge of the natural history of untreated microprolactinomas is incomplete; 90 to 95 percent may remain stable or demonstrate decreased serum prolactin concentrations after 7 years of follow-up. Most patients with "idiopathic hyperprolactinemia" are presumed to harbor small microadenomas. Serum prolactin returns to normal in one-third of patients with idiopathic hyperprolactinemia followed for 5 years without therapy; in two-thirds of patients in whom the basal prolactin is less than 40 ng/mL serum prolactin levels return to normal over this time span.

THERAPY Not all patients with microprolactinomas need therapy. Women with microprolactinomas require therapy when they desire pregnancy, have decreased libido or troublesome galactorrhea, desire regular menses, or are at risk for osteoporosis. Men with microadenomas should be treated for decreased potency or libido or when infertility is a problem. Most patients with macroprolactinomas require therapy.

Dopamine agonist drugs lower prolactin concentrations in virtually all hyperprolactinemic patients (Fig. 321-4). Ovulatory menses and fertility are restored in 90 percent of premenopausal women, underscoring the direct relationship between hyperprolactinemia and amenorrhea. Bromocriptine, an ergot derivative with dopamine agonist actions, is the only effective prolactin-lowering agent licensed in the United States at this time. Bromocriptine should be given twice daily with food or a snack to prevent gastrointestinal irritation. Therapy should begin with 1.25 mg at bedtime to minimize the side effects of nausea, vomiting, fatigue, nasal stuffiness, and postural hypotension. The dosage is gradually increased to an average of 2.5 mg twice daily. However, doses up to 15 mg per day may be required to return the prolactin concentration to normal in some patients with macroprolactinomas. Although the drug is expensive, it is effective in all forms of hyperprolactinemia and often abolishes nonhyperpro-

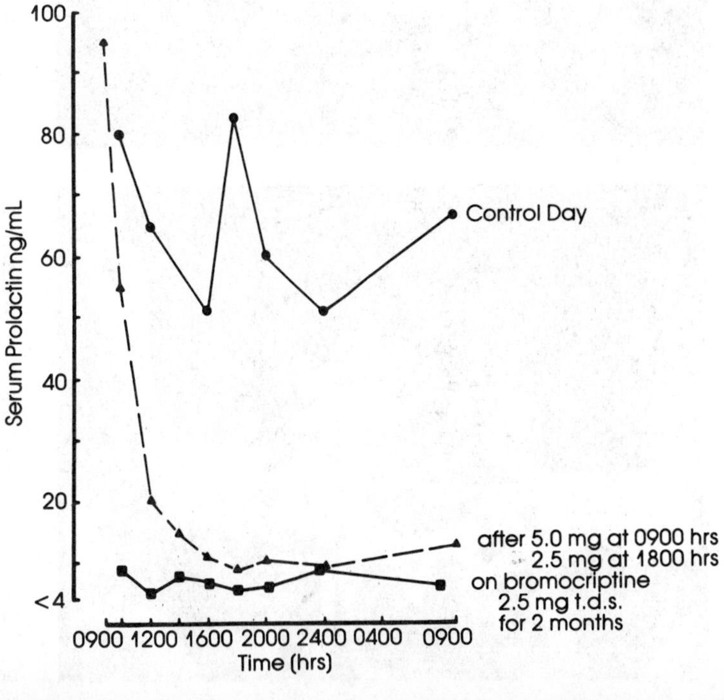

FIGURE 321-4 *Changes in serum prolactin concentration in a woman with "idiopathic" hyperprolactinemia after an initial 5 mg dose of bromocriptine and when maintained on 7.5 mg daily. (From GH Besser and MO Thorner. Postgrad Med J, 52:66, 1976.)*

lactinemic galactorrhea as well. Pergolide, a longer-lasting dopamine agonist, can be administered once daily but is not available in the United States. Although pergolide and bromocriptine have similar side effects, individuals may tolerate one but not the other.

Bromocriptine is the therapy of choice for patients with microprolactinomas who have one of the indications for treatment discussed above. Prolactin concentrations return to normal in almost all who tolerate the medication, usually within days of achieving full therapeutic dosages (Fig. 321-4). Menses usually resume within 2 months but may be delayed up to a year. Since pregnancy may occur without resumption of menses, a barrier contraceptive is recommended until menses become regular. In this way, bromocriptine can be stopped with the first missed period when pregnancy has occurred. Bromocriptine use during pregnancy is not, however, associated with an increased risk of congenital anomalies or fetal wastage. The effects of bromocriptine are usually not permanent, but one-sixth of microprolactinoma patients maintain normal prolactin concentrations after stopping the drug.

In patients with macroprolactinomas, bromocriptine usually lowers the serum prolactin and may cause the tumor mass to shrink. In men testosterone concentrations usually begin to increase after 3 months of therapy and may reach normal levels by 6 to 8 months. Normal sperm counts are achieved in some.

One series of patients with large prolactinomas and suprasellar extension (mean prolactin of 1441 ng/mL in women, 3451 ng/mL in men) is of particular interest. Although prolactin levels fell to 10 percent of baseline in 96 percent of patients, most did not return to the normal range despite bromocriptine dosages of 7.5 to 20 mg per day. Visual field defects improved in 90 percent of those with field cuts. Tumor mass decreased by half or more in 60 percent of patients (see Fig. 321-5). This is a reasonable choice of therapy for patients with small macroprolactinomas. However, for patients with larger tumors who have persistent visual field defects or persistent symptomatic hyperprolactinemia, or in those women with large tumors who desire pregnancy, we do not recommend bromocriptine as the sole form of therapy. In such patients, tumor regrowth is likely when bromocriptine is stopped either inadvertently or for pregnancy or because other medical illnesses preclude its administration. Large nonfunctioning pituitary adenomas associated with hyperprolactinemia due to stalk compression usually do not shrink with bromocriptine therapy, although prolactin concentrations return to normal. Patients with large prolactinomas, refractory to bromocriptine and other modalities of therapy, may partially respond to tamoxifen, an estrogen antagonist.

FIGURE 321-5 *Frontal CT scan of a man with a large prolactin-secreting macroadenoma. Top, pretreatment scan. Bottom, scan after 1 year of treatment with bromocriptine. The upper border of the tumor is shown by arrows. (From Molitch et al.)*

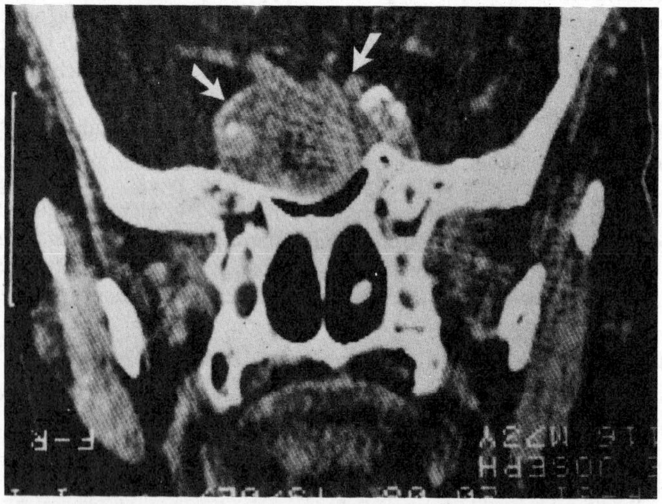

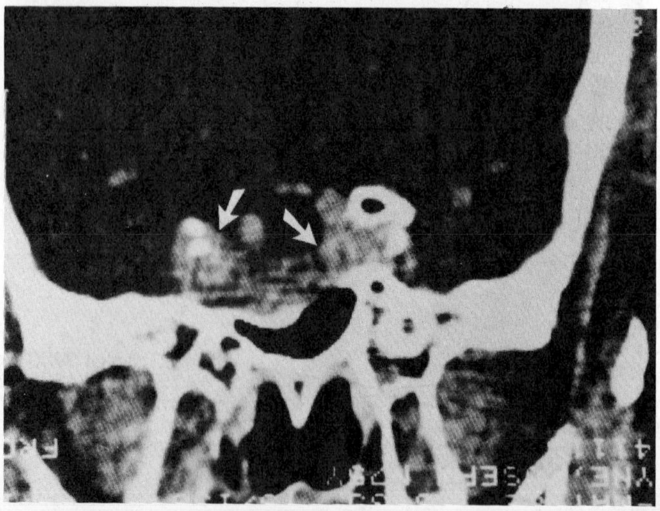

Following transsphenoidal resection of microprolactinomas, serum prolactin concentration returns to normal in up to 80 to 90 percent of patients, usually within 24 h. This procedure has low morbidity and mortality. Unfortunately, recurrence rates average 17 percent after "successful" surgery and may be as high as 40 percent after 6 years of follow-up. Surgery is a reasonable alternative for women with microprolactinomas who desire pregnancy and who cannot tolerate or do not wish to take dopamine agonist drugs.

Surgery, combined with bromocriptine and/or radiation therapy, is indicated in all macroprolactinoma patients with suprasellar extension and persistent visual field defects and particularly in those women desiring pregnancy. However, surgical resection, whether by transsphenoidal or transcranial approach, is rarely curative in patients with macroprolactinomas. Prolactin concentrations return to normal in about 30 percent, but even when they do, recurrence rates of up to 80 percent have been reported. In all patients in whom prolactin levels do not return to normal following surgery, long-term bromocriptine therapy and/or radiation should be given.

Conventional radiation therapy [4500 cGy (4500 rad) over 25 days] for prolactinomas causes a slow decline in serum prolactin concentration. Prolactin concentration returns to normal in about 30 percent of microprolactinoma patients 2 to 10 years post therapy. We do not favor this approach in patients with microprolactinomas because of the risk of their developing hypopituitarism. Radiation therapy is a useful adjunct to surgical or medical therapy in patients with macroprolactinomas; further growth is usually prevented, and shrinkage occurs in about half the patients. This therapy usually prevents tumor growth during subsequent pregnancies, but exceptions have been noted.

Heavy particle therapy with protons or alpha particles may be useful in treatment of macroprolactinomas without suprasellar extension or after surgical debulking of larger tumors. Occasional patients with microprolactinomas opt for this form of therapy. Long-term studies in prolactinoma patients are not available.

PROLACTIN DEFICIENCY Prolactin deficiency is manifested as an inability to lactate. Failure of lactation is often the earliest clue to panhypopituitarism resulting from pituitary destruction during the peripartum period. The lateral wings of the pituitary gland have a precarious blood supply; most lactotrophs reside in this area. During pregnancy, the hypertrophied and hyperplastic lactotrophs are at risk for necrosis. If systemic hypotension develops, as with postpartum hemorrhage, the hypertrophic and hyperplastic lactotrophs may infarct (Sheehan's syndrome). Patients with diabetes mellitus are susceptible to peripartum pituitary infarction even in the absence of significant hemorrhage. Autoimmune pituitary destruction (lymphocytic hypophysitis) may also occur during late pregnancy.

Commercial prolactin radioimmunoassays cannot easily distinguish normal from low concentrations; hence, prolactin stimulation tests are needed to diagnose prolactin insufficiency. After administration of TRH or chlorpromazine, a rise in serum prolactin of less than 200 percent suggests prolactin deficiency. If prolactin deficiency is present, evaluation of other pituitary hormones is necessary as well to define other manifestations of hypopituitarism.

GROWTH HORMONE

PHYSIOLOGY Growth hormone (GH, somatotropin) is secreted by somatotrophs which make up about 50 percent of the anterior pituitary cells. The normal pituitary contains 3 to 5 mg of GH and secretes 500 to 875 μg of GH per day. The gene coding for GH is on chromosome 17; additional GH-related genes are of uncertain significance. Human growth hormone is a single polypeptide chain at 191 amino acids (22,000 mol wt) and contains two intrachain disulfide bonds. A larger (28,000 mol wt) precursor molecule is cleaved to yield GH. GH is stored in cytoplasmic granules in a high-molecular-weight polymeric form.

The structure of GH is similar to that of human placental lactogen (hPL, chorionic somatomammotropin), there being a 92 percent structural homology between the two. GH and hPL genes are found on the same chromosome and appear to have originated by gene duplication.

In the circulation, monomeric GH (22,000 mol wt) predominates. Larger molecular weight forms may represent dimers (i.e., "big" GH, 44,000 mol wt) that appear to be secreted by the pituitary gland into the circulation. Although "big" GH is measured by the GH radioimmunoassay, its biologic activity is reduced. Pulsatile release is characteristic, and circulating levels are low for much of the day. The half-life of the hormone in plasma is 20 to 30 min.

GH is necessary for normal linear growth. Growth hormone deficiency causes short stature; growth hormone excess (prior to epiphyseal closure) leads to gigantism. GH does not appear to be the principal direct stimulator of growth but acts indirectly through serum factors. These factors, known as somatomedins (SM, somatotropin-mediating hormones) or insulin-like growth factors (IGF) are growth hormone–dependent and appear to be responsible for growth stimulation (also see Chap. 322). Somatomedin C (insulin-like growth factor 1, IGF-1/SM-C), the most important somatomedin for growth, is produced in the liver and by other tissues as well. IGF-1/SM-C is a small basic protein (7600 mol wt) which circulates bound to a large carrier molecule (140,000 mol wt). The complex has a half-life of 3 to 18 h, as compared to the half-life of 20 to 30 min for unbound hormone. As a consequence, the concentration of IGF-1/SM-C remains relatively constant throughout the 24 h period, in contrast to the fluctuating levels of GH itself. How the liver integrates GH pulses into somatomedin production is not known. Furthermore, local tissue generation of IGF-1/SM-C may play an important role in mediating growth through paracrine effects.

Somatomedin C and a second somatomedin (somatomedin A) have structural homology with proinsulin, and the somatomedins share some insulin-like actions. Furthermore, GH is a trophic factor for insulin release, facilitating its release in response to various secretagogues, and GH-deficient individuals have impaired insulin release to glucose challenge. Technically, one might consider insulin a somatomedin.

During the prenatal and neonatal period growth is independent of GH, as shown by the normal birth length of GH-deficient children born to GH-deficient mothers. Nevertheless IGF-1/SM-C levels rise during pregnancy, and its concentration correlates with that of hPL, which may regulate somatomedin production. Whether the somatomedins play a physiologic role in utero is uncertain. IGF-1/SM-C levels at birth are about half those of adults and rise gradually during childhood to reach the adult range by age 8 to 10 years. IGF-1/SM-C levels are dependent upon nutritional status, declining in states of malnourishment. Elevated serum IGF-1/SM-C concentrations are present during the pubertal growth spurt, presumably accounting for the growth acceleration during this period. With estrogen deficiency, the pubertal rise of IGF-1/SM-C does not occur.

Although IGF-1/SM-C concentrations correlate with linear growth, the correlation is inexact, and therefore GH may have some direct influence on growth or cause somatomedin generation in target cells.

Other metabolic actions of GH are important. GH is an anabolic hormone that stimulates the incorporation of amino acids into protein. Although most of this action is somatomedin-mediated, GH can directly stimulate amino acid uptake in certain systems. It is not surprising, therefore, that some amino acids, such as arginine, are potent stimuli for GH release.

GH may have a direct effect as an insulin antagonist. Patients with GH deficiency are sensitive to insulin-induced hypoglycemia; patients with GH excess develop insulin resistance. GH is one of the counterregulatory hormones that help restore a low blood sugar to normal (see Chap. 329) and is probably involved in the "dawn" phenomenon in which plasma glucose increases in the early morning in patients with diabetes mellitus. Hypoglycemia is a potent GH stimulus, and an acute rise in blood sugar inhibits GH release. GH causes increased free fatty acid release from adipocytes. The absence of this effect may be responsible for the pudgy appearance of children with GH deficiency. Increased serum free fatty acid concentrations tend to blunt GH release. GH opposes the action of insulin on sugar uptake and fatty acid release and complements the anabolic action of insulin on amino acid uptake.

Serum GH is undetectable much of the day, peaks after meals, and undergoes a sustained rise during sleep. Integrated 24-h GH levels are higher in growing children than in adults.

GH has a dual hypothalamic regulation (Table 321-3). Secretion is stimulated by growth hormone–releasing factor (GRH, somatocrinin) and inhibited by growth hormone release–inhibitory hormone (somatostatin, somatotropin release–inhibitory factor, SRIF). GRH appears to play the more important role, as stalk section leads to failure of GH release. In animals treated with anti-GRH antibodies the GH peaks disappear, and growth ceases; following treatment with antisomatostatin antibodies, the peaks remain, but the baseline values rise. After treatment with both anti-GRH and antisomatostatin antibodies, the peaks disappear but the baseline rises. Although GRH- and somatostatin-containing neurons are separate, their nerve endings interconnect.

TABLE 321-3 Growth hormone regulation

Class of agent	Stimulation	Inhibition
Hypothalamic factors	GRH	Somatostatin
Amines	Alpha-adrenergic stimuli (norepinephrine, clonidine)	Beta-adrenergic stimuli
	Beta-adrenergic blockers (propranolol)	Alpha-adrenergic blockers (phentolamine, dibenzyline)
	Dopaminergic stimuli (levodopa, bromocriptine, apomorphine)	Dopamine blockers (chlorpromazine)
	Serotonergic stimuli (L-tryptophan)	Serotonin blockers (methysergide, cyproheptadine)
Hormones	Decreased IGF-1/SM-C	Increased IGF-1/SM-C (obesity)
	Estrogen	Progestogens
	Vasopressin	Glucocorticoids
	Glucagon	
Fuels	Hypoglycemia*	Increased blood sugar
	Decreased free fatty acids	Increased free fatty acids
	Amino acids (arginine)*	
Others	Exercise*	
	Stress*	
	Sleep	

* *Probably mediated through alpha-adrenergic stimulation.*

Growth hormone–releasing factor GRH was initially isolated from an acromegalic patient with a GRH-secreting adenoma of the pancreatic islet cells. The clue to the diagnosis came from analysis of the pituitary pathology: Somatotroph hyperplasia was present rather than an adenoma that is characteristic for acromegaly. GRH has since been identified in the human hypothalamus.

GRH has 44 amino acids, 29 of which are necessary for full potency. GRH belongs to a family of molecules that includes secretin, glucagon, vasoactive intestinal peptide (VIP), and gastric inhibitory peptide (GIP). The arcuate nucleus of the hypothalamus is the major site of GRH production, although a few neurons are found in the ventromedial nucleus as well. Axons containing the peptide project to the median eminence and terminate on the portal vessels. GRH is also present in normal pancreas.

GRH stimulates GH release in vitro and in vivo, an effect that is calcium-dependent and appears to be mediated by cyclic adenosine monophosphate (cyclic AMP). Intravenous injection of GRH (0.1 to 3.3 μg per kilogram of body weight) produces a peak GH response at 30–60 min with a return to baseline by 2 to 3 h postinjection (Fig. 321-6). The GH response to GRH decreases with age, particularly after age 40.

Somatostatin Somatostatin is a cyclic tetradecapeptide and is the most widely distributed of the hypothalamic releasing hormones. The primary hypothalamic sources are the periventricular and medial preoptic areas of the anterior hypothalamus. Somatostatin is found in neurosecretory granules of axons that terminate in the median eminence. In addition to its function as a hormone, somatostatin is synthesized and distributed throughout the brain and serves as a neurotransmitter in many areas including the spinal cord, brain stem, and cerebral cortex. Somatostatin is also present in the gastrointestinal tract. Specific somatostatin-secreting cells (D cells) of the pancreatic islets participate in the regulation of insulin and glucagon secretion, an example of paracrine regulation by this hormone (see Chap. 327).

Somatostatin is produced by processing of a larger precursor molecule and exists in both 28– and 14–amino acid forms. The 28–amino acid somatostatin has a longer half-life and is a more potent inhibitor of GH and insulin secretion. Somatostatin 14 has a greater affinity for hypothalamic and cortical receptors and is more potent in inhibition of glucagon release. Somatostatin and analogues of somatostatin are being evaluated for efficacy in the therapy of acromegaly, secretory pancreatic tumors, pancreatitis, acute gastric ulcers and stress gastritis.

Somatostatin inhibits GH secretion and decreases the GH response to secretagogues. Somatostatin also lowers serum TSH in normal and hypothyroid individuals and blunts TSH release in response to TRH. Somatostatin probably mediates the secondary hypothyroidism that may develop in GH-deficient children treated with GH. Somatostatin has no significant effect on the release of prolactin, gonadotropins, or ACTH in normal subjects but may lower ACTH concentrations in patients with Nelson's syndrome. Somatostatinomas are rare pancreatic islet-cell or duodenal tumors that secrete somatostatin (see Chap. 329).

Growth hormone release is under complex physiologic control. (Table 321-3) The various mediators appear to act through GRH and somatostatin. IGF-1/SM-C has an important feedback effect on GH secretion. An increased IGF-1/SM-C concentration inhibits GH release both through increased somatostatin production and by a direct action on the pituitary. A decrease in IGF-1/SM-C, as induced by starvation, leads to a compensatory increase in GH release.

A number of neurotransmitters influence GH release:

1 Hypothalamic dopamine, the important prolactin inhibitory factor, stimulates GH through an effect on GRH. Dopamine has a direct but weak inhibitory effect on GH release; this effect is overwhelmed by its hypothalamic stimulation of GRH secretion. Oral administration of dopamine precursors or agonists that cross the blood-brain barrier, such as levodopa, apomorphine, or bromocriptine, causes an increase in serum GH concentration. The effects of these stimuli can be utilized to test the adequacy of GH secretion (GH reserve).

2 Alpha-adrenergic agonists, such as clonidine, stimulate GRH and GH release whereas phentolamine, an alpha blocker, prevents the GH rise. A number of GH stimulators, including insulin hypoglycemia, arginine, and exercise, act through alpha-adrenergic mechanisms. Beta-adrenergic blockers potentiate the GH-stimulatory effect of clonidine (and of many other agents including levodopa), possibly by inhibiting somatostatin secretion.

3 Serotonin agonists stimulate GH release, and the nocturnal surge in GH secretion may be mediated by serotonin, as cyproheptadine (a serotonin antagonist) blocks the sleep-induced GH rise.

Obesity blunts GH release in response to many stimuli, including GRH itself. Weight reduction restores normal GH dynamics. In contrast, malnourished individuals, including women with anorexia nervosa, often have an increased GH concentration, probably as a result of decreased serum IGF-1/SM-C levels. Oral glucose administration decreases serum GH and the GH response to GRH.

A number of hormones influence GH release. Most factors that stimulate GH release are more potent in women than in men, an effect mediated by estrogen. In testing GH reserve in children, estrogen priming may be necessary before adequate GH release can be demonstrated. Although estrogen increases GH concentration, it decreases its biologic effect by blocking somatomedin production. This is similar to the estrogen effect on prolactin in which secretion

FIGURE 321-6 *Response to GRH-44 (1 μg/kg) in eight men and eight women. The shaded area shows the full range of responses at each time point and the error bars indicate the mean ± 1 SD. (From MC Gelato et al, J Clin Endocrinol Metab 59:200, 1984.)*

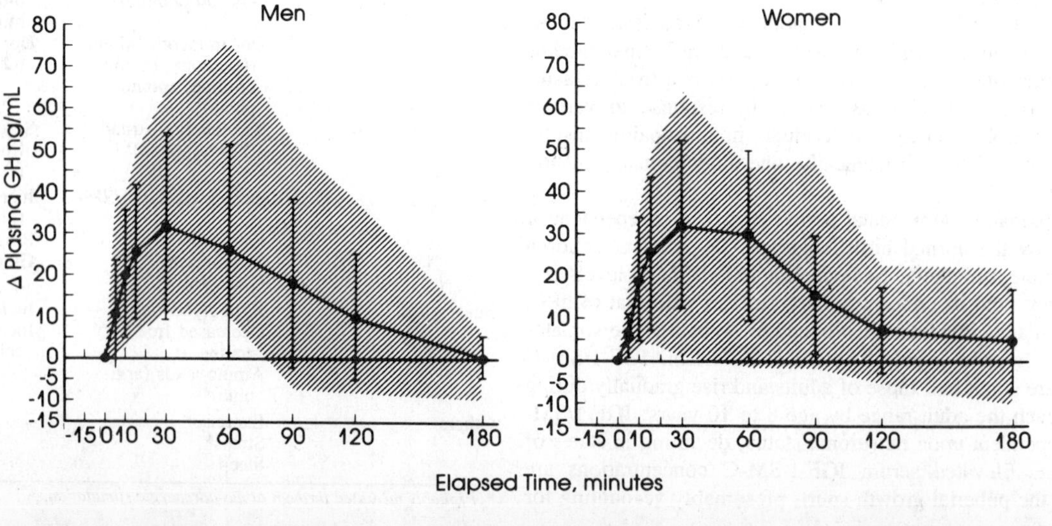

is stimulated, but its action in promoting lactation is inhibited. Glucocorticoids inhibit GH release and may blunt somatomedin action as well, explaining the potent growth-inhibiting effects of these agents in children.

GROWTH HORMONE EXCESS: ACROMEGALY AND GIGANTISM

Clinical features GH excess results in acromegaly, an insidious, chronic debilitating disease associated with bony and soft tissue overgrowth (Table 321-4). Acromegaly occurs most frequently in middle age. It is uncommon with a prevalence of 40 cases per million and an incidence of 3 cases per million per year. When GH excess develops prior to epiphyseal closure in children, increased linear growth and gigantism develop.

Most patients have soft tissue and bone enlargement which results in increased hand, foot, and hat size, prognathism, enlargement of the tongue, wide-spacing of the teeth, and coarsening of facial features. Acromegalics are said to look more like each other than their own family members (Fig. 321-7). Laryngeal hypertrophy and sinus enlargement lead to a hollow-sounding voice. A moist, doughy handshake, increased skin tags, acanthosis nigricans, and oily skin are common.

Acromegaly is more than a cosmetically disfiguring disease. Patients feel weak and tired. The basal metabolic rate increases, which in turn causes increased sweating. Obstructive sleep apnea may be an important cause of hypersomnolence. The majority have neurologic and musculoskeletal symptoms including headaches, paresthesias (often due to carpal tunnel syndrome), muscle weakness, and arthralgias (particularly involving the shoulders, back, and knees). The cartilage hypertrophy and osseous overgrowth often lead to degenerative arthritis. Hypertension occurs in about one-third and is characterized by suppressed renin and aldosterone secretion associated with expansion of plasma volume and total body sodium. Almost all hypertensive acromegalics and about half of nonhypertensive acromegalics have increased left ventricular mass or left ventricular wall thickness. Although it is not established whether a specific cardiomyopathy occurs, acromegalics may develop congestive heart failure in the absence of other known underlying heart disease. Many organs, including the liver and kidneys, increase in size with no evidence of functional impairment. Goiter develops in about one-fourth of patients, and 3 percent are hyperthyroid. Some series report abdominal pain and inguinal hernias each in about one-third of patients. Intracranial aneurysms coexist in 10 percent or less.

Patients with acromegaly have a shortened life expectancy. In older studies, 25 to 50 percent of acromegalics died by age 50 and 65 to 90 percent died by age 60. Increased mortality in men is due mainly to cardiovascular and respiratory disease, whereas mortality in women is principally due to cerebrovascular and respiratory disease. Patients with coexisting diabetes mellitus have increased mortality, as expected, and diabetes may contribute to the atherosclerosis. An increased number of malignancies might be expected in these patients, as acromegaly is associated with increased concentrations of circulating growth factors. However, although increased prevalence of carcinoma has been reported in some series, the differences are not statistically significant. Skin tags correlate with increased prevalence of colonic polyps and possibly with carcinoma of the colon.

Laboratory investigation Insulin resistance occurs in 80 percent, although abnormal glucose tolerance (20 to 40 percent) and clinical diabetes mellitus (13 to 20 percent) are less common. Hypercalciuria is frequent, apparently due to increased levels of circulating 1,25-dihydroxyvitamin D; renal stones occur in about one-fifth of patients. Hypercalcemia, when it occurs, is not due to acromegaly per se but

TABLE 321-4 Acromegaly—Manifestations

Location	Symptoms	Signs
General	Fatigue Increased sweating Heat intolerance Weight gain	
Skin and subcutaneous tissue	Enlarging hands, feet Coarsening facial features Oily skin Hypertrichosis	Moist, warm, fleshy, doughy handshake Skin tags Acanthosis nigricans Increased heel pad
Head	Headaches	Parotid enlargement, frontal bossing
Eyes	Decreased vision	Visual field defects
Ears		Otoscope speculum cannot be inserted
Nose-throat–paranasal sinuses	Sinus congestion Increased tongue size Malocclusion Voice change	Enlarged furrowed tongue Tooth marks on tongue Widely spaced teeth Prognathism
Neck		Goiter Obstructive sleep apnea Enlarged sinuses
Cardiorespiratory system	Congestive heart failure	Hypertension Cardiomegaly Left ventricular hypertrophy
Genitourinary system	Decreased libido Impotence Oligomenorrhea Infertility Kidney stones	
Neurologic system	Paresthesias Hypersomnolence	Carpal tunnel syndrome
Muscles	Weakness	Proximal myopathy
Skeletal system	Joint pains (shoulders, back, knees)	Osteoarthritis

FIGURE 321-7 *Serial photographs of a patient with acromegaly taken at ages 28, 49, 55, and 65 years, 6 months after removal of a GH-secreting adenoma. Note the gradual increase in the size of the nose, lips, and skin folds, particularly the nasolabial skin fold and forehead. (From Reichlin 1982.)*

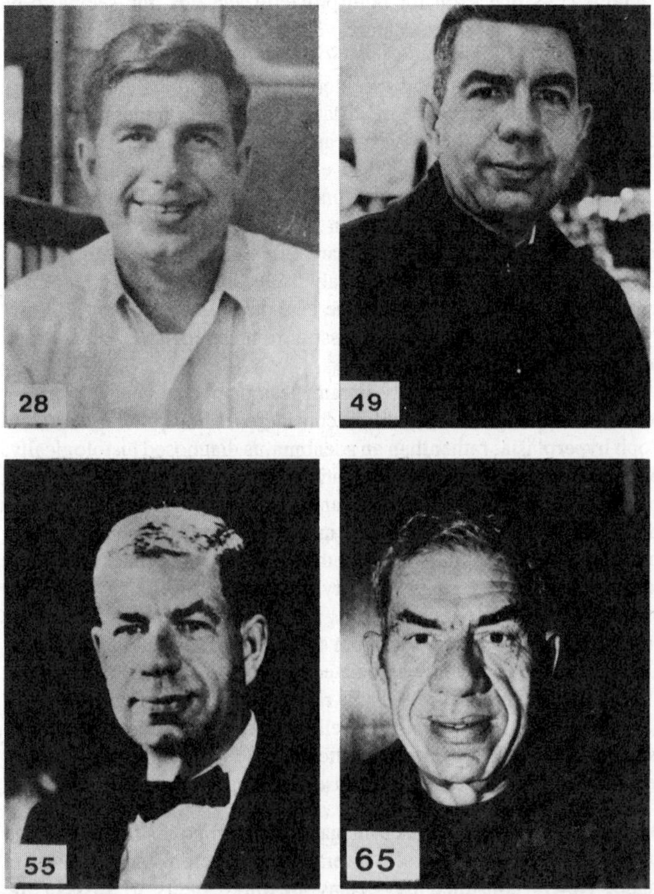

suggests primary hyperparathyroidism as part of the multiple endocrine neoplasia I (MEN I) syndrome (see Chap. 334). GH causes increased renal tubular reabsorption of phosphate by an undefined mechanism. Elevation of serum phosphate occurs in about one-half. Hyperprolactinemia occurs in up to one-half of patients and is responsible for much of the associated galactorrhea, amenorrhea, and decreased libido.

Pathophysiology Well-defined pituitary adenomas are found in almost all patients with acromegaly and gigantism. The tumors tend to occur in the lateral wings of the sella where normal somatotrophs are found in abundance. Occasionally, tumors are found in ectopic locations along the lines of migration of Rathke's pouch, such as the sphenoid sinus or parapharyngeal regions.

GH levels correlate on average with tumor size. Tumors tend to be larger in younger patients, suggesting more rapid growth in this population. At the time of diagnosis 75 percent of somatotroph adenomas are macroadenomas, whereas two-thirds or more of prolactinomas are microadenomas at the time of diagnosis. Aggressive screening for acromegaly on the basis of subtle clinical clues might lead to early diagnosis while tumors are still small.

Immunohistochemical staining and electron microscopy of somatotroph tumors help to predict their behavior. Patients with densely granulated tumors have typical acromegaly, with slow, nonaggressive tumor growth. The sparsely granulated tumors also cause acromegaly but grow more quickly and often invade the sella locally or produce extrasellar extension. Mixed GH- and prolactin-secreting adenomas contain mixtures of somatotrophs and lactotrophs. These mixed cell tumors cause acromegaly, are associated with moderate prolactin elevation, and do not usually demonstrate aggressive growth behavior. In contrast, acidophil stem-cell adenomas, individual cells of which stain for both GH and prolactin, represent poorly differentiated precursors of the somatotrophs and lactotrophs. These tumors grow rapidly, are often invasive, and are associated with marked hyperprolactinemia. Although the cells stain for GH, clinical acromegaly is usually not present. The well-differentiated acidophil adenoma also contains cells that stain for both prolactin and GH and seems to be a slowly growing, more mature variant of the stem-cell adenoma; acromegaly is present with variably elevated prolactin concentrations. Growth hormone–secreting carcinomas are rare and should be diagnosed only in the presence of distant metastases. Tumors that cause local invasion are called invasive adenomas.

Although hypothalamic GRH excess or somatostatin deficiency has been postulated to be the underlying abnormality leading to acromegaly, most acromegalics in fact have primary disease of the pituitary. The evidence for a pituitary etiology includes (1) low serum GRH in patients with acromegaly, (2) absence of somatotroph hyperplasia in the cells outside the adenomas, and (3) return of GH dynamics to normal upon successful removal of the somatotroph adenomas.

GRH-induced acromegaly is rare (less than 1 percent in a recent series). This diagnosis should be considered when pituitary somatotroph hyperplasia, rather than an adenoma, is diagnosed histologically. Bronchial carcinoids and pancreatic islet-cell tumors are the most likely to secrete GRH. Hypothalamic gangliocytomas also produce GRH (as well as somatostatin) and may cause somatotroph hyperplasia and acromegaly. A number of other tumors (including small cell carcinoma of the lung, medullary carcinoma of the thyroid, and thymic carcinoid) contain GRH as shown by immunologic staining, but the amount of secretion from these tumors is unknown. These tumors are also commonly associated with ectopic ACTH production.

Ectopic production of GH is rare but has been described in a patient with a pancreatic islet-cell tumor; the tumor size in this instance (420 g) suggested inefficient GH production since GH-secreting pituitary tumors that cause acromegaly are usually small.

Diagnosis Patients with acromegaly have symptoms for an average of 7 to 8 years and often see several doctors before the diagnosis is made. Newly consulted physicians are more likely to suspect the diagnosis than is a physician or family member who has watched the insidious progress of the disease. When suggestive facial features are noted, a comparison with old pictures may be helpful (Fig. 321-7).

Basal or random GH determinations may be elevated in normal persons, particularly in active women, and should not be used to screen for acromegaly. A physiologic test of the capacity to inhibit GH release must be utilized. The standard screening test is the measurement of serum GH concentrations 60 to 120 min after the oral administration of 100 g glucose. A serum GH concentration of less than 5 ng/mL is usually taken as a normal response, although a postsuppression value of less than 2 ng/mL is a more rigorous criterion. Acromegalics usually have a GH concentration after glucose administration of greater than 10 ng/mL; however, some suppress to values below 5 but rarely below 2 ng/mL.

GH concentrations in acromegaly may vary during the day, although they are never undetectable as in normal persons. After glucose administration to acromegalics the GH concentrations usually are unchanged or increase, but some GH lowering may occur. GH levels increase in response to insulin-induced hypoglycemia and arginine infusion, and the response to GRH is enhanced in most acromegalics. Somatostatin infusion lowers GH concentration but usually not to normal values. In addition, GH-secreting pituitary tumors respond to stimuli that do not affect normal somatotrophs: TRH increases GH in the majority (80 percent), and LHRH increases GH in about 10–15 percent. Dopamine agonists stimulate GH release in normal persons but inhibit GH release in 75 percent of acromegalics. Somatotroph tumors that cosecrete prolactin are most likely to show GH stimulation with TRH and GH inhibition with dopamine agonists.

Measurement of serum IGF-1/SM-C is useful, although clinical experience with this assay is limited; concentrations seem to correlate with disease activity even in patients with basal GH concentrations below 10 ng/mL. Acromegalics usually have IGF-1/SM-C values greater than 2.6 units per milliliter, whereas normal persons have values less than 1.4 units per milliliter. The level does not correlate well with basal GH concentrations but does correlate with heel pad thickness and fasting blood sugar. IGF-1/SM-C is less useful in following acromegalics after therapy.

All patients with large pituitary adenomas should be screened with GH measurements, preferably after glucose ingestion. In rare cases patients with elevated serum GH and IGF-1/SM-C concentrations may have large pituitary tumors, without clinical evidence of acromegaly. This syndrome is unexplained.

Radiologic investigation is necessary once the laboratory tests confirm the clinical suspicion of acromegaly. Conventional skull x-rays or coned-down views of the sella turcica are abnormal in 90 percent of patients with acromegaly. CT scanning or MRI provides better definition of tumor size and is necessary for appropriate therapeutic planning. Additional clues to the diagnosis of acromegaly can be found on conventional skull x-rays and include thickening of the skull with increased bone density, enlargement of the paranasal sinuses and proliferation of the mastoid air cells, and prognathism if the jaw is included. On bone x-rays one may see enlarged vertebral bodies with anterior lipping, tufting of the distal phalanges of the hands and feet, increased thickness and lengthening of the ribs and clavicles, and bowing of the femur, tibia, and fibula. Soft tissue x-rays demonstrate increased thickness of the heel pad (greater than 18 mm in women and 21 mm in men).

Testing of anterior pituitary function for hypopituitarism and for increased prolactin should be performed at some point in the evaluation of all acromegalics. Large somatotrope adenomas commonly cause neurologic abnormalities. In addition, acromegaly may be associated with hyperparathyroidism and pancreatic islet-cell tumors in the MEN I syndrome and rarely with pheochromocytomas or aldosteronomas. The alpha subunit of the glycoprotein hormones may be oversecreted in acromegaly and may serve as an additional marker of tumor regrowth.

Therapy The objectives of therapy are (1) return of GH levels to normal, (2) stabilization or decrease in tumor size, and (3) preservation of normal pituitary function. The available modalities are variably successful in achieving these goals, and none is perfect. Although GH values of less than 5 ng/mL are frequently interpreted as representing cures, a value of less than 2 ng/mL is a better criterion; patients with GH values between 2 and 5 ng/mL may have persistent symptoms and increased IGF-1/SM-C concentrations.

Transsphenoidal surgery has the advantage of producing a rapid therapeutic response and is the procedure of choice. GH concentrations fall to normal with hours, and soft tissue (but not bony) enlargement may melt away, even before the patient has been discharged from the hospital. The success of this procedure depends upon the preoperative GH concentration. In expert hands, apparent cure rates (GH below 5 ng/mL) average 75 percent in patients with preoperative GH levels of less than 40 ng/mL but only 35 percent in those with a GH level greater than 40 ng/mL. The occurrence of tumor regrowth and recurrent acromegaly after successful surgery may be higher than previously appreciated. Persistent GH response to TRH stimulation appears to have predictive value in assessing risk of relapse, even in those patients with normal postoperative GH concentrations. Hypopituitarism may occur in 10 to 20 percent of patients with larger tumors, but up to 10 percent of patients with pituitary insufficiency prior to surgery regain normal function.

Heavy particle pituitary radiation is successful in lowering GH concentrations in acromegaly but is slow in accomplishing this goal. Patients with suprasellar extension of the pituitary adenoma are generally excluded from this therapy. The Harvard cyclotron utilizes the Bragg peak with proton irradiation, achieving up to 12,000 cGy (12,000 rad) to the center of the pituitary adenoma. In patients with mean pretherapy GH concentration of 60 ng/mL, GH concentrations are below 5 ng/mL in 29 percent of patients at 2 years, 40 percent at 4 years, 75 percent at 10 years and 92 percent by 20 years. Hypopituitarism occurs in about 20 percent. The Lawrence Radiation Laboratory at Berkeley uses alpha particles and delivers 9000 cGy (9000 rad) to the adenoma. GH values are less than 5 ng/mL in 30 percent of patient at 1 year and 70 percent by 6 years (mean pretherapy GH of 24 ng/mL).

Conventional pituitary radiation [4500 cGy (4500 rad)] also has its proponents. GH concentrations of less than 5 ng/mL occur in 50 percent of acromegalics at 5 years and in 70 percent at 10 years (mean pretherapy GH 60 ng/mL). Hypopituitarism is a sequela, and up to 50 percent of patients require replacement therapy. The hypopituitarism is most likely due to hypothalamic damage, which is less likely to occur with focused heavy particle radiation. We use heavy particle or conventional radiation in patients who have failed surgery or when surgery is contraindicated or refused by the patient.

Bromocriptine is a useful adjunct to other modalities of therapy but rarely is used alone. Clinical improvement is reported in up to 90 percent of patients when dosages of 20 to 60 mg per day are utilized. Objective decrease in hand and ring size as well as improvement in diabetes mellitus may occur in the absence of decreasing GH values. However, GH concentrations fall to less than 10 ng/mL in only 35 percent, and values of less than 5 ng/mL are achieved in only 15 percent. Those patients who demonstrate GH increase after TRH administration are more likely to respond to bromocriptine. A decrease in tumor size is noted in about 25 percent.

Estrogen administration is an older form of therapy which is empirically successful but is rarely used now. Its clinical efficacy is probably explained by the blockade of somatomedin production by estrogen. Although intravenous somatostatin lowers GH concentration, GH concentrations do not return to normal. Subcutaneous injections of newer long-acting analogues of somatostatin have been effective in lowering GH over the short term. It is not known whether analogues can be developed that suppress GH but not insulin or glucagon.

GH DEFICIENCY AND PITUITARY DWARFISM GH is often the first hormone to be lost in pituitary and hypothalamic disorders. In adults, GH deficiency is often cryptic and can only be diagnosed on the basis of stimulation tests for GH release. GH deficiency is probably responsible for the fine wrinkling of facial skin in patients with hypopituitarism. Diabetics with GH deficiency show a reduction in insulin requirements and may develop hypoglycemia. In children, GH deficiency leads to impaired growth and short stature (see Chap. 322).

GONADOTROPINS

PHYSIOLOGY The gonadotropins, LH and FSH, are secreted by the gonadotrophs (also see Chaps. 330 and 331). These cells, which make up about 10 percent of anterior pituitary cells, are dispersed throughout the anterior lobe, often situated close to the lactotrophs. Most gonadotrophs produce both LH and FSH, although a few cells produce only one hormone.

LH and FSH are glycoprotein hormones of similar size (about 30,000 mol wt), which share a common alpha subunit [also present in TSH and human chorionic gonadotropin (hCG)] but have unique beta subunits. The alpha and beta chains are encoded in separate genes on separate chromosomes, and alpha chains are often produced in excess. The carbohydrate content of the molecules influences the biologic behavior and duration of action and may vary throughout the menstrual cycle. Although both FSH and LH are secreted in pulsatile fashion, the longer FSH half-life (3 to 4 h versus 50 min) means that FSH concentrations fluctuate less throughout the day. FSH and LH regulate ovarian and testicular function.

FSH stimulates the growth of the granulosa cells of the ovarian follicle and controls estrogen formation within these cells. LH stimulates the ovarian theca cells to produce androgens, which diffuse to the granulosa cells where they are converted to estrogens. Estradiol, the principal estrogen, peaks about 1 day prior to the LH surge, which in turn triggers ovulation. Postovulation, LH contributes to corpus luteum formation. Once conception has occurred, pituitary gonadotropin function is no longer necessary to sustain pregnancy.

In the testis LH is primarily responsible for controlling testosterone production in the Leydig cells. FSH, in conjunction with intratesticular testosterone, stimulates the seminiferous tubules to produce sperm. Thus LH and FSH are necessary for normal spermatogenesis, whereas testosterone production requires only LH.

Luteinizing hormone–releasing hormone (LHRH, gonadotropin-releasing hormone), a decapeptide produced by the arcuate nuclei of the hypothalamus, is responsible for the release of both LH and FSH. Extrahypothalamic LHRH is present in other areas of the brain and in the gonads as well. Norepinephrine appears to facilitate, whereas dopamine and the endorphins inhibit, LHRH release.

LHRH interacts with high-affinity pituitary receptors to stimulate LH and FSH production and release, a process mediated through an increase in cytosolic calcium and possibly an effect on cyclic AMP. The pituitary response to LHRH varies greatly throughout life. LHRH and the gonadotropins first appear in the fetus at about 10 weeks of gestation. During the first 3 months after birth, LHRH elicits a brisk gonadotropin rise. The sensitivity to LHRH then declines until the onset of puberty. Before puberty, the FSH response to LHRH is greater than that of LH. With the onset of puberty sensitivity to LHRH increases, and pulsatile LH secretion, first noted during sleep ensues. Later in puberty and during the reproductive years, pulsations are present throughout the day, with LH responsiveness being greater than that of FSH. After the menopause FSH and LH concentrations rise, and postmenopausal FSH levels are higher than those of LH. LHRH may also have direct effects on the gonads, leading to a decreased number of LH, FSH, and prolactin receptors.

Pulsatile LHRH release results in pulsatile LH and FSH release. However, sustained infusion of LHRH and its analogues results in inhibition of LH and FSH release. This phenomenon has been utilized in the successful treatment of gonadotropin-mediated precocious puberty by the sustained administration of LHRH or its analogues. Conversely, in monkeys with experimental hypothalamic defects and in humans with LHRH deficiency, the pulsatile administration of

LHRH can restore a normal menstrual cycle or normal sperm and testosterone production.

The feedback relationship between the gonadal steroids and the hypothalamus and pituitary is detailed in Chaps. 330 and 331. Low doses of estrogens decrease the frequency of LHRH pulses and, more importantly, decrease the pituitary response to LHRH; this phenomenon is seen most clearly in castrated individuals or in postmenopausal women with elevated gonadotropins. However, sustained elevation of estrogens results in a positive feedback signal that stimulates LHRH and LH release; this phenomenon is responsible for the LH surge prior to ovulation. The sensitivity of LHRH to this positive feedback by estrogen increases during mid to late puberty. Progesterone in high concentrations decreases the frequency of LHRH release and to a lesser extent diminishes the pituitary response to LHRH. In castrated men testosterone administration usually suppresses LH to undetectable levels and less often lowers FSH to normal (but not undetectable) concentrations. Inhibin, a peptide produced by the testes and ovaries, is probably the dominant physiologic inhibitor of FSH release. Testosterone decreases the frequency of LH pulsations, probably by a direct effect on LHRH release, and is converted to estradiol which inhibits the pituitary response to LHRH.

Gonadotropin measurements In postmenopausal women and men with primary hypogonadism, gonadal failure results in a marked increase in FSH and LH concentrations, providing an endogenous stimulation test. Such elevated gonadotropin concentrations assure the adequacy of pituitary gonadotroph function. On the other hand, gonadotropin measurements are rarely indicated in a woman with ovulatory menses and in men with normal sperm counts. In evaluating gonadal failure associated with low testosterone concentrations in men or low estradiol levels in women, gonadotropin measurements help separate primary from central (secondary, hypogonadotropic) hypogonadism: high gonadotropin concentrations are indicative of primary gonadal failure; low or normal gonadotropin concentrations suggest hypothalamic or pituitary disease (see Chap. 320).

HYPOGONADOTROPIC (CENTRAL, SECONDARY) HYPOGONADISM Gonadotropin deficiency may be present at birth as a congenital or hereditary disorder. Kallmann's syndrome is inherited as a single gene trait, afflicts men more severely than women, and is characterized by gonadotropin deficiency frequently associated with anosmia and midline anatomic defects. Kallmann's syndrome appears to be due to LHRH deficiency, as most patients secrete gonadotropins in response to LHRH administration after suitable priming. Acquired defects of LHRH production are common: hyperprolactinemic amenorrhea is due to inhibition of LHRH release, possibly mediated by increased hypothalamic dopamine. Anorexia nervosa and starvation inhibit LHRH release as well. Gonadotropin deficiency may be a relatively early defect in patients with large pituitary adenomas. Gonadotropin deficiency also occurs in patients with polyglandular endocrine deficiencies, presumably on an autoimmune basis (see Chap. 334) and in patients with hemochromatosis.

Patients with LHRH deficiency who desire fertility may respond to pulsatile therapy with LHRH or its analogues. When gonadotropin deficiency is due to pituitary disease, injections of FSH (menotropin) and choronic gonadotropin (a hormone with LH-like activity) are necessary to achieve fertility.

ECTOPIC GONADOTROPIN SECRETION AND GONADOTROPIN-SECRETING TUMORS Ectopic gonadotropin production (usually hCG) can be secreted by germinomas of the nonseminoma type (see Chap. 297), lung carcinomas, hepatomas, and other tumors. Children may develop precocious puberty, and men may develop gynecomastia. No distinct clinical syndrome occurs in women. Pituitary gonadotropin-secreting tumors, previously thought to be rare, are now known to be relatively common. Approximately 4 percent of all pituitary adenomas demonstrate gonadotropins or their subunits on immunologic staining; how often these tumors secrete gonadotropins is not clear.

FSH-secreting pituitary adenomas are large tumors, most commonly diagnosed in men with decreased libido, decreased serum testosterone, and normal prolactin levels. The finding of an increased FSH concentration may be misinterpreted as indicating primary hypogonadism if a pituitary adenoma is not suspected. The majority of these tumors overproduce the beta subunit of FSH, and 40 percent demonstrate increased FSH secretion after TRH administration. Normal subjects and patients with primary hypogonadism do not have increased FSH secretion after TRH. Despite the normal or elevated LH concentrations in these patients, testosterone concentrations are low and respond normally to hCG administration. This suggests that the LH measured by radioimmunoassay is biologically inactive or that it represents immunologic cross-reactivity due to subunit overproduction.

LH-secreting pituitary adenomas are usually large tumors and are characterized by increased serum testosterone, elevated LH levels, and normal or low FSH concentrations, often with partial hypopituitarism. It is often difficult to diagnose gonadotropin-secreting pituitary adenomas in postmenopausal women because of the elevated gonadotropins associated with menopause.

THYROTROPIN

PHYSIOLOGY TSH is a glycoprotein hormone (28,000 mol wt) composed of an alpha subunit which it shares with LH, FSH, and hCG and a unique beta subunit that confers specificity (also see Chap. 324). The genes coding for the alpha and beta subunits are on different chromosomes. TSH is produced by thyrotrophs which constitute about 10 percent of the cells of the anterior pituitary. TSH regulates the biosynthesis, storage, and release of thyroid hormones and determines thyroid gland size. TSH first appears in the fetal pituitary at about 10 weeks of gestation. TSH levels in normal subjects average 0.5 to 3.5 μU per milliliter, with a slight increase in the nocturnal hours.

Thyrotropin-releasing hormone (TRH), the major hypothalamic mediator of TSH release, is a tripeptide found in highest concentrations in the medial division of the hypothalamic paraventricular nuclei and in the median eminence. Extrahypothalamic TRH is found in the posterior pituitary, in other parts of the brain and spinal cord, and in the gastrointestinal tract. TRH stimulates TSH secretion by increasing cytoplasmic free calcium; phosphatidylinositol and membrane phospholipids probably participate in TRH-stimulated TSH secretion. TRH stimulates the release of prolactin as well as that of TSH. The prolactin response is enhanced in hypothyroidism and diminished in hyperthyroidism. TRH-induced GH stimulation may occur in acromegaly, renal failure, or depression.

The thyroid hormones thyroxine (T_4) and triiodothyronine (T_3) inhibit TSH production directly at the pituitary level. Both T_3 and T_4 bind to receptors on pituitary nuclei, but T_3 has a 40-fold greater affinity for these receptors than does T_4. Nevertheless, exogenous T_4 is more potent than T_3 in inhibiting TSH release because circulating T_4 is a more effective means of delivering T_3 to the pituitary than is T_3 itself. Half of intrapituitary T_3 is derived from T_4 conversion within the pituitary. The effects of T_4 and T_3 on hypothalamic TRH release are unknown. In hyperthyroidism TSH is suppressed, and the TSH response to TRH is absent; in primary hypothyroidism the basal TSH concentration is elevated, and the response to TRH is exaggerated.

Somatostatin decreases basal TSH release, the TSH response to TRH, and the nocturnal TSH peak. Dopamine and glucocorticoids decrease basal TSH concentration and the TSH response to TRH. Patients with untreated primary adrenal insufficiency may have slightly elevated TSH levels.

TSH concentrations can be interpreted only when serum thyroid hormone concentrations are known (see Chap. 320). In hyperthyroidism, thyroid hormone levels are elevated and TSH release is inhibited. Unfortunately, most TSH assays cannot differentiate between low and normal concentrations. However, since TRH administration causes no rise of serum TSH in hyperthyroidism, a normal TSH response to TRH excludes conventional hyperthyroidism. Low thyroid hormone and elevated serum TSH concentrations are characteristic of primary hypothyroidism. Since the basal TSH concentration is elevated, a TRH stimulation test is superfluous. Low thyroid hormone concentrations with a "normal" or "low" TSH concentration are found in central (secondary) hypothyroidism. The TRH stimulation test is not useful in the diagnosis of secondary hypothyroidism or in differentiating pituitary from hypothalamic disease.

PRIMARY HYPOTHYROIDISM Thyroid gland failure (primary hypothyroidism) leads to compensatory hypertrophy of the thyrotrophs. With thyroid failure of long duration, the pituitary gland and the sella turcica may enlarge. Although TSH-secreting tumors may develop in animals after thyroid gland removal, the increased TSH and pituitary size in human hypothyroidism is not autonomous and decreases with thyroid hormone replacement. Since hyperprolactinemia may also occur in patients with primary hypothyroidism, pituitary enlargement (hyperplasia) may be incorrectly diagnosed as a prolactinoma. Severe primary hypothyroidism may occasionally cause impaired release of GH and ACTH after appropriate stimuli (so-called pituitary myxedema), and hypothyroid children may develop precocious puberty. These abnormalities are all corrected with thyroid hormone therapy.

SECONDARY HYPOTHYROIDISM Hypothyroidism due to pituitary or hypothalamic disease may be difficult to diagnose. With primary hypothyroidism serum TSH commonly rises before thyroid hormone concentrations decline below the normal range. No similar early laboratory clue exists in secondary hypothyroidism. Patients with central hypothyroidism usually do not have goiter, and many have deficiencies of other pituitary trophic hormones.

Some patients with hypothalamic hypothyroidism have mild TSH elevations, rather than normal or low concentrations as expected. Although the TSH elevations rarely exceed 10 μU/mL, they are above the expected range for hypothyroidism due to TSH deficiency. Biologically inactive but immunologically active thyrotropin is present in such cases. After TRH injection, TSH concentration rises, and the biologic potency of the TSH is increased. This suggests an additional role for TRH in controlling the biologic activity of the TSH molecule.

PITUITARY (TSH-INDUCED) HYPERTHYROIDISM Hyperthyroidism is not usually a disease of TSH overproduction. However, two types of TSH-mediated hyperthyroidism are recognized:

1. Pituitary tumors. These are usually macroadenomas with autonomous TSH secretion, unresponsive to thyroid hormone suppression or TRH stimulation. A hallmark of such tumors is overproduction of the glycoprotein hormone alpha subunit (TSH alpha), with a serum molar ratio of alpha to intact TSH of greater than 1:1. The free alpha subunit may be an important tumor marker and differs from the native alpha subunit in that one of its amino acids is carbohydrate-blocked and hence cannot combine with beta subunits. These tumors may produce other pituitary hormones in addition to TSH, most commonly GH.
2. Pituitary resistance to thyroid hormone. In this situation thyroid hormone fails to inhibit TSH secretion appropriately in the absence of a pituitary adenoma. Since TSH secretion is not inhibited, TSH rises and stimulates thyroid hormone overproduction. The peripheral tissues are not resistant to thyroid hormone, and clinical hyperthyroidism results. The pituitary resistance to thyroid hormone is incomplete since TSH can be suppressed with supraphysiologic levels of thyroid hormone and stimulated further with TRH; bromocriptine may lower TSH as well. Pituitary resistance is usually diagnosed after thyroid gland ablation, when TSH cannot be lowered to normal values with the usual therapeutic doses of thyroid hormone. However, once the hyperthyroidism has been treated, pituitary resistance is of no clinical consequence.

ADRENOCORTICOTROPHIC HORMONE

PHYSIOLOGY ACTH is produced by corticotrophs which comprise about 15 percent of anterior pituitary cells, located principally in the central portion. ACTH is synthesized as part of a large precursor molecule termed proopiomelanocortin (POMC, 265 amino acids) (see Chaps. 69 and 325). ACTH contains 39 amino acids, with near complete biologic activity residing in the *N*-terminal 26 amino acids. In the anterior pituitary POMC is cleaved to yield ACTH, β-lipotropin, and an *N*-terminal precursor (see Chap. 325).

ACTH controls the release of cortisol from the adrenal cortex. Although aldosterone is primarily controlled by the renin-angiotensin system, ACTH also stimulates aldosterone release acutely. Other derivatives of the POMC molecule, such as γ-melanocyte-stimulating hormone (γ-MSH), also influence aldosterone production and are found in increased concentrations in the plasma of patients with idiopathic hyperaldosteronism. Patients with ACTH deficiency have near-normal aldosterone production and do not require mineralocorticoid replacement therapy.

Corticotropin releasing hormone (CRH) is the major regulator of ACTH release. CRH contains 41 amino acids on a single polypeptide chain. CRH is produced primarily by neurons of the paraventricular nuclei of the hypothalamus but is also present in other areas of the brain, including the limbic system and cortex, as well as in the pancreas, gut, and adrenal medulla. CRH stimulates cyclic AMP production and increases the concentration of POMC messenger RNA. Vasopressin potentiates the ACTH-releasing properties of CRH through a noncyclic AMP–dependent mechanism and may play a physiologic role in ACTH release. Beta-adrenergic stimuli and oxytocin cause ACTH release as well. Somatostatin blocks CRH-induced ACTH release.

ACTH is released in pulses with an overriding circadian rhythm. With a normal sleeping pattern, ACTH concentration is highest in the early morning (around 4 A.M.) and lowest in late evening. The characteristic diurnal rhythm of plasma cortisol occurs in response to these ACTH changes. In primary adrenal insufficiency (Addison's disease), cortisol concentrations fall and ACTH concentrations rise. This results in hyperpigmentation owing to the melanocyte-stimulating properties of ACTH. Cortisol administration inhibits ACTH release, a phenomenon dependent upon both the rate of rise of cortisol and its absolute concentration. Increased plasma cortisol inhibits CRH-induced ACTH release and may also inhibit CRH release. When supraphysiologic doses of glucocorticoids (e.g., cortisone, prednisone, dexamethasone) are given for prolonged periods, the hypothalamic-pituitary–adrenal cortex axis may remain suppressed for months after the drugs have been stopped, probably as the result of prolonged hypothalamic CRH suppression (see Chap. 325).

Stress, including hypoglycemia, surgery, and psychic distress, stimulates ACTH release, via increased CRH release. With severe illness, the requirements for cortisol may increase tenfold; failure to achieve these levels of cortisol during such periods may result in clinical adrenal insufficiency in subjects with diminished ACTH reserve.

In normal persons ACTH circulates in low concentrations (10 to 80 pg/mL). It is difficult to measure ACTH in plasma and usually not possible to separate low from normal values using commercial assays. Random ACTH measurements have little clinical significance. Tests for adrenal insufficiency and excess rely primarily on measurements of cortisol and its metabolites rather than on measurement of ACTH.

ACTH EXCESS (CUSHING'S DISEASE AND NELSON'S SYNDROME) Clinical features Cortisol excess is characterized by a central distribution of adipose tissue, muscle weakness, purplish striae, hypertension, amenorrhea, osteoporosis, fatigue, and psychiatric abnormalities. This syndrome may be caused by pituitary or ectopic ACTH overproduction, adrenal tumors, or exogenous glucocorticoid administration.

The presence of cortisol excess is established by the finding of increased excretion of urine free cortisol and/or 17-hydroxycorticosteroids that fails to decrease appropriately after low-dose dexamethasone administration (0.5 mg every 6 h for 8 doses). Additional suppression (and occasionally stimulation) tests are required to determine whether the Cushing's syndrome is due to a pituitary lesion. In patients with pituitary ACTH hypersecretion, high-dose dexamethasone administration (2 mg every 6 h for 8 doses) results in suppression of urine 17-hydroxycorticosteroids and free cortisol, usually by greater than 50 percent. Urine 17-hydroxycorticosteroids increase after metyrapone administration in Cushing's disease. Plasma ACTH levels are normal or high-normal and show an exaggerated increase after CRH administration. Pituitary ACTH hypersecretion (Cushing's disease) is caused by a corticotroph microadenoma in 90 percent of patients and by a macroadenoma in most of the rest. Corticotroph hyperplasia has been documented in a few cases. The microadenomas are often small (3 mm or less) and may be missed on CT scanning. Thus pituitary surgery must often be recommended on the basis of dynamic testing along. However, bilateral inferior petrosal sinus catheterizations to localize the site of ACTH production may prove to be useful in patients in whom an adenoma is not radiographically detectable.

Treatment Transsphenoidal microsurgery is successful in treating microadenomas in about 75 percent of patients. When surgery is successful, plasma cortisol concentrations fall almost to zero and often remain low for many months owing to delayed recovery of CRH and ACTH secretion by the hypothalamus and normal remaining pituitary. However, adrenal function eventually returns to normal in most patients. Previously, bilateral adrenalectomy was the therapy of choice for patients with pituitary Cushing's disease. Unfortunately, after this procedure enlarging pituitary adenomas with increased skin pigmentation (Nelson's syndrome) develop in 10 to 30 percent of patients.

Ectopic ACTH production is a relatively common disorder and can cause great difficulty in diagnosis (see Chaps. 303 and 325). When ACTH production by such tumors is of short duration (e.g., when caused by rapidly growing tumors such as oat cell carcinoma of the lung), symptoms of Cushing's syndrome are blunted. Rather, patients often demonstrate hypokalemia, muscle weakness, weight loss, and hyperpigmentation. ACTH concentrations often exceed 300 pg/mL and do not change with dexamethasone administration. When slow-growing tumors such as thymic carcinoids, bronchial carcinoids, medullary carcinoma of the thyroid, and pancreatic islet-cell tumors produce ACTH the typical features of Cushing's syndrome are common. In the latter group ACTH measurements and cortisol response to dexamethasone administration may mimic those found in patients with pituitary adenomas. However, with ectopic ACTH production ACTH concentrations generally do not change after CRH administration. When differentiation between pituitary and ectopic ACTH production is uncertain, bilateral inferior petrosal sinus catheterization is necessary. Production of Cushing's syndrome by ectopic production of CRH itself and by factors that enhance CRH action has also been reported.

ACTH DEFICIENCY (SECONDARY ADRENAL INSUFFICIENCY) ACTH deficiency may be isolated or occur in association with other anterior pituitary hormone deficiencies. Reversible isolated ACTH deficiency is common after long-term glucocorticoid administration. If glucocorticoids are withdrawn suddenly in this situation or continued in physiologic doses when severe illness is present, adrenal insufficiency may occur. Symptoms include nausea, vomiting, fatigue, and dizziness and there may be fever, hypotension, hyponatremia, and hypoglycemia. Although cortisol is necessary for free water excretion, it is not needed for potassium excretion. Hence patients with ACTH deficiency are not hyperkalemic as are patients with primary adrenal insufficiency. Hyperpigmentation also does not occur. These factors make diagnosis of secondary adrenal insufficiency more difficult than that of primary adrenal insufficiency. Isolated ACTH deficiency may occur without prior glucocorticoid therapy.

All patients undergoing pituitary surgery need to be treated with "stress" doses of glucocorticoids until normal adrenal function can be demonstrated postoperatively. All patients with pituitary macroadenomas or hypothalamic disease require testing of the pituitary-adrenal axis but when pituitary surgery is planned, testing can be limited in focus until after surgery is completed.

ENDORPHINS (ENDOGENOUS OPIOIDS)

Endogenous peptides that interact with opioid receptors are termed endorphins, enkephalins, or endogenous opioids (see Chap. 69). In the anterior pituitary the precursor molecule POMC is cleaved to ACTH and β-lipotropin, both of which are secreted into plasma. A small fraction (about 15 percent) of β-lipotropin is cleaved to β-endorphin. In other parts of the brain and in the intermediate pituitary lobe of animals, most POMC is cleaved to β-endorphin. Dynorphin, a potent endogenous opioid, is produced by the same magnocellular neurons of the hypothalamus that synthesize vasopressin and is stored along with vasopressin in the posterior pituitary. Pituitary ablation is successful in relieving pain in about one-third of patients with metastatic carcinoma, independent of any effect on tumor growth. Although the mechanism for this effect is uncertain, most patients who respond to this therapy develop concomitant diabetes insipidus.

Although some endorphins originate in the pituitary and hypothalamus, the role of these compounds in regulating pituitary and hypothalamic function is uncertain. Endorphins appear to inhibit LH and FSH release; naloxone, an opiate antagonist, increase LH and FSH concentrations in men and women. Naloxone can restore LH pulsations to normal in hyperprolactinemic patients with absent LH pulsations. Whereas in trained athletes exogenous opiates (e.g., morphine) stimulate prolactin and GH release, naloxone does not influence basal or stimulated prolactin or GH. Exogenous opioids inhibit ACTH release but endogenous opioids have little influence on ACTH or TSH release.

DISEASES OF THE HYPOTHALAMUS AND PITUITARY

Diseases that affect the hypothalamus and pituitary can have both endocrine and nonendocrine manifestations.

HYPOTHALAMUS The human hypothalamus weighs about 4 g; hypothalamic dysfunction occurs only when disease is bilateral. Tumors in this region are often slow-growing and may achieve large size before symptoms appear. Signs of hydrocephalus or focal cerebral dysfunction may coexist with hypopituitarism and hypothalamic dysfunction and may produce a confusing clinical picture.

The hypothalamus exerts both endocrine and nonendocrine functions. Hypothalamic control of the pituitary gland has already been discussed. Nonendocrine functions that are influenced by the hypothalamus are as follows:

1 Caloric intake and feeding behavior. The basal hypothalamus is necessary for maintenance of a stable weight. The ventromedial nucleus is involved with satiety; the lateral hypothalamus with hunger. Hypothalamic obesity is usually associated with lesions of the ventromedial nucleus; this obesity appears to involve a resetting of the weight set point. Marked hyperphagia, possibly related to rapid gastric emptying, occurs until the new weight set point is reached. Patients often demonstrate decreased activity and finicky eating once the new set point is reached. Lateral hypothalamic lesions may cause aphagia. Other factors that influence eating behavior include hypothyroidism and adrenal insufficiency, both of which can diminish appetite.

2 Temperature regulation. The anterior hypothalamus contains warm- and cold-sensitive neurons that respond to local and environmental thermal gradients. The posterior hypothalamus generates the signals necessary for heat dissipation. The temperature increase associated with infections is generated by the hypothalamus. Phagocytic cells throughout the body produce interleukin 1 (endogenous pyrogen) which stimulates the anterior hypothalamus to produce prostaglandin E_2. Prostaglandin E_2 raises the thermostat set point, leading to heat conservation (e.g., vasoconstriction) and increased heat production (e.g., muscle shivering) until blood and core temperatures match the new hypothalamic set point.

Abnormalities of temperature regulation may occur with hypothalamic disease. Hypothermia is a rare consequence of diffuse hypothalamic disease. Paroxysmal hypothermia with sweating, flushing, and a fall in body temperatures may occur, and sustained hyperthermia without tachycardia is reported with acute pathologic processes such as hemorrhage into the third ventricle. Poikilothermia (a change in body temperature of greater than 1°C with change in environmental temperature) is usually a consequence of posterior hypothalamic disease. Paroxysmal hyperthermia with episodic shaking chills, spiking fevers, and autonomic phenomena is a rare manifestation. It is important to remember that adrenal insufficiency can cause fever or hypothermia and that hypothyroidism may cause hypothermia.

3 Sleep-wake cycle. The anterior hypothalamus contains a sleep center; lesions in this region result in insomnia. The posterior hypothalamus is important for arousal and maintenance of the waking state; posterior hypothalamic destruction due to ischemia, encephalitis, or trauma can result in a hypersomnolent state from which arousal is possible. Larger lesions extending to the reticular formation of the rostral midbrain cause coma (see Chap. 21).

4 Memory and behavior. Lesions of the ventromedial hypothalamus and premammillary region result in loss of short-term memory, often with Korsakoff's syndrome. Longer-term memory is often intact. Hypothalamic lesions may also cause a more typical picture of dementia. Rage reactions may result with ventromedial lesions, and lateral hypothalamic destruction may cause an apathetic state.

5 Thirst. The hypothalamus is the center for AVP production and for the control of thirst by serum osmolality. Impaired thirst may occur with hypothalamic lesions; rarely primary polydipsia without diabetes insipidus is a consequence of hypothalamic lesions.

6 Autonomic nervous system function. Parasympathetic pathways are stimulated by the anterior hypothalamus; sympathetic pathways are stimulated by the posterior hypothalamus. Diencephalic epilepsy is a rare syndrome associated with paroxysms of autonomic hyperactivity.

A diencephalic syndrome in children, characterized by emaciation, hyperkinesis and inappropriate affect, often with a cheerful disposition, is usually associated with invasive tumors of the anterior and basal hypothalamus. Most of these children die by the age of 2 years, but in those who survive the clinical picture changes to one of increased appetite with obesity, irritability, and rage reactions.

In general, slow-growing tumors are more likely to produce dementia, disturbances of food intake (obesity or emaciation), and endocrine dysfunction. Acute destructive processes are more likely to produce coma or disturbances of the autonomic nervous system.

Diseases of the anterior hypothalamus include craniopharyngiomas, gliomas of the optic nerve, sphenoid ridge meningiomas, granulomatous disease (including sarcoidosis), germinomas, and aneurysms of the internal carotid artery. Suprasellar pituitary adenomas and tuberculum sella meningiomas may grow into the hypothalamus as well. Lesions of the posterior hypothalamus include gliomas, hamartomas, ependymomas, germinomas, and teratomas.

Precocious puberty, particularly in males, has often been associated with "pinealomas," leading to the speculation that the pineal is important for gonadotropin regulation. However, these pinealomas actually are germinomas, and the precocious puberty appears to result from the ectopic production of hCG by these tumors rather than from an effect on pituitary gonadotropins.

Craniopharyngiomas Craniopharyngiomas arise from remnants of Rathke's pouch. Most of these tumors are suprasellar, but about 15 percent are intrasellar. The tumors are usually cystic or partially cystic, often contain calcium, and are lined with stratified squamous epithelium. Although craniopharyngiomas are typically thought to be a disease of childhood, 45 percent of patients are over the age of 20, and 20 percent are over the age of 40 at the time of diagnosis.

Children usually present with signs of increased intracranial pressure due to hydrocephalus (80 percent) with headache, vomiting, and papilledema. Visual abnormalities such as loss of vision and field cuts are found in 60 percent. Short stature is sometimes found (7 to 40 percent), but retarded bone age is more common. Delayed sexual development occurs in about 20 percent, and diabetes insipidus may be present.

About 80 percent of adults present with visual complaints and an additional 10 percent have visual abnormalities on careful testing. Papilledema is present in about 15 percent of adults. Headaches (40 percent), mental deterioration or personality change (26 percent), and hypogonadism (35 percent) are relatively common in adults. Hyperprolactinemia is present in one-third to one-half of patients, but prolactin levels rarely exceed 100 to 150 ng/mL. Diabetes insipidus (15 percent), weight gain (15 percent), and panhypopituitarism (7 percent) may occur as well. Rarely, the cyst contents spill into the cerebrospinal fluid, causing a picture of aseptic meningitis.

Suprasellar calcification (see Fig. 321-14) in a flocculent, granular, or curvilinear pattern is present on skull x-rays in most children and in some adults with craniopharyngioma. Calcification is evident on CT scan in most of these adults, however. Hypothalamic germinomas may calcify as well. Skull x-ray abnormalities include calcification, sellar enlargement, and signs of increased intracranial pressure in 90 percent of children and 60 percent of adults.

Therapy of craniopharyngiomas remains controversial. Many advocate total removal whereas others suggest biopsy and partial resection followed by conventional radiation. Tumors less than 3 cm in diameter have a better prognosis.

Germ-cell tumors Germinomas originate in the posterior third ventricle, anterior third ventricle (supra- or intrasellar), or in both locations (also see Chap. 297). Germinomas (also known as atypical teratomas) were previously confused with parenchymal tumors of the pineal (pinealomas); when located in the anterior third ventricle they were known as "ectopic pinealomas." Germinomas often infiltrate the hypothalamus and occasionally metastasize to the CSF or distant sites.

The majority of patients have diabetes insipidus in association with variable anterior pituitary insufficiency. Precocious puberty may occur in males, probably due to hCG production by these tumors. Diplopia, headache, vomiting, lethargy, weight loss, and hydrocephalus are common. The tumors usually begin in childhood but may be diagnosed in young adults. Because germinomas are radiosensitive, early recognition is important. When the tumor is located in the anterior third ventricle, biopsy by the transsphenoidal route is often possible. Tumors in the pineal region are more difficult to biopsy, leading some authors to recommend empirical radiation therapy or chemotherapy, whereas others prefer surgical biopsy or debulking followed by radiation and chemotherapy. Germinomas of the nonseminoma type may produce hCG and/or α-fetoprotein, whereas pure seminomas rarely produce tumor markers (see Chap. 297).

PITUITARY ADENOMAS Pituitary adenomas account for about 10 to 15 percent of all intracranial neoplasms. They can cause anterior pituitary hormonal imbalance, structural problems related to invasion of surrounding structures, or syndromes of hormone excess. Occasionally, the diagnosis is the result of incidental findings during skull x-ray examinations.

Pathology For many years pituitary tumors were classified as basophilic, acidophilic, or chromophobic on the basis of hematoxylin and eosin straining. Corticotroph adenomas are generally basophilic; the more densely granulated prolactin-secreting tumors are acidophilic; the majority of prolactinomas, sparsely granulated GH-secreting tumors, TSH-secreting and gonadotropin-secreting tumors, and non-secreting tumors are all chromophobic. Because this classification provides little specific information about hormone production, it has been abandoned. Many nonfunctioning pituitary tumors are, however, still referred to as ''chromophobes.'' Classification based upon immunohistochemical staining makes it possible to identify and localize specific hormones. Pituitary tumors can also be classified according to hormonal secretion, based upon hormone measurements in serum.

Furthermore, pituitary tumors can be classified according to size and invasive characteristics. Stage I tumors are microadenomas (less than 10 mm in diameter) that may cause hormonal oversecretion but do not cause hypopituitarism and are not associated with structural problems. Stage II tumors are macroadenomas (greater than 10 mm) with or without suprasellar extension. Stage III tumors are macroadenomas that locally invade the floor of the sella and may cause sellar enlargement and suprasellar extension. Stage IV tumors are invasive macroadenomas with diffuse destruction of the sella, with or without suprasellar extension. The difficulty with this system of classification is that not all pituitary tumors fall neatly into one of these categories. For example, it is often difficult to separate thinning of the sellar floor (stage II) from erosion through the floor (stage III).

Endocrine manifestations Anterior pituitary hormone overproduction is suspected on clinical grounds and confirmed by appropriate laboratory evaluation (see Table 321-5). The most common secretory pituitary tumors are prolactinomas. They cause galactorrhea and hypogonadism, including amenorrhea, infertility, and impotence. GH-secreting tumors are the next most common secretory pituitary tumors and cause acromegaly or gigantism. Next in frequency are corticotroph (ACTH-secreting) adenomas which cause cortisol excess (Cushing's disease). Glycoprotein hormone–secreting pituitary adenomas (secreting TSH, LH, or FSH) are the least common. TSH-secreting adenomas are a rare cause of hyperthyroidism. Paradoxically, most patients with gonadotropin-secreting adenomas have hypogonadism.

About 15 percent of patients with tumors that come to surgery have adenomas that secrete more than one pituitary hormone. The most common combination is GH and prolactin, and other common patterns are GH-TSH, GH-prolactin-TSH, and ACTH-prolactin. Most of these tumors have one cell secreting two hormones (unimorphous), but some tumors have two or more cell types, each of which produces a single hormone (polymorphous).

Prolactinomas in women and corticotroph adenomas in both sexes are usually diagnosed while still microadenomas. In contrast, the majority of patients with acromegaly and most men with prolactinomas have macroadenomas at the time of diagnosis. Glycoprotein hormone–secreting tumors are also usually quite large at the time of diagnosis.

About 25 percent of pituitary adenomas that come to surgery are apparently nonsecretory, although some stain immunologically for pituitary hormones. In some cases, particularly in the case of gonadotropin-secreting tumors, hormonal secretion is overlooked. Some of the ''nonfunctioning'' pituitary tumors, as well as some functional ones, secrete part of the glycoprotein hormone molecule, most commonly the alpha subunit. Alpha subunit excess is a frequent finding in patients with TSH-secreting adenomas, and FSH beta may be hypersecreted in patients with gonadotropin-secreting tumors.

Null cell tumors (no specific hormones identified by immunostaining) are generally large when diagnosed, since no hormonal

TABLE 321-5 Pituitary hormone evaluation

Hormone	Excess	Deficiency
Growth hormone	*1* Measurement of plasma growth hormone 1 h following glucose PO *2* Measurement of IGF-1/SM-C	*1* Measurement of plasma growth hormone 30, 60, and 120 min after one of the following: *a* Regular insulin 0.1 to 0.15 unit per kilogram IV *b* Levodopa 10 mg/kg PO *c* L-Arginine 0.5 mg/kg intravenously over 30 min *2* ?Measurement of IGF-1/SM-C
Prolactin	*1* Measurement of basal serum prolactin	*1* Measurement of serum prolactin 10 to 20 min after one of the following: *a* TRH 200 to 500 μg IV *b* Chlorpromazine 25 mg IM
TSH	*1* Measurement of T_4, free T_4 index, T_3, TSH	*1* Measurement of T_4, free T_4, free T_4 index, TSH
Gonadotropins	*1* Measurement of FSH, LH, Testosterone, FSH beta, FSH response to TRH	*1* Measurement of basal LH, FSH in postmenopausal women; no measurements in menstruating, ovulating women *2* Testosterone, FSH, and LH in men
ACTH	*1* Measurement of urine free cortisol* *2* Dexamethasone suppression by one of the following: *a* Measurement of 8 A.M. plasma cortisol after administration of 1 mg dexamethasone at midnight *b* Measurement of 8 A.M. plasma cortisol or 24-h urine 17-hydroxysteroids after 0.5 mg dexamethasone PO q 6 h for 8 doses *3* High-dose dexamethasone suppression by one of the following: *a* Measurement of plasma cortisol after 8 mg dexamethasone PO at midnight *b* Measurement of 8 A.M. plasma cortisol or 24 h urine 17-hydroxysteroids after 2 mg dexamethasone q 6 h for 8 doses *4* Metyrapone response (same protocol as for deficiency testing) *5* Response of plasma ACTH to corticotropin releasing hormone (no standard protocol)	*1* Measurement of serum cortisol at 30 and 60 min following regular insulin 0.1 to 0.15 units per kilogram IV *2* Metyrapone response by one of the following: *a* Measurement of plasma 11-deoxycortisol at 8 A.M. after 30 mg metyrapone at midnight (maximal dose 2 g) *b* Measurement of 24-h urinary 17-hydroxycorticoids day of and day after 750 mg metyrapone q 4 h for 6 doses *c* Measurement of 24-h urinary 17-hydroxycorticoids day of and day after 500 mg metyrapone q 2 h for 12 doses *3* ACTH stimulation test: Measurement of plasma cortisol at 0 and 60 min after IM or IV administration of 0.25 mg cosyntropin
Arginine vasopressin (AVP)	*1* Measurement of serum sodium and osmolality, urine osmolality in presence of normal renal, adrenal, thyroid function *2* Simultaneous measurement of serum osmolality and ADH levels	*1* Comparison of urine osmolality and serum osmolality under conditions of increased AVP secretion† *2* Simultaneous measurement of serum osmolality and AVP levels

* *Tests 1 and 2 establish the diagnosis of Cushing's syndrome. Tests 3, 4, and 5 localize the Cushing's disease to the pituitary gland. Occasionally bilateral inferior petrosal sinus catheterization will be necessary.*

† *May be achieved by water deprivation or saline administration.*

overproduction is present to provide early clues to diagnosis. Oncocytomas are nonsecretory pituitary adenomas with abundant mitochondria, commonly found in older men.

Pituitary adenomas are occasionally part of the multiple endocrine neoplasia (MEN I) syndrome (see Chap. 334). This dominantly inherited disease causes adenomas of the pituitary gland, secretory tumors of the endocrine pancreas, and hyperparathyroidism due to generalized parathyroid hyperplasia. Pituitary adenomas secreting GH or prolactin are common, but nonfunctioning tumors also occur. Insulinomas and gastrinomas are the most common tumors in MEN I. Pancreatic GRH-secreting tumors that cause acromegaly and pituitary hyperplasia may superficially resemble the MEN I syndrome.

Mass effects of pituitary tumors VISUAL FIELD DEFECTS The optic chiasm lies anterior and superior to the pituitary gland and in 80 percent of normal persons overlies the pituitary fossa; in about 10 percent the chiasm is anterior to the tuberculum sella (prefixed), and in another 10 percent it overlaps the dorsum sella posteriorly (postfixed). The chiasm is found at a variable distance above the diaphragma sella, with up to 1 cm of separation in some patients.

The most common visual field defect in patients with pituitary adenomas is a bitemporal hemianopsia, and about 8 percent of patients develop complete loss of vision in one eye with a temporal defect in the opposite eye. Alternatively, patients may demonstrate bitemporal scotomas rather than hemianopsia, particularly with a rapidly growing lesion in association with a prefixed chiasm (see Chap. 13). For this reason careful visual field examinations must assess more than the lateral fields of vision. Of those patients with field defects about 9 percent have a single eye defect, most commonly with a superior temporal defect. Occasionally, there is a monocular field loss such as a central scotoma that mimics nonpituitary lesions. When pituitary adenomas cause visual field defects sellar enlargement is the rule.

OCULOMOTOR PALSIES Pituitary adenomas may extend laterally, invade the cavernous sinuses, and cause oculomotor palsies. When this occurs, visual field defects are usually not present. Involvement of the third cranial nerve is most common and may mimic diabetic third nerve neuropathy in that pupillary reactivity is usually preserved. Additional findings associated with lateral extension of the adenoma may include involvement of the fourth and sixth cranial nerves, pain or numbness in the distribution of the fifth cranial nerve, and compression or obstruction of the carotid artery.

Headaches are common in patients with larger tumors and are also present in the majority of patients with acromegaly. Headaches tend to be dull and annoying and may be exacerbated by coughing. Headaches are thought to be due to stretching of the diaphragma sella and may be referred to several locations, including the vertex of skull and to retroorbital, frontooccipital, frontotemporal, or occipital-cervical areas.

Very large pituitary tumors may invade the hypothalamus and cause hyperphagia, abnormal temperature regulation, loss of consciousness, and loss of hormonal input from the hypothalamus. Obstructive hydrocephalus involving the third ventricle is less common with pituitary adenomas than with craniopharyngiomas. Tumor invasion of the temporal lobe may cause complex partial seizures; invasion of the posterior fossa may be associated with brainstem dysfunction, and invasion into the frontal lobes causes alterations in mental state and frontal release signs.

PITUITARY APOPLEXY Acute hemorrhagic infarction of a pituitary adenoma may cause a dramatic syndrome including severe headache, nausea, vomiting, and depression of consciousness. Ophthalmoplegia, visual and pupillary disturbances, and meningismus may be present. Most of these symptoms are caused by direct pressure from the tumor, whereas meningismus results from blood in the CSF. The syndrome may either evolve slowly over a period of 24 to 48 h or may lead to sudden death.

Pituitary apoplexy is most commonly found in patients with somatotroph or corticotroph adenomas, but it may be the first clinical manifestation of a pituitary tumor. Both anticoagulation and radiotherapy predispose to hemorrhagic infarction. Rarely, pituitary apoplexy produces "autohypophysectomy" with "cure" of clinical acromegaly, Cushing's disease, or hyperprolactinemia. Hypopituitarism is a common sequela; although acute hormonal measurements may be normal during the acute phase, cortisol and gonadal steroid concentrations decline over the ensuing days, and thyroxine concentrations decline over weeks. Diabetes insipidus is rare.

It is important to differentiate between pituitary apoplexy and a leaking aneurysm; angiography is often required in this situation. Acute pituitary apoplexy is generally considered a neurosurgical emergency and may require acute decompression of the pituitary, generally via the transsphenoidal route.

Therapy of pituitary adenomas Ideal therapy for pituitary adenomas would permanently correct hormonal hypersecretion without causing hypopituitarism and would shrink or remove the tumor mass without additional morbidity or mortality. Therapy for microadenomas may achieve both of these goals, whereas therapy for macroadenomas is usually less successful. In considering therapy it is critical to weigh the disability due to the tumor against any disability that may arise from the treatment. Regardless of tumor size the therapy should not be worse than the disease. Potentially lethal diseases such as Cushing's disease or acromegaly may require more aggressive treatment than do prolactinomas.

MEDICAL THERAPY Bromocriptine, a dopamine agonist, is currently the therapy of choice for patients with microprolactinomas who require therapy. Bromocriptine corrects hyperprolactinemia in almost all patients with microprolactinomas; however, when the drug is stopped, prolactin levels usually return to pretreatment levels. It is uncertain if bromocriptine use affects the success of future surgery.

Bromocriptine side effects of nausea, gastric irritation, and postural hypotension can be minimized by initially giving a low dose (1.25 mg) at bedtime with a snack. Other side effects include headache, fatigue, abdominal cramps, nasal congestion, and constipation. The dosage is gradually increased to a twice-daily schedule (most commonly 2.5 mg bid).

Bromocriptine is also effective in larger prolactin-secreting macroadenomas. Bromocriptine lowers prolactin levels by about 90 percent in most patients with large tumors but usually not to normal. Tumor shrinkage of 50 percent or greater occurs in about half the patients, and visual field defects may return to normal. Tumor shrinkage is occasionally accompanied by reversal of hypopituitarism. With giant adenomas, bromocriptine-induced tumor shrinkage may rarely cause a devastating intracranial hemorrhage. Unfortunately macroadenomas usually regrow when bromocriptine is stopped. When pregnancy is desired or when mass effects of the tumor are not reversed with bromocriptine, additional therapy (surgery or radiation) is often necessary.

Bromocriptine is a useful therapeutic adjunct in some patients with acromegaly, particularly in those with coexistent hyperprolactinemia. GH concentrations rarely return to normal, but symptomatic improvement is common and tumor shrinkage may occur. Bromocriptine should be considered in acromegalic subjects whose GH levels remain elevated following surgery or who are waiting for radiation therapy to take effect. Nonfunctioning chromophobe adenomas usually do not shrink in response to bromocriptine, even when high doses are used.

Tamoxifen is occasionally useful as an adjunct in the therapy of large prolactinomas refractory to therapy with dopamine antagonists. Cyproheptadine, a serotonin antagonist, has been reported to induce remissions in occasional patients with corticotroph adenomas.

SURGERY Transsphenoidal surgery of pituitary microadenomas is safe and frequently corrects hormonal oversecretion. Hormonal overproduction is corrected within 24 h in 75 percent of patients with Cushing's disease due to corticotroph microadenomas, acromegaly with GH concentration less than 40 ng/mL, and microprolactinomas associated with serum prolactin concentrations less than 200 ng/mL. The initial success rate varies among institutions, with reported figures ranging from 50 to 95 percent. Unfortunately, after initially successful surgery hyperprolactinemia recurs in about 17 percent of patients followed for 3 to 5 years and possibly in 50 percent after 5 to 10 years. The recurrence rate after initially successful surgery in acromegaly and Cushing's disease is less well-established.

The mortality rate for transsphenoidal surgery of microadenomas is 0.27 percent with a morbidity rate of about 1.7 percent based on 2600 surgical procedures. Major complications include cerebrospinal fluid rhinorrhea, oculomotor palsy, and visual loss.

Pituitary surgery is less successful with larger secretory tumors. In patients with serum prolactin greater than 200 ng/mL or GH greater than 40 ng/mL, hormone concentrations return to normal in only 30 percent following surgery. Surgery is successful in about 60 percent of patients with Cushing's disease due to corticotroph macroadenomas. Recurrence rates with these secretory macroadenomas after a surgery-induced remission are uncertain; in the case at prolactin-secreting tumors, hyperprolactinemia recurs in 10 to 80 percent of patients.

Mass effects of large tumors are also rarely cured with surgery alone; in cases where surgery is the exclusive therapy, the 10-year recurrence of symptoms is 85 percent in patients not treated with radiation and/or bromocriptine. When radiation therapy is used in combination with surgery, the 10-year recurrence is 15 percent.

Surgery for macroadenomas has a mortality rate of around 0.86 percent and a morbidity rate of about 6.3 percent. Hypopituitarism occurs in an additional 10 percent of patients. Transient diabetes insipidus occurs in about 5 percent, and permanent diabetes insipidus occurs in 1 percent. Major complications of surgery for macroadenoma include cerebrospinal rhinorrhea (3.3 percent), permanent visual loss (1.5 percent), permanent oculomotor palsy (0.6 percent), and meningitis (0.5 percent).

RADIATION THERAPY Conventional radiation therapy is effective in preventing tumor growth (70 to 100 percent) but is unsatisfactory in the acute management of pituitary hyperfunction. Therapy consists of delivery of 4500 cGy (4500 rad) over 4.5 to 5 weeks, using rotational techniques. GH values of less than 5 ng/mL can be achieved in half of acromegalics after 5 years and in 70 percent after 10 years. Conventional radiation alone is rarely successful in treating corticotroph adenomas in adults. Long-term efficacy of radiation in patients with prolactinoma is currently being studied. Complications of conventional radiation therapy include hypopituitarism in up to 50 percent of patients.

Heavy particle therapy with proton beam or alpha particles is effective in treating secretory adenomas but response is slow. Tumors with suprasellar extension or tissue invasion are generally excluded from such series. With proton beam therapy at the Harvard cyclotron, radiation doses of up to 14,000 cGy (14,000 rad) can be given safely without damage to surrounding structures. At 2 years, 28 percent of acromegalics achieve GH values of less than 5 ng/mL; the percentages increase to 56 percent at 5 years and 75 percent by 10 years. With Cushing's disease proton beam corrects the hypercortisolism in 55 percent at 2 years and in 80 percent by 5 years. Proton beam therapy effectively lowers ACTH and stops growth of most corticotroph adenomas in patients with Nelson's syndrome with the exception of adenomas that are invasive at the time of therapy. Long-term results for treatment of prolactinomas with proton beam therapy are not available.

Complications of heavy particle therapy include hypopituitarism in at least 10 percent of patients, although the exact long-term prevalence of this complication is uncertain. Visual field defects and oculomotor dysfunction, usually temporary, have been reported in about 1.5 percent of patients. The major draw-back of this form of therapy is the length of time that must elapse before hormonal hypersecretion is corrected.

We generally treat microprolactinomas with bromocriptine. However, we recommend surgery for those patients with microprolactinoma who require therapy and are intolerant of dopamine agonists. Surgery generally does not result in hypopituitarism in this relatively benign disease. Surgery is usually our treatment of choice in patients with acromegaly or Cushing's disease because in most instances rapid reversal of hormonal hypersecretion is essential. Since Cushing's disease and acromegaly are potentially lethal diseases, more extensive surgery that results in hypopituitarism may be required.

Many patients with macroprolactinomas are treated with bromocriptine alone, and a trial of this agent should be given. We recommend transsphenoidal surgery and/or radiation therapy for patients with large prolactinomas who desire pregnancy, show persistent structural abnormalities or symptomatic hyperprolactinemia despite dopamine agonists, and who are intolerant of dopaminergic agents. Patients with nonfunctioning pituitary adenomas with structural abnormalities require transsphenoidal surgery, generally followed by conventional radiation therapy. Heavy particle therapy is an effective alternative to surgery in patients with acromegaly or Cushing's disease who have contraindications to or refuse surgery. Heavy particle or conventional radiation therapy is effective in treating patients with persistent GH elevation after transsphenoidal surgery. Heavy particle therapy is effective in persistent Cushing's disease as well. Proton beam therapy is effective in most patient's with Nelson's syndrome and may be a desirable alternative to conventional radiation therapy in patients with macroprolactinomas and nonsecretory macroadenomas. Transfrontal surgery is occasionally required, particularly in patients with giant adenomas.

TABLE 321-6 Causes of hypopituitarism

A Isolated hormone deficiencies
- *1* Congenital or acquired deficiencies

B Tumors
- *1* Large pituitary adenomas
- *2* Pituitary apoplexy
- *3* Hypothalamic tumors, e.g., craniopharyngiomas, germinomas, chordomas, meningiomas, gliomas, and others

C Inflammatory diseases
- *1* Granulomatous disease, e.g., sarcoidosis, tuberculosis, syphilis, granulomatous hypophysitis
- *2* Histiocytosis X
- *3* Lymphocytic hypophysitis (autoimmune)

D Vascular diseases
- *1* Sheehans post-partum necrosis
- *2* ? Diabetic peripartum necrosis
- *3* Carotid aneurysm

E Destructive-traumatic events
- *1* Surgery
- *2* Stalk section
- *3* Radiation (conventional—hypothalamus; heavy-particle—pituitary)

F Developmental anomalies
- *1* Pituitary aplasia
- *2* Basal encephalocoele

G Infiltration
- *1* Hemochromatosis
- *2* Amyloidosis

H "Idiopathic" causes
- *1* ?Autoimmune disease

HYPOPITUITARISM *Hypopituitarism* refers to deficiency of one or more pituitary hormones and has many etiologies (see Table 321-6). Pituitary hormone deficiency may be congenital or acquired. Isolated GH or gonadotropin deficiency is common. Temporary ACTH deficiency as a consequence of long-term glucocorticoid therapy is also common, but permanent isolated deficiency of ACTH or TSH is rare. Deficiency of any of the anterior pituitary hormones may occur at the level of the pituitary gland or the hypothalamus. When diabetes insipidus is present the primary defect is almost invariably in the hypothalamus or high pituitary stalk, often in conjunction with mild hyperprolactinemia and anterior pituitary hypofunction.

Manifestations of hypopituitarism depend upon the specific pituitary hormones that are lacking. Growth failure due to GH deficiency is a common presenting complaint in children. GH deficiency in adults causes more subtle manifestations such as fine wrinkling around the eyes and mouth and in subjects with diabetes mellitus increased sensitivity to insulin. Complaints related to gonadotropin deficiency include amenorrhea and infertility in women and testosterone deficiency and decreased libido, decreased beard and body hair, and preservation of a youthful scalp hairline in men. TSH deficiency causes hypothyroidism with fatigue, cold intolerance, and puffy skin in the absence of goiter. ACTH deficiency results in cortisol deficiency, manifested by fatigue; decreased appetite; weight loss; decreased skin and nipple pigmentation; abnormal response to stress characterized by fever, hypotension, and hyponatremia; and a high mortality rate. Unlike primary adrenal insufficiency (Addison's disease) ACTH deficiency does not cause hyperpigmentation, hyperkalemia, or salt loss. With combined ACTH and gonadotropin deficiency, axillary and pubic hair may be lost. Children with combined GH and cortisol deficiency often develop hypoglycemia. AVP deficiency causes diabetes insipidus with polyuria and increased thirst. When pituitary adenomas impair anterior pituitary function GH is often the first hormone to be compromised, followed by deficiencies of gonadotropins, TSH, and ACTH.

Etiology Damage to the anterior pituitary is commonly due to a pituitary adenoma (with or without infarction), pituitary surgery, heavy particle pituitary irradiation, or infarction during the postpartum period (Sheehan's syndrome). Postpartum pituitary infarction occurs because the enlarged pituitary gland of pregnancy becomes vulnerable to ischemia; postpartum hemorrhage with systemic hypotension can destroy the pituitary gland. Inability to lactate is the first and most common clinical clue, and other symptoms of hypopituitarism may unfold over months or years. The condition is sometimes diagnosed years after the primary event. Although clinical diabetes insipidus is rare in this setting, a decreased AVP response to appropriate stimuli is common. Patients with diabetes mellitus are also prone to develop hypopituitarism late in pregnancy.

Another cause of hypopituitarism is lymphocytic hypophysitis, a syndrome that usually occurs during pregnancy or in the postpartum period. In this syndrome, a mass lesion is often seen on CT scanning which, when biopsied, consists of lymphocytic infiltration. Lymphocytic hypophysitis is thought to represent autoimmune pituitary destruction and often occurs with other autoimmune diseases such as Hashimoto's (autoimmune) thyroiditis and gastric atrophy (see Chap. 334). Circulating antibodies to prolactin cells have been identified in some of these patients. Although fewer than 20 cases of lymphocytic hypophysitis have been diagnosed, about 7 percent of patients with other autoimmune diseases have prolactin antibodies in serum. It is not yet clear whether autoimmune hypophysitis is a common cause of "idiopathic" hypopituitarism in adults.

Hypothalamic or pituitary stalk damage has many causes (see Table 321-6). Certain lesions in this region, such as sarcoidosis, metastatic carcinoma, germinomas, histiocytosis, and craniopharyngiomas, commonly cause diabetes insipidus along with hypofunction of the anterior pituitary. Pituitary insufficiency, resulting from conventional radiation to the brain or the pituitary, is thought to be largely hypothalamic in origin.

Diagnosis (see Table 321-5) To diagnose GH deficiency, the most reliable GH stimulus is insulin-induced hypoglycemia in which the blood sugar declines to less than 40 mg/dL (Fig. 321-8). A GH concentration of greater than 10 ng/mL after hypoglycemia, levodopa, or arginine effectively excludes GH deficiency. Measuring the basal GH or serum IGF-1/SM-C concentration is less reliable, because GH levels are undetectable in normal persons for much of the day and because IGF-1/SM-C concentrations in patients with GH deficiency may overlap the normal range.

Cortisol deficiency is potentially life-threatening. Basal cortisol function may be preserved in the face of extensive pituitary destruction; consequently, the ability of pituitary ACTH secretion to increase in response to "stress" must be assessed. Either the insulin tolerance test or the metyrapone test can be used to determine the adequacy of ACTH reserve.

The insulin tolerance test is safely performed on an outpatient basis in younger patients without heart disease or diseases predisposing to seizures (Fig. 321-8 and Table 321-5). Both cortisol and GH responses are measured. If hypopituitarism is strongly suspected a lower dose of regular insulin (0.05 to 0.1 units per kilogram of body weight) should be employed. After adequate hypoglycemia, the peak plasma cortisol should be greater than 19 μg/dL, although other criteria have been suggested. Since the metyrapone test can precipitate acute adrenal insufficiency in patients with low basal cortisol secretory rates, it should always be performed in the hospital setting when the 8 A.M. basal plasma cortisol is less than 9 μg/dL. Furthermore, metyrapone administration in most patients should be preceded by a rapid ACTH stimulation test to ensure that the adrenals can respond to ACTH. In patients with an 8 A.M. basal plasma cortisol less than 4 to 5 μg/dL, metyrapone tests should not be performed. A normal response to metyrapone administration (see Table 321-5) is an increase of plasma 11-deoxycortisol to greater than 10 μg/dL and of the urinary 17-hydroxysteroids to at least twofold over baseline, usually to a value greater than 22 mg per 24 h. The plasma cortisol must concomitantly fall to less than 4 μg/dL to ensure that there has been an adequate stimulus for ACTH release. Although ACTH responses to insulin-hypoglycemia and metyrapone have not been well-standardized, a peak ACTH concentration of greater than 200 pg/mL is considered normal.

The rapid ACTH stimulation test (see Table 321-5) may be a safer and more convenient screening test for determining the adequacy of the pituitary-adrenal axis than is insulin tolerance or metyrapone testing. Since the response of the adrenal gland to exogenous ACTH is dependent upon prior endogenous ACTH exposure, patients with profound ACTH deficiency in fact do have a deficient adrenal response to exogenous ACTH stimulation. However, the rapid ACTH stimulation test may be normal in some patients with abnormal insulin tolerance tests and therefore may not detect all who are at risk for stress-induced adrenal insufficiency. Thus, whereas an abnormal

FIGURE 321-8 *The insulin tolerance test. After an intravenous injection of regular insulin (0.1 unit per kilogram of body weight) a fall in blood sugar and rise in plasma GH and cortisol is expected. This test permits evaluation of both GH and ACTH in patients with pituitary disease (After KJ Catt, Lancet 1:933, 1970.)*

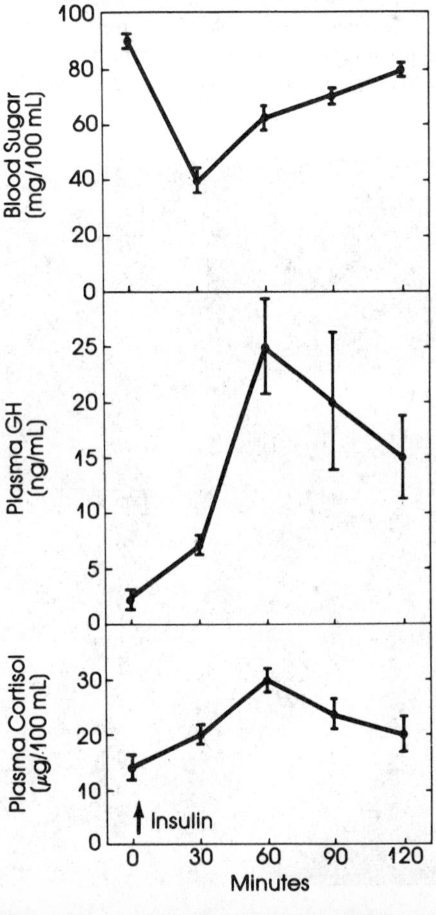

ACTH stimulation test is indicative of an abnormal pituitary-adrenal axis, a normal response in the rapid ACTH stimulation test (cortisol greater than 19 μg/dL) does not always confirm that there is a normal pituitary-adrenal axis.

Gonadotropin function is easier to evaluate. In women with regular menses gonadotropin secretion is normal and gonadotropin measurements are superfluous. Likewise, a man with a normal serum testosterone and normal spermatogenesis need not have gonadotropins measured. In postmenopausal women gonadotropin levels are elevated (an endogenous stimulation test); "normal" levels suggest gonadotropin deficiency. Estrogen deficiency in women and testosterone deficiency in men in the absence of elevated gonadotropins imply gonadotropin deficiency.

To diagnose central hypothyroidism (thyrotropin deficiency), the serum T_4 and free T_4 (or T_3 resin uptake and free T_4 index) should first be measured. If these are in the midnormal range, TSH function is normal. If T_4 and free T_4 are low and the serum TSH is not elevated, central hypothyroidism is present. Mild central hypothyroidism, a consideration in patients with known pituitary disease who have low normal T_4 and free T_4 concentrations, remains a clinical diagnosis. Before considering the diagnosis of isolated TSH deficiency in patients with the biochemical features of central hypothyroidism without evidence of other pituitary hormone deficiency, it is important to exclude the thyroxine-binding globulin (TBG) deficiency syndrome (low T_4, increased T_3 resin uptake, low to low-normal free T_4 index, normal TSH) and the "sick euthyroid" syndrome (low T_4, low free T_4 or free T_4 index, normal TSH) (see Chap. 324).

Several diagnostic tests utilize hypothalamic-releasing hormones to assess pituitary reserve. While these tests are not helpful in assessing the adequacy of anterior pituitary function, they can be useful in certain situations. In GH deficient children documentation of a GH response to GRH may be helpful in deciding which children can be treated with GRH rather than GH. Likewise, in patients with isolated gonadotropin deficiency, the gonadotropin response to LHRH may be useful in predicting which patients will respond to therapy with LHRH analogues. CRH testing may be useful in the differential diagnosis of Cushing's syndrome but does not indicate whether the pituitary-adrenal axis will respond appropriately to stress. TRH stimulation testing is useful in some patients in supporting the diagnosis of hyperthyroidism or of acromegaly and in those cases in which documentation of prolactin deficiency is necessary to support a diagnosis of more generalized anterior pituitary hormone deficiency (e.g., mild central hypothyroidism). TRH testing is not necessary in the evaluation for central hypothyroidism and is not reliable in separating pituitary from hypothalamic hypothyroidism.

Therapy A number of hormones must be replaced in patients with panhypopituitarism, but cortisol replacement is most important. We prefer prednisone for matters of convenience and cost, but many physicians use cortisone acetate. Prednisone (5 to 7.5 mg) or cortisone acetate (20 to 37.5 mg) can be given to some patients as a single morning dosage, whereas others require divided doses (two-thirds at 8 A.M., one-third at 3 A.M.). Hypopituitary patients may require lower daily glucocorticoid dosages than do patients with Addison's disease and do not require mineralocorticoid replacement. In stress situations or when preparing these patients for pituitary or other surgery, higher doses of glucocorticoids should be administered (e.g., for major surgery, hydrocortisone hemisuccinate 75 mg IM/IV every 6 h or methyl prednisolone sodium succinate 15 mg IM/IV every 6 h). Levothyroxine is the therapy of choice in patients with central hypothyroidism (0.1 to 0.2 mg per day). Since thyroxine accelerates the degradation of cortisol and can precipitate adrenal crisis in patients with limited pituitary reserve, glucocorticoid replacement should always precede levothyroxine therapy in subjects with panhypopituitarism. Hypogonadism in women is treated with estrogen/progestogen combinations and in men with testosterone esters by injection. To achieve fertility gonadotropins must be administered by injection in patients with pituitary disease, whereas LHRH or its analogues may be successful in those with hypothalamic disease. GH deficiency is not treated in adults; in children GH administration usually is required, but GRH injections may be effective in those with hypothalamic disease. Diabetes insipidus is treated with nasal desmopressin (usually 0.05 to 0.1 mL twice a day) (see Chap. 323).

RADIOLOGY OF THE PITUITARY Conventional posteroanterior and lateral skull x-rays define the contours of the sella turcica (Fig. 321-9). Abnormalities that may be identified on these films include enlargement, erosions, and calcifications in the region of the sella. CT scanning or magnetic resonance imaging (MRI) is necessary to define further intrapituitary and suprasellar lesions. Angiography is routinely used when an aneurysm or vascular malformation is

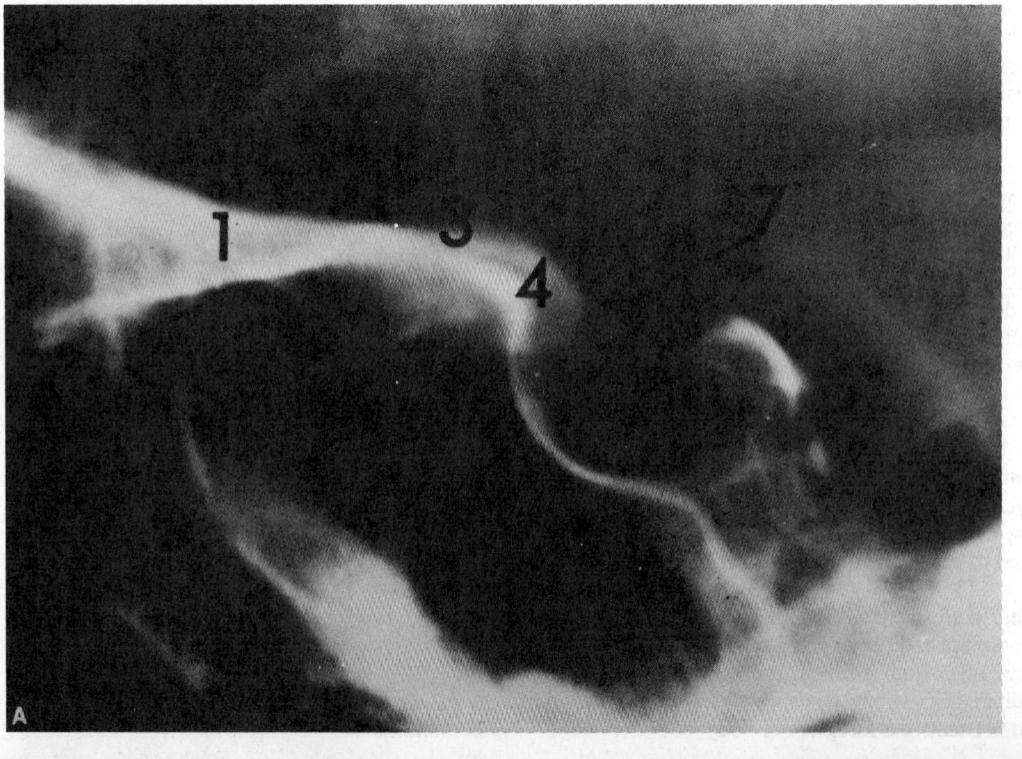

FIGURE 321-9 *X-ray of the sella, lateral view. Note (1) planum sphenoidal, (2) limbus sphenoidal, (3) sulcus chiasmaticus, (4) tuberculum sellae, (5) sella floor with distinct lamina dura, (6) dorsum sella, (7) anterior clinoid, and (8) sphenoid sinus. (From SM Wolpert in Post et al.)*

suspected as the cause of an enlarged sella and is occasionally necessary in patients with large pituitary or hypothalamic tumors. Metrizamide cisternography, in which CT scanning is performed following intrathecal injection of the water-soluble dye metrizamide has largely replaced pneumoencephalography in the delineation of the suprasellar region. Sella tomography is not recommended, as it has a high frequency of false-positive and false-negative findings and exposes the lens of the eye to excessive radiation. MRI may eventually supercede current methods of pituitary evaluation (Fig. 321-10).

The volume of the normal sella turcica (233 to 1092 mm^3, mean 594 mm^3) does not change in patients with pituitary microadenomas. With conventional radiography, pituitary microadenomas may be suspected on the basis of focal erosions or blistering of the floor of the sella, but these findings may also be present in normal individuals. Larger microadenomas may cause the floor of the sella to "tilt" when viewed in the frontal projection and may create the appearance of a double floor on lateral view (Fig. 321-11).

However, since most microadenomas neither affect the volume of the sella nor produce specific radiographic findings, high resolution CT scanning is necessary for localization (Fig. 321-12). On CT scanning the normal pituitary gland has a height of 3 to 7 mm. The upper aspect is flat or concave. The stalk is midline with a maximum

FIGURE 321-10 *Magnetic resonance imaging (MRI) in patient with a large pituitary adenoma. The arrow points to the adenoma which is seen on axial (A), sagittal (B), and coronal (C) views. (From G Gerard et al, Hosp Pract 19:151, 1984.)*

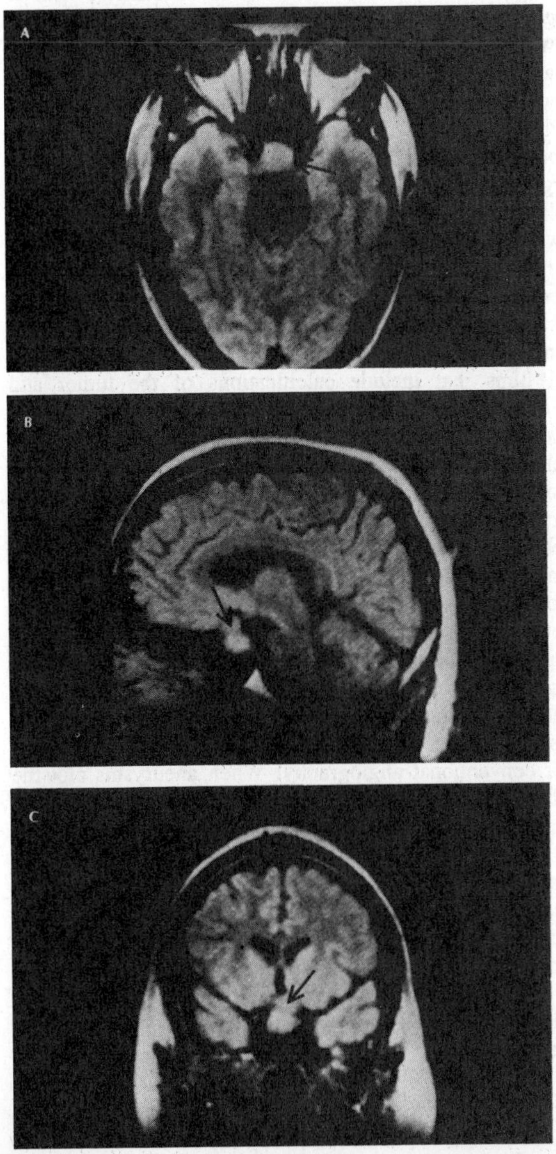

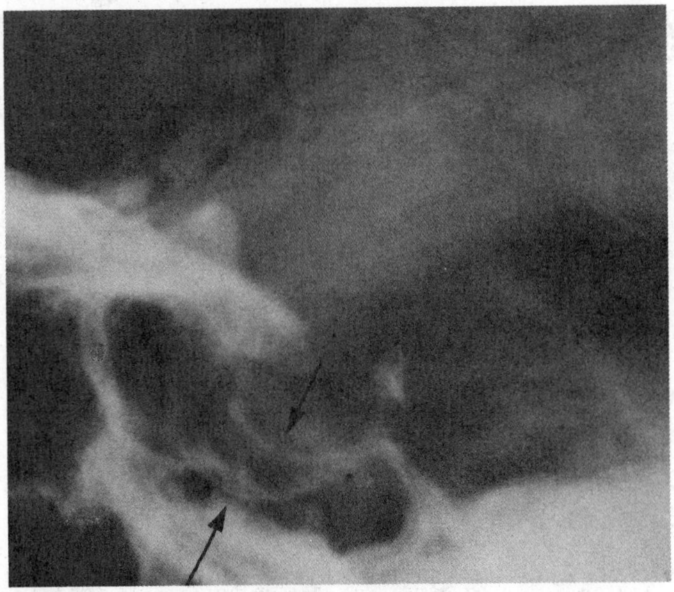

FIGURE 321-11 *Lateral view of the sella turcica demonstrating a "double floor" due to downward displacement by a pituitary adenoma. Top arrow points to normal floor; bottom arrow points to floor displaced by tumor.*

stalk diameter of 4 mm on axial selections. After intravenous contrast administration, the normal pituitary shows homogeneous enhancement in 60 percent of patients and heterogeneous enhancement in 40 percent. Up to 20 percent of normal persons show discrete low-density areas on contrast-enhanced CT scanning. In a random selection of autopsies up to 24 percent of individuals demonstrate small pituitary abnormalities (e.g., microadenomas, cysts, metastatic tumors, pituitary infarcts), but it is unclear whether such abnormalities correspond to the focal abnormal areas on CT scanning.

Microadenomas are best demonstrated on direct coronal views taken in 1 mm sections after rapid infusion of contrast material. The normal pituitary is hyperdense but less so than the cavernous sinus. Microadenomas, particularly microprolactinomas, usually appear to be hypodense using this technique (see Fig. 321-12). Small corticotroph adenomas are particularly difficult to visualize. Larger microadenomas may cause upward convexity of the diaphragma sella and contralateral deviation of the pituitary stalk (Fig. 321-13). If marked intrasellar enhancement is noted angiography is required to exclude an aneurysm or transsellar intercarotid anastamosis.

Pituitary macroadenomas generally cause sella enlargement, with or without bony erosion, seen on conventional radiography. However, the presence of an enlarged sella in itself is not sufficient to diagnose a pituitary adenoma (see below). Additional findings in plain skull x-rays in patients with acromegaly may include prognathism, enlarged paranasal sinuses, hyperostosis of the external occipital protuberance,

FIGURE 321-12 *Sagittal CT scan of sella in patient with small microprolactinoma. The tumor has decreased density, and minimal erosion of the sella floor is demonstrated. Arrow points to tumor.*

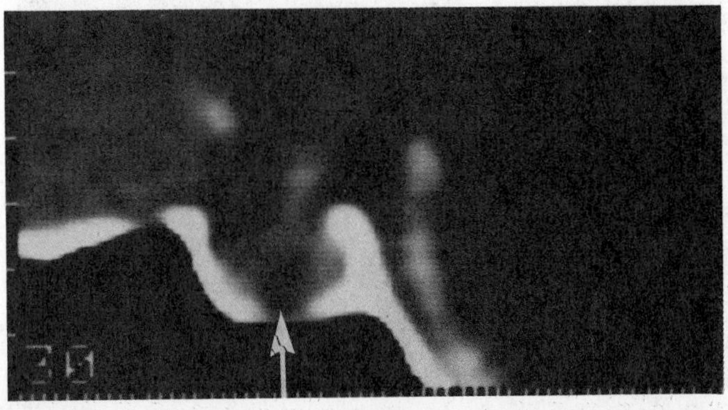

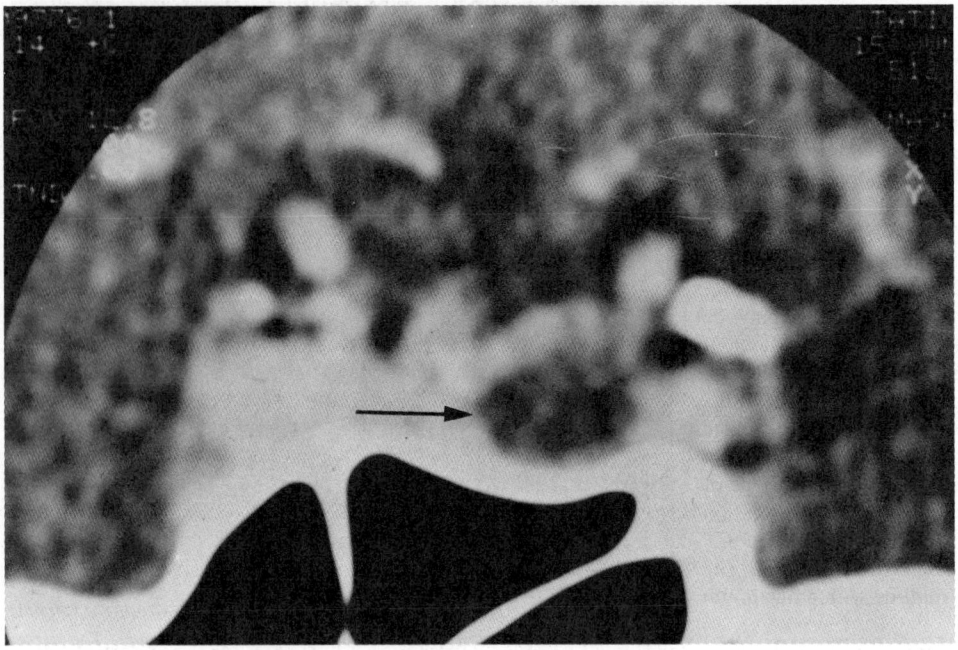

FIGURE 321-13 *Coronal CT scan demonstrating 1.3 cm macroprolactinoma in a 30-year-old woman. Note decreased density of the tumor (arrow). The pituitary stalk is displaced to the left, and the floor of the sella slopes to the left as well.*

increased density of the central bone on the sella, and an enlarged square sella with tapered tuberculum. GH-secreting adenomas may calcify and regress to leave a pituitary calculus or stone. Larger corticotroph adenomas may cause depression of the central floor of the sella.

CT scanning of macroadenomas reveals a mass in the sella that generally enhances after contrast administration (Fig. 321-5). An area of decreased density within an enhancing mass is present in about 20 percent of patients and suggests cystic degeneration of an adenoma. An additional 20 percent of patients with macroadenomas have a partially empty sella with CSF density within the sella (see below). Larger invasive tumors may extend into the cavernous sinus, sphenoid sinus, or any of the cranial fossae. Pituitary hyperplasia (e.g., thyrotroph hyperplasia in primary hypothyroidism) appears on CT as an enlarged, filled sella that does not enhance after contrast administration.

Pituitary apoplexy is caused by a sudden increase in the size of a pituitary macroadenoma due to hemorrhage or infarction. Enlargement of the sella on plain films is almost always evident. In the case of hemorrhage CT scanning reveals a high-density area within the adenoma during the acute phase and a decreased density, with or without marginal enhancement, as the hematoma is resorbed. With infarction low-density areas are seen with or without enhancement.

FIGURE 321-14 *Lateral skull x-ray in a patient with a craniopharyngioma. Note dense calcification in suprasellar region (arrow).*

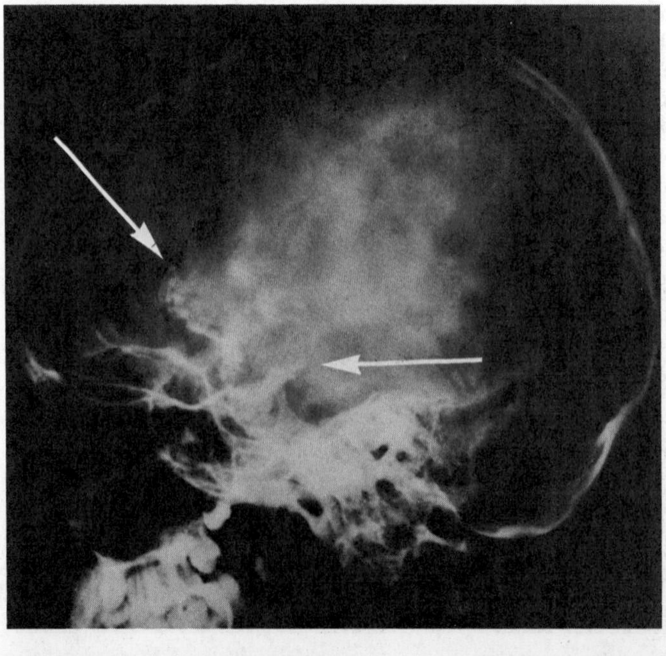

Craniopharyngiomas can often be suspected on plain skull x-rays on the basis of nodular or curvilinear calcification in the suprasellar region (Fig. 321-14). This calcification is visible in 80 to 90 percent of children but in less than 50 percent of adults. Although the sella may be enlarged and ballooned, the cortical bone is usually preserved. With intrasellar craniopharyngiomas, the dorsum sella is often displaced backwards. On CT scanning cystic components are prominent with ring or nodular calcification demonstrable in almost all children and in 80 percent of adults. The noncystic areas show variable enhancement which is usually more prominent in children.

Most meningiomas of the sellar region cause abnormalities on routine skull films that include calcifications of the tumor and hyperostosis of the planum sphenoidale or of the chiasmatic sulcus. Meningiomas may also cause sella enlargement and thereby mimic pituitary adenomas. On CT scanning, meningiomas may give the appearance of an aneurysm because of their dense homogeneous enhancement. Angiography may be required to exclude an aneurysm and to delineate the feeding vessels.

Aneurysms in the region of the sella contain concentric calcifications demonstrable on plain skull films in about 30 percent of patients. Aneurysms may cause sella enlargement, usually with lateral depression and erosion of the sella floor; a "double floor" is therefore seen on lateral films. On CT scanning the aneurysm is hyperdense with homogeneous contrast enhancement. Most patients with hyperdense lesions that enlarge the sella need to be studied with digital subtraction or conventional angiography. When aneurysms clot the CT appearance may change: new clots show no enhancement whereas old clots enhance like adenomas. Complete thrombosis of an aneurysm is sometimes radiologically indistinguishable by radiographic criteria from a pituitary adenoma.

On CT scanning enhancing masses of the suprasellar region include optic chiasm or hypothalamic gliomas, metastases to the hypothalamus or pituitary stalk, germinomas, sarcoid granulomas, histiocytosis, aneurysms, and craniopharyngiomas. Nonenhancing suprasellar masses include dermoid tumors, epidermoid tumors, and arachnoid cysts.

THE ENLARGED SELLA–EMPTY SELLA SYNDROME Enlargement of the sella can be caused by pituitary adenomas, hypothalamic

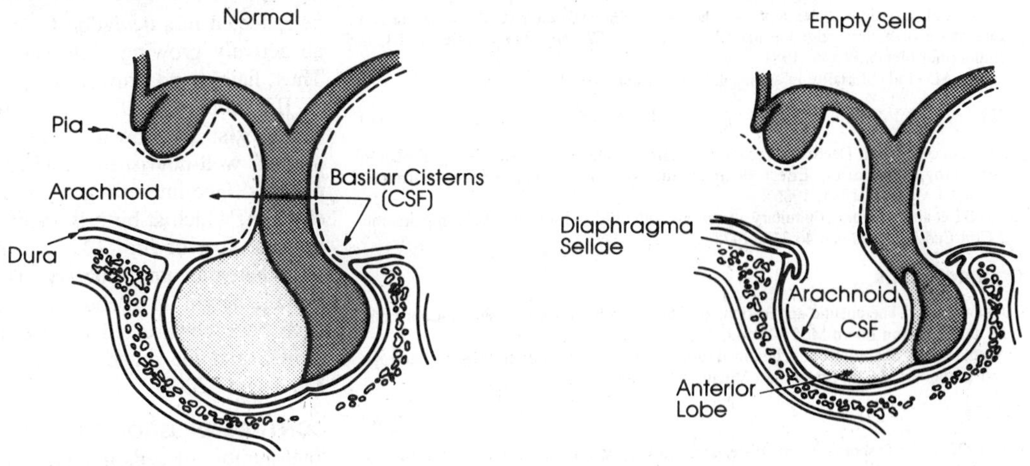

FIGURE 321-15 *The findings in patients with the empty sella syndrome. The left panel shows the normal anatomic relationships. With the empty sella syndrome, right panel, ballooning of the sella results when an arachnoid diverticulum herniates through an incompetent diaphragma sellae. (After Jordan et al.)*

masses and cysts, aneurysms, primary hypothyroidism or hypogonadism, and increased intracranial pressure. It can also occur in patients with the primary empty sella syndrome (Fig. 321-15). In this situation the sella tends to be symmetrically ballooned without evidence of bony erosion. The suprasellar subarachnoid space herniates through an incomplete diaphragma sella (Fig. 321-15) so that the sella becomes filled with CSF within an arachnoid-lined sac. An incomplete diaphragma sella is thought to be a prerequisite for this to occur. It is not clear whether transient or persistent increased CSF pressure is necessary to produce sella enlargement in these patients, but CSF pressure is generally normal when measured. The pituitary gland is flattened and pushed to one side but tends to function normally. The fact that the CSF fills the sella can be demonstrated on metrizamide cisternography, high-resolution CT scanning, or MRI.

It is important to separate the primary empty sella from the enlarged partially empty sella due to a degenerated pituitary adenoma. In the former the pituitary volume is usually normal, in the latter the pituitary volume is generally increased.

The vast majority of patients with the primary empty sella syndrome are obese, multiparous women with headaches; about 30 percent of these women have hypertension. It is of interest that multiparity, obesity, and hypertension are associated with increases in CSF pressure. Selection bias cannot be excluded in case reports since skull x-rays may be obtained in patients with headaches, which in turn uncovers the enlarged sella. Endocrine symptoms are uncommon. Hyperprolactinemia occurs on occasion, possibly due to stalk stretching or coincidental microprolactinomas. GH secretory reserve is often abnormal in these patients, probably the result of obesity. Spontaneous CSF rhinorrhea and pseudotumor cerebri have each been reported in about 10 percent of the cases. CSF rhinorrhea often requires surgical correction. Visual field defects have occasionally been reported and are thought to be caused by herniation of the optic chiasm into the sella turcica. Once the diagnosis of the empty sella syndrome has been established by CT scan, metrizamide cisternography, or MRI further diagnostic studies are superfluous, and the only therapy needed is reassurance.

REFERENCES

General

BESSER GM: The hypothalamus and pituitary. Clin Endocrinol Metab 6:1, 1977

BLACK PMcL et al: *Secretary Tumors of the Pituitary Gland*. New York, Raven Press, 1984

BURROW GN et al: Microadenomas of the pituitary and abnormal sellar tomograms in an unselected autopsy series. N Engl J Med 304:156, 1981

DANIEL PM, PRICHARD MML: The human hypothalamus and pituitary stalk after hypophysectomy or pituitary stalk section. Brain 59:813, 1972

IMURA H (ed): *The Pituitary Gland*. New York, Raven Press, 1985

KRIEGER DT, MARTIN JB: Brain peptides. N Engl J Med 304:876, 1981

MARTIN JB, REICHLIN S: *Clinical Neuroendocrinology*, 2d ed. Philadelphia, FA Davis, 1987

POST KD et al (eds): *The Pituitary Adenoma*. New York, Plenum Medical Book Company, 1980

SCANLON ME: Neuroendocrinology. Clin Endocrinol Metab 12:467, 1983

VANCE ML et al: Bromocriptine. Ann Intern Med 100:78, 1984

Prolactin

CARTER JN et al: Prolactin secreting tumors and hypogonadism in 22 men. N Engl J Med 299:847, 1978

FERRARI C et al: Functional characterization of hypothalamic hyperprolactinemia. J Clin Endocrinol Metab 55:897, 1982

GROSSMAN A et al: Treatment of prolactinomas with megavoltage radiotherapy. Br Med J 288:1105, 1984

KLEINBERG DS et al: Galactorrhea: 235 cases including 48 with pituitary tumor. N Engl J Med 296:589, 1977

KLEINBERG DL et al: Pergolide for the treatment of pituitary tumors secreting prolactin or growth hormone. N Engl J Med 309:704, 1983

KLIBANSKI A et al: Decreased bone density in hyperprolactinemic women. N Engl J Med 303:1511, 1980

MOLITCH ME: Hyperprolactinemia. Med Grand Rounds 1:307, 1982

———: Pregnancy and the hyperprolactinemic woman. N Engl J Med 321:1364, 1985

——— et al: Bromocriptine as primary therapy for prolactin-secreting macroadenomas: Results of a prospective multicenter study. J Clin Endocrinol Metab 60:698, 1985

MORIONDO P et al: Bromocriptine treatment of microprolactinomas: Evidence of stable prolactin decrease after drug withdrawal. J Clin Endocrinol Metab 60:764, 1985

SCHLECTE J et al: Prolactin-secreting pituitary tumors in ammenorrheic women: A comprehensive study. Endocr Rev 1:294, 1980

Growth hormone

ASA SL et al: A case for hypothalamic acromegaly: A clinicopathological study of six patients with hypothalamic gangliocytomas producing growth hormone–releasing factor. J Clin Endocrinol Metab 58:796, 1984

CLEMMONS DR et al: Evaluation of acromegaly by radioimmunoassay of somatomedin-C. N Engl J Med 301:1138, 1979

EASTMAN RC et al: Conventional supervoltage irradiation is an effective treatment for acromegaly. J Clin Endocrinol Metab 48:931, 1979

EDDY RL et al: Human growth hormone release: Comparison of provocative test procedures. Am J Med 56:179, 1974

GELATO MC et al: Effects of a growth hormone releasing factor in man. J Clin Endocrinol Metab 57:674, 1983

——— et al: Effects of growth hormone-releasing factor on growth hormone secretion in acromegaly. J Clin Endocrinol Metab 60:251, 1985

GROSSMAN A et al: Growth hormone releasing factor: Comparison of two analogues and demonstration of hypothalamic defect in growth hormone release after radiotherapy. Br Med J 288:1785, 1984

JADRESIC A: Recent developments in acromegaly. A review. J R Soc Med 76:947, 1983

LAWRENCE JH et al: Successful treatment of acromegaly. Metabolic and clinical studies in 145 patients. J Clin Endocrinol Metab 31:180, 1970

MARTIN, JB: Neural regulation of growth hormone secretion. N Engl J Med 288:1384, 1973

MELMED S et al: Pathophysiology of acromegaly. Endocr Rev 4:271, 1983

——— et al: Acromegaly due to secretion of growth hormone by an ectopic pancreatic islet-cell tumor. N Engl J. Med 312:9, 1985

MOSES AC et al: Bromocriptine therapy in acromegaly. Use in patients resistant to conventional therapy and effect on serum levels of somatomedin C. J Clin Endocrinol Metab 53:752, 1981

PHILLIPS LS, VASILOPOULOU-SELLIN R: Somatomedins. N Engl J Med 302:371, 1980

REICHLIN S: Acromegaly. Med Grand Rounds 1:9, 1982

———: Somatostatin. N Engl J Med 309:1495, 1983

RUDMAN D et al: Children with normal-variant-short stature: Treatment with human growth hormone for six months. N Engl J Med 305:123, 1981

THORNER MO et al: Somatotroph hyperplasia: Successful treatment of acromegaly by removal of a pancreatic islet tumor secreting a growth hormone releasing factor. J Clin Invest 70:965, 1982

——— et al: Extrahypothalamic growth-hormone-releasing factor (GRF) secretion is a rare cause of acromegaly: Plasma GRF levels in 177 acromegalic patients. J Clin Endocrinol Metab 59:846, 1984

WRIGHT AD et al: Mortality in acromegaly. Q J Med 39:1, 1970

TSH

BECK-PECCOZ P et al: Decreased receptor binding of biologically inactive thyrotropin in central hypothyroidism. Effect of treatment with thyrotropin-releasing hormone. N Engl J Med 312:1085, 1985

BIGOS ST et al: Spectrum of pituitary alterations with mild and severe thyroid impairment. J Clin Endocrinol Metab 46:317, 1978

Gonadotropins

CUTLER GB JR: Therapeutic applications of luteinizing-hormone-releasing hormone and its analogs. Ann Intern Med 102:643, 1985

SNYDER PJ et al: Secretion of uncombined subunits of luteinizing hormone by gonadotroph cell adenomas. J Clin Endocrinol Metab 59:1169, 1984

ACTH

BORST GC et al: Discordant cortisol response to exogenous ACTH and insulin-induced hypoglycemia in patients with pituitary disease. N Engl J Med 306:1462, 1982

CHROUSOS GP et al: The corticotropin-releasing factor stimulation test: An aid in the evaluation of patients with Cushing's syndrome. N Engl J Med 310:622, 1984

STREETEN DHP et al: Normal and abnormal function of the hypothalamic-pituitary-adrenal system in man. Endocr Rev 5:371, 1984

Endorphins

MORLEY JE: The endocrinology of the opiates and opioid peptides. Metabolism 30:195, 1981

Alpha Subunits

KLIBANSKI A et al: Pure alpha subunit-secreting pituitary tumors. J Neurosurg 59:585, 1983

Hypothalamus

BRAY GA, GALLAGHER TFJ: Manifestations of hypothalamic obesity in man: A comprehensive investigation of eight patients and a review of the literature. Medicine 54:301, 1974

DINARELLO CA: Interleukin-1 and the pathogenesis of the acute phase response. N Engl J Med 54:301, 1984

———, WOLFF SM: Molecular basis of fever in humans. Am J Med 72:799, 1982

PLUM F, VAN UITERT R: Nonendocrine diseases and disorders of the hypothalamus, in *The Hypothalamus,* S Reichlin et al (eds). New York, Raven Press, 1978, pp 415–473

Craniopharyngiomas

BANNA M: Craniopharyngiomas in adults. Surg Neurol 1:202, 1973

———: Craniopharyngioma: Based on 160 cases. Br J Radiol 49:206, 1976

Hypopituitarism

ASA SL et al: Lymphocytic hypophysitis of pregnancy resulting in hypopituitarism: A distinct clinicopathologic entity. Ann Intern Med 95:166, 1981

BOTTAZZO GF et al: Autoantibodies to prolactin secreting cells of human pituitary. Lancet 2:97, 1975

VELDHUIS JD, HAMMOND JM: Endocrine function after spontaneous infarction of the human pituitary: Report, review, and reappraisal. Endocr Rev 1:100, 1980

Radiology

BRUNETON JN et al: Normal variants of the sella turcica. Radiology 131:99, 1979

HEMINGHY S et al: Computed tomographic study of hormone-secreting microadenomas. Radiology 146:65, 1983

JORDAN RM et al: The primary empty sella syndrome. Analysis of the clinical characteristics, radiographic features, pituitary function, and cerebrospinal fluid adenohypophysial hormone concentrations. Am J Med 62:569, 1977

KENDALL B: Current approaches to hypothalamic-pituitary radiology. Clin Endocrinol Metab 12:535, 1983

WOLPERT SM: The radiology of pituitary adenomas. Semin Roentgenol 19:53, 1984

322 DISORDERS OF GROWTH

RAYMOND L. HINTZ

NORMAL GROWTH Children undergo rapid changes in size over relatively short periods of time, and the physician must be aware of normal standards for growth and development as a function of age. A record of these dynamic changes can be utilized as a sensitive indicator of general health; minimal aberrations in health may initially be reflected in a deviation from the normal growth rate; conversely, an actively growing child seldom has a serious systemic disease. Thus, height and growth rate provide important information.

Both longitudinal and cross-sectional studies indicate that differences exist in growth among different ethnic groups. However, normal well-nourished children have remarkably similar growth patterns. One interesting approximation is that the average length of children, which at birth is about 50 cm, increases by about 25 cm in the first year of life, 12.5 cm in the second year, and 6.2 cm per year thereafter until puberty. This formula can be used to estimate average height up to about 10 years of age. A variety of nomograms have been constructed to give a more accurate picture of average growth and the range of normal deviations from the mean (Figs. 322-1 and 322-2).

CONTROL OF GROWTH Growth involves both an increase in the total number of cells in an organism and the synthesis of macromolecules by individual cells. The relative importance of these processes varies from organ to organ and with age. The control and integration of growth also vary among tissues and with the stage of development. Understanding the control of growth is important to understanding the variations in normal growth patterns as well as the mechanisms of aging and oncogenesis.

Prenatal growth Prenatal development exemplifies the complexities of the integration and control of growth. During this time, a single cell becomes a complex organism with billions of cells working in harmonious concert. The growth rate is astounding; the most rapid growth rate occurs during the second trimester. Prenatal growth may have different control mechanisms from those in the postnatal period. Growth hormone and thyroid hormone have relatively minor effects on growth during prenatal life. Prenatal growth rates are dependent on uterine blood flow and other maternal influences and are less dependent on the factors that determine ultimate stature. At birth the correlation ($r = 0.3$) between body length and adult height is weak; by 2 years of age the correlation with adult height is stronger ($r = 0.7$), indicating that the factors influencing adult stature begin operating early in postnatal life.

Genetic factors Stature is a polygenic trait (see Chap. 57), so that there is no simple method of predicting on the basis of genetic factors the adult height of any given child. However, on average there is a correlation between the mean height of parents and the mean height attained by their children.

Nutrition The next most important factor affecting growth is nutrition. Severe nutritional deprivation, such as in those with marasmus or kwashiorkor (see Chap. 72), severely impairs growth. Selective deficiencies of vitamins and minerals, such as vitamin D, may also cause major abnormalities of growth. In some instances, a subclinical deficiency of a nutrient may retard growth. The trend toward increased adult stature in several countries over the last century may be due to improvement in diet, especially to an increase in protein intake during the growth period.

Hormones GROWTH HORMONE Growth hormone (GH, or somatotropin) plays the central role in the modulation of growth of children from birth until the completion of puberty. In the total absence of GH, linear growth occurs at about half to a third the normal rate. GH may also play a role in the control of body anabolism throughout life.

GH is a member of a family of hormones that includes pituitary prolactin and human placental lactogen (hPL) (see Chap. 321). The most common form of GH in the pituitary and in the circulation is the 22,000-dalton ("22K") form. This is the 191-amino-acid form that was purified and sequenced from human pituitary glands. The second most common form is a 20,000-dalton ("20K") form. This variant is coded by the same gene sequence as the 22K growth hormone, but a segment of an exon (expressed part of the gene) in the growth hormone gene is not transcribed, thus resulting in a shorter

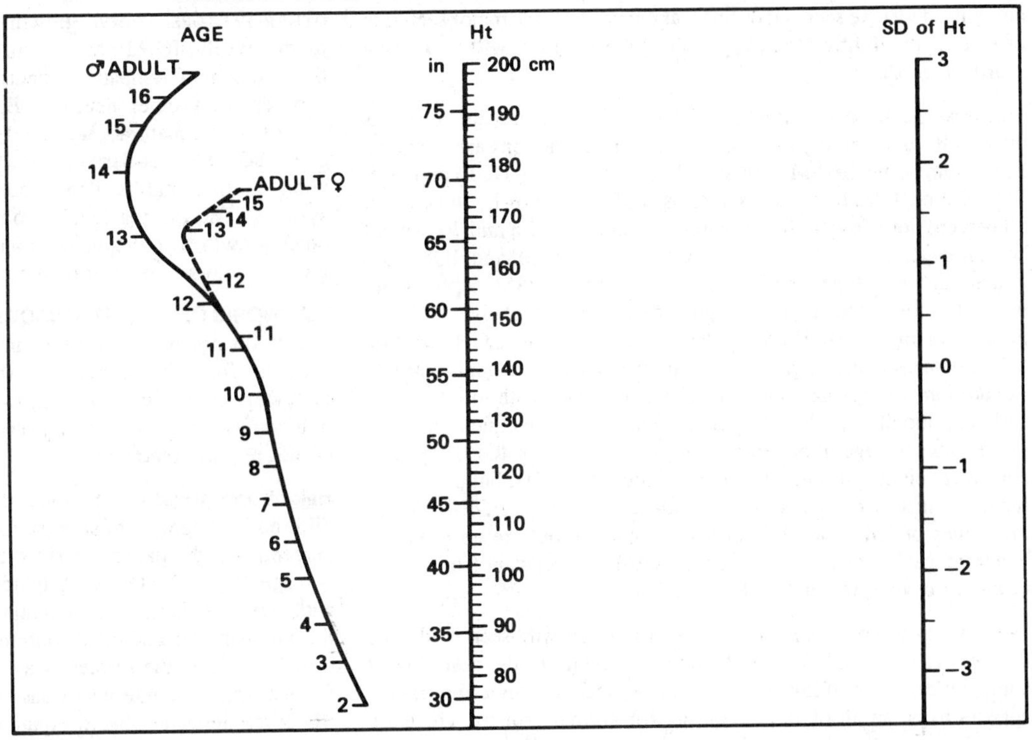

FIGURE 322-1 *Nomogram for height of boys and girls.*

form of growth hormone. Whether this variant fulfills some important metabolic function is not yet clear; the 20K form seems to have equivalent growth promoting activity but may have a lesser effect on carbohydrate function than the 22K form.

GH secretion is under both positive and negative hypothalamic control (see Chap. 321). The somatotropin release–inhibiting factor (somatostatin, SRIF) is a 14-amino-acid peptide that is widely distributed in tissues outside the hypothalamus and is a potent inhibitor of the secretion of other hormones including insulin, glucagon, and gastrin.

The biologic action of GH-releasing hormone (GRH, somatocrinin) is contained in the first 29 amino acids of the 44-amino acid peptide, and the aminoterminal amino acid is crucial for its biologic action. Patients with idiopathic GH deficiency may have a deficiency of GRH rather than an inability to make GH in the pituitary. Indeed, half or more of subjects with GH deficiency respond to prolonged pulsatile administration of GRH with an increase in plasma GH and with an accelerated growth rate.

The secretion of somatostatin and GRH, and hence the release of GH, is under the influence of several factors (Fig. 322-3). Higher centers in the central nervous system have synapses which terminate on hypothalamic cells that secrete somatostatin and GRH and exert both positive and negative influences. In addition, both GH and the GH-controlled somatomedin peptides influence the secretion or action of GRH and somatostatin. The secretion of GH is episodic with a relatively short (10- to 15-min) half-life in plasma. Although small

FIGURE 322-2 *Nomogram for growth rate in boys and girls.*

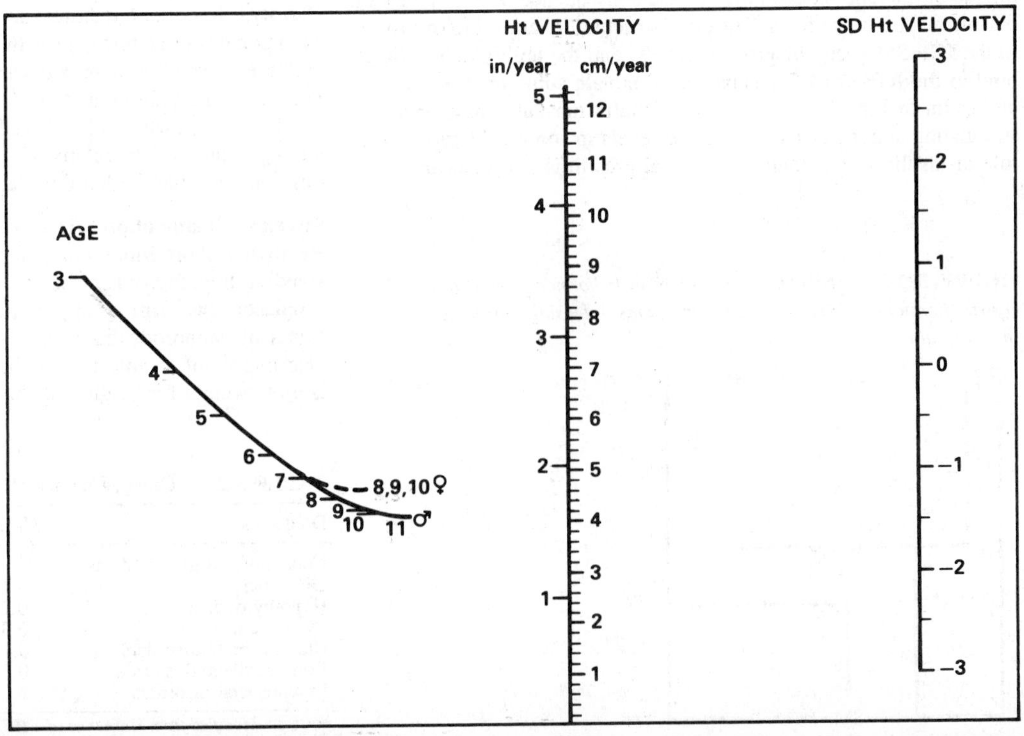

amounts of GH are secreted during waking periods, the major secretion of GH occurs during sleep, especially in association with third- and fourth-stage sleep.

THE SOMATOMEDINS Although GH may exert some direct effects on growth, the majority of its growth-promoting actions are mediated by the somatomedin (SM) or insulin-like growth factor (IGF) peptides. Two IGF peptides from human plasma, IGF-I and IGF-II, show about 50 percent homology to the structure of human insulin and 70 percent homology to each other. Somatomedin C (SM-C) and IGF-I are structurally and functionally equivalent. The IGF/SM peptides are bound tightly to specific plasma proteins and have half-lives of hours rather than minutes. IGF-I/SM-C levels are dependent on GH secretion and are consequently high in acromegaly and low in hypopituitarism. In addition, the normal values are age-dependent, with low levels in early childhood, a peak during adolescence, and a decline in average values after the age of 50 years. The plasma levels of IGF-II are also dependent on the presence of a minimal amount of GH, but pathologic increases in GH do not result in a further increase in IGF-II. Thus, the values of IGF-II are low in hypopituitarism but are not elevated in acromegaly. The average levels of IGF-II are constant from 1 year of age to beyond the eighth decade of life.

THYROID HORMONE Unlike the pattern of growth seen with GH deficiency, the total absence of thyroid hormone leads to an almost complete cessation of linear growth. Thus, adequate thyroid hormone appears to be an absolute prerequisite for normal growth. There are several potential mechanisms for this phenomenon. Thyroid hormones exert direct effects on cell metabolism, and thyroid hormone deficiency results in diminished GH secretion in response to stimulation. Finally, the action of IGF-I/SM-C on cartilage cells may be dependent on thyroid hormone.

GONADAL STEROIDS Androgens and estrogens exert their major role in the stimulation of growth at the time of puberty. Much of the pubertal growth spurt is due to these hormones. Androgens have a direct stimulatory effect on the growth and maturation of bone, cartilage, and muscle. Estrogens appear to have a biphasic action, stimulating growth at low levels and inhibiting growth at high levels.

INSULIN Insulin has strong anabolic actions separate from its effects on carbohydrate metabolism. These actions include stimulation of protein synthesis and cell division. The excessive growth of some infants of diabetic mothers may be the consequence of high levels of plasma insulin in the fetus. The close structural relationship of insulin to the IGF/SM group of growth factors, and the ability of insulin to bind to the IGF-I/SM-C receptor may explain some of these actions of insulin at high levels. However, insulin may also have growth-stimulating actions of its own at low levels in some cells types. The role of insulin in the control of normal growth is still unclear.

FIGURE 322-3 *Feedback control of growth hormone secretion. GH = growth hormone; GRH = growth hormone–releasing hormone; SM = somatomedin.*

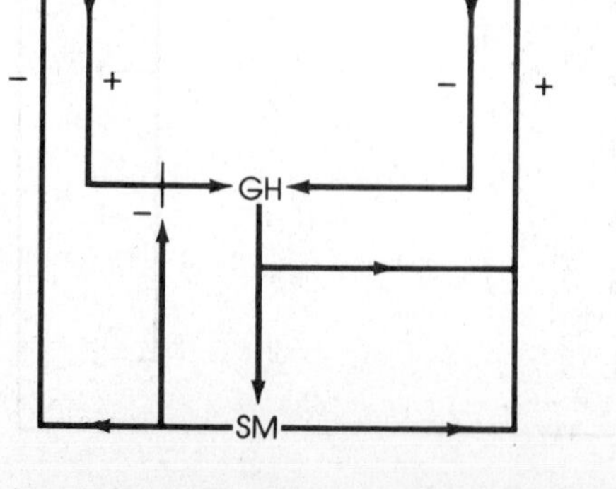

OTHER FACTORS Nerve growth factor which is structurally related to the insulin-IGF-I/SM-C family of peptides has actions on the development of sympathetic neurons and possibly on the maintenance and repair of other neurons. Epidermal growth factor has potent actions on the maturation of epidermal features but also acts on other cell types. Platelet-derived growth factor is released from platelets upon clotting and is also a potent mitogen in many cell culture systems. The plasma levels, control mechanisms, interactions with other growth-stimulating hormones, and physiologic roles of these growth factors remain to be elucidated.

DIAGNOSIS OF GROWTH DISORDERS Most individuals with short stature do not have a disease in the usual sense but exhibit some variation from the normal growth pattern (Table 322-1). Thus, the first step in dealing with growth disorders is to identify those individuals who have a normal variation in stature and who presumably do not require treatment.

Height and growth rate One of the most important factors in the differential diagnosis of short stature is the determination of the height percentile of the patient, derived by a comparison to others of his or her age (Fig. 322-1). A straightedge is placed on the patient's age and present height. The intercept on the right-hand scale estimates the number of standard deviations (SD) from the mean height for age. In general, the further away the patient is from the mean height for age, the more likely a disease is present. A height above the −2-SD level indicates that the patient is likely normal. The patient's growth rate also should be determined, if possible, either from existing growth data or by observation (Fig. 322-2).

Because of the large number of normal children with short stature, clinical judgment plays a large role in the approach to this problem. Individuals with severe short stature (> −3 SD for age) should undergo immediate evaluation, while those with less severe short stature may be serially observed so that the growth rate can be assessed. A consistently low growth rate should lead to further investigation. The diagnosis of constitutional delay is one of exclusion. In general, if the physician has excluded hypothyroidism, GH deficiency, and the more common systemic diseases, it is reasonable to observe the patient. However, the boundaries between "normal" and "disease" may be blurred, and the indications for treatment may change. Furthermore, continued failure to maintain a normal growth rate is an indication for reinvestigation.

History Important features in the history include the weight and gestational age at birth, growth and development in early infancy, and presence of systemic disease. It is also crucial to assess the stature of the parents and first- and second-degree relatives and to review the growth and pubertal development patterns of parents, siblings, and other relatives. A family history or late pubertal development may be helpful diagnostically.

Physical examination The body proportions must be evaluated. Relatively short limbs compared to the trunk suggest either long-standing hypothyroidism or one of the chondrodystrophies. Achondroplastic dwarfism is an extreme example of this, but more subtle forms of chondrodystrophy may elude the casual examination. It is also important to note the height-to-weight ratio. A short child who is underweight for height may have malnutrition or systemic disease.

TABLE 322-1 Causes of short stature

Diagnosis	Usual practice, %	Referral center, %
Constitutional growth delay	98	80
GH deficiency	0.1	10
Hypothyroidism	0.2	4
Systemic disease	0.3	3
Chromosomal disorders	0.1	1
Bone-cartilage dysplasia	0.3	1
Psychosocial disorders	1	1

SOURCE: *Modified from Horner et al., 1978.*

On the other hand, a child who is short but overweight is more likely to have endocrine disease. Patients with Cushing's syndrome, GH deficiency, or hypothyroidism are frequently relatively overweight for their height. Specific physical findings may suggest hypothyroidism, GH deficiency, or other specific syndromes (Table 322-2).

Laboratory evaluation Laboratory tests may either confirm the clinical impression or reveal unsuspected pathology. Assessment of bone age is useful to indicate possible pathology and to estimate final adult height. Because the manifestations of hypothyroidism may be minimal, a serum thyroxine should be obtained routinely. IGF-I/SM-C measurements are also useful screening procedures, since most patients with GH deficiency have low values. There are also syndromes of GH resistance, such as Laron dwarfism, that are characterized by low IGF-I/SM-C levels and high GH levels. Specific chemistries may be ordered to screen for other disease states. Any girl with unexplained short stature should have a chromosomal karyotype. Useful laboratory studies for the evaluation of short stature are summarized in Table 322-3. Abnormalities of these tests should lead to more specific investigations.

TESTING OF GH SECRETION Because GH secretion is episodic and therefore variable, random measurements of plasma GH are not adequate tests of GH deficiency. Some GH stimulation tests for outpatient screening for GH deficiency are summarized in Table 322-4 (also see Chap. 321). Because of the long half-life of IGF-I/SM-C, a random measurement of this hormone during the day is an accurate reflection of the mean plasma concentration. If care is taken to use age-related standards, measurement of IGF-I/SM-C provides a reasonable screen for GH deficiency. Low levels of IGF-I/SM-C should lead to more extensive evaluation. The other tests listed are indirect and largely nonphysiologic ways of provoking the release of GH. In our clinic, a GH level of 7 ng/mL after an exercise or clonidine test is interpreted as a normal response. If that level is not achieved, more definitive testing of GH reserve should be carried out as described in Chap. 321.

TREATMENT WITH GH **GH deficiency** The only established use of human GH is in the treatment of children who are GH-deficient. Only between 1 in 4000 and 1 in 20,000 children have a GH deficiency. About half of these cases are due to idiopathic GH deficiency, and the other half are secondary to tumor and/or radiation therapy. In approximately one-third of the latter cases, only GH is deficient, and in the other two-thirds, there are multiple pituitary hormone deficiencies. If short stature is due to a systemic disease such as renal failure, treatment is directed toward the underlying disease state. Similarly, short stature due to hypothyroidism or cortisol excess is managed by treatment of the primary endocrine disorder. In general, the earlier the disorder is diagnosed and treated, the more successful the growth response will be; if treatment of the underlying disease is delayed until after puberty, little or no improvement in stature can be expected.

Unlike the broad species specificity characteristic of peptide hormones such as insulin, GH exhibits limited species specificity. Human GH stimulates linear growth in children with GH deficiency, whereas the bovine hormone is ineffective in humans. The need for human GH led to the formation of the National Pituitary Agency to facilitate the collection of pituitary glands from autopsy material and the preparation of human GH and other pituitary hormones. This effort did not supply adequate amounts of hormone for the treatment of all children who had GH deficiency, let alone provide sufficient material for the study of GH as a therapeutic agent for other conditions. Furthermore, the distribution of human pituitary GH in the United States and several other countries was discontinued in 1984 because of the development of Creutzfeldt-Jakob disease in four subjects who had been treated with human GH. Since this degenerative central nervous system disease is rare in this age group, the concern is that previous and/or present methods of GH extraction allowed contamination of GH preparations with the causative agent of this disease. The availability since 1985 of synthetic GH produced by recombinant DNA in bacteria has relieved the supply problem. Hormone is again available for patients with GH deficiency, and its relatively unlimited supply will allow the exploration of other therapeutic uses of GH.

Despite the difficulties generated by inadequate supplies, there is an extensive experience with the use of pituitary GH for treating GH deficiency. Most children with GH deficiency respond to GH treatment with an acceleration of growth rate to normal or even above normal

TABLE 322-2 Physical findings in syndromes of short stature

Syndrome	Specific physical findings
GH deficiency	Frontal bossing, central obesity, high-pitched voice
Hypothyroidism	Dry skin, coarse hair, immature facies
Cushing's syndrome	Central obesity, striae, hypertension
Gonadal dysgenesis	Webbed neck, multiple pigmented nevi, shield chest, delayed sexual development
Pseudohypoparathyroidism	Moon facies and obesity, short metacarpals, mental retardation
Bone-cartilage dysplasia	Abnormal proportions, macrocephaly
Russell-Silver dwarfism	Small at birth, "pointed" facies, asymmetry

TABLE 322-3 Screening laboratory investigations in short stature

Test or x-ray	Disorder
Serum thyroxine	Hypothyroidism
IGF-I/SM-C	GH deficiency
Bone age	Constitutional delay, hypothyroidism, GH deficiency
Lateral skull film	Craniopharyngioma or other central nervous system lesion
Serum Ca	Pseudohypoparathyroidism
Serum phosphate	Vitamin D–resistant rickets
Serum bicarbonate	Renal tubular acidosis
Blood urea nitrogen	Renal failure
Complete blood count	Anemia, nutritional disorder
Sedimentation rate	Inflammatory disease of bowel
Chromosomal karyotype	Gonadal dysgenesis or other abnormality

TABLE 322-4 Screening tests for assessing GH secretion

1 IGF-I/SM-C radioimmunoassay
Age-related normals (may vary with method):

Age, years	Range (units/mL)
<1	0.17–0.62
1–5	0.14–1.44
6–11	0.50–2.06
12–17	0.78–3.73
18–25	0.92–2.06
26–40	0.70–2.04

2 Exercise test:
Vigorous exercise (running or stairsteps) for 20 min
20-min rest
Samples for measurement of GH by radioimmunoassay at 0, 20, and 40 min from beginning
Normal response: GH greater than or equal to 7 ng/mL on any sample

3 Clonidine test:
NPO after midnight
Administration of clonidine by mouth

Body weight, kg	Dose, mg
5 to 15	0.05
15 to 25	0.1
25 to 35	0.15
35 to 50	0.2
>50	0.25

Samples for measurement of GH by radioimmunoassay at 0, 60, and 90 min
Side effects: Postural hypotension and somnolence
Keep patient supine until after postural hypotension is gone
Normal response: Greater than or equal to 7 ng/mL on any sample

rates. As with other peptide hormones, there is a dose-response curve to GH. The doses that have been tested range from 0.02 to 0.2 units (0.01 to 0.1 mg) per kilogram of body weight administered as an intramuscular injection three times a week. There is a wide variation in response, but the higher dosages in general result in higher average growth rates. It is possible that in selected clinical circumstances dosages of GH higher than those currently recommended should be administered. Now that synthetic GH is available, treatment should be started at the 0.1 unit per kilogram of body weight dosage, since the majority of GH-deficient patients have a good growth response to this amount of GH. If the patient fails to show an adequate growth rate, the GH dose can be increased until an adequate growth response is obtained or until the upper limit of 0.25 units per kilogram of body weight three times per week is achieved. As doses of GH are increased above this level, the risk of glucose intolerance increases, particularly in children who are prediabetic. An unsettled therapeutic issue is whether daily use of GH results in a greater growth response than with the schedule of three doses a week. Preliminary data suggest that daily subcutaneous injections may lead to better responses. Furthermore, subcutaneous GH may be as effective and safe as when administered intramuscularly.

An alternative method for the treatment of GH deficiency now under study is the use of long-term, subcutaneous infusion of GH-releasing hormone (GRH). Since at least half of children with GH deficiency are able to secrete GH in response to GRH, this approach may ultimately be useful for those patients.

Short stature of other causes IDIOPATHIC SEVERE SHORT STATURE GH hormone treatment has been used for the treatment of some patients with growth failure not due to GH deficiency. Many children with severe short stature (more than 2.5 SD below the mean for age) do not have GH deficiency. Some workers propose that a subgroup of children without GH deficiency but with low IGF-I/SM-C levels are responsive to GH treatment. These patients are believed to have a relatively inactive GH or to have a partial defect in the control of GH secretion. For example, although they do not fulfill the usual criteria for GH deficiency, they may not have normal bursts of GH secretion during certain physiologic circumstances such as sleep. Whatever the etiology, some of these children have a short-term increase in growth rate in response to GH therapy; whether the final height of these children after GH treatment is greater than their predicted height is not established. Furthermore, it is not known whether there are serious side effects associated with the rise of GH levels to the supraphysiologic range. At present such therapy should be undertaken only as part of a research protocol.

GONADAL DYSGENESIS GH may also have a therapeutic role in the treatment of gonadal dysgenesis (see Chap. 60). The majority of women with gonadal dysgenesis have an average adult height between 135 and 142 cm. Androgens can cause a short-term increase in the rate of growth of girls with the disorder but do not result in an increase in final adult stature. The use of GH at modest doses is also associated with a small increase in the rate of growth. Preliminary results of a multicenter group study utilizing a somewhat higher dose of synthetic GH are even more encouraging in terms of initial growth response. However, it is not known whether GH therapy results in an increase in adult stature.

SKELETAL DISORDERS GH hormone has also been used to treat small numbers of subjects with a wide variety of other growth disorders including bone-cartilage dysplasias and other genetic syndromes associated with short stature. It is not clear whether GH is of use in any of these disorders.

REFERENCES

BROWN P: Potential epidemic of Creutzfeldt-Jacob disease from human growth hormone therapy. N Engl J Med 313:728, 1985

FRASIER SD: A review of growth hormone stimulation tests in children. Pediatrics 53:929, 1974

——— et al: A dose response curve for human growth hormone. J Clin Endocrinol Metab 53:1213, 1981

FURLANETTO R et al: Estimation of somatomedin-C levels in normals and patients with pituitary disease by radioimmunoassay. J Clin Invest 60:648, 1977

GERTNER J et al: Prospective clinical trial of human growth hormone in short children without growth hormone deficiency. J Pediatr 104:172, 1984

HINTZ RL: The somatomedins. Adv Pediatr 28:293, 1980

——— et al: Biosynthetic methionyl-human growth hormone is biologically active in adult man. Lancet 1:1276, 1982

HORNER JM et al: Growth deceleration patterns in children with constitutional short stature: An aid to diagnosis. Pediatrics 62:529, 1978

KASTRUP KW et al: Increased growth rate following transfer to daily sc administration from three weekly im injections of hGH. Acta Endocrinol (Copenh) 104:148, 1983

LEWIS UJ et al: Human growth hormone: A complex of proteins. Recent Prog Horm Res 36: 477, 1980

RINDERKNECHT R, HUMBEL RE: Primary structure of human IGF-II. FEBS Lett 89:283, 1978

ROSENFELD RF et al: A prospective, randomized trial of methionyl human growth hormone and/or oxandrolone in Turner's syndrome. Pediatr Res 19:A102, 1985

RUDMAN D et al: Children with normal variant short stature: Treatment with human growth hormone for 6 months. N Eng J Med 305:123, 1981

TANNER JM, ISREALSOHN WJ: Parent-child correlations for body measurements of children between the ages of one month and 7 years. Ann Hum Genet 26:245, 1963

——— et al: Effect of human growth hormone treatment for 1 to 7 years on growth of 100 children with growth hormone deficiency, inherited smallness, Turner's syndrome, and other complaints. Arch Dis Child 46:745, 1971

———, DAVIS PSW: Clinical longitudinal standards for height and height velocity for North American children. J Pediatr 107:317, 1985

THORNER MO et al: Acceleration of growth in two children treated with human growth hormone releasing factor. N Engl J Med 312:4, 1985

VIMPANI OV et al: Prevalence of severe growth hormone deficiency. Br Med J 2:427, 1977

WILSON DM et al: Subcutaneous versus intramuscular growth hormone therapy: Growth and acute somatomedin response. J. Pediatr 76:361, 1985

323 DISORDERS OF THE NEUROHYPOPHYSIS

DAVID H. P. STREETEN / ARNOLD M. MOSES / MYRON MILLER

There are two largely independent hypothalamic-neurohypophyseal systems composed of neurons in the supraoptic and paraventricular nuclei, from which axons extend through the pituitary stalk to the posterior pituitary. Hormones (vasopressin and oxytocin), formed within separate ganglion cells, migrate down the axons as part of precursor proteins that include the neurophysins. They are stored in secretory granules within the nerve terminals in the neurohypophysis. The hormones with their neurophysins are released by exocytosis from the granules into the bloodstream. Vasopressin or antidiuretic hormone (AVP or ADH) is predominantly concerned with the control of water conservation, and its release is coordinated with the activity of the thirst center that regulates fluid intake. Oxytocin stimulates uterine contractions and milk ejection.

VASOPRESSIN RELEASE AND ACTION

CHEMISTRY Arginine vasopressin (AVP) is a nonapeptide composed of six amino acids in a ring attached to a side chain of three amino acids.

ACTIONS Via actions on its V_2 receptors in the distal renal tubules, AVP conserves water and concentrates the urine by enhancing the hydroosmotic flow of water from the luminal fluid through the cells of the collecting tubule of the kidney to the medullary interstitium. This action assists in maintaining constancy of the osmolality and volume of body fluids. High concentrations of AVP acting on V_1 receptors can cause vasoconstriction, as may occur in response to severe hypotension or to infusion of vasopressin for treatment of bleeding esophageal varices.

AVP, perhaps from axons that terminate in the cerebrum, may play a role in learning and memory, and AVP from fibers in the median eminence may influence corticotropin secretion.

NORMAL HORMONE LEVELS AVP concentrations in plasma and urine can be measured by radioimmunoassay. The results may be expressed either as units based on pressor activity in the rat or in terms of weight of purified vasopressin. Arginine vasopressin has a biologic activity of approximately 400 units per milligram (1 μU = 2.5 pg). The human neurohypophysis under conditions of random fluid intake contains approximately 8 units of AVP. Under the same conditions peripheral plasma AVP concentration in humans ranges from 1 to 3 μU/mL. The AVP concentration of blood fluctuates, with a maximum late at night and in the early morning and a minimum in the early afternoon. Under conditions of normal hydration, healthy subjects release approximately 400 to 550 mU from the pituitary and excrete 10 to 35 mU AVP in urine in 24 h. During 24 to 28 h of dehydration the amount released increases three to five times with consequent increases in plasma and urinary levels.

METABOLISM Inactivation of AVP occurs largely in liver and kidneys, a major mechanism being the cleavage of the terminal glycinamide to produce a biologically inactive substance. Approximately 7 to 10 percent of secreted AVP is excreted in the urine as active hormone.

CONTROL OF AVP RELEASE The release of AVP is influenced by a number of stimuli (Fig. 323-1).

Osmoregulation Under normal conditions AVP release is primarily regulated by osmoreceptors in the hypothalamus. Changes in the concentrations of plasma solutes to which the cellular membrane is impermeable cause alterations in the volume of the osmoreceptor cells, which in turn alter the electric activity of the neurons and control AVP release. Osmotic changes that stimulate release also enhance production of AVP. The servomechanism between effective plasma osmolality and AVP release normally maintains plasma osmolality within a very narrow range. The mean plasma osmolality of normal subjects following a water load of 20 mL per kilogram of body weight is 281.7 mosmol/kg, and the osmolality that initiates AVP release following infusion of hypertonic saline solution into water-loaded subjects is 287.3 mosmol/kg. Thus, the increase in plasma osmolality from full diuresis to the initiation of antidiuresis by hypertonic saline solution is only 5.6 mosmol/kg, or 2 percent.

The infusion of hypertonic saline solution at a constant rate into water-loaded subjects causes a linear rise in plasma osmolality with time. After an interval that depends on the infusion rate and the concentration of the saline solution, there is an abrupt, progressive fall in free water clearance without a significant change in solute or creatinine excretion. We have defined the osmotic threshold for AVP release as the plasma osmolality at the onset of antidiuresis under these conditions. In 73 normal subjects, this occurred at a mean plasma osmolality of 287 mosmol/kg.

Volume regulation Decreases in plasma volume, through effects on stretch receptors in the left atrium and perhaps in the pulmonary veins, stimulate the release of AVP by reducing the tonic inhibitory impulses from the left atrium to the hypothalamus. The neural impulses travel via the vagi to the reticular formation of the midbrain and diencephalon and thence to the supraoptic and paraventricular nuclei, where they are integrated with the other stimuli that affect AVP release. Positive pressure breathing, quiet standing, and vasodilatation due to a warm environment may activate this mechanism, which serves to restore plasma volume, even at times overriding osmotic inhibition of AVP release. Following volume contraction, circulating AVP concentrations may reach 10 times the levels induced by hypertonicity. Increased plasma volume inhibits AVP release by the reverse mechanisms, leading to a diuresis and correction of the hypervolemia. Negative pressure breathing, recumbency, lack of gravitational force (as occurs in space travel), submersion in water, and exposure to cold may activate this mechanism.

Baroreceptor regulation Activation of carotid and aortic baroreceptors in response to hypotension causes release. Hypotension due to blood loss is the most potent stimulus and may raise plasma levels of AVP to 1000 μU/mL at times. These concentrations of AVP may cause marked vasoconstriction, which probably plays a role in the restoration of blood pressure.

Neural regulation Neurotransmitters and peptide neuromodulators such as angiotensin II, dopamine, and endorphins may mediate some of the stimulatory and inhibitory input into the hypothalamus and thus alter AVP release. Acetylcholine appears to be the final link connecting neural pathways to the supraoptic neurons involved in AVP release. Both cholinergic and beta-adrenergic stimuli release AVP, while atropine and alpha-adrenergic stimulation inhibit AVP release, apparently by actions on the hypothalamus. Emotional stress, emesis, and pain may overcome a diuresis. A diuresis may follow hypnotic suggestion, psychological conditioning, and inhalation of carbon dioxide.

Aging The aging process is associated with enhanced AVP release in response to a rising plasma osmolality and a progressive increase in plasma AVP concentration. These physiologic changes appear to place the older individual under greater risk of developing water retention and hyponatremia, despite a concomitant decline in maximal renal concentrating capacity in response to AVP, which is usually evident and progressive beyond 60 years of age.

Pharmacologic influences Pharmacologic agents that can stimulate AVP release include nicotine, morphine, vincristine, vinblastine, cyclophosphamide, clofibrate, chlorpropamide, and some of the

FIGURE 323-1 *Schematic representation of control of AVP release and cellular action of AVP. CO, optic chiasma; MB, mamillary body; SON, supraoptic nucleus.*

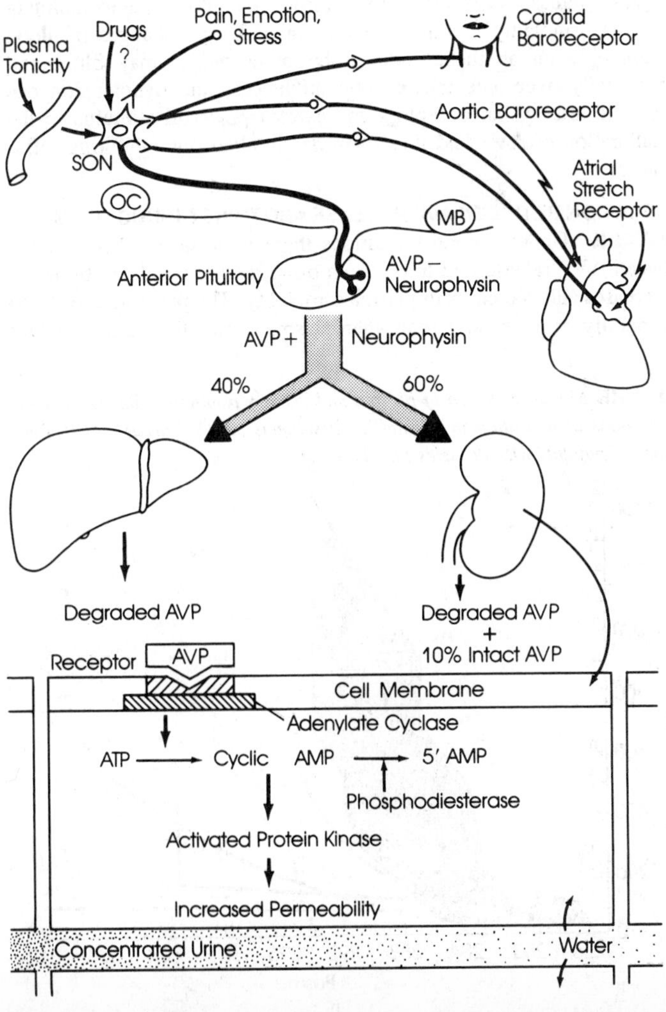

tricyclic anticonvulsants and antidepressants. Ethanol has diuretic properties and inhibits neurohypophyseal function under a variety of conditions. Some narcotic antagonists also inhibit AVP release. Experimentally chlorpromazine, reserpine, and phenytoin all diminish the loss of AVP from the pituitary and the rise in urinary excretion of AVP that result from water deprivation. In humans, phenytoin and chlorpromazine may inhibit AVP release and produce diuresis.

AVP RESPONSE TO WATER DEPRIVATION AND TO WATER LOAD Water deprivation provides both an osmotic and a volume stimulus to vasopressin release by increasing plasma osmolality and decreasing plasma volume. The maximum urinary osmolality after water deprivation varies, depending on renal medullary osmolality and other intrarenal factors. In response to fluid deprivation for 18 to 24 h, in normal individuals, plasma osmolality rarely rises above 292 mosmol/kg. The resultant stimulation of AVP release increases plasma AVP concentration to 6 to 10 μU/mL.

The administration of water lowers plasma osmolality and expands blood volume, inhibiting the release of AVP via both the osmoreceptor and the atrial volume receptor mechanisms. An oral water load of 20 mL/kg in normal adults results in a fall in plasma osmolality to a mean of 281.7 mosmol/kg and causes a maximum diuresis in 1 to 1½ h with free water clearance rising to approximately 12 mL/min and urine osmolality falling to 40 to 60 mosmol/kg. The delay in reaching maximal diuresis is accounted for by the time involved in absorption of water from the gut, in metabolizing previously secreted vasopressin, and in renal recovery from the action of vasopressin.

INTERACTION OF OSMOTIC AND VOLUME INFLUENCES Under conditions of water deprivation and of water loading, volume and osmotic influences act in parallel to influence AVP release. In other circumstances volume and osmotic influences may be competitive, and minor changes in plasma volume can modify hypertonic stimuli to AVP release. Osmotic factors ordinarily predominate to maintain plasma osmolality within a narrow range. Larger changes in blood volume, such as those induced by hemorrhage, may blunt and eventually overcome the osmotic influences, and hypotension can activate arterial baroreceptors and exert a powerful stimulus to the elaboration of AVP and thus override simultaneous inhibiting influences.

RELATION BETWEEN AVP RELEASE AND THIRST-INDUCED WATER INTAKE Under normal conditions there is close coordination between AVP release and thirst, both of which are regulated by small increases and decreases in plasma osmolality. The perception of thirst generally becomes apparent when plasma osmolality rises to values greater than 292 mosmol/kg. Angiotensin II increases thirst and AVP release, at least under experimental conditions. When AVP release is impaired, water losses lead to hypernatremia, which increases thirst and fluid intake to an extent sufficient to restore and maintain normal plasma osmolality. On the other hand, loss of thirst (adipsia) leads to uncorrected fluid losses and hypernatremia despite increased AVP release and excretion of a maximally concentrated urine.

FIGURE 323-2 *Relation of plasma and urinary osmolality during varying conditions of hydration in normal adult subjects (shaded area) and in four types of patients with diabetes insipidus.*

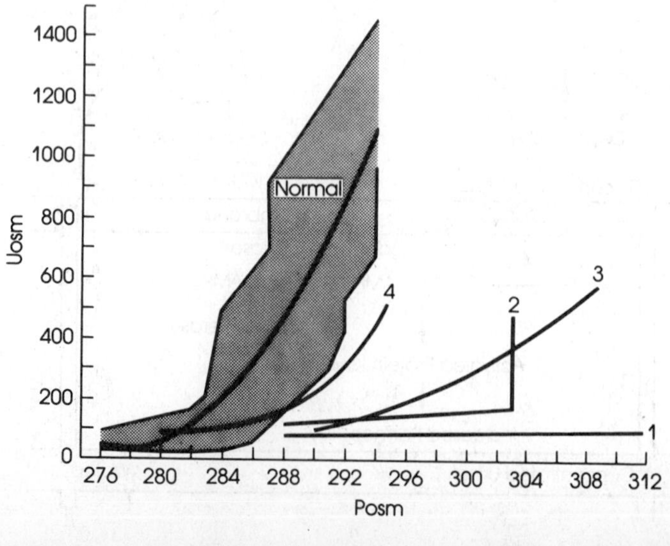

EFFECTS OF GLUCOCORTICOIDS Hormones of the adrenal cortex and the posterior pituitary have antagonist effects on water excretion. Cortisol elevates the osmotic threshold for AVP release elicited by hypertonic saline infusion in water-loaded normal subjects, and glucocorticoids protect against water intoxication and overcome the impaired response to water loading in adrenal insufficiency.

Although the subnormal ability to dilute the urine in patients with adrenal insufficiency may in part be due to excessive circulating AVP, glucocorticoids can also act directly on the renal tubules to decrease water permeability and increase solute-free water in the absence of AVP.

CELLULAR MECHANISM OF AVP ACTIVITY The biochemical basis for the action of AVP on the renal tubule is shown in Fig. 323-1: (1) AVP binds to specific contraluminal V_2 receptor sites; (2) the receptor-hormone complex is coupled to and activates adenylate cyclase in the same contraluminal membrane via a guanine nucleotide regulatory protein (see Chap. 67); (3) the production of cyclic AMP is increased; (4) the cyclic AMP is translocated to the luminal cell membrane where it causes the activation of membrane-bound protein kinase; (5) the activated protein kinase causes the phosphorylation of membrane proteins; and (6) permeability of the luminal membrane to water is increased. The AVP-generated cyclic AMP may be inactivated by a phosphodiesterase that converts cyclic AMP to 5′-AMP. AVP also stimulates prostaglandin E_2 production which, in turn, acts as a feedback inhibitor of adenylate cyclase activation.

The transtubular movement of water depends on the integrity of the microtubular system of the epithelial cells. The above biochemical events lead to the passive flow of water along an osmotic gradient across the collecting tubule. The physiologic action of AVP is accompanied by anatomic changes, including cell swelling, vacuolization, expansion of the medullary interstitium, and widening of the lateral intercellular spaces of the collecting ducts. The latter changes indicate that fluid resorption during AVP-induced antidiuresis occurs in part by way of intercellular channels.

Various cations and drugs can influence the action of AVP. Calcium and lithium inhibit the adenylate cyclase response to vasopressin. Lithium also interferes with a subsequent biochemical action, as does potassium deficiency. Demeclocycline inhibits adenylate cyclase stimulation by AVP and also inhibits the cyclic AMP–dependent protein kinase. In contrast, chlorpropamide increases AVP-induced activation of adenylate cyclase.

DEFICIENCY OF VASOPRESSIN: DIABETES INSIPIDUS

In central diabetes insipidus renal conservation of water is impaired because of deficient AVP release in response to normal physiologic stimuli.

PATHOPHYSIOLOGY Deficiency of vasopressin release in response to the appropriate stimuli may result from lesions at several functional sites in the physiologic chain of events which regulates discharge of the hormone into the bloodstream. For conceptual purposes four types of central diabetes insipidus can be defined. Patients of the first type show very little rise in urine osmolality with increasing plasma osmolality (1, Fig. 323-2) and no evidence of AVP release during hypertonic saline infusion. They are essentially devoid of releasable AVP. In the second type there is an abrupt increase in urine osmolality during dehydration (2, Fig. 323-2), but there is no evidence of an osmotic threshold during saline infusion. These patients have a defective osmoreceptor mechanism but are capable of releasing AVP in response to the hypovolemia of severe dehydration. The third type of patient has some rise in urine osmolality with increasing plasma osmolality (3, Fig. 323-2) and has an elevated osmotic threshold for AVP release. These patients have a sluggish release mechanism and may be said to have a high-set osmoreceptor. In the fourth type of patient, urine and plasma osmolality coordinates are shifted to the right of normal (4, Fig. 323-2). AVP release in these patients is initiated at a normal plasma osmolality but is subnormal in amount.

The second to fourth types of patients may develop a good antidiuresis in response to nausea, nicotine, methacholine, chlorpropamide, or clofibrate, indicating that the synthesis and storage of AVP are sufficient to allow for adequate urinary concentrating ability in the presence of an appropriate stimulus to release. In rare instances patients of the second to fourth types may present with asymptomatic hypernatremia associated with mild or absent evidence of diabetes insipidus.

ETIOLOGY The causes of diabetes insipidus in 100 consecutive patients who satisfied the criteria described under "Diagnostic Tests" (below) and who had had diabetes insipidus for at least 6 months are shown in Table 323-1. Diabetes insipidus frequently starts in childhood or early adult life (median age of onset 21 years) and is more common in males than females. The major causes are as follows: (1) *Neoplastic or infiltrative lesions* of the hypothalamus or pituitary, including chromophobe adenomas, craniopharyngiomas, germinomas, pinealomas, metastatic tumors, leukemia, histiocytosis X, and sarcoidosis, caused diabetes insipidus in 32 patients (in groups 1, 3, 7, and 9 in Table 323-1). In approximately 60 percent of these patients evidence of partial or complete loss of anterior pituitary function was present. (2) *Pituitary or hypothalamic surgery or isotopic ablative therapy* caused diabetes insipidus in 20 patients and almost invariably was associated with anterior hypopituitarism. Surgically induced diabetes insipidus usually develops between 1 and 6 days after surgery and often disappears after a few days and may remain absent or may recur and become chronic after an "interphase" of 1 to 5 days. Removal of the posterior lobe of the pituitary induces permanent diabetes insipidus only if the pituitary stalk is sectioned high enough to induce retrograde degeneration of most of the neurons of the supraoptic nucleus. (3) *Severe head injuries,* usually associated with fractures of the skull, caused diabetes insipidus in 17 patients and were associated with anterior hypopituitarism in only about one-sixth of patients. Spontaneous remissions of traumatic diabetes insipidus occurred in a fourth of patients, presumably because of regeneration of disrupted axons within the pituitary stalk. (4) *Vascular lesions* were a rare cause of diabetes insipidus (4 patients). Three patients had diabetes insipidus associated with cerebral malacia from cardiac asystole followed by resuscitation. (5) *Idiopathic diabetes insipidus* (in 27 patients) usually starts in childhood and is seldom (<20 percent) associated with anterior pituitary dysfunction. This diagnosis can be made only after a careful search has failed to reveal evidence of a tumor, infiltrative lesion, vascular lesion, or other presumptive cause of the AVP deficiency. The presence of anterior hypopituitarism or hyperprolactinemia or radiologic evidence of lesions within or above the sella should stimulate a continuing search for a causative lesion at 3- to 12-month intervals. The diagnosis of idiopathic diabetes insipidus is made with increasing confidence as the duration of negative findings on follow-up increases. A decrease in the number of neurons in the supraoptic and paraventricular nuclei has been reported in idiopathic diabetes insipidus. In rare instances, dominant inheritance has been documented.

CLINICAL MANIFESTATIONS *Polyuria, excessive thirst,* and *polydipsia* are almost invariably present in diabetes insipidus. Characteristically, these symptoms are sudden in onset, both when the disorder first presents itself and whenever the effects of administered vasopressin disappear during long-term therapy. In severe cases the urine is pale in color, and its volume may be immense (up to 16 to 24 liters per day), requiring micturition every 30 to 60 min throughout the day and night. More frequently, however, the urine volume is only moderately increased (2.5 to 6 liters per day), and occasionally it may be less than 2 liters per day, causing no complaints on the part of the patient. Urinary concentration (less than 290 mosmol/kg, specific gravity less than 1.010) is below that of the serum in severe cases but may be higher than that of serum (290 to 600 mosmol/kg) in patients with mild diabetes insipidus.

The slight rise in serum osmolality resulting from hypotonic polyuria stimulates thirst. Large volumes of fluid are imbibed, and cold drinks are preferred, patients often going to great trouble to secure cold fluids. Although thirst is probably secondary to loss of water, the administration of vasopressin often relieves or reduces thirst, even in the absence of fluid intake.

Normal function of the thirst center ensures that polydipsia closely matches polyuria, so that dehydration is seldom detectable except in the mild elevation of serum sodium concentration. However, when adequate replenishment of excreted water is interfered with, dehydration may become severe, causing weakness, fever, psychic disturbances, prostration, and death. These features are associated with a rising serum osmolality and serum sodium concentration, the latter sometimes exceeding 175 meq per liter. Adipsia is not found in idiopathic diabetes insipidus, but it may result from impaired function of the hypothalamic thirst center because of extension of the same abnormality that caused the diabetes insipidus. More frequently, dehydration occurs during unconsciousness produced by surgical anesthesia, head trauma, or other causes. It is particularly hazardous to administer large volumes of isotonic saline solution intravenously or of hyperosmolar protein by nasogastric tube unless adequate amounts of water are administered simultaneously in unconscious patients with untreated diabetes insipidus.

Hydronephrosis is a rare complication of the polyuria, especially in patients who fail to empty their bladders adequately because of bladder atony, uretheral strictures, or other causes.

DIAGNOSTIC TESTS The principle that underlies diagnostic tests for diabetes insipidus is that elevation of the plasma osmolality by fluid deprivation or hypertonic saline infusion elicits subnormal AVP release. This may be documented by plasma or urinary AVP measurements (Fig. 323-3) or by demonstrating that urinary osmolality fails to rise to the extent that occurs when exogenous vasopressin is administered in supramaximal amounts. Measurements of plasma and urinary osmolalities are so simple and reliable that AVP measurements are only occasionally needed, when osmolality measurements are inconclusive.

Assessment of the relation of plasma to urine osmolality The normal relationship between plasma osmolality (assuming no increase

TABLE 323-1 Characteristics of 100 consecutive patients with permanent diabetes insipidus

	Age of onset, years		Total number	Males	Females
	Median*	Range			
1 Histiocytosis X	1.5	1–20	4	2	2
2 Idiopathic causes	12	Infancy–66	27	16	11
3 Primary tumor of brain or pituitary	17.5	3–58	18	15	3
4 Trauma	22	5–48	17	11	6
5 Pituitary surgery	24	6–68	20	7	13
6 Ruptured intracranial aneurysm	39		1		
7 Sarcoidosis	42		1		1
8 Cerebral hypoperfusion	49	37–73	3	1	2
9 Metastatic tumors including leukemia	57	44–71	9	5	3
Totals			100	59	41

* *Median age of onset for all 100 patients = 21.*

NOTE: *Evaluated by authors at SUNY, Upstate Medical Center, Syracuse, New York (arranged in order of increasing median age of onset).*

in blood urea or glucose) and urine osmolality is indicated in Fig. 323-2. If several simultaneously determined plasma and urine osmolalities in a patient with polyuria fall substantially to the right of the shaded area, the patient has central or nephrogenic diabetes insipidus. The latter diagnosis can be made if plasma or urinary AVP concentration is increased or if the response to injected vasopressin is subnormal (see "Dehydration Test" below). The practice of relating plasma to urine osmolality is useful, particularly in postoperative neurosurgical cases or after head trauma, where its use can lead quickly to the differentiation of diabetes insipidus from parenteral fluid excess. In such patients, intravenous hydration can be slowed temporarily, and repeated plasma and urine osmolalities can be obtained and plotted as in Fig. 323-2, to determine whether the relationship is normal.

Dehydration test Comparison of the urinary osmolality after dehydration with that after vasopressin administration is a simple and reliable way of diagnosing diabetes insipidus and of differentiating vasopressin deficiency from other causes of polyuria.

The maximal urinary concentrating capacity varies widely between individuals, and no absolute lower limits of "normal" can be defined in patients with nonspecific illnesses in whom AVP is produced in adequate amounts. It is impossible to distinguish between deficiency and sufficiency of AVP release solely by the level of the urinary osmolality attained after specified periods of water deprivation. On the other hand, if after prolonged dehydration vasopressin administration induces a further rise in urinary osmolality, there is a strong implication that vasopressin deficiency exists.

PROCEDURE

1 Fluids are withheld long enough to result in stable hourly urinary osmolalities (an hourly increase of <30 mosmol/kg for at least three successive hours). This is usually associated with a loss in body weight of at least 1 kg. In patients whose daily urinary volumes exceed 10 liters, the fluid deprivation should begin between 4 A.M. and 6 A.M. so that the patient can be carefully watched and the test terminated if weight loss exceeds 2 kg or the clinical condition deteriorates. In polyuric patients whose urinary volumes are less than 10 liters per day, it is preferable to start fluid deprivation between 6 P.M. and midnight and to continue to withhold fluids until noon the following day.
2 Urine specimens are collected hourly for osmolality measurements from 6 A.M. at least until noon and preferably until the osmolality has been stable for three consecutive hours.
3 At 11 A.M. (if dehydration started at 6 P.M.) or after the third hour of stable urinary osmolalities, the patient is given vasopressin as 5 units aqueous vasopressin or 1 μg desmopressin by subcutaneous injection or 10 μg desmopressin by nasal spray.
4 Plasma osmolality is determined immediately before the injection of vasopressin, and urinary osmolality is measured on the specimen collected during the hour after the injection.

Vital signs should be monitored during the dehydration procedure, but when the test has been performed as described, adverse effects are rare.

INTERPRETATION In subjects with normal pituitary function, urinary osmolality does not rise by more than 9 percent after the injection of vasopressin, whatever the maximal urinary osmolality might be after dehydration alone (Fig. 323-3). In central diabetes insipidus, the rise in urinary osmolality after vasopressin exceeds 9 percent. To ensure adequacy of dehydration, plasma osmolality before the vasopressin injection should be above 288 mosmol/kg. Patients who have polyuria from renal diseases, potassium depletion, or nephrogenic diabetes insipidus (see below) usually show little rise in urinary osmolality with dehydration and no further rise after vasopressin injection. Patients with compulsive water drinking (primary polydipsia) often require prolonged water deprivation before plasma osmolality reaches 288 mosmol/kg and before a plateau in urinary osmolality is reached; urinary osmolality fails to rise by >9 percent after the administration of exogenous vasopressin.

Hypertonic saline infusions Assessment of the renal response to hypertonic saline infusion is required to determine whether AVP deficiency is due to a defect in osmoreceptor function. Urinary and plasma osmolality should be measured before and immediately after the infusion of 5% saline solution to calculate changes in free water clearance and thus obtain conclusive results from the procedure (Fig. 323-4). The test is dangerous in patients who are unable to tolerate a saline load.

PROCEDURE

1 Administer a water load (20 mL/kg by mouth), and subsequently replace the urine voided every 15 min by an equal volume of water by mouth.
2 Infuse 5% sodium chloride solution intravenously into one arm, preferably by infusion pump, at approximately 0.5 mL/min—to replace solute lost in the urine—until urine flow rate is stabilized, usually at 8 to 20 mL/min, for at least four 15-min periods.
3 Increase the rate of infusion of 5% saline solution to 0.05 (mL/kg)/min and continue the infusion until urine flow rate undergoes an abrupt, sustained decrease lasting for at least two 15-min periods, or until ten 15-min periods of the more rapid infusion have elapsed, or until headache, nausea, or other unpleasant symptoms have supervened, whichever comes first.
4 Draw blood through an indwelling cannula or needle in a vein in the other arm every 15 min, starting at least 15 min before the onset of the more rapid rate of infusion.

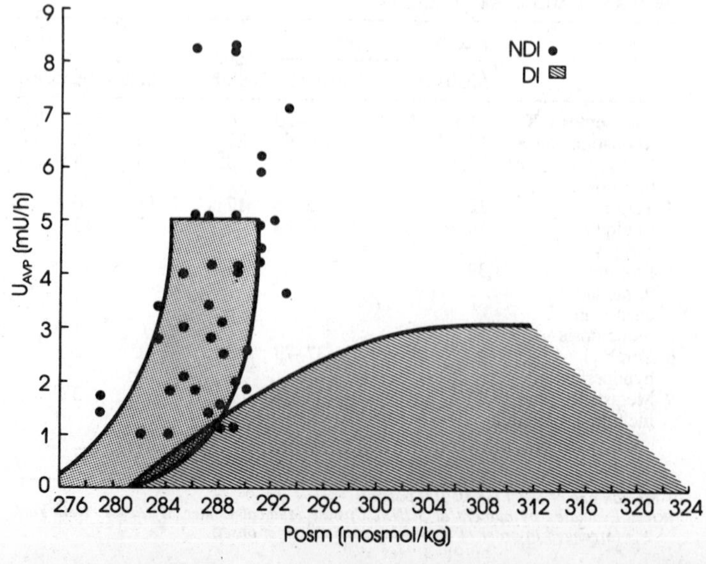

FIGURE 323-3 *Relationship between plasma osmolality (Posm) and urinary AVP excretion (U_{AVP}) in normal subjects (shaded area on left), patients with central diabetes insipidus (shaded area on right), and patients with nephrogenic diabetes insipidus (individual data points). Correlates in patients with SIADH fall to the left of the normal range. [From AM Moses, in P Czernichow and AG Robinson (eds), Frontiers of Hormone Research, vol 13: Diabetes Insipidus in Man, Basel, Karger, 1985.]*

5 Measure urinary and plasma (or serum) osmolality in all specimens. Calculate free water clearances and plot the data.
6 Measurement of plasma AVP concentration in each of the blood samples drawn for plasma osmolality determinations is useful, provided a reliable radioimmunoassay is available.

INTERPRETATION Inspection of the data will show whether a sudden, clear-cut onset of a progressive fall in free water clearance can be identified. The osmotic threshold for AVP release is deduced by interpolation on the best straight line representing plasma osmolality measurements plotted against time, at the onset of the fall in free water clearance (Fig. 323-4). When defined in this way in water-loaded subjects, the osmotic threshold is normally 287.3 ± 3.3 mosmol/kg (mean ± standard deviation). The osmotic threshold may also be computed by plotting plasma AVP against simultaneous plasma osmolality measurements and determining the level of plasma osmolality at which the linear rise in plasma AVP concentration commences. Urinary AVP measurements may be used in the same way. In most patients with diabetes insipidus there is no detectable osmotic threshold, i.e., no fall in free water clearance even after plasma osmolality rises above 300 mosmol/kg (Fig. 323-4). However, some patients may have a high or normal osmotic threshold and yet have diabetes insipidus (3 and 4, Fig. 323-2).

DIFFERENTIAL DIAGNOSIS Diabetes insipidus must be distinguished from other types of polyuria (Table 323-2), in all of which there is loss of the renal tubular response to endogenous vasopressin. The other types of polyuria can, therefore, be recognized by failure of response to administered AVP. Several are recognizable by the history (e.g., recent lithium or mannitol administration, recent surgery under methoxyflurane anesthesia, or recent renal transplantation). In others the physical examination or simple laboratory procedures will indicate the diagnosis (evidence of glycosuria, renal disease, sickle cell anemia, hypercalcemia, or potassium depletion, including primary aldosteronism).

Congenital nephrogenic diabetes insipidus is a rare, usually familial, form of polyuria resulting from unresponsiveness to AVP. It is usually diagnosed from the lack of a reduction in polyuria or rise in urinary osmolality after an injection of vasopressin, as described in the "Dehydration Test" above. These patients can also be distinguished from patients with vasopressin-deficient diabetes insipidus by the familial nature of the disorder (rare in diabetes insipidus) and by lack of the dramatic reduction in daily urine volume when vasopressin or desmopressin is administered to patients with vasopressin-deficient diabetes insipidus. Occasionally patients with nephrogenic diabetes insipidus respond to vasopressin that is injected at the plateau in urinary osmolality with a 40 to 50 percent increase in

TABLE 323-2 Major polyuric syndromes

I Primary disorders of water intake or output
- *A* Excessive water intake
  - *1* Psychogenic polydipsia
  - *2* Hypothalamic disease: histiocytosis X, sarcoidosis
  - *3* Drug-induced polydipsia
    - *a* Thioridazine
    - *b* Chlorpromazine
    - *c* Anticholinergic drugs (dry mouth)
- *B* Inadequate tubular reabsorption of filtered water
  - *1* Vasopressin deficiency
    - *a* Central diabetes insipidus
    - *b* Drug-induced inhibition of AVP release
      - *(1)* Narcotic antagonists
  - *2* Renal tubular unresponsiveness to AVP
    - *a* Nephrogenic diabetes insipidus (congenital and familial)
    - *b* Nephrogenic diabetes insipidus (acquired)
      - *(1)* Several chronic renal diseases, after obstructive uropathy, unilateral renal arterial stenosis, after renal transplantation, after acute tubular necrosis
      - *(2)* Potassium deficiencies, including primary aldosteronism
      - *(3)* Chronic hypercalcemias, including hyperparathyroidism
      - *(4)* Drug-induced: lithium, methoxyflurane anesthesia, demeclocycline
      - *(5)* Various systemic disorders: multiple myeloma, amyloidosis, sickle cell anemia, Sjögren's syndrome

II Primary disorders of renal absorption of solutes (osmotic diuresis)
- *A* Glucose: diabetes mellitus
- *B* Salts, especially sodium chloride
  - *1* Various chronic renal diseases, especially chronic pyelonephritis
  - *2* After various diuretics, including mannitol

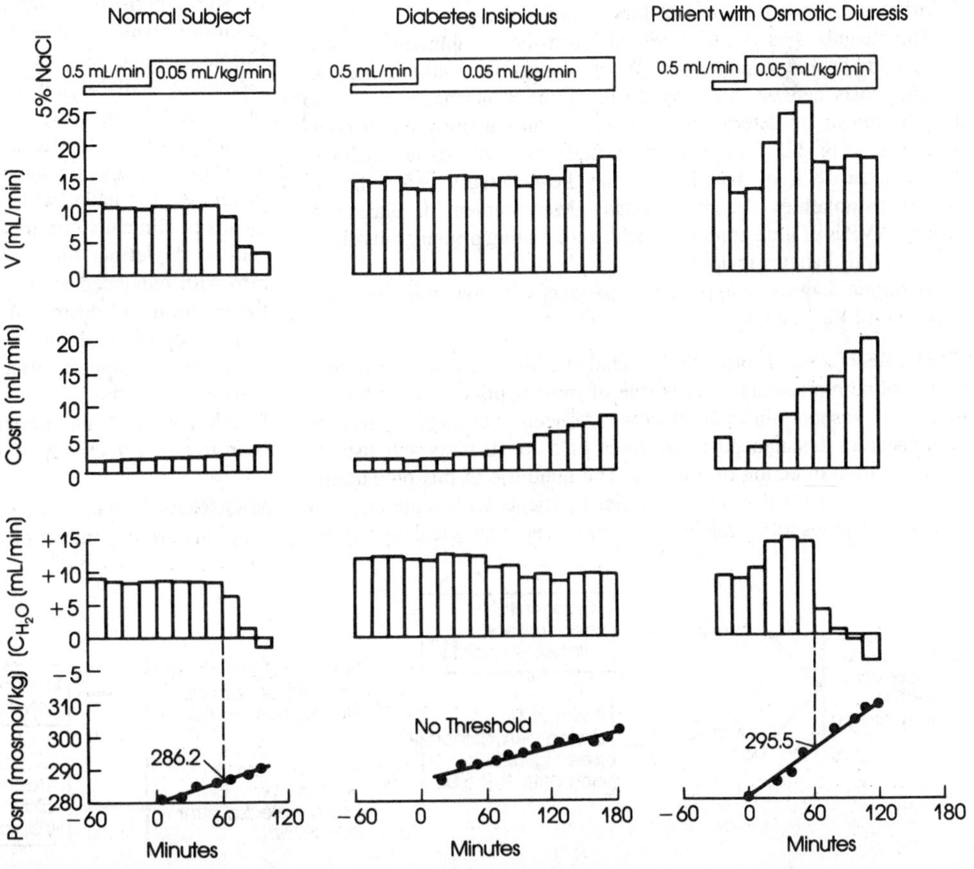

FIGURE 323-4 *Diagnostic use of responses to 5% saline infusion in subjects preloaded with water (20 mL/kg). In the normal subject (left) 5% NaCl, infused at 0.05 (mL/kg)/min, caused a gradual rise in osmolal clearance (Cosm) and an abrupt fall in urine flow rate (V) and free water clearance (C_{H_2O}) when the plasma osmolality (Posm) had been raised to the osmotic threshold for AVP release (286.2 mosmol/kg). In the patient with diabetes insipidus (middle), 5% NaCl infusion failed to cause a fall in V or C_{H_2O} despite elevation of Posm above 300 mosmol/kg. In the third subject (right) 5% NaCl infusion induced a rapid rise in Cosm resulting from osmotic diuresis which prevented a fall in V. This finding might have suggested diabetes insipidus but the fall in C_{H_2O} indicated AVP release at an osmotic threshold (295.5 mosmol/kg) which was elevated because of steroid therapy. (From AM Moses, DHPS Streeten, Am J Med 42:368, 1967.)*

urinary osmolality. This response is intermediate between the responses of patients with mild and severe diabetes insipidus. When nephrogenic and central diabetes insipidus cannot be differentiated with certainty by these procedures, documentation of an appropriately elevated plasma or urinary AVP concentration in relation to plasma osmolality (Fig. 323-3) or of a high AVP concentration in relation to urinary osmolality will establish the diagnosis of nephrogenic diabetes insipidus.

Primary polydipsia Primary or psychogenic polydipsia is occasionally difficult to differentiate from diabetes insipidus and may occur in two forms. Chronic overingestion of water results in hypotonic polyuria and is often confused with diabetes insipidus. Intermittent ingestion of very large volumes of water may also lead to dilutional hyponatremia even though a very dilute urine is excreted.

Polydipsia and polyuria in this disorder are usually somewhat erratic, in contrast to the sustained polydipsia and polyuria of diabetes insipidus. These patients usually have no nocturnal polyuria because polyuria of long duration may result in the development of large bladder capacities and consequently infrequent urination. The patients are often emotionally disturbed. The syndrome may be seen in occasional patients with anorexia nervosa, who may drink huge quantities of water while eating very little. Fluid intake may decrease markedly when food intake increases. Rarely, a patient with chronic fluid overingestion may have a central nervous system lesion, although adipsia or hypodipsia is more common in central nervous system disease.

The intermittent ingestion of large quantities of fluid may lead to water intoxication and dilutional hyponatremia even though there is normal urinary diluting capacity. This phenomenon is rare because normal adults can excrete between 10 and 14 mL/min of solute-free water, and it is an unusual circumstance which results in the ingestion of sufficiently more water than this to cause dilutional hyponatremia. The syndrome of water intoxication with normal diluting capacity has been reported in persons who take large enemas, drink excessive amounts of beer, or are given thioridazine. The phenothiazine drugs have parasympathetic effects and may cause dryness of the mouth, which aggravates tendencies toward compulsive water drinking. Thioridazine may stimulate the thirst center directly.

The diagnosis is usually evident from the combination of low plasma and urinary osmolalities. When plasma osmolality is normal, the diagnosis can be made by documenting a normal response to dehydration or by determining plasma and urinary osmolality coordinates (see Fig. 323-2). However, the patients may be so overhydrated that at least 18 h of dehydration may be necessary before hourly urinary osmolalities become constant. Measurement of plasma or urinary AVP is of little or no value in differentiating primary polydipsia from central diabetes insipidus.

A simple diagnostic approach to patients with hypotonic polyuria is shown in Fig. 323-5.

TREATMENT (See Table 323-3) Diabetes insipidus can be treated by hormone replacement. As is true of most peptides, oral administration of vasopressin is ineffective. Aqueous vasopressin may be administered subcutaneously in doses of 5 to 10 units and usually has a duration of action of 3 to 6 h. The main use of this preparation is in initial management of unconscious patients with acute onset of diabetes insipidus following head trauma or a neurosurgical procedure. Its short duration of action allows recognition of the recovery of neurohypophyseal function and prevents the development of water intoxication in patients receiving intravenous fluids.

Desmopressin has prolonged antidiuretic activity and is almost completely devoid of pressor effects. When used intranasally in amounts between 10 and 20 μg (0.1 to 0.2 mL) or by subcutaneous injection (1 to 4 μg), it has an antidiuretic action for 12 to 24 h in most patients. This analogue is the drug of choice in the treatment of most patients with diabetes insipidus. Lypressin is a nasal spray; a single application may result in an antidiuresis lasting approximately 4 to 6 h. Nasal absorption of both analogues may be decreased in the presence of an upper respiratory infection or allergic rhinitis with edema of the nasal mucosa. In such circumstances and in the unconscious patient with diabetes insipidus, desmopressin should be given by subcutaneous injection.

In the past, patients with an established diagnosis of diabetes insipidus were usually treated with intramuscular injections of vasopressin tannate in oil (2.5 or 5 units), which has an antidiuretic effect for 24 to 72 h. Since this material is a suspension of vasopressin tannate in peanut oil, it is essential that the ampul be warmed and then thoroughly shaken or inverted repeatedly until the brownish deposit of pituitary powder in the ampul is evenly distributed as a slightly cloudy suspension in the oil. A dry syringe should be used.

Patients with diabetes insipidus who have some residual releasable AVP (types 2 to 4) may respond to oral treatment with several nonhormonal agents. Chlorpropamide stimulates AVP release from the neurohypophysis and potentiates the action of submaximal amounts of AVP on the renal tubule, properties that make it of use in many patients with diabetes insipidus. Doses of 200 to 500 mg, usually taken once daily, are sufficient for an antidiuretic response. Its action starts within several hours of administration and usually lasts for 24 h. Chlorpropamide may also restore thirst perception and thus be useful in patients with thirst center defects. Hypoglycemia may occur but can usually be avoided by adherence to a regular schedule of meals. Clofibrate is capable of stimulating AVP release and has also been used in the treatment of diabetes insipidus. Doses of 500 mg four times a day often result in a prompt and sustained antidiuresis. In some patients, combined treatment with chlorpropamide and clofibrate results in complete restoration of water regulation to normal. Carbamazepine has also been observed to produce antidiuresis in patients with diabetes insipidus by stimulation of AVP release. Doses of 400 to 600 mg daily are effective, but the drug is not widely used owing to toxic side effects.

These therapeutic agents are effective only in central diabetes insipidus. In males with nephrogenic diabetes insipidus the only agents of clinical value are thiazides and other diuretics. By producing sodium depletion, the diuretics cause a fall in glomerular filtration rate with enhanced reabsorption of fluid in the proximal portion of the nephron and decreased delivery of sodium to the ascending limb of the loop of Henle and consequently reduced capacity to dilute the urine. The therapeutic effect of diuretics in patients with nephrogenic diabetes insipidus is lost unless sodium intake is restricted. Two female patients with congenital nephrogenic diabetes insipidus have been treated effectively with large doses of desmopressin.

PROGNOSIS The long-term prospects of a patient with diabetes insipidus are dependent primarily upon the underlying cause. In the

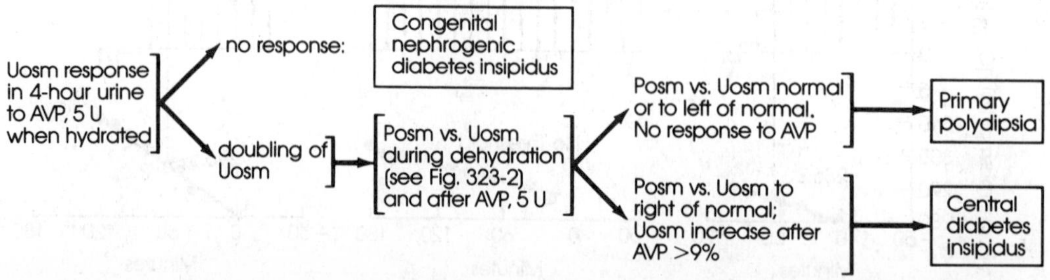

FIGURE 323-5 *Approach to hypotonic polyurias*

TABLE 323-3 Agents used in treatment of diabetes insipidus

	Dose form	Usual dose	Duration of action, h
CENTRAL DIABETES INSIPIDUS			
Hormone replacement:			
Aqueous vasopressin	10 or 20 units/ampul	5–10 units subcutaneously	3–6
Desmopressin	2.5-mL bottle, 0.1 mg/mL	10–20 μg intranasally or 1–4 μg subcutaneously	12–24
Lypressin	5-mL bottle, 50 units/mL	2–4 units intranasally	4–6
Vasopressin tannate in oil	5 units/ampul	5 units intramuscularly	24–72
Nonhormonal agents:			
Chlorpropamide	100- and 250-mg tablets	200–500 mg daily	
Clofibrate	500-mg capsules	500 mg four times daily	
Carbamazepine	200-mg tablets	400–600 mg daily	
NEPHROGENIC DIABETES INSIPIDUS			
Hydrochlorothiazide	50-mg tablets	50–100 mg daily	
Chlorthalidone	50-mg tablets	50 mg daily	

absence of brain tumor or systemic disease, ready access to water and proper treatment of the polyuria usually lead to a normal life and life expectancy. Early recognition and treatment are important to prevent bladder distention, hydroureter, and hydronephrosis which may develop in patients with long-standing polyuria, particularly in patients with nephrogenic diabetes insipidus. The rare patient with adipsia or hypodipsia in association with diabetes insipidus is in danger of developing severe dehydration, which may lead to vascular collapse or central nervous system damage. Similarly severe complications may occur in patients with diabetes insipidus who develop impairment of consciousness. For this reason, all patients with diabetes insipidus should carry identification indicating the presence of the disorder and the necessity for treatment and fluid administration.

SYNDROME OF INAPPROPRIATE AVP SECRETION (SIADH)

The syndrome of inappropriate AVP secretion (known as SIADH) is characterized by hyponatremia that results from water retention attributable to persistent AVP release. In SIADH the vasopressin is released either autonomously or in response to potent stimuli that override the inhibitory influence of hypoosmolality. Since these patients are unable to excrete a dilute urine, ingested fluids are retained, with consequent expansion of the extracellular fluid volume without edema. The continued release of AVP and the consequent elevation of urinary osmolality are considered to be inappropriate only in relationship to the lowered plasma osmolality or sodium concentration.

Water retention can be mediated by AVP through excessive AVP secretion or enhanced renal action of AVP. It can also result from mechanisms unrelated to AVP. A fall in renal blood flow or glomerular filtration rate can increase the percentage reabsorption of sodium and water in the proximal portion of the nephron, with consequent decrease in delivery of sodium and water to the diluting segment. This impairs urinary dilution and leads to water retention.

ETIOLOGY AND PATHOPHYSIOLOGY The various causes of SIADH operate through three pathophysiologic mechanisms (Table 323-4).

In the first of these, AVP is synthesized, stored, and autonomously released from tumor tissue, in amounts that are determined largely by the tumor mass and not by osmolal, volume, pressure, or known chemical stimuli. Small-cell or oat cell carcinoma of the lung accounts for 80 percent of such patients. In prospective studies of patients with oat cell carcinoma, more than half have impaired water excretion and elevated plasma AVP levels, even though many do not have evident hyponatremia. The AVP produced by the neoplasms is identical with arginine vasopressin produced by the normal neurohypophyseal system and may be associated with neurophysin. Other malignancies that can cause SIADH include pancreatic and duodenal carcinomas, lymphosarcoma, reticulum cell sarcoma, Hodgkin's disease, and thymoma.

In the second type of SIADH, nontumorous lung tissue either acquires the capacity to synthesize and release AVP autonomously or reduces left atrial filling which stimulates central AVP release. This type of hyponatremia is a common feature of pulmonary tuberculosis, pneumonias, and other pulmonary or pleural diseases. AVP has been demonstrated in tuberculous lung tissue but not in uninvolved lung or in suspensions of tubercle bacilli.

The third type of SIADH involves release of AVP from the patient's neurohypophysis due to neighboring inflammatory, neoplastic, or vascular lesions (group III, Table 323-4) or of drugs (group IV, Table 323-4), and independently of the normal stimuli.

Chlorpropamide stimulates AVP release, enhances the antidiuretic action of submaximal concentrations of AVP, and can cause water intoxication in patients with diabetes mellitus, particularly in elderly individuals who may be more sensitive to this effect of the drug. The antineoplastic drugs vincristine, vinblastine, and cyclophosphamide produce SIADH by causing release of AVP from the neurohypophysis. The severity of water retention in these patients is aggravated by the

TABLE 323-4 Causes of SIADH

I Malignant neoplasms with autonomous AVP release
- *A* Oat cell carcinoma of lung
- *B* Carcinoma of pancreas
- *C* Lymphosarcoma, reticulum cell sarcoma, Hodgkin's disease
- *D* Carcinoma of duodenum
- *E* Thymoma

II Nonmalignant pulmonary diseases
- *A* Tuberculosis
- *B* Lung abscess
- *C* Pneumonia
- *D* Viral pneumonitis
- *E* Empyema
- *F* Chronic obstructive airways disease

III Central nervous system disorders
- *A* Skull fracture
- *B* Subdural hematoma
- *C* Subarachnoid hemorrhage
- *D* Cerebral vascular thrombosis
- *E* Cerebral atrophy
- *F* Acute encephalitis
- *G* Tuberculous meningitis
- *H* Purulent meningitis
- *I* Guillain-Barré syndrome
- *J* Lupus erythematosus
- *K* Acute intermittent porphyria

IV Drugs
- *A* Chlorpropamide
- *B* Vincristine
- *C* Vinblastine
- *D* Cyclophosphamide
- *E* Carbamazepine
- *F* Oxytocin
- *G* General anesthesia
- *H* Narcotics
- *I* Tricyclic antidepressants

V Miscellaneous causes
- *A* Hypothyroidism
- *B* Positive pressure respiration

common practice of recommending a large fluid intake to prevent formation of uric acid calculi. Carbamazepine can cause water intoxication by stimulating AVP release. Tricyclic compounds can also produce SIADH. Clofibrate is capable of stimulating AVP release but only rarely causes SIADH. Oxytocin possesses inherent antidiuretic activity and, when administered in large amounts to obstetric patients, may cause water intoxication. Patients who have been exposed to general anesthetics or narcotics in association with surgical procedures may release excessive amounts of AVP. Hypothyroidism may produce hyponatremia with all of the features of SIADH by mechanisms involving either increased AVP release or impaired capacity of the kidneys to generate a dilute urine. Elevated plasma AVP concentrations may also occur when AVP release is an appropriate response to hypovolemia, as in sodium depletion (such as after diuretic therapy), adrenal insufficiency, and perhaps congestive heart failure. To consider these conditions as types of SIADH might be technically correct but may lead to the misguided use of fluid restriction.

The excessive AVP release in this syndrome, in the presence of water intake in amounts greater than can be excreted at the existing level of urinary osmolality, results in water retention and extra- and intracellular hypotonicity. Sodium excretion is enhanced because of increased glomerular filtration rate and, probably, suppression of aldosterone secretion. In addition, atrial natriuretic factors may be released by volume expansion and may further contribute to the sodium loss. These urinary losses, which may be profound, aggravate the hypotonicity of body fluids. This combination of factors leads to what many authors describe as a state of euvolemic hyponatremia (in contrast with states of hypovolemic and hypervolemic hyponatremia).

CLINICAL AND LABORATORY FEATURES Patients with SIADH may present with weight gain, weakness, lethargy, and mental confusion, ultimately progressing to convulsions and coma. Edema and hypertension are rare. Laboratory features include low serum levels of BUN, creatinine, uric acid, and albumin. The serum sodium concentration is generally less than 130 meq per liter, and the plasma osmolality is below 270 mosmol/kg. The urine is almost always hypertonic to plasma. Urinary sodium concentration is usually more than 20 meq per liter but may initially be less when chronic sodium depletion is due to poor intake or excessive losses.

DIAGNOSIS SIADH should be suspected in any patient with hyponatremia who excretes urine that is hypertonic relative to plasma. The finding that urinary sodium concentration is greater than 20 meq per liter provides further support for the diagnosis. To make the diagnosis of SIADH it is essential to exclude (1) depletional hyponatremias, especially due to adrenal insufficiency, salt-losing nephritis, diarrhea, and previous diuretic therapy; (2) hyponatremic edema states (congestive heart failure, cirrhosis, nephrosis); (3) pseudohyponatremia (associated with hyperlipemia); (4) severe hyperglycemia; (5) hypothyroidism; (6) primary polydipsia, in which the urine is invariably dilute; and (7) the sick-cell syndrome (essential hyponatremia). In the last disorder the chronic debilitating diseases which it accompanies (congestive heart failure, hepatic cirrhosis, pulmonary tuberculosis, and some malignancies) are thought to reduce osmolality of the intracellular fluid (including that of the hypothalamic osmoreceptors), thereby "setting" the osmoreceptors at a subnormal level. Thus, AVP is released at levels of plasma osmolality below the normal osmotic threshold. These patients show normal renal responses to water loading and deprivation, though the changes occur at subnormal levels of plasma osmolality.

In contrast with patients who have SIADH, patients with depletional hyponatremia are often clearly dehydrated and usually have elevated BUN levels, hemoconcentration, and urinary sodium concentrations below 20 meq per liter (see Chap. 41). Since SIADH is associated with hypervolemia, while primary sodium depletion usually lowers plasma volume, orthostatic hypotension is not a feature of SIADH and is common in depletional hyponatremia. For the same reason, plasma renin activity and plasma aldosterone concentrations are low in SIADH and elevated in sodium depletion except in adrenal insufficiency where plasma renin activity may be high but plasma aldosterone level is usually low. Severe hypertension with hyponatremia may be due to high plasma angiotensin II levels resulting from renovascular stenosis or other forms of angiotensinogenic hypertension, which may increase AVP release. Hypokalemia is uncommon in SIADH.

In patients with the features of SIADH in whom central nervous system disease, pulmonary infections, and the use of drugs capable of causing water retention can be excluded, the possibility of malignancy must be seriously considered, especially oat cell carcinoma of the lung. Water retention and hyponatremia may occur before malignancy can be detected on chest x-ray.

The response to water loading is a useful means of establishing the diagnosis of SIADH. Before water loading is carried out, the serum sodium must be brought to a safe level, generally above 125 meq per liter, by appropriate fluid restriction and sodium administration (if necessary), and the patient must be free of symptoms of hyponatremia. An oral water load of 20 mL per kilogram of body weight is given over a period of 15 to 20 min, and urine is collected hourly for the next 5 h while the patient is recumbent. In normal individuals given such a water load, more than 80 percent of the water is excreted by the end of the fifth hour, and the osmolality of at least one urine specimen, usually in the second hour, falls to less than 100 mosmol/kg (specific gravity 1.005). Patients with hyponatremia who excrete the water load normally may be considered to have essential hyponatremia. In contrast, patients with SIADH have impaired excretion of the water load (often excreting less than 40 percent in 5 h) and fail to dilute the urine to hypotonic levels. When a water load is given to a patient with SIADH, no further water intake should be permitted over the next 24 h or until the serum sodium concentration returns to the pretest value. In this way, production of water intoxication can be avoided. Adrenal insufficiency cannot be distinguished from SIADH by the water load test. A small group of patients with hyponatremia and hypertonic urine demonstrate normal renal excretory and diluting capacity in response to a water load. These individuals should be considered not to have a variant of SIADH but rather to have a downward resetting of their osmoreceptor mechanism so that they dilute and concentrate urine in a normal fashion but around a lowered osmoreceptor set point. In these patients AVP suppresses normally in response to further reduction of plasma osmolality.

Measurements of AVP in patients with SIADH have revealed persistence of inappropriately elevated levels of AVP in plasma and urine when hypoosmolality should normally have inhibited AVP release. In response to further reduction of plasma osmolality after a water load, AVP has remained detectable in plasma and urine, confirming that indeed the secretion is inappropriate relative to plasma osmolality. In SIADH the correlates of plasma osmolality (Posm) versus urinary AVP levels (U_{AVP}) (Fig. 323-3) fall to the left of the values in normal individuals. The initial diagnostic procedures and the more definitive tests for SIADH are summarized in Fig. 323-6.

SIADH cannot be diagnosed with confidence in the presence of severe "stress," pain, hypovolemia, hypotension, and other stimuli that evoke physiologic release of AVP, even in the presence of hypotonicity.

TREATMENT Patients with mild or moderate water intoxication should be treated by restricting fluid intake to about 800 to 1000 mL daily. If water restriction is adequate, a steady increase in serum sodium concentration or osmolality occurs as body weight decreases. Occasional patients with severe water intoxication associated with mental confusion, convulsions, or coma must be treated more vigorously. Intravenous administration of 200 to 300 mL of 5% saline solution is usually sufficient to raise the serum sodium to a level at which the symptoms will improve. This should be accomplished over a period of several hours to avoid the complication of pontine myelinosis, which may result from more rapid increases in serum sodium concentration. When there is the possibility of congestive heart failure due to the fluid overload, the simultaneous administration of large doses of furosemide usually causes a diuresis sufficient to reduce cardiac overload. When furosemide is given, careful attention must be paid to correction of potassium and other electrolyte losses induced by the drug. If, for any reason, intravenous fluid administration is considered necessary when the serum sodium has been raised to an appropriate level, isotonic saline solution and not 5% dextrose solution should be infused slowly to maintain normality of the serum sodium concentration.

Once the initial hyponatremia is improved, careful adherence to a regimen of fluid restriction is necessary to prevent recurrence of water intoxication. Treatment should be directed at the underlying problem. The withdrawal of drugs which might have caused water retention usually results in prompt clearing of SIADH. The SIADH occurring with central nervous system disorders is usually transient and clears with improvement of the underlying disease. In patients with hypothyroidism, correction of the thyroid deficiency by appropriate replacement therapy leads to resolution of hyponatremia. Treatment of pulmonary tuberculosis with appropriate antituberculous therapy results in gradual disappearance of SIADH. Similarly, antibiotic treatment of lung abscess or pneumonia results in resolution of SIADH.

In patients with SIADH due to malignancy, surgical resection, irradiation, or chemotherapy may be successful in alleviating water retention. Sometimes, these measures should be carried out even when there is little likelihood of curing the malignancy, since tumor debulking may correct life-threatening water intoxication and prevent the necessity for rigid fluid restriction. In patients in whom treatment is judged to have been curative, the disappearance of SIADH may confirm the success of treatment. Periodic water load tests may be valuable in following such patients for evidence of recurrence of malignancy.

No drugs are clinically useful in suppressing AVP release from the neurohypophyseal system or from a tumor. Phenytoin inhibits AVP release but is rarely clinically effective. Several opioid agonists, including butorphanol are capable of inhibiting AVP release from the neurohypophysis. Their role in the treatment of SIADH remains to be determined. Drugs capable of blocking AVP effect on the renal tubule may be of value in the chronic management of patients with hyponatremia. Lithium can interfere with the antidiuretic action of AVP on the kidney but is too toxic for use in SIADH. Demeclocycline is effective in interfering with the renal action of AVP. Administration of the drug in doses of 900 to 1200 mg per day to patients with SIADH due to lung malignancy has resulted in diuresis with excretion of an isotonic or hypotonic urine and improvement in hyponatremia. The only untoward effect has been azotemia without other evidence of renal toxicity, which has disappeared promptly on discontinuation of the drug. Thus, demeclocycline may be useful in the management of SIADH when fluid restriction is difficult to accomplish.

PROGNOSIS The prognosis of SIADH depends on the underlying cause of the syndrome. Transient or reversible SIADH as in central nervous system disorders or following use of water-retaining drugs is usually benign as long as proper treatment of acute water intoxication is effectively carried out. SIADH in association with malignancy is ominous, since the malignancies most commonly associated are oat cell carcinoma of the lung and adenocarcinomas of the pancreas, both usually associated with rapid spread and early death.

PARAVENTRICULAR-NEUROHYPOPHYSEAL SYSTEM AND OXYTOCIN

CHEMISTRY AND PHYSIOLOGY Oxytocin, a nonapeptide that differs by two amino acids from vasopressin, is produced predominantly in the cell bodies of the paraventricular nuclei and to a lesser extent in those of the supraoptic nuclei. It is synthesized and transported in neurosecretory granules by way of neuronal axons to the neurohypophysis, where it is stored or released, in conjunction with an oxytocin-specific neurophysin. Oxytocin release is stimulated by nerve impulses originating in the hypothalamus, which cause depolarization of the neurosecretory terminals of the posterior pituitary and subsequent release of oxytocin through a calcium-dependent process, similar to the mechanism for vasopressin. Estrogen stimulates release of oxytocin and its neurophysin. The secretion of oxytocin, as well as of vasopressin, is inhibited by ethanol. Some stimuli such as pain apparently release oxytocin and vasopressin simultaneously, but most stimuli release the two hormones independently. Oxytocin is primarily liberated during suckling, whereas vasopressin is released in much greater quantities than is oxytocin after an osmotic stimulus or hemorrhage. Manipulation or distention of the female genital tract, artificially or during parturition, is a more effective stimulus to oxytocin release than suckling.

Oxytocin acts on the membranes of myometrial and myoepithelial cells and results in an increased force of contraction. Sensitivity of the myometrium to oxytocin increases with the duration of pregnancy, but oxytocin per se probably is not responsible for the initiation and maintenance of labor. Oxytocin may have survival value to the offspring since it may hasten the final stages of birth and lessen the chances of anoxia. Oxytocin also exerts a contractile action on the myometrium post partum and contracts the myoepithelial cells of the mammary alveoli, causing them to expel milk from the secretory tissue to the nipple. Oxytocin is 100 times more potent than vasopressin in its milk-ejecting activity in the human. In contrast, the antidiuretic potency of oxytocin relative to vasopressin is about 1:200. It is unlikely that oxytocin exerts any significant physiologic effect other than on the uterus and breast.

One milligram of purified preparation of oxytocin contains 450 IU of hormone, and the amount of oxytocin in the posterior pituitary ranges from 10 to 15 units. In spite of the fact that there is no known role of oxytocin in the male, the male neural lobe stores oxytocin in amounts similar to those in the female. Plasma oxytocin concentration in both men and women exhibits episodic increases, with values

FIGURE 323-6 *Approach to diagnosis of SIADH in patients with hyponatremia.*

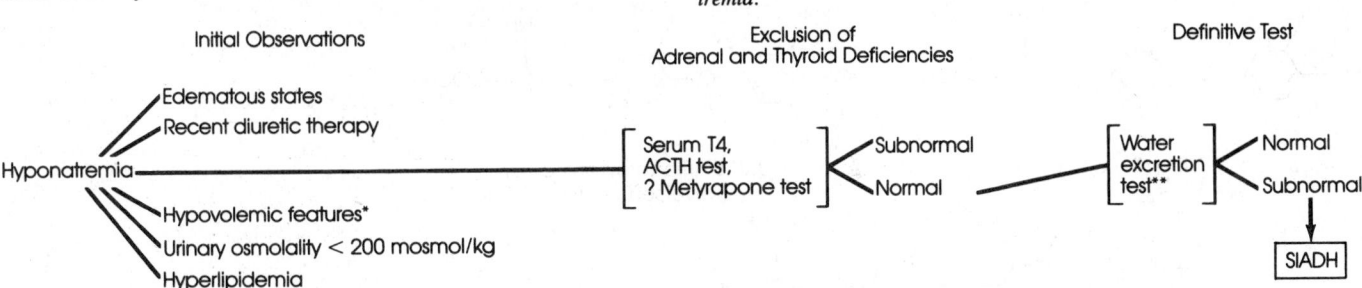

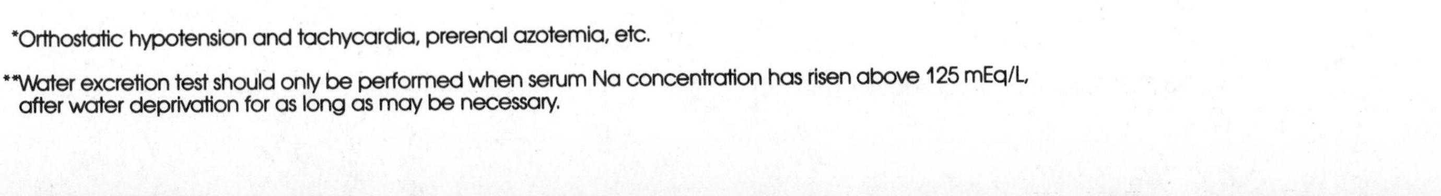

ranging from a low of approximately 0.5 to a high of 2.0 μU/mL but with no diurnal variation. In normal women there is a midcycle increase in plasma oxytocin concentration from a preovulatory value of approximately 1.0 μU/mL to a peak value of 2 to 4 μU/mL at the time of ovulation. During labor, plasma oxytocin concentrations may reach several hundred microunits per milliliter, with a rapid fall to prepartum levels after delivery. During suckling, plasma oxytocin levels of the mother vary but are usually about 5 to 10 μU/mL. The half-life of oxytocin in plasma is about 3 to 5 min. Removal of oxytocin from the circulation is mainly by the kidneys and liver, although the uterus and mammary gland may remove some.

CLINICAL USE OF OXYTOCIN The clinical use of oxytocin is limited to the induction of labor, control of hemorrhage following incomplete abortion and curettage, and treatment of impaired milk ejection. For discussion of the obstetric uses of oxytocin, the reader is referred to textbooks on obstetrics. Care must be taken because oxytocin may cause uterine rupture and fetal death. The antidiuretic action of oxytocin can be elicited with single intravenous doses of as little as 100 mU. Maximal antidiuresis is reached with 40 to 50 mU/min. Since 10 to 40 units of oxytocin per liter of dextrose is often used in obstetric practice, water intoxication may result. The vasodilatory action of oxytocin may cause sudden death of obstetric patients with heart disease because of hypotension, tachycardia, and arrhythmias. Anesthetics may modify the cardiovascular responses to oxytocin. For instance, in patients under cyclopropane anesthesia, oxytocin produces more hypotension but less tachycardia than in unanesthetized subjects. The vasodilatory effect of oxytocin can be blocked by vasopressin.

REFERENCES

BARTTER FC, SCHWARTZ WB: The syndrome of inappropriate secretion of antidiuretic hormone. Am J Med 42:790, 1967

CROSS BA, LENG G: *Progress in Brain Research,* vol 60: *The Neurohypophysis: Structure, Function and Control.* Amsterdam, Elsevier, 1983

KNOBIL E, SAWYER WH (eds): *Handbook of Physiology,* sec 7: *Endocrinology,* vol IV: *The Pituitary Gland—Its Neuroendocrine Control,* part I. Washington, DC, American Physiological Society, 1974

MILLER M et al: Recognition of partial defects in antidiuretic hormone secretion. Ann Intern Med 73:721, 1970

MOSES AM et al: Pathophysiologic and pharmacologic alterations in the release and action of ADH. Metabolism 25:697, 1976

OZERNICHOW P, ROBINSON AE: *Frontiers of Hormone Research,* vol 13: *Diabetes Insipidus in Man.* Basel, Karger, 1985

REICHLIN S: *The Neurohypophysis. Physiological and Clinical Aspects.* New York, Plenum, 1984

ROBERTSON GL: The regulation of vasopressin function in health and disease. Rec Progr Hormone Res 33:333, 1977

SCHRIER RW: *Vasopressin.* New York, Raven, 1985

324 DISEASES OF THE THYROID

SIDNEY H. INGBAR

Normal function of the thyroid gland is directed to the secretion of L-thyroxine (T_4) and 3,5,3′-triiodo-L-thyronine (T_3), iodinated amino acids that are the active thyroid hormones and that influence a diversity of metabolic processes (Fig. 324-1). Diseases of the thyroid gland are manifested by qualitative or quantitative alterations in hormone secretion, enlargement of the thyroid (goiter), or both. Insufficient hormone secretion results in the syndrome of *hypothyroidism* or *myxedema,* in which decreased caloric expenditure (hypometabolism) is a principal feature. Conversely, excessive secretion of active hormone results in hypermetabolism and other features of a syndrome termed *hyperthyroidism* or *thyrotoxicosis.* Enlargement of the thyroid gland (normally 15 to 25 g in adults) may be generalized or focal. Generalized enlargements may not be absolutely symmetric, however, the right lobe tending to enlarge more than the left. They are associated with increased, normal, or decreased hormone secretion, depending upon the underlying disturbance. Truly focal enlargement usually reflects neoplastic disease, either benign or malignant, the former sometimes being responsible for hypersecretion of hormone and hyperthyroidism, the latter very rarely so. Any type of goiter may result in compression of adjacent structures in the neck or mediastinum.

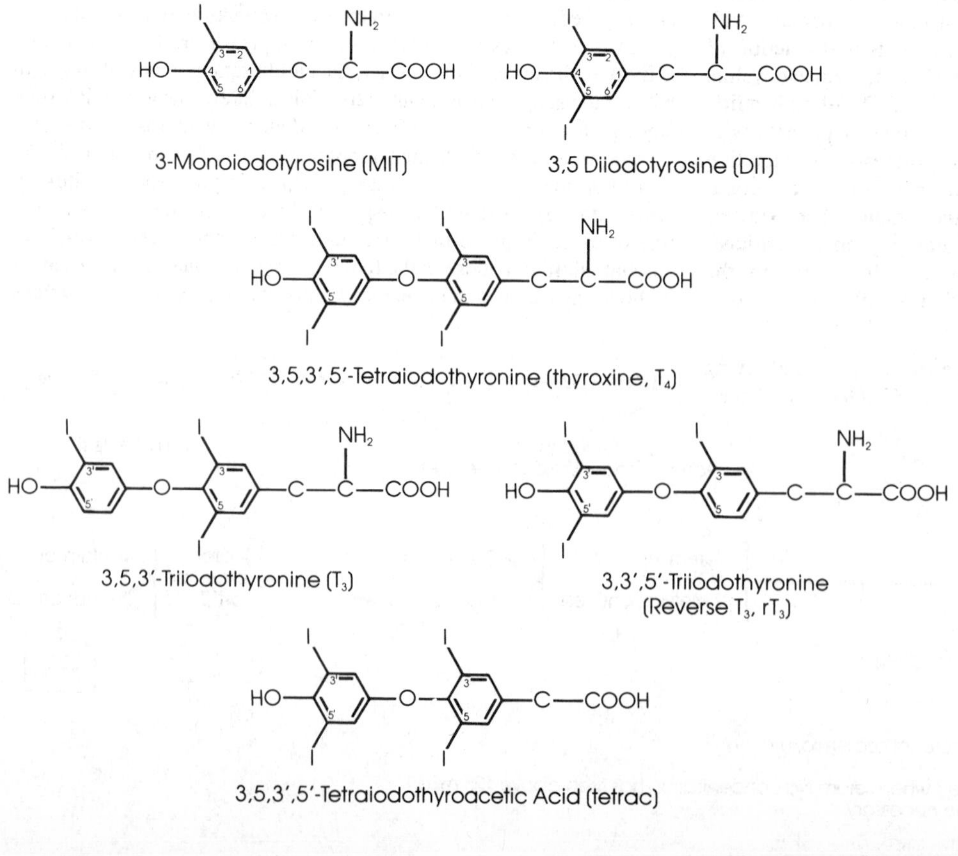

FIGURE 324-1 *Structural formulas of thyroxine, its precursors, and certain of its metabolites.*

EMBRYOLOGY, ANATOMY, AND HISTOLOGY

The human thyroid originates embryologically from an evagination of the pharyngeal epithelium with some cellular contributions from the lateral pharyngeal pouches. Progressive descent of the midline thyroid anlage gives rise to the thyroglossal duct, which extends from the foramen cecum near the base of the tongue to the isthmus of the thyroid. Remnants of tissue may persist along the course of this tract as "lingual thyroid," as thyroglossal cysts or nodules, or as a structure contiguous with the thyroid isthmus called the *pyramidal lobe*. The latter is usually not discernible, except when the remainder of the gland is enlarged. In some individuals, lingual thyroid may be the sole functioning thyroid tissue. In such cases, its secretion may or may not be sufficient to maintain a normal metabolic (euthyroid) state. Thyroid aplasia and functional failure of ectopic thyroid tissue are causes of sporadic neonatal hypothyroidism, an important disorder because of its frequency (1 in every 4000 or 5000 newborns) and its response to early treatment.

The fetal thyroid acquires the capacity to collect and organify iodine at about 10 weeks gestation. Both T_4 and thyroid-stimulating hormone (thyrotropin, TSH) are detectable in the blood soon thereafter and increase in concentration during the second trimester. The increase in serum T_4 is due both to increasing thyroid secretion and to the appearance in plasma of thyroxine-binding globulin (TBG), and the increase in TSH is a reflection of the maturation of the fetal hypothalamus with resulting secretion of thyrotropin-releasing hormone (TRH). Maternal TRH readily crosses the placenta and could play a role in the development of the fetal pituitary-thyroid axis. Maternal TSH, by contrast, does not cross the placenta. T_3 is detectable in the blood later during the second trimester, but its concentration in blood and amniotic fluid remains low until shortly after parturition. By contrast, the concentration of its analogue, 3,3′,5′-triiodo-L-thyronine (reverse T_3, rT_3), is increased in fetal blood and amniotic fluid relative to that in maternal blood (Fig. 324-1). These differences are due to qualitative alterations in T_4 metabolism in the fetus that are discussed below. The low T_3 concentration in fetal blood and amniotic fluid in the face of a high maternal concentration indicates that maternal-fetal transfer of T_3 is minimal, and the same is true of T_4. Hence, T_4 derived from the fetal thyroid is the major thyroid hormone available to the fetus. Except for the possible effect of maternal TRH, therefore, the fetal pituitary-thyroid axis is a functional unit distinct from that of the mother.

The normal adult thyroid contains two lobes joined by an isthmus and lies just anterior and caudad to the cartilages of the larynx. Fibrous septa divide the gland into pseudolobules which, in turn, are composed of vesicles, called *follicles* or *acini,* surrounded by a capillary network. Normally, the follicle walls are composed of cuboidal epithelium. Their lumen is filled with a proteinaceous material termed *colloid,* which contains a protein peculiar to the thyroid, *thyroglobulin,* within the peptide sequence of which T_4 and T_3 are synthesized and stored. The thyroid contains a second population of cells, the C cells. They are the source of calcitonin and give rise to medullary thyroid carcinoma when they undergo malignant transformation.

THYROID HORMONE ECONOMY: NORMAL PHYSIOLOGY

The term *thyroid hormone economy* denotes the complex processes involved in the synthesis of hormones within the thyroid gland; their transport in the circulation; their action and metabolism within the peripheral tissues; and the regulatory mechanisms that maintain a normal supply of thyroid hormones to tissues. This section describes the normal physiology and biochemistry of the thyroid hormone economy. Abnormalities in transport, action, and metabolism are described in the sections dealing with laboratory tests or specific disorders.

HORMONE SYNTHESIS AND SECRETION Thyroid hormone synthesis depends on entry into the thyroid of adequate quantities of iodine, a constituent of the active hormones T_4 and T_3; normality of pathways for iodine metabolism within the gland; and concurrent synthesis of a normal receptor protein for iodine, thyroglobulin. The structure of thyroglobulin favors iodinations and particularly formation of T_4 and T_3. Secretion of normal quantities of hormone, in turn, requires both a normal rate of hormone synthesis and the integrity of processes within the gland by which thyroglobulin is hydrolyzed and the active hormones thereby liberated. Iodine enters the thyroid from the bloodstream in the form of inorganic or ionic iodide whose source is twofold: iodide derived either from the deiodination of thyroid hormones or from iodinated agents that the patient may have received and iodide ingested in food, water, or medication. Formerly, a dietary iodine intake of approximately 200 μg was considered normal within the continental United States, and this was sufficient to sustain a plasma iodide concentration of approximately 0.5 μg/dL. However, owing to iodine contamination of some foods, and to the widespread use of iodine in drugs, vitamin preparations, and antiseptic agents, the average iodine intake has increased to values as high as 1000 μg daily, with corresponding increases in plasma iodide concentration. Iodide is removed from the plasma by the thyroid, kidneys, and salivary and gastrointestinal glands, but since iodide that enters gastrointestinal secretions is reabsorbed, net clearance is effected only by the thyroid and kidneys. In effect, the thyroid and kidneys compete for plasma iodide. Renal clearance is largely a function of glomerular filtration rate and is not influenced by humoral factors or plasma iodide concentration; therefore, the kidney is normally a passive participant in this competition. Hence, adjustments in the rate of entry of iodide into the thyroid relative to the rate of urinary excretion are mediated by changes in thyroid, rather than renal, avidity.

The reactions involved in the synthesis and secretion of the active thyroid hormones can be divided into four sequential steps (Fig. 324-2). The first involves active inward transport of iodide from the

FIGURE 324-2 *Schema depicting pathways in the synthesis and secretion of thyroid hormones and mechanisms for the suprathyroidal and intrathyroidal regulation of thyroid function. Small, solid arrows indicate pathways of iodine metabolism; open arrows indicate stimulation; cross-hatched arrows indicate inhibitory influences. TRH, thyrotropin-releasing hormone; TSH, thyroid-stimulating hormone; IPO, iodide peroxidase; prot., thyroid protease; peptid., thyroid peptidase; MIT, monoiodotyrosine; DIT, diiodotyrosine; T_4, thyroxine; T_3, 3,5,3′-triiodothyronine.*

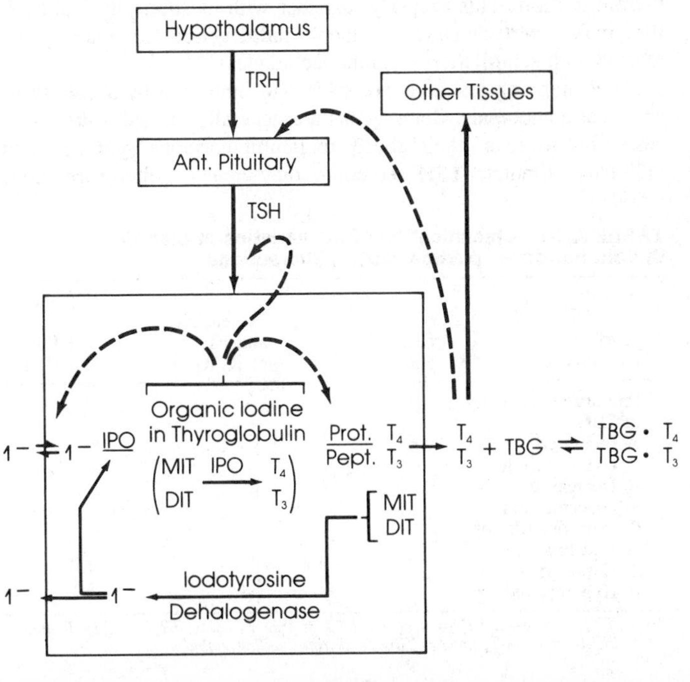

plasma into the thyroid cell and follicular lumen. This occurs at a rate that exceeds passive diffusion of iodide out of the gland, with the result that the thyroid is capable of maintaining concentration gradients for iodide (thyroid/plasma concentration ratios) of substantial magnitude (up to 500, or more, under certain conditions). Energy for iodide transport is phosphate bond–derived and therefore depends upon oxidative metabolism within the gland. The second step in hormone biosynthesis involves oxidation of iodide to a higher valence form that is capable of iodinating tyrosyl residues in thyroglobulin, a glycoprotein of approximately 650,000 mol wt that is synthesized within the follicular cell. Oxidation of iodide is effected by an iodide peroxidase, which utilizes hydrogen peroxide generated during the course of oxidative metabolism within the gland. Organic iodinations occur at the cell-colloid interface, where they take place to a large extent in newly synthesized thyroglobulin undergoing exocytosis into the follicular lumen. They result in the formation of the peptide-bound, hormonally inactive precursors, monoiodotyrosine (MIT) and diiodotyrosine (DIT). Subsequently, these iodotyrosines undergo oxidative condensation, again through the mediation of peroxidase. This coupling reaction occurs within the thyroglobulin molecule and yields a variety of iodothyronines, including T_4 and T_3. Although minute quantities of thyroglobulin are detectable in the blood, most thyroglobulin is retained for a time within the gland, serving as a storage form of thyroid hormone, or "prohormone." Liberation of the active hormones into the blood involves pinocytosis of follicular colloid at the apical margin of the cells to form colloid droplets. Functioning microtubules are necessary for this process. The colloid droplets fuse with thyroid lysosomes to form "phagolysosomes," in which thyroglobulin is hydrolyzed by proteases and peptidases. The final step is release of the free iodothyronines, T_4 and T_3, into the blood. The thyroid gland is the only source of endogenous T_4; in contrast, thyroid secretion normally accounts for only about 20 percent of the T_3 produced, the remainder being generated in extraglandular tissues by the enzymatic removal of the 5′-iodine from the outer ring of T_4. Inactive iodotyrosines liberated by the hydrolysis of thyroglobulin are stripped of their iodine by an intrathyroid enzyme, iodotyrosine dehalogenase. Normally, iodide so liberated is largely reutilized in the synthesis of hormone, but a small proportion is lost into the blood (iodide leak); this proportion may become large in abnormal circumstances.

The thyroid is also capable of concentrating other monovalent anions such as pertechnetate, which is available as the radioactive isotope, sodium [^{99m}Tc]pertechnetate. Unlike iodide, little pertechnetate is organically bound; hence, its duration of stay within the thyroid is short. This property, together with its short physical half-life, makes pertechnetate a valuable radionuclide for imaging the thyroid with scintillation scanning techniques.

The foregoing reactions are subject to inhibition by a variety of chemical compounds. Such agents are generally termed *goitrogens*, since, by virtue of their ability to inhibit hormone synthesis and indirectly stimulate TSH secretion, they induce goiter formation.

TABLE 324-1 Classification of the varieties of disordered thyroid hormone–plasma protein interactions

Type of abnormality	Serum T_4 and T_3	Percent FT_4 and FT_3 or RT_3U	FT_4 and FT_3 or FT_4I and FT_3I
I Primary abnormality in TBG			
A Increased concentration	↑	↓	N
B Decreased concentration	↓	↑	N
II Primary disorder of thyroid function			
A Hypothyroidism	↓	↓	↓
B Hyperthyroidism	↑	↑	↑

NOTE: *FT_4 = free T_4; FT_3 = free T_3; FT_4I = free T_4 index; FT_3I = free T_3 index; RT_3U = resin-T_3 uptake; TBG = thyroid-binding globulin.*

Certain inorganic anions, notably perchlorate and thiocyanate, inhibit the iodide transport mechanism and thereby reduce substrate availability for hormone formation. The goiter and hypothyroidism that follow, however, can be prevented or relieved by doses of iodide sufficiently large to enable adequate quantities to enter the gland by simple diffusion. The commonly employed antithyroid agents, such as the derivatives of thiourea and mercaptoimidazole, exert more complex actions upon hormone biosynthesis. These agents, as well as certain aniline derivatives, inhibit the initial oxidation (organic binding) of iodide, decrease the proportion of DIT relative to MIT, and block coupling of iodotyrosines to form the hormonally active iodothyronines. The latter reaction is the most sensitive. Thus, it is possible for the synthesis of hormonally active iodothyronines to be decreased greatly, although the total incorporation of iodine by the thyroid is inhibited but little. In contrast to the effect of the monovalent anions, the goitrogenic action of inhibitors of organic binding is not overcome by large quantities of iodine. Indeed, certain weak goitrogens, such as sulfonamides and antipyrine, are more potent when given with iodide, an effect not understood. Iodine itself, when given acutely in large doses, is capable of blocking the organic-binding and coupling reactions. This action (Wolff-Chaikoff effect) is normally transient, but in some normal individuals, prolonged administration of iodide is associated with continued inhibition of hormone synthesis and development of goiter, with (iodide myxedema) or without hypothyroidism. Most patients with Graves' disease, especially after treatment with radioiodine or surgery, as well as patients with Hashimoto's disease, are inordinately sensitive to the blocking effect of iodide and develop hypothyroidism when given iodides chronically. The fetal thyroid is similarly sensitive, and consequently pregnant women should not be given iodide in large doses because of the danger of inducing goitrous hypothyroidism in the fetus. Iodide in large doses is capable of inhibiting proteolysis of thyroglobulin and hormone release, an effect that is most readily demonstrable in hyperfunctioning thyroids and that is responsible for the rapid ameliorative action of iodides in most patients with hyperthyroidism. Lithium, which is administered as the carbonate salt in some patients with depressive states, has several effects on intrathyroidal iodine metabolism, one of which is to inhibit hormone release. Dexamethasone in large doses also inhibits hormone release and, in conjunction with iodide, can effect a rapid reduction in the degree of thyrotoxicosis.

HORMONE TRANSPORT AND METABOLISM

HORMONE TRANSPORT In the blood, T_4 and T_3 are almost entirely bound to plasma proteins. T_4 is bound, in decreasing order of intensity, to an inter-alpha globulin, termed thyroxine- or thyronine-binding globulin (TBG), to a T_4-binding prealbumin (TBPA), and to albumin. By virtue of its intense affinity for T_4, TBG is normally the major determinant of overall binding intensity. The interaction between T_4 and its binding proteins conforms to a reversible binding equilibrium in which the majority of the hormone is bound and a small proportion (normally about 0.03 percent) is free. T_3 is not significantly bound by TBPA and is bound less firmly than T_4 by TBG. As a consequence, the normal proportion of free T_3 (approximately 0.3 percent) is 8 to 10 times greater than that of T_4. Only the free or unbound hormone is available to tissues; therefore, the metabolic state correlates more closely with the concentration of free than with the total concentration of hormone in plasma, and homeostatic regulation of thyroid function is directed toward maintenance of a normal concentration of free rather than total hormone. Moreover, the relatively weak binding of T_3 accounts for its failure to contribute materially to the total hormonal iodine concentration in the blood and possibly for its more rapid onset and offset of action. Disturbances of the thyroid hormone–plasma protein interaction are of two general types (see Table 324-1). In the first, the thyroid-pituitary axis is intrinsically normal, and the homeostatic control of thyroid hormone secretion is intact. Under these circumstances, disordered binding interactions result from alterations in thyroid hormone binding. For example, an increase in TBG initially lowers the concentration of free hormone and thus diminishes the quantity of hormone available to tissues. Total hormone concentration in serum then increases until the concentration of free hormone is restored to normal. At this time, the proportions of free T_4 and T_3 are decreased. The increase in total hormone concentration counterbalances the decrease in the free proportion; as a result, the absolute concentration of free hormone is normal, and the metabolic state of the patient is normal. Converse changes occur when the concentration of TBG declines. Table 324-2 summarizes those states associated with primary alterations in the concentration of TBG. Primary disturbances in thyroid hormone binding also occur when other binding proteins in blood are increased, or when abnormal binding proteins appear. These are discussed below.

The second type of disturbance of thyroid hormone–binding interactions results from a primary alteration in the concentration of thyroid hormones in the blood, as in hypothyroidism or thyrotoxicosis. Here, normal homeostatic control of thyroid hormone secretion is lost, either because of disease within the control mechanism itself or because an intact control mechanism is incapable of overcoming the effects of disease elsewhere. Under these circumstances, the concentration of TBG is changed little, if at all, and the concentration of free hormone varies directly with the total concentration of hormone. Since homeostatic mechanisms cannot restore the concentration of free hormone to normal, primary changes in thyroid function are associated with persistent changes in the concentration of total and free hormone, and, consequently, with alterations in the metabolic state. In these disorders, the proportion of free hormone changes in a direction similar to that of the change in hormone supply.

HORMONE METABOLISM Following their penetration into the cell, T_4 and T_3 undergo a variety of reactions that lead ultimately to their excretion or inactivation. Thyroid hormones undergo metabolism mainly through the sequential removal of single iodine atoms (monodeiodinations) that ultimately yields the thyronine nucleus stripped of its iodine content. Deiodinative pathways account for approximately 70 percent of T_4 and T_3 disposal. In the case of T_4, the most important of these is the 5′-monodeiodination that leads to the generation of T_3 (T_3-neogenesis). Since approximately 30 percent of T_4 is converted to T_3 and since T_3 has approximately three times the metabolic potency of T_4, virtually all of the metabolic action of T_4 can be ascribed to the action of the T_3 that it gives rise to. Normally, T_3-neogenesis accounts for about 80 percent of the T_3 in the blood and of overall T_3 production, the remainder coming from direct thyroid secretion. As a consequence, abnormal states and pharmacologic agents that impair T_3-neogenesis lower the serum T_3 concentration (Table 324-3). When patients with thyroid hypofunction are treated with doses of synthetic T_4 (levothyroxine) sufficient to sustain serum T_4 concentrations within or somewhat above the normal range, normal or nearly normal serum T_3 concentrations are maintained. The generalization that the thyroid secretes relatively little T_3 does not apply to states in which the thyroid is hyperfunctioning or under increased stimulation by TSH or when thyroid iodine content is reduced. Under these conditions, the T_3:T_4 ratio of the secretory product and the serum concentration of T_3 relative to that of T_4 are increased. In addition, when T_4 production is decreased, as in early thyroid failure or iodine deficiency, the T_3:T_4 concentration ratio in blood is increased still further by an autoregulatory mechanism that leads to an increase in the efficiency of T_3-neogenesis.

Approximately 40 percent of T_4 disposal is accounted for by monodeiodination at the 5 position of its inner ring to yield 3,3′,5′-triiodo-L-thyronine (reverse T_3,rT_3); this process accounts for nearly all rT_3 produced. rT_3 has little if any metabolic potency; therefore, the relative poise between outer- and inner-ring monodeiodination of T_4 determines the quantity of metabolically active hormone available. Factors that impair T_3-neogenesis almost invariably increase serum rT_3 concentrations. This increase is not due to an increase in the production of rT_3 from T_4, but rather to a decrease in the 5′-monodeiodination of rT_3 to yield 3,3′-diiodothyronine (3,3′T_2), i.e., both the decreased conversion of T_4 to T_3 and the decreased degradation of rT_3 are due to a selective impairment of 5′-monodeiodination.

A second major pathway of metabolism of T_4 and T_3 and of their metabolites is conjugation in the liver, principally with glucuronate and sulfate. Conjugates either undergo deiodination locally or are secreted into the bile, but the magnitude of the enterohepatic circulation in humans is unknown. Reabsorption is incomplete at best, since the fecal excretion of T_4, T_3, and their iodine-containing metabolites accounts for approximately 20 percent of overall T_4 disposal. A small proportion of T_4 and T_3 (approximately 20 percent) undergoes oxidative deamination and decarboxylation of the alanine side chain to yield the acetic acid analogues tetraiodo- and triiodothyroacetic acid (tetrac and triac, respectively).

Under certain circumstances, changes in hormone accumulation and metabolism are the major determinant of changes in the rates of metabolic clearance of T_4 and T_3. Both phenobarbital and phenytoin increase the metabolic clearance of thyroid hormones without increasing the proportion of free hormone in the blood. Indeed, in the case of phenytoin, both total and free T_4 concentrations are diminished. Nevertheless, a normal metabolic state is maintained possibly because of an increase in T_3-neogenesis.

HORMONE ACTION The thyroid hormones influence the growth and maturation of tissues, total energy expenditure, and the turnover of essentially all substrates, vitamins, and hormones, including the thyroid hormones themselves. The primary mechanisms whereby these effects are initiated remain uncertain, but the hormones appear to act in a coordinated manner at the level of the nucleus to alter genomic expression, at the level of the mitochondrion to influence oxidative metabolism, and at the level of the plasma membrane to influence the transcellular flux of substrates and cations.

REGULATION OF THYROID FUNCTION Regulation of thyroid function is effected by two general mechanisms, one suprathyroid and one intrathyroid in locus (Fig. 324-2). The proximate mediator of suprathyroid regulation is thyrotropin (thyroid-stimulating hormone, TSH), a glycoprotein secreted by basophilic (thyrotropic) cells in the anterior pituitary. TSH stimulates thyroid hypertrophy and hyperplasia; accelerates most aspects of intermediary metabolism in the thyroid; enhances synthesis of nucleic acid and protein, including

TABLE 324-2 Circumstances associated with altered concentration of TBG

Increased TBG	Decreased TBG
Pregnancy	Androgenic and anabolic steroids
Newborn state	Large doses of glucocorticoid
Oral contraceptives and other sources of estrogen	Chronic liver disease
Tamoxifen	Severe systemic illness
Infectious and chronic active hepatitis	Active acromegaly
Biliary cirrhosis	Nephrosis
Acute intermittent porphyria	Genetically determined
Perphenazine	Asparaginase
Genetically determined	

TABLE 324-3 States associated with decreased peripheral conversion of T_4 to T_3

I Physiologic
- *A* Fetal and early neonatal life
- *B* ? Old age

II Pathologic
- *A* Fasting
- *B* Malnutrition
- *C* Systemic illness
- *D* Physical trauma
- *E* Postoperative state
- *F* Drugs (propylthiouracil, dexamethasone, propranolol, amiodarone)
- *G* Radiographic contrast agents (Oragrafin, Telepaque)

thyroglobulin; and stimulates all steps in the synthesis and secretion of thyroid hormones. These actions of TSH result from binding of the hormone to specific receptors in the surface of the follicular cell and subsequent activation of the plasma membrane enzyme adenylate cyclase. The resulting increase in the cellular cyclic 3′,5′-adenosine monophosphate (cyclic AMP) concentration initiates most or all of the responses that characterize the action of TSH.

Regulation of TSH secretion, in turn, is effected by two opposing influences at the level of the thyrotropic cell. Thyrotropin-releasing hormone (TRH), a tripeptide of hypothalamic origin, stimulates the secretion and synthesis of TSH, whereas thyroid hormones both inhibit the TSH secretory mechanism directly and antagonize the action of TRH. Thus, homeostatic control of TSH secretion is exerted in a negative-feedback manner by thyroid hormones, and the threshold for feedback inhibition is apparently set by TRH. TRH is synthesized in the ventromedial hypothalamus, reaches the pituitary via the hypophyseal portal blood system, and binds to specific receptors on the plasma membrane of the thyrotropic cell. Either activation of the adenylate cyclase system or a concomitant translocation of extracellular calcium into the cell initiates release of TSH. To what extent, if any, suprahypothalamic centers influence the secretion of TRH is uncertain. The negative-feedback effect of the thyroid hormones appears to take place entirely at the level of the thyrotropic cell. Thyroid hormones do not directly affect the hypothalamic secretion of TRH but reduce the number of TRH receptors on the thyrotrophic cell, thus impairing its responsiveness to TRH. The negative-feedback action of the thyroid hormones is apparently mediated by an inhibitory protein whose synthesis is induced by binding of the hormones to specific receptors in the nucleus of the thyrotrophic cell. The principal arbiter of thyroid hormone action within the pituitary is T_3, both that generated locally from intrapituitary T_4 and that derived from the pool of free T_3 in the plasma. To what extent T_4 itself is effective within the pituitary is uncertain, but other factors modify the secretion of TSH and its response to TRH. Both somatostatin and dopamine appear to be physiologic inhibitors of TRH secretion. Estrogens enhance responsiveness to TRH, whereas glucocorticoids inhibit this function.

Intrathyroid regulation of thyroid function is also important. In some manner, changes in glandular organic iodine content cause reciprocal changes in thyroid iodide transport activity and regulate growth, amino acid uptake, glucose metabolism, and nucleic acid synthesis. These influences are evident in the absence of TSH stimulation and hence may be termed *autoregulatory,* but their most important role is to modify (iodine-enrichment inhibiting and iodine-depletion enhancing) the response to TSH, probably by modifying the generation of cyclic AMP consequent to TSH stimulation.

LABORATORY TESTS

Laboratory tests of thyroid hormone economy can be divided into five major categories: direct tests of thyroid function, tests related to the concentration and binding of thyroid hormones in blood, metabolic indexes, tests of the homeostatic control of thyroid function, and various tests that do not fit into other categories.

DIRECT TESTS OF THYROID FUNCTION Among all tests designed to assess thyroid status, only those that involve in vivo administration of radioactive iodine test glandular function per se, and measurement of the *thyroid radioactive iodine uptake* (RAIU) is the most common. ^{131}I has been used for this purpose for decades, but ^{123}I is preferable because of the lower radiation dose that it delivers. The administered radioiodine mixes uniformly with the endogenous iodide in the extracellular fluid and, in the steady state, can be used to assess what percentage of the iodide entering and leaving the extracellular space per unit time is accumulated by the thyroid. The RAIU is usually measured 24 h after administration of the isotope since it has usually reached a plateau value at this time, but in states of severe thyroid hyperfunction it may peak early. The RAIU varies inversely with the plasma iodide concentration and directly with the functional state of the thyroid. At usual levels of iodine intake in the United States (up to 1000 μg per day), the normal range for the 24-h RAIU is approximately 5 to 30 percent of the administered dose. Consequently, this test discriminates poorly between normal and hypothyroid states. Values above the normal range, however, indicate thyroid hyperfunction and are useful in the diagnosis of hyperthyroidism. The RAIU is also used as part of the thyroid suppression test.

The principal value of the test, however, is in the diagnosis of disorders in which thyrotoxicosis is associated with a low value of the RAIU. These include iodine-induced hyperthyroidism, thyrotoxicosis factitia, and the spontaneously resolving thyrotoxicosis that is associated with painless chronic thyroiditis or subacute thyroiditis.

TESTS RELATED TO HORMONE CONCENTRATION AND BINDING IN BLOOD Measurement of the concentration of one or both thyroid hormones in serum, T_4 and T_3, in conjunction with some assessment of hormone binding, is generally the most reliable means of confirming a diagnosis of hyperthyroidism or hypothyroidism. Highly specific and sensitive radioimmunoassays are used to measure *serum T_4* and *T_3* concentrations and when indicated for measuring *serum rT_3* concentration. The approximate normal ranges are 4 to 12 μg/dL for T_4, 80 to 100 ng/dL for T_3, and 10 to 40 ng/dL for rT_3.

Measurements of serum *protein-bound iodine* (PBI) were once used as an indirect means of assessing serum T_4 concentration. At present, the serum PBI is occasionally measured as a means of detecting release from the thyroid of abnormal iodoproteins, such as occurs in various forms of thyroiditis or as the result of an intrathyroid biosynthetic defect.

As mentioned in a previous section, alterations in the intensity of hormone binding by plasma proteins, as well as alterations in the rate of hormone secretion, influence the concentration of hormone in the blood. However, only alterations in hormone secretion lead to steady-state alterations in the concentration of free hormone. Because they most consistently reflect the rate of hormone production, free hormone concentrations usually correlate better with the metabolic state than do total hormone concentrations. The free T_4 concentration (FT_4) can be measured by equilibrium dialysis of serum enriched with a tracer quantity of labeled T_4. The percent of T_4 that is dialyzable or free is thereby determined, and the product of this value and the total T_4 is the FT_4. However, the dialysis technique is cumbersome; for clinical purposes, the *in vitro uptake test* is simple to perform and usually provides the same information. Here, the serum is enriched with labeled T_4 or labeled T_3 and is then incubated with an insoluble, particulate matter, such as resin or charcoal, that binds free hormone. The percent of labeled hormone taken up by the particulate material varies inversely with both the concentration of unoccupied sites among the serum proteins and their affinity for the particular hormone being used. Labeled T_3 is usually used in preference to labeled T_4, since it is less strongly bound in the serum and hence yields higher, and therefore more nearly accurate, uptake values (resin T_3 uptake, RT_3U). In most clinical conditions, values of the RT_3U are proportionate to those of the percent of FT_4 and percent of FT_3. This proportionality reflects the fact that in normal serum T_4 and T_3 are mainly bound by a common binding site on TBG. Therefore, alterations in binding produced by an excess or deficiency of TBG, or by an excessive or insufficient supply of T_4, do not seriously disturb the relationship between the intensity of T_4 binding and that of T_3. Under these conditions, therefore, one may calculate a *free T_4 index* (FT_4I) and a *free T_3 index* (FT_3I) as the product of the RT_3U and the total T_4 and T_3 concentrations, respectively, and these are proportional to the actual FT_4 and FT_3. (In practice, values of the FT_3 and FT_3I are rarely determined.)

Primary alterations in plasma TBG concentration (Table 324-2) produce changes in the RT_3U that are inverse and approximately proportionate to those in the serum T_4 and serum T_3; as a result, the FT_4I and FT_3I remain normal. By contrast, alterations in T_4 secretion cause changes in the percent FT_4 and RT_3U that are in the same direction as those in serum T_4. As a result, the FT_4 and FT_4I deviate from normal values more markedly than do the percent FT_4 and RT_3U alone. Radioimmunoassay methods for the direct measurement of FT_4 have been developed; some provide reliable results in a wide range of disorders and can replace measurement of the FT_4I in the diagnosis of thyrotoxicosis and hypothyroidism.

As noted earlier, several disorders are characterized by increased plasma binding of T_4 in which, because the protein involved is not TBG, the intensity of T_4 binding relative to that of T_3 is abnormal. Most commonly, binding of T_4 is greatly enhanced, while that of T_3 is increased little, if at all. Included among these disorders is *familial dysalbuminemic hyperthyroxinemia (FDH)*, transmitted by autosomal dominant inheritance, in which the plasma concentration of an albumin variant with an unusually high affinity for T_4 is increased. As a result, the serum T_4 is markedly elevated, but in keeping with the euthyroid state FT_4 is normal. Because the RT_3U does not reflect the increase in the intensity of T_4 binding, calculated values of the FT_4I are greatly increased, often leading to a mistaken diagnosis of thyrotoxicosis. Similar findings occur when there is *increased T_4 binding by TBPA* or when the patient, usually one with autoimmune thyroid disease, develops *circulating antibodies* against T_4 itself.

In the foregoing disorders, in which the serum T_4 is increased owing to an increase in T_4 binding, the FT_4 and the metabolic state are normal. They are therefore classified among the disorders that lead to a state of *euthyroid hyperthyroxinemia,* a term that implies the presence of hyperthyroxinemia not caused by intrinsic thyroid disease (Table 324-4). The mechanism responsible for these findings is variable and in some cases uncertain. Also uncertain is the impact of these increases in FT_4 on the metabolic state, but the clinician should be aware of these causes of euthyroid hyperthyroxinemia lest hyperthyroidism be mistakenly diagnosed.

Some states are associated with an increased thyroid secretion of T_3, at least relative to the secretion of T_4. As a result, the serum T_3 concentration is disproportionately high relative to the prevailing serum T_4 concentration. This is apparently a consequence of hyperfunction of the follicular cell, since it is seen in all varieties of hyperthyroidism and in early thyroid failure, in which the gland is exposed to enhanced stimulation by TSH. Accordingly, the serum T_3 concentration and the derived FT_3I are generally superior to the corresponding values for T_4 in the diagnosis of hyperthyroidism. In *early* hypothyroidism, by contrast, the serum T_3 concentration and FT_3I may be normal despite subnormal values for the serum T_4 concentration and FT_4I.

Measurement of the serum rT_3 concentration is valuable in differentiating the low T_3 syndrome from intrinsic hypothyroidism; in the former state, the serum rT_3 concentration is increased, whereas in the latter it is usually subnormal.

METABOLIC INDEXES Tests in this category assess the metabolic impact of thyroid hormone in the peripheral tissues. Though tests of this type have value in the investigative setting, none of sufficient sensitivity, specificity, and ease of performance is available for routine use. Measurements of oxygen consumption in the basal state (basal metabolic rate, BMR) were once a mainstay in the diagnosis of thyroid disease but are now of historic interest. Serum concentrations of the MM isoenzyme of creatine phosphokinase and, less frequently, lactic dehydrogenase and aspartate aminotransferase are increased in hypothyroidism and may be slightly decreased in hyperthyroidism. The changes are nonspecific, and appreciation of them is important only in avoiding the inference that other diseases that produce similar changes are present. The concentrations in serum of testosterone-binding globulin (TeBG) and of angiotensin-converting enzyme are thyroid hormone–dependent and are, therefore, increased in thyrotoxicosis, but their utility in the diagnosis of thyroid disease has not been demonstrated. Increases in the *serum cholesterol concentration* are common in hypothyroidism of thyroid origin; however, decreases in serum cholesterol are of little value in the diagnosis of thyrotoxicosis. *Systolic time indexes,* such as the preejection period and pulse-wave arrival time, are prolonged in hypothyroidism and shortened in hyperthyroidism. They are of value in monitoring thyroid replacement therapy in elderly patients or in patients with coexisting heart disease.

TESTS OF HOMEOSTATIC CONTROL Measurement of the basal *serum TSH concentration* by radioimmunoassay is useful in the diagnosis of both advanced and subclinical hypothyroidism. The latter state represents a stage in the evolution of hypothyroidism, in which a structural or functional abnormality that impairs hormone synthesis is compensated for by hypersecretion of TSH and activation of the thyroid. The normal TSH level is less than 5 μU/mL. In thyrotoxic states, serum TSH concentration is almost always low or undetectable. This is of little diagnostic value, since most assays cannot distinguish between normal and subnormal values. Serum TSH concentrations are absolutely or inappropriately elevated, relative to serum FT_4 and FT_3 values, in patients with TSH-induced hyperthyroidism. This rare syndrome results either from a TSH-secreting pituitary adenoma or resistance of the TSH secretory mechanism to feedback inhibition by T_4 and T_3. Measurement of serum TSH is the best means of distinguishing between untreated hypothyroidism of thyroid origin, in which the values are invariably increased, and pituitary or hypothalamic hypothyroidism, in which the values are usually undetectable or within the normal range. Occasional patients with hypothyroidism of hypothalamic or pituitary origin secrete a form of TSH that is immunoactive but not bioactive. Here, serum TSH concentrations may be elevated rather than depressed.

TABLE 324-4 States associated with euthyroid hyperthyroxinemia

Disorder	FT_4	FT_4I	T_3	TSH	Comments
I Increased T_4 binding					
A Increased TBG	N	N	↑	N	See Tables 324-1 and 324-2
B FDH	N	↑	N,Sl ↑	N	Autosomal dominant inheritance
C Increased TBPA binding	N	↑	N	N	Increased concentration (islet-cell tumor) or affinity
D Anti-T_4 antibody	N	↑	N	N	Anti-T_3 antibody may be present
II Pituitary and peripheral thyroid hormone resistance	↑	↑	↑	↑	If only pituitary resistant, patient thyrotoxic
III Various disorders					
A Sick euthyroid syndrome	↑	↑	↓	N, ↓	Uncommon; poorly understood
B Acute psychiatric illness	↑	↑	N, ↑	N, ↑	Remits without treatment in several weeks
C Hyperemesis gravidarum	↑	↑	N	↓	Remits in several weeks
IV Drugs					
A Inhibitors of T_3-neogenesis					
1 X-ray contrast agents	↑	↑	↓	↑	Particularly ipodate and iopanoate
2 Propranolol	↑	↑	↓	N, ↑	Especially with large doses
3 Amiodarone	↑	↑	↓	↑	Increased TSH during first several months
B Heparin	↑	↑	N	—	Requires only small intravenous doses
C Levothyroxine therapy	↑	↑	N	↓	Hyperthyroxinemia in about 50% of cases

NOTE: *FT_4 = free T_4 concentration; FT_4I = free T_4 index calculated from an in vitro T_3 uptake test; TSH = basal serum TSH concentration and response to TRH; N = normal; Sl = slightly.*

The *thyrotropin-releasing hormone* (*TRH*) *stimulation test* assesses the functional state of the TSH-secretory mechanism, and has diagnostic value in diverse circumstances. Following the intravenous injection of TRH in normal subjects, the serum TSH begins to increase at 10 min, reaches a maximum between 20 and 45 min, and then rapidly declines. The nature of the pituitary feedback mechanism is such that, when hypothalamic-pituitary function is normal, one would expect an increased response to TRH when the thyrotropic cell senses a deficiency of thyroid hormone, particularly T_3, and a decreased or absent response when there is thyroid hormone excess. Thus, except in the rare instances of pituitary resistance to thyroid hormone, in which responses are usually normal, thyrotoxicosis is invariably accompanied by a blunted or absent TSH response to TRH. Owing to extreme sensitivity of the TSH-secretory mechanism to feedback inhibition, diminished responses to TRH commonly occur in clinically euthyroid patients with autonomously functioning toxic adenomas or toxic multinodular goiters and possibly in some patients with euthyroid Graves' disease. In addition, responses to TRH are often decreased in elderly individuals, especially men. Despite these exceptions, a subnormal or absent response to TRH is an excellent confirmatory test for thyrotoxicosis. TRH tests are of lesser value in the diagnosis of hypothyroidism. Responses are increased in patients with primary hypothyroidism, but the magnitude of increase is generally proportional to the extent of increase in basal serum TSH. Some patients with pituitary hypothyroidism have subnormal responses, and some with TRH deficiency owing to hypothalamic disease have a near normal response, but these expected responses are not seen consistently. Further, in as many as one-fourth of patients with hypothyroidism due to hypothalamic-pituitary disease, basal serum TSH concentrations are normal or slightly elevated, and the response to TRH is exaggerated.

The *thyroid suppression test* is used to assess whether thyroid function is controlled by normal homeostatic mechanisms. Normally, exogenous thyroid hormone suppresses pituitary TSH secretion, resulting in a decrease in the RAIU. Since liothyronine is usually employed (100 μg daily for 10 days), the resulting decline in serum T_4, as well as in the RAIU, can serve as an index of suppression. A normal suppressive response is a decrease of the RAIU to less than half of the control value and a decline of the serum T_4 to low normal or subnormal values. An abnormal suppression test is always present in hyperthyroidism, irrespective of the underlying cause; this indicates either autonomy of thyroid function, the presence of an abnormal stimulator, or unremitting hypersecretion of TSH. A normal suppression test, on the other hand, is incompatible with and excludes a diagnosis of hyperthyroidism. An abnormal suppression test is not pathognomonic of hyperthyroidism, however, since it is seen after treatment of hyperthyroidism in Graves' disease, in about half of the euthyroid patients with the ophthalmopathy of Graves' disease, and in seemingly euthyroid patients in whom autonomous hyperfunctioning adenomas suppress the remainder of the gland.

Because of the risk of adverse effects of exogenous thyroid hormone in elderly patients and in those with cardiovascular disease, and since the TRH test is almost entirely devoid of undesirable side effects, the latter test has almost entirely supplanted the thyroid suppression test as an aid in the diagnosis of hyperthyroidism.

MISCELLANEOUS TESTS Various tests that do not assess thyroid function are of value in defining the nature of the thyroid disorder or in planning therapy. For example, high titers of *antimicrosomal antibodies* or *antithyroglobulin antibodies* are found in the serum of most adults with Hashimoto's disease and in many patients with primary thyroprivic hypothyroidism or Graves' disease. In the latter, the serum also contains antibodies aginst the TSH receptor in the thyroid plasma membrane. In general, these are capable of inhibiting the receptor binding of TSH (TSH-binding inhibitory immunoglobulins, TBII) and of stimulating the production of cyclic AMP therein (thyroid-stimulating immunoglobulins, TSI). The clinical utility of tests for TBII and TSI stems from the fact that the disappearance of the factors from the serum during a course of antithyroid therapy implies the likelihood of a long-term remission of hyperthyroidism when therapy is withdrawn. In some patients, analogous antibodies have no intrinsic stimulatory effect but block the response to endogenous TSH and produce nongoitrous hypothyroidism. Both stimulatory and blocking anti-TSH receptor antibodies have the ability to cross the placenta and, as a consequence, to produce transient hyperthyroidism (neonatal Graves' disease) or hypothyroidism, respectively, in the newborn.

Some patients, most commonly those with autoimmune thyroid disease, develop *circulating antibodies against T_3 or T_4*, or both. In radioimmunoassays for these hormones, because the endogenous antibody competes with the exogenous antibody for binding of the added labeled ligand, spurious values for the concentration of the hormone are obtained. These may be grossly elevated or greatly depressed, depending on the technique of radioimmunoassay used. The true concentration of the hormone, as determined in extracts of the serum, is increased owing to the additional binding sites provided by the antibody, but antibody-bound hormone is unavailable for metabolic action. In the case of anti-T_3 antibodies, which are the more common, values of the RT_3U are low because endogenous antibody competes with the resin for binding of the added labeled T_3. Such antibodies can be detected by adding labeled hormone to serum, separating the immunoglobulins from other serum proteins by any of several techniques, and demonstrating that they bind the labeled hormone.

Along with several other thyroid disorders, differentiated carcinomas of the thyroid release thyroglobulin into the bloodstream. As a consequence, measurements of the *serum thyroglobulin concentration* by radioimmunoassay have value not in the initial diagnosis of thyroid carcinoma but in assessing the adequacy of initial therapy and in monitoring for recurrence or dissemination of the disease. In patients with thyrotoxicosis, subnormal serum thyroglobulin concentrations together with decreased values of the RAIU suggest the presence of thyrotoxicosis factitia.

Imaging by *scintiscanning* permits localization of sites of accumulation of radioiodine or sodium [^{99m}Tc]pertechnetate. This technique is useful for defining areas of increased or decreased function within the thyroid and for detecting retrosternal goiter, ectopic thyroid tissue, hemiagenesis of the thyroid, and functioning metastases of thyroid carcinoma. Ultrasonic examination of the thyroid is also a valuable technique for differentiating cystic nodules from those that are solid. Since ultrasonic scans provide an accurate indication of size, are noninvasive, and apparently have no injurious effects, sequential scans can be employed to assess changes in the size of the thyroid as a whole or of discrete nodules over time or in response to treatment.

SICK EUTHYROID SYNDROME

Severe illness, physical trauma, or physiologic stress can induce changes in one or more aspects of thyroid hormone economy, leading to findings referred to as the sick euthyroid syndrome (SES). Abnormalities in SES include alterations in the peripheral transport and metabolism of the thyroid hormones; the regulation of TSH secretion; and in some cases changes in thyroid function itself. Acting alone or together, these lead to changes in the concentrations of the circulating thyroid hormones, both total and free, that serve to define the several variants of the SES. Because of the frequency of illness in the general population and the nonspecificity of the disorders that cause it, SES is probably a more common cause of abnormalities in the concentration of thyroid hormones in the blood than intrinsic thyroid disease.

NORMAL T_4 VARIANT OF SES Decreased production of T_3 owing to inhibition of the peripheral 5′-monodeiodination of T_4 is a consistent feature of the SES. This is reflected in a decrease in the serum total

T_3 concentration that varies in severity with that of the illness. In moderately ill patients, serum total T_4 concentration is within the normal range. A decrease in the intensity of protein binding, greater for T_4 than T_3, is an additional accompaniment. As a result, values of the RT_3U are moderately increased, and the percent FT_4 is increased to a proportionately greater extent. As a consequence, values of the free T_4 index (FT_4I) and those of the free T_4 concentrations (FT_4) are often increased. Serum rT_3 concentrations are increased, owing to a decrease in the plasma clearance of rT_3 secondary to inhibition of its 5′-monodeiodination. The plasma clearance rate of T_4 is increased, probably as a result of decreased T_4 binding, and this, in the face of normal T_4 concentrations, indicates that the overall rate of T_4 degradation and production is increased. Production rates for T_3 are decreased, and those for rT_3 are normal. Serum TSH concentration and the response of serum TSH to TRH are generally normal, though they may increase to supranormal values and then return to normal as recovery from the illness takes place. Despite the reduction in the serum T_3 concentration, this variant of the SES can be separated from intrinsic thyroid disease because the serum T_4 and TSH are normal and because the serum T_3 is not useful for diagnosing hypothyroidism in any event.

LOW T_4 VARIANT OF SES In more seriously ill patients, T_3 production rates and serum total and free T_3 concentrations decrease still further, and abnormalities in hormone binding increase in severity. As a consequence, serum T_4 concentrations decrease into the hypothyroid range, sometimes markedly so. This is partly but not entirely due to decreased T_4 binding since values of the FT_4 are frequently subnormal. These are probably the result of decreased T_4 production that occurs in the most severely ill patients. Decreased production of T_4 appears to be secondary to decreased secretion of TSH. Serum TSH concentrations appear normal by conventional assay but are low with sensitive TSH assays, and TRH responses may be blunted. Hence, in this variant of the SES, there is an inappropriate hyposecretion of TSH, considering the low serum total and free T_4 and T_3 concentrations; its cause is unknown, but a diagnosis of organic pituitary hypothyroidism may be suggested. Production rates for rT_3 are diminished, owing to the decreased availability of its precursor T_4; nonetheless, serum rT_3 concentrations are increased, owing to retardation of its degradation, and this provides an important means of differentiating the SES from pituitary hypothyroidism, in which serum rT_3 concentrations are low. In patients with primary hypothyroidism who have associated illness, serum TSH concentrations remain elevated, though their concentrations are generally lower than they otherwise would be.

HIGH T_4 VARIANT OF SES An unusual variant of the SES (approximately 1 percent of sick patients) is associated with increased serum total and free T_4 concentrations during acute illness and return to normal thereafter. This variant is most often seen in elderly women, many of whom have received medications that contain iodine. The principal source of diagnostic confusion is with the syndrome of "T_4 toxicosis," i.e., illness superimposed on true thyrotoxicosis, so that serum T_4 concentrations are increased and serum T_3 concentrations are normal. In the latter, however, serum rT_3 concentrations are higher, values of the serum total T_3 and FT_3I are higher, and TRH responses are blunted.

ABNORMALITIES IN HORMONE BINDING IN SES Multiple factors are responsible for the decreased binding of T_4 and, to a lesser extent, T_3 that occurs in the SES. Illness is associated with decreased synthesis of TBPA and a decrease in its serum concentration, but the extent to which this contributes to decreased T_4 binding is uncertain. In chronically ill patients, serum TBG concentration is subnormal. When present, this undoubtedly is a contributory factor. Most often, however, the extent of decreased T_4 binding cannot be explained by decreases in serum TBPA and TBG, and an inhibitor of hormone binding may be responsible. Its nature is uncertain, but it may be one or more fatty acids, which may also be responsible for diminished conversion of T_4 to T_3.

The importance of the SES is that the changes in circulating thyroid hormone concentrations that result should not be confused with those due to intrinsic thyroid or pituitary disease. Unresolved questions are whether the metabolic impact of thyroid hormone in peripheral tissues is decreased in the SES, whether the syndrome is a beneficial or adverse response to illness, and whether some patients would benefit from treatment with thyroid hormones.

SIMPLE (NONTOXIC) GOITER

Endemic goiter implies an etiologic factor or factors common to a particular geographic region. The term has been defined as the presence of generalized or localized thyroid enlargement in more than 10 percent of the population. The connotation of *sporadic* goiter is that goiter arises in nonendemic areas as a result of a stimulus that does not affect the population generally. Since these terms fail to define or distinguish the causes of such goiters and since thyroid enlargement of diverse etiology may exist in both endemic and nonendemic regions, it is prudent to employ a general term such as *simple* or *nontoxic goiter*. This all-inclusive category can be further subdivided into specific etiologic groups as defined by objective procedures. Simple or nontoxic goiter can be defined as any enlargement of the thyroid gland that does not result from an inflammatory or neoplastic process and that is not initially associated with thyrotoxicosis or myxedema.

ETIOLOGY AND PATHOGENESIS Simple goiter is sometimes due to a definable cause of impaired thyroid hormone synthesis, such as iodine deficiency, ingestion of a goitrogen, or a demonstrable defect in a hormone biosynthetic pathway, but in most instances its cause cannot be determined. Whatever the cause, however, the clinical manifestations are thought to reflect the operation of a common pathophysiologic mechanism. Simple goiter occurs when one or more factors impair the capacity of the thyroid gland to secrete quantities of active hormones sufficient to meet the needs of the peripheral tissues. Although this has been presumed to lead to increased secretion of TSH, concentrations of TSH in the serum of patients with established simple goiter are usually normal. Hence, some other mechanism of goitrogenesis may be operative. A likely possibility is that depletion of glandular organic iodine accompanying impaired hormone synthesis increases the responsiveness of thyroid structure and function to levels of TSH that remain within the normal range. The resulting increases in both functioning thyroid mass and cellular activity overcome mild impairment of hormone synthesis; thus, the patient is metabolically normal, though goitrous. When the underlying disorder is severe, compensatory responses, now including hypersecretion of TSH, are inadequate to overcome the impairment, and the patient is both goitrous and hypothyroid. Thus, simple goiter cannot be clearly separated in the pathogenetic sense from goitrous hypothyroidism. Specific causes of simple goiter may exist with or without hypothyroidism (Table 324-5). Defective iodination of thyroglobulin may be an important pathogenetic factor in many patients. The concept that goiter can be due to antibodies that stimulate thyroid growth but not function remains to be fully evaluated.

PATHOLOGY The histopathology of the thyroid in simple goiter varies with the severity of the etiologic factor and the stage at which the examination is made. In its initial stages, the gland exhibits a uniform hypertrophy, hyperplasia, and hypervascularity. As the disorder persists or undergoes repeated exacerbations and remissions, uniformity of thyroidal architecture is lost. Occasionally, the greater part of the gland may display a reasonably uniform degree of involution or hyperinvolution with colloid accumulation. More often such areas are interspersed with patchy areas of focal hyperplasia. Fibrosis may demarcate hyperplastic or involuted nodules. These may resemble true neoplasms (adenomas). Areas of hemorrhage and irregular calcification may be present. The evolution of the multinodular stage is almost always accompanied by the development of functional autonomy. Indeed, heterogeneity of structure and function and a greater or lesser degree of functional autonomy are the hallmarks of the mature stage of this disorder. As a result, hyperthyroidism may ensue spontaneously (toxic multinodular goiter) or be induced by large quantities of iodine (jodbasedow phenomenon).

CLINICAL MANIFESTATIONS In simple goiter the clinical manifestations arise solely from enlargement of the thyroid since the metabolic state is normal. In goitrous hypothyroidism, symptoms caused by thyromegaly are accompanied by signs and symptoms of hormonal insufficiency. Mechanical sequelae include compression and displacement of the trachea or esophagus, occasionally with obstructive symptoms if the goiter becomes sufficiently large. Superior mediastinal obstruction may occur with large retrosternal goiters. Signs of compression can be induced in the case of large retrosternal goiters when the patient's arms are raised above the head (Pemberton's sign); suffusion of the face, giddiness, or syncope may result from this maneuver. Compression of the recurrent laryngeal nerve leading to hoarseness is rare in simple goiter and suggests neoplasm. Sudden hemorrhage into a nodule may lead to an acute, painful swelling in the neck and may produce or enhance compressive symptoms. Hyperthyroidism may supervene in long-standing multinodular goiter (toxic multinodular goiter). In both endemic and sporadic multinodular goiter, the ingestion of excess iodide may result in the development of thyrotoxicosis (jodbasedow phenomenon).

In geographic regions where iodine deficiency is severe, goitrous enlargement may also be associated with varying degrees of hypothyroidism. Cretinism, both goitrous and nongoitrous, occurs with increased frequency in the children of goitrous parents in many countries where goiter is common. Although iodine deficiency is doubtless a necessary factor in the etiology of endemic goiter, the frequency of goiter may differ greatly among areas of equally severe iodine deficiency. In such instances, dietary or waterborne goitrogens appear to be important conditioning factors. In some areas, these goitrogens may be sufficient to cause goiter in the absence of iodine deficiency.

DIAGNOSIS The diagnosis of simple goiter requires, first, demonstration of a euthyroid state and, second, demonstration of normal serum T_4 and T_3 concentrations. The former may be difficult because manifestations of thyrotoxicosis may be subtle or atypical, especially among the elderly (see section on "Toxic Multinodular Goiter"). The latter may be problematic, since serum T_4 and especially T_3 concentrations may be near the upper limit of the normal range. In addition, the fact that serum T_3 concentrations decrease in the euthyroid elderly complicates interpretation of this test. The RAIU is usually normal but may be increased in the presence of iodine deficiency or a biosynthetic defect. Exclusion of thyrotoxicosis is further complicated by the significant functional autonomy and consequent decrease in response to TRH that often accompany long-standing multinodular goiter. Differentiation of nontoxic goiter from Hashimoto's disease is facilitated by the greater frequency of multinodularity in the former and by the presence of high titers of circulating antimicrosomal or antithyroglobulin antibodies in the latter. In some instances, emergence of a strongly dominant nodule may suggest the presence of a carcinoma. This is especially true if bleeding has caused it to increase in size rapidly and to lose the ability to accumulate iodine or pertechnetate.

TABLE 324-5 Classification of the causes of hypothyroidism

I Thyroid
- *A* Thyroprivic
  - *1* Congenital development defect
  - *2* Primary idiopathic
  - *3* Postablative (radioiodine, surgery)
  - *4* Postradiation (lymphoma)
- *B* Goitrous
  - *1* Heritable biosynthetic defects
  - *2* Maternally transmitted (iodides, antithyroid agents)
  - *3* Iodine deficiency
  - *4* Drug-elicited (*p*-aminosalicylic acid, iodides, phenylbutazone, iodoantipyrine, lithium)
  - *5* Chronic thyroiditis (Hashimoto's disease)

II Suprathyroid (trophoprivic)
- *A* Pituitary
- *B* Hypothalamic

III Self-limited
- *A* Following withdrawal of suppressive thyroid therapy
- *B* Subacute thyroiditis and chronic thyroiditis with transient hypothyroidism (usually after a phase of thyrotoxicosis)

TREATMENT The object of treatment is to reduce the size of the goiter, either by relieving external encumbrances to hormone formation or by providing sufficient quantities of exogenous hormone to inhibit TSH secretion and thereby put the thyroid gland almost completely at rest. In disorders characterized by decreased thyroid iodide stores, such as iodine deficiency or impairment of the thyroid iodide-concentrating mechanism, small doses of iodide may prove effective. Occasionally, a known extrinsic goitrogen can be withdrawn. Most commonly, however, no specific etiologic factor can be detected, and suppressive thyroid therapy is required. For this purpose, sodium L-thyroxine (levothyroxine) is the agent of choice. In the younger patient with the early diffuse stage of simple goiter, treatment can be instituted with 100 μg of levothyroxine daily, and the dose is increased over the next month or so to a maximum of 150 or 200 μg daily. Adequacy of suppression can be assessed by measuring the RAIU, which should decrease to less than 5 percent of the administered dose at 24 h. Lesser decreases indicate only partial suppression, reflecting the presence of autonomous foci demonstrable by scanning techniques. In the elderly patient or the patient with long-standing multinodular goiter, a TRH stimulation test should be undertaken before initiating treatment with levothyroxine to determine whether or not significant functional autonomy is present. If such is indicated by diminished or absent TSH responsiveness to TRH, suppressive therapy with levothyroxine is contraindicated since such patients are or will eventually become thyrotoxic. Rather, consideration should be given to radioiodine ablation of the autonomous foci (see later section on "Toxic Multinodular Goiter"). On the other hand, if the TSH response to TRH is normal, excluding significant functional autonomy, treatment with levothyroxine can be initiated. In the elderly patient, the initial dose should not exceed 50 μg daily, and the dosage should be gradually increased, partial rather than complete suppression of the value for the RAIU being the end point. It is the practice to obtain a thyroid scan as part of the initial evaluation of all patients with multinodular goiter and to repeat the RAIU and scan (suppression scan), when practical, in all patients receiving suppressive thyroid hormone therapy.

Reported results of therapy vary widely. There is general agreement that the early diffuse, hyperplastic goiter responds well, with regression or disappearance in 3 to 6 months. In the author's experience, the later, nodular stage responds less favorably, and significant reduction in gland size is achieved only in about one-third of the cases; however, in the remainder, suppressive treatment may forestall further glandular growth. Internodular tissue regresses more often than do nodules themselves. The latter may therefore become more prominent during treatment. After maximum regression of the goiter, suppressive medication may be maintained for prolonged periods, reduced to minimal levels, or at times withdrawn. In an unpredictable manner, goiter in some cases remains relieved while in others it recurs. In the latter instances, suppressive therapy should be reinstituted and continued indefinitely.

In areas of endemic iodine deficiency, the size and prevalence of goiter and the frequency of cretinism can be reduced by the provision of iodized salt or water or the periodic injection of iodized oil.

Surgical therapy of simple goiter is physiologically unsound, but it may occasionally be necessary to relieve obstructive symptoms, especially those that persist after a conscientious trial of medical therapy. Surgical exploration of nodular goiter may be indicated in some individuals when evidence suggests carcinoma. However, the concept that subtotal resection of multinodular nontoxic goiter affords effective prophylaxis against the development of thyroid carcinoma is unsound. If for some reason subtotal thyroidectomy has been performed, levothyroxine in a usual dose of about 150 μg daily is recommended to inhibit regenerative hyperplasia and further goitrogenesis.

HYPOTHYROIDISM

Hypothyroidism can result from any of a variety of structural or functional abnormalities that lead to insufficient synthesis of thyroid hormone. Hypothyroidism dating from birth and resulting in developmental abnormalities is termed *cretinism*. The term *myxedema* connotes severe hypothyroidism in which there is accumulation of hydrophilic mucopolysaccharides in the ground substance of the dermis and other tissues, leading to thickening of the facial features and doughy induration of the skin.

ETIOLOGY AND PATHOGENESIS A classification of the causes of hypothyroidism is presented in Table 324-5. Overall, the thyroid varieties account for approximately 95 percent of cases, only 5 percent or less being suprathyroid in origin. In thyroprivic hypothyroidism, loss of thyroid tissue leads to inadequate synthesis of thyroid hormone, despite maximum stimulation of any thyroid remnant by TSH. The most common cause of thyroprivic hypothyroidism is surgical or radioiodine ablation of the thyroid gland in the treatment of Graves' disease. Thyroprivic hypothyroidism may also occur as a primary idiopathic phenomenon. Primary hypothyroidism is frequently associated with circulating antithyroid antibodies and in some cases may result from the action of antibodies that block the TSH receptor. It may coexist with other diseases in which circulating autoantibodies are found. These diseases include pernicious anemia, systemic lupus erythematosus, rheumatoid arthritis, Sjögren's syndrome, and chronic hepatitis. In addition, hypothyroidism can be one manifestation of a polyglandular endocrine deficiency state in which autoantibodies cause variable insufficiency of thyroid, adrenal, parathyroid, and gonadal function (see Chap. 334). All these diseases, including isolated primary hypothyroidism, are associated with an increased frequency of specific HLA haplotypes and may be diverse reflections of disordered immune regulation. Finally, a developmental defect may result in failure of the gland to function adequately, leading to sporadic nongoitrous cretinism or juvenile hypothyroidism. A self-limited period of hypothyroidism is common in the course of subacute thyroiditis and in the syndrome of "painless thyroiditis," usually after a temporary period of thyrotoxicosis. Owing to a persisting lack of TSH stimulation, intrinsically euthyroid patients from whom chronic suppressive therapy is abruptly withdrawn experience a several-week period of thyroid hypofunction.

Impairment in the ability to synthesize adequate quantities of thyroid hormone leads to hypersecretion of TSH and hence goiter. If this compensatory response is inadequate, goitrous hypothyroidism ensues. The commonest cause of goitrous hypothyroidism in North America is Hashimoto's disease, in which defective organic binding of iodide and abnormal secretion of iodoproteins are frequent abnormalities. Iodide-induced goiter with or without hypothyroidism appears to arise from an intrinsic defect in the organic binding mechanism, which permits a persistent Wolff-Chaikoff effect. Patients with Graves' disease, especially after radioiodine treatment, those with Hashimoto's disease, and the normal fetus are particularly susceptible to iodide-induced goiter. In view of the susceptibility of the fetal thyroid to iodide, with resulting goiter and hypothyroidism, iodine in large doses should not be given during pregnancy. Less common causes of goitrous hypothyroidism are hereditary defects in hormone biosynthesis and ingestion of drugs that induce defects in hormone biosynthesis, such as *p*-aminosalicylic acid and lithium carbonate. Finally, in areas of environmental iodine deficiency, goitrous cretinism and hypothyroidism can occur on an endemic basis. Diminished thyroid reserve occurs as a stage in the evolution of both thyroprivic and goitrous hypothyroidism.

In hypothyroidism of suprathyroid origin, the thyroid is intrinsically normal but is deprived of stimulation by TSH. Deprivation of TSH, most commonly the result of postpartum pituitary necrosis or a tumor of the pituitary or adjacent regions, results in pituitary hypothyroidism. Hypothalamic hypothyroidism is less common and results from inadequate secretion of TRH.

CLINICAL PICTURE The appearance of children with hypothyroidism depends on the age at which the deficiency began and the promptness with which replacement therapy was instituted. Cretinism may be manifested at birth but usually becomes evident within the first several months, depending upon the extent of thyroid failure. Hypothyroidism is present in approximately 1 of every 5000 neonates and manifests itself in abnormally long persistence of physiologic jaundice, hoarse cry, constipation, somnolence, and feeding problems; all neonates should be screened for hypothyroidism with measurements of the serum T_4 or TSH, since clinical diagnosis is difficult and early treatment is crucial for normal intellectual development. In later months, delay in reaching the normal milestones of development becomes evident, and the physical characteristics of the cretin appear. These include short stature, coarse features with protruding tongue, broad flat nose, widely set eyes, sparse hair, dry skin, protuberant abdomen with an umbilical hernia, and impaired mental development. X-ray examination reveals retarded bone age, epiphyseal dysgenesis, and delayed dentition.

In the older child, the clinical manifestations of hypothyroidism are intermediate between those of infantile and adult hypothyroidism. Retardation of linear growth is manifested by shortness of stature, and retardation of sexual maturation results in delay in the onset of puberty. Poor performance at school may call attention to the diagnosis. The manifestations of adult hypothyroidism are present to a variable degree. X-ray examination reveals delayed union of the epiphyses.

In the adult, early symptoms of hypothyroidism are nonspecific and of insidious onset. They may include lethargy, constipation, cold intolerance, stiffness and cramping of the muscles, the carpal tunnel syndrome, and menorrhagia. Over the succeeding months, intellectual and motor activity slows, appetite declines, and weight increases. The hair becomes dry and tends to fall out, and the skin becomes dry. The voice becomes deeper and hoarse, and auditory acuity may deteriorate. Obstructive sleep apnea may occur. Ultimately, the clinical picture of florid myxedema appears, with dull expressionless face, sparse hair, periorbital puffiness, large tongue, and pale, cool skin that feels rough and doughy. Thyroid tissue is not readily palpable, except in the goitrous variety of hypothyroidism. The heart is enlarged owing to both dilation and pericardial effusion; if the heart is small, pituitary hypothyroidism should be considered. Adynamic ileus may occur, producing megacolon or intestinal obstruction. Rarely, psychiatric symptoms or cerebellar ataxia may dominate the clinical picture. The relaxation phase of the deep tendon reflexes is characteristically prolonged, the so-called hung-up reflex. If left untreated, the patient with severe long-standing hypothyroidism may pass into a hypothermic, stuporous state (*myxedema coma*) that is frequently fatal. Respiratory depression is an important component of this state, and hence arterial P_{CO_2} may be increased. Factors that predispose to myxedema coma include cold exposure, trauma, infection, and administration of central nervous system depressants. Dilutional hyponatremia is common and results from impaired water excretion and from disordered regulation of vasopressin secretion.

LABORATORY TESTS A decrease in serum T_4 and in the FT_4I is common to all varieties of hypothyroidism. In the thyroid varieties, the serum T_3 may be decreased to a lesser extent than is the serum T_4, the presumption being that the compensatory hypersecretion of

TSH leads to a relative preponderance of T_3 secretion. In thyroprivic hypothyroidism the decreased RAIU is of limited diagnostic utility because of the low value for the lower limit of the normal range. In goitrous hypothyroidism, the RAIU may be increased or display an abnormal pattern of accumulation or retention. The serum TSH is invariably increased in the thyroprivic and goitrous varieties and is usually normal or undetectable in pituitary or hypothalamic hypothyroidism. In the latter instances, hyposecretion of TSH is usually accompanied by hyposecretion of other pituitary hormones (see Chap. 321).

Frequent manifestations of the hypothyroid state include an increased serum cholesterol in hypothyroidism of thyroid (but not pituitary) origin and increased concentrations in serum of creatine phosphokinase (MM variant), aspartate transaminase, and lactic dehydrogenase. Systolic time intervals are altered in that the preejection period is distinctly prolonged and the ratio of the preejection period to left ventricular ejection time is increased. Electrocardiographic changes include bradycardia, low amplitude QRS complexes, and flattened or inverted T waves. In primary thyroprivic hypothyroidism, overt pernicious anemia occurs in about 12 percent of patients; histamine-fast achlorhydria and circulating antigastric parietal cell antibodies are even more common.

In addition to patients who are clinically hypothyroid, some patients who appear clinically euthyroid display laboratory evidence of early thyroid failure (subclinical hypothyroidism). In mild cases serum TSH and its response to TRH administration are increased while serum T_4 and T_3 concentrations are normal. When there is a greater degree of thyroid failure, serum T_4 concentration is decreased, but the serum T_3 concentration is normal or nearly so owing to TSH-induced hypersecretion of T_3 relative to T_4, and perhaps to more efficient conversion of T_4 to T_3. Subclinical hypothyroidism is most often seen in patients with Hashimoto's disease or those with Graves' disease who have been treated with ^{131}I or surgery and are usually stages in the evolution of frank hypothyroidism.

DIFFERENTIAL DIAGNOSIS Little difficulty will be experienced in diagnosing the classic picture of cretinism or juvenile and adult hypothyroidism. Occasionally, an infant with Down's syndrome may be confused with a cretin. However, the characteristic mongoloid eyes, Brushfield's spots in the iris, hyperextensibility of the joints, and normal skin and hair texture distinguish Down's syndrome from hypothyroid cretinism. Chronic nephritis and the nephrotic syndrome may simulate myxedema, particularly because of the facial puffiness and pallor. The nephrotic patient may also have anemia, hypercholesterolemia, and anasarca. In addition, the serum T_4 concentration may be decreased if there is significant loss of TBG into the urine, but the FT_4I is normal or increased. The serum T_3 concentration is often subnormal, as it might be in any severe systemic illness, owing to impaired peripheral generation from T_4, but the serum TSH concentration is not increased.

TREATMENT Two types of hormone are available for the treatment of hypothyroidism, synthetic hormone and thyroprotein derived from animal thyroids (Table 324-6). Synthetic hormones include L-thyroxine (levothyroxine), L-triiodothyronine (liothyronine), and a combination of the two (liotrix). The preparation of natural origin most commonly used is thyroid extract, USP. Because of their uniform potency, the author prefers the synthetic preparations and specifically levothyroxine. Unlike liothyronine, liotrix, and even thyroid extract, ingestion of levothyroxine does not lead to abrupt increases in serum T_3 concentration, which could be dangerous in the older patient or in the patient with coexisting heart disease. Rather, a stable T_3 concentration is attained through continuous generation from administered T_4.

TABLE 324-6 Approximate therapeutic equivalence of various thyroid hormone preparations

Preparation	Average daily oral maintenance dose	Serum T_4
Thyroid extract, USP	120–180 mg	Normal
Levothyroxine	150 μg	Normal or slightly increased
Liothyronine	50 μg	Decreased
Liotrix (T_4: T_3 = 4:1)	2 units	Normal

In most instances, a normal metabolic state should be restored gradually, especially in the elderly or the patient with heart disease, since sudden increases in metabolic rate may tax cardiac or coronary reserve. In adults, an initial daily dose of 25 μg levothyroxine can be increased by 25- to 50-μg increments at 2- to 3-week intervals, until a normal metabolic state is attained. The dose necessary to sustain a normal metabolic state is usually about 150 μg per day, and this usually results in a serum T_4 at or somewhat above the upper limit of the normal range. The serum T_3 is superior to the serum T_4 as an indicator of the metabolic state in the patient receiving levothyroxine. Because of its long half-life, levothyroxine is generally administered as a single daily dose. The optimum dose for the individual patient should be based on clinical criteria and on measurements of serum TSH or T_3 concentration. Elevations of the former indicate that treatment is insufficient and of the latter that it is excessive.

In neonatal, infantile, and juvenile hypothyroidism it is essential that full replacement therapy be begun as soon as possible; otherwise the chances of normal intellectual development and growth are poor. Infants and children require doses of levothyroxine that are disproportionately large in relation to body size. *In known or strongly suspected pituitary and hypothalamic hypothyroidism, thyroid replacement should not be instituted until treatment with hydrocortisone has been initiated,* since acute adrenocortical insufficiency may be precipitated by an increase in metabolic rate.

In some patients, hypothyroidism should be treated rapidly. This includes patients with myxedema coma and, because of the extreme sensitivity to central nervous system depressants, hypothyroid patients being prepared for emergency surgery. Here, intravenous administration of levothyroxine, in conjunction with the use of hydrocortisone, is indicated.

THYROTOXICOSIS

The term *thyrotoxicosis* denotes the clinical, physiologic, and biochemical findings that result when the tissues are exposed to, and respond to, an excess supply of active thyroid hormone. Rather than a specific disease, thyrotoxicosis is a syndrome that can originate in a variety of ways. In general, three main categories of disorder can produce the thyrotoxic state (Table 324-7). The first, and most important, encompasses those diseases that lead to sustained overproduction of hormone by the thyroid gland itself. Here, hyperfunction

TABLE 324-7 Varieties of thyrotoxicosis

I Disorders associated with thyroid hyperfunction*
- *A* Excess production of TSH (rare)
- *B* Abnormal thyroid stimulator
  - *1* Graves' disease
  - *2* Trophoblastic tumor
- *C* Intrinsic thyroid autonomy
  - *1* Hyperfunctioning adenoma
  - *2* Toxic multinodular goiter

II Disorders not associated with thyroid hyperfunction†
- *A* Disorders of hormone storage
  - *1* Subacute thyroiditis
  - *2* Chronic thyroiditis with transient thyrotoxicosis
- *B* Extrathyroid source of hormone
  - *1* Thyrotoxicosis factitia
  - *2* Ectopic thyroid tissue
    - *a* Struma ovarii
    - *b* Functioning follicular cacinoma

* *Associated with increased RAIU unless body iodine burden is excessive.*
† *Associated with decreased RAIU.*

of the gland variously results from excessive secretion of TSH, a rare cause associated with pituitary tumor or with resistance to thyroid hormone or the pituitary but not in peripheral tissues; the action of an abnormal, homeostatically unregulated thyroid stimulator of extrapituitary origin, as in patients with Graves' disease, patients who develop hyperthyroidism in association with Hashimoto's disease, or patients with trophoblastic tumors; or the development of one or more areas of autonomous hyperfunction within the gland itself. The second category encompasses the thyrotoxic states associated with subacute thyroiditis and the syndrome termed *chronic thyroiditis with spontaneously resolving thyrotoxicosis;* an excess of preformed hormone leaks from the gland owing to the presence of inflammatory disease. New hormone formation is decreased, however, owing to the suppression of TSH secretion by the hormone excess, and in some cases to the inflammatory injury itself. Since the inflammatory disorders are transitory and since stores of preformed hormone are ultimately depleted, the thyrotoxicosis in these disorders is self-limited and is often followed by a transient period of thyroid hormone insufficiency. The third category of thyrotoxic state is one in which the source of excess hormone is outside of the thyroid gland itself, as in thyrotoxicosis factitia, the rare functioning metastatic thyroid carcinoma, or struma ovarii.

Although all of the foregoing disorders are associated with thyrotoxicosis, not all are associated with hyperthyroidism, a term which should be used to denote only those conditions in which sustained hyperfunction of the thyroid leads to thyrotoxicosis. Thus, thyrotoxic states can be classified according to whether or not they are associated with hyperthyroidism. This distinction has practical implications for diagnosis and for treatment. In hyperthyroidism, hyperfunction of the thyroid is reflected in an increased RAIU, whereas in the nonhyperthyroid thyrotoxic states, thyroid function (as reflected in the RAIU) is subnormal. Further, treatment of thyrotoxicosis by means intended to decrease hormone synthesis (antithyroid agents, surgery, or radioiodine) is appropriate in hyperthyroidism but is inappropriate and ineffective in other forms of thyrotoxicosis.

Though the specific diseases that cause thyrotoxicosis each make their own imprint on the clinical picture, the manifestations of the thyrotoxic state are largely the same. In the discussion that ensues, the major diseases that lead to a thyrotoxic state are individually described. Since the first considered and most important is Graves' disease, the common manifestations of thyrotoxicosis are described in relation to Graves' disease.

GRAVES' DISEASE

Graves' disease, also known as Parry's or Basedow's disease, is a disorder of unknown etiology with a triad of major manifestations: hyperthyroidism with diffuse goiter, ophthalmopathy, and dermopathy. Although part of the same disease complex, the three major manifestations need not appear together. Indeed, one or two need never appear, and moreover, the three tend to run courses that are largely independent of one another.

PREVALENCE Graves' disease is a relatively common disorder that occurs at any age but is especially common in the third and fourth decades. The disease is more frequent in women than in men. In nongoitrous areas the ratio of predominance in women may be as high as 7:1. In areas of endemic goiter the ratio is lower. Genetic factors play an important role; there is an increased frequency of haplotypes HLA-B8 and DRw3 in Caucasian, HLA-Bw36 in Japanese, and HLA-Bw46 in Chinese patients with the disease. Not surprisingly, there is a distinct familial predisposition to Graves' disease. In addition, among family members of patients with Graves' disease, a clinical and immunologic overlap exists with respect to Hashimoto's disease, primary thyroprivic hypothyroidism, and pernicious anemia and probably with respect to other diseases in which autoimmune features are prominent. In occasional patients, the disease picture may change from Graves' disease to Hashimoto's disease, or vice versa, and rarely patients with primary myxedema later become hyperthyroid. Thus, it is proper to consider Graves' disease, Hashimoto's disease, and primary myxedema as closely related autoimmune thyroid diseases.

ETIOLOGY AND PATHOGENESIS The cause is unknown. In view of the varied manifestations of Graves' disease and their differing courses, it is possible that no single factor is responsible for the entire syndrome. With respect to hyperthyroidism, the central disorder is a disruption of homeostatic mechanisms that normally adjust hormone secretion to meet the needs of peripheral tissues; if such were able to operate, hyperthyroidism could not be sustained. This homeostatic disruption results from the presence in plasma of an abnormal thyroid stimulator. The existence of such was first recognized when it was shown that the serums of patients with Graves' disease release radioiodine from the prelabeled guinea pig or mouse thyroid. In view of its prolonged duration of action relative to that of TSH in this bioassay system, this material was designated the long-acting thyroid stimulator (LATS). LATS activity is present in one or more immunoglobulins of the class IgG elaborated by lymphocytes of patients with Graves' disease. It soon became apparent, however, that LATS could be detected only in about half of patients with this disorder, and consequently its pathogenetic role was questioned. This failure to detect LATS in all patients with Graves' disease is due to the fact that the stimulator has variable actions in other species and is not uniformly detectable, therefore, in the conventional bioassay. When human thyroid tissue is used as the assay system, however, one or more in vitro responses can be demonstrated in the plasma of most patients. These responses and the corresponding names given to the responsible factors are as follows: prevention of the adsorption of LATS activity by human thyroid particulate fractions (LATS-protector, LATS-p), stimulation of colloid droplet or cyclic AMP generation in thyroid cells, slices, or membranes (thyroid-stimulating immunoglobulins, TSI), and inhibition of the binding of TSH to its receptors in human thyroid tissue (TSH-binding inhibitory immunoglobulins, TBII). The underlying nature of these factors, their number, and their relationship to one another are uncertain, but they are probably antibodies against the thyroid TSH receptor. Activities of this type are also found in serums of some patients with euthyroid ophthalmic Graves' disease, an occasional patient with Hashimoto's disease, and some euthyroid relatives of patients with Graves' disease, though the reason for the absence of thyrotoxicosis in such instances is uncertain. Disappearance of these stimulatory factors from the serum during antithyroid treatment augurs well for long-term remission after treatment is withdrawn. Thus, while the basic cause of Graves' disease is not understood, an immunoglobulin or family of immunoglobulins directed against the TSH receptor mediates the thyroid stimulation of Graves' disease. A heritable abnormality in immune surveillance may permit particular lymphocytes to survive, proliferate, and secrete the stimulatory immunoglobulins in response to some precipitating factors.

The pathogenesis of the ophthalmic component of Graves' disease is even more enigmatic. One proposed mechanism is the development of antibodies against the extraocular muscles. A second postulate invokes lymphatic transport of thyroglobulin from the thyroid to orbital tissues, at which site an immune response is evoked. Nothing is known of the pathogenesis of the dermopathy of Graves' disease.

PATHOLOGY In Graves' disease, the *thyroid gland* is diffusely enlarged, soft, and vascular. The essential pathology is that of parenchymatous hypertrophy and hyperplasia, characterized by increased height of the epithelium and redundancy of the follicular wall, giving the picture of papillary infoldings and cytologic evidence of increased activity. Such hyperplasia is usually accompanied by lymphocytic infiltration that reflects the immune aspect of the disease and that correlates in severity with levels of antithyroid antibodies in the blood. Following iodine medication, there is colloid storage, which sometimes causes enlargement and increased firmness of the gland. Graves' disease is associated with generalized lymphoid hyperplasia and infiltration and occasionally with enlargement of the spleen or thymus. Thyrotoxicosis may lead to degeneration of skeletal muscle fibers, enlargement of the heart, fatty infiltration or diffuse fibrosis of the liver, decalcification of the skeleton, and loss of body tissue (including fat deposits, osteoid, and muscle).

The *ophthalmopathy* of Graves' disease is characterized by an inflammatory infiltrate of the orbital contents, exclusive of the globe, with lymphocytes, mast cells, and plasma cells being the predominant cellular components. The orbital musculature is mainly involved and often is enlarged, largely accounting for the increased volume of the orbital contents that causes the globe to protrude. Muscle fibers show degeneration and loss of striations, with ultimate fibrosis.

The *dermopathy* of Graves' disease is characterized by thickening of the dermis, which is infiltrated with lymphocytes and with hydrophilic, metachromatically staining mucopolysaccharides.

CLINICAL MANIFESTATIONS The manifestations comprise those that reflect the associated thyrotoxicosis and those specifically related to Graves' disease. The former vary in intensity with the severity of the thyrotoxicosis, the age of the patient, and the presence of disease in other organs, such as the heart.

Manifestations of thyrotoxicosis Common manifestations include nervousness, emotional lability, inability to sleep, tremors, frequent bowel movements, excessive sweating, and heat intolerance. Weight loss is usual despite a well-maintained or increased appetite. Loss of strength is often manifested by difficulty in climbing stairs. In premenopausal women, oligomenorrhea and amenorrhea tend to occur. Dyspnea, palpitations, and, in patients over the age of 40, enhancement of angina pectoris or cardiac failure may occur. In general, nervous symptoms dominate the clinical picture in younger individuals, whereas cardiovascular and myopathic symptoms predominate in older subjects.

Usually, the patient appears anxious, restless, and fidgety. The skin is warm and moist with a velvety texture, and palmar erythema is present. Separation of the fingernail from the nailbed (Plummer's nail) is common, especially on the ring finger. The hair is fine and silky. A fine tremor of the fingers and tongue, together with hyperreflexia, is characteristic. *Ocular signs* include a characteristic stare with widened palpebral fissures, infrequent blinking, lid lag, and failure to wrinkle the brow on upward gaze. These signs result from sympathetic overstimulation and usually subside when the thyrotoxicosis is corrected. They are to be distinguished from the *infiltrative ophthalmopathy* characteristic of Graves' disease, discussed below.

Cardiovascular findings include a wide pulse pressure, sinus tachycardia, atrial arrhythmias (especially atrial fibrillation), systolic murmurs, increased intensity of the apical first sound, cardiac enlargement, and, at times, overt heart failure. A to-and-fro, high-pitched sound may be audible in the pulmonic area and may simulate a pericardial friction rub (Means-Lerman scratch).

Manifestations of Graves' disease The three distinctive manifestations of Graves' disease, diffuse hyperfunctioning goiter, ophthalmopathy, and dermopathy, appear in varying combinations and with varying frequency, goiter being the most common. Premature graying of the hair and patchy vitiligo are not specific to Graves' disease per se since they are also common in other autoimmune disorders, whether of the thyroid or other organ systems.

The *diffuse toxic goiter* may be asymmetric and lobular. The presence of a bruit over the gland usually signifies that the patient is thyrotoxic, but it may also rarely be present in other disorders in which the thyroid is markedly hyperplastic. Venous hums and carotid souffles should be distinguished from true thyroid bruits. An enlarged pyramidal lobe of the thyroid may be palpable.

The clinical signs associated with the *ophthalmopathy* of Graves' disease may be divided into two components: the spastic and the mechanical. The former includes the stare, lid lag, and lid retraction that accompany thyrotoxicosis and account for the "frightened" facies and classic eye signs previously described. These findings need not be associated with proptosis and usually return to normal after correction of thyrotoxicosis. The mechanical component includes proptosis of varying degrees with ophthalmoplegia and congestive oculopathy characterized by chemosis, conjunctivitis, periorbital swelling, and the resultant complications of corneal ulceration, optic neuritis, and optic atrophy. When exophthalmos progresses rapidly and becomes the major concern in Graves' disease, it is usually referred to as *progressive,* and if severe, *malignant exophthalmos.* The term *exophthalmic ophthalmoplegia* refers to the ocular muscle weakness that commonly accompanies this disorder and results in strabismus with varying degrees of diplopia. Exophthalmos may be unilateral early in the course of the disorder but usually progresses to bilateral involvement.

The *dermopathy* of Graves' disease usually occurs over the dorsum of the legs or feet and is termed *localized* or *pretibial myxedema.* It occurs in patients with past or present Graves' disease and is not a manifestation of hypothyroidism. About half of cases occur during the active stage of thyrotoxicosis; in the remainder the lesions develop after treatment. The affected area is usually well demarcated from normal skin by the fact that it is raised, thickened, has a *peau d'orange* appearance, and may be pruritic and hyperpigmented. The lesions are usually discrete, assuming a plaquelike or nodular configuration but in some instances becoming confluent. Clubbing of the fingers and toes with characteristic bony changes that differ from those of hypertrophic pulmonary osteoarthropathy may accompany the dermal changes (*thyroid acropachy*). This disorder is usually self-limited.

DIAGNOSIS When severe, Graves' disease presents little difficulty in diagnosis. Florid thyrotoxicosis is manifested by weakness, weight loss despite good appetite, nervous instability, tremor, intolerance to heat, sweating, palpitations, and hyperdefecation. When associated with diffuse thyroid enlargement, often accompanied by a bruit, and particularly when associated with ophthalmopathy, the clinical picture of Graves' disease is virtually unique. In such instances, laboratory tests documenting increased RAIU, serum T_4 and T_3, RT_3U, and FT_4I serve as baselines for evaluation of therapy, rather than necessary diagnostic aids. Occasionally, laboratory tests reveal a normal RAIU, normal serum T_4 and RT_3U, and elevated serum T_3 and FT_3I (T_3 toxicosis).

In less severe cases, particularly when ophthalmopathy is lacking, the diagnosis may be more difficult, since the symptoms of mild thyrotoxicosis are similar to those of other disorders (see "Differential Diagnosis" below). Presence of a goiter makes the diagnosis of hyperthyroidism likely, but careful palpation is necessary to determine whether toxic multinodular goiter, toxic adenoma, or subacute thyroiditis is present, since treatment of these disorders may differ from that of diffuse toxic goiter. Absence of thyroid enlargement makes the diagnosis of Graves' disease unlikely but does not exclude it. In mild cases, confirmatory laboratory tests assume great importance. Unfortunately, mild thyrotoxicosis is often associated with marginal abnormalities in laboratory tests or values within the upper limit of the normal range. In such instances, the TRH stimulation test assumes crucial importance.

In a few patients, the clinical picture may be one of apathy rather than hyperactivity, and evidence of hypermetabolism may be slight. In such patients, myopathic features may be pronounced. More often, cardiovascular manifestations predominate since mild hyperthyroidism may produce severe disability in patients with underlying heart disease. Hence, *all patients with unexplained cardiac failure or irregularities in rhythm, especially if atrial in origin, should be examined for thyrotoxicosis.* Clues to the diagnosis include a relatively rapid circulation time and resistance to the usual doses of digitalis, but laboratory confirmation is required.

DIFFERENTIAL DIAGNOSIS Signs and symptoms in a number of nonthyroid disorders may simulate certain aspects of the thyrotoxic syndrome. Anxiety is a prominent feature of thyrotoxicosis, and there is thus some overlap in the symptomatology of thyrotoxicosis with that of anxiety states of emotional origin. Such symptoms as tachycardia, tremulousness, irritability, weakness, and fatigue are common to both disorders. In anxiety of emotional origin, however, the peripheral manifestations of excessive thyroid hormones are absent; the skin is usually cold and clammy rather than warm and moist. Weight loss, when present in emotional anxiety, is characteristically accompanied by anorexia, whereas in thyrotoxicosis the appetite is generally, but not invariably, increased. Thyrotoxicosis can occasionally be confused with such disorders as metastatic carcinoma, cirrhosis of the liver, hyperparathyroidism, sprue, myasthenia gravis, and muscular dystrophy. Hypokalemic periodic paralysis is more common in thyrotoxic patients, especially in the case of Oriental and Latin American men. Signs and symptoms of thyrotoxicosis may overlap with those of pheochromocytoma, which may cause heat intolerance, excessive perspiration, tachycardia with palpitations, and a severe hypermetabolic state. In all the above disorders, and in other conditions considered in the differential diagnosis, the judicious application of laboratory tests usually makes it possible to differentiate them from thyrotoxicosis.

When bilateral ophthalmopathy is accompanied by goiter and thyrotoxicosis, the origin of the ophthalmopathy in Graves' disease is virtually certain. The presence of unilateral ophthalmopathy, even when associated with thyrotoxicosis, raises the possibility of some other intraorbital or intracranial disease. In the euthyroid patient with either unilateral or bilateral ophthalmopathy other causes must be excluded. These include cavernous sinus thrombosis, sphenoidal ridge meningioma, retrobulbar tumors, including leukemic deposits, and the rare granulomatous disorder, pseudotumor oculi. Exophthalmos may also be seen in certain systemic disorders, such as uremia, accelerated hypertension, chronic alcoholism, chronic obstructive pulmonary disease, superior mediastinal obstruction, and Cushing's syndrome. Ophthalmoplegia in the absence of overt infiltrative manifestations can be confused with that which occurs in diabetes mellitus, myasthenia gravis, and myopathies. When doubt exists about the cause of ophthalmopathy, the demonstration of an abnormal TRH stimulation test or thyroid suppression test suggests that the cause is Graves' disease, though not all patients with "euthyroid Graves' disease" demonstrate abnormal responses. In such cases, ultrasonography or computerized tomography of the orbits is valuable in demonstrating characteristic thickening of the extraocular muscles.

When a thyrotoxic state occurs in a patient lacking the characteristic ophthalmopathy of Graves' disease, other causes of thyrotoxicosis must be considered. Careful palpation of the thyroid and studies with radioactive iodine are important in this regard. A symmetric, diffuse goiter of moderate or large size suggests the diagnosis of Graves' disease, especially if a bruit is present. However, the uncommon patient whose hyperthyroidism is secondary to an excess of TSH (associated with a *pituitary tumor* or resistance to feedback suppression of TSH secretion) or an abnormal stimulator of trophoblastic origin (*hydatidiform mole* or *choriocarcinoma of uterus* or *testis;* see Chap. 303) may present in this way. A single, prominent thyroid nodule or multiple nodules suggest *toxic adenoma* or *toxic multinodular goiter,* respectively. Tenderness of the thyroid associated with firm nodularity strongly suggests *subacute thyroiditis,* while a small, firm, nontender goiter is consistent with the syndrome of chronic thyroiditis with spontaneously resolving thyrotoxicosis. The foregoing disorders are discussed more fully in later sections. Absence of a palpable thyroid gland suggests an extrathyroid source of hormone, such as ectopic thyroid tissue *(struma ovarii)* or, more commonly, self-administration of hormone *(thyrotoxicosis factitia).* Studies with radioactive iodine are also helpful. Except when hormone overproduction is secondary to increased iodine intake, values of the RAIU are increased in all disorders producing hyperthyroidism, and scintillation scanning may aid in differentiating among them. Conversely, thyrotoxicosis that is not the result of hyperthyroidism is characterized by subnormal values of the RAIU. Subacute thyroiditis and chronic thyroiditis with spontaneously resolving thyrotoxicosis are the more common. Ectopic thyroid tissue producing thyrotoxicosis is rare. Here, the RAIU, as measured over the thyroid, is low since TSH secretion is suppressed, but despite this, urinary excretion of the dose of ^{131}I is slowed, owing to accumulation of ^{131}I by the ectopic tissue. Functioning ectopic tissue can be located by direct counting or scintillation scanning. Thyrotoxicosis factitia most frequently occurs in medical or paramedical personnel or in those who have easy access to thyroid hormone preparations. Physiologically, it resembles thyrotoxicosis caused by ectopic thyroid tissue in that the patient's thyroid gland is suppressed. By contrast, however, most of an administered dose of ^{131}I is excreted promptly in the urine. When the disorder is caused by ingestion of preparations containing T_4, such as levothyroxine or thyroid extract, the serum T_4 is increased. On the other hand, when caused by liothyronine, the serum T_4 is subnormal. Irrespective of the preparation, the serum T_3 is increased but more so when liothyronine is the offending agent. Owing to thyroid suppression, serum thyroglobulin concentration is subnormal.

The demonstration of elevated titers of antithyroid antibodies or of TSI or TBII activity in the blood also provides strong evidence that Graves' disease is the cause of thyrotoxicosis.

TREATMENT **Hyperthyroidism** The hyperthyroidism in Graves' disease is often characterized by cyclic phases of exacerbation and remission, each of unpredictable onset and duration. Moreover, long-standing disease may be associated with progressive thyroid failure, probably consequent to chronic thyroiditis, with the result that hypothyroidism or decreased thyroid reserve supervenes. These characteristics of Graves' disease have important implications in the choice of and response to therapy.

The two major approaches to the treatment are directed to limiting the quantity of thyroid hormones the gland can produce. The use of antithyroid agents interposes a chemical blockade to hormone synthesis, the effect of which is operative only as long as the drug is administered or until a spontaneous remission occurs. Thus, the agents can control a given phase of active thyrotoxicity but probably do not prevent exacerbation at some subsequent period. The second major approach is ablation of thyroid tissue, thereby limiting hormone production. This may be achieved either by surgery or by means of radioactive iodine. Since these procedures induce permanent anatomic alterations of the thyroid, they can control the individual active phase and are more likely to prevent a later exacerbation or recurrence. On the other hand, the permanency of the effects of surgery or radiation makes these modes of therapy more likely to lead to hypothyroidism, either shortly after treatment or with the passage of years.

Each therapy has advantages and disadvantages, indications and contraindications. The latter are more often relative than absolute. In general, a trial of long-term antithyroid therapy is desirable in children, adolescents, young adults, and pregnant women but may also be employed in older patients. Indications for ablative procedures include relapse or recurrence following drug therapy, a large goiter, drug toxicity, failure to follow a medical regimen, or failure to return for periodic examinations. Subtotal thyroidectomy may be elected for patients under the age of 40 in whom ablative therapy is required; however, opinions differ, and some authorities employ radioactive iodine in the treatment of patients in the second or third decades. Radioactive iodine is the ablative procedure of choice in older patients, in patients who have had previous thyroid surgery, and in those in whom systemic disease contraindicates elective surgery.

In patients selected for *long-term antithyroid therapy,* satisfactory control can almost always be achieved if sufficient drug is administered. Most patients can be managed with propylthiouracil, 100 to 150 mg every 6 or 8 h. In occasional patients with severe disease, larger doses are required for initial control. Methimazole is at least as effective as propylthiouracil when administered in one-tenth the dosage. However, propylthiouracil has the advantage of inhibiting the peripheral conversion of T_4 to T_3, thereby bringing about more rapid symptomatic improvement. Once euthyroidism is achieved, the daily dosage may be reduced to the smallest doses that control the thyrotoxicosis. In some clinics the initial dose is continued and is supplemented with levothyroxine. By this latter regimen, hypothyroidism from overdosage of antithyroid drugs can be prevented. The undesirable consequences of hypothyroidism, such as enhancement of ophthalmopathy and enlargement of the goiter, may thereby be forestalled. The duration of therapy is difficult to predict in the individual patient and may be a function of the spontaneous course of the disease. If this is the case, the longer the course of therapy, the more likely it is that the patient will remain well when the drug is discontinued. In general a 12- to 24-month course is employed, following which one-third or one-half of patients remain well for a prolonged period or indefinitely. The likelihood of a prolonged remission is increased by a decrease in goiter size, reversion of the thyroid suppression test to normal, or disappearance of Graves' disease–related immunoglobulins (TSI and TBII) from the serum during treatment.

Leukopenia is the principal undesirable side effect of antithyroid drugs. Mild transient leukopenia may occur in approximately 10 percent of patients and is not necessarily an indication for discontinuing therapy. When the absolute number of polymorphonuclear leukocytes reaches 1500 or less, antithyroid medication should be discontinued. Allergic rashes and drug sensitivity occur in a small percentage of patients. These may disappear with antihistamine therapy at the same or reduced dosage of antithyroid agent, but it is probably preferable when sensitivity reactions occur to change to another drug. On rare occasions (in less than 0.2 percent), agranulocytosis occurs. This may be sudden in onset. Hepatitis, drug fever, and arthralgias occur on occasion. In the author's view, severe sensitivity reactions, including agranulocytosis, dictate the abandonment of antithyroid therapy, rather than recourse to an alternate drug.

Iodide inhibits the release of hormones from the hyperfunctioning thyroid gland, and its ameliorative effects occur more rapidly than those of agents that inhibit hormone synthesis. Hence, its main use is in patients with actual or impending thyrotoxic crisis and in patients with severe thyrocardiac disease. The response to iodide is often incomplete and transient. Furthermore, by expanding the thyroid store of hormone, iodide may prolong the latency of response to antithyroid therapy. Therefore, iodide should be used in conjunction with the antithyroid agents. If the clinical course is sufficiently severe to require iodide administration, antithyroid drugs are usually the primary therapeutic agents and should be given in large doses prior to iodide. Since iodide appears to synergize with radiation, it is also useful in controlling thyrotoxicosis following ^{131}I administration, during the period in which the therapeutic effect of radioiodine has not yet taken place. By a poorly understood mechanism, large doses of *glucocorticoids* (2 mg of dexamethasone every 6 h) reduce the serum T_4 concentration and should be added to the regimen when relief of thyrotoxicosis is urgent. The iodinated x-ray contrast agent sodium ipodate has a similar effect. Iodine liberated from this agent inhibits thyroid secretion of T_4 and T_3, and serum T_3 is further reduced by the inhibition by ipodate of peripheral T_3-neogenesis. Daily doses of 1 g orally are effective, but the same precautions concerning the use of iodine therapy are applicable to ipodate as well.

Owing to the pronounced adrenergic component in thyrotoxicosis, various *adrenergic antagonists* have been employed in its management. Of these, propranolol is the agent of choice because of its relative freedom from side effects. In doses of 40 to 120 mg daily, propranolol alleviates such adrenergic manifestations as sweating, tremor, and tachycardia and may reduce to some extent the conversion of T_4 to T_3. However, propranolol should be used only as adjunctive therapy rather than sole therapy, as some have suggested, since the underlying metabolic abnormalities are not affected. Moreover, although the diminution in heart rate and cardiac work may be beneficial, the blocking of adrenergic support of myocardial contractility contraindicates its use in the patient with coexisting heart failure, unless rate- or rhythm-related. As adjunctive therapy, the major usefulness of propranolol is during the period when the response to conventional antithyroid agents or to radioiodine therapy is being awaited and in the management of thyrotoxic crisis. It has been employed as the sole agent in preparation for thyroidectomy, but its use in this setting is not recommended since it does not render the patient euthyroid, with a likely greater risk of surgically induced crisis.

Radioactive iodine (*^{131}I*) affords a relatively simple, effective, and economical means of treating thyrotoxicosis. It can produce the ablative effects of surgery without the immediate operative and postoperative complications. The principal disadvantage of ^{131}I therapy, in the dosage usually employed, is its tendency to produce hypothyroidism with a frequency that increases with time. As many as 40 to 70 percent of patients may develop this complication within 10 years after treatment. Although hypothyroidism is treatable, once diagnosed, the insidious onset may obscure the diagnosis until serious complications have developed. Hence, some recommend that all patients be treated with large doses of ^{131}I to ensure relief of thyrotoxicosis and then placed on permanent physiologic replacement doses of thyroid hormone.

There is no evidence of carcinogenic or leukemogenic effects of radioiodine when it is given to adults in the doses commonly used in treating hyperthyroidism. However, the susceptibility to carcinogenesis may be increased in the thyroids of children. Mutagenic effects have not been reported and would be difficult to document. For these reasons, many physicians prefer to reserve radioiodine therapy for patients over 30 years of age or those unlikely to have children subsequently. Moreover, the longer the life expectancy after ^{131}I therapy, the greater the likelihood that hypothyroidism will develop. Among younger patients, therefore, those with recurrent thyrotoxicosis following surgery, those who refuse surgery, and those with complicating illness that contraindicates surgery are candidates for radioiodine therapy. In elderly patients, treatment with large doses of radioiodine is the general method of choice, so that the undesirable effects of incomplete treatment or recurrence can be avoided. There is general agreement that patients with coexisting cardiac disease should receive ^{131}I in large doses in view of the hazard of recurrent thyrotoxicosis.

The usual therapeutic dose of ^{131}I [approximately 5.92 MBq (160 μCi) per gram of estimated gland weight] has led to the disturbingly high frequency of hypothyroidism. As a result, though continuing to use this dose, some authorities regularly administer prophylactic replacement doses of thyroid hormone. On the other hand, others have administered smaller doses [approximately 2.96 MBq/g (80 μCi/g)]. However, this does not diminish the frequency of late hypothyroidism but merely delays its onset. Moreover, the smaller dose is less likely to relieve thyrotoxicosis within a relatively short period. Antithyroid agents can be employed, however, to speed the attainment of a eumetabolic state, and propranolol can be given to relieve symptoms, while the effect of the ^{131}I is taking hold.

Radiation thyroiditis is an occasional immediate complication of ^{131}I therapy. When present, it commonly appears within 7 to 10 days and is associated with excessive release of hormone into the blood. For this reason, patients with severe hyperthyroidism or underlying heart disease should be rendered eumetabolic with antithyroid agents before ^{131}I is administered. Interruption of antithyroid therapy for several days before and after ^{131}I treatment suffices to permit adequate accumulation and retention of administered ^{131}I. Propranolol may be used as an adjunct both before and after ^{131}I administration but should not be relied upon to provide adequate prophylaxis if given alone. The swelling that accompanies radiation thyroiditis may contraindicate the use of large doses of ^{131}I in patients with large retrosternal goiters.

Before radioactive iodine was introduced, *subtotal thyroidectomy* was the standard form of ablative therapy, and it is still employed in younger patients in whom antithyroid therapy is unsuccessful. Although precise preoperative programs differ, several general principles should be emphasized. Patients should first be rendered fully euthyroid by means of antithyroid agents. Only then should iodide (five drops of Lugol's solution a day for approximately 10 days) be administered concomitantly to effect an involutional response in the gland. Antithyroid drugs should not be discontinued merely because treatment with iodide is instituted. The response of the patient, and not the calendar, should dictate when surgery is performed.

Hazards of subtotal thyroidectomy include immediate complications, such as anesthetic accidents, hemorrhage sometimes leading to respiratory obstruction, and damage to the recurrent laryngeal nerve leading to vocal cord paralysis. Later complications include wound infection, hemorrhage, hypoparathyroidism, or hypothyroidism. Subtotal thyroidectomy should be performed by a surgeon experienced in this procedure; under this condition surgery is effective and relatively safe. Postoperative recurrences are uncommon. However, carefully conducted follow-up studies reveal that hypothyroidism follows surgery more frequently than previously suspected, although not as commonly as following treatment with ^{131}I.

The *treatment of hyperthyroidism during pregnancy* is a subject of some disagreement. Most physicians believe that antithyroid therapy is preferable to surgery, which should not be performed in any event during the first and third trimesters. Antithyroid agents carry less risk to the patient and the pregnancy. Further, since they traverse the placental barrier, they have the theoretical advantage of preventing fetal and neonatal hyperthyroidism when maternal titers of thyroid-stimulating IgG are high. As a clue to the risk of fetal hyperthyroidism, assays of such stimulators should be conducted in pregnant women with a history of Graves' disease, whether treated or not. On the other hand, the major disadvantage of antithyroid therapy is the possibility of inducing hypothyroidism in the fetus. T_4 and T_3 traverse the human placenta from mother to fetus only slowly, if at all, and simultaneous administration of thyroid hormone and antithyroid drugs to the mother will not protect the fetus from developing hypothyroidism. Hence, the cardinal rule in using the antithyroid agents in pregnancy is that the dosage should be the smallest necessary to control hyperthyroidism in the mother. From the laboratory standpoint, the physician should aim to keep the serum FT_4 concentration or the FT_4I within the normal limits, remembering that pregnancy is normally associated with some elevation of the serum total T_4, owing to an increase in serum TBG concentration. Since pregnancy appears to attenuate the severity of hyperthyroidism, control can often be achieved with maintenance doses of 200 mg of propylthiouracil daily or less. At this dose level, fetal goiter or hypothyroidism has not been a problem. Patients who require doses of 300 mg daily or more during the first trimester should probably be treated by subtotal thyroidectomy during the middle trimester. Although some would disagree, the author believes that patients carried through pregnancy on antithyroid agents should not be given propranolol as adjunctive treatment, in view of reports that the agent may cause fetal growth retardation and neonatal respiratory depression. Radioiodine should never be administered to a pregnant woman, and all women of childbearing age who are about to receive ^{131}I should have a pregnancy test performed first.

Ophthalmopathy, dermopathy When severe and progressive, ophthalmopathy is the most difficult component of Graves' disease to treat satisfactorily. Fortunately, in most patients the disorder runs a benign course that is largely independent of the course of the hyperthyroidism. In most instances, the activity of even moderately severe disease declines and disappears with time, although some exophthalmos and ophthalmoplegia may persist. In mild disease, considerable benefit may be obtained from simple measures, such as elevating the head at night, administering diuretics to reduce edema, and providing tinted glasses for protection from sun, wind, and foreign bodies. A 1% solution of methylcellulose or plastic shields may prevent corneal drying in patients unable to oppose the lids during sleep. In more severe cases, as evidenced by progressive exophthalmos, chemosis, ophthalmoplegia, or loss of vision, large doses of prednisone (120 to 140 mg daily) should be administered, since this is usually effective in reducing the edematous and infiltrative components. With improvement, the dosage is reduced to the lowest effective level, since prolonged administration of large doses leads to adverse accompaniments of glucocorticoid excess. Orbital radiation may be helpful in some patients with acute, severe infiltrative manifestations. In cases that progress despite these measures, orbital decompression, i.e., removal of part of the bony orbit to relieve intraorbital pressure, usually halts progression of the disease. The management must always be conducted in concert with an ophthalmologist.

In general, treatment of associated hyperthyroidism should be carried out much as would be the case were ophthalmopathy not present, since the mode of treatment of the hyperthyroidism does not influence the course of the ocular disease. The suggestion that total thyroid ablation by surgery and large doses of ^{131}I is beneficial to the ophthalmic disease has not been borne out. It is agreed, however, that hyperthyroidism should be treated and that hypothyroidism be avoided.

Severe dermopathy can be alleviated by the topical application of glucocorticoids.

TOXIC MULTINODULAR GOITER

Toxic multinodular goiter is an occasional consequence of long-standing simple goiter, although the exact proportion of cases in which this complication arises is uncertain. In areas of nonendemicity, the etiology of nontoxic multinodular goiter is usually indeterminate. Hence, it is unclear whether a specific etiologic factor underlies those cases of nontoxic multinodular goiter that progress to thyrotoxic phase. Common to many nontoxic multinodular goiters, even in areas of iodine sufficiency, is a decrease in the iodine content of thyroglobulin, suggesting either a conditioned deficiency of iodine or an impairment of its normal incorporation into iodinated amino acids. There is no pathologic feature to distinguish the nontoxic from the toxic multinodular goiter. However, the transition from nontoxic to toxic nodular goiter involves the development of a sufficient degree of functional autonomy, i.e., independence from TSH stimulation in one or more areas of the gland. Scattered foci of functional autonomy are present, even early in the disease process. These increase in size and frequency as time passes so that even among seemingly euthyroid patients with nontoxic nodular goiter, approximately a fourth display, as evidence of functional autonomy, subnormal or absent responses to TRH administration. As judged from scintillation scanning studies, functional patterns may be of two types. In the first and more common, iodine accumulation occurs diffusely but in patchy foci throughout the gland. The second, less common, pattern is that of iodine accumulation in one or more discrete nodules within the gland, the remainder appearing to be essentially nonfunctional. Histologic and autoradiographic studies reveal marked heterogeneity of structure and function, the two being poorly correlated. In both endemic and sporadic nontoxic multinodular goiter, administration of iodides may lead to the development of thyrotoxicosis, a complication that is consonant with the functional autonomy that characterizes this disorder.

Because it arises in long-standing simple goiter, toxic multinodular goiter is a disease of the aging or elderly. For this reason and because of the nature of the underlying disease, the clinical presentation differs from that in Graves' disease. Ophthalmopathy is rare and would signal the emergence of Graves' disease superimposed on simple goiter. Some patients have typical thyrotoxicosis. Often, however, the degree of thyrotoxicosis is less severe than that in Graves' disease, although its physiologic impact upon specific organ systems may be great. Notable among these is the cardiovascular system, in which arrhythmias or congestive failure may be precipitated or accentuated by thyrotoxicosis that may be manifested only by subtle findings in other areas (apathetic hyperthyroidism). Weakness and wasting may predominate, frequently with loss of appetite rather than hyperphagia, suggesting the presence of a carcinoma.

In some patients, a definitive diagnosis of toxic nodular goiter is difficult to establish. On the one hand, enlargement or nodularity of the gland may escape detection because the patient has a short neck or is kyphotic or because the thyroid is located substernally. When this is the case and when the clinical findings suggest thyrotoxicosis, RAIU and scintiscan may prove illuminating. On the other hand, even when a nodular goiter is palpable, the presence of mild but clinically significant thyrotoxicosis may be difficult to confirm, since values of the serum total T_4, FT_4, and FT_4I, as well as the serum T_3 concentration, are often only near or slightly above the upper limit of the normal range. For example, a value for the serum T_3 that would be considered normal for a young adult may represent an increase in the elderly patient, since serum T_3 usually declines with age. Despite their value in situations such as this, thyroid suppression tests should not be undertaken in the elderly patient because of the hazard of adverse cardiovascular responses. Unfortunately, although a normal response to TRH would exclude a diagnosis of thyrotoxicosis in a patient with a nodular goiter, subnormal responses do not establish the diagnosis. Responses to TRH decline in the elderly, especially in men, and a high proportion of patients with nodular goiter who otherwise seem euthyroid respond subnormally to TRH as a reflection of at least partial functional autonomy of the thyroid gland. When laboratory findings do not permit a clear diagnosis of thyrotoxicosis but suggestive clinical findings are present, a therapeutic trial of antithyroid drugs is indicated.

Radioactive iodine is the treatment of choice for toxic multinodular goiter. Large doses [740 to 1110 MBq (20 to 30 mCi)] are usually required, owing to the generally lower RAIU and to the variable degree of function throughout the gland. Moreover, the physiologic instability of the elderly patient makes definitive treatment desirable. For the same reason, it is usually wise to initiate therapy with antithyroid agents, withholding radioiodine until a euthyroid state has been achieved and thereby forestalling an exacerbation of thyrotoxicosis, should radiation thyroiditis occur. Unless contraindicated, propranolol is often useful in controlling manifestations of thyrotoxicosis both before and after radioiodine therapy, while its therapeutic effect is awaited. Hypothyroidism is an uncommon consequence of radioiodine treatment of toxic multinodular goiter, owing to the variable activity of differing portions of the gland, which permits previously quiescent areas to replace functionally those that have been destroyed by ^{131}I.

UNUSUAL VARIETIES OF THYROTOXICOSIS

In addition to Graves' disease and toxic multinodular goiter, thyrotoxicosis is seen in other disorders, including follicular adenoma of the thyroid and various forms of thyroiditis, which are discussed in later sections. This section will consider still other infrequent causes of thyrotoxicosis and unusual ways in which thyrotoxicosis may present from the laboratory standpoint.

UNUSUAL CAUSES OF THYROTOXICOSIS Rarely, hyperthyroidism and thyrotoxicosis are the result of sustained hypersecretion of TSH from either a *TSH-secreting pituitary adenoma* or a selective *resistance of the TSH-secretory mechanism* to feedback inhibition by thyroid hormones. The resistance syndrome may be a variant of one in which both the pituitary and peripheral tissues are relatively resistant to thyroid hormones. TSH-secreting pituitary adenomas can be distinguished, in many cases, by radiologic evidence of pituitary tumor, by the fact that the concentration of free alpha subunits of TSH in serum is elevated, and by the fact that the response of the serum TSH to TRH is negligible. In the variant caused by pituitary resistance, subunit concentrations are not grossly elevated, and the TSH response to TRH is usually normal.

Patients with *trophoblastic tumor,* either choriocarcinoma or hydatidiform mole, frequently display elevations, sometimes marked, of serum total and free T_4 and T_3 concentrations. Clinical evidence of thyrotoxicosis may be lacking. Thyroid hyperfunction is caused by a circulating thyroid stimulator of trophoblastic origin, which is probably a variant of human chorionic gonadotropin (hCG), and abnormalities remit promptly after removal of the tumor.

Thyrotoxicosis factitia is a form of thyrotoxicosis without hyperthyroidism and results from purposeful or inadvertent ingestion of supraphysiologic quantities of thyroid hormone. The syndrome is usually a form of malingering and occurs most commonly in women with an underlying psychiatric disorder, usually paramedical personnel, or in patients who have taken thyroid hormones in the past or who have relatives that take thyroid hormones. In such patients, endogenous thyroid function is suppressed, as evidenced by subnormal values of the RAIU and serum thyroglobulin concentration. Both serum T_4 and T_3 concentrations are increased if the patient is taking a preparation that contains T_4, whereas the serum T_3 concentration is elevated and the serum T_4 depressed in patients taking T_3 alone.

Very rarely, thyrotoxicosis with a low RAIU is the result of excess hormone secretion by *ectopic thyroid tissue,* either widespread functioning metastases of thyroid carcinoma or struma ovarii.

Jodbasedow phenomenon refers to the induction of thyrotoxicosis in a previously euthyroid patient as a result of exposure to increased quantities of iodine. It typically occurs in areas of endemic iodine deficiency when measures to increase iodine intake or body iodine stores are implemented. The presumption is that the supplemental iodine permits functionally autonomous thyroid tissue to produce and secrete excessive hormone. A similar phenomenon can occur in patients with nontoxic multinodular goiter who have received large doses of iodide. Since such patients tend to be elderly with the danger of serious cardiovascular manifestations should thyrotoxicosis ensue, large doses of iodine should not be given to those with multinodular goiter. Similarly, in such patients, pharmaceuticals containing iodine, most often x-ray contrast media, should be used only when indicated and with consideration of the possible hazard of inducing the jodbasedow phenomenon. When a contrast study is indicated under these conditions, it may be judicious to administer large doses of propylthiouracil (450 to 600 mg per day) prior to and for a week after the procedure. Some patients may develop hyperthyroidism following exposure to large quantities of iodine despite the fact that after iodine is withdrawn, they recover, their thyroid function appears to be entirely normal, and evidence of functional autonomy is lacking.

UNUSUAL PRESENTATIONS OF THYROTOXICOSIS **T_3 toxicosis** Thyrotoxicosis in which serum T_4 is normal or low in the absence of a deficiency of TBG, while the serum T_3 is increased, is termed T_3 toxicosis. Although the production rate of T_3 is disproportionately increased relative to that of T_4 in all patients with hyperthyroidism, in some this discrepancy is exaggerated. This may occur in association with Graves' disease, multinodular goiter, or hyperfunctioning adenoma. The diagnosis should be suspected in a patient with clinical manifestations of thyrotoxicosis in whom the serum T_4 and FT_4 are normal or low and the RAIU is normal or increased. This, together with the frequently palpable goiter, serves to differentiate this disorder from liothyronine-induced thyrotoxicosis factitia. In contrast to patients with nonthyroidal disorders that mimic thyrotoxicosis, patients with this disorder, as would be expected, demonstrate both nonsuppressibility of thyroid function in response to exogenous T_3 and blunted or absent responses to TRH. In many patients, thyrotoxicosis with increased serum T_3 and normal serum T_4 antecedes emergence of typical increases in both, either during an initial episode of hyperthyroidism or more commonly during recurrence after previous treatment. In some patients in whom symptoms of thyrotoxicosis fail to regress completely during antithyroid therapy despite return of the serum T_4 concentration to normal, the serum T_3 concentration is persistently elevated. Such patients are prone to experience a recurrence of thyrotoxicosis when antithyroid therapy is withdrawn.

T_4 toxicosis In most patients with hyperthyroidism, the serum T_3 is increased to a relatively greater extent than is the serum T_4. This reflects the fact that in hyperthyroidism T_3 generated from T_4 peripherally is supplemented by release of substantial quantities of T_3 from the thyroid. However, thyrotoxicosis may sometimes be associated with a clear elevation of serum T_4 and a seemingly normal serum T_3 concentration. This syndrome of *T_4 toxicosis* occurs most commonly in patients who are elderly, ill, or both, and is, therefore, usually seen in a hospital setting. Presumably, the combination of high serum T_4 and normal serum T_3 concentration reflects inhibition of peripheral T_3 generation from T_4, with persistence of T_3 secretion along with T_4 from the thyroid.

MAJOR COMPLICATIONS OF THYROTOXICOSIS

THYROCARDIAC DISEASE Thyrotoxicosis imposes a variety of burdens upon the heart. Hypermetabolism of the peripheral tissues increases both the metabolic and nonmetabolic (heat-loss) circulatory load, while direct effects of thyroid hormone on the myocardium increase the force, velocity, and rate of ventricular contraction. As a result, cardiac work and cardiac output are increased. Moreover, atrial irritability is enhanced, leading to tachydysrhythmias, most importantly atrial fibrillation. In the patient with a normal heart, these burdens are usually tolerated. In the patient with underlying heart disease, however, cardiac insufficiency may be precipitated or aggravated. As would be expected, this complication is more common in the elderly patient and is common in the patient with toxic multinodular goiter, sometimes as the most prominent manifestation of the thyrotoxic state. In patients with cardiac insufficiency, clues to the presence of thyrotoxicosis include atrial fibrillation, relatively rapid circulation time, increased cardiac output (high-output failure), and resistance to the usual therapeutic doses of digitalis.

Treatment is directed at rapid alleviation of thyrotoxicosis and restoration of cardiac compensation. The former objective is best met by initiation of treatment with large doses of an antithyroid agent, followed by iodine if the clinical situation is urgent. In less severe cases, radioiodine treatment is preceded by antithyroid drug treatment alone. Management of the cardiac decompensation is carried out in the usual manner, employing larger than usual doses of digitalis but with care to avoid digitalis intoxication as thyrotoxicosis is alleviated. Adrenergic antagonists should not be employed in the presence of cardiac failure, unless it is felt that failure is the consequence primarily of disturbance of cardiac rate or rhythm.

THYROTOXIC CRISIS Thyrotoxic crisis or storm causes a fulminating increase in the signs and symptoms of thyrotoxicosis. In the past, this disturbance was most often observed postoperatively in patients poorly prepared for surgery. However, with the preoperative use of antithyroid drugs and iodide and with appropriate measures directed to control of metabolic factors, weight, and nutritional status, postoperative thyrotoxic crisis should not occur. At present, so-called medical storm is more common and occurs in untreated or inadequately treated patients. It is precipitated by surgical emergency or complicating illness, usually sepsis. The syndrome is characterized by extreme irritability, delirium or coma, fever to 41°C or more, tachycardia, restlessness, hypotension, vomiting, and diarrhea. Rarely, the picture may be more subtle, with apathy, prostration, and coma, but with only slight elevation of temperature. Such postoperative complications as sepsis, septicemia, hemorrhage, and transfusion or drug reactions may mimic thyrotoxic crisis. The physiologic factor(s) that initiates thyrotoxic crisis is unknown. It does not appear to be an acute increase in the severity of thyroid hyperfunction.

Treatment consists in providing general supportive therapy while undertaking measures for alleviating thyrotoxicosis as rapidly as possible. Supportive therapy includes treatment of dehydration and the intravenous administration of glucose and saline, vitamin B complex, and glucocorticoids. The latter are indicated because of the increased glucocorticoid requirements in thyrotoxicosis and because adrenocortical reserve is reduced in this disorder. Patients should be placed in a cooled, humidified oxygen tent, and, if hyperpyrexia is present, a cooling blanket should be used. Digitalization is required to control ventricular rate in those with atrial fibrillation. If shock exists, intravenous pressor agents should be employed. Therapy of the hyperthyroidism consists of induction of blockade of hormone synthesis by the immediate and continued administration of large doses of an antithyroid agent (e.g., 100 mg propylthiouracil every 2 h). If the patient is unable to swallow the medication, the tablets should be triturated and given by nasogastric tube, as parenteral preparations are unavailable. Following initiation of antithyroid therapy, inhibition of hormone release is sought through the administration of large doses of iodine intravenously or by mouth. The iodinated x-ray contrast agent sodium ipodate can be administered instead of iodine and has the added action of also inhibiting the peripheral conversion of T_4 to T_3. Doses of 1 g daily are effective. Adrenergic antagonists are an important, and perhaps critical, part of the therapeutic regimen, in the absence of cardiac failure. The beta-adrenergic blocking agent propranolol can be administered in doses of 40 to 80 mg every 6 h. If medications cannot be taken orally, 2 mg of propranolol may be given intravenously, with careful electrocardiographic monitoring. Large doses of dexamethasone (e.g., 2 mg every 6 h) should also be administered, since they inhibit hormone release, impair the peripheral generation of T_3 from T_4, and provide adrenal support. Indeed, with the combined use of propylthiouracil, iodine, and dexamethasone, the serum T_3 concentration generally returns to normal within 24 to 48 h. Antithyroid therapy, iodine, and dexamethasone must be continued until a normal metabolic state is approached, at which time iodine is progressively withdrawn and plans are made for definitive treatment.

THYROIDITIS

Thyroiditis embraces disorders of differing etiology. Two are exceedingly uncommon, *pyogenic thyroiditis* and *chronic fibrosing (Riedel's) thyroiditis*. Pyogenic thyroiditis is usually anteceded by a pyogenic infection elsewhere and is characterized by tenderness and swelling of the thyroid, redness and warmth of the overlying skin, and constitutional signs of infection. Treatment consists of antibiotic therapy and incisional drainage if a fluctuant area within the thyroid should occur. Riedel's thyroiditis is a rare disorder in which intense fibrosis of the thyroid and surrounding structures, leading to induration of the tissues of the neck, may be associated with mediastinal and retroperitoneal fibrosis. The principal importance of this disorder is that it requires differentiation from thyroid neoplasia.

The other forms of thyroiditis, comprising subacute thyroiditis, chronic thyroiditis with transient thyrotoxicosis (CT/TT), and Hashimoto's thyroiditis, are more common. They are notable for their different clinical courses and for the fact that each can be associated, at one time or another, with a euthyroid, thyrotoxic, or hypothyroid state.

SUBACUTE THYROIDITIS This disorder, also termed *granulomatous, giant cell,* or *de Quervain's thyroiditis,* appears to be viral in origin. Symptoms of thyroiditis usually follow those of an upper respiratory infection and include pronounced asthenia, malaise, and symptoms referable to stretching of the thyroid capsule, principally pain over the thyroid or pain referred to the lower jaw, ear, or occiput. Referred pain may predominate. These symptoms may smolder for weeks before the diagnosis is suspected. Less commonly, the onset is acute, with severe pain over the thyroid, accompanied by fever and occasionally symptoms of thyrotoxicosis. Physical findings include exquisite tenderness and nodularity over the thyroid, which may be unilateral but which usually involves other areas of the gland. Although local or referred pain is the commonest symptom, occasional patients have other features typical of the disease but have no pain.

Two laboratory findings are characteristic: a high erythrocyte sedimentation rate (ESR) and a depressed RAIU. Values for the remaining tests depend upon the stage of the disease in which they are obtained. Early, many patients are mildly thyrotoxic owing to leakage of hormone from the gland. The serum T_4 and T_3 are high. Later, as glandular hormone is depleted, the patient may pass through a hypothyroid phase, in which serum T_4 and T_3 are low and TSH increased. Diagnosis of the thyrotoxic phase is especially troublesome in patients with the uncommon, painless variant since the patient may be thought to have Graves' disease or toxic nodular goiter and therapy inappropriate for subacute thyroiditis may be instituted. Demonstration of a low RAIU usually serves to differentiate subacute thyroiditis from these other causes of hyperthyroidism. Differentiation of painless subacute thyroiditis from the syndrome of chronic thyroiditis with transient thyrotoxicosis is discussed below.

The disorder may smolder for months but eventually subsides with a return of normal thyroid function. In mild cases, aspirin suffices to control the symptoms. In more severe cases, glucocorticoid (prednisone, 20 to 40 mg daily) is generally effective. Propranolol can be used to control associated thyrotoxicosis. When the RAIU returns to normal, therapy can be withdrawn without recurrence of symptoms.

CHRONIC THYROIDITIS WITH TRANSIENT THYROTOXICOSIS This term denotes a disorder in which a self-limited episode of thyrotoxicosis is associated with a histologic picture of chronic lymphocytic thyroiditis that differs from that of Hashimoto's disease. This syndrome has been variously designated as painless thyroiditis, silent thyroiditis, hyperthyroiditis, chronic thyroiditis with spontaneously resolving hyperthyroidism, or, as the author prefers, chronic thyroiditis with transient thyrotoxicosis (CT/TT). Designations that imply the existence of hyperthyroidism are inappropriate, since ongoing production of thyroid hormone is negligible and the RAIU is decreased.

The syndrome occurs in patients of any age, and although it occurs mainly in women, the female/male ratio is not as high as in Graves' disease. Manifestations of thyrotoxicosis are usually mild but may be severe. The thyroid is nontender, firm, symmetrical, and enlarged only slightly or moderately. Laboratory features include elevations of the serum T_4 and T_3 concentrations consonant with the thyrotoxicosis and a markedly depressed RAIU. The ESR is normal or only slightly elevated, rarely exceeding 50 mm/h, and antithyroid antibodies, when present, are present in low titer.

The etiology, pathogenesis, and pathophysiology of this disorder are unclear. Viral antibody titers show no characteristic patterns. It is presumed that thyrotoxicosis results from leakage of hormone from the gland, as in subacute thyroiditis. Low values for the RAIU, in turn, reflect suppression of TSH secretion, since urinary iodine excretion is not greatly elevated. Some degree of thyroid malfunction is indicated by failure of the RAIU to respond briskly to exogenous TSH stimulation.

Thyrotoxicosis in CT/TT usually abates within 2 to 5 months. Many patients have recurrent episodes of thyrotoxicosis of similar nature, sometimes following pregnancy. The thyrotoxic phase may be followed in several months by a phase of self-limited hypothyroidism. The latter, which has been noted particularly in the postpartum period, may be the only component of the disease that is diagnosed. In Japan, as many as 5 percent of pregnant women may experience the syndrome post partum.

This disorder, in the thyrotoxic phase, needs differentiation, first from Graves' disease; this can be accomplished by demonstration of a depressed RAIU and absence of increased urinary iodine excretion. The latter serves also to exclude the jodbasedow syndrome. When these data are available, the disorder must be differentiated from other causes of thyrotoxicosis with a low RAIU, principally subacute thyroiditis. Lack of tenderness or nodularity of the thyroid and absence of marked elevation of the ESR tend to exclude the latter diagnosis. Patients with functioning ectopic thyroid tissue and thyrotoxicosis factitia characteristically respond to exogenous TSH stimulation with a brisk increase in RAIU. Definitive diagnosis of CT/TT can be made by thyroid biopsy.

Since the thyroid is not hyperfunctioning in this disorder, measures used in the treatment of hyperthyroidism are useless. Symptomatic treatment with propranolol or mild sedatives is administered until the thyrotoxicosis abates. In patients with frequently recurrent disease, thyroid ablation with ^{131}I during a period of remission followed by long-term replacement therapy has been advocated by some.

HASHIMOTO'S THYROIDITIS This disorder, also termed *lymphadenoid goiter*, is a common chronic inflammatory disease of the thyroid in which autoimmune factors play a prominent role, occurring most frequently in women of middle age. It is also the most common cause of sporadic goiter in children. Evidence of the participation of autoimmune factors includes the lymphocytic infiltration of the gland and the presence in the serum of increased concentrations of immunoglobulins and of antibodies against several components of thyroid tissue. Of these, the most important from the clinical standpoint are the antithyroglobulin antibody detected by the tanned red cell agglutination technique and the antimicrosomal antibody detected by immunofluorescence or complement fixation techniques. This disorder also coexists with some frequency with other diseases of a presumed autoimmune nature, including pernicious anemia, Sjögren's syndrome, chronic active hepatitis, systemic lupus erythematosus, rheumatoid arthritis, nontuberculous Addison's disease, diabetes mellitus, and Graves' disease itself (see Chap. 334). These disorders, as well as Hashimoto's disease itself, also occur frequently in family members of patients with Hashimoto's disease.

Goiter is the outstanding feature. The enlargement involves the entire gland but not necessarily symmetrically. Typically, the consistency is rubbery, the margins are scalloped, and the general outline of the gland is preserved. The pyramidal lobe may be prominent. Early in the disease the patient is metabolically normal; however, even then decreased thyroid reserve is often manifest in an increase in serum TSH. The RAIU may be elevated early in the disease, reflecting the secretion of calorigenically inactive iodoproteins, but the serum T_4 and T_3 are normal and the patient is euthyroid. As the disease progresses, thyroid failure, at first subclinical, gradually supervenes owing to progressive replacement of thyroid parenchyma by lymphocytes or fibrous tissue. The thyroid failure is evident first in a rise in serum TSH concentration. With time, the serum T_4 concentration declines though the serum T_3 remains normal. Eventually, the serum T_3 concentration falls below normal, and the patient is frankly hypothyroid. High titers of antimicrosomal antibody are almost always present. High titers may also occur in other thyroid disorders, particularly primary thyroprivic hypothyroidism and Graves' disease but with lesser frequency. Although the foregoing findings usually suffice to permit a diagnosis, histologic confirmation by needle biopsy may be required. In view of the frequency with which hypothyroidism is either present or eventually develops, treatment with replacement doses of levothyroxine is indicated. In some patients, such therapy is associated with regression of goiter.

Occasional patients present with hyperthyroidism in association with a thyroid gland that is unusually firm and with high titers of circulating antithyroid antibodies, a combination which suggests, probably correctly, the concurrence of Graves' disease and Hashimoto's thyroiditis (''Hashitoxicosis''). In others, hyperthyroidism may supervene in a patient known to have Hashimoto's thyroiditis, presumably due to the emergence of clones of lymphocytes that produce anti-TSH receptor antibodies. Hyperthyroidism in association with Hashimoto's thyroiditis is treated in a conventional manner, but ablative therapy is less commonly employed, since the associated chronic thyroiditis tends to limit the duration of thyroid hyperfunction and also predisposes the patient to the development of hypothyroidism after surgical or radioiodine treatment.

NEOPLASMS

THYROID ADENOMAS True adenomas, as contrasted with localized adenomatous areas, are encapsulated and usually compress contiguous tissue. Adenomas vary in size and histologic characteristics and are often classified into three major types: papillary, follicular, and Hürthle cell. The follicular adenomas can be subdivided according to the size of the follicles into colloid or macrofollicular, fetal or microfollicular, and embryonal varieties. There is variation in physiologic differentiation, as judged by the ability to concentrate radioiodine. The more highly differentiated adenomas (follicular) are the most common and are the most likely to mimic the function of normal thyroid tissue. Though their function may be responsive to TSH stimulation, it differs from that of normal thyroid tissue in being autonomous, i.e., the basal activity is independent of TSH stimulation. Adenomas of this type are usually unifocal, presenting as a single nodule. Often the patient reports that the nodule has grown slowly over many years. Initially, its function is insufficient to disturb hormonal equilibrium though its capacity to accumulate radioiodine is evident in scintiscans as an area of increased density within the still-functioning extranodular tissue (*"warm" nodule*). At this stage, demonstration of the inherent autonomy of the nodule's function requires scintiscanning while the patient is receiving suppressive doses of exogenous thyroid hormone (suppression scan). With time the nodule grows larger, its function increasing until it is sufficient to suppress TSH secretion. Consequently, the remainder of the gland undergoes atrophy and loss of function, and the scintiscan then reveals radioiodine accumulation only in the region of the nodule (*"hot" nodule*). At this time, the patient may or may not be overtly thyrotoxic, but frank thyrotoxicosis usually supervenes eventually (*toxic adenoma*). Relative to its overall rate of occurrence, hyperfunctioning adenoma is a frequent cause of T_3 toxicosis. Hyperfunctioning adenomas are amenable to ablation by surgery or ^{131}I. Large doses of the latter are usually required to bring about prompt cure. Before such treatment it is desirable to administer TSH and demonstrate by scintiscan the latent functional capacity of the extranodular tissue. Although it has been thought that radiation damage would be confined solely to the hyperfunctioning nodule being treated with ^{131}I, the remaining tissue being spared, this may not always be the case, since some patients with hyperfunctioning adenoma become euthyroid after treatment with ^{131}I only to become hypothyroid years later.

Hyperfunctioning nodules are rarely the seat of carcinoma. However, hyperfunctioning adenomas not infrequently undergo hemorrhagic necrosis. The resulting pain and nodularity may suggest subacute thyroiditis. Subsequently, there is loss of function and the appearance of a *"cold" nodule* on scintiscanning, since the remainder of the thyroid will have resumed function. When this happens, the nodule is likely to be mistaken for a carcinoma. Indeed, hypofunctioning, hemorrhagic adenomas and thyroid cysts account for the majority of cold nodules initially suspected of being carcinomas.

THYROID CARCINOMAS Thyroid carcinoma may be classified into two varieties, depending upon whether the lesion arises in thyroid follicular epithelium or whether it arises from the parafollicular or C cells. The latter disorder, medullary thyroid carcinoma, has distinctive physiologic and clinical characteristics and is discussed separately (see Chap. 334). The thyroid may also be the site of one or another of the lymphoproliferative diseases or of carcinoma metastatic from a diagnosed or undiagnosed primary tumor elsewhere.

Carcinomas of follicular epithelium The three general histologic types differ in their clinical course. The least common is *anaplastic carcinoma,* which is histologically undifferentiated, usually afflicts the elderly, and is highly malignant. The lesion is rapidly fatal, owing to extensive local invasion which is refractory to radiation. The second type of tumor, *follicular carcinoma,* is also uncommon and histologically mimics normal thyroid tissue. This lesion usually undergoes early hematogenous spread, and the patient may present with a distant metastasis, usually in lung or bone. Follicular carcinoma or follicular elements in papillary carcinoma are responsible for those instances in which thyroid carcinoma, in situ or in metastases, accumulates significant quantities of ^{131}I. The third and most common type of tumor, *papillary carcinoma,* has a bimodal frequency, peaks occurring in the second or third decades and again in later life. This lesion is slowly growing and typically spreads to the regional lymph nodes, where it may remain indolent for many years. Acceleration of the disease may take place at any time. Follicular elements are usually present in both the primary lesion and its metastases.

DIAGNOSIS AND MANAGEMENT The diagnosis and management of thyroid carcinoma are interwoven with the management of the nodular goiter. In the past, this subject has evoked a wide disparity of views among authorities, stemming from seemingly contradictory data. On the one hand, surgically excised specimens of thyroid nodules, particularly solitary nodules, revealed a high frequency of carcinoma (as much as 20 percent in some series). On the other hand, despite the frequency of nodular goiter in the general population (approximately 4 percent), the frequency of thyroid carcinoma, either newly diagnosed or as a cause of death, is very low. These respective data led either to vigorous or to conservative approaches to the management of nodular goiter. It now appears that this discordance can be explained, by the ability of the physician to select for surgery those patients who are at high risk of harboring thyroid carcinoma, with consequent weighting of statistics from surgical series. This capability has increased, the as yet unrealized aim being to operate on only those patients whose thyroids harbor carcinoma and to avoid surgery in patients whose thyroids do not.

Several features suggest the presence of thyroid carcinoma. Recent growth of a thyroid nodule or mass, especially if rapid and unaccompanied by tenderness and hoarseness, is a source of suspicion. Of particular importance is a history of x-ray to the head or neck or upper mediastinum in infancy or childhood, since this is associated with a high incidence of thyroid disease, including carcinoma, later in life. Nodular disease develops in approximately 20 percent of patients so exposed and may not be apparent until 30 years or more after the radiation exposure. Among patients in this group who have palpable nodules, approximately a third have thyroid carcinoma at surgery, often multicentric and sometimes metastatic.

Skillful palpation of the thyroid provides important information. A nodule in an otherwise normal gland (solitary nodule) creates more suspicion of thyroid tumor than does one nodule among many, since the latter is more likely to be part of a diffuse process, such as simple goiter. In addition, carcinomas are usually firm or hard in consistency and nontender. Fixation to surrounding structures and lymphadenopathy are late features. Since purely cystic lesions, especially those that are less than a few centimeters in diameter, are less likely to reflect malignancy than solid lesions, transillumination is sometimes helpful, and ultrasonograms (see below) are particularly so. Age and sex of the patient also influence the clinical decision. Benign nodular lesions are more common in women than in men, malignant nodular lesions less so. Hence, nodular lesions in men create more suspicion of carcinoma than in women.

Laboratory tests are of little assistance in differentiating between malignant and nonmalignant thyroid nodules. Overall thyroid function is usually normal. Except in patients with medullary thyroid carcinoma, in whom serum calcitonin concentrations may be elevated, tumor markers are of little value. Elevations of serum thyroglobulin are present in many patients with differentiated thyroid carcinoma but are not useful in the initial diagnosis, since they may be elevated in patients with benign adenoma, simple goiter, or Graves' disease. Soft-tissue x-rays of the neck may be of assistance, since finely stippled calcification within the thyroid suggests the presence of psammoma bodies within a papillary carcinoma.

Scintillation scanning is a keystone in the approach to the management of the patient with nodular goiter. Although only approximately 20 percent of nonfunctioning thyroid nodules prove to be malignant, demonstration that a nodule is cold adds substantial weight to the other factors suggesting carcinoma. Nodules that are hyperfunctioning are rarely malignant. Ultrasonograms of the thyroid have value in demonstrating whether nodules are cystic, solid, or a mixture of the two. Cystic nodules can be aspirated, a procedure that is often curative, and their contents should be subjected to cytopathologic examination. Solid or mixed lesions are consistent with tumor but may be either benign or malignant.

At this point in the evaluation, the physician must decide whether to continue to observe the patient; whether to administer suppressive doses of thyroid hormone in the hope that the suspect nodule will shrink or disappear, a hope that in the author's experience is usually unrealized; whether to obtain a closed biopsy; or whether to proceed to excisional biopsy and thyroidectomy. There are some patients in whom the author would choose the latter course. In general, these include patients with a history of radiation to the thyroid and one or more clearly palpable nodules, as well as young men and women with solitary cold nodules, particularly if hard, nontender, and changing rapidly in size. In the remainder, the author recommends either aspiration or cutting-needle biopsy. The former is simpler to learn, free of complications, and applicable to smaller nodules. Optimum application of that technique rests upon the availability of experienced histopathologic interpretation of the specimen obtained. When such is available, aspiration biopsy provides a reliable means of differentiating between benign and malignant nodules in all except highly cellular lesions or follicular lesions, where evidence of vascular invasion may be required to differentiate benign from malignant forms. Despite the occasional occurrence of false-positives and -negatives, the procedure can reduce the number of operations performed for nodules that prove to be benign. Further, a diagnosis of carcinoma permits planning of the surgery to be undertaken preoperatively and is often useful in providing an impetus to surgery when the patient or physician is uncertain if surgery should be performed.

Regardless of the operative procedure planned, surgery for thyroid carcinoma should be performed by a surgeon experienced in the procedure. A several-week period of suppressive therapy with levothyroxine is often recommended preoperatively to facilitate the operative procedure and perhaps to decrease the likelihood of tumor dissemination. In patients in whom a definitive preoperative diagnosis, such as by biopsy, has not been made, the suspected lesion is removed en bloc with a wide margin of surrounding tissue and is examined by frozen section. Opinions vary as to the type of procedure that is preferable when carcinoma is found. For lesions that are not multicentric and that have not metastasized, some recommend ipsilateral lobectomy, isthmectomy, and possibly contralateral partial lobectomy. Despite its higher rate of morbidity, the author prefers that a near-total thyroidectomy be performed, in view of the frequency of seeding of tumor throughout the gland by transglandular lymphatic spread and of evidence that both recurrence rates and subsequent mortality are lower after the more extensive operation. Regional lymph nodes should be explored and removed if there is evidence of involvement, but radical neck dissection is not justified. If permanent sections reveal carcinoma when frozen sections had failed to do so, secondary surgery should be undertaken to remove residual thyroid tissue.

Approximately 3 weeks after surgery, liothyronine (75 to 100 μg daily) is substituted for levothyroxine, since it permits a more rapid return of TSH secretion when withdrawn some 3 weeks later. After an additional 2 or 3 weeks, when the serum TSH concentration has risen to the range of 50 μU/mL, a large scanning dose of ^{131}I [185 to 370 MBq (5 to 10 mCi)] is administered and whole-body scans are obtained at 24, 48, and 72 h. If residual thyroid tissue is found, as is usually the case, a thyroid ablating dose of 1850 MBq (50 mCi) of ^{131}I is administered, and if functioning metastases are present, the dose is doubled. Suppressive therapy with levothyroxine is reinstituted 24 to 48 h later. Approximately 1 week after administration of the second dose of ^{131}I, whole-body scans are repeated, as the larger dose of radioiodine may permit demonstration of functioning metastases not seen after the smaller initial dose. If this proves to be the case, suppressive therapy is withdrawn, an additional 3700 MBq (100 mCi) of ^{131}I is administered, and suppressive therapy with levothyroxine reinstituted.

Patients are reexamined approximately 6 months after the initial operation and at least every 6 months for several years thereafter. At these examinations, the neck is palpated for evidence of recurrence of metastases, which often can be treated with selective surgical removal. Blood is drawn for a serum thyroglobulin measurement, since elevated values in patients receiving suppressive therapy signal the presence of metastatic disease. At the initial 6-month examination, patients in whom metastases had previously been found are prepared for a whole-body scan as described above. Those in whom no metastases had been demonstrated by earlier scans are not rescanned unless the serum thyroglobulin is elevated but are rescanned approximately 1 year after the initial surgery. Patients in whom whole-body scans are positive are reentered into the therapeutic algorithm, as described above. Those in whom scans are negative continue to be reexamined and have measurements of serum thyroglobulin concentrations at regular intervals. If both serum thyroglobulin concentrations and scans are unrevealing, patients are scanned for the last time after approximately 3 years, unless serum thyroglobulin concentrations rise. In some patients, serum thyroglobulin may be elevated despite the absence of demonstrable functioning metastases. Such patients obviously cannot be treated with ^{131}I but should be studied with x-rays and bone scans to ascertain the site of the thyroglobulin-secreting metastases.

A program of this nature, involving near-total thyroidectomy, long-term suppressive therapy, and treatment of functioning metastases with radioiodine reduces the recurrence rate and prolongs survival in patients with papillary carcinoma of the thyroid. Follicular carcinoma should be treated with at least equal vigor, though the results are generally less favorable. Treatment of anaplastic carcinoma is largely palliative; most patients with this disease die within 6 months from the time of diagnosis.

REFERENCES

Beierwaltes WH: The treatment of thyroid carcinoma with radioactive iodine. Semin Nucl Med 8:79, 1978

Bilezekian JP, Loeb JN: The influence of hyperthyroidism and hypothyroidism on the α- and β-adrenergic receptor system and adrenergic responsiveness. Endocr Rev 4:378, 1983

Dunn JT: Choice of therapy in young adults with hyperthyroidism of Graves' disease. Ann Intern Med 100:891, 1984

Fisher DA, Klein AH: Thyroid development and disorders of thyroid function in the newborn. N Engl J Med 304:702, 1981

Ingbar SH, Borges M: Peripheral metabolism of the thyroid hormones, in *Free Thyroid Hormones*, R Ekins et al (eds). Amsterdam, Excerpta Medica, 1979, p 17

Kidd A et al: Immunologic aspects of Graves' and Hashimoto's diseases. Metabolism 29:80, 1980

Mazzaferri EL et al: Papillary thyroid carcinoma: The impact of therapy in 576 patients. Medicine 56:171, 1977

Miller JM et al: Diagnosis of thyroid nodules. Use of fine-needle aspiration and needle biopsy. JAMA 241:481, 1979

Rajatanavin R, Braverman LE: Euthyroid hyperthyroxinemia. J Endocrinol Invest 6:493, 1983

Schneider AB et al: Sequential serum thyroglobulin determinations, ^{131}I scans, and ^{131}I uptakes after triiodothyronine withdrawal in patients with thyroid cancer. J Clin Endocrinol Metab 53:1199, 1981

Sterling K: Thyroid hormone action at the cell level. N Engl J Med 300:117, 173, 1979

Studer H, Ramelli F: Simple goiter and its variants: Euthyroid and hyperthyroid multinodular goiters. Endocr Rev 3:440, 1980

Wartofsky L, Burman KD: Alterations in thyroid function in patients with systemic illness: The "euthyroid sick syndrome." Endocr Rev 3:164, 1982

Witt JR et al: The approach to the irradiated thyroid. Surg Clin N Am 59:45, 1979

Woolf PD: Transient painless thyroiditis with hyperthyroidism: A variant of lymphocytic thyroiditis. Endocr Rev 1:411, 1980

325 DISEASES OF THE ADRENAL CORTEX

GORDON H. WILLIAMS / ROBERT G. DLUHY

BIOCHEMISTRY AND PHYSIOLOGY

STEROID NOMENCLATURE Steroids contain as their basic structure a cyclopentenoperhydrophenanthrane nucleus consisting of three 6-carbon hexane rings and a single 5-carbon pentane ring (D in Fig. 325-1). The carbon atoms are numbered in a sequence beginning with ring A (Fig. 325-1). Adrenal steroids contain either 19 or 21 carbon atoms. The C_{19} steroids have methyl groups at positions C-18 and C-19. C_{19} steroids that have a ketone group at C-17 are termed *17-ketosteroids*. The C_{19} steroids have predominant androgenic activity. The C_{21} steroids have a 2-carbon side chain (C-20 and C-21) attached at position 17 and methyl groups at C-18 and C-19. C_{21} steroids that also possess a hydroxyl group at position 17 are termed *17-hydroxycorticosteroids* or *17-hydroxycorticoids*. The C_{21} steroids have either glucocorticoid or mineralocorticoid properties. *Glucocorticoid* signifies a C_{21} steroid with predominant action on intermediary metabolism; *mineralocorticoid* indicates a C_{21} steroid with predominant action on the metabolism of sodium and potassium.

BIOSYNTHESIS OF ADRENAL STEROIDS Cholesterol, derived from the diet and from endogenous synthesis via acetate, is the starting compound in steroidogenesis. The three major adrenal biosynthetic pathways lead to the production of glucocorticoids (cortisol), mineralocorticoids (aldosterone), and adrenal androgens (dehydroepiandrosterone). Separate zones of the adrenal cortex synthesize specific hormones; this reflects the enzymatic capacity of each zone to carry out certain transformations and hydroxylations (Fig. 325-2). The outer (glomerulosa) zone is mainly involved in aldosterone biosynthesis, and the inner (fasciculata-reticularis) zone is the site of cortisol and androgen biosynthesis.

STEROID TRANSPORT Some steroid hormones, e.g., testosterone and cortisol, circulate to a considerable extent bound to plasma proteins. Cortisol occurs in the plasma in three forms: free cortisol, protein-bound cortisol, and cortisol metabolites. *Free cortisol* refers to that quantity which is physiologically active but not protein-bound and, therefore, represents a form of cortisol acting directly on tissue sites. Normally, less than 5 percent of circulating cortisol is free. The diffusible fraction ranges between 0.7 and 1.0 μg/dL. Only the unbound cortisol and its metabolites are filtrable at the glomerulus. Increased quantities of free steroid are excreted in the urine in states characterized by hypersecretion of cortisol, as the unbound fraction of plasma cortisol rises. *Protein-bound cortisol* is that reversibly bound to circulating plasma proteins. There are two cortisol-binding systems of plasma. One is a high-affinity, low-capacity $alpha_2$ globulin termed *transcortin* or *cortisol-binding globulin* (CBG), and the other is a low-affinity, high-capacity protein, albumin. Cortisol-binding globulin in normal humans can bind approximately 20 to 25 μg of cortisol per deciliter of plasma. When the concentration of cortisol exceeds this level, the excess becomes bound in part to albumin, and a greater proportion circulates unbound. The CBG level is increased in high-estrogen states (e.g., pregnancy, oral contraceptive administration). The rise in CBG is accompanied by a parallel rise in protein-bound cortisol, with the result that the plasma cortisol concentration is elevated. However, the free cortisol levels probably remain normal, and signs and symptoms of glucocorticoid excess are absent. Most synthetic glucocorticoid analogues bind less efficiently to CBG (approximately 70 percent binding). This may explain the propensity of some synthetic analogues to produce cushingoid side effects at low dosage. *Cortisol metabolites* are biologically inactive and bind only weakly to circulating plasma proteins.

Aldosterone is bound to proteins to a smaller extent than either testosterone or cortisol, and an ultrafiltrate of plasma contains as much as 50 percent of the circulating aldosterone. The limited binding of aldosterone by plasma protein is significant in the metabolism of this hormone.

STEROID METABOLISM AND EXCRETION Glucocorticoids The daily secretion of cortisol ranges between 15 and 30 mg, with a pronounced diurnal cycle. Cortisol is distributed in a volume of body fluids approximating the total extracellular fluid space. The total plasma concentration of cortisol in the morning hours is approximately 15 μg/dL, with more than 90 percent in the protein-bound fraction. The plasma concentration of cortisol is determined by the rate of secretion, the rate of inactivation, and the rate of excretion of free cortisol. The liver is the major organ responsible for steroid inactivation, by reduction of ring A and conjugation of the reduced products with glucuronic acid at position C-3 to form water-soluble compounds. The 11-dehydrogenase system converts cortisol to the inactive cortisone and is influenced by the level of circulating thyroid hormone, the oxidative reaction being increased in hyperthyroidism.

Mineralocorticoids In normal subjects on a normal salt intake, the average daily secretion of aldosterone ranges between 50 and 250 μg, and the plasma concentration ranges between 5 and 15 ng/dL. Since aldosterone is only weakly bound to proteins, its volume of distribution is larger than that of cortisol and approximates 35 liters. During a single passage through the liver, more than 75 percent of circulating aldosterone is normally inactivated by ring A reduction and conjugation with glucuronic acid. However, under certain conditions, such as congestive failure, this inactivation is reduced.

From 7 to 15 percent of aldosterone is excreted in the urine as a glucuronide conjugate, from which free aldosterone is released on standing at pH 1. This *acid-labile conjugate* is formed in the liver and in the kidney. For average salt intake, the 24-h urine excretion of the acid-labile conjugate ranges from 2 to 20 μg, that of the reduced derivative from 25 to 35 μg, and that of the nonconjugated, nonreduced free aldosterone from 0.2 to 0.6 μg.

FIGURE 325-1 *Basic steroid structure and nomenclature.*

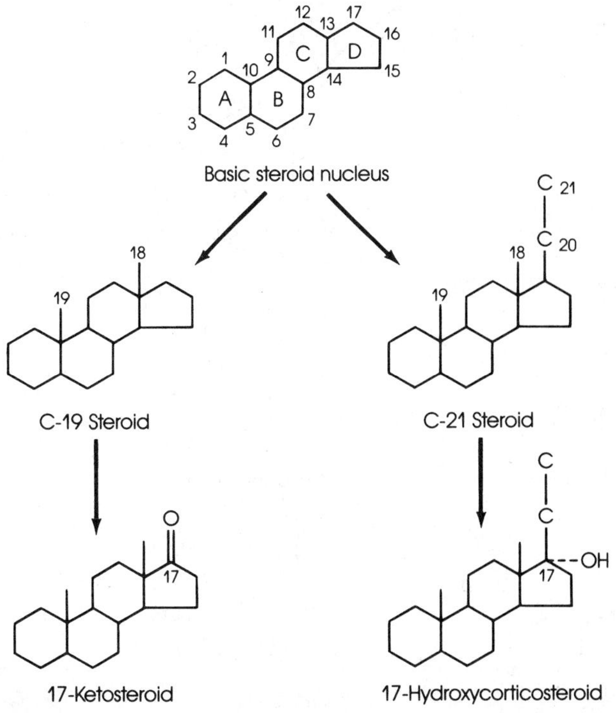

Adrenal androgens The major androgen secreted by the adrenal is dehydroepiandrosterone (DHEA) and its C-3 sulfuric acid ester. From 15 to 30 mg of these compounds is secreted daily. Smaller amounts of Δ^4-androstenedione, 11β-hydroxyandrostenedione, and testosterone are secreted. DHEA is the major precursor of the urinary 17-ketosteroids. Two-thirds of the urine 17-ketosteroids in the male is derived from adrenal metabolites, and the remaining one-third comes from testicular androgens. In the female, almost all urine 17-ketosteroids are derived from the adrenal.

ACTH PHYSIOLOGY Corticotropin (ACTH) (see Chap. 321) is an unbranched polypeptide containing 39 amino acids. ACTH and a number of other peptides (lipotropins, endorphins, and melanocyte-stimulating hormones) are processed from a larger precursor molecule of 31,000 mol wt—pro-opiomelanocortin (POMC) (see Chaps. 69 and 321 and Fig. 325-3). ACTH is synthesized and stored in basophilic cells of the anterior pituitary gland. The basophilic staining of the corticotrophs is the result of the glycosylation of ACTH and related peptides. Much of the potential for the corticotropic actions of ACTH is present in smaller polypeptide fragments; the *N*-terminal 18-amino-acid structure retains full biologic potency, and shorter *N*-terminal fragments exhibit partial biologic activity. Release of ACTH and related peptides from the anterior pituitary gland is governed by a "corticotropin-releasing center" in the median eminence of the

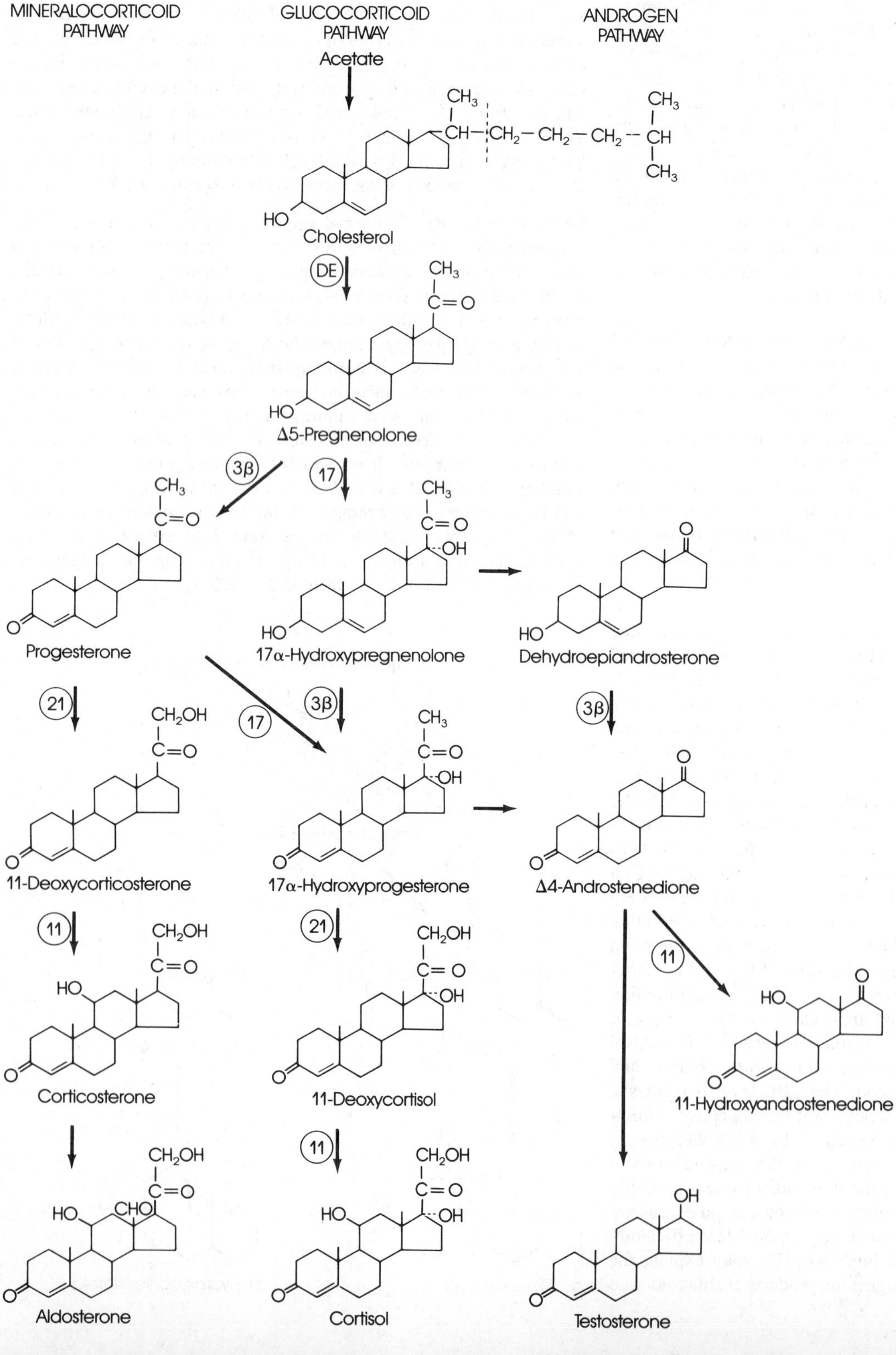

FIGURE 325-2 *Biosynthetic pathways for adrenal steroid production; major pathways to mineralocorticoids, glucocorticoids, and androgens. Circled letters and numbers denote specific enzymes: DE = cholesterol side chain cleavage enzyme; 3β = 3β-ol-dehydrogenase with $\Delta^{4,5}$-isomerase; 11 = C-11 hydroxylase; 17 = C-17 hydroxylase; 21 = C-21 hydroxylase.*

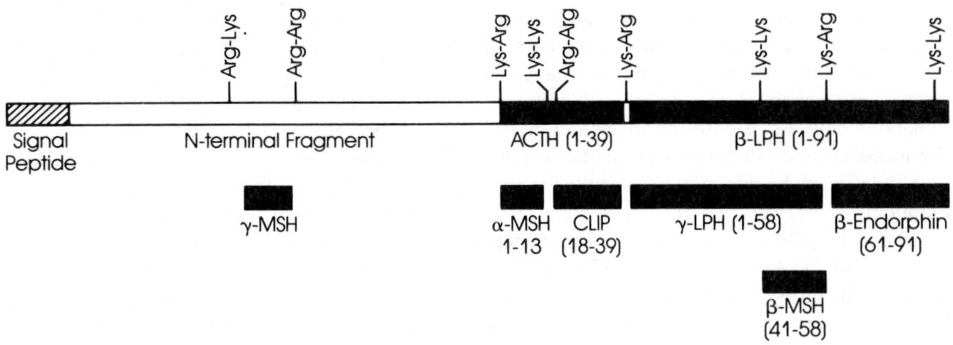

FIGURE 325-3 *Schematic representation of the probable structure of the 31,000–mol wt pro-opiomelanocortin molecule. (From DT Krieger, JB Martin, N Engl J Med 304:880, 1981. By permission of the New England Journal of Medicine.)*

hypothalamus, which upon stimulation releases a peptide with a chain of 41 amino acids (corticotropin-releasing hormone, CRH) that travels via the pituitary-stalk portal bloodstream to the anterior pituitary, where it effects the release of ACTH (Fig. 325-4). Some related peptides such as β-lipotropin (β-LPH) are released in equimolar concentrations with ACTH, suggesting enzymatic cleavage from the parent POMC prior to or concomitant with the secretory process. However, beta endorphin levels may vary disparately with circulating levels of ACTH depending on the nature of the stimulus. The functions and regulation of secretion of the related peptides derived from POMC are not understood.

The major factors controlling ACTH release include CRH, free cortisol concentration in plasma, stress, and the sleep-wake cycle (Fig. 325-4). The plasma level of ACTH varies during the day as a result of its pulsatile secretion but roughly follows a diurnal pattern, with a peak occurring just prior to awaking and a nadir shortly before retiring. After several days on a new sleep-wake cycle, the pattern is altered to conform to the new cycle. ACTH and cortisol levels also increase in response to eating. Stress (e.g., pyrogens, surgery, hypoglycemia, exercise, and severe emotional trauma) can also enhance ACTH release. Stress-related secretion of ACTH abolishes circadian periodicity but is in turn suppressed by prior high-dose glucocorticoid administration. The secretion of ACTH following stress and the normal pulsatile, diurnal ACTH release are regulated by CRH; this is the so-called open feedback loop. CRH secretion, in turn, is influenced by hypothalamic neurotransmitters. For example, serotoninergic and cholinergic systems stimulate the secretion of CRH and ACTH; there is contradictory evidence regarding the inhibitory effects of α-adrenergic agonists and gamma-aminobutyric acid (GABA) on CRH release. In addition, there may be direct pituitary effects of these neurotransmitters. There is also evidence for peptidergic regulation of ACTH release. For example, beta endorphin and enkephalin inhibit and vasopressin and angiotensin II augment the secretion of ACTH. Finally, ACTH release is regulated by the free cortisol level in plasma. Cortisol decreases the responsiveness of adrenal corticotropic cells to CRH; i.e., in the presence of cortisol more CRH is required to produce a given increment of ACTH. Glucocorticoids also inhibit CRH release. This servomechanism establishes the primacy of blood cortisol concentration in the control of ACTH secretion. The inhibition of ACTH occurs in two phases: (1) an early fast feedback, possibly a membrane effect, lasting less than 10 min and dependent on the rate of increase of glucocorticoid levels; and (2) a time-dependent delayed feedback response, probably due to inhibition of synthesis of the precursor protein. The suppression of ACTH secretion that results in adrenal atrophy following *prolonged* glucocorticoid therapy may be primarily related to suppression of hypothalamic CRH release, since exogenous CRH administration in this circumstance still produces a rise in plasma ACTH. Cortisol also exerts feedback on higher brain centers (hippocampus, reticular system, and septum) and perhaps on the adrenal cortex as well (Fig. 325-4).

The biologic half-life of ACTH in the circulation is less than 10 min. The action of ACTH is also rapid; within minutes of its release, the concentration of steroids in the adrenal venous blood increases. ACTH stimulates steroidogenesis via activation of the membrane-bound adenyl cyclase. Adenosine 3′,5′-monophosphate (cyclic AMP) in turn activates protein kinase enzymes, thereby resulting in the phosphorylation of proteins that activate steroid biosynthesis (see Chap. 67).

RENIN-ANGIOTENSIN PHYSIOLOGY (See also Chap. 196) Renin is a proteolytic enzyme that is produced and stored in the granules

FIGURE 325-4 *The hypothalamic-pituitary-adrenal axis. The dominant feedback control of plasma cortisol is on the pituitary gland (1) and on the hypothalamic corticotropin-releasing center (2). Feedback of plasma cortisol may also act on higher nerve centers (3) and/or on the adrenal gland itself (4). There also may be a short feedback inhibition of CRH by ACTH (5). Hypothalamic neurotransmitters influence CRH release; serotoninergic and cholinergic systems stimulate the secretion of CRH and ACTH; alpha-adrenergic agonists and gamma-aminobutyric acid (GABA) probably inhibit CRH release. The opioid peptides, beta endorphin and enkephalin, inhibit and vasopressin and angiotensin II augment the secretion of CRH and ACTH. CRH = corticotropin-releasing hormone; β-LPH = beta lipotropin; POMC = pro-opiomelanocortin.*

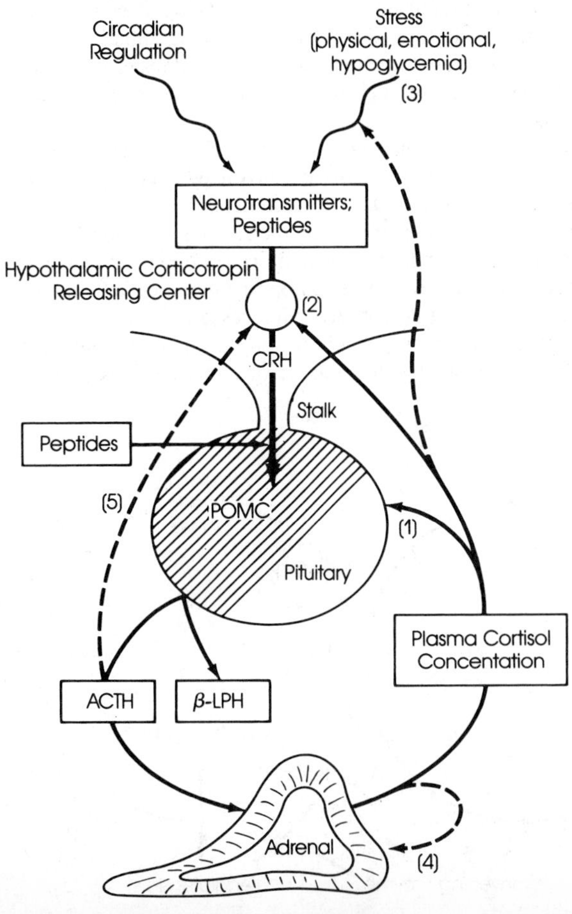

of the juxtaglomerular cells surrounding the afferent arterioles of glomeruli in the kidney. Renin exists both in active and inactive forms. Whether the inactive form is a precursor (''prorenin'') or is a product formed after release is uncertain. The juxtaglomerular apparatus consists of both the juxtaglomerular cells and the cells of the macula densa. Renin acts on the basic substrate angiotensinogen (a circulating alpha$_2$ globulin made in the liver) to form the decapeptide angiotensin I (Fig. 325-5). Angiotensin I is then enzymatically converted by converting enzyme to the octapeptide angiotensin II by splitting off the two *C*-terminal amino acids. Angiotensin II is the most potent pressor compound (on a mole-for-mole basis) made in the body, and it exerts this pressor action by a direct effect on arteriolar smooth muscle. In addition, angiotensin II is a potent stimulus to the production of aldosterone by the zona glomerulosa of the adrenal cortex; the nonapeptide, angiotensin III, may also stimulate aldosterone production. Angiotensinases rapidly destroy angiotensin II (half-life approximately 1 min), while the half-life of renin is more prolonged (10 to 20 min). Other tissues, such as uterus, vascular tissue, brain, and salivary glands, also produce renin-like substances, the significance of these so-called isorenins is not known.

Renin release is controlled by four interdependent factors, and the amount of renin released is a composite of the effects of all four. The *juxtaglomerular cells,* which are specialized myoepithelial cells cuffing the afferent arterioles, act as miniature pressure transducers, sensing renal perfusion pressure and corresponding changes in afferent arteriolar perfusion pressures. For example, under conditions of a reduction in circulating blood volume, there is a corresponding reduction in renal perfusion pressure and, therefore, in afferent arteriolar pressure (Fig. 325-5). This is perceived by the juxtaglomerular cells as a decreased stretch exerted on the afferent arteriolar walls. The juxtaglomerular cells then release increasing quantities of renin within the kidney circulation. This results in the formation of angiotensin I, which is converted in the kidney and peripherally to angiotensin II by a peptidyldipeptide hydrolase (so-called converting enzyme). Angiotensin II stimulates the adrenal cortex to release aldosterone. Increasing plasma levels of aldosterone lead to increasing renal sodium retention and thus result in expansion of extracellular fluid volume, which, in turn, dampens the initiating signal for renin release. Within this context, the renin-angiotensin-aldosterone system subserves volume control by appropriate modifications of renal tubular sodium transport.

A second control mechanism for renin release centers in the *macula densa* cells, a group of distal convoluted tubular epithelial cells in direct apposition to the juxtaglomerular cells. They may function as chemoreceptors, monitoring the sodium (or chloride) load presented to the distal tubule, and such information may be conveyed to the juxtaglomerular cells, where appropriate modifications in renin release take place. Under conditions of increased delivery of filtered sodium to the macula densa, feedback may occur to the juxtaglomerular apparatus, resulting in a release of increasing quantities of renin, which are capable of decreasing glomerular filtration rate, thereby reducing the filtered load of sodium.

The *sympathetic nervous system* regulates release of renin in response to assuming the upright posture. The mechanism is either a direct effect on the juxtaglomerular cell to increase adenyl cyclase activity or an indirect effect on either the juxtaglomerular or the macula densa cells by way of a vasoconstrictive action on the afferent arteriole.

Finally, circulating factors may alter renin release. Increasing dietary *potassium* directly decreases renin release; decreasing potassium intake increases renin release. The significance of this potassium effect is unclear. *Angiotensin II* itself can exert a negative feedback control on renin release independent of alterations in renal blood flow, pressure, or aldosterone secretion. *Atrial natriuretic peptides* also may inhibit renin release. Thus, the control of renin release is complex, consisting of both *intrarenal* (pressor receptor and macula densa) and *extrarenal* (sympathetic nervous system, potassium, angiotensin, etc.) mechanisms. A given level of renin secretion probably reflects all these factors, with the intrarenal mechanism predominating.

GLUCOCORTICOID PHYSIOLOGY The division of adrenal steroids into glucocorticoids and mineralocorticoids is arbitrary in that most glucocorticoids have some mineralocorticoid-like properties, and vice versa. The descriptive term *glucocorticoid* is applied to those adrenal steroids having a predominant action on intermediary metabolism. The principal glucocorticoid is cortisol (hydrocortisone). Cortisol enters the target cell by diffusion, combines with a specific high-affinity cytoplasmic receptor protein, and is transferred to a specific acceptor site on the chromatin tissue of the nucleus, which then produces an increase in RNA synthesis and later in protein synthesis. Thus, an alternative way of defining a glucocorticoid effect is one mediated by a class of high-affinity cytoplasmic receptors (glucorticoid receptors) (see Chap. 320). The physiologic actions of the glucocorticoids on intermediary metabolism include the regulation of protein, carbohydrate, lipid, and nucleic acid metabolism. The actions appear to be mainly catabolic in effect, with an increased protein breakdown and nitrogen excretion. Glucocorticoids increase hepatic glycogen content and promote the hepatic synthesis of glucose (gluconeogenesis). These actions are in large part explained by the mobilization of glycogenic amino acid precursors from peripheral supporting structures, such as bone, skin, muscle, and connective tissue, due to protein breakdown and inhibition of protein synthesis and amino acid uptake. Glucocorticoid-induced hyperaminoacidemia also facilitates gluconeogenesis by stimulating glucagon secretion. Glucocorticoids act directly on the liver to stimulate the synthesis of certain enzymes, such as tyrosine amino transferase and tryptophan pyrrolase. Corticoids inhibit the synthesis of nucleic acids in most body tissues, but in the liver ribonucleic acid (RNA) synthesis is stimulated. Glucocorticoids regulate fatty acid mobilization by enhancing activation of

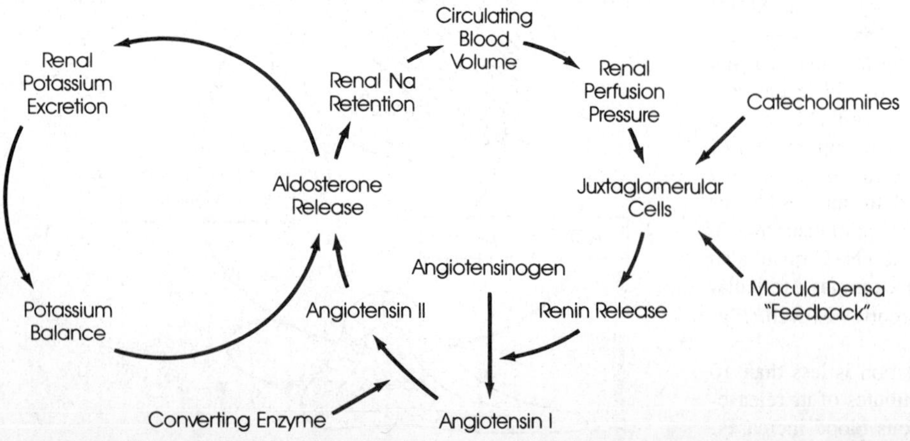

FIGURE 325-5 *The interrelationship of the volume and potassium feedback loops on aldosterone secretion. Integration of signals from each loop determines the level of aldosterone secretion.*

cellular lipase by lipid-mobilizing hormones (e.g., catecholamines and pituitary peptides).

The actions of cortisol on structural protein and on adipose tissue vary in different parts of the body. For example, pharmacologic doses of cortisol may deplete the protein matrix of the vertebral column (trabecular bone), but long bones (primarily compact bone) are affected only minimally; peripheral adipose tissue may diminish, whereas abdominal and interscapular fat may accumulate.

Cortisol levels are responsive within minutes to a variety of physical stresses (trauma, surgery, exercise) and psychological stresses (anxiety, depression). Hypoglycemia and fever are also potent stimuli of ACTH and cortisol secretion. The reasons why elevated glucocorticoid levels protect the organism under stress are not understood, but in their absence such stresses may cause hypotension, shock, and death. For these reasons, glucocorticoid administration should always be increased in individuals with hypofunction of the pituitary-adrenal axis during stress.

Glucocorticoids have anti-inflammatory properties, which are probably related to their actions on the microvasculature as well as to cellular effects. Cortisol maintains normal vascular responsiveness to circulating vasoconstrictor factors and opposes the increase in capillary permeability characteristic of acute inflammation. Glucocorticoids cause a polymorphonuclear leukocytosis; the circulating leukocyte mass is increased due to a release from the bone marrow of mature cells as well as to an inhibition of egress through the capillary wall. Cortisol also inhibits the production of interleukin 2 by macrophages. Reduced adherence of macrophages to vascular endothelium following glucocorticoid administration is probably secondary to antagonism to the action of migration-inhibiting factor (MIF). Glucocorticoids produce a depletion of circulating eosinophils and of lymphoid tissue, specifically T cells or the small lymphocytes derived from the thymus. The mechanism is by redistribution from the circulation into other compartments. Thus, cortisol impairs cellular-mediated immunity. It is probably only at pharmacologic dosages that antibody production is suppressed and stabilization of lysosomal membranes occurs, thereby suppressing the release of proteolytic acid hydrolases stored in these cytoplasmic organelles. Cortisol has a major action on the distribution and excretion of body water. It subserves the extracellular fluid volume by retarding the migration of water into cells. It affects renal water excretion by suppressing the secretion of antidiuretic hormone, increasing the rate of glomerular filtration, and acting directly on the renal tubule, the consequence being to increase solute-free water clearance. Glucocorticoids also have weak mineralocorticoid-like properties, and increasing doses produce renal tubular sodium reabsorption and increased urine potassium excretion. Glucocorticoids can also influence behavior; emotional disorders may occur with either excesses or deficits of cortisol. Lastly, cortisol suppresses the secretion of pituitary ACTH and hypothalamic CRH.

MINERALOCORTICOID PHYSIOLOGY The major mineralocorticoid, aldosterone, has two important activities: (1) It is a major regulator of extracellular fluid volume, and (2) it is a major determinant of potassium metabolism. These effects are mediated by binding of aldosterone to specific, high-affinity mineralocorticoid receptor proteins in target tissues. Volume is regulated through a direct effect on the renal tubular transport of sodium. Aldosterone acts predominantly at the distal convoluted tubule, where it causes a decrease in the excretion of sodium and an increase in excretion of potassium. The reabsorption of sodium ions causes a fall in the transmembrane potential, thus enhancing the flow of positive ions out of the cell into the lumen. The major intracellular singly charged positive ion is potassium. Since its concentration in the cell is forty- to eightyfold greater than in the lumen, potassium passively follows this relative electric gradient to restore the normal positive charge to the lumen. The reabsorbed sodium ions are then transported out of the tubular epithelial cells into the interstitial fluid of the kidney and from there into the renal capillary circulation. Water passively follows the transported sodium.

Hydrogen ion is also abundant in the tubular epithelial cell. Since its concentration is greater in the lumen than in the cell, it is actively secreted, but the reduced intraluminal positivity allows more hydrogen to be secreted with the same amount of energy. Aldosterone and other mineralocorticoids also act on the epithelium of the salivary ducts, sweat glands, and gastrointestinal tract to cause reabsorption of sodium in "exchange" for potassium ions.

When normal individuals are given aldosterone (or deoxycorticosterone acetate), an initial period of sodium retention is followed by a natriuresis, and sodium balance is reestablished after 3 to 5 days. As a result, edema does not develop. This phenomenon is referred to as the "escape phenomenon," signifying an "escape" by the renal tubules from the sodium-retaining action of chronically administered aldosterone.

Three mechanisms control aldosterone release—the renin-angiotensin system, potassium, and ACTH (Table 325-1). The renin-angiotensin system is the major system for control of extracellular fluid volume, via regulation of aldosterone secretion (Fig. 325-5). In effect, the renin-angiotensin system maintains the circulating blood volume constant by causing aldosterone-induced sodium retention during periods registered as volume deficiencies and by decreasing aldosterone-dependent sodium retention under conditions in which volume is registered as being ample.

Potassium ions directly regulate aldosterone secretion independently of the renin-angiotensin system (Fig. 325-5). In normal humans, oral potassium loading increases aldosterone secretion, excretion, and plasma levels. In addition, an increase in serum potassium of as little as 0.1 meq per liter increases plasma aldosterone levels under certain circumstances.

Physiologic amounts of ACTH acutely stimulate aldosterone secretion, but this action is not sustained if ACTH is infused for periods greater than 10 to 12 h. Most studies relegate ACTH to a minor role in the control of aldosterone. For example, subjects on high-dose steroid therapy for several years and with presumably complete suppression of ACTH have normal aldosterone-secretory responses to sodium restriction. Therefore, chronic ACTH deficiency per se does not alter glomerulosa cell responsiveness.

The prior dietary intake of both potassium and sodium can alter the magnitude of the aldosterone response to acute stimulation. Increasing potassium intake or decreasing sodium intake sensitizes the response of the glomerulosa cells to acute stimulation by ACTH, angiotensin II, and/or potassium.

Neurotransmitters (dopamine and serotonin) and some peptides, such as atrial natriuretic factor, γ-melanocyte-stimulating hormone (γ-MSH), beta endorphin, and an unidentified pituitary aldosterone-stimulating factor, also participate in the regulation of aldosterone secretion (Table 325-1). Thus, the control of aldosterone secretion involves both stimulatory and inhibitory factors.

TABLE 325-1 Factors regulating aldosterone biosynthesis

Factors	Effects
I Renin-angiotensin system	Stimulate
II Sodium ion	Inhibit (?physiologic)
III Potassium ion	Stimulate
IV Neurotransmitters	
A Dopamine	Inhibit
B Serotonin	Stimulate
V Pituitary hormones	
A ACTH	Stimulate
B Non-ACTH pituitary hormones (e.g., growth hormone)	Permissive (for optimal response to sodium restriction)
C Unidentified pituitary factors	Stimulate
D Beta endorphin	Stimulate
E γ-MSH	Permissive
VI Natriuretic factors	
A Atrial factors	Inhibit
B Ouabain-like factors	Inhibit

ANDROGEN PHYSIOLOGY Androgens are substances that stimulate male secondary sexual characteristics. They produce these actions by binding to high-affinity cytoplasmic receptors. The secondary sexual characteristics are affected through inhibition of the female characteristics (defeminization) and accentuation of the male characteristics (masculinization). These are seen clinically as hirsutism and virilization in the female with amenorrhea, atrophy of the breasts and uterus, enlargement of the clitoris, deepening of the voice, acne, increased muscle mass, and receding hairline (Chap. 46).

Steroids with predominant androgenic activity have 19 carbon atoms (Fig. 325-1). The principal adrenal androgens are dehydroepiandrosterone (DHEA), androstenedione, and 11-hydroxyandrostenedione. DHEA and its sulfate are *quantitatively* the major androgens secreted by the adrenal; DHEA and androstenedione are weak androgens, and they exert their effects via conversion in extraglandular tissues to the potent androgen, testosterone. The release of adrenal androgens is stimulated by ACTH, not by gonadotropins. With ACTH stimulation, 17-ketosteroids increase but to a lesser extent than do urine 17-hydroxycorticosteroids. It follows that adrenal androgens are suppressed by exogenous glucocorticoid administration.

LABORATORY EVALUATION OF ADRENOCORTICAL FUNCTION

The basic assumption in the measurement of plasma or urinary steroids is that they accurately reflect adrenal *secretory* rates of that steroid. A disadvantage of urine *excretion* values is that they may not truly reflect the secretion rate because of improper collection or altered metabolism. Measurement of the actual adrenal secretory rate of a given steroid would be preferable but is more difficult, involving isotope dilution techniques following administration of a radioactive steroid. Plasma levels reflect the level of secretion only at the time of measurement. The plasma level (PL) is dependent on two factors: the secretion rate (SR) of the hormone and the rate at which it is metabolized, i.e., its metabolic clearance rate (MCR). These three factors can be related mathematically as follows:

$$\mathrm{PL} = \frac{\mathrm{SR}}{\mathrm{MCR}} \quad \text{or} \quad \mathrm{SR} = \mathrm{MCR} \times \mathrm{PL}$$

TABLE 325-2 Range of normal values for tests of adrenal function

Test	Normal value, range
Plasma cortisol, μg/dL:	
8 A.M.	9–24
4 P.M.	3–12
Cortisol secretory rate, mg/24 h	5–25
Urinary free cortisol, μg/24 h	20–100
17-Hydroxycorticoids, mg/24 h	2–10
Plasma testosterone, μg/dL:	
Men	0.3–1.0
Women	0.01–0.1
17-Ketosteroids, mg/24 h:	
Men	7–25
Women	4–15
Plasma dehydroepiandrosterone (DHEA) μg/dL	0.2–0.9
Plasma DHEA sulfate, μg/dL	50–250
Plasma 11-deoxycortisol (S), μg/dL	<1.0
Plasma 17αOH progesterone, ng/dL:	
Women	
Follicular phase	6–110
Luteal phase	50–350
Men	6–300
Plasma aldosterone, ng/dL (100 meq Na, 60–100 meq K, supine, 8 A.M.)	1–5
Aldosterone secretion, μg/24 h (100 meq Na, 600–100 meq K)	50–250
Aldosterone excretion, μg/24 h (100 meq Na, 60–100 meq K)	2–10
Plasma renin activity, (ng/mL)/h (100 meq Na, 60–100 meq K, supine, 8 A.M.)	1–2.5
Plasma angiotensin II, pg/mL (100 meq Na, 60–100 meq K, supine, 8 A.M.)	10–30
Plasma ACTH, pg/mL (8 A.M.)	<80

BLOOD LEVELS (See Table 352-2) **Peptides** ACTH and angiotensin II can be measured by radioimmunoassay, but the measurements are technically difficult because of their low concentrations and their instability in human plasma. In addition, ACTH levels fluctuate from moment to moment, and a circadian rhythm is superimposed on basal ACTH secretion, with lower levels in the early evening than in the morning. Angiotensin II levels also vary diurnally but more importantly are influenced by dietary sodium intake and posture. Both upright posture and sodium restriction elevate angiotensin II levels.

Most clinical determinations of the renin-angiotensin system, however, involve measurements of peripheral "plasma renin activity" (PRA) in which the renin activity is gauged by the generation of angiotensin I during a standardized incubation period. This method depends on the presence of sufficient angiotensinogen in the patient's plasma as substrate. The generated angiotensin I is then measured by radioimmunoassay. Plasma renin activity depends on dietary sodium intake and whether the patient is ambulatory. In normal humans a diurnal rhythm for plasma renin activity is characterized by peak values in the morning with decreases in activity in the afternoon.

Steroids Cortisol and aldosterone are both secreted episodically, and levels generally decline during the day with peak values in the morning and low levels in the evening. In addition, the plasma level of aldosterone, but not of cortisol, is increased by dietary potassium loading, sodium restriction, or assuming the upright posture. Measurement of the sulfate conjugate of DHEA is a useful index of adrenal androgen secretion since little is formed in the gonads and the half-life is prolonged (7 to 9 h).

URINE LEVELS The urine *17-hydroxycorticoids* are determined as Porter-Silber chromogens; this reaction is specific for steroids with a "dihydroxyacetone" C-17 side chain, i.e., with hydroxyl groups on C-17 and C-21 and a ketone group on C-20. Therefore, this determination includes cortisol, cortisone, tetrahydrocortisol, tetrahydrocortisone, and 11-deoxycortisol (Fig. 325-2). Normally, daytime (7 A.M. to 7 P.M.) excretion exceeds night values (7 P.M. to 7 A.M.).

The urine *17-ketosteroids* are those containing a ketone group at C-17 (Fig. 325-1). They originate either in the adrenal gland or the gonad. In normal women, 90 percent or more of total urinary 17-ketosteroids is derived from the adrenal gland, while in men only 60 to 70 percent is of adrenal origin. Urine 17-ketosteroid values are highest in young adults and decline with age.

The determination of urinary free cortisol is perhaps more useful than 17-hydroxysteroid measurements since elevated excretion values correlate with states of hypercortisolism, reflecting changes in the unbound, physiologically active, circulating levels of cortisol.

A carefully timed urine collection is a prerequisite for all excretory determinations. Urinary creatinine should be measured simultaneously to demonstrate the accuracy and adequacy of the collection procedure. Adjustments for body size can be made; e.g., normal subjects excrete 3 to 7 mg of 17-hydroxycorticosteroids per gram of creatinine.

STIMULATION TESTS Stimulation tests are useful in documenting the existence of a hormonal deficiency state. A standardized and specific stimulus for the production and release of a given hormone is applied, and the quantity of the released hormone can then be measured.

Tests of glucocorticoid reserve Within minutes after initiation of an infusion of ACTH, cortisol levels increase in adrenal venous blood. This responsiveness of the adrenal gland to ACTH is utilized as an index of the "functional reserve" of the gland for production of cortisol. Under maximal ACTH stimulation the cortisol secretion increases tenfold to 300 mg per day. Such maximal stimulation can be obtained only with prolonged ACTH infusions. For clinical purposes, the functional adrenal reserve for cortisol production is standardized with a 24-h ACTH infusion. Synthetic α^{1-24}-ACTH (cosyntropin) is usually given in 500 to 1000 mL normal saline solution at a rate of 2 units per hour for 24 h. Normal subjects increase 17-hydroxysteroid excretion rates to at least 25 mg per 24 h, and plasma cortisol levels exceed 40 μg/dL. In patients with secondary adrenal insufficiency, the maximal 17-hydroxysteroid excretion rate is 3 to 20 mg per 24 h, and the plasma cortisol value at 24 h ranges between 10 and 40 μg/dL. Patients with primary adrenal insufficiency have smaller responses.

A rapid screening test is to administer 25 units (0.25 mg) cosyntropin intravenously or intramuscularly and measure plasma cortisol levels before and 30 and 60 min later. An increment of at least 7 μg/dL above base line is observed in normal subjects.

Tests of mineralocorticoid reserve and stimulation of the renin-angiotensin system Stimulation tests utilize protocols of programmed volume depletion, such as sodium restriction, diuretic administration, or upright posture. A simple potent test consists of severe sodium restriction and upright posture. After 3 to 5 days of a 10-meq sodium intake, aldosterone secretion or excretion rates should increase two- to threefold over control. Supine morning plasma aldosterone levels usually increase three- to sixfold. In addition, plasma levels increase two- to fourfold in response to 2 to 3 h of upright posture.

Stimulation tests on normal dietary sodium intake may be carried out by the administration of a potent diuretic, such as 40 to 80 mg furosemide, followed by 2 to 3 h of upright posture. The normal response is a two- to fourfold rise in plasma aldosterone levels.

SUPPRESSION TESTS Suppression tests to document hypersecretion of adrenocortical hormones are based on the demonstration of a decrease in the target hormone following standardized suppression of its tropic hormone.

Tests of pituitary-adrenal suppressibility The ACTH release mechanism is sensitive to the circulating blood level of glucocorticoids. When such blood levels are increased in the normal individual, less ACTH is released from the anterior pituitary, and secondarily, less steroid is produced by the adrenal gland. The integrity of this feedback mechanism can be tested clinically by giving a potent glucocorticoid and judging suppression of ACTH secretion by analysis of urine steroid excretory values and/or plasma cortisol and ACTH levels. A potent glucocorticoid such as dexamethasone is utilized in order that the administered compound can be given in such small amounts that it does not contribute significantly to the steroids to be analyzed.

The best *screening* procedure is the overnight dexamethasone suppression test. This involves the measurement of plasma cortisol levels at 8 A.M. following the oral administration of 1 mg dexamethasone the previous midnight. The 8 A.M. value for plasma cortisol in normal subjects should be less than 5 μg/dL.

The definitive test of adrenal suppressibility is to administer 0.5 mg dexamethasone every 6 h for two successive days while collecting urine over a 24-h period for determination of creatinine, 17-hydroxysteroids and/or free cortisol and/or measuring plasma cortisol levels. In a patient with a normal hypothalamic pituitary ACTH release mechanism, a fall in the urine 17-hydroxycorticoids to less than 3 mg a day on the second day of dexamethasone administration, urinary free cortisol to less than 30 μg per day, or plasma cortisol to less than 5 μg/dL is seen.

Normal responses to either of the suppression tests implies that the ACTH control of the adrenal glands is physiologically normal. However, an isolated abnormal result, particularly when the overnight suppression test is being used, does not in itself imply pituitary and/or adrenal disease.

Tests of mineralocorticoid suppressibility Mineralocorticoid suppression procedures have been devised using saline infusions, oral salt loading, or deoxycorticosterone acetate (DOCA) administration for expansion of the extracellular fluid volume. With expansion of extracellular fluid volume, there is a decrease in renal renin release, a decrease in circulating plasma renin activity, and a decrease in aldosterone secretion and/or excretion. Various tests differ in the rate at which extracellular fluid volume is expanded. One convenient suppression test is the intravenous infusion of 500 mL normal saline solution per hour for 4 h, which normally suppresses plasma aldosterone levels to < 8 ng/dL on a sodium-restricted diet or to < 5 ng/dL on a normal sodium intake. This test should not be performed in potassium-depleted subjects.

TESTS OF PITUITARY-ADRENAL RESPONSIVENESS Stimuli such as insulin hypoglycemia, arginine vasopressin, and pyrogen, cause release of ACTH from the pituitary by an action on higher nerve centers, the hypothalamus, or the pituitary itself. By measuring plasma ACTH or plasma glucocorticoids the status of pituitary ACTH can be evaluated. Insulin-induced hypoglycemia is particularly useful, since the release of growth hormone and of ACTH is stimulated. In this test 0.05 to 0.1 unit of regular insulin per kilogram of body weight is administered intravenously as a bolus to reduce fasting glucose levels at least 50 percent below basal. The normal cortisol response is a rise to more than 18 μg/dL.

Metyrapone is a drug that inhibits 11β-hydroxylase in the adrenal gland. As a result, the conversion of 11-deoxycortisol (compound S) to cortisol is interfered with, and increased amounts of 11-deoxycortisol accumulate while blood levels of cortisol decrease (Fig. 325-2). The hypothalamic-pituitary axis responds to the declining cortisol blood levels by releasing more ACTH. The metabolites of 11-deoxycortisol are excreted in increasing amounts in the urine, where they are measured as 17-hydroxycorticoids. Alternatively, changes in plasma 11-deoxycortisol levels can be measured. *Note that the adrenal glands must be capable of being stimulated by ACTH, since assessment of the response depends both on an intact hypothalamic-pituitary axis and on adrenal steroid production.*

The metyrapone test involves administering orally 750 mg of the drug every 4 h over a 24-h period and comparing the control and the post-metyrapone 17-hydroxysteroid excretion rates and/or plasma 11-deoxycortisol levels. Normal individuals respond with at least a doubling of their basal 17-hydroxysteroid excretion; 11-deoxycortisol levels in the blood should exceed 10 μg/dL following metyrapone administration. The metyrapone test does not accurately reflect ACTH reserve if subjects are ingesting exogenous glucocorticoids or drugs that accelerate the metabolism of metyrapone (e.g., phenytoin).

A direct and selective test of the pituitary corticotrophs can be achieved with the investigational agent corticotropin-releasing hormone (CRH). The bolus injection of 1 μg per kilogam of body weight of ovine CRH stimulates ACTH and beta endorphin secretion in normal human subjects within 60 to 180 min. However, the magnitude of the ACTH response is less than that produced by the insulin tolerance test, which implies that additional factors (such as vasopressin) augment stress-induced increases in ACTH secretion.

A test that distinguishes between primary and secondary adrenal insufficiency takes advantage of the preservation of relatively normal aldosterone secretion in secondary adrenal insufficiency. Twenty-five units of cosyntropin is given intravenously or intramuscularly, and plasma cortisol and aldosterone levels are obtained before and 30 and 60 min later. The cortisol increment is less than 7 μg/dL in both groups, but only patients with primary insufficiency fail to increase aldosterone levels above control by at least 5 ng/dL.

HYPERFUNCTION OF THE ADRENAL CORTEX

Distinct clinical syndromes are produced when excess amounts of the principal adrenocortical hormones are secreted. Thus, excess production of cortisol is associated with Cushing's syndrome, excess production of aldosterone with clinical and chemical signs of aldosteronism, and excess production of adrenal androgens with adrenal virilism. These syndromes do not always occur in the "pure" form but may have overlapping features.

CUSHING'S SYNDROME **Etiology** Cushing described a syndrome characterized by truncal obesity, hypertension, fatigability and weakness, amenorrhea, hirsutism, purplish abdominal striae, edema, glucosuria, osteoporosis, and a basophilic tumor of the pituitary. As awareness of this syndrome increased, the diagnosis of Cushing's syndrome has been broadened into the classification shown in Table 325-3. Regardless of etiology, all cases of endogenous Cushing's syndrome are due to increased production of cortisol by the adrenal gland. Most are due to *bilateral adrenal hyperplasia,* secondary to adrenocortical stimulation by hypersecretion of pituitary ACTH or the production of ACTH by nonendocrine tumors. The incidence of pituitary-dependent adrenal hyperplasia in women is three times that in men, with the most frequent age of onset being the third or fourth decade. The cause of the hypersecretion pituitary ACTH is still unclear, but the primary defect probably resides in the hypothalamus or in higher nerve centers, leading to release of CRH inappropriate to the level of circulating cortisol. Consequently, a higher level of cortisol is required to reduce ACTH secretion to normal. This primary defect leads to hyperstimulation of the pituitary resulting, in some cases, in tumor formation. As the pituitary tumor grows, it may become independent of the regulating influence of central nervous system factors and/or circulating cortisol levels. Thus, individuals with hypersecretion of pituitary ACTH may have a microadenoma (<10 mm) or a macroadenoma (>10 mm) of the pituitary, or diffuse hyperplasia of the corticotropic cells (hypothalamic-pituitary dysfunction). Since microadenomas of the pituitary are often difficult to detect by usual radiologic procedures, the frequency of pituitary adenomas as a cause of Cushing's syndrome is uncertain. Traditionally, only an individual who has an ACTH-producing pituitary tumor has been defined as having *Cushing's disease*. However, in some centers, anyone who has hypersecretion of pituitary ACTH regardless of whether a tumor is present is classified as having Cushing' disease. In this chapter, we will use the traditional definition.

Nonendocrine tumors may secrete polypeptides that are biologically, chemically, and immunologically indistinguishable from either ACTH or CRH and that cause bilateral adrenal hyperplasia (see also Chap. 303). The ectopic production of CRH results in clinical, biochemical, and radiologic features indistinguishable from those caused by hypersecretion of pituitary ACTH. Often, but not invariably, the typical signs and symptoms of Cushing's syndrome are absent with ectopic ACTH production, and hypokalemic alkalosis and glucose intolerance are the prominent manifestations. The majority of these cases are associated with the primitive small-cell (oat cell) type of bronchogenic carcinoma or with tumors of the thymus, pancreas, or ovary, medullary carcinoma of the thyroid, or bronchial adenomas. The onset of Cushing's syndrome may be sudden, particularly in patients with oat cell carcinoma of the lung, and this feature accounts in part for the failure of these patients to exhibit the classic physical findings. On the other hand, patients with carcinoid tumors or pheochromocytomas have longer clinical courses and usually exhibit the typical cushingoid features. The secretion of ACTH by nonendocrine tumors is also accompanied by the accumulation of ACTH fragments in plasma and by elevated plasma levels of ACTH precursor molecules. Since such tumors may produce large amounts of ACTH, baseline urinary steroid values are usually markedly elevated, and increased skin pigmentation is usually present. Indeed, hyperpigmentation in patients with Cushing's syndrome almost always points to an extraadrenal tumor, either in an extracranial location or within the cranium.

Approximately 20 to 25 percent of patients with Cushing's syndrome have primary overproduction of cortisol and other adrenal steroids due to an adrenal neoplasm. These tumors are usually unilateral, and about half are malignant. Occasionally, patients have biochemical features both of hypersecretion of pituitary ACTH and of an adrenal adenoma. These individuals usually have micro- or macro-nodularity of both adrenal glands resulting in *nodular hyperplasia.*

The most common cause of Cushing's syndrome is *iatrogenic* administration of steroids for other reasons. While the clinical features bear some resemblance to those of an individual with an adrenal adenoma, these patients are usually readily distinguishable on the basis of history and initial laboratory studies.

TABLE 325-3 Causes of Cushing's syndrome

I Adrenal hyperplasia
- *A* Secondary to pituitary ACTH overproduction
  - *1* Pituitary-hypothalamic dysfunction
  - *2* Pituitary ACTH-producing micro- or macroadenomas
- *B* Secondary to ACTH or CRH-producing nonendocrine tumors (bronchogenic carcinoma, carcinoid of the thymus, pancreatic carcinoma, bronchial adenoma)

II Adrenal nodular hyperplasia

III Adrenal neoplasia
- *A* Adenoma
- *B* Carcinoma

IV Exogenous, iatrogenic causes
- *A* Prolonged use of glucocorticoids
- *B* Prolonged use of ACTH

Clinical signs, symptoms, and laboratory findings Many of the signs and symptoms of Cushing's syndrome logically follow from the known action of glucocorticoids (Table 325-4). As a result of mobilization of peripheral supportive tissue, muscle weakness and fatigability, osteoporosis, cutaneous striae, and easy bruisability result. The latter two signs are secondary to weakening and rupture of collagen fibers in the dermis. The osteoporosis may be so severe that collapse of vertebral bodies and pathologic fractures of other bones occur. Increased hepatic gluconeogenesis and insulin resistance can cause impaired glucose tolerance. Frank diabetes occurs in less than 20 percent of patients, probably in individuals with a familial predisposition to this disorder. Hypercortisolism promotes the deposition of adipose tissue in characteristic sites, notably in the upper part of the face, the classic "moon" facies; in the interscapular area, the "buffalo" hump; and in the mesenteric bed, where it produces the classic "truncal" obesity (Fig. 325-6). Rarely, there may be episternal fatty tumors and mediastinal widening secondary to fat accumulation. The reason for this peculiar distribution of adipose tissue is not known. The face appears plethoric, even in the absence of any increase in red blood cell concentration. Hypertension is common, and frequently there are profound emotional changes, ranging from irritability or emotional lability to severe depression, confusion, or even frank psychosis. In women, increased adrenal androgen secretion can cause acne, hirsutism, and oligomenorrhea or amenorrhea. The most common signs and symptoms in patients with hypercortisolism, i.e., obesity, hypertension, osteoporosis, and diabetes, are nonspecific and therefore less helpful in diagnosing this condition. On the other hand, easy bruising, typical striae, myopathy, and androgen effects (although less frequent) are, if present, more suggestive of Cushing's syndrome.

Except in iatrogenic Cushing's syndrome, plasma and urine cortisol and urinary 17-hydroxycorticoid levels are variably elevated. Occasionally, hypokalemia, hypochloremia and metabolic alkalosis are present, particularly in individuals who have ectopic production of ACTH.

Diagnosis The diagnosis of Cushing's syndrome depends on the demonstration of increased cortisol production and the failure to suppress endogenous cortisol secretion normally when dexamethasone is administered. Once the diagnosis is established, further testing is

TABLE 325-4 Incidence of signs and symptoms in Cushing's syndrome, percent

Typical habitus	97	Amenorrhea	77
Increased body weight	94	Cutaneous striae	67
Fatigability and weakness	87	Personality changes	66
		Ecchymoses	65
Hypertension (>150/90)	82	Edema	62
		Polyuria, polydipsia	23
Hirsutism	80	Hypertrophy of clitoris	19

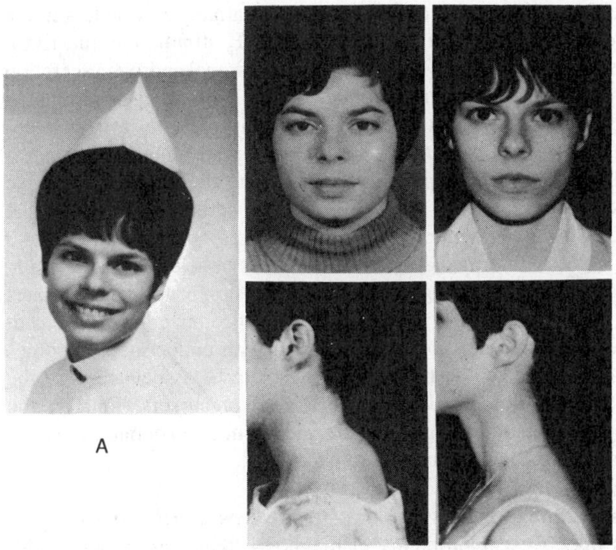

A B C

FIGURE 325-6 *A 20-year-old woman with Cushing's syndrome due to a right adrenal cortical adenoma. A. Two years prior to surgery, age 18. B. One month prior to surgery, age 20. C. One year after surgery, age 21.*

designed to determine the etiology of the hypercortisolism (see Fig. 325-7 and Table 325-5).

For initial screening, the overnight dexamethasone suppression test is recommended (see above). In difficult cases (e.g., in obesity) measurement of a 24-h free cortisol excretion rate can also be used as a screening test. A level greater than 100 μg per day is suggestive

TABLE 325-5 Diagnostic tests to determine the type of Cushing's syndrome

Test	Pituitary macroadenoma	Pituitary-hypothalamic dysfunction or microadenoma	Ectopic ACTH or CRH production	Adrenal tumor
Measurement of plasma ACTH	↑ to ↑↑	N to ↑	↑ to ↑↑↑	↓
Response to high-dose dexamethasone, %	<10	>80	<10	<10
Response to metyrapone, %	>80	>90	<10	<10
Response to CRH, %	>90	>90	<10	<10

NOTE: *N, normal; ↑, elevated; ↓, decreased.*

of Cushing's syndrome. The definitive diagnosis is then established by failure to suppress urinary cortisol to less than 30 μg per day, plasma cortisol to less than 5μg/dL, or 17-hydroxysteroid excretion to less than 3 mg per 24 h after a standard low-dose dexamethasone suppression test (0.5 mg every 6 h for 48 h). Owing to diurnal variability, plasma cortisol and, to a certain extent, ACTH determinations are not meaningful when performed in isolation, but demonstration that the normal fall in bedtime blood levels does not occur may be useful.

Determining the etiology of Cushing's syndrome is complicated by the lack of specificity of all tests available and the spontaneous changes in hormonal secretion, often dramatic, that may occur in the tumors producing this syndrome (periodic hormonogenesis). No test has a specificity greater than 95 percent, and it may be necessary to

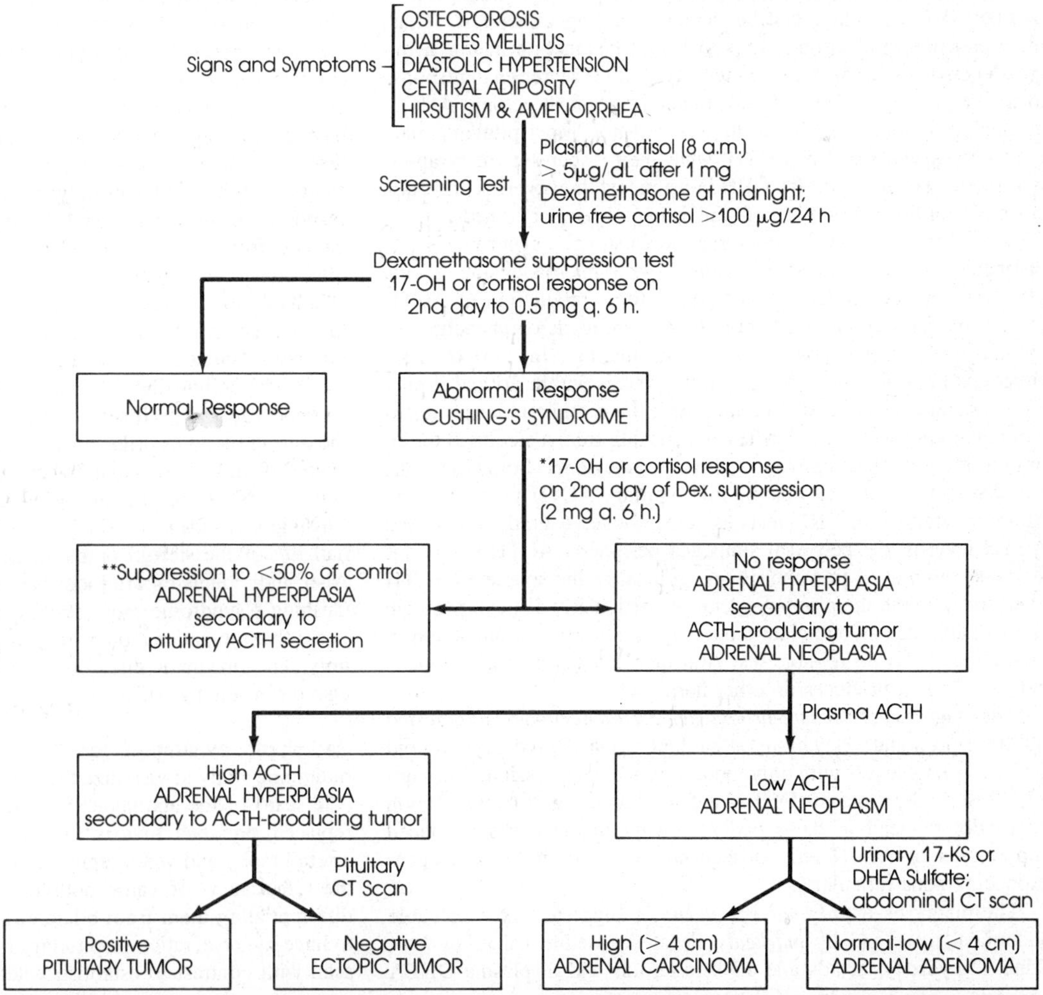

FIGURE 325-7 *Diagnostic flowchart for evaluating patients suspected of having Cushing's syndrome.*

**The 17-hydroxycorticosteroid response to metyrapone (750 mg given orally every 4 h for six doses) may be used as an alternative test to the high-dose dexamethasone test (2 mg given orally every 6 h). Increased urinary 17-hydroxycorticosteroid excretion following metyrapone occurs in the majority of patients with adrenal hyperplasia secondary to pituitary ACTH secretion; no response suggests an adrenal neoplasm or adrenal hyperplasia secondary to a nonendocrine ACTH-producing tumor.*

***This group of patients probably contains subjects with both pituitary-hypothalamic dysfunction and pituitary microadenomas. In some instances, a pituitary microadenoma may be visualized by CT scanning of the sella turcica.*

use a combination of tests to arrive at the correct diagnosis. A particularly useful first step is to determine the response of cortisol output to high-dose dexamethasone administration (2 mg every 6 hours for 2 days). In most series, more than half of the patients so tested have a suppression of urine cortisol and or 17-hydroxysteroid levels to less than 50 percent of basal values. These individuals usually have either an ACTH-secreting pituitary microadenoma or hypothalamic-pituitary dysfunction. Occasionally, in individuals with bilateral nodular hyperplasia and/or ectopic CRH production steroid output is also suppressed. Failure to suppress cortisol production after low- and high-dose dexamethasone administration (see Table 325-5) is usual in patients with adrenal hyperplasia secondary to an ACTH-secreting pituitary macroadenoma or ACTH-producing tumors of nonendocrine origin, and in adrenal neoplasms.

Theoretically, plasma ACTH levels should be useful in distinguishing the various causes of Cushing's syndrome, particularly in separating the ACTH-dependent from the ACTH-independent etiologies of the syndrome. In general, this is true for the ACTH-independent etiologies of the syndrome since most adrenal tumors have low or undetectable ACTH levels. Furthermore, ACTH-secreting pituitary macroadenomas and ACTH-producing nonendocrine tumors usually have elevated ACTH levels. However, at least two problems hinder the utilization of ACTH levels in the differential diagnosis of Cushing's syndrome. First, reliable ACTH assays are still not widely available, and second, ACTH levels may be similar in individuals with hypothalamic-pituitary dysfunction, pituitary microadenomas, ectopic CRH production, and ACTH production from some nonendocrine tumors (especially carcinoid tumors) (Table 325-5).

Because of these difficulties, several additional tests have been advocated, e.g., the metyrapone and the CRH infusion tests. The rationales underlying these tests are similar: Steroid hypersecretion secondary to an adrenal tumor or the ectopic production of ACTH will suppress the hypothalamic-pituitary axis so that inhibition of pituitary ACTH release can be demonstrated by either test. Thus, most patients with pituitary-hypothalamic dysfunction and/or a microadenoma have an increase in steroid or ACTH secretion in response to metyrapone and CRH administration while most ectopic ACTH-producing tumors and adrenal tumors will not. Most pituitary macroadenomas also respond to CRH, while their response to metyrapone is variable. The utility of the CRH infusion test, however, is uncertain since only a limited number of studies have been performed.

The major diagnostic dilemma in Cushing's syndrome is to distinguish between those individuals with microadenoma of the pituitary, ectopic production of CRH, ectopic production of ACTH from some para-endocrine tumors (e.g., carcinoids or pheochromocytoma), and hypothalamic pituitary dysfunction. In most of these situations the CT scan of the pituitary gland is within normal limits. Clinical manifestations are similar unless the ectopic tumor produces other symptoms, such as diarrhea and flushing from a carcinoid tumor or episodic hypertension from a pheochromocytoma. Sometimes one can distinguish between ectopic and pituitary ACTH production by using metyrapone or CRH tests as noted above. A gradient between ACTH level in the petrossal sinus and peripheral ACTH levels has also been employed in some centers to localize the source of ACTH overproduction to the pituitary gland. A particularly difficult problem is to distinguish hypothalamic-pituitary dysfunction from a tumor producing CRH; no reliable test is available if the ectopic tumor is not seen or if it produces no other hormones.

The diagnosis of *cortisol-producing adrenal adenoma* is suggested by disproprotionate elevations in baseline urine 17-hydroxycorticoid or free-cortisol levels with only modest rises or suppression of urinary 17-ketosteroids or plasma DHEA sulfate. Adrenal androgen secretion is usually reduced in these patients owing to the cortisol-induced suppression of ACTH and subsequent involution of the androgen-producing zona reticularis.

The diagnosis of *adrenal carcinoma* is suggested by a palpable abdominal mass and by *markedly* elevated baseline values *both* of urine 17-hydroxysteroids and 17-ketosteroids and of plasma DHEA sulfate. Plasma and urine cortisol levels are variably elevated. Adrenal carcinoma is usually resistant to both ACTH stimulation and dexamethasone suppression. Markedly elevated adrenal androgen secretion often leads to virilization in the female. Feminizing estrogen-producing adrenocortical carcinoma in the male usually presents with gynecomastia. These adrenal tumors secrete increased amounts of androstenedione which is peripherally converted to the estrogens, estrone and estradiol (see Chap. 332). Functioning adrenal carcinomas that produce Cushing's syndrome are most often associated with elevated values for the intermediates of steroid biosynthesis (especially 11-deoxycortisol), suggesting inefficient conversion of the intermediates to the final product. It is also important to recognize that 20 percent of adrenal carcinomas are not associated with endocrine syndromes and are presumed to be nonfunctioning or to be associated with the production of biologically inactive steroid precursors. Finally, the excessive production of gonadal steroids is not detectable in certain situations (e.g., androgens in adult men).

Differential diagnosis PSEUDOCUSHING'S SYNDROME A variety of groups may present problems in diagnosis; these are patients with obesity, chronic alcoholism, depression, and acute illness of any type. Extreme *obesity* is uncommon in Cushing's syndrome; furthermore, with exogenous obesity, the adiposity is generalized, not truncal. On adrenocortical testing, abnormalities in patients with exogenous obesity are usually modest. Basal urine steroid excretion levels in obese patients are either normal or slightly elevated, a finding similar to their cortisol secretory values. Some patients have elevated conversion of secreted cortisol into excreted metabolites. *Urinary* and *blood cortisol* levels are normal, and the diurnal pattern in blood and urine levels is normal. Exogenous obesity may *cause* alterations in the secretion and metabolism of steroids; this points up the secondary nature of altered steroid testing patterns sometimes encountered. Patients with *chronic alcoholism* and *depression* share similar abnormalities in steroid output: elevated urinary 17-hydroxysteroids, absent diurnal rhythm of cortisol levels, and resistance to suppression with dexamethasone (particularly overnight and low dose). In contrast to alcoholic subjects, depressed patients do not have clinical signs and symptoms of Cushing's syndrome. Following discontinuation of alcohol and/or improvement of the emotional status, steroid testing usually returns to normal. A normal cortisol response to insulin-induced hypoglycemia may distinguish these patients from subjects with Cushing's syndrome. *Acutely ill* subjects often have abnormal laboratory tests and fail to suppress with dexamethasone since major stress (such as pain or fever) interrupts the normal regulation of ACTH secretion. *Iatrogenic Cushing's syndrome,* induced by the administration of potent synthetic glucocorticoids, is indistinguishable by physical findings from endogenous adrenocortical hyperfunction. This situation can be distinguished by measuring blood or urine cortisol levels or urinary 17-hydroxysteroid excretion in a basal state where the levels are low secondary to suppression of the pituitary-adrenal axis. The severity of iatrogenic Cushing's syndrome is related to the total steroid dose, to the biologic half-life of the steroid preparation, and to the duration of therapy. Also, individuals on afternoon and evening doses of steroid develop Cushing's syndrome more readily and on smaller total daily steroid doses than do patients on a steroid program limited to morning doses only. The enzymatic disposition and binding of administered steroids also differ among patients.

Radiologic evaluation for Cushing's syndrome The preferred radiologic study to visualize the adrenals is computerized tomography (CT scan) of the abdomen (Fig. 325-8). This procedure has largely replaced previous invasive procedures (such as selective adrenal arteriography and venography) and 19-[^{131}I]iodocholesterol scanning; the CT scan is of value both in localizing adrenal tumors and in differentiating them from bilateral hyperplasia. All patients believed to have hypersecretion of pituitary ACTH should have a pituitary CT scan with contrast to establish whether a pituitary tumor is present.

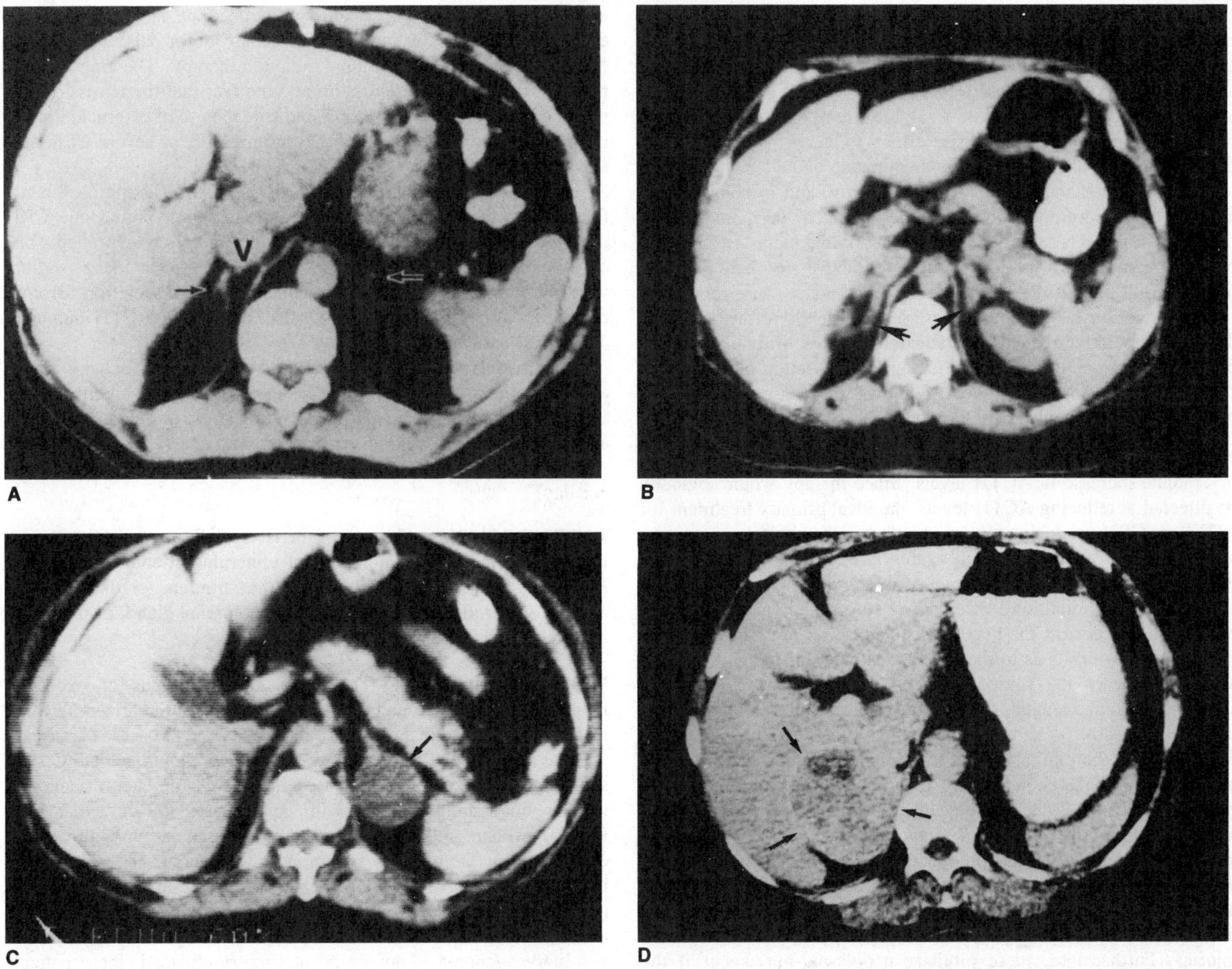

FIGURE 325-8 *Computerized tomography is the preferred method for visualizing the adrenal glands. The adrenal glands are indicated by arrows. A. The normal right adrenal gland is adjacent to the inferior vena cava (V) as it emerges from the liver. Approximately 90 percent of the right adrenal glands appear as linear structures extending posteriorly from the inferior vena cava into the space between the right lobe of the liver and the crus of the diaphragm. The normal left adrenal gland is lateral to the left crus of the diaphragm and below the stomach. The majority of left adrenal glands are shaped like an inverted "V" or "Y." B. Adrenal CT scan of a patient with ectopic ACTH production. Both adrenal glands (arrows) are enlarged (compare with A). In contrast, only 50 percent of patients with bilateral adrenal hyperplasia secondary to pituitary ACTH hypersecretion show enlargement of the adrenals when imaged by CT scan. C. CT scan of a patient with Cushing's syndrome with biochemical evidence only of cortisol overproduction. The left adrenal has been replaced by a racquet-shaped 2-cm tumor (arrow). Attenuation of the tumor is low because of its high lipid content. D. CT scan in a patient with Cushing's syndrome and biochemical evidence of an adrenal carcinoma. In contrast to C, the left-sided mass has a heterogeneous appearance and is larger in size—usual characteristics of an adrenal carcinoma.*

Even with the best CT scanners presently available small microadenomas may be undectable.

Evaluation of asymptomatic adrenal masses With abdominal CT scanning, many incidental adrenal masses are discovered. This is not surprising, since 10 to 20 percent of subjects at autopsy have adrenal cortical adenomas. The first step in evaluating such patients is to determine if the tumor is functioning by appropriate screening tests. However, in 90 percent of the cases tumors detected incidentally at the time of abdominal CT scanning are nonfunctioning. Fortunately, they also are seldom malignant. Yet, nonfunctioning tumors raise difficult therapeutic questions. Since 20 percent of adrenal carcinomas are nonfunctioning, one could argue that all such lesions should be removed. However, the frequency of adrenal carcinomas is low compared with the frequency of benign cortical adenomas (less than 1 percent), and surgery is not indicated in most cases. The size of the tumor sometimes is of value: Adrenal carcinomas are rarely smaller than 3 cm in diameter, and adrenal adenomas are usually smaller than 6 cm (Fig. 325-8). If surgery is not performed, a repeat CT scan in 3 to 6 months is usually required for followup.

Therapy ADRENAL NEOPLASMS When an adenoma or carcinoma is diagnosed, adrenal exploration is performed with excision of the tumor. Because of the possible atrophy of the contralateral adrenal, the patient is treated pre- and postoperatively for total adrenalectomy even when a unilateral lesion is suspected, the routine being similar to that for an Addisonian patient undergoing elective surgery (Table 325-11).

Despite operative intervention, most patients with adrenal carcinoma die within 3 years of diagnosis. Metastases occur most often to liver and lung. The principal antitumor drug used to treat metastatic adrenocortical carcinoma is mitotane (*o,p'*-DDD), an isomer of the insecticide DDT. This drug suppresses cortisol production and decreases plasma and urine steroid levels. Although its cytotoxic action is relatively selective for the glucocorticoid-secreting zone of the adrenal cortex, the zona glomerulosa may also be inhibited.

Because mitotane also alters the extraadrenal metabolism of cortisol, plasma and urinary cortisol levels must be assessed to titrate the effect. The drug is usually given in divided doses three to four times a day, with the dose increased gradually to 8 to 10 g daily. Almost all patients experience gastrointestinal side effects (anorexia, diarrhea, or vomiting) or neuromuscular side effects (lethargy, somnolence, or dizziness). All patients treated with mitotane should be placed on long-term maintenance glucocorticoid therapy, and in some mineralocorticoid replacement should also be instituted. In approximately one-third of patients regression of both tumor and metastases occurs, but long-term survival is limited, as noted above. In many patients, mitotane only inhibits steroidogenesis and does not cause regression of tumor metastases. Osseous metastases are usually refractory to the drug and should be treated with radiation therapy. Mitotane can also be given as adjunctive therapy after surgical resection of an adrenal carcinoma even in the absence of known metastases because the prognosis of this neoplasm is so poor.

BILATERAL HYPERPLASIA Patients with hyperplasia have a relative or absolute increase in ACTH levels. Since therapy would logically be directed at reducing ACTH levels, the ideal primary treatment for ACTH- or CRH-producing tumors, whether in the pituitary or ectopic, is surgical removal. Occasionally, this is not possible because the disease, particularly with ectopic ACTH production, is often far advanced. In this situation "medical" or surgical adrenalectomy may be indicated to correct the hypercortisolism.

Controversy exists as to the proper treatment for bilateral adrenal hyperplasia when the source of the ACTH overproduction is not apparent. In some centers, these patients (especially patients with a positive high-dose dexamethasone suppression test) have surgical exploration of the pituitary via a transsphenoidal approach in anticipation of a microadenoma being found. These explorations prove fruitful in between 20 and 70 percent of the cases, depending on the level of skill of the surgeon and the ability of the radiologist to localize the microadenoma preoperatively. However, in the event that a microadenoma is not found, total hypophysectomy may be needed. Complications of transsphenoidal surgery include rhinorrhea, diabetes insipidus, panhypopituitarism, and optic or cranial nerve injuries. Furthermore, these pituitary neoplasms may recur if the primary abnormality actually resides in the hypothalamus.

In other centers, total adrenalectomy is the treatment of choice. Cure with this procedure is close to 100 percent. The adverse effects include the certain need for lifelong mineralocorticoid as well as glucocorticoid replacement therapy and a 10 to 20 percent probability of a pituitary tumor developing over the next 10 years, many requiring surgical therapy (Nelson's syndrome). It is uncertain whether in these individuals (see Chap. 321) the tumor develops de novo or is present prior to bilateral adrenalectomy but is so small that it is not detected by radiologic procedures. Periodic radiologic evaluation of the pituitary gland by CT scanning and serial ACTH levels should be obtained in any individual who has undergone bilateral adrenalectomy for Cushing's syndrome. Often, such pituitary tumors that become apparent following adrenalectomy become locally invasive and impinge on the optic chiasm or extend into the cavernous or sphenoid sinuses. Thus, an aggressive surgical approach is often followed by postoperative irradiation.

In a few centers, pituitary irradiation is the primary treatment for pituitary ACTH overproduction, with the use of either conventional external or alpha (proton beam) radiation. The latter, while more effective, has a greater incidence of ocular motor palsy and hypopituitarism than does conventional radiation therapy. The long lag time between treatment and remission and the fact that the remission rate is less than 50 percent often contraindicate the use of external pituitary radiation in the presence of rapidly progressive or severe Cushing's syndrome.

Finally, in occasional patients in whom a surgical approach is not feasible, medical therapy directed at reducing hypothalamic CRH release either by administering the serotonin antagonist cyproheptadine or by administering an inhibitor of GABA transaminase, sodium valproate, has been successful in reducing cortisol secretion. Bromocriptine, a dopaminergic agonist, also suppresses ACTH output in occasional patients.

If ACTH levels cannot be successfully lowered by any of the above treatment modalities, then medical or surgical adrenalectomy may be indicated (Table 325-6). Chemical adrenalectomy may be accomplished by the administration of mitotane (2 or 3 g per day) and/or aminoglutethimide (1 g per day) and metyrapone (2 or 3 g per day).

TABLE 325-6 Treatment modalities for patients with adrenal hyperplasia secondary to pituitary ACTH hypersecretion

I Reduce pituitary ACTH production
- *A* Transsphenoidal resection of microadenoma
- *B* Radiation
- *C* Treatment with hypothalamic serotonin antagonist (cyproheptadine) or GABA-transaminase inhibitor (sodium valproate)*

II Reduce or eliminate adrenocortical cortisol secretion
- *A* Bilateral adrenalectomy
- *B* Medical adrenalectomy (metyrapone, mitotane, aminoglutethimide)*

* *Not curative but effective as long as chronically administered in selected patients.*

ALDOSTERONISM Aldosteronism is a syndrome associated with hypersecretion of the major adrenal mineralocorticoid, aldosterone. *Primary* aldosteronism signifies that the stimulus for the excessive aldosterone production resides within the adrenal gland; in *secondary* aldosteronism the stimulus is extraadrenal.

Primary aldosteronism The signs and symptoms of excessive inappropriate aldosterone production were first summarized by Conn in 1956. In the original case and many subsequent cases, the disease was the result of an *aldosterone-producing adrenal adenoma* (Conn's syndrome). The majority of cases involved a unilateral adenoma, usually small and occurring with equal frequency on either side. Rarely, primary aldosteronism occurs in association with adrenal carcinoma. It is twice as common in women as in men, occurs between the ages of 30 and 50, and is present in approximately 1 percent of unselected hypertensive patients. Many cases have clinical and biochemical features characteristic of primary aldosteronism, but a solitary adenoma is not found at surgery. Instead, these patients have *bilateral cortical nodular hyperplasia*. In the literature this disease has been alternatively termed "pseudo" primary aldosteronism, idiopathic hyperaldosteronism, or nodular hyperplasia. The cause is unknown.

SIGNS AND SYMPTOMS The continual hypersecretion of aldosterone increases the renal distal tubular exchange of intratubular sodium for secreted potassium and hydrogen ions, with progressive depletion of body potassium and development of hypokalemia. Most patients have diastolic hypertension, usually not of marked severity, and complain of headaches. The hypertension is probably due to the increased sodium reabsorption and extracellular volume expansion. Potassium depletion is responsible for the muscle weakness and fatigue and is related to the effect of intra- and extracellular potassium ion depletion on muscle membrane. The polyuria results from impairment of concentrating ability and is often associated with polydipsia. Electrocardiographic and roentgenographic signs of left ventricular enlargement are secondary to the hypertension. Electrocardiographic signs of potassium depletion, such as prominent U waves, cardiac arrhythmias, and premature contractions, are common. In the absence of associated congestive heart failure, renal disease, or preexisting abnormalities (such as thrombophlebitis), edema is characteristically absent. In cases of long duration, nephropathy with azotemia may be associated with congestive heart failure and edema.

LABORATORY FINDINGS Laboratory findings are dependent on both the duration and the severity of the potassium depletion. An overnight concentration test often reveals impaired ability to concentrate the urine. Urine pH is neutral to alkaline, because of excessive secretion of ammonium and bicarbonate ions to compensate for a metabolic alkalosis. Tests of glucocorticoid and androgen secretion are within the normal range.

Hypokalemia may be severe (less than 3 meq potassium per liter) and reflects significant body potassium depletion, usually in excess of 300 meq. *Hypernatremia* is due to both sodium retention and a concomitant water loss from polyuria. Metabolic alkalosis and elevation of serum bicarbonate are a result of hydrogen ion loss into the urine and migration into potassium-depleted cells. The alkalosis is perpetuated by potassium deficiency, which increases the capacity of the proximal convoluted tubule to reabsorb filtered bicarbonate. If hypokalemia is severe, serum magnesium levels are also reduced. In the absence of azotemia, serum uric acid is normal.

Total body sodium content and total exchangeable sodium are increased, while total exchangeable body potassium is usually reduced. The expanded extracellular fluid volume may be responsible for the reversed diurnal excretory pattern for salt and water, with predominant salt and water excretion occurring during the night.

DIAGNOSIS The diagnosis is suggested by persistent hypokalemia in a nonedematous patient on a normal sodium intake who is not receiving potassium-wasting diuretics (furosemide, ethacrynic acid, thiazides) or potassium-sparing diuretics (triamterene, spironolactone). If hypokalemia occurs in a hypertensive patient on a potassium-wasting diuretic, the diuretic should be discontinued and the patient should be given potassium supplements. After 1 to 2 weeks the potassium level should be remeasured, and if hypokalemia persists, the patient should be evaluated for a mineralocorticoid excess syndrome (Fig. 325-9).

The criteria for the diagnosis of primary aldosteronism are (1) diastolic hypertension without edema, (2) hyposecretion of renin (as judged by low plasma renin activity levels) that fails to increase appropriately during volume depletion (upright posture, sodium depletion), and (3) hypersecretion of aldosterone that fails to suppress appropriately during volume expansion (salt loading).

Patients with primary aldosteronism characteristically *do not have edema,* since they exhibit an "escape" phenomenon from the sodium-retaining aspects of mineralocorticoids. Rarely, pretibial edema may be present in patients with associated nephropathy and azotemia.

The estimation of plasma renin activity is of limited value in separating patients with primary aldosteronism from those with other causes of hypertension. While the failure of plasma renin activity to rise normally during volume-depletion maneuvers is a criterion for

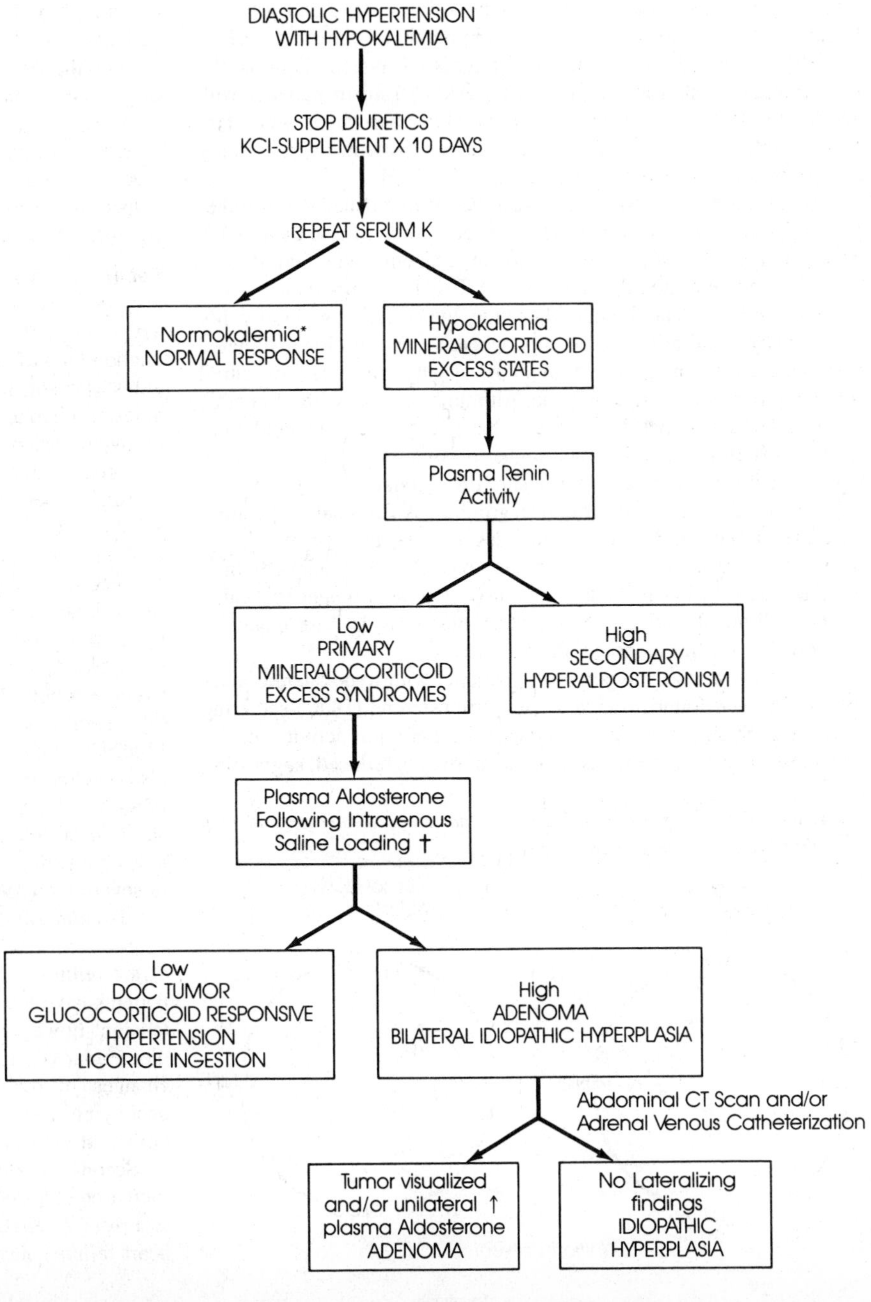

FIGURE 325-9 *Diagnostic flowchart for evaluating patients with suspected primary aldosteronism.*

**Serum K^+ may be normal in some patients with hyperaldosteronism who are taking potassium-sparing diuretics (spironolactone, triamterene) or ingesting low sodium–high potassium intakes.*

†This step should not be taken if hypertension is severe (diastolic pressure >115 mmHg) or if cardiac failure is present. Also, serum potassium levels should be corrected before the infusion of saline solution. Alternative methods producing comparable suppression of aldosterone secretion include oral sodium loading (200 meq per day for 3 days) or 10 mg deoxycorticosterone acetate (DOCA) intramuscularly every 12 h for 3 days.

primary aldosteronism, suppressed renin activity also occurs in about 25 percent of patients with essential hypertension.

Since the determination of plasma renin responsiveness is not sufficient, the demonstration of lack of suppression of aldosterone secretion is necessary to diagnose primary aldosteronism (Fig. 325-9). The autonomy exhibited by aldosterone tumors in these patients refers only to the resistance to suppression of secretion during volume expansion; such tumors can and do respond in normal or supernormal fashion to the stimuli of potassium loading or ACTH infusion.

Once hyposecretion of renin and failure to suppress aldosterone secretion are demonstrated, localization of aldosterone-producing adenomas should be determined preoperatively by abdominal CT scan or by percutaneous transfemoral bilateral adrenal vein catheterization with simultaneous adrenal venography. The latter technique permits radiologic localization, and, in addition, the adrenal vein sampling may demonstrate a two- to threefold increase in plasma aldosterone concentration on the involved side compared with the uninvolved side. In cases of hyperaldosteronism secondary to cortical nodular hyperplasia, no localization is found. It is important for samples to be obtained simultaneously if possible and for cortisol levels to be measured to ensure that false localization does not reflect an ACTH- or stress-induced rise in aldosterone levels.

DIFFERENTIAL DIAGNOSIS Patients with hypertension and hypokalemia may have primary or secondary hyperaldosteronism (see Fig. 325-10). A useful maneuver to distinguish between them is the measurement of plasma renin activity. Aldosteronism patients with accelerated hypertension and secondary aldosteronism is secondary to elevated plasma renin levels; in contrast, patients with primary aldosteronism have suppressed plasma renin levels.

Primary aldosteronism must also be distinguished from other *hypermineralocorticoid states*. The common problem is to distinguish between hyperaldosteronism due to an adenoma and that due to idiopathic bilateral nodular hyperplasia. This is of importance, since hypertension associated with idiopathic hyperplasia is usually not benefited by bilateral adrenalectomy, whereas hypertension associated with aldosterone-producing tumors is usually improved or cured following removal of the adenoma. Although patients with idiopathic bilateral nodular hyperplasia tend to have less severe hypokalemia, lower aldosterone secretion, and higher plasma renin activity than do patients with primary aldosteronism, differentiation is impossible solely on clinical and/or biochemical grounds. An anomalous postural decrease in plasma aldosterone and elevated plasma 18-hydroxycorticosterone levels are present in the majority of patients with a unilateral lesion, but these tests are also of limited diagnostic value in the individual patient. A definitive diagnosis is best made by radiographic studies as noted above.

In a few instances, hypertensive patients with hypokalemic alkalosis have been found to have deoxycorticosterone (DOC)-secreting adenomas. Such patients have reduced plasma renin activity levels, but aldosterone measurements are either normal or reduced, suggesting the diagnosis of mineralocorticoid excess due to a hormone other than aldosterone. Rarely, hypermineralocorticoidism is due to a defect in cortisol biosynthesis, specifically 11- or 17-hydroxylation. ACTH levels are increased, with a resultant increase in the production of the mineralocorticoid 11-deoxycorticosterone. *Hypertension and hypokalemia can be corrected by glucocorticoid administration.* The definitive diagnosis is made by demonstrating an elevation of precursors of cortisol biosynthesis in the blood or urine. Occasionally, glucocorticoid administration produces normotension and normokalemia although a hydroxylase deficiency cannot be identified (Fig. 325-9).

FIGURE 325-10 *Responses of the renin-aldosterone volume control loop in primary versus secondary aldosteronism.*

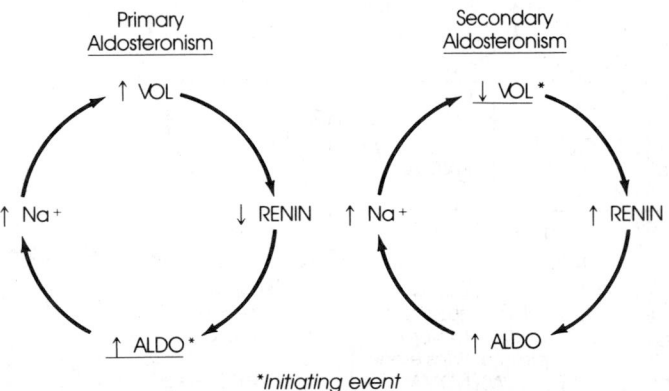

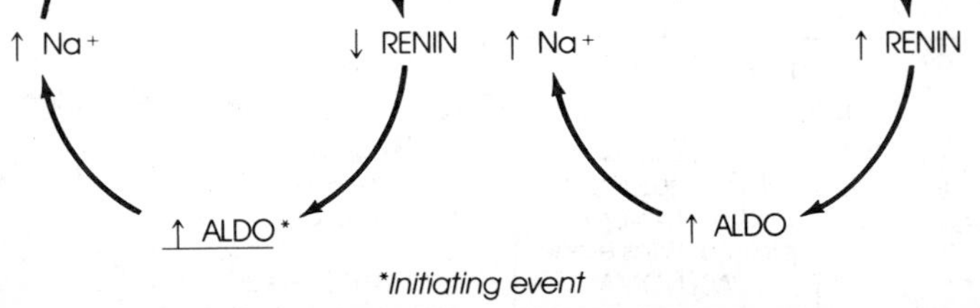

The ingestion of candies or chewing tobacco containing certain forms of licorice produces a syndrome mimicking primary aldosteronism. The sodium-retaining principle in such agents is glycyrrhizinic acid, which causes sodium retention, expansion of the extracellular fluid volume, hypertension, depressed plasma renin levels, and suppressed aldosterone levels. The diagnosis is established or excluded by a careful history.

TREATMENT Primary aldosteronism due to an adenoma is usually treated by surgical excision. However, dietary sodium restriction and the administration of an aldosterone antagonist, spironolactone, are effective in many cases. Hypertension and hypokalemia are usually controlled by doses of 25 to 100 mg spironolactone every 8 h. Some patients have been successfully managed medically for years, but chronic therapy in men is usually limited by the common occurrence of gynecomastia, decreased libido, and impotence.

When bilateral hyperplasia is suspected, surgery is indicated only when significant, symptomatic hypokalemia cannot be controlled with medical therapy, e.g., by spironolactone, triamterene, or amiloride. Hypertension associated with idiopathic hyperplasia is usually not benefited by bilateral adrenalectomy.

Secondary aldosteronism Secondary aldosteronism refers to an appropriately increased production of aldosterone in response to activation of the renin-angiotensin system (Fig. 325-10). The production rates of aldosterone are often higher in patients with secondary aldosteronism than in those with primary aldosteronism. Secondary aldosteronism usually occurs in association with the accelerated phase of hypertension or on the basis of an underlying edema disorder. Secondary aldosteronism in pregnancy is a normal physiologic response to estrogen-induced increases in circulating levels of renin substrate and plasma renin activity, and to the antialdosterone actions of the progestogens.

Secondary aldosteronism in hypertensive states either is secondary to a primary overproduction of renin (primary reninism) or is caused by an overproduction of renin which is secondary to a decrease in renal blood flow and/or perfusion pressure (Fig. 325-5). Secondary hypersecretion of renin can be due to a narrowing of one or both of the major renal arteries either by an atherosclerotic plaque or by fibromuscular hyperplasia. Overproduction of renin from both kidneys also occurs in association with severe arteriolar nephrosclerosis (malignant hypertension) or secondary to profound renal vasoconstriction (accelerated phase of hypertensive disease). The secondary aldosteronism is characterized by hypokalemic alkalosis, moderate to severe increases in plasma renin activity, and moderate to marked increases in aldosterone levels (see Chap. 196).

Secondary aldosteronism with hypertension can also be caused by a rare renin-producing tumor, in so-called primary reninism. These patients have the biochemical characteristics of renal vascular hypertension; however, the primary defect is renin secretion by a juxtaglomerular-cell tumor. The diagnosis can be made by the absence of changes in renal vasculature and/or demonstration of a space-occupying lesion in the kidney by radiographic techniques and unilateral increases in renal vein renin activity.

Secondary aldosteronism is present in many forms of *edema*. Increased aldosterone secretion rates are usual in patients with edema as a result of either cirrhosis or the nephrotic syndrome. In congestive heart failure, elevated aldosterone secretion varies depending on the severity of cardiac decompensation. The stimulus for aldosterone release in these conditions appears to be *arterial hypovolemia* and/or hypotension. Diuretic therapy often exaggerates the secondary aldosteronism via volume depletion; when this happens hypokalemia and on occasion alkalosis can become prominent features.

Secondary hyperaldosteronism rarely occurs without edema or hypertension (Bartter's syndrome). This syndrome is characterized by the signs of severe hyperaldosteronism (hypokalemic alkalosis) with moderate to marked increases in renin activity but normal blood pressure and absence of edema. Renal biopsy shows juxtaglomerular hyperplasia. The pathogenesis may be a defect in the renal conservation of sodium or chloride. The renal loss of sodium is thought to stimulate renin secretion and subsequent aldosterone production. Hyperaldosteronism produces potassium depletion, with the hypokalemia further elevating plasma renin activity. In some cases, the hypokalemia may be potentiated by a defect in renal conservation of potassium. One associated abnormality is an increased production of prostaglandins. (See Chap. 228.)

SYNDROMES OF ADRENAL ANDROGEN EXCESS The syndromes of adrenal androgen excess result from excess production of dehydroepiandrosterone and androstenedione, which are converted to testosterone in extraglandular tissues; the elevated testosterone levels account for most of the androgenic effects. Adrenal androgen excess may be associated with the secretion of greater or smaller amounts of other adrenal hormones and may, therefore, present as "pure" syndromes of virilization or as "mixed" syndromes associated with excessive production of glucocorticoids and some characteristics of Cushing's syndrome.

Clinical signs and symptoms The signs and symptoms of androgen excess can be divided into four areas: hirsutism, oligomenorrhea, acne, and virilization. Clinically, it is important to distinguish between simple hirsutism and hirsutism associated with virilization. In most cases of simple hirsutism, there is no known cause for the increased hair growth. On the other hand, if the patient is virilized as well as hirsute, increased levels of androgens are usually present. Hirsutism, commonly defined as an excess of body hair in a female in a male pattern of distribution (see Chap. 46), may result from androgen excess syndromes either of ovarian or adrenal etiologies or from drug ingestion, or it may be familial or idiopathic. Excess androgen secretion as a cause of hirsutism is probably uncommon in the absence of other signs of increased androgen production.

The four components of virilization are temporal balding, change in body habitus from a female to a male pattern (i.e., loss of pelvic fat and increase in upper torso muscular development), clitoral enlargement, and deepening of the voice. In general, the degree of virilization reflects both the duration and the degree of excess androgen secretion, although significant virilization can result from minimal changes in testosterone production, and a significant increase in testosterone production may be associated with minimal signs of virilization. The occurrence of oligomenorrhea in a hirsute patient increases the probability that an excess secretion of androgens will be found. Thus, the evaluation of the hirsute patient should include a careful history of the onset of menarche, past and present menstrual history, and reproductive capacity and a careful physical examination for signs and symptoms of androgen excess.

Etiology As in other states of adrenocortical hyperfunction, the syndromes associated with androgen excess may result from hyperplasia, adenoma, or carcinoma (the latter two having been discussed above). Adrenal androgen overproduction may also arise from *congenital adrenal hyperplasia,* owing to enzymatic defects. In these patients, increased adrenal androgen production is associated either with excess or decreased secretion of mineralocorticoids or decreased production of glucocorticoids. Since, in humans, cortisol is the principal adrenal steroid regulating ACTH elaboration, and since the ACTH stimulates both cortisol and adrenal androgen production, an enzymatic interference with cortisol synthesis may result in the enhanced secretion of adrenal androgens. In severe congenital virilizing hyperplasia, the adrenal output of cortisol may be so compromised as to cause glucocorticoid deficiency despite anatomic adrenal hyperplasia.

Congenital adrenal hyperplasia is the most common adrenal disorder of infancy and childhood. These children usually have severe enzyme deficiencies (see Chap. 333). The deficiency of enzymes is the result of autosomal recessive mutations. Partial adrenal enzyme deficiencies can be expressed after adolescence, predominantly in women with hirsutism and oligomenorrhea but minimal virilization. Late onset adrenal hyperplasia may account for as many as 25 percent of adult women with hirsutism and oligomenorrhea.

Congenital adrenal hyperplasia is secondary to one of several defects in steroid synthesis. To date, defects have been described in the C-21, C-18, C-17, and C-11 hydroxylase enzymes, as well as in the 3β-ol-dehydrogenase enzyme (see Fig. 325-2). These enzyme deficits usually occur singly. C-21 hydroxylase deficiency has a characteristic histocompatibility leukocyte antigen (HLA) association (HLA-B locus of chromosome 6) so that HLA typing can be used to detect the heterozygous carriers in affected families (see Chap. 63). The clinical expression in the different disorders is variable, ranging from virilization of the female (C-21 deficiency) to feminization of the male (3β-ol-dehydrogenase deficiency). (See also Chap. 333.)

Adrenal virilization in the female at birth is associated with ambiguous external genitalia (*female pseudohermaphroditism*). The onset of virilization is most probably after the fifth month of embryonic development. At birth there may be macrogenitosomia in the male infant, and in the female enlargement of the clitoris, partial or complete fusion of the labia, and sometimes a urogenital sinus. If the labial fusion is nearly complete, the female infant has external genitalia resembling a penis with hypospadias. In the *postnatal* period, congenital adrenal hyperplasia is associated with virilization in the female and isosexual precocity in the male. The excessive androgens result in accelerated growth, with bone age exceeding chronologic age. Since epiphyseal closure is hastened by excessive androgens, growth stops, but truncal development continues, giving the characteristic appearance of a child of short stature with well-developed trunk.

The most common form of congenital adrenal hyperplasia (95 percent of cases) is a result of impairment of *C-21 hydroxylation.* In addition to cortisol deficiency, there is an associated reduction in aldosterone secretion in approximately one-third of the patients. Thus, with C-21 hydroxylase deficiency, adrenal virilization occurs with or without an associated salt-losing tendency due to aldosterone deficiency (see Fig. 325-2).

C-11 hydroxylase deficiency causes a "hypertensive" variant of congenital adrenal hyperplasia. Hypertension and hypokalemia occur because of the impaired conversion of 11-deoxycorticosterone to corticosterone, resulting in the accumulation of 11-deoxycorticosterone, a potent mineralocorticoid. Increased shunting again occurs into the androgen pathway.

The *C-17 hydroxylase* deficiency is characterized by hypogonadism, hypokalemia, and hypertension. This rare deficiency causes decreased production of cortisol and shunting of precursors into the mineralocorticoid pathway with hypokalemic alkalosis, hypertension, and suppressed plasma renin activity. Usually, 11-deoxycorticosterone production is elevated. Because C-17 hydroxylation is required for biosynthesis of adrenal androgens as well as for biosynthesis of gonadal testosterone and estrogen, this defect is associated with sexual immaturity, high urinary gonadotropin levels, and low urinary 17-ketosteroid excretion. Female patients have primary amenorrhea and lack of development of secondary sexual characteristics. Because of deficient androgen production, male patients either have ambiguous external genitalia or a female phenotype (male pseudohermaphroditism). Exogenous glucocorticoids can correct the hypertensive syndrome, and treatment with appropriate gonadal steroids results in sexual maturation.

With 3β-ol-dehydrogenase deficiency, conversion of pregnenolone to progesterone is impaired, with the result that pathways to both cortisol and aldosterone are ''blocked,'' with shunting then occurring into the adrenal androgen pathway via 17α-hydroxypregnenolone to dehydroepiandrosterone. Since dehydroepiandrosterone is a weak androgen and because this enzyme deficiency is also present in the gonad, the genitalia of the male fetus may be incompletely virilized or feminized. Conversely, in the female, overproduction of dehydroepiandrosterone may produce partial virilization.

Diagnosis The diagnosis of *congenital adrenal hyperplasia* should be considered in all infants exhibiting ''failure to thrive,'' particularly those having episodes of acute adrenal insufficiency or salt wasting or showing sustained hypertension. The diagnosis is further suggested by the finding of hypertrophy of the clitoris, fused labia, or urogenital sinus in the female and isosexual precocity in the male. In infants and children with a *C-21 hydroxylation block,* increased urine 17-ketosteroid excretion and plasma DHEA sulfate are typically associated with an increase in the blood levels of 17α-hydroxyprogesterone and the urinary excretion of the metabolite of this steroid, pregnanetriol.

The diagnosis of a *salt-losing form of congenital adrenal hyperplasia* due to defects in C-21 hydroxylase enzyme is suggested by episodes of acute adrenal insufficiency with hyponatremia, hyperkalemia, dehydration, and vomiting. These infants and children often crave salt and exhibit laboratory signs of concomitant deficits in both cortisol and aldosterone secretion.

With the *hypertensive form of congenital adrenal hyperplasia* due to impaired C-11 hydroxylation, 11-deoxycorticosterone and 11-deoxycortisol accumulate. Both urine 17-ketosteroid and 17-hydroxycorticoid excretion may be elevated, since 11-deoxycortisol is included in the analysis of Porter-Silber chromogens. The diagnosis is secured by demonstrating increased levels of 11-deoxycortisol in the blood or increased amounts of tetrahydro-11-deoxycortisol in the urine.

The finding of very high levels of urine dehydroepiandrosterone with low levels of pregnanetriol and of cortisol metabolites in urine is characteristic of patients with 3β-ol-dehydrogenase deficiency. Marked salt wasting may also occur.

Patients with *late onset adrenal hyperplasia* (partial deficiency of C-21 hydroxylase) are characterized by normal or moderately elevated urinary 17-ketosteroids and plasma DHEA sulfate. A high basal level of a precursor of cortisol biosynthesis (such as 17-hydroxyprogesterone) or elevation of the precursor after ACTH stimulation confirms the diagnosis of a partial hydroxylase deficiency. It is uncertain how long the ACTH needs to be infused to unmask the enzyme deficiency. Adrenal androgen output is easily suppressed by the standard low-dose (2 mg) dexamethasone test.

Differential diagnosis The causes of hirsutism can be divided into four broad categories: familial, idiopathic, due to androgen excess, and due to drugs. In general, the first two conditions are not associated with other signs of androgen excess, i.e., oligomenorrhea, significant acne, or virilization. Likewise, drug-induced hirsutism is usually not associated with other signs and symptoms of androgen excess, unless the drug is an androgen. The drugs that produce an increase in body hair include phenothiazines, minoxidil, and phenytoin. Each of these drugs, particularly minoxidil, produces a generalized increase in hair growth, not just an increase in hair growth in androgen target areas. The mechanism may be related to the ability of these drugs to convert vellus into terminal hair follicles.

TABLE 325-7 Causes of hirsutism in women

I Familial
II Idiopathic
III Ovarian
- *A* Polycystic ovaries; hilus-cell hyperplasia
- *B* Tumor: arrhenoblastoma, hilus cell, adrenal rest

IV Adrenal
- *A* Congenital adrenal hyperplasia
- *B* Noncongenital adrenal hyperplasia (Cushing's)
- *C* Tumor: virilizing carcinoma or adenoma

If drugs are excluded, the only known causes of hirsutism amenable to treatment are those secondary to excess production of androgens by either the adrenal or the ovary.

In the female, the differential diagnosis of hirsutism and virilization is between adrenal and ovarian etiologies (Table 325-7). *Sudden onset of progressive hirsutism and virilization* suggests an adrenal or ovarian neoplasm. *Adrenal adenomas and carcinomas* may cause a pure or mixed virilizing syndrome. Since adrenal androgens are weak compared with gonadal androgens, adrenal virilization is characterized by *large increments in urine 17-ketosteroid excretion.* Virilizing adrenal adenomas are rare. *Virilizing adrenal carcinomas,* the most common adrenal tumors causing virilization, are associated with high plasma DHEA sulfate levels and high urinary 17-ketosteroid excretion rates; cortisol levels and 17-hydroxycorticosteroid excretion are normal or moderately elevated. Clinical differentiation between virilizing adrenal adenoma and carcinoma can usually be made preoperatively by CT scanning since carcinomas as a rule exceed 6 cm in size. Failure to reduce 17-ketosteroid levels and plasma DHEA sulfate levels to normal following dexamethasone suppression (0.5 mg given orally every 6 h for 2 days) further supports a diagnosis of virilizing adrenal tumor and excludes congenital adrenal hyperplasia. The most common virilizing *ovarian tumor* is the arrhenoblastoma, but other ovarian tumors, such as adrenal rest tumor, granulosa-cell tumor, hilar-cell tumor, and Brenner tumor, have been associated with virilization. Virilization due to ovarian tumors is usually characterized by normal levels of urinary 17-ketosteroids and DHEA sulfate, since the neoplasm usually secretes the potent androgen testosterone. Occasionally increases in 17-ketosteroid excretion occur in some patients with ovarian neoplasms, but baseline 17-ketosteroid excretion in excess of 30 mg per day is rare with the exception of adrenal rest tumors. Like adrenal neoplasms, ovarian tumors are not suppressed by dexamethasone. With the exception of adrenal rest tumors, these tumors are largely independent of ACTH stimulation. Elevations of plasma testosterone or urinary testosterone excretion do not localize the neoplasm to the ovary, since testosterone can be elevated subsequent to peripheral conversion of adrenal precursors, such as DHEA (see Chap. 331).

The most common ovarian cause of excess androgen production is ovarian hyperplasia or polycystic ovaries (see Chap. 331). As opposed to ovarian or adrenal tumors, virilization is less common with polycystic ovaries, whereas hirsutism is quite frequent. In most cases, the 17-ketosteroid excretion rate is greater than normal. Although the 17-ketosteroid excretion is partially reduced by dexamethasone, the residual level is often greater than in normal subjects. Plasma levels and production rates of androstenedione and to a lesser extent testosterone are usually increased. Follicle-stimulating hormone (FSH) levels tend to be lower than normal, and luteinizing hormone (LH) levels are tonically elevated, leading to the characteristic increased LH/FSH ratio. The laboratory findings in patients with hirsutism-virilizing syndromes are summarized in Table 325-8.

Treatment Treatment of adrenal virilism is dictated by the type of lesion. Patients with *congenital adrenal hyperplasia* have a fundamental defect of cortisol deficiency with resultant excessive ACTH stimulation, producing hyperplasia of the adrenal glands and causing additional ''shunting'' into the adrenal androgen pathway. Therapy in these patients consists of daily administration of glucocorticoids to suppress pituitary ACTH secretion. Because of its cost and intermediate half-life, prednisone is the drug of choice except in infants, when hydrocortisone is usually used. In adult patients with late-onset adrenal hyperplasia, a single bedtime dose of an intermediate-acting glucocorticoid, such as 2.5 or 5 mg of prednisone, suppresses pituitary ACTH secretion. The amount of steroid required by children with congenital adrenal hyperplasia is approximately 1 to 1.5 times the normal cortisol production rate of 12 to 13 mg cortisol per square meter of body surface area per day and is given

TABLE 325-8 Laboratory evaluation of hirsutism-virilizing syndromes

	Ovarian		Adrenal			
	PCO	Ovarian tumor	CAH	Adrenal neoplasm	Cushing's syndrome	Idiopathic
Urinary 17-ketosteroids, plasma DHEA sulfate	N↑	N	N↑	↑↑↑	N↑	N
Plasma testosterone	N↑	↑↑	N↑	N↑	N↑	N
LH/FSH ratio	N↑	N	N	N	N	N
Precursors of cortisol biosynthesis:						
Basal	N	N	N↑	N↑	N	N
Following ACTH infusion	N	N	↑↑	N↑	N	N
Cortisol following overnight dexamethasone suppresion test	N	N	N	↑	↑	N

NOTE: *CAH, congenital adrenal hyperplasia; PCO, polycystic ovary syndrome; N, normal; ↑, elevated.*

in divided doses two or three times per day. The dosage schedule is governed by repetitive analysis of the urinary 17-ketosteroids, plasma DHEA sulfate, and/or precursors of cortisol biosynthesis. Skeletal growth and maturation must also be closely monitored since overtreatment with glucocorticoid replacement therapy retards linear growth.

HYPOFUNCTION OF ADRENAL CORTEX

Adrenocortical hypofunction includes all conditions in which the secretion of adrenal steroid hormones falls below the requirements of the body. Adrenal insufficiency may be divided into two general categories: (1) those associated with primary inability of the adrenal to elaborate sufficient quantities of hormone and (2) those associated with a secondary failure due to a primary failure in the elaboration of ACTH (Table 325-9).

PRIMARY ADRENOCORTICAL DEFICIENCY (ADDISON'S DISEASE) Addison's description of "general languor and debility, remarkable feebleness of the heart's action, irritability of the stomach, and a peculiar change of the color of the skin," summarizes the dominant clinical features of the disease. Advanced cases are usually easy to diagnose, but recognition of the disease in its earlier phases may present a real challenge.

Incidence Primary adrenocortical insufficiency is relatively rare. It may occur at any age and affects both sexes with equal frequency. Because of increasing therapeutic use of exogenous steroids, secondary adrenal insufficiency is relatively common.

Etiology and pathogenesis Addison's disease results from progressive adrenocortical destruction, which must involve more than 90 percent of the glands before signs of adrenal insufficiency appear. The adrenal is a frequent site for chronic granulomatous diseases, predominantly tuberculosis but also histoplasmosis, coccidioidomycosis, and cryptococcosis. In previous years, tuberculosis was found at postmortem examination in 70 to 90 percent of cases; however, the most frequent finding at present is *idiopathic* atrophy, and an autoimmune mechanism is probably responsible. Rarely, other lesions are encountered, such as bilateral tumor metastases, amyloidosis, or sarcoidosis.

The possibility that primary adrenal insufficiency can have an autoimmune basis is strengthened by the finding that half of patients have circulating adrenal antibodies. Some patients also have circulating antibodies to thyroid, parathyroid, and/or gonadal tissue (see also Chap. 334). Cellular immunity may also be altered in patients with idiopathic adrenal insufficiency; for example, the expression of the Ia (immune-associated) antigen on T lymphocytes has been described in patients with recent-onset Addison's disease, probably reflecting activation of the immune system. There is also an increased incidence of chronic lymphocytic thyroiditis (Hashimoto's disease) and an increased incidence of premature ovarian failure, type I diabetes mellitus, Graves' disease, and primary hypoparathyroidism in patients with idiopathic adrenal insufficiency. The occurrence of two or more of these autoimmune endocrine disorders in the same individual defines the polyglandular autoimmune syndrome type II. Additional disorders in these patients include pernicious anemia, vitiligo, alopecia, nontropical sprue, and myasthenia gravis. Within families, multiple generations are affected by one or more of the above diseases. The inheritance of diseases in the type II polyglandular syndrome is associated with the HLA alleles B8 and Dw3.

The combination of parathyroid and adrenal insufficiency and chronic mucocutaneous moniliasis constitutes a distinct familial syndrome (type I polyglandular autoimmune syndrome). Other autoimmune diseases also occur in higher frequency in these patients (e.g., pernicious anemia, chronic active hepatitis, thyroid disease, alopecia, and premature gonadal failure). There is no HLA association; this syndrome is inherited in an autosomal recessive pattern, often with multiple affected siblings within a family. The type I syndrome usually presents during childhood, whereas the peak incidence of expression of the type II syndrome is 20 to 60 years. The mechanisms by which genetic predisposition and/or autoimmunity interact in the pathogenesis of these disease states are unknown.

Clinical signs and symptoms Adrenocortical insufficiency is characterized by an insidious onset of slowly progressive fatigability, weakness, anorexia, nausea and vomiting, weight loss, cutaneous and mucosal pigmentation, hypotension, and occasionally hypoglycemia (Table 325-10). However, the spectrum may vary, depending on the duration and degree of adrenal hypofunction, from a complaint of mild chronic fatigue to the fulminating shock associated with acute

TABLE 325-9 Classification of adrenal insufficiency

- *I* Primary adrenal insufficiency
  - *A* Anatomic destruction of gland (chronic and acute)
    - *1* "Idiopathic" atrophy (autoimmune)
    - *2* Surgical removal
    - *3* Infection (tuberculous, fungous)
    - *4* Hemorrhage
    - *5* Invasion: metastatic
  - *B* Metabolic failure in hormone production
    - *1* Congenital adrenal hyperplasia
    - *2* Enzyme inhibitors (metyrapone)
    - *3* Cytotoxic agents (mitotane)
- *II* Secondary adrenal insufficiency
  - *A* Hypopituitarism due to hypothalamic-pituitary disease
  - *B* Suppression of hypothalamic-pituitary axis
    - *1* Exogenous steroid
    - *2* Endogenous steroid from tumor

TABLE 325-10 Incidence of symptoms and signs in Addison's disease, percent

Weakness	99	Hypotension (<110/70)	87
Pigmentation of skin	98	Abdominal pain	34
Pigmentation of mucous membranes	82	Salt craving	22
Weight loss	97	Diarrhea	20
Anorexia, nausea, and vomiting	90	Constipation	19
		Syncope	16
		Vitiligo	9

massive destruction of the glands in the syndrome described by Waterhouse and Friderichsen.

Asthenia is the cardinal symptom. Early it may be sporadic, usually most evident at times of stress; as adrenal function becomes more impaired, weakness progresses until the patient is continuously fatigued, necessitating bed rest.

Hyperpigmentation may be a striking sign, but its absence does not exclude this diagnosis. It commonly appears as a diffuse brown, tan, or bronze darkening of both exposed and unexposed parts such as elbows or creases of the hand and of areas normally pigmented such as the areolas about the nipples. Bluish-black patches may appear on the mucous membranes. Some patients develop dark freckles, and occasionally irregular areas of vitiligo may appear paradoxically. As an early sign, patients may notice an unusually persistent tanning following exposure to the sun.

Arterial hypotension is frequent, and in severe cases blood pressures may be in the range of 80/50 or less. Postural accentuation of hypotension is common.

Abnormalities of gastrointestinal function often are the presenting complaint. Symptoms may vary from mild anorexia with weight loss to fulminating nausea, vomiting, diarrhea, and ill-defined abdominal pain, which at times may be so severe as to be confused with an acute abdomen. In addition, patients with adrenal insufficiency frequently have marked personality changes, usually in the form of excessive irritability and restlessness. Enhancement of the sensory modalities of taste, olfaction, and hearing is often present and is reversible with therapy. A decrease in axillary and pubic hair is common in women due to loss of adrenal androgen production.

Laboratory findings In the milder forms, there may be no demonstrable abnormalities in the routine laboratory parameters, and even plasma and urinary steroid determinations may indicate values relatively low yet within normal range. However, studies of adrenal stimulation with ACTH show abnormalities even in this stage of the disease. In the more advanced stages, serum sodium, chloride, and bicarbonate are reduced while serum potassium is elevated. The hyponatremia is due to both loss of sodium into the urine (due to aldosterone deficiency) and movement into the intracellular compartment. This extravascular sodium loss depletes extracellular fluid volume and accentuates hypotension. Elevated plasma vasopressin and angiotensin II levels may be contributing factors to hyponatremia through impairment of free water clearance. The hyperkalemia is due to a combination of factors, including aldosterone deficiency, impaired glomerular filtration, and acidosis. Mild to moderate hypercalcemia is seen in 10 to 20 percent of patients; the reason for this is not understood. The electrocardiogram may show nonspecific changes, and the electroencephalogram exhibits a generalized reduction and slowing. There may be a normocytic anemia, a relative lymphocytosis, and usually a moderate eosinophilia.

Diagnosis The diagnosis of adrenal insufficiency should be made only with ACTH stimulation testing to assay the adrenal reserve capacity for steroid production (see above for ACTH test protocols). In *severe adrenal insufficiency* the cortisol secretory rate is markedly decreased, and this may be ascertained indirectly by the finding of low to absent 24-h urine cortisol, 17-hydroxycorticoids, and 17-ketosteroids. With *mild or moderate adrenal insufficiency*, urine steroid excretion values overlap into the normal range; a diagnosis of adrenal insufficiency should never be excluded solely on the basis of normal basal urine steroid determinations. Plasma cortisol values vary from zero to the lower range of normal. Aldosterone secretion is usually low, resulting in salt wasting and secondary rises in plasma renin levels. In primary adrenal insufficiency, plasma ACTH and associated peptides are elevated because of loss of the usual cortisol-hypothalamic-pituitary feedback relationship, whereas in secondary adrenal insufficiency, plasma ACTH values are low, or "inappropriately" normal (Fig. 352-11).

Differential diagnosis Since weakness and fatigue are common complaints, clinical diagnosis of early adrenocortical insufficiency is frequently difficult. However, mild gastrointestinal distress with weight loss, anorexia, and a suggestion of increased pigmentation make mandatory ACTH stimulation testing to rule out adrenal insufficiency, particularly before steroid treatment is begun. Weight loss is useful in evaluating the significance of weakness and malaise. Weight gain associated with lassitude is more characteristic of depressive syndromes. Racial pigmentation in many individuals may be a problem, but a *recent* and progressive *increase* is usually reported by the Addisonian patient. Hyperpigmentation in other diseases may also present a problem, but the appearance and distribution of pigment in Addison's disease are usually characteristic. When doubt exists, measurement of ACTH levels and testing of adrenal reserve with the infusion of ACTH provide clear-cut differentiation.

Treatment All patients with Addison's disease should receive specific hormone replacement. Like diabetics, these patients require careful and persistent education in regard to their disease. Since the adrenal gland elaborates three general classes of hormone, of which two, glucocorticoids and mineralocorticoids, are of primary clinical importance, replacement therapy should correct both deficiencies. Cortisone (or cortisol) is the mainstay of treatment. Cortisone dosage varies from 12.5 to 50 mg daily, with the majority of patients taking 25 to 37.5 mg in divided doses. Cortisol (30 mg daily) or prednisone (7.5 mg daily) in divided doses may also be given for substitution therapy. Because of its effect on gastric mucosa, patients are advised to take their cortisone with meals or, if this is impractical, with milk or an antacid preparation. In addition, the larger proportion of the dose (e.g., 25 mg of cortisone) is taken in the morning and the remainder (12.5 mg of cortisone) in the late afternoon, to simulate the normal diurnal adrenal rhythm. Some patients exhibit insomnia, irritability, and mental excitement after initiation of therapy; in these, the dosage should be reduced. Other indications for smaller amounts of glucocorticoids are hypertension, diabetes, or active tuberculosis.

Since this amount of cortisone or cortisol fails to replace the

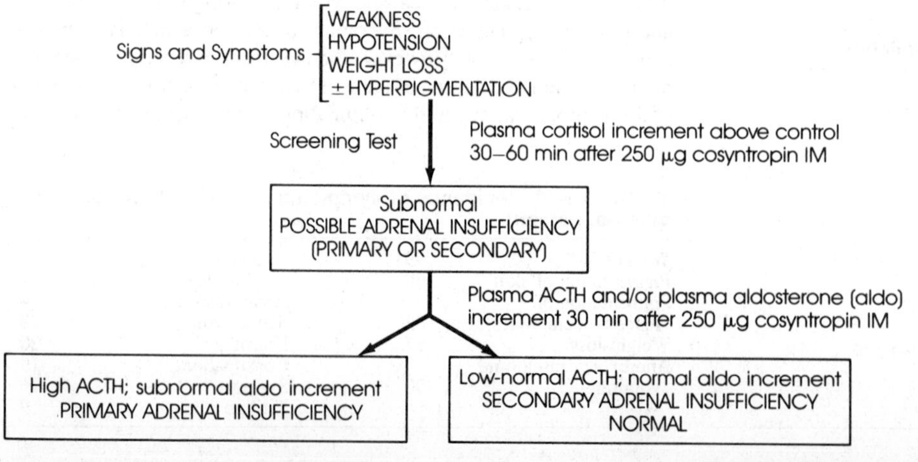

FIGURE 325-11 *Diagnostic flowchart for evaluating patients with suspected adrenal insufficiency. Plasma ACTH levels are low in secondary adrenal insufficiency. In adrenal insufficiency secondary to pituitary tumors or idiopathic panhypopituitarism, other pituitary hormone deficiencies are present. On the other hand, ACTH deficiency may be isolated, as seen following prolonged use of exogenous glucocorticoids.*

Since the isolated blood levels obtained in these screening tests may not be definitive, the diagnosis should always be confirmed by a continuous 24-h ACTH infusion. Normal subjects and patients with secondary adrenal insufficiency may be distinguished by insulin tolerance or metyrapone testing.

mineralocorticoid component of the adrenal gland, supplementary hormone is usually needed. This is accomplished by the daily oral administration of 0.05 to 0.1 mg fludrocortisone. If parenteral administration is indicated, a dosage of 2 to 5 mg deoxycorticosterone acetate in oil may be given every day intramuscularly.

Complications of glucocorticoid therapy, with the exception of gastritis, are *rare* in the dosage used in the treatment of Addison's disease. Complications of mineralocorticoid therapy occur more frequently and include hypokalemia, edema, hypertension, cardiac enlargement, or even congestive failure due to sodium retention. In the management of patients with Addison's disease, periodic measurements of body weight, serum potassium, and blood pressure are useful.

All patients with adrenal insufficiency, including bilaterally adrenalectomized patients, should carry medical identification, should be instructed in the parenteral self-administration of steroids, and should be registered with a national medical alerting system.

Special therapeutic problems During periods of intercurrent illness, the dose of cortisone or cortisol should be increased to 75 to 150 mg per day. When oral administration is not possible, parenteral routes should be employed. Likewise, before surgery or dental extractions, supplemental glucocorticoids should be administered. Patients should also be advised to increase the dose of fludrocortisone and to add excess salt to their otherwise normal diet during periods of excessive exercise with sweating, during extremely hot weather, and with gastrointestinal upsets. For a representative program of steroid therapy for the patient with adrenal insufficiency who is undergoing a major operation, see Table 325-11. This schedule is designed to mimic on the day of surgery the output of cortisol in normal individuals undergoing prolonged major stress (10 mg/h, 250 to 300 mg per 24 h). Thereafter, if the patient is progressing well and is afebrile, the dose of cortisol is tapered by 20 to 30 percent daily. Parenteral mineralocorticoid administration is unnecessary at cortisol doses greater than 100 mg per day because of the mineralocorticoid effects of cortisol at such dosages.

SECONDARY ADRENOCORTICAL INSUFFICIENCY Pituitary ACTH deficiency causes *secondary* adrenocortical insufficiency. ACTH deficiency may be selective, as is seen following prolonged administration of excess glucocorticoids, or may occur in association with multiple pituitary tropic hormone deficiencies (panhypopituitarism) (see Chap. 321). Patients with secondary adrenocortical hypofunction may have many symptoms and signs in common with Addisonian patients but are *characteristically not hyperpigmented* since ACTH and related peptide levels are low. In fact, plasma ACTH levels distinguish between primary and secondary adrenal insufficiency, since they are elevated in the former and decreased to absent in the latter. Patients with total pituitary insufficiency also have signs and symptoms suggestive of multiple hormone deficiencies. An additional feature distinguishing primary from secondary adrenocortical insufficiency is the *near-normal level of aldosterone secretion* seen in the presence of pituitary and/or isolated ACTH deficiencies (Fig. 325-11). Patients with pituitary insufficiency may present with hyponatremia, which may be dilutional or secondary to subnormal increments in aldosterone secretion in response to severe sodium restriction. However, the findings of severe dehydration, *hyponatremia,* and *hyperkalemia* are characteristic of severe mineralocorticoid insufficiency and favor a diagnosis of primary adrenocortical insufficiency.

Patients receiving long-term steroid therapy, despite physical findings of Cushing's syndrome, develop adrenal insufficiency because of prolonged pituitary-hypothalamic suppression and adrenal atrophy secondary to the loss of endogenous ACTH. Thus, these patients have two deficits, a loss of adrenal responsiveness to ACTH and a failure of pituitary ACTH release. These patients are characterized by low blood cortisol and ACTH levels, low baseline steroid excretion, and abnormal ACTH and metyrapone test results. Most patients with steroid-induced adrenal insufficiency eventually recover normal hypothalamic-pituitary-adrenal responsiveness, but individual response time varies from days to months. The rapid ACTH test can be used as a convenient assessment of recovery of hypothalamic-pituitary-adrenal function. Since the plasma cortisol concentrations after injection of cosyntropin and during insulin-induced hypoglycemia correlate closely, the rapid ACTH test assesses the integrated hypothalamic-pituitary-adrenal function. Additional testing to assess endogenous pituitary ACTH reserve includes the standard metyrapone and the insulin tolerance tests.

Substitution glucocorticoid therapy in patients with secondary adrenocortical insufficiency does not differ from that for Addisonian patients. Mineralocorticoid replacement therapy is usually not necessary, since aldosterone secretion is preserved. Otherwise, the same basic principles should be applied to patients with secondary adrenocortical insufficiency.

ACUTE ADRENOCORTICAL INSUFFICIENCY Acute adrenocortical insufficiency may result from several processes. One of these, termed *adrenal crisis,* is a rapid and overwhelming intensification of chronic adrenal insufficiency, usually precipitated by sepsis or surgical stress. Another involves an acute hemorrhagic destruction of both adrenal glands, usually associated with an overwhelming septicemia (Waterhouse-Friderichsen syndrome). Adrenal hemorrhage associated with anticoagulant therapy in patients with increased adrenocortical activity has also been reported, as in the period immediately following a myocardial infarction. Occasionally, adrenal hemorrhage in the newborn results from birth trauma. Hemorrhage also has been observed during pregnancy, following idiopathic adrenal vein thrombosis, and as a complication of venography (e.g., infarction of an adenoma). A third, and probably the most frequent, cause of acute insufficiency results from the rapid withdrawal of steroids from patients with adrenal atrophy secondary to chronic steroid administration. In the presence of severe stress, acute adrenocortical insufficiency may also occur in patients with congenital adrenal hyperplasia and those receiving pharmacologic agents that are capable of inhibiting steroid synthesis (such as mitotane).

TABLE 325-11 Steroid therapy schedule for Addisonian patient undergoing a major operation*

	Cortisone acetate (intramuscularly)		Cortisol infusion, continuous, mg/h	Cortisone acetate (orally)		Fludrocortisone (orally), 8 A.M.
	7 A.M.	7 P.M.		8 A.M.	4 P.M.	
Routine daily medication				25	12.5	0.1
Day before operation		50		25	12.5	0.1
Day of operation	50	50	10			
Postoperative:						
Day 1	50	50	5–7.5			
Day 2	50	50	2.5–5			
Day 3	50	50				
Day 4	50				25	0.1
Day 5				37.5	25	0.1
Day 6				25	25	0.1
Day 7				25	12.5	0.1

* *All steroid doses are given in milligrams.*

Adrenal crisis The long-term survival of patients with Addison's disease largely depends upon prevention and treatment of adrenal crisis. Consequently, the occurrence of infection, trauma (including surgery), gastrointestinal upsets, or other forms of stress requires an immediate increase in hormone. In untreated patients, preexisting symptoms are intensified. Nausea, vomiting, and abdominal pain may become intractable. Fever may be severe or absent. Lethargy deepens into somnolence, and the blood pressure and pulse fail as hypovolemic vascular shock ensues. In contrast, patients previously maintained on chronic glucocorticoid therapy may not exhibit severe dehydration or hypotension until preterminally, since mineralocorticoid secretion is usually preserved. In all patients in crisis, a precipitating cause should be sought. Intercurrent infection associated with omission or failure to increase maintenance therapy is common.

Treatment is primarily directed toward the rapid elevation of circulating glucocorticoid and the replacement of the sodium and water deficits. Hence, an intravenous infusion of 5% glucose in normal saline solution should be immediately started with a bolus intravenous infusion of 100 mg cortisol followed by a continuous infusion of cortisol at a rate of 10 mg/h; 50 mg cortisone acetate should be given intramuscularly in case the infusion becomes infiltrated or inadvertently stopped. Effective treatment of hypotension consists of aggressive repletion of sodium and water deficits. If the crisis was preceded by prolonged nausea, vomiting, and dehydration, several liters of saline solution may be required within the first few hours. Vasoconstrictive agents (such as dopamine) may be indicated in extreme conditions as adjuncts to volume replacement. With large doses of steroid, as for example 100 to 200 mg cortisol, the patient receives a maximal mineralocorticoid effect, and supplementary mineralocorticoid is superfluous. Following improvement, the patient can be offered oral fluids and the steroid dosage is tapered over the next few days to maintenance levels, with reinstitution of supplementary mineralocorticoid if needed (Table 325-11).

HYPOALDOSTERONISM

Isolated aldosterone deficiency accompanied by normal cortisol production occurs in association with hyporeninism, as an inherited biosynthetic defect, postoperatively following removal of aldosterone-secreting adenomas, during protracted heparin or heparinoid administration, in pretectal disease of the nervous system, and in severe postural hypotension.

The feature common to all patients with hypoaldosteronism is the inability to increase aldosterone secretion appropriately during salt restriction. Most patients present with unexplained hyperkalemia often exacerbated by restriction of dietary sodium intake. In severe cases urine sodium wastage occurs on a normal salt intake, whereas in milder forms excessive losses of urine sodium occur only during salt restriction.

Most cases of isolated hypoaldosteronism occur in patients with a deficiency in renin production (so-called hyporeninemic hypoaldosteronism). This syndrome is most commonly seen in adults with mild renal failure and diabetes mellitus in association with hyperkalemia and metabolic acidosis out of proportion to the state of renal impairment. Plasma renin levels fail to rise normally following sodium restriction and postural changes. The pathogenesis is uncertain. Possibilities include renal disease (most likely), autonomic neuropathy, extracellular fluid volume expansion, and a defect in conversion of presumed renin precursors into active renin. Aldosterone levels also fail to rise normally following salt restriction and volume contraction; this is probably related to the hyporeninism since biosynthetic defects in aldosterone secretion cannot usually be demonstrated. In these patients, aldosterone secretion increases promptly following ACTH stimulation, but it is uncertain whether the magnitude of the response is normal. On the other hand, the level of aldosterone appears to be subnormal in relationship to the hyperkalemia.

Hypoaldosteronism can also be associated with high renin levels. In many of these subjects, a biosynthetic defect has been noted where there is an inability to transform the C-18 methyl group of corticosterone to the C-18 aldehyde of aldosterone due to a deficiency of the enzyme 18-hydroxysteroid dehydrogenase. These patients manifest not only low to absent aldosterone secretion and elevated plasma renin levels but also elevated values for the intermediates of aldosterone biosynthesis (corticosterone and 18-hydroxycorticosterone).

Before considering the diagnosis of isolated hypoaldosteronism in a patient with hyperkalemia, "pseudohyperkalemia" (e.g., hemolysis, thrombocytosis) should be excluded by measuring plasma potassium. The next step is to demonstrate a normal cortisol response to ACTH stimulation. Then stimulated (upright posture, sodium restriction) renin and aldosterone levels are obtained. Low renin–low aldosterone levels establish a diagnosis of hyporeninemic hypoaldosteronism. High renin–low aldosterone levels are consistent with an aldosterone biosynthetic defect or a selective unresponsiveness of the glomerulosa to angiotensin II. Finally, elevated renin and aldosterone levels suggest primary renal unresponsiveness to aldosterone, so-called pseudohypoaldosteronism.

Treatment of patients with isolated hypoaldosteronism would logically be to replace the mineralocorticoid deficiency. For practical purposes, the oral administration of fludrocortisone in a dose of 0.1 to 0.2 mg daily should restore electrolyte balance. However, patients with hyporeninemic hypoaldosteronism usually require greater doses of mineralocorticoid to normalize the hyperkalemia. This poses a risk in these patients who usually have hypertension and mild renal insufficiency. Therefore, an alternative approach is to administer furosemide, which can ameliorate the acidosis and the hyperkalemia. Occasionally a combination of these two approaches may be efficacious.

NONSPECIFIC CLINICAL USE OF ADRENAL STEROIDS AND ACTH

The widespread utilization of glucocorticoids and ACTH emphasizes the need for a thorough understanding of the metabolic effects of these agents when used nonspecifically, if optimum effectiveness is to be obtained and if undesirable side reactions are to be minimized. Before instituting adrenal hormone therapy, the gains that can reasonably be expected should be weighed against the potentially undesirable metabolic actions of pharmacologic doses of hormone.

HOW SERIOUS IS THE DISORDER? In a patient whose life is threatened by unexplained shock or in whom other measures have failed, the physician need not hesitate to employ large-dosage steroid therapy. On the other hand, one should exercise restraint in administering steroids to a patient with early rheumatoid arthritis who as yet has not been exposed to the possible benefits of physiotherapy, analgesics, and a well-organized program of general medical care.

HOW LONG WILL GLUCOCORTICOID THERAPY BE REQUIRED? The use of intravenously administered steroids for a period of 24 to 48 h in the treatment of such life-threatening situations as status asthmaticus or pseudotumor cerebri has little or no contraindication, in contrast to the initiation of a program of chronic steroid therapy for asthma, arthritis, or psoriasis. In the latter instances, the almost certain complication of a Cushing's syndrome of some degree must be weighed against the potential benefit. These side effects should be minimized by a careful choice of steroid preparations, alternate-day or interrupted therapy programs, and the judicious use of supplementary adjuvants.

WHICH ADRENAL PREPARATION IS PREFERABLE? At least five considerations need to be taken into account in deciding which steroid preparation to use:

1 The biologic half-life of the compound. The rationale behind every-other-day therapy is to decrease the metabolic effects of the steroids for a significant amount of time over the 2-day period, yet at the same time to produce pharmacologic suppression of sufficient duration to maintain the disease in remission. Too long a half-life would defeat the first purpose, and too short a half-life would defeat the second. In general, the more potent the steroid, the longer its biologic half-life.

2 The importance of the mineralocorticoid effects of the steroid. Synthetic steroids have less mineralocorticoid effect relative to their glucocorticoid effect than do cortisol or cortisone (Table 325-12). This may be an important consideration in certain disease states.
3 The biologically active form of the steroid. Cortisone and prednisone, in contrast to the other glucocorticoids, have to be converted to biologically active equivalents before anti-inflammatory effects can occur. Because of this, in a condition in which steroids are known to be effective and when an adequate dose has been given without response, one should consider substituting cortisol or prednisolone for cortisone or prednisone.
4 The cost of the medication. This is a serious consideration if chronic administration is to be undertaken. Prednisone is the least expensive of available steroid preparations.
5 The variation in the manner in which preparations of glucosteroids are formulated. This factor may modify absorption. Thus, it is advisable for a patient whose steroid dosage has been standardized to continue to utilize the same pharmaceutical preparation to avoid relapse or overdosage.

ACTH VERSUS STEROIDS In general, adrenal steroid therapy is effective by mouth and can be regulated more accurately than ACTH therapy. The amount of steroid produced in response to ACTH varies from day to day, depending on the rate and extent of absorption of ACTH and on the state of the adrenal cortex. ACTH therapy stimulates the secretion of adrenal androgens as well as of hydroxysteroids. Sodium retention with ACTH is often more marked than with cortisone or prednisone therapy.

While some studies imply that ACTH may be superior to oral steroid therapy in the treatment of certain disorders such as dermatomyositis and multiple sclerosis, it is generally believed that the two agents are equally effective (or ineffective). Both ACTH and steroid therapy induce hypothalamopituitary suppression; however, in ACTH therapy adrenal gland size and activity are maintained, in contrast to the adrenal atrophy usually associated with steroid therapy.

EVALUATION OF PATIENT PRIOR TO INITIATING STEROID THERAPY (See Table 325-13) **Chronic infection** Three problems demand attention: (1) Any active infection, particularly tuberculosis, should be identified. If tuberculosis is present, steroid therapy can be employed, if indicated, in conjunction with antituberculous chemotherapy. (2) The chest film and tuberculin test provide baseline information for future comparison. Since high-dosage steroids minimize the tuberculin reaction, serial chest roentgenograms may be indicated. (3) Infection due to ''opportunistic'' low-virulence pathogens should be constantly considered in patients on high steroid dosage, especially when steroid therapy is combined with other immunosuppressive agents.

TABLE 325-12 Glucocorticoid preparations

	Estimated potency†	
Commonly used name*	Glucocorticoid	Mineralocorticoid
SHORT-ACTING		
Cortisol	1	1
Cortisone	0.8	0.8
INTERMEDIATE-ACTING		
Prednisone	4	0.25
Prednisolone	4	0.25
Methylprednisolone	5	±‡
Triamcinolone	5	±
LONG-ACTING		
Paramethasone	10	±
Betamethasone	25	±
Dexamethasone	30–40	±

* *The steroids are divided into three groups according to the duration of biologic activity. Short-acting preparations have a biologic half-life of less than 12 h; long-acting, greater than 48 h; and intermediate, between 12 and 36 h. Triamcinolone has the longest half-life of the intermediate-acting preparations.*
† *Relative milligram comparisons with cortisol, setting the glucocorticoid and mineralocorticoid properties of cortisol as 1. Sodium retention is insignificant in usual doses employed of methylprednisolone, triamcinolone, paramethasone, betamethasone, and dexamethasone.*
‡ ±, *Too low to measure with accuracy.*

TABLE 325-13 A "checklist" for use prior to the administration of glucocorticoids in pharmacologic dosages

1 Presence of tuberculosis or other chronic infection (chest x-ray, tuberculin test)
2 Evidence of glucose intolerance or history of gestational diabetes mellitus
3 Evidence of preexisting osteoporosis (spine x-ray or bone density assessment, if available, in postmenopausal patients)
4 History of peptic ulcer, gastritis, or esophagitis (stool guaiac test)
5 Evidence of hypertension or cardiovascular disease
6 History of psychological disorders

Diabetes mellitus Prolonged glucocorticoid therapy may unmask latent diabetes mellitus or aggravate preexisting disease. The presence of diabetes mellitus or the demonstration of impaired glucose tolerance may affect the decision to institute adrenal hormone therapy.

Osteoporosis All patients receiving long-continued steroid therapy are likely to develop some degree of osteoporosis. Indeed osteoporosis, with vertebral fractures or compression, is one of the most serious potential hazards of long-term steroid therapy. For patients at high risk (postmenopausal women, elderly men, and patients with restricted physical activity) initial films of the thoracolumbar segment of the spine are mandatory. Alternate-day or interrupted steroid therapy minimizes this complication (Table 325-14), and adjunctive therapies may be effective in the therapy of steroid osteoporosis (see Chap. 339).

Peptic ulcer, gastric hypersecretion, or esophagitis In conventional therapeutic doses (equivalent to 15 mg prednisone per day or less) glucocorticoids probably do not cause peptic ulceration; whether higher doses are associated with increased incidence of peptic ulcer disease is not established and probably depends on duration of treatment (as well as dose) and the presence of predisposing factors such as hypoalbuminemia or cirrhosis. However, even in conventional doses patients with a history of ulcer may experience aggravation of symptoms while receiving glucocorticoids. Consequently, all individuals with a positive history or with known risk factors should be given a vigorous ''ulcer combating'' program (antacids, cimetidine) along with glucocorticoids. *The development of anemia in a patient receiving glucocorticoids should suggest gastrointestinal bleeding as a cause, and patients should be cautioned to note black stools.*

Hypertension or cardiovascular disease In general, the sodium-retaining propensity of many adrenal steroid preparations requires

TABLE 325-14 Supplementary measures to minimize undesirable metabolic effects of glucocorticoids

I Monitor caloric intake to prevent weight gain.
II Restrict sodium intake to prevent edema and minimize hypertension and potassium loss.
III Supplement potassium if necessary.
IV Give antacid therapy and/or histamine receptor antagonist therapy.
V Institute alternate-day steroid schedule if possible. Patients on steroid therapy over a prolonged period should be protected by an appropriate increase in hormone level during periods of acute stress. A rule of thumb is to *double* the maintenance dose.
VI Minimize osteopenia by (not proved effective):
  A Estrogen therapy for postmenopausal women; 0.625–1.25 mg conjugated estrogens, may be given ''cyclically.'' Regular Papanicolaou smear and breast examination mandatory (see Chap. 331).
  B Consider supplementary vitamin D and calcium.

that caution be used when they are given to patients with preexisting hypertension or cardiovascular or renal disease. Use of preparations in which sodium-retaining activity is minimal, restriction of dietary sodium intake, and the use of diuretic agents and supplementary potassium salts will minimize the mineralocorticoid actions of steroid therapy. However, hypertension may still be exacerbated by steroid-induced increases in renin substrate and consequently in angiotensin II levels.

Psychological difficulties Steroid therapy may be complicated by minor or severe psychological disturbances. In general, serious psychological disturbances are more closely related to the patient's personality structure than to the actual dose of hormone, although, as might be anticipated, larger doses of hormone are associated with more frequent serious reactions. At present there is no reliable method of determining beforehand a patient's psychological reaction to steroid therapy; moreover, previous tolerance of steroids does not necessarily ensure immunity to subsequent courses of therapy. Likewise, untoward psychological reactions on one occasion do not invariably mean that the patient will respond unfavorably to a second course of treatment; however, prophylactic treatment with lithium may be indicated.

Sleeplessness is a common complication and can be minimized by using the shorter-acting steroids and by prescribing the total dose as a single early-morning medication.

ALTERNATE-DAY STEROID THERAPY The single most effective measure in minimizing the cushingoid effects of glucocorticoid therapy is to administer the total 48-h dose as a *single* dose of *intermediate-acting steroid* in the morning, *every other day*. If symptoms of the underlying disorder can be controlled by this technique, the therapeutic program offers a distinct advantage. Three special considerations deserve mention: (1) The alternate-day schedule may be approached through a series of transition dose schedules that permit the patient an opportunity to adjust to the ultimate program. (2) The physician should provide the patient with supplementary nonsteroid medications, if required, on the "off day" to minimize symptoms of the underlying disorder. (3) The physician and the patient should recognize that many symptoms noted during the off day (e.g., fatigue, joint pain, muscle stiffness or tenderness, and fever) are those of relative adrenal insufficiency, rather than an exacerbation of the underlying disease. Knowing this is of vital importance, since the physician can reassure the patient and avoid giving up the program on the basis of a misconception.

The alternate-day concept capitalizes on the fact that cortisol secretion and plasma levels normally are highest in the early morning and lowest in the evening. The normal pattern is mimicked by administering an intermediate-acting steroid in the morning (7 to 8 A.M.) (Table 325-12).

Initially the steroid program usually requires daily or more frequent doses of steroid to accomplish the desired anti-inflammatory or immunity-suppressing action. *Only after this desired effect has been achieved is an attempt made to switch over to an alternate-day program.* A number of programs may be employed for transferring a patient from a daily to an alternate-day program. The key points to be considered are flexibility in arranging a program and the use of supportive measures on the off day. One may attempt a transition by a series of gradations rather than by an abrupt complete changeover. One approach is to keep the steroid dose constant on one day and gradually reduce the level on the alternate day. Alternatively, the steroid dose can be increased on one day while being reduced on the alternate day. In any case it is important to anticipate that the patient will experience some increase in pain or discomfort between the 36 to 48 h following the last dose of steroid.

The general principles advocated in the long-term use of steroids and in implementing an alternate-day schedule are as follows:

1 Utilize intermediate-acting steroids such as prednisone or prednisolone.
2 Give the total daily steroid as a single morning dose.
3 Begin a transition program as soon as the manifestations of the diseases are under reasonable control.
4 If possible, eliminate steroid medication on the alternate day.

WITHDRAWAL OF CORTICOSTEROIDS FOLLOWING THEIR LONG-TERM USE AS PHARMACOLOGIC AGENTS Complete withdrawal of steroids should be initiated by implementing an alternate-day schedule. Patients on an alternate-day program for a month or more experience less difficulty during a subsequent termination regimen as far as pituitary-adrenal function is concerned. The dosage is gradually reduced and finally discontinued after a normal replacement dosage has been reached (e.g., 5 to 7.5 mg prednisone). Complications rarely ensue unless undue stress is experienced, and patients should understand that for 1 year or longer after the complete withdrawal from long-term high-dosage steroid therapy, they should receive supplementary hormone in the presence of serious infection, operation, or injury.

In patients on high-dose daily steroid therapy, it is frequently advised to reduce total steroid dosage to approximately 20 mg prednisone daily before beginning the transition to every-other-day therapy. If a patient cannot tolerate an alternate-day program, it is debatable as to whether complete discontinuance should be considered. Under these circumstances a daily dose of steroid could be continued, and at some future date another trial of gradual transition to the alternate-day schedule should be attempted. In patients with life-threatening disorders, it may be desirable to consider life-long daily maintenance therapy at an Addisonian replacement dosage. These patients will not require mineralocorticoid therapy, as aldosterone secretion is usually adequate.

REFERENCES

Bloom E et al: Nuclear binding of glucocorticoid receptors: Relations between cytosol binding, activation in the biologic response. J Steroid Biochem 12:175, 1980

Bravo E et al: The changing clinical spectrum of primary aldosteronism. Am J Med 74:641, 1983

Chrousos GP et al: Late onset of 21-hydroxylase deficiency mimicking idiopathic hirsutism or polycystic ovary disease. Ann Intern Med 96:143, 1982

Edelman IS, Marver D: Mediating events in the action of aldosterone. J Steroid Biochem 12:219, 1980

Eisenbarth GS et al: The polyglandular failure syndrome: Disease inheritance, HLA-type and immune function. Ann Intern Med 91:528, 1979

Knox FG et al: Escape from the sodium retaining effects of mineralocorticoids. Kidney Int 17:263, 1980

Krieger DT: Physiopathology of Cushing's disease. Endocr Rev 4:22, 1983

Litra SN et al: Corticotrophin releasing factor: Responses in normal subjects and patients with disorders of the hypothalamus and pituitary. Clin Endocrinol 20:71, 1984

New MI, Levine LS: Recent advances in 21-hydroxylase deficiency. Ann Rev Med 35:649, 1984

Nolan PM et al: Therapeutic problems with transsphenoidal pituitary surgery for Cushing's disease. Clev Clin Q 49:199, 1982

Parrillo JE, Fauci AS: Mechanisms of glucocorticoid action on immune processes. Ann Rev Pharmacol Toxicol 19:179, 1979

Pedersen RC et al: Pro-adrenocorticotropin/endorphin-derived peptides: Coordinated action on adrenal steroidogenesis. Science 208:1044, 1980

Rabinowe SL et al: Ia-positive T lymphocytes in recently diagnosed idiopathic Addison's disease. Am J Med 77:597, 1984

Ross EJ, Lynch DC: Cushing's syndrome—killing disease: Discriminatory value of signs and symptoms aiding early diagnosis. Lancet 2:646, 1982

Schambelan M et al: Prevalence, pathogenesis and functional significance of aldosterone deficiency in hyperkalemic patients with chronic renal insufficiency. Kidney Int 17:89, 1980

Sindler BH et al: The superiority of the metyrapone test vs the high dose dexamethasone test in the differential diagnosis of Cushing's syndrome. Am J Med 74:657, 1983

Thomas JP, Richards SH: Long term results of radical hypophysectomy for Cushing's disease. Clin Endocrinol 19:629, 1983

Weinberger MH: Primary aldosteronism: Diagnosis and differentiation of subtypes. Ann Intern Med 100:300, 1984

Williams GH, Dluhy RG: Control of aldosterone secretion, in *Hypertension*, 2d ed, J Genest et al (eds), New York, McGraw-Hill, 1983, p 320

Williams GH, Dluhy RG: Diagnostic imaging of the adrenal gland, in *Endocrinology*, 2d ed, LG DeGroot et al (eds), Orlando Fla., Grune and Stratton (in press)

326 PHEOCHROMOCYTOMA

LEWIS LANDSBERG / JAMES B. YOUNG

Pheochromocytomas, also known as chromaffin tumors, produce, store, and secrete catecholamines and are derived most often from the adrenal medulla. Pheochromocytomas that develop outside the adrenal arise from chromaffin cells in or about sympathetic ganglia and are known as extraadrenal pheochromocytomas or paragangliomas. Related tumors that secrete catecholamines and produce similar clinical syndromes include chemodectomas derived from the carotid body and ganglioneuromas derived from the postganglionic sympathetic neurons.

The clinical features and morbidity of these tumors are due predominantly to the release of catecholamines. Hypertension is the most common manifestation, and hypertensive paroxysms or crises, often spectacular and alarming, occur in over half the cases.

Pheochromocytoma occurs only in approximately 0.1 percent of the hypertensive population, but it is, nevertheless, an important correctable cause of high blood pressure. Indeed, it is usually curable if properly diagnosed and treated, but may be fatal if undiagnosed or mistreated. Postmortem series indicate that the majority of pheochromocytomas are unsuspected clinically and that in many of these cases the tumor is related to the fatal outcome.

PATHOLOGY **Location and morphology** In adults approximately 80 percent occur as a unilateral solitary lesion, 10 percent are bilateral, and 10 percent are extraadrenal. In children a fourth of tumors are bilateral, and an additional fourth are extraadrenal. Solitary lesions inexplicably favor the right side. Although pheochromocytomas may grow to large size (over 3 kg) most weigh less than 100 g and are less than 10 cm in diameter. The tumors are highly vascular with an arterial supply derived from any of the three arteries that normally supply the adrenal.

The tumors are made up of large, polyhedral, pleomorphic chromaffin cells. Less than 10 percent are malignant. As with other endocrine tumors malignancy cannot be determined by the histologic appearance; local invasion of surrounding tissues or distant metastases indicate malignancy.

FAMILIAL PHEOCHROMOCYTOMA In approximately 5 percent of cases pheochromocytoma is inherited as an autosomal dominant trait either alone or in combination with other abnormalities such as multiple endocrine neoplasia (MEN) type II (Sipple's syndrome) or type III (mucosal neuroma syndrome) (see Chap. 334), von Recklinghausen's neurofibromatosis, or von Hippel–Lindau's retinal cerebellar hemangioblastomatosis. Bilateral adrenal pheochromocytomas are common in the familial syndromes; within MEN kindreds over half with pheochromocytomas have bilateral lesions. A familial syndrome should be suspected in any patient presenting with bilateral pheochromocytomas.

EXTRAADRENAL PHEOCHROMOCYTOMAS Extraadrenal pheochromocytomas have an average weight of 20 to 40 g and are usually less than 5 cm in diameter. Most are located within the abdomen in association with the celiac, superior mesenteric, and inferior mesenteric ganglia. Approximately 1 percent are located within the thorax in relation to the paravertebral sympathetic ganglia, 1 percent are located within the urinary bladder, and less than 1 percent are within the neck, usually in association with the sympathetic ganglia or the extracranial branches of the ninth or tenth cranial nerves.

Catecholamine synthesis, storage, and release Pheochromocytomas synthesize and store catecholamines by processes resembling those of the normal adrenal medulla (Chap. 66). Little is known about the mechanisms of catecholamine release from pheochromocytomas, but changes in blood flow and necrosis within the tumor may be the cause in some instances. These tumors are not innervated, and catecholamine release does not result from neural stimulation.

EPINEPHRINE, NOREPINEPHRINE, AND DOPAMINE Most pheochromocytomas contain and secrete both norepinephrine and epinephrine, and the percentage of norepinephrine is usually greater than in the normal adrenal. Most extraadrenal pheochromocytomas secrete norepinephrine exclusively. Rarely, pheochromocytomas produce epinephrine alone, particularly in association with MEN. Although epinephrine-producing tumors may be associated with a preponderance of metabolic and beta-receptor effects, in general the predominant catecholamine secreted cannot be predicted from the clinical presentation. Increased production of dopamine and homovanillic acid (HVA) is uncommon with benign lesions; the excretion of these precursors is, however, increased in some patients with malignant pheochromocytoma.

CLINICAL FEATURES Pheochromocytoma occurs at all ages but is most common in young to midadult life. Some series show a slight female preponderance. Although the presentation is characteristically unpredictable, most patients come to medical attention as a result of hypertensive crisis, paroxysmal symptoms suggestive of seizure disorder or anxiety attacks, or hypertension that responds poorly to conventional treatment. Less commonly, unexplained hypotension or shock in association with surgery or trauma will suggest the diagnosis.

Hypertension Hypertension is the most common manifestation. In approximately 60 percent of cases the hypertension is sustained, although significant blood pressure lability is usually present and half of patients with sustained hypertension have distinct crises or paroxysms. The other 40 percent have blood pressure elevations only during an attack. The hypertension is often severe, occasionally malignant, and usually resistant to treatment with standard drugs used for therapy of essential hypertension.

Paroxysms or crises The paroxysm or crisis is a typical manifestation, occurring in over half of patients. In an individual patient the symptoms are often similar with each attack. The paroxysms are commonly frequent but may be sporadic at intervals as long as weeks or months. With time the paroxysms usually increase in frequency, duration, and severity.

The attack usually has a sudden onset. It may last from a few minutes to several hours or longer. Headache, profuse sweating, palpitations, and apprehension, often with a sense of impending doom, are common. Pain in the chest or abdomen may be associated with nausea and vomiting. Either pallor or flushing may occur during the attack. The blood pressure is elevated, often to alarming levels, and is usually accompanied by tachycardia.

The paroxysm may be precipitated by any activity that displaces the abdominal contents. In some cases a particular stimulus may reproduce an attack in a characteristic fashion, but no clearly defined precipitating event may be found. Although anxiety may accompany the attacks, mental stress or psychological tension does not usually provoke a crisis.

Other distinctive clinical features Symptoms and signs of an increased metabolic rate, such as profuse sweating and mild to moderate weight loss, are common. Orthostatic hypotension is a consequence of diminished plasma volume and blunted sympathetic reflexes. Both of these factors predispose the patient with unsuspected pheochromocytoma to hypotension or shock during surgery or major trauma.

CARDIAC MANIFESTATIONS Sinus tachycardia, sinus bradycardia, supraventricular arrhythmias, and ventricular premature contractions have all been noted. Angina and acute myocardial infarction may occur even in the absence of coronary artery disease. Catecholamine-induced increase in myocardial oxygen consumption and, perhaps, coronary spasm may be involved in the pathogenesis of these ischemic events. Electrocardiographic changes, including nonspecific ST-T wave changes, prominent U waves, left ventricular strain patterns, and right and left bundle branch blocks may be present in the absence of demonstrable ischemia or infarction. Cardiomyopathy, either congestive with myocarditis and myocardial fibrosis or hypertrophic with concentric or asymmetric hypertrophy, may be associated with heart failure and cardiac arrhythmias.

CARBOHYDRATE INTOLERANCE Over half of patients have impaired carbohydrate tolerance due to suppression of insulin and stimulation of hepatic glucose output. The impaired glucose tolerance almost never requires specific treatment and disappears after removal of the tumor.

HEMATOCRIT Patients may have an elevated hematocrit secondary to diminished plasma volume. Rarely production of erythropoietin by the pheochromocytoma may cause a true erythrocytosis.

PHEOCHROMOCYTOMA OF THE URINARY BLADDER Pheochromocytoma within the wall of the urinary bladder may result in typical paroxysms in relation to micturition. The unique location of these tumors within the bladder wall is responsible for the production of symptoms while the tumors are quite small, and consequently, urinary catecholamine excretion may be normal or only minimally elevated. Hematuria is present in over half, and the tumor can often be visualized at cystoscopy.

Adverse drug interactions Severe and occasionally fatal paroxysms have been induced by opiates, histamine, ACTH, saralasin, and glucagon. These agents appear to release catecholamines directly from the tumor. Indirect-acting sympathomimetic amines, including methyldopa (when administered intravenously), may cause an increase in blood pressure by releasing catecholamines from the augmented stores within nerve endings. Drugs that block neuronal uptake of catecholamines, such as tricyclic antidepressants or guanethidine, may enhance the physiologic effects of circulating catecholamines. These drugs should be avoided in patients with known or suspected pheochromocytoma; indeed all medications should be carefully considered and cautiously administered in such patients.

Associated diseases Pheochromocytoma is associated with medullary carcinoma of the thyroid in the familial MEN syndromes types II and III and with hyperparathyroidism in MEN II (see Chap. 334). Hypercalcemia, resolving after tumor resection, has also been described in patients with pheochromocytoma in the absence of parathyroid disease. Every member of MEN II and III kindreds should be screened periodically for pheochromocytoma by assay of a 24-h urine sample for catecholamines, including measurement of epinephrine. Pheochromocytoma should be excluded or removed before thyroid or parathyroid surgery.

The association of pheochromocytoma and neurofibromatosis is uncommon. Nevertheless, since incomplete forms of neurofibromatosis may be associated with pheochromocytoma, minor manifestations such as five to six café au lait spots, vertebral abnormalities, or kyphoscoliosis should increase the suspicion of pheochromocytoma in a patient with hypertension. The incidence of pheochromocytoma in some kindreds with von Hippel–Lindau disease may be as high as 10 to 25 percent. Many of these are unsuspected clinically and diagnosed postmortem.

The incidence of cholelithiasis is about 15 to 20 percent in patients with pheochromocytoma. Cushing's syndrome is rarely associated with pheochromocytoma, usually a consequence of ectopic secretion of ACTH either by the pheochromocytoma or, less commonly, by a coexistent medullary carcinoma of the thyroid.

DIAGNOSIS The diagnosis is established by the demonstration of increased amounts of catecholamines or catecholamine metabolites in a 24-h urine collection. The diagnosis can usually be made by the analysis of a single 24-h urine sample, provided the patient is hypertensive or symptomatic at the time of collection.

Biochemical tests The determinations employed in the diagnosis include vanillylmandelic acid (VMA), the metanephrines, and unconjugated or "free" catecholamines (Chap. 66). Although much has been written about the relative specificity and sensitivity of the different measurements, they are probably equivalent provided the assays are properly performed. Accuracy of diagnosis is improved when two of the three determinations are employed, although this is not essential as a screening procedure. The following considerations apply to all the urinary tests: (1) Despite claims for the adequacy of determinations made on random urine samples and expressed per milligram of creatinine, analysis of a full 24-h urine sample is preferable. Creatinine should be determined as well to assess the adequacy of collection. (2) Where possible the collection should be obtained when the patient is at rest, on no medication, and without recent exposure to radiographic contrast media. Where it is not practical to discontinue all medications, those drugs known specifically to interfere in the assays (as noted above) should be avoided. (3) The urine collection should be properly acidified and kept cold during and after collection. (4) With specific high-quality assays dietary restrictions are minimal and should be specified by the laboratory performing the analyses. (5) Although the majority of patients with pheochromocytoma excrete increased quantities of catecholamines and catecholamine metabolites each day, in patients with paroxysmal hypertension the yield is increased if a 24-h urine collection is initiated during a crisis.

FREE CATECHOLAMINES The upper limit of normal for total catecholamines is between 100 and 150 μg per 24 h. In most patients with pheochromocytoma values in excess of 250 μg per day are obtained. Specific measurement of epinephrine is often of value since increased epinephrine excretion (over 50 μg per 24 h) is usually due to an adrenal lesion and may be the only abnormality in cases associated with MEN. False-positive increases in catecholamine excretion result from exogenous catecholamines such as methyldopa, levodopa, and sympathomimetic amines, which may elevate catecholamine excretion for up to 2 weeks. Endogenous catecholamines from stimulation of the sympathoadrenal system may also increase urinary catecholamine excretion and result in a false-positive test. The relevant clinical situations include hypoglycemia, strenuous exertion, central nervous system disease with increased intracranial pressure, and clonidine withdrawal.

METANEPHRINES AND VMA In most laboratories the upper limit of normal is 1.3 mg of total metanephrine and 7.0 mg of VMA excretion per 24 h. In most patients with pheochromocytoma the increase in excretion of these metabolites is considerable, often more than three times the normal range. Metanephrine excretion is increased by exogenous and endogenous catecholamines and by treatment with monoamine oxidase inhibitors; propranolol may cause a spurious increase in metanephrine excretion, since a propranolol metabolite interferes in the commonly utilized spectrophotometric assay. VMA is less affected by endogenous and exogenous catecholamines but is spuriously increased by a variety of drugs, including carbidopa. VMA excretion is decreased by monoamine oxidase inhibitors.

PLASMA CATECHOLAMINES Measurement of plasma catecholamines has a limited application in the diagnosis. The care required in obtaining basal catecholamine levels (Chap. 66), the lack of readily available, reliable plasma catecholamine assays, and the satisfactory results obtained with urinary determinations make measurement of plasma catecholamines unnecessary in most cases. Plasma catecholamine levels are affected by the same drugs and physiologic perturbations that increase urinary catecholamine excretion. In addition, alpha- and beta-adrenergic receptor blocking agents may elevate plasma catecholamines by impairing catecholamine clearance.

In occasional patients, when the clinical features suggest pheochromocytoma and the urinary assays are borderline, measurement of plasma catecholamines may be worthwhile. Basal levels of total catecholamines over 2000 pg/mL support the diagnosis, although approximately one-third of patients with pheochromocytoma have basal values below this level. The usefulness of plasma catecholamine determinations may be increased by agents that suppress sympathetic nervous system activity. Clonidine and ganglionic blocking agents (Chap. 66) both markedly reduce plasma catecholamine levels in normal subjects and in patients with essential hypertension. These drugs have little effect on catecholamine levels in patients with pheochromocytoma. In patients with elevated basal plasma catecholamines failure to suppress plasma levels with clonidine supports the diagnosis of pheochromocytoma.

Pharmacologic tests Reliable methods for the measurement of catecholamines and catecholamine metabolites in urine have rendered obsolete both the provocative and adrenolytic tests, which are nonspecific and entail considerable risk. A modified version of the adrenolytic test may be of some use, however, as a therapeutic trial in a patient in hypertensive crisis with features suggestive of pheochromocytoma. A positive response to phentolamine (5-mg bolus following a 0.5-mg test dose) is a reduction in blood pressure of at least 35/25 mmHg that becomes maximal after 2 min and persists for 10 to 15 min. The response to a pharmacologic agent is never diagnostic, and biochemical confirmation must always be obtained. Provocative tests in normotensive patients are potentially dangerous and rarely indicated. However, a glucagon provocative test may be of use in patients with paroxysmal hypertension and basal catecholamine levels below those usually found in patients with pheochromocytoma (less than 1000 to 1500 pg/mL). Glucagon has a negligible effect on blood pressure or on plasma catecholamine levels in normal or hypertensive subjects. In patients with pheochromocytoma, on the other hand, glucagon may substantially increase both blood pressure and circulating catecholamine levels. The elevation in plasma catecholamine concentration, moreover, may occur in patients without a blood pressure response. It must be emphasized, however, that life-threatening pressor crises have occurred after administration of glucagon to patients with pheochromocytoma so that the test should never be performed casually. Careful continuous monitoring of the blood pressure is required, intravenous access must be adequate, and phentolamine must be at hand to terminate the test if a significant pressor reaction enuses.

Differential diagnosis Since the manifestations may be protean, the diagnosis must be considered and excluded in many patients with suggestive clinical features. In patients with essential hypertension and "hyperadrenergic" features such as tachycardia, sweating, and increased cardiac output, and in patients with anxiety attacks associated with blood pressure elevations, analysis of a 24-h urine collection is usually decisive in excluding the diagnosis. Repeated determinations on urine collected during attacks may be necessary, however, before the diagnosis can be excluded with certainty. The clonidine suppression and glucagon stimulation tests may occasionally be helpful in excluding the diagnosis in difficult cases. Pressor crises associated with clonidine withdrawal or the use of monoamine oxidase inhibitors (Chap. 66) may mimic the paroxysms of pheochromocytoma. Factitious crises may be produced by self-administration of sympathomimetic amines in psychiatrically disturbed patients, particularly among those employed in the health care professions.

Intracranial lesions, particularly posterior fossa tumors or subarachnoid hemorrhage, may be associated with hypertension and increased excretion of catecholamines or catecholamine metabolites. While this is most common in patients who have suffered an obvious neurologic catastrophe, the possibility of subarachnoid or intracranial hemorrhage secondary to pheochromocytoma should be considered. Diencephalic or autonomic epilepsy may be associated with paroxysmal spells, hypertension, and increased plasma catecholamine levels. This rare entity may be difficult to distinguish from pheochromocytoma, but an aura, an abnormal electroencephalogram, and a beneficial response to anticonvulsant medications will often suggest the proper diagnosis.

MANAGEMENT Preoperative management The induction of stable alpha-adrenergic blockade is the basis of preoperative management and provides the foundation for successful surgical treatment. Once the diagnosis is established, the patient should be placed on phenoxybenzamine to induce a long-lived, noncompetitive alpha-receptor blockade. The usual initial dose is 10 mg every 12 h with increments of 10 to 20 mg added every few days until the blood pressure is controlled and the paroxysms disappear. Because of the long duration of action the therapeutic effects are cumulative, and the optimal dose must be achieved gradually with careful monitoring of supine and upright blood pressures. Most patients require between 40 and 80 mg of phenoxybenzamine per day although in some cases 200 mg or more may be necessary. Phenoxybenzamine should be administered for at least 10 to 14 days prior to surgery. Over this time the combination of alpha-receptor blockade and a liberal salt intake will restore the contracted plasma volume to normal. Before adequate alpha-adrenergic blockade with phenoxybenzamine is achieved, paroxysms may be treated with intravenous phentolamine. Prazosin, the selective $alpha_1$ antagonist, has been employed in the preoperative management of a small number of patients. Doses in the range of 1.5 to 2.5 mg every 6 h have effectively controlled blood pressure and paroxysms. The role of this agent in the management of pheochromocytoma has not been established; the relatively short duration of action may be a disadvantage compared with phenoxybenzamine. Prazosin may be useful as an antihypertensive agent in patients with suspected pheochromocytoma while workup is in progress, since it is usually better tolerated than phenoxybenzamine and prevents serious pressor crises if pheochromocytoma is present. Nitroprusside is the only other antihypertensive agent that reliably reduces blood pressure in patients with pheochromocytoma and may be useful on occasion.

Beta-adrenergic receptor-blocking agents should be given only after alpha blockade has been established, since administration of such agents by themselves may cause a paradoxic increase in blood pressure by antagonizing beta-mediated vasodilatation in skeletal muscle. Beta blockade is usually initiated when tachycardia develops during the induction of alpha-adrenergic blockade. Low doses often suffice, and a reasonable starting dose is 10 mg propranolol 3 to 4 times per day, increased as needed to control the pulse rate. Beta blockade is effective treatment for catecholamine-induced arrhythmias, particularly those potentiated by anesthetic agents.

Preoperative localization of the tumor Surgical removal of pheochromocytoma is facilitated if the location of the tumor, or tumors, can be established preoperatively. Once pheochromocytoma is diagnosed, localization should be undertaken while the patient is being prepared for surgery by the administration of alpha receptor-blocking agents. Computerized tomography of the adrenals is usually successful in identifying the intraadrenal lesions. Conventional chest roentgenograms and computerized tomography of the chest usually suffice to identify intrathoracic lesions. If these studies are negative, abdominal aortography (once alpha-adrenergic blockade is complete) may be useful in identifying extraadrenal pheochromocytomas within the abdomen, since these lesions are often supplied by a large aberrant artery. If aortography and computerized tomography fail to localize the lesion, venous sampling at different levels of the inferior and superior vena cava may reveal a step-up in catecholamine concentration in the region drained by the tumor; this area may then be restudied by selective angiography or directed scanning by computerized tomography. An additional localization technique involves a radionuclide scintiscan after administration of an investigational radiopharmaceutical ^{131}I-metaiodobenzylguanidine (MIBG). This agent is concentrated by the amine uptake process and produces an external scintigraphic image at the site of the tumor. This type of scanning has no advantages over computerized tomography in the diagnosis of adrenal lesions but may have a role in localizing extraadrenal pheochromocytomas.

Surgery Surgery is best performed in centers with experience in the preoperative, anesthetic, and intraoperative management of pheochromocytoma patients. In experienced hands surgical mortality is below 2 or 3 percent.

Adequate monitoring during the surgical procedure should include continuous recording of arterial pressure, central venous pressure, and electrocardiogram; in the presence of cardiac disease or if congestive failure has been present, pulmonary capillary wedge pressure should be monitored as well. Adequate fluid replacement is crucial. Intraoperative hypotension responds better to volume replacement than to the administration of vasoconstrictors. Hypertension and cardiac arrhythmias are most likely to occur during induction of anesthesia, intubation, and manipulation of the tumor. Intravenous phentolamine is usually sufficient to control the blood pressure, but nitroprusside may be required. Propranolol may be given in the treatment of tachycardia or ventricular ectopy.

PHEOCHROMOCYTOMA IN PREGNANCY Spontaneous labor and vaginal delivery in unprepared patients are usually disastrous for mother and fetus. In early pregnancy it seems reasonable to prepare the patient with phenoxybenzamine and remove the tumor as soon as the diagnosis is confirmed. The pregnancy need not be terminated, but the operative procedure itself may result in spontaneous abortion. In the third trimester, treatment with adrenergic blocking agents should be undertaken; when the fetus is of sufficient size cesarean section followed by extirpation of the tumor may be undertaken. Although the safety of adrenergic blocking drugs in pregnancy has not been established, these agents have been administered in several cases without obvious adverse effect.

UNRESECTABLE TUMOR In cases of metastatic or locally invasive tumor or in patients with intercurrent illness that precludes surgery, long-term medical management is required. When the manifestations of pheochromocytoma cannot be adequately controlled by the chronic administration of adrenergic blocking agents, the concomitant administration of metyrosine may be required. This agent inhibits tyrosine hydroxylase, diminishes catecholamine production by the tumor, and often simplifies chronic management. At present there are no practical ways of destroying the tumor by radiotherapy or chemotherapy.

PROGNOSIS The 5-year survival after surgery is usually over 95 percent, and the recurrence rate is less than 10 percent. After successful surgery catecholamine excretion returns to normal in about 1 week and should be measured to ensure complete tumor removal. In malignant pheochromocytoma the 5-year survival is less than 50 percent.

Complete removal of the pheochromocytoma cures the hypertension in approximately three-fourths. In the remainder hypertension recurs but is usually well controlled by standard antihypertensive agents. In this group either underlying essential hypertension or irreversible vascular damage induced by catecholamines may cause the persistence of the hypertension.

REFERENCES

BRAVO EL, GIFFORD RW: Pheochromocytoma: Diagnosis, localization, and management. N Engl J Med 311:1298, 1984

BROWN MJ et al: Increased sensitivity and accuracy of phaeochromocytoma diagnosis achieved by use of plasma-adrenaline estimations and a pentolinium-suppression test. Lancet 1:174, 1981

ENGELMAN K: Phaeochromocytoma. Clin Endocrinol Metab 6:769, 1977

FUDGE TL et al: Current surgical management of pheochromocytoma during pregnancy. Arch Surg 115:1224, 1980

GLUSHIEN AS et al: Pheochromocytoma: Its relationship to the neurocutaneous syndromes. Am J Med 14:318, 1953

HAMILTON BP et al: Measurement of urinary epinephrine in screening for pheochromocytoma in multiple endocrine neoplasia type II. Am J Med 65:1027, 1978

HORTON WA et al: Von Hippel–Lindau disease: Clinical and pathological manifestations in nine families with 50 affected members. Arch Intern Med 136:769, 1976

JONES DH et al: The biochemical diagnosis, localization and followup of phaeochromocytoma: The role of plasma and urinary catecholamine measurements. Q J Med 49:431, 1980

KHAIRI MRA et al: Mucosal neuroma, pheochromocytoma and medullary thyroid carcinoma: Multiple endocrine neoplasia type 3. Medicine 54:89, 1975

LAURSEN K, DAMGAARD-PEDERSON K: CT for pheochromocytoma diagnosis. AJR 134:277, 1980

MANGER WM, GIFFORD RW JR: *Pheochromocytoma.* New York, Springer-Verlag, 1977

PALUBINSKAS AJ et al: Localization of functioning pheochromocytomas by venous sampling and radioenzymatic analysis. Radiology 136:495, 1980

REMINE WH et al: Current management of pheochromocytoma. Ann Surg 179:740, 1974

ROSS EJ et al: Preoperative and operative management of patients with pheochromocytoma. Br Med J 1:191, 1971

ST JOHN WM, GIFFORD RW JR: Prevalence of clinically unsuspected pheochromocytoma. Mayo Clin Proc 56:354, 1981

SISSON JC et al: Scintigraphic localization of pheochromocytoma. N Engl J Med 305:12, 1981

SJOERDSMA A et al: Pheochromocytoma: Current concepts of diagnosis and treatment. Ann Intern Med 65:1302, 1966

STEINER AL et al: Study of a kindred with pheochromocytoma, medullary thyroid carcinoma, hyperparathyroidism and Cushing's disease: Multiple endocrine neoplasia, type 2. Medicine 47:371, 1968

327 DIABETES MELLITUS

DANIEL W. FOSTER

Diabetes mellitus is the most common of the serious metabolic diseases. The true frequency is difficult to ascertain because of differing standards of diagnosis but probably is around 1 percent. The disease is characterized by metabolic abnormalities; by long-term complications involving the eyes, kidneys, nerves, and blood vessels; and by a lesion of the basement membranes demonstrable by electron microscopy. Patients fulfilling these criteria are not a homogeneous group, and several distinct diabetic syndromes have been delineated.

DIAGNOSIS The diagnosis of symptomatic diabetes is not difficult. When a patient presents with signs and symptoms attributable to an osmotic diuresis and is found to have hyperglycemia, essentially all physicians agree that diabetes is present. There is likewise little disagreement about an asymptomatic patient with persistently elevated fasting plasma glucose concentrations. The problem arises with the asymptomatic patient who for one reason or another is considered to be a potential diabetic but has a normal fasting glucose concentration in plasma. Such patients are often given an oral glucose tolerance test, and, if abnormal values are found, diagnosed as having "chemical" diabetes. There seems to be little question that normal glucose tolerance is strong evidence against the presence of diabetes; the predictive value of a positive test is less certain. Much evidence suggests that the standard oral glucose tolerance test overdiagnoses diabetes to a remarkable degree, probably because a variety of stresses can produce an abnormal response. The operative mechanism is thought to be epinephrine discharge. Epinephrine blocks insulin secretion, stimulates glucagon release, activates glycogen breakdown, and impairs insulin action in target tissues such that hepatic glucose production is increased and the capacity to dispose of an exogenous glucose load is impaired. Even anxiety over venipunctures may generate sufficient epinephrine to produce an abnormal test. Concomitant illness, inadequate diet, and lack of physical exercise also contribute to false-positive examinations.

In an attempt to deal with these problems, the National Diabetes Data Group of the National Institutes of Health in 1979 provided revised criteria for the diagnosis of diabetes following a challenge with oral glucose:

1 Fasting (*overnight*): Venous plasma glucose concentration ≥140 mg/dL on at least two separate occasions.[1]

[1] *Venous whole blood concentrations are 15 percent lower than plasma values. Capillary whole blood, utilized in patient self-monitoring, is equivalent to venous plasma.*

2 *Following ingestion of 75 g of glucose:* Venous plasma glucose concentration ≥200 mg/dL at 2 h and on at least one other occasion during the 2-h test (i.e., *two* values ≥200 mg/dL must be obtained for diagnosis).

If the 2-h value is between 140 and 200 mg/dL and one other value during the 2-h test period is equal to or greater than 200 mg/dL, a diagnosis of "impaired glucose tolerance" is suggested. The interpretation would be that persons in this category are at increased risk for the development of fasting hyperglycemia or symptomatic diabetes but that such progression is not predictable in an individual patient. Most patients (~75 percent) with impaired glucose tolerance never develop diabetes, and subjects diagnosed as having diabetes by the second criterion may never manifest fasting hyperglycemia or symptomatic deterioration. Consequently, the oral glucose tolerance test is rarely indicated in clinical practice although it is useful as a research tool.

CLASSIFICATION A classification of diabetes is given in Table 327-1. The basic categories are those recommended by the National Diabetes Data Group except for division into primary and secondary types. Primary implies that no associated disease is present while in the secondary type some other identifiable condition causes or allows a diabetic syndrome to develop. Insulin dependence in this classification is not equivalent to insulin therapy. Rather, the term means that the patient is at risk for ketoacidosis in the absence of insulin. Many patients classified as non-insulin-dependent require insulin for control of hyperglycemia although they do not become ketoacidotic if insulin is withdrawn.

The term *type 1* has often been used as a synonym for insulin-dependent diabetes (IDDM), and *type 2* diabetes has been considered equivalent to non-insulin-dependent disease (NIDDM). This probably is not ideal since some patients with apparent non-insulin-dependent diabetes may in fact be destined to become fully insulin-dependent and prone to ketoacidosis. The subset of patients in this category are nonobese subjects who carry the HLA-DR3/DR4 phenotype and exhibit islet cell antibodies in the blood (see "Pathogenesis" below). For this reason it has been suggested that the classification shown in Table 327-1 be modified such that the terms *insulin-dependent* and *non-insulin-dependent* describe physiologic states (ketoacidosis-prone and ketoacidosis-resistant, respectively) while the terms *type 1* and *type 2* refer to pathogenetic mechanisms (immune-mediated and non-immune-mediated, respectively). Using such a classification three major forms of primary diabetes would be recognized: (1) type 1 insulin-dependent diabetes, (2) type 1 non-insulin-dependent diabetes and (3) type 2 non-insulin-dependent diabetes. Category 2 can be considered as type 1 insulin-dependent diabetes in evolution; i.e., autoimmune beta-cell destruction occurs slowly rather than rapidly with the result that there is a delay in reaching the ketoacidotic threshold of insulin deficiency.

Secondary forms of diabetes encompass a host of conditions. *Pancreatic disease,* particularly chronic pancreatitis in alcoholics, is a common cause. Destruction of the beta-cell mass is the etiologic mechanism. *Hormonal abnormalities* include pheochromocytoma, acromegaly, and Cushing's syndrome or arise consequent to therapeutic administration of steroid hormones. "Stress hyperglycemia," associated with severe burns, acute myocardial infarctions, and other life-threatening illnesses, is due to endogenous release of glucagon and catecholamines. Mechanisms of hormonal hyperglycemia include varying combinations of impairment of insulin release and induction of insulin resistance. A large number of *drugs* can lead to hyperglycemia, but most simply produce impaired glucose tolerance. Hyperglycemia and even ketoacidosis may occur as a result of abnormalities at the level of the *insulin receptor*. The dysfunction may be due to quantitative or qualitative defects in the receptor itself or to antibodies directed against it. The mechanism is essentially pure insulin resistance. A number of *genetic syndromes* are associated with impaired glucose tolerance or hyperglycemia. The three most common are the lipodystrophies, myotonic dystrophy, and ataxia-telangiectasia. The final category, *other,* is poorly defined and is meant to include any condition which does not fit elsewhere in the etiologic scheme. The appearance of abnormal carbohydrate metabolism in association with any of the secondary causes does not necessarily indicate the presence of underlying diabetes although in some cases a mild, asymptomatic primary diabetes may be made overt by the secondary illness.

TABLE 327-1 Classification of diabetes

A Primary
- *1* Insulin-dependent diabetes mellitus (IDDM, type 1)
- *2* Non-insulin-dependent diabetes mellitus (NIDDM, type 2)
  - *a* Nonobese NIDDM (type 1 IDDM in evolution?)
  - *b* Obese NIDDM
  - *c* Maturity-onset diabetes of the young (MODY)

B Secondary
- *1* Pancreatic disease
- *2* Hormonal abnormalities
- *3* Drug or chemical induced
- *4* Insulin receptor abnormalities
- *5* Genetic syndromes
- *6* Other

PREVALENCE Prevalence of diabetes is difficult to determine because numerous standards, many now no longer acceptable, have been used in diagnosis. As noted above the overall prevalence in western societies is thought to be about 1 percent. Estimates for insulin-dependent diabetes are more reliable than for the non-insulin-dependent form since most patients are diagnosed after the abrupt appearance of symptoms. In England prevalence of the type 1 illness has been estimated to be 0.22 percent by age 16, and a study in the United States suggested a prevalence of 0.26 percent by age 20. If the prevalence of diabetes is actually 1 percent, it follows that about one-fourth of cases have insulin-dependent disease while three-fourths are non-insulin-dependent. The relative frequency of insulin-dependent to non-insulin-dependent diabetes varies with age, being higher if a young population is studied and lower in the older age range.

PATHOGENESIS OF TYPE 1 DIABETES MELLITUS By the time insulin-dependent diabetes mellitus appears, most of the beta cells in the pancreas have been destroyed. The destructive process is almost certainly autoimmune in nature. An overview of the pathogenetic sequence is given in Table 327-2. *First,* genetic susceptibility to the disease must be present. *Second,* an environmental event initiates the process in genetically susceptible individuals. Viral infection is believed to be a common triggering mechanism. The best evidence that an environmental insult is required comes from studies in monozygotic twins, in whom the concordance rate for diabetes is no more than 50 percent. If diabetes were a purely genetic illness, concordance rates would be approximately 100 percent. The *third* step in the sequence is an inflammatory response in the pancreas called "insulitis." The cells that infiltrate the islets are activated T lymphocytes. The *fourth* step is an alteration or transformation of the surface of the beta cell such that it is no longer recognized as "self" but is seen by the immune system as a foreign cell or "nonself." The *fifth* step is the development of an immune response. Because

TABLE 327-2 The pathogenesis of type 1 diabetes mellitus

Step	Event	Agent or response
1	Genetic susceptibility ↓	HLA-DR3, DR4 (T-cell receptor?)
2	Environmental event ↓	Virus (?)
3	Insulitis ↓	Infiltration of activated T lymphocytes
4	Activation of autoimmunity ↓	Self → nonself transition
5	Immune attack on beta cells ↓	Islet cell antibodies, cell-mediated immunity
6	Diabetes mellitus	> 90 percent beta cells destroyed (alpha cells unopposed)

the islets are now considered "nonself," cytotoxic antibodies develop and act in concert with cell-mediated immune mechanisms. The end result is the destruction of the beta cell and the appearance of diabetes.

In the summary, the pathogenetic sequence is genetic predisposition → environmental insult → insulitis → conversion of beta cell from "self" to "nonself" → activation of the immune system → destruction of the beta cell → diabetes mellitus.

Genetics Although insulin-dependent diabetes aggregates in families, the mechanism of inheritance is unclear in mendelian terms. Transmission has been postulated to be autosomal dominant, recessive, and mixed, but none has been proven. The genetic predisposition is probably permissive and not causal.

Analysis of pedigrees shows a low prevalence of direct vertical transmission. In one series of 35 families in which there was a child with classic insulin-dependent diabetes only four of the index cases had a parent with diabetes and two had a diabetic grandparent. Of the 99 siblings of these diabetic children only 6 had overt disease. Overall the chance of a child developing type 1 diabetes when another first-degree relative has the disease is only 5 to 10 percent. The presence of non-insulin-dependent disease in a parent increases the risk for insulin-dependent diabetes in the offspring. It is not known whether the intermixing of IDDM and NIDDM in the same family represents a single genetic trait (i.e., the apparent NIDDM is really type 1 NIDDM) or whether two common genetic predispositions coexist in the same family by chance, each perhaps influencing the expression of the other. Low rates of transmission of IDDM make it difficult to discern mechanisms of inheritance through study of families but are reassuring to diabetic parents who may wish to have children.

One of the susceptibility genes in IDDM likely resides on the sixth chromosome in view of strong associations between diabetes and certain human leukocyte antigens (HLA) coded by the major histocompatibility region on this chromosome (see Chap. 63). Four loci designated by the letters A, B, C, and D are recognized with alleles at each site identified by numbers. Major alleles conferring enhanced risk for IDDM are HLA-DR3, HLA-Dw3, HLA-DR4, HLA-Dw4, HLA-B8, and HLA-B15. The D locus is considered of primary importance with the B and A loci being involved through nonrandom associations with D (*linkage disequilibrium*). When compared with the general population the risk for IDDM imposed by the presence of DR3 or DR4 is 4 to 10 times. If the comparison is made not against a control population but against a subset of persons not bearing the predisposing antigen, relative risks are as high as thirtyfold. However, many persons carrying "high-risk" alleles never develop diabetes. It is likely that further probing of the genes in the D region will sharpen the ability to identify risk; i.e., a particular variant of an HLA-DR or -DQ antigen, not identified by routine screening, may be more tightly associated with diabetes than would be indicated by the mere presence of the antigen. Not all HLA-DR4, for example, may confer risk for diabetes but only a certain subset. It must also be emphasized that diabetes can develop in the absence of HLA determinants shown to be high risk in population studies.

FIGURE 327-1 *A schematic representation of the major histocompatibility complex on chromosome 6. Courtesy of Dr. J. Harold Helderman.*

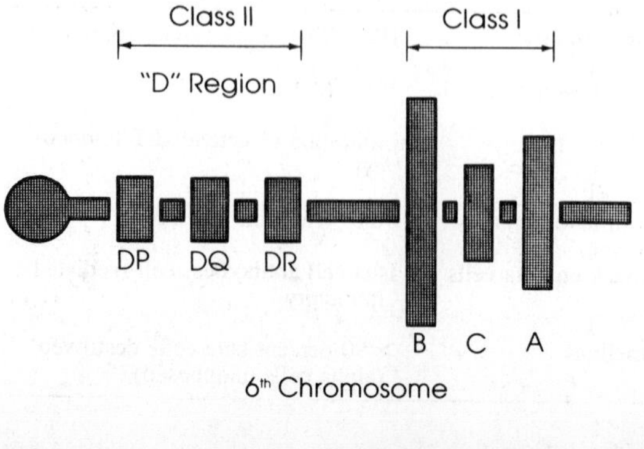

Antigens B7 and DR2 (Dw2) have been called "protective" since they are found with less frequency in diabetic subjects than in the general population. It is likely, however, that they are acutally "low-risk" alleles (rather than protective) because they are present in inverse relationship with DR3/DR4; i.e., if DR2, Dw2 is present, high-risk alleles will be absent.

Current terminology divides the D region into DP, DQ, and DR (Fig. 327-1). (DP was formerly designated SB and DQ was called DC.) The HLA-associated susceptibility gene may be more closely linked to the DQ region than to DR. If so, the relationship to DR3 and DR4 is due to linkage disequilibrium. Many investigators believe that a second susceptibility gene is required for development of diabetes. The second gene might code for an abnormality in the T-cell receptor.

A word is necessary about the function of the cell surface molecules derived from genes in the HLA region. Antigens derived from regions A, B, and C are called class I molecules. They are present on nucleated cells and function primarily in the defense against infections, expecially viruses. D region antigens are called class II molecules. They function in the regulatory (helper/suppressor) T-cell system and in the response to alloantigens (e.g., the rejection of transplanted organs). Class II molecules are normally present only on B lymphocytes and circulating or tissue macrophages.

Class I and II molecules are best considered as recognition/programming signals for initiation and amplification of immune responses in the body. Thus, activation of cytotoxic T lymphocytes to fight a viral infection requires the presence of the same class I molecule on infected cell and cytotoxic T cell; i.e., a "self" class I molecule plus viral antigen yields a recognizable neoantigen to which the T lymphocyte can respond. If exposed to a cell bearing viral antigen but a "nonself" class I HLA antigen, the T cell would not respond. Similarly the helper T cell becomes activated only when exposed to antigen-presenting cells (macrophages) bearing a recognizable class II molecule and an antigen for which it has a correct recognition site.

The appearance of class II molecules on endocrine cells, where they are normally not present, has been thought to play an important role in the autoimmune destructive process that leads to diabetes mellitus and other endocrine conditions such as Hashimoto's thyroiditis. The presence of a "self" class II molecule coupled with a foreign or autoantigen is recognized by a helper T lymphocyte which then initiates activation of the immune system including antibody formation against the cell bearing the class II/foreign (or autologous) antigen combination (see below).

Environmental event As noted earlier, the fact that a significant proportion of monozygotic twins remain discordant for diabetes (one twin with, the other without) has suggested that nongenetic factors are required for expression of diabetes in humans. Similar arguments derive from the fact that HLA haploidentity does not ensure concordance.

The environmental factor in most cases is believed to be a virus capable of infecting the beta cell. A viral etiology was originally suggested by seasonal variations in the onset of the disease and what appeared to be more than a chance relationship between appearance of diabetes and preceding episodes of mumps, hepatitis, infectious mononucleosis, congenital rubella, and coxsackievirus infections. The viral hypothesis gained support from studies showing that certain strains of encephalomyocarditis virus cause diabetes in genetically susceptible mice. The isolation of a coxsackievirus B4 from the pancreas of a previously healthy boy who died following an episode of ketoacidosis and the induction of diabetes in experimental animals inoculated with the isolated virus also suggest that viruses can cause diabetes in humans. A rise in titer of neutralizing antibody to coxsackievirus over the weeks prior to death of the patient indicated that the virus was recently acquired. Further support for the viral theory comes from the observation that congenital rubella is associated with subsequent development of IDDM in about 20 percent of affected individuals in the United States. Presumably viral infections of the pancrease could induce diabetes by two mechanisms: direct inflammatory disruption of islets or induction of an immune response.

Despite its attractiveness, considerable caution should be reserved for the viral theory. Serologic studies seeking evidence of recent viral infection in patients with new-onset insulin-dependent diabetes are inconclusive at best. If viruses are commonly involved, those producing acute disease may not be the major inducers but a slow virus not yet identified.

Insulitis In animals activated T lymphocytes infiltrate the pancreatic islets prior to or simultaneous with development of diabetes. Lymphocytes are also found in the islets of young persons dying from new-onset diabetes, and radioactively labeled lymphocytes localize in the pancrease in humans with IDDM. These findings are in accord with the observation that immune endocrinopathies in general are associated with lymphocytic infiltration of the affected tissue. However, the insulitis might be an epiphenomenon not causally related to the pathogenetic sequence. This follows from the fact that in the low-dose streptozocin model of diabetes in rodents, which is immunologically mediated, loss of beta-cell mass occurs prior to development of insulitis. Moreover, experiments in mice with immune deficiency indicate that T lymphocytes are not necessary for the beta-cell destruction induced by low-dose streptozocin.

Conversion of the beta-cell from "self" to "nonself" and activation of the immune system HLA-DR3 and -B15, known to be associated with immune endocrinopathy, are found with increased frequency in insulin-dependent diabetic subjects. Moreover, there is a frequent coexistence of IDDM and other forms of autoimmune endocrinopathy such as Addison's disease, Hashimoto's thyroiditis, hyperthyroidism, pernicious anemia, vitiligo, myasthenia gravis, and collagen-vascular disease (see Chap. 334). All of these conditions tend to run in families. In addition, islet cell antibodies are found in a high percentage of patients with insulin-dependent diabetes who are examined during the first year after diagnosis. These antibodies are also present in the blood of nonconcordant monozygotic twins or triplets destined to become concordant in the future. The same is true for siblings of patients with insulin-dependent diabetes mellitus. Killer T cells are present in 50 to 60 percent of recently diagnosed diabetic children, a value higher than in control populations. It is noteworthy that diabetes similar to human type 1 disease develops spontaneously in the BB rat. Affected animals exhibit insulitis, thyroiditis, and autoantibodies to pancreatic islets, smooth muscle, thyroid colloid, and gastric parietal cells. Diabetes in these animals can be prevented or reversed by immune modulation.

What causes the autoimmune process? First, there is an increase in the ratio of helper to suppressor T cells in the circulation. This may be a general phenomenon in immune endocrine disease. The increase in this ratio is likely due to a deficiency of suppressor T cells. An unbalanced helper-T-cell population would predispose to exuberant antibody formation on exposure to antigen.

Second, class II HLA molecules appear on the surface of the beta cell. It will be recalled that activation of helper T cells requires the presence of a class II molecule and a foreign or autoantigen. The idea is that the normal islet cell does not express class II molecules but that in response to a virus (probably through the production of γ interferon) the cell develops such molecules, rendering it potentially recognizable as "nonself." Depending on the allele expressed the immune system may be activated. Thus, if HLA-DR2 is present, it would be unlikely that diabetes would develop, as suggested by population studies. Conversely, if HLA-DR3 or -DR4 (or the putative DQ antigen) were present, then the system could be activated. Presumably susceptibility is linked to the fit between newly appearing class II molecules, the requisite membrane antigen (foreign or autologous), and a particular form of the T-cell receptor on the helper T cell. This may account for the appearance of IDDM in the absence of high-risk HLA genes; i.e., in certain cases the class II molecule–T-cell receptor fit occurs even with an ordinarily low-risk allele.

As is true in other immune-mediated endocrinopathies, evidence of an activated immune system may disappear with time. Thus, the islet cell antibodies present in newly diagnosed patients with type 1 IDDM disappear within a year or so. The presence of islet cell antibodies correlates with residual beta-cell mass as assessed in vivo by the capacity to release endogenous insulin in response to a fuel stimulus. As the capacity for endogenous insulin secretion disappears, so do islet cell antibodies. The implication is that as beta cells die, the stimulus to the immune response disappears.

Destruction of beta cells and development of IDDM Because persons developing insulin-dependent diabetes often have a rather abrupt onset of symptomatic hyperglycemia with polyuria and/or ketoacidosis, it was long assumed that beta-cell damage occurred rapidly. In many cases (most?) there may be a slow loss of insulin reserve over many years. This insight came from studies of discordant monozygotic diabetic twins and triplets where one twin or triplet developed diabetes many years after the index case. In the slow course the earliest sign of abnormality is the development of islet cell antibodies at a time when there is no elevation of the blood sugar and glucose tolerance is normal. Insulin responses to a glucose load are intact. A phase then ensues in which the only metabolic abnormality is decreased glucose tolerance. Fasting blood sugar remains normal. In the third stage fasting hyperglycemia develops, but ketosis does not occur even when the diabetes is poorly controlled. The clinical appearance is that of non-insulin-dependent diabetes mellitus. With time, however, insulin dependence and ketoacidosis may develop, especially with stress. Many nonobese patients with non-insulin-dependent diabetes mellitus may have a slow autoimmune form of the disease as mentioned earlier.

The immune-directed destruction of beta cells probably involves both humoral and cell-mediated mechanisms. Initially, antibodies are probably dominant. Two types of antibodies have been identified: cytoplasmic and surface. Usually both are present simultaneously in a given patient, but either can occur alone. Islet cell surface antibodies have the capacity to fix complement and lyse beta cells. Surface antibodies appear to impair insulin release even before the beta cell is physically damaged. They interact with a membrane antigen that has not been precisely characterized. At some point in the course cytotoxic T lymphocytes and antibody-dependent killer T cells participate in and complete the destructive process. By the time overt diabetes appears, most insulin-producing cells have disappeared. In one study pancreatic mass at autopsy averaged 40 g in type 1 diabetes versus 82 g in controls. Endocrine cell mass in subjects with IDDM decreased from 1395 to 413 mg, and beta cells, which averaged 850 mg in normals, were unmeasurable. Since alpha cells remained essentially intact, the ratio of glucagon- to insulin-producing cells approached infinity.

PATHOGENESIS OF TYPE 2 NON-INSULIN-DEPENDENT DIABETES Little progress has been made in understanding the pathogenesis of non-insulin-dependent diabetes mellitus. Although the disease runs in families, modes of inheritance are not known except for the variant known as *maturity-onset diabetes of the young* (MODY). This disease is manifested by mild hyperglycemia in young persons who are resistant to ketosis. Four lines of evidence suggest transmission as an autosomal dominant trait. First, three-generation direct transmission has been demonstrated in over 20 families. Second, a 1:1 ratio of diabetic to nondiabetic children is found when one parent has the disease. Third, about 90 percent of obligate carriers have diabetes. Fourth, direct male-to-male transmission excludes X-linked inheritance.

No HLA relationship has been identified in type 2 NIDDM, and autoimmune mechanisms are not believed to be operative. The 5′ flanking region of the structural gene for insulin, located on the short arm of the eleventh chromosome, is polymorphic in regard to varying number and arrangement of tandemly repeated nucleotides beginning some 363 base pairs before the transcription site (see Chap. 58). It was initially thought that homozygosity for a long insert (>1500 base pairs) correlated with the presence of type 2 NIDDM, but subsequent studies failed to confirm a unique relationship. Alcohol-induced flushing after priming with chlorpropamide has also been suggested as a genetic marker for certain forms of the type 2 illness. Whatever its nature, the genetic influence is powerful, since the concordance rate for diabetes in monozygotic twins with type 2 disease approaches 100 percent. It is likewise thought that risk to offspring and siblings of patients with NIDDM is higher than the risk in type 1 diabetes.

Patients with type 2 NIDDM have two physiologic defects: abnormal insulin secretion and resistance to insulin action in target tissues. The primacy of the secretory defect versus the insulin resistance is not established. Most patients with type 2 diabetes are obese, often massively so, and it has been speculated that obesity-induced insulin resistance leads to exhaustion of the beta cell; i.e., the secretory defect is secondary. On the other hand, many massively obese patients do not have diabetes or glucose intolerance, suggesting that obesity does not lead to diabetes in the presence of normal beta-cell responsiveness. The picture is further complicated by the observations that hyperglycemia per se may induce a beta-cell secretory defect and that relative insulin deficiency can cause insulin resistance. A period of aggressive dietary or insulin therapy leading to return of the blood sugar to normal may partially restore insulin secretory capacity as well as sensitivity to insulin action. Unfortunately this does not help in deciding primacy between a secretory defect and insulin resistance. The author favors the view that an islet cell abnormality is primary and necessary for development of diabetes but that acquired insulin resistance, usually obesity-related, is required for overt hyperglycemia to develop. This view is consistent with the observation that beta-cell mass is intact in type 2 NIDDM, in contrast to the situation with type 1 IDDM.

Although insulin resistance in type 2 NIDDM is associated with decreased numbers of insulin receptors, the bulk of the resistance is postreceptor in type. If experiments in animals apply to humans, the postreceptor defect is likely due to a deficiency of microsome-bound glucose transport units. These units, which facilitate diffusion of glucose across the plasma membrane, are normally rapidly mobilized when insulin binds to its receptor on the plasma membrane. Intracellular stores of the transporter are depleted in rats with either obesity or experimental diabetes and can be restored by weight loss and insulin therapy, respectively.

A rare form of type 2 NIDDM, clinically mild, is due to production of an abnormal insulin that does not bind well to insulin receptors. Such persons respond normally to exogenous insulin.

CLINICAL FEATURES The manifestations of symptomatic diabetes mellitus vary from patient to patient. Most often medical help is sought because of symptoms related to hyperglycemia (polyuria, polydipsia, polyphagia), but the first event may be an acute metabolic decompensation resulting in diabetic coma. Occasionally, the initial expression is a degenerative complication such as neuropathy in the absence of symptomatic hyperglycemia. The metabolic derangements of diabetes are due to a relative or absolute deficiency of insulin and a relative or absolute excess of glucagon. Normally it is a rise in the molar ratio of glucagon to insulin that leads to metabolic decompensation. Changes in this ratio can be caused by a fall in insulin or a rise in glucagon concentration, separately or together. Conceptually alteration in biologic response to either hormone would have the same effect. Thus insulin resistance could cause metabolic effects expected of an elevated glucagon:insulin ratio even though the ratio assessed by immunoassay of the two hormones in plasma was not markedly abnormal or even decreased (the glucagon being biologically active, the insulin relatively inactive). The relationship between metabolic abnormalities and degenerative complications will be discussed subsequently. Typically, the clinical features of IDDM and NIDDM are distinctive.

TABLE 327-3 General characteristics of IDDM and NIDDM diabetes

	IDDM	NIDDM
Genetic locus	Chromosome 6	Chromosome 11 (?)
Age of onset	< 40	> 40
Body habitus	Normal to wasted	Obese
Plasma insulin	Low to absent	Normal to high
Plasma glucagon	High, suppressible	High, resistant
Acute complication	Ketoacidosis	Hyperosmolar coma
Insulin therapy	Responsive	Responsive to resistant
Sulfonylurea therapy	Unresponsive	Responsive

Insulin-dependent diabetes Insulin-dependent diabetes usually begins before the age of 40; in the United States peak incidence is around age 14. Onset of symptoms may be abrupt, with thirst, excessive urination, increased appetite, and weight loss developing over a several-day period. In some cases the disease is heralded by the appearance of ketoacidosis during an intercurrent illness or following surgery. As outlined in Table 327-3, type 1 patients vary from normal weight to wasted, depending on the length of time between onset of symptoms and start of treatment. Characteristically the plasma insulin is low or immeasurable. Glucagon levels are elevated but suppressible with insulin. Once symptoms have developed, insulin therapy is required. Occasionally an initial episode of ketoacidosis is followed by a symptom-free interval (the "honeymoon" period) during which no treatment is required. The likely explanation for this phenomenon is shown in Fig. 327-2.

Non-insulin-dependent diabetes This disorder usually begins in middle life or beyond. The typical patient is overweight. Symptoms begin more gradually than in IDDM, and the diagnosis is frequently made when an asymptomatic person is found to have an elevated plasma glucose on routine laboratory examination. In contrast to insulin-dependent disease, plasma insulin levels are normal to high in absolute terms, although they are lower than predicted for the level of the plasma glucose; i.e., relative insulin deficiency is present. Stated in another way, if plasma glucose concentrations in nondiabetic subjects were raised to levels equivalent to those found in diabetic patients, insulin values would be higher in the normal group. This reflects the previously mentioned insulin secretory defect in NIDDM. Glucagon metabolism in non-insulin-dependent diabetes is complex. While the elevated fasting plasma concentrations can be lowered by large amounts of insulin, the exaggerated glucagon response to

FIGURE 327-2 *Schematic representation of the "honeymoon" period. In this graph insulin secretory capacity is shown gradually decreasing in a patient destined to develop diabetes. At approximately 13½ years insulin would become insufficient to maintain plasma glucose in the normal range. An initial episode of ketoacidosis, for example, in association with acute appendicitis, is shown occurring in the twelfth year. Presumably stress-induced epinephrine release blocks insulin secretion and causes the syndrome. In normal subjects insulin reserve is such that hormone release is adequate, even in the face of stress. Following recovery from the stressful episode insulin secretory capacity returns to the previous level and remains sufficient for an additional year as indicated by the shaded area—the "honeymoon" period.*

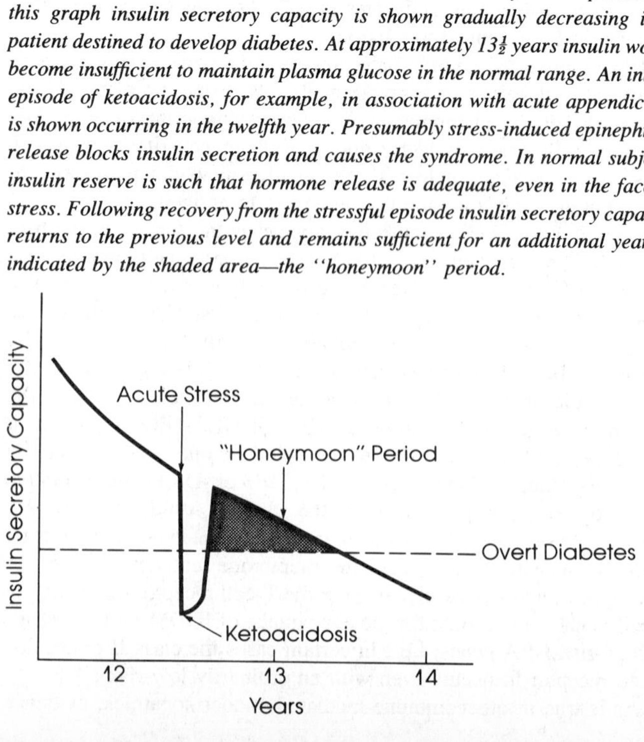

ingested nutrients cannot be suppressed; i.e., alpha-cell function remains abnormal. For unknown reasons non-insulin-dependent diabetics do not develop ketoacidosis. In the decompensated state they are susceptible to the syndrome of hyperosmolar, nonketotic coma. One hypothesis to explain the absence of ketoacidosis during stress is that the liver is resistant to glucagon so that malonyl-CoA levels remain high, inhibiting the fatty acid oxidation–ketogenic pathway (see below). If weight loss can be induced, patients may be managed by diet alone. The majority of patients failing dietary therapy respond to sulfonylureas, but improvement of hyperglycemia in many is not sufficient for control of diabetes. For this reason a high percentage of patients with NIDDM are treated with insulin.

TREATMENT Diet An estimate is made of the total number of calories needed per day based on ideal body weight (determined from life insurance tables). A decision is then made regarding carbohydrate, fat, and protein content, and an appropriate diet is constructed from the exchange system provided by the American Diabetes Association. Caloric recommendations from the Food and Nutrition Board for adults carrying out "average" activity decrease with age and range from 42 kcal per kilogram of body weight in 18-year-old men to 33 kcal per kilogram for 75-year-old women. Intakes slightly less than official recommendations are usually preferable; 36 kcal per kilogram for men and 34 kcal per kilogram for women are reasonable initial values in most patients, but upward or downward adjustments may be necessary to achieve desired weight.

The minimal protein requirement for good nutrition is about 0.9 g per kilogram of body weight per day. Recommended carbohydrate content is 40 to 60 percent of total calories, although fractional intakes as high as 85 percent have been prescribed. Protein and carbohydrate calories are supplemented with sufficient fat to bring caloric intake to the desired level. Although sucrose is ordinarily not allowed in diabetic diets, a number of reports indicate that in moderation ordinary sugar does not exaggerate postprandial hyperglycemia. Currently most diabetic diets emphasize polyunsaturated fats as an antiatherogenic measure. Increased amounts of fiber are also often prescribed.

Once the desirable caloric intake and the fractional distribution between fat, protein, and carbohydrate are decided, a diet is constructed using the exchange lists shown in Table 327-4.[2] For example, a 2200-kcal diet with 50 percent of the calories as carbohydrate and 1 to 1.5 g protein per kilogram of body weight can be met by providing 2 milk exchanges, 7 fruit exchanges, 12 bread exchanges, 8 meat exchanges, 4 fat exchanges, and unlimited type A vegetables (Table 327-5). In practice, precalculated diets of given caloric content prepared by the American Diabetes Association are usually used. Care must be taken to emphasize foods the patient likes and can obtain. Initially it is helpful to weigh and measure foods until visual estimates can be made accurately. As in any dietary regimen it is important to emphasize that it is the long-term, overall dietary pattern which counts. Deviation for one meal or two meals does not matter much. Thus a teenage diabetic may be allowed to eat a dessert, ordinarily forbidden, as a special treat with the understanding that resumption of the diet will be necessary the next day. Even in adults the "treat" technique often ensures better dietary cooperation than more rigid demands. Ideally patients should be trained by dieticians in a formal teaching program. Such classes are available in most large hospitals. If a patient is from a smaller community, it will probably be helpful to refer to a larger center for initial training.

In insulin-requiring diabetics the distribution of calories is also important if hypoglycemia is to be avoided. A typical pattern might include 20 percent of the total calories for breakfast, 35 percent for lunch, 30 percent for dinner, and 15 percent as a late-evening feeding. Occasionally a midafternoon snack is necessary. Different distributions may be required for different lifestyles; i.e., a person employed on a late-evening or night shift would not eat the major meal at noon.

The traditional approach to dietary therapy has come under question as a result of experiments designed to measure actual blood sugar responses to ingested foods. It is now clear that the exchanges are not necessarily equivalent; i.e., foods of the same weight and similar fat, carbohydrate, or protein content may result in different postprandial increases in the plasma glucose. The term *glycemic index* has been coined to express these differences. In calculating a glycemic index the mean plasma glucose is measured over a 2- to 3-h period after ingestion of a test food and compared to the response with a reference standard of defined composition such as bread. Although in principle the approach is attractive because it measures actual glycemic response to foods, its applicability to the general diabetic population is not established. Many foods and combinations must be tested before diets based on glycemic indexes can be compared to standard exchange-based diets under ordinary conditions.

The importance of diet in the management of diabetes varies with type of disease. In insulin-dependent patients, particularly those on intensive insulin regimens, the composition of the diet is not of critical importance since adjustment of insulin can cover wide variations in food ingestion. In non-insulin-dependent patients not treated with exogenous insulin more rigorous adherence to a fixed diet is required since endogenous insulin reserve is limited. Such patients cannot respond to increased demand produced by excess calories or increased intake of rapidly absorbed carbohydrate. Thus diet is of primary importance in non-insulin-dependent subjects.

Insulin Insulin is required for treatment of all type 1 patients and many patients with non-insulin-dependent disease. If the physician does not use oral agents (see below), all diet-unresponsive NIDDM subjects must be given the hormone. It is fairly easy to control the symptoms of diabetes with insulin, but it is difficult to maintain a normal blood sugar throughout 24 h even if one utilizes multiple injections of regular insulin or infusion pumps. It is even more difficult to maintain normal blood sugars utilizing traditional insulin therapy given as one or two injections a day. Nondiabetic subjects maintain the plasma glucose concentration within a narrow range at all times despite episodic food intake. When a meal is eaten, a prompt rise in insulin release occurs such that absorbed carbohydrate is rapidly transported into the liver and other tissues. Even after meals, therefore, the plasma glucose in normal subjects does not rise into the hyperglycemic or glycosuric range. As the plasma glucose

[2] *Copies of* Exchange Lists for Meal Planning *may be ordered from the American Diabetes Association, National Service Center, 1660 Duke Street, P.O. Box 25757, Alexandria, VA 22313, or from any local affiliate of the association.*

TABLE 327-4 Composition of food exchanges*

Exchange	Calories	Carbohydrate, g	Fat, g	Protein, g
Milk	170	12	10	8
Vegetable†	35	7	—	2
Fruit	40	10	—	—
Bread	70‡	15	—	2
Meat	75‡	—	5	7
Fat	45	—	5	—

* *Composition listed for one exchange.*
† *Type A vegetables contain little carbohydrate, fat, or protein and can be eaten in any amount. Exchange values are for type B vegetables.*
‡ *Calculated value for bread exchange is 68 cal and for meat exchange is 73 cal using 4 kcal/g for carbohydrate and protein and 9 kcal/g for fat. The values 70 and 75 cal were adapted to facilitate computations.*

TABLE 327-5 A 2200-cal diabetic diet (50 percent carbohydrate)

Exchange	No.	Calories	Carbohydrate, g	Fat, g	Protein, g
Milk	2	340	24	20	16
Vegetable*		Unlimited amounts of type A vegetables			
Fruit	7	280	70	—	—
Bread	12	840	180	—	24
Meat	8	600	—	40	56
Fat	4	180	—	20	—
Total		2240	274 (50%)	80 (33%)	96 (17%)

* *Type B vegetables include beets, carrots, onions, green peas, pumpkin, rutabagas, winter squash, and turnips. If these are desired, ½ to 1 cup can be substituted for one fruit exchange. All other common vegetables can be eaten as desired.*

falls under the influence of insulin, release of the hormone is damped, and counterregulatory hormones enter the circulation to prevent hypoglycemia, ensuring smooth control of plasma glucose throughout the absorptive process. The diabetic treated with insulin by injection cannot reproduce these physiologic responses. If enough insulin is given to keep the postprandial glucose normal, inevitably too much insulin will be present during the postabsorptive phase and hypoglycemia will result. The same problem exists when insulin infusion pumps or multiple injections of insulin are utilized in an attempt to control diabetes tightly.

Because evidence suggests that some of the complications of diabetes may be prevented or partially reversed by maintenance of normal or near normal plasma glucose concentrations throughout the day, aggressive insulin therapy is frequently prescribed despite these difficulties. Three treatment regimens will be described: conventional, multiple subcutaneous injections (MSI), and continuous subcutaneous insulin infusion (CSII). *Conventional insulin therapy* involves the administration of one or two injections a day of intermediate acting insulin such as zinc insulin (lente insulin) or isophane insulin (NPH insulin) with or without the addition of small amounts of regular insulin. If the newly diagnosed diabetic is not in acute distress, therapy can be started as an outpatient, provided instruction in diet and insulin use and monitoring are adequate, and the physician can be reached by telephone for consultation. Adults of normal weight may be started on 15 to 20 units a day (the estimated daily insulin production rate in nondiabetic subjects of normal size is about 25 units a day). Obese patients, because of insulin resistance, may be started on 25 to 30 units a day. It is preferable to use the same quantity of insulin for several days before changing, the one exception being the hypoglycemic patient, for whom the dose should be immediately decreased unless a nonrecurrent cause of hypoglycemia (such as excessive exercise) is present. Generally changes should be no more than 5 or 10 units per step. It is probable that a single injection of insulin provides adequate control only in patients who have some residual capacity for insulin secretion. Poorly controlled patients should be placed on split therapy with about two-thirds of the total insulin given before breakfast and the remainder before supper. Two injections are almost always used when the total dose reaches 50 or 60 units a day but may be helpful at smaller doses as well since the peak action of intermediate insulins appears to be dose-related; i.e., a low dose may exhibit maximal activity earlier and disappear sooner than a large dose. Many physicians routinely add regular insulin to the intermediate dose even at initiation of therapy. Thus in a single-dose schedule one might begin with 20 units of intermediate and 5 units of regular insulin rather than 25 units of intermediate alone. This practice is based upon the concept that the regular insulin lowers the plasma glucose rapidly after which the more slowly absorbed insulin maintains the lowered level. Most patients on twice-daily insulin injections are also treated with a mixture of intermediate and regular insulin; e.g., 25 units NPH plus 10 units of regular before breakfast and 10 units of NPH plus 5 units of regular before supper. All patients should be taught to decrease insulin when significant extra activity or exercise is anticipated. The proper decrement must be determined by trial and error, although a reduction of 5 to 10 units is a reasonable first step. The blood glucose–lowering effect of excercise is primarily due to increased energy demands in previously non-contracting muscle; enhanced absorption of insulin from depot sites secondary to increased blood flow plays a minor role. Conversely a small amount of extra regular insulin can be taken before a meal that contains extra calories or food ordinarily not allowed (e.g., when the diabetic must eat out at a banquet or the teenager goes out on a date). For patients willing to self-monitor plasma glucose an algorithm for adjusting insulin can be provided. A typical protocol is shown in Table 327-6. Patients with complicated control problems may require hospitalization, where frequent plasma glucose determinations can guide therapy.

The *multiple subcutaneous insulin injection technique* most commonly involves administration of intermediate or long-acting insulin in the evening as a single dose together with regular insulin prior to each meal. Home glucose monitoring by the patient is necessary if the goal is the return of the plasma glucose to normal. One approach to initiation of therapy involves administration of 25 percent of the previous daily insulin dose in the patient's conventional regimen at bedtime as intermediate insulin (NPH or lente) with the other 75 percent given as regular insulin divided such that 40, 30, and 30 percent is given 30 min before breakfast, lunch, and supper, respectively. Alternatively, a three-injection schedule can be designated by omitting the night intermediate insulin and giving a long-acting insulin, such as insulin zinc extended (ultralente insulin) or protamine zinc insulin (PZI insulin), before the evening meal. Adjustments of dosage depend on response of the plasma glucose. A number of different protocols have been utilized, all of which represent sliding scales of insulin based on the plasma glucose. A typical schedule based on home monitoring of plasma glucose is shown in Table 327-7. Individual patients may require different dosages. For specific details the reader should consult one of the published papers utilizing the technique (e.g., Schriffrin and Belmont or the monograph by Schade et al.). MSI can be effective in controlling the plasma glucose and in some studies appears to match goals achieved with CSII.

Continuous subcutaneous insulin infusion involves use of a small battery-driven pump that delivers insulin subcutaneously into the abdominal wall, usually through a 27-gauge butterfly needle. With CSII insulin is delivered at a basal rate continuously throughout the day with increased rates programmed prior to meals. Adjustments in dosage are made in response to measured capillary glucose values in a fashion similar to that used in MSI. Ordinarily about 40 percent of

TABLE 327-6 Adjusting insulin dosage in conventional insulin therapy*

	Regular insulin, units	
Blood sugar, mg/dL	Breakfast (to be mixed with intermediate dosage)	Supper
51–100	8	4
101–150	10	5
151–200	12	6
201–250	14	7
251–300	16	8
>300	20	10

* *Once the patient has most blood sugars in the reasonable range (60–200 mg/dL), a prescription can be written for varying the regular insulin dosage as illustrated. The prescription in this case was for a patient in reasonable control on 25 units of NPH plus 10 units of regular before breakfast and 10 units of NPH plus 5 units of regular before supper. Change in metabolic status may require adjustments in both intermediate insulin and the sliding scale of regular insulin.*

TABLE 327-7 Adjusting insulin dosage in a multiple-injection schedule*

I Initiation of therapy
- *A* 0.6 to 0.7 units insulin per kilogram body weight
- *B* 25% NPH at 9 P.M.; 75% regular in divided doses (40% before breakfast, 30% before lunch, 30% before supper)
- *C* Adjust NPH every 48 h based on fasting blood glucose
  - <60 mg/dL − 2 units
  - >90 mg/dL + 2 units
- *D* Adjust regular insulin every 48 h based on 1-h postprandial glucose
  - < 60 mg/dL − 2 units
  - >140 mg/dL + 2 units

II Daily therapy

Preprandial glucose, mg/dL	Regular insulin, units
<60	−2
61–90	No change
91–120	+1
121–150	+2
151–200	+3
201–250	+4
>250	+6

* *With initiation of therapy insulin dosage is changed until target range is reached (see Table 327-8). After initial stabilization a variable insulin schedule is prescribed to maintain tight control. For example, if the patient after initiation is found to generally require 12 units of regular insulin before breakfast but has a prebreakfast blood sugar of 160 mg/dL, 15 units of regular insulin instead of the usual 12 would be taken.*

SOURCE: *Adapted from Schiffrin and Belmonte.*

the total daily dose is given at the basal rate, the remainder being administered as preprandial boluses. There is little question that CSII can improve diabetic control relative to conventional therapy. Most patients report positive feelings of well-being as control improves. Nevertheless, although insulin infusion pumps have caught the attention of the public and many physicians, they should not be used indiscriminately. The danger of hypoglycemia is real, especially during the night in patients who maintain the plasma glucose consistently below 100 mg/dL. A fall in plasma glucose of 50 mg/dL may not be important if the starting value is 150 mg/dL but may be fatal if it occurs against a steady-state level of 60 mg/dL. Several deaths from hypoglycemia have occurred in pump users. In the author's opinion pumps should be prescribed only in highly disciplined and motivated patients who are followed by physicians with extensive experience in their use. Apart from problems of hypoglycemia, local insulin reactions and abscess formation may occur.

In one or two centers catheters for the insulin infusion pumps have been placed intravenously rather than subcutaneously. While few difficulties have been reported, this procedure appears unwise for routine use. Intraabdominal insulin pumps with reservoirs refillable from outside the body have been tried on experimental protocols. At present no advantage is apparent except that a pump does not have to be worn externally.

Who should be recommended for meticulous control utilizing either MSI or CSII? There are only two absolute indications: pregnancy and renal transplantation. Maintenance of a normal plasma glucose during pregnancy prevents fetal macrosomy and respiratory distress and lowers perinatal mortality. Unfortunately, congenital malformations due to diabetes cannot be prevented by control of the blood sugar after conception occurs. This means that maximal safety for the fetus can only be provided by meticulous treatment of diabetes *prior* to impregnation. Routine treatment of diabetes in pregnancy is not an option, and aggressive treatment should be started at the time pregnancy is planned. Inclusion of patients with renal transplants in the nonoptional category follows from the fact that diabetic nephropathy develops early in normal transplanted kidneys. The hope is that with improved metabolic control the acquired lesions can be slowed or prevented.

Meticulous control is an option for most other patients with insulin-dependent diabetes. Since the treatment schedules require much effort on the part of the patient, reliability and willingness to accept responsibility for self-care must be assessed ahead of time. Glucose monitoring is not inexpensive, and the financial status of the patient also has to be considered. Even if meticulous control does not achieve the goal of preventing late complications, in properly chosen patients it seems worthwhile in and of itself both because patients generally feel better when metabolically normal and because attention to clinical detail provides a sense of self-sufficiency and independence that is otherwise easily lost in diabetes. Meticulous control is rarely appropriate for patients whose life expectancy is shortened because of age, cardiovascular, cerebrovascular, or diabetic complications.

For surgical procedures in diabetic patients, intermediate insulin is omitted, and treatment is carried out with regular insulin alone. An effective method is to add 10 to 20 units of insulin to a liter of 5% glucose in water with infusion at a rate of 100 to 150 mL/h. Measurements of plasma glucose in capillary blood allows change of rate to avoid significant hypo- or hyperglycemia. It is also possible to administer 10 units of regular insulin subcutaneously and infuse 5 or 10% glucose at rates sufficient to avoid major changes in glucose concentration.

Types of insulin A variety of insulins are available for use in the treatment of diabetes. Rapidly acting preparations are used in diabetic emergencies and in CSII and MSI programs. Intermediate preparations are used in conventional and MSI regimens. As noted, long-acting formulations are used in three-injection MSI schedules. Peak effects and duration vary from patient to patient and depend not only on route of administration but on dose. Hypoglycemic effects in insulin-treated diabetics appear to be delayed relative to normal subjects, probably because of the presence of anti-insulin antibodies in plasma. In one study in diabetics, regular insulin given subcutaneously had its onset of action at about 1 h, reached a peak at 6 h, and had measurable effects on average for 16 h, whereas in normal persons onset is within minutes, maximal action is around 2 h, and duration is only 6 to 8 h. With NPH insulin, diabetics exhibited an onset of action at 2.5 h, a peak at 11 h, and a total period of action of 25 h, more closely approximating values in normal subjects.

Commercial insulins are prepared in concentrations of 100 units per milliliter (U100) although higher concentrations can be obtained (e.g., U500). All commercial insulins are now "purified," meaning that they have a contamination with proinsulin <10 parts per million. Some preparations contain as little as 1 part per million. Animal insulins (beef, pork) are still in wide use, but insulin identical to the human molecule is now available. The advantages of purified animal insulins and "human" insulin are that insulin allergy, fat atrophy, and fat hypertrophy occur less frequently than with the older preparations. It is possible that anti-insulin antibody (IgG) formation is slightly less with the "human" hormone. Given equivalent price structure it is appropriate to prescribe "human" insulin routinely. As stated above, the various insulins are available as rapid, intermediate, and long-acting preparations, although not all manufacturers offer all varieties. Lente and NPH insulin are used in most conventional therapy and are roughly equivalent in biologic effects, although lente appears to be slightly more immunogenic and to mix less well with regular insulin than does NPH.

Self-glucose monitoring For many years effectiveness of treatment for diabetes was followed by reviewing symptoms (such as frequency of nocturia) and measurement of glucose in the urine by semiquantitative techniques. Since the renal threshold for glucose in normal persons is in the range of 180 to 200 mg/dL plasma glucose and may increase with the appearance of renal disease, assessment of glycosuria is of little value if the goal of therapy is to maintain the plasma glucose near normal. In consequence most insulin-requiring patients now monitor control and alter therapy based on self-measurement of the capillary blood sugar. In addition to the fact that such measurements are necessary in all treatment schedules utilizing variable insulin dosage the ability to assess the blood glucose as needed has other positive benefits. It bestows a sense of confidence and independence in the patient, has a reinforcing effect on therapeutic goals (for example, the effect of dietary indiscretion can be immediately seen), serves to give early warning of incipient hypoglycemia, and allows documentation of hypoglycemia when suggestive symptoms are present.

Although blood glucose can be estimated visually utilizing reagent strips, it is generally preferable to use an instrument for readings. This is because it is difficult for many patients to extrapolate accurately between the color changes and because subjective wishes may influence the extrapolation. It is harder to ignore a number appearing in a machine. A variety of glucose analyzers are available. The system chosen should be "dry" (i.e., not require washing of the reagent strip). In general, the cost of a machine, spring-driven lancet holder, and lancets is less than $200, and many insurance carriers reimburse for the purchase. The patient needs to have supervised training in the technique, and simultaneous checks of the blood sugar in a laboratory should be done periodically to test accuracy of the self-analysis. Repeated studies show that patients can measure blood glucose accurately using these techniques.

Although urine testing for glucose is now rarely used to follow diabetes, the measurement of ketones in the urine remains important.

Goals of therapy Target levels for glucose control vary amongst diabetologists. The schedule shown in Table 327-8 lists the ranges considered acceptable and ideal by the author. The "acceptable" category would apply in conventional therapy utilizing a two-dose schedule of intermediate and regular insulin. The upper limit of 200 mg/dL postprandially is arbitrary but is based on the finding in the

Pima Indian population that complications of diabetes are rare if the 2-h value in the oral glucose tolerance test is less than 200 mg/dL. The "ideal" column represents values targeted in meticulous control regimens. Although some authors are more stringent and prefer the 1-h postprandial value to be no more than 140 mg/dL, the risk of hypoglycemia is greater under these circumstances. In general avoidance of serious hypoglycemia is more important than avoidance of hyperglycemia because the former has immediate consequences that may threaten the life of the patient or others (e.g., through an automobile accident) while the detrimental effects of hyperglycemia are long-term and less certain.

Hypoglycemia, the Somogyi effect, and the dawn phenomenon (see also Chap. 329) The problem of hypoglycemia is common in insulin-dependent diabetics, particularly when aggressive efforts are made to keep both the fasting plasma glucose and postprandial hyperglycemia within the normal range. Hypoglycemia may be caused by missing a meal or doing unexpected exercise but can occur in the absence of known precipitating events. Daytime episodes of hypoglycemia are usually recognized by adrenergic symptoms, such as sweating, nervousness, tremor, and hunger. Hypoglycemia during sleep may produce no symptoms or cause night sweats, unpleasant dreams, and early-morning headache. In one study of insulin-dependent diabetic children monitored throughout 24 h, 18 percent had asymptomatic nocturnal hypoglycemia. If hypoglycemia is not aborted by the countercurrent regulatory mechanisms or by ingestion of carbohydrate, central nervous system symptoms ensue: confusion, abnormal behavior, loss of consciousness, or convulsions. As diabetes progresses, particularly with the development of neuropathy, epinephrine-induced symptoms may become blunted and lose their effectiveness as warning signals, with the consequence that central nervous system signs predominate. Up to 7 percent of deaths in insulin-dependent diabetic subjects have been attributed to hypoglycemia.

Protection against hypoglycemia is normally provided by two mechanisms as plasma glucose concentrations fall: cessation of insulin release and mobilization of counterregulatory hormones. The latter act to increase hepatic glucose production and decrease glucose utilization in nonhepatic tissues. Glucagon is the primary counterregulatory hormone, and epinephrine (and norepinephrine released from the sympathetic nervous system) serves as the major backup. Epinephrine is not required for maintenance of the plasma glucose provided glucagon is available but becomes critical in its absence. Cortisol and growth hormone do not function acutely but come into play with prolonged fasting or sustained hypoglycemia. Diabetic patients are vulnerable to hypoglycemia because of both insulin excess and counterregulatory failure. Since insulin is given by injection or infusion, the capacity to decrease plasma concentrations of the hormone as glucose levels fall is not available. Very early on the diabetic subject with type 1 insulin-dependent disease loses the capacity to increase glucagon release in response to hypoglycemia. Protection is thus dependent on epinephrine. Unfortunately, many patients also lose the capacity to secrete epinephrine in response to hypoglycemia. In most circumstances the epinephrine deficiency is probably due to diabetic autonomic neuropathy, but the defect may occur in the absence of clinically demonstrable nerve dysfunction. Failure of catecholamine release is usually a late event in diabetes but can occur early. It is thought that beta-adrenergic blocking agents have the same effects as deficiencies of epinephrine, although a prospective clinical trial on the dangers of such agents in producing hypoglycemia under real life circumstances has not been carried out.

TABLE 327-8 Goals for blood glucose in the control of diabetes*

Goal	Acceptable, mg/dL	Ideal, mg/dL
Fasting	60–130	70–100
Preprandial	60–130	70–100
Postprandial (1 h)	<200	<160
3 A.M.	> 65	> 65

* *Values for healthy patients below the age of 65. Goals my be shifted upward in older patients.*

Counterregulatory hormone failure is of particular significance when intensive insulin therapy is prescribed. The incidence of hypoglycemia is inversely related to the mean level of plasma glucose. Unfortunately there is no easy way to predict the occurrence of clinically significant counterregulatory failure. Experimentally an insulin infusion test can be used for this purpose but is probably not practical for routine use. In this test neuroglycopenic symptoms or delay in return of plasma glucose from nadir after infusion of a standard amount of insulin are utilized to identify defects in the response system. Perhaps the best clue to counterregulatory failure is the presence of frequent hypoglycemia not explicable by change in diet or exercise. Of additional concern are reports that intensive insulin therapy (meticulous control) may itself produce abnormal glucose counterregulation.

An important question is whether hypoglycemic symptoms can occur in the absence of low plasma glucose levels, for example, in response to a rapid fall in glucose concentrations. While this question cannot be answered with certainty, the evidence suggests that neither rate nor magnitude of the fall signals counterregulatory release, only a low plasma glucose. Although the triggering level of plasma glucose may vary from patient to patient, counterregulatory hormone release is not induced at normal or elevated levels of glucose. Adrenergic symptoms occurring in the presence of hyperglycemia are likely due to anxiety or cardiovascular mechanisms.

Hypoglycemia can occur in diabetic patients consequent to other mechanisms. Diabetic renal disease is not infrequently accompanied by diminished insulin requirements and may lead to frank hypoglycemia if adjustments in dosage are not made. The mechanism is not known. Although half-times for insulin in plasma are increased in diabetic nephropathy, other factors doubtless play a role.

Hypoglycemia may be due to the development of autoimmune adrenal insufficiency as part of the Schmidt syndrome (see Chap. 334), which is more frequent in diabetics than in the population as a whole. Some patients develop hypoglycemia in association with high levels of circulating insulin antibodies. The exact mechanism has not been established. Occasionally an insulinoma may develop in a diabetic patient. Very rarely, permanent remission of apparently typical diabetes occurs. The reason is not known, but the initial sign may be frequent hypoglycemia in a previously well controlled patient.

It must be emphasized that hypoglycemic attacks are dangerous and if frequent portend a serious or even fatal outcome.

The *Somogyi phenomenon* refers to rebound hyperglycemia following an episode of hypoglycemia due to counterregulatory hormone release. It should be suspected whenever wide swings in the plasma glucose occur over short time intervals even if symptoms are not reported. Such rapid changes contrast with the alterations seen following insulin withdrawal in previously well-controlled diabetic patients in whom hyperglycemia and ketosis develop gradually and smoothly over a 12- to 24-h period. Excessive hunger and weight gain occurring in the context of worsening hyperglycemia are clues that the insulin dosage may be too high, since poor control due to underinsulinization usually results in weight loss (because of osmotic diuresis and glucose wastage). If the Somogyi phenomenon is suspected, the insulin dose should be decreased as a trial, even when specific symptoms of overinsulinization are absent. The Somogyi phenomenon probably occurs less frequently in patients utilizing insulin infusion pumps than in those treated by conventional or multiple injections of insulin as a bolus.

The *dawn phenomenon* refers to an early morning rise in plasma glucose requiring increased amounts of insulin to maintain euglycemia. Although similar early morning hyperglycemia may result from hypoglycemia, as just described, the dawn phenomenon itself is thought to be independent of the Somogyi mechanism. The nocturnal surge of growth hormone release is thought to be a major factor. Increased clearance of insulin also occurs in the early morning hours, but the changes are probably not of major importance. Differentiation between the dawn phenomenon and posthypoglycemic hyperglycemia can usually be accomplished by measuring the blood glucose at 3 A.M. This is important since the Somogyi phenomenon is avoided by decreasing insulin dosages for the critical time period while the dawn phenomenon usually requires increased insulin to maintain glucose in the normal range.

Oral agents Non-insulin-dependent diabetes that cannot be controlled by dietary management often responds to sulfonylureas. The drugs are easy to use and appear to be safe. Fear that sulfonylureas might increase deaths from heart attacks, prompted by reports of the University Group Diabetes Program (UGDP), has largely dissipated because of questions about the design of that study. On the other hand use of the oral drugs has decreased concomitant with the emphasis on better control as a possible means of slowing the development of late complications. While some patients with relatively mild disease have return of plasma glucose to normal on oral drugs, those with significant hyperglycemia tend to improve but do not approach the normal range. Thus a high percentage of non-insulin-dependent diabetics are now treated with insulin.

Sulfonylureas act primarily by stimulating release of insulin from the beta cell. They have the capacity to increase the number of insulin receptors in target tissues, but also enhance insulin-mediated glucose disposal independent of an increase in insulin binding. Since mean levels of plasma insulin do not increase following treatment with sulfonylureas despite significantly improved mean plasma glucose concentrations, extrapancreatic effects of the drugs may be significant. However, the paradox of improved glucose metabolism in the absence of higher steady-state levels of insulin has been resolved by studies which show that elevation of plasma glucose to pretreatment values results in a rise of plasma insulin to levels higher than those seen pretreatment. Thus, the initial action of the drugs is to increase insulin release with lowering of the plasma glucose. As glucose concentrations fall, insulin levels also decrease since plasma glucose is the major stimulus to insulin release, thereby masking the initial stimulation of insulin secretion. The insulinogenic effect can then be unmasked by raising the plasma glucose to the previous elevated levels. The fact that sulfonylureas are ineffective in IDDM, where beta-cell mass is diminished, supports the pancreatic effect as primary, although extrapancreatic mechanisms doubtless play a role.

The characteristics of the sulfonylureas are summarized in Table 327-9. The newer drugs such as glipizide and glyburide are effective in smaller doses but otherwise differ little from agents in long use such as chlorpropamide and tolbutamide. In patients who have significant renal disease it is preferable to treat with tolbutamide or tolazamide since these agents are exclusively metabolized and inactivated by the liver. Chlorpropamide has the capacity to sensitize the renal tubule to antidiuretic hormone. It thus is helpful in some patients with partial diabetes insipidus but may cause water retention in patients with diabetes mellitus. Hypoglycemia is less common with oral agents than with insulin, but when it occurs it tends to be severe and prolonged. Some patients have required massive glucose infusions for days following the last dose of sulfonylurea. For this reason hospitalization is mandatory in patients with sulfonylurea-induced hypoglycemia.

The only other oral agents effective in the treatment of maturity-onset diabetes are the biguanides. They presumably lower plasma glucose by inhibiting gluconeogenesis in the liver although phenformin may increase the number of insulin receptors in some tissues. The drugs are ordinarily used only in combination with sulfonylureas under circumstances in which control is inadequate with sulfonylurea alone. Because of many reports linking phenformin to the appearance of lactic acidosis, the Food and Drug Administration removed the agent from clinical use in the United States except for certain special patients who continue to take it as an investigational drug. Phenformin and other biguanides are still used elsewhere in the world. Biguanides should not be given to patients with renal disease and should be stopped if nausea, vomiting, diarrhea, or any intercurrent illness appears.

Monitoring control of diabetes For those patients who measure blood glucose frequently for adjustment of insulin dosage an estimate of mean ambient glucose concentrations is readily available. For other patients, and as a check on accuracy of the self measurements, most diabetologists now measure hemoglobin A_{1c} to assess long-term control. Hemoglobin A_{1c}, a fast-moving minor hemoglobin component, is present in normal persons but increases in the presence of hyperglycemia. Its enhanced electrophoretic mobility is due to nonenzymatic glycosylation of the amino acids valine and lysine. The reaction is as follows:

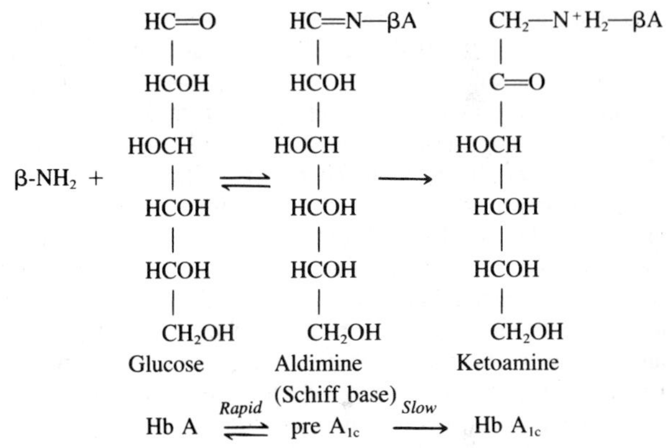

In this scheme β-NH_2 stands for the terminal valine of the β chain of hemoglobin. Aldimine formation is reversible so that pre-A_{1c} is labile while ketoamine formation is irreversible and thus stable. Pre-A_{1c} levels depend on the ambient glucose concentrations and do not reflect long-term control although they are measured in chromatographic methods for determining hemoglobin A_{1c}. Pre-A_{1c} must thus be removed to assess true Hb A_{1c} values accurately. Many laboratories employ high-performance liquid chromatography (HPLC) to make the measurement. A colorimetric method utilizing thiobarbituric acid also does not measure the labile pre-A_{1c} fraction. When properly assayed, the percent of glycosylated hemoglobin gives an estimate of diabetic control for the preceding 3-month period. Normal values must be obtained for each lab; on average nondiabetic subjects have Hb A_{1c} values of around 6 percent, and levels in poorly controlled diabetics may reach 10 to 12 percent. Measurement of glycosylated

TABLE 327-9 The sulfonylureas

Agent	Daily dose, mg	Doses per day	Duration of hyperglycemic action, h	Metabolism/excretion
Acetohexamide	250–1500	1–2	12–18	Liver/kidney
Chlorpropamide	100–500	1	60	Kidney
Tolazamide	100–1000	1–2	12–14	Liver
Tolbutamide	500–3000	2–3	6–12	Liver
Glyburide	1.25–20	1–2	Up to 24	Liver/kidney
Glipizide	2.5–40	1–2	Up to 24	Liver/kidney
Glibornuride	12.5–100	1–2	Up to 24	Liver/kidney

SOURCE: *RH Unger, DW Foster, Diabetes mellitus, in* Williams' Textbook of Endocrinology, *7th ed, JD Wilson, DW Foster (eds), Philadelphia, Saunders, 1985, pp 1018–1080. Adapted from HE Lebovitz and MN Feinglos.*

hemoglobin gives an objective assessment of metabolic control. Discrepancies between reported plasma glucose values and hemoglobin A_{1c} concentrations suggest either that measurement or reporting of the former is not accurate. Measurement of glycosylated albumin, because of its short half-life, can be used to monitor diabetic control over a 1- to 2-week period but clinically is rarely used.

ACUTE METABOLIC COMPLICATIONS In addition to hypoglycemia, diabetics are susceptible to two major acute metabolic complications: diabetic ketoacidosis and hyperosmolar, nonketotic coma. The former is a complication of insulin-dependent diabetes, while the latter usually occurs in the setting of non-insulin-dependent disease. Ketoacidosis rarely, if ever, develops in true type 2 diabetes.

Diabetic ketoacidosis Diabetic ketoacidosis appears to require insulin deficiency coupled with a relative or absolute increase in glucagon concentration. It is often caused by cessation of insulin intake but may result from physical (e.g., infection, surgery) or emotional stress despite continued insulin therapy. In the former case the concentration of glucagon rises secondary to insulin withdrawal, while in stress the operative stimulus is probably epinephrine and/or norepinephrine. In addition to stimulating glucagon secretion epinephrine presumably blocks release of the small amount of residual insulin found in some subjects with IDDM and inhibits insulin-induced glucose transport in peripheral tissues. These hormonal changes have multiple effects, but two are critical: (1) They induce maximal gluconeogenesis and impair peripheral utilization of glucose, causing severe hyperglycemia. Glucagon facilitates gluconeogenesis by inducing a fall in fructose 2,6-bisphosphate, an intermediate that stimulates glycolysis through activation of phosphofructokinase and blocks gluconeogenesis by inhibiting fructose bisphosphatase. When fructose 2,6-bisphosphate concentrations fall, glycolysis is inhibited, and gluconeogenesis is enhanced. The resultant hyperglycemia induces an osmotic diuresis that leads to the volume depletion and dehydration that characterize the ketoacidotic state. (2) They activate the ketogenic process and thus initiate development of metabolic acidosis. For ketosis to occur, changes must be produced in both adipose tissue and the liver. Free fatty acids from adipose stores represent the primary substrate for ketone body formation, and plasma levels of free fatty acids must rise if high rates of ketogenesis are to develop. However, fatty acids delivered to the liver are simply reesterified and stored as hepatic triglyceride or converted into very low density lipoproteins and transported back into the circulation unless the hepatic oxidative machinery for fatty acids is activated. While free fatty acid release is enhanced directly by insulin deficiency, accelerated fatty acid oxidation in the liver is primarily induced by glucagon, via action on the carnitine acyltransferase system of enzymes responsible for the transport of fatty acids into the mitochondria following their esterification to coenzyme A. As shown in Fig. 327-3 carnitine acyltransferase I (carnitine palmitoyltransferase I) transesterifies fatty acyl-CoA to fatty acylcarnitine, which then freely traverses the inner mitochondrial membrane. Reversal of the reaction occurs internally under the influence of carnitine acyltransferase II (carnitine palmitoyltransferase II). In the fed state carnitine acyltransferase I is inactive, and, as a consequence, long-chain fatty acids cannot reach the β-oxidative enzymes for ketone body production. During starvation or uncontrolled diabetes the system is activated; under these circumstances the rate of ketogenesis is a first-order function of the concentration of fatty acids reaching transferase I.

Glucagon (or a change in the glucagon/insulin ratio) activates the transport system in two ways. First, glucagon causes a rapid fall in hepatic malonyl-CoA content. It does so by interrupting the sequence glucose 6-phosphate → pyruvate → citrate → acetyl CoA → malonyl CoA via the previously mentioned decrease in fructose 2,6-bisphosphate. Malonyl-CoA, the first committed intermediate in the synthesis of fatty acids from glucose, is a competitive inhibitor of carnitine acyltransferase I, and a fall in its concentration activates the enzyme. Second, glucagon causes a rise in hepatic carnitine concentration, which then drives the reaction toward fatty acylcarnitine formation by mass action. These events are summarized schematically in Fig. 327-4. At high plasma fatty acid concentrations hepatic uptake of fatty acids is sufficient to saturate both oxidative and esterifying pathways, resulting in fatty liver, hypertriglyceridemia, and ketoacidosis. Overproduction of ketones by the liver is the primary event in ketotic states, but limitation of peripheral utilization also plays a role at high concentrations of acetoacetate and β-hydroxybutyrate.

Clinically ketoacidosis begins with anorexia, nausea, and vomiting, coupled with increased rate of urine formation. Abdominal pain may be present. If untreated, altered consciousness or frank coma may occur. Initial examination usually shows Kussmaul's respiration, together with signs of volume depletion. Rarely the latter is sufficient to cause vascular collapse and renal shutdown. Body temperature is normal or below normal in uncomplicated ketoacidosis, and fever suggests the presence of infection. Leukocytosis, frequently very marked, is a feature of diabetic acidosis per se and may not indicate infection.

The characteristic metabolic abnormalities of diabetic coma are shown in Table 327-10. Several features deserve comment. The metabolic acidosis and anion gap are almost totally accounted for by the elevated plasma levels of acetoacetate and β-hydroxybutyrate, although other acids (e.g., lactate, free fatty acids, phosphates) contribute. Despite initial potassium concentrations that are normal to high, there is a total body potassium deficit of several hundred millimoles. Similarly, initial serum phosphorus may be high despite depletion of body stores. Magnesium deficiency may also be present. The serum sodium concentration tends to be low in the face of modest osmolar concentration because of the hyperglycemia that draws intracellular water into the plasma space. A very low serum sodium (e.g., 110 meq per liter) suggests an artifact due to severe hypertriglyceridemia. The latter is common in ketoacidosis and is the consequence of both impaired activity of lipoprotein lipase (a disposal defect) and the hepatic overproduction of very low density lipoproteins. If a fat meal has been ingested prior to the onset of ketoacidosis, chylomicrons may make up a major portion of the circulating fat. Lipemia is usually visible if triglyceride concentration is above 400 mg/dL. True hyponatremia may occur if the patient has vomited repeatedly and continued to drink water. Prerenal azotemia, reflecting volume

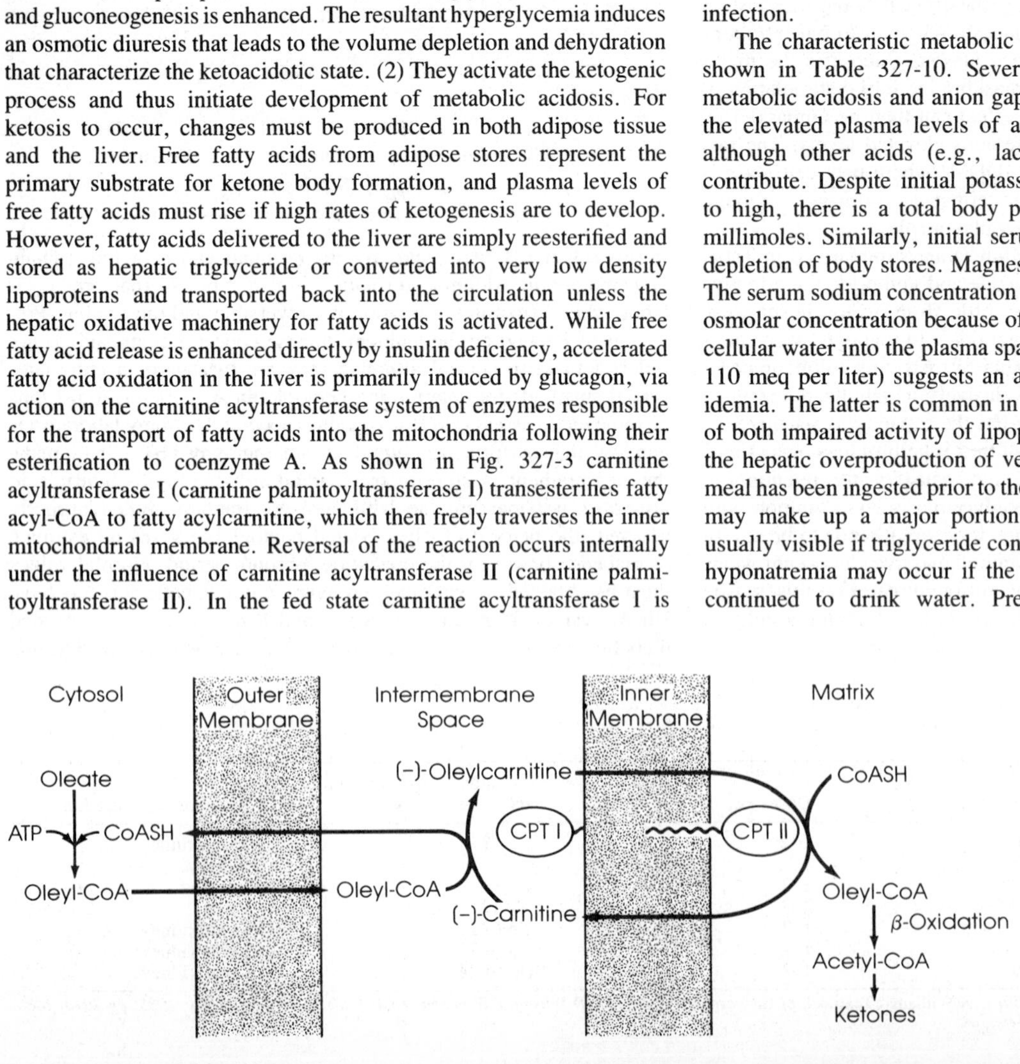

FIGURE 327-3 *The carnitine palmitoyltransferase system for the transfer of long-chain fatty acids into the mitochondria. CPT I-carnitine palmitoyltransferase I; CPT II-carnitine palmitoyltransferase II. (From JD McGarry et al, J Clin Invest 55:1202, 1975. Used by permission.)*

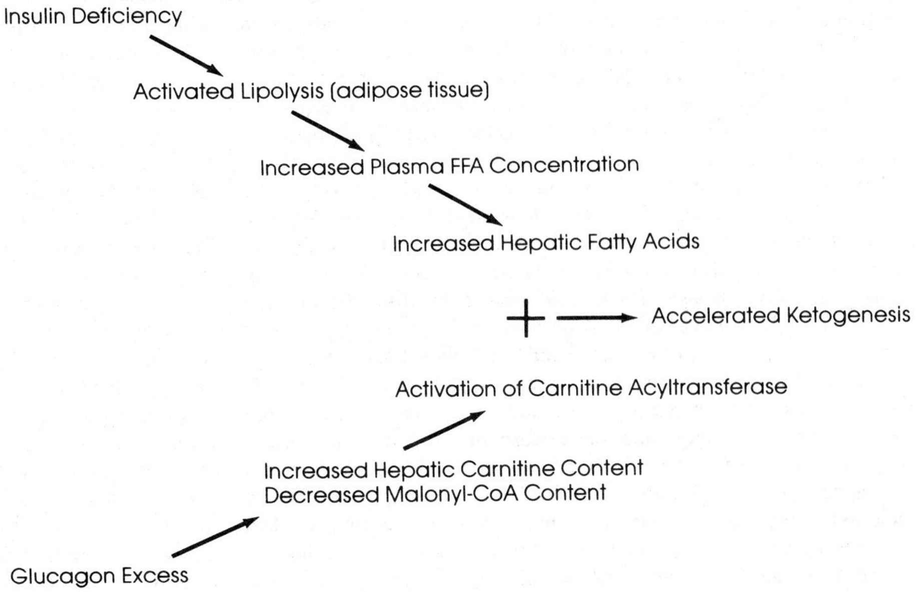

FIGURE 327-4 *The regulation of ketogenesis. Significant production of acetoacetate and β-hydroxybutyrate by the liver requires provision of adequate free fatty acid substrate and activation of fatty acid oxidation. Lipolysis is primarily increased by insulin deficiency while the fatty acid oxidative sequence is activated primarily by glucagon. The immediate signal for oxidation is a fall in malonyl CoA content. (After JD McGarry, DW Foster, Am J Med 61:9, 1976.)*

depletion, is usually modest in degree and reversible with treatment. The serum amylase may be elevated, and frank pancreatitis can occur.

The diagnosis of ketoacidosis in a known diabetic is not difficult. Its appearance in a patient not previously known to have diabetes requires differentiation from the other common causes of metabolic acidosis with an anion gap: lactic acidosis, uremia, alcoholic ketoacidosis, and certain poisonings. The first step is to test the urine for glucose and ketones. If urine ketones are negative, another cause for the acidosis is likely. If positive, plasma examination is required to be certain that something more than starvation ketosis is present. Since quantitative determinations of acetoacetate and β-hydroxybutyrate are not routinely available, semiquantitative tests must be done using ketone reagent strips. Serial dilutions of plasma can be made and tested. A strong test may occur in undiluted plasma owing to starvation alone; a strong reaction beyond 1:1 dilution is presumptive evidence for ketoacidosis. Apart from diabetes the only other common ketoacidotic state is alcoholic ketoacidosis. This syndrome, which by definition occurs in chronic alcoholics, usually follows a debauch, but the patient may not have had alcohol for 24 h or longer. It never occurs in the absence of starvation and frequently is associated with severe vomiting and abdominal pain. Pancreatitis is present in up to 75 percent of patients. A plasma glucose of less than 150 mg/dL was found in three-fourths of cases and in 15 percent was less than 50 mg/dL on arrival at the hospital. Hyperglycemia may occur but is usually mild and rarely, if ever, above 300 mg/dL. Plasma free fatty acid concentrations are higher (mean 2.9 m*M*) than in normal starvation (range 0.7 to 1.0 m*M*), reaching levels seen in diabetic ketoacidosis. Presumably the liver is activated for ketogenesis by starvation in these patients and driven to maximal rates of ketone formation by the high fatty acid levels. Why some alcoholics mobilize fatty acids excessively is not known. In contrast to diabetic acidosis, the syndrome is rapidly reversible by the intravenous administration of glucose. As in all alcoholics given glucose, thiamine should be supplied to avoid precipitation of acute beriberi. (Other water-soluble vitamins, though not as critical, should also be infused.) Insulin is required only if hyperglycemia persists during therapy.

Diabetic ketoacidosis cannot be reversed without insulin. For decades 50 or more units of insulin were given per hour until ketosis was reversed, but now most patients are treated by "low-dose" insulin schedules in which 8 to 10 units of insulin are infused intravenously each hour. Most diabetic acidosis can be reversed adequately with low-dose treatment, but some patients do not respond. Presumably the insulin resistance that is characteristic of diabetic ketoacidosis is more pronounced in these patients than in responsive subjects. The problem is that resistant subjects cannot be identified prospectively. For this reason it is probably preferable to treat ketoacidosis with 25 to 50 units of regular insulin intravenously hourly until the acidosis is reversed. There are no known toxic effects of larger insulin doses, since maximal physiologic response is obtained once insulin receptors are saturated regardless of how much insulin is given. The advantage of the higher dosage schedule is that it ensures saturation of the receptors in the face of competing antibodies or other resistance factors. If physicians choose to use the low-dose insulin schedule, they should be alert to the possibility of resistance. Should acidosis persist unabated after several hours of treatment, larger amounts of insulin are clearly indicated. Ketoacidosis can also be adequately treated with intramuscular (but not subcutaneous) insulin.

Therapy of ketoacidosis also requires intravenous fluids. The usual fluid deficit is 3 to 5 liters, and both salt solutions and free water are needed. One to two liters of isotonic saline or Ringer's lactate should be given rapidly intravenously on arrival, with additional amounts determined by urine output and clinical assessment of the fluid state. When the plasma glucose falls to about 300 mg/dL, 5% glucose solutions should be given, both as a source of free water and as a prophylactic measure to prevent the late cerebral edema syndrome. The latter is a rare complication of ketoacidosis occurring most often in children. It is suspected when the patient remains comatose or lapses into coma following reversal of acidosis.

Potassium replacement is always necessary, but the time of administration will vary. The initial potassium is often high despite a total body deficit because of the severe acidosis. In this case the cation will ordinarily not be needed until 3 to 4 h after initiation of therapy, when reversal of acidosis and the action of insulin cause a

TABLE 327-10 Initial laboratory findings in diabetic ketoacidosis

Series	Dallas*	Los Angeles†	Washington‡
Age	38	36	43
Glucose, mg/dL	475	675	733
Sodium, m*M*	132	131	132
Potassium, m*M*	4.8	5.3	6.0
Bicarbonate, m*M*	<10	6	10
BUN, mg/dL	25	32	42
Acetoacetate, m*M*	4.8	—	—
β-Hydroxybutyrate, m*M*	13.7	—	—
Free fatty acids, m*M*	2.1	—	2.3
Lactate, m*M*	4.6	—	—
Osmolarity, mosmol/liter	310	323	331

* *Eighty-eight consecutive episodes of ketoacidosis at Parkland Memorial Hospital (DW Foster, unpublished observations).*
† *Mean data from 308 episodes of nonfatal ketoacidosis (PM Beigelman, Diabetes 20:490, 1971).*
‡ *Mean data from 10 episodes of ketoacidosis (JE Gerich et al, Diabetes 20:228, 1971).*

shift of K^+ into intracellular water. On the other hand if the admission value is normal or low, potassium should be given early, since plasma concentrations fall rapidly during therapy, predisposing the patient to cardiac arrhythmias. In view of the phosphate depletion of ketoacidosis, potassium should be administered initially as the phosphate salt rather than as potassium chloride.

Bicarbonate therapy is indicated in severely acidotic patients (pH 7.0 or below), especially if hypotension is present (acidosis itself can cause vascular collapse). It is not used routinely in less acutely ill subjects since rapid alkalinization may have detrimental effects on oxygen delivery to tissues. The hemoglobin-oxygen dissociation curve is normal in diabetic ketoacidosis because of the opposing effects of acidosis and deficiency of red blood cell 2,3-diphosphoglycerate (2,3-DPG). If the acidosis is rapidly reversed, the deficiency of 2,3-DPG becomes manifest, increasing the avidity with which hemoglobin binds oxygen and impairing the release of oxygen in peripheral tissues. In a volume-depleted patient with poor tissue perfusion such a change theoretically could predispose to the development of lactic acidosis. If bicarbonate is given, the infusion should be stopped when the pH reaches 7.2 to minimize effects on oxygen binding by hemoglobin and to prevent metabolic alkalosis as circulating ketones are metabolized to bicarbonate with reversal of ketoacidosis.

In following the response to treatment, two points should be emphasized. (1) Plasma glucose invariably falls more rapidly than plasma ketones. Insulin should not be stopped because glucose concentrations approach normal; rather, as mentioned, glucose should be infused and insulin continued until the ketosis has cleared. (2) Plasma ketone values are not very helpful. The testing materials measure acetoacetate and acetone but not β-hydroxybutyrate. Since β-hydroxybutyrate must be oxidized to acetoacetate prior to utilization, it is characteristic for the plasma ketones measured by reagent strip to remain stable or even rise early in therapy at a time when total ketone concentration (acetoacetate plus β-hydroxybutyrate) is steadily falling. Because β-hydroxybutyrate and acetoacetate represent a redox couple in equilibrium with mitochondrial NADH/NAD concentrations, vascular collapse or severe hypoxia may mask the presence of ketoacidosis as acetoacetate is reduced to β-hydroxybutyrate. Under these circumstances the β-hydroxybutyrate/acetoacetate ratio, normally about 3:1, may reach 7:1 or 8:1. Paradoxically, in such a situation, ketosis may seem to worsen as the patient gets better because of conversion of β-hydroxybutyrate to acetoacetate when the circulation is reestablished and tissue oxygenation is restored. The key parameters to follow are the pH and the calculated anion gap since these give a more accurate assessment of therapeutic progress. The usual picture is for the pH to rise and the anion gap to narrow even though the plasma bicarbonate remains low. The persistently low bicarbonate is the consequence of hyperchloremia that develops because of rapid infusion of sodium chloride, the loss of potential bicarbonate from the body in urine as ketones, and exchanges with intracellular buffers.

TABLE 327-11 Clues to complications in diabetic ketoacidosis

Complication	Clues
Acute gastric dilatation or erosive gastritis	Vomiting of blood or coffee-ground material
Cerebral edema	Obtundation or coma with or without neurologic signs, especially if occurring after initial improvement
Hyperkalemia	Cardiac arrest
Hypoglycemia	Adrenergic or neurologic signs; rebound ketosis
Hypokalemia	Cardiac arrhythmias
Infection	Fever
Insulin resistance	Unremitting acidosis after 4–6 h of adequate therapy
Myocardial infarction	Chest pain, appearance of heart failure; appearance of hypotension despite adequate fluids
Mucormycosis	Facial pain, bloody nasal discharge, blackened nasal turbinates, blurred vision, proptosis
Respiratory distress syndrome	Hypoxemia in the absence of pneumonia, chronic pulmonary disease, or heart failure
Vascular thrombosis	Strokelike picture or signs of ischemia in nonnervous tissue

SOURCE: *Adapted from DW Foster, Diabetic ketoacidosis, in* Current Therapy in Endocrinology and Metabolism 1985–1986, *DT Krieger, CW Bardin (eds), Toronto/Philadelphia, Decker, 1985, pp 268–270.*

All patients should be followed with a flow sheet outlining amounts and timing of insulin and fluids together with a record of vital signs, urine volume, and blood chemistries. Without such a record therapy tends to become chaotic.

Most patients with diabetic ketoacidosis recover when properly treated. While mortality in large series is reported to be around 10 percent, the majority of deaths result from late complications rather than from ketoacidosis itself. The major causes are myocardial infarction and infection, particularly pneumonia. Poor prognostic signs on admission include hypotension, azotemia, deep coma, and associated illness. In children, cerebral edema is a common cause of death (less frequent in adults). The cause of the brain swelling is not known. Theories include osmotic disequilibrium between brain and plasma as glucose is rapidly lowered, decreased plasma oncotic pressure due to infusion of large amounts of saline, and insulin-induced ion flux across the blood-brain barrier. Whatever the mechanism, mortality rates are high. Diagnosis is usually made by CT scan. Treatment involves the bolus infusion of 1 g mannitol per kilogram of body weight in the form of a 20% solution. Although of questionable benefit, dexamethasone is also usually given: 12 mg initially then 4 mg every 6 h. If there is no response, hyperventilation to an arterial P_{CO_2} of about 28 mmHg should be carried out by an anesthesiologist or pulmonary specialist.

Other acute complications of ketoacidosis include vascular thrombosis and the adult respiratory distress syndrome. The former is induced by volume depletion, hyperosmolarity, increased viscosity of blood, and changes in clotting factors favoring thrombosis. The cause of the pulmonary lesion is not known; it is probably not related to the metabolic acidosis since respiratory distress syndrome occurs in hyperosmolar coma as well. Acute gastric dilatation is another rare complication. A rare infection associated with ketoacidosis is mucormycosis (see below). Table 327-11 summarizes the complications of diabetic ketoacidosis and its treatment.

Hyperosmolar coma Hyperosmolar nonketotic diabetic coma is usually a complication of non-insulin-dependent diabetes. It is a syndrome of profound dehydration resulting from a sustained hyperglycemic diuresis under circumstances in which the patient is unable to drink sufficient water to keep up with urinary fluid losses. Commonly an elderly diabetic—often living alone or in a nursing home—develops a stroke or infection, which worsens hyperglycemia and prevents adequate water intake. The full-blown syndrome probably does not occur until volume depletion has become severe enough to decrease urine output. Hyperosmolar coma has also been precipitated by therapeutic procedures such as peritoneal dialysis or hemodialysis, tube feeding of high-protein formulas, high-carbohydrate infusion loads, and the use of osmotic agents such as mannitol and urea. Phenytoin, steroids, immunosuppressive agents, and diuretics have also been reported to initiate the disorder.

The absence of ketoacidosis is important in the pathophysiology. When ketoacidosis occurs in an insulin-dependent diabetic, nausea, vomiting, and air hunger bring the patient to the physician before extreme dehydration can occur. Such a protective mechanism is not operative in the ketoacidosis-resistant, maturity-onset diabetic. Interestingly, hyperosmolar coma can occur in insulin-dependent diabetic patients given sufficient insulin to prevent ketosis but insufficient to control hyperglycemia. Although unusual, the same patient may present on one occasion with ketoacidosis and on the next with hyperosmolar coma.

The reason for the absence of ketoacidosis in maturity-onset diabetics is not known. The hepatic ketogenic machinery is not impaired since the patients frequently have ketone concentrations in the starvation range (2 to 4 m*M*). Free fatty acid levels are lower in hyperosmolar coma than in ketoacidosis, and substrate deficiency may limit ketone formation. That this is the sole mechanism seems unlikely since some patients with hyperosmolar coma have high levels of free fatty acids in plasma. A more likely explanation is that insulin concentrations in the portal vein of type 2 diabetics are higher than those of insulin-dependent subjects and prevent full activation of the hepatic carnitine acyltransferase system. Another possibility is that glucagon resistance plays a role.

Clinically patients present with extreme hyperglycemia, hyperosmolality, and volume depletion, coupled with central nervous system signs ranging from clouded sensorium to coma. Seizure activity—sometimes Jacksonian in type—is not unusual, and transient hemiplegia may be seen. Infections, particularly pneumonia and gram-negative sepsis, are common and indicate a grave prognosis. Pneumonia is often due to gram-negative organisms. A high index of suspicion for infection should be maintained, and routine culture of the blood and spinal fluid is indicated. Because of the extreme dehydration plasma viscosity is high, and widespread in situ thrombosis has been found at post mortem. Bleeding, probably the consequence of disseminated intravascular coagulation and acute pancreatitis may accompany the illness.

The laboratory findings in two large series are shown in Table 327-12. Plasma glucose is generally around 1000 mg/dL, about twice the value seen in ketoacidosis. The serum osmolality is extremely high, but because of the hyperglycemia the absolute serum sodium concentration is often not elevated.[3] Prerenal azotemia with marked elevation of BUN and creatinine is characteristic. A mild metabolic acidosis is present, plasma bicarbonate on the average being about 20 meq per liter. The acidosis is due to a combination of starvation ketosis, retention of inorganic acids secondary to the azotemia, and modest elevation of plasma lactate, the latter the consequence of volume depletion. If the bicarbonate is less than 10 meq per liter and plasma ketones are not elevated, it can be assumed that lactic acidosis is present.

The mortality rate in hyperosmolar coma is high (>50 percent). As a consequence immediate treatment is urgent. The most important measure is rapid administration of large amounts of intravenous fluids to reestablish the circulation and urine flow. The average fluid deficit is 10 liters. While free water will ultimately be needed, initial therapy should be with isotonic salt solutions, and 2 to 3 liters should be given over the first 1 to 2 h. Subsequently half-strength saline can be used. As the plasma glucose approaches normal levels, 5% dextrose can be given as a vehicle for free water. While hyperosmolar coma may be reversed by fluids alone, insulin should be given to control the hyperglycemia more rapidly. Many authors recommend small doses of insulin, but larger amounts may be necessary, particularly in the obese patient. Potassium salts are usually required earlier in the treatment of hyperosmolar coma than in ketoacidosis because the intracellular shift of plasma K^+ during therapy is accelerated in the absence of acidosis. If lactic acidosis is present, sodium bicarbonate should be given until tissue perfusion can be reestablished (see Chap. 328). Antibiotics are required if infection complicates the picture.

[3] *Serum osmolality can be estimated from the formula*

Serum osmolality (mosmol/liter)

$$= 2([Na^+] + [K^+]) + \frac{\text{glucose (mg/dL)}}{18} + \frac{\text{BUN (mg/dL)}}{2.8}$$

In practice the contribution of the BUN is often ignored since it contributes to total osmolality but does not reflect the free water deficit. There are situations in clinical medicine in which an increased osmolality is not equivalent to dehydration. Severe alcohol intoxication is the classic example, the ethanol itself providing the measured milliosmoles.

LATE COMPLICATIONS OF DIABETES The diabetic patient is susceptible to a series of complications that cause morbidity and premature mortality. While some patients may never develop these problems and others note their onset early, on the average symptoms develop 15 to 20 years following the appearance of overt hyperglycemia. A given patient may experience several complications simultaneously, or a single problem may dominate the picture.

Circulatory abnormalities Arteriosclerosis of the type seen in nondiabetics occurs more extensively and earlier than in the general population. The cause for this accelerated atherosclerosis is not known, although, as discussed below, nonenzymatic glycosylation of lipoproteins may be important. Atherosclerotic lesions produce symptoms in a variety of sites. Peripheral deposits may cause intermittent claudication, gangrene, and, in men, organic impotence on a vascular basis. Surgical repair of large vessel lesions may be unsuccessful because of the simultaneous presence of widespread disease of the small vessels. Coronary artery disease and stroke are common. Silent myocardial infarction is thought to occur with increased frequency in diabetics and should be suspected whenever symptoms of left ventricular failure appear suddenly. Diabetes may also be associated with the clinical picture of cardiomyopathy, in which heart failure occurs in the face of angiographically normal coronary arteries and the absence of other identifiable causes of heart disease. As in nondiabetic subjects, smoking is a major risk factor for both coronary and peripheral vascular disease and should be avoided.

Retinopathy Diabetic retinopathy is a leading cause of blindness in the United States. On the other hand, most diabetics never become blind. Retinopathic lesions are divided into two large categories, *simple* (background) and *proliferative* (Table 327-13). The earliest sign of retinal change is an increased capillary permeability that is evidenced by leakage of dye into the vitreous humor after fluorescein injection. Occlusion of retinal capillaries follows, with subsequent formation of saccular and fusiform aneurysms. Arteriovenous shunts also occur. The vascular lesions are accompanied by proliferation of lining endothelial cells and a loss of the pericytes that surround and

TABLE 327-12 Initial laboratory findings in hyperosmolar coma

Series	Brooklyn*	Washington†
Age	60	57
Glucose, mg/dL	1166	976
Sodium, m*M*	144	142
Potassium, m*M*	5	5
Chloride, m*M*	99	98
Bicarbonate, m*M*	17	22
BUN, mg/dL	87	65
Creatinine, mg/dL	5.5	—
Free fatty acids, m*M*	0.73	0.96
Osmolarity, mosmol/liter	384	374

* *Mean data from 33 episodes of hyperosmolar coma (AA Arieff, HJ Carroll, Medicine 51:73, 1972).*
† *Mean data from 20 episodes of hyperosmolar coma (JE Gerich et al, Diabetes 20:228, 1971).*

TABLE 327-13 Lesions of diabetic retinopathy

BACKGROUND
Increased capillary permeability
Capillary closure and dilatation
Microaneurysms
Arteriovenous shunts
Dilated veins
Hemorrhages (dot and blot)
Cotton-wool spots
Hard exudates
PROLIFERATIVE
New vessels
Scar (retinitis proliferans)
Vitreal hemorrhage
Retinal detachment

support the vessels. Hemorrhages into the inner retinal areas are dot-shaped, while bleeding into the more superficial nerve fiber layer causes flame-shaped, blot, or linear lesions. Preretinal hemorrhages characteristically have a boat-shaped appearance. Exudates are of two types. Cotton-wool spots can be shown by angiography to be microinfarcts—nonperfused areas surrounded by a ring of dilated capillaries. A sudden increase in the number of cotton-wool spots represents an ominous prognostic sign and may herald the appearance of rapidly advancing retinopathy. Hard exudates are more common than cotton-wool spots and probably represent leakage of protein and lipids from damaged capillaries.

The fundamental characteristics of proliferative retinopathy are new vessel formation and scarring. The stimulus for neovascularization may be hypoxia secondary to capillary or arteriolar occlusion. Two serious complications of proliferative retinopathy are vitreal hemorrhage and retinal detachment. Either may cause a sudden loss of vision in one eye.

The frequency of diabetic retinopathy appears to vary with the age of onset as well as the duration of the disease. Approximately 85 percent of patients eventually develop the complication, but some never develop lesions even after 30 years of disease. Retinopathy appears to develop earlier in older patients, but proliferative retinopathy is less common. Some 10 to 18 percent of patients with simple retinopathy progress to proliferative disease in a 10-year period. About half of patients with proliferative disease progress to blindness within 5 years.

Treatment for diabetic retinopathy is photocoagulation. Such treatment decreases the incidence of hemorrhage and scarring and is always indicated when new vessel formation occurs. Photocoagulation is also useful in treatment of microaneurysms, hemorrhages, and edema even if the proliferative stage has not begun. Panretinal photocoagulation is sometimes used to diminish retinal demands for oxygen in the hope that the stimulus for neovascularization will be decreased. In this technique several thousand lesions are produced over a 2-week period. Complications of photocoagulation are within the acceptable range. Some loss of peripheral vision is inevitable with extensive burns. Another surgical technique, pars plana vitrectomy, is utilized for treatment of nonresolving vitreal hemorrhage and retinal detachment. Postoperative complications are more frequent than with photocoagulation and include retinal tears, retinal detachment, cataracts, recurrent vitreal hemorrhage, glaucoma, infection, and loss of the eye. Hypophysectomy, once widely performed for diabetic retinopathy, is no longer recommended. All patients with diabetic retinopathy should be followed by retinal specialists.

Diabetic nephropathy Renal disease is a leading cause of death and disability in diabetes. One-fourth or more of end-stage renal disease in the United States is now due to diabetic nephropathy. Approximately 40 to 50 percent of patients with insulin-dependent diabetes develop this complication. Prevalence may be somewhat less with the non-insulin-dependent form of the disease, possibly because duration of illness tends to be shorter. However, two-thirds of diabetic Pima Indians (who have non-insulin-dependent diabetes) have diabetic glomerulosclerosis at autopsy.

Diabetic nephropathy involves two distinct pathologic patterns that may or may not coexist: diffuse and nodular. The former, which is more common, consists of widening of the glomerular basement membrane together with generalized mesangial thickening. In the nodular form large accumulations of PAS-positive material are deposited at the periphery of the glomerular tufts, the Kimmelstiel-Wilson lesion. In addition, there may be hyalinization of afferent and efferent arterioles, "drops" in Bowman's capsule, fibrin caps, and occulsion of glomeruli. Deposition of albumin and other proteins occurs in both glomeruli and tubules. The most specific lesions of diabetic glomerulosclerosis are hyalinization of afferent glomerular arterioles and the Kimmelstiel-Wilson nodules. Clinical renal dysfunction in diabetes does not correlate well with the histologic abnormalities.

Diabetic nephropathy may be functionally silent for long periods (~10 to 15 years). At onset of diabetes the kidneys are usually enlarged with "superfunction," i.e., glomerular filtration rates may be 40 percent above normal. The next stage is the appearance of *microproteinuria* (microalbuminuria), the excretion of albumin in the range of 30 to 300 mg per 24 h. Normal persons excrete less than 30 mg per 24 h. Microalbuminuria is not detected by reagent sticks for urinary protein, which generally become positive only when proteinuria is greater than 550 mg per 24 h, a degree of leakage termed *macroproteinuria*. Since microalbuminuria is initially transient and can be induced by mechanisms other than diabetes, diagnosis requires an excretion rate of albumin greater than 20 μg/h (~30 mg per 24 h) in two of three samples collected in a 6-month period. Persistent leakage of protein >50 mg per 24 h is statistically predictive of subsequent macroproteinuria. Once the macroproteinuric phase begins, there is a steady decline in renal function with glomerular filtration rate falling, on average, about 1 mL/min per month. A plot of the reciprocal of the serum creatinine against time usually results in a straight line and allows assessment of the rate of deterioration. Ordinarily azotemia begins about 12 years after diagnosis of diabetes. The nephrotic syndrome may occur prior to azotemia. Progression of renal disease is accelerated by hypertension.

There is no specific treatment for diabetic nephropathy. Meticulous control of diabetes can reverse microalbuminuria in some patients, but there is no evidence that diabetic nephropathy can be prevented by intensive insulin therapy. Hypertension must be treated aggressively whenever present. Low-protein diets may be useful, based on experimental studies in animals, but no prospective study has appeared testing protein restriction in diabetic humans. Once the azotemic phase is reached, treatment does not differ from other forms of renal failure. Chronic dialysis and renal transplantation are routine in patients with renal failure due to diabetes. Hyporeninemic hypoaldosteronism, which is associated with renal tubular acidosis, may require alkalinizing solutions (Shohl's solution) and avoidance of external potassium loads. Rarely, fludrocortisone may be required to control hyperkalemia.

Diabetic neuropathy Diabetic neuropathy may affect every part of the nervous system with the possible exception of the brain. While it is rarely a direct cause of death, it is a major cause of morbidity. Distinct syndromes can be recognized, and several different types of neuropathy may be present in the same patient. The most common picture is that of *peripheral polyneuropathy*. Usually bilateral, the symptoms include numbness, paresthesias, severe hyperesthesias, and pain. The pain, which may be deep-seated and severe, is often worse at night. It is occasionally lancinating or lightning in type, resembling tabes dorsalis (pseudotabes). Fortunately extreme pain syndromes are usually self-limited, lasting from a few months to a few years. Involvement of proprioceptive fibers leads to abnormalities of gait and development of typical Charcot joints, particularly in the feet. Loss of arch with multiple fractures of tarsal bones is a common finding by x-ray. On physical examination absent stretch reflexes and loss of vibratory sense are early signs. Diabetic neuropathy may also cause delay in return of the ankle reflex identical to that seen in hypothyroidism. *Mononeuropathy,* though less common than polyneuropathy, may also occur. Characteristically there is a sudden wrist drop, foot drop, or paralysis of the third, fourth, or sixth cranial nerves. Other single nerves, including the recurrent laryngeal, have been reported to be involved. Mononeuropathy is characterized by a high degree of spontaneous reversibility, usually over a several-week period. *Radiculopathy* is a sensory syndrome in which pain occurs over the distribution of one or more spinal nerves, usually in the chest wall or abdomen. The severe pain may mimic herpes zoster or an acute surgical abdomen. Like mononeuropathy, the lesion is usually self-limited. *Autonomic neuropathy* may present in a variety of ways. The gastrointestinal tract is a prime target, and there may be esophageal dysfunction with difficulty in swallowing, delayed gastric emptying, constipation, or diarrhea. The last is often nocturnal.

Incompetence of the internal anal sphincter may mimic diabetic diarrhea. Patients may suffer from orthostatic hypotension and frank syncope. Cardiorespiratory arrest and sudden death, thought to be due solely to autonomic neuropathy, have been reported. Bladder dysfunction or paralysis is particularly distressing and often leads to the necessity of chronic catheter drainage. Impotence and retrograde ejaculation are additional manifestations in the male. Clues to autonomic neuropathy can be obtained by clinical tests such as measuring response of the heart rate to the Valsalva maneuver or standing. In both tests the subject has an electrocardiograph running for assessment of heart rate. In the former the subject blows against an anaeroid or mercury manometer to 40 mmHg pressure for 15 s. The test is performed three times with a rest period of 1 min in between. Normally the heart rate speeds during Valsalva such that the ratio of the longest interval between beats after release to the shortest interval during the test is >1.2. In autonomic neuropathy involving the parasympathetic system the ratio is <1:1. Similarly the ratio at the thirtieth beat after standing relative to that at the fifteenth beat should be >1.0. It is <1 in autonomic neuropathy. Diabetic *amyotrophy* is likely a form of neuropathy, although atrophy and weakness of the large muscles in the upper leg and pelvic girdle resemble primary muscle disease. Anorexia and depression may accompany amyotrophy.

Treatment of diabetic neuropathy is unsatisfactory in most respects. When pain is severe, it is easy for the patient to become habituated or addicted to narcotics or powerful nonnarcotic analgesics such as pentazocine. If the pain requires something more powerful than aspirin, acetaminophen, or other nonsteroidal anti-inflammatory agents, codeine is the drug of choice. Phenytoin is used by some physicians, but others have not found it helpful. Combination therapy with amitriptyline and fluphenazine causes significant relief of pain in some patients and should always be tried. The recommended dosage is 75 mg amitriptyline at bedtime and 1 mg fluphenazine three times a day. Mononeuropathies and radiculopathies usually require no specific therapy since they are self-limited. Diabetic diarrhea often responds to treatment with diphenoxylate and atropine or loperamide. Orthostatic hypotension is best treated by having the patient sleep with the head of the bed elevated, avoidance of sudden assumption of the upright position, and the use of full-length elastic stockings. Occasionally volume expansion with fludrocortisone is required as in other forms of orthostatic hypotension.

Symptoms of neuropathy may improve following administration of oral myoinositol or an inhibitor of aldose reductase, the enzyme responsible for formation of sorbitol in tissues. These approaches remain experimental at the time of this writing.

Diabetic foot ulcers A special problem in the diabetic patient is the development of ulcers of the feet and lower extremities. The ulcers appear to be primarily due to abnormal pressure distribution secondary to diabetic neuropathy. The problem is accentuated when there is bony distortion in the feet. Callus formation is usually the initial abnormality. Alternatively the ulcer may be initiated by ill-fitting shoes which cause blister formation in patients whose sensory deficits preclude recognition of pain. Cuts and punctures from foreign bodies such as needles, tacks, and glass are common, and a foreign body of which the patient is unaware may be found in the soft tissue. For this reason all patients with ulcers should have x-rays made of the feet. Vascular disease with diminished blood supply contributes to development of the lesion, and infection is common, often with multiple organisms. While no specific therapy is available for diabetic ulcers, aggressive supportive treatment can often lead to salvation of the leg without amputation. One approach is to simply put the patient to bed using frequent foot soaks and debridement to remove nonviable tissue. Others recommend casting the leg with plaster to remove weight bearing and protect the lesion.

All diabetics should be instructed about proper foot care in an attempt to prevent ulcers. Feet should be kept clean and dry at all times. Patients with neuropathy should not be allowed to walk barefoot, even in the home. Properly fitted shoes are essential. This is a particular problem with women, since an adequate shoe for the diabetic is not often stylish. The feet should be carefully inspected daily for callus, infection, abrasions, or blisters and the physician consulted for any potentially troublesome lesion.

What causes diabetes complications? The cause of diabetic complications is not known and may be multifactorial. Major emphasis has been placed on the polyol pathway wherein glucose is reduced to sorbitol by the enzyme aldol reductase. Sorbitol, which appears to function as a tissue toxin, has been implicated in the pathogenesis of retinopathy, neuropathy, cataracts, nephropathy, and aortic disease. The mechanism is perhaps best worked out in experimental diabetic neuropathy where sorbitol accumulation is associated with a decrease in myoinositol content, abnormal phosphoinositide metabolism, and a decrease in $[Na^+ + K^+]$-ATPase activity. In experimental models primacy of the polyol pathway in initiating neuropathy was proven by showing that inhibition of aldol reductase prevented the fall in tissue myoinositol content and the decrease in ATPase activity. Aldol reductase inhibition has also been shown to prevent experimental cataracts and retinopathy. It thus seems possible that neuropathy and retinopathy are primarily due to activation of the polyol pathway. The latter may also play a role in diabetic nephropathy.

A second mechanism of potential pathogenetic importance is nonenzymatic glycosylation of proteins. The effect of such glycosylation on hemoglobin has been mentioned, but multiple proteins in the body are altered in the same way, often with disturbed functions. Examples include plasma albumin, lens protein, fibrin, collagen, lipoproteins, and the glycoprotein recognition system of hepatic endothelial cells. Particularly intriguing is the effect of glycosylation on lipoproteins. Glycosylated low-density lipoprotein (LDL) is not recognized by the normal LDL receptor, and its plasma half-life is increased. Conversely, glycosylated high-density lipoprotein (HDL) turns over more rapidly than native HDL. It has also been reported that glycosylated collagen traps LDL at rates two to three times greater than normal collagen. Conceivably the accelerated atherosclerosis of diabetes might be related to the combined effect of a glycosylated LDL that did not bind normally to LDL receptors but would be trapped to a greater than normal extent in macrophages and glycosylated collagen of blood vessels and other tissues. Dysfunctional HDL could contribute by diminishing cholesterol transport out of affected sites.

Glycosylated collagen is less soluble and more resistant to degradation by collagenase than native collagen. However, it is not clear that this is related either to the basement membrane thickening or the tight, waxy skin syndrome with limited joint mobility (scleroderma-like) seen in some patients with insulin-dependent diabetes (see "Miscellaneous Abnormalities," below). Although it is attractive to presume that nonenzymatic glycosylation of proteins plays a role in some degenerative complications, the evidence is less direct than with the polyol pathway.

Increased blood flow has been postulated to play an initiating role in diabetic complications, possibly by increasing filtration of macromolecules that function as tissue toxins. There is supportive evidence for a role of hyperperfusion in diabetic nephropathy, but the hemodynamic hypothesis does not appear as attractive as the first two.

Can diabetic complications be prevented by meticulous control of diabetes? The critical question in diabetic therapy is whether hyperglycemia or some associated metabolic disorder causes or accelerates the development of the long-term complications just discussed. The alternative possibility is that complications are primarily determined by genetic factors independent of hyperglycemia. Perhaps the strongest evidence that the metabolic environment per se causes complications comes from the observation that kidneys from donors who have neither diabetes nor a family history of diabetes develop characteristic lesions of diabetic nephropathy within 3 to 5 years after transplantation into a diabetic recipient. Diabetic nephropathy did not develop when a kidney was transplanted into a diabetic subject whose disease had been reversed by pancreatic transplantation prior to renal transplantation. It has also been reported that kidneys with the lesions of diabetic nephropathy demonstrated reversal of the lesion when transplanted into normal recipients. All of these findings suggest that hyperglycemia or some other aspect of the abnormal metabolism of diabetes causes or influences the development of complications. On the other hand additional factors, probably genetic, must play a role. This follows from the fact that diabetic subjects with decades of poor control may escape the ravages of the late complications and from the fact that typical diabetic complications may be found in patients at the time of diagnosis of diabetes or even in the absence of hyperglycemia.

Meticulous control with insulin infusion pumps has been reported to decrease microalbuminuria, alter motor nerve conduction velocity, lower plasma lipoproteins, and decrease capillary leakage of fluorescein in the retina. Width of the capillary basement membrane in skeletal muscle has also been decreased. The changes are small in general, however, and of questionable biologic significance. Firm evidence does not exist to show that late complications can be either prevented or reversed by long-term near-normalization of the plasma glucose. Hopefully, definitive answers to this question may be forthcoming from a large multicenter trial now underway under the sponsorship of the National Institutes of Health.

Until the issue is clarified it is prudent to maintain the plasma glucose as near normal as possible in all diabetic patients. About this there appears to be no disagreement. The only question is whether insulin therapy should be routinely aggressive to the point where recurrent hypoglycemia occurs. A mild insulin reaction consisting of nervousness, tremor, hunger, and sweating that is rapidly interrupted by carbohydrate intake is probably not harmful except for the possibility of worsening diabetic control via the Somogyi reaction. Unfortunately, as stated earlier, many diabetics, particularly those with long-standing disease and autonomic neuropathy, do not have or do not recognize the usual warning signals and progress to altered central nervous system function with abnormal behavior, loss of consciousness, or even convulsions. The latter reactions are dangerous for both patient and society. Every effort should be made to control hyperglycemia, but the limit of therapy should be the appearance of hypoglycemic reactions. It does not seem wise to induce a condition that can cause immediate and irreversible damage to a patient in the unproven hope that late complications might be prevented.

Miscellaneous abnormalities of diabetes Diabetes affects almost every system in the body. Space limitations preclude discussion of all associated features, but several deserve comment. *Infections* in diabetics may not occur more frequently than in normal subjects, but they tend to be more severe. This may be due to impaired leukocyte function, a frequent accompaniment of poor control. In addition to common infections of the skin, urinary tract, lungs, and bloodstream, three unusual conditions appear to have specific relationship with diabetes. *Malignant external otitis,* usually due to *Pseudomonas aeruginosa,* tends to occur in older patients and is characterized by severe pain in the ear, drainage, fever, and leukocytosis. Soft tissues around the ear are swollen and tender. A mound of granulation tissue is characteristically present internally at the junction of the osseous and cartilaginous portions of the ear. The facial nerve becomes paralyzed in half the cases, and other cranial nerves may also be involved. Facial nerve paralysis is a poor prognostic sign, and mortality approximates 50 percent in this subset of patients. A 6-week course of ticarcillin or carbenicillin together with tobramycin is the treatment of choice. Surgical debridement is often necessary. *Rhinocerebral mucormycosis* is a rare fungal infection which usually develops in patients during or following an episode of diabetic ketoacidosis. Organisms are from the genera *Mucor, Rhizopus,* and *Absidia.* Onset is sudden with periorbital and perinasal swelling, pain, bloody nasal discharge, and increased lacrimation. The nasal mucosa and underlying tissues become black and necrotic. Cranial nerve palsies are not uncommon. There may be thrombosis of the internal jugular vein or sinuses of the brain. Proptosis, chemosis, and retinal vein engorgement indicate cavernous sinus thrombosis. Untreated, death usually occurs in a week to 10 days. Amphotericin B and aggressive debridement are the indicated therapies. *Emphysematous cholecystitis* tends to affect diabetic men (in contrast to ordinary cholecystitis, a disease predominantly present in women). Gangrene of the gallbladder is 30 times more frequent than in the usual forms, accounting for high rates of perforation and a mortality rate 3 to 10 times higher than in ordinary cholecystitis. Diagnosis is made when gas is seen in the gallbladder wall on plain films of the abdomen. Clostridial species are frequently cultured from bile, but other organisms may be present. Treatment is cholecystectomy coupled with broad-spectrum antibiotics. Clindamycin and an aminoglycoside are adequate coverage until cultures are returned.

Hypertriglyceridemia is common in diabetes and is usually due to insulin deficiency. Both overproduction of very low density lipoproteins in the liver and a disposal defect in the periphery appear to be operative. The latter is a consequence of lipoprotein lipase deficiency, an insulin-dependent enzyme. Some diabetics exhibit hyperlipemia even when diabetic control is adequate, and these patients may have a primary familial hyperlipoproteinemia that is independent of diabetes. Clofibrate is the drug of choice for treatment in subjects unresponsive to diet and insulin therapy.

Some diabetics have *recurrent hyperkalemia* in association with hyperglycemia. Hyperkalemia can occur in the absence of potassium loads, and serum potassium concentrations may rise acutely in response to oral glucose in contrast to normals in whom glucose ingestion produces a fall in potassium levels. The presumption is that potassium shifts from intracellular to extracellular water under these circumstances. Traditionally these patients have been considered to have hyporeninemic hypoaldosteronism although basal renin and aldosterone concentrations may be normal. Since the capacity to increase aldosterone production in response to stimulatory signals is impaired even when basal levels are normal, probably functional hypoaldosteronism plays a central role in the syndrome. With a deficiency of aldosterone, renal secretion of potassium is impaired and disposal of a potassium load is dependent on insulin-mediated transport of the cation into the intracellular space. Administration of potassium salts or triamterene to such patients may be dangerous. Whether potassium transport is directly regulated by insulin or is secondary to glucose movement is not clear.

A variety of skin lesions occur in diabetes. *Necrobiosis lipoidica diabeticorum* is a plaque-like lesion with a central yellowish area surrounded by a brownish border. It is usually found over the anterior surfaces of the legs. Ulceration may occur (see Fig. A1-28). *Diabetic dermopathy* is also usually located over the anterior tibial surface. The lesions are small rounded plaques with a raised border which may crust at the edges and ulcerate centrally. Several plaques may be arranged in linear fashion. Pigmentation is not prominent early, but as the lesion heals a depressed scar occurs with diffuse brown discoloration. A rarer abnormality is *bullosis diabeticorum.* The bullae may be superficial with clear serum or may be mildly hemorrhagic. The cause is unknown. *Infestations of the skin* with *Candida* and dermatophytes are common, and bacterial infections of a variety of types occur. In women *vaginal moniliasis* may be troublesome during hyperglycemic-glycosuric periods. While the symptoms respond to nystatin or gentian violet, recurrence is inevitable unless glycosuria is reversed. *Atrophy of adipose tissue* may occur at the site of insulin injections. The lipoatrophy is said to respond to injection of purified insulin into the atrophic area.

Hyperviscosity occurs in diabetes, and *platelets aggregate abnormally.* The latter may be caused by increased prostaglandin synthesis. *Wound healing* is impaired in experimental diabetes but probably is not a major factor clinically. An interesting accompaniment of insulin-dependent diabetes is the presence of *joint contractures* coupled with *tight, waxy skin* over the dorsum of the hands. The hands resemble those in patients with scleroderma. The cause of the tendon contractures is unknown although alterations of cross-linking in collagen has been proposed. Patients with the joint contracture–waxy skin syndrome appear to have accelerated development of other diabetic complications. *Scleredema* is a common finding in diabetes. The lesion is a thickening of the skin over the shoulders and upper back that resembles scleroderma. The lesion is benign.

Future directions Research aimed at therapy of established diabetes continues. From the pharmacologic standpoint the search for an orally active antiglucagon is ongoing. Likewise development of a somatostatin analogue that would be relatively specific in blocking glucagon release with lesser activity against growth hormone is of high priority. Such an analogue would have to be orally absorbed and have a longer biologic half-life than native somatostatin. Insulin has been successfully given by nasal insufflation, but the clinical usefulness of this approach in the broad spectrum of diabetic patients is uncertain.

Hopes remain that transplantation of islet cells will be possible in humans. Considerable success has been achieved in experimental animals, but human trials have thus far been unpromising. Segmental transplantation of the vascularized whole human pancreas has also been carried out, but overall complication rates have been high. Techniques for islet cell transplantation that remove antigen-presenting cells (such that immunosuppression is not required) may eventually be applicable in humans, but the problem of islet cell supply will be a formidable obstacle. There is also concern that in type 1 patients the transplanted islets will succumb to the same immunologic mechanism that caused diabetes, as mentioned earlier. An alternative approach would be to activate insulin production in cells in which the gene is normally turned off utilizing techniques of molecular biology. This has already been achieved in vitro, but for maintenance of a normal plasma glucose the activated gene would have to be placed in a cell that is fuel-responsive, i.e., releases hormones only in response to substrate signal. Uncontrolled insulin release would mimic an insulinoma.

The possibility of preventing type 1 diabetes by suppression of the immune system prior to destruction of the beta-cell mass has also received attention. In one study treatment with cyclosporine restored insulin secretory capacity and reversed diabetes in about two-thirds of patients treated within the first 6 weeks of diagnosis. Unfortunately, hyperglycemia returned when cyclosporine was stopped, suggesting that immunosuppression must be constant. Continual use of cyclosporine, even at low doses, would appear to be an unacceptable risk, but it might be possible to modulate the immune system with safer drugs and accomplish the same aims. In an ideal program persons at increased risk for developing type 1 diabetes, primarily first-degree relatives of a patient with this disease, would be typed for genetic susceptibility. Persons with haploidentity to the index case would be followed prospectively for appearance of islet cell antibodies and diminution of insulin reserve. At the earliest sign of immune attack against the beta cell, immunosuppression would be started. Careful double-blind trials would be required to prove effectiveness.

INSULIN RESISTANCE Insulin resistance is arbitrarily said to exist when more than 200 units per day are required to control hyperglycemia and prevent ketosis. Relative insulin resistance occurs with lower insulin requirements, but therapy for the resistant state is usually not considered necessary below the 200-unit level. Insulin antibodies of IgG type are present in essentially all diabetics within 60 days of the initiation of insulin therapy. The titer of these antibodies fluctuates for reasons that are not clear. Although the correlation between antibody titer and functional resistance is not close, insulin binding by high levels of antibody is presumed to be the primary mechanism in most cases. Probably less than 0.1 percent of insulin-treated diabetics ever have significant resistance. The problem may appear within a few weeks of the start of therapy or many years later. The onset may be abrupt, resulting in ketoacidosis, but usually is gradual, with uncontrollable hyperglycemia being the major problem. About 20 to 30 percent of patients have concomitant insulin allergy. Therapy of the syndrome requires prednisone in large amounts—80 to 100 mg per day initially. Response often occurs in 48 to 72 h but may take longer. If no improvement has resulted after 3 to 4 weeks it can be assumed that steroids will not be effective. Once insulin requirements begin to fall, prednisone dosage can be rapidly decreased by 10 to 20 mg every 3 to 7 days until a maintenance level of 5 to 10 mg per day is reached. These levels may be required for many months. Whether remission has occurred, allowing cessation of therapy, can only be determined by trial. On rare occasions insulin resistance in diabetics appears to be due to enhanced destruction of the hormone at the subcutaneous injection site. Such patients tend to respond normally to insulin given intravenously or intraperitoneally. In some patients addition of a protease inhibitor (aprotinin) to the insulin mixture has been helpful. When resistance is extreme, U500 regular insulin should be used in order to control the volume of the injection.

Insulin resistance may occur in diseases other than diabetes. The physiologic consequences can be minor or severe. A variety of insulin-resistant syndromes are associated with *acanthosis nigricans,* a brown to black, velvety hyperpigmentation of the skin in the axilla, groin, neck, umbilicus, and other areas. Although acanthosis nigricans may be a sign of occult malignancy, it is not associated with neoplasia in the insulin-resistant states. A classification of insulin resistance based on the absence or presence of acanthosis nigricans is given in Table 327-14. *Obesity* and *antibodies* to insulin are by far the most common causes of insulin resistance, and neither is accompanied by acanthosis. Obesity is associated with diminished insulin receptor number and affinity but also has postreceptor hormone resistance. *Werner's syndrome* is an autosomal recessive illness with a high incidence of hyperglycemia despite elevated concentrations of plasma insulin (see Chap. 334). There is little response to exogenous hormone. Other features include growth retardation, alopecia or premature graying of the hair, cataracts, hypogonadism, leg ulcers, atrophy of muscle, fat, and bone, soft-tissue calcification, and a high frequency of sarcomas and meningiomas.

Of the rare conditions associated with acanthosis nigricans, women with *insulin receptor abnormalities* have attracted the greatest interest. Type A patients are tall young women with a tendency to hirsutism and abnormalities of the reproductive tract who most probably have polycystic ovaries. However, other causes of androgen excess can induce the syndrome. The absolute number of insulin receptors is diminished. Type B subjects are older women with evidence of immunologic disease. The clinical picture includes arthralgias, alopecia, enlarged salivary glands, proteinuria, leukopenia, and antinuclear and anti-DNA antibodies. Insulin resistance in these patients is due to blocking antibodies to the insulin receptor (not to insulin itself). Interestingly, antireceptor antibodies may also cause hypoglycemia. The determinant of agonist (hypoglycemia) or antagonist (insulin resistance) activity presumably depends on the site of binding to the insulin receptor. Both A and B patients have high plasma insulin concentrations.

Generalized and *partial lipodystrophies* are fat depletion syndromes differing primarily in the extent of fat atrophy (see Chap.

TABLE 327-14 Insulin-resistant states

I Insulin resistance without acanthosis nigricans
- *A* Obesity
- *B* Diabetes mellitus with insulin antibodies
- *C* Werner's syndrome

II Insulin resistance with acanthosis nigricans
- *A* Insulin resistance with receptor abnormality
  - *1* Receptor deficiency (type A abnormality)
  - *2* Antibody to insulin receptor (type B abnormality)
- *B* Lipodystrophic states
  - *1* Generalized lipodystrophy (congenital or acquired)
  - *2* Partial lipodystrophy (congenital or acquired)
- *C* Syndrome of familial insulin resistance, somatic abnormalities, and pineal hyperplasia
- *D* The Alström syndrome
- *E* Ataxia-telangiectasia
- *F* Rabson-Mendenhall syndrome

318). In the generalized form essentially all body fat is missing, while the more common partial type exhibits atrophy of fat in the face and trunk with normal or increased adiposity in the lower half of the body. The disease can be either congenital or acquired. Typically the patients develop hyperglycemia at puberty, but ketoacidosis never occurs. Marked hypertriglyceridemia with eruptive xanthoma is a frequent feature. Characteristic features are hepatomegaly, splenomegaly, cardiomegaly, hirsutism, lymphadenopathy, hypertrophy of the external genitalia, varicose veins, and (in the congenital forms) muscle hypertrophy. Mental retardation is common, and renal disease may develop. The term *lipoatrophic diabetes* is synonymous with total lipodystrophy. All patients have elevated plasma insulin levels. Resistance may be due to decreased number of receptors, diminished affinity of the receptor for insulin, or a postreceptor defect.

The *pineal hypertrophy syndrome* is characterized by insulin resistance, early dentition with malformed teeth, dry skin, thick nails, hirsutism, and a peculiar sexual precocity with enlargement of the external genitalia. The latter may reach near adult size by age 3 or 4. The insulin resistance is severe, and ketoacidosis may occur despite high endogenous insulin levels. The *Alström syndrome* is a rare autosomal recessive disease characterized by childhood blindness due to retinal degeneration, nerve deafness, vasopressin-resistant diabetes insipidus, and, in males, hypogonadism with high plasma gonadotropin levels. The patients thus appear to have end organ resistance to multiple hormones. Other features include baldness, hyperuricemia, hypertriglyceridemia, and aminoaciduria. Superficially the patients may resemble subjects with the Lawrence-Moon-Biedl syndrome but can be differentiated on initial exam by the absence of polydactyly and mental deficiency. Insulin resistance in the Alström syndrome is mild. *Ataxia-telangiectasia* is characterized by cerebellar ataxia, telangiectasia, and a variety of abnormalities in the immune system in addition to insulin resistance. The *Rabson-Mendenhall syndrome* consists of dental dysplasia, dystrophic nails, premature puberty, and acanthosis nigricans. The insulin resistance is probably due to an insulin receptor abnormality. Not listed in Table 327-14 is insulin resistance due to hormone excess (acromegaly, Cushing's syndrome), myotonic dystrophy, and leprechaunism. The insulin resistance in these conditions is usually not clinically significant.

INSULIN ALLERGY Insulin allergy is due to IgE antibodies to insulin. Manifestations include immediate reactions with local stinging or itching, delayed local reactions with brawny swelling lasting up to 30 h, and generalized urticaria or frank anaphylaxis. Systemic reactions are usually seen in patients who have stopped insulin therapy for one reason or another and have then resumed treatment. The allergic reaction may occur as early as the second injection on resumption of therapy. Mild reactions can be treated with antihistamines. If the problem is severe, desensitization procedures are required. A 1-day insulin desensitization procedure is shown in Table 327-15. Once the patient is desensitized, insulin therapy should not be interrupted.

TABLE 327-15 Insulin desensitization*

Time, h	Dose, units	Route
0	0.001	Intradermal
0.5	0.002	Intradermal
1	0.004	Subcutaneous
1.5	0.01	Subcutaneous
2	0.02	Subcutaneous
2.5	0.04	Subcutaneous
3	0.1	Subcutaneous
3.5	0.2	Subcutaneous
4	0.5	Subcutaneous
4.5	1	Subcutaneous
5	2	Subcutaneous
5.5	4	Subcutaneous
6	8	Subcutaneous

* *Following desensitization, use 2 to 10 units of regular insulin every 4 to 6 h for 24 to 36 h after the 6-h injection before switching to intermediate-acting insulin.*

SOURCE: *Schedule of JA Galloway. For detailed information see JA Galloway, R Bressler, Med Clin North Amer 62:663, 1978.*

THE EMOTIONAL RESPONSE TO DIABETES Acceptance of the fact that a person has a chronic disease that requires a change in lifestyle is always difficult. This is particularly true in the case of diabetes since patients generally are aware that they are vulnerable to late complications and that life expectancy is shortened. It is not surprising that the emotional response to diabetes often hampers treatment. On the one hand, the primary reaction may be denial with an accompanying refusal to cooperate. At the other extreme is excessive preoccupation with the illness. The physician should make every effort to define a middle ground wherein the patient acknowledges his or her disease and responds prudently without becoming obsessed. The goal is to live with diabetes not for it. Diabetics are no different from other patients in that they may attempt to use their disease manipulatively with both family and physician. The problems are particularly acute with children and adolescents. While the psychiatric aspects of diabetes are not discussed here, most problems can be anticipated and handled if common sense is coupled with sympathy and firmness. It is also appropriate to offer cautious hope that the disease will be handled better in the future than is possible now.

REFERENCES

General review

UNGER RH, FOSTER DW: Diabetes mellitus, in *Williams' Textbook of Endocrinology*, 7th ed, JD Wilson, DW Foster (eds). Philadelphia, Saunders, 1985, pp 1018–1080

Pathophysiology

BOTTAZZO GF: β-Cell damage in diabetic insulitis: Are we approaching a solution? Diabetologia 26:241, 1984

——— et al: In situ characterization of autoimmune phenomena and expression of HLA molecules in the pancreas in diabetic insulitis. N Engl J Med 313:353, 1985

CAHILL GF JR, MCDEVITT HO: Insulin-dependent diabetes mellitus: The initial lesion. N Engl J Med 304:1454, 1981

DEFRONZO RA, FERRANNINI E: The pathogenesis of non-insulin-dependent diabetes: An update. Medicine 61:125, 1982

LERNMARK A: Molecular biology of type 1 (insulin-dependent) diabetes mellitus. Diabetologia 28:195, 1985

WARD WK et al: Diminished β-cell secretory capacity in patients with non-insulin-dependent diabetes. J Clin Invest 74:1318, 1984

Treatment

BANTLE JP et al: Postprandial glucose and insulin responses to meals containing different carbohydrates in normal and diabetic subjects. N Engl J Med 309:7, 1983

CRYER PE, GERICH JE: Glucose counterregulation, hypoglycemia, and intensive insulin therapy in diabetes mellitus. N Engl J Med 313:232, 1985

LEBOVITZ HE, FEINGLOS MN: The oral hypoglycemic agents, in *Diabetes Mellitus: Theory and Practice*, 3d ed, M Ellenberg, H Rifkin (eds). New Hyde Park, Medical Examination Publishing, 1983, pp 591–610

RASKIN P: Treatment of insulin-dependent diabetes mellitus with portable insulin infusion devices. Med Clin North Am 66:1269, 1982

SCHADE DS et al: *Intensive Insulin Therapy*. Princeton, Excerpta Medica, 1983

SCHIFFRIN A, BELMONTE MM: Comparison between subcutaneous insulin infusion and multiple injections of insulin: A one year prospective study. Diabetes 31:255, 1982

SIMONSON DC et al: Intensive insulin therapy reduces counterregulatory hormone responses to hypoglycemia in patients with type 1 diabetes. Ann Intern Med 103:184, 1985

SKYLER JS et al: Algorithms for adjustment of insulin dosage by patients who monitor blood glucose. Diabetes Care 4:311, 1981

WOLEVER TMS et al: Prediction of the relative blood glucose response of mixed meals using the white bread glycemic index. Diabetes Care 8:418, 1985

Acute complications

CARROLL P, MATZ R: Uncontrolled diabetes mellitus in adults: Experience in treating diabetic ketoacidosis and hyperosmolar nonketotic coma with low-dose insulin and a uniform treatment regimen. Diabetes Care 6:579, 1983

FOSTER DW: From glycogen to ketones—and back. Diabetes 33:1188, 1984

———, MCGARRY JD: The metabolic derangements and treatment of diabetic ketoacidosis. N Engl J Med 309:159, 1983

FRANKLIN B et al: Cerebral edema and ophthalmoplegia reversed by mannitol in a new case of insulin-dependent diabetes mellitus. Pediatrics 69:87, 1982

Late complications

BROWNLEE M et al: Nonenzymatic glycosylation and the pathogenesis of diabetic complications. Ann Intern Med 101:527, 1984

DORMAN JS et al: The Pittsburgh insulin-dependent diabetes mellitus (IDDM) morbidity and mortality study: Case-control analyses of risk factors for mortality. Diabetes Care 8 (Suppl 1):54, 1985

GREENE DA et al: Glucose-induced alterations in nerve metabolism: Current perspective on the pathogenesis of diabetic neuropathy and future directions for research and therapy. Diabetes Care 8:290, 1985

LESTRADET H et al: Long-term study of mortality and vascular complications in juvenile-onset (type 1) diabetes. Diabetes 30:175, 1981

LOGERFO FW, COFFMAN JD: Vascular and microvascular disease of the foot in diabetes. N Engl J Med 311:1615, 1984

MOGENSEN CE, CHRISTENSEN CK: Predicting diabetic nephropathy in insulin-dependent patients. N Engl J Med 311:89, 1984

PARVING HH et al: Hemodynamic factors in the genesis of diabetic microangiopathy. Metabolism 32:943, 1983

STEFFES MW et al: Studies of kidney and muscle biopsy specimens from identical twins discordant for type 1 diabetes mellitus. N Engl J Med 312:1282, 1985

VIBERTI G, KEEN H: The patterns of proteinuria in diabetes mellitus. Relevance to pathogenesis and prevention of diabetic nephropathy. Diabetes 33:686, 1984

Future directions

ALEJANDRO R et al: Successful long-term survival of pancreatic islet allografts in spontaneous or pancreatectomy-induced diabetes in dogs. Cyclosporine-induced immune unresponsiveness. Diabetes 34:825, 1985

EISENBARTH GS: Immunotherapy of type 1 diabetes. Diabetes Care 6:521, 1983

FAUSTMAN D et al: Prolongation of murine islet allograft survival by pretreatment of islets with antibody directed to Ia determinants. Proc Natl Acad Sci USA 78:5156, 1981

LAFFERTY KJ, PROWSE SJ: Theory and practice of immunoregulation by tissue treatment prior to transplantation. World J Surg 8:187, 1984

STILLER CR et al: Effects of cyclosporine immunosuppression in insulin-dependent diabetes mellitus of recent onset. Science 223:1362, 1984

Insulin resistance

FLIER JS et al: Acanthosis nigricans in obese women with hyperandrogenism. Characterization of an insulin-resistance state distinct from the types A and B syndromes. Diabetes 34:101, 1985

KAHN CR: Role of insulin receptors in insulin-resistant states. Metabolism 29:455, 1980

KURTZ AB, NABARRO JDN: Circulating insulin-binding antibodies. Diabetologia 19:329, 1980

MISBIN RI et al: Resistance to subcutaneous and intramuscular insulin associated with deficiency of insulin-like growth factor (IGF) 2. Metabolism 32:537, 1983

PAULSEN EP et al: Insulin resistance caused by massive degradation of subcutaneous insulin. Diabetes 28:640, 1979

TAYLOR SI et al: Insulin resistance associated with androgen excess in women with autoantibodies to the insulin receptor. Ann Intern Med 97:851, 1982

328 LACTIC ACIDOSIS

DANIEL W. FOSTER

Lactic acidosis is common. This follows from the fact that lactic acid is produced at accelerated rates in skeletal muscle and other tissues whenever oxygenation is inadequate to supply energy needs. Thus lactic acidosis represents a final common pathway for any disease resulting in circulatory collapse or hypoxia. Lactic acidosis can also occur when tissue hypoxia is not apparent. In most cases an etiology can be established, but in some the lactic acidosis is "idiopathic."

FIGURE 328-1 *Schematic view of aerobic metabolism. Subcellular compartments are not indicated. Glycolysis occurs in the cytosol while enzymes of fatty acid oxidation and the Krebs cycle are located intramitochondrially. The dotted line indicates that glycogenolysis and glycolysis are inactive in the presence of oxygen. (See text.)*

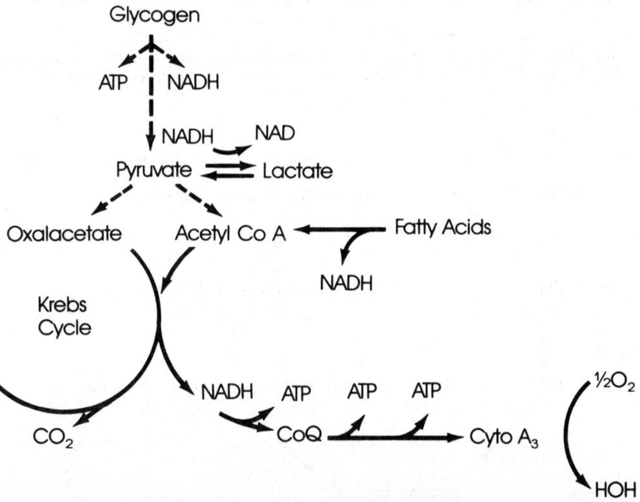

BIOCHEMICAL BACKGROUND In the narrowest sense biologic life can be defined as the capacity to generate high-energy phosphate bonds within the cell. Adenosine triphosphate (ATP) is the most important high-energy compound, but other nucleotides, such as guanosine triphosphate, also play important roles. Structure and function of every tissue in the body are directly or indirectly dependent on ATP or equivalent high-energy nucleotides. During tissue hypoxia ATP cannot be generated in adequate amounts, and lactic acidosis results. The acidosis is the metabolic consequence of activation of a back-up system for the generation of ATP when the primary energy-forming pathway is impaired. The normal mechanism of ATP generation under aerobic conditions is shown in Fig. 328-1. When substrates such as free fatty acids or glucose are oxidized to acetyl CoA, the constituent hydrogen atoms are transferred to nicotinamide adenine dinucleotide (NAD), producing the reduced form of the pyridine nucleotide (NADH). Oxidation of acetyl CoA to CO_2 in the Krebs cycle generates additional NADH. The bulk of NADH is formed intramitochondrially, where fatty acid oxidizing and tricarboxylic acid cycle enzymes are located; cytosolic NADH must be transported into the mitochondria by "shuttle" systems because NADH cannot directly penetrate the inner mitochondrial membrane. In the presence of oxygen, NADH is oxidized by the electron transport chain, the end product being water ("metabolic water"). For each mole of NADH passing through the cytochrome sequence 2 to 3 moles of ATP are formed. When oxygen content of tissues is normal and ATP stores are high, rates of glycogen breakdown and glucose oxidation are low (the *Pasteur effect*). Conversely, when oxygen content is low, ATP stores fall, and glycogen breakdown and glycolysis are activated.

Control of glycolysis is primarily vested in the enzyme phosphofructokinase (PFK). As shown in Fig. 328-2, this enzyme catalyzes the conversion of fructose 6-phosphate to fructose 1,6-bisphosphate. Several allosteric modulators regulate the activity of PFK. In muscle and other tissues ATP is the primary physiologic inhibitor, and AMP is a prominent activator. In liver fructose 2,6-bisphosphate is the major regulator of PFK (see Chap. 327). When fructose 2,6-bisphosphate concentrations are normal, rates of glycolysis (glucose 6-phosphate → pyruvate) are high, and gluconeogenesis (pyruvate → glucose 6-phosphate) is inhibited. Concentrations of fructose 2,6-bisphosphate are low in muscle, and it is not thought to play a primary regulatory role in that tissue. Fructose 2,6-bisphosphate concentrations in the liver fall with hypoxia and thus shift metabolism of the hepatocyte toward gluconeogenesis. This adaptation favors lactate uptake and utilization under circumstances in which lactate production is accelerated in nonhepatic tissues. Muscle contraction causes activation of glycogen breakdown and lactic acid production, but, paradoxically, it also causes a fall in fructose 2,6-bisphosphate concentration. This supports the view that phosphofructokinase ac-

FIGURE 328-2 *Phosphofructokinase and glycolysis. The minus sign indicates inhibition; the plus sign indicates activation. (See text.)*

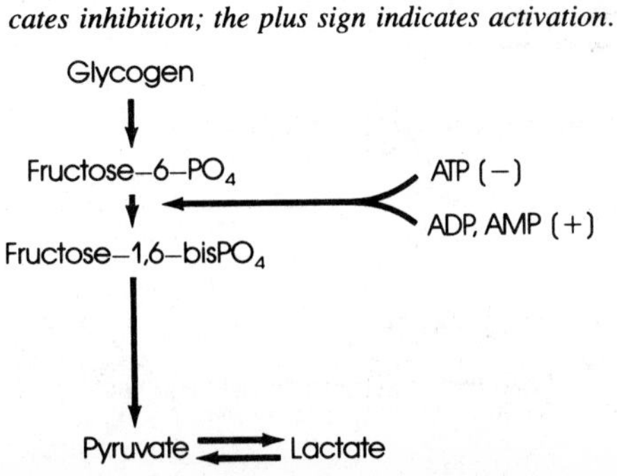

tivity and glycolysis are controlled primarily by the ATP/AMP ratio in muscle and not by fructose 2,6-bisphosphate.

The sequence of events occurring during tissue hypoxia is schematically shown in Fig. 328-3. If blood flow to peripheral tissues is diminished such that oxygen delivery is insufficient to meet metabolic demands, electron flow through the transport chain is impaired or blocked (all cytochromes become reduced). Because of the block, NADH, which for a finite period continues to be generated, cannot be oxidized, resulting in high NADH/NAD ratios in both mitochondrial and cytosolic compartments. As a result all near-equilibrium reactions utilizing NADH as cofactor shift to the reduced side (e.g., oxaloacetate → malate, pyruvate → lactate), slowing substrate flux at a number of critical sites. In addition, ATP cannot be synthesized, and tissue ATP concentrations fall. There is a reciprocal rise in ADP and AMP. As a result, phosphofructokinase is activated, with rapid glycogen breakdown and glucose oxidation. Accelerated glycolysis leads to overproduction of pyruvic acid, which, because of the elevated NADH content of the cell, is reduced to lactic acid. Put simply, the acidosis of tissue hypoxia is due to the conversion of neutral substrate, glycogen/glucose, to a strong acid, pyruvate. It is a lactic acidosis because the high NADH/NAD ratio drives the lactic dehydrogenase reaction to the right. These points are shown schematically in Fig. 328-4.

Even in the fully oxygenated subject lactate is produced by a variety of tissues. This lactate passes to the liver, where it enters the gluconeogenic pathway for conversion to glucose (*Cori cycle*). Diminished hepatic uptake of lactate undoubtedly plays a role in the pathogenesis of lactic acidosis (especially in patients with vascular collapse, severe hepatocellular disease, or enzymic defects in the gluconeogenic pathway), but significant acidosis probably never occurs in the absence of peripheral overproduction. Whether lactate overproduction in lactic acidosis is generalized or limited to specific tissues such as muscle and intestine is not resolved.

Conceptually the accelerated glycolysis induced by hypoxia can be considered an alternative system for the generation of ATP when the normal mitochondrial mechanism is impaired. The glycolytic system is not efficient, however. A mole of glucose derived from glycogen and oxidized completely through the Krebs cycle generates about 37 mol ATP, while the yield from glycogen to pyruvate is only 3 mol. Nevertheless, over the short run, this ATP may be lifesaving.

FIGURE 328-3 *Schematic view of anaerobic metabolism. Diagonally striped boxes indicate metabolic blocks secondary to failure of delivery of oxygen to tissues and high NADH/NAD ratios. Heavy arrows indicate accelerated glycogenolysis, glycolysis, and lactate production. Glycolysis is permitted to continue in the face of high NADH/NAD ratios in the cytosol because one molecule of NAD (required in the glyceraldehyde 3-phosphate dehydrogenase reaction) is produced for each molecule of lactate formed.*

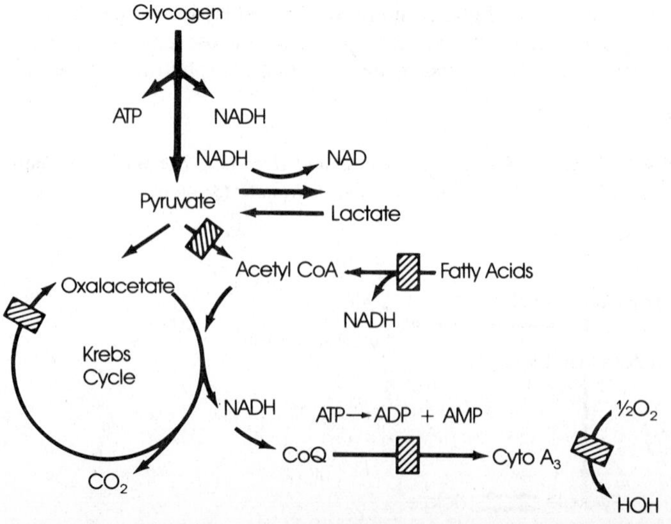

CLINICAL PICTURE Lactic acidosis is usually heralded by the onset of nausea, vomiting, restlessness, and driven respiration of the Kussmaul type. Stupor or coma is sometimes seen. Huckabee, who in 1961 brought the problem of lactic acidosis to the attention of clinicians, recognized that there were two major groups of patients with elevated lactate concentrations in the blood. The first had proportionate increases of lactate and pyruvate and were not considered to be hypoxic. The second group had lactate levels disproportionately elevated when compared with the simultaneously measured pyruvate concentration. Huckabee coined the term "excess lactate" for any increase in lactate that could not be accounted for by a rise in pyruvate concentration and interpreted its presence to mean tissue hypoxia (a high NADH/NAD ratio). The relationship of the lactate/pyruvate concentration to the cytoplasmic NADH/NAD ratio is obvious when the lactate dehydrogenase reaction is rearranged:

$$\text{Pyruvate} + \text{NADH} + \text{H}^+ \rightleftharpoons \text{lactate} + \text{NAD}^+ \quad (1)$$

$$K \times \frac{[\text{NADH}]\,[\text{H}^+]}{[\text{NAD}^+]} = \frac{[\text{lactate}]}{[\text{pyruvate}]} \quad (2)$$

A sample calculation of "excess lactate" is given in Fig. 328-5.

The mean level of lactate in venous blood normally is about 1 m*M* (range 0.6 to 1.5 m*M*), and the pyruvate concentration is about 0.1 m*M* (range 0.05 to 0.15 m*M*)[1]. Accurately determined lactate/pyruvate ratios above 10 to 15 usually mean some degree of hypoxia. In practice pyruvate is usually not measured because instability and low concentrations make assay difficult. As a consequence, excess lactate is rarely quantitated. The concept was seminal, however, in providing the insight that led to understanding of the pathophysiology of lactic acidosis.

Cohen and Woods have suggested a classification of lactic acidosis based on clinical findings rather than on the lactate/pyruvate ratio (Table 328-1). Type A lactic acidosis is associated with poor tissue perfusion or oxygenation. Most patients with lactic acidosis fall into this category. Vascular collapse is the most common cause, and any condition leading to shock (e.g., myocardial infarction, pulmonary embolism, hemorrhage, septicemia, poisoning) can produce the disorder. Hypoxia does not have to be present. Importantly, diminished tissue perfusion may occur in the absence of a measurable fall in the blood pressure. Lactic acidosis occurs physiologically whenever muscular exercise is sufficient to contract an oxygen debt. The pathologic counterpart is lactic acidosis produced by convulsions or hypothermia with prolonged shivering. All type A patients have "excess lactate" in the Huckabee terminology.

Type B patients have elevated blood lactate concentrations without evidence of diminished tissue perfusion. Acidosis may be absent, mild, or severe. Pyruvate and lactate may both be elevated, but high lactate/pyruvate ratios are present when acidosis is severe. Systemic clinical disorders associated with elevations of blood lactate include uncontrolled diabetes mellitus, severe liver disease, leukemia, thiamine deficiency, and metabolic or respiratory alkalosis. Lactic acidosis

[1] *Measurement of lactate and pyruvate requires precautions. The sample should be iced, and red blood cells (which produce lactate) should be separated immediately.*

FIGURE 328-4 *Summary of biochemical mechanisms in lactic acidosis.*

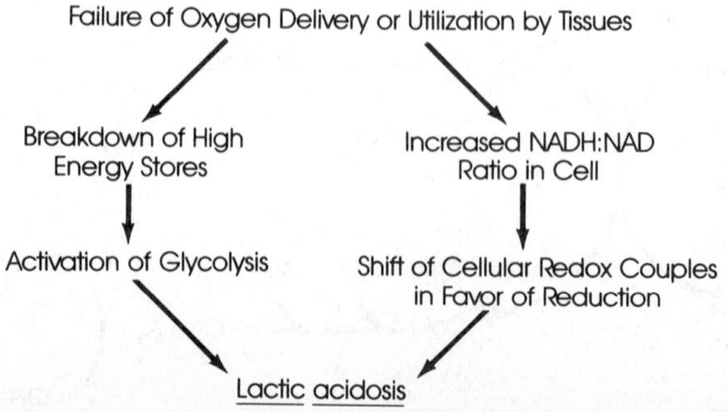

was commonly reported with biguanide therapy of diabetes, and because of this, phenformin was removed from clinical use in the United States by the Food and Drug Administration. The syndrome also occurs with nitroprusside therapy of hypertension, with epinephrine overdosage, and in isolated instances with other drug intoxications. Most of the latter are doubtless associated with hypoxia or shock and rightfully belong in the type A category. Ethanol is often listed as a cause of lactic acidosis but in fact rarely induces the syndrome. The oxidation of ethanol by the liver results in the generation of high NADH/NAD ratios in the cell and presumably blocks the recycling of lactate (and alanine) to glucose. Infants with enzyme defects in the glycolytic-gluconeogenic-tricarboxylic acid pathway appear to be particularly vulnerable to lactic acidosis, and early death is common. Recurrent lactic acidosis occurs in certain primary myopathies characterized by mitochondrial abnormalities. The mitochondrial myopathies typically show "ragged-red fibers" with the modified Gomori trichromic stain and exhibit bizarre-looking mitochondria (see Chap. 355). A variety of defects in the electron transport chain presumably cause lactic acidosis because of inability to generate ATP in the face of increased demand, as in exercise. Subtle mitochondrial disease is likely present in most cases of so-called idiopathic lactic acidosis.

The pathophysiology of lactate accumulation in other forms of type B disease is varied and often incompletely understood. The enzyme defects and alcohol may involve diminished hepatic uptake of lactate as a primary mechanism; i.e., modest increases in lactate production induced by hormones or exercise cause acidosis because of limited capacity for extraction in the liver. Drugs that do not cause perfusion problems probably alter mitochondrial function in some fashion. Hormones such as glucagon and epinephrine raise lactate by stimulating glycolysis. Leukemia probably acts both by direct overproduction of lactate in the white cell mass and through increased blood viscosity that diminishes capillary perfusion.

Most chronic type B conditions cause only mild to moderate hyperlactatemia in themselves, and an additional insult is required for acidosis to develop. The latter might include infection, dehydration, volume depletion, starvation, or unusual exertion. The effect of such an insult would be to add a mild inadequacy of tissue perfusion (insufficient to qualify as type A disease) to the primary abnormality and in combination to cause frank acidosis.

DIAGNOSIS The diagnosis of lactic acidosis requires that a significant metabolic acidosis be present and that the measured lactate concentration be sufficient to account for the bulk of the decrease in plasma bicarbonate content. In general the arterial pH is less than 7.2, and the plasma lactate concentration is greater than 12 m*M*. Unfortunately, in many case reports of "lactic acidosis" plasma lactate concentrations are only modestly elevated (3 to 6 m*M*), and pH values are near normal. There are many causes of elevated plasma lactate levels, but the term *lactic acidosis* should be reserved for situations in which acidosis is present. Confusion also occurs when severe acidosis is present but lactate concentrations do not account for the decrement of bicarbonate (i.e., a mixed acidosis is present). In diabetic ketoacidosis, for example, lactate concentrations of 3 to 6 m*M* are common, but acetoacetate and β-hydroxybutyrate are primarily responsible for the low pH.

FIGURE 328-5 *The concept of excess lactate (XL). The symbols L_t and P_t indicate plasma concentrations of lactate and pyruvate, respectively, in the patient. L_n and P_n refer to mean values in normal subjects.*

$$XL = (L_t - L_n) - (P_t - P_n) \cdot \frac{Ln}{Pn}$$

	Pyruvate	Lactate
Normal	0.1 mM	1.0 mM
Patient	0.3 mM	11.0 mM

$$XL = (11 - 1) - (0.3 - 0.1)\frac{1.0}{0.1} = 8\text{mM}$$

Lactic acidosis should be suspected whenever a metabolic acidosis is associated with an "anion gap" in the absence of an explanation for the unmeasured anions. The anion gap can be calculated in several ways, the simplest of which is $[Na^+] - ([Cl^-] + [HCO_3^-])$. The normal range is 8 to 16 mmol per liter, with the mean about 12. The four most common causes of metabolic acidosis with anion gap are diabetic or alcoholic ketoacidosis, uremic acidosis, lactic acidosis, and acidosis associated with toxin ingestion (salicylates, methanol, ethylene glycol, paraldehyde). Thus if ketoacidosis and uremia are not present and there is nothing to suggest a poisoning, the chances are good that a metabolic acidosis with significant anion gap is due to lactic acid.

TREATMENT If lactic acidosis is caused by shock or hypoxia, reversal of the primary condition cures the secondary acidosis. Traditionally treatment has also involved the infusion of large amounts of sodium bicarbonate intravenously. Questions about this practice have been based on experiments showing a detrimental effect of bicarbonate therapy in dogs with lactic acidosis induced by hypoxia. The applicability of these results to humans is not clear, although bicarbonate therapy is not very effective. Until this issue is clarified, it may be prudent to initiate treatment with 1 to 2 liters of 0.9% saline solution to expand volume and then switch to bicarbonate infusion if improvement is not forthcoming. The recommendation to use bicarbonate follows from the observation that severe and prolonged acidosis in and of itself can cause vascular collapse. If administered, straight bicarbonate solutions should be used. A near isotonic solution can be prepared by adding three 50-mL vials of sodium bicarbonate (1 mmol/mL) to 850 mL of sterile distilled water. Hypertonic (5%) solutions are commercially available and may be required in certain cases.

Because large volumes of bicarbonate are required, the problem of fluid overload often arises, especially in elderly patients and in subjects with impaired renal function. Diuretics should be routinely given with vigorous alkali therapy after it is clear that any volume deficits have been repaired. Occasionally peritoneal dialysis or hemodialysis with hypertonic solutions may be required to prevent pulmonary edema. Dialysis is not indicated as a treatment of lactic acidosis per se.

An experimental drug, dichloroacetate, has been successfully used to reverse lactic acidosis in humans. The drug is thought to stimulate pyruvate/lactate oxidation through activation of pyruvate dehydrogenase. Although the drug causes polyneuropathy, testicular damage,

TABLE 328-1 Some causes of hyperlactatemia

A Hyperlactatemia with hypoxia
- *1* Strenuous muscle exercise (convulsions, hypothermia)
- *2* Inadequate tissue perfusion or oxygenation of any cause*

B Hyperlactatemia without apparent hypoxia
- *1* Systemic clinical disorders
  - *a* Alkalosis (respiratory or metabolic)
  - *b* Uncontrolled diabetes mellitus
  - *c* Leukemia, lymphoma, other cancers
  - *d* Severe liver disease
  - *e* Thiamine deficiency
- *2* Drugs, hormones, toxins
  - *a* Phenformin and other biguanides
  - *b* Salicylates
  - *c* Sodium nitroprusside
  - *d* Ethanol
  - *e* Epinephrine, glucagon
  - *f* Fructose, sorbitol
- *3* Enzyme defects
  - *a* Glucose 6-phosphatase
  - *b* Fructose 1,6-bisphosphatase
  - *c* Pyruvate carboxylase
  - *d* Pyruvate dehydrogenase
  - *e* Unclassified tricarboxylic acid defect
- *4* Certain primary myopathies
- *5* Idiopathic

* *The most common causes of perfusion-oxygenation defects are myocardial infarction, sepsis, hemorrhage, volume depletion, pulmonary embolism, and heart failure. Hypoxia due to severe pulmonary disease, chronic anemia, carbon monoxide inhalation, and cyanide poisoning are much less frequent.*

SOURCE: *After Cohen and Woods, 1976.*

cataracts, and disturbed oxalate metabolism when used chronically, Stacpoole and colleagues observed no serious toxicity with bolus doses at the 50 mg per kilogram of body weight level. The effects of a single dose lasted for a number of hours. Unfortunately, despite improvement in the acidosis, most of the patients went on to die. Such a course would be in accord with the view that lactic acidosis is usually a marker of impending demise from some underlying disease as opposed to being the primary cause of death. Further experience with dichloroacetate will be required before its efficacy can be determined.

REFERENCES

CLAUS TH et al: The role of fructose 2,6-bisphosphate in the regulation of carbohydrate metabolism. Curr Top Cell Regul 23:57, 1984

COHEN RD, WOODS HF: *Clinical and Biochemical Aspects of Lactic Acidosis*. Oxford, Blackwell, 1976

———: Lactic acidosis revisited. Diabetes 32:181, 1983

GABOW PA et al: Diagnostic importance of an increased anion gap. N Engl J Med 303:854, 1980

GRAF H et al: Evidence for a detrimental effect of bicarbonate therapy in hypoxic lactic acidosis. Science 227:754, 1985

HUCKABEE WE: Abnormal resting blood lactate. Am J Med 30:833, 1961

KENNAWAY NG et al: Lactic acidosis and mitochondrial myopathy associated with deficiency of several components of complex III of the respiratory chain. Pediatr Res 18:991, 1984

KREISBERG RA: Lactate homeostasis and lactic acidosis. Ann Intern Med 92:227, 1980

STACPOOLE PW et al: Treatment of lactic acidosis with dichloroacetate. N Engl J Med 309:390, 1983

329 HYPOGLYCEMIA, INSULINOMA, AND OTHER HORMONE-SECRETING TUMORS OF THE PANCREAS

DANIEL W. FOSTER / ARTHUR H. RUBENSTEIN

Maintenance of the plasma glucose concentration within narrow bounds is essential for health. Hypoglycemia is dangerous (in the short run more serious than hyperglycemia) because glucose is the primary energy substrate of the brain. Its absence, like that of oxygen, produces deranged function, tissue damage, or even death if the deficit is prolonged. The vulnerability of the brain to hypoglycemia is due to the fact that it cannot utilize circulating free fatty acids as an energy source in contrast to other tissues of the body. Short-chain metabolites of the free fatty acids, acetoacetic and β-hydroxybutyric acids (the "ketone bodies"), are efficiently oxidized by brain and can protect the central nervous system from damage by hypoglycemia when present at moderate concentrations in plasma. However, development of ketosis requires a number of hours in humans. Ketogenesis is not, therefore, an effective protective mechanism against acute hypoglycemia. Preservation of central nervous system function in the early phases of fasting or during hypoglycemia thus requires a prompt increase in the production of glucose by the liver. At the same time glucose utilization in other tissues is diminished by provision of free fatty acids as alternative substrate. These adaptive mechanisms are hormonally controlled and, under ordinary circumstances, are extremely effective. Occasionally, however, the system breaks down or is overwhelmed, resulting in the clinical syndrome of hypoglycemia.

DEFENSE AGAINST HYPOGLYCEMIA The mechanisms underlying the hypoglycemic states can best be understood by briefly reviewing normal fuel metabolism. Under ordinary circumstances energy needs are met by exogenous substrate derived from food. Oxidation of the constituent molecules of absorbed foodstuffs to carbon dioxide and water is accompanied by the generation of adenosine triphosphate (ATP), the principal high-energy compound of the body. In one sense, life can be defined as the continued ability to generate ATP (and related high-energy nucleotides) for the preservation of cellular integrity in all its manifestations. When caloric intake is greater than immediate oxidative needs, as after the usual meal, excess substrate is stored as fat, structural protein, and glycogen. Substrate flux in this phase of metabolism, called *anabolic,* proceeds from intestine to liver to utilization and storage sites. Insulin is the primary hormone mediating the anabolic phase, during which counterregulatory hormone levels are suppressed.

The *catabolic* phase of metabolism begins about 5 to 6 h after a meal. Normally the only significant period of catabolism is during the overnight fast, but under other circumstances, particularly serious illness, it may be prolonged. During fasting/catabolism a series of metabolic adjustments begin that are designed to maintain the plasma glucose in a safe range for central nervous system metabolism while at the same time providing energy for other tissues in the body. This is accomplished by two mechanisms. First, the liver is activated for glucose production, and second, a lipid economy is established for most other tissues of the body. Initially glucose release from the liver is derived almost exclusively from hepatic glycogen. Because there is only about 70 g of glycogen available in the average human liver, glycogenolysis can only sustain the plasma glucose for a short time, ordinarily 8 to 10 h. Exercise may shorten the protective period significantly, as may the stress of severe illness. To compensate for glycogen depletion gluconeogenesis begins early with flux of substrate from muscle and adipose tissue stores to liver and then to utilization sites. The precursors for glucose synthesis are lactate/pyruvate and amino acids (primarily alanine) derived from muscle and glycerol released from adipose tissue consequent to lipolysis.

The switch to fat metabolism is accomplished by activation of the hormone-sensitive lipase in adipose tissue, which hydrolyzes stored triglycerides to long-chain fatty acids and glycerol. The long-chain fatty acids have two fates. The bulk (normally about 120 g per day) is utilized directly while the remainder (about 40 g per day) is oxidized in the liver to acetoacetic and β-hydroxybutyric acids. The ketones can be utilized efficiently as an energy source by most tissues (liver only minimally), but their primary importance is as backup substrate for the brain, as noted above. The shift of most tissues to lipid metabolism is important since the preferential utilization of free fatty acids and ketones in place of glucose spares the latter for utilization by the central nervous system.

Catabolic metabolism is initiated by a fall in insulin concentration in plasma coupled with secretion of the four counterregulatory hormones glucagon, epinephrine, cortisol, and growth hormone. In addition norepinephrine is released directly in tissues from sympathetic neurons. Glucagon is considered the primary hormone of glucose maintenance with epinephrine playing a backup or secondary role. The latter is particularly important in the defense against hypoglycemia in diabetes mellitus where the glucagon response is lost early (see Chap. 328).

The anabolic and catabolic phases of metabolism are summarized in Table 329-1. Breakdown in any of the adaptive mechanisms can lead to hypoglycemia.

SYMPTOMATOLOGY OF HYPOGLYCEMIA Symptoms of hypoglycemia fall into two main categories: those induced by an *excessive secretion of epinephrine* and those due to *dysfunction of the central nervous system.* Rapid epinephrine release causes sweating, tremor, tachycardia, anxiety, and hunger. Central nervous system symptoms include dizziness, headache, clouding of vision, blunted mental acuity, confusion, abnormal behavior, convulsions, and loss of consciousness. When the onset of hypoglycemia is gradual central nervous system symptoms predominate, and the epinephrine phase may not be recognizable. With more rapid drops in plasma glucose (as in insulin reactions), adrenergic symptoms are prominent. In the diabetic subject adrenergic symptoms may not be manifest if severe neuropathy is present.

CLASSIFICATION It has been traditional to classify hypoglycemia as either *postprandial* (reactive) or *fasting*. Pathologically low plasma

TABLE 329-1 The feeding-fasting cycle

Phase	Primary hormone	Plasma substrates	Substrate flux	Active process
Anabolic*	Insulin	↑ Glucose ↑ Triglycerides ↑ Branched-chain amino acids ↓ Free fatty acids ↓ Ketones	Splanchnic bed → storage and utilization sites	Glycogen storage Protein synthesis Triglyceride formation
Catabolic†	Glucagon	↓ Glucose ↓ Triglycerides ↑ Alanine and glutamine‡ ↑ Free fatty acids ↑ Ketones	Storage sites → liver and utilization sites	Glycogenolysis Gluconeogenesis Proteolysis Lipolysis Ketogenesis

* *Expected findings during the first several hours after ingestion of a mixed meal of fat, carbohydrate, and protein.*
† *The major catabolic phase occurs during the overnight fast, although partial catabolic cycles occur between meals.*
‡ *Arrows indicate plasma concentrations except for alanine and glutamine. While arterial concentrations of these amino acids are relatively constant, uptake by the liver and intestine is increased in the catabolic phase.*

glucose concentrations occur in the former only in response to meals, while in the latter fasting for a few to many hours is necessary to demonstrate the abnormality. Patients with fasting hypoglycemia (particularly those with insulinomas) may exhibit a reactive component, but reactive patients do not have symptoms when food is withdrawn. Fasting hypoglycemia usually means that an identifiable disease process is associated with the lowered plasma glucose, but symptoms suggestive of postprandial hypoglycemia are often found in the absence of recognizable disease.

CAUSES OF HYPOGLYCEMIA **Postprandial hypoglycemia** Some causes of postprandial hypoglycemia are shown in Table 329-2. The most common category is alimentary hyperinsulinism. Patients who have undergone gastrectomy, gastrojejunostomy, pyloroplasty, or vagotomy are subject to hypoglycemia following meals, presumably because of rapid gastric emptying with brisk absorption of glucose and excessive insulin release. Glucose concentrations fall more rapidly than insulin under these circumstances, and the resulting insulin-glucose imbalance leads to hypoglycemia. Ingestion of fructose or galactose induces hypoglycemia in children with fructose intolerance and galactosemia (Chap. 314), respectively. Leucine intake can rarely cause the syndrome in susceptible infants in the absence of insulinoma. Diabetes mellitus in its early phase is usually listed as a cause of reactive hypoglycemia. In our experience symptomatic hypoglycemia as a premonitory symptom of diabetes is uncommon if it occurs at all. Prediabetics, who by definition have normal glucose tolerance, may have a late fall in plasma glucose after oral glucose tolerance testing, but this does not mean hypoglycemia. In fact, this pattern is similar to that frequently present in asymptomatic, healthy individuals (see below).

The fifth cause, idiopathic alimentary hypoglycemia, has in the past been broken down into two categories, *true hypoglycemia* and *nonhypoglycemia.* The former represents a condition in which adrenergic symptoms appear postprandially and are accompanied by a measurably low plasma glucose at the time the symptoms appear spontaneously during everyday life. The symptoms are relieved by ingestion of carbohydrate which raises the plasma glucose. Such patients are extraordinarily rare. The mechanism is unknown, although subtle (nonanatomic) dysfunction of the gastrointestinal tract might be operative. Some patients with true postprandial hypoglycemia turn out to have insulinomas (see below). *Nonhypoglycemia* describes a large number of patients who reproducibly develop adrenergic symptoms suggestive of hypoglycemia 2 to 5 h after a meal but who do not have low plasma glucose concentrations when symptoms appear spontaneously in everyday life. The condition is often self-diagnosed by those who have read the extensive lay-oriented literature that describes hypoglycemia as a common cause of ill health. Further, in almost every community there are physicians who specialize in "hypoglycemia" and make the diagnosis frequently. This is usually based on a 5-h glucose tolerance test that reveals a lower than "normal" plasma glucose between 2 and 5 h.

Two questions have to be asked about nonhypoglycemia. First, what are the symptoms (which may be incapacitating) due to? Second, can a diagnosis of hypoglycemia be made by glucose tolerance test? The symptoms of nervousness, weakness, tremor, tachycardia, dizziness, and sweating reported by these patients are probably due to epinephrine release. Many otherwise normal persons experience similar symptoms at some time in their lives and may even have gained relief by eating. Patients with nonhypoglycemia, on the other hand, develop the symptoms regularly and repetitively. In one study 80 consecutive subjects with reproducible postprandial symptoms by history were studied by 5-h glucose tolerance testing. Hypoglycemia was considered to be present if (1) the plasma glucose fell below 60 mg/dL during the test, (2) symptoms or signs compatible with hypoglycemia were present, and (3) at least a doubling of plasma cortisol occurred 39 to 90 min after the nadir of plasma glucose (suggesting hypoglycemia sufficient to activate the hypothalamic-pituitary-adrenal axis). Only 18 of the 80 (23 percent) who by history were candidates for postprandial hypoglycemia fulfilled these criteria. Twenty-five percent of asymptomatic matched normal controls also met all three criteria. When the patients and controls were tested after a mixed meal, no subject in either group had a plasma glucose below 60 mg/dL, yet 14 of the 18 patients (78 percent) had symptoms typical of those occurring spontaneously and after glucose tolerance testing. The absence of hypoglycemia after mixed meals despite the presence of typical symptoms has been confirmed in other studies. Thus, the syndrome termed *nonhypoglycemia* has been correctly named since the symptoms occur in the absence of chemical hypoglycemia after mixed meals. Most of these patients doubtless have stress and/or anxiety as the primary disorder, with epinephrine released in consequence thereof. However, it is conceivable that some persons discharge epinephrine abnormally in response to meals to account for the syndrome. Sucrose or glucose overfeeding can cause stimulation of the sympathetic nervous system, but in normal subjects it is primarily norepinephrine and not epinephrine that is released. One possibility is that affected subjects have increased sensitivity to the normal postmeal epinephrine secretion. It is suggested that the terms *idiopathic postabsorptive hypoglycemia* and *nonhypoglycemia* be abandoned and the designation *idiopathic postprandial syndrome* be substituted to avoid confusion with true hypoglycemic disorders.

Fasting hypoglycemia The causes of fasting hypoglycemia are many, but in all there is an imbalance between the production of glucose by the liver and its utilization in peripheral tissues. In some, hypoglycemia is due primarily to a defect in glucose production, while in others the problem is due to excess glucose utilization. The two forms can be distinguished by the amount of glucose required to prevent hypoglycemia during a 24-h period. If this is more than 200 g, it can be assumed that overutilization is present. This follows

TABLE 329-2 Causes of postprandial (reactive) hypoglycemia

I	Alimentary hyperinsulinism
II	Hereditary fructose intolerance
III	Galactosemia
IV	Leucine sensitivity
V	Idiopathic

TABLE 329-3 Major causes of fasting hypoglycemia

I Conditions primarily due to underproduction of glucose
- *A* Hormone deficiencies
  - *1* Hypopituitarism
  - *2* Adrenal insufficiency
  - *3* Catecholamine deficiency
  - *4* Glucagon deficiency
- *B* Enzyme defects
  - *1* Glucose 6-phosphatase
  - *2* Liver phosphorylase
  - *3* Pyruvate carboxylase
  - *4* Phosphoenolpyruvate carboxykinase
  - *5* Fructose 1,6-diphosphatase
  - *6* Glycogen synthetase
- *C* Substrate deficiency
  - *1* Ketotic hypoglycemia of infancy
  - *2* Severe malnutrition, muscle wasting
  - *3* Late pregnancy
- *D* Acquired liver disease
  - *1* Hepatic congestion
  - *2* Severe hepatitis
  - *3* Cirrhosis
  - *4* Uremia (probably multiple mechanisms)
- *E* Drugs
  - *1* Alcohol
  - *2* Propranolol
  - *3* Salicylates

II Conditions primarily due to overutilization of glucose
- *A* Hyperinsulinism
  - *1* Insulinoma
  - *2* Exogenous insulin
  - *3* Sulfonylureas
  - *4* Immune disease with insulin antibodies
  - *5* Quinine in falciparum malaria
  - *6* Endotoxic shock
- *B* Appropriate insulin levels
  - *1* Extrapancreatic tumors
  - *2* Systemic carnitine deficiency
  - *3* Deficiency in enzymes of fat oxidation
  - *4* Cachexia with fat depletion

from the fact that hepatic glucose output after an overnight fast is normally about 2 (mg/kg)/min or 196 g per 24 h in a 70-kg person.[1] Since this is sufficient to prevent hypoglycemia, the presence of a low plasma glucose in the face of a 200-g glucose intake strongly suggests enhanced glucose utilization. The diseases that can cause accelerated glucose utilization usually also have an element of underproduction (relative or absolute), and in some cases the latter may predominate. The hepatic response to increased glucose demand may be impaired in conditions of glucose overutilization by several mechanisms, but persistent release of insulin sufficient to blunt the effect of glucagon in the liver is likely of key importance. Other factors include inadequate release of amino acids from muscle (necessary for gluconeogenesis) and/or impairment of fatty acid delivery or oxidation (necessary for maximal rates of gluconeogenesis).

To summarize, if glucose demand is more than 200 g per day, increased glucose flux into peripheral tissues is present. If less than 200 g per day prevents hypoglycemia, no diagnostic implications can be drawn since a condition capable of causing overutilization may, in a given case, function primarily by impairing glucose production. A classification of fasting hypoglycemia based on underproduction or overutilization of glucose is given in Table 329-3. Hypoglycemia occurs in other conditions in isolated fashion.

UNDERPRODUCTION OF GLUCOSE As discussed earlier, the production of glucose by the liver initially involves the breakdown of stored glycogen and subsequently depends on gluconeogenesis, the synthesis of glucose from precursors delivered to the liver from peripheral tissues. The causes of inadequate production of glucose during fasting can be grouped into five general categories: (1) hormone deficiencies, (2) specific defects in glycogenolytic or gluconeogenic enzymes, (3) inadequate substrate delivery, (4) acquired liver disease, and (5) drugs. Hypopituitarism and adrenal insufficiency are the most common of the hormone deficiency states causing hypoglycemia. Defects in catecholamine or glucagon release are rare. Enzymic abnormalities causing hypoglycemia are generally seen in children and not adults. Glucose 6-phosphatase deficiency is the classic example of a defect in glycogen breakdown, but hypoglycemia may occur in young children with deficiencies of hepatic glycogen phosphorylase and in other forms of glycogen storage disease (Chap. 313). The inability to make glycogen because of inadequate glycogen synthetase activity also renders the infant susceptible to fasting hypoglycemia. In addition to glucose 6-phosphatase, three other enzymes are necessary for gluconeogenesis: pyruvate carboxylase, phosphoenolpyruvate carboxykinase, and fructose 1,6-bisphosphatase (fructose 1,6-diphosphatase) (Fig. 329-1). Hypoglycemia can occur with decreased activities of each of these enzymes, often in association with lactic acidosis. Substrate deficiency appears to be one of the mechanisms operative in ketotic hypoglycemia of infancy, since alanine turnover in such patients is low. Inadequate substrate supply may also contribute to hypoglycemia in malnutrition, muscle-wasting states, chronic renal failure, and late pregnancy. Acquired liver disease can cause serious hypoglycemia. Hepatic congestion due to right-sided heart failure is particularly troublesome, but severe viral hepatitis or cirrhosis may also cause symptomatic hypoglycemia. The hypoglycemia of renal failure has been attributed to suppression of hepatic compensatory functions by uremia, but other mechanisms may also play a role.

A number of drugs cause hypoglycemia. By far the most common, apart from insulin and sulfonylureas, is alcohol. Alcohol only induces hypoglycemia after a period of fasting sufficient to deplete liver glycogen stores. In this circumstance hepatic glucose production is dependent on gluconeogenesis. The oxidation of ethanol in the liver is accompanied by generation of high concentrations of NADH, the reduced form of nicotinamide adenine dinucleotide (NAD), in the cytosol of the cell. The increased NADH/NAD ratio diverts oxaloacetate into malate formation, diminishing its availability to the gluconeogenic sequence via the action of phosphoenolpyruvate carboxykinase (Fig. 329-1). The normal pathway of gluconeogenesis from pyruvate is thus blocked, leading to a drop in hepatic glucose output and hypoglycemia. Large amounts of ethanol are not required to produce this syndrome, and plasma alcohol concentrations may be as low as 25 mg/dL at the time symptoms occur. Ethanol-induced hypoglycemia usually occurs in adults but can be seen in children who drink alcohol unknowingly. Salicylates (in children) and pro-

FIGURE 329-1 *Scheme of hepatic carbohydrate metabolism. Only the sequence for gluconeogenesis, glycogen synthesis, and glycogenolysis is shown.*

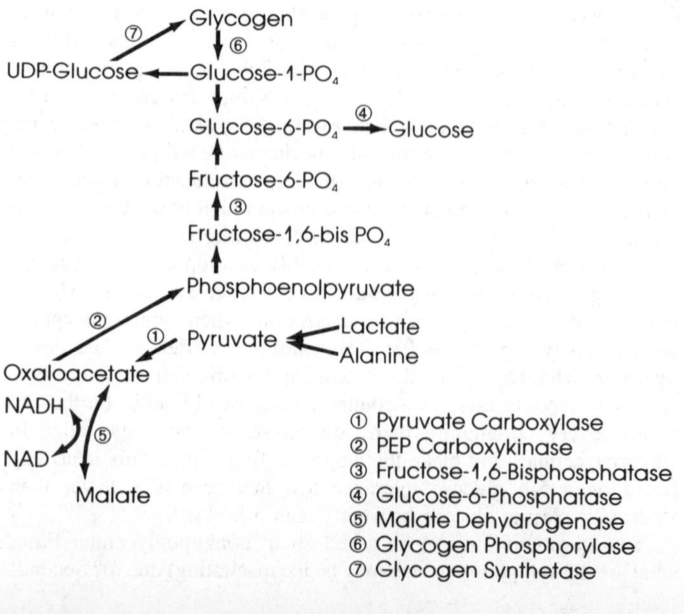

[1] *Much more than 200 g of glucose can be disposed of by normal humans without development of hyperglycemia. Therefore, the rule is valid only if large quantities of glucose are required to avoid hypoglycemia, i.e., if plasma glucose falls below fasting levels and continues at a low concentration despite the infusion of 200 g of glucose per day.*

pranolol are the next most frequently involved drugs. Propranolol presumably causes difficulty in fasting patients or insulin-requiring diabetics by impairing the glycogenolytic response. In diabetes the drug may also prevent recognition of impending hypoglycemia by blunting the symptomatic response to epinephrine release. Other drugs have been reported to cause hypoglycemia in isolated cases, but the relationship is often unproved.

OVERUTILIZATION OF GLUCOSE Overutilization of glucose occurs in two settings. In the first, hyperinsulinism is present, and in the second, plasma insulin concentrations are low. There are basically four causes of hyperinsulinemic hypoglycemia: insulinoma, exogenous insulin administration, sulfonylureas, and a peculiar form of insulin autoimmunity. In areas of endemic malaria some patients develop hyperinsulinemic hypoglycemia when treated with quinine, but this is not a problem elsewhere. Hypoglycemia in a diabetic taking prescribed insulin or oral agents is not a diagnostic problem. The difficulty comes when a nondiabetic subject induces hypoglycemia deliberately and surreptitiously because of psychiatric disturbance, raising the possibility of an insulin-producing tumor. The differential diagnosis between insulinoma and factitious hypoglycemia is considered below. Rarely hypoglycemia with hyperinsulinism occurs in autoimmune disease with antibodies to endogenous insulin. Mechanisms are not well understood, although dissociation of free insulin from hormone-antibody complexes at inappropriate times may play a role. By binding insulin, antibodies may also induce excessive insulin release from the pancreas.

Hypoglycemia in the context of glucose overutilization and appropriately low plasma insulin concentrations occurs in two situations. The first is in association with solid extrapancreatic tumors, usually of large size. The most common are of mesothelial origin and include a variety of fibromas and sarcomas. The syndrome can also be seen with hepatomas, carcinomas of the gastrointestinal tract, and adrenal cancers. The mechanism of the hypoglycemia is not clear, although high levels of insulin-like growth factors (''nonsuppressible insulin-like activity'') may play a role in some.

Symptomatic hypoglycemia due to overutilization may also occur in situations where free fatty acids are not available for oxidation in muscle and other tissues. Patients with *systemic carnitine deficiency* may have severe hypoglycemia. In this condition carnitine, which is necessary to transport fatty acids into mitochondria for oxidation, is low in plasma, muscle, liver, and other tissues. As a consequence, peripheral tissues cannot utilize fatty acids for energy production, and the liver cannot make ketone bodies as alternative substrate. The result is that all tissues become glucose-dependent, exceeding the capacity of the liver to meet the demand. Other features of systemic carnitine deficiency include nausea, vomiting, hyperammonemia, and hepatic encephalopathy. The illness thus constitutes one form of Reye's syndrome. (In *myopathic carnitine deficiency* only muscle is involved, and a polymyositis-like syndrome without hypoglycemia is produced.) Hypoglycemia is less common with deficiency of *carnitine palmitoyltransferase*, the enzyme that transesterifies fatty acyl coenzyme A (CoA) to carnitine for oxidation. Presumably the defect is not complete in most patients, allowing some fatty acid oxidation to occur so that the tendency to hypoglycemia is minimized. The clinical picture is that of an exercise-induced myopathy with myoglobinuria. Nonketotic (or hypoketotic) hypoglycemia may also occur with diminished activity of other enzymes of fatty acid oxidation such as deficiency of medium- or long-chain acyl CoA dehydrogenase. Interestingly, these enzyme deficiencies appear to cause secondary decrease of carnitine levels in tissue and blood. Hypoglycemia also occurs in patients with cachexia due to advanced cancer. At autopsy no recognizable triglyceride stores are present in adipose tissue, suggesting free fatty acid deficiency as the primary mechanism.

DIAGNOSIS Fasting hypoglycemia If a nondiabetic presents with symptoms suggestive of hypoglycemia—particularly if confusion, loss of consciousness, or convulsions are present—the most important rule is to draw blood for simultaneous determinations of plasma glucose and insulin before intravenous glucose is administered, since the critical diagnostic issue will be the presence or absence of hyperinsulinism. Plasma cortisol should be determined at the same time since an elevation demonstrates intact pituitary/adrenal function. In addition to these tests, plasma should be separated and frozen. The stored samples can then be used for drug screening and measurement of insulin, C peptide, proinsulin, counterregulatory hormones, and substrates (e.g., free fatty acids, lactate, carnitine, amino acids) should the diagnosis not be clear after initial workup. Although storage of plasma at the time of spontaneous hypoglycemia is rarely done, it should be routine. *The best time to obtain diagnostic laboratory tests with spontaneous hypoglycemia is at presentation.* Once the patient has become alert (assuming altered mental status is present on arrival) it is important to take a detailed history and carry out a thorough physical examination. Special emphasis should be placed on food intake in the preceding 24 h and the possibility of drug ingestion. Signs of heart failure and hepatic congestion should be sought, and the presence and thickness of the adipose tissue mass should be noted. Pigmentation of the skin may suggest Addison's disease. Workup includes liver function studies and computed tomography (CT) scanning or abdominal sonography (to look for solid tumors in the retroperitoneal space or abdominal cavity). Patients with enzyme defects and rare hormonal deficiencies (epinephrine, glucagon) usually require evaluation in referral centers, since definitive assays for these hormones and enzymes are not routinely available. For reasons cited above it is important to quantitate the amount of glucose required to prevent recurrent hypoglycemia during acute phase therapy.

If the patient has a history compatible with hypoglycemia but does not have symptoms at the time of examination, hospitalization for fasting is generally required. The fast should be carried out for at least 72 h unless symptoms develop. Plasma glucose, insulin, and cortisol should be measured every 6 h. Occasionally quantitation of plasma free fatty acids, glucagon, and total ketones is helpful. (For glucagon, a protease inhibitor such as aprotinin must be added.) Two points are at issue. First, does the patient have fasting hypoglycemia? And second, is the hypoglycemia associated with hyperinsulinism? Neither question is easy to answer. There is no definitive lower limit of plasma glucose that unequivocally defines pathologic hypoglycemia. The mean minimal level of glucose attained during a 72-h fast in one study is shown in Table 329-4. Women usually develop lower levels than men. Another series reported mean minimal levels of 62 mg/dL in men and 52 mg/dL in women during a 72-h fast. However, values as low as 22 mg/dL may occur in normal women without symptoms. On balance, a presumptive diagnosis of hypoglycemia is

TABLE 329-4 Plasma glucose and insulin during fasting

		Hours of fast				
Test	Subjects	0*	24	36	48	72
Glucose, mg/dL	Men	85 ± 1.5	83 ± 3.6	78 ± 3.4	78 ± 3.3	71 ± 2.4
	Women	83 ± 1.3	63 ± 1.6	50 ± 1.7	46 ± 1.7	48 ± 1.4
Insulin, μU/mL	Men	14 ± 0.9	9 ± 0.8	8 ± 1.1	8 ± 0.9	6 ± 0.7
	Women	12 ± 0.8	6 ± 0.4	4 ± 0.5	3 ± 0.4	4 ± 0.5

* *Zero values obtained after overnight fast. Results represent means ± SEM for 20 normal men and 60 normal women.*
SOURCE: *TJ Merimee, JE Tyson, Diabetes 26:161, 1977.*

probably justified if the plasma glucose falls below 50 mg/dL in men and 45 mg/dL in women at any time during the fast, provided typical symptoms are induced. The diagnosis of hypoglycemia is strengthened if symptoms are rapidly relieved by administration of carbohydrate. If symptoms are not produced, the diagnosis of hypoglycemia should be made with caution.

In interpreting plasma insulin concentrations absolute values are not very helpful. In normal subjects when glucose concentrations rise insulin levels also increase, and when plasma glucose concentrations fall insulin release is inhibited. This means that plasma insulin concentrations must be interpreted in the light of the simultaneously determined glucose value. Thus, a "normal" absolute insulin level may be abnormal in the face of hypoglycemia, while high absolute levels may be appropriate if the glucose concentration is elevated. In an attempt to relate the two parameters the concept of the insulin/glucose ratio

$$\frac{\text{Plasma insulin } (\mu\text{U/mL})}{\text{Plasma glucose (mg/dL)}}$$

was developed. In normal persons the ratio is always less than 0.4, while most (but not all) patients with insulinoma have ratios greater than 0.4—often above 1.0. Patients with insulinoma may secrete insulin episodically; the ratio may, therefore, be normal on one occasion and abnormal on another. Multiple sampling is required. The insulin/glucose ratio tends to fall during fasting in normal individuals but increases in patients with insulinoma.

Pancreatic insulin release ceases when the glucose concentration is decreased much below 90 mg/dL, and plasma insulin concentration generally reaches background levels for the assay when the plasma glucose falls below about 80 mg/dL. While some studies have shown lower cutoff points, it is probable that any measurable insulin concentration (>5 to 6 μU/mL) should be considered suspicious if the plasma glucose is below 50 mg/dL in men or 45 mg/dL in women, regardless of the value of the insulin/glucose ratio. If hyperinsulinism is not demonstrated, one of the other causes of fasting hypoglycemia must be sought.

Should hypoglycemia not develop during fasting, an insulinoma or other hypoglycemia-producing organic disease is unlikely, although insulinomas may rarely present solely as postprandial hypoglycemia with no depression of the plasma glucose even during a prolonged fast. Diagnosis usually is suspected in such cases because inappropriate insulin levels are shown during the postmeal episodes. Some authors recommend provocative tests with tolubutamide, glucagon, or leucine in suspected islet-cell tumors, but overlap between normal subjects and patients with insulinoma is so great as to render the tests of little value in a given individual.

Most patients who come to an emergency room with true postabsorptive hypoglycemia have a ready explanation for the problem. In one prospective study in a metropolitan hospital 125 cases of unequivocal hypoglycemia were seen in a 12-month period; 108 had hypoglycemia associated with diabetes or alcohol ingestion or a combination of the two. This experience is in accord with the view that insulinomas and other causes of hypoglycemia are uncommon and that only a minority of patients with hypoglycemia require extensive workup to determine the cause.

Postprandial hypoglycemia In patients presumed to have postprandial hypoglycemia the most widely used test has been a 5-h oral glucose tolerance examination. Since normal persons may have chemical hypoglycemia without symptoms in the glucose tolerance test while subjects with idiopathic postprandial syndrome have symptoms in the absence of hypoglycemia following meal testing, the 5-h glucose tolerance test should be abandoned as a tool for diagnosis. The only unequivocal diagnostic test for true idiopathic postprandial hypoglycemia is the demonstration of a low plasma glucose concentration (less than 50 mg/dL) during spontaneously developed symptoms. Patients with idiopathic postprandial syndrome (anxiety) usually have slightly elevated glucose concentrations during spontaneous attacks because of the hyperglycemic action of epinephrine, the stress hormone that induces the symptoms.

Insulinoma versus factitious hypoglycemia The self-induction of hypoglycemia by the injection of insulin or the ingestion of sulfonylureas is so common as to equal or exceed the incidence of insulinoma. The demonstration of hyperinsulinism during hypoglycemia cannot, therefore, be taken as definitive evidence of the presence of an islet-cell tumor. Factitious disease should always be suspected when hypoglycemic symptoms appear in medical personnel or families of diabetic patients. Several tests are helpful in distinguishing insulinoma from factitious disease once hyperinsulinism has been established. Patients with insulinoma tend to have high concentrations of proinsulin in plasma (>20 percent of total insulin). Plasma proinsulin is not elevated by the administration of commercial insulin preparations or sulfonylureas. Measurement of the insulin connecting peptide (C peptide) will indicate whether the insulin circulating in plasma is of endogenous or exogenous origin. When insulin is cleaved from its precursor proinsulin molecule, C peptide is released into the portal vein in a 1:1 ratio with insulin. Thus, patients with insulinoma should have high C-peptide concentrations which parallel the plasma insulin values. The characteristic pattern in factitious hypoglycemia due to insulin injection would be a high circulating level of insulin with relatively suppressed C-peptide values because exogenous insulin suppresses endogenous insulin release in normal persons, both directly and by inducing hypoglycemia. Suppression does not usually occur in insulinoma. For this reason some investigators recommend a C-peptide suppression test in equivocal situations. In this test 0.1 unit of insulin per kilogram of body weight is infused intravenously over 60 min. C-Peptide concentration should be less than 1.2 ng/mL at the end of the test, provided the plasma glucose has dropped to 40 mg/dL or less. As part of the test counterregulatory hormone response should also be measured 30 min after the nadir of the plasma glucose. Animal and human insulins can be distinguished by some radioimmunoassays and by high performance liquid chromatography. The presence of animal insulin is strong evidence of factitious disease. Antibodies to insulin are helpful if present since they usually indicate chronic insulin injection. Unfortunately sulfonylureas also elevate both the C-peptide and insulin concentrations in plasma. Therefore, factitious hypoglycemia due to oral agents can only be diagnosed by a high index of suspicion coupled with assay of the drug in plasma or urine. The differential characteristics of insulinoma and the two types of factitious hypoglycemia are shown in Table 329-5.

TREATMENT The initial treatment of serious hypoglycemia (producing confusion or coma) is the intravenous administration of a bolus of 25 or 50 g glucose as a 50% solution followed by constant infusion of glucose until the patient is able to eat a meal. The importance of the meal resides in the fact that hepatic glycogen repletion is not effective with small quantities of intravenous glucose. Patients in the overutilization category may require large quantities of intravenous glucose to maintain consciousness. It is not enough to infuse 5% dextrose at a rate of 1 to 2 mL/min and assume the patient is protected (20 to 30% dextrose solutions may be required

TABLE 329-5 Differential diagnosis of insulinoma and factitious hyperinsulinism

Test	Insulinoma	Exogenous insulin	Sulfonylurea
Plasma insulin	High	Very high*	High
Insulin/glucose ratio	High	Very high	High
Proinsulin	Increased	Normal or low	Normal
C peptide	Increased	Normal or low†	Increased
Insulin antibodies	Absent	± Present‡	Absent
Plasma or urine sulfonylurea	Absent	Absent	Present

* *Total plasma insulin in patients with insulinoma is rarely above 200 μU/mL in the basal state and often much lower. Values greater than 1000 μU/mL are highly suggestive of exogenous insulin injection.*

† *C peptide may be normal in absolute terms, but low in relation to the increased insulin value. See text for C-peptide suppression test.*

‡ *Insulin antibodies may not be present if only a few injections have been given, especially with purified insulins.*

in some cases). Frequent measurement of capillary glucose concentrations should be carried out using glucose-sensitive reagent strips to assess effectiveness of glucose infusion rates. Intravenous glucose can usually be stopped once the patient has eaten, but this can only be determined by trial. Adrenergic reactions without central nervous system abnormalities can be treated with oral carbohydrate and do not require parenteral therapy.

Hypoglycemia from sulfonylureas may last for prolonged periods (days), particularly with chlorpropamide (Fig. 329-2). It is common for patients to lapse back into coma if glucose infusions are stopped too soon. The reason for the prolonged effect is not always clear, though drug interactions, hepatic disease, and renal failure may play a role in some cases.

Surgery is the treatment of choice for insulinoma. Localization should be attempted with CT scan or sonography prior to exploration. Arteriography (celiac or superior mesenteric) is less effective. In some centers preoperative or operative sampling of insulin concentrations by selective pancreatic vein catheterization has been performed but appears to be of minimal benefit even if a rapid insulin assay is available. If the tumor cannot be palpated in the pancreas or located in an extrapancreatic site at the time of surgery, stepwise pancreatectomy (from tail to head) should be carried out with frozen sections made of sequential slices. Capillary glucose should be measured frequently (at each stage of the resection if the tumor is not obvious). A rise in plasma glucose may indicate removal of a small, nonpalpable lesion. In general, resection is stopped with an 85 percent pancreatectomy, even if the tumor is not found, to avoid malabsorptive complications. Evaluation of 1012 cases of insulinoma cited in the literature indicated the following outcomes from surgery: operative mortality, 11 percent; cure, 63 percent; postoperative diabetes, 10 percent; and persistent hypoglycemia, 16 percent. Postoperative complications included acute pancreatitis, peritonitis, fistulas, and pseudocyst formation.

Medical treatment is indicated in insulinoma only in preparation for surgery or after failure to find the tumor at operation. The drug of choice is diazoxide, which can be given intravenously or orally in doses of 300 to 1200 mg per day. Because of this drug's salt-retaining properties a diuretic must always be added when diazoxide is administered. Treatment of metastatic insulin-producing carcinomas is unsatisfactory. Streptozocin, plicamycin, and doxorubicin have been tried, but the results are dismal. One multicenter trial reported improved results when streptozocin was combined with fluorouracil. Despite the generally poor prognosis, occasional patients with insulin-producing islet-cell carcinomas survive for long periods.

Therapy of other forms of recurrent hypoglycemia, apart from hormone replacement in pituitary or adrenal insufficiency, is dietary. In most cases avoidance of fasting is all that is required. A high-protein, low-carbohydrate diet is frequently prescribed for patients with the idiopathic postprandial syndrome and often relieves symptoms. With true alimentary hypoglycemia it is probably important to keep the size of the individual meals small. The practice of giving massive amounts of vitamin E, crude adrenocortical extract, and trace metals to patients with the idiopathic postprandial syndrome is useless even if harmless (which has not been proved).

OTHER HORMONE-SECRETING TUMORS OF THE PANCREAS

Tumors of the pancreatic islets can synthesize a variety of hormones other than insulin. Almost all benign tumors are thought to be hormone-secreting, but a fifth or more of islet carcinomas produce no clinically detectable product. Histologically the tumors may be of a single-cell type or of mixed derivation. Despite the capacity of mixed tumors to produce several hormones, one hormone usually predominates so that distinct syndromes result. Tumors are generally named after the primary hormone released. If multiple hormones are produced and none dominates the clinical picture, the tumor is simply classified as "multiple hormone producing." Pancreatic tumors may be part of the multiple endocrine neoplasia syndrome (Chap. 334). This is particularly true of the ulcerogenic islet-cell tumor which is now considered to be a typical manifestation of the multiple endocrine neoplasia type I (MEN I). In addition to insulin, islet-cell tumors have been associated with the production of gastrin, secretin, vasoactive intestinal polypeptide, human pancreatic polypeptide, gastric inhibitory polypeptide, glucagon, ACTH, melanocyte stimulatory hormone, serotonin, neurotensin, enkephalin, and calcitonin. Chorionic gonadotropin and its β subunit may also be elevated in the plasma. A summary of the major tumors is given in Table 329-6.

Ulcerogenic islet-cell tumor (Zollinger-Ellison syndrome, gastrinoma) This is likely the most common of the non-insulin-secreting tumors. The clinical picture is that of intractable ulcer symptoms, hypersecretion of gastric acid, and diarrhea, which may be watery or due to steatorrhea. Complications such as perforation and hemorrhage occur commonly. X-ray frequently shows the stomach to be filled with fluid, and giant gastric rugae are seen. The ulcer may be atypically located in the second or third portion of the duodenum.

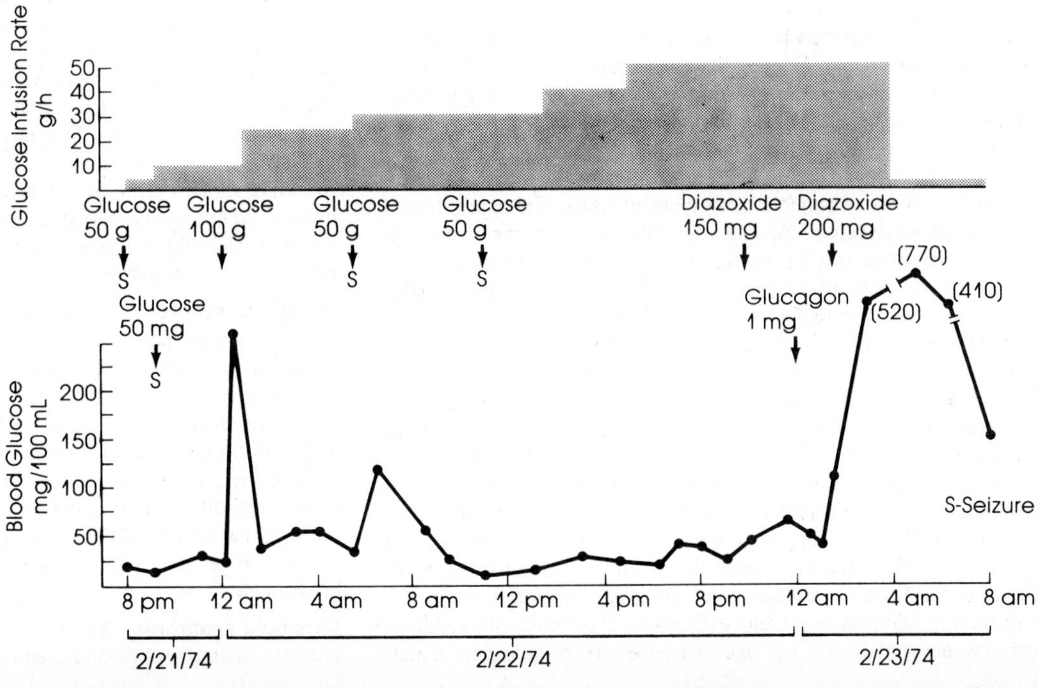

FIGURE 329-2 *Prolonged and refractory hypoglycemia in factitious hypoglycemia due to chlorpropamide in an alcoholic. Note continued hypoglycemia despite the infusion of glucose at rates up to 50 g/h. (From RM Jordan et al, Arch Intern Med 137:390, 1977. Copyright 1977, American Medical Association. Used by permission.)*

TABLE 329-6 Non-insulin-producing tumors of the pancreas

Tumor	Clinical syndrome
Gastrinoma	Severe peptic ulcer disease, secretory diarrhea, steatorrhea, hypersecretion of gastric acid, associated endocrine findings (MEN I)
Vipoma	Secretory diarrhea, hypokalemia, low or absent gastric acid, metabolic acidosis, hypercalcemia, hyperglycemia, dilated gallbladder, flushing
Glucagonoma	Migrating skin rash (necrolytic migratory erythema), sore tongue, cheilosis, weight loss, anemia, mild hyperglycemia, decreased plasma amino acids
Somatostatinoma	Dyspepsia, diarrhea, hyperglycemia, anemia, hypochlorhydria, gallstones, steatorrhea
Corticotropinoma	Cushing's syndrome
Carcinoid tumor	Diarrhea, flushing, tachycardia No asthma
Calcitoninoma	Diarrhea (?)
Parathyrinoma	Hypercalcemia
Neurotensinoma	Esophageal reflux (?)
PP-oma (pancreatic polypeptide)	Asymptomatic

Multiple ulcers may be present. Development of ulcer disease in the very young or very old should always raise suspicion of the Zollinger-Ellison syndrome. Associated endocrine abnormalities of the MEN I syndrome are present in half the patients and in a high percentage of first-degree relatives. Hypercalcemia due to parathyroid adenoma is the most common accompanying abnormality. A careful family history designed to elicit evidence of hypoglycemia, renal stones, and pituitary adenomas is imperative. All first-degree relatives of patients with gastrinomas should be examined by the physician. Multiple lipomas can be a clue to the presence of multiple endocrine neoplasia. Minimal screening should probably include CT scan of the pituitary and measurement of stimulated serum gastrin, cortisol, prolactin, calcium, and phosphorus. If hypercalcemia is present, workup for hyperparathyroidism can be completed. Evaluation for insulinoma is not indicated in the absence of symptoms suggesting hypoglycemia. Details of diagnosis and treatment for the Zollinger-Ellison syndrome are discussed in Chap. 235. Basically patients undergo total gastrectomy followed by treatment with a histamine H-2 receptor–blocking agent (cimetidine or ranitidine). Some authorities believe that gastrectomy is not indicated and that vagotomy plus H-2 blockers gives equally good results.

Diarrheogenic islet-cell tumor (vipoma) The syndrome produced by these tumors has been called pancreatic cholera, the watery diarrhea syndrome, and the WDHA syndrome. The acronym stands for *w*atery *d*iarrhea, *h*ypokalemia, and *a*chlorhydria, major features of the clinical picture. Acid secretion in the basal state may actually be low rather than absent, and stimulation by histamine is intact. About two-thirds of patients have hypercalcemia, and approximately half are hyperglycemic. A dilated gallbladder is characteristic. The secretory diarrhea is often profuse and can produce shock and renal shutdown. It is often nocturnal and persists during fasting. Hypokalemia may be life-threatening. Metabolic acidosis, presumably due to bicarbonate loss but possibly also related to volume depletion, is common. Attacks of flushing occur in about 20 percent of patients.

Considerable confusion has existed about the hormonal cause of the syndrome. Originally secretin was thought to be involved, but subsequently vasoactive intestinal polypeptide (VIP), human pancreatic polypeptide, gastric inhibitory polypeptide, and prostaglandins were all reported to be associated with diarrheogenic islet-cell tumors. It is now almost universally accepted that VIP is the mediator in most cases. The attractiveness of this possibility is enhanced by the fact that the hormone is known to cause hyperglycemia and hypercalcemia in addition to secretory diarrhea. Thus the entire syndrome can be accounted for by one hormone. Hypercalcemia usually disappears after removal of the pancreatic neoplasm and in most cases is not due to concomitant hyperparathyroidism.

Diagnosis requires demonstration of a secretory diarrhea, the presence of a pancreatic tumor, and elevation of plasma VIP levels on more than one occasion. Secretory diarrhea can essentially be ruled out if stool volume is less than 750 mL per 24 h. The diarrheogenic tumors tend to be larger than other islet adenomas and may be more easily localized by CT scan or ultrasonography.

Treatment is surgical removal of the tumor after fluid and electrolyte balance has been restored. Steroids ameliorate the diarrhea in some cases but should be used only if the patient is at risk for life despite conservative management preparatory to surgery. Diarrhea disappears, and gastric acid secretion and potassium concentration return to normal if the tumor is completely removed. Somatostatin analogues may be helpful when the tumor is not resectable.

Glucagonoma Glucagonomas, a high percentage of which appear to be malignant and metastasizing, cause a distinctive skin lesion (necrolytic migratory erythema) on the face, lower abdomen, perineum, buttocks, or distal extremities. The characteristic picture is of multiple crusts, scaly macules and papules, occasional pustules, flaccid bullae, and generalized erythema. Glossitis, stomatitis, and angular cheilosis are common. Spontaneous exacerbations and remissions occur, and hyperpigmentation follows healing. Weight loss and normochromic, normocytic anemia are common. Elevated fasting blood glucose concentrations or abnormal glucose tolerance tests are present in most patients. Plasma amino acid levels are depressed, and hypocholesterolemia may be present. Plasma ketones may be elevated despite normal plasma free fatty acid concentrations. Glucagon levels in plasma are high (5 to 10 times normal) and show abnormal responses to a number of provocative tests. It is of interest that four asymptomatic first-degree relatives of one patient with a proved glucagonoma had persistently elevated glucagon concentrations and abnormal responses to glucose suppression and arginine stimulation. Transmission appeared to follow an autosomal dominant pattern. Whether the asymptomatic subjects had small (undetectable) adenomas or whether the alpha cells were functionally abnormal but not neoplastic is not known. Glucagonomas have also been reported in a family with multiple endocrine neoplasia type I.

Treatment of glucagonoma is surgical removal. Chemotherapy of metastatic disease is unsatisfactory. Experimentally a long-acting somatostatin analogue has been tried and may be of benefit.

Somatostatinoma The secretion of somatostatin by islet-cell tumors causes a picture that includes dyspepsia, diarrhea, weight loss, cholelithiasis with a dilated gallbladder, mild hyperglycemia, anemia, and hypochlorhydria. Steatorrhea and abdominal pain may be present. In addition to a pancreatic mass, liver metastases are usually present at the time of diagnosis. Because somatostatinomas often produce additional hormones, some patients may have hypoglycemia, flushing, or Cushing's syndrome. Diagnosis requires demonstration of high levels of somatostatin in plasma together with a pancreatic tumor. Intestinal somatostatinomas, which histologically are psammomatous tumors, do not release somatostatin into plasma. Treatment is surgical removal. Debulking surgery may be carried out even when complete resection is not possible.

Cushing's syndrome Adrenocorticotropic hormone (ACTH) production by pancreatic islet tumors causes less severe clinical manifestations than are characteristic of other forms of ectopic Cushing's syndrome (see Chap. 325). Pigmentation may be a clue to ectopic ACTH production. Occasionally the tumor produces corticotropin-releasing hormone (CRH) rather than ACTH. Mixed hormone production (insulin, gastrin, serotonin) is common in these tumors. The problem of differentiating between a single islet tumor that produces multiple hormones and the multiple endocrine neoplasia syndrome where two or more adenomas each produce a single hormone may be difficult.

Carcinoid syndrome Serotonin may be synthesized in islet tumors and lead to diarrhea, flushing, and tachycardia. Asthma is not present.

Some of these patients may actually have a diarrheogenic tumor with symptoms primarily due to vasoactive intestinal polypeptide, and serotonin production may represent a second hormone synthesized by a mixed adenoma (see Chap. 299).

General principles of treatment Brief comments about treatment have been made for the major syndromes. It is not always clear what the best therapy might be, especially if metastases to liver are present. A reasonable approach might be the following in all tumors except gastrinoma (which, as noted, requires gastrectomy or vagotomy): (1) resect all primary tumors; (2) resect all primary tumors and follow with partial hepatectomy if the hepatic lesion is localized; (3) utilize antisecretory drugs in inoperable cases or in preparation for surgery if the patient is in poor shape. These would include H-2 receptor antagonists in gastrinoma and somatostatin analogues in vipoma and glucagonoma (somatostatin probably should be tried in all diarrheal forms); (4) reserve chemotherapy for ''last resort'' conditions.

REFERENCES

Hypoglycemia and insulinoma

AVRAM MM et al: Uremic hypoglycemia. A preventable life-threatening complication. NY State J Med 84:593, 1984

BAUMAN WA, YALOW RS: Hyperinsulinemic hypoglycemia. Differential diagnosis by determination of the species of circulating insulin. JAMA 252:2730, 1984

BOLLI G et al: Role of hepatic autoregulation in defense against hypoglycemia in humans. J Clin Invest 75:1623, 1985

CHARLES MA et al: Comparison of oral glucose tolerance tests and mixed meals in patients with apparent idiopathic postabsorptive hypoglycemia. Absence of hypoglycemia after meals. Diabetes 30:465, 1981

CRYER PE: Glucose counterregulation in man. Diabetes 30:261, 1981

———: Glucose homeostasis and hypoglycemia, in *Williams' Textbook of Endocrinology*, 7th ed., JD Wilson, DW Foster (eds). Philadelphia, Saunders, 1985, pp 989–1017

GOLDMAN J et al: Characterization of circulating insulin and pro-insulin-binding antibodies in autoimmune hypoglycemia. J Clin Invest 63:1050, 1979

GORDEN P et al: Hypoglycemia associated with non-islet-cell tumor and insulin-like growth factors. A study of the tumor types. N Engl J Med 305:1452, 1981

HALE DE et al: Long-chain acyl coenzyme A dehydrogenase deficiency: An inherited cause of nonketotic hypoglycemia. Pediatr Res 19:666, 1985

HANSEN IL et al: Differential diagnosis of hypoglycemia in children by responses to fasting and 2-deoxyglucose. Metabolism 32:960, 1983

HOELZER DR et al: Glucoregulation during exercise: Hypoglycemia is prevented by redundant glucoregulatory systems, sympathochromaffin activation, and changes in islet hormone secretion. J Clin Invest 77:212, 1986

HOGAN MJ et al: Oral glucose tolerance test compared with a mixed meal in the diagnosis of reactive hypoglycemia. A caveat on stimulation. Mayo Clin Proc 58:491, 1983

JORDAN RM et al: Sulfonylurea-induced factitious hypoglycemia. A growing problem. Arch Intern Med 137:390, 1977

KLEIN RF et al: High performance liquid chromatography used to distinguish the autoimmune hypoglycemia syndrome from factitious hypoglycemia. J Clin Endocrinol Metab 61:571, 1985

LEV-RAN A, ANDERSON RW: The diagnosis of postprandial hypoglycemia. Diabetes 30:996, 1981

MALOUF R, BRUST JCM: Hypoglycemia: Causes, neurological manifestations, and outcome. Ann Neurol 17:421, 1985

MCGARRY JD, FOSTER DW: Systemic carnitine deficiency. N Engl J Med 303:1413, 1980

MERIMEE TJ, TYSON JE: Hypoglycemia in man. Pathologic and physiologic variants. Diabetes 26:161, 1977

MOERTEL CG et al: Streptozocin alone compared with streptozocin plus fluorouracil in the treatment of advanced islet-cell carcinoma. N Engl J Med 303:1189, 1980

NAYLOR JM, KRONFELD DS: In vivo studies of hypoglycemia and lactic acidosis in endotoxic shock. Am J Physiol 248:E309, 1985

RIZZA RA et al: Pathogenesis of hypoglycemia in insulinoma patients. Suppression of hepatic glucose production by insulin. Diabetes 30:377, 1981

SCARLETT JA et al: Factitious hypoglycemia. Diagnosis by measurement of serum C-peptide immunoreactivity and insulin-binding antibodies. N Engl J Med 297:1029, 1977

SERVICE FJ et al: Insulinoma. Clinical and diagnostic features of 60 consecutive cases. Mayo Clin Proc 51:417, 1976

———: *Hypoglycemia Disorders*, Boston, G. K. Hall, 1983

STEFANINI P: Beta-islet cell tumors of the pancreas: Results of a study on 1067 cases. Surgery 75:597, 1974

Other hormone-secreting islet-cell tumors

CREUTZFELDT W: Endocrine tumors of the pancreas: Clinical, chemical and morphological findings, in *The Pancreas*, PJ Fitzgerald, AB Morrison (eds). Baltimore, Williams & Wilkins, 1980, pp 185–207

FRIESEN SR: Tumors of the endocrine pancreas. N Engl J Med 306:580, 1982

JASPAN JB et al: Clinical features and diagnosis of islet cell tumors, in *Tumors of the Pancreas*, AR Moosa (ed). Baltimore, Williams & Wilkins, 1980, pp 469–504

KREJS GJ: Non-insulin-secreting tumors of the pancreatic islets, in *William's Textbook of Endocrinology*, 7th ed., JD Wilson, DW Foster (eds). Philadelphia, Saunders, 1985, pp 1301–1308

SANTANGELO WC et al: Pancreatic cholera syndrome: Effect of a synthetic somatostatin analog on intestinal water and ion transport. Ann Intern Med 103:363, 1985

STACPOOLE PW et al: A familial glucagonoma syndrome: Genetic, clinical and biochemical features. Am J Med 70:1017, 1981

330 DISORDERS OF THE TESTIS

JAMES E. GRIFFIN III / JEAN D. WILSON

The testis produces sperm and the steroid hormones that regulate male sexual life. Both functions are under complex feedback control by the hypothalamic-pituitary system so that the testis has biosynthetic and regulatory features similar to those of the ovary and the adrenal. Testicular hormones are also responsible for the formation of the basic male phenotype during embryogenesis. The function of the embryonic testis and the disorders that result from abnormalities of testicular function or androgen action during embryogenesis are described in Chap. 333.

PHYSIOLOGY AND REGULATION OF TESTICULAR FUNCTION

The testis consists of two components—a system of spermatogenic tubules for the production and transport of sperm and clusters of interstitial or Leydig cells that produce androgenic steroids.

THE LEYDIG CELL Testosterone synthesis The biochemical pathway by which the 27-carbon sterol cholesterol is converted to androgens and estrogens is depicted in Fig. 330-1. Cholesterol can either be synthesized de novo in the Leydig cell or derived from plasma lipoproteins. Five enzymes or enzyme complexes are required for the conversion of cholesterol to testosterone. In this process the side chain of cholesterol is cleaved in two steps to reduce the size from 27 to 19 carbons, and the A ring of the steroid is converted to the Δ^4-3-keto configuration. The five enzymes are the 20,22-desmolase, the 3β-hydroxysteroid dehydrogenase-$\Delta^{4,5}$-isomerase complex, 17α-hydroxylase, 17,20-desmolase, and 17β-hydroxysteroid dehydrogenase. The first four enzymes are also present in the adrenal.

The rate-limiting reaction in testosterone synthesis is the conversion of cholesterol to pregnenolone by the 20,22-desmolase; luteinizing hormone (LH) from the pituitary regulates the activity of this enzyme and of other enzymes in the pathway. Other steroids including estradiol are synthesized in small amounts in the Leydig cell.

Testosterone secretion and transport Only about 0.02 mg of testosterone is stored in the normal testes so that the total hormone content turns over about 200 times each day to provide the average of 5 to 6 mg that is secreted into plasma in normal young men (Fig. 330-2). Testosterone is transported in plasma bound to protein, largely to albumin and to a specific transport protein, testosterone-binding globulin (TeBG). The bound and unbound fractions in plasma are in dynamic equilibrium, only about 1 to 3 percent being present in the free fraction. The fraction of circulating testosterone available for entry into tissues approximates the sum of the free and albumin-bound fractions or about 40 to 50 percent of the total plasma testosterone in normal men.

Peripheral metabolism of androgens Testosterone serves as a circulating precursor (or prohormone) for the formation of two other types of active metabolites which mediate many of the physiologic processes involved in androgen action (Fig. 330-1). On the one hand, testosterone can be 5α-reducted to dihydrotestosterone, which performs many of the differentiative, growth-promoting, and functional

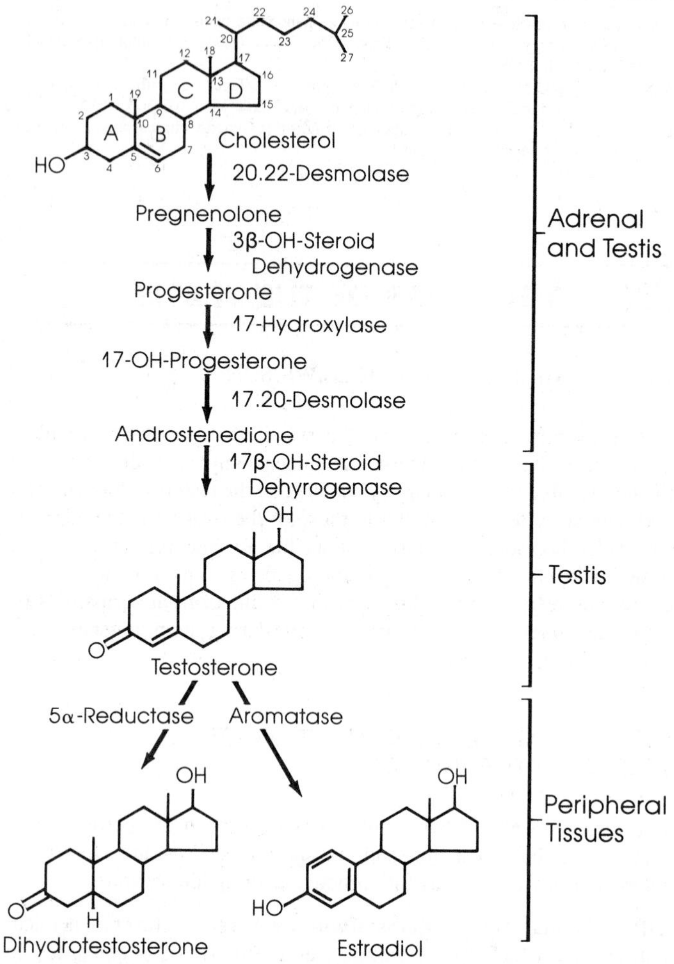

FIGURE 330-1 *Pathways of androgen formation in the testis and the conversion of androgens to other active hormones in peripheral tissues.*

actions involved in male sexual differentiation and virilization. Circulating androgens in both sexes can also be converted to estrogens in extraglandular tissues. In men estrogens act in some instances in concert with androgens but can also have effects independent of or opposite to those of androgens. Thus, the physiologic effects of testosterone are the result of the combined effects of testosterone itself plus those of the active androgen and estrogen metabolites of the parent molecule. (In normal men small amounts of estradiol and dihydrotestosterone are also derived by direct secretion from the testis and indirectly from the weak adrenal androgen androstenedione.)

The quantitative relation between circulating androgens and the formation of estrogen in normal young men is illustrated diagrammatically in Fig. 330-2. The production rates of testosterone and androstenedione average about 6 and 3 mg, respectively, per day. All of estrone production (averaging about 66 μg per day) can be accounted for by formation from circulating precursors. The mean estradiol production rate is about 45 μg per day; about 35 percent of this amount is derived from circulating testosterone, 50 percent is derived from the weak estrogen estrone, and 15 percent is secreted directly into the circulation by the testes. When gonadotropin levels are elevated, the amount of estradiol secretion by the testis is increased.

The 5α-reduced and estrogenic metabolites can exert local (paracrine) actions in the tissues in which they are formed or enter the circulation and act as hormones at other sites. Circulating dihydrotestosterone is formed principally in the androgen target tissues, and estrogen formation takes place in many tissues, the most significant being adipose tissue. The overall rate of extraglandular estrogen formation increases with increasing amounts of adipose tissue and with age.

Plasma testosterone and its active metabolites are converted to inactive metabolites in the liver and excreted predominantly in the urine; approximately half of the daily turnover is excreted in the form of urinary 17-ketosteroids (primarily androsterone and etiocholanolone), and the remainder is excreted as a series of polar compounds (diols, triols, and conjugates).

Gonadotropin regulation and testosterone secretion Testosterone secretion is regulated by pituitary LH (Fig. 330-3). (For the details of pituitary function, see Chap. 321.) Follicle-stimulating hormone (FSH) may also augment testosterone secretion, possibly by inducing maturation of the Leydig cell. Testosterone also regulates the sensitivity of the pituitary to the hypothalamic-releasing factor luteinizing hormone–releasing hormone (LHRH). Although the pituitary can convert testosterone to dihydrotestosterone and to estrogens, testosterone itself is the primary regulator of gonadotropin secretion.

FIGURE 330-2 *Androgen and estrogen production in normal young men. Average production of androstenedione and testosterone are shown in the top boxes, and mean daily production of estrone and estradiol is shown in the lower boxes. Estrogen is formed by extraglandular aromatization (braces) or by direct secretion from the testes. Vertical arrows indicate the rates of extraglandular aromatization of androgens, and the horizontal arrows indicate the interconversion of androgen and estrogens by 17β-hydroxysteroid dehydrogenase. Thus estradiol arises from plasma testosterone, from estrone, and from direct secretion by the testes. (Adapted from PC MacDonald et al.)*

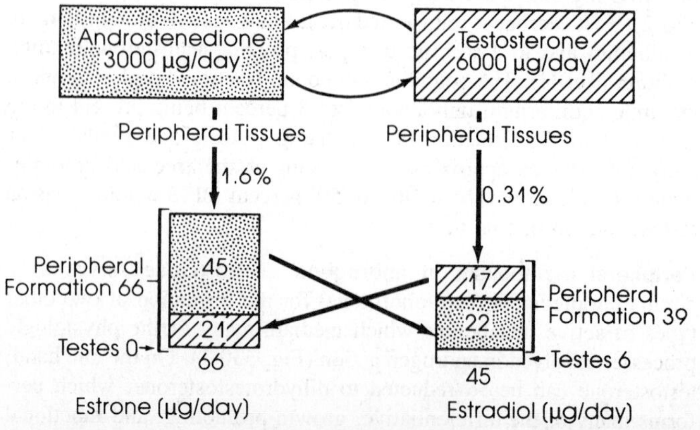

FIGURE 330-3 *Regulation of testosterone and sperm production by LH and FSH. (C, cholesterol; T, testosterone.)*

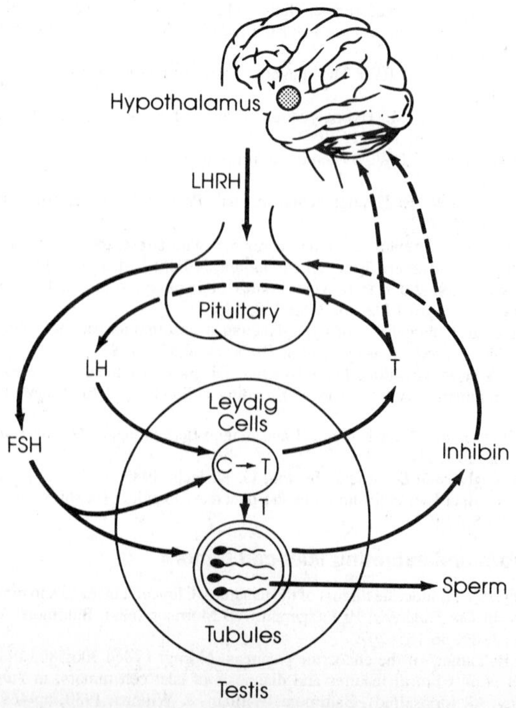

Testosterone also acts in the central nervous system to slow the rate of LHRH formation or secretion and consequently to decrease the frequency of pulsatile LH release. Under ordinary circumstances, LH secretion is exquisitely sensitive to the feedback effects of testosterone, with complete suppression following the administration of amounts of exogenous androgen that approximate the normal daily secretory rate of testosterone (about 6 mg). However, prolonged elevation of plasma LH (as in testicular deficiency) renders the pituitary less sensitive to negative feedback control by exogenous androgen.

Neither the plasma concentration of testosterone nor that of LH is constant, each showing fluctuations of a pulsatile nature that reflect changes in secretory rates (Fig. 330-4). Major sleep-related surges in the pulsatile secretion of both LH and testosterone signal the initiation of male puberty. In the adult the diurnal variation in the magnitude of this episodic secretion of LH and testosterone is minor with peak morning levels only about 10 to 15 percent higher than during the rest of the day.

Androgen action The major functions of androgen are the regulation of gonadotropin secretion, the formation of the male phenotype during sexual differentiation, and the induction of sexual maturation and function following puberty. The cellular mechanisms by which androgens perform these functions are summarized schematically in Fig. 330-5. Testosterone (T) enters the cell by passive diffusion. Inside the cell T can be converted to dihydrotestosterone (D) by the 5α-reductase enzyme. T or D is then bound to the androgen-receptor protein in the cytosol (R). The hormone-receptor complex (TR or DR) is transformed to the DNA-binding state (TR* or DR*) and translocated to the nucleus, where it attaches to specific chromosomal sites; as a result, new messenger RNA is transcribed, and new protein appears within the cytoplasm of the cell.

Although testosterone and dihydrotestosterone bind to the same receptor, their physiologic roles differ. The testosterone-receptor complex regulates gonadotropin secretion and is responsible for the Wolffian stimulation phase of sexual differentiation (see Chap. 333), whereas the dihydrotestosterone-receptor complex is responsible for external virilization during embryogenesis and the major portion of androgen action during sexual maturation and adult sexual life, including the initiation and maintenance of spermatogenesis. The mechanism by which testosterone and dihydrotestosterone mediate these different functions is not known. The mechanisms by which estrogens act to augment or block androgen effects are also not known. It is presumed that estradiol acts by a mechanism similar to that of androgens but involving its own receptor protein (see Chap. 331).

THE SEMINIFEROUS TUBULE AND SPERMATOGENESIS Normal function of the seminiferous tubule is dependent both on the pituitary and on normal function of the adjacent Leydig cells, both FSH and androgen being essential for initiating and maintaining normal spermatogenesis (Fig. 330-3). The major site of FSH action is the Sertoli cell in the seminiferous tubules. The seminiferous tubule also contains specific androgen receptors. Androgen appears to be essential for the initial phase of spermatogenesis, whereas FSH is required for the terminal phases of spermatid development. In the normal adult male this machinery produces more than 200 million sperm per day.

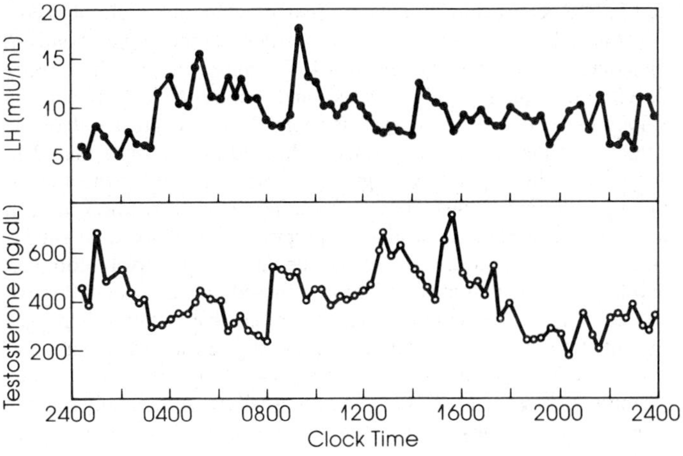

FIGURE 330-4 *Twenty-four-hour pattern of plasma LH and testosterone in a normal man sampled every 20 min. (Reprinted from Griffin and Wilson, 1980.)*

The Sertoli cell cannot synthesize steroid hormones de novo and is dependent on testosterone that diffuses in from adjacent Leydig cells. Sertoli cells can convert testosterone to estradiol and to dihydrotestosterone. The seminiferous tubules also produce the peptide hormone inhibin that regulates the secretion of FSH by the hypothalamic-pituitary axis (Fig. 330-3). Whether inhibin is the primary physiologic regulator of FSH is unclear; testosterone and estradiol also can inhibit FSH secretion, and altered frequency of LHRH pulses can result in selective increases of FSH.

The interlocking system in which two pituitary hormones regulate testicular function provides a precise dual-control mechanism by which plasma testosterone and sperm production feed back upon the hypothalamic-pituitary system to regulate their own rates of production (Fig. 330-3).

ASSESSMENT OF TESTICULAR FUNCTION

LEYDIG CELL FUNCTION History of physical examination The assessment of Leydig cell function and androgen status should include inquiry about the presence at birth of developmental abnormalities of the urogenital tract, the timing and extent of sexual maturation at puberty, the rate of beard growth, and the current libido, sexual function, strength, and energy. Inadequate Leydig cell function or androgen action during embryogenesis may manifest itself by the presence of hypospadias, cryptorchidism, or microphallus. If Leydig

FIGURE 330-5 *Current concepts of androgen action. (T, testosterone; D, dihydrostestosterone; E, estradiol; R, receptor protein; R*, transformed receptor protein; LH, luteinizing hormone; 5α-Red, 5α-reductase.)*

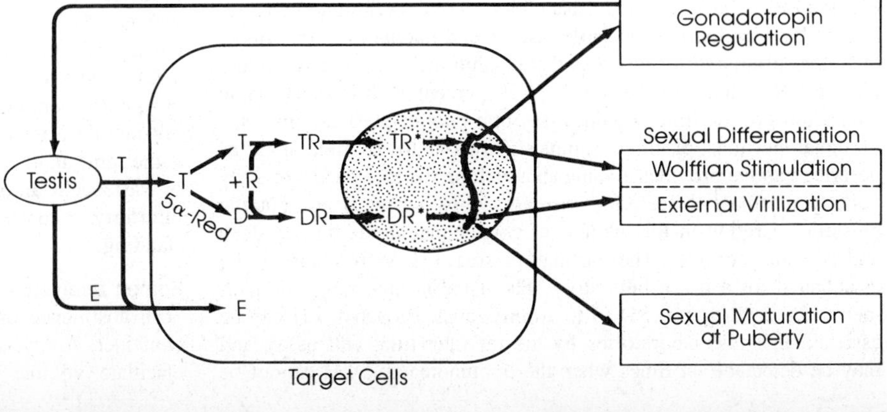

cell failure occurs prior to puberty, sexual maturation will not occur, and the individual will develop the features termed eunuchoidism, including an infantile amount and distribution of body hair, poor development of skeletal muscles, and failure of closure of the epiphyses so that the arm span is more than 2 in greater than the height, and the lower body segment (heel to pubic) more than 2 in longer than the upper body segment (pubic to crown). Detection of Leydig cell failure that commences after puberty requires a high index of suspicion and usually appropriate laboratory assessment. One reason is that decreased sexual function is a relatively common problem among adult men and may be caused by many nonendocrine factors. The second is that certain functions that require androgens for initiation continue unabated when Leydig cell failure occurs, and those functions that eventually regress may do so very slowly. For example, the frequency of shaving may not decrease for many months or even years because of the slow decline in rate of beard growth once established.

Plasma testosterone and dihydrotestosterone levels Plasma testosterone is measured by a specific radioimmunoassay. Testosterone is secreted into plasma in a pulsatile fashion every 60 to 90 min (Fig. 330-4); a single random sample provides a result within ±20 percent of the true mean value only two-thirds of the time while three equally spaced samples 15 to 20 min apart provide a more accurate assessment. The samples do not need to be assayed separately, and aliquots of the three samples can be pooled for a single determination. The range of plasma testosterone in normal adult men is 300 to 1000 ng/dL. In adult men the plasma values vary slightly throughout the day and at different times of the year, but these variations are not as great as those for plasma cortisol and are not significant in routine clinical assessment. Plasma levels of testosterone correlate in general with testosterone secretory rates as measured by isotope infusion. Estimation of TeBG concentration is sometimes useful in the interpretation of total plasma testosterone levels. Such assays can be done either by measuring the binding capacity of radioactive androgen or with a specific radioimmunoassay.

The plasma testosterone value in prepubertal children is statistically higher in boys than girls, the range in both being 5 to 20 ng/dL. The rise in plasma testosterone at the beginning of puberty occurs as a result of sleep-related nocturnal gonadotropin surges so that during the initial phases plasma testosterone and LH are higher at night than during the day. The random daytime levels of plasma testosterone increase gradually as puberty progresses and reach adult levels at about age 17.

Dihydrotestosterone is also measured by radioimmunoassay. In normal young men the plasma dihydrotestosterone level is about one-tenth that of the testosterone value and averages around 50 ng/dL. In older men with benign prostatic hyperplasia, plasma dihydrotestosterone levels are higher and average about 90 ng/dL.

Urinary 17-ketosteroids The measurement of urinary 17-ketosteroids is not a valid way to assess testicular function. Urinary 17-ketosteroids are mainly weak adrenal androgens or their metabolites, and testosterone contributes only about 40 percent of daily 17-ketosteroid production in men.

Plasma LH Plasma LH is measured by specific radioimmunoassay. LH is also secreted in a pulsatile fashion and fluctuates more widely than does plasma testosterone so that in adult men an isolated random plasma LH is likely to be within ±20 percent of true mean value only a third of the time. Again, assay of a pool of plasma comprised of equal portions of three samples drawn 6 to 18 min apart as described above provides a value approaching the true mean. In early puberty plasma LH secretion increases only during sleep, but the pulsatile secretion in the adult is of similar magnitude during sleep and waking periods. The normal plasma LH values should be established for a given laboratory. The usual normal range in adult men is 26 ±18 ng/mL SD (5 to 20 mIU/mL). Bioactive LH can be assessed in some laboratories by the rat interstitial cell assay and may be detectable at times when the immunoreactive LH cannot be measured. A low plasma testosterone concentration can be interpreted correctly only if plasma LH is also measured simultaneously, and likewise the "appropriateness" of a given plasma LH must be interpreted in relation to the plasma testosterone. For example, a low plasma testosterone coupled with a low LH implies hypothalamic or pituitary disease, whereas the finding of a low plasma testosterone and a high LH suggests primary testicular insufficiency (see Chap. 320).

Response to gonadotropin stimulation Leydig cell function is difficult to assess prior to puberty when both LH and testosterone levels are low, and it is common to measure response of plasma testosterone to gonadotropin stimulation as an index of Leydig cell capacity. Normal prepubertal boys respond to 3 to 5 days of injection of 1000 to 2000 IU human chorionic gonadotropin (HCG) with an increase in plasma testosterone to about 200 ng/dL; the magnitude of the response increases with the initiation of puberty and peaks in early puberty.

Response to luteinizing hormone–releasing hormone The response of plasma LH (and/or FSH) to the administration of luteinizing hormone–releasing hormone (LHRH) is utilized in some centers to assess the functional integrity of the pituitary-testicular axis. The responsiveness of the pituitary gland to LHRH changes at the time of puberty. Prior to puberty quantitative responses to LH and FSH are similar. With pubertal development the LH response to acute administration of LHRH increases while the FSH response remains the same. The amount of LH released following acute administration of LHRH probably reflects the amount of stored hormone in the pituitary. When 100 μg of LHRH is given subcutaneously or intravenously to normal men, there is, on average, a four- to fivefold increase in LH with the peak level at 30 min. However, the range of response is broad with some normal men having less than a doubling of LH levels. In general, the peak LH following a single LHRH injection correlates with the basal levels. In patients with primary testicular failure measurement of basal LH is usually sufficient, and measurement of LHRH response adds little to aid the diagnosis. Men who have either pituitary disease or hypothalamic disease may have either a normal or an abnormal LH response to an acute dose of LHRH. Therefore, a normal response is of no diagnostic value, either in determining the presence or absence of disease or in distinguishing hypothalamic from pituitary disease. A subnormal response is of value in determining that an abnormality exists, even though the site is not determined. The LHRH test is most useful in the evaluation of men with secondary hypogonadism and subnormal LH response to an acute dose of LHRH. If daily infusions of LHRH for a week lead to the development of a normal LH response to an acute dose, a hypothalamic etiology is likely.

SEMINIFEROUS TUBULE FUNCTION Examination of the testes Evaluation of the testes is an essential portion of the physical examination. The seminiferous tubules account for about 95 percent of testicular volume. The prepubertal testis measures about 2 cm in length and 2 mL in volume and increases in size during puberty to reach the adult proportions by age 16. When damage to the seminiferous tubules occurs prior to puberty the testes are small and firm, whereas the testes are usually small and soft following postpubertal damage (the capsule, once enlarged, does not contract to its previous size). Testes in adults average 4.6 cm in length (range, 3.5 to 5.5 cm), corresponding to a volume of 12 to 25 mL. Advanced age does not influence testicular size, so that the significance of small testes is the same at all ages in the adult. Because of the frequent occurrence of varicocele among infertile men and its possible causal role in infertility, its presence should be sought by palpation with the patient standing.

Semen analysis Seminal fluid analysis is performed after 24- to 36-h abstinence on samples obtained by masturbation into a glass container. Analysis should be performed within an hour. The normal ejaculate volume is 2 to 6 mL. Immediately after ejaculation, coagulation of the seminal fluid occurs, followed within 15 to 30 min by liquefaction. Estimation of motility should be made on undiluted seminal fluid; more than 60 percent of the sperm should be motile and of normal morphology. The normal range for sperm density is generally considered to be greater than 20 million per milliliter with a total count per ejaculate of more than 60 million, but a major difficulty in the interpretation of a semen analysis is the definition of the minimally adequate ejaculate. Some men with low sperm counts are nevertheless fertile. This uncertainty as to the lower level of sperm density, percent motility, and percent normal forms in fertile semen stems from two issues. First, many factors produce temporary aberrations in sperm count, and in men who present with semen of equivocal quality it is necessary to examine three or more ejaculates to determine whether abnormal findings are permanent or temporary. Second, routine evaluation of the seminal fluid is dependent on tests that do not assess the functional capacity of the sperm. Although methods to measure sperm penetration of bovine cervical mucus and zona-free hamster ova have been developed, they are not sufficiently standardized to permit general use.

Plasma FSH Plasma FSH as measured by specific radioimmunoassay usually correlates inversely with spermatogenesis. In normal adult men, the range of plasma FSH is 102 ±55 ng/mL SD (5 to 20 mIU/mL). Men with intact hypothalamic-pituitary axes have elevations of FSH when damage to the germinal epithelium is severe.

Testicular biopsy Testicular biospy is useful in some patients with oligospermia and azoospermia both as an aid in diagnosis and as an indication of feasibility of treatment. For example, a normal testicular biopsy and a normal FSH in an azoospermic man suggest the presence of obstruction of the vas deferens, which may be surgically correctible. Tissue culture of the biopsy material with subsequent karyotypic analysis is necessary to identify those instances of Klinefelter syndrome secondary to chromosomal mosaicism in which the abnormality is limited to the testes. Testicular biopsy is often followed by a transient decrease in sperm counts, but there are no permanent adverse effects.

ESTROGENIC FUNCTION **Examination of the breasts** Breast enlargement is the most consistent feature of feminizing states in men (see Chap. 332). Gynecomastia, enlargement of the male breast, is due to the proliferation of glandular tissue. The presence of gynecomastia should be sought by examining the patient while he is in the sitting position using the fingers to grasp glandular tissue. Palpation with the flat of the hand while the patient is supine may result in failure to detect early or minimal breast enlargement. In obese men it is important to try to define the edge of the rim of glandular tissue that separates it from adipose tissue of the chest wall.

Plasma estrogen As discussed above, most of the estradiol and all of the estrone produced in normal men is formed by extraglandular aromatization of circulating androgens. Plasma estradiol is usually less than 50 pg/mL in normal men; plasma estrone is somewhat higher but usually less than 80 pg/mL. Elevated estrogen production and elevated plasma levels can be due to elevations in plasma precursors (liver or adrenal disease), to increases in peripheral aromatization (obesity), or to increased production by the testes (testicular tumors or androgen resistance).

PHASES OF NORMAL TESTICULAR FUNCTION

The phases of male sexual life can be defined in terms of the plasma testosterone value (Fig. 330-6). In the male embryo the production of testosterone by the testis commences at about 7 weeks of gestation. Shortly thereafter plasma testosterone attains a high value that is maintained until it falls late in gestation so that at the time of birth plasma testosterone is only slightly higher in males than in females. Shortly after birth, plasma testosterone in the male infant again begins to rise and remains elevated for approximately 3 months, falling to low levels by age 1 year. The concentration then remains low (but slightly higher in boys than girls) until the onset of puberty, when it begins to rise in boys, reaching adult levels by age 17 or thereabouts. The mean plasma level remains more or less constant in the adult until late middle age and then declines slowly during the later decades of life. It is only during the third or adult phase of male sexual life that sperm production becomes sufficient to allow reproduction to take place. The physiologic events that take place during these various phases differ, as do the pathologic consequences of derangements in testicular function at different stages of life. Male sexual differentiation during embryogenesis is considered in Chap. 333. The role of the neonatal surge of testosterone formation during the first year of life is unknown. The focus of this chapter is on testicular pathophysiology during puberty, mature sexual life, and old age.

ABNORMALITIES OF TESTICULAR FUNCTION

PUBERTY The factors that ultimately determine the onset of puberty are poorly understood and may reside in the hypothalamic-pituitary system, the testis, or the adrenal. Prior to the onset of puberty, gonadotropin secretion by the pituitary is low but appears to be under regulatory control by the testis, as prepubertal castration results in a rise in plasma gonadotropin levels. This suggests that prior to puberty the negative feedback control of gonadotropin secretion is exquisitely

FIGURE 330-6 *Phases of male sexual life. (Reprinted from Griffin and Wilson, 1980.)*

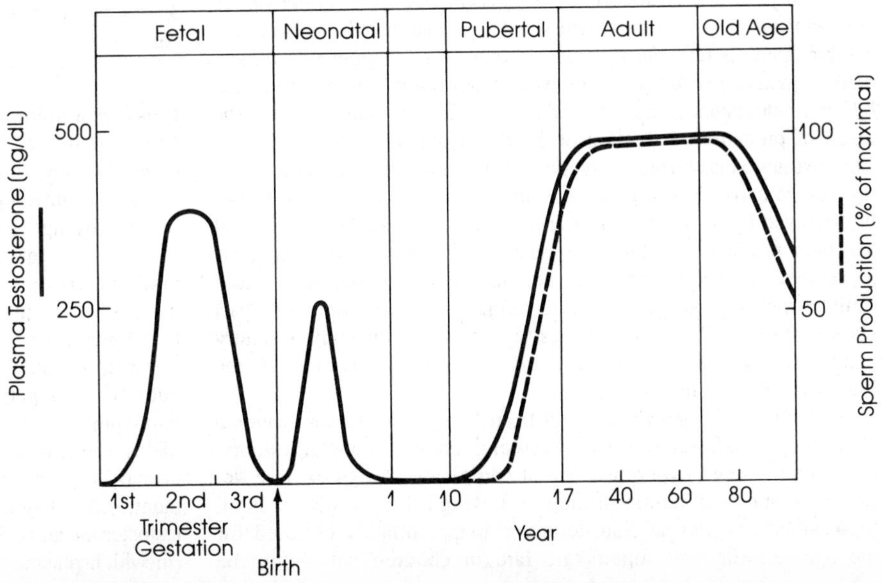

sensitive to the small amount of circulating testosterone. The onset of puberty is heralded by sleep-associated surges in gonadotropin secretion. Later in puberty the rises in LH and FSH persist throughout the day. Thus, with maturation the hypothalamic-pituitary system becomes less sensitive to negative feedback control, and the consequences are a higher mean plasma testosterone, maturation of the testes, and the onset of spermatogenesis. The rise in gonadotropin secretion is believed to be the consequence both of an increase in LHRH secretion and an increased sensitivity of the pituitary to LHRH. Plasma levels of bioactive LH increase even more than those of the immunoreactive hormone. The remaining anatomic and functional changes at the time of puberty are secondary to the rise in plasma testosterone. Maturation of the accessory organs of male reproduction (the penis, the prostate, the seminal vesicles, and the epididymides) accounts for about one-fourth of androgen-mediated nitrogen retention during puberty. The characteristic hair growth of male puberty involves development of mustache and beard, regression of the scalp line, appearance of body, extremity, and perianal hair, and extension of the pubic hair upward into a diamond-shaped pattern. Growth of axillary and pubic hair is initiated under the control of adrenal androgens and promoted by testicular androgens. The larynx enlarges, and the vocal cords become thickened, resulting in a lowering of the pitch of the voice. Linear growth is accelerated and is accompanied by growth of muscle and connective tissue which accounts for the major portion of nitrogen retention at puberty. The principal androgen-sensitive muscles are those of the pectoral region and the shoulder. There is, in addition, an increase in the hematocrit. These various androgen-mediated growth and maturation processes reach some limiting value so that once puberty is completed the administration of pharmacologic doses of androgen has no further effect. The entire process is usually heralded by testicular enlargement at age 11 to 12 and is usually completed within 5 years, although some aspects of virilization, such as growth of the chest hair, may continue over a decade or more.

The events of normal male puberty are variable in onset, duration, and sequence. The central issue in dealing with disorders of puberty is separating instances of true absence or precocity from subjects at the extremes of normal variation. The use of staging criteria that correlate developmental and anatomic landmarks with chronologic age is useful in making this distinction. (See Marshall and Tanner.)

Sexual precocity Those disorders in which the developing sexual characteristics are appropriate for the phenotype, i.e., virilization in boys, are termed *isosexual precocity*. Heterosexual precocity refers to feminizing syndromes occurring in boys with early sexual development.

ISOSEXUAL PRECOCITY Sexual development prior to age 9 in boys is generally considered abnormal. *True precocious puberty* or *complete isosexual precocity* occurs when both premature virilization and spermatogenesis take place, and *precocious pseudopuberty* or *incomplete isosexual precocity* occurs when virilization is unaccompanied by spermatogenesis, indicating that androgen formation is not the result of premature activation of the hypothalamic-pituitary system. This distinction is blurred in practice because pure virilizing syndromes may cause activation of gonadotropin secretion secondarily and thus be followed by development of spermatogenesis. Furthermore, local androgen production in the testis, as in Leydig cell tumors, can cause local areas of spermatogenesis around the tumor and thus cause limited sperm production. We therefore prefer a simple two-part classification: virilizing syndromes (in which hypothalamic-pituitary activity is appropriate for age) and premature activation of the hypothalamic pituitary system.

Virilizing syndromes can result from Leydig cell tumors, human chorionic gonadotropin (hCG)–secreting tumors, adrenal tumors, congenital adrenal hyperplasia (most commonly 21-hydroxylase deficiency), androgen administration, or Leydig cell hyperplasia. In all these situations plasma testosterone is inappropriately elevated for the age. Leydig cell tumors are rare in children but should be suspected when the testes are asymmetric in size (see Chap. 297). Virilizing adrenal tumors are usually associated with the production of large amounts of adrenal androgen (mainly androstenedione and dehydroepiandrosterone, some of which is converted to testosterone) and consequently with elevated 17-ketosteroid secretion. Glucocorticoid administration does not suppress 17-ketosteroid excretion to normal in either testicular or adrenal tumors, in contrast to the prompt decrease that occurs following such treatment in congenital adrenal hyperplasia. Congenital adrenal hyperplasia leads to elevated 17-hydroxyprogesterone levels and as a consequence elevated androgen levels (see Chaps. 325 and 333). In this disorder enhanced gonadotropin secretion can be initiated secondarily so that true precocious puberty can then result.

Gonadotropin-independent sexual precocity in boys may occur as a result of autonomous Leydig cell hyperplasia in the absence of Leydig cell tumor formation. The disorder is inherited as a male-limited autosomal disorder either from father to son or from mothers who are unaffected carriers. Virilization begins usually by age 2. Testosterone levels are elevated, often to the adult male range; however, immunoreactive and bioactive LH levels and the response to LHRH are prepubertal. Many of these boys were mistakenly thought to have true precocious puberty in the past because of the presence of spermatogenesis.

Since sexual precocity is defined as the occurrence of any sign of sexual maturation at an age less than 2 SD below the mean (age 9 in North America), by definition a fraction of normal boys have activation of the hypothalamic-pituitary system before this age. *Premature activation of the hypothalamic-pituitary system* may be "idiopathic" or due to central nervous system tumors, infections, or injuries. Such early hypothalamic-pituitary activation typically is associated with characteristics of normal puberty, i.e., sleep-related gonadotropin secretion, elevated plasma bioactive LH, and enhanced gonadotropin response to LHRH. Since the diagnosis of idiopathic true precocious puberty is one of exclusion, some patients later prove to have been misclassified and to have an identifiable central nervous system abnormality. With improved means of diagnosis, such as CT scans, delays in diagnosis will probably be less frequent.

Management of sexual precocity due to steroid- or gonadotropin-producing tumors, congenital adrenal hyperplasia, or an identified CNS abnormality is directed toward the primary disease. In boys with Leydig cell hyperplasia attempts have been made to lower plasma testosterone with medroxyprogesterone acetate or ketoconazole, but the long-term efficacy and safety of these agents is unknown. Idiopathic true precocious puberty and true precocious puberty due to inoperable CNS lesions are treated with LHRH analogue therapy, resulting in reversal of the pubertal maturation including decreased rate of skeletal development.

HETEROSEXUAL PRECOCITY Feminization in prepubertal boys can result from absolute or relative increases in estrogen due to a variety of causes (see Chap. 332).

Delayed or incomplete puberty The separation of failure of puberty from variants of normal is one of the most difficult problems in endocrinology. Some patients fail to show the normal spurt of growth and sexual development at the usual time but eventually commence puberty by age 16 or older. Adolescence may then either progress rapidly, or there may be a slow development and growth that continues until age 20 to 22. Many men with delayed onset of puberty attain heights within the normal adult range. At times the history reveals that a parent or sibling has shown a similar pattern of development. The major problem is to separate this group of patients with delayed puberty from patients with organic disorders that impair puberty. Panhypopituitarism and hypothyroidism can cause pubertal failure in males (see Chaps. 321 and 324). Absent puberty can also result from primary disease of the testis including defects in testicular development; this diagnosis is suspected on the basis of low plasma testosterone and elevated FSH and LH. Hereditary androgen resistance (in which plasma testosterone and LH are both high) usually results in hereditary male pseudohermaphroditism, but in milder cases may be manifested by absent puberty (see Chap. 333).

The most frequent finding in boys with absent puberty is both low plasma testosterone and low gonadotropin levels; in these patients it is necessary to distinguish those with delayed puberty from those with *hypogonadotropic hypogonadism* (*the Kallman syndrome*). The manifestation of hypogonadotropic hypogonadism varies from boys with eunuchoidal features and testes of prepubertal size to those with partial manifestations of LH and FSH deficiency. Anosmia or hyposmia and cryptorchidism are common. Histologic examination of the testis reveals undifferentiated Leydig cells and immature germinal epithelium similar to a normal prepubertal testis. The disorder is inherited as an X-linked recessive trait or an autosomal dominant trait with variable expressivity. Serum FSH and LH levels are usually below the normal male range, and plasma testosterone levels are low for the age. The secretion of other pituitary hormones is usually normal. The defect appears to be in the synthesis or release of LHRH, and the administration of synthetic LHRH for a sufficient period corrects the endocrine abnormalities and initiates spermatogenesis. If untreated, these patients usually remain in the prepubertal state indefinitely. A prepubertal manifestation of this disorder is microphallus, in which the size of the penis is below the fifth percentile for the age. Indeed, in a fourth or more of prepubertal patients with isolated microphallus the underlying etiology is hypogonadotropic hypogonadism. Distinction between this disorder and delayed puberty is particularly difficult in patients of early or midpubertal age; the presence of microphallus, anosmia, or a family history of hypogonadotropic hypogonadism may make it possible to establish the diagnosis. In the absence of such evidence, differentiation of the two states may become clear only after several years of observation. In some cases the response of plasma LH to LHRH stimulation may be helpful in suggesting that puberty is imminent.

One less severe form of hypogonadotropic hypogonadism is the so-called *fertile eunuch syndrome* in which spermatogenesis is present despite deficient androgen production. Plasma FSH levels are within the normal adult male range, whereas plasma testosterone and plasma LH levels are low. However, LHRH administration to such patients causes an increase in plasma LH as well as FSH. This implies that the defect in this disorder, as in the Kallman syndrome, is defective LH release. *Isolated FSH deficiency* is a rare disorder in which virilization, plasma LH, and plasma testosterone are normal but plasma FSH is persistently low; testicular biopsy in one individual revealed a maturation arrest at the spermatid stage. In some, FSH levels increased following administration of LHRH.

ADULT ABNORMALITIES OF TESTICULAR FUNCTION At the time of the completion of puberty, plasma testosterone levels reach the adult level of 300 to 1000 ng/dL throughout the day, plasma gonadotropins are 5 to 20 mIU/mL each for LH and FSH, and sperm production is sufficient to allow reproduction. The adult set of the complex regulatory system (Fig. 330-3) is sustained in the normal man for more than 40 years. However, the system is subject to a variety of influences, both at the level of the testis and of the hypothalamic-pituitary system. Spermatogenesis is exquisitely sensitive to alterations in temperature, and brief increases either in systemic or local temperature (as in a hot bath) can be followed by temporary decreases in sperm production. The system is likewise subject to influence by diet, drugs, alcohol, environmental agents, and psychological stress, all of which may cause temporary decreases in sperm count.

Persistent abnormalities of testicular function after the time of normal puberty can be due to hypothalamic-pituitary abnormalities (see Chap. 321), testicular defects, or to abnormalities of sperm transport. Certain of these conditions tend to affect Leydig cell function or spermatogenesis selectively, but most influence both aspects of testicular function and cause both underandrogenization and infertility (Table 330-1). The interlocking of defective Leydig cell function with infertility is a consequence of the dependence of spermatogenesis on androgen formation. Even partial decreases in testosterone production can cause infertility. Certain disorders (hyperprolactinemia, radiation, cyclophosphamide therapy, autoimmunity, paraplegia, androgen resistance) can cause either isolated infertility or a combined defect in testicular function in different subjects.

Hypothalamic-pituitary disorders Disorders of the hypothalamus and pituitary can impair secretion of gonadotropins (and cause as a consequence decreased androgen production and defective spermatogenesis) either as an isolated defect (hypogonadotropic hypogonadism) or as a portion of more complex endocrine and systemic manifestations (see Chap. 321). Alternatively, gonadotropin secretion can be altered by factors other than hypothalamic pituitary pathology. For example, elevation of plasma cortisol in the *Cushing syndrome* can depress LH secretion independent of a space-occupying lesion of the pituitary. Some patients with *congenital adrenal hyperplasia* have early activation of gonadotropin secretion and true precocious puberty, while other patients have suppressed gonadotropin secretion and consequent infertility. *Hyperprolactinemia* (either as the consequence of pituitary adenomas or of drugs such as phenothiazines) has been associated with combined Leydig cell and seminiferous tubule dysfunction, presumably the consequence of inhibition of LH

TABLE 330-1 Classification of abnormalities of testicular function in the adult

	Presentation	
Site of defect	Infertility with underandrogenization	Infertility with normal virilization
Hypothalamic-pituitary	Panhypopituitarism	
	Hypogonadotropic hypogonadism	Isolated FSH deficiency
	Cushing's syndrome	Congenital adrenal hyperplasia
	Hyperprolactinemia	Hyperprolactinemia
	Hemochromatosis	
Testicular	Developmental and structural defects:	
	Klinefelter's syndrome*	Germinal cell aplasia
	XX male	Cryptorchidism
		Varicocele
		Immotile cilia syndrome
		Other structural defects of sperm
	Acquired defects:	
	Viral orchitis*	*Mycoplasma* infection
	Trauma	
	Radiation	Radiation
	Drugs (spironolactone, alcohol, ketoconazole, cyclophosphamide)	Drugs (cyclophosphamide)
	Autoimmunity (polyglandular endocrine failure)	Autoimmunity
	Granulomatous disease	
	Associated with systemic diseases:	
	Liver disease	Febrile illness
	Renal failure	Celiac disease
	Sickle cell disease	
	Neurologic diseases (myotonic dystrophy and paraplegia)	Neurologic disease (paraplegia)
	Androgen resistance	Androgen resistance
Sperm transport		Obstruction of the epididymis or vas deferens (cystic fibrosis, diethylstilbesterol exposure, congenital absence)

* *The common testicular causes of underandrogenization and infertility in adults—Klinefelter's syndrome and viral orchitis—are associated with small testes.*

and FSH secretion by prolactin. Occasionally, impaired fertility in hyperprolactinemia is associated with normal gonadotropin and androgen levels and is presumed to result from direct inhibition of spermatogenesis by prolactin. *Hemochromatosis* impairs testicular function most commonly as the result of effects on the pituitary, less often it affects the testis directly (see Chap. 310).

Testicular defects Abnormalities of testicular function in the adult can be grouped into several categories: developmental and structural defects of the testes, acquired testicular defects, and those abnormalities secondary to systemic and/or neurologic disease.

DEVELOPMENTAL ABNORMALITIES The *Klinefelter syndrome* (both the classic and mosaic forms) and the *XX male syndrome* are usually not recognized until after the time of expected puberty (see Chap. 333). Some developmental defects cause infertility in the presence of normal androgen production. These include varicocele, germinal cell aplasia, and cryptorchidism. *Varicocele* is probably the most common treatable cause of male infertility and may be of etiologic importance in as much as one-third of all male infertility. It is caused by retrograde flow of blood into the internal spermatic vein that eventuates in progressive, often palpable dilatation of the peritesticular pampiniform plexus of veins. The incidence of varicocele is about 10 to 15 percent in the general population and 20 to 40 percent in men with infertility. It is thought to result from incompetence of the valve between the internal spermatic vein and the renal vein and is more common on the left (85 percent). Unilateral varicocele increases the blood flow and the temperature of both testes as a result of the extensive anastomoses of the venous systems. The findings on semen analysis are usually nonspecific with all parameters showing some abnormality. The increased scrotal (and testicular) temperature is believed to be the cause of the poor-quality semen and infertility (the testes do not have the usual 2°C lower temperature than that of the abdominal cavity). In some studies, surgical resection results in improved fertility, with the best results (70 percent pregnancy rate) obtained in men whose preoperative sperm counts are over 10 million per milliliter.

Some patients with *germinal cell aplasia* (the Sertoli cell–only syndrome) have a positive family history and may constitute a specific entity in which the germinal epithelium is missing with resulting azoospermia; plasma testosterone and LH values are normal, and plasma FSH levels are elevated. Other patients with identical histologic and clinical findings have androgen resistance or a history of viral orchitis or cryptorchidism. Consequently a variety of conditions are commonly lumped under this term. The syndrome accounts for less than 10 percent of patients with azoospermia.

Unilateral *cryptorchidism,* even when corrected prior to puberty, is associated with abnormal semen in many individuals. This suggests that even in unilateral cryptorchidism the testicular abnormality is usually bilateral.

The *immotile cilia syndrome* is an autosomal recessive defect characterized by immotility or poor motility of the cilia of the airways and of the sperm. Kartagener's syndrome is a subgroup of the immotile cilia syndrome associated with situs inversus. The immotile cilia in the airways result in chronic sinusitis and bronchiectasis, and the immotile sperm cannot fertilize. The structural abnormality leading to impaired motility of cilia can usually be defined by the electron-microscopic appearance. The specific defects that are known to cause the syndrome include defects in the dynein arms, spokes, or microtubule doublets. Cilia from epithelia and sperm tails from the same individual exhibit the same defects, but the pulmonary manifestations may be minor. *Other structural defects of sperm* that are less well understood can apparently lead to immotile sperm without involvement of cilia in the lung.

ACQUIRED TESTICULAR DEFECTS Most acquired testicular failure in the adult results from *viral orchitis*. Mumps is the virus most frequently responsible, although other viruses act in a similar fashion, including echovirus, lymphocytic choriomeningitis virus, and group B arboviruses. The orchitis is due to actual infection of the tissue by virus rather than indirect effects of the infection. Orchitis is the most common complication of mumps in adult men, occurring in as many as one-fourth of men who have the disease. In about two-thirds of the cases it is unilateral, and in the remainder it is bilateral. It usually develops within a few days after the onset of parotitis but may precede it. The testis may return to normal size and function or undergo atrophy. Atrophy is believed to be due both to direct effects of the virus on the seminiferous tubules and to ischemia secondary to pressure and edema within the taut tunica albuginea. Semen analysis returns to normal in three-fourths of men with unilateral involvement and in only one-third of men with bilateral orchitis. Atrophy is usually perceptible within 1 to 6 months after the orchitis subsides, and the degree of atrophy is not necessarily proportional to the severity of the acute orchitis or the development of infertility. Unilateral atrophy occurs in approximately one-third of cases of mumps orchitis, and bilateral atrophy occurs in about one-tenth.

Trauma is the second most common cause of secondary atrophy of the testes. The exposed position of the testis in the scrotum renders it susceptible to both thermal and physical trauma—particularly in individuals with hazardous occupations.

Both the seminiferous tubules and the Leydig cells are sensitive to *radiation damage;* the diminished secretion of testosterone appears to be a consequence of diminished testicular blood flow. Doses higher than 200 mGy (20 rad) cause increases in plasma FSH and LH levels and damage to the spermatogonia. With doses of about 800 mGy (80 rad) oligospermia or azoospermia develops. Higher doses may result in virtual obliteration of the germinal epithelium except for occasional stem and Sertoli cells. Still higher doses [6000 mGy (600 rad)] can cause an increase in the number of Leydig cells. Complete recovery of sperm density to preirradiation levels may require as long as 5 years. Permanent infertility can apparently occur after amounts of radiation used for therapy of malignant lymphoma in spite of shielding the testes. Permanent androgen deficiency in adult men is uncommon from doses of radiation in the therapeutic range; however, most boys receiving direct testicular radiation for acute lymphoblastic leukemia have permanently low plasma testosterone levels.

In general, *drugs* interfere with testicular function in one of four ways—inhibition of testosterone synthesis, blockade of the peripheral action of androgen, enhancement of estrogen levels, or direct inhibition of spermatogenesis. Certain drugs have multiple effects, and agents such as guanethidine that block the sympathetic nervous system can impair sexual function in men whose pituitary-testicular axis is normal.

Spironolactone and ketoconazole block the synthesis of androgen by interfering with the late reactions in androgen biosynthesis. Spironolactone and cimetidine also compete with androgen for the cytoplasmic receptor protein and thus interfere with androgen action in the target cell. Testosterone levels may be low and estradiol levels may be elevated in patients taking large amounts of marijuana, heroin, or methadone, although the exact reasons are unclear. Alcohol, when consumed in excess for prolonged periods, causes decreased plasma testosterone, independent of liver disease or malnutrition. Elevated plasma estradiol levels and decreased plasma testosterone levels have been reported in men taking digitalis.

Antineoplastic and chemotherapeutic agents, especially cyclophosphamide, commonly interfere with spermatogenesis. Cyclophosphamide causes azoospermia or extreme oligospermia within a few weeks after the initiation of therapy. Cessation of drug therapy is followed by a return of spermatogenesis within 3 years in about half of patients. Combination chemotherapy for acute leukemia, Hodgkin's disease, and other malignancies may also impair Leydig cell function. In pubertal boys this is manifested by decreased serum testosterone and elevated LH levels while in adult men testosterone levels do not decline and the impaired Leydig cell function may only be detected by an exaggeration of LH response to LHRH. The alkylating agents in the chemotherapeutic regimens seem to be responsible for the toxic effects on the Leydig cell.

Testicular failure also occurs as a part of a generalized disorder of *autoimmunity* in which multiple primary endocrine deficiencies coexist (Schmidt's syndrome) and in which circulating antibodies to the basement membrane of the testes are present (see Chap. 334). Sperm antibodies are a rare cause of isolated male infertility (less than 1 percent of cases). In some instances such antibodies may be secondary phenomena resulting from duct obstruction or vasectomy. *Granulomatous diseases* can also destroy the testes, the most common such disorder being leprosy. Testicular atrophy occurs in 10 to 20 percent of men with lepromatous leprosy, the result of direct invasion of the tissue by the mycobacteria. The tubules are involved initially, followed by endarteritis and destruction of Leydig cells.

TESTICULAR ABNORMALITIES ASSOCIATED WITH SYSTEMIC DISEASE The common systemic diseases that cause combined underandrogenization and infertility are liver disease and renal failure. In *cirrhosis of the liver* a combined testicular and pituitary lesion leads to decreased testosterone production independent of the direct toxic effects of ethanol. Although plasma LH is elevated, the level may be below the expected range given the degree of androgen deficiency. This is most likely the result of inhibition of LH secretion by the higher estrogen concentrations found in patients with chronic liver disease. Increased estrogen production results from impaired hepatic extraction of adrenal androstenedione and subsequent increased peripheral conversion to estrone and estradiol. In effect there is shunting of estrogen precursors to aromatization sites in peripheral tissues. Testicular atrophy and gynecomastia are present in about half of men with cirrhosis, and many such men are impotent.

In chronic *renal failure* decreased androgen synthesis and diminution of sperm production develop in the setting of elevated plasma gonadotropins. The elevated LH is due to increased production as well as reduced clearance but is incapable of effecting normal testosterone production. In addition, about half of men with chronic renal failure have hyperprolactinemia. Low testosterone levels coupled with normal or increased plasma estrogen levels probably account for the presence of gynecomastia in about half of men on chronic hemodialysis. The role of the hyperprolactinemia in decreasing testosterone production is unclear. About half of men with renal failure on dialysis experience decreased libido and impotence. The etiology of the testicular abnormalities in renal failure is not well understood. Only slight improvement in testosterone production occurs with hemodialysis, but successful transplantation may lead to return of testicular function to normal.

Men with *sickle cell anemia* usually have impaired secondary sexual development, and testicular atrophy is present in one-third. The defect may be either at the testicular or hypothalamic-pituitary level. Abnormalities in Leydig cell function, frequently accompanied by decreased sperm density, have been noted in a variety of chronic systemic diseases including protein-calorie *malnutrtion,* advanced *Hodgkin's disease* and *cancer* prior to chemotherapy, and *amyloidosis*. Most of these disorders cause a lowered plasma testosterone coupled with a normal to increased plasma LH, suggesting combined hypothalamic-pituitary and testicular defects. The low plasma testosterone is not the result of inhibitors that interfere with the binding to TeBG and hence is not analogous to the euthyroid sick syndrome. Similar hormone changes occur following *surgery, myocardial infarction,* and severe *burns,* and thus may be a nonspecific effect of illness.

The temporary decrease in sperm density that occurs following *acute febrile illness* usually occurs in the absence of any changes in testosterone production. Men with *celiac disease* may have infertility associated with a hormonal pattern typical of androgen resistance with elevated testosterone and LH levels on average. The major *neurologic diseases* associated with altered testicular function are myotonic dystrophy and paraplegia. In myotonic dystrophy small testes may be associated with abnormalities of both spermatogenesis and Leydig cell function. Spinal cord lesions resulting in paraplegia lead to a temporary decrease in testosterone levels that tend to return to normal but persistent defects in spermatogenesis; some patients retain the capacity to obtain erection and to ejaculate.

ANDROGEN RESISTANCE Defects of the androgen receptor cause resistance to the action of androgen usually associated with defective male phenotypic development as well as infertility and underandrogenization (see Chap. 333). However, some men with familial Reifenstein's syndrome have a less complete androgen resistance with no abnormalities of phenotypic development except for azoospermia but with endocrine and tissue culture evidence of a defective androgen receptor. An even less severe form of androgen resistance is associated with infertility due to oligo- or azoospermia in otherwise phenotypically normal men; this form of androgen resistance may be the etiology in a significant fraction of men with infertility previously classified as having idiopathic azoospermia.

Impairment of sperm transport Disorders of sperm transport may lead to infertility in as many as 6 percent of infertile men with normal virilization. The obstruction may be unilateral or bilateral, congenital or acquired. In men with unilateral obstruction of sperm transport the infertility may result from antisperm antibodies. Obstructive azoospermia at the level of the epididymis also occurs in association with chronic sinopulmonary infections. Tuberculosis, leprosy, and gonorrhea are rare causes of acquired obstruction of Wolffian duct–derived structures. Congenital defects of the vas deferens can occur as an isolated abnormality associated with absence of the seminal vesicles (and consequently absence of fructose in the ejaculate), in patients with *cystic fibrosis,* or in men whose mothers received *diethylstilbestrol* during pregnancy.

At least 40 percent of infertile men have infertility of unknown etiology; none of the above conditions is found on careful search. The therapy in these patients, as in all infertile men except those with surgically correctable varicocele, vas deferens obstruction, or treatable endocrinopathy, is unsatisfactory. Empirical therapy with androgens or gonadotropins probably has no significant effect on fertility. Although the semen quality may improve with such treatment, the pregnancy rate is usually no greater than in infertile men given no therapy (25 percent fertility in patients followed for a year). This latter fact should be kept in mind, namely that spontaneous resolution may occur in one-fourth of patients with idiopathic infertility followed with no treatment. The extent to which the sperm from men with idiopathic infertility can be used successfully for in vitro fertilization and embryo transfer is unclear (see Chap. 331).

Fertility control in the male Although a variety of approaches to fertility control in men have been tried, the most practical means is ligation of the vas deferens, a procedure that has been utilized successfully in large numbers of men and that can be performed on an outpatient basis. The time required for azoospermia to occur following the operation depends upon the number of sperm in the terminal vas deferens and ejaculatory ducts at the time of surgery but is usually less than 40 days. Azoospermia should be documented in each case to prove effectiveness. No deleterious effects on either testosterone production or the hypothalamic-pituitary axis have been documented. Despite reports of immune-complex-associated accelerated atherosclerosis in vasectomized nonhuman primates, there does not appear to be any association of vasectomy and atherosclerosis in men. Vasectomy should only be recommended for men requesting permanent sterilization. Vasovasostomy for reanastomosis of the vas has a success rate of about 80 to 90 percent as judged by return of sperm to the ejaculate, but only about 30 to 40 percent subsequently achieve fertility. This discrepancy is possibly due to the development of antisperm antibodies as a consequence of the vasectomy.

OLD AGE Beginning at about age 70 mean plasma testosterone concentrations decline. This decrease occurs despite an elevation in TeBG so that the level of free testosterone decreases even more than the total. Though statistically lower than average, both total and free concentrations of testosterone usually remain within the normal range. There is, however, an associated rise in plasma LH and an increase in the rate of conversion of androgen to estrogen in peripheral tissues so that the effective ratio of androgen to estrogen decreases. These endocrine changes in the aging man are believed to be critical for the development of prostatic hyperplasia and probably for development of gynecomastia in aging men (see Chap. 332), but there is no convincing evidence that such changes have any direct bearing on sexual function in the elderly.

Prostatic hyperplasia See Chap. 298.

Cancer of the prostate See Chap. 298.

DISORDERS OF ALL AGES **Testicular tumors** (see Chap. 297) Chorionic gonadotropin is present in normal testes, and it is therefore not surprising that plasma gonadotropins are elevated in testicular tumors. Indeed, an elevated plasma level of the beta subunit of human chorionic gonadotropins (hCG-β) serves as a sensitive and specific marker of tumor activity in some men with germ cell tumors. Plasma levels of the beta subunit are elevated in all patients with choriocarcinoma, in one-third of embryonal carcinomas and teratocarcinomas, and rarely in seminomas. There is a good correlation between change in hCG-β levels and response to therapy.

Elevated estradiol and testosterone production in patients with testicular tumors can arise by at least two mechanisms. In trophoblastic tumors and in tumors of Leydig and Sertoli cells production of both hormones occurs autonomously in the tumor tissue itself; in these instances plasma gonadotropin levels and hormone production by the uninvolved portions of the testes are depressed, and azoospermia is common. However, when gonadotropins are secreted by the tumor, the gonadotropin acts to increase estradiol and testosterone production in the unaffected areas of the testes, and azoospermia is uncommon. When potent estrogens and androgens are formed (directly or indirectly) by the tumors, feminization, virilization, or no obvious change may result, depending on the pattern of hormones produced and the age of the patients involved. Other cellular markers of testicular tumor activity have been described in individual cases, including alpha fetoprotein.

Gynecomastia See Chap. 332.

HORMONAL THERAPY

ANDROGENS **Pharmacologic preparations** Effective androgen therapy requires the use of chemically modified analogues of testosterone. When testosterone itself is administered by mouth, it is absorbed into the portal blood and degraded promptly by the liver so that insignificant amounts reach the systemic circulation; when injected parenterally testosterone is rapidly absorbed from the injection vehicle so that it is difficult to sustain effective levels in the plasma. Therefore, it is necessary to modify the molecule so as to retard the rate of absorption or catabolism, so as to sustain effective blood levels or to enhance the androgenic potency of each molecule, so that full androgenic effects can be achieved at a lower blood level of the drug. Three types of modification of the molecule have received widespread clinical application (Fig. 330-7), namely esterification of the 17β-hydroxyl group, alkylation at the 17α position, and modification of the ring structure, particularly substitutions at the 2, 9, and 11 positions. Esterification serves to decrease the polarity of the molecule. Consequently, the steroid is more soluble in the fat vehicles used for injection, and release of the steroid into the circulation is slowed. Esters cannot be administered by mouth and must be injected parenterally. The more carbon molecules in the acid esterified, the more prolonged the action. Currently available esters such as testosterone cypionate and testosterone enanthate can be injected every 1 to 3 weeks. Because the esters are hydrolyzed before the hormones act, the effectiveness of therapy can be monitored by assaying the plasma level of testosterone with time following administration.

The effectiveness of 17α-alkylated androgens (such as methyltestosterone and methandrostenolone) when given by mouth is due to slower hepatic catabolism than occurs with testosterone itself so that the alkylated derivatives escape degradation by the liver and reach the systemic circulation. For this reason 17α-methyl or -ethyl substitution is a common feature of most orally active androgens. Unfortunately, all 17α-alkylated steroids may cause abnormalities of liver function, and for this reason they have a limited role in medicine.

Other alterations of the ring structure of the androgen molecule have been adopted empirically; in some instances the modification slows the rate of inactivation, in others it enhances the potency of a given molecule, and in still others it alters the conversion to other active metabolites. For example, the potency of fluoxymesterone may be due to the fact that, unlike most androgens, it is a poor precursor for conversion to estrogens in peripheral tissues.

Side effects of androgens All androgens carry the risk of inducing virilization in women. Among the early manifestations are acne, coarsening of the voice, and development of hirsutism. Menstrual irregularities are common. If treatment is discontinued as soon as these effects develop, the manifestations may slowly subside. With prolonged treatment, male-pattern baldness, worsening of the hirsutism and voice changes, and hypertrophy of the clitoris develop and are largely irreversible. There is considerable variation in the frequency and the degree to which these signs develop in women. The variation in response probably results from several factors including individual differences in susceptibility, variability in steady-state blood levels among individuals, and variable duration of therapy. In general, the younger the patient, the more striking the virilizing signs; nevertheless, florid virilization can also occur in adult women.

Retention of a limited amount of sodium is an inevitable consequence of androgen therapy, but in patients with underlying heart disease or renal failure or when androgens are administered in enormous amounts, as in some patients with carcinoma of the breast, the degree of sodium retention may be sufficient to produce edema. Although androgens do not cause malignancy, they may promote growth of and intensify pain from carcinoma of the prostate and from breast carcinoma in men.

Feminizing side effects of androgen therapy in men are poorly

FIGURE 330-7 *Some of the androgen preparations available for pharmacologic use.*

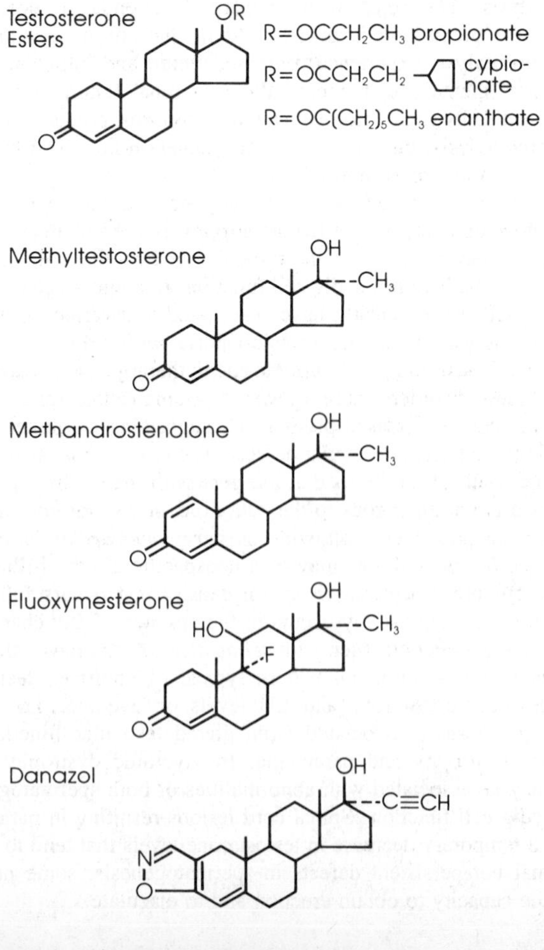

understood. Testosterone itself can be converted (aromatized) in peripheral tissues to estradiol. In contrast, 5α-reduction of the molecule precludes estrogen formation. The commonest manifestation of feminization is development of gynecomastia. Such breast enlargement is common in children given androgens and correlates with an increase in urinary estrogens, possibly because of a greater capacity to convert androgens to estrogens in childhood. The administration of testosterone esters to men results in an increase in plasma estrogen levels. In men with normal liver function, gynecomastia usually develops only after high doses of androgens.

All 17α-alkylated androgens produce sodium sulfobromophthalein retention and frequently cause elevation of plasma alkaline phosphatase and conjugated bilirubin. The incidence of clinically manifest liver disease probably depends upon the previous integrity of the liver, but jaundice may occur even in the absence of preexisting liver disease. 17α-Alkylated drugs also cause an increase in a variety of plasma proteins that are synthesized in the liver. The most serious complications of oral androgen therapy are the development of peliosis hepatis (blood-filled cysts in the liver) and hepatoma. These disorders were initially described in patients with aplastic anemia, many of whom have Fanconi anemia, itself a predisposing factor for the development of malignancy. However, both lesions have also been reported in patients who received oral androgens for a variety of other causes, including use by athletes. There may be a similar increased incidence of hepatocellular neoplasms in women taking oral contraceptives. Although in some individuals these tumors regress and follow a benign course after discontinuation of the drugs, in others the course is rapidly fatal.

One indication for the use of 17α-alkylated androgens is in hereditary angioneurotic edema; in this disorder the desired therapeutic benefit (increase in the level of the inhibitor of the first component of complement) may actually be a side effect of the 17-alkylated steroid rather than an effect of the parent androgen itself. As a consequence, weak androgens such as danazol are effective in this disorder (Fig. 330-7). Another indication for danazol is in the management of endometriosis (see Chap. 43).

Replacement therapy The aim of androgen therapy in hypogonadal men is to restore or bring to normal male secondary sexual characteristics (beard, body hair, external genitalia) and male sexual behavior and to mimic the hormonal effects on somatic development (hemoglobin, muscle mass, nitrogen balance, and epiphyseal closure). Since an assay for plasma testosterone is available for monitoring therapy, the treatment of androgen deficiency is almost universally successful. The parenteral administration of a long-acting testosterone ester such as 100 to 200 mg testosterone enanthate at 1- to 3-week intervals results in a sustained increase in plasma testosterone to the normal male range. Such esters act only through the release of testosterone itself into the circulation. If the hypogonadism is primary and of long duration (as in the Klinefelter syndrome) suppression of plasma LH to the normal range may not occur for many weeks, if at all. Considerable variability exists in the relation between plasma testosterone and male sexual behavior, but in postpubertal testicular failure (even of many years duration) resumption of normal sexual activity is usual following adequate replacement. Androgen does not restore spermatogenesis in hypogonadal states, but the volume of the ejaculate (derived largely from the prostate and seminal vesicles) and male secondary sex characteristics return to normal. The effects of endogenous androgen on hemoglobin, nitrogen retention, and skeletal development are also reproduced.

In patients of all ages in whom hypogonadism developed prior to expected puberty (such as patients with hypogonadotropic hypogonadism), it is appropriate to bring plasma testosterone slowly into the adult range. When therapy is commenced at the time of expected puberty in such patients, the normal events of male puberty proceed in the usual fashion. If therapy is delayed until long after the time of usual puberty, the degree to which normal virilization will occur is variable, but many patients undergo a relatively complete anatomic and functional maturation. Intermittent low-dose androgen therapy is indicated in prepubertal hypogonadal boys with microphallus to bring the external genitalia into the normal range. If such patients are monitored closely and given androgens only for short periods, such therapy usually has no adverse effects on somatic growth.

In boys of pubertal age with either isolated hypogonadotropic hypogonadism or primary testicular deficiency, the usual practice is to institute androgen therapy between the ages of 12 and 14 years, depending on the subjective need for sexual development. The initial administration of small doses of testosterone esters followed by a gradual increase to 100 to 150 mg/m^2 of body surface area every 1 to 3 weeks should result in a normal pubertal growth spurt. The time from the start of treatment to the appearance of secondary sex characteristics is variable. Penile development, deepening of the voice, and other secondary sexual characteristics usually commence during the first year of treatment. In normal boys puberty extends over several years, and treatment designed to replicate normal development does not shorten the process greatly.

Testosterone exerts its full action only in the presence of a balanced hormonal environment and, particularly, in the presence of adequate levels of growth hormone. Consequently, prepubertal patients who have coexisting growth hormone deficiency exhibit a diminished response to androgens both in regard to growth and to the development of secondary sex characteristics unless sufficient growth hormone is given simultaneously.

Pharmacologic uses Androgens have been used for a variety of disorders unassociated with hypogonadism, in the hope that potential benefits from the nonvirilizing actions of the agents (such as increase in nitrogen retention and muscle mass, increased hemoglobin, etc.) would outweigh any deleterious actions of the drugs. The most common nonreplacement uses of androgen have been attempts to improve nitrogen balance in catabolic states, self-administration by athletes in the belief that muscle mass and/or athletic performance will be improved, attempts to enhance erythropoiesis in refactory anemias including the anemia of renal failure, adjuvant therapy in carcinoma of the breast, treatment of hereditary angioneurotic edema and endometriosis, and management of growth retardation of various etiologies. Most expectations of beneficial effects in these disorders have been illusory for two reasons. First, pharmacologic doses of androgens do little if anything in men beyond the normal testicular androgen, and in women the virilizing side effects of all agents are formidable. Second, no androgen has been devised that exhibits only the nonvirilizing effects of the hormone. This is not surprising in view of the fact that all known action of androgens are mediated by a single high-affinity receptor protein in the cytoplasm (Fig. 330-5).

The most pervasive form of androgen abuse is by male athletes in the expectation that muscle development and athletic performance will be improved. In fact, however, in most adequately controlled studies such therapy does not improve performance, and in those rare instances in which it does, such improvement may be the consequence of sodium retention and expansion of the blood volume rather than of an effect on muscle development or strength. Under no circumstances do putative benefits outweigh the risks associated with the use of oral androgens, a practice that cannot be condemned too harshly. At present, the only established indications for androgen therapy outside of male hypogonadism are in selected patients with anemia due to bone marrow failure and in patients with hereditary angioneurotic edema or endometriosis.

Parenteral administration of testosterone esters to normal men results in little effects of any kind, except for the suppression of gonadotropin secretion by the hypothalamic-pituitary system and a consequent decrease in the production of sperm. There is no established contraindication to their administration to men with those disorders (such as short stature) where their use has been advocated, but the efficacy is not yet established. However, the virilizing side effects in women of androgens in usual dosages preclude their use in all except life-threatening situations. Even in potentially fatal diseases in women such as bone marrow failure and carcinoma of the breast great care must be exercised in androgen use.

GONADOTROPINS Treatment with gonadotropins is utilized to establish or restore fertility in patients with gonadotropin deficiency of all causes. Two gonadotropin preparations are available: human menopausal gonadotropins (hMG) (purified from the urine of postmenopausal women) and human chorionic gonadotropin (hCG) (purified from the urine of pregnant women). hMG contains 75 IU FSH and 75 IU LH per vial. hCG has little FSH activity and resembles LH in its ability to stimulate testosterone production by Leydig cells. Because of the expense of hMG, treatment is usually begun with hCG alone, and hMG is added later to stimulate the FSH-dependent stages of spermatid development. A high ratio of LH to FSH activity and a long duration of treatment (3 to 6 months) are necessary to bring about the maturation of the prepubertal testis. Once spermatogenesis has been restored in hypophysectomized patients or initiated in hypogonadotropic hypogonadal men by combined therapy, spermatogenesis can usually be maintained with hCG alone.

Men with oligospermia of unknown etiology have been treated with human gonadotropins; the incidence of fertility in patients so treated is probably no greater than would occur in similar groups of untreated controls.

The dosage of hCG required to maintain a normal testosterone level is variable, ranging from 1000 to 5000 IU weekly. A variety of treatment regimens have been utilized to induce maturation of spermatogenesis. Most involve starting with 2000 IU hCG three or more times a week until most of the clinical parameters, including plasma testosterone, indicate normal adult male development. hMG (usually one ampul) is then added three times a week to complete the development of spermatogenesis. After regression of spermatogenesis has occurred the length of therapy required to bring about restoration of spermatogenesis is variable and may be as long as 12 months.

LUTEINIZING HORMONE–RELEASING HORMONE LHRH (gonadorelin) is now available for endocrine testing. LHRH therapy is now used by some physicians for chronic therapy of the infertility of hypogonadotropic hypogonadism. It is necessary to administer LHRH in frequent boluses (25 to 200 ng/kg of body weight every 2 h), requiring the use of portable infusion pumps or periodic nasal application. The relative efficacies of LHRH and gonadotropin therapy have yet to be defined.

REFERENCES

AIMAN J, GRIFFIN JE: The frequency of androgen receptor deficiency in infertile men. J Clin Endocrinol Metab 54:725, 1982

BAKER HWG et al: Testicular control of follicle-stimulating hormone secretion, in *Recent Progress in Hormone Research,* RO Greep (ed). New York, Academic, 1976, vol 32, pp 429–476

CARR BR, GRIFFIN JE: Fertility control and its complications, in *Williams' Textbook of Endocrinology,* 7th ed, JD Wilson, DW Foster (eds). Philadelphia, Saunders, 1985, pp 452–475

CUTLER GB et al: Therapeutic applications of luteinizing-hormone-releasing hormone and its analogs. Ann Intern Med 102:643, 1985

DAVIS JE: Male sterilization. Clin Obstet Gynaecol 6:97, 1979

DE KRETSER DM: The effects of systemic disease on the function of the testis. Clin Endocrinol Metabol 8:487, 1979

GOLDZIEHER JW et al:Improving the diagnostic reliability of rapidly fluctuating plasma hormone levels by optimized multiple-sampling techniques. J Clin Endocrinol Metab 43:824, 1976

GRIFFIN JE, WILSON JD: Disorders of the testes and male reproductive tract, in *Williams' Textbook of Endocrinology,* 7th ed, JD Wilson, DW Foster (eds). Philadelphia, Saunders, 1985, pp 259–312

MACDONALD PC et al: Origin of estrogen in normal men and in women with testicular feminization. J Clin Endocrinol Metab 49:905, 1979

MARSHALL WA, TANNER JM: Variation in the pattern of pubertal changes in boys. Arch Dis Child 45:13, 1970

MASSEY FJ et al: Vasectomy and health: Results from a large cohort study. JAMA 252:1023, 1984

ROSENBERG E: Gonadotropin therapy of male infertility, in *Human Semen and Fertility Regulation in Men,* ESE Hafez (ed). St Louis, Mosby, 1976, pp 464–475

RYAN AJ: Anabolic steroids are fool's gold. Fed Proc 40:2682, 1981

SHERINS RH et al: Male infertility, in *Campbell's Urology,* 5th ed, PC Walsh et al (eds). Philadelphia, Saunders, 1985, pp 640–699

SNYDER PF, LAWRENCE DA: Treatment of male hypogonadism with testosterone enanthate. J Clin Endocrinol Metab 51:1335, 1980

SPRATT DI, CROWLEY WF: Hypogonadotropic hypogonadism: GnRH therapy, in *Current Therapy in Endocrinology and Metabolism 1985–1986,* DT Krieger, CW Bardin (eds). Toronto, Decker, 1985, pp 155–159

STYNE DM, GRUMBACH MM: Puberty in the male and female: Its physiology and disorders, in *Reproductive Endocrinology: Physiology, Pathophysiology and Clinical Management,* SSC Yen, RB Jaffe (eds). Philadelphia, Saunders, 1978, pp 189–240

WIERMAN ME et al: Puberty without gonadotropins: A unique mechanism of sexual development. N Engl J Med 312:65, 1985

WILSON JD, GRIFFIN JE: The use and misuse of androgens. Metabolism 29:1278, 1980

331 DISORDERS OF THE OVARY AND FEMALE REPRODUCTIVE TRACT

BRUCE R. CARR / JEAN D. WILSON

The ovary is the source of ova for reproduction and of the hormones that regulate female sexual life. The anatomic structure, response to hormonal stimuli, and secretory capacity of the ovary are different at different periods of life. This chapter will review normal ovarian physiology as a background for understanding the abnormalities of the ovary and other tissues of the female reproductive tract.

DEVELOPMENT, STRUCTURE, AND FUNCTION OF THE OVARY

EMBRYOLOGY During the third week of gestation the primordial germ cells arise from the endoderm lining the yolk sac at the caudal end of the embryo. The germ cells migrate to the genital ridge adjacent to the mesonephric kidney by the fifth week of gestation and undergo mitotic divisions. The gonads exist in an undifferentiated state until the seventh week of fetal life, at which time the primitive ovary can be differentiated from the testis (see Chap. 333). Estrogen formation in the ovary commences between weeks 8 and 10, and by 10 to 11 weeks of gestation some oogonia in the developing ovarian cortex begin developing into primary oocytes. The ovary contains a finite number of germ cells, the maximal number of about 7 million oogonia being reached by the fifth to sixth month of gestation. Afterward, the germ cells begin to decrease in number through a process of atresia such that only 1 million remain at birth, 400,000 are present at the time of menarche, and only a few remain at menopause. Two X chromosomes are required for normal development of the ovary; in individuals with a 45,X karyotype ovarian development occurs, but the rate of atresia is accelerated so that only a fibrous streak remains at the time of birth (see Chap. 333).

After the oogonia cease to proliferate, meiosis commences, proceeds until the diplotene stage of the first meiotic division is completed, and then remains stationary until the time of onset of ovulation at puberty. During the fifth month of fetal life, the primordial follicle is formed, consisting of the primary oocyte arrested in meiosis, a single layer of granulosa cells, and a basement membrane that separates the primordial follicle from surrounding stromal (interstitial) tissues.

PUBERTAL MATURATION Final maturation of ovarian follicles commences during puberty. The two major hormones that regulate follicular development are the pituitary gonadotropins—follicle-stimulating hormone (FSH) and luteinizing hormone (LH) (Fig. 331-1). During the second trimester of fetal development the plasma gonadotropins rise to levels equivalent to those at menopause. This peak in gonadotropin levels may be causally related to the simultaneous peak in replication of oocytes. The hypothalamic-pituitary axis (the so-called gonadostat) undergoes maturation and becomes sensitive after the second trimester to negative feedback by circulating steroid hormones, particularly estrogen and progesterone produced in the placenta. The circulating gonadotropins decrease thereafter and are almost undetectable at the time of birth. In the neonate, concomitant with the decrease in estrogen and progesterone levels due to separation from the placenta at birth, there is a rebound increase in gonadotropin secretion that persists for the first few months of life. With continued maturation of the hypothalamic-pituitary system the gonadostat becomes sensitive to negative feedback control by the low levels of circulating steroid hormones, and plasma gonadotropins again decrease.

As the time of puberty nears, a decrease in the sensitivity of the gonadostat allows for increased secretion of FSH and LH, possibly secondary to increased production of luteinizing hormone–releasing hormone (LHRH) by the hypothalamus (see Chap. 321). A sleep-induced, pulsatile pattern of LH secretion then ensues, the first step in the development of a cyclic pattern of gonadotropin secretion (Fig. 331-1). The increase in estrogen secretion subsequently exerts a positive feedback which leads to an exaggeration of the pulsatile release of LH and eventually to ovulation and the menarche, after which mean plasma gonadotropin concentrations reach adult values in which day and night levels are similar. After the menopause plasma gonadotropin levels rise, plateau 5 to 10 years later, and remain fairly constant until the eighth to ninth decade of life when the plasma levels may fall. Although ovarian function is regulated primarily by LH and FSH, the ovary contains receptors for prolactin and LHRH, and both hormones inhibit steroidogenesis in in vitro preparations of human ovary, raising the possibility that they play a role in ovarian pathophysiology.

With the development at puberty of decreased sensitivity of the hypothalamic-pituitary centers to circulating steroid hormones, LHRH release by the hypothalamus increases, gonadotropin secretion by the pituitary is enhanced, ovarian estrogen secretion increases, and the anatomic changes of puberty ensue. At age 10 to 11 the first secondary sexual characteristics begin to appear in girls, namely development of the breast buds (thelarche), followed by the development of pubic hair (pubarche), and later by the development of axillary hair (adrenarche). The appearance of pubic and axillary hair is believed to be the result of an increase in adrenal androgens, commencing at approximately 6 to 8 years of age. A growth spurt ensues, and peak growth rate is attained at a mean age of 12 years.

The culmination of puberty is the onset of predictable, cyclic menses. The average time between the beginning of breast development and the onset of menses (menarche) is 2 years. The age of menarche is variable and is determined in part by socioeconomic as well as by genetic factors and general health. In the United States the mean age of menarche is believed to have decreased at a rate of 3 to 4 months per decade over the last 100 years and is now around 13 years, a decrease believed to be due to an improvement in nutrition in the population at large. A critical body weight of around 48 kg or a critical combination of weight, body water, and body fat is associated with development of hypothalamic insensitivity to circulating steroids that leads to increased secretion of gonadotropins and finally to menarche. Obese girls with a body weight 20 to 30 percent above ideal have earlier menarche than do girls with normal weights. In contrast, participation in certain sports or ballet, malnutrition, and chronic debilitating disease commonly cause delayed menarche.

MATURE OVARY **Morphology** The anatomic components and function of the adult ovary are illustrated schematically in Fig. 331-2. Under the influence of gonadotropins, a group of primary follicles is recruited, and by day 6 to 8 of the menstrual cycle one follicle becomes mature or "dominant," a process characterized by accelerated growth of granulosa cells and enlargement of the fluid-filled antrum. The recruited follicles not destined to ovulate begin to undergo degeneration, similar to the atresia observed in other follicles during embryogenesis. Just prior to ovulation, meiosis resumes in the ova of the dominant follicle, and the first meiotic division is completed with formation of the first polar body. Rapid enlargement of the antrum (up to 10 to 15 mm in size) occurs with an associated increase in follicular fluid, followed by a thinning of the follicular surface and formation of a conical stigma. Ovulation from the dominant follicle occurs some 16 to 23 h after the LH peak or 24 to 38 h after the onset of the LH surge as the result of rupture of the follicular wall at the area of the stigma, followed by expulsion of the ovum together with a mass of surrounding granulosa cells called cumulus cells. The rupture is believed to result from the action of hydrolyzing enzymes on the surface of the follicle, possibly under the control of prostaglandins. The second meiotic division begins after the egg is fertilized by a sperm, and a second polar body is then extruded. Following ovulation, the formation of the corpus luteum begins in the retained remnant of the ovulated follicle; the remaining granulosa and theca cells increase in size and accumulate lipids and a yellow pigment, lutein, to become "luteinized." The basement membrane that separated the granulosa cells from the stroma and blood vessels breaks, and capillaries, fibroblasts, and lymphatics from the theca invade the granulosa cells and reach the central cavity, thereby filling it with blood. After a period of 14 ± 2 days (the functional life of the corpus luteum) regression of vessels and atrophy of the corpus luteum commence and eventuate in replacement of the corpus luteum by a fibrous scar, the corpus albicans. The factors that

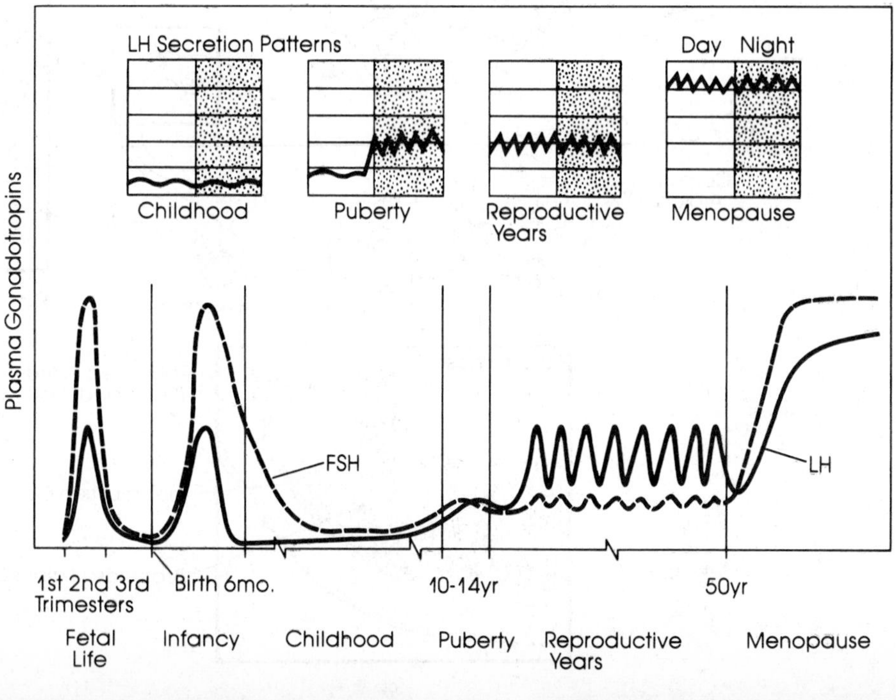

FIGURE 331-1 *Pattern of gonadotropin secretion during different stages of life in women. FSH (follicle-stimulating hormone), LH (luteinizing hormone). The secretory patterns of LH during the waking hours (clear area) and night (stippled area) for each stage are indicated in the upper insets. (After C Faiman et al.)*

limit the life span of the corpus luteum are not known. However, if pregnancy occurs, the corpus luteum persists under the influence of placental or chorionic gonadotropins, and progesterone is produced by the corpus luteum for the support of early pregnancy.

Hormone formation STEROID HORMONES Like other steroid hormones, ovarian steroids are derived from cholesterol (Fig. 331-3). The ovary can synthesize cholesterol de novo from 2-carbon precursors and can also utilize cholesterol from circulating low-density lipoproteins (LDL) as substrate for steroid hormone formation (Fig. 331-4). Virtually all ovarian cells are believed to possess the complete enzymatic complement required for the conversion of cholesterol to estradiol (Fig. 331-3); however, different cell types within the ovary contain different amounts of these enzymes so that the predominant steroids produced differ in the various compartments. For example, the corpus luteum forms progesterone and 17-hydroxyprogesterone predominantly, whereas theca and stromal cells convert cholesterol to the androgens androstenedione and testosterone. Granulosa cells are particularly rich in the aromatase activity responsible for conversion of androgens to estrogen and utilize as substrates for this process androgens synthesized within the granulosa cells and in the adjacent theca cells.

The principal sites of action of LH and FSH are also illustrated in Figs. 331-3 and 331-4. LH acts primarily to regulate the first step in steroid hormone biosynthesis, namely the conversion of cholesterol to pregnenolone, and also induces subsequent enzymes in the pathway. FSH acts to regulate the final process by which androgens are aromatized to estrogens. As a consequence, in the absence of FSH LH enhances substrate flow and the formation of androgens and/or progesterone, whereas FSH action is impeded in the absence of LH because of diminished substrate for aromatization.

Estrogens. Naturally occurring estrogens are 18-carbon steroids characterized by an aromatic A ring, a phenolic hydroxyl group at C-3, and either a hydroxyl group (estradiol) or a ketone (estrone) at C-17 (Fig. 331-3). (For the numbering of the steroid ring see Fig. 330-1.) The principal estrogen secreted by the ovary and the most potent naturally occurring estrogen is estradiol. Estrone is also secreted by the ovary, but the principal source of estrone is from extraglandular conversion of androstenedione in peripheral tissues. Estriol (16-hydroxyestradiol), the most abundant estrogen in urine, arises from the 16-hydroxylation of estrone and estradiol. Catechol estrogens are formed by hydroxylation of estrogens at the C-2 or C-4 position and may act as the intracellular mediators of some estrogen action. Estrogens promote development of the secondary sexual characteristics in women and cause uterine growth, thickening of the vaginal mucosa, thinning of the cervical mucus, and development of the ductular system of the breasts. The mechanism of estrogen action in target tissues is similar to that for other steroid hormones and involves the binding to a specific cytosolic receptor protein, subsequent conformational change and translocation of the hormone-receptor complex to the nucleus, attachment of the complex to DNA, and initiation of the transcription of messenger RNA, which in turn causes increased protein synthesis in the cell cytoplasm (see Chap. 320).

Progesterone. Progesterone, a 21-carbon steroid (Fig. 331-3), is the principal hormone secreted by the corpus luteum and is responsible for progestational effects, namely induction of secretory activity in the endometrium of the estrogen-primed uterus in preparation for implantation of the fertilized egg. Progesterone also induces a decidual reaction in endometrium. Other effects include inhibition of uterine contractions, increased viscosity of cervical mucus, glandular development of the breasts, and increase in basal body temperature (thermogenic effect).

Androgens. The ovary synthesizes a variety of 19-carbon steroids including dehydroepiandrosterone, androstenedione, testosterone, and dihydrotestosterone, principally in stromal and thecal cells. The major ovarian 19-carbon steroid is androstenedione (Fig. 331-3), part of which is secreted into plasma and the remainder of which is converted to estrogen in granulosa cells or to testosterone in the interstitium. In peripheral tissues androstenedione can also be converted to testosterone and to estrogens. Only testosterone and dihydrotestosterone are true androgens with the capacity of interacting with the androgen receptor and thus inducing virilizing signs in women (see Chaps. 46 and 330).

OTHER HORMONES Other ovarian hormones play an uncertain role in human physiology. *Relaxin,* a polypeptide hormone produced by

FIGURE 331-2 *Developmental changes in the adult ovary during a complete 28-day cycle.*

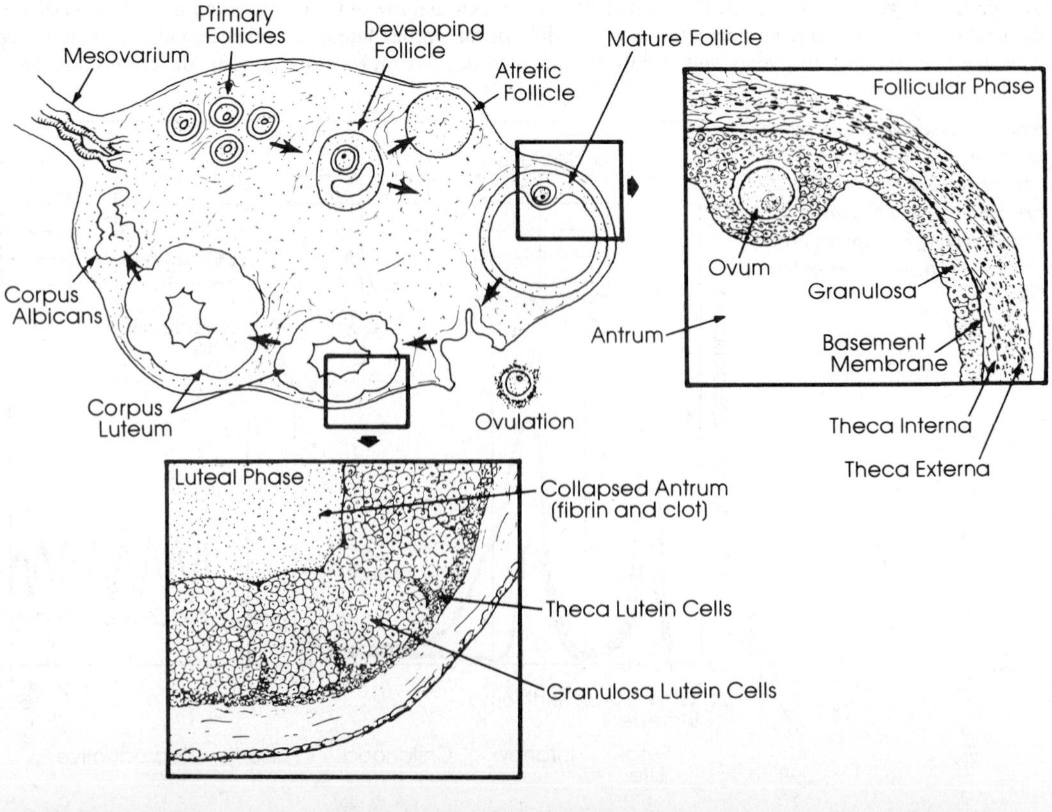

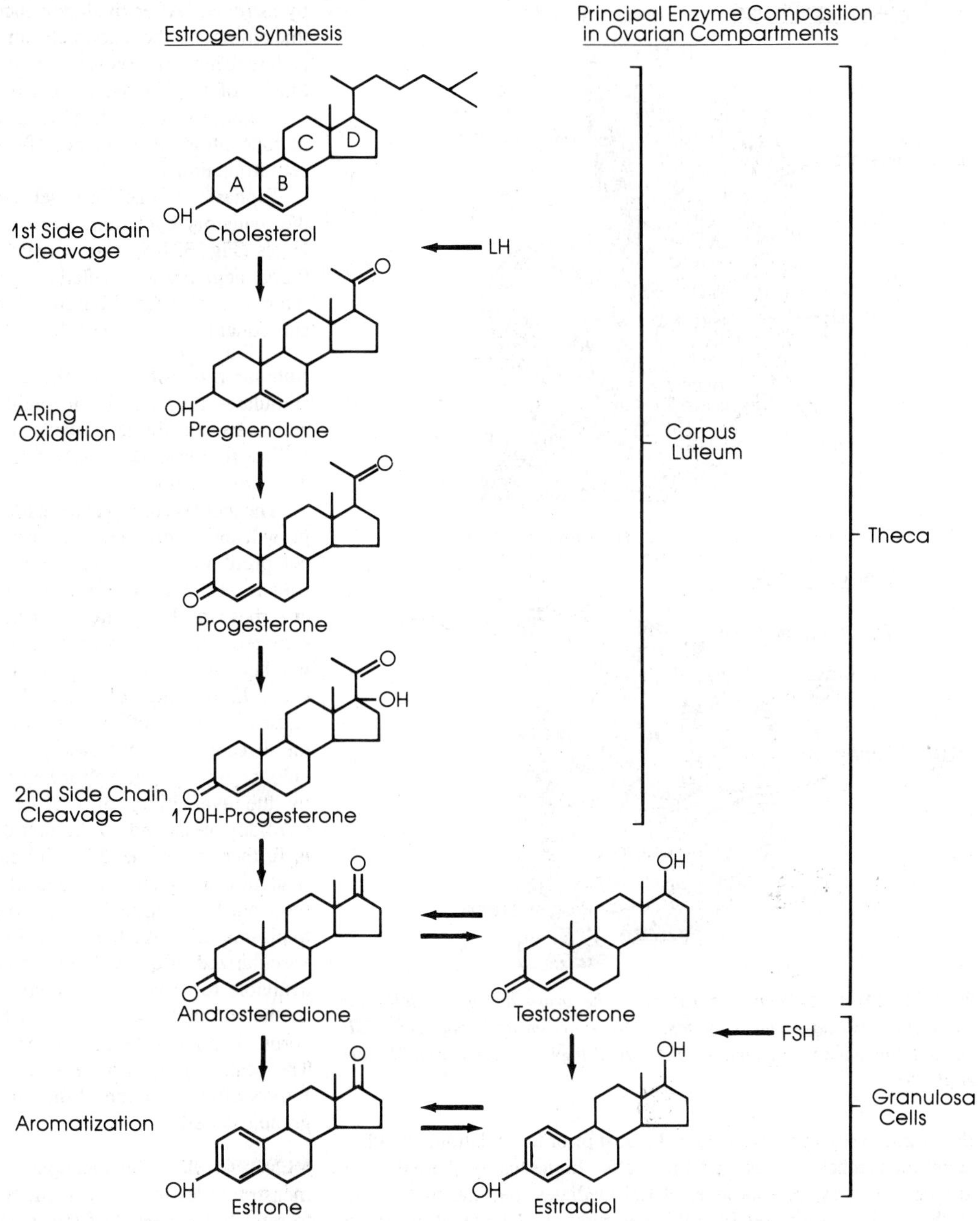

FIGURE 331-3 *The principal pathway of steroid hormone biosynthesis in the ovary. Although every ovarian cell probably contains the complete enzyme complement required for the formation of estradiol from cholesterol, the amounts of the various enzymes and consequently the predominant hormones formed differ among the various cell types. The major enzyme complements for the corpus luteum, stroma, and granulosa cells are shown by the brackets; as a consequence these cells produce predominantly progesterone and 17-OH progesterone, androgen, and estrogen, respectively. The major sites of action of LH and FSH in mediating this pathway are shown in the horizontal arrows.*

the human corpus luteum as well as by the decidua, causes softening of the cervix and loosening of the symphysis pubis in preparation for parturition in animals. *Follicular inhibin* or *folliculostatin* (the equivalent of testicular inhibin) is secreted by the follicle and is believed to regulate the release of FSH by the hypothalamic-pituitary unit. *Follicle regulatory protein* (FRP) of human follicular fluid inhibits granulosa secretion and growth. *Gonadocrinins,* peptides purified from rat follicular fluid, stimulate the release of both FSH and LH from the pituitary in vitro and in vivo. In addition, in the gonads of both sexes a *meiosis-inducing substance* (MIS) triggers the onset of meiosis, an event that occurs earlier in ovarian than in testicular development. In contrast, male fetal testes secrete predominantly a *meiosis-preventing substance* (MPS) that prevents meiosis until the onset of puberty at which time MIS is formed predominantly.

The normal menstrual cycle The menstrual cycle is usually divided into a follicular or proliferative phase and a luteal or secretory phase (Fig. 331-5). The secretion of FSH and LH is fundamentally under negative feedback control by ovarian steroids (particularly estradiol) and probably by inhibin, but the response of gonadotropins to different levels of estradiol varies. FSH secretion is inhibited progressively as estrogen levels increase—typical negative feedback. In contrast, LH secretion is suppressed maximally by estrogen in low amounts and is enhanced in response to a rising and sustained elevation of estradiol—so-called positive feedback control. Negative feedback of estrogen involves both the hypothalamus and pituitary, whereas positive feedback operates primarily at the level of the pituitary.

The length of the normal menstrual cycle is defined as the time from the onset of one menstrual bleeding episode to the onset of the next. In women of reproductive age the menstrual cycle averages 28 ± 3 days, and the mean duration of flow is 4 ± 2 days. Longer menstrual cycles occur at menarche and prior to menopause. At the end of one menstrual cycle and in the face of a waning corpus luteum, plasma levels of estrogen and progesterone fall, and circulating levels of FSH increase concomitantly. Under the influence of increasing levels of FSH, follicular recruitment is initiated to effect development of the follicle that will be dominant during the next cycle.

After the onset of menses, follicular development continues, but FSH levels decrease. Approximately 8 to 10 days prior to the midcycle LH surge, plasma estradiol levels begin to rise as the result of secretion of estradiol by the granulosa cells of the enlarging dominant follicle. During the second half of the follicular phase, LH levels

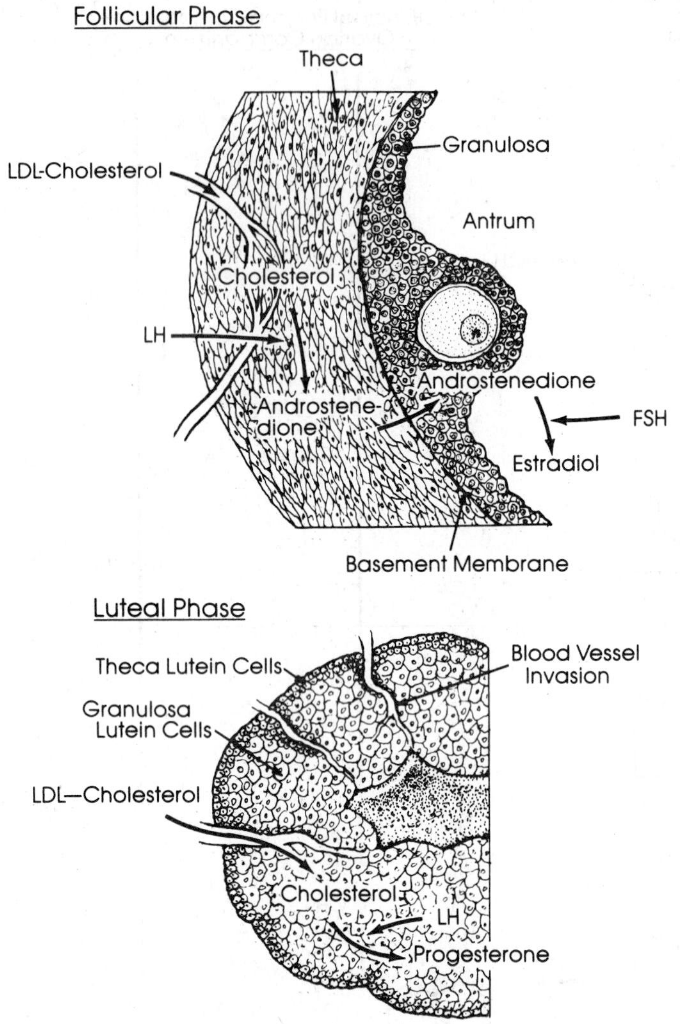

FIGURE 331-4 *Cellular interactions in the ovary during the follicular phase (top) and luteal phase (bottom); LDL (low-density lipoprotein), FSH (follicle-stimulating hormone), and LH (luteinizing hormone). (From BR Carr et al, 1982.)*

also begin to rise (positive feedback). Just prior to ovulation, estradiol secretion reaches a peak and then falls. Immediately thereafter, a further rise in the plasma level of LH mediates the final maturation of the follicle, followed by follicular rupture and ovulation 16 to 23 h after the LH peak. Concomitant with the rise in LH is a smaller increase in the level of plasma FSH, the physiologic significance of which is unclear. Plasma progesterone also begins to rise just prior to midcycle and facilitates the positive feedback action of estradiol on LH secretion.

At the onset of the luteal phase plasma gonadotropins decrease, and plasma progesterone increases. A secondary rise in estrogens causes further gonadotropin suppression. Near the end of the luteal phase progesterone and estrogen levels fall, and FSH levels begin to rise to initiate the development of the next follicle (usually in the contralateral ovary) and the next menstrual cycle.

The endometrium lining the uterine cavity undergoes marked alterations in response to the changing plasma levels of ovarian hormones (Fig. 331-5). Concomitant with the decrease in plasma estrogen and progesterone and the decline of corpus luteum function in the late luteal phase, intense vasospasm occurs in the spiral arterioles supplying blood to the endometrium, followed by an ischemic necrosis, endometrial desquamation, and bleeding. This vasospasm is caused by locally synthesized prostaglandins. The onset of bleeding marks the first day of the menstrual cycle. By the fourth to fifth day of the cycle the endometrium is thin. During the proliferative phase glandular growth of the endometrium is mediated by estrogen. After ovulation increased progesterone leads to further thickening of the endometrium, but the rapid growth slows. The endometrium then enters the secretory phase characterized by tortuosity of the glands, curling of the spiral arterioles, and glandular secretion. As corpus luteum function begins to wane in the absence of conception, the sequence of events leading to menstruation is again set into action.

Biphasic changes in basal body temperature are characteristic of the ovulatory cycle and are mediated by alterations in progesterone levels (Fig. 331-5). An increase in basal body temperature of 0.3 to 0.5°C begins after ovulation, persists during the luteal phase, and returns to the normal baseline (36.2 to 36.4°C) after the onset of the subsequent menses (see Chap. 9).

Cellular interactions in the ovary during the normal cycle LH stimulates thecal cells surrounding the follicle to form androgens, and androstenedione diffuses across the basement membrane of the follicle into granulosa cells where it is aromatized to estrogen (Figs. 331-3 and 331-4).

The increase of FSH late in the preceding menstrual cycle stimulates growth and recruitment of the primary follicles by enhancing granulosa cell proliferation, resulting ultimately in the formation of the dominant follicle. FSH also stimulates activity and amount of aromatizing enzymes in the granulosa cells that convert androstenedione to estrogen. Enhanced secretion of estradiol causes an increase in the number of estradiol receptors and further proliferation of granulosa cells. In the late follicular phase FSH, in concert with estradiol, causes induction of LH receptors on the granulosa cells. LH acts via these receptors to increase progesterone secretion at midcycle. The amount of progesterone formed by the follicle is believed to be limited by the availability of LDL-cholesterol to serve as substrate for steroidogenesis and by the fact that most of the progesterone formed is further metabolized to androstenedione by thecal cells. Prior to ovulation the granulosa cells of the follicle are bathed in follicular fluid but have limited access to circulating blood and consequently to plasma LDL. As depicted in Fig. 331-4, the granulosa cells become vascularized after ovulation, and plasma LDL-cholesterol becomes available to serve as the major substrate for progesterone synthesis by the corpus luteum. Thus, increased progesterone synthesis by the corpus luteum is the consequence of increased substrate availability. The peak in progesterone secretion by the corpus luteum is attained 8 days after ovulation at the time of maximal vascularization of the granulosa cells.

MENOPAUSE The menopause is defined as the final episode of menstrual bleeding in women. However, the term is used commonly to refer to the period of the female climacteric that encompasses the transitional period between the reproductive years up to and beyond the last episode of menstrual bleeding. During this period there is a gradual but progressive loss of ovarian function and a variety of endocrine, somatic, and psychological changes.

The median age of women at the time of cessation of menstrual bleeding is 50 to 51 years. Since the life expectancy in women is now close to 80 years, approximately one-third of life occurs after cessation of reproductive function. Preceding the menopause, the pattern of menstrual cycles is variable, but the interval between menses usually becomes shorter due to a decrease in the length of the follicular phase of the cycle. In addition, there is an increase in the mean levels of plasma FSH and LH, despite the continuation of ovulatory cycles. Thus, the ovary appears to become less responsive to gonadotropins prior to the menopause.

The menopause is the consequence of the exhaustion of ovarian follicles. The decrease in the number of ova begins in intrauterine life; by the time of the menopause few ova remain, and these appear to be nonfunctional. Only a small number of ova are lost as the result of ovulation during reproductive life, the majority of follicles and associated ova being lost by atresia. The cessation of follicular development results in a drop in the production of estradiol and other hormones, which in turn causes a loss of negative feedback on the

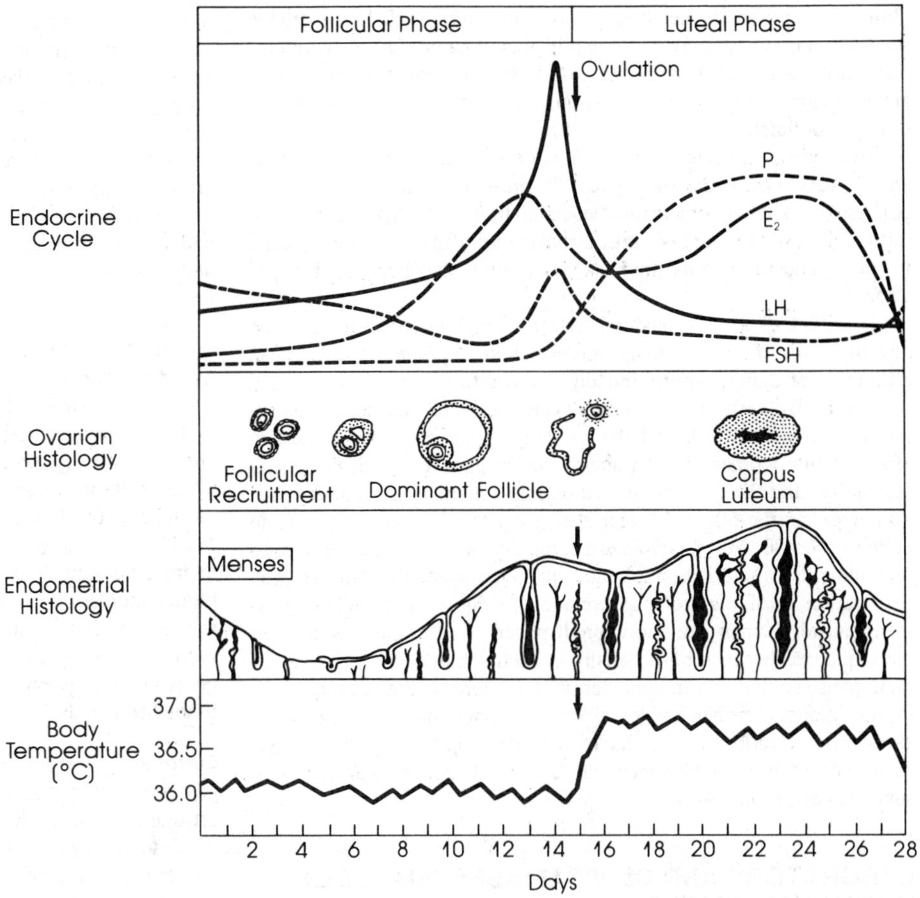

FIGURE 331-5 *The hormonal, ovarian, endometrial, and basal body temperature changes and relationship throughout the normal menstrual cycle.*

hypothalamic-pituitary centers. In turn, the levels of plasma gonadotropins increase with FSH levels rising earlier and to a greater extent than those of LH (Figs. 331-1 and 331-6). The higher concentration of FSH than LH in postmenopausal women may result from the decrease in inhibin secretion by the ovary, from the fact that FSH is cleared from plasma less rapidly than LH due to its higher sialic acid content, and possibly from the loss of positive feedback on LH production by estradiol. Intravenous administration of LHRH to menopausal women results in a pronounced increase in the secretion of both FSH and LH, consistent with the enhanced hypothalamic-pituitary secretory activity in other forms of primary ovarian failure.

The ovaries of postmenopausal women are small, and the residual cells are predominantly stromal in type. Estrogen and androgen levels in plasma are reduced but not absent from the circulation (Fig. 331-6). Prior to the menopause, plasma androstenedione is derived almost equally from the adrenals and the ovaries; after menopause the ovarian contribution ceases so that the plasma levels of androstenedione fall by 50 percent (Fig. 331-6). However, the menopausal ovary continues to secrete testosterone, presumably formed in stromal cells.

Circulating estrogens in the ovulating woman are derived from two sources. Sixty percent of mean estrogen formation during the menstrual cycle is in the form of estradiol formed primarily by ovaries, and the remainder is estrone formed mainly in extraglandular tissues from androstenedione. After menopause, extraglandular estrogen formation becomes the major pathway for estrogen synthesis. Estrogen production by the menopausal ovary is minimal, and subsequent oophorectomy is not followed by any further decrease in estrogen levels. Plasma levels of estradiol, the principal estrogen secreted by the follicle, are lower in postmenopausal women than are the levels of estrone. The rate of peripheral formation of estrone increases somewhat in menopausal women so that estrone production is usually only slightly less than prior to the menopause, despite the fall in plasma androstenedione. Because a major site of extraglandular estrogen production is adipose tissue, peripheral estrogen formation may actually be enhanced in obese postmenopausal women, so that total estrogen production rates may be as great or greater than in premenopausal women. The predominant estrogen formed is estrone rather than estradiol.

The most common menopausal symptoms are those of vasomotor instability (hot flash), atrophy of the urogenital epithelium and skin, decreased size of the breasts, and osteoporosis. Approximately 40 percent of women in the postmenopausal period develop symptoms serious enough to seek medical assistance.

The pathogenesis of the hot flash is uncertain. There is a close temporal relationship between the onset of the hot flash and pulses of LH secretion. Alterations in catecholamine, prostaglandin, endor-

FIGURE 331-6 *Differences in hormone concentration in women during the reproductive years and in women during the menopause. FSH (follicle-stimulating hormone), LH (luteinizing hormone), E_2 (estradiol-17β), E_1 (estrone), Δ^4-A (androstenedione), T (testosterone). (From SSC Yen and RB Jaffe, 1986, and from DR Mishell Jr and V Davajan.)*

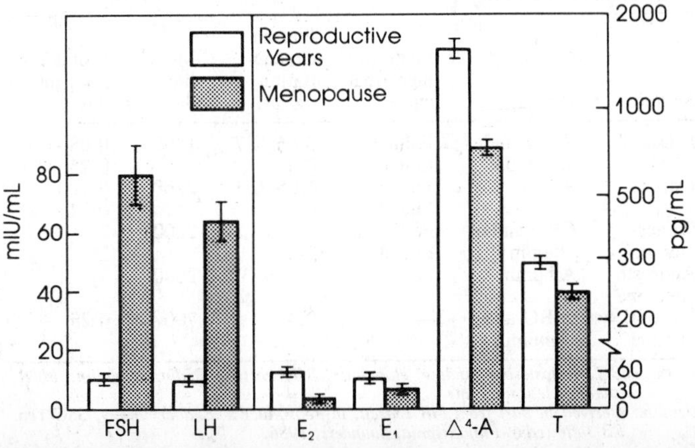

phin, or neurotensin metabolism in conjunction with low estrogen production may also play a role in this phenomenon. Other symptoms commonly associated with the hot flash, including nervousness, anxiety, irritability, and depression, may or may not be due to estrogen deficiency.

The decrease in size of the organs of the female reproductive tract and breasts during the menopause is the consequence of estrogen deficiency. The endometrium becomes thin and atrophic in most (although cystic hyperplasia may occur in one-fifth of postmenopausal women), and the vaginal mucosa and urethra also become thin and atrophic.

There is a close relationship between estrogen deprivation and the development of osteoporosis. Osteoporosis is one of the dread afflictions of aging. Approximately one-fourth of aging women and one-tenth of elderly men sustain a vertebral or hip fracture between the ages of 60 and 90, and the incidence appears to be greatest in elderly white women. Such fractures are a major cause of death and morbidity, and the fracture-related mortality increases from less than 10 percent in the 60- to 64-year age group to 30 percent or more in patients over 80. Many factors affect the development of osteoporosis including diet, activity, smoking, and general health, and estrogen deprivation is of particular importance in this regard. White post-menopausal women are more predisposed to osteoporosis and its consequences because bone density in such subjects is lower prior to menopause so that loss in bone density has more severe consequences in the group. Further evidence that osteoporosis is a disease of estrogen deprivation is suggested by early development of osteoporosis in women with premature menopause due either to natural causes or surgical castration.

LABORATORY AND CLINICAL ASSESSMENT OF HORMONAL STATUS

Assessment of the hormonal status of women can usually be made by obtaining a thorough history and physical examination. In general, presence of secondary sexual characteristics such as normal female breast development indicates adequate estrogen secretion in the past, and the presence of regular, predictable, cyclic menses implies that ovulation and the production of gonadotropins, estrogen, progesterone, and androgens are adequate and that the outflow tract is intact. Such a history may be more valuable than laboratory tests in evaluating ovarian hormone status. However, laboratory tests provide valuable ancillary information in the workup of women with endocrine dysfunction or infertility.

PITUITARY GONADOTROPINS Plasma gonadotropins are assessed by radioimmunoassay. Because both FSH and LH are secreted in pulsatile manner, the results obtained from a single serum sample may be difficult to interpret. Consequently, multiple samples at 20-min intervals for 2 h may be pooled to obtain a mean value. Serum gonadotropin measurements are of most use in evaluating women with suspected ovarian failure and in establishing the diagnosis of polycystic ovarian disease and hypogonadotropic hypogonadism. The normal ranges for serum LH and FSH in ovulating women are 5 to 25 mIU/mL and 5 to 30 mIU/mL, respectively. A persistent FSH above 40 mIU/mL is diagnostic of ovarian failure, and an LH value of less than 5 mIU/mL is suggestive of hypogonadotropic hypogonadism. In practice, however, gonadotropin values may be equivocal and must be interpreted in light of the remainder of the clinical findings.

TABLE 331-1 Concentrations, metabolic clearance rates, and production rates of the major ovarian steroid hormones in blood of ovulatory women

Steroid	Binding	Phase of menstrual cycle	Plasma concentration, ng/mL	MCR, liters/day	Production rate, mg/day
Estradiol	TeBG and albumin	Follicular	0.06–0.7	1400	0.08–1.0
		Luteal	0.2		0.25
Estrone	Albumin	Follicular	0.05–0.3	2200	0.1–0.7
		Luteal	0.1		0.24
Progesterone	CBG and albumin	Follicular	1.0	2200	2
		Luteal	3–25		25
Androstenedione	Albumin	—	1.6	2000	3
Testosterone	TeBG and albumin	—	0.4	700	0.25

NOTE: *TeBG, testosterone-binding globulin; CBG, cortisol-binding globulin; MCR, metabolic clearance rate.*

SOURCE: *Derived in part from MB Lipsett, in Reproductive Endocrinology, SSC Yen, RB Jaffe (eds). Philadelphia, Saunders, 1986.*

OVARIAN HORMONES The mean plasma levels, production rates, and metabolic clearance rates of the principal ovarian hormones are presented in Table 331-1. The metabolic clearance rate of a hormone is that amount of plasma that is cleared of hormone per unit of time and is inversely proportional to the degree of binding to plasma proteins. Testosterone, which is tightly bound to testosterone-binding globulin (TeBG) (also known as sex hormone–binding globulin or SHBG), has a low metabolic clearance rate. Steroids such as androstenedione that are not tightly bound to carrier proteins have higher metabolic clearance rates. The production rate of a hormone is the sum of the amount of hormone produced by direct glandular secretion and by extraglandular conversion of prohormones and can be estimated by multiplying the concentration of hormone in plasma times the metabolic clearance rate of that hormone.

Estrogen Normal secondary sexual characteristics imply that estrogen production was adequate in the past. Indication of the current estrogen status can be obtained by pelvic examination. The presence of a moist, rugated vagina with copious, clear, thin cervical mucus that can be stretched and that exhibits arborization or ferning when spread on a slide is strong evidence of adequate estrogen production. Cytologic demonstration of mature vaginal epithelial cells and abundant cornified squamous epithelial cells with pyknotic nuclei confirms the presence of adequate estrogen levels.

The progesterone-withdrawal test provides a functional assessment of estrogen status. If menses appear within a week to 10 days after the end of a trial of medroxyprogesterone acetate (10 mg by mouth once or twice a day for 5 days) or after a single intramuscular injection of progesterone (100 mg), then prior estrogen priming was adequate to allow withdrawal bleeding.

Due to its variable level in plasma during the normal cycle and the difficulty of estimating the day of the cycle in women with abnormal cycles, the determination of estrogen levels in plasma or urine by radioimmunoassay is of little use in the routine assessment of estrogen status. Plasma estradiol is measured during attempts to induce ovulation with human menopausal gonadotropins to prevent the development of the ovarian hyperstimulation syndrome and is utilized along with ultrasound assessment to monitor follicular growth in women who are to undergo in vitro fertilization.

Progesterone Cyclic, predictable menses also imply that adequate progesterone is secreted during the luteal phase of the menstrual cycle. The indications for specific assay of progesterone are to document ovulation or evaluate the adequacy of the luteal phase in the evaluation of infertile women and to separate subjects with müllerian agenesis from those with the testicular feminization syndrome. Several functional assays of progesterone secretion can be utilized. The least expensive and most useful is the daily measurement of basal body temperature throughout a cycle. Due to the thermogenic properties of progesterone, documentation of the monthly biphasic curve with an elevated temperature for approximately 2 weeks after ovulation is a valid indication of progesterone secretion during the luteal phase (Fig. 331-5). Presence of viscous cervical mucus that does not stretch or fern and the presence of predominant intermediate cells on vaginal cytology or demonstration of a secretory epithelium in an endometrial biopsy during the luteal phase on day 20 to 22 of the cycle provide additional evidence of progesterone secretion. In addition measurement of serum progesterone by radioimmunoassay can be used to estimate progesterone secretion by the corpus luteum.

Androgen Under normal conditions the ovary secretes androstenedione, testosterone, and dehydroepiandrosterone. In conditions of androgen excess, hirsutism and/or virilization are common. The laboratory evaluation of androgen excess is discussed in Chap. 46.

DIAGNOSIS OF PREGNANCY Pregnancy is usually suspected and diagnosed on the basis of the history and findings on physical examination. Namely, a woman with previous cyclic, predictable menses develops amenorrhea accompanied by breast tenderness, malaise, lassitude, and nausea, and on physical examination a softening and enlargement of the uterus is found.

Laboratory assays of placental products excreted in urine facilitate the diagnosis of pregnancy. Human chorionic gonadotropin (hCG) is secreted by the trophoblastic cells of the placenta into the maternal plasma and excreted in the urine. Assays of urinary hCG make it feasible to detect the presence of functioning trophoblasts earlier than can be recognized by clinical assessments. Assays for measurement of hCG content of serum or urine utilize either antibody against hCG or receptor for hCG. With some radioimmunoassays it is possible to detect pregnancies 8 to 10 days after ovulation and before the first missed menstrual period. Radioimmunoassay of the β subunit of hCG in serum or urine makes it possible to differentiate between excess LH and hCG, an important distinction in evaluating women with trophoblastic disease such as hydatidiform mole or choriocarcinoma.

DISORDERS OF OVARIAN FUNCTION

PREPUBERTAL YEARS Puberty is said to be precocious if the onset of breast budding occurs before age 8 or if menarche commences before age 9. Those disorders in which the developing sexual characteristics are appropriate for the genetic and gonadal sex, i.e., feminization in girls or virilization in boys, are termed *isosexual precocity,* whereas *heterosexual precocity* occurs when sexual characters are not in accord with the genetic sex, namely virilization in girls or feminization in boys. Pubertal disorders of boys are described in Chap. 330.

Isosexual precocious puberty Isosexual precocious puberty in girls can be divided into three major categories (Table 331-2).

TRUE PRECOCIOUS PUBERTY True precocious puberty is characterized by an early but otherwise normal sequence of pubertal development, including increased secretion of gonadotropins and ovulatory menstrual cycles. Constitutional or idiopathic precocious puberty comprises 90 percent of cases. In these individuals no cause for the premature maturation of the central nervous system–hypothalamic-pituitary axis can be identified, and the diagnosis is one of exclusion. As many as half of these individuals have abnormal electroencephalograms. Premature appearance of secondary sexual characteristics and of ovulatory cycles with the accompanying risk of fertility may result in significant emotional disturbances. Therefore, prompt initiation of therapy is imperative. The usual treatment is medroxyprogesterone acetate in doses of 100 to 200 mg given intramuscularly every 2 to 4 weeks to suppress gonadotropin secretion. Such a regimen is usually effective in inhibiting ovarian estrogen production and ovulation but does not consistently control bone growth or prevent premature epiphyseal closure and the resultant short stature. LHRH analogues have been utilized to inhibit estrogen synthesis and thus inhibit precocious puberty, and early evidence suggests that they also prevent premature closure of the epiphyses.

About 10 percent of cases are due to organic brain diseases, including brain tumors (hypothalamic gliomas, astrocytomas, ependymomas, germinomas, and hamartomas), encephalitis, meningitis, hydrocephalus, head injury, tuberous sclerosis, and neurofibromatosis. It is essential to separate this group of patients from those with the idiopathic disorder, and patients designated as idiopathic occasionally prove to have such tumors. Fortunately, most patients with organic lesions serious enough to cause precocious puberty have obvious neurologic signs and symptoms. Evaluation of all patients with precocious puberty should include, at a minimum, skull films and computerized tomography scans of the brain. The success of treatment depends upon the nature of the lesion, but surgical and radiation treatment of well-localized tumors is occasionally successful.

A rare cause of isosexual precocity is virilizing congenital adrenal hyperplasia due to 21-hydroxylase deficiency in girls in whom treatment is delayed until 4 to 8 years of age. After initiation of glucocorticoid replacement, such individuals may undergo true isosexual precocious puberty (see Chap. 325).

PRECOCIOUS PSEUDOPUBERTY Precocious pseudopuberty occurs when girls feminize as a consequence of enhanced estrogen formation but do not ovulate or develop cyclic menses. Ovarian cysts or tumors that secrete estrogen (granulosa-theca cell tumors) are the most frequent cause of precocious pseudopuberty. Granulosa-theca-cell tumors associated with intestinal polyps and pigmentation of the mucous membranes occur in the Peutz-Jeghers syndrome. Other ovarian tumors that secrete estrogens (or androgens that can be converted to estrogens at extraglandular sites) include dysgerminomas, teratomas, cystadenomas, and ovarian carcinomas (also see Chap. 296). Ovarian tumors can usually be detected by rectoabdominal examination, and sonography, computerized tomography, and/or laparoscopy may also be of help. Ovarian teratomas and choriocarcinomas and other carcinomas that secrete hCG do not cause precocious puberty in girls unless there is concomitant secretion of estrogen by the tumor (hCG or LH in the absence of FSH does not induce ovarian estrogen production). Rarely, feminizing tumors of the adrenal cause isosexual precocious puberty, either by formation of estrogens directly or by secretion of weak androgens to serve as estrogenic precursors in extraglandular tissues.

Other causes of precocious pseudopuberty include the following: (1) The McCune-Albright syndrome (polyostotic fibrous dysplasia), characterized by café au lait spots, cystic fibrous dysplasia of bones, and sexual precocity. Some of these individuals have increased gonadotropin secretion, but the majority have low gonadotropins and a form of gonadotropin-independent sexual precocity. Occasionally, this disorder leads to true precocious puberty (see Chap. 334). (2) Primary hypothyroidism in which secretion of thyrotropin-releasing hormone (TRH) as well as the secretion of other hypothalamic hormones is enhanced, leading to increased FSH levels and ovarian estrogen secretion, frequently with galactorrhea. (3) The Silver syndrome, or congenital asymmetry associated with short stature and precocious feminization. (4) Estrogen-containing medications including use of estrogen-containing creams for diaper rash or the ingestion of any estrogen by mouth.

INCOMPLETE ISOSEXUAL PRECOCITY This term is used to describe the premature development of a single pubertal event and encompasses

TABLE 331-2 Differential diagnosis of sexual precocity

I Isosexual precocity
- *A* True precocious puberty
  - *1* Constitutional
  - *2* Organic brain disease
  - *3* Congenital adrenal hyperplasia
- *B* Precocious pseudopuberty
  - *1* Ovarian tumors
  - *2* Adrenal tumors
  - *3* McCune-Albright syndrome
  - *4* Hypothyroidism
  - *5* Silver syndrome
  - *6* Estrogen-containing medications
- *C* Incomplete sexual precocity
  - *1* Premature thelarche
  - *2* Premature adrenarche
  - *3* Premature pubarche

II Heterosexual precocity
- *A* Ovarian tumors
- *B* Adrenal tumors
- *C* Congenital adrenal hyperplasia

several entities. The appearance of breast budding prior to the age of 8 (premature thelarche) without other evidence of estrogen secretion and without premature bone maturation is believed to be due to a transient increase in estrogen secretion or a temporary increase in sensitivity to the small amounts of circulating estrogens formed prior to puberty. Usually the disorder is self-limited and resolves spontaneously. Occasionally axillary hair and/or pubic hair (so-called *premature adrenarche* and *pubarche*) appear without any other secondary sexual development. The phenomenon is associated with adrenal androgen secretion in the range of normal puberty and can be distinguished from syndromes of virilization by the absence of clitoromegaly. It requires no treatment, and patients enter puberty at about the average time.

Heterosexual precocity Virilization in a prepubertal female is usually due to congenital adrenal hyperplasia or to androgen secretion by an ovarian or adrenal tumor. The manifestations of virilization are described in Chap. 46. Virilization in girls with congenital adrenal hyperplasia usually takes place in a background of variable sexual ambiguity (see Chap. 333).

Evaluation of sexual precocity The evaluation of sexual precocity involves a careful history and physical examination including rectoabdominal examination, abdominal sonography, determination of bone age, and measurement of gonadotropins (and androgen or estrogen levels when appropriate). Skull films and further diagnostic tests are indicated if a neurologic disorder is suspected and no evidence of ovarian or adrenal tumor is found.

REPRODUCTIVE YEARS Disorders of the menstrual cycle

ABNORMAL UTERINE BLEEDING Between menarche and the menopause, almost every woman experiences one or more episodes of abnormal uterine bleeding, here defined as any bleeding pattern that differs in frequency, duration, or amount from the pattern observed during a normal menstrual cycle. A variety of descriptive terms (such as *menorrhagia, metrorrhagia,* and *menometrorrhagia*) have been used to characterize patterns of abnormal uterine bleeding. A more logical approach is to divide abnormal uterine bleeding into those patterns associated with ovulatory cycles and those associated with anovulatory cycles.

Ovulatory cycles. Normal menstrual bleeding with ovulatory cycles is spontaneous, regular, cyclic, and predictable and frequently associated with discomfort (dysmenorrhea). Deviations from this pattern associated with cycles that are still regular and predictable are most often due to organic disease of the outflow tract. For example, regular but prolonged and excessive bleeding episodes unassociated with bleeding dyscrasias (hypermenorrhea or menorrhagia) can result from abnormalities of the uterus such as submucous leiomyomas, adenomyosis, or endometrial polyps. Regular, cyclical, predictable menstruation characterized by spotting or light bleeding is termed *hypomenorrhea* and is due to obstruction of the outflow tract as from intrauterine synechiae or scarring of the cervix. Intermenstrual bleeding between episodes of regular, ovulatory menstruation is also often due to cervical or endometrial lesions. An exception to the association between organic disease of the uterus and abnormal uterine bleeding is the occurrence of episodes of regular bleeding more frequently than 21 days apart (polymenorrhea). These cycles may be a normal variant.

Anovulatory cycles. Uterine bleeding that is unpredictable with respect to amount, onset, and duration and is usually painless is described as *dysfunctional uterine bleeding*. This disorder is not due to abnormalities of the uterus but rather to chronic anovulation and occurs when there is interruption of the normal progressive sequence of follicular and luteal phases under the influence of a dominant follicle and its resulting corpus luteum. As discussed above normal uterine bleeding in ovulatory cycles is due to progesterone withdrawal and requires that the endometrium first be primed with estrogen (when castrates or postmenopausal women are given progesterone withdrawal bleeding usually does not occur).

Dysfunctional uterine bleeding can occur in women who have a transient disruption of the synchronous hypothalamic-pituitary-ovarian patterns necessary for regular ovulatory cycles, most often at the extremes of the reproductive life, namely in the early menarche and in the perimenopausal period, but also as the secondary consequence of temporary stresses intercurrent illnesses.

On the other hand, primary *dysfunctional uterine bleeding* can result from at least three pathophysiologic mechanisms.

1 *Estrogen withdrawal bleeding* occurs when estrogen is given to a castrate or postmenopausal woman and then withdrawn. As in other types of dysfunctional uterine bleeding, this form of menstrual bleeding is usually painless.
2 *Estrogen breakthrough bleeding* occurs when there is prolonged continuous estrogen stimulation of the endometrium not interrupted by cyclic progesterone secretion and withdrawal. This is the most common type of dysfunctional uterine bleeding and is usually due to anovulation associated with chronic acyclic estrogen production as in women with polycystic ovarian disease. Such women may have histories of irregular, unpredictable menses, oligomenorrhea, or amenorrhea (see below). Alternatively, estrogen breakthrough bleeding can occur in hypogonadal women given estrogens chronically rather than intermittently or in women with estrogen-secreting tumors of the ovary. Estrogen breakthrough bleeding may be profuse and is unpredictable with respect to duration, amount of flow, and time of occurrence. The endometrium is typically thin because its repair between episodes of bleeding is incomplete.
3 *Progesterone breakthrough bleeding* occurs in the presence of abnormally high ratios of progesterone to estrogen, for example, in women on continuous low-dose oral contraceptives.

The approach to a patient with dysfunctional uterine bleeding in the reproductive years begins with a careful history of menstrual patterns and prior hormonal therapy. Since not all bleeding from the urogenital tract is from the uterus, rectal, bladder, and vaginal or cervical sources must be excluded by physical examination. If the bleeding is from the uterus a pregnancy-related disorder such as abortion or ectopic pregnancy must also be excluded. Once the diagnosis of dysfunctional uterine bleeding is established a rational approach to management is as follows. During a first episode of dysfunctional bleeding the patient can simply be observed, provided the bleeding is not copious and no evidence of bleeding dyscrasia is present. If bleeding is moderately severe, control can be achieved with relatively high dose estrogen oral contraceptives for 3 weeks. Alternatively, a regimen of three or four low-dose oral contraceptive pills per day for 1 week followed by tapering to the usual dosage for up to 3 weeks is also effective. If uterine bleeding is more severe, hospitalization, bed rest, and intramuscular injections of estradiol valerate (10 mg) and 17α-hydroxyprogesterone caproate (500 mg) or intravenous or intramuscular conjugated estrogens (25 mg) usually control the bleeding. After initial treatment iron replacement should be instituted, and recurrence can be prevented by cyclic oral contraceptives for 2 to 3 months (or more if pregnancy is not desired). Alternatively, menses should be induced every 2 to 3 months with medroxyprogesterone acetate 10 mg by mouth once or twice a day for 5 days. If hormone therapy fails to control uterine bleeding, an endometrial biopsy or dilatation and curettage may be required for diagnosis and therapy. Indeed, uterine sampling may be indicated prior to hormone therapy in women at risk for endometrial cancer (i.e., in women approaching the age of menopause or in the massively obese); endometrial cancer is rare in ovulatory women of reproductive age.

AMENORRHEA An acceptable definition of amenorrhea is failure of menarche by age 16, irrespective of the presence or absence of secondary sexual characteristics, or the absence of menstruation for 6 months in a woman with previous periodic menses. However, women who do not fulfill these criteria should be evaluated if (1) the subject and/or her family are greatly concerned, (2) no breast development has occurred by age 14, or (3) any sexual ambiguity or virilization is present (Chap. 333). Amenorrhea is usually categorized as either primary (in a woman who has never menstruated) or secondary (in a woman in whom menstruation is present for a variable time and then ceases); some disorders can cause either primary or secondary amenorrhea. For example, most women with gonadal dysgenesis have primary amenorrhea, but occasional such patients have some follicles and ovulate for short periods so that pregnancies may rarely occur. Furthermore, patients with chronic anovulation (polycystic ovarian disease) most often have secondary amenorrhea but occasionally present with primary amenorrhea. For these reasons, categorization of amenorrhea into primary and secondary types is less helpful in the differential diagnosis than a classification based upon the major underlying physiologic derangements: (1) anatomic defects, (2) ovarian failure, and (3) chronic anovulation with or without estrogen present.

Anatomic defects. A variety of anatomic or structural defects of the female genital tract can preclude menstrual bleeding. Starting from the caudal end of the female genital tract, labial agglutination or fusion is often associated with disorders of sexual development, particularly female pseudohermaphroditism (congenital adrenal hyperplasia or exposure to maternal androgens in utero). (See Chap. 333.) Congenital defects of the vagina, imperforate hymen, and transverse vaginal septae can also cause amenorrhea. These women frequently have accumulation of menstrual blood behind the obstruction and may have cyclic, predictable episodes of abdominal pain.

More severe müllerian anomalies include müllerian agenesis (the Mayer-Rokitansky-Küster-Hauser syndrome) (see Chap. 333), second in frequency only to gonadal dysgenesis as a cause of primary amenorrhea. Women with this syndrome have a 46,XX karyotype, female secondary sex characteristics, and normal ovarian function, including cyclical ovulation, but have absence or severe hypoplasia of the vagina. The uterus usually consists of only rudimentary bicornuate cords, but if the uterus contains endometrium, cyclic abdominal pain and accumulation of blood may occur as in other forms of outlet obstruction. One-third of patients have abnormalities of the urogenital tract, and one-tenth have skeletal anomalies, usually involving the spine. The major diagnostic problem is separating müllerian agenesis from complete testicular feminization in which 46,XY genetic males with testes differentiate as phenotypic women with a blind vaginal pouch and an absent uterus. Women with testicular feminization have feminized breasts but a paucity of pubic and axillary hair. The disorder is due to a defect in the intracellular cytoplasmic androgen-receptor protein that results in profound resistance to the action of testosterone (see Chap. 333). Testicular feminization can be diagnosed by demonstrating a male level of serum testosterone or a 46,XY karyotype, whereas the diagnosis of müllerian agenesis is established by demonstrating a 46,XX karyotype, biphasic basal body temperatures characteristic of ovulating women, and elevated levels of progesterone during the luteal phase.

A rare cause of absence of uterus in 46,XY phenotypic women who are sexually infantile is the so-called testicular regression syndrome or testicular agenesis (see Chap. 333).

Other abnormalities of the uterus that cause amenorrhea include obstruction due to scarring or stenosis of the cervix, often resulting from surgery, electrocautery, or cryosurgery. Destruction of the endometrium (Asherman's syndrome) may follow vigorous curettage, usually in association with postpartum hemorrhage or therapeutic abortion complicated by infection. This diagnosis is confirmed by hysterosalpingography or by direct vision of the endometrial scarring or synechiae using a hysteroscope.

Treatment of disorders of the outflow tract is surgical. Repair of vaginal agenesis results in normal menstruation and potential fertility only if an intact uterus is present.

Ovarian failure. Primary ovarian failure is associated with elevated plasma gonadotropins and can result from several causes. The most frequent cause is *gonadal dysgenesis,* in which the germ cells are lacking and the ovary is replaced by a fibrous streak. (Also see Chaps. 60 and 333.) Women with gonadal dysgenesis can be divided into two broad groups on the basis of karyotype. The most common is due to deletion of genetic material in the X chromosomes and accounts for about two-thirds of gonadal dysgenesis. A 45,X karyotype is found in about half, and most have somatic defects including short stature, webbed neck, shield chest, and cardiovascular defects, collectively termed the Turner phenotype. The remainder of patients with identifiable abnormalities of the X chromosome have chromosomal mosaicism with or without associated structural abnormalities of the X chromosome. The most common form of mosaicism is 45,X/46,XX. Gonadal tumors are rare in 45,X patients, but gonadal malignancies have been reported in women with chromosomal mosaicism involving the Y chromosome. Therefore, a chromosomal analysis should be obtained in all cases of amenorrhea associated with ovarian failure, and the streak gonad should be removed if a Y chromosome is present. Approximately 90 percent of individuals with gonadal dysgenesis associated with deletion of genetic material in the X chromosome never have menstrual bleeding, and the remaining 10 percent have sufficient residual follicles to experience menses and, rarely, fertility; the menstrual and reproductive lives of such individuals are invariably brief.

A tenth of subjects with bilateral streak gonads have a normal 46,XX or 46,XY karyotype and are said to have *pure gonadal dysgenesis.* These individuals have either normal or above-average stature due to failure of estrogen-mediated epiphyseal closure in the presence of a normal chromosomal constitution. Pure gonadal dysgenesis does not constitute a phenotypic or chromosomally homogenous disorder. Some are the result of X-linked or autosomal gene defects. Other possible causes include chromosomal mosaicism limited to gonadal tissue and destruction of germinal tissue in utero by environmental or infectious processes. Approximately one-tenth of such individuals with a 46,XY karyotype develop signs of virilization including clitoromegaly and have an increased incidence of tumors in the gonadal streaks; as a consequence gonadal streaks should be removed prophylactically as previously discussed when a Y chromosome is present. Approximately two-thirds of individuals with 46,XX karyotype experience no menses while the remainder have one or more menstrual episodes and are occasionally fertile.

Other causes of ovarian failure and amenorrhea include 17α-hydroxylase or 17,20-desmolase deficiency, premature ovarian failure, the resistant-ovary syndrome, and ovarian failure secondary to chemotherapy or radiation therapy for malignancy. *17α-Hydroxylase deficiency* is characterized by primary amenorrhea, sexual infantilism, and hypertension that is due to increased production of desoxycorticosterone (DOC), whereas women with 17,20-desmolase deficiency have primary amenorrhea and sexual infantilism with normal blood pressure (see Chaps. 325 and 333). The diagnosis of *premature ovarian failure* or *premature menopause* is applied to women who cease menstruating prior to the age of 40. The ovaries are similar to the ovaries of postmenopausal women, namely paucity or absence of follicles as the result of accelerated follicular atresia. Premature ovarian failure due to ovarian antibodies may be one component of polyglandular failure together with adrenal insufficiency, hypothyroidism, and other autoimmune disorders (see Chap. 334). A rare form of ovarian failure is the *resistant-ovary syndrome* in which the ovaries contain many follicles arrested in development prior to the antral stage, possibly because of resistance to the action of FSH in the ovary. To differentiate this disorder from the 46,XX variety of pure gonadal dysgenesis, both of which are associated with sexual immaturity, it is necessary to perform ovarian biopsy. However, such a distinction is not clinically useful since the treatment of infertility in both conditions is usually unsuccessful.

Chronic anovulation. At least 80 percent or more of gynecologic endocrine problems result from chronic anovulation. Women with chronic anovulation fail to ovulate spontaneously but may ovulate with appropriate therapy. The ovaries of such women do not secrete estrogen in a normal cyclic pattern; it is clinically useful to differentiate those women who produce sufficient estrogen to have withdrawal bleeding after progesterone therapy from those who fail to produce enough estrogen to have progesterone withdrawal bleeding and who often have hypothalamic-pituitary dysfunction.

Chronic anovulation with estrogen present. Women with chronic anovulation who experience withdrawal bleeding after progesterone administration are said to be in a state of "estrus" due to the acyclic production of estrogen, largely estrone, by extraglandular aromatization of circulating androstenedione. The most common term for this disorder is *polycystic ovarian disease* (PCOD), a syndrome characterized by infertility, hirsutism, obesity, and amenorrhea or oligomenorrhea. When spontaneous uterine bleeding occurs in subjects with PCOD, it is unpredictable with respect to time of onset, duration, and amount, and on occasion the bleeding can be severe. The dysfunctional uterine bleeding is usually due to estrogen breakthrough (see above).

The disorder, which may be transmitted as an autosomal dominant or X-linked trait, was originally described by Stein and Leventhal as characterized by enlarged, polycystic ovaries, but the syndrome and its accompanying endocrine abnormalities are now known to be associated with a variety of pathologic findings in the ovaries, only some of which result in enlargement of the ovaries and none of which are pathognomonic. The most common finding is a white, smooth, sclerotic ovary with a thickened capsule, multiple follicular cysts in various stages of atresia, a hyperplastic theca and stroma, and rare or absent corpora albicans. Other ovaries have hyperthecosis in which the ovarian stroma is hyperplastic and may contain lipid-laden luteal cells. Thus, the diagnosis of PCOD is a clinical one, based upon the coexistence of chronic anovulation and varying degrees of androgen excess.

In most women with PCOD menarche occurs at the expected time, but uterine bleeding is unpredictable in onset, duration, and amount. Amenorrhea ensues after a variable time, although primary amenorrhea occurs in some women. Signs of androgen excess (hirsutism) usually become evident around the time of menarche. One formulation suggests that this disorder originates as an exaggerated adrenarche in obese girls (Fig. 331-7). The combination of elevated adrenal androgens and obesity would result in increased formation of extraglandular estrogen and lead to an acyclic positive feedback on LH secretion and negative feedback on FSH secretion so that the characteristic LH/FSH ratios in plasma would be greater than 2. The increased LH levels could then lead to hyperplasia of the ovarian stroma and theca cells and increased androgen production, which in turn would provide more substrate for peripheral aromatization and perpetuate the chronic anovulation. In the advanced state the ovary is the major site of androgen production, but the adrenal may continue to secrete excess androgen as well. The greater the obesity, the more this sequence would be perpetuated because adipose tissue stromal cells aromatize androgens to estrogens, which in turn exaggerates inappropriate LH release by positive feedback.

Thus, the fundamental defect in PCOD is viewed as one of inappropriate signals to the hypothalamus and pituitary. In fact, the hypothalamic-pituitary axis responds appropriately to high levels of estrogen, and ovulation can be induced with antiestrogens such as clomiphene citrate. Increased levels of plasma endorphins and inhibin may contribute to the perpetuation of the defect. The concept that the fundamental defect is one of inappropriate signals is supported by the findings in the ovary itself. Ovarian follicles from women with PCOD have low aromatase activity, but normal aromatase can be induced when the follicles are treated with FSH. In short, the anovulation is not due to an intrinsic abnormality in the ovary itself but rather the result of FSH deficiency and LH excess. An association exists between PCOD or hyperthecosis, acanthosis nigricans, and diabetes mellitus due to insulin resistance. The meaning of this association is not clear.

Treatment of PCOD is directed toward interrupting this self-perpetuating cycle and can be accomplished in several ways, including decreasing ovarian androgen secretion (wedge resection or oral contraceptive agents), decreasing peripheral estrogen formation (weight reduction), enhancing FSH secretion [administration of clomiphene, human menopausal gonadotropin (hMG), or LHRH (gonadorelin) by portable infusion pump]. The choice of therapy depends on the clinical findings and the needs of the patient. Attempt at weight reduction is appropriate in all who are obese. If the woman is not hirsute and does not desire pregnancy, periodic withdrawal menses can be induced with medroxyprogesterone acetate every 2 to 3 months; such treatment prevents development of endometrial hyperplasia. If the woman is hirsute but does not desire pregnancy, the ovarian (and possibly the adrenal) component of androgen production can be suppressed with combined estrogen-progestogen oral contraceptive agents. Combined oral contraceptives are also indicated if prolonged or excessive menstrual bleeding is present. Once androgen excess is controlled, treatment of previously existing hair growth by shaving, depilatories, or electrolysis may be indicated (see Chap. 46). If the

FIGURE 331-7 *Proposed mechanism for the initiation and perpetuation of chronic anovulation in polycystic ovarian disease (PCOD). This cycle may be entered or initiated via adrenal androgen excess or obesity, both of which result in enhanced extraglandular formation of estrogens. The therapy of PCOD involves interruption of the cycle at various sites. (From SSC Yen and RB Jaffe, 1986, and from U Goebelsmann in DR Mishell Jr and V Davajan.)*

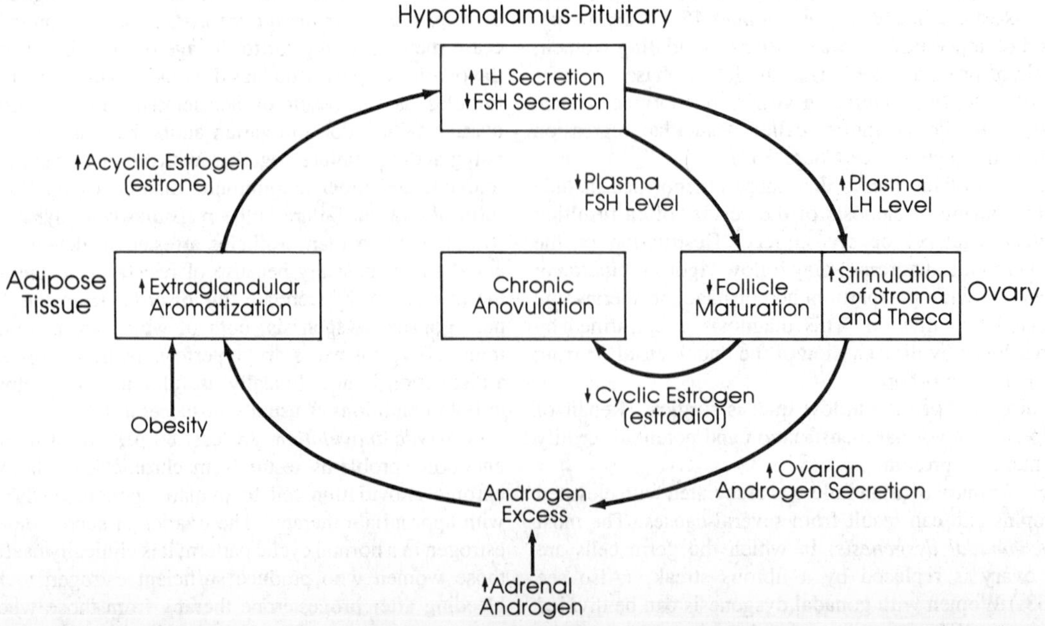

woman wants to become pregnant, induction of ovulation is necessary. The drug of choice for this purpose is clomiphene, which promotes ovulation in three-fourths of cases, and treatment with hMG, gonadorelin, or wedge resection of the ovaries may be successful in the remainder.

Chronic anovulation with estrogen present may also occur with tumors of the ovary. These include granulosa-theca cell tumors, Brenner tumors, cystic teratomas, mucous cystadenomas, and Krukenberg tumors (also see Chap. 296). These tumors can either secrete excess estrogen themselves or produce androgens that can then be aromatized in extraglandular sites. As a result, chronic anovulation and the clinical features of PCOD are produced. Occasionally areas of the ovary not involved with tumors show the characteristic histologic changes of PCOD. Other causes of chronic anovulation with estrogen present include adrenal production of excess androgen and various thyroid disorders.

Chronic anovulation with estrogen absent. Women with chronic anovulation who have low or absent estrogen production and do not experience withdrawal bleeding after progestogen treatment usually have hypogonadotropic hypogonadism due either to pituitary disease or to any of several organic or functional disorders of the central nervous system.

Isolated hypogonadotropic hypogonadism associated with defects of smell (olfactory bulb defects) is known as the Kallman syndrome (see Chaps. 321 and 330). Affected women are sexually infantile with a eunuchoid habitus and appear to have a defect in either the synthesis or release of LHRH. A variety of rare hypothalamic lesions can also impair LHRH production and cause hypogonadotropic hypogonadism; these include craniopharyngioma, germinoma (pinealoma), glioma, Hand-Schüller-Christian disease, teratomas, endodermal-sinus tumors, tuberculosis, sarcoidosis, and metastatic tumors that cause suppression or destruction of the hypothalamus. Central nervous system trauma and radiation can also cause hypothalamic amenorrhea and deficiencies in secretion of growth hormone, ACTH, and thyroid hormone.

More commonly, gonadotropin deficiency leading to chronic anovulation is believed to arise from functional disorders of the hypothalamus or higher centers. A history of a stressful event in a young woman is frequent. For example, chronic anovulation can begin suddenly in a woman who leaves home for the first time or experiences the death of a loved one. Gonadotropin and estrogen levels are in the low to low-normal range as compared to normal women in the early follicular phase of the cycle. In addition, rigorous exercise such as jogging or ballet and diets that result in excessive weight loss may lead to the development of chronic anovulation particularly in girls with a history of prior menstrual irregularity. The amenorrhea in these women does not appear to be due to weight loss alone but to a combination of a decrease in the percentage of body fat and chronic stress. An extreme form of weight loss with chronic anovulation is seen in anorexia nervosa. Anorexia nervosa is characterized by the development in a young woman of amenorrhea with associated severe weight loss, distorted attitudes toward eating and weight gain, self-induced vomiting, extreme emaciation, and distorted body image. Amenorrhea in anorexia nervosa can precede, follow, or appear coincidently with the loss in body weight (see Chap. 73). During successful therapy gonadotropin changes recapitulate those observed during normal puberty (Fig. 331-1).

In addition, chronic debilitating diseases such as end-stage kidney disease, malignancy, or the malabsorption syndrome are believed to lead to development of hypogonadotropic hypogonadism via a hypothalamic mechanism.

Treatment of chronic anovulation due to hypothalamic disorders includes reversal of the stressful situation, reducing exercise, or correction of weight loss if appropriate. These women appear to be susceptible to the development of osteoporosis, and estrogen replacement therapy to induce and maintain normal secondary sexual characteristics and prevent bone loss is recommended in those who do not desire pregnancy, and gonadotropin or gonadorelin therapy is indicated when pregnancy is desired (see therapy section). When appropriate, therapy is directed at the primary disease of the hypothalamus.

Disorders of the pituitary can lead to the estrogen-deficient form of chronic anovulation by at least two mechanisms—direct interference with gonadotropin secretion by lesions that either obliterate or interfere with the gonadotropic cells (chromophobe adenomas, Sheehan's syndrome) or inhibition of gonadotropin secretion in association with excess prolactin (prolactinoma). *Pituitary tumors* make up approximately 10 percent of all intracranial tumors and may secrete no hormone, one hormone, or more than one hormone (see Chap. 321). In the past most pituitary tumors were assumed to be nonfunctional chromophobe adenomas, but prolactin levels are elevated in 50 to 70 percent of cases, either because of prolactin secretion by the tumor (prolactinomas) or interference by tumor mass with the normal inhibitory influence of the hypothalamus on prolactin secretion.

Prolactinomas can be divided into microadenomas (less than 10 mm in diameter) and macroadenomas (greater than 10 mm). Prolactin excess associated with low levels of LH and FSH constitutes a specific subgroup of hypogonadotropic hypogonadism. One-tenth or more of amenorrheic women have increased levels of serum prolactin, and more than half of women with both galactorrhea and amenorrhea have elevated prolactin levels. The amenorrhea in this disorder is most often associated with decreased or absent estrogen production, but prolactin-secreting tumors may on occasion be associated with normal ovulatory menses or chronic anovulation with estrogen present. Most prolactin-secreting adenomas grow slowly, and some cease growth after attainment of a certain size. The increased frequency of diagnosis of prolactin-secreting adenomas is probably due to several factors, including increased awareness, improved radiographic detection methods, and availability of radioimmunoassays for prolactin. However, since in older autopsy series a 9 to 23 percent prevalence of pituitary adenomas was observed in asymptomatic women, the clinical and prognostic significance of small microadenomas remains to be established. When tumors of any size are associated with symptoms of amenorrhea or galactorrhea, however, therapy should be considered, and when visual field defects or severe headaches are present bromocriptine therapy or neurosurgical evaluation is mandatory. The evaluation, differential diagnosis, and management of hyperprolactinemia is described in Chap. 321. In the latter half of pregnancy, prolactin-secreting pituitary tumors may expand, leading to headaches, compression of the optic chiasm, and blindness. Therefore, prior to induction of ovulation for the purposes of achieving pregnancy, it is mandatory to exclude the presence of a pituitary tumor.

Large pituitary tumors such as chromophobe adenomas—whether or not hyperprolactinemia is present—are likely to be associated with deficiency of hormones in addition to gonadotropins (Chap. 321).

Craniopharyngiomas, thought to arise from remnants of Rathke's pouch, account for 3 percent of intracranial neoplasms, occur most frequently in the second decade of life, and may extend into the suprasellar region. A large percentage of these tumors calcify and can be diagnosed by conventional skull films. Patients often present with sexual infantilism, delayed puberty, and amenorrhea due to gonadotropin deficiency. Craniopharyngioma may also result in impaired secretion of TSH, ACTH, growth hormone, and vasopressin.

Panhypopituitarism may occur spontaneously, result from surgical or radiation treatment of pituitary adenomas, or develop after postpartum hemorrhage (Sheehan's syndrome). The latter patients exhibit characteristic clinical manifestations including failure to lactate or ovulate, loss of genital and axillary hair, hypothyroidism, and adrenal insufficiency (see Chap. 321).

Evaluation of amenorrhea. A general schema for the evaluation of women with amenorrhea is given in Fig. 331-8. In the initial physical examination, special attention should be given to three features: (1) degree of maturation of the breasts, the pubic and axillary hair, and the external genitalia; (2) the current estrogen status; and (3) the presence or absence of a uterus. All women with amenorrhea should be assumed to be pregnant until proven otherwise. Even when history and physical examination are not suggestive, it is prudent to exclude pregnancy by a suitable screening test. Once this is done, the cause of amenorrhea can frequently be diagnosed by history and physical examination. For example, Ashermans syndrome is suggested by a history of curettage in a woman who previously menstruated; in women with primary amenorrhea and sexual infantilism the essential differential diagnosis is between gonadal dysgenesis and hypopituitarism, and, in addition, the diagnosis of gonadal dysgenesis (Turner's syndrome) or of anatomic defects of the outflow tract (müllerian agenesis, testicular feminization, and cervical stenosis) is frequently suggested on the basis of physical findings. When a specific cause is suspected, it is appropriate to proceed directly to confirm the diagnosis (such as obtaining a chromosomal karyotype or measurement of plasma gonadotropins). It is also useful to measure serum prolactin level during the initial evaluation.

Estrogen status is evaluated by determining if the vaginal mucosa is moist and rugated and if the cervical mucus can be stretched and shown to fern upon drying. If these criteria are indeterminate a progestational challenge is indicated, most often administration of 10 mg of medroxyprogesterone acetate by mouth once or twice daily for 5 days or 100 mg of progesterone in oil intramuscularly. (It should be emphasized that progestogen should never be administered until pregnancy is excluded.) If estrogen levels are adequate (and the outflow tract is intact) menstrual bleeding should occur within 1 week of ending the progestogen treatment. If withdrawal bleeding occurs, the diagnosis is chronic anovulation with estrogen present, usually polycystic ovarian disease.

If no withdrawal bleeding occurs, the nature of the subsequent workup is dependent on the results of the initial prolactin assay. If plasma prolactin is elevated or if galactorrhea is present, radiography of the pituitary should be undertaken. When the plasma prolactin is normal in the anovulatory woman with estrogen absent, plasma gonadotropins should be measured. If the gonadotropin levels are elevated, the diagnosis is ovarian failure. If the gonadotropins are in the low or normal range, the diagnosis is either hypothalmic-pituitary disorder or anatomic defect of the outflow tract. As indicated previously, the diagnosis of outflow tract disorder is usually suspected or established on the basis of the history and physical findings. When the physical findings are not clear-cut, it is useful to administer cyclic estrogen plus progestogen (1.25 mg of oral conjugated estrogens per day for 3 weeks with 10 mg of medroxyprogesterone acetate added for the last 5 to 7 days of estrogen treatment) followed by 10 days of observation. If no bleeding occurs, the diagnosis of Asherman's syndrome or other anatomic defect of the outflow tract is confirmed by hysterosalpingography or hysteroscopy. If withdrawal bleeding occurs following the estrogen-progestogen combination, the diagnosis of chronic anovulation with estrogen absent (functional hypothalamic amenorrhea) is suggested. Radiologic evaluations of the pituitary-hypothalamic areas may be indicated in the latter cases—irrespective of the prolactin level—because of the danger of overlooking a pituitary-hypothalamic tumor and because the diagnosis of functional hypothalamic amenorrhea is one of exclusion (see Chap. 321).

Infertility Infertility, the failure to become pregnant after 1 year of unprotected intercourse, affects approximately 10 to 15 percent of couples and is one of the common complaints for which women seek gynecologic assistance. Male factors account for 40 percent of infertility problems (see Chaps. 44 and 330). In women, failure of ovulation accounts for 30 percent, pelvic factors such as tubal disease and endometriosis account for half, and a cervical factor is implicated in about one-tenth of infertility evaluations. In 10 to 20 percent of infertile women no etiology is found. An immunologic cause may explain a large fraction of infertility in these couples. Finally, infertility in women may be due to *luteal phase dysfunction* in which ovulation is assumed to occur but progesterone formation is insufficient to allow preparation of the endometrium for implantation; the disorder is believed to be due to inadequate FSH secretion or action and consequent inadequate estrogen formation by the dominant follicle during the follicular phase.

The first diagnostic step in evaluation of the infertile couple is to determine whether the man or woman is the infertile partner, ordinarily by first obtaining a semen analysis in the man (see Chap. 330) and demonstration of presumed ovulation in the woman. Documentation of ovulatory cycles is obtained by daily measurement of basal body temperatures throughout the month. Occasionally, accurate basal body temperature records are not obtained, and demonstration of elevated serum progesterone levels during the luteal phase may be used as evidence of ovulation. Dating of endometrium by histologic examination of a biopsy sample is also useful for establishing ovulation or luteal phase dysfunction.

If the infertility is associated with amenorrhea, then the workup is that described in Fig. 331-8. If anovulation due to polycystic ovarian disease is the basis for infertility, ovulation can be induced

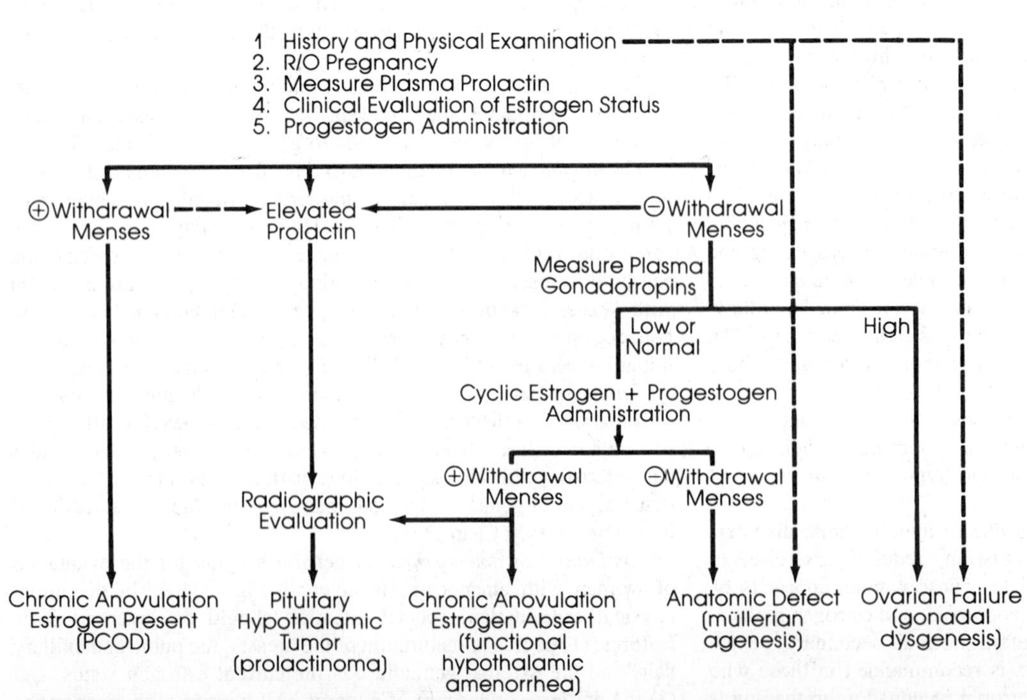

FIGURE 331-8 *Flow diagram for the evaluation of women with amenorrhea. The most common diagnosis for each category is shown in parenthesis. The dotted lines indicate that in some instances a correct diagnosis can be reached on the basis of history and physical exam alone.*

utilizing clomiphene, human menopausal gonadotropins, gonadorelin, or, on occasion, wedge resection of the ovaries. Bromocriptine is used to induce ovulation in cases of hyperprolactinemia. In the presence of prolactinomas the appropriate therapy prior to induction of ovulation remains controversial. Recommended therapies in this situation include observation, reinstitution of bromocriptine therapy, radiation therapy, or surgical resection of the tumor (see Chap. 321).

Hysterosalpingograms may be obtained to evaluate the fallopian tubes and uterine cavity. Further evaluation of tubal and ovarian disease is obtained by diagnostic laparoscopy and the demonstration of dye spillage from the fimbria after transcervical injection of dye during laparoscopy. Microsurgical repair of damaged or previously ligated fallopian tubes has resulted in an apparent increase in pregnancy rates. Removal of peritubular and fimbrial adhesions utilizing laser beam surgery is another treatment mode. Endometriosis can be diagnosed by laparoscopy, and treatment of endometriosis associated with infertility includes surgical resection of the endometrial implants or temporary gonadotropin suppression utilizing danazol (400 to 800 mg orally in divided doses for 4 to 6 months), LHRH analogues given by nasal spray or subcutaneous injection, or continuous low-dose oral contraceptive agents to promote regression of the implants.

The cervical factor in infertility is evaluated by study of cervical mucus at an appropriate time after coitus. The test is preferably performed just prior to ovulation (day 12 to 13) when cervical mucus is thin and stretches and provides information as to the penetration and survival of the sperm in the female genital tract. Treatment of infertility due to such abnormality is often unsuccessful.

When other treatment modalities are unsuccessful, in vitro fertilization and embryo transfer (IVF-ET) may be tried. Indications for the use of IVF-ET in infertile couples include tubal obstructive disease, cervical factors, endometriosis, oligospermia, and unexplained infertility. Multiple follicles are induced with clomiphene and/or hMG, and follicles are obtained by laparoscopy or transabdominal or transvaginal aspiration with ultrasound monitoring. After fertilization and cleavage, embryos are transferred to the uterine cavity. Although pregnancy rates vary, successful pregnancy has been reported in as high as 30 percent of cases after IVF-ET. A modification of IVF-ET, known as gamete-intrafallopian transfer (GIFT) in which a mixture of sperm and ova are introduced into the end of the fallopian tube at laparoscopy, has resulted in successful pregnancies.

Medical aspects of pregnancy The possibility of pregnancy should be considered in all women of reproductive age who are evaluated for medical illness or considered for surgery. Procedures such as x-ray exposure, drugs, and anesthetics may be harmful to the developing fetus, and a variety of medical problems may worsen during pregnancy, including hypertension; diseases of the heart, lungs, kidney, and liver; and metabolic and endocrine disorders. Indeed, all women who present with abnormal vaginal bleeding or amenorrhea during the reproductive years should be assumed to have a complication of pregnancy, such as incomplete abortion, ectopic pregnancy, or trophoblastic disease (hydatidiform mole or choriocarcinoma). Women who present with these complications of pregnancy often have histories of abdominal pain and vaginal bleeding and may have evidence of intraabdominal hemorrhage.

Choriocarcinoma is a particular problem because of its protean manifestations. Half of these malignancies follow pregnancies complicated by hydatidiform mole, and the remainder occur after spontaneous abortion, ectopic pregnancy, or normal deliveries. Patients may present with intraabdominal bleeding due to rupture of the uterus, liver, or ovary, with pulmonary manifestations (cough, hemoptysis, pleuritic pain, dyspnea, and respiratory failure), or with gastrointestinal symptoms, usually chronic blood loss or melena. In addition, patients can present with cerebral metastases or renal involvement. The diagnosis can be established by demonstrating an elevated level of the β subunit of hCG in plasma. Treatment and cure are possible with chemotherapeutic agents (actinomycin D and/or methotrexate). (For manifestations of choriocarcinoma in men see Chap. 297.)

Ovarian tumors See Chap. 296.

TREATMENT

PROGESTOGENS The major use of progestogen is in conjunction with estrogen to ensure the full maturation of the endometrium, both in combination birth control pills and in the therapy of hypogonadal states. In certain circumstances, however, progestogen therapy is appropriate by itself—to induce a progestational effect on the estrogen-primed endometrium (diagnostic tests for the evaluation of amenorrhea), to inhibit pituitary gonadotropins (precocious puberty in girls, and the progestogen-only birth control pill), for prophylaxis to prevent hyperplasia in PCOD, and for palliation in endometrial and breast carcinoma or treatment of endometriosis. Even when a direct progestational effect is desired, the available oral drugs substitute a synthetic derivative for the naturally occurring hormone. Oral progestogens include medroxyprogesterone acetate, megestrol acetate, norethindrone, and norgestrel. Parenteral agents include progesterone in oil, medroxyprogesterone acetate suspension, and 17-hydroxyprogesterone caproate.

The most common undesirable side effect is breakthrough bleeding, which occurs when progestogens are used continuously. Other complications include nausea, vomiting, and hirsutism. Abnormal liver function is a side effect of those derivatives with alkyl substitution in the 17α position. Progestogens are contraindicated if pregnancy is known or suspected because of the risk of birth defects.

ESTROGENS Estrogenic drugs are used for three purposes—the treatment of gonadal failure, control of fertility, and in the management of dysfunctional uterine bleeding and carcinoma of the breast. (The use of estrogens in management of carcinoma of the breast is discussed in Chap. 295.) However, none of the presently available orally active or parenteral hormones replaces the pattern of concentration of estradiol characteristic of the normally cycling, premenopausal woman (Fig. 331-5). Estrogens that can be given by mouth are either nonsteroidal agents (such as diethylstilbestrol) that mimic the action of estradiol, estrogen conjugates that must be hydrolyzed before they become active (estrogen sulfates, predominantly estrone sulfate from pregnant mare's urine), or estrogen analogues that cannot be metabolized to estradiol (mestranol, quinestrol) (Fig. 331-9). Even when micronized estradiol is given orally, it is rapidly converted in the body to estrone. Because oral therapy neither replaces nor mimics the daily secretory pattern of the lost hormone, such therapy must be viewed as a pharmacologic substitution rather than a physiologic replacement. Likewise, the use of parenteral estrogens rarely mimics the physiologic situation. Parenteral preparations of conjugated estrogens, like the oral derivatives, are poor precursors of estradiol, and estradiol esters (estradiol benzoate and valerate) rarely cause plasma estradiol levels that mimic the normal monthly secretory pattern of the hormone. Transdermal estrogen results in constant levels of blood estrogen and is effective in the treatment of menopausal symptoms. The side effects of estrogen substitution differ at various times of life.

Hypoestrogenism In women with decreased estrogen production, whether due to disease of the ovaries (gonadal dysgenesis) or to hypogonadotropic hypogonadism, treatment with cyclic estrogens should be instituted at the time of expected puberty for development and maintenance of female secondary sexual characteristics and prevention of osteoporosis. The most commonly used medications are conjugated estrogens (0.625 to 1.25 mg per day by mouth) or ethinyl estradiol or its precursors (0.02 to 0.05 mg by mouth). The addition of medroxyprogesterone acetate (5 to 10 mg daily) is recommended by most physicians during the last several days of monthly estrogen treatment to prevent development of endometrial

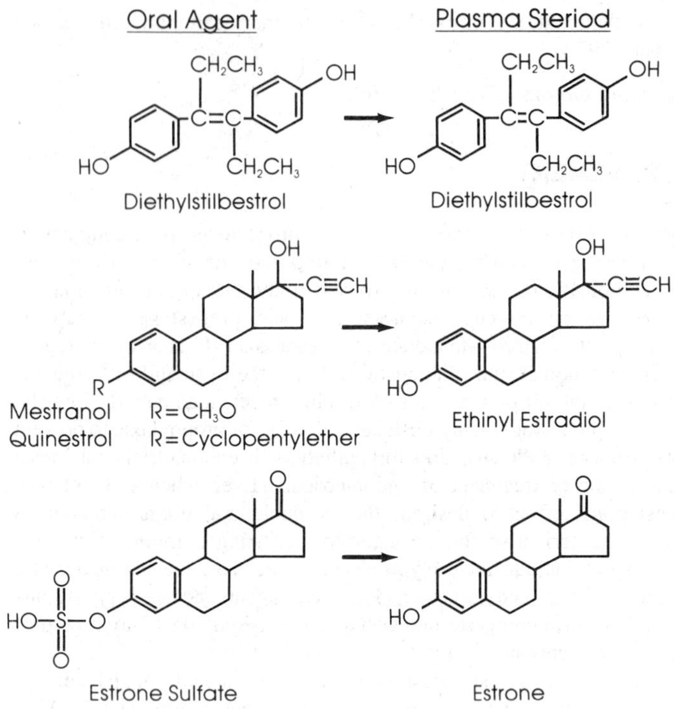

FIGURE 331-9 *The circulating forms of administered estrogenic drugs.*

hyperplasia during long-term estrogen treatment. Abnormal bleeding in women receiving estrogen replacement requires histologic evaluation of the endometrium. Such substitution therapy or the use of oral contraceptives (see below) may also be used for the purpose of suppressing pituitary gonadotropins, as in women with PCOD in whom the major therapeutic aim is suppression of ovarian androgen production prior to the time when fertility is desired.

Temporary administration of estrogens in larger quantities (up to two times the usual adult maintenance dose) may be necessary to induce full development of secondary sexual characteristics in girls and for the control of menopausal symptoms. Even larger doses of parenteral estrogens (10 mg of estradiol valerate or 25 mg of conjugated estrogen) in conjunction with progestogen may be required in some instances of dysfunctional uterine bleeding. Estrogen replacement (100 ng/kg) stimulates growth in women with gonadal dysgenesis, but at high doses (400 ng/kg) has no effect on growth. In addition to the potential long-term side effects of all estrogens (see below), these dosages may cause specific problems including nausea, vomiting, and edema.

Fertility control Since the use of all contraceptive methods is associated with diverse side effects, an understanding of the use, methods of actions, and consequences of these agents is important to all physicians. Furthermore, since pregnancy may aggravate a variety of chronic illnesses, fertility control should be recommended in many patients.

To be effective, fertility control requires patient acceptance and compliance. The most widely utilized methods include (1) rhythm and withdrawal techniques; (2) barrier methods including the condom, jellies, foam, suppositories, and diaphragms; (3) intrauterine devices (IUD); (4) hormonal contraceptives; (5) sterilization; and (6) abortion.

The rhythm and withdrawal technique and the barrier methods are effective if used correctly and consistently but in actual practice result in high failure rates because of imperfect compliance. Nevertheless, these methods carry the lowest incidence of side effects, and the side effects, when produced, are minor except for local allergic reactions. Their use should be recommended when there is a relative or absolute contraindication to other therapy.

The most widely utilized nonsurgical methods of contraception, the IUD and birth control pills, are effective but associated with significant side effects.

IUD The success rates of most IUDs are 95 to 98 percent. These devices are available in a variety of shapes and sizes, but the 7- or T-shaped devices cause minimal pain at insertion and are associated with low expulsion rates. Some IUDs contain copper, which enhances their effectiveness, and some contain slow-release progestational drugs, which makes replacement necessary at 1- to 3-year intervals. The IUD is believed to prevent pregnancy by the induction of a chronic inflammatory reaction in the endometrium, resulting in an unfavorable environment for the implantation of the blastocyst.

Once the IUD is inserted, it is necessary to check periodically to be certain that the device is in place. Both minor and serious side effects can occur. Intermenstrual spotting and increased bleeding and pain or cramps at the time of menses are frequent causes of discontinuation of the IUD. In addition, the device may be expelled spontaneously during a menstrual period without the subject being aware of its loss. The most serious side effect is pelvic infection, occasionally leading to the development of tuboovarian abscess and subsequent infertility. For this reason, use in nulligravida women is not advocated by many gynecologists. In addition, pregnancy with an IUD in place is more likely to be ectopic since intrauterine but not extrauterine pregnancies are inhibited. Because of the increased incidence of spontaneous and septic abortions when IUDs are in place, the device should be removed if pregnancy is detected. Any user who develops persistent, severe bleeding, lower abdominal pain, fever, or discharge should have the IUD removed.

ORAL CONTRACEPTIVES Oral contraceptive agents have been used by over 200 million women worldwide and by 1 out of 4 women in the United States under the age of 45. These agents are popular because of ease of administration, low pregnancy rate (less than 1 percent), and a relatively low incidence of side effects.

The most widely utilized oral contraceptive pills are either combination tablets or biphasic or triphasic formulations. A list of oral contraceptives marketed in the United States is given in Table 331-3. Combination oral contraceptive tablets contain one of two synthetic estrogens (mestranol or ethinyl estradiol) and one of five synthetic progestogens (norethindrone, norethindrone acetate, norethynodrel, norgestrel, or ethynodiol diacetate). The combination or biphasic or triphasic tablets are taken for 21 consecutive days followed by 7 days' rest. Progestogen-only tablets are taken continuously on a daily basis. Presumably, the ideal contraceptive contains the lowest amount of steroid to minimize side effects but an amount that is at the same time sufficient to prevent pregnancy or breakthrough bleeding. The triphasic tablets containing 30 μg of estrogen and a progestogen come closest to this goal.

Oral contraceptives inhibit ovulation by suppressing FSH and LH secretion. As a consequence, the secretion of all ovarian steroids is also suppressed, including estrogen, progesterone, and androgen (Fig. 331-10). These agents also exert minor direct inhibitory effects on the reproductive tract, altering the cervical mucus and thereby decreasing sperm penetration and decreasing the motility and secretions of the fallopian tubes and uterus.

The death rates associated with oral contraceptives and other forms of birth control are summarized in Table 331-4. Up to age 40 the mortality rates in women using oral contraceptives and IUDs are lower than in women using no form of contraception (this difference is because of the increased risk of death associated with pregnancy). The decrease in death rate below age 40 is even more striking in nonsmokers than in smokers using contraceptives. In fact, the death rates in nonsmoking women age 15 to 24 who use oral agents are lower than those with other forms of fertility control. The increased death rates in women using rhythm or barrier techniques probably results from the higher failure rate and the consequent risk of pregnancy in such women. Oral contraceptive agents are not recommended for smoking women after age 35, all women after age 40, and women of all ages who are at increased risk for myocardial infarction.

Despite the overall safety of these agents, users are at risk for several serious side effects. In most retrospective and prospective studies an increased incidence has been found for *deep vein thrombosis* and *pulmonary embolism*. The relative increased risk varies from two- to twelvefold and is greater for women taking tablets containing more than 50 μg estrogen. The use of oral contraceptives is also associated with an increased risk of thromboembolism after surgery, and for this reason these agents should be discontinued at least 1 month prior to elective surgery. There is a 3- to 9-times increased risk for *thromboembolic stroke* and a twofold greater risk for *hemorrhagic stroke* in users of oral contraceptives. Therefore, the drugs should be discontinued in women who experience visual complaints or severe headaches. Smoking and age increase the risk for stroke as well as the frequency of death from complications of deep venous thrombosis, pulmonary emboli, and myocardial infarction.

A small rise in blood pressure while taking oral contraceptives is common, and 5 percent of women develop significant *hypertension* (blood pressure greater than 140/90) after 5 years of continuous use. Estrogens induce the synthesis of a variety of proteins by the liver including the renin substrate angiotensinogen. The resulting increased formation of angiotensin is believed to be involved in the development of hypertension. In most cases, blood pressure returns to normal when oral contraceptives are discontinued.

Serum lipids and lipoproteins are altered in women on oral contraceptives, the nature of the change depending on the specific components of the oral contraceptives. In general, estrogens increase serum high-density (HDL) and very low density lipoproteins (VLDL). Progestogens depress the concentration of HDL.

A few women taking oral contraceptives develop *impairment of glucose tolerance* as manifested by abnormal glucose levels and elevated plasma insulin after an oral glucose load, both of which usually return to normal after discontinuing the agents. Consequently, oral contraceptives are contraindicated in women with adult-onset diabetes. Because juvenile-onset diabetes may be associated with increased incidence of cardiovascular disease, it is also preferable to utilize other forms of contraception in these individuals.

Oral contraceptives should not be used by women with abnormal liver function tests or in women with acute or chronic liver disease. A rare complication linked to the long-term use of oral contraceptives is the development of peliosis hepatis, which can cause death due to

TABLE 331-3 Composition of oral contraceptives

Name	Estrogen	μg	Progestogen	mg
COMBINATION-TYPE				
Fixed type				
Estrogen content > 50 μg:				
Enovid E	Mestranol	100	Norethynodrel	2.5
Enovid 5	Mestranol	75	Norethynodrel	5.0
Ovulen	Mestranol	100	Ethynodiol diacetate	1.0
Norinyl 2	Mestranol	100	Norethindrone	2.0
Norinyl 1/80	Mestranol	80	Norethindrone	1.0
Ortho-Novum 2	Mestranol	100	Norethindrone	2.0
Ortho-Novum 1/80	Mestranol	80	Norethindrone	1.0
Estrogen content = 50 μg:				
Ortho-Novum 1/50	Mestranol	50	Norethindrone	1.0
Norinyl 1/50	Mestranol	50	Norethindrone	1.0
Ovcon 50	Ethinyl estradiol	50	Norethindrone	1.0
Ovral	Ethinyl estradiol	50	Norgestrel	0.5
Demulen	Ethinyl estradiol	50	Ethynodiol diacetate	1.0
Norlestrin 2.5/50	Ethinyl estradiol	50	Norethindrone acetate	2.5
Norlestrin 1/50	Ethinyl estradiol	50	Norethindrone acetate	1.0
Estrogen content <50 μg:				
Ortho-Novum 1/35	Ethinyl estradiol	35	Norethindrone	1.0
Norinyl 1+35	Ethinyl estradiol	35	Norethindrone	1.0
Modicon	Ethinyl estradiol	35	Norethindrone	0.5
Brevicon	Ethinyl estradiol	35	Norethindrone	0.5
Ovcon 35	Ethinyl estradiol	35	Norethindrone	0.4
Demulen 1/35	Ethinyl estradiol	35	Ethynodiol diacetate	1.0
Loestrin 1.5/30	Ethinyl estradiol	30	Norethindrone acetate	1.5
Loestrin 1/20	Ethinyl estradiol	20	Norethindrone acetate	1.0
Nordette	Ethinyl estradiol	30	Levonorgestrel	0.15
Lo-Ovral	Ethinyl estradiol	30	Norgestrel	0.3
Biphasic type				
Ortho-Novum 10/11	Ethinyl estradiol	35	Norethindrone	0.5
First 10 days	Ethinyl estradiol	35	Norethindrone	1.0
Next 11 days				
Triphasic type				
Ortho-Novum 7/7/7				
First 7 days	Ethinyl estradiol	35	Norethindrone	0.5
Second 7 days	Ethinyl estradiol	35	Norethindrone	0.75
Third 7 days	Ethinyl estradiol	35	Norethindrone	1.0
Tri-Norinyl				
First 7 days	Ethinyl estradiol	35	Norethindrone	0.5
Next 9 days	Ethinyl estradiol	35	Norethindrone	1.0
Next 5 days	Ethinyl estradiol	35	Norethindrone	0.5
Triphasil				
First 6 days	Ethinyl estradiol	30	Levonorgestrel	0.05
Second 5 days	Ethinyl estradiol	40	Levonorgestrel	0.075
Third 10 days	Ethinyl estradiol	30	Levonorgestrel	0.125
Tri-Levein				
First 6 days	Ethinyl estradiol	30	Levonorgestrel	0.05
Second 5 days	Ethinyl estradiol	40	Levonorgestrel	0.075
Third 10 days	Ethinyl estradiol	30	Levonorgestrel	0.125
PROGESTOGEN ONLY				
Micronor	None		Norethindrone	0.35
Nor Q.D.	None		Norethindrone	0.35
Ovrette	None		Norgestrel	0.075

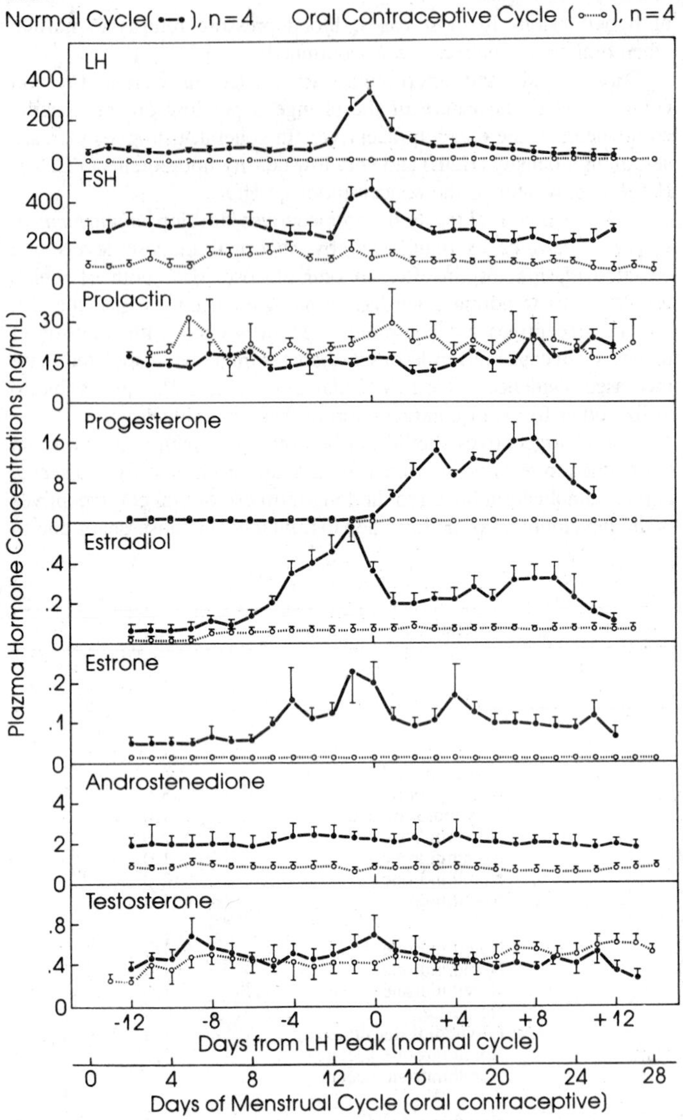

FIGURE 331-10 *The mechanism of action of the birth control tablet. Mean daily plasma hormone concentrations during the ovarian cycle are shown for four ovulating women and four women treated with combination-type oral contraceptives. Data for the normal ovarian cycle are presented in relationship to the day of the LH peak; day 1 of the contraceptive cycle corresponds to the first day of uterine bleeding. The values are the mean ± SE obtained from four women. (From BR Carr et al, 1979.)*

sudden rupture and hemorrhage of the liver. Cholestatic jaundice may occur in those women predisposed to the development of the syndrome of recurrent jaundice of pregnancy.

Oral contraceptives cause an increased concentration of cholesterol in the bile, which is probably the cause for the twofold increase in *cholelithiasis* and cholecystitis in women on oral contraceptives.

Estrogens induce elevation of a variety of proteins secreted by the liver including cortisol-binding globulin (CBG), testosterone-binding globulin (TeBG), and thyroxine-binding globulin (TBG). Consequently, various laboratory tests of adrenal and thyroid function may be altered and must be interpreted with caution (see Chaps. 320 and 324). Oral contraceptives also lower morning plasma ACTH levels, possibly due to an inhibitory effect on ACTH secretion or cortisol catabolism. Finally, serum prolactin levels are slightly elevated in women on oral contraceptives, but such treatment is not believed to play a role in the development of pituitary prolactinomas.

Other effects of oral contraceptive pills include minor dyspepsia, breast discomfort, weight gain, development of pigmentation of the face (chloasma), which is augmented by exposure to the sun, and a variety of psychological effects, such as depression and changes in libido. There is no convincing evidence that oral contraceptives are associated with an increased incidence of cancer of the uterus, cervix, or breast. In fact, oral contraceptives have many beneficial effects including control of dysmenorrhea and anovulatory bleeding, prevention of sexually transmitted diseases, and decreased incidence of endometrial and ovarian cancer.

The absolute contraindications to the use of oral contraceptives include previous thromboembolic disorders, cerebral vascular or coronary artery disease, known or suspected carcinoma of the breast or estrogen-dependent neoplasia, undiagnosed abnormal genital bleeding, or known or suspected pregnancy. Relative contraindications must be weighed against the risk/benefit ratio of the oral contraceptive pills and include hypertension, migraine headaches, diabetes mellitus, uterine leiomyomas, sickle cell anemia, hyperlipemia, and elective surgery.

OTHER STEROID CONTRACEPTIVES Types of steroid contraception other than the conventional oral contraceptives include (1) postcoital contraception and (2) injectable steroids. Use of high-dose estrogen for 5 days during the fertile part of the cycle (the morning-after pill) is an effective method of contraception, but is associated with significant side effects, particularly nausea. Administration of progestogens by injection, implants, or vaginal rings is used infrequently in the United States.

Estrogen treatment of the menopause The use of estrogens in postmenopausal women with osteoporosis is based on the belief that such therapy may relieve many of the disorders of the menopause and indeed of aging itself. In some parts of the United States by the mid-1970s as many as half of women in the menopausal age group used one or more forms of estrogen replacement for a median period of 5 years, accounting for more than 30 million prescriptions per year.

The menopause is not associated with a simple state of estrogen deprivation since some estrogens continue to be produced but is instead a state of altered estrogen metabolism; the predominant estrogen becomes estrone formed by extraglandular conversion of prehormone rather than estradiol secretion by the ovary. As is true for all estrogen therapy, the estrogen treatment of the menopause is actually a pharmacologic substitution of one or another estrogen analogue for the physiologic estradiol rather than a physiologic replacement of the missing steroid. Estrogens available for replace-

TABLE 331-4 Annual death rates associated with fertility control per 100,000 women

Contraceptive techniques	Age group 15–19	20–24	25–29	30–34	35–39	40–44
None (birth-related)	7.0	7.4	9.1	14.8	25.7	28.2
Oral contraceptives						
Smokers	2.4	3.6	6.8	13.7	51.4	117.6
Nonsmokers	0.5	0.7	1.1	2.1	14.1	32.0
IUD	1.3	1.1	1.3	1.3	1.9	2.1
Abortion	0.5	1.1	1.3	1.9	1.8	1.1
Barrier methods (birth-related)	1.5	1.4	1.0	0.8	1.3	7.6

SOURCE: *Adapted from HW Ory, Fam Plan Perspect 15:57, 1983.*

ment therapy include conjugated estrogens, estrogen substitutes (diethylstilbestrol), synthetic estrogen (ethinyl estradiol or derivatives), micronized estradiol, estrogen-containing vaginal creams, and estrogen-containing dermal patches. Regimens associated with low risk of complications include (1) cyclic estrogen therapy in the lowest effective dose for 21 to 25 days per month, and (2) cyclic estrogens plus the addition of progestogen during the last 10 days of estrogen therapy.

The most clear-cut benefit of estrogen therapy in the menopause is the relief of vasomotor instability (hot flashes) and of atrophy of the urogenital epithelium and skin. Estrogen therapy ameliorates these symptoms in the majority of cases. When estrogen therapy is designed to treat hot flashes alone, such therapy should be continued for only a few years since hot flashes tend to diminish after 3 to 4 years in untreated women.

Several lines of evidence indicate that routine estrogen therapy is beneficial in preventing the complications of menopausal osteoporosis, especially in high-risk women (i.e., thin white women). First, in women undergoing premature menopause the incidence and complication rates of osteoporosis are increased, and long-term estrogen replacement appears to be beneficial. Second, estrogen therapy has short-term positive effects on calcium balance and long-term beneficial effects on bone density. Third, in women given combination estrogen and calcium therapy, the incidence of fractures is decreased.

Of the potential side effects, the possibility of an increased risk of endometrial carcinoma is perhaps most worrisome. The relative risk of developing endometrial adenocarcinoma in estrogen users is between 6 and 8. The risk is increased with duration and dosage of estrogen but is decreased in women given combination estrogen-progestogen therapy.

Despite the large body of evidence linking endometrial carcinoma and estrogen use, two types of doubt have been raised about the clinical significance of the association. First, some epidemiologists have argued that the increased risk associated with estrogens has been exaggerated because of problems inherent in obtaining adequate controls in retrospective analyses. Second, in spite of an increased incidence of endometrial carcinoma in the United States, there was no concomitant increased mortality from this disease. Indeed the increased incidence apparently involves low-grade malignancies which may be difficult to distinguish histologically from various forms of hyperplasia. These forms of malignancy have little effect on life expectancy.

Apprehension concerning worsening of hypertension and thromboembolic disease appears to be due to reports of the effects of estrogen-progesterone oral contraceptive pills during the reproductive years and not to estrogen use in menopausal women. There is no documented evidence that low-dose estrogen therapy in the menopause enhances the development or the severity of thromboembolic disease, breast cancer, or hypertension. Low-dose estrogen treatment in the menopause does not appear to influence the development of atherosclerosis, myocardial infarction, or stroke. There is a slightly increased risk for the development of gallbladder disease with estrogen use in the menopause.

A reasonable approach to the use of estrogens in the menopause is as follows: (1) For long-term use, estrogens should be given in the minimal effective doses (0.625 mg conjugated estrogen or 0.01 to 0.02 mg ethinyl estradiol per day). Except when hot flashes preclude intermittent use, the agents should be prescribed for 25 days each month followed by a rest period. (For women with an intact uterus it is the practice in some clinics to give estrogens alone for 15 days, estrogen plus a daily progestogen for an additional 10 days, and nothing for a week.) (2) Such replacement therapy is indicated routinely in women undergoing premature menopause (surgically induced or spontaneous) at least until the age of normal menopause. (3) Estrogen therapy is also indicated routinely in women of all ages who have severe hot flashes or symptomatic atrophy of the urogenital epithelium. Hot flashes rarely persist for longer than 4 years, so that if given for this purpose the duration of therapy can be limited. (4) In women who have had prior hysterectomy potential benefits of treatment appear to outweigh the dangers. Whether estrogens should be given routinely to all women with intact uteri is unsettled, but the authors prescribe it routinely in the absence of contraindications in hopes of ameliorating osteoporosis (in combination with calcium or fluoride). (5) Each woman receiving estrogens must be monitored indefinitely and frequently.

DRUGS TO INDUCE OVULATION The most common treatment for ovulation induction in women with PCOD is *clomiphene*. This antiestrogen is believed to act by binding to estrogen receptors in the hypothalamus and allowing FSH to rise to stimulate follicular development and ultimately result in ovulation. Clomiphene therapy is usually begun in a dose of 50 mg by mouth daily for 5 days commencing on the fifth day of progestin-induced uterine bleeding. If ovulation does not occur, the dose may be increased to 100 or 150 mg per day. Such treatment results in ovulatory cycles in 60 percent of women with PCOD. Additional regimens include clomiphene in combination with human menopausal gonadotropins (hMG), estrogen, glucocorticoids, or human chorionic gonadotropin (hCG).

The most commonly used gonadotropins for induction of ovulation are hMG and hCG. These agents are indicated in women who fail to ovulate on clomiphene and in women with hypogonadotropic hypogonadism. The usual treatment regimen requires 1 to 3 ampuls of hMG per day over an 8- to 12-day period to achieve adequate follicular stimulation and growth, followed by a single injection of 10,000 units of hCG 12 to 24 h after the last injection of hMG. Ovulation is successful in 90 percent of women, and pregnancy rates exceed 50 to 60 percent. Measurement of daily estrogen levels and frequent evaluation of ovarian size by ultrasound are indicated to prevent ovarian hyperstimulation. Ovarian hyperstimulation syndrome results from excessive stimulation of ovarian follicles with resultant enlargement of the ovaries and may progress to the development of ascites, hypotension, and shock. Therapy using hMG and hCG also carries a 20 percent risk of multiple pregnancies.

Bromocriptine is a dopamine agonist that is effective in inducing ovulation in women with elevated prolactin levels. Treatment is instituted at a usual dosage of 2.5 mg by mouth two or three times a day. Treatment should be discontinued as soon as pregnancy is diagnosed. The management of prolactin-secreting pituitary tumors is discussed in Chap. 321.

Luteinizing hormone–releasing hormone (LHRH, gonadorelin) and analogues Gonadorelin has been used successfully to induce ovulation in infertile women. The agent is infused subcutaneously or intravenously by a portable infusion pump which administers pulses at 90- to 120-min intervals for 10 to 20 days. After ovulation has occurred hCG is given to maintain corpus luteum function.

LHRH analogues that block ovulation have been used to treat a variety of gynecologic disorders; ovulation and ovarian steroidogenesis are inhibited due to down-regulation of LHRH receptors with a resultant decreased release of gonadotropins. Conditions in which these agents are under trial include fertility control, true precocious puberty, endometriosis, and uterine leiomyomas.

OTHER DISORDERS OF THE FEMALE REPRODUCTIVE TRACT

VULVA Most disorders of the vulva are due to venereal disease, most commonly syphilis (painless chancre), condyloma acuminata (venereal warts), and herpes vulvitis (painful ulcers) (see Chap. 90). All other lesions of the vulva, particularly in older women, must be biopsied. Early biopsy of cancer of the vulva is mandatory, because when it becomes symptomatic (pruritus and bleeding), it has often progressed to an advanced stage.

VAGINA Infections of the vagina usually present as vaginal discharge and pruritis. The most frequent organisms are *Trichomonas, Candida* *albicans*, and *Gardnerella vaginalis* (also see Chap. 90). The diagnosis is made by microscopic examination of the discharge, and appropriate therapy can be instituted utilizing vaginal or oral antibiotics.

Abnormalities of the vagina and cervix in female offspring of women given diethylstilbestrol during pregnancy include adenosis of the vagina as well as structural abnormalities of the vagina, cervix, and uterus; the risk of developing a rare form of vaginal cancer (adenocarcinoma, clear cell type) is increased (2 per 10,000 exposed women). Periodic examination of women at risk should commence at age 12 to 14, and reevaluation should be undertaken after any episode of abnormal bleeding.

CERVIX Preinvasive lesions of the cervix (also known as cervical intraepithelial neoplasia) as well as invasive carcinoma of the cervix can be detected reliably by obtaining a Papanicolaou smear (Pap smear). Current recommendations by the American Cancer Society are that a Pap smear be obtained every 3 years after 2 negative Pap smears were obtained at yearly intervals in all women between the ages of 20 to 65 and in sexually active women below the age of 20. However, many gynecologists recommend yearly Pap smears especially in patients with more than one sexual partner.

UTERUS Only 40 percent of endometrial adenocarcinoma is detected by Pap smears. In women at high risk for endometrial carcinoma (obesity, history of chronic anovulatory cycles, diabetes, hypertension, estrogen treatment), yearly endometrial sampling should be performed. Low-dose oral estrogen therapy rarely causes breakthrough or withdrawal bleeding in menopausal women. Therefore, irrespective of whether the patient is on estrogen therapy, occurrence of postmenopausal bleeding makes it mandatory to obtain a tissue diagnosis to exclude endometrial cancer either by endometrial sampling or by curettage.

One of the most common disorders of the uterus and the most frequent tumor of women (1 of 4 women affected) is the uterine leiomyoma, or fibroid tumor. Three-fourths of women with leiomyoma are asymptomatic, and the diagnosis is made on routine pelvic examination. When associated with excessive menstrual blood loss, excessive size or rapid growth, or significant pelvic pain (see Chap. 43), the preferred treatment is surgical removal by hysterectomy if there is no desire for further childbearing. In young women myomectomy may on occasion be indicated when infertility or repeated fetal wastage is a manifestation or where future childbearing is desired.

FALLOPIAN TUBES AND OVARIES Infectious pelvic inflammatory disease is a common disorder of the fallopian tubes and usually becomes symptomatic after a menstrual period; the symptoms include fever, chills, abdominal pain, and vaginal discharge, and pelvic tenderness on physical examination is common. The initiating organism most often is *chlamydia trachomatis* or *Neisseria gonorrhoeae*, but tuboovarian abscess and sterility are probably caused by mixed aerobic and anaerobic superinfections and require wide-spectrum antibiotic treatment (see Chap. 91).

Endometriosis is a benign disorder characterized by the presence and proliferation of endometrial tissue (stroma and glands) outside the endometrial cavity. The clinical manifestations are variable. Endometriosis occurs most commonly between the ages of 30 to 40 and is found incidentally at the time of surgery in approximately one-fifth of all gynecologic operations. The fertility rate is significantly reduced in affected women. The disorder usually involves the posterior cul-de-sac or the ovaries and can give rise to ovarian enlargement (endometriomas), although it may also involve sites distant to the pelvis (lung, umbilicus). The most significant symptom is pelvic pain, characteristically dysmenorrhea (see Chap. 43). However, the frequency and degree of pelvic symptomatology correlate poorly with the extent of disease. Other symptoms include dyspareunia, pain with defecation, and infertility. The characteristic physical findings are multiple tender nodules palpable along the uterosacral ligament at the time of rectal-vaginal examination, a posteriorly fixed uterus, or enlarged cystic ovaries. The diagnosis can only be confirmed by direct visualization, usually at diagnostic laparoscopy. Treatment depends on the degree of involvement and the desires of the patient and includes observation for mild disease with no associated infertility or pain, hormonal suppressive therapy (see infertility), conservative surgery if fertility is desired, or removal of the uterus, tubes, and ovaries in severe disease. Endometriosis is rarely found after the menopause.

Any adnexal mass that persists for more than 6 weeks or is larger than 6 cm must be evaluated. Although ovarian cysts and neoplasms compose the largest group of pelvic adnexal masses (see above), tumors of the fallopian tubes, uterus, gastrointestinal tract or urinary tract should also be considered. Sonography or radiographic evaluation is often helpful in identifying the nature of the adnexal mass prior to surgical exploration.

REFERENCES

CARR BR, GRIFFIN JD: Fertility control and its complications, in *Williams' Textbook of Endocrinology*, JD Wilson, DW Foster (eds). Philadelphia, Saunders, 1985, pp 452–475

——— et al: Plasma levels of adrenocorticotropin and cortisol in women receiving oral contraceptive steroid treatment. J Clin Endocrinol Metab 49:346, 1979

——— et al: Plasma lipoprotein regulation or progesterone biosynthesis by human corpus luteum tissue in organ culture. J Clin Endocrinol Metab 52:875, 1981

——— et al: The role of lipoproteins in the regulation of progesterone secretion by human corpus luteum. Fertil Steril 38:303, 1982

D'ARMIENTO M et al: McCune-Albright syndrome: Evidence for autonomous multiendocrine hyperfunction. J Pediatr 102:584, 1983

DIZEREGA GS, HODGEN GD: Folliculogenesis in the primate ovarian cycle. Endocrinol Rev 2:27, 1981

——— et al: The possible role for a follicular protein in the intraovarian regulation of steroidogenesis. Semin Reprod Endocrinol 1:309, 1983

DMOWSKI WP: Endocrine properties and clinical applications of danazol. Fertil Steril 31:237, 1979

ERICKSON GF et al: Functional studies of aromatase activity in human granulosa cells from normal and polycystic ovaries. J Clin Endocrinol Metab 49:514, 1979

FAIMAN C et al: Patterns of gonadotropins and gonadal steroids throughout life. Clin Obstet Gynaecol 3:467, 1976

FRASIER SD: *Pediatric Endocrinology*. New York, Grune & Stratton, 1980

FUTTERWEIT W: *Polycystic Ovarian Disease*. New York, Springer-Verlag, 1984

GEMZELL C, WANG CF: Outcome of pregnancy in women with pituitary adenoma. Fertil Steril 31:363, 1979

GLUCKMAN PD et al: The human fetal hypothalamus and pituitary gland, in *Maternal-Fetal Endocrinology*, D Tulchinksy, KJ Ryan (eds). Philadelphia, Saunders, 1980

GOLD JJ et al: *Gynecologic Endocrinology*. Hagerstown, Harper & Row, 1980

GOLDZIEHER JW: Polycystic ovarian disease. Fertil Steril 35:371, 1981

HAMMOND MG, TALBERT LM: *Infertility*. Chapel Hill, Health Sciences Consortium, 1981

HATCHER RA et al: *Contraceptive Technology 1980–1981*. New York, Irvington, 1980

JUDD HL et al: Estrogen replacement therapy: Indications and complications. Ann Intern Med 98:195, 1983

KAPLAN NM: Complications of the birth control pill, in *Update I: Harrison's Principles of Internal Medicine*, KJ Isselbacher et al (eds). New York, McGraw-Hill, 1981, p 57

KASE N, WEINGOLD A: Principles and practice of clinical gynecology. New York, Wiley, 1983

KELCH RP: Management of precocious puberty. N Engl J Med 312:1057, 1985

MISHELL DR JR, DAVAJAN V (eds): *Reproductive Endocrinology, Infertility, and Contraception*. Philadelphia, Davis, 1979

PIEPER DR et al: Ovarian gonadatropin-releasing hormone (GnRH) receptors: Characterization, distribution, and induction by GnRH. Endocrinology 108:1148, 1981

PRITCHARD JA et al: *William's Obstetrics*. New York, Appleton-Century-Crofts, 1985

RIGGS BL et al: Effect of the fluoride/calcium regimen on vertebral fracture occurrence in postmenopausal osteoporosis. N Engl J Med 306:446, 1982

ROMNEY SL et al: *Gynecology and Obstetrics: The Health Care of Women*. New York, McGraw-Hill, 1980

ROSS GT: Disorders of the ovary and female reproductive tract, in *Williams' Textbook of Endocrinology*, JD Wilson, DW Foster (eds). Philadelphia, Saunders, 1985, pp 206–258

ROSS JL et al: A preliminary study of the effect of estrogen dose on growth in Turner's syndrome. N Engl J Med 309:1104, 1983

SHEARMAN RP (ed): *Clinical Reproductive Endocrinology*, Edinburgh, Churchill Livingston, 1985

SCULLY RE: Ovarian tumors: A review. Am J Pathol 87:686, 1977

SITTERI PK, MACDONALD PC: Role of extraglandular estrogen in human endocrinology, in *Handbook of Physiology*, sec 7, *Endocrinology*, SR Geiger et al (eds). Washington, DC, American Physiological Society, 1973, p 615

SPEROFF L: Menopause. Semin Reprod Endocrinol 1:1, 1983

——— et al: The ovary, in *Endocrinology and Metabolism*, P Felig et al (eds). New York, McGraw-Hill, 1981, p 669

——— et al: *Clinical Gynecologic Endocrinology and Infertility*, 3d ed. Baltimore, Williams & Wilkins, 1983

STEINGOLD KA et al: Treatment of hot flashes with transdermal estradiol administration. J Clin Endocrinol Metab 61:627, 1985

STYNE DM, GRUMBACH MM: Puberty in the male and female: Its physiology and disorders, in *Reproductive Endocrinology*, SSC Yen, RB Jaffe (eds). Philadelphia, Saunders 1978 pp 189–240

WALLACH EE, KEMPERS RD: *Modern Trends in Infertility and Contraception Control*, vol 3. Baltimore, Williams & Wilkins, 1985

YEN SSC: Neuroendocrine regulation of the menstrual cycle. Hosp Prac 14:84, 1979

———: Clinical application of gonadotropin-releasing hormone and gonadotropin-releasing hormone analogs. Fertil Steril 39:257, 1983

———, JAFFE RB (eds): *Reproductive Endocrinology*, 2d ed. Philadelphia, Saunders, 1986

YING SY et al: Gonadocrinins: Peptides in ovarian follicular fluid stimulating the secretion of pituitary gonadotropins. Endocrinology 108:1206, 1981

332 ENDOCRINE DISORDERS OF THE BREAST

JEAN D. WILSON

Examination of the breasts is an important part of the physical examination. The breasts are the site of fatal and preventable disease in women and frequently provide clues to underlying systemic disease in both men and women. The internist frequently does not examine the male breast and in the evaluation of women is apt to refer this task to a gynecologist. It is the duty of every physician to distinguish the abnormal from the normal at the earliest possible stage and to call for assistance if there is any doubt. (For cancer of the breast see Chap. 295.)

ENDOCRINE CONTROL OF THE BREAST There is no histologic or functional difference in the breasts of boys and girls prior to the onset of puberty, but a profound sexual dimorphism in breast development ensues at the time of puberty. The endocrine control of female breast development is illustrated in Fig. 332-1. The development of the normal nonlactating female breast is dependent primarily upon the action of estradiol, which induces the growth, division, and elongation of the tubular duct system and maturation of the nipples. In men the administration of estrogen is equally effective in this regard. To produce true alveolar development at the ends of the ducts, however, the synergistic action of progesterone is required, a ratio of estrogen to progesterone of 1:20 to 1:100 being optimal. Once the anatomic development of the ducts and alveoli is complete, the continued action of estrogen and progesterone does not appear to be required for lactation itself.

The endocrine control of milk formation by the differentiated breast is complex, requiring in addition to appropriate priming by estrogen and progesterone specific lactogenic hormone and the permissive action of glucocorticoid, insulin, thyroxine, and in some species growth hormone. There are two lactogenic hormones. Human placental lactogen (hPL or chorionic somatomammotropin) is secreted in large amounts by the placenta during the latter phases of gestation and prepares the breast for milk production. It disappears from the fetal (and maternal) circulation shortly after termination of pregnancy. Prolactin, a peptide hormone synthesized in the pituitary (see Chap. 321), plays the critical role in the initiation and maintenance of normal as well as inappropriate lactation. The plasma level of prolactin rises during pregnancy; during late pregnancy and lactation 60 to 80 percent of the anterior pituitary may consist of prolactin-secreting cells.

Unlike most pituitary hormones, the predominant regulation of prolactin secretion is negative, i.e., under ordinary basal condition the hypothalamus secretes one or more inhibitory hormones, the most important being dopamine, which are delivered to the pituitary via the hypothalamic portal system and inhibit the release of prolactin into the blood (see Chap. 321). Most factors that influence prolactin release do so by affecting the synthesis or release of the inhibiting factors. Basal prolactin levels fall following delivery, but prolactin secretion is enhanced by stimulation of the breasts such as the act of nursing (the so-called sucking reflex), a phenomenon that is probably mediated by the reflex release of oxytocin. In the postgestational state the normal woman is capable of forming about a liter of milk per day containing 38 g fat, 70 g lactose, and 12 g protein. Normal lactation can be suppressed by the administration of estrogens or diethylstilbestrol, which inhibit milk production by direct effects on the breast, or by the administration of bromocriptine, which inhibits prolactin secretion by the pituitary. Alternatively, if a woman does not nurse or empty her breasts post partum, lactation usually ceases of its own accord in 1 to 2 weeks.

GALACTORRHEA Exactly what constitutes nonpuerperal or inappropriate lactation is not always clearly defined in the literature. According to the studies of Friedman and Goldfein, it is not possible to demonstrate any breast secretion whatsoever in normal, regularly menstruating nulligravid women, but breast secretions can be demonstrated in a fourth of normal women who have been pregnant in the past; thus, breast secretions may be of no clinical significance in these instances. Spontaneous leakage of milk from the breasts is usually of more concern than milk that must be expressed. A second problem is related to the composition of the breast secretions. When the secretion is milky or white, it is safe to assume that it contains casein and lactose and is in fact milk; however, when the secretion is brown or greenish in color, it rarely contains normal milk constituents and consequently may not result from an underlying

FIGURE 332-1 *Endocrine control of female breast development and function at various stages of life.*

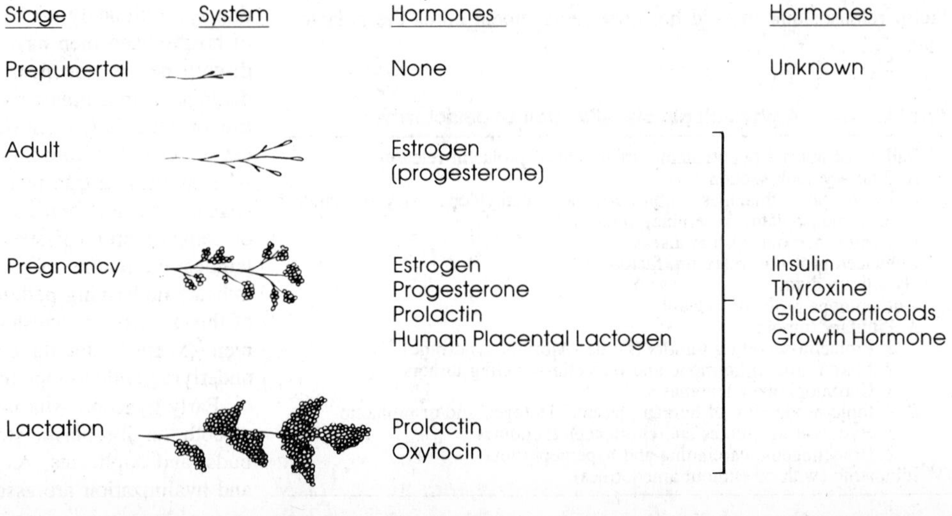

endocrinopathy. Furthermore, upon repeated sampling, the composition of milk carbohydrates and proteins may increase in a given individual from low, colostrum-like values to those typical of milk. Milky discharges must also be distinguished from blood or bloody secretions that may be present with neoplasms of the breast (see Chap. 295).

With these problems in mind galactorrhea can be defined as an inappropriate production of milk that is persistent or worrisome to the patient, recognizing that in some instances no underlying pathology will be demonstrated.

Since the action of a lactogenic hormone is a necessary requirement for the initiation of milk production, it is logical to consider galactorrhea as a manifestation of deranged prolactin physiology. However, as indicated above, a complex endocrinologic milieu is necessary for lactation, and in many instances in which prolactin is elevated both in women who have not been appropriately primed and in men, no production of milk takes place. As a consequence, hyperprolactinemia is more common than galactorrhea. Furthermore, although enhanced prolactin secretion is necessary for the initiation of milk formation, production can be maintained in the presence of minimally elevated or intermittently elevated prolactin levels so that basal plasma prolactin levels are not always elevated in patients with galactorrhea. For example, repeated stimulation of the nipples of women who have previously been pregnant can cause galactorrhea with minimal elevations of basal prolactin (the wet nurse phenomenon) similar to that in the normal nursing mother. Perhaps the strongest evidence that prolactin is always involved in galactorrhea is the fact that administration of bromocriptine, which suppresses plasma prolactin levels, causes a disappearance of galactorrhea even when the basal plasma prolactin levels are normal.

Differential diagnosis It is thus appropriate to consider galactorrhea as the result of a failure of the normal hypothalamic inhibition of prolactin release, of enhanced prolactin-releasing factor, or of autonomous prolactin secretion by tumors (Table 332-1). Pituitary stalk section in humans results in a striking increase in prolactin secretion, as the result of the inhibition of the delivery of prolactin inhibitory factors to the pituitary. Likewise, many drugs that influence the central nervous system (including virtually all psychotropic agents, methyldopa, reserpine, and antiemetics) result in enhanced prolactin release, presumably by inhibiting synthesis or release of dopamine or other prolactin inhibitory factors. Estrogens enhance prolactin levels by an uncertain mechanism. Extrapituitary central nervous system diseases can cause galactorrhea, presumably by interfering with delivery of the inhibitory factors to the pituitary (central nervous system sarcoidosis, craniopharyngioma, pinealoma, encephalitis, meningitis, hydrocephalus, hypothalamic tumors).

The existence of a physiologic prolactin-releasing factor is still a matter of controversy, but in at least one pathologic state, primary hypothyroidism, galactorrhea results from enhanced prolactin-releasing activity. Thyrotropin-releasing hormone (TRH) stimulates prolactin release, and thyroid hormone replacement cures the galactorrhea.

TABLE 332-1 A physiologic classification of galactorrhea

I Failure of normal hypothalamic inhibition of prolactin release
- *A* Pituitary stalk section
- *B* Drugs (phenothiazines, butyrophenones, methyldopa, tricyclic antidepressants, opiates, reserpine, verapamil)
- *C* Central nervous system disease

II Enhanced prolactin-releasing factor
- Hypothyroidism

III Autonomous prolactin release
- *A* Pituitary tumors
  - *1* Prolactin-secreting tumors (Forbes-Albright syndrome)
  - *2* Mixed growth hormone and prolactin-secreting tumors
  - *3* Chromophobe adenomas
- *B* Ectopic production of human placental lactogen and/or prolactin
  - *1* Hydatidiform moles and chorionephitheliomas
  - *2* Bronchogenic carcinoma and hypernephroma

IV Idiopathic (with or without amenorrhea)

Enhanced prolactin release can also occur from pituitary or nonpituitary tumors. Three types of pituitary tumors (see Chap. 321) may be associated with galactorrhea: pure prolactin-secreting tumors (micro- or macroadenomas), mixed tumors that secrete both growth hormone and prolactin and result in acromegaly with galactorrhea, and some chromophobe adenomas. The latter may either secrete prolactin or interfere with the delivery of inhibitory factors to the pituitary. Prolactin can also be secreted on occasion by other malignancies such as bronchogenic carcinoma, and hydatidiform moles and choriocarcinomas may secrete placental lactogen.

The known etiologies account for only a part of the cases of galactorrhea. In four published series totaling more than 500 carefully studied patients, a pituitary tumor was identified in about one-fourth of the patients, other known causes could be identified in another fourth or fifth, and the remaining half fall into the unknown category. Many patients may prove ultimately to have prolactin-secreting pituitary tumors, some probably have subtle disorders of hypothalamic function, and in others a drug-related cause may have been missed, but the fact remains that no satisfactory diagnosis is reached in half or more of patients. When normal menses and galactorrhea coexist, the likelihood of establishing a diagnosis is poor.

Galactorrhea is unusual in men, even in the presence of profound elevations of plasma prolactin; when it does occur, it is usually upon the background of a feminizing state (see below).

Diagnostic evaluation If hyperprolactinemia is present, the workup is fundamentally that of a pituitary tumor once drug causes and hypothyroidism are excluded (see Chap. 321). Even when a specific cause cannot be identified and a diagnosis of idiopathic galactorrhea is made by exclusion, it is necessary to remember that pituitary tumors may subsequently become manifest. The higher the prolactin values and the more persistent the galactorrhea, the greater the likelihood of such a development.

Treatment The aim of treatment is to remove the source of the elevated prolactin, and resection of pituitary tumor, cessation of causative drugs, or correction of hypothyroidism is often followed by the disappearance of galactorrhea. Two other forms of therapy may have some usefulness. Breast binders can be effective in some patients with mild galactorrhea of unknown etiology, presumably by preventing stimulation of the nipple and the consequent perpetuation of lactation. Bromocriptine, which suppresses plasma prolactin, has been used to treat patients with idiopathic hyperprolactinemia as well as patients with prolactin-secreting tumors of the pituitary. This drug not only suppresses lactation but may also cause resumption of normal menstrual cycles (and even fertility) in patients in whom amenorrhea accompanies galactorrhea.

GYNECOMASTIA A central issue in the evaluation of breast tissue in adult men is the separation of the normal from the abnormal. Whereas in autopsy data the incidence of active gynecomastia is between 5 and 9 percent, Nuttall and his colleagues have reported that approximately 40 percent of normal men and up to 70 percent of hospitalized men have palpable breast tissue. The reason for this discrepancy is not clear. On the one hand, it may be difficult to distinguish true breast tissue from masses of adipose tissue without true breast enlargement (lipomastia); in such cases true gynecomastia can be separated from lipomastia by mammography or by sonography. Alternatively, a true increase in the incidence of gynecomastia may have taken place, or the autopsy data may underestimate the frequency of palpable breast tissue. Regardless, we are left with major uncertainties; the finding of gynecomastia (in contrast to lipomastia) could indicate underlying pathology or a normal variant. For the purposes of this discussion, we shall assume that any palpable breast tissue in men (except for the three so-called physiologic states) may reflect an underlying endocrinopathy and deserves a limited evaluation.

Early gynecomastia is characterized by proliferation in the breast of both the fibroblastic stroma and the duct system, which elongates, buds, and duplicates. As gynecomastia persists, progressive fibrosis and hyalinization are associated with regression of epithelial proliferation. Eventually the number of ducts decreases. Resolution occurs by reduction in size and epithelial content with gradual disappearance of the ducts, leaving hyaline bands that eventually disappear.

Growth of the breast in men, as in women, is mediated by estrogen and results from disturbances of the normal ratio of active androgen to estrogen in plasma or within the breast itself. As described in Chap. 330 estradiol formation in the normal man occurs principally by the conversion of circulating androgens to estrogens in peripheral tissues; the normal ratio of production of testosterone to estradiol in adult men is approximately 100:1 (6 mg versus 45 μg), and the normal ratio of the two hormones in plasma is about 300:1. Feminization results when there is a significant decrease in this effective ratio, as the result of diminished testosterone production or action, enhanced estrogen formation, or both processes occurring simultaneously. The predominant manifestation of feminization in men is enlargement of the breasts.

Enlargement of the male breast can occur as a normal physiologic phenomenon at certain stages of life or as the result of a variety of pathologic conditions (Table 332-2).

Physiologic gynecomastia In the *newborn* transient enlargement of the breast results from the action of maternal and/or placental estrogens. The enlargement ordinarily disappears in a few weeks but may persist longer. *Adolescent* gynecomastia occurs in many boys at some time during puberty. The median age of onset is 14; it is often asymmetric, occasionally unilateral for a portion of its course, and frequently tender, and it regresses so that by age 20 only a small number of men have palpable vestiges of gynecomastia in one or both breasts. Although the origin of the excess estrogen has not been identified, the onset of gynecomastia correlates with transient elevations of plasma estradiol prior to the completion of puberty so that the androgen/estrogen ratio is altered. *Gynecomastia of aging* also occurs in otherwise healthy men. Forty percent or more of aged men have gynecomastia, as the result of true increase in frequency. A likely explanation is the elevation in plasma estrogen as the result of an increase with age in the conversion of androgens to estrogens in extraglandular tissues. Since abnormal liver function or drug therapy may be contributing causes to gynecomastia in such men, the significance of this finding in the aging man is uncertain.

Pathologic gynecomastia Pathologic gynecomastia can result from one of three basic mechanisms: deficiency in testosterone production or action (with or without a secondary increase in estrogen production), increase in estrogen production, or drugs (Table 332-2). Most of the individual disorders that cause primary and secondary testicular failure have been discussed in Chap. 330. The fact that a deficiency in testosterone production per se can cause gynecomastia is illustrated by the syndrome of congenital anorchia in which normal (or slightly low) estradiol production in the presence of profoundly decreased testosterone production results in florid gynecomastia. Such is the case in some patients with Klinefelter syndrome. In the inherited syndromes of androgen resistance, such as testicular feminization, deficient androgen action and increased testicular estrogen production are both present, although diminished androgen action is the more critical in inducing gynecomastia.

A primary increase in estrogen production can result from a variety of causes. Increased testicular estrogen secretion may result from elevations in plasma gonadotropins, for example, in cases of aberrant production of chorionic gonadotropin by testicular tumors or by bronchogenic carcinoma, from the ovarian elements in the gonads of men with true hermaphroditism, or as the result of direct secretion by testicular tumors (particularly interstitial cell and Sertoli cell tumors). Increased conversion of androgen to estrogens in peripheral tissues can either be due to increased availability of substrate for extraglandular estrogen formation or to increased amount of the enzymes of estrogen formation in peripheral tissues. Increased substrate availability for extraglandular conversion can result from increased production of androgens such as androstenedione (congenital adrenal hyperplasia, hyperthyroidism, and most feminizing adrenal tumors) or because of diminished catabolism of androstenedione by the usual pathways (liver disease). Increased amount of extraglandular aromatase can occur as the result of a rare hereditary abnormality or in tumors of the liver or adrenal gland.

The ingestion of drugs can cause gynecomastia by several mechanisms. Many drugs either act directly as estrogens or cause an increase in plasma estrogen activity, for example, in men receiving diethylstilbestrol for prostatic carcinoma and in transsexuals in preparation for sex-change operations. Boys and young men are particularly sensitive to estrogen and can develop gynecomastia after the use of dermal ointments containing estrogen or after the ingestion of milk or meat from estrogen-treated animals. The gynecomastia of digitalis ingestion is usually attributed to an estrogen-like side effect of the drug, but in the experience of the author it is usually associated with abnormal liver function tests. A second mechanism by which drugs can induce gynecomastia is illustrated by gonadotropin, such as from human chorionic gonadotropin (hCG)–secreting tumors, which causes enhanced testicular secretion of estrogen. Other drugs cause gynecomastia by interfering with testosterone synthesis (ketoconazole and alkylating agents) and/or testosterone action, for instance by blocking the binding of androgen to its cytosol receptor protein in target tissues (spironolactone and cimetidine). Finally, drugs that cause gynecomastia by mechanisms which have not been defined include busulfan, ethionamide, isoniazid, methyldopa, tricyclic antidepressants, penicillamine, and diazepam, marijuana, and heroin. In some instances the feminization is due to effects of the drugs on liver function.

Diagnostic evaluation The evaluation of patients with gynecomastia should include the following procedures: (1) a careful drug history; (2) measurement and examination of the testes (if both are small, a chromosomal karyotype should be obtained; if they are asymmetric, an evaluation for testicular tumor should be instituted); (3) an evaluation of liver function; (4) an endocrine evaluation to include measurement of serum androstenedione or 24-h urinary 17-ketosteroids (usually elevated in feminizing adrenal states), measurement of plasma estradiol (helpful if elevated but usually normal), and measurement of plasma luteinizing hormone (LH) and testosterone. If LH is high and testosterone is low, the diagnosis is usually testicular

TABLE 332-2 Differential diagnosis of gynecomastia

PHYSIOLOGIC GYNECOMASTIA
Newborn
Adolescence
Aging
PATHOLOGIC GYNECOMASTIA
Deficient production or action of testosterone:
Congenital anorchia
Klinefelter syndrome
Androgen resistance (testicular feminization and Reifenstein syndrome)
Defects in testosterone synthesis
Secondary testicular failure (viral orchitis, trauma, castration, neurologic and granulomatous diseases, renal failure)
Increased estrogen production:
Estrogen secretion:
True hermaphroditism
Testicular tumors
Carcinoma of the lung
Increased substrate for peripheral aromatase:
Adrenal disease
Liver disease
Starvation
Thyrotoxicosis
Increase in peripheral aromatase
Drugs:
Estrogens (diethylstilbestrol, birth control pills, digitalis)
Gonadotropins
Inhibitors of testosterone synthesis and/or action (ketoconazole, alkylating agents, spironolactone, cimetidine)
Unknown mechanisms (busulfan, ethionamide, isoniazid, methyldopa, tricyclic antidepressants, penicillamine, diazepam, marijuana, heroin)
Idiopathic

failure; if LH and testosterone are both low, the diagnosis is most likely increased primary estrogen production (for example, a Sertoli cell tumor of the testis); and if both LH and testosterone are elevated, the diagnosis is either an androgen-resistance state or a gonadotropin-secreting tumor.

Using these various tests a satisfactory diagnosis can be made in only half or fewer of the patients referred for gynecomastia. This implies either that the diagnostic techniques are not sufficiently refined to recognize mild disturbances, that many causes of gynecomastia are as yet undefined, that the causes may be transient and difficult to diagnose, or, as suggested by Nuttall, that gynecomastia may in some instances be normal rather than due to a pathologic state. Because of the problem of separating the normal from the pathologic, gynecomastia should probably be routinely worked up only if the drug history is negative, if the breast is tender (indicating rapid growth), or if the breast mass is larger than 4 cm in diameter. In other instances a decision to perform an endocrine evaluation depends on the clinical context. For example, all gynecomastia associated with signs of underandrogenization should be evaluated.

Treatment When the primary cause of the overestrogenization can be identified and corrected, the breast enlargement usually subsides promptly and eventually disappears. However, if the gynecomastia is of long duration (and fibrosis has replaced the original ductal hyperplasia), correction of the primary defect may not be followed by improvement. In such instances and when the primary cause cannot be corrected, surgery is the only effective therapy. Indications for surgery include several psychologic and/or cosmetic problems, continued growth, or a suspected malignancy. Although the relative risk of carcinoma of the breast is increased in men with gynecomastia, it is rare nevertheless. Prophylactic radiation of the breasts prior to the institution of diethylstilbestrol therapy is effective in preventing gynecomastia and has a low complication rate in elderly men. In rare patients who have painful gynecomastia and who are not candidates for other therapy, treatment with antiestrogens such as tamoxifen may be indicated.

REFERENCES

Galactorrhea

ADLER RA: The evaluation of galactorrhea. Am J Obstet Gynecol 127:569, 1977

CHOTINER HC et al: Lactose and casein content of nonpuerperal breast secretion. J Reprod Med 22:267, 1979

DAVAJAN V: The significance of galactorrhea in patients with normal menses, oligomenorrhea, and secondary amenorrhea. Am J Obstet Gynecol 130:894, 1978

FRANTZ AG, WILSON JD: Endocrine disorders of the breast, in *Williams' Textbook of Endocrinology*, 7th ed, JD Wilson, DW Foster (eds): Philadelphia, Saunders, 1985, pp 402–421

FRIEDMAN S, GOLDFEIN A: Breast secretions in normal women. Am J Obstet Gynecol 104:846, 1969

GOMEZ F et al: Nonpuerperal galactorrhea and hyperprolactinemia. Am J Med 62:648, 1977

KLEINBERG DL et al: Galactorrhea: A study of 235 cases, including 48 with pituitary tumors. N Engl J Med 296:589, 1977

KULSKI JK et al: Changes in the milk composition of nonpuerperal women. Am J Obstet Gynecol 139:597, 1981

PARKES D: Bromocriptine. N Engl J Med 301:873, 1979

TOLTS G: Prolactin: Physiology and pathology. Hosp Prac February 1980, p 85

TURKSOY RN et al: Diagnostic and therapeutic modalities in women with galactorrhea. Obstet Gynecol 56:323, 1980

Gynecomastia

ANDERSON JA, GROOM JB: Male breast at autopsy. Acta Pathol Microbiol Immunol Scand 90:191, 1982

CARLSON HE: Gynecomastia. N Engl J Med 303:795, 1980

CIMORA GA et al: Percutaneous oestrogen-induced gynecomastia: A case report. Br J Plast Surg 35:209, 1982

FRANTZ AG, WILSON JD: Endocrine disorders of the breast, in *Williams' Textbook of Endocrinology*, 7th ed, JD Wilson, DW Foster (eds). Philadelphia, Saunders, 1985, pp 402–421

GAGNON JD et al: Pre-estrogen breast irradiation for patients with carcinoma of the prostate: A critical review. J Urol 121:182, 1979

JEFFREYS DB: Painful gynecomastia treated with tamoxifen. Br Med J, April 1979, p 1119

NIEWOEHNER CV, NUTTAL FQ: Gynecomastia in a hospitalized male population. Am J Med 77:633, 1984

NUTTAL FQ: Gynecomastia as a physical finding in normal men. J Clin Endocrinol Metab 48:338, 1979

PORT A et al: Ketoconazole blocks testosterone synthesis. Arch Intern Med 142:2137, 1982

SATIANI B et al: Cancer of the male breast: A thirty-year experience. Am Surg 44:86, 1978

333 DISORDERS OF SEXUAL DIFFERENTIATION

JEAN D. WILSON / JAMES E. GRIFFIN III

Sexual differentiation is a sequential and ordered process. *Chromosomal sex,* which is established at the moment of fertilization, determines *gonadal sex,* and *gonadal sex* in turn causes the development of *phenotypic sex* in which the male or female urogenital tract is formed (Table 333-1). A disturbance during embryogenesis of any step in this developmental process may result in a disorder of sexual differentiation. Known causes of abnormalities in sexual development include environmental insults as in the ingestion of a virilizing drug during pregnancy, nonfamilial aberrations of the sex chromosomes as in 45,X gonadal dysgenesis, developmental birth defects of multifactorial etiology as in most cases of hypospadias, and hereditary disorders resulting from single gene mutations as in the testicular feminization syndrome.

Limitations of knowledge make it necessary to make empiric assignments as to the nature of the physiologic derangement in certain disorders. Nevertheless, a specific diagnosis can usually be made as the result of combined genetic, phenotypic, and chromosomal assessment. As a consequence appropriate gender assignment can be made, even in extreme instances of ambiguous genitalia, and tailoring of the phenotype can be undertaken when appropriate.

NORMAL SEXUAL DIFFERENTIATION

The first process in sexual differentiation is the establishment of chromosomal sex, the heterogametic sex (XY) being male and the homogametic sex (XX) female. The embryos of both sexes then develop in an identical fashion until approximately 40 days of gestation. The second phase of sexual differentiation is the conversion of the indifferent gonad into a testis or an ovary. The differentiation of the indifferent gonad into a testis is mediated by gene(s) on the Y chromosome, one of which is either identical to or closely linked to a gene that specifies the HY antigen. The final process, the translation of gonadal sex into phenotypic sex, is the direct consequence of the type of gonad formed and the endocrine secretions of the fetal gonads.

TABLE 333-1 Classification of disorders of sexual development in human beings

Disorders of chromosomal sex:
- Klinefelter syndrome
- XX male
- Gonadal dysgenesis
- Mixed gonadal dysgenesis
- True hermaphroditism

Disorders of gonadal sex:
- Pure gonadal dysgenesis
- Absent testis syndrome

Disorders of phenotypic sex:
- Female pseudohermaphroditism:
  - Congenital adrenal hyperplasia
  - Nonadrenal female pseudohermaphroditism
  - Developmental disorders of müllerian ducts
- Male pseudohermaphroditism:
  - Abnormalities in androgen synthesis
  - Abnormalities in androgen action
  - Persistent müllerian duct syndrome
  - Development defects of male genitalia

The development of phenotypic sex results in the formation of the male and female urogenital tracts.

The internal genitalia are derived from the wolffian and müllerian ducts that exist side by side in early embryos of both sexes (Fig. 333-1*A*). In the male the wolffian ducts give rise to the epididymides, vasa deferentia, and seminal vesicles, and the müllerian ducts disappear. In the female the fallopian tubes, uterus, and upper vagina are derived from the müllerian ducts, and the wolffian ducts regress. The external genitalia and urethra in the two sexes develop from common anlage—the urogenital sinus and the genital tubercle, folds, and swellings (Fig. 333-1*B*). The urogenital sinus gives rise to the prostate and prostatic urethra in the male and to the urethra and a portion of the vagina in the female. The genital tubercle is the origin of the glans penis in the male and clitoris in the female. The urogenital swellings become the scrotum or the labia majora, and the genital folds develop into the labia minora or fuse to form the male urethra and the shaft of the penis.

In the absence of the testis, as in the normal female or in the male embryo castrated prior to the onset of phenotypic differentiation, the development of phenotypic sex proceeds along female lines. Thus, masculinization of the fetus is the positive result of action of hormones from the fetal gonad, whereas female development does not require the presence of a gonad. Development of the sexual phenotype normally conforms to the chromosomal sex. That is, chromosomal sex determines gonadal sex, and gonadal sex in turn controls phenotypic sex.

The formation of the male phenotype is vested in the action of three hormones. Two—müllerian-inhibiting substance and testosterone—are secretory products of the fetal testis. Müllerian-inhibiting substance is a protein hormone that acts to suppress the müllerian ducts and consequently prevents development of the uterus and fallopian tubes in the male. Testosterone acts directly to stimulate differentiation of the wolffian duct derivatives and is the precursor for the third fetal hormone, dihydrotestosterone (see Chap. 330).

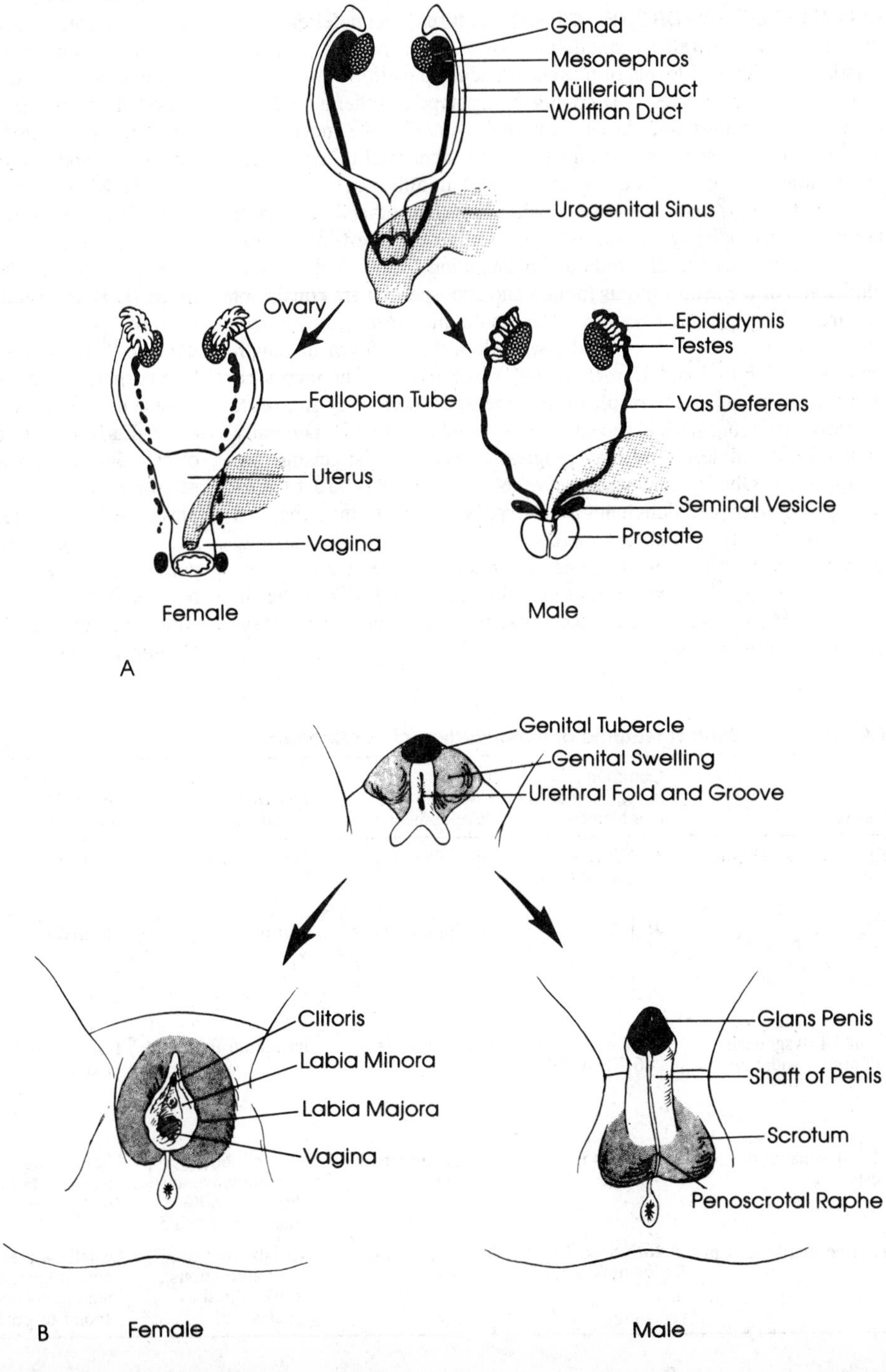

FIGURE 333-1 *Normal sexual differentiation. A. Internal genitalia. B. External genitalia.*

Dihydrotestosterone, which is formed from circulating testosterone, acts to induce formation of the male urethra and prostate and to cause formation of the penis and scrotum. Thus, testosterone and dihydrotestosterone function during fetal life to induce formation of the accessory organs of male reproduction by the same intracellular machinery by which they act in differentiated tissues (Chap. 330).

The secretion of testosterone by the fetal testis approaches a maximum by the eighth to tenth week of gestation, and formation of the sexual phenotypes is largely completed by the end of the first trimester. During the latter phases of gestation ovarian follicular development and maturation of the vagina occur in the female, and descent of the testes and growth of the external genitalia take place in the male.

DISORDERS OF CHROMOSOMAL SEX

Disorders of chromosomal sex (Table 333-2) occur when the number or structure of the X or Y chromosomes is abnormal (see Chap. 60).

KLINEFELTER SYNDROME Clinical features Klinefelter syndrome is characterized by small, firm testes, azoospermia, gynecomastia, and elevated levels of plasma gonadotropins in men with two or more X chromosomes. The common karyotype is either a 47,XXY chromosomal pattern (the classic form) or 46,XY/47,XXY mosaicism. The disorder is the most frequent major abnormality of sexual differentiation, the incidence being around 1 in 500 men.

Prepubertally, patients have small testes but otherwise appear normal. After puberty the disorder is manifest as infertility, gynecomastia, or occasionally underandrogenization (Table 333-3). Hyalinization of the seminiferous tubules and azoospermia are consistent features of the 47,XXY variety. The small, firm testes are characteristically less than 2.0 cm and always less than 3.5 cm in length (corresponding to 2 and 12 mL volume, respectively). The increased mean body height is the result of an increased lower body segment. Gynecomastia ordinarily appears during adolescence, is generally bilateral and painless, and may progress to become disfiguring (see Chap. 332). Obesity and varicose veins occur in one-third to one-half, and mild mental deficiency, social maladjustment, abnormalities of thyroid function, diabetes mellitus, and pulmonary disease may be more common than in the general population. The risk of breast cancer is 20 times that of normal men (but only about a fifth that in women). Most have a male psychosexual orientation and function sexually as normal men.

The mosaic variant comprises about 10 percent of the patients, as estimated by chromosomal karyotypes on peripheral blood leukocytes. The frequency of this variant may be underestimated since chromosomal mosaicism may be present only in the testes in subjects whose peripheral leukocyte karotype is normal. The mosaic form is usually not as severe as the 47,XXY variety, and the testes may be normal in size (Table 333-3). The endocrine abnormalities are also less severe, and gynecomastia and azoospermia are less common. Indeed, occasional patients with mosaicism may be fertile. In some the diagnosis may not even be suspected because of the minor degree of the physical abnormalities.

Approximately 30 additional karyotypic varieties of Klinefelter syndrome have been described, including those with uniform cell lines (such as XXYY, XXXY, and XXXXY) and a variety of mosaicisms of the X chromosome with or without associated structural abnormalities of the X. In general, the greater the degree of chromosomal abnormality (and in mosaic forms the more cell lines that are abnormal), the more severe the manifestations.

Pathophysiology The classic form is due to meiotic nondisjunction of the chromosomes during gametogenesis (Fig. 333-2). About 40 percent of the responsible meiotic nondisjunctions occur during spermatogenesis, and 60 percent occur during oogenesis. Advanced maternal age is a predisposing factor. The mosaic form is thought to result from chromosomal mitotic nondisjunction after fertilization of the zygote and can take place either in a 46,XY zygote (Fig. 333-2) or a 47,XXY zygote. The latter defect or double nondisjunction (meiotic and mitotic) may be the usual cause and thus explain why the mosaic form is less frequent than the classic disorder.

Plasma follicle-stimulating hormone (FSH) and luteinizing hormone (LH) are usually high; FSH shows the best discrimination, and little overlap occurs with normals, a consequence of the consistent damage to the seminiferous tubules. The plasma testosterone averages half normal, but the range of values overlaps the normal range. Mean plasma estradiol levels are elevated, the cause of which is not entirely clear. Early in the course, the testes may secrete increased amounts of estradiol in response to the elevated plasma LH, but the testicular secretion of estradiol (and testosterone) eventually declines. Elevated plasma estradiol late in the course is probably due to a combination of a decreased metabolic clearance rate and an increased rate of conversion of testosterone to estradiol in extraglandular tissues. The net result both early and late is a variable degree of insufficient androgenization and enhanced feminization. The feminization, including gynecomastia, depends on the ratio of circulating estrogen

TABLE 333-2 Clinical features of the disorders of chromosomal sex

Disorder	Common chromosomal complement	Gonadal development	External genitalia	Internal genitalia	Breast development	Comment
Klinefelter syndrome	47,XXY *or* 46,XY/47,XXY	Hyalinized testes	Normal male	Normal male	Gynecomastia	Most common disorder of sexual differentiation; tall stature.
XX male	46,XX	Hyalinized testes	Normal male	Normal male	Gynecomastia	Shorter than normal men; increased incidence of hypospadias. Similar to Klinefelter syndrome. May be familial.
Gonadal dysgenesis (Turner syndrome)	45,X *or* 46,XX/45,X	Streak gonads	Immature female	Hypoplastic female	Immature female	Short stature and multiple somatic abnormalities. May be 46,XX with structurally abnormal X chromosome.
Mixed gonadal dysgenesis	46,XY/45,X *or* 46,XY	Testis and streak gonad	Variable but almost always ambiguous; 60% reared as female	Uterus, vagina, and one fallopian tube	Usually male	Second most common cause of ambiguous genitalia in the newborn; tumors common.
True hermaphroditism	46,XX *or* 46,XY *or* mosaics	Testis and ovary or ovotestis	Variable but usually ambiguous; 60% reared as males	Usually a uterus and urogenital sinus; ducts correspond to gonad	Gynecomastia in 75%	May be familial.

TABLE 333-3 Characteristics of patients with classic versus mosaic Klinefelter syndrome*

	47,XXY, %	46,XY/47,XXY, %
Abnormal testicular histology	100	94†
Decreased length of testis	99	73†
Azoospermia	93	50†
Decreased testosterone	79	33
Decreased facial hair	77	64
Increased gonadotropins	75	33†
Decreased sexual function	68	56
Gynecomastia	55	33†
Decreased axillary hair	49	46
Decreased length of penis	41	21

* *Table based on 519 XXY patients and 51 XY/XXY patients.*
† *Significantly different at p <.05 or better.*
SOURCE: *After Gordon et al.*

to androgen (relative or absolute), and subjects with lower plasma testosterone and higher plasma estradiol levels are more likely to develop gynecomastia (see Chap. 332). The increase in plasma gonadotropins after the administration of luteinizing hormone–releasing hormone (LHRH) is exaggerated after the age of expected puberty, and the normal feedback inhibition of testosterone on pituitary LH secretion is diminished. Subjects with untreated Klinefelter syndrome may have "reactive pituitary abnormalities" in the form of enlarged or abnormal sella turcicas, presumably secondary to the persistent lack of gonadal feedback and hypertrophy of the gonadotrophes in response to stimulation by LHRH. It is not known whether actual adenoma formation occurs.

Management No method is available for reversing the infertility, and surgical removal is the only means for effective treatment of the gynecomastia. Some underandrogenized patients benefit from supplemental androgen, but such treatment may paradoxically worsen the gynecomastia, presumably by providing increased androgen substrate for the conversion to estrogens in the peripheral tissues. Androgen should be administered in the form of testosterone cypionate or testosterone enanthate. Following the administration of testosterone, plasma LH returns to normal only after several months, if at all.

XX MALE SYNDROME The incidence of a 46,XX karyotype in phenotypic males is approximately 1 in 20,000 to 24,000 male births. Affected individuals have absence of all female internal genitalia and male psychosexual identification. Indeed, the findings resemble those in the Klinefelter syndrome: the testes are small and firm (generally less than 2 cm), gynecomastia is frequent, the penis is normal to small in size, azoospermia and hyalinization of the seminiferous tubules are usual, mean plasma testosterone is low, plasma estradiol is elevated, and plasma gonadotropin levels are high. Affected individuals differ from typical Klinefelter patients only in that average height is less than in normal men, the incidence of mental deficiency is not increased, and the incidence of hypospadias is increased.

Four theories have been proposed to explain the pathogenesis of this disorder: (1) translocation of a portion of a Y chromosome to the X chromosome, (2) mosaicism for a Y chromosome in some cell lines or early loss of a Y chromosome, (3) mutation of an autosomal gene, or (4) deletion of genetic material on X chromosome that normally has a negative regulatory effect on testis development. Although some evidence has been marshalled to support each of these four possibilities in individual XX males, no unifying hypothesis can explain the disorder. While mosaicism appears to be unlikely in most cases, the other listed explanations remain possible. The etiology may be heterogeneous. The management of the disorder is similar to that of Klinefelter syndrome.

GONADAL DYSGENESIS (TURNER SYNDROME) Clinical features Gonadal dysgenesis is characterized by primary amenorrhea, sexual infantilism, short stature, multiple congenital anomalies, and bilateral streak gonads in phenotypic women with any of several defects of the X chromosome. This condition should be distinguished from (1) mixed gonadal dysgenesis in which a unilateral testis and a contralateral streak gonad are present; (2) pure gonadal dysgenesis in which bilateral streak gonads are associated with a normal 46,XX or 46,XY karyotype, normal stature, and primary amenorrhea; and (3) the Noonan syndrome, an autosomal dominant disorder of males and females characterized by webbed neck, short stature, congenital heart disease, cubitus valgus, and other congenital defects despite normal karyotypes and normal gonads.

The incidence is estimated at 1 in 2500 newborn females. The diagnosis is either made at birth because of the associated anomalies or more frequently at puberty when amenorrhea and failure of sexual development are noted in conjunction with the associated anomalies. Gonadal dysgenesis is the most common cause of primary amenorrhea, accounting for a third of such patients. The external genitalia are unambiguously female but remain immature, and there is no breast development unless the patient is treated with exogenous estrogen. The internal genitalia consist of infantile fallopian tubes and uterus and bilateral streak gonads located in the broad ligaments. Primordial germ cells are present transiently during embryogenesis but disappear as the result of an accelerated rate of atresia (see Chap. 331). After the age of expected puberty these streaks lack identifiable follicles and ova but contain fibrous tissue that is indistinguishable from normal ovarian stroma.

The associated somatic anomalies primarily involve the skeleton and connective tissue. Lymphedema of the hands and feet, webbing of the neck, low hair line, redundant skin folds on the back of the neck, a shield-like chest with widely spaced nipples, and a low birth weight are features that suggest the diagnosis in infancy. In addition, the facies may be characterized by micrognathia, epicanthal folds, prominent low-set or deformed ears, a fishlike mouth, and ptosis. Short fourth metacarpals are present in half, and 10 to 20 percent have coarctation of the aorta. In adults the average height rarely exceeds 150 cm. Associated conditions include renal malformations, pigmented nevi, hypoplastic nails, tendency to keloid formation, perceptive hearing loss, unexplained hypertension, and autoimmune disorders. Frank hypothyroidism is present in 20 percent.

Pathophysiology About half have a 45,X karyotype, approximately one-fourth have mosaicism with no structural abnormality (46,XX/45,X), and the remainder have a structurally abnormal X chromosome with or without mosaicism (see Chap. 60). The 45,X variety may result from chromosome loss during gametogenesis in either parent or a mitotic error during one of the early cleavage divisions of the fertilized zygote (Fig. 333-2). Short stature and other somatic features result from loss of genetic material on the short arm of the X chromosome. Streak gonads result when genetic material is missing from either the long or short arm of the X. In individuals with mosaicism or with structural abnormalities of the X, phenotypes on average are intermediate in severity between that seen in the 45,X variety and the normal. In some patients with hypertrophy of the clitoris, there is an unidentified fragment of a chromosome present in addition to the X chromosome, assumed to be an abnormal Y. Rarely, familial transmission of gonadal dysgenesis can be the result of a balanced X-autosome translocation (see Chap. 60).

Assessment of sex chromatin was previously utilized as a means of screening for abnormalities of the X chromosome. Sex chromatin (the Barr body) in normal women is the result of inactivation of one of two X chromosomes, and women with a 45,X chromosome composition like normal men are said to be chromatin-negative. However, only about half of patients with gonadal dysgenesis (those with 45,X and those with the most extreme mosaicism and structural abnormalities) are chromatin-negative, and analysis of chromosomal karotype is necessary to establish the diagnosis and to identify the fraction with Y chromosomal elements and a high chance of developing malignancy in the streak gonads.

Sparse pubic and axillary hair develop at the time of expected puberty, the breasts remain infantile, and no menses occur. Serum FSH is elevated in infancy, falls during midchildhood to the normal range, and increases to castrate levels at the age of 9 or 10. At this time, serum LH is also elevated, and plasma estradiol levels are low (<10 pg/mL). Approximately 2 percent of 45,X subjects and 12 percent of mosaic subjects have sufficient residual follicles to allow some menstruation. Indeed, occasional pregnancy has been reported in minimally affected individuals; the reproductive life in such individuals is brief.

Management At the anticipated time of puberty replacement therapy with estrogen should be instituted to induce maturation of the breasts, labia, vagina, uterus, and fallopian tubes (see Chap. 331). Linear growth and bone maturation rates are approximately doubled during the first year of treatment with estradiol, but the eventual height of patients rarely approaches the predicted height (see Chap. 331). Treatment with growth hormone has not been helpful.

Gonadal tumors are rare in 45,X patients but have occurred in several patients with mosaicism involving the Y chromosome; consequently, streak gonads should be removed in any patient with evidence of virilization or a Y-containing cell line.

MIXED GONADAL DYSGENESIS **Clinical features** Mixed gonadal dysgenesis is an entity in which phenotypic males or females have a testis on one side and streak gonad on the other. Most have 45,X/46,XY mosaicism, but the clinical entity is not confined to that chromosomal pattern. The incidence is unknown, but in most hospitals it is the second most common cause of ambiguous genitalia in the neonate after congenital adrenal hyperplasia.

About two-thirds are reared as females, and most phenotypic males are incompletely virilized at birth. The majority have ambiguous genitalia, including some degree of phallic enlargement, a urogenital sinus, and varying degrees of labioscrotal fusion. In most the testis is located intraabdominally; individuals with a testis in the inguinal or scrotal position are usually reared as males. A uterus, vagina, and at least one fallopian tube are almost invariably present.

The prepubertal testis appears relatively normal. The postpubertal testis contains abundant mature Leydig cells, but the seminiferous tubules lack germinal elements and contain only Sertoli cells. The streak gonad, a thin, pale, elongated structure located either in the broad ligament or along the pelvic wall, is composed of ovarian stroma. At puberty the testis secretes androgen, and virilization and phallic enlargement both occur. Feminization is rare; when it occurs, estrogen secretion from a gonadal tumor should be suspected.

Approximately a third exhibit the somatic features of 45,X gonadal dysgenesis, i.e., low posterior hairline, shield chest, multiple pigmented nevi, cubitus valgus, webbing of the neck, and short stature (height less than 150 cm).

Virtually all are chromatin-negative. In one series, two-thirds had the 45,X/46,XY karyotype, and in the remainder a 46,XY karyotype was present but mosaicism might have gone undetected or been limited to certain cell lines. The origin of 45,X/46,XY mosaicism is best explained by the loss of a Y chromosome during an early mitotic division of an XY zygote similar to the postulated loss of the X chromosome in the 46,XY/47,XXY mosaicism shown in Fig. 333-2.

Pathophysiology It has been assumed that the 46,XY cell line stimulates testicular differentiation whereas the 45,X stem leads to the development of the contralateral streak gonad, but actual comparisons between karyotype and phenotypic expression have failed to substantiate such a relationship. Furthermore, no clear correlation has been found between the percentage of cells cultured from blood or skin containing 45,X or 46,XY and the degree of gonadal development or of somatic anomalies.

Both masculinization and müllerian duct regression in utero are incomplete. Since Leydig cell function is normal at puberty, inadequate virilization in utero may be the result of delayed development of a testis that is ultimately capable of normal Leydig cell function. Alternatively, the fetal testis may simply be incapable of synthesizing adequate amounts of müllerian-inhibiting substance and androgen.

Management For the older child or adult in whom gender is fixed prior to diagnosis, the central issue in management is the possibility of tumor development in the gonads. The overall incidence of gonadal tumors is about 25 percent. Seminomas occur more frequently than gonadoblastomas, and the tumors may occur prior to puberty. The tumors occur most frequently in patients with a female phenotype who lack the somatic features typical of 45,X gonadal dysgenesis and are more common in intraabdominal testes than in the streak gonad. When the diagnosis is established in phenotypic females, early exploratory laparotomy and prophylactic gonadectomy should be undertaken both because gonadal tumors may occur in childhood and because the testis secretes androgen at puberty and thus causes virilization. Such subjects, like those with gonadal dysgenesis, are then given estrogen to induce and maintain feminization.

When the diagnosis is established in phenotypic males during late childhood or in adults the management is more complicated. Phenotypic males with mixed gonadal dysgenesis are infertile (no germinal elements are present in the testes) and also have a high risk of developing gonadal tumors. Which testes can be safely conserved? In general the following observations apply: (1) tumors develop in scrotal streak gonads but not in scrotal testes, (2) tumors that develop in intraabdominal testes are always associated with ipsilateral müllerian duct structures, and (3) tumors in streak gonads are always associated with tumors in the contralateral abdominal testis. Based on these observations, it is recommended that (1) all streak gonads should be removed, (2) scrotal testes should be preserved, and (3) intraabdominal testes should be excised unless they can be

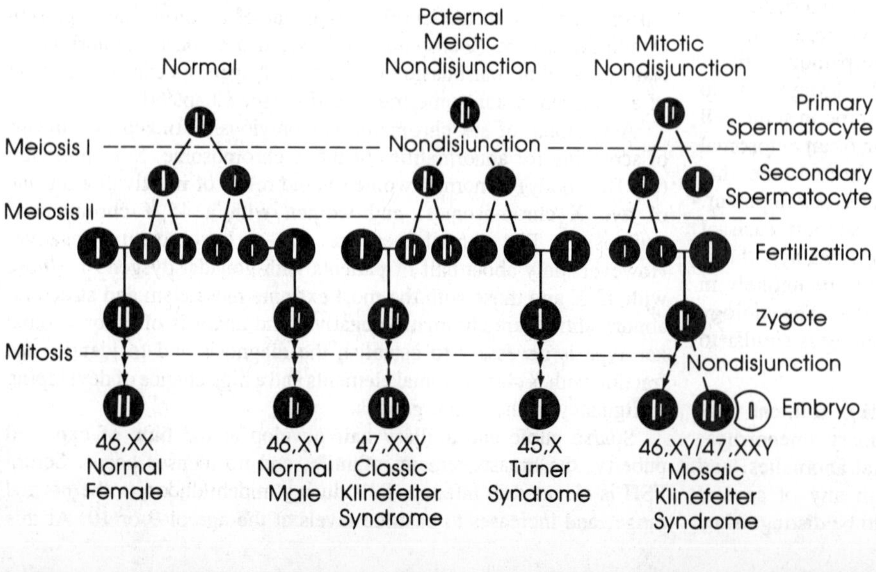

FIGURE 333-2 *Schema for normal spermatogenesis and fertilization showing effects of meiotic and mitotic nondisjunction leading to classic Klinefelter syndrome, Turner syndrome, and mosaic Klinefelter. The schema would be similar if the abnormal events took place during oogenesis.*

relocated in the scrotum and are not associated with ipsilateral müllerian duct structures. Decisions as to reconstructive surgery of the phallus depend upon the nature of the defect.

When the diagnosis is established in early infancy and the genitalia are ambiguous, gender assignment is usually female. Resection of the enlarged phallus and gonadectomy can then be accomplished in infancy, usually in one procedure. If the decision is for male gender assignment, the same criteria apply as to which testes should be removed in infants as in older males.

TRUE HERMAPHRODITISM Clinical features True hermaphroditism is a condition in which both an ovary and a testis or a gonad with histologic features of both (ovotestis) is present. To justify the diagnosis there must be histologic documentation of both types of gonadal epithelium, the presence of ovarian stroma without oocytes not being sufficient. The incidence is unknown, but more than 400 cases have been reported. Three categories are recognized: (1) one-fifth are bilateral—testicular and ovarian tissue (ovotestes) on each side, (2) two-fifths are unilateral—an ovotestis on one side and an ovary or a testis on the other, and (3) the remainder are lateral—a testis on one side and an ovary on the other.

The external genitalia display all gradations of the male-to-female spectrum. Two-thirds are sufficiently masculinized to be reared as males. However, less than one-tenth have normal male external genitalia; most have hypospadias, and more than half have incomplete labioscrotal fusion. Two-thirds of phenotypic females have an enlarged clitoris, and most have a urogenital sinus. Differentiation of the internal ducts usually corresponds to the adjacent gonad. Although an epididymis usually develops adjacent to a testis, development of the vas deferens is complete in only one-third. Of the patients with an ovotestis, three-fourths have an epididymis, two-thirds have a fallopian tube, one-tenth have a vas deferens, and one-tenth have both a vas deferens and a fallopian tube. A uterus is usually present although it may be hypoplastic or unicornuate. The ovary usually occupies the normal position, but the testis or ovotestis may be found at any level along the route of embryonic testicular descent, frequently associated with an inguinal hernia. Testicular tissue is present in the scrotum or the labioscrotal fold in one-third, in the inguinal canal in one-third, and in the abdominal area in one-third.

Variable feminization and virilization develop at puberty, three-fourths develop gynecomastia, and about half menstruate. In phenotypic men menstruation presents as cyclic hematuria. Ovulation occurs in approximately one-fourth and is more common than spermatogenesis. In men ovulation may present as testicular pain. Fertility has been reported in women following removal of an ovotestis and in a man who fathered two children. Congenital malformations of other systems are rare.

Pathophysiology About two-thirds of subjects have a 46,XX karyotype, a tenth have a 46,XY karyotype, and the remainder are chromosomal mosaics in which a Y cell line is present. The mechanism responsible for the gonadal development is unknown. Even if not demonstrable with conventional karyotyping methods, it is assumed that sufficient genetic material derived from the Y chromosome is present (as the result of translocation, nondisjunction, or mutation) to induce the development of testicular tissue. In rare instances multiple sibs with a 46,XX karyotype are affected, possibly the result of an autosomal recessive gene or a common translocation.

Because corpora lutea are present in the ovaries of more than one-fourth of subjects, it can be deduced that a female neuroendocrine axis is present and functions normally in such individuals. Feminization (gynecomastia and menstruation) is the result of secretion of estradiol by the ovarian tissue present. In masculinized patients secretion of androgen predominates over secretion of estrogen, and some produce sperm.

Management When the diagnosis is made in a newborn or early infant, gender assignment depends upon the anatomic findings. In older children and adults gonads and internal duct structures that are contradictory to the predominant phenotype (and the gender of rearing) should be removed, and when necessary the external genitalia should be modified appropriately. Although gonadal tumors are rare in true hermaphroditism, a gonadoblastoma has been reported in an individual with an XY cell line. Consequently, the possibility of future tumor development must be taken into account when the decision regarding conservation of gonadal tissue is made.

DISORDERS OF GONADAL SEX

Disorders of gonadal sex result when chromosomal sex is normal, but for one of several reasons differentiation of the gonads is abnormal. Thus, chromosomal sex does not correspond to gonadal and phenotypic sex.

PURE GONADAL DYSGENESIS Clinical features Pure gonadal dysgenesis is a disorder in which phenotypic females with gonads and genitalia identical to those with gonadal dysgenesis (bilateral streaks, infantile uterus and fallopian tubes, and sexual infantilism) have normal height, few if any congenital anomalies, and either a normal 46,XX or 46,XY karyotype. This disorder is only about one-tenth as common as gonadal dysgenesis. On genetic grounds this can be considered a separate disorder from gonadal dysgenesis, but it cannot be distinguished clinically from those instances of gonadal dysgenesis associated with minimal somatic abnormalities. The height is normal or greater than normal, some subjects being over 170 cm. Estrogen deficiency varies from profound deficiency typical of 45,X gonadal dysgenesis to some breast development and appearance of menses that terminate in an early menopause. About 40 percent have some feminization. Axillary and pubic hair are scanty, and the internal genitalia consist of müllerian derivatives only.

Tumors may develop in the streak gonads, particularly dysgerminoma or gonadoblastoma in the 46,XY disorder. Such tumors are frequently heralded by the development of virilizing signs or a pelvic mass.

Pathophysiology Although chromosomal mosaicisms have been described under this nosology, the designation here is restricted to subjects with uniform 46,XX or 46,XY karyotypes. (Those with mosaicism are variants of gonadal dysgenesis or mixed gonadal dysgenesis as described above.) The rationale for this restricted definition is based upon the fact that both the XX and XY varieties can result from single gene mutations. Several sibships have been reported in which more than one individual is affected with the 46,XX type of the disorder, frequently the result of consanguineous matings, suggesting an autosomal recessive pattern of inheritance. Familial occurrence of the 46,XY variety has also been described; in some the mutation appears to be inherited in an X-linked recessive pattern, while in other families the occurrence is compatible with a male-limited autosomal recessive inheritance. In both the 46,XX and the 46,XY forms the mutation prevents differentiation of ovary or testis, respectively, by an uncertain mechanism; the development of the female phenotype is the consequence of the failure of gonadal development. As in all individuals with nonfunctional gonads, gonadotropin secretion is elevated and estrogen secretion is low.

Management The management of the estrogen deficiency is identical to that in gonadal dysgenesis, namely appropriate estrogen replacement therapy is initiated at the time of expected puberty and maintained in adult life (see Chap. 331). Because of the high frequency of gonadal tumors in the 46,XY variety, exploratory surgery and removal of the streak gonads should be undertaken once the diagnosis is made. The development of virilizing signs is indication for immediate surgery. The natural history of the gonadal tumors in this disorder is uncertain, but the prognosis after surgical removal is usually good.

THE ABSENT TESTES SYNDROME (ANORCHIA, TESTICULAR REGRESSION, GONADAL AGENESIS, AGONADISM) Clinical features A spectrum of phenotypes has been described in 46,XY males with absent or rudimentary testes but in whom unequivocal evidence exists that endocrine function of the testis (e.g., invariable müllerian duct regression and variable testosterone synthesis) was present at some time during embryonic life. This rare disorder can be distinguished from pure gonadal dysgenesis in which no evidence can be inferred for gonadal function during embryonic development. The disorder varies in its manifestations from complete failure of virilization through varying degrees of incomplete virilization of the external genitalia to otherwise normal males with bilateral anorchia.

The purest form is represented by 46,XY phenotypic females with absent testes, sexual infantilism, and absence of both müllerian duct derivatives and accessory organs of male reproduction. Such individuals differ from the 46,XY form of pure gonadal dysgenesis in that no gonadal remnant whatsoever can be identified, including no streak gonad, and in the absence of müllerian derivatives. Testicular failure must have occurred between the onset of formation of müllerian-inhibiting substance and the secretion of testosterone, that is, after development of the seminiferous tubules but before the onset of Leydig cell function.

In others the clinical features indicate that testicular failure occurred later in gestation, and these individuals may constitute problems in gender assignment. In some, failure of müllerian regression occurs to a greater extent than the failure of testosterone secretion, but none exhibit complete müllerian development. In those with more extensive virilization the external genitalia are phenotypically male, but rudimentary oviducts and vasa deferentia may coexist internally.

At the final extreme is the syndrome of bilateral anorchia in phenotypic men with absence of müllerian structures and gonads but male development of the wolffian system and external genitalia. Microphallus implies that failure of androgen-mediated growth occurred during late embryogenesis after anatomic development of the male urethra is complete. Persistent gynecomastia may or may not develop after the time of puberty.

Pathophysiology The pathogenesis is not understood. The testicular regression could be the result of mutant genes, teratogen, or trauma. Multiple instances of agonadism in the same family have been reported, some of whom have unilateral and others bilateral disease.

The quantitative dynamics of gonadal steroid production have been studied in only a few patients. In two phenotypic females who had primary amenorrhea, sexual infantilism, and no internal genital structures, androgen and estrogen kinetics were similar to those in gonadal dysgenesis; production rates of estrogen were low, and no glandular secretion of testosterone was found, confirming the functional as well as anatomic absence of the testes. In one phenotypic male with bilateral anorchia testosterone and estrogen production was accounted for by peripheral conversion from plasma androstenedione. However, some subjects in whom no testes can be identified at laparotomy have blood testosterone values clearly above the castrate range, presumably derived from remnant testes.

Management The management of the two extremes is clearcut. Sexually infantile, phenotypic females should be treated like patients with gonadal dysgenesis, namely given adequate estrogen to ensure appropriate breast and female somatic development, and any coexisting vaginal agenesis should be treated by surgical or medical means. Likewise, phenotypic males with anorchia should be given adequate androgen replacement to allow normal male secondary sexual development. The cases with incomplete virilization or ambiguous development of the external genitalia are more complex and require individual assessment as to whether surgical therapy is appropriate in addition to hormonal therapy at the time of expected puberty.

DISORDERS OF PHENOTYPIC SEX

FEMALE PSEUDOHERMAPHRODITISM Congenital adrenal hyperplasia CLINICAL FEATURES The pathways by which glucocorticoids are synthesized in the adrenal gland and androgens are formed in the testis and adrenal are summarized in Fig. 333-3. Three enzymes are common to the formation of glucocorticoids and androgens (20,22-desmolase, 3β-hydroxysteroid dehydrogenase, and 17α-hydroxylase); deficiency of any of these enzymes results in deficiency of glucocorticoid and androgen synthesis and consequently in both congenital adrenal hyperplasia (due to enhanced ACTH levels) and defective virilization of the male embryo (male pseudohermaphroditism). Two enzymes are involved exclusively in androgen synthesis (17,20-desmolase and 17β-hydroxysteroid dehydrogenase); deficiency in either results in pure male pseudohermaphroditism with normal glucocorticoid synthesis. Deficiency of either of the terminal two enzymes of glucocorticoid synthesis (21-hydroxylase and 11β-hydroxylase) results in defective formation of hydrocortisone; the compensatory increase in ACTH secretion causes adrenal hyperplasia and a secondary increase in androgen formation that results in virilization in the female or precocious masculinization in the male.

The *adrenal insufficiency* in these disorders may produce equally severe and life-threatening problems in both sexes and is described

FIGURE 333-3 *Pathways of glucocorticoid and androgen synthesis.*

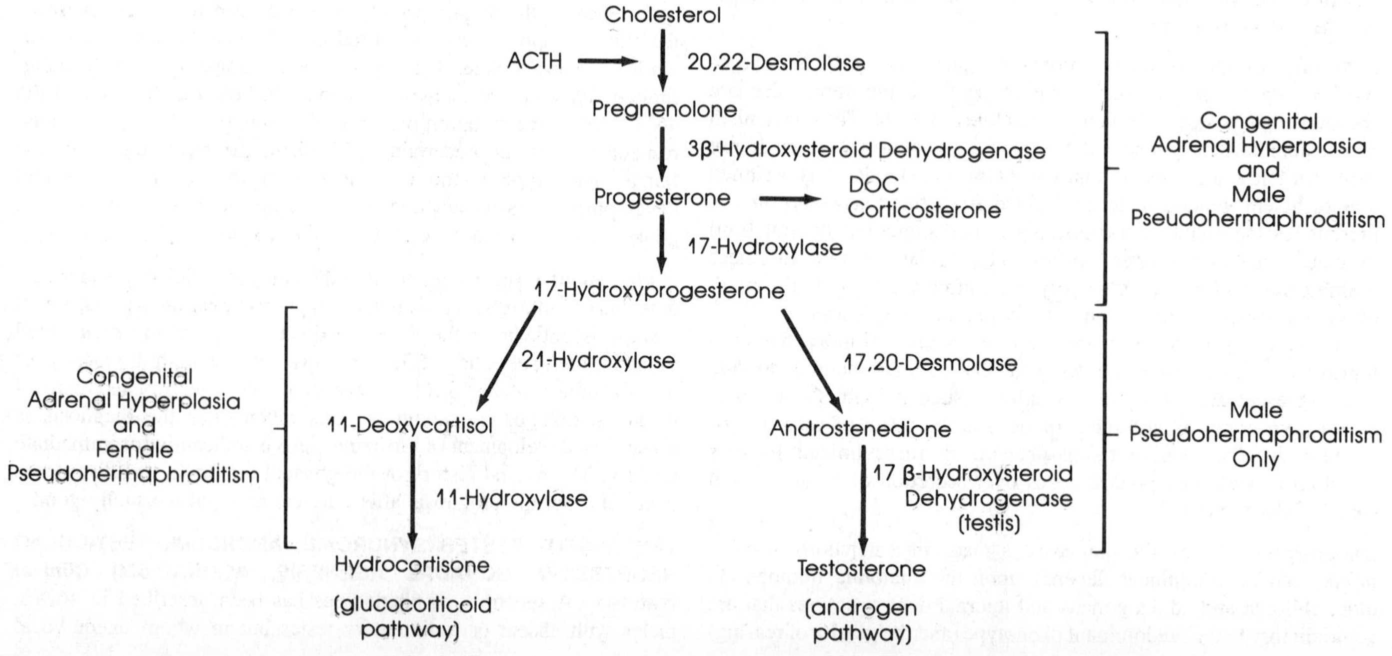

in detail in Chap. 325. The major features of the different forms of congenital adrenal hyperplasia are listed in Table 333-4. From the standpoint of *abnormal sexual development* it is helpful to consider separately those enzyme defects in steroidogenesis that result in female pseudohermaphroditism and those that cause male pseudohermaphroditism. (One disorder, 3β-hydroxysteroid dehydrogenase deficiency, can cause either male or female pseudohermaphroditism, but since the more common genital defect is incomplete virilization of the male, it will be discussed as an abnormality of male phenotypic differentiation.)

Congenital adrenal hyperplasia due to 21-hydroxylase deficiency is the most common cause of ambiguous genitalia in the newborn, with an incidence of between 1:5000 and 1:15,000 in Europe and the United States. Virilization is usually apparent at birth in the female and within the first 2 to 3 years of life in the male. Manifestations in females include hypertrophy of the clitoris associated with ventral binding (chordee), partial fusion of the labioscrotal folds, and variable virilization of the urethra. The internal female structures and ovaries remain unaltered, and the wolffian ducts regress normally, probably because the onset of adrenal function occurs relatively late in embryogenesis. The external appearance of affected females is similar to that of a male with bilateral cryptorchidism and hypospadias. The labioscrotal folds are bulbous and rugated and resemble a scrotum. Rarely the virilization is so severe that development of a complete male penile urethra and prostate results in errors in sex assignment at birth. Radiography following the injection of radiopaque dye into the external genital orifice is helpful in demonstrating the presence of a vagina, uterus, and sometimes even fallopian tubes. In a few cases virilization of the female is slight or absent at birth and becomes evident in later infancy, adolescence, or adulthood, presumably as the result of allelic variation of the mutant genes (the so-called late-onset or adult form of the disorder). The untreated female grows rapidly during the first year of life and has progressive virilization. At the time of expected puberty there is a failure of normal female sexual development and absence of menstruation. In both sexes rapid somatic maturation results in premature epiphyseal closure and a short adult height.

Since male phenotypic differentiation is normal, the condition is usually not recognized in the male at birth in the absence of overt adrenal insufficiency. However, early growth and maturation of the external genitalia, appearance of secondary sex characteristics, coarsening of the voice, frequent erections, and excessive muscular development are noticeable in the first few years of life. Virilization in the male can follow either of two patterns. Excessive adrenal androgens can inhibit gonadotropin production so that the testes remain infantile in size despite the acceleration of masculinization. Such untreated adult men are capable of erection and ejaculation but have no spermatogenesis. Alternatively, adrenal androgen secretion can activate a premature maturation of the hypothalamic-pituitary axis and initiate a true precocious puberty including early maturation of spermatogenesis (see Chap. 330). The untreated male is also subject to the development of ACTH-dependent "tumors" of the testis composed of adrenal rest cells.

In 21-hydroxylase deficiency, which accounts for about 95 percent of congenital adrenal hyperplasia, there is a reduced activity of the 21-hydroxylase enzyme which leads to decreased production of hydrocortisone and consequently to increased release of ACTH, enlargement of the adrenal glands, and partial or complete compensation of the defect in the secretion of hydrocortisone. In about half the enzyme defect appears to be partial, and cortisol secretion is normal. This form is termed "simple virilizing" or "compensated." In the remainder there seems to be a more complete deficiency of the enzyme; the enlarged adrenal fails to produce adequate amounts of cortisol and aldosterone leading to severe salt wastage with anorexia, vomiting, volume depletion, and collapse within the first few weeks of life, the so-called salt-losing form of 21-hydroxylase deficiency. In all untreated patients overproduction of the cortisol precursors prior to the 21-hydroxylase step occurs, leading to increase in plasma progesterone and 17-hydroxyprogesterone. These act as weak aldosterone antagonists at the receptor level and in the compensated form result in greater than normal aldosterone production to maintain normal sodium balance.

Female pseudohermaphroditism may also occur in 11β-hydroxylase deficiency. In this disorder a block in hydroxylation at the 11 carbon results in the accumulation of 11-deoxycortisol and deoxycorticosterone (DOC), a potent salt-retaining hormone that causes hypertension rather than salt loss. The clinical features that stem from glucocorticoid deficiency and androgen excess are similar to those in 21-hydroxylase deficiency.

PATHOPHYSIOLOGY Both disorders are due to autosomal recessive mutations. The carrier frequency for 21-hydroxylase deficiency is about 1 in 50. At least three forms of 21-hydroxylase deficiency have been identified, all involving mutations of a gene on the sixth chromosome close to the HLA-B locus: the common type, which acts like an ordinary autosomal recessive enzyme mutation; a cryptic allele, which is clinically silent in homozygous form but which causes typical disease when present as a genetic compound with the common variety; and a late-onset variant. Carriers of the disorder (as well as homozygotes) within a given family can be identified on the basis of the HLA haplotype. In 11β-hydroxylase deficiency there is no known linkage of the mutation to the HLA system.

TABLE 333-4 Forms of congenital adrenal hyperplasia

Deficiency	Cortisol	Aldosterone	Degree of virilization of females	Failure of virilization in males	Dominant steroid secreted	Comment
21-Hydroxylase, partial (simple virilizing or compensated)	Normal	↑	+ + + +	0	17-Hydroxyprogesterone	Most common type (~95% of total); from one- to two-thirds salt losers
Severe (salt-losing)	↓	↓	+ + + +	0	17-Hydroxyprogesterone	
11β-Hydroxylase (hypertension)	↓	↓	+ + + +	0	11-Deoxycortisol and 11-deoxycorticosterone	Hypertension
3β-Hydroxysteroid dehydrogenase	0	0	+	+ + + +	Δ^5-3β-OH compounds (dehydroepiandrosterone)	Probably second most common, usually salt loss
17α-Hydroxylase	↓	↓	0	+ + + +	Corticosterone and 11-deoxycorticosterone	No feminization of female, hypertension
20,22-Desmolase (lipoid adrenal hyperplasia)	0	0	0	+ + + +	Cholesterol(?)	Rare, usually salt loss

For discussion of the endocrine pathology see Chap. 325. In brief, excretion of ketosteroids is elevated, as is the excretion of the major metabolites that accumulate proximal to the enzymatic blocks. Plasma ACTH is elevated in untreated patients. In 21-hydroxylase deficiency, 17-hydroxyprogesterone accumulates in blood and is excreted predominantly as pregnanetriol. In 11-hydroxylase deficiency 11-deoxycortisol accumulates in blood and is excreted predominantly as tetrahydrocortexolone.

MANAGEMENT Gender assignment should correspond to the chromosomal and gonadal sex, and appropriate surgical correction of the external genitalia should be undertaken as early as possible. This is of importance because appropriately treated men and women are capable of fertility. However, if the correct diagnosis is made late (after 3 years of age) gender assignment should be changed only after careful consideration of the psychosexual background.

Medical treatment with appropriate glucocorticoids prevents the consequences of hydrocortisone deficiency, arrests the rapid virilization, and prevents premature somatic advancement and epiphyseal maturation. The suppression of the abnormal steroid secretion results in cure of the hypertension in patients with 11β-hydroxylase deficiency and allows normal onset of menses and development of female secondary sex characteristics in both disorders. In males glucocorticoid therapy suppresses adrenal androgens and results in normal gonadotropin secretion, testicular development, and spermatogenesis. Measurements of plasma 17-hydroxyprogesterone, androstenedione, ACTH, and renin have all been used to assess adequacy of replacement therapy. In severe forms of 21-hydroxylase deficiency associated with salt loss or with elevated plasma renin activity treatment with mineralocorticoids is also indicated. In such patients the monitoring of plasma renin activity is useful for determining the adequacy of mineralocorticoid replacement.

Nonadrenal female pseudohermaphroditism Nonadrenal causes of female pseudohermaphroditism are rare. In the past, the administration to pregnant women of progestational agents with androgenic side effects (such as 17α-ethinyl-19-nor-testosterone) to prevent abortion resulted in masculinization of female fetuses. Female pseudohermaphroditism may also occur in babies born to mothers who have virilizing tumors (e.g., arrhenoblastomas or luteomas of pregnancy) and, rarely, under circumstances in which no etiology can be determined.

Developmental disorders of müllerian ducts (congenital absence of the vagina, müllerian agenesis) CLINICAL FEATURES Congenital hypoplasia or absence of the vagina in combination with some form of abnormal or absent uterus (the Mayer-Rokitansky-Kuster-Hauser syndrome) is second only to gonadal dysgenesis as a cause of primary amenorrhea. Most patients are ascertained after the time of expected puberty because of failure to menstruate. The height and intelligence are normal, and the breasts, axillary and pubic hair, and habitus are feminine in character. The uterus may vary from almost normal, lacking only a conduit to the introitus, to the more characteristic rudimentary bicornuate cords with or without a lumen. In some patients cyclical abdominal pain indicates that sufficient functional endometrium is present to result in retrograde menstruation and/or hematometra.

About one-third have abnormal kidneys, most commonly agenesis or ectopy. Fused kidneys of the horseshoe type and solitary ectopic kidneys located in the pelvis also occur. Skeletal abnormalities are present in one-tenth; two-thirds involve the spine, and limb and rib abnormalities account for the remainder. Specific bone abnormalities include wedge vertebrae, fusions, rudimentary or asymmetric vertebral bodies, and supernumerary vertebrae. The Klippel-Feil syndrome (congenital fusion of the cervical spine, short neck, low posterior hairline, and painless limitation of cervical movement) is a frequent association.

PATHOPHYSIOLOGY The karyotype is 46,XX. Most are believed to be sporadic in nature, but several instances of familial occurrence have been described. The pattern of inheritance in most familial disease is consistent with a sex-limited autosomal dominant mutation. It is not known whether the sporadic cases represent new mutations of the type responsible for the familial disorder or are multifactorial in etiology. In the familial cases variable expressivity is common; some affected family members have skeletal or renal abnormalities only, while others have other abnormalities of müllerian derivatives such as a double uterus. Bilateral renal aplasia in stillborn infants is also commonly associated with absence of the uterus and vagina. Thus, the family histories should be probed for instances of isolated skeletal and renal abnormalities and for stillbirths that might result from congenital absence of both kidneys.

Documentation of ovulatory peaks of plasma LH and biphasic temperature curves during the cycle suggest that ovarian function is normal, and successful pregnancies have been reported following corrective vaginal surgery in patients who have normal uteri.

MANAGEMENT Vaginal agenesis can be treated by surgical or nonsurgical means. Surgical repair generally utilizes a split-thickness skin graft around a solid rubber mold for the creation of an artificial vagina. Medical treatment consists of the repeated application of pressure against the vaginal dimple with a simple dilator to cause development of adequate vaginal depth. In view of the overall complication rate of around 5 to 10 percent in surgical series, medical treatment should be tried in most, and surgery should be reserved for patients in whom a well-formed uterus is present and the possibility of fertility exists. Continued coitus or instrumental dilatation is probably essential for maintaining the neovagina formed by either technique.

MALE PSEUDOHERMAPHRODITISM Defective virilization of the male embryo (male pseudohermaphroditism) can result from defects in androgen synthesis, defects in androgen action, defects in müllerian duct regression, and uncertain causes. Four-fifths of male pseudohermaphrodites have normal androgen synthesis.

Abnormalities in androgen synthesis CLINICAL FEATURES Five enzymatic defects are known to result in defective testosterone synthesis (Fig. 330-3) and cause incomplete virilization of the male embryo during embryogenesis (Tables 330-4 and 330-5). Each of the enzymes catalyzes a step in the conversion of cholesterol to testosterone. Three (20,22-desmolase, 3β-hydroxysteroid dehydrogenase, and 17α-hydroxylase) are common to the synthesis of other adrenal hormones as well; consequently, their deficiency results in congenital adrenal hyperplasia (Table 333-4) as well as male pseudohermaphroditism. The other two (17,20-desmolase, and 17β-hydroxysteroid dehydrogenase) are unique to the pathway of androgen synthesis, and their deficiency results only in male pseudohermaphroditism. Since androgens are obligatory precursors of estrogens, it likewise follows that in all but the terminal defect (17β-hydroxysteroid dehydrogenase deficiency) synthesis of estrogen is also low in affected individuals of both sexes.

The adrenal dysfunction in the three relevant disorders is described in Chap. 325, and the present discussion concerns the abnormal sexual development. In 46,XY subjects there is usually no trace of uterus or fallopian tubes, indicating that the müllerian-inhibiting function of the testis takes place normally during embryogenesis. The masculinization of the wolffian ducts, urogenital sinus, and urogenital tubercle and the degree of virilization at puberty vary from almost normal to absent, and therefore, the clinical picture spans the range from phenotypic men with mild hypospadias to phenotypic women who prior to puberty resemble patients with complete testicular feminization. This extreme variability is the consequence of varying severity of the enzymatic defects in different patients and of varying effects of the steroids that accumulate proximal to the metabolic blocks in the different disorders. In patients with partial defects and in whom plasma testosterone is normal the diagnosis can only be made by measuring the steroids that accumulate proximal to the metabolic block in question.

20,22-Desmolase deficiency (lipoid adrenal hyperplasia) is a form of congenital adrenal hyperplasia in which virtually no urinary steroids (either 17-ketosteroids or 17-hydroxycorticoids) can be detected. The defect is prior to the formation of pregnenolone and is assumed to involve one or more of the enzymes of the 20,22-desmolase complex responsible for the conversion of cholesterol to pregnenolone. The syndrome is associated with salt wasting and profound adrenal insufficiency, and most affected individuals die during infancy. At autopsy the adrenals and testes are enlarged and infiltrated with lipid. Affected males are incompletely masculinized whereas affected female infants have normal genital development.

3β-Hydroxysteroid dehydrogenase deficiency is the second most common cause of congenital adrenal hyperplasia. In male infants it causes varying degrees of hypospadias or complete failure of masculinization associated with presence of a vagina. Female infants may be modestly virilized at birth due to the weak androgenic potency of dehydroepiandrosterone, the major steroid secreted. If the enzyme is absent in both the adrenal and testis, no urinary steroids contain a Δ^4-3-keto configuration, whereas in patients in whom the defect is partial or affects only the testis, the urine may contain normal or even elevated levels of Δ^4-3-ketosteroids. Most patients have marked salt wasting and profound adrenal insufficiency, and long-term survival in untreated cases occurs only in states of partial deficiency. Affected males may experience an otherwise normal male puberty except for profound gynecomastia. In these individuals a low-normal blood testosterone level is accompanied by elevated Δ^5 precursors. The enzyme in different tissues must be under complex control since deficiency of the enzyme in the testis may be less severe than in the adrenal and since enzyme activity in the liver may be normal in the face of profound deficiency in the adrenal and testis. Individuals with normal liver enzymes can be mistakenly identified as having 21-hydroxylase deficiency if urinary Δ^5-pregnenetriol is not documented to be greater than urinary pregnanetriol.

17α-Hydroxylase deficiency characteristically results in hypogonadism, absence of secondary sex characteristics, hypokalemic alkalosis, hypertension, and virtually undetectable hydrocortisone secretion in phenotypic women. The secretion of both corticosterone and desoxycorticosterone (DOC) by the adrenal is elevated, and urinary 17-ketosteroids are low. Aldosterone secretion is low, presumably as the result of high plasma DOC and depressed angiotensin levels, and returns to normal after suppressive doses of hydrocortisone are administered. In 46,XX subjects amenorrhea, absent sexual hair, and hypertension are common, but, since gonadal steroids are not required for female development during embryogenesis, the phenotype is that of a normal prepubertal woman. In males, however, the enzyme deficiency results in defective virilization that varies from complete male pseudohermaphroditism to ambiguous genitalia with perineoscrotal hypospadias. In males with partial enzyme deficiency pathologic gynecomastia may develop at puberty. Subjects with this disorder do not develop adrenal insufficiency, since the secretion of both corticosterone (a weak glucocorticoid) and DOC (a mineralocorticoid) is elevated. The hypertension and hypokalemia that are prominent features of the disorder (even in the neonatal period) remit after suppression of the DOC secretion by adequate glucocorticoid replacement.

17,20-Desmolase deficiency has been described in several families. Affected males have a 46,XY chromosome pattern, normal adrenocortical function, and a variable pattern of male pseudohermaphroditism. In the majority there is genital ambiguity at birth with some virilization at the time of expected puberty. However, two 46,XY patients have had a female phenotype and no virilization at the time of expected puberty. The disorder has been recognized in one 46,XX woman with sexual infantilism.

17β-Hydroxysteroid dehydrogenase deficiency involves the final step in androgen biosynthesis, reduction of the 17-keto group of androstenedione to form testosterone. This disorder is the most common of the enzymatic defects in testosterone synthesis. Affected 46,XY males usually have a female phenotype with a blind-ending vagina and absence of müllerian derivatives, but inguinal or abdominal testes and virilized wolffian duct structures are present. At the time of expected puberty, both virilization (with phallic enlargement and development of facial and body hair) and a variable degree of female breast development take place. In some untreated patients reversal of gender behavior from female to male occurs at puberty. Androgen and estrogen dynamics have not been elucidated in detail, but the 17-keto reduction of estrone to estradiol by the gonads is also low. 17β-Hydroxysteroid dehydrogenase is normally present in many tissues besides the gonads, and only the gonadal enzyme appears to be defective in this disorder. Plasma testosterone may be in the low-normal range, making it essential to document elevation in plasma androstenedione to make the diagnosis.

PATHOPHYSIOLOGY The available data for the 17α-hydroxylase and 3β-hydroxysteroid dehydrogenase defects are compatible with autosomal recessive inheritance. The limited family data for 17,20-desmolase deficiency and 17β-hydroxysteroid dehydrogenase deficiency are compatible either with autosomal recessive or X-linked recessive mutations, and insufficient data are available for the 20,22-desmolase defect to warrant any conclusions as to the pattern of inheritance.

The pattern of steroid secretion and excretion depends on the site of the various metabolic blocks (Fig. 333-3). In general, gonadotropin secretion is high, and as a consequence many individuals with incomplete defects are able to compensate so that the steady-state concentration of end products such as testosterone may be normal or almost normal.

In some cases of male pseudohermaphroditism testosterone formation is deficient for reasons other than a single enzyme defect in androgen synthesis. These include disorders in which Leydig cell agenesis (possibly due to absence of the LH receptor) or the secretion of a biologically inactive LH molecule has been thought to be the primary defect. In addition, as described above, a spectrum of defects in testicular development has been characterized, including familial XY gonadal dysgenesis, sporadic dysgenetic testes, and the absent testis syndrome in which deficient testosterone production is secondary to the underlying disorder of gonadal development.

MANAGEMENT Replacement therapy with glucocorticoids and in some instances mineralocorticoids is indicated in those disorders causing adrenal hyperplasia. The decision as to the management of the genital abnormalities depends upon the individual case. Fertility has not been reported, and its consideration does not enter into the decision of sex assignment. In genetic females there is no problem (except in diagnosis) in that affected individuals are raised appropriately as females, and suitable estrogen replacement is indicated at the time of expected puberty to promote development of normal female secondary sex characteristics. The decision as to whether affected newborn males with ambiguous genitalia should be raised as males or females depends upon the anatomic defect; in general the more severely affected should be raised as females, and corrective surgery of the genitalia and removal of the testes should be undertaken as early as possible. In subjects raised as females estrogen therapy is also indicated at the appropriate age to allow development of normal female secondary sex characteristics. In individuals raised as males, corrective surgery is indicated for any coexisting hypospadias, and careful monitoring of plasma androgens and estrogens should be undertaken at the time of expected puberty to determine whether long-term supplemental testosterone therapy is appropriate.

Abnormalities in androgen action Several disorders of male phenotypic development result from abnormalities of androgen action. The spectrum of phenotypes is illustrated in Fig. 333-4 and described in Tables 333-4 and -5. In these disorders testosterone formation and müllerian regression are normal, but male development is impaired to a variable degree as a result of resistance to androgen action in the target cells.

5α-REDUCTASE DEFICIENCY This autosomal recessive form of male pseudohermaphroditism is characterized by (1) severe perineoscrotal

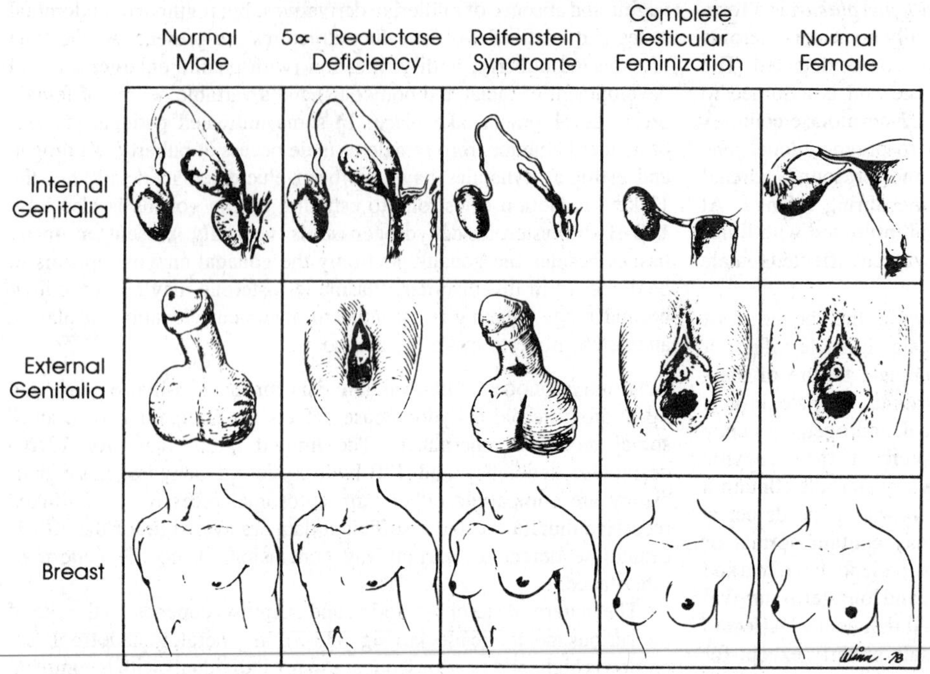

FIGURE 333-4 *Schema of the different appearance of the internal and external genitalia and breast development in androgen-resistance syndromes.*

hypospadias with a hooded prepuce, a ventral urethral groove, and opening of the urethra at the base of the phallus; (2) a blind vaginal pouch of variable size opening either into the urogenital sinus or onto the urethra immediately behind the urethral orifice; (3) well-developed testes with normal epididymides, vasa deferentia, and seminal vesicles, and termination of the ejaculatory ducts into the blind-ending vagina; (4) a female habitus without female breast development but with normal axillary and pubic hair; (5) the absence of female internal genitalia; (6) normal male plasma testosterone; and (7) masculinization to a variable degree at the time of puberty.

The fact that the defective virilization during embryogenesis is limited to the urogenital sinus and the anlage of the external genitalia provided insight into the nature of the fundamental abnormality. Testosterone, the androgen secreted by the fetal testis, is the intracellular mediator for differentiation of the wolffian duct into the epididymis, the vas deferens, and the seminal vesicle, whereas dihydrotestosterone mediates virilization of the urogenital sinus and the external genitalia. Consequently, in a male embryo with normal testosterone synthesis and normal androgen receptors a failure of dihydrotestosterone formation would be expected to result in the phenotype observed in this disorder, normal male wolffian duct derivatives with defective masculinization of the structures originating

TABLE 333-5 Anatomic, genetic, and endocrine profile of hereditary male pseudohermaphroditism

		Phenotype				
Disorder	Inheritance	Müllerian ducts	Wolffian ducts	Spermatogenesis	Urogenital sinus	External genitalia
DEFECTS IN TESTOSTERONE SYNTHESIS						
Five enzyme deficiencies	Autosomal or X-linked recessive	Absent	Variable development	Normal or decreased	Variable from male to female	Generally female
DEFECTS IN ANDROGEN ACTION						
5α-Reductase deficiency	Autosomal recessive	Absent	Male	Normal or decreased	Female	Clitoromegaly
Receptor disorders:						
Complete testicular feminization	X-linked recessive	Absent	Absent	Absent	Female	Female
Incomplete testicular feminization	X-linked recessive	Absent	Male	Absent	Female	Clitoromegaly and posterior fusion
Reifenstein syndrome	X-linked	Absent	Variable development	Absent	Variable from male to female	Incomplete male development
Infertile male syndrome	Probably X-linked recessive	Absent	Male	Absent or decreased	Male	Male
Receptor-positive resistance	Uncertain	Absent	Variable	Absent or decreased	Variable	Female to male
DEFECTS IN MÜLLERIAN REGRESSION						
Persistent müllerian duct syndrome	Autosomal or X-linked recessive	Rudimentary uterus and fallopian tubes	Male	Normal	Male	Male

from the urogenital sinus, genital tubercle, and genital swellings. Since testosterone itself regulates LH secretion (see Chap. 330), plasma LH is usually only minimally elevated. As a result testosterone and estrogen production rates are those of normal men, and gynecomastia does not develop.

The fact that the 5α-reductase enzyme is deficient in this disorder was established by direct enzymatic assay in biopsied tissues and fibroblasts cultured from affected individuals. In most subjects the 5α-reductase is either profoundly deficient or functionally absent, and in others the enzyme protein is synthesized at a normal rate but is structurally abnormal. It is not clear why virilization at puberty appears to be more normal than the virilization that takes place during sexual differentiation.

RECEPTOR DISORDERS Disorders of the androgen receptor may result in several distinct phenotypes. Despite differences in clinical presentation and molecular pathology these disorders are similar in regard to endocrinology, genetics, and basic pathophysiology. The major clinical features of the disorders will be considered first and followed by a discussion of the similar endocrinology and pathophysiology.

Clinical features. Complete testicular feminization is the most common form of male pseudohermaphroditism; estimates of frequency vary from 1 in 20,000 to 1 in 64,000 male births. It is the third most common cause of primary amenorrhea in phenotypic women after gonadal dysgenesis and congenital absence of the vagina. The features are characteristic. Namely, a woman is seen by the physician either because of inguinal hernia (prepubertal) or primary amenorrhea (postpubertal). The development of the breasts after puberty, the general habitus, and the distribution of body fat are female in character so that many patients have a truly feminine appearance. Axillary and pubic hair are absent or scanty, but slight vulval hair is usually present. Scalp hair is that of a normal woman, and facial hair is absent. The external genitalia are unambiguously female, and the clitoris is normal or small. The vagina is short and blind-ending and may be absent or rudimentary. All internal genitalia are absent except for undescended testes that contain normal Leydig cells and seminiferous tubules without spermatogenesis.

Breast	Endocrine profile relative to normal male		
	Testosterone production	Estrogen production	LH
Usually male	Normal to decreased	Variable	High
Male	Normal	Normal	Normal or increased
Female	High	High	High
Female	High	High	High
Female	High	High	High
Usually male	Normal or high	Normal or high	Normal or high
Variable	Normal or high	Normal or high	Normal or high
Male	Normal	Normal	Normal

The testes may be located in the abdomen, along the course of the inguinal canal, or in the labia majora. Occasionally, remnants of müllerian or wolffian duct origin are present in the paratesticular fascia or in fibrous bands extending from the testis. Patients tend to be rather tall, bone age is normal, and intelligence is normal. The psychosexual development is unmistakably female in regard to behavior, outlook, and maternal instincts.

The major complication of undescended testes in this disorder as in other forms of cryptorchidism (Chap. 330) is the development of tumors. Since affected individuals undergo a normal pubertal growth spurt and feminize successfully at the time of expected puberty and since testicular tumors rarely develop until after puberty in patients with intraabdominal testes, it is usual to delay castration until after the time of expected puberty. Surgical intervention is indicated prepubertally if the testes are present in the inguinal region or the labia majora and result in discomfort or hernia formation. (If hernia repair is indicated prepubertally most physicians prefer to remove the testes at the same time so as to limit the number of operative procedures.) If the testes are removed prepubertally, estrogen therapy is required at the appropriate age to ensure normal growth and breast development. When castration is performed postpubertally menopausal symptoms and other evidences of estrogen withdrawal supervene, and suitable estrogen replacement is indicated (see Chap. 331).

Incomplete testicular feminization is about one-tenth as frequent as the complete form. In the incomplete disorder there is a minor virilization of the external genitalia (partial fusion of the labioscrotal folds and some degree of clitoromegaly), normal pubic hair, and some virilization as well as feminization at the time of expected puberty. The vagina is short and blind-ending, but in contrast to the complete form, the wolffian duct derivatives are often partially developed. The family history is usually uninformative, but in some instances multiple family members are affected in a pattern compatible with X-linkage. The management of patients with the complete and incomplete forms of testicular feminization differs. Since patients with the incomplete disorder virilize at the time of expected puberty, gonadectomy should be performed before the expected time of puberty in prepubertal patients with clitoromegaly or posterior labial fusion.

Reifenstein syndrome is the term applied to forms of incomplete male pseudohermaphroditism initially described by a number of eponyms (Reifenstein syndrome, Gilbert-Dreyfus syndrome, Lubs syndrome). Each of these phenotypes was originally assumed to be a distinct entity, but since families have now been described in which affected members exhibit variable manifestations that span the phenotypes described under these terms, these syndromes are now thought to constitute variable manifestations of a single mutation. The most common phenotype is a man with perineoscrotal hypospadias and gynecomastia, but the spectrum of defective virilization in such families ranges from men with azoospermia to phenotypic women with pseudovaginas. Axillary and pubic hair are normal, but chest and facial hair are minimal. Cryptorchidism is common, the testes are small, and azoospermia is present. Some have defects in wolffian duct derivatives such as absence or hypoplasia of the vas deferens. Since the psychological development in most is unequivocally male, the hypospadias and cryptorchidism should be corrected surgically. The only successful form of treatment of the gynecomastia is surgical removal.

The *infertile male syndrome* is the most common disorder of the androgen receptor and is not actually a form of male pseudohermaphroditism. Some such individuals are minimally affected subjects in families with Reifenstein syndrome with only azoospermia as a manifestation of the receptor abnormality. More commonly, the individuals present with male infertility and have negative family histories; indeed a disorder of the androgen receptor may be present in a fifth or more of men with idiopathic azoospermia. There is no treatment for the infertility in any of these disorders.

Pathophysiology. The karyotype is 46,XY, and the mutant gene is X-linked. The frequency of a positive family history varies from about two-thirds of patients with testicular feminization and Reifenstein syndrome to only occasional patients with the infertile male syndrome. The patients with a negative family history are believed to be the result of new mutations.

Hormone dynamics are similar in all disorders of the androgen receptor. Plasma testosterone levels and rates of testosterone production by the testes are normal or higher than normal. The elevated rate of testosterone production is caused by the high mean plasma level of LH, which in turn is due to defective feedback regulation caused by resistance to the action of androgen at the hypothalamic-pituitary level. Elevated LH concentration is probably responsible also for the increased estrogen production by the testes (see Chap. 330). (In normal men most estrogen is derived from peripheral formation from circulating androgens, but when plasma LH is elevated the testes secrete significant amounts of estrogen into the circulation.) Thus, resistance to the feedback regulation of LH secretion by circulating androgen results in elevated plasma LH levels, and this in turn results in the enhanced secretion of both testosterone and estradiol by the testes. Gonadotropin levels rise even higher (and menopausal symptoms may develop) when the testes are removed, indicating that gonadotropin secretion is under partial regulatory control. Presumably, in the steady state and in the absence of an androgen effect, estrogen alone regulates LH secretion, a control that is purchased at the expense of an elevated plasma estrogen concentration for a male. The hormonal changes in the infertile male syndrome are similar to those in the other receptor disorders but less marked. Some men with this syndrome do not have an elevation of plasma LH or plasma testosterone.

Feminization in these disorders is the result of two interlocking phenomena. First, androgens and estrogens have antagonistic effects at the peripheral level, and virilization occurs in normal men when the ratio of androgen to estrogen is 100 to 1 or greater; in the absence of androgen action the cellular effect of estrogen is unopposed. Second, the production of estradiol is greater than that of the normal male (although less than that of the normal female). Variable degrees of androgen resistance coupled with variably enhanced estradiol production result in different degrees of defective virilization and enhanced feminization in the four clinical syndromes.

Each of these four syndromes is the result of an abnormality of the androgen receptor. Initially fibroblasts cultured from the skin of some subjects with complete testicular feminization were shown to have a near absence of high-affinity dihydrotestosterone binding. Subsequently, other individuals with complete testicular feminization as well as subjects with incomplete testicular feminization, Reifenstein syndrome, and the infertile male syndrome have been found to have either a decreased amount of an apparently normal receptor or a qualitatively abnormal androgen receptor.

Receptor-positive resistance. A category of androgen resistance that does not appear to involve either the 5α-reductase or the androgen receptor was first identified in a family with the syndrome of testicular feminization. Subsequent patients have been described with a variety of phenotypes ranging from incomplete testicular feminization to findings similar to those in the Reifenstein syndrome. The hormonal profile is similar to that seen in the receptor disorders. The site of the molecular abnormality in these patients is unclear. It could be due to defects of the androgen receptor too subtle to be detected by the usual assay. If the defect is truly distal to the receptor, there could be failure of generation of specific messenger RNA or an abnormality of RNA processing. Indeed, the disorder may represent a heterogeneous group of molecular abnormalities. Management depends on the phenotype.

Persistent müllerian duct syndrome Men with this disorder have normal penile development but have in addition bilateral fallopian tubes, a uterus, and an upper vagina, and variable development of the vas deferens. The subjects commonly present with inguinal hernias which contain the uterus, and cryptorchidism is common. Most have uninformative family histories, but several pairs of siblings have been described in whom the condition must be inherited either as an autosomal recessive or an X-linked recessive mutation. Because the external genitalia are well developed and the patients masculinize normally at puberty, it is assumed that during the critical stage of embryonic sexual differentiation the fetal testes produced a normal amount of androgen. However, müllerian regression does not occur for one of three possible reasons: failure of the fetal testis to produce müllerian-inhibiting substance, poor timing of the release of müllerian-inhibiting substance, or failure of the tissues to respond to this hormone. To minimize the chance of tumor development and to maintain virilization, a primary or staged orchiopexy should be performed. Malignancy in the uterus or vagina has not been described, and because the vasa deferentia are closely associated with the broad ligaments, the uterus and vagina should be left in place to avoid disruption of the vasa deferentia during removal and consequently to preserve possible fertility.

Developmental defects of the male genitalia HYPOSPADIAS Hypospadias is a congenital anomaly in which the urethra terminates in an abnormal position along the midline of the ventral surface of the penis at some site between the normal urethral meatus and the perineum. This malformation is often associated with some degree of ventral contraction and bowing of the penis (chordee). The disorder occurs in 0.5 to 0.8 percent of male births in the United States. It is common to categorize hypospadias as glandular (involving the glans penis), penile, or perineoscrotal. Since penile development is mediated by androgens, it is assumed that hypospadias results from some defect in earlier androgen formation or androgen action during embryogenesis. Indeed hypospadias occurs in most disorders of male sexual differentiation. A rare cause of hypospadias is maternal ingestion of progestational agents early in pregnancy. However, the known causes (single gene defects, chromosomal abnormalities, and maternal drug ingestion) at best can account for only about one-fourth of cases, and the etiology of most remains unknown. The management is surgical.

CRYPTORCHIDISM The normal descent of the testis is perhaps the most poorly understood portion of male sexual differentiation, both in regard to the nature of the forces that result in the movement and to the hormonal factors that regulate the process. In anatomic terms testicular descent can be divided into three phases: (1) transabdominal movement of the testis from its site of origin above the kidney to the inguinal ring, (2) formation of the opening in the inguinal canal (processus vaginalis) through which the testis exits the abdominal cavity, and (3) actual movement of the testis through the inguinal canal to its permanent site in the scrotum. This entire process occurs over a 6- to 7-month period during gestation, beginning at about the sixth week and not completed in some normal individuals until after birth. Whatever its involvement, androgen is probably not the sole hormone responsible for normal descent. Failure of any of the above anatomic events can be responsible for the failure of descent of one or both testes that occurs in 3 percent of full-term males and 30 percent of premature male infants. Cryptorchidism can be classified as intraabdominal, retractile (intermittently in the groin), obstructed (permanently in the groin), and high scrotal. Most are retractile and descend permanently by 6 weeks to 3 months of age so that the incidence of failure of descent in late teenagers is only 0.6 to 0.7 percent. It is this latter category that requires intervention.

The cryptorchid testis functions poorly after puberty, but the extent to which maldescent is the result of an abnormality of the testis or the cause of abnormal function is unknown. Two general theories have been advanced as to the etiology—inadequate intraabdominal pressure and deficient endocrine function of the testis either because of deficient testosterone synthesis or inadequate formation of müllerian-inhibiting substance. Indeed, hereditary defects that result in inadequate development of intraabdominal pressure or inadequate development of the testes themselves can cause cryptorchidism. As is true for hypospadias, however, the known causes of cryptorchidism constitute only a small fraction of the cases, and the etiology in most remains to be identified. Two complications of cryptorchidism are important; spermatogenesis cannot occur at the temperature of the abdominal cavity, and it is therefore necessary to correct the process as early as possible to allow possible fertility. However, the fact that infertility is common in men who have been treated for unilateral as well as bilateral cryptorchidism suggests that maldescent is usually the consequence rather than the cause of the testicular malfunction. There is also a greater frequency of malignancy in undescended testis, and all should be surgically corrected for this reason (see Chap. 297).

REFERENCES

De La Chapelle A: The etiology of maleness in XX men. Hum Genet 58:105, 1981

Donahoe PK et al: Mixed gonadal dysgenesis, pathogenesis and management. J Pediatr Surg 14:287, 1979

Edman CD et al: Embryonic testicular regression: A clinical spectrum of XY agonadal individuals. Obstet Gynecol 49:208, 1977

George FW, Wilson JD: Sexual differentiation, in *Campbell's Textbook of Urology*, 5th ed, PC Walsh et al (eds). Philadelphia, Saunders, 1986, pp 1804–1818

Gordon DL et al: Pathologic testicular findings in Klinefelter's syndrome. 47,XXY vs 46,XY/47,XXY. Arch Intern Med 130:726, 1972

Griffin JE et al: Congenital absence of the vagina. The Mayer-Rokitansky-Kuster-Hauser syndrome. Ann Intern Med 85:224, 1976

———, Wilson JD: Disorder of sexual differentiation, in *Campbell's Textbook of Urology*, 5th ed, PC Walsh et al (eds). Philadelphia, Saunders, 1986, pp 1819–1855

Grumbach MM, Conte FA: Disorders of sexual differentiation, in *Williams' Textbook of Endocrinology*, 7th ed, JD Wilson, DW Foster (eds). Philadelphia, Saunders, 1985, pp 312–401

Leonard JM et al: The classification of Klinefelter's syndrome, in *Genetic Mechanism of Sexual Development*, HL Vallet, IH Porter (eds). New York, Academic, 1979

McDonough PG et al: Phenotypic and cytogenetic findings in eighty-two patients with ovarian failure-changing trends. Fertil Steril 28:638, 1977

New M et al: Congenital adrenal hyperplasia and related conditions, in *Metabolic Basis of Inherited Disease*, 5th ed, JB Stanbury et al (eds). New York, McGraw-Hill, 1983, pp 973–1000

Simpson JL: *Disorders of Sexual Differentiation*. New York, Academic, 1976, p 466

———: Gonadal dysgenesis and sex chromosome abnormalities: Phenotypic-karyotypic correlations, in *Genetic Mechanisms of Sexual Development*, HL Vallet, IH Porter (eds). New York, Academic, 1979

——— et al: XY gonadal dysgenesis: Genetic heterogeneity based upon clinical observations, H-Y antigen status and segregation analysis. Hum Genet 58:91, 1981

Van Niekerk WA: True hermaphroditism. Pediatr Adolesc Endocrinol 8:80, 1981

Wilson JD et al: The androgen resistance syndromes: 5α-Reductase deficiency, testicular feminization and related disorders, in *The Metabolic Basis of Inherited Disease*, 5th ed, JB Stanbury et al (eds). New York, McGraw-Hill, 1983, pp 1001–1026

Zah W et al: Mixed gonadal dysgenesis. A case report and review of the world literature. Acta Endocrinol Suppl 197:3, 1975

334 DISORDERS AFFECTING MULTIPLE ENDOCRINE SYSTEMS

R. NEIL SCHIMKE

Multiple endocrine gland hyper- or hypofunction can result from mechanisms other than a primary abnormality in the hypothalamic-pituitary axis. While not common, certain of the conditions that affect multiple endocrine systems are inherited and thus have significance out of proportion to their frequency.

SYNDROMES WITH MULTISYSTEM HYPERFUNCTION

MULTIPLE ENDOCRINE NEOPLASIA, TYPE I (MEN I) This disorder, also termed the *Wermer syndrome*, comprises tumors or hyperplasia of the parathyroids, pancreatic islet cells, pituitary, adrenal cortex, and thyroid. The clinical presentation is variable, depending on which of the potentially affected glands is hyperfunctioning at the time of diagnosis. About two-thirds of patients have adenomas of two or more endocrine systems, and one-fifth develop tumors of three or more systems.

The majority of affected subjects present with one of the following problems: (1) peptic ulcer and its complications, (2) hypoglycemia, (3) hypercalcemia and/or nephrocalcinosis, (4) complaints referable to pituitary dysfunction such as headaches, visual field defects, and secondary amenorrhea, and (5) multiple lipomas of the skin. A minority (probably <10 percent) come to medical attention with acromegaly, Cushing's syndrome, nonfunctional thyroid adenomas, hyperthyroidism, hepatomegaly (due to metastatic liver disease), or flushing (associated with the carcinoid syndrome).

Parathyroid involvement in MEN I may be asymptomatic for prolonged periods, although most patients eventually show some signs of hyperparathyroidism. Tumors of the islet cells may elaborate excessive insulin or gastrin. Insulinomas cause hypoglycemia (Chap. 329), whereas excess gastrin secretion causes the Zollinger-Ellison syndrome with its multifocal or atypically located ulcers and massive hypersecretion of gastric acid. Symptoms may be identical with those of ordinary peptic ulcer, but there is a higher incidence of complications, including perforation, bleeding, and obstruction. Diarrhea is frequent, often with steatorrhea. Radiographic findings include giant gastric rugae, duodenal nodularity, ectopic ulcers in the esophagus, lower duodenum, and jejunum, and intestinal hyperperistalsis. Associated endocrine abnormalities consistent with the MEN syndrome are present in over one-quarter of patients with the Zollinger-Ellison syndrome and in half of the first-degree relatives of such patients. MEN I should be considered in a patient with the Zollinger-Ellison syndrome even when no other endocrine abnormalities are apparent.

Islet-cell tumors may also produce glucagon, vasoactive intestinal polypeptide (VIP), prostaglandins, adrenocorticotropic hormone (ACTH), parathyroid hormone, antidiuretic hormone (ADH), serotonin, somatostatin, calcitonin, and pancreatic polypeptide (also see Chap. 329). Glucagonomas cause hyperglycemia, weight loss, stomatitis, and a peculiar skin rash called *necrotizing migratory erythema*. VIP and prostaglandins have been implicated in the watery diarrhea (pancreatic cholera) syndrome sometimes seen in MEN I. Cushing's syndrome may be due to an adrenal adenoma or may occur as a consequence of ectopic ACTH production by an islet tumor or a thymic carcinoid. Some adrenal adenomas produce aldosterone or adrenal androgens. Involvement of the thyroid gland is uncommon in MEN I, but goiter, simple adenoma, and thyroiditis have all been reported. Other features of MEN I include small-intestinal and bronchial carcinoid tumors, schwannomas, thymomas, multiple lipomas, inclusion cysts, and cutaneous leiomyomas.

Patients with MEN I may develop symptoms at any age, but the condition presents rarely in childhood or after the age of 60. Affected individuals may demonstrate multiple endocrine system involvement simultaneously, or months to years may elapse between the discovery of one adenoma and the appearance of the next. Once the diagnosis is established, the patient must be surveyed periodically for appearance of new facets of the syndrome. By the same token, all first-degree relatives should be studied. A reasonable approach for screening relatives at risk is as follows: (1) review history for symptoms of peptic ulcer disease, hypoglycemia, renal calculi, lipomas, or hypopituitarism; (2) examine for multiple lipomas; (3) assay serum calcium, phosphorus, prolactin, and gastrin. Upper gastrointestinal series and sella turcica x-rays have proved of no value as screening tests. Serum pancreatic polypeptide determinations may be useful in centers where the assay is available.

The fundamental lesion in MEN I is unknown. Some have considered the basic abnormality to be in the islet cells with their extensive capability for hormone synthesis, attributing changes in the other glands to secondary effects of islet hormone hypersecretion. Others have classified MEN I as a neurocrestopathy implicating faulty differentiation or regulation of the embryonic neural crest, which is the anlage of at least part of the endocrine system. The endocrine components of the neural crest have been classified into a subsystem of APUD cells, so named because of their capacity for amine precursor uptake and decarboxylation. The evidence supporting the contention that all APUD cells are derived from neural crest is not strong; instead, cells of diverse origin probably develop similar characteristics; i.e., they represent a structural-functional convergence.

The pituitary and parathyroid tumors in MEN I are usually benign, but pancreatic tumors are frequently malignant. Surgical removal of the affected gland is the usual therapy, although standard radiation techniques may be employed for the pituitary tumors, and homergocryptine is useful in prolactinomes. Hyperparathyroidism may be due to a single adenoma, but diffuse hyperplasia of more than one gland is more common. In some centers selective venous catheterization with measurement of serum parathyroid hormone levels can be used to differentiate between those possibilities. Since new adenomas may arise in normal glands left after removal of an adenoma (and since second operations are difficult because of scar formation), some have advocated removal of all the parathyroid glands with transplantation of extirpated fragments into the thigh or forearm, where they can be easily removed should hyperparathyroidism recur. Successful transplantation obviates the need for long-term therapy of hypoparathyroidism. In hypergastrinemia due to islet-cell lesions, total gastrectomy has been used to prevent recurrent peptic ulcers, and in rare cases distant metastases have regressed after this procedure. Histamine-2-receptor antagonists are efficacious in controlling the hyperacidity and diarrhea seen with hypergastrinemia.

MULTIPLE ENDOCRINE NEOPLASIA, TYPE II (MEN II OR IIA) MEN II, also known as the *Sipple syndrome,* consists of pheochromocytoma (frequently bilateral and occasionally extraadrenal), medullary thyroid carcinoma (MTC), and, in about half of the reported cases, parathyroid hyperplasia. MEN II can be related more directly to abnormal neural crest development than can MEN I, since both the adrenal medulla and the parafollicular or C cells of the thyroid originate in neural crest. However, there is no evidence that the parenchymal component of the parathyroid glands are so derived. The parafollicular cell elaborates calcitonin, the primary marker of medullary carcinoma of the thyroid. MTC is not common, comprising less than 10 percent of thyroid malignancies. At least 10 percent of MTC cases are familial, usually appearing as a component of MEN II or MEN III (see below). Medullary carcinoma may also occur in families without other associated endocrine dysfunction; this form is also transmitted as an autosomal dominant trait. MTC may present as a thyroidal mass or be clinically silent and undetectable by palpation or radioiodine scanning. The diagnosis is usually established by immunoassay of serum calcitonin, provided ectopic sites of calcitonin production can be excluded, e.g., breast, lung, and pancreatic islet-cell tumors. Occasionally, basal serum calcitonin levels are borderline in at-risk individuals, and measurement of plasma levels after calcium-pentagastrin infusion can be used to establish the diagnosis. MTC may on occasion secrete substances other than calcitonin, including ACTH, prolactin, serotonin, VIP, histamine, and various prostaglandins, resulting in a confusing array of symptoms.

The pheochromocytoma of MEN II may produce the classic signs of catecholamine excess as described in Chap. 326 or be asymptomatic. Approximately 7 percent of patients who present with pheochromocytomas also have MTC. Symptoms of hyperparathyroidism rarely bring the patient with MEN II to initial clinical attention.

Examination of cells from both the MTC and the pheochromocytoma components of MEN II using X-linked gene markers has led to the conclusion that the inherited defect produces multiple clones of abnormal cells; tumors then develop from a second mutation in the abnormal clone, accounting for the appearance of varying clinical patterns. Other tumors in MEN II include gliomas, glioblastomas, and meningiomas, all of which may be derived from the neural crest.

The age of the patient at the time of diagnosis varies from 2 to 67 years. C-Cell hyperplasia of the thyroid may precede development of malignancy by many years, making early screening studies for calcitonin elevation mandatory in all family members at risk. The only effective therapy for MTC is surgical removal of the entire thyroid, as the tumor is probably always multifocal in origin. Limited node dissection is often indicated since the cancer may progress slowly despite an aggressive histologic appearance, and prolonged survival is seen in patients with known metastatic disease. Serum calcitonin levels can be used to assess completeness of surgical removal of the tumor and in concert with selective venous catheterization may be utilized to locate distant metastases that are surgically accessible. Neither standard radioiodine nor x-ray therapy is helpful in disseminated medullary thyroid cancer, and chemotherapy has been of limited value (see Chap. 324). The pheochromocytomas are usually benign and are also treated surgically. Unresectable malignant pheochromocytoma requires long-term sympathetic blockade. A new radiopharmaceutical, *meta*-iodobenzyl guanidine, shows promise as both a diagnostic and a therapeutic agent.

MULTIPLE ENDOCRINE NEOPLASIA, TYPE III (MEN III OR IIB) MEN III also consists of medullary thyroid carcinoma and pheochromocytoma, but affected individuals have striking dysmorphic features such as neuromas of the conjunctival, labial, and buccal mucosa, the tongue, the larynx, and the gastrointestinal tract; hence the alternate designation of the condition as the *mucosal neuroma syndrome*. Other physical findings include enlarged corneal nerves, "blubbery" lips, soft-tissue prognathism, and a habitus resembling that seen in the Marfan syndrome with hypotonia, lax joints, kyphoscoliosis, genu valgus, and pes cavus. The patients may have café au lait spots or a diffuse lentiginous type of skin pigmentation along with cutaneous neuromas or neurofibromas. Megacolon may occur.

MEN III and MEN II appear to be distinct syndromes. For example, both parathyroid hyperplasia and production of hormones other than calcitonin by MTC are rare in MEN III. The mean survival of patients with MEN III is around 30 years compared with 60 years for those with MEN II, suggesting a more malignant course in the former disorder, although histologically the thyroid tumors appear to be identical. As with MEN II treatment of the medullary carcinoma is surgical. The unusual physical features of MEN III should immediately suggest the diagnosis of underlying thyroid malignancy. MTC has been documented in asymptomatic children with MEN III, and C-cell hyperplasia has been found at operation as early as 15 months of age. Clinically, the associated pheochromocytomas behave as expected (Chap. 326).

McCUNE-ALBRIGHT SYNDROME This condition is characterized by the triad of polyostotic fibrous dysplasia, café au lait spots, and isosexual precocity, the latter occurring predominantly but not exclusively in females. The isosexual precocity may be hypothalamic in origin, but gonadotropin-independent ovarian function has been implicated in some cases (see Chap. 331). Cushing's syndrome, gigantism or acromegaly, and hyperprolactinemia may also occur in affected patients. The Cushing's syndrome may result from abnormal ACTH production or adrenal adenomas. Nodular toxic goiter and pheochromocytoma have also been reported. The bone lesion resembles that seen in hyperparathyroidism, and parathyroid hyperplasia has been described histologically but not clinically. The condition is usually sporadic, but pedigrees compatible with autosomal dominant inheritance have been seen. The cause of the condition is unknown (see Chap. 339).

SYNDROMES WITH MULTISYSTEM HYPOFUNCTION

POLYGLANDULAR DEFICIENCY SYNDROME (SCHMIDT SYNDROME) (See also Chaps. 324 and 325) The prototype of a polyglandular deficiency state is the Schmidt syndrome, originally described as the presence of both Addison's disease and lymphocytic thyroiditis in a single patient. This syndrome has subsequently been expanded to include any combination of adrenal insufficiency, lymphocytic thyroiditis, hypoparathyroidism, and gonadal failure. Diabetes mellitus is a frequent accompaniment. The manifestations may be so extensive as to simulate panhypopituitarism; rarely, true pituitary deficiency has been described. The first evidence of endocrinopathy generally appears in adult life. The most significant laboratory feature, in addition to the low levels of circulating hormones, is the presence of antibodies to one or more endocrine glands. The antibodies may be directed against a clinically normal gland, but with time hypofunction usually supervenes. Additional evidence for an immune pathogenesis is provided by the increased frequency of antibodies to parietal cells of the stomach, with or without overt achlorhydria or pernicious anemia, and the presence of other disorders felt to have an autoimmune basis such as sprue, vitiligo, myasthenia gravis, pure red cell aplasia, and antibody-mediated immunoglobulin A deficiency. Hyperthyroidism may complicate the clinical picture.

The majority of affected individuals are female, and most cases are sporadic. A few reports have noted multiple affected family members, suggesting a genetic basis. Members of these families who show no endocrine disability frequently have serologic abnormalities indicative of a disturbance in immune function. Many of the component endocrine disorders in this syndrome are associated with the presence of certain HLA antigens, notably HLA-B8 and -Dw3 (in white populations). Other racial groups show different associations, e.g., hyperthyroidism with HLA-Bw35 in the Japanese. Because of this association it has been postulated that the basic lesion may reside in a mutation of an inherited immunologic mechanism. For example, a selective immunodeficient state might render an individual unduly susceptible to certain environmental antigens (e.g., viruses) that have a predilection for the endocrine system. Cell lysis or damage could result in release of intracellular contents and lead to development of autoantibodies. Such autoantibodies would not necessarily be pathogenic but could represent secondary phenomena, important as markers of potential clinical disease. Alternatively, the defect could reside in a genetically determined defect in suppressor T cells and with consequent inadequate suppression of antibody synthesis. The syndrome is probably etiologically heterogeneous, and several pathogenetic mechanisms may be operative. At present, treatment is confined to providing hormone replacement.

CANDIDIASIS-ENDOCRINOPATHY SYNDROME An autoimmune pathogenesis has also been invoked in the candidiasis-endocrinopathy syndrome. Features that differentiate this condition from the Schmidt syndrome include childhood onset and extensive mucocutaneous monilial infection that becomes evident shortly after birth. Hypoparathyroidism is common, and adrenal insufficiency may develop acutely. Diabetes is rare. Organ-specific antibodies against a variety of endocrine glands may be detected early, and pernicious anemia, sprue, chronic active hepatitis, and membranoproliferative glomerulonephritis have been seen. Defective cellular immunity to *Candida albicans* is present; some have more generalized anergy. A cause-and-effect relationship between the monilial infection and the endocrinopathy has not been established. The disorder has occurred in sibs, occasionally from consanguineous unions, and the disease may be inherited as an autosomal recessive trait. No association with the HLA system has been demonstrated, but affected individuals may have a deficiency of immunoglobulin A and hypergammaglobulinemia. Suppressor T-cell function may be defective, but the immune profile can be variable even in sibs. The fungal infection is usually refractory to conventional chemotherapeutic drugs, although partial remission has been reported with a combination of ketoconazole and transfer factor. Amelioration of the candidiasis in no way affects the endocrinopathy, and conventional replacement therapy is required.

LIPODYSTROPHIC SYNDROMES The lipodystrophic syndromes are described in Chap. 318. Insulin-resistant diabetes mellitus is common and may be associated with elevated growth hormone levels and with an increased incidence of polycystic disease of the ovaries, acromegaly, and Cushing's disease.

TABLE 334-1 Disorders with common polyglandular manifestations

		Type of endocrine involvement						
Condition	Clinical feature	Hypothalamic-pituitary	Thyroid	Parathyroid	Pancreas	Adrenal	Gonads	Inheritance
Ataxia-telangiectasia	Early ataxia Oculocutaneous telangiectasia Immunologic deficiency	?Variably decreased pituitary reserve			Diabetes mellitus	Cortical hypoplasia	Dysgenetic ovaries; gonadoblastomas later	Autosomal recessive
Pseudohypoparathyroidism	Short stature Short metacarpals and metatarsals Round facies Ectopic calcification	Variable deficiency of all pituitary hormones, including prolactin	Hypo- or hyperthyroidism	Elevated parathyroid hormone levels with either normo- or hypocalcemia	Diabetes mellitus		Ovarian failure	Probable X-linked dominant; heterogeneous
Myotonic dystrophy	Muscular dystrophy Premature baldness Mental retardation	Gonadotropin, growth hormone abnormalities, related to central integrative defect (?)	Hypothyroidism		Diabetes mellitus		Primary failure	Autosomal dominant
Noonan syndrome	Short stature Ptosis Webbed neck Pulmonary stenosis	Gonadotropin deficiency	Thyroiditis				Primary failure	Autosomal dominant
Fanconi syndrome	Short stature Bone marrow hypoplasia Abnormal skin pigmentation Radius malformations	Panhypopituitarism			Diabetes mellitus	Adrenal atrophy	Gonadal atrophy	Autosomal recessive
Werner syndrome	Premature aging of all organ systems Atrophic skin Cataracts Early osteoporosis		Papillary carcinoma		Diabetes mellitus		Gonadal atrophy	Autosomal recessive

DIABETES MELLITUS, DIABETES INSIPIDUS, AND OPTIC ATROPHY This clinical triad has been noted in sibs and likely constitutes a rare autosomal recessive defect. Nerve deafness, usually mild, may also occur. The diabetes mellitus is of the early-onset insulin-dependent type. The diabetes insipidus usually appears prior to age 20. The varying manifestations are difficult to reconcile, and treatment requires replacement of the missing hormones.

OBESITY-HYPOGONADISM SYNDROMES A number of seemingly discrete entities share obesity, generally with frank diabetes mellitus, and hypogonadism that may be either primary or secondary. The *Biedl-Bardet syndrome* features retinitis pigmentosa, polydactyly, mental retardation, and renal anomalies along with obesity, hypogonadotropic hypogonadism, and in some patients, diabetes mellitus. There is sufficient resemblance between this syndrome and the *Alström syndrome* (retinitis pigmentosa, nerve deafness, diabetes mellitus, and primary gonadal failure) to cause frequent diagnostic confusion. Both are autosomal recessive disorders. However, polydactyly and mental retardation do not occur in the Alström syndrome. A similar condition is the *Biemond syndrome* in which obesity, diabetes mellitus, secondary hypogonadism, and postaxial polydactyly are combined with iris colobomata rather than pigmentary retinopathy. Patients with the *Prader-Willi syndrome* (obesity, hypogonadism, hypotonia, mental retardation) also have diabetes mellitus of the maturity-onset type. A genetic basis has not been established for the Biemond or the Prader-Willi syndromes. A small deletion of chromosome 15 is present in some patients with the latter disorder.

CHROMOSOMAL DISORDERS WITH ENDOCRINE DEFICIENCY (See also Chaps. 60 and 333) Patients with Turner syndrome have hypogonadism and an increased incidence of diabetes mellitus and thyroiditis, thought to be on an autoimmune basis. In the Klinefelter syndrome an increased frequency of diabetes mellitus may occur along with gonadal failure. In the Down syndrome hypogonadism is probably universal in males, and menstrual irregularities and early menopause are common in women; in addition, increased prevalences of lymphocytic thyroiditis and diabetes mellitus have been reported.

OTHER CONDITIONS WITH MULTISYSTEM MANIFESTATIONS There are a number of other rare conditions in which involvement of more than one endocrine gland has been recorded often enough to constitute a significant facet of the syndrome. Some, like neurofibromatosis (von Recklinghausen's disease) and tuberous sclerosis, may show either hypo- or hyperfunction of endocrine glands because of interference with central regulatory mechanisms caused by the brain tumors characteristic of the diseases. By the same token, pheochromocytomas may occur in neurofibromatosis because the adrenal medulla is derived from the same embryonic source.

Table 334-1 lists some conditions in which disorders of multiple endocrine systems have been seen. It is noteworthy that both primary and secondary failures have been reported within the diagnostic confines of the same syndrome. For example, both gonadotropin deficiency and primary testicular atrophy have been documented in patients with the Noonan syndrome and in unaffected members of the same families. Whenever a clinical condition like diabetes mellitus occurs in such distinct entities as myotonic dystrophy and ataxia-telangiectasia, the molecular mechanisms underlying the disease are probably heterogeneous. A better understanding of the genetic defect would provide insight into the function of the endocrine system.

REFERENCES

FARID N, BEAR JC: The human major histocompatibility complex and endocrine disease. Endocr Rev 2:50, 1981

NEUFELD M et al: Two types of autoimmune Addison's disease associated with different polyglandular autoimmune syndromes. Medicine 60:355, 1981

RIMOIN DL, ROTTER JI: Genetic syndromes associated with diabetes mellitus and glucose intolerance, in *The Genetics of Diabetes Mellitus*, J Kobberling, R Tattersall (eds). New York, Academic, 1982, pp 149–181

SCHIMKE RN: Syndromes with multiple endocrine gland involvement. Prog Med Genet 3:143, 1979

———: Genetic aspects of multiple endocrine neoplasia. Ann Rev Med 35:25, 1984

YAMAGUCHI K et al: Multiple endocrine neoplasia type I. Clin Endocrinol Metab 9:261, 1980

PART ELEVEN DISORDERS OF BONE AND MINERAL METABOLISM

335 CALCIUM, PHOSPHORUS, AND BONE METABOLISM: CALCIUM-REGULATING HORMONES

MICHAEL F. HOLICK / STEPHEN M. KRANE / JOHN T. POTTS, JR.

BONE STRUCTURE AND METABOLISM (See also Chap. 337) Bone is a dynamic tissue, constantly remodeling itself throughout life. The skeleton is highly vascular and receives about 10 percent of the cardiac output. The arrangement of compact and cancellous bone provides a combination of strength and density suitable for mobility. In addition, bone provides calcium, magnesium, phosphorus, sodium, and other ions necessary for the support of homeostatic functions.

The properties of bone are a function of its extracellular components. The structure consists of a solid mineral phase in close association with an organic matrix of which 90 to 95 percent is type I collagen (see Chap. 319). The noncollagenous portion of the organic matrix contains proteins derived from serum (albumin and α_2-HS glycoproteins), an α-carboxyglutamic acid (GLA)–containing protein (called *bone GLA-protein* or *osteocalcin*), a glycoprotein called *osteonectin*, a bone proteoglycan, and other glycoproteins, phosphoproteins, and sialoproteins. Some of these proteins may function in initiating mineralization and in binding of the mineral phase to the matrix. The mineral phase is made up of calcium and phosphate, best characterized as a poorly crystalline hydroxyapatite, although the calcium/phosphate molar ratio is less than the 1.67 of hydroxyapatite [empiric formula, $Ca_{10}(PO_4)_6(OH)_2$]. In addition, other ions are present, predominantly in the surface layers. The mineral phase of bone is deposited in intimate relation to the collagen fibrils and is found largely in specific locations within the "holes" of the collagen fibrils that result from the manner in which the collagen molecules are packed. This architectural organization of mineral and matrix results in a two-phase material uniquely suited to withstand mechanical stresses. The formation and the localization of the inorganic phase are probably determined in part by the organic matrix.

Bone is formed by cells of mesenchymal origin that synthesize and secrete the organic matrix. Mineralization of the matrix, particularly in *osteons* (haversian systems), begins soon after it is secreted (primary mineralization) but is not completed until after several weeks (secondary mineralization). As an *osteoblast* secretes matrix which is then mineralized, this cell becomes surrounded by matrix and becomes an *osteocyte,* still connected with its blood supply through a series of canaliculi. Resorption of bone is carried out mainly by *osteoclasts*. Osteoclasts are multinucleated cells formed by fusion of precursor cells derived from a hematopoietic stem cell related to the mononuclear phagocyte series. Resorption of bone takes place in scalloped spaces (Howship's lacunae) where the osteoclasts are attached to the bone matrix through a ring of contractile proteins (clear zone) and form a specialized ruffled border. Mineral and matrix are removed in this space where the ruffled border is folded and is in contact with the bone. Proteins such as a proton pump ATPase are found in the ruffled border membrane, which contributes to the production of a unique acid environment in the enclosed extracellular compartment and results in solubilization of the mineral phase. Osteoblasts are involved in synthesis and secretion of most of the organic matrix and regulate the mineralization of the matrix. The alkaline phosphatase of bone is localized to the osteoblasts. The active principle that eventually results in formation of bone has been termed *bone morphogenetic protein.* Additional factors can stimulate growth and/or matrix synthesis by osteoblast-related cells (several bone-derived growth factors, somatomedins, transforming growth factor beta).

In the embryo and in the growing child, bone develops either by remodeling and replacing previously calcified cartilage (endochondral bone formation), or it is formed without a cartilage matrix (intramembranous bone formation). New bone, whether in embryos or infants or that formed in adults during repair, has a relatively high ratio of cells to matrix and is characterized by coarse fiber bundles of collagen that are interlaced and randomly dispersed (woven bone). In adults, the more mature bone is organized with fiber bundles regularly arranged in parallel or concentric sheets (lamellar bone). In long bones, the lamellar bone is deposited in a concentric arrangement around blood vessels and forms the haversian systems. Growth in length of bones is dependent upon proliferation of cartilage cells and on the endochondral sequence at the growth plate. Growth in width and thickness is accomplished by formation of bone at the periosteal surface and by resorption at the endosteal surface with the rate of formation exceeding that of resorption. In adults, after the epiphyses close, growth in length and endochondral bone formation cease, except for some activity in the cartilage cells beneath the articular surface. However, even in adults, remodeling of bone (remodeling of haversian systems as well as trabecular bone) continues through life, as can be shown by microradiographic studies utilizing radioisotopes or fluorescence of tetracyclines fixed in bone in regions of new mineralization. Quantitative histomorphometric techniques demonstrate that newly forming surfaces are characterized by smooth character, by uptake of tetracycline, and by relatively low mineral density. Actively forming surfaces are covered by active osteoblasts. The osteoid seam that results from the relative lag in mineralization of the newly formed organic matrix is normally no greater than about 12 μm. An index of the rate of bone formation can be obtained by examination of undemineralized sections of bone biopsies obtained from individuals who have received tetracycline for two periods separated by a drug-free interval. The distance between the fluorescent bands on the sections reflects the new bone formed. Resorption areas are characterized by their irregular configurations and the presence of osteoclasts (Fig. 335-1). Resorption precedes formation and is more intense, but it does not persist as long as formation. In adults, approximately 4 percent of the surface of trabecular bone (such as iliac crest) is involved in active resorption, whereas 10 to 15 percent of trabecular surfaces is covered with osteoid. Kinetic studies using isotopes such as radioactive calcium (^{47}Ca) provide estimates that as much as 18 percent of the total skeletal calcium may be deposited and removed each year. Thus, bone is an active metabolizing tissue, with its cells dependent upon an intact blood supply. The remodeling of bone occurs in a manner somehow related to the continuous mechanical stresses to which it is subjected. Bone also serves as an important reservoir of mineral ions, particularly calcium, which are critical for a variety of processes.

The response of bone to injuries, such as fractures, infection, interruption of blood supply, and to expanding lesions is relatively limited. Dead bone must be resorbed, and new bone must be formed, a process carried out in association with new blood vessels growing into the involved area. In injuries that disrupt the organization of the tissue, such as a fracture in which apposition of fragments is poor and motion exists at the fracture site, the osteoprogenitor stromal cells differentiate into cells with functional capacities other than those of osteoblasts, and repair is accompanied by formation of varying amounts of fibrous tissue and cartilage. When there is good apposition with fixation and little motion at the fracture site, repair occurs predominantly by formation of new bone without other scar tissue. Remodeling of this bone occurs along lines of force determined by mechanical stresses that are somehow translated into biologic response.

Expanding lesions in bone, such as tumors, induce resorption at the surface in contact with the tumor. A bowing deformity causes increased new bone formation at the concave surface and resorption at the convex surface, all seemingly designed to produce the strongest mechanical structure. Even in a disorder as architecturally disruptive as Paget's disease, remodeling is dictated by mechanical forces. Thus, the plasticity of bone is due to the response of cells interacting with each other and with the environment.

Mechanisms of bone formation and resorption Bone formation is an orderly process in which inorganic mineral is deposited in relation to an organic matrix. The mineral phase is composed of calcium and phosphorus, and the concentration of these ions in the plasma and extracellular fluid influences the rate at which the mineral phase is formed. In vitro, mineralization can proceed, and crystals of hydroxyapatite can grow at concentrations of calcium and phosphorus similar to those in an ultrafiltrate of plasma. However, the concentration of these ions at the sites of mineralization is unknown, and the cells involved (osteoblasts, osteocytes) may somehow regulate the local concentration of calcium, phosphorus, and other ions. Collagens from a variety of sources can catalyze the nucleation of a mineral phase of calcium and phosphorus from solutions of these ions, and the initial mineral phase is deposited in specific locations in the holes produced by the particular packing arrangement of the collagen molecules. The organization of collagen probably influences the amount and type of mineral phase formed in bone. There is one gene for each of the two $\alpha 1$ chains and the single $\alpha 2$ chain that make up type I collagen. The primary structures of type I collagen in skin and bone tissues are similar. There are differences, however, in posttranslational modifications of type I collagen such as hydroxylation, glycosylation, and the type, number, and distribution of intermolecular cross-links. In addition, the "holes" in the packing structure of the collagen are larger in normally mineralized collagen of bone and dentin than in unmineralized collagens such as tendon. The noncollagenous organic components such as the bone-GLA protein or osteonectin may also play a role in the formation of the mineral phase of bone. Alkaline phosphatase is a marker for osteoblasts, and cellular levels of this enzyme correlate with mineralization potential of osteoblasts. Although mineralization defects occur in individuals with decreased levels of alkaline phosphatase (hypophosphatasia), the function of alkaline phosphatase in the mineralization process is not completely understood. To explain how collagens from tissues that are normally not mineralized can catalyze nucleation of an inorganic phase from solutions similar to normal extracellular fluid, regulation of mineralization by inhibitory substances has been suggested. Inorganic pyrophosphate is a potent inhibitor of mineralization at concentrations below those necessary to bind calcium ions. Since alkaline phosphatase, present in osteoblasts and other cells, can catalyze the hydrolysis of inorganic pyrophosphate at neutral pH, this enzyme could regulate mineralization by controlling the concentrations of pyrophosphate. In addition, macromolecular inhibitors such as the proteoglycan aggregates may also influence the rate and extent of mineralization. In cartilage undergoing calcification, membrane-bound vesicles containing mineral are present outside the cells, and it has been suggested that this is the initial mineral phase.

FIGURE 335-1 *Schematic representation of bone remodeling surfaces in trabecular bone. Most bone surfaces in adults are involved in neither formation nor resorption. Such surfaces are usually smooth, have no osteoid seam, and are covered either by no visible cells or by flattened cells. Active formation surfaces are smooth and covered by osteoblasts which have an osteoid seam (clear), normally no thicker than 12 μm. The calcification front is located at the junction of the osteoid seam and mineralized bone (stippled). Inactive forming surfaces are not covered by osteoblasts but by only a few flattened cells. Active resorbing surfaces are irregular or scalloped and contain multinucleated osteoclasts. The latter are not seen on inactive resorbing surfaces.*

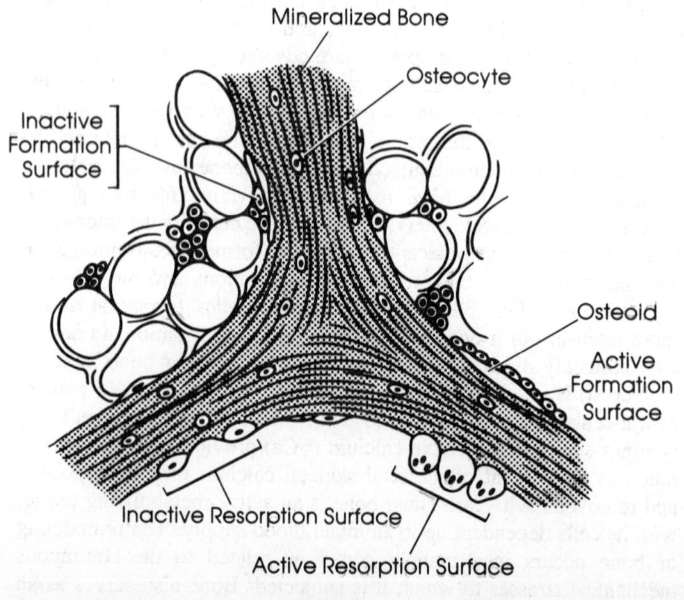

In bone, the calcium phosphate solid phase at the inception of mineralization is brushite ($CaHPO_4 \cdot 2H_2O$). As mineralization progresses, the solid phase is a poorly crystalline hydroxyapatite with a relatively low (~ 1.2) calcium/phosphate molar ratio. With age and maturation, the degree of crystal perfection increases as does the calcium/phosphate ratio. Fluoride ions, when incorporated into the mineral phase, decrease the proportion of amorphous calcium phosphate and increase crystallinity.

There is a limit for the concentration of calcium and phosphorus ions in the extracellular fluid below which mineralization will not occur. A "solubility product" for bone mineral is difficult to calculate since the mineral phase itself is of variable composition and the true nature of species in solution governing this solubility product is not known. Nevertheless, when the concentrations of calcium and phosphorus in extracellular fluid are excessive, a mineral phase may be formed in areas that are not normally mineralized.

When bone is resorbed, calcium and phosphorus ions from the solid phase are released into the extracellular fluid, and the organic matrix is subsequently resorbed. It is not entirely clear how these processes occur. A decrease in pH, the presence of a chelating substance, and the operation of a cellular pump mechanism to shift the equilibrium between solids and solution may explain mineral release. The fact that bone resorption takes place in the region of the osteoclast adjacent to the bone surface, where the extracellular pH is low, lends support to the concept that this unique acid environment is required for solubilization of the bone mineral. Although osteoclasts are rich in tartrate-resistant acid phosphatase, a specific function for this enzyme has not been established. Whereas the activity of alkaline phosphatase in osteoblasts may be increased in serum when osteoblast number or function is increased, no such spillover from acid phosphatase is observed. The matrix is resorbed through the action of proteinases released by the osteoclasts. Matrix proteins in bone cannot be degraded, however, until the mineral phase is first removed. The rate of bone resorption is modulated by hormones such as parathyroid hormone and $1,25(OH)_2$ vitamin D and by local factors such as prostaglandins, heparin from mast cells, and various cytokines that augment the activity of osteoclasts already present or that enhance their differentiation from hematopoietic precursors. Some of these factors affect the osteoclast directly, and some act indirectly through effects on other cells such as osteoblasts or stromal fibroblasts. For example, parathyroid hormone receptors are present on osteoblasts but not on osteoclasts; therefore, parathyroid hormone effects on increasing bone resorption are mediated by the osteoblasts.

Interleukin 1, a monokine which increases bone resorption in vitro, also acts on the osteoclasts through osteoblasts or stromal fibroblasts. Interleukin 1 has been found to be an osteoclast-activating factor. Other such factors may be products of B or T lymphocytes. The bone-resorbing effects of ligands such as transforming growth factor alpha may in some bones be mediated through stimulation of prostaglandin synthesis and release. On the other hand, a major inhibitor of bone resorption, calcitonin, acts directly through receptors on osteoclasts. The cellular site of action of other inhibitors of bone resorption such as interferon gamma has not yet been elucidated.

CALCIUM METABOLISM There is about 1 to 2 kg calcium in the average adult human body, of which over 98 percent is in the skeleton. The calcium of the mineral phase at the surface of the crystals is in equilibrium with ions of the extracellular fluid, but only a minor proportion of the total calcium (about 0.5 percent) is exchangeable. The calcium in the extracellular fluid is critical for a variety of functions, and it is remarkably constant. In normal adults, the range of plasma concentration is 8.8 to 10.4 mg/dL (2.2 to 2.6 m*M*). The calcium in plasma is in three forms: as free ions, bound to plasma proteins, and, to a small extent, as diffusible complexes. The concentration of free calcium ions influences neuromuscular irritability and other cellular functions and is subjected to tight hormonal control, especially through parathyroid hormone, as described below. The concentration of serum proteins is an important factor in determining the concentration of calcium ions; most of the protein binding is to albumin. One formula that approximates the amount of calcium bound to proteins is

$$\% \text{ protein-bound Ca} = 8 \times \text{albumin (g/dL)} + 2 \times \text{globulin (g/dL)} + 3$$

Another correction is to subtract 1 mg/dL from the serum calcium concentration for every 1.0 g/dL serum albumin lower than 4.0 g/dL. Thus the concentration of ultrafiltrable calcium is usually about half the total calcium. In most laboratories only total calcium is determined, and knowledge of the concentration of proteins is essential to estimate concentration of calcium ions. Free ions can be measured with the use of calcium-specific electrodes.

The concentration of calcium ions in the extracellular fluid is kept constant by the interaction of processes that constantly feed calcium into and withdraw calcium from the extracellular fluid. Calcium enters the plasma via absorption from the intestinal tract and by resorption of ions from the bone mineral. Calcium leaves the extracellular fluid via secretion into the gastrointestinal tract, urinary excretion, deposition in bone mineral, and, to a minor extent, via losses in sweat. Resorption and formation are usually tightly coupled, approximately 0.5 g calcium entering and leaving the skeleton daily (Fig. 335-2).

The average diet in the United States provides about 0.6 to 1 g calcium daily, mostly in the form of dairy products. However, in adults less than half of the calcium in the diet is absorbed. Calcium absorption increases during periods of rapid growth in children, in pregnancy, and in lactation and decreases with advancing age. If adequate vitamin D is available and vitamin D metabolism is normal, more dietary calcium is absorbed (adaptation). Most of the calcium is absorbed in the proximal small intestine, and the efficiency of absorption decreases in the more distal intestinal segments. Both active transport and diffusion-limited absorption are involved; the former is more important in the upper, and the latter is more important in the lower, intestine. Both are influenced by vitamin D through the action of its metabolites. All forms of calcium in the diet may not be equally absorbed; even with defined salts, calcium as the chloride is probably absorbed more efficiently than that in other preparations.

Calcium is also secreted into the lumen of the gastrointestinal tract. When isotopes of radioactive calcium are administered intravenously, radioactivity appears in the feces, making possible calculations of *endogenous fecal calcium* (Fig. 335-2). Higher estimates of calcium losses in intestinal juices have been made by other approaches. Secretion of calcium into the intestinal lumen is constant and independent of absorption. If calcium availability in the diet is low (less than 500 mg per day), positive calcium balance requires an efficiency of absorption greater than 30 to 40 percent if intestinal uptake is sufficient to exceed losses via intestinal secretion and to match calcium losses through renal calcium excretion.

The urinary calcium excretion of normal adults on average calcium intakes ranges between 100 and 400 mg per day. When the dietary calcium is below 200 mg daily, urinary calcium excretion is usually less than 200 mg per day. However, in most normal individuals the level of dietary intake over a wide range has relatively little effect on the urinary excretion of calcium. Hence, in individuals on diets low in calcium, this relative inefficiency of renal calcium conservation leads to negative calcium balance unless calcium absorption is maximally efficient (Fig. 335-2).

FIGURE 335-2 *Calcium homeostasis. Schematic illustration of calcium content of extracellular fluid (ECF) and bone as well as of diet and feces; magnitude of calcium flux per day as calculated by various methods is shown at sites of transport in intestine, kidney, and bone. Ranges of values shown are approximate and chosen to illustrate certain points discussed in text. In intestine, absorption efficiency varies inversely with dietary calcium (chronic adaptation). This is reflected in typical quantities absorbed and excreted in feces; with 0.5-g intake, 50 percent absorption is depicted to occur (0.25 g), but at 1.5 g only 30 percent (0.5 g). Endogenous fecal calcium, the 0.1 to 0.2 g secreted into the intestinal lumen daily, is constant and does not vary with calcium intake or absorption. Quantities of calcium depicted as filtered, reabsorbed, and excreted at the kidney are chosen arbitrarily to indicate that at lower rates of filtration of calcium (expected at lower glomerular filtration rates), most is reabsorbed (e.g., 5.85 of 6 g), leading to urinary excretion of 150 mg; at higher rates of filtration (at high dietary calcium intake), slightly less is reabsorbed (e.g., 9.7 of 10 g), leading to a higher urinary excretion, 300 mg. In all situations, renal calcium reabsorption exceeds 95 percent of filtered load. Urinary calcium excretion is seen, therefore, to increase by only 150 mg despite a 1-g increase in dietary intake. In conditions of calcium balance, rates of calcium release from and uptake into bone are equal.*

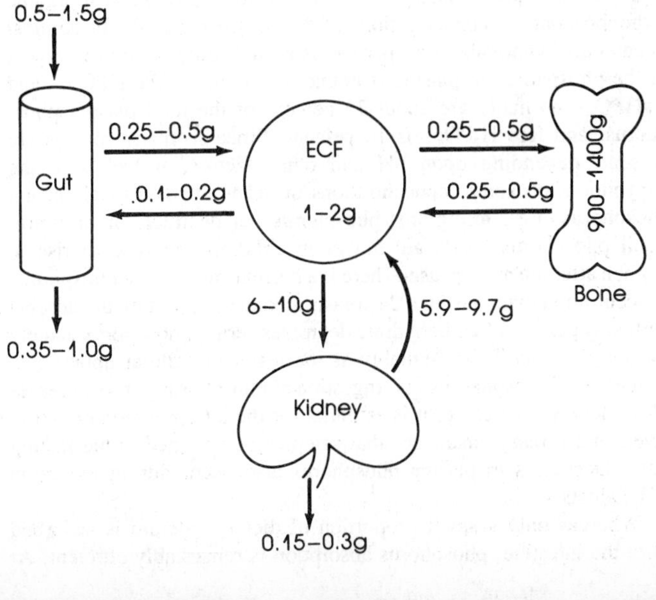

The amount of calcium in the urine is minute compared with that filtered through the glomerulus (about 6 to 10 g per day), but it is not certain whether some non-protein-bound, nonionic forms of calcium (e.g., calcium citrate) are cleared at rates considerably greater than others. The excretion of other electrolytes also affects the urinary excretion of calcium. For example, urinary calcium is usually proportional to urinary sodium; other ions, such as sulfate, also increase calcium excretion.

Maintenance of calcium balance (Fig. 335-2) is dependent upon the efficiency of intestinal absorption. Deficiency of parathyroid hormone or vitamin D, intestinal disease, or severe dietary calcium deprivation may provide challenges to calcium homeostasis that cannot be compensated adequately by renal calcium conservation, resulting in negative calcium balance. Increased bone resorption may protect against extracellular fluid calcium depletion even in states of chronic negative calcium balance but only at the expense of progressive osteopenia.

Pathophysiology Decrease in the concentration of free calcium ions in plasma results in increased neuromuscular irritability and the syndrome of tetany. This syndrome is characterized, when fully expressed by peripheral and perioral paresthesias, carpal spasm, pedal spasm, anxiety, seizures, bronchospasm, laryngospasm, Chvostek's, Trousseau's, and Erb's signs, and lengthening of the QT interval of the electrocardiogram. In infants tetany may be manifested only by irritability and lethargy. The level of calcium ions that determines which features of tetany will be manifested varies among individuals. The occurrence of tetany is also influenced by the concentration of other components of the extracellular fluid. For example, hypomagnesemia and alkalosis lower the threshold for tetany, whereas hypokalemia and acidosis raise the threshold.

Increases in total serum calcium are usually accompanied by increases in calcium ions and may be associated with manifestations including anorexia, nausea, vomiting, constipation, hypotonia, depression, and occasionally lethargy and coma. Persistent hypercalcemia, especially when accompanied by normal or elevated levels of serum phosphate, may result in deposition of a solid phase of calcium and phosphate in abnormal sites such as walls of blood vessels, connective tissue about the joints, gastric mucosa, cornea and renal parenchyma. Hypercalcemia per se alters renal function in addition to the pathologic effects of calcium-phosphate deposits in the lumen of renal tubules and in the interstitial areas of the kidney.

PHOSPHORUS METABOLISM Phosphorus is a major component of bone and is among the most abundant constituents of all tissues and in some form is involved in almost all metabolic processes. The total amount of phosphorus in the normal adult is about 1 kg, of which about 85 percent is in the skeleton.

In fasting plasma most of the phosphorus is present as inorganic orthophosphate in concentrations of 2.8 to 4.0 mg P/dL. In contrast to calcium, where about 50 percent is bound, only about 12 percent of the phosphorus in plasma is bound to proteins. Free HPO_4^{2-} and $NaHPO_4^-$ normally are about 75 percent of the total plasma phosphorus, and free $H_2PO_4^-$ is 10 percent. Since so many species are present, depending upon pH and other factors, it has been the convention to express concentrations in terms of mass of elemental phosphorus, i.e., milligrams phosphorus per deciliter, or molarity. Total phosphorus levels are higher in children and tend to rise in women after the menopause. There is a diurnal variation of phosphorus concentration even during a 24-h fast, mediated in part by the adrenal cortex. Ingestion of carbohydrate depresses serum phosphorus acutely by 1 to 1.5 mg/dL, presumably as the result of cellular uptake and formation of phosphate esters. Ingestion of phosphorus per se increases serum levels. Therefore, it is essential for the interpretation of serum levels and urinary clearances that samples be obtained in the fasting state. Decreases in plasma phosphorus also occur during induction of alkalosis.

Whereas only a small proportion of dietary calcium is absorbed from the intestine, phosphorus absorption is remarkably efficient. At low levels of dietary intake (less than 2 mg per kilogram of body weight per day) 80 to 90 percent of ingested phosphorus is absorbed. Even with the higher levels of intake (greater than 10 mg per kilogram of body weight per day) in the form of dairy products, cereals, eggs, and meat, absorption is about 70 percent. Hypophosphatemia due to deficient intestinal absorption is unusual except when excessive quantities of nonabsorbable antacids are consumed; the antacids bind phosphorus and prevent absorption from the intestinal lumen.

The major control of phosphorus economy is exerted at the level of the kidney. Phosphorus filtered through the glomerulus is largely reabsorbed in the proximal tubule (there is homeostatically important distal reabsorption as well) so that normally only about 10 to 15 percent of the filtered load is excreted. When filtered loads of phosphorus decrease, proximal tubular reabsorption increases. Conversely, when phosphorus loads are increased, tubular reabsorption decreases, and clearance rises. Thus, the urinary excretion of phosphorus normally reflects dietary intake, and conservation or elimination of excessive amounts of the ion depends upon adequate renal handling (Fig. 335-3). There is no good evidence for renal tubular phosphate secretion. Proximal reabsorption of phosphorus is dependent upon parallel sodium reabsorption, but whereas the sodium rejected by the proximal tubule may be reabsorbed distally, the rejected phosphorus is not. Therefore, the effects of volume expansion and decreased sodium reabsorption are to increase phosphorus clearance; similarly, diuretics such as acetazolamide, which act proximally, are phosphaturic parallel to the degree to which they are natriuretic.

Pathophysiology No direct symptoms result from hyperphosphatemia. However, when high levels are maintained for long periods, the driving force for mineralization is increased, and calcium phosphate may be deposited in abnormal sites. Severe, acute hypophosphatemia may or may not be accompanied by symptoms such as anorexia, dizziness, bone pain, proximal muscular weakness, and waddling gait. In severe hypophosphatemia (which may be aggravated, after hospitalization, by administration of nutrients to alcoholics or with therapy of diabetic ketoacidosis), elevations in serum creatine phosphokinase (CPK) suggest that rhabdomyolysis may be superimposed on myopathy. This sequence of events also occurs in experimental phosphate depletion in animals. Severe congestive cardiomyopathy has also been noted with chronic hypophosphatemia; restoration of phosphorus deficits leads to prompt reversal of the abnormalities. The bone pain and waddling gait are attributed to the osteomalacia which develops as a result of phosphate depletion. The muscular weakness may be due either to direct effects of hypophosphatemia on nerves and muscle or, in some instances, to the effects of hyperparathyroidism (either primary or secondary) which may have a role in the etiology of the hypophosphatemia. Defective growth in children may also be due to phosphate depletion. Hypophosphatemia results in decreased levels of 2,3-diphosphoglyceric acid and adenosine triphosphate (ATP) in erythrocytes which in turn alter the dissociation of oxyhemoglobin so that less oxygen is delivered in the periphery. Hemolytic anemia may be produced as the result of impairment of the ability of erythrocytes to deform in small vessels.

Negative phosphorus balance (Fig. 335-3) is rarely caused by inadequate phosphorus absorption in the intestine, and maintenance of normal phosphorus balance is dependent upon efficiency of renal excretion or conservation. In severe renal failure, hyperphosphatemia results from inadequate renal phosphorus clearance; heritable or acquired renal tubular defects may lead to hypophosphatemia due to inadequate renal conservation of phosphorus.

VITAMIN D

Vitamin D is a hormone, not a vitamin. With adequate exposure to sunlight, no dietary supplements are needed. The active principle of vitamin D is synthesized under metabolic control via successive hydroxylations in the liver and kidney and is transported through the blood to its target tissues (the small intestine and bone) to help maintain calcium homeostasis. Calcium and phosphate ions, parathyroid hormone, and possibly other peptide and steroid hormones play major roles directly or indirectly in the regulation of the renal metabolism of vitamin D. Analysis of hereditary and acquired defects in these metabolic processes have provided new insights into the pathophysiology of several disorders involving calcium, phosphorus, and bone metabolism. These discoveries have been the impetus for several advances, including the chemical synthesis of active vitamin D metabolites and analogues, the clinical use of 1α,25-dihydroxyvitamin D_3 [1,25$(OH)_2D_3$] in many vitamin D–resistant disorders, the development and application of assays for measuring vitamin D metabolites in blood to define suspected abnormalities in vitamin D metabolism, and a growing interest in developing more potent vitamin D analogues for clinical use.

PHOTOBIOGENESIS OF VITAMIN D Vitamin D_3 is a derivative of 7-dehydrocholesterol (provitamin D_3), the immediate precursor of cholesterol. When skin is exposed to sunlight or certain artifical light sources, the ultraviolet radiation enters the epidermis and causes a variety of photobiochemical events. Among them is the transformation of 7-dehydrocholesterol to vitamin D_3. Wavelengths between 290 and 315 nm are absorbed by the conjugated double bonds at C_5 and C_7 of 7-dehydrocholesterol that result in the fragmentation of the B ring between C_9 and C_{10} to yield a 9,10-secosterol (*seco* means "split"), previtamin D_3 (Fig. 335-4). Previtamin D_3 is biologically inert but is thermally labile and spontaneously undergoes a temperature-dependent molecular rearrangement of its conjugated triene system (three double bonds) to form the thermally stable 9,10-secosterol, vitamin D_3 (Fig. 335-4). At body temperature it takes approximately 3 days for previtamin D_3 to convert completely into vitamin D_3. Large changes in the temperature of the surface of the skin do not affect the rate of this conversion because the process occurs in the actively growing layers of the epidermis where the temperature is relatively constant; changes in the core body temperature also have little effect on this reaction. Once vitamin D_3 is synthesized, it is translocated from the epidermis into the circulation by the vitamin D–binding protein. Thus, vitamin D_3 is made in the skin from previtamin for days after a single sun exposure (Fig. 335-4). Although melanin in the skin competes with 7-dehydrocholesterol for ultraviolet photons and thus can limit the synthesis of previtamin D_3, the photochemical isomerization of previtamin D_3 to two biologically inert products (lumisterol$_3$ and tachysterol$_3$) appears to be more important in preventing excessive production of previtamin D_3 during prolonged exposure to the sun (Fig. 335-4).

Aging decreases the capacity of the skin to produce vitamin D_3; greater than twofold reduction occurs after the age of 70 years. Topical sunscreens reduce cutaneous vitamin D_3 production by absorbing the solar radiation that is responsible for vitamin D_3 synthesis in the skin. Other factors that affect the cutaneous synthesis of vitamin D_3 include altitude, geographical location, time of day, and area of exposure. When the entire body is exposed to sufficient sunlight to cause mild erythema, the increase in the blood vitamin D is equivalent to consuming an oral dose of 10,000 international units (1 IU = 0.025 μg) of vitamin D_3. Only when skin radiation is insufficient to produce the required quantities of vitamin D_3 is there a need for dietary supplementation to prevent skeletal mineralization defects. Fish liver oils, a natural source of vitamin D, were used widely for the treatment of rickets early in this century. Crystalline vitamin D_2 (Fig. 335-4) or vitamin D_3 is now added to milk and cereals. Such supplementations prevent rickets and osteomalacia. The National Research Council of the United States recommends an intake of 400 IU per day.

Once vitamin D enters the circulation, either by its absorption from the diet or through the skin, it is transported to the liver bound to a specific alpha$_1$ globulin (vitamin D–binding protein).

FIGURE 335-3 *Phosphate homeostasis. Schematic illustration of inorganic phosphorus content (termed here phosphate) in extracellular fluid (ECF) and bone as well as diet and feces; magnitude of phosphorus flux per day as estimated by various methods is shown at transport sites in intestine, kidney, and bone. Range of values shown illustrates special features of phosphorus metabolism discussed in text. Intestinal phosphorus absorption is highly efficient, 85 percent at a lower intake (0.5 g of a 0.6-g intake) and 70 percent at a higher intake (1.4 g of a 2.0-g intake). Estimates of magnitude of endogenous fecal phosphate are less well established than for calcium. Contribution of at least 0.15 g is estimated to be added to the nonabsorbed phosphorus to provide a total of 0.2 g fecal phosphorus at the low intake level. At high phosphorus dietary intakes, no correction for endogenous fecal phosphate is calculated. Higher quantities of phosphorus are excreted in urine at all levels of dietary intake than for corresponding intakes of calcium; quantities excreted match closely the quantities absorbed, thereby maintaining phosphorus balance (no correction in this illustration is made for endogenous fecal phosphorus). Note that renal phosphorus reabsorption, in contrast to high and relatively invariant renal calcium reabsorption, varies from a low of 75 percent of filtered load to greater than 85 percent. The compartment labeled ICF refers to intracellular phosphorus, both organic and inorganic; rapid shifts of phosphorus into cells (and corresponding, possibly slower, efflux of phosphorus from cells) contribute to changes in ECF phosphorus. These shifts between ECF and ICF and phosphorus release from and uptake by bone are equal in conditions of phosphorus balance.*

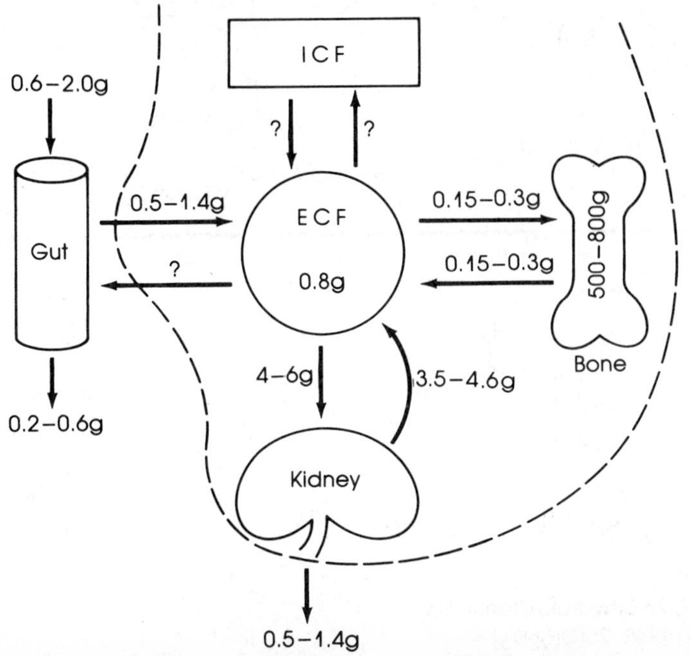

METABOLISM OF VITAMIN D In the liver, vitamin D is metabolized to 25-hydroxyvitamin D [25(OH)D] by hepatic mitochondrial and/or microsomal enzyme(s) (Fig. 335-4). 25(OH)D is one of the major circulating metabolites of vitamin D, and its half-life is estimated to be about 21 days. The concentration of 25(OH)D and some of its metabolites in the serum is measured using competitive binding assays. The normal circulating concentration of 25(OH)D varies among different laboratories from 5 to 80 ng/mL. Individuals exposed to excessive sunlight may have concentrations of 25(OH)D up to 150 ng/mL without adverse effects on calcium metabolism. Assays that employ chromatographic separation prior to binding analysis often have a lower normal range, possibly because other vitamin D metabolites simulate 25(OH)D in this assay. The normal range, apparently independent of method, is lower in Great Britain than in the United States; in Great Britain dietary supplements of vitamin D are not routine, and exposure to sunlight is less than in most regions of the United States. The serum 25(OH)D levels routinely measured reflect both 25-hydroxyvitamin D_2 [25$(OH)D_2$] and 25-hydroxyvitamin D_3 [25$(OH)D_3$]. The ratio of these two 25-hydroxylated derivatives depends on the relative amounts of vitamins D_2 or D_3 present in the diet and the amount of previtamin D_3 produced by exposure to sunlight.

The hepatic 25-hydroxylation of vitamin D is regulated by a product feedback mechanism. This regulation, however, is not tight; an increase in dietary intake or endogenous production of vitamin D_3 is reflected by elevations in 25(OH)D concentration levels in the serum. The levels can rise to greater than 500 ng/mL when the intake of vitamin D is increased. Serum 25(OH)D concentration levels are reduced in severe chronic parenchymal and cholestatic liver disease (Table 335-1).

25(OH)D is not biologically active at physiologic levels in vivo but is active in vitro at high concentrations. Normally, after formation in the liver, 25(OH)D is bound by the high-affinity vitamin D–binding protein that is synthesized in the liver and transported to the kidney for an additional stereospecific hydroxylation on either C_1 or C_{24} (Fig. 335-4). The kidney plays a pivotal role in the metabolism of 25(OH)D to the biologically active metabolite. The renal mitochondrial 25(OH)D-1α-hydroxylase activity is enhanced by hypocalcemia so that the rate of conversion of 25(OH)D to $1,25(OH)_2D$ increases. However, hypocalcemia may not control this hydroxylation

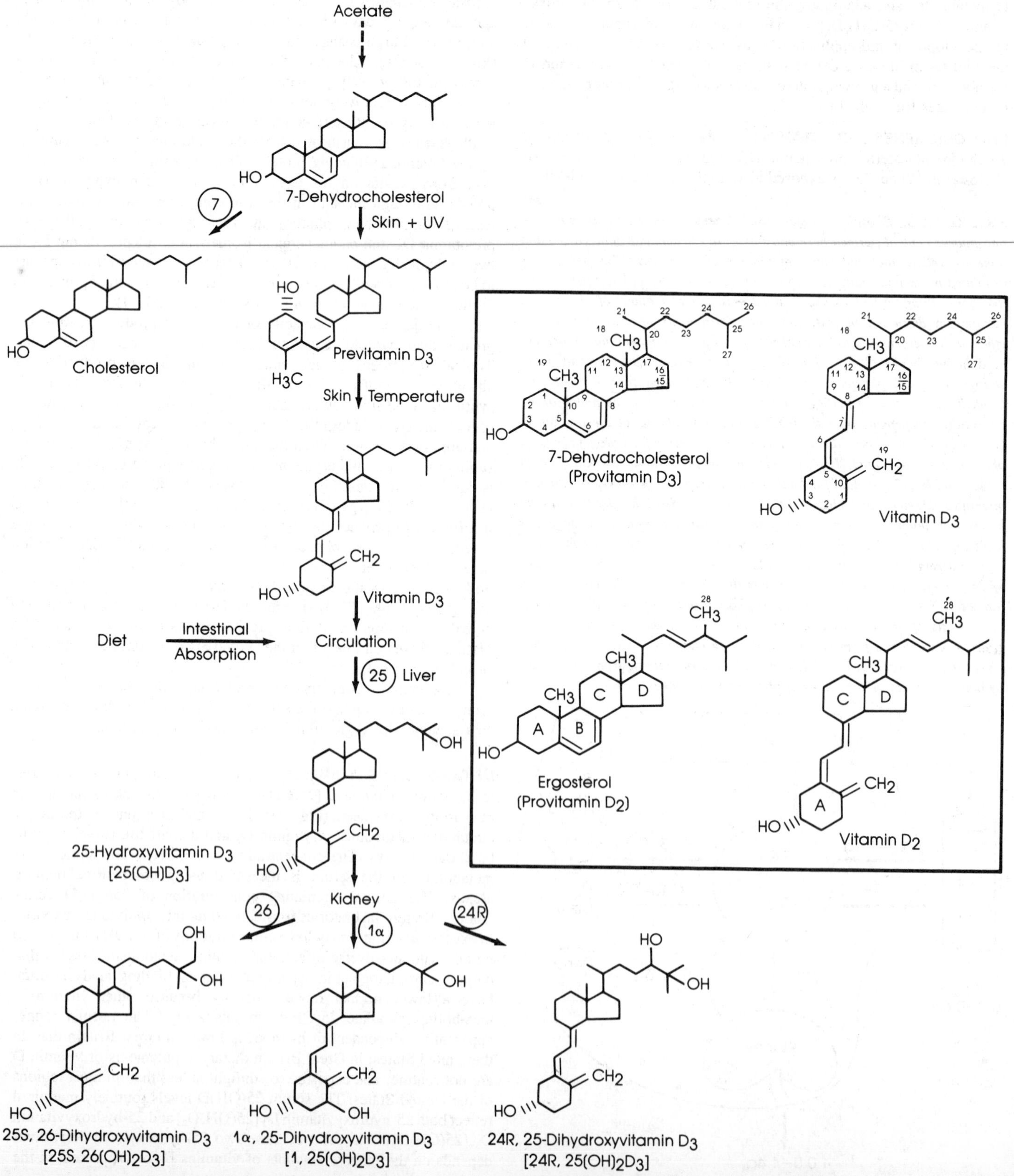

directly. Any decrease in the serum concentration of calcium below normal is a stimulus for increased secretion of parathyroid hormone. Parathyroid hormone acts physiologically as a tropic hormone to increase the synthesis of $1,25(OH)_2D$ in the renal proximal convoluted tubule. The mechanism by which parathyroid hormone exerts its influence on the renal metabolism of 25(OH)D is not established; however, the renal production of $1,25(OH)_2D$ correlates with the effects of parathyroid hormone in lowering circulating concentrations (and presumably renal intracellular concentrations) of phosphate. $1,25(OH)_2D$ also influences the renal metabolism of 25(OH)D by diminishing 25(OH)D-1α-hydroxylase activity and enhancing the metabolism of 24R,25-dihydroxyvitamin D [$24,25(OH)_2D$].

$24,25(OH)_2D$ is a circulating metabolite of 25(OH)D normally present in serum at a concentration of 0.5 to 5.0 ng/mL. $24,25(OH)_2D$ is also a substrate for renal 25(OH)D-1α-hydroxylase and is converted to 1α,24R,25-trihydroxyvitamin D [$1,24,25(OH)_3D$]. This trihydroxy metabolite is less potent than $1,25(OH)_2D$ in stimulating intestinal calcium transport; whether it has a physiologic role in maintaining calcium homeostasis is unclear. Cultured chondrocytes, skin fibroblasts, intestinal cells, and pituitary cells are among the cell types that also metabolize 25(OH)D to $24,25(OH)_2D$. $24,25(OH)_2D$ may play a role in the expression of vitamin D action, especially on the skeleton. There is no agreement, however, concerning the biologic importance of $24,25(OH)_2D$ per se as distinct from actions resulting from its conversion to $1,24,25(OH)_3D$.

The kidney also metabolizes 25(OH)D to 25S,26-dihydroxyvitamin D [$25,26(OH)_2D$]. $25,26(OH)_2D$, like $24,25(OH)_2D$, is metabolized by the kidney to 1α,25S,26-trihydroxyvitamin D [$1,25,26(OH)_3D$]. $1,25,26(OH)_3D$ is less active than $1,25(OH)_2D$ in inducing intestinal calcium transport, and the physiologic function of this metabolite remains to be defined.

$1,25(OH)_2D$ is a substrate for the 25(OH)D–24R-hydroxylase and is metabolized to $1,24,25(OH)_3D$, but this conversion is not believed to be important for the expression of biologic activity of $1,25(OH)_2D$.

FIGURE 335-4 *Photobiogenesis and metabolic pathways for vitamin D production and metabolism. Circled letters and numbers denote specific enzymes: (7) = 7-dehydrocholesterol reductase; (25) = vitamin D-25-hydroxylase; (1α) = 25(OH)D-1α-hydroxylase; (24R) = 25(OH)D-24R-hydroxylase; (26) = 25(OH)D-26-hydroxylase. The insert denotes the basic $\Delta^{5,7}$-diene steroid structures for the precursors of vitamin D_2 (ergosterol) and vitamin D_3 (7-dehydrocholesterol) and the 9,10-secosteroid structures of vitamin D_2 (ergocalciferol) and vitamin D_3 (cholecalciferol). Historically, the subscripts for vitamin D are related to the order in which the compounds were isolated and characterized. What was originally called vitamin D_1 is a mixture of compounds, and the term is no longer used. The next two vitamin D compounds, vitamin D_2 and vitamin D_3, were isolated, respectively, from the irradiation products of ergosterol (a $\Delta^{5,7}$-diene steroid found primarily in plants) and 7-dehydrocholesterol (a $\Delta^{5,7}$-diene steroid precursor of cholesterol present in animal tissues, including humans). Vitamin D_2 and D_3 differ in their side chains; the side chain for vitamin D_2 contains a Δ^{22} and a C_{24}-methyl group. Even though vitamin D_3 is the only endogenous form of vitamin D in skin, both vitamins D_2 and D_3 are metabolized identically and have equivalent biologic potencies in most mammals; in the absence of subscript the term vitamin D may refer to either compound.*

In steroid nomenclature, substituents on the steroid ring skeleton that are spatially oriented below the plane of the molecule (drawn as a broken line) are called α substituents, *and those substituents spatially oriented above the plane of the molecule (drawn as a solid line) are called* β substituents. *Because vitamin D is a structural derivative of a $\Delta^{5,7}$-diene steroid, by convention the numbering of the carbon atoms and the stereochemical designation of the functional groups remain the same as for the parent steroid. During the transformation $\Delta^{5,7}$-diene→previtamin D→vitamin D, the geometric position of ring A is altered, thereby changing the stereochemical orientation of its substituents; nonetheless, the original designation(s) of the hydroxyl function(s) on ring A of the steroid precursor are retained. The R,S notation, as in 24R,25-dihydroxy-vitamin D_3, specifies the spatial configuration of a substituent at an asymmetric carbon center.*

More than twenty metabolites of vitamin D have been identified. All of the metabolites originate from 25(OH)D or $1,25(OH)_2D$. Most of the metabolites may be degradation products. Of particular interest is the metabolic sequence that results in the inactivation of $1,25(OH)_2D$ by the oxidative cleavage of the side chain between C_{23} and C_{24} to yield a biologically inert and water-soluble product, 1α-hydroxyvitamin D–23-carboxylic acid.

PHYSIOLOGY OF VITAMIN D $1,25(OH)_2D$, produced by the kidney and during pregnancy by the placenta, is the only known important metabolite of vitamin D; the potential roles of other metabolites have not been clarified. $1,25(OH)_2D$ bound to a vitamin D–binding protein is delivered to the intestine, where the free form is taken up by the cells and transported to a specific nuclear receptor protein. The interaction of $1,25(OH)_2D$ with its specific nuclear receptor results in the phosphorylation of the receptor complex, and subsequent interaction with the chromatin activates transcription of genes whose products stimulate calcium and phosphate transport from the small intestinal lumen into the circulation. Under physiologic conditions the action of $1,25(OH)_2D$ is believed to be synergistic with that of parathyroid hormone on bone resorption. However, effects on bone resorption of physiologic concentrations of $1,25(OH)_2D$ independent of parathyroid hormone are not established. $1,25(OH)_2D$ can, however, mobilize bone mineral independently at supraphysiologic levels by inducing differentiation of precursor mononuclear cells to osteoclasts. Whether $1,25(OH)_2D$ has direct effects on the renal handling of calcium and phosphorus is also uncertain.

Cytoplasmic receptors for $1,25(OH)_2D_3$ are present in bone, in renal tubular cells, and in tissues and cells that have not classically been recognized as target organs for this hormone, including skin, breast, pituitary gland, parathyroid glands, beta cells of the pancreatic islets, gonads, brain, skeletal muscle, circulating monocytes, and activated B and T lymphocytes. Although the physiologic role of $1,25(OH)_2D$ in these cells remains to be determined, $1,25(OH)_2D_3$ in vitro inhibits human fibroblast proliferation, stimulates terminal differentiation of human keratinocytes, induces monocytes to produce interleukin 1 and mature into macrophages and osteoclast-like cells, inhibits interleukin 2 production by T lymphocytes, and induces synthesis and secretion of thyroid-stimulating hormone (TSH) by pituitary cells. In addition, a variety of tumor cell lines including breast carinomas, melanomas, and promyeloblasts possess receptors for $1,25(OH)_2D$.

Cultured tumor cell lines that possess receptors for this hormone respond to the hormone by decreasing the rate of proliferation and by enhancing differentiation. For example, when malignant, receptor-positive human promyelocytic cells (HL-60) are exposed to $1,25(OH)_2D_3$, the cells mature into functioning macrophages within 1 week. Although the mechanism of $1,25(OH)_2D_3$ induction of maturation is unknown, $1,25(OH)_2D_3$ decreases the expression of c-*myc* oncogene coincident with decreasing replication. This effect, however, is not a lasting one; when the metabolite is removed from maturing HL-60 promyelocytes, the cells revert to their original malignant state, and expression of c-*myc* oncogene is no longer suppressed.

The importance of $1,25(OH)_2D$ in the regulation of differentiation and immunoregulation is unknown. Patients with vitamin D–dependent rickets type II who are unable to respond to physiologic concentrations of $1,25(OH)_2D_3$ (because of insufficient or defective receptors for this hormone) appear to have no demonstrable in vivo

TABLE 335-1 Serum concentrations of 25(OH)D in disorders of calcium, phosphorus, and bone metabolism

Disease states	Serum 25(OH)D
Vitamin D deficiency	↓
Intestinal malabsorption syndromes	↓
Liver disorders (chronic and severe)	↓
Nephrotic syndrome	↓
Osteopenia in the aged	N or ↓
Vitamin D intoxication	↑

NOTE: ↓ = *decreased;* N = *normal;* ↑ = *increased.*

defects in their cellular immune response. $1,25(OH)_2D_3$ may play a role in inducing differentiation of stem cells in the bone marrow to osteoclasts.

Most measurements of circulating $1,25(OH)_2D$ in humans in various physiologic or pathologic states utilize a receptor/competitive binding assay (Table 335-2). Serum concentrations of vitamin D and 25(OH)D vary with the seasons and with vitamin D intake. Serum concentrations of $1,25(OH)_2D$, however, appear to be unaltered by seasonal variation, by increases in dietary vitamin D, or by exposure to sunlight; as long as vitamin D supplies and circulating concentrations of 25(OH)D are sufficient, metabolic influences operate on the renal 25(OH)D-1α-hydroxylase to ensure a closely regulated circulating concentration of $1,25(OH)_2D$. The serum concentration of $1,25(OH)_2D$ ranges from 25 to 75 pg/mL. The serum half-life of $1,25(OH)_2D_3$ is from 3 to 6 h.

When the serum calcium falls below normal, secretion of parathyroid hormone is enhanced, resulting in increased production of $1,25(OH)_2D$. The principal physiologic regulation of the production of $1,25(OH)_2D$ appears to involve changes in serum calcium concentrations that result in reciprocal changes in secretion of parathyroid hormone, the latter controlling, possibly through actions on serum or tissue phosphorus concentrations, the rate of $1,25(OH)_2D$ production. Other factors that enhance $1,25(OH)_2D$ production in animals include estrogen, prolactin, and growth hormone. Humans adapt to increased calcium requirements during growth, pregnancy, and lactation by increasing the efficiency of intestinal calcium absorption, possibly by enhancing 25(OH)D-1α-hydroxylase activity. During the first two trimesters of pregnancy the concentrations of $1,25(OH)_2D$ increase proportional to increases in the concentrations of the vitamin D–binding protein; concentrations of free $1,25(OH)_2D$ do not change. During the last trimester when maximal mineralization of the fetal skeleton takes place, the increased demand for calcium is met by an increase in the free concentrations of $1,25(OH)_2D$, which in turn enhance maternal intestinal calcium absorption.

PATHOPHYSIOLOGY OF DISORDERS OF VITAMIN D NUTRITION AND METABOLISM *Hypovitaminosis D* results from inadequate endogenous production of vitamin D_3 in the skin, insufficient dietary supplementation, and/or the inability of the small intestine to absorb adequate amounts of vitamin D from the diet. Disease states equivalent to hypovitaminosis D result from (1) effects of drugs that antagonize vitamin D action, (2) alterations in the metabolism of vitamin D, or (3) deficient or defective cellular receptors for vitamin D metabolites. Hypovitaminosis D results in (1) disturbances of mineral ion metabolism and secretion of parathyroid hormone and (2) mineralization defects in the skeleton (e.g., rickets in children, osteomalacia in adults). The changes in the skeleton are described in Chap. 337. With regard to calcium metabolism, lack of vitamin D action leads to deficient intestinal calcium absorption and to hypocalcemia. The latter stimulates compensatory secondary hyperparathyroidism; the increased secretion of parathyroid hormone, which enhances calcium release from bone and decreases calcium clearance by the kidney, tends to blunt the hypocalcemia. (Late in the course of untreated hypovitaminosis D, severe hypocalcemia develops.) Hypophosphatemia is more marked than hypocalcemia, especially in early stages of vitamin D deficiency. The efficiency of intestinal phosphate absorption, similar to that of calcium absorption, decreases with severe vitamin D deficiency. The increased secretion of parathyroid hormone, although partially effective in minimizing hypocalcemia, leads to urinary phosphate wasting through decreases in renal tubular reabsorption. This latter effect may be the most significant factor in causing hypophosphatemia. With an adequate glomerular filtration rate, the predominant changes in blood are severe hypophosphatemia, moderate or slightly low levels of calcium, and increased levels of parathyroid hormone. Blood levels of 25(OH)D are low (Table 335-1). As discussed in Chap. 337 defects in skeletal mineralization may accompany these disturbances in mineral ion metabolism.

TABLE 335-2 Serum concentrations of $1,25(OH)_2D$ in disorders of calcium, phosphorus, and bone metabolism

Disease states	Serum $1,25(OH)_2D$
Vitamin D deficiency	↓*
Renal failure:	
GFR > (30 mL/min)/1.7 m²	↓ or N
GFR < (30 mL/min)/1.7 m²	↓
Hypoparathyroidism	↓ or N
Pseudohypoparathyroidism	↓ or N
Vitamin D–dependent rickets:	
Type I	↓ or N
Type II	↑ or N
X-linked vitamin D–resistant rickets	↓ or N
Tumor-induced osteomalacia	↓
Oncogenic hypercalcemia	↓
Some lymphomas	↑
Hyperparathyroidism	↑
Sarcoidosis, tuberculosis, silicosis	↑
Idiopathic hypercalciuria	N or ↑
Williams' syndrome	↑
Vitamin D intoxication	↓ or N

* *Serum $1,25(OH)_2D$ concentrations are normal or elevated in occasional patients with biopsy-proven osteomalacia and undetectable or low circulating concentrations of 25(OH)D. These patients also have secondary hyperparathyroidism, and they may represent a partially treated state; if a small amount of vitamin D is obtained from the diet or generated in the skin in these patients, the vitamin is efficiently converted to $1,25(OH)_2D$. The net effect is low or undetectable circulating concentrations of 25(OH)D along with normal or elevated concentrations of $1,25(OH)_2D$. However, in extreme vitamin D deficiency, circulating concentrations of $1,25(OH)_2D$ are low or undetectable.*

NOTE: ↓ = *decreased*; N = *normal*; ↑ = *increased*; *GFR* = *glomerular filtration rate.*

Although the conversion of vitamin D to 25(OH)D is impaired in liver disease, there is no strong correlation between low serum 25(OH)D levels and osteopenia; multiple effects of the primary disease state seem to affect skeletal metabolism as well. There is a relation between chronic anticonvulsant therapy and the development of osteomalacia or rickets; mineralization defects are worse in patients on multiple drug therapy and where vitamin D intake or exposure to sunlight is inadequate. These drugs have multiple and complex effects on calcium metabolism. Phenobarbital induces hepatic microsomal enzymes, alters the kinetics of the vitamin D–25-hydroxylase and stimulates bile secretion, which results in decreased serum concentrations of vitamin D and 25(OH)D. Both phenytoin and phenobarbital influence calcium metabolism by inhibiting intestinal calcium transport and bone mineral mobilization, independent of effects of vitamin D metabolism.

Glucocorticoids in high doses cause disturbances in calcium metabolism and osteoporosis, but osteomalacia and rickets per se are not a consequence of glucocorticoid therapy. Actions of glucocorticoids on vitamin D–mediated calcium metabolism include a direct inhibitory effect of vitamin D–mediated intestinal calcium absorption and bone mineral mobilization and an enhancement of the sensitivity of $1,25(OH)_2D_3$ on bone cells either by stabilizing the $1,25(OH)_2D_3$ receptor or by increasing the affinity or number of receptors. Patients receiving glucocorticoids chronically may have depressed serum $1,25(OH)_2D$ concentrations; the mechanism(s) is unknown.

A genetic defect in the hepatic 25-hydroxylation of vitamin D has not been described. However, in one inherited disorder of calcium and bone metabolism renal production of $1,25(OH)_2D$ may be defective. In the syndrome of pseudovitamin D–deficient rickets (also known as vitamin D–dependent rickets, type I; see Chap. 337), low serum $1,25(OH)_2D$ concentrations and a normal therapeutic response to physiologic doses of $1,25(OH)_2D_3$ (calcitriol) (0.25 to 1.0 μg per day) have been attributed to an inherited deficiency in renal 25(OH)D-1α-hydroxylase activity. In addition, patients with a similar phenotype, pseudovitamin D–resistant rickets (vitamin D–dependent rickets, type II), appear to have a lack of (or defective) receptors for $1,25(OH)_2D$ rather than defective metabolism of the vitamin. Individuals with this defect have high serum $1,25(OH)_2D$ concentrations; therapeutic responses to high-dose vitamin D therapy are associated with a further increase in the serum $1,25(OH)_2D$ concentrations.

In patients with X-linked hypophosphatemic rickets, serum concentrations of $1,25(OH)_2D$ are normal or low. Since hypophosphatemia is a potent stimulus for the renal 25(OH)D-1α-hydroxylase, the serum $1,25(OH)_2D$ concentrations should be high. Thus, even a normal serum $1,25(OH)_2D$ concentration suggests a functional defect in the 25(OH)D-1α-hydroxylase system. In some cases, the combination of calcitriol and phosphate supplements offers a therapeutic advantage to phosphate therapy by itself (Chap. 337). In patients with mild to moderate chronic renal failure (glomerular filtration rate >30 mL/min) and decreased phosphate clearance, hyperphosphatemia and acidosis play important roles in suppressing the renal production of $1,25(OH)_2D$ despite high circulating concentrations of parathyroid hormone. As the destruction of the renal cortex progresses, the reserves of the 25(OH)D-1α-hydroxylase are depleted to a point at which the kidney is unable to produce sufficient quantities of $1,25(OH)_2D$ to maintain calcium homeostasis, even when serum phosphorus concentrations are normal. Under these circumstances replacement therapy with calcitriol is most beneficial (Chap. 337).

Patients with hypoparathyroidism and pseudohypoparathyroidism have lower than normal mean serum concentrations of $1,25(OH)_2D$ although individual values overlap with the normal range. In these hypocalcemic patients favorable response to small replacement doses of calcitriol (0.25 to 1.0 μg per day; see Chap. 336) occur even when the serum 25(OH)D concentrations are higher than normal. These observations are consistent with the concept that patients with hypoparathyroidism or pseudohypoparathyroidism due to absent or ineffective action of parathyroid hormone have defective function of renal 25(OH)D-1α-hydroxylase. It is not known to what extent serum $1,25(OH)_2D$ concentrations would be restored toward normal if the hyperphosphatemia were adequately controlled.

Patients with tumor-induced (oncogenous) osteomalacia have low serum phosphorus and $1,25(OH)_2D$ levels. These tumors presumably secrete a substance(s) that causes renal phosphorus wasting and inhibits the formation of $1,25(OH)_2D$; after removal of the tumor the serum phosphorus and $1,25(OH)_2D$ levels return to normal.

In disease states equivalent to hypervitaminosis D such as sarcoidosis (and other chronic granulomatous disorders), lymphomas, idiopathic hypercalciuria, and Williams' syndrome there is an abnormality in the metabolism of 25(OH)D to $1,25(OH)_2D$ (Table 335-2). Hypercalcemia in sarcoidosis is associated with elevated circulating concentrations of $1,25(OH)_2D$; sarcoid granulomas metabolize 25(OH)D to $1,25(OH)_2D$ in an unregulated manner, and pulmonary alveolar macrophages from patients with sarcoidosis synthesize $1,25(OH)_2D$. In addition, normal pulmonary macrophages can be induced to metabolize 25(OH)D to $1,25(OH)_2D$ in vitro when exposed either to lipopolysaccharides from the cell wall of gram-negative bacteria or to gamma interferon. Most patients with tumor-induced hypercalcemia have low circulating concentrations of $1,25(OH)_2D$ (Table 335-2). The exceptions are patients with several types of lymphoma (including T-cell, mixed histiocytic-lymphocytic, and B-cell immunoblastic lymphomas) whose hypercalcemia is associated with elevated concentrations of $1,25(OH)_2D$. In one report, surgical excision of a solitary splenic lymphoma resulted in rapid return of elevated serum $1,25(OH)_2D$ and calcium levels to normal suggesting that the lymphoma cells metabolize 25(OH)D to $1,25(OH)_2D$ in an unregulated manner. There is a direct association between elevated circulating concentrations of $1,25(OH)_2D$ in patients with primary hyperparathyrodisim, hypercalciuria, and renal stones. Similarly, in some instances of idiopathic hypercalciuria, intestinal calcium absorption is inappropriately increased. Approximately one-third of these patients have elevated circulating $1,25(OH)_2D$. These findings are consistent with the hypothesis that excessive $1,25(OH)_2D$ production is responsible for the hyperabsorption of calcium by the small intestine. Infants with hypercalcemia associated with supravalvular aortic stenosis, mental retardation, and elfin facies (*Williams' syndrome*) also have elevated serum $1,25(OH)_2D$ concentrations. It is not clear whether the increased levels result from abnormal synthesis or degradation of $1,25(OH)_2D$.

PHARMACOLOGY OF VITAMIN D AND ITS METABOLITES A variety of over-the-counter vitamin preparations contain 400 IU of either vitamin D_2 or vitamin D_3. More potent forms of vitamin D (calciferol) are available in capsule and tablet form (50,000 IU) as well as in oil (500,000 IU/mL) and in oral solution 8000 IU/mL). A single oral dose of 50,000 IU of vitamin D_2 increases the circulating concentrations of vitamin D from less than 10 ng/mL to 50 to 100 ng/mL within 12 to 24 h; the plasma half-life is about 2 days. Serum concentrations of 25(OH)D and $1,25(OH)_2D$ are not changed. For treatment of vitamin D deficiency, 50,000 IU of vitamin D twice a week for several weeks raises the circulating concentration of 25(OH)D into the normal range; in the presence of secondary hyperparathyroidism the circulating concentrations of $1,25(OH)_2D$ increase to supranormal levels (up to 250 pg/mL). $25(OH)D_3$ (calcifediol) is available in capsules containing either 20 or 50 μg. This drug may be useful in treating vitamin D deficiency [low 25(OH)D concentrations] in patients with severe liver dysfunction. Pharmacologic doses are used to treat disorders of 25(OH)D metabolism; in pharmacologic doses $25(OH)D_3$ is believed to be effective through its interaction with the receptor for $1,25(OH)_2D$. $1,25(OH)_2D_3$ (calcitriol) is available in capsules containing 0.25 or 0.5 μg. Calcitriol is efficacious in therapy of a variety of calcium metabolic disorders (see Chap. 341). 1α-Hydroxyvitamin D_3 [$1(OH)D_3$] is also a potent $1,25(OH)_2D_3$ agonist. The structure of this analogue is identical to that of the natural renal hormone with the exception that it lacks a C_{25}-OH (Fig. 335-5). In humans, this analogue is rapidly metabolized by the liver to $1,25(OH)_2D_3$. This analogue is used in Europe and Japan.

When vitamin D is chemically manipulated to rotate the A ring through 180 degrees, the C_3-β-OH assumes a geometric position that mimics the C_1-α-OH (Fig. 335-5). These compounds, called pseudo-1α-hydroxyvitamin D analogues, include dihydrotachysterol and 5,6-*trans*-vitamin D_3. These analogues are less effective in stimulating intestinal calcium transport on a weight basis than either vitamin D or $1,25(OH)_2D_3$. However, because the pseudo-1α-hydroxyvitamin D analogues do not require a renal 1α-hydroxylation to be active on intestinal calcium transport, they are 3 to 10 times more potent than vitamin D in disease states that adversely affect the renal 25(OH)D-1α-hydroxylase, such as hypoparathyroidism and chronic renal failure. These analogues are efficiently metabolized in the liver to the corresponding 25-hydroxy derivatives, which are the biologically active forms.

PARATHYROID HORMONE Physiology The function of parathyroid hormone is to maintain extracellular fluid calcium concentration. The hormone acts directly on bone and kidney and indirectly on intestine through its effects on synthesis of $1,25(OH)_2D_3$ to increase serum calcium; in turn, parathyroid hormone production is closely regulated by the concentration of serum ionized calcium. This feedback system is one of the most important homeostatic mechanisms for the close regulation of extracellular fluid calcium concentration. Any tendency toward hypocalcemia, as might be induced by calcium-deficient diets, is counteracted by an increased rate of secretion of parathyroid hormone. This in turn (1) acts to increase the rate of dissolution of bone mineral, thereby increasing the flow of calcium from bone into blood, (2) reduces the renal clearance of calcium, returning more of the calcium filtered at the glomerulus into extracellular fluid, and (3) increases the efficiency of calcium absorption in the intestine. The relative physiologic importance of these three actions of parathyroid hormone, stimulation of calcium transport in bone, kidney, and intestine, is not clear. Most evidence suggests that rapid changes in blood calcium are due to effects of the hormone on bone and, to a lesser extent, on renal calcium clearance; maintenance of calcium balance, on the other hand, is probably due to the effects of the hormone on $1,25(OH)_2D_3$ levels and hence on the efficiency of intestinal calcium absorption. Evidence from calcium kinetic studies indicates that as much as 500 mg calcium is transferred between extracellular fluid and bone each day (a large amount in relation to the total extracellular fluid calcium pool), and parathyroid hormone has a major effect on this transfer. The action of the hormone tends to preserve calcium concentration in blood acutely at the cost of bone destruction and bone mineral release. However, the action

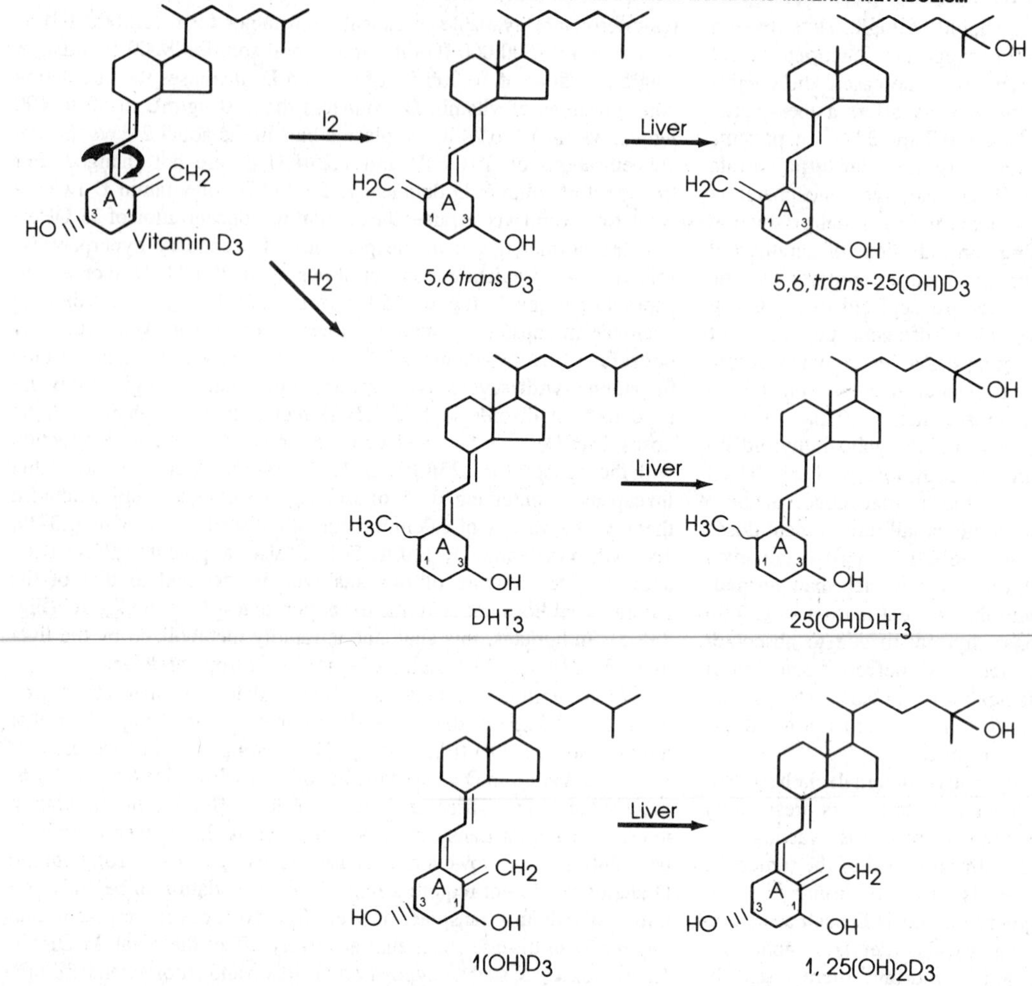

FIGURE 335-5 *When vitamin D is treated with I_2 or reduced with H_2, ring A of the vitamin D molecule rotates 180° to reorient spatially the 3β-OH in a pseudo-1α-OH position. These analogues, 5,6-trans-vitamin D_3 and dihydrotachysterol, (DHT_3), are called pseudo-1α-hydroxy analogues. $1(OH)D_3$ is a synthetic analogue of $1,25(OH)_2D_3$ that lacks a C_{25}-OH. $1(OH)D_3$, 5,6-trans-vitamin D_3, and DHT_3 all undergo a hepatic C_{25}-hydroxylation before they are biologically active.*

of parathyroid hormone on kidney to preserve calcium by increasing the reabsorption of filtered calcium may also be important in rapid regulation of blood calcium concentration.

Parathyroid hormone has a dual action on bone, the *calcium replacement* and the *bone remodeling* effects. There is an increased rate of release of calcium from bone into blood within minutes of the administration of parathyroid hormone, but a rapid efflux of calcium out of blood, presumably into bone cells, precedes the release of calcium. On the other hand, the more chronic effects of parathyroid hormone, mainly an increase in the number and activity of osteoclasts and a general increase in the remodeling of bone, are apparent only hours after the hormone is given. These latter actions, which involve increased protein synthesis, persist for hours after parathyroid hormone has been given. It is not clear whether the two effects of parathyroid action on bone represent a continuous spectrum with a common initiating biochemical event or whether they are separate actions. Only osteoblastic cells and not osteoclasts are believed to have receptors for parathyroid hormone.

Chemistry The complete amino acid sequences of the major forms of parathyroid hormone from cow, pig, rat, and human have been defined. The peptides consist of a single-chain structure composed of 84 amino acids. The molecules lack cysteine or cystine; the sequences of the three forms of the hormone are similar, as is illustrated in Fig. 335-6.

The structural requirements for the binding of the hormone to receptors and hence for its biologic activity have been defined. Synthetic fragments containing the amino-terminal sequence exert the known biologic actions of the hormone on mineral ion transport in kidney and bone and by stimulating the renal 25-hydroxyvitamin D-1α-hydroxylase also exert the capacity of the hormone to stimulate intestinal calcium absorption. Since osteoblasts and fibroblasts but not osteoclasts have receptors for parathyroid hormone, the effects of parathyroid hormone on stimulating osteoclastic bone resorption are indirect.

Fragments shortened at the amino terminus lose binding affinity more slowly than capacity to stimulate biologic response. The peptide 7-34 is a competitive inhibitor of the binding of active hormone to receptors in vitro and serves as a competitive inhibitor of the renal responses to the hormone, including the increased excretion of cyclic AMP and the enhanced clearance of phosphate. Rapid mobilization of calcium from bone is also blocked in certain test systems in vivo.

Any fragment of parathyroid hormone, to be biologically active on bone and kidney, must consist of the continuous peptide sequence beginning with residue 2, valine, and extending as far as residue 26, lysine.

These observations are of particular interest because the biosynthesis and peripheral metabolism of parathyroid hormone are complex.

Biosynthesis, secretion, metabolism, and mode of action Several larger molecular forms have been identified in the biosynthetic sequence leading from gene transcription and translation to final packaging of the 84-amino acid peptide in secretory granules prior to secretion (Fig. 335-7). The earliest detected precursor form, termed *preproparathyroid hormone,* consists of 115 amino acids; this molecular form is converted to an intermediate form of 90 amino acids termed *proparathyroid hormone*. The details of intracellular regulation of biosynthesis are unknown. Parathyroid hormone shares, with other polypeptides and proteins destined for secretion from cells, this complex pattern of initial synthesis as a larger molecule which is then reduced in size by several cleavages prior to secretion. The hydrophobic regions of the preproparathyroid hormone are similar to preprotein-specific regions of other cell-secreted proteins and may serve a role in guiding transport of the polypeptide from sites of synthesis on polyribosomes through the cytoskeleton to secretory granules. The genes for bovine, rat, and human parathyroid hormone have been cloned, and their structures have been determined. There are considerable homologies in the gene structures as well as in the proteins from these two species.

Blood calcium concentration controls the secretion of parathyroid hormone, and the ionized fraction of blood calcium is the important determinant of hormone secretion. Hormone secretion increases steeply to a maximum value of fivefold above basal rates of secretion whenever calcium concentration falls from normal to the range of 7.5 to 8.0 mg/dL (measured as total calcium). Beta-adrenergic agonists such as epinephrine and histamine-2 agonists may also increase hormone secretion, but the physiologic significance of these secretagogues is not established. Furthermore, drugs such as propranolol or cimetidine do not reproducibly decrease circulating parathyroid hormone levels.

Magnesium may influence hormone secretion in the same direction as calcium. It is unlikely that physiologic variations in magnesium concentration affect parathyroid secretion, but severe intracellular magnesium deficiency is associated with defective hormone secretion.

The hormone secreted in vivo from normal bovine and human parathyroid glands and from parathyroid adenomas is indistinguishable by immunologic criteria and by molecular size from the 84-amino acid peptide (molecular weight 9500) extracted from glands. However, much of the immunoreactive material found in the peripheral circulation of humans and animals (cow, dog) is smaller than the extracted or secreted hormone. The principal circulating fragments of immunoreactive hormone (approximate molecular weight 7000) lack a portion of the critical amino-terminal sequence required for biologic activity and, hence, are biologically inactive hormonal fragments.

Cleavage of the native peptide by an endopeptidase would be expected to result in formation of a second fragment, molecular weight 2000 to 3000, representing the amino-terminal, biologically active, portion of the hormone. There is uncertainty concerning the presence or absence of such a circulating amino-terminal fragment. It is also unclear (1) whether peripheral metabolism accounts for the circulating fragment(s) of hormone or whether fragments as well as intact hormone can also be secreted by the gland and (2) whether peripheral metabolism is a purely catabolic process concerned only with hormone destruction or whether the peripheral cleavage results in formation of a metabolically active amino-terminal fragment of parathyroid hormone. Present evidence suggests that the liver and kidney are the principal sites at which peripheral metabolism of hormone occurs. Cleavages in these organs may regulate the concentration of hormonally active polypeptides in the circulation (Fig. 335-5). Peripheral metabolism, in turn, may be affected by pathologic processes, such as renal failure or severe hepatic dysfunction.

The rate of clearance of the secreted 84-amino acid peptide from blood is more rapid than the rate of clearance of the smaller, biologically inactive fragment(s) that result from peripheral metabolism. Hence, measurements of parathyroid hormone in blood by most immunoassays provide only an overall index of parathyroid gland activity rather than a direct measure of biologically active hormone,

FIGURE 335-6

Model illustrating the sequence of human, cow, rat, and pig parathyroid hormone.

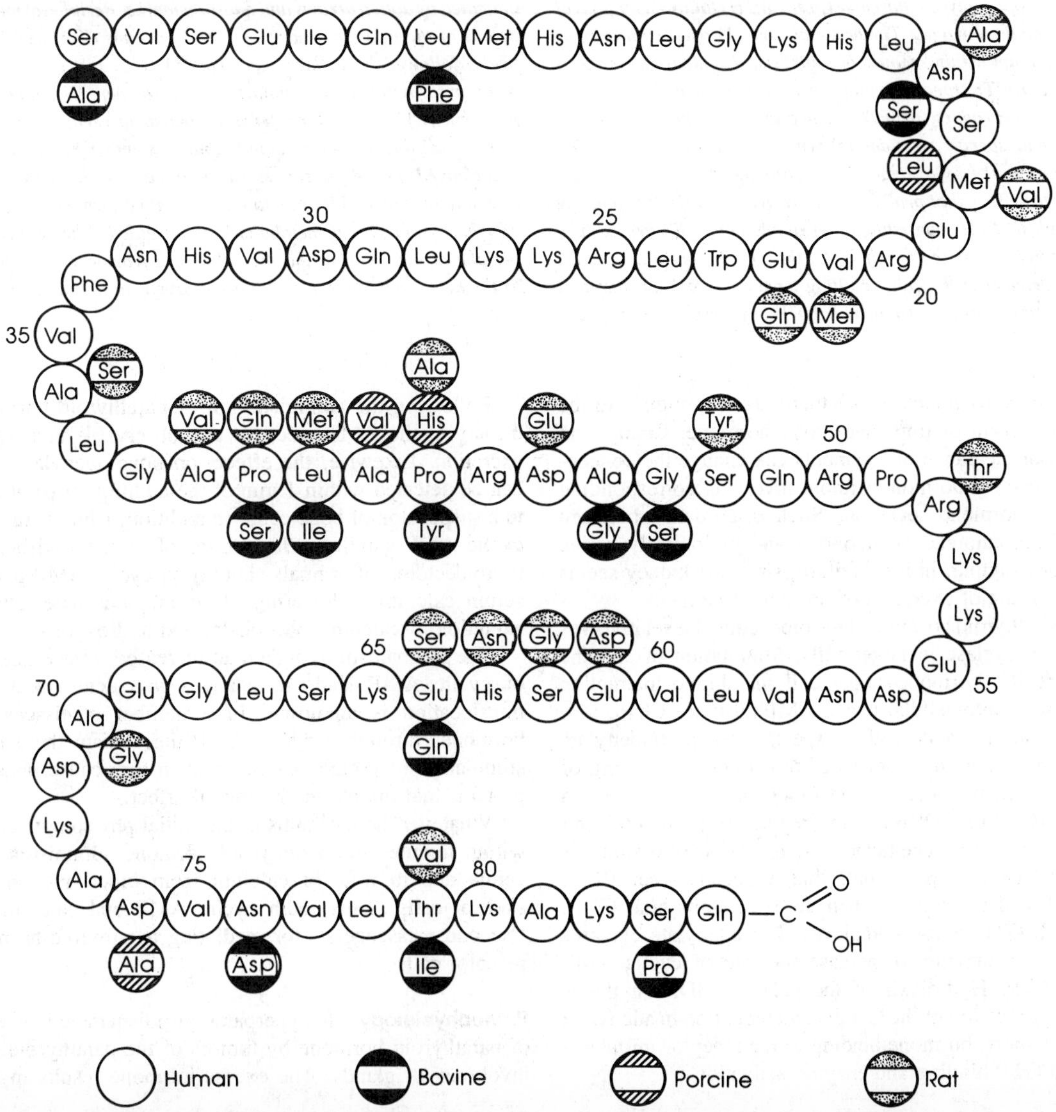

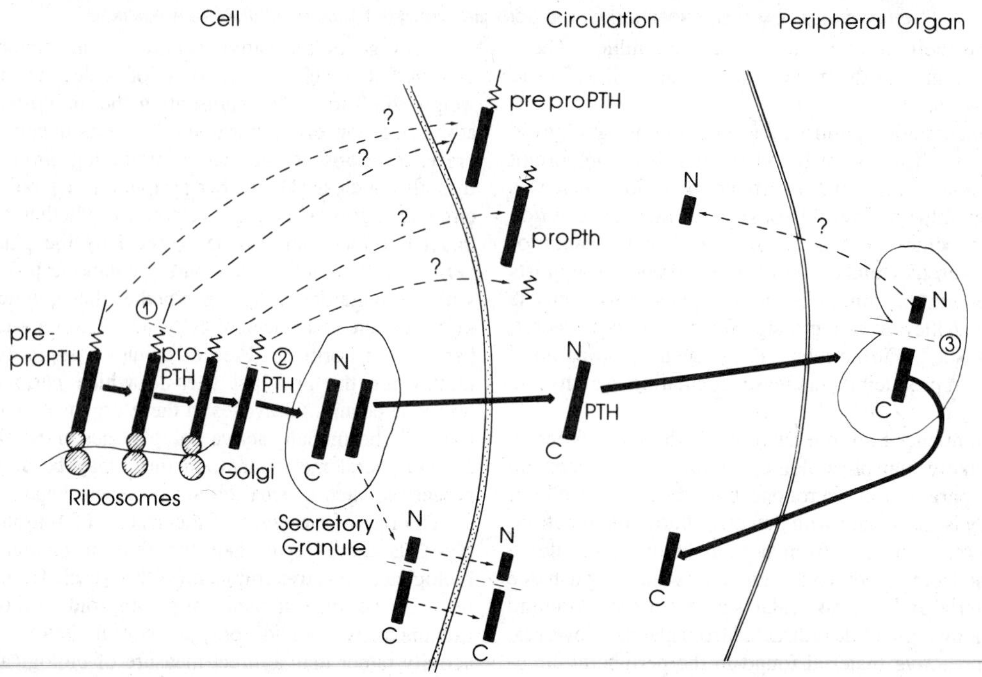

FIGURE 335-7 *Schematic model of the biosynthesis, secretion, and peripheral metabolism of parathyroid hormone, as well as contributions of these processes to the heterogeneity of circulating, immunoreactive parathyroid hormone (see text for details). Biosynthesis involves initial translation of parathyroid hormone–specific messenger RNA (mRNA) into a polypeptide of 115 amino acids, preproparathyroid hormone (preproPTH) followed by several specific posttranslational cleavages. The first cleavage (1) occurs on or near the endoplasmic reticulum within seconds of synthesis; this cleavage removes the 25-amino acid preproPTH-specific peptide, or leader sequence (represented by a straight line). The product, proPTH, a peptide of 90 amino acids, is converted by a second specific peptidase(s) with removal of the proPTH-specific peptide (represented by a jagged line), forming PTH. (An alternate possibility, not illustrated, is that proPTH is converted to PTH after packing into secretory granules.) PTH, consisting of 84 amino acids (illustrated as a heavy bar with N indicating amino terminus, C, the carboxy terminus), is the principal secretory product of the cell, resulting from exocytosis of secretory granules containing the hormone (indicated by heavy arrow). Some have reported that there is an alternate secretory pathway in which amino-terminal fragments (N) and carboxy-terminal fragments (C) of the molecule are formed by further proteolytic processing within the cell followed by release into the circulation (dotted arrows). Speculations concerning release of precursor forms, or fragments (not yet proved), from the cell into the circulation are indicated by dotted arrows and question marks. Peripheral metabolism involves uptake of the intact hormone by certain organs (liver and kidney being most likely) followed by a third cleavage (3). This last cleavage is presumed to result in formation of an amino-terminal fragment (N) and a carboxy-terminal fragment (C). The carboxy-terminal fragment reenters the circulation, from which it disappears more slowly than the intact hormone, and is taken up and cleaved; hence the concentration of carboxy-terminal fragment is higher than that of intact PTH. The fate of the amino-terminal fragment, presumably derived by peripheral metabolism, is unsettled. The relative contribution of peripheral metabolism and the release of fragments directly from the gland to the heterogeneity of circulating parathyroid hormone awaits clarification.*

since biologically inert fragments rather than intact hormone are the principal circulating form of immunoreactive hormone. Changes in rate of production or clearance of fragments can change the concentration of immunoreactive hormone without involving corresponding changes in rate of hormone secretion. Such discordance between concentrations of immunoreactive hormone and biologically active peptide occurs, for example, in renal failure, since the kidney seems to be the principal route of excretion of hormone fragments.

The action of parathyroid hormone at the biochemical level involves effects on adenylate cyclase in target cells. Stimulation of enzyme activity during specific hormone–target cell membrane interaction leads to an increase in intracellular cyclic AMP (also see Chap. 67). Parathyroid hormone interacts with a specific receptor/adenylate cyclase complex on plasma membranes of target cells consisting of hormone receptor, enzyme catalytic unit (adenylate cyclase), and a guanyl nucleotide (GTP or GDP)–binding regulatory protein (G unit or N protein) (see Chap. 67). The latter protein consists of α subunits that bind GTP or GDP and β subunits that dissociate when the α subunits bind GTP and reassociate when the α subunits bind GDP. The α subunit with GTP bound complexes with adenylate cyclase, thereby activating the enzyme to increase the rate of cyclic AMP production from ATP. Hydrolysis of the GTP to GDP on the α subunit leads to reassociation of the G units and reduction in adenylate cyclase activity. In short, hormone binding to the receptor initiates a cycle of α subunit/GTP binding and enzyme activation.

Following the administration of parathyroid hormone the rise in urinary cyclic AMP precedes any observable increase in phosphate excretion. Likewise, the effects on bone adenylate cyclase activity can be detected within 1 min of the addition of parathyroid hormone to a suspension of bone cells. In addition, administration of dibutyryl cyclic AMP simulates the actions of parathyroid hormone in parathyroidectomized animals. Dibutyryl cyclic AMP leads to a rise in serum calcium, a lowering of serum phosphate, and an increased excretion of calcium, phosphate, and hydroxyproline in urine.

The mechanism by which an increased intracellular concentration of cyclic AMP leads to changes in calcium and phosphate ion translocation is unknown. In a number of tissues responsive to hormones through a cyclic AMP mechanism there is evidence for stimulation of protein kinases that in turn cause phosphorylation of proteins that initiate the hormonal effect.

Whatever the mechanism, the initial physiologic effect (occurring within minutes) of parathyroid hormone administration is hypocalcemia due to flow of calcium from blood into cells, apparently skeletal cells. Thus, both cyclic AMP and calcium may serve as "second messengers" for mediating parathyroid hormone effects in receptor cells.

Pathophysiology In hyperparathyroidism there is an overproduction of parathyroid hormone by tumors of the parathyroid or hyperplasia involving all glands. The excess hormone results in hypercalcemia secondary to increased intestinal calcium absorption [increased synthesis of $1,25(OH)_2D_3$] and reduced renal calcium clearance. In many patients there is also increased bone resorption; bone turnover increases in all patients, with resorption exceeding formation in many. Individual patients respond to the excess hormone variably at intestinal, renal, and bone target sites; the factors influencing the variable response from patient to patient are not known (see Chap. 336).

Hypophosphatemia results from the actions of the excessive parathyroid hormone on renal tubular phosphate reabsorption. Hypophosphatemia in turn aggravates the hypercalcemia in part by increasing the synthesis of $1,25(OH)_2D_3$ and by increasing the sensitivity of the bone to resorption. The hypophosphatemia may also interfere with the normal mineralization of bone leading to a mixed picture of both increased resorption and deficient mineralization in adjacent skeletal sites.

Hypoparathyroidism causes hypocalcemia and hyperphosphatemia, a reversal of the response seen with hormone excess (see Chap. 336).

CALCITONIN (See also Chap. 334) Calcitonin is the potent hypocalcemic, hypophosphatemic peptide hormone that, in many ways, acts as the physiologic antagonist to parathyroid hormone. Calcitonin reduces bone resorption and has opposing effects to parathyroid hormone on the kidney in that it increases renal calcium clearance. Calcitonin exerts its effects through stimulation of membrane-bound adenylate cyclase in receptor cells in kidney and bone. There is a variable hormonal responsiveness of renal tubular cells to calcitonin, parathyroid hormone, and vasopressin. In some portions of the nephron, cells respond to all three hormones, whereas in others the response is restricted to one or two. In bone, osteoclasts possess calcitonin receptors.

The thyroid gland is the major source of the hormone in mammalian species, and the cells involved in calcitonin synthesis arise from neural crest tissue. During embryogenesis these cells migrate into the ultimobranchial body. The latter body or gland arises from the last branchial pouch, hence the name *ultimobranchial body*. In submammalian vertebrates the ultimobranchial body remains as a discrete organ, anatomically separate from the thyroid gland. In mammals the ultimobranchial gland fuses with and is incorporated into the thyroid gland. Calcitonin is found in all vertebrate classes.

The naturally occurring calcitonins consist of a peptide chain of 32 amino acids. There is a considerable amount of variability in sequence among species. The entire chain of 32 amino acids appears to be required for biologic activity in the whole animal, although fragments function in in vitro systems. The factors that regulate the synthesis of calcitonin are not known. Calcitonin from salmon is 25 to 100 times more potent by weight in lowering serum calcium in animals than are other forms of calcitonin. For example, the salmon hormone is at least 10 times more potent in humans than human calcitonin. Slow turnover may explain in part the greater biologic potency of salmon calcitonin, but the hormone binds more strongly to receptor sites as well. Calcitonin is synthesized as a precursor molecule, the parent molecule being four times larger than calcitonin itself. Analysis of the sequence of the coding portions of the gene for rat calcitonin indicates that at least two peptides flank calcitonin from which they are separated by basic residues. It is likely (in analogy with the common precursor for ACTH and endorphin) that these peptides are released with calcitonin and have actions that, for example, might explain certain pathophysiologic features in syndromes associated with excess calcitonin production. There are two calcitonin genes, α and β, located on chromosome 11 in the general region of the beta globin and parathyroid hormone genes. The transcription of the calcitonin gene is complex. Two different messenger RNA molecules are transcribed from the α gene; one is translated into the precursor for calcitonin, and the other message is transcribed into an alternate product, calcitonin-gene-related peptide (CGRP). CGRP is synthesized wherever the calcitonin message is expressed, for example, in medullary carcinoma of the thyroid. The β gene is transcribed into the messenger RNA for CGRP in the central nervous system in animals. CGRP may serve a neurotransmitter role; the expression of the β gene in human beings, as distinct from animals, has not been shown but is presumed to occur.

The secretion of calcitonin is under the direct control of blood calcium: an increase in calcium causes an increase and a decrease in calcium causes a decrease in calcitonin levels. Once secreted, calcitonin disappears rapidly from the circulation with a half-life of 2 to 15 min.

The concentration of calcitonin in the peripheral blood of normal humans is lower than in many other species. Basal and stimulated immunoreactive calcitonin levels are lower in women than in men and tend to decrease with age to a greater extent in women.

The physiologic role of calcitonin is incompletely understood. In animals calcitonin acts to lower both blood calcium and blood phosphate; the principal action is inhibition of bone resorption. The importance of calcitonin in increasing urinary calcium and phosphate clearance is synergistic with its effects on bone resorption. The actions of calcitonin on kidney and bone are in turn modulated by the regulation of calcitonin production by serum calcium. The view that calcitonin serves to protect against hypercalcemia is thus explained by the hypocalcemic effects of calcitonin triggered in response to hypercalcemia.

The role of calcitonin, if any, however, in normal adult humans is unknown. Changes in calcium and phosphate metabolism are not seen in humans despite extremes of variation in hormone production; there are no definite effects attributable to calcitonin deficiency (totally thyroidectomized patients replaced only with thyroxine) or excess (patients with the calcitonin-secreting tumor, medullary carcinoma of the thyroid). Patients with the latter disorder suffer multiple deleterious consequences of their malignancy (see Chap. 334), but no abnormalities in calcium or bone metabolism are recognized, perhaps because they become refractory to the skeletal effects of calcitonin.

Medical interest in calcitonin, therefore, at present is centered principally upon its use as a therapeutic agent and its usefulness, when deployed in radioimmunoassays, for detection of medullary carcinoma (Chap. 334). The use of calcitonin in the treatment of Paget's disease of bone is established (Chap. 338).

REFERENCES

ADAMS JS et al: Isolation and structural identification of 1,25-dihydroxyvitamin D_3 produced by cultured alveolar macrophages in sarcoidosis. J Clin Endocrinol Metab 60:960, 1985

AVIOLI LV, KRANE SM: *Metabolic Bone Disease*. New York, Academic, 1977 and 1978, vols I and II

BRINGHURST FR, POTTS JT JR: Calcium and phosphate distribution, turnover, and metabolic actions, in *Endocrinology*, vol 2, LJ DeGroot (ed). New York, Grune & Stratton, 1979, p 551

BROADUS AE et al: The importance of circulating 1,25-dihydroxyvitamin D in the pathogenesis of hypercalcemia and renal stone-formation in primary hyperparathyroidism. N Engl J Med 302:421, 1981

BURGER EH et al: Osteoclast formation from mononuclear phagocytes: Role of bone-forming cells. J Cell Biol 99:1901, 1984

CENTRELLA M, CANALIS E: Local regulators of skeletal growth: A perspective. Endocrinol Rev 6:544, 1985

CHAMBERS TJ, DUNN CJ: Pharmacological control of osteoclastic motility. Calcif Tissue Int 35:566, 1983

DELUCA HF: The vitamin D system in the regulation of calcium and phosphorus metabolism. Nutr Rev 37:161, 1979

EIL C et al: A cellular defect in hereditary vitamin D-dependent rickets type II. Defective nuclear uptake of 1,25-dihydroxyvitamin D in culture skin fibroblasts. N Engl J Med 304:1588, 1981

FRAME B, POTTS JT JR: *Clinical Disorders of Bone and Mineral Metabolism*. Amsterdam Excerpta Medica, 1983

GRAY TK et al: Vitamin D and pregnancy: The maternal-fetal metabolism of vitamin D. Endocrinol Rev 2:264, 1981

KEUTMANN HT et al: Rat parathyroid hormone (1–34) fragments: Renal adenyl/cyclase activity and receptor binding properties in vitro. Endocrinology, 117:1230, 1985

KRANE SM, SCHILLER AL: Metabolic bone disease: Introduction and classification, in *Endocrinology*, vol 2, LJ DeGroot (ed). New York, Grune & Stratton, 1979, p 839

MACLAUGHLIN J, HOLICK MF: Aging decreases the capacity of human skin to produce vitamin D_3. J Clin Invest 76:1536, 1985

NORMAN AW et al (eds): *Vitamin D: Chemical, Biochemical and Clinical Update*

(*Proceedings 6th Workshop on Vitamin D, Merano, Italy*). New York, de Gruyter 1985
PARFITT AM: The coupling of bone formation to bone resorption: A critical analysis of the concept and of its relevance to the pathogenesis of osteoporosis. Metab Bone Dis Relat Res 4:1, 1982
———: The cellular basis of bone remodeling: The quantum concept reexamined in light of recent advances in the cell biology of bone. Calcif Tissue Int 36:S37, 1984
POTTS JT JR et al: Parathyroid hormone: Chemistry, biosynthesis, and mode of action, in *Advances in Protein Chemistry*, CB Afinsen et al (eds). New York, Academic, 1982, vol 35
RAISZ LG, KREAM BE: Regulation of bone formation. N Engl J Med 309:29, 83, 1983
ROBEY PG, TERMINE JD: Human bone cells in vitro. Calcif Tissue Int 37:453, 1985
RODAN GA, MARTIN TJ: Role of osteoblasts in hormonal control of bone resorption—A hypothesis. Calcif Tissue Int 33:349, 1981
ROSENFELD MG et al: Production of a novel neuropeptide encoded by the calcitonin gene via tissue-specific RNA processing. Nature 304:129, 1983
ROSENTHAL N et al: Elevations in circulating 1,25-dihydroxyvitamin D in three patients with lymphoma-associated hypercalcemia. J Clin Endocrinol Metab 60:29, 1985
SCRIVER CR et al: Serum 1,25-dihydroxyvitamin D levels in normal subjects and in patients with hereditary rickets or bone disease. N Engl J Med 299:976, 1978
TALMAGE RV et al: *The Physiological Significance of Calcitonin in Bone and Mineral Research, Annual 1*, WA Peck (ed). Amsterdam, Excerpta Medica, 1983
URIST MR et al: Bone cell differentiation and growth factors. Science 220:680, 1983

336 DISEASES OF THE PARATHYROID GLAND AND OTHER HYPER- AND HYPOCALCEMIC DISORDERS

JOHN T. POTTS, JR.

HYPERCALCEMIA

Management of hypercalcemia is a particular problem when the patient is asymptomatic. The number of patients recognized with asymptomatic hypercalcemia has increased severalfold in the last two decades; the hypercalcemia is usually found after use of screening tests during annual physical examinations. If the patient is asymptomatic, does the hypercalcemia always require further evaluation? What are the most probable causes of hypercalcemia, and how can they be diagnosed? Can asymptomatic patients be followed, or is definitive therapy to eliminate the hypercalcemia the optimal medical management?

There is a consensus that whenever hypercalcemia is confirmed, a definitive diagnosis must be established. Although hyperparathyroidism, a frequent cause of asymptomatic hypercalcemia, is a chronic disorder in which manifestations, if any, may be expressed only over months or years, hypercalcemia can also be the earliest clue to the presence of malignancy, the second most common cause of hypercalcemia in the adult. In Table 336-1 the causes of hypercalcemia have been grouped into five categories based upon the pathophysiologic mechanism involved.

Before undertaking an evaluation of hypercalcemia it is essential to ensure that true hypercalcemia is actually present, not a false-positive laboratory test. Hypercalcemia is a chronic problem, and it is cost-effective to obtain several serum calcium measurements; these tests need not be in the fasting state. False-positive calcium tests are usually the result of inadvertent hemoconcentration during blood collection or elevation in serum proteins, particularly albumin. Measurement of ionized calcium in technically feasible, but there is no advantage, except in research applications, to measurement of ionized rather than total calcium.

TABLE 336-1 Classification of causes of hypercalcemia

Parathyroid-related: *1* Primary hyperparathyroidism *a* Solitary adenomas *b* Multiple endocrine neoplasia *2* Lithium therapy *3* Familial hypocalciuric hypercalcemia	Vitamin D-related *1* Vitamin D intoxication *2* ↑ $1,25(OH)_2D$; sarcoidosis and other granulomatous diseases *3* Idiopathic hypercalcemia of infancy
Malignancy-related: *1* Solid tumor with metastases (breast) *2* Solid tumor with humoral mediation of hypercalcemia (lung, kidney) *3* Hematologic malignancies (multiple myeloma, lymphoma, leukemia)	Associated with high bone turnover: *1* Hyperthyroidism *2* Immobilization *3* Thiazides *4* Vitamin A intoxication Associated with renal failure: *1* Severe secondary hyperparathyroidism *2* Aluminum intoxication *3* Milk alkali syndrome

All causes of hypercalcemia other than hyperparathyroidism and malignancy account for less than 10 percent of hypercalcemia. Hypercalcemia in an adult who is asymptomatic is usually due to primary hyperparathyroidism, but the problem of differentiating primary hyperparathyroidism from occult malignancy can occasionally present a problem in differential diagnosis. In most cases of malignancy-associated hypercalcemia the disease is not occult; rather, symptoms of the underlying malignancy bring the patient to the physician, and hypercalcemia is discovered during the workup. In patients with malignancy the interval between detection of hypercalcemia and death is often less then 6 months. Accordingly, if an asymptomatic individual has had hypercalcemia or some manifestation of hypercalcemia, such as kidney stones, for more than 1 or 2 years, it is unlikely that malignancy is the cause.

Hypercalcemia not due to hyperparathyroidism or malignancy can result from excessive vitamin D action, high bone turnover from any of several causes, or renal failure (Table 336-1). The sensitivity and specificity of various diagnostic tests for the differential diagnosis are not optimal. The radioimmunoassays for measurement of parathyroid hormone and $1\alpha,25$-dihydroxyvitamin D ($1,25(OH)_2D$), the active metabolite of vitamin D, are useful in distinguishing certain broad categories of disease associated with hypercalcemia, for example, primary hyperparathyroidism from malignancy-associated hypercalcemia. Dietary history and a history of ingestion of vitamins and drugs are often helpful in recognizing some of the less frequent causes. Except in malignancy-associated hypercalcemia, acute management of the hypercalcemia is usually easy to accomplish prior to the institution of definitive therapy. The type of treatment is based on the severity of the hypercalcemia and the nature of associated symptoms.

Hypercalcemia from any cause can result in fatigue, depression, mental confusion, anorexia, nausea, vomiting, constipation, reversible renal tubular defects, increased urination, alteration in the electrocardiogram (a short QT interval), and, in some patients, cardiac arrhythmias. There is a variable relation between the severity of hypercalcemia and the presence or absence of symptoms from one patient to the next. Generally, symptoms are more common at calcium levels above 11.5 to 12.0 mg/dL, but some patients, even at this level, are asymptomatic. When calcium exceeds 13 mg/dL, renal insufficiency and calcification in kidneys, skin, vessels, lungs, heart, and stomach may occur, particularly if blood phosphate levels are normal or elevated due to impaired renal function. Severe hypercalcemia, usually defined as 15 mg/dL or above, is a medical emergency. When serum calcium is 15 to 18 mg/dL or higher, coma and cardiac arrest can occur.

PARATHYROID-RELATED HYPERCALCEMIA Primary hyperparathyroidism NATURAL HISTORY AND INCIDENCE Primary hyperparathyroidism is a generalized disorder of calcium, phosphate, and bone metabolism that results from an increased secretion of parathyroid hormone. The excessive concentration of circulating hormone usually leads to hypercalcemia and hypophosphatemia. There is great variation in the clinical presentation. Patients may present with multiple signs and symptoms, including recurrent nephrolithiasis, peptic ulcers, mental changes, and, less frequently, extensive bone resorption. However, with greater awareness of the disease and wider use of multiphasic screening tests, including blood calcium, the diagnosis is frequently made in patients who have no symptoms and minimal, if any, signs of the disease other than hypercalcemia and elevated levels of parathyroid hormone. If the frequency of diagnosis in referral centers reflects the incidence of the disease, hyperparathyroidism is more common than previously appreciated. In fact, the *incidence* of primary hyperparathyroidism may approximate *1 case per 1000 per year* in men over the age of 60, and *2 per 1000* in women 60 years of age older. This incidence is greater than earlier estimates of *1 case per 10,000 persons per year* which were based on evaluation of patients with symptoms, such as calcium-containing kidney stones. The clinical manifestations may be subtle, and the disease may have a benign course for many years or a full lifetime. Rarely, the disease seems to appear abruptly, and patients may exhibit severe complications, such as marked dehydration and coma, so-called hypercalcemic parathyroid crisis. The disease most commonly occurs in adults, with peak incidence between the third and fifth decades but it has been detected in young children and in the elderly.

ETIOLOGY AND PATHOLOGY *Solitary adenomas* Disease in a single gland occurs in approximately 85 percent (81 percent adenoma, 4 percent carcinoma), and hyperplasia of all glands is present in approximately 15 percent of cases (usually chief-cell hyperplasia). Rarely, adenomas are present in more than one gland with the other glands normal. The finding that either one gland only is abnormal or that all glands are abnormal is helpful to the surgeon in planning exploration of the neck. Resection of a single adenoma usually cures the disease.

Adenomas are most often located in the inferior parathyroid glands, but they are found in unusual locations in 6 to 10 percent of patients; such parathyroid adenomas may be located in the thymus, the thyroid, the pericardium, or behind the esophagus. Adenomas are usually 0.5 to 5 g in size, but may be as large as 10 to 20 g (normal glands are 25 mg in weight on average). Chief cells are predominant in both hyperplasia and adenoma. The adenoma is sometimes encapsulated by a rim of normal tissue. Chief-cell hyperplasia is especially common in familial cases of hyperparathyroidism and those that are part of the multiple endocrine neoplasia syndromes (see Chap. 334). Cells of a different histologic appearance such as oxyphil cells are occasionally present. The distinction between hyperplasia and adenoma can sometimes be difficult to establish. With hyperplasia the enlargement may be so asymmetric that some involved glands appear normal grossly. In this case, histologic examination reveals a uniform pattern of chief cells and disappearance of fat even in the absence of an increase in gland weight. Thus, microscopic examination of biopsy specimens of several glands is essential to interpret findings at surgery. When an adenoma is present, the other glands are normal and contain a normal distribution of all cell types (rather than only chief cells) and normal amounts of fat.

Parathyroid carcinoma is usually not aggressive in character. Long-term survival without recurrence is common if at initial operation the entire gland is removed without rupture of the capsule. Even recurrent parathyroid carcinoma is usually slow-growing with local spread in the neck, and surgical correction of recurrent disease may be feasible. Occasionally, parathyroid carcinoma is more aggressive in character with distant metastases (lung, liver, and bone) found at the time of initial operation. It may be difficult initially to decide if the primary tumor is carcinoma; increased numbers of mitotic figures and increased fibrosis of the gland stroma may precede invasive features. Hyperparathyroidism from a parathyroid carcinoma may be clinically indistinguishable from other forms of primary hyperparathyroidism; a potential clue to the diagnosis, however, is provided by the degree of calcium elevation. Calcium values of 14 to 15 mg/dL are frequent with carcinoma.

Multiple endocrine neoplasia Hyperparathyroidism may occur in a familial pattern without other endocrinologic abnormality. More often, however, hereditary hyperparathyroidism is part of a multiglandular endocrinopathy (see Chap. 334). There are several distinct syndromes of multiple endocrine neoplasia (MEN). The type I disorder (MEN I, Wermer's syndrome) consists of hyperparathyroidism and tumors of the pituitary and pancreatic islet cells, often associated with peptic ulcer and gastric hypersecretion (the Zollinger-Ellison syndrome). Another distinct constellation of endocrinologic abnormalities consists of hyperparathyroidism associated with pheochromocytoma and medullary carcinoma of the thyroid (MEN II). The pattern of inheritance is autosomal dominant. Tumors of the thyroid and adrenal medulla are not found in patients with MEN I, and pancreatic and pituitary tumors are not found in patients with MEN II. Since the different endocrine tumors can develop at widely separated intervals, hyperparathyroidism and the related endocrine disorders should be carefully and repeatedly searched for in kindreds afflicted with the MEN syndromes.

SIGNS AND SYMPTOMS Half or more of patients with hyperparathyroidism are asymptomatic. These patients are either followed without therapy or are operated upon, eliminating the disease state. Specific signs or symptoms of hyperparathyroidism involve primarily the kidneys and the skeletal system. Kidney involvement, due either to deposition of calcium in the renal parenchyma or to recurrent nephrolithiasis, was present in 60 to 70 percent of patients prior to 1970. With the increased frequency of detection of asymptomatic individuals, the incidence of renal complications is lower.

Renal stones are usually composed of either calcium oxalate or calcium phosphate. Repeated episodes of nephrolithiasis or the formation of large calculi may lead to urinary tract obstruction and infection, and may result in loss of renal function. Nephrocalcinosis may also cause decreased renal function and phosphate retention. Nephrolithiasis and nephrocalcinosis rarely occur in the same patient.

The unique bone involvement in hyperparathyroidism is osteitis fibrosa cystica. Several decades ago, an incidence of osteitis fibrosa cystica of 10 to 25 percent or even higher was reported in patients with hyperparathyroidism. Histologically the pathognomonic features include a reduction in the number of trabeculae, an increase in the giant multinucleated osteoclasts in scalloped areas on the surface of the bone (Howship's lacunae), and a replacement of the normal cellular and marrow elements by fibrous tissues. Other bone changes include resorption of the phalangeal tufts and a replacement of the usually sharp cortical outline of the bone in the digits by an irregular outline (subperiosteal resorption). Loss of the lamina dura of the teeth is less specific. Tiny, "punched-out" lesions may be present in the skull, producing the so-called salt-and-pepper appearance.

At the present time osteitis fibrosa cystica is not common, even though there may be a long history of manifestations of the disease. The reduced frequency has not been explained. Other manifestations of bone disease, however, are still common. Histomorphometric analyses of biopsied bone reveal an abnormality in bone turnover in most patients, even in those who do not evidence progressive loss of net bone mass; in such patients, rate of bone formation and bone restoration may be increased but balanced. In many patients, however, who do not have symptomatic bone disease or osteitis fibrosa cystica, rates of formation and resorption are not balanced so that a progressive loss of bone mineral mass causes osteopenia, indicating the need for surgery. There are no pathognomonic criteria to separate unequivocally parathyroid-dependent osteopenia from "high-turnover" osteoporosis as occurs in patients who are not hyperparathyroid.

Improved techniques are now available for monitoring bone mineral density. Computer tomography of the spine provides reproducible quantitative estimates (within a few percent) of spinal bone density. Similar, highly reproducible quantitation is also possible by photon densitometry for measurement of cortical bone density in the extremities, and dual beam photometry can be used to estimate bone density in the spine. These techniques can provide an early indication of progressive osteopenia through serial measurements. In some patients surgery is recommended because of progressive loss of bone, with the presumption that the progressive osteopenia is parathyroid hormone–dependent and hence treatable by correction of the hyperparathyroidism. Some patients have been followed for periods of several years, on the other hand, without any evidence of loss of bone mass.

Hence, bone disease in association with primary hyperparathyroidism can be quite variable.

Symptoms attributable to the central nervous system, peripheral nerve and muscle function, the gastrointestinal tract, and the joints are the next most common manifestations of hyperparathyroidism after those attributable to the skeleton and the genitourinary tract. An awareness of the signs and symptoms of advanced disease may be the initial clue to diagnosis. In patients with serum calcium above 12 mg/dL, central nervous system manifestations and gastrointestinal disorders are more common; even more severe hypercalcemia may supervene in such patients with dehydration. It is not apparent why some patients with hyperparathyroidism have no symptoms, while others, with an equal degree of biochemical abnormality, develop symptomatic disease.

FIGURE 336-1 *The relation between blood calcium and iPTH in normal subjects (panel A) and subjects with 2° hyperparathyroidism (panel B). This is a model of secondary hyperparathyroidism associated with an increased mass of parathyroid tissue. The heavy line represents normal secretory patterns and the lighter line the exaggerated secretion (steeper slope) typical of secondary hyperparathyroidism [secretion represented as hormone concentration (PTH) plotted against blood calcium]. When calcium level in blood is raised or lowered by EDTA or calcium infusion, and multiple measurements of PTH and calcium are made, some portion of hormone secretion in normals or hyperparathyroid subjects is constant despite high calcium levels in blood (nonsuppressible secretion) and is higher in hyperparathyroidism. An elevation of blood calcium from low levels (8 mg/100 mL, X) to higher levels (9 mg/100 mL, ●) results in a reduction in PTH in both normal and hyperparathyroid individuals, but true involution of secondary hyperparathyroidism with improved treatment can be confirmed only by showing a return of the exaggerated response curve to a normal response.*

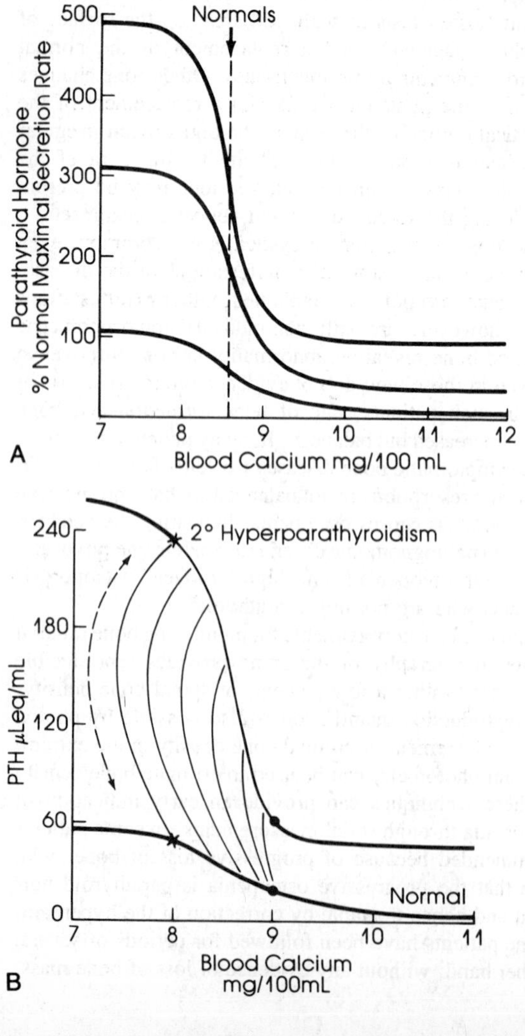

Central nervous system manifestations range from mild personality disturbance to severe psychiatric disorders to mental obtundation or coma. In some instances, multiple vague complaints can be mistaken for psychoneurosis. It must be emphasized, however, that mild depression, a common problem in the absence of hyperparathyroidism, cannot be the sole clinical criterion for parathyroid surgery.

Neuromuscular manifestations include proximal muscle weakness, easy fatigability, and atrophy of muscles. The electromyogram is abnormal, and muscle fibers atrophy without myopathic changes. The clinical signs may be so striking as to suggest a primary neuromuscular disorder. The distinguishing feature is the complete regression of neuromuscular disease after surgical correction of the hyperparathyroidism.

Gastrointestinal manifestations are sometimes subtle and include vague abdominal complaints and disorders of the stomach and pancreas. Duodenal ulcers occur more frequently than in the general population. In MEN I patients with hyperparathyroidism, duodenal ulcer is a result of the associated pancreatic tumors that secrete excessive quantities of gastrin (the Zollinger-Ellison syndrome). Pancreatitis has been reported in association with hyperparathyroidism, but the incidence and the mechanism are not established.

Chondrocalcinosis and pseudogout are said to be seen in sufficiently frequent association with hyperparathyroidism that screening of such patients is warranted. Occasionally, pseudogout is the initial manifestation.

DIAGNOSIS The diagnosis is made primarily on clinical grounds. The immunoassay for parathyroid hormone (PTH) is of value as a diagnostic test, but there are many problems in interpretation of assay results. Characteristically, immunoreactive PTH levels are frankly elevated or inappropriately normal for the degree of hypercalcemia (Fig. 336-1). Since hypercalcemia can be the presenting evidence for malignancy or other serious disease, a thorough evaluation of possible etiologies, including hyperparathyroidism, is indicated even in asymptomatic subjects. If the diagnosis of hyperparathyroidism is suspected after such an evaluation, a decision may be made to follow the patient for a time rather than recommend surgery.

Hypercalcemia is the most common manifestation, either sustained hypercalcemia or intermittent hypercalcemia. Careful consideration must be given to the justification for surgical exploration in the absence of hypercalcemia. So-called normocalcemic hyperparathyroidism, that is, patients with surgically proven hyperparathyroidism who have normal calcium but elevated values of immunoreactive PTH (iPTH), is rare in the absence of renal failure or gastrointestinal disease. If the patients have coexisting conditions that interfere with the calcium-elevating actions of PTH, such as chronic renal failure, severe malabsorption, or vitamin D deficiency, then the lack of calcium elevation need not argue against the presence of true hyperparathyroidism. Confusing situations can arise, however, in patients with recurrent kidney stones who are suspected of having hyperparathyroidism because of elevated iPTH levels but who have normal serum calcium. These patients may represent true normocalcemic hyperparathyroidism. In such situations where the symptoms call for an early definitive diagnosis, it may be useful to search for postabsorptive hypercalcemia (detectable in certain patients when fasting hypercalcemia is absent) or to use a provocative test with benzothiadiazides (see below).

Hypercalciuria is common in hyperparathyroidism. However, PTH actually reduces calcium clearance, and the daily excretion of calcium in urine is lower than in patients with equivalent degrees of hypercalcemia from nonparathyroid causes.

Serum phosphate is usually low but may be normal, especially if renal failure has developed. Hypophosphatemia is a less stringent diagnostic criterion than hypercalcemia for two reasons. One, phosphate levels are influenced by dietary intake, diurnal variations, and other factors; to be useful samples must be obtained in the morning under fasting conditions. Two, patients with severe hypercalcemia of all causes may have a low serum phosphate.

Other electrolyte abnormalities are not sufficiently specific to be of diagnostic value. Serum magnesium levels tend to be low, serum chloride and citrate are often elevated, and serum bicarbonate is reduced. The combination of elevated chloride and low phosphate (reflecting the acidosis and renal phosphate wasting, respectively) can be a diagnostic clue.

Blood alkaline phosphatase (of bone origin) and urinary hydroxyproline concentrations are elevated when bone involvement is significant. Renal involvement can be reflected by a decreased concentrating ability, by specific tubular defects such as renal tubular acidosis, or by frank renal failure with azotemia.

Assessing the response of serum calcium to glucocorticoid administration can be useful in differentiating the hypercalcemia of hyperparathyroidism from that associated with sarcoidosis, multiple myeloma, vitamin D intoxication, and some malignant diseases with osseous metastases. In these diseases, administration of hydrocortisone at 100 mg per day (or an equivalent dose of prednisone) for 10 days often results in a lowering of the serum calcium, whereas calcium does not usually decrease in hyperparathyroidism. Occasional false-positive and false-negative results occur. The mechanism of the glucocorticoid effect in hypercalcemic states may reflect the physiologic antagonism between glucocorticoids and vitamin D action in vitamin D intoxication and sarcoidosis and the tumor-suppressive action of glucocorticoids in some forms of malignancy.

A variety of tests of parathyroid function are based on the known effects of the hormone on the renal handling of phosphate, namely PTH decreases tubular resorption of phosphate. Phosphate clearance is determined by standard techniques over 1- to 2-h periods. Normal phosphate clearance is 10.8 ± 2.7 mL/min; values 50 percent or more above this figure may occur in hyperparathyroidism. In normal subjects the tubular resorption of phosphate exceeds 85 percent; in hyperparathyroidism tubular resorption of phosphate may be as low as 50 to 60 percent.

Measurements of nephrogenous cyclic AMP are useful in diagnosis. The test requires timed urine collections and measurements of plasma and urinary cyclic AMP. The test is limited in applicability, not only by technical difficulties, but also by problems of specificity. For example, patients with the humoral hypercalcemia of malignancy may have elevated nephrogenous cyclic AMP values in the range seen in primary hyperparathyroidism. In other studies, nephrogenous cyclic AMP correlates poorly with the presence or absence of hypercalcemia, and urinary cyclic AMP levels may be elevated in some cancer patients, independent of whether skeletal metastases or hypercalcemia is present.

TREATMENT *Medical treatment* The medical treatment of hyperparathyroidism involves two separate issues. If hypercalcemia is severe and symptomatic, then the calcium must be lowered (the measures are described subsequently in the general section of the medical management of hypercalcemia of any cause). Hypercalcemia is not symptomatic in most patients with hyperparathyroidism, and it is usually not difficult to control the hypercalcemia. Simple hydration will suffice to lower the calcium concentration to values below 11.5 mg/dL. There have been some discussions in the past about whether chronic management of the hypercalcemia of hyperparathyroidism should be undertaken with oral phosphate therapy. Although the calcium concentration is lowered by phosphate in most patients, this is accompanied by an increase in iPTH levels in blood. It is unclear whether the increased PTH levels would cause more or less organ deterioration. There have been no systematic trials to evaluate effects of specific medical therapy for hypercalcemia.

Rather, the usual issue is to decide whether surgical intervention is required in a particular patient. If not, medical management consists of following the patient without specific therapy, but monitoring bone and renal function periodically to ensure that silent osseous and renal deterioration does not occur. If undesirable signs or symptoms occur, surgical intervention can then be recommended.

The natural history of the disease has been studied in several centers. Several hundred patients have been followed in attempts to afford a rational explanation for the benefits of surgery or the risks of medical observation. Large-scale randomized prospective clinical trials have not been undertaken, however. Rather, the long-term effects of hyperparathyroidism have been assessed in patients who do not have kidney stones, osteitis fibrosa cystica, or other clear-cut symptoms. Of principal concern is the possibility of progressive loss of bone density, a worrying problem in women who face the problem of age-dependent and estrogen-deficient bone loss in the absence of hyperparathyroidism. The concern is that such patients, even though asymptomatic, will suffer a degree of bone loss due to PTH excess that will lead to acceleration of symptomatic osteoporosis. No generalization can be made in this regard other than that some patients, followed with noninvasive techniques for measuring bone density, show no evidence of substantial bone loss. Others show bone loss that is progressive. The reproducibility of the available noninvasive techniques for assessing bone density is 1 to 2 percent, and if progressive bone loss becomes significant, for example, a loss of 10 percent of skeletal mass, most physicians recommend surgery to prevent further bone loss. Such decisions are arbitrary in that the loss of bone, particularly in an older patient, may not be due to the hyperparathyroidism, and bone loss may not cease once the patient is rendered euparathyroid. It is not that one can guarantee that parathyroidectomy will arrest progressive bone loss but rather that one cannot afford, except in a very elderly patient, to run the risk that persistent hyperthyroidism may accelerate skeletal disease.

There are no indexes that help in predicting whether bone loss will be progressive or whether skeletal mass will remain stable. Hence, if patients wish to avoid surgery, bone mass must be monitored systematically at intervals of 6 months to 1 year. Loss of renal function does not usually occur in the absence of kidney stones or infection.

No uniform recommendation can be made regarding medical (nonsurgical) management of patients with hyperparathyroidism. Decisions must be made in the light of the age of the patient and social and psychological factors. Most physicians believe it is appropriate to operate on young persons to avoid lifelong monitoring with time-consuming and expensive studies, particularly since surgical treatment is usually successful and does not carry a significant risk of mortality or morbidity. In patients over the age of 50 conservative evaluation without surgery is reasonable if the patient prefers and if progressive bone loss is not seen. The operation can be recommended in any patient in whom progressive bone loss is documented or in whom other symptoms of the disease appear, or if the stress of long-term follow-up is greater than the commitment to surgical "cure."

Surgical treatment Parathyroid exploration should be undertaken only by an experienced surgeon with the help of an experienced pathologist. Certain clinical features help in predicting the pathology; for example, in familial cases, multiple abnormal glands are likely. However, some critical decisions regarding management can be made only during the operation. The examination of tissue removed at surgery by frozen section should direct the subsequent course of the operation. The usual procedure recommended by the author's colleagues is as follows: if an abnormal gland is identified, remove it and search for at least one additional gland. If the second gland is normal in size and normal histologically (frozen section), the hyperparathyroidism is likely due to a single adenoma, and exploration is stopped. Some surgeons have argued that several glands are usually involved and that subtotal parathyroidectomy is the procedure of choice. The risk of the former approach is lack of cure or early recurrence; the risk of the latter is hypoparathyroidism. It is our belief that single gland removal leads in most patients to long-term cure.

Hyperplasia involves even more difficult questions of surgical management. Once a diagnosis of hyperplasia has been established, it is necessary to identify all the glands. It usually is recommended that three glands be totally removed and that the fourth gland be partially excised; care should be taken to leave a good blood supply for the remaining gland. Some surgeons advocate transplantation of a portion of the removed, minced tissue into the muscles of the forearm to avoid late vascular failure of residual parathyroid tissue in the neck. When parathyroid carcinoma is encountered, the tissue should be widely excised; care must be taken to avoid rupture of the capsule to prevent local seeding of the tumor.

If no glandular abnormalities are found in the neck, the issue of further neck exploration must be decided. There are documented cases of five or six parathyroid glands and of unusual locations for adenomas. A variety of techniques have been developed to aid in the preoperative localization of the abnormal parathyroid tissue. The early techniques featured either selective intraarterial angiography or selective venous catheterization of the thyroid venous plexus and adjacent areas coupled with radioimmunoassay for PTH. The techniques were often successful, but the frequency of detection was too low in comparison with the rate of success of an experienced parathyroid surgeon in finding the abnormal tissue at the first operation to warrant the morbidity and complications of the procedures. Subsequently, noninvasive techniques were introduced, particularly ultrasound, computerized tomography of the neck and mediastinum, differential scanning after simultaneous radiothallium and technetium administration, and intraarterial digital angiography. These techniques, with the possible exception of ultrasonography, should be used only when the initial parathyroid exploration is unsuccessful.

Ultrasound is reported to detect abnormal parathyroid tissue in 60 to 70 percent of cases but is most useful for lesions in the vicinity of the thyroid and less successful for lesions in the anterior mediastinum. The technique may assist the surgeon even in the initial operation by directing the surgery to the side of the neck where the abnormal gland is located. Computerized tomography has a similar success rate and is more helpful in anterior mediastinal lesions. Caution is appropriate in that false-positives are encountered in the anterior mediastinum. Needle biopsy with radio immunoassay for PTH in aspirated tissue fluid can be coupled with computerized tomography prior to a second parathyroid exploration. The subtraction of the technetium image, which targets the thyroid, from the radiothallium image, which targets both thyroid and parathyroid, has led to successful preoperative localization in approximately half of patients undergoing a second exploration.

Several generalizations are warranted. Localization and removal of a single abnormal parathyroid gland at the first operation is usually successful, depending upon the experience of the surgeon (greater than 90 percent success for experienced surgeons). Preoperative localization techniques should be reserved for patients in whom initial exploration is unsuccessful. If a second exploration is indicated, ultrasound, computerized tomography, and thallium-technetium scanning should probably be combined with selective digital arteriography in one of the centers specializing in these techniques. At one center, there has been experience with angiographic ablation of mediastinal adenomas with reports of long-term cure using selective embolization or deliberate excessive injection of contrast material into the end-arterial circulation feeding the parathyroid tumor. Such procedures and the continual intraoperative monitoring of urinary cyclic AMP as a marker for successful removal of abnormal parathyroid tissue may serve as adjuncts in the management of patients with unsuccessful initial operations.

A decline in serum calcium occurs within 24 h after successful surgery; usually blood calcium falls to low normal values for 3 to 5 days until the remaining parathyroid tissue resumes hormone secretion. Severe postoperative hypocalcemia is likely if osteitis cystica is present or if injury to the normal parathyroid glands occurs during surgery.

In general, patients with good renal and gastrointestinal function, who do not have symptomatic bone disease and a large deficit in bone mineral, have few problems with postoperative hypocalcemia. The extent of the postoperative hypocalcemia varies with the surgical approach. If all glands are biopsied, hypocalcemia may be more prolonged and may be transiently symptomatic. Symptomatic hypocalcemia is more likely to occur after second parathyroid explorations, when normal parathyroid tissue may have been removed at the unsuccessful initial operation and when the manipulation and/or biopsy of the remaining normal gland has been more extensive in the search for the missing adenoma. Patients with hyperparathyrodism have efficient intestinal calcium absorption due to the increased levels of $1,25(OH)_2D$ stimulated by parathyroid excess. Once hypocalcemia signifies successful surgery, patients can be put on a high calcium intake or be given oral calcium supplements. Despite manifestations of mild hypocalcemia, most patients do not require parenteral therapy and do not experience severe symptoms. If the serum calcium falls below 8 mg/dL, in particular if the phosphate level rises, the possibility of more extensive hypoparathyroidism must be considered. Coexistent hypomagnesemia should be checked for, as it interferes with PTH secretion, and causes a relative hypoparathyroidism. Parenteral calcium replacement at a low level should be instituted if symptomatic hypocalcemia supervenes, such as a general sense of anxiety and positive Chvostek and Trousseau signs coupled with serum calcium consistently below 8 mg/dL. For parenteral therapy, calcium (gluconate or chloride) solutions are prepared at a concentration of 1 mg/mL in 5% dextrose in water. The rate and duration of intravenous therapy are determined by the severity of the symptoms and the response of the serum calcium. A rate of infusion of 0.5 to 2 (mg/kg)/h or 30 to 100 mL/h of a 1-mg/mL solution usually suffices to relieve symptoms. Generally, parenteral therapy is required for only a few days. If symptoms become severe or if the need for parenteral calcium continues for more than 2 to 3 days, replacement therapy with vitamin D and/or oral calcium (2 to 4 g per day) should be started (see section on treatment of hypocalcemia). It is cost-effective to use calcitriol (doses of 0.5 to 1.0 μg per day) because of the rapidity of onset and rapidity of cessation of action in contrast to vitamin D per se (see below). A sudden rise in blood calcium after several months of vitamin D replacement may indicate restoration of parathyroid function to normal.

Magnesium deficiency may also complicate the postoperative course. Magnesium deficiency impairs the secretion of PTH, and, therefore, hypomagnesemia should be corrected whenever detected. Magnesium chloride is effective by mouth, but this compound is not widely available. Accordingly, repletion is usually parenteral. Only a fraction of body magnesium is present in extracellular fluid, but total-body magnesium deficiency is reflected by hypomagnesemia. Since the depressant effect of magnesium on central and peripheral nerve functions does not occur below 4 meq per liter (normal range, 1.5 to 2 meq per liter) parenteral replacement can be given rapidly. A cumulative dose as great as 1 to 2 meq per kilogram of body weight can be administered if severe hypomagnesemia is present; often, however, doses of 25 to 30 meq total are sufficient. The magnesium is given either as an intravenous infusion over 8 to 12 h or in divided doses intramuscularly (magnesium sulfate, USP).

Lithium therapy Lithium, employed in conventional doses for extended periods in the management of bipolar depression and other psychiatric disorders, causes hypercalcemia in approximately 10 percent of patients. The parathyroids appear to participate in mediation of the hypercalcemia. In some, elevated PTH levels have been documented; levels of vitamin D metabolites and of urinary cyclic AMP have not been reported. The hypercalcemia is dependent on continued lithium treatment, remitting and recurring when lithium is stopped and restarted, yet when the patients are explored, parathyroid adenomas are found. The histologic findings in the other parathyroids have not been described in the reported series.

The frequency with which hypercalcemia occurs is sufficiently high to make it unlikely that the association is fortuitous; a causal relationship is supported by the dependence of the hypercalcemia on the continuation of the lithium, but the presence of hypercalcemia does not correlate with plasma lithium level. Long-term follow-ups have not been reported; most patients are continued on lithium because of its importance in the management of psychiatric problems. These patients are presumably best managed according to the principles used in asymptomatic hypercalcemia, independent of lithium administration. If troubling symptoms or unfavorable signs, such as progressive bone demineralization or kidney stones, develop, it may be necessary to remove the abnormal parathyroid tissue so that the therapy can be continued.

Familial hypocalciuric hypercalcemia Familial hypocalciuric hypercalcemia (familial benign hypercalcemia, FHH) is transmitted as an autosomal dominant trait. Recognition of the disorder is important because affected individuals are frequently ascertained because of asymptomatic hypercalcemia; surgical exploration of the parathyroids is never indicated because it does not cure the disorder. It is, therefore, important to recognize such patients as differing from those with primary hyperparathyroidism.

The pathophysiology is not understood, and there is no single biochemical marker to distinguish these patients from patients with primary hyperparathyroidism. Nonetheless, the aggregate evidence serves to separate FHH from primary hyperparathyroidism. Few clinical signs or symptoms are present in patients with FHH. Unlike the MEN syndromes, other endocrine abnormalities are not present. The hypercalcemia may be detectable in the first decade of life, whereas hypercalcemia rarely occurs in the MEN syndrome patients under the age of 10 years. The iPTH values may be elevated in FHH, but the values are usually lower than in patients with primary hyperparathyroidism. Renal calcium reabsorption is high. The majority of patients with primary hyperparathyroidism have less than 99 percent calcium reabsorption, and most patients with FHH exceed 99 percent reabsorption. Serum magnesium levels are higher in FHH than in primary hyperparathyroidism.

Most patients are detected as a result of family screening after the diagnosis has been made in one member of the kindred. Unfortunately, the initial patient is frequently operated upon without reversal of the hypercalcemia. At operation, a moderate degree of hyperplasia of all parathyroid glands is seen. No patient has had reversal of hypercalcemia by surgery unless all of the parathyroid tissue is inadvertantly removed, rendering the patient hypoparathyroid, a most undesirable result. The high renal calcium reabsorption and the prompt recurrence of excessive parathyroid secretion, as long as any parathyroid tissue remains, are consistent with some abnormality in the ratio of extracellular to intracellular calcium concentration or with some abnormal sensing mechanisms in cell membranes of parathyroid and renal tubular epithelium. The nature of this disorder and the proper long-term management are not clear. By no means is surgery to be advocated, nor is medical treatment needed to lower the calcium, in view of the lack of symptoms.

MALIGNANCY-RELATED HYPERCALCEMIA Clinical syndromes and mechanisms of hypercalcemia Hypercalcemia due to malignancy is common (as frequent as 10 to 15 percent in certain types of tumor such as lung carcinoma), often severe and difficult to manage, confusing as to etiology, and sometimes difficult to distinguish from primary hyperparathyroidism. Traditionally, hypercalemia in malignancy was thought to be due to a local invasion and destruction of bone by tumor cells or, in a minority of cases, to the elaboration by the malignant cells of humoral mediators of hypercalcemia.

Although the presence of malignancy is often clinically obvious, hypercalcemia can occasionally be due to an occult tumor. With occult malignancy, diagnosis and definitive treatment must be accomplished quickly if the patient is to be protected from the complications of the underlying malignancy.

Pseudohyperparathyroidism (humoral hypercalcemia of malignancy is the term used to define the syndrome of hypercalcemia in patients with malignancies), especially of lung and kidney, in which bone metastases are minimal or not detectable, the clinical picture resembles primary hyperparathyroidism (hypophosphatemia accompanies hypercalcemia), and cure or remission of the primary tumor leads to disappearance of the hypercalcemia. Ectopic production by the tumor of PTH or material resembling PTH was initially felt to be the mechanism of the hypercalcemia, but the disease mechanisms are more complicated than simple ectopic production of PTH by the malignant tissue.

Investigations employing multiple diagnostic procedures, tests of serum and urinary mineral ion metabolism, hormone assays, and measurements of cyclic AMP excretion have clarified the issue in part. The level of iPTH is not elevated in most cases of hypercalcemia associated with malignancy, although most laboratories report detectable, rather than suppressed levels. If PTH were the mediator produced ectopically by tumor tissue, elevated levels of iPTH would be expected unless altered forms of hormone were secreted. On the other hand, if parathyroid function is normal and nonparathyroid-related humoral factors are responsible, undetectable iPTH levels would be expected. The low levels of iPTH may represent false-positive signals in the assay or altered forms of the hormone in the circulation.

Many patients with hypercalcemia and malignancy, generally of the type classified as pseudohyperparathyroidism, have elevated urinary nephrogenous cyclic AMP excretion, hypophosphatemia, and increased urinary phosphate clearance, findings compatible with the actions of a humoral agent that emulates PTH action. On the other hand, these same patients have barely detectable iPTH levels in multiple immunoassays, high, rather than low, renal calcium clearance, and low to normal levels of $1,25(OH)_2D$, suggesting mediation by humoral factors distinct from PTH.

The importance of skeletal metastases in the genesis of the hypercalcemia of malignancy has been reevaluated. The histologic character of the tumor is more important than the extent of skeletal metastases in predicting hypercalcemia. Small cell carcinoma (oat cell) and adenocarcinoma of lung, although the most common lung tumors associated with skeletal metastases, rarely cause hypercalcemia. By contrast, as many as 10 percent of patients with squamous cell carcinoma of the lung develop hypercalcemia. Histologic studies of bone in patients with squamous cell or epidermoid carcinoma of the lung, in sites invaded by tumor as well as areas remote from tumor invasion, reveal bone remodeling, including osteoclastic and osteoblastic activity. In contrast, minimal evidence of metabolic activation is seen despite extensive skeletal metastases of small cell (oat cell) carcinoma.

The cumulative findings suggest that agents other than PTH must be responsible for hypercalcemia and that only certain tumor types produce these factors. Two mechanisms of hypercalcemia are suspected. Some solid tumors associated with hypercalcemia, particularly squamous cell tumors and renal tumors, produce cellular growth factors that are believed to cause increased bone resorption and mediate the hypercalcemia through *systemic* actions on the skeleton as a whole, by stimulation of bone resorption. Substances produced by cells involved in the marrow response to hematologic malignancies resorb bone through *local* destruction and may be identical or analogous to some of the known lymphokines and cytokines.

Classification of the hypercalcemia of malignancy is arbitrary (Table 336-2). Multiple myeloma and other hematologic malignancies involving the bone marrow probably cause bone destruction and hypercalcemia through local mechanisms. Breast carcinoma also usually causes hypercalcemia through localized osteolytic destruction, probably mediated by locally secreted tumor products different from those involved in multiple myeloma or lymphoma. Finally, the category of pseudohyperparathyroidism (humoral mediation) can probably result from more than one distinctive mediator (Table 336-2).

In addition to the multiplicity of bone-resorbing factors elaborated by malignant cells in patients with hypercalcemia of malignancy, there is a variable synergism and antagonism between the bone-active agents secreted by the tumors. In the humoral hypercalcemia of malignancy, osteoclastic resorption is generalized, and there is an absence of an osteoblastic or bone-forming response to the surge of bone resorption, implying some inhibition of the normal coupling of formation and resorption. Cooperativity and anatagonism in the skeletal actions of cytokines may include blockade of cytokine-induced bone resorption by interferon, both of which may be produced by the same tumor cells. Thus, the interaction of more than one substance may determine whether hypercalcemia develops with a particular tumor rather than whether or not a particular factor is secreted.

Several distinctive hormones, hormone analogues, specific cytokines, and/or growth factors have been implicated through clinical assays or in vitro tests. In some lymphomas there is an increased blood level of $1,25(OH)_2D$. It is not clear whether the increased $1,25(OH)_2D$ is produced by stimulation of the renal 1α-hydroxylase or whether the metabolite is produced ectopically by lymphocytes. The principal interest in etiologic mechanisms in hematologic malignancies has focused on the production of bone-resorbing factors by activated normal lymphocytes and by myeloma and lymphoma cells. This factor(s), termed osteocyte activation factor (OAF), now appears to represent the biologic action of several different cytokines, including interleukin 1 and possibly lymphotoxin and tumor necrosis factor, two closely related cytokines.

In most instances, breast carcinoma is believed to cause hypercalcemia by local stimulation of osteoclasts directly by products secreted by the metastatic breast carcinoma cells and associated inflammatory cells. Breast carcinoma cells produce and secrete prostaglandins of the E series which are potent local stimulators of bone-resorbing cells.

More than one factor may be responsible for humorally mediated hypercalcemia in patients with solid tumors. Fractions partially purified from extracts of human tumors stimulate cyclic AMP production in in vitro assays, cause bone resorption in vitro, and induce hypercalcemia in nude mice. In other studies, extracts of tumors have given positive results in the cytochemical bioassay for PTH, and the cyclic AMP stimulation and cytochemical bioassay response given by these factors is blocked by a competitive inhibitor of PTH. On the other hand, the tumor extracts that act like PTH do not react with antiserum to the hormone, nor is their action blocked by neutralizing anti-PTH antibody. The active principle is believed, therefore, to be a substance with a distinct amino acid sequence that acts through the PTH receptor. The lack of identity with PTH probably explains the differences in the biologic actions of the tumor substance(s) and those of authentic PTH.

Another line of investigation points to the importance of cellular growth factors in the genesis of tumor hypercalcemia. Tumor-derived growth factors, believed to play a central role in maintaining the transformation and growth of tumor cells by acting as autocrine regulators, are also potent bone-resorbing agents in vitro. Among other actions, they stimulate production of prostaglandins of the PGE_2 type. Epidermal growth factor (EGF) and tumor-derived growth factor cause bone resorption in vitro, acting through the same receptor, and in some systems bone resorption by tumor extracts can be blocked by antibodies to the EGF receptor. Platelet-derived growth factor (PDGF), also a frequent product of tumors, also stimulates bone resorption in vitro. Further work is needed to clarify the role of the growth factors, cytokines, and PTH-like principles in the hypercalcemia of malignancy.

TABLE 336-2 Classification of tumor hypercalcemia

I Hematologic malignancies	
A Multiple myeloma, lymphomas:	
*OAF, lymphokines—*local bone destruction*	
B Certain lymphomas:	
*↑ $1,25(OH)_2$—*systemic mediation*	
II Solid tumors with *local bone destruction*	
A Breast carcinoma:	
*Prostaglandin, E series	
III Solid tumors, *humorally mediated bone resorption*	
A Lung (squamous cell)	*Tumor-derived growth factors (transforming growth factors); adenyl cyclase stimulating factors (PTH-like); other humoral agents
B Kidney	
C Urogenital tract	
D Other squamous cell tumors	

* *Indicates a factor or hormone identified as present in human tumors, active on bone resorption in vitro, and putative etiologic agent in tumor hypercalcemia.*

Diagnostic issues and treatment Ordinarily, the diagnosis of hypercalcemia secondary to tumor is not difficult to make because the tumor symptoms are prominent at the time the hypercalcemia is detected. Indeed, the hypercalcemia may be noted incidentally during the work-up of a patient with known malignancy. Patients with malignancy and hypercalcemia may have a coexistent parathyroid adenoma, some reports suggesting an incidence as high as 10 percent. Laboratory testing becomes critical when occult carcinoma is suspected. Levels of iPTH are not uniformly undetectable in tumor hypercalcemia, as would be expected with the mediation of the hypercalcemia due to a nonparathyroid agent (the hypercalcemia suppressing the normal parathyroid glands), but are lower than in patients with primary hyperparathyroidism.

Hypercalcemia in association with truly occult malignancy is rare. Clinical suspicion that malignancy is the cause of the hypercalcemia is heightened when weight loss, fatigue, muscle weakness, unexplained skin rash, symptoms associated with the paraneoplastic syndromes, or symptoms specific for a particular tumor are present. Tumors of the so-called squamous cell phenotype are most frequently associated with hypercalcemia, and the organs most frequently involved are the lung, kidney, and urogenital tract. X-ray examinations can focus on these areas. Bone scans with technetium-labeled diphosphonate are useful for detection of osteolytic metastases; the sensitivity is high, but it is of low specificity and must be confirmed by conventional x-rays to be certain that areas of increased uptake are due to osteolytic metastases per se. Bone marrow biopsies are helpful in patients with anemia or abnormal peripheral blood smears.

Treatment of the hypercalcemia of malignancy must be considered in the perspective of the history and presumed course of the individual patient. Control of the tumor is the principal objective, and reduction of tumor mass is usually also the key to satisfactory control of the hypercalcemia. If a patient has severe hypercalcemia, yet has an excellent chance for effective tumor therapy, treatment of the hypercalcemia should be vigorous. If hypercalcemia, on the other hand, is an accompaniment of the late stages of a tumor that is resistant to therapy, the treatment of the hypercalcemia should not be vigorous, as hypercalcemia can have a mild sedating effect. Standard therapies for hypercalcemia are applicable to patients with malignancy.

VITAMIN D–RELATED HYPERCALCEMIA Hypercalcemia related to abnormal vitamin D action can be due to *excessive ingestion* of vitamin D or *abnormal metabolism* of the vitamin. Abnormal metabolism of the vitamin is usually acquired in association with some widespread granulomatous disorder, but one rare hereditary form of vitamin D sensitivity in infants is associated with other developmental anomalies. As discussed in Chap. 337, vitamin D metabolism is carefully regulated, particularly the activity of the renal 1α-hydroxylase responsible for the production of $1,25(OH)_2D$. Many details of the regulation of 1α-hydroxylase remain unclarified, but the normal feedback suppression by $1,25(OH)_2D$ on the enzyme seems to work less well in infants than in adults and operates poorly, if at all, in ectopic sites, as distinct from the renal tubule.

There are difficulties in the clinical interpretion of assays for vitamin D metabolites, particularly at low levels of the metabolites. Nevertheless, with the above limitations in mind, a working model can be formulated for the pathophysiology of the several disorders associated with hypercalcemia and excessive vitamin D action.

Vitamin D intoxication The chronic ingestion of large doses of vitamin D, usually at least 50 to 100 times the normal physiologic requirement (doses in excess of 50,000 to 100,000 units per day) are required to produce hypercalcemia in normal individuals. In animals, vitamin D intoxication causes increased bone resorption and increased intestinal calcium absorption. In humans excessive vitamin D action leads to an increase in intestinal calcium absorption, but it is not known whether increased bone resorption occurs.

The immediate mechanism for the hypercalcemia is presumed to be an excessive production of $1,25(OH)_2D$ that occurs as a consequence of an increase in the substrate for the renal 1α-hydroxylase, namely, 25(OH)D. 25(OH)D production is less tightly regulated than is the production of the active metabolite, $1,25(OH)_2D$. Hence, concentrations of 25(OH)D average 5 to 10 times above normal in patients on high-dose vitamin D, whether therapeutically, as in hypoparathyroidism, or accidentally, as in vitamin D intoxication. 25(OH)D has low biologic activity in intestine and bone. Hence, part of the excessive vitamin D action may be attributable to the high levels of 25(OH)D themselves, as well as supernormal levels of $1,25(OH)_2D$. Because of the infrequency of vitamin D intoxication, there have been few reports of the actual level of $1,25(OH)_2D$ in patients with vitamin D intoxication. Presumably, the presence of normal renal function and parathyroid reserve would lead to higher rates of formation of $1,25(OH)_2D$ than would occur in patients, for example, with impaired renal function or absence of PTH secretion in whom high doses of vitamin D may be given to counter calcium deficiency.

The diagnosis is substantiated by measurement of 25(OH)D, confirming concentrations in excess of the upper limit of normal. Hypercalcemia is usually controlled by restriction of dietary calcium intake and appropriate attention to hydration. These measures, plus discontinuation of vitamin D, usually lead to satisfactory management, but vitamin D stores in fat may be substantial and vitamin D intoxication may persist for weeks after vitamin D ingestion is terminated. Such patients are sensitive to glucocorticoids, which in doses of 100 mg of hydrocortisone or its equivalent return calcium levels to normal over several days.

Sarcoidosis and other granulomatous diseases Normal relations between 25(OH)D and the product, the active metabolite $1,25(OH)_2D$, are not maintained in patients with sarcoidosis and other granulomatous diseases. There is a positive correlation between 25(OH)D levels (reflecting vitamin D intake) and the circulating concentrations of $1,25(OH)_2D$ [normally, there is no increase in the active metabolite with increasing 25(OH)D levels]. In patients with sarcoidosis the site of synthesis of $1,25(OH)_2D$ is presumed to be in macrophages or other cells associated with the granulomatous deposits. Hypercalcemia has been reported in an anephric sarcoidosis patient in association with increased $1,25(OH)_2D$ levels. Macrophages obtained from granulomatous tissue form $1,25(OH)_2D$ at an increased rate when 25(OH)D is provided as substrate. Thus, the usual regulation of active metabolite production by calcium or PTH is circumvented in these patients, and high calcium intakes do not lead to a reduction in the blood levels of $1,25(OH)_2D$ in patients with sarcoidosis. Production of $1,25(OH)_2D$ was normal in one patient with sarcoidosis and hypoparathyroidism. Clearance of $1,25(OH)_2D$ from blood may be decreased as well.

Even normocalcemic patients with sarcoidosis have unregulated production of $1,25(OH)_2D$ in response to vitamin D loading. Exposure to sunlight, as in summer months, or administration of as little as 9000 units of vitamin D daily is followed by increased levels of the active metabolite. Treatment with moderate doses of steroids leads to a reversal, not only of the hypercalcemia as in other cases of excessive vitamin D actions such as vitamin D intoxication, but also to the reversal of the abnormal responsiveness of $1,25(OH)_2D$ levels to vitamin D challenge. Presumably, steroid administration causes multiple effects in the disease, and both excessive production of the metabolite and the responsiveness to it in target organs are blocked.

Variation in frequency of hypercalcemia in sarcoidosis (between 10 and 60 percent) is probably explained in part by the moderating influence of steroids used to control pulmonary complications and other manifestations of the granulomatous disease per se. Lytic lesions also occur in bone so that increased bone resorption could play a role in some cases. In most, however, hypercalcemia is directly related to an increased intestinal calcium absorption. Clinically, hypercalcemia is usually a manifestation of disseminated disease. Hence, pulmonary involvement is usual; chest x-ray may reveal a diffuse fibronodular infiltrate and/or prominent hilar adenopathy. Blood gamma globulin may also be elevated. The most useful diagnostic procedure is demonstration on noncaseating granulomas in liver or lymph node biopsy. The hypercalcemia of sarcoidosis can present a difficult problem in differential diagnosis, especially when many of the typical features of the disease are lacking (see Chap. 270).

Management of the hypercalcemia in these patients can be accomplished by avoiding excessive sunlight exposure and by limiting vitamin D and calcium intake; glucocorticoids in the equivalent of 100 mg of hydrocortisone per day or less are sufficient to control hypercalcemia when it occurs. Presumably, however, the abnormal sensitivity to vitamin D and abnormal regulation of $1,25(OH)_2D$ synthesis will persist as long as the disease is active. PTH levels are usually suppressed and $1,25(OH)_2D$ levels elevated, but primary hyperparathyroidism and sarcoidosis may occur in some patients.

Idiopathic hypercalcemia of infancy This unusual disorder, sometimes referred to as Williams' syndrome, consists of multiple congenital developmental defects, including supravalvular aortic stenosis, mental retardation, and an elfin facies, in association with hypercalcemia due to abnormal sensitivity to vitamin D. The syndrome was first recognized in England after the introduction of vitamin D fortification of milk. Hypercalcemia develops with vitamin D intakes as small as 2000 to 4000 units per day. Levels of $1,25(OH)_2D$ are elevated, ranging from 150 to 500 pg/mL. The mechanism of the abnormal sensitivity to vitamin D and of the increased circulating levels of $1,25(OH)_2D$ is unclear. The children become hypercalcemic because of excessive intestinal calcium absorption. The abnormality in vitamin D metabolism and the increased sensitivity to vitamin D intake are not seen after the first year of life. Treatment is restriction of calcium intake. Occasionally, the hypercalcemia can be severe, and calcium values above 16 mg/dL are recorded. Treatment with glucocorticoids in the doses used for vitamin D intoxication or sarcoidosis, adjusted for body weight, rapidly reverses the hypercalcemia.

HYPERCALCEMIA ASSOCIATED WITH HIGH BONE TURNOVER

Hyperthyroidism Mild elevation of serum calcium is common in patients with hyperthyroidism, and hypercalciuria is even more common. As many as 20 percent of patients show high normal or mildly elevated serum calcium concentrations. The hypercalcemia seems due to increased bone turnover with bone resorption exceeding bone formation; direct effects of thyroid hormone on the skeleton seem to be responsible. Severe calcium elevations are not typical, however, and the presence of such suggests a concomitant disease such as hyperparathyroidism. Indeed, patients with thyrotoxicosis are more sensitive to the hypercalcemic effects of PTH.

Usually, the hyperthyroidism is obvious, and the hypercalcemia is managed by specific therapy of the hyperthyroidism. Signs of hyperthyroidism may occasionally be occult, particularly in the elderly.

Immobilization Immobilization in adults is rarely associated with hypercalcemia in the absence of an associated disease but may cause hypercalcemia in children and young adolescents, particularly after spinal cord injury and paraplegia or quadriplegia. Upon ambulation the hypercalcemia in children usually returns to normal spontaneously.

The mechanism appears to involve a disproportion between rates of bone formation and bone resorption that result from the sudden loss of weight bearing. Hypercalciuria and mobilization of skeletal calcium can be seen in normal volunteers subjected to extensive bed rest, although hypercalcemia does not usually occur. An underlying disease associated with high bone turnover, such as Paget's disease, may cause hypercalcemia with immobilization.

Thiazides Administration of benzothiadiazines (thiazides) can cause hypercalcemia in patients with high rates of bone turnover, such as patients with hypoparathyroidism treated with high doses of vitamin D. Traditionally, thiazides are associated with aggravation of hypercalcemia in primary hyperparathyroidism and have been used as a provocative test to bring out hypercalcemia that is borderline in patients suspected of having hyperparathyroidism. However, the effect can be seen in other high bone turnover states as well. The mechanism of action of the drugs is complex, but the overall result seems to be to impose a challenge to calcium homeostasis by actions on renal calcium excretion, on bone-calcium turnover, and on the efficiency of parathyroid action per se. Thiazide administration to normal individuals causes a transient increase in blood calcium, usually within the normal range, which reverts to preexisting levels after a week or more of continued administration. If normal hormonal function and calcium and bone metabolism are present, homeostatic controls are reset to counteract the calcium-elevating effect of the thiazides. In the presence of hyperparathyroidism or increased bone turnover from another cause, homeostatic mechanisms cannot be reset. Thiazides are categorized as a cause of hypercalcemia in association with high bone turnover rather than parathyroid-related per se because thiazides aggravate but do not really cause hypercalcemia in primary hyperparathyroidism. The abnormal effects of the thiazide on calcium metabolism disappear within days of cessation of the drug.

Many aspects of the action of the thiazides in normal subjects and in patients with hyperparathyroidism remain unclear. Chronic thiazide administration leads to reduction in urinary calcium excretion. In hypoparathyroid patients the actions of the drug cannot be an augmentation of PTH's biologic actions. At the same time, the drug clearly augments PTH responsiveness of bone and renal tubule. The hypocalciuric effect of the drug appears to reflect the enhancement of proximal tubular resorption of sodium and calcium in response to sodium depletion and is more pronounced in subjects with parathyroid secretion, whether normal or increased. Nevertheless, the substantial hypocalciuric effect in hypoparathyroid patients on high-dose vitamin D and oral calcium replacement is the rationale for the use of thiazides as an adjunct to therapy in such patients.

Vitamin A intoxication Vitamin A intoxication is a rare cause of hypercalcemia. Most vitamin A intoxication results from experiments with nutritional supplements. Calcium levels can be elevated into the 12 to 14 mg/dL range after the ingestion of 50,000 to 100,000 units of vitamin A daily (10 to 20 times the minimum daily requirement). The patients have typical features of severe hypercalcemia that include fatigue and anorexia. They also have severe muscle pain and sometimes diffuse bone pain. The excess vitamin A intake is presumed to increase bone resorption.

Diagnosis can be established by history and by confirmatory measurements of vitamin A levels in serum, which may be increased severalfold above normal. Occasionally, skeletal x-rays reveal periosteal calcifications, particularly in the hands. Withdrawal of the vitamin is usually associated with the prompt disappearance of the hypercalcemia and reversal of the skeletal changes. As in vitamin D intoxication, administration of 100 mg of hydrocortisone or its equivalent per day leads to a rapid return of the serum calcium to normal.

HYPERCALCEMIA ASSOCIATED WITH RENAL FAILURE **Severe secondary hyperparathyroidism** Secondary hyperparathyroidism is the state in which excessive production of PTH is due to partial resistance to the metabolic actions of the hormone. Parathyroid gland hyperplasia with resultant increased secretion of PTH occurs because resistance to the normal level of the hormone leads to hypocalcemia which, in turn, is a stimulus to enlargement of the parathyroid glands. This concept is based on animal and human studies, the former involving experimental renal failure with phosphate retention and the latter involving treatment of patients with diphosphonates which acutely block skeletal resorptive response. Figure 336-1*A* and 1*B* illustrates the consequences of these changes. When the parathyroid secretory reserve is tested by deliberately lowering blood calcium, the extent of rise in PTH for each milligram of decrement of plasma calcium is greater with parathyroid hyperplasia than with the normal gland. There is, therefore, a higher concentration of hormone at any given level of calcium concentration. Since a portion of PTH secretion by each individual parathyroid cell is not suppressible by any degree of elevation of blood calcium concentration, larger glands (more cells) have a higher concentration of hormone output at the hypercalcemic end of the dose-response curve.

Secondary hyperparathyroidism occurs in patients with renal failure, osteomalacia (vitamin D deficiency), and pseudohypoparathyroidism (deficient response to PTH at the level of the receptor). The clinical manifestations of secondary hyperparathyroidism vary in these states. Hypocalcemia seems to be the common denominator of secondary hyperparathyroidism. Primary and secondary hyperparathyroidism can be distinguished by the autonomous nature of the growth of the parathyroid glands in primary hyperparathyroidism (presumably irreversible) and the adaptive increase in parathyroid gland size in secondary hyperparathyroidism (presumably reversible). In fact, reversal from an abnormal pattern of secretion, presumably accompanied by an involution of parathyroid gland mass to a normal pattern of function, has been shown following treatment with diphosphonate (Fig. 336-1*B*).

In progressive kidney disease, the initial tendency to hypocalcemia seems attributable to two causes: phosphate retention that develops because of the reduced renal capacity to excrete phosphate and reduced concentrations of $1,25(OH)_2D$ concomitant with progressive renal damage. The two disturbances reduce skeletal responsiveness to PTH. The deficient $1,25(OH)_2D$ also interferes with the absorption of calcium from the intestine, already impaired in uremia. The ultimate pathophysiologic consequences in chronic renal failure represent the divergent effects of stimuli that cause parathyroid gland hyperplasia and those that modify the hormonal responsiveness of the end organs—bone, gut, and residual renal tubules. Development of secondary hyperparathyroidism must be an imbalance between the rate of increased PTH secretion due to parathyroid hyperplasia versus a restoration of normal responsiveness to the peripheral action of the hormone. In a few patients with severe secondary hyperparathyroidism, hypercalcemia and hyperphosphatemia develop due to a sudden increase in bone resorption; parathyroid hypersecretion "overshoots" the degree of resistance to hormone action.

In addition to hypercalcemia and hyperphosphatemia, patients may develop bone pain, ectopic calcification, and pruritus. The bone disease in patients with secondary hyperparathyroidism and renal failure is usually termed *renal osteodystrophy*. Concomitant osteomalacia (vitamin D deficiency) and osteitis fibrosa cystica (excessive PTH action) may be seen. In fact, osteitis fibrosa cystica is now more common in untreated renal failure than in primary hyperparathyroidism.

Judicious medical therapy, which includes reduction of excessive blood phosphate by dietary phosphate restriction plus the use of nonabsorbable antacids and careful, selective addition of vitamin D metabolites in the form of 0.25 to 2.0 μg per day of calcitriol may reverse severe secondary hyperparathyroidism. Somewhat paradoxically, serum calcium and phosphate levels may return to normal despite the administration of increased amounts of the vitamin D metabolite and calcium supplements. As illustrated in Fig. 336-1*B*, involution of the parathyroids presumably occurs with reduction of increased cellular mass, and consequently the exaggerated secretory response returns to a normal rate of responsiveness. The level of PTH at any given level of blood calcium is now more appropriate, and excessive parathyroid action is reversed.

Aluminum intoxication Aluminum intoxication occurs in patients on chronic dialysis; manifestations include acute dementia and unresponsive, severe osteomalacia. Bone pain, multiple nonhealing fractures, particularly of the ribs and pelvis, and a proximal myopathy may occur. Hypercalcemia occurs when attempts are made to treat these patients as in renal osteodystrophy and renal failure, namely, administration of vitamin D or calcitriol. Apparently, acute hypercalcemia develops with administration of vitamin D because of impaired skeletal responsiveness. Aluminum is present at the site of osteoid mineralization, and osteoblastic activity is minimal. Presumably, these patients are unable to incorporate the increased blood calcium into the skeleton. Prevention is accomplished by avoidance of aluminum excess in the dialysis regimen; treatment involves mobilizing aluminum through the use of the chelating agent deferoxamine. Aluminum is mobilized from bone and, being tightly bound to the chelating agent, can be removed via dialysis. After aluminum toxicity has been reversed, patients may show typical features of renal osteodystrophy and secondary hyperparathyroidism. They can then be managed like other patients with secondary hyperparathyroidism with renal disease. A failure to recognize the syndrome is associated with persistence of the disabling bone disease and a fatal course due to progressive fractures or to hypercalcemia inadvertently induced by treatment with vitamin D.

Milk-alkali syndrome The milk-alkali syndrome can cause several clinical presentations—acute, subacute, and chronic—all of which feature hypercalcemia, alkalosis, and renal failure. The syndrome is due to an excessive ingestion of calcium and absorbable antacids such as milk or calcium carbonate. The disorder is less frequent since nonabsorbable antacids and H-2 receptor antagonists such as cimetidine and ranitidine became available for the treatment of peptic ulcer disease.

Individual susceptibility must be important in pathogenesis since many patients are treated with calcium carbonate without developing the syndrome. One important variable is the fractional calcium absorption as a function of calcium intake. Some individuals absorb a high fraction of calcium, even with intakes as high as 2 g and more of elemental calcium per day, instead of reducing calcium absorption with high intake, as occurs in most normal subjects. Resultant, mild hypercalcemia after meals in such patients may be the critical factor in the generation of alkalosis. Most individuals are resistant to the development of alkalosis after the ingestion of large quantities of non-calcium-containing alkali such as sodium bicarbonate. However, with the development of hypercalcemia, mild increased sodium excretion and some depletion of total body water occurs. This phenomenon and perhaps, additionally, some suppression of endogenous PTH secretion would lead to increased bicarbonate reabsorption. This bicarbonate retention then leads to alkalosis in the face of continued calcium carbonate ingestion. Alkalosis, per se, results in selective enhancement of calcium reabsorption in the distal nephron, thus aggravating the hypercalcemia. The cycle, mild hypercalcemia → bicarbonate retention → alkalosis → renal calcium retention → severe hypercalcemia, thus perpetuates and aggravates hypercalcemia and alkalosis as long as calcium and absorbable alkali are ingested.

Acute hypercalcemia and alkalosis within days of beginning calcium and alkali, *acute milk-alkali syndrome,* is manifested by weakness, myalgia, irritability, and apathy. The impairment of renal function, including reduced renal concentrating ability, tubular dysfunction, and hypercalcemia and alkalosis, reverses rapidly upon stopping the intake of calcium and alkali.

The far advanced milk-alkali syndrome, sometimes referred to as *Burnett's syndrome,* represents the results of long-standing calcium and alkali ingestion; severe hypercalcemia, irreversible renal failure, and phosphate retention may be accompanied by ectopic calcification. Some improvement may result when calcium and alkali ingestion is reduced, but prior to the availability of renal dialysis renal failure led to death. There is an intermediate or subacute form in which the renal failure is reversible over a period of weeks after withdrawal of excessive calcium and alkali intake.

DIFFERENTIAL DIAGNOSIS: SPECIAL TESTS Differential diagnosis in hypercalcemic disorders is best achieved by using clinical criteria (Fig. 336-2 and Table 336-3). While helpful, when several laboratory tests are applied simultaneously, they lack adequate sensitivity and/or specificity when considered individually. The points that deserve major emphasis in arriving at a correct diagnosis are the presence or absence of symptoms or signs and evidence of chronicity. If one discounts fatigue or depression, which is common in the population, patients with *asymptomatic hypercalcemia* have primary hyperparathyroidism in well over 90 percent of the instances; symptoms of malignancy are usually present when hypercalcemia is due to cancer. Disorders other than hyperparathyroidism and malignancy are estimated to cause no more than 10 percent of all cases of hypercalcemia, and some of the nonparathyroid causes are associated with manifestations such as renal failure, the signs or symptoms of which are evident on initial routine laboratory test screening.

Chronicity is the second most important clinical point. If hypercalcemia has been manifest for more than a year, malignancy can usually be excluded as the cause of hypercalcemia on clinical grounds alone. A striking feature of malignancy-associated hypercalcemia is the rapidity of the course, whereby signs and symptoms relatable to the underlying malignancy are evident within months of the first detection of hypercalcemia. Hyperparathyroidism is the likely diagnosis in patients with *chronic hypercalcemia.* Diseases other than hyperparathyroidism, such as sarcoidosis, are rare, alternative causes of chronic hypercalcemia. A careful *history* of dietary supplements and drug use will often readily reveal intoxication with vitamin D or A or the use of thiazides.

Although clinical considerations are helpful in arriving at the correct diagnosis of the cause of hypercalcemia, appropriate laboratory testing is essential for diagnosis. Theoretically, the radioimmunoassay for PTH should separate hyperparathyroidism from all other causes of hypercalcemia, those with hyperparathyroidism having elevated

FIGURE 336-2 *Schematic illustrating simultaneous measurements of immunoreactive parathyroid hormone (PTH RIA) and serum calcium in normal subjects (N), patients with tumor hypercalcemia (TH), hypoparathyroidism (HP), pseudohypoparathyroidism (PHP), chronic renal failure with secondary hyperparathyroidism [CRF (2° HPTH)], and primary hyperparathyroidism (1° HPTH). Enclosed areas indicate the range of values typical for each class of subject measured; note overlap of regions and interrupted scales (see text for details).*

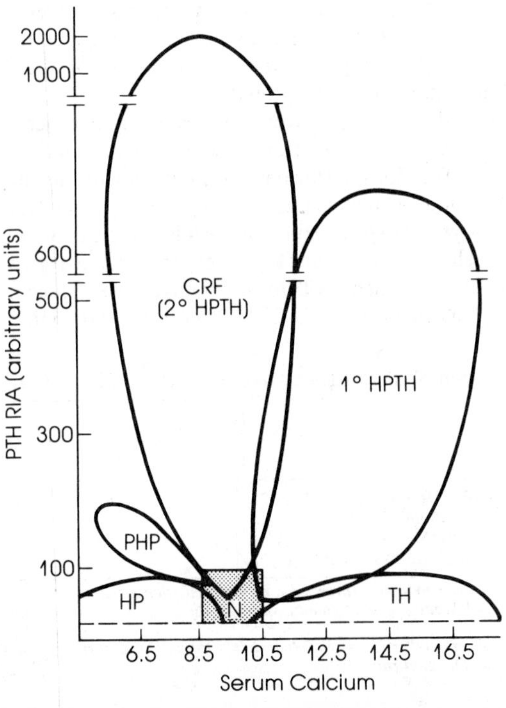

levels of iPTH despite hypercalcemia and patients with malignancy and the other causes of hypercalcemia (except those related to primary hyperparathyroidism, such as lithium-induced hypercalcemia and familial hypocalciuric hypercalcemia) having levels of hormone below normal or undetectable. $1,25(OH)_2D$ levels would be expected to be elevated in primary hyperparathyroidism as a secondary event and also increased in states of vitamin D intoxication, particularly sarcoidosis. In other disorders associated with hypercalcemia, concentrations of $1,25(OH)_2D$ would be expected to be low or, at the most, normal. Such clear distinctions in laboratory findings are not the rule in differential diagnosis of hypercalcemia, however.

Circulating iPTH is heterogeneous, as discussed in Chap. 335. Thus, what is measured may vary from one assay to another, depending on the region of the molecule recognized by different antiserums directed against the hormone. Furthermore, the concentration of PTH fragments may rise in the presence of renal failure, without implying a corresponding increase in the level of biologically active, intact hormone.

As illustrated in Fig. 336-2, the most useful clinical interpretation of PTH radioimmunoassays is achieved by covariant analysis [(iPTH) × (Ca^{2+})], plotting results of iPTH concentration in each patient against the simultaneously measured calcium concentration and then contrasting the individual test results with the results found in clinical correlation studies utilizing the particular immunoassay. A rectangular domain, in this type of plotting, includes the values found for many normal control individuals; the domain is bounded laterally by the upper and lower limits of serum calcium and vertically by the lower limit of assay detection, and the highest range of normal iPTH concentration.

Those patients with surgically documented hyperparathyroidism whose concentration of iPTH overlaps the upper limit of normal values can usually (especially with several repeated assays) be discerned as abnormal because iPTH level should be undetectable due to hypercalcemia if the parathyroids are normally responsive. Some overlap occurs between the values in patients with various types of hypercalcemia and much of the normal range. In some assays, more of an elevation of the PTH levels occurs in patients with tumor hypercalcemia than shown in Fig. 336-2.

Assays based on exclusive recognition of the amino terminal portion of the molecule obviate the difficulties inherent in detection of fragments. In general, however, all PTH radioimmunoassays must operate close to the limits of detectability to encompass all values found in normal subjects. Under these conditions, the assays are prone to interference by factors present in plasma, especially in renal failure and in malignancy. These problems appear to account for many false-positive and false-negative values. The assay for $1,25(OH)_2D$ is also hampered by technical problems.

A certain fraction of surgically proven hyperparathyroid patients have PTH concentrations in the upper limit of normal (false-negative immunoassay results) (Fig. 336-2). Hormone concentration in patients with the hypercalcemia of malignancy is normal or even moderately increased in most assays (false-positives). Fortunately, the parathyroid radioimmunoassay values in malignancy are lower for the same degree of calcium elevation than in patients with hyperparathyroidism. Hence, the more severe the hypercalcemia, the more useful the parathyroid immunoassay result in distinguishing between primary hyperparathyroidism and the hypercalcemia of malignancy. $1,25(OH)_2D$ levels are normal or low in these patients, as distinct from the evelated levels in most patients with primary hyperparathyroidism.

PTH levels are elevated in chronic renal failure, a part of which reflects accumulation of fragments secondary to renal failure rather than true parathyroid oversecretion and part of which is due to true secondary hyperparathyroidism. Patients with sarcoidosis have low or undetectable levels of iPTH. No systematic surveys have been reported concerning PTH radioimmunoassay results in many of the other non-parathyroid-related causes of hypercalcemia shown in Table 336-1, largely because of the infrequency with which the disorders are encountered.

In summary, iPTH values are elevated in >90 percent of parathyroid-related causes of hypercalcemia, normal or moderately elevated in malignancy-related hypercalcemia, increased to varying degrees (and therefore not usually helpful) in disorders associated with renal failure, and normal or undetectable in vitamin D–related and high bone turnover–related causes of hypercalcemia (although there is a paucity of data for these latter categories).

Measurements of nephrogenous cyclic AMP are of limited value in distinguishing the two major causes of hypercalcemia, primary hyperparathyroidism vs. malignancy. Elevation of nephrogenous cyclic AMP occurs in some patients with malignancy and in essentially all patients with primary hyperparathyroidism. Several other laboratory tests are of utility in confirming the diagnosis of particular disorders.

Table 336-3 summarizes laboratory findings among primary hyperparathyroidism, malignancies with local bone destruction (osteolytic metastases) and humorally related tumor hypercalcemia, or pseudohyperparathyroidism. It is evident by inspection of expected values for iPTH and $1,25(OH)_2D$ levels that laboratory testing may not be definitive in separating primary hyperparathyroidism from malignancy-related hypercalcemia. However, on the average, iPTH values are elevated in primary hyperparathyroidism and normal in malignancy-associated hypercalcemia; the same general tendency to separate groups is seen with measurements of $1,25(OH)_2D$.

Some general recommendations can be made as to the differential diagnosis of hypercalcemia. If a specific disease traditionally associated with hypercalcemia (Table 336-1) is clinically evident, it is reasonable to assume that the disease is responsible for the hypercalcemia. The hypercalcemia can be managed initially by general measures, if necessary, and the suspected disease can be treated by specific measures. If the hypercalcemia disappears in response to specific therapy, as with surgery for hyperparathyroidism, for example, or after reduction of excessive intake of fat-soluble vitamins or alkali and calcium, as in the case of vitamin D intoxication or milk-alkali syndrome, respectively, then there is no need to search for other causes of hypercalcemia. If specific treatment does not lead to a reversal of the hypercalcemia, a search for an additional cause, such as primary hyperparathyroidism, must be undertaken. Signs suggestive of malignancy may be evident, and initial phases of evaluation will focus on arriving at a diagnosis of the malignancy.

When no clues are evident as to the diagnosis, either because the patient is asymptomatic or chronic illness obscures symptoms or

TABLE 336-3 Differential diagnosis of hypercalcemia: clinical criteria

Disease	Blood*				Urine†		
	Ca†	P_i	$1,25(OH)_2D$	iPTH	NcAMP	Ca†	TMP/GFR
Primary hyperparathyroidism	↑	↓	↑	↑ (↔)	↑	↔ ↑	↓
Malignancy-associated hypercalcemia:							
Humorally mediated (HHM)	↑ ↑	↓	↓,↔	↔, ↓,(↑)	↕	↑ ↑	↓
Local destruction (osteolytic metastases)	↑	↔	↓,↔	↔, ↓	↕	↑ ↑	↔

* *Symbols in parentheses refer to values rarely seen in the particular disease.*
† *Some report cyclic AMP values in malignancy vary greatly ↑, ↓, ↔ independent of systemic versus locally mediated bone resorption or even presence or absence of hypercalcemia.*
NOTE: *P_i = inorganic phosphate; iPTH = immunoreactive parathyroid hormone; NcAMP = nephrogenous cyclic AMP; TMP = tubular maximal for phosphate reabsorption; GFR = gomerular filtration rate.*

signs that might provide a clue to the presence of malignancy, the following general approach can be used. If the patient is *asymptomatic* and if there is evidence by history of *chronicity* to the hypercalcemia, hyperparathyroidism is almost certainly the cause of the hypercalcemia. If iPTH levels on several occasions are elevated along with the typical features of hyperparathyroidism mentioned above, little other evaluation is necessary. Hyperparathyroidism is never confirmed until abnormal parathyroid tissue is surgically removed, correcting the hypercalcemia, but patients with asymptomatic hypercalcemia who have the presumptive diagnosis on the basis of elevated concentrations of iPTH can be followed, as described above, or recommended for surgery with reasonable confidence of cure. If in such patients there is a family history suggestive of other endocrine abnormality, more detailed screening for multiple endocrine neoplasia should be undertaken in the patient and family.

If the patient does not have clear-cut symptoms and there is only a short history or no clue to the duration of the hypercalcemia, *occult malignancy* must be considered with more care than if the hypercalcemia is known to be chronic. Even if the iPTH levels in such an asymptomatic patient are increased convincingly, it is probably useful to obtain values of $1,25(OH)_2D$ as well and follow the patient with the presumed diagnosis of primary hyperparathyroidism with less confidence.

If such patients have systemic symptoms and/or the iPTH levels are not elevated, then a thorough survey must be undertaken for malignancy, including chest x-ray, computerized tomography of chest and abdomen, and bone scan. Attention should also be paid to clues for underlying hematologic disorders such as anemia, increased plasma globulin, and abnormal serum immunoelectrophoresis; bone scans can be negative in patients with multiple myeloma. If no signs of a tumor are evident, the patient may have hyperparathyroidism with equivocal elevation in iPTH, and with time, the diagnosis of hyperparathyroidism may become more clear-cut.

Finally, if a patient is asymptomatic with chronic hypercalcemia but iPTH values are not elevated, it is useful to search for other chronic illnesses that cause hypercalcemia but may be atypical in presentation, such as occult sarcoidosis.

MEDICAL TREATMENT OF HYPERCALCEMIA The acute treatment of hypercalcemia is usually successful. The serum calcium concentration can be decreased by 3 to 9 mg/dL in 24 to 48 h in most patients, enough to relieve acute symptoms, prevent death from hypercalcemia crisis, and permit diagnostic evaluation. However the chronic medical management of hypercalcemia is usually unsatisfactory unless the underlying cause can be corrected because the available therapies are inconvenient or toxic.

Hypercalcemia develops because skeletal calcium release is excessive, intestinal calcium absorption is increased, or renal calcium excretion is inadequate. Understanding the particular pathogenesis helps guide therapy. For example, hypercalcemia in patients with osteolytic metastases or acute immobilization is primarily due to excessive skeletal calcium release and is, therefore, minimally affected by restriction of dietary calcium. On the other hand, patients with vitamin D hypersensitivity or vitamin D intoxication have excessive intestinal calcium absorption, and restriction of dietary calcium is beneficial. Decreased renal function or extracellular fluid depletion decreases urinary calcium excretion. If additional abnormalities, such as increased bone breakdown, are present, hypercalcemia will develop. This may happen, for example, when patients with resorptive bone disease become dehydrated. In such situations, rehydration may rapidly cure the hypercalcemia, even though excessive bone resorption and increased urinary calcium excretion continue.

Hydration, increased salt intake, mild and forced diuresis The first principle of treatment is to restore *normal hydration*. Many hypercalcemic patients are dehydrated because of vomiting, inanition, or hypercalcemia-induced defects in urinary concentrating ability. The resultant drop in glomerular filtration rate is accompanied by an additional decrease in renal tubular sodium and calcium clearance. Restoring a normal extracellular fluid volume corrects these abnormalities and increases urine calcium excretion by 100 to 300 mg (2.5 to 7.5 mmol) per day. Increasing urinary sodium excretion to 400 to 500 meq per day increases urinary calcium excretion even further than simple rehydration. Finally, after full benefits of simple rehydration have been achieved saline can be administered, or conventional doses of furosemide or ethacrynic acid can be given twice daily to depress the tubular reabsorptive mechanism for calcium (unless the diuretic is allowed to provoke dehydration). The combined use of these therapies can increase urinary calcium excretion to 400 mg per day or higher in most hypercalcemic patients. Since this is a substantial percentage of the exchangeable calcium pool, the serum calcium concentration usually falls 1 to 3 mg/dL (0.25 to 0.75 mmol per liter) within 24 h. The combination of fluids (by mouth), sodium, and furosemide or ethacrynic acid is also adaptable to chronic outpatient treatment, if necessary, using sodium chloride tablets. Precautions should be taken to prevent potassium and magnesium depletion during chronic therapy; calcium-containing renal calculi are a potential complication.

Under life-threatening circumstances, the above therapy can be pursued more aggressively, giving 6 liters of isotonic saline (900 meq sodium) daily plus furosemide in doses up to 100 mg every 1 to 2 h or ethacrynic acid in doses to 40 mg every 1 to 2 h. Urinary calcium excretion may exceed 1000 mg (25 mmol) per day, and the serum calcium may decrease by 4 mg/dL or more within 24 h. Severe potassium and magnesium depletion is inevitable unless replacements are given; pulmonary edema can be precipitated. The potential complications can be averted by careful monitoring of central venous pressure and plasma or urine electrolytes. A bladder catheter is usually necessary after the first day to allow the patient to sleep.

Plicamycin For the acute management of hypercalcemia plicamycin (mithramycin) which inhibits bone reabsorption, is a useful therapeutic agent. Plicamycin must be given intravenously, either as a bolus injection or by slow infusion. The usual dose is 25 μg per kilogram of body weight. Given once or twice a week, 10 μg/kg can be effective for chronic therapy in some patients; treatment should not be repeated until hypercalcemia recurs because the toxicity of the drug is dependent on the frequency of treatment and the total dosage.

Careful monitoring is needed if repeated doses are used. The major side effects are thrombocytopenia, hepatocellular necrosis with increased lactic acid dehydrogenase (LDH) and aspartate aminotransferase (AST) levels, and decreased levels of clotting factors with resultant epistaxis, bruising, hemorrhage, and bleeding gums. Azotemia, proteinuria, and hypocalcemia may occur. Hypophosphatemia and hypokalemia may also develop, as may nausea, vomiting, stomatitis, and facial swelling. Toxicity is rare when only one or two doses are used and can be minimized by repeating single doses only when hypercalcemia recurs. Toxic effects other than hemorrhage can usually be reversed by stopping the drug.

Other therapies Glucocorticoids increase urinary calcium excretion and decrease intestinal calcium absorption when given in pharmacologic doses (e.g., 40 to 200 mg prednisone daily in divided doses), but they also cause negative skeletal calcium balance. In normal subjects and in patients with primary hyperparathyroidism, glucocorticoids neither increase nor decrease the serum calcium concentration. In patients with hypercalcemia due to certain osteolytic malignancies, however, glucocorticoids may be effective as a result of antitumor effects. The malignancies in which hypercalcemia responds to glucocorticoid are usually hematologic malignancies such as multiple myeloma, leukemia, Hodgkin's disease, and other lymphomas; carcinoma of the breast may also respond, at least early in the course of the disease. Glucocorticoids are effective in treating hypercalcemia due to vitamin D intoxication or vitamin D hypersensitivity of sarcoidosis. The mechanism of action in the latter circumstances is unclear. In all the above situations, the hypocalcemic effect develops over several days, and the usual glucocorticoid dosage is 40 to 100 mg prednisone (or its equivalent) daily in four divided doses. The side effects of chronic glucocorticoid therapy may be acceptable in some circumstances.

The hormonal mediator of hypercalcemia secondary to malignancies that cause excessive bone breakdown without actually metastasizing to bone may be a prostaglandin of the E series in some patients. Since prostaglandin synthesis can be blocked by indomethacin or aspirin, these drugs sometimes correct the hypercalcemia in such patients. The analytical methods necessary to define prostaglandin excess are not widely available, and a therapeutic trial is the accepted diagnostic maneuver. Indomethacin, 25 mg every 6 h, or aspirin in sufficient doses to produce a serum salicylate level of 20 to 30 mg/dL generally lowers the serum calcium concentrations over several days if prostaglandin excess is the cause.

Hypercalcemia complicated by severe renal failure is difficult to manage; dialysis is often the treatment of choice. Peritoneal dialysis can remove 500 to 200 mg (12.5 to 50 mmol) of calcium in 24 to 48 h and lower the serum calcium concentration by 3 to 12 mg/dL (0.75 to 3.0 mmol per liter), if calcium-free dialysis fluid is used. Large quantities of phosphate are lost during dialysis, and serum inorganic phosphate concentrations usually fall, thus aggravating hypercalcemia. Therefore, the serum inorganic phosphate concentration should be measured after dialysis, and phosphate supplements should be added to the diet or to dialysis fluids if necessary.

Calcitonin decreases the skeletal release of calcium, phosphorus, and hydroxyproline within minutes of its intravenous injection. The subsequent changes in serum calcium and phosphorus depend upon the initial magnitude of skeletal resorption: subjects with the most rapid bone turnover show the greatest reduction in serum calcium concentration. Calcitonin also increases the renal clearance of calcium and phosphorus (and sodium). The most impressive results are seen in patients with hypercalcemia due to immobilization, thyrotoxicosis, or vitamin D intoxication, situations characterized by a high rate of bone turnover. Surprisingly, calcitonin is less effective than phosphate or plicamycin in patients with hypercalcemia due to malignancy or hyperparathyroidism, conditions in which bone turnover is also high. Escape from drug action occurs in patients and animals invariably after 12 to 24 h of high-dose therapy or after several days of continuous therapy with calcitonin. The mechanism of escape is unknown; there have been reports that coadministration of glucocorticoids and calcitonin prevents escape. This promising lead deserves further clinical evaluation since calcitonin would be advantageous due to its minimal toxicity. Calcitonin is effective by intravenous, intramuscular, or subcutaneous injection; doses used are 25 to 50 units every 6 to 8 h, usually in the form of salmon calcitonin.

Phosphate Patients with primary hyperparathyroidism are frequently hypophosphatemic, and hypercalcemia of other causes may also be complicated by hypophosphatemia. Hypophosphatemia decreases the rate of calcium uptake into bone, increases intestinal calcium absorption, and directly and indirectly stimulates bone breakdown. These effects aggravate hypercalcemia, and correcting hypophosphatemia lowers the serum calcium concentration. The usual treatment is 1 to 1.5 g of phosphate phosphorous per day for several days, given in four divided doses to minimize the chances of developing hyperphosphatemia. Such therapy has been administered for prolonged periods in selected patients. It is generally believed but not established that toxicity will not occur if the phosphate therapy is limited to restoring serum inorganic phosphate concentrations to normal rather than making them supranormal.

Raising the serum inorganic phosphate concentration above normal further decreases serum calcium levels. Intravenous phosphate is one of the most dramatically effective treatments available for severe hypercalcemia. A dose of 1500 mg phosphate phosphorus or more intravenously over 6 to 8 h leads to a prompt decrease in serum calcium of 2 to 10 mg/dL in patients with initially normal serum inorganic phosphate concentrations. However, this therapy should be employed only in extreme emergencies for two reason. First, fatal hypocalcemia can be produced by excessive dosage; frequent serum calcium determinations are necessary if intravenous phosphate is administered. Second, unlike sodium chloride, sodium phosphate does not remove calcium from the body. In fact, urine calcium generally declines, and fecal calcium declines or remains the same. The decline in serum calcium reflects a redistribution of calcium within the body. There is a rapid efflux of calcium with no change in calcium influx to the circulation, findings indicative of precipitation of calcium phosphate salt. The calcium precipitates in bone, and metastatic calcification has also been reported in patients receiving oral or intravenous phosphate therapy for hypercalcemia. Indeed, hyperphosphatemia can cause metastatic calcification in normocalcemic animals. Thus, administration of intravenous phosphate is justifiable only as an emergency treatment.

Inorganic phosphate is commercially available for oral use in liquid, powder, and capsule form and as a liquid for intravenous use. It is important to calculate doses in terms of phosphate phosphorous (see Table 336-4).

Summary The various therapies for hypercalcemia are listed in Table 336-5. The choice depends upon the underlying disease, the severity of the hypercalcemia, the serum inorganic phosphate level, and the patient's renal, hepatic, and bone marrow function. Mild hypercalcemia (12 mg/dL or 3 mmol per liter) can usually be managed by hydration, sodium chloride, and small doses of furosemide or ethacrynic acid. Severe hypercalcemia (15 mg/dL or 3.75 mmol per liter) requires rapid correction. Aggressive sodium-calcium diuresis with large doses of furosemide and ethacrynic acid works rapidly but should only be undertaken if appropriate monitoring is available and cardiac function is adequate. Plicamycin is often the drug of choice, since it has the advantages of effectiveness and simplicity of use; the principal contraindication is its potential for toxicity. Renal, hepatic, or bone marrow disease may preclude its use.

Since continuation of intravenous therapy is usually impracticable and long-term use of plicamycin may increase chances of toxicity, there is a role for oral phosphate therapy for chronic management of hypercalcemia. Phosphate supplements should never be administered if hyperphosphatemia is present. Severe dietary calcium restriction should be employed if intestinal absorption is enhanced. Glucocorticoids and prostaglandin-synthesis inhibitors, even when effective in a particular disease, work slowly over several days and should not be relied upon as the sole treatment for life-threatening hypercalcemia. Dialysis should be reserved for hypercalcemia complicating acute or chronic renal failure.

The only satisfactory therapy for chronic use is a combination of dietary calcium restriction, administration of sodium chloride with or without furosemide and ethacrynic acid, and moderate-dose oral phosphate (the patient is kept normophosphatemic). The more effective remedies (plicamycin, glucocorticoids, high-dose oral phosphate) have significant toxicity when used chronically. There may be a role for calcitonin combined with glucocorticoids, but more experience is needed.

TABLE 336-4 Commercially available phosphate preparations

	1000 mg P	meq Na	meq K
Oral phosphate preparations:			
Neutraphos (1250-mg capsule	4 caps	28.5	28.5
Neutraphos-K (1450-mg capsule)	4 caps	—	57
Phos-Tabs (860-mg tablet)	6 tabs	—	51
Fleets Phospho-Soda (liquid)	6.7 mL	40	—
Intravenous phosphate preparations:			
In-Phos	40 mL	65	8
Hyper-Phos-K	15 mL	—	50

SOURCE: *After Neer and Potts (with permission).*

TABLE 336-5 Summary of useful treatments for hypercalcemia

Therapy	Therapeutic details	Indications	Complications	Precautions
MOST GENERALLY USEFUL THERAPIES				
Hydration	2 liters or more	Universal	—	—
High salt intake	Achieve urine Na of 300 meq/day or more	Universal	Edema	—
Furosemide or ethacrynic acid	40–160 mg/day 50–200 mg/day	Universal	↓K and ↓Mg	Measure serum K and Mg
Forced diuresis	4–6 liters fluid IV/day containing 600–900 meq Na plus furosemide every 1-2 h, plus at least 60 meg K/day, plus at least 60 meq Mg/day	Universal	Pulmonary edema; ↓K and ↓Mg	Intensive monitoring, including venous pressure and serum Mg and K
Oral phosphate	250 mg P every 6 h PO	Universal if serum P < 3 mg/dL	Ectopic calcification	Keep serum P below 5–6 mg/dL
Plicamycin	10–25 μg/kg IV, repeat prn	Increased bone resorption	Liver; kidney; marrow toxicity	Monitor platelets CBC, BUN, SCOT
Prednisone or equivalent	5–15 mg every 6 h	Breast cancer, lymphomas, leukemias, multiple myeloma, vitamin D poisoning, sarcoidosis	Cushing's syndrome if chronic Rx	Alternate-day Rx for chronic use
SPECIAL THERAPIES FOR PARTICULAR USES				
IV phosphate	1500 mg P every 12 h until P 6 mg/dL	Severe hypercalcemia; diuresis or mithramycin contraindicated	Ectopic calcification: severe hypocalcemia	Monitor serum Ca and P closely
Calcitonin	2 units every 4 h subcutaneously	Adjunct when ↑bone reabsorption; paralysis; immobilization	—	—
Indomethacin	25 mg every 6 h PO	Certain types of pseudo-hyperparathyroidism	Na retention: GI bleeding; headache	Careful clinical monitoring
Dialysis	Low-Ca bath	Acute renal failure	Multiple	Monitor serum P after dialysis

HYPOCALCEMIA

PATHOPHYSIOLOGY OF HYPOCALCEMIA: CLASSIFICATION BASED ON MECHANISM Chronic hypocalcemia is less common than hypercalcemia; causes include chronic renal failure, hereditary and acquired hypoparathyroidism, and hypomagnesemia. Critically ill patients may have *transient hypocalcemia* in association with disorders such as severe sepsis, burns, and acute renal failure or after extensive transfusions with citrated blood. In many instances, however, the hypocalcemia is more apparent than real. Although as many as half of patients in intensive care settings are reported to show calcium concentrations below 8.5 mg/dL, less than 10 percent have a reduction in ionized calcium. Often, hypoalbuminemia is the cause of the reduced total calcium concentration. In addition, however, alkalosis may tend to increase calcium binding to proteins, and in this setting direct measurements of ionized calcium should be made.

Medications such as protamine, heparin, and glucagon may cause transient hypocalcemia. These forms of hypocalcemia, apparent or real, are usually not associated with tetany and resolve with improvement in the overall medical condition. The transient hypocalcemia after repeated transfusions of citrated blood also usually resolves quickly.

Subacute hypocalcemia may also occur. Patients with acute *pancreatitis* have hypocalcemia which persists during the acute inflammation and varies in severity with the severity of the pancreatitis. The cause of the hypocalcemia in pancreatitis remains unclear. Parathyroid hormone (PTH) values may be low, normal, or elevated, and both resistance to PTH and impaired PTH secretion have been reported, leaving no clear view as to the principal mechanism. There are also occasional reports of a chronic low total blood calcium in elderly patients, with documented reduction in ionized calcium concentration but without obvious cause and with a paucity of symptoms of hypocalcemia.

Neuromuscular or neurologic symptoms are the most common manifestations of untreated chronic hypocalcemia. Patients may show muscle spasms, carpopedal spasm, facial grimacing, and in extreme cases, laryngeal spasm and convulsions. Respiratory arrest may occur. Increased intracranial pressure occurs in some patients with long-standing hypocalcemia, often in association with papilledema. Other chronic mental changes include irritability, depression, and psychosis. The QT interval on the electrocardiogram is prolonged, in contrast to its shortening with hypercalcemia. Arrhythmias are reported, and digitalis may be ineffective. Intestinal cramps and chronic malabsorption may occur. Chvostek's or Trousseau's signs can be used to confirm latent tetany.

The classification of hypocalcemia shown in Table 336-6 is based on the premise that PTH is responsible for minute-to-minute regulations of plasma calcium concentration within narrow limits and, therefore, that the occurrence of hypocalcemia must mean a failure of the homeostatic action of PTH. This can occur if PTH is simply absent due to hereditary or acquired gland failure, if the hormone is rendered ineffective by any of several mechanisms that interfere with its action at target organs, or if the action of the hormone to raise blood calcium is simply overwhelmed by the loss of calcium from the extracellular fluid at a rate faster than it can be replaced.

PTH ABSENT Hypoparathyroidism, whether hereditary or acquired, has a number of common components. Acute and chronic symptoms that result from untreated hypocalcemia are shared by the two disorders, although typically the onset of hereditary hypoparathyroidism is more gradual and although acquired hypoparathyroidism often does not cause abnormalities in the teeth. Traditionally, acquired hypoparathyroidism secondary to surgery in the neck was more common than hereditary hypoparathyroidism, but the frequency of surgically induced parathyroid failure has diminished with the recognition of the importance of parathyroid gland preservation and the use of nonsurgical approaches to treatment of hyperthyroidism. Basal ganglia calcification and extrapyramidal syndromes occur in both hereditary and acquired hypoparathyroidism but are more common and earlier in onset in hereditary hypoparathyroidism. Pseudohypoparathyroidism, an example of ineffective PTH action rather than a failure of parathyroid gland production, shares several features with hypoparathyroidism. Both disorders exhibit the extraosseus calcification and extrapyramidal syndromes, the latter including choreoathetoic movements and dystonia. Papilledema and raised intracranial pressure occur in both states, as do lenticular cataracts and chronic changes in fingernails and hair, the latter usually reversible with treatment of hypocalcemia. Certain skin manifestations, including alopecia and candidiasis, are seen exclusively in hereditary hypoparathyroidism.

Hypocalcemia associated with hypomagnesemia is associated both with deficient PTH release and impaired responsiveness to the hormone. Patients with hypocalcemia secondary to hypomagnesemia have absent or low levels of circulating iPTH, indicative of diminished hormone release despite maximum physiologic stimulus by hypocalcemia. Plasma PTH levels return to normal with correction of the hypomagnesemia. Thus, hypoparathyroidism, associated with low levels of PTH in blood, can be due to hereditary gland failure, acquired gland failure, or acute, but reversible, gland dysfunction (hypomagnesemia). Patients with acquired or hereditary hypoparathyroidism also have hyperphosphatemia and absent or very low levels of $1,25(OH)_2D$.

Hereditary hypoparathyroidism Hypoparathyroidism can occur as an isolated entity without other endocrine or dermatologic manifestations or, more typically, in association with other organ deficiencies, such as defective development of the thymus, adrenal insufficiency, and ovarian insufficiency.

One rare form of hypoparathyroidism due to congenital aplasia of the parathyroid glands is manifested shortly after birth. The hereditary patterns are unclear with no simple pattern established. A linkage between defective development of the thymus and the parathyroid glands is recognized in the *DiGeorge syndrome,* which is also associated with congenital cardiovascular and other developmental defects. Most patients die in early childhood.

Hypoparathyroidism can occur as part of a more complex autoimmune syndrome involving failure of the adrenals, the ovaries, and the parathyroids in association with recurrent mucocutaneous candidiasis, alopecia, vitiligo, and pernicious anemia (see Chap. 334). In many cases, antibodies to endocrine organs are present. The inheritance appears to be autosomal recessive, and some unaffected family members show antibodies to endocrine tissue without evidence of endocrine failure. The disorder is usually referred to as autoimmune polyglandular deficiency. There is a failure of cell-mediated immunity.

Hereditary hypoparathyroidism occurs also as an isolated entity. The disease is usually manifest in the first decade but may occur much later, including in adult life. The mechanism of inheritance is unclear.

Treatment of hereditary hypoparathyroidism is similar to that for acquired hypoparathyroidism and pseudohypoparathyroidism, although specific features of each disease lead to additional treatment considerations. Replacement therapy with vitamin D or the active metabolite $1,25(OH)_2D$ combined with a high oral calcium intake usually suffices to regulate blood calcium and phosphate levels satisfactorily. Care must be taken to avoid excessive urinary calcium excretion; oral calcium and vitamin D therapy restores the overall calcium-phosphate balance but does not reverse the lowered urinary calcium clearance typical of hypoparathyroidism. Kidney stones may form due to excessive urinary calcium excretion during vitamin D and calcium replacement therapy in hypoparathyroidism. Thiazide diuretics will lower urine calcium by as much as 100 mg per day in hypoparathyroid patients on vitamin D, and calcium replacement therapy has been adopted by many in the management of hypoparathyroid patients. The approach seems to be of benefit in preventing severe hypercalciuria and in improving the management of certain patients (see "Treatment" section below).

TABLE 336-6 Functionally based classification of hypocalcemia (excluding neonatal conditions)

I PTH absent
- *A* Hereditary hypoparathyroidism
- *B* Acquired hypoparathyroidism
- *C* Hypomagnesemia

II PTH ineffective
- *A* Chronic renal failure
- *B* Active vitamin D lacking
  - *1* ↓ dietary intake or sunlight
  - 2 Defective metabolism:
    - Anticonvulsant therapy
    - Vitamin D dependent rickets—type I
- *C* Active vitamin D ineffective
  - *1* Intestinal malabsorption
  - *2* Vitamin D–dependent rickets—type II
- *D* Pseudohypoparathyroidism

III PTH overwhelmed
- *A* Severe, acute hyperphosphatemia
  - *1* Tumor lysis
  - *2* Acute renal failure
  - *3* Rhabdomyolysis
- *B* Osteitis fibrosa after parathyroidectomy

Acquired hypoparathyroidism Acquired, chronic hypoparathyroidism is usually the result of inadvertent surgical removal of all the parathyroid glands; in some instances, not all of the tissue is removed but the gland undergoes compromise of vascular supply secondary to fibrotic changes in the neck after surgery. Historically, the most frequent cause of acquired hypoparathyroidism was encountered in the surgical management of hyperthyroidism. Chronic hypoparathyroidism is now more often encountered following surgery for chief cell hyperplasia of the parathyroids where the surgeon, facing the dilemma of removing too little tissue and thus not curing the hyperparathyroidism, removes too much, with consequent hypoparathyroidism.

Parathyroid function is not totally absent in all patients with postsurgical hypoparathyroidism. Presumably, the persistence of some residual parathyroid activity reduces the amount of replacement therapy that is necessary, but therapy varies greatly from patient to patient irrespective of the type of hypoparathyroidism or the question of residual parathyroid activity.

There are other rare causes of acquired chronic hypoparathyroidism, such as radiation-induced damage subsequent to radioiodine therapy of hyperthyroidism or glandular damage in patients with hemochromatosis or with hemosiderosis after repeated blood transfusions. Other chronic infectious diseases, although they may involve one or more of the parathyroids, usually do not cause permanent hypoparathyroidism because all four glands are not usually involved.

Transient hypoparathyroidism is frequent following surgical exploration for hyperparathyroidism, particularly in patients in whom more than one exploration is required and in patients with multiple gland disease in which all glands must be identified and biopsied. Often, after a variable period of hypoparathyroidism, normal parathyroid function returns with hypertrophy of remaining tissue. Occasionally, recovery occurs months after surgery. The management of transient, postoperative hypoparathyroidism is discussed under the surgical treatment of hyperparathyroidism. The treatment of chronic, acquired hypoparathyroidism is similar to that used with idiopathic hypoparathyroidism—replacement with vitamin D and oral calcium.

Hypomagnesemia Hypomagnesemia, of a severe degree, is associated with severe hypocalcemia, and restoration of the total-body magnesium deficits leads to rapid reversal of the hypocalcemia. There are at least two separate causes, impaired secretion of PTH and reduced peripheral responsiveness to hormone action.

Hypomagnesemia is generally classified as primary or secondary; primary hypomagnesemia is due to hereditary defects in intestinal absorption or renal reabsorption of magnesium. Secondary hypomagnesemia, a more common condition, occurs on a nutritional basis or as a result of acquired intestinal or renal disorders. The most common causes of the secondary disorder are intestinal malabsorption syndromes, chronic alcoholism with poor nutritional intake, and parenteral nutrition in which magnesium replacement is omitted.

In experimental animals magnesium in extracellular fluid has effects similar to that of calcium on secretion of PTH; hypermagnesemia suppresses and hypomagnesemia stimulates PTH secretion.

Effects of magnesium on hormone secretion are normally of little physiologic significance, however, because the effects of calcium dominate. Greater change in magnesium than in calcium is needed to influence hormone secretion. Nonetheless, hypomagnesemia, if it influences hormone secretion at all, might be expected to increase hormone secretion. It is, therefore, surprising to find that severe hypomagnesemia is associated with blunted secretion of PTH. The explanation for the paradox is that severe, chronic hypomagnesemia is a marker of total-body magnesium deficiency; severe magnesium deficiency intereferes with normal secretory mechanisms and normal peripheral responses to PTH, both of which involve function of adenyl cyclase in glandular and target tissues. This chronic change, reduced intracellular stores, completely obscures any effects that might be brought about by acute changes in extracellular fluid magnesium in a magnesium-replete individual.

Severe hypocalcemia is often seen when serum magnesium is substantially below normal. Normal serum magnesium is 2 to 3 mg/dL or 1.5 to 2.5 meq per liter. In the majority of the cases in which hypomagnesemia is associated with hypocalcemia, serum magnesium has been below 0.8 meq per liter or 1.0 mg/dL.

Immunoreactive PTH (iPTH) levels are usually undetectable or inappropriately low despite the extreme stimulus of severe hypocalcemia. Even when iPTH levels are elevated, acute repletion of magnesium leads to a further increase in iPTH concentration. The overall data are interpreted to mean that PTH secretion is blunted in virtually all patients with severe hypomagnesemia; thus, absolute or relative acute hypoparathyroidism seems to be the rule in patients with hypocalcemia secondary to hypomagnesemia.

Diminished peripheral responsiveness to administered PTH can be shown in some patients with severe hypomagnesemia in addition to defects in hormone secretion. Some clinical reports document normal response in urinary phosphorus and urinary cyclic AMP excretion after administration of exogenous PTH to patients who are hypocalcemic and who have diminished PTH secretion. Both blunted PTH secretion and lack of renal response to administered PTH can occur in the same patient. Blunted skeletal responses have been claimed in many, but by no means all, patients studied with the hypomagnesemia-hypocalcemia syndrome. When acute magnesium repletion is undertaken, the restoration of PTH concentrations to normal or supranormal levels, precedes by several days the restoration of serum calcium.

Overall, blunted PTH secretory response in hypomagnesemia is probably the more important cause of the hypocalcemia. The variable defect in peripheral responsiveness, particularly renal responses, may indicate that an even greater degree of magnesium deficiency is required to induce end organ resistance than for impairment of hormone secretion.

Several other features have been noted. The brisk response in hormone secretion following magnesium repletion, sometimes demonstrable within minutes of giving a large parenteral dose of magnesium, indicates that hormone biosynthesis is not impaired, only secretion. Serum phosphate levels are not elevated as they often are in patients with hypoparathyroidism, probably because phosphate deficiency is a frequent accompaniment of the nutritional deficiencies that cause hypomagnesemia. There have been a few reports of magnesium-wasting chronic renal disease; although magnesium is elevated in acute renal failure, increases in magnesium concentration are an infrequent accompaniment of chronic renal failure.

Repletion of magnesium is the cure of the condition, and attention must be given to restoring the intracellular deficiency which may be considerable. After intravenous magnesium, serum magnesium may return to the normal range, but unless replacement therapy is continued, it will rapidly fall to subnormal levels again. A sometimes useful indicator of restoration of magnesium deficiency is the urinary magnesium excretion; magnesium retention by the kidney is usually seen until magnesium deficiencies are repleted. Intracellular deficits can be as great as 100 meq or more, but in many of the reported cases parenteral administration of approximately 25 meq magnesium seemed to reverse the signs of magnesium deficiency. Depending on the associated condition which caused the hypomagnesemia, treatment may have to be administered chronically to prevent recurrence.

PTH INEFFECTIVE PTH can be considered ineffective when the hormone's action to promote calcium absorption from the diet is interfered with because of a primary deficiency of vitamin D, because of a condition in which vitamin D is ineffective, or in chronic renal failure in which the calcium-elevating action of PTH is opposed by several different processes. With diverse pathophysiologic mechanisms, these conditions center around but are not limited to the unavailability of vitamin D as a cofactor for the hormone and are usually associated with mild hypomagnesemia. Typically, hypophosphatemia is more severe than hypocalcemia due to the increased secretion of PTH which, while ineffective to elevate blood calcium, still promotes renal phosphate excretion. Varying degrees of bone disease featuring impaired mineralization and/or frank osteomalacia are the more frequent and harmful consequences of chronic renal failure or inadequate or ineffective vitamin D action.

Pseudohypoparathyroidism, on the other hand, is distinct from the other disorders classified under ineffective PTH action. Pseudohypoparathyroidism resembles conditions in which there is a true absence of PTH synthesis and secretion and is manifested, in the untreated state, by severe hypocalcemia and hyperphosphatemia. The cause of the disease, however, is inadequate peripheral response to PTH involving any of several defects in the biochemical events involving hormone binding to the receptor, activation of guanyl nucleotide binding proteins, and stimulation of adenyl cyclase to increase intracellular cyclic AMP.

Chronic renal failure Severe abnormalities in mineral ion and bone metabolism occur in chronic renal failure. Even prior to the initiation of extensive programs of dialysis, however, improved medical management of chronic renal failure and/or a more indolent course of the renal disease allowed many patients to survive for a sufficiently long period that renal osteodystrophy, the mixed bone disease associated with renal failure, often became an important feature.

After the initiation of chronic dialysis programs, many of the impairments in mineral and bone metabolism became even more apparent. Now the roles of phosphate retention and impaired production of $1,25(OH)_2D$ are recognized as the principal factors responsible for inducing calcium deficiency, secondary hyperparathyroidism, and a picture of often severe bone disease. Less clearly, the uremic state appears to be associated with impairment of intestinal absorption by factors other than impairment in vitamin D metabolism. Nonetheless, replacement of physiologic levels of $1,25(OH)_2D$ usually leads to satisfactory calcium absorption, suggesting it is the lack of the vitamin D rather than intrinsic defects in intestinal cellular function that is the more important cause of the impaired mineral metabolism in chronic renal failure.

Hyperphosphatemia per se tends to lower blood calcium concentration by several actions; these include extraosseous deposition of calcium and phosphate, impaired sensitivity of the skeleton to the bone-resorbing action of PTH, reduced $1,25(OH)_2D$ production by surviving renal tissue, and reduction in calcium absorption due to trapping of calcium in insoluble form as calcium phosphate complexes. In animals prevention of hyperphosphatemia by dietary means can block the development of secondary hyperparathyroidism, emphasizing the importance of phosphate retention in the pathogenesis of secondary hyperparathyroidism and the associated disorders of mineral and bone metabolism. The low levels of $1,25(OH)_2D$ also play an important role, particularly in chronic renal failure.

Therapy of chronic renal failure (discussed elsewhere in this text) features careful medical management of patients prior to dialysis as well as careful adjustment of dialysis regimens once this becomes necessary. At various stages of the development of the renal failure, attention should be paid to restriction of phosphate in the diet, use of phosphate-binding antacids such as those based on aluminum hydroxide, provision of an adequate calcium intake by mouth, usually

1 to 2 g per day, and supplementation with calcitriol in doses from 0.25 to 1.0 μg per day. Each patient must be monitored closely. The aims of therapy are to restore a normal calcium balance to prevent osteomalacia and the development of secondary hyperparathyroidism. Renal osteodystrophy, as discussed above, is the principal disabling feature of chronic renal failure related to calcium metabolism. Reduction of hyperphosphatemia and restoration of normal intestinal calcium absorption by the use of supplemental calcitriol can lead to an improvement in blood calcium concentration and a concomitant reduction in secondary hyperparathyroidism.

Active vitamin D lacking DEFICIENT DIETARY INTAKE AND/OR SUNLIGHT Vitamin D deficiency is more common in the United States at the present time than previously recognized. Biopsies of bone in elderly patients with hip fracture and evaluation of patients with regard to concentrations of vitamin D metabolites, PTH, and mineral ions themselves have revealed that vitamin D deficiency may occur in as many as 25 percent of elderly patients, particularly in areas where there is little ambient sunlight. Concentrations of 25-(OH)D are at the lower limits of normal or well below normal in these patients. Quantitative histomorphometry on bone biopsy specimens reveals widened osteoid seams consistent with osteomalacia. Again, the bone disease is the serious problem. Hypocalcemia is modest in degree at best. PTH hypersecretion compensates for a tendency of the blood calcium level to fall but at the consequence of inducing renal phosphate wasting and a combined mineral ion abnormality that results in osteomalacia.

The genesis of the vitamin D deficiency is impaired intake of dairy products that are enriched with vitamin D, lack of vitamin supplementation in the elderly, and reduced sunlight exposure, particularly in winter in northern parts of the country.

Treatment involves the administration of vitamin D and provision of 1 to 1.5 g of calcium in the diet. Vitamin D supplementation should aim to provide several times the recommended daily requirement in younger people, which is probably a safe recommendation; 1000 to 2000 units of vitamin D per day would be satisfactory. Vitamin D is usually not available in multiple-dose forms. Hence, the administration of a capsule containing 50,000 units of vitamin D once monthly is safe in elderly patients who have osteomalacia. The increased awareness of the importance of calcium supplementation, particularly in women, even without supplementation of vitamin D, may lessen the frequency of this problem. It should be emphasized that severe hypocalcemia is rarely seen in the moderately severe vitamin D deficiency of the elderly but needs to be considered in the differential diagnosis of mild hypocalcemia.

DEFECTIVE VITAMIN D METABOLISM *Anticonvulsant therapy* Anticonvulsant therapy with any of several agents induces a state of acquired vitamin D deficiency by increasing the turnover of vitamin D into inactive compounds. The more marginal the degree of vitamin D intake in the diet, the more likely it is that anticonvulsant therapy will lead to abnormalities in mineral and bone metabolism. The syndrome in its extreme case involves severe rickets with bone fractures, hypocalcemia, and hypophosphatemia. Occasionally, a severe proximal myopathy is reported. More often, frank hypocalcemia is not detected, and mild osteomalacia is the only clinical symptom. In other patients on long-term anticonvulsant therapy, no symptoms or signs are present, but bone density is lower than normal and responds favorably to vitamin D supplementation.

Anticonvulsants stimulate the hepatic microsomal mixed-oxidase enzymes and hence increase the rate of clearance of vitamin D and its metabolites. Phenytoin also impairs intestinal calcium absorption independent of effects on vitamin D; the drug also has deleterious effects on bone cell function in vitro including inhibition of collagen synthesis. The syndrome can be reversed with adequate vitamin D supplementation.

Although $1,25(OH)_2D$ levels are lower for the degree of vitamin D intake in patients treated with chronic anticonvulsants than in the normal population, there is a great deal of variation. The greater prevalence of the disorder in some European populations and in children in homes for the mentally retarded probably reflects the lower vitamin D intake of those groups. Restoration of bone mineral mass and reversal of hypocalcemia, when seen, can be accomplished with vitamin D replacement plus added oral calcium. Adjustments in dose are indicated depending on the age and body size of the patient, but approximately 50,000 units of vitamin D weekly plus 1 g of elemental calcium per day for several months are usually sufficient. Alternatively, administration of one 50,000-unit capsule of vitamin D once monthly may be preventative if the anticonvulsant therapy must be given chronically.

Vitamin D–dependent rickets type I Rickets can be due to *resistance* to the *action* of vitamin D as well as to vitamin D deficiency. Vitamin D–dependent rickets type I, previously termed pseudo-vitamin D–dependent rickets, differs from vitamin D–resistant rickets in that it is less severe and in that the biochemical and radiographic abnormalities can be reversed with large doses of the vitamin.

Clinical features include hypocalcemia, often with tetany or convulsions, hypophosphatemia, secondary hyperparathyroidism, and osteomalacia, often associated with skeletal deformities and increased alkaline phosphatase. Doses of vitamin D or 25(OH)D, 100 to 1000 times above the usual amounts, are required to heal the bone disease, whereas physiologic amounts of calcitriol cure the disease. The disorder, an autosomal recessive trait, is due to a defect in conversion of 25(OH)D to $1,25(OH)_2D$. Plasma levels of $1,25(OH)_2D$ are low or undetectable even after administration of large doses of vitamin D or 25(OH). Response to high doses of vitamin D or 25(OH)D is probably due to direct actions of high levels of 25(OH)D. Treatment requires careful adjustment of calcitriol dose, particularly during growth periods.

ACTIVE VITAMIN D INEFFECTIVE *Intestinal malabsorption* Mild hypocalcemia, secondary hyperparathyroidism, severe hypophosphatemia, and a variety of nutritional deficiencies occur with gastrointestinal diseases. Hepatocellular dysfunction can lead to reduction in 25(OH)D levels, as in portal or biliary cirrhosis of the liver. Malabsorption of vitamin D and its metabolites, including calcitriol, may occur in a variety of intestinal diseases, hereditary or acquired. Hypocalcemia itself can lead to steatorrhea, due to deficient production of pancreatic enzymes and bile salts. Depending on the disorder, vitamin D or its metabolites can be administered parenterally, thereby guaranteeing adequate blood levels of active metabolites.

Vitamin D–dependent rickets type II Pseudo-vitamin D–dependent rickets can be due to defective response as well as to defective production of $1,25(OH)_2D$. This disorder, vitamin D–dependent rickets type II, results from any of several types of end organ resistance to the active metabolite, including absence or qualitative defects of the cytosolic receptor protein for the hormone and postreceptor blocks in hormone action. The clinical features are similar to those with the type I disorder and include hypocalcemia, hypophosphatemia, secondary hyperparathyroidism, and rickets. Plasma levels of $1,25(OH)_2D$ are elevated at least three times above normal, in keeping with the refractoriness of the end organs. Severe alopecia totalis may commence early in life. Patients with this disorder usually require higher dose of vitamin D or vitamin D metabolites than in the type I disorder.

Pseudohypoparathyroidism Pseudohypoparathyroidism (PHP) is a hereditary disorder characterized by symptoms and signs of hypoparathyroidism, typically in association with distinctive skeletal and developmental defects. The hypoparathyroidism is due to a deficient end organ response to PTH. Excessive secretion of PTH is the consequence of hyperplasia of the parathyroids, a response to the resistance to hormone action. The entity is actually a syndrome in which various individuals and kindreds exhibit different aberrancies in hormone-receptor complex response.

A working classification of the various forms of pseudohypoparathyroidism is given in Table 336-7. The classification scheme is based on the signs of ineffective parathyroid hormone action (low calcium and high phosphate), urinary cyclic AMP response to exogenous PTH, the presence or absence of Albright's hereditary osteodystrophy (AHO), and assays of the concentration of the G_s subunits of the adenylate cyclase enzyme (see Chap. 67). Using these criteria there are four types: pseudohypoparathyroidism (PHP) type I, subdivided into a and b categories; PHP-II; and pseudopseudohypoparathyroidism (PPHP). Individuals with PHP-I, the most common of the disorders, show a deficient response in urinary cyclic AMP following administration of exogenous parathyroid hormone. Pseudohypoparathyroidism type II refers to patients with hypocalcemia and hyperphosphatemia who have a normal urinary cyclic AMP response to PTH. These patients are assumed to have a defect in the response to PTH at a locus beyond that of cyclic AMP production. Patients with the PHP-I syndrome are divided into type a with reduced activity of the stimulatory G protein subunit (G_s) in in vitro assays and type b with normal amounts of G_s in erythrocytes. Subjects with PHP-Ia also have shortened metacarpals and metatarsals and the other features of Albright's hereditary osteodystrophy (AHO) syndrome and commonly show resistance to hormones in addition to PTH. Patients with PHP-Ib have a normal phenotype without the AHO syndrome and do not show resistance to any hormones other than parathyroid hormone. Fibroblasts cultured from the skin of some patients with PHP-Ib show a much reduced response of cyclic AMP accumulation to agents that stimulate adenylate cyclase such as prostaglandins, forskolin, and PTH, consistent with the presence of a defective receptor. A subset of these patients, however, have a normal response to cyclic AMP production in fibroblasts in vitro.

Patients with PPHP have typical features of the hereditary osteodystrophy syndrome despite normal serum calciums and normal response of urinary cyclic AMP to exogenous PTH. Some such individuals are first degree relatives of patients with PHP-Ia, and patients initially classified as having PPHP have subsequently developed mild hypocalcemia. Patients with PPHP on average have levels of G_s subunits that are half normal. These various features suggest that PPHP is a mild variant of PHP-Ia and illustrate the heterogeneity of the defect in PTH responsiveness. Further studies will be necessary to clarify the pathogenesis of these disorders.

Little is known about the pathophysiology of the skeletal defects. The AHO syndrome includes round facies, short stature, obesity, brachydactyly, and heterotopic calcification. Mental deficiency is frequent.

The mode of inheritance in these various disorders is uncertain and may itself be heterogeneous. In some families the disorder may be an X-linked dominant defect, whereas in others the disorder appears to result from an autosomal dominant mutation with variable expressivity.

The mineral deposits in ectopic sites may include true bone, whereas bone formation in ectopic sites never occurs in idiopathic hypoparathyroidism. Amorphous deposits of calcium and phosphate are found in the basal ganglia in about half of patients. The defects in metacarpal and metatarsal bones are sometimes accompanied by abnormal phalanges as well, possibly reflecting premature closing of the epiphyses. The typical findings are abnormally short fourth and fifth metacarpals and metatarsals. The defects are usually bilateral. Exostoses are frequent, as is radius curvus. Impairments in olfaction and taste and unusual dermatoglyphic abnormalities have been reported. There is little improvement in mental status even after adequate therapy with calcium and vitamin D.

The diagnosis can usually be made without difficulty. Positive family history for developmental defects and/or the presence of developmental defects characteristic of PHP-Ia, including brachydactyly, in association with the signs of hypoparathyroidism, low calcium, and high phosphate, essentially make the diagnosis on clinical grounds. On the other hand, patients with PHP-Ib or PHP-II do not have phenotypic abnormalities. In PHP-Ib, administration of exogenous parathyroid hormone can lead to detection of the blunted cyclic AMP response; such tests are usually used to confirm the diagnosis even in PHP-Ia. Low levels of G_s subunits in erythrocyte membranes can also distinguish patients with PHP-Ia from those with PHP-Ib. Patients in both categories have elevated serum PTH, particularly if they are hypocalcemic. The diagnosis of PHP-II is more complex, in that cyclic AMP responses in urine are, by definition, normal. Since vitamin D deficiency itself can result in dissociation between phosphaturic and urinary cyclic AMP responses to exogenous PTH, vitamin D deficiency must be excluded before diagnosis of PHP-II can be made. PHP-II is separated from hypoparathyroidism by finding of elevated PTH levels; this finding per se, however, does not distinguish between secretion of abnormal PTH and a post-cyclic AMP receptor defect. Some patients with the PHP-II phenotype may actually have hypoparathyroidism secondary to secretion of an abnormal, biologically inactive PTH.

Treatment of PHP and PPHP is similar to that of hypoparathyroidism, except that the dose of vitamin D and calcium is usually lower than that required in true hypoparathyroidism. Variations in individual responses make it necessary to establish the optimal therapeutic program for each patient, based on maintaining the appropriate blood calcium concentration and urinary calcium excretion.

PTH Overwhelmed Occasionally, loss of calcium from the extracellular fluid (ECF) is so severe that PTH cannot compensate. Such situations include severe, acute hyperphosphatemia, often in association with renal failure, and rapid loss of calcium from the ECF, as in acute pancreatitis. Severe hypocalcemia can occur quickly; PTH rises in response to hypocalcemia but does not return blood calcium to normal. The chance of hypocalcemia is enhanced when there is some degree of compromise of the target tissues, as when renal failure occurs.

Severe, acute hyperphosphatemia Severe hyperphosphatemia occurs in situations associated with extensive tissue damage or cell destruction. The combination of an increased release of phosphate from muscle and an impaired ability to excrete phosphorous secondary to the renal failure causes moderate to severe hyperphosphatemia. Calcium loss from the blood results in hypocalcemia of mild to moderate severity; hypocalcemia is usually reversed with tissue repair and restoration of renal function as phosphorus and creatinine values return to normal. There may even be a mild hypercalcemic period in the oliguric phase of recovery of renal function. This sequence, severe hypocalcemia followed by mild hypercalcemia, reflects widespread deposition of calcium in muscle with subsequent redistribution of some of the calcium to the ECF after restoration of phosphate levels to normal.

Other causes of hyperphosphatemia that lead to hypocalcemia include hypothermia, massive hepatic failure, and hematologic malignancies, either because of high cell turnover as part of the malignancy or because of cell destruction when chemotherapy is instituted.

TABLE 336-7 Classification of pseudohypoparathyroidism (PHP) and pseudopseudohypoparathyroidism (PPHP)

Type	Hypocalcemia, hyperphosphatemia	Response of Urinary cAMP to PTH	Serum PTH	G_s subunit deficiency	AHO	Resistance to hormones in addition to PTH
PHP-Ia	Yes	↓	↑	Yes	Yes	Yes
PHP-Ib	Yes	↓	↑	No	No	No
PHP-II	Yes	Normal	↑	No	No	No
PPHP	No	Normal	Normal	Yes	Yes	±

NOTE: ↓ = *decreased;* ↑ = *increased; AHO = Albright's hereditary osteodystrophy.*

Treatment is directed toward lowering of blood phosphate by the administration of phosphate-binding antacids or dialysis, often needed for the management of renal failure. Although calcium replacement may be necessary if hypocalcemia is severe and symptomatic, calcium administration during the hyperphosphatemic period may increase extraosseous cellular calcium deposition, thereby aggravating ultimate tissue damage. Although the levels of 1,25$(OH)_2$D may be low during the hyperphosphatemic phase and may return to normal during the oliguric phase of recovery, mineral ion imbalance per se seems to be the principal pathophysiologic mechanism.

Osteitis fibrosa after parathyroidectomy Severe hypocalcemia after parathyroid surgery is less common now that osteitis fibrosa cystica is an infrequent manifestation of hyperparathyroidism. When osteitis fibrosa cystica is severe, however, bone mineral deficits can be large, and after parathyroidectomy, blood calcium levels can fall to the hypocalcemic range and remain depressed for days if calcium replacement is inadequate. The mechanism of the hypocalcemia is complex. Increased cellularity of bone in severe osteitis fibrosa cystica involves both osteoblastic and osteoclastic cells. High levels of PTH enhance bone-blood exchange, with resorption favored over formation; an abrupt decrease in PTH levels with surgery promotes bone formation. Calcium loss from blood is increased, and temporarily hyporesponsiveness of bone to the bone-resorbing actions of PTH hormone may add to the imbalance between bone resorption and bone formation. Treatment may require parenteral administration of calcium; addition of calcitriol and oral calcium supplementation may hasten the ability to withdraw parenteral calcium supplementation and/or reduce the amount needed.

DIFFERENTIAL DIAGNOSIS Care must be taken to ensure that true hypocalcemia is present; in addition, acute transient hypocalcemia can be a manifestation of a variety of severe, acute illnesses as discussed above. *Chronic hypocalcemia,* however, can usually be ascribed to a few disorders associated with an absence of PTH or its ineffectiveness. Important clinical criteria include the duration of the illness, signs or symptoms of associated disorders, and the detection of features that suggest an hereditary abnormality in calcium and bone metabolism. A nutritional history can be helpful in detecting a low intake of vitamin D and calcium in the elderly, and a history of excessive alcohol intake can be the clue to magnesium deficiency.

Hypoparathyroidism and pseudohypoparathyroidism are life-long illnesses; hence, a recent onset of hypocalcemia in an adult will rarely prove to be due to hypoparathyroidism and is more likely due to nutritional deficiencies, renal failure, or intestinal disorders that result in vitamin D deficiency or ineffective vitamin D action. A history of seizure disorder raises the issue of anticonvulsive medication. Neck surgery, even in the past, can be associated with a delayed onset of postsurgical hypoparathyroidism. Developmental defects, particularly in childhood and adolescence may point to the diagnosis of pseudohypoparathyroidism. Rickets and a variety of neuromuscular syndromes and deformities may indicate ineffective vitamin D action, usually due in the United States to hereditary defects in vitamin D metabolism rather than to vitamin D deficiency.

A pattern of *low calcium* with *high phosphorus* in the absence of renal failure or massive tissue destruction almost invariably means hypoparathyroidism or pseudohypoparathyroidism. A *low calcium* with a *low phosphorus* points to absent or ineffective vitamin D, thereby rendering the action of PHT on calcium metabolism ineffective. The relative ineffectiveness of PTH in vitamin D deficiency, anticonvulsant therapy, gastrointestinal disorders, and hereditary defects in vitamin D metabolism leads to secondary hyperparathyroidism as a compensation. The relatively unopposed action of the excess PTH on renal tubule phosphate transport, less dependent on vitamin D sufficiency than calcium transport, accounts for renal phosphate wasting and hypophosphatemia.

Exceptions to these patterns may occur. Most forms of hypomagnesemia are due to long-standing nutritional deficiency, and, despite the fact that the hypocalcemia is due principally to an acute absence of PTH, phosphate levels are usually low rather than elevated as in hypoparathyroidism. Chronic renal failure is often associated with hypocalcemia and hyperphosphatemia, despite secondary hyperparathyroidism.

Diagnosis is usually established by application of the PTH radioimmunoassay, tests for vitamin D metabolites, and measurements of the urinary cyclic AMP response to exogenous PTH. In hereditary and acquired hypoparathyroidism and severe hypomagnesemia, PTH is either undetectable or in the normal range. The latter finding may reflect in some instances a false-positive assay result, as in the case of tumor hypercalcemia, but the result in a hypocalcemic patient is supportive of hypoparathyroidism, as distinct from ineffective PTH action, in which even mild hypocalcemia is associated with clearly elevated PTH levels. Hence, a failure to detect elevated PTH levels establishes the diagnosis of hypoparathyroidism; elevated levels suggest the presence of secondary hyperparathyroidism as found in many of the situations in which the hormone is ineffective due to associated abnormalities in vitamin D action. Assays for 25(OH)D and 1,25$(OH)_2$D can be quite helpful. Low or low normal 25(OH)D indicates vitamin D deficiency due to lack of sunlight, inadequate vitamin D intake, or intestinal malabsorption. A low level of 1,25-$(OH)_2$D in the presence of elevated concentrations of PTH suggests ineffective PTH action, including chronic renal failure, severe vitamin D deficiency, vitamin D–dependent rickets type I, and pseudohypoparathyroidism. Recognition that mild hypocalcemia, rickets, and hypophosphatemia are due to chronic anticonvulsant therapy is made by history.

TREATMENT OF HYPOCALCEMIA The chronic management of hypoparathyroidism or pseudohypoparathyroidism, chronic renal failure, and hereditary defects in vitamin D metabolism all feature the use of vitamin D or vitamin D metabolites and calcium supplementation. Vitamin D itself is the least expensive form of vitamin D replacement and is frequently used in the management of uncomplicated hypoparathyroidism and disorders associated with ineffective vitamin D action. When vitamin D is used prophylatically, as in the elderly or in those with chronic anticonvulsant therapy, there is a wider margin of safety than with the more potent metabolites. On the other hand, most of the conditions in which vitamin D is used for chronic management of hypocalcemia require the use of 50 to 100 times the daily replacement doses, because the formation of 1,25$(OH)_2$D is deficient. In such situations, vitamin D is no safer than the active metabolite because with high-dose vitamin D therapy, intoxication does occur. Calcitriol is more rapid in onset of action and also has a short biologic half-life; in high doses vitamin D is stored in body tissues and is cleared slowly.

One to five micrograms per day of vitamin D or calcifediol [25-$(OH)D_3$] and slightly lower doses of calcitriol (0.25 to 1.0 μg per day) are required to prevent rickets. In contrast, 500 to 3000 μg of vitamin D_2 or D_3 are typically required in hypoparathyroidism; doses of calcifediol are also high (several hundred micrograms per day) compared with doses required in euparathyroid individuals. The dose of calcitriol is unchanged in hypoparathyroidism since the defect is in hydroxylation by the 1α-hydroxylase.

The slightly greater therapeutic efficacy of calcifediol than vitamin D_3 in conditions in which the metabolism of the vitamin is impaired may be due to superior metabolic availability for the renal 1α-hydroxylase or to direct action directly by 25(OH)D at receptors in target tissues. Vitamin D is metabolized to a variety of compounds other than the principal product, 25(OH)D. Calcifediol bypasses these alternate pathways and is directly available for metabolism to 1,25$(OH)_2$D. In hypoparathyroidism and in hereditary defects in renal hydroxylase, the efficiency of formation of 1,25$(OH)_2$D from 25(OH)D is low, but some formation does occur with high substrate levels. Calcifediol has about 1 percent of the potency of calcitriol in in vivo and in vitro tests of vitamin D responsiveness.

Unless a loading dose is given, 2 to 4 weeks or even longer are required to achieve the maximum calcium replacement action of vitamin D or calcifediol; again, the onset of action of calcifediol is slightly more rapid. Calcitriol can be given for hypoparathyroidism at the same dose required for the prevention of rickets in euparathyroid individuals, 0.2 to 1.0 μg per day. Its onset of action is days rather than weeks. When vitamin D or calcifediol is withdrawn, weeks are required for the disappearance of the biologic effects but only a few days for calcitriol.

Patients with hypoparathyroidism should be given 2 to 3 g of elemental calcium by mouth each day. The two agents, vitamin D or vitamin D metabolites and oral calcium, can be varied independently. Higher doses of vitamin D or its metabolites increase the efficiency of intestinal calcium absorption; higher intakes of oral calcium permit adequate calcium assimilation despite a lower efficiency of intestinal calcium absorption. In the event of hypercalcemia during the treatment of chronic hypocalcemia, the withdrawal of the supplemental oral calcium is effective in lowering calcium within 24 h, even more rapidly than withdrawal of calcitriol. Most patients with hypoparathyroidism can be managed with high-dose vitamin D therapy combined with 2 to 3 g of oral calcium per day. If hypocalcemia alternates with episodes of hypercalcemia, then substitution of calcitriol will often make management easier.

The administration of thiazide diuretics in the usual antihypertensive doses to patients with hypoparathyroidism lowers urinary calcium excretion. This hypocalciuric effect allows the calcium and vitamin D supplementation to be reduced. The treatment also may protect against the development of kidney stones, a potential complication of the long-term management of hypoparathyroidism. If on dialysis, patients with chronic renal failure and hypocalcemia can have adjustments in dialysate calcium concentration as an alternative to vitamin D and calcium supplementation. The doses of vitamin D and calcium required for the management of pseudohypoparathyroidism are usually lower than those required for hypoparathyroidism, reflecting incomplete resistance to the action of PTH in pseudohypoparathyroidism. The acute treatment of hypomagnesemia is discussed above; the use of magnesium chloride by mouth may be sufficient to restore blood magnesium.

REFERENCES

AKITA Y et al: The stimulatory and inhibitory guanine nucleotide-binding proteins of adenylate cyclase in erythrocytes from patients with pseudohypoparathyroidism type 1. J Clin Endocrinol Metab 61:1012, 1985

BELL NH: Vitamin D endocrine system. J Clin Invest 76:1, 1985

DREZNER M et al: Pseudohypoparathyroidism type II: A possible defect in the reception of the cyclic AMP signal. N Engl J Med 289:1056, 1973

GARABEDIAN M et al: Elevated plasma 1,25-$(OH)_2D$ concentrations in infants with hypercalcemia and elfin facies. N Engl J Med 312:948, 1985

HEUBI JE et al: Hypocalcemia and steatorrhea: Clues to etiology. Dig Dis Sci 28:124, 1983

KNOCHEL JP: Editorial: Serum calcium derangements in rhabdomyolysis. N Engl J Med 305:161, 1981

LEVINE MA et al: Activity of the stimulatory guanine nucleotide-binding protein is reduced in erythrocytes from patients with pseudohypoparathyroidism and pseudopseudohypoparathyroidism: Biochemical, endocrine, and genetic analysis of Albright's hereditary osteodystrophy in six kindreds. J Clin Endocrinol Metab 62:497, 1986

LIBERMAN UA et al: Resistance to 1,25-$(OH)_2D$. Association with heterogenous defects in cultured skin fibroblasts. J Clin Invest 71:192, 1983

MUNDY GR et al: Tumor products and the hypercalcemia of malignancy. J Clin Invest 76:391, 1985

——— et al: The hypercalcemia of cancer: Clinical implications and pathogenetic mechanisms. N Engl J Med 310:1718, 1984

NAGANT DE DEUXCHAISNES C et al: Dissociation of parathyroid hormone bioactivity and immunoreactivity in pseudohypoparathyroidism type I. J Clin Endocrinol Metab 53:1105, 1981

NEER RM, POTTS JT JR: Medical management of hypercalcemia and hyperparathyroidism, in *Endocrinology*, LJ DeGroot et al (eds). New York, Grune & Stratton, 1979, vol 2

NEUFELD M et al: Two types of autoimmune Addison's disease associated with different polyglandular autoimmune (PGA) syndromes. Medicine 60:355, 1981

ORWOLL ES: The milk-alkali syndrome: Current concepts. Ann Intern Med 97:242, 1982

RAO DS et al: Dissociation between effects of endogenous parathyroid hormone on adenosine 3′5′-monophosphate generation and phosphate reabsorption in hypocalcemia due to vitamin D depletion: An acquired disorder resembling pseudohypoparathyroidism type II. J Clin Endocrinol Metab 61:285, 1985

RUDE RK et al: Parathyroid hormone secretion in magnesium deficiency. J Clin Endcrinol Metab 47:800, 1978

SILVE C et al: Selective resistance to parathyroid hormone in cultured skin fibroblasts from patients with pseudohypoparathyroidism type Ib. J Clin Endocrinol Metab 62:640, 1986

ZALOGA GP, GHERNOW B: Stress-induced changes in calcium metabolism. Semin Respir Med 7:52, 1985

337 METABOLIC BONE DISEASE

STEPHEN M. KRANE / MICHAEL F. HOLICK

OSTEOPOROSIS

GENERAL CONSIDERATIONS *Osteoporosis* is the term used for diseases of diverse etiology that are characterized by a reduction in the mass of bone per unit volume to a level below that required for adequate mechanical support function. The reduction in mass is not accompanied by a significant reduction in the ratio of the mineral to the organic phase, nor by any known abnormality in the structure of the mineral or the organic matrix. Histologically, osteoporosis is characterized by a decrease in cortical thickness and in the number and size of the trabeculae of cancellous bone with normal width of the osteoid seams. Osteoporosis is the most common of the metabolic bone diseases (disorders in which all the skeleton is involved, presumably as a result of systemic factors acting on the skeleton) and is an important cause of morbidity in the elderly.

The remodeling of bone (its formation and resorption) is a continuous process. Any combination of changes in the rates of formation and resorption which results in bone resorption exceeding bone formation can cause a decrease in bone mass. In osteoporosis the bone mass *is* decreased, indicating that the rate of bone resorption must exceed that of bone formation. Osteoporosis is a heterogeneous disorder. In most series rates of bone formation are normal or low, although rates may be high in some patients, consistent with an absolute increase in bone resorption (high-turnover osteoporosis). For many years after closure of the epiphyses and after longitudinal growth has ceased, in normal individuals skeletal mass remains constant, and the rates of bone formation and resorption are relatively low and approximately equal. Resorption and formation of bone are normally tightly coupled. However, the rate of remodeling is not uniform throughout the skeleton after epiphyseal closure. Most of the bone surfaces are "inactive" and not involved at any given time either in formation or resorption. Active surfaces may be randomly distributed, but formation and resorption are locally coupled as units. Resorption areas are covered by osteoclasts if active; bone formation surfaces are characterized by the presence of osteoid seams and are covered by active osteoblasts. Resorption precedes formation and is probably more intense, but it does not last as long as formation. As a consequence, there are normally more sites of active formation than of resorption. Bone turnover is high when there are many units active and low when there are few. Unless formation compensates for resorption, bone mass decreases. After the age of 40 to 50 skeletal mass begins to decline, at a faster rate in women than in men, and at different rates in different parts of the skeleton. The loss has been documented in selected regions using techniques such as single- and dual-photon absorptiometry of the wrist, femoral neck, and spine, quantitative computerized tomography of the vertebral bodies of the lumbar spine, and neutron activation analysis. For example, the rate of loss is greater in the metacarpals, in the femoral neck, and in the vertebral bodies than in the midshaft of the femur, the tibia, and the skull. Over the succeeding three or four decades the total loss in skeletal mass may be 30 to 50 percent of that present at age 30 or 40. Kinetic studies (using radioactive isotopes of calcium and strontium) and quantitative microradiography (which includes both cortical and cancellous bone) indicate that in most older subjects the resorption rate is high, whereas the bone formation rate remains at a level similar to that of younger adults.

The fact that bone resorption is low in some osteoporotic subjects, especially in cancellous bone, is further evidence for the heterogeneity of the disorder and indicates that no single etiologic factor accounts for all cases. At some critical point if the difference between rates of formation and resorption is maintained, loss of bone substance may become so marked that the bone can no longer resist the normal mechanical forces to which it is subjected, and fracture results. Osteoporosis is then evident as a clinical problem. The level of reduction in bone mass sufficient to result in fractures after minimal trauma is variable. The strength of bones such as the vertebrae may depend upon additional factors such as adequacy of ligamentous support and the age-related changes in the intervertebral disks. The normal trabecular architecture is also disturbed. For example, the horizontal trabeculae of the vertebral bodies are preferentially lost in osteoporosis. Microfractures are also frequent.

In the process of remodeling of lamellar bone in adults, most of the net resorption occurs at the corticoendosteal surface. The abnormal remodeling in osteoporosis follows the same pattern; the bone loss includes cancellous bone, cortical bone at the endosteal surface, and intracortical bone, resulting in enlargement of the medullary cavity and thinning of the cortex. Since bone formation at the periosteum continues at a very slow rate, the diameter of the bone does not decrease, and the periosteal surface retains its smooth configuration. In addition, the cancellous bone also undergoes progressive resorption, with some trabeculae being resorbed at rates faster than others, particularly those vertebral trabeculae with horizontal orientation.

Although the loss of bone that accompanies advancing age is universal, it begins earlier and proceeds more rapidly in women than in men, and there is a trend toward acceleration of bone loss in the perimenopausal years in women. All of the reasons for this age-associated bone loss are not known, although several risk factors have been identified in those individuals whose bone loss is sufficient to predispose to fracture with minimal trauma. In general, white women have a greater risk than black women, and white men have a greater risk than black men. One explanation for these population differences is that the bone mass at skeletal maturity is one determinant of the bone mass at subsequent ages. Blacks tend to have a higher bone mass at maturity than whites. Osteoporotic subjects are frequently less muscular and have lower average body weight than their nonosteoporotic controls. Exercise may have a beneficial effect in maintaining bone mass. The facts that accelerated bone loss accompanies the menopause in some women and that premature osteoporosis occurs when bilateral oophorectomy is performed prior to the age of normal menopause suggest that estrogens play a major role in preventing bone loss. Furthermore, osteoporotic women as a group may have an earlier menopause than age-matched nonosteoporotic women. Osteoporotic women also have a higher incidence of smoking; cigarette smoking might directly affect bone remodeling or have secondary effects on ovarian function. Dietary calcium intake and the efficiency of intestinal calcium absorption may also influence bone mass. Inability to synthesize normal amounts of 1α,25-dihydroxyvitamin D [1,25$(OH)_2$D] may play a role in the decreased calcium absorption, possibly because of decreased parathyroid hormone levels or impaired activity of the renal 25(OH)D 1α-hydroxylase.

A contributing role of the cytokines that alter either bone resorption or bone formation in the genesis of osteoporosis has yet to be established. Although osteoporosis is associated with Cushing's syndrome, there is no established role of adrenal steroids in the pathogenesis of the osteoporosis associated with the menopause or advancing age.

Another factor implicated in bone loss is the possibility that excessive acid intake, particularly in the form of high-protein diets, results in "dissolution" of bone in an attempt to buffer the extra acid. Prolonged use of heparin as an anticoagulant is also associated with osteoporosis, and heparin potentiates bone resorption in vitro. Patients with osteoporosis have increased numbers of mast cells, presumably capable of producing heparin, in their bone marrow. Circumscribed and diffuse areas of osteoporosis occur in patients with systemic mastocytosis.

As mentioned earlier, the remodeling of bone is responsive to mechanical forces of many types. The early response to immobilization in the normal skeleton is an increase in bone resorption while bone formation remains normal or is decreased; later there is a compensatory increase in bone formation. In osteoporosis, immobilization tends to aggravate the defect by increasing the gap between formation and resorption. It is, therefore, possible that a sedentary life in an individual with poor musculature reduces mechanical forces exerted on the skeleton and increases the tendency to bone loss.

TABLE 337-1 Classification of osteoporosis

I Common forms of osteoporosis of unknown cause unassociated with other disease
A Idiopathic osteoporosis (juvenile and adult)
B Type I osteoporosis
C Type II osteoporosis
II Disorders or conditions in which osteoporosis is a common feature or pathogenesis partially understood
A Hypogonadism
B Hyperadrenocorticism
C Thyrotoxicosis
D Malabsorption
E Scurvy
F Calcium deficiency
G Immobilization
H Chronic heparin administration
I Systemic mastocytosis
J Adult hypophosphatasia
K Associated with other metabolic bone diseases
III Osteoporosis as a feature of heritable disorders of connective tissue
A Osteogenesis imperfecta
B Homocystinuria due to cystathionine synthase deficiency
C Ehlers-Danlos syndrome
D Marfan's syndrome
IV Disorders in which osteoporosis is associated but pathogenesis not understood
A Rheumatoid arthritis
B Malnutrition
C Alcoholism
D Epilepsy
E Diabetes
F Chronic obstructive pulmonary disease
G Menkes' syndrome

CLASSIFICATION (See Table 337-1) In some instances osteoporosis is a well-defined feature of another disease such as Cushing's syndrome. A skeletal disorder that could also be considered osteoporosis (decreased bone mass with normal mineralization) is the major characteristic of certain heritable diseases of connective tissue such as forms of osteogenesis imperfecta (see Chap. 319). In most instances of osteoporosis, however, no other disease is apparent. This category of osteoporosis can be conveniently considered to comprise several forms. One form occurs in children or young adults of both sexes and with normal gonadal function. This form is frequently termed *idiopathic osteoporosis,* although most of the other forms are in fact also of unknown pathogenesis. So-called *type I osteoporosis* is found in a relatively small subset of postmenopausal women who are between 51 and 65 years of age and is characterized by an accelerated and disproportionate loss of trabecular bone as contrasted with cortical bone. In these individuals fractures of vertebral bodies and the distal forearm are the most common complications. Decreased parathyroid gland function in this group of individuals may be compensatory to increased bone resorption. So-called *type II osteoporosis* is found in a large proportion of women and men over the age of 75. Fractures of the femoral neck, proximal humerus, proximal tibia, and pelvis are most common in this group. These skeletal sites contain both cortical (compact) and trabecular bone. In these individuals circulating levels of parathyroid hormone tend to be higher than normal. Although both groups may have decreased mean circulating levels of 1,25$(OH)_2$D compared to age-matched controls, levels are often in the normal range.

GENERAL CLINICAL FEATURES Although osteoporosis is a generalized disorder of the skeleton, its major clinical manifestations result from fractures of the vertebrae, wrist, hip, humerus, and tibia, depending upon the pattern of the disease (type I or II osteoporosis) as described above. The most frequent symptoms that result from vertebral body fractures are pain in the back and deformity of the spine. Pain usually results from collapse of the vertebrae especially in the lower dorsal and upper lumbar regions, is typically acute in onset, and often radiates anteriorly around the flank into the abdomen. Such episodes frequently occur after sudden bending, lifting, or jumping movements which may seem to have been trivial; on some occasions they cannot be related to trauma. The pain may be increased even with slight movements such as turning in bed or by the Valsalva maneuver. Rest in bed in one position may relieve the pain temporarily, but it then may recur in spasms of variable duration. Radiation of pain down one leg is uncommon, and symptoms or signs of spinal cord compression are rare. The acute episodes of pain may also be accompanied by abdominal distention and ileus, thought to be due to retroperitoneal hemorrhage, but the use of narcotics at this stage also contributes to the ileus. Loss of appetite and apparent muscular weakness, which is probably due to fear of reproducing pain, may also be present. Episodes of pain usually subside after several days to a week, and by 4 to 6 weeks patients may be fully ambulatory and able to resume their normal activities. Although the acute pain may be minimal, many patients continue to have nagging, deep, dull, uncomfortable sensations localized to the area of fracture and brought about by straining or sudden changes in position. They may be unable to sit up in bed and have to arise by rolling over on their sides and then propping themselves up. Most patients have disappearance or marked diminution of pain between episodes of vertebral body collapse. Others never have acute episodes but complain of backache often made worse by standing or moving suddenly. Tenderness over involved areas of the spinous processes or rib cage is common. The collapse fractures of the vertebral bodies are usually anterior, producing a wedge-shaped deformity and contributing to loss in height. This is particularly common in the middorsal region where collapse may be unassociated with pain but result in a dorsal kyphosis and exaggerated cervical lordosis described as a "dowager's" or "widow's" hump. Postural slumping with increase in existing curves also contributes to the loss of height. Scoliosis is also common in women with osteoporosis. Generalized skeletal pain is uncommon, and between fractures most patients are free of pain. Although recurrent episodes of collapse fractures of vertebral bodies, increasing spine deformity, and loss of height are common in osteoporosis, the course of the disorder in any one subject is not predictable, and there may be intervals of several years between fractures.

RADIOLOGIC FEATURES Prior to fracture and collapse the osteoporotic vertebral body shows a decrease in mineral density, an increase in prominence of vertical striations due to a relatively greater loss of the horizontally oriented trabeculae, and prominence of the end plates. The bodies may become increasingly biconcave because of weakening of the subchondral plates and expansion of the intervertebral disks, resulting in the so-called codfish vertebrae. When collapse occurs, most frequently in lower dorsal and upper lumbar spine, it usually produces a decrease in the anterior height of the vertebral body and irregularity in the anterior cortex (Fig. 337-1). Older compression fractures may show reactive changes and osteophytes about the anterior margins. Although the cortices of long bones may be thin because of excessive endosteal resorption, the outer margins are sharp in contrast to the typical effects of the subperiosteal resorption of hyperparathyroidism. Pseudofractures or Looser's zones are not present in osteoporosis in the absence of osteomalacia, but distinguishing osteoporosis from osteomalacia may be impossible on radiologic grounds alone. In the absence of fractures standard roentgenograms are insensitive indicators of bone loss since as much as 30 percent decrease in bone mass may not be appreciated. Other procedures are required to establish whether a given individual has a sufficient decrease in bone mass to be at risk for fracture. These include single- and dual-photon absorptiometry, quantitative computerized tomography, or neutron activation analysis of total-body calcium.

LABORATORY FINDINGS The concentrations of calcium and inorganic phosphorus in the blood are usually normal in patients with osteoporosis; slight hyperphosphatemia is present in women who are past the menopause. The alkaline phosphatase in uncomplicated instances is normal, although slight increases may be seen after fractures. About 20 percent of postmenopausal women with osteoporosis have significant hypercalciuria. Urinary excretion of peptides containing hydroxyproline, an index of bone resorption, is usually normal or slightly increased.

DIFFERENTIAL DIAGNOSIS Since decrease in skeletal mass is an age-associated finding, it is difficult to evaluate asymptomatic decreased bone density in older women, especially when unaccompanied by marked increase in biconcavity of vertebral bodies or fractures. In the presence of bone pain with or without fracture or deformity, it is important to establish the presence or absence of known causes of osteoporosis as listed in Table 337-1 and to be certain that osteoporosis in the broad sense is the correct diagnosis. Malignancies of various types, particularly *multiple myeloma, lymphoma, leukemia,* and *carcinomatosis,* may result in diffuse loss of bone, especially the trabecular bone of the vertebral column, even in the absence of hypercalcemia. The absence of anemia, elevated erythrocyte sedimentation rate, abnormal electrophoretic patterns of serum proteins, and Bence Jones proteinuria is helpful in eliminating the possibility of multiple myeloma. However, needle bone biopsy or marrow aspiration is frequently recommended in instances of severe osteoporosis with fractures. It is necessary to perform histomorphometry, usually on biopsies taken from the iliac crest, to quantitate bone mass and rule out osteomalacia, but the technique is not widely available.

Radiologic osteoporosis is common in patients with primary *hyperparathyroidism,* who may not have osteitis fibrosa (discrete lytic lesions of varying size and subperiosteal resorption) or elevation

FIGURE 337-1 *Lateral views of the lumbar spine of a 54-year-old man with idiopathic osteoporosis. A typical anterior compression fracture is indicated by the arrow.*

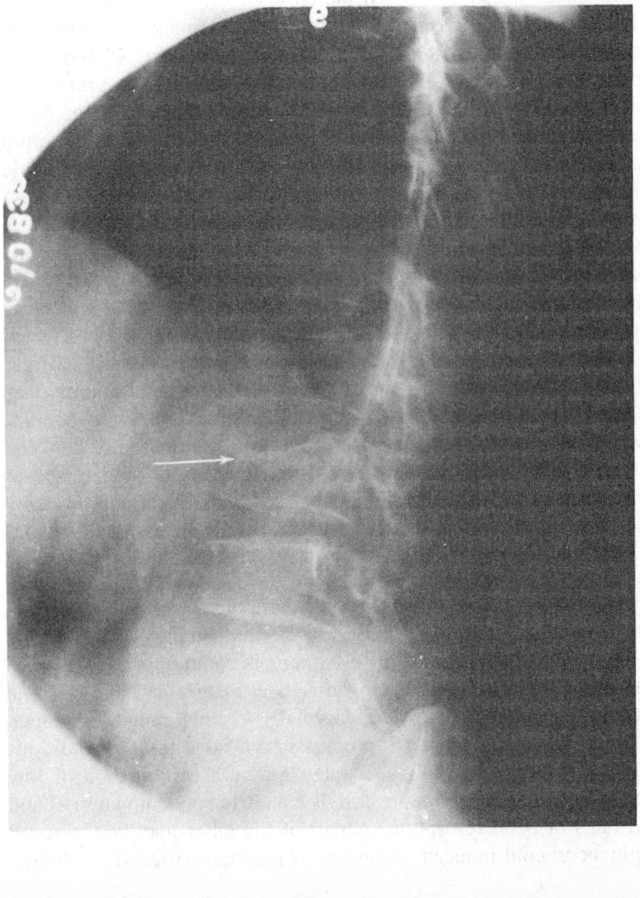

of serum alkaline phosphatase. Although hyperparathyroidism could accelerate osteoporosis and contribute to it, it is not clear that excessive secretion of parathyroid hormone is the sole cause of the bone disease, even in these cases, rather than an associated finding. Repeated determinations of fasting serum calcium and phosphorus levels are therefore necessary. An element of secondary hyperparathyroidism may be present in some elderly patients with type II osteoporosis and in others in whom there is impairment of renal function, inadequate oral calcium intake, or decrease of intestinal calcium absorption. Increased numbers of osteoclasts may be present in bone biopsy specimens from such patients.

Osteomalacia may mimic osteoporosis or coexist with it, yet specific radiologic signs of osteomalacia may not always be present. Although the presence of abnormalities such as low or undetectable circulating levels of 25-hydroxyvitamin D [25(OH)D] and/or hypophosphatemia would suggest the possibility of osteomalacia, these abnormalities too may be absent in some cases of osteomalacia, and bone biopsy may be essential for diagnosis, as discussed below. Since osteomalacia is more responsive to specific therapy than the usual case of osteoporosis, such diagnostic procedures are often warranted and provide, in addition, adequate specimens for examination for the presence of malignant cells.

In an occasional patient with *Paget's disease* the radiologic features may be almost purely lytic and be confused with osteoporosis. However, high alkaline phosphatase levels and moderately or markedly increased urinary excretion of hydroxyproline-containing peptides are clues to the presence of Paget's disease. Scanning procedures with bone-seeking isotopes are not helpful in differential diagnosis if fractures are present, because in any disease fractures demonstrate preferential uptake of isotope. However, in the absence of fracture, "hot spots" suggest presence of tumor or early Paget's disease, particularly if present in the appendicular skeleton.

IDIOPATHIC OSTEOPOROSIS *Idiopathic osteoporosis* is the term used to describe the disorder in younger men or in premenopausal women in whom no other etiologic factor is detected. It is likely that these patients have a number of different disorders with superficial resemblances. In some women the onset of the disease and deterioration of bone appear to be related to pregnancy and may represent a transient failure in homeostatic mechanisms such as failure to increase circulating levels of $1,25(OH)_2D$ and hence to protect the maternal skeleton from the stresses of childbirth (see Chap. 335). Some patients with idiopathic osteoporosis have low levels of serum alkaline phosphatase, though not low enough to fulfill diagnostic criteria for *hypophosphatasia*. Estrogens are ineffective in therapy. Losses of calcium and phosphorus are probably excessive, and it is unwise to permit women with osteoporosis to breast-feed their infants since additional calcium losses via lactation are appreciable. Some patients have a disorder similar to mild forms of osteogenesis imperfecta, although such features as family history, blue scleras, and deafness are lacking. The course is variable; although recurrent episodes of fractures are characteristic, progressive deterioration does not occur in all patients, and in some the clinical problem is benign. Juvenile osteoporosis is a rare disorder with onset usually between the ages of 8 and 14 years and is characterized by the abrupt appearance of bone pain and fractures after minimal trauma. In many cases the disorder is self-limited, and recovery takes place spontaneously within 4 or 5 years.

GLUCOCORTICOID EXCESS Glucocorticoid excess does not appear to be involved in osteoporosis of the idiopathic variety or in the type I or II disorder. However, osteoporosis commonly accompanies Cushing's syndrome, both endogenous and exogenous, and in some instances is rapidly progressive, especially in children and in women over the age of 50. The rapid progression of bone loss in conditions of glucocorticoid excess is accounted for by a combination of low rates of bone formation (depressed osteoblastic oppositional rate) and high rates of bone resorption. A part of the latter may be the result of glucocorticoid-induced secondary hyperparathyroidism, although increases in circulating immunoreactive parathyroid hormone have not been found regularly using a variety of radioimmunoassays. Glucocorticoids, however, potentiate the effects of parathyroid hormone and $1,25(OH)_2D$ on isolated populations of bone cells. Glucocorticoids depress collagen synthesis in organs other than bone, as evidenced by delayed wound healing, thinning of the dermis, striae, and tendency to blue scleras. In some disorders in which glucocorticoids are administered in pharmacologic doses such as rheumatoid arthritis, a tendency to thin skin and osteoporosis is initially present, and the skeletal effects of the glucocorticoids may become particularly apparent. Even low dosages of glucocorticoids may accelerate bone loss in postmenopausal women with rheumatoid arthritis. Glucocorticoid excess also results in alteration in the metabolism of vitamin D; blood levels of 25(OH)D are normal or only slightly decreased, and blood levels of $1,25(OH)_2D$ are low in some patients, particularly in children. Part of the defect in calcium absorption is explainable by a vitamin D–dependent mechanism, but glucocorticoids also inhibit intestinal calcium absorption by a direct, vitamin D–independent action on the intestine. Osteomalacia is not observed histologically, despite possible abnormalities in vitamin D metabolism. Once osteoporosis develops in adults with Cushing's syndrome, the abnormality may persist indefinitely following alleviation of the glucocorticoid excess. In children, however, cure of the Cushing's syndrome may result in striking improvement in the appearance of the spine due to new endochondral bone formation around the less dense, older osteoporotic bone. This does not occur in adults since endochondral bone formation has ceased. Withdrawal of glucocorticoids or decrease of the dose by alternate-day schedule may be the only way to halt progression of the osteoporosis. Anabolic steroids are not effective in this regard. The defect in intestinal calcium absorption may be helped by administering vitamin D in doses of 50,000 IU two times weekly plus supplemental oral calcium of 1 to 1.5 g per day. The use of vitamin D metabolites such as 25(OH)D may be more effective. When large doses of vitamin D are used, it is important to monitor serum and urinary calcium and serum 25(OH)D levels at intervals of 2 to 4 months, especially if glucocorticoid dosages are lowered. In Cushing's syndrome, spontaneous, symptomless fractures may occur in bones such as ribs and pubic and ischial rami even in the absence of marked osteoporosis of the spine. These fractures often heal partially with an exuberant calcified callus surrounding a radiolucent zone of nonunion, which superficially resembles the pseudofractures of osteomalacia. If they appear in the thorax superimposed upon the lungs, they may be confused with nodules suggesting primary or metastatic tumor.

GONADAL DEFICIENCY Estrogen lack is present in the postmenopausal woman with osteoporosis, and the administration of estrogen to such an individual reduces the negative calcium balance and decreases urinary hydroxyproline excretion as is consistent with a decrease in bone resorption. Estrogens are particularly useful in retarding the bone loss in women who have oophorectomy at an early age. Bone mass is also decreased in women athletes who are amenorrheic, such as marathon runners. Such women are particularly prone to tibial stress fractures. In patients of either sex castrated at an early age, the adult skeleton is smaller to begin with, and therefore age-related losses are more significant.

THYROTOXICOSIS In many patients with hyperthyroidism, there is excessive bone resorption, occasionally marked in degree and far exceeding that in the usual patient with osteoporosis, associated with increased excretion of calcium and phosphorus in urine and feces. The excessive bone resorption is usually accompanied by a compensatory increase in bone formation. Parathyroid hormone secretion is decreased, and levels of $1,25(OH)_2D$ are normal or low. If the hyperthyroidism is of short duration, skeletal losses are inconsequential. However, in patients with chronic hyperthyroidism, especially in women after the menopause, this accelerated bone loss becomes clinically significant, and it is important to eliminate hyperthyroidism as a contributing cause of osteoporosis. Although typical osteitis fibrosa (resorption lacunae containing osteoclasts and a fibrous stroma) may be seen on biopsy, even in these cases the skeletal lesions have the appearance of osteoporosis when examined radiologically.

ACROMEGALY Hypercalciuria and overall net negative calcium balance occur in acromegaly, and occasionally osteoporosis is an associated finding. The panhypopituitarism secondary to a pituitary adenoma and the associated gonadal insufficiency may be factors in production of the osteoporosis. In adult animals growth hormone decreases endosteal resorption and stimulates bone formation, and it is therefore unlikely that excessive secretion of growth hormone in itself produces osteoporosis.

DIABETES MELLITUS Individuals with juvenile or adult-onset diabetes mellitus have a decreased bone mass. In some series the incidence of hip fractures has been increased, but studies of large groups of diabetic subjects have not revealed abnormal calcium metabolism or bone disease specifically attributable to the diabetes.

CALCIUM DEFICIENCY AND MALABSORPTION Although calcium deficiency may be a factor in some instances of osteoporosis, it cannot be the sole or major cause in idiopathic, senile, or postmenopausal osteoporosis. Osteoporosis is an associated finding in a significant number of cases of steatorrhea, prolonged obstructive jaundice, and lactose intolerance and in patients following gastrectomy. Other patients may have a specific defect in calcium absorption or a failure to adapt adequately to a low-calcium diet either by increasing the percentage of dietary calcium absorbed or by decreasing urinary calcium excretion. Presumably, vitamin D is adequate in these instances to prevent osteomalacia.

HERITABLE DISORDERS OF CONNECTIVE TISSUE In the strict sense, the bone disease of osteogenesis imperfecta is osteoporosis (see Chap. 319). *Osteogenesis imperfecta* is a heterogeneous disorder. The most common form is transmitted as an autosomal dominant trait and is associated with blue scleras and later with deafness. The bone disease in this form tends to be relatively mild, and the tendency toward fractures may decrease after puberty. Another form, which itself is likely autosomal recessive, is usually detected shortly after birth and is progressive with recurrent fractures of long bones and kyphoscoliosis. Sclerae are white, and deafness is uncommon. A lethal perinatal type (autosomal recessive) is also seen. The organization of the collagen in bone and skin is abnormal, and in some instances defects in the synthesis of type I collagen in bone and skin have been defined. It is possible that some cases of idiopathic osteoporosis represent unrecognized osteogenesis imperfecta. Osteoporosis also occurs in patients with *homocystinuria* due to cystathionine synthase deficiency, an autosomal recessive trait, associated with ectopia lentis, various deformities of the extremities, mental retardation, decreased pigmentation of hair and skin, and thromboembolism. The diagnosis is established by the finding of homocystine in urine. The osteoporosis may be due to the effect of homocysteine or other metabolites in interfering with the cross-linking of collagen.

THERAPY Before considering treatment of osteoporosis, it should be emphasized that one is dealing with a group of disorders rather than a single entity. Even in patients within the same category, e.g., those with idiopathic osteoporosis, the etiologies may be different. It is also difficult to predict the course of the disease in any patient, especially when seen initially because of pain and collapse-fracture. Many patients in the idiopathic, postmenopausal (type I), and senile (type II) groups have a few episodes of vertebral body collapse with symptom-free intervals of months or years but then go for many years without symptoms or further loss in height. Furthermore, the acute pain associated with vertebral body fracture tends to subside in a matter of weeks, and *any* treatment administered at that time might be considered efficacious. Therapy for this condition is far from ideal, despite claims to the contrary.

General measures Patients with acute pain secondary to fracture of vertebral bodies frequently require hospitalization with rest in bed in a position of maximum comfort, local heat, adequate analgesics, and avoidance of constipation. Use of traction or plaster jacket splints is not indicated. As soon as pain permits, the patient should attempt to move out of bed, slowly at first, perhaps with support of a walker or crutches. The patient should not become too fatigued when starting ambulation. Braces of various types are commonly employed, but their efficacy in preventing progression of spinal deformity has not been established. A well-made corset may provide support and comfort. Exercises to correct postural deformity and increase muscle tone are useful. Patients should be taught to avoid sudden painful movements such as jumping and how to lift and carry objects with minimal back strain. After the fractures have healed, a supervised exercise program which includes daily walking may be helpful in preventing further skeletal losses.

Estrogens and androgens The use of estrogens in postmenopausal women with osteoporosis causes a decrease in urinary calcium and hydroxyproline excretion, especially during the first few months of treatment (see Chap. 331). Estrogens decrease the rate of bone resorption, but bone formation does not increase and eventually usually decreases. Although still within the normal range, the mean level of circulating $1,25(OH)_2D$ is lower in osteoporotic subjects than in controls and is brought to the normal mean level by estrogen therapy. Thus, estrogens produce significant, although modest, calcium retention, decrease the difference between formation and resorption, and therefore tend to retard the progress of osteoporosis, but they are not capable of restoring skeletal mass. The magnitude of calcium retention also tends to decrease with continuous therapy. Therefore, it is not surprising that there is no change in radiologic features of the osteoporosis with such therapy. The major role of estrogens is in preventing osteoporosis in menopausal women rather than treating clinical disease already developed, although they may also be effective in the woman with mild or moderate disease within the first 5 to 6 years following cessation of ovarian function. Testosterone preparations are useful in treatment of osteoporotic men with gonadal deficiency, but there are no convincing reports of their efficacy in men with normal gonadal function. There is also no proven advantage to combinations of estrogens and androgens.

Calcium preparations Use of oral calcium preparations in doses of 1.0 to 1.5 g elemental calcium per day increases calcium retention in some osteoporotic subjects and decreases bone resorption. The elemental calcium content of available preparations varies, depending upon the accompanying anion and the composition (Table 337-2). However, as with the use of estrogens, this eventually results in decrease in bone formation and tends to arrest rather than ''cure'' the osteoporosis. Calcium preparations may be of greater use in patients with normal gonadal function and relatively mild disease. In patients with malabsorption, calcium may be effective in addition to vitamin D given orally in doses of 50,000 IU once weekly. The use of more active metabolites of vitamin D may prove more efficacious. Therapy with $1,25(OH)_2D$ (calcitriol), 0.25 μg daily, results in improved intestinal calcium absorption and suppression of bone resorption. Levels of serum calcium, 25(OH)D, $1,25(OH)_2D$, and urinary calcium excretion should be monitored at intervals of several months to be certain that hypercalcemia and hypercalciuria do not result. Thiazide diuretics are useful in patients with high-turnover

TABLE 337-2 Elemental calcium content in various oral calcium preparations

Calcium preparation	Elemental calcium content per unit weight or volume
Calcium citrate	40 mg/300 mg
Calcium carbonate	400 mg/g
Calcium lactate	80 mg/600 mg
Calcium gluconate	40 mg/500 mg
Calcium carbonate + 5 μg vitamin D_2 (Os−Cal 250)	250 mg/tablet

osteoporosis associated with hypercalciuria and secondary hyperparathyroidism. In the absence of secondary hyperparathyroidism the thiazide diuretics lower urinary calcium excretion, suppress parathyroid gland function, inhibit synthesis of 1,25$(OH)_2D$, and reduce intestinal calcium absorption.

Fluoride Fluoride ions are deposited in the skeleton where they become incorporated into the crystal lattice of hydroxyapatite, substituting for hydroxyl ions. This process results in a mineral phase of greater crystallinity. Fluoride ions in chronic high doses also increase new bone formation and produce a form of hyperostosis with dense bones, exostoses, neurologic complications due to bony overgrowth, and ligamentous calcification. Experimental treatment with fluoride has not resulted in uniformly satisfactory results, possibly because of variations in dosage of fluoride ion, retention of absorbed ion, and calcium intake while on fluoride. The stimulation of new bone formation, a desirable effect not seen with the other agents mentioned previously, unfortunately causes the production of bone that is poorly mineralized and also, presumably, structurally unsound. If the dose of fluoride ion is moderate (25 mg per day) and calcium supplements are given in doses of at least 1 g daily plus vitamin D, 50,000 IU twice weekly, considerable new bone may be produced associated with decreased incidence of fractures, particularly if combined with estrogen therapy. Significant toxicity is absent, although weight-bearing pain, especially in ankles and knees, may occur and disappears when fluoride is discontinued. It is likely that the use of fluoride to treat osteoporosis will soon be approved.

Other measures Although calcitonin therapy has been advocated, this therapy probably does not produce benefits greater than attained with supplemental calcium and vitamin D. Oral phosphates (greater than 1 g elemental phosphorus per day in divided doses) may decrease urinary calcium excretion and improve calcium tolerance in patients with marked hypercalciuria. However, phosphate is of no value in patients with postmenopausal osteoporosis who have normal levels of serum phosphorus.

RICKETS AND OSTEOMALACIA

The terms *rickets* and *osteomalacia* describe disorders in which mineralization of the organic matrix of the skeleton is defective (Table 337-3). In *rickets* the growing skeleton is involved; defective mineralization occurs not only in bone but also in the cartilaginous matrix of the growth plate. The term *osteomalacia* is usually reserved for the disorder of mineralization of the adult skeleton in which the epiphyseal growth plates are closed. A number of conditions result in rickets and/or osteomalacia such as inadequate dietary intake of vitamin D, inadequate exposure to ultraviolet radiation to form endogenous vitamin D, intestinal malabsorption of vitamin D, acquired and inherited disorders of vitamin D metabolism, inherited defects in the receptors for 1,25$(OH)_2D$ in target tissues, chronic acidosis, renal tubular defects which produce hypophosphatemia or acidosis, and chronic administration of anticonvulsants. In the renal tubular disorders rickets and osteomalacia develop in the presence of normal intestinal function and are not cured by treatment with doses of vitamin D adequate to cure deficiency rickets. Thus the term *vitamin D–resistant* (or *–refractory*) *rickets* has been applied in these instances. Renal insufficiency, especially in children, is also associated with rickets or osteomalacia.

PATHOGENESIS AND HISTOPATHOLOGY For mineralization of skeletal tissues, sufficient calcium and phosphate must be present at the mineralization sites. Other conditions required for normal mineralization include intact metabolic and transport functions of osteoblasts and chondrocytes, adequate collagen matrix, possibly phosphorylation or other modifications of matrix components, and low concentrations of inhibitory substances such as proteoglycan aggregates or inorganic pyrophosphate. A specific function in the mineralization process for the γ-carboxyglutamic acid–containing proteins synthesized by bone cells has not been demonstrated, although they bind calcium ions. In cartilage the initial mineral phase is in membrane-bound extracellular vesicles. If the osteoblast continues to produce matrix components which cannot be adequately mineralized, rickets and osteomalacia result. If calcification continues to be inadequate, the production of organic matrix (osteoid) also gradually decreases. In bone there will be an increase in the fraction of the forming surface covered by incompletely mineralized osteoid, an increase in osteoid volume and thickness (the latter normally less than 12 to 14 μm), and a decrease in the calcification or mineralization front. The latter is detected in undemineralized sections by the fluorescence of previously ingested tetracycline or by special stains. There is a marked

TABLE 337-3 Classification of rickets and osteomalacia

- *I* Vitamin D deficiency
  - *A* Dietary deficiency
  - *B* Deficient endogenous synthesis
- *II* Gastrointestinal
  - *A* Small-intestinal diseases with malabsorption
  - *B* Partial or total gastrectomy
  - *C* Hepatobiliary disease
  - *D* Chronic pancreatic insufficiency
- *III* Disorders of vitamin D metabolism
  - *A* Hereditary: pseudovitamin D deficiency or vitamin D dependency, types I and II
  - *B* Acquired
    - *1* Anticonvulsants
    - *2* Chronic renal failure
- *IV* Acidosis
  - *A* Distal renal tubular acidosis (classic or type I)
  - *B* Secondary forms of renal acidosis
  - *C* Ureterosigmoidostomy
  - *D* Drug-induced disease
    - *1* Chronic acetazolamide ingestion
    - *2* Chronic ammonium chloride ingestion
- *V* Chronic renal failure
- *VI* Phosphate depletion
  - *A* Dietary: low phosphate intake plus ingestion of nonabsorbable antacids
  - *B* Impaired renal tubular phosphate reabsorption
    - *1* Hereditary
      - *a* X-linked hypophosphatemic rickets (vitamin D–resistant rickets)
      - *b* Adult-onset vitamin D–resistant hypophosphatemic osteomalacia
    - *2* Acquired
      - *a* Sporadic hypophosphatemic osteomalacia (phosphate diabetes)
      - *b* Tumor-associated (oncogenous) rickets and osteomalacia
      - *c* Neurofibromatosis
      - *d* Fibrous dysplasia
- *VII* Generalized renal tubular disorders (Fanconi's syndrome)
  - *A* Primary renal
  - *B* Associated with systemic metabolic abnormality
    - *1* Cystinosis
    - *2* Glycogenosis
    - *3* Lowe's syndrome
  - *C* Systemic disorder with associated renal disease
    - *1* Hereditary
      - *a* Inborn errors
        - (*1*) Wilson's disease
        - (*2*) Tyrosinemia
      - *b* Neurofibromatosis
    - *2* Acquired
      - *a* Multiple myeloma
      - *b* Nephrotic syndrome
      - *c* Transplanted kidney
    - *3* Intoxications
      - *a* Cadmium
      - *b* Lead
      - *c* Outdated tetracycline
- *VIII* Primary mineralization defects
  - *A* Hereditary: hypophosphatasia
  - *B* Acquired
    - *1* Diphosphonate (disodium etidronate) treatment
    - *2* Fluoride treatment
- *IX* States of rapid bone formation with or without a relative defect in bone resorption
  - *A* Postoperative hyperparathyroidism with osteitis fibrosa cystica
  - *B* Osteopetrosis
- *X* Defective matrix synthesis: fibrogenesis imperfecta ossium
- *XI* Miscellaneous
  - *A* Magnesium-dependent conditions
  - *B* Axial osteomalacia
  - *C* Parenteral alimentation
  - *D* Aluminum intoxication

decrease in the rate of apposition of mineralized bone. A variety of methods are available to measure the thickness of the osteoid seams and the calcification front. In routine histologic sections stained with hematoxylin and eosin, the more heavily mineralized areas tend to appear violet or blue, whereas the osteoid seams appear pink. Subtle degrees of osteomalacia may not be appreciated with routine preparations, and undecalcified, thin sections (3 to 5 μm) stained, for example, with Goldner's trichrome method are necessary to establish its presence (Fig. 337-2). Rickets is also characterized by inadequate mineralization of the matrix of cartilage in the growing epiphyseal plate. Calcification in the interstitial regions of the hypertrophic zone is defective, the growth plate increases in thickness, the columns of cartilage cells (usually highly ordered) are disorganized, and there is a variable cupping of the epiphyses. The rachitic bones are often incapable of withstanding usual mechanical stresses and tend to undergo bowing deformities. If rickets is untreated, growth at the epiphyseal plates is slowed, and the eventual length of the long bones is diminished.

It has not been established whether vitamin D, through one of its metabolites, has a major direct effect on mineralization. Its primary roles after metabolic conversion to 25(OH)D and $1,25(OH)_2D$ are to regulate and enhance absorption of calcium ions from the intestinal lumen and, possibly, to enhance differentiation of stem cells to form osteoclasts. Insufficiency of the active metabolites of vitamin D leads to decreased intestinal absorption of calcium and decreased mobilization of calcium from bone, resulting in hypocalcemia. This stimulates increased synthesis and secretion of parathyroid hormone (PTH) and hyperplasia of the parathyroid glands. The increased circulating concentration of PTH tends to raise plasma calcium concentrations but also stimulates increased renal phosphate clearance, which, in turn, produces hypophosphatemia. When the concentration of phosphorus in the extracellular fluid falls below a critical level, mineralization cannot proceed normally. In severe vitamin D lack, normal levels of serum calcium cannot be maintained, and the driving force for mineralization is further decreased. The absence of some critical metabolite of vitamin D that acts directly on the skeleton may also play a role in the defective mineralization of rickets and osteomalacia.

Phosphate depletion alone can produce osteomalacia as in patients consuming large amounts of nonabsorbable antacids and in patients with excessive renal loss of phosphate due to decreased tubular reabsorption. Secondary hyperparathyroidism is usually not present in these patients. Hypophosphatemia per se produces mineralization defects despite its effect on increasing the activity of the renal 25(OH)D-1α-hydroxylase, but it cannot account for the osteomalacia in all the disorders listed in Table 337-3. In chronic renal failure, for example, plasma phosphate levels are not decreased and usually are increased. Similarly, plasma phosphorus levels are not depressed in infants and children with osteomalacia secondary to hypophosphatasia, a hereditary deficiency in alkaline phosphatase. Osteomalacia in some patients with chronic renal failure is associated with accumulation of aluminum in bone, and the aluminum probably plays a role in production of the mineralization defect.

FIGURE 337-2 *Photomicrograph of an undemineralized section stained with Goldner method of an iliac crest bone biopsy from a 45-year-old man with chronic renal failure maintained on hemodialysis. Almost the entire surface is covered by osteoid (O) readily distinguished from mineralized bone (MB). The thickness of the osteoid seams exceeds 100 μm in several areas.*

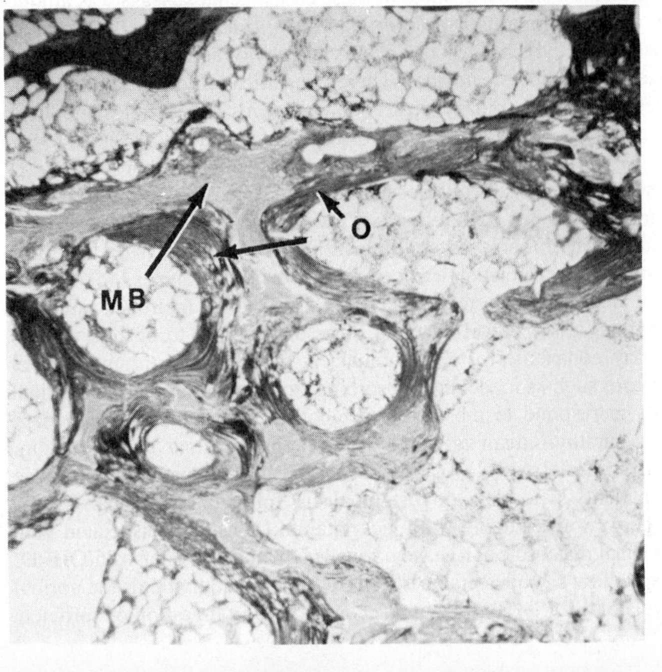

CLINICAL FINDINGS The clinical manifestations of rickets are the result of skeletal deformities, susceptibility to fractures, weakness and hypotonia, and disturbances in growth. In extreme instances of vitamin D–deficiency rickets, hypocalcemia may be sufficient to produce tetany which, when severe, may be accompanied by laryngeal spasm and convulsive seizures.

In infants and young children features include listlessness, irritability, and often profound hypotonia and muscular weakness. As the disorder progresses, children become unable to walk without support. Abnormal parietal flattening and frontal bossing develop in the skull. The calvaria are softened (craniotabes), and widening of sutures may be evident. Prominence of the costochondral junctions is called the "rachitic rosary," and the indentation of the lower ribs at the site of attachment of the diaphragm is known as *Harrison's groove*. If untreated, progressive deformities of the pelvis and extremities result, with bowing particularly common in the tibia, femur, radius, and ulna. Fractures are frequent, dental eruption is often delayed, and enamel defects are common.

The presentation of osteomalacia in adults usually is not as dramatic as in infants and children. The skeletal deformities may be overlooked, and the features of the underlying disorder may dominate, as, for example, in the vitamin D loss associated with adult celiac disease. Symptoms, when they occur, include diffuse skeletal pain and bony tenderness. Pain may be especially prominent about the hips and result in an antalgic gait. Muscular weakness is also common, although it may be difficult to distinguish from hesitancy to move because of skeletal pain. Proximal weakness may mimic that of primary muscle disorders and contribute to the waddling gait. Pain and weakness may be sufficient to cause patients to be confined to bed and chair. Many factors, including the secondary hyperparathyroidism, contribute to the myopathy. Clinical improvement in the myopathy usually results from specific therapy such as vitamin D repletion in nutritional osteomalacia, phosphate replacement in renal hypophosphatemia, or correction of acidosis. Fractures of involved bones may occur with minimal trauma. When the ribs are involved, severe deformities may develop in the thoracic cage, and the collapse of vertebral bodies may produce loss of height.

RADIOLOGIC FEATURES Radiologic changes in the skeleton in rickets and osteomalacia reflect the pathologic changes. In rickets the alterations are most evident at the epiphyseal growth plate which is increased in thickness, cupped, and hazy at the metaphyseal border due to decreased calcification of the hypertrophic zone and inadequate mineralization of the primary spongiosa. The trabecular pattern of the metaphyses is abnormal, the cortices of the diaphyses may be thinned, and the shafts may be bowed.

In osteomalacia decrease in bone density is usually associated with loss of trabeculae and variable thinning of the cortices. The radiologic changes may be indistinguishable from those in osteoporosis. Trabecular patterns may be blurred, producing a homogeneous ground glass appearance. The specific finding that suggests osteomalacia is the presence of radiolucent bands ranging from a few millimeters to several centimeters in length, usually perpendicular to the surface of the bones. They are particularly common at the inner aspects of the femur, especially near the femoral neck, in the pelvis, in the outer edge of the scapula, in the upper fibula, and in the metatarsals (Figs. 337-3 and 337-4). These radiolucent bands, called *pseudofractures* or *Looser's zones,* occur most often at sites where major arteries cross the bones, and are thought to be due to the mechanical stress of the pulsation of these vessels. Subperiosteal erosions along the diaphyseal cortices are sometimes seen in patients with secondary hyperparathyroidism.

Increased rather than decreased density of bones may be observed in patients with renal tubular disorders rather than with vitamin D deficiency and may produce a striking thickening of the cortices and trabeculae of spongy bone. Despite the increase in mass of bone per unit volume, the trabeculae are covered with thickened osteoid seams typical of osteomalacia. Similar findings may occur in patients with chronic renal failure. The reason for the hyperostosis is unknown; the bone is architecturally abnormal and subject to fracture with minimal trauma.

LABORATORY FINDINGS Changes in serum concentrations of calcium, inorganic phosphorus, 25(OH)D, and $1,25(OH)_2D$ vary with the different disorders (see Chap. 325). In vitamin D deficiency, whether due to dietary lack, inadequate sunlight exposure, or intestinal malabsorption, serum calcium levels are normal or low, whereas phosphorus and 25(OH)D levels are characteristically low, the latter usually < 5 ng/mL depending upon the assay. In contrast, levels of $1,25(OH)_2D$ may not be low due to secondary hyperparathyroidism (Table 327-2). In adults the lower limit of serum phosphorus concentration is around 2.8 mg/dL; in children the lower limit of normal is closer to 4.0 to 4.5 mg/dL. In *severe* vitamin D depletion, hypocalcemia may be sufficient to produce tetany. Mild acidosis and generalized aminoaciduria also result from secondary hyperparathyroidism. As a rule, patients with renal tubular disorders maintain normal serum calcium levels, while hypophosphatemia is characteristic. Other laboratory findings such as glucosuria, aminoaciduria, acidosis, and hypouricemia reflect variable degrees of disturbance of proximal tubular function or features of the underlying disease (e.g., low plasma ceruloplasmin in Wilson's disease or abnormalities of immunoglobulins in multiple myeloma). In chronic renal failure hyperphosphatemia and some degree of hypocalcemia are usually accompanied by normal 25(OH)D and low $1,25(OH)_2D$ levels. In nephrotic syndrome serum 25(OH)D levels can be low due primarily to urinary losses of protein-bound 25(OH)D. Serum phosphorus levels are also normal or elevated in hypophosphatasia. Increased excretion of hydroxyproline-containing peptides occurs in those conditions in which secondary hyperparathyroidism and excessive bone resorption are associated with the defect in mineralization. Alkaline phosphatase levels in plasma are usually elevated in rickets or osteomalacia, but typical and even severe osteomalacia, especially that due to renal tubular disorders, may be accompanied by normal or only borderline elevations. Levels may increase during the early phases of therapy.

FIGURE 337-3 *Radiographs of the scapula of a 58-year-old woman with phosphate diabetes. The presence of a pseudofracture or Looser's zone is indicated by the arrow.*

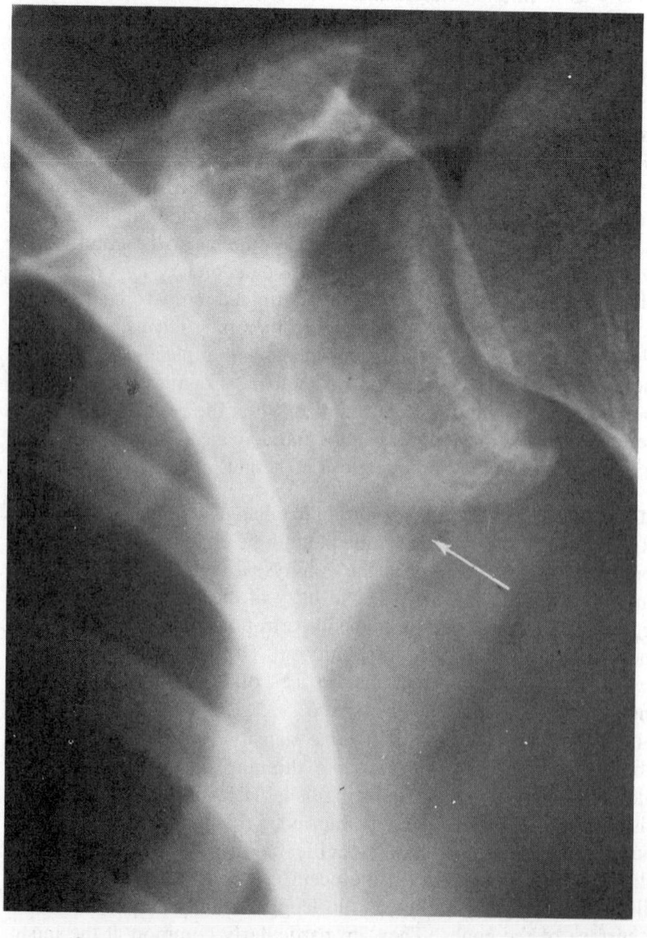

DIETARY VITAMIN D DEFICIENCY AND INADEQUATE ENDOGENOUS SYNTHESIS Most foods unfortified with vitamin D contain insufficient amounts of the vitamin to prevent rickets in growing children or osteomalacia in adults living in temperate-zone cities. As discussed in Chap. 335, in the absence of supplements, vitamin D must be formed endogenously through the ultraviolet irradiation of precursor 7-dehydrocholesterol in the skin. Many factors decrease the formation of vitamin D_3 from its precursor: increased melanin pigmentation, hyperkeratosis, sunscreens, limited exposure of the body, short days of sunlight, oblique angle of ultraviolet irradiation, and factors in the atmosphere, such as smog, which prevent adequate penetration of ultraviolet radiation. Since fortification of dairy products and routine use of vitamin D supplements for infants have been in effect, deficiency rickets is unusual in the United States. Poor, dark-skinned infants living in crowded northern cities are most susceptible. However, osteomalacia due to vitamin D deficiency still occurs in adults, especially in elderly individuals who tend to remain indoors and whose dietary intake of vitamin D is inadequate (probably less than 70 to 100 IU per day) because of avoidance of milk due to lactose intolerance.

VITAMIN D LOSS AND INTESTINAL MALABSORPTION Osteomalacia may be seen in patients with intestinal malabsorption such as in adult celiac disease and regional enteritis. Prior to the discovery of gluten sensitivity in some of these cases, celiac disease was among the more common disorders underlying osteomalacia. Vitamin D absorption, which normally occurs via chylomicrons, is impaired in diseases causing steatorrhea where emulsification of fat is disturbed, such as chronic biliary obstruction. Patients with cholestatic liver disease or extrahepatic biliary obstruction may have low serum levels of 25(OH)D and osteomalacia, due not only to poor vitamin D absorption but also to decreased hepatic production of 25(OH)D and disruption of its enterohepatic circulation. Osteomalacia is less frequent in chronic pancreatic insufficiency. Patients who have had gastric surgery for peptic ulcer disease or gastric bypass for obesity may also develop osteomalacia, possibly due to malfunction of the proximal small bowel. Factors other than failure to absorb vitamin D may contribute to the osteomalacia in patients with small-bowel disease, such as inadequate absorbing surface and failure of intestinal cells to respond to the active metabolites of vitamin D. Secondary hyperparathyroidism is usually present in intestinal malabsorption, as it is in dietary lack of vitamin D and may be particularly severe in patients who develop osteomalacia following intestinal bypass surgery. Some patients who lack vitamin D, usually associated with intestinal malabsorption, have normal circulating levels of $1,25(OH)_2D$, despite low or undetectable 25(OH)D. In these individuals the normal levels of $1,25(OH)_2D$ may be accounted for by ingestion of sufficient

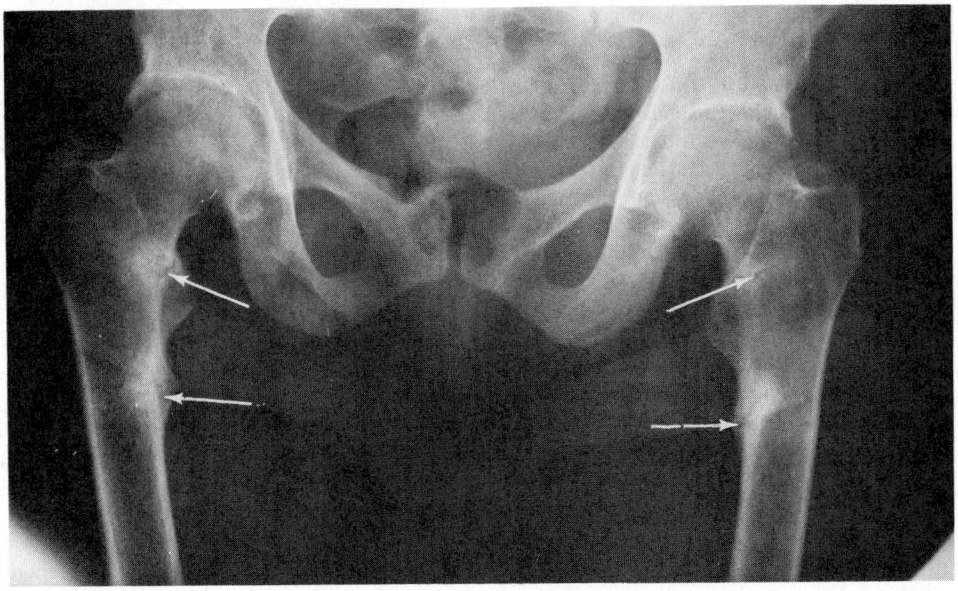

FIGURE 337-4 *Radiograph of the femurs of a 47-year-old woman with Fanconi's syndrome of adult onset. The presence of multiple pseudofractures is indicated by the arrows.*

vitamin D in hospital diets to produce substrate 25(OH)D for 1α-hydroxylation by the renal enzyme that is increased in activity due to secondary hyperparathyroidism. In other patients, circulating $1,25(OH)_2D$ levels may not reflect levels at critical target cells.

ABNORMAL METABOLISM OF VITAMIN D Serum 25(OH)D levels are reduced in some instances of parenchymal and obstructive liver disease, but these findings have not yet been correlated with quantitative histologic studies of bone. Patients consuming anticonvulsant drugs such as phenobarbital, phenytoin or carbamazepine may develop rickets or osteomalacia. For a given intake of vitamin D, patients receiving chronic anticonvulsant drugs have lower serum levels of calcium and 25(OH)D. Consumption of anticonvulsants may be especially important in individuals whose intake of vitamin D is marginal, who are nonambulatory and confined indoors, who have chronic recurrent infections, or in whom mild intestinal malfunction exists as in the postgastrectomy state. As discussed in Chap. 335 the anticonvulsant drugs have multiple actions on calcium homeostasis.

A syndrome superficially resembling vitamin D–resistant rickets has been termed *pseudovitamin D deficiency*. Because these patients respond to pharmacologic doses of vitamin D, this disease is also termed *vitamin D–dependent rickets* (also see Chap. 336). These patients have rickets or osteomalacia, a tendency to hypocalcemia but normal or only slightly depressed serum phosphorus levels, a response to moderate doses of vitamin D that is usually excellent and complete, and an autosomal recessive inheritance. No other renal tubular abnormalities are found. These patients also respond to small doses of $1,25(OH)_2D$ (calcitriol). Most patients have low serum $1,25(OH)_2D$ levels, suggesting a defect in the renal production of $1,25(OH)_2D$; these have been classified as having vitamin D–dependent rickets, type I. Vitamin D–dependent rickets, type II, results from an impaired responsiveness of target tissues to $1,25(OH)_2D$ since skin fibroblasts cultured from most affected subjects have abnormalities in the amount or function of $1,25(OH)_2D$ receptors. In these subjects elevated serum $1,25(OH)_2D$ levels are elevated and increase further when large doses of vitamin D are administered.

Other individuals with rickets unresponsive to 25(OH)D (calcifediol) or calcitriol have low circulating levels of $24,25(OH)_2D$ and have return of serum calcium concentrations to normal when synthetic $24,25(OH)_2D$ is administered.

Osteomalacia may also occur in patients on long-term total parenteral nutrition. Some of these individuals have hypoparathyroidism but this cannot account for the osteomalacia. Serum levels of 25(OH)D are normal although levels of $1,25(OH)_2D$ may be low. Aluminum has been detected in increased amounts in plasma, urine, and bone and may play a role in genesis of the osteomalacia similar to that postulated in patients with renal failure on chronic hemodialysis.

RENAL TUBULAR DISORDERS Rickets and osteomalacia occur in association with a variety of disorders of proximal renal tubular function. These disorders have in common increased renal clearance of inorganic phosphorus and hypophosphatemia with normal or near normal glomerular filtration rate. Increased phosphate clearance with resultant hypophosphatemia is usually an isolated defect with no other abnormalities except for increase in urinary glycine excretion (hyperglycinuria). X-linked hypophosphatemia (*phosphate diabetes* and *vitamin D–resistant rickets* are terms applied to these cases especially when the disorder presents in early childhood) is characterized by progressively severe skeletal deformities, dwarfism, and X-linked dominant inheritance. Many of these individuals have a unique disorder of tendons, ligaments, and joint capsules characterized by calcification or, more probably, ossification of insertions of tendons and ligaments and joint capsules. In some patients spontaneous remissions may be followed by recurrences in adult life associated, for example, with pregnancy and lactation. Serum levels of 25(OH)D are normal, and levels of $1,25(OH)_2D$ are in the low-normal range. The latter may be inappropriately low with respect to the hypophosphatemia (although the low levels of $1,25(OH)_2D$ do not account for the renal tubular defect in phosphate transport), and therefore high concentrations of $1,25(OH)_2D$ would be required to heal the osteomalacia. Similar mechanisms have been proposed to account for renal tubular and skeletal abnormalities. Combined therapy with calcitriol and inorganic phosphorus reverses the osteomalacia of trabecular bone surfaces and corrects the microscopic periosteocytic mineralization defects as well. Sporadic cases of hypophosphatemia have also been described in adults in whom family histories are negative and where proximal muscle weakness is a prominent feature. These patients also are best treated with a combination of calcitriol and inorganic phosphorus. As mentioned above, in most untreated patients with renal tubular disorders associated with rickets and osteomalacia, secondary hyperparathyroidism is not present.

In other patients the disorder in tubular function may be more widespread, involving (besides phosphorus) glucose, potassium, amino acids, and uric acid; the various combinations are termed the de Toni-Debré-Fanconi syndrome. The more complete renal tubular defects may occur sporadically or in families. In some instances the lesion is simply part of a more widespread disorder as in Wilson's disease and cystinosis. The acidosis of proximal tubular defects also plays a role in development of osteomalacia, possibly by altering metabolism of vitamin D or altering renal handling of calcium and phosphorus. In this regard osteomalacia has accompanied the hyperchloremic acidosis of ureterocolic anastomosis.

TUMOR-ASSOCIATED (ONCOGENOUS) OSTEOMALACIA Osteomalacia and hypophosphatemia with high renal phosphate clearance have been associated with a variety of mesenchymal tumors. The latter have included giant cell tumors (benign or malignant), reparative granulomas, hemangiomas, fibromas, and other mesenchymal neoplasms. A similar syndrome occurs in patients with prostatic carcinoma. In some instances, removal of the tumor resulted in return of renal phosphorus clearance to normal, rise in serum phosphorus levels, and healing of the osteomalacia (or the rickets in children). Serum $1,25(OH)_2D$ levels are low or undetectable, although chronic administration of sufficient calcitriol to raise circulating levels of this metabolite to normal does not alter renal phosphorus clearance or serum phosphorus concentrations. Some renal toxin released by the tumor may impair proximal tubular functions such as 1α-hydroxylation of 25(OH)D *and* phosphate transport; removal of the tumor results in a return of circulating levels of $1,25(OH)_2D$ and serum phosphorus levels to normal.

CHRONIC RENAL FAILURE Osteomalacia is common in patients with chronic renal failure; it often tends to be the predominant type of renal osteodystrophy in younger patients and is more frequent in those with the lower plasma levels of calcium and phosphorus. A component of secondary hyperparathyroidism and osteitis fibrosa almost always accompanies the defect in mineralization. The defect itself probably involves a decreased conversion of 25(OH)D to $1,25(OH)_2D$ either because of insufficient viable renal cortical tissue or the inhibitory effect of hyperphosphatemia on renal 25(OH)D-1α-hydroxylase activity. In addition, there may be a primary defect in intestinal calcium absorption. Part of the secondary hyperparathyroidism may also be due to decreased phosphate clearance and subsequent hyperphosphatemia. Under circumstances of near-normal plasma concentration of calcium and hyperphosphatemia, the presence of inhibitors probably accounts for the defective mineralization. In some patients the osteomalacia responds to large doses of vitamin D or dihydrotachysterol or to small doses of calcitriol or calcifediol. However, some patients with renal osteodystrophy do not respond to pharmacologic doses of vitamin D or improve when given small amounts of calcitriol. Accumulation of aluminum in the bone of some of these subjects accounts for the vitamin D–refractory osteomalacia. These individuals have deposits of aluminum at the mineralization fronts and decreased mineralization rates. They can be recognized by the extent to which the plasma aluminum levels are increased following a standard infusion of the chelating agent deferoxamine. Deferoxamine can mobilize aluminum from bone and other tissues and is effective therapy of the aluminum osteodystrophy. In some patients with renal osteodystrophy the total bone mass may be increased (osteosclerosis), resulting in increased density of bone. This is particularly evident in the spine, where a characteristic appearance is that of dense bone at the superior and inferior margins of the vertebral bodies with more radiolucent central portions ("rugger jersey sign"). Histologically, although there is more bone per unit area, each trabecula is covered by an abnormally wide osteoid seam.

HYPOPHOSPHATASIA Rickets is a feature of a deficiency of alkaline phosphatase in infants and children which is inherited as an autosomal recessive trait. The disorder that affects adults, however, is probably distinct from the infantile and childhood forms and is inherited as an autosomal dominant trait with variable expressivity. The precise defects are not known, although the fundamental abnormality relates to deficient circulating and tissue activity of the tissue nonspecific alkaline phosphatase isoenzyme. Despite the presence of osteomalacia serum phosphorus levels are not reduced. Phosphoryl ethanolamine is excreted in excessive amounts in the urine, and circulating levels of pyridoxal 5′-phosphate are elevated, although it is not clear how these findings are related to the inadequate skeletal mineralization. There is a direct correlation between plasma alkaline phosphatase and inorganic pyrophosphatase. Since patients with hypophosphatasia are also deficient in pyrophosphatase, concentrations of inorganic pyrophosphate, a potent inhibitor of mineralization, may be too high to allow normal mineralization at formation sites. Elevated levels of inorganic pyrophosphate in this disorder could also account for the occurrence of arthropathy associated with chondrocalcinosis. Bone disease in adult hypophosphatasia may be due to a generalized defect in osteoblasts or other alkaline phosphatase–producing cells or to a qualitative defect in the alkaline phosphatase molecule.

OTHER DISORDERS ASSOCIATED WITH DEFECTIVE MINERALIZATION Disturbances in mineralization may be seen in patients consuming high doses of fluoride ion and in patients with Paget's disease treated with etidronate. Some decrease in mineralization of newly forming matrix, increase in surface covered by osteoid, and increase in the width of the osteoid seams occur in conditions that are not usually considered as osteomalacia except by these criteria. Biopsies in some of these conditions show a normal calcification front. Examples include patients with the osteitis fibrosa of hyperparathyroidism in the weeks to months following surgical cure. In these circumstances there is a temporary imbalance between the rate at which mineral is supplied to bone and the rate at which bone matrix is formed. Wide osteoid seams and hypophosphatemia are also seen in children with osteopetrosis in whom there is inadequate resorption of bone and calcified cartilage but active bone formation.

A condition that resembles osteomalacia and is associated with a coarsened, mottled bony trabecular pattern, pseudofractures, and bone pain but normal plasma levels of calcium and phosphorus is *fibrogenesis imperfecta ossium*. The bone has a distinctive histologic appearance, with wide osteoid seams and a distortion of the birefringent pattern of normal bone suggesting an abnormality in the collagen recently deposited. The nature of the abnormality is not known.

TREATMENT OF RICKETS AND OSTEOMALACIA In rickets and osteomalacia due to dietary absence of vitamin D or inadequate exposure to sunlight, vitamin D_2 (cholecalciferol) or vitamin D_3 (ergocalciferol) is given orally in doses of 2000 to 4000 IU (0.05 to 0.1 mg) daily for 6 to 12 weeks, followed by daily supplements of 200 to 400 IU, which are adequate to prevent the development of the disorder in otherwise normal subjects. In infants and children such treatment causes improvement in muscle tone and strength, increase in serum calcium and phosphorus, and fall in alkaline phosphatase levels after several weeks. Radiologic evidence of healing is first noted within weeks and may be complete by a few months. Calcium supplements and larger initial doses of vitamin D may be necessary in infants and children with tetany. In adults with nutritional osteomalacia healing of pseudofractures may be evident within 3 to 4 weeks after therapy with as little as 2000 IU (0.05 mg) vitamin D daily. Healing is complete usually by 6 months.

Patients with osteomalacia due to intestinal malabsorption do not respond to the relatively small doses of vitamin D that can cure osteomalacia due to dietary absence or inadequate sunlight. In the presence of active steatorrhea, daily oral doses of vitamin D of 50,000 to 100,000 IU (1.25 to 2.5 mg) and large doses of calcium (e.g., 15 g calcium lactate or 4 g calcium carbonate orally per day) may be required. In some instances oral vitamin D is ineffective, and the parenteral route is required (e.g., 10,000 IU intramuscularly per day). Another approach is the use of ultraviolet irradiation in addition to supplemental calcium. Small doses of calcitriol (0.5 to 1.0 μg daily) are usually effective in this form of osteomalacia. Inorganic phosphate therapy is not indicated either in deficiency or in intestinal malabsorption of the vitamins, since hypocalcemia will develop and intestinal calcium absorption will remain inadequate. In all patients in whom large doses of vitamin D are used, periodic monitoring of serum calcium and 25(OH)D levels is essential. Semiquantitative urinary calcium measurements alone are inadequate.

In patients on anticonvulsants, it is usually necessary to continue the drugs while adding supplemental vitamin D and monitoring levels of serum calcium and serum 25(OH)D until a therapeutic response (evidence of radiologic healing, improvement in symptoms) is obtained. Doses varying from 4000 to 40,000 IU daily have been recommended.

Treatment of rickets and osteomalacia in the presence of renal tubular disorders is more difficult. The X-linked form of hypophosphatemic osteomalacia is usually treated with large doses of vitamin D (from 50,000 to several hundred thousand IU or more daily). The use of dihydrotachysterol, a pseudo-1α(OH)D analogue, 0.2 to 0.6 mg, or calcitriol, 0.5 to 2.0 μg (see below) orally per day, in place of vitamin D has the advantage of shorter onset and duration of action and more consistent skeletal healing. With vitamin D therapy alone radiologic evidence of healing in many patients is incomplete; some hypophosphatemia persists, linear skeletal growth remains abnormally slow, and bony deformities continue to develop. In addition, hypercalcemia and its consequences are potential hazards. The addition of oral supplements of inorganic phosphate in divided doses of 1.0 to 3.6 g phosphorus daily has improved the clinical and radiologic response, allowed the use of smaller doses of vitamin D or calcitriol, and improved the rate of linear growth in many younger subjects. In some adults, therapy with inorganic phosphate alone abolishes muscle weakness and bone pain and produces radiologic and histologic healing. The addition of calcitriol improves calcium balance and helps decrease secondary hyperparathyroidism and maintain a sufficient level of serum phosphorus to permit complete healing. In some patients there may be temporary increase in bone pain and rise in serum alkaline phosphatase during the early phases of treatment. In the osteomalacia associated with the chronic acidosis of renal tubular disorders, the use of alkali may be of value in supplementing therapy with phosphate and calcitriol. In patients with ureterosigmoidostomy, oral sodium bicarbonate has reversed acidosis, improved serum phosphate level, and healed the bone disease; with maintenance doses of alkali, recurrence of symptoms has been prevented.

Patients with nephrotic syndrome and low serum 25(OH)D levels benefit from modest vitamin D supplementation. In chronic renal failure high doses of vitamin D, similar to those needed to treat osteomalacia of renal tubular disorders, are used. Dihydrotachysterol at doses of 0.2 to 1.0 mg daily is effective in treating hypocalcemia and osteodystrophy resulting from chronic renal failure. Calcitriol in small doses is equally effective in most cases of renal osteodystrophy. The recommended initial dose is 0.25 μg per day. If after 2 to 4 weeks on this dose the biochemical parameters are unaltered, the dose is increased by 0.25 μg per day every 2 to 4 weeks until a satisfactory clinical biochemical response (including elevation of serum calcium levels and decrease in PTH levels) is obtained. The usual dose is 0.5 to 1.0 μg per day. Because there are no regulatory mechanisms to control the biological responses to calcitriol, there is a high incidence of transient hypercalciuria and hypercalcemia, especially initially. Thus, serum calcium should be monitored frequently during the first 1 to 2 months of therapy and less frequently once a stable dose has been established. Since calcitriol has a short duration of action and is not stored in fat depots, hypercalcemia usually resolves in 2 to 7 days after the dose is discontinued or decreased. Phosphate supplements are, of course, contraindicated in the usual patient with chronic renal failure. Occasionally, however, hypophosphatemia may result from the excessive use of nonabsorbable antacids in addition to excessive removal of phosphate through hemodialysis.

In patients who have had rickets in childhood, the abnormal mechanical stress of severe deformities may contribute to the development of degenerative joint disease, particularly in hips and knees. Osteotomies at the proper time after healing may prevent this complication and more extensive arthroplasties later in life.

REFERENCES

Osteoporosis

AVIOLI LV: Osteoporosis: Pathogenesis and therapy, in *Metabolic Bone Disease*, LV Avioli, SM Krane (eds). New York, Academic, 1977, vol 1, p 307

ALOIA JF et al: Risk factors for postmenopausal osteoporosis. Am J Med 78:95, 1985

BROWN JP et al: Serum bone GLA-protein: A specific marker for bone formation in postmenopausal osteoporosis. Lancet 1:1091, 1984

CHRISTIANSEN C et al: Bone mass in postmenopausal women after withdrawal of oestrogen/gestagen replacement therapy. Lancet 1:459, 1981

DELMAS PD et al: Increase in serum bone γ-carboxyglutamic acid protein with aging in women. J Clin Invest 71:1316, 1983

DRINKWATER BL et al: Bone mineral content of amenorrheic and eumenorrheic athletes. N Engl J Med 311:277, 1984

Editorial: Fluoride and the treatment of osteoporosis. Lancet 1:547, 1984

Editorial: Risk factors in postmenopausal osteoporosis. Lancet 1:1370, 1985

GALLAGHER JC et al: Epidemiology of fractures of the proximal femur in Rochester, Minnesota. Clin Orthopaed Rel Res 150:163, 1980

GRUBER HE et al: Long-term calcitonin therapy in postmenopausal osteoporosis. Metabolism 33:295, 1984

HARRISON JE et al: Three-year changes in bone mineral mass of postmenopausal osteoporotic patients based on neutron activation analysis of the central third of the skeleton. J Clin Endocrinol Metab 52:751, 1981

HEATH H III: Athletic women, amenorrhea, and skeletal integrity (editorial). Ann Intern Med 102:258, 1985

HORSMAN A et al: The effect of estrogen dose on postmenopausal bone loss. N Engl J Med 309:1405, 1983

JENSEN J et al: Cigarette smoking, serum estrogens, and bone loss during hormone-replacement therapy early after menopause. N Engl J Med 313:973, 1985

KANIS JA: Treatment of osteoporotic fracture. Lancet 1:27, 1984

KLIBANSKI A et al: Decreased bone density in hyperprolactinemic women. N Engl J Med 303:1511, 1980

KRØLNER B et al: Physical exercise as prophylaxis against involutional vertebral bone loss: A controlled trial. Clin Sci Mol Med 64:541, 1983

LANE JM et al: Treatment of osteoporosis with sodium fluoride and calcium: Effects on vertebral fracture incidence and bone histomorphometry. Orthop Clin North Am 15:729, 1984

LINDSAY R et al: Prevention of spinal osteoporosis in oophorectomised women. Lancet 2:1151, 1980

NEED AG et al: 1,25-Dihydroxycalciferol and calcium therapy in osteoporosis with calcium malabsorption: Dose response relationship of calcium absorption and indices of bone turnover. Mineral Electrolyte Metab 11:35, 1985

PARFITT AM: Dietary risk factors for age-related bone loss and fractures. Lancet 2:1181, 1983

——— et al: Relationships between surface, volume, and thickness of iliac trabecular bone in aging and in osteoporosis: Implications for the microanatomic and cellular mechanisms of bone loss. J Clin Invest 72:1396, 1983

PROCKOP DJ: Mutations in collagen genes: Consequences for rare and common diseases. J Clin Invest 75:783, 1985

RECKER RR et al: Effect of estrogens and calcium carbonate on bone loss in postmenopausal women. Ann Intern Med 87:649, 1977

RIGGS BL, MELTON J III: Evidence for two distinct syndromes of involutional osteoporosis. Am J Med 75:899, 1983

——— et al: Effect of the fluoride/calcium regimen on vertebral fracture occurrence in postmenopausal osteoporosis: Comparison with conventional therapy. N Engl J Med 306:446, 1982

——— et al: Changes in bone mineral density of the proximal femur and spine with aging: Differences between the postmenopausal and senile osteoporosis syndromes. J Clin Invest 70:716, 1982

SAKHAEE K et al: Postmenopausal osteoporosis as a manifestation of renal hypercalciuria with secondary hyperparathyroidism. J Clin Endocrinol Metab 61:368, 1985

SEEMAN E et al: Risk factors for spinal osteoporosis in men. Am J Med 75:977, 1983

SILLENCE D: Osteogenesis imperfecta: An expanding panorama of variants. Clin Orthopaed Rel Res 159:11, 1981

SMITH R et al: Osteoporosis of pregnancy. Lancet 1:1178, 1985

SPENCER H et al: Chronic alcoholism: Frequently overlooked cause of osteoporosis in men. Am J Med 80:393, 1986

STEWART AF et al: Calcium homeostasis in immobilization: An example of resorptive hypercalciuria. N Engl J Med 306:1136, 1982

WAHNER HW et al: Assessment of bone mineral. J Nucl Med 25:1241, 1984

WEINSTEIN MC: Estrogen use in postmenopausal women—costs, risks, and benefits. N Engl J Med 303:308, 1980

Osteomalacia

CHARHON SA et al: Effects of parathyroidectomy on bone formation and mineralization in hemodialyzed patients. Kidney Int 27:426, 1984

FRAME B, PARFITT AM: Osteomalacia: Current concepts. Ann Intern Med 89:966, 1978

GODSALL JW et al: Vitamin D metabolism and bone histomorphometry in a patient with antacid-induced osteomalacia. Am J Med 77:747, 1984

GOLDRING SR, KRANE SM: Disorders of calcification: Osteomalacia and rickets, in *Endocrinology*, LJ DeGroot (ed). New York, Grune & Stratton, 1979, vol 2, p 853

HARRELL RM et al: Healing of bone disease in X-linked hypophosphatemic rickets/osteomalacia: Induction and maintenance with phosphorus and calcitriol. J Clin Invest 75:1858, 1985

HOCHBERG Z et al: 1,25-Dihydroxyvitamin D resistance, rickets, and alopecia. Am J Med 77:805, 1984

HODSMAN AB et al: Bone aluminum and histomorphometric features of renal osteodystrophy. J Clin Endocrinol Metab 54:439, 1982

——— et al: Vitamin D–resistant osteomalacia in hemodialysis patients lacking secondary hyperparathyroidism. Ann Intern Med 94:629, 1981

HOIKKA V et al: Carbamazepine and bone mineral metabolism. Acta Neurol Scand 70:77, 1984

KLEIN GL, COBURN JW: Metabolic bone disease associated with total parenteral nutrition. Adv Nutr Res 6:67, 1984

KUMAR R: Hepatic and intestinal osteodystrophy and the hepatobiliary metabolism of vitamin D. Ann Intern Med 98:662, 1983
LYLES KW et al: Hypophosphatemic osteomalacia: Association with prostatic carcinoma. Ann Intern Med 93:275, 1980
MANKIN HJ: Rickets, osteomalacia and renal osteodystrophy. J Bone Joint Surg (AM) 56A:101,352, 1974
MARIE PJ, GLORIEUX FH: Relation between hypomineralized periosteocytic lesions and bone mineralization in vitamin D–resistant rickets. Calcif Tissue Int 35:443, 1983
MILLINER DS et al: Use of deferoxamine infusion test in the diagnosis of aluminum-related osteodystrophy. Ann Intern Med 101:775, 1984
PARFITT AM et al: Metabolic bone disease with and without osteomalacia after intestinal bypass surgery: A bone histomorphometric study. Bone 6:211, 1985
PIKE JW et al: D_3–resistant fibroblasts have immunoassayable 1,25-dihydroxyvitamin D_3 receptors. Science 224:879, 1984
POLISSON RP et al: Calcification of entheses associated with X-linked hypophosphatemic osteomalacia. N Engl J Med 313:1, 1985
RYAN EA, REISS E: Oncogenous osteomalacia: Review of the world literature of 42 cases and report of two new cases. Am J Med 77:501, 1984
STEINBACH HL, NOETZLI M: Roentgen appearance of the skeleton in osteomalacia and rickets. Am J Roentgenol 91:955, 1964
SWEET RA et al: Vitamin D metabolite levels in oncogenic osteomalacia. Ann Intern Med 93:279, 1980
WHYTE MP et al: Markedly increased circulating pyridoxal-5′-phosphate levels in hypophosphatasia. J Clin Invest 76:752, 1985
——— et al: Adult hypophosphatasia with chondrocalcinosis and arthropathy: Variable penetrance of hypophosphatasemia in a large Oklahoma kindred. Am J Med 72:631, 1982

338 PAGET'S DISEASE OF BONE

STEPHEN M. KRANE

Paget's disease of bone (osteitis deformans) is usually focal, but occasionally it may be widespread. The initial event is excessive resorption of bone by cells such as osteoclasts, followed by the replacement of normal marrow by vascular, fibrous connective tissue. At some stage and to a variable degree, the resorbed bone is replaced by coarse-fibered, dense trabecular bone organized in haphazard fashion. The irregular and often rapid deposition of this new bone, to a great extent still lamellar, causes an increase in the number of prominent, irregular cement lines which gives the bone its characteristic "mosaic" pattern. Most lesions show evidence of both excessive resorption and the chaotic new bone formation.

INCIDENCE The prevalence is difficult to determine since it is often asymptomatic and is frequently detected when roentgenograms are obtained for other reasons. On the basis of autopsy examination, the incidence has been estimated to be about 3 percent in individuals over the age of 40; there is increased likelihood of occurrence with increasing age. The incidence varies in different parts of the world. Figures based on radiological surveys indicate less than a 1 percent frequency in the adult population in the United States, Great Britain, and Australia. In India, Japan, the Middle East, and Scandinavia, the disease is rare.

ETIOLOGY The etiology of Paget's disease is unknown. No convincing evidence of endocrine abnormality has been produced. Likewise, although pagetic bone can be exceedingly vascular, it has not been established that the vascular abnormality is primary. Some of the manifestations of the disease can be suppressed with the use of glucocorticoids, salicylates, and cytotoxic drugs, but there is not sufficient information to support the hypothesis that the fundamental lesion is inflammatory. Intranuclear inclusions have been found by electron microscopy in osteoclasts in pagetic bone but not in osteoclasts or any other cells in bone from normal persons or patients with various bone diseases with the exception of pyknodysostosis. Some of the inclusions are morphologically similar to nucleocapsids of viruses belonging to the measles group. Indirect immunofluorescence and immunoperoxidase studies support the suggestion that the inclusions are indeed measles virus nucleocapsids. Other evidence suggests that the inclusions are due to respiratory syncytial virus. In one area of England ownership of dogs is more common in pagetic subjects than in controls, suggesting that a canine virus (for example, canine distemper) might be a primary infective agent. Thus, different viral agents might be responsible for Paget's disease in different instances.

PATHOPHYSIOLOGY The characteristic feature is increased resorption of bone accompanied by an increase in bone formation, which is usually adequate to compensate. In the early phase bone resorption predominates (for example, in the variant, *osteoporosis circumscripta*), and the bones are exceedingly vascular. This has been termed the *osteoporotic, osteolytic,* or *destructive phase* of disease in which the external calcium balance may be negative. Commonly the excessive resorption is followed closely by formation of new pagetic bone. In this so-called mixed phase of the disease, the rate of bone formation is so geared to that of bone resorption that the magnitude of the increase in bone turnover is not reflected in the overall calcium balance.

As the activity decreases, a progressive decrease in resorptive rate may occur, eventually leading to the occurrence of hard, dense, less vascular bone (the so-called *osteoplastic* or *sclerotic* phase) and a positive external calcium balance. The rates of bone turnover may be increased enormously in patients with active Paget's disease, occasionally more than 20 times normal. Quantitative histomorphometry of pagetic bone biopsies confirms the extent of remodeling with findings of marked increase in resorption surfaces with deep scalloped lacunae containing giant osteoclasts with numerous nuclei. Resorption surfaces are also increased, and increased numbers of osteoblasts line the edges. The calcification rate is also increased. The normal hematopoietic marrow is replaced by a loose stroma which may be highly vascular. The magnitude of the increase in turnover varies with the extent as well as the activity of the disease. The increase correlates with the increased plasma levels of bone alkaline phosphatase, which are higher in Paget's disease than in any other condition with the exception of hereditary hyperphosphatasia. Although increased bone resorption enhances release of calcium and phosphate ions from bone, utilization of these ions for new bone formation and, presumably, feedback control of parathyroid hormone secretion usually maintain the concentration of calcium ions in the plasma at normal levels. The concentration of phosphate in the plasma is normal or slightly elevated. When marked imbalance between bone formation and resorption occurs in favor of resorption, as after prolonged immobilization or fractures, urinary calcium excretion may be increased, and rarely hypercalcemia may occur. If, on the other hand, bone formation exceeds resorption (relatively uncommon), circulating levels of parathyroid hormone may be increased. Resorption involves the organic phase of bone as well as the mineral phase. While the inorganic ions of the mineral phase are reutilized for bone formation, amino acids such as hydroxyproline and hydroxylysine are released during resorption of the collagen matrix of bone and are not reutilized for collagen biosynthesis. The urinary excretion of small peptides containing hydroxyproline is increased, reflecting the increased bone resorption. Peptides of about 1500 to 2000 mol wt containing hydroxyproline and other amino acids in proportions characteristic of collagen are also excreted in increased amounts in the urine and are correlated with increased bone formation. Other markers for increased matrix synthesis include elevated levels of osteocalcin (bone-GLA protein) (see Chap. 335) and procollagen extension fragments in plasma.

RADIOLOGIC CHANGES The radiologic findings reflect the underlying pathology and the phase of the disease that predominates at the time of the examination. The pelvic bones are most commonly involved, followed by the femur, skull, tibia, lumbosacral spine, dorsal spine, clavicles, and ribs in that order; small bones are not as frequently diseased. The lytic phase of the disease may be overlooked except when it occurs in the skull as *osteoporosis circumscripta,* with areas of sharply demarcated radiolucency in the frontal, parietal, and occipital bones. In the long bones the lytic areas are usually first seen at one end, from which they progress toward the other end with a V-shaped advancing edge. The lesion may produce expansion of the cortex and exhibit other features which suggest malignancy. Usually the lytic area is followed by a zone of increased density, representing the new bone formation of the mixed phase of the disease. In general, the bone shows enlargement with irregularly widened cortex in a coarse, striated pattern and increased density, occasionally focal in distribution. Perpendicular lines of radiolucency (cortical infractions) are frequent and occur on the convex side of bowed long bones, particularly the femur and tibia. Transverse fractures may also occur, some initiated at the sites of these cortical infractions. The remodeling of the pagetic bone usually follows the lines of stress produced by muscle pull or gravity, accounting for the characteristic lateral bowing of the femur or anterior bowing of the tibia and the tendency for most of the dense bone to be deposited on the concave side of the bowed bone. In the skull, in the mixed stage, there is enlargement and thickening, especially of the outer table, with irregular areas of increased density, often spotty (Fig. 338-1). Basilar invagination is common with involvement of the base of the skull. The changes in the pelvis also consist of the combination of bone resorption and new bone formation and are frequently accompanied by a characteristic thickening of the pelvic brim. In the sclerotic phase of the disease, the bone may show uniform increase in density, often in the absence of striations. This is common in the facial bones but is occasionally seen as well in the vertebrae where a homogeneous, dense pattern gives an "ivory" appearance similar to that typical of Hodgkin's disease, although the involved vertebrae are not enlarged in Hodgkin's disease.

CLINICAL PICTURE The clinical presentation is variable and is a function of the extent of the disease, the particular bones involved, and the presence of associated complications. Many patients are asymptomatic. In these individuals the disorder is discovered during the course of radiologic examination of the pelvis or spine for an unrelated disease or complaint, or because of the finding of an elevated level of plasma alkaline phosphatase. Other individuals may gradually become aware of a swelling or deformity of a long bone or develop a disturbance in gait due to unequal length of and change in the distribution of mechanical forces in the lower extremities. Enlargement of the skull is often not noticed by the patients, or they may be aware of increasing hat size. Pain in the face and headache are initial complaints in some; backache and pain in the lower extremities are common. The pain is usually dull but may be shooting or knifelike. Back pain is most common in the lumbar region and may radiate into the buttocks or lower extremities. This pain is probably due to the pagetic process itself and to distortion of articular facets and secondary osteoarthritis. Pain in the lower extremities may be associated with the transverse cortical infractions along the convex lateral surface of the femur or the anterior surface of the tibia. Often the new lytic lesions detected on bone scan are the most painful. Pain may also be due to involvement of the hip joint resembling degenerative joint disease and characterized by narrowing of the joint space, bony lipping at the margin of the acetabulum, and deepening of the acetabulum. Angioid streaks may be present in the retina. Hearing loss is due to direct pagetic involvement of the ossicles of the inner ear or of bone in the region of the cochlea or to impingement on the eighth cranial nerve by pagetic bone narrowing the auditory foramen. More serious neurologic complications can result from overgrowth of pagetic bone at the base of the skull (platybasia) due to compression of the brainstem. Compression of the spinal cord with paraplegia has been observed, particularly with involvement of the middorsal spine. Pathologic fractures of vertebrae may also produce spinal cord lesions.

COMPLICATIONS Blood flow may be markedly increased in extremities involved with Paget's disease. There is proliferation of blood vessels in pagetic bone, but anatomic and functional studies have not confirmed the presence of arteriovenous fistulas. Although blood flow in the bone itself is increased, there is also cutaneous vasodilatation in the pagetic extremities, which accounts for the increased warmth noted clinically. When the disease is widespread, involving over one-third of the skeleton, the increased blood flow may be associated with *high cardiac output*. In the rare patient so-called high-output heart failure may result. However, heart disease in pagetic individuals is usually accounted for by the same conditions that occur in other patients of similar age. *Pathologic fracture* may occur in bones involved in the destructive phase of the disease. In the weight-bearing bones fractures are often incomplete, multiple, and on the convex side of the bone. They may occur spontaneously or follow only slight trauma; the lesions are painful but heal spontaneously with no major disability. More serious fractures may also occur. Complete fractures are often transverse as if the bone were snapped like a piece of chalk. Under these circumstances the fracture may upset the delicate balance between bone formation and resorption in favor of resorption. At this stage the imbalance may be reflected by increased urinary calcium excretion, and in rare instances the serum calcium level may rise to dangerous levels.

There is no characteristic level of urinary calcium excretion, although calcium excretion tends to be higher when the resorptive phase predominates. This may be a factor which accounts for the somewhat higher incidence of *urinary stone* in these patients, although many of the urinary calculi reported may be unrelated to the pagetic process. Secondary changes in the cartilage of the hip joint and in bones about the knees may result in articular symptoms. Hyperuricemia and gout commonly occur in men with Paget's disease, and calcific periarthritis may occur.

Sarcoma is the most dreaded complication. The incidence is probably no greater than 1 percent, although higher incidence has been noted in some series which include many patients with polyostotic involvement. The sarcomas most frequently arise in the femur, humerus, skull, face, and pelvis, and rarely in the vertebrae. In about 20 percent the tumors are multicentric. Histologically, they are usually osteosarcomas, although fibrosarcomas and chondrosarcomas have also been found. Increase in pain and swelling are the most common complaints that lead to recognition of the sarcomas. The level of alkaline phosphatase in the serum of patients with sarcomas usually reflects the activity and extent of the Paget's disease. In occasional patients an "explosive rise" of the phosphatase level may accompany the growth of the sarcoma, whereas in patients with limited Paget's disease, phosphatase levels may be only slightly elevated and give no clue to the development of the malignant lesion. The prognosis is poor following the development of sarcomas, and ablative surgery

FIGURE 338-1 *Lateral roentgenogram of the skull from a 58-year-old woman with Paget's disease of bone.*

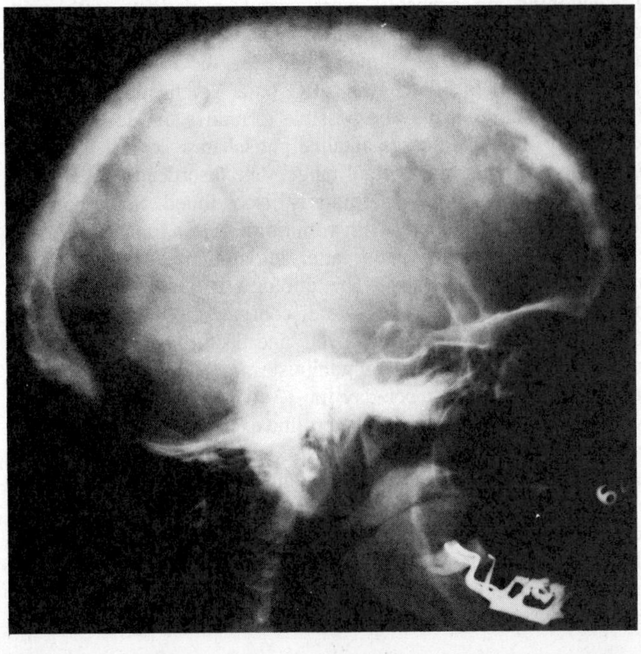

is rarely successful. Reparative granulomas closely resembling giant cell tumors may be locally destructive, but they do not metastasize.

THERAPY Most patients require no treatment, since the disease is localized and does not cause symptoms. Indications for therapy include persistent pain in involved bones, neural compression, rapidly progressive deformity resulting in disabling disturbance of posture and/or gait, high-output congestive heart failure, hypercalcemia, severe hypercalciuria with or without formation of renal stones, repeated fractures or nonunion in pagetic bone, and preparation for major orthopedic surgery. *Aspirin* is an effective analgesic, and if it can be tolerated in large enough doses (3.6 to 4.0 g per day) for months or years, disease activity may be suppressed, as shown by decreases in the level of plasma alkaline phosphatase and urinary hydroxyproline excretion. Nonsteroidal anti-inflammatory drugs such as *indomethacin,* 25 mg three or four times daily, may also relieve pain, especially in the presence of hip involvement. *Glucocorticoids* suppress the disease but only in large doses (greater than 60 mg prednisone per day) which are usually not tolerated and, therefore, are not recommended. It is of interest that the high cardiac output of some patients may be reduced significantly after only a few days of glucocorticoid treatment. Orthopedic procedures also have a role in the management of selected cases. Total hip replacement may be indicated in the patient with severe hip involvement, and osteotomy is useful to correct marked bowing deformities, particularly of the tibia. In patients with fractures or orthopedic procedures or in patients immobilized for any reason, urinary and serum calcium levels should be measured at intervals to anticipate the development of hypercalciuria and hypercalcemia. Early ambulation and adequate fluid intake are essential. Preparations of inorganic phosphate may reduce hypercalciuria under these circumstances (5 to 6 g neutral sodium phosphate daily in divided doses).

Several agents reduce the excessive bone resorption of Paget's disease and are of possible therapeutic value. Porcine, salmon, and human *calcitonins* have been administered subcutaneously for prolonged periods to pagetic patients, accompanied by a decrease in plasma alkaline phosphatase levels and in urinary hydroxyproline excretion. Treatment with calcitonin causes variable decrease in bone pain, improvement in neurologic symptoms, and decrease in elevated cardiac output. Some patients have not continued to respond to porcine and salmon calcitonins, possibly because of the development of neutralizing antibodies. These individuals usually continue to exhibit a satisfactory response to human calcitonin. In others in whom diminution in response is not associated with development of antibodies, the development of secondary hyperparathyroidism has been postulated, although this cannot account for resistance in all cases. The calcitonins are probably most useful in patients with pain corresponding to areas of pagetic involvement, not due to associated joint disease. The dose of salmon calcitonin (the form available in the United States) is 50 to 100 MRC units given subcutaneously daily. In some cases it may be possible to reduce the dose to three times weekly. In severe cases alkaline phosphatase levels, although reduced, do not reach the normal range. The disorder relapses after weeks or months when the calcitonin is discontinued. Some patients develop nausea, occasionally with vomiting, 30 min to several hours after injection. This may occur after initiating treatment or after months or years of therapy. The etiology is unknown, but the symptoms may be severe enough to discontinue the medication.

Cytotoxic drugs such as plicamycin and dactinomycin are potent agents in the disorder. Parenteral administration of plicamycin, 10 to 25 μg/kg of body weight per day for 10 to 14 days, has produced striking decrease in urinary hydroxyproline excretion with subsequent decreases in plasma alkaline phosphatase level and clinical improvement. The indexes of active disease again become abnormal within weeks to months following completion of plicamycin therapy. Maintenance therapy may be administered as a weekly intravenous bolus. With doses of less than 15 μg/kg of body weight per week toxicity is low despite potential risks.

Etidronate, a diphosphonate compound, given orally in doses up to 20 mg/kg of bodyweight per day has also been effective in reducing bone resorption in almost all and producing clinical improvement in some. In contrast to the calcitonins, etidronate often brings biochemical abnormalities to normal even in severe cases. Serum alkaline phosphatase and urinary hydroxyproline excretion remain decreased for several months after withdrawal of the drug and only gradually return to pretreatment levels. In doses of 20 mg/kg of body weight per day for periods of 6 months or longer mineralization of new bone may be inhibited and predispose to fracture. Some patients develop disabling pain over pagetic lesions within weeks or months of starting treatment that may be severe enough to warrant discontinuing the drug. Radiographs in some instances show an increase in bone lysis. This heals when the drug is stopped. It is therefore recommended that doses of 5 mg or occasionally 10 mg/kg of body weight per day be used for 6-month periods. Treatment could be reinstituted within 3 to 12 months if biochemical relapse occurs.

Other diphosphonate compounds such as the dichloromethylidene, 3-amino-1-hydroxypropylidine, aminohexane, or aminobutane derivatives have been introduced for therapy in Europe. Their onset is rapid and they do not inhibit mineralization. The use of these agents for brief periods (weeks) can cause remission that persists for months or even years. Although the diphosphonates and calcitonins act primarily to decrease bone resorption, the rate of new bone formation subsequently falls. As a result, the state of high bone turnover is shifted to a state of lower turnover, where rates of formation and resorption are still apparently geared to each other. In this lower turnover state, collagen fibers of the bone matrix are deposited in a more orderly fashion similar to normal bone.

REFERENCES

ALTMAN R, SINGER FR (eds.): Proceedings of the Kroc Foundation Conference on Paget's Disease of Bone, Arthritis Rheum 23:1073, 1980

BOYCE BF et al: Focal osteomalacia due to low-dose diphosphonate therapy in Paget's disease. Lancet 1:821, 1984

EVANS RA: Treatment of Paget's disease of bone. Med J Aust 1:159, 1983

HOSKING DJ: Paget's disease of bone. Br Med J 283:686, 1981

KRANE SM: Etidronate disodium in the treatment of Paget's disease of bone. Ann Intern Med 96:619, 1982

NAGANT DE DEUXCHAISNES C, KRANE SM: Paget's disease of bone: Clinical and metabolic observations. Medicine 43:233, 1964

O'DRISCOLL JB, ANDERSON DC: Past pets and Paget's disease. Lancet 2:919, 1985

SINGER FR et al: Paget's disease of bone, in *Metabolic Bone Disease,* vol 2, LV Avioli, SM Krane (eds). New York, Academic, 1978

———, MILLS BG: Evidence for a viral etiology of Paget's disease of bone. Clin Orthop 178:245, 1983

UPCHURCH KS et al: Giant cell reparative granuloma of Paget's disease of bone. A unique clinical entity. Ann Int Med 98:35, 1983

WALLACH S (ed): Paget's Disease. Clin Orthop 127:1, 1977

YATES AJP et al: Intravenous clodronate in the treatment and retreatment of Paget's disease of bone. Lancet 1:1474, 1985

339 HYPEROSTOSIS, NEOPLASMS, AND OTHER DISORDERS OF BONE AND CARTILAGE

STEPHEN M. KRANE / ALAN L. SCHILLER

HYPEROSTOSIS

A number of disease states have in common an increase in the mass of bone per unit volume (hyperostosis) (Table 339-1). Such increase in bone mass is detected radiologically as increased density of the bone, often associated with a variable disturbance in the architecture of the tissue. In the absence of quantitative histomorphometric data, it is usually not possible to distinguish between an increase in bone mass due to excessive formation of new bone or decreased resorption of bone already formed. When bone deposition is rapid, the new

TABLE 339-1 Causes of hyperostosis

1 Endocrine disorders
- *a* Primary hyperparathyroidism
- *b* Hypothyroidism
- *c* Acromegaly

2 Radiation osteitis

3 Chemical poisoning
- *a* Fluoride
- *b* Elemental phosphorus
- *c* Beryllium
- *d* Arsenic
- *e* Vitamin A intoxication
- *f* Lead
- *g* Bismuth

4 Osteomalacic disorders
- *a* Renal tubular osteomalacia (vitamin D resistance or phosphate diabetes)
- *b* Chronic renal glomerular failure

5 Osteosclerosis (localized) associated with chronic infection

6 Osteosclerotic phase of Paget's disease

7 Osteosclerosis associated with carcinomatous metastases, malignant lymphoma, and hematologic disorders (myeloproliferative disorders, sickle cell disease, leukemia, multiple myeloma, systemic mastocytosis)

8 Osteosclerosis of erythroblastosis fetalis

9 Osteopetrosis
- *a* Infantile (malignant, autosomal recessive form)
- *b* Adult (benign, dominant form)
- *c* Intermediate form with carbonic anhydrase II deficiency and renal tubular acidosis

10 Unclassified diseases
- *a* Pyknodysostosis
- *b* Osteomyelosclerosis
- *c* Hyperostosis corticalis generalisata
- *d* Hyperostosis generalisata with pachydermia
- *e* Hereditary hyperphosphatasia
- *f* Progressive diaphyseal dysplasia (osteopathia hyperostotica multiplex infantilis; Camurati-Engelmann disease)
- *g* Melorheostosis
- *h* Osteopoikilosis
- *i* Hyperostosis frontalis interna

bone may be of the woven type, but if the process is more chronic, true lamellar bone is formed. The additional bone may be located at the periosteum, within the compact bone of the cortex, or in the trabeculae of the cancellous regions. In the medullary area, the new bone is deposited on and between the trabeculae and encroaches upon the medullary spaces. Typical examples of such responses are seen in areas adjacent to tumors or in association with infection. In some diseases the increase in bone mass may be spotty, as in osteopoikilosis, whereas in others most of the skeleton may be involved, as in the malignant form of osteopetrosis in children. The increase in mass is usually not due to an excessive amount of mineral relative to matrix, except in disorders such as osteopetrosis where islands of calcified cartilage may persist. (The mineral density of calcified cartilage is greater than that of bone.) In some diseases such as the osteosclerosis of renal insufficiency, the bone mass and radiodensity may be increased, even though the new bone formed is poorly mineralized and contains widened osteoid seams.

Several of these conditions are discussed in more detail in other chapters, although some generalizations are pertinent. Bone that is denser than normal may be seen occasionally in the osteitis fibrosa associated with active hyperparathyroidism. When the hyperparathyroidism is successfully treated, the rate of bone resorption decreases abruptly out of proportion to the rate of bone formation; this imbalance may lead to the production of areas of bone density greater than in the surrounding skeleton, especially in the healing of brown tumors. In hypothyroidism, the rates of both bone formation and resorption may be decreased, but when the balance is in favor of formation bones are of increased density but normal architecture. Increased bone density also occurs in some instances of osteomalacia associated with disturbances in renal tubular function. The increased mass of bone occurs together with widened osteoid seams, as in chronic renal glomerular insufficiency. In the vertebral bodies the bone appears denser in transverse bands at the upper and lower margins, with a relatively radiolucent center. This "sandwich" appearance is similar to that seen in some patients with osteopetrosis and has been termed by the British the *rugger jersey sign*.

OSTEOPETROSIS Osteopetrosis (marble bone disease) is clinically, biochemically, and genetically heterogeneous. The most severe form in infants can be ascribed to defects in differentiation and/or function of osteoclasts. Several different types of hereditary osteopetrosis which resemble the infantile human disease have been described in rodents, and in some the disorder can be cured by engraftment of hematopoietic cells from a normal donor. In humans infantile osteopetrosis is manifested in utero and progresses after birth with marked anemia, hepatosplenomegaly, hydrocephalus, cranial nerve involvement, and death, often due to infection. Some attempts to transplant bone marrow from normal donors to provide normal osteoclast precursor cells have been successful, and osteopetrotic bone has been repopulated with functioning osteoclasts of donor origin and radiologic and/or bone biopsy evidence of bone resorption. In some individuals with osteopetrosis, defects have also been recognized in peripheral blood monocyte function. In other cases of osteopetrosis, clinical improvement has been obtained using high doses of calcitriol.

The less fulminant adult form is inherited as an autosomal dominant trait, and the anemia is not as severe, neurologic abnormalities are not as frequent, and recurrent pathologic fractures are the main feature. Although most cases are in infants and children, many are discovered first in adult life when roentgenograms are obtained because of fractures or unrelated diseases. There is no particular predilection for either sex.

In kindreds where it has been associated with renal tubular acidosis and cerebral calcification, osteopetrosis is inherited as an autosomal recessive defect, is compatible with long survival, and is associated with a deficiency of one of the isoenzymes of carbonic anhydrase (carbonic anhydrase II). Disturbances in bone resorption may result from failure to secrete hydrogen ions at sites of bone resorption.

Both bone formation and resorption are depressed, particularly resorption. Islands of unresorbed calcified cartilage are frequently encased in bone. The defect in remodeling results in disorganization of bone structure with thickened cortices and lack of funnelization of metaphyses. Despite its increased density, the bone is abnormal mechanically and fractures readily. Osteomalacia or rickets is sometimes a component of the osteopetrosis in children (Fig. 339-1).

The histologic changes are reflected in the roentgenograms (Fig. 339-2), which reveal uniformly dense, sclerotic bone often without distinction between the cortical and cancellous regions. There is

FIGURE 339-1 *Lateral roentgenogram of the thorax of a 9-month-old boy with the "malignant" form of osteopetrosis. Note the uniform increase in mineral density of the vertebral bodies and the marked flaring of the ends of the ribs (arrows), indicative of rickets.*

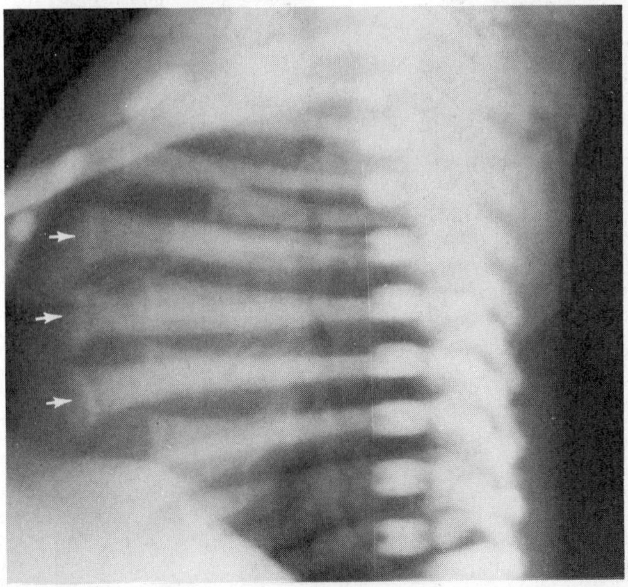

persistence of the primary spongiosa with central calcified cartilage cores surrounded by woven bone. Osteoclasts are often increased in number but apparently do not function properly. Osteoclasts may be morphologically normal or have loss of their ruffled borders suggesting that a spectrum of changes may occur. The variability may reflect heterogeneity in this syndrome, as in the osteopetrosis that occurs spontaneously in rodents. The long bones are usually involved, with increased density along the entire shaft. Foci of increased density may be seen in the epiphyses corresponding to regions of unresorbed calcified cartilage. The metaphyses have a characteristic clubbed or splayed appearance. Horizontal bandings of increased density alternating with zones of decreased density in the long bones and vertebrae suggest that the defect may be intermittent during periods of growth. The skull, pelvis, ribs, and other bones may also be involved. The phalanges and the distal humerus may appear normal when the disease is not severe.

Encroachment of bone upon the marrow cavity is associated with anemia of the myelophthisic type with foci of extramedullary hematopoiesis in liver, spleen, and lymph nodes and enlargement of these organs. In the malignant form of the disease the abundant osteoclasts may crowd out the hematopoietic marrow. Neurologic abnormalities are associated with encroachment on cranial nerves, which may result in optic atrophy, nystagmus, papilledema, exophthalmos, and impairment of extraocular motility. Facial paralysis and deafness are frequent; trigeminal lesions and anosmia have also been described. In infants with severe disease, macrocephaly, hydrocephalus, and convulsions may occur. Infections such as osteomyelitis are frequent in these children. Renal tubular acidosis is also a feature of the form of osteopetrosis associated with a deficiency in carbonic anhydrase II.

In the milder dominant osteopetrosis, about half of the patients have no symptoms, and the disorder is discovered incidentally on roentgenograms. Other such patients present because of fractures, bone pain, osteomyelitis, and cranial nerve palsies.

Fractures are a common complication even with trivial trauma.

FIGURE 339-2 *Roentgenogram of the spine and pelvis of a 55-year-old man with the more benign, dominant form of osteopetrosis.*

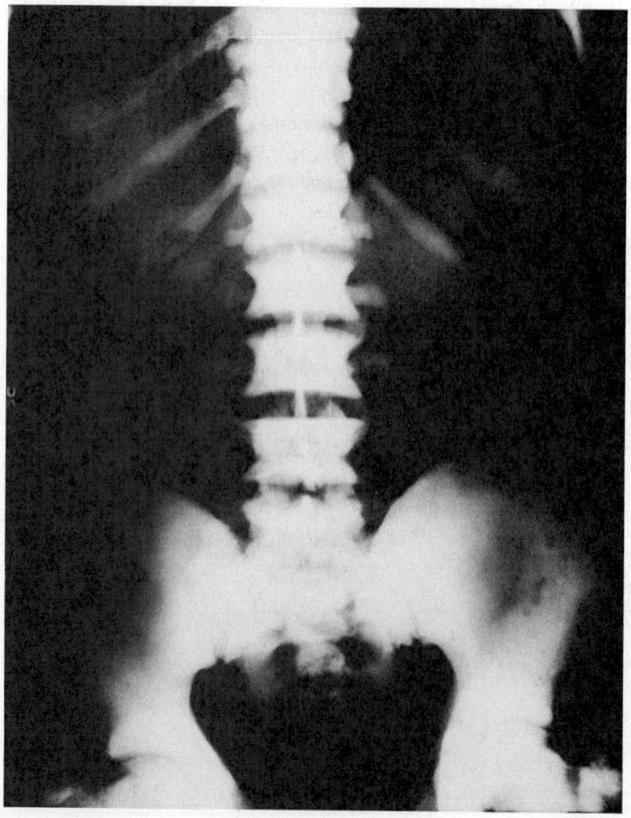

Healing of such fractures is usually satisfactory, although delayed union may occur. When the disease is manifested first in adult life, fractures may be the only clinical problem. Levels of calcium and alkaline phosphatase in the plasma are usually normal in adults, although in children hypophosphatemia and, occasionally, moderate hypocalcemia have been noted. Serum acid phosphatase levels are usually increased.

The skeletal defect is not the same in all forms of osteopetrosis, and within a clinical subtype genetic and biochemical heterogeneity is common. As mentioned, several children with severe osteopetrosis have received bone marrow transplants from HLA-identical siblings which resulted in histologic and radiologic increases in bone resorption, accompanied by improvement in anemia, vision, hearing, and growth and development. In one report, donor (male) nuclei were identified by Y-chromosome analysis in recipient (female) osteoclasts.

Unfortunately, it is not always possible to find appropriate donors for bone marrow transplantation, or patients may not be good candidates to receive transplants. Patients with the lethal forms have been treated with calcitriol. This therapy is associated with appearance of osteoclasts with normal ruffled borders and other evidence for increased bone resorption.

PYKNODYSOSTOSIS *Pyknodysostosis* resembles osteopetrosis but is usually a more benign condition not associated with hepatosplenomegaly, anemia, or cranial nerve involvement. In addition to a generalized increase in bone density, features include short stature, separated cranial sutures, hypoplasia of the mandible, persistence of deciduous teeth, and progressive acroosteolysis of the terminal phalanges. Life span is usually unaffected, and the patient usually presents because of frequent fractures. Pyknodysostosis is inherited as an autosomal recessive trait. In one case levels of plasma calcitonin were intermittently elevated, and the response of the plasma calcitonin to infusions of calcium and glucagon was exaggerated. The gene that causes this disorder may be located on the short arm of a small acrocentric chromosome.

OSTEOMYELOSCLEROSIS *Osteomyelosclerosis* is a disorder in which the marrow cells are replaced by diffuse fibroplasia, occasionally accompanied by osseous metaplasia. When the latter is prominent, increased skeletal density is seen on roentgenograms. In early stages woven bone may be found in intratrabecular locations whereas in more advanced stages woven bone is observed in the medulla. The disorder is probably a phase in the course of the myeloproliferative disorders and is characteristically accompanied by extramedullary hematopoiesis.

Hyperostosis corticalis generalisata (van Buchem's disease) is characterized by osteosclerosis of the skull (base and calvaria), lower jaw, clavicles, and ribs, and thickening of the diaphyseal cortices of the long and short bones. Alkaline phosphatase levels in the serum are elevated, and the disorder may be due to increased formation of bone of normal structure. The major manifestations are due to neural compression and consist of optic atrophy, facial paralysis, and perception deafness. In *hyperostosis generalisata with pachydermia* (Uehlinger), the sclerosis is due to increased formation of subperiosteal spongy bone and involves the epiphyses, metaphyses, and diaphyses. Pain, swelling of joints, and thickening of the skin of the lower arms are common.

HEREDITARY HYPERPHOSPHATASIA This disorder is characterized by severe structural deformities of the skeleton with increase in thickness of the calvaria, large homogeneous areas of increased density at the base of the skull, and widening and loss of normal architecture of the shafts and the epiphyses of the long and short bones. There is a failure to deposit normal bone, with haphazard orientation of lamellae suggesting active remodeling. Plasma alkaline phosphatase levels and urinary excretion of hydroxyproline peptides and other collagen degradation products are markedly increased. The disorder is apparently inherited as an autosomal recessive trait. Calcitonin therapy may be of value in some of these patients.

PROGRESSIVE DIAPHYSEAL DYSPLASIA A disorder in which a symmetric thickening and increased diameter of the diaphyses of long bones occurs, particularly in femurs, tibias, fibulas, radii, and ulnas, has been termed *progressive diaphyseal dysplasia* (Camurati-Engelmann disease). Pain over affected areas, fatigue, abnormal gait, and muscle wasting are the major manifestations. Serum alkaline phosphatase levels may be elevated and, on occasion, hypocalcemia and hyperphosphatemia may be found. Other abnormalities include anemia, leukopenia, and elevated erythrocyte sedimentation rate. Clinical and biochemical improvement may result from the use of glucocorticoids.

MELORHEOSTOSIS This rare condition usually begins in childhood and is characterized by areas of sclerosis in the bones of one limb. All segments of the bone may be involved, with sclerotic areas that have a ''flowing'' distribution. The involved limb is often extremely painful.

OSTEOPOIKILOSIS This benign disorder is usually discovered by chance and is not associated with symptoms. It is characterized by dense spots of trabecular bone less than a centimeter in diameter, usually of uniform density, that are located in the epiphyses and adjacent parts of the metaphyses. All bones may be involved except the skull, ribs, and vertebrae.

HYPEROSTOSIS FRONTALIS INTERNA *Hyperostosis frontalis interna* is an abnormality of the inner table of the frontal bones of the skull consisting of smooth, rounded enostoses covered by dura and projecting into the cranial cavity. These enostoses are usually less than 1 cm at their greatest diameter and usually do not extend posteriorly beyond the coronal suture. The abnormality is found almost exclusively in women, who are frequently obese, hirsute, and who have a variety of neuropsychiatric complaints (Morgagni-Stewart-Morel syndrome). However, hyperostosis frontalis interna also occurs in women with no obvious illness or particular associated disease. The finding in the skull may be a manifestation of a generalized metabolic disorder.

NEOPLASMS OF BONE

Primary neoplasms of the skeletal system reflect in their histology the cellular and extracellular components of the skeleton. However, it is not always possible to prove that a tumor arises from the same type of tissue that it produces. The precursor cells of bone tissue are probably derived from distinct cell lines in which the osteoclasts arise from hematopoietic cells and the osteoblasts arise from the stromal cell system. The primitive stromal cell could differentiate into chondroblasts and fibroblasts as well as osteoblasts. Neoplasms can arise from all these cell types. Each of these cells can produce its characteristic extracellular matrix, and neoplasms arising from them may thus be recognized. Primary neoplasms of bone can arise also from other hematopoietic, vascular, and neural elements.

PATHOPHYSIOLOGY Neoplasms in bone induce resorption of skeletal tissue. This bone resorption results from production by the tumor cells of factors that stimulate osteoclast function and/or recruitment and differentiation of the osteoclast hematopoietic precursor cells. Some of these factors are ''parathyroid hormone–like'' but immunologically and chemically different from the normal hormone. These factors, whose structures have not yet been elucidated, interact with the parathyroid hormone receptor or a similar receptor. Other resorption-inducing factors are related to transforming growth factors alpha and beta, platelet-derived growth factor, or interleukin 1. What has been termed ''osteoclast-activating factor'' includes interleukin 1 and other polypeptides produced by T lymphocytes. Prostaglandin production by some tumors may also mediate bone resorption. T lymphocytes infected with some viruses can metabolize circulating 25(OH)D to $1,25(OH)_2D$, which may also stimulate bone resorption. Tumors may also alter blood supply to bone by obstructing vessels or inducing angiogenesis. Tumors may also produce reaction in surrounding bone and alter the normal contour. The epiphyseal plate, articular cartilage, cortex, and periosteum of bone often offer a barrier to the spread of neoplastic tissue. Alteration of the contour of the cortex is not due to ''expansion'' but to remodeling of the bone in the area and formation of new bone with the new contour. Some tumors induce primarily an osteoblastic or sclerotic reaction in surrounding bone, which results in increased radiodensity. Primary neoplasms may be less radiopaque than surrounding bone or more radiopaque, depending upon the degree of calcification or ossification of the matrix and the density of the tissue. Bone tumors may be recognized because of (1) the presence of a mass in the soft tissues, (2) deformity of a bone, (3) pain and tenderness, or (4) pathologic fractures. Tumors of bone may also be detected incidentally on roentgenograms obtained for other reasons. Although it is usually possible to classify bone tumors as benign or malignant, prediction of the clinical outcome on histologic and radiologic criteria is not always possible.

The extent of the lesions should be defined by standard and computerized tomographic techniques and magnetic resonance imaging, if available. Lesions can also be assessed by bone scans utilizing ^{99m}Tc polyphosphonate. There are numerous pitfalls in the clinical diagnosis and interpretation of histologic features of tumors of bone. However, proper evaluation and selection of therapy require evaluation of both radiographic and histologic features. Management, therefore, requires cooperation of the orthopedist, oncologist, radiologist, radiotherapist, and pathologist.

BENIGN TUMORS The most common benign tumors are *osteochondromas* (exostoses) and *endochondromas* (which may be multiple in Ollier's disease), *benign giant cell tumors, unicameral bone cysts, osteoid osteomas,* and *nonossifying fibromas* (fibrous cortical defects). As a rule benign tumors are not painful except for osteoid osteomas, benign chondroblastomas, and benign chondromyxoidfibroma. The usual clinical problem is that of slowly progressing mass, pathologic fracture, or deformity. Treatment is usually accomplished by resection or curettage and bone grafting. When wide resection of tissue is necessary, insertion of metal and plastic prostheses or allograft transplantation may preserve limb function.

MALIGNANT TUMORS The most common malignant tumor of bone is multiple myeloma (see Chap. 258). Primary lymphoma may also arise locally in bone. Malignant tumors of nonhematopoietic origin include osteosarcomas, chondrosarcomas, fibrosarcomas, and Ewing's tumor. Giant cell tumors may be included here since they may metastasize and are locally destructive. *Osteogenic sarcomas* are presumed to arise from osteoprogenitor cells and have a wide variation in histopathology, with at least six histologic types. These tumors always contain woven bone at least in small foci, and may contain in addition cartilaginous and fibrous elements. They are most common in the second and third decades and are less common under the age of 10 and over the age of 40. When they occur in older individuals, some predisposing cause is usually present such as Paget's disease, prior exposure to ionizing radiation, or a bone infarct. In primary osteogenic sarcomas the lesions usually arise in the metaphyseal region of long bones, especially in the distal femur, proximal tibia, and proximal humerus. The most common symptoms are pain and swelling which may be present for weeks or months. The roentgenographic features of osteosarcomas depend upon the degree of bone destruction, the extent to which mineralized bone is formed by and within the tumor, and the type of reaction in the surrounding bone. Thus, the lesions may vary from purely lytic lesions to dense areas containing radiopaque lumps, clouds, or spicules of tumor bone in varying patterns of organization. Discontinuities may occur in the cortex surrounding the lesion. In other cases, hyperostotic periosteal reactions may involve grossly layered bone. If the tumor grows rapidly, it may destroy the cortex and penetrate the soft tissue surrounding the bone; it leaves only a cuff of periosteal new bone at the peripheral margin of the tumor, just at the point of penetration (Codman's triangle). High plasma alkaline phosphatase levels in those sarcomas that are predominantly osteogenic parallel the course of the tumor. When lesions are adequately treated by amputation, chemotherapy, or radiation, the level of alkaline phosphatase falls, and when metastases appear, the level rises again, often reaching values higher than those present initially. When values are initially high, the course is often rapidly fatal. Metastases occur primarily by the hematogenous route especially to the lung.

The prognosis of osteosarcoma was very poor prior to development of effective chemotherapy, with radiologic evidence of pulmonary metastases usually occurring within a year following surgical amputation that was potentially curative. The course varies with the type of tumor; for example, a ''telangiectatic'' variant has a very poor prognosis, unless treated with aggressive chemotherapy, whereas the less common low-grade intramedullary type has a better prognosis. In the typical intramedullary type of osteosarcoma, death occurs within 6 months from the onset of detectable pulmonary metastases, suggesting that the lesions in the lungs were present at the time of amputation or that cells were shed from the tumor during the operation.

Several chemotherapeutic programs are efficacious. The disease-free and overall survival rates of patients with nonmetastatic disease have increased from about 20 percent when the programs were first developed to 60 to 80 percent in 1985. Chemotherapeutic agents include high-dose methotrexate with leukovorum rescue, doxorubicin, cisplatin, and the combination of bleomycin, cyclophosphamide, and dactinomycin. Survival is also improved by resection of pulmonary metastases. Additional approaches include limb-sparing surgical resection and attempts to resect lesions such as pelvic osteosarcomas which were previously considered to be unresectable. Surgery of osteosarcomas, primarily amputation, still has an important place in therapy.

Chondrosarcomas are distinguishable from osteogenic sarcomas. In contrast to the latter, chondrosarcomas usually arise in adulthood and old age, with the peak incidence in the fourth, fifth, and sixth decades. Most are located in the pelvic girdle, ribs, and diaphyseal portions of the femur and humerus; distal portions of the extremities are involved rarely. Chondrosarcomas probably arise by malignant transformation in enchondromas and more rarely in the cartilaginous cap of osteochondromas. As a rule, chondrosarcomas are slow growing and slow to recur. Radiographically the lesions appear destructive, with mottled increases in radiodensity which reflect the variable degree of calcification of cartilaginous matrix and ossification. Radical excision is the treatment of choice. Histologic grading of the tumor can be valuable for predicting prognosis and determining appropriate surgical therapy.

Ewing's tumor This is a malignant sarcoma composed of small, round cells that occurs most frequently in the first three decades of life. Most are located in the long bones, although any bone may be involved. Ewing's sarcoma is highly malignant with a low incidence of cure by ablative surgery with or without radiation. However, combined radiation therapy and chemotherapy with doxorubicin, cyclophosphamide, vincristine, and dactinomycin improves survival of patients with Ewing's sarcoma, including some with metastatic disease.

TUMORS METASTATIC TO BONE The skeleton is a common site for metastases from carcinomas and occasionally even from sarcomas. Skeletal metastases may be silent or produce symptoms by the same mechanisms as primary tumors, i.e., pain, swelling, deformity, encroachment on hematopoietic tissue in the marrow, compression of spinal cord or nerve roots, and pathologic fractures. In addition, rapidly lytic skeletal metastases can result in hypercalcemia. The bones involved most commonly are the vertebrae, proximal femur, pelvis, ribs, sternum, and proximal humerus, in that order of frequency. The carcinomas that most frequently metastasize to bone arise in prostate, breast, lung, thyroid, kidney, and bladder. Malignant cells reach the skeleton via the bloodstream. Those that survive may proliferate and distort the normal architecture, probably by production of substances that cause dissolution of both mineral phase and organic matrix.

Osteolysis most often results from modulation of osteoprogenitor cells to osteoclasts in the surrounding bone. Some mediators involved in induction of osteoclasts were described earlier in this section. Some carcinoma cells may also act directly to resorb bone. Carcinomatous metastases (which are usually predominantly osteolytic) arise from thyroid, kidney, and lower bowel. Other tumors induce *osteoblastic* response in which the new bone does not arise from the tumor itself, but is induced from normal skeletal cells by some product(s) of the tumor cells. The resulting lesion may be more dense than the surrounding tissue. Occasionally the increase in radiodensity is uniform, simulating osteosclerosis. Carcinoma of the prostate characteristically produces osteoblastic metastases. Carcinoma of the breast can cause both osteolytic and osteoblastic metastases. Malignant carcinoid tumors arising from the embryonic foregut and hindgut metastasize to bone with high frequency, producing an osteoblastic reaction. Hodgkin's disease in bone also produces an osteoblastic response both focal and diffuse. More malignant lymphomas in bone produce predominantly destructive lesions. As a rule, osteolytic metastases are the ones associated with hypercalcemia, hypercalciuria, and increased excretion of hydroxyproline-containing peptides (reflecting matrix destruction); they are usually associated with normal or only slightly increased levels of serum alkaline phosphatase. Osteoblastic metastases, on the other hand, may cause more marked elevations of serum alkaline phosphatase and may be associated with hypocalcemia. With some metastases (as in carcinoma of the breast) there may be phases in which osteolysis predominates (with hypercalciuria, hypercalcemia, and normal alkaline phosphatase levels) alternating with phases in which alkaline phosphatase levels rise and the skeletal lesions become more sclerotic.

Treatment of skeletal metastases is usually palliative. In slowly growing localized lesions (as in some instances of carcinoma of the thyroid or occasionally in carcinoma of the kidney), local radiation is useful to relieve pain or reduce compression of surrounding structures. Many patients with carcinomas of breast or prostate survive for years even after extensive skeletal metastases are recognized. Castration and estrogen therapy or receptor antagonists may slow the progress of the lesions in patients with metastatic prostatic carcinoma (see Chap. 298). When patients with mammary cancer are treated with estrogens or androgens, the character of the reaction to the metastases may temporarily shift from a predominantly osteoblastic to a lytic phase with resultant hypercalcemia (see Chap. 295). Plicamycin, which inhibits osteoclast function and is effective in treating hypercalcemia associated with malignant disease, may also be useful in palliation of osteolytic metastases. Etidronate, which has been used to decrease bone resorption in Paget's disease, also decreases the bone resorption secondary to malignant disease. The bone pain in patients with metastatic carcinoma may be relieved by the use of levodopa. Hypercalcemia in patients with malignant tumors is not due solely to skeletal metastases, although this is the most common cause. Production of circulating stimulators of osteoclast activity by extraosseous neoplasms is one cause of the humoral hypercalcemia of malignancy. Hypercalcemia per se, whether spontaneous or induced by therapy, may produce anorexia, polyuria, polydipsia, depression, and eventually coma. In addition, nephrocalcinosis can result from hypercalcemia, and death may result from renal insufficiency.

OTHER DISORDERS OF BONE AND CARTILAGE

FIBROUS DYSPLASIA (ALBRIGHT'S SYNDROME) This syndrome is characterized by osteitis fibrosa disseminata, areas of pigmentation, and endocrine dysfunction, with precocious puberty in females. The bony lesions, called *fibrous dysplasia,* may occur in the absence of the other features. The fundamental nature of the disorder is unknown; the disease does not appear to be heritable, although it has been

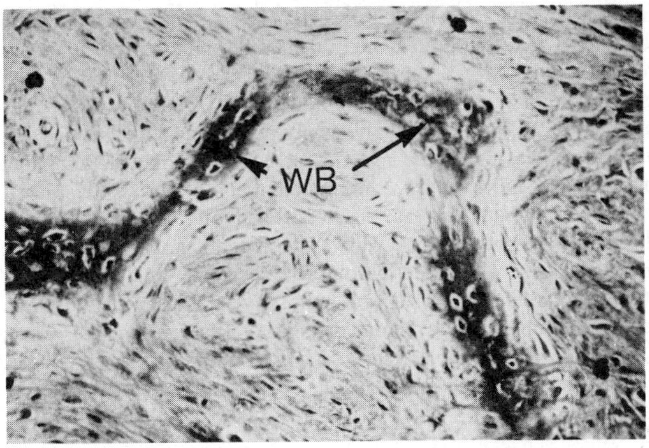

FIGURE 339-3 *Photomicrograph of the lesion of fibrous dysplasia. Note spicules of dark-staining woven bone (WB) surrounded by loose fibroblastic tissue.*

reported to affect monozygotic twins. The disease occurs with equal frequency in both sexes.

Incidence The disease may be divided into three main categories: (1) monostotic, (2) polyostotic, and (3) Albright's syndrome and its variants. The monostotic form is the most common. It can be asymptomatic or lead to a pathologic fracture. The majority of the lesions are in the ribs or in the craniofacial bones, especially the maxillas. Many other bones may be affected, however, such as metaphyseal or diaphyseal portions of the proximal femurs or tibias. Monostotic fibrous dysplasia is most often diagnosed between 20 and 30 years of age. There are usually no associated skin lesions. Approximately a quarter of the individuals with the polyostotic form have more than half the skeleton involved by disease. One side of the body may be affected, and the lesions may be distributed segmentally in a limb, particularly in the lower extremities. Craniofacial lesions are present in approximately half of patients with the polyostotic form. Whereas the monostotic form is usually detected in young adults, fractures and skeletal deformities occur in childhood in the polyostotic form; the disease is generally more severe and deforming with early clinical onset. Lesions, especially monostotic lesions, may become quiescent around the time of puberty and may worsen during pregnancy. Albright's syndrome is more common in females. Short stature is ascribed to premature closure of the epiphyses. The most frequent extraskeletal manifestations are the skin lesions.

Pathology All forms of fibrous dysplasia have an identical histologic appearance, although cartilage is more commonly involved in the polyostotic form. The marrow cavity is filled by gritty, gray-pink, rubbery tissue that replaces the normal cancellous bone. Often, the endosteal cortical surface is scalloped. Histologically, the lesions contain benign-appearing fibroblastic tissue arranged in a loose whorled pattern (Fig. 339-3). The grittiness is due to irregularly arranged woven bone spicules, most of which lack osteoblastic palisading or rimming, which are embedded in the fibrous tissue. These bone spicules may also have prominent cement lines. In approximately 10 percent of cases, islands of hyaline cartilage are present, and more rarely, myxoid tissue may predominate in young patients. Examination by polarized light and with the use of special stains indicates a contiguity of collagen fibers of the osseous and marrow tissue. In the polyostotic form cystic degeneration may be characterized by the presence of hemorrhage with hemosiderin-containing macrophages and osteoclast-type giant cells in the periphery of the cyst. Malignant degeneration into a sarcoma (osteosarcoma, chondrosarcoma, fibrosarcoma) occurs rarely, and in most instances these sarcomas arise in previously radiated lesions. Ossifying fibroma of long bones is a peculiar fibroosseous cortical lesion which may be a variant of fibrous dysplasia. It is most common in the tibial shaft of teenagers. Although benign, the lesion has a tendency to recur if not adequately excised.

Radiologic changes The roentgenographic appearance of the lesions is that of a radiolucent area with a well-delineated, smooth or scalloped border, typically associated with focal thinning of the cortex of the bone (Fig. 339-4). Fibrous dysplasia and Paget's disease of bone are two disorders that can cause a bone to become larger than normal. The lesions of fibrous dysplasia are not usually cysts in the strict sense, since they are not fluid-filled cavities. They occasionally appear multiloculate. The so-called ground glass appearance reflects the content of the thin spicules of calcified, woven bone. Frequently, deformities are present such as coxa vara, shepherd's-crook deformity of the femur, bowing of the tibia, Harrison's grooves, and protrusio acetabuli. Involvement of facial bones, usually with lesions of increased radiodensity, may create a leonine appearance (leontiasis ossea) superficially resembling leprosy. Fibrous dysplasia of the temporal bones can cause progressive loss of hearing and obliteration of the external ear canal. Advanced skeletal age in females is correlated with sexual precocity but may also be seen in males without sexual precocity. The lesions tend to spare the epiphyseal regions before puberty, but in older individuals fibrous dysplasia may develop in the epiphyses. Occasionally, a focus of fibrous dysplasia may undergo cystic degeneration with an enormous distortion of the shape of the bone, and mimic the so-called aneurysmal bone cyst.

Clinical picture The clinical course is highly variable. Skeletal lesions are usually detected because of deformity or fractures. Symptoms ascribable to bone involvement are headache, seizures, cranial nerve abnormalities, hearing loss, narrowing of the external

FIGURE 339-4 *Roentgenogram of the upper extremity from a 33-year-old woman with fibrous dysplasia of bone. Typical lesions involve the entire humerus as well as the scapula and proximal ulna.*

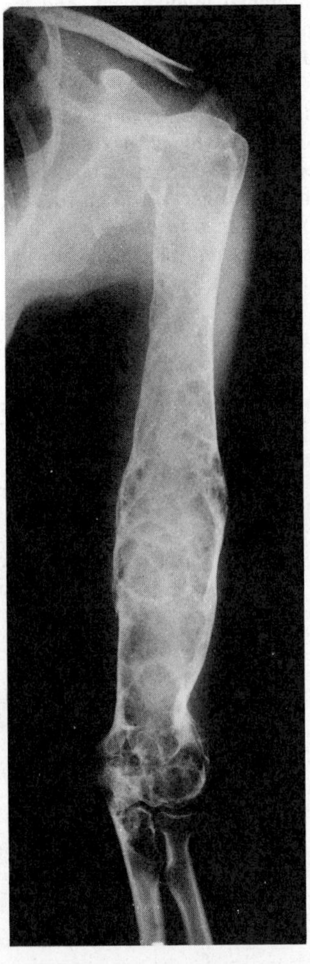

ear canal, or even spontaneous scalp hemorrhages if there is craniofacial bone disease. In some females and even less commonly in males sexual precocity is the presenting complaint, occasionally before the appearance of skeletal symptoms. Serum calcium and phosphorus values are usually normal. In approximately one-third of patients levels of serum alkaline phosphatase may be elevated to high values, and urinary hydroxyproline excretion is often increased. In some subjects, high cardiac output similar to that in extensive Paget's disease may be found. In general, patients with extensive involvement have widespread disease when symptoms first appear, whereas when disease is mild at the onset extensive disease does not usually develop.

The cutaneous pigmentation in most patients with Albright's syndrome consists of isolated dark-brown to light-brown macules which tend to remain on one side of the midline (Fig. 339-5). The border is usually, although not always, irregular or jagged ("coast of Maine") in contrast to the smooth borders of the pigmented macules of neurofibromatosis ("coast of California"). As a rule there are fewer than six of the lesions, which range in size from 1 cm to those covering very large areas, particularly the back, buttocks, or sacral regions. When the lesions are present in the scalp, the overlying hair may be more deeply pigmented than that over the remainder of the scalp. Localized alopecia is associated with osteomas of the skin, and such lesions tend to have concordance with the skeletal lesions. The pigmentation tends to be on the same side as the skeletal lesions and actually overlie them.

The sexual precocity of unknown cause is found in females and rarely in males (see also Chaps. 330 and 331). Premature vaginal bleeding and development of axillary and pubic hair and of breasts are the main features. In the few ovaries that have been examined, no corpora lutea have been seen. The cause of the precocious sexuality is still not clear. In the few cases where measurements have been reported, the girls have high estrogen levels and low or undetectable gonadotropins. In one studied case gonadotropin levels did not respond to luteinizing hormone–releasing hormone (LHRH). Precocious sexuality is not limited to patients with cranial involvement, and the characteristic pigmented macules are usual but not invariable. Another endocrine abnormality with increased frequency is hyperthyroidism. Rarer associations include Cushing's syndrome, acromegaly, possibly hypogonadotropic hypogonadism, and soft tissue myxomas. Hypophosphatemic osteomalacia may also accompany fibrous dysplasia and resembles the disorder associated with other skeletal and nonskeletal tumors. As mentioned, sarcomatous degeneration may rarely occur in fibrous dysplasia. Sarcomatous changes are found only in a focus of preexisting fibrous dysplasia, are more common in the polyostotic forms, and have usually been associated with previous radiation of the lesions.

Although the lytic lesions of fibrous dysplasia resemble the brown tumors of hyperparathyroidism, the age of the patient, normal calcium levels, increased density of bone in the skull, and areas of cutaneous pigmentation identify the former condition. However, fibrous dysplasia and hyperparathyroidism may coexist. Neurofibromas may involve bone and produce cutaneous pigmentation as well as nodules in the skin. The pigmented macules of neurofibromatosis are more numerous and more widely distributed than in fibrous dysplasia, usually have smooth borders, and tend to involve areas such as the axillary folds. Other lesions which have roentgenographic features similar to those of isolated fibrous dysplasia are unicameral bone cysts, aneurysmal bone cysts, and nonossifying fibromas. Leontiasis ossea is most often due to fibrous dysplasia, although other disorders may also produce this appearance such as craniometaphyseal dysplasia, hyperphosphatasia, and, in adults, Paget's disease.

Treatment Fibrous dysplasia is not curable. The symptoms, however, can be managed using a variety of orthopedic procedures such as osteotomy, curettage, and bone grafting. Indications for such procedures include progressive deformity, nonunion of fractures, and pain unresponsive to conservative treatment. Calcitonin may be effective in treatment of widespread disease associated with bone pain and high serum alkaline phosphatase levels (see Chap. 338).

DYSPLASIAS AND CHONDRODYSTROPHIES A variety of diseases of bone and cartilage have been called *dystrophies* or *dysplasias*. The underlying defect is not usually known. It is possible that a biochemical lesion, such as the defect in the metabolism of the mucopolysaccharides in Hunter's and Hurler's syndromes, will also be found in a number of these disorders and permit more than a descriptive classification. However, a useful scheme has been proposed by Rubin based on the consideration of errors in modeling of bone and cartilage (Table 339-2). Other clinical and genetic features form the basis of a classification by Rimoin. Pathologic processes in the skeletal dysplasias may be expressed as a deficiency (hypoplasia) or excess (hyperplasia) in relation to normal development.

Spondyloepiphyseal dysplasia The spondyloepiphyseal dysplasias are disorders in which abnormalities of growth occur in various bones including the vertebrae, pelvis, carpal and tarsal bones, and the epiphyses of tubular bones. On the basis of roentgenographic findings, this group can be divided into (1) those with generalized platyspondyly, (2) those with multiple epiphyseal dysplasias, and (3) those with epiphysometaphyseal dysplasias. *Morquio's syndrome,* a mucopolysaccharidosis inherited as an autosomal recessive trait and associated with corneal opacities, dental defects, variable disturbances in intellect, and increased urinary excretion of keratosulfate, belongs in the first group. Other forms of spondyloepiphyseal dysplasias show no abnormality in mucopolysaccharide metabolism and are sometimes

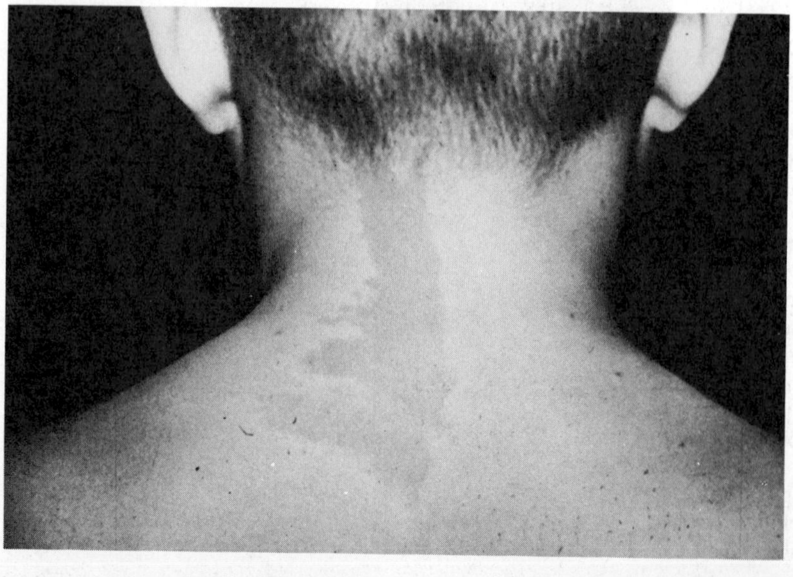

FIGURE 339-5 *Typical pigmented café au lait lesion of the skin in an 11-year-old boy with polyostotic fibrous dysplasia. The border has the jagged "coast of Maine" appearance that is characteristic of Albright's syndrome. Note that the lesion is limited to one side (left) of the body.*

TABLE 339-2 Working classification of bone dysplasias

I Epiphyseal dysplasias
- *A* Epiphyseal hypoplasias
  - *1* Failure of articular cartilage: spondyloepiphyseal dysplasia, congenita and tarda
  - *2* Failure of ossification of center: multiple epiphyseal dysplasia, congenita and tarda
- *B* Epiphyseal hyperplasia
  - *1* Excess of articular cartilage: dysplasia epiphysialis hemimelica

II Physeal (growth plate) dysplasias
- *A* Cartilage hypoplasias
  - *1* Failure of proliferating cartilage: achondroplasia, congenita and tarda
  - *2* Failure of hypertrophic cartilage: metaphyseal dysostosis, congenita and tarda
- *B* Cartilage hyperplasias
  - *1* Excess of proliferating cartilage: hyperchondroplasia
  - *2* Excess of hypertrophic cartilage: enchondromatosis

III Metaphyseal dysplasias
- *A* Metaphyseal hypoplasias
  - *1* Failure to form primary spongiosa: hypophosphatasia, congenita and tarda
  - *2* Failure to absorb primary spongiosa: osteopetrosis, congenita and tarda
  - *3* Failure to absorb secondary spongiosa: craniometaphyseal dysplasia, congenita and tarda
- *B* Metaphyseal hyperplasia
  - *1* Excessive spongiosa: familial exostosis

IV Diaphyseal dysplasias
- *A* Diaphyseal hypoplasias
  - *1* Failure of periosteal bone formation: osteogenesis imperfecta, congenita and tarda
  - *2* Failure of endosteal bone formation: idiopathic osteoporosis
- *B* Diaphyseal hyperplasias
  - *1* Excessive periosteal bone formation: Engelmann's disease
  - *2* Excessive periosteal bone formation: hyperphosphatasia

not recognized until late in childhood. Flat vertebral bodies are associated with other abnormalities in shape and alignment. The disordered development of the capital femoral epiphyses leads to irregularities in shape and flattening of the femoral heads and early onset of osteoarthritis of the hips.

Achondroplasia *Achondroplasia* is a physeal dysplasia in which dwarfism results from decrease in the proliferation of cartilage in the growth plate. This disorder is among the more common types of dwarfism and is inherited as an autosomal dominant trait. Histologic sections through the growth plate show a thin zone of cartilage cells with absence or abbreviation of the normal columnar arrangement and zone of provisional calcification, although endochondral ossification may not be completely disorganized. Formation of the primary spongiosa is reduced since there is often a transverse bar of bone sealing off the plate from further endochondral ossification. However, formation and maturation of the secondary ossification centers and articular cartilage are not disturbed. Appositional growth at the metaphysis continues, with resulting flare in this region of the bone; intramembranous bone formation at the periosteum is normal. The abnormal proliferation at the growth plate, leaving other areas relatively unaffected in the tubular bones, causes production of short bones that are proportionately thick. However, the length of the spine is almost always normal. The appearance of short limbs with a normal trunk is characteristically accompanied by a large head, saddlenose, and an exaggerated lumbar lordosis. The disease is usually recognized at birth. Those who survive the period of infancy usually have normal mental and sexual development, and life span may be normal. However, spinal deformity may lead to cord compression and nerve root encroachment, especially in those with kyphoscoliosis. Homozygous achondroplasia is a more serious disorder and a cause of neonatal death.

Enchondromatosis (dyschondroplasia, Ollier's disease) This is also a disorder affecting the growth plate in which the hypertrophic cartilage is not resorbed and ossified in a normal fashion. It results in masses of cartilage with disorderly arrangement of the chondrocytes showing variable proliferative and hypertrophic changes. These masses are located in the metaphyses in close association with the growth plate in very young patients but often are diaphyseal in teenagers and young adults. The disorder is usually recognized in childhood by the appearance of deformities or retardation in growth. The most common sites of involvement are the ends of long bones, usually in the region where rate of growth is most marked. The pelvis is often involved, but ribs, sternum, and skull are seldom affected. There is also a tendency toward unilateral involvement. Chondrosarcoma develops occasionally in the enchondromata. The association of enchondromatosis and cavernous hemangiomata in the soft tissues including the skin is known as Maffucci's syndrome.

Multiple exostoses (diaphyseal aclasis or osteochondromatosis) This is a disorder of the metaphysis, inherited as an autosomal dominant character, in which areas of the growth plate become displaced, presumably by growing through a defect in the perichondrium or so-called ring of Ranvier. The spongiosa forms within the mass as vessels invade the cartilage. Therefore, the diagnostic radiographic finding is the direct continuity of the mass to the marrow cavity of the parent bone with absence of underlying cortex. Usually the growth of these exostoses ceases when growth of the adjacent plate ceases. The lesions may be solitary or multiple and are usually located in the metaphyseal areas of long bones with the apex of the exostosis directed toward the diaphysis. Often the lesions produce no symptoms, but occasionally interference with the function of a joint or tendon or compression of nerves may result. Dwarfism may occur. The metacarpals may be shortened, resembling those seen in Albright's hereditary osteodystrophy. Multiple exostoses are sometimes seen in patients with pseudohypoparathyroidism.

An exostosis may suddenly begin to enlarge long after growth should have ceased, and rarely chondrosarcomas may develop from the cartilage cap of an exostosis. Pregnancy may stimulate growth of an exostosis that clinically may mimic malignancy. However, the lesion merely undergoes exuberant endochondral ossification and cartilage hyperplasia without malignant changes.

RELAPSING POLYCHONDRITIS See Chap. 278.

TIETZE'S SYNDROME (COSTOCHONDRAL SYNDROME) See Chap. 278.

REFERENCES

Hyperostosis

CANALIS E et al: Dynamic bone morphology and studies on the effects of serum on bone metabolism in vitro in a case of pycnodysostosis. Metab Bone Dis Rel Res 2:99, 1981

CHAN Y-L et al: Dialysis osteodystrophy: A study involving 94 patients. Medicine 64:296, 1985

COCCIA PF et al: Successful bone-marrow transplantation for infantile malignant osteopetrosis. N Engl J Med 302:701, 1980

———: Cells that resorb bone. N Engl J Med 310:456, 1984

COINDRE JM et al: Histomorphometric analysis of sclerotic bone from idiopathic myeloid metaplasia (nine cases). J Pathol 144:163, 1984

CRISP AJ, BRENTON DP: Engelmann's disease of bone—a systemic disorder? Ann Rheum Dis 41:183, 1982

ELMORE SM et al: Pycnodysostosis, with a familial chromosome anomaly. Am J Med 40:273, 1966

GENANT HK et al: Osteosclerosis in primary hyperparathyroidism. Am J Med 59:104, 1975

JACOBSON HG: Dense bone—too much bone: Radiological considerations and differential diagnosis. Part II. Skeletal Radiol 13:97, 1985

JAFFE HL: *Metabolic, Degenerative and Inflammatory Disease of Bones and Joints*. Philadelphia, Lea & Febiger, 1972

JOHNSON CC et al: Osteopetrosis: A clinical, genetic, metabolic and morphologic study of the dominantly inherited benign form. Medicine 47:149, 1968

KEY L et al: Treatment of congenital osteopetrosis with high-dose calcitriol. N Engl J Med 310:409, 1984

LORIA-CORTES R et al: Osteopetrosis in children: A report of 26 cases. J Pediatr 91:43, 1977

MANZKE E et al: Skeletal remodelling and bone-related hormones in two adults with increased bone mass. Metabolism 31:25, 1982

SHELDON J et al: Engelmann's disease (progressive diaphyseal dysplasia): A review and presentation of two cases with abnormal phosphate retention. Metab Bone Dis Rel Res 2:307, 1981

SLY WS et al: Carbonic anhydrase II deficiency in 12 families with the autosomal recessive syndrome of osteopetrosis with renal tubular acidosis and cerebral calcification. N Engl J Med 313:139, 1985

SMITH R et al: Clinical and biochemical studies in Engelmann's disease (progressive diphyseal dysplasia). Q J Med 46:273, 1977
SORELL M et al: Marrow transplantation for juvenile osteopetrosis. Am J Med 70:1280, 1981
THOMPSON RC JR et al: Hereditary hyperphosphatasia. Am J Med 47:209, 1969
VAN BUCHEM FSP et al: Hyperostosis corticalis generalisata. Am J Med 33:387, 1962

Neoplasms of Bone

CHARHON SA et al: Parathyroid function and vitamin D status in patients with bone metastases of prostatic origin. Mineral Electrolyte Metab 11:117, 1985
DOUGLAS DL et al: Effect of dichloromethylene diphosphonate in Paget's disease of bone and in hypercalcemia due to primary hyperparathyroidism or malignant disease. Lancet 1:1043, 1980
ETTINGER LJ et al: Adjuvant adriamycin and cisplatin in newly diagnosed, nonmetastatic osteosarcoma of the extremity. J Clin Oncol 4:353, 1986
FECHNER RE et al: A symposium on the pathology of bone tumors. Pathol Ann 19(Part 1):125, 1984
GOORIN AM et al: Osteosarcoma: Fifteen years later. N Engl J Med 313:165, 1985
HAN M-T et al: Aggressive thoracotomy for pulmonary metastatic osteogenic sarcoma in children and young adolescents. J Pediatr Surg 16:928, 1981
JAFFE HL: *Tumors and Tumorous Conditions of the Bones and Joints*. Philadelphia, Lea & Febiger, 1958
LICHTENSTEIN L: *Bone Tumors*. St. Louis, Mosby, 1972
MANKIN HJ: Current concepts. Advances in diagnosis and treatment of bone tumors. N Engl J Med 300:543, 1979
——— et al: Massive resection and allograft transplantation in the treatment of malignant bone tumors. N Engl J Med 294:1247, 1976
MINTON JP: The response of breast cancer patients with bone pain to L-dopa. Cancer 33:358, 1974
MOSELEY JE: *Bone Changes in Hematologic Disorders*. New York, Grune & Stratton, 1963
MUNDY GR et al: Tumor products and the hypercalcemia of malignancy. J Clin Invest 76:391, 1985
ROSEN G et al: Curability of Ewing's sarcoma and considerations for future therapeutic trials. Cancer 41:888, 1978
——— et al: Primary osteogenic sarcoma: The rationale for preoperative chemotherapy and delayed surgery. Cancer 43:2163, 1979
——— et al: Preoperative chemotherapy for osteogenic sarcoma: Selection of postoperative adjuvant chemotherapy based on the response of the primary tumor to preoperative chemotherapy. Cancer 49:1221, 1982
SCHILLER AL: Diagnosis of borderline cartilage lesions of bone. Semin Diag Pathol 2:42, 1985
SIRIS ES et al: Effects of dichloromethylene diphosphonate on skeletal mobilization of calcium in multiple myeloma. N Engl J Med 302:310, 1980
SUTOW WW et al: Survival after metastasis in osteosarcoma. Natl Cancer Inst Monogr 56:227, 1981
UNNI KK et al: Conditions that simulate primary neoplasms of bone. Pathol Ann 15(Part 1):91, 1980
YUNIS EJ, BARNES L: The histologic diversity of osteosarcoma. Pathol Ann 21(Part 1):121, 1986

Other Disorders of Bone and Cartilage

AKESON WH et al: *Symposium on Heritable Disorders of Connective Tissue*. St. Louis, Mosby, 1982
ALBRIGHT FA et al: Syndrome characterized by osteitis fibrosa disseminata, areas of pigmentation and endocrine dysfunction, with precocious puberty in females: Report of five cases. N Engl J Med 216:727, 1937
BENEDICT PH: Endocrine features in Albright's syndrome (fibrous dysplasia of bone). Metabolism 11:30, 1962
——— et al: Melanotic macules in Albright's syndrome and in neurofibromatosis. JAMA 205:618, 1968
DENT CE, GERTNER JM: Hypophosphatemic osteomalacia in fibrous dysplasia. Q J Med 45:411, 1976
GRABIAS SL, CAMPBELL CJ: Fibrous dysplasia. Orthoped Clin North Am 8:771, 1977
GRAF CJ, PERRET GE: Spontaneous recurrent hemorrhage as an unusual complication of fibrous dysplasia of the skull. J Neurosurg 52:570, 1980
HARRIS RI: Polyostotic fibrous dysplasia with acromegaly. Am J Med 78:539, 1985
HARRIS WH et al: The natural history of fibrous dysplasia: An orthopaedic, pathological and roentgenographic study. J Bone Joint Surg (Br) 44A:207, 1962
LICHTENSTEIN L: Polyostotic fibrous dysplasia. Arch Surg 36:874, 1938
NAGER GT et al: Fibrous dysplasia: A review of the disease and its manifestations in the temporal bone. Ann Otol Rhinol Laryngol 91(suppl 92):1, 1982
RIMOIN DL: The chondrodystrophies. Adv Hum Genet 5:1, 1975
RUBIN P: *Dynamic Classification of Bone Dysplasias*. Chicago, Year Book, 1964
SILLENCE DO et al: Neonatal dwarfism. Pediatr Clin North Am 25:431, 1978
STEENDIJK R: Metabolic bone disease in children, in *Metabolic Bone Disease*, LV Avioli, SM Krane (eds). New York, Academic, 1978, vol II, p 633

340 OSTEOMYELITIS

JAN V. HIRSCHMANN

DEFINITION *Osteomyelitis* denotes infection of bone. While many types of microorganisms, including viruses and fungi, may cause osteomyelitis, it is usually bacterial in origin.

PATHOGENESIS Organisms reach the bone to cause infection by one of three routes: (1) hematogenous spread, (2) extension from a contiguous site of infection, and (3) direct introduction of organisms into bone by trauma, including surgery.

Acute hematogenous osteomyelitis usually involves bone with rich, red marrow; in children the long bones, especially the femur and tibia, are most frequently affected. The infection begins in the metaphyseal sinusoidal veins, where sluggish blood flow and a paucity of phagocytes favor the growth of organisms. In adults acute hematogenous infection rarely involves the long bones, where adipose tissue has largely replaced the red marrow. Instead, hematogenous osteomyelitis most commonly occurs in the vertebrae, where cellular marrow and an abundant vascular supply exist. The organisms reach the spine directly through the nutrient branches of the posterior spinal artery or, probably less commonly, from retrograde flow through the valveless paravertebral venous plexus of Batson, which drains the vertebral bodies, body wall, and the pelvis. Infection usually begins in the vertebral body near the anterior longitudinal ligament and may spread to adjacent vertebrae by direct extension through the disk space or by a system of freely communicating venous channels. Because the disk in adults possesses no vascular supply, disk space infection in *hematogenous* infections is always secondary to osteomyelitis in an adjacent vertebra.

Osteomyelitis caused by extension from a contiguous site of infection may occur with soft tissue suppuration resulting from trauma, necrosis of a malignant tumor, radiation therapy, burns, pressure sores, or other causes. In patients with vascular insufficiency from diabetes mellitus or atherosclerosis, organisms commonly enter the soft tissues through a cutaneous ulcer, usually in the foot, causing cellulitis and subsequently osteomyelitis. Osteomyelitis of the skull bones may result from underlying sinus or dental infections.

Direct introduction of organisms into bone may occur with open fractures, the open surgical reduction of closed fractures, or penetrating trauma by bullets or other foreign bodies. Osteomyelitis may also occur from perioperative contamination of bone during surgery for nontraumatic orthopedic disorders. Most infections of joint prostheses arise in this way. Because the causative organisms, usually flora like *Staphylococcus epidermidis,* are often not very virulent, clinical manifestations may not appear for months after surgery.

PATHOLOGY Pathologic findings during the acute phase include neutrophilic inflammation, edema, and vascular congestion. Because of the bone's rigidity, increased intramedullary pressure develops, compromising the blood supply and causing ischemia, cell death, and vascular thrombosis. After several days, the suppurative and ischemic injury may cause the bone to fragment into devitalized segments called *sequestra*. The inflammation spreads via the haversian and Volkmann canals to reach the periosteum, beneath which abscesses may form or through which the purulent material may penetrate to form soft tissue abscesses or sinus tracts.

With persistent infection, chronic inflammatory cells—lymphocytes, histiocytes, and plasma cells—may join the neutrophils. Fibroblastic proliferation and new bone formation also occur. Osteogenesis from the periosteum may surround the inflammation to form a bony envelope or *involucrum*. Occasionally, a dense fibrous capsule confines the infection to a localized area of suppuration, called *Brodie's abscess*. Rarely, exuberant osteogenesis may result in a sclerotic, nonpurulent osteomyelitis (Garré's sclerosing osteomyelitis).

MANIFESTATIONS Hematogenous osteomyelitis The bacteremia causing hematogenous osteomyelitis may be from a urinary infection, bacterial endocarditis, a distant soft tissue infection, or another location. Frequently, the original site is not apparent. Intravenous drug abusers, in whom *Pseudomonas aeruginosa* is the most common infecting organism, and patients receiving chronic hemodialysis are especially at risk for hematogenous osteomyelitis, presumably because of frequent bacteremias. Diabetes mellitus also seems to be a predisposing condition, perhaps because of impaired neutrophil function and frequent infections of the skin and urinary tract, sites from which bacteremias frequently originate.

Vertebral osteomyelitis may occasionally begin abruptly with back pain and systemic signs of infection, but usually the onset is insidious and the course gradually progressive. Persistent back pain, exacerbated by movement and commonly unrelieved by heat, analgesics, or bed rest, is the predominant symptom. Fever is usually minimal or absent. Physical examination typically reveals tenderness to percussion and palpation over the affected vertebrae, guarding and splinting on movement, and paravertebral muscle spasm.

Leukocytosis is usually absent, but the erythrocyte sedimentation rate is almost always increased. The earliest roentgenographic changes are erosion of the subchondral bony plate, narrowing of the intervertebral disk space, and involvement of the adjacent vertebra. Bony destruction follows, sometimes with loss of vertebral height, usually anteriorly. Anterior osteogenesis with coarse bony density and sclerosis may occur. Soft tissue densities, representing paravertebral abscesses, may lie adjacent to the vertebrae. The lumbar vertebrae are most frequently involved, the cervical vertebrae least. While roentgenographic changes may not develop for several weeks following infection, radionuclide scans with technetium pyrophosphate are positive early.

Complications of vertebral osteomyelitis include anterior extension to cause retropharyngeal abscesses, mediastinitis, empyema, pericarditis, subdiaphragmatic abscess, psoas muscle abscess, or peritonitis, depending upon the vertebrae involved. Posterior extension by pus (epidural abscess), bony fragments, or inflammatory tissue can cause spinal cord compression; if infection penetrates the dura to enter the subarachnoid space, meningitis results.

Acute hematogenous osteomyelitis occurring in sites other than the vertebrae is unusual in adults. When it does develop in such locations as the clavicle or the long bones of the extremities, its typical features are pain and evidence of soft tissue infection over the affected bone.

Hematogenous osteomyelitis acquired in childhood may present in adults as intermittent or persistent drainage from sinus tracts communicating with the involved bone—usually the femur, tibia, or humerus—or as a soft tissue infection overlying it. Signs of infection may recur after months or years of quiescence. Roentgenographic changes include bony destruction with radiolucent areas, radiopaque sequestra, and formation of an involucrum. A roentgenogram of contrast material injected into a sinus tract (sinogram) or computed tomography may help define the location and extent of involvement.

Posttraumatic osteomyelitis and osteomyelitis from a contiguous infection The clinical features of these forms of osteomyelitis are a varying combination of local pain, draining sinuses, and heat, swelling, tenderness, and erythema over the involved bone. Patients often are afebrile. Leukocytosis and an elevated erythrocyte sedimentation rate are present in a minority of patients. Radiographic changes are similar to those in chronic hematogenous osteomyelitis. With plates, nails, screws, pins, or prostheses there is frequently evidence of loosening of the appliance. Radionuclide scans with technetium pyrophosphate are nearly always positive. Since increased uptake in these scans depends in part on bone hyperemia, which may occur with adjacent inflammation alone, there may be difficulty in distinguishing early osteomyelitis from cellulitis or a subcutaneous abscess when the roentgenograms do not show bony destruction.

Infection of joint prostheses may become evident shortly after surgery, especially if the infecting organism is virulent. Erythema, warmth, and draining at the operative site are common findings. More frequently, the onset is later, with persistent pain and loosening of the prosthesis developing 3 to 12 months after surgery. Local signs of infection are typically absent, and the white cell count and erythrocyte sedimentation rate are often normal. Distinction from noninfectious mechanical loosening of the prosthesis can be very difficult and depends on isolation of an organism from the joint by arthrocentesis (although in up to 15 percent of infections the aspirate is sterile), or culture of material obtained at surgery.

DIAGNOSIS While radiographic or radionuclide studies may be helpful, definitive diagnosis requires isolation of the responsible organism. If blood cultures are negative (they usually are), patients with suspected vertebral osteomyelitis should undergo needle aspiration of the intervertebral disk space if it appears infected, percutaneous needle biopsy of the infected bone, or open bone biopsy at surgery. Although *Staphylococcus aureus* is the most common cause, aerobic gram-negative bacilli, typically arising from a previous or concurrent urinary infection, are also frequent. Moreover, pyogenic vertebral osteomyelitis is often impossible to differentiate from tuberculous or fungal vertebral osteomyelitis.

In patients with chronic hematogenous osteomyelitis, posttraumatic osteomyelitis, or osteomyelitis from a contiguous infection, the diagnosis is best established by careful cultures, both aerobic and anaerobic, of bone, tissue, or pus from a deep abscess obtained during surgery. These infections are often polymicrobial and sometimes include anaerobic bacteria; precise bacteriologic identification is necessary for appropriate antimicrobial therapy. Cultures of material obtained from draining sinuses are generally unreliable, even if only a single organism grows, because the tracts may become colonized by bacteria present on the skin surface but absent in the infected bone.

TREATMENT Bed rest and appropriate parenteral antimicrobial agents given for 4 to 6 weeks cure most cases of vertebral osteomyelitis.

The antibiotic(s) used in the treatment of osteomyelitis depend on the result of culture and sensitivity tests; the appropriate drugs are detailed in Chap. 88. In general, the first several weeks of therapy should be parenteral in order to achieve adequate levels of antibiotic in bony tissue. If no organisms are culturable, the choice of the antimicrobial must be based on cultures from other sites or, if these are negative, on the clinician's best estimate of the infecting pathogen. When staphylococcal infection is suspected, a penicillinase-resistant penicillin or a cephalosporin should be used.

External stabilization by traction or brace is indicated for an unstable cervical spine but is unnecessary for most patients with thoracic or lumbar osteomyelitis. Surgery is usually necessary only to drain paravertebral or spinal epidural abscesses. With successful therapy, bony bridging and spontaneous fusion of adjacent vertebral bodies occur, and the erythrocyte sedimentation rate returns to normal.

The main treatment of chronic hematogenous osteomyelitis, posttraumatic osteomyelitis, and osteomyelitis from a contiguous infection is surgery, with antimicrobial therapy an important adjunct. Antibiotics alone rarely cure these infections. The major surgical principles are thorough removal of all necrotic bone and tissue and the elimination of dead space. Rigid bone, unlike soft tissue, does not collapse around a site evacuated of pus; the resultant cavity provides an area for blood, debris, and organisms to collect. This dead space may be obliterated by (1) open packing of the wound, allowing the slow process of granulation to fill the defect, (2) packing the cavity with potentially viable grafts from cancellous bone, (3) transfer of a pedicle of skeletal muscle into the cavity, (4) skin grafting directly onto the granulating bone surface, or (5) constant irrigation to keep the cavity free of debris, followed by one of the methods mentioned above. These surgical measures are accompanied by appropriate parenteral antimicrobial therapy for 3 to 6 weeks. Since there are no controlled studies, the optimal choice and duration of antibiotics are unknown, but antimicrobial therapy is clearly doomed to failure unless the surgical debridement is thorough. Sometimes the location or extent of osteomyelitis makes surgical cure short of amputation impossible. In these patients, if amputation is not performed, treatment is given only for acute exacerbations, such as the formation of overlying soft tissue abscesses, where surgical drainage and a short course of antibiotics help control the acute manifestations.

Osteomyelitis associated with a prosthesis generally requires removal of the appliance, thorough debridement, and appropriate antimicrobial therapy. With either quiescent or low-grade infection, a new prosthesis may be implanted at the same operation as the removal of its predecessor; otherwise, the therapeutic choices are excision arthroplasty or replacement of the prosthesis later when the infection subsides.

Osteomyelitis associated with plates, screws, rods, or pins used for the open reduction of fractures also requires removal of the appliance, thorough debridement, and antimicrobial therapy if union of the fracture has occurred. In infected fractures with nonunion, the principles of treatment are the establishment of rigid bony stability and debridement of infected material to permit union to occur. Screws, plates, pins, and rods that have not loosened are left in place, and the wound is treated with open irrigation. If the hardware is loose and fails to provide rigid stability, it is removed, and stability is attained by other means, such as external fixation with pins above and below the fracture site. When the infection is controlled, bone grafts may be necessary for union to occur, but some fractures will unite without them.

In osteomyelitis associated with vascular insufficiency, cure is seldom possible without amputation. With single bone involvement removal of the infected bone may suffice. When many bones are affected, as is common in osteomyelitis of the feet in diabetics, a below-knee amputation is usually necessary.

REFERENCES

BONEAKDAR-POUR A, GAINES VD: The radiology of osteomyelitis. Orthop Clin North Am 14:21, 1983

BURRI C: *Posttraumatic Osteomyelitis*. Bern, Hans Huber, 1975

FITZGERALD RH, KELLY PJ (eds): Musculoskeletal sepsis. Orthop Clin North Am, July 1984

GRISTINA AG, KOLKIN J: Total joint replacement and sepsis. J Bone Joint Surg 65-A: 128, 1983

LEWIS RP et al: Bone infections involving anaerobic bacteria. Medicine 57:279, 1978

MACKOWIAK PA et al: Diagnostic value of sinus tract cultures in chronic osteomyelitis. JAMA 239:2772, 1978

SUGARMAN B et al: Osteomyelitis beneath pressure sores. Arch Intern Med 143:683, 1983

WALDVOGEL FA et al: Osteomyelitis: A review of clinical features, therapeutic considerations, and unusual aspects. N Engl J Med 282:198, 260, 316, 1970

———, VASEY H: Osteomyelitis: The past decade. N Engl J Med 303:360, 1980

PART TWELVE DISORDERS OF THE CENTRAL AND PERIPHERAL NERVOUS SYSTEM

section 1 Disorders of the central nervous system

341 DIAGNOSTIC METHODS IN NEUROLOGY

KEITH H. CHIAPPA / JOSEPH B. MARTIN / ROBERT R. YOUNG

The analysis and interpretation of data elicited by a careful history and examination may prove to be adequate for diagnosis in clinical neurology; special laboratory tests can then do no more than corroborate the initial impression. But more often the final conclusion of the nature of the disease is not reached by simple case study. The possibilities may be reduced to two or three, but the correct diagnosis cannot be determined. Under these conditions, one resorts to one or several of the laboratory tests outlined below.

It must be stressed that laboratory procedures should follow rather than precede clinical case study, except in emergencies when the disease threatens life and time does not allow detailed clinical observation. Laboratory procedures are but a part of the clinical method outlined in Chap. 10. Because many of the procedures are costly, time-consuming, and occasionally dangerous or painful, they should be undertaken only for the specific purpose of obtaining certain otherwise unavailable data that can shed light on the clinical problem.

LUMBAR PUNCTURE AND EXAMINATION OF CEREBROSPINAL FLUID The information yielded by the examination of the cerebrospinal fluid (CSF) is often of crucial importance.

Indications for lumbar puncture Lumbar puncture is performed for the following reasons:

1 To obtain pressure measurements and to secure a sample of CSF for cellular, chemical, and bacteriologic examination.
2 To aid in therapy by the administration of spinal anesthetics and occasionally antibiotics or antitumor agents.
3 To inject air for air contrast myelography or, rarely, for pneumoencephalography; a radiopaque substance (Pantopaque) or a water-soluble contrast medium for myelography; or a radioactive substance [e.g., indium or radioactive iodinated serum albumin (RISA)] for the study of CSF dynamics and to aid in the diagnosis of hydrocephalus or CSF leak.

Lumbar puncture carries a risk if the CSF pressure is high (evidenced by headache and papilledema), for it increases the possibility of fatal cerebellar or tentorial herniation. In doubtful cases, it is wise first to obtain a computerized tomography (CT) or magnetic resonance imaging (MRI) scan to exclude a mass lesion before proceeding to perform a lumbar puncture. However, if it seems important in a given case of suspected increased intracranial pressure to have the information yielded by CSF examination, the lumbar puncture may be performed with a fine-bore (no. 22 or 24 gauge) needle as the last part of the clinical study. (Note that if the pressure is over 400 mmHg, one should obtain the necessary sample of fluid, remove the needle, and then, according to the suspected clinical disease and patient's condition, administer a unit of urea or mannitol.) Dexamethasone (Decadron) should be started in a dose of 4 to 6 mg every 6 h in cases of tumor, cerebral trauma, hemorrhage, and certain types of encephalitis (acute hemorrhagic leukoencephalitis, herpes simplex encephalitis).

Cisternal puncture and lateral cervical puncture (C1–C2), although safe in the hands of the expert, are too hazardous to entrust to those without experience. The lumbar puncture is to be preferred except in obvious instances of spinal block requiring a sample of cisternal fluid or myelography above the lesions, or in rare instances where infection of the skin or subcutaneous tissue render needle penetration dangerous.

Experience teaches the importance of meticulous technique. Lumbar puncture should always be done under sterile conditions. If procaine is injected in and beneath the skin, the procedure should be painless. Failure to enter the lumbar subarachnoid space after two or three trials can usually be corrected by doing the puncture with patients in the sitting position and then assisting them to lie on their side for pressure measurements and fluid removal. The "dry tap" is more often due to an improperly placed needle than to a pathologic obliteration of subarachnoid space by compressive lesion of the spinal cord or chronic adhesive arachnoiditis. A bloody tap due to transfixation of a meningeal vessel may result in hopeless confusion of the diagnosis if it is falsely interpreted as indicating hemorrhage in the subarachnoid spaces and ventricles. Lumbar puncture should be undertaken with particular care in patients with thrombocytopenia or disorders of blood coagulation because serious hemorrhage into the extradural or intradural space may occur.

Examination procedures Once the lumbar puncture is successful, some or all of the following aspects of the CSF should be studied: (1) pressure and "dynamics"; (2) gross appearance of CSF including centrifugation, if blood is present, to examine the supernatant for xanthochromia; (3) number and type of cells and presence of microorganisms; (4) protein, sugar, and, in special instances, analysis of pigments; (5) exfoliative cytology using Millipore filters; (6) Wassermann reaction and appropriate serologic precipitation reactions; (7) protein immunoelectrophoresis for determination of gamma globulin levels, and other special biochemical tests (for NH_3, pH, CO_2, enzymes, etc.); and (8) bacteriologic cultures and virus isolation. See the appendix for normal values of CSF.

RADIOLOGIC EXAMINATION OF SKULL AND SPINE Plain x-rays of the skull or spinal column, according to the nature of the symptoms, constitute an indispensable part of the thorough study of traumatic,

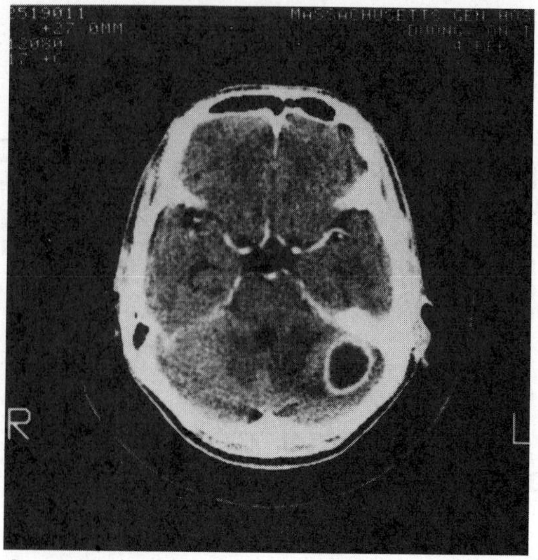

A

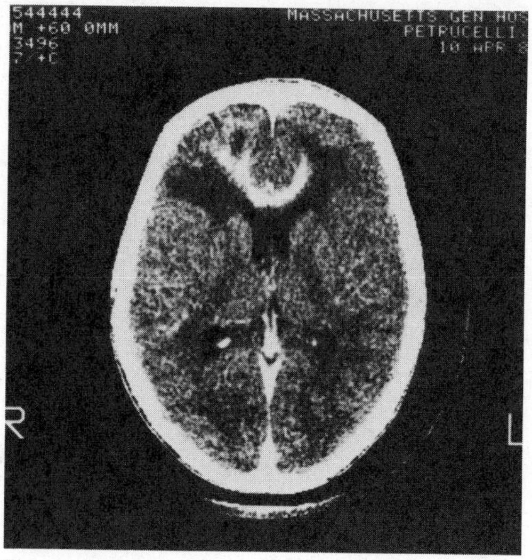

B

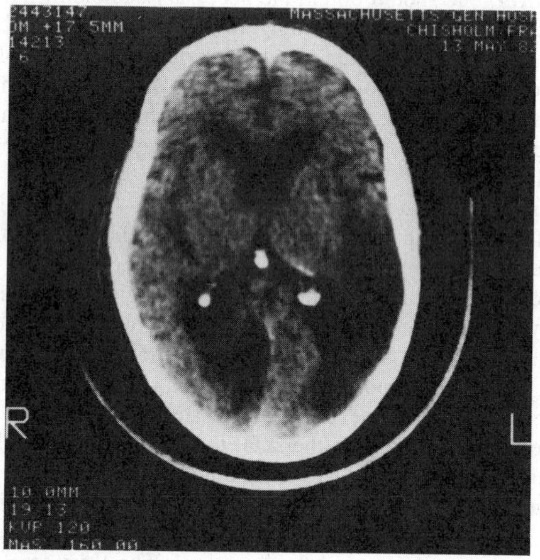

C

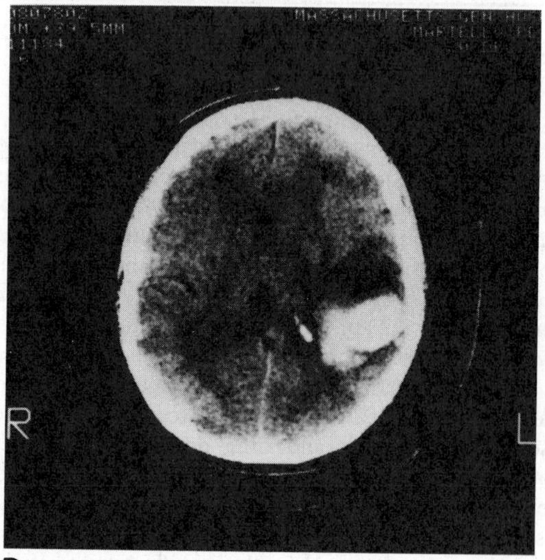

D

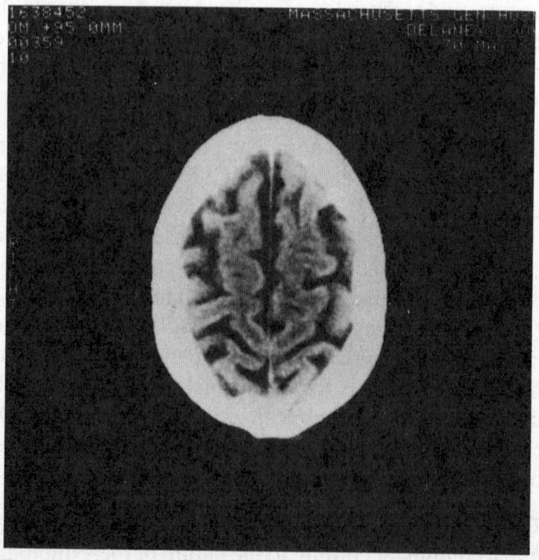

E

FIGURE 341-1 *Computerized tomography scans in disease. Frontal lobes above; right hemisphere to viewer's left. A. Left cerebellar abscess arising as a complication of mastoid sinus infection. Typical "ring" enhancement is evident in contrast-enhanced scan. B. Malignant astrocytoma infiltrating corpus callosum and bifrontal white matter. Edema surrounding tumor in frontal lobes is shown. C. Large cerebral infarcts, bilateral. Infarct on right is in distribution of posterior cerebral artery, that on left in distribution of middle cerebral artery. D. Intracerebral hematoma in left parietal lobe. Blood in hemorrhage is evident without administration of contrast media. E. Cerebral cortical atrophy in Alzheimer's disease.*

spondylitic, and neoplastic diseases but are of relatively little value in others. The procedure is relatively simple, and the findings are interpretable by most general radiologists. Space does not permit an illustration of such common findings as fractures, bone erosion, intracerebral calcifications, premature closure or separation of sutures, or alterations of skull configuration.

Of more specific value in neurology and neurosurgery are six special radiologic procedures which now permit the visualization of most parts of the brain and spinal cord and their vessels.

Computerized tomography (CT scan) This radiologic procedure, which computerizes the absorption offered by brain, CSF, and skull to more than thirty thousand 2- to 4-mm beams of x-ray and permits

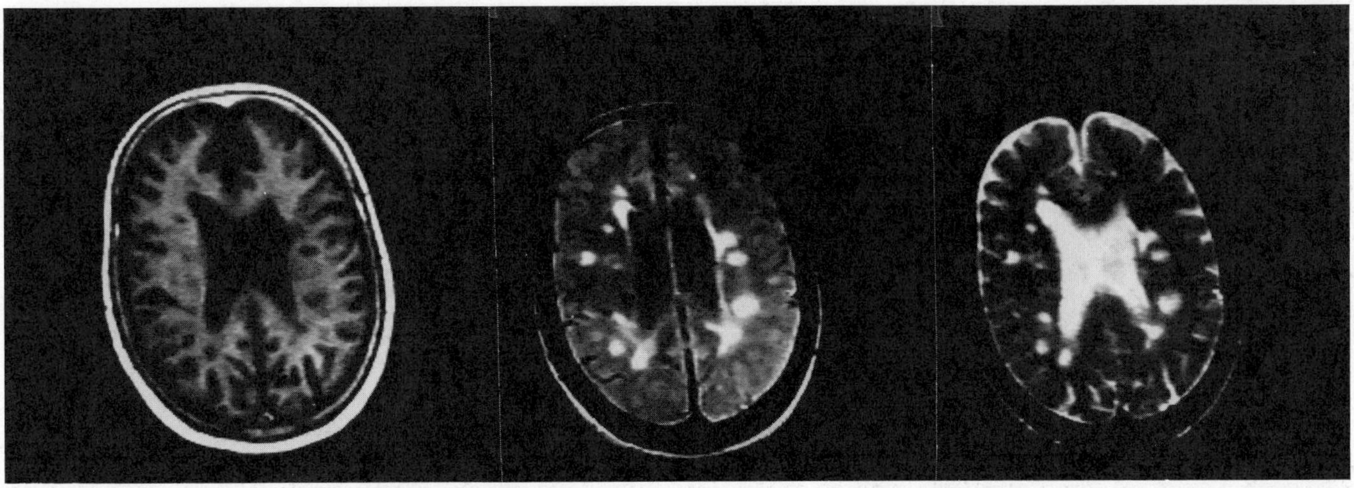

A B C

FIGURE 341-2 *Multiple sclerosis (MS) demonstrated by magnetic resonance imaging (MRI). Multiple foci of abnormally prolonged T1 and T2 relaxation times are evident in the white matter. In T1 MRI (A), MS plaques show decreased density. In T2 weighted images (B and C), plaques show increased signal intensity. A mild degree of brain atrophy is best noted in (C), where cerebrospinal fluid signal is brightest. Although the frequency, location, and distribution of such lesions in large numbers of patients with multiple sclerosis strongly suggest that the foci of abnormal relaxation may represent plaques, there has been a dearth of pathological confirmation. A. IR study: TR = 1500, TI = 450, TE = 20. B. SE study: TR = 2000, TE = 60. C. As in B, but TE = 120.*

visualization of the ventricles, subarachnoid space, and the major cisternal fissures and sulci in several horizontal planes (Fig. 341-1*A* to *E*), has become available in most medical centers and has replaced plain x-rays and most of the other contrast procedures such as pneumoencephalography and arteriography. It differentiates epidural, subdural, and intracerebral hemorrhages and deformities of the ventricular system from "mass" lesions, and demonstrates tumors, abscesses, granulomas [when done after an intravenous injection of meglumine diatrizoate (Renografin) or other contrast medium], as well as areas of brain edema and infarction, hydrocephalus, and brain atrophy. The simplicity of this noninvasive procedure, its low risk to patients with expanding lesions, and the low exposure to x-ray have virtually revolutionized diagnostic neurology and neurosurgery.

Magnetic resonance imaging The recent application of magnetic resonance imaging (MRI) has permitted the visualization of cerebral lesions not evident on CT scans (Figs. 341-2 to 341-4). MRI is noninvasive and does not involve exposure to ionizing radiation. The technique permits delineation of tissues without administration of contrast-enhancing agents, and because bone elicits no interference, it is particularly useful for visualizing structures at the brain-bone interface, i.e., in the posterior cranial fossa. MRI has already greatly improved neuroradiologic diagnostic abilities and promises, in the future, to permit measurement of brain metabolites by spectroscopic application. The high resolution of MRI in delineating white and gray matter has resulted in its widespread use in localizing lesions in the white matter, such as those caused by demyelination. Its use has been extended to visualize the spinal cord, which can be displayed in either sagittal or cross-sectional planes.

Angiography This has been developed over the last 30 years to the point where it is a relatively safe and extremely valuable method in the diagnosis of occluded arteries, aneurysms, and vascular malformations, tumors, abscesses, and intracranial hemorrhages. Its use has diminished greatly since the advent of CT and MRI scans. Following local anesthesia, a needle or cannula can be placed percutaneously

FIGURE 341-3 *MRI: Right carotid occlusion, with resultant right parieto-temporal infarction. T1-weighted inversion recovery study (IR), with repetition time of 1500 ms and inversion time of 450 ms (A) shows areas of prolonged T1 (dark) in the infarcted zones; in addition, small foci of prolonged relaxation times are also noted in the posterior frontal parietal and temporal areas of the coronae radiatae bilaterally. The T2-weighted studies (B and C) show the affected areas to also possess prolonged T2 characteristics (bright signals); the later echo (TE = 120 ms) shows some heterogeneity of signal, but it is undetermined whether the areas of longer T2 (brightest zones) represent infarct or edema. (Spin echo sequences: TR = 2000, TE = 60 in B and 120 in C.)*

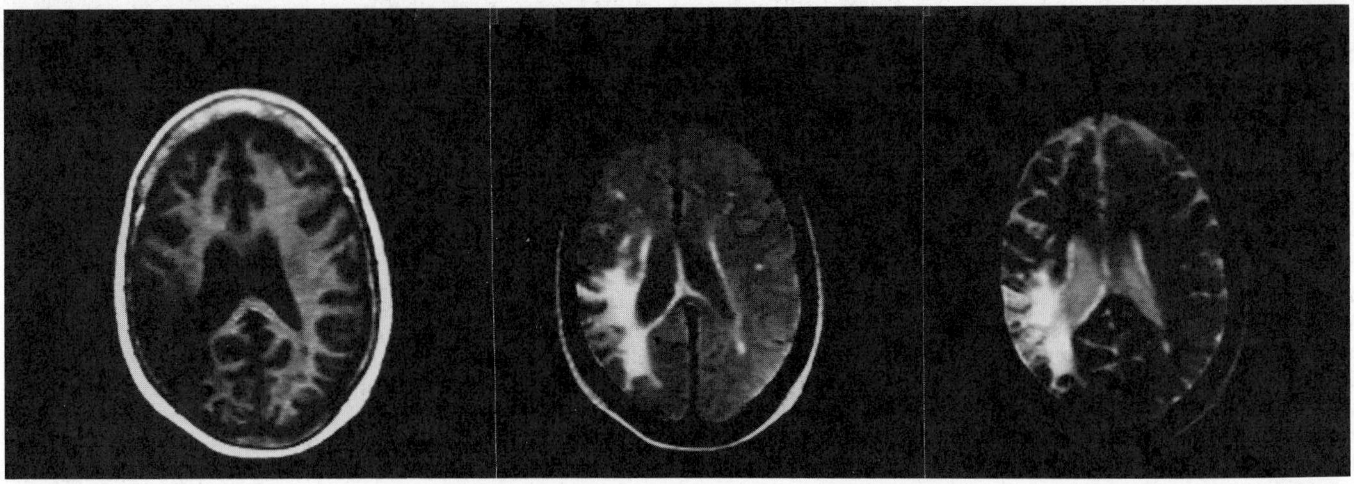

A B C

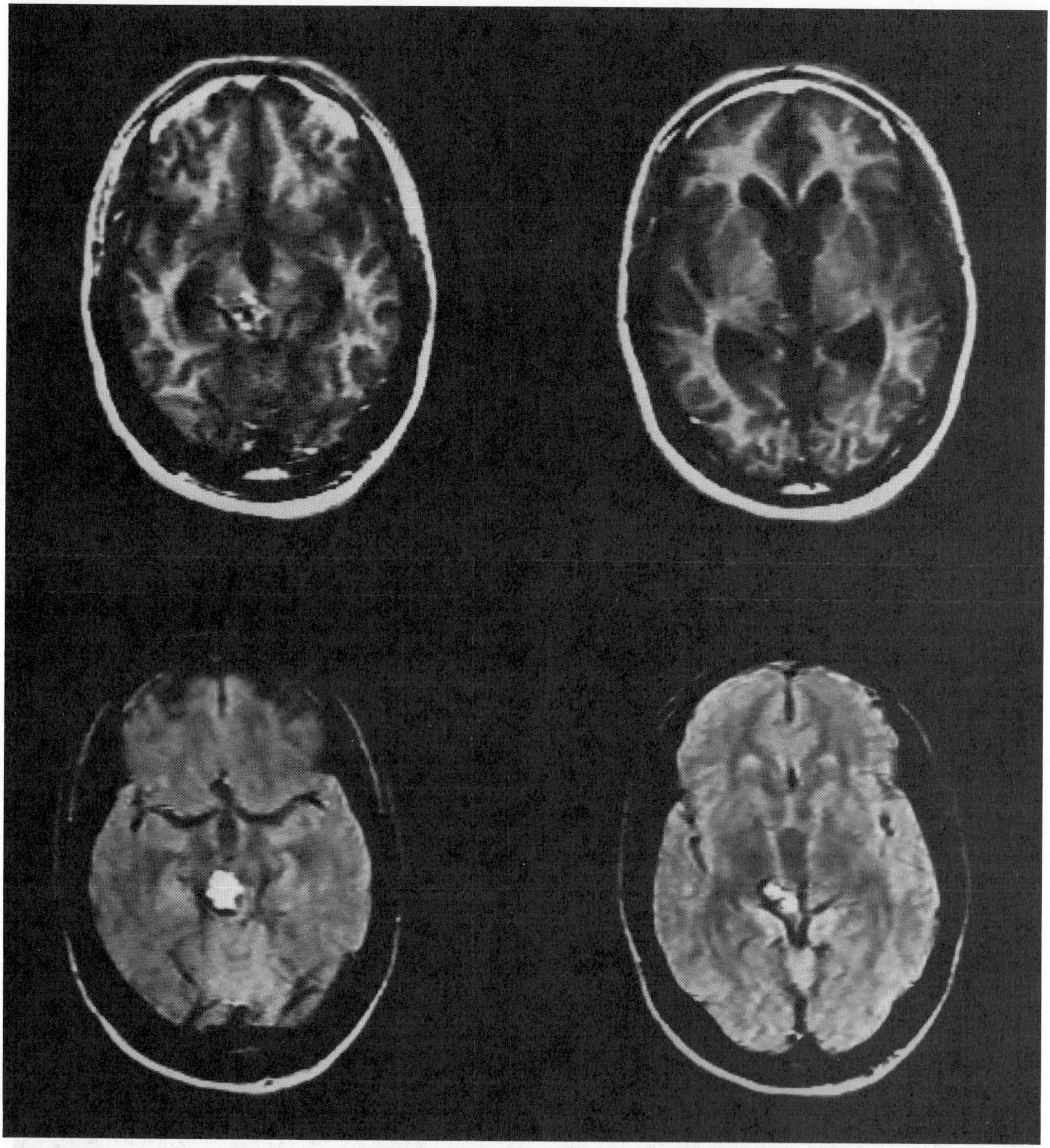

FIGURE 341-4 *Arteriovenous malformation. Thrombosed AVM involving the right posterior subthalamic and upper mesencephalic areas. Dark areas within the AVM on the IR study probably represent foci of abnormal brain with prolonged T1 rather than ''flow void'' effects; compare with the middle cerebral arteries. Bright zones on the IR study possess short T1; these areas also possess long T2 values; this combination is seen in subacute or chronic hemorrhages, in some fatty lesions, and metastases from melanoma. (Above: IR study, TR = 1500, TI-450, TE = 45; below: SE study, TR = 2000, TE = 60.)*

into the lumen of a brachial or femoral artery and a catheter can be introduced and threaded along the aorta to cannulate the major arteries in the cervical region. Radiopaque contrast media can be injected to visualize the arch of the aorta, the origins of carotid and vertebral systems and their extent through the neck into the cranial cavity, and when indicated, the spinal cord arteries. It is possible to show with clarity cerebral arteries down to about 0.1 mm lumen diameter under optimal conditions, as well as small veins of comparable size, vascular abnormalities (angiomas, aneurysms), occluded arteries, delayed circulation from increased intracranial pressure as with masses or occlusion of dural sinuses and veins, displacement of vessels by mass lesions, or complete failure of intracranial vascular filling with cerebral death. *Digital subtraction venous angiography,* which requires pressure injection of contrast dye into a brachial vein, is commonly used as an alternative or adjunct to arterial angiography, particularly for initial study of the lumen diameters of the large extracranial arteries.

Pneumoencephalography and ventriculography Injection of air into the lumbar subarachnoid space with the patient in the sitting position permits visualization in considerable detail of the size and position of the ventricles, the subarachnoid space (upper spinal and cerebral), and, indirectly, the structures which lie between the ventricles and the meninges. This technique is now rarely used. Air myelography to demonstrate cavities within the spinal cord (syringomyelia) has now been largely replaced by injection of metrizamide. Ventriculography, accomplished by injection of air or contrast material directly into the lateral ventricles, is also largely of historic interest. CT scan and MRI have largely replaced both pneumoencephalography and ventriculography.

Iophendylate (pantopaque) myelography and ventriculography By injecting 5 to 15 mL iophendylate through a lumbar puncture needle and then tipping the patient on a tilt table, the entire spinal subarachnoid space and portions of the posterior cranial fossa may be visualized. The procedure is almost as harmless as the lumbar puncture, provided that the iophendylate is afterward removed through the needle. Ruptured lumbar and cervical disks and spinal cord tumors can be diagnosed accurately. Intraventricular injection of iophendylate is occasionally done to visualize the third and fourth ventricles and the aqueduct of Sylvius in tumors of the posterior fossa. Water-soluble contrast media (e.g., metrizamide) that are self-absorbing are now commonly used. Metrizamide injected in the lumbar CSF affords the additional advantage of assessing the subarachnoid space with a body CT scan. The body CT scan with or without metrizamide allows accurate visualization of the spinal canal and the spinal cord. It reveals tumors, ruptured disks, etc., that compress or displace the spinal canal and roots and also destructive lesions of the vertebrae. The latter may also be evident in bone scans.

Radioactive isotopes Radioactive isotopes, such as technetium (brain scan), are occasionally used for the visualization of tumors, inflammatory masses, viral encephalitis, and some vascular lesions such as "watershed" infarcts that are difficult to demonstrate otherwise. Since this is a simple, noninvasive procedure, the only limitation in its use is the expense. The more the lesion disrupts the blood-brain barrier, the more consistent its demonstration by these methods. Ultrasound can also be used to show displacement of central structures of the brain by a mass lesion.

POSITRON EMISSION TOMOGRAPHY Positron emission tomography (PET) is an experimental investigative technique currently available in only a few centers. The procedure involves the systemic administration of positron-emitting radionuclides of oxygen or ^{18}F 2-deoxyglucose (^{18}FDG) combined with computerized tomography. The latter permits three-dimensional localization of the disintegrating positrons with a tissue resolution of 0.5 to 1 cm. Administration of labeled O_2, CO_2, and ^{18}FDG provides regional quantitation of oxygen uptake, blood flow, and glucose utilization, respectively. Studies in patients with cerebrovascular diseases, seizure disorders, and degenerative conditions have been undertaken. In stroke, PET imaging is useful in acute studies to discriminate viable from nonviable tissue. In patients with seizure disorders interictal ^{18}FDG studies may show localized areas of decreased glucose metabolism in and around a seizure focus, with increased glucose metabolism evident during a seizure. Metabolic studies with ^{18}FDG have also shown decreased glucose uptake in the striatum in patients with Huntington's disease who have normal CT scans. Although these studies show great promise in the biochemical analysis of brain functions, the cost of the instrumentation and the technology required to produce isotopes will restrict PET scanning to major medical centers.

ELECTROMYOGRAPHY (EMG) This examination supplements the clinical study of patients with neurologic diseases which affect the neuromuscular apparatus or with primary or secondary diseases of the skeletal musculature. It is described in relation to muscle diseases (see Chap. 354). Newer EMG techniques ("central EMG") permit quantitative analysis of motor system function.

ELECTROENCEPHALOGRAPHY (EEG) The electroencephalographic examination is part of the clinical study of a patient suspected of having a cerebral disease; it is also used in the evaluation of the central nervous system (CNS) effects of many medical diseases.

In addition to the resting record, a number of so-called activating procedures are usually carried out.

1 The patient is requested to breathe deeply 20 times a minute for 3 min. The resulting alkalosis and cerebral vasoconstriction may activate characteristic seizure patterns or other abnormalities.
2 A powerful light (a stroboscope) is placed over the patient's face and flashed at frequencies from 1 to 20 per s with the patient's eyes opened and closed. The EEG may then show abnormal discharges in photosensitive patients.
3 The EEG is recorded after the patient is allowed to fall asleep naturally or following sedative drugs given by mouth or by vein. Procedures 1 and 2 are more commonly employed, but sleep is extremely helpful in bringing out abnormalities, especially where temporal lobe epilepsy and certain other seizures are concerned. Sleep deprivation the night prior to the study is a common adjunct to a sleep EEG.

Certain preparations are necessary if electroencephalography is to be most useful. The patient should not be sedated and should not have been for a long time without food, for both sedative drugs and relative hypoglycemia modify the normal EEG pattern. The same may be said of mental concentration, extreme nervousness, or drowsiness, all of which tend to suppress the normal alpha rhythm and increase muscle artifacts. When dealing with patients suspected of having epilepsy who are already being treated for it, most physicians prefer to record the first EEG while the patient continues to receive drugs.

Types of normal recordings The normal EEG in adults shows somewhat asymmetric 8- to 12-Hz, 50-μV sinusoidal *alpha* waves in both occipital and parietal regions. These waves wax and wane spontaneously and usually disappear promptly when patients open their eyes or fix their attention on something. Faster waves than 13 Hz of lower amplitude (10 to 20 μV), called *beta* waves, are also seen symmetrically in the frontal regions. Very slow waves (*delta* waves), sharp waves, or other unusual patterns are absent in a normal record. When normal subjects fall asleep, the rhythm slows symmetrically, and characteristic waveforms (vertex sharp waves and sleep spindles) appear; if the sleep is induced by barbiturates or benzodiazepines, an increase in the fast frequencies is seen and is considered to be normal (see Chap. 20). Excessive fast activity should raise the possibility that a patient is receiving one of these classes of compounds.

An occipital response to each flash may be seen in the normal EEG during stroboscopic stimulation and is called the evoked response, or, at faster repetition rates, photic "driving." The clinical utility of this evoked occipital response has increased the scope of electroencephalography in several ways: (1) one can be reasonably sure that a person with such a response can at least perceive light; (2) when this evoked response is absent on one side of the head but present on the other, there is physiologic evidence of a lesion interfering with normal transmission between the thalamus and the occipital lobe on this side; and (3) when the flashing light produces abnormal waves, there is evidence of increased excitability. Actual seizure patterns may be produced in the EEG if the activation procedure is continued (a "photoparoxysmal" response); if the sensitivity is still greater, frank myoclonic jerks of face or arms, or, rarely, major convulsions may occur. This finding is to be differentiated from the purely muscular response, also myoclonic, produced normally in contracting scalp muscles and often visible in routine EEGs (photomyoclonus).

Types of abnormal recordings The most pathologic finding of all is the disappearance of the EEG pattern and its replacement by "electrocerebral silence," which means that the electrical activity of the cortical mantle, measured at the scalp, is below 2 μV and probably absent. Acute intoxication with anesthetic levels of drugs, such as barbiturates, and extreme hypothermia (<70°F) can produce this sort of isoelectric EEG. However, in the absence of CNS depressants or extreme hypothermia, a record which is "flat" (except for artifacts) all over the head is almost always a result of cerebral hypoxia, ischemia, or widespread cortical destruction. Such a patient, without EEG activity, reflexes, spontaneous respiration, or muscular activity of any kind for 6 h or more, is said to be in "irreversible coma." The brain of such patients is largely necrotic. There is no chance for neurologic recovery, and the patient may be considered dead, despite the preservation of vegetative (cardiovascular) functions supported by mechanical means, such as respirators. There has been no exception to this statement in more than 900 patients examined at the Massachusetts General Hospital in the past 18 years.

Localized regions with absence of EEG activity may rarely be seen when there is a large area of infarction or an extensive surface tumor or clot lying between the cerebral cortex and the electrodes. The localization of this abnormality is precise, but of course the nature of the lesion cannot be ascertained by EEG. Most such lesions, however, are too small, relative to the recording arrangement, to be visible, and the EEG may then record abnormal waves arising from functional, though deranged, brain at the borders of the lesion. These abnormal waves are slower and of higher amplitude (50 to 350 μV) than normal. Those which are less than 4 Hz are called *delta* waves; those from 4 to 7 Hz are called *theta* waves; and the higher-voltage, faster waves are known as *spikes* or *sharp waves*. These fast and slow waves may be combined, and when a series of them suddenly interrupts relatively normal EEG patterns in a paroxysmal fashion, they are highly suggestive of epilepsy. The ones associated with *petit mal* (absence) spells are 3-Hz spike-and-wave complexes that characteristically appear in all leads of the EEG at the same time and disappear almost as suddenly at the end of the seizure.

Neurologic conditions with abnormal EEG In the following groups of neurologic disorders, the EEG may be of considerable help in reaching the correct diagnosis.

EPILEPSY All types of generalized epileptic seizures (grand mal and petit mal) are associated with some abnormality in the EEG, provided it is being recorded at the time. The EEG is also often abnormal during the more restricted types of seizure activity (complex partial, myoclonic, focal, and Jacksonian) (see Chap. 342). One exception is certain deep temporal lobe foci where the discharge fails to reach the scalp in sufficient amplitude to be seen against the background activity of the normal EEG, particularly if there is a strong alpha rhythm. A zygomatic or sphenoidal lead may localize an epileptic focus in the medial temporal lobe, but rarely does it provide the only EEG evidence of epileptic activity. Other exceptions in which, on occasion, no EEG abnormality may be recorded during a seizure include some of the patients with other focal seizures (sensory, Jacksonian, myoclonic, and epilepsia partialis continua). This fact presumably means that the neuronal discharge is too deep, discrete, fast, or asynchronous to be transmitted by volume conduction through the skull and recorded via the EEG electrode, which is some 2 cm from the cortex. The petit mal, certain myoclonic, and grand mal patterns correlate closely with the clinical seizure type and may be present in the interictal EEG. The artifact produced by motor activity during a "seizure" usually cannot be distinguished from brain electrical activity. The differentiation of psychogenic from true seizures requires careful inspection of the EEG at seizure onset where a typical pattern of fast frequency activity may be seen, or immediately following cessation of motor activity, when postictal slowing or suppression is the rule if consciousness has been affected. A normal alpha pattern postictally in an "unresponsive" patient suggests a psychogenic pseudoseizure.

A fact of importance is that between seizures as many as 20 percent of patients with petit mal and 40 percent with grand mal epilepsy show a normal EEG. Anticonvulsant therapy also tends to diminish the EEG abnormalities. The records of another 30 to 40 percent of epileptics, though abnormal between seizures, are nonspecifically so, and therefore the diagnosis of epilepsy can be made only by correct interpretation of the clinical data in relation to the EEG abnormality.

BRAIN TUMOR, ABSCESS, AND SUBDURAL HEMATOMA Clinically significant intracranial space-occupying lesions are characteristically associated with abnormalities in the EEG, depending on their type and location, in some 90 percent of patients. In addition to diffuse changes, the classic abnormalities are focal or localized slow waves (usually delta), or, occasionally, seizure activity and decreased amplitude and synchronization of normal rhythms. As a rule, those lesions which expand more rapidly (abscess, some metastases, glioblastoma), especially when situated supratentorially, have the greatest frequency of EEG abnormalities (90 to 95 percent of the latter two and virtually 100 percent of abscesses). Slower growing tumors (astrocytomas) and particularly those outside the cerebral hemispheres (meningiomas, pituitary tumors) often produce no change in the EEG, though they may be very evident clinically. The EEG abnormality has the correct lateralization in as many as 75 to 90 percent of patients with supratentorial tumors or abscesses. The EEG may be focally abnormal at a time when a cerebral metastasis is not yet visible on a CT scan. A normal EEG and CT scan together almost exclude the presence of a supratentorial brain tumor or abscess. The EEG may be normal, however, in 20 to 25 percent of patients with infratentorial tumors.

CEREBROVASCULAR DISEASE Both the diffuse and localized EEG changes produced by vascular lesions such as cerebral infarcts and intracranial hemorrhages depend on their location and size rather than their type. The EEG has been shown to be useful in the differential diagnosis of vascular hemiplegia. If the lesion responsible is in the internal carotid or a major cerebral artery, an area of decreased normal activity and excessive slowing is practically always seen acutely in the appropriate region. If the hemiplegia is due to small vessel disease, i.e., a lacunar infarction deep in the cerebrum or brainstem (Chap. 343), the EEG should be normal. Large hemispheral lesions associated with acutely depressed levels of consciousness also produce widespread, diffuse, slow-wave activity of a nonspecific type as is seen with stupor or coma from any cause. Resolution begins after a few days, cerebral edema subsides, and focal activity may then be seen (slow-wave activity or suppression of normal background rhythms). Smaller infarctions are associated with acute focal abnormalities which lateralize the lesion well but do not localize it precisely. In contrast with tumors, further resolution continues, and after 3 to 6 months roughly 50 percent of patients with cerebrovascular accidents have a normal EEG despite the persistence of clinical abnormalities. Under these circumstances the prognosis for further recovery is poor. Persistence of moderate- to high-voltage EEG abnormalities after this time period, particularly if spikes or sharp waves are present, suggests the presence of abnormally functioning tissue, which might be epileptogenic. The EEG may be of lateralizing value in acute subarachnoid hemorrhage, depending upon the extent to which the adjacent cerebrum is affected.

BRAIN INJURY Cerebral contusion or laceration produces EEG changes similar to those described for cerebrovascular disease. Diffuse changes often give way to focal ones, especially if the lesions are on the lateral or superior surface of the brain, and these in turn usually disappear over a period of weeks or months unless seizures supervene. Sharp waves or spikes sometimes emerge as the focal slow-wave abnormality resolves. These or failure of the EEG to "normalize" usually precede the occurrence of posttraumatic epilepsy. Following head injury, therefore, serial EEGs may be of prognostic value as regards the prospect of epilepsy.

DISEASES WHICH CAUSE COMA AND STATES OF IMPAIRED CONSCIOUSNESS The EEG is abnormal in almost all conditions in which there is some impairment of consciousness. With hypothyroidism the rhythms are normal in configuration but are usually slow.

In general, the more profound the change in consciousness, the more abnormal the EEG recording. In these latter situations slow waves (delta) are bilateral, are of high amplitude, and tend to be more conspicuous over the frontal regions. This pertains to such differing conditions as acute meningitis or encephalitis, severe disorders of blood gases, glucose, electrolyte and water balance, uremia, diabetic coma, liver coma, or impairment of consciousness accompanying the large cerebral lesions discussed above. In hepatic coma, the degree of abnormality in the EEG corresponds with the degree of confusion, stupor, or coma. Moreover, paroxysms of bilaterally synchronous large, sharp "triphasic waves" are characteristic, though they may also be seen with other metabolic encephalopathies associated with renal or pulmonary failure. Diffuse degenerative diseases (e.g., Alzheimer's disease) affecting the cerebral cortex are accompanied by relatively slight degrees of diffuse, slow-wave abnormality in the theta (4- to 7-Hz) range. Certain more rapidly progressive ones, such as subacute sclerosing panencephalitis (SSPE), Creutzfeldt-Jakob disease, and to a lesser extent the cerebral lipidoses, have, in addition, very characteristic, almost pathognomonic EEG changes consisting of recurring complex bursts of sharp and slow activity. A normal EEG in a patient who is apathetic, slow, depressed, or forgetful is a point in favor of the diagnosis of an affective disorder or schizophrenia.

An EEG may also assist the physician in caring for a comatose patient when the pertinent history is unavailable. It may point to such otherwise unexpected causes as hepatic encephalopathy (bilaterally synchronous triphasic waves), intoxication with barbiturates or benzodiazepines (excess fast activity), clinically inapparent continuous epileptic discharges, a large space-occupying lesion, or diffuse anoxia-ischemia ("burst-suppression" pattern with repetitive generalized complexes separated by periods with very little EEG).

OTHER DISEASES OF THE CEREBRUM There are many disorders of nervous function that cause little or no alteration in the EEG. Multiple sclerosis and other demyelinating diseases are examples, though as many as 50 percent of advanced cases will have an abnormal record. Delirium tremens, Wernicke-Korsakoff disease, and withdrawal seizures, despite the dramatic nature of the clinical picture, cause little or no changes in the EEG. Some degree of slowing usually accompanies confusional states which have been designated elsewhere as hypokinetic delirium. Interestingly, neuroses and psychoses, such as manic-depressive disorders or schizophrenia, abnormal states due to hallucinogenic drugs such as LSD, and the majority of cases of mental retardation are associated with no important modification of the normal record or with nonspecific abnormalities.

Special applications of the EEG Because the EEG provides information about the status and function of the cerebrum, it is useful as a monitor in the operating room to ensure the presence of a viable brain during the increasingly extensive procedures of modern cardiovascular surgery. EEG apparatus has long been available for indicating the level of anesthesia, and such simple equipment should eventually be used by the anesthetist to monitor both the cardiac and cerebral status of all patients during surgical anesthesia.

It is routine practice now for the EEG to be monitored continuously during carotid endarterectomies, a procedure performed in carefully selected patients suffering from stenotic or ulcerative carotid artery disease. Characteristic EEG changes (particularly marked voltage attenuation) signal the need for a temporary bypass shunt to maintain sufficient cerebral blood flow to preclude ischemic cerebral damage during surgery.

In the neurosurgical operating room the EEG can be recorded from exposed brain *(electrocorticogram),* and seizure patterns can be localized more precisely than from the scalp so that resection of such physiologically abnormal tissue may be undertaken.

The routine EEG can be of value in the diagnosis of hysterical blindness. Similarly, a response evoked by noise during light sleep can be of help in confirming the presence of hearing in a patient who feigns total deafness. These responses may also be helpful in evaluating hearing and vision in infants.

EVOKED RESPONSES An *evoked response* (sometimes termed an *evoked potential*) is the record of electrical activity produced by groups of neurons within the cord, brainstem, thalamus, or cerebral hemispheres following stimulation of one or another sensory system by means of visual, auditory, or tactile input. The amplitude of these potentials, as recorded from the scalp using ordinary EEG electrodes, ranges from less than 0.5 to 20 μV. Because of their extremely small size, they can rarely be recognized on the ink-written EEG record with the background of ongoing EEG activity, which itself is usually 50 μV or more in amplitude. Therefore, special techniques, requiring simple computers, must be used to extract the evoked response waveform that one is interested in, from the continuous background EEG activity. These techniques are called "averaging" because the process involves repeating 100 to 1000 precisely timed stimuli and recording the electrical activity during a certain brief interval following each stimulus. The random ongoing EEG activity which, at any given point in time following the stimulus, is sometimes negative and at other times positive in polarity, tends to cancel out with sufficient repetition. The evoked response, on the other hand, is time-locked to the stimulus, and at a given time following the stimulus always has the same electrical sign as well as shape. The evoked response thus grows larger with repetition while the background averages out and becomes smaller. It is important to have special amplifiers, to apply the electrodes to the surface of the scalp with great care, and to time stimuli precisely with a minimum of accompanying electrical artifact. These evoked responses provide sensitive, objective extensions of the clinical neurologic examination of the related sensory system, but they are no more specific etiologically.

Visual evoked responses *Visual evoked responses* produced by a pattern shift (PSVER) have the longest history of clinical usefulness. During this test, patients are asked to watch an alternating black and white checkerboard pattern which is projected on a screen. When patients watch this pattern shift, it produces a characteristic waveform which can be recorded from the scalp over the posterior portion of the head. Under normal circumstances, this triphasic wave has a distinctive positive peak at 95 to 115 ms latency (usually called P100; see Fig. 341-5) from the time of pattern reversal. This latency, the duration of the response, and the amplitude of the peak are measured; the latency is the most important parameter clinically. Each eye is tested independently. A purely monocular abnormality indicates that the conduction defect is anterior to the chiasm.

Many disease processes affecting the optic nerve fibers in their intraocular, orbital, or intracranial portions produce abnormalities of this potential. Glaucoma, compression of the optic nerve, chiasm, or tract by various space-occupying lesions, and degenerative disease of this system often produce a reduction in amplitude and/or prolonged latency of the PSVER. If the visual system is sufficiently affected, no response may be recorded by stimulation of one or both eyes. In a general hospital setting, however, the most common cause of abnormality in this response is optic neuritis, frequently associated with multiple sclerosis. Demyelination of the optic nerve fibers, as a primary demyelinating disease or due to one of the lesions listed above, slows conduction in the nerve fibers so that the latency of the positive peak of the PSVER is prolonged (115 to 200 ms). In fact, almost all patients with optic neuritis, even after the visual acuity has returned to normal, continue to show distinct abnormalities in this PSVER at a time when detailed ophthalmologic evaluations reveal no abnormality. In multiple sclerosis, if the PSVER is normal, the neuroophthalmologic examination is always normal. We have found no exceptions to this rule in more than 200 patients. When the PSVER is abnormal, the visual fields, visual acuity, pupillary reactions, and optic fundus examination are normal in a considerable number of patients.

Approximately one-half of the patients with multiple sclerosis who have never had visual symptoms also show abnormalities, and this accounts for one of the most useful aspects of the test. If a patient presents with what appears to be the first episode of a neurologic illness in which the lesion is in the brainstem or spinal cord, a demonstration by means of an abnormal PSVER of another clinically unsuspected lesion in a different part of the central nervous system (the optic nerves) makes the diagnosis of multiple sclerosis more likely and may spare the patient certain neuroradiologic procedures.

Abnormalities in visual acuity have no effect on the PSVER unless the acuity is so poor that the patient cannot see the checkerboard pattern—patients with acuity of 20/200 or better are suitable for testing. The only other requirement is that the patient be cooperative enough to sit still for 20 min and watch the pattern. Infants and children can also be tested by using special techniques.

Brainstem auditory evoked responses *Brainstem auditory evoked responses* (BAERs) are more difficult to obtain than PSVERs because BAERs are much smaller, of the order of 0.5 μV. These are produced by clicks transmitted to one of a patient's ears through earphones. The patient may be alert or comatose and need not be particularly cooperative except that excess movement or muscle artifact makes the response even more difficult to obtain. BAERs of essentially normal appearance can be recorded from infants and children. BAERs consist of a series of seven waves which appear within the first 10 ms after the click (Fig. 341-5). These (named I to VII) are considered to represent successive activation of the auditory nerve (I) and the brainstem auditory pathways (cochlear nucleus, II; superior olivary complex, III; lateral lemniscus, IV; inferior colliculus, V; and higher auditory centers, VI, VII). A lesion at or between any of these levels either obliterates or delays the appearance of waves from successively higher levels. Multiple sclerosis can, for example, also produce slow conduction between any of the levels in this test. The same is true of other lesions affecting the brainstem, such as small vascular lesions, central pontine myelinolysis, hypoxic damage, and so on. The waves which arise from structures caudal to the lesion are perfectly normal in latency, whereas those arising from structures cranial to the lesion are either obliterated or delayed. This allows one to pinpoint quite accurately the level of the lesion within the brainstem auditory pathways and provides a very neat opportunity for correlation of clinical observations with neurophysiologic and occasionally pathologic data. This test is useful as a screening test for patients with acoustic neuromas (who always show an abnormality), for patients suspected of having multiple sclerosis, for comatose patients in whom the level of lesion within the central nervous system is not clear, and for other patients in whom documentation of brainstem lesions is important. Hearing loss can often be recognized in this test, since changes in the latency of the first (and, therefore, subsequent) waves are produced, and these must be taken into consideration in the evaluation of the results obtained. Interwave latencies, which are the parameters used to measure central conduction, are not affected by hearing loss or stimulus intensity. The test is also useful in screening high-risk infants for hearing defects.

Somatosensory evoked responses *Somatosensory evoked responses* (SERs) are produced by small painless electrical stimuli administered to large sensory fibers in mixed nerves of the hand or leg. The afferent valley is recorded at many levels as it ascends the somatosensory pathways, and a series of waves can be recorded which reflect activity in peripheral nerve trunks, tracts in the spinal

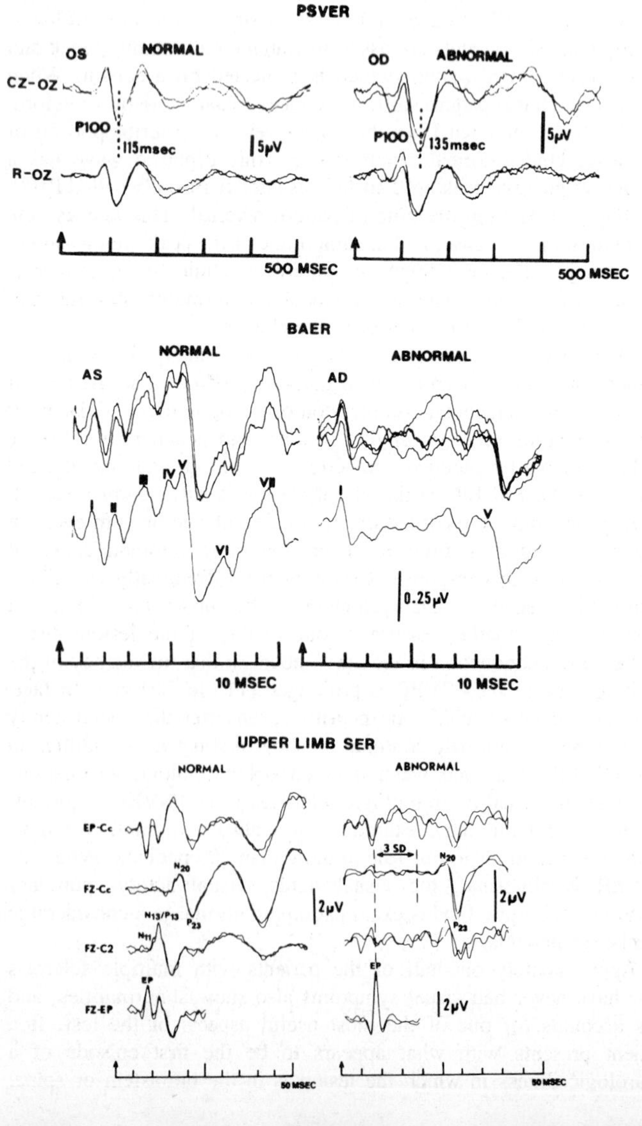

FIGURE 341-5 *Evoked responses (ER). PSVER. Pattern-shift visual ER recorded from a patient with multiple sclerosis showing a monocular latency abnormality. Latency of the occipital response (P100) following stimulation of the left eye (OS) was normal at 115 ms; right response (OD) was abnormal because the latency of the P100 peak was delayed at 135 ms. Relative positivity at G2 causes a downward trace deflection. Electrode locations; CZ = vertex, OZ = midline occipital, R = linked ears. [From EB Brooks, KH Chiappa, Clinical applications of evoked potentials, in Neurology, J Courjoun et al (eds), New York, Raven Press, 1982.]*

BAER. Brainstem auditory ERs from a patient with multiple sclerosis showing the marked asymmetry which can be present with monaural click stimulation. The responses following left ear (AS) stimulation are normal. The right ear (AD) responses are missing wave III (lower pons) and have a markedly abnormal I–V (cochlear nerve to midbrain) separation of 6.7 ms, evidence of a conduction defect in the pontine auditory tracts on the right. Left ear responses for superimposed trials (above) are produced by N = 1024 clicks each; in the right ear N = 2048 clicks each. The single trace below each is the grand average of the superimposed trials. Recording is from vertex to earlobe of stimulated ear; relative positivity at the vertex produces an upward trace deflection. (Reprinted from KH Chiappa et al, Ann Neurol 7:135, 1980.)

Upper limb SER. Short-latency somatosensory ERS produced by stimulation of the median nerve at the wrist. The left set of responses is from a normal subject; the right set is from a patient with multiple sclerosis who had no sensory symptoms or signs. In the patient, note preservation of the brachial plexus component (EP) and absence of cervical cord (N11) and lower medullary components (N13-P13). The latency of thalamocortical components (N20-P23) was prolonged markedly above the normal mean plus 3 standard deviations for the separation of N20 from the brachial plexus potential. Unilateral stimulation at 5 per second. Each trace is the averaged response to 1024 stimuli, with the superimposed trace a repetition following 1024 stimuli to demonstrate waveform consistency. Recording electrode locations: FZ = midfrontal, EP = Erb's point (supraclavicular), C2 = middle back of neck over C2 cervical vertebra, and Cc = scalp overlying sensoriparietal cortex contralateral to limb stimulated.

cord, gracile and cuneate nuclei, pontine and/or cerebellar structures, thalamus, thalamocortical radiations, and primary sensory fields of the cortex (see Fig. 341-5). Lesions of the pathways at any level affect the subsequent waves, thus providing localizing and confirmatory data in a similar fashion to the BAER.

Evoked responses can be used for a single evaluation of patients (looking for lesions in the various pathways discussed) or as a quantitative method for following a patient's course to document functional improvement or deterioration as time passes, following therapy, and so on. They also prove useful for on-line monitoring of function in optic nerve, brainstem, or spinal cord during neurosurgical procedures that involve manipulation of those structures. Since BAERs and SERs are unaffected by general anesthesia and high-dose barbiturates, they also can be used to follow CNS function in comatose patients. Longer latency auditory and somatosensory evoked responses have been studied for a number of years. These are largely cortically produced responses, dramatically affected by drowsiness, inattention, and other poorly controllable variables, and have not proved to be clinically useful. Neither have most visual evoked responses produced by stroboscopic flashes. They are very useful in evaluation of visual pathways in infants and young children who are not cooperative enough to watch the checkerboard pattern and in adults during surgery or when comatose. Under other circumstances, pattern-shift PSVERs afford a much more reliable and reproducible response.

PSYCHOMETRY, PERIMETRY, AUDIOMETRY, AND TESTS OF LABYRINTHINE FUNCTION These methods are of utility in quantitating and defining the nature of psychic or sensory deficits produced by disease of the nervous system. Limitations of space do not permit a description of them here. The precise indications for doing these tests are (1) to obtain confirmation of a functional disorder in particular parts of the nervous system and to ascertain its nature, and (2) to quantitate the disorder to determine, by subsequent examinations, the course of the underlying illness (see Chap. 23).

BIOCHEMICAL TESTS With advances in the biochemistry of metabolic diseases, a number of highly specific tests of serum, CSF, and circulating red and white blood cells have become available. These will be presented in relation to the metabolic diseases of which they are diagnostic.

REFERENCES

BUONANNO FS et al: Applications of proton nuclear magnetic resonance imaging in neurology, in *Harrison's Principles of Internal Medicine, Update V*, RG Petersdorf et al (eds). New York, McGraw-Hill, 1984

CHIAPPA KH: *Evoked Potentials in Clinical Neurology*. New York, Raven Press, 1983

———, ROPPER AH: Evoked potentials in clinical medicine. N Engl J Med 306:1136, 1982

KLASS DW, DALY DD (eds): *Practice of Clinical Electroencephalography*. New York, Raven Press, 1981

NEWTON TH, POTTS DG (eds): *Radiology of the Skull and Brain*, vol 3. St. Louis, Mosby, 1977

NIEDERMEYER E, LOPES DA SILVA F (eds): *Electroencephalography*. Baltimore, Urban & Schwarzenberg, 1982

PYKETT IL: NMR imaging in medicine. Sci Am 246(5):78, 1982

REMOND A: *Handbook of Electroencephalography and Clinical Neurophysiology*, vols 1–15. Amsterdam, Elsevier/North-Holland, 1976–1978

SPEHLMANN R: *EEG Primer*. Amsterdam, Elsevier/North-Holland, 1981

STALBERG E, YOUNG RR (eds): *Clinical Neurophysiology*. London, Butterworths, 1981

TAVERAS J, WOOD EH: *Diagnostic Neuroradiology*, 2d ed, *Golden's Diagnostic Radiology Series*, sec 1. Baltimore, Williams & Wilkins, 1976

WERNER SS et al: *Atlas of Neonatal Electroencephalography*. New York, Raven Press, 1977

342 THE EPILEPSIES AND CONVULSIVE DISORDERS

MARC A. DICHTER

The *epilepsies* are a group of disorders characterized by chronic, recurrent, paroxysmal changes in neurologic function caused by abnormalities in the electrical activity of the brain. They are common neurologic disorders, estimated to affect between 0.5 and 2 percent of the population, and can occur at any age. Each episode of neurologic dysfunction is called a *seizure*. Seizures may be *convulsive* when they are accompanied by motor manifestations, or may be manifested by other changes in neurologic function (i.e., sensory, cognitive, emotional events). Epilepsy can be acquired as a result of neurologic injury or a structural brain lesion and can also occur as a part of many systemic medical diseases. Epilepsy also occurs in an *idiopathic* form in an individual with neither a history of neurologic insult nor other apparent neurologic dysfunction. Isolated, nonrecurrent seizures may occur in otherwise healthy individuals for a variety of reasons, and, under these circumstances, the individual is not said to have epilepsy.

CLASSIFICATION OF SEIZURES

The neurologic manifestations of epileptic seizures are varied, ranging from a brief lapse of attention to a prolonged loss of consciousness with abnormal motor activity. The proper classification of the kinds of seizures which an individual is experiencing is important for an appropriate diagnostic workup, prognostic evaluation, and selection of therapy. The classification of epileptic seizures provided in this chapter is based on the International Classification of Epileptic Seizures developed in 1969 and subsequently modified in 1981. It emphasizes the clinical seizure type and ictal (seizure-associated) and interictal (between seizures) electroencephalographic pattern (Table 342-1), whereas etiology, anatomic substrate, and pathways of spread are not major considerations. The older terminology of grand mal, petit mal, and psychomotor or temporal lobe epilepsy has been integrated into the current scheme.

The major underlying premise of this classification is that some seizures (partial or focal seizures) start in a localized area of brain (cortex) and either remain localized or secondarily generalize (that is, spread throughout the brain), whereas other seizures appear to be generalized from their earliest manifestation.

PARTIAL OR FOCAL SEIZURES Partial or focal seizures begin with the activation of neurons in one localized area of cortex. The

TABLE 342-1 Classification of epileptic seizures

1 Partial or focal seizures
- *a* Simple partial seizures (with motor, sensory, autonomic, or psychic signs)
- *b* Complex partial seizures (psychomotor or temporal lobe seizures)
- *c* Secondary generalized partial seizures

2 Primary generalized seizures
- *a* Tonic-clonic (grand mal)
- *b* Tonic
- *c* Absence (petit mal)
- *d* Atypical absence
- *e* Myoclonic
- *f* Atonic
- *g* Infantile spasms

3 Status epilepticus
- *a* Tonic-clonic status
- *b* Absence status
- *c* Epilepsia partialis continua

4 Recurrence patterns
- *a* Sporadic
- *b* Cyclic
- *c* Reflex (photomyoclonic, somatosensory, musicogenic, reading epilepsy)

specific clinical symptoms depend on the area of cortex involved and imply dysfunction in a localized area of cortex. The lesion may be due to birth injury, postnatal trauma, tumor, abscess, infarction, vascular malformation, or some other structural abnormality. The abnormal area of cortex underlying the seizure activity can be identified by the specific neurologic phenomena observed during the focal seizure. Partial seizures are classified as *simple* if there is no alteration of consciousness or awareness of the environment and *complex* if there is such a change.

Simple partial seizures Simple partial seizures can occur with motor, sensory, autonomic, or psychic symptoms. A simple partial seizure with motor signs consists of recurrent contractions of the muscles of one part of the body (finger, hand, arm, face, etc.) without loss of consciousness. Each muscular contraction is caused by the discharge of neurons in the corresponding area of the contralateral motor cortex.

The muscle activity of a partial seizure (*ictus*) may remain confined to one area or may spread from the affected area to involve contiguous ipsilateral body parts (i.e., right thumb to right hand to right arm to right side of face). This "Jacksonian march," named after Hughlings Jackson who first described it, is caused by a demonstrable progression of epileptiform discharges in the contralateral motor cortex and may occur over seconds or minutes. The EEG manifestations of this form of seizure are often very striking and consist of regularly occurring spike discharges in the appropriate area of (frontal) motor cortex. Between seizures (interictal period) this region may give rise to irregular spike discharges in the EEG.

Simple partial seizures may have other behavioral manifestations if the seizure discharges occur in other cortical regions. Thus, sensory symptoms (paresthesias, vertiginous feelings, simple auditory or visual hallucinations) occur with epileptiform discharges in the contralateral sensory cortex, and autonomic and psychic symptoms [i.e., the sensation of having experienced something before (déjà vu), unwarranted sense of fear or anger, illusions, and even complex hallucinations] occur with discharges in temporal and frontal lobes.

Complex partial seizures (temporal lobe or psychomotor seizures) Complex partial seizures are episodic changes in behavior in which an individual loses conscious contact with the environment. The onset of these seizures may consist of any of a variety of auras: an unusual smell (as of burning rubber), a feeling that the current experience has happened before (déjà vu), a sudden intense emotional feeling, a sensory illusion such as that of objects growing smaller (*micropsia*) or larger (*macropsia*), or a specifically formed sensory hallucination. Patients may come to recognize these as heralding their seizures, or the memory of the aura may be lost in the postictal amnesia which often occurs if the seizure becomes generalized. During complex partial seizures there may be a cessation of activity with some minor motor activity, such as lip smacking, swallowing, walking aimlessly, or picking at one's clothes (*automatisms*). Complex partial seizures may also be accompanied by the unconscious performance of highly skilled activities such as driving a car or playing complicated musical pieces. When the seizure ends, the individual is amnesic for events which took place during the seizure and may take minutes or hours to recover full consciousness.

Patients with complex partial seizures have EEGs which exhibit unilateral or bilateral spikes or slow wave discharges over temporal or frontotemporal regions both interictally and during seizures. Most of these seizures originate from epileptiform activity in the temporal lobes—especially the hippocampus or amygdala—or other parts of the limbic system, but others have been shown to originate from mesial parasagittal or orbital frontal regions. These seizures are also referred to as *temporal lobe epilepsy* and *psychomotor epilepsy* in older classification schemes.

Although often showing spike discharges or focal slowing during complex partial seizures, exceptionally the surface EEG may be normal. Nasopharyngeal or sphenoidal electrodes may record the abnormal discharges, but in some cases only depth electrodes in the amygdaloid nuclei or other limbic structures will show seizure discharges. The occasional discrepancy between surface and depth electrophysiologic events is a particularly difficult problem when trying to use the surface EEG to determine the nature of an abnormal behavior in an individual suspected of having complex partial seizures. (See "Differential Diagnosis of Seizures" below.)

Secondary generalization of partial seizures Simple or complex partial seizures can progress to generalized seizures with loss of consciousness and often with convulsive motor activity. This may occur immediately or after many seconds or a minute or two. In addition, many patients with focal seizures have generalized seizures without an obvious initial focal component which are difficult to distinguish from primary generalized seizures. The presence of an aura or the observation of any focal feature (twitching of one extremity, aphasia, tonic eye deviation) at the onset of the generalized seizure or the presence of a postictal focal neurologic deficit (Todd's paralysis) is an important clue to a focal origin to the seizure.

PRIMARY GENERALIZED SEIZURES Tonic-clonic (grand mal) One of the most common kinds of epileptic paroxysms is the generalized tonic-clonic seizure. Some of these appear to be primary generalized seizures, and others are the result of secondary generalization from partial seizures. In either case, the seizures follow a common pattern. The primary generalized seizures usually start without warning, although some individuals sense a vague, nonspecific sense of the impending event. The onset is heralded by a sudden loss of consciousness, a *tonic* contraction of the muscles, a loss of postural control, and a cry produced by a forced expiration caused by contraction of the respiratory muscles. The individual falls to the floor in an opisthotonic posture, often sustaining injury, and remains rigid for many seconds. There may be cyanosis as respiration is inhibited. Soon a series of rhythmic contractions of all four limbs occurs. This *clonic* phase can last for a variable period of time and ends when the muscles relax. The individual remains unconscious and unarousable for a period of minutes or longer. There is usually a gradual return to consciousness and often a period of disorientation during recovery. The patient may even be combative if restrained. During the seizure, urinary or fecal incontinence and tongue biting may occur. Postictally there is amnesia for the seizure, and sometimes a retrograde amnesia as well. Headache and drowsiness are common sequelae, and the individual may not return to baseline functioning for days.

The EEG in patients with tonic-clonic seizures shows low-voltage fast (10 Hz or more) activity during the tonic phase, which converts gradually to slower, larger sharp waves throughout both hemispheres. During the clonic phase there are bursts of sharp waves associated with the rhythmic muscular contractions and slow waves coincident with the pauses. Often the excessive muscular activity of the seizure causes artifacts which interfere with ictal EEG recordings. Interictally, the EEG is usually abnormal with polyspike (or spike) and wave or occasionally sharp and slow wave discharges.

Tonic seizures Tonic seizures are a less common form of primary generalized seizure which consist of the sudden occurrence of a rigid posturing of the limbs or torso, often with deviation of the head and eyes toward one side. They are not followed by a clonic phase and are often of shorter duration than tonic-clonic seizures.

Absence seizures (petit mal) Pure absence seizures consist of the sudden cessation of ongoing conscious activity without convulsive muscular activity or loss of postural control. Such seizures may be so brief as to be inapparent. Usually they last for seconds or minutes. The brief lapses of consciousness or awareness may be accompanied by minor motor manifestations such as eyelid fluttering, small chewing movements of the mouth, or mild shaking of the hands. During longer absences, automatisms may occur which may be difficult to distinguish from complex partial seizures. At the end of the absence seizure, the patient regains awareness of the environment very quickly, and there is usually no period of postictal confusion.

Absence seizures almost always begin in young children (6 to 14 years of age) and rarely appear for the first time in adults. These brief seizures may occur hundreds or more times per day and go on for weeks or months before it is recognized that the child is having seizures. In fact, it is not uncommon for these to be first recognized when the child begins having problems with learning.

The EEG is pathognomonic in this form of seizure disorder. During the seizures there are 3-Hz spike-and-wave discharges which appear synchronously throughout all the leads. The EEG is usually normal during the interictal periods. Often the EEG demonstrates that the child is having more seizures than was thought from clinical observation alone.

Absence seizures usually occur in otherwise neurologically normal children. These seizures are usually sensitive to anticonvulsants (see below). Children with this condition often do quite well once it is treated. Approximately one-third outgrow the seizure disorder, one-third continue to have only absence seizures, and one-third have occasional concomitant generalized tonic-clonic seizures.

Absence seizures can be differentiated from absencelike attacks, which occasionally occur in complex partial seizures, by the lack of aura, immediate recovery from the absence, and typical 3-Hz spike-and-wave EEG pattern.

Atypical absence seizures Atypical absence seizures are similar to absence seizures but coexist with other forms of generalized seizures, such as tonic seizures, myoclonic seizures, or atonic seizures (see below). The EEG is more heterogeneous, containing spike-and-wave discharges at 2 or 4 Hz during the absence attacks and poorly developed background with spike or polyspike activity during interictal periods.

Atypical absence seizures commonly occur in children with some other form of underlying neurologic dysfunction and tend to be resistant to medication. In the most severe form of this disorder, the Lennox-Gastaut syndrome, children have several kinds of generalized seizures and often have intellectual impairment.

Myoclonic seizures Myoclonic seizures are sudden, brief, single or repetitive muscle contractions involving one body part or the entire body. In the latter case, the seizure is accompanied by a violent fall, without a loss of consciousness. Myoclonic seizures often coexist with other seizure types but may occur alone. The EEG shows polyspike-and-wave discharges or sharp and slow waves, both ictally and interictally. Although often idiopathic, myoclonic seizures occur as a major neurologic symptom in a variety of medical conditions including uremia, hepatic failure, Creutzfeldt-Jakob disease, subacute leukoencephalopathies, and a hereditary degenerative condition, Lafora body disease.

Atonic seizures Atonic seizures are brief losses of consciousness and postural tone not associated with tonic muscular contractions. The individual may simply drop to the floor without apparent cause. Atonic seizures usually occur in children and are often accompanied by other forms of seizures. The EEG contains polyspikes and slow waves. The "drop attacks" of atonic seizures need to be distinguished from cataplexy seen in narcolepsy (where the patient remains conscious), transient brainstem ischemia, or sudden rises in intracranial pressure.

Infantile spasms or hypsarrhythmia This form of primary generalized seizure occurs in infants between birth and approximately 12 months of age and consists of brief synchronous contractions of the neck, torso, and both arms (usually in flexion). Infantile spasms often occur in children with underlying neurologic diseases, such as anoxic encephalopathy or tuberous sclerosis, but can rarely occur in an otherwise apparently normal infant. The prognosis for children with this form of seizure disorder is grave, and approximately 90 percent develop mental retardation in addition to their seizures. The EEG is characterized by a very disorganized background, random high-voltage slow waves, spikes and burst suppression (hypsarrhythmia). The spasms and hypsarrhythmia tend to disappear over the first 3 to 5 years of life, only to be replaced by other forms of generalized seizures.

STATUS EPILEPTICUS Prolonged or repetitive seizures without a period of recovery between attacks can occur with all forms of seizures and is defined as *status epilepticus*. When tonic-clonic seizures are involved, this state can be life-threatening (see "Treatment of Seizures"). Absence status, on the other hand, may proceed for some time before it is recognized because the patient does not lose consciousness or have convulsive movements. Status epilepticus of partial seizures is called *epilepsia partialis continua* and may occur with partial motor, sensory, or visceral seizures. Complex partial seizures may also present as status epilepticus.

RECURRENCE PATTERNS All classes of recurrent seizures can occur sporadically or randomly, with no apparent triggering event, or can occur cyclically, i.e., in concert with the sleep-waking cycle or the menstrual cycle (*catamenial epilepsy*). Epileptic seizures can also occur as evoked reactions to a specific stimulus (*reflex epilepsy*), although this is relatively infrequent. Examples are seizures triggered by photic stimulation (*photomyoclonic or photoconvulsive epilepsy*), specific musical compositions (musicogenic epilepsy), tactile stimulation (somatosensory induced epilepsy), or reading (reading or language epilepsy). The latter usually consists of brief myoclonic jerks of the jaw, cheek, and tongue which occur during silent or oral reading and may progress to generalized tonic-clonic seizures.

PATHOPHYSIOLOGY OF EPILEPSY

Epileptic seizures can be induced in any normal human (or vertebrate) brain with a variety of different electrical or chemical stimuli. The ease and rapidity with which these seizures can occur, and the stereotyped nature of the seizures produced suggest that the normal brain, particularly the cerebral cortex, contains within its fine anatomic and physiologic structure a mechanism which is inherently unstable and which can be influenced in many different ways to produce a seizure. Thus, many kinds of metabolic abnormalities and anatomic lesions of brain can produce seizures, and conversely, there is no pathognomonic lesion of the epileptic brain.

The hallmark of the altered physiologic state of epilepsy is a rhythmic and repetitive hypersynchronous discharge of many neurons in a localized area of the brain. A reflection of this hypersynchronous discharge can be observed in the electroencephalogram (EEG). The EEG records the integrated electrical activity generated by synaptic potentials in neurons in the superficial layers of a localized area of cortex. Normally, the EEG records unsynchronized activity during periods when the mind is actively working, or mildly synchronized activity when the mind is in a restful state (i.e., alpha waves during relaxation with closed eyes) or during various stages of sleep. In the epileptic focus, neurons in a small area of the cortex are activated in an unusually synchronized manner, and this produces a larger, sharper waveform in the EEG—the *spike discharge*. If the neuronal hypersynchrony is large, a focal, simple seizure follows; if it spreads through the brain and lasts for seconds or minutes, a complex partial or generalized seizure (the *ictus*) will occur and the EEG can have a variety of appearances, depending on which areas of brain are involved and how the primary discharging areas project to the superficial cortex. During the seizure, the EEG may display low-voltage fast activity or high-voltage *spikes* or *spike-and-wave* discharges throughout both hemispheres.

During the interictal spike discharge, the neurons in the epileptic focus undergo a large membrane depolarization (the *depolarizing shift*, or DS) accompanied by action potential generation. After the DS, the neurons hyperpolarize and stop firing for several seconds. In areas around the discharging focus, the neurons are also inhibited but do not first have the large DS. Thus, it appears as if the epileptic discharge is limited to a localized area of cortex by a ring of inhibition around the focus and slightly delayed inhibition within the focus.

When the epileptic focus undergoes a transition from the isolated discharges to a seizure, the post-DS inhibition disappears and is replaced by a depolarizing potential. Neurons in contiguous areas and in synaptically connected distant areas are then recruited into the seizure and become activated. Local cortical circuits, long association pathways (including callosal), and subcortical pathways are all utilized for the spread of the discharges. Thus, a focal seizure can spread locally or generalize throughout the brain. Widely ramifying thalamocortical pathways are likely to be responsible for the rapid generalization of some forms of epilepsy, including absence seizures.

A number of metabolic events occur within the brain during the epileptic discharges which may contribute to the development of the focus, to the transition to seizures, or to postictal dysfunction. During the discharges, extracellular potassium concentration increases and extracellular calcium concentration decreases. Both of these changes have profound effects on neuronal excitability and neurotransmitter release and on neuronal metabolism. Neurotransmitters and neuropeptides are also released in unusually large amounts during seizure discharges. Some of these substances can have prolonged actions on central neurons and may be responsible for prolonged postictal phenomena such as Todd's paralysis. In addition to the ionic effects, seizures produce increases in cerebral blood flow to the primary involved areas, increases in glucose utilization, and alterations in oxidative metabolism and local pH. It is possible that these events are not just consequences of the seizures but actually contribute to the development of the seizure activity and that manipulation of such factors could become an effective means for controlling seizures.

There are many mechanisms by which seizures can develop in either normal or pathologic brains. One of the most common methods for producing epilepsy in experimental animals is to block inhibitory mechanisms. For example, agents which antagonize the inhibitory neurotransmitter γ-aminobutyric acid (GABA) are potent convulsants, both in animals and in human beings. A diminution of inhibition may also be involved in some forms of chronic focal epilepsy, as it has been demonstrated that inhibitory terminals on neurons in areas around cortical gliotic lesions are reduced. This reduction of inhibition may allow excess excitation to develop. It has been postulated that some forms of generalized epilepsy could also be due to an abnormality in the GABA-inhibitory system, but this has not yet been established. At least two antiepileptic drugs, including phenobarbital and the benzodiazepines, can enhance GABA-mediated inhibition in the brain, and this effect is likely to contribute to their antiepileptic actions. Whether other antiepileptic drugs also enhance inhibition is not yet established.

Electrical stimulation is another mechanism by which seizures can easily be produced in a normal brain. At certain current strengths and stimulus frequencies seizure discharges are produced and become self-sustaining beyond the original stimulus. Generalized tonic-clonic seizures result. At lower stimulus parameters, seizure afterdischarges may not occur. However, if a stereotyped subthreshold stimulus is repeated at regular intervals (which may even be as infrequent as one stimulation per day), there is a gradual buildup of response until generalized seizures occur to the same stimulus which was originally subthreshold. Eventually spontaneous seizures may occur without any further electrical stimulation. This phenomenon has been called *kindling*. Its relationship to the pathophysiology of posttraumatic epilepsy or to the issue of whether the occurrence of seizures themselves tends to foster the continued development of a seizure focus in human beings has not been resolved.

THE CAUSES OF EPILEPSY

The likely etiology of a given seizure depends upon the age of the patient and the type of seizure (see Table 342-2). In young infants, anoxia or ischemia before or during birth; intracranial birth injury; metabolic disturbances, such as hypoglycemia, hypocalcemia, and hypomagnesemia; congenital malformations of the brain; and infections are the most common causes of seizures. In the young child, trauma and infections are common causes of epilepsy, although idiopathic seizures account for the majority of patients.

Genetic factors can influence the development of epilepsy and have also been shown to affect EEG patterns in general. Patients with primary generalized seizures, especially absence seizures, have a higher familial incidence of epilepsy than is found in the normal population, and relatives of such patients have higher incidences of dysrhythmic EEGs, even when they do not have seizures. The mode of inheritance of susceptibility to epilepsy appears complicated and probably represents multiple genes with variable penetrance. Even in the highest risk group, however, the chance of a sibling or a child of an individual with generalized seizures also having epilepsy is below 10 percent.

Young children also frequently (approximately 2 to 5 percent of the population) develop seizures with febrile illnesses. These febrile convulsions are short, generalized tonic-clonic convulsions which occur during the early phases of a febrile illness in children between the ages of 3 months and 5 years. Febrile seizures must be distinguished from seizures that are triggered by central nervous system infections which coincidentally produce fever (meningitis or encephalitis). There is minimal likelihood that the child will develop epilepsy or any neurologic impairment from the febrile convulsion if the seizure lasts less than 5 min, is generalized rather than focal, and is not associated with any interictal EEG abnormalities or abnormalities on neurologic exam. There may be a family history of febrile seizure. Febrile seizures of this kind are probably best treated with quick and relatively vigorous attempts to keep children from developing excessive fevers during various childhood illnesses but without specific antiepileptic medication. Some pediatricians prefer to maintain children susceptible to febrile convulsions on chronic phenobarbital medication. On the other hand, if the febrile convulsion is prolonged or focal or is associated with an abnormal EEG, or if the child has a neurologic abnormality, there is a significant risk of subsequent epilepsy. These children should be treated with chronic antiepileptic therapy. Intermittent antiepileptic medication given at the onset of a febrile illness is ineffective and should be avoided.

In adolescents and young adults, head trauma is a major cause of focal epilepsy. Epilepsy can be caused by any kind of serious head injury, with the likelihood of developing recurrent seizures being proportional to the extent of the damage. Injuries which either cause dural penetration or produce posttraumatic amnesia of more than 24-h duration may result in a 40 to 50 percent incidence of later epilepsy, while the incidence with closed head injuries with cerebral contusion varies from 5 to 25 percent. Brief concussive illnesses or nonpenetrating head injuries without loss of consciousness are not epileptigenic. Seizures which occur immediately or within the first

TABLE 342-2 The causes of seizures

Infant (0–2 years)	Paranatal hypoxia and ischemia Intracranial birth injury Acute infection Metabolic disturbances (hypoglycemia, hypocalcemia, hypomagnesemia, pyridoxine deficiency) Congenital malformation Genetic disorders
Child (2–12 years)	Idiopathic Acute infection Trauma Febrile convulsion
Adolescent (12–18 years)	Idiopathic Trauma Drug, alcohol withdrawal Arteriovenous malformations
Young adult (18–35 years)	Trauma Alcoholism Brain tumor
Older adult (over 35 years)	Brain tumor Cerebrovascular disease Metabolic disorders (uremia, hepatic failure, electrolyte abnormality, hypoglycemia) Alcoholism

24 h of injury are not associated with a poor prognosis, whereas seizures occurring after the first day and within the first 2 weeks indicate a high likelihood of posttraumatic epilepsy. Most recurring seizures develop by 2 years after the injury, although longer intervals may occur. Approximately 50 percent of patients with posttraumatic seizures spontaneously recover, 25 percent have medically controllable seizures, and 25 percent have seizures that are much more intractable to antiepileptic medication. The effectiveness of prophylactic anticonvulsant medication after head trauma still requires adequate documentation, although many physicians treat such patients (and other postoperative neurosurgical patients) with phenytoin or phenobarbital to attempt to prevent the development of posttraumatic seizures.

In the adolescent or young adult age group, generalized tonic-clonic seizures tend to be idiopathic or are associated with drug (especially barbiturate) or alcohol withdrawal. Arteriovenous malformations may present as focal seizures in this age group. Between ages 30 and 50, brain tumors become more common causes of seizures and may be present in 30 percent of patients with new focal seizures. In general, the incidence of seizures is higher with slowly growing brain tumors involving the cerebrum, such as meningiomas or low-grade gliomas, than with the more malignant types. However, seizures can occur in individuals with any kind of central nervous system mass lesion, including highly malignant metastatic tumors or completely benign vascular malformations.

Above age 50, cerebrovascular disease is the most common cause of focal or generalized seizures. Seizures can occur acutely in patients with an embolus, hemorrhage, or, more rarely, a thrombosis but more often as a late sequel to these lesions. Seizures can also result from "silent" cerebral infarctions in patients with no known cerebrovascular disease. Brain tumors, either primary or metastatic, also present with seizures in the older age group.

At any age, a variety of medical diseases can produce metabolic disturbances which may present as seizures. Uremia, hepatic failure, hypo- or hypercalcemia, hypo- and hyperglycemia, or hypo- and hypernatremia may be associated with myoclonic seizures or generalized tonic-clonic seizures.

EVALUATION OF THE PATIENT WITH A SEIZURE

Individuals with seizures present to physicians either in an emergency room setting during the acute attack or in an office setting days after the epileptic event. In the former case, the seizure may be the presenting symptom of a serious central nervous system disorder which requires immediate diagnosis and therapy. In the latter case, the seizure may be a symptom of a more chronic neurologic dysfunction and a different approach is warranted.

Initial emergency evaluation is directed toward ensuring adequate ventilation and perfusion and stopping the seizure (see "Treatment"). Once the patient is medically stable, the investigation is directed at determining the cause of the seizure. Often a careful history (either from the patient, if recovered, or from a friend or relative), a physical examination, and a few blood studies can provide the diagnosis.

A history suggesting a recent febrile illness accompanied by headaches, change in mental status, or confusion suggests an acute central nervous system (CNS) infection (either meningitis or encephalitis) and indicates the need for urgent examination of the cerebrospinal fluid. In this context, a complex partial seizure may be the presenting symptom of herpes simplex encephalitis. A history of headache and/or change in mental functioning preceding the seizure, coupled with either signs of increased intracranial pressure or a focal neurologic deficit suggests an underlying mass lesion (tumor, abscess, arteriovenous malformation) or a chronic subdural hematoma. Seizures with a clear focal onset or aura are especially worrisome in this regard. A computerized tomography (CT) scan should be performed for a more definitive diagnosis.

The general physical examination may provide important etiologic information. Gum hyperplasia is usually the result of chronic phenytoin therapy. Exacerbation of a chronic seizure disorder due to intercurrent infection, alcohol, or cessation of therapy is a common cause of patients presenting to an emergency room. Skin examination may reveal the port-wine facial stain of Sturge-Weber disease (with cerebral calcifications being detectable on skull x-ray), or the stigmata of tuberous sclerosis (adenoma sebaceum and shagreen patches) or neurofibromatosis (subcutaneous nodules, café au lait spots). Body or limb asymmetries may indicate hypotrophic somatic development contralateral to a congenital or infantile cerebral lesion.

The history or physical examination may also reveal evidence of chronic alcoholism. Heavy alcohol users commonly have seizures for any of several reasons—alcohol withdrawal *(rum fits),* old cerebral contusion (from falls or fights), chronic subdural hematoma, or metabolic derangements of undernutrition and liver disease. Withdrawal seizures usually occur between 12 and 36 h after cessation of drinking and are brief, generalized tonic-clonic seizures. They occur singly or in a flurry of two or three. After the period of epileptic activity, the seizures do not have to be treated since they are usually self-limiting. Seizures in alcoholics which occur at other times should be treated, but this group of patients presents a particular challenge because of lack of compliance and metabolic problems which complicate drug therapy.

Routine blood studies will indicate if the seizure was caused by hypoglycemia, hypo- or hypernatremia, or hypo- or hypercalcemia. These biochemical abnormalities should be corrected and the cause determined. In addition, other less common causes of seizures which can be sought with the appropriate tests are thyrotoxicosis, acute intermittent porphyria, and lead or arsenic intoxication.

In the older patient, a seizure may indicate an acute cerebrovascular accident or may be a delayed effect of an old cerebral infarct (even a silent one). The manner in which further evaluation proceeds is dictated by the patient's age, cardiovascular status, and accompanying symptoms.

Generalized tonic-clonic seizures can occur in neurologically normal individuals after moderate sleep deprivation. Such seizures can be seen in individuals working double shifts, in college students around examination time, and in soldiers returning from short leaves of absence. After the first seizure, if all investigations are normal, such individuals do not require further treatment.

If the patient's history, physical examination, and blood chemistries are all normal after a seizure, it is likely that the seizure was *idiopathic* and was not caused by a serious underlying CNS lesion. However, tumors or other mass lesions may be entirely asymptomatic except for the seizure and further investigation of such cases is mandatory.

The EEG is important in relation to the differential diagnosis of the seizure, the determination of the cause of the seizure, and the proper classification of the seizure. When the diagnosis of a seizure is in doubt, as, for example, when trying to distinguish seizures from syncope, the presence of a paroxysmal EEG abnormality supports the diagnosis of epilepsy. For this purpose, special activation procedures (sleep recording, photic stimulation, or hyperventilation) or special EEG leads (nasopharyngeal, nasoethmoidal, sphenoidal) for recording from deep structures or prolonged monitoring even on an ambulatory basis, can be employed. The EEG can also reveal focal abnormalities (spikes, sharp waves, or focal slow waves) which would indicate the possibility of a focal neurologic lesion even if the seizure symptomatology appeared generalized from the outset.

The EEG is also used to help classify seizures. It can distinguish focal seizures with secondary generalization from primary generalized seizures and is especially useful in the differential diagnosis of brief lapses of consciousness. Absence seizures are always accompanied by bilateral spike-and-wave discharges, whereas complex partial seizures are accompanied by either focal paroxysmal spikes or slow waves or by a normal surface EEG. In cases of absence seizures, the EEG may reveal that the patient is having many more small seizures than was clinically apparent and may help in monitoring antiepileptic drug therapy.

Until very recently, lumbar puncture, skull x-rays, arteriography, and pneumoencephalography were important adjuncts to the evaluation of the seizure patient. Lumbar puncture is still employed in those situations where acute or chronic CNS infections or subarachnoid hemorrhage are suspected. CT scan and magnetic resonance imaging (MRI) can now provide more definite information about anatomic lesions than the older, invasive techniques. All adults with a new onset seizure disorder should have a diagnostic CT scan both without and with contrast enhancement. In initial studies are normal, continued difficulties with a focal seizure disorder warrant repeat evaluation at 6 to 12 months. MRI appears particularly useful early in the evaluation of a focal seizure disorder when it can demonstrate low-grade abnormalities better than the CT scan. Arteriograms are still performed if the suspicion of an arteriovenous malformation is high, even in the presence of a normal CT, or for the delineation of the vascular pattern in a lesion detected by noninvasive techniques.

DIFFERENTIAL DIAGNOSIS OF SEIZURES

SYNCOPE VERSUS SEIZURE Sudden loss of consciousness, usually without convulsive movements, presents a common diagnostic problem in both children and adults (see Chap. 12). Faints are often preceded by a feeling of lightheadedness, of the room spinning, of a flush, and are often, but not always, precipitated by an environmental stimulus such as prolonged standing in a hot, crowded area, the sight of blood, a fright, etc. In older people, pure syncope is most often secondary to cardiovascular problems, such as Stokes-Adams attacks, tachyarrhythmias, or orthostatic hypotension, and these may occur with or without a warning. A clear focal onset of the event (i.e., abnormal smell, head turning, staring, etc.) favors seizure as the cause. In addition, convulsive muscular contractions, tongue biting, or incontinence commonly accompany seizures but are much less common with fainting spells. Occasionally vasovagal or other types of fainting episodes can be accompanied by either clonic movements or brief generalized tonic-clonic seizures. If the original loss of consciousness can be ascribed to a clearly nonepileptic cause (e.g., the patient was having blood drawn or a dental procedure at the time), it is not necessary to regard the episode as a manifestation of epilepsy, and antiepileptic drug therapy is not indicated.

When the origin of a syncopal episode is in doubt, the patient should undergo a complete cardiovascular evaluation and an EEG with sleep recording and, if available, a prolonged ambulatory EEG monitoring. If the EEG shows paroxysmal activity (which is often brought out by drowsiness and sleep onset), and the patient has no signs of cardiac arrhythmia with ECG monitoring or of valvular disease on echocardiogram, it is likely that the syncopal episode represented a seizure and the patient should be evaluated and treated accordingly.

TRANSIENT ISCHEMIC ATTACKS AND MIGRAINE Transient ischemic attacks (TIAs) and migraine episodes can present as a transient alteration in neurologic function (usually without loss of consciousness) which may be confused diagnostically with focal seizures. Neurologic dysfunction due to ischemia (TIA or migraine) is often a negative symptom (i.e., loss of feeling, numbness, visual field deficit, paralysis), whereas deficits due to focal seizure activity are often positive (twitching, paresthesias, visual distortion, or hallucination), although this distinction is not absolute. Brief stereotyped episodes which conform to dysfunction in a single vascular territory in an individual with either known vascular disease, heart disease, or with risk factors for vascular disease (diabetes, hypertension) are more likely TIAs. However, since cerebral infarcts are a common cause of subsequent seizures in older patients, a paroxysmal EEG focus should be sought.

Classic migraine headaches with a visual aura, unilateral headache, and gastrointestinal upset are usually easy to distinguish from seizures. However, some migraine patients have only "migraine equivalents" such as a hemiparesis, numbness, or aphasia and may not have subsequent headache. These episodes, especially when they occur in older individuals, are hard to distinguish from TIAs, but may also represent focal seizures. The presence of loss of consciousness after some forms of vertebrobasilar migraine and the common occurrence of headaches after seizures makes this differential diagnosis more difficult. The slower development of neurologic dysfunction in migraine (often occurring over minutes) is the most helpful point. Nevertheless, occasionally such patients need to be investigated for all three problems with a CT scan, cerebral angiography, and specialized EEG procedures before a diagnosis can be made. In some cases, a therapeutic trial with antiepileptic drugs (which, interestingly, can prevent migraines as well as seizures in some patients) will be necessary for the final diagnosis.

PSYCHOMOTOR VARIANTS AND "HYSTERICAL" SEIZURES As remarked above, patients with complex partial seizures often have bizarre behavioral manifestations of their seizures. These may consist of abrupt changes in personality, feelings of impending doom or of undirected fear, abnormal bodily sensations, episodic forgetfulness, or brief repetitive motor activities such as picking at one's clothes or stamping a foot. Many of these patients also have personality disorders, and a significant proportion have had psychiatric intervention. It is common, especially if these patients do not have tonic-clonic seizures or loss of consciousness and when these patients appear emotionally disturbed, for such episodes of psychomotor seizures to be called psychopathic fugues or hysterical seizures. This incorrect diagnosis is often reinforced by a "normal EEG" interictally, or even during one of the episodes. It must be emphasized that seizures can arise from foci deep in temporal lobe structures with *no* surface EEG manifestations. This has been repeatedly demonstrated with depth electrode recordings. Moreover, deep temporal seizures can be manifested only by the kinds of phenomena described above and may be free of the usual seizure phenomena of motor convulsions and loss of consciousness.

In a small number of cases, individuals present with seizurelike events which upon investigation turn out to be hysterical "pseudoseizures" or frank malingering. Often these individuals have had true seizures in the past or are acquainted with an individual with epilepsy. Such pseudoseizures can be quite difficult to distinguish from true seizures. Hysterical seizures are characterized by nonphysiologic events such as a progression of twitching from one hand to the other without spread to subjacent ipsilateral face or leg areas, twitching of all four extremities without loss of consciousness (or with surreptitious loss of consciousness), or careful attention to avoiding injury by moving away from a wall or bed edge while having motor convulsions. In addition, hysterical seizures, especially in adolescent girls, may have frankly sexual overtones, with pelvic thrusting or genital manipulation. While many forms of temporal lobe seizures can occur with normal surface EEGs, generalized tonic-clonic seizures always produce abnormal EEGs both during and after the seizure. Most generalized tonic-clonic seizures and many complex partial seizures of moderate duration are accompanied by rises in serum prolactin (during the immediate 30-min postictal period), whereas hysterical seizures are not. Although not an absolute distinguishing point, such measurements, especially if positive, can be very helpful in characterizing the origin of a given "spell."

TREATMENT OF SEIZURES

Treatment of the patient with a seizure disorder is directed at eliminating the cause of the seizures, suppressing the expression of the seizures, and dealing with the psychosocial consequences which may occur as a result of the neurologic dysfunction underlying the seizure disorder or from the presence of a chronic disability.

If the seizure disorder is a result of a metabolic disturbance, such as hypoglycemia or hypocalcemia, restoration of normal metabolic function is usually accompanied by cessation of the seizures. If the seizures are caused by a structural brain lesion, such as a brain tumor, arteriovenous malformation or cerebral cyst, removal of the offending lesion may eliminate the seizures. However, long-standing lesions, even nonprogressive ones, can result in gliosis and other denervation changes. These changes may lead to chronic epileptic foci which will not be eliminated by the subsequent removal of the original lesion. In such cases, surgical extirpation of the epileptic brain regions may be necessary for control of the epilepsy (see "Neurosurgical Treatment of Epilepsy" below).

There is a complex interrelationship between the limbic system and neuroendocrine function which may have significant implications for patients with epilepsy. Normal hormonal fluctuations may influence the frequency of seizures, and epilepsy can cause changes in neuroendocrine function. For example, some women will have a marked change in the pattern of their seizures during particular parts of the menstrual cycle (catamenial epilepsy), while others may have changes in seizure frequency in response to oral contraceptives or pregnancy. In general, estrogens tend to exacerbate seizures, while progesterones tend to be protective. On the other hand, some patients with epilepsy, especially complex partial seizures, may also have an associated reproductive endocrine dysfunction. Disorders in sexual interest, especially hyposexuality, are frequently observed. In addition, women may have polycystic ovary disease and men may have disturbances in potency. Some patients with these endocrine disorders have not had clinical seizures but have abnormal EEGs (often with temporal discharges). Whether the epilepsy causes the endocrine and/or behavioral dysfunction or whether the two conditions are separate manifestations of a common underlying neuropathologic process is not known. However, endocrine manipulation can sometimes be useful in controlling some forms of seizures, and antiepileptic medication may be a useful adjunct for treating some forms of endocrine dysfunction.

PHARMACOLOGIC CONTROL OF EPILEPSY The fundamental modality for the treatment of epilepsy is pharmacologic therapy. The goal is to protect the patient from having seizures without interfering with normal cognitive function (or, in the child, with development of normal intellectual function) and without producing harmful systemic side effects. If possible, the individual should be treated with the lowest possible dose of a single anticonvulsant medication. Precise knowledge of the kind of seizure the patient is having, the spectrum of action of the available anticonvulsant medications, and a few basic pharmacokinetic principles can result in the complete control of approximately 60 to 75 percent of patients with epilepsy. Many patients appear to be resistant to medications or develop unnecessary side effects because the medications chosen are not appropriate for the kind(s) of seizure or are not administered in the optimum doses.

The availability of serum levels of anticonvulsant drugs makes it possible to optimize dosage regimens for individual patients and to monitor drug compliance. Thus, patients can be placed on a medication and after a suitable equilibration period (usually several weeks, but at least five *half-lives*), the amount of medication in the serum can be determined and compared to standard *therapeutic ranges* established for each drug. Utilizing blood levels to adjust doses can compensate for individual patient variability in absorption or metabolism of drugs.

Many anticonvulsant drugs are bound by serum proteins, and it is the unbound, or *free*, drug which is in equilibrium with extracellular spaces within the brain; this level correlates best with seizure control. However, *total* drug is measured in the serum by conventional assays. Under most circumstances, this is adequate for determining if the anticonvulsant is in the therapeutic range. Occasionally, serum anticonvulsant levels will be high, yet the patient continues to have seizures without any pharmacologic side effects of the anticonvulsant. In these cases, it is possible that serum protein binding is higher than expected and that the patient is undermedicated in relation to the free drug available. "Free" levels can be determined by measurements of drug concentrations in saliva. Increase in dose may produce control without any untoward side effects (despite a blood level above therapeutic range). Similarly, individuals with impaired liver or renal function may have low serum proteins or circulating "toxins" which reduce drug binding. In this case, toxicity may appear at unusually low serum levels because of a relatively higher free level of drug.

Intensive long-term EEG and video monitoring has demonstrated that careful characterization of seizures and selection of anticonvulsant drugs can significantly increase seizure control in many patients whose seizures had previously been considered intractable to conventional antiepileptic drugs. In fact, often these patients can have one or more of their multiple drugs removed while still achieving better control.

INDICATIONS FOR USE OF SPECIFIC DRUGS **Generalized tonic-clonic seizures (grand mal)** There are three medications which are of proven value in this very common form of seizure—phenytoin (or diphenylhydantoin), phenobarbital (and other long-acting barbiturates), and carbamazepine (see Table 342-3). Most patients will be controlled by adequate doses of any one of these, although individual patients may respond better to one or another. The choice among them often relates to minimizing undesirable side effects. Phenytoin is probably the drug of choice producing effective control with no sedation and very little, if any, intellectual impairment. However, phenytoin does produce gum hyperplasia in some individuals and can produce mild hirsutism, which is especially unpleasant for young women. Prolonged use can produce coarsening of facial features. Phenytoin may produce lymphadenopathy and, in very high doses, may be toxic to the cerebellum. Carbamazepine is equally effective and does not have many of the side effects seen with phenytoin. Cognitive function appears as well or even better preserved than with phenytoin. However, carbamazepine can cause gastrointestinal upset and may cause bone marrow depression with mild to moderate falls in peripheral white count (3.5 to 4 $\times$ 10^3 per milliliter) which can occasionally become severe and which must be watched carefully. In addition, carbamazepine can produce hepatotoxicity. For these reasons, a complete blood count and liver function tests should be performed before starting carbamazepine and at 2-week intervals for a period after initiating therapy.

Phenobarbital is also effective against tonic-clonic seizures and has none of the side effects mentioned above. It can cause sedation and a dulling of intellect, however, especially early in its use, and this may lead to poor compliance. The sedation is dose-dependent and may limit the amount of drug which can be given to achieve complete control. However, if control can be achieved with nonsedative doses of phenobarbital, it may be the safest chronic regimen. Primidone is a barbiturate which is metabolized to phenobarbital and phenylethylmalonamide (PEMA) and may be more effective than phenobarbital alone because of its active metabolite. In children, the barbiturates can produce a state of hyperactivity and hyperirritability which will limit their usefulness.

In addition to their systemic side effects, all three classes of drugs have neurologic toxicities at higher doses. Nystagmus is common at therapeutic blood levels, but ataxia, dizziness, tremor, intellectual dulling, forgetfulness, confusion, and even stupor may occur with increasing blood concentrations. These are reversible when blood levels fall back to therapeutic levels.

Partial seizures, including complex partial seizures (temporal lobe epilepsy) The same drugs which are useful for tonic-clonic seizures are also effective for partial seizures. Although not definitely established, it may be that carbamazepine and phenytoin are slightly more effective than the barbiturates for these seizures. In general, complex partial seizures are difficult to control, and patients with these seizures often require more than one medication (i.e., carbamazepine and primidone or phenytoin and primidone or any one of the primary drugs and high doses of methsuximide) and may become candidates for neurosurgical intervention. These are the kinds of seizures for which many epilepsy centers are conducting trials of new antiepileptic drugs.

TABLE 342-3 Commonly used antiepileptic drugs

Generic name	Trade name	Principal uses	Dosage	Half-life
Phenytoin (diphenylhydantoin)	Dilantin	Tonic-clonic (grand mal) Focal Complex partial	300–400 mg/day (3–5 mg/kg—adult; 4–7 mg/kg—child)	24 h (with wide variation)
Carbamazepine	Tegretol	Tonic-clonic Focal Complex partial	600–1200 mg/day (20–30 mg/kg—child)	13–17 h
Phenobarbital	Luminol	Tonic-clonic Focal	60–200 mg/day (1–5 mg/kg—adult; 3–6 mg/kg—child)	90 h (shorter in children)
Primidone	Mysoline	Tonic-clonic Focal Complex partial	750–1000 mg/day (10–25 mg/kg)	Primidone—8 h PEMA—24–48 h Phenobarbital—90 h
Ethosuximide	Zarontin	Absence (petit mal)	750–1250 mg/day (20–40 mg/kg)	60 h (adult) 30 h (child)
Methsuximide	Celontin	Absence	600–1200 mg/day	
Clonazepam	Clonopin	Absence Atypical absence Myoclonic	1–12 mg/day (0.1–0.2 mg/kg)	24–48 h
Sodium valproate	Depakene	Absence Atypical absence (Tonic clonic)	750–1250 mg/day (30–60 mg/kg)	6–20 h 15 h
Trimethadione	Tridione	Absence Atypical absence (Use only with intractable seizures)	900–2100 mg/day (20–60 mg/kg)	6–13 days (for dimethadione)

Primary generalized absence seizures (petit mal, atypical petit mal) These seizures respond to different classes of medications than either tonic-clonic or focal seizures. For simple absence, ethosuximide is the drug of choice. Side effects include gastrointestinal upset, behavior changes, dizziness, and lethargy, but are not often troublesome. For more difficult to control atypical absence seizures and for myoclonic seizures, valproic acid is the drug of choice. (It may also be useful in primary generalized tonic-clonic seizures.) Valproic acid can cause gastrointestinal irritation, bone marrow suppression (especially thrombocytopenia), hyperammonemia, and hepatic dysfunction (including rare instances of fatal progressive hepatic failure which appear to be idiosyncratic rather than dose-related). A complete blood count with platelet count and liver function tests should be performed before beginning therapy and at biweekly intervals after initiating therapy for a suitable period until the safety of the drug is established in the individual patient. Clonazepam (a benzodiazepine) can also be used for atypical absence and myoclonic seizures. It can cause drowsiness and irritability, but usually it does not cause other systemic side effects. Trimethadione was one of the first antiabsence drugs but is now rarely used because of its potential toxicity.

Approximately one-third of children who present with "pure" absence seizures also have tonic-clonic seizures at some later time. The question of whether these children should be treated prophylactically with an anti-tonic-clonic seizure medication has not been resolved. Since valproic acid has actions against both classes of seizures, its use has been increasing in children with absence. The concurrent use of phenobarbital with antiabsence drugs for this purpose should be avoided as it may interfere with therapy for the absence.

Status epilepticus Generalized tonic-clonic status epilepticus is a life-threatening medical emergency, but overzealous and incautious treatment can produce more harm than good. Patients are in danger from hyperpyrexia and acidosis (from prolonged muscle activity) and less commonly, hypoxia or compromise of respiratory function. Immediate treatment for status is protection of the airway, protection of the tongue (with a soft object, large enough not to be swallowed, between the clenched teeth), protection of the head, and then establishment of a secure parenteral (intravenous) access. A bolus of 50% glucose in water (after blood is drawn for analysis), even if hypoglycemia is not expected, may stop the seizures. All further intravenous medication should be given after preparation for respiratory and circulatory support is available.

Phenytoin, 500 to 1500 mg (13 to 18 mg/kg) in a slow intravenous "push" (*not* 5% dextrose in water—phenytoin precipitates in this low pH solution)—no faster than 50 mg/min—is one of the drugs of choice. It does not depress respiration but may produce mild AV block and, if given too rapidly, can cause a fall in blood pressure.

The benzodiazepines, diazepam 10 mg or lorazepam 4 mg (followed by another dose if necessary), are also effective in stopping status epilepticus when administered intravenously. However, these drugs may depress respiratory function (or even cause respiratory arrest), and measures for respiratory support should be available before they are administered. The use of a benzodiazepine after phenobarbital administration carries a particular risk. The benzodiazepines are short-acting drugs, and after they are administered, a second, longer-acting anticonvulsant such as phenytoin is usually required to prevent recurrence of seizures.

Phenobarbital, in a dose of 10 to 20 mg/kg (up to 1 g), divided into two to four doses at 30- to 60-min intervals, can also be administered for status epilepticus. Phenobarbital also causes respiratory depression and should not be used immediately after treatment with intravenous diazepam.

After stopping the seizures it is imperative to determine the cause of the status epilepticus in order to prevent its recurrence. In approximately two-thirds of adults the cause can be determined and is usually tumor, vascular disease, infection, cerebral damage, or precipitous withdrawal from alcohol or antiepileptic medication. In children, the incidence of idiopathic status is higher (approximately

Therapeutic range	% Protein-bound	Toxic effects: Neurologic	Toxic effects: Systemic	Drug interactions
10–20 μg/ml	90	Ataxia Incoordination Confusion	Gum hyperplasia Lymphadenopathy Hirsutism Osteomalacia Skin rash Altered folate metabolism	Level increased by INH, dicumeral, sulfonamides Level decreased by carbamazepine, phenobarbital Folate interferes with effects
4–12 μg/ml	80	Ataxia Dizziness Diplopia Vertigo	Bone marrow suppression Gastrointestinal irritation Hepatotoxicity	Level decreased by phenobarbital, phenytoin
10–50 μg/ml	40–60	Sedation Ataxia Confusion Dizziness	Skin rash	Level increased by valproate, phenytoin
2–10 μg/ml	Small for primidone or PEMA	Same as phenobarbital	Same as phenobarbital	
40–100 μg/ml	Small	Ataxia Lethargy	Gastrointestinal irritation Skin rash Bone marrow suppression	
	Small	Ataxia Lethargy	Same as ethosuximide	
5–70 ng/ml	50	Ataxia Sedation Lethargy	Anorexia	May precipitate absence status if given with valproic acid
50–100 μg/ml	80–94	Ataxia Sedation	Hepatotoxicity Bone marrow suppression Gastrointestinal irritation Weight gain Transient alopecia	May precipitate absence status if given with clonazepam
700 μg/ml (for dimethadione)	Small	Sedation Blurred vision	Skin rash Bone marrow suppression Nephrosis Hepatitis	

50 percent), and the remaining cases are divided between acute brain illnesses such as purulent meningitis, encephalitis, and dehydration with electrolyte disturbances, and chronic encephalopathies. Tonic-clonic status epilepticus is a dangerous condition; the mortality rate may be over 10 percent with another 10 to 30 percent of patients being left with permanent neurologic sequelae.

NEUROSURGICAL TREATMENT OF EPILEPSY If a structural lesion (i.e., tumor, cyst, abscess, etc.) is causing recurrent seizures, the removal of that lesion and nearby diseased brain will often eliminate the seizures or make them easier to control. Some patients, however, have uncontrollable seizures without a demonstrable structural lesion. These are often complex partial seizures with ictal and interictal EEG abnormalities emanating from one or both temporal lobes. Many surgical series have shown that if the epileptogenic lesion can be clearly localized to one temporal lobe, neurosurgical removal of that temporal lobe can result in significant improvement in 60 to 80 percent of the patients. Localization often depends on intensive EEG monitoring and even depth electrode recordings from the temporal lobes. In a high percentage of cases the removed temporal lobe can be shown to have microscopic pathology, such as *hippocampal* (or *Ammon's horn*) *sclerosis* (loss of pyramidal cells in the hippocampus), a hamartoma, or cortical ectopia.

Some individuals with complex partial seizures also develop a psychiatric illness characterized most often as a borderline personality with certain specific behavioral manifestations including hypergraphia, hyperreligiosity, lack of sense of humor, and disordered sexuality. The psychiatric aspects of this illness may result from the epilepsy or may be independently produced by the same underlying brain lesion which produces the epilepsy. The personality disorder may not significantly change after epilepsy surgery, even if the seizures are controlled.

TREATMENT OF A SINGLE SEIZURE Some individuals present with a single, brief generalized tonic-clonic seizure and, after complete evaluation, are found to have a normal EEG and no underlying cause for the seizure. Some of these individuals go on to have recurrent seizures, but an unknown proportion do not. The decision to treat such a patient with several years (at least) of antiepileptic medication must be made on an individual basis, considering the patient's lifestyle, risks from a sudden loss of consciousness, and feelings about medications.

CESSATION OF ANTIEPILEPTIC DRUG THERAPY Many patients with epilepsy require antiepileptic drug therapy for life. However, a large proportion of epileptic patients become seizure-free on appropriate medication, and approximately half of such patients can eventually stop their medications and remain seizure-free. The patient who has had no seizures for 4 years, who has had relatively few seizures before control was attained, who only required a single medication, who has a normal neurologic exam and no structural lesion causing the seizures, and who has a normal EEG at the end of the therapeutic period has the best chance of remaining seizure-free if medication is slowly tapered (over 3 to 6 months). An abnormal EEG is not a contraindication to discontinuing medication. When considering the discontinuance of antiepileptic therapy, the consequences of the recurrence of seizures must be carefully considered. One inopportune seizure in a previously well controlled patient who is not used to taking precautions may be a life-threatening event, or lead to loss of a driver's license or loss of employment. Nevertheless, since all medications carry some risk of toxicity and since medication compliance in a healthy individual is often variable, it is worth a careful trial of medication tapering in individuals who meet the above criteria and are willing to accept the risk.

EPILEPSY AND PREGNANCY Most women with epilepsy can undergo uneventful pregnancies and deliver healthy babies—even those taking anticonvulsant medications. During the pregnant state, however, body metabolism changes and close attention must be given to antiepileptic drug levels. Sometimes relatively high doses have to be given to ensure therapeutic levels. Most women who are well controlled before pregnancy will remain so during pregnancy and delivery. Women whose seizures are not under good control before becoming pregnant are at higher risk for having increased difficulties during the pregnancy.

One of the most serious complications of pregnancy, toxemia, often presents as a generalized tonic-clonic convulsion in the third trimester. This seizure is a symptom of a severe neurologic disturbance and is not a manifestation of epilepsy, nor is it more common in epileptic women. The toxemic state must be treated in order to control the seizures.

There is a two- to threefold higher incidence of fetal malformations in offspring of epileptic women, and this is likely due to a combination of the low incidence of medication-induced malformation and of genetic predisposition in this population. Among those malformations which do occur, a *fetal-hydantoin syndrome* consisting of cleft lip and palate, heart defects, digital hypoplasia, and nail dysplasia has been identified.

Although it would be ideal for women contemplating pregnancy to have their antiepileptic drugs discontinued, it is likely that for a large number of women this would result in recurrence of seizures which would, in the long run, be more harmful for both mother and baby. If patients meet the criteria for discontinuance of medication, this should be done with a suitable interval before pregnancy is to occur. Other patients should be tapered to a minimal effective dosage and, if possible, be maintained on only one medication. There are no clear data indicating differences in safety for phenobarbital, phenytoin, or carbamazepine when used alone. Less experience is available for valproate. Phenobarbital, primidone, or phenytoin can cause transient and reversible deficiency in vitamin K–dependent clotting factors in the neonate, and these should be promptly treated. Babies exposed to chronic barbiturates in utero are often transiently sluggish, hypotonic, jittery, and often show signs of barbiturate withdrawal. These babies should be considered at risk for neonatal problems and should be slowly withdrawn from barbiturates and closely observed in the nursery during the neonatal period.

DRIVING AND EPILEPSY Each state has its own regulations for determining when an individual with epilepsy can obtain a driver's license, and several states have laws about the physician's obligations in either reporting epileptic patients to the registry or informing the patients of their responsibilities to do so. In general, patients can drive after a seizure-free interval (on or off medications) which ranges from 6 months to 2 years. In some states there is no fixed interval, but the individual is required to have a physician's letter attesting to seizure control. It is the physician's responsibility to warn the epileptic patient of the risks of driving when seizures are not under control.

SOCIAL AND EDUCATIONAL REHABILITATION Most people with epilepsy attain adequate control of their seizures and are able to attend school, obtain employment, and live a relatively normal life. Children with epilepsy tend to have more problems in school than their peers, but every effort should be made to keep these children integrated into the mainstream of the educational process while supplying additional help in the form of academic tutoring or psychological counseling.

REFERENCES

Aird R et al: *The Epilepsies: A Critical Review.* New York, Raven Press, 1984

Browne TR, Feldman RG (eds): *Epilepsy: Diagnosis and Management.* Boston, Little Brown, 1983

Commission on Classification and Terminology of the ILAE: Proposal for revised clinical classification of epileptic seizures. Epilepsia 22:489, 1981

Emerson R et al: Stopping medication in children with epilepsy. N Engl J Med 304:1125, 1981

Engel J Jr et al: Recent Developments in the Diagnosis and Therapy of Epilepsy. Ann Intern Med 97:584, 1982

Laidlaw J, Richens A (eds): *A Textbook of Epilepsy,* 2d ed. London, Churchill Livingstone, 1982

Leppik IE: Drug treatment of epilepsy in *Current Therapy in Neurologic Disease,* RT Johnson (ed). Philadelphia, BC Decker Inc, 1986, pp 41–46

Solomon G et al: *Clinical Management of Seizures.* Philadelphia, Saunders, 1983

Thurston J et al: Prognosis in childhood epilepsy. N Engl J Med 306:831, 1982

Woodbury D et al (eds): *Antiepileptic Drugs,* 2d ed. New York, Raven Press, 1982

343 CEREBROVASCULAR DISEASES

J. PHILIP KISTLER / ALLAN H. ROPPER / JOSEPH B. MARTIN

Cerebrovascular disease is the third leading cause of death after heart disease and cancer in developed countries. More importantly, in adults, it is the most lethal and disabling of the neurologic diseases. It has an overall prevalence of 794 per 100,000. Five percent of the population over 65 has at one time in their lives had a stroke. In the United States it is estimated that more than 400,000 patients are discharged each year from hospitals after a stroke. The removal of these patients from the work force and the extended hospitalization they require make the economic impact of this disease one of the most devastating in medicine.

PATHOGENESIS OF STROKE Cerebrovascular disease implicates one or more of the blood vessels of the brain in a pathologic process. The process may be intrinsic to the vessel, as it is in atherosclerosis, lipohyalinosis, inflammation, amyloid formation, dissection (traumatic or spontaneous), developmental malformation, or aneurysmal dilatation; or the process may start at a remote site, as occurs when an embolus from the heart or extracranial circulation lodges in an intracranial vessel, or when decreased perfusion pressure or increased blood viscosity results in inadequate blood flow through a vessel. A vascular lesion tends to be silent until it causes critical narrowing with ischemia, or embolises, occludes, or ruptures. A *stroke* is defined as a neurologic injury occurring as a result of one of these pathologic processes. A thrombus, atheroma, or embolus may critically narrow or block a vessel and produce ischemia with infarction; or a vessel may rupture and give rise to intracerebral or subarachnoid hemorrhage. Other symptoms may occur secondary to vascular disease, such as pressure on cranial nerves from an aneurysm, vascular headache (migrainous or with arteritis or hypertension), or increased intracranial pressure accompanying a venous thrombosis.

CEREBRAL METABOLISM AND INFARCTION To function normally, the brain must receive a moment-to-moment supply of oxygenated blood, but even a reduced supply may suffice to forestall infarction for an indeterminate period. Cardiac arrest results in unconsciousness within 10 s; and in animal experiments, total cessation of blood flow produces irreversible cerebral infarction within 3 min. However, reduced flow allows the brain to remain ischemic but viable for prolonged periods before it either infarcts or recovers as flow returns toward normal. For example, patients who suffer cerebral embolism, or cerebral vasospasm following subarachnoid hemorrhage, often recover partially or completely. Such recovery suggests that focal areas of brain can remain functionless and ischemic for hours, even days, yet revive. This has led to the notion of an ischemic zone (penumbra or halo) that surrounds an infarct. The extent to which recovery can occur after ischemia remains uncertain. What is clear is that once brain cells become infarcted, cell membrane integrity is lost, the blood-brain barrier is disrupted, and mitochondrial high-energy phosphate metabolism ceases.

PATHOLOGY An infarcted brain is pale initially. Within hours to days, the gray matter, in particular, may become congested with engorged, dilated blood vessels and minute petechial hemorrhages (hemorrhagic infarction). The cause of such hemorrhagic infarction is uncertain, but is usually considered to result from an embolus blocking a major vessel, e.g., middle cerebral artery stem (Figs.

343-1 and 343-2) or one of its major branches; the embolus migrates, lyses, and disperses within hours, allowing recirculation into the infarcted area. The recirculation may cause the hemorrhagic infarction and possibly aggravate the subsequent edema formation after the blood-brain barrier has broken down. A primary intracerebral hemorrhage, on the other hand, damages the brain by disrupting tissue at the site of the hemorrhage and by compressing the surrounding tissue.

Once an ischemic stroke or intracerebral hemorrhage has occurred, or when transient spells of cerebral ischemia occur, the prelude to adequate therapy is a precise diagnosis. It must include definition of the character and location of the lesion, the vascular pathologic process producing the symptoms, and knowledge of the anatomy of any spared collateral circulation to the ischemic area. The brain repairs itself only by forming fibrogliotic scar tissue at the site of an infarction or hemorrhage; therefore, therapeutic efforts can only be preventive. Such efforts should attempt to protect both the normal and ischemic brain from either initial or recurrent pathologic processes, as well as from the secondary effects of the stroke itself, e.g., brain compression from intracranial hemorrhage or edema. Broadly, such preventive therapy has three goals: to prevent stroke by reducing risk factors, thus attenuating the pathologic process; to prevent initial or recurrent stroke by removing the underlying pathologic process—for example, by performing a carotid endarterectomy; and to prevent

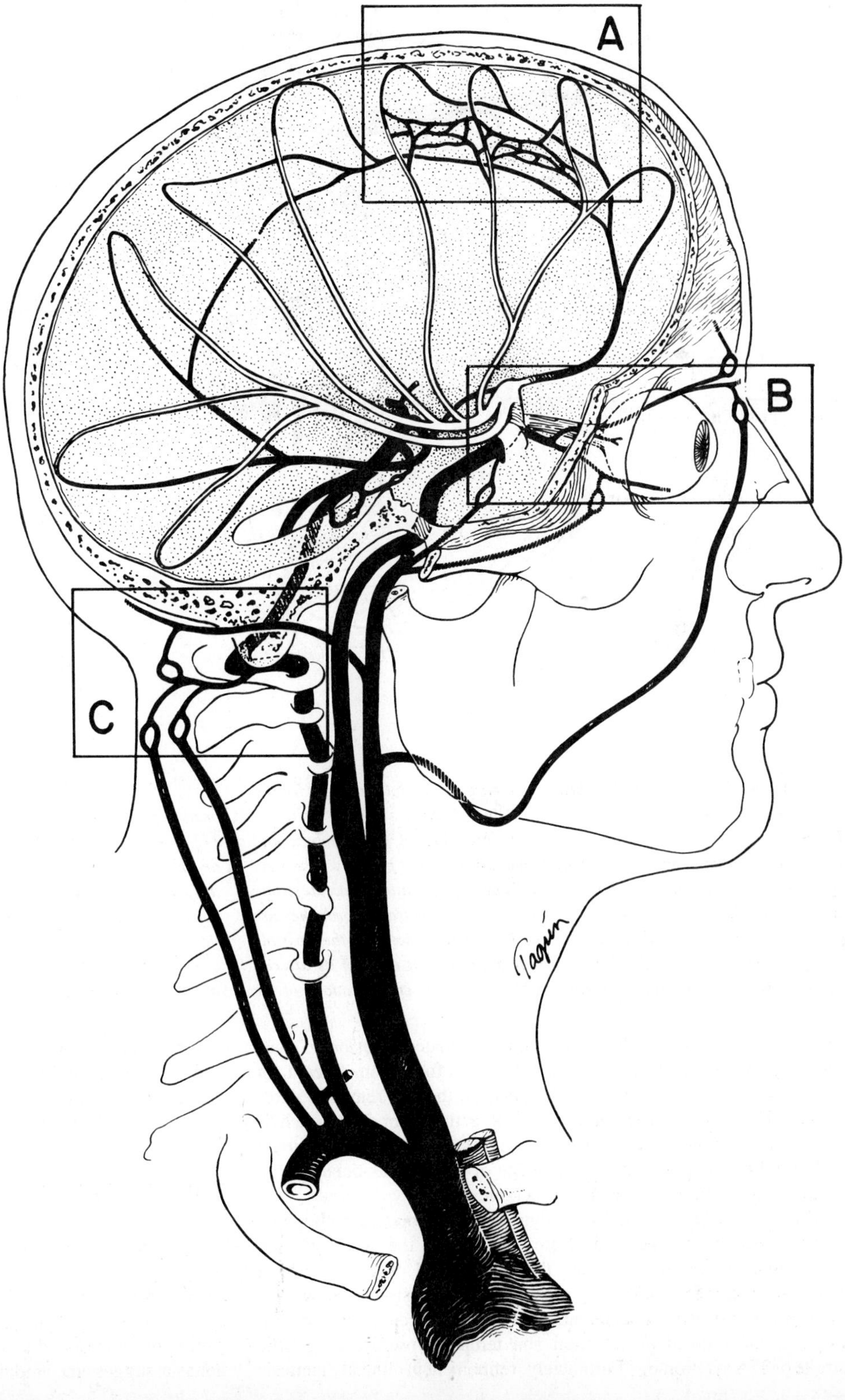

FIGURE 343-1 *Arrangement of the major arteries of the right side carrying blood from the heart to the brain. Also shown are vessels of collateral circulation that may modify the effects of cerebral ischemia (A,B,C). Not shown is the circle of Willis which also provides a source for collateral circulation. A. The anastomotic channels between the distal branches of the anterior and middle cerebral artery, termed borderzone or watershed anastomotic channels. Note that they also occur between the posterior and middle cerebral arteries and the anterior and posterior cerebral arteries. B. Anastomotic channels occurring through the orbit between branches of the external carotid artery and the ophthalmic branch of the internal carotid artery. C. Wholly extracranial anastomotic channels between the muscular branches of the ascending cervical arteries and muscular branches of the occipital artery that anastomose with the distal vertebral artery. Note that the occipital artery arises from the external carotid artery, thereby allowing reconstitution of flow in the vertebral from the carotid circulation. (Courtesy of C.M. Fisher, M.D.)*

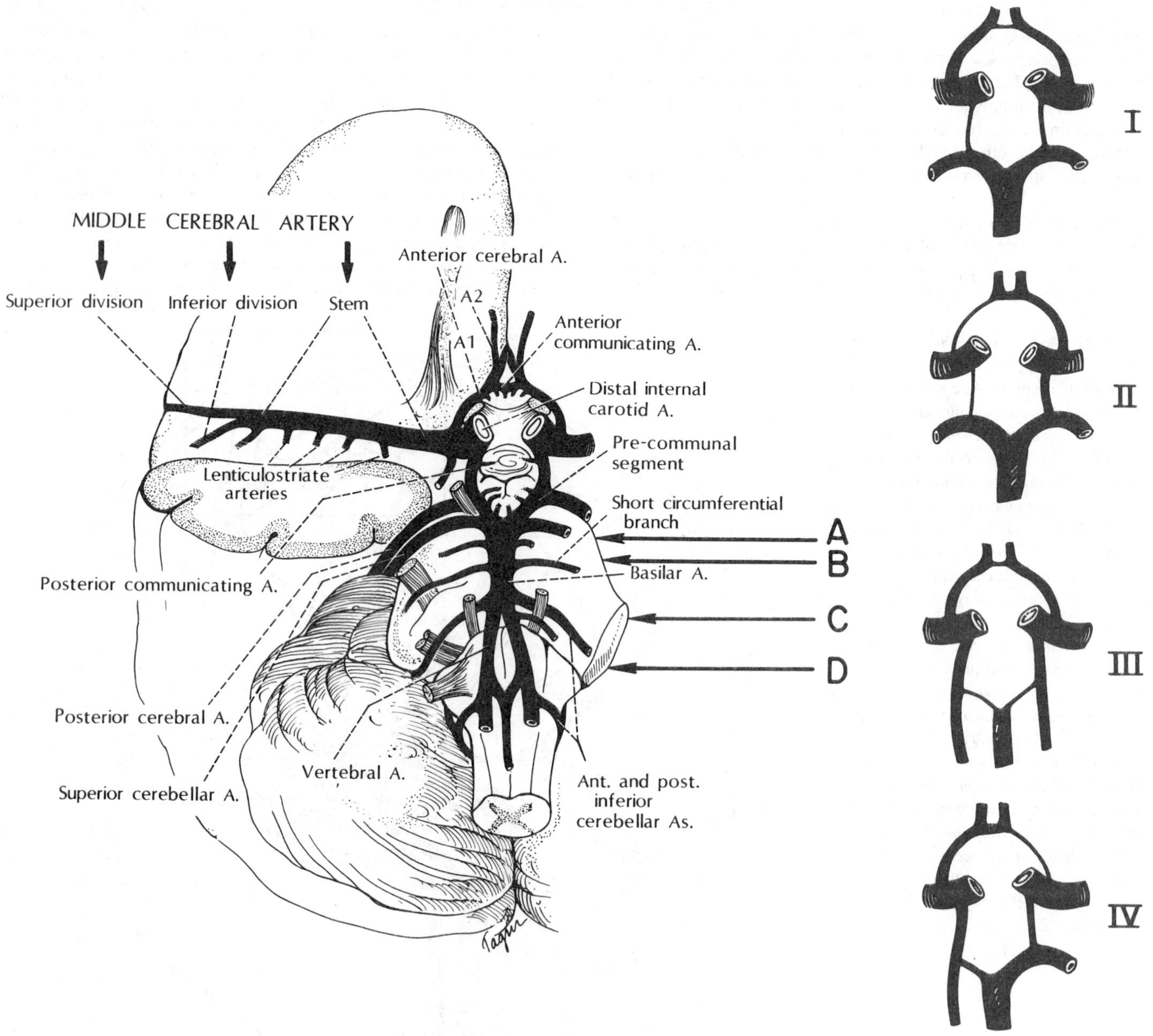

FIGURE 343-2 *Diagram of the brainstem, cerebellum, inferior right frontal lobe, and temporal lobe transected. Principal branches of the vertebral basilar arterial system are pictured. Small branches of the vertebral and basilar artery that penetrate the medulla and pons are not pictured. The stem of the middle cerebral artery with its small, deep penetrating lenticulostriate arteries and the circle of Willis with its small, deep penetrating branches are pictured. Roman numerals I, II, III, and IV represent some of the possible variations of the Circle of Willis due to atresia of one or more of its arterial components. A, B, C, and D arrows point to the four cross-sections of the brainstem diagrammed below (D = Fig. 343-7, A = Fig. 343-8, B = Fig. 343-9, C = Fig. 343-10). Although typical vascular syndromes of the pons and medulla have been designated by the shaded areas in Figs. 343-7 to 10, the shading is arbitrary. Great variability in infarct size and location occurs when the basilar or vertebral arteries, or one of their penetrating branches, occludes because of variation in arterial anatomic location and available collateral circulation. Thus the stroke syndromes produced are often atypical, incomplete, or merge with one another. (Courtesy of C.M. Fisher, M.D.)*

secondary brain damage by maintaining adequate perfusion to marginally ischemic areas and by reducing edema formation. Except for the elimination of risk factors, all aspects of therapy remain controversial. Established proof of efficacy of a therapeutic approach is lacking in many instances; hence, current therapy is largely empirical and based on the physician's knowledge of the risks associated with various diagnostic procedures and therapies.

Strokes can be classified according to their proposed pathophysiologic mechanism. The clinical presentation and the diagnostic and therapeutic options for each can then be defined. The single most important factor in establishing a precise pathophysiologic diagnosis of stroke or transient ischemic attack (TIA) is an accurate assessment of its initial clinical presentation and temporal profile, i.e., "the stroke or TIA syndrome." Fortunately, refinement in clinical diagnosis and neuroradiologic techniques can now allow diagnosis of the type and location of strokes and their concomitant vascular lesions with considerable frequency and accuracy, making a more focused approach to therapy both possible and mandatory.

THE STROKE SYNDROME

The characteristics of the mode of onset, together with the specific neurologic symptoms and signs, suggest the lesion's location and its cause. In most cases, the abrupt, dramatic onset of focal neurologic symptoms stamps the process as a stroke, particularly when the symptoms correspond to a specific vascular territory: hemiparesis and aphasia suggest the middle cerebral artery territory of the dominant hemisphere; a sudden disturbance in a visual field suggests the territory of the posterior cerebral artery; or a pure motor hemiparesis suggests a small "lacunar" stroke in the internal capsule or basis pontis corresponding to the territory of the small penetrating branches of the middle cerebral or basilar arteries, respectively. The initial symptoms may be minimal or maximal at onset, or the deficit may fluctuate, improving or worsening in a stepwise manner. It is this temporal profile that first suggests whether a lesion is thrombotic, embolic, or hemorrhagic. For example, sudden deep coma can accompany either basilar artery embolism, subarachnoid hemorrhage, or hypertensive hemorrhage in the basis pontis. To define the nature of the lesion causing the coma, both the neurologic deficits found on examination and details of the subsequent neurologic course are needed. Frequently, the precise details of the early temporal course are difficult to delineate. The patient may not remember until prompted; or the location of a deficit may preclude awareness, as it does when anosognosia occurs in lesions of the nondominant hemisphere. Often the family is the best source of important historical details in cases of acute stroke or suspected transient cerebral ischemia.

The stroke syndrome, therefore, is recognized chiefly by its temporal profile and its characteristic pattern of symptoms and signs.

In hemorrhagic strokes, the location and size of the hemorrhage and its type (subarachnoid vs. intracerebral) determine the characteristic stroke syndrome. However, in ischemic stroke, the stroke syndrome is determined not only by the pathologic process and the size and location of the occluded vessel but also by the availability of collateral circulation. Often, there is sufficient collateral flow to prevent infarction or reduce the size of infarction significantly, altering the evolution of the stroke syndrome.

Collateral flow may be sufficient for a major arterial trunk to be entirely occluded without symptoms or visible damage to the brain parenchyma. In other cases, occlusion of major vessels may lead to softening throughout their entire arterial territory. Between these two extremes countless variations in the size, shape, and completeness of an infarct depend on the availability of collateral flow (Fig. 343-1). In addition, collateral flow depends on vascular anatomy, the speed of occlusion, and the level of the systemic blood pressure. These factors and possibly others such as altered physical state of the blood (viscosity, polycythemia, abnormal red blood cells) may at times operate adversely to produce ischemia in the territory of partially occluded vessels.

The only vessels not subject to collateral flow are the small, deep penetrating vessels that arise from the stem of the middle cerebral arteries (lenticulostriate arteries), the distal vertebral arteries, the basilar artery, and the arteries of the circle of Willis (Figs. 343-2 and 343-3). They supply deep white and gray matter in the brainstem, thalamus, basal ganglia, and corona radiata. Occlusion of one of these small penetrating vessels, either by atherothrombotic or lipohyalinotic disease or embolism, produces a small "lacunar" infarction.

The terms *stroke in evolution* (also called *progressive stroke*) and *completed stroke* need special mention. Stroke in evolution refers to a neurologic deficit that progresses or fluctuates while the patient is under observation, whereas completed stroke implies that no further deterioration will occur. Several mechanisms have been attributed to stroke in evolution, among them progressive narrowing of an artery by thrombus, development of cerebral edema, thrombus propagation obliterating collateral branches to the ischemic brain, and systemic factors, e.g., arterial hypotension. Although these may have a role in some cases, it is more likely that fluctuating neurologic deficits are the result of emboli propagating, migrating, lysing, and dispersing, or are caused by recurrent artery-to-artery embolization, fluctuating collateral flow through the circle of Willis, through border zone anastomotic channels, or through orbital or cervical-vertebral collaterals (Figs. 343-1*A*, *B*, and *C*, and 343-2).

RISK FACTORS IN STROKE Certain types of cerebrovascular disease suggest themselves not only by their stroke syndromes but also by their association with risk factors. An atherothrombotic stroke often suggests that the patient has silent or symptomatic cardiovascular and peripheral vascular disease; conversely, severe atherothrombotic disease anywhere in the body suggests an atherothrombotic process as the cause of an ischemic stroke. Since atrial fibrillation, valvular heart disease, myocardial infarction, and bacterial endocarditis are sources of emboli, their presence suggests embolism as the diagnosis. Severe hypertension is invariably linked to small vessel lipohyalinotic

FIGURE 343-3 *Diagram of a cerebral hemisphere in coronal section, showing the territories of the major cerebral vessels. (Courtesy of C. M. Fisher, M.D.)*

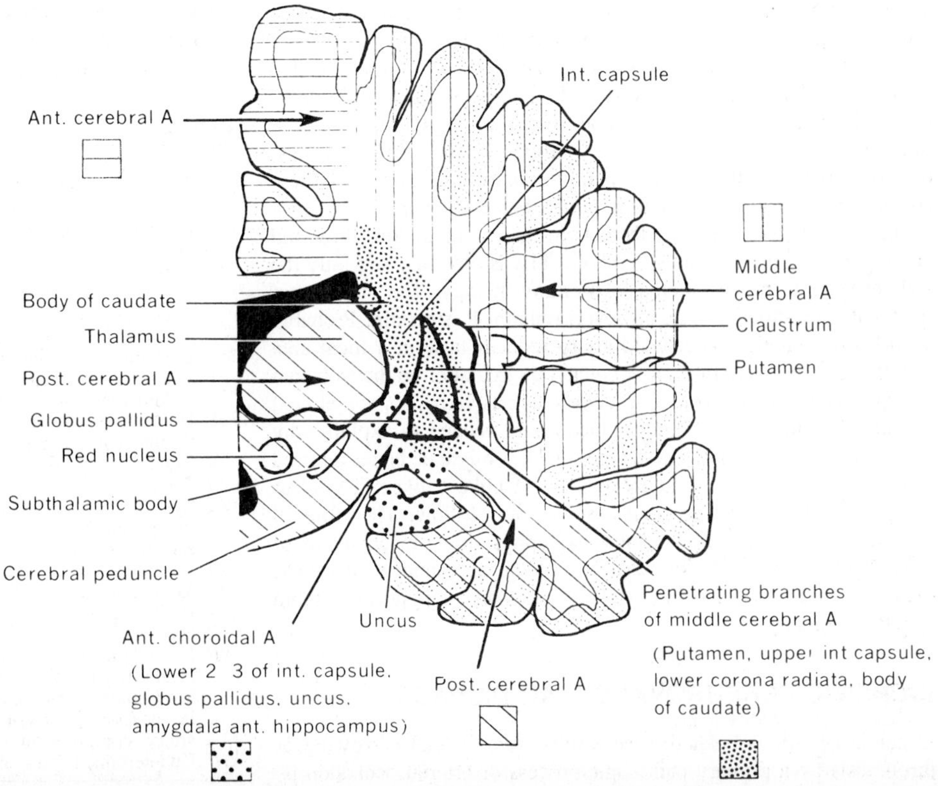

disease, lacunar strokes, and the formation of atherothrombotic lesions at the carotid bifurcation, in the middle cerebral artery stem, and in the vertebral-basilar system. Hypertension also predisposes to deep intracerebral hemorrhages. Some argue that the advent of antihypertensive therapy is the principal factor accounting for the declining incidence of stroke. Smoking and familial hyperlipidemia, although less important than hypertension, are associated with an increased risk of atherothrombotic disease in general, and ischemic cerebrovascular disease in particular.

TIA SYNDROME

In the TIA syndrome, the character, duration, and repetitiveness of a transient neurologic dysfunction suggest its pathophysiologic cause; that is, the clinical symptoms and signs and the temporal profile of a TIA suggest the nature and location of the underlying arterial pathophysiology. The term *transient ischemic attack* has usually been applied to any sudden focal neurologic deficit that clears completely in less than 24 h. This definition is too broad, because it includes too many syndromes, some of which are not necessarily caused by ischemia, e.g., a focal epileptic manifestation or migraine attack with neurologic symptoms. Furthermore, ischemic symptoms that persist longer than an hour suggest that some of the tissue may have become infarcted.

The specific symptoms of a TIA point to the particular arterial territory involved [carotid, middle cerebral, vertebral-basilar, or small vessel penetrating artery (lacunar TIA)]. Furthermore, the duration, stereotypic nature, and frequency of repetitive spells suggest a pathophysiologic mechanism. For example, repetitive (up to 5 to 10 per day), short-lived (15 min or less), stereotypic spells of hand and arm weakness with or without speech difficulty suggest that proximal arterial narrowing or occlusion and inadequate collateral circulation have produced transient focal ischemia (''low flow'') in the contralateral cortex. On the other hand, a single spell of speech difficulty with or without hand and arm and face weakness lasting 12 h suggests an embolic ischemic event probably with some degree of infarction in the left frontal lobe. A transient short-lived episode of pure motor hemiparesis—face, arm, leg, and foot—occurring *without* dysphasia or hemineglect suggests transient ischemia in the internal capsule, i.e., in the territory supplied by one of the small penetrating arteries arising from the stem of the middle cerebral artery (lenticulostriate arteries). Should a stroke evolve in this setting, it would be less than 1 cm in size, i.e., a lacune. Such a transient episode could be called a ''lacunar TIA.'' TIA in the vertebral-basilar system, when it is the result of proximal basilar or bilateral, distal vertebral artery stenosis, often presents with short-lived, repetitive episodes of dizziness, diplopia, and dysarthria. The repetitive, short-lived nature of these spells suggests transient low flow rather than embolism.

In general, TIAs evolve from two causes: focal low flow and embolism. The mechanism of embolic TIA is obvious, and only the source needs to be considered in deciding therapy. The mechanism for focal ''low-flow'' TIAs, however, remains less certain. Probably a critically stenotic or occluded artery reduces flow in a focal area of normal brain. Certainly, poor collateral circulation to the ischemic area plays a prominent role, but factors such as viscosity, vessel wall compliance, and other unknown factors are needed to explain why the reduction is transient. These types of TIAs might be better referred to as true TIAs, i.e., not embolic events. Unlike stroke, TIAs clear completely, but they warn that a stroke may follow. Therefore, it becomes important to consider the pathophysiologic mechanisms of stroke and TIA together. In essence, a physician cannot treat a TIA, only the cause of it. TIA, like stroke, is a syndrome requiring a more specific diagnosis.

ISCHEMIC CEREBROVASCULAR DISEASE

Ischemic cerebrovascular disease results from arterial narrowing or thrombosis by a primary pathologic process or arterial occlusion by embolism. Most of this section will be devoted to cerebral thrombosis and its various pathologic causes. Cerebral embolism causes many of the same symptoms and signs as thrombosis. Where the symptomatology differs, it will be discussed in the section on cerebral embolism.

THROMBOSIS WITH ATHEROSCLEROSIS Of the many causes of cerebral thrombosis listed in Table 343-1, thrombosis with atherosclerosis accounts for most cases. Atherosclerosis affects each of the extra- and intracranial arteries at specific locations. In general, atheromatous plaques tend to form at branchings and curves of large vessels, and thrombosis is likely to occur where plaque narrows the lumen most.

The details of the process which superimposes thrombosis on atherosclerosis are poorly understood (see Chap. 195). The atheromatous lesion itself lies between the intima and media of the vessel. It penetrates and disrupts the media. The plaque is composed of hyaline connective tissue, fibroblasts, macrophages, and smooth muscle cells. It is spotted with focal deposits of cholesterol crystals. Presumably, thrombosis forms when the underlying atherosclerotic formation fragments the endothelial lining of the vessel wall, establishing a nidus for platelet accumulation and mural thrombus formation. Occasionally, blood from the lumen dissects into an atheromatous plaque. This penetration may be the mechanism by which an ulcer crater forms and becomes a nidus for the production of a mural thrombus. Less often, hemorrhage into a plaque further narrows the lumen. The atheromatous narrowing of the lumen usually resembles an hourglass whose narrowest segment is only 1 to 2 mm long. A mural thrombus may form at this segment or proximal or distal to it. Thrombotic occlusion usually occurs when atheroma narrows the lumen to a point where distal blood flow is impeded.

It is difficult to predict the damage atherosclerotic thrombosis may cause to the brain. Available collateral flow, the speed of thrombotic occlusion, and the occurrence of embolism distal to the thrombosis may alter the clinical picture. Inevitably, the picture resulting from occlusion of a particular artery differs from one patient to another, and most syndromes are partial. The following descriptions apply to infarction and ischemia in specific arteries due to thrombosis, recognizing that similar clinical pictures may occur after embolism. Occasionally, hemorrhage within these vascular territories also may give rise to similar symptoms and signs.

ATHEROTHROMBOTIC DISEASE OF THE INTERNAL CAROTID ARTERY AND ITS BRANCHES Pathophysiology In the carotid artery system atherosclerosis and superimposed atherothrombosis that

TABLE 343-1 Causes of cerebral thrombosis

I	Atherosclerosis
II	Cerebral thrombophlebitis: secondary to infection of ear, paranasal sinus, face, etc.; with meningitis and subdural empyema; debilitating states, postpartum, postoperative; cardiac failure; hematologic disease (polycythemia, sickle cell disease), and of undetermined cause
III	Arteritis
	A Meningovascular syphilis, arteritis secondary to pyogenic and tuberculous meningitis, rare types [typhus, schistosomiasis mansoni, malaria (?), trichinosis (?), mucormycosis, etc.]
	B Connective tissue diseases: polyarteritis (necrotizing, granulomatous, allergic, Wegener's), temporal arteritis, Takayasu's disease, granulomatous arteritis of aorta, lupus erythematosus
IV	Hematologic disorders: polycythemia, sickle cell disease, thrombotic thrombocytopenic purpura, etc.
V	Trauma to carotid
VI	Dissecting aortic aneurysm
VII	Systemic hypotension: ''simple faint,'' acute blood loss, myocardial infarction, Stokes-Adams syndrome, traumatic and surgical shock, sensitive carotid sinus, severe postural hypotension
VIII	Complications of arteriography
IX	Migrainous aura with persistent deficit
X	With tentorial, foramen magnum, and subfalcial herniation
XI	Hypoxia
XII	Miscellaneous: radioactive or x-ray radiation, lateral pressure of intracerebral hematoma, unexplained middle cerebral infarction in closed head injury, pressure of unruptured saccular aneurysm, mural thrombus in fusiform aneurysm, local dissection of carotid or middle cerebral artery, complication of contraceptive medication
XIII	Undetermined cause as in childhood

lead to TIA or stroke most commonly occur at its origin and less often at the siphon (s-shaped portion of the internal carotid artery in the cavernous sinus) or at the proximal segment (stem) of the middle or anterior cerebral arteries. Rarely, it occurs at the origin of the common carotid artery. The natural history of atherosclerotic stenosis or ulcerated lesions at these locations that have not yet become symptomatic is unknown. Presumably, in most instances the disease is progressive.

INTERNAL CAROTID ARTERY ORIGIN Atherosclerosis in the proximal internal carotid artery is usually most severe in the first 2 cm and is located on the posterior wall; often it extends downward into the distal common carotid artery. Disease in this area is usually (50 to 80 percent of cases) heralded by a minor stroke or TIA caused by a ''low-flow'' hemodynamic crisis or embolism from the carotid artery to its intracranial branches. Clinical experience and pathologic examination suggest that emboli rather than low flow cause most strokes from carotid disease. Embolism from an atherosclerotic plaque at the origin of the internal carotid artery may cause TIAs, but when they are repetitive, short-lived, and stereotyped, a hemodynamic cause seems likely.

CEREBRAL ISCHEMIA CAUSED BY LOW FLOW Low arterial blood flow can cause cerebral infarction or TIA in the border zone or watershed areas where the cortical surface branches of the middle cerebral artery anastomose with the branches of the anterior and posterior cerebral artery (Fig. 343-1*A*). Two conditions contribute to this complication. First, blood pressure may be reduced distal to the carotid artery stenotic lesion if there is more than 80 percent reduction in carotid lumen diameter, or, equivalently, the residual lumen diameter is less than 1.5 to 2 mm. Second, impaired collateral circulation to the region may occur. Impairment generally results from an incomplete circle of Willis secondary to congenital atresia of the initial (A1) portion of the anterior cerebral artery or the anterior or posterior communicating arteries (Fig. 343-2*B*). Less often, impairment results from occlusion of either the contralateral carotid artery or the basilar artery—conditions that limit flow into the circle of Willis. Occasionally enough flow can be obtained through the external carotid ophthalmic collaterals (Fig. 343-1*B*) or cortical surface border zone collaterals (Fig. 343-1*A*) to ensure adequate flow or minimize the ischemic area, even if the circle of Willis is inadequate. It is this variation in collateral flow that is responsible for the variable location of low-flow stroke or TIA in the carotid territory.

Other explanations of the pathophysiology of low-flow TIAs have been given. It has been suggested that severely stenotic lesions at the carotid bifurcation may intermittently occlude the vessel due to spasm. On rare occasions, systemic hemodynamic factors, i.e., abnormal blood viscosity or arterial hypotension, may reduce flow to a critical level across a tightly stenotic lesion. Alternatively, regional circulation in the hemisphere may be altered to accommodate diminished carotid blood flow, and transient decompensation of this mechanism may cause TIAs. Other factors, including polycythemia vera, thrombocythemia, and cardiac arrhythmia, may rarely cause recurrent ''low-flow''-type TIAs.

EMBOLISM When emboli arise from a stenotic or ulcerated atherosclerotic lesion at the origin of the internal carotid artery (*local embolism* or *artery-to-artery embolus*), symptoms usually relate to occlusion of the ophthalmic artery, the middle cerebral artery stem or one or more of its branches, or occasionally to the anterior cerebral artery or its branches. The size of an embolus determines which vessel is occluded. Small platelet emboli may occlude only the very distal vessels of the middle cerebral artery or ophthalmic artery, causing only transient monocular blindness (*amaurosis fugax*) or small asymptomatic infarctions in the cerebral arterial watershed. But larger emboli composed of platelet-fibrin clot may occlude the primary and secondary branches of the middle cerebral artery where discrete neurologic syndromes suggest the area involved. Some emboli are large enough to occlude the proximal ''stem'' of the middle cerebral artery, leading to devastating ischemia of the entire middle cerebral territory (deep white matter, lenticular nuclei, and cortical surface). Other emboli large enough to occlude the middle cerebral stem may cause only deep infarction because collateral flow through the cortical surface is sufficient (Fig. 343-1*A*). Large emboli that occlude a major vessel may migrate or lyse and disperse. If this dispersion occurs early, the neurologic deficit may fluctuate or resolve.

In a few symptomatic patients, an ulcerated plaque may be the only lesion in the carotid bifurcation, but far more often there is a stenotic lesion with a residual luminal diameter of less than 2 mm. The incidence of large embolic strokes resulting from an ulcerated lesion alone is undetermined. It is probably low and mostly associated with large ulcers (4 mm or greater). *A nonstenotic or minor stenotic carotid lesion in conjunction with a stroke or a single prolonged TIA suggests the heart as the source of the embolus.* Atheromatous lesions at the origin of the great vessels in the aortic arch can also produce cerebral emboli that cause transient ischemia or infarction, but the incidence of this mechanism is also undetermined.

Internal carotid artery occlusion at its origin may be entirely asymptomatic if collateral circulation through the circle of Willis is adequate. On the other hand, if collateral circulation is inadequate, low flow may induce a stroke or TIA. In addition, a clot may propagate upward from the occlusion through the siphon to the origin of the middle or anterior arteries and cause a stroke. More often, a fresh embolus breaks off from the thrombotic material and lodges in the middle or anterior cerebral artery or one of its branches. Some authorities postulate that emboli can arise from the proximal stump of the internal carotid artery and travel through the external carotid collateral circulation to reach the intracranial internal carotid artery and its branches (Fig. 343-1*B*). This process is probably rare.

The cause of a delayed stroke—one occurring months after complete carotid occlusion—is often unclear, and the incidence has not been established. One study suggests it is as high as 5 percent per year. Yet that seems high by clinical experience. Most embolism from carotid occlusion occurs within the first year, although it can occur up to 2 years later. Strokes caused by low flow tend to occur earlier, usually within the first few weeks after carotid occlusion.

INTRACRANIAL INTERNAL CAROTID ARTERY The carotid siphon is less commonly involved with atherosclerosis than the proximal internal carotid. Lesions in the siphon can cause strokes and TIAs whose pathophysiologic and clinical features duplicate those discussed above. The natural history of siphon stenosis is undetermined. In general, one should not consider siphon stenosis as symptomatic until the atheromatous process has reduced the residual lumen to 1.5 mm or less. Only angiography can diagnose accurately carotid siphon stenosis distal to the ophthalmic artery. The effect of collateral flow around the circle of Willis undoubtedly influences the natural history of these lesions and their response to medical or surgical therapy.

MIDDLE CEREBRAL ARTERY Atheromatous lesions in the middle cerebral stem may cause ischemic symptoms either by narrowing the artery or occluding the origin of one or more of the lenticulostriate arteries supplying the deep white matter and basal ganglia. Symptomatic atheroma rarely occurs distal to the first bifurcation of the middle cerebral artery. Because the circle of Willis is proximal to the origin of the middle cerebral artery, collateral blood flow to the middle cerebral artery territory must arise from small cortical-surface border zones and anastomotic vessels of the anterior and posterior cerebral arteries. Existing evidence indicates that before infarction develops, TIAs in the middle cerebral artery territory usually warn of vessel narrowing prior to thrombotic occlusion. Symptoms resemble those due to low-flow hemodynamic TIAs occurring with a tightly stenotic lesion of the internal carotid artery. In contrast to the internal carotid artery, the middle cerebral stem or one or more of its major branches is usually occluded by embolus (artery-to-artery, cardiac, or unknown source).

ANTERIOR CEREBRAL ARTERY Atheromatous deposits in the proximal segment of the anterior cerebral artery rarely cause symptoms because the occlusion is circumvented by collateral circulation through the anterior communicating artery. However, if this source of collateral circulation is congenitally atretic or if the atheromatous lesion occurs more distally in the anterior cerebral artery, TIAs and stroke become more likely.

Clinical syndromes MIDDLE CEREBRAL ARTERY The cortical branches of the middle cerebral artery supply the lateral surface of the hemisphere except for (1) the frontal pole, (2) a strip along the superomedial border of the frontal lobe supplied by the anterior cerebral artery, and (3) the lowest temporal convolutions, which are in the territory of the posterior cerebral artery (Figs. 343-3 to 343-5).

The middle cerebral artery's area includes the cortex and white matter of the lateral and inferior aspects of the frontal lobe, the motor cortex (areas 4 and 6, the centers for contraversive eye movements, and in the dominant hemisphere the motor speech area of Broca), the cortex and white matter of the lateral parietal lobe (sensory cortex, angular and supramarginal convolutions), the lateral and superior parts of the temporal lobe, and the insula (Figs. 343-3 and 343-4). The penetrating branches of the middle cerebral artery supply the putamen, outer globus pallidus, the posterior limb of the internal capsule above the plane of the upper border of the globus pallidus, the adjacent part of the corona radiata, the body of the caudate nucleus, and the superior and lateral portion of the head of the caudate nucleus (Fig. 343-3).

The middle cerebral territory is the region most frequently affected in embolic and thrombotic cerebrovascular disease. The entire artery may be occluded at its stem, blocking both penetrating branches to the deep white and gray matter as well as the major branches to the cortical surface. The classic picture of this lesion is contralateral hemiplegia and hemianesthesia. If the dominant hemisphere is involved, global or total sensorimotor aphasia also is present. If the nondominant hemisphere is affected, apractagnosia and anosognosia are added to the clinical syndrome (Fig. 343-4). While there may be dysarthria, dysphasia is absent.

Complete middle cerebral territory syndromes occur most often when an embolus occludes the stem of the artery. Effective cortical surface arterial collateral flow requires some time to develop (Figs. 343-1 and 343-4), but it is responsible for the development of partial syndromes when atherothrombosis occludes the stem of the middle cerebral artery. Partial middle cerebral territory syndromes also occur due to embolism. An embolus may enter the middle cerebral stem, progress distally, lodge in a distal branch, and lyse. Symptoms and signs then fluctuate accordingly (Fig. 343-4). Partial syndromes resulting from embolic occlusion of a single branch include hand or arm and hand weakness alone (brachial syndrome) or facial weakness

FIGURE 343-4 *Diagram of a cerebral hemisphere, lateral aspect, showing the branches and distribution of the middle cerebral artery and the principal regions of cerebral localization. Note the bifurcation of the middle cerebral artery into a superior and inferior division. (Courtesy of C.M. Fisher, M.D.)*

Signs and symptoms	*Structures involved*
Paralysis of the contralateral face, arm, and leg; sensory impairment over the contralateral face, arm, and leg (pinprick, cotton touch, vibration, position, two-point discrimination, stereognosis, tactile localization, barognosis, cutaneographia)	*Somatic motor area for face and arm and the fibers descending from the leg area to enter the corona radiata and corresponding somatic sensory system*
Motor aphasia	*Motor speech area of the dominant hemisphere*
Central aphasia, word deafness, anomia, jargon speech, alexia, agraphia, acalculia, finger agnosia, right-left confusion (the last four comprise the Gerstmann syndrome)	*Central, suprasylvian speech area and parietooccipital cortex of the dominant hemisphere*
Conduction aphasia	*Central speech area (parietal operculum)*
Apractognosia of the minor hemisphere (amorphosynthesis), anosognosia, hemiasomatognosia, unilateral neglect, agnosia for the left half of external space, dressing "apraxia," constructional "apraxia," distortion of visual coordinates, inaccurate localization in the half field, impaired ability to judge distance, upside-down reading, visual illusions (e.g., it may appear that another person walks through a table)	*Nondominant parietal lobe (area corresponding to speech area in dominant hemisphere); loss of topographic memory is usually due to a nondominant lesion, occasionally to a dominant one*
Homonymous hemianopsia (often homonymous inferior quadrantonopsia)	*Optic radiation deep to second temporal convolution*
Paralysis of conjugate gaze to the opposite side	*Frontal contraversive field or fibers projecting therefrom*

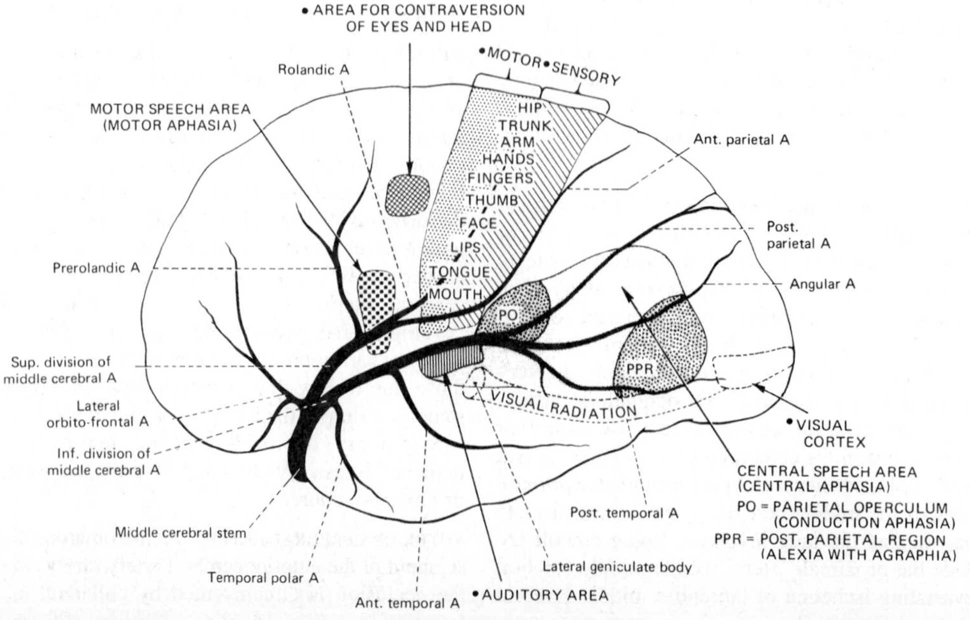

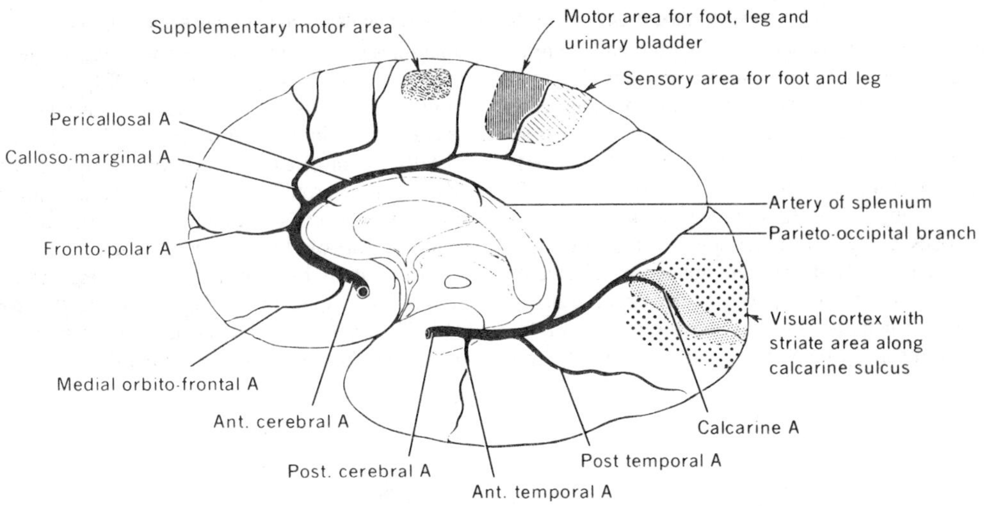

FIGURE 343-5 *Diagram of a cerebral hemisphere, medial aspect, showing the branches and distribution of the anterior cerebral artery and the principal regions of cerebral localization. (Courtesy of C.M. Fisher, M.D.)*

Signs and symptoms	*Structures involved*
Paralysis of opposite foot and leg	*Motor leg area*
A lesser degree of paresis of opposite arm	*Involvement of arm area of cortex or fibers descending to corona radiata therefrom*
Cortical sensory loss over toes, foot, and leg	*Sensory area for foot and leg*
Urinary incontinence	*Sensorimotor area in paracentral lobule*
Contralateral grasp reflex, sucking reflex, gegenhalten (paratonic rigidity)	*Medial surface of the posterior frontal lobe (?) supplemental motor area*
Abulia (akinetic mutism): slowness, delay, intermittent interruption, lack of spontaneity, whispering, motor inaction, reflex distraction to sights and sounds	*Uncertain localization—probably cingulate gyrus and medial portion of parietal and temporal lobes*
Impairment of gait and stance (gait apraxia)	*Frontal cortex near leg motor area*
Dyspraxia of left limbs, tactile aphasia in left limbs	*Corpus callosum*

with motor aphasia with or without arm weakness (frontal opercular syndrome). A combination of sensory disturbance, motor weakness, and motor aphasia suggests that the origin of the superior division branch has been embolized (Fig. 343-4). If receptive aphasia occurs without weakness, the inferior division of the middle cerebral artery is probably involved, for it supplies the posterior sensory part of the dominant hemisphere (Fig. 343-4). Sudden difficulty with hemineglect or spatial agnosia without weakness indicates that the inferior division of the middle cerebral artery in the nondominant hemisphere is involved.

ANTERIOR CEREBRAL ARTERY The anterior cerebral artery is divided into two segments: the precommunal (A1) circle of Willis, or stem segment, which connects the internal carotid artery to the anterior communicating artery, and the postcommunal (A2) segment beginning at the junction of the A1 segment and the anterior communicating artery (Fig. 343-2). The A2 segment of the anterior cerebral artery, through its cortical branches, supplies the anterior four-fifths of the medial part of the orbital surface of the frontal lobe, the frontal pole, a strip of the cortical surface along the superomedial border, and the anterior seven-eighths of the corpus callosum (Fig. 343-5). The A1 segment of the anterior cerebral artery, on the other hand, gives rise to many deep penetrating branches, which run chiefly to the anterior limb of the internal capsule, the anterior perforate substance, amygdala, anterior hypothalamus, and the inferior part of the head of the caudate nucleus (Fig. 343-3).

Infarction in the territory of the anterior cerebral artery is uncommon. Occlusion of the stem or A1 segment of the anterior cerebral artery proximal to the anterior communicating artery is usually well tolerated, since collateral flow is possible from the opposite side. The greatest disturbance occurs when both anterior cerebral arteries arise from a single anterior cerebral stem, occlusion of which then results in a devastating infarction of the anterior cerebral territory of both hemispheres. The clinical signs include bilateral pyramidal signs with paraplegia and profound mental symptoms due to bilateral frontal lobe damage. The components of the typical syndrome resulting from occlusion of one anterior cerebral artery distal to the circle of Willis are indicated in the legend of Fig. 343-5.

ANTERIOR CHOROIDAL ARTERY This artery arises from the internal carotid artery and supplies the posterior limb of the internal capsule and the white matter posterolateral to it through which pass some of the geniculocalcarine fibers. This territory, however, is also supplied by penetrating vessels of the middle cerebral stem (lenticulostriate arteries), penetrating vessels of the posterior communicating artery, and the posterior choroidal artery. As a consequence, the complete clinical syndrome of contralateral hemiplegia, hemianesthesia (hypesthesia), and homonymous hemianopsia may not occur; instead syndromes with minimal deficits may be found. Indeed, cases of surgical occlusion of the artery for treatment of symptoms of Parkinson's disease have produced no deficit in some patients. Patients who initially have the full syndrome frequently recover in part or totally, presumably because of adequate collateral circulation.

INTERNAL CAROTID ARTERY The clinical picture of internal carotid occlusion varies depending upon whether the cause of ischemia is propagated thrombus, embolism, or low flow. Occlusion can be entirely asymptomatic. Less often an infarction is massive, involving the deep gray and white matter and cortical surface, as when an occlusive thrombus propagates up the internal carotid artery and projects into the middle cerebral stem and anterior cerebral arteries, or when a thrombotic fragment breaks off and embolizes the middle or anterior artery. Symptoms are identical to middle cerebral stem occlusion (see above). When both the anterior and middle cerebral arteries are involved, stupor is often seen in addition to the hemiplegia, hemianesthesia, and aphasia or anosognosia. When the posterior cerebral artery arises from the internal carotid artery (fetal posterior cerebral artery), it also may become occluded by the above processes and give rise to symptoms referable to its peripheral territory (Figs. 343-5 and 343-6).

No matter what the cause of ischemia in symptomatic internal carotid atherothrombotic disease, the middle cerebral territory alone is most often affected. Low-flow infarction tends to involve the territory of the distal cortical branches of the middle cerebral artery, giving rise to transient or stepwise hip, shoulder, or arm weakness. Ocasionally, transient ischemic episodes of dysphasia or hand and arm weakness occur, lasting 10 to 15 min before improving. As many as 5 to 10 episodes a day have been noted in this setting. If the dominant hemisphere is involved, transient aphasia or dyscalculia may occur. If the nondominant hemisphere is involved, transient hemineglect can ensue. When the inferior division of the middle cerebral artery in the dominant hemisphere is involved, fluent jargon aphasia is prominent, and written or oral language is incomprehensible (Wernicke's aphasia) (see Chap. 22). Even in artery-to-artery embolism symptoms often fluctuate because the embolus may not totally occlude the middle cerebral stem or branch, or it may lyse and move distally. In most cases, symptoms lasting a prolonged time but less than 24 h are probably embolic. But if a symptom is transient, lasting only a few seconds or minutes, it is often difficult to decide between embolism or low flow as the etiology.

In addition to supplying the brain, the internal carotid artery supplies the optic nerve and retina via the ophthalmic artery (Fig. 343-1). In about 25 percent of cases of symptomatic internal carotid occlusion, transient monocular blindness (TMB or amaurosis fugax)

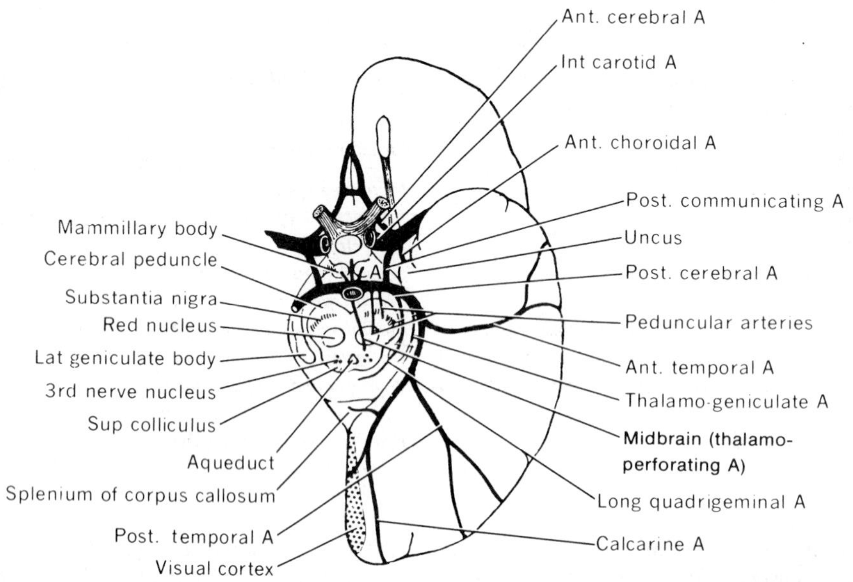

FIGURE 343-6 *Inferior aspect of the brain with the branches and distribution of the posterior cerebral artery and the principal anatomic structures shown. (Courtesy of C.M. Fisher, M.D.)*

Signs and symptoms	*Structures involved*
Peripheral territory (see also Fig. 343-5)	
Homonymous hemianopsia (often upper quadrantic)	*Calcarine cortex or optic radiation nearby*
Bilateral homonymous hemianopsia, cortical blindness, awareness or denial of blindness; tactile naming, achromatopsia (color blindness), failure to see to-and-fro movements, inability to perceive objects not centrally located, apraxia of ocular movements, inability to count or enumerate objects, tendency to run into things which the patient sees and tries to avoid	*Bilateral occipital lobe with possibly the parietal lobe involved.*
Verbal dyslexia without agraphia, color anomia	*Dominant calcarine lesion and posterior part of corpus callosum*
Memory defect	*Hippocampal lesion bilaterally or on the dominant side only*
Topographic disorientation and prosopagnosia	*Usually with lesions of nondominant, calcarine, and lingual gyrus*
Simultagnosia, hemivisual neglect	*Dominant visual cortex, contralateral hemisphere*
Unformed visual hallucinations, metamorphopsia, teleopsia, illusory visual spread, irreminiscence, paliopsia, distortion of outlines, central photophobia	*Calcarine cortex*
Complex hallucinations	*Usually nondominant hemisphere*
Central territory	
Thalamic syndrome: sensory loss (all modalities), spontaneous pain and dysesthesias, choreoathetosis, intention tremor, spasms of hand, mild hemiparesis	*Posteroventral nucleus of thalamus; involvement of the adjacent subthalamus body or its afferent tracts*
Thalamoperforate syndrome: crossed cerebellar ataxia with ipsilateral third nerve palsy (Claude's syndrome)	*Dentatothalamic tract and issuing third nerve*
Weber's syndrome: third nerve palsy and contralateral hemiplegia	*Third nerve and cerebral peduncle*
Contralateral hemiplegia	*Cerebral peduncle*
Paralysis or paresis of vertical eye movement, skew deviation, sluggish pupillary responses to light, slight miosis and ptosis (retraction nystagmus and "tucking" of the eyelids may be associated)	*Supranuclear fibers to third nerve, interstitial nucleus of Cajar nucleus of Darkschewitsch, and posterior commissure*
Contralateral rhythmic, ataxic action tremor; rhythmic postural or "holding" tremor (rubral tremor)	*Dentatothalamic tract (?)*

occurs intermittently to warn of the onset. Describing the event, patients may say that a shade seemed to sweep up, down, or across the field of vision or that the periphery of vision faded away. They may also complain that their vision was blurred in that eye or that the upper or lower half of vision disappeared. In most cases, these symptoms last only a few minutes. Rarely, ophthalmic or central retinal artery occlusion develops at the time of stroke.

COMMON CAROTID ARTERY All the neurologic symptoms and signs of internal carotid occlusion may also be present with occlusion of the common carotid artery. Both common carotid arteries may be occluded at their origin as in "pulseless disease" or the aortic arch syndrome (see Chap. 197). The following manifestations give a clue to this condition: absence of pulsation in carotid and radial arteries, faintness on arising from the horizontal position, recurrent loss of consciousness, headache, neck pain, transient blindness (unilateral or bilateral), dimness of vision with exercise, premature cataracts, retinal atrophy and pigmentation, atrophy of the iris, leukomas, peripapillary arteriovenous anastomoses, optic atrophy, and/or claudication of the jaw muscles. An incomplete aortic arch syndrome consisting of various combinations of carotid, subclavian, or innominate stenosis or occlusion is not uncommon (see below).

Laboratory evaluation A variety of diagnostic techniques are available for evaluating patients with a carotid bruit, carotid-territory stroke, or TIA. Auscultation of a bruit over the bifurcation of the common carotid artery in the neck, or over the eye, and palpation of the arteries in the neck and over the face and forehead in conjunction with the compression of the preauricular artery (dynamic facial palpation) often provide suggestions about the presence and nature of disease at the bifurcation of the common and proximal internal carotid artery. High-pitched bruits that fade into diastole suggest a tightly stenotic lesion at the origin of the internal carotid. However, only trained experience can judge the duration and pitch of a bruit or assess subtle changes in pulse intensity during dynamic facial palpation. Therefore, several noninvasive tests have been developed to determine more reliably the severity and location of carotid atherothrombotic disease.

NONINVASIVE CAROTID TESTS Ophthalmodynamometry, oculoplethysmography, and directional supraorbital Doppler examination indirectly assess pressure in the internal carotid artery. These tests are most helpful when the residual luminal diameter of the atheromatous lesion at the origin of the internal carotid artery is more than 2 mm and the tests are normal, or when the residual diameter is less than 1 mm and pressure distally is greatly reduced, rendering the tests abnormal.

Two types of noninvasive tests study the bifurcation of the common carotid artery directly. *Ultrasound techniques* include real-time B-mode ultrasound imaging and analysis of the Doppler-shift signal of the returning echo of flowing blood. Unfortunately, ultrasound imaging has limited resolution, because calcification in a plaque prevents penetration of the ultrasound beam, and a soft thrombus has approximately the same density as flowing blood. However, it reliably identifies atheromatous lesions at the common carotid bifurcation. Since blood flowing through an atherosclerotic stenotic lesion changes from laminar flow with uniform velocity to streamline flow with high velocity and then to turbulent flow with a broad range of velocities immediately distal to the stenosis, this change can be detected by continuous-wave (cw) or range-gated pulsed-Doppler techniques. It appears as a spectral broadening of the returning echoes of the Doppler-shift signal. Duplex ultrasound scanning combines B-mode images of the artery with range-gated pulsed-Doppler analysis of flowing blood at each point in the image. A second technique, *quantitative spectral phonoangiography*, analyzes the audible frequency-intensity components of the bruit of the turbulent blood flow. It estimates the residual luminal diameter of the internal carotid artery, and it differentiates between a bruit originating at the carotid bifurcation and one radiating from the base of the heart. External carotid artery bruits may, however, be mistaken for more serious internal carotid artery sounds. This test tends to be most accurate when the bruit arises from a stenotic lesion with a residual luminal diameter between 0.9 and 2.5 mm. Therefore, it is most useful in the range of stenoses where other noninvasive tests are least accurate.

Experience suggests that an optimal set of noninvasive tests should include direct assessment of the bifurcation of the common carotid artery by duplex Doppler examination or B-mode ultrasound imaging combined with spectral analysis of the Doppler-shift signal. Quantitative phonoangiography should be used when a bruit is present. Oculoplethysmography is used in most laboratories to measure indirectly the pressure in the internal carotid artery and to assess more accurately the hemodynamic importance of the lesion. These tests help most in three clinical settings: assessing the bifurcation of the common carotid artery when an ischemic stroke or TIA of uncertain cause occurs in the territory fed by the internal carotid artery; following the progress of a known carotid stenosis; and evaluating an asymptomatic bruit. All noninvasive tests are subject to some error (10 percent in experienced hands). Furthermore, they cannot distinguish complete carotid occlusion from extremely tight stenosis at the origin of the internal carotid artery. Hence, they are less valuable when a patient who has had a minor stroke or TIA needs appropriate prompt therapy to prevent further stroke, in which case there is frequently no substitute for angiography. Most recently range-gated pulsed-Doppler analysis has been extended to examine the vertebral artery flow and flow in the large intracranial arteries, i.e., the middle cerebral stem, and anterior and posterior cerebral arteries. Efficacy of such analysis in documenting disturbed flow with constrictive lesions has yet to be demonstrated.

CEREBRAL ANGIOGRAPHY Cerebral angiography performed by selective extracranial injection after transfemoral catheterization remains the most reliable method of assessing the cerebrovascular system. It can detect ulcerative lesions, severe stenosis, and formation of a mural thrombus at the carotid bifurcation, and it can visualize directly carotid artery dissections and atherothrombotic disease in the siphon and intracranial vessels. It can demonstrate collateral circulation around the circle of Willis and on the cortical surface and embolic occlusion of cerebral branch vessels. Although angiography cannot measure blood flow directly, it records certain features that indicate compromised flow in the internal carotid system. For example, the intracranial circulation may fill more slowly than the external carotid artery. Cerebral angiography, therefore, allows the physician to evaluate many of the factors that are relevant to an understanding of the pathophysiologic nature of the stroke.

However, the advantages of selective cerebral angiography must be seen in the context of its risks. According to various reviews, complications range from 1.3 to 12 percent. The risks that have attracted the most comment are aortic dissection and embolic stroke. Although some find angiography to be particularly risky for patients with a tightly stenotic lesion at the carotid bifurcation, others find it to be relatively safe in all settings if performed by experienced angiographers. Simply preventing dehydration and hypotension during and after angiography can often prevent cerebral ischemic complications. Patients with recurrent headaches or a history of migrainous phenomena have been given corticosteroids before angiography, but the medication's value in preventing ischemic complications has not been established. At times, the less risky technique of brachial artery injection offers as much relevant information as selective intracranial angiography from transfemoral catheterization.

INTRAVENOUS DIGITAL SUBTRACTION ANGIOGRAPHY Intravenous digital subtraction angiography is a computer-reconstruction method developed to circumvent problems inherent in arterial catheterization. It demonstrates carotid occlusion or severe stenosis, but often leaves the degree of stenosis uncertain. It may miss a near occlusion with a threadlike lumen, and it fails to delineate adequately either intracranial arterial lesions or patterns of collateral blood flow. Digital subtraction angiography requires breath holding, cessation of swallowing, and a brisk cardiac output—all of which may be difficult for patients who have had a stroke. Furthermore, the large volume of contrast agent may precipitate angina, congestive heart failure, and renal failure. Arterial injection of the contrast agent used in digital angiography may offer some advantages over the intravenous method, but it has risks similar to those of conventional angiography. Usually, the local institutional experience will determine which technique is the safest for a particular patient.

CEREBRAL IMAGING Methods that study the extent and location of infarcted brain tissue have all hinged on the development of computerized axial tomography (CT), positron-emission tomography, and magnetic resonance imaging. The latter two are currently in developmental phases. CT scanning provides an estimate of the extent and location of supratentorial cerebral infarction, including small 0.5-cm lacunar infarctions. In addition, it can detect surrounding edema, and less consistently, hemorrhagic infarction. CT, however, cannot differentiate early ischemic tissue from normal tissue, *nor can it detect most cerebral infarctions for at least 48 h.* Furthermore, when infarction occurs in the brainstem—i.e., in the vertebral or basilar territories—CT is less reliable because of bone and motion artifacts and the small size of many infarcts.

Xenon blood flow techniques and positron-emission tomography with use of labeled carbon dioxide and oxygen provide qualitative and quantitative tomographic assessment of cerebral blood flow. These methods are not in routine clinical use and are not used in guiding therapy. Proton magnetic resonance imaging (MRI) has been used to identify accurately the extent and location of infarcted tissue within hours of infarction. With the introduction of magnets of high-field strength (1.5 to 4 tesla), it may be possible to obtain in vivo a regional nuclear magnetic resonance spectrum of high-energy phosphate compounds and therefore to judge the viability of tissue. Once developed, this technology may permit moment-to-moment assessment of the response of brain tissue to therapy.

Therapy for carotid territory transient ischemic attacks ANTICOAGULANT THERAPY When impending carotid or middle cerebral occlusion is suspected as the cause of a TIA, then acute anticoagulation with heparin is an option. Given the suggested pathophysiologic mechanism of stroke in this setting, a cogent argument can be made for such therapy. But in the absence of published proof of efficacy vs. hazard, it must be considered empirical.

The use of chronic anticoagulant therapy with sodium warfarin is even more controversial and problematic. Most studies of efficacy of chronic anticoagulant therapy to prevent stroke or to decrease TIAs are difficult to appraise for a number of reasons—e.g., lack of randomization, small number of patients, and lack of uniformity in the diagnosis of the cause of the TIA. In some studies, inclusion of TIAs not due to atheromatous disease of the internal carotid artery or inclusion of transient neurologic symptoms that were not related to ischemia have further complicated assessment of the results. Many believe that chronic anticoagulation therapy benefits patients with carotid-territory TIAs who are not candidates for surgery either for medical reasons or because the lesion is surgically inaccessible (carotid siphon or middle cerebral stem). Because of the often devastating effect of middle cerebral artery occlusions, anticoagulation is recommended when patients present with TIAs or minor strokes from a tightly stenotic lesion in the stem of the middle cerebral artery. To minimize the bleeding complications of warfarin sodium, the prothrombin time should generally not exceed $1\frac{1}{2}$ times control value. Contraindications to anticoagulant therapy have been well defined and include the presence of an actively bleeding ulcer, malignant hypertension, uremia, hepatic failure, or poor patient compliance. Relative contraindications are old age, systolic blood pressure above 190 mmHg, or a history of bleeding ulcer or bleeding diathesis. Heparin may be useful in the short term in stemming additional TIAs and preventing complete occlusion of a tightly stenotic lesion while the patient is awaiting angiography, surgery, or oral anticoagulation.

ANTIPLATELET THERAPY Studies of the effect of antiplatelet agents on the natural histroy of TIAs and minor strokes can be criticized for the same reasons as the anticoagulation studies. Aspirin is the agent most widely investigated in the prevention of stroke. Eight randomized trials have considered either aspirin alone or aspirin in combination with another antiplatelet agent. The two largest have suggested that aspirin alone may be beneficial in preventing further TIAs and strokes in symptomatic patients. Another study, in which angiography was performed routinely, suggested that aspirin benefited patients who had TIAs associated with a lesion in the internal carotid artery but not those who had a single TIA and no carotid lesion—i.e., those thought to have emboli from the heart. In these studies, aspirin at best reduced the stroke risk over 3 years from approximately 19 to 12 percent, the latter risk being considerably higher than the risk of endarterectomy. Most physicians agree that aspirin may help, but it is not the treatment of choice for TIAs resulting from atherothrombotic disease of the internal carotid artery. It is often used when transient ischemic symptoms appear in association with tightly stenotic carotid siphon lesions or with minor degrees of stenosis at the origin of the internal carotid artery, carotid siphon, or stem of the middle cerebral artery.

There are theoretical reasons to avoid the excessive use of aspirin. Paradoxically, aspirin inhibits platelet formation of thromboxane A_2, a platelet-aggregating, vasoconstricting prostaglandin, but also inhibits the formation of prostacyclin, and antiaggregating, vasodilating prostaglandin derived from endothelial cells. Aspirin in low doses predominantly inhibits the production of thromboxane A_2; therefore, many physicians recommend aspirin in small doses of 300 mg or less per day.

Dipyridamole acts by inhibiting platelet phosphodiesterase, which is responsible for breakdown of cyclic adenosine monophosphate. The resulting elevation in platelet cyclic AMP level inhibits aggregation of platelets. However, there is no compelling clinical evidence to suggest that dipyridamole prevents recurrent TIAs or stroke in patients with symptomatic atherothrombotic cerebrovascular disease. Sulfinpyrazone inhibits the platelet-release reaction and interferes with platelet adhesion to subendothelial tissues. It does prolong platelet survival in patients with prosthetic heart valves. There is no evidence that proves that sulfinpyrazone or other antiplatelet agents such as clofibrate or ibuprofen have any benefit over aspirin alone in preventing TIAs or stroke.

CAROTID ENDARTERECTOMY Carotid endarterectomy remains the usual therapy for TIAs caused by carotid stenosis. First introduced in 1954, the procedure has been associated with a morbidity ranging from 1 to 20 percent, depending on the patient population and the experience of the team of surgeons and physicians. Although many studies suggest that this procedure is effective in preventing additional TIAs or strokes, its value has yet to be confirmed by a well-designed, controlled, randomized clinical trial. *Unless the combined complication rate of angiography and surgery is less than 3 percent, performing surgery is likely to be more dangerous than no treatment.*

Patients with a tightly stenotic lesion in one carotid artery and either an occlusion of the contralateral carotid artery or an inadequate circle of Willis are at somewhat higher risk of intraoperative stroke during endarterectomy. However, intraoperative electroencephalographic monitoring can detect cerebral ischemia during the procedure and warn the surgeon to take steps to improve circulation.

Most patients who undergo endarterectomy have hypertensive arteriosclerotic cardiovascular disease and peripheral vascular disease. Active coronary diseases, such as unstable angina, recent myocardial infarction (within 6 months), or congestive heart failure, are contraindications to surgery. Severe hypertension is often corrected before surgery, but excessive lowering of the blood pressure should be avoided with tight carotid artery stenosis because it has been implicated in progression to total occlusion and stroke.

Stenosis can recur after surgery, although it seldom does. Poor surgical technique, excessive scar formation, and active arteriosclerotic disease have been implicated. Within the first year, the underlying pathologic process appears to be largely the proliferation of fibrous tissue; after the first year, of fibrous tissue and atherosclerosis. When restenosis gives rise to symptoms, surgery, although feasible, becomes more difficult technically.

Tandem lesions of the internal carotid artery—i.e., one at the carotid bifurcation and one at the carotid siphon—require special consideration. If the siphon stenosis has a residual luminal diameter of more than 2 mm and the lower carotid a diameter of less than 2 mm, then endarterectomy can be recommended. If the siphon narrowing is more severe, the value of endarterectomy is less certain. Anticoagulant or antiplatelet therapy may be preferable. But there is no consensus about the efficacy of either therapy in this setting.

EXTRACRANIAL/INTRACRANIAL BYPASS SURGERY Anastomosis of a superficial temporal branch of the external carotid artery to a cortical surface branch of the middle cerebral artery can provide collateral flow to the middle cerebral territory. Such surgery has been considered in patients with an occluded carotid artery or a tightly stenotic lesion of the carotid siphon or middle cerebral stem who present with recurrent TIAs or minor strokes. However, the results of a worldwide randomized study failed to prove greater efficacy of surgical compared to anticoagulation or antiplatelet therapy in these conditions.

Therapy for carotid territory stroke The severity of a recent stroke in the territory of the internal carotid artery is an important factor in the decision about therapy. If there is a complete hemiplegia, severe aphasia, or anosognosia, indicating involvement of the major portions of the middle cerebral territory, the prevention of additional strokes in that arterial distribution becomes less urgent. Instead, careful attention to maintenance of adequate blood pressure and prevention of delayed cerebral edema becomes important. There is little evidence to support the use of anticoagulant therapy once a "completed" or static major stroke deficit exists. However, if marked clinical improvement occurs during the first hours after onset or the deficit is small, some evidence suggests that short-term anticoagulation (heparin) prevents further damage, i.e., benefits "stroke in evolution." Many authors now recommend that a fluctuating or progressing deficit be treated with heparin. Given the pathophysiologic mechanisms of carotid stroke, many physicians use short-term anticoagulation in a patient with a slight stroke from a recently occluded or tightly stenotic internal carotid artery, hoping to prevent a second, possibly more devastating, event. In such cases, small ischemic infarcts could become hemorrhagic but rarely do. For this reason, the timing and benefit of early heparinization remains controversial.

Even though no controlled studies exist, endarterectomy is recommended for patients with tightly stenotic internal carotid lesions who present with a minor stroke in the territory distal to the lesion. The risk of surgery in experienced hands may be as low as 2 percent if no medical contraindications exist. When the contralateral carotid artery is tightly stenotic or occluded, endarterectomy of the ipsilateral carotid artery has a higher morbidity. Comparison of the natural history of cases of symptomatic tight carotid stenosis with surgical results has not been made. Experience suggests that additional strokes develop in more than 3 percent of patients who are treated nonsurgically.

Hemorrhage into a cerebral infarct is an extremely rare event following internal carotid endarterectomy and probably is no more common than without surgery if postoperative hypertension is avoided. Nevertheless, after stroke, a 2- to 6-week delay of carotid endarterectomy has been recommended. Although it seems reasonable to allow patients to stabilize before surgery, undue delay can be disastrous. Early surgery, although controversial, may be preferable when the neurologic deficit is small or transient.

Surgery has also been performed in some cases of acute carotid artery occlusion, usually less than 8 h old, but the results are generally unsatisfactory when a major neurologic deficit is present. Hence, surgery should be reserved for patients with a mild neurologic deficit. For most patients with a mild to moderate stroke and demonstrated occlusion of the internal carotid artery, alternative therapies include the use of anticoagulants or antiplatelet agents or neither. Some physicians anticoagulate for 6 months in hopes of preventing embolization of the propagated thrombus. Occasionally, endarterectomy of the external carotid artery or the contralateral stenotic internal carotid artery may be considered, depending on the findings of angiography and the nature of the recurrent clinical symptoms. The probable cause of an ischemic event determines the appropriate therapy. An embolism from an occluded carotid artery suggests the use of anticoagulation therapy, whereas recurrent symptoms suggestive of low flow in a hemisphere isolated from collateral sources of blood supply warrant consideration of surgery.

The appropriate therapy for stenosis of the carotid siphon or the middle cerebral stem associated with stroke or recurrent TIAs can be considered together. Because of the failure of external carotid/internal carotid (EC/IC) bypass surgery to reduce risks of ischemic stroke, antiplatelet therapy (aspirin) or anticoagulant therapy (sodium warfarin) is recommended in most cases. In the absence of randomized studies to indicate which is more efficacious, antiplatelet therapy is recommended initially for carotid siphon stenosis followed by anticoagulation if recurrent symptoms occur. Because of the potentially devastating effects of middle cerebral artery occlusion, anticoagulation with sodium warfarin is recommended for symptomatic middle cerebral stem stenosis. In cases where recurrent symptoms occur in spite of this therapy, lowering of the blood viscosity may be helpful. Often, with time, however, recurrent symptoms diminish despite the choice of treatment.

The unusual case of atherothrombotic stenosis or occlusion of the proximal anterior cerebral artery may cause intermittent symptoms involving the contralateral leg. Antiplatelet or anticoagulation therapy has been recommended, but no studies have documented the natural history of atherothrombotic disease at this location, and no surgical procedure protects the distal territory of the anterior cerebral artery from ischemia caused by proximal stenosis.

Although much attention has been directed toward the investigation of the opioid-like substance naloxone in the treatment of acute ischemic infarction, it has yet to be shown to be efficacious. Whole-blood viscosity reduction is a more promising innovative therapy for ischemic stroke. If the blood pressure remains constant, whole-blood viscosity reduction through lowering hematocrit and/or serum fibrinogen results in increased flow through a stenotic lesion. In theory, this form of therapy is expected to increase flow to the ischemic zone (penumbra) that lies between infarcted and normal brain. The size of the penumbra, however, is unknown for each individual stroke. The therapy has little risk.

ASYMPTOMATIC CAROTID BIFURCATION STENOSIS THAT CAUSES A BRUIT The natural history of a bruit caused by an atherosclerotic lesion of the carotid bifurcation that has not yet caused a TIA or stroke is unknown. The available studies have examined small populations and most failed to localize and quantitate the severity of the stenotic lesion. The studies of asymptomatic patients with cervical bruits who are about to undergo major surgical procedures have the same deficiencies. In most studies, patients with cervical bruits were found to be at increased risk of heart disease, stroke, and death. The strokes, however, did not necessarily occur in the vascular territory of the carotid bruit. Given these facts, there is little reason to operate on the carotid artery in patients with asymptomatic carotid stenosis, either routinely or before surgery.

However, patients with a tightly stenotic lesion at the origin of the internal carotid artery (1.5 mm or less) that reduces flow in the distal internal carotid artery may be at higher risk of thrombotic occlusion. Even though these patients have reduced flow in the distal internal carotid artery, they are asymptomatic because of adequate collateral flow across the anterior circle of Willis to the ipsilateral middle and anterior cerebral arteries. Stroke, therefore, should occur only by subsequent artery-to-artery embolism. The bruit associated with a tightly stenotic lesion at the origin of the internal carotid artery is high-pitched and prolonged, often fading into diastole. The bruit becomes fainter as the stenosis progresses and flow is further slowed, and finally disappears when occlusion is imminent. Noninvasive carotid testing that includes B-mode ultrasound imagery, Doppler analysis of flow immediately distal to the stenosis, quantitative spectral analysis of the bruit itself, and measurement of the oculosystolic pressure by oculoplethysmography can identify these tightly stenotic lesions. In the absence of a randomized trial of the efficacy of endarterectomy vs. antiplatelet therapy for this type of lesion, the physician has an option for either. In most cases, antiplatelet therapy is recommended. Only when signs of progressive narrowing are documented and the residual lumen diameter is 1.5 mm or less is surgery considered an option at our institution. Surgical morbidity should be less than 2 percent. However, no evidence suggests that surgery is more efficacious than medical therapy, and a randomized trial is needed.

ATHEROTHROMBOTIC DISEASE OF THE VERTEBRAL-BASILAR–POSTERIOR CEREBRAL ARTERY SYSTEM The two vertebral arteries join to form the basilar artery at the pontomedullary junction. The basilar artery divides into two posterior cerebral arteries in the interpeduncular fossa (Fig. 343-2). Each of these major arteries gives rise to large long and short circumferential branches and small deep penetrating branches that supply the cerebellum, medulla, pons, midbrain, subthalamus, thalamus, hippocampus, and medial temporal and occipital lobes. Atherosclerosis has a predilection for certain parts of the vertebral, basilar, and posterior cerebral arteries. Most frequently it occupies the origin of both vertebral arteries, the distal segments of both vertebral arteries, and the proximal basilar artery. In addition, atheroma tends to form at the origin of the major and minor branches of the vertebral, basilar, or posterior cerebral arteries. Predictably, atheromatous disease at each site carries its unique natural history, produces its own clinical syndromes, and has its own specific therapeutic implications.

POSTERIOR CEREBRAL ARTERY **Pathophysiology** In 70 percent of cases, both posterior cerebral arteries come from the bifurcation of the top of the basilar artery; in 22 percent, one or the other comes from the ipsilateral internal carotid artery; in 8 percent, both come from the ipsilateral internal carotid artery (Fig. 343-2*B*). When the latter occurs, the posterior communicating arteries are large and become the origin of the posterior cerebral arteries; the precommunal segment (mesencephalic portion, A1 segment, or stem) of the true posterior cerebral artery is atretic (Fig. 343-2*B*).

Atheroma occurring at the top of the basilar artery or along the precommunal segment of the posterior cerebral artery may block or symptomatically narrow one or more of the small brainstem-penetrating branches (Figs. 343-2 and 343-6*A*). These important branches supply the middle portion of the cerebral peduncles, the ipsilateral substantia nigra, red nucleus, oculomotor nuclei, midbrain reticular formation, subthalamic nucleus of Luys, decussation of superior cerebellar peduncles, the medial longitudinal fasciculus, and the medial lemniscus. The artery of Percheron, i.e., the posterior thalamosubthalamoparamedial artery, is a single artery arising from either the right or the left medial precommunal (mesencephalic) segment of the posterior cerebral artery. It divides in the subthalamus to supply bilaterally the inferior medial and the anterior portions of the thalamus and subthalamus. The thalamic thalamogeniculate branches, also originating in the precommunal portion of the posterior cerebral artery, supply the dorsal, dorsomedial, anterior, and inferior thalamus and the medial geniculate body. These branches include the medial and lateral posterior choroidal arteries. The medial posterior choroidal artery supplies the superior dorsomedial and dorsal anterior thalamus and the medial geniculate body in addition to the tela choroidea of the third ventricle. The lateral posterior choroidal artery supplies the choroid plexus of the lateral ventricle. Both posterior choroidal arteries send branches that anastomose with branches of the anterior choroidal artery. But the other small branches of the precommunal segment of the posterior cerebral artery end without anastomosing.

Atheromas occurring in the posterior cerebral artery distal to the junction with the posterior communicating artery (Fig. 343–6*B*) may symptomatically occlude the small circumferential branches that course around the midbrain to supply the lateral part of the cerebral peduncles, medial lemniscus, tegmentum of the midbrain, superior colliculi, lateral geniculate body, and posterior lateral nucleus of the thalamus, choroid plexus, and hippocampus. On the rare occasions when atheromas occur more distally in the posterior cerebral artery (Fig. 343-6*C*), a symptomatic occlusion may produce ischemia and infarction in the medial inferior temporal lobe, parahippocampal and hippocampal gyri, and occipital lobe—including the calcarine cortex and the visual association areas 18 and 19.

Clinical syndromes The location of atheromatous disease in the posterior cerebral artery or at the origin of one of its branches and the degree of narrowing usually determine the onset, severity, and nature of the clinical syndrome. Other factors, including the collateral circulation via the posterior communicating artery or over the cortical surface and serum viscosity, play significant but less important roles. However, even when atheroma is present in the posterior cerebral artery, embolic occlusion of it or one of its branches is usually the mechanism responsible for the stroke. The pathologic anatomy of the posterior cerebral artery generates syndromes that divide into two groups: first, midbrain, subthalamic, and thalamic syndromes due to atheromatous narrowing or atherothrombotic or embolic occlusion of either the proximal precommunal segment of the posterior cerebral artery or the origin of its penetrating branches; second, those cortical syndromes due to atheromatous narrowing or atherothrombotic or embolic occlusion of the postcommunal segment of the posterior cerebral artery.

PROXIMAL PRECOMMUNAL SYNDROMES (THE CENTRAL TERRITORY) If the stem of the posterior cerebral artery is occluded, infarction occurs in the subthalamus and medial thalamus, extending either ipsilaterally or bilaterally, and in the ipsilateral cerebral peduncle and midbrain, producing concomitant signs (Fig. 343-6). Obviously, if the posterior communicating artery is not functional (i.e., atretic), the peripheral territory supplied by the postcommunal segment of the posterior cerebral artery will become symptomatic as well (Fig. 343-6). Unless the origin of the posterior cerebral artery is completely occluded, hemiplegia secondary to infarction of the cerebral peduncle rarely occurs. Partial proximal syndromes suggest but do not prove mesencephalic thalamic perforant branch occlusion. A superior syndrome, one including involvement of the red nucleus and/or dentatorubro-thalamo tract, can produce a gross contralateral ataxia. An inferior syndrome can produce a third nerve palsy and a contralateral ataxia (Claude's syndrome), or a third nerve palsy and a contralateral hemiplegia (Weber's syndrome). When the subthalamic nucleus of Luys is involved, contralateral hemiballismus may occur. Occlusion of the artery of Percheron produces paresis of upward gaze and drowsiness. It is often associated with abulia or a euphoric state giving way to abulia. CT scan and MRI may detect bilateral butterfly lesions in the subthalamus and medial inferior thalamus. Extensive infarction in the midbrain or subthalamus occurring with bilateral posterior cerebral stem occlusion is usually secondary to embolism. Deep coma, bilateral pyramidal signs, and "decerebrate rigidity" occur in this setting.

Atheromatous occlusion of the penetrating branches of the thalamic and thalamogeniculate group at their origin produces smaller thalamo and thalamocapsular lacunar syndromes. The *thalamic syndrome of Déjerine and Roussy* is the best known. Its main feature is contralateral hemisensory loss of both superficial sensation (pain and temperature) and deep sensation (touch and proprioception). Occasionally, it may affect only pain and temperature or vibration and joint position sense. Most often it affects face, arm, hand, trunk, leg, and foot; occasionally, only one extremity. Hyperpathia may occur; and after a few weeks or months, an agonizing, searing pain may develop in the affected areas. Patients describe it as tight, drawing, icy, and knifelike. It is devastatingly persistent and responds poorly to analgesics. Occasionally, anticonvulsants are beneficial. If the posterior limb of the internal capsule is involved, hemiparesis or hemiplegia may occur with the hemisensory syndrome. Other associated motor signs include hemiballismus, choreoathetosis, intention tremor, incoordination, and posturing of the hand and arm, particularly while walking.

POSTCOMMUNAL SYNDROMES (THE PERIPHERAL OR CORTICAL TERRITORY) (Figs. 343-6*B* and *C*) Infarction in the pulvinar of the thalamus may result from occlusion of a posterior thalamic thalamogeniculate penetrating branch of the postcommunal posterior cerebral artery. Occlusion in the peripheral posterior cerebral artery itself most often infarcts the cortical surface of the medial temporal and occipital lobe. Contralateral homonymous hemianopsia is the usual manifestation. If the visual association areas are spared and only the calcarine cortex is involved, the patient is acutely aware of visual defects. Occasionally, only the upper quadrant of the visual field is involved. Central vision may be spared if middle cerebral artery branches supply the tip of the occipital pole. Medial temporal lobe and hippocampal involvement may cause an acute disturbance in memory, particularly if it occurs in the dominant hemisphere, but the defect usually clears because memory has bilateral representation. If the dominant hemisphere is affected and the infarct extends laterally into the deep white matter involving the splenium of the corpus callosum, alexia without agraphia may occur. Visual agnosia for faces, objects, mathematical symbols, and colors and anomia with paraphasic errors (amnestic aphasia) may also occur in this setting even without callosal involvement. When the ipsilateral internal carotid is occluded, tight stenosis or occlusion of the ipsilateral posterior cerebral artery can reduce flow in the watershed territory between the posterior and middle cerebral arteries. Often, visual agnosia, visual neglect, and inability to enumerate objects in a contralateral visual field follow. Occlusion of the posterior cerebral artery can produce peduncular hallucinosis (visual hallucinations of brightly colored scenes and objects), but the exact location of the infarct remains uncertain.

Bilateral infarction in the distal posterior cerebral artery territory produces cortical blindness. The patient is often unaware that vision is gone and the pupil reacts normally to light. Even if the defect is complete on one or both sides, tiny islands of vision may persist; and the patient will report that vision fluctuates, as images are still captured in the preserved islands. Rarely, only peripheral vision is lost and central vision is spared; then the patient reports gun-barrel vision. Optic ataxia (inability to visually guide limb movements), ocular ataxia (inability to direct eyes to a precise point in the visual field), inability to enumerate objects in a picture or project meaning from a picture, and inability to avoid objects seen in one's path can occur with bilateral visual association area lesions. Such a constellation of symptoms has been termed Balint's syndrome. It is most often seen with bilateral infarctions, presumably secondary to low flow in the distal posterior and/or middle cerebral "watershed" territories as occurs in cardiac arrest cases. Finally, occlusion of the top of the basilar artery, most often due to embolism, can produce a clinical picture which includes any or all of the central or peripheral territory symptoms. Its hallmark is suddenness of onset and bilaterality of symptoms.

Laboratory evaluation Infarction in the peripheral territory of the posterior cerebral artery can be easily documented by CT scan. However, infarction in the central territory of the posterior cerebral artery, especially infarction secondary to occlusive disease of the penetrating branches of the posterior cerebral artery, is not reliably detected by CT scanning. MRI can detect infarctions greater than 0.5 cm in this area. Angiography remains the only certain method of documenting atheromatous disease or embolic disease of the posterior cerebral artery. No form of angiography, however, can detect occlusive disease in the small penetrating branches. Thus, the diagnosis rests mainly on clinical grounds corroborated by MRI.

Therapy When infarction occurs in the territory of the posterior cerebral artery, it is usually secondary to embolism from lower segments of the vertebral-basilar system or the heart. Anticoagulants to prevent further embolic events are appropriate. Atheromatous occlusion of the posterior cerebral artery, on the other hand, requires no special therapy. Transient ischemic symptoms in the territory of the posterior cerebral artery may result from atherothrombotic stenosis of its proximal portion or one of its penetrating branches (lacunar TIA). The natural history of such atheromatous disease is unknown. Thus, the efficacy of anticoagulants vs. antiplatelet therapy vs. no medication is still uncertain. In general, antiplatelet therapy seems safest in this setting.

VERTEBRAL AND POSTERIOR INFERIOR CEREBELLAR ARTERIES Pathophysiology The vertebral artery, which arises from the innominate artery on the right and the subclavian artery on the left, divides into four anatomic segments. The first segment extends from its origin to its entrance into the sixth or fifth transverse vertebral foramen. The second is the vertical segment through the C6 to the C2 vertebral foramen. The third is the horizontal segment through the transverse foramen, circling around the arch of the atlas to pierce the dura at the level of the foramen magnum. The fourth begins as it penetrates the dura and courses up to join the other vertebral artery to form the basilar artery. The fourth segment gives rise to small penetrating branches that supply the medial and lateral medulla and to a large branch, the posterior inferior cerebellar artery: the latter's proximal segments supply the lateral medulla; its distal branches, the inferior surface of the cerebellum. Anastomotic channels exist among the ascending cervical arteries, thyrocervical arteries, the occipital artery (branch of the external carotid artery), and the second segment of the vertebral artery (Fig. 343-1). In 10 percent of patients, one vertebral artery is too small (atretic) to contribute significant blood to the brainstem.

Atherothrombotic lesions have a predilection for the first and fourth segments of the vertebral artery. Although the atheromatous narrowing in the first segment (the origin) may be significant, it seldom produces brainstem ischemic strokes. Collateral flow from the contralateral vertebral artery or the ascending cervical and ascending thyrocervical or occipital arteries is usually sufficient (Fig. 343-1*D*). When one vertebral artery is atretic and atherothrombotic lesion threatens the origin of the other, the only avenues for collateral circulation are through the ascending cervical artery, the thyrocervical artery, and the occipital artery, or by retrograde flow down the basilar artery via the posterior communicating artery (Figs. 343-2 and 343-6). In this setting, low flow in the vertebral-basilar system exists and TIAs occur. In addition, incipient thrombosis in the distal basilar proximal vertebral system may occur. If the subclavian is blocked proximal to the origin of the vertebral artery, exercise of the left arm may draw blood from the vertebral-basilar system to the arm, sometimes causing symptoms of vertebral-basilar insufficiency, *subclavian steal.* It rarely leads to significant vertebral-basilar ischemia.

Atheroma in the fourth segment of the vertebral artery can occur proximal to the origin of the posterior inferior cerebral artery, at the origin of the posterior inferior cerebral artery or distal to it, and at the junction with the other vertebral artery to form the basilar artery. When it is proximal to the origin of the posterior inferior cerebral artery, a critical narrowing can threaten the lateral medulla and posterior inferior surface of the cerebellum.

Although atheromatous disease rarely narrows the second and third segments of the vertebral artery, they are subject to dissection lesions, fibromuscular dysplasia, and rare encroachment by osteophytic arthritic changes in the vertebral foramens.

Clinical syndromes Transient cerebral ischemic attacks resulting from vertebral artery insufficiency cause dizziness or vertigo, numbness of the ipsilateral face and contralateral limbs, diplopia, hoarseness, dysarthria, and dysphagia. Hemiparesis is exceedingly rare. These TIAs are usually short (up to 10 to 15 min) and repetitive (up to many times a day).

When infarction ensues, it most often affects the lateral medulla with or without the posterior inferior cerebellum (Wallenberg's syndrome). Its features are listed in Fig. 343-7. In 80 percent of the cases, the syndrome occurs after vertebral occlusion; in 20 percent, it results from posterior inferior cerebellar artery occlusion. Atherothrombotic occlusion of the medullary penetrating branches of the vertebral or posterior inferior cerebellar artery results in partial syndromes of the ipsilateral lateral or medial medulla.

Rarely, a medial syndrome occurs in which the medullary pyramid becomes infarcted causing a contralateral hemiparesis of the arm and leg, sparing the face. If the medial lemniscus and emerging hypoglossal nerve fibers are involved, contralateral loss of joint position sense and ipsilateral tongue weakness occur.

Cerebellar infarction with edema formation can lead to sudden respiratory arrest due to raised intracranial pressure in the posterior fossa. Drowsiness, Babinski signs, dysarthria, and bifacial weakness may be absent or present only briefly before respiratory arrest ensues. Gait unsteadiness, dizziness, nausea, and vomiting may be the only early symptoms and signs and should arouse suspicion of this impending complication.

Laboratory evaluation When TIAs occur in the territory of the lateral medulla, it becomes important to determine the adequacy of blood flow in the distal vertebral artery and the posterior inferior

FIGURE 343-7 *(Courtesy of C.M. Fisher, M.D.)*

Signs and symptoms	*Structures involved*
1 Medial medullary syndrome (occlusion of vertebral artery or of branch of vertebral or lower basilar artery)	
On side of lesion:	
Paralysis with atrophy of half the tongue	*Ipsilateral twelfth nerve*
On side opposite lesion:	
Paralysis of arm and leg sparing face; impaired tactile and proprioceptive sense over half the body	*Contralateral pyramidal tract and medial lemniscus*
2 Lateral medullary syndrome (occlusion of any of five vessels may be responsible—vertebral, posterior inferior cerebellar superior, middle, or inferior lateral medullary arteries)	
On side of lesion:	
Pain, numbness, impaired sensation over half the face	*Descending tract and nucleus fifth nerve*
Ataxia of limbs, falling to side of lesion	*Uncertain—restiform body, cerebellar hemisphere, cerebellar fibers, spinocerebellar tract (?)*
Nystagmus, diplopia, oscillopsia, vertigo, nausea, vomiting	*Vestibular nucleus*
Horner's syndrome (miosis, ptosis, decreased sweating)	*Descending sympathetic tract*
Dysphagia, hoarseness, paralysis of palate, paralysis of vocal cord, diminished gag reflex	*Issuing fibers ninth and tenth nerves*
Loss of taste	*Nucleus and tractus solitarius*
Numbness of ipsilateral arm, trunk, or leg	*Cuneate and gracile nuclei*
On side opposite lesion:	
Impaired pain and thermal sense over half the body, sometimes face	*Spinothalamic tract*
3 Total unilateral medullary syndrome (occlusion of vertebral artery): Combination of medial and lateral syndromes	
4 Lateral pontomedullary syndrome (occlusion of vertebral artery): Combination of lateral medullary and lateral inferior pontine syndromes	
5 Basilar artery syndrome (the syndrome of the lone vertebral artery is equivalent): A combination of the various brainstem syndromes plus those arising in the posterior cerebral artery distribution	
Bilateral long tract signs (sensory and motor; cerebellar and peripheral cranial nerve abnormalities)	*Bilateral long tract; cerebellar and peripheral cranial nerves*
Paralysis or weakness of all extremities, plus all bulbar musculature	*Corticobulbar and corticospinal tracts bilaterally*

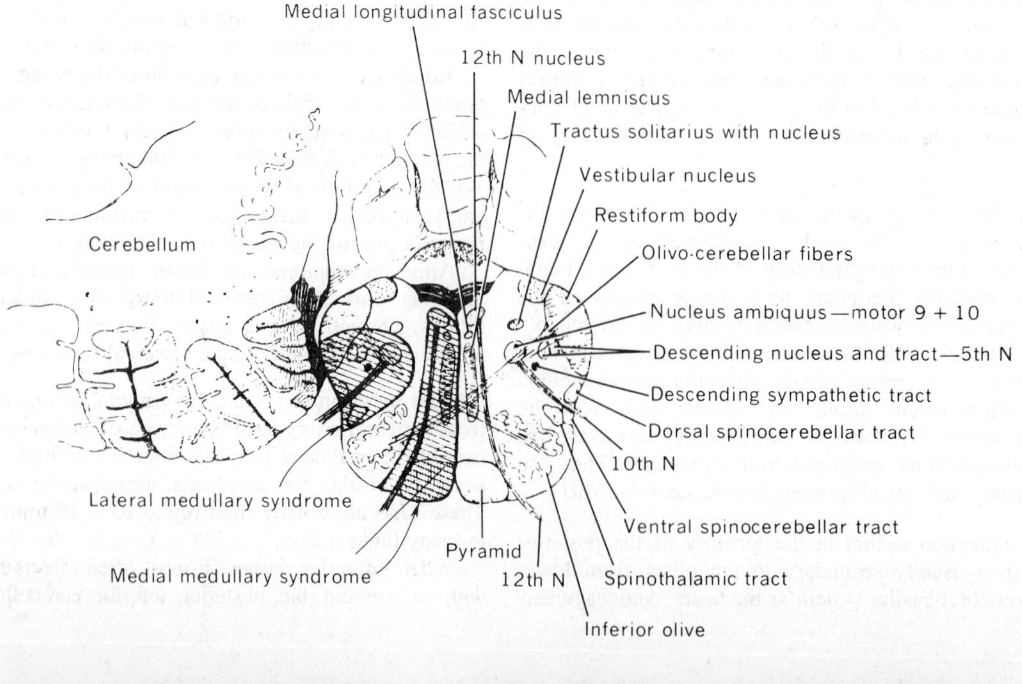

cerebellar artery. Angiography is therefore indicated. CT scanning may detect a large cerebellar infarction in the territory of the posterior inferior cerebellar artery. MRI can detect cerebellar infarction earlier and, with refinement in technique, may be able to detect lateral medullary infarction. Even now it has been able to image the fourth segment of the vertebral artery if it contains flowing blood. It is anticipated that with the further development of MRI technology it may be possible to image atherothrombotic material in the vertebral and basilar arteries and determine if they are patent or occluded, and supplant the need for angiography.

Therapy Four important therapeutic issues arise when dealing with a patient with ischemia or infarction in the territory of the vertebral or posterior inferior cerebellar artery. First, in vertebral or posterior inferior cerebellar artery occlusion, the posterior inferior cerebellum and sometimes the lateral medulla may be infarcted. The ensuing cerebellar edema can be treated with osmotic agents (mannitol), but surgical decompression may be necessary. Second, when the fourth segment of the vertebral artery becomes thrombosed, clot may propagate into the basilar artery or embolize up the basilar and lodge at the top or in one of its branches. Thus, in cases of lateral medullary infarction, symptoms or signs of basilar insufficiency may ensue. Acute anticoagulation with heparin is advocated in such cases. Some physicians argue for its prophylactic use in acute vertebral artery occlusion, although there is little support for chronic sodium warfarin anticoagulation. Third, when one vertebral artery is symptomatic with atheromatous disease and the contralateral vertebral is congenitally atretic or already occluded, basilar ischemia may ensue and proximal basilar thrombosis may develop. Acute anticoagulation with heparin followed by chronic sodium warfarin anticoagulation is recommended. Fourth, when the same circumstance occurs but the symptomatic vertebral atherothrombotic lesion lies immediately proximal to the posterior inferior cerebellar artery, occipital-to-posterior-inferior bypass grafting has been recommended. The efficacy of this surgery is unproven, and it should be considered only after anticoagulation therapy has failed.

BASILAR ARTERY Pathophysiology The basilar artery is formed by the union of the vertebral arteries at the pontomedullary junction. After coursing under the surface of the basis pontis, it ends in the interpeduncular fossa, where it bifurcates, forming the posterior cerebral arteries (Figs. 343-2 and 343-6). Branches of the basilar artery supply the basis pontis and superior cerebellum. The branches of the basilar divide into three groups: (1) paramedians, 7 to 10 in number, supply a wedge of pons on either side of the midline; (2) short circumferential branches, 5 to 7 in number, supply the lateral two-thirds of the pons and the middle and superior cerebellar peduncles; and (3) two bilateral long circumferential arteries (superior cerebellar and anterior/inferior cerebellar arteries) course around the pons to supply the cerebellar hemispheres.

Atheromatous lesions can occur anywhere along the basilar trunk, but are most often in the proximal basilar and distal vertebral segments. Typically, lesions occlude either the proximal basilar and one or both distal vertebral arteries. The clinical picture varies depending on the availability of retrograde collateral flow from the posterior communicating arteries.

Atherothrombosis occasionally occludes the top of the basilar artery; more often, an embolus from the heart or proximal vertebral or basilar segments occludes it. Such artery-to-artery emboli may also occlude one of the smaller basilar branches or one of the posterior cerebral arteries.

Clinical symptoms—basilar artery vs. basilar branch Because the brainstem contains so many different neuronal systems in close approximation, many clinical syndromes can emerge when it becomes ischemic. The most important symptom-producing systems include the corticospinal tracts, corticobulbar tracts, medial and superior cerebellar peduncles, spinothalamic tracts, and the cranial nerve nuclei. Figures 343-8 to 343-10 outline some of the vascular syndromes, including some which await clinicopathologic definition.

Unfortunately, the symptoms of transient ischemia or stroke in the territory of the basilar artery often do not indicate whether it is the basilar artery or one of its branches that is diseased, yet the difference has important implications for therapy. The complete picture of basilar insufficiency, however, is easy to recognize. A combination of bilateral long tract signs (sensory and motor) and signs of cranial nerve and cerebellar dysfunction suggest the diagnosis. A locked-in state of quadriplegia occurs with bilateral basis pontis infarction. Coma due to dysfunction of the reticular activating system and quadriplegia with cranial nerve signs suggest complete and devastating pontine and midbrain infarction. The goal, however, is to recognize impending basilar occlusion long before such a devastating infarction occurs. Thus a series of TIAs or a slowly progressive, fluctuating stepwise stroke becomes extremely significant when they herald an atherothrombotic occlusion of the distal vertebral or proximal basilar artery.

TRANSIENT ISCHEMIC ATTACKS When transient ischemic spells herald occlusion of the proximal basilar, the medulla as well as the pons may be involved. Patients often say they are ''dizzy''; when asked to describe what they mean, they may use the words ''swimming,'' ''swaying,'' ''moving,'' ''unsteady,'' or ''light-headed.'' They may complain that the room is upside down or that the floor seems to move or come toward them. As such, dizziness is the most common symptom of transient basilar territory ischemia, but is usually associated with other symptoms before a basilar thrombosis produces an infarction (see Chap. 14). Thus, transient ''dizziness'' associated with diplopia, dysarthria, facial or circumoral numbness, and hemisensory symptoms indicates the presence of transient vertebral-basilar insufficiency. Usually, hemiparesis indicates the basilar artery is involved whether or not the vertebral is involved. Most often TIAs, whether due to impending occlusion of either the basilar artery or a basilar branch, are short-lived (5 to 30 min) and repetitive, occurring several times a day. The pattern suggests intermittent reduction of flow rather than recurrent embolism. In general, symptoms of basilar branch TIAs affect one side of the brainstem, whereas symptoms of basilar artery TIAs usually affect both sides.

STROKE Atherothrombotic occlusion of the basilar artery with stroke usually causes bilateral brainstem signs. Sometimes, only gaze paresis or internuclear ophthalmoplegia associated with ipsilateral hemiparesis, i.e., a particular combination of cranial nerve and long tract (sensory and/or motor) deficits, signifies bilateral brainstem ischemia. More often, bilateral basis pontis signs coexist with unilateral or bilateral pontine tegmental signs.

When atherothrombotic occlusion of a basilar branch artery becomes symptomatic, it generates unilateral symptoms and signs involving motor, sensory, and cranial nerves. Occlusions of the long circumferential branches of the basilar artery produce specific clinical syndromes (see below and ''Lacunar Disease'').

SUPERIOR CEREBELLAR ARTERY Occlusion of the superior cerebellar artery results in severe ipsilateral cerebellar ataxia (middle and/or superior cerebellar peduncles), nausea and vomiting, dysarthria, and contralateral loss of pain and temperature sensation over the extremities, body, and face (spino- and trigeminothalamic tract). Partial deafness, ataxic tremor of the ipsilateral upper extremity, Horner's syndrome, and palatal myoclonus may rarely occur. Partial syndromes occur frequently.

ANTERIOR INFERIOR CEREBELLAR ARTERY Occlusion of the anterior inferior cerebellar artery produces variable degrees of infarction, because the size of this artery and the territory it supplies vary inversely with those of the posterior inferior cerebellar artery. The principal symptoms include ipsilateral deafness, facial weakness, true vertigo (whirling dizziness), nausea and vomiting, nystagmus, tinnitus and cerebellar ataxia, Horner's syndrome, and paresis of conjugate lateral gaze. The opposite side of the body loses pain and temperature sensation. An occlusion close to the origin of the artery may cause corticospinal tract signs.

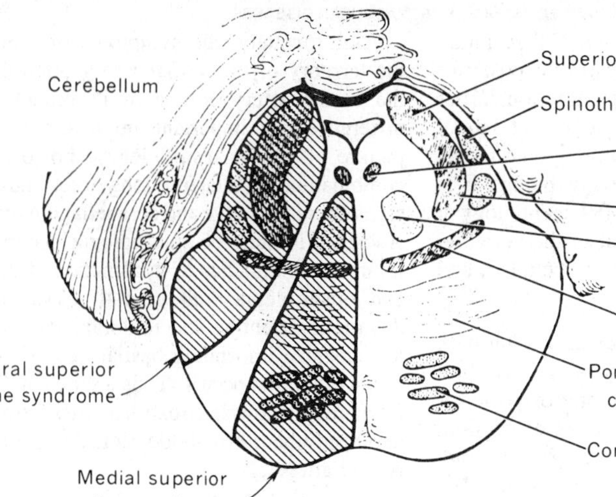

FIGURE 343-8 *(Courtesy of C.M. Fisher, M.D.)*

Signs and symptoms	*Structures involved*
1 Medial superior pontine syndrome (paramedian branches of upper basilar artery)	
On side of lesion:	
Cerebellar ataxia (probably)	*Superior and/or middle cerebellar peduncle*
Internuclear ophthalmoplegia	*Medial longitudinal fasciculus*
Myoclonic syndrome, palate, pharnyx, vocal cords, respiratory apparatus, face, oculomotor apparatus, etc.	*Localization uncertain—central tegmental bundle (?), dentate projection (?), inferior olivary nucleus (?)*
On side opposite lesion:	
Paralysis of face, arm, and leg	*Corticobulbar and corticospinal tract*
Rarely touch, vibration, and position are affected	*Medial lemniscus*
2 Lateral superior pontine syndrome (syndrome of superior cerebellar artery)	
On side of lesion:	
Ataxia of limbs and gait, falling to side of lesion	*Middle and superior cerebellar peduncles, superior surface of cerebellum, dentate nucleus*
Dizziness, nausea, vomiting; horizontal nystagmus	*Vestibular nucleus*
Paresis of conjugate gaze (ipsilateral)	*Pontine center for conjugate lateral gaze*
Skew deviation	*Uncertain*
Miosis, ptosis, decreased sweating over face (Horner's syndrome)	*Descending sympathetic fibers*
Static tremor reported in one case	*Dentate nucleus (?), superior cerebellar peduncle (?)*
On side opposite lesion:	
Impaired pain and thermal sense on face, limbs, and trunk	*Spinothalamic tract*
Impaired touch, vibration, and position sense, more in leg than arm (there is a tendency to incongruity of pain and touch deficits)	*Medial lemniscus (lateral portion)*

Occlusion of one of the five to seven short circumferential branches of the basilar artery renders ischemic a specific area in the lateral two-thirds of the pons and/or middle or superior cerebellar peduncle, whereas occlusion of one of the seven to ten paramedian branches of the basilar artery renders ischemic a specific wedge-shaped area on either side of the medial pons (Figs. 343-8 to 343-10).

Many syndromes of brainstem lesions have been described and given eponyms, e.g., Weber, Claude, Benedict, Foville, Raymond-Cestan, Millard-Gubler. The pons contains so many neuronal structures that minor variations in the territory supplied by each arterial branch and variations in the overlap among vascular territories modify the clinical picture. For instance, dysarthria associated with a clumsy hand suggests a small basis pontis infarct. However, hemiparesis alone does not differentiate basis pontis ischemia from ischemia in the corticospinal tract above the tentorium, i.e., posterior limb of the internal capsule.

Hemiparesis coexisting with ipsilateral sensory loss suggests the stroke lies supratentorially. Dissociated sensory loss (pain and temperature only) over the face or half of the body suggests brainstem ischemia. On the other hand, sensory loss involving all modalities, i.e., pain and temperature as well as touch and joint position sense, suggests a lesion in the ventral posterior thalamus or in the deep parietal white matter and cortical surface adjacent to it. Findings indicative of cranial nerve dysfunction, i.e., deafness, peripheral seventh nerve weakness, sixth nerve weakness, or third nerve palsy, are extremely helpful in locating a segmental level of the pons or midbrain.

Laboratory evaluation Although CT scanning localizes most supratentorial strokes after 48 h, it is less reliable for detection and localization of stroke in the posterior fossa. Bone artifact often obscures details. Partial volume artifacts and plane restrictions further account for its poor resolution of infarcts in the brainstem. MRI eliminates many of these drawbacks. It reliably detects small (lacunar) infarcts in the basis pontis resulting from occlusion of paramedian basilar branches as well as larger infarcts resulting from disease of the larger basilar branches or the basilar artery itself. In addition, MRI can detect ischemic infarction earlier than CT scanning. On the other hand, CT scanning detects small pontine hematomas better than MRI and thus differentiates them from acute ischemic strokes. MRI is more sensitive for defining a pontine glioma or plaque of multiple sclerosis and can often differentiate them from infarction.

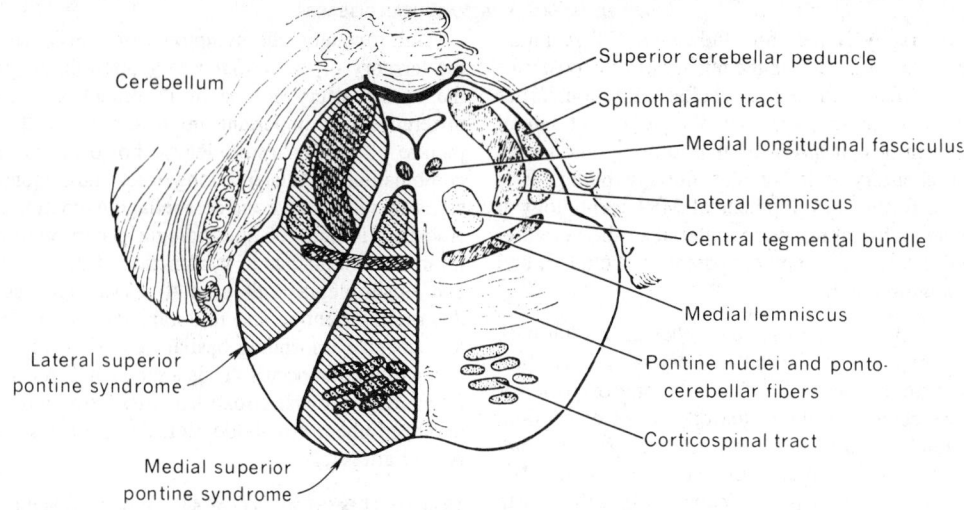

Only selective cerebral arteriography can document atherothrombotic disease of the basilar artery. Since arteriography entails potential morbidity and may precipitate the very stroke one is seeking to prevent, it must be recommended only when the information provided will assist in the management of the patient (see below). Occasionally, injection of angiographic dye in the posterior circulation precipitates a delirious state sometimes associated with cortical blindness. This state can last up to 24 to 48 h, and rarely several days. Arterial digital angiography may provide sufficient resolution to diagnose atheromatous narrowing at the distal vertebral and basilar arteries; intravenous digital angiography does not provide adequate resolution.

Therapy Suspected impending basilar occlusion causing transient or fluctuating symptoms should be treated with short-term anticoagulation with intravenous heparin, after a CT scan has excluded hemorrhage. Angiography is considered if the diagnosis is uncertain only after the patient's condition is stable. When basilar artery stenosis or occlusion is associated with minor or improving stroke, long-term anticoagulation with sodium warfarin is recommended. If, on the other hand, basilar branch disease is the cause, then the rationale for using sodium warfarin is uncertain. While embolism from the heart or atheroma in the distal vertebral system may occlude a penetrating basilar branch, this is unlikely. Therefore, chronic control of blood pressure and antiplatelet therapy are recommended as preventive measures in the management of small vessel basilar branch disease. Because of the long-term accumulative risk of anticoagulant therapy, it is generally reserved for larger vessel atherothrombotic disease, i.e. distal vertebral or proximal basilar disease.

LACUNAR DISEASE The term *lacunar disease* refers to atherothrombotic and lipohyalinotic occlusive disease of the penetrating branches of the circle of Willis, middle cerebral stem, and vertebral and basilar arteries.

Pathophysiology The middle cerebral artery stem, the arteries comprising the circle of Willis (A1 segment of the anterior cerebral artery, anterior and posterior communicating arteries, and precommunal segment of the posterior cerebral arteries), the basilar, and the vertebral arteries all give rise to 100- to 400-μm branches that penetrate the deep gray and white matter of the cerebrum or brainstem (Fig. 343-2). Each of these small branches can be thrombosed either by atherothrombotic disease at its origin (basilar or middle cerebral stem branch disease) or by the development of lipohyalinotic thickening of its wall more distally. When they become thrombosed, small (less than 2-cm) infarcts occur and are referred to as *lacunes*. Many may be as small as 3 to 4 mm. Hypertension is invariably a risk factor for such small vessel disease. These infarcts represent 10 percent of strokes.

Clinical syndromes The clinical picture resulting from lacunes are called lacunar syndromes. Often transient symptoms (lacunar TIAs) herald a lacunar infarct. Such TIAs may occur many times a day, but last only a few minutes. When infarction occurs, it may present with a sudden deficit or evolve in a progressive fashion over a few days. Recovery often begins within hours or days after the infarct, although in some cases significant disability persists. Recovery over weeks or months may be complete or result in minimal residual deficit.

Many neurologic or lacunar syndromes occur and many more await documentation. The most common syndromes are the following:

1 Pure motor hemiparesis from an infarct in the posterior limb of the internal capsule or basis pontis. Here, the face, arm, leg, foot, and toes are almost always involved. The weakness may be intermittent (TIA), progress in a stepwise manner, or appear abruptly. The weakness may progress to plegia, then commonly improve. In many cases, recovery is almost complete.

2 Pure hemisensory syndromes from a thalamic infarct.

FIGURE 343-9 *(Courtesy of C.M. Fisher, M.D.)*

Signs and symptoms	*Structures involved*
1 Medial midpontine syndrome (paramedian branch of midbasilar artery)	
On side of lesion:	
Ataxia of limbs and gait (more prominent in bilateral involvement	*Middle cerebellar peduncle*
On side opposite lesion:	
Paralysis of face, arm, and leg	*Corticobulbar and corticospinal tract*
Variable impaired touch and proprioception when lesion extends posteriorly	*Medial lemniscus*
2 Lateral midpontine syndrome (short circumferential artery)	
On side of lesion:	
Ataxia of limbs	*Middle cerebellar peduncle*
Paralysis of muscles of mastication	*Motor fibers or nucleus of fifth nerve*
Impaired sensation over side of face	*Sensory fibers or nucleus of fifth nerve*
On side opposite lesion:	
Impaired pain and thermal sense on limbs and trunk	*Spinothalamic tract*

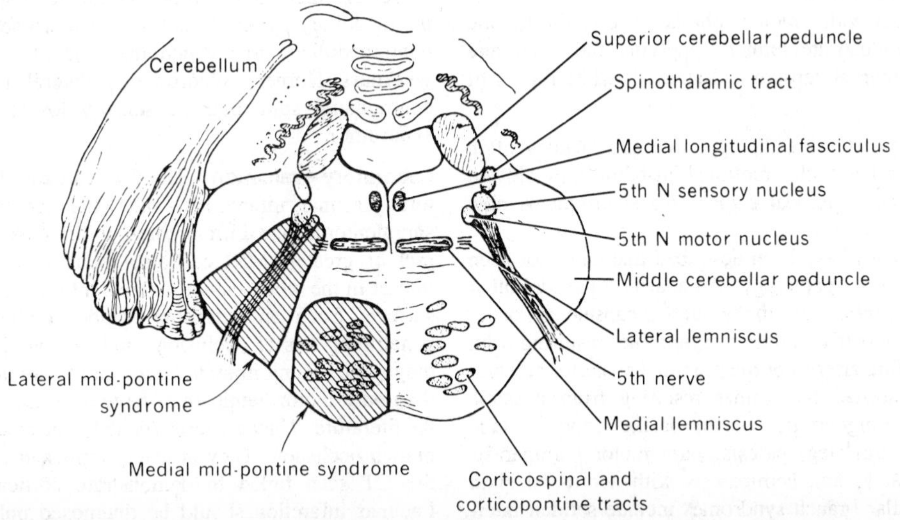

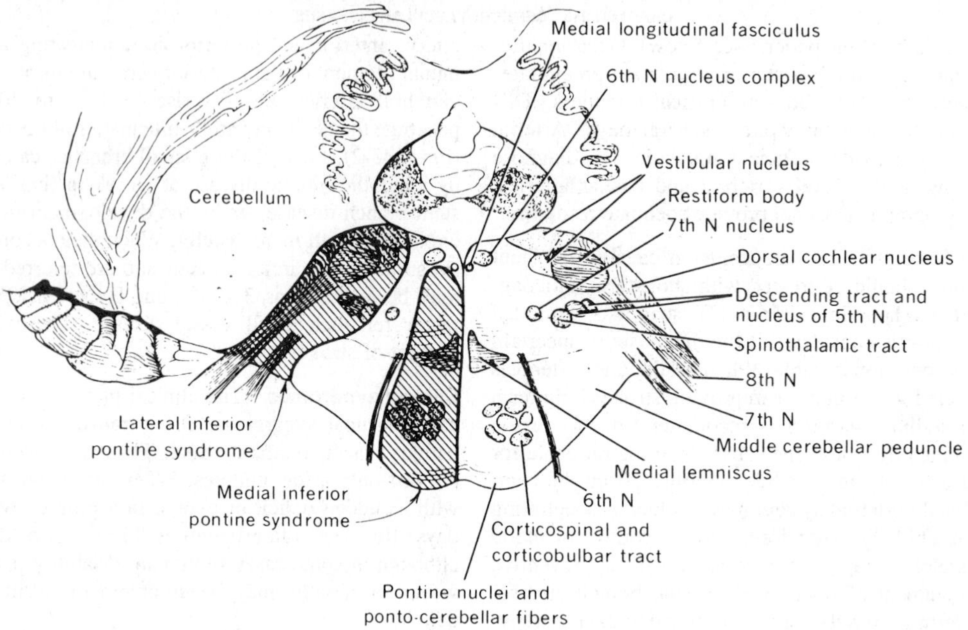

FIGURE 343-10 *(Courtesy of C.M. Fisher, M.D.)*

Signs and symptoms	*Structures involved*
1 Medial inferior pontine syndrome (occlusion of paramedian branch of basilar artery)	
On side of lesion:	
Paralysis of conjugate gaze to side of lesion (preservation of convergence)	*"Center" for conjugate lateral gaze*
Nystagmus	*Vestibular nucleus*
Ataxia of limbs and gait	*Middle cerebellar peduncle (?)*
Diplopia on lateral gaze	*Abducens nerve*
On side opposite lesion:	
Paralysis of face, arm, and leg	*Corticobulbar and corticospinal tract in lower pons*
Impaired tactile and proprioceptive sense over half of the body	*Medial lemniscus*
2 Lateral inferior pontine syndrome (occlusion of anterior inferior cerebellar artery)	
On side of lesion:	
Horizontal and vertical nystagmus, vertigo, nausea, vomiting, oscillopsia	*Vestibular nerve on nucleus*
Facial paralysis	*Seventh nerve*
Paralysis of conjugate gaze to side of lesion	*"Center" for conjugate lateral gaze*
Deafness, tinnitus	*Auditory nerve or cochlear nucleus*
Ataxia	*Middle cerebellar peduncle and cerebellar hemisphere*
Impaired sensation over face	*Descending tract and nucleus fifth nerve*
On side opposite lesion:	
Impaired pain and thermal sense over half the body (may include face)	*Spinothalamic tract*

3 True ataxic hemiparesis from a basis pontis infarct, and dysarthria with a clumsy hand or arm due to infarction in the basis pontis or the genu of the internal capsule.

4 Pure motor hemiparesis with "motor aphasia" due to thrombotic occlusion of a lenticulostriate branch supplying the genu and anterior limb of the internal capsule and adjacent white matter of the corona radiata.

Before the advent of hypertensive therapy, multiple lacunes often induced pseudobulbar palsy with emotional instability, a slowed abulic state, and bilateral pyramidal signs. This syndrome is now uncommon.

Other lacunar syndromes have been described that have not been correlated with actual arterial pathology. An anarthric pseudobulbar syndrome due to bilateral infarctions in the internal capsule can occur from disease in the lenticulostriate arteries. Syndromes resulting from occlusion of the penetrating arteries of the proximal posterior cerebral artery were discussed above. Syndromes resulting from possible occlusion of the penetrating arteries of the basilar artery include ipsilateral ataxia and crural (leg) paresis, pure motor hemiparesis with horizontal gaze palsy, and hemiparesis with a crossed sixth nerve palsy. Lower basilar branch syndromes include sudden internuclear ophthalmoplegia, horizontal gaze palsy, and appendicular cerebellar ataxia. Syndromes resulting from possible vertebral branch occlusions include pure motor hemiparesis sparing the face involving the medullary pyramid, and those syndromes that involve the lateral pontomedullary area which may include vertigo, vomiting, facial weakness, Horner's syndrome, ipsilateral trigeminal numbness, and contralateral spinothalamic sensory loss (partial lateral medullary syndrome).

Laboratory evaluation The CT scan can document most supratentorial lacunar infarctions, and MRI successfully documents both supratentorial and infratentorial infarctions when the lacunes are 7 mm or greater. MRI can also reliably document whether a small infarct in the white matter extends into the gray matter of the cortical surface. Such an extension implies embolism rather than small penetrating vessel occlusion, and lacunar infarction should not be diagnosed. Many infarcts larger than 2 cm and associated with more than pure motor hemiparesis have been incorrectly called lacunes in the literature. They are too large to be the result of a single penetrating branch occlusion. They probably represent embolic infarction where the CT scan failed to demonstrate cortical surface involvement. Lacunar infarction should be diagnosed only when the size of the infarct is less than 2 cm and its location attributable to occlusion of a small penetrating branch of one of the major arteries at the base of the brain. Larger deep white matter infarcts in the territory of the middle cerebral artery are probably due to embolism. The electroencephalogram (EEG) is usually normal in contrast to cortical surface infarction. If the EEG is normal early after the onset of symptoms, it suggests the infarct is in the deep white matter.

Therapy The best therapy for small vessel disease is prevention, i.e., careful control of hypertension. However, during stroke evolution, a reduction in blood pressure may worsen the symptoms. Antihypertensive therapy is begun after the patient's symptoms become stable. The value of anticoagulant or antiplatelet agents to patients with lacunar TIAs and fluctuating stroke is unknown. Some suggest that thalamic lacunes secondary to lipohyalinosis may be associated with minor hemorrhage. Hemosiderin-laden macrophages are sometimes seen at autopsy in such infarctions. This condition precludes use of heparin. On the other hand, some patients with fluctuating hemiparesis from atherothrombotic disease of a basilar branch or of the middle cerebral stem lenticulostriate arteries may improve coincident with heparin administration. Lacunar stroke does not require long-term anticoagulant therapy; it requires, instead, careful control of hypertension to prevent progression of vascular disease.

OTHER CAUSES OF CEREBRAL INFARCTION **Venous thrombosis** Lateral or sagittal sinus thrombosis or thrombosis of small cortical veins occurs in relation to sepsis, intracranial infections (meningitis), or conditions associated with hypercoagulable states such as polycythemia, sickle cell anemia, or during pregnancy or administration of oral contraceptives. Venous thromboses may cause an increase in intracranial pressure, headaches, focal seizures, and focal neurologic signs. Massive cerebral infarction with secondary edema may be fatal.

Systemic hypotension Systemic hypotension from Stokes-Adams attacks or other causes may, on rare occasions, result in ischemia distal to a stenotic lesion. Usually infarction does not occur unless hypotension is prolonged, as it is in cardiac arrest. Infarction tends to occur in distal segments of the major intracranial arteries, i.e., the distal middle cerebral, anterior cerebral, or posterior cerebral territory, causing a border zone lesion between the middle and anterior or middle and posterior cerebral arteries (watershed infarction) (Fig. 343-1*A*). Here proximal weakness and distal parietal deficits suggest the diagnosis.

Dissection of the cervicocerebral arteries Dissection of the large extracranial arteries may cause cerebral infarction and is a frequent cause of stroke in children and young adults. The dissection divides the media of the vessel or separates the intima from the media. TIAs and infarction can occur when the vessel occludes or when dissection causes emboli. Trauma, either severe or trivial, accounts for a substantial proportion of cases. Spontaneous dissection also occurs in atheromatous lesions or as a complication of fibromuscular dysplasia, and in patients with homocystinuria or arteritis. Dissection of the internal carotid artery is the most common, but it may also occur in the vertebral and basilar arteries and in the stems of the middle and anterior cerebral arteries. Dissection of the internal carotid artery produces an oculosympathetic palsy (Horner's syndrome) in over half of the cases, and a self-audible bruit. Tenderness over the carotid bulb may be present. The above symptoms and signs and transient monocular blindness or TIAs often precede embolic or "low-flow" watershed carotid territory infarction; this leaves time for therapeutic intervention. However, the natural history of dissection lesions is so uncertain that proper management remains problematic. Therapeutic options for cervical carotid dissection include surgical exploration and removal of the dissection clot and intima with a Fogarty catheter or medical treatment with anticoagulation or antiplatelet agents. When the patient has only oculosympathetic palsy, TIAs, or a minor stroke, anticoagulation with heparin is preferable. Surgical exploration is only considered for patients with increasingly severe TIAs or a mild stroke that is worsening. After the patient's symptoms have stabilized, anticoagulation with sodium warfarin is recommended for 6 months.

Patients with symptomatic vertebral, middle cerebral, or posterior cerebral artery dissection may also be managed in the acute phase with heparin and later with warfarin.

Fibromuscular dysplasia of the cervical vessels Fibromuscular dysplasia of the cervical vessels occurs mainly in young women. The carotid and/or vertebral arteries show multiple rings of segmental narrowing alternating with dilatation. Occlusion is usually incomplete. The process is often asymptomatic, but occasionally is associated with an audible bruit, TIAs, and stroke. Hypertension, if present, may be the result of renal artery stenosis. The cause and natural history of fibromuscular dysplasia is unknown (see Chap. 227). Caution should be used in attributing transient ischemic symptoms and/or embolic stroke to this disease when the residual lumen diameter of the narrowed portion of the artery is greater than 2 mm. Surgical dilatation of the cervical internal carotid artery is possible in symptomatic cases, but is associated with considerable morbidity. Anticoagulation may be more successful than surgery in patients with TIAs of increasing severity.

Arteritis Arteritis due to bacterial or syphilitic infection is no longer a common cause of cerebral thrombosis. The other arteritides are rare, yet any can cause cerebral thrombosis (see below and Chap. 269). *Necrotizing* or *granulomatous arteritis,* occurring alone or in association with generalized polyarteritis nodosa or Wegener's granulomatosis, involves the distal small branches (less than 1-mm diameter) of the main intracranial arteries and produces small ischemic infarcts in the brain, optic nerve, or spinal cord. The disease, although rare, is relentlessly progressive. In some cases, steroid therapy (prednisone, 40 to 60 mg per day) has been helpful, and recently, immunosuppressive drugs have been used with some success (see Chap. 269). *Idiopathic giant cell arteritis* involving the great vessels arising from the aortic arch (Takayasu's syndrome) may, on rare occasions, cause carotid or vertebral thrombosis. It is an infrequent cause of the aortic arch syndrome in the western hemisphere (see Chap. 195).

Temporal arteritis (cranial arteritis) (see Chap. 269) This is a relatively common affliction of elderly persons in which the external carotid system, particularly the temporal branches, is the site of a subacute granulomatous inflammation with an exudate of lymphocytes, monocytes, neutrophilic leukocytes, and giant cells. Usually the most severely affected parts of the artery become thrombosed. Headache or head pain is the chief complaint. Systemic manifestations include anorexia, loss of weight, malaise, and polymyalgia rheumatica. The inflammatory nature of the illness is indicated by some one or several of the following: fever, slight leukocytosis, increased erythrocyte sedimentation rate, and anemia. Occlusion of branches of the ophthalmic artery results in blindness in one or both eyes in over 25 percent of patients, and occasionally an ophthalmoplegia due to involvement of ocular nerves occurs. An arteritis of the aorta and its major branches, including carotid, subclavian, coronary, and femoral arteries, has been found at postmortem examination in some cases. Significant inflammatory involvement of intracranial arteries is rare, but strokes occur occasionally on the basis of occlusion of the internal carotid, middle cerebral, or vertebral arteries. The diagnosis depends on the finding of a tender thrombosed or thickened cranial artery and the demonstration of the lesion in a biopsy specimen. Corticosteroids bring striking subjective relief and often prevent blindness. Prednisone is most often used. It is generally started in large daily doses of 80 to 120 mg and is then tapered using the erythrocyte sedimentation rate as a guide.

Moya moya disease Moya moya disease is a poorly understood occlusive disease involving large intracranial arteries, especially the internal carotid artery and the stem of the middle and anterior cerebral artery. The lenticulostriate arteries develop a rich source of collateral flow around the middle cerebral occlusive lesion which, on cerebral angiography, gives the impression of a puff of smoke (*moya moya*). Other collaterals include transdural anastomosis between the cortical surface branches of the middle cerebral artery and the scalp arteries. This disease mainly occurs in the Oriental population, but should be suspected when TIAs or stroke occur in children or young adults. Its etiology is unknown. Few pathologic studies have been made; they suggest that hyalinotic fibrous-type material is associated with the arterial narrowing. Because of the occurrence of subarachnoid hemorrhage from rupture of the transdural anastomotic channels, anticoagulation is to be considered with caution in symptomatic cases. Extracranial/intracranial (EC/IC) bypass grafting has been recommended in some cases, but its efficacy is not established. The craniotomy needed for bypass grafting may disrupt the transdural anastomosis and theoretically could cause worsening of the deficit. In addition, EC/IC bypass grafting could precipitate proximal middle cerebral artery occlusion.

Oral contraceptive agents Oral contraceptive agents have been associated with an increased incidence of stroke in young women (13.2/100,000 among women who take oral contraceptives compared to 2.8/100,000 among those who do not). In most cases, the suspected artery of involvement appears open on angiography; or if it appears occluded, it is found to be open later, a circumstance suggesting embolism as the primary cause of the stroke. The source of the embolus, however, is uncertain. The rare instances of pathologic examination found the affected arteries and the cardiac system normal. Migraine and cigarette smoking have been associated with such strokes in young women and suggest that a hypercoagulable state promotes thrombosis formation and embolization.

Polycythemia, thrombotic thrombocytopenic purpura, idiopathic thrombocytosis, hyperproteinemia, and sickle cell anemia These diseases have been associated with ischemic infarction. Presumably, this is due to thrombosis formation with embolization in patients who because of these diseases have a hypercoagulable state (see Chaps. 279 and 280).

Binswanger's disease Binswanger's disease (*chronic progressive subcortical encephalopathy*) is a rare condition in which the subcortical white matter (sparing the U fibers) becomes infarcted. The CT scan detects areas of periventricular low x-ray absorption. Lipohyalinosis invariably develops in the small arteries of the deep white matter, as it does in hypertension. Binswanger's disease may represent border zone ischemic infarction in the deep white and gray matter between the penetrating arteries of the circle of Willis and of the cortex. Unfortunately, the pathophysiologic basis of the disease, even its basic pathology, remains unknown. It is one of the causes of gait disability and abulia in the elderly.

TABLE 343-2 Causes of cerebral embolism

I Cardiac origin
- *A* Atrial fibrillation and other arrhythmias (with rheumatic, atherosclerotic, hypertensive, or congenital heart disease)
- *B* Myocardial infarction with mural thrombus
- *C* Acute and subacute bacterial endocarditis
- *D* Heart disease without arrhythmia or mural thrombus (mitral stenosis, etc.)
- *E* Complications of cardiac surgery
- *F* Valve prostheses
- *G* Nonbacterial thrombotic (marantic) endocardial vegetations
- *H* Paradoxical embolism with congenital heart disease
- *I* Trichinosis

II Noncardiac origin
- *A* Atherosclerosis of aorta and carotid arteries (mural thrombus, atheromatous material)
- *B* From sites of cerebral artery thrombosis (basilar, vertebral, middle cerebral)
- *C* Thrombus in pulmonary veins
- *D* Fat
- *E* Tumor
- *F* Air
- *G* Complications of neck and thoracic surgery

III Undetermined origin

CEREBRAL EMBOLISM Pathophysiology Cerebral embolism is the most common cause of ischemic stroke; the heart, the most common source of embolic material. Artery-to-artery embolism, usually arising from an atherothrombotic lesion in either the carotid or vertebral-basilar system, occurs somewhat less frequently (see above). Other causes (Table 343-2) (thrombus in the pulmonary vein, fat emboli, tumor emboli, marantic endocarditis, air emboli, paradoxical emboli, and complications of neck or thoracic surgery) occur occasionally. Frequently, however, embolic cerebral infarction occurs without an obvious source.

"Unknown source" cerebral embolism poses one of the most perplexing problems in cerebrovascular disease. Granted, patients with an altered, heightened state of coagulation due to oral contraceptive agents, chronic illness, or metastatic tumor may develop sudden cerebral embolism. Sometimes physical diagnosis may not disclose a cardiac sound such as the opening snap of mitral stenosis or may miss an arrhythmia such as intermittent atrial fibrillation. Nevertheless, many patients, especially those in the second to fifth decade, suffer sudden embolic strokes that leave no clue to their etiology.

The size, site, and to some extent the pathologic nature of the fragment determines the size, location, and character of the ensuing infarct. Emboli large enough to occlude the stem of the middle cerebral artery (2 to 3 mm) lead to a large stroke, one that involves both deep gray and white matter as well as the cortical surface and its underlying white matter. A smaller stroke ensues if the embolus is small enough to occlude a small cortical surface branch or a small penetrating branch arising from the middle cerebral artery stem or basilar artery. Furthermore, embolic material composed of platelet fibrin clot characteristically has a tendency to migrate, lyse, and disperse, accounting for fluctuations in symptoms and, in some cases, complete recovery of the ischemic deficit. The location and size of an infarct also depends on the extent of any spared collateral circulation.

If collateral flow around the circle of Willis or through the other vertebral artery is sufficient, an embolic fragment lodging in the distal internal carotid artery, proximal A1 segment of the anterior cerebral artery, or distal vertebral artery may not result in brain ischemia or infarction. Similarly, emboli may block a cortical surface middle cerebral artery branch—or even the stem of the middle cerebral artery—and lead to no more than patchy infarction in the cortical surface or underlying white matter of the cerebral hemisphere if collateral flow occurs through the cortical surface border zone anastomotic channels from the anterior or posterior cerebral artery to the middle cerebral artery territory. The same holds true for cerebellar infarction. Because emboli migrate and lyse, recirculation into the infarcted brain often occurs. Here, bland infarcted tissue becomes laden with petechial hemorrhages 1 to 2 mm in size (hemorrhagic infarction). On rare occasions, petechial hemorrhages coalesce to form a significant hemorrhagic mass (hemorrhage into infarction). This is more likely to occur when the stem of the middle cerebral artery is occluded, and large areas of deep gray and white matter infarction develop before recirculation occurs. When the heart is the source of an embolus, it lodges in the middle cerebral artery 80 percent of the time, in the posterior cerebral artery 11 percent, and in the vertebral or basilar artery or their branches in the remainder.

Heart disease of many types may produce cerebral emboli. For conceptual purposes, they may be divided into arrhythmic and structural causes.

Cardiac arrhythmias of any type have been associated with symptomatic cerebral and systemic embolism. Of particular concern is the frequency of embolism associated with sick sinus syndrome and atrial fibrillation. The high incidence of cerebral embolism associated with atrial fibrillation in patients with rheumatic valvular disease is firmly established. In this setting it is accepted practice to institute chronic anticoagulation therapy with sodium warfarin to prevent embolic events. Recently it has been documented that patients with atrial fibrillation, of whatever cause, are at increased risk of symptomatic embolization. Indeed, the incidence of cerebral embolism in patients with atrial fibrillation from nonvalvular causes is estimated to approach 4 to 7 percent per year, and in most cases, the initial stroke causes severe disability.

Mural thrombus formation with embolism occurs relatively frequently in patients with arteriosclerotic cardiovascular disease and myocardial infarction, whether or not papillary muscle dysfuntion, congestive heart failure, or a ventricular aneurysm is present.

SURGERY Intracardiac surgery and prosthetic valve surgery have an especially high risk of embolism. (Starr-Edwards and Bjork-Shiley valves have been particularly implicated in cerebral embolism.) Thoracic surgery (pulmonary vein embolism) and head-and-neck surgery (aortic or carotid artery-to-artery emboli) have an uncommon but definite association with cerebral embolism. Long bone fracture and thoracic surgery or angiography are associated with cerebral fat embolism and air embolism, both of which give rise to multiple areas of petechial hemorrhage. The principal complication of the use of artificial hearts is heart-to-brain embolism.

Congenital septal defects may give rise to paradoxical embolism. Material (thrombus, tumor, infective or fibrous marantic vegetation) accumulating on an endocardial surface, either valvular or chamber, may become displaced. Vegetations on the aortic and mitral valves from rheumatic or marantic endorcarditis are associated with systemic or cerebral emboli and can be diagnosed by a combination of history, physical examination, and laboratory tests. Typically flat vegetations under the mitral and, to a lesser extent, aortic valve leaflets have been noted in patients with systemic lupus erythematosus (Libman-Sacks vegetations). These may give rise to cerebral embolism, but more often are a nidus for bacterial endocarditis. The *vegetations of acute and subacute bacterial endocarditis* give rise to septic embolism (see Chap. 188). These emboli can cause large areas of infarction not different from noninfective embolic infarction if they occlude a major intracranial artery. Alternatively, they may be responsible for tiny septic infarcts with microscopic abscesses. Large brain abscesses, however, are not associated with embolization from subacute bacterial endocarditis. Mycotic aneurysms caused by septic embolism give rise to subarachnoid or intracerebral hemorrhage. The diagnosis of endocarditis should always be considered and ruled out when cerebral embolism is suspected.

Atrial myxoma results in tumor emboli arising from the endocardial surface. Here, physical signs of pulmonary hypertension or a high ESR and signs of systemic illness (fever, malaise) may help with the differential diagnosis. *Mitral valve prolapse* with mural thrombus formation has been associated with cerebral embolism, but insufficient data exist on the natural history of this abnormality to predict the incidence of recurrent embolism. It is presumably low. Echocardiography is valuable in establishing this diagnosis.

Clinical syndromes When embolism is the cause, the onset of the neurologic deficit is sudden and most often maximal. But the neurologic deficit may not be complete; and after its sudden onset, it may change significantly. In one instance, the deficit may wax and wane, lasting only a few minutes or hours then disappear, i.e., an embolic TIA. In another instance, a mild deficit may progress to complete major arterial territory infarction. In any case, the nature of the neurologic deficit corresponds to the location of the embolus in a specific territory either of the large extracerebral arteries or of the small penetrating arteries. The resulting deficits resemble those caused by either large vessel or small vessel disease. (See sections on atherothrombosis and lacunar stroke.) Obviously, the size of an embolus determines the size of the vessel it will occlude. Some neurologic syndromes strongly suggest embolism as their mechanism. In the middle cerebral artery territory these include (1) the frontal opercular syndrome, in which the face droops and severe aphasia and dysarthria are present; (2) the brachial or hand plegia syndrome, in which the entire arm and hand, the arm and hand from the elbow down, or just the hand is paralyzed with or without cortical sensory abnormalities, depending on whether the sensory cortex is involved along with the motor cortex; (3) the syndrome of Broca's or Wernicke's aphasia alone, when the dominant hemisphere is involved; or (4) the syndrome of left visual neglect, when the nondominant parietal lobe is involved. A sudden hemianopic field defect fully realized by the patient suggests a posterior cerebral territory embolus, whereas a sudden foot incoordination or weakness suggests an anterior cerebral territory embolus. Sudden gait unsteadiness may suggest a cerebellar embolus. It is more difficult to determine whether an embolus or atherothrombotic or lipohyalinotic occlusion has caused a small vessel stroke. Most often it is one of the latter two. However, sudden sleepiness and an inability to look up, associated with bilateral ptosis, suggest embolus to the top of the basilar artery, specifically to the artery of Percheron (the small vessel supplying both sides of the medial subthalamus and thalamus arising from the top of the basilar artery).

Septic embolism with endocarditis or fat embolism often presents with nonfocal symptoms such as confusion, agitation, or delirium. Cardiac surgery may be associated with a particular neurologic syndrome in which the patient wakes slowly and when awake, thinks slowly, is disoriented, and possibly is agitated and combative. Poor memory is invariable and visual hallucinations are common. Most symptoms resolve within a week, but often a persistent visual perceptive deficit suggests a parietal occipital middle cerebral territory watershed infarct, presumably secondary to hypotension or multiple small emboli.

Seizures following cerebral infarction occur most often after embolic infarction and are not associated with deep white matter lacunar infarction. They are associated with supratentorial cortical surface infarction but never as the heralding event. Many cases of idiopathic epilepsy in the elderly are the result of silent cortical surface chronic infarction that can easily be treated with phenytoin.

Laboratory evaluation Before beginning anticoagulation therapy, a CT scan should be obtained to rule out the possibility of a small lobar hemorrhage masquerading as embolic stroke. Lumbar puncture is not necessary to detect red blood cells, unless dysarthria or clumsy hand syndrome or other posterior fossa syndromes suggest a small (possibly hemorrhagic) pontine infarct. Because of bone artifact, the CT scan may miss an occult hemorrhage masquerading as a small infarct in this area. Proton MRI can distinguish between acute vs. chronic hemorrhage vs. infarction and may be more reliable than CT in the early detection of infarction.

When a definitive diagnosis of cerebral artery embolism and its suspected arterial source is essential for management, cerebral angiography is justified. However, after 24 h, the embolus may have migrated, lysed, or dispersed, and evidence for embolism as the cause of an ischemic stroke becomes inferential. Intravenous digital subtraction angiography does not have adequate resolution to detect cerebral embolism.

Therapy Therapy of patients with embolic cerebral infarction consists of managing the stroke itself, in both the acute and chronic phases, and in prevention of further embolic strokes. When cerebral embolism is suspected, the immediate goal is to keep cerebral perfusion in the ischemic area as adequate as possible. The blood pressure should not be lowered even if hypertension is found unless it is malignant hypertension (see Chap. 196). If the blood pressure is low, raising it is a consideration. Caution is essential, however, for an excessive rise may aggravate edema formation. Once infarction becomes evident, edema seldom becomes problematic until the second or third day but can then remain for up to 10 days. Although there is some suggestion that recirculation in infarcted tissue due to lysis of the embolus contributes to the severity of edema formation, two rules governing the morbidity of the edema associated with cerebral embolism seem to apply. First, in instances of supratentorial embolic infarction, the larger the area of infarct, the more likely that edema formation will become a problem. Emboli that lodge in the middle cerebral artery stem are much more likely to cause symptomatic edema formation that could lead to coma and death from temporal lobe herniation than are emboli that lodge in a branch of the middle cerebral artery. Second, small amounts of edema formation in the cerebellum following embolic infarction, usually in the territory of the posterior inferior cerebellar artery (inferior cerebellum), can lead to an acute increase in intracranial pressure in the posterior fossa. The resulting compression of the brainstem may result in sudden coma and respiratory arrest requiring emergency surgical decompression. Water restriction and agents that raise the osmotic pressure should be considered early in both instances. Intravenous mannitol is most frequently used to raise the serum osmolality to 300 to 310 mosmol per liter; it is given as often as every 2 to 4 h. The acute management of artery-to-artery embolus, in either the carotid or vertebral territory, is discussed above (see Ischemic Cerebrovascular Disease).

The suspicion that fragments of clot from the heart or an unknown source are the embolic material raises the question of anticoagulation. Concern about developing hemorrhagic infarction and, more importantly, hemorrhage into infarction, makes timing of anticoagulation controversial. A conservative argument notes that reembolization seldom occurs in the first few days; therefore, anticoagulation can generally be delayed 3 to 4 days. However, another argument notes that serious hemorrhage into infarction is extremely rare and usually occurs in large infarcts involving the basal ganglia like those produced by middle cerebral stem emboli. Therefore, it may not be prudent to withhold anticoagulation for a few days unless the infarcted territory seems large. Certainly septic embolization contraindicates both immediate and delayed anticoagulation because of the threat of intracerebral or subarachnoid hemorrhage from mycotic aneurysm.

Except for marantic, septic, or tumor (myxoma) embolization, mural thrombus formation causes all cardiac embolization. It may be microscopic in the left atrial appendage, as in the case of atrial fibrillation, or large on the ventricular surface adjacent to an infarcted area, or it may occur in a ventricular aneurysm or on the mitral or aortic valve. Mural thrombus formation and embolization should be treated with chronic anticoagulation until the threat of reembolization is remote. In the setting of an acute myocardial infarction, 6 months of anticoagulation is considered sufficient; in the setting of chronic or intermittent atrial fibrillation, medication should be continued indefinitely. Although now rare, atrial fibrillation associated with rheumatic valvular disease indicates need for chronic lifelong anticoagulation even if embolization has not occurred. Patients with asymptomatic atrial fibrillation due to ischemic or other types of heart disease also have a higher incidence of cerebral embolism than age-matched controls. Here, however, controversy exists as to whether chronic anticoagulation is worth the risk. Most physicians agree that only a randomized, controlled study will settle the issue. When chronic anticoagulation is prescribed in any type of heart disease or cerebral embolism of unknown source, low-dose warfarin therapy is usually recommended. The prothrombin time should be no greater than 1½ times the control, and all of the known contraindications to warfarin therapy apply (see Chap. 281). Finally, there are no reliable guidelines for the duration of anticoagulation therapy for patients with cerebral embolus of unknown source. But if the patient is under 50, anticoagulation for 6 months to 1 year seems appropriate.

INTRACRANIAL HEMORRHAGE

Although there are many causes of intracranial hemorrhage (Table 343-3), four are particularly common: hypertensive and lobar intracerebral hemorrhages, ruptured aneurysm (saccular), and ruptured arteriovenous malformation. Less common are hemorrhage associated with a bleeding disorder and rupture of a mycotic aneurysm. Rare causes include idiopathic brain purpura, brainstem (Duret) hemorrhages associated with brainstem torsion during uncal herniation, and small multifocal hemorrhages associated with hypertensive encephalopathy. These rarely simulate a stroke.

HYPERTENSIVE INTRACEREBRAL HEMORRHAGE Pathophysiology Hypertensive hemorrhage typically occurs in four sites: (1) putamen and adjacent internal capsule, often extending into the central white matter (50 percent of cases), (2) thalamus, (3) pons, and (4) cerebellum. Hypertensive hemorrhage rarely originates in the central white matter. The vessel involved is generally one of the penetrating arteries arising from the middle cerebral artery stem, basilar artery, or circle of Willis, i.e., precisely the vessels involved with segmental lipohyalinosis as a consequence of hypertension.

The hemorrhage begins as a small oval mass, then spreads by dissection, growing in volume, displacing and compressing adjacent brain tissue. In these types of hemorrhage, rupture or seepage into the ventricular system almost always occurs, yet rupture from the white matter through the cortical surface gray matter is very rare. Only when the hemorrhage is small (1 to 2 cm) will it be confined to the central gray and white matter and not gain access to the CSF via the ventricular system. Large hemorrhages may compress the ventricular system and displace midline structures to the opposite side, leading to stupor, coma, and death.

Most hypertensive intracerebral hemorrhages develop in a few minutes, but some evolve over 30 to 60 min, and others, particularly those associated with anticoagulant therapy, evolve for as long as 24 to 48 h. In contrast to ruptured saccular aneurysm, once the bleeding stops, it generally does not start again. However, edema forms in the compressed tissue around the hemorrhage, leading to a greater mass effect and, in some cases, worsening the clinical status. Within 48 h, macrophages begin to phagocytize the hemorrhage at its outer surface. After 1 to 6 months, the hemorrhage mass is generally resolved to a slitlike orange cavity lined with astroglial scar tissue and hemosiderin-laden macrophages.

Clinical syndromes Although hypertensive intracerebral hemorrhage may occur in anyone with hypertension, it is most common in those with sustained essential hypertension. Although not particularly associated with exertion, hypertensive intracerebral hemorrhage almost always occurs while the patient is awake. Unlike the sudden onset of embolism, these strokes evolve over a few minutes with the neurologic signs and symptoms dependent on the site and size of the extravasation.

The most common picture is that associated with a *putaminal hemorrhage,* in which the adjacent internal capsule is damaged. When these hemorrhages are large, the patient lapses within a few moments into a coma with hemiplegia. More often, however, the patient complains of something going awry within the head. In a few minutes the face sags on one side, speech becomes slurred or aphasic, the arm and leg gradually weaken, and the eyes tend to deviate away from the side of the paretic limbs. The history often documents that these events occurred gradually over a period of 5 to 30 min. This type of evolution is strongly suggestive of intracerebral bleeding.

TABLE 343-3 Causes of intracranial hemorrhage

I	Hypertensive intracerebral hemorrhage
II	Lobar hemorrhage of undetermined cause and intracerebral hemorrhage associated with congophilic angiopathy (analyzed)
III	Ruptured saccular aneurysm, giant aneurysm, or mycotic aneurysm
VI	Ruptured angioma
V	Hemorrhagic disorders: leukemia, aplastic anemia, thrombocytopenic purpura, liver disease, complication of anticoagulant therapy, hyperfibrinolysis, hypofibrinogenemia, hemophilia, Christmas disease
VI	Trauma, including posttraumatic apoplexy
VII	Hemorrhage into primary and secondary brain tumor
VIII	Hemorrhagic infarction, arterial or venous
IX	Inflammatory disease of the arteries and veins
X	Miscellaneous rare types: after vasopressor drugs, upon exertion, during arteriography, during painful urologic examination, as a late complication of early life carotid occlusion, complication of carotid-cavernous arteriovenous fistula, with anoxemia, migraine, teratomatous malformations (Acute inclusion body encephalitis produces xanthochromia and up to 2000 red blood cells or more in the cerebrospinal fluid; acute necrotizing hemorrhagic encephalopathy may be associated with up to 100 red blood cells in the cerebrospinal fluid; tularemia and snake venom poisoning may cause bloody cerebrospinal fluid.)

The paralysis worsens until the affected limbs become flaccid. Pinprick is then not appreciated, a Babinski sign appears, speaking becomes impossible (dominant hemisphere), and drowsiness gives way to stupor. In the worst cases, signs of upper brainstem compression appear. Coma ensues accompanied by deep, irregular, or intermittent respiration, a dilated and fixed ipsilateral pupil, bilateral Babinski signs, and decerebrate rigidity. When progressive deterioration occurs 12 to 72 h after the initial deficit, it is due to edema formation in adjacent brain rather than rerupture.

Thalamic hemorrhage of moderate size also produces a hemiplegia or hemiparesis from pressure on or dissection through the adjacent internal capsule. The sensory deficit is prominent and includes hemisensory abnormalities of pain and temperature as well as proprioception and touch. Dysphasia, often with preserved repeating aloud, may be present with lesions of the dominant side and apractagnosia with lesions of the nondominant. A homonymous field defect if present usually clears in a few days. Thalamic hemorrhage by virtue of its extension medially and inferiorly into the subthalamus causes a series of ocular disturbances, including paralysis of vertical gaze, forced deviation of the eyes downward, inequality of pupils with absence of light reaction, skew deviation with the eye opposite the hemorrhage being displaced downward and medially, ipsilateral ptosis and miosis, absence of convergence, an assortment of lateral gaze abnormalities (paresis or pseudoparesis of the sixth nerve), retraction nystagmus, and tucking in of the eyelids. Neck retraction may be present. Hemorrhage into the nondominant thalamus may produce mutism.

In *pontine hemorrhage,* deep coma usually ensues in a few minutes, and the clinical picture includes quadriplegia, prominent decerebrate rigidity, and small (1-mm) pupils that react to light. Reflex horizontal eye movements, evoked by head turning (doll's-head maneuver) or irrigation of the ears with cold water, are impaired (see Chap. 20). Hyperpnea, severe hypertension, and hyperhidrosis are common. Death usually occurs within a few hours, but there are rare exceptions where consciousness is retained and the clinical manifestations indicate a small lesion in the tegmentum of the pons, e.g., disturbances of lateral ocular movements, profound dysarthria, crossed sensory or motor disturbances, small pupils, cranial nerve palsies, and bilateral signs of pyramidal tract involvement.

Cerebellar hemorrhage usually develops over a period of several hours, and loss of consciousness at the onset is rare. Repeated vomiting with inability to walk or stand are the hallmarks of cerebellar hemorrhage. They occur early and must raise suspicion of the diagnosis to allow timely consideration of surgery. Occipital headache and vertigo are also prominent symptoms. There is a paresis of conjugate lateral gaze of the eyes to the side of the hemorrhage, forced deviation of the eyes to the opposite side, or an ipsilateral sixth nerve weakness. In the acute phase there may be little or no evidence of cerebellar disease, and only a minority of cases show nystagmus or cerebellar ataxia of the limbs. Other ocular signs include blepharospasm, involuntary closure of one eye, and skew deviation. Ocular bobbing, generally thought to be a sign of pontine disease, may be noted late when coma is present. Vertical eye movements remain, and small pupils continue to react until very late in the illness. A mild ipsilateral facial weakness and a diminished corneal reflex are common. Dysarthria and dysphagia may be prominent. Contralateral hemiplegia and contralateral facial weakness do not occur. Occasionally at the onset there is a quadriplegia with preservation of consciousness or a spastic paraparesis. The plantar reflexes are flexor early, extensor late. As the hours pass, and occasionally with unanticipated suddenness, the patient becomes stuporous, then comatose as a result of brainstem compression, at which point reversal of the syndrome, even by surgical therapy, is seldom successful.

Ocular signs are important in the localization of intracerebral hemorrhages. In putaminal hemorrhage, the eyes are deviated to the side opposite the paralysis; in thalamic hemorrhage, the eyes are deviated downward and the pupils may be unreactive; in pontine hemorrhage, the reflex lateral eye movements are impaired and the pupils tiny yet reactive; and in cerebellar hemorrhage, the eyes are deviated laterally (to the side opposite the lesion) in the absence of paralysis.

Headache is not an invariable finding associated with hypertensive intracerebral hemorrhage. It occurs in about half of the cases, while vomiting occurs in almost all cases. The patient need not be comatose, and if the hematoma is small, the patient may be fully alert even if the hemorrhage extends into the ventricular system. Seizures are uncommon, occurring in less than 10 percent of cases. In most instances, the correct diagnosis is suggested by the constellation of symptoms and signs. If, however, the patient is fully awake, confusion may exist between ischemic infarct and intracerebral hemorrhage. The CT scan allows precise differentiation and localization, especially with the more difficult small hemorrhages.

Laboratory evaluation The CT scan has revolutionized the diagnosis of intracerebral hemorrhage. It reliably detects all hemorrhages in the cerebral or cerebellar hemispheres of 1 cm or more in diameter if they are studied in the first 2 weeks. Because x-ray attenuation values of clotted blood diminish over time, intracranial hematoma may appear isodense after 2 weeks and may be missed if not associated with surrounding edema or mass effect. In some cases a rim of contrast-enhancing tissue appears after 2 to 4 weeks and may persist for months. Rarely, small pontine hemorrhages may not be identified because of motion and possibly bone artifact. MRI scans may prove more reliable than CT scanning for detecting either small pontine or medullary hematomas or hematomas in which the clot has become isodense. Here, however, precise pulse sequencing is required in order to differentiate acute hematomas, less than 3 days old, from chronic hematomas that are older than 3 days. The development of CT and MRI scanning minimizes the need for lumbar puncture except when a small pontine hemorrhage is in question. Such a hematoma could gain access to the cerebrospinal fluid without being visualized because of CT artifact. Lumbar puncture in a patient with intracerebral hemorrhage involves considerable risk, because it may aggravate temporal lobe herniation if the hematoma is large and located in a supratentorial area. However, when CT and MRI are not available, lumbar puncture may be necessary to establish the diagnosis if specific therapeutic measures are contemplated. When intracerebral hematoma occurs in the temporal lobe and appears near the sylvian cistern, rupture of an aneurysm at the bifurcation of the middle cerebral artery must be considered. Because of that and because temporal lobe swelling around the hematoma could occur and result in temporal lobe herniation, the etiology of the hemorrhage must be documented by angiography. Then, if temporal lobe edema threatens to cause herniation, it can be evacuated with knowledge that an aneurysm is or is not present. Angiography is also indicated if an intracerebral hematoma is not in one of the four classic locations for hypertensive hemorrhage, i.e., putamen, thalamus, pons, or cerebellum. Then surgically treatable arteriovenous malformations (AVM) may be responsible (see below). Angiography cannot completely exclude the possibility until the hematoma has been fully absorbed. A CT scan done without and with contrast may suggest that an AVM is the cause of intracerebral hematoma, but a negative result does not exclude this possibility. MRI may document an AVM once the hematoma resolves, for blood flowing in the malformation does not contribute to the MRI signal. The scan reveals the large vascular channels of an AVM as black. Chest x-ray and electrocardiogram often suggest cardiac hypertrophy secondary to chronic hypertension and provide a clue as to the etiology of the intracerebral hemorrhage.

The size of the hematoma, in many cases, determines the prognosis. Supratentorial hematomas greater than 5 cm in diameter have a guarded prognosis, and infratentorial pontine hematomas greater than 3 cm in size are almost invariably fatal. The formation of edema for up to a week after the intracerebral hemorrhage often worsens the prognosis. However, in intracerebral hematomas, the tissue surrounding the hematoma is displaced and compressed but not necessarily infarcted. Hence, after the resolution of the hematoma, considerable improvement can result, as the tissue regains its function. Careful management of the patient during the critical phase of the cerebral hematoma can lead to considerable recovery.

Therapy Surgical removal of the clot in the acute stage is rarely indicated. However, surgical evacuation of a supratentorial clot may prevent temporal lobe herniation in comatose patients who still have reflex eye movements. Surgical evacuation of acute cerebellar hemorrhage is usually the treatment of choice because it is often lifesaving and offers an excellent prognosis for recovery of function. If patients are alert without focal brainstem signs and if the cerebellar hematoma is small, the physician may elect against acute surgical removal. It must be remembered, however, that deterioration of the clinical state can be rapid. The option for acute surgery must always be available.

Mannitol and other osmotic agents reduce edema around an intracerebral hemorrhage. Steroids are of uncertain value in curtailing edema from intracerebral hematoma. Monitoring of the intracranial pressure may help to assess medical therapy. Both excessive hypo- and hypertension should be avoided. Dramatic reduction in blood pressure to "stop the hemorrhage" is not helpful, because most intracerebral hemorrhages have stopped bleeding by the time the patient is examined. Toxemia of pregnancy and malignant hypertension should be detected early and treated cautiously to avoid excessive or precipitous lowering of the blood pressure.

LOBAR INTRACEREBRAL HEMORRHAGE As control of hypertension in the general population improves, the relative proportion of hemorrhages outside the basal ganglia and thalamus increases. These "lobar hemorrhages" appear on CT scan as oval or circular clots in the subcortical white matter. The role of chronic hypertension in their genesis is controversial, but many occur without a history of increased blood pressure. A number of other underlying conditions are established in almost half the cases. The most common is arteriovenous malformation. Others are bleeding diathesis, often associated with warfarin administration; hemorrhages into tumor, often a melanoma; aneurysms of the circle of Willis that point upward and bleed into brain substance; and a large number whose causes remain undetermined even after extensive study including arteriography.

Among the latter, the most common is *amyloid angiopathy,* which can only be diagnosed at postmortem examination with demonstration that the vessels stain positive with Congo red. Amyloid is deposited in the walls of the cerebral arteries; the angiopathy is unassociated with amyloid deposition elsewhere in the body. The condition seems to account for many lobar hemorrhages among the elderly. Often patients suffer multiple hemorrhages, although months may elapse between occurrences.

Most lobar hemorrhages are small enough to cause a restricted clinical syndrome that simulates an embolus to a vessel supplying one lobe. Larger hemorrhages, associated with stupor or coma, cause larger deficits and affect two or more lobes. Most patients experience focal headaches: occipital hemorrhage afflicts the area around or over the ipsilateral eye; temporal hemorrhage, the area around or anterior to the ipsilateral ear; frontal hemorrhage, the forehead or diffusely in the frontal quadrant; and parietal hemorrhage, the temple region. At the onset, stiff neck or seizures are uncommon, but more than half the patients vomit or are drowsy. The neurologic syndrome appears suddenly, over one to several minutes, not instantaneously as it does in embolus. The clinical syndrome corresponds to the location of the hematoma: the major neurologic deficit of occipital hemorrhage is hemianopsia; of left temporal hemorrhage, aphasia and delirium; of parietal hemorrhage, thalamic-like hemisensory loss; of frontal hemorrhage, arm weakness. The region of hemorrhage adds other but less prominent signs to these.

Treatment depends upon the underlying condition. Angiography should be performed in most cases, but immediate angiography may not reveal a small vascular malformation. If a vascular malformation is still suspected, angiography should be performed again after 2 to 4 months, when the vessels adjacent to the clot may have decompressed. In awake or drowsy patients, surgical evacuation offers little benefit over medical management with fluid restriction, corticosteroids, and small doses of an osmotic agent if necessary. But stuporous or comatose patients not responding rapidly to medical therapy for raised intracranial pressure should have the clot evacuated immediately.

SACCULAR ANEURYSM AND SUBARACHNOID HEMORRHAGE

Rupture of an intracranial saccular aneurysm is the most common cause of subarachnoid hemorrhage. In comparison, rupture of an intracranial arterial mycotic or myxomatous aneurysm is rare. Rupture of an arteriovenous malformation is the second most frequent cause of subarachnoid hemorrhage. Although autopsy studies estimate that 5 percent of the population harbor aneurysms, the incidence of ruptured saccular aneurysms is about 4/100,000 per year. It is a devastating disease; as many as 25 percent of patients die during the first day, and nearly half succumb in the first 3 months. Of those who survive, more than half are left with major neurologic deficits as a result of the initial hemorrhage or of a delayed complication, such as rerupture, symptomatic cerebral vasospasm, or hydrocephalus. More than half of those patients discharged home after neurosurgical treatment of the aneurysm never achieve the quality of life they enjoyed prior to the rupture. Given these alarming figures, it becomes evident that the major therapeutic emphasis should be placed on prevention, i.e., preventing the initial rupture and, if rupture occurs, preventing the direct complications that ensue.

Pathophysiology Saccular aneurysms occur at the bifurcations of the large arteries at the base of the brain and rupture into the subarachnoid space of the basal cisterns (Fig. 343-11). Mycotic aneurysms, on the other hand, occur at distal branch points of the middle, anterior, or posterior cerebral, vertebral, or basilar arteries. They rupture into the subarachnoid space over the cortical surface rather than into the basal cisterns. These differences determine the clinical features of saccular aneurysms, distinguishing them from mycotic aneurysms. The common sites of saccular aneurysms include the junction of the anterior communicating artery with the anterior cerebral artery, the junction of the posterior communicating artery and the internal carotid artery, the bifurcation of the middle cerebral artery, the top of the basilar artery, the junction of the basilar artery and the superior cerebellar artery or the anterior inferior cerebellar artery, or the junction of the vertebral artery and the posterior inferior cerebellar artery (Fig. 343-11). Approximately 85 percent of cases occur in the anterior circulation; 12 to 31 percent have multiple aneurysms; 9 to 19 percent have bilateral identical locations.

As an aneurysm develops, it often displays a neck with a dome. The length of the neck and the size of the dome vary greatly, factors that are important in planning microsurgical obliteration. The internal elastic lamina disappears at the base of the neck. The media thins, and connective tissue replaces smooth muscle cells. At the site of rupture, most often the dome, the wall thins to less than 0.3 mm, and the rent is often no more than 0.5 mm long.

It is not possible to determine which aneurysms are likely to rupture, but limited data suggest that size is an important variable and that those larger than 7 mm may warrant prophylactic microsurgical obliteration.

Clinical symptoms, evolution, and management PRODROMAL SYMPTOMS Prodromal symptoms may betray the location of an unruptured aneurysm and, at times, suggest progressive enlargement. The onset of a third nerve palsy, particularly when associated with pupillary dilation, loss of light reflex, and focal pain above and behind the eye, point to an expanding aneurysm at the junction of the posterior communicating artery and the internal carotid artery. In order for a third nerve palsy to occur, the aneurysm at the origin of the posterior communicating artery has to be 7 mm or greater and be expanding. Hence, prompt consideration of surgery is indicated. Sixth nerve palsy may indicate a cavernous sinus aneurysm, and visual field defects can occur with an expanding supraclinoid carotid

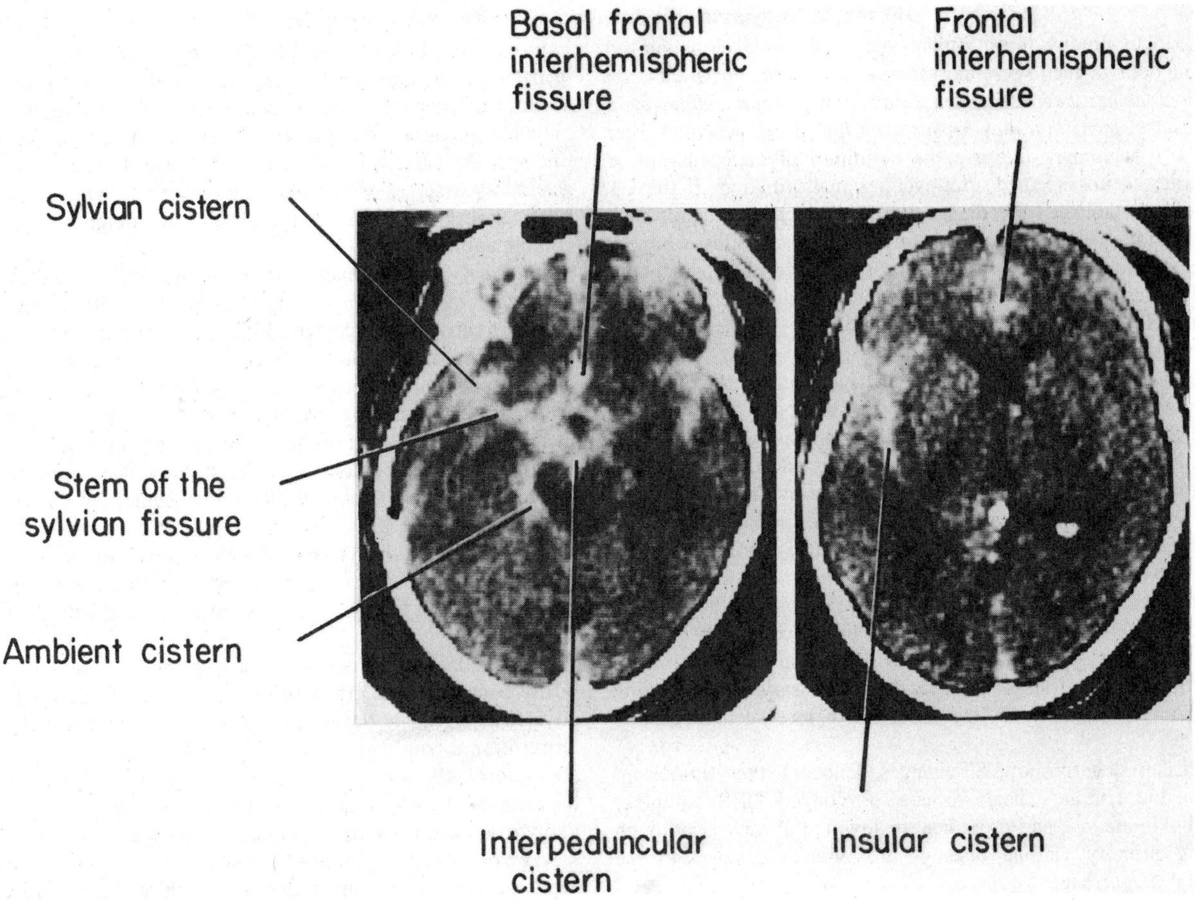

FIGURE 343-11 *Blood in the basal cisterns of the subarachnoid space. The main subarachnoid cisterns and fissures are labeled.*

aneurysm. Occipital and posterior cervical pain may signal a posterior/inferior cerebellar artery (PICA) or anterior/inferior cerebellar artery (AICA) aneurysm. Pain in or behind the eye and in the low temple can occur with an expanding middle cerebral aneurysm.

Whether an aneurysm can cause small, intermittent leakage of blood into the subarachnoid space is an unresolved issue. However, the importance of documenting the clinical correlates of the smallest aneurysmal rupture or leak is undeniable. Sudden unexplained headache at any location should rouse suspicion of subarachnoid hemorrhage and be investigated by a CT scan to look for blood in the basal cisterns. Often a small subarachnoid hemorrhage will not be detected by CT scan, necessitating a lumbar puncture to examine for subarachnoid blood.

INITIAL CLINICAL PRESENTATION: ACUTE MAJOR SUBARACHNOID HEMORRHAGE For the brief moment of aneurysmal rupture, when acute major subarachnoid hemorrhage occurs, intracranial pressure approaches the mean arterial pressure and cerebral perfusion pressure falls. This may account for the sudden transient loss of consciousness which occurs in 45 percent of cases. The sudden loss of consciousness may be preceded by a brief moment of excruciating headache, but most patients first complain of headache upon regaining consciousness. In 10 percent of cases, aneurysmal bleeding may be severe enough to cause loss of consciousness for several days. In about 45 percent of cases, severe headache, usually associated with exertion, but without loss of consciousness, occurs as the presenting complaint. The headache is often called by the patient "the worst headache of my life." Words like "explode" or "burst" may be used. Often it is described as "all over" or "in the back of the head and neck." Whatever the onset, vomiting is a prominent symptom, and vomiting with sudden headache should always raise the question of acute subarachnoid hemorrhage.

Although sudden severe headache in the absence of focal neurologic symptoms is the hallmark of aneurysmal rupture, not infrequently neurologic deficits emerge. Unilateral third nerve palsy strongly suggests a posterior communicating artery aneurysm. Sixth nerve palsy is common but does not have great significance as a localizing sign, although it often corresponds to an infratentorial aneurysmal rupture. Anterior communicating artery aneurysms or a middle cerebral bifurcation aneurysm may rupture into the subdural space or into the basal cisterns of the subarachnoid space and form a clot that is large enough to produce a localized mass effect. The common deficits that result include hemiparesis, aphasia of the dominant hemisphere, anosognosia (hemineglect) of the nondominant hemisphere, memory loss, and abulia. An aneurysm, especially one located at the bifurcation of the middle cerebral artery, may rupture into the sylvian cistern, into the temporal lobe, or up into the frontal and parietal lobes. It may therefore present as a mass and be mistaken for an intracerebral hemorrhage. Cerebral edema often follows, resulting in progressive deterioration, sometimes requiring emergency surgical intervention.

Occasionally, acute unilateral hemispheric swelling and associated focal neurologic signs and stupor occur immediately following aneurysmal rupture. The reasons for such swelling are uncertain. The possibility exists that transient interruption of the cerebral circulation in a given arterial territory occurs, possibly secondary to acute vascular spasm of the stem of the artery. Often there is no adequate explanation for the initial neurologic deficits, and in most cases they gradually improve over a matter of days.

Careful documentation of the initial neurologic deficit, attempting to establish its cause, and closely following its course is of utmost importance for management of the patients and in timing the onset and evolution of delayed neurologic deficit.

INITIAL EVALUATION Over 75 percent of cases exhibit evidence of subarachnoid clot on a noncontrast CT scan if the scan is obtained within the first 48 h after aneurysmal rupture (Fig. 343–11). The extent and location of subarachnoid blood may help locate the aneurysm and identify the cause of the initial neurologic deficit. It may also help predict those patients destined to develop delayed neurologic deficits due to cerebral vasospasm. *A noncontrast CT scan should be done first because contrast may show arterial enhancement in the basal cisterns that may be mistaken for clotted blood.* A later contrast CT scan may improve the definition of an aneurysm or demonstrate an unsuspected arteriovenous malformation. If the CT scan neither establishes the diagnosis of subarachnoid hemorrhage nor demonstrates a mass lesion or obstructive hydrocephalus, a lumbar puncture should be done to establish the presence of subarachnoid blood. The only indication for lumbar puncture prior to CT scanning is if the CT scan is not available at the time of the suspected subarachnoid hemorrhage.

If the diagnosis of subarachnoid hemorrhage from ruptured saccular aneurysm has been firmly established, then angiography is delayed until the time of surgery. Cerebral angiography is usually planned immediately prior to surgery to localize and characterize the anatomy of the aneurysm and to document the presence or absence of focal cerebral vasospasm. If an arteriovenous malformation or mycotic aneurysm is suspected because of the presence of intraparenchymal blood or subarachnoid blood located over the hemisphere rather than in the basal cisterns, then angiography should be done without delay. Another indication for acute angiography is an intracerebral hematoma secondary to aneurysmal rupture which with cerebral edema formation may make emergency surgical evacuation necessary. Documenting the location and anatomy of the aneurysm before such surgery is imperative.

The ECG frequently shows ST changes identical to those associated with ischemic coronary heart disease. Prolonged QRS complex, increased QT interval, and prominent or inverted T waves, although suggesting primary cardiac disease, are often secondary to the intracranial hemorrhage.

Serum electrolytes are obtained because hyponatremia may develop secondary to inappropriate antidiuretic hormone (ADH) secretion with volume expansion or because of unknown factors that cause salt and water loss with subsequent volume depletion.

INITIAL MANAGEMENT Following subarachnoid hemorrhage, a stuporous or comatose patient may have increased intracranial pressure. Care is required to maintain adequate cerebral perfusion pressure while avoiding excessive elevation of mean arterial pressure. Frequent arterial blood-gas determinations are helpful to assess alveolar ventilation. If hypercapnia exists, mechanically assisted ventilation is necessary. If a subdural or intracerebral hematoma mass is causing neurologic deterioration, its surgical removal and, if feasible, obliteration of the aneurysm become more compelling options.

Because of the threat of rebleeding, all patients are put on bed rest in a quiet, preferably darkened room and are given adequate bowel softeners to prevent constipation. Excessive sensory deprivation can lead to agitation, so the patient is permitted to read, listen to the radio, and visit with the family. If headache or neck pain is severe, mild sedation and analgesics are prescribed. Aspirin, an antiplatelet agent, is inappropriate, but acetaminophen or meperidine and phenobarbital or other sedatives may be used. Heavy sedation is avoided because it can obscure the assessment of initial or delayed neurologic deficits.

Seizures are uncommon at the onset of aneurysmal rupture. The quivering, jerking, and extensor posturing that usually accompany loss of consciousness are probably related to the sharp rise in intracranial pressure. However, phenytoin, 300 mg a day, or phenobarbital, 30 mg three times a day, are sometimes given as prophylactic therapy, since a grand mal seizure risks rerupture.

Steroids may help reduce the head-and-neck ache caused by the irritative effect of blood in the subarachnoid space, but there is no evidence to suggest they help in treatment of the cerebral edema that is sometimes seen in patients immediately after a subarachnoid hemorrhage.

DELAYED NEUROLOGIC DEFICITS There are three major causes of delayed neurologic deficits (i.e., those following stabilization or improvement of the initial neurologic symptoms and signs): *rerupture*, *hydrocephalus*, and *cerebral vasospasm*. Recognizing the onset and severity of each of these delayed neurologic deficits depends upon knowing precisely the cause and extent of the initial neurologic findings. An early CT scan (24 to 48 h after the hemorrhage) which accurately assesses ventricular size and the extent and location of subarachnoid blood is invaluable in the diagnosis of the three complications.

Rupture. The incidence of rerupture in the first 3 weeks following subarachnoid hemorrhage ranges from 10 to 30 percent. Because rerupture carries significant morbidity and mortality, numerous clinical investigations of the effects of antifibrinolytic agents have been carried out. Despite their widespread use, evidence of efficacy in preventing rebleeding is conflicting. Moreover, they may be associated with an increased incidence of ischemic stroke presumably from cerebral vasospasm. A prospective randomized study that correlates the extent and location of subarachnoid blood documented by CT scan with the incidence of rerupture and of symptomatic vasospasm is needed. Those patients destined to develop cerebral vasospasm severe enough to cause stroke because of the effect and location of blood in the basal cistern will probably do so whether or not antifibrinolytic agents are used.

Despite lack of evidence that antifibrinolytic therapy is unequivocally beneficial, the effect of rerupture is so devastating that many physicians advocate the use of epsilon aminocaproic acid, administering it as a continuous intravenous infusion of 30 g per day from admission until surgery, but not for longer than 3 weeks. In some of the centers where it is used, it is withheld in those patients who seem likely to develop severe symptomatic vasospasm.

Hydrocephalus. After aneurysmal rupture, communicating hydrocephalus with dilatation of the lateral, third, and fourth ventricles can occur at any time but usually between 4 and 20 days. There is no clinical or laboratory method to predict which patient is in jeopardy of developing hydrocephalus or how severe it might be. However, extensive subarachnoid blood in the ambient and suprasellar cisterns is ominous. Hydrocephalus may cause no detectable neurologic change or may lead to profound stupor developing over minutes to hours. Mild drowsiness, urinary incontinence, and inability to move the eyes above the mid position are associated with early, mild-to-moderate communicating hydrocephalus. Often, hydrocephalus is transient and requires no surgery; but if significant neurologic deterioration occurs, ventricular drainage or ventricular atrial shunting may be required. Knowledge of the precise site and location of the aneurysm is important before inserting a ventricular catheter.

Cerebral vasospasm. It is now clearly established that narrowing of the caliber of the arteries at the base of the brain following subarachnoid hemorrhage from ruptured saccular aneurysm (*cerebral vasospasm*) can lead to cerebral ischemia and infarction (*symptomatic cerebral vasospasm*).

Symptomatic cerebral vasospasm is the major cause of delayed morbidity or death, occurring in approximately 30 percent of patients. Most patients seem to improve or are stable during the period between the aneurysmal rupture and the onset of symptomatic vasospasm. Signs usually appear 4 to 14 days after the initial subarachnoid hemorrhage, peaking at 7 days. The new neurologic deficits are usually recognizable if the initial deficit and clinical course are clearly delineated. The new deficits correspond to ischemia in specific arterial territories, and the severity of vasospasm determines whether cerebral infarction will develop.

Cerebral vasospasm is a focal phenomenon related to the presence of blood in the cerebrospinal fluid, but why it occurs is not known. Laboratory studies have suggested that chemical substances such as serotonin, prostaglandins, and catecholamines can produce arterial narrowing. However, all these compounds break down rapidly in vivo, and only large amounts produce spasm in vitro. More sustained arterial vasospasm has been produced by experiments with incubated whole blood and erythrocyte breakdown products.

Clinical evidence suggests that the extent and location of clotted blood, seen on CT scans, in the basal cisterns and fissures of the subarachnoid space can be used to predict the incidence, location, and severity of cerebral vasospasm in patients after subarachnoid hemorrhage. In these studies, a high incidence of symptomatic cerebral vasospasm was found in patients whose early CT scans showed globular subarachnoid clots larger than 5 × 3 mm in the basal cisterns or layers of blood 1-mm thick or greater in the cerebral fissures. In addition, the location of the clot in the subarachnoid space as seen on CT scan correlated almost perfectly with the location of the spasm in the artery lying in the subarachnoid space. While these studies demonstrated that CT scans reliably predict the location and severity of vasospasm in the anterior and middle cerebral arteries, they provide less precision in the vertebral, basilar, or posterior cerebral arteries. The CT scan cannot reliably detect significant clot in the posterior fossa. Furthermore, for the prediction to be accurate, the CT scan should be obtained between 24 and 96 h following subarachnoid hemorrhage. Blood appearing on CT scan within the first hours following subarachnoid hemorrhage can disappear on a scan obtained after 24 h, presumably because it "washed away." With the further passage of time, x-ray attenuation values of clotted blood diminish so that its full extent and location may not be reliably detected after 96 h.

Because of the close relationship between the location of cerebral vasospasm and clotted blood surrounding the vessel, any hypothesis concerning the mechanism of vasospasm must take into account the prolonged effect of such a clot. The best current hypothesis suggests that a clot encases the artery; then after a few days spasmogenic hemoglobin breakdown products induce spasm. Once the vessel is in spasm, high-energy phosphate metabolism becomes impaired, due to the surrounding clot preventing cerebrospinal fluid from nourishing the vessels. (Vasa vasorum are not present in the vessels at the base of the brain or over the cortical surface.) This insulation may then prevent the artery from relaxing because that requires energy.

CLINICAL SYNDROMES OF SYMPTOMATIC CEREBRAL VASOSPASM Clinically symptomatic severe cerebral vasospasm presents with symptoms referable to the specific arterial territories involved. For example, if the middle cerebral stem or its main branches are involved, contralateral hemiparesis and/or dysphasia (dominant hemisphere) or anosognosia or apractagnosia (nondominant hemisphere) may be present. But even severe vasospasm may not produce ischemic symptoms if sufficient collateral blood flow develops through border zone anastomotic channels (Fig. 343-1*A*). The ischemic symptoms of anterior cerebral territory involvement are an abulic state in which the patient lies quietly awake, eyes either open or closed, responsive to commands but with a delay. Such a patient may offer no spontaneous conversation but answer questions in short, whispered phrases. Food is chewed for a long time and often held between the cheek and the gum. Severe vasospasm of the posterior cerebral artery may produce homonymous field defects. Severe spasm of the basilar or vertebral arteries occasionally produces focal brainstem ischemia. All of these focal neurologic symptoms may develop over a few days or present abruptly, peaking within minutes to an hour.

If the entire middle cerebral artery territory becomes ischemic and infarcted, cerebral edema may ensue and cause a fatal rise in intracranial pressure. An early CT scan predicts this outcome when it demonstrates a large clot in the stem of the sylvian fissure and/or sylvian cistern and a second significant clot in the basal frontal interhemispheric fissure. Simultaneous clots in these areas correlate well with severe symptomatic spasm in the middle and anterior cerebral artery. In this setting, cortical surface collaterals over the cortical surface from the anterior cerebral artery fail to relieve ischemia in the middle cerebral artery territory.

Treatment TREATMENT OF SYMPTOMATIC SEVERE CEREBRAL VASOSPASM Therapeutic efforts to prevent or treat symptomatic cerebral vasospasm have been universally disappointing. Reserpine and kanamycin to reduce serum serotonin levels, isoproterenol or aminophylline to indirectly increase cyclic AMP, or nitroprusside to directly dilate the arteries have all failed.

The failure to find a satisfactory therapy for cerebral vasospasm has prompted a search for prophylactic measures to prevent or minimize its occurrence. In one study, treatment with the calcium channel–blocking agent nemodipine was reported to have beneficial effects, but patients in both the treated and untreated groups developed symptomatic vasospasm. Confirmation of this study and trials of other dilating agents are in progress. Because patients with symptomatic cerebral vasospasm have increased blood volume and many have cerebral edema, the small further rise in intracranial volume occurring with vasodilating agents may be detrimental. Therefore, vasodilating agents are not recommended once severe symptomatic vasospasm has become established.

The commonly accepted form of therapy for symptomatic cerebral vasospasm is to increase the cerebral perfusion pressure by increasing the mean arterial pressure through plasma volume expansion together with judicious use of pressor agents, ordinarily phenylephrine or dopamine. Dopamine is given in dosages of 3 to 6 μg/kg per minute. Therapy to raise the perfusion pressure has been associated with symptomatic improvement in some patients, but high arterial pressure entails the theoretical risk of rebleeding. This therapy requires information about the cerebral perfusion pressure and cardiac output, necessitating direct measurement of the central venous pressure, arterial pressure, and, in severe cases, the intracranial and pulmonary artery wedge pressure.

Severe edema formation in patients with symptomatic cerebral vasospasm may increase the intracranial pressure enough to reduce cerebral perfusion pressure sharply. This requires that the serum osmolality be raised with mannitol while maintaining an adequate intravascular volume and mean arterial pressure: 125 mL of 20% mannitol every 4 h is administered until the plasma osmolality is raised to between 300 to 310 mosmol per liter. As a last resort, barbituate coma has been used to reduce intracranial pressure. Although it is effective in lowering intracranial pressure in some patients, it has not been proven to have significant clinical benefit.

In conclusion, there is no proven, effective therapy for preventing or treating symptomatic cerebral vasospasm following subarachnoid hemorrhage. If further studies demonstrate that the CT scan reliably predicts those patients in jeopardy of developing cerebral vasospasm, early operation to remove the spasmogenic clot as well as the prophylactic use of vasodilators or prostaglandin agonists can be evaluated more accurately.

MEDICAL COMPLICATIONS OF SUBARACHNOID HEMORRHAGE Complications following subarachnoid hemorrhage include thrombophlebitis with pulmonary embolism, perforated stress-induced duodenal ulcer, and ECG changes suggestive of myocardial infarction or ischemia. Subarachnoid hemorrhage causes overactivity of the sympathetic nervous system resulting in focal myofibrillar degeneration of the myocardium. Cardiac arrhythmias can develop. Beta-adrenergic blocking agents are useful but should be given cautiously, especially if an atrioventricular block is present. An additional complication is hyponatremia, occurring either from inappropriate ADH secretion or from secretion of a natriuretic hormone. Restriction of free water, while maintaining adequate intravascular volume, is the recommended treatment.

SURGICAL TREATMENT OF THE ANEURYSM The advent of the operating microscope has made microsurgical obliteration of a ruptured aneurysm a safe and effective means of preventing disastrous rerupture. Most neurosurgeons delay surgery for at least 10 to 14 days. Operation is undertaken when the patient is clinically stable. Delayed surgery allows cerebral swelling from the initial rupture time to resolve, and minimizes the risk of symptomatic vasospasm in the postoperative period.

The wisdom of delaying surgery has been questioned, especially if the patient is neurologically intact. Surgery within the first 48 h eliminates the problem of rebleeding and can remove potentially spasmogenic clots from the basal cisterns, theoretically preventing vasospasm from occurring at that site. While it is technically possible to remove local clots and obliterate aneurysms early, some subarachnoid clots are too extensive for safe, complete removal. The timing of surgery should therefore be tailored to the individual patient. If a CT scan finds no threatening subarachnoid clot or if the location of a potentially dangerous clot permits its safe and effective removal, early surgery may be appropriate.

GIANT ANEURYSMS Giant aneurysms larger than 2 cm in diameter occur at the same sites as small aneurysms. The three most common locations are the intracranial internal carotid, middle cerebral bifurcation, and top of the basilar artery. Although they can rupture, they usually cause symptoms by compressing the brain as they expand. Edema formation in the compressed brain can be relentless and lead to major brain compression and death. This progression is particularly likely if a giant aneurysm occurs at the bifurcation of the middle cerebral artery. Surgical decompression remains the only adequate thereapy, but it is extremely difficult technically and entails a high morbidity in the presence of edema.

MYCOTIC ANEURYSMS When an aneurysm is located distal to the first bifurcation of the arteries of the circle of Willis, a mycotic aneurysm must be suspected. Bacterial endocarditis with embolization should be assumed and appropriate blood cultures taken. Because of their location more distal in the arterial tree (cerebellar hemisphere, cortical surface), they rarely leave significant amounts of clotted blood in the basal cisterns. Severe cerebral vasospasm almost never occurs. Mycotic aneurysms, however, are subject to rerupture. Although antibiotic therapy may decrease the threat of rebleeding, surgical obliteration remains the definitive treatment. It should be undertaken while the patient is receiving antibiotics for presumed or actual bacterial endocarditis.

OTHER CAUSES OF INTRACRANIAL HEMORRHAGE **Arteriovenous malformation** An angioma, or hemangioma, consists of a tangle of abnormal vessels forming an abnormal communication between the arterial and venous systems. In reality, it is an arteriovenous fistula that is a developmental abnormality where the constituent vessels enlarge and grow with the passage of time. Angiomas vary in size from a small blemish a few millimeters in diameter lying in the cortex or white matter to a huge mass of tortuous channels composing an arteriovenous shunt of sufficient magnitude to raise the cardiac output. Hypertrophic dilated arterial "feeders" approach the main lesion, disappear below the cortex, and break up into a network of thin-walled blood vessels which connect directly with draining veins. These often form huge, dilated, pulsating channels, carrying away arterial blood. The blood vessels forming the tangle interposed between arteries and veins are usually abnormally thin and do not have the normal structure of arteries or veins. Angiomas occur in all parts of the brain, brainstem, and spinal cord, but the larger ones are more frequently found in the posterior half of the hemispheres, commonly forming a wedge-shaped lesion extending from the cortex to the ventricular lining.

Angiomas predominate in males over females in a ratio of about 2:1. They may occur in more than one member of a family in the same or successive generations. Although the lesion is present from birth, the onset of complaints is most common between the ages of 10 and 30, but occasionally it is delayed as late as the fifties.

The chief clinical symptoms and signs are headache, seizures, and those associated with rupture or ischemia. When headache occurs, it may be hemicranial and throbbing or diffuse. It may mimic migraine. Occasionally it may be associated with hemiplegia and resemble hemiplegic migraines. Focal seizures that become generalized occur in about 30 percent of cases and are usually well managed with anticonvulsants. In half the cases, arteriovenous malformations herald their onset with intracerebral hemorrhage. In most of these cases, the hemorrhage is intraparenchymal to a greater extent than subarachnoid. Blood is usually not deposited in the basal cistern, and symptomatic cerebral vasospasm in the arteries in the cisterns rarely occurs. The threat of rerupture in the first 3 weeks is low so that there is no need to consider the use of antifibrinolytic agents. The hemorrhage may be massive, leading to death acutely, or may be as small as 1 cm in diameter, leading to minor focal symptoms or no deficit. In either case, the hemorrhage mass may mask the arteriovenous malformation so completely that acute angiography cannot detect it. Hence, when arteriovenous malformation (AVM) is suspected, angiography is best postponed until the hematoma has completely resolved, i.e., after 2 to 4 months. Rarely, the angioma may be large enough to steal blood away from adjacent normal brain tissue, rendering the surrounding brain ischemic. This deprivation is most often seen when large AVMs in the middle cerebral–posterior cerebral system or middle cerebral–anterior cerebral system extend from the cortical surface to the ventricular system. Hydrocephalus may result when the vein of Galen is involved.

Large AVMs of the carotid–middle cerebral system may be associated with a systolic and diastolic bruit heard over the eye, forehead, or neck where a bounding, forceful carotid pulse may be perceived. At the time of rupture, the blood pressure may be normal and should suggest that an AVM, hemorrhage into a brain tumor, or a ruptured saccular aneurysm has occurred. Headache at the onset of AVM rupture is not as prominent or as common as it is with a ruptured saccular aneurysm. Vomiting, on the other hand, is common in any intracranial hemorrhage. Both MRI and contrast CT scan offer the opportunity to detect the channels of an arteriovenous malformation prior to rupture.

Although many AVMs eventually rupture, definitive surgical therapy is usually reserved until after the first rupture; the threat of rerupture is 3 percent per year thereafter. When surgery is not feasible because of the location and size of AVMs, other therapeutic options include artificial embolization and focused proton beam radiation.

Trauma Trauma may result in intracerebral (especially temporal lobe and inferior frontal) hematoma and infratentorial hematomas, subarachnoid bleeding, acute and chronic subdural hematoma formation, and acute epidural hematoma formation. It must be considered in any patient with an unexplained acute neurologic deficit (hemiparesis, stupor, or confusion), particularly if the strokelike deficit occurred in the context of a fall. CT scan and even angiography should be used without hesitation if such a diagnosis is suspected. Surgical intervention in these cases is often lifesaving. The diagnosis should not be missed. These entities and their distinction from spontaneous hemorrhage are discussed more fully in Chap. 344.

Hematologic disorders Intracerebral hemorrhage associated with hematologic disorders (leukemia, aplastic anemia, thrombocytopenic purpura) can occur at any intracranial site and may present as multiple intracerebral hemorrhages. Skin and mucous membrane bleeding is usually evident and offers a diagnostic clue. Intracerebral hemorrhage associated with anticoagulant therapy can occur at any location intracerebrally and may evolve slowly over 24 to 48 h. Fresh frozen plasma should be given immediately. When intracerebral hemorrhage is associated with aspirin, fresh platelet transfusions may be required to stop the oozing.

Brain tumors Hemorrhage into brain tumors may be the first manifestation of neoplasm. Choriocarcinoma, malignant melanoma, renal cell carcinoma, and bronchogenic carcinoma are among the most common metastatic tumors associated with intracerebral hemorrhage. Glioblastoma multiforme in adults and medulloblastoma in children are among the most common primary intracranial tumors that lead to intracerebral hemorrhage.

Other causes Occasionally hemorrhage of unknown origin occurs. This is most often associated with small angiomas or amyloid angiopathy. Primary intraventricular hemorrhage is rare. When it is suspected, it is usually secondary to a hemorrhage that begins intraparenchymally and dissects into the ventricular system immediately without leaving sign of intraparenchymal hemorrhage.

Hemorrhagic encephalitis consists of small petechial hemorrhages through the cerebral white matter. In this setting blood is not found in the spinal fluid, and this condition should not be confused with a stroke. Gram-negative sepsis is generally the cause. Herpes simplex encephalitis may also result in red blood cells in the CSF.

Brainstem hemorrhages occur with temporal lobe herniation when there is torsion of the brainstem. These occur as coma ensues and do not present as a stroke.

Inflammatory disease of the arteries and veins, especially polyarteritis nodosa and lupus erythematosus, can produce hemorrhage into the central nervous system. Most of the time it is associated with hypertension.

Other types of hemorrhage are noted (Table 343-3) and are self-explanatory. Hemorrhages into the spinal cord are usually the result of an arteriovenous malformation or metastatic tumor. Epidural spinal hemorrhage usually compresses the cord rapidly and should be diagnosed without hesitation if surgery is to effect the cure and prevent paraplegia (see Chap. 353).

HYPERTENSIVE ENCEPHALOPATHY (See Chap. 196)

This term refers to an acute syndrome in which severe hypertension is associated with headache, nausea, vomiting, convulsions, confusion, stupor, and coma. Focal or lateralizing neurologic signs, either transitory or lasting, may occur but are infrequent and always suggest some other form of vascular disease (hemorrhage, embolism, or atherosclerotic thrombosis). By the time neurologic manifestations appear, the hypertension has usually reached the malignant state, with retinal hemorrhages, exudates, papilledema (hypertensive retinopathy grade IV), and evidence of renal and cardiac disease. In many, but not all cases, the cerebrospinal fluid pressure and the protein values are both elevated, the latter sometimes to over 100 mg/dL. The hypertension may be essential or due to chronic renal disease, acute glomerulonephritis, acute toxemia of pregnancy, pheochromocytoma, Cushing's syndrome, or ACTH toxicity. Lowering of the blood pressure with hypotensive drugs may reverse the picture in a day or two. If the hypertension cannot be controlled, the outcome is fatal. Neuropathologic examination may reveal a rather normal-looking brain, but usually cerebral swelling and/or hemorrhages of various sizes from massive to petechial will be found. A cerebellar pressure cone reflects increased volume of brain tissue and increased pressure in the posterior fossa, and in some instances lumbar puncture may have precipitated a fatality. Microscopically there are, in addition to small hemorrhages, clusters of microglial cells, minute cerebral infarcts, and necrosis of arterioles.

The term *hypertensive encephalopathy* should be reserved for the above syndrome and not used to refer to chronic recurrent headaches, dizziness, epileptic seizures, recurrent TIAs, or small strokes which often occur in association with high blood pressure.

INFLAMMATORY DISEASES OF BRAIN ARTERIES

Inflammatory diseases of the vessels of the brain have been mentioned on several occasions in the preceding paragraphs, and here they are discussed briefly.

Meningovascular syphilis, formerly one of the most frequent causes of occlusive vascular disease in patients of all ages, has become a rarity since the introduction of penicillin therapy. Tuberculous meningitis, fungal meningitis, and the subacute forms of bacterial meningitis (*Haemophilus,* streptococcal, pneumococcal) may also be accompanied by vascular disorders of the occlusive type, in either the cerebral arteries or veins. Occasionally in tuberculous meningitis, a stroke may be the first clinical sign of meningitis; more often it develops after the meningeal symptoms are established.

Typhus, schistosomiasis mansoni, mucormycosis, malaria, and *trichinosis* are rare types of infective inflammatory diseases of the arteries and, unlike the above, are not secondary to meningeal inflammation. In typhus and other rickettsial diseases, capillary and arteriolar changes and perivascular inflammatory cells are found in the brain, and presumably they underlie the convulsions, acute psychoses, and coma which reflect the central nervous system involvement. They do not cause strokes, however. The internal carotid artery may be occluded in diabetic patients during orbital and cavernous sinus infections with mucormycosis. In trichinosis, the sudden onset of convulsions, aphasia, hemiplegia, and coma may either accompany or, as happens more often, follow the systemic and muscular symptoms. The cause of the cerebral symptoms has not been established. Parasites have been found in the brain; in one case, the cerebral lesions were produced by bland emboli arising in the heart and related to a severe myocarditis. Malaria of the malignant or falciparum variety is frequently attended by a clinical state known as cerebral malaria, in which convulsions, coma, and sometimes focal symptoms appear to be due to blockage of capillaries and precapillaries by masses of parasitized red blood corpuscles.

The *arteritides of obscure origin* include polyarteritis nodosa, disseminated lupus erythematosus, granulomatous arteritis, giant cell arteritis, temporal (cranial) arteritis, and rheumatic arteritis (see above and Chap. 269). In addition, herpes zoster and acquired immunodeficiency syndrome (AIDS) have been associated with cerebral arteritis.

Lupus erythematosus causes cerebral symptoms in over 50 percent of cases. Seizures and psychoses are common. Small cerebral infarcts lead to widespread focal deficits. Accompanying hypertension may precipitate hemorrhage or hypertensive encephalopathy, or endocarditis may cause cerebral embolism.

Thromboangiitis obliterans of cerebral vessels (Winiwarter-Buerger disease) has not been included in the foregoing list. Despite the large volume of literature on the subject, the pathology is so dubious that it does not merit further exposition. All the patients that have been well studied proved to have had either atherosclerosis of the carotid or cerebral arteries with "stasis thrombosis" of more distant cerebral branches. Buerger's disease of the legs has an equally uncertain status.

DIFFERENTIATION OF CEREBROVASCULAR DISEASE FROM OTHER NEUROLOGIC ILLNESSES

It has already been stated that the diagnosis of a vascular lesion rests solely on recognizing the stroke syndrome. Otherwise, the diagnosis always remains in doubt. Three useful criteria in the identification of stroke have already been emphasized: (1) the tempo of the clinical syndrome, (2) evidence of focal brain disease, and (3) the clinical setting. The temporal profile can usually be defined by means of a clear history of premonitory phenomena, the mode of the onset, and the evolution of the neurologic disturbance taken in relation to the medical status at the time of examination. If these data are lacking, the course may still be determined by extending the period of observation for a few more days or weeks. An inadequate history is probably the most frequent cause of diagnostic errors.

Few other neurologic illnesses mimic cerebrovascular disease. When the details of the history are missing, however, subdural hematoma, brain tumor, brain abscess, and senile dementia may lead to diagnostic difficulties.

REFERENCES

AUSMAN JI et al: Vertebrobasilar insufficiency: A review. Arch Neurol 42:803, 1985

BARNETT HJM: Heart in ischemic stroke: A changing emphasis. Neurol Clin 1:291, 1983

BOUGHNER DR, BARNETT HJM: The enigma of the risk of stroke in mitral valve prolapse. Stroke 16:175, 1985

BOUSSER MG et al: "AICLA" controlled trial of aspirin and dipyridamole in the secondary prevention of athero-thrombotic cerebral ischemia. Stroke 14:5, 1983

CANADIAN COOPERATIVE STUDY GROUP: A randomized trial of aspirin and sulfinpyrazone in threatened stroke. N Engl J Med 299:53, 1978

CAPLAN LR: "Top of the basilar" syndrome. Neurology 30:72, 1980

———: Vertebrobasilar disease: Time for a new strategy. Stroke 12:111, 1981

——— et al: Occlusive disease of the middle cerebral artery. Neurology 35:975, 1985

CEREBRAL EMBOLISM STUDY GROUP: Immediate anticoagulation of embolic stroke: Brain hemorrhage and management options. Stroke 15:779, 1984

DUNCAN GW et al: Concomitants of atherosclerotic carotid artery stenosis. Stroke 8:665, 1977
EC/IC BYPASS STUDY GROUP: Failure of extracranial-intracranial arterial bypass to reduce the risk of ischemic stroke: Results of an international randomized trial. N Engl J Med 313:1191, 1985
FISHER CM: Occlusion of the internal carotid artery. Arch Neurol Psychiatry 65:346, 1951
———: Occlusion of the carotid arteries: Further experiences. Arch Neurol Psychiatry 72:187, 1954
——— et al: Lateral medullary infarction: The pattern of vascular occlusion. J Neuropathol Exp Neurol 20:323, 1961
———: The arterial lesions underlying lacunes. Acta Neuropathol (Berl) 12:1, 1969
———: Cerebral ischemia: Less familiar types. Clin Neurosurg 18:267, 1971
———: Clinical syndromes in cerebral thrombosis, hypertensive hemorrhage, and ruptured saccular aneurysm. Clin Neurosurg 22:117, 1975
———: The natural history of carotid occlusion, in *Microneurosurgical Anastomoses for Cerebral Ischemia*, GM Austin (ed). Springfield, Ill, Charles C Thomas, 1976, pp 194–201
——— et al: Atherosclerosis of the carotid and vertebral arteries—extracranial and intracranial. J Neuropathol Exp Neurol 24:455, 1965
——— et al: Cerebral vasospasm with ruptured saccular aneurysm: The clinical manifestations. Neurosurg 1:245, 1977
——— et al: Spontaneous dissection of cervico-cerebral arteries. Can J Neurol Sci 5:9, 1978
——— et al: The correlation of cerebral vasospasm and the amount of subarachnoid blood detected by computerized cranial tomography after ruptured aneurysm. Neurosurg 6:1, 1980
———: Late-life migraine accompaniments as a cause of unexplained transient ischemic attacks. Can J Neurol Sci 7:9, 1980
———: Lacunar strokes and infarcts: A review. Neurology 32:871, 1982
GENTON E et al: Cerebral ischemia: The role of thrombosis and of antithrombotic therapy. Study group on antithrombotic therapy. Stroke 8:150, 1977
HINTON RC et al: Influence of etiology of atrial fibrillation on incidence of systemic embolism. Am J Cardiol 40:509, 1977
——— et al: Symptomatic middle cerebral artery stenosis. Ann Neurol 5:152, 1979
KISTLER JP: Cardiac embolic cerebrovascular disease. Primary Care 6:745, 1979
——— et al: The relation of cerebral vasospasm to the extent and location of subarachnoid blood visualized by CT scan: A prospective study. Neurol 33:424, 1983
——— et al: Vertebral basilar territory stroke. Delineation by proton nuclear magnetic resonance imaging. Stroke 15:417, 1984
——— et al: Therapy of ischemic cerebral vascular disease due to atherothrombosis. N Engl J Med 311:27, 100, 1984
MOHR JP: Valvular disease, cardiac arrest, systemic hypotension, and cardiac surgery, in *Handbook of Clinical Neurology*, GW Bruyn, PJ Vinken (eds). Amsterdam, North-Holland, 1978
——— et al: The Harvard Cooperative Stroke Registry: A prospective registry. Neurology 28:754, 1978
———: Lacunes. Stroke 13:3, 1982
ROPPER AH, DAVIS KR: Lobar cerebral hemorrhages: Acute clinical syndromes in 26 patients. Ann Neurol 8:141, 1980
TOOLE JF, YUSON CP: Transient ischemic attacks with normal arteriograms: Serious or benign prognosis. Ann Neurol 1:100, 1977
WILKINS RH: Natural history of intracranial vascular malformation: A review. Neurosurg 16:421, 1985
WOLF PA et al: Epidemiologic assessment of chronic atrial fibrillation and risk of stroke. Neurol 28:973, 1978
——— et al: Asymptomatic carotid bruit and risk of stroke: The Framingham study. JAMA 245:1442, 1981

344 TRAUMA OF THE HEAD AND SPINAL CORD

ALLAN H. ROPPER

Head injuries are frequent in industrialized countries, affecting many patients in the prime of life. To appreciate the medical and social magnitude of this problem it needs only to be recognized that almost 10 million Americans have head injuries yearly, about 20 percent serious enough to cause brain damage. Among men under 35 years old, accidents, usually motor vehicle collisions, are the chief cause of death, and over 70 percent of these involve head injury. Minor head injuries are so common that almost all physicians encounter patients requiring immediate care or suffering from various sequelae. Traumatic spinal cord injuries often occur in conjunction with head injury. The two are best considered together in the context of trauma to the nervous system.

In the last decade, declining mortality from head and spinal cord injuries can be attributed mainly to public health measures, such as use of seat belts and motorcycle helmets, and the development of ambulance systems with trained personnel. A systematic approach to the evaluation of patients with head and spine trauma, beginning at the scene of the accident, has improved outcome. An understanding of the pathologic lesions produced by trauma is essential for diagnosis and to provide a framework for management.

TYPES OF HEAD INJURIES

SKULL FRACTURES A blow to the skull causes fractures if the elastic tolerance of the bone is exceeded. Significant intracranial lesions accompany two-thirds of skull fractures, and the presence of a skull fracture increases manyfold the chances of an underlying subdural or epidural hematoma. Consequently, fractures assume importance primarily as markers of the site and severity of injury. They also cause cranial nerve injuries and produce entry pathways to the cerebrospinal fluid (CSF) for bacteria (meningitis) and air (pneumocephalus), or for leakage of CSF. Fractures are classified as linear, basilar, compound, or depressed; linear fractures account for 80 percent of all skull fractures and are most often associated with subdural or epidural hematomas. Linear fractures usually extend from the point of impact toward the base of the skull.

Basilar skull fractures are often extensions of adjacent fractures over the convexity of the skull but may occur independently due to stresses on the floor of the middle cranial fossa or occiput. They are usually located parallel to the petrous bone or along the sphenoid bone toward the sella turcica and ethmoidal groove. Most are uncomplicated, but they may cause CSF leak, pneumocephalus, or cavernous-carotid fistula. Fractures of the basal skull bones are often accompanied by signs of hemotympanum (blood behind the tympanic membrane), delayed ecchymosis over the mastoid process (Battle's sign), or periorbital ecchymosis (''racoon sign''). Because routine x-ray examination can fail to disclose basilar fractures, they should be suspected in the presence of these clinical signs. Cerebrospinal fluid may also leak through the cribriform plate or the adjacent sinus and present as a watery discharge from the nose (CSF rhinorrhea). Persistence of rhinorrhea or recurrent meningitis is an indication for a surgical repair of torn dura underlying the fracture. The site of the leak is often difficult to determine, but metrizamide instillation into the CSF with subsequent computerized tomography (CT) scans, or radionuclide or fluorescein injection into the CSF followed by assessment of uptake by absorptive nasal pledgets, are useful diagnostic tests. The site of intermittent leaks is rarely delineated; most resolve spontaneously. Sellar fractures can also be radiologically occult, although they are sometimes associated with serious neuroendocrine dysfunction. Occasionally, fractures of the dorsum sella cause sixth or seventh nerve palsies or optic nerve damage. An air-fluid level in the sphenoid sinus suggests a fracture of the sellar floor.

About 20 percent of petrous bone fractures, usually along the long axis of the bone, are associated with facial palsy. Disruption of ear ossicles and CSF otorrhea are other complications. Transverse petrous fractures are less common, almost always damaging the cochlea or labyrinths and often the facial nerve. External bleeding from the ear can result from petrous bone fractures, though local laceration of the external canal from abrasions is more common. Frontal bone fractures are often depressed, involving the frontal and paranasal sinuses and the orbits; anosmia frequently follows if the olfactory filaments in the cribriform plate are disrupted.

Depressed skull fractures are often compound but are commonly asymptomatic, except for amnesia due to concussions, because the impact energy is dissipated in breaking the bone. Some cause brain contusions and focal neurologic signs appropriate to the underlying cortical area. Surgical repair and bone elevation with exploration of the dura is required in most cases. Delayed or incomplete debridement of the wound leads to a high incidence of infection. If the skin is lacerated over a skull fracture and the underlying meninges are torn, or if the fracture passes through the posterior wall of a nasal sinus, bacteria or air may enter the cranial cavity resulting in meningitis, abscess formation, or pneumocephalus.

CRANIAL NERVE INJURIES Cranial nerves liable to injury with basilar skull fractures are the olfactory, optic, oculomotor, trochlear, and first and second branches of the trigeminal, facial, and auditory. Anosmia and an apparent loss of taste (actually a loss of perception of aromatic flavors, with elementary tastes retained) occurs in approximately 10 percent of serious head injuries, particularly with falls on the back of the head. This results from displacement of the brain and shearing of the olfactory nerve filaments. Recovery is usual with residual hyposmia, but if bilateral anosmia persists for several months, the prognosis is poor. Fractures of the sphenoid bone may bruise or transect the optic nerve, resulting in unilateral partial or complete blindness, and an unreactive pupil usually equal in size to the other side, with a preserved consensual light response. Partial optic nerve injuries from closed trauma result in blurring of vision, central or paracentral scotomas, or sector defects. Recovery of vision varies widely. Direct orbital injury may cause short-lived blurred vision for close objects because of reversible iridoplegia. Oculomotor nerve injury causes the globe to turn outward with loss of adduction and vertical movement and a fixed dilated pupil; vision is preserved. Diplopia only on looking down suggests trochlear nerve damage from fracture of the lesser sphenoid wing. It is not uncommon as an isolated problem from minor injury and may be delayed in appearance for several days. Patients report correction of the diplopia by tilting the head away from the affected eye. Direct facial nerve injury by a basal fracture is present immediately in 3 percent of severe injuries or may also be delayed 5 to 7 days. Petrous fractures, particularly the less common transverse type, are liable to produce this injury. Delayed facial palsy has a good prognosis; its mechanism is not known. Injury to the eighth cranial nerve with fractures of the petrous bone causes loss of hearing, vertigo, and nystagmus immediately after injury; the nystagmus is frequently positional. Deafness due to nerve injury must be distinguished from rupture of the eardrum, blood in the middle ear, or disruption of the ossicles from fracture through the middle ear. A high-tone hearing loss occurs with direct cochlear concussion.

CONCUSSION Concussion refers to an immediate but transient loss of consciousness often described as dazed or "star-struck" and associated with a short period of amnesia. It typically occurs after blunt impact or deceleration of the frontal or occipital areas that creates sudden movement of the brain within the skull. In severe cases autonomic symptoms and signs such as facial pallor, bradycardia, faintness with mild hypotension, or sluggish pupillary reaction may occur, but most patients are neurologically normal. Higher primates are particularly susceptible to concussion; billy goats, rams, and woodpeckers, for example, can tolerate impact velocity and deceleration a hundred times greater than that experienced by humans. The mechanism of loss of consciousness in concussion is believed to be transient electrophysiologic dysfunction of the reticular activating system in the upper midbrain caused by rotation of the cerebral hemispheres on the relatively fixed brainstem. The mechanism of amnesia is not known. Gross and light microscopic changes in the brain are usually absent after concussion, but biochemical and ultrastructural changes such as mitochondrial ATP depletion and local disruption of the blood-brain barrier suggest that complex changes occur. The CT scan is normal, and there are usually no red blood cells in the CSF as occurs with more severe injuries.

Amnesia after concussion typically follows a few moments of unresponsiveness after impact. Rarely there is no loss of consciousness. The memory loss spans the time of, and moments before, mild impact injuries but may encompass previous weeks (rarely months) in more severe trauma. Any anterograde amnesia is usually brief and disappears rapidly in alert patients. The extent of retrograde amnesia has been suggested as a coarse measure of the severity of injury. Improvement usually occurs in an orderly progression from most distant to recent memories, with islands of amnesia occasionally remaining in severe cases. Hysterical posttraumatic amnesia is not uncommon. It should be suspected when abnormalities of behavior occur, such as a tendency to recount events that cannot be recalled on later testing, bizarre affect, a person forgetting his or her own name, disproportionate or selective memory loss, or exaggerated anterograde deficit in comparison to the degree of injury.

CONTUSION, BRAIN HEMORRHAGES, AND SHEARING LESIONS
Hemispheral lesions Contusions on the surface of the brain and deeper hemorrhages result from mechanical forces that move the hemispheres relative to the skull. Deceleration of the brain against the inner skull causes contusions, either under a point of impact (coup lesion) or in the antipolar area (contrecoup lesion). Trauma sufficient to cause prolonged unconsciousness beyond concussion usually produces contusions varying from small superficial cortical petechiae to hemorrhagic and necrotic destruction of large portions of a hemisphere. Because the motion of the hemispheres brings them into contact with the prominences of the sphenoid and other frontal basal bones, blunt impact, as from an automobile dashboard, typically causes contusions on the orbital surfaces of the frontal lobes and the anterior and basal portions of the temporal lobes. The anterior corpus callosum may also be bruised from striking the falx. With lateral forces, as from the doorframe of a car, contusions occur on the convexity of the hemispheres.

Contusions are visible on CT scan, appearing early as smudged hyperlucencies from scattered cortical and subcortical blood and a mass that distorts adjacent structures, most prominently the lateral ventricles (Fig. 344-1*C*). After several hours the surrounding edematous tissue appears as a ring of lower density. Confluent, roughly spherical contusions can be distinguished from spontaneous cerebral hemorrhages because the former characteristically extend to the cortical surface. After a week some contusions have a surrounding ringlike contrast-enhancing density that may be mistaken for tumor or abscess. Glial and macrophage reactions begin within 2 days, years later resulting in scarred hemosiderin-stained depressions on the surface (*plaques jaune*) that are one source of posttraumatic epilepsy. Large single hemorrhages after minor trauma are found in patients with a bleeding diathesis or in the elderly, sometimes related to cerebrovascular amyloidosis.

The clinical signs produced by contusions vary with their location and size; most often a hemiparesis or gaze preference is seen, similar to a middle cerebral artery stroke. Bilateral large contusions produce coma with extensor posturing; when contusions are limited to the frontal lobes, an abulic-taciturn state or inappropriate jocularity and indifference occur. Contusions of the temporal lobes cause an aggressive combative syndrome, described below. With large contusions the secondary effect of progressive edema is the most threatening aspect of the injury. Coma and signs of secondary brainstem compression (pupillary enlargement) then dominate the examination. Seizures soon after trauma are rare with contusions, as indeed they are for several weeks after most acute head injuries.

Deep hemorrhages in the central white matter may result from confluent contusions in the depths of a sulcus. However, ganglionic, diencephalic, and other deep hematomas due to torsion or shearing forces in the brain often occur independently of surface damage. The areas around these hematomas may become edematous, resulting in enlargement of the affected region and progressively raised intracranial pressure.

Another type of white matter, or "shearing," lesion consists pathologically of widespread acute disruption of axons. Axonal shearing occurs at, or soon after, impact. The affected areas of white matter are replaced with glial proliferation over a period of several months. There are characteristically small areas of tissue disruption in the corpus callosum and dorsolateral pons. Widespread axonal shearing lesions in the deep white matter of both hemispheres may explain persistent coma or vegetative state, but hemorrhages in the midbrain and diencephalon are as often the cause. Shearing lesions are not usually visualized by CT scanning, but in severe cases small hemorrhages of the corpus callosum and centrum semiovale are seen.

On occasion head trauma causes diffuse brain swelling within a few hours after injury. Most instances are due to widespread contusion though CT scanning fails to reveal significant focal lesions or hemorrhage. The edema creates a mass effect with disastrous consequences. This problem is encountered in children and young adults who may develop a virtually instantaneous generalized edema probably due to microvascular disruption, hypertension, and greatly increased cerebral blood flow.

Deep cerebral hemorrhages may occur several days after severe injury. Sudden neurologic deterioration, often in already comatose patients, or a sustained and unexplained rise in intracranial pressure should prompt a CT scan to detect delayed hemorrhage.

Brainstem hemorrhages A syndrome with coma, midposition or larger pupils unreactive to light, and impaired or absent oculocephalic reflex eye movements results from small linear or oval-shaped hemorrhages in the high midbrain, visible on CT scan, though often delayed in appearance. Though extensor posturing occurs with stimulation, the limbs are otherwise flaccid. This clinical syndrome should be suspected even in the initial absence of a hemorrhage on CT scan. These acute midbrain hemorrhages may be the result of primary injury from rotational forces in the upper midbrain. They also occur from secondary compression of the brainstem by supratentorial hematomas and lateral tissue shifts or pressure from the adjacent temporal lobes. In pathologic material from severe, acutely fatal injuries, small linear and oval hemorrhages are found in the low thalamic and subthalamic regions and throughout the midline of the brainstem (termed *Duret hemorrhages*).

Residual symptoms and signs of primary or secondary brainstem hemorrhages or ischemic lesions include tremor, pupillary enlargement, eye movement abnormalities, or the "locked-in" syndrome (see Chap. 21). Midbrain or diencephalic hemorrhages are the only well-defined traumatic brainstem lesions responsible for coma. Most other cases of coma without fixed pupils and unexplained by CT scan are probably due to diffuse axonal shearing injuries in the cerebral hemispheres.

SUBDURAL AND EPIDURAL HEMATOMAS In severe head injury, hemorrhages beneath the dura (subdural) or between the dura and skull (epidural) may be combined with contusions and other injuries, making it difficult to determine their relative contribution to the clinical state. However, subdural and epidural hematomas often occur as the primary lesion, each with a characteristic clinical and CT scan appearance. Because the mass effect of the hemorrhage and rise in intracranial pressure may be life-threatening, it is important to make an immediate diagnosis and carry out surgical evacuation.

Acute subdural hematoma Acute subdural hematomas become symptomatic in minutes to hours after injury. Up to one-third of patients have a lucid interval before coma supervenes, but the majority are drowsy or comatose from the moment of injury. Arousable patients complain of unilateral headache and frequently have a slightly enlarged pupil on that side. Stupor or coma with unilateral pupillary enlargement are the major signs in larger hematomas. Pupillary dilation is ipsilateral in most, but 5 to 10 percent are contralateral to the hematoma. Lateralizing signs such as a hemiparesis are helpful in only a few patients and may be ipsilateral to the clot. Acute seizures or isolated hemianopsias are uncommon. The CT scan shows the clot, allowing early evacuation (Fig. 344–1*A*). Angiography with oblique projections can also outline subdural hematomas and has been used if CT scanning is unavailable. In an acutely deteriorating patient with rapidly diminishing alertness and pupillary enlargement, burr holes or an emergency craniotomy are appropriate without prior radiographic confirmation of subdural hematoma. A subacute syndrome is seen in alcoholics and in the elderly, with drowsiness, headache, confusion, or mild hemiparesis occurring days to 2 weeks after injury.

FIGURE 344-1 *Computerized tomographic (CT) scans from patients with head trauma. A. Acute subdural hematomas with compression of adjacent brain tissue. B. Chronic subdural hematoma, less dense than brain tissue. C. Contusion–traumatic hemorrhage of the frontal and parietal lobes. D. Epidural hematoma in relation to a fracture and tearing of the middle meningeal artery. The lenticular shape of the hemorrhage is typical. E. Skull fractures in the path of a bullet trajectory. By manipulating the windows on the CT scan, fractures and radiodense objects are shown to advantage and appear similar to plain radiographs.*

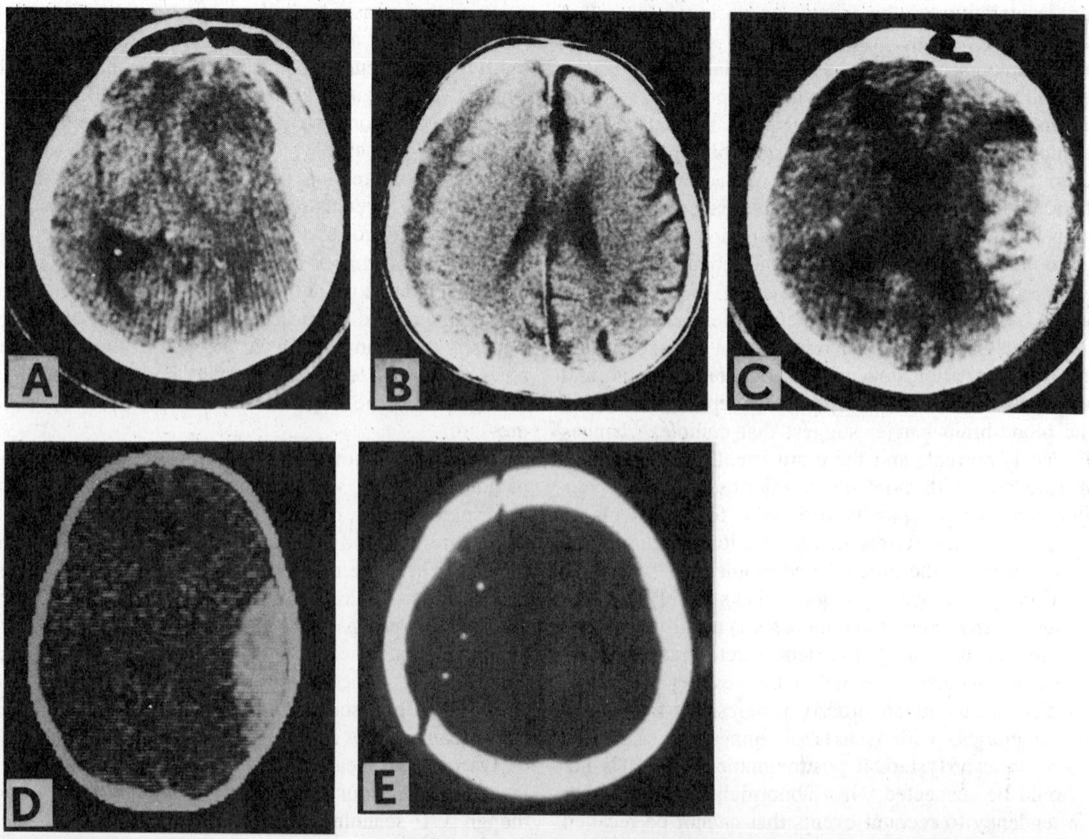

Direct trauma or surface contusions are not required for the formation of acute subdural hemorrhage; acceleration forces alone, as from whiplash, are adequate especially in the elderly. Most subdural hematomas are small crescentic collections over the hemispheral convexity, adjacent to variable degrees of surface hemorrhagic contusions. Larger clots are thought to be primarily venous in origin, though additional arterial bleeding sites are often found, and some appear to be exclusively arterial when explored surgically. Most are located over the frontotemporal region, less often in the inferior middle fossa or over the occipital poles. Less common instances of interhemispheric, posterior fossa, or bilateral convexity clots are difficult to diagnose clinically, although drowsiness and the signs expected for each region can be detected. Small subdural hematomas may be asymptomatic and usually do not require therapy.

Acute epidural hematoma Epidural hematomas evolve more rapidly and therefore can be more treacherous. They occur in 1 to 3 percent of all head injuries and in up to 10 percent of severe ones. They are less often associated with underlying cortical damage than subdural hematomas. The majority of patients are unconscious when first seen, often with associated injuries of subdural clot and contusion. A "lucid interval" of several minutes to hours before coma supervenes is said to be most characteristic of epidural hemorrhage, though it is not common and by no means the only cause of this temporal profile. The findings of drowsiness progressing to coma, pupillary enlargement, and focal hemispheral signs are similar in some respects to subdural hematoma, but occur more rapidly.

The location of epidural hematomas is explained by their origin from torn dural vessels, most commonly the middle meningeal artery. Epidural clots therefore overlie the lateral temporal convexity. The majority of patients have fractures of the squamous portion of the temporal bone, through the path of the torn vessel. Frontal, inferior temporal, or occipitoparietal epidural hematomas are less frequent, occurring when fractures disrupt branches of the middle meningeal artery. Dural laceration over the sagittal or lateral sinuses or rupture of small diploic veins can rarely cause venous epidural hemorrhages. Epidural hematomas strip the tightly attached dura from the inner table of the skull, producing a characteristic lenticular-shaped clot on CT scan (Fig. 344–1*D*). They may be relatively less frequent in the elderly because of the tighter attachment of dura to skull that occurs with aging. Posterior fossa epidural hematomas are rare and difficult to detect clinically; most result from surgery such as resection of an acoustic neuroma.

Chronic subdural hematoma In chronic subdural hematoma, a preceding traumatic cause is less often clear; 20 to 30 percent of patients fail to give a history of injury. Elderly patients or those with a bleeding diathesis seemingly form clots spontaneously. The causative injury may be trivial (striking the head against the branch of a tree, a sudden stop in a car with lurching forward, or striking the head during a fall or faint) and is often forgotten because it was remote in time. A period of weeks, or even months, follows when headaches (common but not invariable), slowed thinking, confusion, changes in personality, seizures, or a mild hemiparesis are the main findings. Fluctuation in the severity of the headache is typical, often with positional changes. Many chronic subdural hematomas are bilateral and give particularly misleading clinical syndromes. The initial clinical impression is often a stroke, brain tumor, drug intoxication, or a depressive, senile, or other type of dementia, the latter because disturbances of consciousness (drowsiness, inattentiveness, incoherence of thought) are more prominent than focal or lateralizing signs such as hemiparesis. Hemianesthesia or hemianopsia are seldom observed, probably because the anatomic structures subserving these functions are deep and not easily compressed. The diagnosis should be considered in dementias of apparently rapid onset, particularly if headache is present. The condition does not always progress. When it does, the patient may become comatose with fluctuations of alertness and pupillary dilation as occurs in acute subdural hematoma. Acute bleeding is superimposed on the chronic hematoma in these cases. Occasionally patients present with "spells" of hemiparesis or aphasia typically lasting more than 10 min, indistinguishable from transient ischemic attack. Patients with undetected small bilateral subdural hematoma seem to tolerate surgery, anesthesia, and nervous system depressive drugs poorly, often remaining drowsy or confused for long periods postoperatively.

Skull x-rays are usually normal except for a shift of a calcified pineal body to one side or an occasional unexpected fracture. The CT scan without contrast infusion typically shows a low-density mass over the convexity of the hemisphere (Fig. 344-1*B*), but may show only a shift of the midline structures and compression of the lateral ventricles because the clot becomes isodense to adjacent brain after 2 to 6 weeks. Bilateral chronic hematomas are often missed because of the absence of lateral tissue shifts. A "hypernormal" CT scan with absent cortical sulci and small ventricles in an older patient should suggest the diagnosis of bilateral isodense hematomas. Contrast infusion demonstrates the chronic fibrous capsule in some cases. Radionuclide brain scans with anterior projections are often the most successful method of confirming the diagnosis. The CSF may be clear, bloody, or xanthochromic, depending on the presence or absence of recent or old contusion and subarachnoid hemorrhage, and the pressure is usually elevated. However, lumbar puncture is not recommended for diagnosis because of risk of worsening tissue shifts. Chronic subdural hematomas can gradually expand, and then behave clinically like a tumor. Treatment with corticosteroids alone is sufficient in some cases, but surgical evacuation is most often successful. Fibrous membranes (pseudomembranes) grow from the dura and encapsulate the region. Craniotomy and removal of the membranes is required if there is recurrent fluid accumulation. Small hematomas are largely resorbed, and only the organizing membranes remain, becoming calcified after many years.

PENETRATING INJURIES, COMPRESSIONS, AND LACERATIONS Tangential scalp wounds from bullets can produce neurologic signs or delayed seizures due to small hemorrhages or contusions, even in the absence of missile penetration. Bullets entering the brain cause considerable damage because of tremendous kinetic energy. A cylindrical area of necrosis surrounds the bullet track. Injuries differ with varying projectiles; soft civilian bullets typically shatter on impact and leave a track of metallic fragments with disporportionately less parenchymal damage (Fig. 344-1*E*). Military bullets, because of high velocity and energy, disrupt tissue at great distances from the track and produce massive brain destruction.

Penetrating bullet injuries cause a rapid increase in intracranial pressure for several minutes followed by a drop depending on the volume of secondary hemorrhage and the degree of developing edema. Infection is a risk mainly from shell fragments, shrapnel, grenades, and mines, because such small projectiles carry surface bacteria and dirt into the brain. Nevertheless, most neurosurgeons administer systemic antibiotics prophylactically and perform local debridement in all types of penetrating injuries. Traumatic aneurysms can form due to disruption of vessel walls from the shock wave of the projectile; facial-orbital entrance wounds have the highest incidence. The aneurysms have an unpredictable course; most that rupture do so in the first month. The prognosis for survival after missile injuries is good if consciousness is preserved and poor if coma is present from the outset.

Other intracranial foreign bodies from knives, picks, studguns, or high-speed tool bits may be missed unless skull x-rays are taken after minor penetrating injuries. Surgical removal, debridement, and extensive exploration for hemorrhage and necrotic tissue is required. Simply removing a protruding object is not sufficient.

TRAUMATIC VASCULAR OCCLUSION AND DISSECTION Minor, sometimes unnoticed, neck trauma can produce dissection (stripping of the intima or the media) of the internal carotid or vertebral arteries. Chiropractic neck manipulation accounts for some cases. Severe blunt trauma to the neck can initiate a dissection several centimeters above the origin of the internal carotid artery. In awake patients there is usually local neck pain over the internal carotid artery, a Horner's syndrome, and headache over the ipsilateral anterior cranium. Some patients with carotid dissection subsequently have large middle cerebral artery strokes with hemiplegia, visual field and sensory deficits, and if the dominant hemisphere is affected, aphasia. In drowsy or comatose patients evidence of dissection or subsequent stroke is difficult to discern but is suggested by unexplained hemiplegia, unilateral miosis, or the appearance of cerebral infarction on CT scan. Angiography demonstrates either the typical "string sign" characterized by an elongated narrowed lumen extending over 5 to 10 cm, or complete occlusion of the carotid artery beginning several centimeters distal to the bifurcation, sometimes accompanied by a distal embolus in the middle cerebral artery. On rare occasion, basilar skull fractures cause carotid dissection beginning at the point of entry of the artery into the skull. Traumatic "false" aneurysms of the cervical carotid artery result from deep penetrating, and occasionally from nonpenetrating, blunt trauma of the neck. A pulsatile mass and bruit over the artery establish the diagnosis and mandate surgical repair. Traumatic vertebral artery dissection can produce vertigo, vomiting, suboccipital or supraorbital headache, and other signs of lateral medullary ischemia. These symptoms are frequently attributed to vestibular concussion. In drowsy or comatose patients the only indication of vertebral artery occlusion may be inferior cerebellar infarction on CT scan.

Intracranial vascular damage is rare except in penetrating injuries. High-velocity projectiles, as discussed above, disrupt vessel walls, leading to aneurysms of large vessels in the vicinity of the wound, usually a surface branch of the middle cerebral artery. Preexisting saccular aneurysms may rupture after basilar skull fractures, and this diagnosis should be considered if subarachnoid hemorrhage is profuse and inadequately explained by accompanying subdural blood on CT scan. Vasospasm from traumatic subarachnoid blood may be involved in the development of infarction after head injury.

Cavernous sinus arteriovenous fistulas are serious complications in patients surviving severe head injury. They are first evident as a self-audible bruit (many are also audible to the examiner), proptosis, conjunctival injection, or visual impairment. Angiography shows early filling of the cavernous sinus and its draining tributaries. The fistula generally enlarges, causing increasingly severe local changes around the eye and orbit and decreased chances of visual recovery. About 10 percent, mostly small fistulas, resolve spontaneously. Many surgical approaches have been tried including ligation of the carotid artery, direct obliteration of the fistula or cavernous sinus, and angiographic guided balloon embolization. A detachable balloon technique has proved successful in many cases. The inability to tolerate therapeutic carotid occlusion (because of an incomplete circle of Willis) can be remedied by a superficial temporal artery to middle cerebral artery anastomosis performed prior to correcting the fistula.

INTRACRANIAL PRESSURE AND CEREBRAL BLOOD FLOW

The pathophysiology of intracranial pressure (ICP) regulation and its relationship to cerebral blood flow (CBF), which is applicable to many pathologic processes including cerebral hemorrhage, encephalitis, and brain edema after stroke, is best understood in the context of head trauma. The components of the intracranial compartment are brain, CSF, and blood. Because the skull limits total intracranial content, the volume of these compartments is compromised by expanding lesions within the cranial cavity. The brain is virtually incompressible; therefore CSF and blood serve as the main buffers of increasing intracranial volume. The relationship between increments in intracranial volume and the associated rises in ICP, termed *compliance,* approximates an exponential function after the volume buffering capacity of CSF and blood are exceeded. ICP is normally between 2 and 12 torr. Raised ICP in the range 15 to 40 torr, while not harmful by itself, can rapidly result in secondary damage, either by precipitously decreasing global cerebral perfusion when ICP exceeds blood pressure in the cranium, or by associated shifts of brain tissue that damage the thalamus and brainstem. The global damage from increased ICP is therefore ischemic in nature and related to the arithmetic difference between ICP and blood pressure in the major cerebral arteries. This difference is termed *cerebral perfusion pressure,* or CPP. Cerebral perfusion pressure below 40 to 60 torr is considered detrimental to nerve cells; therapy is therefore directed toward maintaining perfusion above this range. The rationale for keeping CPP even higher (i.e., bringing ICP below 15 to 20 torr) is to afford a margin of safety should transient increases in ICP occur. Physiologic changes or medications that increase blood pressure do not necessarily improve CPP because increased vascular pressures exacerbate brain edema in damaged areas and induce plateau waves (see below), resulting in further increases in ICP that ultimately lower perfusion.

The most important secondary complication of head injury is raised intracranial pressure arising from the added volume of contusions, hematomas, and the progressive edema surrounding them. A close relationship exists between clinical outcome and ICP in patients with closed head injury. At least 50 percent of patients who die as a result of head injury do so solely because of uncontrolled rises in ICP, and outcome is inversely related to the level of ICP after acute injury. Aggressive treatment of raised ICP in modern intensive care units is believed by many workers to improve survival after severe head injury. The role of direct monitoring of ICP to guide therapy is controversial.

Resting ICP, CPP, and compliance are spontaneously interrupted by rises in ICP termed *plateau waves.* They often are precipitated by iatrogenic maneuvers such as suctioning, physical therapy, excess fluid administration, or pain. Such plateau waves (lasting 1 to 10 min, and ranging from 25 to 60 torr) are most pronounced in patients with diminished intracranial compliance. They are best observed on continuous recordings of ICP. Plateau waves are probably due to a loss of cerebrovascular tone with a resultant increase in cerebral blood volume. Signs of apparent transtentorial herniation such as pupillary enlargement may occur after plateau waves (they more often do not), and occasionally brain death ensues. The proximate cause of deterioration is probably a reflex rise in blood pressure, part of the Cushing reflex (hypertension and bradycardia), greatly increasing intracranial blood volume and cerebral edema.

There is little consensus about the importance of alterations in cerebral blood flow caused by head injury. For several minutes to an hour after acute head injury, cerebral blood flow may increase in some patients although metabolic demands and oxygen consumption are diminished. Autoregulation, the ability of the cerebral vasculature to keep blood flow constant in response to decreased or increased perfusion pressure, is also impaired in damaged regions. The increased cerebral blood flow enhances already increased ICP by raising blood volume. The blood-brain barrier also becomes more permeable after head injury and may disappear in badly damaged regions, making edema formation more likely.

There is a complex relationship between raised ICP and clinical signs such as coma and pupillary enlargement that accompany supratentorial masses. ICP represents the accommodation of intracranial contents to additional mass; clinical signs are a parallel barometer of tissue shifts, particularly affecting structures around the tentorial opening. Raised ICP per se does not cause signs (including coma) until it reaches levels that preclude cerebral perfusion; it then causes global ischemia in a fashion similar to acute hypotension. Coma and other secondary signs resulting from tissue shifts in the region of the tentorial opening are described in Chap. 21. It has been our experience that horizontal midline shift at the level of the pineal body is most closely related to the level of consciousness with acute lesions.

Other secondary phenomena after severe head injury cause brain damage and alter outcome. Hypoxia, for example, is common from a number of causes, and when severe, is associated with a poorer outcome.

CLINICAL SYNDROMES AND TREATMENT OF HEAD INJURY

MINOR INJURY A fully alert and attentive patient presenting after head injury with one or more symptoms of headache, faintness, nausea, a single episode of emesis, difficulty with concentration, or slight blurring of vision has a good prognosis with little risk of subsequent deterioration. Focal signs of brain injury are absent. Such patients have sustained a concussion or have been dazed, and have a brief amnestic epoch surrounding the moment of impact. Occasionally vasovagal syncope occurs several minutes to an hour after the injury and causes concern. Constant generalized or frontal headache is common in the days following trauma; it is often throbbing or hemicranial in nature, like migraine. The majority of patients with a minor syndrome do not have a skull fracture on skull x-ray, or hemorrhage on CT scan. The decision to obtain these tests depends largely on the availability of CT scanning and clinical signs suggesting that the impact was severe (e.g., prolonged concussion, periorbital or mastoid hematoma, repeated vomiting, etc). Children and young adults are particularly prone to drowsiness, vomiting, and irritability, sometimes delayed for several hours after apparently minor injuries. After a period of observation for an hour or so, arrangements may be made for the patient to be accompanied home to be observed by family or friends.

Persistent severe headache and repeated vomiting in the context of normal alertness and no focal neurologic signs are usually benign, but CT scanning and/or skull x-rays should be obtained. Skull fractures increase the likelihood of a subdural or epidural hematoma. Patients with these exaggerated signs, even if they follow minor injury, deserve observation in the hospital for 24 h. Clinical judgment, the presence of associated noncranial injuries, the availability of others at home, and the examiner's certainty of a normal neurologic examination should guide the need for further surveillance.

INJURY OF INTERMEDIATE SEVERITY Patients who are not comatose but who have persistent confusion, behavioral changes, less than normal alertness, extreme dizziness, or focal neurologic signs such as hemiparesis should be admitted to the hospital and have a CT scan. The clinical syndromes most common in this group, in addition to postconcussive headache and dizziness, unsteadiness, photophobia, and vomiting of minor injury, include (1) delirium with a disinclination to be examined or moved, expletive speech, and resistance if disturbed, most often associated with anterior temporal lobe contusions; (2) a quiet, disinterested, slowed mental state (abulia) with dull facial appearance and slight irascibility if bothered, the patient lying quietly with eyes closed when undisturbed, sometimes with inappropriate jocularity (*witzelsucht*), seen with inferior and frontopolar frontal contusions (usually without grasp responses); (3) severe memory loss with poor retrograde and anterograde performance, headache, and photophobia, with medial temporal lobe contusions or diffuse injury; (4) a focal deficit such as aphasia or mild hemiparesis (hemianopsia is rare as an isolated posttraumatic finding), suggesting subdural hematoma or convexity contusion; (5) global confusion with inattention, poor performance on simple mental tasks, fluctuating or slightly erroneous orientation, associated with several types of injuries including the first two described above as well as medial frontal contusions and interhemispheric subdural hematoma; (6) repetitive vomiting, nystagmus, drowsiness, and unsteadiness, usually from a labyrinthine concussion but occasionally due to a posterior fossa subdural hematoma or vertebral artery dissection; (7) drowsiness alone or with muteness, often unassociated with significant CT scan abnormalities; and (8) diabetes insipidus with or without a frontal-temporal lobe syndrome, from damage to median eminence or pituitary stalk and adjacent medial cortex.

The syndromes of intermediate severity are usually preceded by brief loss of consciousness and many are associated with skull fractures. A CT scan is required to exclude surgically remediable subdural or epidural hematomas and to define areas of contusion that later enlarge with edema, or coalesce to form intraparenchymal hemorrhages. Paroxysmal or rhythmic EEG abnormalities, in contrast to acute convulsions, are common over the region of a large contusion. Many intermediate injuries are complicated by drug or alcohol intoxication making toxic screening important.

Close clinical observation in a well-staffed setting is advisable in order to detect increasing drowsiness, change in respiratory pattern or pupillary enlargement, and to ensure fluid restriction. Fully awake or slightly drowsy patients with small subdural hematomas may be treated with corticosteroids and fluid restriction; larger clots, especially with fluctuating or worsening alertness, require surgery. Epidural hematomas causing compression of adjacent brain should be evacuated in patients who have a good chance of recovery from other injuries. Free water intake must be limited, allowing serum osmolarity to rise spontaneously toward 290 to 305 mosmol per liter. Fever must be treated assiduously with antipyretics or a cooling blanket, and its source must be identified (usually aspiration). So-called central fever is rare. The routine, acute administration of phenytoin is controversial. About half of neurosurgeons advocate its use, particularly in children and young adults, in the belief that it may reduce the incidence of posttraumatic epilepsy. Corticosteriods may be useful if there is a contusion, hemorrhage, or edema on the CT scan; otherwise they complicate management and should be omitted. The possibility of associated cervical spine injuries should be considered in all patients with syndromes of intermediate severity. The neck should be immobilized, and adequate x-rays of the spine should be obtained.

The majority of patients with intermediate injury improve over 1 to 6 weeks. During the first week alertness, irascibility, memory, and mental performance fluctuate. Behavioral changes such as agitation are most evident at night and sometimes seem to be worsened by large doses of corticosteroids or CNS-depressant drugs. Haloperidol is useful when used sparingly. Subtle abnormalities of intellectual function particularly attention, spontaneity, and memory, tend to return to normal later, and frequently do so abruptly.

SEVERE HEAD INJURY AND COMA Patients who are stuporous or comatose from the outset require immediate neurologic attention and often, resuscitation. There is usually pupillary enlargement or asymmetry. Persistent unresponsiveness is a grave sign. After the patient is intubated and the blood pressure is stabilized, attention is given to life-threatening noncranial injuries, followed by a survey neurologic examination.

The possibility of cervical injuries should not be overlooked, and the cervical spine must be immobilized during the initial assessment. The depth of coma and the size of the pupils are most important. Most severely injured patients hyperventilate. Extensor limb posturing and bilateral Babinski signs, combined with apparently purposeful movements, are common. Asymmetry in limb posture, limb movement, or gaze perference suggest a subdural or epidural hematoma or a large contusion.

As soon as vital functions permit, the patient should be taken to a critical care unit; cervical spine x-rays and a CT scan are obtained. The finding of an epidural or subdural hematoma or large intracerebral hemorrhage are usually indications for surgery and intracranial decompression. In one large series the time between injury and evacuation of acute subdural hematomas was the major determinant of outcome. If such lesions are not present and the patient is still comatose and critically ill, attention is directed toward treating raised ICP. Patients with abnormal CT scans showing contusions, hemorrhages, or tissue shifts are the best candidates for ICP monitoring. Since the lumbar CSF pressure does not accurately reflect the intracranial pressure and may increase the risk of brain herniation, the practice in most head injury treatment centers is to use a subarachnoid screw device with a hollow bore, an epidural monitor, or a ventricular catheter to measure ICP. The pressure can be monitored continuously, disturbances in compliance and falling CPP can be identified, and appearance of plateau waves can be noted.

The treatment of raised ICP is best guided by direct measurement but may proceed on a presumptive basis using clinical status and CT scan as guides. All potentially exacerbating factors must be eliminated.

Hypoxia, hyperthermia, hypercarbia, awkward head positions, and high mean airway pressures from mechanical ventilation all increase cerebral blood volume and ICP. Many, but not all, patients will have lower ICPs when the head and trunk are elevated approximately 60° than when supine. Active management of raised ICP includes induced hypocarbia to an initial level of 28 to 33 torr P_{CO_2} and hyperosmolar dehydration with 20% mannitol (0.25 to 1 g/kg every 3 to 6 h), preferably using directly measured ICP as a guide. Otherwise, a serum osmolality of 305 to 315 mosmol per liter is desirable, as is ventricular or subarachnoid fluid drainage when it is possible.

Persistently raised ICP after inception of this conservative therapy generally indicates a poor outcome, but the addition of high-dose barbiturates may further lower ICP and salvage a small number of patients. In many instances there is a parallel reduction in ICP and blood pressure without resulting net improvement in cerebral perfusion. The beneficial effects of barbiturates, aside from their sedative and anticonvulsant activities, are not established, and they can cause disastrous hypotension. Further details of treatment of raised ICP are given in Chap. 21. Systolic blood pressure should be maintained above 100 torr by vasopressor agents, if necessary, but when pressors are required to support barbiturate use, there is usually little improvement in CPP. Mean blood pressure levels above 110 to 120 torr exaggerate brain edema and are associated with plateau waves; hypertension should be treated with diuretics and beta-adrenergic blocking agents. Fluid and electrolytes must be administered cautiously, and free water administration should be limited. Administration of phenytoin or phenobarbital to prevent seizures is recommended by many neurosurgeons. Cimetidine, 300 mg IV every 4 h, or hourly antacids by nasogastric tube to keep gastric pH above 3.5 is the usual prophylaxis to prevent gastrointestinal bleeding. The use of large doses of corticosteroids in severe head injury is controversial, but some patients appear to benefit, particularly those less severely injured. If the patient remains comatose, it is worthwhile to repeat the CT scan to exclude a delayed surface or intracerebral hemorrhage. Intensive care salvages some critically ill head-injured patients by concentrating efforts on simple treatments that avoid medical complications and preventable increases in ICP. Whether more assiduous control of ICP and CPP will produce better results remains to be proved.

ASSOCIATED DERANGEMENTS OCCURRING WITH SEVERE HEAD TRAUMA Injuries outside the cranium should be searched for at the outset, because they are likely to be forgotten if not initially noted. In particular, associated spinal, long bone, and abdominal injuries may cause delayed difficulties in management. However, medical complications dominate the intermediate-term intensive care of head trauma patients.

Fluids and electrolytes Over half of patients who persist in coma for 24 h after head injury develop abnormalities of electrolytes or fluid balance. Frequently these are a consequence of therapy, but the metabolic responses to head trauma are similar to those produced by trauma elsewhere and are important in planning treatment. Daily input-output records and body weights, when possible, are important in management. Water restriction and osmotic agents render most patients hyperosmolar and hypovolemic, requiring monitoring of serum osmolality and sodium concentrations. Diabetes insipidus should be suspected if urine output increases and urine specific gravity is low. Replacement of water losses suffices for mild cases, but vasopressin may be required in persistent cases. Serum osmolality above approximately 325 mosmol per liter should be avoided because of the associated decrease in cardiac output.

Aldosterone and antidiuretic hormone (ADH) secretion in response to stress favor sodium and free water retention, respectively. The latter usually predominates, leading to mild hypervolemic hyponatremia in untreated patients, but is obscured by concomitant administration of osmotic agents. Severe hyponatremia results from excessive ADH secretion, which may occur with raised ICP, basilar skull fractures, and after prolonged mechanical ventilation. Potassium is lost in head injury because of trauma-induced aldosterone hypersecretion, therapeutic osmotic diuresis, and corticosteroids. Because potassium is predominantly an intracellular ion, hypokalemia is frequently manifested as a hypochloremic alkalosis with normal or minimally depressed serum potassium and requires adequate replacement therapy with KCl.

Respiratory complications Some patients with head injuries have hypoxia acutely after injury without obvious pulmonary pathology. Aspiration pneumonia presents a great risk; acid burn injury from aspirated gastric contents, infection, and atelectasis may combine to produce the adult respiratory distress syndrome (ARDS) and severe arteriovenous shunting. ARDS can also occur due to disseminated intravascular coagulopathy, fat embolism, or rarely ''neurogenic'' pulmonary edema. Treatment is similar to other cases of ARDS with positive end-expiratory pressure (PEEP) to allow lowered inspired oxygen concentrations and to prevent further atelectasis. The effect of PEEP on ICP is complex, but PEEP should not be withheld if necessary for oxygenation.

Atelectasis is common in all poorly responsive patients and is treated with chest physical therapy and adequate ventilator tidal volumes. Pulmonary embolism is also a major threat to bedridden patients, and intermittent pneumatic calf compression or modest doses of subcutaneous heparin may be useful prophylaxis. The latter has not predisposed to intracerebral or gastrointestinal bleeding. Early recognition of deep leg vein thrombosis and aggressive treatment by occlusion of the inferior vena cava may prevent later emboli.

Gastrointestinal hemorrhage The majority of patients with severe head injuries develop gastric erosions, but only a few have clinically significant hemorrhages. Gastrointestinal bleeding usually occurs in the first days to 1 week. Unlike most patients in shock or with stress ulceration, head-trauma patients often have elevated gastric acidity. The synergistic effect of corticosteroids in causing upper tract hemorrhage has been questioned, but the incidence of viscus perforation, particularly of the cecum, is elevated. Prophylactic treatment with cimetidine or with frequent antacid administration to keep gastric pH high (above 3.5) reduces gastric hemorrhage in other stress states and is commonly used in head trauma.

Fat embolism Patients with severe long bone injuries are subject to widespread cerebral fat embolism. This complication is seen less often than previously, perhaps due to better fluid replacement. In the typical case, head injury is a minor part of the overall trauma; in a few, severe cranial injury masks the syndrome. Several days after the bone fractures, restlessness, delirium, or drowsiness progressing to coma in severe cases, seizures, generalized brain edema, and respiratory insufficiency develop. About half have retinal and conjunctival punctate hemorrhages or visible fat in retinal vessels. A petechial rash, prominent in the anterior axillary folds and supraclavicular fossae, diffuse interstitial infiltrates on the chest x-ray, fat in the urine, or renal failure occur in some patients. Severe reduction in arterial oxygen content is common from widespread lung injury (ARDS). Cerebral fat embolism causes cerebral purpura, mainly in the white matter, due to capillary occlusion by fat globules. There is evidence that cases recognized and treated early have a better prognosis. Massive doses of corticosteroids, reduction of ICP, and administration of positive-pressure ventilation with high end-expiratory pressures have been useful. Heparin or intravenous alcohol are no longer recommended.

Cardiovascular changes Acute head trauma may cause transient apnea and cardiac arrest. In the absence of overwhelming brain damage recovery from the arrest is the rule. Subsequently, raised ICP may cause systemic hypertension, either with the classically associated bradycardia (Cushing response) or, almost as frequently, with tachycardia. Cardiac arrhythmias are common, most notably sinus bradycardia, supraventricular tachycardias, nodal rhythm, and heart block. T-wave inversion and alterations in the ST segment may simulate subendocardial ischemia.

Neurogenic pulmonary edema is a form of ARDS in which the alveoli fill with fluid as they would in congestive heart failure but left ventricular end-diastolic pressure (measured by pulmonary capillary wedge pressure) is normal. A pulmonary vascular leak may be produced when a sudden shift of intravascular volume occurs from the systemic to pulmonary circulation as occurs transiently with suddenly raised ICP. Once the pulmonary vasculature has been damaged, an alveolar capillary leak may continue despite return of blood pressure to normal. The result is pulmonary edema with normal central venous and wedge pressures after the initial injury.

Hematologic complications A large number of patients demonstrate a mild coagulopathy, and 5 to 10 percent have various degrees of disseminated intravascular coagulation. A correlation may exist between the severity of injury and the level of increased fibrin degradation products in blood. The cause of the coagulopathy is thought to be the release of highly thromboplastic material into the systemic circulation from the damaged brain.

PROGNOSIS Extensive work by Jennet's group in Glasgow has provided data on the outcome in severe head injury (Table 344-1). Verbal output, eye opening, and the best motor response are important predictors of ultimate outcome. Eighty-five percent of patients with aggregate Glasgow Coma Scale scores of 3 or 4 die 24 h after injury. Yet a number of patients with a poor initial prognosis, including absent pupillary light responses, survive, suggesting that aggressive management is justified in virtually all patients. Patients below approximately 20 years of age, particularly children, may make remarkable recoveries after grave early neurologic signs.

Evoked potentials have prognostic value in head injury, and their accuracy probably exceeds clinical observations and ICP measurements. Somatosensory evoked potentials are the most useful, with bilaterally absent cortical potentials (with more caudal potentials present) are predictive of death or a vegetative state in 85 to 95 percent of patients. Prediction of a good functional outcome in the presence of normal or mildly abnormal tests is less certain.

TABLE 344-1 Glasgow Coma Scale for head injury

Eye opening (E):	
Spontaneous	4
To loud voice	3
To pain	2
Nil	1
Best motor response (M):	
Obeys	6
Localizes	5
Withdraws (flexion)	4
Abnormal flexion posturing	3
Extension posturing	2
Nil	1
Verbal response (V):	
Oriented	5
Confused, disoriented	4
Inappropriate words	3
Incomprehensible sounds	2
Nil	1

NOTE: *Coma score = E + M + V. Patients scoring 3 or 4 have an 85 percent chance of dying or remaining vegetative, while scores above 11 indicate 5 to 10 percent likelihood of death or vegetative state and 85 percent chance of moderate disability or good recovery. Intermediate scores correlate with proportional chances of patients recovering.*

SPINAL CORD TRAUMA

Approximately 10,000 patients a year in the United States, mostly young and otherwise healthy, become paraplegic or quadriplegic because of spinal cord injuries. There are an estimated 200,000 quadriplegics in the country. The majority of cord injuries in civilian life result from damage to the surrounding vertebral column, from fracture, dislocation, or both. Vertical compression with flexion is the main mechanism of injury in the thoracic cord, and hyperextension or flexion is the main cause of injury in the cervical cord. Preexisting spondylosis, a congenitally narrowed spinal canal, hypertrophied ligamentum flavum (see Chap. 353), or instability of the apophyseal joints of adjacent vertebrae from diseases such as rheumatoid arthritis, predispose to severe spinal cord damage after minor degrees of injury.

PATHOPHYSIOLOGY AND PATHOLOGY OF CORD INJURY Much damage to the spinal cord is due to secondary phenomena in the minutes and hours following injury. Even when a complete transverse myelopathy is evident immediately after impact, some secondary changes are avoidable, and the resultant damage may be reversible. The immediate injury causes pericapillary hemorrhages that coalesce and enlarge, particularly in the gray matter. Infarction of gray matter and early white matter edema are evident within 4 h of experimental blunt injury. Eight hours after injury there is global infarction at the injured level, and only at this point does necrosis of white matter and paralysis below the level of the lesion become irreversible. The necrosis and central hemorrhages enlarge to occupy one or two levels above, and below, the point of primary impact. Gliosis in these regions results in necrotic areas over several months and may cavitate causing a progressive syringomyelic syndrome.

The early phases of injury are associated with reduced regional blood flow from direct capillary damage and a more prolonged secondary ischemia. A number of interventions including opiate antagonists, thyrotropin-releasing hormone, local cord cooling, dextran infusion, adrenergic blockade, corticosteroids, and hyperbaric oxygen are of uncertain clinical usefulness. More importantly, the critical factor for recoverable function is the time from injury to institution of therapy. Complete axonal disruption from the immediate trauma or secondary phenomena precludes recovery.

TYPES OF SPINAL CORD INJURY AND THEIR MANAGEMENT Any patient with severe head injury potentially has an associated instability of the spinal column. The care of such patients begins at the scene of the accident. The neck should be immobilized to prevent cord damage, and care should be taken during transport and during the physical and radiologic examinations to avoid neck extension or rotation and to prevent torsion-rotation of the thoracic spine. Blood pressure, respiratory status, and systemic injuries are attended to rapidly. Most patients can be intubated, if necessary, by blind nasotracheal technique without neck extension. High thoracic or cervical cord trauma regularly cause mild hypotension and bradycardia because of functional sympathectomy (often corroborated by bilateral ptosis and miosis—Horner's syndrome) that responds to infusion of crystalloid or colloid.

The neurologic examination in the awake patient focuses on neck or back pain, diminished limb power, a sensory level on the trunk, and deep tendon reflexes, usually absent below the level of an acute cord injury. Injuries above C5 cause quadriplegia and respiratory failure. At C5 and C6 the biceps are also weak, and at C4 and C5 the deltoid and supra- and infraspinatus are weak. C7 injuries cause weakness of the triceps, wrist extensors, and forearm pronators. Injuries at T1 and below cause paraplegia; the precise level can be determined from the level of sensory loss. Compression in the low thoracic and lumbar region causes a conus medullaris or cauda equina syndrome (see Chap. 353). Cauda equina injuries are usually incomplete, involving peripheral nerves rather than spinal cord, and therefore are surgically remediable for longer periods after injury than spinal cord compression. In a comatose patient absent reflexes should be sought in the legs, or in all the extremities, associated in the latter case with small pupils or paradoxical breathing from high cervical cord injury.

The next priority is to exclude a surgically remediable and potentially reversible cord compression due to dislocation of a vertebral body. Many traumatic myelopathies have no clearly associated fracture or dislocation. If x-rays suggest any aberration in the position of vertebrae, then reduction should be quickly undertaken. The role of myelography is controversial, but many neurosurgeons instill a few drops of Pantopaque into the spinal subarachnoid space to demonstrate a block to the flow of CSF. At present, examination by CT and magnetic resonance imaging scanning may be more useful. Decompression within 2 h of severe injury may lead to some recovery of cord function. With incomplete myelopathies, especially if the limbs are becoming progressively weaker, early decompression is strongly recommended, even many hours after injury. Surgical approaches to decompressing the spinal column depend upon the specific nature of the injury. In complete transverse myelopathies beyond 6 to 12 h in duration, decompressive laminectomies are usually unsuccessful in restoring function.

The concerns with spinal column fractures, with or without myelopathy, are threefold: (1) detection of vertebral dislocations causing cord compression, (2) instability caused by fractures that will lead to misalignment and cord compression in the future, and (3) the proper treatment of fractures through the pedicles, facets, or vertebral bodies. Some fractures heal with immobilizaton and time, usually 2 to 3 months; others require surgical fusion to ensure stability.

Atlantoaxial dislocations can cause immediate death from respiratory failure, an event that may occur with no neurologic signs. Rheumatoid arthritis predisposes to this injury. Atlantooccipital dislocations occur predominantly in children and are almost always fatal. "Jefferson's fractures" are burst fractures of the ring of the atlas resulting from a force descending on the vertex of the skull as in diving accidents; they are usually asymptomatic. "Hangman's fractures" are produced by hyperextension and longitudinal distraction of the upper cervical spine, as occurs with penal hanging or striking the chin on a steering wheel in head-on collisions. These are usually fractures through the pedicles of C2 with subluxation anteriorly of C2 on C3. Traction reduction and immobilization allow proper healing.

Hyperflexion dislocation of the cervical vertebrae commonly causes traumatic quadriplegia. Occasionally, a markedly displaced injury is unassociated with neurologic dysfunction, presenting only with neck pain. In most cases, however, minor subluxation is associated with a severe neurologic deficit. Ligamentous disruption presumably allows compression of the cord at the moment of impact, but the vertebral bodies return closer to their original stations afterward. Therefore, any degree of subluxation must be treated as potentially unstable.

Compression fractures of the cervical spine can cause neurologic damage if a bone fragment is driven backward (burst fracture) into the spinal cord. "Teardrop fractures" with crushing of a vertebral body, leaving a fragment of bone anteriorly, are usually associated with ligamentous disruption and spinal instability. Single compression fractures of the thoracic spine are usually stable because the thoracic cage provides support, but they may be associated with anterior cord compression and require decompression and stabilization with the insertion of metal rods.

Mild hyperextension injuries may cause only disruption of supporting ligamentous structures and be well tolerated. More severe injuries cause vertebral displacement and cord compression. The "central cord syndrome" is produced by brief compression of the cord and disruption of the central gray matter usually occurring in patients with an already narrow spinal canal, either congenitally or from cervical spondylosis. There is weakness of the arms, often with pinprick loss over the arms and shoulders, and relative sparing of leg power and sensation on the trunk and legs. Abnormality of bladder function is variable. The prognosis for recovery is good.

Thoracolumbar fractures are produced by impact in the high or midback, usually while the patient is bent over. Impingement on the spinal canal results in a complex combination of cauda equina and conus medullaris dysfunction. Pure lumbar fractures produce cauda equina compression. Myelography or CT scan allows precise localization, and surgical decompression is usually recommended, even with complete deficits, because the potential for recovery of peripheral nerves is great.

The subsequent care of patients with spinal cord injury is best undertaken in specialized centers. General principles of medical and urologic management are discussed in Chap. 353.

REFERENCES

ADAMS JH et al: Diffuse brain damage of the immediate impact type. Brain 100:489, 1977

BAKAY L, GLASSAUER FE: *Head Injury*. Boston, Little, Brown, 1980

BECKER DP et al: Outcome from severe head injury with early diagnosis and intensive management. J Neurosurg 47:491, 1977

DAVIS KR et al: Computed tomography in head trauma. Semin Roentgenol 12:53, 1977

JENNET B et al: Predicting outcome in individual patients after head injury. Lancet 1:1081, 1976

LANGFITT TW, GENARELLI TA: Can the outcome from head injury be improved? J Neurosurg 56:19, 1982

MARSHALL LF et al: The outcome with aggressive treatment in severe head injury. I: The significance of intracranial pressure monitoring. II: Acute and chronic barbiturate administration in the management of head injury. J Neurosurg 50:20, 1979

ROPPER AH et al (eds): *Neurological and Neurosurgical Intensive Care*. Baltimore, University Park Press, 1983

———, MILLER D: Acute traumatic midbrain hemorrhages. Ann Neurol 18:80, 1985

ROWBOTHAM GF: *Acute Injuries of the Head*, 4th ed. Baltimore, Williams & Wilkins, 1964

345 NEOPLASTIC DISEASES OF THE CENTRAL NERVOUS SYSTEM

FRED HOCHBERG / AMY PRUITT

Tumors of the brain, of its meningeal coverings, and of the spinal cord are estimated to cause the death of 90,000 patients in the United States each year. Of these tumors, more than three-quarters are metastases occurring in patients undergoing treatment for systemic cancer. Primary tumors arising within the meninges or the parenchyma of the brain or spinal cord are common at all ages of life. Brain neoplasms claim a disproportionate share of hospital beds, diagnostic tests, and other medical resources. One-fourth of the annual $4 billion cost for care of cancer patients in the United States is allocated to patients with neoplasms of the central nervous system (CNS).

Although the specialized care of such patients is usually delegated to the neurosurgeon, radiotherapist, or neurooncologist, with the advent of new imaging techniques the internist is increasingly involved in the initial diagnosis. Late in the course of the disease, such patients again may come under the care of a general physician. The proper care of patients with primary or metastatic tumors of the central nervous system requires a systematic approach that enables the physician to (1) distinguish tumor from other causes of neurologic dysfunction such as infection, metabolic derangement, pseudotumor cerebri, or subdural hematoma; (2) make proper use of sophisticated diagnostic techniques such as computerized tomography (CT) and magnetic resonance imaging (MRI) and of more invasive tests such as arteriography; (3) provide early therapy to control cerebral edema and seizure activity; (4) exclude systemic malignancy prior to referring the patient for a biopsy; and (5) recognize the medical complications of the tumor and of its therapy.

APPROACH TO THE PATIENT WITH CENTRAL NERVOUS SYSTEM TUMORS

CLASSIFICATION OF TUMORS Tumors of the CNS may originate in the brain or spinal cord (primary tumors) or may spread from systemic sites of cancer (metastatic tumors). Both benign and malignant primary CNS tumors are capable of producing neurologic impairment. Primary tumors arise from glial cells (astrocytoma, oligodendroglioma, glioblastoma), ependymal cells (ependymoma), or supporting tissue (meningioma, schwannoma, papilloma of the choroid plexus). In childhood, tumors arise from more primitive cells (medulloblastoma, neuroblastoma, chordoma). Malignant astrocytoma or glioblastoma is the most common type of primary tumor in adults over age 20. A classification of intracranial tumors is given in Table 345-1.

CLINICAL MANIFESTATIONS OF INTRACRANIAL TUMOR Intracranial tumors may be located within the brain substance (intraaxial) or in close proximity to the brain (extraaxial). The latter produce symptoms by compression or infiltration of brain. Many of the symptoms caused by intracranial masses reflect tumor expansion within a fixed bony vault into space normally occupied by brain, blood, and cerebrospinal fluid (CSF). The nature and severity of these symptoms depend on the location of the tumor and the rate of its growth. Although brain tissue can accommodate the presence of slowly growing tumors, masses larger than 3 cm in diameter compress the brain, its blood supply, and CSF pathways. This compression is increased by peritumoral edema (vasogenic cerebral edema). Neurologic deterioration occurs as tumor infiltrates or displaces normal brain structures; as the tumor develops areas of hemorrhage, necrosis or cyst formation; or as the tumor obstructs the normal flow of CSF, producing hydrocephalus.

Papilledema, or choking of the optic nerve head, emerges in the setting of impaired retinal venous return or axoplasmic flow along the optic nerve. Increasing intracranial pressure caused by a mass in one hemisphere may displace the medial temporal lobe (uncus) through the tentorial notch. As the uncus is forced inferiorly (*uncal herniation*) the midbrain is displaced and the third cranial nerve is compressed. The clinical signs of a unilateral third-nerve palsy—fixed, dilated pupil followed shortly thereafter by depression of consciousness, dilation of the opposite pupil, and hemiparesis on the opposite side of the original pupillary abnormality—should alert the physician to uncal herniation. A mass located more centrally in the supratentorial region produces a less specific picture called *central herniation*. In this situation the patient develops depression of consciousness as supratentorial structures compress the diencephalon and upper midbrain. Cheyne-Stokes respiration develops, but there is preservation of pupillary activity until late in the course of the deterioration.

Cerebellar masses may cause the cerebellar tonsils to herniate into the foramen magnum. As the tonsils are pushed inferiorly, the medulla and portions of the cervical spinal cord are compressed or infarcted. Abnormalities of cardiovascular regulation ensue. The resulting bradycardia and hypertension are followed by irregularity or cessation of respiration. Posterior fossa lesions of small size may produce early hydrocephalus by obstruction of CSF flow at the level of the fourth ventricle or aqueduct of Sylvius.

Symptoms of intracranial tumor may develop in patients with previously diagnosed systemic cancer or in those not known to harbor a malignancy. Patients with intracranial tumor usually present with one or more of the following groups of symptoms: (1) headache with or without evidence of increased intracranial pressure; (2) progressive generalized decline in cognitive abilities or impairment of specific neurologic functions affecting speech and language, gait, or memory; (3) adult-onset seizures or increased frequency or severity of previously documented seizure activity; or (4) focal neurologic symptoms reflecting the particular anatomic site of the tumor, such as those caused by acoustic schwannoma (neuroma) in the cerebellopontine angle or by meningioma of the olfactory groove, sella, or parasellar areas.

Headache is the initial symptom in half of patients with brain tumors. Traction on the dura, blood vessels, or cranial nerves results from local compression, elevation of intracranial pressure, edema, or hydrocephalus. In most patients with supratentorial tumor, pain radiates to the side of the tumor mass, whereas patients with posterior fossa masses describe retroorbital, retroauricular, or occipital pain. Emesis, often without nausea, signals development of increased intracranial pressure and is especially common in patients with masses located beneath the tentorium.

Tumors of the frontal lobes may attain considerable size before symptoms develop, and then symptoms often are nonspecific. Subtle, progressive disturbances of mentation, slowness of comprehension, loss of acuity in business affairs, memory disorders, or apathy, lethargy, and drowsiness may be reported. Spontaneity of thought and activity is lost. Incontinence of urine and disordered gait may be seen by family members. The development of a true dysphasia and/or motor weakness signal progression of the tumor or its associated edema into motor cortex and speech areas of the frontoparietal region.

Masses in the temporal lobes are associated with personality changes which may resemble psychotic thought disorders. Various combinations of auditory hallucinations, abrupt shifts in mood, and altered sleep, appetite, and sexual functions are soon interspersed with complex partial seizures possibly accompanied by visual field defects in the superior quadrants contralateral to the tumor.

Disorders of communication and vision characterize parietooccipital masses. Receptive aphasia with contralateral hemianopsia characterizes left parietal tumors, while a combination of spatial disorientation, constructional apraxia, and left homonymous hemianopsia bespeaks right parietal tumors.

Tumors of the diencephalon often present with a combination of failure of pupillary constriction to light, failure of upward gaze, and neuroendocrine abnormalities. Hydrocephalus due to obstruction to CSF flow at the level of the third ventricle leads to headache. Syndromes suggesting tumors of diencephalon or posterior fossa origin are more fully discussed in the section of this chapter devoted to neoplasms of these regions.

Cerebellar and brainstem lesions lead to a combination of cranial nerve palsies and incoordination of limbs or gait with or without accompanying signs of hydrocephalus. (See Chap. 352 for discussion of cranial nerve symptoms and signs.)

Seizures occur as the initial symptom in 20 percent of patients with brain tumors. Patients with new onset of epilepsy after the age of 35 must be evaluated for brain tumor. Similar high-risk groups of new seizure patients include those with previously diagnosed systemic cancer, longstanding neurologic diseases (including such neuroectodermal disorders as von Recklinghausen's disease and tuberous sclerosis), or acute or atypical psychiatric disorders. A carefully obtained history may uncover "complex partial" (temporal lobe) seizures or personality changes that antedate the diagnosis by years. Occasionally, the first symptom simulates a transient ischemic attack with no residual deficit or discernible seizure, but more commonly the pattern of clinical seizures provides localizing information. Thus, the "Jacksonian march" of tonic-clonic seizure points to frontal tumors and a sensory march characterizes tumors of the sensory parietal cortex. Metastatic tumors, occupying the junction of gray and white matter, are more likely than are primary tumors to produce acute symptoms evolving in days to weeks. Even more rapid onset of symptoms reflects hemorrhage in tumors of lung, melanoma, renal cell, choriocarcinoma, or thyroid origins. In contrast, with the exception of malignant astrocytoma, primary brain tumors are unlikely to hemorrhage.

TABLE 345-1 Classification of intracranial tumors

Type of tumor	Percent of total	
Glioma:	40	
Glioblastoma		20
Astrocytoma grades I and II		10
Ependymoma		6
Medulloblastoma		2
Oligodendroglioma		1
Papilloma of choroid plexus		1
Metastases	23	
Meningioma	17	
Pituitary adenoma	5	
Schwannoma	5	
Lymphoma	3	
Miscellaneous (congenital tumors, PNETs*)	7	

* *Primitive neuroectodermal tumors.*

PHYSICAL EXAMINATION OF THE PATIENT WITH SUSPECTED CNS TUMORS When the physician examines a brain tumor suspect who is not previously known to have a systemic cancer, the general examination should include (1) a survey of the skin for stigmata of neurocutaneous syndromes or melanoma, (2) a search for enlarged lymph nodes, (3) an examination of the abdomen for hepatic or splenic enlargement, (4) a rectal examination with stool guaiac test, (5) a breast examination in female patients, and (6) a cardiopulmonary examination.

The neurologic examination of the patient with suspected brain tumor should focus first on an evaluation of the mental status. The examiner should look for evidence of specific localizing cognitive deficits, such as dysphasia, dyspraxia, or memory loss, in addition to gleaning a sense of any personality change which has occurred. The patient is examined for increased intracranial pressure (papilledema or sixth cranial nerve paresis) and for other cranial nerve abnormalities. Asymmetries of strength, sensation, visual fields, and reflex activity should be sought. Attention should be paid to the constellation of signs suggestive of tumors in specific supratentorial, diencephalic or posterior fossa sites (see above). Combinations of cranial nerve abnormalities and corticospinal or lumbosacral radicular signs raise suspicion of leptomeningeal metastases (see below).

INVESTIGATION OF THE PATIENT WITH INTRACRANIAL TUMOR Advances in neuroradiology have contributed greatly to the diagnosis and management of patients with suspected neoplastic disease of the central nervous system. A plan for appropriate diagnostic studies based on the initial CT or MRI scan results is outlined in Table 345-2. The language of neurooncology differs from that of medical oncology, familiar terms such as "benign," "malignant," and "metastasizing" taking on different connotations when the tumor involves the CNS. Benign and malignant tumors are not differentiated in the scheme of Table 345-2 because the initial clinical approach is identical. Although many primary CNS tumors exhibit characteristics classifiable as "benign" because they are well-differentiated histologically and grow slowly, they are, nevertheless, incurable. Tumors of identical histology may have very different prognoses, depending upon their location and amenability to resection. Secondary CNS tumors are malignant in the conventional sense, since they represent metastases and invade normal tissue. Both benign and malignant tumors may produce profound, irreversible neurologic impairment. Primary brain tumors, with rare exceptions, do not metastasize outside the CNS; however, virtually all primary brain tumors are capable of diffuse seeding to the leptomeninges. Thus, the approach to *all* intracranial tumors, summarized in Table 345-2, relies on the clinical history and physical examination and on information provided by CT scan and MRI.

The laboratory evaluation of intracranial tumors Contrast-enhanced CT scanning and MRI have now largely replaced the combination of skull x-ray, electroencephalogram, radionuclide brain scan, and arteriography as the principal tests for the evaluation of patients with suspected brain tumor. The universal use of CT and MRI is unlikely to be altered substantially by the introduction of other techniques such as computer-analyzed EEG, venous or arterial digital subtraction angiography, or brain scanning using radiolabeled monoclonal antibodies directed against specific tumor types.

CT SCAN Contrast-enhanced CT imaging delineates intracranial masses as small as 0.5 cm in diameter. Certain tumors whose density exceeds that of normal brain parenchyma, including meningioma, melanoma, and primary lymphoma, and tumors with spontaneous hemorrhage can be visualized without contrast enhancement. Reconstructions in coronal and sagittal planes and magnification of focal regions allow detection of 95 percent of intracranial masses and definition within 1 cm of the histologic border of the tumor. Tumors commonly appear as homogeneous or ring-enhancing masses surrounded by variable amounts of edema. Although not a substitute for biopsy diagnosis, the CT often correctly predicts the histology of the tumor (Fig. 345-1).

Initial CT studies may show no abnormality in meningeal carcinomatosis, small metastases, primary brain lymphoma, or some glial tumors; repeat CT scanning, utilizing single or double doses of contrast, 4 to 6 weeks later usually provides tumor detection. The clinician should be wary of attributing all CT scan masses to tumor, as ring-like enhancement may occur in abscesses, in recent cerebral infarctions, in the plaques of multiple sclerosis, and in certain vascular malformations with or without hemorrhage. Asymptomatic menin-

TABLE 345-2 Evaluation following CT or MRI scan of the patient with suspected neoplastic disease of the CNS

Clinical setting	Possible diagnoses	Pretreatment evaluation	Primary treatment	Secondary treatment
SOLITARY MASS ON CT OR MRI SCAN				
No known systemic cancer	Nonneoplastic disease Primary or secondary tumor Benign or malignant tumor	Metastatic evaluation Arteriogram Surgical opinion	Steroids Surgery	Radiation, chemotherapy as indicated Steroids as needed
Known systemic cancer	Radioresistant or radiosensitive tumor Unrelated tumor (second primary)	Double-dose contrast CT scan Metastatic evaluation Surgical opinion*	Steroids, radiation if radiosensitive tumor or active systemic disease found	Steroids as needed
			Steroids, surgery if radioresistant tumor or quiescent systemic disease found	Postoperative radiation Steroids as needed
MULTIPLE MASSES ON CT OR MRI SCAN				
No prior known systemic cancer	Nonneoplastic disease Primary or secondary tumor	Metastatic evaluation	Steroids, radiation if systemic tumor identified	Steroids as needed
			Steroids, biopsy, radiation if no systemic tumor found	Steroids as needed
Known systemic cancer	Metastases	None	Steroids, radiation	Steroids as needed
NEGATIVE† CT OR MRI SCAN				
No focal deficits on examination	Infection Metabolic abnormality	Lumbar puncture Exclude infection or metabolic problem	See text	——
Focal deficits on examination	Vascular disease Carcinomatous meningitis Seizure, paraneoplastic syndrome, complication of therapy	Lumbar puncture Follow-up CT 4–6 weeks	See text	——

* *Posterior fossa mass with hydrocephalus.*
† *Patient with cancer and neurologic signs.*

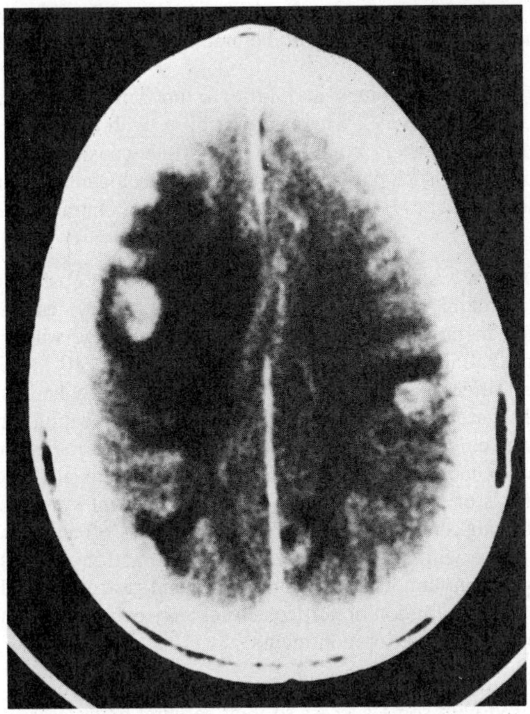

FIGURE 345-1 *Contrast-enhanced CT scan showing three metastatic brain tumors. Note extensive edema surrounding lesion in right frontal lobe with associated transfalcial herniation.*

giomas and aneurysms are often incidentally detected during the evaluation of a patient for intracranial mass.

Brainstem, cerebellar, and spinal cord masses can be defined further by combination of CT and subarachnoid administration of metrizamide. Because of the risk of seizures after instillation of metrizamide, patients should be treated prophylactically with phenobarbital.

MAGNETIC RESONANCE IMAGING Magnetic resonance imaging (MRI, nuclear magnetic resonance) delineates most metastatic and primary tumors and distinguishes surrounding edema (see Chap. 341). It is an important adjunct to CT, particularly for lesions located in close proximity to bone at the skull base. Tumors of the brainstem and spinal cord are also visualized, and advances in surface coil technology will reduce the need for contrast myelography. Recent observations show that MRI cannot at present distinguish radiation necrosis from recurrent tumor or edema secondary to chemotherapy from edema due to tumor growth. However, with intravenous gadolinium diethylenetriamine pentaacetic acid (DPTA) paramagnetic contrast, the MRI of the brain indicates defects in patterns quite similar to those observed with the use of organic iodides in CT. The combination of this paramagnetic agent and higher energy units may provide better separation of tumor from nontumor tissue.

ANGIOGRAPHY Transfemoral arteriography provides selective visualization of internal carotid and vertebral arteries and their branches. Vessels of malignant tumors are characterized by an angiographic "blush" with enlarged, early draining veins, features not seen in association with an intracerebral hemorrhage, infarction, or abscess. Preoperative neurosurgical planning is often aided by knowledge of the vascular anatomy. In some cases, sufficient detail is revealed after intravenous administration of contrast using digital subtraction angiography.

MANAGEMENT OF INTRACRANIAL TUMORS **Surgery: biopsy and resection** Surgical exploration allows tumor identification in patients with either solitary or multiple intracranial masses. Surgical exploration may be necessary to obtain a diagnosis in patients with multiple CT masses in whom a thorough systemic evaluation, including hemogram, liver function studies, carcinoembryonic antigen, chest x-ray, sputum cytology, radionuclide bone and liver scans, and perhaps intravenous pyelography is unrewarding. Of patients with multiple CNS metastatic lesions, 20 percent have no evidence of systemic cancer.

Tumor biopsy is performed through an open craniotomy or with CT-guided stereotaxic techniques. The establishment of a diagnosis is important to determine prognosis and treatment. *Resection* is undertaken and may be curative for some primary tumors such as meningioma, ependymoma, oligodendroglioma, and low-grade astrocytoma (see below) in nondominant, frontal, anterior temporal, or occipital locations or in the ventricular system. *Partial resection* improves patient symptoms, often including better seizure control; by diminishing cerebral edema, it reduces dependence on corticosteroids. Although resection offers little to the patient with multiple intracranial lesions, it may be of value for solitary metastases. Resection of a *solitary tumor* in patients with known systemic cancer may be considered if: there is a greater than 2-year interval without known residual systemic malignancy; relief of specific symptoms such as hydrocephalus is required; the tumor is known to be radioresistant as in the case of melanoma, sarcoma, and renal or colonic carcinomas; symptomatic tumor recurs after radiation; and the patient's systemic disease is under good control and the cerebral tumor is the limiting factor in quality of survival. For selected patients, this approach offers survival free of neurologic disease of more than 1 year.

Acute treatment of intracranial tumors Clinical evidence of acute or subacute deterioration, such as stupor, focal neurologic signs, or evidence of transtentorial herniation, requires aggressive management. Treatment is directed to reducing cerebral edema, lowering intracranial pressure and reducing the risk of seizures. Treatment with daily doses of dexamethasone 30 to 60 mg or methylprednisolone 120 to 200 mg in four to six divided doses reduces cerebral edema and associated surgical morbidity. Corticosteroids may not control symptoms caused by obstruction of the ventricular system, and emergency ventricular drainage may be required. Anticonvulsant medications are usually prescribed for patients with seizures, though many physicians administer them prophylactically when intracranial tumor has been diagnosed.

SYSTEMIC CANCER AND THE CENTRAL NERVOUS SYSTEM

CEREBRAL METASTASES The most common CNS tumors are metastatic. The following section discusses the approach to patients who present with a CNS tumor where systemic cancer must be considered.

Pathogenesis and pathology Cerebral metastases occur in one-quarter of patients with systemic cancer. Spread to the calvarium, brain parenchyma, and subarachnoid space occurs through several mechanisms. *Hematogenous tumor embolism* from intermediate sites such as lung and liver is the most common mechanism in solid tumors of the breast and lung, and in melanoma. Spread into the spinal canal via the *perivertebral venous system* occurs with uterine, colonic, and prostatic tumors. *Direct extension* of tumors originating in the head and neck may occur through the base of the skull. *Paraspinal direct* infiltration may occur with lymphoma and with prostate and breast carcinomas. *Tumor passage into the eye* or through the choroid plexus to the brain and subarachnoid space occurs in lymphoma and leukemia.

Clinical manifestations Sixty percent of cerebral metastases occur in the setting of diagnosed systemic cancer. Cancers of lung in men and of breast in women account for the largest percentage, although melanoma is the tumor with highest likelihood of spread to the CNS. Of patients with a cerebral metastasis (most often arising in the lung) 20 percent develop neurologic symptoms before discovery of the primary malignancy. At some point after diagnosis of systemic cancer, 25 percent of patients with lung carcinoma, 6 to 20 percent of patients with breast carcinoma, and about 50 percent of those with melanoma (when this last tumor has already metastasized to a site outside the CNS) develop tumors in brain or spinal cord. Patients with recurrent sarcoma or ovarian or colorectal cancer who survive beyond 3 years after the original diagnosis face a heightened risk of neurologic involvement. These tumors rarely accounted for cerebral metastases in the past. In the majority of patients, cerebral metastases occur with systemic relapse (Table 345-3). An exception occurs in patients with lung cancer, where the CNS is frequently either the initial site of presentation or of first demonstrated recurrence in otherwise apparently well-controlled disease. As systemic treatment continues to improve survival, the incidence of CNS involvement can be expected to rise for virtually all tumors.

Diagnosis of cerebral metastases More often than is the case with primary brain tumors, those of metastatic origin occur in a setting of seizure activity, increasingly severe head pain, and motor weakness. These difficulties often evolve in days to weeks. Contrast-enhanced CT scan is the procedure of choice for evaluating patients with known systemic cancer and new neurologic symptoms (Table 345-2). Tumors appear as multiple ring-enhancing lesions or solitary masses with equal frequency. Three categories of patients without neurologic symptoms or signs are initially evaluated by CT scanning. First, patients with lung carcinoma for whom attempted cure with pulmonary lobectomy is planned should have a CT scan preoperatively, since 5 percent of such patients will have clinically unsuspected cerebral metastases. Second, prophylactic brain radiation for small cell carcinoma of the lung should be preceded by a CT scan. Third, patients with widely disseminated cancer due to breast or testicular tumors, sarcoma, or melanoma who are about to receive systemic chemotherapy should have a CT scan to stage the disease.

Ten percent of patients with cancer develop neurologic difficulties in the absence of an intracranial mass on CT scan. Focal motor or cranial nerve symptoms, headache, or impaired intellectual performance may reflect cerebrovascular lesions known to be associated with systemic cancer, unwitnessed seizures, meningeal carcinomatosis, paraneoplastic syndromes, or complications of tumor therapy (Table 345-4).

Patients with systemic neoplasms can develop several types of cerebrovascular disease (see Graus et al.). Multiple cerebral infarctions are the most frequent in patients with solid tumors; those with lymphoma or leukemia may develop diffuse encephalopathic difficulties from infarcts due to disseminated intravascular coagulation or from hemorrhage in the setting of clotting abnormalities, or from thrombocytopenia.

Focal deficits in patients with negative CT scans may result from seizures due to undetectable metastatic disease or may be manifestations of meningeal carcinomatosis or paraneoplastic syndromes (see Chap. 304). Repeat CT scan in 4 to 6 weeks often discloses the tumor if present. A lumbar puncture with cytologic examination is mandatory in such patients both to exclude infection and to search for leptomeningeal tumor (see below). CSF pleocytosis with mild elevation of protein may be found with paraneoplastic disorders.

Treatment The common assumption that brain metastases represent a uniform disease has been proved invalid. Therapeutic decisions must be based on the type, extent, and radiosensitivity of the primary tumor, the morbidity produced, and the number and location of metastases.

Patients with solitary lesions and little or no active systemic disease may require surgery, whereas for those with advanced, widespread systemic cancer, comfort is the prime consideration. Steroids may be used in such patients to maximize neurologic function and to reduce headache (see "Acute Treatment of Intracranial Tumors").

RADIATION THERAPY After acute symptoms are treated, most patients with multiple cerebral metastases or unresectable solitary lesions receive radiation therapy. A common approach is palliative whole-brain radiation totaling about 30 Gy (3000 rad) given in 10 to 15 equal fractions. Three-quarters of patients improve clinically and by CT; over one-half are able to discontinue their steroid medication for a time. However, only 30 percent of patients who complete radiation therapy survive 6 months and fewer than 20 percent are alive at 1 year. Two-thirds of the latter patients die from recurrent systemic tumor and not from cerebral disease. Treatment is less effective in the elderly, in those with advanced systemic cancer, and in patients with radiation-resistant tumors such as melanoma and gastrointestinal and lung tumors. Reinstitution of corticosteroids may be useful when progressive neurologic deterioration recurs.

CHEMOTHERAPY Systemic (intravenous or intraarterial) chemotherapy has been used with some success to treat cerebral metastases of lung (small cell), breast, and testicular origin. Anecdotal reports of brain metastases of breast origin responding to tamoxifen or other systemic chemotherapy have appeared.

LEPTOMENINGEAL METASTASES Pathogenesis and pathology Eight percent of patients with cancer develop diffuse infiltration of the meninges. The cranial and spinal nerve roots are usually affected. Tumors that commonly invade the meninges include non-Hodgkin's lymphoma, leukemia, melanoma, and adenocarcinoma of breast, lung, or gastrointestinal origin.

Clinical manifestations The common symptoms are headache, alteration in mentation, cranial nerve abnormalities, and lumbosacral radiculopathies. Patients may also present with seizures. The CT scan usually is normal, but it may reveal enlarged ventricles and diffuse enhancement of the meninges over the cerebral hemispheres and at the base of the brain.

A lumbar puncture is required for diagnosis. Three-quarters of patients show a modest CSF mononuclear pleocytosis of 5 to 100 cells. Elevation of protein and lowered glucose content may occur, but demonstration of malignant cells is required to confirm the diagnosis. Repeat lumbar punctures may be necessary to obtain positive cytology. Myelography is often done in such patients because of back pain and radicular symptoms; it may disclose multiple small nodules on the nerve roots. Larger lesions can be detected and treated with radiation.

Treatment Treatment of meningeal carcinomatosis usually requires a combination of cranial radiation and intrathecal administration of chemotherapeutic agents. Chemotherapy is given either into the lumbar subarachnoid space or (more effectively) into a reservoir

TABLE 345-3 Interval between diagnosis of cancer and occurrence of brain metastases

Tumor	Patients with brain metastases, percent: At diagnosis of primary	Sometime during course of tumor growth	At autopsy	Interval from diagnosis of primary tumor to diagnosis of brain metastasis
Lung tumor	10–15	22–30	15–30	90 after 3 months
Breast tumor	1	6–20	15–30	90 after 1 year
Melanoma	6	50	40–80	80 after 1 year
Renal tumor	4	11–13	8–20	90 after 1 year
Colorectal tumor	1	—	1	75 after 2 years
Sarcoma	1	36	—	90 after 1 year

SOURCE: *Weiss et al., Deutsch et al.*

connected to the lateral ventricle. Agents commonly used include methotrexate, triethylenethiophosphoramide (thio-TEPA), and cytosine arabinoside either alone or in combination.

About one-half of patients with breast carcinoma respond initially to these treatments, but the median survival is only 7 months. The prognosis is particularly grave for meningeal carcinomatosis of melanoma or lung tumor origin; few responses are seen. A much better prognosis is expected in patients with lymphoma or leukemia with control for 2 or more years being common. Treatment failures reflect tumor drug resistance, poor circulation of drug within the subarachnoid space, and complications arising from chemotherapy and radiation (see Table 345-4).

TOXIC EFFECTS OF CANCER TREATMENT Chemotherapy Chronic corticosteroid therapy may induce insulin-dependent diabetes mellitus, myopathy, and aseptic necrosis of the hip and may predispose to thrombophlebitis. In the early stages the muscle changes reverse with steroid taper and intensive physical therapy. Administration of anticonvulsants is associated with cutaneous allergies. Anticonvulsant doses may need to be adjusted in patients receiving corticosteroids. Allergy to an anticonvulsant may be masked while the patient receives corticosteroids and revealed later when the steroid medication is tapered. Table 345-4 summarizes the neurologic toxicities of currently used *chemotherapeutic agents.*

TABLE 345-4 Complications of chemotherapy

Neurologic problem	Drug(s)	Route
Encephalopathy	Steroids	PO/IM/IV
	L-Asparaginase	IV
	Procarbazine	PO/IV
	Nitrosoureas	PO/IV/IA/HDIV
	Cytosine arabinoside	HDIV
Leucoencephalopathy	Methotrexate	HDIV/IT
Cerebral edema	Cisplatin	IA
	Nitrosoureas	IA/HDIV
Optic nerve damage	Nitrosoureas	IA/HDIV
Cerebellar ataxia	5-Fluorouracil	IV
	Cytosine arabinoside	IT
Cranial neuropathy	Vincristine	IV
	Cisplatin*	IV/IA
Myelopathy/radiculopathy	Thio-TEPA	IT
	Methotrexate	HDIV/IT
	Cystosine arabinoside	HDIV/IT
Peripheral neuropathy	Vincristine†	IV
	Cisplatin	IV
Myopathy	Steroids	PO/IM/IV
	Vincristine	IV

* *Ototoxicity and vestibular toxicity.*
† *Autonomic neuropathy may be seen as well.*
NOTES: *IA = intraarterial; IM = intramuscular; IV = intravenous; PO = per os; IT = intrathecal; HDIV = high dose intravenous.*
SOURCE: *Modified from Young.*

Radiation therapy Radiation therapy may cause toxic effects on the CNS. Acute changes in mental status or exacerbation of previous symptoms and signs may develop within 1 to 2 weeks of its initiation. These effects are usually attributable to worsening cerebral edema and are best treated with increased doses of corticosteroids. Subacute changes that develop between 3 and 18 months after treatment are ascribed to radiation-induced demyelination and are unresponsive to steroids. These changes include the reappearance of previous neurologic impairment and the appearance of a mass which is indistinguishable from recurrent tumor on CT scan. Patients who have received spinal radiation may develop Lhermitte's phenomenon with tingling in the back and legs following flexion of the neck.

Between 18 and 60 months after radiation, still other less reversible changes occur. These include retarded growth rate and impaired intellectual development in children who have received more than 30 Gy (3000 rad) of whole-brain radiation. At doses above 50 Gy (5000 rad), adults may exhibit cortical atrophy, communicating hydrocephalus, and hypothalamic dysfunction with elevated prolactin levels and amenorrhea or impotence. Dementia resulting from these changes is irreversible and in the case of hydrocephalus is usually unimproved by ventricular shunting.

The peripheral nervous system can also be affected by radiation therapy. Localized dysfunction of the brachial or lumbosacral plexus may follow radiation in excess of 40 Gy (4000 rad), usually appearing more than 1 year after treatment (see Chap. 355). Unlike peripheral nerve problems due to tumor invasion, radiation plexopathy is commonly painless. Additional tests, including CT scan, may be necessary to distinguish tumor invasion from radiation toxicity. Corticosteroids may afford some benefit.

PRIMARY BRAIN TUMORS

In the following section, the most common primary brain tumors in adults are discussed by histologic type. Other tumors which occur in characteristic locations and whose presenting symptoms therefore reflect site rather than specific histology are then discussed by location. These include tumors located in the diencephalon-third ventricle, the posterior fossa, and the skull base.

MALIGNANT ASTROCYTOMA (GLIOBLASTOMA) Definition Malignant astrocytoma or glioblastoma (also known as malignant glioma or grade 3 or 4 astrocytoma) and the less malignant anaplastic astrocytoma account for about one-quarter of the 5000 intracranial gliomas diagnosed yearly in the United States; 75 percent of gliomas in adults are of this category. Because of its profound and uniform morbidity, it contributes more to the cost of cancer on a per capita basis than does any other tumor. The patient, commonly stricken in the fifth decade of life, enters a cycle of repetitive hospitalizations and operations while experiencing the progressive complications associated with relatively ineffective treatments of radiation and chemotherapy.

Pathogenesis and pathology Epidemiologic studies offer few clues to the etiology of malignant astrocytoma. Some tumors arise in patients with longstanding seizure disorders or personality disorders resulting from temporal lobe dysfunction and in scars incurred from head trauma, suggesting that in certain instances the malignant cells emerge from a more benign glial proliferation. There are rare instances of malignant tumors occurring in families, suggesting a genetic propensity. At least four human viral oncogenes (*sis, myc, src, n-myc*) have been identified in cell lines derived from primary brain tumors. Small clusters of tumors have appeared in certain occupational settings, notably in the petroleum processing industry. The tumor has an appearance similar to that produced by a variety of viral agents inoculated into animals. Examined by the naked eye, normal brain is distorted and infiltrated by yellow tumor tissue containing areas of necrosis, cysts, and hemorrhage. Microscopic examination reveals a highly cellular composite of heterogeneous glial cells with elongated or rounded astrocytes whose processes stain for glial fibrillary acidic protein. Giant cells may be seen along with mitotic figures and the proliferation of small capillaries.

Clinical manifestations Patients commonly present with a subacute progressive neurologic deficit exhibiting either focal signs or personality changes. Prior mental changes or seizures may antedate tumor diagnosis by months to years. Clinical symptoms may occur abruptly with seizures or with sudden deficits secondary to tumor hemorrhage. The CT scan reveals a heterogeneous pattern of tumor enhancement interspersed with hypodense foci presumably corresponding to tumor necrosis and edema. Multiple tumors can occur but are uncommon. MRI scans often define more extensive tumor involvement than is indicated on the CT scan (Fig. 345-2).

Malignant astrocytoma can arise in the brainstem, cerebellum, or spinal cord in addition to the more common locations within the white matter of the cerebral hemispheres. The prognosis for any site, unfortunately, has not changed greatly in the last 20 years. Following treatment, less than 6 months of useful function can be expected for most patients before progression of symptoms signals recurrent tumor.

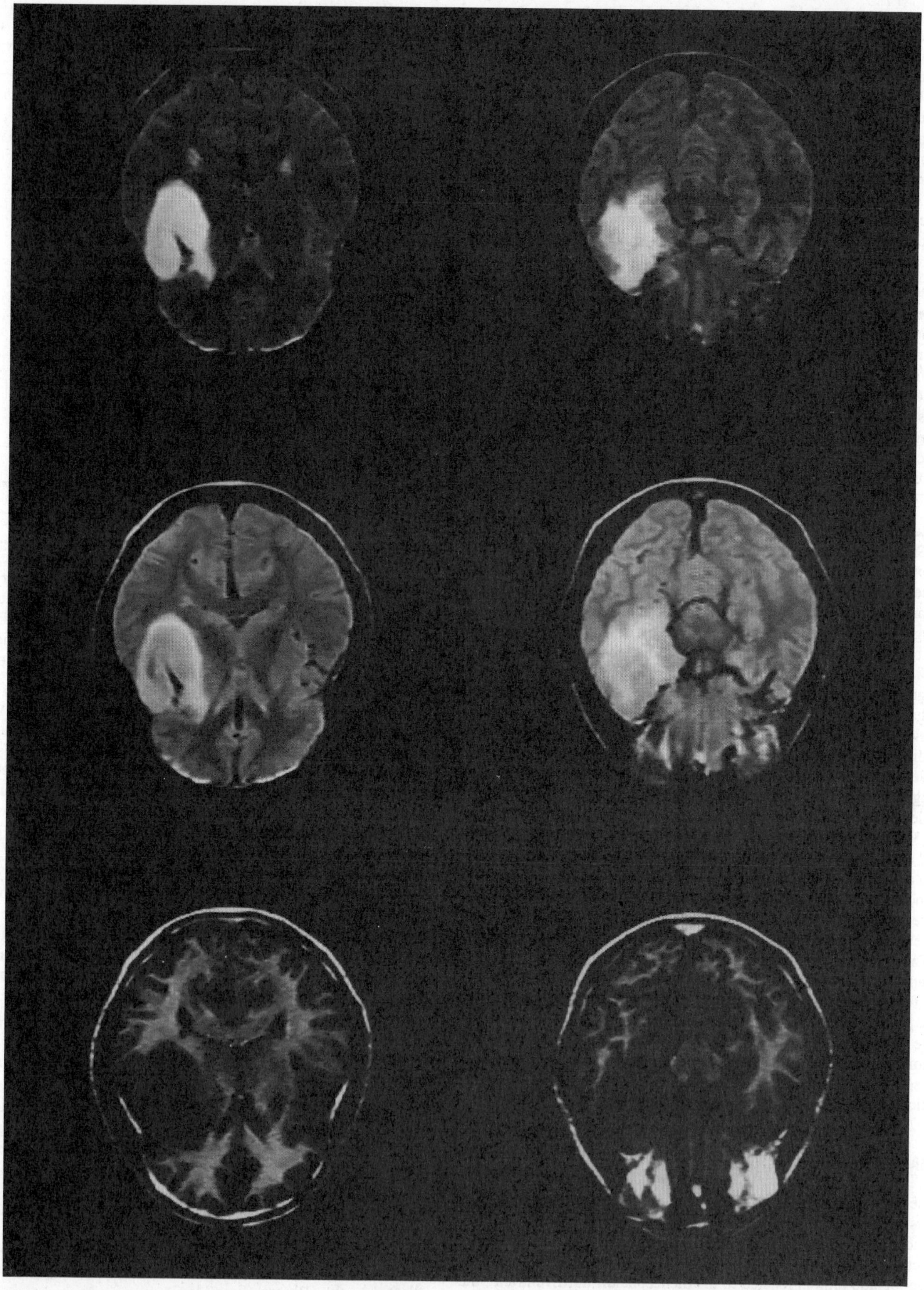

FIGURE 345-2 *MRI scans of glioblastoma multiforme. A large lesion is evident involving the anterior left temporal pole and operculum, with a central zone of markedly prolonged relaxation times (dark on IR sections, above, and bright on SE sections, below). This area is surrounded by a thin rim of moderately prolonged T1 (gray appearance) and T2 (brighter on earlier echo, middle row, and less bright on later echo, bottom row). It is thought, but not proven by histologic study, that the central area represents tumoral mass, with a greatly prolonged T2, surrounded by a thin rim of edema or compressed brain (moderately prolonged relaxation times). (Top row: IR study; TR = 1500, TI = 450, TE = 45 ms. Middle row: SE study; TR = 2000, TE = 60 ms. Bottom row: SE study; TR = 2000, TE = 120 ms.)*

Death results in 80 percent of patients from tumor recurrence within 6 to 12 months. Progressive neurologic deterioration is followed by stupor and coma. In patients who survive over 1 year, often young adults, CNS dissemination can occur to the meninges or the ventricular ependyma. Metastasis outside the CNS is extremely rare.

Treatment Confirmation of histology by biopsy should be performed in most patients; debulking of tumor is recommended if the tumor is located in an area that permits an extensive operation.

Therapeutic modalities are not highly effective. The average life expectancy of 17 weeks for untreated patients is improved by postoperative external beam radiation alone to 47 weeks and by radiation combined with chemotherapy to 62 weeks. A subgroup of young patients under age 50 obtains significant improvement in quality and duration of life. Such patients have a 20 percent 2-year survival after cranial radiation of 55 to 60 Gy (5500 to 6000 rad) combined with adjunctive chemotherapy with the nitrosoureas carmustine (BCNU) or lomustine (CCNU).

Efforts to improve prognosis for this malignancy include radiotherapy trials of implanted radiation sources (brachytherapy). Current chemotherapeutic trials are based on the localized nature of the tumor and of its recurrence and involve local arterial infusions of carmustine or cisplatin prior to radiation or at the time of tumor recurrence. Experimental approaches include the use of interferon or monoclonal antibodies.

ASTROCYTOMA Definition Low-grade astrocytomas occur throughout the brain and spinal cord. The subcortical white matter is the most common site in adults. In children and young adults astrocytomas arise in the optic nerves, cerebellum (cystic, juvenile, pilocytic astrocytoma), and brainstem (pontine glioma). These tumors are also associated with neurofibromatosis and tuberous sclerosis and are found in 20 percent of patients undergoing temporal lobectomy for control of chronic seizure disorders.

Pathogenesis and pathology The tumors are avascular without necrosis and contain homogeneous populations of well-differentiated astrocytes. In cerebellar locations and, less commonly, in supratentorial sites, the tumor may consist of a small nodule of astrocytes accompanied by a much larger cyst. Calcification is uncommon.

Clinical manifestations The tumors evolve slowly over several years, producing symptoms by displacement of normal brain or by invasion of white matter tracts. Optic nerve gliomas cause progressive, monocular or bitemporal visual field defects leading eventually to blindness and sometimes proptosis. Hypothalamic compression may cause endocrine dysfunction. Hydrocephalus is rare. In the brainstem, such tumors typically involve several cranial nerves (often the abducens, facial, and trigeminal) and later impinge on corticospinal fibers and medial lemniscal and spinothalamic tracts. These symptoms must be distinguished from those caused by multiple sclerosis, arteriovenous malformations, cysts of cysticercosis and echinococcal origin, and extramedullary tumors such as schwannomas or meningiomas. Cerebellar astrocytomas cause progressive incoordination and gait ataxia combined with abnormalities of eye movements. In supratentorial locations, these tumors may produce seizures before any focal abnormality appears on clinical examination or on CT scan.

The characteristic CT appearance is an indistinct mass which is hypodense with respect to surrounding brain and which exhibits little or no contrast enhancement or evidence of edema. MRI often demonstrates white matter abnormalities in patients with normal CT scans and is becoming the preferred procedure for early diagnosis and follow-up. A stable clinical course is common and repeat radiologic studies may show little change. In an extreme form this process of slow infiltration of white matter, known as *gliomatosis cerebri,* causes diffuse panhemispheric infiltration by atypical individual astrocytes without evidence of localized tumor. Malignant degeneration of astrocytomas is heralded by rapid progression of symptoms and signs, evidence of growth on CT, development of peritumoral edema, and contrast enhancement.

Treatment Surgical excision can be curative for some cerebellar, optic nerve, and lobar astrocytomas. Cyst drainage and partial resection are feasible for many. Biopsy should be obtained for supratentorial tumors but is less frequently considered for brainstem or spinal cord gliomas. Exceptions to the latter are tumors that have a cystic or extraaxial component. Postoperative radiation is recommended for incompletely resected tumors. Its role in the treatment of excised tumors is less clear. The timing of radiation therapy should be carefully weighed against the known long natural course of the astrocytoma, particularly those in supratentorial locations. Radiation is recommended when symptoms and signs progress or enlargement on CT or MRI is observed. Radiation may be safely delayed for several years in apparently totally resected tumors because of the accuracy of MRI and CT scans. The judicious use of corticosteroids during radiation or when symptoms recur improves function. The median life expectancy is 67 months for supratentorial tumors and 89 months for cerebellar tumors. Average survivals of 15 months after radiation are reported for patients with brainstem tumors. However, the 5-year survival is only 30 percent. Chemotherapy, currently under investigation for brainstem tumors, may offer some improvement in survival.

OLIGODENDROGLIOMA Definition This tumor of oligodendroglial origin may develop in isolation or may be mixed with other glial cells. An uncommon tumor, it represents less then 10 percent of all gliomas.

Pathology Microscopic examination discloses rounded cells containing darkly staining nuclei with poorly staining cytoplasm, the "fried egg" appearance. The tumor is prone to spontaneous hemorrhage.

Clinical manifestations Presentation is most commonly in the third or fourth decade and tumors are most frequently in the frontal lobes or within the ventricles. CT reveals a well-defined, low-attenuation mass with fine speckled calcium deposits and small cysts.

Treatment Although the oligodendroglioma is histologically "benign," resection is curative in only one-third of patients. The role of postoperative radiation is uncertain; it is recommended only for unresectable tumors or those with features suggesting malignant change, such as contrast enhancement or radiographically proven tumor growth. Prospective studies of postoperative radiation have not been performed. Chemotherapy is not effective. Approximately one-third of patients survive 5 years after diagnosis.

MENINGIOMA Definition Meningiomas account for 20 percent of brain tumors. They can arise in either the cranium or the spinal canal. They occur more frequently at all sites in women. They are commonly found as asymptomatic tumors at postmortem. When symptomatic they usually present in the fifth or sixth decades.

Pathogenesis and pathology Meningiomas arise from cells of the pia-arachnoid. Common sites include the midline along the falx cerebri and the lateral cerebral convexity, the olfactory groove and along the sphenoid ridge, the tuberculum sellae, foramen magnum, and tentorium of the cerebellum. They also arise on occasion within the ventricles, where on radiographic examination they are indistinguishable from a papilloma of the choroid plexus. Meningiomas may coexist with schwannomas in patients with the central form of neurofibromatosis. They occur more frequently in women with breast cancer; some meningiomas contain estrogen and progesterone receptors.

On the basis of microscopic characteristics, meningiomas are divided into seven categories: syncytial, transitional, fibroblastic, microcystic, psammomatous, angioblastic, and malignant meningiomas. Malignant tumors display mitoses, invade normal brain, and occasionally develop CNS and extraneural metastases. Angioblastic and malignant forms are more likely than the other types to recur.

Clinical manifestations The clinical presentation reflects the slow expansion of tumor in the characteristic locations within the skull and spine, with neurologic deficits evolving over many years. Tumors of the parasellar region produce a combination of second, third, fourth, fifth, and sixth cranial nerve deficits. Cerebellopontine tumors may produce a syndrome similar to that of acoustic schwannomas (see "Tumors of the Posterior Fossa" below). Early hearing loss is not a typical finding in meningioma. Parasagittal and frontal tumors may produce seizures or may be entirely asymptomatic, often growing to enormous size before they are discovered. Parasagittal lesions that attain sufficient size may cause spastic paraparesis and incontinence. Falx meningioma should be considered in the differential diagnosis of gait disorders in the middle-aged and elderly. In all locations, meningiomas must be distinguished from similar-appearing dural metastases from breast, prostate, and lung.

Treatment Tumor site, rather than histology, is the major determinant of outcome. Intraventricular or parasagittal tumors are usually resectable and recurrence is rare. Those in the olfactory groove, sphenoid ridge, and parasellar locations are more difficult to resect completely and are prone to recur. Tumors of the foramen magnum may be totally removed with microneurosurgical techniques (see "Spinal Tumors" below). Radiation is advocated for malignant meningiomas and for incompletely excised symptomatic tumors of other histologic subtypes.

PAPILLOMA OF THE CHOROID PLEXUS **Definition** Neoplasms derived from choroid plexus epithelium are rare, representing only 0.5 percent of all intracranial tumors.

Pathogenesis and pathology In children most such tumors occur in the lateral ventricles, whereas in adults the fourth ventricle is the most common site. The histologic structure resembles normal choroid plexus, with a connective tissue core covered by a single layer of cuboidal epithelium.

Clinical manifestations Very rare examples of malignant transformation have been described. Metastases to the leptomeninges may occur. The tumor may secrete excessive CSF leading to communicating hydrocephalus.

Treatment Surgery is the treatment of choice and is usually highly successful.

LIPOMA Lipoma can develop anywhere within the brain or spinal cord, though the corpus callosum is the most common location. The association of lipomas with partial or complete agenesis of this structure and with other dysplastic or hamartomatous anomalies such as ectopias, colloid cysts, and epidermoids supports the theory that they are the result of disorders of development. Intraspinal lipomas are most common in the thoracic region and are associated with spina bifida in one-third of cases. All lipomas can be easily demonstrated by MRI. The treatment of symptomatic cranial and spinal lipomas is excision.

DERMOID AND EPIDERMOID TUMOR **Definition** The distinction between dermoid tumors and epidermoids (true cholesteatomas) is often difficult. Both result from inclusion of ectodermal tissue at the time of closure of the neural groove and soon thereafter.

Pathology and pathogenesis Cholesteatomas are slowly growing tumors that most often afflict young adults, occurring commonly in lateral or midline locations within the skull, i.e., the cerebellopontine angle, the suprasellar region, the fourth ventricle, the pineal region, and over the hemispheres. No clear relationship has been established between cholesteatoma of the cerebellopontine angle and middle ear infection. Dermoid tumors, which are frequently cystic, occur largely in the posterior fossa or in the lumbosacral region. Rarely they are found in suprasellar or pineal regions.

Clinical manifestations Symptoms vary according to the location of these tumors, the general pattern being slow evolution of defects attributable to the specific area with seizures interspersed when the tumor occupies cortical regions.

Treatment Treatment of the cholesteatoma is total surgical removal of the tumor together with its capsule. Dermoid tumors similarly are curable if total surgical excision is possible.

PRIMARY LYMPHOMA OF THE CENTRAL NERVOUS SYSTEM **Definition** Primary lymphomas are now recognized to be relatively common in the CNS. Before 1972, fewer than 25 cases had been identified at the Massachusetts General Hospital over a 50-year period. Since 1977, 10 cases per year have been diagnosed. Primary lymphoma is distinguished from the more frequent secondary involvement of the meninges that occurs in patients with poorly differentiated non-Hodgkin's lymphomas.

Pathogenesis and pathology The tumor is uncommon in patients without immunologic compromise. It is usually seen in patients with mixed humoral and cellular immune deficits. Three such disorders are recognized: inherited disorders of immunity such as combined immunodeficiency disease, selective IgM deficiency, or selective IgA abnormalities seen with ataxia-telangiectasia and Wiskott-Aldrich syndrome; acquired immunodeficiency syndrome (AIDS); and therapeutic immunosuppression following organ transplantation or treatment of autoimmune disorders. The demonstration of Epstein-Barr virus (EBV) DNA within primary lymphoma and of elevated titers of anti-EBV antibodies in affected patients raises the possibility that this agent plays a role in the pathogenesis of this disease.

The tumor may be focal or multicentric in the subcortical white matter, the walls of the ventricles, or the subarachnoid space. Tumor cells are always found in a perivascular distribution. At biopsy, tumor cells are often indistinguishable from normal lymphocytes, leading to an erroneous early diagnosis of "encephalitis" or "nonspecific perivascular inflammation." The cells may be characterized as malignant by monoclonal antibodies to immunoglobulin surface proteins. The tumors contain cells defined histologically as diffuse histiocytic or poorly differentiated lymphocytes by the Rappaport system and as follicular center cells and small cleaved cells by the Lukes-Collins system (see Chaps. 293 and 294). Burkitt-type lymphomas are rarely reported.

Clinical manifestations A history of personality change, focal deficits, or seizures evolving over several weeks in an immunosuppressed patient should raise the suspicion of cerebral lymphoma. Obviously, in these circumstances infection must be excluded. The CT scan typically reveals multiple periventricular masses which enhance with contrast (Fig. 345-3). A characteristic feature, rarely observed with other types of intracranial tumor, is the marked reduction or disappearance of lesions after a few weeks of high-dose corticosteroid therapy (dexamethasone 6 to 10 mg four times daily). When both symptoms and CT abnormalities resolve after corticosteroids, remissions lasting several months are common, and steroids can be tapered. Spontaneous remissions without corticosteroid therapy have been described. The usual clinical course is recurrence after 4 to 6 months, with resistance to steroid administration. The tumor may seed the meninges in one-quarter of patients. Systemic lymphoma is found in less than 10 percent of patients and occurs late in the course of the disease. However uveitis or vitreitis may occur at the time of presentation or early in the evolution of the disease; when present, it is helpful in the initial diagnosis.

Treatment After biopsy or diagnosis by CSF cytology, the recommended treatment is corticosteroids and radiation. The median survival is 17 months. Increasingly used is chemotherapy before radiation and at recurrence of tumor. High-dose methotrexate administered parenterally at 3.5 gm/m^2 followed by citrovorum factor rescue has been demonstrated to achieve therapeutic drug levels in brain parenchyma and most importantly, in the CSF. When methotrexate is administered prior to radiation, there is a reduced risk of radiation-drug white matter damage.

TUMORS OF THE THIRD VENTRICLE AND PINEAL REGION Several categories of tumors occur in close proximity to the diencephalon,

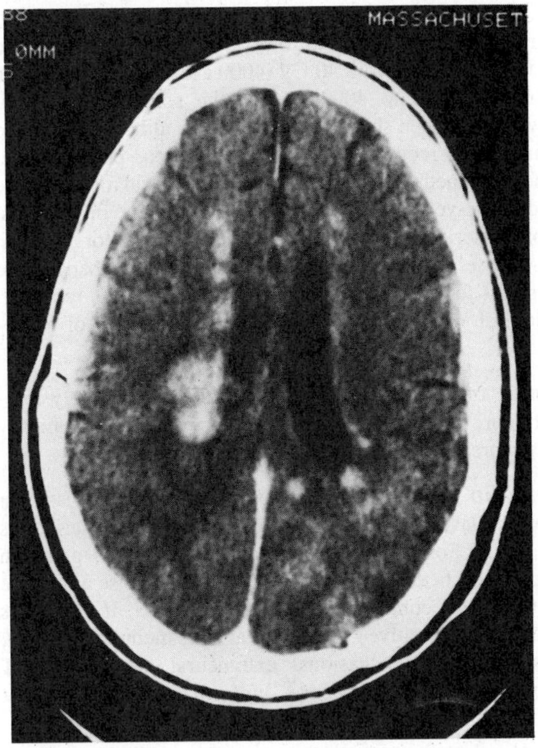

FIGURE 345-3 *Contrast-enhanced CT scan showing periventricular enhancement in a young man with primary CNS lymphoma. Note absence of surrounding edema.*

hypothalamus, and third ventricle; these are pituitary adenoma, craniopharyngioma, germ-cell neoplasms, pineal tumors, and glial, meningeal, or metastatic tumors.

Uncommon tumors of the pineal region include *astrocytomas, glioblastomas, meningiomas,* and *metastases*. Nonneoplastic masses occurring in this region include colloid cysts of the third ventricle (see "Colloid Cysts" below) and parasitic cysts (cysticercosis).

Pituitary adenomas These tumors are described in Chap. 321.

Craniopharyngiomas These tumors arise from remnants of Rathke's pouch, derived from the primitive stomatodeum. They are usually suprasellar in location and cause symptoms related to neuroendocrine dysfunction or visual compromise (see also Chap. 321).

Germ-cell tumors DEFINITION Germ-cell tumors, which account for half of all pineal region neoplasms, arise primarily during childhood or early adolescence and include germinoma, teratoma, embryonal carcinoma, endodermal sinus tumor, and choriocarcinoma.

CLINICAL MANIFESTATIONS The most common of these germ-cell tumors is the germinoma. It may occur in the pineal region or at the base of the hypothalamus. It occurs more frequently in males, who present with findings of diabetes insipidus and other neuroendocrine deficiences, bitemporal visual field defects, paralysis of upward gaze (see Chap. 13), and sometimes hydrocephalus. The typical features of pineal masses occur more commonly with nongerminomatous germ-cell tumors. Findings include Parinaud's syndrome—a failure of upward gaze and pupillary dilatation with deficiencies in response to light. Rarely, other signs such as nystagmus retractorius or brainstem signs due to compression may occur. Diagnosis may be assisted by the finding of elevated serum and CSF levels of alphafetoprotein (AFP) and of human chorionic gonadotropin (hCG) in germinomas.

TREATMENT Germinomas are radiosensitive; up to 80 percent are cured by well-tolerated doses of radiation. Other histologic subtypes have poorer prognoses and recurrence is common, often with seeding of the cranial nerves and meninges. Recurrences sometimes respond to drug treatment with etoposide, cisplatin, and doxorubicin, which are beneficial in testicular tumors of similar histology.

Pineoblastoma and pineocytoma These tumors account for 20 percent of growths in the pineal region.

PATHOGENESIS AND PATHOLOGY Pineoblastoma and pineocytoma arise from pineal organ cells. The pineoblastoma is a primitive malignant tumor of childhood and early adult life and is indistinguishable from primitive neuroectodermal tumors that arise elsewhere in the CNS. The tumor may contain astrocytic or neuronal elements. Recurrence is invariable and dissemination through the ventricular system and subarachnoid space is frequent.

TREATMENT Brain and neuraxis radiation are recommended, and chemotherapy as outlined above for germ-cell tumors has been successful in producing remissions in a few patients. The pineocytoma is a more slowly growing tumor which is often well-demarcated and resembles the normal structure of the pineal. Although histologically benign, it tends to recur, probably because of incomplete removal. It is resistant to radiation.

Colloid cysts PATHOGENESIS AND PATHOLOGY Colloid cysts arise within the anterior third ventricle and are considered to develop from the anlage of the paraphysis, a component of the third ventricle, or possibly from the ependyma itself. The cysts are well-encapsulated and consist of a layer of connective tissue covered with columnar ciliated cells. The cyst is filled with glycoproteinaceous material which stains with periodic acid Schiff (PAS).

CLINICAL MANIFESTATIONS Symptoms occur usually in adults and may be dramatic, with episodes of headache, weakness of the limbs, and loss of consciousness. These symptoms are attributed to intermittent acute hydrocephalus due to blockage of the foramen of Monro by the mobile cyst. Diagnosis cannot be made with certainty prior to operation; treatment is removal of the cyst.

TUMORS OF THE POSTERIOR FOSSA Tumors of the posterior fossa pose special problems in diagnosis and treatment. Rapidly growing tumors may cause obstructive hydrocephalus, and even small mass lesions in the posterior fossa may result in vomiting, lethargy, headache, and papilledema. Slowly growing tumors give rise to progressive signs which are recognized by rather specific syndromes. These include progressive unilateral hearing loss, facial weakness, pain or numbness, and a unilateral sixth nerve deficit occurring with tumors in the cerebellopontine angle. Gait ataxia and unilateral cerebellar signs occur with hemangioblastoma, medulloblastoma, or cystic astrocytoma of the cerebellum. Progressive diplopia, cranial nerve abnormalities, and crossed corticospinal tract and reflex abnormalities occur in brainstem glioma. Nuchal and occipital pain are common with all tumors of the posterior fossa. Corticospinal signs develop with further tumor enlargement and encroachment on the brainstem.

Acoustic schwannoma DEFINITION The acoustic schwannoma (synonymous with acoustic neuroma) is composed of myelin-forming Schwann cells that cover the acoustic nerve fibers. Schwann cells normally replace oligodendroglia as the nerve leaves the brain stem to enter the internal auditory meatus.

PATHOGENESIS AND PATHOLOGY Schwannomas are slow-growing masses that compress rather than invade normal tissue. When bilateral, they represent an inherited form of schwannoma which is diagnostic of "central" neurofibromatosis. Other CNS tumors associated with neurofibromatosis or von Recklinghausen's disease are schwannomas of spinal and other cranial nerves, intracranial and spinal meningiomas, gliomas, and ependymomas (see Chap. 351).

CLINICAL MANIFESTATIONS AND TREATMENT Early detection of acoustic schwannomas at a time of minimal hearing deficit and minimal facial motor difficulty is essential, as hearing may be spared by microneurosurgical intervention while the tumor is still restricted to the canal. Brainstem auditory-evoked responses, CT and MRI studies, and metrizamide cisternography have greatly enhanced the physician's ability to detect these tumors in their early stages.

Hemangioblastoma DEFINITION The cerebellar hemangioblastoma is an uncommon tumor which may be solitary but is frequently multiple. When the tumors are multiple, they are considered part of von Hippel-Lindau disease. This frequently familial syndrome typically consists of retinal, cerebellar, and spinal hemangioblastomas and visceral lesions, usually renal and/or pancreatic tumors or cysts. Polycythemia may be present.

PATHOGENESIS AND PATHOLOGY Hemangioblastomas are well-circumscribed and often cystic. The tumor may consist solely of a small nodule attached to the wall of a large cyst. The lesion is usually highly vascular and may be mistaken for an arteriovenous malformation. The microscopic appearance is one of numerous capillary vessels separated by sheets of clear cells with an abundance of intracytoplasmic vacuoles. The tumors are probably derived from capillary endothelial cells.

CLINICAL MANIFESTATIONS Dizziness, ataxia of gait or of the limbs, and symptoms of raised intracranial pressure are characteristic features of the cerebellar hemangioblastoma. The tumors may bleed spontaneously, resulting in a paroxysmal onset of headache and neurologic deficit.

TREATMENT Craniotomy with opening of the cerebellar cyst and excision of the mural tumor may be curative. Though the tumor is histologically benign, postoperative recurrences and the appearance of less operable spinal lesions worsen the prognosis. Patients with the von Hippel-Lindau syndrome should have periodic ophthalmologic evaluation for the appearance of retinal angiomas and general medical follow-up for early detection of renal tumors.

Ependymoma PATHOGENESIS AND PATHOLOGY These are glial tumors that occur chiefly in childhood and young adulthood, with a typical cranial location in the fourth ventricle. The tumor is composed of uniform ependymal cells surrounding a central lumen. Spinal ependymomas, which are more common, arise within the dura of the lumbar spine and represent more than half of spinal intramedullary gliomas. In this location, the prognosis is excellent.

TREATMENT Resection and radiation to the tumor site results in 5-year survival in excess of 80 percent for spinal cord lesions and between 30 percent and 50 percent for posterior fossa tumors. The role of chemotherapy in the treatment of local recurrences and of seeding within the subarachnoid space is not established.

PRIMITIVE NEUROECTODERMAL TUMORS (PNET) Several histologic varieties of tumor arise from primitive neuroectodermal tumors (PNET) which contain cells with a capacity to differentiate into medulloblasts, astrocytes, oligodendrocytes, ependyma, ganglion cells, or skeletal muscle. Some tumors have several cell types, but all PNETs share a propensity for local invasion, subarachnoid dissemination, and extraneural metastases. The initial evaluation should include CT scan and myelography with CSF cytology.

Medulloblastoma DEFINITION The *medulloblastoma* is the most common variety of PNET. It accounts for 25 percent of childhood brain tumors. However, one-fourth of medulloblastomas occur in patients over age 20.

PATHOGENESIS AND PATHOLOGY The tumor is usually located in the midline, in the inferior portion of the vermis of the cerebellum. It is composed of small, densely staining cells which elicit a brisk glial response. Invasion of the meninges, ventricles, and subarachnoid space is common.

CLINICAL MANIFESTATIONS The common presentation is occipital headache, vomiting, and trunkal ataxia. Hydrocephalus is frequent. With enlargement of the tumor other signs of brainstem compression emerge.

TREATMENT Resection of the tumor by resection is usually attempted, followed by radiation in doses of 45 to 50 Gy (4500 to 5000 rad) to the posterior fossa, together with 40 Gy (4000 rad) to the whole brain and 35 to 40 Gy (3500 to 4000 rad) to the spinal cord. Initial chemotherapy has not been shown to be effective, although it is used with some success in recurrent tumors. Nitrosourea, procarbazine, and vincristine combined with prednisone and intrathecal methotrexate are advocated. Five-year survival is nearly 75 percent in the most recently reported series. A pessimistic outlook exists for children under 3 years, those with large tumors, and those with subarachnoid spread. Metastases to lung, liver, vertebrae, and pelvis are reported. Some medulloblastomas may take on features reminiscent of neuroblastoma.

Neuroblastoma DEFINITION The neuroblastoma, a relatively common adrenal tumor, can rarely occur as a primary CNS tumor. Eighty percent of cases present during the first decade of life.

PATHOGENESIS AND PATHOLOGY Microscopically, neuroblastoma resembles medulloblastoma because of its dense small cells. Variations in pathology occur. Some tumors show differentiation to ganglion cells but do not have a better prognosis. The tumor can arise anywhere in the CNS but is most common in the posterior fossa. It resembles in its clinical behavior primitive glial tumors and the medulloblastoma, with neuraxis spread and occasional extraneural metastases. CT reveals a hypodense mass with dense, uniform enhancement after contrast administration, as well as variable hemorrhage and calcification.

TREATMENT Treatment of neuroblastoma consists of radical excision with postoperative radiation, though definitive evidence that radiation increases survival is lacking. Because of the frequency of local recurrence and CSF metastases, prophylactic spinal radiation may be justified. Chemotherapeutic trials have involved few patients and a variety of regimens. Long-term follow-up is incomplete, but with a greater than 30 percent 5-year survival, prognosis may be better than that of other primitive CNS tumors.

TUMORS OF THE SKULL BASE Tumors in this region produce characteristic clinical presentations which pose unique diagnostic difficulties even with advanced neuroradiologic procedures. Meningiomas, tumors of bone (including epidermoid and dermoid tumors and osteomas), chordomas, schwannomas (neurofibromas) of the cranial nerves, nasopharyngeal carcinoma, and metastases may all present with pain localized to the lower face, ear, or occiput and with involvement of one or more cranial nerves making exit from the skull. Metastases arise commonly from the lung, breast, nasopharynx, testicle, and prostate. Multiple myeloma and occasionally lymphoma may appear at this site. The mass may be palpable or may be visualized on polytomography, CT scan, or MRI; however, even a combination of all three studies may be negative. These studies usually differentiate successfully other erosive processes of the skull base, including fibrous dysplasia, Paget's disease, xanthomatosis, and osteitis fibrosa cystica. Enlargement of specific cranial nerve foramens may be the first evidence of schwannomas or of *glomus* tumors of the chromaffin cells in the jugular bulb. These last tumors invade temporal and occipital bone and produce hearing abnormalities and lower cranial nerve deficits.

Chordomas arise from remnants of the notochord. Of these, 60 percent are localized in the clivus, 30 percent in the sacral region, and the remaining 10 percent along the extent of the spine and skull base. They are highly invasive, expanding along the skull base and causing serial cranial nerve compression, sometimes with invasion of the nasopharynx. Up to one-third may metastasize via the subarachnoid space. A cauda equina syndrome (see "Spinal Tumors") results from sacral tumors. Clivus tumors may be difficult to visualize adequately on CT scan but are clearly delineated by MRI. Complete removal is rarely feasible and postoperative radiation therapy is recommended.

Metastases to the skull base are treated with radiation therapy. In the presence of characteristic patterns of pain and cranial nerve deficit, radiation may be considered to treat presumptive metastases in patients with known systemic malignancy even when radiographic examinations are inconclusive.

SPINAL TUMORS Pathogenesis and pathology Tumors of the spinal canal and of the cord are only one-quarter as common as are intracranial tumors. Spinal neoplasms arise from the same types of cells as their counterparts in the cerebrum. They are classified according to location as intramedullary (within the substance of the spinal cord), extramedullary (or intradural), and extradural. Some tumors, such as schwannomas, may be both extradural and intradural. The most frequent location for all types of spinal neoplasms is in the thoracic cord, presumably reflecting its greater total length. These tumors arise from cells of the spinal cord, nerve roots, meninges, vascular structures, or the vertebral column. Tumors of the spinal cord parenchyma are relatively infrequent compared to lesions arising outside the substance of the cord. In one large series, nerve sheath tumors (schwannomas) accounted for 29 percent of all spinal tumors, meningiomas for 25.5 percent, gliomas for 22 percent, and sarcomas for 12 percent. Metastatic lesions represent about 13 percent of all spinal tumors, but as with intracranial tumors, these figures reflect neurosurgical service statistics and metastases are likely underrepresented.

Clinical manifestations Any lesion that narrows the spinal canal sufficiently to encroach on neural structures can give rise to neurologic symptoms. Dysfunction may arise from direct compression of the spinal cord and its nerve roots or from interference with blood supply. The rapid growth of metastatic lesions leads to motor and sensory symptoms over a period of days to weeks, whereas slowly growing astrocytomas and ependymomas produce symptoms over a period of months to years.

Extramedullary tumors (both intradural and epidural) cause symptoms by compressing the spinal cord or nerve roots. The initial symptoms are usually focal back pain and paresthesias followed by sensory loss below the level of the pain, weakness, and bladder and bowel dysfunction. Intramedullary lesions usually extend over several spinal cord segments, and their symptoms and signs are more varied than those of extramedullary tumors. A common pattern is dissociated sensory loss, with pain and temperature sensation impairment in the segments of tumor origin and with sparing of posterior column sensory function. Later, as the tumor grows peripherally, spinothalamic tracts may be involved. Since, in the thoracic and cervical regions, the sacral pain and temperature fibers lie superficial to those fibers representing more rostral regions, the sacral segments may be spared. Atrophy in the appropriate segments due to anterior horn cell involvement may combine with corticospinal tract signs.

These clinical presentations are not diagnostic of spinal cord neoplasm. Transverse myelitis from multiple sclerosis or other causes can lead to rapid onset of spinal cord dysfunction associated with pain, paresthesias, and weakness (see Chap. 353). A similar syndrome can occur as a paraneoplastic process, resulting from a necrotic myelopathy (see Chap. 304). Syringomyelia can produce a chronic syndrome indistinguishable from that produced by intramedullary neoplasms. Other diseases that can lead to a progressive spinal cord syndrome include combined system degeneration due to vitamin B_{12} deficiency, amyotrophic lateral sclerosis, cervical spondylosis, arachnoiditis, vascular anomalies, meningeal carcinomatosis, and spinal stenosis due to a combination of degenerative disk disease and hypertrophy of the ligamentum flavum (see Chap. 353).

Additional specific clinical syndromes occur in two other locations within the spinal canal. *Foramen magnum tumors* may extend into the cervical region or rostrally into the posterior fossa. A combination of signs and symptoms referrable to lower cranial nerves, sensory loss in the distribution of the second cervical segment, posterior headache, and asymmetric sensory and motor involvement of the limbs leads to the suspicion of such a tumor, most commonly a meningioma. *Tumors of the conus medullaris or cauda equina* produce pain in the back, rectum, and/or both legs and may mimic lumbosacral disk disease. With tumor growth, muscle atrophy in the legs associated with sphincter dysfunction and reflex changes usually point to the correct site of involvement.

Diagnosis of spinal cord tumors Extradural metastastic spinal tumors cause changes in x-rays of the affected area in about 80 percent of cases. Lytic destructive lesions are the most common. Lymphomas less frequently show bony abnormalities. Radiographs aid in the diagnosis in only about 15 percent of primary spinal neoplasms, whether intradural or intramedullary in location. Findings include: changes in contour, separation of the pedicles, or enlargement of neural foramens which occur with schwannomas; proliferation of bone with meningiomas; and distortion of paraspinal tissues with masses that have grown into the spinal canal from extraneural sites. CT scans and MRI of the spine can demonstrate soft tissue masses encroaching on the canal and can visualize the bony structures; instillation of metrizamide is sometimes required to define the canal deformities of intraspinal tumor. When contrast medium flows into the cord, a diagnosis of syringomyelia may be established.

Magnetic resonance imaging (MRI) is now rapidly evolving as a useful diagnostic method for spinal cord tumor. Both intramedullary and extramedullary neoplasms are well seen with this technique and otherwise difficult to visualize regions such as the cervicomedullary junction are clearly evident. Meningeal carcinomatosis may also be suggested by MRI.

Myelography remains an important procedure for localizing and defining the level and extent of involvement. A small amount of contrast instilled at the beginning of the procedure can demonstrate whether a complete block is present; the rostral limit of the tumor can be defined by instillation of more dye through a lateral cervical puncture. Extramedullary lesions deform the contrast column on its outer surface, while intramedullary lesions widen the cord and displace the contrast laterally (see Chap. 353).

Cerebrospinal fluid removed at the time of myelography should be analyzed for cell count, protein content, and cytology. A specimen stained with Wright's stain should be analyzed and cells examined further after cytocentrifugation. The cell count is usually normal in spinal tumors unless there is meningeal tumor, but protein content is increased in virtually all cases of high-grade spinal cord block. The CSF glucose is usually normal unless there is meningeal tumor invasion.

Treatment Once the diagnosis of spinal cord tumor is established, rapid treatment is mandatory to maximize neurologic recovery. Extramedullary primary neoplasms are treated with microneurosurgery, and complete resection is usually possible. The most common intramedullary tumors, ependymomas and astrocytomas, usually can only be partially resected and are likely to recur. The role of radiation therapy for slowly growing tumors of this class is not well established; for high-grade astrocytomas a course of postoperative radiation is recommended. Corticosteroids may improve function temporarily. There is no established role for chemotherapy of spinal neoplasms.

EPIDURAL CANCER: THE PATIENT WITH CANCER AND BACK PAIN Spinal epidural cancer should be suspected in patients with back pain and known systemic malignancy even in the absence of neurologic signs. Progressive paraparesis with bladder dysfunction and development of a sensory deficit may be avoided by early intervention. High doses of steroids (up to 100 mg dexamethasone per day) are administered immediately and radiation therapy is usually recommended. The results of treatment in the large series of patients with epidural cancer reported by Gilbert has led to the conclusion that radiation therapy is as effective as surgery in the relief of symptoms. The clinical condition of the patient at the time of diagnosis is the most important factor in prognosis; only 3 percent of patients paraplegic at the time of treatment, regardless of type of therapy, regain ambulation. Reconsideration is being given to surgical decompression as a primary mode of treatment in patients with radioresistant malignancies such as melanoma and lung, prostatic, and colonic cancers and in the setting of paraparesis of recent onset.

PSEUDOTUMOR—BENIGN INTRACRANIAL HYPERTENSION Symptoms of increased intracranial pressure may occur in the absence of demonstrable parenchymal or leptomeningeal tumor or hydrocephalus. However, little distinguishes the symptomatic presentation of true tumor from that of pseudotumor, which includes headache, papilledema, visual blurring and obscurations with enlargement of the blind spot, diplopia, nausea, and vomiting. Pseudotumor usually afflicts young, often obese women; it occurs most often in the absence of systemic cancer and focal neurologic difficulties. The marked increases in intracranial pressure may reflect impaired venous drainage within the brain or skull or may accompany the hormonal alterations of pregnancy, oral contraceptive use, or obesity. Less-common predisposing endocrinologic illnesses include both hypo- and hyperthyroidism, adrenal insufficiency, and both endogenous and exogenous excess of adrenocorticoids. A variety of drugs have been implicated, including supplemental vitamin A, tetracycline, nalidixic acid, nitrofurantoin, and sulfa preparations. The diagnosis is confirmed by the exclusion of an intracranial mass lesion or meningeal cancer. In the presence of a normal or small ventricular system on CT scan, lumbar puncture carries no risk for brain herniation. Cerebrospinal fluid is invariably under increased pressure but is otherwise unremarkable. Treatment is aimed at prevention of visual deficits and lasting symptoms by reducing the CSF volume by repetitive lumbar punctures. The removal of an offending drug or metabolic cause will reverse symptoms within 1 week's time. Patients refractory to this may benefit from acetazolamide, furosemide, or short-term corticosteroid therapy. Lumboperitoneal shunting and surgical decompression are reserved for patients with progressive visual impairment who have failed medical therapy. The outlook for most patients is excellent—fully 80 percent respond to conservative therapy, but as many as 10 percent experience permanent or recurrent visual deficits.

REFERENCES

DEUTSCH M et al: Radiotherapy for intracranial metastases. Cancer 34:1607, 1974

GILBERT RW et al: Epidural spinal cord compression from metastatic tumor: Diagnosis and treatment. Ann Neurol 3:40, 1978

GRAUS F et al: Cerebrovascular complications in patients with cancer. Medicine (Baltimore) 64(1):16, 1985

HART R et al: Acoustic tumors: Atypical features and recent diagnostic tests. Neurology (NY) 33:211, 1983

HELLE TL et al: Primary lymphoma of the central nervous system: J Neurosurg 60:94, 1984

HOCHBERG FH et al: Central nervous system lymphoma related to Epstein-Barr virus. N Engl J Med 309:745, 1983

JENNINGS MT et al: Intracranial germ cell tumors: Natural history and pathogenesis. J Neurosurg 63:155, 1985

LAWS ER et al: Neurosurgical management of low grade astrocytomas of the cerebral hemispheres. J Neurosurg 61:665, 1984

SUNDAESAN N, GALICICH JH: Surgical treatment of brain metastases: Cancer 55:1382, 1985

WALKER MD (ed): *Cancer Treatment and Research Series, Oncology of the Nervous System.* WL McGuire, (series ed). Boston, Martinus Nijhoff, 1983

——— et al: Randomized comparison of radiation therapy and nitrosoureas for the treatment of malignant glioma of the brain. N Engl J Med 303:1323, 1980

WARA WM: Radiation therapy for brain tumors. Cancer 55:2291, 1985

WASSERSTROM WR: Diagnosis and treatment of leptomeningeal metastases from solid tumors. Cancer 49:759, 1982

WEISS L et al: *Brain Metastases,* Boston, Hall, 1980

YOUNG DP: Neurological complications of chemotherapy, in *Neurological Complications of Therapy,* A Silverstein (ed). Mount Kisco, NY, Futura Publishing Co, 1982, pp 57–113

346 PYOGENIC INFECTIONS OF THE CENTRAL NERVOUS SYSTEM

DONALD H. HARTER / ROBERT G. PETERSDORF

Pyogenic infections of the cranial contents originate in one of two ways, by hematogenous spread or by extension from surface structures, paranasal sinuses, osteomyelitic foci in the skull, penetrating cranial injuries, congenital sinus tracts, or following neurosurgical procedures.

ACUTE BACTERIAL MENINGITIS

DEFINITION Bacterial meningitis may be defined as an inflammation of the pia-arachnoid and the fluid residing in the space which it encloses and also that in the ventricles of the brain. Since the subarachnoid space is continuous around the brain, spinal cord, and the optic nerves, an infective agent (or tumor cells or blood) gaining entry to any one part of it may extend immediately to all of it, even its most remote recesses; therefore, meningitis is always *cerebrospinal.* It also reaches the ventricles, either directly or by reflux through the basal foramens of Magendie and Luschka.

PATHOLOGY The effect of bacteria or other organisms in the subarachnoid space is to cause an inflammatory reaction in the pia and arachnoid and in the cerebrospinal fluid (CSF); in pyogenic meningitis, pus accumulates in this space. The infective agent or its toxin, if allowed sufficient time to act, injures those structures which lie within the subarachnoid space (cranial and spinal roots) or ventricles (choroid plexuses) and adjacent to it (pial arteries and veins, underlying cerebral and cerebellar cortices, subpial white matter of the spinal cord, peripheral fibers of optic nerves, ependymal and subependymal tissues). In addition, purulent material may interfere with the flow of CSF from the ventricles or along the subarachnoid space over the brainstem, with resulting obstructive hydrocephalus. Although the outer arachnoidal membrane proves to be a remarkably effective barrier to the extension of infection, some reaction in the cranial subdural space and even in the inner surface of the dura and the spinal epidural space may occur. This happens more often in infants, approximately 15 percent of whom develop subdural effusions in response to meningitis, than in adults.

The most immediate clinical effects of acute subarachnoid suppuration, distinguishing it from infections in other parts of the body, are severe headache, vomiting, drowsiness, stupor, or coma, and, occasionally, convulsions. The one clinical sign of importance is stiffness of the neck (resistance to passive movement) on forward bending. Kernig's and Brudzinski's signs are of the same nature but less reliable.

ETIOLOGY The causes of bacterial meningitis vary with age as follows:

1 *Streptococcus pneumoniae* (see Chap. 93) causes 30 to 50 percent of cases in adults, 10 to 20 percent in children, and up to 5 percent of cases in infants.
2 *Neisseria meningitidis* (see Chap. 103) causes from 10 to 35 percent of cases in adults and from 25 to 40 percent in children up to age 15. It is a rare cause in infants.
3 *Haemophilus influenzae,* type B (see Chap. 109) is responsible for 40 to 60 percent of cases in children, but for only 1 to 3 percent in adults and for virtually none in infants.

Also important in the etiology of meningitis are *Staphylococcus aureus* and *Staph. epidermidis;* the latter accounts for 75 percent of infections associated with shunting procedures for hydrocephalus. Other causative organisms include group B streptococci, particularly in infants; anaerobic or microaerophilic streptococci and gram-negative bacilli, usually in association with brain abscess, epidural abscess, head trauma, neurosurgical procedures, or cranial thrombophlebitis; *Escherichia coli* and other Enterobacteriaceae such as *Klebsiella-Enterobacter, Proteus, Citrobacter, Pseudomonas,* and *Acinetobacter calcoaceticus,* usually as a consequence of head trauma, neurosurgical procedures, spinal anesthesia, lumbar puncture, or shunting procedures to relieve hydrocephalus. Heretofore, gram-negative bacilli were associated most often with neonatal meningitis, but the spectrum has shifted to adults with debilitating diseases and other predisposing causes. Almost one-fifth of bacterial meningitis cases occurring in persons 50 years of age or older are due to gram-negative enteric bacteria. The outcome in this group has been notoriously poor. Rare meningeal pathogens include *Salmonella, Shigella, Clostridium perfringens,* and *Neisseria gonorrhoeae.*

The changing etiology of bacterial meningitis is reflected by the appearance of *Listeria monocytogenes* as a major pathogen, particularly in elderly, debilitated patients or in those with immunosuppression secondary to transplantation, receiving therapy for cancer, or with connective tissue diseases. Alcoholism and high-dose steroids also appear to be predisposing factors. *Listeria* meningitis accounts for approximately 2 percent of all reported cases of bacterial meningitis in the United States. The mortality rate in the adult group with severe underlying disease is 70 percent.

EPIDEMIOLOGY AND CLINICAL SETTING The incidence of bacterial meningitis is between 4.6 and 10 cases per 100,000 persons per year. *H. influenzae* is the most frequent cause, followed by *N. meningitidis* and *S. pneumoniae.* About 70 percent of all cases occur in children under the age of 5. Pneumococcal, *H. influenzae,* and meningococcal infections have a worldwide distribution, tending to occur more often in males and during the fall, winter, and spring. *H. influenzae* meningitis is the most frequent meningeal infection in children between 2 months and 3 years of age. Meningococcal infections occur most often in children and adolescents, but they are also encountered throughout most of adult life with a sharp decline after age 50. Meningococcal meningitis differs from other forms of meningitis because it may occur in epidemics. Pneumococcal meningitis predominates in adults over 40 years of age.

A variety of factors apart from age predispose to the development of certain types of acute bacterial meningitis. Acute otitis media and mastoiditis occur in about 25 percent of patients with pneumococcal meningitis, and pneumonia occurs in another 25 percent. Recent head injury is recorded in 10 to 20 percent of patients with pneumococcal meningitis and may give rise to recurrent meningitis because of persistent cerebrospinal fluid rhinorrhea. Pneumococcal meningitis also occurs in patients with sickle cell disease, Hodgkin's disease, or multiple myeloma; in urban general hospitals many adults who develop pneumococcal infections suffer from chronic alcoholism. Immunoglobulin deficiency (whether congenital or acquired), splenectomy, and renal or bone marrow transplantation also predispose patients to pneumococcal infection. Adults who develop *H. influenzae* meningitis should be suspected of harboring an anatomic defect (dermal sinus tract, old skull fracture) or abnormality of immune defenses, diabetes mellitus, or alcoholism. Meningitis caused by *Staph. aureus* usually follows neurosurgical procedures or a penetrating cranial wound. This organism and *Staph. epidermidis* account for the majority of cerebral ventricular shunt infections and occasionally neonatal omphalitis and meningitis. Gram-negative bacillary infections also complicate neurosurgical operations and other nosocomial diseases; they are assuming progressively greater importance in meningitis in adults. Bacterial meningitis can also occur by extension from an abscess of the psoas muscle.

PATHOGENESIS The three common meningeal pathogens are invasive and depend upon antiphagocytic capsular or surface antigens for survival in the tissues of the infected host; all express their pathogenicity largely in the form of extracellular proliferation. All three are inhabitants of the nasopharynx in a significant part of the population. It is evident from the frequency with which the carrier state is detected that nasal colonization is not a sufficient explanation for infection of the meninges. The factors which predispose the colonized patient to bloodstream invasion, which is the usual route by which bacteria reach the meninges, are obscure but include antecedent viral infections of the upper respiratory passages or, as in the case of the pneumococcus, infections in the lung. Once bloodborne, the factors which lead to meningeal localization of bacteria are unknown, but it has been postulated that pneumococci, *H. influenzae,* and meningococci possess a unique predilection for the meninges. Other possibilities are that the entry of bacteria into the subarachnoid space is facilitated by disruption of the blood-CSF barrier by trauma, circulating endotoxin, or an initial viral infection of the meninges.

Avenues other than the bloodstream by which bacteria can gain access to the meninges include congenital neuroectodermal defects, craniotomy sites, diseases of the middle ear and paranasal sinuses, and cranial trauma, notably skull fractures. Occasionally brain abscesses may rupture into the subarachnoid space or ventricles, infecting the meninges. The isolation of anaerobic streptococci, *Bacteroides* spp., or *Actinomyces* or of a mixture of microorganisms in the CSF should suggest the possibility of a brain abscess occurring as an antecedent to meningitis.

SYMPTOMATOLOGY Fever, headache, seizures, vomiting, impairment of consciousness, and stiff neck and back are common to bacterial meningitis irrespective of its etiology. When the initial symptoms are pain in the neck or abdomen, a confusional state, or delirium, the diagnosis is much more difficult. Three patterns of onset have been documented. In approximately 25 percent of patients, meningitis has a fulminant onset and patients become seriously ill within 24 h, usually without antecedent respiratory tract infections. In over 50 percent, meningitis develops over 1 to 7 days and is associated with respiratory symptoms. Slightly less than 20 percent have meningeal symptoms after 1 to 3 weeks of respiratory symptoms.

In children, the onset is often nonspecific. Fever and vomiting are more frequent than headache. There is a higher incidence of seizures, and the error of misinterpreting seizures as febrile convulsions is greater. The classic signs of meningitis may often be minimal in elderly, debilitated patients where low-grade fever and changes in mental status may occur without headache or nuchal rigidity.

There are certain special clinical features that correlate with particular types of meningitis. Meningococcal meningitis should always be suspected in epidemics of meningitis; when the evolution is extremely rapid; when the onset is attended by a morbilliform, petechial, or purpuric skin eruption, larger ecchymoses, and lividity of skin of lower parts of the body; and if circulatory collapse has occurred. Since a rash accompanies approximately 50 percent of meningococcal infections, its presence should dictate immediate institution of therapy for a neisserial infection, even though similar rashes may be observed with echovirus type 9 meningitis and rarely with staphylococcal, *H. influenzae,* and streptococcal meningitis. Recurrent systemic infections should lead to the suspicion of complement deficiency. A family history of fulminant meningococcal disease in males in skipped generations suggests properdin deficiency. Pneumococcal meningitis is usually preceded by an infection in the lungs, ears, and sinuses, and the heart valves may be affected. In addition a pneumococcal etiology should be suspected in patients suffering from alcoholism, sickle cell disease, and basal skull fracture and following splenectomy or organ transplantation. *H. influenzae* meningitis usually follows upper respiratory and ear infections in young children.

The signs of meningeal irritation—stiff neck or positive Kernig's and Brudzinski's signs—may be absent in the very young, the very old, or the severely obtunded. Signs of focal cerebral disease, although seldom prominent, are more frequent in pneumococcal and influenzal meningitis and are associated with a comparatively poor prognosis. Seizures are encountered most often in infants with *H. influenzae* meningitis. In some instances they are caused by hypoglycemia or penicillin neurotoxicity, especially the latter if they are preceded by myoclonus of the face and extremities. Some of the more transitory focal cerebral signs may represent postictal phenomena (Todd's paralysis); stable, local, cerebral lesions are probably the result of vasculitis and occlusion of cerebral veins with infarction of cerebral tissue, or they may connote localization of pus as occurs in brain abscess or subdural empyema. Abnormalities involving the third, fourth, and sixth as well as other cranial nerves are particularly frequent with pneumococcal meningitis.

LABORATORY FINDINGS The alterations of the cerebrospinal fluid are diagnostic. The *number of leukocytes* in the CSF ranges between 1000 and 100,000 per milliliter but averages between 5000 and 20,000. Cell counts above 50,000 per milliliter raise suspicion of the possibility of a brain abscess having ruptured into the ventricle (ventricular empyema). Neutrophilic leukocytes generally predominate, but an increasing proportion of mononuclear cells are found in the exudate as the infection continues, especially in partially treated meningitis. CSF lymphocytosis occurs in about one-third of bacterial meningitis patients with CSF cell counts of 1000 per milliliter or less. In the early stages careful cytologic examination may reveal some of the mononuclear cells to be myelocytes or young neutrophils. Later, as treatment takes effect, the proportions of lymphocytes, plasma cells, and histiocytes steadily increase.

The CSF *pressure* is so consistently elevated (above 180 mmH_2O) that a normal or low pressure on the initial lumbar puncture in a case of suspected bacterial meningitis should raise the possibility that the needle was partially occluded or that the spinal arachnoid space was blocked.

The *protein levels* of CSF are higher than 45 mg/dL in 90 percent of cases, and most determinations fall in the range of 150 to 500 mg/dL.

The *sugar concentration* of CSF is depressed, usually to a level lower than 40 mg/dL or less than 40 percent of the blood sugar concentration (measured concomitantly), provided the latter is less than 250 mg/dL. However in atypical or "culture-negative cases," other conditions associated with a depressed CSF glucose should be considered. These include hypoglycemia from any cause, sarcoidosis of the central nervous system, meningeal carcinomatosis or gliomatosis, fungal or tuberculous meningitis, and subarachnoid hemorrhage. In acute cases of pyogenic meningitis, the CSF glucose concentration often approaches zero.

Gram stain of sedimented CSF permits identification of the causative agent in most cases of bacterial meningitis; it will be positive in about three-fourths of patients with untreated bacterial meningitis. Pneumococci and *H. influenzae* are identified more readily than are meningococci. Small numbers of gram-negative diplococci present within leukocytes may be indistinguishable from nuclear material which may also be gram-negative and of the same shape. In such cases a thin film of uncentrifuged CSF may lend itself more readily to morphologic interpretation than will a smear of sedimented CSF. The commonest errors in reading Gram-stained smears of CSF are misinterpretation of precipitated dye or debris as gram-positive cocci and confusion of pneumococci with *H. influenzae*. *Haemophilus* organisms may stain heavily at the poles so that they resemble gram-positive diplococci, and older pneumococci often lose their capacity to take a gram-positive stain. *Listeria monocytogenes* may be misidentified as a "diphtheroid" or hemolytic streptococcus in the microbiology laboratory. Staining with acridine orange and examination under a fluorescence microscope may demonstrate bacteria not observed with the Gram stain.

Cerebrospinal fluid cultures are positive in 70 to 80 percent of cases. When brain abscess is suspected, anaerobic cultures should be made, and meningococci should be cultured under 10% CO_2 (see Chap. 83). Partially treated meningitis poses a most difficult problem in diagnosis because cultures are often negative. The measurement of bacterial antigen in the CSF by latex agglutination tests or countercurrent immune electrophoresis (CIE) to determine the presence of a specific capsular polysaccharide associated with *H. influenzae* type B, *S. pneumoniae*, and meningococcal serogroups A, B, C, and Y has been helpful. It has limited value in *E. coli* and streptococcal group B infections. Latex agglutination appears the more sensitive of the two procedures. Detection of antigen in the serum or urine of bacterial meningitis patients is not a sensitive diagnostic method. The concentration of bacterial antigen diminishes as treatment progresses. Failure to detect antigen does not rule out bacterial meningitis.

The *Limulus* amebocyte gelation assay for endotoxin may be of diagnostic help, particularly in meningitis with trauma or following neurosurgery, where infection with *N. meningitidis* and *H. influenzae* (which also give a positive result) are uncommon causes. Measurements of the CSF C-reactive protein, lactic acid concentration, and lactic dehydrogenase (LDH) activity and isoenzyme pattern have been reported to be of help in differentiating bacterial from viral meningitis. The accuracy and usefulness of these tests are limited because elevated levels have been observed in a variety of conditions other than meningitis. Repeat CSF examination may provide an answer when the diagnosis is in question.

In addition to CSF cultures, *blood cultures* should always be obtained because they are positive in 40 to 60 percent of patients with *H. influenzae* and with meningococcal and pneumococcal meningitis and may provide the only definitive clue to the causative agent (if CSF cultures are negative). Routine cultures of the pharynx or external ear are as often misleading as helpful because pneumococci, *H. influenzae,* and meningococci are such common inhabitants of these locations. However, culture of pus from the middle ear or sinuses is often helpful.

The *blood leukocyte count* is generally elevated, and usually there is a shift to the left. Most patients with meningitis are sufficiently ill to require determination of blood urea nitrogen and serum electrolytes. These may be abnormal because of severe dehydration and may reveal inappropriate secretion of antidiuretic hormone (AVP) with resultant hyponatremia.

ROENTGENOGRAPHIC STUDIES Patients with bacterial meningitis should have x-rays of the chest, skull, and sinuses as soon as possible after admission. Chest x-rays are particularly important because they may reveal a silent area of pneumonitis or abscess. Sinus and skull films may provide clues to the presence of cranial osteomyelitis, paranasal sinusitis, or skull fracture. Computerized tomography (CT scan) is usually not necessary in bacterial meningitis and is normal early in most infections. In severe cases there may be evidence of cerebritis, vascular occlusions, and encephalomalacia. Later in the course, CT will detect hydrocephalus, brain abscess, and subdural effusions or subdural empyema. If bacterial meningitis is suspected and the patient does not have papilledema or focal neurologic findings, lumbar puncture should not be delayed while waiting for a CT scan to be done.

COMPLICATIONS OF BACTERIAL MENINGITIS The longer the duration of meningitis and the less effective the treatment, the greater the chances that complications and neurologic residua will develop. The cranial nerve palsies, usually third, sixth, seventh, and eighth nerves, which occur in some 10 to 20 percent of cases usually disappear within a few weeks. Approximately 10 percent of infants and children who have bacterial meningitis will be left with persistent unilateral or bilateral sensory hearing loss. The cochlea may be damaged by infection as it passes from the meninges along the cochlear duct. Deafness is especially frequent with pneumococcal and meningococcal meningitis. If focal and lateralizing neurologic signs last for some days or occur late in the course of meningitis, they are usually indicative of a vasculitis and cerebral infarction. Such lesions are most extensive in children with *H. influenzae* meningitis who are inadequately treated. If these lesions are extensive, they may leave the child retarded and epileptic. Persistent coma is more common in pneumococcal meningitis in adults. In infants or very young children with bacterial meningitis (particularly due to *H. influenzae*), prolonged alteration in state of consciousness or increased intracranial pressure (ICP) should raise the suspicion of obstructive hydrocephalus and subdural effusions.

DIFFERENTIAL DIAGNOSIS The diagnosis of bacterial meningitis is not difficult, providing a high index of suspicion is maintained. All febrile patients with lethargy, headache, or confusion of sudden onset, even if only low-grade fever is present, should be subjected to lumbar puncture. It is particularly important to consider meningitis in febrile, confused alcoholic patients. Too often the symptoms are mistakenly ascribed to inebriation, delirium tremens, or hepatic encephalopathy until the CSF reveals a meningitis.

Bacterial meningitis can be diagnosed definitively only by examination of the CSF. Viral meningoencephalitis and tuberculous, leptospiral, and fungal meningitides often enter into the differential diagnosis. Also to be considered are Behçet's syndrome, a disease characterized by recurrent oral and genital ulcers along with meningitis, and Mollaret's meningitis, which consists of recurrent episodes of fever, headache, and meningeal irritation accompanied by a leukocytosis in the CSF.

The diagnosis of other intracranial suppurative diseases is detailed below.

PROGNOSIS The case fatality rate for bacterial meningitis in the United States approximates 14 percent; it is highest for gram-negative and miscellaneous causes of meningitis. Of the three common forms of meningitis, pneumococcal meningitis is the most lethal. The triad of pneumococcal meningitis, pneumonia, and endocarditis has a particularly high fatality rate. The case fatality rate of *H. influenzae* or meningococcal meningitis has remained fixed at 5 to 15 percent for many years. Also in meningococcal infection, because of the fulminating nature of the disease and the often complicating adrenocortical necrosis (Waterhouse-Friderichsen syndrome), the mortality rate remains significant. Old age, infancy, abrupt onset, bacteremia, coma, seizures, and a variety of concomitant diseases including alcoholism, diabetes mellitus, multiple myeloma, and head trauma all worsen the prognosis.

It is often impossible to explain the death of the patient or at least to trace it to a single specific mechanism. Bacteremia with hypotension or brain swelling and bilateral temporal and/or cerebellar herniation are clearly implicated in the deaths of some patients during the initial 48 h. These events may occur in bacterial meningitis of any etiology; however, some observations suggest that they are more important in meningococcal infection. There is experimental evidence that acute centrally mediated respiratory failure (rather than circulatory collapse) is the major mechanism of early death. Deaths occurring later during the course of illness may be attributed to necrosis of brain tissue and respiratory failure, often consequent to aspiration pneumonia.

TREATMENT Antimicrobials Bacterial meningitis is a medical emergency; the rapid destruction of bacteria in the meninges and in the CSF is essential to survival. For this reason, bactericidal drugs should be used where possible. The following therapeutic regimens are recommended:

1 For adults with *pneumococcal* or *meningococcal meningitis*, penicillin G, 20 to 24 million units intravenously each day in four to six divided doses, is recommended; for children the dose of penicillin G should be 300,000 units per kilogram of body weight; and for neonates, up to one month of age, 150,000 to 200,000 units per kilogram of body weight. Chloramphenicol, 4 to 6 g given intravenously in divided doses, is an alternative treatment regimen in adults.
2 For children over 2 months of age with *H. influenzae* or uncomplicated meningitis of unknown etiology, ampicillin, 300 to 400 mg per kilogram of body weight intravenously in divided doses, plus chloramphenicol, 100 to 200 mg/kg per day intravenously, should be given. The reason for the use of two drugs is that 15 to 25 percent of *H. influenzae* isolates are resistant to ampicillin; a few strains of chloramphenicol-resistant *H. influenzae* have also been reported. In order to avoid interference between the two drugs, ampicillin should be given 30 min before chloramphenicol. Once the etiologic organism and its sensitivity have been determined, chloramphenicol can be discontinued if the organism is sensitive to ampicillin. In adults with *H. influenzae* meningitis, the doses of ampicillin (12 to 18 g daily) and chloramphenicol (4 to 6 g daily) are administered intravenously either as a constant infusion or in divided doses.
3 In adult patients with any of these types of bacterial meningitis who may be allergic to the penicillins, chloramphenicol in a dosage of 4 to 6 g per day intravenously may be used. The cephalosporins are questionable alternates for pneumococcal meningitis, and there have been some failures also in *H. influenzae* and meningococcal meningitis; hence, chloramphenicol is preferred in infections due to these organisms.
4 In community-acquired meningitis due to a gram-negative enteric bacillus, the organism is usually susceptible to third-generation cephalosporins; therapy should begin with either cefotaxime or moxalactam (2 g every 4 h). If gram-negative enteric meningitis is acquired in the hospital or follows head trauma or neurosurgery, *Pseudomonas aeruginosa* and *Acinetobacter calcoaceticus* are also likely pathogens and cefotaxime or moxalactam is given in combination with tobramycin intravenously (5 mg/kg daily) and intrathecally (8 to 10 mg daily). The antibiotic regimen can be modified when the bacterial species has been identified and its sensitivity to antimicrobials determined. Trimethoprim-sulfamethoxazole (TMP-SMX) may provide a useful alternative for gram-negative meningitis when the causative agent is resistant to cephalosporins such as cefotaxime.
5 Meningitis due to *Staphylococcus aureus* should be treated with a penicillinase-resistant penicillin rather than penicillin G because over 80 percent of isolates are penicillin-resistant. Nafcillin or oxacillin in daily doses of 12 to 18 g can be used alone or in combination with rifampin, 600 mg each day, in adult patients. Patients allergic to penicillin can be given vancomycin, 2.0 mg intravenously in divided doses.
6 When the etiology of meningitis is unknown, the drugs of choice are as follows: in adults, ampicillin 12 g per day in divided doses; in children, ampicillin 400 mg/kg and chloramphenicol 100 mg/kg over 24 h; and in neonates, ampicillin 100 to 200 mg/kg per day and an aminoglycoside, usually gentamicin (5 mg/kg per day), are recommended.
7 Foci of infection in the paranasal sinuses or mastoids, in an infected shunt, or in cranial osteomyelitis should be identified so that appropriate drainage may be carried out when the acute episode of meningitis has subsided.
8 In most patients bacterial meningitis need not be treated for longer than 10 days except when there is a persistent parameningeal focus of infection. Antibiotics should be administered in full doses parenterally (preferably intravenously) throughout the period of treatment. Treatment failures with several drugs, notably ampicillin, are attributable to oral or intramuscular administration, resulting in inadequate concentration in the CSF.
9 Repeated lumbar punctures are not necessary to follow the course of therapy as long as the patient is doing well. The CSF sugar may remain low for a number of days after cultures become negative and should occasion concern only if bacteria are present. Likewise, persistent but steadily diminishing mononuclear pleocytosis, following pyogenic meningitis, is the rule. CSF examination at the end of treatment for bacterial meningitis in patients who have recovered clinically is not useful because it may lead to unnecessary detention in the hospital or fail to identify patients who need further treatment.

Adrenocortical steroids The few controlled studies available have demonstrated that steroids exert no beneficial effects in pyogenic meningitis. These drugs should not be used except possibly in overwhelming meningococcal sepsis or as an adjunct to intravenous mannitol in severe cerebral edema.

Other forms of therapy Intrathecal administration of enzymes to lyse excessive subarachnoid cellular exudate which may be associated with spinal block or hydrocephalus in the subacute stages of bacterial meningitis is of no value. There is also no evidence to support the therapeutic efficacy of repeated drainage of CSF. In fact, increased CSF pressure in the acute phases of bacterial meningitis is largely a consequence of cerebral edema, and lumbar puncture may predispose to temporal lobe or cerebellar herniation and death. Mannitol and urea have been employed apparently successfully in some cases of severe brain swelling with unusually high initial CSF pressures (>400 mmH_2O). Either should be accompanied by dexamethasone in relatively high doses. An adequate but not excessive amount of parenteral fluids should be given, and phenytoin should be given to control seizures. In children care should be taken to avoid hyponatremia and water intoxication—a cause of brain swelling. Subdural effusions should be drained repeatedly by subdural taps; if they persist after the infection has subsided, surgical removal may become necessary.

RECURRENT MENINGITIS

Recurrent attacks of bacterial meningitis usually follow in the wake of trauma. The interval between the traumatic episode and the initial bout of posttraumatic meningitis may be as long as several years. *S. pneumoniae* is the usual bacterial pathogen. Often it proves to be one of the higher serologic types, reflecting the predominance of such strains in nasal carriers. *Cerebrospinal fluid rhinorrhea* is present in most of these patients but may be transient. The patient with recurrent meningitis of inapparent origin should always be suspected of having a fistulous connection between the nasal sinuses and the subarachnoid space. The fistula is usually traumatic (old basal skull fracture), and the site is the frontal or ethmoid sinuses or the cribriform plate. The rhinorrhea may be difficult to demonstrate except by injection of a radioactive tracer into the CSF and watching for its appearance in nasal secretions. Cerebrospinal fluid rhinorrhea may also be detected by measuring the glucose concentration of nasal secretions. The usual mucous secretions contain little glucose, but in CSF rhinorrhea the amount approximates that in CSF. The prognosis in recurrent meningitis is remarkably benign, and the mortality is much lower than in ordinary pneumococcal meningitis. Nevertheless, vaccination of these patients with pneumococcal vaccine is indicated, and long-term prophylactic chemotherapy with penicillin V should be considered. Treatment of recurrent meningitis is similar to that for first bouts. Attempts to demonstrate CSF rhinorrhea should be made only after the acute infection has subsided; if evidence of a fistula is found, surgical repair should be considered.

Other causes of recurrent meningitis include congenital bony abnormalities of the inner ear, congenital dermal sinus tract, and tumors at the base of the skull.

SUBDURAL EMPYEMA

DEFINITION Subdural empyema is a suppurative process in the cranial subdural space between the inner surface of the dura and the outer of the arachnoid. The proper term for this condition is not *abscess* but *empyema,* indicating suppuration in a preformed space. Subdural empyema accounts for approximately one-fifth of all localized intracranial infections. About three-fourths of cases are unilateral, and the remainder bilateral, usually in the parafalcial region.

ETIOLOGY The infection usually gains entry to the subdural space from the frontal or ethmoid sinuses or, less often, from the mastoid cells. These cases are termed *primary* subdural empyema. The subdural space may also become infected by extension of bacteria from a contiguous site of osteomyelitis or from a brain abscess. Septic thrombophlebitis and venous drainage of bacteria to the subdural space may be important in its development. Rarely has it been observed with bloodstream infections. Secondary subdural empyema usually follows neurosurgical drainage of a chronic subdural hematoma.

The bacterial flora in subdural empyema closely resembles that seen in chronic sinusitis and brain abscess; it may be polymicrobial. Isolates in order of decreasing frequency include aerobic streptococci, staphylococci, microaerophilic and anaerobic streptococci, aerobic gram-negative rods, and other anaerobes.

PATHOLOGY A collection of subdural pus in quantities of a few milliliters to 100 to 200 mL lies over the cerebral hemisphere. It is often mistaken for meningitis. The arachnoid, when cleared of exudate, is cloudy, and thrombosis of meningeal veins may be seen. The underlying cerebral hemisphere is depressed, and in fatal cases there is often an ipsilateral temporal lobe pressure cone. Microscopic studies demonstrate various degrees of organization of the exudate on the inner surface of the dura and infiltration of the underlying pia with small numbers of neutrophilic leukocytes, lymphocytes, and mononuclear cells. There is superficial thrombophlebitis; the thrombi in cerebral veins appear to begin on the outer side (toward the empyema). The thrombosis extends to other dural sinuses, and the superficial layers of the cerebral cortex undergo ischemic necrosis, which probably accounts for the unilateral seizures and signs of disordered cerebral function.

SYMPTOMATOLOGY AND LABORATORY FINDINGS The usual history includes chronic sinusitis or otitis with a recent flare-up and evidence of local pain and increase in purulent nasal or aural discharge. The illness is severe and progressive. Generalized headache, fever, vomiting, and a depressed sensorium are the first indications of intracranial spread. They are followed within a few days by localizing signs including focal motor seizures, hemiplegia, hemianesthesia, and aphasia. Papilledema is present in one-half of the patients at the time of diagnosis. Stupor or coma develops rapidly as the cerebral symptoms progress. Fever is usually present, but the neck is not always stiff. There is a leukocytosis and increased erythrocyte sedimentation rate. Lumbar puncture poses a distinct risk because it may precipitate transtentorial herniation. It is generally contraindicated if the diagnosis of subdural empyema is suspected. When the CSF is examined, increased pressure, a raised white blood cell count in the range of 50 to 1000 per milliliter including both neutrophils and lymphocytes, elevated protein (75 to 300 mg/dL), and normal sugar values are the usual findings. Unless subdural empyema is complicated by bacterial meningitis, no bacteria can be recovered from the CSF. In the type of subdural empyema that follows drainage of a chronic subdural hematoma, the onset is more indolent, fever is lower, and there is usually a local wound infection.

DIAGNOSIS Skull films may show involvement of the sinus or mastoid. CT scanning is the method of choice for establishing the diagnosis and location of a subdural empyema. The usual CT scan appearance is a crescentic or elliptical hypodense area lying directly below the cranial vault or adjacent to the falx cerebri. After administration of contrast, the CT scan may demonstrate an intense line of enhancement between the subdural collection and cerebral cortex. False-negative CT scans have been reported. When there is question about the diagnosis after CT scanning, cerebral angiography may be required to define the lesion. In secondary empyemas, CT scan is invariably positive. Four conditions need to be distinguished clinically from subdural empyema: cerebral thrombophlebitis, brain abscess, viral encephalitis, and acute hemorrhagic encephalitis (see Chap. 347).

TREATMENT Drainage of pus is the single most important part of treatment. In particular, it is important to institute drainage early because delaying it sharply increases the mortality rate. Specimens of pus obtained at surgery should be transported to the laboratory in oxygen-free containers and cultured both aerobically and anaerobically. Appropriate empiric antibiotic therapy consists of 20 million units of penicillin per day plus chloramphenicol, 4 g per day, administered intravenously. Without such massive antimicrobial therapy and surgery, most patients will die, usually within 7 to 14 days, often while the unsuspecting physician and surgeon are waiting for better localization of an assumed cerebral abscess, the most commonly mistaken diagnosis. Antibiotic therapy can be made optimally when final culture and sensitivity results are available. It should be continued for 3 to 6 weeks. Drugs to reduce cerebral edema and to prevent seizures should be given. Mortality in subdural empyema is now between 10 and 20 percent. Long-term sequelae include seizures, hemiparesis, and dysphasia.

CRANIAL EXTRADURAL ABSCESS

This condition is almost invariably associated with osteomyelitis in a cranial bone which originates from an infection in the ear or paranasal sinuses. Pus and granulation tissue accumulate on the outer surface of the dura, separating it from the cranial bone. Symptomatically, the effects are those of a local inflammatory process: frontal or auricular pain, purulent discharge from the sinuses or ear, and fever and local tenderness. Unrelenting headache is a frequent complaint. Focal neurologic signs are uncommon. A cranial epidural abscess characteristically enlarges too slowly to cause sudden neurologic abnormalities. The CSF is usually clear and under normal pressure but may contain a few lymphocytes and neutrophils (20 to 100 per milliliter) and slightly raised protein concentration. CT scan is the diagnostic procedure of choice. False-negative scans have been reported; the diagnosis can then be made by contrast-enhanced CT scan or angiography. Treatment consists of prompt surgical drainage of the epidural space and appropriate systemic antibiotics. The primary sinusitis or mastoiditis, from which the extradural infection has arisen, may also require surgical drainage.

SPINAL EPIDURAL ABSCESS

This type of abscess possesses unique clinical features and constitutes an important neurologic and neurosurgical emergency. It is discussed in Chap. 353.

INTRACRANIAL THROMBOPHLEBITIS

The lateral, cavernous, and superior longitudinal sinuses are relatively uncommon sites of infection. Usually there is evidence that the intracranial process has extended from the middle ear and mastoid cells, the paranasal sinuses, and skin around the upper lip, nose, and eyes.

LATERAL SINUS THROMBOPHLEBITIS In lateral sinus thrombophlebitis, which usually follows otitis media and mastoiditis, the earache and mastoid tenderness are succeeded, after a period of days to a few weeks, by fever, headache, nausea, and vomiting due to increased ICP. There may be swelling over the mastoid region, distention of veins, and tenderness of the jugular vein in the neck. With jugular vein involvement, there may be neck pain and restriction of movement. Drowsiness and coma are common. Papilledema (unilateral in some patients) is seen in about one-half of cases. Convulsions occur, but focal neurologic findings are infrequent. Abducens nerve paralysis and trigeminal nerve involvement (Gradenigo's syndrome) are found when there is spread to the inferior petrosal sinus.

CAVERNOUS SINUS THROMBOPHLEBITIS In this condition, which is usually secondary to oculonasal infections, the clinical syndrome is one of orbital edema, chemosis, venous congestion, and evidence of palsy of the third, fourth, ophthalmic fifth, and sixth cranial nerves. Later spread through the circular sinus to the opposite cavernous sinus results in bilateral symptoms and signs. The posterior part of the cavernous sinus may be infected via the superior and inferior petrosal veins without the occurrence of orbital edema or ophthalmoplegia. The patient appears acutely ill with high fever, headache, nausea, and vomiting. There is eye pain and the orbits are tender to pressure. Chemosis, edema, and cyanosis of the upper face are present; the bulbs are proptosed. Sensorium may remain clear until late in the infection. Ophthalmoplegia, pupillary changes, retinal hemorrhages, papilledema, and sensory changes in the ophthalmic division of the trigeminal nerve may be present. The CSF is usually normal unless there is associated meningitis or subdural empyema. The only effective therapy in the fulminant variety, associated with thrombosis of the anterior portion of the sinus, has been antimicrobial therapy usually aimed at coagulase-positive staphylococci (see Chap. 94) and occasionally gram-negative pathogens as well. Anticoagulants have been used occasionally, but their value has not been proved. Cavernous sinus thrombosis must be differentiated from mucormycosis which may cause a similar clinical picture in uncontrolled diabetics or in immunosuppressed patients (see Chap. 147).

SUPERIOR LONGITUDINAL SINUS THROMBOPHLEBITIS The superior sagittal sinus may become infected by spread from the lateral or cavernous sinuses or by extension from the nasal cavities, from a focus of osteomyelitis, or from epidural or subdural infection. General signs include fever, headache, and papilledema. Edema of the forehead and anterior part of the scalp occur. The typical neurologic picture is one of unilateral convulsions and hemiplegia, first on one side of the body, then on the other, because of extension into the superior cerebral veins. The paralysis may be predominantly monoplegic and involve mainly the legs.

Cerebral angiography with particular attention to the late filling of venous sinuses is the most specific diagnostic test. Digital subtraction angiography has been useful in the diagnosis of sagittal sinus thrombosis. CT scans show normal or small ventricles, hemorrhages, low-density lesions, and a high-density lesion in the involved sinus. Postcontrast CT scan may demonstrate a filing defect in the involved sinus. Radionuclide dynamic and static scans may indicate termination of isotope activity in the midportion of the sinus.

All types of thrombophlebitis, especially those related to ear and paranasal sinus infection, may be complicated by other forms of intracranial suppuration including bacterial meningitis, subdural empyema, or brain abscess. The proper treatment of major sinus thrombosis due to infection is the systemic administration of appropriate antibiotics in high dosage and surgical drainage of infected bone and tissues. The initiating focus should be brought under control by surgery if necessary, once the patient's condition permits such a procedure. To operate on the primary focus before medical treatment is instituted is to court disaster. The better plan is to institute antibiotic therapy; surgery on the ears or sinuses should be decided upon only after the infection is controlled. In general, anticoagulants should be avoided because brain hemorrhage may be produced. Residual neurologic deficits are frequent, but the prognosis for recovery is good when optimal treatment is given early in the illness.

ASEPTIC THROMBOSIS OF INTRACRANIAL VENOUS SINUSES This may develop after sinus and ear infections and may lead to an obscure increase in intracranial pressure because of the occlusion of one lateral or superior sagittal sinus. The more common conditions which may be accompanied by aseptic thrombosis are postpartum and postoperative states, which are often characterized by thrombocytosis and hyperfibrinogenemia; use of oral contraceptive drugs; congenital heart disease and marasmus in infants; systemic cancer; Behçet's disease; sickle cell disease; primary or secondary polycythemia; disseminated intravascular coagulation; and cryofibrinogenemia.

MALIGNANT EXTERNAL OTITIS

This paracranial infection is found in elderly patients with diabetes mellitus. Beginning in the external auditory canal, it spreads from the outer ear to the soft tissues below the temporal bone and invades the parotid gland, temporomandibular joint, masseter muscle, and temporal bone. *Pseudomonas aeruginosa* is responsible for the infection. The high mortality rate (initially reported at 40 percent) led to the term *malignant* for the condition; the adjective *necrotizing* or *invasive* may be preferable.

Symptoms and signs include pain in the ear with or without a purulent discharge, swelling of the parotid gland, trismus, and paralysis of the sixth to twelfth cranial nerves. Death is usually due to the development of meningitis. CT scan findings include obliteration of the normal fat planes in the subtemporal area and patchy destruction of the bony cortex of the mastoid. Radionuclide scans using Tc 99m or Ga67 citrate are helpful in the initial identification of the disease and in following the course of the infection.

Prolonged intravenous administration of tobramycin and carbenicillin is used to treat the condition. Surgical debridement may also be indicated. Antibiotics should be given for 6 weeks or for at least 2 weeks after all symptoms have resolved; treatment for basilar skull involvement may need to last as long as 3 months.

BRAIN ABSCESS

PATHOGENESIS Most of the focal suppurative intracranial processes of this type are linked to chronic ear and sinus or pulmonary infections. The majority of brain abscesses are due to disease of the middle ear, mastoids, or paranasal sinuses. Infection spreads to the brain directly across bone and dura mater or through vascular channels by septic thrombophlebitis or arteritis.

With frontal or ethmoid sinusitis, the abscess forms in the frontal lobe; with middle ear or mastoid infection, the abscess localizes to the temporal lobe or cerebellum. Of the remaining cases, a small portion are due to contaminated penetrating wounds or postoperative infections; the rest are metastatic. Of these, about half are traceable to pleuropulmonary disease—usually bronchiectasis, empyema, lung abscess, or bronchopleural fistula. In the rest, the source of infection may be skin, bone, teeth, or heart. In about 10 percent of cases, the source cannot be ascertained. Brain abscess is seldom a consequence of bacterial meningitis. Brain abscess also occurs in patients whose immune systems are defective or suppressed. In these instances, nonbacterial causes such as fungi, protozoans, and helminths may be recovered from the abscess.

Brain abscess is particularly frequent in congenital heart disease with right-to-left shunts (e.g., tetralogy of Fallot) and may also complicate arteriovenous vascular abnormalities of the lung, as in cases of familial telangiectasia (Osler-Rendu-Weber syndrome). When brain abscess is associated with a right-to-left cardiac shunt, it is frequently single. With cranial trauma, the location of the abscess will depend on the site of the penetrating wound. In contrast to the otogenic and rhinogenic abscesses, abscesses of hematogenous origin are frequently multiple and may occur anywhere in the brain.

Bacterial endocarditis rarely gives rise to brain abscess. Instead, the picture is one of focal embolic encephalitis with or without signs of embolic vascular disease elsewhere (see Chap. 188). In subacute endocarditis the emboli are sterile and cause only infarction and mycotic aneurysms. The CSF may contain a small number of neutrophilic leukocytes, lymphocytes, and red blood cells; the protein level may be elevated, but cultures are sterile and sugar values remain normal. In acute bacterial endocarditis, miliary abscesses and purulent meningitis may develop. There may be infarcts and there may be subarachnoid or intracerebral hemorrhages secondary to rupture of a mycotic aneurysm. Rarely do the miliary abscesses progress to large ones. Rapidly evolving cerebral signs in endocarditis are nearly always caused by embolic infarction or hemorrhage.

ETIOLOGY (See Chap. 102) Streptococci, including *S. milleri* (a member of the viridans group), other viridans and nonhemolytic streptococci, enterococci, β-hemolytic streptococci, and peptostreptococci are the most commonly isolated group of microorganisms. Next in order of frequency are members of the *Bacteroides* group, Enterobacteriaceae (*Proteus, Escherichia coli, Klebsiella*) and *Staphylococcus aureus*. Pneumococci, meningococci, and *Haemophilus influenzae* rarely cause brain abscess. In addition to *Bacteroides* and anaerobic streptococci, anaerobic actinomyces, veillonellae, and fusobacteria have been isolated. Bacterial species vary with the site of the abscess—staphylococcal abscesses are usually a consequence of penetrating head trauma or bacteremia; enteric organisms are almost always associated with ear infections; anaerobic streptococci are commonly metastatic from the lung. Two or more species of bacteria are often identified in a single abscess, and mixtures of aerobes and anaerobes may be found.

PATHOLOGY The location of brain abscess in decreasing order of frequency is in frontal, parietal, temporal, and occipital lobes, followed by cerebellum and basal ganglia. Abscesses rarely occur in the pituitary gland or brainstem. Localized inflammatory necrosis and edema, septic thrombosis of vessels, and aggregates of degenerating leukocytes (suppurative encephalitis) represent the early reaction of bacterial invasion of the brain. This is followed by encapsulation of the liquefied brain and of accumulated pus. the lesion becomes encapsulated by fibroblasts and newly formed vessels, and the capsule thickens over a period of weeks. The meninges adjacent to the abscess, especially near the point of entry of infection, are infiltrated by neurotrophils, lymphocytes, and plasma cells. Cerebral edema associated with the abscess and products of bacterial metabolism (such as an aerobically produced gas) result in increased ICP. The evolution of cerebral abscess can be divided into four stages: early cerebritis (1 to 3 days), late cerebritis (4 to 9 days) early capsule formation (10 to 13 days) and late capsule formation (14 days and later).

CLINICAL MANIFESTATIONS Most patients have symptoms for less than 2 weeks. Characteristically the clinical presentation is more like that of an expanding intracranial mass lesion than an infectious process. In patients with chronic ear, sinus, or pulmonary infections, a recent reactivation of the infection usually precedes the onset of cerebral symptoms. In a number of patients, evidence of CNS invasion is acute, and headache, vomiting, increasing obtundation, seizures, and a variety of localizing neurologic signs appear within a few days. In other patients, bacterial invasion of the brain substance may be asymptomatic or may be attended only by a transitory focal neurologic disorder. Sometimes stiff neck accompanies generalized headache, suggesting the diagnosis of meningitis. Early symptoms may subside or appear to respond to antimicrobials. Within a week or two, recurrent headache, slowness in mentation, focal or generalized convulsions, and obvious signs of increased intracranial pressure provide evidence of a mass in the brain. At this stage, the symptoms of infection are not conspicuous. Fever is present in less than half of the patients. Symptoms are usually progressive in their intensity. The majority of patients will have altered consciousness with lethargy, irritability, confusion, or coma.

Hemiplegia is the most common focal finding. Seizures, either focal or generalized, occur in about one-third of patients; papilledema and neck stiffness are present in about one-quarter of patients.

Patients demonstrate focal neurologic signs related to location of the abscess as described below.

Frontal lobe abscess Headache, drowsiness, inattention, and general impairment of mental function are prominent. Hemiparesis with unilateral motor seizures and expressive aphasia are the most frequent neurologic signs.

Temporal lobe abscess Headache is usually on the side of the abscess and is localized to the frontotemporal region. If the abscess lies in the dominant hemisphere, there is aphasia and anomia (inability to name objects). A homonymous upper quadrantic field defect may also be demonstrable owing to interruption of the inferior portion of the optic radiation. This may be the only sign in abscess of the right temporal lobe. Contralateral motor or sensory defects in the limbs tend to be minimal, though weakness of the lower face is often observed.

Cerebellar abscess Headache in the postauricular or suboccipital region is usually the first symptom and may at first be ascribed to infection in the mastoid cells. Coarse nystagmus and gaze weakness to the side of the lesion and a cerebellar ataxia of the ipsilateral arm and leg are present in most patients. As a rule, the signs of increased ICP are more prominent than those of focal cerebral disease. Mild contralateral or bilateral pyramidal signs may provide evidence of ipsilateral brainstem compression.

DIAGNOSIS The diagnosis of a brain abscess depends on (1) a demonstrated source of infection in the ears, sinuses, or lungs or the presence of a right-to-left cardiac shunt, (2) evidence of increased ICP, and (3) focal cerebral or cerebellar signs. Clues to the origin of the abscess are often present on initial evaluation. They include chronic ear disease with discharge, sinus infection, orbital cellulitis, pharyngitis, infected skin wound, and chest infection.

Lumbar puncture in suspected brain abscess is potentially dangerous, particularly when the ICP is obviously elevated, and the information to be derived is not specific enough to justify the risk. Routine x-rays of the skull may demonstrate gas in an abscess cavity. The electroencephalogram (EEG) is usually abnormal with focal changes.

The CT scan is the most valuable procedure for visualizing brain abscess(es). It also demonstrates ventricular distortion, surrounding edema of white matter, and the thickness of the capsule; it enables close follow-up of therapy. Injection of iodine-containing contrast material will enhance the selectivity of the CT scan and will permit the visualization of an abscess from the early stage of focal cerebritis to a densely encapsulated mass demonstrated as a ''ring'' that is sharply demarcated both internally and externally with a homogenous central area of decreased attenuation. Generally only a CT scan is required to make the diagnosis. Peripheral ring enhancement may also be found in tumor, cerebral infarction, resolving hematoma, radiation necrosis, and recent surgery; these conditions may enter into the differential diagnosis of the CT scan findings. Experience with magnetic resonance imaging (MRI) of brain abscess is limited, but no specific features identifying the infectious nature of the mass lesion have been described. If CT scanning is not available, radionuclide brain scan is a reliable method for localizing brain abscess. If both CT and radionuclide scans are negative, there is little likelihood of cerebral abscess. Scanning procedures have supplanted arteriography in most instances.

When the typical clinical picture is present and CT scan corroborates the presence of a mass lesion, the diagnosis is easy. If there is no source of infection and there are only signs and symptoms of a mass lesion, the diagnosis may be difficult. Sometimes only surgical exploration will settle the issue.

TREATMENT During the stage of acute suppurative cerebritis, intracranial operation accomplishes little and probably causes only additional trauma and swelling of brain tissue. There is good evidence that many brain abscesses visible by CT scanning can be cured at this stage by the administration of adequate doses of antimicrobials. Since the bacteriologic diagnosis must be presumptive, the most widely used regimen for adults consists of 20 to 40 million units of penicillin G and 4 to 6 g of chloramphenicol, both drugs being given intravenously in divided doses. This choice of antimicrobial agents is based on the preponderance of anaerobic streptococci and *Bacteroides* that are usually isolated from brain abscess. Metronidazole (500 mg every 6 h) with cefotaxime (12 gm daily) is an alternative method of treatment. Treatment should be continued for 6 to 8 weeks, and if there is clinical improvement and recovery during the course of therapy, surgical intervention can be withheld.

Selection of specific antimicrobials requires recovery of the responsible microorganism(s). Pus from the abscess cavity can be obtained by needle puncture at the time of craniotomy or by CT-guided percutaneous stereotactic operation. The specimen should be sent to the laboratory for Gram stain and for routine and anaerobic bacteriologic cultures. Specimens must be handled in a way that will not kill fastidious bacteria. They cannot be kept for too long a time in too small a volume of material or in the presence of preoperatively administered inhibitory antimicrobials. Pus can be delivered to the laboratory in a capped sterile syringe from which all the air has been removed. Once the infecting bacteria have been identified and their sensitivities determined, the appropriate antibiotic regimen can be chosen.

Serial CT scanning and prompt, aggressive antibiotic treatment has avoided surgical intervention in many cases. The instances for medical management include presence of multiple abscess, abscesses located in deep brain structures, concomitant meningitis or ependymitis, the presence of a ventricular shunt, and an underlying debilitating disease.

ICP monitoring is important in the management of brain abscess patients. Initial elevation of ICP and threatening temporal lobe or cerebellar herniation should be managed by the prompt intravenous injection of urea, mannitol, or dexamethasone. Persistence or progression of high ICP manifested by deepening coma mandates operation, regardless of the stage of the abscess. Likewise, clear-cut evidence of a mass lesion that is not improving with antimicrobial therapy is an indication for surgery. Gas-containing abscesses should be surgically excised. The usual methods of treatment are unroofing and drainage by aspiration. If the abscess is superficial and encapsulated, total excision is sometimes attempted; if deep, aspiration and the injection of antimicrobial agents into the abscess are the only possible treatment methods, and they may have to be repeated.

PROGNOSIS With the availability of CT scanning, more effective antimicrobials, and ICP monitoring, abscesses have been treated earlier and more effectively. Mortality has fallen to approximately 10 percent. Neurologic abnormalities, particularly focal epilepsy, are sometimes troublesome sequelae to brain abscess surgery. Following successful treatment of cerebral abscess in patients with congenital heart disease, correction of the cardiac anomaly is indicated to prevent recurrence.

REFERENCES

ANON JB, MILLER GW: Malignant external otitis. South Med J 77:1541, 1984

BLAQUIÈRE RM: The computed tomographic appearances of intra- and extracerebral abscesses. Br J Radiol 56:171, 1983

CHERUBIN CE, ENG RHK: Experience with the use of cefotaxime in the treatment of bacterial meningitis. Am J Med 80:398, 1986

DURACK DT: Prevention of central nervous system infections in patients at risk. Am J Med 76(5A):231, 1984

FEIGIN RD, DODGE PR: Bacterial meningitis: Newer concepts of pathophysiology and neurologic sequelae. Pediatr Clin North Am 23:541, 1976

GARVEY G: Current concepts of bacterial infections of the central nervous system: Bacterial meningitis and bacterial brain abscess. J Neurosurg 59:735, 1983

GORDON JJ et al: Meningitis due to *Staphylococcus aureus*. Am J Med 78:965, 1985

GORSE GJ et al: Bacterial meningitis in the elderly. Arch Intern Med 144:1603, 1984

HARRISON MJG: The clinical presentation of intracranial abscess. Q J Med 204:461, 1982

KAUFMAN DM et al: Subdural empyema: Analysis of 17 recent cases and review of the literature. Medicine 54:485, 1975

LEFROCK JL et al: Gram-negative bacillary meningitis. Med Clin North Am 69:243, 1985

MARTON KI, GEAN AD: The spinal tap: A new look at an old test. Ann Intern Med 104:840, 1986

MAYHALL CG et al: Ventriculostomy-related infections: A prospective epidemiological study. N Engl J Med 310:553, 1984

POLLOCK SS et al: Infection of the central nervous system by *Listeria monocytogenes:* A review of 54 adult and juvenile cases. Q J Med 211:331, 1984

RAO KCVG et al: Computed tomographic findings in cerebral sinus and venous thrombosis. Radiology 140:391, 1981

SCHLECH WF III et al: Bacterial meningitis in the United States, 1978 through 1981: The national bacterial meningitis surveillance study. JAMA 253:1749, 1985

347 VIRAL DISEASES OF THE CENTRAL NERVOUS SYSTEM: ASEPTIC MENINGITIS AND ENCEPHALITIS

DONALD H. HARTER / ROBERT G. PETERSDORF

Viruses can affect the central nervous system (CNS) in a variety of ways. Although much is known about the nature and replication of viruses, the correlation between viral properties and the type of the neurologic disease produced is inadequate or incomplete. Viruses that differ widely in their morphology, chemical composition, and replication can provoke identical clinical and pathologic changes in the CNS.

It is helpful to consider the time between the patient's first exposure to the viral agent and the appearance of disease, that is, to distinguish between CNS infections of a "fast" or "slow" nature. In fast or acute viral disease, neurologic changes occur very shortly after the patient first becomes infected by the virus. The illness follows a course of one to several weeks. In slow viral disease, the neurologic changes appear months to years after viral invasion, are insidious in development, and progress slowly.

ACUTE VIRAL CNS DISEASE

GENERAL CONSIDERATIONS Most viral CNS infections are the end result of preceding infection in other tissues and organs. There is usually a phase of extraneural viral replication before the nervous system becomes involved. Acute viral CNS infections are classified according to the clinical findings presented by the patient or, more indirectly, by the part of the nervous system involved by the disease process. In these terms, acute viral CNS disease is defined as meningitis, encephalitis, or myelitis, depending on the patient's symptoms and signs and the location of the infection. It is often difficult, however, to arrive at a single satisfactory localization on the basis of clinical findings alone. This leads to the use of compound terms such as meningoencephalitis or encephalomyelitis to describe the disease. This manner of classification is less than satisfactory because it gives no clear idea about the virus causing the condition.

Viruses vary in size, morphology, chemical composition, and effect on the host. Their common characteristics include a genome, which is either RNA or DNA surrounded by a protective protein shell; the fact that they multiply only inside the cell; and the fact that the initial step in replication involves separation of the genome from its protective shell. They are divided into two broad categories on the basis of their nucleic acid content and then into major families and genera (Table 347-1). Certain common properties of viruses are important determinants of the disease they produce. Herpesviruses have a tendency to remain latent in cells. Togaviruses and bunyaviruses are transmitted by insect vectors. Enteroviruses replicate in the gastrointestinal tract and are transmitted by the oral-fecal route. Myxoviruses contain a segmented genome which is prone to genetic recombination. Selection of the most effective methods of virus isolation depends in great measure on the virus's properties. Knowledge of a virus's biochemical composition is of help in determining whether antiviral therapy can be used. Understanding the biologic features of viruses within the major families and genera permits associations which are impossible when the location of the disease process is considered alone (see Chap. 128).

TABLE 347-1 Viruses of vertebrates

RNA-containing	DNA-containing
Picornavirus:*	Parvovirus:
Enterovirus*	Parvovirus
Cardiovirus	Dependovirus
Rhinovirus	Papovavirus:*
Aphthovirus	Papillomavirus
Calicivirus	Polyomavirus*
Reovirus:	Adenovirus:
Reovirus	Mastadenovirus
Orbivirus	Aviadenovirus
Rotavirus	Iridovirus
Togavirus:*	Herpesvirus:*
Alphavirus*	Alphaherpesvirus*
Flavivirus*	Betaherpesvirus*
Rubivirus*	Gammaherpesvirus*
Pestivirus	Poxvirus:
Orthomyxovirus:	Orthopoxvirus
Influenza virus	Parapoxvirus
Influenza C virus	Avipoxvirus
Paramyxovirus:*	Capripoxvirus
Paramyxovirus*	Leporipoxvirus
Morbillivirus*	Suipoxvirus
Pneumovirus	
Rhabdovirus:*	
Lyssavirus*	
Vesiculovirus	
Retrovirus:*	
Oncovirus	
Spumavirus	
Lentivirus*	
Bunyavirus:*	
Bunyavirus*	
Phlebovirus	
Nairovirus	
Uukuvirus	
Arenavirus*	
Coronavirus	

* *Virus families and groups of neurologic importance.*

ASEPTIC OR VIRAL MENINGITIS Etiology The term *aseptic meningitis* designates a disease characterized by an acute onset, meningeal symptoms, fever, cerebrospinal fluid (CSF) pleocytosis, and bacteriologically sterile cultures. The illness has a relatively benign clinical course of short duration, and recovery is the rule. With the introduction of more refined methods of viral isolation and the use of new culture techniques to define other microorganisms, it has become clear that aseptic meningitis is a syndrome of multiple etiologies. When viral infection produces the syndrome, the condition should be referred to as viral meningitis.

Epidemiology Aseptic meningitis affects between 9000 and 12,000 persons in the United States every year. Although all ages are involved, more than 90 percent of the patients are under age 30. The peak incidence of aseptic meningitis is in the late summer. The majority of cases seen in the summer are due to picornaviruses other than polioviruses, such as the coxsackie- and echoviruses. Mumps meningitis occurs more often in the winter and late spring. Both sexes are affected equally by enteroviruses, but there is a 2:1 or 3:1 male predominance in the meningitis produced by mumps.

Clinical picture The symptoms and signs of viral meningitis are similar irrespective of the particular virus involved. The onset of illness is acute. There may be a prodromal "flulike" illness before the onset of meningitis, as in lymphocytic choriomeningitis. This biphasic pattern of illness also may be observed in young children with poliomyelitis or in illness due to other insect-borne viruses (see Chaps. 143 and 144). CNS involvement is manifested by an intense frontal or retroorbital headache. Malaise, nausea and vomiting, listlessness, and photophobia may be present. As a rule, there is little impairment of consciousness. The patient may be drowsy and slightly confused but is usually oriented and rational. Stupor and coma occur rarely. The temperature is usually elevated in the range of 38 to 40°C. There is neck stiffness on forward flexion. Kernig's and Brudzinski's signs are present in most cases but may be absent in patients with minimal meningeal irritation. Stiffness of the spine may be such that a child will sit with the head retracted and the arms extended posteriorly in the form of a tripod. Signs of focal damage to the central nervous system are rarely present. Occasionally, strabismus or diplopia, asymmetry of tendon reflexes, and an inconstant extensor plantar response may be found.

Clinical findings outside the nervous system may provide clues to the virus involved in the infection. Parotitis in association with viral meningitis suggests mumps. Skin rash has been a prominent feature of coxsackievirus or echovirus infections (see Chap. 139). Blotchy or punctate maculopapular rashes which involve the extremities and which occur chiefly in the summertime are commonly due to echovirus. Herpangina (large, painful vesicles in the posterior one-third of the oropharynx) are usually caused by coxsackieviruses. Sharp pains in the chest aggravated by deep respiration or coughing suggest the pleurodynia seen with Coxsackie B viruses.

Laboratory findings The lumbar CSF is usually under increased pressure and clear or slightly turbid in appearance. Slight turbidity can be demonstrated by holding a tube containing CSF to the light and agitating the fluid with a gentle finger tap. CSF usually contains 10 to 100 cells per cubic millimeter. At times, the cell count rises to levels of 3000 per cubic millimeter or greater. The cells are usually more than three-fourths lymphocytes or mononuclear cells. Polymorphonuclear cells may predominate in the early phases of aseptic meningitis. The CSF protein and sugar concentrations are usually normal. Isolated instances of depressed CSF sugar in patients with infections due to mumps or herpes simplex virus (HSV) have been reported but are rare. If the patient presents with a spinal fluid which contains less sugar than expected, meningitis due to bacteria, mycobacteria, or fungi should receive first attention. Oligoclonal IgG bands may be found in the CSF of patients with viral meningitis. In viral meningitis, Gram stain and india ink preparations fail to identify an organism; bacterial and fungal cultures are negative. Although certain viruses (such as mumps virus) can be recovered from CSF with relative ease, in most cases of viral meningitis, it is usually impossible to recover the responsible viral agent from the patient's CSF. The white cell count in the blood is usually normal, but leukopenia is present in about one-third of patients.

The specific viral diagnosis can usually be made by performing serologic tests on acute and convalescent serums and by attempting to isolate viruses from feces, urine, and throat washings. Attempts to isolate the agent from blood are usually unsuccessful.

Differential diagnosis The syndrome of viral or aseptic meningitis can be caused by a number of different infectious and noninfectious agents. The majority of cases of viral origin are due to picornaviruses, togaviruses, herpesviruses, paramyxoviruses, and arenaviruses. The list of nonviral infectious causes of the aseptic meningitis syndrome is extensive. It includes intracranial infections located near the meninges (otitis, mastoiditis, vertebral osteomyelitis); brain abscess; partially treated bacterial meningitis; and fungal, rickettsial, protozoan, or helminthic infections.

Also, there are a number of infrequently encountered neurologic diseases in which the CSF findings resemble viral meningitis. These include (1) Behçet's disease, characterized by uveitis, genital and oral ulcers, and focal neurologic abnormalities; (2) Vogt-Koyanagi and Harada's diseases, which combine uveitis, depigmentation of the hair and skin about the eyes, loss of eyelashes, and deafness; (3) Mollaret's meningitis; and (4) Lyme disease.

Noninfectious causes of the aseptic meningitis syndrome include the intrathecal introduction of drugs and agents for diagnostic tests and tumors in close proximity to the cerebral ventricles or that invade the subarachnoid space. Cytologic examination of cells in the CSF will distinguish neoplastic meningeal infiltration from viral meningitis. Systemic diseases such as sarcoidosis, disseminated lupus erythematosus, and infective endocarditis may be associated with aseptic meningitis.

Treatment The treatment of viral meningitis is symptomatic. Antiviral agents are not indicated in uncomplicated cases. Fever and other symptoms resolve in 3 to 5 days, and patients are usually entirely well within 2 weeks. CSF abnormalities are most pronounced from the fourth to sixth day, but the CSF white blood cell count may remain elevated for several weeks in patients who are otherwise asymptomatic. Initial therapy with antimicrobial agents may be appropriate if the initial elevation is not completely typical for viral infection. In most instances, patients recover from viral meningitis without sequelae. A limited number of patients may develop muscular weakness and other forms of motor disability. A very small number of patients may have recurrent attacks of viral meningitis; the multiple episodes are often due to different viruses.

Prognosis It is important to recognize that viral meningitis is an acute and self-limited illness and to realize that it may mimic life-threatening CNS infections which are potentially treatable. Most important to appreciate is the similarity between viral meningitis and partially treated bacterial meningitis, tuberculous meningitis, or fungal meningitis. If the CSF changes are not completely characteristic of viral meningitis or if the patient's clinical response is atypical, it is important to perform repeated lumbar punctures and to reexamine the CSF within a relatively brief period of time, until the clinical picture becomes clear.

VIRAL ENCEPHALITIS Definition The term *encephalitis* is used when there is clinical and/or pathologic evidence of involvement of the cerebral hemispheres, brainstem, or cerebellum by the infectious process. It is customary to divide viral encephalitis into primary and postinfectious or parainfectious forms and to consider whether the disease is sporadic or epidemic. The *primary* form of the disease occurs when the encephalitis is the presenting form of the disease and is due to direct invasion and replication of virus within the CNS. The term *postinfectious* or *parainfectious* is used to describe an encephalitis which follows or occurs in combination with other viral illnesses or administration of certain vaccines. The cause of the encephalitis in such cases is believed to be a hypersensitivity reaction. The pathologic picture is typical of multifocal perivenous demyelination. The virus cannot be recovered from the CNS. If the inflammatory condition extends into the spinal cord, the term encephalomyelitis is used.

Clinical picture When encephalitis is the primary illness, such as with togaviruses and herpesviruses, there may be a minor illness consisting of such systemic symptoms as headache, myalgia, malaise, and upper respiratory symptoms. These nonspecific symptoms may occur several days before neurologic complaints and signs are recognized.

The onset of neurologic symptoms is abrupt. There is alteration in the patient's state of consciousness with lethargy, drowsiness, or stupor. The patient's behavior may be abnormal as a consequence of confusion, disorientation, and hallucinations. A convulsion or series of convulsions may occur at the start of the illness, and seizures may be the sole presenting symptom. The patient usually complains of headache, nausea, and vomiting. Fever is usually present, and there may be stiffening of the neck on forward bending. Focal neurologic abnormalities are found, depending on the portion of the nervous system involved by the inflammatory process. Involvement of the cerebral hemispheres may result in aphasia, signs of corticospinal and corticobulbar tract lesions, involuntary movements, ataxia, sensory defects, and loss of retentive memory.

Laboratory examinations General laboratory tests are usually of little help in the diagnosis of encephalitis. They may provide evidence of systemic disease, such as abnormal lymphocytes in infectious mononucleosis, cells in the urinary sediment with inclusions characteristic of cytomegalovirus infection, and elevated amylase and transaminase levels in mumps and certain picornavirus infections.

Lumbar puncture, followed by examination of the CSF, is the most important diagnostic test. The CSF is usually under normal or slightly elevated pressure, clear or slightly turbid, and contains an increased number of white cells (in the range of 50 to 500 per cubic millimeter), a slight-to-moderate elevation of protein content, and a normal glucose level. There may be a predominance of polymorphonuclear leukocytes in the early phase of the illness. The protein content will often rise as the total cell count diminishes. In HSV encephalitis, the CSF may be slightly bloody or xanthochromic and contain a significant number of red blood cells. This reflects the sometimes hemorrhagic nature of HSV encephalitis. Occasionally a viral encephalitis may exist without CSF abnormalities, which makes the diagnosis even more difficult.

The electroencephalogram (EEG) may be of diagnostic help in suspected encephalitis. Diffuse or bilateral abnormalities can be defined by the EEG in patients who present with focal or unilateral neurologic deficits. A number of EEG changes may be seen, but the most common pattern is a diffuse slow wave activity with disruption of normal rhythms, punctuated at times with periodic high-amplitude bursts and spike-and-wave complexes. Computerized tomography (CT), magnetic resonance imaging (MRI), and radionuclide scans may be helpful in demonstrating intracranial mass lesions or localized foci of infection about or within the brain. The cerebral cortex may be enhanced diffusely.

Diagnosis When presented with a patient with suspected viral encephalitis, it is important to exclude nonviral infections for which potential treatment is available. A number of conditions can mimic viral encephalitis (Table 347-2). It is imperative to consider these alternative causes when the patient is first evaluated. Once the diagnosis of primary viral encephalitis is secure, it is important to determine if the illness is occurring as part of an epidemic or as an isolated sporadic event. Knowledge of the seasonal, geographic, and age group occurrence of the disease can often furnish enough information to make an informed guess about the correct viral etiology. During the summer and early fall, togaviruses, bunyaviruses, and picornaviruses may prevail. Some of these viruses may produce milder disease than others; some, such as western equine and California encephalitis viruses, affect a predominantly young age group. In the winter, epidemic encephalitis is more often associated with paramyxovirus, varicella-zoster (V-Z), Epstein-Barr (EB), or rubella virus infection. HSV is responsible for more cases of nonepidemic sporadic encephalitis cases than any other virus.

The course of viral encephalitis is variable. It may be a short-lived, benign illness or a devastatingly severe one which leaves the patient with pronounced impairment of cerebral functions. Severe sequelae may be associated with certain viruses (HSV, eastern equine encephalitis, Japanese encephalitis, and St. Louis encephalitis). Other viruses cause milder disease (California encephalitis, western equine encephalitis). The acute phase of the disease usually lasts a few days to a week. Resolution can be abrupt or gradual. The disease may be complicated by a salt-wasting syndrome resulting from hypothalamic involvement and/or alterations in temperature or respiratory control centers owing to brainstem involvement. These events may occur rapidly and require prompt recognition and correction. Neurologic defects may continue to improve over a period of weeks to months.

In most instances of epidemic encephalitis, the viral diagnosis is made by serologic tests of acute and convalescent phase serums. Three major serologic tests are employed: complement-fixation, hemagglutination-inhibition, and neutralization. Because the serologic test is crucial for viral diagnosis, it is imperative to obtain an acute-phase serum as soon as the diagnosis of viral encephalitis is suspected. In vector-transmitted encephalitis which does not result in fatality, the blood is the most likely tissue source of viral isolation. Isolation of virus from blood is difficult, however, because viremia is usually brief and occurs before the onset of neurologic symptoms. In fatal cases, the virus can often be isolated from brain and spinal cord by inoculation of susceptible animals and tissue culture cells.

When HSV encephalitis is suspected, greater urgency is required in arriving at a viral diagnosis because there is a definite advantage in initiating antiviral therapy as quickly as possible (see Chap. 136). A number of patients with HSV encephalitis present with fever and neurologic findings compatible with a bilateral space-occupying lesion of the medial parts of the temporal and the orbital parts of the frontal lobes. A severe retentive memory defect is a frequent sequela. HSV can be best demonstrated in brain tissue obtained by biopsy. Examination of the tissue by light, electron, and immunofluorescence microscopy and inoculation of a brain homogenate into cell cultures and animals permit a specific diagnosis of HSV early in the course of the patient's illness. However, many neurologists object to biopsy as a diagnostic procedure because the risks and sequelae outweigh the dangers of treatment. Moreover, enhanced CT scans and radionuclide brain imaging often reveal the temporal lobe lesions which, when added to the clinical picture and a CSF pleocytosis, make the diagnosis fairly certain and permit treatment without brain biopsy.

Encephalitis may present as an infrequently encountered manifestation of a systemic disease such as measles, varicella, or neoplasia. When this is the case, the encephalitis occurs after the more characteristic features of the disease have become evident. Rarely, the systemic disease may appear after the diagnosis of encephalitis has been established.

TABLE 347-2 Nonviral conditions mistaken for acute viral encephalitis

Infection:	
Bacterial	Early or imperfectly treated meningitis Brain abscess Parameningeal infections Illness due to mycobacteria, spirochetes, *Mycoplasma*
Fungi	*Cryptococcus, Coccidioides immitis, Histoplasma, Candida, Nocardia, Blastomyces*
Rickettsia	Rocky Mountain spotted fever
Protozoa	"Fresh water" amebiasis, malaria, toxoplasmosis
Metazoa	Cysticercosis, trichinosis, and others
Intoxication	Salicylates, barbiturates, heavy metals, tick paralysis
Endocrine and metabolic disorders	Acute sodium, calcium, or carbohydrate imbalance; porphyria, pheochromocytoma
Systemic diseases	Sarcoidosis, hyperglobulinemia, collagen disease, neoplasms, endocarditis with embolization
Acute psychotic disorders	

SOURCE: *After Brown.*

UNUSUAL FORMS OF VIRAL ENCEPHALITIS *Acute cerebellar ataxia* may be associated with a number of different viruses (picornaviruses, V-Z, and EB virus). The illness usually afflicts children between the ages of 1 and 5 years. The majority of patients have had a preceding mild infectious illness a week or so before the onset of neurologic signs. The onset of the illness is characteristically abrupt with prominent ataxia of the trunk and limbs. Complete recovery is the rule, but a permanent cerebellar deficit may ensue in patients when ataxia is profound in the early stages of the illness. In some instances of V-Z infection, the cerebellar lesions are of the parainfectious, demyelinating type (see Chap. 348).

Acute hemorrhagic leukoencephalitis is an infrequently encountered hyperacute disease of cerebral white matter which is often preceded by some form of systemic viral illness, most often an upper respiratory tract infection. The disease is marked by an acute onset, progressively deepening disturbance of consciousness, fever, seizures, and focal cortical abnormalities. Cerebral involvement is frequently unilateral. The course is rapid and usually fatal. There is a peripheral leukocytosis, and the CSF frequently contains mononuclear and polymorphonuclear leukocytes. The presence of mass effect or increased absorption coefficient on CT scan within the first 3 days of encephalitis should suggest this diagnosis. The cause of the disease is unknown. It has not been linked to infection by a specific virus or group of viruses and may well be allergic in nature. A virus has not been recovered from brain tissue. Treatment includes vigorous control of intracranial pressure and seizures and aggressive use of corticosteroids in high dosage (see Chap. 348).

Limbic encephalitis is a form of encephalitis localized to the temporal and frontal lobes—the limbic part of the brain. It is encountered as a remote effect of malignancy—most commonly carcinoma of the lung. A viral etiology has been suspected but never proved. Patients with limbic encephalitis have marked impairment of recent memory manifested by a confabulatory-amnestic state, and generalized seizures. The patient's CSF often contains a limited number of lymphocytes and mononuclear cells. The EEG is characterized by paroxysmal and/or slow waves over one or both temporal lobes. Pathologic changes are most pronounced in the hippocampal formation and amygdaloid nuclei. Encephalitis with predilection for the brainstem has also been reported as a remote effect of tumor.

Encephalitis lethargica (von Economo's disease) first occurred during and for about 10 years after World War I. A causative viral agent was never identified, but the clinical and pathologic features were those of a viral infection of the thalamus and midbrain. The disease was characterized by pronounced somnolence and ophthalmoplegia. A high proportion of survivors developed a parkinsonian syndrome months or years after the encephalitis. Sporadic case reports of patients with the clinical features of encephalitis lethargica appear even to the present time.

MYELITIS Viral infection of the central nervous system may localize in the parenchyma of the spinal cord producing myelitis. Poliovirus infection with damage to spinal motor neurons is the prototype of a viral infection localized chiefly to the spinal cord. Vaccination has markedly reduced but not eliminated poliomyelitis because patients who have not been vaccinated remain susceptible. Progressive muscular weakness, fasciculations, and atrophy occur in some patients many years after an acute episode of poliomyelitis. The cause of this "postpolio" syndrome is still uncertain; it may be a recrudescence of viral activity.

Spinal paralytic disease has also been described with other enteroviruses (coxsackieviruses and echoviruses). The illness is characterized by an asymmetric flaccid paralysis of the limbs; it is usually less severe and has a higher rate of recovery from muscular weakness than poliomyelitis.

Other viruses have also been reported to affect the spinal cord directly. Herpesvirus infection in the genital and perineal region has been associated with paralysis of sphincter function, probably indicative of direct viral involvement of the sacral spinal cord. Myelitis due to V-Z virus (aside from the ganglionitis and unilateral poliomyelitis) is another very rare cause of a leukomyelitis resulting in bilateral weakness of the legs with occasional ankle clonus or extensor plantar responses. Sphincter disturbances are present in two-thirds of patients and a sensory level in about one-half of patients. The CSF contains from 25 to 125 cells per cubic millimeter; the protein content may be normal or elevated. Recovery of function is the rule.

There may also be delayed involvement of the white matter of the spinal cord following viral infection. This is a parainfectious demyelinative process that interrupts sensory and motor tracts at one level and is termed an acute transverse myelitis. It begins with the abrupt onset of bilateral weakness of the legs and concomitant involvement of ascending sensory pathways. Urinary bladder and bowel functions are usually disturbed early in the course of the illness. An exanthem or respiratory infection not uncommonly precedes neurologic symptoms. Acute myelitis in the absence of encephalitis has been described in association with measles, V-Z, echovirus, HSV, and infectious mononucleosis. It has also been observed after rabies and smallpox vaccination. Virus isolation from CSF has been unsuccessful. A small proportion of patients with acute transverse myelitis will later develop multiple sclerosis. Acute spinal epidural abscess should be considered and excluded in patients who present with an acute nontraumatic transverse spinal cord syndrome.

TREATMENT Of the various viruses that cause acute encephalitis, HSV is the most responsive to antiviral chemotherapy. The drug of choice is acyclovir, given intravenously. Details of therapy are given in Chap. 136 and Table 136-1.

CNS DISEASES DUE TO SLOW VIRUS INFECTION

In slow virus infections, a protracted period, often on the order of months or years, passes between the introduction of the infectious agent and the appearance of clinical illness. Once neurologic disease is established, it may progress slowly over many months or years. The reasons why a certain virus will cause acute illness in one patient and slow infection in another are still largely unknown. Viruses causing slow infections do not appear to share any common features. No single virus property can be correlated with the slow virus disease process. The factors invoked to explain slow virus infections include (1) a defect in the composition of the virus; (2) a change in the virus's antigenicity; (3) an altered or defective host immune response; (4) a special property of the virus which permits it to remain latent or to become integrated in the host cell's genome; or (5) a yet incompletely understood and possibly unique method of replication.

Slow virus CNS diseases affect the parenchyma of the cerebral hemispheres and, in some instances, the cerebellum, brainstem, and spinal cord. These infections are not grouped by their topography, i.e., the part of the nervous system that they damage, or by their clinical presentation. Some slow viruses provoke a mild conventional inflammatory response during the time they are clinically silent; others are able to reside within cells for long periods without causing detectable cytopathic changes. The role of immunity in slow virus infection is largely unknown. Some slow virus infections occur in the presence of elevated levels of circulating antibodies; in others, there may be no detectable immune response.

Because infective agents causing some human slow CNS diseases have not been demonstrated to contain nucleic acid, the slow viral CNS infections are divided into those due to conventional viruses and those due to unconventional agents whose viral nature has not been fully established (Table 347-3). There are currently eight well-defined neurologic diseases caused by slow viruses. No consistently effective therapy is now available for any of them. Conventional viruses have been recovered from the CNS of patients with subacute sclerosing panencephalitis (SSPE), progressive multifocal leukoencephalopathy (PML), progressive rubella encephalitis, and persistent viral infection in immunodeficient patients. Each of these is based on an inflammatory reaction in the CNS. Kuru, Creutzfeldt-Jakob disease (CJD), and Gerstmann-Sträussler-Scheinker (GSS) disease share common neuropathologic features which are noninflammatory. They produce fine vacuolation of nervous tissue and hence are referred to as the subacute spongiform virus encephalopathies. Although these diseases have been shown to be of infectious etiology by the transmission of neurologic illness to higher primates, their causative agents remain incompletely characterized. They are classified as the slow virus infections due to unconventional agents.

The best studied of the unconventional transmissible agents is scrapie, a neurologic disease of sheep. The nature of the scrapie agent has not been defined. Concentrated and partially purified scrapie agent contains a sialoglycoprotein of 27,000 to 30,000 mol wt, designated PrP 27-30. Because of this association, the term *prion* was introduced as an operational name for the putative infectious agent. Prion is defined as a small proteinaceous infectious particle which is resistant to inactivation by most procedures that modify nucleic acids. PrP 27-30 is the product of a single gene; specific messenger RNA for PrP 27-30 is found in normal as well as infected tissues. Scrapie prion preparations aggregate into amyloid-like bifringent rods. In addition, filamentous structures, called scrapie-associated fibrils (SAF), have been found by electron microscopy of membrane fractions from scrapie-infected brain. These observations further testify to the unusual nature of the scrapie agent, but they do not fully exclude the possibility that the scrapie agent contains nucleic acid.

SUBACUTE SCLEROSING PANENCEPHALITIS (SSPE) This progressive and ultimately fatal disease of children and adolescents had been suspected to be of viral origin since its initial description as inclusion body encephalitis. Measles virus or a virus very closely related to measles virus has been recovered from the brains of patients with the disease. The disorder may be considered to be a slow form of measles encephalitis (see Chap. 132).

SSPE occurs in patients between the ages of 4 and 20; 80 percent are under 11. The disease affects boys 3 to 10 times as frequently as girls. Mean annual incidence rates have fallen rapidly in the last two

TABLE 347-3 Slow virus diseases of the CNS

Conventional viruses	Subacute sclerosing panencephalitis (SSPE) Progressive multifocal leukoencephalopathy (PML) Progressive rubella encephalitis Persistent infection in immunodeficiency: Congenital or primary Acquired or induced
Unconventional viruslike agents	Kuru Creutzfeldt-Jakob disease (CJD) Gerstmann-Sträussler-Scheinker disease (GSS)

decades; the drop in incidence roughly parallels the decline in the number of measles cases diagnosed since the introduction of live attenuated measles vaccine. Most patients are from rural areas or small towns. Characteristically, they are entirely well until the disease begins. The onset of usually insidious mental deterioration, often expressed by a decline in the patient's schoolwork, is the presenting symptom. Incoordination, ataxia, and myoclonic jerks develop within a few months along with abnormalities of the pyramidal and extrapyramidal motor systems. Cortical blindness, papilledema, and optic atrophy may be present; focal chorioretinitis has been described. A few cases have occurred in association with infectious mononucleosis.

The patient becomes bedridden within 6 to 9 months. Death results from superimposed pulmonary or urinary tract infections or from decubiti. Signs of meningeal irritation are absent. The differential diagnosis includes cerebral storage diseases, nonstorage poliodystrophies, leukodystrophies, and demyelinating diseases of childhood.

The CSF gamma-globulin level, as determined by electrophoresis, quantitative immunochemical assay, or colloidal gold curve, is elevated, but the fluid is otherwise normal. The EEG typically shows a "burst suppression" pattern characterized by synchronous and symmetrical spike and high-voltage slow wave activity followed by electrical inactivity. Elevated levels of measles antibody are found in the serum and CSF. CT scan abnormalities correlate with the stage and duration of the disease. They include lateral ventricular dilatation, cortical atrophy, low parenchymal attenuation, and brainstem and cerebellar atrophy.

Pathologic findings include lymphocyte and mononuclear infiltrations about small cerebral arteries and veins, intranuclear and intracytoplasmic inclusions in neurons and glial cells, and varying degrees of destruction of medullated nerve fibers. The lesions occur in the cerebral gray and white matter, brainstem, and cerebellum.

Measles virus is the etiologic agent. Electron-microscopic studies show that the intranuclear inclusions in brain cells are composed of hollow tubular filaments resembling the internal nucleocapsid component of a paramyxovirus. Staining of brain tissue from patients with the disease demonstrates measles virus antigen in the inclusions. An agent serologically identical with measles virus and having the properties of measles virus has been recovered from brain by cocultivating cell cultures originating from brain tissue with established laboratory cell lines.

Attempts to transmit the disease to animals have met with variable results. Ferrets inoculated with suspensions of brain from patients with the disease develop a nonfatal neurologic disorder with EEG changes.

There is evidence that SSPE patients have clinical measles at an unusually early age, but SSPE appears many years after the patient's initial rubeola infection. A few reported cases may have been related to measles vaccination. The risk of SSPE following measles vaccination is far less, however, than the risk of encephalitis or SSPE following natural measles.

SSPE patients lack antibody to one of the measles virus proteins (the M or matrix protein) despite high titers of antibodies to the other viral proteins. Extracts of SSPE-infected brain lack significant quantities of M antigen. The M protein is a nonglycosylated protein localized to the inner surface of the viral membrane; it is important in the assembly of the virus particle at the cell surface. SSPE brain cells do not appear capable of synthesizing the M protein even in normal amounts. The molecular reasons for the absence of M polypeptide in terminal SSPE may involve decreased transcription and translation of M messenger RNA.

Isoprinosine[1] has been reported by some to affect the course of the disease favorably in an open therapeutic trial, but there is controversy about the drug's effectiveness. Other forms of treatment (including interferon and plasmapheresis) have been ineffective.

PROGRESSIVE MULTIFOCAL LEUKOENCEPHALOPATHY (PML) This rare neurologic condition that usually occurs in patients who have leukemia, malignant lymphoma, carcinomatosis, acquired immunodeficiency syndrome (AIDS), or a variety of other chronic disease processes, or who are involved with immunosuppressive therapy. The disease is consistently associated with disorders of cell-mediated immunity with which deficits in humoral antibody response may or may not coexist.

The disease affects adults of both sexes, and its duration from onset of symptoms to death is 1 to 6 or more months. The neurologic signs and symptoms reflect a diffuse, asymmetric involvement of the cerebral hemispheres. Hemiplegia, hemianopsia, aphasia or dysarthria, and organic mental changes are frequent; visual field abnormalities and complete or incomplete transverse myelitis may develop. Headache and convulsive seizures are rare, but EEG abnormalities consisting of diffuse or focal abnormalities are often present. Lesions in the white matter may be recognized on CT scans. MRI is helpful in demonstrating white matter destruction. CSF is normal. Specific diagnosis can be made by brain biopsy.

The pathologic changes consist of multiple areas of demyelination with little or no perivascular infiltration and abnormal mitotic figures in astrocytes. The presence of distinctive intranuclear inclusions in oligodendrocytes first suggested that the disease was of a viral etiology. Electron-microscopic observations show the intranuclear inclusion bodies to be composed of closely packed spheres, which have the physical dimensions and properties of the polyomavirus genus of the papovaviruses.

By employing tissue cultures derived from human fetal brain, it has been possible to recover a new human polyomavirus serotype (JC virus) from the brains of PML patients. Abundant virus particles are present in brain. Rapid identification of the virus in brain is possible using fluorescent antibody staining or electron-microscopic agglutination with monospecific hyperimmune rabbit serum. Serologic diagnosis using the patient's serum is unreliable. The virus has not been demonstrated in tissues other than brain; the disease has not been transmitted to animals. There are isolated reports of clinical remission with cytosine arabinoside, but no cures. Death usually occurs within 6 months of onset.

PML may result from the activation of a polyomavirus which has been latent in brain or other tissues since childhood infection. Alternatively, there may be certain individuals who fail to acquire immunity in childhood and have their first encounter with the virus when a disease which interferes with cell-mediated immunity develops. The demyelination which occurs may be related to virus-induced damage of oligodendroglia, cells which appear to be required for the normal maintenance of myelin.

PROGRESSIVE RUBELLA ENCEPHALITIS A chronic progressive encephalitis developing in boys with the typical stigmata of the congenital rubella syndrome (Chap. 133) and sharing some of the features of SSPE was first described in 1974. Fewer than 20 patients have been reported.

The illness begins in the second decade and is characterized by dementia, cerebellar ataxia, spasticity, and seizures. The CSF has an increased cell count, and the protein and IgG levels are elevated. High titers of antibody to rubella virus can be detected in both the serum and CSF. Rubella virus has been recovered from the brain by use of the cocultivation technique.

Unlike SSPE, patients with rubella panencephalitis have the stigmata of congenital rubella before the onset of progressive disease. Myoclonus is less constant, and the EEG does not show the burst suppression observed in SSPE. Histologic examination of the brain shows mineralization of old lesions and an inflammatory reaction, but not the inclusion bodies characteristically found in SSPE.

The clinical picture of progressive rubella encephalitis also resembles the rare case of juvenile paresis which may occur in patients with congenital syphilis. The immune status of patients with rubella encephalitis has not been fully defined, and the pathogenesis of the disease remains obscure.

PERSISTENT VIRAL DISEASE IN IMMUNODEFICIENT PATIENTS Persistent or chronic neurologic infections of the nervous system may

[1] *This drug has not been approved by the Food and Drug Administration at the time of publication.*

occur in immunodeficient patients. The immunodeficiency state may be congenital (primary) or acquired. Enteroviruses may be recovered from the CSF of patients with primary agammaglobulinemia over a period of many years, during which time there is a persistent CSF pleocytosis. A chronic or subacute encephalitis has also been described in children with congenital hypogammaglobulinemia. A specific virus has not been associated with this disorder.

NEUROLOGIC CONDITIONS RELATED TO THE ACQUIRED IMMUNODEFICIENCY SYNDROME (AIDS) Involvement of the CNS in AIDS may produce complex clinical findings. Evidence is accumulating that the human immunodeficiency viruses (HIV) responsible for AIDS [human T-cell leukemia virus (HTLV III), lymphadenopathy-associated virus (LAV), or AIDS-associated retrovirus (ARV)] may produce a primary neurotropic disorder as well as furnish the immunologic compromise that permits other viruses to replicate in and damage nerve tissue.

The immunocompromised AIDS patient is susceptible to a variety of infectious agents that can attack the CNS. The most common viral agents that assert themselves belong to the herpesvirus and papovavirus groups, i.e., viruses that may remain latent until there is dysfunction of normal immunologic processes. The most commonly isolated viruses from these groups include herpes simplex virus (HSV), cytomegalovirus, and the PML agent (JC virus). Infection with these viruses in the AIDS patient can produce a variety of neurologic conditions—most notably atypical aseptic meningitis, acute or subacute encephalitis, PML, and viral myelitis. In addition to viral encephalitis and PML, the AIDS patient may also develop toxoplasma brain abscess and primary CNS lymphomas. Differentiation from PML is often difficult solely on the basis of CT scan and other laboratory tests. Because treatment for these conditions varies, it is often necessary to perform a brain biopsy and obtain a specimen of the cerebral lesion to make the correct diagnosis.

The AIDS patient may also develop a number of different conditions of the spinal cord. These include a vacuolar myelopathy that most severely affects the lateral and posterior columns of the thoracic cord, an acute viral myelitis usually due to HSV, and an ascending myelitis. AIDS can also affect peripheral nerves producing a neuropathy.

There is evidence that HTLV III can replicate in brain. Injection of brain suspension from AIDS patients into chimpanzees produced seroconversion in the animals; virus could be isolated from the chimpanzee's leukocytes. Seroconversion for anti-HTLV III has been associated with the appearance of acute encephalopathy in AIDS patients. HTLV III DNA and RNA have been found in the brains of both children and adults with AIDS, and HTLV III has been directly isolated from CSF and neural tissues of AIDS patients. HTLV III–specific IgG has been found to a higher measure in the CSF than in the blood in AIDS patients with neurologic symptoms, suggesting IgG synthesis within the CNS. The HTLV III agent has also been recovered from the spinal cord and sural nerve, suggesting that the AIDS myelopathy and peripheral neuropathy also may be caused by infection with this retrovirus.

AIDS dementia, a subacute dementia accompanied by motor system abnormalities, has been described in AIDS patients. This condition may well be a direct manifestation of HTLV III infection of the brain. The dementia is insidious in onset and progresses gradually. The early manifestations include an inability to recall, loss of capacity to concentrate, and difficulty in performing complex sequential tasks. There is slowing of verbal and motor responses; spontaneity and animation are reduced. The condition may be difficult to differentiate from depression. As the disease advances, there may be gait unsteadiness, leg weakness, impaired handwriting, and tremor. In the advanced stage, there is global cognitive impairment and pronounced psychomotor slowing. The CT scan may show cortical atrophy and enlargement of the ventricles. MRI demonstrates patchy multifocal areas of increased signal in the central white matter in T2 weighted images. The spinal fluid may contain mononuclear cells and have mildly elevated protein content.

The brains of patients with AIDS demonstrate moderate to marked cerebral atrophy and histologic changes involving the white matter and subcortical structures; the cortical gray matter is largely spared. The microscopic findings include multifocal perivascular rarefaction and focal vacuolation of the white matter with perivascular and parenchymal collections of macrophages and multinucleated giant cells. Neuronal loss is present only in the most severe cases.

There is no effective treatment for AIDS dementia.

KURU Kuru, or "trembling with fear," is a progressive and fatal neurologic disorder which occurs exclusively among natives of the New Guinea highland. The disease is rare and seems to be disappearing; its elucidation represented a major hallmark in microbiology.

Difficulty in walking is usually the first sign of kuru. This usually progresses from a minor disturbance in gait to marked ataxia with lurching and staggering. Eventually, ambulation becomes so incoordinated that patients are unable to walk independently or to use their limbs because of intention tremor. Patients display an inability to perform rapid alternating movements, hypotonia, and abnormal involuntary movements which take the form of myoclonus, athetosis, or chorea. Slurring of speech and convergent strabismus appear as the disease progresses. There are no abnormalities in the blood or CSF. Dementia develops in the later phases of the disease. The illness terminates fatally in 4 to 24 months, usually from decubitus ulcers or bronchopneumonia. Kuru was common in male and female children and in adult women, but rare in adult men. The incubation period may be longer than 20 years in older patients.

Pathologic changes are limited to the CNS and include widespread neuronal loss, intense astrocytosis and microglial proliferation, loss of myelinated fibers, and the presence of plaquelike bodies. Perivascular cuffing by lymphocytes and mononuclear cells is rarely present.

It was the close similarity between the neuropathologic and clinical findings found in kuru and in scrapie that suggested the possibility that kuru might be caused by a virus or some closely related infectious agent. The infectious origin of kuru was confirmed subsequently by the transfer of a kurulike syndrome in chimpanzees 10 to 82 months after intracerebral inoculation of suspensions of brain from human cases. Disease has also been produced in chimpanzees by inoculation of tissues other than brain. The clinical illness in chimpanzees appears 3 to 11 months after inoculation. The disease has also been successfully transmitted to a number of new world and old world monkeys as well as to other animals. The specific agent responsible for the disease has not been fully characterized.

Cannibalism is the probable mode of transmission of kuru. Native custom in New Guinea dictated that bone marrow, viscera, and brain be cooked and eaten. The agent may be introduced by conjunctival, nasal, or skin contamination during the practice of ritual cannibalism. The marked predilection of kuru for the adult female may be explained by the observation that cannibalism appears more prevalent among women and that males who practice cannibalism seldom eat the bodies of women. The recent influx of foreign settlers into the kuru area has led to increasing rejection of cannibalistic practices and this in turn may be responsible for the progressive decline in the number of cases of kuru since 1960. Oral feeding of kuru agent to squirrel monkeys has been reported to produce the disease.

CREUTZFELDT-JAKOB DISEASE (CJD) CJD is an invariably fatal degenerative disease of the CNS that afflicts persons between the ages of 55 to 75 years and presents as a rapidly evolving dementia with myoclonus. Unlike kuru, the disease is not geographically limited and has been reported from over 50 countries around the world. The annual incidence is about one case per million inhabitants in metropolitan areas. The majority of cases occur between the ages of 55 and 75, but patients as young as 16 and as old as 80 have been reported. The peak incidence is in the early 1960s.

Although CJD may have diverse clinical presentations, it usually begins with gradually progressive mental deterioration in the form of memory loss, mood changes, and errors in judgment. Disturbances of stance, gait, and motor control, visual disturbances, and dizziness and vertigo may be prominent in the early stages of the disease. Some patients complain of headache. The patient may experience distortions in the shape and appearance of objects. Higher cortical function deficits, such as aphasia or apraxia, may occur. Hallucinations, delusional ideas, and confusion may appear as the disease progresses. In certain patients, cerebeller signs and visual abnormalities may predominate and may be confused initially with cerebrovascular insufficiency. As the condition worsens, the patient becomes mute, stuporous, spastic, and rigid. Myoclonic jerks and other abnormal movements become more prominent as the disease progresses. Visual deterioration may advance to cortical blindness. Disturbances of oculomotor control and of the autonomic nervous system have been noted.

The disease progresses rapidly; the mean duration of illness is about 8 months, but about 5 to 10 percent of cases will have an illness lasting 2 years or more. The majority of patients die within 6 months, most often 2 to 3 months after the onset of their disease.

Only rarely has a second member of a family been affected. Fifteen percent of CJD patients have a family history of the disease consistent with an autosomal dominant transmission; the onset of the illness in familial cases is earlier than in sporadic cases. A family history of presenile dementia can be obtained in about 10 percent of CJD patients.

The EEG can often be helpful in making the correct diagnosis. During the early stages, it may only show mild, excessive generalized slowing more marked over one hemisphere or even focal. As the disease progresses, distinctive repetitive sharp waves with a characteristic interval of 0.5 to 1.0 s are seen. The sharp waves may first be unilateral, resembling periodic lateralized epileptiform discharges (PLEDS), but eventually they become bilateral and synchronous. In the final stages of the disease, all background EEG activity becomes progressively slower and of lower amplitude, sometimes with the persistence of period complexes. Repetitive sharp waves are also occasionally seen in the EEGs of patients with dementia due to other illnesses such as Alzheimer's disease or Binswanger's subcortical encephalopathy, but not with the regular rate that they are found in CJD patients. Serial EEG tracings are helpful in questionable cases.

A CT scan of the brain is usually normal, but sulcal widening, ventricular enlargement, and moderate cortical atrophy may be visualized. Rapid progressive atrophic changes on serial CT scans may suggest the diagnosis. MRI scanning demonstrates bilateral cortical atrophy without apparent white matter changes. Positron emission tomography (PET) has demonstrated temporal lobe hypometabolism with hemispheric asymmetry. The CSF is usually normal except for a slight elevation in the protein content. No immunologic response, either humoral or cellular, to the CJD agent has been demonstrated in the blood.

The cerebrum and cerebellum are affected predominantly. The brain may show cerebral atrophy. Microscopic examination demonstrates widespread status spongiosus, nerve cell loss, and intensive gliosis. Vacuoles are located within the neuropil, i.e., within axons, dendrites, and glial fibers. There is no inflammatory reaction.

Electron-microscopic observations in CJD have disclosed membrane fragments in vacuoles. Abnormal fibrils similar in appearance to the serum accelerator factor (SAF) have been observed in CJD brain fractions. The exact composition of these fibrils is unclear. CJD brains have been shown to contain protease-resistant proteins with molecular weights ranging from 10,000 to 50,000. These CJD proteins reacted with antibodies raised against the scrapie PrP 27-30. Immunological identification by Western blots provides a diagnostic adjunct to neuropathological examination and animal transmission experiments. Protein polymers from CJD brain exhibit the staining properties of amyloid. The SAF and protease-resistant proteins present in CJD brain resemble those observed in other naturally occurring and experimentally induced spongiform encephalopathies of humans and other animals. It is uncertain if they represent a form of the infectious agent or modified pathologic products.

Sixty percent of patients with kuru and CJD demonstrate an autoimmune antibody directed against 10-nm neurofilaments. The antibody usually appears late in the disease. It can occasionally be found in normal subjects. The significance of this antibody is unclear.

CJD may be mistaken for Alzheimer's disease with myoclonus. In this situation, the presence of cerebellar signs provides strong evidence against the possibility of Alzheimer's disease. At times, CJD can be confused with multi-infarct dementia, alcoholic or nutritional deficiency syndromes, or primary brain tumors. The hallmarks of the disorder (mental deterioration, multisystem neurologic signs, myoclonus, and typical EEG changes) evolving over a period of months in a middle-aged patient usually secures the diagnosis.

The CJD agent has been found in lymph nodes, liver, kidney, spleen, lung, cornea, and CSF of patients with the disorder. The way the disease is acquired naturally is unknown. Incubation periods as long as 20 years may occur in natural transmission. The higher incidence of CJD among Israelis of Libyan origin who eat sheep's eyeballs has led to speculation that the disease may be naturally transmitted by the ingestion of scrapie-infected meat. There is an unexpectedly high incidence of previous brain or eye operations among CJD patients. Human-to-human transmission has occurred by corneal transplantation, by the implantation of contaminated stereotactic electroencephalographic electrodes, and by the parenteral administration of growth hormone prepared from cadaveric human pituitary glands. Transmission of CJD has not been linked to blood transfusion.

There is no evidence of an increased risk among spouses, friends, and medical or nursing personnel caring for CJD patients. The patient's CSF and blood should be considered, however, as potential sources of infection. Precautions should be taken to avoid autoinoculation with needles, scalpels, or other instruments that have been contaminated by the patient's tissues. Maximum care should be taken to avoid accidental percutaneous exposure to blood, CSF, or tissue. Contaminated skin can be disinfected by a 5- to 10-min exposure to 1 *N* sodium hydroxide followed by extensive washing with water. Contaminated material should be steam-autoclaved for 1 h at a temperature of at least 132°C or immersed for 1 h in 1 *N* sodium hydroxide or a 10% sodium hypochlorite solution. More detailed guidelines for the handling of materials from patients with these disorders have been developed by the Centers for Disease Control. These should be applied to all patients who have evidence of rapid intellectual deterioration, particularly when it is associated with myoclonus.

There is no effective treatment for CJD. Claims that amantadine hydrochloride is effective have not been substantiated.

GERSTMANN-STRÄUSSLER-SCHEINKER (GSS) DISEASE GSS disease is a familial illness characterized by spinocerebellar ataxia with dementia and plaquelike deposits of amyloid in the brain. Inoculation of brain tissue from GSS disease produces spongiform encephalopathy in nonhuman primates. The usual onset of the disease is in the fifth decade. GSS disease follows a lengthy course, usually on the order of 2 to 10 years. Ataxia is prominent in the early phase of the illness; dementia follows later. The patient's symptoms and signs are reminiscent of olivopontocerebellar atrophy. Pathologic changes include spinocerebellar and corticospinal tract degeneration, extensive amyloid deposits, and spongiform degeneration. Like other human spongiform encephalopathies, there is no effective treatment for GSS disease.

There have been isolated reports that brain tissues for a restricted number of patients with familial Alzheimer's disease induced neurologic disease and spongiform changes in chimpanzees. Numerous other transmission attempts from patients with both familial and nonfamilial Alzheimer's disease have been negative. At present, there is no direct evidence to indicate that Alzheimer's disease is caused by a slow virus.

REFERENCES

Bockman JM et al: Creutzfeldt-Jakob disease prion proteins in human brains. N Engl J Med 312:73, 1985

Brown P: Acute viral encephalitis, in *Current Diagnosis 7*, RB Conn (ed). Philadelphia, Saunders, 1985, p 918
Dyken PR: Subacute sclerosing panencephalitis. Current status. Neurol Clin 3:179, 1985
Gajdusek DC: Unconventional viruses and the origin and disappearance of kuru. Science 197:943, 1977
———: Unconventional viruses causing subacute spongiform encephalopathies, in *Virology*, BN Fields et al (eds). New York, Raven Press, 1985, p 1519
Griffith JF, Ch'ien LT: Herpes simplex virus encephalitis. Diagnostic and treatment considerations. Med Clin North Am 67:991, 1983
Ho DD, Hirsch MS: Acute viral encephalitis. Med Clin North Am 69:415, 1985
——— et al: Isolation of HTLV-III from cerebrospinal fluid and neural tissues of patients with neurologic syndromes related to the acquired immunodeficiency syndrome. N Engl J Med 313:1493, 1985
Hudson AJ et al: Gerstmann-Sträussler-Scheinker disease with coincidental familiar onset. Ann Neurol 14:670, 1983
Kennard C, Swash M: Acute viral encephalitis. Its diagnosis and outcome. Brain 104:129, 1981
Levy RM et al: Neurological manifestations of the acquired immunodeficiency syndrome (AIDS). Experience at UCSF and review of the literature. J Neurosurg 62:475, 1985
Price RW et al: AIDS encephalopathy. Neurol Clin 4:285, 1986
Ratzan KR: Viral meningitis. Med Clin North Am 69:399, 1985
Richardson EP: Progressive multifocal leukoencephalopathy. N Engl J Med 265:815, 1961
Rosenberg RN et al: Precautions in handling tissues, fluids, and other contaminated materials from patients with documented or suspected Creutzfeldt-Jakob disease. Ann Neurol 19:75, 1986
Walker DL: Progressive multifocal leukoencephalopathy, in *Handbook of Clinical Neurology*, JC Koetsier (ed). Amsterdam, Elsevier Science Publishers 1985, vol 3(47), p 503
Weil ML et al: Chronic progressive panencephalitis due to rubella virus simulating subacute sclerosing panencephalitis. N Engl J Med 292:994, 1975
Wilfert CM et al: Persistent and fatal central-nervous-system echovirus infections in patients with agammaglobulinemia. N Engl J Med 296:1485, 1977

348 DEMYELINATING DISEASES

JACK P. ANTEL / BARRY G. W. ARNASON

The demyelinating diseases comprise a group of neurologic disorders important both because of the frequency with which they occur and the disability which they cause. Demyelinating diseases have in common the pathologic feature of focal or patchy destruction of myelin sheaths in the central nervous system accompanied by an inflammatory response. Some degree of axonal damage may occur as well, but demyelination always predominates. No cause has been determined for any of the demyelinating diseases. Current opinion holds that autoimmunity or viral infection is likely to be implicated in their pathogenesis.

Myelin loss occurs in other conditions as well, but in these others an inflammatory response is lacking. Included are genetically determined defects in myelin metabolism, exposure to toxins such as carbon monoxide, and opportunistic viral infection of oligodendrocytes (e.g., progressive multifocal leukoencephalopathy) against a background of immune incompetence. These entities, which are usually not classified as demyelinating diseases, are discussed in Chaps. 347 and 350.

Three demyelinating diseases can be distinguished on the basis of clinical history, examination, and pathologic findings: (1) multiple sclerosis, (2) acute disseminated encephalomyelitis (including postinfectious and postvaccinal encephalomyelitis), and (3) acute necrotizing hemorrhagic encephalomyelitis.

MULTIPLE SCLEROSIS

This disease usually presents in the form of recurrent attacks of focal or multifocal neurologic dysfunction, reflecting lesions within the central nervous system (CNS). Attacks occur, remit, and recur, seemingly randomly over many years. The disease begins most commonly in early adult life. The frequency of flare-ups is greatest during the first 3 to 4 years of disease, but a first attack, which may have been so mild as to escape medical attention and can barely be recalled, may not be followed by another attack for 10 to 20 years. During typical episodes, symptoms worsen over a period of a few days to 2 to 3 weeks and then remit. Recovery is usually rapid over a period of weeks, although at times it may extend over several months. The extent of recovery varies markedly between patients and from one attack to the next in the same person. Remission may be complete, particularly after early attacks; often, however, remission is incomplete and as one attack follows another, a stepwise downward progression ensues with increasing permanent deficit.

In perhaps as many as one-third of cases the disease declares itself as a slowly but inexorably progressive illness. This is particularly likely to be the case if onset is after age 40. Although occasional patients die within the first few years of disease onset, most do not, and the average survival from multiple sclerosis (MS) is better than 30 years after onset of disease.

Multiple sclerosis is pleomorphic in its presentations. The clinical picture is determined by the location of foci of demyelination within the CNS. Classic features include impaired vision, nystagmus, dysarthria, decreased perception of vibration and position sense, ataxia and intention tremor, weakness or paralysis of one or more limbs, spasticity, and bladder problems.

Criteria which must be satisfied to establish a diagnosis of clinically definite MS include a reliable history of at least two episodes of neurologic deficit and objective clinical signs of lesions at more than one site within the CNS. Demonstration of a second lesion by laboratory tests (e.g., evoked potentials, computerized tomography, magnetic resonance imaging, or urologic studies), in concert with one objective clinical lesion, also fulfills the criteria. A finding of increased cerebrospinal fluid immunoglobulin with oligoclonal bands supports the diagnosis but will not substitute for the above criteria. Clinically probable MS is defined as either two attacks with clinical evidence of one lesion or one attack with clinical evidence of two lesions (or one clinical and one paraclinical lesion). Follow-up studies of probable MS patients indicate considerable diagnostic imprecision in this category. When signs pointing to damage of white matter tracts in optic nerves, brainstem, and spinal cord are present together and more than one attack is known to have occurred, a diagnosis of multiple sclerosis can be made with greater than 95 percent certainty. In the early years of the disease, when few relapses have occurred and fixed deficits are mild, the diagnosis may prove difficult, and single or multiple focal lesions due to other causes must be excluded.

PATHOLOGY Many scattered, discrete areas of demyelination, termed *plaques*, are the pathologic hallmark of multiple sclerosis. Macroscopically, plaques appear as gray-pink sharply defined areas which stand out against the surrounding white matter of the central nervous system. Lesions may extend into gray matter, although nerve cell bodies are seen to be preserved on microscopic examination. Plaques vary in size from a few millimeters to several centimeters; larger ones form by coalescence of smaller ones and by expansion of their margins. Plaques may be found anywhere in the white matter but typically occur in the paraventricular areas of the cerebrum and subpially, and within the brainstem and spinal cord. Their topography conforms to that of the venous drainage of the brain and spinal cord, and no particular anatomic structures are respected. The peripheral nervous system is not affected. The number of plaques found at autopsy invariably exceeds the number expected on the basis of physical signs. Many plaques, therefore, are clinically silent; this establishes that substantial impulse conduction occurs across regions of demyelination. In fact, autopsy studies indicate that 20 percent of multiple sclerosis cases are clinically silent during life.

The microscopic features of multiple sclerosis lesions depend on their age. Typically lesions of different ages and evidence of new activity about the margins of old lesions are encountered. Active multiple sclerosis lesions feature T-lymphocyte and monocyte-macrophage accumulations about venules and at plaque margins where myelin is being destroyed. The invasion of white matter by inflammatory cells is held responsible for the myelin breakdown. Macrophages (microglia) are believed to be the vectors of myelin breakdown.

They also function as scavengers of myelin debris; fat-laden macrophages may persist for months, perhaps for years, after the acute inflammatory response has subsided. Plasma cells accumulate within plaques and are usually found at or near their centers.

An astroglial response at or just beyond the margins of acutely demyelinating lesions is characteristic. In established, inactive plaques, a thick mat of fibrillary gliosis throughout the demyelinated regions is usual, and only a few residual perivascular macrophages are found. Oligodendrocyte number has been said to be normal or increased at the plaque margin. Yet, oligodendrocyte number is reduced within plaques, indicating that ultimately, this cell type is lost in multiple sclerosis. Indeed, damage to oligodendrocytes may be the primary event.

Only limited regeneration of myelin occurs in multiple sclerosis. The reason for this is unclear but may relate to loss of oligodendrocytes. At the pial margins of spinal cord plaques remyelination by peripheral nerve Schwann cells that have invaded the CNS may be encountered. Despite assiduous search, viral inclusions have not been detected in multiple sclerosis lesions. Mechanisms responsible for recovery from an MS attack are likely multiple. Resolution of edema, as documented by CT scan, and of inflammation may permit return of saltatory conduction along partially demyelinated axons (shadow plaque). Restoration of conduction, may also relate, in part, to insertion of K^+ channels along the length of denuded axonal segments rather than exclusively at the nodes of Ranvier as is the situation in myelinated nerve.

Axons within plaques tend to be spared, although in acute lesions frank necrosis with loss of axons sometimes occurs. At least 10 percent of multiple sclerosis plaques show marked axonal loss, and ultrastructural studies indicate that loss of axons may be more general than can be appreciated by routine histology. All gradations of pathologic change between the extremes described above are encountered.

The pathologic features of MS fail to account for the hour-to-hour and day-to-day waxings and wanings in function so characteristic of the disease. Conduction of impulses through demyelinated nerve is compromised and is further altered by transient changes in the internal milieu such as alterations in temperature and in electrolyte balance or by stress. Fever, or even minor increases in body temperature, such as may follow a hot bath or exercise, may cause a failure of conduction through demyelinated regions and lead to evanescent symptoms and signs. The mechanism of this axonal fatigability is unknown, but some type of conduction block is assumed to occur. It is important to distinguish transient fluctuations in symptomatology of the type just described from attacks of disease.

ETIOLOGY The cause or causes of MS remain unknown. A role for immune-mediated or infectious factors has been proposed, but data to support these postulates are fragmentary and indirect.

Epidemiology Epidemiologic studies have established several facts which will ultimately have to be incorporated into any coherent theory of the disease. Average age of onset of the first clinical episode of MS falls within the third and fourth decades. Females account for 60 percent of cases. For disease to begin in childhood or beyond the sixth decade is uncommon but not unknown.

In general, incidence in temperate climatic zones exceeds that in tropical zones; but variations within regions with similar climates do exist; hence the effect is not simply one of latitude or temperature. The incidence of MS in northern Europe, Canada, and the northern United States is approximately 10 new cases each year per 100,000 persons between the ages of 20 and 50. The incidence in Australia, New Zealand, and the southern United States is one-third to one-half of that; in Japan, elsewhere in the Orient, and in Africa MS is rare. Some epidemiologic evidence also suggests that persons migrating from high- to low-risk regions as children may be partially protected from MS. The data are consistent with the existence of an environmental factor, possibly a virus, and perhaps geographically restricted, that influences development of MS.

Genetic factors The incidence of MS among American Indians and blacks is lower than among whites living in the same regions. This suggests that genetic factors also influence disease susceptibility. Blood relatives of MS patients (parents, siblings) have an eightfold increased risk of developing MS. This could reflect an interplay of several genetic factors, shared exposure to an environmental factor, or a combination of the two. A study of MS in identical twins has revealed concordance for MS to be markedly greater than for fraternal twins; concordance among identical twins exceeds 50 percent. Family studies have failed to reveal any predictable genetic pattern but do argue persuasively for a genetically determined predisposition to disease.

Certain histocompatibility antigens (HLA) are overrepresented in patients with MS. Among whites with the disease the HLA-B7 and -DW2 alleles occur with increased frequency. Most illnesses with which an HLA association has been shown are autoimmune or infectious in nature, a finding in keeping with current thought about the etiology of MS. Many American blacks with MS express the DW2 allele; this allele is rare in blacks in Africa, among whom MS is virtually unknown. It follows that an HLA-linked genetic factor which predisposes to MS exists, but inasmuch as the vast majority of persons bearing B7 or DW2 do not develop the disease, additional genetic or environmental factors must play a role. Paradoxically, siblings concordant for MS have concordance rates for HLA haplotypes little above those expected by chance. The HLA-B12 allele is less frequent in MS than in the population at large. This finding suggests that genetically determined protective factors may operate in MS.

Autoimmune factors The lesions of MS are mimicked by those of experimental allergic encephalomyelitis (EAE), an autoimmune disease induced in animals by immunization with myelin. Lesions of EAE are demyelinating, perivenular, plaque-like, occur in chronic and recrudescent forms, and have an inflammatory infiltrate composed of lymphocytes, macrophages, and plasma cells. In EAE, T-lymphocyte sensitivity to a single antigen known as myelin basic protein can be shown to be the cause of the disease; yet in MS, sensitivity to myelin basic protein cannot be demonstrated. This indicates that should MS prove to be an autoimmune process, as the clinical and histologic parallels with EAE might suggest, the antigen is something other than myelin basic protein. Attempts to find any antigen to which only MS patients react have failed.

Attacks of MS are associated with changes in peripheral blood monocyte and lymphocyte properties. Reported changes include heightened prostaglandin secretion by macrophages (which may in turn influence lymphocyte properties), reduced suppressor cell function, an increased number of activated T cells as evidenced by expression of surface antigens characteristic of activated cells, heightened T cell–dependent in vitro immunoglobulin secretion, deficient interferon secretion, and possibly reduced natural killer (NK) cell function. Whether these changes relate to the etiology of MS is not known.

Within the cerebrospinal fluid (CSF), T-cell activation is apparent during active disease. Excessive IgG production within the CNS is characteristic of MS at all stages of disease; whether this reflects the presence of some stimulator of B cells in the brain in MS or is the result of a defect in immune regulation is not known. Viral infection of brain remains a possible cause of MS, despite the fact that all attempts to isolate, rescue, or ''passage'' a virus from MS brains or to visualize a virus within them have failed.

Precipitating factors Various infections, injury, and even emotional upsets have been claimed to precipitate a first attack of MS. Evidence in support of these claims remains anecdotal and nonpersuasive. The probability that an attack of MS will occur during the first 6 months after pregnancy is greater than chance would predict, but this observation is counterbalanced by a decreased risk of an attack during the second and third trimesters of pregnancy. In established cases, trauma, including lumbar puncture, myelography, and surgery, has not been shown to relate to attacks or to progression of disability nor has emotional turmoil been shown to alter the tempo at which the disease evolves. Experience has also shown that vaccinations do not provoke attacks of MS.

CLINICAL MANIFESTATIONS The first attack of MS may declare itself as a single symptom or sign (45 percent) or as more than one (55 percent). Approximately 40 percent of MS patients will have an episode of optic neuritis, either as their first difficulty or at some point along the course of their disease. Optic neuritis presents as loss of vision, partial or total, usually in one eye, seldom in both, and is often associated with pain on movement of the eye. Macular vision tends to be most affected (central scotoma), but a wide range of field defects may occur. Disturbances of color perception sometimes provide an early indication of mild disease. Fewer than half of optic neuritis patients will show evidence of an inflamed optic nerve head (papillitis); most show no changes in the optic disc at the outset, indicating that the demyelinating lesion is developing some distance behind the nerve head (retrobulbar neuritis). Both forms of optic neuritis will be followed by optic nerve atrophy, detected as pallor of the optic disc.

It is important to recognize that most cases of optic neuritis occur as an isolated event. At most, 40 percent of individuals with optic neuritis subsequently go on to develop MS; unfortunately it is difficult to predict who will and who will not develop the disease, although presence of oligoclonal bands in the CSF is seemingly an unfavorable finding. Whether optic neuritis occurring alone and for unknown reasons constitutes a forme fruste of MS with but a single attack is not known. Approximately one-third of patients with optic neuritis recover completely, one-third partially, and one-third little or not at all. Visual evoked response testing reveals prolonged latencies of the evoked potential in the occipital cortex in more than 80 percent of established cases of MS; less than half of these can describe an antecedent optic neuritis. Clearly subclinical involvement of the optic pathways is common.

Symptoms and signs of neurologic dysfunction arising from brainstem, cerebellar, and spinal cord lesions are frequent in MS. Diplopia may occur either because the third, fourth, or sixth cranial nerve pathways are damaged along their course within the CNS or because an internuclear ophthalmoplegia (INO) has developed (see Chap. 13). An INO reflects involvement of the medial longitudinal fasciculus. The sign consists of an inability to adduct one eye on attempted lateral gaze together with full abduction of the other eye, which shows horizontal nystagmus. Bilateral INO in a young adult is virtually diagnostic of MS, although a few instances of bilateral INO in systemic lupus erythematosus are on record. Another clinical feature of brainstem involvement is either facial hypesthesia or tic douloureux (fifth cranial nerve). When tic douloureux occurs in a young adult, the possibility of underlying MS should be seriously entertained. Bell's palsy or hemifacial spasm (seventh cranial nerve), vertigo, vomiting, and nystagmus (vestibular connections of the eighth cranial nerve) are also frequent; less commonly there is complaint of deafness. Involvement of cerebellar connections or of spinocerebellar pathways results in ataxia which can affect speech (scanning), head or trunk (titubation), limbs (intention tremor), and stance and gait. Cerebellar ataxia may be combined with sensory ataxia due to involvement of the spinal cord.

Spinal cord lesions produce a myriad of motor and sensory problems. Corticospinal tract interruption results in the classical features of upper motor neuron dysfunction (weakness, spasticity, hyperreflexia, clonus, Babinski response, loss of abdominal skin reflexes). Posterior column lesions cause loss, or diminution, of joint-position and vibration senses as well as the frequently encountered complaints of tingling or tightness of the extremities and of bandlike sensations about the trunk. Less often pain and temperature sensations are lost or diminished, reflecting spinothalamic tract involvement. Partial lesions of sensory tracts or of the root entry zones of sensory nerves can produce painful dysesthesias as well as interruption of reflex arcs. On occasion, spinal cord lesions will result in paroxysmal symptoms including tonic spasms which can be painful.

Symptoms of bladder dysfunction, including hesitancy, urgency, frequency, and incontinence, are common features of spinal cord involvement. Equally common is bowel dysfunction, particularly constipation. Males with MS, if questioned, often complain of sexual impotence; methods exist to distinguish physical from psychogenic causes. Patients with MS may experience an electric shock-like sensation on flexion of the neck, called Lhermitte's sign.

Severe spinal cord lesions can result in loss of function, sometimes total, below the level of the lesion; less complete lesions can result in the hemicord syndrome of Brown-Séquard (see Chap. 353). When either of these events occurs, it is referred to as a transverse myelitis. A single episode of transverse myelitis not followed by subsequent progression of disease may, as with an isolated episode of optic neuritis, represent a forme fruste of MS, although less than 10 percent of acute transverse myelitis cases develop MS. Again as with optic neuritis, approximately one-third of patients with transverse myelitis recover completely, one-third partially, and one-third not at all. It must be stressed that spinal cord involvement is the predominating feature in most advanced cases of MS.

Cerebral symptoms may occur in MS due to extensive involvement of subcortical and central white matter. With extensive lesions of brain, intellect may suffer, sometimes disastrously. By far the most frequent emotional feature of MS is depression. Euphoria, when it occurs, indicates widespread cerebral disease and is often associated with dementia and pseudobulbar palsy. Three to five percent of patients (twice the expected rate) will have one or more epileptic seizures, presumably because of extension of plaques into gray matter. Focal neurologic signs of cerebral origin, such as hemiparesis, homonymous hemianopsia, and dysphasia, while seen in MS, are rare.

Neuromyelitis optica and MS An ill-defined symptom complex known as Devic's syndrome, or neuromyelitis optica, is considered by some to be an entity distinguishable from MS. The complex is characterized by acute optic neuritis, usually bilateral, which is followed, or less frequently preceded, within hours to weeks by transverse myelitis. The cerebrospinal fluid may show a pleocytosis with polymorphonucler cells and a protein content that is higher than is usual for MS. Pathologic examination in fatal cases reveals more tissue destruction and cavitation than is expected in MS, although this may bespeak no more than the intensity of the process.

COURSE OF ILLNESS AND PROGNOSIS The clinical course of MS is unpredictable. In general, symptoms which appear acutely and those referable to sensory paths and the cranial nerves have a more favorable prognosis than those developing insidiously or involving motor and especially cerebellar function. According to McAlpine, 80 percent of patients who have a purely exacerbating and remitting disease have unrestricted function after 10 years. Of cases in which exacerbations and remissions are superimposed on a progressive tempo of evolution, 50 percent are disabled after 10 years. In cases that have a purely progressive course from the outset (in these the brunt of the disease usually falls on the spinal cord) long-term prognosis for ambulation is poor.

Rarely MS may be fulminant and fatal within weeks to months. Such cases, which are referred to as acute MS, show intense inflammatory responses within the plaques. Onset in such patients may be with headache, vomiting, delirium, convulsions, even coma, plus an array of signs indicating severe compromise of cortical, brainstem, optic nerve, and spinal cord function. Distinction from acute disseminated encephalomyelitis may be difficult in life; at autopsy the lesions are larger and more like those of MS.

DIFFERENTIAL DIAGNOSIS The diagnosis of MS becomes secure when signs referable to multiple lesions of CNS white matter have developed and remitted at different times. Particularly in the early phases of disease, the neurologic symptoms may suggest discrete dysfunction of the nervous system, and other causes of focal disease must be excluded. An excellent clinical rule is that MS should not be diagnosed when all the patient's symptoms and signs can be explained by a single lesion. A common aphorism is that MS presents with symptoms in one leg and signs in both.

Conditions to be excluded vary depending on the sites of the lesions. Abrupt monocular loss of vision may result from impaired vascular supply to the optic nerve, including embolic and thrombotic occlusion of the carotid, ophthalmic, or central retinal arteries, or as an accompaniment of migraine. When monocular visual loss is more gradual, compressive lesions affecting the optic nerve or an optic nerve glioma need to be considered.

In patients presenting with acute or progressive spinal cord disease, the presence of focal lesions affecting the cord and of degenerative-nutritional diseases which selectively affect spinal cord tracts should be considered (see Chaps. 349 and 353). Patients with progressive spastic paraplegia should be evaluated for the presence of intrathecal or extradural neoplasm and for cervical spondylosis. Such evaluation often requires a CT body scan, magnetic resonance imaging (MRI), or myelography. Hereditary ataxias can present as degeneration of multiple CNS tracts, with or without involvement of the peripheral nervous system. Degeneration of posterior columns and corticospinal and spinocerebellar tracts is common in these disorders. Hereditary ataxias are slowly progressive and feature stereotyped symmetric involvement as well as a family history consistent with autosomal dominant, or recessive, inheritance. Amyotrophic lateral sclerosis (ALS) usually presents with prominent lower motor neuron signs (atrophy, weakness, and fasciculations) in addition to pyramidal signs (spasticity, hyperreflexia) and without sensory abnormalities. Subacute combined degeneration of the cord can be excluded by symmetry of spinal symptoms and by a normal serum vitamin B_{12} level, a normal bone marrow, and a normal Schilling test.

When progressive brainstem dysfunction occurs, posterior fossa tumor as well as brainstem encephalitis should be excluded. Single cranial nerve palsies, particularly Bell's palsy, trigeminal sensory neuropathy, or tic douloureux may occur as part of the MS picture, but evidence of multifocal disease must be present before they can be ascribed to MS. When vertigo is the complaint and nystagmus is detected, inner ear disease should be considered as well as the possibility that barbiturates or phenytoin have been taken.

There are several multifocal and recrudescent diseases of the central nervous system which may mimic MS. Systemic lupus erythematosus and other vasculitides may cause scattered and recurring lesions within brain, brainstem, and spinal cord. Behçet's disease is characterized by recurrent episodes of focal brain disease, CSF pleocytosis, oral and genital ulcers, and uveitis. Other disorders to be excluded include meningovascular syphilis, cryptococcosis, toxoplasmosis, other chronic nervous system infections, and sarcoidosis.

When complaints are vague and findings minimal, a diagnosis of conversion reaction (hysteria) may come to mind. This diagnosis should always be made on the basis of positive criteria for hysteria and never as a "diagnosis by exclusion." Early in its course, MS is mislabeled as hysteria with distressing frequency. Patients with MS may develop superimposed hysterical phenomena adding to the complexity of the clinical syndrome.

A few patients present with pain as their principal symptom. Awareness of its occurrence in MS and careful attention to a thorough examination will usually clarify the diagnosis.

A firm diagnosis of MS should only be made when the evidence is unequivocal. Aside from the distress that such a diagnosis causes, it will serve to explain almost any subsequent neurologic event and may divert attention away from other possibly treatable diseases.

LABORATORY TESTS Although the diagnosis of MS continues to depend on its clinical features, laboratory aids have become increasingly useful as supports for the diagnosis. In the vast majority of patients with MS, one or more tests will be abnormal, although normal results do not rule out the diagnosis.

The CSF in MS patients typically reveals only a slight or no increase in cell number. Ninety percent of patients show fewer than 10 cells per cubic millimeter in their CSF; cell counts greater than 50 are rare. The cells in the CSF are predominantly T lymphocytes, although rare plasma cells may be found. Some correlation exists between the extent of pleocytosis and disease activity. Higher cell counts also are more typical in early stages of disease. Evidence that the lymphocytes in the CSF are activated not only during exacerbations of disease but also during seeming remission has been presented; this indicates that disease activity smolders at all times, even though neither the physician nor the patient may be able to detect changes. T-cell lines specifically reactive with various viral and nonviral antigens can be derived from the CSF of MS patients, again suggesting that a heterogeneous immune response is ongoing (see discussion of oligoclonal bands below). The CSF of 90 percent of patients contains less than 60 mg/dL of total protein; protein of greater than 100 mg/dL should raise questions about whether the diagnosis is correct.

The most characteristic CSF finding in MS is an increase in immunoglobulin G (IgG) which contrasts with relatively normal total protein and albumin concentrations. IgG levels are increased in 80 percent of MS patients; the increase is greatest in long-standing cases with severe neurologic deficits. Early in the disease, when the diagnosis is most in doubt, IgG values can be normal. IgG levels do not change in any meaningful way with relapses and remissions. Most of the IgG in the CSF is synthesized within the central nervous system. The increased IgG fraction in the CSF explains the first-zone abnormality of the colloidal gold curve, a test of historical interest.

When the CSF IgG from MS patients is subjected to electrophoresis or isoelectric focusing, it fractionates into a restricted number of bands (termed oligoclonal bands). Oligoclonal banding of IgG has also been found in the CSF in a number of acute and chronic central nervous system infections; in subacute sclerosing panencephalitis cases, these bands have been shown to be antibodies to the infective agent. In MS, the IgG bands have not been shown to be directed against any single viral or intrinsic brain antigen; more likely they represent a heterogeneous group of antibodies directed against many antigens. The number of bands in the CSF is greater in those with longer disease duration. It has also been suggested that high levels of IgG and many oligoclonal bands are associated with a severe course. The overall IgG shows further restrictions in its heterogeneity, with the IgG_1 being mainly of the $G1m_1$ allotype. Rare cases of MS without increased CSF IgG synthesis or oligoclonal bands have been documented at autopsy.

Within CSF, myelin debris as well as myelin basic protein appears during attacks of disease. Myelin basic protein levels can be measured by radioimmunoassay; the level seems to reflect the extent of myelin breakdown since levels also increase in other disorders associated with white matter breakdown such as stroke.

Conduction of nerve impulses along axons denuded of their myelin is slowed. Evoked response testing provides a sensitive means to detect slowed conduction of visual, auditory, or somatosensory impulses. Such tests employ repetitive sensory stimuli and utilize computer averaging techniques to record the electric responses evoked during the conduction of these stimuli along visual, auditory, or somatosensory afferent pathways. In normal subjects, the pattern of the evoked responses and time for conduction are highly predictable. One or more of the evoked response tests will reveal slowing of conduction in 80 percent of MS patients; in 30 to 40 percent of patients, abnormal evoked responses are detected without any clinical symptoms or signs in the involved pathway being apparent. Evoked response testing may confirm the presence of additional sites of disease in suspected cases with only a single clinically detectable lesion (see Chap. 341).

Computerized tomography (CT) of the brain may reveal low-density lesions within white matter, usually in a paraventricular or subcortical distribution. The incidence of such abnormalities discovered by CT scanning is reported to range from 10 to 50 percent and may reflect either active or chronic lesions as determined by pathologic criteria. Similar lesions may be noted in optic nerves and brainstem. At times, enhancement may be revealed by iodine infusion, particularly when coupled with use of high dosage of dye and delayed scanning. This finding indicates the presence of acute lesions and a disruption of the blood-brain barrier. Enhancement may disappear as the clinical symptoms resolve. Cortical atrophy with enlarged ventricles is also found in some patients.

Magnetic resonance imaging (MRI) provides an even more sensitive means to detect lesions corresponding to the low-density lesions found on CT scans. MRI scanning detects more lesions than CT scanning but fails to distinguish enhancing lesions with the sensitivity of the CT infusion scan.

Elevated CSF IgG, abnormal evoked responses, and lesions on CT scans and MRI provide useful adjuncts in evaluation of the patient with suspected MS; however, the clinical findings remain paramount in establishing the diagnosis.

TREATMENT OF MS No effective treatment for MS is known. Therapeutic efforts are directed toward (1) amelioration of the acute episode, (2) prevention of relapses, and (3) relief of symptoms.

In acute flare-ups of disease, glucocorticoid treatment may lessen the severity of symptoms and speed recovery; however, ultimate recovery is not improved by this drug nor is the extent of permanent disability altered. Glucocorticoids likely act chiefly via mechanisms other than modulation of the immune response. They may improve the ability of demyelinated nerve to conduct and reduce edema and inflammation within plaques. Usual regimens utilize either ACTH, to stimulate endogenous glucocorticoid synthesis, or prednisone. ACTH is preferred by many clinicians since the only controlled trials that demonstrated the efficacy of glucocorticoid therapy in flare-ups of MS and in acute optic neuritis were performed with this drug. ACTH is commonly given in a dose of 80 units daily intravenously for 3 to 7 days, followed by intramuscular injections in periodically decreasing doses over the next 2 to 3 weeks. Prednisone, 15 mg qid, is sometimes given rather than ACTH, again over 3 to 7 days with gradually tapering doses over the next 2 to 3 weeks. Since prednisone is taken by mouth, the treatment is simpler than with ACTH, and an admission to the hospital may sometimes be avoided. Use of long-term daily or alternate-day steroids is not advised.

Immunosuppressive agents such as azathioprine have been claimed to reduce the number of relapses in several series, but there is no consensus about the efficacy of this drug. Although the question of efficacy remains unresolved, the abnormal B-cell response seen in the blood in MS returns to normal levels with azathioprine treatment. Results from clinical trials with plasmapheresis and interferon have been equivocal. High-dose intravenous cyclophosphamide appears to transiently benefit a proportion of patients with the progressive form of MS. The above therapies and others including antithymocyte serum, total lymphoid irradiation, cyclosporine A, and copolymer I remain under active investigation.

Symptomatic treatment should address both the physical and psychological needs of patients. Patients should avoid excess fatigue and extremes of temperature and eat a balanced diet. Diets containing low levels of saturated fats have been advocated. The use of belladonna alkaloids and bethanechol chloride can help bladder dysfunction. Periodic checks for urinary tract infection should be performed. Bowel training can alleviate disorders of bowel function. Drugs available for the treatment of spasticity include diazepam, baclofen, and dantrolene sodium. Painful dysesthesias, facial twitching, tic douloureux, and tonic spasms may respond to carbamazepine or phenytoin. Occasionally trigeminal root injection is required to relieve tic douloureux (see Chap. 352).

ACUTE DISSEMINATED ENCEPHALOMYELITIS

Acute disseminated encephalomyelitis (ADEM) may be defined as a monophasic encephalitis or myelitis of abrupt onset characterized by symptoms and signs indicative of damage chiefly of the white matter of the brain or spinal cord. The process may be severe, and even fatal, or mild and evanescent. Pathologic features are those of innumerable minute foci of perivenular lymphocyte and mononuclear cell infiltration with demyelination. The topography of the demyelination corresponds to that of the inflammatory infiltrates. The condition most commonly follows vaccinations against rabies or smallpox or acute infectious illnesses, especially measles, but may occur without any obvious antecedent. The cause is uncertain but is believed by some to represent a hypersensitivity, perhaps to myelin basic protein, and to be the human counterpart of experimentally induced EAE.

ETIOLOGY The entity has been described after two types of vaccination: after rabies vaccination with the Semple vaccine, which contains brain tissue, now seldom used, and after vaccination against smallpox, now seldom performed.

Shortly after introduction of rabies vaccination by Pasteur, it became evident that neuroparalytic accidents could follow this procedure. After a course of injections a sudden encephalitic or myelitic catastrophe might occur coincident with hypersensitivity-type reactions at the sites of vaccine injection. The process clearly involved hypersensitivity to nervous system antigens. The incidence was variously reported as between 1 in 1000 and 1 in 5000 persons vaccinated. An identical syndrome has followed inoculation with noninfected brain material, indicating that killed rabies virus was not the cause; with the introduction of duck embryo killed rabies virus vaccine (which is free of myelinated nervous tissue), the condition has markedly decreased in incidence, although rare cases continue to be reported. Neuroparalytic accidents were most frequent in young adults, the peak age of occurrence corresponding to that of onset of MS.

Smallpox vaccination was also followed by an incidence of ADEM averaging perhaps 1 case per 5000 persons vaccinated but with marked differences between vaccination programs. The complication almost always occurred in conjunction with a primary take rather than a booster-type response. The encephalitis usually followed the peak of the vaccination response by a few days to a week or more but on occasion preceded it. The complication was unknown in children less than 2 years of age; in infants, smallpox vaccination was sometimes associated with an encephalopathy with brain swelling, i.e., toxic encephalopathy.

One case of measles in 1000 is followed by neurologic complications, which are often severe. The mortality rate averages 20 percent, and half the survivors are left with residual damage. The syndrome usually follows the rash by a few days. It bears no relationship to the severity of measles itself. Systemic lymphocyte sensitivity to myelin basic protein has been demonstrated in some patients. All attempts to isolate a virus have failed. Abnormal CSF and changes in the electroencephalogram are observed in perhaps half the children who contract measles, suggesting that subclinical neurologic involvement may be much more widespread than is usually appreciated. A subtle decline in performance and changes in behavior following measles may reflect this inapparent nervous system involvement. Measles vaccination has drastically reduced the frequency of this complication.

An identical clinical picture was seen formerly as a complication of smallpox and is still encountered during or following chickenpox and extremely rarely as a complication of rubella. Demyelinating encephalomyelitis is very rare in mumps; instead there is often a true viral meningitis. A clinical picture identical to postinfectious encephalomyelitis has been described after mycoplasma infections. Despite its striking association with measles, the occurrence of the same clinical picture after several different infections fits better with the postulate that the basic process involves hypersensitivity rather than a direct viral infection of the brain and spinal cord. All attempts to isolate a virus have failed.

CLINICAL MANIFESTATIONS The disease usually begins abruptly. Headache and delirium may give way to lethargy and coma. Coma has an ominous prognosis. Seizures at the onset or shortly thereafter are not infrequent. There may be stiffness of the neck, other signs of meningeal irritation, and fever. Focal signs may be engrafted on this picture, and spinal cord involvement with flaccid paralysis of all four limbs is particularly common. Monoparesis and hemiplegia are also seen. Tendon reflexes may be lost initially only to become hyperactive later; extensor plantar responses are the rule, and sphincter control is generally lost. Sensory loss is variable but may be extensive and severe. Brainstem involvement may be reflected by nystagmus, ocular palsies, and pupillary changes. Some cases may present as a purely spinal cord syndrome and in mild instances with minor signs such as a facial palsy. Chorea and athetosis are rare. Cerebellar signs may predominate, particularly in cases associated with chickenpox. Involvement of motor and sensory peripheral nerves can be documented clinically and electromyographically in some patients. The CSF almost always shows an increase in protein (50 to 100 mg/dL) and lymphocytes (10 to several hundred cells); rarely it is normal. The mortality is 20 percent, and perhaps half the survivors have residual deficits. Recurrences are almost unknown.

The diagnosis is not difficult if there is a history of rabies or smallpox vaccination or of measles. In cases without such a history, distinction from viral encephalitis may be difficult and at times not possible. Reye's syndrome (see Chap. 347) may be difficult to distinguish from acute disseminated encephalomyelitis. Vomiting at onset, a normal CSF, hyperammonemia, and raised intracranial pressure should suggest Reye's syndrome; frequent convulsions and focal signs argue against it. A distinction from acute MS may not be possible.

PREVENTION AND TREATMENT Since smallpox has been eradicated, there is no longer reason to vaccinate against it. Use of duck embryo and human diploid vaccine in rabies prophylaxis has almost eliminated neuroparalytic accidents, and measles vaccination has drastically reduced what used to be the largest group of postinfectious encephalomyelitides.

Administration of high doses of glucocorticoids every 4 to 6 h is the treatment of choice though controlled trials have not been carried out.

ACUTE NECROTIZING HEMORRHAGIC ENCEPHALOMYELITIS

Acute necrotizing hemorrhagic encephalomyelitis is a rare tissue-destructive disease of the CNS which occurs with explosive suddenness within a few days of an upper respiratory infection. The pathologic findings are distinctive. On sectioning the brain, much of the white matter of one or both hemispheres is seen to be destroyed almost to the point of liquefaction. The involved tissue is pink or yellowish-gray and flecked with multiple small hemorrhages. Sometimes similar changes are localized to the brainstem or spinal cord. On histologic examination the core lesion resembles that of acute disseminated encephalomyelitis in showing perivenular foci of demyelination, all of like age. As in acute disseminated encephalomyelitis lymphocytes and macrophages are present in the regions of myelin loss, but superimposed on and dominating the picture is an intense polymorphonuclear infiltrate, in keeping with the necrotizing nature of the process. The vessels themselves are partially necrotic; they may contain platelet or fibrin thrombi within their lumens and fibrin deposits beyond their walls. Multiple small hemorrhages at sites of vessel damage are an invariable feature as is a violent inflammatory reaction in the meninges. Large necrotic foci form by coalescence of smaller lesions in the hemispheres, brainstem, or spinal cord.

The clinical course of the illness resembles that of acute disseminated encephalomyelitis save for its apoplectiform onset and rapidity of progress, sometimes leading to death within 48 h. Neurologic signs are frequently unilateral, reflecting disease in one cerebral hemisphere, but may be bilateral. It is probable that certain patients showing an explosive myelitic illness are suffering from a necrotizing myelitis of similar type, but pathologic evidence in support of this view has been difficult to obtain. The CSF examination discloses a more intense reaction than in other demyelinating diseases. Often a polymorphonuclear pleocytosis of up to 2000 cells and a considerable increase in amount of protein are detected. In cases of slower evolution the cell counts are lower and cells are mainly of the mononuclear type.

The etiology of this disease is not established; however, the entire clinical-pathologic entity bears a close resemblance to a hyperacute form of EAE which can be induced in animals by administration of endotoxin, pertussis vaccine, or its histamine sensitizing factor coincident with or shortly after injection of myelin in adjuvant. The lesions in this experimental disease can perhaps be considered as those of a Sanarelli-Schwartzman reaction within the brain superimposed on an acutely demyelinating process. Rarely a lesion like acute necrotizing hemorrhagic encephalomyelitis occurs in MS.

The differential diagnosis of this disorder includes acute encephalitis, particularly those types causing tissue necrosis (herpes simplex, arbovirus), acute bacterial cerebritis, septic embolic occlusion of an artery, thrombophlebitis, and suppurative brain abscess. The similarity of acute necrotizing hemorrhagic encephalomyelitis to acute disseminated encephaloymyelitis suggests that steroid therapy may be beneficial.

REFERENCES

Ebers GC, Paty D: HLA typing in multiple sclerosis sibling pairs. Lancet 1:88, 1982
Johnson RT et al: Measles encephalomyelitis: Clinical and immunological studies. N Engl J Med 310:137, 1984
McAlpine D et al: *Multiple Sclerosis: A Reappraisal*. London, Churchill Livingston, 1972
McFarlin DE, McFarland ME: Multiple sclerosis. N Engl J Med 307:1183 and 1246, 1982
Poser CM et al: *The Diagnosis of Multiple Sclerosis*. New York, Thieme-Stratton, 1984
Scheinberg L, Raine CS: *Multiple Sclerosis—Experimental and Clinical Aspects*. New York, Annals of The New York Academy of Sciences, 1984, vol 436
Waxman SG: Membranes, myelin, and the pathophysiology of multiple sclerosis. N Engl J Med 306:1529, 1982

349 NUTRITIONAL AND METABOLIC DISEASES OF THE NERVOUS SYSTEM

MAURICE VICTOR / JOSEPH B. MARTIN

Included under the title of this chapter is a large and diverse number of neurologic disorders which fall readily into two distinct types—acquired and inherited. In this chapter, emphasis will be on the *acquired* diseases, insofar as they are essentially disorders of adult life and a major source of concern to internist and neurologist alike. In fact, no other category of disease so clearly exemplifies the interdependence of these two medical disciplines. The *inherited* metabolic and nutritional diseases, on the other hand, are predominantly disorders of infancy and childhood, and are more appropriately considered in a textbook of pediatrics. However, a small proportion of the inherited diseases permit survival to adolescence or early adult life or may even have their onset during these periods. These latter instances, which need to be differentiated from certain degenerative and acquired metabolic diseases, are discussed here briefly and in other chapters of this book to which the reader will be referred.

DISEASES DUE TO NUTRITIONAL DEFICIENCY

The general aspects of deficiency disease have been presented in Chap. 76, which should be reviewed as an introduction to the discussion of deficiency diseases of the nervous system. The term *deficiency* will be used here in its strictest sense, to designate those diseases or syndromes which result from the *lack of an essential nutrient in the diet or from a conditioning factor which increases the need for that nutrient*. The neurologic diseases which belong in this category are the following:

1 Wernicke's disease and Korsakoff's psychosis
2 "Alcoholic" cerebellar degeneration
3 Nutritional polyneuropathy (neuropathic beriberi)
4 Pellagra
5 Deficiency amblyopia (nutritional optic neuropathy)
6 The syndrome of amblyopia, painful neuropathy, and orogenital dermatitis (Strachan's syndrome)
7 Subacute combined degeneration of the spinal cord (vitamin B_{12} deficiency)
8 Vitamin E deficiency

A number of general principles are applicable to all of the diseases under consideration. Of the known vitamin deficiencies, it is essentially those of the B group which are of importance in neurologic disease [vitamin E deficiency due to cholestasis is a rare cause of central nervous system (CNS) disease in young children]. Thiamine chloride, nicotinic acid, pyridoxine, pantothenic acid, and riboflavin all play a role in carbohydrate metabolism, upon which the CNS depends for its principal source of energy. These vitamins function as coenzymes in the Krebs tricarboxylic acid cycle; in addition, thiamine is involved in the hexose-monophosphate shunt. Vitamin B_{12} is required for the conversion of methylmalonyl to succinyl coenzyme A and for the conversion of homocystine to methionine.

Except for subacute combined degeneration of the spinal cord and other manifestations of vitamin B_{12} deficiency, it is not possible to relate the deficiency diseases in humans to the lack of one particular vitamin. For example, polyneuropathy may result from any one of several vitamin deficiencies [thiamine chloride (vitamin B_1), pyridoxine (vitamin B_6), pantothenic acid, and probably B_{12}]. Moreover, pellagra, beriberi, and Strachan's syndrome are probably related to a deficiency of several vitamins. These generalizations should not obscure the fact that certain manifestations of deficiency disease are related to the lack of a specific nutrient (e.g., the ocular signs of Wernicke's disease to a deficiency of thiamine).

In the western world the deficiency diseases of the nervous system are observed most often in the alcoholic population of large urban centers. Alcohol acts mainly by displacing food in the diet, but it also increases the demand for B vitamins, which are necessary to metabolize the carbohydrate furnished by alcohol itself, and it may impair the gastrointestinal absorption of vitamins. Dietary faddism, impaired absorption of dietary nutrients (as occurs in sprue or following plication of the stomach or resection of stomach and small bowel), and the use of certain drugs (e.g., isoniazid and hydralazine, which interfere with the enzymatic function of pyridoxine) account for a relatively small number of cases of deficiency disease.

Each of the deficiency diseases may occur in pure form and will be so described. More often they occur in various combinations. Stated in another way, it is usual for deficiency diseases to involve both the central and peripheral nervous systems, an attribute which they share with few other categories of disease. Also, the examination of patients with deficiency disease frequently discloses nonneurologic signs of malnutrition such as general wasting, lesions of the skin and mucous membranes, and circulatory abnormalities.

WERNICKE'S DISEASE OR ENCEPHALOPATHY In 1881, Carl Wernicke described an illness of acute onset characterized by mental disturbance, paralysis of eye movements, and ataxia of gait. Swelling of the optic discs and retinal hemorrhages were also said to be present. In all three of Wernicke's patients there was a progressive depression of the state of consciousness, leading to death, so that a fatal outcome was at one time thought to be a universal feature of this disease. Wernicke described focal vascular lesions, affecting the gray matter around the third and fourth ventricles and aqueduct of Sylvius. He regarded the disease as inflammatory in nature and suggested the name *acute superior hemorrhagic polioencephalitis*. Since Wernicke's time, views regarding this disease have undergone considerable modification.

Symptoms and signs The most readily recognized abnormalities are the ocular motor signs, and it is difficult to make the diagnosis without them. The usual ocular abnormality is a weakness or paralysis of abduction (6th nerve palsy) which is invariably bilateral though rarely symmetric and is accompanied by horizontal diplopia, internal strabismus, and nystagmus. Three types of nystagmus may occur, conjugate horizontal or vertical gaze–evoked nystagmus being the most frequent. Rarely, one sees a primary position upbeat or downbeat nystagmus with oscillopsia. An asymmetric horizontal gaze–evoked nystagmus in the abducting eye is characteristic of internuclear ophthalmoplegia. The latter disorder may be present alone, but far more often a constellation of signs of disordered motility are present, including supranuclear paralysis of gaze. Horizontal gaze palsy, unilateral or bilateral, is more frequently seen than vertical gaze palsy. Rarely an isolated paralysis of downgaze occurs, or isolated paralysis of convergence or divergence. The vestibular responses to caloric stimulation are characteristically impaired. In advanced stages of the disease there may be complete loss of ocular movement, and the pupils, which ordinarily are spared, may become miotic and nonreacting. Ptosis and retinal hemorrhages are observed rarely. It is noteworthy that intravenous vitamin therapy in the early stages of the disease can result in dramatic recovery of the eye movement disorders although nystagmus may persist.

The *ataxia* affects stance and gait predominantly. It may be so severe initially that the patient is unable to stand or walk without support. With specific treatment the disorder of equilibrium improves, and the patient is left with a wide-based, uncertain gait. The mildest degree of ataxia is brought out only by heel-to-toe walking. In contrast to the gross disorder of locomotion, an intention (cerebellar) tremor of the limbs is relatively infrequent. The latter abnormality, when present, affects the legs more than the arms. Scanning speech is present only in isolated cases.

A derangement of mental function is found in about 90 percent of patients and takes one of several forms: (1) The most common is a *global confusional-apathetic state,* characterized by profound listlessness, inattentiveness, indifference to the surroundings, and disorientation. Unconsciousness or deep stupor as the initial abnormality is distinctly rare, but mild drowsiness is common. Spontaneous speech is minimal. Many questions directed to the patient go unanswered, or the patient may fall asleep while being questioned, a state from which he or she can be readily aroused, however. Whatever questions the patient answers betray disorientation in time and place, misidentification of those nearby and an inability to grasp the meaning of the illness or immediate situation. Many of the patient's remarks are irrational and show no consistency from one moment to another. Under these circumstances a more extensive evaluation of intellectual function is seldom possible. (2) Some patients, at the time they are first seen, already show a disproportionate disorder of retentive memory, i.e., Korsakoff's amnesic state (see Chap. 23 and later in this chapter). (3) A relatively small number of patients (less than 20 percent in our series) show the symptoms of alcohol withdrawal, either delirium tremens or a variant thereof.

The symptoms of Wernicke's disease may all appear simultaneously and rather acutely, but more often the ophthalmoplegia and/or ataxia precede the mental signs by a few days and sometimes by a week or more.

Wernicke's disease is usually associated with other nutritional disorders, both neurologic and nonneurologic. In more than 80 percent of patients, a *polyneuropathy* of varying degrees of severity is evident. Rarely, *amblyopia* or *spinal spastic ataxia* may be added to the clinical picture. Many patients in the chronic stage of the disease demonstrate impaired olfactory discrimination, a defect that is most likely related to the diencephalic lesions (see below).

Full-blown beriberi heart disease is rarely observed in association with Wernicke's disease, although indications of *disordered cardio-*

vascular function such as tachycardia, exertional dyspnea, postural hypotension, and minor ECG abnormalities are common. Occasionally patients may die suddenly, the mode of death suggesting "cardiovascular collapse." It has been shown that Wernicke's disease is characterized by a state of high cardiac output which is out of proportion to the oxygen consumption. This is probably due to an abnormal state of peripheral vasodilatation, which in turn may be related to thiamine deficiency. Postural hypertension and syncope are related to impaired function of the automatic nervous system, more specifically to a defect in sympathetic regulation.

Ancillary findings Vestibular function, as measured by the response to standard caloric testing, is always impaired bilaterally and more or less symmetrically in the acute stages of Wernicke's disease (*vestibular paresis*). The cerebrospinal fluid (CSF) is normal or shows only a modest elevation of protein content; protein values above 100 mg/dL or a pleocytosis should always suggest the presence of a complicating illness. In untreated cases of Wernicke's disease, there is invariably an elevation of the *blood pyruvate,* and a marked reduction in the *blood transketolase* (a thiamine-dependent enzyme of the hexose monophosphate shunt). Diffuse slowing of the EEG, mild to moderate in degree, occurs in about one-half of the patients. On the other hand, total cerebral blood flow and cerebral oxygen and glucose consumption may be greatly reduced in the acute stages of the disease and may persist for several weeks after the institution of treatment.

Course of the illness Death occurs in 15 to 20 percent of hospitalized patients and is usually due to a complicating infection (pneumonia, pulmonary tuberculosis, and septicemia being the most common) or to hepatic failure.

Patients who recover do so in a characteristic manner. Ocular palsies may *begin to improve* within hours after the administration of thiamine and practically always within several days. Failure of the patient to respond in this manner should raise doubts about the diagnosis of Wernicke's disease. Sixth nerve palsies, ptosis, and vertical gaze palsies recover completely, within a week or two in most cases, but gaze–evoked vertical nystagmus may occasionally persist for several months. Horizontal gaze palsies recover completely as a rule, but in more than half the patients a fine horizontal gaze–evoked nystagmus remains as a permanent sequela of the disease.

Ataxia improves somewhat more slowly than the ocular motor abnormalities. Approximately half the patients recover incompletely and are left with a slow, shuffling, wide-based gait and inability to walk tandem. The residual gait disturbance and horizontal nystagmus provide a means of identifying obscure and chronic cases of dementia as alcoholic-nutritional in origin. Vestibular function, as measured by caloric testing, improves at about the same rate as the ataxia of stance and gait, i.e., over a period of weeks or months, and recovery is usually but not always complete.

The symptoms of apathy, drowsiness, and confusion recede gradually, and as they do, the *defect in retentive memory and learning (Korsakoff's psychosis; see Chap. 23)* stands out more clearly. It is important to emphasize that in the alcoholic, nutritionally deficient patient Wernicke's disease and Korsakoff's psychosis are not separate diseases, but the changing ocular and ataxic signs and the transformation of the global confusion state into an amnesic syndrome are successive stages in the recovery of a single disease process. Stated in another way, Korsakoff's psychosis is the psychic component of Wernicke's disease. Hence the symptom complex should be called Wernicke's disease when the amnesic state is not evident and the Wernicke-Korsakoff syndrome when both the ocular-ataxic and amnesic symptoms can be recognized.

The outcome of Korsakoff's psychosis varies. Complete or almost complete recovery occurs in less than 20 percent of patients. In the remainder recovery is slow and incomplete. Depending on the severity of the residual symptoms, the patient may or may not be able to lead a supervised existence out of a hospital. The residual mental state is characterized by large gaps in memory, without confabulation, and an inability of the patient to sort out events in their proper temporal sequence. This late stage of the disease, when the ocular and ataxic signs have receded or are not recognized, is often loosely referred to as "alcoholic deteriorated state" or "alcoholic dementia."

Pathologic changes Postmortem examination of patients who die in the acute stages of Wernicke-Korsakoff disease discloses symmetrically placed lesions in the paraventricular regions of the thalamus and hypothalamus, the mamillary bodies, the periaqueductal region of the midbrain, the floor of the fourth ventricle, and the anterior-superior folia of the cerebellum, particularly of the vermis. Lesions are invariably found in the mamillary bodies and less consistently in the other areas. Microscopically, the principal change consists of varying degrees of necrosis of parenchymal structures. Many nerve cells and fibers are destroyed; others remain intact and are seen against a background of reactive glial elements, both astrocytes and microgliocytes. The blood vessels are prominent, owing to adventitial and endothelial proliferation. Hemorrhagic lesions are present in a small proportion of cases and usually give the appearance of being of recent origin. The oculomotor and vestibular nuclei are regularly involved, but to a lesser degree.

Clinical-pathologic correlations The ocular motor signs are attributable to lesions in the brainstem affecting the abducens nuclei and eye movement centers in the pons and rostral midbrain (see Chap. 13). The lesions of the vestibular nuclei are probably responsible for the loss of caloric responses and gross abnormality of equilibrium that characterize the initial stage of the disease. The lack of significant destruction of nerve cells in these lesions accounts for the rapid improvement in oculomotor and vestibular function.

The persistent ataxia of stance and gait is related to the loss of neurons in the superior vermis of the cerebellum; extension of the lesion into the anterior parts of the anterior lobes accounts for the ataxia of individual movements of the legs. These cerebellar lesions are indistinguishable from those of so-called *alcoholic cerebellar degeneration* (see below).

The amnesic defect is related to lesions in the diencephalon, more specifically to those in the medial dorsal nuclei of the thalami. Lesions in the mamillary bodies are probably not critical in respect to memory function since they are found in patients with Wernicke's disease who had shown no disorder of memory during life.

Etiology and pathogenesis Nutritional deficiency is now established as the causal factor. Wernicke's disease has been encountered in prisoners-of-war and in patients with wasting diseases of varied origin, i.e., circumstances in which alcohol played no part. The specific factor that is responsible for most, if not all, of the symptoms of the Wernicke-Korsakoff syndrome is a deficiency of thiamine. The marked sensitivity of the ocular abnormalities to the administration of thiamine accounts for their rapid abatement after the ingestion of a meal or two. The quality of prompt reversibility suggests that the ocular signs are due to a biochemical abnormality and not to irreversible structural changes. On the other hand, the slow and incomplete recovery of the memory defect suggests that this symptom is due to irreversible structural changes, presumably in the medial dorsal nuclei.

The selective vulnerability of certain periventricular regions to a deficiency of thiamine is not understood. McEntee and Mair have pointed out that the lesions lie in the monoamine-containing pathways and have presented evidence that 3-methoxy-4-hydroxyphenylglycol (MHPG), the primary brain metabolite of norepinephrine, is decreased in the CNS of patients with Korsakoff's psychosis; moreover, the administration of clonidine, an $alpha_2$ adrenergic agonist, seemed to improve the memory disorder in these patients. These authors theorized that damage to the ascending norepinephrine-containing neurons in the brainstem and diencephalon may be the basis for the amnesia.

The topography of the lesions caused by thiamine deficiency has been studied in rhesus monkeys. Witt and Goldman-Rakic found that the severity and number of brain nuclei affected are related to the duration and number of bouts of thiamine deficiency. Blass and Gibson have suggested that a genetically determined defect in transketolase may be operative in the pathogenesis of Wernicke's disease. They found that transketolase in cultural fibroblasts from patients with this disease bound thiamine pyrophosphate (TPP) less avidly than did the transketolase from control lines. This defect in transketolase would presumably be insignificant if the diet were adequate, but would be harmful if the diet were low in thiamine. These findings may explain why only a small proportion of alcoholics develop Wernicke-Korsakoff disease.

Treatment of the Wernicke-Korsakoff syndrome Wernicke's disease represents a medical emergency, and its recognition demands the immediate administration of thiamine. A delay of a few hours may be crucial in determining whether the patient with ocular and ataxic signs will be prevented from developing Korsakoff's psychosis and whether the patient with early Korsakoff's changes will be restored to a state of mental competency. Although 2 to 3 mg of thiamine may modify the ocular signs, much larger doses are needed to replenish the thiamine stores—50 mg intravenously and 50 mg intramuscularly, the latter dose being repeated each day until the patient resumes a normal diet. The other B vitamins may be given by mouth in the dosages outlined in Chap. 76. If the patient cannot or will not eat, parenteral feeding and administration of B vitamins become necessary.

A particular danger attends the treatment of the severely depleted alcoholic patient with intravenous glucose solutions. Such infusions may exhaust the patient's reserve of B vitamins and either precipitate Wernicke's disease in a previously unaffected patient or cause a rapid worsening of an early form of the disease. For this reason, B vitamins must be administered to all alcoholic patients requiring parenteral glucose. If there are signs of cardiac failure, rapid digitalization should be undertaken. Since these patients are confused and forgetful, they must be supervised continually, preferably on a medical ward.

A special problem in management arises when the patient recovers from the acute phase of the illness and the amnesic psychosis becomes prominent. The disposition of the patient to family, nursing home, or mental institution should be undertaken on the basis of the severity of the mental illness as well as the capacity of the family unit and social circumstances.

"ALCOHOLIC" CEREBELLAR DEGENERATION This is the term applied to a common, stereotyped, nonfamilial form of cerebellar ataxia which occurs on a background of prolonged ingestion of alcohol. Usually the symptoms evolve in subacute fashion, i.e., over several weeks or months, sometimes more rapidly. In some patients the symptoms are present in mild but stable form and worsen after an attack of pneumonia or delirium tremens.

The signs are those of cerebellar dysfunction, affecting stance and gait predominantly. The legs are involved more severely than the arms, and nystagmus and speech disturbances occur relatively infrequently. Once established, the signs change very little, although some improvement of gait may follow the cessation of drinking, due probably to improvement in general nutrition and recovery from an associated polyneuropathy.

The pathologic changes consist of degeneration of varying severity of all the neurocellular elements of the cerebellar cortex, particularly of the Purkinje cells, with a striking topographic restriction to the anterior and superior aspects of the vermis and adjacent parts of the anterior lobes of the cerebellum. The disorder of stance and gait is related to the lesion in the vermis, and the ataxia of the limbs to the involvement of the anterior lobes. A similar clinical-pathologic syndrome is observed occasionally in nutritionally depleted nonalcoholic patients.

NUTRITIONAL POLYNEUROPATHY (See also Chaps. 76 and 355) In the United States, nutritional polyneuropathy is essentially a disease of the alcoholic population. As mentioned above, it is present in more than 80 percent of patients with the Wernicke-Korsakoff syndrome, but it also occurs frequently as the only manifestation of deficiency disease. The peripheral neuropathy of alcoholics ("alcoholic polyneuropathy") does not differ in any fundamental way from that of beriberi. The clinical features of nutritional polyneuropathy and its identity with beriberi are discussed in Chaps. 76 and 355. A deficiency of thiamine chloride, pyridoxine, pantothenic acid, vitamin B_{12}, and perhaps folic acid has been demonstrated in individual cases to cause nutritional polyneuropathy. In the alcoholic patient it is usually not possible to incriminate any particular one of these vitamins.

Central nervous system toxicity to alcohol not associated with vitamin deficiency Alcohol-related brain lesions not attributable to nutritional deficiency or trauma are now recognized to occur. There is an increased incidence of hypertension in alcoholics and probably of strokes, both ischemic infarction and spontaneous subarachnoid hemorrhage. Alcoholics as a group also show dilatation of the lateral ventricles and widening of sulci on CT scanning compared to controls. The nature of these changes is obscure. They do not represent cerebral atrophy insofar as partial and sometimes complete reversal occur with sustained abstinence. The notion that alcohol can cause intellectual deterioration separate from effects due to nutritional deficiency is constantly reiterated in medical writings, but the entity of "alcoholic dementia" has never been established on the basis of clinical and neuropathologic studies. A syndrome of progressive myelopathy occurring in alcoholics has also been described clinically. Such patients show no evidence of nutritional deficiency (B_{12} or folic acid) or of liver disease (Sage et al.). The nature of the spinal cord disease is unknown, and a causal relationship to the toxic effects of alcohol remains to be established.

PELLAGRA This disease is described in Chap. 76. The comments here are concerned only with the neurologic manifestations, which in themselves are quite diverse. Pellagra is essentially an encephalopathy, although involvement of the spinal cord and peripheral nerves may occur. The early mental symptoms—insomnia, fatigue, anxiety, nervousness, irritability, and feelings of depression—may be mistaken for those of a psychiatric disorder. However, careful examination as the disease advances will reveal slowing and inefficiency of mental processes and impairment of memory. Pellagra may not only be the cause of psychiatric manifestations but occasionally may result from them because certain mental illnesses, including alcoholism, are accompanied by anorexia and dietary deficiency.

The spinal cord affection in pellagra has not been clearly delineated, perhaps because the mental state of the patients has precluded accurate testing. In general, there is evidence of both posterior and lateral column involvement, predominantly the former. Neuropathic signs are frequent and difficult to distinguish from other types of nutritional polyneuropathy. Other manifestations such as tremor, extrapyramidal rigidity, suck and grasp reflexes, and coma (referred to in the past as "nicotinic acid–deficiency encephalopathy") have indiscriminately been included in the pellagrous syndrome, as have various disorders of the special senses.

A *spastic paretic syndrome*, apart from the other symptoms and signs of pellagra, may be a rare manifestation of the deficiency. The chief clinical signs are spastic weakness of the legs with absent abdominal and increased tendon reflexes, clonus, and extensor plantar responses. These signs are usually accompanied by other manifestations of nutritional deficiency, such as Wernicke's disease, amblyopia, and peripheral neuropathy.

Pathologic features The distinctive neuropathologic changes in pellagra are most readily discerned in the large Betz cells of the motor cortex, although the same changes are seen to a lesser extent in the smaller pyramidal cells of the cerebral cortex and cells of the basal ganglia, cranial motor and dentate nuclei, and anterior horns of the spinal cord. The affected cells appear swollen and rounded with eccentric nuclei and loss of Nissl staining. This *central neuritis of pellagra*, as it is called, appears to represent a primary affection of the whole motor cell. The spinal cord lesions take the form of a symmetric degeneration of the dorsal columns, especially the fasciculus gracilis, and to a lesser extent of the corticospinal tracts. The posterior column degeneration is probably secondary to degeneration of specific dorsal root ganglion cells.

DEFICIENCY AMBLYOPIA (NUTRITIONAL OPTIC NEUROPATHY, TOBACCO-ALCOHOL AMBLYOPIA) These terms refer to a characteristic form of visual impairment that complicates nutritional disease and is due to a lesion in the optic nerve, more or less confined to the zone of the papillomacular bundle. The cornea and other parts of the refractive mechanism are uninvolved, hence the term *amblyopia*.

The main symptoms are dimness or blurring of vision for near and distant objects and impairment of color vision which worsens progressively and insidiously for several days or weeks. In addition to a reduction in visual acuity, examination discloses the presence of bilateral and roughly symmetric central or centrocecal scotomas, which are larger for colored than for white test objects. Pallor of the temporal portion of the optic disc is observed in some cases. Untreated, this condition progresses to irreversible optic atrophy.

Deficiency amblyopia was a common occurrence during the second World War and the Korean War. Although this form of amblyopia had previously been described in association with beriberi (due to thiamine deficiency) and pellagra (due to niacin deficiency), the peak incidence among prisoners coincided with neither of these syndromes but with the syndrome of orogenital dermatitis and "burning feet" (see below, "Strachan's syndrome").

In the United States, most, if not all, of the cases of retrobulbar neuropathy attributed to the toxic effects of alcohol or tobacco—so-called tobacco-alcohol amblyopia—are of nutritional origin. Although optic neuropathy may occur as the only manifestation of vitamin deficiency, more often it is combined with other evidence of nutritional deficiency, such as peripheral neuropathy and the Wernicke-Korsakoff syndrome.

Although the nutritional origin of this type of amblyopia has been established, the specific vitamin deficiency can rarely be determined. Observations in both humans and experimental animals indicate that a deficiency of thiamine (vitamin B_1), vitamin B_{12}, or perhaps riboflavin may cause lesions in the optic nerves. Heavy smokers with vitamin B_{12} deficiency appear to be particularly vulnerable to optic neuropathy. Two causative mechanisms for the pathogenesis of tobacco amblyopia have been offered: (1) chronic cyanide (generated in tobacco smoke) poisoning; and (2) alterations of fatty acid metabolism resulting from derangement of proprionate metabolism in the central nervous system. The notion that cyanide or other substances in tobacco smoke have a toxic effect upon the optic nerves is not supported by experimental data. And, since fatty acids take part in the formation and preservation of myelin, it is conceivable that the biochemical consequences of vitamin B_{12} deficiency are sufficient in themselves to account for both ophthalmologic and neurologic involvement.

Treatment consists of the administration of a balanced diet, supplemented with B vitamins, and the interdiction of alcohol and smoking where this is a factor.

SYNDROME OF AMBLYOPIA, PAINFUL NEUROPATHY, AND OROGENITAL DERMATITIS (STRACHAN'S SYNDROME) Beginning with the observations of Strachan, in 1888 and 1897, there have been many reports from diverse sources concerning a neurologic syndrome which is undoubtedly nutritional in origin but which cannot be forced into the boundaries of the classic deficiency diseases, beriberi and pellagra. Strachan attributed the disorder to malaria. Originally known as "Jamaican neuritis," the syndrome was soon recognized among the undernourished population of many other tropical countries. Large numbers of patients with this syndrome were observed also in the beseiged population of Madrid during the Spanish Civil War and later during World War II among prisoners of war in the Middle and Far East. In the United States, patients with this syndrome are found occasionally in the alcoholic population.

Strachan's syndrome is essentially a disorder of the peripheral and optic nerves. The peripheral nerve disorder is characterized mainly by sensory symptoms and signs (paresthesias and painful hyperesthesia of the feet, loss of superficial and deep sensation, and ataxia). On the other hand, foot drop and muscle weakness occur very rarely. A frequently associated disorder is failing vision, which may go on to complete blindness and pallor of the optic discs. Deafness and vertigo are rare additional complications, but in some outbreaks among prisoners of war these symptoms were so prominent as to earn the epithet "camp dizziness." In all these respects the syndrome differs from beriberi. Along with the neurologic signs there may be varying degrees of stomatoglossitis, corneal degeneration, and genital dermatitis. These mucocutaneous lesions are spoken of together as the *orogenital syndrome* and are quite distinct from the dermal changes of pellagra.

There have been only a few pathologic studies of this syndrome. Aside from the damage to the papillomacular bundle in the optic nerve, the most consistent abnormality has been a loss of myelinated fibers in posterior columns (fasciculus gracilis) of the spinal cord. This indicates a systematized degeneration of the central processes of the bipolar large sensory neurons of the lumbosacral spinal ganglia. The loss of pain and temperature sensation is thought due to an axonopathy. There are no reliable data concerning the specific vitamin deficiencies that cause this disease.

SUBACUTE COMBINED DEGENERATION (SCD) OF THE SPINAL CORD (See Chap. 76) This term designates the spinal cord disease that is due to vitamin B_{12} deficiency. The brain, optic nerves, and peripheral nerves may also be affected but far less often than the spinal cord. The neurologic manifestations of vitamin B_{12} deficiency and the hematologic ones (pernicious anemia) are distinctive insofar as they are caused not by a lack of vitamin B_{12} in the food but by an inability to transfer minute amounts of this nutrient across the intestinal mucosa—aptly characterized by Castle as "starvation in the midst of plenty." Such a nutritional disorder is referred to as a *conditioned deficiency,* since it depends upon the lack of an intrinsic factor in the gastric secretions (see Chap. 285). Rarely neurologic symptoms due to vitamin B_{12} deficiency occur in patients with disease of the distal small intestine (Crohn's disease, lymphoma) or after surgical resection.

Clinical manifestations Neurologic symptoms are present in the majority of patients with vitamin B_{12} deficiency. The patient first notices general weakness and paresthesias, consisting of tingling, "pins-and-needles" feelings, or other vaguely described sensations in the distal parts of the limbs; the lower extremites may be involved before the upper ones or vice versa. The paresthesias tend to be constant, to progress steadily, and to be the source of much distress. As the illness progresses, the gait becomes unsteady, and movements of the limbs, especially the legs, become stiff and awkward.

Early in the course of the illness, when only paresthesias are present, there may be no objective signs. Later, the neurologic examination discloses a disorder of the posterior and lateral columns of the spinal cord, predominantly the former. Loss of vibration sense is by far the most consistent sign; it is more pronounced in the legs than in the arms, and frequently it extends over the trunk. Position sense is involved somewhat less frequently. The motor defects are usually limited to the legs and include loss of power, spasticity, changes in the tendon reflexes, clonus, and extensor plantar responses. At first the patellar and Achilles reflexes are found to be diminished as frequently as they are increased, and they may even be absent. With treatment, the reflexes may return to normal or become hyperactive. The gait at first is predominantly ataxic, later ataxic and spastic. If the disease remains untreated, an ataxic paraplegia with variable degrees of spasticity and contracture may develop.

A loss of superficial sensation below a segmental level on the trunk, implicating the spinothalamic tracts, occurs rarely, but such a finding should always suggest the possibility of some other disease of the spinal cord. More often the sensory defect takes the form of a blunting of tactile, painful, and thermal sensation over the distal segments of the lower limbs, implicating the peripheral nerves, but such findings are also uncommon.

The nervous system involvement in vitamin B_{12} deficiency is characteristically, though not perfectly, symmetric. A definite asymmetry of motor or sensory findings, maintained over a period of weeks or months, should always cast doubt on the diagnosis.

Mental signs are frequent, ranging from irritability, apathy, somnolence, suspiciousness, and emotional instability to a marked confusional or depressive psychosis, or even to intellectual deterioration. Optic neuropathy with impaired acuity and cecocentral scotoma has been reported with virtually all causes of vitamin B_{12} deficiency including postsurgical malabsorption syndrome and pernicious anemia. In all cases, variable improvement in acuity has occurred once systemic vitamin B_{12} has been administered. Pathologic studies in the setting of vitamin B_{12} deficiency optic neuropathy and subacute combined degeneration of the spinal cord have shown patchy demyelination of the optic nerves. If involvement of the optic nerve is severe, optic atrophy may occur. Although dementia and amblyopia are relatively uncommon occurrences, each may occasionally be the initial manifestation of the disease.

Pathology and pathogenesis The pathologic process takes the form of a diffuse, though uneven, degeneration of the white matter of the spinal cord and sometimes of the brain. At first there is swelling of myelin sheaths, characterized by separation of myelin lamellae and formation of intramyelinic vacuoles. This is followed by a coalescence of small foci of tissue destruction into larger ones, giving the tissue a vacuolated appearance. The myelin sheaths and the axis cylinders are both affected, the former perhaps earlier and to a greater extent than the latter. Astrocyte gliosis is minimal in the early lesions, but in the more chronic ones gliosis is pronounced. The changes begin in the posterior columns of the lower cervical and upper thoracic cord and spread from this region up and down the cord, as well as forward into the lateral columns. The lesions are not limited to specific systems of fibers within the posterior and lateral funiculi but are scattered irregularly through the white matter.

The *pathogenesis* of the nervous system lesions in vitamin B_{12} deficiency is not well understood. Impairment of DNA synthesis probably accounts for the hematologic abnormalities and the production of megaloblasts; however, since neurons do not divide, this mechanism cannot be invoked to explain the central nervous system changes. One of the better-understood functions of vitamin B_{12} is its role as a coenzyme in the methylmalonyl CoA mutase reaction. Impairment of this metabolic step may lead to the production of abnormal fatty acids, which are important building blocks of cell membranes and of myelin. Conceivably, this biochemical abnormality may in some way be responsible for the nervous system lesions.

Diagnosis and treatment The chief obstacle to early diagnosis is the lack of parallelism between the hematologic and neurologic signs. This is particularly true of patients who have received folic acid, which serves to maintain a hematologic remission for an indefinite period while the neurologic signs worsen, often to an irreversible stage. Under these circumstances the most reliable diagnostic procedures are the measurement of the serum B_{12} concentration and the two-stage Schilling test (see Chap. 285).

The treatment of the neurologic manifestations of vitamin B_{12} deficiency differs in no way from the treatment of the hematologic ones. Patients whose vitamin B_{12} stores have been depleted require large doses of cobalamin—1000 μg intramuscularly each day during hospitalization, then weekly for a month, and then monthly for the remainder of the patient's life.

The most important factor influencing the *response to treatment* is the duration of the neurologic disease. Recovery may be complete if therapy is instituted within a few weeks of the onset of symptoms. For this reason SCD and the other neurologic complications of vitamin B_{12} deficiency represent medical emergencies. If symptoms have been present for longer than a month or two, only partial recovery can be expected, and in long-standing cases the best that can be expected is the arrest of progression of the symptoms.

Although many patients with vitamin B_{12} deficiency secondary to gastrointestinal disease also have folic acid deficiency, the contribution of the latter, if any, to neurologic symptoms and signs remains unsettled.

VITAMIN E DEFICIENCY Children or adults with chronic liver disease (biliary atresia) or malabsorption syndromes may present with neurologic dysfunction. The clinical features include dysarthria, cerebellar ataxia, diminution of vibration and position sense, sensory polyneuropathy, and absent deep tendon reflexes. Ophthalmoplegia occurs in some patients. Intellectual processes are usually preserved. Neuropathologic examination in two adults disclosed loss of large-diameter myelinated axons in the sural nerves with axonal degeneration. Nerve cell loss was evident in dorsal root ganglia with degeneration of the posterior columns and the cuneate and gracile nuclei. The condition shows improvement if treated early with vitamin E supplementation.

NEUROLOGIC SYNDROMES CAUSED BY HYPERVITAMINOSIS Acute toxicity with vitamin A causes symptoms of headache, dizziness, irritability, and drowsiness. Chronic hypervitaminosis A can give rise to chronic increased intracranial pressure (pseudotumor cerebri) (see Chap. 76).

Excess ingestion of pyridoxine in amounts in excess of 2 g daily can cause a sensory neuropathy characterized clinically by progressive ataxia, impairment of position and vibration sense, and loss of deep tendon reflexes. Motor strength is preserved. The syndrome is reversible with discontinuation of pyridoxine.

ACQUIRED (SECONDARY) METABOLIC DISEASES OF THE NERVOUS SYSTEM

In this important category of neurologic disease, a disturbance of cerebral function is usually consequent upon disease in some other organ system—heart (and circulation), lungs (and respiration), kidneys, liver, pancreas, and endocrine glands. Each of these visceral diseases affects the nervous system in a somewhat different way.

ANOXIC ISCHEMIC ENCEPHALOPATHY This common and often disastrous condition is caused by a lack of oxygen to the brain, resulting from hypotension or respiratory failure. Sometimes both are responsible, and one cannot say which predominates—hence, the ambiguous allusion in clinical records to "cardiorespiratory failure." The conditions which most often lead to anoxic/ischemic encephalopathy are (1) myocardial infarction; (2) cardiac arrest from whatever cause; (3) hemorrhage, with shock and circulatory collapse; in these situations vascular supply to the brain is compromised before respiration; (4) infective and traumatic shock; (5) suffocation (from drowning, strangulation, aspiration of vomitus or blood, compression of the trachea by hemorrhage or a surgical pack, or a foreign body in the trachea); (6) diseases which paralyze the muscles of respiration or compromise the central nervous system respiratory drive (trauma, vascular disease of the brain, epilepsy) with respiratory failure followed by cardiac failure; and (7) carbon monoxide (CO) poisoning, in which respiration fails first and then cardiovascular functions. Experimental studies support clinical observations that hypoxia alone may induce different clinicopathologic states than a combination of hypoxia and hypoperfusion (ischemia).

Clinical manifestations Mild degrees of hypoxia induce inattentiveness, impaired judgment, and motor incoordination but have no lasting effects. With severe hypoxia or anoxia, as occurs with cardiac arrest, consciousness is lost within seconds, but recovery will be complete if breathing, oxygenation of blood, and cardiac action are restored within 3 to 5 min. If anoxia persists beyond this time, there is serious and permanent injury to the brain, particularly to those parts in which the efficiency of circulation is marginal (globus pallidus, cerebellum, hippocampus, and the ''borderzone regions'' of the parietooccipital lobes). Clinically, it is difficult to judge the precise degree of hypoxia/ischemia since slight heart action or an imperceptible blood pressure may serve to maintain the circulation to some extent. Hence some individuals have made an excellent recovery after cerebral anoxia that allegedly lasted 8 to 10 min or longer. *An important clinical rule is that degrees of hypoxia which at no time abolish consciousness rarely if ever cause permanent damage to the nervous system.* P_{O_2} as low as 20 mmHg is well tolerated if it develops gradually and blood pressure is normal. Also, generally speaking, subjects who demonstrate intact brainstem function (as indicated by normal ciliospinal, oculovestibular, and pupillary light responses, and intact doll's-head eye movements) when the acute hypoxic event has terminated tend to have a better outlook for recovery of consciousness and perhaps all of their faculties. Conversely, absence of these reflex activities and the presence of pupils persistently fixed to light suggest a grave prognosis.

Extreme or sustained global ischemia causes brain death (see Chap. 21). Immediately after resuscitation from cardiorespiratory arrest, the signs may indicate brain death (dilated, unresponsive pupils, absent brainstem reflexes and respiration, and isoelectric EEG), yet full recovery may occur. However, persistence of the unresponsive state for more than an hour or two invariably carries a poor prognosis (see Chap. 21). The diagnosis of brain death must be made with caution because anesthesia, drug intoxication, and hypothermia may also cause deep coma, absent brainstem reflexes, and an isoelectric EEG, but permit recovery. Cases of brain death have been brought increasingly to public attention because of ethical and moral issues that surround the question of discontinuing supportive medical therapy (see Chap. 21). Issues of management are most difficult in the patient who has suffered severe but lesser degrees of cerebral anoxia.

Patients who suffer a severe degree of anoxic encephalopathy that falls short of causing ''brain death'' often stabilize breathing and heart action. Neurologic evaluation shows the patient to be profoundly comatose, with eyes slightly divergent and motionless but with reactive pupils, and flaccid or intensely rigid limbs, and diminished tendon reflexes. Within a few minutes after cardiac action and breathing have been restored, generalized convulsions and isolated or grouped twitches of muscles (myoclonus) may supervene. Decerebrate or decorticate postures may be present or occur upon pinching the limbs, and bilateral Babinski signs can be evoked. In the first 24 to 48 h death may terminate this state in a setting of rising temperature, deepening coma, and circulatory collapse. Or, with somewhat lesser degrees of injury, where the cerebral and cerebellar cortices are partly or completely destroyed but brainstem-spinal structures remain intact, the individual may survive in a state referred to as ''irreversible coma'' or ''persistent vegetative state'' (see Chap. 21). These patients remain mute, unresponsive, and unaware of their environment for weeks, months, or years. Criteria to predict accurately the outcome of this condition early in the comatose period have been developed (see Chap. 21). If intoxication can be excluded, the presence of fixed dilated pupils and paralysis of eye movement for 24 to 48 h, along with marked slowing of the EEG, usually signifies irreversible cerebral damage. Deep coma of this type, lasting more than a few days, is rarely attended by full recovery.

Patients with still lesser degrees of injury improve after a period of coma. Consciousness is regained, and then various degrees of confusion, visual agnosia, extrapyramidal rigidity, or movement disorder (action or intention myoclonus, choreoathetosis) become manifest. Some of these patients quickly pass through this acute hypoxic phase and proceed to make full recovery; others are left with permanent neurologic sequelae. The *posthypoxic syndromes* observed most frequently are (1) *persistent coma or stupor;* and, with lesser degrees of cerebral injury, (2) *dementia,* with or without extrapyramidal signs; (3) *visual agnosia;* (4) *parkinsonism;* (5) *choreoathetosis;* (6) *cerebellar ataxia;* (7) *intention or action myoclonus;* and (8) *Korsakoff's amnesic state. Seizures* may continue to be a problem, but are uncommon.

A relatively uncommon and unexplained phenomenon is *delayed postanoxic encephalopathy.* Initial improvement, which appears to be complete, is followed after a variable period of time (1 to 4 weeks in most cases) by a relapse, characterized by apathy, confusion, irritability, and occasionally agitation or mania. A few patients have recovered from this second episode, but in most of them there has been progression of the neurologic syndrome, with shuffling gait, diffuse rigidity and spasticity, coma, and death after 1 to 2 weeks. Postmortem examination of these patients has shown the major abnormality to be widespread cerebral demyelination. Exceptionally, there occurs yet another delayed syndrome, in which a period of hypoxia is followed by a slow, deteriorating state, affecting basal ganglia more than cerebral cortex and white matter and progressing for weeks to months until the patient is mute, rigid, and helpless.

The essential *mechanism* in hypoxic encephalopathy is a lack of oxygen and an arrest of all aerobic metabolic processes necessary to sustain the Krebs tricarboxylic cycle and the electron transport system. Lactic acid accumulates in the tissues. The pathophysiology of delayed progression is not understood.

Diagnosis This depends on (1) the history of a hypoxic ischemic event and evidence of reduced oxygenation of arterial blood (P_{O_2}<40 mmHg), CO intoxication (the latter is indicated by its spectroscopic band or cherry-red color of the skin for a few minutes to hours after the episode), blood pressures below 70 mmHg systolic, or cardiac arrest; and (2) as outlined above, the typical clinical sequence of events after a possible hypoxic/ischemic episode has terminated. Renal damage (anuria) and myocardial infarction may also have occurred and provide corroborative evidence of hypoxia.

Treatment The treatment of anoxic encephalopathy is directed mainly at the prevention of a critical degree of hypoxic injury. After a clear airway is secured, artificial respiration, external thoracic cardiac massage, the use of a cardiac defibrillator or pacemaker, and open chest surgery all have their place, and every second counts in their prompt utilization. Once cardiac and pulmonary function are restored, there is no evidence that any pharmacologic treatment will benefit recovery. Barbiturates, corticosteroids, hypothermia, dimethylsulfoxide, and benzodiazepines have been given without proof of benefit. A small, unpredictable proportion of patients develop secondary complications of diffuse brain swelling after cardiac arrest; this condition is more common in children. This is detected by compression of lateral ventricles and cisterns on CT scan, or by very high lumbar CSF pressure. Treatment is detailed in Chap. 21. Seizures should be controlled by anticonvulsants. Posthypoxic myoclonus may respond to oral administration of 5-hydroxytryptophan.

HYPERCAPNIC ENCEPHALOPATHY Chronic emphysema, chronic fibrosing lung disease, and in rare instances, an inadequacy of central respiratory drive lead to chronic respiratory acidosis, with an elevation of P_{CO_2} and a reduction in arterial P_{O_2}. Secondary polycythemia and cor pulmonale often accompany these diseases of the lungs, and pulmonary infection may be superimposed.

Clinical Manifestations The clinical syndrome consequent upon hypercapnia (and hypoxia) comprises generalized or bilateral frontal or occipital headache, often intense and persistent for hours; papilledema; mental dullness, drowsiness, confusion, stupor, and coma; a fast-frequency action tremor and coarse twitching of all muscles, which are in a state of sustained contraction; and an ability to maintain a fixed posture or interruption of a voluntary movement because of brief lapses of sustained muscle contraction (asterixis). Intermittent drowsiness, indifference and inattention to the environment, reduction of psychomotor activity, imperception of the sequence of events, and forgetfulness constitute the more subtle manifestations of this syndrome.

In fully developed cases, the cerebrospinal fluid (CSF) is under increased pressure, P_{CO_2} may exceed 75 mmHg, and oxygen saturation of the arterial blood ranges from 85 to 40 percent. The EEG reveals slow activity, in the delta and theta range, sometimes bilaterally synchronous. The mechanism of the cerebral disorder is said to be CO_2 narcosis, but the biochemical details are not known. The danger of administering morphine or sedatives, which blunt the respiratory drive (already depressed by the CO_2 retention), or inhaled O_2, which removes the sole stimulus (low P_{O_2}) to the respiratory center, is now widely recognized.

Treatment Forced ventilation with an intermittent positive-pressure respirator, treatment of heart failure with digitalis and diuretics, venesection to reduce the viscosity of the blood, and antibiotics to combat pulmonary infection are the most effective therapeutic measures. If stupor or coma persists, the arterial O_2 level should be rechecked; it may be critically reduced, and needs to be raised by controlled O_2 administration to a point (50 to 55 mmHg) where consciousness is improved but the stimulus to respiratory drive is not removed. Also, the pH of the CSF may be very low, in the range of 7.15 to 7.25. In CO_2 narcosis, correction of the acidosis of blood is easier than that of CSF, which tends to lag. Aminophylline administration is the initial treatment in chronic obstructive pulmonary disease because it improves both airway resistance and diaphragm contractility. Hypokalemia may complicate the rapid correction of CO_2 and pH abnormalities.

Differential diagnosis Unlike pure hypoxic encephalopathy, hypercapnia rarely causes prolonged coma, and is not a cause of irreversible brain damage. Papilledema and asterixis (the latter is also characteristic of liver failure, uremia, and rarely other metabolic disorders) are important diagnostic features. The syndrome of hypercapnia is apt to be mistaken for brain tumor, a confusional psychosis of nondescript type, or a disease causing myoclonus or chorea. In the latter instance, it must be distinguished from a chronic extrapyramidal syndrome.

HYPOGLYCEMIC ENCEPHALOPATHY (See also Chaps. 327 and 329) This condition is a relatively infrequent but important cause of episodic confusion, convulsions, coma, and sometimes focal neurologic signs, i.e., hemiparesis. The essential biochemical abnormality is a critical lowering of the blood glucose concentration to less than 25 to 30 mg/dL (lower in infants), which, if it lasts for many minutes leads to exhaustion of cerebral glucose reserve. As cerebral oxidation proceeds without exogenous glucose, the lipid and protein components of neurons are metabolized, and irreversible damage occurs. The severely hypoglycemic patient becomes deeply comatose before permanent damage occurs. Consequently prompt treatment is important.

Etiology The most common causes of hypoglycemic encephalopathy are (1) the accidental or deliberate overdose of insulin or an oral antidiabetic agent, (2) an islet cell, insulin-secreting tumor of the pancreas, or retroperitoneal sarcoma, (3) rarely, a prolonged drinking spree associated with depletion of liver glycogen, (4) acute, nonicteric hepatic encephalopathy of childhood (Reye's syndrome), (5) glycogen storage disease in infancy, and (6) an idiopathic syndrome occurring in the neonatal period. In the past, hypoglycemic encephalopathy was a rather frequent complication of "insulin shock" therapy of schizophrenia. Postprandial and fasting hypoglycemia are never of sufficient duration or severity to damage the central nervous system.

Clinical manifestations As the concentration of blood glucose decreases to about 30 mg/dL, the initial symptoms appear—nervousness, hunger, flushed facies, headache, palpitation, anxiety, sweating, and trembling—and these gradually give way to confusion, drowsiness, focal neurologic signs, and occasionally excitement or overactivity. In the next stage, forced sucking, grasping, motor restlessness, muscular spasms, and finally decerebrate rigidity occur, in that sequence. Myoclonic twitching and convulsions may develop in some patients. Blood levels of approximately 10 mg/dL are associated with deep coma, dilatation of pupils, pallor, shallow respirations, bradycardia, and hypotonicity of limb musculature—the so-called medullary phase of hypoglycemia. If glucose is administered before the medullary phase is reached, the patient is restored to normalcy, retracing the aforementioned steps in reverse order with recovery within a few minutes. Once the medullary phase appears, and particularly if it persists for a time before the hypoglycemia is corrected, neurologic recovery is delayed for a period of days or weeks and may be incomplete.

A huge dose of insulin that produces severe hypoglycemia, even of relatively brief duration (30 to 60 min), is more dangerous than a series of less severe hypoglycemic episodes from smaller doses of insulin, possibly because the former impairs or exhausts essential enzymes. This condition cannot then be overcome by large quantities of glucose given intravenously.

Pathology The major *neuropathologic effect* is on the cerebral cortex; nerve cells degenerate and are replaced by microgliocytes and astrocytes. The distribution of lesions is similar though not identical to that in hypoxic encephalopathy (the cerebellar cortex is relatively spared in hypoglycemic encephalopathy). The sequelae of the two disorders are also much alike.

Chronic episodes of hypoglycemia may give rise to two other syndromes, both relatively uncommon. One, termed *subacute hypoglycemia,* is characterized by drowsiness and lethargy, diminution in psychomotor activity, deterioration of social behavior, and confusion. Oral or intravenous glucose will immediately alleviate the symptoms. In the other, more *chronic syndrome,* there is gradual deterioration of intellectual function, raising the question of a presenile dementia, and in some reported instances there have been tremor, chorea, rigidity, cerebellar ataxia, and rarely signs of lower motor neuron involvement ("hypoglycemic amyotrophy"). These subacute and chronic forms of hypoglycemia have been observed with islet cell hypertrophy or tumor, carcinoma of the stomach, fibrous mesothelioma, carcinoma of the cecum, and hepatoma. An insulin-like substance is elaborated by these nonpancreatic tumors.

Differential diagnosis The major clinical differences between hypoglycemia and hypoxia are in the clinical setting and mode of evolution of the neurologic disorder. Hypoglycemia usually disturbs cerebral function more slowly than hypoxia, over a period of 30 to 60 min rather than in a few seconds or minutes. The recovery phase and sequelae of the two conditions are much the same. *Recurrent hypoglycemia,* as occurs with an islet cell tumor, may masquerade for some time as an episodic confusional psychosis or convulsive illness, and diagnosis awaits a period of demonstrably low blood glucose or hyperinsulinism (see Chap. 329).

The correction of the hypoglycemia at the earliest moment is the obvious therapy. It is not known whether hypothermia or other measures will increase the safety period in hypoglycemia or alter the outcome.

HYPERGLYCEMIC COMA Two hyperglycemic syndromes have been described, mainly in the diabetic: (1) hyperglycemia with ketoacidosis and (2) hyperosmolar nonketotic hyperglycemia. These are described in Chap. 327.

ACUTE HEPATIC ENCEPHALOPATHY Chronic hepatic insufficiency with portacaval shunting of blood is often punctuated by episodes of stupor, coma, and other neurologic symptoms, a state referred to as hepatic coma or portal-systemic encephalopathy. Also, there are a number of hereditary hyperammonemic syndromes of infancy which may lead to episodic coma with or without seizures. A special type of nonicteric hepatic encephalopathy (Reye's syndrome) occurs in children, presenting as acute brain swelling, in conjunction with rapid enlargement of the liver, fine droplets of fat in hepatocytes, high serum glutamic oxaloacetic transaminase (SGOT) and other liver enzymes, and very high levels of serum ammonia (see Chap. 251).

Clinical features The central feature of acute hepatic encephalopathy occurring in the adult is a derangement of consciousness, presenting first as mental confusion with increased or decreased psychomotor activity, followed by progressive drowsiness, stupor, and coma. The confusional state that occurs before coma intervenes is frequently combined with characteristic lapses of sustained muscle contraction (asterixis) and an EEG abnormality consisting of paroxysms of bilaterally synchronous delta waves, characteristically triphasic and prominent in the frontal regions which at first are interspersed with alpha activity and which later, as the coma deepens, displace all normal activity. A variable, fluctuating rigidity of the trunk and limbs, grimacing, suck and grasp reflexes, exaggeration or asymmetry of tendon reflexes, Babinski signs, and focal or generalized seizures round out the clinical picture.

The syndrome of acute hepatic encephalopathy usually evolves over a period of days to weeks and often terminates fatally. At times it does not advance beyond the stage of mild mental dulling and confusion with asterixis and EEG changes. This relatively mild form needs to be differentiated from other acute confusional psychoses and deliria. If the metabolic disorder persists for months and years, a mild dementia and a disorder of posture and movement may gradually appear (grimacing, tremor, dysarthria, ataxia of gait, choreoathetosis), and the condition must then be distinguished from the other dementing and extrapyramidal syndromes (see further on in this chapter).

Pathology and pathogenesis The striking *neuropathologic finding* in patients who die in a state of hepatic coma is a diffuse increase in the number and size of the protoplasmic astrocytes (Alzheimer type II astrocytes) in the deep layers of the cerebral cortex and in the lenticular nuclei, with little or no visible alteration in the nerve cells or other parenchymal elements.

The *pathogenesis* of hepatic encephalopathy is not fully understood. The most plausible theory relates it to an abnormality of nitrogen metabolism, wherein ammonia or other amines, which are formed in the bowel by the action of urease-containing organisms on dietary protein and are carried to the liver in the portal circulation, fail to be converted into urea, either because of hepatocellular disease or portal-systemic shunting of blood, or both. As a result, these substances reach the systemic circulation, where they interfere with cerebral metabolism in some obscure way. Other theories of causation have related hepatic coma to the synergistic action of certain fatty acids and possibly methyl mercaptan with ammonia, or to the excess production of false neurotransmitters (e.g., octopamine), or to an increase in the inhibitory neurotransmitter γ-aminobutyric acid (GABA) (see Chap. 249). These and other theories have recently been reviewed by Victor (1986).

Treatment Despite an incomplete understanding of the role of disordered nitrogen metabolism in the genesis of hepatic coma, an awareness of this relationship has provided the most effective means of treating this disorder: restriction of dietary protein; mechanical cleansing of the colon; oral administration of neomycin or kanamycin, which suppresses or eliminates urease-producing organisms in the bowel; and the use of lactulose, an inert sugar that acidifies the colonic contents. Should these measures not control the protein intolerance, surgical exclusion of the bowel may be undertaken, but this operation carries a high risk of mortality. More recent methods of treatment, the practicality of which remain to be established, include the use of keto analogues of essential amino acids (which theoretically should supply a nitrogen-free source of essential amino acids) and bromocriptine, a dopamine agonist which is thought to enhance dopaminergic transmission (see Chap. 249).

In acute hepatitis, delirious, confusional, and comatose states also occur, but their mechanisms are not understood. Blood ammonia levels are usually elevated, but of unclear significance, because of other associated metabolic abnormalities.

CHRONIC HEPATIC ENCEPHALOPATHY (ACQUIRED HEPATOCEREBRAL DEGENERATION) Clinical manifestations Patients who survive an episode or several episodes of hepatic coma are occasionally left with residual neurologic abnormalities, such as tremor of the head or arms, asterixis, grimacing, choreatic twitching of the limbs, dysarthria, ataxia of gait, or impairment of intellectual function, and these symptoms may worsen with repeated attacks of stupor and coma. In other patients with hepatic failure, these neurologic abnormalities become manifest in the absence of discrete episodes of hepatic coma. In either event, patients thus afflicted deteriorate neurologically over a period of months or years. As the condition evolves, a rather characteristic dysarthria, mild ataxia, wide-based, unsteady gait, and choreoathetosis, mainly of the face, neck, and shoulders, are joined in a common syndrome. Mental function is slowly altered—a simple dementia with lack of concern and indifference to the illness evolves. A coarse rhythmic tremor of the arms, appearing with certain sustained postures, mild corticospinal tract signs, and diffuse EEG abnormalities complete the clinical picture. Other less frequent signs are muscular rigidity, grasp reflexes, tremor in repose, nystagmus, asterixis, and action or intention myoclonus. Many of the neurologic abnormalities that occur as part of acute hepatic encephalopathy may also be observed in patients with chronic hepatocerebral degeneration, the only difference being that the abnormalities are evanescent in the former and irreversible in the latter.

The chronic cerebral symptoms, like the transient ones, may occur with all varieties of chronic liver disease. Portacaval shunts are always present; jaundice, ascites, and esophageal varices are manifest in most of the cases.

Pathology Chronic hepatocerebral degeneration, like hepatic coma, is characterized by a widespread hyperplasia of protoplasmic astrocytes in the deep layers of the cerebral and cerebellar cortices as well as in the thalamic and lenticular nuclei and many other nuclear structures of the brainstem. In addition, in the chronic disease, medullated fibers and nerve cells are destroyed in the affected areas, and polymicrocavitation is prominent at the corticomedullary junction, in the striatum (particularly in the superior pole of the putamen), and in the cerebellar white matter. Protoplasmic astrocytic nuclei contain periodic acid Schiff (PAS)–positive glycogen granules. Nerve cells may appear swollen and chromatolyzed, accounting for the so-called Opalski cells. The similarity of the neuropathologic lesion in the familial (Wilson's) and acquired forms of liver disease suggests a common hepatogenesis.

UREMIC ENCEPHALOPATHY Episodic confusion and stupor and other neurologic symptoms may accompany any form of severe renal disease. In addition, a number of neurologic syndromes complicate chronic hemodialysis and kidney transplantation. Chronic polyneuropathy, the most common neurologic complication of renal failure, is discussed in Chap. 355.

Acute uremic encephalopathy The initial cerebral symptoms attributable to uremia consist of apathy, fatigue, inattentiveness, and irritability; later, confusion, disturbances of sensory perception, hallucinations, and stupor supervene. These later symptoms are practically always associated with twitching of the muscles and myoclonic jerks, and the patient may convulse. Similar twitch-convulsive phenomena occur in association with a variety of diseases, such as widespread neoplasia, delirium tremens, diabetes with necrotizing pyelonephritis, and lupus erythematosus, all when associated with renal failure. Elevated blood urea nitrogen is sometimes accompanied by subnormal serum calcium and magnesium levels.

The prognosis of uremic encephalopathy, if associated with irreversible and progressive renal disease, is poor and can only be managed with dialysis or renal transplantation. Convulsions, which occur in about one-third of cases, often preterminally, respond to relatively low plasma concentrations of phenytoin and phenobarbital.

The brains of patients with uremic encephalopathy and the twitch-convulsive syndrome show hyperplasia of protoplasmic astrocytes in some cases, but never to the degree observed in hepatic encephalopathy. Cerebral edema is notably absent. Restoration of renal function corrects the neurologic syndrome, attesting to a biochemical rather than a structural abnormality. Whether this is caused by the retention of organic acids, elevation of phosphate in the CSF, or by the action of other toxins has never been settled.

"Disequilibrium syndrome" and dialysis encephalopathy These terms refer to syndromes that commonly complicate hemodialysis or peritoneal dialysis. Under *disequilibrium syndrome* are included headaches, nausea, muscular cramps, nervous irritability, agitation, drowsiness, and convulsions. The headache develops in approximately 70 percent of patients, while the other symptoms are observed in 5 to 10 percent, usually in those undergoing rapid dialysis or in the early stages of a dialysis program. The symptoms tend to occur in the third to fourth hour of dialysis and last for several hours. Sometimes the symptoms appear 8 to 48 h after completing dialysis. Originally these symptoms were attributable to the rapid lowering of serum urea, leaving the brain with a higher concentration of urea than the serum and resulting in a shift of water into the brain to equalize the osmotic gradient ("reverse urea syndrome"). Now the condition is attributed to a shift of water into the brain, analogous to the volume expansion due to water intoxication and inappropriate secretion of antidiuretic hormone.

Dialysis encephalopathy or dialysis dementia is an unusual and now uncommon complication of chronic hemodialysis. It begins with stuttering and dysarthria, coupled with a predominantly motor aphasia, to which are added facial and generalized myoclonus, focal and generalized seizures, personality changes and psychotic episodes, intellectual decline, progressive aphasic disorder, and EEG abnormalities. The latter consist of bisynchronous predominantly frontal or multifocal bursts of slow wave discharges, associated with spikes and sharp waves. The CSF is usually normal. At first these symptoms are intermittent, occurring during or immediately after dialysis and lasting for only a few hours, but gradually they become more persistent and eventually permanent. Once established, the syndrome is usually steadily progressive over a 1- to 15-month period (average survival of 6 months in 42 cases analyzed by Lederman and Henry). A few patients have a waxing and waning course and survive for several years. In some patients the myoclonus and seizures subside for several months under the influence of clonazepam or diazepam.

The neuropathologic changes are subtle and consist of a mild microcavitation of the upper layers of the cerebral cortex. Although the changes are diffuse, the left (dominant) hemisphere is affected more than the right, and the left frontotemporal operculum more than other parts of the cortex (Winkelman). The predominant affection of the operculum would explain the striking disturbance of speech and language. Current concepts of the etiology center on the role of aluminum. Alfrey and his associates found that the cerebral gray matter of patients who died with dialysis encephalopathy contained a much greater amount of aluminum than analogous tissue from dialysis patients without encephalopathy. The aluminum is derived from both the dialysate and orally administered aluminum gels. These authors suggested that dialysis encephalopathy represents a form of aluminum intoxication, a view that is supported by the observations that (1) the frequency of dialysis dementia was related to the concentrations of aluminum in the dialysate, and (2) deionization of the water used in the dialysate prevented the occurrence of new cases. The possibility that other trace elements contribute to the syndrome has not been entirely excluded.

Kidney transplantation involves an increased risk of developing primary cerebral lymphoma, Wernicke's encephalopathy, and central pontine myelinolysis. Systemic fungal infections are found at autopsy in about 45 percent of patients who have had renal transplants and long periods of immunosuppressive treatment, and in about one-third of these patients there has been involvement of the central nervous system. *Cryptococcus, Listeria, Aspergillus, Candida, Nocardia,* and *Histoplasma* are the usual organisms. Other central nervous system infections that complicate transplantation are toxoplasmosis and cytomegalic inclusion disease.

ENCEPHALOPATHIES DUE TO ELECTROLYTE AND ENDOCRINE DISTURBANCES Brief reference to these important groups of metabolic encephalopathies is given here. More detailed accounts are found in the cross-referenced chapters.

Metabolic acidosis (arterial pH$<$7.30, $P_{CO_2}<35$, $HCO_3<10$ meq per liter) due to diabetes mellitus, renal failure, lactic acidosis, or poisoning with an acid substance produces a syndrome characterized by drowsiness, stupor, and coma with dry skin and Kussmaul breathing, described in Chap. 42. Extreme degrees of *hyperosmolality* of the blood may develop in the course of diabetes mellitus (blood glucose$>$400 mg/dL) and in *hypernatremic dehydration,* resulting in both instances in tremulousness, convulsions, and coma. In some instances the movement disorder resembles chorea or the myoclonic twitching of uremia. *Hypokalemia* is characterized by extreme muscular weakness associated with a stuporous-confusional state, and sometimes by striking changes in personality and behavior (see Chap. 42).

Hyponatremia, usually with water intoxication, is another cause of episodic coma, especially in infants. Among the many causes, the syndrome of inappropriate secretion of antidiuretic hormone (SIADH) is of special importance, since it commonly complicates neurologic diseases of many types—head trauma, bacterial meningitis and encephalitis, cerebral infarction and subarachnoid hemorrhage, neoplasm, and sometimes Guillain-Barré disease (see Chap. 323). The diagnosis of SIADH should be suspected in any critically ill neurologic or neurosurgical patient who excretes urine that is hypertonic relative to the plasma. As the hyponatremia develops, there is a decrease in alertness, which progresses through stages of confusion to coma, often with convulsions. Lack of recognition of this state may allow the serum Na^+ to fall to dangerously low levels, 100 meq per liter or lower. Treatment is described in Chap. 323. Replacement with intravenous NaCl in severe cases must be done cautiously because vigorous and rapid correction of severe hyponatremia has been incriminated in the pathogenesis of central pontine myelinolysis (CPM) and related brainstem, cerebellar, and cerebral syndromes (Laureno). Ayus and colleagues emphasize the risks of persistent severe hyponatremia and recommend the following therapeutic guidelines: serum Na^+ above 120 meq per liter does not require immediate correction. If Na^+ is $>$105 meq per liter, it can be safely corrected to a level of 125 to 130 meq per liter at a rate of administration of Na^+ of 2 meq per liter. If serum Na^+ is less than 105 meq per liter, it is corrected by 20 meq per liter at a rate of 2 meq per liter and then permitted to return slowly to normal.

In children more than adults, cholera being an exception, extremely *severe diarrhea* may be attended by an encephalopathy. Irritability, weakness, headache, seizures, stupor, and coma may develop over a period of 2 to 3 days and carry a grave prognosis unless promptly relieved. Presumably this is a metabolic encephalopathy due to loss of fluids and electrolytes and can be corrected by their replacement. In the more protracted illness of *typhoid fever,* approximately half the patients develop a delirium, and a small number will exhibit meningism and become comatose with twitching and seizures or spasticity and hyperactive reflexes, all of which are transitory.

In the *endocrine encephalopathies* the clinical phenomena are even more abstruse. Confusional states may be combined with agitation, hallucinations, delusions, anxiety, and depression. And the time course of the illness may be in terms of weeks and months, rather than days. Derangement of higher nervous function may follow the *administration of ACTH or corticosteroid agents,* and the same symptoms have been reported in *Cushing's disease* (see Chap. 325). The neurology of *thyrotoxicosis* has proved to be peculiarly elusive. Allusions to thyrotoxic psychosis are widely recorded in the medical literature; mental confusion, seizures, manic or depressive attacks, delusions, and chorea occur in various combinations with muscular weakness and atrophy, periodic paralysis, and myasthenia (see Chap. 324). Treatment of the hyperthyroidism gradually restores the patient to a normal mental state. *Myxedematous patients* may show slow mentation and depression, but only in a small proportion is there a major change in cerebral function, taking the form of drowsiness or extreme somnolence, inattentiveness, and apathy. These symptoms can be reversed within a few weeks by thyroid medication. The association of myxedema and cerebellar ataxia is well documented. The neuropathologic basis of this disorder remains unclear, as does the pathogenesis. In *hyperparathyroidism,* when the serum calcium levels reach 15 mg/dL or higher, the patient sinks into a quiet state of inattentiveness, lethargy, and confusion. Stupor, coma, and death may be caused by extreme degrees of hypercalcemia such as occur occasionally in cases of excessive vitamin D administration and metastatic tumors of the bones. Chronic *hypoparathyroidism,* either idiopathic or following thyroid or parathyroid resection may rarely give rise to intracranial calcifications and an extrapyramidal motor syndrome. *Addison's disease* (adrenal insufficiency) may be attended by episodic confusion, stupor, or coma, without special identifying features. Hypoglycemia, hypotension, and hyponatremia with diminished cerebral circulation are thought to be the underlying mechanisms, and measures which correct them appear to be beneficial.

The term *pancreatic encephalopathy* describes a syndrome of agitation and confusion, sometimes with hallucinations and clouding of consciousness, dysarthria, and changing rigidity of the limbs, in association with acute pancreatic disease. The status of this entity is uncertain. A uniform neuropathologic change has not been discerned. We agree with Pallis and Lewis who suggest that before such a diagnosis can be seriously entertained in a patient with acute pancreatitis, one should exclude delirium tremens, the cerebral effects of shock, renal or hepatic failure, hypoglycemia, diabetic acidosis, hyperosmolality, hypokalemia, hypo- or hypercalcemia, any one of which may complicate the underlying disease(s).

D-*Lactic acidosis* can cause encephalopathy in patients who undergo jejunoileostomy for treatment of morbid obesity. Up to 10 percent of such patients report episodes of confusion, ataxia, and slurred speech. D-Lactate, an isomer not normally found in the blood, is present in serum, urine, and stool in these patients. D-Lactate, a product of intestinal bacteria, causes encephalopathy by interfering with pyruvate metabolism. The symptoms are similar to those of thiamine deficiency. Diagnosis is dependent upon recognition of metabolic acidosis associated with hyperchloremia and measurement of elevated D-lactate (see Dahlquist; Cross).

HEREDITARY METABOLIC DISEASES OF LATE ONSET

Inherited metabolic disorders affecting amino acid metabolism (Chaps. 306 and 307), lysosomal enzyme functions (Chap. 316), and cerebral lipids (Chap. 316) are generally rare disorders that first are manifest during infancy or childhood. The salient features of these conditions are summarized in Chaps. 306, 307, and 316. In this chapter are described a small number of hereditary metabolic disorders which may have their onset in late adolescence and adulthood and which may present diagnostic problems because of the similarity of their clinical presentation to other more common acquired and degenerative diseases of the nervous system. Noteworthy attributes of these diseases are their chronicity and progressive nature.

METACHROMATIC LEUKODYSTROPHY (See Chap. 316) Probably the most common member of this category is *adult metachromatic leukodystrophy (MLD).* While the majority of cases appear in early childhood, approximately 25 percent manifest their first symptoms beyond the twenty-first year of life. Cases among men have outnumbered those in women 2:1. The mode of inheritance is autosomal recessive in almost all instances. The onset is insidious and the course protracted, over 20 or more years.

Mental symptoms tend to dominate the clinical picture. Failing scholastic performance, forgetfulness, and irrationality occur early in the illness but may be obscured by peculiarities of personality, such as suspiciousness, delusional thinking, and bizarre actions. These latter qualities may raise the question of schizophrenia or immature ("borderline") personality development. Sooner or later a mild cerebellar ataxia presenting as awkwardness and falling, mild pyramidal signs, masked facies, and bizarre postures stamp the illness as neurologic. Eventually the patient's mental processes deteriorate to the point where he or she is totally helpless, demented, mute, incontinent of sphincteric control, and bedfast.

Specific diagnostic tests include (1) the demonstration of a diminished arylsulfatase A activity in white blood cells, serum, and urine, (2) increased excretion of sulfatides in urine, (3) slowed conduction velocity in nerves, and (4) deposits of metachromatic material in nerve biopsies.

No treatment is presently available.

ADRENOLEUKODYSTROPHY In *adrenoleukodystrophy* either bronzing of the skin and Addison's disease or cerebral symptoms may be the initial manifestation. The cerebral lesions may present as a homonymous hemianopsia, cortical blindness, hemiparesis, aphasia, or dementia. Usually the signs are asymmetric at first and progress intermittently. A relatively pure polyneuropathic and myelopathic form has also been described. The diagnosis is usually settled by the finding of a low blood cortisol level in a male with cerebrospinal demyelinating disease, although recently a purely spinal type, taking the form of a progressive spastic paraparesis, has been described in the heterozygote (female carrier). Increased urinary concentration of C22-C26 fatty acids is diagnostic. Corticosteroid replacement therapy helps the Addison's disease but has no effect on the neurologic disorders. The latter progress intermittently over a few years, and usually the outcome is fatal.

ADULT LIPID STORAGE DISEASES G_{M2} *gangliosidosis* (hexosaminidase A deficiency) has been observed in young adults. Many are from non-Jewish families, and males and females in the same generation are equally affected. Generalized seizures may mark the beginning of a cerebral disorder that later is evidenced by alterations of behavior and intellectual decline. A progressive ataxia and mild signs of corticospinal disease, the combination of which interferes with independent locomotion, clarifies the diagnosis. The fundi and visual function are normal in most cases, but typical cherry-red macular spots are seen occasionally. The liver and spleen are normal or slightly enlarged. The CSF protein is normal. CT scans reveal a modest ventricular enlargement. A slowly developing dementia, cerebellar ataxia, polymyoclonus, and failing vision may characterize the clinical picture in some cases. In yet others, the presenting syndrome has consisted of prominent motor neuron involvement accompanied by muscle cramps, suggesting a diagnosis of spinal muscular atrophy or amyotrophic lateral sclerosis (see Chap. 350). G_{M2} ganglioside is shown to be increased by thin-layer chromatography of tissue obtained by cerebral biopsy. Membranous cytoplasmic bodies are visualized by electron microscopy of rectal, appendicular, and cortical neurons. Gaucher's and Niemann-Pick diseases are yet other storage diseases that may present in adult life.

Ceroid lipofuscinosis The Kufs type of *ceroid lipofuscinosis* is another form of lipid storage disease that only becomes evident in adolescence or early adult life. Usually the disease begins with mental deterioration, followed by seizures, ataxia, increasing rigidity, athetotic posturing, and corticospinal signs. Skin and conjunctival biopsies (electron-microscopic examination) showed lipofuscin storage material in fibroblasts and endothelial cells.

LEIGH'S DISEASE Some cases of Leigh's subacute necrotizing encephalomyelopathy only begin in adolescence, and take the form of a progressive polymyoclonus with seizures and cerebellar ataxia and relatively mild impairment of intellectual function.

SUMMARY One should at least consider some of these rare forms of hereditary metabolic diseases whenever an adolescent or young adult becomes demented, shows a psychiatric syndrome with decline in cognitive functions, has seizures (especially with polymyoclonus), failing vision, and cerebellar ataxia in combination with corticospinal signs or a progressive polyneuropathy.

REFERENCES

ADAMS RD, FOLEY JM: The neurological disorder associated with liver disease of the nervous system. Proc Assoc Res Nerv Ment Dis 32:198, 1953

———, VICTOR M: *Principles of Neurology,* 3d ed. New York, McGraw-Hill, 1985

ALFREY AC et al: The dialysis encephalopathy syndrome: Possible aluminum intoxication. N Engl J Med 294:184, 1976

AYUS JC et al: Changing concepts in treatment of severe symptomatic hyponatremia. Am J Med 78:897, 1985

BLASS JP, GIBSON GE: Abnormality of a thiamine-requiring enzyme in patients with Wernicke-Korsakoff syndrome. N Engl J Med 297:1367, 1977

BRAIN RESUSCITATION CLINICAL TRIAL I STUDY GROUP. Randomized clinical study of thiopental loading in comatose survivors of cardiac arrest. N Engl J Med 314:397, 1986

CARDINALE GJ et al: Effect of methylmalonyl coenzyme A: A metabolite which accumulates in vitamin B_{12} deficiency on fatty acid synthesis. J Biol Chem 245:3771, 1970

CREMER GM et al: Myxedema and ataxia. Neurology 19:37, 1969

CROSS SA, CALLOWAY WC: D-Lactic acidosis and selected cerebellar ataxias. Mayo Clin Proc 59:202, 1984

DAHLQUIST NR et al: D-Lactic acidosis and encephalopathy after jejunoileostomy: Response to overfeeding and to fasting in humans. Mayo Clin Proc 59:141, 1984

FRASER CL, ARIEFF AI: Hepatic encephalopathy. N Engl J Med 313(14):865, 1985

HARDING AE et al: Spinocerebellar degeneration secondary to chronic intestinal malabsorption: A vitamin E deficiency syndrome. Ann Neurol 12:419, 1982

KLATSKY AL et al: Alcohol consumption and blood pressure. N Engl J Med 296:1194, 1977

KOLODNY EH, BOUSTANY RM: Storage diseases of the reticuloendothelial system, *Hematology of Infancy and Childhood,* 3d ed, D Nathan, F Oski (eds). Philadelphia, Saunders, 1986

LAURENO R: Central pontine myelinolysis following rapid correction of hyponatremia. Ann Neurol 13:232, 1983

LEDERMAN RS, HENRY CE: Progressive dialysis encephalopathy. Ann Neurol 4:199, 1978

MCENTEE WJ, MAIR RG: Memory enhancement in Korsakoff's phychosis by clonidine: Further evidence for a nonadrenergic deficit. Ann Neurol 7:466, 1980

MARKS R, ROSE FC: *Hypoglycemia.* Oxford, Blackwell, 1965

MOSER HW et al: Adrenoleukodystrophy: Studies of the phenotype, genetics and biochemistry. John Hopkins Med J 147:217, 1980

NADEL AM, WILSON WP: Dialysis encephalopathy: A possible seizure disorder. Neurology 26:1130, 1976

O'HARE JA: Dialysis encephalopathy: Clinical, electroencephalographic, and interventional aspects. Medicine 62:129, 1983

PALLIS CA, LEWIS PD: *The Neurology of Gastrointestinal Disease.* Philadelphia, Saunders, 1974

PLUM F (ed): *Brain Dysfunction in Metabolic Disorders.* New York, Raven, 1974

———, POSNER JB: *Diagnosis of Stupor and Coma,* 3d ed. Philadelphia, Davis, 1980

POTTS AM: Tobacco amblyopia. Surv Ophthalmol 17:313, 1973

RASKIN NH, FISHMAN RA: Neurologic disorders in renal failure. N Engl J Med 294:143, 204, 1976

ROTHERMICH NO, VON HAAM E: Pancreatic encephalopathy. J Clin Endocrinol 1:872, 1941

SAGE JI et al: Alcoholic myelopathy without substantial liver disease. A syndrome of progressive dorsal and lateral column dysfunction. Arch Neurol 41:999, 1984

SCHAUMBURG HH et al: Sensory neuropathy from pyridoxine abuse. A new megavitamin syndrome. N Engl J Med 309:445, 1983

SHIMOJYO S et al: Cerebral blood flow and metabolism in the Wernicke-Korsakoff syndrome. J Clin Invest 46:849, 1967

VICTOR M: Polyneuropathy due to nutrional deficiency and alcoholism, in *Peripheral Neuropathy,* 2d ed, PJ Dyck et al (eds). Philadelphia, Saunders, 1984, pp 1899–1940

———: The neurologic complications of hepatic and gastrointestinal disease, in *Textbook of Neurology,* A Asbury et al (eds). Philadelphia, Saunders, 1986

———, ADAMS RD: On the etiology of the alcoholic neurologic diseases: With special reference to the role of nutrition. Am J Clin Nutr 9:379, 1961

——— et al: A restricted form of cerebellar degeneration occurring in alcoholic patients. Arch Neurol 1:577, 1959

——— et al: Deficiency amblyopia in the alcoholic patient: A clinicopathologic study. Arch Ophthalmol 64:1, 1960

——— et al: The acquired (nonwilsonian) type of chronic hepatocerebral degeneration. Medicine 44:345, 1965

——— et al: *The Wernicke-Korsakoff Syndrome. A Clinical and Pathological Study of 245 Patients, 82 with Postmortem Examinations.* Philadelphia, Davis, 1971

WILKINSON DS, PROCKOP LD: Hypoglycemia: Effects on the nervous system, in *Handbook of Clinical Neurology,* PJ Vinken, BW Bruyn (eds). Amsterdam, North-Holland, 1976, vol 27, pp 53–78

WINKELMAN MD, RICANATI ES: The neuropathology of dialysis encephalopathy. Hum Pathol (in press)

WITT ED, GOLDMAN-RAKIC PS: Intermittent thiamine deficiency in the rhesus monkey. I. Progression of neurological signs and neuranatomical lesions. Ann Neurol 13:376, 1983

350 DEGENERATIVE DISEASES OF THE NERVOUS SYSTEM

EDWARD P. RICHARDSON, JR. / M. FLINT BEAL / JOSEPH B. MARTIN

In classifying the diseases of the nervous system, it has long been customary to designate a group of them as *degenerative,* indicating that they are characterized by gradually evolving, relentlessly progressive neuronal death occurring for reasons that are still entirely unknown. The identification of these diseases depends upon careful, thoroughgoing exclusion of such possible causative factors as infections, metabolic derangements, and intoxications. Experience shows that a considerable proportion of the disorders that are classed as degenerative are associated with genetic predisposition, resulting in a pattern of dominant or recessive inheritance. Others, however, while not differing in any fundamental way from the hereditary disorders, occur only sporadically—as isolated instances in a given family.

Since by definition, classification of the degenerative diseases cannot be based upon any exact knowledge of their cause or pathogenesis, their subdivision into individual syndromes rests on descriptive criteria based largely upon pathologic anatomy but also taking into account clinical aspects. In practice, this group of diseases presents itself in the form of several clinical syndromes, the recognition of which can assist the clinician in arriving at a diagnosis. Apart from the individual differences that serve to allow distinction of one syndrome from another, there are some general attributes that typify the entire class of disorders under discussion.

GENERAL CONSIDERATIONS It is characteristic of the degenerative disorders that they begin insidiously and run a gradually progressive course that can extend over many years. As a rule, the course is more protracted than that of the hereditary metabolic diseases of the nervous system (see Chap. 349). The earliest changes may be so subtle that it often is impossible to assign any precise time of onset. At times the patient or the family may give a history suggesting an abrupt onset of disability—particularly when an injury or some other dramatic event in the patient's life has occurred, to which illness might conceivably be related. By careful questioning, it still may be possible to discern that the patient or family under these circumstances has suddenly become aware of a condition which had, in fact, already been present but had passed unnoticed.

The family history is of great importance, but denial of familial occurrence of a disorder cannot always be taken at face value. One reason is that patients or their relatives may be ashamed to disclose that a neurologic disease afflicts the family. Another is that the extent of the disease affecting other family members may be so slight that the patient or family may be unaware of its presence—as may occur, for instance, in the group of the hereditary ataxias. Moreover, small sibships in a family may prevent well-established hereditary diseases from being recognized. Familial occurrence, of course, does not always mean that a disease is hereditary; it may indicate instead that there has been a common exposure to an infective or toxic agent.

Another general aspect of the degenerative nervous system diseases is that their progressive course is in the long run uninfluenced by attempted therapeutic measures. Caring for a patient with an illness of this kind is often, therefore, an anguishing experience for all concerned. Yet symptoms can often be alleviated, sometimes remarkably so (as in Parkinson's disease), by wise and skillful management, and the physician's kindly interest may be of great help even when curative measures cannot be offered.

A noteworthy feature of this group of diseases is that the changes brought about by them tend to have a bilaterally symmetric distribution. This aspect alone may help to distinguish a disorder of this class from many other varieties of neurologic disease. It is true, nevertheless, that in the early stages, one side of the body, or one limb, may become involved in the presence of normal findings elsewhere. Sooner or later, though, despite the asymmetric beginning, the inherently bilateral nature of the process generally asserts itself.

It is a striking fact that many of the disorders classed as degenerative involve, almost selectively, particular anatomically or physiologically related systems of neurons while leaving others entirely intact. This is clearly exemplified in amyotrophic lateral sclerosis, in which the disease process is limited to cerebral and spinal motor neurons, and in some forms of progressive ataxia in which the Purkinje cells of the cerebellum are alone affected. In Friedreich's ataxia and some other syndromes, the disease process affects multiple neuronal systems.

In this respect these degenerative neuronal diseases resemble some disease processes of known cause, particularly intoxications, which likewise can result in similarly circumscribed effects on the nervous system. Diphtheria toxin, for example, produces selective breakdown of peripheral nerve myelin, triorthocresyl phosphate affects the corticospinal tracts in the spinal cord together with the peripheral nerves, and, as will be brought out later, the newly discovered neurotoxin 1-methyl-4-phenyl-1,2,5,6-tetrahydropyridine (MPTP) brings about localized nerve cell death in the substantia nigra. Selective involvement of particular neuronal systems is not, to be sure, characteristic of all of the degenerative diseases; some are characterized by pathologic changes that are diffuse and unselective. These exceptions nevertheless do not detract from the importance of affection of particular neuronal systems as a distinguishing feature of many of the diseases under discussion.

Typically, the pathologic process in the nervous system is one of slow involution of nerve cell bodies or their prolongations as nerve fibers, unaccompanied by any intense tissue reaction or cellular response, although the loss of neurons and fibers is accompanied by a reactive hyperplasia of fibrillary astrocytes (gliosis). The cerebrospinal fluid (CSF) thus shows little if any change—at most a slight elevation of protein, without abnormalities in specific proteins, cell count, or in other constituents. Moreover, since these diseases invariably result in tissue loss, rather than in new tissue formation, radiographic visualization of the brain, the ventricular system, or subarachnoid space shows either no change or an enlargement of the CSF compartments. These negative laboratory findings thus help to distinguish the degenerative disorders from the other large classes of progressive diseases of the nervous system—tumors and infections.

CLASSIFICATION Since etiologic classification is impossible, subdivision of the degenerative diseases into individual syndromes rests on descriptive criteria based largely on pathologic anatomy, but to some extent on clinical aspects as well. In the terms used to designate many of these syndromes, the names of a number of distinguished neurologists and neuropathologists are commemorated. A useful way of keeping in mind the various disease states is to group them according to the outstanding clinical features that may be found in an actual case. The classification outlined in the following table (Table 350-1) and described below is based on such a plan.

SYNDROMES IN WHICH PROGRESSIVE DEMENTIA PREDOMINATES

In the disease entities about to be discussed, the clinical picture is dominated by gradual loss of intellectual capacities, i.e., by dementia. Other neurologic abnormalities, except in the terminal stages, are absent or relatively insignificant. (For further discussion of dementia, including its clinical evaluation, Chaps. 10, 11, and 23 should be consulted.)

ALZHEIMER'S DISEASE Alzheimer's disease is perhaps the most important of all the degenerative diseases because of its frequent occurrence and devastating nature. It is the commonest cause of dementia in the elderly, with all that this implies in the way of distress for patients and families, and economic loss in the form of the costs entailed in the long-term care of patients totally disabled by the disease. Historically, the term *Alzheimer's disease* was applied to progressive dementia coming on in late middle life but preceding the senile period, following the original description by Alois Alzheimer in 1907, in which the illness of a woman dying at the age of 55 was depicted clinically and pathologically. It became usual to classify cases of this kind under the heading of *presenile dementia*. Meanwhile, it became increasingly apparent that very old people dying with progressive mental deterioration, generally referred to as *senile dementia*, showed cerebral lesions that were identical to those found in cases of presenile dementia as described by Alzheimer. Consequently, to designate cases of this kind, the category of *senile dementia of the Alzheimer type* has been suggested. All evidence indicates that the disease process is the same, no matter what the age of occurrence may be. At the same time, it clearly is age-related. It is extremely uncommon in young people and rare in middle age; as age advances, however, it is increasingly frequent, such that its prevalence in persons over 80 years old is estimated at more than 20 percent (Ball, 1982). Advancing age is unmistakably a predisposing factor, and aging itself is accompanied by neuronal loss in the cerebral cortex, but it would be erroneous to consider Alzheimer's disease as the inevitable accompaniment of aging because, as general experience shows, there are many old people who remain mentally unimpaired to the end. Genetic predisposition to Alzheimer's disease does not emerge as a clear-cut pattern. In most instances, the disorder appears sporadically; there are well-documented familial cases, however,

TABLE 350-1 Clinical classification of the degenerative diseases of the nervous system

I Disorders characterized by progressive dementia in the absence of other prominent neurologic signs
- *A* Alzheimer's disease
- *B* Senile dementia of the Alzheimer type
- *C* Pick's disease (lobar atrophy)

II Syndromes combining progressive dementia with other prominent neurologic abnormalities
- *A* Mainly in adults
  - *1* Huntington's disease
  - *2* Multiple system atrophy combining dementia with ataxia and/or manifestations of Parkinson's disease
  - *3* Progressive supranuclear palsy (Steele-Richardson-Olszewski)
- *B* Mainly in children or young adults
  - *1* Hallervorden-Spatz disease
  - *2* Progressive familial myoclonic epilepsy

III Syndromes of gradually developing abnormalities of posture and movement
- *A* Paralysis agitans (Parkinson's disease)
- *B* Striatonigral degeneration
- *C* Progressive supranuclear palsy (see *II, A, 3* above)
- *D* Torsion dystonia (torsion spasm; dystonia musculorum deformans)
- *E* Spasmodic torticollis and other restricted dyskinesias
- *F* Familial tremor
- *G* Gilles de la Tourette syndrome

IV Syndromes of progressive ataxia
- *A* Cerebellar degenerations
  - *1* Cerebellar cortical degeneration
  - *2* Olivopontocerebellar atrophy (OPCA)
- *B* Spinocerebellar degenerations (Friedreich's ataxia and related disorders)

V Syndrome of central autonomic nervous system failure (Shy-Drager syndrome)

VI Syndromes of muscular weakness and wasting without sensory changes (motor neuron disease)
- *A* Amyotrophic lateral sclerosis
- *B* Spinal muscular atrophy
  - *1* Infantile spinal muscular atrophy (Werdnig-Hoffmann)
  - *2* Juvenile spinal muscular atrophy (Wohlfart-Kugelberg-Welander)
  - *3* Other forms of familial spinal muscular atrophy
- *C* Primary lateral sclerosis
- *D* Hereditary spastic paraplegia

VII Syndromes combining muscular weakness and wasting with sensory changes (progressive neural muscular atrophy; chronic familial polyneuropathies)
- *A* Peroneal muscular atrophy (Charcot-Marie-Tooth)
- *B* Hypertrophic interstitial polyneuropathy (Déjerine-Sottas)
- C Miscellaneous forms of chronic progressive neuropathy

VIII Syndromes of progressive visual loss
- *A* Pigmentary degeneration of the retina (retinitis pigmentosa)
- *B* Hereditary optic atrophy (Leber's disease)

some following an autosomal dominant pattern of inheritance. An exception to the statement that Alzheimer's disease is rare in young people occurs in the instance of Down's syndrome (trisomy 21), which leads to the development of the characteristic lesions of Alzheimer's disease in the majority of the patients after 30 years of age.

Pathology The outstanding pathologic feature is death and disappearance of nerve cells in the cerebral cortex. This leads ultimately to extensive convolutional atrophy, especially in the frontal and medial temporal regions. There is a corresponding enlargement of the ventricular system, but this is not extreme unless there is a concomitant hydrocephalus.

Two kinds of microscopic lesions are distinctive for the disease. The first, originally described by Alzheimer, consists of intracytoplasmic accumulations within neurons of a filamentous material in the form of loops, coils, or tangled masses—now often referred to as *Alzheimer neurofibrillary tangles*. The nature of these filaments is now under active investigation, because the neuropathologic evidence strongly suggests that these fibrillar masses are of major importance in bringing about the death of neurons. Electron microscopy shows them to be accumulations of paired helical filaments that clearly differ from the normal intracytoplasmic neurofilaments and tubules. Moreover, Rasool and Selkoe have produced evidence that the Alzheimer filaments differ antigenically from the normal neurofilaments. Apparently, therefore, these neurofibrillary tangles represent deposition of a pathologic substance rather than an overaccumulation of any normal cytoplasmic constituents. Neurofibrillary tangles tend to be most abundant, together with the most extreme degrees of neuronal loss, in the hippocampus and adjacent parts of the temporal lobe—structures that have been found to be of greatest importance in the faculty of retentive memory.

The other histopathologic change that characterizes Alzheimer's disease is the presence of intracortical foci of clustered thickened neuronal processes, both axons and dendrites (collectively referred to as *neurites*), generally in the form of an irregular ring surrounding a usually spherical deposit of amyloid fibrils. These lesions, which had already been recognized before Alzheimer's description of the neurofibrillary change, for many years were termed *senile plaques*. Recent elucidation of their structure has led to their currently being designated as *neuritic plaques*. The neuritic components of these plaques have been shown to contain paired helical filaments identical to those found in the perinuclear cytoplasm of the diseased neurons. The nature and origin of the amyloid component are being intensively studied. It is now evident that amyloid, identified by its staining reactions and ultrastructural features, is not a uniform substance; instead, its tinctorial and morphologic character depends upon a particular molecular spatial configuration (beta-pleated sheet fibrils) that can be brought about with various proteins, some of immunologic origin, some not. According to Glenner, the cerebral amyloid protein may be derived from an abnormal circulating protein (of as yet undetermined origin) which takes on the properties of amyloid as a result of the underlying pathologic process that is intrinsic to the disease. As far as can be determined, the earliest change in the development of the plaques is the production of the abnormal neurites; the amyloid deposition appears to be secondary.

There is another aspect to the problem of cerebral amyloidosis in Alzheimer's disease. In many, but not all, cases identical amyloid deposits may be found in the walls of small meningeal and intracortical arteries, and the question has arisen as to whether this cerebrovascular amyloidosis (often called *cerebral amyloid angiopathy* or *congophilic angiopathy* because of the characteristic staining of amyloid with the dye Congo red) has a close relationship, perhaps even causative (as suggested by Glenner), to plaque amyloidosis. At present, plaque amyloidosis and cerebrovascular amyloidosis are perhaps best considered as concomitant, or significantly interrelated, rather than interdependent; at any rate, experience shows that either one can be found in the brain independently of the other.

On the biochemical side, it is of interest that choline acetyltransferase, the key enzyme required for the synthesis of acetylcholine, is decreased in the cerebral cortex in Alzheimer's disease, as well as acetylcholinesterase. Recent studies have indicated that the major source of neocortical cholinergic innervation is a group of neurons situated in the basal part of the forebrain just beneath the corpus striatum—the nucleus basalis of Meynert. Careful pathoanatomic investigations have shown that in Alzheimer's disease, this nucleus is a site of major neuronal loss and of frequent Alzheimer neurofibrillary tangles. These studies suggest that impairment of cholinergic transmission may play a part in the clinical expression of the disease. However, attempted therapy with cholinomimetic agents has been largely unsuccessful. Less consistent reductions in cortical norepinephrine and serotonin appear to be caused by neuronal loss in the locus coeruleus and raphe nucleus, respectively. Loss of neurons in cerebral cortex is also associated with reduced cortical concentrations of somatostatin. Reduction in CSF concentrations of somatostatin is also reported.

It is to be hoped that the ongoing active investigations of the nature of these cerebral lesions will lead ultimately to an understanding of their causation. The remarkable discovery that one form of progressive dementia, Creutzfeldt-Jakob disease, is the result of infection with a transmissible virus-like agent has led to the question as to whether Alzheimer's disease and other neuronal degenerations might be due to a similar form of infectious agent. All attempts to transmit Alzheimer's disease have failed, however, so that currently an infective basis is thought unlikely. The fact, demonstrated by Perl and Brody, that neurofibrillary tangles contain aluminum is of interest, but its etiologic significance remains unclear.

Clinical manifestations The onset is insidious and subtle, with changes most noticeable first in memory for recent happenings and in other aspects of mental activity. Emotional disturbances such as depression, anxiety, or odd, unpredictable quirks of behavior, may be salient features in the early stages. Progression is usually slow and gradual, and unless other medical conditions supervene, it may smolder on for 10 or more years.

In the milder cases, including those of the senile period, the noteworthy features are those of simple dementia, as described in Chap. 23. More unusual disorders of thought and intellect, including aphasia, apraxic disturbances, and abnormalities of space perception, may be seen, especially in the presenile group. Exceptionally, and only in the advanced stages of the disease, extrapyramidal signs appear; the patient walks in a shuffling manner with short steps, and there is a generalized stiffness of the musculature with slowness and awkwardness of all movements. In some patients, sudden jerklike contractions of various muscles (myoclonus) may occur in the presence of otherwise typical Alzheimer's disease, but this is unusual and should immediately raise the suspicion of Creutzfeldt-Jakob disease (Chap. 347). Terminally the patient may become nearly decorticate, losing all ability to perceive, think, speak, or move. This is sometimes called "the late vegetative phase." Laboratory investigations, including the usual blood and CSF determinations, do not yield any conclusive or pertinent data. There is a diffuse slowing in the electroencephalogram in the more advanced stages of the disease. The enlargement of the ventricular system and subarachnoid space resulting from the diffuse brain atrophy can be demonstrated by computerized tomography (CT) scan and by magnetic resonance imaging (MRI). These imaging procedures, however, are not decisive for making the diagnosis, especially in the earlier stages, because the degree of cerebral atrophy demonstrated may be no more than that seen in patients of a similar age group who are functioning normally. During the course of the illness, occasional convulsive seizures may occur, but they are relatively rare and should raise suspicion of other diseases. Terminally, the patient dies from intercurrent disease, in a state of total helplessness. Institutional care is usually necessary long before the end.

Differential diagnosis The physician must be alert to the fact that what at first may appear to be dementia of the Alzheimer type, and hence be untreatable, may instead be mimicked by another disorder for which effective therapeutic measures are available. Evidence of space-occupying lesions, such as chronic subdural hematoma or slowly growing frontal neoplasms (for instance, meningioma or glioma) should be sought. CT and MRI scanning usually demonstrate mass lesions of these kinds, as well as an unsuspected hydrocephalus, which, when treated by a shunt procedure for ventricular decompression, may lead to dramatic improvement in the patient's state. Other treatable conditions producing a dementia-like state include metabolic derangements (as with liver disease), vitamin B_{12} (cyanocobalamin) deficiency, and hypothyroidism. Moreover, elderly people may be unusually susceptible to the sedative effects of medications, so that chronic drug intoxication may need to be considered. Cerebrovascular disease is not ordinarily a cause of uncomplicated dementia, but when, during study of a case, multiple small infarcts are disclosed on CT or MRI scanning, this poses a major problem in differential diagnosis and raises the possibility of multi-infarct dementia. Another disorder that can mimic dementia is depression, particularly in the elderly, in whom it may be all too easy to attribute deficits in thinking, motivation, and memory to an irreversible cerebral disease (see Chaps. 11 and 23). When due to depression—as may occur—these abnormalities may show a most gratifying response to appropriate treatment (see Chap. 360).

The evidence that cholinergic innervation may be impaired in Alzheimer's disease has led to attempts to correct the deficiency pharmacologically, much as is done in Parkinson's disease by giving L-dopa, but so far none of these has proved to be consistently effective.

Practical measures that may help in the management of cases of Alzheimer's disease are suggested in Chaps. 11 and 23, which are concerned with the delirious and demented patient.

PICK'S DISEASE (LOBAR ATROPHY) This remarkable form of cerebral disease, which is characterized by the circumscription of the atrophy (lobar sclerosis), was first described by Arnold Pick at the turn of the century. In the differential diagnosis of dementia in the presenile period, it is often mentioned in the same breath with Alzheimer's disease. It is, however, an extremely rare condition as compared with diffuse cerebral atrophy of the Alzheimer type. Moreover, hereditary transmission (as a dominant trait) is more frequent in Pick's disease, and women are more frequently affected than men. The age distribution is similar in both of these varieties of progresive dementia.

Pathology So striking are the gross pathologic changes in the brain that in typical cases the diagnosis can be made at a glance. Severe atrophy of the anterior portions of the frontal and temporal lobes occurs, and there is a curiously sharp line of demarcation between the atrophied portions and the remainder of the brain, which appears normal or nearly so. In some cases, the frontal atrophy is more prominent; in others, the temporal lobes are more severely involved; in general, both regions are affected. Rarely, the disorder has a predominantly unilateral localization—as in cases described originally by Pick. Characteristically, there likewise are atrophic changes in a number of subcortical structures: caudate nucleus, putamen, thalamus, and substantia nigra, and in the descending frontopontine fiber system. In the diseased regions, the local destruction of central and convolutional white matter may be out of proportion to the degree of loss of nerve cell bodies in corresponding areas of the cortex. In many cases (20 of 32 in the well-studied series of Tissot et al.), there are striking changes in nerve cells in the affected regions. These consist of fibrillary deposits within the cytoplasm—masses of straight fibrils, differing from the paired helical filaments of Alzheimer's disease. In some neurons, densely packed spherical aggregates (Pick bodies) can be seen with special staining techniques, such as silver-impregnation methods. In the other affected neurons, the fibrils are more widely dispersed, and the neuronal cytoplasm takes on a rounded, distended appearance, forming ballooned cells. Recent evidence suggests that despite the morphologic differences, these neuronal changes are biochemically related to those in Alzheimer's disease, as indicated by common antigenic properties. In the cases in which these cytopathologic changes are found, other pathologic features are identical to those seen in cases in which they are present: extreme neuronal loss and gliosis in the affected lobes and concomitant lobar atrophy of white matter. In rare instances of Alzheimer's disease, disproportionate atrophy of the frontal and temporal lobes may suggest Pick's disease, but in such cases the distinguishing feature is the presence of the characteristic plaques and neurofibrillary tangles, which are not found in Pick's disease.

Clinical manifestations If Pick's disease has any distinctive clinical features, they consist of unusually severe signs of frontal lobe or temporal lobe dysfunction (see Chap. 24). Typical early manifestations are a general impoverishment of mental function, changes in behavior patterns, and a striking lack of insight. The later phases of the disease are characterized by loss of retentive memory (with temporal lobe involvement), loss of all language functions, and, when the frontal lobes are mainly affected, prominent grasp and sucking reflexes. In CT and MRI scans the shrinkage of the cortex and the low density of the white matter in the affected lobes may be diagnostic. Progression, as in Alzheimer's disease, is slow and relentless, the average duration being about 7 years. In the late stages, rigidity, dystonic postures, and perhaps tremor may be prominent features; these can be ascribed to extension of the disease process into the basal ganglia.

Differential diagnosis The considerations already noted with regard to Alzheimer's disease apply to Pick's disease as well.

SYNDROMES COMBINING DEMENTIA WITH OTHER NEUROLOGIC SIGNS

HUNTINGTON'S DISEASE This disorder, which is characterized by a combination of choreoathetotic movements and progressive dementia usually beginning in midadult life, is transmitted from generation to generation as an autosomal dominant disease. Recent genetic studies have shown that the determining gene is located on the short arm of chromosome 4. The classic description is that of George Huntington, who, together with his father and grandfather, both physicians, made clinical observations on familial cases living near their home on Long Island, New York. Huntington, writing in 1872, entitled his paper "On Chorea"; subsequently the disorder described by him came to be known as *Huntington's chorea*. The more general term used in this chapter—Huntington's disease—is preferable, since the disease state comprises more than abnormal movements, and the motor abnormalities often are more complex than would be implied by the unqualified term *chorea*.

Because of its distressing and incapacitating nature, and its implications for members of any family in which it appears (50 percent risk in all children of an affected parent), the disease has attracted attention in recent years and has been found to be considerably more frequent and widely distributed than once was thought. In virtually all cases that come to the notice of a physician, there is a family history of the disease, although very occasionally a new case may turn up as the result of an apparent genetic mutation; however, no proven case of a new mutation has occurred. An apparently negative family history may be obtained in a few cases of late onset, often classified as senile chorea, where family members have died of other causes before the disease became manifest.

Pathology Distinctive for Huntington's disease is atrophy of the caudate nucleus, and, to a lesser extent, other structures of the basal ganglia (putamen and globus pallidus), out of proportion to any other changes in the brain. The degree of atrophy is directly related to the severity and duration of the disease. In the late stages, the caudate nucleus, which normally forms a convexly rounded eminence in the lateral wall of the lateral ventricle, takes on instead a flattened or concave appearance. As the result of the tissue loss, the ventricular system becomes correspondingly widened, especially the frontal horns. Along with these changes in the basal ganglia, there characteristically is diffuse gyral atrophy, most severe over the convex aspect of the brain.

The atrophy of the caudate nucleus and putamen is seen microscopically to be due to extensive loss of neurons, which stands out in contrast to the intactness of adjacent structures such as the nucleus accumbens septi, the nucleus basalis of Meynert (so strikingly involved in Alzheimer's disease), and the thalamus.

There are no morphologically distinctive or characteristic cytopathologic alterations in the neurons in Huntington's disease such as occur in Alzheimer's and some other diseases. Neurochemical studies have shown a striking decrease of γ-aminobutyric acid (GABA) and of its synthesizing enzyme, glutamic acid decarboxylase (GAD) in the caudate nucleus, putamen, globus pallidus, and pars reticulata of the substantia nigra, and some decrease also in choline acetyltransferase (CAT) in the caudate nucleus. The loss of GABA can be attributed to depletion of the abundant medium-sized *spiny* neurons within the striatum. Spiny neurons are characterized in Golgi studies by a large number of dendritic spines and have been shown to constitute the projection neurons of the striatum. They provide efferents to both the globus pallidus and substantia nigra. In contrast *aspiny* neurons, with few dendritic spines, are striatal interneurons with locally arborizing axons. In addition to GABA, other neurotransmitters contained within striatal spiny neurons, including substance P, enkephalins, and dynorphin, are similarly depleted in the striatum and its sites of projection.

Recent observations indicate that the peptide neurotransmitter somatostatin is relatively increased in the caudate nucleus and putamen in Huntington's disease, and cells identifiable as somatostatin neurons (*aspiny* neurons) are selectively preserved—in striking contrast to the loss of other neurons in the same regions. The pathophysiologic meaning of this sparing is not clear as yet; in any event, its occurrence further emphasizes the fact that in Huntington's disease, as well as in other neuronal-system degenerations, there is selective vulnerability of some neurons in a particular region and preservation of others. The nature of the resistance of particular neuronal groups is unknown but its investigation may provide clues to the underlying disease process. Another interesting point is that the disease informs us of the presence of a diversity of functions of seemingly identical-appearing small neurons in the striatum.

The progressive dementia of Huntington's disease is still not well characterized neuropathologically. It has generally been attributed to neuronal loss in the cerebral cortex, but we have had great difficulty in discerning abnormalities in the cortex in comparison with appropriately chosen control material. Recent biochemical studies, however, are consistent with a mild neuronal loss, particularly in frontal cortex. Further correlative biochemical and neuropathologic studies, using careful quantitative methods, will be needed to resolve this issue.

Clinical aspects The disorder has a prevalence in Europe and North America of 7 to 10 per 100,000 population. The movement disorder generally makes its appearance in early to middle adult years (average age of onset about 35 to 40 years). It is characteristic of the disease that younger patients, with onset of symptoms in the age group of 15 to 40 years, suffer a more severe form of the disorder than older patients, with onset in the 50s and 60s, and the neuropathologic changes in the brain are correspondingly more extensive and severe in the younger as compared with the older patients. There also is evidence that paternal transmission results in a more severe form of the disease than maternal transmission. Huntington's disease is occasionally manifest in childhood (even before the age of 4). Such cases are rare and tend to be characterized more by rigidity than by chorea and by other atypical features such as convulsive seizures and cerebellar ataxia (Westphal's variant).

The involuntary movements (bizarre grimacing, respiratory irregularity, faulty articulation of speech, and irregular, arrhythmic, unpatterned movements of the limbs, imparting to the gait a peculiar dancing quality) tend to be less quick and more athetoid than in Sydenham's chorea (see Chap. 15). Some reported cases which on genealogic and pathologic grounds must be classified with Huntington's chorea have shown progressive rigidity rather than choreiform movements, even in the adult. As a general rule, dementia runs parallel with the motor disorder. Occasionally it may appear before or after chorea; very rarely it may be slight or lacking altogether. Neuropsychiatric manifestations of depression, erratic behavior, and emotional outbursts often seriously handicap the patient before dementia or the movement disorder are severe. The advance of the disease is slow. There is increasing disability because of both involuntary movements and mental changes, terminated after many years by death from intercurrent infection or, not rarely, by suicide.

Differential diagnosis There is no difficulty in the recognition of typical cases. The relatively late onset, the slowly progressive course, the prominent dementia, and lack of association with rheumatic fever help to exclude Sydenham's chorea. Patients with Parkinson's disease when overdosed with L-dopa may develop a widespread chorea or choreoathetosis, and this, combined with the early dementia that occurs in some patients, can reproduce the picture of Huntington's disease. Phenothiazine drugs may induce generalized chorea, unassociated with dementia, and the movement disorder may persist for months or years after the medication is discontinued (tardive dyskinesia). Finally, there is a form of self-limited chorea which, like other localized dyskinesias, may appear in older persons without identifiable cause. Hepatolenticular degeneration (Wilson's disease) and nonfamilial forms of hepatocerebral degeneration may display clinical abnormalities resembling those of Huntington's disease, but the specific changes characteristic of these disorders, including liver disease, corneal Kayser-Fleischer rings (in Wilson's disease), and the typical biochemical abnormalities, are absent in Huntington's disease (see Chap. 311). Choreoathetosis appearing during the second postnatal year and lasting throughout life is due to hypoxic birth injury or kernicterus. Sporadic cases of choreiform movements beginning in middle or late life may present a difficult problem in exact diagnosis. The occasional cases of violent choreiform movements produced by vascular lesions, classically in the subthalamic region, are characterized by sudden onset, unilateral distribution (hemiballismus), and a tendency to improve after a period of initial severity. A few cases of acute choreoathetosis have accompanied hyperthyroidism. Virus encephalitis may occasionally be associated with choreiform movements; acute development, fever, and pleocytosis in the CSF help in recognition of such cases. Hereditary acanthocytosis is a rare condition which can mimic Huntington's disease.

Treatment No form of treatment has as yet been devised that halts the relentless progression of this disease, and therapeutic attempts to alleviate the abnormal movements have generally been unsatisfactory. Dopamine receptor antagonists (butyrophenones or phenothiazines) may partially ameliorate the chorea, but the side effects characteristic of this class of drugs limit their use. The application of molecular genetic probes for presymptomatic and prenatal discovery of the gene is currently under evaluation.

MULTIPLE SYSTEM ATROPHY General experience has indicated that cases of multiple affection of neuronal systems may occur in which progressive dementia is combined with varying degrees of ataxia, dysarthria, and parkinsonian dyskinesia, depending upon the pattern of anatomic distribution of the pathologic changes. For cases of this kind, the general term *multiple system atrophy or degeneration* has been applied. In some, loss of neurons in the cerebellar cortex and in the pontine nuclei and inferior olivary nuclei results in the predominating picture of *olivopontocerebellar degeneration,* to be discussed below as one of the syndromes of progressive ataxia. These changes may be combined with similar neuronal loss in the substantia nigra (and in the striatum in striatonigral degeneration), resulting in parkinsonian features (discussed below under "Parkinson's Disease"). Pathologically, the disease process is characterized by death and disappearance of the affected cells and an accompanying reactive gliosis, without intracellular inclusions or other distinctive features. The cerebral cortex generally shows little discernible change, so that it may be difficult to ascribe a definite pathoanatomic basis for the dementia, which, for this reason, is sometimes designated as *subcortical.* Typically multiple system atrophy is a disorder of late adult life, occurring sporadically in some instances and genetically transmitted in others. Further details of individual syndromes are given in later sections.

PROGRESSIVE SUPRANUCLEAR PALSY (STEELE-RICHARDSON-OLSZEWSKI SYNDROME) This disorder is discussed below among the syndromes characterized by gradually developing abnormalities of posture and movement. It is mentioned here because progressive dementia may accompany the other neurologic abnormalities, although it appears late in the course and generally is not severe.

HALLERVORDEN-SPATZ DISEASE This unusual disorder, often affecting several siblings in a family in a manner suggesting an autosomal recessive trait, is associated with a rather variable clinical picture in which abnormalities of posture and muscle tone, involuntary movements, and progressive dementia predominate. Pathologically, there are characteristic abnormalities in the basal ganglia, suggesting a localized disorder of metabolism. The features of the condition were classically described in an affected family by Hallervorden and Spatz (1922).

Pathology Distinctive for this condition is the accumulation of large amounts of pigmented material in the globus pallidus and pars reticulata of the substantia nigra, resulting in grossly visible brownish discoloration of these regions. Microscopically, there are irregular pigmented, ferruginous concretions and granules of varying brownish or greenish hues, depending on the stains used. Although much of this pigment contains iron, serum iron and ferritin are normal, and there is no systemic disorder of iron metabolism. There also is loss of nerve cell fibers. Another feature of the disease is the presence of focal swelling of axons, most probably in their terminal portions; this is especially pronounced in the regions affected by the pigmentary disorder, but typically can be found at all levels of the central nervous system, including the cerebral cortex. This neuroaxonal change may link the disease with childhood neuroaxonal dystrophy.

Clinical aspects The disorder typically makes its appearance in childhood or adolescence, with abnormalities in muscle tone and movements, such as rigidity and choreoathetosis. Abnormal postures of the trunk characteristic of torsion spasm (dystonia) may be seen, or the clinical picture may be reminiscent of parkinsonism. Cerebellar ataxia is also present in some instances. Speech becomes indistinct, and there is progressive intellectual impairment. Eventually, the involuntary movements give way to increasing generalized rigidity, and death comes as a rule about 10 years after onset. A few cases of late onset have shown a parkinsonian syndrome.

Differential diagnosis No feature of the clinical picture serves to distinguish this particular disorder from other conditions showing dementia with extrapyramidal motor abnormalities. Wilson's disease must be excluded by appropriate laboratory tests. The clearly progressive course sets this condition apart from clinically similar abnormalities resulting from accidents or illnesses at birth or in the neonatal period. It has lately been demonstrated that following intravenous injection of labeled ferrous citrate, there is a selective uptake of radioactive iron in the region of the basal ganglia; possibly a study of this kind would be helpful in diagnosis. In an advanced case, CT scanning may show extreme atrophy of the brain, especially including the structures of the basal ganglia, but the pigmented deposits do not show any increased radiographic density. In some cases there is lucency in the putamen and globus pallidus. At present no effective treatment is known. Treatment with a chelating agent, deferoxamine mesylate, has not shown definite benefit, and L-dopa and other antiparkinsonian medications, tryptophan, and megavitamin therapy have been of only temporary and questionable help.

PROGRESSIVE FAMILIAL MYOCLONIC EPILEPSY There are several neurologic disorders that can result in a syndrome of convulsive seizures, myoclonic jerklike contractions of the musculature, and progressive dementia. Those most frequently encountered in practice are subacute sclerosing panencephalitis in children, adolescents, and young adults (Chap. 347), and subacute spongiform encephalopathy (Creutzfeldt-Jakob disease) in older adults (Chap. 347). The syndrome can also occur in some of the rare forms of metabolic familial disorders: neuraminidase deficiency associated with macular cherry-red spots (Chap. 316) and ceroid-lipofuscinosis (Chap. 318). When these and other disorders of known cause can be excluded from consideration, there remain some clinicopathologic entities which can appropriately be considered under the heading of the hereditary degenerative diseases. Several families presenting this syndrome have been carefully studied in northern Europe (Sweden and Finland), but there is no specific geographical distribution.

Lafora's disease This variety of recessively inherited progressive myoclonic epilepsy is characterized by distinctive intracytoplasmic inclusions in cerebral neurons, called Lafora bodies following their original description by Gonzalo Lafora (1911). These have been found to be composed of polymers of glucose (polyglucosans) and thus indicate a disorder of carbohydrate metabolism, but the biochemical defect that leads to their accumulation is unknown. The Lafora bodies are widely distributed, but most numerous in the thalamus, substantia nigra, and dentate nucleus of the cerebellum. Subsequent to Lafora's reports, similar polysaccharide deposits have been found in myocardial and skeletal muscle fibers and in the liver, and it is now possible to establish the diagnosis in the presymptomatic phase by liver biopsy.

The disorder characteristically makes its appearance during childhood or adolescence in the form of recurrent seizures (generalized or restricted), or uncontrollable myoclonic jerks, or combinations of the two. With the passage of time, the myoclonic phenomena become increasingly severe, and there is deterioration of all intellectual functions. Death from intercurrent infection generally occurs before the age of 25. Anticonvulsive treatment may help in controlling the seizures, but there currently is no effective treatment for the underlying disease.

Other varieties of myoclonic epilepsy When Lafora's disease and the metabolic and infective disorders mentioned above have been excluded, there remains a rather heterogeneous group of progressive neurologic illnesses having in common autosomal recessive inheritance, myoclonic phenomena, convulsive seizures, and mild dementia. Ataxia of stance, gait, and limb movements is a prominent feature in most cases—so much so that the term introduced by Ramsay Hunt, *dyssynergia cerebellaris myoclonica,* is often applied. In a few cases, including some of those originally described by Hunt, there is an overlap with Friedreich's ataxia, or with chronic sensorimotor neuropathies (see Chaps. 353 and 355). The neuropathologic changes in the few cases that have come to postmortem examination have varied from case to case. In some, atrophy of the dentate nucleus and its fiber projections has been prominent; in others, there has been loss of neurons, especially Purkinje cells, in the cerebellar cortex; in still others, changes have been confined to long-tract degeneration (posterior columns and spinocerebellar tracts) in the spinal cord; a few patients have had cortical, basal-ganglionic, or retinal lesions. Variations also occur in the age of onset and the rate of progression. Until more is known about the biochemistry and genetics of this group of disorders, no satisfactory classification is possible. For further details of these syndromes, general reference works on neurology, such as that of Adams and Victor, should be consulted.

Treatment with appropriate anticonvulsant medications has been helpful in some mild cases, but phenytoin is contraindicated. L-Tryptophan and carbidopa or valproic acid have ameliorated myoclonus in a few cases.

SYNDROMES OF ABNORMAL POSTURE, TREMOR, AND INVOLUNTARY MOVEMENT

PARALYSIS AGITANS (PARKINSON'S DISEASE) This is a common condition first named and described by James Parkinson in 1817. His remarkably complete account gives this definition:

Involuntary tremulous motion, with lessened muscular power, in parts not in action and even when supported; with a propensity to bend the trunk forward, and to pass from a walking to a running pace, the senses and intellects being uninjured.

Typically, paralysis agitans is a disorder of middle or late life, with very gradual progression and a prolonged course. Although it has been seen to occur in families (the estimated familial incidence is 1 to 2 percent), it usually is sporadic. It is well recognized, however, that the epidemic encephalitis of von Economo, which occurred in a worldwide distribution in the years following World War I, was followed by a syndrome clinically almost indistinguishable from paralysis agitans. It is usual in such instances to speak of postencephalitic parkinsonism, whereas the term *Parkinson's disease* should be reserved for true paralysis agitans of unknown cause. Paralysis agitans bears no consistent relation to any known disease process such as arteriosclerosis, trauma, or intoxication (except for MPTP, see below), although such conditions have often been invoked as etiologically significant and may at times produce somewhat similar clinical manifestations.

Pathology Despite the general medical familiarity with the condition and an extensive literature on the subject, it cannot be said that the pathologic changes of paralysis agitans are yet fully understood. The most regularly observed changes have been in the aggregates of melanin-containing nerve cells in the brainstem (substantia nigra, locus coeruleus), where there are varying degrees of nerve cell loss with reactive gliosis (most pronounced in the substantia nigra) along with distinctive eosinophilic intracytoplasmic inclusions (called Lewy bodies, after their description by F.H. Lewy in 1913). Similar changes are seen in the nucleus basalis of Meynert, to which reference is already made in the discussion of Alzheimer's disease. In the older literature, cell loss was also described in other structures of the basal ganglia, but these changes turn out not to be clearly different in nature or degree from what may be encountered in other patients of similar age without extrapyramidal motor disorders. Lesions in these same pigmented nuclei, but without Lewy bodies, characterize the pathologic findings in postencephalitic parkinsonism, in striatonigral degeneration, and in the Shy-Drager syndrome (discussed below).

Biochemical studies which show a decrease of dopamine in the caudate nucleus and putamen—an alteration consistently found in experimental ablation of the substantia nigra—emphasize the possibility that Parkinson's disease can be considered an example of neuronal system disease, involving mainly the nigrostriatal dopaminergic system.

Further confirmation of the importance of disease of the nigrostriatal dopaminergic system in Parkinson's disease comes from the accidental intoxication of drug users by self-injection with MPTP, which selectively destroys the pigmented (dopaminergic) neurons of the substantia nigra and produces the typical clinical manifestations of the disease. The pathologic features of MPTP-induced Parkinson's disease, however, differ from those of idiopathic cases in the absence of Lewy bodies and the lack of neuronal loss in the locus coeruleus. Although MPTP lesions do not exactly mimic those of idiopathic Parkinson's disease, the mechanism by which the drug kills substantia nigra neurons is under active investigation and may provide new insights about the pathogenesis of the idiopathic illness.

Clinical apsects In its fully developed form, this disorder cannot be mistaken for any other. The stooped posture, the stiffness and slowness of movement, the fixity of facial expression, and the rhythmic tremor of the limbs which subsides on active willed movement or complete relaxation are familiar to every clinician. Although symmetric in the later stages, the disorder typically begins asymmetrically, e.g., as a slight tremor of the fingers of one hand or in one leg. Also typical are more or less general hypokinesia and stiffness of the musculature so that even where tremor is inapparent, the disease may betray itself by a somewhat staring and immobile facial expression, a monotonous voice, a general slowness and diminution of all motor activity, and a curious lack of the little spontaneous movements of postural adjustment that are so characteristic of the normal individual. When tremor is minimal, patients often are able to alleviate it by relaxation or by movement or to hide it by keeping their hands in their pockets. The tremor is generally most pronounced in the hands but may involve the legs (and thus secondarily the trunk), lips, tongue, and neck muscles, and is easily seen in the eyelids when they are lightly closed. Its frequency is 4 to 5 per second, but another faster (action) tremor (7 to 8 per second) predominates in some patients. There is never total paralysis, although this is implied by the name of the disease; nevertheless, general enfeeblement of voluntary movement is characteristic of the fully developed disorder. Generally accompanying the stooped attitude is the typical festinating gait, whereby the patient, prevented by the abnormality of postural tone from making the appropriate reflex adjustments required for effective walking, progresses with quick shuffling steps at an accelerating pace as if to catch up with the body's center of gravity. Clinical examination of the tendon and plantar reflexes discloses no abnormalities. There are no sensory changes, although deep aching in joints and muscles is common. Eventually, patients may become so incapacitated by rigidity and tremor as to be helpless in caring for themselves. It has often been observed, however, that even severely disabled patients may, when excited or under great emotional stress, perform complex motor acts quickly and efficiently. Although the temporary alleviation under extreme provocation can never be long maintained, it is nevertheless true that the severity of the symptoms is considerably influenced by emotional factors, being aggravated by anxiety, tension, and unhappiness, and minimal when the patient is in a contented frame of mind. Despite the inherently progressive nature of the condition, much can be achieved with good medical management, and patients may continue for years to live effective, happy lives in spite of this affliction.

Although intellectual deterioration is not a consistent feature of early Parkinson's disease, dementia has been increasingly recognized to be a feature of advanced Parkinson's disease. It eventually afflicts up to one-third of all cases. The dementia is typically insidious in onset and may be heralded by disorientation at night. In advanced cases patients may suffer from vivid auditory and visual hallucinations often precipitated by levodopa therapy.

Differential diagnosis In typical cases, this is not difficult. The extrapyramidal syndromes associated with most diseases of known cause or established nature, such as cerebrovascular disease, cerebral hypoxia (including carbon monoxide asphyxia), or metallic poisoning, differ from paralysis agitans in a number of respects, such as atypical behavior or tremor, presence of signs of corticospinal tract deficit, or early onset of dementia. The differentiation from postencephalitic parkinsonism may be impossible; a clear history of an attack of epidemic encephalitis (prolonged somnolence, disturbance of consciousness, diplopia) and relatively early age of onset of the disorder and the presence of tics, localized spasms, and oculogyric crises may be the only clues to this diagnosis. A neurologic disorder similar to some degree to Parkinson's disease occurs with the prolonged administration of large amounts of reserpine and phenothiazine drugs, as the result of their blocking action on dopaminergic transmission. This drug-induced syndrome usually subsides on discontinuation or decrease in the dosage of the drug, but it may continue indefinitely in the syndrome of *tardive dyskinesia*. MPTP-induced parkinsonism persists because of the destructive effects of the drug on the nigral dopaminergic neurons. Parkinsonism very rarely is produced by cerebral neoplasms or other focal lesions, but then only when the nigrostriatal system has been largely destroyed, with relative sparing of the corticospinal projections.

Some Parkinson-like postural and motor abnormalities may be seen following the repeated blows to the head sustained by boxers—in the "punch drunk" syndrome, in which lesions of the substantia nigra are one of the neuropathologic components. In this condition, dementia, ataxia, dysarthria, and inappropriate behavior are prominent, and neuronal cell loss with neurofibrillary tangles is evident in cerebral coretex.

Multiple bilateral infarcts in the corticospinal pathways and central structures of the brain may induce a syndrome that in some ways resembles paralysis agitans (so-called arteriosclerotic parkinsonism), but careful clinical assessment of the history and findings, particularly the reflex status, serves to distinguish this disorder from true Parkinson's disease. Striatonigral degeneration is a rare syndrome which can be clinically indistinguishable from Parkinson's disease but which does not respond to dopaminergic agents (see below).

Treatment Although there is no treatment that is known to halt or reverse the neuronal degeneration that presumably underlies Parkinson's disease, methods are now available which can bring about a considerable degree of relief from symptoms in many patients. An important part of any therapeutic program is the maintenance of optimum general health and neuromuscular efficiency by planned programs of exercise, activity, and rest; expert physical therapy may be of great help in achieving these ends. In addition, the patient often needs much emotional support in meeting the stress of the illness, in comprehending its nature, and in carrying on courageously in spite of it. Along with these general supportive measures, which are applicable to many chronic illnesses, patients generally require a carefully thought-out program of treatment specifically aimed at counteracting the pathophysiologic disorder that produces their disabilities.

The principles of medical treatment are those that have been presented by Growdon. According to his suggestions, the drug therapy should be adapted to the patient's needs, which vary with the stage of the disease and the predominant manifestation(s). Usually anticholinergic drugs are most effective in suppressing tremor at rest, and propranolol or primidone is best for action tremor. L-Dopa improves akinesia and postural imbalance; anticholinergic drugs have little effect on these two abnormalities.

The decision about whether to treat with a drug and the choice of drug(s) are influenced by the stage of the disease. The scale of Hoehn and Yahr is recommended:

Stage I: Unilateral involvement.
Stage II: Bilateral involvement but no postural abnormalities.
Stage III: Bilateral involvement with mild postural imbalance; the patient leads an independent life.
Stage IV: Bilateral involvement with postural instability; the patient requires substantial help.
Stage V: Severe, fully developed disease; the patient is restricted to bed and chair.

For patients with mild disease (stages I and II), no medication may be required, or only an anticholinergic drug, or amantadine (a dopamine agonist), or a combination of both. Levodopa is required for stages III, IV, and V. In each instance, one uses the lowest dose that gives satisfactory benefit; this decreases the chances of unwanted side effects such as dyskinesias, the on-off phenomenon, and mental confusion, as well as of loss of efficacy of the drug.

The anticholinergic drugs in use share the capacity to block muscarinic receptors and thereby to reduce cholinergic transmission. They are effective not only in relieving the rest tremor of mild Parkinson's disease but also may be combined with levodopa in the treatment of the severe forms of the disease. The anticholinergic drugs also reverse the dystonia and parkinsonian symptoms of neuroleptic drugs.

Currently available anticholinergic drugs are trihexyphenidyl, benztropine, biperiden, and procyclidine. The usual dose of trihexyphenidyl is 1 to 2 mg qid. Benztropine has both anticholinergic and antihistaminic properties; the usual dose is 0.5 to 1.0 mg tid. The optimal dose of all these medications varies for each patient and often needs adjusting. Low doses of these drugs cause dry mouth but few if any other side effects. Larger doses should be given with caution for in the elderly they may cause confusion, visual and tactile hallucinations, narrow-angle glaucoma, and urinary retention. Anticholinergic drugs may exacerbate dementia and should be withdrawn when dementia becomes clinically evident.

Propranolol, a beta-adrenergic antagonist, is helpful in suppressing the fast-frequency action tremor in Parkinson's disease and in the hereditary tremor syndrome. The usual dose is 40 to 80 mg tid. In large doses, it may slow the heart rate and lower blood pressure, which are disadvantages in patients with a tendency to orthostatic hypotension. Metoprolol, a specific beta-adrenergic antagonist, is also effective and is safer in patients with suspected asthma. Primidone in a dose of 50 mg at bedtime has also been shown to be effective. If the tremor is not improved after 1 week, the dose can be increased up to 250 mg daily. Many clinicians now initiate therapy with this regimen.

Amantadine was found by accident to be helpful in Parkinson's disease. Its effect is achieved by its capacity to release stored dopamine from presynaptic terminals; thus it is efficacious in the earlier stages of the disease, before the majority of the dopaminergic neurons in the midbrain have degenerated. It tends to be especially beneficial for tremor. The usual dosage is 100 mg bid; larger doses may produce side effects such as skin changes (livido reticularis), ankle edema, and mental confusion. In some patients, the addition of amantadine to levodopa achieves better results then either medication alone.

Levodopa, which increases the dopamine levels in the striatum and restores neurotransmitter balance between dopamine and acetylcholine, improves akinesia and postural disorders (and sometimes rest tremor) in 75 percent of patients. Levodopa is now given in combination with a dopa-carboxylase inhibitor (carbidopa) which prevents destruction of levodopa in the bloodstream and peripheral tissues but does not pass the blood-brain barrier. This combination therefore makes it possible to achieve optimum effects with a smaller dosage of levodopa than would otherwise need to be used. In this way, some of the side effects of levodopa, particularly nausea and vomiting, can be greatly reduced. The combination (Sinemet) is available in ratios of 1:4 carbidopa to levodopa (25 mg/100 mg) or 1:10 (10/100, 25/250). A total dosage of levodopa from 300 to 2000 mg daily can be used; the relative amounts of carbidopa and levodopa, and the timing of the medications, should be adjusted according to the needs of the individual patient. Although levodopa now is the cornerstone of therapy, it can be combined with an anticholinergic drug, with amantandine, or with bromocriptine.

Bromocriptine is a dopamine agonist which acts directly upon dopamine receptors, unlike levodopa, which requires enzymatic transformation into dopamine within the brain. It has been found to be helpful in the treatment of Parkinson's disease, generally in combination with levodopa. When used alone, patients with mild early disease will often respond to doses of 15 to 30 mg daily. However, more advanced patients may need a dosage range of 50 to 100 mg daily. When given in combination with other drugs, smaller quantities should be used, beginning with 2.5 mg tid. Doses of bromocriptine ranging from 20 to 30 mg daily have been effective as an adjunct to levodopa therapy. Whether or not to use bromocriptine and the dosage are matters that must be decided on the basis of what seems best for an individual patient. The side effects are much the same as those with levodopa.

It must be said that although the modern treatment of Parkinson's disease is more successful than any that was available before the introduction of levodopa, including stereotactic surgery, there are still many problems. Underlying much of the difficulty undoubtedly is the fact that none of these therapeutic measures has an affect on the underlying disease process, which consists of neuronal degeneration. Ultimately a point seems to be reached where pharmacotherapy can no longer compensate for the loss. The major difficulties consist of fluctuations or sudden variations in the response to the drugs used (the on-off response), the development of weakness or immobility (akinesia), and dyskinesias, which increasingly become a problem as the years go by. The dyskinesias consist of choreiform or choreoathetotic movements, which in the late stages of the disease alternate with paralyzing akinesia depending upon a very narrow dosage variation (50 to 100 mg) of levodopa. Interference with absorption of levodopa may be partially responsible since continuous intravenous infusions of levodopa result in a stable clinical state. Loss of therapeutic efficacy also occurs: a single dose which at one time was effective for 5 to 6 h may last only an hour or so. Giving smaller amounts of medication more frequently is sometimes efficacious. In addition, agents acting directly on the postsynaptic receptor, such as bromocriptine, are sometimes more effective. It has recently been shown that temporary levodopa withdrawal, advocated as a method of dealing with the long-term complications of Parkinson's disease, carries some risk and does not result in improved efficacy of levodopa.

Progressive dementia, which eventually overtakes one-third to one-half of the patients in later years, may render them less tolerant to medication. Visual and tactile hallucinations are especially prominent in this group of patients.

As many as one-half of patients with Parkinson's disease have depressive symptoms. They should be treated along the lines suggested in Chap. 360.

The introduction of stereotaxic surgery, with the placement of precisely localized focal lesions in central structures in the brain—mainly the ventrolateral thalamus, or globus pallidus contralateral to the side of the major symptoms—was an important advance in the attempt to relieve the symptoms of Parkinson's disease. The success that has been achieved with levodopa has supplanted these procedures, which, although very beneficial in well-chosen cases, were not without risk and at times were followed by severe disability. Neurosurgical treatment of this kind can still be recommended for the very occasional patient who is relatively young and in good general health and who has a severe unilateral disabling or disfiguring tremor.

STRIATONIGRAL DEGENERATION This rare syndrome closely resembles Parkinson's disease clinically, but clearly differs from it pathologically. The classic clinicopathologic description is that of Adams, van Bogaert, and Vander Eecken, who encountered the disorder in four middle-aged patients with no family history of similar disease. Three of the patients showed the typical clinical picture of Parkinson's disease; orthostatic hypotension was observed in one of them, and cerebellar ataxia in another.

The principal neuronal cell loss is in the striatum and substantia nigra. There is an association in some cases with a progressive ataxic disorder resembling olivopontocerebellar degeneration, and in others with degeneration of spinal cord neurons of the autonomic nervous system, similar to the Shy-Drager syndrome, in which postural hypotension is a major component (see below). The degree to which parkinsonian symptoms occur probably depends on the extent of the nigral lesions as balanced against those in the cerebellum and its connections. Cases of this kind represent examples of multiple system degeneration as described above.

The disorder characteristically occurs in late middle age. Treatment with anti-Parkinson's disease medications has usually not been successful. For measures which control hypotension see under "Shy-Drager Syndrome" (below and Chap. 12).

PROGRESSIVE SUPRANUCLEAR PALSY (STEELE-RICHARDSON-OLSZEWSKI SYNDROME) This disorder, first clearly described in 1963 by Richardson, Steele, and Olszewski, occurs in elderly individuals in approximately the same age period as paralysis agitans. Moreover, it is among the group of parkinsonian patients that most of the examples of this disease are to be found.

Pathology A loss of neurons and gliosis are found on postmortem examination in the tectum and tegmentum of the midbrain, the subthalamic nuclei of Luys, the vestibular nuclei, and to some extent the ocular nuclei. A characteristic finding is the presence of neurofibrillary tangles similar to those of Alzheimer's disease on light-microscopic examination, but differing from them on electron microscopy in that they are composed of straight rather than paired helical filaments. The cause of the disease is unknown. A slow virus has been suspected, but attempts to transfer it to monkeys by the intracerebral inoculation of brain tissue have failed.

Clinical manifestations The clinical features are quite distinctive: disturbances of balance and gait with unexpected falls; rigidity of the neck and other trunk muscles, resembling Parkinson's disease; "masking" of the face; reduction in the volume of the voice; extreme flexion or extension dystonia of the neck; and difficulty in looking down—all these are early symptoms and any one of them may first bring the patient to a physician. Ophthalmoplegia has been regarded as the cardinal clinical sign of the disease. Typically there is initial impairment of vertical saccadic movements and a loss of the fast component of optokinetic nystagmus usually affecting downward more than upward gaze. With progression of the disease horizontal eye movements are affected, with oculovestibular reflexes preserved. Symptoms progress over months and years, until the patient becomes virtually anarthric with total loss of voluntary control of eye movements, and severe cervical and truncal rigidity. Dementia is usually mild with forgetfulness, slowing of thought processes, apathy and impaired ability to manipulate acquired knowledge. There are no impairments of vision, hearing, somatic sensation, or voluntary power, and signs of corticospinal involvement are minimal or absent. The diagnosis should be considered whenever an elderly patient begins to fall repeatedly and inexplicably and has extrapyramidal symptoms with a rigid neck and paralysis of conjugate or vertical gaze.

Treatment Treatment has been unsuccessful. Relatively little benefit comes from the administration of the antiparkinsonian group of drugs, although they should be tried. Occasionally levodopa, or a combination of levodopa with an anticholinergic drug, has helped to diminish some of the symptoms.

NORMAL-PRESSURE HYDROCEPHALUS Normal-pressure hydrocephalus (NPH) is a syndrome of communicating hydrocephalus in which intracranial hypertension is either absent or not recognized. It is discussed here because of the common association of the condition with dementia and abnormalities of gait.

Pathology and pathophysiology Although it is recognized that delayed hydrocephalus can occur after meningitis, head injury, or subarachnoid hemorrhage, the majority of patients presenting with NPH give no history of such an illness. Studies of isotope cisternography indicate that NPH is a communicating hydrocephalus presumed to be due to partial obliteration of the subarachnoid space with defective CSF reabsorption through the arachnoid villi. Whether episodes of increased intracranial pressure occur during the course of the illnes is debated. Some patients monitored continuously show fluctuations in CSF pressure including so-called plateau waves.

Clinical manifestations Typically, the patient or family describe a subacute onset, over weeks, months, or sometimes years, of progressive intellectual deterioration accompanied by slowness and restriction of movements, particularly of gait. No single diagnostic gait disorder occurs (see description, Chap. 16). A broad-based stance with hesitant initiation of walking is common. In some patients ataxic features are present. Hyperreflexia in the legs and extensor plantar responses may be found. Urinary incontinence is noted in less than one-half of patients.

Differential diagnosis Parkinson's disease can be differentiated by its clinical features and the response to Sinemet. Bifrontal disease due to tumor (butterfly glioma), metastases, or cerebral infarction can be identified by CT or MRI. Multi-infarct dementia with gait disorder can be recognized by focal, often asymmetric, neurologic signs and by CT changes. Aqueductal stenosis may present occasionally in late adulthood with hydrocephalus, headaches, dementia, and incontinence. The CT or MRI usually will demonstrate an enlarged third ventricle with normal fourth ventricle.

Treatment The diagnosis can be difficult because of the common association of ventricular enlargement and gait disorder in patients with degenerative brain conditions, particularly Alzheimer's disease. CSF pressure in NPH is usually in the normal range of 80 to 150 mmH_2O. Isotope cisternography demonstrating reflux into the ventricular system may be helpful in some cases. However, the finding of ventricular reflux has not proved to determine reliably which patients are likely to improve following a surgical shunt. Temporary benefit in the gait disorder after removal of 25 to 30 mL of CSF has been noted in some patients. When the history of dementia and gait disorder is subacute in onset and accompanied by considerable ventricular dilatation, surgical shunting is warranted. Ventricular-peritoneal shunting is the procedure most commonly performed. Between 40 and 70 percent of patients show benefit after surgery. The gait disorder tends to show a better response to shunting than the dementia (see Black et al. for review).

TORSION DYSTONIA (TORSION SPASM; DYSTONIA MUSCULORUM DEFORMANS) This is a clinical term denoting a state characterized by nonrhythmic, relatively slow involuntary movements that produce abnormal, at times bizarre, postures of the limbs and trunk. Eventually these postures become more or less fixed. Underlying the clinical disorder may be any of several pathologic conditions, such as the lesions of neonatal hypoxia, Wilson's disease, the pigmented lesions of Hallervorden-Spatz disease (described above), GM_1 gangliosidosis, ataxia-telangiectasia, or kernicterus. There is, in addition, an important group of cases with a variable pattern of genetic transmission. Occasionally, a similar disorder occurs sporadically in late adult life. It is to these cases, both hereditary and sporadic, that the term *torsion dystonia* (torsion spasm, dystonia musculorum deformans) is correctly applied. In these conditions, the course tends to be progressive, and the cause and pathogenesis remain unknown.

Pathology Few cases of dystonia musculorum deformans not due to one of the definable disease processes indicated above have been adequately studied neuropathologically. Reported results from these cases has led to uncertainty as to what the pathologic-anatomic basis of the clinical state might be, although it was generally assumed that the basal ganglia were diseased. A careful study by Zeman and Dyken which included comparison of the findings in patients with the disease with control material, failed to demonstrate any neuropathologic abnormality to which the clinical changes could reasonably be attributed. These negative findings, which are perhaps surprising, must not be interpreted as indicating that there is "no disease" in the brain, but rather that the pathologic state is not one that can be disclosed by the usual histopathologic techniques. It may well be that more careful quantitative assessments of certain populations of neurons and studies of the pathophysiology of neurotransmitters will result in further elucidation of this disease.

Clinical manifestations The motor abnormalities are described in Chap. 15. In the early stages, the involuntary muscular contractions are intermittent and variable in location and severity, but typically interfere with motor performance by superimposing an unwanted posture upon parts in use. One leg may briefly be pulled into a flexed or extended position or one shoulder elevated. Later the lingual, pharyngeal, neck, and thoracic muscles participate, and grimacing may occur. These latter may also be the first and only signs of disease for several years. Progression may be relatively rapid in cases with onset during early childhood, but is slow in those beginning in late childhood or adult life. The end result is extreme disability, with grossly distorted postures of the trunk and contractures of the limbs. Affection of face and tongue muscles results in faulty articulation of speech, which eventually becomes incomprehensible. The tendon and plantar reflexes are normal.

The most severe type, which occurs almost exclusively in Ashkenazi Jews, characteristically makes its appearance in childhood after a preceding period of normalcy. Typically it becomes first evident in the lower limbs and then evolves, sometimes relatively rapidly, into the generalized state of severe incapacity described above. The manner of genetic transmission—whether autosomal recessive or dominant with variable penetrance—is still not wholly settled. In the recognized autosomal dominant type, which occurs mainly in non-Jewish populations, the disorder comes on later (often in midadult life) and takes a milder form. It tends to appear first in the upper limbs and to remain more restricted in its extent than the early-onset variety, and progression is less relentless. The late-life sporadic cases are generally similar in character to those of the autosomal dominant form; here, the possibility of dominant transmission with incomplete penetrance cannot always be excluded.

FOCAL DYSTONIAS In addition to the generalized dystonias noted above, there is a group of focal or segmental dystonias which appear sporadically in adult life. Their clearly involuntary nature, and lack of susceptibility to willed control by the patient, distinguish them from the common tics, habit spasms, and mannerisms described in Chap. 15. They have often been erroneously interpreted as manifestations of hysteria. If the muscle contraction is frequent and prolonged, aching pain accompanies it—for which the spasm may mistakenly be blamed.

The most frequent and familiar type of focal dystonia is *spasmodic torticollis*. This is a disorder of adults that afflicts women somewhat more frequently than men. It consists of an involuntary turning of the head to one side—intermittent at first, then gradually worsening to the point of being more or less continuous. In some cases, torticollis is the first manifestation of a generalized dystonia, but more usually it remains focal and segmental.

Another frequent focal dystonia of adults is exemplified by *writer's cramp*, in which the dystonic postures and movements occur only during the performance of specific acts, to the extent that carrying out the act in the usual way, such as writing with a pen or pencil, becomes impossible, while other motor activities using the same musculature are unimpaired. An analogous disorder sometimes afflicts musicians.

The combination of blepharospasm and oromandibular dystonia—*cranial dystonia*—is sometimes referred to as Meige's syndrome. When the throat and respiratory muscles are involved, this interferes with speech production, resulting in spastic dysarthria. The muscles of the neck are variably affected. It should be recalled that similar dystonic states (facial-cervical and more extreme dyskinesias) can result from the use of phenothiazine and similar drugs. This sometimes persists after discontinuation of the medication as *tardive dyskinesia*—a troublesome condition that may resist all forms of treatment.

Differential diagnosis Hepatolenticular degeneration (Wilson's disease) should be seriously considered in any case presenting these motor symtoms and appropriate measures should be undertaken for its investigation (see Chap. 311). The progressive course, and possibly the family history, differentiate the degenerative group from the "symptomatic" dystonias resulting from infections or metabolic disorders occurring at birth or later. Hallervorden-Spatz disease, however, cannot be distinguished on clinical grounds alone. Rare instances of GM_1 gangliosidosis or other lipid storage diseases may begin in adult life with a dystonic syndrome, and drug-induced (tardive) dyskinesia must be considered in all cases of focal or generalized dystonia in adults, especially if they have or have had a psychiatric illness.

Treatment This is extremely difficult and often unsatisfactory. In the generalized dystonias, pharmacotherapy should certainly be attempted and, in most patients, needs to be individualized. Marsden and Fahn, whose experience with this disorder is extensive, suggest beginning with an anticholinergic agent such as trihexyphenidyl or ethopropazine and very gradually increasing the dosage until either benefit ensues or intolerable side effects appear. They found that the response in children (who may be able to take as much as 80 mg per day of trihexyphenidyl) was better than in adults, who tolerated the high doses less well, generally because of mental disturbances. In their experience, the next best group of drugs for ameliorating dystonic spasms are the benzodiazepines (such as diazepam) which likewise are used in high dosage after a very gradual introduction and increase (up to 80 mg of diazepam daily). Again, children are more tolerant of the side effects (mainly drowsiness). A combination of anticholinergics and benzodiazepines may work out best. Other drugs—both dopaminergic agonists and antagonists—have been used, occasionally with success.

Stereotaxic surgical operations have been used in the past to treat generalized dystonias, with insufficient benefit to counterbalance the risks. Cervical cord stimulation, a less hazardous procedure, has helped some patients; referral to a neurosurgeon with experience in the technique should be considered when medical treatment has failed.

The symptoms of the focal dystonias, if not severe, may be more acceptable to the patient than prolonged trials with various drugs or surgical intervention. Biofeedback techniques are sometimes helpful. Denervative surgical procedures may at times be beneficial if only a very restricted group of muscles is involved (as in torticollis). Blepharospasm has recently been successfully treated temporarily with local injection of botulinum toxin into the orbicularis oculi muscles. Growdon suggests that neuroleptics (dopamine-antagonists) such as haloperidol or perphenazine may be useful in the treatment of focal dystonias. Here again, the program of management must be adapted to the individual patient's needs.

FAMILIAL TREMOR One of the commonest hereditary disorders of the human nervous system is that which gives rise to a fast-frequency (6 to 8 per second) action tremor. This may appear at any age but more often during adolescence and adult years; once started, it lasts throughout life. The heredity is dominant. Probably all cases are not the same, for some patients have tremors of slower frequency, looking more like those of Parkinson's disease, but lacking the slowness of movement, rigidity, and flexed postures of that disorder. In patients of advanced age it is called *senile tremor*. Consumption of alcohol suppresses the fast-frequency forms, as does a beta-adrenergic blocking agent (propranolol) in doses of 20 to 40 mg three times daily. The slightly slower rhythmic action tremors with frequencies of approximately 6 per second do not consistently respond to propranolol or alcohol. Primidone 50 mg at bedtime has recently been found to be effective and has been advocated for use as initial therapy. If there is no response after 1 week the dose should be increased gradually up to 250 mg at bedtime. Usually the tremor is the only abnormality, but in a few patients a cerebellar ataxia or an extrapyramidal syndrome may appear years later. The pathologic basis is unknown.

GILLES DE LA TOURETTE SYDROME This condition, of unknown cause and uncertain pathology, presents with multiple tics, associated with snorting, sniffing, and involuntary vocalizations. It begins in childhood, usually as isolated tics, which are at first difficult to distinguish from habit spasms. Progression occurs over years, and other behavioral findings appear; compulsive touching of others, repeating of words or phrases, and explosive utterance of obscenities (coprolalia). Careful attention to other members of the family has given evidence that the disease is hereditary, with the pattern of transmission uncertain, although autosomal recessive inheritance appears likely in some pedigrees.

The course of the illness is unpredictable. In some cases associated mild neurologic abnormalities are found with hyperactivity, disorders of attention, and abnormal psychologic tests. Dementia does not occur. In some patients the condition abates, in others it progresses, leading to serious disability. Treatment is only partially satisfactory. Haloperidol has received the most clinical attention, but should be used only in severe cases, and in the smallest effective dosage: 0.25 to 0.5 mg daily. Clonidine has proved effective in some cases.

SYNDROMES OF SLOWLY DEVELOPING ATAXIA

These conditions are distinguished clinically by progressive unsteadiness in standing and walking, along with impaired coordination of the limbs. Pathologically, they are characterized by degeneration of the cerebellum and/or its related fiber systems, and thus constitute classic examples of the system diseases. Although sporadic instances occur, hereditary transmission is an outstanding feature in most cases; as a result, this group of disorders is often referred to as the *hereditary ataxias*. Their subdivision into more or less separate entities is largely arbitrary, with pathologic changes of varying distribution underlying clinically indistinguishable symptom complexes. As yet, not enough is known about the underlying basis for the pathophysiologic alterations for a more satisfactory classification to be established.

Attempts to establish a classification on a genetic basis, on the presumption that a defective gene expressed as a progressive ataxia would produce a distinctive clinicopathologic picture have not been successful. Instead, the phenotypic expression of the genetic abnormality commonly varies widely among affected members of an individual family. Because of these difficulties, the most that a clinician can do when confronted with a case is to exclude infective, toxic, metabolic, or neoplastic diseases for which there might be effective treatment, to search for evidence of genetic factors, and to assess the state of the patient as precisely as possible. There are now indications that some of the hereditary ataxic disorders may be associated with an identifiable biochemical abnormality though at present it is not possible to make use of this information in a way that would correct the abnormality and benefit the individual patient.

Nevertheless, if one takes a broad view of the whole group of hereditary ataxias, it turns out that there are certain clinicopathologic groupings that allow a very simplified descriptive classification. According to this principle, three main categories may be emphasized: (1) *cerebellar cortical degeneration,* (2) *olivopontocerebellar atrophy,* and (3) *spinocerebellar degenerations,* including *Friedreich's ataxia*.

CEREBELLAR CORTICAL DEGENERATION In this disorder, the principal neuropathologic feature is loss of neurons (mainly of Purkinje cells) in the cerebellar cortex. Cases of this kind characteristically occur in late adult life. Although the condition can occur sporadically, in the majority it is inherited as an autosomal dominant trait.

Pathology The loss of Purkinje cells tends to be most severe in the superior vermis and adjacent parts of the cerebellar cortex, but can be more extensive. The granule neurons are less affected. In longstanding cases, there is an associated atrophy of neurons in the olivary nuclei of the medulla, apparently representing a transsynaptic retrograde degeneration resulting from the loss of Purkinje cells, to which the olivocerebellar fibers project. In advanced cases atrophy of the cerebellar cortex can be readily demonstrated by CT scanning. In the purest forms of this disorder, as exemplified by the cases of late onset, slow progression, and dominant inheritance, other neuronal systems remain relatively intact.

Clinical manifestations Incoordination first appears in the legs, resulting in abnormal stance and an unsteadiness of gait of a wavering, lurching character typical of cerebellar ataxia (see Chap. 16). This gait disturbance is a consequence of degenerative changes in the superior vermis of the cerebellum and adjacent parts of the cerebellar cortex. With more extensive cerebellar involvement, a disturbance in articulation and rhythm of speech occurs and the arms become ataxic. There may be nystagmus. The illness progresses gradually often extending over two or three decades, without appreciably curtailing the life span. Dementia tends not to be a feature of this circumscribed cerebellar atrophy of late life. However, cerebellar cortical degeneration with very similar features may occur as a component in many of the ataxic disorders.

In addition to this slowly evolving, relatively circumscribed form of cerebellar cortical degeneration, there is a subacutely developing diffuse cerebellar cortical degeneration that affects all parts of the cerebellar cortex indiscriminately, often in association with some inflammatory changes. This disorder occurs in the presence of malignant neoplastic diseases of various kinds and is referred to as *carcinomatous cerebellar degeneration* (see Chap. 304). It is now apparent that this is one of a number of interrelated neurologic degenerative syndromes that occur on the background of malignant disease but do not result from any direct effect of the neoplasm on the nervous system such as invasion or metastasis. These so-called paraneoplastic disorders are etiologically unclarified; an immunologic or viral attack on neural structures has been postulated, but never proven. Paraneoplastic cerebellar degeneration produces a striking clinicopathologic syndrome that tends to stand out as a particular entity (see Chap. 304).

OLIVOPONTOCEREBELLAR ATROPHY (OPCA) Grouped under this category are a number of similar disorders characterized by a combination of cerebellar cortical degeneration, atrophy of the inferior olivary nuclei secondary to this, and degeneration and disappearance of the neurons of the pontine nuclei and their fiber projections in the basis pontis and middle cerebellar peduncles. Konigsmark and Weiner distinguished five varieties on the basis of differences in the form of hereditary transmission and in the extent of other abnormalities both within and outside of the nervous system. Most instances of OPCA can now be considered to represent various forms of multiple system degeneration in which admixtures of parkinsonism, dementia, spasticity, choreoathetosis, retinal degeneration, myelopathy, and peripheral neuropathy may be encountered, sometimes obscuring the ataxic component. For present-day views of the classification of OPCA and the features of the various forms of disease brought under this heading, the monograph edited by Duvoisin and Plaitakis may be usefully consulted. The introduction of the new techniques of imaging—CT and MRI—now make it possible to visualize clearly the pontocerebellar lesions and some of the other atrophic changes in the central nervous system.

Autosomal dominant inheritance characterizes an important group of cases, and several families—most notably the Schut family, on which information extending over five generations has been obtained, and the families of Portuguese ancestry, mainly from the Azores, who manifest the various syndromes that have been brought together under the heading of Joseph's disease—have been extensively studied. These families illustrate with striking clarity the varied phenotypic expression of what seems to be a particular genetic abnormality.

Recessively transmitted OPCA has on the whole been less distinctly established than the dominant (or sporadic) forms, but of particular interest is a group of families with an autosomal recessive disorder and late-adult onset of neurologic symptoms, in whom the disease is characterized by multiple system degeneration, including a prominent OPCA component, and in which deficiency of glutamic acid dehydrogenase (GDH) has been demonstrated in leukocytes and cultured fibroblasts from affected family members (Plaitakis, in Duvoisin and Plaitakis monograph). Glutamate, among its other functions, acts as an excitatory neurotransmitter and is involved in the excitatory input to the Purkinje cells from the granule cells of the cerebellar cortex. In excess, this transmitter has neurotoxic effects, which might be the basis of the Purkinje cell degeneration that is so prominent in OPCA. These observations, and other biochemical leads that have opened up in connection with some of the dominant forms of OPCA, suggest a promising field of research that may give new etiologic and pathophysiologic insights into a wide group of neuronal degenerative diseases and may ultimately suggest avenues for therapeutic approach.

Pathology OPCA and the disorders related to it exemplify clearly the phenomenon of selective premature neuronal death, and of affection of particular, vulnerable neuronal systems with sparing of others. The distribution of neuronal lesions that characterizes OPCA as distinct from other neuronal system degenerations has already been indicated. The neuronal changes are in no way distinctive or specific in OPCA. Rather, it is the particular location of the neuronal loss that determines the clinicopathologic picture. Still not fully clarified in this group of disorders is what determines the dementia that so often accompanies them. It has been generally assumed that abnormalities occur in the cerebral cortex, but examination of the cortex in typical cases discloses insufficient pathology to account for the cognitive and behavioral alterations. On the other hand, the lesions of the cerebellum and related systems provide a reasonable explanation for the incoordination (ataxia) that is observed; the lesions in the basal ganglia and substantia nigra (equivalent to striatonigral degeneration) underlie the features of parkinsonism and of other postural and movement disorders that are so frequently seen as manifestations of OPCA; and involvement of the peripheral motor neurons, similar to what occurs in the motor neuron disease group to be discussed later, produces the severe muscular weakness and atrophy that may be encountered. The disturbances of ocular motility that typify some cases still are in need of further anatomic elucidation.

Clinical manifestations There is great clinical variation among cases of OPCA. Some present a picture of a relatively pure cerebellar ataxia indistinguishable from that seen in cases with atrophy of the cerebellar cortex (and secondarily of the inferior olivary nuclei) alone. Others are characterized by parkinsonian features. Superimposed is an evolving dementia. For accounts of these varied forms of clinical expression, general neurologic reference works and specialized monographs (such as that edited by Duvoisin and Plaitakis) should be consulted.

SPINOCEREBELLAR DEGENERATIONS (FRIEDREICH'S ATAXIA) This group of ataxic disorders is characterized by degeneration of long ascending and descending fiber systems in the spinal cord, including the spinocerebellar tracts, and concomitant degeneration of peripheral axons and myelin sheaths in the form of chronic peripheral neuronopathy.

The classic form of hereditary ataxia, first clearly depicted by Nikolaus Friedreich of Heidelberg in 1863, constitutes a relatively distinct symptom complex which generally runs true to form, although it overlaps other heredodegenerative syndromes, particularly other types of spinocerebellar atrophy. In some families, the disorder occurs with dominant inheritance; usually it is a recessive trait.

Pathology The principal changes are cell loss in the dorsal root ganglia and secondary degeneration in the posterior columns and spinocerebellar tracts of the cord and in the peripheral nerves. Degeneration is also evident in the corticospinal tracts in most cases. The cerebellum is variably affected. In addition to these neuropathologic changes there is in some cases a peculiar form of myocardial degeneration resulting in fiber loss and fibrosis. There are no other associated visceral lesions.

Clinical manifestations As with other progressive ataxias, the disorder first appears in the legs, affecting the individual during late childhood. The patient, previously healthy, begins to stagger and lurch in walking and is unsteady on standing. Clumsiness and cerebellar tremor of the hands and arms appear later along with dysarthria and abnormal rhythm (scanning) of speech. These symptoms result from changes in the dorsal root ganglia, the spinocerebellar tracts, and cerebellum; it is not easy to ascertain the relative contribution of lesions in each structure to the ataxia. The limbs, in addition to being ataxic, generally show considerable weakness. Examination usually discloses nystagmus and skeletal deformities: kyphoscoliosis, the basis of which is not certain, and a peculiar foreshortening of the feet (pes cavus) with cocking of the toes, best ascribed to atrophy and contractures of the musculature of the feet at a time when the bones of the feet are malleable. Typically, there is the unusual combination of total absence of tendon reflexes with extensor plantar reflexes (Babinski sign). This results from the presence of degeneration of the corticospinal tracts together with the involvement of peripheral sensory neurons that relay afferent signals from muscle spindles. Impairment of position and vibration sense in the extremities is prominent and, in some patients, sensation of pain, temperature, and light touch is diminished in a distal and roughly symmetric distribution consistent with an axononeuropathy affecting small nerve fibers. Mentation is usually preserved, though a few of the patients have been of low intelligence or have become demented late in the course of the disease. Survival beyond early adult life is rare, with death frequently the result of associated cardiomyopathy.

Occasionally very mild or fragmentary forms of the disorder (such as pes cavus and absent or hyperactive tendon reflexes) may be encountered with little if any disability or progression. Such abnormalities are most likely to be seen in other members of the family of a patient afflicted with the fully developed form of the disease. A related syndrome, the Roussy-Lévy syndrome, shows similarities to Friedreich's ataxia and to peroneal muscular atrophy. Mild ataxia, pes cavus, absent ankle and knee tendon jerks, and atrophy of lower leg muscles occur. In some well-documented cases the peripheral nerves show hypertrophy due to proliferation of Schwann cells (see Chap. 355). Chronic familial polyneuropathies are particularly difficult to distinguish since they also give rise to sensory ataxia, but signs of pyramidal tract disease are absent (see Chap. 355). Hereditary forms of cerebellar ataxia with corticospinal signs (hyperactive tendon reflexes) and sensory disturbances are also known to occur in the adolescent or adult. Familial spastic paraplegia with or without optic atrophy (Behr's syndrome) is another closely related disease. In the absence of a family history, and with atypical clinical findings, further diagnostic studies to exclude congenital malformation, spinal cord compression, foramen magnum tumor, and multiple sclerosis will be necessary.

No treatment is of proven value. Earlier reports of disturbed pyruvate metabolism have not been confirmed.

DIFFERENTIAL DIAGNOSIS OF THE ATAXIAS The slow but relentless progression in the absence of abnormalities in other parts of the nervous system and in the CSF distinguishes the hereditary group from other diseases and other forms of cerebellar ataxia such as may occur with hereditary metabolic diseases, or with neoplastic, infectious, or demyelinative disease, or with drug intoxications (e.g., phenytoin) or with hyperpyrexia. The degenerative disorders under discussion tend to develop slowly over many years in a setting of otherwise good general health, and in the absence of other neurologic symptoms and signs; this, together with the other clinical differences, distinguishes them from such hereditary metabolic diseases as juvenile Gaucher's disease, juvenile Niemann-Pick disease, and juvenile hexosaminidase deficiency and from alcoholic cerebellar ataxia or nutritional deficiency disease, with or without Wernicke-Korsakoff syndrome. Alcoholic cerebellar degeneration usually develops over a few days to weeks, and then may remain more or less unchanged for the remainder of the patient's life (Chap. 349).

In the cases associated with carcinoma, the tempo of evolution of the process is relatively rapid, with severe disability coming on within a period of months. Vertigo, diplopia, and nausea may be prominent. In an occasional patient, the neurologic symptoms have appeared before there was any obvious evidence of carcinoma. Opsoclonus (rapid side-to-side jerking of the eyes) and oscillopsia (movement back and forth of objects seen) may be conjoined. In contrast to the consistently normal CSF findings in the forms of cerebellar degeneration noted above, the CSF in paraneoplastic degeneration may show increased lymphocytes and protein.

TREATMENT No specific treatment is available for any of the progressive ataxias, although encouragement to remain active is beneficial to health in general. Gait training is of relatively little value in enabling patients to compensate for their disability. In cases where parkinsonian features are prominent, antiparkinsonian medications should be tried (see above), but the response in the group of multiple system degenerations is generally unsatisfactory. Trauner has reported that baclofen in high dosage may help control involuntary movements in some cases of OPCA, but the ataxia is not benefited. Initial reports of benefit with thyrotropin-releasing hormone have not been confirmed.

IDIOPATHIC AUTONOMIC FAILURE (IDIOPATHIC ORTHOSTATIC HYPOTENSION, SHY-DRAGER SYNDROME)

Abnormalities of central autonomic nervous system functions manifest principally by failure to maintain blood pressure and by urinary incontinence are now recognized to be caused in some cases by a progressive degenerative disorder of the CNS that affects several systems; in some patients the peripheral nervous system is also involved (postganglionic sympathetic neurons). Bradbury and Eggleston in 1925 called attention to the combination of postural hypotension, incontinence, impotence, and abnormality of sweating (anhidrosis). Symptoms of central neurologic origin develop later in many of these patients consisting predominantly of extrapyramidal or cerebellar dysfunction.

PATHOGENESIS AND PATHOLOGY The cause of the disorder is unknown. In 1960 Shy and Drager described neuropathologic changes in the brainstem and basal ganglia, and subsequently others showed a prominent loss of neurons in central regions of the autonomic nervous system, affecting in particular the cells of the intermediolateral column of the thoracic spinal cord. Abnormalities have also been found in peripheral autonomic ganglia (cell loss). In the brainstem and basal ganglia there is widespread symmetric neuronal degeneration affecting the caudate nucleus, substantia nigra, locus coeruleus, olivary nuclei, dorsal vagal nuclei, and in some cases affecting the cerebellum. Cell loss is accompanied by gliosis; Lewy bodies typical of Parkinson's disease are present in some cases. For these reasons many neurologists consider the Shy-Drager syndrome to be a unique form of multisystem degeneration resembling but distinct from either Parkinson's disease or OPCA.

Clinical manifestations The onset is insidious, usually in the sixth or seventh decade. Men are more frequently affected than women. Disturbances of urinary bladder function, including hesitancy and incontinence, postural dizziness and syncope, impotence, and decreased sweating are the presenting manifestations. Later symptoms of extrapyramidal dysfunction resembling parkinsonism or cerebellar findings may emerge. The condition becomes severely disabling over the course of 5 to 7 years in most patients. The hallmark of the condition is postural hypotension, defined as a fall in blood pressure greater than 30/20 mmHg on standing upright from a supine position (see Chap. 12). Despite this fall in blood pressure there is usually a total failure of compensatory tachycardia, the pulse rate remaining unchanged. Autonomic signs of pupillary asymmetry, partial Horner's syndrome, or partial parasympathetic denervation occur in some patients. Anhidrosis is common and can be demonstrated by placing the individual in a warm room after application of a starch-iodine mixture to the skin. The parkinsonian manifestations may be identical to those of idiopathic parkinsonism, although in many patients rigidity and bradykinesia are more prominent than tremor. Cerebellar gait ataxia and mild limb ataxia may be evident. Other findings include laryngeal paralysis and sleep apnea.

Treatment The treatment is symptomatic. The postural hypotension is usually the most disabling initial symptom. Antigravity stockings to minimize pooling of venous blood in the legs are recommended. Pharmacologic agents are given to expand blood volume and to enhance vascular responsivity. Increased NaCl intake combined with fludrohydrocortisone 0.05 to 0.2 mg twice daily is usually beneficial (see Chap. 12). In severe cases, adrenergic drugs such as ephedrine, levodopa, or amphetamine may improve the disability. The parkinsonism symptoms often respond initially to Sinemet or bromocriptine, but later in the course most patients become refractory to these agents. Centrally acting alpha agonists (e.g., yohimbine or clonidine) may also be beneficial.

SYNDROMES OF MUSCULAR WEAKNESS AND WASTING WITHOUT SENSORY CHANGES: MOTOR NEURON DISEASE

AMYOTROPHIC LATERAL SCLEROSIS (ALS) ALS is the most frequently encountered form of progressive motor neuron disease, and it presents a clinical syndrome that is generally familiar to physicians who see patients with neurologic diseases. It is characteristically a disorder of late middle age. Most patients are older than 50 when they become aware of symptoms. The disease rarely develops before the third decade, and patients whose symptoms begin in the late teenage years often seem to have an inherited variant of the disorder. Men are more frequently affected than women. Because of its restriction to motor neurons of the central nervous system, ALS represents another prime example of a neuronal system disease. It occurs sporadically in most instances. Familial occurrence, with transmission as an autosomal dominant trait, is observed in about 10 percent of cases and differs in some clinical and pathologic aspects (Table 350-2).

Pathology The disease is characterized by progressive loss of motor neurons, both in the cerebral cortex and in the anterior horns of the spinal cord, together with their homologues in some motor nuclei of the brainstem. It typically affects both upper and lower motor neurons, although variants may predominantly involve only particular subsets of motor neurons, particularly early in the course of the illness. Thus, in bulbar palsy and spinal muscular atrophy (or progressive muscular atrophy) the lower motor neurons of brainstem and spinal cord, respectively, are most severely involved while pseudobulbar palsy and primary lateral sclerosis affect upper motor neurons innervating the brainstem and spinal cord. The loss of motor neurons is not accompanied by any distinctive or unique cytopathologic features. The affected cells undergo shrinkage, often with some excessive accumulation of the pigmented lipid (lipofuscin) that normally develops in these cells with advancing age, and they eventually disappear. Focal enlargement of proximal motor axons is frequently seen; ultrastructurally, these "spheroids" are composed of accumulations of neurofilaments. Beyond some astroglial proliferation, which is the inevitable accompaniment of all disintegrative processes in the central nervous system, the interstitial and supportive tissues and the macrophage system remain largely inactive, and there is no inflammation. The death of the peripheral motor neurons in the brainstem and spinal cord leads to denervation and consequent atrophy of the corresponding muscle fibers. Histochemical and electrophysiologic evidence indicate that in the early phases of the illness denervated muscle can be reinnervated by sprouting of nearby distal motor nerve terminals, although reinnervation in this disease is considerably less extensive than in most other disorders affecting motor neurons (e.g., poliomyelitis, peripheral neuropathy). As denervation progresses, there is shrinkage of the musculature and a fiber atrophy that is readily recognized in muscle biopsies. It is this muscular atrophy that is designated by the term *amyotrophy,* which appears in the common name for the disease. The loss of motor neurons in the cortex results in disappearance of the long axons and their myelin sheaths that make up the corticospinal tracts, which travel via the internal capsule and extend through the brainstem, including the pyramids of the medulla oblongata, to the lateral (and a portion of the anterior) white matter columns of the spinal cord. The loss of fibers in the lateral columns, together with the fibrillary gliosis which imparts a particular firmness (sclerosis) to the affected tissues, makes up the lateral sclerosis component of the disease. The fact that the nerve fiber loss is more extensive in the distal parts of the affected tracts in the lower spinal cord rather than the more proximal parts, such as the internal capsule, suggests that the affected neurons first undergo disintegration at their distal terminals and the disease process proceeds in a centripetal direction until ultimately the parent cell body dies, a phenomenon referred to as "dying back." The disease clearly affects the large pyramidal neurons (Betz cells) of the motor cortex in the precentral gyrus, but in some cases the extent of degeneration in the long projection pathways provides evidence that many other neurons involved in voluntary movement, both in the cortex and in subcortical nuclei, are also affected.

A remarkable feature of the disease is the selectivity of neuronal cell death. The entire sensory apparatus, the regulatory mechanisms for the control and coordination of movement, and the components of the brain that are needed for intellect and thinking, remain intact. There is also some consistent selectivity in motor system involvement. The motor neurons required for ocular motility remain unaffected as do the parasympathetic neurons in the sacral spinal cord (the nucleus of Onufrowicz, or Onuf) which innervate the sphincters of the bowel and bladder.

Clinical manifestations The first evidence of the disease is manifest as insidiously developing asymmetric weakness, usually first apparent in one of the limbs. Fatigue and easy cramping of affected muscles can be prominent. The weakness is accompanied by visible wasting and atrophy of the muscles involved; particularly in the early stages of the disease, affected muscles may display focal twitchings—fasciculations—when not concealed by overlying adipose tissue. Virtually any muscle group may be the first to show signs of the disease, but as time passes, more and more muscles become involved until ultimately the disorder takes on a symmetric distribution in all regions, including the muscles of chewing, swallowing, and movements of the face and tongue. Early involvement of the muscles of respiration may lead to death before the disease is far advanced elsewhere; otherwise the disorder generally is terminated by pulmonary infection secondary to the profound generalized weakness.

The corticospinal component of the disease becomes apparent in the form of hyperactivity of the muscle-stretch reflexes (tendon jerks) and, often, spastic resistance to passive movements of the affected limbs. With corticospinal involvement the plantar reflex will be upgoing (the Babinski sign) until—as often occurs—lower motor neuron dysfunction in the legs advances sufficiently that extensor movement of the great toes is impossible. The disease process in the corticobulbar projections innervating the brainstem results in dysarthria and exaggeration of the motor expressions of emotion leading to involuntary weeping or laughter (so-called pseudobulbar affect), or strange admixtures of both. Ocular motility is spared, even when other brainstem functions are greatly impaired. Throughout the evolution of the disease, awareness and intellectual abilities typically remain intact. Dementia is not usually a component of ALS; when it occurs, it is due to the superimposition of another disease process.

The course is relentlessly progressive and leads ultimately to

TABLE 350-2 Categories of degenerative motor neuron diseases

I Amyotrophic lateral sclerosis
- *A* Spinal muscular atrophy
- *B* Bulbar palsy
- *C* Primary lateral sclerosis
- *D* Pseudobulbar palsy

II Heritable motor neuron diseases
- *A* Autosomal recessive spinal muscular atrophy (SMA)
  - *1* Type I: Werdnig-Hoffmann, acute
  - *2* Type II: Werdnig-Hoffmann, chronic
  - *3* Type III: Kugelberg-Welander
  - *4* Type IV: Adult onset
- *B* Familial amyotrophic lateral sclerosis
- *C* Familial ALS with dementia or Parkinson's disease (Guam)
- *D* Other
  - *1* Arthrogryposis multiplex congenita
  - *2* Progressive juvenile bulbar palsy (Fazio-Londe)
  - *3* Neuroaxonal dystrophy

III Associated with other degenerative disorders
- *1* Olivopontocerebellar atrophies
- *2* Peroneal muscular atrophy

death, but the total duration of the illness is variable. In recent studies approximately 50 percent of patients can be expected to die within 3 to 5 years from the onset of the disease; some may live considerably longer. Very rarely, what seems to be ALS may become stabilized, or even regress to the point of recovery.

Differential diagnosis Because the underlying process in ALS is currently untreatable, it is imperative that potentially remediable causes of motor neuron dysfunction be excluded (see Table 350-3), particularly in atypical cases. Compression of the cervical cord or cervicomedullary junction from tumors in the cervical region or at the foramen magnum, or from cervical spondylosis with osteophytes projecting into the vertebral canal, can at times give rise to weakness, wasting, and fasciculations in the upper limbs and spasticity in the legs, thus closely resembling ALS. The absence of cranial nerve involvement may be helpful in differentiation, although some compressive lesions in the foramen magnum may implicate the twelfth cranial (hypoglossal) nerve, with resulting affection of the tongue. Absence of pain or of sensory changes, normal function of bowels and bladder, normal roentgenographic studies of the spine, and absence of changes in the composition or dynamics of the cerebrospinal fluid are all points in favor of ALS against spinal cord compression. Where doubt exists, CT scans and contrast myelography should be performed in order to visualize the cervical spinal cord.

Other treatable disorders that occasionally can mimic ALS are chronic lead poisoning and thyrotoxicosis. These may be suggested by the patient's social or occupational history or by unusual clinical features. When the family history is positive, inherited enzyme disorders such as hexosaminidase A or α-glucosidase deficiency must be excluded (see Chap. 349). These can readily be identified by appropriate laboratory tests. Benign fasciculations are occasionally a source of concern because on inspection they resemble the fascicular twitchings that accompany motor neuron degeneration. The absence of weakness or atrophy, and of denervation phenomena on electrophysiologic examination, excludes ALS or other serious neurologic disease. Poliomyelitis is now recognized to result in a delayed progressive deterioration of motor neurons which presents clinically with progressive weakness, atrophy, and fasciculations. Its cause is unknown but is thought to reflect prior sublethal injury to motor neurons by the poliovirus.

Treatment There is no treatment that has influence on the underlying pathologic process in any form of motor neuron disease. Modern rehabilitative measures, including mechanical aids of various kinds, can do much in helping patients to overcome the effects of their disabilities and often, with respiratory support, to survive longer than would otherwise have been the case. Recent observations (reviewed by Tandan and Bradley) suggest that intravenous (or intrathecal) infusions of thyrotropin-releasing hormone (TRH) result in transitory improvement of motor functions in some patients with ALS, for reasons that are not well understood. Whether TRH will have any long-term effect on the course of the disease is still unknown.

SPINAL MUSCULAR ATROPHY (SMA) In the varieties of motor neuron disease that are grouped under this heading, the peripheral motor neurons are affected without evidence of involvement of the corticospinal motor system (Table 350-2). In comparison with ALS, SMA in general occurs in a younger age group, runs a slower, more protracted course (except in the infantile form), and tends to be hereditary (usually autosomal recessive) rather than sporadic. The SMA group undoubtedly includes several distinct disease processes that differ from one another genetically and phenotypically.

Infantile SMA (Werdnig-Hoffmann disease) This rapidly fatal disorder is characterized by autosomal recessive transmission. Not infrequently, this severe form of infantile SMA (sometimes also referred to as SMA type I) is apparent even before birth, as indicated by decreased fetal movements in comparison with what normally would be expected. The afflicted infants are weak and floppy (hypotonic), though alert, and muscle-stretch reflexes are absent. Weakness progresses relatively rapidly, and death ensues generally within the first year of life; rarely, the child survives to 3 years of age.

Neuropathologically, Werdnig-Hoffmann disease is characterized by extensive loss of the large motor neurons. Sections of the muscles show extreme degrees of denervation atrophy. During life, the diagnosis is made by electrophysiologic studies and by muscle biopsy, which shows the characteristic denervational pattern rather than an intrinsic myopathy or inflammatory disease of muscle. There is no effective treatment, but a family that has had an affected infant may be helped by genetic counseling.

There is another form of infantile muscular atrophy, also characterized by autosomal recessive inheritance, which appears to be distinct from Werdnig-Hoffmann disease in that the evolution is considerably slower, with survival into preadolescence or even into adult life. This disorder, which has been called *chronic childhood SMA*, or SMA type II, is considerably rarer than Werdnig-Hoffmann disease.

These motor neuron diseases can be distinguished from benign congenital hypotonia, which is nonprogressive form of myopathy, by electrophysiologic assessment and by muscle biopsy.

Juvenile SMA (Wohlfart-Kugelberg-Welander disease) This disorder, also referred to as SMA type III, manifests itself during late childhood and runs a slow, indolent course. Typically the muscles of the trunk and the proximal parts of the limb are earliest and most severely involved—a picture that closely resembles that of progressive muscular dystrophy, even to the presence of pseudohypertrophy of

TABLE 350-3 Etiology and investigation of secondary motor neuron disorders

Diagnostic categories	Investigations
I Structural lesions	
A Parasagittal or foramen magnum tumors	MRI/CT scan—head, spine including foramen magnum
B Cervical spondylosis	
C Chiari malformation or syrinx	MRI/CT scan or myelogram
D Spinal cord arteriovenous malformation	
II Infections	
A Bacterial—tetanus	CSF exam
B Viral—poliomyelitis, herpes zoster	Antibody titers
III Intoxications, physical agents	
A Toxins—lead, aluminum, other metals	24-h urine for lead, mercury arsenic, thallium, aluminum
B Drugs—strychnine, phenytoin, dapsone	
C Electric shock	
D X-irradiation	Serum lead and aluminum
IV Immunologic mechanisms	
A Plasma cell dyscrasias	Complete blood count, sedimentation rate
B Autoimmune polyradiculoneuropathy	Immunoprotein electrophoresis, Antinuclear antibody (ANA), cryoglobulins (+/−) bone marrow biopsy
V Paraneoplastic	
A Paracarcinomatous	
B Paralymphomatous; Hodgkin's	
VI Metabolic	
A Hypoglycemia	Fasting blood sugar (FBS)
B Hyperparathyroidism	Routine chemistries including calcium, magnesium, phosphate
C Hyperthroidism	Thyroid functions
D Vitamin B_{12}, Vitamin E deficiency	Vitamin B_{12}, folate, vitamin E levels
E Malabsorption	Stool fat (72-h; spot), carotene, prothrombin time (PT)
VII Hereditary biochemical disorders	
A Hexosaminidase A deficiency	Lysosomal enzyme screen
B α-Glucosidase deficiency (Pompe's)	
C Hyperlipidemia	Lipid electrophoresis
D Hyperglycinuria	Urine and serum amino acids
E Methylcrotonylglycinuria	CSF amino acids

the calf muscles in some cases. Electrophysiologic and biopsy evidence of denervation in the affected muscles serves to distinguish this disease from any of the myopathic syndromes.

Other genetically determined varieties of SMA In individual families, other syndromes characterized by SMA in varying patterns have been described. An infantile variety involving mainly the musculature innervated by the brainstem is referred to as the *Fazio-Londe syndrome*. In some juvenile cases, the distribution is distal, rather than proximal, as in the Wohlfart-Kugelberg-Welander variety. In addition, there is a slowly evolving adult form of SMA, sometimes called SMA type IV (Table 350-2). Depending upon the family, autosomal dominant, autosomal recessive, or X-linked recessive patterns of heredity may be discerned.

A component of SMA may also be found in some of the multiple system degenerations that have already been referred to, e.g., in Joseph's disease and in some of the syndromes characterized by olivopontocerebellar degeneration. Some of the recognized familial metabolic disorders also present a striking picture of progressive symmetric muscular weakness and atrophy, for instance, adult hexosaminidase A deficiency (the enzymopathy that results in Tay-Sachs disease in infancy) and adrenomyeloneuropathy. For details and more extensive discussions of these disorders, specialized monographs (such as that edited by Rowland), reviews (Tandan and Bradley), and general reference works on neurology (Adams and Victor) should be consulted.

Primary lateral sclerosis (PLS) It might be thought that this is a variant of ALS in which the amyotrophic component is lacking, but the few cases of this disorder that have been described have been encountered in remarkably pure form. It occurs as a sporadic disease of late life, affecting the same age group that is prone to develop ALS. The course may be similar to that of ALS with approximately 3 years from onset to death. Clinically, the illness is characterized by progressive spastic weakness of the limbs, preceded or followed by spastic dysarthria and dysphagia, indicative of corticobulbar tract involvement. Fasciculations, amyotrophy, and sensory changes are absent. On neuropathologic examination, there is selective loss of large pyramidal cells in the precentral gyrus and degeneration of the corticospinal and corticobulbar projections; the peripheral motor neurons and other neuronal systems are spared.

It may be necessary to consider PLS in the differential diagnosis of late-life progressive spastic paresis of the limbs, but obviously it is necessary, by appropriate studies of CSF and radiographic investigations, to exclude treatable disorders such as parasagittal intracranial tumors, neoplasms of the spinal cord, cervical spondylosis, or inflammatory diseases.

HEREDITARY SPASTIC PARAPLEGIA This is a very rare disorder which differs from PLS in several respects. Instead of occurring sporadically, it is characterized by genetic transmission—as an autosomal dominant trait in the majority of cases. Several families are on record in which it has appeared in many successive generations. It appears at a younger age, usually in the fourth decade and the course is very slowly progressive, to the extent that patients often live out a full life span. The condition is probably genetically heterogeneous; the group with onset in childhood or adolescence can be distinguished from those in whom the disease does not appear until the age of 35 years or older; as might be expected, there is considerable overlap between these groups. In a few families, a clinically indistinguishable disorder shows a pattern of autosomal recessive inheritance.

Pathology Neuropathologically, there is degeneration of the corticospinal (pyramidal) tracts, which appear almost normal at brainstem levels but become increasingly atrophic as they descend through the spinal cord. In addition, the ascending tracts in the posterior columns and the spinocerebellar tracts show some loss of fibers so that the picture resembles to some degree the findings in Friedreich's ataxia. In fact, some individual cases of what seems to be a fairly pure spastic paraparesis may actually represent an incomplete form of Friedreich's ataxia. In such families spastic paraparesis is the outstanding phenotypic expression of Friedreich's ataxia.

Clinical manifestations As the name implies, the lower limbs are affected earliest and most severely. The major cause of disability is spasticity rather than weakness. There is concomitant exaggeration of the muscle stretch reflexes. Late in the course, urinary urgency and incontinence, and sometimes fecal incontinence, may occur; sexual potency tends to be preserved. In pure forms of the disorder, ataxia and amyotrophy are absent or minimal. In some patients, minor sensory changes (in the form of impaired vibration and position sense) may be observed in the late stages.

It is important in cases of otherwise unexplained progressive spastic paraparesis, despite a negative family history, to examine as many family members as possible. Members of a family with minimal degrees of the disease may be asymptomatic and unaware of its presence, even though they can be shown on examination to have spasticity and hyperreflexia.

SYNDROMES COMBINING MUSCULAR WEAKNESS AND WASTING WITH SENSORY CHANGES

PROGRESSIVE NEURAL MUSCULAR ATROPHY The degenerative disorders characterized by progressive weakness and wasting of skeletal muscles combined with sensory changes are usually chronic diseases of peripheral nerves, often occurring as hereditary conditions. Although clinical and pathologic subvarieties exist, there is no sharp dividing line between them, and they are best considered together under the designation given above, in which the term *neural* emphasizes the peripheral nerve affection. Chronic peripheral neuropathy is an associated disorder in some of the hereditary ataxias and is regularly encountered in the classic form of Friedreich's ataxia. It is also a component of adrenomyeloneuropathy and other leukodystrophies (see Chap. 316). In some cases of progressive neural muscular atrophy other genetically determined CNS diseases may occur such as progressive optic atrophy or pigmentary degeneration of the retina. The peripheral neuropathy begins distally and progresses in a centripetal fashion with the feet and legs first affected, and involvement of the hands and more proximal parts only after a considerable interval, usually several years.

The two most frequent forms of hereditary polyneuropathy, *peroneal muscular atrophy* (Charcot-Marie-Tooth disease) and *hypertrophic interstitial polyneuropathy* (Déjerine-Sottas disease), are described in Chap. 355. Brief reference is also made there to a rare condition known as *Refsum's disease*.

Although no specific treatment is available (except in Refsum's disease, as indicated in Chap. 355), patients whose disease is of slow progression and in whom conditions are otherwise favorable may be greatly helped by measures to ensure a stable walking surface, such as corrective shoes, braces to prevent foot drop, and even orthopedic procedures to stabilize the joints.

SYNDROMES OF PROGRESSIVE VISUAL LOSS Although the preceding discussion of the various hereditary progressive nervous system disorders categorized as degenerative has emphasized the intellectual, motor, and peripheral sensory derangements that result from these, many of these syndromes are accompanied by concomitant loss of the neural structures subserving vision. The hereditary ataxias, including Friedreich's, and hereditary spastic paraplegia stand out as examples. The pathologic changes, viewed broadly, take on two forms: selective degeneration of retinal ganglion cells with secondary optic atrophy, and a more diffuse degenerative process involving all retinal components, with subsequent migration of the melanin-containing cells of the pigment epithelium into the superficial retinal layers, resulting in the picture of *pigmentary degeneration of the retina* (formerly, but erroneously—since there is no inflammation—called retinitis pigmentosa). Occasionally, the peripheral visual system is the major, or only, site of disease resulting in progressive blindness without other neurologic defects. The major entities of this kind, including Leber's *hereditary optic atrophy,* are described in Chap. 352. A more complete review, with references to the pertinent literature, is given by Adams and Victor.

REFERENCES

General

ADAMS RD, VICTOR M: *Principles of Neurology,* 3d ed. New York, McGraw-Hill, 1985
——— et al: Striatonigral degeneration. J Neuropathol Exp Neurol 23:584, 1964
GILMAN S et al: *Disorders of the Cerebellum.* Philadelphia, Davis, 1981
Greenfield's Neuropathology, 4th ed, JH Adams et al (eds). New York, Wiley, 1984
MARSDEN CD, FAHN S (eds): *Movement Disorders.* London, Butterworth, 1982
ROSENBERG RN: *Neurogenetics: Principles and Practice.* New York, Raven, 1986

Alzheimer's disease

BALL MJ: Alzheimer's disease: A challenging enigma. Arch Pathol Lab Med 106:157, 1982
CANDY JM et al: Pathological changes in the nucleus of Meynert in Alzheimer's and Parkinson's diseases. J Neurol Sci 59:277, 1983
GLENNER GG: On causative theories in Alzheimer's disease. Human Pathol 16:433, 1985
HYMAN BT et al: Alzheimer's disease: Cell-specific pathology isolates the hippocampal formation. Science 225:1168, 1984
KATZMAN R: Alzheimer's disease. N Engl J Med 314:964, 1986
PERL DP, BRODY AR: Alzheimer's disease: X-ray spectrometric evidence of aluminum accumulation in neurofibrillary tangle-bearing neurons. Science 208:297, 1980
RASOOL CG, SELKOE DJ: Sharing of specific antigens by degenerating neurons in Pick's disease and Alzheimer's disease. N Engl J Med 312:700, 1985
WHITEHOUSE PJ et al: Alzheimer's disease and senile dementia: Loss of neurons in the basal forebrain. Science 215:1237, 1982

Huntington's disease

FERRANTE RJ et al: Selective sparing of a class of striatal neurons in Huntington's disease. Science 230:561, 1985
HAYDEN MR: *Huntington's Chorea.* Berlin, Springer-Verlag, 1981
MARTIN JB: Huntington's disease: New approaches to an old problem. Neurology 34:1059, 1984
VON SATTEL JP et al: Neuropathological classification of Huntington's disease. J Neuropathol Exp Neurol 44:559, 1985

Parkinson's disease

FAHN S et al (eds): *Recent Advances in Parkinson's Disease.* New York, Raven, 1986
GROWDON JH: Medical treatment of extrapyramidal diseases, in *Update III: Harrison's Principles of Internal Medicine,* KJ Isselbacher et al (eds). New York, McGraw-Hill, 1982
HOEHN MM, YAHR MD: Parkinsonism: Onset, progression and mortality. Neurology 17:427, 1967
LANGSTON JW et al: Chronic parkinsonism in humans due to a product of meperidine-analog synthesis. Science 219:979, 1983
MAYEUX R et al: Reappraisal of temporary levodopa withdrawal ("drug holiday") in Parkinson's disease. N Engl J Med 313:724, 1985
MCGEER PL, MCGEER EG: Amino acid neurotransmitters, in *Basic Neurochemistry,* GJ Siegel et al (eds). Boston, Little, Brown, 1981, pp 233–253
NUTT JG et al: The "on-off" phenomenon in Parkinson's disease: Relation to levodopa absorption and transport. N Engl J Med 310:438, 1984
SOURKES TL: Parkinson's disease and other disorders of the basal ganglia, in *Basic Neurochemistry,* GJ Siegel et al (eds). Boston, Little, Brown, 1981

Cerebellar degeneration

DUVOISIN RC, PLAITAKIS A (eds): *Advances in Neurology,* vol 41, *The Olivopontocerebellar Atrophies.* New York, Raven, 1984
KONIGSMARK BW, WEINER LP: The olivopontocerebellar atrophies: A review. Medicine 49:227, 1970
TRAUNER DA: Olivopontocerebellar atrophy with dementia, blindness, and chorea. Arch Neurol 42:757, 1985

Motor neuron disease

ROWLAND LP (ed): *Advances in Neurology,* vol 36, *Human Motor Neuron Diseases.* New York, Raven, 1982
TANDAN R, BRADLEY WG: Amyotrophic lateral sclerosis: Part 1, Clinical features, pathology, and ethical issues in management. Ann Neurol 18:271, 1985
———, ———: Amyotrophic lateral sclerosis: Part 2, Etiopathogenesis. Ann Neurol 18:419, 1985

Miscellaneous

BAUMANN RJ et al: Lafora disease: Liver histopathology in presymptomatic children. Ann Neurol 14:86, 1983
BEAL MF et al: Somatostatin: Alterations in the central nervous system in neurological diseases, in *Neuropeptides in Neurologic and Psychiatric Disease,* ARNMD vol 64, JB Martin, J Barchas (eds). New York, Raven, 1986, pp 25–258
BLACK PM et al: CSF shunts for dementia, incontinence and gait disturbance. Clin Neurosurg 32:632, 1985
BØGESEN S, GJERRIS F: The predictive value of conductance to outflow of CSF in normal pressure hydrocephalus. Brain 105:65, 1982
HARDING AE: Hereditary "pure" spastic paraplegia: A clinical and genetic study of 22 families. J Neurol Neurosurg Psychiatry 44:871, 1981
HENSON RA, URICH H: *Cancer and the Nervous System.* Blackwell Scientific, 1982
IIVANAINEN M, HIMBERG J-J: Valproate and clonazepam in the treatment of severe progressive myoclonus epilepsy. Arch Neurol 39:236, 1982
LOGIGIAN EL et al: Myoclonus epilepsy in two brothers: Clinical features and neuropathology of a unique syndrome. Brain (in press)
MUNOZ-GARCIA D, LUDWIN SK: Classic and generalized variants of Pick's disease: A clinicopathological, ultrastructural, and immunocytochemical study. Ann Neurol 16:467, 1984
O'BRIEN MD et al: Benign familial tremor treated with primidone. Br Med J 282:178, 1981
STEEL JC: Progressive supranuclear palsy. Brain 95:693, 1972
TISSOT R et al: *La Maladie de Pick.* Paris, Masson et Cie, 1975
ZEMAN W, DYKEN P: Dystonia musculorum deformans: Clinical, genetic and pathoanatomical studies. Psychiatr Neurol Neurochir 70:77, 1967

351 DEVELOPMENTAL AND CONGENITAL ABNORMALITIES OF THE NERVOUS SYSTEM

G. ROBERT DeLONG / RAYMOND D. ADAMS

This chapter discusses diseases traceable to insults or defects of development of the nervous system which have persisting effects into adult life, and which thus are likely to be of concern to the general physician and internist.

Specific diagnostic and therapeutic considerations arise in such developmental diseases—examples would be visceral tumors occurring in the neurocutaneous syndromes, or leukemia in Down's syndrome. A knowledge of these disorders is important to understanding the patient in the broader context of medical care: physical and mental limitations, ability to understand and comply with diagnostic and treatment programs, and genetic and familial issues. Finally, in the full cycle of life it is important for physicians caring for adults—especially for those who may become parents—to be aware of ways in which general medical disease and treatment, as well as genetic disorders, may affect the neurologic development of offspring.

Developmental abnormalities of the nervous system can conveniently be divided into those which are associated with recognizable somatic malformations, and those which are confined only to the nervous system (60 percent of all congenital malformations affect the nervous system). They may also be usefully classified as those determined by acquired or environmental factors, and those of genetic origin. In some cases, of course, there may be complicated interactions between genetic and environmental factors.

INFLUENCES ON NERVOUS SYSTEM DEVELOPMENT The effects of insults to brain during development are a complex function of the severity of the insult, its duration, the specific biologic impact of the insulting agent, and the precise stage in developmental time at which the insult is sustained. Environmental causes of developmental abnormalities of the nervous system are particularly important because they are potentially preventable.

Maternal toxins pose an important source of damage to developing brain and nerves. The fetal alcohol syndrome, an important cause of mental retardation, results from excessive exposure of the fetus to maternally ingested alcohol. Maternal exposure to other medications, especially anticonvulsants, may affect fetal brain development. Trimethadione produces severe fetal anomalies. Valproic acid has been implicated as causing spina bifida. Maternal use of phenytoin in the first months of pregnancy produces generally mild but identifiable effects on brain and somatic development. Isotretinoin, a preparation for acne, has been associated with congenital abnormalities of the brain. Organic mercury toxin in Minimata Bay, Japan, produced severe fetal brain abnormalities. Radiation and radiomimetic agents during the first trimester of pregnancy can produce microcephaly and mental retardation.

Maternal disease during gestation may damage the developing fetal brain. Examples include congenital infections (maternal rubella, toxoplasmosis, cytomegalic inclusion disease, syphilis, and herpes simplex); maternal diabetes; prolonged maternal hyperthermia causing anomalies of central nervous system development and microcephaly; severe maternal iodine deficiency causing endemic cretinism; and maternal hypoxia, shock, or carbon monoxide poisoning producing hypoxic-ischemic injury to fetal brain. Prolonged and severe fetal malnutrition, whether from placental insufficiency or maternal protein-calorie malnutrition, may permanently curtail brain and somatic growth and mental development. Isoimmunization by fetal Rh or ABO blood factors may result in erythroblastosis fetalis, hyperbilirubinemia, and kernicterus.

Diseases of the uteroplacental unit and of parturition are important causes of injury to the developing nervous system. The result is often hypoxic-ischemic insults of brain, either pre- or perinatally, resulting in impaired brain growth, ischemic necrosis, cerebral infarction, and porencephaly. Associated with this complex of insults is germinal matrix and intraventricular hemorrhage, seen in premature infants with respiratory distress and cardiovascular instability. These insults, depending on severity, result in sensory, mental, and motor deficits.

Genomic defects, whether point mutations or chromosomal anomalies, may profoundly affect central nervous system development. To review the hundreds of specific entities, often rare or even restricted to a single family, the reader is referred to a textbook on human genetics. Chromosomal abnormalities almost invariably impair brain development and function; they include some of the commonest and most important forms of mental retardation. Among these are Down's syndrome (caused by chromosome 21 trisomy or translocation); the fragile X syndrome, manifested by somatic signs (large ears, large testes), mental retardation, and language deficits (associated with a fragile site, revealed by culture in folate deficient media, on the X chromosome); Prader-Willi syndrome, characterized by hypotonia in infancy, pathologic obesity, and moderate psychomotor retardation (caused by a deletion on chromosome 15); and sex chromosome anomalies (XO, XXY, XYY, XXX, etc.), associated with mild or moderate somatic and mental aberrations. Genetic disorders affecting the nervous system are further discussed below, under neurocutaneous syndromes and mental retardation, and in the chapters on metabolic, hereditary, and degenerative diseases of the nervous system (Chaps. 349 and 350).

Neurodevelopmental abnormalities demonstrate complex and instructive interactions between genetic and environmental influences. Women with phenylketonuria invariably bear children with microcephaly and severe psychomotor retardation, not because of genetic transmission but because high maternal blood levels of phenylalanine are toxic to the developing fetal brain. In another example, offspring of mothers with myotonic dystrophy may suffer a double insult: They may inherit the autosomal dominant genetic trait, which may affect brain as well as muscle, and they may suffer perinatal asphyxia because of uterine dystocia that results in failure of normal progress of labor, caused by the maternal muscular dystrophy.

Spina bifida is an important example of a condition with interactive genetic and environmental determinants. Evidence for a genetic factor includes its high incidence in certain ethnic populations (especially in the United Kingdom where the incidence approximates 1 in 500 births) and a familial risk of recurrence of approximately 5 percent, many times higher than the population incidence. Data suggesting environmental factors include the decline in incidence (by about 50 percent) in both the United Kingdom and the United States in the past 40 years, and more recently, data implicating a nutritional factor. Controlled studies demonstrate a significant decrease in recurrence of spina bifida in offspring of women who received vitamin supplements, especially folic acid, during pregnancy.

Neurodevelopmental defects, primarily familial and genetic but also acquired, are being recognized in more subtle childhood developmental disorders which primarily affect intellect, language, behavior, and emotion. Examples include dyslexia, attention deficit disorder with hyperactivity, autism, and affective disease (major depression and manic depression).

Adult disorders of the nervous system that originate in early life may be classified under the following headings:

1 Congenital malformations of head, spine, and other structures, including dwarfism
2 Hereditary diseases which begin during childhood and persist throughout life, some progressing
3 Diseases which retard motor, speech, and intellectual development
4 Epilepsy

CONGENITAL MALFORMATIONS

MALFORMATIONS OF CRANIUM, SPINE, AND LIMBS Certain alterations in the size and shape of the head observed in the adult can be assumed to have had their origin prenatally or in early childhood. Beyond the first 4 to 5 years the brain approximates adult size, and the cranial sutures are so firmly closed that disease acquired later will have relatively little effect on the skull. Enlargement of the head is due either to *macrocephaly* with enlargement of brain (ventricles not enlarged significantly) or to *hydrocephalus*. Macrocephaly may be an incidental finding, often familial, in persons entirely normal neurologically, or it may be associated with neurologic disorders as in neurofibromatosis and the syndrome of cerebral gigantism (macrocephaly, tall stature, mental dullness, and seizures).

Microcephaly is related to lack of brain growth or to a destructive lesion of brain early in life. There are several rare forms of genetically determined microcephaly. In addition, microcephaly may result from chromosomal disorders, congenital infections, asphyxia, or any of the noxious insults detailed in the preceding section. In general, mental disability parallels the degree of microcephaly.

Unusual shape of head is usually caused by craniosynostosis. If the sagittal suture fuses too early, the head is long and narrow (scaphocephaly) with prominent brow and occiput; if the coronal suture closes prematurely, the head is wider than long (brachycephaly). Closure of all sutures produces a characteristic tower skull (turricephaly), shallow orbits, and bulging eyes. The last condition, if it is not recognized early and the suture lines excised, may prevent brain growth and raise intracranial pressure. Apert's syndrome (craniosynostosis with "mitten hands" or syndactyly) is associated often with enlarged ventricles and mental retardation. In achondroplasia true megalencephaly occurs, and disproportion between the base of the skull and the brain results in internal hydrocephalus in some cases.

Hydrocephalus of infancy and early childhood causes frontal bossing and variable degrees of cranial enlargement (usually over 60 cm, which is above the 97th percentile). In about 50 percent of cases the underlying condition is a congenital malformation, such as an Arnold-Chiari malformation, which is followed in frequency by meningeal fibrosis around the brainstem from subarachnoid or neonatal periventricular hemorrhage or meningitis, aqueductal stenosis, Dandy-Walker syndrome (cystic expansion of the fourth ventricle due to failure of foramens of Magendie and Luschka to open), or posterior fossa arachnoid cyst. Hydrocephalic states may arrest, only to present at a later age period with headache, spasticity, optic atrophy, and behavioral, emotional, and intellectual changes. Occult asymptomatic hydrocephalus may be destabilized in adulthood by seemingly minor head injury.

The main point to be remembered is that the cranial circumference is a valuable index of cerebral volume, and it reflects disease originating in the early period of life.

ABNORMALITIES OF THE SPINE A remarkable variety of lifelong neurologic syndromes are associated with abnormality of the vertebral column. Some of these, such as hemivertebra, platybasia, fusion of the atlas and occiput or of cervical vertebrae, or congenital dislocation of the atlas, are the consequence of a malformation of the spine itself, and the enclosed spinal cord may or may not be involved. Others, such as spina bifida occulta, spinal meningocele or myelomeningocele, or dysraphism, involve the whole neural tube, including spinal cord, investing meninges, vertebral bodies, and even the overlying skin and subcutaneous tissues. Finally there is a group of hereditary metabolic diseases that alter the spine progressively during childhood and adolescence (e.g., the mucopolysaccharidoses).

Primary malformations of vertebrae These are most frequent in the upper cervical region. The *Klippel-Feil deformity* consists of maldevelopment and fusion of two or more cervical vertebrae, resulting in a short neck of limited mobility. The hairline is low, often at the level of the first thoracic vertebra. There may or may not be associated neurologic symptoms or signs. The importance of the spinal deformity lies in its frequent association with other abnormalities, especially those of platybasia and syringomyelia, the symptoms of which may not become manifest until adolescence or adult life (see Chap. 353).

Deformity of the craniocervical junction or instability of the atlantoaxial joint may cause compression of the cervical spinal cord. Atlantoaxial dislocation may result from maldevelopment of the odontoid, seen with Down's syndrome, Morquio's syndrome, and spondyloepiphyseal dysplasia.

Platybasia and basilar impression This is a rare maldevelopment in which either the base of the skull is flattened or the occiput and upper cervical spine are invaginated into the posterior fossa. Often the foramen magnum itself is imperfectly developed, or the atlas and occiput are fused. Basilar impression may be caused by a group of diseases with biochemical and structural bony abnormalities of genetic origin. The conditions may be asymptomatic, but often there is "crowding," distortion, or compression of the spinal cord, medulla, and lower cranial and cervical spinal nerves. An acquired form of basilar impression occurs with rickets and Paget's disease. It is usually asymptomatic but sometimes involves the lower cranial nerves and may cause normal-pressure hydrocephalus.

The resulting clinical picture is variable. Symptoms may be present from early life or may begin in late childhood, adolescence, or even adult years. Early symptoms consist of "dizzy" or "weak" spells and downward nystagmus on tilting the head; evidences of increased intracranial pressure such as headache; occipital neuralgia; vomiting; transient paresthesias in the occipital region, neck, or arms; facial paresthesias, deafness, nasal voice, and dysphagia; cerebellar ataxia; and spastic weakness of the legs. The symptoms may first be intermittent and at any time in the course of the illness may be aggravated by straining, moving the head, or placing the head and neck in certain positions. Inspection alone provides a clue to diagnosis. The whole configuration of the head and neck is abnormal. The neck is short; the ears and hairline are low; the neck movements are obviously restricted; and the normal cervical lordosis is lost or greatly exaggerated, sometimes to the extent that the occiput lies almost on the upper dorsal spine and shoulders.

Platybasia and these related anomalies of the spine should be suspected in all cases presenting progressive cerebellar, brainstem, and cervical cord syndromes. Many of these cases have been misdiagnosed as multiple sclerosis or spinocerebellar degeneration. Others present a typical syringomyelic syndrome and have been so labeled. The clinical suspicion of platybasia and other spine anomalies can be confirmed by a true lateral roentgenogram of the skull.

Arnold-Chiari malformation This condition, in which the medulla and inferior-posterior portions of the cerebellar hemispheres project caudally through the foramen magnum, often to the level of the second cervical vertebra, is a common cause of hydrocephalus. It is often associated with a spinal myelomeningocele or meningocele, and usually there are deformities of the cervical spine and cervicooccipital junction. The symptoms of hydrocephalus dominate the clinical picture in infants. In milder cases, there may develop during adolescence or adult years any one of the several syndromes described above in the section "Platybasia and Basilar Impression." A second type of Arnold-Chiari malformation in patients who have no meningomyelocele is often associated with syringomyelia.

The treatment of platybasia and the Arnold-Chiari malformation has not been entirely satisfactory. If clinical progression is slight or uncertain, no treatment is warranted. If progression is certain and disability is increasing, upper cervical laminectomy and enlargement of the foramen magnum are indicated. Often this procedure halts the course of the illness or results in improvement. The surgical procedure must be done cautiously, however, for extensive manipulation of these structures may aggravate the symptoms or even cause death.

Malformations associated with a defect in closure of the neural arch These take the forms of craniorachischisis totalis, craniocele, spinal meningocele, meningomyelocele, spina bifida occulta, and sinus tracts. Since these conditions seldom figure in adult neurology, only some of the late complications are mentioned here.

Sinus tracts in lumbosacral or occipital regions are of importance, for at any age they may be sources of bacterial meningitis. They are often indicated by a small dimple in the skin or by a tuft of hair along the posterior surface of the body in the midline located high, above the buttocks. They may be associated with dermoid cysts at the central part of the tract. Evidence of such tracts should be sought in every instance of meningitis, especially when infection has recurred. The pilonidal sinus, which is found lower down, should not be included in this group.

There are, in addition, other congenital cysts (dermoids) and benign tumors (lipomas) which may produce progressive symptoms and signs by compressing the spinal cord or by implicating nerve roots. So-called tethering of the spinal cord is caused by a stout filum terminale exerting downward traction on the cord; the traction may cause ischemic injury to the conus medullaris and lower spinal segments. Diastematomyelia is a form of dysraphism characterized by a bony midline spur associated with partial duplication of the spinal cord at the same level; it may cause spinal symptoms by impingement on the cord.

Several clinical syndromes of delayed progressive disease (in the adolescent or adult) have been delineated in patients who have had an asymptomatic or symptomatic spina bifida, meningocele, or spinal dysraphism:

1 Progressive spastic weakness of some of the already weakened muscles of the legs.
2 An acute cauda equina syndrome following some unusual activity or incident, e.g., rowing, or a fall in a sitting position. The implicated sensory and motor roots are believed to be injured by sudden or repeated stretching. Weakness of bladder control, impotence (in the male), and numbness of feet and legs or footdrop compose the clinical syndrome.
3 Progressive cauda equina syndrome in the lumbosacral region.
4 Syringomyelia (see Chap. 353).

MALFORMATIONS OF THE EXTREMITIES These malformations include syndactylism, clinodactyly along with broad hand and transverse palmer (simian) line (common with Down's syndrome), club feet, and arthrogryposis multiplex. They are rarely of concern to internists.

DWARFISM IN RELATION TO NEUROLOGIC DISEASE It is noteworthy that the majority of mentally retarded individuals fall below normal in statural growth, and dwarfism is part of many special syndromes. Persons with Down's syndrome and with most of the other chromosomal abnormalities are examples, and there are others in which an inherited or acquired metabolic defect blights brain and skeletal growth (e.g., cretinism and mucupolysaccharidoses). Microcephaly characterizes many of the dwarfs with cerebral diseases.

The 30 or 40 neurologic syndromes with statural underdevelopment and neurologic disease are described and illustrated in the atlas of mental retardation by Holmes et al.

HEREDITARY DISEASES

THE PHAKOMATOSES This is a unique group of diseases, usually hereditary, in which neurologic abnormalities are combined with congenital defects of skin, retina, and other organs. The terms *congenital ectodermal dysplasias, congenital neurocutaneous syndromes,* or *phakomatoses* (Greek *phakos,* "lentil," "mole," or "freckle") are used frequently to designate this general class of disorders. The major syndromes include neurofibromatosis, tuberous sclerosis, encephalotrigeminal syndrome, and rarely, ataxia telangiectasia, cerebelloretinal hemangioblastomatosis, and the Klippel-Trénaunay-Weber syndrome. Osler-Rendu-Weber disease, an autosomal dominant disease with vascular anomalies affecting skin, mucous membranes, and the gastrointestinal and genitourinary tracts, occasionally has angiomas in either spinal cord or brain, where they may produce bleeding (see Chap. 185). Cerebral abscess formation is another complication of this condition involving the central nervous system.

Neurofibromatosis (von Recklinghausen's disease) This is an autosomal dominant disease, in which spots of increased skin pigmentation are combined with multiple neurofibromas. Its incidence is 1 per 3000; about 50 percent of cases are apparently sporadic. It has been characterized as a maldevelopment of cells of neural crest origin. The pigmented spots are irregular in shape with relatively even borders, vary in size from a few millimeters to several centimeters, and are of brownish coffee color (café au lait). They are most prominent over the trunk, in the axilla (axillary freckles), and about the pelvis. Similar lesions occur in individuals without neurofibromatosis, but in such instances they are generally smaller than 1.5 cm in diameter and fewer than five in number. The tumors arise from the neurilemmal sheath (Schwann cells) of the peripheral nerve. They are usually multiple and vary in size from minute lesions to large tumors several centimeters in diameter. The majority are smoothly rounded or lobulated, soft or firm, and can sometimes be seen or felt along the course of a peripheral nerve. Often they sink into the subcutaneous fat on gentle pressure. Like the pigmented lesions, the tumors are more frequent over the trunk than on the extremities. Both the pigmented areas, because of giant melanosomes in pigment epithelial cells, and also the tumors of nerve sheaths become increasingly apparent with age. Most of the tumors are asymptomatic; occasionally, if they attain a large size or occupy an unusual position, they may produce pressure upon contiguous structures. Tumors of the spinal nerve roots may compress the spinal cord and at the same time extend through the intervertebral foramens to form a large mass in the posterior mediastinum (dumbbell tumors). Acoustic neurinomas, usually bilateral in patients with neurofibromatosis, may produce deafness and other symptoms and signs of a cerebellopontine angle lesion (Chap. 345); this form apparently represents a distinct variant. Such patients almost always lack any peripheral neurocutaneous signs of neurofibromatosis. Other histopathologic types of tumor (meningioma, glioma) are encountered more often in neurofibromatosis than in the general population. Diffuse overgrowth of Schwann cells and fibroblasts may also occur, giving rise to plexiform neuromas. They may cause hideous deformities, often with overgrowth of underlying bone. Bone cysts may also form. Most of these associated tumors are rare in infancy and childhood, though glioma of the optic nerve and chiasm is an exception to the clinical rule. The latter condition should always be considered in the differential diagnosis of unilateral (rarely bilateral) blindness, proptosis, and extraocular muscle paralysis in childhood, especially if there are signs of von Recklinghausen's disease. Diagnosis is evident by computed tomography (CT) scan. Pulsating exophthalmos resulting from congenital absence of part of the sphenoid bone is an infrequent but characteristic lesion of neurofibromatosis. Pheochromocytoma is a rare accompaniment of the disease. In about 5 to 10 percent of cases of neurofibromatosis one of the tumors will become sarcomatous.

Fibrous dysplasia, congenital vertebral anomalies, local gigantism of an extremity, subperiosteal bone cysts, and pseudoarthrosis of the tibia may be associated with neurofibromatosis. Scoliosis is a common skeletal deformity in children with this disease, so that neurofibromatosis must be added to the list of neurogenic and myogenic kyphoscolioses (the others are syringomyelia, Friedreich's ataxia, progressive muscular dystrophy, and poliomyelitis). Stenosis of the aqueduct of Sylvius with obstructive hydrocephalus is at times observed in neurofibromatosis. Also there may be a mild degree of mental retardation, related presumably to developmental abnormalities of the cerebral cortex. Spina bifida, hypospadias, glaucoma, and elephantiasis are occasionally seen. An association of vascular stenoses (renal, cerebral, or pulmonic) and neurofibromatosis has been recognized.

About one-third of cases of neurofibromatosis are discovered accidentally on routine examination, there being no complaints. Another third of these patients come seeking advice about the cosmetic aspects of the disease. The remainder have neurologic syndromes. Those with prominent neurologic signs may have few cutaneous lesions. There is no treatment for the disease other than excision of symptomatic tumors.

Tuberous sclerosis This autosomal dominant disease is manifested by the clinical triad of convulsive seizures, mental deficiency, and adenoma sebaceum. The latter are fine, wart-like lesions distributed predominantly in a butterfly distribution over the cheeks, nose, and forehead. The individual adenomas vary in size from 0.1 to 1.0 cm and are elevated and pinkish or pinkish yellow in color. In addition, the skin over the lower part of the back may be thick, rough, and of yellowish color, like sharkskin or pigskin (shagreen patch). Actually the earliest lesions are ash-leaf-shaped hypopigmented spots ("white spots") over the trunk and limbs, which are seen most clearly under ultraviolet light (Wood's lamp). They are distinguishable on the basis of size, shape, and character from avascular nevi and vitiligo, and are highly diagnostic, often providing the earliest clue to the etiology of mental retardation or infantile epilepsy. The mental deficiency may be relatively stationary or progressive. The seizures are usually generalized but may be focal. Retinal tumors and other visible malformations may be conjoined.

Patients with the most advanced form of tuberous sclerosis are severely mentally retarded, but not all are so disabled. In general hospital clinics it is not unusual to see such patients with average intelligence and only seizures and a few skin lesions. Occasionally a focal cerebral syndrome will prove at biopsy to have a typical "tuber" or an associated glioma as its basis in a patient not known to have this disease. Family history is frequently unhelpful—approximately one-half of cases are sporadic, presumably due to mutation.

Pathologically, the lesions of the skin are fibromas and not true adenomas. Some are rather vascular and suggest telangiectasia. The brain lesions consist of areas of malformed cortex with extensive astrogliosis and a peculiar mixture of glioblasts and monster nerve cells. Calcification may or may not be present. Masses of subependymal glial tissue account for the nodules projecting into the walls of the ventricles that are often seen in computerized tomography. Most cases of rhabdomyoma of heart muscle are associated with tuberous sclerosis. Tumorous malformations may occur in the kidney, liver, adrenal glands, and pancreas.

The diagnosis is aided by CT scans. Calcified nodules occur, particularly in the temporal lobes and adjacent to the ventricles. If large, they may obstruct the foramen of Monro, causing a unilateral or bilateral hydrocephalus. The center of the nodule tends to be more densely radiopaque than the periphery. Hypodense areas may appear at the cortical junction with the white matter. The electroencephalogram is usually abnormal but without specific pattern. The cerebrospinal fluid may be normal; rarely, the total protein level is elevated.

Treatment is symptomatic, with excision of tumors as necessary. The prognosis for life beyond the third decade is poor. Death is usually due to seizures, associated tumors, or intercurrent diseases. Genetic counseling is an obligation of the physician.

Cerebelloretinal hemangioblastomatosis (von Hippel–Lindau syndrome) As the name implies, the syndrome consists of vascular malformations of the retina and cerebellum. The retinal lesions are capillary angiomas, usually multiple, causing progressive loss of vision; the cerebellar lesion consists of a slowly growing hemangioblastoma, frequently multiple, with a large cystic component, lending itself to surgical removal; spinal and medullary hemangioblastomas also occur. The clinical symptoms and signs consist of progressive cerebellar ataxia, headache, and papilledema. Seldom is a vascular bruit audible over the head. Polycythemia, possibly related to the production of erythropoietin, has been observed in many cases and has in a few instances disappeared after excision of the tumor. The disease is transmitted as an autosomal dominant trait, but many cases are sporadic. Rarely do these tumors appear before adolescence. One should consider this diagnosis in all patients with a cerebellar tumor syndrome (see Chap. 345). Not all have a retinal lesion—the von Hippel part of the disease. The hemangioblastoma of the cerebellum is usually but one part of a constellation of abnormalities including angiomas and cysts of the liver, pancreas, and kidneys and tumors of the epididymis and kidney, the last named being the cause of death in some cases. Pheochromocytomas have been described in this and in other of the phakomatoses. Syringomyelia has been observed in a few cases, and if a careful search is made, a hemangioblastoma can often be found in relation to the syrinx at some level.

The cerebellar hemangioblastoma demands surgical treatment, and if the nodule of the tumor is found in the wall of the cyst and is excised, the results can be excellent; if the tumor cannot be operated on because of size or multiplicity, radiation may be tried. The retinal lesions, when small, can be arrested by photocoagulation.

Encephalotrigeminal syndrome (Sturge-Weber disease) This disease consists of capillary or cavernous hemangiomas, within but not always limited to the cutaneous distribution of the trigeminal nerve unilaterally, and of a predominantly venous hemangioma of the leptomeninges over the occipital, parietal, or frontal lobe on the same side. The intracranial and cutaneous lesions may occur separately. The disease is usually sporadic; familial occurrence is exceptional.

Pathologically, the cortex subjacent to the abnormal meningeal vessels is progressively destroyed, owing probably to stagnation of blood flow and consequent hypoxia, and in some cases a band of calcium develops within the lesion. This band, following the convolutional pattern as it does, is responsible for the characteristic "railroad track" roentgenographic picture. Deeply situated arteriovenous malformations rarely coexist.

The first neurologic symptom is usually a focal seizure on the side opposite the skin lesion. Transient postictal (Todd's) paralysis or permanent paralysis may follow the seizure. Sensorimotor paralysis or permanent visual field defect, the most frequent findings, may be either of insidious onset with slow progression or apoplectic. Blindness in the eye on the side of the nevus is frequent and is nearly always due to glaucoma. Most patients with this malformation survive for many years, often with residual mental defects and hemiparesis.

The lesions are usually too extensive to be treated surgically, though hemispherectomy has been advised by some surgeons for intractable epilepsy. Anticonvulsant medication is indicated, but the seizures may be difficult to control.

Hemangioma of the trunk or upper or lower extremity may be associated with a spinal cord vascular malformation (Klippel-Trénaunay-Weber syndrome). The extremity may be hypertrophied. The cord lesion may bleed into or cause infarction in the nervous tissue, producing a spinal sensorimotor paralysis. Surgical exploration and decompression are seldom beneficial.

Ataxia telangiectasia (see Chap. 256) This condition has attracted considerable interest because of theoretical implications of its apparent cause and pathogenesis. Inherited as a recessive trait, the disease is characterized neurologically by a progressive cerebellar ataxia, apraxia of ocular movement, and choreoathetosis beginning during the early years of life. Not all neurologists classify this condition as a phakomatosis because of its progressive nature and associated immunologic defects. Telangiectases of bulbar conjunctivas and skin, especially about the ears, neck, and in flexor creases at the elbows and knees, appear somewhat later in childhood or adolescence. Recurring pulmonary and sinus infections have been prominent in many cases, and a deficiency in the IgA globulins and a defect of delayed cellular hypersensitivity are found. The diagnosis can be supported by the finding of abnormal humoral and cell-mediated immunity and of raised levels of alpha fetoprotein and cytogenetic abnormalities. Fibroblasts and lymphocytes from patients with this disease have enhanced in vitro radiosensitivity, attributed to deficiencies in enzyme systems that repair DNA. The associated pathologic changes consist of an extensive loss of Purkinje cells of the cerebellum and possibly degeneration of the neurons in other parts of the basal ganglia. Dysplasia of the thymus has been well documented, and death usually occurs by the second or third decade of life from infection or a reticuloendothelial tumor.

Familial dysautonomia (Riley-Day syndrome) This disease is characterized by autonomic instability (abnormal sweating, loss of vasomotor control, labile hypertension), impaired taste with absence of fungiform papillae, diminished pain and temperature sensation, hyporeflexia, episodic fever, vomiting attacks, lack of lacrimation (alacrima), and corneal anesthesia and ulceration. Familial dysautonomia is an autosomal recessive disease limited to Ashkenazi Jews.

The clinical manifestations become apparent soon after birth with difficulty in feeding (dysphagia) and motor functions which becomes increasingly evident in childhood. A few patients reach adult years, but the mortality rate is high because of recurrent pulmonary infections with inappropriate autonomic responses. Emotional instability presents a problem in most patients. Although intelligence has been within normal limits in some patients, in others it has been subnormal. Growth seems to be delayed for unclear reasons, and the natural tendency is to undernutrition and scoliosis. Neuropathic (Charcot) joints due to lack of pain and related injury have been reported.

Proof of the disturbance of the autonomic nervous system comes from special tests such as absence of skin flare after histamine and skin stroking (loss of axonal reflex), and hypersensitivity to both cholinergic and adrenergic agents. Nerve conduction velocities are decreased. Quantitative pathologic studies of peripheral and autonomic nervous systems have shown marked depletion of small-caliber axons in peripheral nerves (which could account for the deficit in pain and temperature appreciation) and decreased numbers of small neurons in the dorsal root ganglia, in sympathetic ganglia, and in the ciliary ganglia (which could account for some of the dysautonomic features). A primary enzymatic defect has not been demonstrated. Intermediolateral cell columns of the spinal cord are normal, as is the rest of the central nervous system.

In the differential diagnosis one must consider other forms of small-fiber polyneuropathy with analgesia and dysautonomia (including congenital indifference to pain and amyloidosis) (see Chap. 355), as well as the Shy-Drager syndrome (a degenerative disease of lateral horn cells and basal ganglia) (see Chap. 350).

Bethanechol may control vomiting attacks, increase tearing, and reduce the risk of pulmonary aspiration. Orthopedic measures are needed to stabilize neuropathic joints. Injury must be avoided and wounds treated carefully.

DISEASES THAT RETARD DEVELOPMENT

ABNORMALITIES OF MOTOR FUNCTION (CEREBRAL PALSY) In this category of neurologic defect a major disturbance of motor function, usually nonprogressive, has been present since infancy or childhood. The popular term for these conditions is *cerebral palsy*. Cerebral palsy may be used as a generic term defining a nonprogressive static disturbance of motor function, present from birth or early life, caused by a discrete encephaloclastic insult to the central nervous system during gestation, the perinatal period, or infancy. Most cases result from ischemic-hypoxic insults, but infection, hemorrhage, or trauma may occasionally have a similar outcome. Familial/genetic, metabolic, and degenerative diseases should be excluded from this classification.

Forms of cerebral palsy are designated according to the pattern of motor disturbance. Spastic diplegia (referring to spasticity in paired limbs but in practice referring to spasticity predominant in the legs) is the commonest form (accounting for 50 percent of cerebral palsy) and generally the mildest. Only about 8 percent of spastic diplegics are mentally retarded; most become ambulatory. The stiff, awkward movements of the legs, maintained in an extended, adducted posture, do not usually attract attention until several weeks or months after birth. Seizures occur in some cases, and it is not uncommon to observe a delay in all normal developmental sequences, especially those which depend on the motor system. Once walking is attempted, usually much later than in the normal child, the characteristic stance and gait become manifest. The legs are advanced stiffly in short steps, each describing an arc of a circle; adduction is often so strong as to lead to actual crossing (scissors gait), with lower legs slightly splayed out and the feet flexed and turned in, the heels not touching the ground. In the adolescent and adult, the legs tend to be short and small, but the muscles are not markedly atrophic. Passive manipulation of the limbs reveals marked spasticity in the extensors and adductors and also slight shortening of the calf muscles. The hands and arms may be affected only slightly, if at all; there may be awkwardness and stiffness of the fingers. In a few, pronounced weakness and spasticity are noted. Speech may be well-articulated or noticeably slurred, and in some instances the face is set in a spastic smile. The deep-tendon reflexes are exaggerated, those in the legs more so than those in the arms, and the plantar reflexes are extensor. Usually there is no disturbance of spincteric function, though delay in acquiring voluntary control is usual. Athetotic postures and movements of the face, tongue, and hands are present in some patients and may actually conceal the pyramidal weakness. Ataxic and hypotonic forms also exist.

The condition must be distinguished from familial types of spastic paraparesis, which are well-recognized clinical entities (Chap. 353).

Spastic quadriplegia, the term referring to spasticity of all four extremities (generally with legs more severely affected than arms) accounts for 30 percent of cerebral palsy; children so affected are generally markedly retarded and nonambulatory. Spastic hemiplegia accounts for 10 percent of cerebral palsy; it can be divided roughly into two groups: two-thirds to three-quarters have normal intelligence; one-third have seizures; and about one-quarter are mentally retarded. These two features tend to be correlated; i.e., patients with congenital hemiplegia with seizures have lower intelligence scores. Other forms of cerebral palsy together account for 10 percent. These include choreoathetotic, ataxic, dystonic, and atonic forms; these forms may be mixed, including features of spasticity and mental retardation. In patients with a combination of cerebral diplegia and ataxia, difficulty in standing and walking cannot be attributed to spasticity or paralysis. Incoordination, similar to that seen in cerebellar disease, and hypotonia are the principal findings. The motor defect may be so great that the individual is never able to sit or stand; the muscles are of normal size, and voluntary movements, though weak, are possible in all the limbs. In less severe cases, sitting, standing, and walking are merely delayed, and with advancing years cerebellar ataxia and tremor become manifest. Relative improvement may occur in later years. The tendon reflexes are present, and the plantar reflexes are either flexor or extensor. Many of these patients suffer a severe degree of amentia and retardation of speech development. Pure choreoathetotic cerebral palsy may be associated with striking preservation of intelligence. At the opposite extreme, atonic cerebral palsy is uniformly accompanied by profound developmental deficit.

A rare condition, infantile quadriplegia without involvement of intellect or bulbar musculature, may result from a high cervical cord lesion. Although this may occasionally result from cysts, tumors, and other malformations, it is usually produced in the infant by a rupture of the cervical cord induced by traction during a difficult breech delivery. Similarly, in paraplegia, with weakness or paralysis limited to the legs, the lesion may be either a cerebral form of diplegia or a spinal one. Sphincteric disturbances and a definite loss of somatic sensation below a certain level on the trunk always favor a spinal localization. Congenital cysts including rare spinal arachnoid cysts, tumors, and diastematomyelia are more frequently the cause of paraplegia than of quadriplegia. An additional cause of infantile paraplegia is spinal infarction from thrombotic complications of umbilical artery catheterization.

The lesions associated with cerebral palsy are predominantly caused by ischemic-hypoxic insults to the immature brain because of asphyxia. Asphyxia has been estimated to occur antenatally in 50 percent of cases, intrapartum in 40 percent, and postpartum in 10 percent. Modern obstetric practice has reduced the incidence of perinatal asphyxia from 4 percent to 0.5 percent. The type of cerebral palsy which results depends on the pattern and severity of hypoxic-ischemic insult. Spastic diplegia probably results from ischemic-hypoxic necrotic lesions localized near the dorsolateral surfaces of the lateral ventricles, thought to be an end-arterial zone in preterm infants. More extensive ischemic-hypoxic insults produce extensive cystic destruction of central white matter of the hemispheres (deep lesion), a lesion associated with quadriplegia and mental deficiency. Hypoxic-ischemic insult in term infants tends to affect the parasagittal and parietooccipital cortex watershed zone, hippocampus, thalamus, and cerebellar hemispheres (superficial lesion). Congenital hemiplegia results from arterial occlusion in the middle cerebral artery territory (probably secondary to hypoxia and ischemia) resulting in a porencephalic lesion of the hemisphere, or from a more diffuse and partial hemispheral insult. Cohen and Duffner have shown that if a subsequent CT scan shows damage to the cerebral cortex, the likelihood of seizures and subnormal intelligence is increased.

Choreoathetotic cerebral palsy usually results from intrapartum asphyxia and hypoxia. It correlates with the pathologic finding of status marmoratus, a partial lesion of the basal ganglia characterized by neuronal loss, gliosis, and condensation of myelinating fibers.

Ataxic cerebral palsy is commonly associated with sclerotic lesions of the cerebellum. Other lesions of the cerebral hemispheres, as described above, may also be present.

Clinical pictures similar to those described above may result from postnatal disease states, including meningitis, herpes simplex encephalitis, seizures, trauma, subdural hematomas, or vascular insults. In the premature infant, ischemia followed by hyperperfusion may result in hemorrhage into the periventricular germinal matrix zones, lateral ventricles, and parenchyma of the hemispheres. This intraventricular hemorrhage (IVH), occurring in about 40 percent of premature infants with respiratory distress syndrome and requiring respiratory assistance, may result in hydrocephalus and delayed psychomotor development. Hypoxic-ischemic injury, independent of the hemorrhage, appears to play a role in the neurologic outcome of these infants.

Kernicterus is a special form of neonatal insult that can be considered with cerebral palsy. Its distinctive clinical picture includes choreoathetosis, deafness, failure of upward gaze, and sometimes mental retardation. The degree of involvement ranges from mild to severe. Either athetosis or ataxia may be present, and a few have also shown rigid limbs and a picture not too different from that of cerebral spastic diplegia with involuntary movements. The neuropathologic changes in these surviving patients consist of symmetrically distributed nerve-cell loss and gliosis in the subthalamic nucleus of Luys, the globus pallidus, thalamus, and oculomotor and cochlear nuclei. These lesions result from hyperbilirubinemia. In the newborn, unconjugated bilirubin can pass through the poorly developed blood-brain barrier into these central and brainstem nuclei, where it is directly toxic. Acidosis and hypoxia exacerbate the effect.

MENTAL RETARDATION Mentally retarded individuals pose special problems for physicians not only in childhood but also in adulthood. They are unable to give an adequate medical history; one must rely more on objective signs of disease than on subjective complaint. Often they cannot cooperate in diagnostic studies or independently manage treatment regimens. Then, too, the reactions of such patients to drugs and fever may be extreme and unpredictable. Recognition of the etiology of mental retardation also becomes important in genetic counseling for other members of the family.

Mental retardation poses a great challenge for the physician. Responsibilities may include the recognition and prevention of factors—both genetic and environmental—apt to cause mental retardation, diagnosis of mental retardation itself, genetic counseling, treatment of conditions causing mental retardation, treatment of intercurrent illnesses in the mentally retarded, advising about the social and educational management of the retarded, and treatment of behavioral disorders which may accompany mental deficiency. The task of differentiating mental retardation from deafness, from disorders of language or motor development, and from other medical illnesses falls largely to the pediatrician. Genetic counseling increasingly becomes the province of specialized geneticists. Neuropsychopharmacology may contribute greatly to the well-being of some mentally retarded persons with behavioral and emotional dyscontrol or with epilepsy.

The clinical manifestations of mental retardation are relatively easy to perceive. Dull or silly behavior and inability to give a sensible account of the medical problem constitute one useful datum. Slowness in motor development, inability to learn and poor school progress, lack of a concept of time or space, and inability to secure and hold a job or to perform more than the menial tasks of society are other useful indexes.

The differentiation of the various classes of mental retardation by clinical criteria is facilitated if the framework of reference in Table 351-1 is used. In spite of the wide spectrum of specific disease entities causing mental retardation, perhaps half of all mentally retarded persons cannot presently be classified in terms of specific etiology by clinical criteria. They probably represent the consequence of a wide variety of genetic and acquired insults impairing brain development. Many of the known noxious agents acting during gestation and early life have been described above. Many cases are familial, the patients coming from families in which other members are retarded or have important mental disorders, and the heritable factors may be polygenic. There also appears to be another group of disorders, due to single gene defects affecting only the brain, which have been poorly defined clinically and pathologically; included are several types of maldevelopment of the cerebral cortex. An important and varied group of X-linked recessive disorders causing mental retardation in males has recently come to medical attention. One subgroup of these affected males has physical stigmata including macroorchidism, prognathism, large ears, and dolichocephaly; an identifiable abnormality of the X chromosome, called the *fragile X*, appears when their cells are grown in folate-deficient media.

Within the spectrum of types of mental retardation, even within a group of persons of similar intelligence quotients (IQ), there are vast differences and contrasts in overall behavioral functioning. Some mentally retarded persons are pleasant and amiable and achieve a rather satisfactory social adjustment; this is especially true of simple mental retardates. At the opposite extreme is the ill-understood syndrome of autism, associated with varying degrees of retardation, in which the child or older person fails to manifest interpersonal social contact—including communicative language—and demonstrates a limited and bizarre interest primarily in inanimate objects (see "Autism" below). It is impossible to list all variations of mental retardation here, but the point should be made that all aspects of intellectual life and personality are touched in differing degrees. Many retarded individuals are dull, apathetic, and underactive. Others display an incessant hyperactivity, characterized by a very short attention span, a restless and inquisitive searching of the environment, and low frustration tolerance. They may be destructive or recklessly fearless, and may seem strangely impervious to injury. Some display a peculiar anhedonia and are indifferent to either punishment or reward. Improvement in these children can often be achieved by using amphetamines. Other aberrant types of behavior, such as violent aggressiveness and even self-mutilation, are not uncommon. Rhythmic rocking, rolling, head banging, and bouncing movements are features of the motor activities of some severely retarded persons and may be performed hour after hour without fatigue, often to the accompaniment of vocal ejaculations. Here the abnormality is not the appearance of rhythmic movements of the body, which are to be observed at one period in the development of many normal children, but their persistence and exaggeration.

It is apparent that the clinical and behavioral characteristics of

TABLE 351-1 Clinical classification of nonprogressive types of mental retardation

I Mental defect with associated developmental abnormalities in nonnervous structures
- *A* Those affecting cranioskeletal structures
  - *1* Microcephaly
  - *2* Macrocephaly
  - *3* Hydrocephalus (including myelomeningocele with Arnold-Chiari malformation and associated cerebral anomalies)
  - *4* Down's syndrome (mongolism)
  - *5* Cretinism (congenital hypothyroidism)
  - *6* Mucopolysaccharidoses (Hurler, Hunter, and Sanfilippo types)
  - *7* Acrocephalosyndactyly (craniosynostosis)
  - *8* Arthrogryposis multiplex congenita (some cases)
  - *9* Rare specific syndromes: e.g., Rubinstein-Taybi
  - *10* Dwarfism, short stature: Seckel's bird-headed dwarf, Cockayne-Neel dwarf, etc.
  - *11* Hypertelorism, median facial cleft syndromes, agenesis of corpus callosum
- *B* Those affecting nonskeletal structures
  - *1* Neurocutaneous syndromes: tuberous sclerosis, Sturge-Weber syndrome, neurofibromatosis
  - *2* Congenital rubella syndrome (deafness, blindness, congenital heart disease, small stature)
  - *3* Chromosomal disorders: Down's syndrome, some cases of Klinefelter's syndrome (XXY), Turner's (XO) syndrome (occasionally), fragile X syndrome
  - *4* Laurence-Moon-Biedl syndrome (retinitis pigmentosa, obesity, polydactyly)
  - *5* Eye disorders: toxoplasmosis (chorioretinitis), galactosemia (cataract), congenital rubella (chorioretinitis)
  - *6* Prader-Willi syndrome (obesity, hypogenitalism)

II Mental defect without developmental anomalies in nonnervous structures but with focal cerebral and other neurologic abnormalities
- *A* Cerebral spastic diplegia and quadriplegia
- *B* Cerebral hemiplegia, unilateral or bilateral
- *C* Congenital choreoathetosis or ataxia
  - *1* Kernicterus
  - *2* Status marmoratus
- *D* Congenital atonic diplegia
- *E* Posthypoglycemic, posttraumatic, postmeningitic, and postencephalitic states
- *F* Those associated with other neuromuscular abnormalities (muscular dystrophy, Friedreich's ataxia, etc.)
- *G* Cerebral degenerative diseases (lipidoses)
- *H* Lesch-Nyhan syndrome (choreoathetosis and self-mutilation)

III Mental defect without signs of other developmental abnormality or neurologic disorder (epilepsy may or may not be present)
- *A* Simple mental retardation, familial mental retardation
- *B* Some cases of encephaloclastic disease (hypoxia, hypoglycemia)
- *C* Infantile autism
- *D* Those associated with inborn errors of metabolism (phenylketonuria, other aminoacidurias, organic acidurias)
- *E* Congenital infections (some cases of congenital syphilis, cytomegalic inclusion disease)
- *F* Epileptic encephalopathies

individuals with retarded development cannot be adequately described by a single parameter, the IQ. There are many other factors which determine the social success of retarded children and which should give direction to their education and training. These include specific sensory or motor handicaps, such as blindness and deafness as well as athetosis or hemiplegia; specific language or speech deficits; behavioral disturbances, such as autism, aggressiveness, or hyperactivity; and the presence of seizures. Measures can be taken, including pharmacologic treatment, physical therapy, and behavior training, to help the handicapped person compensate for these deficiencies. These become primary considerations in functional diagnosis and in guiding the parents or guardians.

The least severely retarded individual (IQ of 50 to 70) grows and develops in many ways not different from normal ones, and he or she can be taught useful occupational skills. A few of these persons can work under careful supervision. All scholastic pursuits are relatively unsuccessful, and vocational training is of more value than other types of education.

Special varieties of mental retardation Several of the special types of mental retardation are discussed in other chapters (see Chaps. 305, 306, 307, and 316). In the following sections are presented only those with special features likely to be seen in adults.

DOWN'S SYNDROME This unique condition, although accounting for only about 1 percent of all mental defectives, accounts for nearly one-third of the admissions to state schools for the mentally retarded. The degree of mental retardation varies from mild to severe and is associated with a curious facial configuration and a dwarfed physical stature. Many stigmata of Down's syndrome can be recognized in the neonatal period. The head tends to be small and round, with sloping forehead. The ears are set low and are oval, with small lobules. The eyes slant slightly upward and outward owing to the presence of a medial epicanthal fold, which partly covers the angle of the palpebral fissure. The bridge of the nose is generally absent or poorly developed. The mouth tends to hang open, and the tongue is usually enlarged, heavily fissured, and protruding. Gray-white specks of depigmentation are seen in the iris (Brushfield's spots). The little fingers are often short and curved inward (clinodactyly), owing to a hypoplastic middle phalanx. The hands are broad and short, with a single transverse palmar crease. Lenticular opacities and congenital heart lesions (septal defects) are found in some cases. At birth these children are of average size, but at later periods of life they are characteristically small.

The brain shows a rather rounded shape which conforms to that of the skull, a subnormal weight, and a relatively simple convolutional pattern, with particular smallness of the frontal lobes and superior temporal convolutions.

The mortality rate is high in the first years of life, death usually being due to respiratory infections, cardiac disease, or leukemia. Of the patients who survive to adult life, many then suffer a premature form of Alzheimer's cerebral degeneration (onset in the majority before age 40).

Older mothers are more apt to have Down's syndrome babies than are young mothers. The mean age of the mother at the time of birth of these children is 37. Down's syndrome is caused by trisomy of chromosome 21 or translocation of parts of this chromosome. It is diagnosable in utero by amniocentesis.

CRETINISM AND CHILDHOOD HYPOTHYROIDISM True endemic cretinism, along with endemic goiter, is an iodine deficiency disorder, occurring widely in remote areas of the world where severe iodine deficiency is not corrected. Cretins born of iodine-deficient mothers have irreversible deaf-mutism, mental retardation, and a spastic and rigid posture and gait.

This disorder is determined in utero by maternal iodine deficiency, which affects fetal brain development through a combination of failure of maternal provision of thyroxine to the fetus and failure of fetal thyroxine production because of iodine deficiency. In the neurologic form, thyroid function may be normal by the time of birth, but neurologic deficits persist. In the myxedematous form, severe hypothyroidism persists after birth.

Sporadic cretinism occurs in infants suffering a congenital disorder of thyroid function. The latter occurs in about 1 in 4000 births. Symptoms of hypothyroidism may be evident at birth or later. If untreated, hypothyroidism impairs brain development causing mental retardation. This form may be detected by neonatal screening programs. With prompt treatment (within the first weeks of life), children with sporadic cretinism may develop normally, with virtually no permanent neurologic or intellectual impairment. If treatment is withheld or delayed, permanent mental retardation results.

Childhood hypothyroidism and myxedema resemble the adult forms of the diseases described in Chap. 324.

MUCOPOLYSACCHARIDOSES AND PHENYLKETONURIA (PHENYLPYRUVIC OLIGOPHRENIA) These conditions are discussed in Chaps. 307 and 316.

AUTISM Autism is a syndrome of pervasive developmental disorder of personality, characterized by failure of the young child to develop normal social interaction or communicative language and by a bizarre obsessiveness, preoccupation, perseveration, resistance to change, and stereotypic actions. Language, if it develops, is characterized by a pragmatic and semantic deficit. Islands of preserved or precocious function may be evident. Autism is now considered a disorder of brain development, though etiologies are unclear; evidence has been put forward of genetic determinants and also of gestational and perinatal risk factors. The autistic syndrome may probably result from any of several disparate disease processes.

CT scans or pneumoencephalograms have shown abnormalities in some cases, implicating the medial temporal regions or enlargement of lateral ventricles. A recent detailed histopathologic study of one case by Bauman and Kemper disclosed abnormalities of cell growth in hippocampus and amygdala bilaterally, and in neocerebellum. No consistent biochemical abnormality has been discovered. Electroencephalograms are nonspecific, although temporal lobe discharges are occasionally seen, and up to 30 percent of autistic children eventually manifest epilepsy. The ultimate prognosis depends largely on the child's IQ. Those high-functioning children who develop communicative language by age 5 and have a normal IQ may exhibit certain exceptional talents, as in mathematics, though they remain socially stiff and incompetent. Most autistic children prove to be retarded, and in adult life they retain the same characteristics. There is no effective treatment, though psychotropic medications may have useful benefits in some cases.

SIMPLE MENTAL RETARDATION Although presented last, this category includes the great number of cases of defective mentality of indeterminate etiology in which neither somatic nor neurologic abnormality is exhibited. The degree of mental impairment tends to be mild (educable) or moderate (trainable). This group of retardates constitutes 25 percent of institutionalized individuals, and of course those who are in institutions represent only the more severely damaged individuals in our society. Their physical appearance is usually not strikingly abnormal, yet many of the aforementioned characteristics of the mentally retarded individual are to be observed. Seizures occur in a significant number, being several times more frequent than in a normal population. Within the limits of their intelligence, the success of these individuals in learning to look after themselves is often determined by how effectively their parents and teachers have inculcated or reinforced good work habits and stable personality traits. The brighter ones can profit to some extent from formal education. Those less well endowed may be trained to care for their personal wants and needs and may profit from special occupational training. Special schools and classes are of great help. Later in life, supervised work situations are possible solutions to their occupational needs.

EPILEPSY

The majority of adult patients with recurrent seizures acquire the tendency toward seizures during childhood. The seizures may represent the sequelae of disease processes which impinged on the brain in the distant past, or they may represent a familial genetic etiology. Seizures are generally much more common in childhood, and most childhood seizures disappear before adulthood. Certain types are peculiar to the earlier periods of life, depending on the occurrence of special diseases in these periods and the level of development of the nervous system. Others are identical in child and adult. The latter are discussed in Chaps. 12 and 342.

REFERENCES

ADAMS RD: Neurocutaneous diseases, in *Dermatology in General Medicine,* 3d ed, TB Fitzpatrick et al (eds). New York, McGraw-Hill, 1986

BAUMAN ML, KEMPER TL: The brain in infantile autism: A histoanatomic case report. Neurology 34(suppl 1):275, 1984

COHEN MF, DUFFNER PK: Prognostic indicators in hemiparetic cerebral palsy. Ann Neurol 9:353, 1981

COOPER IS: *Involuntary Movement Disorders.* New York, Hoeber-Harper, 1969

DOBBING J (ed): *Prevention of Spina Bifida and Other Neural Tube Defects.* London, Academic, 1983

GREENBERG AD: Atlantoaxial dislocations. Brain 91:655, 1968

HOLMES LB et al: *Mental Retardation: An Atlas of Disease with Associated Physical Abnormalities.* New York, Macmillan, 1972

McCUSICK VA: *Mendelian Inheritance in Man,* 6th ed. Baltimore, Johns Hopkins, 1983

MYERS RE: A unitary theory of causation of anoxic and hypoxic brain pathology. Adv Neurol 26:195, 1979

RICCARDI VM: Von Recklinghausen neurofibromatosis. N Engl J Med 305:1617, 1981

RITVO ER et al: Concordance for the syndrome of autism in 40 pairs of afflicted twins. Am J Psychiatry 142:1, Jan 1985

ROSENBERG RN: *Neurogenetics: Principles and Practice.* Raven Press, New York, 1986

SALAM M, ADAMS RD: Arnold-Chiari malformation, in *Handbook of Clinical Neurology.* Amsterdam, North-Holland, 1978

SWAIMAN KF, WRIGHT FS: *The Practice of Pediatric Neurology,* 2d ed., St. Louis, Mosby, 1982, 2 vols

352 DISEASES OF THE CRANIAL NERVES

MAURICE VICTOR / JOSEPH B. MARTIN

The cranial nerves are susceptible to disorders that rarely affect the spinal peripheral nerves, and for this reason deserve to be considered separately. This chapter describes the principal syndromes of disordered function and the diseases that cause them. Cranial nerve disorders of taste and smell, vision and ocular movement, and vertigo and deafness are also discussed in Chaps. 13, 14, and 19.

OLFACTORY NERVE

SYNDROME OF ANOSMIA AND AGEUSIA AND RELATED DISORDERS OF OLFACTION (See Chap. 19)

OPTIC NERVE

SYNDROME OF TRANSIENT MONOCULAR BLINDNESS (AMAUROSIS FUGAX) (See also Chap. 343)

Definition Amaurosis fugax is the name applied to an attack of transient, painless loss of vision in one eye. Frequently it is recurrent. (The term *amaurosis* refers to blindness from any cause, in distinction to *amblyopia,* which refers to a loss of vision from disease of structures other than the eye itself.)

Clinical manifestations Amaurosis fugax is a common clinical symptom indicative of transient retinal ischemia, usually associated with ipsilateral internal carotid artery stenosis or to embolism of the retinal arteries. In some cases the basis for the symptom cannot be discerned.

Typically, the episode of blindness evolves swiftly, in a matter of 10 to 15 s, and is described as a shade that falls smoothly and painlessly over the field until the eye is completely blind. Or, a similar obliteration of the visual field may occur from below. The blindness lasts for a few seconds or minutes, sometimes longer, then clears slowly and uniformly, the patient's vision returning in the reverse direction from that in which it was lost. Sometimes there is only a generalized dimness of vision, rather than a complete loss, or only a segment of the visual field may be involved. Many patients who experience amaurosis fugax on the basis of carotid stenosis also have transient attacks of contralateral hemiparesis, but it is uncommon for the eye and ipsilateral cerebral hemisphere to be clinically involved simultaneously. This is presumably due to the fact that showers of microemboli occur and block pial-size hemispheral vessels without causing clinical symptoms or signs. An abnormal EEG immediately after an attack of amaurosis fugax may be found.

Differential diagnosis The transient visual loss that accompanies migraine is of a different type. Often it begins with unformed flashes of light (photopsia) or dazzling zigzag lines (fortification spectra or terchopsia), which move across the visual field for several minutes, leaving scotomatous or hemianopic defects. The patient with migraine may complain of blindness in one eye, but examination usually shows the defects to be bilateral and homonymous, i.e., they occupy corresponding halves of both visual fields. The latter symptoms point to an origin in the visual cortex of one occipital lobe. In so-called vertebrobasilar migraine, in which the neurologic symptoms are referable to the territory of the basilar artery, the transient visual disturbances may occupy the whole of both visual fields.

Treatment Amaurosis fugax is most commonly a manifestation of ipsilateral internal carotid artery disease. Attention should be directed to carotid bruits, and noninvasive tests for carotid blood flow and lumen diameter should be carried out in every case. The decision of when to proceed to angiography is discussed in Chap. 343. Definitive treatment is dependent upon the results of these investigations. In the absence of carotid disease investigations should be directed toward excluding another source of emboli (cardiac or aorta). Amaurosis fugax may herald occlusion of the central retinal artery or anterior ischemic optic neuropathy due to giant cell arteritis or to nonarteritic (arteriosclerotic) disease. The sedimentation rate is usually elevated in giant cell arteritis (Chap. 269).

SYNDROME OF RETROBULBAR OPTIC NEUROPATHY OR NEURITIS **Definition** This syndrome is characterized by the rapid development over hours or days of impaired vision in one or both eyes. In the latter case the eyes may be affected either simultaneously or sequentially. The visual loss in idiopathic cases (i.e., when other causes of optic nerve lesions have been ruled out) is the result of acute demyelination of optic nerve fibers.

Clinical manifestations The most frequent setting is one in which a child, adolescent, or young adult notes a rapid diminution of vision in one eye (as though a veil or haze covered every object seen). The condition may progress to severe loss of vision (<20/100) within a few days but complete blindness is rare. The optic disc and retina may appear normal, but in some patients the optic disc is hyperemic and elevated with blurring of the disc margins (papillitis). Peripapillary hemorrhages are infrequently seen, and the veins are not engorged. *Papillitis* is distinguished from *papilledema* due to increased intracranial pressure by the acute and often marked reduction of visual acuity that accompanies the former. In retrobulbar neuropathy, characterized by a normal disc on initial examination, there is often pain on movement of the eye or on pressure on the globe. After a few days or weeks the other eye may become similarly involved, with loss, typically, of central vision but with some preservation of peripheral vision. The pupillary light reflex is impaired. In a high percentage of patients, no cause can be found, and after days or weeks there is spontaneous recovery of vision. In the majority of patients the visual acuity returns to normal or near normal within months of the attack. Sometimes a small central scotoma persists. The optic disc later becomes slightly pale due to atrophy, often most prominent in the temporal region. The CSF may be normal or may contain from 10 to 20 lymphocytes, and the protein content, particularly the gamma globulin portion, may be increased. Oligoclonal bands are found in some patients.

A considerable number of such patients (15 to 40 percent) will develop other symptoms and signs consistent with multiple sclerosis within 10 to 15 years, and even more will do so if the patients are observed for longer periods (see Chap. 348). Less is known about children with retrobulbar neuropathy, but the prognosis for them is considerably better than that for adults. Multiple sclerosis is the most common cause of a *unilateral retrobulbar neuritis*. Bilateral optic neuritis may occur a few days or weeks in advance of an attack of transverse myelitis. This combination is called neuromyelitis optica or Devic's disease (Chap. 348). Other causes of unilateral optic neuropathy include postinfectious or disseminated encephalomyelitis, posterior uveitis (sometimes with reticulum cell sarcoma), vascular lesions of the optic nerve, tumors (glioma of optic nerve, von Recklinghausen's neurofibromatosis, meningioma, metastatic carcinoma), and fungus infections.

Differential diagnosis *Anterior ischemic optic neuropathy* (*AION*) is a condition caused by interruption of blood supply to the optic nerve secondary to atherosclerotic or inflammatory disease of the ophthalmic artery or its branches. It presents clinically as acute, painless, visual loss in one eye, usually accompanied by an altitudinal visual field defect. In severe cases visual loss is complete and permanent. The fundus shows a pale swollen optic disc surrounded by splinter-shaped peripapillary hemorrhages. Occasionally only a section of the disc is pale and swollen. The macula and the retina are normal (see Fig. A4-6).

Investigations are directed toward excluding temporal arteritis (see Chap. 269). Rarely, microemboli can cause occlusion of the posterior ciliary arteries and AION; for example, following open heart or coronary artery bypass surgery.

Central retinal artery occlusion (*CRAO*) also presents with sudden blindness. In this entity the optic disc initially appears normal. The retina is infarcted and appears pale with accentuation of the macular cherry-red spot (see Fig. A4-2).

Treatment Acute optic neuropathy due to demyelination usually resolves without specific treatment. Severe visual loss is commonly treated with prednisone 40 to 80 mg daily in divided doses for 7 to 10 days with gradual tapering over a few days. Some physicians recommend ACTH treatment. Neither form of treatment has been proven to be more beneficial than no treatment.

TOXIC-NUTRITIONAL OPTIC NEUROPATHY Simultaneous impairment of vision in the two eyes, with central or centrocecal scotomas, occurring over a period of days or weeks, is usually due to a toxic or nutritional disorder rather than to a demyelinative process (see Chap. 349). Impairment of vision due to *methyl alcohol intoxication* is abrupt in onset and is characterized by large symmetric central scotomas, as well as by symptoms of systemic disease and acidosis (see Chap. 171). Here the lesion is in the optic nerve and the outer segments of the retina, the rods, and cones. Treatment is directed mainly to correction of the acidosis. Other drugs with proven but less devastating toxic effects on the optic nerve include chloramphenicol, ethambutol, isoniazid, streptomycin, sulfonamides, digitalis, ergot, disulfiram, and heavy metals.

Degenerative diseases may affect the retina or the optic nerves, taking the form of optic atrophy. There are several types of hereditary optic atrophy, the most frequent being the Leber type, which is sex-linked, occurring in males (see Chap. 350). An autosomal dominant form of congenital or early infantile optic atrophy and optic atrophy with diabetes mellitus and deafness are described. Senile macular degeneration and various forms of retinitis pigmentosa may cause visual loss (see Chap. 13).

SYNDROME OF BITEMPORAL HEMIANOPSIA This type of visual disorder is usually related to suprasellar extension of a pituitary adenoma (often with an enlarged sella), but may also be due to a craniopharyngioma, saccular aneurysm of the circle of Willis, meningioma of the tuberculum sellae (normal sella or thickened tuberculum by radiography), and rarely sarcoidosis, metastatic carcinoma, and Hand-Schüller-Christian disease (see Chap. 321). The lesion involves the decussating nasal fibers from each retina.

SYNDROMES OF HOMONYMOUS HEMIANOPSIA (See Chap. 13)

SYNDROME OF VISUAL AGNOSIA (See Chap. 24)

OCULOMOTOR, TROCHLEAR, AND ABDUCENS NERVES

SYNDROME OF OPHTHALMOPLEGIA The acute development of a sixth or third nerve palsy on one side is a relatively common occurrence in the adult, the former being about twice as common as the latter. An isolated sixth nerve palsy frequently proves to be due to diabetes mellitus, neoplasm, or increased intracranial pressure. Involvement of the third, fourth, and sixth cranial nerves may occur with lesions affecting their nuclei or fibers of exit in the pons or mesencephalon, or in the course of the nerves through the subarachnoid space, the cavernous sinus, and the superior orbital fissure. Different syndromes occur with lesions at each of these sites (Table 352-1). Pontine glioma in children and metastatic tumor from the nasopharynx in adults may cause isolated sixth nerve lesions. Tumor at the base of the brain (primary, metastatic, meningeal carcinomatosis) is an important cause of isolated third nerve palsies. Other causes of sixth and third nerve palsies are trauma, ischemic infarction of nerve, and aneurysms of the circle of Willis. An acute palsy of the fourth nerve is relatively uncommon; usually it is due to trauma. In all cases of isolated ocular motor paralysis, exophthalmic ophthalmoplegia (Graves' disease) and myasthenia gravis must be ruled out. In third nerve lesions due to compression by aneurysm, tumor, or temporal lobe herniation, enlargement of the pupil is an early sign because of the peripheral location of the pupilloconstrictor fibers. Infarction of the third nerve, associated with pain in or around the eye, as occurs in diabetes mellitus or, rarely, in cranial arteritis, usually spares the pupil. In cases of undetermined cause, continued observation is essential to confirm recovery or to prompt reinvestigation.

Rarely, children or adults may have one or more attacks of ocular palsy in conjunction with an otherwise typical migraine (*migrainous ophthalmoplegia*). The muscles innervated by the oculomotor nerve, less often by the abducens nerve, are affected. Presumably, intense vascular spasm affecting the nutrient artery to the nerve causes transitory ischemia. Arteriograms, done after the onset of the palsy, usually reveal no abnormality. Recovery is the rule.

Combined unilateral ocular palsies of painful type (Tolosa-Hunt syndrome) is most often indicative of parasellar granuloma. An acute onset of unilateral or bilateral ophthalmoplegia and drowsiness occurs in pituitary apoplexy. Visual loss and signs of chiasmal compression may be associated. The slow development of a complete ophthalmoplegia on one side is most often due to an enlarging aneurysm (it may also be of acute onset), tumor, or inflammatory process in the cavernous sinus or at the superior orbital foramen. This is known as the *syndrome of Foix* (see Table 352-1). Such a syndrome frequently presents first with affection of the sixth nerve.

Gaze palsies or mixed ophthalmoplegia and gaze palsies, due usually to vascular, demyelinative, or neoplastic processes in the brainstem, are discussed in Chap. 13.

TRIGEMINAL NERVE

The trigeminal nerve supplies sensation to the skin of the face and half of the vertex of the skull and motor innervation to the masseter and pterygoid masticatory muscles.

SYNDROME OF PAROXYSMAL FACIAL PAIN (TRIGEMINAL NEURALGIA, TIC DOULOUREUX) Definition The most striking disorder of the trigeminal nerve is tic douloureux, a condition consisting of excruciating paroxysms of pain in the lips, gums, cheek, or chin, and, very rarely, in the distribution of the ophthalmic division of the fifth nerve. The disorder occurs almost exclusively in middle-aged and elderly persons. The pain seldom lasts more than a few seconds or a minute or two but may be so intense that the patient winces, hence the term *tic*. The paroxysms recur frequently, both day and night, for several weeks at a time. Another characteristic feature is the initiation of pain by obvious stimuli applied to certain areas on the face, lips, or tongue (the so-called trigger zones) or by movement of these parts. Sensory loss cannot be demonstrated. In studying the relations between stimuli applied to the trigger zone and the paroxysm of pain, it is found that the adequate stimulus for precipitating an attack is a tactile one and possibly tickle, rather than a noxious or thermal stimulus. Usually a spatial and temporal summation of impulses is necessary to trigger an attack, which is followed by a refractory period of up to 2 or 3 min.

The diagnosis of this disorder rests upon these strict clinical criteria, and the condition must be distinguished from other forms of facial and cephalic neuralgia and pain arising from diseases of the jaw, teeth, or sinuses. Tic douloureux is usually without assignable cause; occasionally it is a manifestation of multiple sclerosis when it appears in younger adults and may be bilateral. Very rarely it may occur with herpes zoster or a tumor. To a degree that remains uncertain and controversial, pain of tic douloureux may be caused by a redundant or torturous artery in the posterior fossa, causing an irritative lesion of the nerve or its root. Usually, however, space-occupying lesions, such as aneurysms, neurofibromas, or meningiomas affecting the nerve, produce a loss of sensation (trigeminal neuropathy).

TABLE 352-1 Cranial nerve syndromes

Site	Cranial nerves involved	Eponymic syndrome	Usual cause
Sphenoid fissure (superior orbital)	III, IV, first division V, VI	Foix	Invasive tumors of sphenoid bone, aneurysms
Lateral wall of cavernous sinus	III, IV, first division V, VI, often with proptosis	Foix Tolosa-Hunt	Aneurysms or thrombosis of cavernous sinus, invasive tumors from sinuses and sella turcica, sometimes benign granuloma responsive to steroids
Retrosphenoid space	II, III, IV, V, VI	Jacod	Large tumors of middle cranial fossa
Apex of petrous bone	V, VI	Gradenigo	Petrositis, tumors of petrous bone
Internal auditory meatus	VII, VIII		Tumors of petrous bone (dermoids, etc.), infectious processes, acoustic neuroma
Pontocerebellar angle	V, VII, VIII, and sometimes IX		Acoustic neuroma, meningioma
Jugular foramen	IX, X, XI	Vernet	Tumors and aneurysms
Posterior laterocondylar space	IX, X, XI, XII	Collet-Sicard	Tumors of parotid gland, carotid body, and metastatic tumor
Posterior retroparotid space	IX, X, XI, XII and Horner syndrome	Villaret Mackenzie Tapia	Tumors of parotid gland, carotid body, metastatic tumor, lymph node tumors, tuberculous adenitis

Treatment The initial treatment of tic douloureux is pharmacologic. Carbamazepine is the drug of choice and is effective initially in 75 percent of patients. Unfortunately, up to one-third cannot tolerate the drug in the doses required to alleviate pain. Carbamazepine should be started gradually, 100 mg with food, as a single dose, and increased to 200 mg qid. Doses greater than 1200 to 1600 mg provide no additional benefit.

If drug treatment fails, surgical therapy should be offered. The two primary operations are gangliolysis and suboccipital craniectomy with decompression of the trigeminal nerve. Gangliolysis is a minor surgical procedure performed by transcutaneous injection, usually under local anesthesia. Glycerol or alcohol injection or radiofrequency lesions have been widely used. Glycerol injections have proved beneficial in many patients, but onset of effect is slow and pain may recur. Radiofrequency lesions abolish pain in 80 percent of cases for 1 year and 60 percent for 5 years. The procedure results in partial numbness of the face and carries a risk of corneal denervation with secondary keratitis when used for first division trigeminal neuralgia.

Suboccipital craniectomy is a major procedure requiring about 1 week of hospitalization. It has an 80 percent efficacy but is accompanied by a 5 percent major complication rate. Not all patients operated upon have a demonstrated vascular or other compression lesion of the trigeminal nerve. The most troublesome complication of all surgical treatments is the development of anesthesia dolorosa or denervation hypersensitivity. This condition responds poorly to treatment. Tricyclic antidepressants or phenothiazines are usually given with only partial success in alleviating the discomfort.

TRIGEMINAL NEUROPATHY A variety of rare causes of trigeminal neuropathy in addition to those mentioned above may be found. Most present with sensory loss on the face or with weakness of the jaw muscles. Deviation of the jaw on opening indicates weakness of the pterygoids of the side to which the jaw deviates. Tumors of the middle cranial fossa (meningiomas), of the trigeminal nerve (schwannomas), or of the base of the skull (metastatic) may cause a combination of motor and sensory signs. Lesions in the cavernous sinus can affect the first and second divisions of the trigeminal nerve, and lesions of the superior orbital fissure can affect the ophthalmic first division. The accompanying corneal anesthesia increases the risk of ulceration (neurokeratitis).

Anesthesia and analgesia of the face have been reported after treatment with stilbamidine (formerly used in the treatment of kala azar and multiple myeloma). Pain and itching may occur during recovery. Rarely, an idiopathic form of trigeminal neuropathy is observed. It is characterized by feelings of numbness and paresthesias, sometimes bilaterally, and loss of sensation but without weakness of the jaw. Recovery is the rule, but the symptoms may be troublesome for many months, or even years. Leprosy may involve the trigeminal nerves.

Tonic spasm of the masticatory muscles, known as *trismus*, is symptomatic of tetanus. It may also occur as an idiosyncratic reaction in patients treated with phenothiazine drugs; lesser degrees may be associated with disease of the pharynx, temporomaxillary joint, teeth, and gums.

FACIAL NERVE

SYNDROMES OF FACIAL PALSY AND FACIAL SPASM The seventh cranial nerve supplies all the muscles concerned with facial expression. The sensory component is small (the nervus intermedius of Wrisberg); it conveys taste sensation from the anterior two-thirds of the tongue and probably cutaneous impulses from the anterior wall of the external auditory canal. The motor nucleus of the seventh nerve lies anterior and lateral to the abducens nucleus. After leaving the pons the seventh nerve enters the internal auditory meatus with the acoustic nerve. The nerve continues its course through the middle ear to exit from the skull via the stylomastoid foramen. It then passes through the parotid gland and subdivides to supply the facial muscles.

A complete interruption of the facial nerve at the stylomastoid foramen paralyzes all muscles of facial expression. The corner of the mouth droops, the creases and skin folds are effaced, the forehead is unfurrowed, and the eyelids will not close. Upon attempted closure of the lids, the eye on the paralyzed side is seen to roll upward (Bell's phenomenon). The lower lid sags also, and the punctum falls away from the conjunctiva, permitting tears to spill over the cheek. Food collects between the teeth and lips, and saliva may dribble from the corner of the mouth. The patient complains of a heaviness or numbness in the face, but no sensory loss is demonstrable and taste is intact.

If the lesion is in the middle ear portion, taste is lost over the anterior two-thirds of the tongue on the same side. If the nerve to the stapedius is interrupted, there is hyperacusis (painful sensitivity to loud sounds). Lesions in the internal auditory meatus may also affect the adjacent auditory and vestibular nerves, causing deafness, tinnitus, or dizziness. Intrapontine lesions that paralyze the face usually affect the abducens nucleus and often the corticospinal and sensory tracts.

If the peripheral facial paralysis has existed for some time and recovery of motor function has begun but is incomplete, a kind of contracture (actually a continuous diffuse contraction) of facial muscles may appear (hemifacial spasm). The palpebral fissure becomes narrowed and the nasolabial fold deepens. With the passage of time, the face and even the tip of the nose become pulled to the unaffected side. Attempts to move one group of facial muscles result in contraction of all of them (associated movements, or *synkinesis*). Facial spasms may develop and persist indefinitely, being initiated by every facial movement (see below). Anomalous regeneration of the seventh nerve fibers may result in other curious disorders. If fibers originally connected with the orbicularis oculi come to innervate the orbicularis oris, closure of the lids may cause a retraction of the mouth; or if fibers originally connected with muscles of the face later innervate the lacrimal gland, anomalous tearing (crocodile tears) may occur with any activity of the facial muscles, such as eating. Yet another unusual facial synkinesia is one in which jaw opening causes a closure of the eyelids on the side of the facial palsy (jaw-winking).

BELL'S PALSY **Definition** The most common form of facial paralysis is idiopathic, i.e., *Bell's palsy*. The incidence rate of this disorder is about 23 per 100,000 annually, or about 1 in 60 or 70 persons in a lifetime. The pathogenesis of the paralysis is unknown. The few autopsied cases of this disease have shown only nondescript changes in the facial nerve and not inflammatory changes, as is commonly presumed.

Clinical manifestations The onset of Bell's palsy is fairly abrupt, maximum weakness being attained by 48 h as a general rule. Pain behind the ear may precede the paralysis for a day or two. Occasionally taste sensation is lost, and hyperacusis may be present. In some cases there is mild CSF pleocytosis. Fully 80 percent of patients recover within a few weeks or months. Electromyographic evidence of denervation after 10 days indicates that there has been axonal degeneration and that there will be a long delay before regeneration occurs, and that it may be incomplete. Electromyography may be of value in distinguishing a temporary conduction defect from a pathologic interruption in the continuity of nerve fibers. The presence of incomplete paralysis in the first week is the most favorable prognostic sign.

Treatment Protection of the eye during sleep, massage of the weakened muscles, and a splint to prevent drooping of the lower part of the face are the measures generally employed in the management of such cases. A course of prednisone beginning with 60 to 80 mg daily during the first 5 days and then tapered over the next 5 days may be beneficial. Unroofing of the facial nerve in the facial canal has been suggested, but there is no evidence that this measure is helpful, and it may be harmful.

Differential diagnosis There are many other causes of facial palsy. Tumors which invade the temporal bone (carotid body, cholesteatoma, dermoid) may produce a facial palsy, but the onset is insidious and the course progressive. The *Ramsay Hunt syndrome,* presumably due to herpes zoster of the geniculate ganglion, consists of a severe facial palsy associated with a vesicular eruption in the pharynx, external auditory canal, and other parts of the cranial integument; often the eighth cranial nerve is affected as well. Acoustic neuromas frequently involve the facial nerve by local compression (see Chap. 345). Infarcts and tumors are the common pontine lesions which may interrupt the facial nerve fibers. Bilateral facial paralysis (facial diplegia) occurs in acute inflammatory polyradiculoneuritis (Guillain-Barré disease) and in a variety of sarcoidosis known as *uveoparotid fever* (*Heerfordt's syndrome*). The *Melkersson-Rosenthal syndrome* consists of a rarely encountered triad of recurrent facial paralysis, recurrent—and eventually permanent—facial (particularly labial) edema, and less constantly, plication of the tongue. Many causes of this syndrome have been suggested, but none has been established. Leprosy frequently involves the facial nerve.

A puzzling disorder is the *facial hemiatrophy of Romberg*. It occurs mainly in females and is characterized by a disappearance of fat in the dermal and subcutaneous tissues on one side of the face. It usually begins in adolescence or early adult years and is slowly progressive. In its advanced form the face is gaunt and the skin is thin, wrinkled, and rather brown. The facial hair may turn white and fall out, and the sebaceous glands become atrophic. The muscles and bones are not involved as a rule. Sometimes the atrophy becomes bilateral. The condition is a form of lipodystrophy, and the localization within a dermatome suggests a disorder of some neural trophic factor of unknown nature. The treatment is transplantation of skin and subcutaneous fat by a plastic surgeon.

The facial muscles on one side may be affected by irregular clonic contractions of varying degree (*hemifacial spasm*). This condition may represent a transient or permanent sequela to a Bell's palsy but may also appear de novo, as a benign phenomenon in adults. Hemifacial spasm may also be due to an irritative lesion of the facial nerve (e.g., an acoustic neuroma, an aberrant artery which compresses the nerve and is relieved by surgery, or a basilar artery aneurysm). However, in the most common form of hemifacial spasm, the cause and pathology are unknown. A fine fibrillary activity of the facial muscles (*facial myokymia*) may be caused by a plaque of multiple sclerosis. An involuntary recurrent spasm of both eyelids (*blepharospasm*) may occur in elderly persons as an isolated phenomenon or with varying degrees of spasm of the facial muscles. Relaxant and sedative drugs are of little help, although in many patients this disorder subsides spontaneously. In very severe and persistent cases, an effective treatment has been differential facial nerve section of selected branches of the nerve or nerve decompression (from vessels) intracranially. More recently, cases have been successfully treated by local injection of botulinum toxin into the eyelids.

Abnormalities of taste are discussed in Chap. 19.

All these forms of nuclear or peripheral facial palsy must be distinguished from the supranuclear type. In the latter the frontalis and orbicularis oculi muscles are involved less than those of the lower part of the face, since the upper facial muscles are innervated by corticobulbar pathways from both motor cortices, whereas the lower facial muscles are innervated only by the opposite hemisphere. In supranuclear lesions there may be a dissociation of emotional and voluntary facial movements, and often some degree of paralysis of the arm and leg or an aphasia (in dominant hemisphere lesions) is conjoined.

VESTIBULAR NERVE

The eighth cranial nerve has two components, vestibular and auditory. Symptoms and signs of involvement of the vestibular portion are discussed in Chap. 14 and in this section. The auditory nerve and its disorders are discussed in Chap. 19.

SYNDROME OF BENIGN RECURRENT VERTIGO **Ménière's syndrome** DEFINITION AND CLINICAL MANIFESTATIONS Ménière's disease, or Ménière's syndrome, is the name applied to recurrent vertigo accompanied by tinnitus and deafness. The latter symptoms may be absent during the initial attack(s) of vertigo, but they invariably appear as the disease progresses and are increased in severity during an acute attack. With milder forms of the syndrome the patient may complain more of head discomfort, slight instability, and difficulty in concentration than of vertigo and may be considered to be anxious or depressed. Provided that deafness is not complete, the recruitment phenomenon can be demonstrated (see Chap. 19).

Ménière's disease has its onset most frequently in the fifth decade of life, though younger adults and the elderly are not spared. The pathologic changes are said to consist of a dilatation of the endolymphatic system which leads to a degeneration of the delicate vestibular and cochlear hair cells. The relation of these pathologic changes to the paroxysmal disorder of labyrinthine function is unknown.

TREATMENT During an acute attack, rest in bed is the most effective treatment, since the patient can usually find a position in which vertigo is minimal. Dimenhydrinate, cyclizine, or meclizine in doses of 25 to 50 mg tid is useful in the more protracted cases. A low-salt diet is still used in treatment, but its value is difficult to judge. Mild sedative drugs may help the anxious patient between attacks. Usually the deafness is unilateral and progressive, and when it is complete, the vertiginous attacks cease. However, the course is variable, and if the attacks persist in a severe manner, permanent relief can be obtained by surgical destruction of the labyrinth or section of the vestibular portion of the eighth nerve intracranially.

Benign positional vertigo Another disorder of labyrinthine function is characterized by the occurrence of paroxysmal vertigo and nystagmus with the assumption of certain critical positions of the head. This is the positional vertigo of Bárány, of the so-called benign paroxysmal type (see Chap. 14). In refractory cases, in which attacks continue, vestibular exercises, as outlined by Lee, may be beneficial.

Differential diagnosis of vertigo There are many other causes of acute vertigo, such as purulent labyrinthitis complicating meningitis, serous labyrinthitis due to infection of the middle ear, "toxic labyrinthitis" due to drug intoxication (e.g., with alcohol, quinine, streptomycin, gentamicin, and other antibiotics), motion sickness, trauma, and hemorrhage into the internal ear. In these instances the attacks of vertigo tend to last longer than in the recurrent form, but in other respects the symptoms are similar. Streptomycin or gentamicin may damage the fine hair cells of the vestibular end organs and cause a permanent disorder of equilibrium (as well as hearing), especially in older patients.

There has been described a dramatic clinical syndrome, characterized by the abrupt onset of severe vertigo, nausea, and vomiting, without tinnitus or hearing loss. The vertigo persists for several days or weeks, and labyrinthine function is permanently ablated on one side. Occlusion of the labyrinthine division of the internal auditory artery would logically explain this syndrome, but pathologic or angiographic confirmation of this hypothesis has so far not been obtained.

Vertigo of vestibular nerve origin may occur with diseases that involve the nerve in the petrous bone or the cerebellopontine angle. Except that it is less severe and is less frequently paroxysmal, it has many of the characteristics of labyrinthine vertigo. The adjacent auditory division of the eighth cranial nerve may also be affected, which explains the frequent association of vertigo with tinnitus and deafness. The function of the eighth cranial nerve may be disturbed by tumors of the lateral recess (especially acoustic neuroma), less frequently by meningeal inflammation in this region and rarely, by an abnormal vessel which compresses the nerve.

Vestibular neuronitis and *benign recurrent vertigo* are the names that have been applied to a clinical syndrome which occurs mainly in middle-aged and young adults (sometimes in children) and is characterized by the abrupt onset of vertigo, nausea, and vomiting, without impairment of hearing. The attacks are brief and leave the patient for some days with a mild positional vertigo. They may occur only once or recur in varying degrees of severity. The cause is unknown. The medical treatment is the same as for Ménière's disease.

A particular variety of paroxysmal vertigo affects children. The attacks occur in a setting of good health and are of sudden onset and brief duration. Pallor, sweating, and immobility are prominent manifestations, and occasionally vomiting and nystagmus occur. No relation to posture or movement of the head has been observed. The attacks are recurrent but tend to cease spontaneously after a period of several months or years. The outstanding abnormal finding is demonstrated by caloric testing, which shows impairment or loss of vestibular function, bilateral or unilateral, frequently persisting after the attacks have ceased; cochlear function is unimpaired, however. The pathologic basis of this disorder has not been determined.

Cogan has described a peculiar syndrome in young adults, in which an interstitial keratitis is associated with vertigo, tinnitus, nystagmus, and rapidly progressive deafness. The prognosis for life and vision is good, but the deafness is usually permanent. The cause or pathogenesis of this disease is not understood, although several patients have later developed aortitis and a vasculitis that resembles periarteritis nodosa.

GLOSSOPHARYNGEAL NERVE

SYNDROME OF GLOSSOPHARYNGEAL NEURALGIA Glossopharyngeal neuralgia resembles trigeminal neuralgia in many respects. The pain is intense and paroxysmal; it originates in the throat, approximately in the tonsillar fossa. In some cases the pain is localized in the ear or may radiate from the throat to the ear, because of implication of the tympanic branch of the glossopharyngeal nerve (Jacobson's nerve). Spasms of pain may be initiated by swallowing. There is no demonstrable sensory or motor deficit. Cardiac symptoms of bradycardia with hypotension are reported. A trial of carbamazepine or phenytoin is the recommended therapy, but if this is unsuccessful, division of the glossopharyngeal nerve near the medulla is the definitive treatment.

Very rarely, herpes zoster may involve the glossopharyngeal nerve. Glossopharyngeal neuropathy in conjunction with vagus and accessory nerve palsies may occur due to a tumor or aneurysm in the posterior fossa or in the jugular foramen. Hoarseness due to vocal cord paralysis, some difficulty in swallowing, deviation of the soft palate to the intact side, anesthesia of the posterior wall of the pharynx, and weakness of the upper part of the trapezius and sternocleidomastoid muscles make up the syndrome (see Table 352-1, jugular foramen syndrome).

VAGUS NERVE

SYNDROME OF DYSPHAGIA AND DYSPHONIA Complete interruption of the intracranial portion of one vagus nerve results in a characteristic paralysis. The soft palate droops ipsilaterally and does not rise in phonation. There is loss of the gag reflex on the affected side, as well as the "curtain movement" of the lateral wall of the pharynx, whereby the faucial pillars move medially as the palate rises in saying "ah." The voice is hoarse, slightly nasal, and the vocal cord lies immobile in the cadaveric position, i.e., midway between abduction and adduction. There may also be a loss of sensibility at the external auditory meatus and back of the pinna. Usually no change in visceral function can be demonstrated.

Complete interruption of both vagi is said to be incompatible with life, and this is probably true if the nuclei are involved in the medulla by poliomyelitis or some other disease. However, in the cervical region, both vagi have been blocked with procaine (Novocain) for the treatment of intractable asthma, without mishap. The pharyngeal branches of both vagi may be affected in diphtheria; the voice has a nasal quality, and regurgitation of liquids through the nose occurs during the act of swallowing.

The vagus nerve may be implicated at the meningeal level by neoplastic and infectious processes and within the medulla by tumors and vascular lesions, e.g., the lateral medullary syndrome of Wallenberg, and by motor neuron disease. This nerve may be involved by the inflammatory lesion of herpes zoster. Polymyositis and dermatomyositis, which cause hoarseness and dysphagia by direct involvement of laryngeal and pharyngeal muscles, may be confused with diseases of the vagus nerves. Also dysphagia is a symptom in some patients with myotonic dystrophy (see Chap. 32 for discussion of nonneurologic forms of dysphagia).

The recurrent laryngeal nerves, especially the left, are most often damaged as a result of intrathoracic disease. Aneurysm of the aortic arch, an enlarged left atrium, and tumors of the mediastinum and bronchi are much more frequent causes of an isolated vocal cord palsy than are intracranial disorders.

When confronted with a case of laryngeal palsy, the physician must attempt to determine the site of the lesion. If it is intramedullary, there are usually other signs, such as ipsilateral cerebellar dysfunction, loss of pain and temperature sensation over the ipsilateral face and contralateral arm and leg, and an ipsilateral Horner's syndrome. If the lesion is extramedullary, the glossopharyngeal and spinal accessory nerves are frequently involved (see discussion of the jugular foramen syndrome above). If it is extracranial in the posterior laterocondylar or retroparotid space, there may be a combination of ninth, tenth, eleventh, and twelfth cranial nerve palsies and a Horner's syndrome. Combinations of these lower cranial nerve palsies have a variety of eponymic designations, listed in Table 352-1. If there is no sensory loss over the palate and pharynx and no palatal weakness or dysphagia, the lesion is below the origin of the pharyngeal branches, which leave the vagus nerve high in the cervical region; the usual site of disease is then the mediastinum.

HYPOGLOSSAL NERVE

The twelfth cranial nerve supplies the ipsilateral muscles of the tongue. Lesions affecting the motor nucleus may occur in the brainstem (tumor, poliomyelitis, or motor neuron disease) during the course of the nerve in the posterior fossa, or in the hypoglossal canal. Isolated lesions of unknown cause can occur. Atrophy and fasciculation of the tongue develop weeks to months after interruption of the nerve.

MULTIPLE CRANIAL NERVE PALSIES

Several cranial nerves may be affected by the same disease process. In this situation, the main clinical problem is to determine whether the lesion lies within the brainstem or outside of it. Lesions that lie on the surface of the brainstem are featured by involvement of adjacent cranial nerves (often occurring in succession) and late and rather slight involvement of the long sensory and motor pathways and segmental structures lying within the brainstem. The opposite is true of intramedullary, intrapontine, and intramesencephalic lesions. The extramedullary lesion is more likely to cause bone erosion or enlargement of the foramens of exit of cranial nerves. The intramedullary lesion involving cranial nerves often produces a crossed sensory or motor paralysis (cranial nerve signs on one side of the body and tract signs on the opposite side).

Involvement of multiple cranial nerves outside the brainstem is frequently the result of trauma (sudden onset), localized infections such as herpes zoster (acute onset), granulomatous disease such as Wegener's granulomatosis (subacute onset), Behçet's disease, or tumors and enlarging saccular aneurysms (chronic development). Of the tumors, neurofibromas, meningiomas, chordomas, cholesteatomas, carcinomas, and sarcomas have all been observed to implicate a succession of lower cranial nerves. Owing to their anatomic relationships, the multiple cranial nerve palsies form a number of distinctive syndromes, listed in Table 352-1. Sarcoidosis has been found to be the cause of some cases of multiple cranial neuropathy, and chronic glandular tuberculosis (scrofula) the cause of a few others. Malignant granuloma of the nasopharynx may also affect mutilple cranial nerves, as do nasopharyngeal tumors, platybasia, and basilar invagination of the skull, and the Arnold-Chiari malformation that becomes evident in adult life. A purely motor disorder without atrophy always raises the question of myasthenia gravis (see Chap. 358). Guillain-Barré syndrome commonly affects the facial nerves bilaterally (facial diplegia). In the Miller Fisher variant of the Guillain-Barré syndrome oculomotor paresis occurs with ataxia and areflexia in the limbs. Wernicke's encephalopathy can cause a severe ophthalmoplegia combined with brainstem signs (see Chap. 349).

A benign idiopathic form of multiple cranial nerve involvement on one or both sides of the face is occasionally seen. The disease may recur over a period of years with variable degrees of recovery between attacks. The condition is called *polyneuritis cranialis multiplex*.

REFERENCES

ADAMS RD, VICTOR M: *Principles of Neurology*, 3d ed. New York, McGraw-Hill, 1985

ALEXANDER GE, MOSES H: Carbamazepine for hemifacial spasm. Neurology 32:286, 1982

BRODAL A: The cranial nerves, in *Neurological Anatomy in Relation to Clinical Medicine*, 3d ed. New York, Oxford, 1980, chap 7, pp 448–577

BROWNSTONE PK et al: Bilateral superior laryngeal neuralgia. Arch Neurol 37:525, 1980

COGAN DG: *Neurology of the Ocular Muscles*, 2d ed. Springfield, Ill, Charles C Thomas, 1956

———: *Neurology of the Visual System*. Springfield, Ill, Charles C Thomas, 1966

DURELLI L et al: The Melkersson-Rosenthal syndrome: A case with increased CNS IgG synthesis. Ann Neurol 18:623, 1985

EISEN A, BERTRAND G: Isolated accessory nerve palsy of spontaneous origin: A clinical and electromyographic study. Arch Neurol 27:496, 1972

GLASER JS: Heredofamilial disorders of the optic nerve, in *Genetic and Metabolic Eye Diseases*, MF Goldberg (ed). Boston, Little, Brown, 1974

———: *Neuro-ophthalmology*. Hagerstown, Harper & Row, 1978

GROVES J: Bell's (idiopathic) facial palsy, in *Scientific Foundations of Otolaryngology*, R Hinchcliffe, D Harrison (eds). London, Heinemann, 1976, pp 446–459

HAUSER WA et al: Incidence and prognosis of Bell's palsy in the population of Rochester, Minnesota. Mayo Clin Proc 46:258, 1971

KARNES WE: Diseases of the seventh cranial nerve, in *Peripheral Neuropathy*, 2d ed, PJ Dyck et al (eds). Philadelphia, Saunders, 1984, chap 55, pp 1266–1299

KAYE AH, ADAMS CBT: Hemifacial spasm: A long-term follow-up of patients treated by posterior fossa surgery and nerve wrapping. J Neurol Neurosurg Psychiatry 44:1100, 1981

LIEBOLD JE: Drugs having a toxic effect on the optic nerve. Intern Ophthalmol Clin 11:137, 1970

LOESER J: Trigeminal and glossopharyngeal neuralgia, in *Current Therapy in Neurologic Disease*, RT Johnson (ed). Philadelphia, BC Decker, 1985/1986, pp 86–89

ZEE D: Vertigo, in *Current Therapy in Neurologic Disease*, RT Johnson (ed). Philadelphia, BC Decker 1985/86, pp 8–13

353 DISEASES OF THE SPINAL CORD

ALLAN H. ROPPER / JOSEPH B. MARTIN

Diseases of the spinal cord are frequently devastating, causing permanent and severe neurologic disability. Small lesions can produce quadriplegia, paraplegia, and sensory deficits far beyond the damage they would inflict elsewhere in the nervous system because the spinal cord contains, in a small cross-sectional area, almost the entire motor output and sensory input systems. Many diseases, particularly extrinsic cord compression, are reversible, making acute spinal cord lesions among the most critical of neurologic emergencies.

The spinal cord is organized in a stereotyped fashion, innervating the limbs and trunk segmentally through 31 pairs of spinal nerves, making anatomic diagnosis relatively straightforward. A sensory level, paraplegia, or other typical syndromes usually permit recognition of a spinal cord process. Full assessment of cord disease requires a careful examination supplemented by laboratory tests, including magnetic resonance imaging (MRI), computerized tomography (CT) scanning, often myelography, analysis of cerebrospinal fluid (CSF), and somatosensory evoked responses. Most deficiencies in evaluating patients with signs of spinal cord disease result from cursory physical examination or inadequate x-rays. Computerized tomography and MRI are replacing conventional myelography because of their ease of performance and better resolution; MRI gives particularly valuable information about intrinsic cord structure.

SPINAL COLUMN AND SPINAL CORD ANATOMY RELEVANT TO CLINICAL SIGNS The spinal cord is organized in a uniform somatotopic fashion throughout its length giving rise to easily identifiable syndromes (see Chaps. 3, 15, and 18). The longitudinal location of lesions is established by the uppermost level of sensory and motor dysfunction. However, the relationship between the vertebral bodies of the spinal column (or their surface markers, the vertebral spines) and the cord segments that underline them complicates anatomic interpretation of signs of spinal cord diseases. Spinal cord syndromes are described according to the spinal cord segment affected rather than the surrounding vertebrae. During embryologic development the growth of the cord lags behind that of the spinal column, so that the cord ends behind the first lumbar vertebral body and nerve roots must take an increasingly oblique downward course to exit near their targets in the limbs or viscera. A useful rule is that the cervical roots (except C8) exit from neural foramina above their respective vertebral bodies, while thoracic and lumbar roots exit below each body. The upper cervical cord segments lie behind the same numbered vertebral body, whereas the lower cervical segments are located one above each corresponding vertebral body, the upper thoracic cord two segments higher, and the lower thoracic cord three segments higher. The lumbar and sacral cord segments, the latter forming the conus medullaris, are located behind the ninth thoracic to first lumbar vertebrae. In judging encroachment by various extrinsic masses, particularly spondylosis, careful measurement of the sagittal diameters of the spinal canal is important; they are normally 16 to 22 mm in the cervical and thoracic spine, 15 to 23 mm from L1 to L3, and 16 to 27 mm below.

CLINICAL SYNDROMES OF SPINAL CORD DISEASE The principal clinical signs of spinal cord damage are loss of sensation below a circumferential horizontal line on the trunk, a "sensory level," and weakness in the extremities innervated by the descending corticospinal fibers. Sensory symptoms, particularly paresthesias, may begin in the feet (or in one foot) and ascend, giving the impression early on of a polyneuropathy before a static sensory level is apparent. Lesions that disrupt descending corticospinal and bulbospinal tracts at a single cord level cause paraplegia or quadriplegia, with the characteristics of increased muscle tone, exaggerated deep tendon reflexes, and Babinski signs. A careful examination often also elicits segmental signs such as a band of altered sensation at the rostral extent of the sensory level (hyperalgesia or hyperpathia), and flaccidity, atrophy, or isolated diminished deep tendon reflexes. The sensory level and segmental signs are approximate indicators of the location of a transverse lesion. Midline back pain is often an accurate localizing sign, particularly in the thoracic region, where interscapular pain may be the first sign of cord compression. Radicular pain that marks the primary site of a more laterally placed spinal lesion may also occur. Pain from lower cord (conus medullaris) lesions is often referred to the low back.

Early in the course of an acute transverse lesion there may be flaccidity of the limbs rather than spasticity, due to so-called spinal shock. This state may last for several weeks and be mistaken for extensive segmental damage, but the reflexes later become increased. Brief clonic or myoclonic limb movements often precede paralysis in acute transverse lesions, particularly those due to infarction. Autonomic dysfunction, mainly urinary retention, is another prominent sign in transverse spinal lesions and should call attention to cord disease if it occurs in conjunction with spasticity or a sensory level.

Much is made of the clinical distinction between intramedullary (within the cord) and extramedullary compressive lesions, but most rules are approximations, not distinguishing dependably one from the other. Features said to favor extramedullary lesions include radicular pain; a Brown-Séquard hemicord syndrome (see below); lower motor neuron signs in one or two segments, often asymmetric; early corticospinal signs; marked sacral sensory loss; and early, prominent CSF abnormalities. On the other hand, poorly localized burning pain, dissociated loss of pain sensation with sparing of joint position sensation, sparing of sensation in the perineal and sacral areas, late and less prominent corticospinal signs, and normal or minimally altered CSF generally favor an intramedullary lesion. "Sacral sparing" refers to the preservation of pinprick and temperature sensation in the sacral dermatomes, usually S3 to S5 with rostral areas up to the sensory level affected. This is usually a dependable sign of intrinsic cord disease damaging the innermost fibers of the spinothalamic tracts while sparing those placed more laterally which subserve sacral sensation. The *Brown-Séquard syndrome* is an eponym given to a hemicord syndrome consisting of ipsilateral mono- or hemiplegia, accompanied by joint position and vibration sense loss, associated with contralateral pain and temperature (spinothalamic) sensory loss. The segmental level for pain and temperature loss is sometimes one or two levels below the anatomic lesion, a result of the course of sensory fibers which ascend and cross to the opposite spinothalamic tract after synapsing in the dorsal horn. Segmental signs, such as radicular pain, muscle atrophy, or decreased tendon reflexes when they occur, are often unilateral.

Lesions limited to, or primarily occurring within, the central portion of the cord preferentially damage gray matter neurons and segmental tracts crossing at that level. Traumatic contusion, developmental syringomyelia, tumors, and vascular lesions in the territory of the anterior spinal artery are the most common lesions localized to the central cord. In the cervical cord, the central cord syndrome gives arm weakness out of proportion to leg weakness, and a "dissociated" sensory loss signifying analgesia (loss of pin sensation)—in a cape distribution over the shoulders and lower neck—without anesthesia (loss of touch sensation) or pallanesthesia (loss of vibration sense).

Lesions located in the region of the first lumbar vertebral body or below compress the spinal nerves of the cauda equina and cause a flaccid, areflexic, asymmetric paraparesis usually accompanied by bladder and bowel dysfunction. A sensory level is found in a saddle distribution up to L1, corresponding to the roots carried in the cauda equina. The Achilles and patellar reflexes are diminished or absent. Pain is common and projected to the perineum or thighs. With conus medullaris lesions pain is less prominent than in cauda equina lesions, and bladder and prominent bowel symptoms occur earlier; only the Achilles reflex is diminished. Compressive lesions may involve both the cauda and conus causing a combined syndrome of lower motor neuron signs and some hyperflexia or a Babinski sign.

The classic syndrome of the foramen magnum is weakness of the shoulder and arm followed by weakness of the ipsilateral leg, then contralateral leg, and finally, contralateral arm. Masses in this region sometimes produce suboccipital pain spreading to the neck and shoulders. A Horner's syndrome is another clue to a high cervical cord lesion; it does not occur with lesions below T2. A few diseases are capable of producing sudden "strokelike" myelopathy without preceding symptoms. They include epidural hemorrhage, hematomyelia, cord infarction, nucleus pulposus embolism, and compression by spinal subluxation.

SPINAL CORD COMPRESSION **Tumors of the spinal cord** Tumors in the spinal canal may be primary or metastatic, and are classified as extradural ("epidural") or intradural, and the latter as intra- or extramedullary (see Chap. 345). The majority are epidural arising from metastases to the adjacent spinal column. Neoplasms originating in the prostate, breast, and lung, and lymphoma and plasm cell dyscrasias are particularly common, though virtually every malignant tumor has been reported to cause metastatic epidural cord compression. The initial symptom in epidural compression is usually local back pain, often worse in the recumbent position, and causing the patient to awaken at night. Radiating radicular pain exacerbated by coughing, sneezing, or straining may be an accompaniment. Pain and local tenderness often precede other symptoms by many weeks. Neurologic signs commonly evolve over several days to a few weeks. The cord syndrome begins with progressive weakness, eventually acquiring all the hallmarks of a transverse myelopathy with paraparesis and a sensory level. A plain radiograph may show lytic or blastic changes, or a compression fracture at the level appropriate to the cord syndrome; radionuclide bone scans are more frequently positive. CT scan, MRI, or myelography remain the optimal way of demonstrating cord compression. A horizontally and symmetrically widened and flattened cord from extrinsic compression is seen at the margins of the subarachnoid block, and the adjacent vertebral body is usually abnormal (Fig. 353-1).

In the past, emergency laminectomies were considered necessary to treat extrinsic cord compression, but recent treatment with high-dose corticosteroids and rapid, fractionated radiation therapy has been as successful. Outcome is most closely related to the tumor type and its radiosensitivity. Paraparesis frequently improves within 48 h of the administration of corticosteroids. Some incomplete or early transverse cord syndromes may still be better treated surgically, but each case must be analyzed individually taking into account the radiosensitivity of the tumor, distribution of other metastases, and the patient's general medical condition. Whichever therapy is chosen, it is wise to proceed quickly and use corticosteroids as soon as the diagnosis of cord compression is suspected.

Intradural, extramedullary tumors are a less frequent cause of spinal cord compression and evolve more slowly than extradural lesions. Meningiomas and neurofibromas are most common; hemangiopericytomas and other tumors of meningeal origin are rare.

FIGURE 353-1 *Sagittal section MRI showing compression deformity of the T12 vertebral body from metastatic adenocarcinoma (below arrows), and compression and displacement of the spinal cord. (Courtesy of Greg Shoukimas, M.D., Department of Radiology, Massachusetts General Hospital.)*

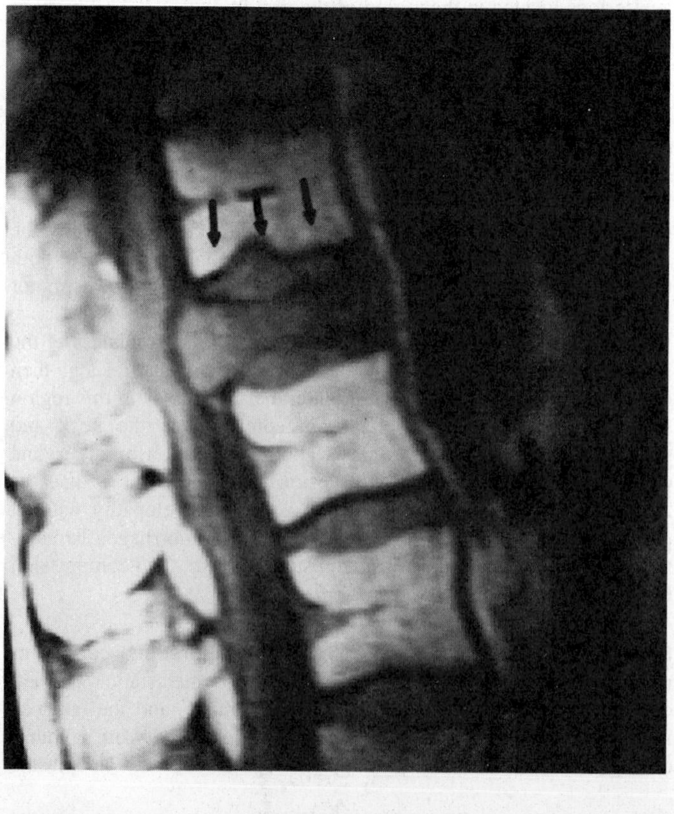

Symptoms usually begin with radicular sensory changes and an asymmetric syndrome. The CT and myelogram have a typical appearance with dislocation of the cord to one side and outline of the tumor within the subarachnoid space. Primary intramedullary tumors of the spinal cord are discussed in Chap. 345.

Neoplastic compressive myelopathies of all types initially cause minimal elevation of CSF protein, but with complete block of the subarachnoid space CSF protein concentration rises to the 100 to 1000 mg/dL range due to impediment of CSF circulation from the caudal sac to the intracranial subarachnoid space. There are usually few or no cells, cytology for malignant cells is often negative, and CSF glucose concentration remains normal unless there is accompanying widespread carcinomatous meningitis (see Chap. 345).

Epidural abscess This is a treacherous lesion, often misdiagnosed at first (see Chap. 346). The predisposing clinical settings are furunculosis of the back or scalp, bacteremia, or minor back injury. The condition can occur as a complication of operation or lumbar puncture. Spinal osteomyelitis acts as the nidus for the abscess formation which subsequently enlarges to compress the cord. The osteomyelitis is usually small and not often evident on plain radiographs. For several days to 2 weeks there may be only unexplained fever and mild spinal ache with local tenderness; later, radicular pain occurs. As the abscess expands, it rapidly causes cord compression with a transverse and usually complete transection syndrome. The proper treatment is rapid decompression by laminectomy and drainage, followed by appropriate antibiotics determined from culture of the purulent material. Incomplete drainage is not uncommon resulting in a chronic granulomatous and fibrous reaction that may be sterilized with antibiotics but continues to act as a compressing mass. Tuberculous pyogenic abscess formation, more common in the past, still occurs in developing countries.

Spinal epidural hemorrhage and hematomyelia An acute transverse myelopathy evolving over minutes or hours accompanied by severe pain may be produced by hemorrhage into the spinal cord (hematomyelia), subarachnoid, or epidural space. Although these may originate from an arteriovenous malformation, or from hemorrhage into a tumor during anticoagulation with warfarin, more commonly they are spontaneous. Those in an epidural location may occur in the setting of minor trauma, lumbar puncture, warfarin anticoagulation, or secondary to hematologic disorders. Back pain, with associated radicular pain, can precede weakness by several minutes to hours, and be so severe that patients may be perceived to act in a peculiar, exaggerated fashion. Lumbar epidural hematoma results in loss of both knee and ankle reflexes, whereas retroperitoneal hematomas usually cause only absence of the knee reflexes. A myelogram defines the mass; computerized tomography is sometimes normal because the clot cannot be distinguished from adjacent bone. Subdural and subarachnoid clots are particularly painful and may occur spontaneously or under circumstances similar to those causing epidural hemorrhages. The CSF with epidural hemorrhage is usually clear or contains a few red blood cells; in subarachnoid or subdural hemorrhage the CSF is grossly bloody at first and later becomes discolored to a deep yellow-brown characteristic of blood pigments present in the CSF. There may be, in addition, a pleocytosis and lowered CSF glucose, giving the impression of bacterial meningitis.

Acute disk protrusion Lumbar disk herniation, a common disorder, is discussed in Chap. 7. Thoracic or cervical disk protrusion is less often a cause of spinal cord compression, usually occurring after direct trauma to the spinal column. Degeneration of cervical disk spaces with adjacent osteoarthritic hypertrophy causes a subacute spondylytic-compressive myelopathy in the cervical region, discussed below. Embolism from nucleus pulposus material causing acute spinal cord infarction is also described below.

Other unusual compressive lesions Patients with iatrogenic or primary Cushing's syndrome have a tendency to form increased epidural fat tissue that rarely can reach a size large enough to compress the thoracic cord. Extramedullary hematopoiesis has caused cord compression in a number of hematologic diseases. Eroding aortic aneurysms, echinococcal or other parasitic cysts, gummas, lymphomatoid-granulomatosis, mucopolysaccharidoses, and other rare lesions can also compress the cord.

Arthritic diseases of the spine occur in two clinical forms: a lumbar or cauda equina compression from ankylosing spondylitis, or cervical cord compression from destruction of the cervical apophyseal or atlantoaxial joints in rheumatoid arthritis. Spinal complications arising as one component of severe generalized joint disease in rheumatoid arthritis are often overlooked. Forward subluxation of cervical vertebral bodies, or of the atlas on the axis, can cause a devastating, even fatal, acute cord compression after minor trauma such as whiplash, or it may present as a chronic compressive myelopathy similar to cervical spondylosis. Separation of the odontoid process from the axis may narrow the upper spinal canal compressing the cervicomedullary junction, particularly in flexion movements.

NONCOMPRESSIVE NEOPLASTIC MYELOPATHIES Intramedullary metastasis, paracarcinomatous myelopathy, and radiation myelopathy In the context of known cancer most myelopathies are compressive. However, when radiologic studies fail to show a block, there is often difficulty distinguishing between several less common entities: intramedullary metastasis, paracarcinomatous myelopathy, and radiation myelopathy. In a patient with known metastatic cancer and a progressive myelopathy shown to be noncompressive by myelography, CT scan, or MRI, intramedullary metastasis is the most likely diagnosis; paraneoplastic myelopathy is rarer (see Chap. 304). Back pain is the most common initial symptom with intramedullary metastasis, though it is not invariable, followed by progressive spastic paraparesis and less often paresthesias. Dissociated sensory loss or sacral sparing, though more characteristic of intrinsic than extrinsic compression, is uncommon, and asymmetric paraparesis and incomplete sensory loss is the rule. Myelography, CT scan, or MRI show a swollen cord without extrinsic compression; in almost half of patients CT or myelography are normal; MRI is more successful in outlining a metastatic mass or primary intramedullary tumor (Fig. 353-2). Intramedullary metastases usually arise from bronchogenic carcinoma and less often from breast cancer and other solid tumors (see Chap. 304). Metastatic melanoma, an uncommon cause of extrinsic cord compression, more often presents as an intramedullary mass. The pathology of the metastasis is usually a single eccentrically placed nodule that seeds hematogenously. Radiation therapy may be helpful in appropriate circumstances.

Carcinomatous meningitis, a common form of CNS invasion in malignancy, does not cause a myelopathy unless there is extensive subpial infiltration from adjacent roots causing nodules with secondary compression or infiltration of the cord. An incomplete, painless cauda equina syndrome can result from carcinomatous root infiltration (see Chap. 345). Headache is common, and repeated CSF examinations eventually reveal malignant cells, an elevated protein, and, in some cases, reduced CSF glucose concentration.

A progressive necrotic myelopathy associated with a paucity of inflammation can occur as a remote effect of cancer, usually with solid tumors. The myelogram and CSF are normal or there may be slightly elevated protein. A subacute progressive spastic paraparesis evolves over days or weeks, usually asymmetrically, with distal paresthesias ascending to establish a sensory level, and late bladder dysfunction. Several adjacent segments of cord are involved.

Radiation produces a delayed subacute progressive myelopathy due to microvascular hyalinization and vascular occlusion (see Chap. 345). It frequently presents a differential diagnostic problem when the cord lies within radiation portals used to treat other structures such as the mediastinal lymph nodes. Differentiation from paracarcinomatous myelopathy or intramedullary metastasis is difficult except by circumstantial history of prior radiation.

INFLAMMATORY MYELOPATHIES Acute myelitis, transverse myelitis, and necrotic myelopathy These are a group of related diseases marked by intrinsic inflammation of the cord and a clinical syndrome evolving over several days to 2 or 3 weeks. There may be a transverse or virtually complete spinal syndrome (transverse myelitis) or incomplete variants such as a posterior column myelopathy with ascending paresthesias and a sensory level for vibration; ascending, predominantly spinothalamic findings; or a Brown-Séquard syndrome with leg paresis and contralateral spinothalamic-type sensory changes. Many cases follow a viral illness. The most common presenting findings in transverse myelitis are back pain; progressive paraparesis; and asymmetric ascending paresthesias in the legs, later affecting the hands if the disease progresses, creating confusion with Guillain-Barré syndrome. Radiologic studies are necessary to exclude a compressive lesion. The CSF contains 5 to 50 lymphocytes per cubic millimeter in most patients; occasionally more than 200 cells per cublic millimeter are found, and rarely, polymorphonuclear cells predominate. The inflammatory process is most common in the mid and low thoracic regions, but any level of the cord may be affected. A chronic progressive cervical myelitis has been described, predominantly in older women, and is believed to be a form of multiple sclerosis (see Chap. 348).

In some cases necrosis is profound and may progress intermittently for several months to involve contiguous portions of the cord, reducing much of it to a thin gliotic ribbon. The term *progressive necrotic myelopathy* has been given to this condition. Exceptional cases of necrotic myelopathy progress to involve virtually the entire cord (necrotic panmyelopathy). When a transverse necrotic lesion occurs before or shortly after optic neuritis, it has been termed Devic's disease or neuromyelitis optica. All of these processes appear to be related to, and many are variants of, multiple sclerosis. Systemic lupus erythematosis and other autoimmune disorders have been associated with myelitis. The postinfectious demyelinating disorders are usually monophasic and only rarely recur, though fluctuation of symptoms related to a single level of the cord is common (see Chap. 347).

FIGURE 353-2 *Sagittal MRI showing intrinsic fusiform enlargement of the cervical spinal cord from an intramedullary tumor. The tumor displays a low-density signal (arrows). (Courtesy of Greg Shoukimas, M.D., Department of Radiology, Massachusetts General Hospital.)*

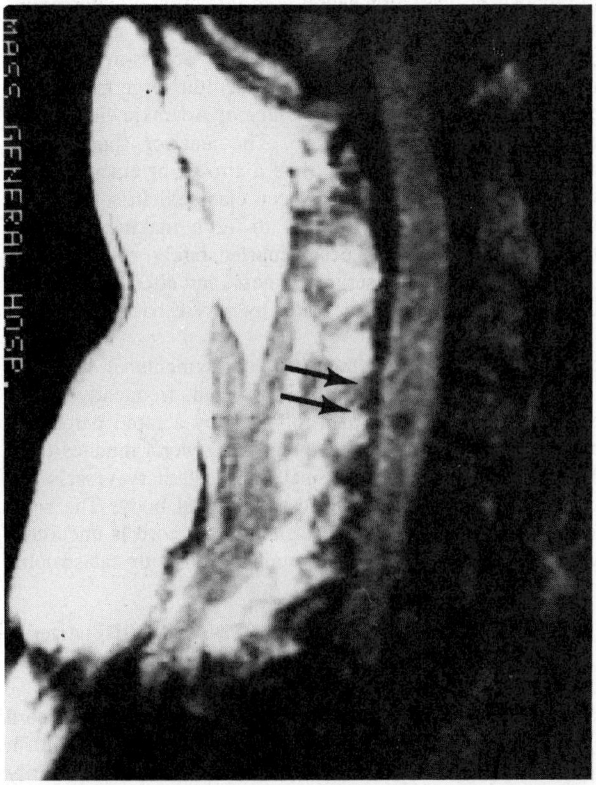

Infectious myelopathy Direct viral infection of the cord produces specific types of myelitis. In the past, the most common form was poliomyelitis. Herpes zoster, preceded by radicular symptoms, is presently the most common cause of viral myelitis. The pathologic process is not restricted to the gray matter as is polio. Lymphocytes are always found in the CSF. Intramedullary cord abscesses caused by bacteria or mycobacteria arising in the context of systemic infection have been reported. Chronic meningitic lesions due to syphilis may produce a secondary subpial myelitis and radiculitis that evolve slowly (see below). An intense granulomatous, necrotic, and inflammatory myelitis is peculiar to infestation by *Schistosoma mansoni,* caused by a local response to tissue-digesting enzymes produced by ova from the parasite.

Toxic myelopathy A toxic noninflammatory myelopathy, sometimes with optic atrophy, has been reported, mainly in Japan, and linked to ingestion of iodochlorhydroxyquinoline. Most patients have recovered, but many have persistent paresthesias.

Arachnoiditis This is a nonspecific term referring to inflammation, scarring, and fibrous thickening of the arachnoid membrane capable of compressing nerve roots or rarely the spinal cord. It is usually a postoperative complication or results from instillation of radiographic dye, antibiotics, or noxious chemicals into the subarachnoid space. The CSF contains many cells and an elevated protein concentration soon after the inciting event, but the inflammation then subsides. There may be slight fever in acute cases. Bilateral asymmetric radicular limb pain is the most prominent feature, with additional signs of root compression, such as reflex loss. Back pain and radicular symptoms are attributed to lumbar arachnoiditis, perhaps more often than justified; nor is arachnoiditis often responsible for cord compression (see Chap. 7). Treatment is controversial; laminectomy has led to improvement in some patients. Multiple meningeal cul-de-sacs, or arachnoid cysts, along nerve roots, occur as a congenital process that may produce severe radicular pain in midadulthood when the cysts enlarge and distort or exert traction on spinal nerve roots or ganglia.

SPINAL CORD INFARCTION Because the anterior or posterior spinal arteries are not usually involved by atherosclerosis, and only occasionally are affected by angiitis or emboli, most infarctions of the spinal cord are due to ischemia due to distant vascular occlusions. Aortic thrombosis or dissection causes cord infarction by interrupting the entire radicular and direct arterial supply to the anterior and posterior spinal arteries. The infarction typically occurs in a vascular watershed region of the thoracic cord between the large tributary to the spine arising from the aorta, the artery of Adamkiewicz below, and the anterior spinal artery above. The anterior spinal artery syndrome usually appears abruptly, like a stroke, or emerges postoperatively if the proximal aorta has been clamped. In some cases, however, symptoms progress over 24 to 72 h making diagnosis difficult. Spinal infarction has been reported rarely with systemic arteritis, immune reactions of serum sickness, and after intravascular contrast injection, heralded in the latter by severe back pain at the time of injection.

Cord infarction caused by microscopic fragments of herniated nucleus pulposus may occur after minor trauma, frequently during athletics. There is sharp local pain followed by a rapid paraplegia and a transverse cord syndrome evolving over several minutes to an hour. Pulposus tissue is found in small intramedullary vessels and often within the marrow of the adjacent vertebral body. The route from the disk space to marrow and thence to the cord is uncertain. This entity should be suspected in young adults with catastrophic transverse cord syndromes.

VASCULAR MALFORMATION OF THE SPINAL CORD Arteriovenous malformations (AVM) of the spinal cord are among the most difficult lesions to detect because of their great clinical variability. They may simulate multiple sclerosis, transverse myelitis, spinal cord stroke, or neoplastic compression. AVMs are most often found in the low thoracic or lumbar cord in middle-aged men. The majority begin with an incomplete progressive cord syndrome that may advance subacutely or episodically, like multiple sclerosis, producing bilateral corticospinal, spinothalamic, and posterior column symptoms and signs in any combination. Almost all patients are paraparetic and unable to walk within several years. About one-third have an abrupt syndrome with a single acute transverse myelopathy from bleeding, which simulates acute myelitis; others present with several acute exacerbations. About half have back or radicular pain, a few have a claudication syndrome similar to lumbar canal stenosis, and rare patients describe an acute onset with severe, localized back pain. Fluctuation of pain or neurologic signs with exercise, posture, or menses is helpful in suspecting the diagnosis. Bruits over the lesion are rare but should be sought at rest and after exercise. Most patients have mild elevation of CSF protein and a few show CSF pleocytosis. Bleeding into the cord or CSF may occur. Myelography or CT shows a lesion in 75 to 90 percent of cases if the dorsal subarachnoid space is examined by placing the patient in the supine position. The anatomic details of most AVMs can be demonstrated with selective spinal angiography, a procedure requiring experience for safe performance and completeness.

The pathogenesis of the myelopathy caused by AVMs (that have not bled) is incompletely understood, but appears to be a necrotic noninflammatory process consistent with ischemia. A dorsal AVM with a prominent progressive intramedullary syndrome has been reported with necrotic myelopathy. Since any necrotic process within the cord may give rise to neovascularization and thick-walled vessels, the pathologic basis of this vascular malformation remains controversial.

CHRONIC MYELOPATHIES Spondylosis This is a general term for several related degenerative changes of the spine giving rise to compression of the cervical cord and adjacent roots. The cervical form is primarily a disease of older patients, affecting men more often than women, and consisting of a combination of (1) narrowing of intervetebral disk spaces with nucleus pulposus herniation or annulus bulging, (2) osteophytic spur formation on the dorsal aspect of the vertebral bodies, (3) partial subluxation of vertebrae, and (4) hypertrophy of the dorsal spinal ligament and dorsolateral facet articulations (see Chap. 7). The bony changes are reactive in nature, but there is no true arthritis. The most important feature causing spinal cord symptoms and signs is a "spondylitic bar" formed by osteophytes arising from the dorsal surfaces of adjacent vertebral bodies resulting in a horizontal compression of the ventral cord (Fig. 353-3*A* and *B*). Extension of the bar laterally accompanied by articulatory hypertrophic changes or encroachment on the neural foramina often causes additional radicular symptoms. The sagittal diameter of the spinal canal may be narrowed further by actual disk protrusion, or by hypertrophy or buckling of the dorsal spinal ligament, particularly during neck extension. Though the radiographic findings of spondylosis are common in the elderly, only a few patients develop myelopathy or radiculopathy, often dependent upon a congenitally narrow canal.

Neck and shoulder pain with stiffness are early symptoms; pressure on nerve roots is associated with radicular arm pain, most often in a C5 or C6 distribution. Compression of the cervical cord produces a slowly progressive spastic paraparesis, at times asymmetric, and often accompanied by paresthesias in the feet and hands. Vibratory sense is substantially diminished in the legs in most patients, and occasionally there is a sensory level for vibration on the upper thorax. Coughing or straining often produces leg weakness or radiating arm or shoulder pain. Dermatomal sensory loss in the arms, atrophy of intrinsic hand muscles, increased deep tendon reflexes in the legs, and asymmetric Babinski signs are common. Urinary urgency or incontinence do not occur unless the process is well-advanced. The reflexes in the arms are often diminished at some level, notably the biceps, corresponding to C5–C6 cord compression or root involvement. Either radicular, myelopathic, or combined signs may predominate. The diagnosis should be considered in cases of progressive cervical myelopathy, paresthesias of feet or hands, or wasting of the hands. Spondylosis is also one of the most common causes of gait difficulty in the elderly often causing an unexplained increase in leg reflexes or Babinski signs.

Plain radiographs demonstrate spondylitic bars, intervertebral narrowing and subluxations, reversal of the normal cervical spine curvature, and reduction of the sagittal diameter of the canal to less than 11 mm, or to 7 mm with neck extension (Fig. 353-3*A*). The CSF is usually normal or shows a slightly elevated protein concentration. Somatosensory evoked potentials can be very helpful by demonstrating normal conduction in peripheral large sensory fibers and a delay in central conduction in the mid or high cervical cord.

Cervical spondylosis is both an under- and overdiagnosed disease. Many patient with intrinsic cord processes, particularly amyotrophic lateral sclerosis, multiple sclerosis, and subacute combined degeneration, have had cervical laminectomies in the belief that spondylosis was responsible. Often there is temporary improvement suggesting that there was an element of spondylolytic compression, but the underlying intrinsic myelopathy soon progresses. On the other hand, mild progressive gait disorder with sensory symptoms in the feet and hands caused by cervical spondylosis may be incorrectly attributed to peripheral neuropathy.

Rest and cervical immobilization with a soft collar are helpful in minor cases, traction may be helpful in others, but an operation is advisable if there are advanced symptoms of gait difficulty, severe hand weakness, or bladder difficulty, or if there is a virtually complete myelographic or CT spinal block.

Lumbar stenosis (also discussed in Chap. 7) is an intermittent and chronic compression of the cauda equina usually based on congenital narrowing of the lumbar spinal canal, which is further compromised by disk protrusion or spondylitic changes. Exercise brings about an aching pain in the buttocks, thighs, and calves, frequently sciatic in distribution, ceasing with rest and thereby simulating vascular-induced claudication. During the peak of pain, deep tendon reflexes and sensation may be reduced as compared to the resting state, and vascular studies are normal. Lumbar stenosis and cervical spondylosis commonly occur together, the former probably explaining occasional lower extremity fasciculations in cervical spondylosis.

Degenerative and inherited myelopathies The prototype of the inherited disorders causing spinal cord syndromes is Friedreich's ataxia, a progressive, recessively inherited, leg and truncal ataxia of late childhood onset. Intention tremor, clumsiness of the arms, and, later dysarthria occur. Kyphoscoliosis and pes cavus are common. Areflexia, Babinski signs, and severely impaired vibratory and joint position sense loss are found on examination. Fragmentary or milder forms of the illness occur and overlap with other syndromes including spastic paraparesis (Strümpell-Lorrain form), cerebellar cortical degeneration with ataxia, and olivopontocerebellar atrophy.

Amyotrophic lateral sclerosis (motor neuron disease) must be considered in patients presenting with symmetric spastic paraparesis without sensory findings. It causes a pure motor syndrome with combined corticospinal, corticobulbar, and anterior horn cell involvement. Clinical or electromyographic evidence of muscle fasciculations and denervation indicating motor neuron degeneration confirms the diagnosis (see Chaps. 350 and 354).

Subacute combined degeneration due to vitamin B_{12} deficiency This treatable myelopathy causes a progressive spastic and ataxic paraparesis and neuropathy, usually with prominent distal paresthesias of the feet and hands. It should be considered in cases simulating cervical spondylosis, late-onset degenerative myelopathies, and symmetric late-onset spinal multiple sclerosis. The disease can also involve the peripheral and optic nerves, and the brain. The diagnosis is confirmed by low B_{12} serum concentration and a positive Schilling test. This entity and related nutritional degenerations are discussed in Chap. 349. Whether folate or vitamin E deficiencies can produce a similar syndrome is controversial. Rarely, multiple sclerosis and B_{12} deficiency myelopathy are found in the same patient.

Syringomyelia Syringomyelia is a progressive myelopathy characterized pathologically by cavitation of the central spinal cord. It is often idiopathic or developmental (see Chap. 351) but may result from trauma, primary intramedullary tumors, extrinsic compression with central cord necrosis, arachnoiditis, hematomyelia, or necrotic myelitis. The developmental type usually begins in the midcervical cord and extends upward to the medulla or downward as low as the lumbar cord. It commonly takes an eccentric position often causing unilateral long tract signs or reflex asymmetries. Many cases occur in association with craniovertebral abnormalities, most commonly the Arnold-Chiari malformation, but also including myelomeningocele, basilar skull impression (platybasia), atresia of the foramen of Magendie, or Dandy-Walker cysts (see Chap. 351).

The cardinal clinical signs of syringomyelia correspond to a central high cervical cord syndrome and depend on the extent of the syrinx and associated abnormalities such as the Arnold-Chiari malformation.

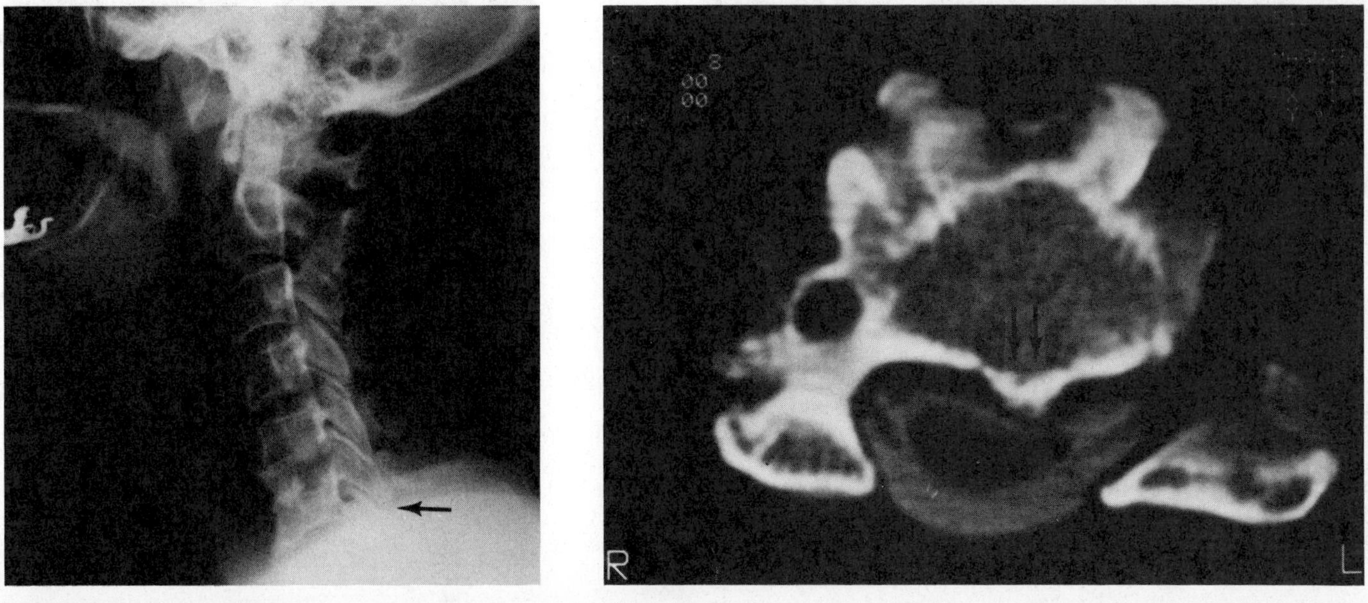

FIGURE 353-3 *A. Lateral x-ray of the cervical spine showing spondylitic ''bar'' formation from the junction of adjacent osteophytes at C6–C7 (arrow). B. Horizontal CT section at C6 from patient shown in A, after instillation of water-soluable dye into the subarachnoid space. A spur of the bony osteophyte compresses and distorts the spinal cord (arrows).*

The classic presentation is (1) sensory loss, usually of a dissociated type (loss of pain and temperature and preservation of touch and vibration senses), which is ''suspended'' over the nape of the neck, shoulders, and upper arms (cape distribution), and eventually extends to the hands, (2) wasting of muscles in the lower neck, shoulders, arms, and hands, with asymmetric or absent reflexes, and (3) high thoracic kyphoscoliosis. The majority begin asymmetrically with unilateral sensory loss. A number of patients develop loss of pin sensation on the face attributed to damage to the descending tract of the trigeminal nerve in the upper cervical cord. Cough-induced headache and neck pain are common with associated Arnold-Chiari malformations.

Symptoms in idiopathic cases begin in adolescence or early adulthood, progress irregularly, and frequently arrest for several years. A few patients escape major disability, but over half become wheelchair-bound. Analgesia leads to injuries, burns, and trophic ulcers in the fingertips. Charcot joints in the shoulders, elbows, or knees are common in advanced cases. Prominent lower extremity weakness or hypereflexia suggest an associated abnormality at the craniovertebral junction. Syringobulbia results from extension of the cavity into the medulla, or rarely the pons, usually occupying the lateral medullary tegmentum. Palatal and vocal cord paralysis, dysarthria, nystagmus, episodic dizziness, tongue weakness, and Horner's syndrome may occur.

Slow enlargement of the cavity may create a narrowing or complete block of the subarachnoid space. The cavity is separate from the central canal but usually communicates with it. The diagnosis can be made dependably from the clinical features, confirmed by finding an enlarged cervical cord on myelography or on delayed CT images several hours after subarachnoid instillation of metrizamide or another water-soluble contrast material (Fig. 353-4*A*). Syrinx cavities are shown to greatest advantage by magnetic resonance imaging (MRI) (Fig. 353-4*B*). The cervicomedullary junction should be examined for associated developmental abnormalities.

Therapy is directed at decompressing the cavity to prevent progression of damage and decompressing the spinal canal if the cord is distended. Laminectomies and suboccipital decompression are advisable when an Arnold-Chiari malformation accompanies an enlarged cervical cord.

Tabes dorsalis Tabes and meningovascular syphilis of the spinal cord are presently rare but at one time had to be considered in the differential diagnosis of most spinal cord syndromes. The most common symptoms of tabes are characteristic fleeting and repetitive, lancinating pains occurring mostly in the legs, less commonly in the back, thorax, abdomen, arms, and face. Severe gait and leg ataxia due to loss of position sense occurs in half of patients. Paresthesias, bladder disturbances, and acute abdominal pain with vomiting (visceral crisis) occur in 15 to 30 percent. The cardinal signs of tabes are loss of reflexes in the legs, impaired position and vibratory sense, Romberg's sign, and bilateral abnormalities of the pupils, Argyll Robertson pupils that fail to constrict to light but react with accommodation.

Traumatic spinal cord lesions and compression of the cord secondary to orthopedic disorders are discussed in the chapter on cranial and spinal injury (Chap. 344).

GENERAL CARE OF THE PATIENT WITH ACUTE PARAPLEGIA OR QUADRIPLEGIA Protection from secondary damage to the urinary tract is a high priority in the acute stages of paraplegia. The bladder is areflexic, retains urine, and the patient is unaware of bladder distention, making damage to the detrusor muscle form overdistention possible. Urologic rehabilitation requires bladder drainage and avoidance of urinary infection. This is best accomplished by intermittent catheterization by trained personnel. Continuous closed system urinary drainage, which is associated with a higher infection rate than intermittent catheterization, or suprapubic drainage are alternatives. Patients with acute lesions, especially those causing spinal shock, frequently need special cardiovascular care because of paroxysmal hypertension or hypotension often requiring fluids to correct volume aberrations. Ileus and gastric stress ulcers are other potential acute medical problems in patients with complete transverse cord lesions. Cimetidine and ranitidine may be useful in these circumstances.

High cervical cord lesions cause varying degrees of mechanical respiratory failure requiring artificial ventilation. In cases of incomplete respiratory failure with forced vital capacities of 10 to 20 mL/kg, chest physical therapy is useful, and a negative pressure cuirass may be used to alleviate atelectasis and fatigue, particularly if the major lesion is below C4. With severe respiratory failure, tracheal

FIGURE 353-4 *A. Horizontal CT section 1 h after subarachnoid instillation of water-soluble contrast medium showing the cervical spinal cord surrounded by contrast and dye in a large intramedullary syrinx cavity (arrow). B. Sagittal MRI of same patient shown in A showing the syrinx cavity and enlargement of the spinal cord (arrows). (Courtesy of Greg Shoukimas, M.D., Department of Radiology, Massachusetts General Hospital.)*

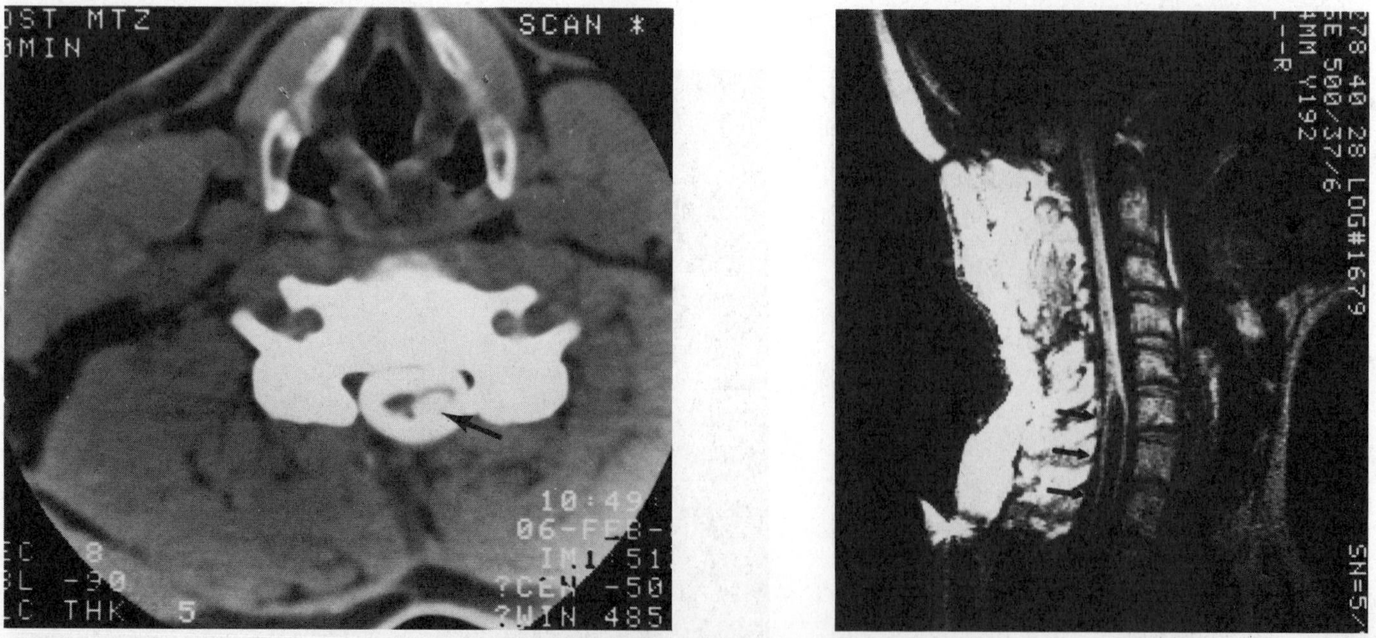

intubation (performed over an endoscope if the spine is unstable), followed by tracheostomy, provides tracheal access for ventilation and suctioning. A promising new technique is phrenic nerve pacing in patients with lesions at C5 or above.

As clinical signs stabilize, attention should be directed to the psychological state of the patient and the development of a rehabilitation plan framed by realistic expectations. An aggressive program is often remarkably successful with younger and middle-aged patients allowing return to home and a productive lifestyle.

Chronic nursing care problems can be handled by patients with varying degrees of assistance. The major issues are related to immobilization: skin breakdown over pressure points, urinary sepsis, and autonomic instability, and the potential for pulmonary embolism. Early care includes frequent repositioning, application of skin emollients and soft bed coverings. Specialized beds turn the patient or distribute body weight evenly rather than predominantly on bony prominences. If the sacral cord segments are undamaged, then a large degree of automatic voiding can be entrained. Patients initially void reflexly between catheterizations and later learn to induce voiding with various maneuvers. If residual urinary volumes lead to infection, surgical procedures or an indwelling catheter may be necessary. Bowel regimens and disimpaction are necessary in most patients to ensure at least biweekly evacuation and avoid colonic distention or obstruction.

Severe hypertension and bradycardia occur in response to noxious superficial stimuli, bladder or bowel distention, or surgery, particularly in patients with cervical and high thoracic cord lesions. Flushing and diaphoresis above the level of the lesion may accompany the hypertension. The mechanism of this dysautonomia is not well understood. A potent antihypertensive agent may be necessary, particularly during surgery, but beta-blocking drugs should probably be avoided. Some patients become severely bradycardic with tracheal suctioning; this can be prevented with small doses of atropine. Pulmonary embolism due to immobilization is a grave early risk occurring in approximately one-third of patients after acute cord trauma.

Detailed aspects of the physical therapy, rehabilitation, and orthotics related to severe spinal cord diseases may be found in specialized texts. The orthopedic stabilization of the spine in relation to cord trauma is discussed in Chap. 344.

REFERENCES

Adams CBT, Logue V: Studies in cervical spondylitic myelopathy. Brain 94:579, 1971

Aminoff MJ, Logue V: Clinical features of spinal vascular malformations. Brain 97:197, 1974

Auld AW et al: Metastatic spinal epidural tumors: An analysis of 50 cases. Arch Neurol 15:100, 1966

Baker AS et al: Spinal epidural abcess. N Engl J Med 293:463, 1975

Barnett HJM et al: *Syringomyelia*. Philadelphia, Saunders, 1973

Brain WR et al: The neurological manifestations of cervical spondylosis. Brain 75:188, 1952

Edelson R et al: Intramedullary spinal cord metastasis. Neurology 22:1222, 1972

Gilbert et al: Epidural cord compression from metastatic tumor: Diagnosis and treatment. Ann Neurol 3:40, 1978

Greenberg HS et al: Epidural spinal cord compression from metastatic tumor: Results with a new treatment protocol. Ann Neurol 8:361, 1980

Hardy AG, Rossier AB: *Spinal Cord Injuries: Orthopedic and Neurological Aspects*. Stuttgart, Thieme, 1975

Logue V: Angiomas of the spinal cord: Review of the pathogenesis, clinical features, and results of surgery. J Neurol Neurosurg Psychiatr 42:1, 1979

———, Edwards MR: Syringomyelia and its surgical treatment. J Neurol Neurosurg Psychiatr 44:273, 1981

McIlroy WJ, Richardson JC: Syringomyelia: A clinical review of 75 cases. J Can Med Assoc 93:731, 1965

Ropper AH, Poskanzer DC: Prognosis of acute and subacute transverse myelopathy based on early signs and symptoms. Ann Neurol 4:51, 1978

Rossier AB et al: Posttraumatic cervical syringomyelia. Brain 108:439, 1985

Srigley et al: Spinal cord infarction secondary to intervertebral disc embolism. Ann Neurol 9:296, 1981

section 2 Diseases of nerve and muscle

354 APPROACH TO THE PATIENT WITH NEUROMUSCULAR DISEASE

ROBERT C. GRIGGS / WALTER G. BRADLEY / BHAGWAN T. SHAHANI

The neuromuscular diseases are disorders of the *motor unit* and of the sensory and autonomic peripheral nerves. Each motor unit consists of (1) the *motor neuron* cell body, located in either the anterior horn (for muscles innervated by the spinal cord) or a cranial nerve nucleus (for ocular, facial, and bulbar musculature); (2) *the axon* of the motor neuron in the peripheral nerve; (3) the *neuromuscular junction*; and (4) the *muscle fibers* innervated by the motor neuron. The sensory peripheral nerves comprise (1) the *sensory neuron* cell body in the posterior root ganglion; (2) the *central axon* passing to the spinal cord in the posterior root; (3) the *distal* axon in the peripheral nerve; and (4) the *sensory nerve terminal* in skin, muscle, joint capsule, etc. The autonomic nerves are divided into *sympathetic* and *parasympathetic* nerves. The sympathetic preganglionic fibers arise from cell bodies in the intermediolateral column of the spinal cord and enter the sympathetic ganglia, from whence postganglionic fibers arise to innervate blood vessels or viscera. The parasympathetic preganglionic neurons lie in the brainstem and sacral spinal cord, and axons terminate in the viscera, which contain the postganglionic neurons and their nerve terminals.

The major symptoms of diseases of the motor unit are muscle weakness, fatigue, cramps, pain, or stiffness. Symptoms of peripheral nerve disease include, in addition, decreased sensation (hypesthesia or hypalgesia), abnormal sensations (paresthesias), or painful sensations (dysesthesias) (see Chap. 18). Symptoms of autonomic nervous system disease include postural dizziness, abnormal cardiac, visceral, and ocular function, and changes in sweating.

CLINICAL ASSESSMENT

History and physical examination will lead to a diagnosis in a majority of patients with neuromuscular disease. Failure to arrive at a diagnostic impression before routine and sophisticated laboratory studies are done often leads to diagnostic inaccuracy and confusion. Few of the biochemical, histologic, and electrodiagnostic studies used to evaluate patients with neuromuscular disease are pathognomonic, since nerve and muscle can respond in only a limited number of ways to disease processes.

CLINICAL HISTORY **Weakness and fatigue** (see Chap. 15) The patient with weakness, particularly of gradual onset, may not recognize it; this emphasizes the useful axiom that "signs of muscle weakness precede symptoms of weakness." Words such as numbness, deadness, tiredness, or fatigue may be used by a patient unfamiliar with what is taking place. On the other hand, some complaints of "weakness" result from systemic rather than neuromuscular disease. In such patients, strength is often normal or only mildly reduced, since the complaint is usually loss of stamina and endurance. The patient with fatigue should be asked to distinguish between true weakness and the less specific symptoms of lassitude and asthenia. If the patient is unable to perform a normal activity, true weakness is suggested. Objective evidence of weakness is established if symptoms exceed the bounds of normal variation (e.g., double vision, drooping eye lids, difficulty in swallowing, or aspiration of food or liquids into the airway) as opposed to the more subjective complaints of inability to lift, carry, or push an object.

The time course and severity of weakness must be quantitated by questions concerning alterations in functional abilities: for the legs, difficulty in rising from a chair or commode, rising from a squatting position, or climbing and descending stairs and a history of frequent tripping, stumbling, or falling; for the trunk, difficulty in sitting up in bed; or for the arms, difficulty in washing the hair, opening jars, fastening buttons, or raising objects onto a shelf.

Abnormalities of sensation (see Chaps. 18 and 355) Sensory symptoms suggest peripheral nerve disease although, as with weakness, sensory abnormalities can occur with disease at any level of the nervous system. The characteristics and localization of sensory symptoms in the various peripheral nerve syndromes and diseases are discussed in Chap. 18. In contradistinction to weakness, it is axiomatic that "sensory symptoms precede objective sensory signs."

Muscle pain (see Chap. 17) Muscle aches and pains may suggest inflammatory or metabolic muscle disease but are far more common in bone, joint, and nerve disease. Persistent muscle pain with normal strength usually results from a cause other than myopathy. Intermittent muscle pain, on the other hand, particularly when precipitated by exercise, suggests a substrate utilization defect such as a glycogen or lipid storage myopathy or the purine nucleotide cycle disorder, myoadenylate deaminase deficiency. It is important to determine if other factors, such as fasting, precipitate pain and then to inquire about associated findings such as dark urine, which may indicate myoglobinuria.

Autonomic dysfunction The most common complaint is of "dizziness," or "blackouts," which prove to be precipitated by standing up. Loss of male potency, explosive diarrhea, cyclic diarrhea-constipation or partial urinary retention may also occur.

PHYSICAL EXAMINATION **Strength testing** Reliable testing of strength requires that the examiner have an adequate frame of reference for normal strength and that the patient be motivated and able to cooperate with testing. As with history taking, it is helpful to quantitate the ability to perform tasks of daily living. The legs are particularly easy to test by observing the following: walking on heels and toes; rising from a chair, noting whether there is a need to use the arms; rising from a squat; and stepping up onto a chair. It is useful to examine the legs for a *knee extension lag*, the inability to fully extend the leg against gravity. This sign is an indication of quadriceps weakness; patients with even a minor extension lag almost invariably report frequent tripping and falling. Trunk and neck muscles can be tested by having the patient sit up; extending the head over the edge of an examining table is a sensitive method of detecting neck weakness. The arms are not as easily evaluated with function testing; inspection of shoulders for scapular winging as the arms are elevated and observation of the patient lifting the arms above the head test shoulder girdle function. Hand strength can be judged by determination of the degree of difficulty in extraction of two fingers from the grip of the patient and by the ability of the patient to blanch the knuckles when making a tight fist. When the lesion affects a specific region, e.g., the brachial plexus or the ulnar nerve, it is essential to test each individual muscle of the arm or hand.

Formal muscle testing, assigning a numeric grade to muscle strength, is usually based on the MRC (Medical Research Council of Great Britain) 0 to 5 scale:

5 — normal
4 — able to oppose gravity plus resistance
3 — able to move fully against gravity but not resistance
2 — able to move when gravity is eliminated
1 — trace movement
0 — no movement

Other scales expand the ratings to 10, allowing for greater precision in the ranges of 3 to 5 (or 6 to 10).

An important distinction to be made with any scale is whether a muscle is indeed *weaker than might be expected,* with allowances for age, male-female differences, inactivity, or generalized illness. If there is a limited time for the testing of muscle strength, the assessment of function is likely to be of more value than formal muscle testing.

Muscle bulk Muscle atrophy and hypertrophy are often difficult to recognize because of wide variation among normal persons. The problem is accentuated in young children and in obese patients because of overlying adipose tissue. Atrophy is easier to appreciate when asymmetric. Muscle enlargement or hypertrophy is a normal accompaniment of physical training. It is occasionally a sign of disease in patients with long-standing spasticity or myotonic disorders. So-called pseudohypertrophy, in which the muscles become enlarged by replacement with connective tissue or fat, may be prominent in certain of the muscular dystrophies but is also seen with spinal muscular atrophy and other denervating conditions. Actual hypertrophy of muscle fibers may also be present in these patients. Muscle enlargement may also be caused by infiltration with substances such as amyloid or by parasitic infestation (e.g., cysticercosis).

LOCALIZED ENLARGEMENT OF MUSCLE Focal muscle swelling may be due to inflammatory infiltrates, calcium deposits, or tendon rupture. Preservation of some parts of a muscle, while other parts atrophy, may occur in spinal muscular atrophy and some forms of muscular dystrophy, giving an appearance of a focal swelling during muscle contraction. Single or multiple muscle masses in a patient without weakness may indicate a neoplastic process. Other causes of muscle enlargement include focal myositis, sarcoidosis, ectopic ossification, and tendon rupture.

Pathologic fatigue Patients with disorders of neuromuscular transmission such as myasthenia gravis can usually be shown on examination to fatigue. Sustained upward gaze produces gradual ptosis of the eyelids (curtain sign); eye movements become disconjugate on sustained horizontal gaze; the voice may become hoarse, slurred, or nasal with prolonged speech; a smile may rapidly become a sneer when the patient cannot maintain facial muscle activity. The inability of the patient to sustain limb activity is less easily quantitated since patients who are weak from any cause may have decreased endurance.

Sensory testing Patients with peripheral neuropathy usually have sensory loss. The distribution of sensory disturbance as well as the modalities affected are often of diagnostic importance (see Chaps. 18 and 355).

Autonomic testing A fall of systolic blood pressure of more than 20 mmHg from lying to standing indicates impaired autonomic control of peripheral blood vessels. A greater fall often occurs with exercise in the erect position. The pulse rate does not increase normally in response to this hypotension if there is an autonomic neuropathy. Similarly, there is no slowing of the heart rate following a sustained Valsalva maneuver.

TABLE 354-1 Presenting clinical features of the neuromuscular diseases

Site of involvement	Anterior horn cell	Peripheral nerve	Neuromuscular junction	Muscle
Example	Spinal muscular atrophy	Nutritional neuropathy	Myasthenia gravis	Polymyositis
Distribution of weakness	Asymmetric limb or bulbar	Symmetric distal	Extraocular, bulbar, proximal limb	Symmetric proximal limb, bulbar
Atrophy	Marked and early	Moderate	None	Slight
Sensory involvement	None	Paresthesias, hypesthesia	None	Aching
Characteristic features	Fasciculations, cramps, tremor		Diurnal fluctuation	
Reflexes	Variable	Decreased out of proportion to weakness	Normal	Parallel strength

Other findings Myotonia, fasciculations, myokymia, and other spontaneous activity (Chap. 17) should be looked for. Certain disorders such as myotonic dystrophy and facioscapulohumeral dystrophy have distinctive and virtually pathognomonic facial features. Less characteristic but significant facial weakness is found in other myopathies and in myasthenia gravis. Joint contractures, particularly of the Achilles tendons and the hips, and scoliosis may indicate that weakness is of long duration.

DIFFERENTIAL DIAGNOSIS The portion of the motor unit involved by a disease process is usually evident from clinical findings (Table 354-1). Motor neuron diseases (Chap. 350) are suggested in the patient whose weakness is accompanied by prominent atrophy, fasciculations, and lack of sensory involvement. The reflexes may be depressed if anterior horn cell disease alone is present and may be pathologically increased if there is coexistent upper motor neuron disease, as in amyotrophic lateral sclerosis. Peripheral neuropathy (Chap. 355) is suggested by the findings of distal weakness associated with sensory loss. Patients with peripheral neuropathy usually have depressed tendon reflexes; preservation of reflexes combined with significant weakness suggests another cause for the dysfunction. Neuromuscular junction disorders (Chap. 358) come to mind if ocular and bulbar weakness is prominent, particularly if there is *diurnal variation,* with the patient becoming weaker as the day progresses. Pathologic fatigue can usually be demonstrated. Reflexes are preserved in most neuromuscular junction disorders, particularly myasthenia gravis.

Myopathy versus other neuromuscular disease Clinical features which suggest myopathy in contrast to other motor unit diseases include a proximal distribution of weakness, relative preservation or increase of muscle bulk, and the preservation of reflexes. Table 354-2 presents a classification of primary muscle diseases. Many patients with muscle symptoms, however, have disorders that do not fit into this classification because evaluation discloses disease in another portion of the motor unit or in another system (see Chap. 15). For example, a patient with a denervation produced by nerve root damage from a lumbar disk protrusion may have muscle cramps, pain, and weakness in muscles innervated by those nerve roots. Furthermore, fatigue, weakness, and pain are common accompaniments of derangements of cardiac, hematologic, gastrointestinal, pulmonary, renal, or hepatic function. The expectation of strength and endurance in such patients is diminished since the patient is acutely or chronically ill. Despite complaints of weakness and fatigue and the finding of atrophy, patients with pulmonary or cardiac disease are rarely mistaken for those with primary muscle disease.

Proximal weakness, although characteristic of most myopathies, can also occur in acute or chronic inflammatory polyneuropathy, in neuromuscular junction disorders, and in anterior horn cell diseases. Many disorders are termed "myopathies" solely on the basis of proximal weakness, including the weakness associated with hyperthyroidism, corticosteroid administration, and hyperparathyroidism. However, the underlying pathophysiology of these muscle disorders has not been defined.

Acute generalized weakness Weakness developing over the course of less than an hour is usually caused by a metabolic or toxic disorder affecting either the neuromuscular junction or the muscle. A sudden alteration in circulating potassium, calcium, sodium, magnesium, or phosphate may result in partial or complete paralysis of muscle. Acute failure of neuromuscular junction transmission may occur with botulism and other toxins, hypermagnesemia, and with aminoglycoside antibiotics and other medications. Weakness developing over the course of 24 h may occur in electrolyte, metabolic, and toxic disorders; in periodic paralysis (Chap. 359); and in acute inflammatory myopathies, particularly those related to viral and parasitic infection (Chap. 356) and certain acute polyneuropathies (Chap. 355). Occasionally, patients with more chronic disorders first realize that they are weak when the insidious progression of their weakness produces an abrupt change in function.

Subacute weakness Weakness developing over days is more common in peripheral nerve or neuromuscular junction diseases than in muscle or anterior horn cell disease. Acute inflammatory polyneuropathy (Guillain-Barré syndrome) and porphyric, diphtheritic, and toxic neuropathies are of subacute onset. Myasthenia gravis and other neuromuscular junction diseases must also be considered in the differential diagnosis. Subacute weakness can occur in severe polymyositis and dermatomyositis. Weakness from endocrine disorders and certain muscle toxins (Table 354-2) may also develop subacutely (Chap. 357). Of the anterior horn cell disorders only infections with poliomyelitis and other viruses evolve subacutely.

Slowly progressive weakness *Slowly progressive proximal weakness* evolving over weeks to months may be caused by polymyositis or dermatomyositis or by an unsuspected endocrinopathy. When the course has extended for a year or more, however, one of the muscular dystrophies, spinal muscular atrophy, or a neuromuscular junction

TABLE 354-2 Classification of primary muscle diseases

I Hereditary
- *A* Muscular dystrophy (Chap. 357): Duchenne, myotonic, facioscapulohumeral, limb-girdle, oculopharyngeal, scapuloperoneal, congenital, distal, ocular
- *B* Congenital myopathies (Chap. 357): Central core, nemaline, centronuclear, fiber-type disproportion
- *C* Metabolic myopathies (Chap. 357):
  - *1* Glycogen: Deficiencies of phosphorylase, phosphofructokinase, phosphoglyceromutase, acid maltase, others
  - *2* Lipid: Defective synthesis or transport of carnitine; deficiency of carnitine palmityl transferase
  - *3* Purine nucleotide cycle: Deficiency of myoadenylate deaminase
- *D* Myotonia (Chap. 357); Congenita, paramyotonia
- *E* Periodic paralysis (Chaps. 17 and 359): Hypokalemic, hyperkalemic

II Inflammatory (Chap. 356)
- *A* Collagen disease: Systemic lupus erythematosus, rheumatoid arthritis, scleroderma, mixed-connective tissue
- *B* Sarcoidosis, carcinoid, neoplastic disease
- *C* Infections: Numerous, especially viral (influenza B), protozoal (toxoplasmosis), parasitic (trichinosis)
- *D* Idiopathic: Polymyositis, dermatomyositis

III Endocrine and metabolic (Chap. 357)
- *A* Electrolyte abnormalities: Calcium, phosphate, magnesium, sodium, potassium
- *B* Endocrine abnormalities: Hypo- and hyperfunction of thyroid, adrenal, parathyroid, pituitary

IV Toxic (Chap. 357): Alcohol, opiates, pentazocine, clofibrate, others

V Tumors and masses: Primary and metastatic neoplasms, infection, sarcoidosis, myositis ossificans, calcinosis, muscle rupture and hemorrhage defect such as myasthenia gravis may be present. Neuropathies are seldom proximal, the major exceptions being acute and chronic inflammatory polyneuropathy, porphyric neuropathy, and diabetic proximal mononeuropathy. *Slowly progressive distal weakness* is more characteristic of anterior horn cell or peripheral nerve disorders than of disorders of muscle or the neuromuscular junction. The only commonly encountered distal myopathy is myotonic dystrophy. Less common disorders such as distal muscular dystrophy, nemaline and centronuclear myopathies (see Chap. 357), and a variant of polymyositis known as *inclusion body myositis* may present with distal weakness (Chap. 356). Prominent distal lower limb weakness is also present in the facioscapulohumeral and scapuloperoneal muscular dystrophies, but more proximal involvement is invariably also present in such patients. *Slowly progressive bulbar weakness* is more typical of anterior horn cell or neuromuscular junction disorders than of myopathies. Bulbar weakness (difficulty in speaking, coughing, and swallowing) occurs commonly in motor neuron disease (especially amyotrophic lateral sclerosis) and neuromuscular junction disorders. It is also seen in oculopharyngeal dystrophy, myotonic dystrophy, and polymyositis or dermatomyositis. *Ocular muscle weakness and ptosis* do not occur in motor neuron disease and are uncommon in peripheral neuropathy. Ophthalmoparesis is typical of myasthenia gravis and may occur in myotonic and oculopharyngeal dystrophies. Weakness limited to or predominantly of an ocular location (*progressive external ophthalmoplegia*) occurs in disorders such as the Kearns-Sayre syndrome (Chap. 357).

LABORATORY ASSESSMENT

Patients with impaired strength merit thorough diagnostic study. Hematologic, renal, and hepatic function and serum electrolytes should be evaluated. In many instances thyroid, adrenal, and other endocrine studies may be indicated. Other useful diagnostic tests are the serum creatine kinase test, nerve conduction studies, electromyography, and in many instances muscle biopsy. Nerve conduction studies should be obtained when the history and examination suggest peripheral neuropathy. Nerve biopsy is a more specialized technique with a relatively small number of specific indications (see Chap. 355). Repetitive stimulation of nerve with recording from muscle should be obtained when a neuromuscular junction defect is suspected. In requesting each diagnostic test it is important to consider what information is being sought in order to prevent the accumulation of misleading data. For example, creatine kinase may be elevated after minor muscle trauma such as that caused by electromyography. Electromyography and muscle biopsy obtained from a muscle affected by past nerve root disease (e.g., from a herniated disk) may show neuropathic abnormalities unrelated to a new disease process. Muscle biopsy from a muscle that has been recently injured, even by the minor trauma of an injection or electromyogram, may mislead the unwary into a diagnosis of myositis.

If a patient complains of weakness and fatigue but is not found on examination to have weakness, the indications for diagnostic studies are less definite. Depending on other clinical assessment, complaints of long duration and severity usually warrant diagnostic evaluation. When the history is suggestive of a metabolic myopathy (Chap. 357) further metabolic testing may be indicated.

ANATOMIC AND PHYSIOLOGIC BASIS OF HISTOPATHOLOGY AND ELECTROPHYSIOLOGY

The motor unit is the final common pathway for motor activity of the nervous system, and muscle is the final effector of the motor unit. All movement, posture, and reflex activity result from integrated discharge of large numbers of motor units by spinal and supraspinal mechanisms. The strength of a muscle contraction depends upon the number of motor units recruited, the frequency of motor unit discharge, the speed of contraction of muscle fibers in the motor unit, and the nature of the motor unit (whether fatigue-resistant or fatigue-prone). The number of motor units varies greatly between muscles, ranging from approximately 100 in the intrinsic muscles of the hands to several thousand in leg muscles. The number of muscle fibers per motor unit varies between as few as 10 in the extraocular muscles to nearly 2000 in leg muscles such as the gastrocnemius. The number of muscle fibers per muscle varies nearly a thousandfold, from 1000 in extraocular muscles to over 1 million in large leg muscles. An understanding of the organization of motor units and their patterns of firing is important in the interpretation of clinical and laboratory findings in normal and diseased muscle. The muscle fibers of the motor unit are dispersed randomly within a muscle, and fibers innervated by the same anterior horn cell are generally not contiguous.

Motor units differ both in size and in the biochemical and physiologic properties of their muscle fibers. On the basis of these properties, muscle fibers are subdivided into two types. The ATPase stain identifies two major types of fibers: type I fibers that stain lightly and type II fibers, which appear dark. This differentiation of histologic type is often useful in the interpretation of muscle pathology, since certain muscle diseases are characterized by preferential abnormalities of a single fiber type. Type II fibers are diminished in many congenital myopathies, whereas in myotonic dystrophy, type I fibers are often atrophic.

All muscle fibers within a motor unit are probably of identical histochemical type. Cross-innervation experiments in animals in which all of the muscle fibers of certain muscles are of the same histochemical type (as opposed to human muscle, where the fibers are dispersed in a random pattern throughout the muscle) have shown that muscle fibers change their histochemical, biochemical, and physiologic properties in response to changing innervation. The basis for the neurogenic control of muscle fiber characteristics is probably related to the characteristics of the firing pattern, since experimental chronic electric stimulation of nerves can change the biochemical and physiologic properties of muscle. A similar change in muscle fiber type in man can be induced by endurance exercise training, where an increase in type I (aerobic) muscle fibers is observed.

The physiologic characterization of the muscle fibers relate importantly to the exercise capacity of muscle. Motor units with type I, slow-twitch muscle fibers are designed for continuous and prolonged activity, since their energy supply for ATP generation is derived from substrate metabolism through the oxidative pathways of mitochondria. The muscle fibers of these motor units are activated (*recruited*) by small, low-threshold, slowly conducting motor neurons which are activated by low intensity exertion. Higher-intensity effort, such as the lifting of a heavy weight, recruits larger, higher-threshold, more rapidly conducting motor neurons which innervate type II muscle fibers.

The physiologic properties of motor units and their response to voluntary contraction are such that there is a stereotyped pattern of recruitment for each muscle with an orderly sequence of activation of muscle units. Certain motor units are activated only with intense activity. This fact underlies in part the ability of muscles to gain size and strength with repeated heavy exertion. An increase in the myofibril content of muscle fibers and possibly a small increase in the number of muscle fibers occurs with repeated heavy exertion. The lack of activation of some motor units except with vigorous training may underlie the weakness common in many sedentary persons and explain the response to physical therapeutic maneuvers in such patients.

As muscles relax, the cessation of firing of individual motor units occurs in a groupwise fashion so that a patient exerting an inadequate effort owing to functional weakness (e.g., malingering), lack of motivation, or pain will frequently have a ratchet-like or "give-way" quality on muscle testing which permits the distinction between true and feigned weakness.

ELECTROMYOGRAPHY The measurement of electric activity arising from muscle fibers is usually performed by inserting a needle electrode percutaneously into muscle. The electric activity from this electrode is then displayed on a cathode-ray oscilloscope and can be made audible by inserting a loudspeaker into the circuit.

Skeletal muscles are numerous and often large. As a result, electrode studies provide only an average picture of the electric activity of muscle. Since many neuromuscular diseases are restricted to selected muscles, normal electric activity in one area does not exclude the possibility of pathologic phenomena close by. Accurate physiologic analysis requires that fine concentric needle electrodes be placed within carefully selected muscles so as to register the activity of only a small number of motor units and muscle fibers in those muscles.

The action potential As an electric impulse travels from the center toward either end of the muscle fiber, current flows outward through the normally polarized region of the muscle membrane (sarcolemma) toward the depolarized zone (Fig. 354-1). The recording electrode initially becomes slightly positive relative to the reference electrode. When the depolarized region moves under the recording electrode, a negative deflection occurs. As the active region moves away from the electrode, the membrane under the electrode slowly becomes repolarized. The net result is a *triphasic action potential* recorded on the oscilloscope (Fig. 354-1).

Recording of motor unit activity Triphasic action potentials result from the activity of single muscle fibers. In normal muscle, excitation is initiated by motor nerves supplying many muscle fibers so that all muscle fibers of one motor unit are activated by one impulse from the motor neuron. The number of muscle fibers in a single motor unit varies, and muscle fibers differ in diameter, length, and shape and in spatial orientation with regard to the electromyogram (EMG) electrode. Muscle fibers of one motor unit are not clustered tightly together but are dispersed in a region of the muscle, interspersed with fibers of adjacent motor units. Therefore, muscle activation produces complex motor unit potentials, resulting from the summation of individual action potentials.

The normal electromyogram Normal muscle is electrically silent when at rest. Once *insertional activity,* produced by the trauma of placing the needle, has died down, electrodes record no action potentials. When a muscle is voluntarily contracted, action potentials appear; with increasing strength of contraction, second or third units are recruited. As the contraction becomes stronger, action potentials of more and larger motor units appear, until with full contraction, a disorderly array of action potentials varying at rates of up to 20 to 50 Hz appears. Individual motor unit potentials can no longer be distinguished, and a *complete recruitment* (*interference*) *pattern* is produced. In disease of the central or peripheral nervous system, the recruitment pattern produced by maximal voluntary effort is reduced because fewer motor units are activated with voluntary effort. In patients with muscle disease, the recruitment pattern with maximal effort remains complete; however, the peak-to-peak amplitude of the recruitment pattern is reduced. *A complete recruitment pattern of reduced amplitude in a weak muscle is one of the most characteristic EMG findings in muscle disease.*

The abnormal electromyogram Findings of pathologic significance include (1) the occurrence of spontaneous activity during relaxation (fibrillations, positive sharp waves, and fasciculations); (2) abnormalities in the amplitude, duration, and shape of single motor unit potentials; (3) decrease in the number of motor units which can be recruited; (4) demonstration of myotonia, coupling (tetany), bizzare repetitive potentials, or the occurrence of electric silence during shortening of the muscle (contracture).

SPONTANEOUS ACTIVITY DURING COMPLETE RELAXATION Persistent insertional activity occurs in myotonic disorders, in polymyositis, and in denervated muscles. Spontaneous activity of part of or an entire motor unit is called a *fasciculation,* and spontaneous activity of single muscle fiber is called a *fibrillation*. Fibrillations appear with destruction of the motor neuron or its axon and in muscle diseases where a portion of a muscle fiber is separated from its innervated portions by segmental necrosis. When a motor neuron is destroyed by disease or when its axon is severed, the distal part of the axon degenerates over a period of several days. Muscle fibers formerly innervated by the branches of the dead axon are disconnected from the nervous system. The chemosensitive region of the sarcolemma at the motor end plate spreads after denervation to involve the entire surface of the muscle fiber. This, together with the lowered resting membrane potential of denervated muscle fibers, results in the development of spontaneous activity in denervated muscle fibers 7 to 25 days after the death of the axon (depending upon the distance of the denervated muscle fibers from the site of the lesion). This spontaneous activity is similar to that found in the sinoatrial node of the heart; that is, each fiber contracts at its own rate without relation to the activity of adjacent fibers. The denervated muscle has a random conglomeration of brief, triphasic fibrillation potentials and diphasic *positive sharp waves*. Fibrillation and positive sharp wave activity continue until muscle fibers are reinnervated by the outgrowth of new axons, either from the proximal end of the damaged nerve or from nearby healthy nerve fibers, or until the muscle fibers are replaced over a period of months or years by connective tissue. *Fasciculations* are the involuntary single contractions of a part of or an entire motor unit. Since a large number of muscle fibers contract together, visible dimpling or twitching of the skin occurs, though ordinarily not enough power is exerted to move a joint. The form of the accompanying EMG potential, like that of an ordinary motor unit, is relatively constant for any one fasciculating unit. It usually has three to five phases (polyphasic), a duration of 5 to 15 ms, and an amplitude of several hundred microvolts. In the *benign fasciculations* seen in many normal subjects, the same unit tends to contract at a regular rate, which indicates a rhythmic activation of muscle fibers innervated by a particular axon. The EMG appearance of benign fasciculations is

FIGURE 354-1 *The triphasic muscle action potential. The shaded area represents the zone of the action potential, which is negative to all other points on the fiber surface. It is shown at three points in its course (from left to right) along the fiber. At each point, the correspondingly lettered portion of the triphasic muscle action potential displayed on the cathode ray oscilloscope (CRO) reflects the potential difference between the active (vertical arrow) and reference (Ref.) electrodes. Polarity in this and subsequent figures is negative upward as depicted. The time calibration is on the CRO screen. (For further details see text.)*

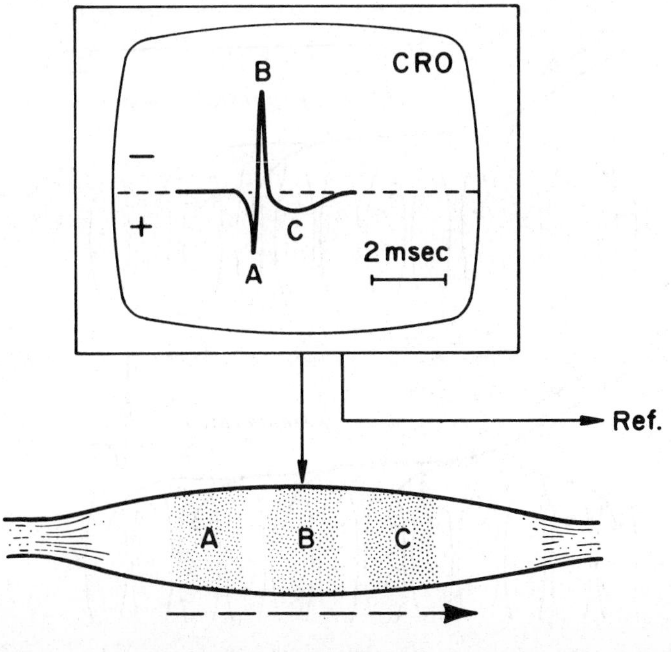

similar to that of normal motor unit potentials, and their rate of firing is usually faster than that of fasciculations indicative of disease.

The fasciculations seen with slowly progressive disease of the anterior horn cells, such as amyotrophic lateral sclerosis and progressive spinal muscular atrophy, are numerous, of relatively prolonged duration, and of high amplitude. Such fasciculations also occur with compressive nerve root lesions, in some motor neuropathies, and early in the course of acute inflammatory polyneuropathy. With nerve root lesions such as those caused by a herniated nucleus pulposus (ruptured disk), large numbers of axons may be affected, producing prominent fasciculations. In these cases the damaged neuron seems to be "irritated" by the disease process, fires repetitively, and in doing so, produces activity in muscle fibers innervated by it. Fasciculations may also follow traumatic peripheral nerve lesions, giving way to fibrillations upon death of the axon. Fasciculations in the calves and hands occur in many normal persons.

ABNORMALITIES IN MOTOR UNIT POTENTIALS Motor unit potentials may show abnormalities in *amplitude, number, duration,* and *shape.* *Increased amplitude* Early in the course of denervation, motor units with functional connection to the spinal cord remain normal, but the number of motor unit potentials appearing during contraction is reduced. In time, the remaining motor unit potentials may increase in amplitude to as much as two to three times normal, become longer in duration, and become polyphasic (more than 4 phases). Such large potentials (greater than 5 mV) arise from motor units (Fig. 354-2*C*) that contain an increased number of muscle fibers distributed through an enlarged territory within the muscle. These enlarged motor units arise when new nerve twigs sprout from undamaged axons and reinnervate previously denervated fibers, adding them to their own motor units. These reinnervated units may produce polyphasic and prolonged action potentials, a finding pathognomonic of reinnervation. These units must be differentiated from the polyphasic potentials of normal duration that occur in normal muscles, particularly in the end-plate zone, and brief polyphasic potentials seen with muscle disease.

FIGURE 354-2 *Motor unit potentials. The shaded muscle fibers are functional members of one motor unit; the axon, which enters from the upper left, branches terminally to innervate the appropriate muscle fibers. The motor unit action potential produced by each motor unit is seen in the upper right; its duration is measured between the two small vertical lines. The normal-appearing but unshaded fibers belong to other motor units. A. The normal situation, with five muscle fibers in the active unit. B. In this myopathic unit, only two fibers remain active; the other three (shrunken) have been affected by a muscle disease. C. Four fibers which belonged to other motor units and had been denervated have now been reinnervated by terminal axon sprouting from the healthy motor unit. Both the motor unit and its action potential are now larger than normal. Note that only under these abnormal circumstances do fibers in the same unit lie next to one another.*

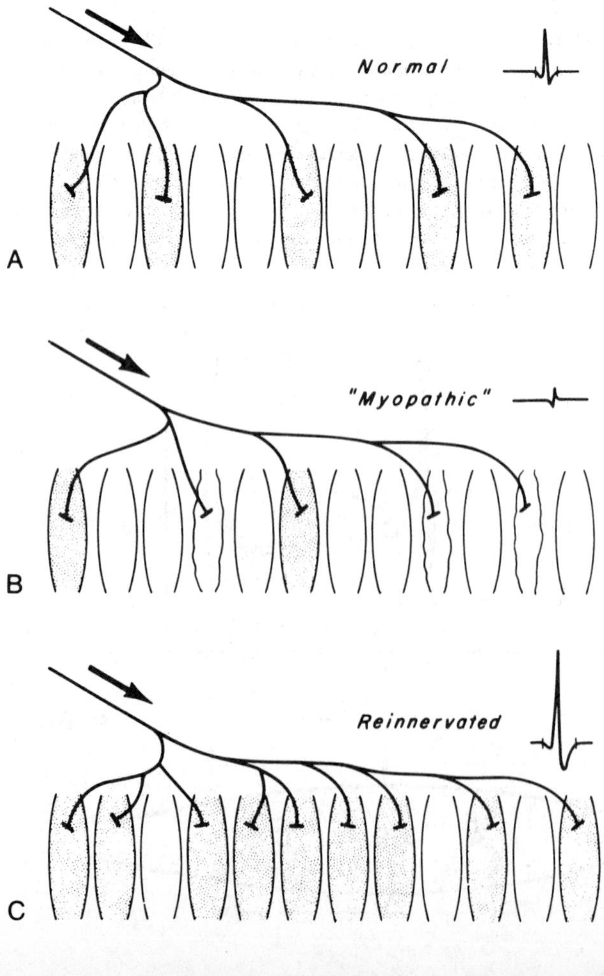

Reduced amplitude and duration Diseases such as polymyositis, the muscular dystrophies, and other myopathies that destroy scattered fibers within a motor unit (Fig. 354-2*B*), reduce the population of fibers per motor unit. When such a unit is activated, its potential is of lower amplitude and shorter duration than normal and may appear polyphasic since individual muscle fiber potentials are visible. When most of the muscle fibers within a motor unit are affected, the action potentials may be difficult to differentiate from fibrillation, and when destruction of all fibers is completed, electric activity ceases. The small, brief action potentials cause characteristic high-pitched crackling sounds from the loudspeaker.

In myasthenia gravis and other disorders where the transmission of impulses fails progressively at one neuromuscular junction after another, the EMG potential of that unit may be normal at first and become more myopathic as fatigue develops. Action potentials from weak muscles in myasthenia gravis are therefore proportionately myopathic. As shown in Fig. 354-2*B*, motor unit potentials appear equally "myopathic" whether the disease process directly affects single muscle fibers within the unit, as in a muscular dystrophy, or disturbs neuromuscular transmission at single junctions, as in myasthenia gravis.

Decrease in the number of motor units Diseases that reduce the number of lower motor neurons or motor axons within the peripheral nerve decrease the number of motor units which can be recruited in affected muscles. The number of motor units available for activation in denervated muscles varies in proportion to the strength of maximum voluntary contraction, and the action potential appears no longer as a complete recruitment (interference) pattern but rather as a *single unit pattern* or *mixed pattern* with maximum voluntary effort.

Decrease in number of muscle fibers In muscle diseases such as muscular dystrophy or other myopathies, where individual muscle fibers are affected, there is little or no reduction in the number of motor units available for recruitment even though each unit has fewer muscle fibers than normal. Maximum voluntary effort produces a normal full recruitment pattern despite marked weakness. Because fewer muscle fibers are active, however, the amplitude of the pattern is reduced from normal. *A full recruitment pattern of less than normal amplitude, in the face of significant clinical weakness, is the hallmark of a so-called myopathic EMG.*

Variation in the shape of action potentials In certain neuromuscular junction disorders, such as myasthenia gravis and Lambert-Eaton syndrome, there is abnormal variation in the shape and amplitude of single motor unit potentials with sustained voluntary activity. This variation of motor unit potentials results from an intermittent block of conduction at individual neuromuscular junctions.

Other abnormalities In *myotonia,* the sarcolemmal membrane is irritable, and repeated muscle depolarization and contraction occur despite voluntary attempts at relaxation (Chap. 17). Such patterns occur in myotonia congenita, myotonic dystrophy, and hyperkalemic periodic paralysis. On EMG, myotonia causes high-frequency repetitive discharges which wax and wane in amplitude and frequency, producing a "dive bomber" or "motorcycle" sound on the loud speaker. Myotonia occurs with percussion or movement of the needle electrode or following voluntary contraction of the muscle. Motor unit potentials appear normal but are not followed by the silence which normally occurs on relaxation. Instead there is a burst of rapid activity which may take as long as several minutes to subside. Some of the potentials of this prolonged discharge have the duration, amplitude, and form of single-fiber activity, while others have characteristics of motor unit potentials.

Bizarre, repetitive high-frequency discharges without waxing and waning are seen in hypothyroidism and other disorders affecting peripheral nerve or muscle. High-frequency *coupling* of action potentials into doublets, triplets, or higher multiples of single units occurs in tetany and hemifacial spasm and indicates instability in repolarization of the nerve fiber. Electric silence characterizes *contracture,* as in McArdle's disease or malignant hyperthermia.

Single-fiber EMG and macro EMG In addition to conventional EMG with concentric needle electrodes, specialized techniques permit the recording of the EMG of single muscle fibers or of the entire motor unit (macro EMG). Single fiber techniques, by recording *jitter,* can measure accurately, within microseconds, the performance of individual neuromuscular junctions. Characteristic quantitative abnormalities are found in patients with myasthenia gravis and other disorders of neuromuscular transmission. Single-fiber EMG studies are also used to calculate *fiber density,* the number of single muscle fiber action potentials belonging to one motor unit within the recording area of the single-fiber EMG electrode (approximately 200 μm). Fiber density values are increased after denervation-reinnervation processes.

Macro EMG techniques measure all fibers belonging to a motor unit and allow estimation of true motor unit size. The amplitude and area of macro EMG motor unit potentials is increased in reinnervation and decreased in primary muscle diseases that cause reduction in the number of muscle fibers per motor unit.

NERVE CONDUCTION STUDIES Stimulation of the larger peripheral motor and sensory nerves permits the recording of their action potentials and provides objective quantitative data of *latency* and *conduction velocity.* The technique is performed by stimulating the nerve with surface electrodes placed on the skin over the nerve. The resulting *compound action potential* is recorded by electrodes—over the nerve proximally in the case of large sensory fibers; over the muscle distally in the case of motor fibers in a mixed motor-sensory nerve (Fig. 354-3). The conduction time from the most distal stimulating electrode, measured in milliseconds from the stimulus artifact to the onset of the response, is termed the *distal* or *peripheral* latency. If a second stimulus is applied to a mixed nerve, more proximally (or if recording electrodes are placed more proximally in the case of sensory fibers), a new and longer conduction time can be measured. When the distance (in millimeters) between the two sites of stimulation of motor fibers or recording of sensory fibers is divided by the difference in conduction times (in milliseconds), a *maximal conduction velocity* (in meters per second) is obtained. It describes the velocity of propagation of the action potentials in the largest and fastest nerve fibers. These velocities in normal subjects vary roughly from 40 or 45 m/s, depending upon which nerve is studied, to 75 or 80 m/s. Values are lower in newborn infants (approximately half of the adult values) and reach the adult range by 3 to 4 years of age. Normal values also exist for peripheral latencies from the most distal site on various mixed nerves to the appropriate muscles. When one stimulates the median nerve at the wrist, for example, the latency for conduction through the carpal tunnel to the abductor pollis brevis muscle is usually less than 4.5 ms in normal subjects. Tables of similar normal values have been compiled for conduction velocity and distal latencies that vary with the distance. It is important to maintain normal body temperature during nerve conduction studies because subnormal temperatures cause slower conduction velocity. Nerve conduction velocity is related to fiber diameter and to the degree of demyelination. Unmyelinated and small-diameter fibers have slower conduction velocities than large-diameter, myelinated fibers. Fibers with segmental demyelination have decreased conduction velocities. When motor fibers in the mixed peripheral nerve are stimulated and when each nerve fiber is in functional continuity with its many muscle fibers, the large *compound muscle action potential* arising from many firing muscle fibers can be recorded from skin electrodes over the muscle. Sensory action potentials, recorded from nerve fibers themselves, lack the "amplification" provided by muscle fibers; hence, more electronic amplification is required. In abnormal nerves, sensory potentials may be small or absent, and sensory conduction measurements may be impossible to record. In contrast, reliable measurement of motor conduction velocities is usually possible even though only one functional nerve fiber remains intact.

Nerve conduction velocity measurements reflect the status of the best surviving nerve fibers and, if even a few fibers are unaffected by the disease process, may be normal despite extensive nerve degeneration. After incomplete transection of nerve by a sharp object, the maximum motor conduction velocity may be normal in the few remaining fibers although the muscle involved is almost totally paralyzed. The axon is the primary site of pathology in alcoholic, nutritional, uremic, and diabetic neuropathy. The axons which remain intact conduct impulses normally, so that when the larger fibers are affected, the remaining smaller-diameter fibers, which normally conduct more slowly, account for a slightly slower maximum motor conduction velocity.

Nerve conduction velocity in many neuropathies is often normal or only slightly below normal. Ordinary nerve conduction studies

FIGURE 354-3 *Measurement of nerve conduction velocity. The median nerve is stimulated through the skin at the wrist (1) or in the antecubital fossa (2), and the resultant compound muscle action potential is recorded as the potential difference between a surface electrode over the thenar eminence (vertical arrow) and a reference electrode (Ref.) more distally. Sweep 1′ on the cathode ray oscilloscope (CRO) depicts the stimulus artifact (moment of stimulation at 1) followed by the muscle potential. The distal latency is the time A′ on the CRO sweep (3.0 ms, for example) which corresponds to conduction over distance A in the hand. The same is true for sweep 2′, where stimulation is at point 2 and the time from artifact to response is A′ + B′. The maximal motor conduction velocity from point 2 to point 1 is obtained by dividing distance B by time B′.*

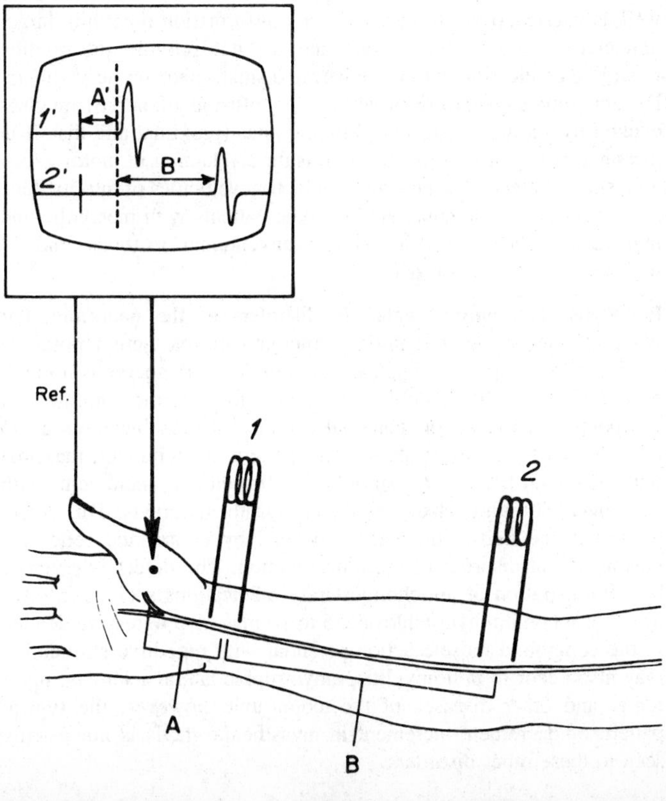

can usually, therefore, be used to document the presence of neuropathy only by comparison of recorded values with those from an adequate control group of the same age and sex.

Although many diseases of peripheral nerves do not cause reduction in nerve conduction velocity, disorders such as acute idiopathic polyneuropathy (Guillain-Barré syndrome), diphtheria, metachromatic leukodystrophy, and the hypertrophic neuropathies cause slowed velocities because they affect Schwann cells primarily and produce segmental demyelination. Focal compressions of nerve, as in entrapment syndromes, produce localized slowing of conduction because of narrowing of axons and demyelination at the site of compression. The demonstration of such localized slowing of conduction is useful in confirming nerve entrapment. A comparison of the peripheral (terminal) latency of one median nerve with the other median nerve or with an ulnar nerve may provide evidence for compression of the median nerve in the carpal tunnel. Normal conduction times do not, however, exclude an entrapment syndrome.

Other techniques for evaluation of nerve conduction Methods for study of conduction in more proximal segments of nerve include measurements of latencies for *F responses, H reflexes,* and *blink reflexes.* These techniques determine conduction velocity in nerves going from the periphery (of a limb or the face) to the central nervous system (spinal cord or brainstem) and back again. The *F response* measures the time required for a stimulus applied to the axon of an alpha motor neuron to pass antidromically to the anterior horn of the spinal cord and then to return orthodromically down the same axon. The *H reflex* measures the time required for orthodromic conduction up the nerve via group IA sensory fibers, through the spinal monosynaptic connection with the alpha motor neuron, and then orthodromically down the motor axon. Thus, conduction along proximal sensory and motor nerves and spinal roots can be measured. The application of these techniques to the measurement of proximal nerve conduction has increased the likelihood of recognition of abnormal conduction velocity in patients with peripheral neuropathy to 80 to 90 percent. The *blink reflexes* measure conduction in branches of the trigeminal and facial nerves. The blink reflex evoked by electric stimulation of the supraorbital branches of the trigeminal nerve permits localization of lesions in the distribution of facial or trigeminal nerves.

The nerve conduction studies described above, conventional as well as late-response studies, only give information regarding large-diameter fast-conducting axons and do not provide information regarding conduction in intermediate and small-diameter nerve fibers. By applying physiologic principles of collision of nerve impulses evoked by stimulation to two different sites (proximal and distal) in the same nerve, it is possible to measure conduction in motor axons with small diameters. Abnormal conduction velocities of intermediate size fibers can be demonstrated in some patients with metabolic and nutritional neuropathies in whom conventional methods and F-response studies are normal.

Repetitive stimulation tests In disorders of the neuromuscular junction, the size of the initial compound muscle action potential produced by a supramaximal electric stimulus to the nerve is normal; however, after a few stimuli at rates of 2 to 3 Hz the amplitude of compound muscle action potential declines; it then increases again after the fourth or fifth stimulus. This pattern of decrement, maximal with the fourth or fifth stimulus, followed by increment with subsequent stimuli is characteristic of myasthenia gravis. This defect resembles the partial blockade produced by curare and reflects a postjunctional disorder of synaptic function. The defect is reversed by administration of anticholinesterase medications such as intravenous edrophonium hydrochloride (5 to 10 mg). A progressive decline in the compound muscle action potential with repetitive stimulation may also occur in poliomyelitis, amyotrophic lateral sclerosis, myotonia, and other diseases of the motor unit; however, the typical pattern of decrement-increment in myasthenia gravis is not usually seen in these other disorders.

In the Lambert-Eaton (myasthenic) syndrome, repetitive stimulation causes a facilitation of transmission. Rapid stimulation of nerve (20 to 30 Hz) results in a progressive increase in muscle action potentials, which are small or virtually absent at the first stimulus, to a nearly normal amplitude. This facilitation response is not affected by anticholinesterase drugs but may be reversed by guanidine hydrochloride (10 to 30 mg/kg per day in divided doses). The neuromuscular transmission defect of this "reversed" myasthenic syndrome is prejunctional and is the result of a defective release of acetylcholine; a similar defect results from botulinum toxin or from the paralysis produced by the aminoglycoside antibiotics (see Chap. 358).

EMG IN DISORDERS OF THE CENTRAL NERVOUS SYSTEM The application of EMG and nerve conduction studies to evaluation of function of the central nervous system is termed *central EMG.* Since the motor unit is the final common path for all nerve impulses controlling skeletal muscles, the disorders of motor control produced by lesions of the central nervous system result in abnormal discharge patterns of motor neurons that can be documented by electrophysiologic techniques. For example, surface EMG recordings from pairs of antagonistic muscles, analysis of single motor unit recruitment patterns, and microneurographic studies are useful in evaluating different types of tremor, including rest tremor of Parkinson's disease, essential familial tremor, and physiologic tremor. Cerebellar ataxia can usually be separated from other tremors and from sensory ataxia. Asterixis can be distinguished from tremor, and different types of myoclonus can be documented. Studies of proprioceptive and exteroceptive reflexes are helpful in the differential diagnosis of movement disorders and in differentiating spasticity from other types of rigidity. Studies of the H reflex and F responses provide information regarding the excitability of the motor neuron pool. The effect of vibration on the H reflex has been used to evaluate presynaptic inhibition in different neurologic disorders. Silent-period studies have been used to evaluate function of proprioceptive input from muscle spindles. Mismatching of information from muscle spindles and joint receptors can result in an apparent "cerebellar" ataxia in patients with acute inflammatory polyneuropathy (Fisher syndrome) due to a lesion in the peripheral nervous system. EMG recordings and blink reflexes are useful in documenting clinically inapparent lesions of the brainstem in multiple sclerosis and in localizing early compressive lesions of trigeminal and facial nerves produced by small posterior fossa tumors.

HISTOPATHOLOGY OF MUSCLE AND NERVE *Muscle biopsy* is useful in (1) distinguishing between neurogenic and myopathic processes; (2) recognizing specific disorders of muscle such as muscular dystrophy or the congenital myopathies; (3) identifying specific metabolic defects of muscle by histochemical or biochemical techniques; and (4) diagnosing diseases of connective tissue and blood vessels, such as polyarteritis nodosa, and infections such as trichinosis or toxoplasmosis.

Muscle biopsy is performed under local anesthesia. In children and in adults with chronic conditions, an adequate specimen can often be obtained by needle biopsy. Open biopsy may be necessary to diagnose focal, patchy processes such as myositis or vasculitis. In all instances the muscle chosen for sampling must be appropriate for the condition suspected, and the specimen must be handled by a laboratory skilled in the evaluation of muscle. If the biopsy is taken from a muscle that has recently been traumatized by an EMG needle or that has been affected by a preexisting disease (e.g., coincidental nerve root compression), misleading information will be obtained.

Normal muscle histology Transverse sections of normal muscle show large numbers of muscle fibers grouped into areas (or fascicles) by connective tissue septa (perimysium), which may contain nerve bundles and blood vessels. The individual muscle fibers lie surrounded by thin collagen sheaths (endomysium) and by capillaries. The range of muscle fiber diameter is 40 to 80 μm in adult limb muscles, and the distribution of diameters is unimodal. Each fiber consists of myofibrils surrounded by and interspersed with cytoplasm containing glycogen, mitochondria, and sarcotubular systems. The muscle fiber is surrounded by a plasmalemma (sarcolemma) and a basal lamina. Multiple muscle nuclei are present in each fiber (which is a syncitium) and are almost all restricted to the subsarcolemmal region. A few stem cells or satellite cells are located between the basal lamina and the plasmalemma of the muscle fiber, and these provide the major source of myoblasts for regeneration of damaged muscle fibers. The histochemical separation of fibers into types I and II has been described above.

Muscle has a relatively limited number of pathologic reactions.

DENERVATION, REINNERVATION A denervated muscle fiber undergoes atrophy, and in the initial stages myofibrils are lost to a greater degree than is sarcoplasm containing the mitochondria, so that muscle fibers appear ''super dark'' with stains for oxidative enzymes (Fig. 354-4). Such denervated fibers are squeezed by adjacent innervated fibers and therefore become angulated and atrophic. In the initial stages of denervation, because of the overlap of many motor units in the same area, denervated atrophic fibers are distributed randomly throughout the muscle. Remaining motor axons sprout to reinnervate such fibers, eventually producing fiber type grouping (Fig. 354-2*C*). With subsequent death of such enlarged motor units, grouped fiber atrophy occurs. The typical appearance of a denervated and reinnervated muscle is shown in Fig. 354-4. The fiber diameter distribution in chronically denervated and reinnervated muscle is bimodal, with the atrophic denervated fibers making up one population and the normal size (or hypertrophied) innervated fibers making up the other population. It is generally difficult to make a specific diagnosis or determine a specific etiology from the muscle biopsy in cases of muscle denervation and reinnervation.

MUSCLE FIBER NECROSIS AND REGENERATION Damage of the sarcolemma of the muscle fiber allows entry of calcium at the high extracellular concentration into the low-calcium environment of the sarcoplasm. Calcium entry activates a neutral protease, thereby initiating proteolysis. Calcium also poisons mitochondrial function and causes cell death. Invading macrophages phagocytose the muscle fibers. Satellite cells, which provide the basis for regeneration of muscle fibers, are spared in most of the processes that damage muscles. They proliferate and fuse to produce multinuclear myotubes leading to regeneration of the muscle fiber. Characteristically, regenerating fibers are small, are basophilic owing to an increased concentration of RNA, and have large vesicular internal nuclei. The distribution of muscle fiber diameters in a typical chronic myopathy is broad and unimodal—very different from the bimodal diameter distribution of denervated and reinnervated muscle.

Muscle fiber necrosis and regeneration are common responses to damage, including damage caused by trauma, Duchenne's dystrophy, polymyositis, and dermatomyositis. Eventually, if the necrosis is sufficiently chronic, regeneration may fail, causing progressive loss of muscle fibers and replacement with fat and fibrous tissue. A chronic myopathy, Duchenne's dystrophy, is illustrated in Fig. 354-5. Differences in the extent and tempo of these processes allow histologic distinction between the muscular dystrophies, inflammatory myopathies, and acute rhabdomyolysis.

STRUCTURAL CHANGES IN MUSCLE FIBERS Degeneration of muscle fibers without frank necrosis produces structural alteration of individual muscle fibers; disorganization of myofibrils and sarcoplasm produces target fibers (Fig. 354-4), ringbinden (appearance of a portion of a fiber wrapped around another), central cores, cytoid bodies, and nemaline bodies. In one condition the fibers resemble

FIGURE 354-4 *A. Normal skeletal muscle biopsy stained for myosin ATPase (pH 9.4). Type I fibers are light, type II dark. B. Chronic denervation-reinnervation showing fiber type grouping. (Myosin ATPase, pH 9.4.) C. Chronic denervation-reinnervation in amyotrophic lateral sclerosis, preparation stained for mitochondrial enzyme, NADH-TR. There are groups of reinnervated type II fibers (light) and of denervated angulated atrophic fibers, many of them ''superdark'' and showing target fiber changes. D. Type II fiber atrophy. (Myosin ATPase, pH 9.4.)*

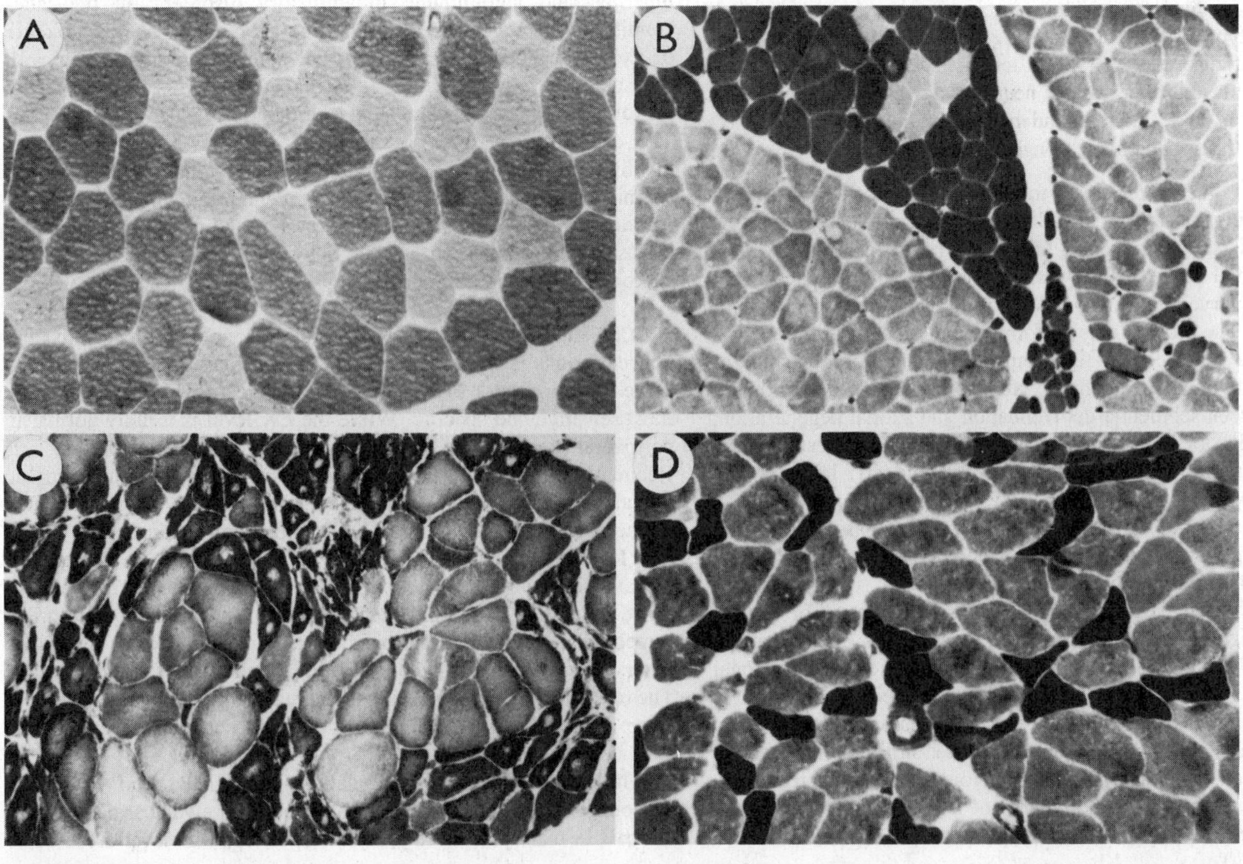

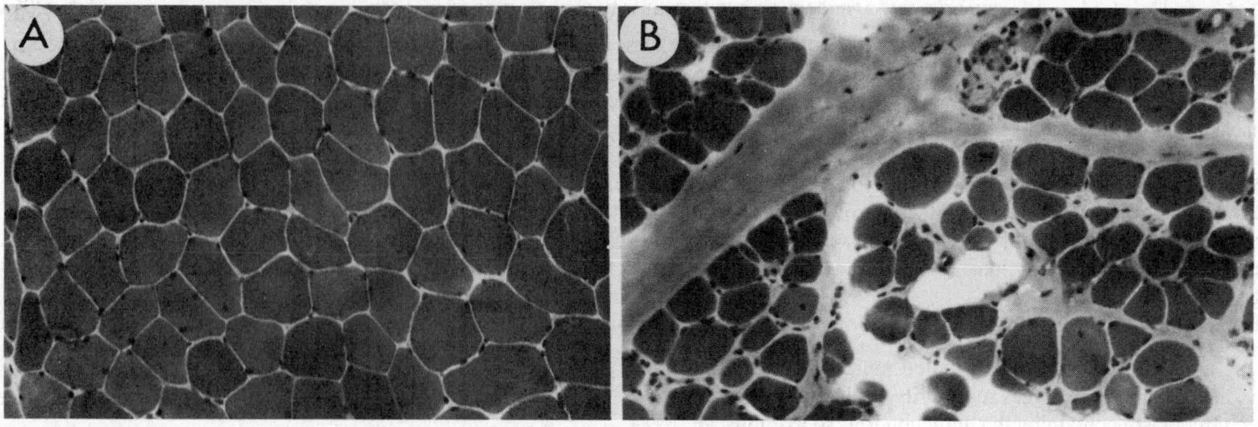

FIGURE 354-5 *A. Normal muscle (Hematoxylin-eosin.) B. Duchenne's muscular dystrophy, showing hypertrophy and atrophy of fibers, fiber degeneration, loss of fibers and fibrosis. (Hematoxylin-eosin.)*

myotubes (centronuclear myopathy). In others, abnormal mitochondria suggest an abnormality of mitochondrial biochemistry, while the presence of vacuoles suggests a disturbance of glycogen or lipid metabolism. Rimmed vacuoles (accumulations of degenerating phospholipid material between myofibrils) occur particularly in oculopharyngeal muscular dystrophy and inclusion body myositis.

INFLAMMATORY CHANGES Perivascular and interstitial inflammatory cell infiltration with lymphocytes is characteristic of polymyositis and dermatomyositis. Necrosis and regeneration of muscle fibers are also present. In some instances, atrophy of the fibers located on the periphery of muscle fasciculi (perifascicular atrophy) is prominent and can be an indicator of inflammatory myopathy, even though a focus of inflammation is not present in the muscle taken at biopsy. Muscle biopsy may show vasculitis in patients with collagen diseases or granulomas in patients with sarcoidosis.

CHANGES SPECIFIC TO FIBER TYPE Pathologic changes may be restricted to one fiber type in the muscle. The most common such condition is type II fiber atrophy (Fig. 354-4), which occurs in a wide range of disorders that limit activity such as disuse, muscle pain, joint pain, and upper motor neuronal dysfunction. Atrophy of type I fibers is less frequent and occurs in myotonic dystrophy, rheumatoid arthritis, and some congenital myopathies.

NERVE BIOPSY *Nerve biopsy* is more difficult and more traumatic than muscle biopsy and is useful in a limited number of specific circumstances (see Chap. 355). The sural nerve in the leg or the superficial radial nerve at the wrist are the usual biopsy sites. Both are sensory nerves and may show no changes in pure motor neuropathies. The procedure is performed under local anesthesia, and specimens are obtained for light and electron microscopy and for teasing of individual nerve fibers. Nerve biopsy aids in (1) distinguishing between segmental demyelination and axonal degeneration; (2) identification of inflammatory neuropathies; and (3) establishing specific diagnoses such as amyloidosis, sarcoidosis, leprosy, and several metabolic neuropathies. Full evaluation of the nerve biopsy requires the facilities of a laboratory with special interest and experience in peripheral nerve disease. There are two basic pathologic processes seen in nerve biopsies.

Light microscopic examination of biopsied nerves is of limited value, showing only gross changes such as vasculitis, inflammation, infiltration by granuloma or amyloid, loss of axons, and axonal degeneration. More information is obtained by electron microscopy and studies of single, teased nerve fibers. Some diseases affect specific fiber types; large myelinated fibers are affected in Friedreich's ataxia and unmyelinated fibers in familial amyloidosis. Quantitative morphometry (measurement of the number of fibers and the distribution of their diameters) is of additional help.

SEGMENTAL DEMYELINATION Diseases may attack either myelin or the Schwann cell, causing the myelin sheath to undergo degeneration but leaving the axon essentially unchanged. Healing of this segmental demyelination proceeds through a phase of abnormally thin myelin sheaths, which may eventually return to normal thickness. However, even after apparent recovery of segmental demyelination, single, teased nerve fiber studies demonstrate short and variable lengths of the internodes (distance between the nodes of Ranvier). If this process is progressive, ''onion-bulb'' formation occurs with thinly remyelinated fibers lying at the center of concentric lamellae of redundant Schwann cell cytoplasm.

AXON DEGENERATION Death of the nerve cell body or section of the axon at any level will lead to degeneration of the distal parts of the axon with secondary degeneration of the myelin sheath. If the nerve cell body remains intact proximally there is attempted axonal regeneration with sprouting. Such nerve sprouts (clusters) are characteristic of an axonal, degenerating and regenerating neuropathy.

Axonal degeneration is most common in toxic, inherited, traumatic, and ischemic diseases. Segmental demyelination may occur in the inherited and autoimmune inflammatory disorders; in the latter condition inflammatory cell infiltration may be seen. A mixed picture of axonal degeneration and segmental demyelination, together with a vasculopathy, is characteristic of diabetes mellitus. Some specific pathologic changes may indicate the probable etiology of a neuropathy. The deposition of IgM on the myelin-associated glycoprotein of myelin in IgM gammopathies can be detected by immunofluorescence techniques and leads to an increase in myelin periodicity in the nerve. Amyloid fibrils are present in nerve in amyloid neuropathy. Specific inclusions may be seen in the Schwann cells in metachromatic leukodystrophy and adrenomyeloleukodystrophy.

BIOCHEMICAL EVALUATION Certain enzymes that occur in high concentrations in the sarcoplasm of muscle may leak into blood and serve as an indicator of muscle damage. Creatine kinase (CK) is the most sensitive and specific. While the CK level is usually normal in peripheral neuropathies and neuromuscular junction disorders, it is frequently mildly elevated in spinal muscular atrophy, amyotrophic lateral sclerosis, and other motor neuron disorders. Serum aspartate aminotransferase (AST, SGOT), alanine aminotransferase (ALT, SGPT), lactic dehydrogenase (LDH), and aldolase levels may be elevated in the serum of a patient with active muscle destruction. Since several of these enzymes are determined during routine office screening, it is not uncommon for a patient with muscle disease to be first identified by an unexpected elevation in one of these enzymes. The reason for the disproportionate increase in CK level is not entirely clear. For evaluating a patient with neuromuscular disease, only the CK need be studied.

Three isoenzymes of CK occur—MM, MB, and BB. MM predominates in skeletal muscle, MB occurs mainly in cardiac muscle, and BB is mainly in brain. Elevations of CK-MB level are used to indicate the presence of myocardial damage. CK level elevation caused by acute muscle injury is usually due to the MM isozyme. However, in patients with long-standing muscular diseases, in athletes, and in others who have a chronic elevation in CK level, the proportion of MB in skeletal muscle rises and in consequence the proportion of CK-MB in blood is elevated. A greater than tenfold elevation of CK level usually indicates the presence of muscle destruction. Lesser elevations of CK level can occur in many neuromuscular diseases as well as from minor muscle trauma, such as that after electromyography, in psychotic or alcoholic patients, in hypothyroidism or hypoparathyroidism, in individuals with muscle hypertrophy, and in the carrier state of certain genetic myopathies. Strenuous exercise or muscle trauma can elevate the level of CK in normal individuals. This elevation occurs 6 h or more following exercise.

Muscle composition and mass Computerized tomography and magnetic resonance imaging can differentiate between muscle fibers, fat, and connective tissue and may show distinctive differences between muscular dystrophy and other forms of muscle disease. The high cost, the limitations in terms of the number of cross sections of a limb that can be examined, and the nonspecificity of the findings suggest that the role of these techniques is limited. Estimations of total muscle mass are of some importance in metabolic studies. A simple decline in muscle mass without weakness is indicative of a process other than a neuromuscular disease, for example, aging, neoplasm, malnutrition, or renal or hepatic disease. The 24-h urine creatinine excretion is the most widely available technique used to estimate muscle mass; creatinine excretion is decreased in patients with wasting from any cause. Patients with wasting neuromuscular diseases have decreased serum creatinine levels, with values as low as 0.2 to 0.5 mg/dL. In patients with muscle wasting this reduction results in a disproportionately low serum creatinine level despite impaired renal function; patients with active muscle destruction have a correspondingly *increased* serum creatinine level.

Metabolic and endocrine studies Hypo- and hyperkalemia, hypernatremia, hypo- and hypercalcemia, hypophosphatemia, and hypermagnesemia can all cause severe, usually acute, weakness. Serum potassium levels are labile and subject to rapid shifts induced by acidosis or alkalosis. The intracellular concentration of potassium is high, so that hemolysis during blood collection may spuriously elevate the potassium level. Acute muscle damage producing rhabdomyolysis may produce a true hyperkalemia. Such elevations in serum potassium are not greater than 0.1 meq per liter, however, unless the serum is stained with hemoglobin, as occurs with hemolysis, or the urine with myoglobin, as in the case of rhabdomyolysis. Chronic endocrine disorders, either hypo- or hyperfunction of thyroid, adrenal, or parathyroid glands, may cause weakness. Thyroid and parathyroid disorders may cause muscle weakness in the absence of other clinical evidence of endocrinopathy. Rheumatoid arthritis, systemic lupus erythematosus, scleroderma, and the polymyalgia rheumatica syndrome may present with or be complicated by muscle weakness. Tests for these diseases are usually indicated in the evaluation of unexplained muscle pain and weakness. The weakness in most of these disorders is related to disuse atrophy and joint pain; muscle inflammation and evidence of muscle destruction are relatively uncommon.

Exercise testing (see Chap. 357) Patients with substrate utilization defects characteristically have decreased exercise tolerance and muscle pain and weakness during or following exercise. Most defects in the enzymatic pathways of glycolysis result in the failure of muscle to generate adenosine triphosphate (ATP) from glycogen and a diminished or absent production of lactic acid. Patients with these disorders can be evaluated with a forearm exercise test evaluating the level of venous lactic acid. Patients with disturbance of fatty acid metabolism (such as carnitine palmityl tranferase deficiency, in which long-chain fatty acids cannot be transferred into mitochondria for beta oxidation) generate lactic acid normally. Patients with myoadenylate deaminase deficiency generate lactate in normal or increased amounts but fail to produce ammonia in the exercise test (Chap. 357). Measurement of other muscle metabolites and specific enzymes can define the cause of the disorder.

Myoglobinuria Acute muscle destruction, *rhabdomyolysis* associated with myoglobinuria, occurs with acute toxic, metabolic, infectious, and traumatic muscle damage (Chap. 356). The molecular weight of myoglobin is lower than that of hemoglobin so that the urine rather than the serum changes color in extensive rhabdomyolysis. Lesser degrees of myoglobinuria can cause positive urine tests for blood in the absence of urinary erythrocytes. Confirmatory testing for myoglobin is possible with a specific immunoassay.

GENERAL THERAPEUTIC CONSIDERATIONS Cardiac disease Most disorders of skeletal muscle also involve cardiac muscle. Clinical cardiac dysfunction is relatively uncommon, perhaps because the limited exercise capacity of the patient with weakness decreases demand on cardiac performance. Relatively specific electrocardiographic abnormalities occur in Duchenne's dystrophy and infantile acid maltase deficiency. Cardiac conduction disorders including complete heart block occur in patients with myotonic dystrophy. An electrocardiogram should be obtained in all patients with neuromuscular disease, particularly in patients with myopathies.

Respiratory disease Diminished pulmonary function in patients with acute or chronic neuromuscular disease may progress to ventilatory failure. The earliest manifestation of respiratory muscle weakness is a decrease in maximum expiratory and inspiratory pressures. Diaphragmatic weakness, in particular, may be significant in patients with neuromuscular disease; diaphragmatic function should be evaluated by examining pulmonary function both while the patient is supine and sitting. The patient with diaphragmatic weakness has a greater impairment of pulmonary function in the supine position than in the erect position, as well as having paradoxical abdominal movements. Patients with chronic respiratory failure may be maintained with home respiratory support.

Physical therapy Physical therapy is of greatest value in patients with muscle weakness when joint contractures are developing and when enforced immobility, such as due to an injury, results in decreased activity. Exercises may increase strength in muscles weakened by disease just as it does in normal persons, but there is little convincing evidence that exercise improves functional abilities. On the other hand, therapeutic standing in patients with marginal leg and trunk function has considerable pyschological benefit and may help to preserve bone mineralization and cardiovascular reflexes.

Dietary modification Dietary restriction is often necessary in patients with muscle weakness since caloric expenditure is decreased because of immobility and loss of muscle mass. Development of obesity further compromises already reduced mobility, worsens pulmonary function, and may depress ventilatory drive. Unless there is specific evidence for malabsorption of vitamin B_{12} or vitamin E, neither these nor any other vitamin has a specific role in the treatment of neuromuscular disease. Certain vitamins are hazardous in excessive doses, including vitamins B_6, A, and D (see Chaps. 76 and 336).

Bracing In patients with distal leg weakness, particularly of foot dorsiflexion, ankle-foot orthoses can restore gait to nearly normal. With more proximal weakness, however, leg braces diminish mobility and are of value only in enabling patients who are unable to walk to perform therapeutic standing. In most adults, even this use of braces is impractical because such standing in braces usually requires assistance.

Scoliosis Spinal deformity may complicate neuromuscular diseases that occur before puberty. Duchenne's dystrophy, spinal muscular atrophy, and congenital myopathies are particularly liable to this complication. Once full long-bone growth has been achieved, many of these patients have surgical correction of the scoliosis. Severely impaired pulmonary function is a contraindication to such therapy, and patients with limited life expectancy should probably be spared the pain and risks of the procedure.

Genetic evaluation and counseling (see also Chap. 357) Management of the patient with hereditary muscle disease should include family pedigree analysis and genetic counseling. The family history may initially be negative in many patients with autosomal dominant diseases such as Charcot-Marie-Tooth disease, myotonic dystrophy, and facioscapulohumeral dystrophy because of the variable expressivity of the disorders. The availability of chromosomal markers for linkage analysis has made carrier detection, antenatal diagnosis, and early diagnosis of disease feasible in several hereditary neuromuscular diseases (e.g., in Duchenne's and myotonic dystrophy). The availability of therapy for disorders such as periodic paralysis, myotonia, and certain metabolic myopathies and of preventive measures in disorders such as malignant hyperthermia provides a strong impetus for early diagnosis. History is inadequate for family evaluation. Physical examination of, or inspection of photographs of, family members may provide clues to the characteristic facial or other features of the disorder and will often identify mildly afflicted individuals.

REFERENCES

BRADLEY WG: *Disorders of Peripheral Nerves*. Oxford, Blackwell, 1974

BROOKE MH: *A Clinician's View of Neuromuscular Disease*, 2d ed, Baltimore, Williams and Wilkins, 1986

BUCHTHAL F, SIMPSON JA (eds): *Handbook of Electroencephalography and Clinical Neurophysiology*, vol 16: *Electromyography*, Part A: *Nervous and Muscular Evoked Potentials;* Part B: *Neuromuscular Disease*. Amsterdam, Elsevier, 1973

CARPENTER S, KARPATI G: *Pathology of Skeletal Muscle*. New York, Churchill Livingston, 1984.

DYCK PJ et al (eds): *Peripheral Neuropathy*. Philadelphia, Saunders, 1984

ENGEL AG, BANKER BQ (eds): *Myology*. New York, McGraw-Hill, 1986

KIMURA J: *Electrodiagnosis in Diseases of Nerve and Muscle: Principles and Practice*, Philadelphia, Davis, 1983

LANG H, WURZBURG U: Creatine kinase, an enzyme of many forms. Clin Chem 28:1439, 1982

SHAHANI BT: *Electromyography in Central Nervous System Disorders: Central Electromyography*. Boston, Butterworth, 1984

SCHAUMBURG HH et al: *Disorders of Peripheral Nerves*. Philadelphia, Davis, 1983

355 DISEASES OF THE PERIPHERAL NERVOUS SYSTEM

ARTHUR K. ASBURY

Peripheral neuropathy is a general term indicating a disorder of peripheral nerve of any cause; therefore, the knowledge that a peripheral neuropathy is present in a particular patient should instigate a search for its basis.

The basic processes affecting nerve and muscle and the approach to diseases of nerve and muscle are fully set forth in Chap. 354. The first purpose here is to build upon that base by providing an overview of the wide array of peripheral neuropathies which afflict humans. Disorders of peripheral nerve exhibit such a bewildering and complex set of manifestations that it is difficult for the physician to know where to begin and how to proceed. Therefore the second purpose here is to develop a logical approach and assessment scheme (summarized in Fig. 355-1) which will guide the examiner to correct diagnoses and management decisions.

GENERAL DESCRIPTION OF NEUROPATHIC SYNDROMES The prototypical picture of polyneuropathy occurs with acquired toxic or metabolic neuropathic states. From a symptom standpoint, the first noticeable features tend to be sensory and consist of tingling, prickling, burning, or bandlike dysesthesias in the balls of the feet or tips of the toes, or in a general distribution over the soles. Symmetry of symptoms and findings in a distal graded fashion is the rule, but occasionally dysesthesias appear in one foot a brief time before the other or may be more pronounced in one foot. Some care and judgment must be exercised here to avoid confusion with mononeuropathy multiplex. If the polyneuropathy remains mild, no objective motor or sensory signs may be detectable.

With progression, a definite pansensory loss is usually found over both feet, ankle jerks will be lost, and a weakness of dorsiflexion of the toes, best demonstrated in the great toe, may be present. In some instances, the process begins with weakness in the feet, usually dorsiflexion of the toes and feet without subjective sensory symptoms. As worsening occurs, sensory loss moves centripetally in a graded "stocking" fashion, and the patient may complain that the feet have a numb or "wooden" feeling or may say "I feel as though I'm walking on stumps." Patients experience difficulty walking on their heels during examination and their feet may slap while walking. Later, the knee jerk reflex disappears and foot drop becomes more apparent. By the time sensory disturbance has reached the upper shin, dysesthesias are generally noticed in the tips of the fingers. The degree of spontaneous pain varies, but is often considerable. Light stimuli to hypesthetic areas, once perceived, may be experienced as extremely uncomfortable (hyperpathia). Unsteadiness of gait may be out of proportion to muscle weakness because of proprioceptive loss.

Worsening proceeds in a centripetal, symmetrically graded manner with muscle atrophy, pansensory loss, and areflexia and with motor weakness that is usually greater in the extensor muscles than in corresponding flexor groups. When the sensory disturbance reaches mid thigh, generally a tent-shaped area of hypesthesia on the lower abdomen may be demonstrated. This will grow broader, and the apex will extend rostrally toward the sternum as the neuropathy worsens. By this time, patients generally cannot stand or walk or hold objects in their hands.

In the most extreme cases, ventilatory capacity may be impaired along with sphincteric function. Hypesthesia at the crown of the scalp may be present and spreads radially into both the trigeminal and C2 distribution. In considering this entire sequence of events, it becomes apparent that nerve fibers are affected according to length of axon without regard to root or nerve trunk distribution—hence, the aptness of the term "stocking-glove" to describe the pattern of sensory deficit. In general, the motor deficit is also graded, distal, and symmetric.

Variations on the general sequence outlined above are manifold. They include the rate of evolution of symptoms; fluctuations in the course; the eventual degree of severity; the presence or absence of positive motor and sensory symptoms; the symmetry of features and their distribution in terms of proximal versus distal, arms versus legs, and motor versus sensory; the relative proportion of dysfunction attributable to large fiber deficit and to small fiber deficit; and the determination, mainly by electrodiagnostic examination, of axonal versus demyelinating processes.

ASSESSMENT AND DIAGNOSIS OF NEUROPATHY Taking the first step Clues to the diagnosis of specific peripheral neuropathies often lie in unnoted or readily forgotten events occurring weeks or months prior to the onset of symptoms. Inquiry should be made about recent viral illnesses; other systemic symptoms; institution of new medications; potentially toxic exposures to solvents, pesticides, or heavy metals; the occurrence of similar symptoms in family members or coworkers; habits concerning alcohol; and the presence of known preexisting medical disorders. It is also useful to ask patients if they would otherwise feel well if free of their neuropathic symptoms, to obtain an idea of the presence or absence of an underlying systemic illness.

It is important to learn how symptoms first appeared. Even with distal polyneuropathies, symptoms may appear in the sole of one foot a few days or a week before the other, but usually the patient will

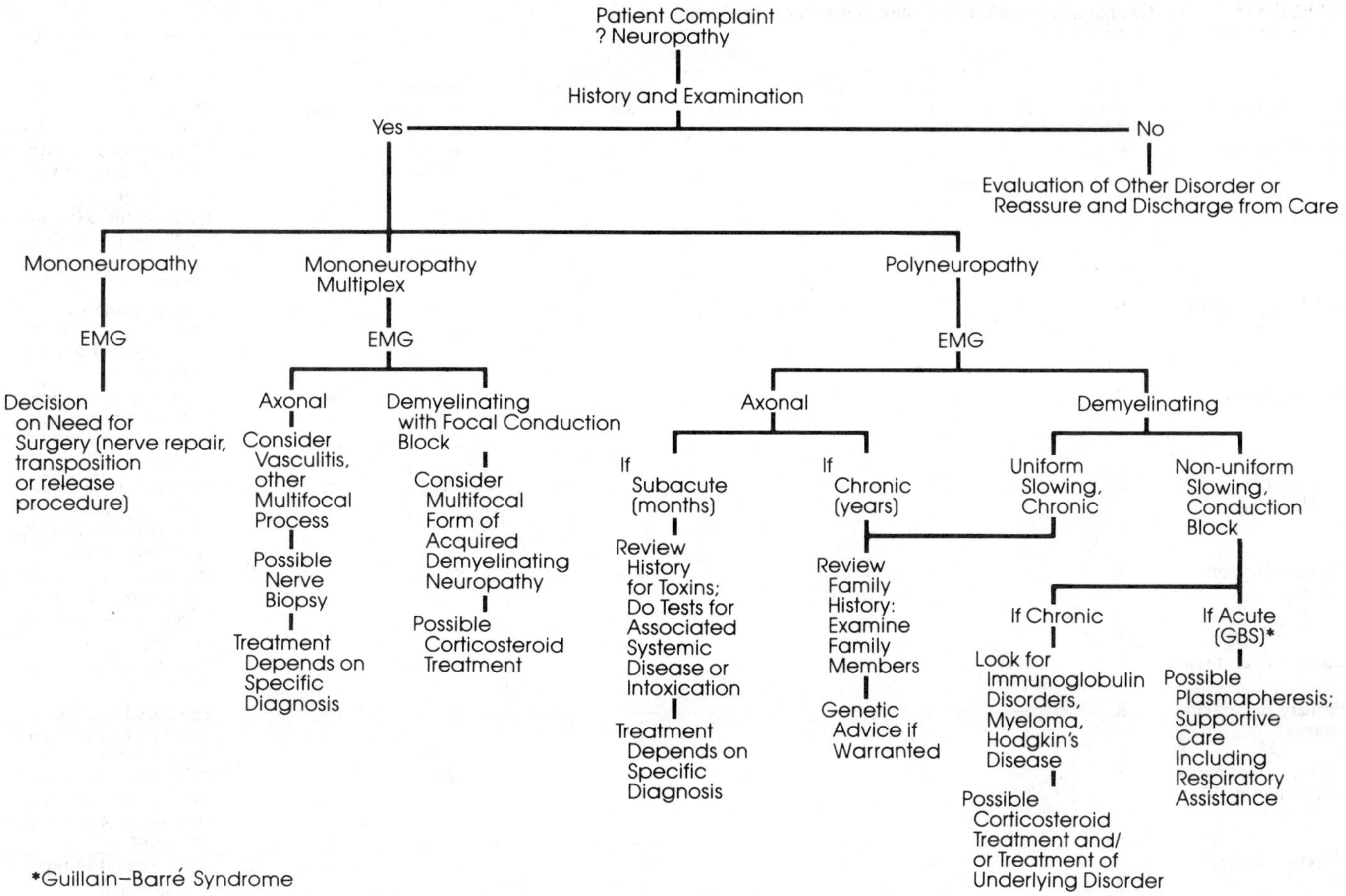

FIGURE 355-1 *Flowchart approach to the evaluation of peripheral neuropathies. (After Asbury, 1983.)*

describe a distal graded disturbance that moves evenly and symmetrically in centripetal fashion. Tingling dysesthesias will appear in the fingertips only when similar symptoms have reached the level of the knees. It is most important to determine whether symptoms first appeared in the distribution of individual digital nerves involving only one-half of a digit at a time and then gradually spread to become coalescent. This pattern of onset raises strong suspicions of a multifocal process (mononeuropathy multiplex) such as might be encountered with a systemic vasculitis or cryoglobulinemia.

The evolution of neuropathy ranges from rapid worsening over a few days to an indolent process extending many years. Polyneuropathies with a slowly progressive course lasting more than 5 years are most likely to be genetically determined, particularly if the major manifestations are distal atrophy and weakness with few or no positive sensory symptoms. Exceptions are diabetic polyneuropathy and paraproteinemic neuropathies in which the progression may be insidious over 5 to 10 years. Axonal degenerations of toxic or metabolic origin tend to evolve over several weeks to a year or more, and the rate of progression of demyelinating neuropathies is highly variable, ranging from a few days in Guillain-Barré syndrome to many years in others.

Major fluctuations in the course of neuropathy bring to mind two possibilities: (1) relapsing forms of neuropathy, or (2) repeated toxic exposures. A slow fluctuation in symptoms taking place over weeks or months (reflecting changes in the activity of neuropathy) should not be confused with day-to-day variation or diurnal undulation of symptoms. The latter are common to all neuropthic disorders. An example is carpal tunnel syndrome in which dysesthesias may be prominent at night but absent during the day.

In polyneuropathies, the findings can be expected to be quite symmetric on both sides of the body. If only one foot slaps when the patient walks, the process is not symmetric and the possibility of a multifocal process is raised. In addition, in acquired symmetric polyneuropathies, the muscles of extension and abduction tend to be weakened to a greater extent than the muscles of flexion and adduction. Hence, a weakness in lower legs often affects the peronei and anterior tibial muscles, with attendant foot drop, more than the gastrocnemius group or foot inverters. In most polyneuropathies the legs are more severely affected than the arms and the distal muscles more than the proximal ones. There are exceptions to this rule, as in lead neuropathy, in which manifestations of bilateral wrist drop may predominate, and occasionally in porphyric neuropathy, in which arms may be more affected than legs and proximal muscles more than distal.

Palpation of the nerve trunk to detect enlargement is a frequently forgotten part of the neurological examination. In mononeuropathies, the entire course of the nerve trunk in question should be explored manually for focal thickening; the presence of neurofibroma, point tenderness, or Tinel's phenomenon (generation of a tingling sensation in the sensory territory of the nerve by tapping along the course of the nerve trunk); and elicitation of pain by putting the nerve trunk on stretch. In leprous neuritis, fusiform thickening of nerve trunks is frequent, and beading of nerve trunks may be encountered in amyloid polyneuropathy. Certain genetically determined neuropathies of the hypertrophic variety may be attended by uniform thickening of all nerve trunks, often to the caliber of a clothes line or larger.

Most neuropathies involve nerve fibers of all sizes, but on occasion selective damage restricted to large or to small fibers predominates. In a polyneuropathy affecting mainly small fibers, diminished pinprick and temperature sensation, often with burning painful dysesthesias, may predominate along with autonomic dysfunction but with relative sparing of motor power, balance, and tendon jerks. Selected cases of amyloid and distal diabetic polyneuropathies fall into this category. In contrast, large-fiber polyneuropathy is characterized by areflexia, imbalance, relatively minor cutaneous sensory deficit, and variable but often severe motor dysfunction.

In addition to taking a history and doing a physical examination that bears in mind the emphases described above, certain other measures can be undertaken routinely in the evaluation of a patient

TABLE 355-1 Polyneuropathy associated with systemic diseases

Systemic disease	Occurrence*	Axonal† Acute	Axonal† Subacute	Axonal† Chronic	Demyelinating† Acute	Demyelinating† Subacute	Demyelinating† Chronic	Sensory vs. motor‡	Autonomic†	Comment
Diabetes mellitus	C	—	±	+	—	±	+	S, SM, rarely M	± to +	Mixed axonal-demyelination often seen; see Table 355-4
Uremia	S	±	+	+	—	—	—	SM	±	Controllable with proper dialysis; curable with successful renal transplant
Porphyria (3 types)	R	+	±	—	—	—	—	M	± to +	May be proximal > distal and may have atypical proximal sensory deficits
Hypoglycemia	R	±	+	±	—	—	—	M	—	Usually with insulinoma; arms often > legs; ? anterior horn cells affected
Vitamin deficiency, exclude B_{12}	S	—	+	+	—	—	—	SM	±	Involves at least thiamine, pyridoxine, folate, pantothenic acid; probably others
Vitamin B_{12} deficiency	S	—	±	+	—	—	—	S	—	Peripheral nerve involvement variable; often overshadowed by myelopathy
Chronic liver disease	S	—	—	—	—	—	+	S or SM	—	Usually mild or subclinical
Primary biliary cirrhosis	R	—	±	+	—	—	—	S	—	Epineurial and subperineurial xanthomatous deposits
Primary systemic amyloidosis	R	—	±	+	—	—	—	SM	+	Also seen with amyloidosis associated with myeloma or macroglobulinemia
Hypothyroidism	R	—	—	—	—	±	+	S	—	May respond to thyroid replacement
Chronic obstructive lung disease	R	—	±	+	—	—	—	S or SM	—	Few reports; a questionable entity
Acromegaly	R	—	—	+	—	—	—	S	—	Carpal tunnel syndrome also frequent
Malabsorption (sprue, celiac disease)	S	—	±	+	—	—	—	S or SM	±	Basis for neuropathy unclear; deficiency suspected
Carcinoma (sensory)	R	—	+	+	—	—	—	Pure S	—	Carcinomatous sensory neuropathy; due to gangliitic neuronopathy; mostly breast carcinoma; paraneoplastic; relatively rare

with neuropathy. Electrodiagnostic examination is a key procedure in all patients. For patients with polyneuropathy or mononeuropathy multiplex, standard tests should include a complete blood count and erythrocyte sedimentation rate, urinalysis, chest x-ray, postprandial blood glucose, and serum protein electrophoresis. Further tests should be dictated by the formulation arrived at via the combined history and physical and electrodiagnostic examination (see Fig. 355-1).

Taking the next step The next step is electrodiagnostic examination. It is not generally possible to make the distinction between axonal versus demyelinating disorders on clinical examination alone, and it is in this category that electrodiagnostic analysis is particularly useful. Electrodiagnostic features of demyelination are slowing of nerve conduction velocity (NCV), dispersion of evoked compound action potentials (CAPs), conduction block (major decrease in amplitude of muscle CAP upon proximal stimulation of its nerve as compared to distal stimulation), and marked prolongation of distal latencies. In contrast, axonal neuropathies are characterized by a reduction in amplitude of evoked CAPs with relative preservation of NCV. The distinction between a primarily demyelinating neuropathy from one which is primarily axonal is crucial because of the differing approaches to diagnosis and management. If in a particular instance of progressive polyneuropathy or subacute or chronic evolution the electrodiagnostic findings are those of an axonopathy, a long list of metabolic states and exogenous toxins come into consideration (see Tables 355-1 and 355-2). If the course is protracted over several years, it raises the likelihood of the neuronal (axonal) form of peroneal muscular atrophy (HMSN-II); family members must be examined and additional attention given to the family history.

Alternatively, if the electrodiagnostic findings are more indicative of primary demyelination of nerve, the approach is entirely different. The possibilities then include acquired demyelinating neuropathy, thought to be immunologically mediated, and genetically determined neuropathies, some of which are marked by uniform and drastic slowing of nerve conduction velocities.

With these considerations in hand, a flowchart can be constructed (Fig. 355-1) which summarizes the clinical and electrodiagnostic approach to the evaluation and management of a neuropathic disorder. Using this scheme, the clinician determines for each patient the tempo, distribution, severity, and functional impairment, and other features previously discussed, making a clinical judgment as to whether the problem represents a mononeuropathy, a mononeuropathy multiplex, or a polyneuropathy. Often this distinction is obvious. With the sum of clinical and electrodiagnostic information in hand,

TABLE 355-1 Polyneuropathy associated with systemic diseases *(continued)*

		Axonal†			Demyelinating†					
Systemic disease	Occurrence*	Acute	Subacute	Chronic	Acute	Subacute	Chronic	Sensory vs. motor‡	Autonomic†	Comment
Carcinoma (sensorimotor)	S	—	+	+	—	—	—	SM	±	Sensorimotor axonal neuropathy; mostly with lung carcinoma; more common than pure sensory, but still infrequent
Carcinoma (late)	C	—	+	+	—	—	—	S>M	±	Mild, late axonal neuropathy, probably related to weight loss and wasting
Carcinoma (demyelinating)	S	—	—	—	+	+	±	SM	—	Acute or relapsing demyelinating neuropathy sometimes seen with carcinoma
Lymphoma including Hodgkin's	S	—	+	+	+	+	±	See above	±	Same as carcinomatous types, although pure sensory type is even rarer
Polycythemia vera	R	—	±	+	—	—	—	S	—	Also many CNS manifestations; often shooting pains in limbs
Multiple myeloma lytic type	S	—	±	+	—	—	—	S, M, or SM	±	Symptomatic neuropathy uncommon, subclinical neuropathy frequent
Multiple myeloma§: osteosclerotic or solitary plasmacytoma	S	—	—	±	—	±	+	SM	—	Although may show severe slowing of nerve conduction velocity recent work suggests this is secondary demyelination
Benign monoclonal gammopathy:	S									
IgA		—	±	+	—	—	—	SM	—	IgM_{κ} (or occasionally IgM_{λ}) may bind to myelin-associated glycoprotein or glycolipids
IgG		—	±	+	—	—	—	SM	—	
IgM		—	—	—	—	±	+	SM	—	
Macroglobulinemia	R	—	—	±	—	—	+	SM	—	Usually but not always axonal
Cryoglobulinemia	R	—	±	+	—	—	—	SM	—	May be mononeuropathy multiplex in presentation

* *R = rare; S = sometimes; C = common.*
† *± = sometimes; + = usual.*
‡ *S = sensory; M = motor; SM = sensorimotor.*
§ *Some cases associated with POEMS syndrome (see text).*

the differential diagnostic possibilities and management options will have been narrowed to only a few. The remainder of this chapter deals with the details of this formulation.

Electrodiagnosis As seen in Fig. 355-1, electrodiagnosis is a key part of the evaluation of any neuropathy. See Chap. 354 for details of technique and interpretation. For example, electrodiagnosis helps one to be certain about the presence or absence of a sensory deficit when this is not clear by clinical examination alone. It provides information about the distribution of subclinical findings, thus sharpening the diagnostic focus. A listing of the general questions which may be posed by the clinician to the electrodiagnostician includes

1 The distinction between disorders primary to nerve or to muscle.
2 The distinction between root involvement and more distal nerve trunk involvement.
3 The distinction between generalized polyneuropathic processes and widespread multifocal nerve trunk affection.
4 The distinction between upper and lower motor neuron weakness.
5 The distinction, in a given generalized polyneuropathic process, between a primary demyelinating neuropathy and axonal degeneration.
6 The assessment, in both primary axonal and demyelinating neuropathies, of many factors bearing on the nature, activity, and likely prognosis of the neuropathy.
7 The assessment, in mononeuropathies, of the site of the lesion and its major effect on nerve fibers, especially the distinction between demyelinating conduction block and wallerian degeneration.
8 The characterization of disorders of the neuromuscular junction.
9 The identification, often in muscle of normal bulk and strength, of chronic partial denervation, fasciculations, and myotonia.
10 The analysis of cramp, and its distinction from physiologic contracture.

Nerve biopsy The sural nerve at the ankle is the preferred site for cutaneous nerve biopsy. There are only a few indications to employ this invasive technique. The main one is in asymmetric and multifocal neuropathic disorders producing a clinical picture of mononeuropathy multiplex, the basis of which is still unclear after other laboratory investigations are complete. Diagnostic considerations include vasculitis, amyloidosis, leprosy, and occasionally sarcoidosis. Nerve biopsy is also helpful when one or more cutaneous nerves are palpably enlarged. Another clinical application is in establishing the diagnosis in some genetically determined pediatric disorders such as metachromatic leukodystrophy, Krabbe's disease, giant axonal neuropathy, and infantile neuroaxonal dystrophy. In all of these recessively inherited diseases, both the central nervous system (CNS) and the peripheral nervous system (PNS) are affected.

There is a tendency to carry out sural nerve biopsy in distal symmetric polyneuropathies of subacute or chronic evolution. This practice is discouraged because it is a low-yield measure. Nerve biopsy in this situation is only useful as part of an approved research

TABLE 355-2 Polyneuropathy associated with drugs or environmental toxins

	Axonal*			Demyelinating*			Sensory vs. motor†	Auto-nomic*	CNS*	Comment
	Acute	Subacute	Chronic	Acute	Subacute	Chronic				
DRUGS										
Amiodarone (antiar-rhythmic)	—	—	+	—	—	+	SM	—	—	Dose-dependent neuropathy, reversible by decreasing dose; lysosomal dense body accumulation
Aurothioglucose (anti-rheumatic)	±	±	—	+	+	—	SM	—	—	Idiosyncratic reaction, ? immune-mediated
cis-Platinum (antineo-plastic)	—	+	+	—	—	—	S	—	—	Severe sensory neuropathy, ? neuronopathy; also ototoxicity; dose-related
Dapsone (dermatologic including leprosy)	—	±	+	—	—	—	M	—	—	Dose-related pure motor neuropathy
Disulfiram (antialcohol)	±	+	+	—	—	—	SM	—	±	Usually occurs after months of treatment
Hydralazine (antihyper-tensive)	—	±	+	—	—	—	S>M	—	—	A pyridoxine antagonist; only rarely neurotoxic
Isoniazid	—	±	+	—	—	—	SM	±	—	A pyridoxine antagonist; neurotoxic in slow acetylators
Metronidazole (antiproto-zoal	—	—	±	—	—	—	S	—	+	Dose-related central-peripheral distal axonopathy
Misonidazole (radiosen-sitizer)	—	±	+	—	—	—	S	—	+	Neurotoxicity is the limiting factor
Perhexilene (antiar-rhythmic)	—	—	±	—	—	+	SM	±	—	Dose-related neuropathy; lysosomal dense body accumulation
Phenytoin (anticonvul-sant)	—	—	+	—	—	—	S>M	—	—	Large-fiber neuropathy, mild, after 20–30 years of phenytoin use
Thalidomide (anti-leprous)	—	—	+	—	—	—	S>M	±	+	Red skin and brittle nails; also teratogenic; recovery from neuropathy poor
Vincristine (antineoplas-tic)	—	+	+	—	—	—	S>M	—	—	Mild sensory neuropathy is nearly universal, hands>feet; motor signs should prompt cessation of treatment

protocol when the biopsy will provide crucial information not otherwise obtainable.

POLYNEUROPATHY Although this term connotes a widespread symmetric process, usually distal and graded, polyneuropathies present a high degree of diversity because of the extreme variability of tempo, severity, mix of sensory and motor features, and presence or absence of positive symptoms. The patient with a fulminant, severely dysesthetic sensory neuropathy and alopecia who is in the early phases of thallium intoxication bears little similarity to the patient with a 40-year history of insidiously progressive clumsiness of gait whose findings are foot drop, lower leg atrophy, pes cavus, and minimal asymptomatic distal sensory deficit (i.e., peroneal muscular atrophy, either type I or II; see Table 355-3). These two patients fall near opposite ends of the spectrum of polyneuropathy.

The classification of peripheral neuropathies has become increasingly complex as the capacity to discriminate new subgroups and identify new associations with toxins and systemic disorders improves. Further, our grasp of the pathophysiologic basis for the clinical phenomena observed in neuropathy has increased rapidly (see Chap. 354). But these advances are primarily descriptive, little or no progress has been made in illuminating the fundamental pathogenetic events in nervous tissue which eventuate in any one of the polyneuropathies.

The important features of each major grouping of polyneuropathies are summarized below and key aspects of specific polyneuropathies may be found in Tables 355-1 to 355-4.

Acute axonal polyneuropathy In this setting the term acute means evolution over days, making these neuropathies relatively uncommon. Included are porphyric neuropathy and massive intoxications, often suicidal or homicidal in intent. For example, an individual receiving a large dose of arsenic (e.g., 100 mg of arsenous oxide) will become violently ill in a few hours with vomiting, diarrhea, and circulatory collapse. In 1 to 3 days serious renal and liver failure will ensue, and between 14 and 21 days polyneuropathy will appear, often as the systemic disorder abates. Progression occurs for 2 or 3 weeks, but following a plateau, recovery requires months.

Subacute axonal polyneuropathy Subacute, meaning to evolve in weeks, characterizes many instances of toxic and metabolic polyneuropathy, but perhaps even more of these are chronic in evolution (months). Scanning the appropriate columns in Tables 355-1 and 355-2 provides many possibilities. Management in almost all instances involves removing from contact the offending agent or treating the associated systemic order.

Chronic axonal polyneuropathy This category includes many more types of polyneuropathy, in part because the term chronic subsumes neuropathies which have progressed over a period as short as 6 months to as long as 60 years. As a rough approximation, a slow worsening for more than 5 years, an absence of positive symptoms, mainly motor deficit, and an absence of systemic disorder all favor a genetically determined neuropathy. Although these are mostly autosomal dominant in inheritance pattern, recessively inherited and X-linked varieties also occur, including a form phenotypically resembling dominantly inherited peroneal muscular atrophy (HMSN-II) and also adrenomyeloneuropathy (see Table 355-3). To complete the picture, an array of rare autosomal recessive neuropathies occur in childhood.

TABLE 355-2 Polyneuropathy associated with drugs or environmental toxins *(continued)*

	Axonal*			Demyelinating*						
	Acute	Subacute	Chronic	Acute	Subacute	Chronic	Sensory vs. motor†	Autonomic*	CNS*	Comment
Nitrofurantoin (urinary antiseptic)	—	±	+	—	—	—	SM	—	—	Generally total dose-related; presence of renal failure may enhance toxicity
TOXINS										
Acrylamide (flocculant; grouting agent)	—	±	+	—	—	—	S>M	±	+	Large-fiber neuropathy; sensory ataxia
Arsenic (herbicide; insecticide)	±	+	+	—	—	—	SM	±	±	Skin changes and Mees' lines in nails; if acute intoxication, many systemic effects
Buckthorn (toxic berry)	—	—	—	+	+	—	SM	—	—	Only occurs where berries grow; may mimic GBS
Carbon disulfide, CS_2 (industrial)	—	—	+	—	—	+	SM	—	+	Neurofilamentous accumulation in axons; demyelinating features are secondary
Diphtheria	—	—	—	+	+	—	SM	—	—	Clinically very rare now; can be confused with GBS
Dimethylamino propionitrile (industrial)	—	—	+	—	—	—	S>M	+	—	Small-fiber neuropathy with prominent bladder symptoms and impotence in males
γ-Diketone hexacarbons (solvents)	—	±	+	—	—	+	SM	±	+	Same features as CS_2; these solvents now in restricted use
Inorganic lead	—	—	+	—	—	—	M>S	—	±	Selective motor neuropathy with prominent wrist drop
Organophosphates	—	±	+	—	—	—	SM	—	+	Brain and spinal cord are also affected, the latter irreversibly
Thallium (rat poison)	—	+	+	—	—	—	SM	—	+	Also alopecia, Mees' lines in nails; ? selective damage to neural mitochondria
Pyridoxine (vitamin)	—	±	+	—	—	—	S	—	—	Occurs with megadose intake; >1 g per day

* ± = *sometimes*, + = *usual.*
† *S = sensory; M = motor; SM = sensorimotor.*

Acute demyelinating polyneuropathy For all practical purposes, this category is synonymous with Guillain-Barré syndrome (GBS). This acute, frequently severe and fulminant polyneuropathy occurs at a rate of one case per million population per month, or approximately 3500 cases per year in the United States and Canada. In over two-thirds, a viral infection, either clinically overt or evidenced by serum titer rise, precedes the onset of neuropathy by 1 to 3 weeks. Herpes infections [cytomegalovirus, Epstein-Barr virus (EBV)] account for a large proportion of virus-triggered cases. Another 5 to 10 percent of cases occur within 1 to 4 weeks of a surgical procedure. GBS occurs on a background of lymphoma, including Hodgkin's disease, and in lupus erythematosus more frequently than can be attributed to chance alone. Although the weight of evidence suggests that GBS is immune-mediated, the immunopathogenesis remains obscure. In 1976 to 1977, a flurry of some 500 cases followed in the wake of the national swine flu vaccination program in the United States. This exceeded by severalfold the baseline incidence expected in this period among the vaccines. The epidemiologic features of this outbreak resembled a point-source epidemic with an ''incubation'' period of 1 to 6 weeks.

The clinical features of GBS typically include areflexic motor paralysis with mild sensory disturbance coupled with an acellular rise of total protein in the cerebrospinal fluid by the end of the first week of symptoms. Most patients with GBS require hospitalization, and about one-fourth will need ventilatory assistance at some point during the illness. The prognosis is good; approximately 85 percent of patients make a complete or nearly complete recovery. The mortality rate is 3 to 4 percent. Management is generally supportive care, but plasmapheresis also has a role. A large, multicenter, controlled trial in North America has demonstrated a beneficial effect of plasmapheresis, expecially when initiated in the first 2 weeks of illness. In contrast, corticosteroid treatment is generally not considered to be effective.

Other acute demyelinating polyneuropathies are rare and include buckthorn berry intoxication and diphtheritic polyneuritis (see Table 355-2).

Subacute demyelinating polyneuropathy Neuropathies in this category are heterogeneous in origin, although all are acquired. Most common is a relapsing and remitting neuropathy which has many clinical features in common with GBS, but differs from GBS in tempo, course, and absence of discernible triggering events. Previously mentioned toxins (buckthorn berry, diphtheria toxin, aurothioglucose) may also induce a picture of widespread subacute demyelination of peripheral nerves (see Table 355-2).

Chronic demyelinating polyneuropathy Although more common than the subacute neuropathies, chronic polyneuropathy with demyelinating features encompasses a wide diversity of disorders, including hereditary neuropathies, inflammatory neuropathies, and other acquired neuropathies associated with diabetes mellitus, dysproteinemias, other metabolic states, and some chronic intoxications. To complicate matters, many of these disorders present an electrodiagnostic picture of mixed axonal-demyelinative findings. Frequently it is difficult to determine which process, axonal degeneration or demyelination is the primary event. Aspects of many of these

TABLE 355-3 Genetically determined neuropathies

Genetic disorder	Inheritance pattern	Age of onset	Basic process	Other features*	Other systems involved	Metabolic defect	Comment
Peroneal muscular atrophy (HMSN-I)†	Dominant	Decades 2–3	Demyelinating	Hypertrophic change with onion bulb formation; marked ↓ NCV	Some families—Duffy locus linkage	Unknown	Pes cavus, congenital hip problems, motor deficit predominates
Peroneal muscular atrophy (HMSN-II)†	Dominant	Decades 3–5	Axonal	Marked ↓ NAP; NCV sl. decreased	—	Unknown	Same as HSMN-I
Hereditary amyloid neuropathies	Dominant	Decades 3–4	Axonal	Small fiber involvement; endoneurial amyloid deposition	Some families—cornea	Prealbumin is major protein of amyloid fibril	Dysautonomia may be prominent
Hereditary sensory neuropathy (HSN-I)	Dominant	Decades 1–3	Neuronopathic	DRG neurons selectively involved	Sensorineural deafness, some families	Unknown	Frequent distal mutilation—hands and feet
Porphyric neuropathy	Dominant	Adult life	Axonal	Neuropathy part of attacks; may be recurrent	Widespread cellular abnormality	Enzyme defects in porphyrin pathway	Acute intermittent porphyria, variegate porphyria, and erythropoietic porphyria
Hereditary liability to pressure palsy	Dominant	Decades 2–3	? Demyelinating	Tomaculous changes in myelin	—	Unknown	Ulnar, peroneal, and brachial plexus involvement particularly
Fabry's disease	X-linked	Young males	Neuronopathic	Sensory neuronopathy, small DRG neurons	Kidney, skin, lung	Accumulation of ceramide-trihexoside	Neuropathy painful; often die of renal failure
Peroneal muscular atrophy (Phillips et al., 1985)	X-linked	Infancy to 2d decade	Axonal or demyelinating	Heterozygote females may have symptoms		Unknown	Localizes to long arm of X chromosome
Adrenomyeloneuropathy	X-linked	Young males	? Axonal	Mild neuropathy, spastic paraparesis, baldness, hypogonadism	Adrenal cortex, cerebral white matter, spinal cord	Accumulation of very long chain fatty acids	Phenotypic variant of adrenoleukodystrophy; dietary therapy possible
Hereditary sensory neuropathy (HSN-II)	Recessive	Decades 1–3	Neuronopathic	DRG neurons selectively involved	—	Unknown	May be less severe than HSN-I

neuropathies are included in Tables 355-1 to 355-3 and in the sections below.

SPECIAL CATEGORIES OF NEUROPATHY **Hereditary neuropathies** The major characteristics of this highly variegated group of disorders are summarized in Table 355-3. With the exception of the porphyric neuropathies, the onset of neuropathic dysfunction is insidious and progression is indolent over years or decades. Most of these diseases are quite rare with the striking exception of the dominantly inherited peroneal muscular atrophies (HMSN-I and HMSN-II; see Table 355-3). In peroneal muscular atrophy, phenotypic expression is often variable, so that affected family members of a propositus may have no symptoms and minimal neurologic findings but (in HMSN-I) may still show severe reduction of nerve conduction velocity.

Neuropathies with inflammation Acquired inflammatory demyelinating neuropathies fall into two major groups, the acute form called Guillain-Barré syndrome (GBS) and more chronic forms. The entire group of acquired inflammatory demyelinating neuropathies constitutes a significant proportion of all cases of polyneuropathy and shares a distinctive clinical, electrophysiologic, and pathologic pattern. The diagnosis rests upon recognition of the clinical pattern and of other features, including elevated cerebrospinal fluid protein level, electrophysiologic changes (marked slowing of conduction velocities, delayed late responses, prolonged distal latencies, dispersion of evoked responses, and frequent evidence of conduction block), and pathologic changes of low-grade inflammation and demyelination-remyelination of peripheral nerves. The course of GBS is acute and monophasic, whereas the more chronic forms pursue either a slowly progressive or a relapsing course. Cases with an intermediate course occur frequently enough to blur the diagnostic delimitation of GBS from the more chronic types of acquired inflammatory demyelinating neuropathy.

Pathogenetically, this group of inflammatory neuropathies is generally agreed to be immune-mediated, but the specific antigens involved and the crucial events of the immune response and why it is activated are uncertain.

Management of chronic, acquired inflammatory neuropathies involves a judicious mix of corticosteroid therapy, other immunosuppressants, and plasmapheresis. These powerful agents are used only if the disorder is severe enough to threaten walking.

Diabetic neuropathies Classifications of the neuropathies of diabetes are found in Table 355-4. Although this provides a satisfactory frame of reference, the limitations inherent in classifying diabetic neuropathies should be understood. The most serious limitation is that most patients will not fit neatly into any single category, but rather will have overlapping clinical features of several. For instance, many diabetics with distal, primarily sensory polyneuropathy also can be shown to have autonomic dysfunction, usually in the form of vasomotor disturbance in the limbs and abnormalities of sweating. Similarly, patients who develop a proximal motor syndrome may have dysautonomic features (including sexual impotence in males) and some degree of distal sensory polyneuropathy. To compound matters, such patients appear at risk to develop a cranial mononeuropathy.

TABLE 355-3 Genetically determined neuropathies *(continued)*

Genetic disorder	Inheritance pattern	Age of onset	Basic process	Other features*	Other systems involved	Metabolic defect	Comment
Déjerine-Sottas neuropathy (HMSN-III)	Recessive	1st decade	Demyelinating	Hypertrophic change with onion bulb formation	May be mentally retarded	Unknown	Marked nerve trunk enlargement
Refsum's disease	Recessive	1st or 2d decade	Demyelinating	Hypertrophic change with onion bulb formation	Retinitis pigmentosa, ichthyosis, sensorineural deafness	Defect in α-oxidation of β-methylated fatty acids	Low phytanate diet, plasmapheresis therapy
Ataxia-telangiectasia	Recessive	Decade 1 or 2	Axonal	Neuropathy moderate	Cell nuclear aneuploidy, skin and scleral telangiectasia, cerebellar atrophy, immunopathy	Basic defect unknown	High incidence of early neoplasia
Abetalipoproteinemia	Recessive	Decade 1 or 2	Neuronopathic	Large DRG neurons	Retinitis pigmentosa, acanthocytosis of red blood cells	Absence of all lipoprotein-containing apo B	Proprioceptive disturbance marked, minimal small fiber deficit
Giant axonal neuropathy	Recessive	1st decade	Axonal	Massive segmented accumulation of neurofilaments in axons	Slowly progressive encephalopathy with Rosenthal fibers	Generalized disorder of 10-nm filaments	Intermediate filament masses in other cell types
Metachromatic leukodystrophy	Recessive	1st decade	Demyelinating	Schwannopathy with cerebroside accumulation	Cerebral white matter disease predominates	Defect of arylsulfatase A	Infantile, juvenile, and adult onset forms
Globoid cell leukodystrophy	Recessive	1st decade	Demyelinating	Schwannopathy with galactocerebroside accumulation	Cerebral white matter disease predominates	Defect of β-galactosidase	Characteristic clefts in Schwann cell cytoplasm
Friedreich's ataxia	Recessive	1st decade	Axonal	Spinocerebellar and corticospinal tracts involved; also 1° sensory neuron	Cardiomyopathy; usual cause of death	Controversial	Ataxia is both sensory and cerebellar

* *DRG, dorsal root ganglia; NAP, nerve action potential; sl, slightly; HMSN, hereditary motor-sensory neuropathy; HSN, hereditary sensory neuropathy.*
† *Both forms are also collectively referred to as Charcot-Marie-Tooth neuropathy.*

Classifying the diabetic neuropathies does not reveal any knowledge of the basis or pathogenesis of the neuropathic lesion. Rather, attempts at classification represent an educated guess at identifying the apparent anatomic sites of disorder and the critical clinical features. Pain is a frequent feature of diabetic neuropathies (see Table 355-4) but is variable in incidence and degree and is subjective in nature. The term diabetic amyotrophy should be avoided because of its ambiguity.

Diabetic neuropathies tend to occur in the setting of long-standing hyperglycemia (decades) whether insulin-dependent or not. By far the most common neuropathies related to diabetes are the diffuse sensory and autonomic types (categories 1 and 2 under "Symmetric" in Table 355-4). Sensory and autonomic polyneuropathy, chronic and indolent in evolution, may first be noticed in the third or fourth decade in patients with juvenile-onset diabetes but tends to occur after age 50 in patients with adult-onset diabetes. Focal and multifocal types of neuropathy are less common but quite dramatic (categories 1, 2, and 3 under "Asymmetric" in Table 355-4). They rarely occur before the age of 45 and are usually subacute or acute in onset. Cranial mononeuropathies refer to isolated sixth or third nerve palsies. The latter spares the pupil in three-fourths of cases, and some local pain or headache occurs in one-half. Truncal, or thoracoabdominal, neuropathy is painful, involves one or more intercostal or lumbar nerves unilaterally, and frequently coexists with the asymmetric proximal motor neuropathy. Femoral and obturator nerve innervated-muscles (quadriceps femoris, iliopsoas, adductor magnus) and loss of knee jerk on that side are the most evident features of asymmetric proximal motor neuropathy. Sensory deficit is minor, but pain in the hip and anterior thigh may predominate. Common to all of these multifocal and focal neuropathies is the strong likelihood for subsidence of pain within weeks to a year and partial or complete recovery of function. The same is true of symmetric proximal motor neuropathy (category 3 under "Symmetric" in Table 355-4).

Focal and multifocal diabetic neuropathies are considered to be ischemic in origin, but the basis for symmetric polyneuropathies is thought to involve abnormality of nerve metabolism as well as the possibility of ischemia.

Management of diabetic neuropathies is directed toward optimal control of hyperglycemia and symptomatic pain suppression. Entrapment neuropathies are frequently amenable to surgical decompression procedures.

Neuropathies with dysproteinemia An association between polyneuropathy and both multiple myeloma and macroglobulinemia has been recognized for many years. With commonly encountered multiple myeloma (MM) having either lytic or diffuse osteoporotic bone

TABLE 355-4 Classification of diabetic neuropathies

A Symmetric
- *1* Distal, primarily sensory polyneuropathy
  - *a* Mainly large fibers affected
  - *b* Mixed*
  - *c* Mainly small fibers affected*
- *2* Autonomic neuropathy
- *3* Chronically evolving proximal motor neuropathy*†

B Asymmetric
- *1* Acute or subacute proximal motor neuropathy*†
- *2* Cranial mononeuropathy†
- *3* Truncal neuropathy*†
- *4* Entrapment neuropathy in the limbs

* *Often painful.*
† *Recovery, partial or complete, is likely.*

lesions, clinically overt polyneuropathy is relatively infrequent, occurring in approximately 5 percent of patients. These neuropathies are sensorimotor, may be severe, and generally do not reverse with successful suppression of the myeloma. In most cases, electrodiagnostic and pathologic features are consistent with a process of axonal degeneration.

In contrast, myeloma with osteosclerotic features, although representing only 3 percent of all myelomas, is associated with a polyneuropathy in almost one-half of cases. These neuropathies, which may also occur with solitary plasmacytoma, seem to be different from these linked to MM in that they (1) often respond to radiation or removal of the primary lesion, (2) are more frequently demyelinating in character, (3) are associated with different monoclonal proteins and light chains (almost all lambda as opposed to mostly kappa in MM), and (4) frequently occur in association with other systemic findings. These include skin thickening, hyperpigmentation, hypertrichosis, organomegaly, endocrinopathy, anasarca, papilledema, and clubbing of fingers. (POEMS syndrome: *p*olyneuropathy, *o*rganomegaly, *e*ndocrinopathy, *m* protein, and *s*kin changes.) A great deal of attention has been paid to this curious syndrome in Japan where it is prevalent, but the underlying mechanism remains unknown.

Benign monoclonal gammopathy with an IgM serum spike, and usually with kappa light chains, is described in association with demyelinating polyneuropathy that often follows a protracted course and indolent progression. In about one-quarter of cases, the monoclonal serum protein binds to normal human peripheral myelin, specifically to myelin-associated glycoprotein. Immunocytochemical studies show binding of IgM to nerve obtained at biopsy or autopsy of these patients, but in a pattern different from that seen following incubation of sections of nerve with the IgM serum. Incubated nerves show uniform staining of the entire expanse of compact myelin sheath, but in vivo deposited IgM can be demonstrated to localize more selectively, probably at sites of myelin splitting, the latter being a phenomenon which occurs characteristically in most dysglobulinemic neuropathies. Whether the IgM bound to nerve in vivo plays a role in damaging nerve is unresolved.

Autonomic neuropathy The autonomic nervous system regulates the visceral organs and vegetative functions. Many pharmacologic agents modify specific autonomic functions, but autonomic neuropathy (dysautonomia) with structural changes in pre- and postganglionic neurons can also occur. Usually autonomic neuropathy is a manifestation of a more generalized polyneuropathy also affecting somatic peripheral nervous function, as in diabetic neuropathy, GBS, and alcoholic polyneuropathy, but occasionally syndromes of pure pandysautonomia are encountered. Symptoms of dysautonomia are mainly negative (i.e., loss of function) and include postural hypotension with faintness or syncope, anhidrosis, hypothermia, bladder atony, obstipation, dry mouth and dry eyes from failure of salivary and lachrymal glands to secrete, blurring of vision from lack of pupillary and ciliary regulation, and sexual impotence in males. Positive phenomena (hyperfunction) may also occur and include episodic hypertension, diarrhea, hyperhidrosis, and either tachycardia or bradycardia.

Miscellaneous causes of neuropathy Ischemia of nerve severe enough to produce clinical symptoms has as its basis the widespread compromise of blood flow in the vasa nervorum. Typically, this is the result of small-vessel disease involving the vasa nervorum directly, as occurs with vasculitis, rather than large-vessel disease, such as atherosclerosis. Clinically, widespread disease of the vasa nervorum produces mononeuropathy multiplex, which electrodiagnostically has the features of a patchy axonal process.

Cold exerts deleterious effects on peripheral nerve directly without an intermediate step of ischemia being necessary. Cold injury to nerve occurs after prolonged exposure, usually of a limb, to moderately low temperatures, as with immersion of the feet in seawater; actual freezing of tissue is not required. Axonal degeneration of myelinated fibers is the pathologic expression of cold injury. Frequently limbs affected by cold injury to nerve show sensory deficit and dysesthesias, cutaneous vasomotor instability, pain, and marked sensitivity to minimal cold exposure, which persist for many years. The pathophysiology of these phenomena is uncertain.

TROPHIC CHANGES IN SEVERE NEUROPATHY The array of observable changes in completely denervated muscle, bone, and skin, including hair and nails, is well known, if incompletely understood. It is unclear what portion of the changes is due purely to denervation versus that caused by disuse, immobility, lack of weight bearing, and particularly recurrent, unnoticed, painless trauma. Considerable evidence favors the view that ulceration of skin, poor healing, tissue resorption, neurogenic arthropathy, and mutilation are the result of repeated heedless injury to insensitive parts. This sequence of events is avoidable with proper attention to and care of the insensitive parts by both patient and physician.

RECOVERY FROM NEUROPATHY In contrast to axons in the central nervous system, peripheral nerve fibers have an excellent capability to regenerate under proper circumstances. The process of regeneration following axonal degeneration may take from 2 months to more than a year, depending on the severity of the neuropathy and the length of regeneration required. Whether regeneration takes place depends upon the subsidence of the initial basis for neuropathy. This could be removal from contact with a neurotoxic substance or correction of an abnormal metabolic state. A deficit secondary to demyelination may recover rapidly since intact axons may remyelinate in just a few weeks. For example, a patient with GBS, in whom demyelination but no secondary axonal degeneration has occurred, may recover to normal strength from bedfastness and paralysis of arms and legs in as little as 3 to 4 weeks.

MONONEUROPATHY MULTIPLEX (MULTIFOCAL NEUROPATHY) This term means simultaneous or sequential involvement of individual noncontiguous nerve trunks, either partially or completely, evolving over days to years. Since the disease process underlying mononeuropathy multiplex involves peripheral nerves in a multifocal and random fashion, there is a tendency, as worsening occurs, for the neurologic deficit to become less patchy and multifocal and more confluent and symmetric. Some patients present initially with a distal symmetric neuropathy. Attention to the pattern of early symptoms is therefore important in making the judgment that a particular neuropathy is indeed a mononeuropathy multiplex.

Once that issue is settled, the next question is whether the process is primarily axonal or demyelinating. Almost one-third of all adults with the clinical syndrome of mononeuropathy multiplex have a clear-cut picture of a demyelinating disorder usually with multiple foci of persistent conduction block by electrodiagnostic examination. More intensive study of this subgroup suggests that the multifocal demyelinating neuropathy represents part of the spectrum of chronic acquired demyelinating neuropathy, also known as chronic inflammatory demyelinating polyradiculoneuropathy (CIDP). Management of this multifocal subgroup is the same as for CIDP.

The remaining two-thirds of patients with mononeuropathy multiplex have a picture by electrodiagnostic examination of axonal involvement that is heterogeneously distributed. Although ischemia would be suspected as the basis for neuropathy in these patients, only about one-half can be shown to have a process, usually vasculitis, affecting the vasa nervorum. The others remain undiagnosed even on follow-up, and the basis for their mononeuropathy multiplex is uncertain. Management in this group is conservative, but the management of those with proven vasculitis of vasa nervorum is the same as treatment for systemic vasculitis (see Chap. 269).

In individuals in whom vasculitic change in vasa nervorum can be demonstrated, any one of a large number of underlying disorders may be responsible. The primary vasculitides of the polyarteritis nodosa group constitute the most frequent basis, followed closely by the vasculitis syndrome occurring in the course of other connective tissue disorders. In descending order of frequency, the latter are rheumatoid arthritis, systemic lupus erythematosus, and mixed connective tissue disease. Other rarer causes of mononeuropathy multiplex due to nerve ischemia from occlusion of vasa nervorum include mixed cryoglobulinemia, Sjögren's syndrome, Wegener's granulomatosis, progressive systemic sclerosis, Churg-Strauss allergic granulomatosis, and hypersensitivity angiitides. Management of the neuropathy in each instance is predicated upon the appropriate treatment of the responsible disease.

Mononeuropathy multiplex syndrome may also be seen as a manifestation of leprosy, sarcoidosis, certain types of amyloidosis, hypereosinophilia syndrome, cryoglobulinemia, and multifocal types of diabetic neuropathy.

MONONEUROPATHY Mononeuropathy means focal involvement of a single nerve trunk and therefore implies a local causation. Direct trauma, compression, and entrapment are the usual causes. Ulnar neuropathies, due to lesions either at the ulnar groove or in the cubital tunnel, and median neuropathy due to compression in the carpal tunnel constitute the great majority of mononeuropathies encountered in clinical practice. In the absence of a history of trauma to the nerve trunk, factors favoring conservative management include sudden onset, no motor deficit, few or no sensory findings even though pain and sensory symptoms might be present, and no evidence of axonal degeneration by electrodiagnostic criteria. Factors favoring surgical intervention include chronicity and worsening neurologic deficit on examination, particularly if motor, and electrodiagnostic evidence that the lesion has produced a degree of Wallerian degeneration.

Ulnar nerve This nerve is derived from the eighth cervical and first thoracic roots. It innervates the ulnar flexor of the wrist, the inner half of the deep finger flexors, the adductors and abductors of the fingers, the adductor of the thumb, the two medial lumbricals, and the muscles of the hypothenar eminence. It is the sensory nerve to the fifth and ulnar half of the fourth fingers and the ulnar border of the hand. Complete ulnar paralysis results in a characteristic claw-hand deformity owing to wasting of the small hand muscles and hyperextension of the fingers at the metacarpophalangeal joints and flexion at the interphalangeal joints. The flexion deformity is most pronounced in the fourth and fifth fingers. Sensory loss occurs over the fifth finger, the ulnar aspect of the fourth finger, and the ulnar border of the palm. The ulnar nerve is most commonly injured at the elbow because of fracture or dislocation involving the joint. Delayed ulnar palsy may occur many years after an injury to the elbow joint which has resulted in a cubitus valgus deformity of the joint. Because of the deformity, the nerve is stretched in its course over the ulnar condyle. The superficial location of the nerve at the elbow makes it a common site of pressure palsy. The ulnar nerve may also become entrapped just distal to the elbow in the cubital tunnel formed by the aponeurotic arch linking the two heads of the flexor carpi ulnaris. Prolonged pressure on the base of the palm may result in damage to the deep palmar branch of the ulnar nerve, causing weakness of the small hand muscles but no sensory loss.

Median nerve This nerve is derived from the sixth cervical to the first thoracic root and is formed by the union of two heads from the medial and lateral cords of the brachial plexus. It innervates the pronators of the forearm, long finger flexors, and abductor and opponens muscles of the thumb and is a sensory nerve to the palmar aspect of the hand. Complete median nerve paralysis results in wasting of the affected muscles and inability to pronate the forearm, weakness of wrist flexion, paralysis of flexion of the index finger and terminal phalanx of the thumb, weakness of flexion of the remaining fingers, weakness of abduction and opposition of the thumb, and sensory impairment over the radial two-thirds of the palmar aspect of the hand and over the distal phalanges of the dorsum of the index and third fingers. The nerve may be injured in the axilla by shoulder dislocation and in any part of its course by laceration, stab, or gunshot wounds. The wrist is the most common site of external injury, particularly in association with Colles' fractures of the wrist. Compression of the nerve at the wrist (carpal tunnel syndrome) may be secondary to prolonged occupational pressure, tenosynovitis with arthritis, or local infiltration, for example, by a thickening of connective tissue and deposit of amyloid with multiple myeloma or one of the mucopolysaccharides. Other systemic diseases associated with an increased incidence of carpal tunnel syndrome are acromegaly, hypothyroidism, rheumatoid arthritis, and diabetes mellitus. The treatment of carpal tunnel syndrome is surgical section of the carpal ligament. Incomplete lesions of the median nerve between the axilla and wrist may result in causalgia (a particularly severe type of burning pain; see Chap. 3).

Radial nerve This nerve is derived from the fifth to eighth cervical roots and is the termination of the posterior cord of the brachial plexus. It innervates the triceps muscle and the supinator and extensor muscles of the forearm and hand. Complete radial paralysis results in the inability to extend the elbow, paralysis of supination of the forearm, and complete wrist and finger drop. Sensation is impaired over the posterior aspect of the forearm and a small area over the radial aspect of the dorsum of the hand. The nerve may be injured in the axilla, for example, in "crutch" palsy, but most common trauma occurs in the midarm where the nerve winds around the humerus. Common types of injury at this site are fractures and pressure palsies incurred during sleep, or during coma in association with intoxications.

Musculocutaneous nerve This nerve is derived from the fifth and sixth cervical roots and is a branch of the lateral cord of the brachial plexus. It innervates the biceps and brachialis anticus muscles. Lesions of the nerve result in weakness of elbow flexion. It is rarely injured alone.

Axillary nerve This nerve arises from the posterior cord of the brachial plexus and supplies the teres minor and deltoid muscles. It may be involved in injuries resulting from fractures of the neck of the humerus, serum neuritis, or brachial neuritis. The anatomic localization depends on the recognition of paralysis of abduction of the arm, wasting of the deltoid, and a patch of impaired sensation over the outer aspect of the shoulder.

Suprascapular nerve This nerve is derived from the fifth and sixth cervical roots and supplies the supra- and infrasinatus muscles. Lesions may be diagnosed by the presence of weakness of abduction and external rotation of the arm and atrophy of the supra- and infraspinatus muscles. The nerve may be injured by blows on the top of the shoulder, fracture dislocations of the shoulder joint, or by entrapment in the suprascapular notch.

Long thoracic nerve This nerve is derived from the fifth, sixth, and seventh cervical roots and supplies the serratus magnus muscle. Paralysis of the serratus magnus muscle results in an inability to raise the arm over the head from a forward position, and there is winging of the medial border of the scapula on pushing forward against resistance. It is injured most commonly by pressure on the shoulder, from either a sudden blow or prolonged pressure from carrying heavy weights. It is also involved at times in diabetic patients and as a manifestation of brachial and serum neuritides.

Brachial plexus Brachial plexus lesions, which are usually unilateral, are relatively common and readily distinguishable on clinical grounds from upper limb mononeuropathies. The usual causes are direct trauma to the plexus, stretch injury, cervical rib or bands, infiltration or compression by malignancy, brachial neuritis (neuralgic amyotrophy), and damage due to therapeutic radiation. As an approximation, injury to the upper plexus, which arises from C5 to C6 roots, results from particular types of trauma (arm jerked downward), brachial neuritis, and radiation damage. The muscles affected are the biceps, deltoid, brachialis anticus, supinator longus, supra- and infraspinatus, and the rhomboids. The arm hangs at the side, internally rotated, with the elbow extended. The forearm is pronated. Hand motion is unaffected. The prognosis for spontaneous recovery is generally good, especially in cases of birth injury.

Findings localizing to the lower plexus, which arises from C8 to T1 roots, are likely to be due to malignant infiltration, other types of trauma (arm jerked upward), and cervical rib or bands. There is paralysis and wasting of the small muscles of the hand and a characteristic claw-hand deformity. Sensory loss is limited to the ulnar border of the hand and inner side of the forearm, and there may be an associated paralysis of the cervical sympathetic nerve with Horner's syndrome (ptosis and meiosis) if the first thoracic motor root is involved. Involvement of the brachial plexus by malignancy is more likely to present with pain, Horner's syndrome, and a subacute course, whereas radiation damage to the brachial plexus is more likely to result in paresthesias without pain, indolent progression, and more prominent electrodiagnostic findings.

Lesions of the cords of the brachial plexus The lateral and medial cords are most commonly affected. Dislocation of the head of the humerus, pressure of the cervical ribs, and stab wounds are the most frequent causes. Injury to the lateral cord results in paralysis of the biceps and coracobrachialis muscles and all muscles supplied by the median nerve except the intrinsic hand muscles. There is some loss of sensation over the radial aspects of the forearm. Involvement of the medial cord, as may occur in compression by a cervical rib, results in paralysis of the muscles supplied by the ulnar nerve together with the median-innervated intrinsic muscles of the hand and sensory loss over the ulnar aspect of the hand and forearm. Sternum-splitting operations may compress the lower brachial plexus by displacement of the clavicle. Usually it is the medial cord of the brachial plexus that is affected.

Lumbosacral plexus lesions The lumbosacral plexus is subject to a number of disease processes, mostly secondary. Disease of the upper plexus produces a unilateral weakness in the flexion and adduction of the hip, extension of the knee, and sensory loss over the anterior thigh and leg; those of the lower plexus cause a weakness of the posterior thigh, leg, and foot muscles with the loss of sensation over the fifth lumbar and first and second sacral roots. The diseases that affect the plexus are carcinoma of the cervix and prostate, retroperitoneal tumors, iliopsoas hemorrhages from a ruptured aneurysm or hemophilia, lumbosacral plexitis, abdominal and thoracolumbar operations, and diabetes mellitus.

Lateral femoral cutaneous nerve This nerve is derived from the second and third lumbar roots. It is a sensory nerve supplying the lateral aspect of the thigh. The nerve enters the thigh beneath the lateral end of the inguinal ligament and then enters the fascia lata, where it may become constricted. Compression of the nerve results in uncomfortable paresthesias in its cutaneous distribution and in sensory impairment. The condition is called *meralgia paresthetica*. The definitive treatment is surgical, usually decompression of the nerve at the inguinal ligament, but this is seldom necessary.

Obturator nerve This nerve is derived from the second, third, and fourth lumbar roots. It supplies the adductor muscles of the thigh, and injury to the nerve results in almost complete paralysis of adduction of the thigh. The nerve is most frequently injured during the course of a difficult labor and also as a result of dislocation of the hip or an obturator hernia. It may be affected in diabetes, polyarteritis nodosa, osteitis pubis, and retroperitoneal and pelvic malignant tumors.

Femoral nerve This nerve is derived from the second, third, and fourth lumbar roots. It supplies the iliopsoas muscles (hip flexion) and the quadriceps femoris muscles (knee extension) and conveys cutaneous sensation from the anterior thigh and medial side of the lower leg (saphenous nerve). Following injury to the nerve, there is paralysis of extension of the knee, with wasting of the quadriceps muscle and also some weakness of hip flexion. The knee jerk is abolished. The nerve may be involved in fractures and dislocation of the hip, in fractures of the pelvis, and in attempts to catheterize the femoral artery. It may be affected in diabetes, in polyarteritis nodosa, and in retroperitoneal, pelvic, or abdominal lesions such as a tumor, psoas abscess, or retroperitoneal hemorrhage. Because the femoral artery may also be severed, wounds in the femoral triangle may be fatal.

Sciatic nerve This nerve is derived from the fourth and fifth lumbar and first and second sacral roots. It provides the motor innervation of the hamstring muscles and all those below the knee; it carries sensory impulses from the posterior aspect of the thigh and posterior and lateral aspects of the leg and entire sole. In complete sciatic paralysis, the knee cannot be flexed and all muscles below the knee are paralyzed. The sciatic nerve is commonly injured in fractures of the pelvis or femur, in gunshot wounds of the buttock and thigh, by lying or sitting insensate and compressing the nerve in the lower buttock area, and by inadvertent intraneural injections. It may also be involved by pelvic tumors and in both diabetes mellitus and polyarteritis nodosa. Cryptogenic forms also occur and are actually more frequent than those with an identifiable cause. A ruptured lumbar disk often simulates sciatic neuropathy. Incomplete lesions of the sciatic nerve occasionally result in causalgia.

Common peroneal nerve This nerve is one of the terminal divisions of the sciatic nerve in the popliteal fossa. It supplies the dorsiflexors of the foot and toes, the everters of the foot, and sensation to the dorsum of the foot and lateral aspect of the lower half of the leg. These functions are lost with lesions which completely interrupt the nerve. Pressure or sleep palsy is one of the most frequent types of injury, the compression being of that part of the nerve which passes over the head of the fibula. It is also commonly involved by fractures involving the upper end of the fibula and in diabetic neuropathy, polyarteritis nodosa, and operations on the knee.

Tibial nerve This nerve is the other of the two terminal divisions of the sciatic nerve in the popliteal fossa. It supplies all the calf muscles and the flexors of the foot. Complete paralysis of the nerve results in a calcaneovalgus deformity of the foot, which no longer can be plantar-flexed. There is loss of sensation over the plantar aspect of the foot.

OTHER FOCAL NEUROPATHIES **Peripheral nerve tumors** These are mostly benign and can arise on any nerve trunk or twig. Although peripheral nerve tumors occur anywhere in the body including the spinal roots and cauda equina, many are subcutaneous in location and present as a soft swelling, sometimes with a purplish discoloration of the skin. Two major categories of peripheral nerve tumors are recognized: neurilemmoma (Schwannoma) and neurofibroma. Neurilemmomas are usually solitary and grow within the nerve sheath, rendering the tumor relatively easy to dissect free. In contrast, neurofibromas tend to be multiple, grow within the endoneurial substance, rendering them difficult to dissect, may undergo malignant changes, and are the hallmark of von Recklinghausen's neurofibromatosis. This disease is characterized by an autosomal dominant inheritance pattern, any number of neurofibromas from one to thousands, five or more café au lait–pigmented skin lesions greater than 1.5 cm (80 percent of patients), axillary freckles (93 percent of patients), and an increased incidence of seizure disorder and mental retardation (see Chap. 351).

Herpes zoster This is a sensory neuritis of viral cause characterized by acute inflammation of one or more dorsal root ganglia, due to varicella-zoster virus infection. Lancinating pain and hyperalgesia over the skin surface supplied by affected roots occur for 3 to 4 days, followed by the appearance of herpetic eruption in the same segment characterized by painful raised blisters on reddened bases. If the inflammatory process spreads to involve adjacent motor roots of anterior horns of the cord, segmental motor weakness and wasting appear. Paralysis of the oculomotor nerves may occur in conjunction with ophthalmic division involvement of the trigeminal ganglion (ophthalmoplegic zoster). Facial paralysis may occur with involvement of the geniculate ganglion and herpetic eruption on the ipsilateral tympanic membrane or external ear canal (Ramsay Hunt syndrome).

Leprous neuritis This is a major worldwide cause of neuropathy. *Mycobacterium lerae* organisms readily invade Schwann cells in cutaneous nerve twigs, particularly those associated with unmyelinated nerve fibers. Two major forms of leprous neuritis are recognized, tuberculoid and lepromatous, which actually represent the far ends of a spectrum of disease, the middle of which is called dimorphous leprosy (patchy and multifocal involvement of skin and nerve). Tuberculoid (high-resistance) leprosy is restricted to a single patch of hypesthetic or anesthetic skin in any location. The skin patch is frequently thickened, reddened, or hypopigmented. If a superficially placed nerve trunk, typically a cutaneous nerve, courses just beneath the area of affected skin, it may be engulfed in the inflammatory reaction, resulting in an associated mononeuropathy. Such a nerve may be palpably enlarged and beaded. Lepromatous (low-resistance) leprosy is marked by immunologic tolerance and widespread skin thickening, cutaneous anesthesia, and anhidrosis, sparing only the warmest parts of the body, notably the axilla, groin, and beneath the scalp hair. Motor signs (focal weakness and atrophy) result from damage to mixed nerves lying close to the skin, particularly the median, ulnar, peroneal, and facial nerves.

Bell's palsy This is due to inflammation of the facial nerve in the facial canal, the basis for which remains obscure. Edema may play a part leading to compression of nerve fibers, with resulting acute unilateral paralysis of facial muscles (see Chap. 352).

Sarcoidosis This may involve single or multiple peripheral nerves, producing asymmetric mononeuritis or polyneuritis. Unilateral or bilateral facial paralysis is common in association with parotitis and uveitis (Heerfordt's syndrome).

Polyneuritis cranialis This is a relapsing and remitting mononeuropathy multiplex restricted to cranial nerves. It is usually associated with indolent tuberculous cervical adenitis (scrofula) or sarcoidosis. Treatment of the underlying condition will halt the cranial nerve palsies.

Acknowledgment

Portions of this section also appear in substantially the same form in Asbury AK: Diseases of peripheral nerve, in *Diseases of the Nervous System,* AK Asbury, GM McKhann, WI McDonald (eds), by arrangement with the publishers, Philadelphia, Saunders, 1986, and London, Heinemann, 1986.

REFERENCES

Asbury AK: New aspects of disease of the peripheral nervous system, in *Harrison's Textbook of Internal Medicine, Update IV.* McGraw-Hill, New York, 1983, 211–229

———, Gilliatt RW: *Peripheral Nerve Disorders: A Practical Approach.* London, Butterworth, 1984

——— et al: Criteria for diagnosis of Guillian-Barré syndrome. Ann Neurol 3:565, 1978

Dawson DM et al: *Entrapment Neuropathies.* Boston, Little, Brown, 1983

Dyck PJ et al (eds): *Peripheral Neuropathy,* 2d ed. Philadelphia, Saunders, 1984

Layzer RB: *Neuromuscular Manifestations of Systemic Disease,* vol 25: *Contemporary Neurology Series.* Philadelphia, Davis, 1984

Schaumburg HH et al: *Disorders of Peripheral Nerves,* vol 24: *Contemporary Neurology Series.* Philadelphia, Davis, 1983

Spencer PS, Schaumburg HH (eds): *Experimental and Clinical Neurotoxicology.* Baltimore, Williams & Wilkins, 1980

Sumner AJ (ed): *The Physiology of Peripheral Nerve Disease.* Philadelphia, Saunders, 1980

356 DERMATOMYOSITIS AND POLYMYOSITIS

WALTER G. BRADLEY

Dermatomyositis and polymyositis are conditions of unknown etiology in which the skeletal muscle is damaged by a nonsuppurative inflammatory process dominated by lymphocytic infiltration. The term *polymyositis* is applied when the condition spares the skin and the term *dermatomyositis* when polymyositis is associated with a characteristic skin rash. One-third of cases are associated with various connective tissue disorders, such as rheumatoid arthritis, lupus erythematosus, mixed connective tissue disorder, and scleroderma and one-tenth with a malignancy.

ETIOLOGY The cause of these diseases is unknown. The two main theories are that the diseases are due to a viral infection of the skeletal muscle or to an autoimmune disorder (Chap. 269). Experimental viral myositis can be induced in animals by Coxsackie virus. A mild inflammatory myopathy can occur with influenza. The numerous electron-microscope observations of virus-like particles in muscle fibers in dermatomyositis or polymyositis have not been confirmed by virus isolation, rising titers of antiviral antibodies have not been demonstrated, and the disease has not been passed into animals by injection of extracts of affected muscles. One-third of cases have elevated serum antibodies to toxoplasma, but the disease does not generally respond to therapy against toxoplasmosis. A disease resembling polymyositis has been reported in laboratory animals injected with sterile muscle extracts together with Freund's adjuvant (experimental allergic myositis). Circulating lymphocytes reactive against skeletal muscle antigens and the lymphocytic infiltration of affected muscles suggest the presence of cell-mediated immunity. A small proportion of patients have deposition of immunoglobulins on intramuscular blood vessels, suggesting that circulating antibodies may play some role in the disease. The close association of polymyositis and diseases of connective tissue favors the notion of a common autoimmune etiology or pathogenesis. In older patients dermatomyositis is frequently associated with a malignancy. Thus dermatomyositis-polymyositis is a syndrome which probably has a number of different causes.

CLASSIFICATION The classification of the dermatomyositis-polymyositis group which is most widely used is given in Table 356-1. This classification is not based on known differences in etiology and has a number of drawbacks, as noted below. Other uncommon associations of polymyositis are sarcoidosis, giant cell myositis with thymoma, and myositis in systemic infections due to viruses or toxoplasma. A focal infective myositis due to streptococcal or staphylococcal infection is mostly seen in the tropics. Focal nodular myositis is a variant of polymyositis where focal areas of myositis cause hot, often painful, multifocal muscle masses. Inclusion body myositis is an inflammatory myopathy with characteristic clinical and pathologic features (see below).

INCIDENCE Current estimates that the annual incidence of the inflammatory myopathies is about five per million of the population are probably too low.

TABLE 356-1 Classification of polymyositis-dermatomyositis

Group I:	Primary idiopathic polymyositis
Group II:	Primary idiopathic dermatomyositis
Group III:	Dermatomyositis (or polymyositis) associated with neoplasia
Group IV:	Childhood dermatomyositis (or polymyositis) associated with vasculitis
Group V:	Polymyositis (or dermatomyositis) with associated collagen-vascular disease

SOURCE: *Classification suggested by Bohan et al.*

CLINICAL MANIFESTATIONS Group I: Primary idiopathic polymyositis This group comprises about one-third of all cases of inflammatory myopathy. It is insidiously progressive over weeks, months, or even years. Rarely the disease is acute, producing severe muscle weakness in a matter of days. The disease may develop at any age and in either sex. Females outnumber males two to one.

The patients first become aware of weakness of the proximal limb muscles, especially the hips and thighs, and find difficulty in arising from the squatting or kneeling position and in climbing or descending stairs. When shoulder girdle muscles are involved, placing an object on a high shelf or combing the hair becomes difficult. Occasionally the disease is more restricted, affecting only the neck, the shoulder, or the quadriceps muscles. Pain of an aching type in the buttocks, thighs, and calves is experienced in about 10 percent of the cases, and tenderness on palpation in another 20 percent. Early symptoms of dysphagia and weakness of extensor muscles of the neck in a patient with a chronic myopathy suggest the diagnosis of polymyositis.

When the patient is first seen, there may be weakness of the muscles of the trunk, the upper and lower limb girdles, the upper arms and thighs, the posterior and anterior neck, and the pharynx. Ocular muscles are almost never affected except in a rare association with myasthenia gravis. The distal muscles are spared in about 75 percent of cases. Muscle atrophy, contractures, and diminished tendon reflexes are rare in early myositis and never as pronounced as in muscular dystrophies and denervating conditions. When the reflexes are disproportionately reduced, carcinoma with polymyositis and polyneuropathy or the Lambert-Eaton syndrome should be considered. Occasionally, the reflexes may be paradoxically brisk in dermatomyositis-polymyositis, perhaps due to irritation of muscle spindle receptors by the inflammation.

At presentation about 25 percent of patients have dysphagia, about 5 percent have significant respiratory impairment, and 5 percent are unable to walk. Dysphagia is due to involvement of striated muscles of the pharynx and upper esophagus. At some time in the course of the disease cardiac abnormalities are observed in about 30 percent of cases; these include ECG changes, arrhythmias, and heart failure secondary to myocarditis. About half of the fatal cases have pathologic evidence of cardiac disease with necrosis of myocardial fibers, usually with only modest inflammatory reaction. The frequency of myocardial infarction may be increased in those treated for long periods with corticosteroids. In a few cases there is dyspnea due to pulmonary fibrosis. Arthralgia, Raynaud's phenomenon, and rarely low-grade fever may also be present.

Group II: Primary idiopathic dermatomyositis This group comprises about one-quarter of all cases of myositis. The skin changes may precede or follow the muscle syndrome and include a localized or diffuse erythema, maculopapular eruption, scaling eczematoid dermatitis, or rarely an exfoliative dermatitis. The classic lilac-colored (heliotrope) rash is on the eyelids, bridge of the nose, cheeks (butterfly distribution), forehead, chest, elbows, knees and knuckles, and around the nailbeds. Itching may be troublesome in some cases. The skin lesions may be subtle and easily overlooked. Periorbital edema is frequent, particularly in acute cases. The skin lesions may occasionally ulcerate. Subcutaneous calcification may occur, especially in children.

The typical rash and myositis allow a diagnosis of dermatomyositis, and such cases may be placed in this category (group II, Table 356-1) if idiopathic and into groups III, IV, and V if there are other features, namely malignancy, vasculitis in children, and an established collagen-vascular disease. About 40 percent of all patients with myositis have dermatomyositis. Most patients over the age of 60 with dermatomyositis have an underlying malignancy.

Group III: Polymyositis or dermatomyositis with neoplasia This syndrome, which comprises about 8 percent of all cases of myositis, is categorized separately, although muscle and skin changes are indistinguishable from those in the other groups. The malignancy may antedate or postdate the onset of the myositis by up to 2 years. The incidence of this paraneoplastic syndrome is higher in patients with dermatomyositis over the age of 55; therefore, in such patients the search for an underlying malignancy is mandatory. The most common malignancies are lung, ovary, breast, gastrointestinal tract, and myeloproliferative disorders. The myositis is a paraneoplastic syndrome, the cause of which may lie in an altered immune status or an occult viral infection of the muscle.

Group IV: Childhood polymyositis and dermatomyositis associated with vasculitis This group comprises about 7 percent of all cases of myositis. Inflammatory myopathy in childhood is frequently associated with skin involvement and clinical or pathologic evidence of vasculitis in skin, muscles, gastrointestinal tract, and other organs. There are degeneration and loss of capillaries in a perifascicular distribution in the skeletal muscles; often necrotizing lesions of the skin; and ischemic infarction of kidneys, gastrointestinal tract, and rarely brain. Consequently, authors of some reports on series of cases have reported mortality rates of up to one-third in childhood dermatomyositis, though most have found that the prognosis is better than it is in adult dermatomyositis-polymyositis. One limitation of the classification of Bohan et al is that it is not clear whether or not all cases of childhood myositis should be included in group IV. Subcutaneous calcification is frequently present in the childhood form of dermatomyositis.

Group V: Polymyositis or dermatomyositis with an associated connective tissue disorder This "overlap group" comprises about one-fifth of all cases of myositis. Rheumatoid arthritis, scleroderma, mixed connective tissue disease, and lupus erythematosus are the most common associated conditions; polyarteritis nodosa and rheumatic fever are more rarely associated. Criteria for placement in the overlap group combine the demonstration of the appropriate clinical and laboratory abnormalities required for the diagnosis of the connective tissue disorder together with clinical and laboratory evidence of myositis. The diagnosis of myositis is often difficult in patients with connective tissue disorders producing arthritis, since this may often produce muscle weakness with type II fiber atrophy. Moreover, perivascular inflammatory foci are common in muscle in connective tissue disorders. Demonstration of increased serum creatine kinase (CK), electromyography (EMG), and muscle biopsy are often required to make this diagnosis. Though patients in this overlap group respond to corticosteroid therapy, the prognosis for recovery of function is poorer than it is in pure dermatomyositis-polymyositis. Dysphagia in group V patients with scleroderma is often due to involvement of the smooth muscle of the distal third of the esophagus.

Other disorders associated with myositis SARCOIDOSIS AND POLYMYOSITIS The skeletal muscle contains noncaseating granulomas with Langhans-type multinuclear giant cells in at least one-quarter of patients with sarcoidosis. Symptomatic polymyositis is, however, uncommon. Regenerating multinuclear myoblasts resemble Langhans' giant cells, which has led to misdiagnosis in many of the cases reported in the literature to have "sarcoid myositis." A giant cell or granulomatous polymyositis, sometimes associated with myasthenia gravis, has been recorded in patients with thymomas.

FOCAL NODULAR MYOSITIS A syndrome of acutely developing and painful focal inflammatory nodules, sometimes occurring sequentially in different muscles, has been termed *focal nodular myositis*. The pathologic appearance and response to therapy are similar to those in generalized polymyositis. The differential diagnosis includes, when single, a muscle tumor (sarcoma or rhabdomyosarcoma) and, when multiple, muscle infarcts such as can occur in polyarteritis nodosa.

INFECTIOUS POLYMYOSITIS Rare cases of polymyositis have clearcut evidence of being due to known pathogens such as toxoplasmosis (Chap. 157) and Coxsackie virus infection (Chap 139). Antibody screening will suggest the diagnosis in such cases. Trichinosis may be confused with idiopathic polymyositis, particularly if the history of raw pork ingestion is not obtained. The symptoms of trichinosis are variable and depend upon the parasitic load. Low-grade fever, muscle pain of variable degree, conjunctival and periorbital edema, and fatigue are frequent. Weakness is generally mild. Heavy infestation is often associated with central nervous system symptoms of delirium, coma, or focal neurologic deficit. The frequent myocardial involvement is manifested by tachycardia and ECG changes. The diagnosis is made by the history of ingestion of undercooked pork, marked eosinophilia, sensitivity to intradermal *Trichina* antigen, and the appearance of serum antibodies to *Trichina* during the course of the disease. Occasionally the diagnosis is not recognized until a muscle is biopsied. Pyomyositis, a suppurative inflammation of muscle due to staphylococcus or streptococcus, is mainly seen in the tropics. The presentation is that of a diffuse abscess of the muscle.

INCLUSION BODY MYOSITIS The clinical features of this condition are similar to those of chronic idiopathic polymyositis, except that distal muscle involvement is more frequent. Muscle biopsy shows interstitial and perivascular inflammatory infiltration, necrosis, and regeneration of muscle fibers, but in addition there are "rimmed vacuoles" in the fibers. Electron microscopy reveals paramyxovirus-like filaments in the nuclei and sarcoplasm. A recent study suggests these are mumps virus. This disorder responds poorly to immunosuppressive therapy, and the prognosis is poor.

LABORATORY FINDINGS In all forms of polymyositis there may be elevated serum levels of the enzymes present in skeletal muscle, such as CK, aldolase, serum glutamic oxaloacetic transaminase (SGOT), lactic acid dehydrogenase (LDH), and serum glutamic pyruvate transaminase (SGPT). The degree of rise decreases from the first to the last in this series of enzymes, and the pattern is the reverse of that seen in liver disease. Tests for circulating rheumatoid factor and antinuclear antibodies are positive in less than one-half of the cases. Myoglobin can be found in the urine when muscle destruction is acute and extensive; rarely, acute polymyositis causes the full syndrome of rhabdomyolysis and myoglobinuria. The erythrocyte sedimentation rate is elevated in about two-thirds of cases. Most other hematologic indices are normal. In about 40 percent of cases the electromyogram reveals a markedly increased insertional activity (muscle irritability), together with the typical myopathic triad of motor unit action potentials which are of low amplitude, are polyphasic, and have an abnormally early recruitment. In a further 40 percent of the patients only myopathic changes are present. The ECG is abnormal in about 5 to 10 percent of the cases at presentation. The muscle biopsy should be taken from two clinically affected muscles, and muscles recently used for EMG or intramuscular injection must be avoided. In about two-thirds of cases, the biopsies will demonstrate the typical pathologic changes of myositis. Since the lesions have a patchy distribution, it is recommended that skip serial sections of all the specimens be studied. Despite this, about 10 percent of cases have a normal muscle biopsy.

Skeletal muscle pathology The principal changes in muscle consist of infiltrates of inflammatory cells (lymphocytes, macrophages, plasma cells, and rare eosinophils and neutrophils) and destruction of muscle fibers with a phagocytic reaction. Perivascular (usually perivenular) inflammatory cell infiltration is the hallmark of polymyositis. Interstitial inflammatory cell infiltration is also a prominent feature of the disease, but lesser degrees of it may be seen in other conditions as a secondary reaction (e.g., in facioscapulohumeral and Becker's muscular dystrophy). Evidence of muscle fiber degeneration and regeneration is almost invariably present. Many of the residual muscle fibers are small, with increased numbers of sarcolemmal nuclei. Either the degeneration of muscle fibers or the infiltration of inflammatory cells may predominate in any given biopsy specimen. Perifascicular atrophy of muscle fibers, type II muscle fiber atrophy, and muscle infarcts may also be found.

DIAGNOSIS Patients with dermatomyositis with the characteristic skin rash, muscle weakness, and evidence of muscle damage by EMG and elevation of serum CK may not require a muscle biopsy to confirm the diagnosis. In the case of idiopathic polymyositis, however, a firm diagnosis must be based on the presence of a typical clinical picture, a typical EMG, elevation of serum CK, and a diagnostic muscle biopsy. All four criteria are required to be certain of the diagnosis, since inflammatory changes may occasionally occur in other myopathies (e.g., facioscapulohumeral muscular dystrophy) and in other connective tissue disorders without clear muscle weakness. However, in less than one-third of cases of polymyositis are *all* these criteria satisfied. It may be particularly difficult to obtain a diagnostic muscle biopsy because of the patchy nature of the disease. Thus, a therapeutic trial of corticosteroids should be given when full investigation of a patient with significant disability leaves a diagnosis of "possible polymyositis," usually because of a nondiagnostic muscle biopsy.

DIFFERENTIAL DIAGNOSIS The clinical picture of skin rash and proximal or diffuse muscle weakness has few causes other than dermatomyositis. However, proximal muscle weakness without skin involvement can be due to many conditions other than polymyositis and necessitates detailed investigation to establish the correct diagnosis.

Subacute or chronic progressive muscle weakness This may be due to denervating conditions such as the spinal muscular atrophies or amyotrophic lateral sclerosis. Upper motor neuron signs in the latter in addition to the muscle weakness aid in the diagnosis. The muscular dystrophies, such as those of Duchenne and Becker and the limb-girdle and facioscapulohumeral types, may appear similar to polymyositis (Chap. 357). However, the muscular dystrophies usually develop more slowly, rarely present after the age of 30, usually involve the pharyngeal and posterior neck muscles only in their later course, and have a pattern of muscle involvement which is selective, involving some muscles such as the biceps and brachioradialis early in the course of the disease, and sparing others, such as the deltoid. Nevertheless, in rare patients it may be difficult, even with a muscle biopsy, to distinguish chronic polymyositis from a rapidly advancing muscular dystrophy. This is particularly true of facioscapulohumeral muscular dystrophy, where interstitial inflammatory cell infiltration is commonly found early in the disease. Such doubtful cases should always be given an adequate trial of corticosteroid therapy. Dystrophia myotonica produces a characteristic facies with ptosis, facial myopathy, temporalis muscle wasting, and grip myotonia (Chap. 357). Some of the metabolic myopathies, including glycogen storage disease due to myophosphorylase deficiency and the lipid storage diseases due to carnitine and carnitine palmityltransferase deficiency, produce exertional cramps, rhabdomyolysis, and muscle weakness; diagnosis rests upon biochemical studies of the muscle biopsy (Chap. 357). Glycogen storage disease due to acid maltase deficiency also requires muscle biopsy for diagnosis. The endocrine myopathies such as those due to hypercorticosteroidism and hyper- and hypothyroidism require the appropriate laboratory investigations for diagnosis. Toxic myopathies (e.g., those due to aminocaproic acid or emetine) have a different pathology from polymyositis and require a careful drug history for diagnosis. Muscle wasting in patients with an underlying neoplasm may be true polymyositis, but it can be due to a protein-wasting state (cachexia), a paraneoplastic neuropathy, or type II fiber atrophy.

Muscle weakness with marked exercise-induced fatigue Fatigue without much muscle wasting may be due to the neuromuscular junction disorders, myasthenia gravis, or the Lambert-Eaton syndrome. Repetitive nerve stimulation studies aid in the diagnosis of these conditions (Chap. 358).

Acute muscle weakness This may be caused by an acute neuropathy such as that due to the Guillain-Barré syndrome or a neurotoxin. When combined with painful muscle cramps, rhabdomyolysis, and myoglobinuria, it may be due to known metabolic disorders including some of the glycogen storage diseases such as myophosphorylase deficiency (McArdle's disease), carnitine palmityltransferase deficiency, and myoadenylate deaminase deficiency. Acute viral infections may cause a similar syndrome. In other cases investigation reveals no etiology, and these may be due to a true acute autoimmune polymyositis or to an as yet undiscovered metabolic defect.

Pain on movement and muscle tenderness Patients with muscle pain and little or no weakness may be thought to be neurotic or hysterical. A number of conditions including *polymyalgia rheumatica* (Chap. 269) and arthritic disorders of adjacent joints enter into the differential diagnosis of polymyositis. The muscle biopsy either is normal or discloses type II fiber atrophy, but in polymyalgia rheumatica the temporal artery biopsy may show giant cell arteritis (Chap. 269). *Fibrositis* and *fibromyalgia* are syndromes which frequently enter into the differential diagnosis of polymyositis. Patients complain of focal or diffuse muscle tenderness, aching, and weakness, which is sometimes poorly separated from joint pain. In other patients there may be minor signs of a collagen-vascular disorder, such as an increased erythrocyte sedimentation rate, antinuclear antibody (ANA), or rheumatoid factor, and occasionally there is slight elevation of the serum CK. The muscle biopsy occasionally shows a few interstitial inflammatory cells. Where there is a focal "trigger point," biopsy may show inflammatory infiltration of the connective tissue. Rarely does this syndrome develop into frank polymyositis, and the prognosis is therefore more benign than that of polymyositis (see below). Many such patients show some response to nonsteroidal anti-inflammatory agents, though most continue to have indolent complaints.

TREATMENT Corticosteroids in high dosage are the accepted treatment for severe dermatomyositis-polymyositis, though there is no controlled trial to prove their effectiveness. The best results are obtained from the use of prednisone, starting at a dose of 1 to 2 mg per kilogram of body weight per day (60 to 100 mg per day for adults). Improvement may begin within 1 to 4 weeks, though in some patients treatment may need to be continued for 3 months before improvement occurs. When there is significant improvement in the weakness, the dose may be reduced every 4 weeks by 5 mg per day. Repeated manual muscle testing and serum CK determinations should be performed to ensure that the myositis does not relapse. At about 40 mg per day, the schedule is changed gradually to 80 mg every other day in order to reduce the incidence of corticosteroid side effects. Children and patients with acute to subacute dermatomyositis-polymyositis tend to improve more rapidly than those with chronic polymyositis. If the dose is reduced too rapidly, or to too low a level, relapse will occur, necessitating return to high dosage. Prednisone therapy may have to be continued for several years, but an attempt should be made every year to withdraw the therapy from patients who are clinically stable in order to determine if the disease is still active.

Cytotoxic drugs should be tried when the disease is severe, when the response to corticosteroids is inadequate, or when relapses are frequent. Azathioprine (2.5 to 3.5 mg per kilogram of body weight per day in divided doses) is the most commonly used cytotoxic drug in this disease. Cyclophosphamide and methotrexate have also been used with benefit. The aim of cytotoxic therapy is to lower the total lymphocyte count to about 750 per cubic millimeter, while maintaining the hemoglobin level above 12 g/dL, the total white cell count above 3000 per cubic millimeter, and the platelet count above 125,000 per cubic millimeter. Weekly blood counts are required to monitor the cytotoxic drug therapy. The combined use of prednisone and a cytotoxic drug usually allows a lower dose of prednisone to be used. Bed rest has been recommended in the acute phase of the disease but is harmful in the long term. Physiotherapy and rehabilitative devices are important in the long-term treatment of patients with dermatomyositis-polymyositis.

Elderly patients, particularly those with dermatomyositis, should be investigated at yearly intervals for a malignancy. If a malignant lesion is found, it should be treated, since the muscle weakness may disappear if the neoplasm is eradicated. However, a response to corticosteroids can usually be obtained even in patients with polymyositis associated with a malignancy.

The serum CK activity is useful for following patients during reduction of immunosuppressant therapy, since a rise in level generally indicates an incipient clinical relapse. However it cannot be used to indicate initial response in patients being treated with prednisone for dermatomyositis-polymyositis, since this drug lowers the serum CK activity in a way which is not fully understood, but which is not related to the suppression of muscle inflammation.

Side effects of high-dose corticosteroid therapy (Chap. 325) are relatively common in patients treated for polymyositis, and these may limit therapy. When patients who have been stable on a static dose of prednisone develop increasing muscle weakness, this may be due to either a relapse of the myositis or to corticosteroid myopathy. An EMG, serum CK measurement, and rarely muscle biopsy may help in differentiating these two conditions if the changes of myositis are present. However, often the only way to separate them is to reduce the dose of prednisone slowly; if corticosteroid myopathy is the cause of the weakness, it will improve; if a relapse of the myositis is responsible, the weakness will increase.

Side effects of cytotoxic drugs include marrow suppression, alopecia, gastrointestinal tract disorders, damage to the testes and ovaries (including potential genetic damage), and disorders of chronic immunosuppression.

PROGNOSIS The overall mortality rate of individuals with dermatomyositis-polymyositis is about four times that of the general population; death is due usually to pulmonary, renal, and cardiac complications. Females and blacks have a worse prognosis. Nevertheless, the 5-year survival rate is about 75 percent overall, and is better than this in children. The majority of patients improve with therapy. Many patients make a full functional recovery, though some weakness of the shoulders and hips, usually not disabling, remains at the conclusion of treatment. Relapse may occur at any time. Corticosteroids should not be discontinued too soon, for the relapse which may follow is often more difficult to treat than the original presentation. About one-half of the patients with this disease recover and can discontinue therapy within 5 years after the onset of the symptoms; about 20 percent still have active disease requiring continued therapy. The remaining 30 percent have inactive disease but residual muscle weakness.

REFERENCES

BOHAN A et al: A computer-assisted analysis of 153 patients with polymyositis and dermatomyositis. Medicine 56:255, 1977

BRADLEY WG: Inflammatory diseases of muscle, in *Textbook of Rheumatology*, 2nd ed., WN Kelley et al (eds). Philadelphia, Saunders, 1984, chap 79

CARPENTER S, KARPATI G: *Pathology of Skeletal Muscle*. New York, Churchill Livingstone, 1984, pp 515–592

CURIE S.: Inflammatory myopathies, Part I: Polymyositis and related disorders, in *Disorders of Voluntary Muscle*, 4th ed., JN Walton (ed). London, Churchill Livingstone, 1981, chap 15

DEVERE R, BRADLEY WG: Polymyositis: Its presentation, mortality, and morbidity. Brain 98:637, 1975

ENGEL AG, BANKER BQ (eds): *Myology*. New York, McGraw-Hill, 1986

MASTAGLIA FL, OJEDA VJ: Inflammatory myopathies. Ann Neurol 17:215, 317, 1985

357 MUSCULAR DYSTROPHY AND OTHER CHRONIC MYOPATHIES

JERRY R. MENDELL / ROBERT C. GRIGGS

Most myopathies (see Table 354-2) including the hereditary, inflammatory, endocrine, metabolic, and toxic disorders can result in chronic weakness. The approach to differential diagnosis of these disorders is summarized in Chap. 354.

HEREDITARY MYOPATHIES

MUSCULAR DYSTROPHIES *Muscular dystrophy* refers to a group of disorders that have little in common except for their name and the fact that they are inherited. Each type of muscular dystrophy has unique phenotypic and genetic differences (Table 357-1).

Duchenne's muscular dystrophy This disorder was first described by Edward Meryon (1852) but the disease bears the name of the French neurologist Duchenne. Duchenne dystrophy is an X-linked recessive disorder affecting males almost exclusively. Estimates of incidence range from 13 to 33 per 100,000 live-born males. In one-third or more of cases the family history is negative, suggesting that many are due to new mutations.

Careful studies of rare females with the Duchenne phenotype have provided information about the localization of the Duchenne gene on the chromosome. Translocations and deletions have been consistently found on the short arm of the X chromosome at the Xp21 site. Confirmation of a close proximity of the Duchenne locus to the Xp21 site has been accomplished through genetic linkage studies employing restriction endonucleases. The further development of a specific DNA probe will permit identification of fetuses at risk and provide a direct and definitive carrier detection test. Heterozygous female carriers of the trait often manifest some features of the disease, but current methods of detection using the serum levels of creatine kinase (CK), pyruvate kinase, and lactic dehydrogenase or other methods fail to identify half of such carriers.

Clinical manifestations usually begin at 3 to 5 years of age. The boys fall frequently and have difficulty keeping up with their friends when playing. Running, jumping, and hopping are invariably abnormal. Motor milestones may be delayed even before age 2, but if there is no family history the diagnosis is often not suspected.

By age 5 muscle weakness is obvious by manual muscle testing or by observing the inability to run, jump, or hop. On getting up from the floor the patient must use his hands to climb up himself (Gowers' maneuver). In younger children the calf muscles are usually enlarged from muscle hypertrophy; later, calf enlargement is appropriately called *pseudohypertrophy* since muscle is replaced by fat and connective tissue.

Contractures of heel cords and iliotibial bands become apparent by age 7 to 8, when toe walking is associated with a lordotic posture. Loss of muscle strength is progressive with predilection for proximal limb muscles and the neck flexors; leg involvement is more severe than arm involvement. Between ages 8 and 10 walking usually requires the use of braces; joint contractures and limitation of hip flexion and knee, elbow, and wrist extension are made worse by prolonged sitting. By age 12 most patients are confined to a wheelchair. Contractures become fixed and a progressive scoliosis often develops which may be associated with considerable discomfort. The chest deformity associated with scoliosis further impairs pulmonary function which is already diminished by the muscle weakness. By age 14 to 18 patients may develop serious, even fatal, pulmonary infections. Other causes of death include aspiration of food and acute gastric dilatation.

A cardiac cause of death is uncommon despite the existence of a cardiomyopathy in almost all patients. Congestive heart failure seldom occurs except with severe stress such as pneumonia. Cardiac arrhythmias are rare. The typical ECG shows an increased net RS in lead V_1; deep narrow Q waves in the lateral precordial leads; and RSR′ or polyphasic R waves in V_1.

TABLE 357-1 Progressive muscular dystrophies

Type	Usual inheritance	Clinical features	Other organ systems involved
Duchenne's (pseudohypertrophic)	X-linked recessive	Onset by age 5 Progressive weakness of girdle muscles Inability to walk after age 12 Kyphoscoliosis Respiratory failure in second to third decade	Cardiomyopathy Mental impairment
Becker's (benign pseudohypertrophic)	X-linked recessive	Onset in early to late childhood Slowly progressive weakness of girdle muscles Ability to walk after age 5 Respiratory failure after fourth decade	Cardiomyopathy
Myotonic	Autosomal dominant	Onset any decade Slowly progressive weakness of eyelids, face, neck, distal limb muscles Myotonia	Cardiac conduction defects Mental impairment Cataracts Frontal baldness Gonadal atrophy
Facioscapulohumeral	Autosomal dominant	Onset second to fourth decade Slowly progressive face, shoulder girdle, foot dorsiflexion weakness	Hypertension
Limb-girdle (may include several disorders)	Autosomal recessive	Onset early childhood to adult Slowly progressive weakness of shoulder and hip girdle muscles	Cardiomyopathy
Oculopharyngeal	Autosomal dominant (French-Canadian or Hispanic background)	Onset fifth to sixth decade Slowly progressive weakness of extraocular, eyelid, face, and pharyngeal muscles Cricopharyngeal achalasia	
Less well-characterized forms of muscular dystrophies:			
Congenital (may include several disorders)	Autosomal recessive	Onset at birth Hypotonia, contractures and delayed milestones Early respiratory failure in some; others have static course	
Distal (may include several disorders)	Autosomal recessive	Onset second to third decade Slowly progressive weakness of legs beginning with foot drop	
Scapuloperoneal (may include several disorders)	Autosomal dominant	Onset third to fifth decade Progressive shoulder girdle and foot dorsiflexor weakness	Cardiomyopathy

Intellectual impairment is common in Duchenne's dystrophy. One-third of patients have intelligence quotients below 75 and the mean is estimated at 85. The intellectual impairment is not the result of weakness since verbal skills are impaired before weakness is severe; its basis is not known. In contrast to the muscle disease, intellectual impairment is nonprogressive.

Laboratory confirmation includes assessment of serum CK level, which is invariably elevated twentyfold and may be as high as 100 times normal. The levels are abnormal at birth, making it possible to diagnose an affected boy early in life. Serum CK activity remains high until late in the disease, when levels decline because of inactivity and loss of muscle mass.

Myopathy can be demonstrated by electromyography (EMG). The muscle biopsy shows muscle fibers of varying size as well as small groups of necrotic and regenerating fibers. Connective tissue and fat replaces lost muscle fibers.

Becker's muscular dystrophy This less severe form of X-linked recessive muscular dystrophy was described by Becker and Keiner in 1955. It is often called the benign form of pseudohypertrophic muscular dystrophy. The presentation is similar to that of Duchenne's dystrophy except that the time course is slow. The incidence of Becker's dystrophy is approximately one-tenth that of the Duchenne type. The condition is not usually recognized before age 5 and walking continues well beyond age 15, sometimes into the fourth decade. Calf muscle enlargement is prominent. Death from complications similar to those of Duchenne's dystrophy may occur after age 40.

The fact that the Becker and Duchenne genes are at or near the same locus on the X chromosome suggests that the disorders may be allelic. Carrier detection methods are identical for Duchenne's and Becker's dystrophies, and both suffer the same shortcomings. Unlike Duchenne's dystrophy, Becker patients reach child-bearing age; while none of their sons will be affected, the daughters of the Becker patient will all be carriers.

Laboratory confirmation of Becker's dystrophy is the same as that for Duchenne's dystrophy in that high serum CK levels are present early in the course and then gradually decline. The EMG and muscle biopsy changes are similar to those of Duchenne's dystrophy.

Facioscapulohumeral muscular dystrophy This slowly progressive, relatively mild disorder is usually inherited as an autosomal dominant disorder, affecting males and females equally. It is extremely variable in severity and may start at any age, commonly in the third or fourth decade. Patients may, however, remain asymptomatic throughout life. As the name implies, there is characteristic weakness of facial, shoulder girdle, and proximal arm muscles. Scapular winging and sloping shoulders reflect weakness of the serratus anterior, trapezius, and rhomboid muscles; later, the biceps and triceps muscles are affected; the deltoid muscles are usually relatively spared. Facial involvement often produces a lifelong inability to whistle, an expressionless face, and a sullen appearance. Foot drop may occur early in the disease from peroneal and anterior tibial muscle weakness. Leg weakness may eventually progress to loss of ambulation.

Other systems are usually unaffected in facioscapulohumeral dystrophy. Cardiac disease and respiratory compromise are rare, and their occurrence usually suggests a coincidental illness. Patients frequently appear to have exophthalmos but thyroid function is normal; a mild but labile hypertension is common. Intellectual function is intact and life span is often normal.

Diagnostic studies may be unnecessary in typical cases, particularly when a family history is present. CK level may be normal or slightly elevated; EMG and muscle biopsy tend to have mixed features of myopathy and neuropathy and may be misleading. No specific treatment is available; ankle-foot orthoses are occasionally helpful for foot drop. Scapular stabilization procedures improve scapular winging but may not improve function.

Limb-girdle dystrophy This term encompasses more than one disorder, and since inheritance is usually by autosomal recessive transmission, cases are often sporadic. Proximal muscle weakness may begin in either the legs or the arms but usually progresses to all extremities. Weakness may begin before age 5 or as late as the third decade and may be associated with pseudohypertrophy of calves and other muscles. Ambulation continues for over 20 years after the disease first appears. In some patients cardiac involvement results in congestive heart failure or arrhythmias; occasional patients may present with a cardiomyopathy. Respiratory failure ensues after 30 or more years of disease. Intellectual function remains normal. Diagnosis requires the exclusion of inflammatory and metabolic myopathies as well as the phenotypically similar spinal muscular atrophies. The serum CK level is elevated in limb-girdle dystrophy although the values are usually lower than in Duchenne's and Becker's dystrophies; the EMG pattern is that of a myopathy. The muscle biopsy shows active myopathy but is not specific.

Myotonic dystrophy This autosomal dominant disorder affects muscle and numerous other tissues. The incidence is estimated to be 1 per 10,000 and may be higher since many cases escape recognition. Associated features include intellectual impairment, hypersomnia, cardiac disease, cataracts, gonadal atrophy, respiratory failure, and gastrointestinal disease. Weakness initially involves eyelid, temporalis, facial, and neck flexor muscles, as well as the distal extremity muscles. Myotonia is demonstrable in hand grip or by percussion of the tongue, the wrist extensors, or the thenar eminence. Disease onset is usually in the second and third decade, but affected individuals may remain free of signs or symptoms throughout life. A severe form of the disease, *congenital myotonic dystrophy,* occurs in some infants of affected mothers and is characterized by severe facial and bulbar weakness; neonatal respiratory insufficiency may occur but is usually self-limited. Affected infants are frequently intellectually impaired.

Diagnosis is often self-evident because of the distinctive facial appearance; the characteristic pattern of weakness and the abnormalities cause the typical narrow, ''hatchet'' face; premature frontal balding is frequent. The presence of distal weakness and myotonia confirm the diagnosis. Laboratory studies are often unnecessary and may be misleading. The CK activity is normal or slightly elevated. EMG of distal hand muscles usually shows myotonia and myopathic features. Muscle biopsy often shows distinctive type I fiber atrophy; severely involved muscles may have a characteristic appearance including ring fibers, sarcoplasmic masses, and numerous central nuclei.

Cardiac involvement most commonly affects the conduction system; first-degree heart block is present in a majority, and complete heart block may require pacemaker implantation. Since sudden death may occur, patients must be monitored carefully for conduction disturbances, though precise criteria for the timing of pacemaker implantation are lacking. Tachyarrhythmias and congestive failure are less frequent. Respiratory muscle weakness may be severe even in patients with minor limb weakness. Impaired ventilatory drive and hypersensitivity to the depressant effects of small doses of opiates and sedatives may result in sudden ventilatory failure, particularly in the pre- or postoperative setting. Sleep apnea may occur on both a central and peripheral basis (Chap. 215). Chronic hypoxia may lead to cor pulmonale and is the usual cause of heart failure.

Myotonia is seldom disabling enough to require treatment; phenytoin is the therapy of choice since the other antimyotonia agents, quinine and procainamide, may worsen cardiac conduction.

Myotonic dystrophy is transmitted by a mutant gene on chromosome 19 which is linked to the genes for secretor substance, the Lutheran blood group, peptidase D, and the third component of complement. Early disease detection and antenatal diagnosis are now possible in selected families using linkage techniques. Furthermore, prior to the onset of symptoms affected family members can frequently be identified by clinical and EMG evaluation for myotonia and by slit-lamp examination for the characteristic posterior subcapsular cataracts.

Myotonia congenita This disorder occurs in autosomal dominant (Thomsen) and autosomal recessive forms (Chap. 17). Patients with the autosomal recessive form may develop slight weakness; patients with the dominant form do not develop weakness. Myotonia can be markedly alleviated by antimyotonia agents including quinine, procainamide, phenytoin, or acetazolamide. These patients have no cardiac involvement.

Oculopharyngeal dystrophy The term *progressive external ophthalmoplegia* describes disorders characterized by slowly progressive ptosis and limitation of eye movements with the sparing of pupil and accommodation muscles. Patients usually do not complain of diplopia, in contrast to conditions with a more acute onset of ocular muscle weakness. *Oculopharyngeal dystrophy* is an autosomal dominant disorder in which ophthalmoplegia appears in the fifth or sixth decade. Many patients are of French-Canadian or Hispanic ancestry. Pharyngeal weakness leads to cricopharyngeal achalasia, progressive difficulty in swallowing, and frequent, often asymptomatic, aspiration. Severe malnutrition may develop but can be alleviated by surgical correction of cricopharyngeal achalasia.

Additional types of *ocular myopathies* are associated with mitochondrial abnormalities in muscle (see discussion of metabolic myopathies below).

Congenital muscular dystrophy This rare disorder may represent more than one disease. The usual picture is infantile hypotonia and muscle wasting associated with joint contractures of limbs. Serum CK level is usually elevated and the muscle biopsy shows features typical of muscular dystrophy. The condition is relatively nonprogressive, but many patients are not able to walk. Respiratory failure may occur in the first or second decade. Hypomyelination of the deep white matter of the brain can be detected in some cases by computerized tomography (CT), but it has no known clinical manifestations.

Distal muscular dystrophy This rare disorder has at least three separate variants. The most frequent is an autosomal recessive or sporadic disorder that presents with distal leg weakness in the second or third decade. Slow progression to more proximal muscles occurs. The CK level is markedly elevated. Other distinct forms of a distal myopathy include an autosomal dominant Scandinavian form (Welander) which begins in the hands, and a late-onset (fourth to fifth decade) autosomal dominant disorder that begins in the legs and in which cardiomyopathy is frequent.

Scapuloperoneal dystrophy Several forms of neuromuscular disease cause foot drop and winging of the scapulas. An autosomal dominant form presents in the third to fifth decade and is variable in its progression; respiratory failure is uncommon, but cardiomyopathy may occur. An X-linked recessive form (Emery-Dreifuss) begins in early childhood and is associated with prominent joint contractures and cardiac conduction disorders. Certain cases of facioscapulohumeral dystrophy may lack facial weakness and resemble scapuloperoneal dystrophy.

CONGENITAL MYOPATHIES These rare disorders are distinguished from muscular dystrophies by the presence of specific histochemical and structural abnormalities in muscle. A nonprogressive course is common but not invariable. The typical infant has hypotonia and delayed motor milestones. Pectus excavatum, kyphoscoliosis, hip dislocation, and pes cavus are common. The diagnosis is important, since the long-term prognosis and management differ from that of the muscular dystrophies.

Four major forms of congenital myopathies have been described: central core disease, nemaline (rod) myopathy, myotubular (centronuclear) myopathy and congenital fiber-type disproportion.

Central core disease This disease, the first congenital myopathy described, was identified by Shy and Magee in 1956. The disorder is inherited as an autosomal dominant disorder but sporadic cases also occur. In infancy hypotonia and delayed motor milestones are typical, but the diagnosis may come to attention in an adult with muscle weakness or skeletal abnormalities.

Short, slender stature and skeletal abnormalities including congenital hip dislocation, scoliosis, pes cavus, and pectus excavatum are characteristic. Weakness of the muscles of the face and limbs, particularly the legs, is mild. The muscle biopsy is diagnostic; it shows fibers with single or multiple central or eccentric discrete zones (cores) devoid of oxidative enzymes. Other laboratory studies are less helpful since the serum CK and the EMG may be normal. Patients with this disorder may be predisposed to develop malignant hyperthermia (Chap. 8).

Nemaline myopathy This disorder, also called rod myopathy, was described by Shy and colleagues in 1963. Inheritance is usually as an autosomal dominant trait but it may be recessive or sporadic. Infantile hypotonia is frequent, and death may occur from respiratory failure. The skeletal abnormalities are striking; they include a long face, high arched palate, and slender musculature. Kyphoscoliosis, pectus excavatum, and pes cavus may be present. Muscle weakness affects the face, palate, and limb muscles. The prognosis is variable, with some patients progressing to wheelchair confinement or respiratory failure while in others the disease does not progress.

Muscle histology shows clusters of small rod or nemaline (thread-like) bodies for which the condition was named. Rods, derived from Z-band material, are usually found in type I fibers, and the muscle often shows type I predominance. The serum CK level may be normal or mildly elevated, and the EMG usually shows myopathy.

Myotubular myopathy This disorder was described by Spiro, Shy, and Gonatas in 1966. The histologic abnormality in myotubular myopathy resembles the embryonic or developmental myotube stage of a muscle fiber. Others have preferred to call the disease *centronuclear myopathy,* arguing that the fibers are not embryonic. The condition is usually sporadic, but inheritance may be as an autosomal dominant, recessive, or X-linked recessive trait. Infantile hypotonia and weakness are common and may cause death. Presentations at an older age include features similar to nemaline myopathy with a long narrow face, pes cavus, and scoliosis. Muscle bulk is reduced, and proximal and distal weakness is of varying severity. The feature that separates these patients from those with other congenital myopathies is the presence of external ophthalmoplegia. The course may or may not be progressive.

Serum CK activity is normal or slightly elevated. The EMG is usually abnormal with excessively recruited small motor unit potentials associated with fibrillations and positive sharp potentials. Muscle biopsy shows muscle fibers with rows of central nuclei often surrounded by a perinuclear clear zone. Type I fibers may be preferentially affected and may be atrophic.

Congenital fiber-type disproportion Clinical features of this disorder include hypotonia, weakness, delayed milestones, and skeletal deformities similar to those of other congenital myopathies. The diagnosis is established by the muscle biopsy which shows an increased number of small type I fibers and normal or hypertrophied type II fibers. The pathogenesis is poorly understood. The prognosis is generally good, with most patients showing improvement with age although some residual motor impairment commonly persists; occasional patients may have progressive weakness.

DISORDERS OF MUSCLE ENERGY METABOLISM Skeletal muscle utilizes two principal sources of energy—fatty acids and glucose. Abnormalities in either glucose or lipid utilization can be associated with distinct clinical features. The more dramatic feature is an acute muscle pain syndrome which can evolve into severe rhabdomyolysis and myoglobinuria. The other is progressive muscle weakness simulating muscular dystrophy. The explanation for the different clinical syndromes is often unknown.

Glycogen storage and glycolytic defects There are four disorders of glycogen metabolism (types II, III, IV, and V) and four disorders of glycolysis (types VII, IX, X, and XI) associated with significant skeletal muscle manifestations (also see Chap. 313).

ACID MALTASE DEFICIENCY (TYPE II GLYCOGENOSIS) Acid maltase is a lysosomal enzyme, an acid hydrolase, having α-1,4- and α-1,6-glucosidase activity which breaks down glycogen to glucose; however, the enzyme has no well-defined role in carbohydrate metabolism. Three clinical forms of acid maltase deficiency are each inherited as autosomal recessive traits. The biochemical basis for the different clinical presentations is not understood.

In infancy, acid maltase deficiency has features of a generalized glycogenosis. No abnormalities are noted at birth, but shortly thereafter severe muscle weakness, cardiomegaly, hepatomegaly, and tongue enlargement develop. Glycogen accumulation in motor neurons of the spinal cord and brainstem contribute to the muscle weakness. Death usually occurs by 1 year of age.

In children and adults, the picture resembles muscular dystrophy. The childhood form is associated with delayed developmental milestones, proximal limb muscle weakness, and calf enlargement and may progress to respiratory failure and death before the end of the second decade. Cardiac involvement may be present, but hepatomegaly and macroglossia are infrequent.

The adult form begins in the third or fourth decade and may be misdiagnosed as limb-girdle dystrophy or polymyositis. Respiratory failure from diaphragmatic weakness may be the initial manifestation of the disease. The heart, liver, and tongue are not involved. The diagnosis is suggested by muscle biopsy which shows vacuoles containing glycogen and the lysosomal enzyme, acid phosphatase. By electron miscroscopy, membrane-bound and free tissue glycogen are found. Definitive diagnosis is established by muscle biochemistry. Acid maltase activity is also reduced in the urine. Serum CK level may be as high as ten times normal. EMG distinguishes acid maltase deficiency from muscular dystrophy by the occurrence of bizarre high-frequency and myotonic discharges accompanying short-duration motor unit potentials, fibrillations, and positive sharp potentials.

DEBRANCHER ENZYME DEFICIENCY (TYPE III GLYCOGENOSIS) Muscle weakness is uncommon in debrancher enzyme deficiency. This mild disease of childhood is dominated by hepatomegaly, growth retardation, and hypoglycemia. These findings usually diminish or disappear after puberty, and muscle weakness and wasting associated with decreased exercise tolerance may develop. Diagnosis is suggested by a failure of lactic acid level to rise following exercise of the forearm. The serum CK level is elevated. EMG shows myopathy which may be accompanied by membrane irritability with myotonic discharges. Muscle biopsy shows a vacuolar myopathy with increased glycogen. Definitive diagnosis requires muscle biochemistry.

BRANCHER ENZYME DEFICIENCY (TYPE IV GLYCOGENOSIS) Brancher enzyme deficiency is a severe fatal disorder of infancy in which skeletal muscle manifestations are relatively minor in the face of the chronic liver failure. The muscle hypotonia and wasting may, however, suggest the possibility of a primary muscle disease or spinal muscular atrophy.

MUSCLE PHOSPHORYLASE DEFICIENCY (TYPE V GLYCOGENOSIS) Exercise intolerance is the dominant feature of muscle phosphorylase deficiency, first described in 1951 by McArdle. The disorder, usually inherited as an autosomal recessive trait, has an unexplained predilection for males. Painful muscle cramps and fatigue after intense exercise such as running or lifting heavy objects usually develops after adolescence. Early infantile and late onset variants have been described. Many patients report a "second wind" phenomenon if they rest briefly or slow down during exercise, which allows them to continue an activity for a longer period of time. Overexertion may lead to rhabdomyolysis and myoglobinuria, and renal failure can result. Persistent weakness and wasting of muscle is rare, and examination of the patient between attacks is usually normal. Other organs are not affected.

Serum CK levels fluctuate widely and may be elevated even during symptom-free periods. The forearm exercise test shows no rise in lactic acid. The EMG is often normal except when taken following an episode of rhabdomyolysis. Muscle biopsy often shows subsarcolemmal blebs containing glycogen. Muscle phosphorylase deficiency can be recognized by a histochemical stain and confirmed by biochemistry. Patients can remain moderately active once they establish their limitations. Dietary supplementation with either glucose or fructose has not alleviated symptoms.

PHOSPHOFRUCTOKINASE DEFICIENCY (TYPE VII GLYCOGENOSIS) This disorder resembles muscle phosphorylase deficiency and is also an autosomal recessive trait with a male predominance. The precipitating events and the laboratory features also resemble phosphorylase deficiency. A histochemical stain for phosphofructokinase (PFK) can demonstrate the deficiency. Definitive diagnosis requires biochemical analysis of muscle enzymes. Some patients with PFK deficiency have mild hemolysis, increased reticulocyte count, and elevated bilirubin because of a deficiency of a PFK subunit shared by muscle and red blood cells.

NEW GLYCOLYTIC ENZYME DEFICIENCY SYNDROMES Since 1981 deficiencies of three additional glycolytic enzymes have been identified: phosphoglycerate kinase (PGK) deficiency (type IX), phosphoglycerate mutase (PGAM) deficiency (type X) and lactate dehydrogenase deficiency (LDH) (XI). The clinical pictures of the three are similar. In each, episodic myoglobinuria and myalgias precipitated by intense exercise begin in childhood or adolescence. Autosomal recessive inheritance is probable in each disorder. Serum CK level may be elevated during and between episodes. In PGAM and LDH deficiencies, the rise in lactic acid following forearm exercise is lower than normal. PGK deficiency shows no rise in lactate and closely resembles muscle phosphorylase and PFK deficiencies. The muscle histology is unremarkable in these disorders with little evidence of glycogen storage. Diagnosis requires muscle biochemistry.

Disorders of lipid metabolism Lipid is an important muscle energy source during rest and prolonged, moderately intense exercise (Fig. 357-1).

CARNITINE DEFICIENCY Carnitine deficiency occurs in myopathic and systemic forms.

Myopathic carnitine deficiency is associated with generalized muscle weakness, usually beginning in childhood. The clinical features overlap with muscular dystrophy and polymyositis. Most cases are sporadic, but the inheritance pattern is thought to be autosomal recessive. Cardiomyopathy may be present. Serum CK level is mildly elevated, and the EMG shows myopathy. The muscle biopsy shows striking lipid accumulation. Serum carnitine is normal. The cause for decreased muscle carnitine is not understood. A defect of transport into muscle has been postulated. Some patients respond to oral carnitine supplements; this should be tried in all cases. Other patients have responded to prednisone for unknown reasons. A diet substituting medium-chain for long-chain triglycerides has been helpful in some cases. Rare patients have also responded to riboflavin.

Systemic carnitine deficiency, an autosomal recessive disease of infancy and early childhood, is characterized by progressive weakness and episodes of hepatic encephalopathy with nausea, vomiting, confusion, coma, and early death. The low *serum* carnitine level distinguishes this condition from the myopathic form. No single cause has been identified to explain the low serum carnitine level. Decreased synthesis explains some cases while increased urinary excretion is seen in others. Serum CK level may be slightly elevated. The muscle biopsy shows lipid storage. In some cases the liver, heart, and kidney also show increased lipid. Treatment with oral carnitine supplements or corticosteroids has helped some but not all patients.

CARNITINE PALMITYLTRANSFERASE DEFICIENCY Deficiency of carnitine palmityltransferase (CPT) presents with recurrent myoglobinuria. It is not known if CPT I or CPT II activities are selectively deficient; the deficiency apparently results from disordered regulatory properties of an abnormal enzyme. Rhabdomyolysis may follow prolonged exercise such as soccer, football, or a long hike, but at times no precipitating cause can be found. Initial symptoms often commence in childhood. In contrast to defects in glycolysis where muscle cramps follow short intense bursts of exercise, limiting the amount of exercise and protecting the patient, in CPT deficiency muscle pain does not occur until the limits of energy utilization have been exceeded and muscle breakdown has begun. Episodes of rhabdomyolysis may produce severe weakness, and some patients require ventilatory assistance. In contrast to carnitine deficiency, strength is normal between attacks and the muscle biopsy does not show lipid accumulation. The diagnosis requires direct measurement of muscle CPT. Treatment consists of increasing carbohydrate intake before exercise or of substituting medium-chain for long-chain triglycerides in the diet. Neither has been entirely satisfactory.

Myoadenylate deaminase deficiency The enzyme adenylate deaminase converts 5′-adenosine monophosphate (5′-AMP) to inosine monophosphate (IMP) with liberation of ammonia and may play a role in regulating adenosine triphosphate (ATP) levels in muscle. In 1978 a group of patients with myalgias and exercise intolerance were found to be deficient in the muscle isoenzyme, myoadenylate deaminase. The deficiency, however, occurs in as many as 1 percent of the population and can be detected by histochemical staining of muscle tissue as well as by biochemical analysis. Muscle ammonia production is decreased following forearm exercise. Since the original description, a less consistent clinical picture has emerged. Patients with other neuromuscular disorders including anterior horn cell disease, muscular dystrophy, and myasthenia gravis occasionally have the same enzyme deficiency. The full clinical significance of myoadenylate deaminase deficiency is not established.

Mitochondrial myopathies A heterogeneous group of disorders is characterized by abnormal mitochondria in "ragged-red fibers," named for their appearance in the trichrome stain of biopsied muscle. The *Kearns-Sayre syndrome* is a sporadic disorder beginning in childhood in which progressive external ophthalmoplegia is accompanied by cardiac conduction defects that often culminate in complete heart block. Retinal degeneration, short stature, and gonadal defects also occur. A familial disorder with progressive external ophthalmoplegia and proximal weakness may be difficult to distinguish from the Kearns-Sayre syndrome. Another disorder recently assigned the acronym *MERRF syndrome,* because of its myolonic epilepsy and ragged-red fibers, presents between the first and fifth decades with generalized seizures, myoclonus, dementia, hearing loss, and ataxia. A third disorder, the *MELAS syndrome*, is a slowly progressive disease characterized by mitochondrial myopathy, encephalopathy, lactic acidosis, stroke-like episodes including alternating hemiparesis, hemianopsia or cortical blindness, and focal or generalized seizures. The cause of the mitochondrial myopathies is unknown but there is evidence that familial cases may be transmitted by mitochondrial as opposed to chromosomal DNA.

INFLAMMATORY MYOPATHIES

Polymyositis and dermatomyositis (Chap. 356) develop slowly over the course of months. The presence of a characteristic skin rash usually makes the diagnosis of dermatomyositis straightforward. Chronic polymyositis, with slowly progressive proximal weakness, may be impossible to separate on clinical grounds from sporadic cases of limb-girdle dystrophy. Even with detailed EMG and biopsy studies it may prove difficult to establish the diagnosis of polymyositis with confidence. A subgroup of subacute or chronic inflammatory myopathy has been identified and is termed *inclusion body myositis* because of distinctive cytoplasmic membranous inclusions and nuclear inclusions consisting of abnormal filaments. Inclusion body myositis does not respond to corticosteroid therapy. Chronic myositis may also occur with all of the collagen-vascular diseases and with sarcoidosis.

ENDOCRINE AND METABOLIC MYOPATHIES

Many endocrine disorders cause weakness. Muscle fatigue is more common than true weakness. The cause of weakness in these disorders is not well-defined. It is not even clear that weakness results from

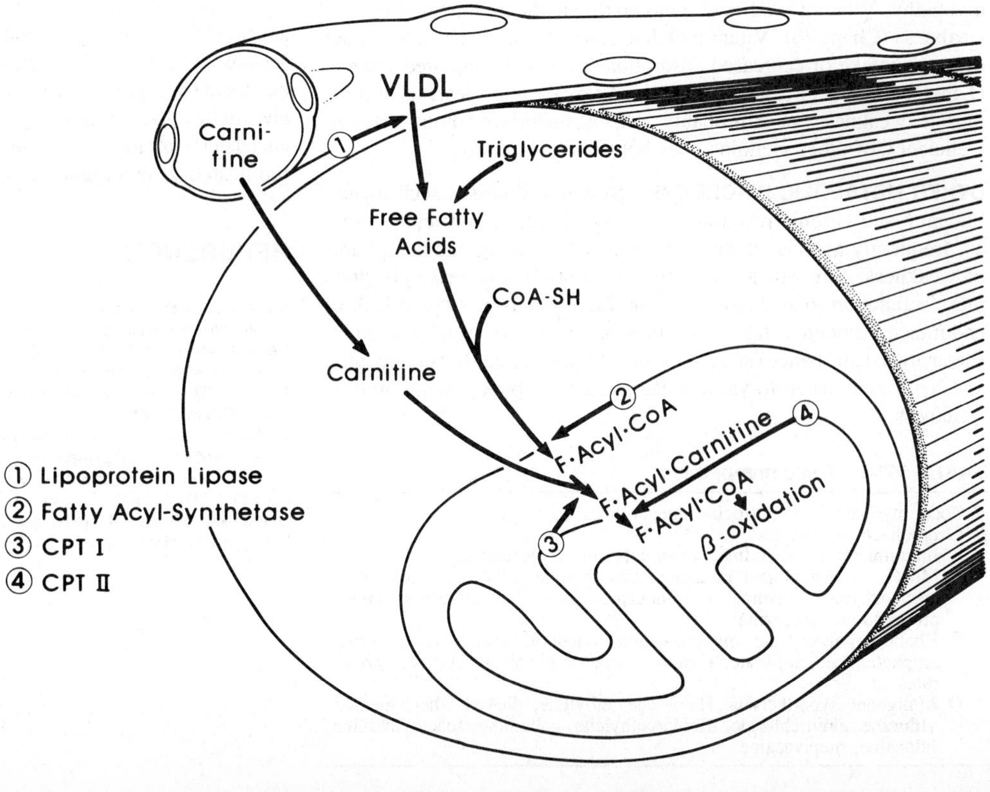

FIGURE 357-1 *Free fatty acids for muscle energy are derived from triglycerides stored in muscle and from circulating very low density lipoproteins (VLDL) which are broken down by endothelial lipoprotein lipase (1) in the capillary. Carnitine, an essential substrate for lipid metabolism, is made in the liver and transported to muscle. In muscle, free fatty acids combine with coenzyme A (CoA SH) through the action of fatty acylsynthetase (2) found in the outer mitochondrial membrane forming fatty acylcoenzyme A (F acyl CoA). Transport through inner mitochondrial membrane requires transfer to carnitine by carnitine palmityltransferase I (CPT I) bound to the outer surface of the inner mitochondrial membrane (3). Inside the mitochondrion, fatty acylcarnitine (F acyl carnitine) is regenerated by CPT II (4) bound to the inner surface of the inner mitochondrial membrane. The fatty acylcoenzyme A then proceeds to beta oxidation.*

disease of muscle as opposed to another part of the motor unit since the CK level is often normal and the muscle histology is characterized by atrophy rather than by destruction of muscle fibers. Nearly all respond to appropriate endocrine management.

THYROID DISORDERS (See Chap. 324) *Hyperthyroidism* may occasionally present as muscle weakness, and the majority of patients are weak. *Hypothyroidism* commonly presents with muscle weakness and pain. The serum CK is often elevated and levels as high as 100 times normal may occur even with minimal clinical evidence of muscle disease. Adult patients may have muscle hypertrophy with cramps (Hoffmann's syndrome) and in children with cretinism a distinctive myopathy with muscle hypertrophy may occur (Kocher-Debré-Sémélaigne syndrome).

PARATHYROID DISORDERS (See Chap. 336) *Hyperparathyroidism* is often associated with muscle weakness and atrophy and may be accompanied by "muscle" pain which is probably from associated bone disease. *Hyperreflexia* is characteristic. *Hypoparathyroidism* frequently presents with neurologic involvement. The neuromuscular manifestations are usually those of tetany, but since the serum CK level is often elevated such patients are occasionally considered to have polymyositis. Hyporeflexia or areflexia is usually present despite the presence of Chvostek's and Trousseau's signs.

ADRENAL DISORDERS (See Chap. 325) Endogenous elevations of corticosteroids may produce severe muscle weakness and wasting. Adrenal insufficiency is frequently associated with lassitude and weakness although there is usually little objective reduction in strength.

PITUITARY DISORDERS (See Chap. 321) Acromegaly is occasionally associated with muscle enlargement. Myopathic weakness may occur, but weakness usually results from associated endocrine abnormalities or from neuropathy. The weakness of panhypopituitarism is probably due to coexisting adrenal or thyroid insufficiency.

DIABETES (See Chap. 327) Proximal weakness in the patient with diabetes is usually the result of neuropathy. The finding of evidence on EMG or biopsy for myopathy or of a markedly elevated serum CK level usually suggests coincidental illness.

VITAMIN DEFICIENCY Severe malabsorption, particularly when it occurs in early childhood, may lead to a vitamin E deficiency myopathy. Vitamin E otherwise has no role in the treatment of muscle weakness (Chap. 76). Vitamin D deficiency (Chap. 337), from either decrease intake or decreased absorption, as well as impaired vitamin D metabolism such as occurs in renal disease may lead to chronic muscle weakness; pain probably reflects underlying bone disease. Deficiency of other vitamins does not cause myopathy.

OTHER METABOLIC DISORDERS Systemic illnesses such as malignancy and chronic respiratory, cardiac, hepatic, and renal failure are frequently associated with severe muscle wasting and complaints of weakness. Strength testing often demonstrates surprisingly good muscle function in such patients, and the problem is often a lack of endurance. Evidence for active muscle disease is usually lacking. Electrolyte disturbances such as chronic hypokalemia, hypercalcemia, and hypocalcemia from various causes may produce chronic muscle weakness.

TABLE 357-2 Toxic myopathies

I Focal myopathies: Pentazocine, meperidine
II Generalized myopathies
- *A* Inflammatory: Cimetidine, D-penicillamine, procainamide
- *B* Muscle weakness and myalgias: Chloroquine, clofibrate, colchicine, corticosteroids, emetine, ϵ-aminocaproic acid, labetalol, perhexilene, propranolol, vincristine
- *C* Rhabdomyolysis and myoglobinuria: Alcohol, azathioprine, heroin, amphetamine, clofibrate, ϵ-aminocaproic acid, phencyclidine, barbiturates
- *D* Malignant hyperthermia: Halothane, ethylene, diethyl ether, methoxyflurane, ethyl chloride, trichloroethylene, gallamine, succinylcholine, lidocaine, mepivacaine

TOXIC MYOPATHIES

A classification of toxic myopathies is shown in Table 357-2. Drugs and chemicals may produce focal or generalized damage of skeletal muscle.

The most common cause of focal damage is the injection of narcotic analgesics. Two agents in particular, pentazocine and meperidine, may cause a severe fibrotic reaction in muscle. Common injection sites include deltoid, triceps, gluteus maximus and quadriceps muscles. The muscles become indurated and hard and may have local abscess formation. Cutaneous ulcerations and depressions may occur. Severe joint contractions may develop.

Other drugs may induce generalized muscle weakness, particularly affecting the proximal muscles. In most cases the exact mechanism of drug toxicity is poorly understood. D-Penicillamine induces a condition simulating the clinical and pathologic picture of dermatomyositis and polymyositis. A similar condition has been reported with cimetidine. Procainamide may cause myositis as part of a systemic lupus-like reaction. After many months of treatment, chloroquine produces a distinctive vacuolar myopathy that may involve the heart. Clofibrate is associated with muscle pain and weakness either shortly after the start or following several months of treatment. Serum CK elevation may be the only clofibrate-induced abnormality. Emetine hydrochloride (used for treatment of amebiasis), ϵ-aminocaproic acid (an antifibrolytic agent), and perhexilene (used for angina pectoris) have all been observed to cause weakness and muscle fiber necrosis following several weeks of therapy.

Drug-induced myopathy accompanied by proximal weakness occurs with corticosteroid therapy. Those fluorinated in the 9α-position, such as triamcinolone, dexamethasone, and betamethasone, are most likely to cause weakness, but chronic administration of all corticosteroids including prednisone also causes weakness. Divided-dose as opposed to single-morning-dose therapy produces more severe weakness. A single-dose, alternate-day regimen has the greatest muscle-sparing effect (Chap. 325). The clinical diagnosis of steroid-induced muscle weakness can be difficult if the medication is being used to treat an underlying inflammatory myopathy. The presence of a normal serum CK level, minimal or no changes of myopathy on EMG, and type II muscle fiber atrophy on biopsy are helpful in suggesting corticosteroid-induced weakness.

In some instances toxic myopathy may be more catastrophic, causing rhabdomyolysis and myoglobinuria (Chap. 376). A very serious drug-induced condition, *malignant hyperthermia* (Chap. 8), occurs in susceptible individuals following exposure to certain general anesthetics and depolarizing muscle relaxants (Table 357-2). In local anesthesia, amides including lidocaine and mepivacaine have been implicated as precipitating agents.

REFERENCES

BAKKER et al: Prenatal diagnosis and carrier detection of Duchenne muscular dystrophy with closely linked RFLPs. Lancet 1:655, 1985

BENDER AN: Congenital myopathies, in *Handbook of Clinical Neurology*, PJ Vinken, GW Bruyn (eds). New York, North-Holland, 1979, vol 41

BROOKE MH: *A Clinician's View of Neuromuscular Disease*, 2d ed. Baltimore, Williams and Wilkins, 1985

DIMAURO S et al: Disorders of lipid metabolism in muscle. Muscle Nerve 3:369, 1980

———: Mitochondrial myopathies. Ann Neurol 17:521, 1985

ENGEL AG et al: The spectrum and diagnosis of acid maltase deficiency. Neurology (NY) 2:395, 1973

GRIGGS RC, MOXLEY RT (eds): Metabolic Myopathies. Semin Neurol, 3:225, 1983

WALTON JN, MASTALGIA FL (eds): The Muscular Dystrophies. Br Med Bull 36:105, 1980

358 MYASTHENIA GRAVIS AND OTHER DISORDERS OF NEUROMUSCULAR TRANSMISSION

ANDREW G. ENGEL

Disorders of neuromuscular transmission are genetic or acquired diseases associated with abnormal weakness and fatigability on exertion. In each disorder the generation of an end-plate potential that is of sufficient amplitude to trigger a propagated muscle fiber action potential is compromised by one or more specific mechanisms. Table 358-1 shows a classification of currently recognized disorders of neuromuscular transmission.

MYASTHENIA GRAVIS

DEFINITION Myasthenia gravis (MG) is an acquired autoimmune disorder associated with acetylcholine receptor (AChR) deficiency at the motor end plate. The number of acetylcholine (ACh) quanta released from the nerve terminal by a nerve impulse and the probability of quantal release are normal, but the lack of available receptors to bind ACh reduces the amplitude of the end-plate potential. The response to single ACh quanta released from the nerve terminal during rest, the miniature end-plate potential, is also reduced. The disease involves the external ocular muscles selectively or is generalized. The symptoms are improved by rest and anticholinesterase drugs. Circulating AChR antibodies are present in 80 to 90 percent of the cases, and immune complexes (IgG and complement components) are deposited on the postsynaptic membrane of the motor end plate.

CLINICAL FEATURES The incidence of the disease is 2 to 5 per year per million and its prevalance is 13 to 64 per million. The ratio of female to male patients is 6:4. The disease may present at any age, but the incidence in females peaks in the third decade and in males in the sixth or seventh decade.

The symptoms may fluctuate from hour to hour, day to day, or over longer periods. They are provoked or worsened by exertion, exposure to extremes of temperature, viral or other infections, menses, and excitement. Ocular muscle involvement is usually bilateral, asymmetric, and typically is associated with ptosis and diplopia. Weakness of other muscles innervated by cranial nerves results in loss of facial expression, everted lips, a smile that resembles a snarl, jaw drop, nasal regurgitation of liquids, choking on foods and secretions, and a slurred, hypernasal speech of a reduced volume. Abnormal fatigability of the limb muscles causes difficulty in combing the hair, lifting objects repeatedly, climbing stairs, walking, or running. Depending on the severity of the disease, dyspnea appears on moderate or mild exertion or is present even at rest. The abnormal fatigability can be demonstrated by asking the patient to look up without closing the eyes for 1 min, count loudly from 1 to 100, hold the arms abducted to the horizontal position for 1 min, or perform repeated deep knee bends. The deep tendon reflexes are normally active even in weak muscles. Atrophy of masseter, temporal, facial, or tongue muscles, and less often of other muscles, occurs in about 15 percent of the patients.

The natural history of the disease During the first month after the onset, the symptoms are purely ocular in 40 percent of patients, generalized in 40 percent, involve only the extremities in 10 percent, and involve only the bulbar or bulbar and eye muscles in 10 percent. With progression from mild to more severe disease the weakness spreads from ocular to facial to lower bulbar muscles and then to torso and limb muscles, but this sequence may vary. Proximal limb muscles are more affected than distal ones, but in the most advanced cases the weakness is universal. By the end of the first year, the ocular muscles are affected in nearly all patients. The symptoms remain ocular in only 16 percent. In nearly 90 percent of those patients in whom the disease becomes generalized, this occurs within the first year. Progression is most rapid within the first 3 years, and more than half of the deaths stemming from the disease occur in that period. Spontaneous remissions lasting from weeks to years can occur, but long spontaneous remissions are uncommon and most remissions occur during the first 3 years.

Two-thirds of MG patients have thymic hyperplasia, and 10 to 15 percent have thymoma. A few with thymoma also develop myocarditis and/or giant cell myositis. In about 10 percent the MG is associated with another autoimmune disease, such as hyperthyroidism, polymyositis, systemic lupus erythematosus, Sjögren's syndrome, rheumatoid arthritis, ulcerative colitis, pemphigus, sarcoidosis, pernicious anemia, and Lambert-Eaton myasthenic syndrome.

Clinical types of myasthenia gravis A classification proposed by Osserman, based on the distribution and severity of symptoms, is as follows:

Group 1, ocular symptoms
Group 2A, mild generalized symptoms
Group 2B, moderately severe generalized symptoms
Group 3, acute fulminating symptoms
Group 4, late severe symptoms

An alternative classification is related to thymoma and age of onset:

Type 1, *MG with thymoma:* The disease is usually severe and the AChR antibody level is high. There is no association either with sex or HLA antigen.
Type 2, *no thymoma, onset before age 40:* The AChR antibody level is intermediate. There is female preponderance and an increased association with HLA-A1, HLA-B8, and HLA-DRw3 antigens (HLA-B12 in Japan).
Type 3, *no thymoma, onset after age 40:* The AChR antibody level tends to be low. There is male preponderance, and increased association with HLA-A3, HLA-B7, and HLA-DRw2 antigens (HLA-A10 in Japan).

Striated-muscle antibodies are found in 90 percent, 5 percent, and 45 percent in the three types, respectively. The association with other autoimmune disease is highest in type 3 and lowest in type 1.

Transient neonatal myasthenia gravis Circulating AChR antibodies can be detected in most infants born to myasthenic mothers, but only 12 percent of infants develop myasthenic symptoms. The disease usually presents during the first few hours of life and its mean duration is 18 days. The principal findings are feeding difficulty, generalized weakness, respiratory difficulty, feeble cry, facial weakness, and ptosis. There is no relation between the severity of symptoms in the mother and the infant. The disease is caused by the passive transfer of AChR antibodies or the adoptive transfer of immunocytes from mother to infant, or perhaps fetal AChR damaged by maternal antibodies triggers a transient immune response in the infant.

TABLE 358-1 Classification of disorders of neuromuscular transmission

Autoimmune:
Myasthenia gravis
Lambert-Eaton syndrome
Congenital:
Familial infantile myasthenia*
End-plate acetylcholinesterase deficiency†
Slow-channel syndrome‡
End-plate acetylcholine receptor deficiency*
Toxic:
Botulism
Drug-induced disorders

* *Autosomal recessive inheritance*
† *Autosomal or X-linked recessive inheritance*
‡ *Autosomal dominant inheritance*

IMMUNOPATHOGENESIS The autoimmune character of MG and the pathogenic role of AChR antibodies has been established by several measures. These include (1) the demonstration that animals immunized with AChR develop a syndrome which in many respects resembles human MG; (2) the detection of circulating AChR antibodies in most patients; (3) the passive transfer with IgG of several features of the disease from human to mouse; (4) the localization of immune complexes on the postsynaptic membrane; and (5) the beneficial effects of plasmapheresis. That AChR deficiency occurs at the end plate in MG was established by autoradiographic, ultrastructural, and radiochemical studies in which α-bungarotoxin, a molecule that binds with high affinity to AChR, was used to quantitate end-plate AChR. Further, the AChR decrease in myasthenic muscles can be correlated with the decrease of the miniature end-plate potential amplitude.

Antibodies bound to end-plate AChR induce AChR deficiency by two major mechanisms—complement attack and modulation. Complement fixation and activation of the lytic phase of the complement reaction sequence causes focal destruction of the junctional folds and loss of AChR into the synaptic space. Modulation is the accelerated internalization and destruction of AChRs cross-linked by antibody. AChR depletion occurs if synthesis and membrane insertion of new AChR cannot keep up with the loss of AChR. Further, lysis of the junctional folds by complement reduces the membrane surface available for insertion of new AChR and enhances the subsequent AChR depletion by both modulation and complement. Some AChR antibodies may also interfere with AChR function by blocking the binding of ACh to AChR. Blocking antibodies account for only a minor fraction of all AChR antibodies.

The frequent thymus gland abnormalities and the beneficial effects of thymectomy implicate the thymus in the pathogenesis of MG. It has been postulated that lymphocyte sensitization to AChR occurs in the thymus and that antigen-specific T-helper cells are subsequently exported from the gland to other antibody-producing sites.

DIAGNOSIS This is based on the characteristic history, physical examination, anticholinesterase tests, and laboratory studies. The latter include electromyographic studies, serologic tests, and, in selected cases, in vitro microelectrode studies of neuromuscular transmission and ultrastructural and cytochemical studies of the end plate.

Anticholinesterase tests Edrophonium given intravenously acts within a few seconds and its effects last for a few minutes. An amount of 0.1 to 0.2 mL out of 10 mg/mL is injected intravenously over 15 s. If there is no response in 30 s, 0.8 to 0.9 mL of the drug is injected. The evaluation of the response requires objective assessment of one or more signs such as degree of ptosis, range of ocular movements, and the force of the hand grip. Possible side effects of the drug include fasciculations, flushing, lacrimation, abdominal cramps, nausea, vomiting, and diarrhea. The drug must be given cautiously to patients with cardiac disease, for it may cause sinus bradycardia, atrioventricular block, and rarely cardiac arrest. Atropine is used to reverse toxicity. Intramuscular neostigmine, 0.5 to 1.0 mg, acts maximally in about 30 min and its effects last up to 2 h allowing a more leisurely evaluation of changes in clinical status.

Electromyography In MG supramaximal stimulation of a motor nerve at 2 to 3 Hz results in a 10 percent or greater decrement of the amplitude of the evoked compound muscle action potential from the first to the fifth response. The test is positive in nearly all patients provided that two or more distal and two or more proximal muscles are examined. The decrement is caused by a normally occurring decrease in the number of quanta released from the nerve terminal, and hence in the amplitude of the end-plate potential, at the beginning of low-frequency stimulation. In MG, the end-plate potential amplitude is already reduced by the AChR deficiency, and the additional decrease during stimulation results in blocking of transmission at an increasing number of end plates. The transmission defect improves for a few seconds after a 15- to 30-s period of maximal voluntary contraction and becomes worse a few minutes later. These phenomena also reflect normally occurring presynaptic mechanisms that increase or decrease the quantal content of the end-plate potential and hence the safety margin of neuromuscular transmission. Single-fiber electromyography compares the timing of action potentials between pairs of closely adjacent muscle fibers in the same motor unit. In MG the low amplitude and prolonged rise time of the end-plate potentials cause abnormally long interpotential intervals and intermittent blocking of action potential generation at some fibers.

Serologic tests The AChR antibody test is positive in nearly all patients with moderately severe or acute severe MG, in 80 percent with mild generalized MG, in 50 percent with ocular MG, but in only 25 percent of those in remission. The antibody titer correlates only loosely with disease severity in a series of patients, but in individual patients a greater than 50 percent decrease in titer for more than 12 months is nearly always associated with sustained clinical improvement. Striated-muscle antibodies also occur in MG patients. Their role in MG remains unknown, but their association with thymoma is clinically relevant.

Other diagnostic studies Immune complexes can be localized at the MG end plate in cryostat sections even when circulating AChR antibodies cannot be detected. The technically easiest and most convenient way to confirm the suspected diagnosis is by C3 localization. To date, immune complexes have not been demonstrated by light microscopy at the end plate in other neuromuscular diseases. In vitro electrophysiologic studies of neuromuscular transmission can distinguish between atypical cases of MG, the Lambert-Eaton myasthenic syndrome, and some of the congenital myasthenic syndromes.

DIFFERENTIAL DIAGNOSIS This includes consideration of neurasthenia, oculopharyngeal dystrophy, the progressive external ophthalmoplegias with or without associated weakness of other cranial or limb muscles, intracranial mass-lesions compressing cranial nerves, drug-induced myasthenic syndromes, and other disorders of neuromuscular transmission (Table 358-1). Neurasthenia is recognized by giving way on muscle testing and by the lack of objective clinical and laboratory findings. In those myopathies involving the ocular muscles the weakness does not fluctuate, diplopia is seldom a symptom, the muscle biopsy may show distinct morphologic abnormalities, and pharmacologic and laboratory tests for MG are negative. Drug-induced and other myasthenic syndromes are considered in subsequent sections.

TREATMENT Anticholinesterases, alternate-day prednisone treatment, azathioprine, thymectomy, and plasmapheresis are currently used forms of therapy for MG.

Anticholinesterases are useful in all clinical forms of the disease. Pyridostigmine bromide (60-mg tablets) acts for 3 to 4 h and neostigmine bromide (15-mg tablets) for 2 to 3 h. Because pyridostigmine bromide acts longer and has fewer muscarinic side effects than does neostigmine bromide, it is the more widely used drug. One-half to four tablets of pyridostigmine bromide are given every 4 h in the daytime. Pyridostigmine bromide is also available in 180-mg "timespan" tablets for use at bedtime and as a syrup for children and patients requiring nasogastric feeding. If the muscarinic side effects are significant, these can be treated with 0.4 to 0.6 mg atropine given orally two to three times daily. Postoperatively or in critically ill patients, intramuscularly injectable pyridostigmine bromide (dose = 1/30 of oral dose) and neostigmine methyl sulfate (dose = 1/15 of oral dose) can be used.

Progressive weakness with increasing amounts of anticholinesterases usually signals the onset of a myasthenic or cholinergic crisis. Cholinergic crises are associated with muscarinic effects such as abdominal cramps, nausea, vomiting, diarrhea, miosis, lacrimation, increased bronchial secretions, diaphoresis, and bradycardia. The crisis is myasthenic rather than cholinergic if muscarinic effects are not conspicuous and if 2 mg of edrophonium given intravenously improves rather than worsens the weakness. In practice, however, the two types of crises are difficult to distinguish, and overmedication of a myasthenic crisis can convert it into a cholinergic crisis. Therefore, patients with increasing difficulty with respiration, feeding, or handling secretions and not responding to relatively high doses of anticholinesterases are best treated by drug withdrawal, tracheal intubation or tracheostomy, support with a respirator, and intravenous feeding. Refractoriness to drug therapy usually disappears after a few days.

In patients with generalized disease not responding adequately to modest doses of anticholinesterases, other forms of therapy must be employed. Thymectomy increases the remission rate and improves the clinical course of MG. Although controlled clinical studies of thymectomy according to age, sex, and severity of disease have never been carried out, there is general agreement that the best response occurs in young women with hyperplastic thymus glands and high antibody titer. Thymoma represents an absolute indication for thymectomy because the tumor is often locally invasive. Chest x-rays combined with linear tomography detect most thymomas. Computerized tomography of the mediastinum is a sensitive screening test, but may also yield false-positive results.

Alternate-day prednisone treatment induces remission or significantly improves the disease in more than half of the patients. The treatment is relatively safe provided that the usual precautions for patients taking corticosteroid therapy are instituted. With an average dose of 70 mg on alternate days, the average time for significant improvement is 5 months. After the improvement reaches a plateau the dose must be lowered over several months to establish the minimum maintenance dose.

Azathioprine in doses of 150 to 200 mg per day also induces remissions or significantly improves the disease in more than half of patients, but some responding patients have also received concurrent prednisone treatment or have had thymectomy. The minimum time for improvement is 3 months. Surveillance to detect side effects (pancytopenia, leukopenia, serious infection, and hepatocellular injury) must be maintained during therapy.

Plasmapheresis is indicated in severe generalized or fulminating MG refractory to other forms of treatment. Daily exchanges of 2 liters of plasma result in objective improvement and lower the AChR antibody titer in a few days. However, plasmapheresis itself does not confer greater long-term protection than do immunosuppressants alone.

LAMBERT-EATON MYASTHENIC SYNDROME

This is an acquired autoimmune disease associated with a reduced probability of quantal release from the nerve terminal by nerve impulse. Presynaptic ACh stores and the postsynaptic response to ACh quanta are normal.

The male/female ratio is close to 1:1. Carcinoma is present in 72 percent of males and 32 percent of females, but is uncommon under age 40. More than 80 percent of the tumors are small cell carcinomas of the lung. The syndrome may present up to 3 years before the tumor can be detected. In one-third of the patients the syndrome is nonneoplastic and occurs at any age.

Patients have weakness and fatigability of proximal limb and torso muscles with relative sparing of extraocular and bulbar muscles. The lower limbs are more severely involved than the upper ones. On maximal voluntary contraction, the force produced by a weak muscle increases for a few seconds and then again decreases. The tendon reflexes are hypoactive or absent in most patients. Autonomic manifestations (dry mouth, impotence, decreased sweating, orthostatic hypotension, or altered pupillary reflexes) occur in one-half of the patients.

On electromyography, the amplitude of the compound muscle action potential evoked by a single nerve stimulus from rested muscle is abnormally small. Repetitive stimulation at 2 Hz induces a further decrement, but stimulation at frequencies higher than 10 Hz or voluntary exercise for a brief period markedly facilitates the response so that the evoked potential attains normal amplitude.

Freeze fracture electron microscopy reveals a paucity and disorganization of presynaptic membrane active zones and active zone particles. These particles are topographically related to quantal release and are thought to be the voltage-sensitive calcium channels of the presynaptic membrane. The reduced quantal release by nerve impulse is attributed to reduced ingress of calcium into the nerve terminal.

Evidence for the autoimmune origin of the syndrome rests on its responsiveness to immunosuppressants and plasmapheresis, association of nonneoplastic cases with other autoimmune disorders and organ-specific autoantibodies, and the passive transfer of the electrophysiologic and morphologic features of the disease from human to mouse with IgG. The presynaptic membrane active zone particles are direct or indirect targets of the pathogenic autoantibodies.

Anticholinesterases have only a slight beneficial effect. Guanidine hydrochloride (10 mg/kg per day) or 3,4-diaminopyridine (1 mg/kg per day) increase quantal release from the nerve terminal and relieve the symptoms. However, the former drug has severe toxic side effects and the latter is not yet available in clinical practice. Optimal treatment of nonneoplastic cases consists of modest doses of alternate-day prednisone and 2 mg/kg per day of azathioprine.

CONGENITAL MYASTHENIC SYNDROMES

FAMILIAL INFANTILE MYASTHENIA This is an autosomal recessive disorder characterized by fluctuating ophthalmoparesis since birth, feeding difficulty during early infancy, weakness after exercise, and attacks of apnea precipitated by crying, vomiting, or fever. The symptoms tend to improve with age. A decremental electromyographic response is present in muscles weak when examined. Weakness can be induced in some, but not all, muscles by exercise or repetitive stimulation at 10 Hz for a few minutes. In contrast to autoimmune MG, the postsynaptic region is intact and there is no AChR deficiency. The miniature end-plate potential amplitude is normal in rested muscle but decreases to abnormally low values after 10-Hz stimulation for a few minutes. This suggests a presynaptic defect in ACh resynthesis or in ACh packaging into synaptic vesicles. Weakness, when present, responds to small or modest doses of anticholinesterases. Parenteral anticholinesterase therapy is indicated in crises. Parents of young patients must be taught to use a hand-assisted ventilatory device and to inject appropriate doses of neostigmine intramuscularly during crises.

CONGENITAL END-PLATE ACETYLCHOLINESTERASE DEFICIENCY Sporadic cases of the disorder, occurring only in males, have been observed to date. Weakness and a decremental electromyographic response are present in all voluntary muscles from birth. The symptoms are refractory to anticholinesterases and cause severe disability. The basic abnormality is total absence of acetylcholinesterase from the end-plate. ACh-AChR interaction and the duration of the end-plate potential are prolonged, so that a single stimulus applied to a motor nerve evokes two or more compound muscle action potentials. The motor nerve terminals are abnormally small and contain a reduced number of releasable ACh quanta. Smallness of the nerve terminals is not as constant as, and is probably secondary to, the enzyme deficiency. AChR is preserved or reduced at the end-plate. The AChR loss, if present, is caused by degenerative changes in the junctional folds, which can be accounted for by the ACh excess, but this itself is mild because ACh release is also reduced. The safety margin of neuromuscular transmission is compromised by lack of releasable ACh quanta and by AChR deficiency.

SLOW-CHANNEL SYNDROME This is an autosomal dominant disorder with high penetrance and variable expressivity. It presents in infancy or later life with selective weakness, fatigability, and atrophy of cervical, shoulder girdle, and forearm muscles. There is variable involvement of extraocular, other cranial, trunkal, or limb muscles.

The tendon reflexes are normal or hypoactive. Anticholinesterases are usually ineffective. A decremental electromyographic response appears in clinically affected muscles. The basic abnormality is an abnormally slow closure of the AChR ion channel. This prolongs the duration of the end-plate potential, causes a stimulus-linked repetitive compound action potential in all muscles, and allows abnormal accumulation of calcium in the postsynaptic region. The calcium excess results in destruction of the junctional folds, loss of AChR, and myopathic changes near the end plates. The safety margin of neuromuscular transmission is compromised by the AChR deficiency.

CONGENITAL END-PLATE AChR DEFICIENCY This is an autosomal recessive disorder that presents during infancy. The symptoms and electrophysiologic abnormalities resemble those in autoimmune MG and respond to anticholinesterases. Circulating AChR antibodies are absent and no immune complexes are found at the end plate. The cause of the AChR deficiency has not been established. It could stem from decreased synthesis, impaired membrane insertion, or accelerated degradation of AChR or from abnormal ACh-AChR interaction.

BOTULISM

Botulinum toxin, described in Chap. 100, interferes with the mechanism by which calcium facilitates the release of ACh quanta from the nerve terminal. *Food botulism in adults* follows the ingestion of food that already contains the toxin. The food originally contained *Clostridium botulinum* spores that had germinated into toxin-producing bacilli. *Food botulism in infants* is caused by ingestion of food that contains viable bacilli that produce toxin in the intestine. The contaminated food usually remains unidentified. *Wound botulism* occurs after open injuries that allow the growth of anaerobic bacilli in devitalized tissues.

In adults, the illness may begin with nausea, vomiting, diarrhea, abdominal cramps, and a dry, painful throat. Blurred vision, loss of accommodation, and dilated pupils can occur at this stage. The external ocular and other cranial muscles are affected early, and in severe cases this progresses to generalized paralysis. The deep tendon reflexes may or may not be preserved, and there may be a slight response to anticholinesterases. In infants, the syndrome is associated with constipation, hypotonia, multiple cranial nerve palsies, descending muscle weakness, and sudden apnea or progressive respiratory failure.

The electromyographic findings resemble those in the Lambert-Eaton syndrome but may not be present early in the disease and may occur in one but not another extremity. The diagnosis is confirmed by detection of the toxin in serum and/or feces. The paralysis improves with the gradual elimination of the toxin, and with guanidine or 3,4-aminopyridine. Respiratory support may be needed.

DRUG-INDUCED MYASTHENIC SYNDROMES

These are uncommon in clinical practice. Tetracycline, polymyxin and aminoglycoside antibiotics, antiarrhythmic agents (procainamide, quinidine), β-adrenergic blockers (propranolol, timolol), phenothiazines, lithium, trimethaphan, methoxyflurane, and magnesium, given parenterally or in cathartics, reduce the safety margin of neuromuscular transmission. However, overt myasthenic symptoms do not usually appear unless an overdose of the drug is administered or the renal or hepatic elimination of the drug is impaired. The same drugs also can potentiate neuromuscular blocking agents used during surgical procedures and both may worsen or unmask preexisting disorders of neuromuscular transmission. Treatment of these syndromes is reviewed by Swift.

Poisoning with insecticides containing long-acting anticholinesterases causes ACh accumulation at central, muscarinic, and nicotinic cholinergic synapses. The intoxication is associated with alterations in sensorium, severe muscarinic effects, and muscle weakness from desensitization of AChR at the neuromuscular junction. Therapy consists of respiratory support, large doses of atropine (2 to 4 mg intramuscularly, repeated as necessary), and pralidoxime (1 g intravenously, repeated in 20 min if necessary).

Penicillamine induces autoimmune MG in a small proportion of patients who receive the drug for another autoimmune disease. The MG gradually disappears when the drug is discontinued.

REFERENCES

ENGEL AG: Myasthenia gravis and myasthenic syndromes. Ann Neurol 16:519, 1984

GROB D et al: The natural course of myasthenia gravis and effect of therapeutic measures. Ann NY Acad Sci 377:652, 1981

LAMBERT EH, ELMQVIST D: Quantal components of end-plate potentials in the myasthenic syndrome. Ann NY Acad Sci 183:183, 1971

LANG B et al: Autoimmune etiology for myasthenic (Eaton-Lambert) syndrome. Lancet 2:224, 1981

LEWIS GE JR (ed): *Biomedical Aspects of Botulism*. New York, Academic, 1981

LINDSTROM J et al: Antibody to acetylcholine receptor in myasthenia gravis. Neurology 26:1054, 1976

SWIFT TR: Disorders of neuromuscular transmission other than myasthenia gravis. Muscle Nerve 4:344, 1981

359 PERIODIC PARALYSIS

ROBERT C. GRIGGS

Disorders that cause patients of normal strength to become weak intermittently are not common. In contrast, the complaint of intermittent weakness is frequently encountered. The evaluation of such symptoms is challenging because the examination is often normal between attacks and because reliance on history is crucial for diagnosis. This chapter considers the primary periodic paralyses. Other disorders that cause episodic weakness are considered elsewhere (see Chap. 17).

All primary periodic paralyses have some features in common. In most patients the disorders are inherited as autosomal dominant traits. Symptoms usually begin early in life and rarely commence after age 25. Attacks typically follow rest or sleep and almost never occur in the midst of vigorous activity, although antecedent exercise frequently provokes weakness. Patients remain alert during the attacks. Early in the course of these disorders interattack strength is normal, but after years of attacks progressive weakness may develop. All forms of periodic paralysis are amenable to treatment, and progressive weakness can be prevented and even reversed.

Diagnosis is based upon patient history and confirmed by appropriate evaluation of serum electrolytes during attacks and on evaluating the response of strength to provocative testing with glucose, insulin, potassium, and cold.

HYPOKALEMIC PERIODIC PARALYSIS This disorder occurs as an autosomal dominant condition in two-thirds of cases and as sporadic cases in one-third. Males are more frequently and more severely affected. Attacks of weakness characteristically begin in adolescence but may commence in the first decade. Onset after age 25 is rare; the new onset of episodic paralysis in older individuals is almost never due to periodic paralysis.

Attack frequency varies from daily to yearly. Attacks last from 3 to 4 h to as long as a day or more. Meals high in carbohydrate or high in sodium may provoke attacks. Paralysis involves limb muscles, usually proximal more than distal; rarely ocular, bulbar, or respiratory muscles are weakened, and bulbar and respiratory involvement may prove fatal. Reflexes become hypoactive, and cardiac arrhythmias may occur during attacks. Patients may develop persistent proximal weakness after years of attacks. Examination during attack-free intervals is otherwise normal except for the frequent presence of eyelid myotonia.

Diagnosis is established by demonstrating a low serum potassium during a paralytic attack and by excluding secondary causes of hypokalemia (Chap. 17). Electrocardiograms during attacks show characteristic features of hypokalemia. Electromyography is not helpful in diagnosis, but muscle biopsy often shows the presence of single or multiple centrally placed vacuoles. Patients whose attacks are so infrequent as to preclude the study of a spontaneous attack require provocative testing with glucose and insulin administration. Such tests are potentially hazardous, and patients must be carefully monitored during their performance. Since these disorders are rare such testing is most appropriately carried out in referral centers.

Pathogenesis The pathogenesis of paralytic attacks is incompletely understood. Patients with hypokalemic periodic paralysis do not have a decrease in total body potassium. There is no increased excretion of potassium in the urine before or during attacks, but there is excessive flux of potassium from blood into muscle, possibly owing to an abnormality of muscle membrane that causes muscle to become electrically inexcitable. Muscle from these patients is abnormally sensitive to the effect of insulin on potassium uptake; the significance of this increased sensitivity is not known since weakness is often severe at levels of serum potassium that do not affect normal individuals. Moreover, attacks may occur when insulin levels are low. Therefore, factors other than hypokalemia per se are important in the induction of weakness.

Treatment ACUTE ATTACKS The acute paralysis improves following the administration of potassium salts. Oral KCl (0.2 to 0.4 meq/kg) should be given to patients with severe weakness and repeated at 15 to 30 min intervals depending on the response of the electrocardiogram, serum potassium, and muscle strength. Milder attacks usually resolve spontaneously; resolution of weakness is hastened by exercising affected muscles. When patients are unable to swallow or are vomiting, intravenous therapy may be necessary. Small, repeated bolus therapy with KCl (0.1 meq/kg) may be administered over 5 to 10 min with careful monitoring of the electrocardiogram and serum potassium. If potassium is administered as a dilute solution (20 to 40 meq per liter) in 5% glucose or in physiologic saline solution, serum potassium may decline, and weakness may worsen. Mannitol is the preferred vehicle for administering intravenous potassium in such situations, since it facilitates rapid return of serum potassium to normal and avoids the hazard of lowering of serum potassium as may occur when glucose or saline solution are given.

PREVENTION OF ATTACKS The goal of therapy is the elimination of attacks, which also prevents interattack weakness and may improve interattack weakness after it has developed. Prior to availability of effective means of attack prevention, chronic progressive interattack weakness frequently caused serious disability. Prophylactic administration of potassium salts, even in large dosage, does not prevent attacks but acetazolamide (125 to 1000 mg per day in divided dosage) abolishes attacks in the majority of cases. The mechanism of action of acetazolamide is not fully understood, but it may block the flux of potassium from serum into muscle. The metabolic acidosis that it produces may underlie its beneficial effect. Paradoxically, acetazolamide lowers serum potassium through kaliuresis; to achieve an adequate response in some patients it may be necessary to give supplementary potassium along with acetazolamide and to avoid high-carbohydrate meals. Chronic acetazolamide treatment may be associated with renal calculi, and patients should be monitored for this complication. In occasional patients attacks may not respond to or may even be worsened by acetazolamide. In such patients triamterene (25 to 100 mg per day or spironolactone 25 to 100 mg per day) may prevent attacks.

THYROTOXIC PERIODIC PARALYSIS Attacks of hypokalemic periodic paralysis can occur in subjects with thyrotoxicosis, most commonly in young Latin American or oriental men where up to 10 percent of thyrotoxic patients may have periodic paralysis. In many patients thyrotoxicosis has also been overlooked for many months; periodic paralysis has also occurred with T_3-toxicosis and with exogenous thyroid hormone administration. The usual age of onset of the disorder is that of thyrotoxicosis; otherwise the clinical features resemble familial hypokalemic periodic paralysis. Acute attacks respond to potassium administration. Treatment of underlying thyrotoxicosis abolishes attacks, and β-adrenergic blocking agents reduce the frequency and severity of attacks while measures to control thyrotoxicosis are being instituted. Acetazolamide is not helpful in preventing attacks.

HYPERKALEMIC PERIODIC PARALYSIS This disorder differs from hypokalemic periodic paralysis in that attacks are usually brief (1 to 2 h or less) and more frequent; clinical or electromyographic myotonia is often demonstrable. Attacks are usually precipitated by fasting or by rest following exercise. The disease onset is usually at an earlier age than is the case for hypokalemic periodic paralysis, and attacks or myotonia may be evident in the first year of life. The disorder is usually transmitted as an autosomal dominant defect; rare sporadic cases occur.

The name "hyperkalemic" is misleading, since patients are often normokalemic during attacks. It is the fact that attacks are *precipitated by potassium administration* that best defines the disorder. "Potassium-sensitive" periodic paralysis is probably preferable terminology. Moreover, the serum potassium is often slightly elevated when patients are not having attacks of weakness. Attacks are characterized by limb weakness predominantly, though cranial and respiratory muscle involvement may occur. Cardiac arrythmias occur occasionally. Paresthesias and muscle pain are present during many attacks, and Chvostek's sign is often present during attacks.

Diagnosis is suggested by a modest elevation of serum potassium during attacks in nearly half of patients; at times, however, the serum potassium is normal or even low. Intravenous glucose-insulin loading does not precipitate weakness but potassium-loading tests (0.05 to 0.15 g/kg) will provoke weakness in such patients. Myotonia may be increased. Potassium-loading tests are potentially hazardous and are contraindicated in patients with renal disease and diabetes. Random serum potassium measurements may suggest the diagnosis, since potassium elevations are frequent during attack-free intervals. Electromyographic evidence of myotonia and the finding of vacuoles on muscle biopsy provide supporting data.

Pathogenesis Hyperkalemia during attacks of hyperkalemic periodic paralysis seldom reaches levels that would be expected to produce paralysis. Furthermore, serum potassium may remain within the normal range. Factors other than hyperkalemia are clearly important in the pathogenesis of attacks. An abnormality of the sarcolemma may cause spontaneous depolarization of the muscle cell and lead both to myotonia and to paralysis. A decreased activity of the sodium-potassium pump may be involved in the spontaneous depolarization.

Treatment Attacks of weakness are seldom severe enough to require emergency treatment and are never fatal. Oral glucose or other carbohydrate hastens recovery. Since interattack weakness may develop after repeated attacks, prophylactic treatment is usually indicated. Remarkably, acetazolamide (125 to 1000 mg per day), the treatment of choice for hypokalemic periodic paralysis, was first found to be beneficial for hyperkalemic periodic paralysis, possibly because of its kaliopenic effect. Thiazide diuretics (e.g., chlorothiazide, 250 to 1000 mg per day) are usually more effective and have fewer side effects.

NORMOKALEMIC PERIODIC PARALYSIS Most subjects with periodic paralysis in whom potassium is normal during attacks behave like those with typical "hyperkalemic" periodic paralysis, since they are similarly sensitive to potassium administration. In fact, the so-called hyperkalemic and normokalemic forms of this disorder may be one entity.

Rarely, patients with episodic normokalemic paralysis are not potassium sensitive, but they usually show evidence of muscle destruction or other features suggesting that they should not be classified with the primary periodic paralyses.

PARAMYOTONIA WITH PERIODIC PARALYSIS Attacks of paralysis may occur in the paramyotonias, either provoked by cold or spontaneously. Paramyotonia congenita is characterized by paradoxical myotonia (i.e., myotonia worsening with activity), cold provocation, spontaneous attacks, and a family history compatible with an autosomal dominant defect. The cold provocation of weakness distinguishes this disease from other periodic paralyses. A therapeutically useful subclassification of the paramyotonias has been proposed as follows: (1) paramyotonia congenita, in which spontaneous attacks of weakness are associated with a lowering of serum potassium and in which measures that decrease serum potassium provoke weakness; and (2) paralysis periodica paramyotonica, in which spontaneous attacks may be associated with hyperkalemia and may be provoked by oral potassium administration. This potassium sensitivity has led in the past to the incorrect classification of this disorder as a variant of hyperkalemic or normokalemic periodic paralysis.

Diagnosis depends upon the provocation of weakness with cold. Glucose and insulin loading and potassium challenges aid in the subclassification of the disorder and provide assistance in the choice of medication for treatment.

Pathogenesis The two types of paramyotonia probably have different etiologies. In paramyotonia congenita cooling of muscle results in an abnormal depolarization, leading first to myotonia and then to inexcitability. Sodium and potassium conductance become abnormal with cooling of muscle. An abnormality of sodium channels may account for this alteration in conductance.

Treatment Spontaneous attacks of periodic paralysis in paramyotonia congenita are relatively infrequent. Many patients do not require prophylactic treatment for prevention. In the case of paramyotonia congenita, patients with severe and frequent attacks of weakness may respond to spironolactone, and subjects with paralysis periodica paramyotonica may respond to acetazolamide or thiazides. Acetazolamide may provoke weakness in paramyotonia congenita, whereas myotonia in paramyotonia congenita may improve with either acetazolamide or tocainide; the latter may work by blocking abnormal sodium channels.

REFERENCES

GRIGGS RC et al: Intravenous treatment of hypokalemic periodic paralysis. Arch Neurol 40:539, 1983

MARTIN AR, LEVINSON SR: Contribution of the Na^+-K^+ pump to membrane potential in familial periodic paralysis. Muscle Nerve 8:359, 1985

RESNICK JS et al: Acetazolamide prophylaxis in hypokalemic periodic paralysis. N Engl J Med 278:582, 1968

RIGGS JE et al: The diagnosis and treatment of the periodic paralyses. Clin Neuropharmacol 4:123, 1979

PART THIRTEEN PSYCHIATRY

section 1 Psychiatric disorders

360 MAJOR AFFECTIVE DISORDERS

LEWIS L. JUDD / LEIGHTON Y. HUEY

For centuries it has been recognized that extremes in mood are inherent in the human condition, but distinguishing mood alterations that are pathologic from those that are not has been an elusive problem until recently. The realization that major mental disorders are psychobiologic phenomena resulting from abnormal brain mechanisms together with the development of a more empirically based diagnostic classification scheme has now made it possible for clinicians to distinguish consistently between abnormal mood states and the normal evanescent changes in feeling tones that are a part of everyday life.

Recent surveys indicate that 5 to 6 percent of the adult population in this country is suffering from clinically significant mood or affective disorders. The major affective disorders are a heterogenous group of mental disorders characterized by extreme exaggerations and disturbances of mood and affect which also affect cognitive and psychomotor functions. There is a marked tendency to periodicity and recurrence throughout the patient's lifetime, in which diagnosable affective episodes appear and remit and are followed by symptom-free periods (euthymia) lasting weeks, months, or years. The two most prevalent and important diagnostic syndromes among the major affective disorders are *major depression* and the *bipolar disorders*.

To reduce diagnostic heterogeneity, the major affective disorders are divided into those depressed patients with a history of manic episodes (bipolar) and those who manifest episodes of depression only (unipolar). The *unipolar-bipolar* distinction is a useful dichotomization in regard to clinical characteristics, life course, and treatment. Evidence continues to accumulate indicating that unipolar and bipolar depressions are, in all likelihood, psychobiologically different but very closely related disorders. An additional diagnostic dichotomization which has also been helpful in reducing heterogeneity among those disorders is the *primary-secondary* distinction. The rationale behind this is that affective disorders occurring in a pure form are likely to be more similar than affective disorders which coexist with other psychiatric or medical conditions. A major affective disorder is *primary* when the affective episode (manic or depressive) is the first-appearing psychiatric illness in a patient's lifetime and is not associated with other psychiatric or medical illnesses. Conversely, an affective disorder is classified as *secondary* when it appears in conjunction with other psychiatric or medical conditions. For example, depressive episodes can be observed in conjunction with virtually every mental disorder, for example, schizophrenia, alcoholism, dementia, and personality disorders. Affective disorders can also be associated with medical diseases and occur during treatment with commonly prescribed medications. The diseases associated with depressive disorders include the following: endocrinopathies (Cushing's disease, hyper- or hypothyroidism), collagen diseases (systemic lupus erythematosus), cardiovascular diseases (congestive heart failure, myocardial infarction), neurologic diseases (multiple sclerosis), infections (hepatitis, influenza), malignancies (pancreatic adenocarcinoma), metabolic disorders (porphyria), and vitamin deficiencies (vitamin B_1 deficiency, nicotinic acid deficiency). In addition, the chronic administration of the following medications can also precipitate an affective episode: corticosteroids, alpha-methyldopa, propranolol, benzodiazepines, reserpine derivatives, and L-dopa. It should be noted, however, that even though an affective episode may be classified as being secondary, it can be the most important and compelling aspect of a patient's clinical picture requiring immediate and specific therapeutic intervention (see also Chap. 11).

A conceptual overview of the major affective disorders is presented in Table 360-1. In this classification the relationships and interaction of the unipolar-bipolar and primary-secondary dichotomizations are clearly demonstrated.

DIAGNOSTIC CATEGORIES OF AFFECTIVE DISORDERS The diagnosis of a clinically significant affective episode is based upon the criteria contained in the third edition of the Diagnostic and Statistical Manual (DSM-III). This method of diagnostic classification has been developed and approved by the American Psychiatric Association and is the standard diagnostic system in use in this country today. There are two general types of affective episodes which manifest in patients: major depressive episodes and manic episodes. The diagnostic criteria for *major depressive episodes* and *manic episodes* are included in Tables 360-2 and 360-3. Most experienced clinicians require that the dysphoric mood or the euphoric, expansive, or irritable mood be persistently present for at least 1 week before these two diagnoses are considered.

Major depression The diagnosis of major depression is made when the patient presents with the necessary signs and symptoms of a major depressive episode (see Table 360-2). The diagnostic category of major depression represents the unipolar form of the major affective disorders, in which patients manifest only the single pole of affect, that of depression. The diagnosis of *recurrent major depression* is made when major depressive episodes are repeated throughout a patient's lifetime and is synonymous with the term *recurrent unipolar depression*. Following the first episode, between 50 and 80 percent of patients will have at least one more major depressive episode. Approximately 10 to 15 percent will have a subsequent manic episode, at which point the patient is then reclassified as having a bipolar disorder. Major depression is approximately twice as common in

TABLE 360-1 Major affective disorders

Primary affective disorder:
Unipolar depression (major depressive episodes only)
Bipolar depression (manic and major depressive episodes)
Secondary affective disorder:
Disorder occurring with medical diseases
Disorder secondary to medications
Disorder occurring with other mental disorders

TABLE 360-2 Diagnostic criteria for a major depressive episode

A Dysphoric mood or loss of interest or pleasure in all or almost all usual activities and pastimes. The dysphoric mood is characterized by symptoms such as the following: patient is depressed, sad, blue, hopeless, low, down in the dumps, irritable. The mood disturbance must be prominent and relatively persistent but is not necessarily the most dominant symptom and does not include momentary shifts from one dysphoric mood to another dysphoric mood (e.g., anxiety to depression to anger) such as are seen in states of acute psychotic turmoil

B At least four of the following symptoms have each been present nearly every day for a period of at least 2 weeks:

1 Poor appetite or significant weight loss (when not dieting) or increased appetite or significant weight gain
2 Insomnia or hypersomnia
3 Psychomotor agitation or retardation (not merely subjective feelings of restlessness or being slowed down)
4 Loss of interest or pleasure in usual activities or decrease in sexual drive (not limited to a period when delusional or hallucinating)
5 Loss of energy; fatigue
6 Feelings of worthlessness, self-reproach, or excessive or inappropriate guilt (may be delusional)
7 Complaints or evidence of diminished ability to think or concentrate, such as slowed thinking or indecisiveness (not associated with marked loosening of associations or incoherence)
8 Recurrent thoughts of death, suicidal ideation, desire to be dead, or suicide attempt

women as men. The point prevalence in the adult population ranges from 4.5 to 9.3 percent for women and 3.2 percent for men. The peak onset for first episodes in women is from 35 to 45 years; it decreases with age until 55, when the risk increases. The risk for younger men is lower but appears to increase steadily with age. Most natural-course studies indicate that unipolar patients average two to three major depressive episodes during their lifetimes, although some patients have only single episodes and others have many more. The average duration of an untreated depressive episode is 8 to 9 months with a range of 5 to 13 months. There is no established relationship between risk for major depression and socioeconomic class, race, education, or occupation.

Not all clinically significant depressive phenomena present as classic major depressions. The diagnostic categories of *dysthymic disorder* and *atypical depression* are clinical manifestations of depression without the full features of a major affective disorder. There is a high degree of heterogeneity and overlap between these two diagnostic categories. Patients who have some of the signs and symptoms of a depressive episode and who feel chronically dysphoric but do not meet full criteria for major depression are categorized here. Continued research has gradually identified a more homogeneous patient population with atypical features. Patients with atypical depression may have initial insomnia rather than early morning awakening and often may be hypersomniac. Their mood is frequently worse in the evening rather than the morning, and they also complain of a generalized dysphoria combined with fatigue, low energy, irritability, tension, and anxiety. Rather than being unreactive to environmental changes, as is usually seen in major depressive episodes, they often can be temporarily cheered up by specific environmental changes. Further, they are often not anorexic and may be hyperphagic and crave carbohydrates. Some experts have suggested that patients with atypical depression should be classified in a new diagnostic category entitled *mood reactive depression*.

TABLE 360-3 Diagnostic criteria for a manic episode

A One or more distinct periods with a predominantly elevated, expansive, or irritable mood. The elevated or irritable mood must be a prominent part of the illness and relatively persistent, although it may alternate or intermingle with depressive mood

B Duration of at least 1 week (or any duration if hospitalization is necessary), during which, for most of the time, at least three of the following symptoms have persisted (four if the mood is only irritable) and have been present to a significant degree:

1 Increase in activity (socially or at work) or physical restlessness
2 More talkativeness than usual or pressure to keep talking
3 Flight of ideas or subjective experience that thoughts are racing
4 Inflated self-esteem (grandiosity, which may be delusional)
5 Decreased need for sleep
6 Distractibility (attention too easily drawn to unimportant or irrelevant external stimuli)
7 Excessive involvement in activities that have a high potential for painful consequences which is not recognized (buying sprees, sexual indiscretions, foolish business investments, reckless driving)

Bipolar disorders Bipolar disorders are diagnosed using the criteria for both manic and major depressive episodes. In this category of major affective disorder, both the affective poles of mania and depression are present. Bipolar disorders are diagnosed as bipolar disorder, manic, if the current episode meets criteria for a manic episode and as bipolar disorder, depressed, if the episode meets criteria for a major depressive episode. Bipolar patients who have more rapid cycling, with manic and depressive episodes alternating every few days or weeks, are classified as bipolar disorder, mixed. Bipolar depression is more frequent in women than men in a ratio ranging from 1.2:1 to 2:1. Men have significantly more manic than depressive episodes, whereas women have significantly more depressive than manic episodes. The age of risk for bipolar disorder extends from as early as 6 or 7 years to over 65, but the peak age of onset in both men and women for the first attack is in the early thirties, with a mean age of onset of 32.5 years. About two-thirds of first episodes are manic and 60 percent of these patients will have a predominantly manic course, while the remaining 25 to 30 percent manifest primarily depressive episodes. Most natural-course studies of untreated bipolar patients generally agree that they will average nine diagnosable affective episodes during their lifetimes (range 1 to more than 20). The pattern is that the cycle length, which is measured from the onset of one episode to the onset of the next, will decrease and the number of episodes will increase over time. For example, in untreated bipolar patients the time between the first and second episode averages from 3.5 to 4 years, between the second and third episodes about 2 years, and between episodes three and four somewhere between 12 and 18 months. Episode duration is from 4 to 13 months, and the average is about 8.5 months. Attempts have been made to categorize affective episodes in the bipolar patient based on how often the episodes occur in juxtaposition to those of opposite polarity. The vast majority of episodes are uniphasic, i.e., a manic or depressive episode is preceded by a symptom-free period; however, approximately 10 or 15 percent are biphasic with a depressive episode more often preceding the manic.

There is a small but distinct group of bipolar patients who manifest very *rapid cycling* patterns (bipolar disorder, mixed). The rapid cycler is a patient who presents with more than four or five episodes in 1 year, but there are patients who have considerably more episodes and there are case reports of patients cycling every 24 h. The rapid-cycling bipolar patient has eight times the number of affective episodes in his or her lifetime in comparison to slow cyclers. Eighty percent of rapid cyclers are women, and the appearance of rapid cycling is sometimes related to impaired thyroid function. Although it is still controversial, there is evidence that rapid cycling may be induced by a course of tricyclic antidepressants and can only be effectively controlled after the patient is euthyroid and removed from tricyclics.

The life-long intensity of illness in bipolar disorder, even among the slow cyclers, is much more extreme than it is in unipolar disorder. Bipolar patients have significantly more episodes of illness, more hospitalizations, and spend more total time in the hospital during their lifetimes.

ETIOLOGY AND PATHOPHYSIOLOGY OF THE MAJOR AFFECTIVE DISORDERS Considerable progress has been made in identifying and characterizing the etiologic factors in major affective disorders, but a comprehensive and detailed understanding of the etiology of these disorders has yet to be achieved. Tremendous advances in knowledge during the past 20 years have provided excellent leads for focused scientific inquiry into the causes of these disorders; these leads, in turn, have led to the development of very specific and effective treatments. Like many other human diseases, the affective disorders are the result of interactions between the patient's genetic makeup and the environment. Evidence continues to mount that significant genetic factors are involved in these disorders, but the genetic components do not appear to be so overwhelming that the disorder is manifested without any environmental challenges. In general, the causality of a major affective episode can effectively be conceptualized by using an interactional model of two intersecting continua both with progressive intensities. One involves the patient's inherited constitutional predisposition to develop affective episodes; this interacts with the second continuum of the environmental stresses and life events to which the patient is exposed. Thus, there are those individuals with very high genetic predispositions for affective psychopathology in whom the disorder will be manifested seemingly without identifiable precipitating events. In contrast, there are patients with lower genetic predisposition in whom the disorder is manifested only when the patient is exposed to more serious precipitating life events and cumulative life stresses.

Genetic factors Data derived from virtually every methodologic strategy in human genetics strongly suggest significant genetic influences in the major affective disorders, but as yet the mode of genetic transmission has not been established. The degree of genetic expression varies considerably from patient to patient and in some patients marked and predictable genetic factors are present; in others genetic expression appears to be significantly less influential. The *twin studies* have been one of the major research strategies used by psychiatric geneticists to attempt to quantify genetic loading in various psychiatric diseases. Twin studies in affective disorders have reported concordance rates among monozygotic (MZ) twins ranging from 33.3 to 75 percent, with an average of 65 percent. In contrast, the concordance rates for dizygotic (DZ) twins range from 9 to 23 percent, averaging 15 percent. The difference in concordance rates between MZ and DZ twins strongly suggests inherited genetic vulnerability. Further, there is evidence that even the polarity of the disorder may be genetically controlled, since there is an 80 percent concordance for bipolar and 59 percent concordance for unipolar disorders in MZ twins. In an attempt to separate the "nature" and "nurture" contributions to the development of affective disorders, the *adoption study* strategy has also been used. Unfortunately, because of methodologic problems and the paucity of subjects studied, no definitive answers are available. There is, however, a trend indicating that adoptees with affective disorders have a greater incidence of affective illness in their biologic parents than in their adopted parents. A large number of *family studies* have been conducted in the affective disorders. The standard paradigm is to make independent and blind diagnoses in the first-degree relatives of affective disorder patients, anticipating that if genetic components are present, the consanguineous relatives will manifest an increased risk for affective illness. First-degree relatives of bipolar patients have a morbidity risk for bipolar disorder ranging from 2.8 to 17.7 percent and a risk of 0 to 22.4 percent for unipolar depression. The first-degree relatives of unipolar patients have a risk of 6.4 to 17 percent for unipolar depression and of 0.3 to 29 percent for bipolar disorder. Thus, bipolar patients have both unipolar and bipolar disorders among their blood relatives, whereas unipolar patients have increased incidence for unipolar, but not bipolar, disorders in their relatives. Modern studies of *genetic transmission* combine careful family pedigree studies with molecular genetics in an attempt to identify the linkage between the specific gene markers and manifestation of major affective disorder in an afflicted or informative family. At present, no clear dominant or recessive inheritance pattern has been identified. It appears that genetic heterogeneity is present, which suggests a multiple threshold model in order to account for the varying degrees of genetic variability in the affective disorders. Genetic marker surveys in informative families have been conducted, including studies which have used genetically regulated markers that are etiologically significant in affective illness, such as the concentrations of dopamine β-hydroxylase, monoamine oxidase A, monoamine oxidase B, and lithium red blood cell (RBC)/plasma ratio. No marker has yet been found which segregates to the presence of affective disorder. There is however, a small subgroup of bipolar patients who do manifest a linkage of protan-deutan (red-green) color blindness and the Xg blood group with the presence of bipolar disorder. Unfortunately this very interesting genetic linkage pattern has not been present in other families similarly afflicted with major affective disorder.

In summary, the genetic studies strongly indicate the inheritance of a vulnerability to affective illness, but the genetic expression is heterogeneous and the degree of vulnerability varies significantly. There is evidence that the genetic factors are stronger in bipolar disorder than in unipolar depression. There are currently several large-scale surveys combining molecular and pedigree methodologies which are either in progress or in the final stages of implementation, and it is possible that the gene(s) coding for affective disorders will be identified and cloned in the foreseeable future.

Neurotransmitter systems The most consistent search for etiologic mechanisms in the affective disorders has involved studies of the various neurotransmitter systems in the brain. The original *biogenic amine hypothesis* focused primarily on the central nervous system (CNS) neurotransmitters norepinephrine, serotonin, and dopamine, attributing depression and mania, respectively, to the deficiency or excess of these neurotransmitters at important synaptic sites in the brain. This hypothesis has stimulated and directed research in the field for many years, and data consistent with the hypothesis continue to emerge. Urinary and cerebrospinal fluid (CSF) studies of norepinephrine, its metabolite 3-methoxy-4-hydroxyphenethyleneglycol (MHPG), and the catalytic enzyme dopamine β-hydroxylase have been consistently reported as being increased or decreased in the predictable direction during depressed and manic episodes. More recently, increases in norepinephrine have been described in both mania and depression. Alterations in serotonin and its metabolites have also been identified in patients during depressive episodes. In addition, 5-hydroxyindole acetic acid (5HIAA), a serotonin metabolite, has been found to be reduced in the CSF of depressed patients who make frequent and aggressive suicide attempts. Deficits in other neurotransmitters such as dopamine and gamma-aminobutyric acid (GABA) have also been identified in some patients with major depression. Finally, another neurotransmitter hypothesis which has directed research in the affective disorders is the *cholinergic hypothesis,* which postulates increased central cholinergic tone in depression, decreased cholinergic tone in mania, and an imbalance between the cholinergic and adrenergic neurotransmitter systems as being a central pathophysiologic mechanism in affective disorders.

Within the last 5 years, there has been a shift of research focus from the neurotransmitter biosynthetic, storage, and release mechanisms in the presynaptic neuron to the study of receptors on postsynaptic neurons. There is growing evidence that postsynaptic receptor kinetics and activity are predictibly and consistently altered during affective episodes and by the psychotropic medications known to ameliorate these disorders. Future research in the pathophysiology of the affective disorders will be concentrated on the role of *postsynaptic receptor systems* and the cascade of intraneuronal biochemical events in the postsynaptic neuron which follow the binding of the neurotransmitter to the receptor.

In summary, there is a general agreement in the large number of studies which have been conducted to date that the relative paucity of a neurotransmitter or the inactivation or down-regulation of postsynaptic receptors has often been correlated with depressive episodes, but the reciprocal changes which one would predict have not been consistently identified in manic episodes.

Environmental factors There is little systematic data available indicating what role environmental stresses and untoward life events play or what types of stressors might be etiologically significant in the development of major affective episodes. Attempts have been made, for example, to relate early childhood loss and parental separation as predisposing factors for the future development of an affective illness, but the data are inconsistent. In general, studies have shown an overall temporal relationship between stressful and negative life events and the subsequent appearance of affective episodes. Research attempting to characterize qualitative differences in the impact of life stress have been disappointing, although serious life events such as the death of a child or a spouse, job loss, marked changes in social status, and even severe assaults on self-esteem have been linked to affective episodes. While the relationship between environmental stresses and the appearance of affective episodes has not always been demonstrated, generally speaking most experts agree that a single severe or multiple severe adverse events in life can interact with the constitutional predisposition of a patient and result in the triggering of an affective episode.

In further support of the influence of environmental events are the studies which have been conducted in higher primates. In these studies, phenomena which resemble or are analogous to the depressive states in humans are seen in monkeys following both mother/infant and peer separation paradigms. Furthermore, the monkey's "despair" response to the separation paradigms can be predictably enhanced by drugs known to specifically alter central concentrations and metabolism of various relevant CNS neurotransmitters (e.g., norepinephrine, dopamine).

Biologic rhythms The marked tendency of major affective disorders to periodic manifestation and possibly to seasonal variations has stimulated hypotheses which suggest that the dysregulation of biologic rhythms may be centrally involved in the pathophysiology of affective disorders. There are reports of dysynchronization of circadian rhythms in some bipolar patients in which these patients manifested both rapid free-running circadian rhythms (e.g., 23- versus 24-hour rhythms) and a phase delay in their rhythms. There is also a specific subgroup of patients with major depression in which the depressive episodes are manifested seasonally during the wintertime. These patients, while residing in more northern latitudes, experience major depressive episodes during the winter when days are significantly shorter and periods of darkness more prolonged; they do not experience depression of this type when residing in latitudes where the environmental light/dark cycle is not as extreme.

BIOLOGIC CORRELATES AND LABORATORY STUDIES Neurohormonal correlates For a number of years probes into the pathophysiologic mechanisms of the affective disorders have used various neurohormones whose secretion is regulated by one or more of the CNS neurotransmitters. One consistent finding from these studies has been that a significant subpopulation of patients with major depression hypersecrete cortisol and have abnormal cortisol circadian secretion patterns. In addition, even though it is now somewhat controversial, the *dexamethasone suppression test* (*DST*) has been useful in both diagnosis and monitoring of treatment. The standard DST used in psychiatry involves the administration of 1 mg of dexamethasone at 2300 hours with subsequent cortisol determinations at 1600 and 2300 hours the following day. The nonsuppression of cortisol is an abnormal or positive response (>5 μg/dL cortisol concentration in the 1600 or 2300 sample). Initial studies reported that up to 50 percent of patients with serious major depression were nonsuppressors on the DST. Further investigations indicate that DST nonsuppression is most likely a state marker, which is positive during the depressive episode but returns to normal after successful resolution of the episode. False positives on the DST can occur in patients with alcoholism, malnutrition, obesity, pregnancy, major physical illnesses, and in patients over 65 years and this has eroded the usefulness of the test. In addition, more recently a number of studies have appeared in the literature reporting a much smaller percentage of DST nonsuppressors associated with major depressive episodes and an increased percentage in many other psychiatric illnesses. The range of DST nonsuppression among depressed patients has now been reported as low as 10 to 15 percent to as high as 50 percent. While the status of this diagnostic marker is still controversial, it is useful in monitoring treatment efficacy in DST-positive depressives, since the DST response reverts to normal when the episode remits.

Other neuroendocrine markers have also been explored, but none as widely as the DST. In major depression, between 25 and 30 percent of patients respond to thyrotropin releasing hormone (TRH) with blunted *thyroid stimulating hormone* (*TSH*) responses. TSH blunting is not specific to depressive episodes and the use of this test for diagnostic purposes has been abandoned. Small subgroups of depressed patients have manifested blunted *growth hormone* responses to the following challenge agents: clonidine, amphetamine, L-dopa, 5-hydroxytryptophan, and hypoglycemia (insulin tolerance test). Even though 15 to 25 percent of depressed patients have blunted growth hormone responses, it has not proved to be diagnostically useful. More recently, blunted *prolactin* responses to both TRH and opiate alkaloid challenges have also been reported in subpopulations of depressed patients; while these findings may be of interest in terms of pathophysiologic mechanisms, they are not useful diagnostically.

Sleep studies The disruption of sleep patterns is present in virtually every patient with major affective disorder, and polysomnographic studies of sleep in these patients have proved to be of interest. In 25 to 45 percent of cases of major depression there is a significantly shortened time period between the onset of sleep and the appearance of the first rapid eye movement (REM) (i.e., decreased REM latency). In addition, the density of the REM epoch, measured by the number of eye movements, is increased, there is a tendency for the REM epoch to be increased in duration, and there is a shift of REM activity to an earlier part of the night. These findings from all-night EEG sleep recordings have remained among the most consistent biologic markers for major depression, although they lack specificity, since short REM latency has also been reported in anorexia nervosa, obsessive-compulsive disorders, schizoaffective schizophrenia, and narcolepsy.

Neurotransmitter metabolites The neurotransmitter hypotheses of affective disorders have stimulated a number of studies correlating biogenic amine metabolites with manic and depressive episodes. The data are inconsistent and have not been useful either diagnostically or therapeutically. The one possible exception is MHPG, a metabolite of norepinephrine. Some workers have reported low MHPG excretion as predicting a positive therapeutic response to the antidepressants imipramine, desipramine, etc., and high MHPG excretion as predicting a response to amitriptyline, nortriptyline, etc. While these data are of interest and with further study may result in the identification of biochemical subtypes in major depression, these findings have not been consistently replicated in other laboratories.

TREATMENT OF THE MAJOR AFFECTIVE DISORDERS Important advances have been made in the treatment of the major affective disorders, and the majority of these patients can now be treated with a high degree of specificity and success. The most important discoveries have been in the development of potent psychotropic medications for both major depression and the bipolar disorders. The central therapeutic tools in the treatment of the major affective disorders are the antidepressants and lithium. The use of these psychotropic medications is covered in much greater detail in Chap. 364.

Because major affective disorders have strong tendencies for recurrence, an important aspect of the patient's treatment is the comprehensive education of patients and their families about the disorder. It should be emphasized to the patient that these are psychobiologic disorders which involve altered biochemical states in the brain, and that episodes can be triggered by adverse events and stresses in the environment but may occur spontaneously as well. Each patient should be urged to become an expert on his or her own disorder, concentrating on how it manifests and what early signs and symptoms may herald an impending manic or depressive episode. The patient and the family must be urged to take on the responsibility for the early recognition of the impending episode, since the earlier a patient presents for treatment, the easier it is to remediate the episode. The absolute necessity of medication compliance must be emphasized, and the patient must understand thoroughly the need to take the medications as prescribed and to be aware of side effects and of the potential medical sequelae from the medications.

The counseling and therapeutic techniques the physician uses in dealing with patients who are suffering acute manic or depressed episodes are simple and relatively straightforward. During the acute phase of these episodes, patients respond better to short (10 to 20 min) visits one to three times per week. During these visits the general focus is on monitoring the medication and side effects, but it is also essential that the physician be very reassuring and supportive to the patient. Because patients are functioning essentially in an altered state secondary to the depressive or manic episode, the treatment must be sustained by the physician's optimism and knowledge that with time these episodes can be treated if the right medication and dose are prescribed. Virtually all the mood-stabilizing and -ameliorating psychotropic medications have a significant delay between the time the patient begins the medication and the time of achieving full therapeutic benefits. It is during this time that supportive reassurance and encouragement from the physician is particularly important in sustaining the patient in treatment.

There are approximately 25,000 suicides a year in this country, and clinical surveys have indicated that approximately 30 percent of these patients have major affective disorders. Suicidal ideation is one of the important symptoms which accompany major depression, in both bipolar and unipolar disorders; considerations of suicidal lethality are significant components of the management of these patients. Although it is not possible to distinguish precisely between patients who will attempt suicide and those who will not, there are some factors which should be considered. Generally speaking, many experts agree that patients who have given detailed thought to the method of suicide, who have concomitant alcoholism, and who are socially isolated with few (if any) social supports, in addition to elderly males and patients with terminal medical illnesses, have a greater potential risk for suicide. On the other hand, all of the characteristics lack true specificity in the assessment of suicidal risk.

Once the acute depressive or manic episode is under control, the switch from supportive to more insight-oriented psychotherapy is a useful adjunct to the pharmacotherapy. Recent studies have established that the combination of psychotherapy with pharmacotherapy is significantly better than either of these two modalities alone. There is also evidence that specific types of psychotherapy (e.g., cognitive therapy) can be successfully used in the treatment of mild to moderate depressive disorders, but learning to become a competent psychotherapist requires considerable effort and time to achieve results comparable to that of the relatively simple administration of an antidepressant. It is, therefore, recommended that the nonpsychiatric physician rely primarily on the antidepressants or lithium (depending upon the disorder being treated) in combination with educational and supportive psychotherapeutic approaches in the management of patients with major affective disorders (see Chap. 364).

REFERENCES

BALDESSARINI RJ: Biological hypotheses in psychiatry, in *Chemotherapy in Psychiatry*. Cambridge, Mass, Harvard, 1985, pp 9–12

———: *Biomedical Aspects of Depression*. Washington, DC, APA Press, 1982, pp 1–83

CLAYTON PJ, BARRETT JE (eds): *Treatment of Depression: Old Controversies and New Approaches*. Raven, New York, 1983

Diagnostic and Statistical Manual of Mental Disorders (3d ed). American Psychiatric Association, Washington, DC, 1980

KLERMAN GL: History and development of modern concepts of affective illness, in *Neurobiology of Mood Disorders*, RM Post, RC Ballenger (eds). Baltimore, Williams & Wilkins, 1984, pp 1–19

MARTIN JB, REICHLIN S: *Clinical Neuroendocrinology*, 2d ed. Davis, Philadelphia, 1987

POST RM, BALLENGER JC (eds): *Neurobiology of Mood Disorders*. Williams & Wilkins, Baltimore, 1984, vol 1

ROBINS LN et al: Lifetime prevalence of specific psychiatric disorders in three sites. Arch Gen Psychiat 41:949, 1984

361 ANXIETY DISORDERS

KAREN THATCHER BRITTON / S. CRAIG RISCH / J. CHRISTIAN GILLIN

Anxiety is a common emotion and as such is often a normal response to the vicissitudes of life. In its mild forms, anxiety may be adaptive. A little anxiety, for example, helps a student prepare for examinations. In its extreme forms, however, anxiety is incapacitating or terrifying. High anxiety may cause the same student to lose concentration, memory, or even his or her voice.

Physicians observe anxiety most commonly in patients experiencing an acute external stress. Although short-term treatment with antianxiety or sedative drugs, such as benzodiazepines, has a place in the management of such patients, physicians often can offer more help by their presence, reassurances, and attitude. Anxiety states often resolve spontaneously with time, although clinicians should be aware that acute stress can lead to chronic anxiety or posttraumatic stress disorder.

The word *anxiety* has more precise diagnostic meaning in psychiatry. It refers to both *paroxysmal* and *persistent* psychological feelings (dread, irritability, ruminations) and physiologic changes (dyspnea, sweating, insomnia, trembling) which endure over time and impair normal functioning. These are often chronic disorders in which symptoms persist in the absence of obvious contemporaneous external stresses or in which the degree of symptoms seems out of proportion to the degree of external stress. Anxiety disorders were formerly lumped together under the term "anxiety neurosis." It is now recognized that a number of relatively distinct clinical syndromes exist under the general rubric of anxiety disorders, as reflected in the diagnostic criteria in the third edition of the Diagnostic and Statistical Manual (DSM-III) (Table 361-1).

PANIC DISORDER **Definition** The cardinal feature of panic disorder is the sudden, unexpected, and often overwhelming feeling of terror and apprehension accompanied by somatic symptoms in multiple organ systems such as dyspnea, palpitations, and faintness. The symptoms and signs of panic disorder are similar to those occurring during intense physical exertion or in a life-threatening situation.

Incidence and epidemiology Panic disorder is estimated to occur in 1 to 2 percent of the population, with women outnumbering men two to one. The most frequent age of onset of panic attack is the late teen years and early twenties. Panic disorders tend to be familial, and both panic disorder and affective disorder often coexist in the same family. If an individual has a diagnosed panic disorder, up to 18 percent of first-degree relatives also will have panic disorder. Furthermore, twin studies demonstrate a greater incidence in monozygotic twins, suggesting that panic anxiety may have a genetic basis.

Clinical features A typical panic attack often begins abruptly and without warning while a patient is involved in a relatively nonthreatening and nonstressful activity, like entering a store, driving a car, or sitting at a desk working. The patient becomes flushed, lightheaded, and sweaty and is overwhelmed by feelings of terror, apprehension, and impending doom. Dyspnea may occur with a subjective sense of choking or smothering, and palpitations or chest pain are often so

TABLE 361-1 Classification of anxiety disorders

Anxiety states:
Panic disorder
Generalized anxiety disorder
Obsessive-compulsive disorder
Posttraumatic stress disorder
Phobic disorders:
Agoraphobia (with and without panic attacks)
Social phobia
Simple phobia

severe that patients believe they are having a heart attack or are dying. The symptoms of panic attacks usually peak in less than 10 min and resolve in 20 to 30 min. Most patients experiencing their first panic attack obtain help, sometimes going to a doctor's office or emergency room, but the fear has usually subsided by this time. Fatigue or exhaustion frequently follows a panic attack, and the patient may sleep.

The DSM-III criteria for diagnosis of panic disorder are listed in Table 361-2.

Complications After repeated panic attacks, most patients develop some degree of anticipatory anxiety and try to avoid those situations that have been paired with panic attacks in the past. Some patients develop *agoraphobia*—an irrational fear of being alone or in public places. Without effective treatment, the course of panic attacks and agoraphobia leads to an increasingly restricted life-style marked by preoccupation with avoiding those situations that might trigger an attack. Cases of severe panic disorder with agoraphobia may result in patients remaining house-bound for one or more decades, convinced that leaving the house will induce an attack.

Other complications of panic disorder include major depressive syndrome, higher death rates from both suicide and cardiovascular disease, and drug and alcohol dependency. Losses from unemployment and health care costs are estimated to exceed $100 million a year.

Laboratory findings Lactate infusions precipitate panic attacks in vulnerable individuals, although at present this is only used as a test in research paradigms. One study employing positron emission tomography demonstrated a decreased rate of blood flow in the left parahippocampus during panic attacks.

Differential diagnosis Many patients with panic disorder complain of chest pain, cardiac extrasystoles, and palpitations. The diagnostic challenge is to differentiate anxiety with cardiovascular symptoms from the organic diseases it mimics. Because there may be an increased prevalence of mitral valve prolapse in patients with panic disorder this condition should be investigated; however, in the vast majority of patients wtih panic disorder, no significant cardiac pathology is ever found.

Other diagnostic possibilities include both hyperthyroidism and hypothyroidism, a catecholamine-secreting pheochromocytoma, complex partial seizures, and hypoglycemia. Drug ingestions (amphetamine, cocaine, caffeine, sympathomimetic nasal decongestants) and drug withdrawal (alcohol, barbiturates, opiates, minor tranquilizers) may produce symptoms that simulate panic attacks.

Etiology and pathophysiology The etiology of panic disorders is uncertain and involves an interplay of multiple psychological and biologic determinants.

PSYCHOLOGICAL FACTORS In the psychodynamic model, anxiety is considered to be a response to the threatened emergence into consciousness of painful, unacceptable thoughts, impulses, or desires, i.e., psychological conflicts from the past and present. The anxiety response is an attempt to mobilize and ward off danger to the self.

PHYSIOLOGIC FACTORS Clinical and experimental evidence point to the involvement of noradrenergic neurons, particularly those projecting rostrally from the locus coeruleus in the upper brainstem, in the pathophysiology of panic disorder. Three lines of evidence suggest that hyperactivity of noradrenergic pathways may play a role in the pathogenesis of panic. First, the clinical manifestations of panic attacks are similar to those induced by sudden, massive stimulation of beta-adrenergic receptors. Second, isoproterenol hydrochloride, a beta agonist, and yohimbine, an alpha-adrenergic receptor antagonist that increases noradrenergic function, produce signs and symptoms that mimic panic attacks. Third, clinical studies support a role for noradrenergic beta blockers, such as propranolol, in successful treatment of pathologic anxiety.

Another avenue of investigation is based on the finding that infusions of sodium lactate into patients with a history of panic disorder often provoke a panic attack indistinguishable from a spontaneous one. Normal subjects without a history of panic disorder are unaffected. In addition, patients whose panic attacks are controlled by antidepressants are protected against lactate-induced panic attacks. Although the mechanism of lactate's effect is unclear, the findings appear to have diagnostic usefulness and provide a good model of anxiety for further clinical investigation.

Overall, the evidence suggests that the main contribution to panic disorder may be a genetic vulnerability to a biologic disease state. Over time, panic attacks may become associated with environmental events that by themselves are able to elicit symptoms. The particular constellation of environmental stimuli that precipitate panic attack may be influenced by past experience or particular psychological conflicts. A full understanding of the etiology of anxiety probably will require knowledge of a combination of genetic, biologic, and psychological factors.

Treatment A comprehensive treatment program combines both pharmacologic and psychotherapeutic approaches. The first step is to block the attacks pharmacologically, usually with tricyclic antidepressants or monoamine oxidase inhibitors (see Chap. 364). These drugs have 80 to 90 percent effectiveness in the treatment and prevention of spontaneous panic attacks. New antianxiety medications such as alprazolam given in high dose are as effective as antidepressants, have fewer side effects, and work within 1 or 2 days. Other benzodiazepines have not proved efficacious. Antidepressant medication may take 4 to 6 weeks before being effective. Beta blockers, e.g., propranolol or atenolol, may block the peripheral manifestations of the panic attacks but have proved ineffective in preventing the psychic fear or panic and may also predispose to or worsen depressive symptomatology. Clonidine may also block panic manifestations, but its efficacy is usually only transient. Relapse is common on discontinuance of pharmacotherapy.

For some patients with panic disorder, particularly those with debilitating agoraphobia, psychotherapy is indicated. The exact form of psychotherapy needed is controversial, but approaches that seek to understand the anxiety and encourage the patient to confront the feared situations are the most effective.

GENERALIZED ANXIETY DISORDER **Definition** Unlike patients with panic disorders whose symptoms come on suddenly, patients with generalized anxiety disorder experience persistent diffuse anxiety, without the specific symptoms that characterize phobic disorders, panic disorders, or obsessive-compulsive disorders. Although the symptoms and signs of anxiety vary from individual to individual, common signs are motor tension, autonomic hyperactivity, apprehensive expectation, and vigilance. Patients with generalized anxiety disorder do not report acute fluctuations in anxiety level and autonomic arousal characteristic of panic disorder.

Incidence and epidemiology The prevalence of generalized anxiety disorder has been estimated at 2 to 3 percent, but precise epidemiologic

TABLE 361-2 Diagnosis of panic disorder

A At least three panic attacks within a 3-week period in circumstances other than during marked physical exertion or in a life-threatening situation. The attacks are not precipitated only by exposure to a circumscribed phobic stimulus

B Panic attacks are manifested by discrete periods of apprehension or fear, and at least four of the following symptoms appear during each attack:

1 Dyspnea
2 Palpitations
3 Chest pain or discomfort
4 Choking or smothering sensations
5 Dizziness, vertigo, or unsteady feelings
6 Feelings of unreality
7 Paresthesias (tingling in hands and feet)
8 Hot and cold flashes
9 Sweating
10 Faintness
11 Trembling or shaking
12 Fear of dying, going crazy, or doing something uncontrolled during an attack

TABLE 361-3 Diagnosis of generalized anxiety disorder

A Generalized, persistent anxiety is manifested by symptoms from three of the following four categories:
  1 Motor tension: shakiness, jitteriness, jumpiness, trembling, tension, muscle aches, fatigability, inability to relax, eyelid twitch, furrowed brow, strained face, restlessness, easy startle
  2 Autonomic hyperactivity: sweating, heart pounding or racing, cold and clammy hands, dry mouth, dizziness, light-headednesss, paresthesias (tingling in hands or feet), upset stomach, hot or cold spells, frequent urination, diarrhea, discomfort in the pit of the stomach, lump in the throat, flushing, pallor, high resting pulse and respiration rate
  3 Apprehensive expectation: anxiety, worry, fear, rumination, and anticipation of misfortune to self or others.
  4 Vigilance and scanning: hyperattentiveness resulting in distractibility, difficulty in concentrating, insomnia, feeling "on edge," irritability, impatience.

B The anxious mood has been continuous for at least 1 month

C Patient is at least 18 years of age

data are lacking because of variations in definition and case acquisition. In patients who seek professional help for anxiety, women outnumber men by two to one. There is no evidence to support the popular belief that anxiety is related to the stresses of modern society. In contrast to panic disorder, studies showing a familial or genetic basis for generalized anxiety disorder are inconclusive.

The diagnostic criteria for generalized anxiety disorder are listed in Table 361-3.

Complications In contrast to panic disorder, generalized anxiety disorder has a more chronic course and favorable outcome. However, the symptoms are persistent and can lead to secondary depression and alcohol and drug abuse, especially of benzodiazepines.

Differential diagnosis Symptoms and signs resembling anxiety may occur with a number of medical disorders including coronary artery disease, thyroid disease, and drug intoxication or withdrawal. Anxiety may be present in other psychiatric disorders such as depression, schizophrenia, and organic mental states. Diagnosis of these conditions is essential, since the treatment of them is different from that of the anxiety disorders. Because patients with generalized anxiety may abuse alcohol or antianxiety medications to reduce or block anxiety, a careful history of drug use is important. Although the overall degree of psychosocial or occupational impairment is generally less than that noted for the other anxiety disorders, chronic anxiety is an uncomfortable emotion that can restrict a person's ability to enjoy a normal life.

Etiology and pathophysiology One approach to understanding the etiology of anxiety has been to delineate the mechanisms by which antianxiety drugs exert their therapeutic effects. High affinity, stereospecific receptors for benzodiazepines have been discovered which appear to be coupled to the receptor for the inhibitory neurotransmitter gamma-aminobutyric acid (GABA). Considerable evidence supports the hypothesis that the anxiolytic actions of the benzodiazepines are mediated through this receptor.

These findings have several implications. First, the characterization of a benzodiazepine receptor complex implies the existence of a natural (endogenous) ligand for the receptor. Conceivably, the levels of this substance might correlate with individual differences in anxiety or emotionality or tolerance to stress. Second, pharmacologic antagonists of this receptor block the effects of benzodiazepines and may induce anxiety, a finding which implicates these mechanisms in pathologic anxiety. Third, new *anxiolytic* compounds that influence benzodiazepine receptor binding are being discovered that have fewer and potentially less serious side effects. The possibility exists that *anxiogenic* substances may also be found in the brain. Though major questions remain to be answered, these advances have opened new avenues for understanding the origins and management of anxiety.

Treatment Because feelings of anxiety are normal human emotions with adaptive value, a decision must be made before any treatment or medication is considered concerning whether or not the manifestations of anxiety are within the normal range. There is no justification for the use of anxiolytic drugs in anxiety if it is considered to be within the normal limits of human experience.

Once a decision is made to treat, consideration should be given first to modalities of nonpharmacologic intervention, including supportive or intensive psychotherapy. These approaches may modify maladaptive life-styles, cognition, and avoidance behaviors. Behavior therapy aims at teaching the patient practical means to reduce anxiety and includes techniques like relaxation training, biofeedback, and desensitization. These techniques are of at least temporary benefit for many people.

When generalized anxiety is severe enough to warrant treatment with drugs, benzodiazepines are the agents of choice. In many patients, short courses of anxiolytic drugs (5 to 7 days) are effective, following which the drug should be discontinued. Patients should be warned about the possibility of dependence with long-term use, and the physician should make regular assessments of the need for continuation of medications.

POSTTRAUMATIC STRESS DISORDER Definition Acute and chronic psychological distress following traumatic events have long been recognized. The diagnostic criteria for posttraumatic stress disorders (PTSD), according to DSM-III, are listed in Table 361-4.

PTSD is classified as either acute or chronic (or delayed). In the former, onset of symptoms begin within 6 months of the trauma, or the duration of the symptoms persist less than 6 months. In the latter, symptoms persist more than 6 months (chronic) or start more than 6 months after the trauma (delayed).

Etiology Whether or not PTSD develops appears to depend upon the nature of the trauma, the characteristics of the individual, and the context in which these events take place. The trauma can be anticipated or not, acute or chronic, constant or repetitive, due to natural events (e.g., an earthquake) or malevolence (e.g., rape, child abuse, torture). PTSD can develop in individuals who were apparently healthy, successful, and well-adjusted prior to the traumatic experiences. Among the factors which influence the development of PTSD are (1) the extent to which the individual's life-space is affected, (2) the duration of the impact, (3) the extent to which the individual perceives human malevolence behind the traumatic event (e.g., a fire attributed to arson will probably be more traumatic than one attributed to lightning), and (4) social isolation.

Epidemiology It is difficult to gauge the extent of PTSD following a traumatic event because the studies that have been done have often followed subjects for only a short period of time, and the nature of the events is often so situation-specific. About 15 percent or more of the civilian population may experience mental distress severe enough to require treatment following a major natural disaster. For example,

TABLE 361-4 Diagnosis of posttraumatic stress disorder

A Existence of a recognizable stressor that would evoke significant symptoms of distress in almost everyone

B Reexperiencing of the trauma as evidenced by at least one of the following:
  1 Recurrent and intrusive recollections of the event
  2 Recurrent dreams of the event
  3 Sudden acting or feeling as if the traumatic event were recurring, because of an association with an environmental or ideational stimulus

C Numbing of responsiveness to or reduced involvement with the external world, beginning some time after the trauma, as shown by at least one of the following:
  1 Markedly diminished interest in one or more significant activities
  2 Feeling of detachment or estrangement from others
  3 Constricted affect

D Presence of at least two of the following symptoms that were not present before the trauma:
  1 Hyperalertness or exaggerated startle response
  2 Sleep disturbance
  3 Guilt about surviving when others have not, or about behavior required for survival
  4 Memory impairment or trouble concentrating
  5 Avoidance of activities that arouse recollection of the traumatic event
  6 Intensification of symptoms by exposure to events that symbolize or resemble the traumatic event

in a study that followed survivors of a shipboard fire for $3\frac{1}{2}$ to $4\frac{1}{2}$ years, one-third were found to be unable to return to sea because of psychological symptoms. Following extreme prolonged harsh conditions such as combat, prisoner-of-war camps, or Nazi death camps, a higher incidence of both acute and delayed PTSD is likely. Some evidence, based on follow-up of World War II veterans 20 years after the war, indicates an increasing incidence of new patients seeking psychiatric care for war-associated symptoms. The vicissitudes of normal aging may unmask a latent traumatic stress disorder.

Complications Anxiety, depression, alcoholism, drug abuse, impaired marital and occupational activities, and perhaps increased physical morbidity and mortality have been blamed on various forms of PTSD.

Differential Diagnosis In adjustment disorder, symptoms such as reexperiencing the trauma are absent. Other considerations include major depressive disorder, generalized anxiety disorder, phobic disorder, organic mental disorders, and other conditions such as "compensation neurosis" and "postconcussion syndrome."

Prophylaxis Military experience suggests that PTSD can be prevented partially if soldiers are taught that a degree of fear and anxiety are normal concomitants of battle rather than signs of cowardice or mental illness. Furthermore, the development of chronic PTSD can often be prevented if the soldier with acute PTSD is seen close to the battle front under the principles of immediate treatment, expectancy of return to normal duties, and brevity of treatment contact.

Treatment The treatment goals of PTSD are reduction of target symptoms, prevention of chronic disability, and occupational and social rehabilitation. An important therapeutic issue is the extent to which the victim of acute PTSD should be allowed to leave the traumatic situation, to regress, and to enjoy the secondary gains of the patient role. The caretakers' unthinking natural sympathy, nurturing instincts, admiration, and, indeed, gratitude (for example, in the case of soldiers who are protecting the homeland) may be as detrimental as an unreasonably cynical, suspicious distrust of someone who is seen as trying to get attention and avoid responsibilities or hoping to collect money from the consequences of the traumatic experience. Successful treatment involves a combination of psychosocial support systems, psychotherapy, behavioral and conditioning techniques, and medications. Group therapy with others who have shared similar experiences may be beneficial.

OBSESSIVE-COMPULSIVE DISORDER Definition The major characteristics are recurrent *obsessions* (persistent intrusive thoughts) and *compulsions* (intrusive behaviors) which the patient experiences as involuntary, senseless, or repugnant. The DSM-III diagnostic criteria for obsessive-compulsive disorder are listed in Table 361-5.

Common obsessions include thoughts of violence (e.g., killing a loved one), obsessive slowness, fears of germs or contamination, and doubt (e.g., a priest who worries excessively that he had not said his prayers properly). Examples of compulsions include repeated checking to be assured that something was done properly, hand washing, extreme neatness, and counting rituals, as in numbering steps while walking.

Obsessions and compulsions do not invariably coexist in the same individual. The relationship of the obsessive-compulsive disorder to obsessive or compulsive characterologic traits remains controversial.

Etiology and pathophysiology The etiology of the obsessive-compulsive state is uncertain, but it can be viewed from psychodynamic, psychosocial, and biologic perspectives. Obsessions and compulsions often seem to symbolize unconscious wishes, impulses, and fears and to reflect dynamic adaptations to unwanted aggressive or sexual urges. Biologic factors are suggested by reports of an increased incidence of obsessive compulsive disorder in monozygotic twins and first-degree relatives of probands, of biologic markers associated with the disorder, and of favorable response to certain tricyclic antidepressants and monoamine oxidase inhibitors.

Epidemiology The lifetime prevalence of obsessive compulsive disorder, based upon interviews of the general population 18 years and older, varies between 1.9 and 3.0 percent. The prevalence tends to be slightly higher in females than males but does not vary significantly by race, education, or urbanization of area of residence.

Clinical manifestations These disorders usually begin in adolescence or young adulthood, with about 65 percent of cases beginning before age 25. They are rarely seen in children. Clear precipitants are reported in up to 60 percent of cases. Long term prognosis appears to be variable. Some patients (perhaps 10 percent) show a chronic, unremitting course; some show periods of complete remission; the majority show an episodic course with periods of incomplete remission.

Complications Depression is probably the most common secondary problem but anxiety, avoidant behavior, alcoholism, abuse of sleeping pills and tranquilizers, and impairment of social, marital, and occupational life can be marked.

Laboratory findings No pathognomonic pathologic or laboratory abnormalities have been found.

Differential diagnosis Repetitive self-destructive behaviors, such as gambling, drinking, drug abuse, and overeating, should not be diagnosed as "obsessive-compulsive" disorder since the individual normally derives pleasure from the activity. Stereotyped behavior is also common in schizophrenia, Tourette's syndrome, and depression.

Treatment Controlled studies have shown that both behaviorally oriented psychotherapy and psychopharmacology can be helpful in these disorders. Compulsions and rituals probably respond more than do obsessions and ruminations to behavior therapy. The tricyclic antidepressant drugs and monoamine oxidase inhibitors are relatively effective but require chronic administration. In severe unresponsive cases of obsessional-compulsive disorder cingulotomy or modified frontal leukotomy is reported to be helpful.

PHOBIC DISORDERS Phobic disorders comprise a group of disorders having in common persistently recurring, irrational severe anxiety of specific objects, activities, or situations with secondary avoidance behavior of the phobic stimulus. Phobias are relatively commonplace, and the diagnosis of a phobic disorder is made only when fear or avoidance behavior is a significant source of distress to the individual or interferes with social or occupational functioning.

The phobic disorders listed in DSM-III include three separate disorders—agoraphobia, social phobia and simple phobia.

Agoraphobia DEFINITION Agoraphobia, the fear of being alone or in public places (see Table 361-6), may occur rarely in the absence of panic disorder, but it is almost invariably preceded by that condition.

Social phobias DEFINITION Social phobias are persistent irrational fears and the need to avoid any situation where one might be exposed

TABLE 361-5 Diagnosis of obsessive-compulsive disorder

A Either obsessions or compulsions are present:

1 Obsessions: Recurrent, persistent ideas, thoughts, images, or impulses that are ego-dystonic, i.e., they are not experienced as voluntarily produced, but rather as thoughts that invade consciousness and are experienced as senseless or repugnant. Attempts are made to ignore or suppress them.

2 Compulsions: Repetitive and seemingly purposeful behaviors that are performed according to certain rules or in a stereotyped fashion. The behavior is not an end in itself but is designed to produce or prevent some future event or situation. However, either the activity is not connected in a realistic way with what it is designed to produce or prevent or it may be clearly excessive. The act is performed with a sense of subjective compulsion coupled with a desire to resist the compulsion (at least initially). The individual generally recognizes the senselessness of the behavior (this may not be true for young children) and does not derive pleasure from carrying out the activity, although it provides a release of tension.

B The obsessions or compulsions are a significant source of distress to the individual or interfere with social or role functioning.

TABLE 361-6 Diagnosis of agoraphobia

A The individual has marked fear of and thus avoids being alone or being in public places from which escape might be difficult or help not available in case of sudden incapacitation, e.g., crowds, tunnels, bridges, public transportation.
B There is increasing constriction of normal activities until the fear or avoidance behavior dominates the individual's life.

to scrutiny by others and potentially be embarrassed or humiliated. Even the possibility of such a situation evokes anticipatory anxiety. The individual is aware that this fear is excessive. Common examples are excessive fear of public speaking and anxiety induced by eating in restaurants or by any public performance. The resulting anxiety may actually impair performance and thereby potentiate the phobic disorder.

EPIDEMIOLOGY AND PATHOGENESIS Social phobias are relatively rare, and there is no evidence for a genetic or familial transmission. Social phobias presumably arise from stressful life events occurring during early development. The disorder usually begins in late childhood or early adolescence and tends to be chronic and to wax and wane in severity.

COMPLICATIONS Complications are rare and the disorder is not often incapacitating; it may lead to sedative or hypnotic drug and alcohol abuse and addiction, and to problems in professional advancement.

TREATMENT Treatment of social phobia is primarily behavioral, with use of such techniques as relaxation therapy, systematic desensitization, and related techniques. Pharmacotherapy with beta blockers, i.e., propranolol or atenolol and/or alprazolam, may also be helpful.

Simple phobia DEFINITION Simple phobias are persistent irrational fears and avoidance of specific objects or situations.

CLINICAL FEATURES The individual experiences significant distress when confronted with the phobic stimulus or even the possibility of confrontation with the phobic stimulus and also recognizes this fear and anxiety as irrational and excessive. When confronted with the phobic stimulus the individual may experience symptoms identical to those of panic attacks. Common examples include fear of heights (acrophobia), fear of closed spaces (claustrophobia), and fear of animals. Fear of the possibility of exposure to the phobic stimulus will often cause the individual to attempt to elicit significant information, e.g., if the party or restaurant is at the top of a high-rise building; if they have a dog.

Age of onset is variable, but the disorder often begins in childhood. Simple phobias that begin in childhood may disappear without treatment, but may persist into adulthood. Although phobias are relatively common in the general population, they rarely result in significant impairment and individuals rarely seek treatment. Simple phobias are more common in women. Treatment, if required, is behavioral using relaxation therapy and systematic desensitization.

REFERENCES

CHARNEY DS et al: Noradrenense function in panic anxiety. Arch Gen Psychiat 41:75, 1984

LECKMAN JF et al: Panic disorder and major depression, alcoholism, panic, and phobic disorders in families of depressed patients with panic disorder. Arch Gen Psychiat 40:1055, 1983

LIEBOWITZ MR et al: Lactate provocation of anxiety attacks. Arch Gen Psychiat 41:764, 1984

ROSENBAUM JF: Current concepts in psychiatry. The drug treatment of anxiety. N Engl J Med 306:401, 1982

ROTH M: Agoraphobia, panic disorder and generalized anxiety disorder: Some implications of recent advances. Psychiat Dev 2:31, 1984

TALLMAN JF et al: Receptors for the age of anxiety. Pharmacology of the benzodiazepines. Science 207:274, 1984

362 SCHIZOPHRENIC DISORDERS

DAVID L. BRAFF

Schizophrenic disorders are serious mental illnesses that have a duration of 6 months or more and cause significant social, vocational, and personal disability and suffering. The schizophrenic patient often appears to be bizarre, inappropriate, and mentally impaired. Despite its stereotypic presentation, perhaps no other psychiatric disorder has proved as vexing and difficult to define, identify, and treat.

Schizophrenia has a lifetime prevalence rate of about 1 percent across all cultures. In the United States alone there are perhaps 2 million affected individuals who often become ill in their late teenage years and in the third decade of life. Poor outcome frequently leads to extensive disability, and schizophrenia accounts for a staggering estimated $20 billion per year of lost productivity. Most patients with schizophrenic disorders also cause major perturbations for family and social support systems, adding to the economic losses and the toll of human misery.

DEFINITION AND CLINICAL MANIFESTATIONS In 1919, Emil Kraepelin first made the distinction between dementia praecox, a psychotic illness with progressive deterioration, and manic depressive psychosis. Kraepelin's emphasis on deteriorating outcome was a new thrust in the largely descriptive nineteenth century psychiatric literature. Kraepelin noted, however, that about 13 percent of patients with dementia praecox did not have an inevitably deteriorating outcome, and this favorable outcome has significantly increased owing to the development and use of antipsychotic medications. Eugen Bleuler concentrated on the putative underlying psychological splitting of personality functions in his classic paper on the "group of schizophrenias." Bleuler's emphasis was on the "four As" of schizophrenia: *a*utism, flattened *a*ffect, loose *a*ssociations, and *am*bivalence. Other authors have focused on specific symptoms of schizophrenia, such as the sense of being influenced by others and feelings of being controlled by outside forces. To date, research has yet to identify specific and inevitably pathognomonic signs or symptoms of the schizophrenic disorders.

According to the third edition of the Diagnostic and Statistical Manual of the American Psychiatric Association (DSM-III), after the first and most central criterion of psychotic symptoms is met (see Table 362-1), the schizophrenic individual must show deterioration from a previous level of functioning in such areas as work, social relations, and self-care. Finally, continuous signs of the illness should be present for 6 months at some point during the individual's life with some signs of illness at the time of diagnosis. There may be prodromal, active, and/or residual phases of the illness that are not always clearly demarcated. Prodromal or residual symptoms are quite characteristic of the schizophrenic illness and may consist of isolation; marked psychosocial impairment; peculiar behavior; impaired personal

TABLE 362-1 Diagnosis of schizophrenia disorders

A Presence of certain psychotic symptoms during the active phase of the illness before the patient is 45 years old
B Psychotic features must last at least 6 months and include at least one of the following:
1 Bizarre delusions
2 Somatic, grandiose, religious, nihilistic or other delusions without persecutory or jealous content
3 Delusions with persecutory or jealous content
4 Delusions with persecutory or jealous content if accompanied by hallucinations
5 Auditory hallucinations in which a voice maintains a running commentary or two or more voices converse
6 Auditory hallucinations on several occasions with content of more than one or two words
7 Incoherence, marked loosening of associations, markedly illogical thinking, or poverty of speech content associated with either blunted or inappropriate affect, delusions, hallucinations, or catatonic or other grossly disorganized behavior

hygiene and grooming; blunted, flat, or inappropriate affect; digressive, vague, over-elaborate, circumstantial, or metaphorical speech; odd or bizarre ideation or magical thinking; and unusual perceptual experiences.

The DSM-III lists four major types of schizophrenic disorders: *disorganized, catatonic, paranoid,* and *undifferentiated.* This emphasis on subtypes carries forward Bleuler's notion of the "group of schizophrenias." There is moderate support for a paranoid/nonparanoid dichotomy as being important in schizophrenia. In an attempt to reduce diagnostic heterogeneity, Crow (1980) and other researchers have identified "type I" schizophrenic patients with a predominance of "positive" symptoms (e.g., hallucinations, paranoid ideation), normal cerebral ventricular size, and symptoms that respond to the hypothesized dopaminergic-blocking effects of antipsychotic drugs. In contrast, "type II" schizophrenic patients seem similar to Kraepelin's dementia praecox patients. Type II patients show a predominance of "negative" symptoms (e.g., anhedonia, social withdrawal, asociality), neuropsychological impairment, and possibly increased cerebral ventricular volume; they do not respond well to antipsychotic medications.

DIFFERENTIAL DIAGNOSIS Schizophrenic patients have no unique or pathognomonic signs and symptoms; at times, this makes the diagnosis difficult. DSM-III separates psychotic illnesses by a durational criterion into *brief reactive psychoses* lasting 2 weeks or less, *schizophreniform* disorders lasting between 2 weeks and 6 months, and *schizophrenic disorders* lasting more than 6 months. While these distinctions are practical and heuristic, the scientific basis for such a durational criterion is poorly documented. In addition, an acute manic patient may be difficult to distinguish from the schizophrenic patient, especially on a cross-sectional as opposed to longitudinal basis. To complicate matters further, the initial clinical appearance of a patient intoxicated with phencyclidine (PCP) or amphetamines may also be indistinguishable from that of the schizophrenic patient. It appears then that many functional and organic states may lead to a final common pathway of psychotic symptoms. The diagnosis can only be established reliably by a broad-based multifactorial approach utilizing neurobiologic data (e.g., toxicologic screens, genetic history) and psychosocial data (e.g., premorbid adjustment status) obtained both acutely and over time. Despite these problems, the DSM-III criteria for schizophrenic disorders have undergone extensive and successful field trials for reliability and validity. In general, clinicians using the DSM-III criteria can accurately and consistently diagnose schizophrenia.

PREDISPOSING, PRECIPITATING, AND SUSTAINING FACTORS IN SCHIZOPHRENIA Factors that contribute to the development of schizophrenia can be analyzed in terms of predisposing, precipitating, and sustaining factors. These factors may be anlayzed in terms of neuroanatomic and biochemical factors and neurophysiologic, psychophysiologic, intrapsychic, interpersonal, social, and socioeconomic factors. In a complex, multifactorial disorder such as schizophrenia, these neurobiologic and psychosocial factors should be seen as interactive rather than as competing or mutually exclusive. This approach is analogous to comprehensive analyses of diabetes mellitus or hypertension, which also have contributions based on genetics, receptor physiology, and physiologic, familial, psychosocial, and a myriad of other conceptually diverse factors. Within this context, predisposing factors are limited to etiologic variables, precipitating factors are related to pathophysiology, and sustaining factors are linked to outcome variables.

Etiology (predisposing factors) GENETIC FACTORS It is clear from twin, family, and adoptive studies that schizophrenia has a significant genetic basis. Monozygotic twins have roughly a 65 percent or greater concordance rate for schizophrenia, whereas dizygotic twins have a 12 percent concordance rate. Other family studies show that the morbid risk for developing schizophrenia is 5 to 10 percent if one parent is schizophrenic. This figure rises to 46 percent or more if both parents are schizophrenics. Second-degree relatives of schizophrenics run a 2 to 4 percent risk of developing the illness compared to a risk of 1 to 2 percent in the general population.

Adoption studies reveal that these risk factors are largely genetically linked and are not primarily due to the "schizophrenogenic" psychosocial environment of certain families. Still, these figures are fraught with methodologic complexities. For example, reflecting the probable complex mode of inheritance, 89 percent of schizophrenics do not have a parent who is schizophrenic. Eighty-one percent of schizophrenics do not have either a schizophrenic sibling or parent. The appropriate model with which to explain these figures is complex and may include a weighted polygenic model or other sophisticated interpretations of genetic theory.

The *stress-diathesis model* hypothesizes that there is a vulnerability which is inherited in schizophrenia-prone individuals. These vulnerable individuals are at high risk for developing schizophrenia under certain stressful circumstances. Studies of high-risk children with one or two schizophrenic parents indicate that such children may have a significantly increased incidence of morbidity in utero, at birth, and in the perinatal period. In addition, these infants and children may have psychophysiologic lability, attentional dysfunction, and specific motor disturbances. A number of human and animal studies suggest that such labile attentional mechanisms may result partly or largely from instabilities and increased activity of the mesolimbic dopaminergic system that has significant connections to the frontal cortex. The literature on neurophysiologically labile and vulnerable children seems to tie the genetic, dopaminergic, and attentional dysfunction hypotheses together. According to the stress-diathesis model, a host of stressful factors may precipitate a psychotic state in a high-risk individual. These factors include intoxication with PCP or amphetamines as well as more nonspecific factors such as medical illnesses with concomitant general stress. Further, specific hallucinogens such as lysergic acid diethylamide (LSD) may precipitate a psychotic episode that is ultimately indistinguishable from a schizophrenic disorder. Lastly, there have been a number of hypotheses that a viral vector may be important as an etiologic agent in at least some cases of schizophrenic disorders.

PSYCHOSOCIAL FACTORS There are many psychosocial hypotheses concerning creation of a predisposition or vulnerability to developing schizophrenia. Empirical support for most of these hypotheses is variable and far from definitive.

In the vulnerable individual, schizophrenia is seen as having its onset in a critical developmental period. The teenager may attempt to leave home and separate from family members for school or work reasons. The onset is often, but not invariably, insidious. In terms of psychosocial approaches to schizophrenia, there is felt to be a developmental or intrapsychic deficit in the vulnerable individual. Once set into motion, the psychosis passes through a series of stages leading to the final common pathway of a psychotic state.

Despite much theorizing, there is no inevitable schizophrenia-prone personality type, although at least a small but significant percentage of schizoid, paranoid, and schizotypal personality-disordered individuals do seem to be vulnerable to developing schizophrenic disorders. In the 1960s, a more family-systems-oriented view emerged. An example of this approach is the hypothesis of Bateson and coworkers who analyzed the formal communications patterns in "schizophrenogenic" families. In this view, communications content is less important than the frequently conflicting and self-contradictory form of communications style of schizophrenic patients' families. It remains unclear whether these familial factors are a cause or a result of having a schizophrenic child in the family. As the importance of biologic factors in schizophrenia have become clearer, family psychosocial factors have been seen more as secondary or epiphenomenal factors.

Psychosocial researchers have also examined the importance of socioeconomic factors in schizophrenia. Lower socioeconomic status correlates with a higher incidence of schizophrenia. There are two possible interpretations of these data. First, there may be a "social drift'' of vulnerable individuals to lower socioeconomic status. The second hypothesis is more etiologic—socioeconomic stresses may precipitate schizophrenic episodes, especially in vulnerable individuals.

Pathophysiology (precipitating factors) NEUROTRANSMITTERS AND NEUROPEPTIDES A number of neurobiologic factors have been correlated with schizophrenic episodes. Which neurobiologic systems underlie the acute psychotic symptoms? Currently, the predominant neurotransmitter hypothesis explaining the pathophysiology of schizophrenic disorders involves dopaminergic overactivity. Evidence supporting the *dopamine hypothesis* comes from several sources. First, the potency of all antipsychotic medications can be roughly predicted by their dopaminergic-blocking capacity. Second, mesolimbic dopamine plays a role in attentional mechanisms and stimulus filtering. When stimulus-filtering mechanisms break down, there is a collapse of the information-processing capacity of the individual, with resulting sensory inundation, cognitive fragmentation, and symptoms of thought disorder. Despite this support, the dopamine theory of schizophrenia is fraught with complexities when compared with the catecholamine theory of the affective disorders. Affective disorders hypothetically (and oversimplistically) reflect a decrease in norepinephrine tone in hypothalamic nuclei leading to a final common pathway of neurovegetative symptoms. In schizophrenia, there seems to be increased dopamine tone in mesolimbic-frontal cortical pathways leading to a final common pathway of cognitive fragmentation, thought disorder, and clinical impairment, but the impairment and the clinical symptoms are quite complex and highly variable. In this framework, affective disorders may be seen as impinging on the diencephalic ''core'' of the brain, whereas schizophrenia is conceptualized as a disorder of the mesolimbic-frontal cortical mantle. It is doubtful if any ''one neurotransmitter'' theory of any psychiatric disorder can reflect the interactive complexity of various neurobiologic and psychosocial systems, although such theories may be heuristically useful.

The hypothesis of dopamine overactivity in schizophrenia is generally characterized as a static theory. In reality, dopamine tone is related in a dynamic and variable manner to gamma-aminobutyric acid, serotonin, and other neurotransmitters that are functionally arrayed in important brain systems. Longer-term correlates of schizophrenia may also involve alterations of neuropeptides with their longer latency and response effects on behavior. At an electrophysiologic level, it has been hypothesized that the initial disturbance in schizophrenia is an aberrant temporal lobe focus that perturbs the homeostasis of the dopamine system. All of these theories are receiving critical experimental scrutiny.

NEUROPATHOLOGIC CHANGES The use of computerized tomography (CT) and magnetic resonance imaging (MRI) has been widely employed in studies of schizophrenic patients. Initial reports indicated that a minority of schizophrenic patients had abnormally increased ventricular brain ratios, reflecting increased ventricular fluid volume associated with brain atrophy. Subsequent studies have been less dramatic but the presence of increased ventricular brain ratios, mostly in type II schizophrenic patients, has supported the type I–type II dichotomy and stimulated further interest in ''Kraepelinian'' schizophrenia. It is quite possible that these type II patients have a disorder that is distinct and associated with poor medication response and poor clinical outcome. Positron emission tomography (PET) data reveal patterns of decreased frontal lobe activity in schizophrenia (hypofrontality) that seem important, especially in view of the close relationship of dopamine activity and frontal lobe function. Future PET studies utilizing new ligands will undoubtedly add to the knowledge of dopamine and other neurotransmitters in the schizophrenic disorders.

PSYCHOPHYSIOLOGY AND INFORMATION PROCESSING Important insights into the pathophysiology of schizophrenia have also been generated by psychophysiologic and information-processing studies. Individuals at high risk for developing schizophrenia and patients with a schizophrenic disorder are frequently psychophysiologically labile and vulnerable to being inundated by stimuli. The proposed mechanism for such vulnerability is an impairment in an individual's ability to screen out irrelevant stimuli and an associated inability to habituate to externally and internally generated cues. Ultimately, this dysfunction, which has been linked to dopamine overactivity in humans and animals, leads to an information-processing overload. The affected person becomes inundated with stimuli and displays cognitive fragmentation and thought disorder. Using attentional tasks, skin conductance habituation, and other measures, investigators have increasingly underscored the importance of these dysfunctions in the schizophrenic disorders.

Treatment and outcome (sustaining factors) NEUROBIOLOGIC FACTORS Five-year follow-up studies show that 60 percent of schizophrenic individuals have social recovery and half of those are employed. Thirty percent are handicapped and 10 percent remain hospitalized. This pattern of outcome seems still to be generally accurate. Which factors determine the outcome of the schizophrenic disorders are not clear. It is commonly stated that the outcome of schizophrenia is better when disorientation, affective symptoms, and acute onset are present. The outcome of schizophrenic disorders is thought to be poorer when the patient is well-oriented and has fewer affective symptoms and when the onset is insidious.

The outcome of schizophrenic disorders has been greatly improved by the use of potent and efficacious antipsychotic medications, such as the phenothiazines (see Chap. 364). Studies indicate that antipsychotic medications (often expressed in terms of chlorpromazine equivalents) act selectively against specific target symptoms that are similar to the ''positive'' symptoms of type I schizophrenia, which include hallucinations and psychotic agitation. In contrast to these responsive target symptoms, antipsychotic medications may not necessarily improve ''negative'' symptoms such as anhedonia and social withdrawal. The primary treatment modalities for the acute schizophrenic disorders are antipsychotic medication along with psychosocial therapies. The typical schizophrenic patient usually requires at least the equivalent of 600 to 800 mg per day of chlorpromazine, although higher doses are sometimes necessary. Maintenance doses of antipsychotic medications are often required to prevent relapse.

Antipsychotic medications alter dopaminergic-cholinergic balance in nigrostriatal structures (via dopamine blockade) so that acute extrapyramidal side effects are induced (e.g. dystonia, motor restlessness). These side effects can be treated with anticholinergic medications that restore dopaminergic-cholinergic balance. Aliphatic phenothiazines (such as chlorpromazine) with inherent anticholinergic properties cause fewer extrapyramidal side effects but induce more anticholinergic side effects, such as hypotension or blurred vision. Additionally, blood dyscrasias, liver toxicity, and other idiosyncratic reactions can occur. Also, the long-term use of antipsychotic medications may induce tardive dyskinesia, a long-lasting and potentially disabling motor syndrome (see Chaps. 15 and 364).

PSYCHOSOCIAL FACTORS The outcome of schizophrenic patients can be divided into the semiindependent axes of symptoms, rehospitalization, social function, and vocational function. It is possible to treat the specific psychotic symptoms of a schizophrenic individual (affecting the symptomatic axis of outcome), but the patient may be left with major psychosocial deficits (the social axis of outcome). Antipsychotic medications should thus be combined with sensitive psychosocial management including, where appropriate, individual psychotherapy, family counseling, and vocational rehabilitation in order to maximize therapeutic outcome and to restore the patient to the premorbid level of adjustment. For example, returning an acutely treated schizophrenic patient to a home filled with anger and turmoil (the so-called high-expressed-emotion family) without the benefit of family therapy is poor psychosocial management and may lead to relapse and poor outcome. Family counseling is often a critical determinant of therapeutic outcome in the schizophrenic disorders.

Antipsychotic medication alone cannot reverse years of psychosocial deficits and poor premorbid adjustment. Consequently, a large part of the therapeutic variance in outcome is accounted for by psychosocial factors. The range of outcome for schizophrenic patients is broad, and the clinician should use a broad multifactorial therapeutic approach.

REFERENCES

BATESON G et al: Towards a theory of schizophrenia. Behav Sci 1:251, 1956

BLEULER E: *Dementia Praecox or the Group of Schizophrenias*, J Zinkin (trans). New York, International Universities Press, 1950

BRAFF DL: Attention, information processing, and habituation in psychiatric disorders. *Psychiatry, III*. Philadelphia, Lippincott, 1985

BROWN GW et al: Influence of family life on the course of schizophrenic disorders: A replication. Br J Psychiatry 11:241, 1972

CARLSON G, GOODWIN F: The stages of mania. Arch Gen Psychiatry 28:221, 1973

CROW TJ: Molecular pathology of schizophrenia: More than one disease process? Br Med J 280:66, 1980

DOCHERTY JP et al: Stages of onset of schizophrenic psychosis. Am J Psychiatry 135:420, 1978

GOTTESMAN II, SHIELDS J: *Schizophrenia: The Epigenetic Puzzle*. New York, Cambridge, 1982

KRAEPELIN E: *Dementia Praecox*, RM Barclay (trans). Edinburgh, ES Livingstone Ltd, 1919

ROSENBAUM CP: *The Meaning of Madness*. New York, Science House, 1970

ROSENTHAL D, KETY S: *The Transmission of Schizophrenia*. New York, Pergamon, 1968

SNYDER SH: Dopamine receptors, neuroleptics, and schizophrenia. Am J Psychiatry 138:460, 1981

Special issue: Negative symptoms in schizophrenia. Schizophr Bull 11, 1985

STRAUSS JS, CARPENTER WT: *Schizophrenia*. New York, Plenum Medical Book Company, 1981

SWERDLOW NR, BRAFF DL, et al: Central dopamine hyperactivity in rats mimics abnormal sensory gating of the acoustic startle response in schizophrenics. Biol Psychiatry 21:23, 1986

WALKER E et al: Environmental factors related to schizophrenia in psychophysiologically labile high-risk males. J Abnorm Psychol 90:313, 1981

ZUBIN J, SPRING B: Vulnerability: A new view of schizophrenia. J Abnorm Psychol 86:103, 1977

363 PERSONALITY DISORDERS

IGOR GRANT

Personality denotes characteristic ways of thinking, feeling, behaving, and reacting to the environment. When this "psychological signature" strikes a useful balance between consistency and adaptive flexibility, we speak of personality *traits*. A personality *disorder* is said to exist when a person chronically uses certain mechanisms of coping in an inappropriate, stereotyped, and maladaptive fashion.

DIAGNOSIS OF PERSONALITY DISORDERS The *Diagnositc and Statistical Manual* of the American Psychiatric Association (DSM-III) recognizes 11 distinctive personality disorders. These are grouped into three thematic clusters. *Paranoid, schizoid,* and *schizotypal* personality disorders are characterized by oddness or eccentricity. *Histrionic, narcissistic, antisocial,* and *borderline* personality disorders share a dramatic presentation along with self-centeredness, emotionality, and erratic behavior. Anxiety and fear underlie *avoidant, dependent, compulsive,* and *passive-aggressive* personalities.

The DSM-III diagnostic classification scheme stipulates specific inclusion and exclusion criteria for diagnosis of each disorder. Since the number of criteria for individual disorders ranges from 3 to 24, the descriptions in this chapter are highlights rather than complete expositions. The reader is referred to the DSM-III for the detailed listing of the necessary signs and symptoms required to make the diagnosis of the various personality disorders.

Paranoid personality disorder People with this disorder are suspicious and hypersensitive to perceived slights and injuries. They are hypervigilant to the possibility that someone might trick or harm them and tend to be guarded and secretive and to blame others. They may be jealous and concerned with hidden meanings. They tend to exaggerate difficulties and to take offense and become hostile easily. Their affective range is limited, and they are often perceived as cold, unemotional, and humorless.

Schizoid personality disorder Schizoid individuals are loners who seem to have little need for others. They appear emotionally cold and aloof and indifferent to praise and criticism; they lack close friendships, and may be social recluses.

In earlier nomenclatures eccentric thinking was sometimes added to the schizoid picture. DSM-III, however, has split off a second category, schizotypal, to describe persons whose principal difficulties are cognitive rather than interpersonal.

Schizotypal personality disorder Schizotypal persons share with schizophrenics certain eccentricities of thinking, perception, speech, and interpersonal interaction; however, the degree and pervasiveness of such "schizophrenic-like" symptomatology is not sufficient to meet diagnostic criteria for schizophrenia. Odd speech (e.g., vague, circumstantial, metaphorical), ideas of reference (inappropriately inferring that neutral events have some special relevance to the person), magical thinking, and suspiciousness can be prominent. Many schizotypal persons are also socially isolated, and this can lead to confusion with schizoid personality.

Borderline personality disorder Borderline persons have been described as having "stable instability," characterized by chronic difficulty in regulating mood and interpersonal attachments and in maintaining a consistent self-image. Borderline persons can manifest impulsive behavior, some of it self-damaging (e.g., self-mutilation, suicidal behavior). Their mood is unpredictable. Some have brief outbursts of anger, irritability, sadness, and fear. Others suffer from a chronic emptiness. Despite having chaotic interpersonal relationships punctuated by intense love and hate, borderline persons generally are intolerant of being alone. The defense mechanism of "splitting" (regarding persons and events either as "all good" or "all bad") can be prominent.

Histrionic personality disorder People with a histrionic personality have seemingly intense but actually superficial relationships. They present in a dramatic, engaging, but self-centered fashion. There is an exaggerated expression of emotions, attention seeking, craving for excitement, and a tendency to overreact. While superficially warm and charming, histrionic persons are generally perceived as shallow, inconsiderate, self-indulgent, vain, demanding, dependent, and manipulative. Some make frequent suicidal threats or attempts.

Narcissistic personality disorder The narcissistic person has an inflated sense of self-importance, and may be preoccupied with being unique, powerful, and gifted. The patient exaggerates his or her talents and contributions, seeks admiration, and uses others to achieve a better position, while being indifferent to their feelings and needs. A rejection can produce excessive rage, inferiority, shame, or humiliation. The narcissistic person has difficulty seeing others in a realistic light, tending either to overidealize or devalue them.

Antisocial personality disorder Antisocial behavior is characterized by unconcern with the rules and expectations of society and repeated violation of the rights of others. The diagnosis is limited to adults (persons under 18 with antisocial features are classified as having conduct disorder) and requires a history of antisocial behaviors which have their onset before age 15. Such behaviors include truancy, delinquency, running away from home, lying, precocious sexuality, troubles with the law, and alcohol or drug abuse. Beyond such historical considerations, the antisocial diagnosis requires current evidence of certain deviant behaviors which include irresponsibility in work, as a parent, in financial matters, and in personal behavior (e.g., recklessness, driving while intoxicated). Additionally, antisocial persons will usually commit multiple illegal acts, lie and deceive, manifest an inability to maintain a long-term attachment to a sexual partner, and exhibit irritability and agressiveness. Alcohol or other substance abuse is common.

Avoidant personality disorder People who are inappropriately concerned with rejection or humiliation, and for this reason avoid close ties with others, are classified as having an avoidant personality disorder. Despite being withdrawn, they give evidence for wishing that they did have intimate relations with others. In contrast with the narcissistic individual, the avoidant person tends to manifest low self-esteem and a tendency to exaggerate his or her shortcomings.

Dependent personality disorder Dependent people allow others to assume responsibility for major aspects of their life and decision making. Because they see themselves as helpless or inept, they are willing to subordinate their needs and wishes to those of others in order to avoid taking personal responsibility.

Passive-aggressive personality disorder Passive-aggressive people resent responsibility, either social or work-related. Rather than expressing their opposition directly, they tend to procrastinate, dawdle, behave stubbornly, work inefficiently, and "forget." As a consequence, they fail to achieve their potential.

Compulsive personality disorder This disorder, which is equivalent to the term *obsessive-compulsive personality*, describes people who tend to be preoccupied with rules, procedures, and detail. They are often stubbornly insistent on certain things being done a particular way, yet at other times may become indecisive to the point of ineffectiveness. Compulsives tend to value their work and possessions more than their interpersonal relationships. They have difficulties expressing warm and tender feelings toward others and are sometimes seen as stiff, cold, and awkward.

Atypical, mixed, or other personality disorder This residual DSM-III category accommodates personality disturbances that do not fit neatly into any of the categories listed above. The most commonly used is *mixed personality disorder,* which indicates that an individual's behavior fulfills the criteria for more than one personality disorder, e.g., passive-aggressive and dependent. *Atypical personality disorder* is used when a personality disorder is suspected but there is not sufficient information to make a clear classification. *Other personality disorder* indicates presence of a personality disturbance not specifically included in *DSM-III*, e.g., masochistic, impulsive, or immature personality (which are concepts from other diagnostic schemes). One increasingly recognized disorder is *adult attention deficit disorder (ADD)*, a residual form of childhood ADD (hyperkinesis). As adults, such individuals continue to have problems in attending and manifest labile mood, explosive temper, impulsivity, stress intolerance, and inability to complete tasks. They may also manifest a paradoxical (calming) reaction to central nervous system (CNS) stimulants.

RELIABILITY OF PERSONALITY DISORDER DIAGNOSES Despite continued research efforts to improve interclinician agreement through specification of diagnostic criteria, reliability is problematic for most personality disorder diagnoses. While trained clinicians tend to agree whether or not some form of personality disorder is present, this reliability breaks down when specific diagnoses are attempted. Best agreement is reported for antisocial and paranoid personality disorders.

DIFFERENTIAL DIAGNOSIS **Major mental disorders** In its early phases, *schizophrenia* can be mistaken for schizoid, schizotypal, paranoid, and borderline personality disorders. *Affective disorders* can mimic some features of borderline, histrionic, and compulsive personality disorders. *Anxiety disorders* can share features with compulsive, histrionic, and avoidant personalities. *Alcohol and substance abuse disorders* may need to be differentiated from antisocial, borderline, and histrionic personalities. *Paranoid disorders* can sometimes be difficult to differentiate from paranoid, schizotypal, and borderline personalities. Differential diagnostic points are that the major mental disorders tend to have a definite time of onset, that the symptomatology is more severe and causes greater disturbance in everyday functioning, and that specific diagnostic features will be present that transcend the criteria for personality disorders.

Additional personality disorders DSM-III criteria for personality disorders sometimes overlap. "Schizophrenic-like" phenomena, including eccentricity and psychotic experiences, can form part of the picture of paranoid, schizoid, schizotypal, and borderline personalities. Dramatic presentation, emotional outbursts, and erratic behavior can lead to confusion among antisocial, borderline, narcissistic, and histrionic personalities. Impulsivity is found in antisocial, borderline, and histrionic personalities; while anxiety and fearfulness can be part of avoidant, passive-aggressive, dependent, and compulsive behavior.

Medical conditions Medical and neurologic conditions can mimic personality disorders. For example, persons with complex partial seizures with foci in the left temporal lobe can present with excessive orderliness, religiosity, and "viscosity" which might be confused with compulsive personality. Alternatively, they can develop paranoid features or fuzzy thinking suggestive of paranoid or schizotypal personality. Rigid, orderly, and ritualistic behavior mirroring compulsive personality can be part of a dementing process or a sequel of head injury, while irritability, dysregulation of affect, and inappropriate interpersonal behavior in such patients can be confused with borderline personality. Beyond these specific examples, virtually any disease affecting the brain can cause behavioral change suggestive of a personality disorder. The key differential points are that there is a relatively sudden onset and that there are neuropsychological changes indicative of compromised brain function.

ETIOLOGY AND PATHOPHYSIOLOGY It was commonly held that the personality disorders reflected the warping effect of adverse early social environment. Now there is mounting evidence that personality is, in great measure, biologically determined. Both genetic and constitutional (i.e., intrauterine and early physical developmental) factors may be important.

Genetic factors Although not all personality disorders have been examined, for the majority there is a severalfold increase in concordance between monozygotic twins compared with dizygotic twins.

Some of the most careful work has been with antisocial personality. Here it is noted that prevalence among men is three- to fourfold higher than in women, and that first-degree relatives of persons diagnosed as antisocial show increased prevalence of antisocial personality, alcoholism, and somatization disorder (Briquet's syndrome). The latter is characterized by intractable multiorgan system complaints in women who often have a histrionic personality. The association of these two disorders in the same pedigrees has led to suggestions that Briquet's syndrome and antisocial disorder are expressions in women and men of a common biogenetic substrate.

The operation of genetic factors in antisocial personality is further demonstrated by the finding that biologic offspring of antisocial and alcoholic parents have a higher risk of developing antisocial personality disorder even if they are raised by adoptive parents who do not have any antisocial traits. The converse has also been demonstrated: children adopted by antisocial parents tend not to develop antisocial disorder themselves unless they have antisocial personality or alcoholism in their blood relatives.

The XYY chromosomal abnormality was once thought to be related to antisocial personality disorder. More recent studies indicate that although XYY might be overrepresented in certain prison populations, the vast majority of XYY men are not antisocial.

The schizotypal, borderline, and schizoid diagnoses evolved orginally from the notion that there ought to be a "preclinical" form of schizophrenia characterized by lesser severity or fewer numbers of the cognitive and interpersonal symptons of that disorder. Thus, the schizotypal personality might, theoretically, embody earlier forms of the disturbance in thinking, perception, and attention that occur in schizophrenia; whereas the schizoid personality would represent the interpersonal awkwardness inherent in that disorder. Genetic studies have confirmed that there is some increase in schizotypal (but not schizoid) personality in relatives of diagnosed schizophrenics.

The borderline personality is genetically heterogeneous. Up to 50 percent of borderline patients have a family history of affective disorder. Borderline disorder itself, as well as other personality disorders, are also more common in first-degree relatives of borderline patients, but schizophrenia is not consistently related.

There is increased schizophrenia in the families of patients with paranoid personality. For compulsive disorder, twin studies indicate increased concordance for obsessional traits in monozygotic versus dizygotic twins. There is also some evidence that orderliness and rigidity run in families.

The other personality disorders have not been studied carefully from a biogenetic standpoint.

Constitutional factors Although there is good evidence that infants are born with certain temperamental characteristics (e.g., high versus low activity level; long versus short attention span), there is little evidence that these temperamental characteristics persist into adolescence. Infant temperament does not appear to predict later personality disorder with the exception that the "difficult child" (irritable, hard to console, irregular rhythms) tends to exhibit more behavioral disturbances. Low intelligence quotient and poor physical health as a child have been noted more frequently in the histories of persons with personality disorders.

Neurophysiologic and neuroendocrine correlates Several neurophysiologic and biochemical changes may be associated with personality disorders. Abnormal slow waves and spikes have been reported in the EEGs of antisocial persons. For borderline patients, patterns suggestive of periodic limbic epileptiform discharges have sometimes been noted.

Some observers suggest that a common neurophysiologic feature of both antisocial and hysterical disorders is reduced cortical arousal to cortical stimulation, secondary to increased inhibition from lower brain regions. This may be coupled with motor disinhibition in antisocial persons and autonomic disinhibition in hysterics.

The schizotypal personality disorder has been associated with disturbance in smooth pursuit eye movement (SPEM). Since many schizophrenics are also poor trackers, it may be that schizotypals share with schizophrenics decreased neural effectiveness in "centering." Some schizophrenics and schizotypals have lowered platelet monoamine oxidase (MAO) levels. It has been suggested that lowered MAO activity could be related to inefficient degradation of certain biologically active amines, leading to accumulation of substance with psychotomimetic properties.

Cortisol escape from dexamethasone suppression and shortened rapid eye movement (REM) latency (REM latency is the time between falling asleep and first REM episode) are associated with affective disorder. Both phenomena have also been observed in borderline and obsessive-compulsive personalities, suggesting a link among the affective, borderline, and obsessive-compulsive disorders.

There are no specific data on biologic correlates of the other personality disorders.

Environmental factors Early social environment has proved to be an inconsistent predictor of late personality disorder. For example, one study found that 30 percent of men with personality disorders who were investigated reported lack of maternal warmth as children, but so did 24 percent of controls. Multiple problems in the early environment were found in 16 percent of personality-disordered men and 10 percent of those without disorders. Being abused as a child is associated with violence in later life.

The relative weakness of both temperamental and environmental factors as predictors of future personality disorder has led to a "goodness of fit" hypothesis. This theory suggests that later behavioral disorders are more likely when there is a severe mismatch between a child's temperament and childrearing practices and environmental circumstances.

EPIDEMIOLOGY The prevalence of personality disorders ranges from 5 to 23 percent. Antisocial personality is diagnosed more commonly in men than women, whereas borderline and histrionic personalities are diagnosed more commonly in women.

There is increased prevalence of personality disorder in inner cities, prisons, and areas of social disintegration. Personality disorders are three times as common in the lowest social classes as compared to the highest. These sociodemographic patterns are particularly striking for antisocial personality disorder.

NATURAL HISTORY AND PROGNOSIS Compared to controls, a disproportionate number of persons with personality disorders are found to have emotional problems as children. The prevalence of most personality disorders declines with age, the peak being in the age group 20 to 29. This trend is especially prominent for antisocial personality disorder. It is possible that slowly evolving maturational processes during adulthood account for these age effects.

Although only about 20 percent of persons with personality disorders seek psychiatric treatment, the majority evidence long-standing difficulties in maintaining stable employment, marriages, and friendships.

With regard to psychiatric complications, about one-third of persons with personality disorders have significant depression or anxiety. Alcohol abuse is related to personality disorder, with the association being particularly striking for men, whose rate of alcohol problems approaches 50 percent.

TREATMENT Persons with personality disorders generally do not recognize the inner source of their difficulties. They tend to blame others and their environment and make those around them feel badly. Only 20 percent of persons with personality disorders actually seek psychiatric treatment.

Treatment usually consists of psychotherapy in some form. In some specific instances psychopharmacology has been used. Success has been claimed for various types of psychotherapy. Individual, group, couples, and family treatments all have been employed. Despite differences in techniques and orientations, most psychotherapists emphasize the importance (and initial difficulty) of establishing a trusting relationship. The goals tend to be to identify inner sources of maladaptive behavior. From a psychodynamic standpoint this means that the painful feelings which are being avoided need to be identified and their causes traced. Cognitive-behavioral therapists will try to identify the faulty assumptions, lack of foresight regarding consequences of behavior, and ineffectiveness of the existing coping repertoire, with an eye to teaching more useful behavior.

As a broad generalization patients with "dramatic" presentations (borderline, antisocial, histrionic, narcissistic) tend to require a more intrusive, confrontative, limit-setting posture by the therapist. More specifically, antisocial personality probably cannot be treated in an outpatient setting and requires a containing enviroment (e.g., prison, inpatient unit). In such a setting groups emphasizing mutual interdependence and confrontation appear to produce some success. Regarding the treatment of borderline persons, psychiatrists are divided as to whether a supportive "here and now" versus intensive exploration work best. In either instance, treatment is often punctuated by prolonged periods in which the patient expresses negative feelings toward the therapist, makes suicide attempts, or undergoes psychotic decompensation requiring hospitalization.

In contrast to this more intrusive posture, patients whose personalities fit into the "fearful" and "odd" clusters may benefit from a more gentle, accepting, and clarifying approach.

Psychotherapy tends to be a long-term enterprise, lasting many years. Therapists can expect to feel frustrated, angry, helpless, and inadequate at times. Clinical reports of major improvements are many, but controlled outcome studies are practically nonexistent. This reflects continuing problems in achieving reliable diagnoses and in general methodologic issues in outcome research, especially in prospective studies spanning many years.

There is increasing evidence that psychopharmacologic intervention may be helpful for some of the personality diagnoses. Borderline patients, particularly those with coexisting mood disorder, have benefited from tricyclic antidepressants and MAO inhibitors. Other groups of borderline patients in whom mood dysregulation and impulsiveness are prominent have responded to lithium. Still others with explosive outbursts have benefited from carbamazepine. A few such patients have had EEG abnormalities suggestive of epileptic foci in limbic structures. Both borderline and schizotypal patients undergoing cognitive disorganization can improve with low doses of neuroleptic drugs.

Persons with compulsive personality disorder who have obsessional ruminations may benefit from the tricyclic clomipramine (unavailable in the United States). Clomipramine may have specific antiruminative effects which go beyond its antidepressive activity. The utility of other antidepressants for this disorder has not been established, although the MAO inhibitors show promise in compulsives who also experience anxiety or panic attacks.

Methylphenidate may improve inattention and reduce motor overactivity, affective lability, and impulsivity in persons whose personality difficulties are related to adult attention deficit disorder.

REFERENCES

American Psychiatric Association: *Diagnostic and Statistical Manual of Mental Disorders*, 3d edition. Washington, DC, APA Press, 1980

Drake RE, Vaillant GE: A validity study of Axis II of DSM-III. Am J Psychiatry, 142:555, 1985

Frosch JP: The psychosocial treatment of personality disorders, in *Current Perspectives on Personality Disorders*, JP Frosch (ed). Washington, DC, APA Press, 1983, pp 96–112

Grant I: *Behavioral Disorders: Understanding Clinical Psychopathology*, New York, Spectrum, 1979

Gunderson JG: DSM-III diagnoses of personality disorders, in *Current Perspectives on Personality Disorders*, JP Frosch (ed). Washington, DC, APA Press, 1983, pp 20–39

Liebowitz MR: Psychopharmacological intervention in personality disorders, *Current Perspectives on Personality Disorders*, JP Frosch (ed). Washington DC, APA Press, 1983, pp 68–93

Lion JR: *Personality Disorders: Diagnosis and Management (Revised for DSM-III)*, 2d ed. Baltimore, Williams, & Wilkins, 1981

Millon T: *Disorders of Personality, DSM-III, Axis II*, New York, Wiley, 1981

Siever LJ et al: Biogenetic factors in personalities, in *Current Perspectives on Personality Disorders*, JP Frosch (ed). Washington, DC, APA Press, 1983, pp 42–65

Waldinger RJ: *Psychiatry for Medical Students*. Washington, DC, APA Press, 1984

Wender PH et al: A controlled study in the treatment of attention deficit disorder, residual type, in adults. Am J Psychiatry, 142:547, 1985

364 THE THERAPEUTIC USE OF PSYCHOTROPIC MEDICATIONS

LEWIS L. JUDD

Perhaps no other area of pharmacology has experienced the rapid development that has occurred in psychopharmacology during the past two decades. An almost bewildering array of specific and effective psychotropic agents are currently available, with new medications appearing with great frequency. This chapter presents an overview of the major classes of psychopharmacologic drugs to provide the reader with a pragmatic understanding of these potent medications. The most clinically meaningful classification schema is based upon the therapeutic use in patients, as follows: antidepressant medications, lithium and other mood stabilizing medications, anxiolytic or antianxiety medications, and antipsychotic or neuroleptic medications.

ANTIDEPRESSANT MEDICATIONS The successful search for new and better antidepressant medications has resulted in the two generations of antidepressants that are currently available. The first-generation antidepressants include the tricyclic (TCA) and the monoamine oxidase (MAO) inhibitor antidepressants. To date, no newly developed drug has greater efficacy than the antidepressants in these two major classes. The MAO inhibitors are clinically effective and recently have experienced a resurgence in clinical use, but the problems of drug-drug and drug-food interactions have made these the second-line medications in the treatment of depressive disorders. In contrast, the TCAs imipramine and amitriptyline have emerged as the standards for antidepressant efficacy.

No antidepressant is ideal, and all currently available drugs have at least one of the following undesirable characteristics: delayed onset of therapeutic action (7 to 28 days), significant anticholinergic side effects, sedation, cardiotoxicity, weight gain, the possible induction of manic episodes in patients with bipolar disorders, or other equally problematic side effects. Therefore, the developmental goal of the second-generation antidepressants has been to increase efficacy and eliminate side effects, but the search has not met with notable success.

Mechanisms of action The primary brain mechanism originally hypothesized for the TCA antidepressants was the capacity to increase synaptic concentrations of central nervous system (CNS) monoaminergic neurotransmitter substances (e.g., norepinephrine, serotonin, and dopamine) by blocking their reuptake by presynaptic monoaminergic neurons. While this is still valid, the focus now is on the regulation of postsynaptic receptor activity in monoaminergic neurons, and down-regulation of neurotransmitter receptors has been identified with the antidepressant effect. Most of the proven antidepressants fit the mechanisms hypothesized, but some newer antidepressants do not. At present, therefore, there is a great deal of information available about how antidepressants may ameliorate the pathophysiologic mechanisms of depressive disorders, but no precise central mechanism(s) has been identified by which all drugs with antidepressant properties work.

Clinical conditions in which antidepressant medications are used Antidepressants are very effective in treatment of major depression (Chap. 360) but do not affect the vicissitudes of mood inherent in normal human behavior nor do they make unhappy people into happy ones. Chronic low-grade depression or dysthymic disorders (neurotic depression) do not respond well to antidepressants, but patients with major depression are very likely to respond. Antidepressants are not often prescribed for patients who become temporarily depressed over difficult and stressful life situations (situational depression).

There is, however, growing evidence that antidepressants are effective in the treatment of some anxiety disorders (Chap. 361). TCA and the MAO inhibitor antidepressants are the drugs of choice for agoraphobia, simple phobias, and panic disorder. Patients with phobic or panic disorders have concomitant anxiety about the recurrence of these attacks; this "anticipatory" anxiety may not respond to antidepressants but often requires treatment with antianxiety medication. There may also be a potentially broader role for the antidepressants in the management of pure anxiety disorders, but this requires further study.

Clinical use of the antidepressants Table 364-1 lists the more commonly used first-generation antidepressants and the oral doses needed for therapeutic efficacy in the typical patient. Currently imipramine and amitriptyline are the standards for antidepressant potency. Amitriptyline is more sedative while imipramine is more energizing. Because of the undesirable side effects observed in these original TCAs, during the past decade there has been a gradual shift among experienced clinical psychopharmacologists to the secondary tricyclic amines of desipramine and nortriptyline. The advantage of desipramine is that it has relatively fewer anticholinergic side effects, and nortriptyline appears to have a clearer relationship between plasma levels and clinical efficacy.

Before antidepressants are prescribed, a patient's physical health must be evaluated by a physical examination and the patient should show normal values on baseline complete blood count (CBC), urinalysis, liver function tests, and (if over 45 years) an electrocardiogram (ECG). Patients are started on low doses in a twice daily regimen for 1 day (e.g., 25 mg desipramine bid) and checked for idiosyncratic reactions (e.g., postural hypotension). The dose is then raised quickly over a few days to that needed for a full therapeutic response. The minimum daily dose for clinical response is the low figure in the ranges listed in Table 364-1, but often higher doses are needed. Physicians inexperienced in psychopharmacology should not exceed the upper dosage limits listed in the table. From 7 to 28 days are required for a full therapeutic effect to be present. Changes in the depressive symptoms are often noted by friends and family before the patient reports feeling subjectively better. A therapeutic trial of an antidepressant requires at least 28 days at the upper end of the dose range. Patients are maintained on antidepressants for approximately 8 months after the depressive symptoms disappear. Medications can be given in a single dose an hour before bedtime once an appropriate dose for a given patient has been established. The advantages of this procedure are improved medication compliance; that the sedative side effects induce sleep in depressed patients, who are often insomniac; and that the troublesome side effects occur while the patient is asleep. Some patients cannot tolerate the single bedtime dose, and in these patients a daytime twice daily or three times daily schedule is necessary.

Plasma levels of the tricyclic antidepressants are routinely available, but unfortunately the relationship of plasma levels to clinical response has been inconsistent. Linear relationships between plasma levels and therapeutic response exist for imipramine, desipramine and amitriptyline, while nortriptyline may have a curvilinear plasma level–response relationship, implying a therapeutic window. Plasma levels may be useful in treatment-resistant patients to evaluate compliance and to see if the dose is sufficient to maintain concentrations above the threshold necessary for response (e.g., imipramine > 180 ng/mL; desipramine > 125 ng/mL; amitriptyline > 95 ng/mL; and nortriptyline 60 to 140 ng/mL).

After a number of months of treatment with antidepressants, it is recommended that the drug be withdrawn gradually over a 3- to 4-week period rather than that it be stopped suddenly. Should depressive symptoms reemerge, restoration of the antidepressant treatment is necessary for several more months, and then the withdrawal attempt can be repeated.

TABLE 364-1 Commonly used first-generation antidepressants

Antidepressant	Daily oral therapeutic dose range, mg
Tricyclic derivatives:	
Amitriptyline (Elavil, etc.)	150–300
Nortriptyline (Aventyl, etc.)	50–150
Imipramine (Tofranil, etc.)	150–300
Desipramine (Norpramin)	150–250
Doxepin (Sinequan, etc.)	150–300
Monoamine oxidase inhibitors:	
Phenelzine (Nardil)	45–90
Tranylcypromine (Parnate)	10–30
Isocarboxazid (Marplan)	10–30

TABLE 364-2 More common side effects of tricyclic antidepressants

- Anticholinergic (atropine-like) responses:
  - Dry mouth*
  - Nausea and vomiting*
  - Constipation
  - Urinary retention
  - Blurred vision (mydriasis and cycloplegia)
- Cardiovascular effects:
  - Postural hypotension*
  - Tachycardia
  - Cardiotoxic side effects—can induce an arrhythmia
- Obstructive jaundice—more rare—is reversible when drug is removed
- Drowsiness and sleepiness—may want to avoid driving a car until this diminishes*
- Fine rapid tremor*
- Dizziness, ataxia
- Hematologic effects:
  - Leukopenia

* *Side effects seen most commonly*

TABLE 364-3 Selected second-generation antidepressants

Antidepressant	Daily oral therapeutic dose range, mg
Tricyclic derivatives:	
Trimipramine (Surmontil)	100–250
Amoxapine (Asendin)	150–300
Tetracyclic derivatives:	
Mianserin (Bolvidon)	50–150
Maprotiline (Ludiomil)	150–300
Derivatives of other chemical classes:	
Trazodone (Desyrel)	100–600
Alprazolam (Xanax)	0.75–4

Side effects and interactions with other drugs Listed in Table 364-2 are some of the more common side effects from the tricyclic antidepressants; they include dry mouth, sedation, a fine tremor of the hands, and mild constipation. More serious are the effects on the cardiovascular system, where tachycardia and postural hypotension are the most common. The TCAs, especially imipramine, have a quinidine-like action, can induce cardiac arrhythmias, and have been associated with sudden death in a few patients (see section below on overdose). Patients with preexisting cardiac illness, especially those with heart block, should be treated cautiously with the TCAs, or drugs with milder cardiac effects should be considered. The most bothersome symptoms are from the anticholinergic effects; while rarely serious, they do cause discomfort and compliance problems.

Some preexisting medical conditions increase the risk of using TCAs in certain depressed patients. Tricyclics can produce tachycardia, which may push some patients from asymptomatic congestive failure into symptomatic heart failure. TCAs lower the seizure threshold and should be used cautiously in patients with seizures. The anticholinergic effects preclude TCAs in patients with glaucoma, and men with mild to moderate prostatic hypertrophy can develop urinary retention. Finally, the use of tricyclic antidepressants in patients with bipolar disorders may act to shorten the cycle length between affective episodes and may induce an acute manic episode in some patients.

The tricyclics, especially amitriptyline, imipramine, and doxepin, potentiate the effects of other CNS-depressant medications (e.g., ethanol, benzodiazepines) and patients should be cautioned about ethanol use while on antidepressants. Patients should either not drink or reduce their usual ethanol dose by one-half during tricyclic treatment. Other drug interactions include the potentiation of other anticholinergic agents (e.g., antihistamines, antiparkinsonian agents), which can result in severe constipation, urinary retention, and even paralytic ileus. This combination in the elderly can produce a serious anticholinergic blockade (e.g., paralytic ileus, fecal impaction) and not uncommonly has been the cause of frank delirium and confusional states in geriatric patients. Therefore this combination should be used with caution in the elderly.

Despite the problems, the risk/benefit ratio is overwhelmingly in favor of the antidepressants, and literally hundreds of thousands of patients have been treated with these compounds safely and effectively.

The newer antidepressant medications The development of new antidepressant medications has proceeded rapidly and many second-generation drugs are now available. Table 364-3 lists the more prominent second-generation drugs for which some evidence of antidepressant efficacy exists. Unfortunately, many of the clinical trials in which these drugs were studied are sufficiently flawed that the antidepressant potency of the new antidepressants has not been fully established. How these drugs will fare over time under more rigorous scrutiny is unknown. An example of the unforeseen problems which arise when promising new drugs are given broader exposure is the experience with zimelidine. This relatively selective serotonin uptake blocker was originally reported to be an effective antidepressant with milder anticholinergic side effects. With increased study it has been associated with Guillain-Barré syndrome in several patients and has now been withdrawn pending further investigation. This new generation of psychotropic medications is promising and may eventually lead to drugs that offer additional benefits.

One of the first of the new medications developed is *trimipramine*, a tricyclic derivative. It has proved to be similar in its antidepressant potency and clinical spectrum to imipramine and amitriptyline. It is quite sedative and may actually have specific anxiolytic characteristics. The potential advantage of this drug is that patients may report fewer anticholinergic symptoms, even though the drug has anticholinergic properties.

Amoxapine is also a tricylic derivative with clinical efficacy equal to that of the original antidepressants. It has been claimed that this compound may have earlier onset of action (within the first week), although its clinical efficacy at the endpoint of treatment is identical to that of the original TCAs. This compound has the interesting feature that one of its metabolites (7-hydroxyamoxapine) is a neuroleptic which has been associated with the unwanted side effects seen with the antipsychotic drugs (e.g., extrapyramidal syndrome). Other side effects from amoxapine appear to be similar to those of the original tricyclics although a disproportionate number of seizures was found in some retrospective studies. It is claimed, but not yet established, that it is less cardiotoxic.

Clomipramine, a tricyclic antidepressant commonly used in Europe and Canada but not approved for use in the United States, has been shown in controlled studies to be an effective drug in the treatment of depression and to be perhaps uniquely effective in obsessive-compulsive disorders.

Mianserin is a tetracyclic derivative, but there are very few placebo-controlled studies in the United States establishing its antidepressant efficacy. There is one unpublished controlled study indicating that it is similar in its antidepressant effects to amitriptyline, but many of the studies involving mianserin have been open studies which are of dubious value in assessing its therapeutic spectrum and potency. The advantage of this drug is that it has virtually no anticholinergic side effects and little if any cardiotoxicity, but it does produce considerable sedation.

Maprotiline is also a tetracyclic derivative which is equal in antidepressant potency to the original tricyclics. It is reported to have fewer anticholinergic side effects. Originally it was offered as a promising drug for use in patients with cardiovascular problems, but this has not been established and it is not recommended for this purpose. Initially it was also felt to have less effect on the seizure threshold but it has now been reported to have caused grand mal seizures in several patients. Moreover, its use has been associated with more than the expected incidence of blood dyscrasias.

Nomifensine, a potentially interesting antidepressant related to a nonanalgesic opiate derivative, has now been withdrawn from the market worldwide because of serious hypersensitivity reactions.

Trazodone is a triazolopyridine derivative and is the first of its type to be used as an antidepressant. There is considerable controversy whether or not this drug has the same antidepressant efficacy and spectrum as the original tricyclics. The advantage of this drug is that it has few if any anticholinergic side effects. It is reported to be a potentially useful drug in patients with cardiac illness, but this has not been established. The major problems with trazodone include an unacceptable level of sedation and increased risk of priapism.

Alprazolam, a benzodiazepine derivative with proven anxiolytic efficacy, has been reported to be an effective antidepressant. It has not been established that it is as potent as the original TCAs in the treatment of major depressive disorders. It is likely to have a place in the treatment of mixed anxiety and depressive syndromes, and it has the added advantage of a more rapid onset. It has no anticholinergic effects but does cause sedation and lethargy. Since it is a benzodiazepine, withdrawal symptoms may appear after prolonged use in high dose. This is a promising new drug, which may herald the development of other benzodiazepines with antidepressant properties.

Bupropion initially appeared to be a promising antidepressant, but its tendency to cause seizures in some patients has resulted in its removal from the market for further study.

Clinical management of tricyclic overdosage Antidepressants are the fourth most common cause of drug overdose seen in emergency departments in the United States and the third most frequent cause of drug-related death (after alcohol-drug combinations and heroin). Of the antidepressants, tricyclics were the primary cause of death. In the California study (Callaham and Kassel) the annual incidence of fatal tricyclic overdose was 1.3 per 100,000 of population. More than two-thirds were women. Amitriptyline, desipramine, and nortriptyline were the most frequently implicated.

The first 6 h after an overdose of a tricyclic antidepressant are crucial. CNS depression and seizures, respiratory arrest, and cardiovascular arrhythmias are the principal causes of death. ECG changes showing QRS prolongation are early signs of toxicity, and ventricular fibrillation is a common complication. ECG changes are a more sensitive measure for monitoring patients than are blood levels of the drug.

LITHIUM AND OTHER MOOD-NORMALIZING MEDICATIONS The most important psychotropic medication in this group is lithium. Although lithium possesses some antidepressant properties, it is not, strictly speaking, an antidepressant. Lithium's effectiveness in the treatment of patients with bipolar disorders (see Chap. 360) and other disorders of mood has revolutionized the practice of psychiatry. Since lithium's approval by the FDA in 1969, there has been an explosion of basic and clinical research focused on its pharmacologic mechanisms and clinical use.

Mechanism of action of lithium Considerable progress has been made in advancing our understanding of its clinical use, but the underlying mechanism by which lithium works is largely unknown. Lithium exerts effects on the brain's monoaminergic neurotransmitter concentrations at the synapse, and there is agreement that, in part, this mediates its clinical effects. Lithium has strong effects on biologic membranes, and this has been offered as an additional mechanism of action in the CNS. Lithium is unique since it both attenuates the frenetic agitation of mania and controls depression in bipolar disorders. However, the central mechanisms by which lithium exerts its clinical effects on extremes of mood are not fully understood.

Conditions in which lithium is used Lithium is the drug of choice of acute manic/hypomanic episodes and for the prevention of recurrent episodes of mania and depression in bipolar depression. Although evidence exists that lithium is a low-grade antidepressant, especially in depressions seen in bipolar disorders, it is not a drug of choice for depression per se. Lithium may also be an effective agent in the prophylaxis of recurrent unipolar depressive disorders. It has been successfully used in conjunction with neuroleptics in schizoaffective schizophrenia; there may be a subpopulation of schizophrenics responsive to lithium, although most workers feel that lithium responders are atypical bipolar patients and not schizophrenics. Finally, there are reports that lithium may be useful in alcoholism; while this is of interest, it has not been established.

Clinical use of lithium Lithium is a very safe drug with an excellent risk/benefit ratio when it is used knowledgeably. The only genuine contraindication to lithium's use is seriously compromised renal function. The following baseline studies should be obtained before prescribing lithium: CBC, routine urinalysis with a concentration test, total thyroxine (T_4), serum creatinine, electrolytes, and (for those over 40) an ECG.

Serum lithium levels peak 1 to 3 h after an oral dose, and the biologic half-life is 24 h, but this varies with age. Elderly patients frequently have a drug half-life over 30 h (requiring lower doses) and adolescent patients less than 20 h (requiring higher doses). Lithium is monitored by serum levels, which are most informative approximately 10 h after the last dose. Therapeutic efficacy in acute mania is achieved at levels between 0.8 and 1.5 meq per liter. There is rarely a necessity for patients to be treated at serum levels above 1.5 meq per liter. Lithium is always administered orally, and the oral dose range is from 600 mg to 3000 mg qd. A general rule of thumb equates a 0.2 meq per liter rise in serum level with each additional 300-mg tablet of lithium. Unless sustained release tablets are used, lithium is usually administered in a two or three times daily regimen, allowing for smooth, sustained 24-h serum levels. There is a 7- to 10-day delay between starting lithium and achieving full therapeutic effects, which often necessitates the addition of antipsychotic medications during the early phase of treating a manic patient. Patients during acute manic episodes often tolerate relatively higher doses of lithium, but once the manic episode remits it is necessary to quickly reduce the dose to prevent toxicity. When an isolated acute manic/hypomanic episode is being treated, it is common practice to maintain the patient on lithium for 6 to 8 months following symptom disappearance. The drug is tapered gradually over 3 to 4 weeks.

Because of medical complications, clinicians have become increasingly conservative about long-term maintenance on lithium unless it is clearly justified. Generally, for maintenance therapy, the patient should have had a total of three diagnosed and treated episodes of mania and/or depression, with two of the episodes occurring within a 2-year period and the next episode during the following 2 years. In other words, the clinician should be convinced that the patient is experiencing frequent, serious, and disruptive episodes. The current maintenance strategy is to seek the lowest possible serum levels that will prevent relapse. Previously, higher serum levels were used, but now maintenance levels range from 0.4 to 1.0 meq per liter with recent evidence indicating that the relapse rate is significantly increased only when serum levels fall below 0.4 meq per liter.

Lithium's excretion rate is very stable within each patient; as a result patients can be maintained on the same dose day in and day out, with relative certainty that stable levels are present. Patients during maintenance are seen every 3 to 6 months, and serum lithium, sodium, potassium, T_4, TSH, and creatinine are monitored along with urinalysis with a concentration test. The lithium excretion pattern is altered by conditions which change sodium concentrations, and patients on thiazide diuretics or low-salt diets should be monitored more frequently.

TABLE 364-4 Common lithium side effects

Severity	Side effect
SIDE EFFECTS COMMONLY SEEN	
Very mild	Thirst Nausea (particularly during first few days of treatment) Fine tremor of hands
Mild to moderate	Anorexia Vomiting Diarrhea "Upset stomach" or "abdominal pain" Polydipsia and/or polyuria Muscular weakness and fatigue
SIDE EFFECTS INDICATING TOXICITY	
	Muscle hyperirritability with twitching, muscle fasciculation, or chronic movements Sedation, sluggishness, languidness, drowsiness, giddiness Coarse tremor Ataxia
Moderate to severe	Hypertonic muscles Hyperactive deep tendon reflexes Hyperextension of arms and legs with grunts and gasping Chorea, athetotic movements Impairment of consciousness Somnolence, confusion, stupor Seizures Transient focal neurologic signs Dysarthria Cranial nerve signs
Very severe	Coma Complications of coma Death

Side effects and interactions with other drugs Lithium's side effects are listed in a continuum ranging from those seen relatively commonly to those which indicate lithium toxicity (see Table 364-4). Many of these are minor side effects, which appear early and disappear as time passes, but some may persist throughout treatment. As a general rule the rapid escalation of serum levels often induces side effects, especially those involving the gastrointestinal tract, and therefore smoother, more gradual serum lithium increases are desirable.

Usually the first signs of lithium toxicity are increases in the deep tendon reflexes and muscle fasciculations. Unusual degrees of sedation and cognitive disruption also may herald lithium toxicity. Lithium toxicity mimics barbiturate intoxication, and when death occurs it is secondary to respiratory depression and its complications. The treatment involves good supportive care and excellent hydration; and since lithium's half-life is 24 h, this treatment sustains the patient while awaiting the kidney's elimination of lithium at the predictable rate. Various methods have been tried to improve the treatment of lithium toxicity, such as increasing lithium excretion by aminophylline or alkalinizing the urine, but all have been disappointing. For life-threatening cases, the last resort is renal dialysis, but toxicity rarely progresses to the point where this intervention is needed.

Lithium's interactions with other drugs primarily involve its reciprocal relationship with the sodium ion. Diuretics, which increase sodium excretion, can increase lithium toxicity. There have also been reports that combined neuroleptic and lithium therapy has resulted in a reversible neurotoxicity in a small number of middle-aged and older patients. Clinical observations indicate that this combination is safe and effective provided that the antipsychotic drug and lithium are used in low to moderate doses and are carefully monitored, and that the combination treatment is discontinued as soon as the lithium effect is sufficiently present for the patient to be managed without it.

Medical sequelae of lithium's use Several medical complications can develop during lithium treatment. Because of its effect on adenylate cyclase activity, lithium inhibits the secretory function of the thyroid gland; nontoxic goiters and hypothyroidism can develop, which can be readily corrected during lithium therapy by thyroid supplement. Lithium may induce the following ECG changes especially in older patients: T-wave depression, sinus node dysfunctions, and very rarely sinoatrial block and ventricular irritability.

The most important sequelae are the renal complications. About 25 percent of patients develop some degree of antidiuretic hormone–resistant nephrogenic diabetes insipidus with polyuria and polydipsia. The lithium inhibition of adenylate cyclase activity is responsible for the disruption of renal tubular transport. These symptoms are usually completely reversible by lithium withdrawal and often can be ameliorated by reduction in serum level. The most economic and accurate method of monitoring changes in renal function during lithium treatment is by the urine concentration test and serum creatinine level. Urine concentration levels below a specific gravity of 1.025 indicate an early renal effect, and a creatinine clearance test should be obtained. If creatinine clearance is abnormal, the patient's clinical condition is reevaluated and termination of the lithium treatment should be considered. There have been reports of renal focal necrosis and interstitial fibrosis in a few long-term lithium patients, and there is evidence, by biopsy, for an increased basal rate of renal pathology among patients with affective disorders. Nonetheless, this nonspecific renal lesion does appear with a higher degree of frequency in patients receiving long-term lithium. Therefore, many experienced clinicians do not maintain patients on lithium for more than 5 years without a drug-free trial.

Evidence has emerged linking the more serious renal complications to increased episodes of lithium toxicity and possibly to prolonged combined use of lithium and neuroleptics. While good clinical practice should obviate lithium toxicity, it may be equally important to avoid extremes of high and low serum lithium levels during the day. Despite these concerns, lithium remains one of the most important and effective psychotropic agents with an excellent risk/benefit ratio.

Carbamazepine and other mood-stabilizing medications The anticonvulsant *carbamazepine* has, in controlled trials, been used successfully in the treatment of manic and, to a lesser extent, depressive episodes in bipolar patients. There is also growing evidence that a significant number of bipolar patients who do not respond to lithium benefit from carbamazepine treatment, and that the combination of lithium and carbamazepine may be therapeutically additive. The drug regimen for bipolar disorders is initated beginning with 200 mg bid administered orally increasing to 600 to 1600 mg daily in divided doses with the therapeutic blood levels ranging from 8 to 12 mg/dL. Carbamazepine is not a completely benign drug; side effects include nausea, blurred vision, and ataxia, and more importantly there have been cases of aplastic anemia reported. Patients treated with carbamazepine must be monitored for renal, liver, and bone marrow functions during the time they are on the medication. There are also reports of reversible CNS toxicity when this drug is combined with lithium, therefore patients on this combination should be monitored carefully. *Valproic acid,* the drug of choice in certain seizure disorders, has also been reported to prevent recurrence of manic episodes in a small number of bipolar patients. The development of this new class of psychotropic compounds is very promising and may herald the future development of a new and useful group of medications.

ANTIANXIETY OR ANXIOLYTIC MEDICATIONS The development of the benzodiazepines has been a great advance in the pharmacologic management of anxiety. They have also replaced barbiturates as the sedative-hypnotic drugs of choice. The benzodiazepines, unlike the barbiturates, are not complete CNS depressants and even at high doses are rarely associated with lethal respiratory depression or vasomotor collapse. True addiction to benzodiazepine compounds is also very rare. In addition, depending upon the drug, benzodiazepines possess anticonvulsant and muscle relaxant properties as well.

Mechanisms of action There is growing evidence that gamma-aminobutyric acid (GABA), an inhibitory amino acid neurotransmitter, may play a central role in the brain mechanism(s) of anxiety. Benzodiazepines selectively, but indirectly, enhance GABA neurotransmission, possibly by increasing neuronal receptor sensitivity to GABA. Also, a close interaction has been described between GABA and benzodiazepine receptor binding, which involves the neuronal chloride ionophore channel. Despite these observations, the specific mechanism by which benzodiazepines mediate their clinical effects is not completely understood.

Clinical conditions in which anxiolytic medications are used The antianxiety medications are most effective in the management of relatively short-lived reactive states of tension and anxiety and are the drugs of choice in the treatment of generalized anxiety disorders (see Chap. 361). The anxiolytic benzodiazepines are useful in treating panic disorders but are not the drugs of choice, although alprazolam at higher doses (4 to 10 mg) can block panic attacks. Rather, it is the TCA and MAO inhibitor antidepressants which are the drugs of choice to suppress symptoms of panic disorder (see Chap. 361). However, the anxiolytics may have a role in the treatment of anticipatory anxiety, which is almost always present in patients with panic disorders. Sometimes, both a TCA and a benzodiazepine anxiolytic may be necessary in the treatment of panic disorder. The anxiolytics are also useful in the treatment of anxiety symptoms that accompany phobic disorders.

Clinical use of the antianxiety medications Clinically the benzodiazepines are divided on the basis of their use as either primarily anxiolytics or sedative-hypnotics. The more commonly prescribed drugs are listed in Table 364-5 along with the usual oral dose ranges. The pharmacokinetic characteristics of many of the benzodiazepines are complicated by long drug elimination half-lives and the metabolic conversion of parent compounds to active metabolites (see Table 364-5). Diazepam is converted to the active metabolite desmethyldiazepam (nordiazepam) which, in turn, can be hydroxylated to yield oxazepam, also a potent benzodiazepine. This metabolic pathway extends the activity half-life of diazepam threefold. The hypnotic flurazepam is converted to its active metabolite N-1-desalkylflurazepam, whose half-life is more than 48 h; hence, repetitive daily doses given in excess of a week or two can result in the accumulation of the active metabolites of the drug. Prazepam has metabolic compounds identical to those of diazepam and has a similar drug elimination half-life. Oxazepam and lorazepam, both of which undergo glucuronide conjugation, have no active metabolites and therefore have the advantage of a shorter half-life. The benzodiazepines temazepam, triazolam, and alprazolam also have the advantage of shorter half-lives and to date, no long-acting active metabolites have been identified.

Diazepam has been the standard against which all anxiolytic drugs are measured, and no other anxiolytics have demonstrated better antianxiety potency. The newly developed benzodiazepines appear equally effective and have eliminated certain of the undesirable side effects. Specifically, lorazepam, oxazepam, and alprazolam are without active metabolites and cumulative effects of daytime sedation are less noticeable.

Treatment regimens usually last 4 weeks or less and medications are prescribed continually for 7 to 10 days followed by a 2- to 3-day drug holiday; then this sequence is repeated. This helps avoids the development of tolerance to the anxiolytic effects. The shorter-acting medications (lorazepam, alprazolam, etc.) are prescribed in a three or four times daily regimen, and the longer-acting drugs (diazepam, etc.) are given in a single dose or a twice daily regimen. For example, it is common practice to prescribe one dose of diazepam at bedtime, since it will both promote sleep and reduce anxiety levels during the following day.

In prescribing the anxiolytic benzodiazepines clinicians should avoid the possibility of habituating patients to chronic benzodiazepine use. One of the earliest signs is the development of tolerance, where the patient repeatedly requests escalations in drug dose. Since benzodiazepines do produce mild euphoria and a sense of well-being, anxious patients often want to preserve this feeling and request additional medication. On the other hand, clinical surveys of prescription practices have shown that clinicans are aware of the problems of benzodiazepine habituation and sometimes respond by being too cautious and by unnecessarily undertreating patients. The use of the drug holiday treatment regimen described above and the physician's resistance to repetitively increasing dosage will help to minimize the problem of drug habituation.

In addition to its role as an anxiolytic, diazepam is also the drug of choice in this class for muscle relaxation and for the treatment of alcohol withdrawal syndromes. It is the benzodiazepine of choice for intractable seizures. Oxazepam, because of the nonaccumulation of active metabolites, is a good choice for anxiolysis in the elderly.

TABLE 364-5 More commonly used benzodiazepines

Benzodiazepines	Daily oral dose range, mg	Half-life, h*
Anxiolytics:		
Chlordiazepoxide (Librium)	20–100†	7–28*
Diazepam (Valium)	5–40†	20–90*
Lorazepam (Ativan)	1–10‡	10–12
Oxazepam (Serax)	30–120‡	3–20
Prazepam (Centrax)	20–60†	40–70*
Alprazolam (Xanax)	0.75–10.0‡	12–15
Sedative-hypnotics:		
Flurazepam (Dalmane)	15–30§	24–100*
Temazepam (Restoril)	30§	8–10
Triazolam (Halcion)	0.5–1.0§	2–5

* *Indicates long-acting active metabolites.*
† *Prescribed in a daily or twice daily regimen.*
‡ *Prescribed in a three or four times daily regimen.*
§ *Prescribed in a daily or bedtime regimen.*

Side effects and interactions with other drugs The most important adverse effect of the benzodiazepines is the discomfort caused by the withdrawal syndrome, which can occur after chronic treatment. While there is very little risk of physiologic dependence on these drugs when used appropriately, the withdrawal symptoms do contribute to the development of psychological habituation. Between 40 and 50 percent of patients develop minor withdrawal symptoms after cessation of chronic benzodiazepine treatment. Symptoms include muscle aches, agitation, restlessness, insomnia, and generalized anxious dysphoria. In some patients more serious CNS withdrawal symptoms may appear, including confusional and delirium states and, more rarely, grand mal seizures. Rebound anxiety can also be seen in patients with anxiety disorders but is less prevalent when benzodiazepines with long-acting metabolites are used and less frequent if the drug is gradually discontinued. Risk for withdrawal increases with the length of the treatment and is reported with much greater frequency (e.g., more than 90 percent) among patients who have been treated for 1 year or more. Withdrawal symptoms occur within the first 24 to 48 h after cessation of drug use in the short-acting benzodiazepines, but in those benzodiazepines with long-acting metabolites (e.g., diazepam, chlordiazepoxide), the withdrawal symptoms can occur 4 to 6 days and even longer after drug cessation. With the usual recommended dosage regimens and the gradual withdrawal technique (e.g., over 3 to 4 weeks), the appearance of a withdrawal syndrome in patients can be minimized significantly. While there is little true addiction potential, patients should be on these medications for only as long as necessary.

The most common minor side effects are daytime sedation, mild cognitive impairment, motor clumsiness and, with some drugs, specific memory decrements (e.g., lorazepam). Another rare but troublesome side effect from some benzodiazepines is paradoxical emotional responses, primarily manifested as aggressive and impulsive behavior.

Unlike barbiturates, the benzodiazepines do not noticeably induce hepatic microsomal enzyme activity and therefore do not affect the metabolism of other medications. Their primary interaction with other drugs is their additive effects with other CNS depressants. The cross-tolerance with ethanol has made the benzodiazepines ideal medications for the treatment of alcohol withdrawal syndromes. Patients should be cautioned that ethanol is potentiated by benzodiazepines and this combination ought to be avoided.

The newer anxiolytic medications It has been established that certain beta-adrenergic blocking agents, such as *propranolol*, can dampen the peripheral physiologic symptoms of anxiety. Initially, it was felt that these drugs might be better nonsedative anxiolytic compounds, but this has not held up in controlled studies. While propranolol does attenuate somatic manifestations of anxiety (e.g., palpitations, tremor), it appears to have lesser effects on the psychological components (e.g., intense fearfulness). Although propranolol has been used in the treatment of severe cases of fear of public speaking and in musicians (oral dose 40 to 320 mg qd), it is not a comprehensively effective anxiolytic. It is possible that with additional study other peripheral blocking agents may prove to be more effective.

A new class of anxiolytic drugs, the azaspirodecanediones, has been developed. One of the first compounds studied clinically is *buspirone*. It has little structural similarity to other anxiolytics or even to other psychotropics. It is not anticonvulsant, does not interact with the putative benzodiazepine receptor, is not cross-tolerant to other CNS depressants, and no abstinence syndrome has yet been described. In several controlled trials it has proved to be an effective anxiolytic with relatively less sedation and decrements in psychomotor performance. To date it has not been extensively studied and it is possible that efficacy problems and as yet unidentified side effects may be associated with its use.

In addition to their efficacy in panic and phobic disorders, there are controlled studies reporting that *tricyclic antidepressants* are anxiolytics as effective as the benzodiazepines in generalized anxiety disorders. It is possible that continued investigations will identify a broader role for TCAs in the treatment of the full spectrum of anxiety disorders.

ANTIPSYCHOTIC OR NEUROLEPTIC MEDICATIONS The antipsychotics have the capacity to sedate, tranquilize, blunt emotional expression, attenuate aggressive and impulsive behavior, and cause disinterest in the environment and lack of initiative. Unique features of the drugs are that higher intellectual functions are left relatively intact and yet they act to specifically ameliorate the agitation and bizarre behavior and thinking of psychotic patients. Unfortunately no antipsychotic medication currently available even approaches what an ideal drug in this group should be. Virtually all have prominent anticholinergic side effects and produce a wide variety of dystonias and extrapyramidal symptoms. Of greater concern is the fact that these agents cause tardive dyskinesia (see Chap. 15), a seriously disabling movement disorder that is often irreversible. Nonetheless, the antipsychotics, primarily used in schizophrenia, have reduced enormously the patient populations in mental hospitals and have allowed for maintenance in the community of chronic mentally ill patients who before the advent of neuroleptics would have been lifelong residents of hospitals.

Mechanism of action of the antipsychotics With few exceptions, antipsychotics have notable effects on the brain's dopaminergic neurotransmitter system. Specifically, antipsychotics antagonize the effects of the neurotransmitter dopamine in the basal ganglia and in the limbic portions of the forebrain. Since one of the central characteristics of neuroleptics is their capacity to block dopaminergic neurotransmission, this has led researchers to postulate that abnormalities in the CNS dopaminergic neurotransmitter systems are one of the central underlying pathophysiologic mechanisms in the etiology of schizophrenia. While specific aspects of the brain mechanism(s) by which the antipsychotics mediate their effects have been well-established, the full and detailed understanding of how these drugs actually work is not yet available.

Clinical conditions in which the antipsychotic medications are used Because the risk of tardive dyskinesia is significant, antipsychotics should only be used when necessary and in those conditions for which they are the drug of choice. Antipsychotics are drugs of choice in the treatment of schizophrenic disorders (see Chap. 362), in combination with lithium for acute manic episodes (see Chap. 360), and in combination with antidepressants for psychotic and agitated depressions. They are also used in Tourette's syndrome and Huntington's disease. There is a relatively narrow spectrum of mental disorders for which the antipsychotics should be used, although these disorders, in terms of sheer numbers of patients, make up a significant majority of patients with serious and chronic mental illness.

Clinical use of the antipsychotics The more commonly used antipsychotics from each of the pharmacologic classes and their average daily oral doses are given in Table 364-6. Chlorpromazine, one of the first drugs of this class developed, is the prototype antipsychotic drug and is the potency standard for the others. Dose equivalency for the antipsychotics is calculated on a ratio of the effect of that particular drug compared to the effect of 100 mg of chlorpromazine. For example, 5 mg of trifluoperazine or 2 mg of haloperidol is equivalent in potency to 100 mg of chlorpromazine. Using this ratio as a reference point, acutely psychotic patients usually require an accumulated dose of 500 to 800 mg orally of a chlorpromazine equivalent during the first 24 to 36 h. Following control of the acute agitation, the oral dose is increased over the next week to the chlorpromazine equivalent of between 600 and 1500 mg a day in divided doses. It is uncommon for therapeutic benefits to be measurably increased by exceeding the daily dose equivalent of 1500 mg of chlorpromazine, although it may be necessary to go to two and three times this level in some patients.

Schizophrenia is a chronic disorder and patients need long-term maintenance on antipsychotics to prevent relapse. In controlled studies as many as 60 percent of schizophrenics relapse within 6 months

TABLE 364-6 Some of the more commonly used antipsychotic medications

	Average daily oral dose range, mg	Potency ratio compared to 100 mg of chlorpromazine
Phenothiazines:		
Aliphatics:		
Chlorpromazine (Thorazine)	400–800	1:1
Piperazines:		
Fluphenazine (Prolixin)	4–20	1:50
Fluphenazine enanthate or decanoate	25–100*	
Perphenazine (Trilafon)	8–32	1:10
Trifluoperazine (Stelazine)	6–20	1:20
Piperidines:		
Thioridazone (Mellaril)	200–600	1:1 (approx)
Butyrophenones:		
Haloperidol (Haldol)	8–32	1:50
Thioxanthenes:		
Chlorprothixene (Taractan)	400–800	1:1
Thiothixene (Navane)	15–30	1:25
Oxoindoles:		
Molindone (Moban, Lidone)	40–200	1:10
Dibenzoxazepines:		
Loxapine (Loxitane, Daxolin)	60–100	1:10

* *Intramuscular injection, long acting, every 1–3 weeks*

after discontinuing drug therapy. Patients are maintained on the lowest dose possible that will prevent reemergence of symptoms. This is usually in the range of 20 percent of the peak dose level needed to ameliorate the acute phase of the psychotic symptoms. Compliance is difficult to achieve in this chronically disordered group of patients, and it is often therapeutically advantageous for the clinician to use parenteral long-acting fluphenazine enanthate or decanoate, which can be administered by injection every week or two. Previously it was recommended that drug holidays be used, but this has not prevented tardive dyskinesia and there are few if any advantages to this technique, which is now rarely used.

Side effects and interactions with other drugs Initially patients are sedated, lethargic, and drowsy, but within days they develop tolerance to these effects. All of the antipsychotics have anticholinergic action, which may produce dry mouth, cycloplegia, postural hypotension, constipation, and urinary retention. Obstructive jaundice, retinal pigmentation, lenticular opacities, skin pigmentation and hypersensitivity to sunlight, and male impotence are also side effects seen with antipsychotics.

It is the extrapyramidal side effects that are the most bothersome. During the first five days of treatment patients may develop acute muscular dystonic reactions but the extrapyramidal Parkinson-like syndrome is the most common. Both the dystonias and the parkinsonism respond well to antiparkinsonian medications (benztropine mesylate, 1 to 2 mg bid or tid; trihexyphenidyl, 2 to 5 mg bid or tid, etc.). Another common side effect is akathisia, a motor restlessness in which patients feel compelled to move their extremities and to move about. It is not uncommon to mistake akathisia for psychotic agitation and increase the antipsychotic dose, exacerbating the problem. Akathisia may respond to antiparkinsonian agents but more often requires decreasing the dose of the antipsychotic. It is rarely necessary to continue antiparkinsonian drug treatment beyond the first 3 months of antipsychotic maintenance.

The most serious side effect of the antipsychotics is *tardive dyskinesia,* which has been seen with virtually every neuroleptic. The specter of tardive dyskinesia has altered the risk/benefit ratio of the antipsychotics so that exposure to these drugs should be reserved for those disorders in which these compounds are clearly the drugs of choice. Usually the symptoms of tardive dyskinesia appear late and consist of involuntary, repetitive movements of the lips, tongue (tongue thrusting, lip smacking, etc.) and not infrequently, of the extremities and trunk. Patients over 60 and those with preexisting CNS pathology are at a higher risk for this disorder, but no other risk factors have been identified. Further, no method of prevention or effective treatment for this frequently irreversible disorder has been developed. Mild to moderate tardive dyskinesia has been found in 10 to 20 percent of chronically hospitalized schizophrenics.

The *malignant neuroleptic syndrome*, a rare complication of neuroleptic drugs, is discussed in Chap. 8.

Newer antipsychotic drugs The newer antipsychotic drugs offer, at best, only slight improvements in the side effect profile over the older drugs and achieve little or no improvement in clinical effectiveness. Two of the more promising new antipsychotics are *clozapine* and *sulpiride,* but they are not routinely available in the United States. Each has a different molecular structure from the other neuroleptics, which may herald the development of new classes of safer and better antipsychotics.

REFERENCES

Appleton WS, Davis JM: *Practical Clinical Psychopharmacology,* 2d ed. Baltimore, Williams & Wilkins, 1980

Baldessarini RJ: *Chemotherapy in Psychiatry.* Cambridge, Mass., Harvard, 1985, pp 1–354

Boehnert MT, Lovejoy FH Jr: Value of the QRS duration versus the serum drug level in predicting seizures and ventricular arrhythmias after an acute overdose of tricyclic antidepressants. N Engl J Med 313:474, 1985

Callaham M, Kassel D: Epidemiology of fatal tricyclic antidepressant ingestion: Implications for management. Ann Emerg Med 14:1, 1985

Clark WG, del Guidice J (eds): *Principles of Psychopharmacology,* 2d ed. New York, Academic, 1978

Cooper TB et al (eds): *Lithium: Controversies and Unresolved Issues,* Amsterdam, Excerpta Medica, 1979

Gilman AG, Goodman LS (eds): *The Pharmacological Basis of Therapeutics,* 7th ed. New York, MacMillan, 1985

Guzé BH, Baxter LR Jr: Current concepts: Malignant neuroleptic syndrome. N Engl J Med 313:163, 1985

Haneston PD: *Drug Interactions,* 3d ed. Philadelphia, Lea & Febiger, 1975

Hippuis H, Winokur G (eds): Part 2, clinical psychopharmacology, in *Psychopharmacology 1.* Amsterdam, Excerpta Medica, 1983

Hollister, LE: *Clinical Pharmacology of Psychotherapeutic Drugs.* New York, Churchill Livingston, 1978

Iverson LL, Snyder SS (eds): *Handbook of Psychopharmacology.* New York, Plenum, 1977

Jarvik ME: *Psychopharmacology in the Practice of Medicine.* New York, Appleton-Century-Crofts, 1977

Klein DF et al: *Diagnosis and Drug Treatment of Psychiatric Disorders: Adults and Children,* 2d ed. Baltimore, Williams & Wilkins, 1980

Post RM, Ballenger JC (eds): Neurobiology of mood disorders, in *Frontiers of Clinical Neuroscience.* Baltimore, Williams & Wilkins, 1984, vol 1

Shader RI: *Psychiatric Complications of Medical Drugs.* New York, Raven Press, 1972

section 2 Alcoholism and drug dependency

365 ALCOHOL AND ALCOHOLISM

MARC A. SCHUCKIT

Ninety percent of people drink alcohol, 40 to 50 percent of men have temporary alcohol-induced problems, and 10 percent of men and 3 to 5 percent of women develop pervasive and persistent alcohol-related problems (alcoholism). Even light drinking may adversely interact with other medications, temporary heavier drinking can exacerbate most medical illnesses, and alcoholism can masquerade as many different medical disorders and psychiatric syndromes. The following sections describe the pharmacology and clinical effects of alcohol and identify circumstances where drinking may cause a major medical or psychiatric problem or exacerbate a preexisting disorder. While these comments apply to the hypothetical "average" person, there is considerable individual variability depending on genetic vulnerability, concomitant drug use and prior unrelated pathology or disease.

PHARMACOLOGY OF ETHANOL: ABSORPTION AND METABOLISM Ethanol is a weakly charged molecule that moves easily through cell membranes, rapidly equilibrating between blood and tissues. The effects of drinking depend in part on the amount of ethanol consumed per unit of body weight; the level of alcohol in the blood is expressed as milligrams or grams of ethanol per deciliter (e.g., 100 mg/dL or 0.1000 g/dL). In round figures, 12 oz of beer, 4 oz of nonfortified wine, and 1.5 oz (a shot) of 80-proof beverage each contain approximately 10 g of ethanol; 1 pint of 86-proof beverage contains approximately 160 g and 1 liter of wine contains approximately 80 g of ethanol. Congeners found in alcohol beverages may contribute to body damage with heavy drinking; these include low-molecular-weight alcohols (e.g. methanol and butanol), aldehydes, esters, histamine, phenols, tannins, iron, lead, and cobalt.

Ethanol is a central nervous system (CNS) depressant that decreases activity of neurons, although some behavioral stimulation is observed at low blood levels. This drug has cross-tolerance and shares a similar pattern of behavioral problems with other brain depressants, including the benzodiazepines, barbiturates, and other sedatives and hypnotics. Alcohol is absorbed from mucus membranes of the mouth and esophagus (in very small amounts), from the stomach and large bowel (in modest amounts), and from the proximal portion of the small intestine (the major site). The rate of absorption *increases* with rapid gastric emptying; the absence of proteins, fats, or carbohydrates (which interfere with absorption); the absence of congeners; dilution to a modest percentage of ethanol (maximum absorption is seen at about 20 percent by volume); and carbonation (champagne).

Between 2 percent (at low blood alcohol concentrations) and about 10 percent (at high blood alcohol concentrations) of ethanol is excreted directly through the lungs, urine, or sweat, but the greater part is metabolized to acetaldehyde in the liver. At least two metabolic routes, each with different optimal concentrations of ethanol (K_m), result in the metabolism of approximately one drink per hour. The *first* and clinically most important pathway occurs in the cell cytosol via alcohol dehydrogenase (ADH) with a K_m of about 2 mmol. This reaction produces acetaldehyde which is then rapidly destroyed by aldehyde dehydrogenase (ALDH) in the cytosol and mitochondria. Each of these steps requires nicotinamide adenine dinucleotide (NAD) as a cofactor, and it is the increased ratio of the reduced cofactor (NADH) to NAD (NADH:NAD) that is responsible for many of the metabolic derangements observed after drinking. *Second,* microsomes of the smooth endoplasmic reticulum (the microsomal ethanol-oxidizing system or MEOS) with a K_m of about 10 mmol may be responsible for 10 percent or more of ethanol oxidation at high blood alcohol concentrations. Increased activity of this system can be induced after repeated exposure to ethanol.

All pathways result in the production of acetaldehyde, which is oxidized to acetate. The clinical significance of acetaldehyde is not known, but accumulation in liver, brain, or other body tissues may cause organ damage.

BEHAVIORAL EFFECTS, TOLERANCE, AND DEPENDENCE The behavioral and physiologic effects of any drug depend upon the dose, its rate of increase in plasma, the concomitance of other drugs or medical problems, and the past experience with the agent. With alcohol, one must also consider whether observation is during rising (where the effects are more intense) or falling blood alcohol levels.

Even though "legal intoxication" requires a blood alcohol concentration of at least 80 to 100 mg/dL (0.1 g/dL), behavioral, psychomotor, and cognitive changes are seen at levels as low as 20 to 30 mg/dL (i.e., after one to two drinks). Narcosis or deep sleep is induced in many people at twice the legal intoxication level, and even in the absence of concomitant medications, death can occur with levels between 300 and 400 mg/dL. Ethanol, either alone or in combination with agents such as benzodiazepines, is probably responsible for more toxic overdose deaths than any other agent.

The mechanisms of action of ethanol on nervous tissues are not fully understood because even modest doses simultaneously change many neurotransmitters and increase the fluidity of neuronal cell membranes. After repeated exposure to the drug, the body compensates in at least three ways to tolerate higher ethanol levels. *First,* after 1 to 2 weeks of daily drinking the liver can increase the metabolic rate of ethanol in humans by as much as 30 percent; i.e., there is *metabolic or pharmacokinetic tolerance,* an adaptation that disappears almost as rapidly as it develops. *Second,* cellular or *pharmacodynamic tolerance* probably occurs through complex neurochemical adaptations or changes in cell membranes with subsequent altered ion flow—changes that may contribute to physical dependence. *Third,* even at the same blood alcohol concentrations and neuronal adaptation, organisms can learn to adapt behavior and to function better than expected under drug influence (*behavioral tolerance*). For example, practicing driving while intoxicated might result in a psychomotor performance which (*while still impaired*) is better than that observed before practice.

Once the cells have adapted to chronic ethanol exposure, the structural or biochemical changes may not return to normal for several weeks or more. In the face of these adaptations, the neurons require ethanol to function optimally; i.e., the person is physically addicted or drug-dependent. This physical condition is distinct from psychological dependence, a poorly defined concept indicating that the person is psychologically uncomfortable without the drug.

NUTRITIONAL FACTORS One gram of ethanol has approximately 7.1 kcal, and a drink contains between 70 and 100 kcal from ethanol and other carbohydrates. Therefore, 8 to 10 drinks can yield over 1000 kcal per day, but these are "empty" of nutrients such as minerals, proteins, and vitamins.

Any vitamin absorbed through the small intestine by active transport or stored in the liver can be deficient in alcoholics. These include folate (folacin or folic acid), pyridoxine (B_6), thiamine (vitamin B_1), nicotinic acid or niacin (B_3), and vitamin A. Thiamine deficiency causes Wernicke's and Korsakoff's syndromes (see Chap. 349).

Low blood potassium, magnesium, calcium, zinc, and phosphorous can occur as a consequence of dietary deficiency and acid-base imbalances during excess alcohol ingestion or withdrawal. Hypokalemia can lead to periodic muscle paralysis and areflexia. Deficiencies in magnesium can add to a clouded sensorium and other neurologic symptoms; hypocalcemia can cause tetany and weakness; low levels of zinc are speculated to contribute to gonadal dysfunction, anorexia, problems with wound healing, and immune deficiencies; and low phosphate levels can contribute to myocardial failure, brain dysfunction, weakness of muscles (including those of respiration), and white blood cell and platelet dysfunction.

An ethanol load in a fasting, healthy individual is likely to produce transient hypoglycemia within 6 to 36 h, secondary to the acute actions of ethanol on gluconeogenesis. This impairment is exacerbated by poor diet and by liver and pancreatic disease. As a result, glucose intolerance may be marked until the alcoholic has been abstinent for 2 to 4 weeks. Alcohol ketoacidosis, probably reflecting a decrease in fatty acid oxidation coupled with poor diet or recurrent vomiting, should not be misdiagnosed as diabetic ketosis. With the former, patients show an increase in serum ketones along with a mild increase in glucose but a large anion gap, a mild to moderate increase in serum lactate, and a β-hydroxybutyrate/lactate ratio of between 2:1 and 9:1 (with normal being 1:1).

THE EFFECTS OF ETHANOL ON BODY SYSTEMS

This overview of acute and chronic effects of alcohol on body systems outlines signs and symptoms that can aid in the recognition of the hidden alcoholic. It emphasizes the interactions between drinking and medications and the effects of alcohol on chronic medical conditions.

CENTRAL NERVOUS SYSTEM In addition to acute behavioral effects, an evening of heavy drinking can result in an alcoholic *"blackout,"* i.e., an episode of forgetting all or part of what occurred during drinking. This problem is experienced by 30 to 40 percent of men in their late teens and early 20s, most of whom do not go on to develop more serious and pervasive alcohol-related problems. Even after only a few drinks, alcohol acutely decreases *sleep* latency (helping people to fall asleep) and depresses rapid eye movement (REM) sleep early in the night, sometimes followed by later REM rebound associated with bad dreams. The consequence is to "fragment" sleep, causing a more rapid than normal alternation between sleep stages and a deficiency in deep sleep.

Chronic intake of high doses of ethanol can cause *peripheral neuropathy* in 5 to 15 percent of alcoholics (see Chaps. 349 and 355). This syndrome probably results from both thiamine deficiency and direct effects of ethanol and/or acetaldehyde. Patients complain of bilateral limb numbness, tingling, and parasthesias, more pronounced distally than proximally. Although these symptoms can be incapacitating, more often the pain and numbness are mild to moderate in severity. The treatment is abstinence and thiamine supplementation.

Wernicke's and Korsakoff's syndromes are important problems in alcoholics (see Chap. 349). Thiamine deficiency is the major cause in vulnerable individuals (possibly interacting with a genetic transketolase deficiency). Classically, patients with Korsakoff's syndrome present with profound anterograde and retrograde amnesia along with possible impairment in visuospatial, abstract, and conceptual reasoning but with a normal intelligence quotient (IQ). In general, the level of recent memory loss is out of proportion to the global level of cognitive impairment. While most patients demonstrate an acute onset of Korsakoff's syndrome in association with the neurologic stigmata seen with Wernicke's syndrome (e.g., sixth nerve palsy and ataxia), some individuals may have a more gradual development of symptoms probably secondary to repeated bouts of thiamine deficiency. Wernicke's syndrome responds rapidly to oral thiamine replacement of 50 to 100 mg followed by 50 to 100 mg per day. However, only one-quarter of Korsakoff's patients are likely to achieve full recovery, one-half experience partial recovery, and one-quarter show no improvement with thiamine even after many months of supplementation.

About 1 percent of alcoholics with long histories of associated malnutrition develop *cerebellar degeneration,* a syndrome of progressive unsteady stance and gait often accompanied by mild nystagmus (see Chap. 349). Cerebellar atrophy is seen on computerized tomography (CT) scans but the cerebrospinal fluid is usually normal. While ethanol or acetaldehyde might contribute to the problem, the major cause is probably nutritional, and identical symptoms can be seen with some forms of severe malnutrition alone. Treatment consists of abstinence and multiple vitamin supplementation.

Alcoholics can show severe *cognitive* problems and impairment in recent and remote memory for weeks to months after an alcoholic binge. Cortical functioning (e.g., psychomotor performance and short-term memory) tends to improve with abstinence, but long-term memory problems, perhaps reflecting subcortical damage, may persist. Increased size of the brain ventricles and cerebral sulci are seen in up to 50 percent of chronic alcoholics. These changes are partially reversible, returning toward normal after a year or more of abstinence. Permanent CNS impairment (*alcoholic dementia*) may supervene. Up to 20 percent of chronically demented patients may have had prior alcoholism. There is no single alcoholic dementia syndrome; rather, this label is used to describe patients who have apparently irreversible cognitive changes (possibly from diverse causes) in the midst of chronic alcoholism (see also Chap. 349).

Finally, to borrow a phrase from the past, alcohol could be termed "the great mimicker" because almost every psychiatric syndrome can be seen during heavy drinking or subsequent withdrawal. This includes intense *sadness* lasting for days to weeks in the midst of heavy drinking, severe *anxiety* during alcoholic withdrawal and remaining for many months after cessation of drinking, *psychoses* during the severe form of the alcohol abstinence syndrome, and auditory *hallucinations* and/or *paranoid delusions* in the absence of any obvious signs of withdrawal—a state called alcoholic hallucinosis or alcoholic paranoia. Whatever the cause, the treatment of alcohol-induced psychopathology includes abstinence and supportive care, with the likelihood of full recovery within several days or weeks. Another alcohol-related psychiatric syndrome is *pathologic intoxication* or alcohol idiosyncratic intoxication, a state of severe agitation, confusion, and violence lasting minutes to hours which is seen after a very low dose of ethanol (e.g., one to two drinks) and for which the individual is amnestic. This extremely rare phenomenon, seen almost exclusively in individuals with severe preexisting brain damage, is sometimes invoked erroneously for the purposes of legal defense.

THE GASTROINTESTINAL SYSTEM Esophagus and stomach Acute alcoholic intake can result in inflammation of the esophagus (possibly secondary to reflux of gastric contents) and stomach (resulting from damage to the gastric mucosal barrier). Esophagitis can cause epigastric distress, and gastritis, the most frequent cause of gastrointestinal bleeding in heavy drinkers, can present with anorexia and abdominal pain. Chronic heavy drinking, if associated with violent vomiting, can produce a longitudinal tear in the mucosa at the gastroesophageal junction—a Mallory-Weiss lesion. Although many gastrointestinal problems are reversible, two complications of chronic alcoholism, esophageal varices secondary to cirrhosis-induced portal hypertension and atrophy of gastric cells, may be irreversible (see Chaps. 234 and 236).

Small bowel The greater part of the ethanol is absorbed from the proximal small bowel, where it may interfere with absorption of B vitamins and other nutrients. Acutely, ethanol can cause hemorrhagic lesions of the duodenal villi and diarrhea secondary to increased small-bowel motility and decreased water and electrolyte absorption.

Chronic alcoholism can contribute to diarrhea through its effects on the pancreas (see Chaps. 237 and 255).

Pancreas Alcoholics commonly develop acute or chronic pancreatitis (see Chap. 255).

Liver Ethanol absorbed from the small bowel is carried directly to the liver, where it becomes the preferred fuel; NADH accumulates and oxygen utilization escalates, gluconeogenesis is impaired (with a resulting fall in the amount of glucose produced from glycogen), lactate production increases, and there is a decreased oxidation of fatty acids in the citric cycle with an increase in fat accumulation within liver cells. In the healthy individual taking no medications these changes are reversible, but with repeated exposure to ethanol more severe changes in liver functioning are likely to occur. These include, in overlapping stages, fatty accumulation, alcohol-induced hepatitis, and cirrhosis (see Chap. 249).

Increased cancer risk Cancer is the second leading cause of death in alcoholics (after cardiovascular disease), who have a rate of carcinoma 10 times higher than that expected in the general population. The sites with the greatest increase over expected rates include the head and neck, esophagus, cardia of the stomach, liver, and pancreas.

HEMATOPOIETIC SYSTEM Ethanol exerts multiple reversible acute and chronic effects on all blood cells. Alcohol alters acutely the production of red blood cells (RBC), which reaches clinical significance after days to weeks of heavy drinking. The most common finding is an increase in RBC size (mean corpuscular volume, MCV) with a mild anemia. If this is accompanied by folic acid deficiency, there can also be hypersegmented neutrophils, reticulocytopenia, and hyperplastic bone marrow. Other forms of anemia, including sideroblastic changes, can occur concomitantly, especially in the presence of severe malnutrition.

Chronic heavy drinking can also decrease production of most white blood cells (WBC), decrease granulocyte mobility and adherence, and impair the delayed hypersensitivity response to new antigens (with a possible false-negative tuberculin skin test). While the changes in WBCs themselves are usually temporary, they may contribute to the risk of infections, liver damage, and perhaps to the increased risk of cancers in alcoholics. Alcohol can also cause toxic granulocytosis.

Many alcoholics present with mild thrombocytopenia (rarely associated with hemorrhage) due to a decrease in platelet survival and altered function; hypersplenism may occur as a complication of cirrhosis. Alcohol may decrease platelet aggregation and inhibit release of thromboxane A_2. These problems usually return toward normal within a week of abstinence.

CARDIOVASCULAR SYSTEM Modest doses of alcohol can have both deleterious and beneficial effects in individuals with normal cardiovascular status who take no medications. Ethanol decreases myocardial contractility and causes peripheral vasodilatation resulting in a mild drop in blood pressure and a compensatory increased heart rate and cardiac output. Exercise-induced increases in cardiac oxygen consumption are higher after alcohol. On the other hand, one to two drinks per day over long periods may decrease the risk of cardiovascular death, perhaps through an increase in high density lipoprotein cholesterol (HDL) or changes in clotting mechanisms.

Although ethanol in low doses causes a mild acute drop in blood pressure, the consumption of three or more drinks per day results in a dose-dependent increase in blood pressure which returns to normal within weeks of abstinence. Chronic heavy drinking can cause cardiomyopathy with symptoms ranging from unexplained arrhythmias in the presence of left ventricular impairment to heart failure with dilatation of all four heart chambers and hypocontractility of heart muscle. Mural thrombi can form in the left atrium or ventricle, while heart enlargement exceeding 25 percent can cause mitral regurgitation. Finally, there is an association between cerebrovascular accidents and alcoholism, especially within 24 h of heavy drinking. Atrial or ventricular arrhythmias, especially paroxysmal tachycardia, can also occur after a binge in individuals showing no other evidence of heart-disease—a syndrome known as the "holiday heart."

GENITOURINARY SYSTEM CHANGES, SEXUAL FUNCTIONING, AND FETAL DEVELOPMENT Acutely, modest ethanol doses (e.g., blood alcohol concentrations of 100 mg/dL or even less) increase sexual drive in men. However, modest ethanol doses may simultaneously decrease erectile capacity. Even in the absence of liver impairment, a significant minority of chronic alcoholic men may show irreversible testicular atrophy with concomitant shrinkage of the seminiferous tubules and loss of sperm cells (see Chap. 330).

The repeated administration of ethanol to women can result in amenorrhea, a decrease in ovarian size, an absence of corpora lutea with associated infertility, and spontaneous abortions. Heavy drinking during pregnancy results in the rapid placental transfer of both ethanol and acetaldehyde, which may have serious consequences for fetal development. The *fetal alcohol syndrome* can include a mixture of any of the following: facial changes with epicanthal eye folds, poorly formed concha, and small teeth with faulty enamel; cardiac atrial or ventricular septal defects; an aberrant palmar crease and limitation in joint movement; and microcephaly with mental retardation. More severe syndromes occur with heavy and persistent drinking, although the specific amount of ethanol and/or specific time of vulnerability during pregnancy have not been defined. Considering the possibility that one to two drinks per day might increase the risk for mild aspects of this syndrome, it is advisable for pregnant women to abstain completely.

OTHER EFFECTS OF ETHANOL Heavy drinking can produce an acute *alcoholic myopathy* characterized by painful and swollen muscles, high levels of serum creatine phosphokinase (CK), and rarely myoglobinemia and myoglobinuria. Effects on the *skeletal system* include alterations in calcium metabolism with an increased risk for fractures and osteonecrosis of the femoral head. *Hormonal* changes include an increase in cortisol levels, which can remain elevated during heavy drinking; inhibition of vasopressin secretion at rising blood alcohol concentrations and the opposite at falling blood alcohol concentrations, with the final result that most alcoholics are likely to be slightly overhydrated; a modest decrease in serum thyroxine (T_4); and a more marked decrease in serum triiodothyronine (T_3). After weeks of abstinence, T_4 and T_3 levels usually return to normal.

ALCOHOLISM

Because many drinkers occasionally imbibe to excess, temporary alcohol-related pathology is common in nonalcoholics. The time of heaviest drinking is usually the late teens to the late twenties when between one-third and one-half of male drinkers experience some isolated (although potentially dangerous) alcohol-related social, occupational, or driving difficulty. These include alcohol-related blackouts, a single drunk driving arrest, arguments with friends, and so on. This prevalent alcohol-related morbidity, however, is temporary and a separate problem from alcoholism. The following sections describe diagnostic criteria for alcoholism, offer suggestions for identifying the usual (i.e., middle-class) alcoholic in everyday medical practice, review evidence that alcoholism is a biologic and genetically influenced disorder, and offer advice on confrontation, detoxification, and rehabilitation of alcoholics.

DEFINITIONS AND EPIDEMIOLOGY The original version of the Third Diagnostic and Statistical Manual of the American Psychiatric Association (DSM-III) divides alcoholism into alcohol abuse and alcohol dependence, but this distinction may not be clinically relevant. *Alcohol abuse* indicates psychological dependence, i.e., the need for alcohol for adequate functioning, along with occasional heavy consumption, and continuation of drinking despite social or occupational problems. *Alcohol dependence* encompasses similar impairment *along* *with* evidence of increased ethanol tolerance or physical signs on withdrawal from alcohol.

A modified approach to a definition of alcoholism is easier to apply in clinical settings. The diagnosis of *alcoholism* is made when an individual ignores the early warning signs that alcohol is causing problems in marriage and goes on to an alcohol-related marital separation or divorce; *or* when alcohol-related problems on the job actually result in the patient being fired or laid off; *or* when there are two or more arrests related to alcohol; *or* when there is physical evidence that alcohol has harmed health (e.g., cardiomyopathy, cirrhosis, alcoholic hepatitis), including signs of alcoholic withdrawal.

It is important to distinguish between *primary and secondary alcoholism*. For example, serious alcohol-related problems occurring during the course of mania or a preexisting antisocial personality disorder (i.e., secondary alcoholism) might be symptomatic of the primary diagnosis, and the course is likely to be that of the primary disorder, not alcoholism. The information on alcoholism offered in this chapter is relevant for *primary alcoholism*. This diagnosis applies to the majority of alcoholics (70 to 80 percent) who develop major life problems from alcohol *before* they fulfill criteria for any other major psychiatric illness.

Using this or similar criteria, the lifetime risk for primary alcoholism in most western countries is about 10 percent for men and 3 to 5 percent for women. Alcoholism is seen in all races, ethnic groups, and socioeconomic strata and, therefore, the average alcoholic (just as the average person) is a blue-collar or white-collar worker or housewife. The homeless or skid row alcoholic represents only 5 percent or less of alcoholics.

GENETICS OF ALCOHOLISM There is strong evidence that alcoholism is a multifactorial disorder in which biologic and genetic factors interact. The importance of genetic factors in alcoholism is supported by family, twin, and adoption studies. Close relatives of primary alcoholics have an approximate fourfold increased risk for the disorder but are not significantly more vulnerable for other psychiatric illnesses. The probability that the familial nature of the problem is in part a consequence of genetic factors is supported by twin research, where the risk for the identical twin of an alcoholic is about 60 percent while the concordance rate for fraternal twins is only about 30 percent. Finally, adoption studies reveal that the fourfold increased risk for children of alcoholics is true even if they were adopted away at birth and raised without knowledge of the problems of their biologic parents.

The evidence supporting genetic influences in alcoholism has stimulated numerous studies of children of alcoholics. The goal is to identify possible trait markers of a vulnerability toward the disorder before alcoholism appears. For example, some studies suggest that these children become significantly less intoxicated at a given blood alcohol concentration than do controls, even before alcoholism develops. After modest alcohol doses, the sons of alcoholics report less intense subjective feelings of intoxication, show less alcohol-related impairment in cognitive and psychomotor tests, and have less intense changes in prolactin and cortisol secretion than do controls. However, after heavy alcohol intake the differences between the two groups are less marked. These data may indicate that men at high future risk for alcoholism may be less able than controls to tell when they are beginning to become intoxicated. Taken as a whole these data underscore the probability that alcoholism is biologically influenced and not related to a lack of "moral fiber." It is not surprising that the average alcoholic may continue to work, has a family, and may be difficult to identify if the physician persists with old stereotypes.

NATURAL HISTORY For the "average" alcoholic, the age of first drink and first minor problems (e.g., an argument with a friend while drunk or an alcoholic blackout) are similar to those in the general population. However, by the mid to late twenties, most men and women moderate their drinking (perhaps learning from minor problems), whereas difficulties for alcoholics are likely to escalate, with the first major life problem from alcohol appearing in the late twenties to early forties. Once established, the course of alcoholism is likely to be one of exacerbations and remissions; the alcoholic becomes frightened when a problem develops and abstains for a period of days to months before experimenting with controlled drinking; this step almost inevitably results in escalation of drinking and problems. The course is not hopeless because a fifth or more achieve permanent abstinence without formal treatment or aid from self-help groups such as Alcoholics Anonymous (AA). However, should the alcoholic continue to drink, the life span is shortened by an average of 15 years with the leading causes of death, in decreasing order, being heart disease, cancer, accidents, and suicide.

IDENTIFICATION AND CONFRONTATION OF THE ALCOHOLIC The physician should recognize that any patient may have alcoholism and must therefore pay attention to physical findings and laboratory tests that are likely to be abnormal in the alcoholic. These include a high normal or slightly elevated MCV, γ-glutamyl transferase (GGT) (35 to 40 or more units), serum uric acid (greater than 7 mg/dL), and triglycerides (180 mg/dL or more). Mild and fluctuating levels of hypertension (e.g., 140/95), repeated infections such as pneumonia, and otherwise unexplained cardiac arrhythmias all suggest that the patient might be an alcoholic. Certain specific clinical findings also should raise suspicions, including cancer of the head and neck, esophagus, or cardia of the stomach as well as cirrhosis, unexplained hepatitis, pancreatitis, bilateral parotid gland swelling, and peripheral neuropathy.

Once the likelihood of alcoholism is established, only a few moments are needed to gather the history of alcohol-related life problems. The patient *and spouse* should be asked about patterns of accidents, marital difficulties, problems on the job, and driving-related difficulties, after which the role played by alcohol should be identified. All physicians should be able to take the time needed to gather such information. In addition, a simple 25-item form to be answered by the patient, the Michigan Alcohol Screening Test (MAST), or the CAGE questionnaire (see Ewing) are available to aid in identifying the alcoholic.

After an alcoholic is identified, he or she should be confronted with the diagnosis. The presenting complaint can be used as an entrée to the alcohol problem. For instance, the patient complaining of insomnia or hypertension could be told that these are clinically important symptoms and that laboratory tests and physical findings indicate that alcohol appears to have contributed to the complaints and is increasing the risk for further medical and psychological problems. The physician should share information about the course of alcoholism and explore possible avenues of attacking the problem.

The process of confrontation is rarely accomplished in one session. It is helpful to let patients know that they are responsible for their own actions and that the decision to quit drinking rests with them. For the person who refuses to stop drinking at the first confrontation, a logical step is to "keep the door open," establishing future meetings so that help is available as problems escalate. In the meantime the family may benefit from counseling or referral to self-help group such as Alanon (the Alcoholics Anonymous group for family members) and Alateen (for teenage children of alcoholics).

Those patients who refuse to stop but who want to "cut down" should be reminded that the average alcoholic successfully cuts back scores of times but that sooner or later drinking again escalates. The patient who refuses to stop might be offered a guideline of drinking no more than two drinks (4 oz of wine, 12 oz of beer, or 1.5 oz of 80-proof beverage amounts to one drink) in any 24-h period, but it is very unlikely that this will be effective for an extended period of time. This is another way of keeping the door open in the hope that the patient will return as drinking escalates.

TREATMENT OF THE ALCOHOL-RELATED WITHDRAWAL SYNDROME **The clinical syndrome** In the presence of ethanol-induced cellular tolerance, any sudden decrease in ethanol may lead to symptoms of withdrawal from the CNS-depressant effects. As with most syndromes, most patients do not develop every symptom and the usual clinical picture is mild. Features include a tremor of the hands (shakes or jitters); autonomic nervous sytem dysfunction such as mild increases in pulse, respiratory rate, and body temperature; insomnia, possibly accompanied by bad dreams; feelings of generalized anxiety or panic attacks; and gastrointestinal upset. Symptoms begin within 5 to 10 h of decreasing ethanol intake (addicted patients are likely to awaken in the morning with some signs of withdrawal), peak in intensity on day two or three, and disappear by day four or five. Anxiety, insomnia, and mild levels of autonomic dysfunction may persist for 6 months or more. These continuing phenomena may contribute to the tendency to return to drinking.

About 5 percent of alcoholics show evidence of severe withdrawal symptoms. These include a state of confusion sometimes accompanied by visual, tactile, or auditory hallucinations. These psychotic symptoms are likely to disappear as the mental state becomes clearer over a period of several days and are distinct from the chronic alcoholic auditory hallucinosis with a clear sensorium described earlier in this chapter. A small percentage of alcoholics also demonstrate one or two generalized seizures (''rum fits''), usually within 48 h of stopping drinking. These are rarely focal in nature (unless there is underlying neuropathology) and electroencephalographic abnormalities are mild and usually return to normal within several days. There is no evidence that withdrawal seizures represent ''latent'' epilepsy.

The diagnosis of delirium tremens (DTs) is made when the course progresses beyond the usual symptoms of withdrawal to include confusion (with associated delusions and hallucinations), severe agitation, and generalized seizures. The likelihood of developing severe withdrawal symptoms increases with concomitant infections or medical problems, a prior history of withdrawal seizures or DTs, and higher quantity and frequency of drinking. Most periods of severe withdrawal begin and end abruptly, rarely lasting longer than 3 to 5 days. The mortality risk is less than 5 percent but increases with preexisting medical illnesses or organ system failure.

Treatment of withdrawal The *first* and most important step is to perform a *thorough* physical examination in all alcoholics who are considering stopping drinking and in those patients who might be undergoing withdrawal. It is necessary to evaluate organ systems likely to be impaired by heavy drinking, including searching for evidence of liver failure, gastrointestinal bleeding, cardiac arrhythmia, and glucose or electrolyte imbalance.

The *second* step in treating withdrawal is to give patients adequate nutrition and rest. All patients should be administered multiple B vitamins, including 50 to 100 mg of thiamine daily for a week or more. Most patients enter withdrawal with normal levels of body water or mild levels of overhydration, and intravenous fluids should be avoided unless there is evidence of hypotension or a history of recent excessive bleeding, vomiting, or diarrhea. Usually medications can be administered orally.

The *third* step in treatment is to recognize the symptoms due to CNS dysfunctions caused by removal of the brain-depressant effect of ethanol. Symptoms can be alleviated by administering another CNS depressant and gradually decreasing the levels of the drug over a 3- to 5-day period. While many CNS depressants are effective, the *benzodiazepines* have the highest margin of safety and are, therefore, the preferred class of drugs in the treatment of alcohol withdrawal. Benzodiazepines with short half-lives (see Chap. 364) are especially useful for patients with serious liver impairment or evidence of preexisting encephalopathy or brain damage. On the other hand, short half-life benzodiazepines, e.g., oxazepam or lorazepam, result in rapidly changing drug blood levels; administration every 4 h is required to avoid abrupt fluctuations in blood levels that may increase the risk for seizures. Therefore, most clinicians use drugs with longer half-lives, like diazepam or chlordiazepoxide. The goal is to administer sufficient drug on day one to alleviate most of the symptoms of withdrawal and then to decrease the dose by 20 percent on successive days over a period of 3 to 5 days. The dose is increased if signs of withdrawal escalate, and the medication is withheld if the patient is sleeping or shows signs of increasing orthostatic hypotension. The average patient requires 25 to 50 mg of chlordiazepoxide or 10 mg of diazepam given orally every 4 to 6 h on the first day.

The most effective treatment of more *severe withdrawal* including delirium tremens remains controversial. Most clinicians use benzodiazepines, but despite as much as 300 mg or more per day of chlordiazepoxide the patient may still remain awake and agitated. Since it is probable that the confused, agitated state will persist for 3 to 5 days regardless of the pharmacologic intervention used, drugs are given to control behavior rather than to change the course of the syndrome. Antipsychotic medications like thioridazine or haloperidol have no place in the treatment of mild withdrawal symptoms and should only be used for treatment of psychotic patients with delusions and hallucinations.

The generalized seizures or ''rum fits'' rarely require aggressive pharmacologic intervention beyond that given to the usual patient undergoing withdrawal, i.e., adequate doses of benzodiazepines. There is little evidence that phenytoin is effective in drug withdrawal seizures, and the risk of seizures usually has passed by the time effective drug levels are reached. The rare patient with status epilepticus can be treated initially with intravenous diazepam. If anticonvulsants are used for alcohol withdrawal seizures, they should be stopped within 5 to 7 days unless a cause for a persisting seizure disorder is documented.

While alcohol withdrawal is usually treated in a hospital, efforts at reducing health care costs have resulted in experimentation with outpatient detoxification for alcoholics with mild abstinence syndromes. This is appropriate for patients in good physical condition who demonstrate mild signs of withdrawal despite low blood alcohol concentrations and for those without prior history of DTs or withdrawal seizures. Such individuals still require careful physical examination, evaluation of blood tests, treatment with vitamin supplementation, and appropriate doses of benzodiazepines. The latter are given *in a 1- to 2-day supply* to be administered to the patient by a spouse four times a day. Patients are asked to *return daily* for evaluation of vital signs, and the patient's family or friends are told to bring him or her to the emergency room if signs and symptoms of withdrawal escalate.

THE TREATMENT OR REHABILITATION OF ALCOHOLICS After completing alcoholic rehabilitation, 60 percent or more of middle-class alcoholics maintain abstinence for at least a year, many for a lifetime. There is no single best way to rehabilitate the alcoholic, and therapeutic approaches center on general supports which meet commonsense guidelines. Considering the lack of evidence for superiority of any specific treatment type, it is best to keep interventions as simple, safe, and inexpensive as possible.

Maneuvers in rehabilitation fall into two general categories. *First* are attempts to help the alcoholic achieve and maintain a high level of motivation toward abstinence. This includes educating the patient about alcoholism, educating family and/or friends to stop protecting the alcoholic from the problems caused by alcohol, and the use of disulfiram to help the physically healthy alcoholic avoid returning to drinking on the spur of the moment. The *second* series of maneuvers help the patient to readjust to life without alcohol and to reestablish a functional life-style through personal counseling, vocational rehabilitation, family support, and sexual counseling.

There is no convincing evidence that inpatient rehabilitation is more effective for the average primary alcoholic than is outpatient care. The decision to hospitalize can be made if (1) the patient has medical problems that are difficult to treat outside a hospital; (2) depression, confusion, or psychosis interfere with outpatient care; (3) the patient has such a severe life crisis that it is difficult to get his or her attention as an outpatient; (4) outpatient treatment has failed; or (5) the patient lives too far from the treatment center. If inpatient care is needed, free-standing treatment programs, units that are divisions of general hospitals, and those in psychiatric hospitals are equally effective. The characteristics of the patient predict outcome more than any specific attribute of the program.

Whether the treatment begins in an inpatient or an outpatient setting, subsequent contact should be maintained for a minimum of 6 months after abstinence is achieved. Counseling with an individual physician or through groups focuses on day-to-day living—emphasizing areas of improved functioning in the absence of alcohol (i.e., why it is a good idea to continue to abstain) and helping the patient to deal with free time without alcohol, develop a nondrinking peer group, and handle stresses on the job without alcohol.

The physician serves an important role in identifying the alcoholic, treating medical or psychiatric syndromes associated with alcoholism, carrying out detoxification, referring to rehabilitation programs, and counseling alcoholics in an inpatient or outpatient setting. The physician must also regulate drug treatment during alcoholism rehabilitation. Once acute detoxification is complete (an average of 3 to 5 days), there is *no place* for hypnotics or antianxiety drugs in the treatment of most alcoholics. The patient has already demonstrated an inability to moderate the use of one brain depressant, alcohol, and is at considerable risk for abusing sleeping pills or tranquilizers. Anxiety and insomnia can be treated with behavior modification such as relaxation training, meditation, and exercise or through increased activity in hobbies or religion.

One medication which has been used in alcohol rehabilitation is disulfiram. This drug inhibits aldehyde dehydrogenase, causing very high levels of acetaldehyde to accumulate after alcohol is consumed. The height and timing of the acetaldehyde level (usually peaking $\frac{1}{2}$ h after drinking) depend upon the dose of ethanol and its rate of intake. The disulfiram-ethanol reaction includes tremor, hypertension or hypotension, nausea and possibly severe vomiting, and diarrhea. Disulfiram must not be given to persons for whom such a reaction could be dangerous, including patients with portal hypertension, diabetes mellitus, heart disease, or a history of stroke. For healthy individuals for whom no contraindication for disulfiram exists, patients can be given 250 mg per day, with instructions to take the medication at the same time daily, preferably in the presence of someone else, so that there can be no "forgetting" to take the drug. There are no data about how long disulfiram should be continued, but many experienced physicians suggest giving the drug for a period of 6 to 12 months. All drugs have their dangers, and the physician is advised to read carefully about disulfiram and be fully aware of the potential, although rare, serious adverse reactions that can occur. Many physicians experienced in the treatment of alcoholics now aovid its use entirely or prescribe it for only short periods of time. Patients should be warned of the dangers of taking disulfiram and should sign a form acknowledging that mixing disulfiram with ethanol can result in a lethal reaction.

Finally, an inexpensive, readily available, and dedicated additional support for all alcoholics is available in almost every community. Alcoholics Anonymous (AA) is a self-help group of recovering alcoholics (men and women who have stopped drinking, perhaps many years ago) which offers an effective model showing that abstinence can be achieved, provides a sober peer group, and makes crisis intervention available when the drive to drink escalates. No matter what type of rehabilitation program is planned, the alcoholic should be offered the option of joining Alcoholics Anonymous.

REFERENCES

Adams KM, Grant I: Failure of nonlinear models of drinking history variables to predict neuropsychological performance in alcoholics. Am J Psychiatry 141:663, 1984

Altura BM (ed): Alcohol, stroke, hypertension, and the heart. Proceedings of the Symposium of the American Medical Society on Alcoholism, April 13, 1984. Alc: Clin Exp Res 1:319, 1984

Blass JP, Gibson GE: Abnormality of a thiamine-requiring enzyme in patients with Wernicke-Korsakoff syndrome. N Engl J Med 297:1367, 1977

Brandt J et al: Cognitive loss and recovery in long-term alcohol abusers. Arch Gen Psychiat 40:435, 1983

Cicero TJ: Neuroendocrinological effects of alcohol. Ann Rev Med 32:123, 1981

Deykin D, Janson P: Ethanol potentiation of aspirin-induced prolongation of the bleeding time. N Engl J Med 306:852, 1982

Dreyfus PM: Diseases of the nervous system in chronic alcoholics, in *The Biology of Alcoholism*, B Kissin, H Begleiter (eds). New York, Plenum, 1974, vol 3 p 265

Ewing JA: Detecting alcoholism. JAMA 252:1905, 1984

Frank D, Raicht RF: Alcohol-induced liver disease. Alc: Clin Exp Res 9:66, 1985

Geokas MC: Ethanol, the liver, and the gastrointestinal tract. Ann Intern Med 95:198, 1981

Goldstein DB: *Pharmacology of Alcohol*. New York, Oxford University Press, 1983

Goodwin DW, Guze SB: *Psychiatric Diagnosis*, 2nd ed. New York, Oxford University Press, 1979

Greenspon AJ, Schaal SF: The "holiday heart": Electrophysiologic studies of alcohol effects in alcoholics. Ann Intern Med 98:135, 1983

Haglund RMJ, Schuckit MA: The epidemiology of alcoholism, in *Alcoholism: Development, Consequences, and Intervention*, N Estes et al (eds). St. Louis, Mosby, 1981

Lieber C: *Metabolic Aspects of Alcoholism*. Lancaster, England, MTP Press, 1977

———: To drink (moderately) or not to drink? N Engl J Med 310:846, 1984

Lishman WA: Cerebral disorder in alcoholism: Syndromes of impairment. Brain 104:1, 1981

Meagher RC et al: Suppression of hematopoietic-progenitor-cell proliferation by ethanol and acetaldehyde. N Engl J Med 307:845, 1982

Mello NK, Bree MP: Alcohol self-administration disrupts reproductive function in female macaque monkeys. Science 221:677, 1983

Mendelson JH, Mello NK: Biologic concomitants of alcoholism. N Engl J Med 301:912, 1979

Potter JF, Beevers DG: Pressor effect of alcohol in hypertension. Lancet: 1:119, 1984

Schuckit MA: Genetic and clinical implications of alcoholism and affective disorder. Am J Psychiatry 143:140, 1986

———: *Drug and Alcohol Abuse: A Clinical Guide to Diagnosis and Treatment*, 2d ed. New York, Plenum, 1984

———: Studies of populations at high risk for alcoholism. Psychiatr Dev 3:31, 1985

———: Genetics and the risk for alcoholism. JAMA 254:2614, 1985

Sellers EM, Kalant H: Alcohol intoxication and withdrawal. N Engl J Med 294:757, 1976

Streissguth AP, Landesman-Dwyer S: Teratogenic effects of alcohol in humans and laboratory animals. Science 209:353, 1980

Vaillant GE: *The Natural History of Alcoholism*. Cambridge, Mass., Harvard, 1983

Van Thiel DH: Gastrointestinal and hepatic manifestations of chronic alcoholism. Gastroenterology 81:594, 1981

Victor M et al: *The Wernicke-Korsakoff Syndrome*. Philadelphia, Davis, 1971

366 OPIOID DRUG USE

MARC A. SCHUCKIT / DAVID S. SEGAL

The principal effects of the opioids (opiate-like drugs) are a significant damping of pain perception along with modest levels of sedation and euphoria. Tolerance to any one drug is likely to generalize to the others (i.e., cross-tolerance is likely) and all share a similar pattern of drug-related problems. Each of these substances is capable of producing physical addiction (and thus they all have some legal restrictions), and the abstinence syndrome from any one of the substances can be treated with administration of any of the others.

PHARMACOLOGY The prototypic opiates, morphine and codeine (3-methoxymorphine), are taken directly from the milky juice of the poppy, *Papaver somniferum*. The semisynthetic drugs produced from the morphine or thebane molecules include hydromorphone, codeine, diacetylmorphine (heroin), and oxycodone. The purely synthetic opioids, sharing many of the basic properties of opium and morphine, include meperidine, propoxyphene, diphenoxylate, methadone, and pentazocine. Despite claims to the contrary, all of these substances (including almost all prescription analgesics) are capable of producing euphoria as well as psychological and physical dependence when taken in high enough doses over prolonged periods of time.

The opioids interact with opiate receptors throughout the body including the central nervous system (CNS). Endogenous opioid peptides (i.e., enkephalins, endorphins, and dynorphin) have been identified. These appear to be natural ligands for opiate receptors and possess many of the same pharmacologic properties as the opiate alkaloids. Substances capable of antagonizing some actions of both the endogenous and exogenous opioids include nalorphine, levallorphan, cyclazocine and pentazocine, each of which have mixed agonist and antagonist properties, as well as naloxone and naltrexone, which are pure opiate antagonists. Mixed agonist-antagonist drugs, for example pentazocine, if administered to a patient addicted to other narcotics may precipitate opiate withdrawal symptoms.

Opiate tolerance, dependence, and withdrawal are considered to be related phenomena with common underlying mechanisms. A number of neurochemical systems and psychological processes are implicated in these effects which emerge with chronic administration of morphine or related opiates. Among the possible biochemical mechanisms, the endogenous opioid system has received the most attention. The results of this research to date have been somewhat disappointing; there is little consistent evidence for changes in opioid receptors or in the levels of endogenous opioid peptides corresponding to the development of tolerance and dependence. The discrepant findings may reflect methodologic differences as well as the complexity introduced by the apparent multiplicity of the opioid systems and the difficulties in accurately measuring indices of the activity of these peptides (i.e., turnover and biosynthesis). Other biochemical systems that might contribute to the development of tolerance and dependence include changes in intracellular modulators such as adenyl nucleotides, calcium and related substances, as well as alterations in neurotransmitters, including acetylcholine, serotonin, and the catecholamines, norepinephrine and dopamine. Evidence also implicates environmental and learning factors. For example, clinical observations suggest that classic conditioning plays a role in maintaining dependence in at least some addicts and that conditioning extinction procedures may be useful when integrated into a comprehensive treatment program for opioid addiction. Further research into these phenomena and efforts to elucidate neurochemical mechanisms could significantly facilitate the development of more effective approaches to treatment and prevention.

All of the opioid drugs are easily absorbed from the gastrointestinal (GI) system, the lungs, and the muscles. The most rapid and pronounced effects occur following intravenous administration, and the least intense actions are seen after absorption from the digestive tract, at least in part because some of the oral drug is metabolized before it passes into the general circulation. Most of the metabolism of opiates occurs in the liver, primarily through conjugation with glucuronic acid, and only small amounts are excreted directly in the urine or feces. The plasma half-lives of these drugs range from 2.5 to 3 h for morphine to more than 22 h for methadone and even longer for methadyl acetate.

Street heroin typically contains only 5 to 10 percent of the opiate. The remainder consists of materials such as lactose and fruit sugars, quinine, powdered milk, phenacetin, caffeine, antipyrine, and strychnine which are used to "cut" the drug and increase the margin of profit.

THE ACUTE AND CHRONIC EFFECTS OF OPIOID DRUGS ON BODY SYSTEMS With the exception of overdose conditions and changes associated with physical addiction, most opiate actions are relatively benign and rapidly reversible.

Effects on body systems Acute changes in the *GI system* are the result of decreased GI motility with resulting constipation and anorexia. Chronic GI problems in opiate addicts typically occur as a consequence of impaired liver function resulting from concomitant administration of other drugs and from the development of hepatitis B from shared "dirty" needles.

The direct effects on opiate receptors in the *CNS* can result in nausea and vomiting (medulla), decreased pain perception (spinal cord, thalamus, and periaqueductal grey region), euphoria (limbic system), and sedation (reticular activating system and striatum). The adulterants added to street drugs may contribute to some of the more permanent nervous system damage, including peripheral neuropathy, amblyopia, myelopathy, and leucoencephalopathy, while use of contaminated needles can produce abscesses in the CNS. Acute opiate administration results in decreases in luteinizing hormone (LH), with a subsequent decrease in testosterone which might contribute to the decreased sex drive reported by most opiate addicts. Other hormonal changes include a decrease in the release of thyrotropin as well as increases in prolactin and possibly in growth hormone (see Chap. 321).

Acute changes in the *respiratory system* include respiratory depression, which results from a decreased response of the brainstem to carbon dioxide tension, a component of the drug overdose syndrome described below. At even low drug doses, this effect can be clinically significant in individuals with compromised lung activity. *Cardiovascular* changes tend to be relatively mild with no direct opiate effect on heart rhythm or myocardial contractility, but there is a potential problem from orthostatic hypotension, probably secondary to dilatation of peripheral vessels. Bacterial infections of both the lungs and heart valves can occur from contaminated needles.

The toxic reaction or overdose syndrome High doses of opiates taken intentionally (in a suicide attempt) or by the street user who has misjudged the potency of the injected substance can result in a toxic reaction or overdose syndrome with a potentially lethal consequence. The typical syndrome, which occurs immediately with intravenous (IV) overdose, includes shallow respirations of two to four per minute, pupillary miosis (with mydriasis once brain anoxia develops), bradycardia, a decrease in body temperature, and a general absence of responsiveness to external stimulation. If this medical emergency is not treated rapidly, symptoms can progress to cyanosis, and death can ensue from respiratory depression and cardiorespiratory arrest. Postmortem examination reveals few specific changes except for diffuse cerebral edema. An "allergic-like" reaction to adulterants can also occur and is characterized by decreased alertness, a frothy pulmonary edema, and an elevation in the blood eosinophil count.

The preferred treatment for the typical opiate overdose is the narcotic antagonist naloxone, given in an initial dose of 0.4 mg (1 mL) or 0.01 mg/kg intramuscularly (IM) or IV, which can be repeated in 3 to 10 min if no response occurs. Because the effects of this drug diminish within 2 to 3 h, it is important to monitor the individual for at least 24 h after a heroin overdose and 72 h after an overdose of longer-acting drugs such as methadone. Patients who are also physically addicted to an opioid are likely to experience a precipitous onset of an abstinence syndrome within 2 to 8 h after administration of the opioid antagonist, but aggressive treatment of this syndrome is not appropriate until all vital signs are relatively stable.

As with any drug overdose, treatment of either the typical or the "allergic" type of opiate toxic reaction often requires support of vital signs until the body detoxifies the substance. Patients may require a respirator (especially one using oxygen and positive pressure breathing for the "allergic" type of overdose), IV fluids perhaps accompanied by pressor agents to support blood pressure, and gastric lavage to remove any remaining drug, with care taken to use a cuffed endotracheal tube to prevent aspiration if the patient is not alert. Cardiac arrhythmias and/or convulsions, especially likely to be seen with codeine, propoxyphene, or meperidine, also need to be treated.

THE OPIATE ABUSER The medical abuser Two groups of individuals are at high risk for abusing analgesics. First, evidence suggests that a majority of people with *chronic pain syndromes* (e.g., back, joint, and muscle disorders) may misuse their prescribed drugs at various times. If physical dependence is established, abstinence syndromes can then intensify the pain, promoting continued drug intake. A few precautions can help the physician to avoid contributing to physical dependence in chronic pain patients, particularly those who have demonstrated a propensity to misuse opioids: (1) the goal is to minimize the debilitating effects of pain with the understanding that discomfort may not be completely eliminated; (2) all possible efforts must be taken to reinforce the need for the patient to become actively involved in and committed to improvement; (3) analgesic medication should be only one component of treatment and limited to oral administration of the least potent analgesic required to take the "edge off" the pain (e.g., propoxyphene); all such drugs should be coordinated through one physician; (4) behavior modification techniques can include muscle relaxation and meditation, while carefully selected exercises can help increase function and decrease pain; (5) nonmedicinal approaches including electrical transcutaneous neurostimulation for muscle and joint disease can be applied (see also Chap. 3).

The second group at high risk are *physicians, nurses, and pharmacists,* primarily because of their easy access to substances of abuse. Physicians may begin to use opiates to help them sleep or to reduce stress or physical aches and pains. A family history of substance abuse (including alcoholism) probably helps to identify the physician at exceptionally high risk. Because of the growing awareness of these problems, impaired physician programs have been established in many hospitals and by most state medical societies. These groups attempt to identify and aid substance-impaired physicians, giving them peer support and education so as to achieve abstinence before problems escalate to the point of licensure revocation. In general, doctors are advised to never prescribe opiates for themselves or for members of their family—physicians deserve the same level of care and protection from future problems as their patients.

The street abuser Some opiate addicts satisfy criteria for the antisocial personality disorder as evidenced by serious antisocial problems beginning prior to age 15 and before the first major life problem from drugs (see Chap. 363). However, the majority of opiate addicts have a relatively high level of premorbid functioning. The usual street abuser begins using opiates occasionally, often after experimenting with tobacco, then alcohol, then marijuana, and then brain depressants or stimulants. Occasional opiate use, or "chipping," might continue for some time, and some individuals probably never escalate their intake to the point of developing serious problems. Another pattern of temporary or intermittent abuse is represented by the experiences of Vietnam soldiers, most of whom had little or no prior experience with opiates and who found themselves in a situation of high stress and readily available drugs. Under these circumstances, as many as one-half tried opiates and, although many became physically addicted, those who had not misused drugs before Vietnam tended to return to drug-free status when back in their home communities.

Once persistent opiate use is established, the outcome is often extremely serious. At least 25 percent of such opiate abusers are likely to die within 10 to 20 years of active abuse, with death from suicide, homicide, accidents, and infectious diseases such as tuberculosis or serum hepatitis. As many as 50 percent of male and 25 percent of female addicts turn to alcohol when their primary drug is not available, and many of these people meet the criteria for secondary alcohol abuse. The prevalence of alcohol misuse is higher in drug treatment dropouts than in those who stay with therapy, and abuse is more likely in individuals with a history of alcohol problems before they developed opiate-related difficulties.

PHYSICAL ADDICTION AND THE OPIATE ABSTINENCE SYNDROME **The symptoms of withdrawal** The time to onset as well as the intensity and duration of the acute abstinence syndrome are influenced by a number of factors including the drugs' half-life, its dose, and the chronicity of administration. The withdrawal symptoms tend to be opposite to the acute effects of the drug and include nausea and diarrhea, coughing, lacrimation, rhinorrhea, profuse sweating, twitching muscles, and piloerection or "goose bumps"; mild elevations in body temperature, respiratory rate, and blood pressure are also observed. In addition, sensations of diffuse body pain, insomnia, and yawning occur with intense drug craving. Drugs with a short half-life, such as morphine or heroin, cause symptoms typically within 8 to 16 h of the last dose (thus, many addicts awake in mild withdrawal every morning); peak effects are apparent within 36 to 72 h after discontinuation of the drug, and the acute syndrome disappears within 5 to 8 days. However, a protracted abstinence phase of mild symptoms (e.g., slight changes in pupillary size, autonomic dysfunction, changes in sleep pattern) may persist for 6 or more months.

Treatment of the withdrawal syndrome Patients *must* receive a thorough physical examination which includes an assessment of liver and neurologic function as well as identification of local and systemic infections, especially abscesses. Proper nutrition and rest must be initiated as soon as possible.

Effective treatment of withdrawal, however, also requires readministration of sufficient opiate medication on day one to decrease symptoms, followed by a more gradual withdrawal of the drug, usually over 5 to 10 days. Any opiate will work (they all have some level of cross-tolerance) but for ease of administration many physicians prefer to use a long-acting drug like methadone. In estimating the first day's dose from the patient's history, 1 mg of methadone is approximately equivalent to 3 mg of morphine, 1 mg of heroin, or 20 mg of meperidine. Most patients require between 10 and 25 mg of methadone orally given twice on day one, with higher doses given if prominent symptoms of withdrawal are not damped. After several days of a stabilized drug dose, the opiate is then decreased by 10 to 20 percent of the original day's dose each day.

Most states have restrictions on the prescription of opiates to addicts, and in the absence of special permits, detoxification with opiates is usually limited to 1 month or less. One relatively successful nonopiate approach to the treatment of withdrawal is the use of the alpha$_2$-adrenergic agonist, clonidine, used in part to decrease sympathetic nervous system overactivity. Given at doses of approximately 5 μg/kg (up to 0.3 mg given two to four times a day), clonidine causes most patients undergoing opiate withdrawal to experience a decrease in autonomic nervous system dysfunction. Opiates, however, are more effective in relieving discomfort and pain, and clonidine is often not well tolerated because it produces high levels of sedation and orthostatic hypotension. Therefore, under most circumstances opiates are the treatment of choice.

A special case of opiate withdrawal is seen in the newborn, passively addicted by the mother's drug misuse during pregnancy. Some level of addiction develops in 50 to 90 percent of children of heroin-dependent mothers, and the withdrawal syndrome carries a mortality of between 3 and 30 percent if not treated when prominent signs are apparent. In distinction to street addicts, as few as 25 percent of infants of methadone-maintenance-addicted mothers show clinically relevant withdrawal symptoms. The syndrome consists of irritability, crying, a tremor (in 80 percent), increased reflexes, increased respiratory rate, diarrhea, hyperactivity (in 60 percent), vomiting (40 percent), and sneezing/yawning/hiccuping (in 30 percent). The child usually has a low birth weight but may be otherwise unremarkable until the second day, when symptoms are likely to begin.

The treatment follows the same general steps used in the treatment of the physically addicted adult. The child must be carefully evaluated to rule out medical problems such as hypoglycemia, hypocalcemia, infections, and trauma; general supports in a warm, quiet environment and regulation of electrolytes and glucose are also required. The infant with moderate to severe symptoms can be treated with any of the following: paregoric (0.2 mL orally every 3 to 4 h); methadone, (0.1 to 0.5 mg/kg per day); phenobarbital (8 mg/kg per day); or diazepam (1 to 2 mg/kg every 8 h). Medication should be given in decreasing levels for 10 to 20 days. It is also possible to treat the addicted infants of mothers on methadone maintenance by having them breast feed while the mothers continue to take methadone.

REHABILITATION OF OPIATE ADDICTS Despite some differences in demographics, the same general rules for rehabilitation apply to the opiate abuser and to the alcoholic. The basic strategy includes beginning detoxification and general family support. It is also important to establish realistic patient goals and a program of counseling and education to increase motivation toward abstinence. A long-term commitment to rebuilding a life-style without the substance is essential for preventing recidivism.

Identifying and confronting the patient The first step in treatment requires identification of the opiate abuser—an especially difficult problem with the middle-class street abuser and the medical patient or physician with an iatrogenic addiction. An important step is to gather a clinical history which includes the patterns of opiate usage, information regarding the possible existence of an antisocial personality disorder, or a history of chronic pain. Blood and urine screens can be used to identify opiates in patients in whom misuse is suspected, and clinicians should search for physical stigmata of misuse (e.g., needle marks). One potentially important diagnostic procedure (which should be used carefully because it can precipitate an intense withdrawal) is the opiate antagonist challenge. A 0.4 mg dose of naloxone is given subcutaneously or slowly IV over a 5-min period, and the patient is observed for signs of withdrawal over the next several hours. This challenge test should only be carried out in the presence of a physician and it is important to be prepared to begin treating withdrawal if needed.

After identifying the opiate addict, the next step is confrontation. The need for active treatment of the abstinence syndrome can be presented, and the availability of help in establishing a drug-free life-style can be emphasized. The final decision, of course, rests with the patient.

Rehabilitation Most rehabilitation approaches have common elements. Patients are educated about their responsibility for improving their lives and *motivation for abstinence* is increased by providing information about the medical and psychological problems that can be expected if addiction continues. Patients and families are helped to *establish an opiate-free life-style* by being educated about dealing with chronic pain and developing realistic vocational planning (e.g., this applies to pharmacists, physicians, and nurses). The addict should also be encouraged to establish a drug-free peer group and to participate in self-help groups such as Narcotics Anonymous (NA). Much of this advice and counseling can be given by the physician, but many clinicians refer patients to more formal drug programs, including methadone maintenance clinics, programs using narcotic antagonists, and therapeutic communities. Long-term follow-up of treated patients shows that approximately one-third of addicts are completely drug free in the year before the follow-up interview, and that a total of 60 percent are off opiates, although some may be abusing other substances. Individuals who stay in methadone maintenance or in therapeutic communities show significant decreases in police and social problems and increases in job functioning. In general, the best prognosis for rehabilitation is for those who are employed, who have higher levels of school completion, and who remain in treatment for at least 2 months.

METHADONE MAINTENANCE Methadone and methadyl acetate maintenance should only be used along with education and counseling. It is important to note that drug maintenance is not aimed at "curing" opiate addiction; rather it provides a substitute drug that is legally accessible. The goal is to help the addict who has failed in drug-free programs to improve functioning within the family and job, to decrease legal problems, and to improve health.

Methadone is a long-acting opiate that possesses almost all the physiologic properties of heroin. The addict who has been carefully screened to rule out prior psychiatric disorders may be maintained on a relatively low dose (e.g., 30 to 40 mg per day); a higher dosage schedule (100 to 120 mg per day) can also be used and may be more effective in blocking heroin-induced euphoria. Although the results are not definite, there is some evidence that the higher methadone doses may result in greater retention in treatment and consequently lower levels of arrest and readdiction to street drugs. Methadone is administered in an oral liquid given once a day at the program center, with weekend portions taken by the patient at home. The longer acting analogues, such as methadyl acetate, can be given in lower doses (e.g., 20 to 30 mg) two or three times a week, with levels increased to as high as 80 mg three times a week if needed.

After a period of maintenance (usually 6 months to 1 year or longer), the clinician should work closely with the patient to regulate the rate of drug decrease (by about 5 percent per week). The British have used heroin maintenance with similar goals and following similar guidelines as those used for methadone. There is no evidence that heroin maintenance has any advantages over methadone maintenance, but the heroin approach does add the risk that the drug will be sold on the streets.

OPIATE ANTAGONISTS The opiate antagonists (e.g., naloxone) compete with heroin and other opiates for opioid receptors, reducing the effects of the opiate agonists. Administered over long periods of time in order to block the "high" produced if the patient takes opiates, these drugs can be useful as part of an overall treatment approach which includes counseling and support. Cyclazocine was the first antagonist tested, but its blockade of receptors is incomplete and the level of side effects (including a drunken feeling) are unacceptable. Naloxone is an excellent narcotic antagonist with no agonistic properties, but it has such a short period of action (2 to 3 h) that it is of little use in rehabilitation. The most widely used antagonist in rehabilitation is naltrexone, which is effective for about 24 h with few side effects. An amount of 50 mg of naltrexone per day will block 15 mg of heroin for 24 h, and higher doses (125 to 150 mg) are capable of blocking the effects of 25 mg of IV heroin for up to 3 days. Naltrexone is free of agonist properties, there are no known withdrawal symptoms when the medication is stopped, and side effects tend to be mild. Patients started on this antagonist should be free of opiates for a minimum of 5 days. In addition they must be given a thorough physical examination and should be challenged with 0.4 or 0.8 mg of the shorter-acting naloxone to be certain that they are able to tolerate the long-acting antagonist. Following this procedure, a test dose of 10 mg of naltrexone can be given, with the expectation that any withdrawal symptoms will be seen in ½ to 2 h. Over the next 10 days, the daily dose should be increased to about 100 mg on Mondays and Wednesdays and 150 mg on Fridays. Unfortunately, despite the apparent advantages of this treatment approach, patients demonstrate great resistance to continuing care. In one study, only about 60 percent of the patients completed 6 days of naltrexone induction, and only 10 percent remained in the program at the end of 6 months.

DRUG-FREE PROGRAMS Most existing half-way houses and recovery centers for the opiate abuser utilize the therapeutic community (TC) approach. This is an exception to the general preference for short-term inpatient rehabilitation, as care lasts up to a year while the addict is taken out of the street culture and given a new life within the group. In this structure members, including addict leaders, frequently confront participants in an attempt to help them gain insights into more successful life-styles for coping with problems.

REFERENCES

CHARNEY DS et al: The clinical use of clonidine in abrupt withdrawal from methadone. Arch Gen Psychiat 38:1273, 1981

CROUGHAN JL et al: Alcoholism and alcohol dependence in narcotic addicts: A prospective study with a five-year follow-up. Am J Drug Alcohol Abuse 8:85, 1981

CROWLEY T et al: Naltrexone-induced dysphoria in former opioid addicts. Am J Psychiatry142:1081, 1985

GREENSTEIN RA et al: Naltrexone: A short-term treatment of opiate dependence. Am J Drug Alcohol Abuse 8:291, 1981

HARTNOLL RL et al: Evaluation of heroin maintenance in controlled trial. Arch Gen Psychiat 37:877, 1980

JAFFE JH, MARTIN WR: Opiate analgesics and antagonists, in *The Pharmacological Basis of Therapeutics,* AG Gilman et al (eds). New York, Macmillan, 1980, pp 494–534

JASINSKI D et al: Clonidine in morphine withdrawal. Arch Gen Psychiat 42:1063, 1985

KLEBER HK, RIORDAN CE: The treatment of narcotic withdrawal: A historical review. J Clin Psychiatry 43:30 1982

MCCUE JD: The effects of stress on physicians and their medical practice. N Engl J Med 306:458, 1982

MIRIN SM et al: Opiate use and sexual function. Am J Psychiatry 137:909, 1980

O'BRIEN CP, WOODY GE: Long-term consequences of opiate dependence. N Engl J Med 304:1098, 1981

O'BRIEN CP et al: Classical conditioning is opiate dependence, in *Problems of Drug Dependence,* LS Harris (ed). NIDA Research, Monograph 49, pp 35–46. Washington, DC, US Government Printing Office, 1984

OLIVERIO A et al: Psychobiology of opioids. Int Rev Neurobiol 25:277, 1984

REDMOND DE JR, KRYSTAL JH: Multiple mechanisms of withdrawal from opioid drugs. Annu Rev Neurosci 7:443, 1984

Rounsaville BJ et al: Identifying alcoholism in treated opiate addicts. Am J Psychiatry 140:764, 1983
Schuckit MA: *Drug and Alcohol Abuse: A Clinical Guide to Diagnosis and Treatment*, 2d ed. New York, Plenum, 1984
Simon E: Recent studies on opioid receptors: Heterogeneity and isolation, in *Problems of Drug Dependence*, LS Harris (ed). NIDA Research Monograph 49, pp 5–13. Washington, DC, US Government Printing Office, 1984
Simpson DD et al: Six-year follow-up of opioid addicts after admission to treatment. Arch Gen Psychiat 39:1318, 1982
Vaillant GE: A 20-year follow-up of New York narcotic addicts. Arch Gen Psychiat 29:237, 1973
Wallot H, Lambert J: Characteristics of physician addicts. Am J Drug Alcohol Abuse 10:53, 1984

367 COMMONLY ABUSED DRUGS

JACK H. MENDELSON / NANCY K. MELLO

Drug abuse in America appears to be an increasing public health problem. In 1984, the largest and most comprehensive survey of noninstitutionalized persons in the United States (the National Institute of Mental Health's Epidemiologic Catchment Area Surveys) showed that drug abuse and dependence was the third most frequently reported psychiatric disorder by men aged 18 to 65. Among young women (aged 18 to 24), drug abuse was the second most frequent psychiatric disorder. The initiation and continuation of drug abuse is determined by a complex interaction of the pharmacologic properties and relative availability of each drug, the personality and expectancy of the user, and the environmental context in which the drug is used. Over the years, drugs of choice have changed; marijuana superceded heroin as the focus of drug abuse concern during the 1970s while expensive "boutique" drugs such as cocaine have achieved extraordinary popularity and widespread abuse during the 1980s.

Polydrug abuse, the concurrent use of several drugs with different pharmacologic effects, is increasingly common among individuals from all socioeconomic strata. Sometimes the goal is to attenuate one drug effect with another, e.g., alcohol is used to modulate the cocaine "high," sometimes one drug is used to enhance the effects of another, as with benzodiazepines and methadone. Toxic drug interactions associated with polydrug abuse are likely to further increase the health impact of drug abuse. This chapter discusses marijuana, cocaine, two hallucinogens (PCP and LSD), and polydrug abuse.

MARIJUANA AND CANNABIS COMPOUNDS *Cannabis sativa* contains over 400 compounds in addition to the psychoactive substance, delta-9-tetrahydrocannabinol (THC). Marijuana cigarettes are prepared from the leaves and flowering tops of the plant, and a typical marijuana cigarette contains 0.5 to 1 g of plant material. Although the usual THC concentration varies between 5 and 20 mg, concentrations as high as 100 mg per cigarette have been detected. Hashish is prepared from concentrated resin of *Cannabis sativa* and contains a THC concentration of between 8 to 12 percent by weight. "Hash oil," a lipid-soluble plant extract, may contain a THC concentration of 25 to 60 percent, and it may be added to marijuana or hashish to enhance their THC concentration. Smoking is the most common mode of marijuana or hashish self-administration. During pyrolysis, over 150 compounds in addition to the THC are released in the smoke. Although most of these compounds do not have psychoactive properties, they do have potential physiologic effects.

THC is quickly absorbed from the lungs into blood and is then rapidly sequestered in tissues. It is metabolized primarily in the liver where it is converted to 11-hydroxy-THC, a psychoactive compound, and more than 20 other metabolites. Most THC metabolites are excreted through the feces at a rate of clearance that is relatively slow in comparison to that of most other psychoactive drugs.

Prevalance of marijuana use A 1983 National Household Survey on Drug Abuse indicated that 64 percent of young adults (aged 18 to 25) stated that they used marijuana. This represents a 59 percent increase in marijuana use over a decade; in 1972, a similar survey found that only 5 percent of young adults had tried the drug. The rate of increase in marijuana use by males appeared to have stabilized by 1985 but marijuana use among women continues to increase. A recent detailed evaluation of social and behavioral concomitants of marijuana use (published in 1984) found that young marijuana users also reported significant use of other psychoactive substances and are likely to become polydrug abusers. Survey data also report that although adolescents and young adults are aware of the potential health hazards of marijuana use, this information does not effectively deter use by many individuals.

Acute and chronic marijuana intoxication Acute intoxication from marijuana and cannabis compounds is related to both THC dose and route of administration. THC is absorbed more rapidly from marijuana smoking than from orally ingested cannabis compounds. The most frequent form of acute intoxication consists of a subjective perception of relaxation and mild euphoria resembling mild to moderate alcohol intoxication. This condition is usually accompanied by some impairment in thinking, concentration, and perceptual and psychomotor functions. Higher doses of cannabis may produce behavioral effects analogous to severe alcohol intoxication. Although the effects of acute marijuana intoxication are relatively benign in normal users, the drug can precipitate severe emotional disorders in individuals who have antecedent psychotic or neurotic problems. As with other psychoactive compounds both set (user's expectancy) and setting (environmental context) are important determinants of the type and severity of behavioral intoxication.

As is true of alcoholics, *chronic* marijuana abusers may lose interest in common socially desirable goals and devote progressively more time to drug acquisition and use. However, it should be emphasized that THC does not cause a specific and unique "amotivational syndrome." The range of symptoms sometimes attributed to marijuana use are difficult to distinguish from mild depression and the maturational dysfunctions often associated with protracted adolescence. Chronic use of marijuana has also been reported to increase the probability of exacerbation of psychotic symptoms in individuals with a past history of schizophrenia.

Physical effects of marijuana Conjunctival injection and tachycardia are the most frequent immediate physical concomitants of smoking marijuana. Tolerance for marijuana-induced tachycardia develops rapidly among regular users; angina may be precipitated by marijuana smoking in persons with a history of coronary insufficiency. Exercise-induced angina may be increased after marijuana use to a greater extent than after tobacco cigarette smoking. Patients with cardiac disease should be strongly advised not to smoke marijuana or use cannabis compounds.

Significant decrements in pulmonary vital capacity have been found in regular daily marijuana smokers. Because marijuana smoking typically involves deep inhalation and prolonged retention of marijuana smoke, marijuana smokers may develop pulmonary disease such as chronic bronchial irritation. Impairment of single-breath carbon monoxide diffusion capacity (DL_{CO}) is greater in persons who smoke both marijuana and tobacco than in tobacco smokers. At present, there is no direct evidence that marijuana smoking induces lung cancer that is comparable to the well-documented association between tobacco smoking and lung cancer, although it should be emphasized that heavy marijuana use among Americans may be of too brief duration for detection of this problem.

Although marijuana has also been associated with adverse effects on a number of other systems, many of these studies await replication and confirmation. For example, the reported correlation between marijuana use and decreased testosterone levels in males has not been confirmed. Decreased sperm count and motility and abnormalities of morphology of spermatozoa following marijuana use have also been reported. Administration of high doses of marijuana to female rhesus monkeys has revealed significant marijuana-induced suppression of pituitary gonadotrophins and gonadal steroids. Carefully conducted prospective studies demonstrated a significant correlation between impaired fetal growth and development and heavy marijuana use during pregnancy. Marijuana also has been implicated in derangements of the immune response system, in chromosomal abnormalities, and in inhibition of DNA, RNA, and protein synthesis, but these findings have not been confirmed or related to any specific physiologic effect of marijuana in humans. One report of cannabis-induced brain atrophy in young adults has not been confirmed in studies of computerized tomography with young men who had documented histories of heavy marijuana smoking.

Tolerance and physical dependence Habitual marijuana users rapidly develop tolerance to the psychoactive effects of marijuana, often smoking more frequently and trying to secure more potent cannabis compounds. Tolerance for physiologic effects of marijuana develops at different rates; e.g. tolerance for marijuana-induced tachycardia develops rapidly, but tolerance for marijuana-induced conjunctival injection develops more slowly. Tolerance to both behavioral and physiologic effects of marijuana decreases rapidly upon cessation of marijuana use.

Mild to moderate withdrawal signs and symptoms have been reported in chronic cannabis users, with severity of symptoms related to dosage and duration of use. These include tremor, sweating, nausea, vomiting, diarrhea, irritability, anorexia, and sleep disturbances. Withdrawal signs and symptoms observed in chronic marijuana users are usually relatively mild in comparision to those observed with heavy opiate or alcohol users and rarely require medical or pharmacologic intervention. Somewhat more severe and protracted abstinence syndromes may occur after sustained use of high potency cannabis compounds for long periods.

COCAINE Cocaine is a stimulant and a local anesthetic with potent vasoconstrictor properties. Leaves of the coca plant (*Erythroxylon coca*) contain 1 to 1.5 percent cocaine. The drug is marketed illicitly in the form of a white crystalline powder, usually adulterated with lactose or glucose to 50 percent purity. Frequently cocaine is adulterated with other local anesthetics such as lidocaine, procaine, and tetracaine. Cocaine's biologic effects result from alteration and blockade of cellular membrane transport, particularly prevention of the reuptake of biogenic amines, an effect shared with the tricyclic antidepressants.

Prevalence of cocaine use Cocaine is expensive in comparison to most other illicit drugs and has attained the reputation of a "status" drug in western industrialized societies. The actual extent of illicit cocaine use is unknown, but there is evidence of a recent escalation in the United States. The Drug Abuse Warning Network (DAWN) reported that emergency room mentions of cocaine abuse increased by 75 percent from 1981 through the fourth quarter of 1983. During the first quarter of 1984, approximately 2000 cocaine mentions were reported, a number equal to all the cocaine mentions for the full year of 1978. A National Household Survey conducted in 1982 revealed that 21.6 million persons had tried cocaine at least once, a dramatic increase from the 5.4 million who reported at least one use of cocaine during 1974. The most prevalent pattern of use in America appears to be occasional, sporadic intake of relatively low doses of cocaine.

Acute and chronic cocaine intoxication The most common mode of cocaine self-administration is by inhalation or "snorting," where the drug is rapidly absorbed from the nasal mucosa and produces a brief, dose-related stimulation and enhancement of mood. Cardiac rate and blood pressure also increase in a dose-related manner. An increase in body temperature usually occurs following cocaine administration, and high doses of cocaine may induce lethal pyrexia or hypertension. Because cocaine inhibits reuptake of catecholamines at adrenergic nerve endings, the drug potentiates sympathetic nervous system activity. During recent years smoking of coca paste (a product produced by extracting cocaine preparations with flammable solvents) has become increasingly popular. Administration of the drug via intravenous injection also occurs more frequently. Cocaine has a short plasma half-life of approximately 1 h. In humans, cocaine is primarily metabolized by plasma esterases, and cocaine metabolites are excreted in urine. The very short duration of euphorigenic effects of cocaine observed in chronic abusers is probably due to both acute and chronic tolerance. Frequent self-administration of the drug (2 to 3 times per hour) is often reported by chronic cocaine abusers. Modulation of both the cocaine "high" and the abrupt dysphoric disappearance of cocaine's effects with alcohol is often reported.

The prevalent assumption that cocaine use is relatively safe is challenged by reports of death from respiratory depression, cardiac arrhythmias, and convulsions after cocaine snorting and intravenous administration. Severe pulmonary disease may develop in individuals who smoke coca paste; this is attributed both to the direct effects of cocaine and to residual solvent contaminants in the smoked material. Numerous clinical reports, dating from the late nineteenth century, strongly suggest that protracted cocaine abuse may induce paranoid ideation and visual and auditory hallucinations, a state which resembles alcoholic hallucinosis. Psychological dependence upon cocaine, as manifested by inability to abstain from frequent compulsive use, has also been reported. Although occurrence of withdrawal syndromes involving psychomotor agitation and autonomic hyperactivity remains controversial, severe depression ("crashing") may be a concomitant of drug withdrawal.

Treatment of cocaine intoxication and abuse Treatment of cocaine overdose is a medical emergency which involves resuscitation in an intensive care unit. Cocaine toxicity produces hypertension, tachycardia, tonic-clonic seizures, dyspnea, and ventricular arrhythmias. Intravenous diazepam in doses up to 0.5 mg/kg administered over an 8-h period has been shown to be effective for control of seizures. The systemic concomitants of a hypermetabolic state produced by cocaine toxicity with concurrent ventricular arrhythmias have been managed successfully by administration of 0.5 to 1.0 mg of propranolol intravenously. Since many instances of cocaine-related mortality have also been associated with concomitant use of other illicit drugs (particularly heroin), the physician must be prepared to institute effective emergency treatment for multiple drug toxicity.

Treatment of chronic cocaine abuse requires combined efforts by family physicians, psychiatrists, and psychosocial care providers. Early abstinence from cocaine use is often complicated by symptoms of depression and guilt, insomnia, and anorexia, which may be as severe as those observed in major affective disorders. Individual and group psychotherapy, family therapy, and peer group assistance programs are often useful for inducing prolonged remission from drug use. Preliminary reports suggest that both lithium treatment and tricyclic antidepressant medication may be of value for the long-term treatment of cocaine abuse, even when affective disorder or depression are not present. In fact, depressive illness does not appear to be a frequent antecedent of cocaine abuse.

LYSERGIC ACID DIETHYLAMIDE (LSD) The serendipitous discovery of psychedelic effects of LSD in 1947 culminated in an epidemic of LSD abuse during the 1960s. Imposition of stringent legal and regulatory constraints on the manufacture and distribution of LSD (classified as a Schedule I substance by the FDA), as well as public recognition that psychedelic experiences induced by LSD were a health hazard, has resulted in a significant reduction in LSD abuse. During 1984, relatively few instances of LSD abuse were reported, but the drug still retains some popularity among adolescents and young adults.

LSD is a very potent drug; oral doses as low as 20 μg may induce profound psychological and physiologic effects. Tachycardia, hypertension, pupillary dilation, tremor, and hyperpyrexia occur within minutes following LSD in oral doses of 0.5 to 2 μg/kg. A variety of bizarre and often conflicting perceptual and mood changes, including visual illusions, synesthesias, and extreme lability of mood states, occur within one-half hour after LSD intake. The action of LSD can persist for 12 to 18 h even though the half-life of the drug is only 3 h.

Tolerance develops rapidly for LSD-induced changes in psychological function when the drug is used one or more times per day over a course of 4 days or more. Abrupt abstinence following continued use does not produce withdrawal signs or symptoms. To date there have been no clinical reports of death caused by the direct effects of LSD.

The most frequent acute medical emergency associated with LSD use is panic episodes which may persist up to 24 h ("the bad trip"). Management of this problem is best accomplished by supportive reassurance ("talking down") and, if necessary, administration of small doses of anxiolytic drugs. Adverse consequences of chronic LSD use include enhanced risk for schizophreniform psychosis and derangements in memory function, problem solving, and abstract thinking. Treatment of these disorders is best carried out in specialized psychiatric facilities.

PHENCYCLIDINE (PCP) Phencyclidine, a cyclohexylamine derivative, is widely used in veterinary medicine to briefly immobilize large animals and is sometimes described as a *dissociative anesthetic*. PCP is easily synthesized and is abused, primarily by young people and polydrug users. The true extent of PCP abuse is unknown, but recent national surveys indicate an increase in frequency of use.

Phencyclidine is taken orally, by smoking, or by intravenous injection. It is also used as an adulterant in illicit sales of THC, LSD, amphetamine, or cocaine. The most common street preparation, "angel dust," is a white granular powder which contains 50 to 100 percent of the drug. Low doses (5 mg) produce agitation, excitement, impaired motor coordination, dysarthria, and analgesia. Users may have horizontal or vertical nystagmus, flushing, diaphoresis, and hyperacusis. Behavioral changes include distortions of body image, disorganization of thinking, and feelings of estrangement. Higher doses of PCP (5 to 10 mg) may produce hypersalivation, vomiting, myoclonus, fever, stupor, or coma. PCP doses of 10 mg or more cause convulsions, opisthotonus, and decerebrate posturing which may be followed by prolonged coma.

The diagnosis of PCP overdose is difficult because the patient's initial symptoms may suggest an acute schizophrenic reaction. Confirmation of PCP use is possible by determination of PCP levels in serum or urine. PCP analysis is currently available at most toxicologic centers. Large quantities of PCP remain in urine for 1 to 5 days following high-dosage PCP intake.

PCP overdose requires prompt life support measures including treatment of coma, convulsions, and respiratory depression in a hospital intensive care unit (see Chap. 21). There is no specific antidote or antagonist for PCP. PCP excretion from the body can be enhanced by acidification of urine and gastric lavage (see Chap. 171). Death from PCP overdose may occur as a consequence of some combination of pharyngeal hypersecretion, hyperthermia, respiratory depression, severe hypertension, seizures, hypertensive encephalopathy, and intracerebral hemorrhage.

Acute psychosis associated with PCP use should be considered a psychiatric emergency since patients may be at high risk for suicide or extreme violence toward others. *Phenothiazines should not be used for treatment of acute PCP psychosis because these drugs potentiate PCP's anticholinergic effects.* Haloperidol (5 mg intramuscularly) has been administered on an hourly basis to induce suppression of psychotic behavior. PCP, like LSD and mescaline, produces vasospasm of cerebral arteries at relatively low doses. Chronic PCP use has been shown to induce insomnia, anorexia, severe social and behavioral changes, and, in some cases, chronic schizophrenia.

POLYDRUG ABUSE Although drug abusers often report a preference for a particular drug, such as alcohol or opiates, the concurrent use of other drugs is common. Multiple drug use often involves substances which may have different pharmacologic effects from the preferred drug. Concurrent use of such dissimilar compounds as stimulants and opiates or stimulants and alcohol is not unusual. The diversity of reported drug use combinations suggests that achieving some perceptible change in state, rather than any particular direction of change (stimulation or sedation), may be the primary reinforcer in polydrug use and abuse.

A practical determinant of polydrug use patterns is the relative availability and cost of the drugs. There are many examples of situationally determined drug use patterns, including the fact that soldiers who became dependent on heroin in Vietnam seldom continued heroin use after separation from military service. However, a significant number of Vietnam heroin addicts abused alcohol and became alcohol-dependent when they returned to the United States. Alcohol abuse, with its attendant medical complications, is one of the most serious problems encountered in former heroin addicts participating in methadone maintenance programs.

The physician must recognize that perpetuation of polydrug abuse and drug dependence is not necessarily a symptom of an underlying emotional disorder. Neither alleviation of anxiety nor reduction of depression accounts for initiation and perpetuation of polydrug abuse. Severe depression and anxiety are as frequently the consequences of polydrug abuse as they are the antecedents. There is also evidence that some of the most adverse consequences of drug use may be reinforcing and contribute to the continuation of polydrug abuse.

Adequate treatment of polydrug abuse, as well as other forms of drug abuse, requires innovative and eclectic programs of intervention. The first step in successful treatment is detoxification, a process which may be difficult because the patient has abused several drugs with different pharmacologic actions (e.g. alcohol, opiates, and cocaine). Since patients may not recall or may deny simultaneous multiple drug use, diagnostic evaluation should always include urinalysis for qualitative detection of psychoactive substances and their metabolites. Treatment of polydrug abuse requires hospitalization or inpatient residential care during detoxification and the initial phase of drug abstinence. When possible, specialized facilities for the care and treatment of chemically dependent persons should be used. Outpatient detoxification of polydrug abuse patients is likely to be ineffective and may be dangerous.

As in the treatment of alcohol abuse, no single therapeutic modality has been shown to be uniquely effective in inducing remission. Polydrug abuse is a chronic disorder with an unpredictable pattern of remission and recrudescence. Therapeutic management of chronic disorders such as cardiac or neoplastic disease should serve as a model for helping the person with polydrug abuse problems. Even temporary remissions with attendant physical, social, and psychological improvements are preferable to the continuation or progressive acceleration of polydrug abuse and its related adverse medical and interpersonal consequences. In polydrug abuse, as in most chronic disorders, definitive "cures" rarely occur. The concerned physician should continue to assist polydrug abuse patients throughout the cyclic oscillations of this complex behavior disorder, recognizing that resumption of drug use may be the rule rather than the exception.

REFERENCES

ABEL EL: *Marihuana: The First Twelve Thousand Years*, New York, Plenum, 1980

BERNSTEIN JG: Medical consequences of marihuana use, in *Advances in Substance Abuse, Behavioral and Biological Research*, NK Mello (ed). Greenwich, JAI Press, 1980, vol 1, pp 255–258

DOMINO EF (ed): *PCP (Phencyclidine): Historical and Current Perspectives*. Ann Arbor, NPP Books, 1981

GRABOWSKI J (ed): *Cocaine: Pharmacology, Effects, and Treatment of Abuse*, NIDA Research Monograph 50, DHEW Publication (ADM) 84–1325. Washington DC, US Government Printing Office, 1984

JAFFE JH: Drug addiction and drug abuse, in *The Pharmocological Basis of Therapeutics*, 4th ed, AG Gilman et al (eds). New York, Macmillan, 1980, pp 535–584

KANDEL D: Marihuana users in young adulthood. Arch Gen Psychiat 41:200, 1984

MELLO NK: A behavioral analysis of the reinforcing properties of alcohol and other drugs in man, in *The Pathogenesis of Alcoholism, Biological Factors*, B Kissin and H Begleiter (eds). New York, Plenum, 1983, vol 7, pp 133–198

MENDELSON JH: Chronic effects of cannabis on human brain function and behavior, in *Cannabis and Health Hazards. Proceedings of an ARF/WHO Scientific Meeting on Adverse Health and Behavioral Consequences of Cannabis Use*, KO Fehr and H

Kalant (eds). Toronto, Alcohol and Drug Addiction Research Foundation, 1983, pp 475–500

MENDELSON JH, MELLO NK (eds): *The Diagnosis and Treatment of Alcoholism*, 2d ed. New York, McGraw-Hill, 1985

PETERSEN RC, STILLMAN RD (eds): *Phencyclidine (PCP) Abuse: An Appraisal*, NIDA Research Monograph 21, DHEW Publication (ADM) 78–728. Washington, DC, US Government Printing Office, 1978

VAN DYKE C, BYCK R: Cocaine use in man, in *Advances in Substance Abuse, Behavioral and Biological Research*, NK Mello (ed). Greenwich, JAI Press, 1983, vol 3, pp 1–24

APPENDIX LABORATORY VALUES OF CLINICAL IMPORTANCE

INTRODUCTORY COMMENTS

Since *Principles of Internal Medicine* is a textbook used internationally, in preparing the Appendix the editors have taken into account the fact that the system of international units (SI, système international d'unités) has been adopted by many laboratories. To this end, where possible and appropriate, common laboratory values are expressed in terms of both traditional units and SI units. *Values in SI units appear in brackets* after values in traditional units. The use of SI units in medicine was endorsed by the Thirtieth World Health Assembly (May 1977) with the purpose of implementing an international language of measurement.[1] The SI *base* units, SI *derived* units, other units of measurement referred to in this Appendix, and SI prefixes are listed in Tables A-1 to A-3. These and other tables of laboratory values are to be found at the end of the Appendix.

ASCITIC FLUID

See Table 39-1, page 190.

BODY FLUIDS AND OTHER MASS DATA

Body fluid, total volume: 50 percent (in obese) to 70 percent (lean) of body weight
- Intracellular: 30 to 40 percent of body weight
- Extracellular: 20 to 30 percent of body weight

Blood:
- Total volume:
  - Males: 69 mL per kilogram of body weight
  - Females: 65 mL per kilogram of body weight
- Plasma volume:
  - Males: 39 mL per kilogram of body weight
  - Females: 40 mL per kilogram of body weight
- Red blood cell volume:
  - Males: 30 mL per kilogram of body weight (1.15 to 1.21 liters per square meter of body surface area)
  - Females: 25 mL per kilogram of body weight (0.95 to 1.00 liters per square meter of body surface area)

$$\text{meq/liter} = \frac{\text{mg/dL} \times 10 \times \text{valence}}{\text{atomic weight}}$$

$$\text{mg/dL} = \frac{\text{meq/liter} \times \text{atomic weight}}{10 \times \text{valence}}$$

CEREBROSPINAL FLUID[2]

Osmolarity	292–297 mosmol per liter
Electrolytes:	
Sodium	137–145 meq per liter
Potassium	2.7–3.9 meq per liter
Calcium	2.1–3.0 meq per liter
Magnesium	2.0–2.5 meq per liter
Phosphorus	1.2–2.0 mg/dL
Chloride	116–122 meq per liter
Bicarbonate	20–24 meq per liter
P_{CO_2}	45–49 mmHg
pH	7.31–7.34
Glucose	40–70 mg/dL
Lactate	10–20 mg/dL
Pyruvate	0.078–0.081 meq per liter
Lactate/pyruvate ratio	26.0
Total protein:	20–45 mg/dL
Prealbumin	2–6%
Albumin	56–75%
Alpha$_1$ globulin	2–7%
Alpha$_2$ globulin	4–12%
Beta globulin	8–16%
Gamma globulin	3–12%
IgG	1.0–1.4 mg/dL
IgA	0.1–0.3 mg/dL
IgM	0.01–0.12 mg/dL
IgG synthesis rate	(−) 9.9 to (+) 3.3 mg per day
Ammonia	25–80 μg/dL
Urea	4.4–4.8 mmol per liter
Creatinine	0.5–1.9 mg/dL
Uric acid	0.23–0.27 mg/dL
Putrescine	130–230 pmol/mL
Spermidine	110–190 pmol/mL
Cyclic AMP	3–30 nmol per liter
HVA (homovanillic acid)	35–85 μg/mL
5-HIAA (5-OH indoleacetic acid)	0.03–0.05 μg/mL
MHPG (3-methoxy-4-hydroxy-phenylethyleneglycol)	13.0–17.0 mg/dL
Myelin basic protein	<4 ng/mL
CSF pressure	50–180 mmH_2O
CSF volume (adult)	100–160 mL
Leukocytes:	
Total	<4 per cubic millimeter
Differential:	
Lymphocytes	60–70%
Monocytes	30–50%
Neutrophils	1–3%

CHEMICAL CONSTITUENTS OF BLOOD

See also "Function Tests," especially "Metabolic and Endocrine."

Acetoacetate, plasma: <1.0 mg/dL [<0.1 mmol per liter]
Albumin, serum: 3.5 to 5.5 g/dL [35 to 55 g per liter]
Aldolase: 0 to 8 units per liter [0 to 130 nmol/s per liter]
Alpha$_1$ antitrypsin, serum: 85–213 mg/dL [0.85–2.13 g per liter]

[1] *The SI for the Health Professions, Geneva, World Health Organization, 1977.*

[2] *Since cerebrospinal fluid concentrations are equilibrium values, measurement of blood plasma obtained at the same time is recommended.*

α-Amino nitrogen, plasma: 3.0 to 5.5 mg/dL [2.1 to 3.9 mmol per liter]
Alpha fetoprotein (adult), serum: <30 mg/mL
Aminotransferases, serum:
Aspartate (AST, SGOT): 10 to 40 Karmen units per milliliter; 6 to 18 units per liter [100 to 300 μmol/s per liter]
Alanine (ALT, SGPT): 10 to 40 Karmen units per milliliter; 3 to 26 units per liter [50 to 430 μmol/s per liter]
Ammonia, whole blood, venous: 80 to 110 μg/dL [47 to 65 μmol per liter]
Amylase, serum: 60 to 180 Somogyi units per deciliters; 0.8 to 3.2 units per liter [13 to 53 nmol/s per liter]
Arterial blood gases:
[HCO_3^-]: 21 to 28 meq per liter [21 to 28 mmol per liter]
P_{CO_2}: 35 to 45 mmHg [4.7 to 6.0 kPa]
pH: 7.38 to 7.44
P_{O_2}: 80 to 100 mmHg [11 to 13 kPa]
Ascorbic acid (vitamin C), serum: 0.4 to 1.0 mg/dL [23 to 57 μmol per liter]
Leukocytes: 25 to 40 mg/dL [1420 to 2270 μmol per liter]
Barbiturates, serum: nondetectable
Phenobarbital, "potentially fatal" level (Schreiner): approximately 9 mg/dL [390 μmol per liter]
Most short-acting barbiturates: 3.5 mg/dL [150 μmol per liter]
Base, total, serum: 145 to 155 meq per liter [145 to 155 mmol per liter]
β-Hydroxybutyrate, plasma: <3mg/dL [<0.3 mmol per liter]
Bilirubin, total, serum (Malloy-Evelyn): 0.3 to 1.0 mg/dL [5.1 to 17 μmol per liter]
Direct, serum: 0.1 to 0.3 mg/dL [1.7 to 5.1 μmol per liter]
Indirect, serum: 0.2 to 0.7 mg/dL [3.4 to 12 μmol per liter]
Bromides, serum: nondetectable
Toxic levels: >17 meq per liter; 150 mg/dL [17 mmol per liter]
Bromsulphalein, BSP (5 mg per kilogram of body weight, intravenously): 5 percent or less retention after 45 min
C-reactive protein, serum: 7–820 μg/dL
Calciferols (vitamin D), plasma:
1,25-dihydroxyvitamin D [1,25$(OH)_2$D]. 20 to 60 pg/mL [48 to 144 nmol per liter]
25-hydroxyvitamin D [25(OH)D]. 8 to 42 ng/mL [20 to 100 μmol per liter]
Calcium, ionized: 2.3 to 2.8 meq per liter; 4.5 to 5.6 mg/dL [1.1 to 1.4 mmol per liter]
Calcium, plasma: 4.5 to 5.5 meq per liter; 9 to 10.5 mg/dL [2.2 to 2.6 mmol per liter]
Carbon dioxide-combining power, serum (sea level): 21 to 28 meq per liter; 50 to 65 volume percent [21 to 28 mmol per liter]
Carbon dioxide content, plasma (sea level): 21 to 30 meq per liter; 50 to 70 volume percent [21 to 30 mmol per liter]
Carbon dioxide tension, arterial blood (sea level): 35 to 45 mmHg [4.7 to 6.0 kPa]
Carbon monoxide content, blood: nondetectable symptoms with over 20 percent saturation of hemoglobin
Carcinoembryonic antigen (CEA): 0 to 2.5 ng/mL (in healthy nonsmokers) [0 to 2.5 μg per liter]
Carotenoids, serum: 50 to 300 μg/dL [0.9 to 5.6 μmol per liter]
Ceruloplasmin, serum: 27 to 37 mg/dL [1.8 to 2.5 μmol per liter]
Chlorides, serum (as Cl^-): 98 to 106 meq per liter [98 to 106 mmol per liter]
Cholesterol: see Table A-4
Complement, serum:
Total hemolytic (CH_{50}): 150 to 250 units per milliliter
C3: 55 to 120 mg/dL [0.55 to 1.20 g per liter]
C4: 20 to 50 mg/dL [0.20 to 0.50 g per liter]
Copper, serum (mean ± 1 SD): 114 ± 14 μg/dL [17.9 μmol per liter]
Creatine phosphokinase, serum (total):
Females: 10 to 70 units per millimeter [0.17 to 1.18 mmol/s per liter]
Males: 25 to 90 units per milliliter [0.42 to 1.51 mmol/s per liter]
Isoenzymes, serum: fraction 2 (MB) <5 percent of total
Creatinine, serum: <1.5 mg/dL [<133 μmol per liter]
Digoxin serum:
Therapeutic level: 1.2 ± 4 ng/mL [1.54 ± 0.5 nmol per liter]
Toxic level: >2.4 ng/mL [>3.2 nmol per liter]
Ethanol, blood:
Mild to moderate intoxication: 80 to 200 mg/dL [17 to 43 mmol per liter]
Marked intoxication: 250 to 400 mg/dL [54 to 87 mmol per liter]
Severe intoxication: >400 mg/dL [>87 mmol per liter]
Fatty acids, free (nonesterified), plasma: <18 mg/dL [<0.7 mmol per liter]
Ferritin, serum: 15 to 200 ng/mL [15 to 200 μg per liter]
Fibrinogen, plasma: see "Platelets and Coagulation"
Fibrinogen split products: see "Platelets and Coagulation"
Folic acid, serum: 6 to 15 ng/mL [14 to 34 nmol per liter]
Folic acid, red cell: 150 to 450 ng per milliliter of cells [340 to 1020 nmol per liter cells]
γ-Glutamyl transferase (transpeptidase), serum: 4 to 60 units per liter [0.07 to 1.00 μmol/s per liter]
Gastrin, serum: 40 to 200 pg/mL [40 to 200 ng per liter]
Globulins, serum: 2.0 to 3.0 g/dL [20 to 30 g per liter]
Glucose (fasting), plasma:
Normal: 75 to 115 mg/dL [4.2 to 6.4 mmol per liter]
Diabetes mellitus: >140 mg/dL (on more than one occasion) [>7.8 mmol per liter]
Glucose, 2 h postprandial, plasma:
Normal: <140 mg/dL [<7.8 mmol per liter]
Impaired glucose tolerance: 140 to 200 mg/dL [7.8 to 11.1 mmol per liter]
Diabetes mellitus: >200 mg/dL [>11.1 mmol per liter] (on more than one occasion)
Hemoglobin, blood (sea level):
Males: 14 to 18 g/dL [8.7 to 11.2 mmol per liter]
Females: 12 to 16 g/dL [7.4 to 9.9 mmol per liter]
Hemoglobin A_{1c}: up to 6 perrcent of total hemoglobin
Immunoglobulins, serum:
IgA: 90 to 325 mg/dL [0.9 to 3.2 g per liter]
IgD: 0 to 8 mg/dL [0 to 0.08 g per liter]
IgE: <0.025 mg/dL [<0.00025 g per liter]
IgG: 800 to 1500 mg/dL [8.0 to 15.0 g per liter]
IgM: 45 to 150 mg/dL [0.45 to 1.5 g per liter]
Iron, serum:
Males and females (mean ± 1 SD): 105 ± 35 μg/dL [19 ± 6 μmol per liter]
Iron-binding capacity, serum (mean ± 1 SD): 305 ± 32 μg/dL [55 ± 6 μmol per liter]
Saturation: 20 to 45 percent
Ketones, total: 0.5 to 1.5 mg/dL [5.0 to 15.0 mg per liter]
Lactate dehydrogenase, serum:
200 to 450 units per milliliter (Wrobleski)
60 to 100 units per milliliter (Wacker)
25 to 100 units per liter [0.4 to 1.7 μmol/s per liter]
Lactic dehydrogenase isoenzymes, serum (agarose):
Fraction 1 (% of total): 14–26
Fraction 2: 29–39
Fraction 3: 20–26
Fraction 4: 8–16
Fraction 5: 6–16
Lactate, venous plasma: 5 to 15 mg/dL [0.6 to 1.7 mmol per liter]
Lead, serum: <20 μg/dL [<1.0 μmol per liter]
Lipase, serum: 1.5 units (Cherry-Crandall)
Lipids: see Table A-4
Lipids, triglyceride, serum: see Table A-4
Lipoprotein: see Table A-4
Lithium, serum:
Therapeutic concentration: 0.6 to 1.2 mmol per liter
Toxic concentration: >2 mmol per liter [>2 mmol per liter]

Magnesium, serum: 1.3 to 2.1 meq per liter; 2 to 3 mg/dL [0.8 to 1.3 mmol per liter]
Nitrogen, nonprotein, serum: 15 to 35 mg/dL [0.15 to 0.35 g per liter]
5′-Nucleotidase, serum: 0.3 to 2.6 Bodansky units per deciliter [27 to 233 nmol/s per liter]
Osmolality, plasma: 285 to 295 mosmol per kilogram of serum water
Oxygen content:
Arterial blood (sea level): 17 to 21 volume percent
Venous blood, arm (sea level): 10 to 16 volume percent
Oxygen percent saturation (sea level):
Arterial blood: 97 percent [0.97 mol/mol]
Venous blood, arm: 60 to 85 percent [0.60 to 0.85 mol/mol]
Oxygen tension, blood: 80 to 100 mmHg ob11 to 13 kPa]
pH, blood: 7.38 to 7.44
Phenytoin, plasma:
Therapeutic level: 10 to 20 μg/mL [40 to 79 μmol per liter]
Toxic level: >30 μg/mL [>119 μmol per liter]
Phosphatase, acid, serum:
Bessey-Lowry method: 0.10 to 0.63 units [28 to 175 nmol/s per liter]
Bodansky method: 0.5 to 2.0 units
Fishmann-Lerner (tartrate sensitive): <0.6 units per deciliter (up to 0.15 units per deciliter)
Gutman method: 0.5 to 2.0 units
International units: 0.2 to 1.8 [3 to 30 nmol/s per liter]
King-Armstrong method: 1.0 to 5.0 units
Phosphatase, alkaline, serum:
Bessey-Lowry method: 0.8 to 2.3 units (3.4 to 9 units[3])
Bodansky method: 2.0 to 4.5 units (3.0 to 13.0 units[3]) [0.18 to 0.40 nmol/s per liter]
Gutman method: 2.0 to 4.5 units (3.0 to 13.0 units[3])
International units: 21 to 91 per liter at 37°C [0.4 to 1.5 μmol/s per liter]
King-Armstrong method: 4.0 to 13.0 units (10.0 to 20.0 units[3])
Phospholipids, serum: 150 to 250 mg/dL (as lecithin) [48 to 81 mmol per liter]
Phosphorus, inorganic, serum: 1 to 1.5 meq per liter; 3 to 4.5 mg/dL [1.0 to 1.4 mmol per liter]
Potassium, serum: 3.5 to 5.0 meq per liter [3.5 to 5.0 mmol per liter]
Proteins, total, serum: 5.5 to 8.0 g/dL [55 to 80 g per liter]
Protein fractions, serum:
Albumin: 3.5 to 5.5 g/dL (50 to 60 percent) [35 to 55 g per liter]
Globulin: 2.0 to 3.5 g/dL (40 to 50 percent) [20 to 35 g per liter]
Alpha_1: 0.2 to 0.4 g/dL (4.2 to 7.2 percent) [2 to 4 g per liter]
Alpha_2: 0.5 to 0.9 g/dL (6.8 to 12 percent) [5 to 9 g per liter]
Beta: 0.6 to 1.1 g/dL (9.3 to 15 percent) [6 to 11 g per liter]
Gamma: 0.7 to 1.7 g/dL (13 to 23 percent) [7 to 17 g per liter]
Pyruvate, venous, plasma: 0.5 to 1.5 mg/dL [0.06 to 0.17 mmol per liter]
Quinidine, serum:
Therapeutic range: 1.5 to 3 μg/mL [4.6 to 9.2 μmol per liter]
Toxic range: 5 to 6 μg/mL [15.4 to 18.5 μmol per liter]
Salicylate, plasma: 0 mmol per liter
Therapeutic range: 20 to 25 mg/dL [1.4 to 1.8 mmol per liter]
Toxic range: >30 mg/dL [2.2 mmol per liter]
Sodium, serum: 136 to 145 meq per liter [136 to 145 mmol per liter]
Steroids: see "Metabolic and Endocrine" under "Function Tests"
Transaminase, serum glutamic oxaloacetic (SGOT, AST): 10 to 40 Karmen units per milliliter; 6 to 18 units per liter [100 to 300 μmol/s per liter]
Transaminase, serum glutamic pyruvic (SGPT, ALT): see Aminotransferases, serum
Transferase, γ-glutamyl, serum: 4 to 60 units per liter [0.07 to 1.00 μmol/s per liter]
Triglycerides: see Table A-4

[3] *Values in parentheses are those found in children.*

Urea nitrogen, serum: 10 to 20 mg/dL [3.6 to 7.1 mmol per liter]
Uric acid, serum:
Men: 2.5 to 8.0 mg/dL [0.15 to 0.48 mmol per liter]
Women: 1.5 to 6.0 mg/dL [0.09 to 0.36 mmol per liter]
Vitamin A, serum: 20 to 100 μg/dL [0.7 to 3.5 μmol per liter]
Vitamin B_{12}, serum: 200 to 600 pg/mL [148 to 443 pmol per liter]
Zinc, serum (mean $\pm$ 1 SD): 120 $\pm$ 20 μg/dL [18 $\pm$ 3 μmol per liter]

FUNCTION TESTS

Circulation

Arteriovenous oxygen difference: 30 to 50 mL per liter
Cardiac output (Fick): 2.5 to 3.6 liters per square meter of body surface area per minute
Contractility indexes:
Maximum left ventricular *dp/dt:* 1650 $\pm$ 300 mmHg/s
Maximum *(dp/dt)/p:* 44 $\pm$ 8.4 s^{-1}
(dp/dt)/DP at DP = 40 mmHg: 37.6 $\pm$ 12.2 s^{-1} (DP = diastolic press.)
Mean normalized systolic ejection rate (angiography): 3.32 $\pm$ 0.84 end-diastolic volumes per second
Mean velocity of circumferential fiber shortening (angiography) 1.66 $\pm$ 0.42 circumferences per second
Ejection fraction, stroke volume/end-diastolic volume (SV/EDV):
Normal range: 0.55 to 0.78; average: 0.67
End-diastolic volume: 75 $\pm$ 15 mL/m^2
End-systolic volume: 25 $\pm$ 8 mL/m^2
Left ventricular work:
Stroke work index: 30 to 110 (g·m)/m^2
Left ventricular minute work index: 1.8 to 6.6 [(kg·m)/m^2]/min
Oxygen consumption index: 110 to 150 mL per liter
Pressures, intracardiac and intraarterial: see Table A-5
Pulmonary vascular resistance: 20 to 120 (dyn·s)/cm^5 [2 to 12 kPa·s per liter]
Systemic vascular resistance: 770 to 1500 (dyn·s)/cm^5 [77 to 150 kPa·s per liter]
Systolic time intervals: see Table A-6

Gastrointestinal See also "Stool."

Absorption tests:
D-Xylose absorption test: After an overnight fast, 25 g xylose is given in aqueous solution by mouth. Urine collected for the following 5 h should contain 5 to 8 g [33 to 53 mmol] (or >20 percent of ingested dose). Serum xylose should be 25 to 40 mg per 100 mL 1 h after the oral dose [1.7 to 2.7 mmol per liter].
Vitamin A absorption test: A fasting blood specimen is obtained and 200,000 units of vitamin A in oil is given by mouth. Serum vitamin A levels should rise to twice fasting level in 3 to 5 h.
Bentiromide test (pancreatic function): 500 mg bentiromide (chymex) orally; *p*-aminobenzoic acid (PABA) measured in plasma and/or urine
Plasma: >3.6 ($\pm$1.1) μg/mL at 90 min
Urine: >50 percent recovered as PABA in 6 h
Gastric juice:
Volume:
24 h: 2 to 3 liters
Nocturnal: 600 to 700 mL
Basal, fasting: 30 to 70 mL/h
Reaction:
As pH: 1.6 to 1.8
Titratable acidity of fasting juice: 15 to 35 meq/h [4 to 10 μmol/s]
Acid output:
Basal:
Females (mean $\pm$ 1 SD): 2.0 $\pm$ 1.8 meq/h [0.6 $\pm$ 0.5 μmol/s]
Males (mean $\pm$ 1 SD): 3.0 $\pm$ 2.0 meq/h [0.8 $\pm$ 0.6 μmol/s]

Maximal [after subcutaneous histamine acid phosphate 0.004 mg/kg and preceded by 50 mg promethazine (Phenergan); or after betazole (Histalog) 1.7 mg/kg or pentagastrin 6μg/mg]:
Females (mean ± 1 SD): 16 ± 5 meq/h [4.4 ± 1.4 μmol/s]
Males (mean ± 1 SD): 23 ± 5 meq/h [6.4 ± 1.4 μmol/s]
Basal acid output/maximal acid output ratio: 0.6 or less
Gastrin, serum: 40 to 200 pg/mL [40 to 200 ng per liter]
Secretin test (pancreatic exocrine function): 1 unit per kilogram of body weight, intravenously
Volume (pancreatic juice): >2.0 mL/kg in 80 min
Bicarbonate concentration: >80 meq per liter [>80 mmol per liter]
Bicarbonate output: >10 meq in 30 min [>10 mmol in 30 min]

Metabolic and endocrine

ACTH, plasma, 8 A.M.: <80 pg/mL [<80 ng per liter]
Adrenal cortex function tests: see Chap. 325
Adrenal medulla function tests: see Chap 326
Adrenal steroids, plasma:
Aldosterone, 8 A.M.: <8.5 ng/dL [<0.24 nmol per liter] (patient supine, 100 meq Na and 60 to 100 meq K intake)
Cortisol:
8 A.M.: 5 to 25 μg/dL [138 to 691 nmol per liter]
4 P.M.: 3 to 12 μg/dL [82 to 331 nmol per liter]
Dehydroepiandrosterone (DHEA): 0.2 to 0.9 μg/dL [7 to 31 nmol per liter]
Dehydroepiandrosterone sulfate (DHEA sulfate): 50 to 250 μg/dL [1.3 to 6.5 μmol per liter]
11-Deoxycortisol (compound S): <1 μg/dL [<30 nmol per liter]
17-Hydroxyprogesterone:
Women: follicular phase, 20 to 100 ng/dL [0.6 to 3 nmol per liter]; luteal phase, 50 to 350 ng/dL [1.5 to 10.6 nmol per liter]
Men: 6 to 300 ng/dL [1.8 to 9.0 nmol per liter]
Adrenal steroids, secretion rates:
Aldosterone: 50 to 250 μg per day [138 to 690 nmol per day]
Cortisol: 8 to 24 mg per day [22 to 69 μmol per day]
Adrenal steroids, urinary excretion:
Aldosterone: 5 to 19 μg per day [14 to 53 nmol per day]
Cortisol, free: 20 to 100 μg per day [54 to 276 nmol per day]
17-Hydroxycorticosteroids: 2 to 10 mg per day [5.4 to 28 μmol per day]
17-Ketosteroids:
Men: 7 to 25 mg per day [24 to 88 μmol per day]
Women: 4 to 15 mg per day [14 to 52 μmol per day]
Angiotensin II, plasma, 8 A.M.: 10 to 30 pg/mL [10 to 30 nmol per liter]
Arginine vasopressin (AVP), plasma:
Random fluid intake: 1 to 3 pg/mL [1 to 3 ng per liter]
Fluid deprivation, 18 to 24 h: 6 to 12 pg/mL [6 to 12 ng per liter]
Calcitonin, plasma: <50 pg/mL [<50 ng per liter]
Catecholamines, urinary excretion:
Free catecholamines: <100 μg per day [<590 nmol per day]
Epinephrine: <50 μg per day [295 nmol per day]
Metanephrines: <1.3 mg per day [<6.2 μmol per day]
Vanillylmandelic acid (VMA): <8 mg per day [<40 μmol per day]
Gastrin, plasma: <120 pg/mL [<120 ng per liter]
Glucagon, plasma: 50 to 100 pg/mL [14 to 29 pmol per liter]
Gonadal function tests: see Chaps. 330 and 331
Gonadal steroids, plasma:
Androstenedione:
Women: 110 to 190 ng/dL [3.9 to 6.6 nmol per liter]
Men: 80 to 130 ng/dL [2.9 to 4.6 mmol per liter]
Estradiol:
Women: 20 to 60 pg/mL [0.07 to 0.22 nmol per liter], higher at ovulation
Men: <50 pg/mL [<0.18 nmol per liter]
Progesterone:
Men, prepubertal girls, preovulatory women, and postmenopausal women: <2 ng/mL [<6 nmol per liter]
Women, luteal, peak: >5 ng/mL [>16 nmol per liter]
Testosterone:
Women: <100 ng/dL [<3.5 nmol per liter]
Men: 300 to 1000 ng/dL [10 to 35 nmol per liter]
Prepubertal boys and girls: 5 to 20 ng/dL [0.17 to 0.7 nmol per liter]
Gonadotropins, plasma:
Women, mature, premenopausal, except at ovulation:
FSH: 5 to 20 mU/mL [5 to 20 U per liter]
LH: 5 to 25 mU/mL [5 to 25 U per liter]
Ovulatory surge:
FSH: 12 to 30 mU/mL [12 to 30 U per liter]
LH: 25 to 100 mU/mL [25 to 100 U per liter]
Postmenopausal women:
FSH: >50 mU/mL [>50 U per liter]
LH: >50 mU/mL [>50 U per liter]
Men, mature:
FSH: 5 to 20 mU/mL [5 to 20 U per liter]
LH: 5 to 20 mU/mL [5 to 20 U per liter]
Children of both sexes, prepubertal:
FSH: <5 mU/mL [<5 U per liter]
LH: <5 mU/mL [<5 U per liter]
Growth hormone, after 100 g glucose by mouth: <5 ng/dL [<50 ng per liter]
Human chorionic gonadotropin, β subunit (β-hCG), plasma:
Men and nonpregnant women: <3 mIU/mL [<3 IU per liter]
Insulin, serum or plasma, fasting: 6 to 26 μU/mL [43 to 186 pmol per liter]
Insulin-like growth factor I (somatomedin C, IGF-1/SM C): see Chap. 322
Oxytocin, plasma:
Men and preovulatory women: 0.5 to 2 μU/mL [2 to 4 mU per liter]
Lactating women: 5 to 10 μU/mL [5 to 10 mU per liter]
Pancreatic islet function tests: Chap. 327
Parathyroid function tests: see Chap. 336
Pituitary function tests: see Chaps. 321 to 323
Pregnancy tests: see Chap. 331
Prolactin, serum: 2 to 15 ng/mL [2 to 15 μg per liter]
Renin-angiotensin function tests: see Chap. 325
Semen analysis: see Chap. 330
Thyroid function tests:
Dynamic tests of thyroid function: see Chap. 324
Radioactive iodine uptake, 24 h: 5 to 30 percent (range varies in different areas due to variations in iodine intake)
Resin T_3 uptake: 25 to 35 percent (varies among laboratories; for calculation of indexes of resin T_3 uptake, see Chap. 324)
Reverse triiodothyronine (rT_3), plasma: 10 to 40 ng/dL [0.15 to 0.61 nmol per liter]
Thyroid-stimulating hormone (TSH): <5 μU/mL [<5 mU per liter]
Thyroxine (T_4), serum radioimmunoassay: 5 to 12 μg/dL [64 to 154 nmol per liter]
Triiodothyronine (T_3), plasma: 70 to 190 ng/dL [1.1 to 2.9 nmol per liter]

Pulmonary See Tables A-9 and A-10.

Arterial blood gas measurements in normal subjects (sea level):
P_{CO_2}, seated (mean ± 1 SD): 38.0 ± 2.9 mmHg (no change with age) [5.0 kPa]
P_{O_2}:
Seated (mean ± 1 SD): (104.2 ± 0.27 mmHg) × age in years [13.8 kPa]
Supine (mean ± 1 SD): (103.5 ± 0.42 mmHg) × age in years [13.8 kPa]

Renal

Clearances (corrected to 1.72 m^2 body surface area):
  Measures of glomerular filtration rate:
    Inulin clearance (C1):
      Males (mean ± 1 SD): 124 ± 25.8 mL/min [2.1 ± 0.4 mL/s]
      Females (mean ± 1 SD): 119 ± 12.8 mL/min [2.0 ± 0.2 mL/s]
    Endogenous creatinine clearance: 91 to 130 mL/min [1.5 to 2.2 mL/s]
    Urea: 60 to 100 mL/min [1.0 to 1.7 mL/s]
  Measures of effective renal plasma flow and tubular function:
    p-Aminohippuric acid clearance (Cl_{PAH}):
      Males (mean ± 1 SD): 654 ± 163 mL/min [10.9 ± 2.7 mL/s]
      Females (mean ± 1 SD): 594 ± 102 mL/min [9.9 ± 1.7 mL/s]
Concentration and dilution test:
  Specific gravity of urine:
    After 12-h fluid restriction: 1.025 or more
    After 12-h deliberate water intake: 1.003 or less
Phenosulfonphthalein:
  After intravenous injection:
    Excretion in urine in 15 min: 25 percent or more
    Excretion in urine in 2 h: 55 to 75 percent
Protein excretion, urine: <150 mg in 24 h [<0.15 g per day]
  Males: 0 to 60 mg in 24 h [0 to 0.06 g per day]
  Females: 0 to 90 mg in 24 h [0 to 0.09 g per day]
Specific gravity, maximal range: 1.002 to 1.028
Tubular reabsorption, phosphorus: 79 to 94 percent of filtered load

HEMATOLOGIC EXAMINATIONS

See also "Chemical Constituents of Blood."

Bone marrow See Table A-11.

Erythrocytes and hemoglobin See also Table A-12.

Carboxyhemoglobin:
  Nonsmoker: 0 to 2.3 percent
  Smoker: 2.1 to 4.2 percent
Erythrocyte "life span":
  Normal survival: 120 days
  Chromium-labeled, half-life ($t_{½}$): 28 days
  Glucose 6-phosphate dehydrogenase: 12.1 ± 2 IU/gHb (WHO)
Ham's test (acid serum): negative
Haptoglobin, serum (mean ± 2 SD): 128 ± 15 mg/dL [1.3 ± 0.2 g per liter]
Heinz body stain: negative
Hemoglobin, plasma: 1 to 5 mg/dL [0.03 to 0.05 g per liter]
Hemoglobin A_2 (HbA_2): 1.5 to 3.5 percent
Hemoglobin, fetal (HbF): <2 percent
Hemoglobin H prep: negative
Methemoglobin: <1.7 percent
Nitroblue tetrazolium (chronic granulomatous disease): normal
Osmotic fragility:
  Slight hemolysis: 0.45 to 0.39 percent
  Complete hemolysis: 0.33 to 0.30 percent
Plasma iron turnover: 20 to 42 mg per 24 h [0.47 mg/kg]
Protoporphyrin, free erythrocyte (FEP): 16 to 36 μg per deciliter of red blood cells [0.28 to 0.64 μmol per liter]
Red cell distribution width (Coulter): 13 ± 1.5 percent
Sedimentation rate:
  Westergren, <50 years of age:
    Males: 0 to 15 mm/h
    Females: 0 to 20 mm/h
  Westergren, >50 years of age:
    Males: 0 to 20 mm/h
    Females: 0 to 30 mm/h
  Wintrobe:
    Males: 0 to 9 mm/h
    Females: 0 to 20 mm/h
Sucrose hemolysis: negative

Leukocytes See Table A-13.

Platelets and coagulation

Alpha$_2$ antiplasmin: 70 to 130 percent
Antithrombin III: 80 to 120 percent
Bleeding time:
  Ivy method, 5-mm wound: <9 min
  Duke method: <4 min
  Simplate: <7 min
Clot retraction, qualitative: apparent in 60 min, complete <24 h, usually <6 h
Euglobulin lysis time: >2 h
Factor II: 60 to 100 percent
Factor V: 60 to 100 percent
Factor VII: 60 to 100 percent
Factor IX: 60 to 100 percent
Factor X: 60 to 100 percent
Factor XI: 60 to 100 percent
Factor XII: 60 to 100 percent
Factor XIII: clot stable in urea
Fibrinogen: 200 to 400 mg/dL
Fibrin split products: <10 μg/mL
Plasminogen: 2.4 to 4.4 CTA U/mL
Protein C (antigenic assay): 58 to 148 percent
Protein S (antigenic assay): 58 to 148 percent
Partial thromboplastin time (activated PTT): comparable to control
Prothrombin time (quick one-stage): control ± 1 s
Protamine paracoagulation (3P) test: negative
Platelets: 130,000 to 400,000 per cubic millimeter
Thrombin time: control ± 3 s
von Willebrand's antigen: 60 to 150 percent

Miscellaneous

Leukocyte alkaline phosphatase (LAP): 13 to 100
Lysozyme (muramidase), serum: 5 to 25 μg/dL
Lysozyme, urine: <2 μg/mL
Schilling test: excretion in urine of orally administered radioactive vitamin B_{12}: 7 to 40 percent
Viscosity, plasma: 1.7 to 2.1
Viscosity, serum: 1.4 to 1.8

STOOL

Bulk:
  Wet weight: <197.5 (115 ± 41) g per day
  Dry weight: <66.4 (34 ± 16) g per day
Alpha$_1$ antitrypsin: 0.98 (±0.17) mg per gram of dry weight stool
Coproporphyrin: 400 to 1000 μg in 24 h [610 to 1500 nmol per day]
Fat (on diet containing at least 50 g fat): <6.0 (4.0 ± 1.5) g per day when measured on a 3-day (or longer) collection
  Percent of dry weight: <30.4 (13.3 ± 8.07)
  Coefficient of fat absorption: >95 percent
Fatty acid:
  Free: 1 to 10 percent of dry matter
  Combined as soap: 0.5 to 12 percent of dry matter
Nitrogen: <1.7 (1.4 ± 0.2) g per day
Protein content: minimal
Urobilinogen: 40 to 280 mg in 24 h [67 to 470 μmol per day]
Water: approximately 65 percent

URINE

See also "Metabolic and Endocrine" under "Function Tests."

Acidity, titratable: 20 to 40 meq in 24 h [20 to 40 mmol per day]
α-Amino nitrogen: 0.4 to 1.0 g in 24 h [28 to 71 mmol per day]
Ammonia: 30 to 50 meq in 24 h [30 to 50 mmol per day]
Amylase: 35 to 260 Somogyi units per hour
Amylase/creatinine clearance ratio [$(Cl_{am}/Cl_{cr}) \times 100$]: 1 to 5
Bentiromide (pancreatic function): 50 percent excreted in 6 h as *p*-amino benzoic acid (PABA) after 500 mg oral bentiromide
Calcium (10 meq or 200-mg calcium diet): <7.5 meq in 24 h; <150 mg in 24 h [<3.8 mmol per day]
Catecholamines: <100 μg in 24 h
Copper: 0 to 25 μg in 24 h [0 to 0.4 μmol per day]
Coproporphyrins (types I and III): 100 to 300 μg in 24 h [150 to 460 nmol per day]
Creatine, as creatinine:
Adult males: <50 mg in 24 h [<0.38 mmol per day]
Adult females: <100 mg in 24 h [<0.76 mmol per day]
Creatinine: 1.0 to 1.6 g in 24 h [8.8 to 14 mmol per day]
Glucose, true (oxidase method): 50 to 300 mg in 24 h [0.3 to 1.7 mmol per day]
5-Hydroxyindoleacetic acid (5-HIAA): 2 to 9 mg in 24 h [10 to 47 μmol per day]
Ketones, total (mean ± 1 SD): 50.5 ± 30.7 mg in 24 h
Lactic dehydrogenase: 560 to 2050 units in 8-h urine
Lead: <0.08 μg/mL; <120 μg in 24 h [0.39 μmol per liter]
Protein: <150 mg in 24 h [<0.05 g per day]
Porphobilinogen: none
Potassium: 25 to 100 meq in 24 h (varies with intake) [25 to 100 mmol per day]
Sodium: 100 to 260 meq in 24 h (varies with intake) [100 to 260 mmol per day]
Urobilinogen: 1 to 3.5 mg in 24 h [1.7 to 5.9 μmol per day]
Vanillylmandelic acid (VMA): <8 mg per day [<40 μmol per day]
D-Xylose excretion: 5 to 8 g within 5 h after oral dose of 25 g [33 to 53 mmol in 5 h]

TABLE A-1 SI and other units

Quantity	Name of unit	Symbol for unit	Derivation of units
SI BASE UNITS			
Length	meter	m	
Mass	kilogram	kg	
Time	second	s	
Thermodynamic temperature	Kelvin	K	
Amount of substance	mole	mol	
SI DERIVED UNITS			
Force	newton	N	$(m \cdot kg)/s^2$
Pressure	pascal	Pa	$N \cdot m^2$
Work, energy	joule	J	$N \cdot m$
Celsius temperature	degree Celsius	°C	K
OTHER UNITS RETAINED FOR USE			
Time	minute	min	
	hour	h	
	day	d	
Volume	liter	L	

TABLE A-2 Radiation derived units

Quantity	Old unit	SI unit	Name for SI unit (and abbreviation)	Conversion
Activity	curie (Ci)	Disintegrations per second (dps)	becquerel (Bq)	1 Ci = 3.7×10^{10} Bq 1 mCi = 37 mBq 1 μCi = 0.037 MBq or 37 GBq 1 Bq = 2.703×10^{-11} Ci
Absorbed dose	rad	joule per kilogram (J/kg)	gray (Gy)	1 Gy = 100 rad 1 rad = 0.01 Gy 1 mrad = 10^{-3} cGy
Exposure	roentgen (R)	coulomb per kilogram (C/kg)	—	1 C/kg = 3876 R 1 R = 2.58×10^{-4} C/kg 1 mR = 258 pC/kg
Dose equivalent	rem	joule per kilogam (J/kg)	sievert (Sv)	1 Sv = 100 rem 1 rem = 0.01 Sv 1 mrem = 10 μSv

TABLE A-3 SI prefixes and their symbols

Factor	Prefix	Symbol for prefix
10^9	giga	G
10^6	mega	M
10^3	kilo	k
10^2	hecto	h
10^1	deka	da
10^{-1}	deci	d
10^{-2}	centi	c
10^{-3}	milli	m
10^{-6}	micro	μ
10^{-9}	nano	n
10^{-12}	pico	p
10^{-15}	femto	f
10^{-18}	alto	a

TABLE A-4 Plasma lipid concentration in normal subjects*

	Total plasma cholesterol, mg/dL		Plasma LDL-cholesterol, mg/dL		Plasma HDL-cholesterol, mg/dL		Plasma triglyceride, mg/dL	
Age	Men	Women	Men	Women	Men	Women	Men	Women
19	113–197	120–203	62–130	59–137	30–63	35–74	37–148	39–132
29	133–244	130–229	70–165	71–164	31–63	37–83	46–249	40–172
39	146–270	141–245	81–189	75–172	29–62	34–82	54–321	41–194
49	158–276	152–268	98–202	79–186	30–64	34–87	58–327	47–228
59	156–276	169–294	88–203	89–210	28–71	37–91	58–286	56–257
69	158–274	171–297	98–210	92–221	30–78	35–98	57–267	60–241
70+	151–270	167–288	80–186	96–206	31–75	33–92	58–258	60–235

* *5th and 95th percentiles not ideal ranges for white men and women; data are too fragmentary to ascertain whether these values apply to other groups.*
SOURCE: *The Lipid Research Clinics Population Studies Data Book, vol 1, The Prevalence Study, NIH Publication No 80-1529, Bethesda, National Institutes of Health, July 1980.*

TABLE A-5 Hemodynamic values

Pressures (mmHg):	
Systemic arterial:	
Peak systolic/end-diastolic	100–140/60–90
Mean	70–105
Left ventricle:	
Peak systolic/end-diastolic	100–140/3–12
Left atrium (or pulmonary capillary wedge):	
Mean	2–12
a wave	3–10
v wave	3–15
Pulmonary artery:	
Peak systolic/end-diastolic	15–30/4–14
Mean	9–17
Right ventricle:	
Peak systolic/end-diastolic	15–30/2–7
Right atrium:	
Mean	2–6
a wave	2–8
v wave	2–7
Resistances [(dyn·s)/cm⁵]:	
Systemic vascular resistance	700–1600
Total pulmonary resistance	100–300
Pulmonary vascular resistance	20–130
Flows:	
Cardiac index (liters per minute per square meter)	2.4–3.8
Stroke index (milliliters per beat per square meter)	30–65
Oxygen consumption (liters per minute per square meter)	110–150
Arteriovenous oxygen difference (milliliters per liter)	30–50

TABLE A-6 Systolic time intervals in normal individuals (in milliseconds)

Regression equation	SD of index
QS_2 (M) = −2.1 HR + 546	14
QS_2 (F) = −2.0 HR + 549	14
PEP (M) = −0.4 HR + 131	13
PEP (F) = −0.4 HR + 133	11
LVET (M) = −1.7 HR + 413	10
LVET (F) = −1.6 HR + 418	10

NOTE: *QS_2 = total electromechanical systole, PEP = preejection phase, LVET = left ventricular ejection time, HR = heart rate, M = male, F = female, SD = standard deviation of the systolic time interval index. Systolic ejection period = 220–320 ms per beat; diastolic filling period = 380–500 ms per beat.*

SOURCE: *AM Weissler, CL Garrard, Mod Concepts Cardiovasc Dis 40:1, 1971.*

TABLE A-7 Normal values of echocardiographic measurements in adults*

	Range, cm	Mean, cm	Number of subjects
Age (years)	13 to 54	26	134
Body surface area (m^2)	1.45 to 2.22	1.8	130
RVD—flat	0.7 to 2.3	1.5	84
RVD—left lateral	0.9 to 2.6	1.7	83
LVID—flat	3.7 to 5.6	4.7	82
LVID—left lateral	3.5 to 5.7	4.7	81
Posterior LV wall thickness	0.6 to 1.1	0.9	137
Posterior LV wall amplitude	0.9 to 1.4	1.2	48
IVS wall thickness	0.6 to 1.1	0.9	137
Mid IVS amplitude	0.3 to 0.8	0.5	10
Apical IVS amplitude	0.5 to 1.2	0.7	38
Left atrial dimension	1.9 to 4.0	2.9	133
Aortic root dimension	2.0 to 3.7	2.7	121
Aortic cusps' separation	1.5 to 2.6	1.9	93
Percentage of fractional shortening†	34 to 44%	36%	20
Mean rate of circumferential shortening (Vcf)‡, or mean normalized shortening velocity	1.02 to 1.94 circ/s	1.3 circ/s	38

* *RVD = right ventricular dimension; LVID = left ventricular internal dimension; d = end diastole; s = end systole; LV = left ventricle; IVS = interventricular septum.*

† $\frac{\text{LVIDd} - \text{LVIDs}}{\text{LVIDd}}$

‡ $\frac{\text{LVIDd} - \text{LVIDs}}{\text{LVIDd} \times \text{ejection time}}$

SOURCE: *From H Feigenbaum, Echocardiography, in Heart Disease—A Textbook of Cardiovascular Medicine, E Braunwald (ed), Philadelphia, Saunders, 1980.*

TABLE A-8 Amplitude of Q, R, S, and T waves in scalar electrocardiogram of 100 normal adults*

	I	II	III	aV_R	aV_L	aV_F	V_1	V_5	V_6
Patients with Q wave	38%	41%	50%	—	38%	40%	0%	60%	75%
Q amplitude:									
Mean	0.4	0.6	0.9	—	0.4	0.7	0	0.3	0.3
Range	0 to 0.10	0 to 1.6	0 to 2.3	—	0 to 1.1	0 to 1.7	0	0 to 1.8	0 to 1.8
R amplitude:									
Mean	5.6	8.9	4.5	1.3	3.4	6.0	1.9	12.6	10.2
Range	1.0 to 10.0	2.0 to 16.9	1.0 to 12.1	0 to 2.9	0 to 8.2	0 to 13.8	1.0 to 6.0	7.0 to 21.0	5.0 to 18.0
S amplitude:									
Mean	2.0	2.1	2.4	7.0	2.6	—	8.0	2.5	1.3
Range	0 to 5.0	0 to 3.7	0 to 6.4	2.2 to 11.8	0 to 5.8	—	3.0 to 13.0	0 to 5.0	0 to 2.0
T amplitude:									
Mean	1.9	2.3	1.0	—	0.3	1.7	1.0	3.3	1.0
Range	1.0 to 3.0	1.0 to 4.0	−2.0 to 2.0	—	−1.0 to 2.0	0 to 4.0	−2.0 to 2.0	2.0 to 7.0	1.0 to 4.0

* *Values of Q, R, S, and T amplitudes are in millimeters (1 mm = 0.1 mv).*

SOURCE: *From J D Cooksey et al, Clinical Vectorcardiography and Electrocardiography, 2d ed, Chicago, Year Book Medical Publishers, 1977. Used by permission.*

TABLE A-9 Summary of values useful in pulmonary physiology

	Symbol	Typical values: Men	Women
PULMONARY MECHANICS			
Spirometry—volume-time curves:			
Forced vital capacity	FVC	≥4.0 liters	≥3.0 liters
Forced expiratory volume in 1 s	FEV_1	>3.0 liters	>2.0 liters
FEV_1/FVC	$FEV_1\%$	>60%	>70%
Maximal midexpiratory flow	MMF (FEF 25–27)	>2.0 liters per second	>1.6 liters per second
Maximal expiratory flow rate	MEFR (FEF 200–1200)	>3.5 liters per second	>3.0 liters per second
Spirometry—flow-volume curves:			
Maximal expiratory flow at 50% of expired vital capacity	$\dot{V}_{max}$ 50 (FEF 50%)	>2.5 liters per second	>2.0 liters per second
Maximal expiratory flow at 75% of expired vital capacity	$\dot{V}_{max}$ 75 (FEF 75%)	>1.5 liters per second	>1.0 liters per second
Resistance to airflow:			
Pulmonary resistance	RL (R_L)	<3.0 cmH_2O/s per liter	
Airway resistance	Raw	<2.5 cmH_2O/s per liter	
Specific conductance	SGaw	>0.13 cmH_2O/s	
Pulmonary compliance:			
Static recoil pressure at total lung capacity	Pst TLC	25 ± 5 cmH_2O	
Compliance of lungs (static)	CL	0.2 L/cmH_2O	
Compliance of lungs and thorax	C(L + T)	0.1 L/cmH_2O	
Dynamic compliance of 20 breaths per minute	C dyn 20	0.25 ± 0.05 liters per cmH_2O	
Maximal static respiratory pressures:			
Maximal inspiratory pressure	MIP	> 90 cmH_2O	> 50 cmH_2O
Maximal expiratory pressure	MEP	>150 cmH_2O	>120 cmH_2O
LUNG VOLUMES			
Total lung capacity	TLC	6–7 liters	5–6 liters
Functional residual capacity	FRC	2–3 liters	2–3 liters
Residual volume	RV	1–2 liters	1–2 liters
Inspiratory capacity	IC	2–4 liters	2–4 liters
Expiratory reserve volume	ERV	1–2 liters	1–2 liters
Vital capacity	VC	4–5 liters	3–4 liters
GAS EXCHANGE (SEA LEVEL)			
Arterial O_2 tension	Pa_{O_2}	95 ± 5 mmHg	
Arterial CO_2 tension	Pa_{CO_2}	40 ± 2 mmHg	
Arterial O_2 saturation	Sa_{O_2}	97 ± 2%	
Arterial blood pH	pH	7.40 ± 0.02	
Arterial bicarbonate	HCO_3^-	24 + 2 meq per liter	
Base excess	BE	0 ± 2 meq per liter	
Diffusing capacity for carbon monoxide (single breath)	DL_{CO}	25 mL CO/min/mmHg	
Dead space volume	VD	50 ± 25 mL	
Physiologic dead space: dead space-tidal volume ratio (rest)	VD/VT	≤35% VT	
(exercise)		≤20% VT	
Alveolar-arterial difference for O_2	A-a D_{O_2}	≤20 mmHg	

TABLE A-10 Prediction equations for spirometric tests, lung volumes, and gas exchange in adults

Variable	Sex	Age (A)	Height (H)	Weight (W)	Constant (C)	Standard deviation (SD)
PULMONARY MECHANICS						
Spirometry—volume-time curves* (H in inches):						
FVC	M	−0.025	+0.148	—	−4.241	0.74
	F	−0.024	+0.115	—	−2.852	0.52
FEV_1	M	−0.032	+0.092	—	−1.260	0.55
	F	−0.025	+0.089	—	−1.932	0.47
MEFR	M	−0.047	+0.109	—	+2.010	1.66
(FEF 200–1200)	F	−0.036	+0.145	—	−2.532	1.19
MMF	M	−0.045	+0.047	—	+2.513	1.12
(FEF 25–75)	F	−0.030	+0.060	—	+0.551	0.80
Spirometry—flow-volume curves† (H in centimeters):						
$\dot{V}_{max}$ 50	M	−0.015	+0.069	—	−5.400	1.422
(FEF 50%)	F	−0.013	+0.035	—	−0.444	1.22
$\dot{V}_{max}$ 75	M	−0.012	+0.044	—	−4.143	1.026
(FEF 75%)	F	−0.014	—	—	+3.042	0.936
Lung volumes‡ (H in meters; W in kilograms):						
TLC	M	—	+6.92	−0.017	−4.30	0.67
	F	−0.015	+6.71	—	−5.77	0.48
FRC	M	+0.015	+5.30	−0.037	−3.89	0.56
	F	—	+5.13	−0.028	−4.50	0.41
RV	M	+0.022	+1.98	−0.015	−1.54	0.38
	F	+0.007	+2.68	—	−3.42	0.32
VC	M	−0.020	+4.81	—	−2.81	0.50
	F	−0.022	+4.04	—	−2.35	0.40
Gas exchange§ (H in meters; W in kilograms):						
DL_{CO}	M	−0.20	+32.5	—	−17.6	5.1
	F	−0.16	+21.2	—	− 2.66	3.6

NOTE: *Answer = (A × age) + (H × height) + (W × weight) + C ± 2 SD. Example: The normal value and lower limit for the FEV_1 are sought in a man, age 40 years, height 183 cm, and weight 91 kg. The following equation gives the normal value:*
FEV_1 = (−0.032 × 40) + (0.092 × 72) + (−1.260) = 4.08 liters
The lower limit of normal:
4.08 − (2 × SD) = 4.08 − (2 × 0.55) = 2.98 liters
Only 2.5% of a normal population will fall below this value (2 SD below the mean).
For other abbreviations, see Table A-9.

* *Morris et al, Am Rev Respir Dis 103:57, 1971.*
† *Knudson et al, Am Rev Respir Dis 113:587, 1976.*
‡ *Grimby G, Söderholm B, Acta Med Scand 173:199, 1963.*
§ *Coates, JE, Lung Function and Application in Medicine, Davis, 1965.*

TABLE A-11 Differential nucleated cell counts of bone marrow

	Normal, mean%*	Range, %†
Myeloid:	56.7	
Neutrophilic series:	53.6	
Myeloblast	0.9	0.2–1.5
Promyelocyte	3.3	2.1–4.1
Myelocyte	12.7	8.2–15.7
Metamyelocyte	15.9	9.6–24.6
Band	12.4	9.5–15.3
Segmented		
Eosinophilic series	3.1	1.2–5.3
Basophilic series	<0.1	0–0.2
Erythroid:	25.6	
Pronormoblasts	0.6	0.2–1.3
Basophilic normoblasts	1.4	0.5–2.4
Polychromatophilic normoblasts	21.6	17.9–29.2
Orthochromatic normoblasts	2.0	0.4–4.6
Megakaryocytes	<0.1	
Lymphoreticular:	17.8	
Lymphocytes	16.2	11.1–23.2
Plasma cells	2.3	0.4–3.9
Reticulum cells	0.3	0–0.9

* *Frm MM Wintrobe et al, Clinical Hematology, 8th ed, Philadelphia, Lea & Febiger, 1981.*

† *Range observed in 12 healthy men.*

TABLE A-12 Erythrocytes and hemoglobin: Normal values at various ages

Age	Red blood cell count,* millions/mm³	Hemoglobin,* g/dL	Vol. packed RBCs,* mL/dL	Corpuscular values: MCV, fl	MCH, pg	MCHC, g/dL	MCD, μm
Days 1–13	5.1 ± 1.0	19.5 ± 5.0	54.0 ± 10.0	106–98	38–33	36–34	8.6
Days 14–60	4.7 ± 0.9	14.0 ± 3.3	42.0 ± 7.0	90	30	33	8.1
3 months to 10 years	4.5 ± 0.7	12.2 ± 2.3	36.0 ± 5.0	80	27	34	7.7
11–15 years	4.8	13.4	39.0	82	28	34	
Adults:							
Females	4.8 ± 0.6	14.0 ± 2.0	42.0 ± 5.0	90 ± 7	29 ± 2	34 ± 2	7.5 ± 0.3
Males	5.4 ± 0.9	16.0 ± 2.0	47.0 ± 5.0	90 ± 7	29 ± 2	34 ± 2	7.5 ± 0.3

* *The range of values represents almost the extremes of observed variations (93 percent or more) at sea level. The blood values of healthy persons should fall well within these mean ± SD figures.*

NOTE: *MCV = mean corpuscular volume, MCH = mean corpuscular hemoglobin, MCHC = mean corpuscular hemoglobin concentration, MCD = mean corpuscular diameter.*

SOURCE: *MM Wintrobe et al, Clinical Hematology, 8th ed, Philadelphia, Lea & Febiger, 1981.*

TABLE A-13 Normal leukocyte count, differential count, and hemoglobin concentration at various ages

Age	Leukocytes, total	Neutrophils: Total	Band	Segmented	Eosinophils	Basophils	Lymphocytes	Monocytes	Hemoglobin, g/dL blood
12 mo	11.4(6.0–17.5)	3.5(1.5–8.5)	0.35	3.2	0.3(0.05–0.7)	0.05(0–0.20)	7.0(4.0–10.5)	0.55(0.05–1.1)	11.6(9.0–14.6)
		31	3.1	28	0.4	0.4	61	4.8	
4 yr	9.1(5.5–15.5)	3.8(1.5–8.5)	0.27(0–1.0)	3.5(1.5–7.5)	0.25(0.02–0.65)	0.05(0–0.20)	4.5(2.0–8.0)	0.45(0–0.8)	12.6(9.6–15.5)
		42	3.0	39	2.8	0.6	50	5.0	
6 yr	4.3(1.5–8.0)	0.25(0–1.0)	4.0(1.5–7.0)	4.0(1.5–7.0)	0.23(0–0.65)	0.05(0–0.20)	3.5(1.5–7.0)	0.40(0–0.8)	12.7(10.0–15.5)
		51	3.0	48	2.7	0.6	42	4.7	
10 yr	8.1(4.5–13.5)	4.4(1.8–8.0)	0.24(0–1.0)	4.2(1.8–7.0)	0.20(0–0.60)	0.04(0–0.20)	3.1(1.5–6.5)	0.35(0–0.8)	13.0(10.7–15.5)
		54	3.0	51	2.4	0.5	38	4.3	
21 yr	7.4(4.5–11.0)	4.4(1.8–7.7)	0.22(0–0.7)	4.2(1.8–7.0)	0.20(0–0.45)	0.04(0–0.20)	2.5(1.0–4.8)	0.30(0–0.8)	♂15.8 (14.0–18.0)
		59	3.0	56	2.7	0.5	34	4.0	♀13.9 (11.5–16.0)

NOTE: *Values are expressed as "cells × 10³/μL." The numbers underlined are percentages.*

SOURCE: *WJ Williams et al (eds), Hematology, 3d ed, New York, McGraw-Hill, New York, 1983. By permission.*

INDEX

INDEX

(Page numbers in **boldface** indicate major discussions.)